Anne Fielding
April 24, 1996

PDR MEDICAL DICTIONARY

FIRST EDITION

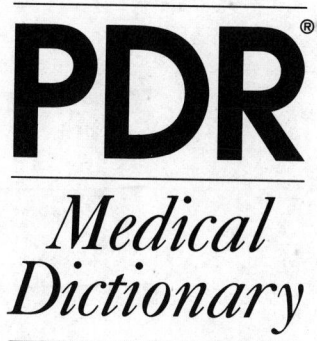

PDR®
Medical Dictionary

PDR MEDICAL DICTIONARY

FIRST EDITION

PDR®

Medical Dictionary

MEDICAL ECONOMICS

MONTVALE, NEW JERSEY

Editor: Marjory Spraycar
Senior Editor: Elizabeth Randolph
Editorial Assistant: Maureen Barlow Pugh
Copy Editors: Christopher Muldor, Jane Sellman, Barbara Werner
On-Line Editors: Kathryn J. Cadle, Barbara L. Ferretti, Catherine N. Kelly, Leslie Simpson
Editorial Proofreaders: Peter W. Binns, Jolanta Obrebska, Carol Sorgen
Medical Proofreaders: Alfred Jay Bollet, M.D.; John H. Dirckx, M.D.; Thomas W. Filardo, M.D.; Robert Hogan, M.D.; Edward Stim, M.D.
Database Programmers: Dennis P. Smithers, Dave Marcus, Lexi-Comp Inc., Hudson, OH
Production Coordinator: Paula K. Huber
Printing Coordinator: Brian Smith
Illustration Planning: Wayne J. Hubbel
Design: Robert C. Och, Dan Pfisterer
Cover Design: Sharon Reuter, Reuter & Associates

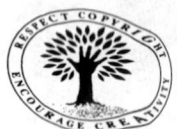

CONTENTS

PREFACE

Welcome to the newest volume in PDR's ever-expanding library of medical references. This unique resource combines PDR's unparalleled database of pharmaceutical names and manufacturers with an exhaustive new dictionary of medical terminology. It sets a new standard in convenience, range of coverage, and up-to-the-minute information.

The rapid growth of knowledge in fast-paced specialties such as biotechnology, biochemistry, genetics, embryology, epidemiology, radiology, and neurology has spawned an equally explosive expansion of the medical lexicon. The *PDR Medical Dictionary* fully reflects these dynamic developments. Of the more than 100,000 medical terms in this volume, no less than 12,000 have entered the language within the last 5 years.

This state-of-the-art dictionary offers you a host of other thoughtful features, many of them new to the field of medical lexicography.

High Profile Terms Some terms have so profoundly altered the way medicine is practiced and delivered that they warrant more than the standard dictionary definition. The consultants who contributed to this work identified 125 high profile terms, which appear with expanded definitions. They are in the A-Z section of the book, highlighted between two green horizontal rules to make them easy to locate.

Nomina Anatomica The dictionary also reflects the latest trend in anatomical nomenclature–the vocabulary that plays such an important part in the language of medicine. Faculty and students today are moving away from Latin (Nomina Anatomica), substituting English translations of terms instead. In keeping with this movement, the definitions are located where readers are most likely to look–under English translations of the Latin terms. Although the Latin terms are listed as well, they simply direct readers to their English equivalents. Arthur F. Dalley, II, Professor of Anatomy and Director of Medical Gross Anatomy in the Department of Biomedical Sciences at Creighton University of Medicine, spent nearly a year accomplishing this mammoth shift from Latin to English.

Color and Graphics Graphics are playing an ever more important role in the delivery of information everywhere, and in no discipline are they more crucial than in medicine. The *PDR Medical Dictionary* boasts more than 1,000 color illustrations, photographs, and tables reproduced from the *Roche Lexikon Medizin,* a dictionary that serves the German-language market.

The use of color in the *PDR Medical Dictionary* is by no means limited to these illustrations, either. It is used strategically throughout the text to help readers find information faster.

Green Means Go Many entries do not have definitions; instead they present synonyms that point readers to the main term where the definition is found. These synonyms are printed in green, signaling readers to look up the word in green to find the definition.

♻ **Means Recycle** About 1,200 Greek and Latin word parts account for about 90 percent of technical scientific language, so learning these word parts can be a boon in the study of medical language. In the A-Z section of this dictionary, these suffixes, prefixes, and combining forms are marked with the universal symbol for recycling. They've also been collected for convenient reference in a list.

Precision Thumb Tabs On every page is a green thumb tab with the first two letters of the last word on that page. This strategic thumb index lets you know exactly where you are in the alphabet whenever you open the book. This is another way that makes it easier to get into the dictionary, get the information you need, and get back out.

A.D.A.M. Anatomical Art Near the center of the book–between the letters L and M–are 29 images of color anatomical illustrations. They were created by A.D.A.M., publishers of the computer-based anatomy program of the same name. The illustrations are richly labeled, and the book includes a complete index to each of the labels that appear on the plates.

Easy-to-find Subentries To assist you in finding the exact information you need as quickly as possible, the dictionary starts each subentry on a new line. Although this may seem like a minor matter, it is this sort of detail that makes a dictionary truly easy to use.

WordFinder You will find a long list of multiple-term entries in the front part of the book. Its purpose is to identify where in the dictionary a multiple-term entry is defined -- the main challenge in a dictionary organized, as this one is, in main entry-subentry format. All the definitions involving the word "cochlear," for example, are not found at cochlear, but as subentries of these other, organizing entries:

> aqueduct; area; canal; canaliculus; duct; implant; joint; labyrinth; nerve; nucleus; part; prosthesis; recess; root; window.

More information about using WordFinder can be found on page WF 1, the section immediately following the Guide to Pharmaceutical Names.

Appendices You'll see an extensive collection of ready-reference tables, reflecting the fact that good tabular matter enables easy access to information.

Consultants The *PDR Medical Dictionary* is written and reviewed by a group of 40 consultants who are physicians, researchers, and academicians. They represent all the traditional medical specialties, plus such disciplines as biotechnology, nursing, statistics/epidemiology, neurosurgery and neuropathology.

Working Dictionary This is a working dictionary, a record of a living language, and words are formed, spelled, pronounced, and defined as they are actually used. Every dictionary contains words that by philological standards are misformed, misspelled, mispronounced, or misused. A dictionary may suggest standards, but it cannot enforce them. The *PDR Medical Dictionary,* therefore, serves as a guide for those who wish to speak and write more precisely and to coin new terms more accurately.

Acknowledgements

Editing a dictionary is by its very nature a collective endeavor. Directed by Marjory Spraycar, Editor, a large group of consultants, editors, database experts, publishing experts, and artists are responsible for this massive work.

Also indispensable in the development of any truly useful reference tool is another large group–the thousands of users whose comments, suggestions, additions, and corrections guide the evolution of the work. We invite your recommendations for further improvements. Please feel free to call us, toll-free at 1-800-232-7379 or fax us at 201-573-4956.

CONSULTANTS

Donald Allison, Ph.D.   **Biochemistry**
Associate Scientist, Department of Biochemistry & Molecular Biology, University of Florida College of Medicine, Gainesville, FL

William K. Beatty   **History/Biography**
Professor of Medical Bibliography, Northwestern University Medical School, Chicago, IL

David A. Bloom, M.D.   **Urology and Urologic Surgery**
Chief, Pediatric Urology, Professor, Surgery, University of Michigan & Mott Children's Hospital, Ann Arbor, MI

Alfred Jay Bollet, M.D.   **Internal Medicine**
Clinical Professor of Medicine, Yale University School of Medicine, New Haven, CT

David G. Bostwick, M.D.   **Pathology**
Consultant in Pathology and Associate Professor of Pathology, Department of Laboratory Medicine and Pathology, The Mayo Clinic, Rochester, MN

Michael J. Burridge, BVM&S, MPVM, Ph.D.   **Veterinary Medicine**
Professor, Department of Infectious Diseases, College of Veterinary Medicine, University of Florida, Gainesville, FL

John E. Chimoskey, M.D.   **Physiology**
Department of Physiology, Michigan State University, East Lansing, MI

Helen Cox, R.N., C., Ed.D., F.A.A.N.   **Nursing**
Executive Associate Dean and Professor, Texas Tech University Health Sciences Center, School of Nursing, Lubbock, TX

Arthur F. Dalley II, Ph.D.   **Gross Anatomy**
Professor of Anatomy, Director of Medical Gross Anatomy, Department of Biomedical Sciences, Creighton University School of Medicine, Omaha, NE; President, Anatomical Board of the State of Nebraska; Associate Editor, *Clinical Anatomy*

John H. Dirckx, M.D.   **Etymology**
Director, University of Dayton Health Center, Dayton, OH

William Droegemueller, M.D.   **Obstetrics and Gynecology**
Robert A. Ross Distinguished Professor and Chairman, Department of Obstetrics and Gynecology, University of North Carolina School of Medicine, Chapel Hill, NC

Paul J. Friedman, M.D.   **Radiology**
Professor of Radiology and Dean for Academic Affairs, School of Medicine, University of California, San Diego, CA

Robert M. Goldwyn, M.D.   **Plastic & Reconstructive Surgery**
Clinical Professor of Surgery, Harvard Medical School, Head, Division of Plastic Surgery, Beth Israel Hospital, Boston, MA

Nicholas M. Greene, M.D.   **Anesthesiology**
Professor Emeritus of Anesthesiology, Yale University School of Medicine, New Haven, CT

Steven I. Gutman, M.D., M.B.A.   **Laboratory Medicine**
Medical Officer, Division of Clinical Laboratory Devices, Office of Device Evaluation, Food and Drug Administration, Rockville, MD

Duane E. Haines, Ph.D.   **Neuroanatomy**
Professor of Anatomy and Chairman, Department of Anatomy, University of Mississippi Medical Center, Jackson, MS

Donald Heyneman, Ph.D.   **Parasitology**
Professor of Parasitology Emeritus, Associate Dean for Health and Medical Sciences Emeritus, School of Public Health, University of California, Berkeley/University of California, San Francisco, Joint Medical Program

Steven E. Hyler, M.D.   **Psychiatry**
Associate Professor of Clinical Psychiatry, Columbia University, New York State Psychiatric Institute, New York, NY

Iain Kalfas, M.D., FACS   **Neurosurgery**
Head, Section of Spinal Surgery, Department of Neurosurgery, Cleveland Clinic Foundation, Cleveland, OH

John M. Last, M.D., FRACP, FRCPC   **Medical Statistics and Epidemiology**
Professor Emeritus, Department of Epidemiology and Community Medicine, University of Ottawa, Ottawa, Ontario, Canada

Stanley S. Lefkowitz, Ph.D.   **Immunology/Virology**
Professor, Department of Microbiology and Immunology, Texas Tech University Health Sciences Center, Lubbock, TX

Alan T. Marty, M.D., FACS, FCCP, FACC, FCCM   **Thoracic Surgery**
Consultant, Indiana University Medical School, Evansville, IN

Joseph P. Matarazzo, Ph.D.   **Psychology**
Professor of Medical Psychology, Chairman, Department of Medical Psychology, Oregon Health Sciences University, Portland, OR

David N. Menton, Ph.D.   **Histology**
Associate Professor of Anatomy, Washington University School of Medicine, St. Louis, MO

Edmond A. Murphy, M.D.   **Genetics**
Professor Emeritus, The Johns Hopkins University School of Medicine, Baltimore, MD

Martin L. Nusynowitz M.D.   **Nuclear Medicine**
Professor, Radiology, Internal Medicine, and Pathology, University of Texas Medical Branch at Galveston, Galveston, TX

Thomas Poirier, M.D., Ph.D.   **Bacteriology**
Division of Infectious Disease, College of Medicine, University of Florida; Florida Infection Physicians, Gainesville, FL

Richard Prayson, M.D.   **Neuropathology**
Department of Anatomic Pathology, The Cleveland Clinic Foundation, Cleveland, OH

Arthur Raines, Ph.D.   **Pharmacology & Toxicology**
Professor of Pharmacology and Neurology, Department of Pharmacology, Georgetown
University Medical Center, Washington, DC

Alvin L. Rogers, Ph.D.   **Mycology**
Professor Emeritus, Medical Mycology, Michigan State University, East Lansing, MI

Clarence T. Sasaki, M.D.   **Otorhinolaryngology**
Charles W. Ohse Professor of Surgery and Chief, Section of Otolaryngology, Yale School of
Medicine, New Haven, CT

George S. Schuster, D.D.S., M.S., Ph.D.   **Dentistry**
Ione and Arthur Merritt Professor and Acting Chairman, Department of Oral Biology, Medical
College of Georgia School of Dentistry, Augusta, GA

Donald P. Speer, B.S., M.D.   **Orthopaedics**
Professor of Surgery and Anatomy, Associate Head for Academic Affairs, Department of
Surgery, University of Arizona College of Medicine, Tucson, AZ

David H. Spodick M.D., D.Sc.   **Cardiology**
Professor of Medicine, University of Massachusetts Medical School; Lecturer in Medicine,
Tufts University School of Medicine; Lecturer in Medicine, Boston University School of
Medicine; Director of Clinical Cardiology and Director of Cardiovascular Fellowship Training,
St. Vincent Hospital, Worcester, MA.

Sheldon M. Schuster, Ph.D.   **Biotechnology**
Professor, Biochemistry and Molecular Biology, Program Director, Biotechnology Program,
University of Florida, Gainesville, FL

Martha E. Sucheston, Ph.D.   **Embryology**
Associate Professor, Cell Biology, Neurobiology, and Anatomy; Powelson Professor of
Medicine; Director MEDPATH, Ohio State University College of Medicine, Columbus, OH

Michael L. Steer, M.D.   **General Surgery**
Professor of Surgery, Harvard Medical School; Chief of General Surgery and Associate
Surgeon-In-Chief, Beth Israel Hospital, Boston, MA

H. Stanley Thompson, M.D.   **Ophthalmology**
Professor of Ophthalmology, University of Iowa College of Medicine, Iowa City, IA

Asa J. Wilbourn, M.D.   **Neurology**
Director, EMG Laboratory, The Cleveland Clinic Foundation and Associate Clinical Professor
of Neurology, Case-Western Reserve University School of Medicine, Cleveland, OH

Colin Wood, M.D.   **Dermatology**
Professor Emeritus of Pathology, University of Maryland School of Medicine, Baltimore, MD

CONTRIBUTORS

Gladys Alonsozana, M.D., Department of Pathology, University of Maryland School of Medicine, Baltimore, MD. Contributing editor, Laboratory Reference Range Values

Audrey K. Brown, M.D., Professor of Pediatrics, Suny Health Science Center, Brooklyn, NY. Contributing editor, hematology and pediatrics

Show-Hong Duh, Ph.D., D.A.B.C.C., Department of Pathology, University of Maryland School of Medicine, Baltimore, MD. Contributing editor, Laboratory Reference Range Values

Thomas W. Filardo, M.D., Evendale, OH. Contributing editor and proofreader

James Michael Hall, D.D.S., Department of Oral Pathology, Medical College of Georgia. Contributing editor, dentistry

Robert Hogan, M.D., Director, Southern California Permanente Medical Group, El Cajon, CA. Contributing editor and proofreader

Doris L. Lefkowitz, Ph.D., Associate Professor, Department of Biological Sciences, Texas Tech University, Lubbock, TX. Contributing editor, immunology/virology

Gerald H. Malsbary, Ph.D., Assistant Professor of Classics, St. Charles Borromeo Seminary, Wynnewood, PA. Translator of figures and tables from the *Roche Lexikon Medizin*

Gina Maranto, Miami Beach, FL. Contributing editor, High Profile Terms

John Moulds, President and Chief Operating Officer, Gamma Biologicals, Houston, TX. Contributing editor, Blood Group appendix

James T. McDonough, Jr., Ph.D., Bala Cynwyd, PA. Contributing editor, etymology revisions to the 25th Edition

Albert Pawlina, M.D., Assistant Scientist, Department of Anatomy and Cell Biology, University of Florida College of Medicine. Contributing editor, anatomy image labels

Edward Stim, M.D., Yokohama, Japan. Contributing editor and proofreader

ILLUSTRATION CREDITS

All illustrations, photographs, and tables that appear in the A-Z section of this book originally appeared in the *Roche Lexikon Medizin*, 3. Auflage, Urban & Schwarzenberg, Munich, Germany.

The color anatomy plates that follow the letter L were developed by A.D.A.M. Software, Inc., Atlanta, Georgia, using A.D.A.M.® Software Program. All A.D.A.M. images ©1995 A.D.A.M. Software Inc., all rights reserved.

Both collections are used with permission.

ILLUSTRATIONS IN THIS EDITION

amino acid	abortion	accommodation of eye	acupuncture
adrenergic receptors	Abrams' heart reflex	acinar carcinoma	acute hemorrhagic
abdominal reflexes	absolute temperature	acne conglobata	pancreatitis
abdominal regions	absorption	acrodermatitis chronica	adaptation
abdominal pressure	acarid	atrophicans	adaptive enzyme
abdominal pulse	accessory placenta	active transport	adductor

successive contrast
superior sagittal sinus
supernumerary kidney
swallow
synapse
syndesmophyte
syphilis
systemic circulation
Taenia
talipes
talipes cavus
taxonomy
temperature
temporal arteritis
temporal bone
tenodesis
tension pneumothorax
testis
tetany
tetralogy of Fallot
thalamus
thalidomide
thrombocyte
thromboelastogram
thrombus
thyroid
thyrotropin-releasing
   hormone stimulation test

tinea pedis
TNM staging
tongue
tooth
total lung capacity
Toxoplasma gondii
toxoplasmosis
trace elements
trachoma
transcription
transitional cell carcinoma
transmission
transposition of the great
   vessels
transverse presentation
Treponema pallidum
Treponema
triacylglycerol
tricarboxylic acid cycle
Trichosporon
tricuspid atresia
tricuspid
trigeminal nerve
trilogy of Fallot
trisomy
trochlear nerve
trophoblast
Trypanosomatidae

tuberculous spondylitis
tumor marker
twin
ulcer
ulcerative colitis
ulnar nerve
ultrasound
umbilical artery
urachus
ureterocele
ureterocystoscope
ureterostenosis
urine
urogenital system
uropoietic system
uterus
vaccine
vagotomy
varicella
varicose veins
varicosis
vasopressin
vectorcardiogram
vegetative endocarditis
vein stripper
Velpeau's bandage
vena
venous pulse

venous angle
ventricular septal defect
ventriculography
vermicular pulse
vertebra
viral hepatitis type B
viral hepatitis
virion
virus
visual field
vitamin
Volkmann's contracture
vomiting
vulva
Watson-Crick helix
Wigand maneuver
worm
x-ray
xeroderma
yeast
Z-plasty
Zahn's infarct
zoster
Zygomycetes

HIGH PROFILE TERMS IN THIS EDITION

AIDS
allele
Alzheimer's disease
anneal
antioncogene
assisted reproductive
   technology
atherosclerosis
background radiation
base pair
capture-recapture method
carcinoma
CD4/CD8 count
cell determination
clinical epidemiology
clinical trial
cloning
cochlear implant
colposcopy
computed tomography
crack cocaine
cumulative trauma disorders
cytogenetics

cytokine network
dental implants
diabetes mellitus
diabetic neuropathy
diabetic retinopathy
Diagnostic and Statistical
   Manual
DNA fingerprinting
Doppler color flow
Doppler ultrasonography
drug abuse
drug resistance
endogenous depression
epidemiology
free radical
gene therapy
growth factors
hairy leukoplakia
health
hepatitis
histocompatibility complex
HMO

hormone replacement
   therapy
Human Genome Project
human papilloma virus
immunotherapy
laparoscopic-assisted
   vaginal hysteroscopy
laparoscopy
laser iridotomy
laser trabeculoplasty
leishmaniasis
Loop excision
low-fat diet
Lyme disease
lymphoma
magnetic resonance imaging
mammography
managed care
melanoma
monoclonal antibody
mood disorders
nitric oxide
nuclear medicine

nurse practitioner
palatopharyngoplasty
pelvic inflammatory disease
perimenopause
polymerase chain reaction
positron emission
   tomography
premenstrual syndrome
prion
probe
prostate-specific antigen
psychopharmacology
radiation risks
radionuclide
refractive keratotomy
retinoid
retrovirus
schizophrenia
silicone
snowball sampling
sports medicine
surveillance
uvulopalatoplasty

HOW TO USE THIS DICTIONARY

ORGANIZATION OF THE VOCABULARY

Main Entry-Subentry Format

Entries are organized as subentries under governing single-word noun main entries.

To find	Look under
hemorrhagic fever	
paratyphoid fever	fever
Q fever	
myocardial infarction	infarction
carcinoid tumor	
giant cell tumor of bone	tumor
Wilms' tumor	

Verbs, adjectives, adverbs, combining forms, prefixes, abbreviations, and symbols follow the general rules of indexing and thus are located as main entries.

Compound words or chemical and drug terms may deviate from the standard main entry-subentry format

Compound words that usually are written closed up as one word or that are hyphenated are located as main entries rather than as subentries under the portion of the term that would otherwise represent the main entry. For example, "aftercontraction" is located in the A's rather than under contraction; "self-hypnosis" is located in the S's rather than under hypnosis.

Multiple-word chemical and drug terms generally are located at the first word of a term, unless the term includes a general noun that would be considered a kind or type. For example:

To find	Look under
adrenergic blocking agent (type of agent)	agent
Agent Orange (a specific compound)	Agent Orange
bile acid (a type of acid)	acid
acid red (a stain that is neither an acid nor red)	acid red
ribonucleic acid (a molecule rather than an acid)	ribonucleic acid

Tips on Finding Multiple-word Terms

- Look in the WordFinder, immediately preceding the A-Z section
- Look at the alphabetical location of the specific words making up the term
- Look under another main entry that is similar to the term you are looking for
- Look at cross-references

To find	Look under
a surgical procedure	operation
	technique
	method
a disease	syndrome

ALPHABETIZATION
Main Entries

Main entries are alphabetized letter by letter as spelled, rather than word by word as in a telephone directory:

blood	cross
blood bank	crossbreed
bloodletting	cross-cylinder
blood purple	crossing-over of genes
bloodstream	cross-matching
blood vessel	crossway

Exceptions

- ***Disregarded are***   Prepositions, conjunctions, articles, apostrophes of possessive eponyms, spaces, punctuation, Greek letters (e.g., α, β, γ), numbers, configurational characters (e.g., D-, +, -), italicized forms (e.g., *p*-, *N*-, *cis*-), whether as prefixes or as interior components in compound chemical terms.

- ***Included are***   Prepositional phrases, especially Latin expressions:

To find	Look in
ante cibum	the A's
in vitro	the I's

- Spelled-out Greek letters and configurational forms are considered in alphabetization:

To find	Look in
α-naphthylurea	the N's
alpha-blocker	the A's
L-dopa	the D's
levodopa	the L's

- Capitalized words (proper nouns) precede lower case words (common nouns):

Streptococcus	appears before streptococcus
Down	appears before down

Subentries

Subentries are alphabetized letter by letter following the same rules given above for main entries, but with some additional significant differences.

To save space, a subentry is represented by its initial letter, if it is singular; by addition of apostrophe and s, if it is a regular plural; or by a spelled-out form, if it is an irregular plural or a plural Latin word. Regardless of its form, the main entry word is disregarded in alphabetization of subentries, as also are prepositions, conjunctions, articles, and possessive forms used in eponymic terms:

crest	gyrus
gluteal c.	angular g.
c. of greater tubercle	gyri breves insulae
inguinal c.	central gyri
c's of nail bed	g. dentales
nasal c.	short gyri of insula
c. of neck rib	gyri temporales transversi

SPELLING

For alphabetizing letter by letter, spelling disregards spaces, punctuation, Greek letters, numbers, configurational characters, italicized forms.

Alternative spellings, especially those of prefixed combining forms, are given as main entries with cross-references to the various spellings:

chilitis (ki-li´tis) Cheilitis

hem-, hema- [G. haima, blood]. Combining forms meaning blood. See also hemat-, hemato-, hemo-.

kyto- See cyto-.

Alternative spellings that have been superseded are also given as main entries with cross-references to the currently used spellings:

oari-, oario- [G. oarion, a small egg, dim. of oon, egg]. Obsolete combining forms denoting ovary. See oo-, oophor-, ovario-.

pleio- Rarely used alternative spelling for pleo-.

Differences in British and American spellings, particularly those at or near the beginning of a word, are handled by prefix main entries that are cross-referenced from the British spelling to the American spelling:

ae- For words so beginning and not found here, see under e-.

oe- For words so beginning and not found here, see e-.

British spellings within compound words may also change the alphabetical location of some entries:

	British	American
ae* for e	aetiology	etiology
	faeces	feces
	orthopaedic	orthopedic
oe for e	coeliac	celiac
	oedema	edema
	diarrhoea	diarrhea
our for or	tumour	tumor
re for er	fibre	fiber

* Ae in the combining form aero- is accepted spelling in both usages, as in aerosol, anaerobe, and other words derived from the G. aer, air; aeroplane/airplane is a well-known exception.

Surnames, used as biographical main entry cross-references to associated eponymic terms, are also alphabetized by their most commonly used spellings. Users should keep in mind spelling variations such as a/ae, o/oe, u/ue, and Mac/Mc. For names beginning with prefixes, such as Van, van der, von, de, and which may be used with or without the prefix, cross-reference main entries have been provided to direct the user to the proper entry location. Regardless of the form of a surname (e.g., Crohn, Bence Jones, d'Herelle, von Willebrand, Loeffler), the name is alphabetized letter by letter as spelled.

ORGANIZATION OF ENTRIES AND CROSS-REFERENCES

The definition is given at only one location for two or more synonymous terms. Entries for the other synonymous terms are cross-referenced to the term where the definition is to be found. This system is also used for obsolete or outmoded terms, for spelling variations, or when there is a definite preference dictated by its usage. The practice of placing a definition at only one location primarily serves to focus all of the information concerning a term at a single place, rather than strictly as an indicator of preference. It also keeps the size of *Stedman's* manageable by avoiding duplication of definitions.

Main Entries

Defined main entries usually are constructed as follows: (1) boldface entry word followed by its abbreviation or symbol (if any) in parentheses, (2) pronunciation in parentheses, (3) the definition proper, and (4) derivation in brackets

> **electrocardiogram (ECG, EKG)** (ē-lek-trō-kar′dē-ō-gram). Graphic record of the heart's integrated action currents obtained with the electrocardiograph. [electro- + G. *kardia*, heart, + *gramma*, a drawing]

If the entry of the word is used in the definition, it is abbreviated to its first letter or to its accepted abbreviation, e.g., b. for bone, DNA for deoxyribonucleic acid, Hb for hemoglobin.

When there is more than one definition, each definition is indicated by a boldface number; however, the numerical sequence of the definitions is not necessarily an indication of importance or of preference:

> **mesocardia** (mez̄ō-kar′dē-ă). **1.** Atypical position of the heart in a central position in the chest, as in early embryonic life. **2.** Plural of mesocardium. [meso- + G. *kardia*, heart]

Synonyms follow the final definition if a term and are preceded by SYN.

Synonyms appearing in green. If an entry or a subentry is followed by a synonym and no other definition, synonyms appear in green, signaling readers to move to the term in green to find the definition.

> **nephropathy** (ne-frop′a-the). Any disease of the kidney. SYN renopathy

> **analgesic n.,** SYN analgesic nephrins

Systematic names of defined trivial or generic chemical and drug terms are likewise placed at the beginning of the definition, along with the molecular formula:

> **acetone** (as´e-ton) Dimethyl ketone; CH3COCH3; a colorless, volatile, inflammable liquid; extremely small amounts are. . . .
>
> **aspirin** (as´pi-rin) Acetylsalicylic acid; C6H4(OCOCH3)COOH; a widely used analgesic, antipyretic, and anti-inflammatory.

Subentries

Defined subentries are organized much like main entries, as described above. Pronunciation and derivation are provided when the principal words making up the subentry term are not provided as main entries in the vocabulary.

Multiple definitions are distinguished by boldface numbers in parentheses, but their numerical sequence is not necessarily indicative of importance or preference:

> **age**
> **developmental a. (DA), (1)** fetal a.; a. estimated by anatomic development since implantation; **(2)** a. of an individual estimated from the degree of anatomic, physiologic, mental, and emotional maturation.

In the definition, the main entry word, whenever used, is abbreviated to its first letter or to its accepted abbreviation as a space-saving device:

Cross-references

Cross-references may be main entries or subentries or may be part of a main entry or subentry definition. They may serve to direct the user to a defined entry or to an entry where additional or related information can be found. The following types of cross-references are used in *Stedman's*:

Synonym   A word that has the same meaning as the entry. When a synonym occurs at a term without a definition, it appears in green after **SYN**:

> **boil** (boyl) **SYN** furuncle. [A.S. byl, a swelling]

When the relevant synonym is a multiple-word term located as a subentry, the governing main entry word under which it will be found is italicized, as in the following example:

> **candle-power** (kan´dl-pow´er). **SYN** Luminous *intensity*.

When the synonym cross-reference is from one subentry to another subentry under the same main entry, the main entry word is abbreviated, as in the following example:

> **calculus**
> **arthritic c. SYN** gouty tophus.
> **biliary c. SYN** gallstone.
> **dendritic c. SYN** staghorn c.

SEE

Refers to a term with a meaning similar to the entry.

SEE ALSO

Refers to a term with further information about entry.

Cf. *(L. confer, compare)* **and q.v.** *(L. quod vide, which see)*

Refers to comparative or related information, but with a less direct relationship than a **SEE ALSO** reference.

Obsolete term for

Term no longer widely used. Refers to term in current use.

Eponyms

These are terms that are named after people. A brief biography appears at a person's name, along with a cross-reference to the eponym. These cross-references are not necessarily to the defined entry, since a synonymous descriptive term may be the defined term; if this is the case, a cross-reference to the defined term is provided:

> **Hoffman,** Johann, German neurologist, 1857-1919. See H.'s muscular *atrophy, phenomenon, reflex, sign*; Werdnig-H. *disease.*
>
> **Sylvius,** (DuBois, de le Boe), Franciscus (Francois), Dutch physician, anatomist, and physiologist, 1614-1672. See sylvian *angle, aqueduct, fissure, line, point, valve, ventricle*; fossa of S.; vallecula sylvii.
>
> **Wilms,** Max, German surgeon, 1867-1918. See W.'s *tumor.*

Note that the abbreviated possessive form of the surname in the cross-reference is apostrophe and s regardless of whether the spelled-out possessive form is apostrophe and s or s and apostrophe.

Traditionally, the possessive form has been appended to the name of the discoverer or describer of, for example, a disease (Wilms' tumor) but not to the name of the person having the disease (Christmas disease, Job syndrome **but**, Lou Gehrig's disease), a compound name (Bence Jones proteinuria, Niemann-Pick disease), or the name of the location where the disease was first found to occur (Lyme disease, Pontiac fever). In recent years, this rule of thumb has not been followed consistently (Legionnaires disease, Legionnaire's disease, Legionnaires' disease). The use of the possessive form is increasingly less common, particularly in certain specialties.

User's Guide

Abbreviations and Symbols

Abbreviations and symbols, as well as acronyms and other contractions, are included in the vocabulary if they are accepted usage as opposed to ad hoc creations. They are located as main entries, generally as cross-references to the spelled-out terms where they are cited parenthetically in boldface immediately after the boldface entry word(s):

> **Cyt** Symbol for cytosine
>
> **PET** Abbreviation for positron emission *tomography*
>
> **stat.** Abbreviation for L. *statim*, at once, immediately.
>
> **cytosine** (Cyt) (si´to-sen). 4-Amino-2(1H)-pyrimidinone; a. . . .
>
> **tomography**
>   **positron emission t. (PET),** tomographic imaging of local. . . .

Some abbreviations and symbols are self-explanatory or are more appropriately defined at their entries than at a contrived entry for the spelled-out terms:

> **APUD** [amine precursor uptake, decarboxylase] Proposed designation
>   for a group of cells in different organs secreting polypeptide hor-
>   mones. Cells in this group have certain biochemical. . . .
>
> **b.i.d.** Abbreviation for L. *bis in die*, twice a day.
>
> **FUO** Abbreviation for fever of unknown origin.
>
> **M.D.** Abbreviation of *Medicinae Doctor*, Doctor of Medicine.
>
> **PUVA** Abbreviation for oral administration of psoralen and subsequent
>   exposure to long wavelength ultraviolet light (uv-a); used to treat pso-
>   riasis.
>
> **QCO2** Symbol for the microliters STPD of CO_2 given off per mil-
>   ligram of tissue per hour.

Abbreviations may appear with or without periods. Some nomenclature conventions have eliminated the period from certain types of abbreviations. In general, use of periods with most abbreviations is progressively declining, but in some instances periods are retained to avoid confusion.

PRONUNCIATION

Conventions Used

Phonetic spelling for pronunciation is given in parentheses immediately after the boldface entry word(s). Pronunciation is provided in main entries except where it would be redundant because the phonetic spelling is the same as the spelling of the boldface entry word(s). Pronunciation is not given for subentry words unless they are foreign words or they do not appear as pronounced main entries. For Latin boldface subentry words, a prime (´) is used to indicate the stressed syllable.

The phonetic system used is a basic one and has only a few conventions:

- Two diacritical marks are used; the macron (¯) for long vowels; and the breve (˘) for short vowels.

- Principal stressed syllables are followed by a prime (´); monosyllables do not have a stress mark.

- Other syllables are separated by hyphens.

The following pronunciation key provides examples and consonant sounds encountered in the phonetic system. No attempt has been made to accommodate the slurred sounds common in speech or regional variations in speech sounds. Note that a vowel with a breve (˘) is used for the indefinite vowel sound of the schwa (e). Native pronunciation of foreign words is approximated as closely as possible.

Pronunciation Key

Vowels

ā   day, mate, care, dairy, aorta, ape, ate, face, way, sail, air, aero, behave, gauge, heir, beige, eight, their, they, suede

a   mat, hat, plaid, act, para, damage, banana

ă   abortion, media, banana, about, alone, aorta, para, hepatitis, cephalo, damage, mountain, equal

ah   father, hurrah, wasp, wander, yacht

ar   far, artery, guard, cart, heart

aw   fall, cause, taught, tall, talk, calm, raw, thaw, lawyer, saw, auto

ē   be, bee, meet, deer, bleed, equal, key, fetal, even, perineo, prosthesis, team, ear, beat, bacteria, anterior, pity, busy, -logy, meridian, machine

ĕ   taken, system, synthesis, genesis

er   term, err, merry, operation, father, earn, learn, firm, thirst, myrtle

ī   pie, pine, fire, high, side, ice, bite, height, buy, hyper, deny, pylon

i   pit, mirror, tip, fit, differ, habit, easily, perineo, -ism, archi-, sieve, build, pyramid, physical, women, walking

ĭ   pencil

ō   no, note, fore, for, so, toe, open, bone, phone, perineo, thorus, road, boat, owe, snow, soul, four, sew

o   not, rotten, box, bother, cot, on, oncology, ought, fought, broad

ŏ   occult, lemon, collect, love, son, ton, flood, does, rough

ow   cow, brow, power, plow, now, out, bough, hour, loud, thou

oy   boy, troy, toy, void, mastoid, oil, coin, buoy, Freud ū   food, ooze, pool, to, too, tool, prove, move, canoe, rule, lupus, June, fruit, acoustic, dew, new, grew

u   wood, foot, wool, took, wolf, would, pull, put

ŭ   but, sun, bud, cup, up, humdrum, fudge, lupus, occult, adjust, us, couple, traction, adjust, uterus

yū   dispute, pure, unit, union, curable, future, uterus, youth, beauty, cue, feud, fuse, few, view

Consonants

b	bad, table, tab		n	no, sunset, on
ch	child, teacher, much		ng	single, ring
d	dog, ladder, led		p	pan, upper, top
dh	this, rhythm, smooth		r	rot, hurry, near
f	fit, differ, if, rough, phone		s	so, passing, miss, cent, dancing
g	got, bigger, leg		sh	should, tension, plantation
h	hit, behave		t	ten, button, cat
j	jade, adjust, germ, edge		th	thin, ether, with
k	cat, action, kept, wake, book, chronic		v	very, liver, gave
			w	we, away
ks	exquisite, excellent, tax		y	yes, lawyer
kw	exquisite, acquire, quit		z	zero, maze, those, braces, says, browse
l	law, alone, all			
m	me, simple, him		zh	azure, measure

In some words the initial sound is not that of the initial letter(s), or the initial letter(s) is not sounded or has a different sound, as in the following examples:

aerobe (ar´ob)	phthalein (thal´e-in)
eimeria (ime´re-a)	pneumonia (nu-mo´ne-a)
gnathic (nath´ik)	psychology (si-kol´o-je)
knuckle (nuk-l)	ptosis (to´sis)
oedipism (ed´i-pizm)	xanthoma (zan-tho´ma)

MEDICAL ETYMOLOGY

Background

When it was time to revise the 25th edition of *Stedman's*, we asked readers about etymologies: are they important, should they be more complete, should they be provided for every entry in the book? Readers said they thought etymologies were interesting, but they shouldn't get in the way of finding the meaning of a term. Responding to this information, we have moved etymologies to follow definitions.

Our etymology consultant, John H. Dirckx, M.D., concurred with this move. "The etymology of a medical term is often its most interesting and least useful feature," he said. "Most interesting because it puts us in touch with the history of medicine, of human ideas, and of the human struggle to understand the forces of nature that determine destiny and mortality. It also yields fascinating insights into human psychology. Least useful because change is the very essence of language, and just when a pattern seems to be emerging with perfect clarity and consistency, words veer off on a tangent, creating exceptions so that most etymologies give only approximate indications of meaning; many give entirely misleading cues."

Organization

The origin or etymology of a boldface entry term is given in brackets [ ] at the end of an entry. Of necessity, derivations are brief and as simple as possible to facilitate memory and promote association with similar derivatives. The information provided has three basic components: (1) the abbreviation of the language to which the original word(s) belongs; (2) in italics, the original word(s) from which the term is derived; and (3) the English translation of the word(s). For Greek and Latin verbs, the first person singular present form, rather than the infinitive, is used because the root word is more readily recognized in the former form; however, the English translation is given in the infinitive:

> **diphtheria** (dif-thēr´ē-a). Diphtheritis; a sep. . . . [G. *diphthera*, leather]

> **graph** (graf). A line or tracing. . . . [G. *grapho*, to write]

> **union** (yūn´yŭn). 1. The joining or amalgamation. . . . [L. *unus*, once]

When the boldface entry term has the same or approximately the same meaning and/or spelling as the word(s) from which it is derived, the redundant material is not included in the derivation, as in the following examples:

> **fascia,** pl. **fasciae** (fash´ē-a, -e-e) [L. a band or fillet]

> **idea** (i-dē´a). Any mental image or concept. [G. *semblance*]

Derivations frequently include additional components, especially when a derivation involves compound words or more than one word from one or more languages. A Greek or Latin verb may be hyphenated to indicate that the second part of the word exists as a simple verb with the same or approximately the same meaning, qualified by the addition of an adjectival or adverbial prefix; if the simple verb undergoes a change when forming part of a compound, that change is also shown:

> **apocrine** (ap´ō-krin). Denoting a mechanism of glandular secretion in which the apical portion of secretory cells is shed and incorporated into the secretion. **SEE ALSO** a. *gland*. [G. *apo-krino*, to separate]

> **component** (kom-pō´nent) . An element forming a part of the whole. [L. *com-pono*, pp. *-positus*, to place together]

When words originating from more than one language are part of a derivation, the language of each word and the word's English translation are given; when the words are from the same language, the language is indicated only for the first word:

> **apicectomy** (ap-i-sek´tō-mē). 1. Opening and exenteration of air cells. . . . [L. *apex*, summit or tip, + G. *ektome*,excision]

> **gonarthrotomy** (gon-ar-throt´ō-mē). Incision into the knee joint. [G. *gony*, knee, + *arthron*, joint, + *tome*, incision]

Prefixes and Suffixes

Combining forms used as prefixes or within compound words are listed in the vocabulary as boldface main entries with their own bracketed derivations and full definitions and full definitions. They are preceded by the ⟁ symbol. When used in bracketed derivations of other boldface entry terms, which follow alphabetically in the vocabulary, their language of origin and English translation are not given:

> ⟁ **neur-, neuri-, neuro-.** Combining forms denoting a nerve or relating to the nervous system. [G. *neuron*, nerve]

> **neuralgia** (nu-ral´je-a). Pain of a severe, throbbing, or stabbing character in the course or distribution of a nerve. **SYN** neurodynia. [neur- + G. *algos*, pain]

> **neuritis**, pl. **neuritides** (nuri´tis, nu-rit´i-dez) . 1. Inflammation of a nerve. **SYN** neuropathy. [neuri- + G. *-itis*, inflammation]

Word parts—prefixes, suffixes, and combining forms—are also listed in the vocabulary as boldface main entries with their own bracketed derivations and full definitions. They are also marked with the universal symbol of recycling, which appears in green: ♻. When used in bracketed derivations of other boldface entry items, the language of origin is indicated (only if different from the preceding word), and the English translation is given:

> **-osis,** pl. **-oses** [G.]. Suffix, properly added only to words formed from G. roots, meaning a process, condition, or state, usually abnormal or diseased. It denotes. . . .

ABBREVIATIONS AND SYMBOLS USED IN THE DICTIONARY

The abbreviations and symbols listed below are used in the derivations and definitions of entries in the dictionary. They should be distinguished from the abbreviations and symbols given as entries in the vocabulary or accompanying the spelled-out entry words that they represent, as discussed above.

acc.	accusative	i.e.	L. id est, that is
adj.	adjective	Ind.	Indian
Am. Ind.	American Indian	It.	Italian
Ar.	Arabic	Jap.	Japanese
A.S.	Anglo-Saxon	L.	Latin
c., ca	L. circa, about	L.L.	Late Latin
cf.	L. confer, compare	masc.	masculine
Ch.	Chinese	M.E.	Middle English
char.	character	Med. L.,	Medieval Latin
C.I.	Colour Index	Mediev. L.	Mediev. L.
D.	Dutch	Mod. L.	Modern Latin
dial.	dialect	myth.	mythological
dim.	diminutive	N.A.	Nomina Anatomica
EC	Enzyme Commission	neut.	neuter
e.g.	L. exempli gratia, for example	N.G.	New Guinea
Eng.	English	ntr.	neuter
etym.	etymology	obs.	obsolete
fem.	feminine	O.E.	Old English
Fr.	French	O.Fr.	Old French
fr.	from	O.H.G.	Old High German
fut.	future	O.N.	Old Norse
G.	Greek	p.	participle
Gael.	Gaelic	Pers.	Persian
gen.	genitive	Pg.	Portuguese
Ger.	German	pl.	plural
Hind.	Hindu	pp.	past participle
Ice.	Icelandic	priv.	privative, negative
pr. p.	present participle	US	United States
q.v.	L. quod vide, which see	W. Af.	West African
Sansk.	Sanskrit	Sc.	Scandinavian
sing.	singular	Sp.	Spanish
Sw.	Swedish	thr.	through

* In biographical data, denotes year of birth when year of death is not given.
† In biographical data, denotes year of death when year of birth is not given.

BUILDING BLOCKS OF MEDICAL LANGUAGE

Medical Prefixes, Suffixes, and Combining Forms

a- not, without, less

ab- from, away from, off

abs- from, away from, off

ad- increase, adherence, motion toward; very

-ad toward, in the direction of; -ward

alge- pain

algesi- pain

algio- pain

algo- pain

ambi- around, on (both) sides, on all sides, both

amyl- starch, polysaccharide nature or origin

amylo- starch, polysaccharide nature or origin

an- not, without, -less

ana- up, toward, apart

ante- before

anti- 1 against, opposing; **2** curative; **3** an antibody

apo- separated from, derived from

arteri- artery

arterio- artery

arthr- a joint, an articulation

arthro- a joint, an articulation

-ase an enzyme

-ate a salt or ester of an "-ic" acid

aut- self, same

auto- self, same

bacteri- bacteria

bacterio- bacteria

bi- twice, double

bio- life

blasto- budding by cells or tissue

bronch- bronchus

bronchi- bronchus

broncho- bronchus

carcin- cancer

carcino- cancer

cardi- 1 the heart; **2** esophageal opening of stomach

cardio- 1 the heart; **2** esophageal opening of stomach

cata- down

cephal- the head

cephalo- the head

chem- chemistry

chemo- chemistry

chlor- 1 green; **2** chlorine

chloro- 1 green; **2** chlorine

chol- bile

chondrio- 1 cartilage; **2** granular; **3** gritty

chondro- 1 cartilage; **2** granular; **3** gritty

chrom- color

chromat- color

chromo- color

-cidal killing, destroying

-cide killing, destroying

cis- on this side, on the near side

co- with, together, in association, very, complete

col- with, together, in association, very, complete

com- with, together, in association, very, complete

con- with, together, in association, very, complete

cor- with, together, in association, very, complete

crani- cranium

cranio- cranium

cry- cold

cryo- cold

cycl- 1 a circle, a cycle; **2** the ciliary body

cyst- the bladder; the cystic duct; a cyst

cysti- the bladder; the cystic duct; a cyst

cysto- the bladder; the cystic duct; a cyst

cyt- cell

-cyte cell

cyto- cell

dactyl- the fingers, the toes

dactylo- the fingers, the toes

de- away from, cessation

derm- skin

derma- skin

dermat- skin

dermato- skin

dermo- skin

dextr- right, toward or on the right side

dextro- right, toward or on the right side

di- separation, taking apart, reversal, not, un-

dif- separation, taking apart, reversal, not, un-

dir- separation, taking apart, reversal, not, un-

dis- separation, taking apart, reversal, not, un-

duodeno- the duodenum

-dynia pain

dynamo- force, energy

dys- bad, difficult

ect- outer, on the outside

ecto- outer, on the outside

encephal- the brain

encephalo- the brain

end- within, inner

endo- within, inner

enter- the intestines

entero- the intestines

epi- upon, following, subsequent to

ergo- work

erythr- red, redness

erythro- red, redness

esthesio- sensation, perception

eu- good, well

ex- out of, from, away from

exo- exterior, external, outward

extra- without, outside of

ferri- the presence in a compound of a ferric ion

ferro- metallic iron, the divalent ion Fe^{2+}

fibr- fiber

fibro- fiber

-form in the form or shape of

galact- milk

galacto- milk

-gen 1 producing, coming to be; **2** precursor of

gen- 1 producing, coming to be; **2** precursor of

gloss- the tongue

glosso- the tongue

gluco- glucose

glyco- sugars

gnath- the jaw

gnatho- the jaw

-gram a recording

granul- granular, granule

granulo- granular, granule

-graph a recording instrument

gyn- woman

gyne- woman

gyneco- woman

gyno- woman

hem- blood

hema- blood

hemat- blood

hemato- blood

hemi- one-half

hemo- blood

hepat- the liver

hepatico- the liver

hepato- the liver

hidr- sweat

hidro- sweat

hist- tissue

histio- tissue

histo- tissue

hydr- water; hydrogen

hydro- water; hydrogen

hyper- excessive, above normal

hypo- beneath; diminution, deficiency; the lowest

hyster- 1 uterus; hysteria; **2** late, following

hystero- 1 uterus; hysteria; **2** late, following

-ia a condition

-iasis a condition, a state

-ic pertaining to

-ics organized knowledge, practice, treatment

ileo- the ileum

infra- below

inter- between, among

intra- within

irid- the iris

irido- the iris

ischi- the ischium

ischio- the ischium

-ism 1 condition, disease; **2** practice, doctrine

-ismus spasm; contraction

iso- 1 equal, like; **2** "isomer of"; **3** sameness

-ite the nature of, resembling

-ites -y, -like

-itides plural of -itis

-itis inflammation

karyo- nucleus

kerat- the cornea

kerato- the cornea

kin- movement

kine- movement

kinesi- motion

kinesio- motion

kineso- motion

kino- movement

lact- milk

lacti- milk

lacto- milk

laryng- the larynx

laryngo- the larynx

latero- lateral, to one side, a side

-lepsis a seizure

-lepsy seizure

lepto- light, slender, thin, frail

leuk- white

leuko- white

linguo- the tongue

lip- fat, lipid

lipo- fat, lipid

lith- a stone, calculus, calcification

litho- a stone, calculus, calcification

-log speech, words

log- speech, words

-login 1 study of; **2** collecting

logo- speech, words

-logy 1 study of; **2** collecting

lymph- lymph
lympho- lymph
lys- lysis, dissolution
lyso- lysis, dissolution
macr- large; long
macro- large; long
mast- breast
masto- breast
meg- 1 large, oversize; 2 one million
mega- 1 large, oversize; 2 one million
megal- large
megalo- large
-megaly, large
melan- black
melano- black
mening- meninges
meningo- meninges
mes- 1 middle, mean, intermediacy; 2 mesentery
meso- 1 middle, mean, intermediacy; 2 mesentery
meta- 1 after, behind; 2 joint action, sharing
micr- 1 smallness; 2 one-millionth; 3 microscopic
micro- 1 smallness; 2 one-millionth; 3 microscopic
mon- single
mono- single
morph- form, shape, structure
morpho- form, shape, structure
myx- mucus
myxo- mucus
necr- death, necrosis
necro- death, necrosis
nephr- the kidney
nephro- the kidney
neur- a nerve, the nervous system
neuri- a nerve, the nervous system
neuro- a nerve, the nervous system
oculo- eye, ocular
odont- tooth
odonto- tooth
odyn- pain
odyno- pain
-oid resemblance to
olig- few, little
oligo- few, little
-oma tumor, neoplasm
-omata plural of -oma
oncho- onco-
onco- tumor, bulk, volume
-one a ketone (–CO–) group
onych- fingernail, toenail
onycho- fingernail, toenail
oo- egg, ovary
oophor- ovary
oophoro- ovary
ophthalm- the eye
ophthalmo- the eye

orchi- testis
orchido- testis
orchio- testis
-oses plural of -osis
-osis process, condition, state
ossi- bone
osseo- bony
ost- bone
oste- bone
osteo- bone
ovari- ovary
ovario- ovary
ovi- egg
ovo- egg
oxa- the presence or addition of oxygen atom(s)
oxo- addition of oxygen
oxy- sharp; acid; acute; shrill; quick; oxygen
pachy- thick
pan- all, entire
pant- all, entire
panto- all, entire
para- 1 abnormal; 2 involvement of two like parts
path- disease
patho- disease
-pathy disease
ped- 1 child; 2 foot
pedi- 1 child; 2 foot
pedo- 1 child; 2 foot
-penia deficiency
per- through, thoroughly, intensely
peri- around, about
-pexy fixation, usually surgical
phaco- 1 lens-shaped; 2 relation to a lens
-phage eating, devouring
-phagia eating, devouring
phago- eating, devouring
-phagy eating, devouring
pharmaco- drugs, medicine
pharyng- the pharynx
pharyngo- the pharynx
phleb- vein
phlebo- vein
phon- sound, speech
phono- sound, speech
phor- carrying, bearing; a carrier, a bearer; phoria
phoro- carrying, bearing; a carrier, a bearer; phoria
phos- light
phot- light
photo- light
phren- 1 diaphragm; 2 the mind; 3 phrenic
phreni- 1 diaphragm; 2 the mind; 3 phrenic
-phrenia of mind
phrenico- 1 diaphragm; 2 the mind; 3 phrenic
phreno- 1 diaphragm; 2 the mind; 3 phrenic

physi- 1 physical; 2 natural; 3 the science of physics
physio- 1 physical; 2 natural; 3 the science of physics
physo- 1 tendency to swell or inflate; 2 air, gas
phyt- plants
phyto- plants
-plasia formation
plasma- plasma
plasmat- plasma
plasmato- plasma
plasmo- plasma
-plegia paralysis
pleur- rib, side, pleura
pleura- rib, side, pleura
pleuro- rib, side, pleura
pluri- several, more
-pnea breath, respiration
pneo- breath, respiration
pneum- 1 air, gas; 2 the lungs; 3 breathing
pneuma- 1 air, gas; 2 the lungs; 3 breathing
pneumat- 1 air, gas; 2 the lungs; 3 breathing
pneumato- 1 air, gas; 2 the lungs; 3 breathing
pod- foot, foot-shaped
-pod foot, foot-shaped
podo- foot, foot-shaped
-poiesis production
poly- 1 multiplicity; 2 "polymer of"
post- after, behind, posterior
pre- anterior, before
pro- 1 before, forward; 2 precursor of
proct- the anus, the rectum
procto- the anus, the rectum
psych- the mind
psyche- the mind
psycho- the mind
pyel- (renal) pelvis
pyelo- (renal) pelvis
pyo- suppuration, an accumulation of pus, pus
pyreto- fever
pyro- fire, heat, fever
rachi- the spine
rachio- the spine
radio- 1 radiation, chiefly x-ray; 2 radius
re- again, backward
rect- the rectum
recto- the rectum
retro- backward, behind
rhin- the nose
rhino- the nose
-rrhagia discharge
-rrhaphy surgical suturing
-rrhea a flowing, a flux
salping- a tube
salpingo- a tube
sarco- muscular substance, flesh-like
schisto- split, cleft

schiz- split, cleft, division
schizo- split, cleft, division
scler- hardness (induration), sclerosis, the sclera
sclero- hardness (induration), sclerosis, the sclera
-scope an instrument for viewing
-scopy the use of an instrument for viewing
semi- one-half; partly
sial- saliva, the salivary glands
sialo- saliva, the salivary glands
sigmoid- sigmoid, the sigmoid colon
sigmoido- sigmoid, the sigmoid colon
sito- food, grain
somat- the body, bodily
somato- the body, bodily
somatico- the body, bodily
spasmo- spasm
spermato- semen, spermatozoa
spermo- semen, spermatozoa
sperma- semen, spermatozoa
splanchn- the viscera
splanchni- the viscera
splanchno- the viscera
splen- the spleen
spleno- the spleen
staphyl- a grape, a bunch of grapes; staphylococci
staphylo- a grape, a bunch of grapes; staphylococci
-stat an agent to prevent changing or moving
steno- narrowness, constriction
stheno- strength, force, power
stom- mouth
stoma- mouth
stomat- mouth
stomato- mouth
sub- beneath, less than normal, inferior
super- in excess, above, superior, in the upper part
sy- together
syl- together
sym- together
syn- together
sys- together
thel- the nipples
thelo- the nipples
therm- heat
thermo- heat
thorac- the chest, the thorax
thoracico- the chest, the thorax
thoraco- the chest, the thorax
thromb- blood clot
thrombo- blood clot
thyr- the thyroid gland

thyro- the thyroid gland
toco- childbirth
-tome 1 a cutting instrument;
  2 a segment, section
-tomy a cutting operation
tono- tone, tension, pressure
top- place, topical
topo- place, topical
tox- a toxin, a poison
toxi- a toxin, a poison
toxico- a toxin, a poison

toxo- a toxin, a poison
trache- the trachea
tracheo- the trachea
trans- across, through,
  beyond
trich- the hair, a hairlike
  structure
trichi- the hair, a hairlike
  structure
-trichia the hair, a hairlike
  structure

tricho- the hair, a hairlike
  structure
-trophic food, nutrition
tropho- food, nutrition
-trophy food, nutrition
-tropic turning toward,
  affinity
uri- uric acid
uric- uric acid
urico- uric acid
vas- a duct, a blood vessel

vasculo- a blood vessel
vaso- a duct, a blood vessel
vesic- a vesica, a vesicle
vesico- a vesica, a vesicle
xanth- yellow, yellowish
xantho- yellow, yellowish
zo- an animal, animal life
zoo- an animal, animal life
zym- fermentation, enzymes
zymo- fermentation, enzymes

GUIDE TO PHARMACEUTICAL NAMES

Whether you need to check a spelling, locate brand-name drugs containing a particular generic ingredient, or identify a product's manufacturer, this convenient compilation of brand and generic drug names will provide the answer you seek. The section is organized alphabetically, with brand and generic entries integrated throughout. Brand names are shown in upper and lower case, followed in parentheses by the manufacturer. Generic names are shown underlined and in upper case. Below each generic name you'll find a list of brands containing the ingredient. Additional information on any of the listed brands and their manufacturers can be found in *Physicians' Desk Reference*.

A

ACES Antioxidant Soft Gels
  (J. R. CARLSON LABORATORIES, INC.)
APAP Drops
  (BARRE-NATIONAL INC.)
APAP-Elixir (ALRA LABORATORIES, INC.)
APAP Elixir-Cherry or Grape
  (BARRE-NATIONAL INC.)
A.P.L. (WYETH-AYERST LABORATORIES)
ATP (Enteric Adenosine Triphosphate)
  (TYSON AND ASSOCIATES, INC.)
A/T/S 2% Acne Topical Gel and Solution
  (HOECHST-ROUSSEL PHARMACEUTICALS INC.)
AVC Cream (MARION MERRELL DOW INC.)
AVC Suppositories (MARION MERRELL DOW INC.)
Abbokinase (ABBOTT LABORATORIES)
Abbokinase Open-Cath (ABBOTT LABORATORIES)
Abbo-Pac (ABBOTT LABORATORIES)
Accupril Tablets (PARKE-DAVIS)
Accutane Capsules (ROCHE LABORATORIES)

ACEBUTOLOL HYDROCHLORIDE
  Sectral Capsules
Acel-Imune Diphtheria and Tetanus Toxoids and Acellular Pertussis Vaccine Adsorbed
  (LEDERLE LABORATORIES)

ACETAMINOPHEN
  APAP Drops
  APAP-Elixir
  APAP Elixir-Cherry or Grape
  Acetaminophen and Codeine Phosphate Oral Soln.
  Acetaminophen and Codeine Phosphate Tablets
  Acetaminophen Oral Solution (Cherry)
  Acetaminophen Tablets and Caplets, USP
  Actifed Plus Tablets and Caplets
  Actifed Sinus Daytime/Nighttime Caplets and Tablets
  Anexsia 5/500 Tablets
  Anexsia 7.5/650 Tablets
  Axocet
  Bancap HC Capsules
  Benadryl Allergy/Sinus Headache Caplets
  Benadryl Cold/Flu Tablets
  Bupap Tablets
  Capital And Codeine Suspension
  Co-Gesic Tablets
  Allergy-Sinus Comtrex Multi-Symptom Allergy Sinus Formula Tablets & Caplets
  Comtrex Maximum Strength Multi-Symptom Cold Reliever Tablets/Caplets/Liqui-Gels/Liquid
  Non-Drowsy Comtrex Maximum Strength Caplets
  DHCplus Capsules
  Darvocet-N 50 Tablets

  Darvocet-N 100 Tablets
  Duadacin Cold & Allergy Capsules
  Duradrin Capsules
  Esgic-Plus Tablets
  Esgic Tablets & Capsules
  Aspirin Free Excedrin Analgesic Caplets
  Excedrin Extra-Strength Analgesic Tablets & Caplets
  Excedrin P.M. Analgesic/Sleeping Aid Tablets and Caplets
  Femcet Capsules
  FEVERALL Children's Suppositories
  FEVERALL Infant's Suppositories
  FEVERALL Junior Strength Suppositories
  FEVERALL Sprinkle Caps Powder
  Fioricet Tablets
  Fioricet with Codeine Capsules
  Gelpirin Tablets
  Gelpirin CCF Tablets
  Hyco-Pap Capsules
  Hydrocet Capsules
  Hydrocodone Bitartrate and APAP Tablets
  Hydrocodone with APAP Tablets
  Lorcet Plus
  Lorcet-HD
  Lorcet 10/650
  Lortab 2.5/500 Tablets
  Lortab 5/500 Tablets
  Lortab 7.5/500 Tablets
  Lortab Elixir
  Lurline PMS Tablets
  Medigesic Capsules
  Midrin Capsules
  Migralam Capsules
  Neopap Suppositories
  Norel Plus
  Pacaps Capsules
  Panacet 5/500 Tablets
  Percocet Tablets
  Phenaphen with Codeine Capsules
  Phrenilin Forte Capsules
  Phrenilin Tablets
  Propoxyphene Hydrochloride & Acetaminophen Tablets
  Propoxyphene Napsylate/Acetaminophen Tablets
  Propoxyphene Napsylate & Acetaminophen Tablets
  Protid Tablets
  Redutemp
  Repan Tablets and Capsules
  REPAN-CF Tablets
  Roxicet 5/500 Caplets (Oxycodone & Acetaminophen)
  Roxicet Tablets & Oral Solution (Oxycodone & Acetaminophen)
  Sedapap Tablets 50 mg/650 mg
  Sine-Aid Maximum Strength Sinus Headache Gelcaps, Caplets and Tablets
  Sinulin Tablets

  Sinutab Maximum Strength Sinus Allergy Tablets
  Sinutab Sinus Maximum Strength Without Drowsiness Tablet
  Sinutab Regular Strength Without Drowsiness Tablet
  Sudafed Cold & Cough Liquid Caps
  Sudafed Severe Cold Formula Tablets
  Talacen
  Tencon Capsules
  TYLENOL acetaminophen Children's Chewable Tablets & Elixir
  TYLENOL acetaminophen Children's Suspension Liquid
  TYLENOL Allergy Sinus NightTime Caplets
  Tylenol with Codeine Elixir
  Tylenol with Codeine Phosphate Tablets
  Children's TYLENOL Cold Multi-Symptom Liquid Formula and Chewable Tablets
  Children's TYLENOL Cold Multi-Symptom Plus Cough Liquid Formula and Chewable Tablets
  TYLENOL Flu NightTime, Maximum Strength, Gelcaps
  TYLENOL Cold Hot Medication Packets
  TYLENOL Cold Medication No Drowsiness Formula Gelcaps and Caplets
  TYLENOL Extended Relief Caplets
  TYLENOL, Extra Strength, acetaminophen Adult Liquid Pain Reliever
  TYLENOL, Extra Strength, acetaminophen Gelcaps, Geltabs, Caplets, Tablets
  TYLENOL, Extra Strength, Headache Plus Pain Reliever with Antacid Caplets
  TYLENOL, Infants' Drops and Infants' Suspension Drops
  TYLENOL, Junior Strength, acetaminophen Coated Caplets, Grape and Fruit Chewable Tablets
  TYLENOL Maximum Strength Allergy Sinus Medication Gelcaps and Caplets
  TYLENOL Maximum Strength Allergy Sinus Nighttime Medicine
  TYLENOL Cough Multi-Symptom Medication
  TYLENOL Cough Multi-Symptom Medication with Decongestant
  TYLENOL Flu Maximum Strength Gelcaps
  TYLENOL Cold Multi-Symptom Formula Medication Tablets and Caplets
  TYLENOL, Maximum Strength, Sinus Medication Geltabs, Gelcaps, Caplets and Tablets
  TYLENOL Flu NightTime, Maximum Strength, Hot Medication
  TYLENOL, Regular Strength, acetaminophen Caplets and Tablets
  TYLENOL PM, Extra Strength Pain Reliever/Sleep Aid Caplets, Gelcaps, Geltabs, Tablets
  Tylox Capsules

Unisom With Pain Relief-Nighttime Sleep Aid
  and Pain Reliever
Vicodin Tablets
Vicodin ES Tablets
Wygesic Tablets
Acetaminophen and Codeine Phosphate Oral
  Soln. (BARRE-NATIONAL INC.)
Acetaminophen and Codeine Phosphate Tablets
  (ROXANE LABORATORIES, INC.)
Acetaminophen Oral Solution (Cherry)
  (ROXANE LABORATORIES, INC.)
Acetaminophen Tablets and Caplets, USP
  (WARNER CHILCOTT LABORATORIES)
Acetasol (BARRE-NATIONAL INC.)
Acetasol HC (BARRE-NATIONAL INC.)
ACETAZOLAMIDE
  Diamox Parenteral
  Diamox Sequels (Sustained Release)
  Diamox Tablets

ACETIC ACID
  Acetasol
  Acetasol HC
  Aci-Jel Therapeutic Vaginal Jelly
  Otic Domeboro Solution
  Otic Tridesilon Solution 0.05%
  VōSoLä Otic Solution
  VōSoL Otic Solution

ACETOHYDROXAMIC ACID
  Lithostat

ACETYL SULFISOXAZOLE
  Gantrisin Pediatric Suspension
  Gantrisin Syrup
  Pediazole

ACETYLCYSTEINE
  Acetylcysteine Solution, USP
  Mucosil Acetylcysteine Solution
Acetylcysteine Solution, USP
  (CHIRON THERAPEUTICS)
Achromycin V Capsules
  (LEDERLE STANDARD PRODUCTS)
Achromycin 3% Ointment
  (LEDERLE STANDARD PRODUCTS)
Achromycin Ophthalmic Ointment 1%
  (LEDERLE LABORATORIES)
Achromycin Ophthalmic Suspension 1%
  (LEDERLE LABORATORIES)
Acid Mantle Creme
  (SANDOZ PHARMACEUTICALS/ CONSUMER
  DIVISION)
Aci-Jel Therapeutic Vaginal Jelly
  (ORTHO PHARMACEUTICAL CORPORATION)
Aclovate Cream (GLAXO DERMATOLOGY)
Aclovate Ointment (GLAXO DERMATOLOGY)

ACRIVASTINE
  Semprex-D Capsules
  Semprex-D
Acthar
  (RHONE-POULENC RORER PHARMACEUTICALS INC.)
ActHIB (CONNAUGHT LABORATORIES, INC.)
Actidose with Sorbitol
  (PADDOCK LABORATORIES, INC.)
Actidose-Aqua (PADDOCK LABORATORIES, INC.)
Actifed Allergy Daytime/Nighttime Caplets
  (WARNER WELLCOME)
Actifed Plus Tablets and Caplets
  (WARNER WELLCOME)
Actifed with Codeine Cough Syrup
  (BURROUGHS WELLCOME CO.)
Actifed Sinus Daytime/Nighttime Caplets and
  Tablets (WARNER WELLCOME)
Actifed Syrup (WARNER WELLCOME)
Actifed Tablets (WARNER WELLCOME)
Actigall Capsules (SUMMIT PHARMACEUTICALS)

Actimmune (GENENTECH, INC.)
Actinex Cream (REED & CARNRICK)
Activase (GENENTECH, INC.)
Acular (ALLERGAN, INC.)
Acular
  (FISONS CORPORATION PRESCRIPTION PRODUCTS)
ACUPRIN 81 Adult Low Dose Aspirin
  (RICHWOOD PHARMACEUTICAL COMPANY, INC.)
Acutrim 16 Hour Steady Control
  Appetite Suppressant
  (CIBA CONSUMER PHARMACEUTICALS)
Acutrim Late Day Strength Appetite Suppressant
  (CIBA CONSUMER PHARMACEUTICALS)
Acutrim II Maximum Strength
  Appetite Suppressant
  (CIBA CONSUMER PHARMACEUTICALS)

ACYCLOVIR
  Zovirax Capsules
  Zovirax Ointment 5%
  Zovirax Suspension
  Zovirax Tablets
  Zovirax Suspension

ACYCLOVIR SODIUM
  Zovirax Sterile Powder
Adagen (pegademase bovine) Injection
  (ENZON, INC.)
Adalat Capsules (10 mg and 20 mg)
  (MILES INC. PHARMACEUTICAL DIVISION)
Adalat CC
  (MILES INC. PHARMACEUTICAL DIVISION)
Adapin Capsules
  (LOTUS BIOCHEMICAL CORPORATION)
Adderall Tablets
  (RICHWOOD PHARMACEUTICAL COMPANY, INC.)
Adeflor M Tablets (KENWOOD LABORATORIES)
Adenocard Injection (FUJISAWA USA, INC.)

ADENOSINE
  Adenocard Injection

ADENOSINE TRIPHOSPHATE
  ATP (Enteric Adenosine Triphosphate)
Adipex-P Tablets and Capsules
  (TEVA PHARMACEUTICALS)

ADRENOCORTICOTROPIC HORMONE
  Acthar
  Cortrosyn
  HP Acthar Gel
Adriamycin PFS
  (PHARMACIA ADRIA PHARMACIA INC.)
Adriamycin RDF
  (PHARMACIA ADRIA PHARMACIA INC.)
Advera Specialized Complete Nutrition
  (ROSS PRODUCTS DIVISION)
Children's Advil Suspension
  (WYETH-AYERST LABORATORIES)
AeroBid Inhaler System
  (FOREST PHARMACEUTICALS, INC.)
Aerobid-M Inhaler System
  (FOREST PHARMACEUTICALS, INC.)
AeroChamber with Mask
  (FOREST PHARMACEUTICALS, INC.)
Aerolate Jr. T.D. Capsules
  (FLEMING & COMPANY)
Aerolate Liquid (FLEMING & COMPANY)
Aerolate Sr. T.D. Capsules
  (FLEMING & COMPANY)
Aerolate III T.D. Capsules
  (FLEMING & COMPANY)
Aeroseb-Dex Topical Aerosol Spray
  (ALLERGAN HERBERT)
Aeroseb-HC Topical Aerosol Spray
  (ALLERGAN HERBERT)

Aflaxen Tablets
  (INTERNATIONAL ETHICAL LABS.)
Agoral Liquid (WARNER WELLCOME)
AH-CHEW Chewable Tablets
  (WE PHARMACEUTICALS, INC.)
AH-CHEW D Chewable Tablets
  (WE PHARMACEUTICALS, INC.)
Airet Solution for Inhalation
  (ADAMS LABORATORIES, INC.)
Akne-mycin Ointment
  (HERMAL PHARMACEUTICAL LABORATORIES, INC.)
Akineton Injection
  (KNOLL PHARMACEUTICAL COMPANY)
Akineton Tablets
  (KNOLL PHARMACEUTICAL COMPANY)
Albatussin SR Caplets (RICO PHARMACAL)

ALBUMIN (HUMAN)
  Albumin (Human), USP 5% Solution,
    Albumarc 5%
  Albumin (Human) 5%
  Albumin (Human), USP 25% Solution,
    Albumarc 25%
  Albumin (Human) 25%
  Albuminar-5, Albumin (Human) U.S.P. 5%
  Albuminar-25, Albumin (Human) U.S.P. 25%
  Albutein 5% Albumin (Human)
  Albutein 25% Albumin (Human)
  Buminate 5%, Albumin (Human), USP,
    5% Solution
  Buminate 25%, Albumin (Human), USP,
    25% Solution
Albumin (Human), USP 5% Solution,
  Albumarc 5% (AMERICAN RED CROSS)
Albumin (Human) 5% (IMMUNO-U.S., INC.)
Albumin (Human), USP 25% Solution,
  Albumarc 25% (AMERICAN RED CROSS)
Albumin (Human) 25% (IMMUNO-U.S., INC.)
ALBUMINAR-5, ALBUMIN (HUMAN) U.S.P. 5%
  (ARMOUR PHARMACEUTICAL COMPANY)
Albuminar-25, Albumin (Human) U.S.P. 25%
  (ARMOUR PHARMACEUTICAL COMPANY)
Albutein 5% Albumin (Human)
  (ALPHA THERAPEUTIC CORPORATION)
Albutein 25% Albumin (Human)
  (ALPHA THERAPEUTIC CORPORATION)

ALBUTEROL
  Albuterol Tablets
  Proventil Inhalation Aerosol
  Ventolin Inhalation Aerosol and Refill

ALBUTEROL SULFATE
  Airet Solution for Inhalation
  Albuterol Sulfate Inhalation Solution
  Albuterol Sulfate Syrup
  Albuterol Sulfate Tablets
  Albuterol Sulfate Tablets
  Albuterol Sulfate Tablets
  Albuterol Sulfate Tablets, 2 + 4 mg
  Proventil Repetabs Tablets
  Proventil Solution for Inhalation 0.5%
  Proventil Inhalation Solution 0.083%
  Proventil Syrup
  Proventil Tablets
  Ventolin Inhalation Solution
  Ventolin Nebules Inhalation Solution
  Ventolin Rotacaps for Inhalation
  Ventolin Syrup
  Ventolin Tablets
  Volmax Extended-Release Tablets
Albuterol Sulfate Inhalation Solution
  (DEY LABORATORIES)
Albuterol Sulfate Syrup
  (WATSON LABORATORIES, INC.)
Albuterol Tablets
  (BIOCRAFT LABORATORIES, INC.)

Albuterol Sulfate Tablets
  (LEDERLE STANDARD PRODUCTS)
Albuterol Tablets
  (MYLAN PHARMACEUTICALS INC.)
Albuterol Sulfate Tablets
  (WARNER CHILCOTT LABORATORIES)
Albuterol Sulfate Tablets, 2 + 4 mg
  (NOVOPHARM, USA INC.)

ALCLOMETASONE DIPROPIONATE
  Aclovate Cream
  Aclovate Ointment
Alconefrin 12 Drops
  (POLYMEDICA PHARMACEUTICALS (U.S.A.), INC.)
Alconefrin 25 Drops
  (POLYMEDICA PHARMACEUTICALS (U.S.A.), INC.)
Alconefrin 50 Drops
  (POLYMEDICA PHARMACEUTICALS (U.S.A.), INC.)
Alconefrin 25 Spray
  (POLYMEDICA PHARMACEUTICALS (U.S.A.), INC.)
Aldactazide (G.D. SEARLE & CO.)
Aldactone (G.D. SEARLE & CO.)

ALDESLEUKIN
  Proleukin for Injection
Aldoclor Tablets (MERCK & CO., INC.)
Aldomet Ester HCl Injection
  (MERCK & CO., INC.)
Aldomet Oral Suspension (MERCK & CO., INC.)
Aldomet Tablets (MERCK & CO., INC.)
Aldoril Tablets (MERCK & CO., INC.)
Aleve (PROCTER & GAMBLE)
Alfenta Injection (JANSSEN PHARMACEUTICA INC.)

ALFENTANIL HYDROCHLORIDE
  Alfenta Injection
Alferon N Injection
  (THE PURDUE FREDERICK COMPANY)

ALGLUCERASE
  Ceredase Injection
**Alimentum Protein Hydrolysate Formula
  With Iron** (ROSS PRODUCTS DIVISION)
**AlitraQ Specialized Elemental Nutrition With
  Glutamine** (ROSS PRODUCTS DIVISION)
Alka-Mints Chewable Antacid
  (MILES INC. CONSUMER HEALTHCARE PRODUCTS)
Alka-Seltzer Effervescent Antacid
  (MILES INC. CONSUMER HEALTHCARE PRODUCTS)
**Alka-Seltzer Effervescent Antacid
  and Pain Reliever**
  (MILES INC. CONSUMER HEALTHCARE PRODUCTS)
**Alka-Seltzer Extra Strength Effervescent Antacid
  and Pain Reliever**
  (MILES INC. CONSUMER HEALTHCARE PRODUCTS)
**Alka-Seltzer Lemon Lime Effervescent Antacid
  and Pain Reliever**
  (MILES INC. CONSUMER HEALTHCARE PRODUCTS)
Alka-Seltzer Plus Cold Medicine
  (MILES INC. CONSUMER HEALTHCARE PRODUCTS)
Alka-Seltzer Plus Cold & Cough LiquiGels
  (MILES INC. CONSUMER HEALTHCARE PRODUCTS)
Alka-Seltzer Plus Cold & Cough Medicine
  (MILES INC. CONSUMER HEALTHCARE PRODUCTS)
Alka-Seltzer Plus Liqui-Gels
  (MILES INC. CONSUMER HEALTHCARE PRODUCTS)
Alka-Seltzer Plus Night-Time Cold Medicine
  (MILES INC. CONSUMER HEALTHCARE PRODUCTS)
Alka-Seltzer Plus Night-Time Liqui-Gels
  (MILES INC. CONSUMER HEALTHCARE PRODUCTS)
Alka-Seltzer Plus Sinus Medicine
  (MILES INC. CONSUMER HEALTHCARE PRODUCTS)
Alkeran for Injection
  (BURROUGHS WELLCOME CO.)

Alkeran Tablets (BURROUGHS WELLCOME CO.)

ALLANTOIN
  Herpecin-L Cold Sore Lip Balm Stick
  Woun' dress, Natural Collagen Hydrogel Wound
    Dressing
**All-Flex Arcing Spring Diaphragm (See Ortho
  Diaphragm Kit)**
  (ORTHO PHARMACEUTICAL CORPORATION)
Alomide (ALCON LABORATORIES, INC.)

ALLOPURINOL
  Allopurinol Tablets
  Allopurinol Tablets
  Allopurinol Tablets
  Zyloprim Tablets
Allopurinol Tablets
  (MYLAN PHARMACEUTICALS INC.)
Allopurinol Tablets
  (PAR PHARMACEUTICAL, INC.)
Allopurinol Tablets
  (WARNER CHILCOTT LABORATORIES)

ALOE
  Hydrocortisone Acetate 0.5% Cream w/Aloe

ALOE VERA
  Dermaide Aloe Cream
Alophen Pills (WARNER WELLCOME)
Alpha Keri Moisture Rich Body Oil
  (BRISTOL-MYERS PRODUCTS)
Alpha Keri Moisture Rich Cleansing Bar
  (BRISTOL-MYERS PRODUCTS)
AlphaNine-SD Coagulation Factor IX (Human)
  (ALPHA THERAPEUTIC CORPORATION)

$ALPHA_1$ -PROTEINASE INHIBITOR (HUMAN)
  Prolastin $Alpha_1$ -Proteinase Inhibitor (Human)
Alphatrex Cream, Ointment & Lotion
  (SAVAGE LABORATORIES)

ALPRAZOLAM
  Alprazolam Tablets
  Alprazolam Tablets
  Alprazolam Tablets
  Alprazolam Tablets, .25 mg
  Alprazolam Tablets, .5 mg
  Alprazolam Tablets, 1 mg
  Alprazolam Tablets 0.25 mg
  Alprazolam Tablets 0.5 mg
  Alprazolam Tablets 1 mg
  Xanax Tablets
Alprazolam Tablets
  (LEDERLE STANDARD PRODUCTS)
Alprazolam Tablets
  (MYLAN PHARMACEUTICALS INC.)
Alprazolam Tablets
  (ROXANE LABORATORIES, INC.)
Alprazolam Tablets, .25 mg
  (NOVOPHARM, USA INC.)
Alprazolam Tablets, .5 mg
  (NOVOPHARM, USA INC.)
Alprazolam Tablets, 1 mg
  (NOVOPHARM, USA INC.)
Alprazolam Tablets 0.25 mg
  (PAR PHARMACEUTICAL, INC.)
Alprazolam Tablets 0.5 mg
  (PAR PHARMACEUTICAL, INC.)
Alprazolam Tablets 1 mg
  (PAR PHARMACEUTICAL, INC.)

ALPROSTADIL
  Prostin VR Pediatric Sterile Solution
Alramucil Instant Mix, Orange
  (ALRA LABORATORIES, INC.)
Alramucil Instant Mix, Regular
  (ALRA LABORATORIES, INC.)

Altace Capsules
  (HOECHST-ROUSSEL PHARMACEUTICALS INC.)

ALTEPLASE, RECOMBINANT
  Activase
ALternaGEL Liquid
  (JOHNSON & JOHNSON • MERCK CONSUMER)

ALTRETAMINE
  Hexalen Capsules
Alu-Cap Capsules (3M PHARMACEUTICALS)
Aludrox Oral Suspension
  (WYETH-AYERST LABORATORIES)
Alumina and Magnesia Oral Suspension
  (ROXANE LABORATORIES, INC.)
**Alumina, Magnesia, and Simethicone Oral
  Suspension I** (ROXANE LABORATORIES, INC.)

ALUMINUM ACETATE
  Otic Domeboro Solution

ALUMINUM CARBONATE GEL
  Basaljel Capsules
  Basaljel Suspension
  Basaljel Tablets

ALUMINUM CHLORHYDROXIDE
  Pedi-Pro Topical Powder

ALUMINUM CHLORIDE
  Drysol
  Xerac AC

ALUMINUM CHLOROHYDRATE
  Ostiderm Roll On

ALUMINUM HYDROXIDE
  ALternaGEL Liquid
  Alumina and Magnesia Oral Suspension
  Alumina, Magnesia, and
    Simethicone Oral Suspension I
  Gelusil Liquid
  Gelusil Tablets
  Maalox Antacid Plus Anti-Gas
  Extra Strength Maalox Antacid
    Plus Anti-Gas Suspension
  Maalox TC Suspension Antacid

ALUMINUM HYDROXIDE GEL
  Alu-Cap Capsules
  Aludrox Oral Suspension
  Aluminum Hydroxide Gel Concentrated
  Aluminum Hydroxide Gel
  Aluminum Hydroxide Gel
  Alu-Tab Tablets
  Amphojel Suspension
  Amphojel Suspension without Flavor
  Amphojel Tablets
  Arthritis Pain Ascriptin
  Regular Strength Ascriptin Tablets
  Dialume Capsules
  Extra Strength Maalox Antacid
    Plus Anti-Gas Tablets
  Mylanta Liquid
  Mylanta Tablets
  Mylanta Double Strength Liquid
  Mylanta Double Strength Tablets
Aluminum Hydroxide Gel Concentrated
  (ROXANE LABORATORIES, INC.)
Aluminum Hydroxide Gel
  (ROXANE LABORATORIES, INC.)
Aluminum Hydroxide Gel (BARRE-NATIONAL INC.)

ALUMINUM SULFATE
  Pedi-Boro Soak Paks
Alupent Inhalation Aerosol
  (BOEHRINGER INGELHEIM PHARMACEUTICALS, INC.)
Alupent Inhalation Solution
  (BOEHRINGER INGELHEIM PHARMACEUTICALS, INC.)

UNDERLINE DENOTES GENERIC NAME

Alupent Syrup
(BOEHRINGER INGELHEIM PHARMACEUTICALS, INC.)
Alupent Tablets
(BOEHRINGER INGELHEIM PHARMACEUTICALS, INC.)
Alu-Tab Tablets (3M PHARMACEUTICALS)

AMANTADINE HYDROCHLORIDE
   Amantadine Capsules
   Amantadine HCl Capsules
   Amantadine HCl Syrup 50 mg/5 mL
Amantadine Capsules
(DURAMED PHARMACEUTICALS, INC.)
Amantadine HCl Capsules
(WARNER CHILCOTT LABORATORIES)
Amantadine HCl Syrup 50 mg/5 mL
(BARRE-NATIONAL INC.)
Ambenyl Cough Syrup
(FOREST PHARMACEUTICALS, INC.)

AMCINONIDE
   Cyclocort Topical Cream 0.1%
   Cyclocort Topical Lotion 0.1%
   Cyclocort Topical Ointment 0.1%
Ambien Tablets (G.D. SEARLE & CO.)
Amen Tablets (CARNRICK LABORATORIES, INC.)
Americaine Anesthetic Lubricant
(FISONS CORPORATION PRESCRIPTION PRODUCTS)
Americaine Otic Topical Anesthetic Ear Drops
(FISONS CORPORATION PRESCRIPTION PRODUCTS)
Amicar Syrup, Tablets, and Injection
(IMMUNEX CORPORATION)
Amidate (ABBOTT LABORATORIES)

AMIKACIN SULFATE
   Amikacin Sulfate Injection, USP
   Amikin Injectable
Amikacin Sulfate Injection, USP
(ELKINS-SINN, INC.)
Amikin Injectable (APOTHECON)

AMILORIDE HYDROCHLORIDE
   Amiloride Hydrochloride and
      Hydrochlorothiazide Tablets
   Amiloride Hydrochloride and
      Hydrochlorothiazide Tablets
   Amiloride Hydrochloride and
      Hydrochlorothiazide Tablets, U.S.P.
   Amiloride HCl and Hydrochlorothiazide Tablets
   Midamor Tablets
   Moduretic Tablets
Amiloride Hydrochloride and
Hydrochlorothiazide Tablets
(BIOCRAFT LABORATORIES, INC.)
Amiloride Hydrochloride and
Hydrochlorothiazide Tablets
(MYLAN PHARMACEUTICALS INC.)
Amiloride Hydrochloride and
Hydrochlorothiazide Tablets, U.S.P.
(WEST POINT PHARMA)
Amiloride HCl and Hydrochlorothiazide Tablets
(WARNER CHILCOTT LABORATORIES)
Amin-Aid Instant Drink
(R&D LABORATORIES, INC.)

AMINO ACID PREPARATIONS
   Amin-Aid Instant Drink
   Amino-Cerv
   Aminolete Capsules
   Aminomine Capsules
   Aminoplex Capsules
   Aminostasis Capsules
   Aminotate Capsules
   Aminovirox Capsules
   L-Carnitine 250mg and 500mg Tablets
   Marlyn Formula 50 Capsules
   Nephramine
   Pro-Hepatone Capsules

AMINOSALICYLIC ACID
   PASER Granules

AMINOBENZOATE POTASSIUM
   Potaba

AMINOCAPROIC ACID
   Amicar Syrup, Tablets, and Injection
   Aminocaproic Acid Injection
Aminocaproic Acid Injection (ELKINS-SINN, INC.)
Amino-Cerv (MILEX PRODUCTS, INC.)

AMINOGLUTETHIMIDE
   Cytadren Tablets

AMINOHIPPURATE SODIUM
   Aminohippurate Sodium Injection
Aminohippurate Sodium Injection
(MERCK & CO., INC.)
Aminolete Capsules
(TYSON AND ASSOCIATES, INC.)
Aminomine Capsules
(TYSON AND ASSOCIATES, INC.)

AMINOPHYLLINE
   Aminophylline Oral Liquid-Dye Free 105 mg/5 mL
   Aminophylline Tablets & Oral Solution
   Mudrane Tablets
   Mudrane GG-2 Tablets
Aminophylline Oral Liquid-Dye Free 105 mg/5 mL
(BARRE-NATIONAL INC.)
Aminophylline Tablets & Oral Solution
(ROXANE LABORATORIES, INC.)
Aminoplex Capsules
(TYSON AND ASSOCIATES, INC.)
Aminostasis Capsules
(TYSON AND ASSOCIATES, INC.)
Aminotate Capsules
(TYSON AND ASSOCIATES, INC.)
Aminovirox Capsules
(TYSON AND ASSOCIATES, INC.)
Aminoxin Tablets (Coenzymatic B$_6$)
(TYSON AND ASSOCIATES, INC.)

AMIODARONE HYDROCHLORIDE
   Cordarone Tablets

AMITRIPTYLINE HYDROCHLORIDE
   Amitriptyline Hydrochloride Tablets
   Amitriptyline Hydrochloride Tablets
   Amitriptyline Hydrochloride Tablets
   Chlordiazepoxide & Amitriptyline
      Hydrochloride Tablets
   Elavil Injection
   Elavil Tablets
   Endep Tablets
   Etrafon-A Tablets (4-10)
   Etrafon Forte Tablets (4-25)
   Etrafon 2-10 Tablets (2-10)
   Etrafon Tablets (2-25)
   Limbitrol DS Tablets
   Limbitrol Tablets
   Perphenazine & Amitriptyline
      Hydrochloride Tablets
   Perphenazine/Amitriptyline HCl Tablets
   Triavil Tablets
Amitriptyline Hydrochloride Tablets
(BIOCRAFT LABORATORIES, INC.)
Amitriptyline Hydrochloride Tablets
(MYLAN PHARMACEUTICALS INC.)
Amitriptyline Hydrochloride Tablets
(ROXANE LABORATORIES, INC.)

AMLODIPINE BESYLATE
   Norvasc Tablets

AMMONIATED MERCURY
   Unguentum Bossi

AMMONIUM ALUM
   Massengill Powder

AMMONIUM LACTATE
   Lac-Hydrin 12% Lotion

AMOXAPINE
   Amoxapine Tablets
   Amoxapine Tablets, USP
   Asendin Tablets
Amoxapine Tablets
(WARNER CHILCOTT LABORATORIES)
Amoxapine Tablets, USP
(WATSON LABORATORIES, INC.)

AMOXICILLIN
   Amoxil Capsules and Chewable Tablets
   Amoxil Pediatric Drops, Powder for Oral
      Suspension

AMOXICILLIN TRIHYDRATE
   Amoxicillin Capsules
   Amoxicillin Capsules
   Amoxicillin Capsules, Oral Suspension
   Amoxicillin Capsules USP and Oral Suspension,
      Caps 125, 250, O.S. 125/5 mL, 250/5 mL
   Amoxicillin for Oral Suspension
   Amoxicillin for Oral Suspension
   Amoxicillin Tablets (Chewable)
   Amoxicillin Trihydrate Capsules & for Oral
      Suspension
   Augmentin Powder for Oral Suspension
   Augmentin Tablets and Chewable Tablets
   Moxilin Capsules
   Moxilin O/S
   Wymox Capsules
   Wymox for Oral Suspension
Amoxicillin Capsules
(BIOCRAFT LABORATORIES, INC.)
Amoxicillin Capsules
(WARNER CHILCOTT LABORATORIES)
Amoxicillin Capsules, Oral Suspension
(LEDERLE STANDARD PRODUCTS)
Amoxicillin Capsules USP and Oral Suspension,
Caps 125, 250, O.S. 125/5 mL, 250/5 mL
(NOVOPHARM, USA INC.)
Amoxicillin for Oral Suspension
(WARNER CHILCOTT LABORATORIES)
Amoxicillin for Oral Suspension
(BIOCRAFT LABORATORIES, INC.)
Amoxicillin Tablets (Chewable)
(BIOCRAFT LABORATORIES, INC.)
Amoxicillin Trihydrate Capsules
& for Oral Suspension
(MYLAN PHARMACEUTICALS INC.)
Amoxil Capsules and Chewable Tablets
(SMITHKLINE BEECHAM PHARMACEUTICALS)
Amoxil Pediatric Drops, Powder
for Oral Suspension
(SMITHKLINE BEECHAM PHARMACEUTICALS)

AMPHETAMINE ASPARTATE
   Adderall Tablets

AMPHETAMINE RESINS
   Biphetamine Capsules

AMPHETAMINE SULFATE
   Adderall Tablets
Amphojel Suspension
(WYETH-AYERST LABORATORIES)
Amphojel Suspension without Flavor
(WYETH-AYERST LABORATORIES)
Amphojel Tablets
(WYETH-AYERST LABORATORIES)

AMPHOTERICIN B
   Fungizone Intravenous

AMPICILLIN
   Ampicillin Capsules
   Ampicillin Capsules
   Ampicillin for Oral Suspension

Ampicillin for Oral Suspension
Ampicillin-Probenecid for Oral Suspension
Omnipen Capsules
Omnipen for Oral Suspension
Ampicillin Capsules
(BIOCRAFT LABORATORIES, INC.)
Ampicillin Capsules
(WARNER CHILCOTT LABORATORIES)
Ampicillin for Oral Suspension
(BIOCRAFT LABORATORIES, INC.)
Ampicillin for Oral Suspension
(WARNER CHILCOTT LABORATORIES)
Ampicillin-Probenecid for Oral Suspension
(BIOCRAFT LABORATORIES, INC.)

AMPICILLIN SODIUM
Omnipen-N Injection
Unasyn

AMPICILLIN TRIHYDRATE
Ampicillin Trihydrate Capsules, Oral Suspension
Ampicillin Trihydrate Capsules
& for Oral Suspension
Ampicillin Trihydrate Capsules, Oral Suspension
(LEDERLE STANDARD PRODUCTS)
**Ampicillin Trihydrate Capsules & for Oral
Suspension** (MYLAN PHARMACEUTICALS INC.)

AMRINONE LACTATE
Inocor Lactate Injection
AMYLASE
CREON 10 Capsules

AMYLOLYTIC ENZYME
Arco-Lase Tablets
Cotazym
Kutrase Capsules
Ku-Zyme Capsules
Ku-Zyme HP Capsules
Anadrol-50 Tablets
(SYNTEX PUERTO RICO, INC.)
Anafranil Capsules (BASEL PHARMACEUTICALS)
Ana-Kit Anaphylaxis Emergency Treatment Kit
(MILES INC., PHARMACEUTICAL DIVISION
ALLERGY PRODUCTS)
Analgesic Balm (BARRE-NATIONAL INC.)
Analgesic Balm-Greaseless (BARRE-NATIONAL INC.)
Analpram-HC Rectal Cream 1% and 2.5%
(FERNDALE LABORATORIES, INC.)
Anaplex HD Cough Syrup
(ECR PHARMACEUTICALS)
Anaprox and Anaprox DS Tablets
(SYNTEX PUERTO RICO, INC.)
Anaspaz Tablets (B. F. ASCHER & COMPANY, INC.)
Anatuss DM Syrup
(MAYRAND PHARMACEUTICALS, INC.)
Anatuss DM Tablets
(MAYRAND PHARMACEUTICALS, INC.)
Anatuss LA Tablets
(MAYRAND PHARMACEUTICALS, INC.)
Ancef Injection
(SMITHKLINE BEECHAM PHARMACEUTICALS)
Ancobon Capsules (ROCHE LABORATORIES)
Android Capsules, 10 mg
(ICN PHARMACEUTICALS, INC.)
Android-10 Tablets
(ICN PHARMACEUTICALS, INC.)
Android-25 Tablets
(ICN PHARMACEUTICALS, INC.)
Anectine Flo-Pack (BURROUGHS WELLCOME CO.)
Anectine Injection (BURROUGHS WELLCOME CO.)
Anestacon Jelly
(POLYMEDICA PHARMACEUTICALS (U.S.A.), INC.)
Anexsia 5/500 Tablets
(BOEHRINGER MANNHEIM PHARMACEUTICALS)
Anexsia 7.5/650 Tablets
(BOEHRINGER MANNHEIM PHARMACEUTICALS)

ANISTREPLASE
Eminase
Anolor 300 (BLANSETT PHARMACAL)
Ansaid Tablets (THE UPJOHN COMPANY)
Antabuse Tablets
(WYETH-AYERST LABORATORIES)

ANTERIOR PITUITARY HORMONES
Acthar
HP Acthar Gel

ANTHRALIN
Drithocreme 0.1%, 0.25%, 0.5%, 1.0% (HP)
Dritho-Scalp 0.25%, 0.5%
Anti-Fungal Cream (BARRE-NATIONAL INC.)

ANTIHEMOPHILIC FACTOR (HUMAN)
Antihemophilic Factor (Human), Method M,
Monoclonal Purified
Hemofil M, Antihemophilic Factor (Human),
Method M, Monoclonal Purified
Humate-P, Antihemophilic Factor (Human),
Pasteurized
Koāte-HP Antihemophilic Factor (Human)
Monoclate-P Factor VIII:C, Pasteurized,
Monoclonal Antibody Purified Antihemophilic
Factor (Human)
Profilate OSD Antihemophilic Factor (Human)
**Antihemophilic Factor (Human), Method M,
Monoclonal Purified** (AMERICAN RED CROSS)

ANTIHEMOPHILIC FACTOR (PORCINE)
HYATE: C Antihemophilic Factor (Porcine)

ANTIHEMOPHILIC FACTOR (RECOMBINANT)
Bioclate, Antihemophilic Factor (Recombinant)
Helixate, Antihemophilic Factor (Recombinant)
KOGENATE Antihemophilic Factor
(Recombinant)

ANTI-INHIBITOR COAGULANT COMPLEX
Autoplex T, Anti-Inhibitor Coagulant Complex,
Dried, Heat Treated
Antilirium Injectable
(FOREST PHARMACEUTICALS, INC.)
ANTIOX Capsules
(MAYRAND PHARMACEUTICALS, INC.)

ANTIPYRINE
Auralgan Otic Solution
Auroto Otic Solution
Tympagesic Ear Drops

ANTITHROMBIN III
THROMBATE III Antithrombin III (Human)
Antivenin (Black Widow Spider)
(MERCK & CO., INC.)
Antivenin (Crotalidae) Polyvalent
(WYETH-AYERST LABORATORIES)

ANTIVENIN (CROTALIDAE) POLYVALENT
Antivenin (Crotalidae) Polyvalent
Antivenin (Micrurus fulvius)
(WYETH-AYERST LABORATORIES)

ANTIVENIN (MICRURUS FULVIUS)
Antivenin (Micrurus fulvius)
**Antivert, Antivert/25 Tablets, & Antivert/50
Tablets** (ROERIG DIVISION)
Antrocol Elixir (ECR PHARMACEUTICALS)
Anturane Capsules
(CIBA PHARMACEUTICAL COMPANY)
Anturane Tablets
(CIBA PHARMACEUTICAL COMPANY)
Anusol Hemorrhoidal Ointment
(WARNER WELLCOME)
Anusol HC-1 Ointment (WARNER WELLCOME)
Anusol-HC Cream 2.5% (PARKE-DAVIS)
Anusol-HC Suppositories (PARKE-DAVIS)
Anusol Suppositories (WARNER WELLCOME)

Apatate Liquid/Tablets
(KENWOOD LABORATORIES)
Apatate Liquid with Fluoride
(KENWOOD LABORATORIES)
Apatate Forte Liquid (KENWOOD LABORATORIES)
Aphrodyne (STAR PHARMACEUTICALS, INC.)
Apresazide Capsules
(CIBA PHARMACEUTICAL COMPANY)
Apresoline Hydrochloride Tablets
(CIBA PHARMACEUTICAL COMPANY)
Aquachloral Supprettes Suppositories
(POLYMEDICA PHARMACEUTICALS (U.S.A.), INC.)
AquaMEPHYTON Injection (MERCK & CO., INC.)
Aquanil Lotion (PERSON & COVEY, INC.)
Aquaphor Healing Ointment (BEIERSDORF INC)
Aquaphor Healing Ointment, Original Formula
(BEIERSDORF INC)
Aquasol A Vitamin A Capsules, USP
(ASTRA USA, INC.)
Aquasol A Parenteral, USP (ASTRA USA, INC.)
AquaTar Therapeutic Tar Gel
(ALLERGAN HERBERT)
Aquatensen Tablets (WALLACE LABORATORIES)
Aralen Hydrochloride Injection
(SANOFI WINTHROP PHARMACEUTICALS)
Aralen Phosphate Tablets
(SANOFI WINTHROP PHARMACEUTICALS)
Aramine Injection (MERCK & CO., INC.)
Arco-Lase Plus Tablets
(ARCO PHARMACEUTICALS, INC.)
Arco-Lase Tablets
(ARCO PHARMACEUTICALS, INC.)
Arduan (ORGANON INC.)
Aredia for Injection
(CIBA PHARMACEUTICAL COMPANY)
Arfonad Ampuls (ROCHE LABORATORIES)
Aristocort Suspension (Forte Parenteral)
(FUJISAWA USA, INC.)
Aristocort Suspension (Intralesional)
(FUJISAWA USA, INC.)
Aristocort Tablets (FUJISAWA USA, INC.)
Aristocort A Topical Cream
(FUJISAWA USA, INC.)
Aristocort A Topical Ointment
(FUJISAWA USA, INC.)
Aristospan Suspension (Intra-articular)
(FUJISAWA USA, INC.)
Aristospan Suspension (Intralesional)
(FUJISAWA USA, INC.)
Armour Thyroid Tablets
(FOREST PHARMACEUTICALS, INC.)
Aromatic Cascara Fluidextract
(ROXANE LABORATORIES, INC.)
Artane Elixir (LEDERLE LABORATORIES)
Artane Sequels (LEDERLE LABORATORIES)
Artane Tablets (LEDERLE LABORATORIES)
Asacol Delayed-Release Tablets
(PROCTER & GAMBLE PHARMACEUTICALS, INC.)
Asbron G Elixir
(SANDOZ PHARMACEUTICALS CORPORATION)
Asbron G Inlay-Tabs
(SANDOZ PHARMACEUTICALS CORPORATION)
Arthritis Pain Ascriptin
(RHONE-POULENC RORER PHARMACEUTICALS INC.)
Maximum Strength Ascriptin
(RHONE-POULENC RORER PHARMACEUTICALS INC.)
Regular Strength Ascriptin Tablets
(RHONE-POULENC RORER PHARMACEUTICALS INC.)
Asendin Tablets (LEDERLE LABORATORIES)

ASPARAGINASE
Elspar

ASPIRIN
ACUPRIN 81 Adult Low Dose Aspirin
Alka-Seltzer Effervescent Antacid and Pain
Reliever

UNDERLINE DENOTES GENERIC NAME

Alka-Seltzer Extra Strength Effervescent Antacid and Pain Reliever
Alka-Seltzer Lemon Lime Effervescent Antacid and Pain Reliever
Arthritis Pain Ascriptin
Regular Strength Ascriptin Tablets
Aspirin Tablets
Aspirin 15gr Delayed Release Tablets
Axotal
Azdone Tablets
Arthritis Strength Bufferin Analgesic Caplets
Extra Strength Bufferin Analgesic Tablets
Bufferin Analgesic Tablets and Caplets
Carisoprodol and Aspirin Tablets
Damason-P
Darvon Compound-65 Pulvules
Easprin
Ecotrin Enteric Coated Aspirin Low Strength Tablets
Ecotrin Enteric Coated Aspirin Maximum Strength Tablets and Caplets
Ecotrin Enteric Coated Aspirin Regular Strength Tablets and Caplets
Empirin Tablets
Empirin with Codeine Tablets
Equagesic Tablets
Excedrin Extra-Strength Analgesic Tablets & Caplets
Fiorinal Capsules
Fiorinal with Codeine Capsules
Fiorinal Tablets
Gelpirin Tablets
Halfprin
Lortab ASA Tablets
Methocarbamol and Aspirin Tablets
Norgesic Forte Tablets
Norgesic Tablets
PC-CAP Propoxyphene Hydrochloride Compound, USP
Panasal 5/500 Tablets
Percodan Tablets
Robaxisal Tablets
Roxiprin Tablets (Oxycodone & Aspirin)
Soma Compound w/Codeine Tablets
Soma Compound Tablets
Synalgos-DC Capsules
Talwin Compound
Aspirin-Free Cream (BARRE-NATIONAL INC.)
Aspirin Tablets
  (WARNER CHILCOTT LABORATORIES)
Aspirin 15gr Delayed Release Tablets
  (DURAMED PHARMACEUTICALS, INC.)

ASPIRIN BUFFERED
  Arthritis Pain Ascriptin
  Regular Strength Ascriptin Tablets
  Arthritis Strength Bufferin Analgesic Caplets
  Extra Strength Bufferin Analgesic Tablets
  Bufferin Analgesic Tablets and Caplets

ASPIRIN, ENTERIC COATED
  Ecotrin Enteric Coated Aspirin Low Strength Tablets
  Ecotrin Enteric Coated Aspirin Maximum Strength Tablets and Caplets
  Ecotrin Enteric Coated Aspirin Regular Strength Tablets and Caplets

ASTEMIZOLE
  Hismanal Tablets
Astramorph/PF Injection, USP (Preservative-Free) (ASTRA USA, INC.)
Atabrine Hydrochloride Tablets
  (SANOFI WINTHROP PHARMACEUTICALS)
Atamet (ATHENA NEUROSCIENCES, INC.)
Atarax Tablets & Syrup (ROERIG DIVISION)

ATENOLOL
  Atenolol and Chlorthalidone Tablets
  Atenolol Tablets
  Atenolol Tablets
  Atenolol Tablets 50 + 100
  Atenolol Tablets
  Tenoretic Tablets
  Tenormin Tablets and I.V. Injection
Atenolol and Chlorthalidone Tablets
  (MYLAN PHARMACEUTICALS INC.)
Atenolol Tablets
  (LEDERLE STANDARD PRODUCTS)
Atenolol Tablets
  (MYLAN PHARMACEUTICALS INC.)
Atenolol Tablets 50 + 100
  (NOVOPHARM, USA INC.)
Atenolol Tablets
  (DURAMED PHARMACEUTICALS, INC.)
Atgam Sterile Solution (THE UPJOHN COMPANY)
Ativan Injection
  (WYETH-AYERST LABORATORIES)
Ativan Tablets (WYETH-AYERST LABORATORIES)
Ativan in Tubex (WYETH-AYERST LABORATORIES)

ATOVAQUONE
  Mepron Tablets
Atrac-Tain, Moisturizing Cream
  (SWEEN CORPORATION)

ATRACURIUM BESYLATE
  Tracrium Injection
Atrohist Pediatric Suspension
  (ADAMS LABORATORIES, INC.)
Atrohist Plus Tablets
  (ADAMS LABORATORIES, INC.)
Atrohist Sprinkle Capsules
  (ADAMS LABORATORIES, INC.)
Atromid-S Capsules
  (WYETH-AYERST LABORATORIES)

ATROPINE SULFATE
  Antrocol Elixir
  Arco-Lase Plus Tablets
  Atrohist Plus Tablets
  Atropine Sulfate Injection
  Atropine Sulfate Injection, USP
  Bellatal Tablets
  Diphenoxylate Hydrochloride & Atropine Sulfate Tablets
  Diphenoxylate Hydrochloride & Atropine Sulfate Tablets & Oral Solution
  Donnatal Capsules
  Donnatal Elixir
  Donnatal Extentabs
  Donnatal Tablets
  Enlon-Plus Injection
  Lomotil Liquid
  Lomotil Tablets
  Motofen Tablets
  Rexatal Tablets
  Ru-Tuss Tablets
  Urised Tablets
Atropine Sulfate Injection (ELKINS-SINN, INC.)
Atropine Sulfate Injection, USP (ASTRA USA, INC.)
Atrovent Inhalation Aerosol
  (BOEHRINGER INGELHEIM PHARMACEUTICALS, INC.)
Atrovent Inhalation Solution
  (BOEHRINGER INGELHEIM PHARMACEUTICALS, INC.)

ATTAPULGITE
  Parepectolin Suspension
Attenuvax (MERCK & CO., INC.)
Augmentin Powder for Oral Suspension
  (SMITHKLINE BEECHAM PHARMACEUTICALS)
Augmentin Tablets and Chewable Tablets
  (SMITHKLINE BEECHAM PHARMACEUTICALS)
Auralgan Otic Solution
  (WYETH-AYERST LABORATORIES)

AURANOFIN
  Ridaura Capsules
Aureomycin Ophthalmic Ointment 1.0%
  (LEDERLE LABORATORIES)

AUROTHIOGLUCOSE
  Solganal Suspension
Auroto Otic Solution (BARRE-NATIONAL INC.)
Autoplex T, Anti-Inhibitor Coagulant Complex, Dried, Heat Treated
  (BAXTER HEALTHCARE CORPORATION)
Axid Pulvules (ELI LILLY AND COMPANY)
Axocet (SAVAGE LABORATORIES)
Axotal (SAVAGE LABORATORIES)
Aygestin Tablets (ESI PHARMA, INC.)
Ayr Saline Nasal Drops
  (B. F. ASCHER & COMPANY, INC.)
Ayr Saline Nasal Mist
  (B. F. ASCHER & COMPANY, INC.)
Azactam for Injection
  (BRISTOL-MYERS SQUIBB COMPANY)

AZATADINE MALEATE
  Trinalin Repetabs Tablets

AZATHIOPRINE
  Imuran Injection
  Imuran Tablets
Azdone Tablets
  (CENTRAL PHARMACEUTICALS, INC.)

AZITHROMYCIN
  Zithromax Capsules
Azmacort Oral Inhaler
  (RHONE-POULENC RORER PHARMACEUTICALS INC.)
Azo Gantanol Tablets (ROCHE LABORATORIES)
Azo Gantrisin Tablets (ROCHE LABORATORIES)
Azo-Standard Tablets
  (POLYMEDICA PHARMACEUTICALS (U.S.A.), INC.)

AZTREONAM
  Azactam for Injection
Azulfidine Tablets and EN-tabs
  (PHARMACIA ADRIA PHARMACIA INC.)

B

BCG, LIVE (INTRAVESICAL)
  TheraCys BCG Live (Intravesical)

BCG VACCINE
  BCG Vaccine, USP (Tice)
  Tice BCG, USP
BCG Vaccine, USP (Tice) (ORGANON INC.)
B & O No. 15A & No. 16A Supprettes
  (POLYMEDICA PHARMACEUTICALS (U.S.A.), INC.)

BACAMPICILLIN HYDROCHLORIDE
  Spectrobid Tablets

BACITRACIN
  Bacitracin Ointment 500 units/g
Bacitracin Ointment 500 units/g
  (BARRE-NATIONAL INC.)

BACITRACIN ZINC
  Cortisporin Ointment
  Cortisporin Ophthalmic Ointment Sterile
  Neosporin Original Ointment
  Neosporin Plus Maximum Strength Ointment
  Neosporin Ophthalmic Ointment Sterile
  Polysporin Ointment
  Polysporin Ophthalmic Ointment Sterile
  Polysporin Powder
Backache Caplets (BRISTOL-MYERS PRODUCTS)

UNDERLINE DENOTES GENERIC NAME

BACLOFEN
Baclofen Tablets
Baclofen Tablets
Lioresal Intrathecal
Lioresal Tablets
Baclofen Tablets
(BIOCRAFT LABORATORIES, INC.)
Baclofen Tablets
(WARNER CHILCOTT LABORATORIES)
Bactine Antiseptic/Anesthetic First Aid Liquid
(MILES INC. CONSUMER HEALTHCARE PRODUCTS)
Bactine First Aid Antibiotic Plus Anesthetic Ointment
(MILES INC. CONSUMER HEALTHCARE PRODUCTS)
Maximum Strength Bactine Hydrocortisone Anti-Itch Cream 1.0%
(MILES INC. CONSUMER HEALTHCARE PRODUCTS)
Bactocill Capsules
(SMITHKLINE BEECHAM PHARMACEUTICALS)
Bactrim DS Tablets (ROCHE LABORATORIES)
Bactrim I.V. Infusion (ROCHE LABORATORIES)
Bactrim Pediatric Suspension
(ROCHE LABORATORIES)
Bactrim Tablets (ROCHE LABORATORIES)
Bactroban Ointment
(SMITHKLINE BEECHAM PHARMACEUTICALS)

BALANCED SALT SOLUTION
Eye-Stream Eye Irrigating Solution

BALSAM PERU
Granulex
Bancap HC Capsules
(FOREST PHARMACEUTICALS, INC.)

BARIUM SULFATE
Barotrast
Esophotrast Cream
Oratrast
Barotrast
(RHONE-POULENC RORER PHARMACEUTICALS INC.)
Basaljel Capsules
(WYETH-AYERST LABORATORIES)
Basaljel Suspension
(WYETH-AYERST LABORATORIES)
Basaljel Tablets
(WYETH-AYERST LABORATORIES)
Bebulin VH Immuno (IMMUNO-U.S., INC.)

BECLOMETHASONE DIPROPIONATE
Beclovent Inhalation Aerosol
Beclovent/Beconase Inhalation Aerosol Refill
Beconase AQ Nasal Spray
Beconase Inhalation Aerosol
Vancenase AQ Nasal Spray 0.042%
Vancenase PocketHaler Nasal Inhaler
Vanceril Inhaler
Beclovent Inhalation Aerosol
(ALLEN & HANBURYS)
Beclovent/Beconase Inhalation Aerosol Refill
(ALLEN & HANBURYS)
Beconase AQ Nasal Spray (ALLEN & HANBURYS)
Beconase Inhalation Aerosol
(ALLEN & HANBURYS)
Beelith Tablets (BEACH PHARMACEUTICALS)

BEE POLLEN
Urokin

BELLADONNA ALKALOIDS
B & O No. 15A & No. 16A Supprettes
Bellergal-S Tablets
Donnatal Capsules
Donnatal Elixir
Donnatal Extentabs
Donnatal Tablets
Bellatal Tablets
(RICHWOOD PHARMACEUTICAL COMPANY, INC.)

Bellergal-S Tablets
(SANDOZ PHARMACEUTICALS CORPORATION)
Benadryl Allergy Liquid (WARNER WELLCOME)
Benadryl Allergy/Sinus Headache Caplets
(WARNER WELLCOME)
Benadryl Capsules (PARKE-DAVIS)
Benadryl Cold/Flu Tablets (WARNER WELLCOME)
Benadryl Cream (WARNER WELLCOME)
Benadryl Cream Maximum Strength
(WARNER WELLCOME)
Benadryl Decongestant Liquid
(WARNER WELLCOME)
Benadryl Decongestant Tablets
(WARNER WELLCOME)
Benadryl Dye-Free Allergy Liqui-Caps
(WARNER WELLCOME)
Benadryl Dye-Free Allergy Liquid
(WARNER WELLCOME)
Benadryl Itch Relief Stick
(WARNER WELLCOME)
Benadryl Kapseals (PARKE-DAVIS)
Benadryl Kapseals (WARNER WELLCOME)
Benadryl Parenteral (PARKE-DAVIS)
Benadryl Spray Maximum Strength 2%
(WARNER WELLCOME)
Benadryl Spray Regular 1% (WARNER WELL-COME)
Benadryl Steri-Vials, Ampoules, and Steri-Dose Syringe
(PARKE-DAVIS)
Benadryl Tablets (WARNER WELLCOME)

BENAZEPRIL HYDROCHLORIDE
Lotensin Tablets
Lotensin HCT
Benemid Tablets (MERCK & CO., INC.)
Benoquin Cream 20%
(ICN PHARMACEUTICALS, INC.)
Bensulfoid Cream (ECR PHARMACEUTICALS)
Bentyl 10 mg Capsules
(MARION MERRELL DOW INC.)
Bentyl Injection (MARION MERRELL DOW INC.)
Bentyl Syrup (MARION MERRELL DOW INC.)
Bentyl 20 mg Tablets
(MARION MERRELL DOW INC.)
Benylin Adult Formula (WARNER WELLCOME)
Benylin Expectorant (WARNER WELLCOME)
Benylin Multi-Symptom (WARNER WELLCOME)
Benylin Pediatric (WARNER WELLCOME)
Benzac 5 & 10 Gel
(GALDERMA LABORATORIES, INC.)
Benzac AC 2¹/₂%, 5%, and 10% Water-Base Gel
(GALDERMA LABORATORIES, INC.)
Benzac AC Wash 2¹/₂%, 5%, 10% Water-Base Cleanser (GALDERMA LABORATORIES, INC.)
Benzac W Wash 5 & 10 Water-Base Cleanser
(GALDERMA LABORATORIES, INC.)
Benzac W 2¹/₂, 5 & 10 Water-Base Gel
(GALDERMA LABORATORIES, INC.)
5 Benzagel (DERMIK LABORATORIES, INC.)
10 Benzagel (DERMIK LABORATORIES, INC.)

BENZALKONIUM CHLORIDE
Amino-Cerv
Cetylcide Germicidal Concentrate
Benzamycin Topical Gel
(DERMIK LABORATORIES, INC.)
BenzaShave Medicated Shave Cream 5% and 10% (MEDICIS DERMATOLOGICS, INC.)

BENZETHONIUM CHLORIDE
Critic-Aid, Antimicrobial Skin Paste
Puri-Clens, Wound Deodorizer and Cleanser
Sween Cream

BENZOCAINE
Americaine Anesthetic Lubricant
Americaine Otic Topical Anesthetic Ear Drops

Auralgan Otic Solution
Auroto Otic Solution
Cetacaine Topical Anesthetic
Hurricaine Topical Anesthetic Aerosol Spray, 2 oz (wild cherry flavor)
Hurricaine Topical Anesthetic Spray Kit
Hurricaine Topical Anesthetic Gel, 1 oz Wild Cherry, Pina Colada, Watermelon, ¹/₈ oz Wild Cherry, Watermelon
Hurricaine Topical Anesthetic Liquid, .25 gm, 1 oz Wild Cherry and Pina Colada .25 ml Dry Handle Swab Wild Cherry, ¹/₈ oz Wild Cherry
Otocain
Tympagesic Ear Drops

BENZOIC ACID
Urised Tablets

BENZONATATE
Benzonatate Capsules, USP
Tessalon Perles
Benzonatate Capsules, USP
(WARNER CHILCOTT LABORATORIES)

BENZOYL PEROXIDE
Benzac 5 & 10 Gel
Benzac AC 2¹/₂%, 5%, and 10% Water-Base Gel
Benzac AC Wash 2¹/₂%, 5%, 10% Water-Base Cleanser
Benzac W Wash 5 & 10 Water-Base Cleanser
Benzac W 2¹/₂, 5 & 10 Water-Base Gel
5 Benzagel
10 Benzagel
Benzamycin Topical Gel
BenzaShave Medicated Shave Cream 5% and 10%
Brevoxyl Gel
Brevoxyl Cleansing Lotion
Desquam-E 2.5 Emollient Gel
Desquam-E 5 Emollient Gel
Desquam-E 10 Emollient Gel
Desquam-X 2.5 Gel
Desquam-X 5 Gel
Desquam-X 10 Gel
Desquam-X 10 Bar
Desquam-X 5 Wash
Desquam-X 10 Wash
PanOxyl 5 Acne Gel
PanOxyl 10 Acne Gel
PanOxyl AQ 2¹/₂ Acne Gel
PanOxyl AQ 5 Acne Gel
PanOxyl AQ 10 Acne Gel
Persa-Gel (benzoyl peroxide)
Persa-Gel W (benzoyl peroxide)
Sulfoxyl Lotion Regular
Sulfoxyl Lotion Strong

BENZPHETAMINE HYDROCHLORIDE
Didrex Tablets

BENZQUINAMIDE HYDROCHLORIDE
Emete-con Intramuscular/Intravenous

BENZTHIAZIDE
Exna Tablets

BENZTROPINE MESYLATE
Benztropine Mesylate Tablets
Benztropine Mesylate Tablets
Cogentin Injection
Cogentin Tablets
Benztropine Mesylate Tablets
(DURAMED PHARMACEUTICALS, INC.)
Benztropine Mesylate Tablets
(PAR PHARMACEUTICAL, INC.)

BEPRIDIL HYDROCHLORIDE
Vascor (200, 300 and 400 mg) Tablets

UNDERLINE DENOTES GENERIC NAME

BERACTANT
　Survanta Beractant Intratracheal Suspension
Berocca Plus Tablets (ROCHE LABORATORIES)
Berocca Tablets (ROCHE LABORATORIES)

BETA CAROTENE
　ACES Antioxidant Soft Gels
　ANTIOX Capsules
　Beta-Carotene Super D. Salina
　Carotene-E Forté Capsules
　Carotene Health Packs
　Centrum Singles Beta Carotene
　Glutathione Health Packs
　Glutofac Caplets
　Performance Packs
　Performance Packs-Light
　Protegra Antioxidant Vitamin
　　& Mineral Supplement
　Solatene Capsules
Beta-Carotene Super D. Salina
　(J. R. CARLSON LABORATORIES, INC.)
Betadine Disposable Medicated Douche
　(THE PURDUE FREDERICK COMPANY)
Betadine First Aid Cream
　(THE PURDUE FREDERICK COMPANY)
Betadine Medicated Douche
　(THE PURDUE FREDERICK COMPANY)
Betadine Medicated Gel
　(THE PURDUE FREDERICK COMPANY)
Betadine Medicated Vaginal Suppositories
　(THE PURDUE FREDERICK COMPANY)
Betadine Ointment
　(THE PURDUE FREDERICK COMPANY)
Betadine Pre-Mixed Medicated
　Disposable Douche
　(THE PURDUE FREDERICK COMPANY)
Betadine Skin Cleanser
　(THE PURDUE FREDERICK COMPANY)
Betadine Solution
　(THE PURDUE FREDERICK COMPANY)
Betadine Surgical Scrub
　(THE PURDUE FREDERICK COMPANY)

BETAMETHASONE ACETATE
　Celestone Soluspan Suspension

BETAMETHASONE DIPROPIONATE
　Alphatrex Cream, Ointment & Lotion
　Betamethasone Dipropionate Cream, USP 0.05%
　Betamethasone Dipropionate Cream, Lotion, and
　　Ointment, USP 0.05%
　Diprolene AF Cream
　Diprolene Gel 0.05%
　Diprolene Lotion 0.05%
　Diprolene Ointment 0.05%
　Lotrisone Cream
Betamethasone Dipropionate Cream, USP 0.05%
　(TARO PHARMACEUTICALS U.S.A., INC.)
Betamethasone Dipropionate Cream, Lotion, and
　Ointment, USP 0.05%
　(BARRE-NATIONAL INC.)

BETAMETHASONE SODIUM PHOSPHATE
　Celestone Soluspan Suspension

BETAMETHASONE VALERATE
　Betamethasone Valerate Cream, USP 0.1%
　Betamethasone Valerate Cream, Lotion, and
　　Ointment, USP 0.1%
　Betatrex Cream, Ointment & Lotion
Betamethasone Valerate Cream, USP 0.1%
　(TARO PHARMACEUTICALS U.S.A., INC.)
Betamethasone Valerate Cream, Lotion, and
　Ointment, USP 0.1%
　(BARRE-NATIONAL INC.)
Betapace Tablets (BERLEX LABORATORIES)
Betasept Surgical Scrub
　(THE PURDUE FREDERICK COMPANY)

Betaseron for SC Injection
　(BERLEX LABORATORIES)
Betatrex Cream, Ointment & Lotion
　(SAVAGE LABORATORIES)

BETAXOLOL HYDROCHLORIDE
　Betoptic Ophthalmic Solution
　Betoptic S Ophthalmic Suspension
　Kerlone Tablets

BETHANECHOL CHLORIDE
　Myotonachol
　Urecholine Injection
　Urecholine Tablets
Betoptic Ophthalmic Solution
　(ALCON LABORATORIES, INC.)
Betoptic S Ophthalmic Suspension
　(ALCON LABORATORIES, INC.)
Biavax II (MERCK & CO., INC.)
Biaxin Granules (ABBOTT LABORATORIES)
Biaxin Tablets (ABBOTT LABORATORIES)
Bichloracetic Acid Kahlenberg
　(GLENWOOD, INC.)
Bicillin C-R Injection
　(WYETH-AYERST LABORATORIES)
Bicillin C-R in Tubex
　(WYETH-AYERST LABORATORIES)
Bicillin C-R 900/300 Injection
　(WYETH-AYERST LABORATORIES)
Bicillin C-R 900/300 in Tubex
　(WYETH-AYERST LABORATORIES)
Bicillin L-A Injection
　(WYETH-AYERST LABORATORIES)
Bicillin L-A in Tubex
　(WYETH-AYERST LABORATORIES)
Bicitra (BAKER NORTON PHARMACEUTICALS, INC.)
BiCNU
　(BRISTOL-MYERS SQUIBB ONCOLOGY DIVISION)
BiCozene Creme
　(SANDOZ PHARMACEUTICALS/ CONSUMER DIVISION)
Biltricide Tablets
　(MILES INC. PHARMACEUTICAL DIVISION)
Biocef Capsules and Oral Suspension
　(INTERNATIONAL ETHICAL LABS.)
Bioclate, Antihemophilic Factor (Recombinant)
　(ARMOUR PHARMACEUTICAL COMPANY)

BIOFLAVONOIDS
　Peridin-C Tablets
Bio-Tab Tablets (INTERNATIONAL ETHICAL)

BIOTIN
　d-Biotin Capsules
　Mega-B
　Megadose
d-Biotin Capsules (R&D LABORATORIES, INC.)

BIPERIDEN HYDROCHLORIDE
　Akineton Injection
　Akineton Tablets
Biphetamine Capsules
　(FISONS CORPORATION PRESCRIPTION PRODUCTS)

BISACODYL
　Bisacodyl Suppositories
　Dulcolax Suppositories
　Dulcolax Tablets
　Fleet Bisacodyl Enema
　Fleet Prep Kits
Bisacodyl Suppositories
　(BARRE-NATIONAL INC.)

BISMUTH SUBSALICYLATE
　Pepto-Bismol Liquid, Tablets and Caplets
　Maximum Strength Pepto-Bismol Liquid

BISOPROLOL FUMARATE
　Zebeta Tablets
　Ziac

BITOLTEROL MESYLATE
　Tornalate Inhalation Solution, 0.2%
　Tornalate Metered Dose Inhaler

BLACK WIDOW SPIDER ANTIVENIN (EQUINE)
　Antivenin (Black Widow Spider)
Blenoxane
　(BRISTOL-MYERS SQUIBB ONCOLOGY DIVISION)

BLEOMYCIN SULFATE
　Blenoxane
Bleph-10 Ophthalmic Ointment 10%
　(ALLERGAN, INC.)
Bleph-10 Ophthalmic Solution 10%
　(ALLERGAN, INC.)
Blephamide Liquifilm Sterile Ophthalmic
　Suspension (ALLERGAN, INC.)
Blocadren Tablets (MERCK & CO., INC.)
Bluboro Powder Astringent Soaking Solution
　(ALLERGAN HERBERT)
Blue Gel (BARRE-NATIONAL INC.)
Bonamil Infant Formula with Iron, Powder
　(WYETH-AYERST LABORATORIES)
Bonine Tablets
　(PFIZER CONSUMER HEALTH CARE)
Bontril PDM Tablets
　(CARNRICK LABORATORIES, INC.)
Bontril Slow-Release Capsules
　(CARNRICK LABORATORIES, INC.)

BORIC ACID
　Boric Acid Ointment
Boric Acid Ointment
　(BARRE-NATIONAL INC.)
Borofax (WARNER WELLCOME)
BOTOX (Botulinum Toxin Type A) Purified
　Neurotoxin Complex (ALLERGAN, INC.)

BOTULINUM TOXIN TYPE A
　BOTOX (Botulinum Toxin Type A) Purified
　　Neurotoxin Complex
Breezee Mist Antifungal Foot Powder
　(PEDINOL PHARMACAL INC.)
Brethaire Inhaler (GEIGY PHARMACEUTICALS)
Brethine Ampuls (GEIGY PHARMACEUTICALS)
Brethine Tablets (GEIGY PHARMACEUTICALS)

BRETYLIUM TOSYLATE
　Bretylium Tosylate Injection (Preservative-Free)
　Bretylium Tosylate Injection
Bretylium Tosylate Injection (Preservative-Free)
　(ELKINS-SINN, INC.)
Bretylium Tosylate Injection (ASTRA USA, INC.)
Brevibloc Injection (OHMEDA PHARMACEUTICAL
　PRODUCTS DIVISION INC.)
Brevicon 21-Day Tablets
　(SYNTEX PUERTO RICO, INC.)
Brevicon 28-Day Tablets
　(SYNTEX PUERTO RICO, INC.)
Brevital Sodium Vials
　(ELI LILLY AND COMPANY)
Brevoxyl Gel (STIEFEL LABORATORIES, INC.)
Brevoxyl Cleansing Lotion
　(STIEFEL LABORATORIES, INC.)
Brexin L.A. Capsules (SAVAGE LABORATORIES)
Bricanyl Injection (MARION MERRELL DOW INC.)
Bricanyl Tablets (MARION MERRELL DOW INC.)
Bromanate DC Cough Syrup
　(BARRE-NATIONAL INC.)
Bromanate DM (BARRE-NATIONAL INC.)
Bromanate Elixir (BARRE-NATIONAL INC.)
Bromanyl Cough Syrup
　(BARRE-NATIONAL INC.)
Bromarest DX Cough Syrup
　(WARNER CHILCOTT LABORATORIES)
Bromfed Capsules (Extended-Release)
　(MURO PHARMACEUTICAL, INC.)
Bromfed Syrup (MURO PHARMACEUTICAL, INC.)
Bromfed Tablets (MURO PHARMACEUTICAL, INC.)

UNDERLINE DENOTES GENERIC NAME

Bromfed-DM Cough Syrup
(MURO PHARMACEUTICAL, INC.)
Bromfed-PD Capsules (Extended-Release)
(MURO PHARMACEUTICAL, INC.)

BROMOCRIPTINE MESYLATE
Bromocriptine Mesylate Tablets and Capsules
Parlodel Capsules
Parlodel SnapTabs
Bromocriptine Mesylate Tablets and Capsules
(ATHENA NEUROSCIENCES, INC.)

BROMODIPHENHYDRAMINE HYDROCHLORIDE
Ambenyl Cough Syrup

BROMPHENIRAMINE MALEATE
Bromarest DX Cough Syrup
Bromfed Capsules (Extended-Release)
Bromfed Tablets
Bromfed-DM Cough Syrup
Bromfed-PD Capsules (Extended-Release)
Dallergy-JR Capsules
Dimetane-DC Cough Syrup
Dimetane-DX Cough Syrup
E.N.T. Tablets
HISTINEX DM
Lodrane LD Capsules
Lodrane Liquid
Poly-Histine CS
Poly-Histine DM Syrup
Touro A&H Capsules
ULTRABROM Capsules
ULTRABROM PD Capsules
Broncholate Softgels
(BOCK PHARMACAL COMPANY)
Broncholate Syrup (BOCK PHARMACAL COMPANY)
Brondelate Elixir (BARRE-NATIONAL INC.)
Bronkometer Aerosol
(SANOFI WINTHROP PHARMACEUTICALS)
Bronkosol Solution
(SANOFI WINTHROP PHARMACEUTICALS)
Brontex
(PROCTER & GAMBLE PHARMACEUTICALS, INC.)

BUDESONIDE
Rhinocort Nasal Inhaler
Arthritis Strength Bufferin Analgesic Caplets
(BRISTOL-MYERS PRODUCTS)
Extra Strength Bufferin Analgesic Tablets
(BRISTOL-MYERS PRODUCTS)
Bufferin Analgesic Tablets and Caplets
(BRISTOL-MYERS PRODUCTS)
Bufferin AF Nite Time Analgesic/Sleeping Aid
Caplets (BRISTOL-MYERS PRODUCTS)
Bugs Bunny Complete Children's Chewable
Vitamins + Minerals with Iron and Calcium
(Sugar Free)
(MILES INC. CONSUMER HEALTHCARE PRODUCTS)
Bugs Bunny With Extra C Children's Chewable
Vitamins (Sugar Free)
(MILES INC. CONSUMER HEALTHCARE PRODUCTS)
Bugs Bunny Plus Iron Children's Chewable
Vitamins (Sugar Free)
(MILES INC. CONSUMER HEALTHCARE PRODUCTS)

BUMETANIDE
Bumex Injection
Bumex Tablets
Bumex Injection (ROCHE LABORATORIES)
Bumex Tablets (ROCHE LABORATORIES)
Buminate 5%, Albumin (Human), USP, 5%
Solution (BAXTER HEALTHCARE CORPORATION)
Buminate 25%, Albumin (Human), USP, 25%
Solution (BAXTER HEALTHCARE CORPORATION)
Bupap Tablets (ECR PHARMACEUTICALS)

BUPIVACAINE HYDROCHLORIDE
Marcaine Hydrochloride with Epinephrine
1:200,000

Marcaine Hydrochloride Injection
Marcaine Spinal
Sensorcaine with Epinephrine Injection
Sensorcaine Injection
Sensorcaine-MPF with Epinephrine Injection
Sensorcaine-MPF Spinal
Buprenex Injectable
(RECKITT & COLMAN PHARMACEUTICALS, INC.)

BUPRENORPHINE HYDROCHLORIDE
Buprenex Injectable

BUPROPION HYDROCHLORIDE
Wellbutrin Tablets
Buro-Sol Astringent Packets
(DOAK DERMATOLOGICALS)

BUROW'S SOLUTION
Buro-Sol Astringent Packets
BuSpar (BRISTOL-MYERS SQUIBB COMPANY)

BUSPIRONE HYDROCHLORIDE
BuSpar

BUSULFAN
Myleran Tablets

BUTABARBITAL
Axocet

BUTABARBITAL SODIUM
Butabarbital Sodium Elixir USP 30 mg/5 mL
Butisol Sodium Elixir & Tablets
Butabarbital Sodium Elixir USP 30 mg/5 mL
(BARRE-NATIONAL INC.)

BUTALBITAL
Axotal
Bupap Tablets
Esgic-Plus Tablets
Esgic Tablets & Capsules
Femcet Capsules
Fioricet Tablets
Fioricet with Codeine Capsules
Fiorinal Capsules
Fiorinal with Codeine Capsules
Fiorinal Tablets
Medigesic Capsules
Pacaps Capsules
Phrenilin Forte Capsules
Phrenilin Tablets
Repan Tablets and Capsules
REPAN-CF Tablets
Sedapap Tablets 50 mg/650 mg
Tencon Capsules
Butisol Sodium Elixir & Tablets
(WALLACE LABORATORIES)

BUTOCONAZOLE NITRATE
Femstat Prefill Vaginal Cream 2%
Femstat Vaginal Cream 2%

BUTORPHANOL TARTRATE
Stadol Injection
Stadol NS Nasal Spray

BUTYL AMINOBENZOATE
Cetacaine Topical Anesthetic

C

Cafergot Suppositories
(SANDOZ PHARMACEUTICALS CORPORATION)
Cafergot Tablets
(SANDOZ PHARMACEUTICALS CORPORATION)

CAFFEINE
Cafergot Suppositories
Cafergot Tablets
DHCplus Capsules
Darvon Compound-65 Pulvules
Esgic-Plus Tablets
Esgic Tablets & Capsules
Aspirin Free Excedrin Analgesic Caplets
Excedrin Extra-Strength Analgesic Tablets &
Caplets
Femcet Capsules
Fioricet Tablets
Fioricet with Codeine Capsules
Fiorinal Capsules
Fiorinal with Codeine Capsules
Fiorinal Tablets
Gelpirin Tablets
Medigesic Capsules
Migralam Capsules
No Doz Maximum Strength Caplets
Norgesic Forte Tablets
Norgesic Tablets
PC-CAP Propoxyphene Hydrochloride
Compound, USP
Pacaps Capsules
Repan Tablets and Capsules
Synalgos-DC Capsules
Wigraine Tablets & Suppositories
Caladryl Clear Lotion (WARNER WELLCOME)
Caladryl Cream For Kids (WARNER WELLCOME)
Caladryl Lotion (WARNER WELLCOME)

CALAMINE
Caladryl Cream For Kids
Caladryl Lotion
Calan SR Caplets (G.D. SEARLE & CO.)
Calan Tablets (G.D. SEARLE & CO.)
Calcet (MISSION PHARMACAL COMPANY)
Calcet Plus (MISSION PHARMACAL COMPANY)
Calcibind (MISSION PHARMACAL COMPANY)
Calci-Chew Tablets (R&D LABORATORIES, INC.)

CALCIFEDIOL
Calderol Capsules

CALCIFEROL
Calciferol Drops
Calciferol in Oil Injection
Calciferol Tablets
Calciferol Drops (SCHWARZ PHARMA)
Calciferol in Oil Injection (SCHWARZ PHARMA)
Calciferol Tablets (SCHWARZ PHARMA)
Liquid Cal-600 Capsules
(J. R. CARLSON LABORATORIES, INC.)
Calcijex Calcitriol Injection
(ABBOTT LABORATORIES)
Calcimar Injection, Synthetic
(RHONE-POULENC RORER PHARMACEUTICALS INC.)
Calci-Mix Capsules (R&D LABORATORIES, INC.)

CALCIPOTRIENE
Dovonex Ointment 0.005%

CALCITONIN-SALMON
Calcimar Injection, Synthetic
Miacalcin Injection

CALCITRIOL
Calcijex Calcitriol Injection
Rocaltrol Capsules

CALCIUM
Casamin

CALCIUM ACETATE
Pedi-Boro Soak Paks
PhosLo Tablets

CALCIUM CARBONATE
Arthritis Pain Ascriptin

Regular Strength Ascriptin Tablets
Calcet
Calcet Plus
Calci-Chew Tablets
Calci-Mix Capsules
Calcium Carbonate Tablets & Oral Suspension
Calel-D
Caltrate PLUS
Caltrate 600
Caltrate 600 + D
Centrum Singles Calcium
Gerimed Tablets
Materna Tablets
Mission Prenatal
Mission Prenatal H.P.
Mylanta Gelcaps Antacid
Mylanta Soothing Lozenges
Nephro-Calci Tablets
Nu-Iron V Tablets
Performance Packs-Light
Pramilet FA
Prenate 90 Tablets
TYLENOL, Extra Strength, Headache Plus Pain
    Reliever with Antacid Caplets
Calcium Carbonate Tablets & Oral Suspension
   (ROXANE LABORATORIES, INC.)

CALCIUM CASEINATE
Promote High Protein Liquid Nutrition

CALCIUM CHLORIDE
Calcium Chloride 10% Injection, USP
Calcium Chloride 10% Injection, USP
   (ASTRA USA, INC.)

CALCIUM CITRATE
Citracal
Citracal Caplets+D
Citracal Liquitab
Glusamin
NutraVescent

CALCIUM DISODIUM EDETATE
Calcium Disodium Versenate Injection
Calcium Disodium Versenate Injection
   (3M PHARMACEUTICALS)

CALCIUM GLUBIONATE
Neo-Calglucon Syrup

CALCIUM GLUCONATE
Calcet
Calcium Gluconate Tablets
Mission Prenatal
Mission Prenatal H.P.
Calcium Gluconate Tablets
   (ROXANE LABORATORIES, INC.)

CALCIUM GLYCEROPHOSPHATE
Calphosan

CALCIUM IODIDE
Norisodrine with Calcium Iodide Syrup

CALCIUM LACTATE
Calcet
Calphosan
Mission Prenatal
Mission Prenatal H.P.

CALCIUM PANTOTHENATE
Eldercaps
Mega-B
Performance Packs-Light

CALCIUM PHOSPHATE, DIBASIC
Dical-D Tablets & Wafers
Gerimed Tablets

CALCIUM POLYCARBOPHIL
FiberCon Tablets

CALCIUM SODIUM ALGINATE FIBER
Kaltostat Wound Dressing
Calderol Capsules (ORGANON INC.)
Calel-D
   (RHONE-POULENC RORER PHARMACEUTICALS INC.)
Calphosan (GLENWOOD, INC.)
Caltrate PLUS (LEDERLE LABORATORIES)
Caltrate 600 (LEDERLE LABORATORIES)
Caltrate 600 + D (LEDERLE LABORATORIES)
Cama Arthritis Pain Reliever
   (SANDOZ PHARMACEUTICALS/ CONSUMER DIVISION)

CAMPHOR
Nephro-Derm Cream
Panalgesic Gold Liniment
Capastat Sulfate Vials
   (ELI LILLY AND COMPANY)
Capital And Codeine Suspension
   (CARNRICK LABORATORIES, INC.)
Capitrol Shampoo
   (WESTWOOD-SQUIBB PHARMACEUTICALS INC.)
Capoten (BRISTOL-MYERS SQUIBB COMPANY)
Capozide (BRISTOL-MYERS SQUIBB COMPANY)

CAPREOMYCIN SULFATE
Capastat Sulfate Vials

CAPSAICIN
Zostrix
Zostrix-HP Topical Analgesic Cream

CAPTOPRIL
Capoten
Capozide
Carafate Suspension
   (MARION MERRELL DOW INC.)
Carafate Tablets (MARION MERRELL DOW INC.)

CARBAMAZEPINE
Carbamazepine Chewable Tablets, USP
Tegretol Chewable Tablets
Tegretol Suspension
Tegretol Tablets
Carbamazepine Chewable Tablets, USP
   (WARNER CHILCOTT LABORATORIES)

CARBENICILLIN INDANYL SODIUM
Geocillin Tablets

CARBETAPENTANE TANNATE
Rynatuss Pediatric Suspension
Rynatuss Tablets

CARBIDOPA
Atamet
Carbidopa and Levodopa Tablets, USP
Sinemet Tablets
Sinemet CR Tablets
Carbidopa and Levodopa Tablets, USP
   (WATSON LABORATORIES, INC.)

CARBINOXAMINE MALEATE
Rondec Oral Drops
Rondec Syrup
Rondec Tablet
Rondec-DM Oral Drops
Rondec-DM Syrup
Rondec-TR Tablet
Tussafed Drops & Syrup
Carbocaine Hydrochloride Injection
   (SANOFI WINTHROP PHARMACEUTICALS)

CARBOHYDRATES
SMA Lo-Iron Infant Formula, Concentrated,
   Ready-To-Feed and Powder

CARBOPLATIN
Paraplatin for Injection
Cardec-DM Drops and Syrup
   (BARRE-NATIONAL INC.)
Cardec-S Syrup (BARRE-NATIONAL INC.)
Cardene Capsules (SYNTEX PUERTO RICO, INC.)

Cardene I.V. (WYETH-AYERST LABORATORIES)
Cardene SR Capsules
   (SYNTEX PUERTO RICO, INC.)
Cardilate Oral/Sublingual Tablets
   (BURROUGHS WELLCOME CO.)
Cardioquin Tablets
   (THE PURDUE FREDERICK COMPANY)
**Cardizem CD Capsules-120 mg, 180 mg, 240 mg
and 300 mg** (MARION MERRELL DOW INC.)
Cardizem SR Capsules-60 mg, 90 mg and 120 mg
   (MARION MERRELL DOW INC.)
Cardizem Injectable (MARION MERRELL DOW INC.)
Cardizem Tablets-30 mg, 60 mg, 90 mg and 120 mg
   (MARION MERRELL DOW INC.)
Cardura Tablets (ROERIG DIVISION)

CARISOPRODOL
Carisoprodol and Aspirin Tablets
Soma Compound w/Codeine Tablets
Soma Compound Tablets
Soma Tablets
Carisoprodol and Aspirin Tablets
   (PAR PHARMACEUTICAL, INC.)
Carmol 10 (DOAK DERMATOLOGICALS)

CARMUSTINE (BCNU)
BiCNU
L-Carnitine Capsules (R&D LABORATORIES, INC.)
L-Carnitine Capsules
   (TYSON AND ASSOCIATES, INC.)
L-Carnitine 250mg and 500mg Tablets
   (VITALINE CORPORATION)
Carnitor Injection
   (SIGMA-TAU PHARMACEUTICALS, INC.)
Carnitor Tablets and Solution
   (SIGMA-TAU PHARMACEUTICALS, INC.)
Carotene-E Forté Capsules
   (HEALTH MAINTENANCE PROGRAMS, INC.)
Carotene Health Packs
   (HEALTH MAINTENANCE PROGRAMS, INC.)
Carpuject Sterile Cartridge-Needle Unit
   (SANOFI WINTHROP PHARMACEUTICALS)

CARTEOLOL HYDROCHLORIDE
Cartrol Tablets
Cartrol Tablets (ABBOTT LABORATORIES)
Casamin (VITALINE CORPORATION)

CASANTHRANOL
Docusate Sodium with Casanthranol Capsules
   (D-S-S Plus)

CASCARA SAGRADA
Aromatic Cascara Fluidextract
Milk of Magnesia-Cascara Suspension
   Concentrated
Castellani Paint Modified
   (PEDINOL PHARMACAL INC.)

CASTOR OIL
Castor Oil
Castor Oil, Aromatic
Fleet Flavored Castor Oil Emulsion
Fleet Prep Kits
Granulex
Hydrisinol Creme & Lotion
Neoloid Emulsified Mint Castor Oil
Castor Oil (ROXANE LABORATORIES, INC.)
Castor Oil, Aromatic
   (ROXANE LABORATORIES, INC.)
Cataflam (GEIGY PHARMACEUTICALS)
Catasod (VITALINE CORPORATION)
Catapres Tablets
   (BOEHRINGER INGELHEIM PHARMACEUTICALS, INC.)
Catapres-TTS
   (BOEHRINGER INGELHEIM PHARMACEUTICALS, INC.)
Catemine Enteric Tablets (Tyrosine)
   (TYSON AND ASSOCIATES, INC.)
Catrix (SAVAGE LABORATORIES)

UNDERLINE DENOTES GENERIC NAME

Ceclor Pulvules & Suspension
  (ELI LILLY AND COMPANY)
CeeNU
  (BRISTOL-MYERS SQUIBB ONCOLOGY DIVISION)
CEFACLOR
  Ceclor Pulvules & Suspension
CEFADROXIL MONOHYDRATE
  Duricef
CEFAMANDOLE NAFATE
  Mandol Vials, Faspak & ADD-Vantage
CEFAZOLIN SODIUM
  Ancef Injection
  Kefzol Vials, Faspak & ADD-Vantage
CEFIXIME
  Suprax for Oral Suspension
  Suprax Tablets
Cefizox for Intramuscular or Intravenous Use
  (FUJISAWA USA, INC.)
CEFMETAZOLE SODIUM
  Zefazone I.V. Solution
  Zefazone Sterile Powder
Cefobid Intravenous/Intramuscular
  (ROERIG DIVISION)
**Cefobid Pharmacy Bulk Package - Not for Direct
  Infusion** (ROERIG DIVISION)
Cefol Filmtab (ABBOTT LABORATORIES)
CEFONICID SODIUM
  Monocid Injection
CEFOPERAZONE SODIUM
  Cefobid Intravenous/Intramuscular
  Cefobid Pharmacy Bulk Package - Not for Direct
    Infusion
Cefotan (STUART PHARMACEUTICALS)
Cefotan Injection (STUART PHARMACEUTICALS)
CEFOTAXIME SODIUM
  Claforan Sterile Injection
CEFOTETAN DISODIUM
  Cefotan
  Cefotan Injection
CEFOXITIN SODIUM
  Mefoxin
  Mefoxin Premixed Intravenous Solution
CEFPODOXIME PROXETIL
  Vantin for Oral Suspension and Vantin Tablets
CEFPROZIL
  Cefzil Tablets and Oral Suspension
CEFTAZIDIME
  Ceptaz
  Fortaz
  Tazicef for Injection
  Tazidime Vials, Faspak & ADD-Vantage
Ceftin for Oral Suspension
  (GLAXO PHARMACEUTICALS)
Ceftin Tablets (GLAXO PHARMACEUTICALS)
CEFTIZOXIME SODIUM
  Cefizox for Intramuscular or Intravenous Use
CEFTRIAXONE SODIUM
  Rocephin Injectable Vials, ADD-Vantage
CEFUROXIME AXETIL
  Ceftin for Oral Suspension
  Ceftin Tablets
CEFUROXIME SODIUM
  Kefurox Vials, Faspak & ADD-Vantage
  Zinacef
Cefzil Tablets and Oral Suspension
  (BRISTOL-MYERS SQUIBB COMPANY)

Celestone Soluspan Suspension
  (SCHERING CORPORATION)
CELLULOSE, OXIDIZED REGENERATED
  INTERCEED* (TC7) Absorbable Adhesion
    Barrier
  SURGICEL* Absorbable Hemostat
  SURGICEL* NU-KNIT Absorbable Hemostat
CELLULOSE SODIUM PHOSPHATE
  Calcibind
Celluvisc Lubricant Ophthalmic Solution
  (ALLERGAN, INC.)
Celontin Kapseals (PARKE-DAVIS)
Centrum (LEDERLE LABORATORIES)
Centrum, Jr. (Children's Chewable) + Extra C
  (LEDERLE LABORATORIES)
**Centrum, Jr. (Children's Chewable) + Extra
  Calcium** (LEDERLE LABORATORIES)
Centrum, Jr. (Children's Chewable) + Iron
  (LEDERLE LABORATORIES)
Centrum Liquid (LEDERLE LABORATORIES)
Centrum Silver (LEDERLE LABORATORIES)
Centrum Singles Beta Carotene
  (LEDERLE LABORATORIES)
Centrum Singles Calcium
  (LEDERLE LABORATORIES)
Centrum Singles Vitamin C
  (LEDERLE LABORATORIES)
Centrum Singles Vitamin E
  (LEDERLE LABORATORIES)
Ceo-Two Rectal Suppositories (BEUTLICH L.P.)
CEPHALEXIN
  Biocef Capsules and Oral Suspension
  Cephalexin Capsules
  Cephalexin Capsules USP and Oral Suspension
    250, 500
  Cephalexin Capsules and for
    Oral Suspension, USP
  Cephalexin Capsules, Tablets, Oral Suspension
  Cephalexin for Oral Suspension
  Cephalexin Tablets
  Keflex Pulvules & Oral Suspension
Cephalexin Capsules
  (BIOCRAFT LABORATORIES, INC.)
**Cephalexin Capsules USP and Oral Suspension
  250, 500** (NOVOPHARM, USA INC.)
**Cephalexin Capsules and for Oral Suspension,
  USP** (WARNER CHILCOTT LABORATORIES)
Cephalexin Capsules, Tablets, Oral Suspension
  (LEDERLE STANDARD PRODUCTS)
Cephalexin for Oral Suspension
  (BIOCRAFT LABORATORIES, INC.)
Cephalexin Tablets
  (BIOCRAFT LABORATORIES, INC.)
CEPHALEXIN HYDROCHLORIDE
  Keftab Tablets
CEPHRADINE
  Cephradine Capsules
  Cephradine Capsules
  Cephradine Capsules, USP
  Cephradine for Oral Suspension
Cephradine Capsules
  (BIOCRAFT LABORATORIES, INC.)
Cephradine Capsules
  (LEDERLE STANDARD PRODUCTS)
Cephradine Capsules, USP
  (WARNER CHILCOTT LABORATORIES)
Cephradine for Oral Suspension
  (BIOCRAFT LABORATORIES, INC.)
Ceptaz (GLAXO PHARMACEUTICALS)
Ceredase Injection (GENZYME CORPORATION)
Cerose-DM (WYETH-AYERST LABORATORIES)
Cerubidine (WYETH-AYERST LABORATORIES)

Cerumenex Drops
  (THE PURDUE FREDERICK COMPANY)
Cetacaine Topical Anesthetic
  (CETYLITE INDUSTRIES, INC.)
Cetaphil Gentle Cleansing Bar
  (GALDERMA LABORATORIES, INC.)
Cetaphil Skin Cleanser
  (GALDERMA LABORATORIES, INC.)
CETYL ALCOHOL
  Aquanil Lotion
  Cetaphil Skin Cleanser
  Exosurf Neonatal for Intratracheal Suspension
CETYL DIMETHYL ETHYL AMMONIUM BROMIDE
  Cetylcide Germicidal Concentrate
Cetylcide Germicidal Concentrate
  (CETYLITE INDUSTRIES, INC.)
CHARCOAL, ACTIVATED
  Actidose with Sorbitol
  Actidose-Aqua
CHEMET (succimer) Capsules
  (MCNEIL CONSUMER PRODUCTS COMPANY)
Cheracol-D Cough Formula
  (ROBERTS PHARMACEUTICAL CORPORATION)
Cheracol Nasal Spray Pump
  (ROBERTS PHARMACEUTICAL CORPORATION)
Cheracol Plus Cough/Cold
  (ROBERTS PHARMACEUTICAL CORPORATION)
Cheracol Sore Throat Spray
  (ROBERTS PHARMACEUTICAL CORPORATION)
Chibroxin Sterile Ophthalmic Solution
  (MERCK & CO., INC.)
**Children's Vicks Chloraseptic Sore Throat
  Lozenges** (PROCTER & GAMBLE)
Children's Vicks Chloraseptic Sore Throat Spray
  (PROCTER & GAMBLE)
Children's Vicks DayQuil Allergy Relief
  (PROCTER & GAMBLE)
Children's Vicks NyQuil Cold/Cough Relief
  (PROCTER & GAMBLE)
Chlor-3 Condiment (FLEMING & COMPANY)
CHLORAL HYDRATE
  Aquachloral Supprettes Suppositories
  Chloral Hydrate Capsules & Syrup
Chloral Hydrate Capsules & Syrup
  (ROXANE LABORATORIES, INC.)
CHLORAMBUCIL
  Leukeran Tablets
CHLORAMPHENICOL
  Chloromycetin Kapseals
  Elase-Chloromycetin Ointment
CHLORAMPHENICOL SODIUM SUCCINATE
  Chloromycetin Sodium Succinate
CHLORCYCLIZINE HYDROCHLORIDE
  Mantadil Cream
CHLORDIAZEPOXIDE
  Chlordiazepoxide & Amitriptyline
    Hydrochloride Tablets
  Libritabs Tablets
  Limbitrol DS Tablets
  Limbitrol Tablets
**Chlordiazepoxide & Amitriptyline Hydrochloride
  Tablets** (MYLAN PHARMACEUTICALS INC.)
CHLORDIAZEPOXIDE HYDROCHLORIDE
  Librax Capsules
  Librium Capsules
  Librium Injectable
Chloresium Ointment (RYSTAN COMPANY, INC.)
Chloresium Solution (RYSTAN COMPANY, INC.)

UNDERLINE DENOTES GENERIC NAME

CHLORHEXIDINE GLUCONATE
Betasept Surgical Scrub
Hibiclens Antimicrobial Skin Cleanser
Hibistat Germicidal Hand Rinse
Hibistat Towelette
Peridex

CHLORMEZANONE
Trancopal Caplets

CHLOROETHANE
Ethyl Chloride, U.S.P.
Chloromycetin Kapseals (PARKE-DAVIS)
Chloromycetin Sodium Succinate (PARKE-DAVIS)

CHLOROPHYLL PREPARATIONS
Chloresium Ointment
Chloresium Solution
Derifil Tablets
Panafil Ointment

CHLOROPHYLLIN COPPER COMPLEX
Chloresium Ointment
Chloresium Solution
Derifil Tablets
PALS Internal Deodorant
Panafil Ointment

CHLOROPROCAINE HYDROCHLORIDE
Nesacaine Injections
Nesacaine-MPF Injection

CHLOROQUINE HYDROCHLORIDE
Aralen Hydrochloride Injection

CHLOROQUINE PHOSPHATE
Aralen Phosphate Tablets
Chloroquine Phosphate Tablets
Chloroquine Phosphate Tablets
(BIOCRAFT LABORATORIES, INC.)

CHLOROTHIAZIDE
Aldoclor Tablets
Chlorothiazide Tablets
Chlorothiazide Tablets, U.S.P.
Diupres Tablets
Diuril Oral Suspension
Diuril Tablets
Reserpine & Chlorothiazide Tablets
Chlorothiazide Tablets
(MYLAN PHARMACEUTICALS INC.)
Chlorothiazide Tablets, U.S.P.
(WEST POINT PHARMA)

CHLOROTHIAZIDE SODIUM
Diuril Sodium Intravenous

CHLOROXINE
Capitrol Shampoo

CHLOROXYLENOL
Cortic Ear Drops
Gordochom Solution
Pedi-Pro Topical Powder

CHLORPHENIRAMINE MALEATE
AH-CHEW Chewable Tablets
Ana-Kit Anaphylaxis Emergency Treatment Kit
Anaplex HD Cough Syrup
Atrohist Plus Tablets
Atrohist Sprinkle Capsules
Brexin L.A. Capsules
Codimal-L.A. Capsules
Codimal-L.A. HALF Capsules
Comhist LA Capsules

Allergy-Sinus Comtrex Multi-Symptom Allergy
Sinus Formula Tablets & Caplets
Comtrex Maximum Strength Multi-Symptom
Cold Reliever Tablets/Caplets/Liqui-
Gels/Liquid
D.A. Chewable Tablets
Dallergy Caplets, Syrup, Tablets
Deconamine SR Capsules, Tablets, Syrup
Donatussin Drops
Duadacin Cold & Allergy Capsules
Dura-Tap/PD Capsules
Dura-Vent/A Capsules
Dura-Vent/DA Tablets
Endal-HD
Extendryl Chewable Tablets
Extendryl Sr. & Jr. T.D. Capsules
Extendryl Syrup
Fedahist Gyrocaps
Fedahist Timecaps
Gelpirin CCF Tablets
HISTALET FORTE Tablets
HISTINEX HC
HISTINEX PV Syrup
Histussin HC
Kronofed-A Kronocaps
Kronofed-A-Jr. Kronocaps
Nolamine Timed-Release Tablets
Novahistine DH (+)
OMNIHIST L.A. Tablets
Ornade Spansule Capsules
P-V-TUSSIN Syrup
PediaCare Cold-Allergy Chewable Tablets
PediaCare Cough-Cold Chewable Tablets
PediaCare Cough-Cold Liquid
PediaCare NightRest Cough-Cold Liquid
Pediacof Cough Syrup
Protid Tablets
Rescon Capsules
Rescon Liquid
Rescon-DM Liquid
Rescon-ED Capsules
Rescon JR Capsules
Ru-Tuss Tablets
Sinulin Tablets
Sinutab Maximum Strength Sinus Allergy Tablets
Sudafed Plus Liquid
Sudafed Plus Tablets
Tussar DM
Children's TYLENOL Cold Multi-Symptom
Liquid Formula and Chewable Tablets
Children's TYLENOL Cold Multi-Symptom Plus
Cough Liquid Formula and Chewable Tablets
TYLENOL Cold Hot Medication Packets
TYLENOL Maximum Strength Allergy Sinus
Medication Gelcaps and Caplets
TYLENOL Cold Multi-Symptom Formula
Medication Tablets and Caplets
Vanex Forte Caplets
Vanex-HD Liquid

CHLORPHENIRAMINE POLISTIREX
Tussionex Pennkinetic Extended-Release
Suspension

CHLORPHENIRAMINE TANNATE
Atrohist Pediatric Suspension
R-Tannate Tablets and Pediatric Suspension
Ricobid Tablets and Pediatric Suspension
Rynatan Tablets
Rynatan-S Pediatric Suspension
Rynatuss Pediatric Suspension
Rynatuss Tablets
Triotann Pediatric Suspension
Triotann Tablets

CHLORPROMAZINE
Thorazine Suppositories

**Chlorpromazine HCl Oral Concentrate
100 mg/mL** (BARRE-NATIONAL INC.)
CHLORPROMAZINE HYDROCHLORIDE
Chlorpromazine HCl Oral Concentrate
100 mg/mL
Chlorpromazine Hydrochloride Injection
Chlorpromazine HCl Tablets
Thorazine Ampuls
Thorazine Concentrate
Thorazine Multi-dose Vials
Thorazine Spansule Capsules
Thorazine Syrup
Thorazine Tablets
Chlorpromazine Hydrochloride Injection
(ELKINS-SINN, INC.)
Chlorpromazine HCl Tablets
(GENEVA PHARMACEUTICALS, INC.)

CHLORPROPAMIDE
Chlorpropamide Tablets
Chlorpropamide Tablets
Diabinese Tablets
Chlorpropamide Tablets
(LEDERLE STANDARD PRODUCTS)
Chlorpropamide Tablets
(MYLAN PHARMACEUTICALS INC.)

CHLORTETRACYCLINE HYDROCHLORIDE
Aureomycin Ophthalmic Ointment 1.0%

CHLORTHALIDONE
Atenolol and Chlorthalidone Tablets
Chlorthalidone Tablets
Clonidine HCl and Chlorthalidone Tablets
Clonidine Hydrochloride & Chlorthalidone
Tablets
Combipres Tablets
Demi-Regroton Tablets
Hygroton Tablets
Regroton Tablets
Tenoretic Tablets
Thalitone
Chlorthalidone Tablets
(MYLAN PHARMACEUTICALS INC.)

CHLORZOXAZONE
Chlorzoxazone Tablets
Paraflex Caplets
Parafon Forte DSC Caplets
Remular-S
Chlorzoxazone Tablets
(PAR PHARMACEUTICAL, INC.)
Cholac Lactulose Syrup
(ALRA LABORATORIES, INC.)
Choledyl Tablets (PARKE-DAVIS)
Choledyl SA Tablets (PARKE-DAVIS)

CHOLERA VACCINE
Cholera Vaccine
Cholera Vaccine (WYETH-AYERST LABORATORIES)

CHOLESTYRAMINE RESIN
Questran Light
Questran Powder
Questran Tablets

CHOLINE BITARTRATE
Mega-B
Megadose

CHOLINE MAGNESIUM TRISALICYLATE
Tricosal Tablets
Trilisate Liquid
Trilisate Tablets

CHORIONIC GONADOTROPIN
A.P.L.
Pregnyl
Profasi (chorionic gonadotropin for injection,
USP)
Chromagen Capsules (SAVAGE LABORATORIES)

UNDERLINE DENOTES GENERIC NAME

CICLOPIROX OLAMINE
Loprox 1% Cream and Lotion
Ciloxan Ophthalmic Solution
(ALCON LABORATORIES, INC.)

CIMETIDINE
Cimetidine Tablets
Cimetidine Tablets
Cimetidine Tablets, 200 mg
Cimetidine Tablets, 300 mg
Cimetidine Tablets, 400 mg
Cimetidine Tablets, 800 mg
Cimetidine Tablets
Tagamet Tablets
Cimetidine Tablets
(LEDERLE STANDARD PRODUCTS)
Cimetidine Tablets
(MYLAN PHARMACEUTICALS INC.)
Cimetidine Tablets, 200 mg
(NOVOPHARM, USA INC.)
Cimetidine Tablets, 300 mg
(NOVOPHARM, USA INC.)
Cimetidine Tablets, 400 mg
(NOVOPHARM, USA INC.)
Cimetidine Tablets, 800 mg
(NOVOPHARM, USA INC.)
Cimetidine Tablets
(WARNER CHILCOTT LABORATORIES)

CIMETIDINE HYDROCHLORIDE
Tagamet Injection
Tagamet Liquid
Cinobac (OCLASSEN PHARMACEUTICALS, INC.)

CINOXACIN
Cinobac
Cinoxacin Capsules
Cinoxacin Capsules
(BIOCRAFT LABORATORIES, INC.)
Cipro I.V.
(MILES INC. PHARMACEUTICAL DIVISION)
Cipro I.V. Pharmacy Bulk Package
(MILES INC. PHARMACEUTICAL DIVISION)
Cipro Tablets
(MILES INC. PHARMACEUTICAL DIVISION)

CIPROFLOXACIN
Cipro I.V.
Cipro I.V. Pharmacy Bulk Package

CIPROFLOXACIN HYDROCHLORIDE
Ciloxan Ophthalmic Solution
Cipro Tablets

CISAPRIDE
Propulsid

CISPLATIN
Platinol
Platinol-AQ Injection
Citracal (MISSION PHARMACAL COMPANY)
Citracal Caplets+D
(MISSION PHARMACAL COMPANY)
Citracal Liquitab
(MISSION PHARMACAL COMPANY)

CITRIC ACID
Alka-Seltzer Effervescent Antacid
Alka-Seltzer Effervescent Antacid and
Pain Reliever
Alka-Seltzer Extra Strength Effervescent Antacid
and Pain Reliever
Bicitra
Polycitra Syrup
Polycitra-K Crystals
Polycitra-K Oral Solution
Polycitra-LC
Renacidin Irrigation
Citrocarbonate Antacid
(ROBERTS PHARMACEUTICAL CORPORATION)

Citrolith Tablets (BEACH PHARMACEUTICALS)

CLADRIBINE
Leustatin
Claforan Sterile Injection
(HOECHST-ROUSSEL PHARMACEUTICALS INC.)

CLARITHROMYCIN
Biaxin Granules
Biaxin Tablets

CLAVULANATE POTASSIUM
Augmentin Powder for Oral Suspension
Augmentin Tablets and Chewable Tablets
Timentin for Injection
Claritin (SCHERING CORPORATION)
**Clear Eyes ACR Astringent/Lubricating Eye
Redness Reliever Drops**
(ROSS PRODUCTS DIVISION)
**Clear Eyes Lubricating Eye Redness
Reliever Drops** (ROSS PRODUCTS DIVISION)

CLEMASTINE FUMARATE
Clemastine Fumarate Syrup 0.5 mg/5 mL
Clemastine Tablets
Tavist Syrup
Tavist Tablets
Clemastine Fumarate Syrup 0.5 mg/5 mL
(BARRE-NATIONAL INC.)
Clemastine Tablets
(GENEVA PHARMACEUTICALS, INC.)
Cleocin HCl Capsules (THE UPJOHN COMPANY)
Cleocin Pediatric Flavored Granules
(THE UPJOHN COMPANY)
Cleocin Phosphate IV Solution
(THE UPJOHN COMPANY)
Cleocin Phosphate Sterile Solution
(THE UPJOHN COMPANY)
Cleocin T Topical Gel (THE UPJOHN COMPANY)
Cleocin T Topical Lotion (THE UPJOHN COMPANY)
Cleocin T Topical Solution
(THE UPJOHN COMPANY)
Clinda-Derm (PADDOCK LABORATORIES, INC.)

CLIDINIUM BROMIDE
Librax Capsules
Quarzan Capsules

CLINDAMYCIN HYDROCHLORIDE
Cleocin HCl Capsules
Clindamycin Hydrochloride Capsules
Cleocin Vaginal Cream (THE UPJOHN COMPANY)
Clindamycin Hydrochloride Capsules
(BIOCRAFT LABORATORIES, INC.)

CLINDAMYCIN PALMITATE HYDROCHLORIDE
Cleocin Pediatric Flavored Granules

CLINDAMYCIN PHOSPHATE
Cleocin Phosphate IV Solution
Cleocin Phosphate Sterile Solution
Cleocin T Topical Gel
Cleocin T Topical Lotion
Cleocin T Topical Solution
Clinda-Derm
Cleocin Vaginal Cream
Clindamycin Phosphate Injection
Clindamycin Phosphate Injection
Clindamycin Phosphate Injection, USP
Clindamycin Phosphate Topical Soln. USP 1%
Clindamycin Phosphate Injection
(ELKINS-SINN, INC.)
Clindamycin Phosphate Injection
(LEDERLE STANDARD PRODUCTS)
Clindamycin Phosphate Injection, USP
(ASTRA USA, INC.)
**Clindamycin Phosphate Topical Soln. USP
1%**(BARRE-NATIONAL INC.)
Clinoril Tablets (MERCK & CO., INC.)

CLOBETASOL PROPIONATE
Temovate Cream
Temovate Emollient Cream
Temovate Gel
Temovate Ointment
Temovate Scalp Application

CLOCORTOLONE PIVALATE
Cloderm
Clocream Skin Cream
(ROBERTS PHARMACEUTICAL CORPORATION)
Cloderm
(HERMAL PHARMACEUTICAL LABORATORIES, INC.)

CLOFAZIMINE
Lamprene Capsules

CLOFIBRATE
Atromid-S Capsules
Clofibrate Capsules USP, 500 mg
Clofibrate Capsules USP, 500 mg
(NOVOPHARM, USA INC.)

CLOMIPHENE CITRATE
Serophene (clomiphene citrate tablets, USP)

CLOMIPRAMINE HYDROCHLORIDE
Anafranil Capsules

CLONAZEPAM
Klonopin Tablets

CLONIDINE
Catapres-TTS

CLONIDINE HYDROCHLORIDE
Catapres Tablets
Clonidine HCl Tablets, USP
Clonidine HCl Tablets
Clonidine HCl and Chlorthalidone Tablets
Clonidine Hydrochloride Tablets
Clonidine Hydrochloride & Chlorthalidone
Tablets
Combipres Tablets
Clonidine HCl Tablets, USP
(WARNER CHILCOTT LABORATORIES)
Clonidine HCl Tablets
(LEDERLE STANDARD PRODUCTS)
Clonidine HCl and Chlorthalidone Tablets
(PAR PHARMACEUTICAL, INC.)
Clonidine Hydrochloride Tablets
(MYLAN PHARMACEUTICALS INC.)
**Clonidine Hydrochloride & Chlorthalidone
Tablets** (MYLAN PHARMACEUTICALS INC.)

CLORAZEPATE DIPOTASSIUM
Clorazepate Dipotassium Tablets
Clorazepate Dipotassium Tablets
Clorazepate Dipotassium Tablets
Gen-XENE Tablets
Tranxene T-TAB Tablets
Tranxene-SD Half Strength Tablets
Tranxene-SD Tablets
Clorazepate Dipotassium Tablets
(MYLAN PHARMACEUTICALS INC.)
Clorazepate Dipotassium Tablets
(WATSON LABORATORIES, INC.)
Clorazepate Dipotassium Tablets
(WARNER CHILCOTT LABORATORIES)
Clorpactin WCS-90 (GUARDIAN LABORATORIES)

CLOTRIMAZOLE
Clotrimazole Cream, USP 1% (Rx)
Clotrimazole Cream, USP 1% (OTC)
Clotrimazole Vaginal Cream USP 1%
Lotrimin Cream 1%
Lotrimin Lotion 1%
Lotrimin Solution 1%
Lotrisone Cream
Mycelex OTC Cream Antifungal
Mycelex OTC Solution Antifungal

UNDERLINE DENOTES GENERIC NAME

Mycelex Troches
Mycelex-7 Vaginal Cream Antifungal
Mycelex-7 Vaginal Inserts Antifungal
Mycelex-G 500 mg Vaginal Tablets
Clotrimazole Cream, USP 1% (Rx)
(TARO PHARMACEUTICALS U.S.A., INC.)
Clotrimazole Cream, USP 1% (OTC)
(TARO PHARMACEUTICALS U.S.A., INC.)
Clotrimazole Vaginal Cream USP 1%
(BARRE-NATIONAL INC.)

CLOXACILLIN SODIUM
Cloxacillin for Oral Suspension
Cloxacillin Sodium Capsules
Cloxacillin Sodium Capsules, USP
Cloxacillin Sodium for Oral Solution
Cloxacillin for Oral Suspension
(WARNER CHILCOTT LABORATORIES)
Cloxacillin Sodium Capsules
(BIOCRAFT LABORATORIES, INC.)
Cloxacillin Sodium Capsules, USP
(WARNER CHILCOTT LABORATORIES)
Cloxacillin Sodium for Oral Solution
(BIOCRAFT LABORATORIES, INC.)
Cloxapen Capsules
(SMITHKLINE BEECHAM PHARMACEUTICALS)

CLOZAPINE
Clozaril Tablets
Clozaril Tablets
(SANDOZ PHARMACEUTICALS CORPORATION)

COAL TAR
DHS Tar Gel Shampoo
DHS Tar Shampoo
Doak Tar Distillate
Doak Tar Lotion
Doak Tar Oil
Doak Tar Shampoo
Fototar Cream
Ionil T Plus Shampoo
Pentrax Anti-dandruff Shampoo
Zetar Emulsion

COCAINE HYDROCHLORIDE
Cocaine Hydrochloride Topical Solution
Cocaine Hydrochloride Topical Solution
Cocaine Hydrochloride Viscous Topical Solution
Cocaine Hydrochloride Topical Solution
(ASTRA USA, INC.)
Cocaine Hydrochloride Topical Solution
(ROXANE LABORATORIES, INC.)
Cocaine Hydrochloride Viscous Topical Solution
(ROXANE LABORATORIES, INC.)
Codamine Pediatric Syrup (BARRE-NATIONAL INC.)
Codamine Syrup (BARRE-NATIONAL INC.)

CODEINE PHOSPHATE
Acetaminophen and Codeine Phosphate Oral
Soln.
Acetaminophen and Codeine Phosphate Tablets
Actifed with Codeine Cough Syrup
Ambenyl Cough Syrup
Brontex
Capital And Codeine Suspension
Codeine Phosphate Injection
Codeine Phosphate in Tubex
Codimal PH Syrup
Deconsal C Expectorant Syrup
Deconsal Pediatric Syrup
Dimetane-DC Cough Syrup
Empirin with Codeine Tablets
Fioricet with Codeine Capsules
Fiorinal with Codeine Capsules
Isoclor Expectorant
Novahistine DH (+)
Novahistine Expectorant (+)
Nucofed Expectorant
Nucofed Pediatric Expectorant

Nucofed Syrup and Capsules
Pediacof Cough Syrup
Phenaphen with Codeine Capsules
Phenergan with Codeine
Phenergan VC with Codeine
Poly-Histine CS
Promethazine VC with Codeine
Robitussin A-C Syrup
Robitussin-DAC Syrup
Soma Compound w/Codeine Tablets
Triaminic Expectorant with Codeine
Tussar-2
Tussar SF
Tussi-Organidin NR Liquid and S NR Liquid
Tylenol with Codeine Elixir
Tylenol with Codeine Phosphate Tablets
Codeine Phosphate Injection
(ELKINS-SINN, INC.)
Codeine Phosphate in Tubex
(WYETH-AYERST LABORATORIES)

CODEINE SULFATE
Codeine Sulfate Tablets
Codeine Sulfate Tablets
(ROXANE LABORATORIES, INC.)
Codiclear DH Syrup
(CENTRAL PHARMACEUTICALS, INC.)
Codimal DH Syrup
(CENTRAL PHARMACEUTICALS, INC.)
Codimal DM Syrup
(CENTRAL PHARMACEUTICALS, INC.)
Codimal PH Syrup
(CENTRAL PHARMACEUTICALS, INC.)
Codimal-L.A. Capsules
(CENTRAL PHARMACEUTICALS, INC.)
Codimal-L.A. HALF Capsules
(CENTRAL PHARMACEUTICALS, INC.)

COENZYME Q-10
Coenzyme Q10 200mg & 100mg Chewable
Wafers with Vitamin E and Tablets 200mg,
60mg & 25mg
**Coenzyme Q10 200mg & 100mg Chewable
Wafers with Vitamin E and Tablets 200mg,
60mg & 25mg** (VITALINE CORPORATION)
Cogentin Injection (MERCK & CO., INC.)
Cogentin Tablets (MERCK & CO., INC.)
Co-Gesic Tablets
(CENTRAL PHARMACEUTICALS, INC.)
Cognex Capsules (PARKE-DAVIS)
ColBENEMID Tablets (MERCK & CO., INC.)

COLCHICINE
ColBENEMID Tablets
Colchicine Ampoules
Colchicine Ampoules (ELI LILLY AND COMPANY)
Colestid Granules (THE UPJOHN COMPANY)
Flavored Colestid Granules
(THE UPJOHN COMPANY)

COLESTIPOL HYDROCHLORIDE
Colestid Granules
Flavored Colestid Granules

COLFOSCERIL PALMITATE
Exosurf Neonatal for Intratracheal Suspension

COLISTIMETHATE SODIUM
Coly-Mycin M Parenteral

COLISTIN SULFATE
Coly-Mycin S Otic w/Neomycin &
Hydrocortisone

COLLAGEN
INSTAT* Collagen Absorbable Hemostat

COLLAGEN, BOVINE
INSTAT* MCH Microfibrillar Collagen
Hemostat

COLLAGENASE
Collagenase Santyl Ointment
Collagenase Santyl Ointment
(KNOLL PHARMACEUTICAL COMPANY)
Collyrium for Fresh Eyes
(WYETH-AYERST LABORATORIES)
Collyrium Fresh (WYETH-AYERST LABORATORIES)
Coly-Mycin M Parenteral (PARKE-DAVIS)
**Coly-Mycin S Otic w/Neomycin &
Hydrocortisone** (PARKE-DAVIS)
Colyte and Colyte flavored (REED & CARNRICK)
Combipres Tablets
(BOEHRINGER INGELHEIM PHARMACEUTICALS, INC.)
Comhist LA Capsules
(ROBERTS PHARMACEUTICAL CORPORATION)
Compazine Injection
(SMITHKLINE BEECHAM PHARMACEUTICALS)
Compazine Multi-dose Vials
(SMITHKLINE BEECHAM PHARMACEUTICALS)
Compazine Prefilled Disposable Syringes
(SMITHKLINE BEECHAM PHARMACEUTICALS)
Compazine Spansule Capsules
(SMITHKLINE BEECHAM PHARMACEUTICALS)
Compazine Suppositories
(SMITHKLINE BEECHAM PHARMACEUTICALS)
Compazine Syrup
(SMITHKLINE BEECHAM PHARMACEUTICALS)
Compazine Tablets
(SMITHKLINE BEECHAM PHARMACEUTICALS)
Complete Allergy Cream 1%
(BARRE-NATIONAL. INC.)
Complete Allergy Cream 2%
(BARRE-NATIONAL INC.)
**Allergy-Sinus Comtrex Multi-Symptom Allergy
Sinus Formula Tablets & Caplets**
(BRISTOL-MYERS PRODUCTS)
Day-Night Comtrex (BRISTOL-MYERS PRODUCTS)
**Comtrex Maximum Strength Multi-Symptom
Cold Reliever Tablets/Caplets/Liqui-
Gels/Liquid** (BRISTOL-MYERS PRODUCTS)
**Non-Drowsy Comtrex Maximum Strength
Caplets** (BRISTOL-MYERS PRODUCTS)
**Conceptrol Contraceptive Gel,
Single Use Contraceptive**
(ORTHO PHARMACEUTICAL CORPORATION)
Conceptrol Contraceptive Inserts
(ORTHO PHARMACEUTICAL CORPORATION)
Condylox (OCLASSEN PHARMACEUTICALS, INC.)
**Congespirin For Children Aspirin Free Chewable
Cold Tablets** (BRISTOL-MYERS PRODUCTS)
Congess Jr. T.D. Capsules (FLEMING & COMPANY)
Congess Sr. T.D. Capsules (FLEMING & COMPANY)
Constilac Lactulose Syrup
(ALRA LABORATORIES, INC.)
Constulose (BARRE-NATIONAL INC.)
**Contac Continuous Action
Decongestant/Antihistamine Capsules**
(SMITHKLINE BEECHAM CONSUMER HEALTHCARE, L.P.)
**Contac Maximum Strength Continuous Action
Decongestant/Antihistamine Caplets**
(SMITHKLINE BEECHAM CONSUMER HEALTHCARE, L.P.)
Contac Severe Cold and Flu Formula Caplets
(SMITHKLINE BEECHAM CONSUMER HEALTHCARE, L.P.)
Contac Severe Cold & Flu Nighttime
(SMITHKLINE BEECHAM CONSUMER HEALTHCARE, L.P.)

COPPER
Caltrate PLUS
ParaGard T380A Intrauterine
Copper Contraceptive
Cordarone Tablets
(WYETH-AYERST LABORATORIES)
Cordran Lotion
(OCLASSEN PHARMACEUTICALS, INC.)
Cordran Ointment
(OCLASSEN PHARMACEUTICALS, INC.)

UNDERLINE DENOTES GENERIC NAME

Cordran SP Cream
(OCLASSEN PHARMACEUTICALS, INC.)
Cordran Tape
(OCLASSEN PHARMACEUTICALS, INC.)
CORNSTARCH
Perative Specialized Liquid Nutrition
Promote High Protein Liquid Nutrition
Cortane B OTIC (BLANSETT PHARMACAL)
CORTENEMA (SOLVAY PHARMACEUTICALS, INC.)
Cortic Ear Drops (EVERETT LABORATORIES, INC.)
Cortifoam (REED & CARNRICK)
CORTISONE ACETATE
Cortone Acetate Sterile Suspension
Cortone Acetate Tablets
Cortisporin Cream (BURROUGHS WELLCOME CO.)
Cortisporin Ointment
(BURROUGHS WELLCOME CO.)
Cortisporin Ophthalmic Ointment Sterile
(BURROUGHS WELLCOME CO.)
Cortisporin Ophthalmic Suspension Sterile
(BURROUGHS WELLCOME CO.)
Cortisporin Otic Solution Sterile
(BURROUGHS WELLCOME CO.)
Cortisporin Otic Suspension Sterile
(BURROUGHS WELLCOME CO.)
Cortone Acetate Sterile Suspension
(MERCK & CO., INC.)
Cortone Acetate Tablets (MERCK & CO., INC.)
Cortrosyn (ORGANON INC.)
Cosmegen Injection (MERCK & CO., INC.)
Cotazym (ORGANON INC.)
Cotazym-S (ORGANON INC.)
Cough-X Lozenges
(B. F. ASCHER & COMPANY, INC.)
Coumadin Tablets (DUPONT PHARMA)
CREON 10 Capsules
(SOLVAY PHARMACEUTICALS, INC.)
CREON 20 Capsules
(SOLVAY PHARMACEUTICALS, INC.)
Critic-Aid, Antimicrobial Skin Paste
(SWEEN CORPORATION)
CROMOLYN SODIUM
Cromolyn Sodium Inhalation USP
Gastrocrom Capsules
Intal Capsules
Intal Inhaler
Intal Nebulizer Solution
Nasalcrom Nasal Solution
Cromolyn Sodium Inhalation USP
(DEY LABORATORIES)
CROTAMITON
Eurax Cream & Lotion
Crystodigin Tablets (ELI LILLY AND COMPANY)
Cuprimine Capsules (MERCK & CO., INC.)
Cutivate Cream (GLAXO DERMATOLOGY)
Cutivate Ointment (GLAXO DERMATOLOGY)
CYANOCOBALAMIN
Apatate Liquid/Tablets
Apatate Liquid with Fluoride
Chromagen Capsules
Cyanocobalamin in Tubex
Cyanocobalamin (Vit. B_{12}) Injection
Eldertonic
Ener-B Vitamin B_{12} Nasal Gel
Dietary Supplement
Fetrin Capsules
May-Vita Elixir
Niferex-150 Forte Capsules
Trinsicon Capsules
Vitamin B_{12} (Cyanocobalamin) in Tubex
Cyanocobalamin in Tubex
(WYETH-AYERST LABORATORIES)
Cyanocobalamin (Vit. B_{12}) Injection
(ELKINS-SINN, INC.)

CYCLOBENZAPRINE HYDROCHLORIDE
Cyclobenzaprine HCl Tablets
Cyclobenzaprine Hydrochloride Tablets
Cyclobenzaprine Hydrochloride Tablets, U.S.P.
Cyclobenzaprine Tablets
Cyclobenzaprine Hydrochloride Tablets
Cyclobenzaprine Hydrochloride Tablets, USP
Flexeril Tablets
Cyclobenzaprine HCl Tablets
(GENEVA PHARMACEUTICALS, INC.)
Cyclobenzaprine Hydrochloride Tablets
(MYLAN PHARMACEUTICALS INC.)
Cyclobenzaprine Hydrochloride Tablets, U.S.P.
(WEST POINT PHARMA)
Cyclobenzaprine Tablets
(WARNER CHILCOTT LABORATORIES)
Cyclobenzaprine Hydrochloride Tablets
(DURAMED PHARMACEUTICALS, INC.)
Cyclobenzaprine Hydrochloride Tablets, USP
(WATSON LABORATORIES, INC.)
Cyclocort Topical Cream 0.1%
(FUJISAWA USA, INC.)
Cyclocort Topical Lotion 0.1%
(FUJISAWA USA, INC.)
Cyclocort Topical Ointment 0.1%
(FUJISAWA USA, INC.)
CYCLOPHOSPHAMIDE
Cytoxan for Injection
Cytoxan Tablets
NEOSAR Lyophilized/Neosar
CYCLOSERINE
Seromycin Pulvules
CYCLOSPORINE
Sandimmune I.V. Ampuls for Infusion
Sandimmune Oral Solution
Sandimmune Soft Gelatin Capsules
Cycrin Tablets (ESI PHARMA, INC.)
Cyklokapron Tablets and Injection
(PHARMACIA ADRIA PHARMACIA INC.)
Cylert Chewable Tablets
(ABBOTT LABORATORIES)
Cylert Tablets (ABBOTT LABORATORIES)
CYPROHEPTADINE HYDROCHLORIDE
Cyproheptadine HCl Syrup USP 2 mg/5 mL
Cyproheptadine HCl Tablets
Periactin Syrup
Periactin Tablets
Cyproheptadine HCl Syrup USP 2 mg/5 mL
(BARRE-NATIONAL INC.)
Cyproheptadine HCl Tablets
(PAR PHARMACEUTICAL, INC.)
Cystospaz Tablets
(POLYMEDICA PHARMACEUTICALS (U.S.A.), INC.)
Cystospaz-M Capsules
(POLYMEDICA PHARMACEUTICALS (U.S.A.), INC.)
Cytadren Tablets
(CIBA PHARMACEUTICAL COMPANY)
CYTARABINE
Cytosar-U Sterile Powder
CytoGam (MEDIMMUNE, INC.)
CYTOMEGALOVIRUS IMMUNE GLOBULIN
CytoGam
Cytomel Tablets
(SMITHKLINE BEECHAM PHARMACEUTICALS)
Cytosar-U Sterile Powder
(THE UPJOHN COMPANY)
Cytotec (G.D. SEARLE & CO.)
Cytovene Sterile Powder
(SYNTEX PUERTO RICO, INC.)
Cytoxan for Injection
(BRISTOL-MYERS SQUIBB ONCOLOGY DIVISION)
Cytoxan Tablets
(BRISTOL-MYERS SQUIBB ONCOLOGY DIVISION)

D

D.A. Chewable Tablets
(DURA PHARMACEUTICALS, INC)
DDAVP Injection
(RHONE-POULENC RORER PHARMACEUTICALS INC.)
DDAVP Nasal Spray
(RHONE-POULENC RORER PHARMACEUTICALS INC.)
DDAVP Rhinal Tube
(RHONE-POULENC RORER PHARMACEUTICALS INC.)
DHA (DOCOSAHEXAENOIC ACID)
Super Omega-3 Fatty Acids Soft Gels
DHCplus Capsules
(THE PURDUE FREDERICK COMPANY)
D.H.E. 45 Injection
(SANDOZ PHARMACEUTICALS CORPORATION)
DHS Conditioning Rinse
(PERSON & COVEY, INC.)
DHS Shampoo (PERSON & COVEY, INC.)
DHS Clear Shampoo (PERSON & COVEY, INC.)
DHS Tar Gel Shampoo
(PERSON & COVEY, INC.)
DHS Tar Shampoo (PERSON & COVEY, INC.)
DHS Zinc Dandruff Shampoo
(PERSON & COVEY, INC.)
DHT (Dihydrotachysterol) Tablets & Intensol
(ROXANE LABORATORIES, INC.)
DMH-Syrup (ALRA LABORATORIES, INC.)
DML Facial Moisturizer with Sunscreen
(PERSON & COVEY, INC.)
DML Forte Cream (PERSON & COVEY, INC.)
DML Moisturizing Lotion
(PERSON & COVEY, INC.)
DPH-Elixir, USP (ALRA LABORATORIES, INC.)
DTIC-Dome
(MILES INC. PHARMACEUTICAL DIVISION)
DACARBAZINE
DTIC-Dome
DACTINOMYCIN
Cosmegen Injection
Dalalone D.P. Injectable
(FOREST PHARMACEUTICALS, INC.)
Dalgan Injection (ASTRA USA, INC.)
Dallergy Caplets, Syrup, Tablets (LASER, INC.)
Dallergy-JR Capsules (LASER, INC.)
Dalmane Capsules (ROCHE PRODUCTS INC.)
Damason-P (MASON PHARMACEUTICALS, INC.)
DANAZOL
Danocrine Capsules
Danex Dandruff Shampoo (ALLERGAN HERBERT)
Danocrine Capsules
(SANOFI WINTHROP PHARMACEUTICALS)
Dantrium Capsules
(PROCTER & GAMBLE PHARMACEUTICALS, INC.)
Dantrium Intravenous
(PROCTER & GAMBLE PHARMACEUTICALS, INC.)
DANTROLENE SODIUM
Dantrium Capsules
Dantrium Intravenous
DAPSONE
Dapsone USP
Dapsone USP
(JACOBUS PHARMACEUTICAL CO., INC.)
Daranide Tablets (MERCK & CO., INC.)
Daraprim Tablets (BURROUGHS WELLCOME CO.)
Darvocet-N 50 Tablets
(ELI LILLY AND COMPANY)
Darvocet-N 100 Tablets
(ELI LILLY AND COMPANY)
Darvon Compound-65 Pulvules
(ELI LILLY AND COMPANY)
Darvon Pulvules (ELI LILLY AND COMPANY)

UNDERLINE DENOTES GENERIC NAME

Darvon-N Suspension & Tablets
(ELI LILLY AND COMPANY)

DAUNORUBICIN HYDROCHLORIDE
  Cerubidine
Daypro Caplets (G.D. SEARLE & CO.)
Debrox Drops
(SMITHKLINE BEECHAM CONSUMER HEALTHCARE, L.P.)
Decadron Elixir (MERCK & CO., INC.)
Decadron Phosphate Injection (MERCK & CO., INC.)
Decadron Phosphate Respihaler
(MERCK & CO., INC.)
Decadron Phosphate Sterile Ophthalmic
  Ointment (MERCK & CO., INC.)
Decadron Phosphate Sterile Ophthalmic Solution
(MERCK & CO., INC.)
Decadron Phosphate Topical Cream
(MERCK & CO., INC.)
Decadron Phosphate Turbinaire
(MERCK & CO., INC.)
Decadron Phosphate with Xylocaine Injection,
  Sterile (MERCK & CO., INC.)
Decadron Tablets (MERCK & CO., INC.)
Decadron-LA Sterile Suspension
(MERCK & CO., INC.)
Deca-Durabolin (ORGANON INC.)
Decaspray Topical Aerosol (MERCK & CO., INC.)
Declomycin Tablets (LEDERLE LABORATORIES)
Decofed Liquid (BARRE-NATIONAL INC.)
Deconamine SR Capsules, Tablets, Syrup
(KENWOOD LABORATORIES)
Deconsal Sprinkle Capsules
(ADAMS LABORATORIES, INC.)
Deconsal C Expectorant Syrup
(ADAMS LABORATORIES, INC.)
Deconsal Pediatric Syrup
(ADAMS LABORATORIES, INC.)
Deconsal II Tablets
(ADAMS LABORATORIES, INC.)
D-FEDA II Tablets
(WE PHARMACEUTICALS, INC.)

DEFEROXAMINE MESYLATE
  Desferal Vials
Delatestryl Injection
(BTG PHARMACEUTICALS CORP.)
Delfen Contraceptive Foam
(ORTHO PHARMACEUTICAL CORPORATION)
Delsym Cough Formula
(FISONS CORPORATION PRESCRIPTION PRODUCTS)
Deltasone Tablets (THE UPJOHN COMPANY)
Demadex Tablets and Injection
(BOEHRINGER MANNHEIM PHARMACEUTICALS)

DEMECARIUM BROMIDE
  Humorsol Sterile Ophthalmic Solution

DEMECLOCYCLINE HYDROCHLORIDE
  Declomycin Tablets
Demerol Hydrochloride Carpuject
(SANOFI WINTHROP PHARMACEUTICALS)
Demerol Hydrochloride Injection
(SANOFI WINTHROP PHARMACEUTICALS)
Demerol Hydrochloride Syrup
(SANOFI WINTHROP PHARMACEUTICALS)
Demerol Hydrochloride Tablets
(SANOFI WINTHROP PHARMACEUTICALS)
Demerol Hydrochloride Uni-Amp
(SANOFI WINTHROP PHARMACEUTICALS)
Demi-Regroton Tablets
(RHONE-POULENC RORER PHARMACEUTICALS INC.)
Demser Capsules (MERCK & CO., INC.)
Demulen 1/35-21 (G.D. SEARLE & CO.)
Demulen 1/35-28 (G.D. SEARLE & CO.)
Demulen 1/50-21 (G.D. SEARLE & CO.)
Demulen 1/50-28 (G.D. SEARLE & CO.)
Depakene Capsules (ABBOTT LABORATORIES)

Depakene Syrup (ABBOTT LABORATORIES)
Depakote Sprinkle Capsules
(ABBOTT LABORATORIES)
Depakote Tablets (ABBOTT LABORATORIES)
Depen Titratable Tablets
(WALLACE LABORATORIES)
Depo-Medrol Single-Dose Vial
(THE UPJOHN COMPANY)
Depo-Medrol Sterile Aqueous Suspension
(THE UPJOHN COMPANY)
Depo-Provera Contraceptive Injection
(THE UPJOHN COMPANY)
Depo-Provera Sterile Aqueous Suspension
(THE UPJOHN COMPANY)
DEPO-Testosterone Sterile Solution
(THE UPJOHN COMPANY)
Deponit NTG Transdermal Delivery System
(SCHWARZ PHARMA)
Derifil Tablets (RYSTAN COMPANY, INC.)
Dermacin Creme (PEDINOL PHARMACAL INC.)
Dermaide Aloe Cream
(DERMAIDE RESEARCH CORPORATION)
Derma-Smoothe/FS Topical Oil
(HILL DERMACEUTICALS, INC.)
Dermatop Emollient Cream 0.1%
(HOECHST-ROUSSEL PHARMACEUTICALS INC.)
DermUspray (WARNER CHILCOTT LABORATORIES)
Desferal Vials (CIBA PHARMACEUTICAL COMPANY)

DESFLURANE
  Suprane

DESIPRAMINE HYDROCHLORIDE
  Desipramine HCl Tablets
  Desipramine Tablets
  Norpramin Tablets
Desipramine HCl Tablets
(GENEVA PHARMACEUTICALS, INC.)
Desipramine Tablets
(WARNER CHILCOTT LABORATORIES)

DESMOPRESSIN ACETATE
  DDAVP Injection
  DDAVP Nasal Spray
  DDAVP Rhinal Tube
  Desmopressin Acetate Rhinal Tube
  Stimate (desmopressin acetate)
    Nasal Spray, 1.5 mg/mL
Desmopressin Acetate Rhinal Tube
(FERRING LABORATORIES, INC.)
Desogen Tablets (ORGANON INC.)

DESOGESTREL
  Desogen Tablets
  Ortho-Cept Tablets

DESONIDE
  Desonide Cream, USP
  DesOwen Cream, Ointment and Lotion
  Otic Tridesilon Solution 0.05%
  Tridesilon Cream 0.05%
  Tridesilon Ointment 0.05%
Desonide Cream, USP
(TARO PHARMACEUTICALS U.S.A., INC.)
DesOwen Cream, Ointment and Lotion
(GALDERMA LABORATORIES, INC.)

DESOXIMETASONE
  Desoximetasone Cream, USP 0.25% and 0.05%
  Topicort Emollient Cream 0.25%
  Topicort Gel 0.05%
  Topicort LP Emollient Cream 0.05%
  Topicort Ointment 0.25%
Desoximetasone Cream, USP 0.25% and 0.05%
(TARO PHARMACEUTICALS U.S.A., INC.)

DESOXYRIBONUCLEASE
  Elase Ointment
  Elase Vials
  Elase-Chloromycetin Ointment

Desoxyn Gradumet Tablets
(ABBOTT LABORATORIES)
Despec Caplets (INTERNATIONAL ETHICAL LABS.)
Despec Liquid (INTERNATIONAL ETHICAL LABS.)
Despec SF (INTERNATIONAL ETHICAL LABS.)
Desquam-E 2.5 Emollient Gel
(WESTWOOD-SQUIBB PHARMACEUTICALS INC.)
Desquam-E 5 Emollient Gel
(WESTWOOD-SQUIBB PHARMACEUTICALS INC.)
Desquam-E 10 Emollient Gel
(WESTWOOD-SQUIBB PHARMACEUTICALS INC.)
Desquam-X 2.5 Gel
(WESTWOOD-SQUIBB PHARMACEUTICALS INC.)
Desquam-X 5 Gel
(WESTWOOD-SQUIBB PHARMACEUTICALS INC.)
Desquam-X 10 Gel
(WESTWOOD-SQUIBB PHARMACEUTICALS INC.)
Desquam-X 10 Bar
(WESTWOOD-SQUIBB PHARMACEUTICALS INC.)
Desquam-X 5 Wash
(WESTWOOD-SQUIBB PHARMACEUTICALS INC.)
Desquam-X 10 Wash
(WESTWOOD-SQUIBB PHARMACEUTICALS INC.)
Desyrel and Desyrel Dividose (APOTHECON)
Detussin Expectorant and Liquid
(BARRE-NATIONAL INC.)
Dexacort Phosphate in Respihaler
(ADAMS LABORATORIES, INC.)
Dexacort Phosphate in Turbinaire
(ADAMS LABORATORIES, INC.)

DEXAMETHASONE
  Aeroseb-Dex Topical Aerosol Spray
  Decadron Elixir
  Decadron Tablets
  Decaspray Topical Aerosol
  Dexamethasone Elixir USP 0.5 mg/5 mL
  Dexamethasone Tablets
  Dexamethasone Tablets, Oral Solution & Intensol
  Hexadrol Tablets
  TobraDex Ophthalmic Suspension and Ointment
Dexamethasone Elixir USP 0.5 mg/5 mL
(BARRE-NATIONAL INC.)
Dexamethasone Tablets
(PAR PHARMACEUTICAL, INC.)
Dexamethasone Tablets, Oral Solution & Intensol
(ROXANE LABORATORIES, INC.)

DEXAMETHASONE ACETATE
  Dalalone D.P. Injectable
  Decadron-LA Sterile Suspension

DEXAMETHASONE SODIUM PHOSPHATE
  Decadron Phosphate Injection
  Decadron Phosphate Respihaler
  Decadron Phosphate Sterile
    Ophthalmic Ointment
  Decadron Phosphate Sterile Ophthalmic Solution
  Decadron Phosphate Topical Cream
  Decadron Phosphate Turbinaire
  Decadron Phosphate with Xylocaine
    Injection, Sterile
  Dexacort Phosphate in Respihaler
  Dexacort Phosphate in Turbinaire
  Dexamethasone Sodium Phosphate Injection
  Hexadrol Phosphate Injection
  NeoDecadron Sterile Ophthalmic Ointment
  NeoDecadron Sterile Ophthalmic Solution
  NeoDecadron Topical Cream
Dexamethasone Sodium Phosphate Injection
(ELKINS-SINN, INC.)
Dexedrine Spansule Capsules
(SMITHKLINE BEECHAM PHARMACEUTICALS)
Dexedrine Tablets
(SMITHKLINE BEECHAM PHARMACEUTICALS)

DEXPANTHENOL
  May-Vita Elixir

UNDERLINE DENOTES GENERIC NAME

DEXTRAN I
Promit

DEXTRAN 40
Rheomacrodex

DEXTRAN 70
Hyskon Hysteroscopy Fluid
Tears Naturale II Lubricant Eye Drops
Tears Naturale Free

DEXTRANS (LOW MOLECULAR WEIGHT)
Rheomacrodex

DEXTROAMPHETAMINE
Biphetamine Capsules

DEXTROAMPHETAMINE SACCHARATE
Adderall Tablets

DEXTROAMPHETAMINE SULFATE
Adderall Tablets
Dexedrine Spansule Capsules
Dexedrine Tablets
Dextroamphetamine Sulfate Tablets
DextroStat Dextroamphetamine Tablets
Dextroamphetamine Sulfate Tablets
(REXAR PHARMACAL)

DEXTROMETHORPHAN HYDROBROMIDE
Albatussin SR Caplets
Anatuss DM Syrup
Anatuss DM Tablets
Benylin Adult Formula
Benylin Expectorant
Benylin Multi-Symptom
Benylin Pediatric
Bromarest DX Cough Syrup
Bromfed-DM Cough Syrup
Codimal DM Syrup
Comtrex Maximum Strength Multi-Symptom
   Cold Reliever Tablets/Caplets/
   Liqui-Gels/Liquid
Non-Drowsy Comtrex Maximum Strength
   Caplets
Dimetane-DX Cough Syrup
Fenesin DM
HISTINEX DM
Humibid DM Sprinkle Capsules
Humibid DM Tablets
PediaCare Cough-Cold Chewable Tablets
PediaCare Cough-Cold Liquid
PediaCare NightRest Cough-Cold Liquid
Phenergan with Dextromethorphan
Poly-Histine DM Syrup
Rescon-DM Liquid
Rondec-DM Oral Drops
Rondec-DM Syrup
Safe Tussin 30
Sudafed Cold & Cough Liquid Caps
Sudafed Cough Syrup
Sudafed Severe Cold Formula Tablets
Touro DM Caplets
Tuss-DA RX
Tussafed Drops & Syrup
Tussar DM
Tussi-Organidin DM NR Liquid and DM-S NR
   Liquid
Children's TYLENOL Cold Multi-Symptom Plus
   Cough Liquid Formula and Chewable Tablets
TYLENOL Cold Hot Medication Packets
TYLENOL Cold Medication No Drowsiness
   Formula Gelcaps and Caplets
TYLENOL Cough Multi-Symptom Medication
TYLENOL Cough Multi-Symptom Medication
   with Decongestant
TYLENOL Flu Maximum Strength Gelcaps
TYLENOL Cold Multi-Symptom Formula
   Medication Tablets and Caplets

DEXTROSE
Dextrose 50% Injection, USP
Emecheck
Emetrol Solution - Cherry
Emetrol Solution - Lemon-Mint
Glutose 15, Glutose 45 (Oral Glucose Gel)
Glutose Tablets
Xylocaine 1.5% Solution with Dextrose 7.5%
Dextrose 50% Injection, USP (ASTRA USA, INC.)
DextroStat Dextroamphetamine Tablets
   (RICHWOOD PHARMACEUTICAL COMPANY, INC.)
Dey-Pak (DEY LABORATORIES)
Dey-Vial (DEY LABORATORIES)

DEZOCINE
Dalgan Injection
DiaBeta Tablets
   (HOECHST-ROUSSEL PHARMACEUTICALS INC.)
Diabinese Tablets (PFIZER LABS DIVISION)
Dialose Tablets
   (JOHNSON & JOHNSON • MERCK CONSUMER PHAR-
   MACEUTICALS CO.)
Dialose Plus Tablets
   (JOHNSON & JOHNSON • MERCK CONSUMER PHAR-
   MACEUTICALS CO.)
Dialume Capsules
   (RHONE-POULENC RORER PHARMACEUTICALS INC.)
Diamox Parenteral (LEDERLE LABORATORIES)
Diamox Sequels (Sustained Release)
   (LEDERLE LABORATORIES)
Diamox Tablets (LEDERLE LABORATORIES)
Diaper Rash Ointment (BARRE-NATIONAL INC.)
Diapid Nasal Spray
   (SANDOZ PHARMACEUTICALS CORPORATION)

DIAZEPAM
Diazepam Injection
Diazepam Injection, Tablets
Diazepam Tablets
Diazepam Oral Solution
Valium Injectable
Valium Tablets
Valrelease Capsules
Diazepam Injection (ELKINS-SINN, INC.)
Diazepam Injection, Tablets
   (LEDERLE STANDARD PRODUCTS)
Diazepam Tablets
   (MYLAN PHARMACEUTICALS INC.)
Diazepam Oral Solution
   (ROXANE LABORATORIES, INC.)

DIAZOXIDE
Hyperstat I.V. Injection
Proglycem Capsules
Proglycem Suspension
Dibenzyline Capsules
   (SMITHKLINE BEECHAM PHARMACEUTICALS)

DIBUCAINE
Dibucaine Ointment USP 1%
Dibucaine Ointment USP 1%
   (BARRE-NATIONAL INC.)
Dical-D Tablets & Wafers
   (ABBOTT LABORATORIES)

DICHLORALPHENAZONE
Duradrin Capsules
Midrin Capsules

DICHLOROACETIC ACID
Bichloracetic Acid Kahlenberg

DICHLORODIFLUOROMETHANE
Fluori-Methane

DICHLOROTETRAFLUOROETHANE
Fluro-Ethyl

DICHLORPHENAMIDE
Daranide Tablets

DICLOFENAC POTASSIUM
Cataflam

DICLOFENAC SODIUM
Voltaren Tablets

DICLOXACILLIN SODIUM
Dicloxacillin Sodium Capsules
Dicloxacillin Sodium Capsules
Dicloxacillin Sodium Capsules, USP
Pathocil Capsules
Pathocil for Oral Suspension
Dicloxacillin Sodium Capsules
   (BIOCRAFT LABORATORIES, INC.)
Dicloxacillin Sodium Capsules
   (LEDERLE STANDARD PRODUCTS)
Dicloxacillin Sodium Capsules, USP
   (WARNER CHILCOTT LABORATORIES)

DICYCLOMINE HYDROCHLORIDE
Bentyl 10 mg Capsules
Bentyl Injection
Bentyl Syrup
Bentyl 20 mg Tablets

DIDANOSINE
Videx Tablets, Powder for Oral Solution, &
   Pediatric Powder for Oral Solution
Didrex Tablets (THE UPJOHN COMPANY)
Didronel I.V. Infusion (MGI PHARMA, INC.)
Didronel Tablets
   (PROCTER & GAMBLE PHARMACEUTICALS, INC.)

DIENESTROL
Ortho Dienestrol Cream

DIETARY SUPPLEMENT
Hepacolin
Neurochol Dietary Supplement

DIETHYLSTILBESTROL
Diethylstilbestrol Tablets

DIETHYLSTILBESTROL DIPHOSPHATE
Stilphostrol Tablets and Ampuls
Diethylstilbestrol Tablets
   (ELI LILLY AND COMPANY)

DIFENOXIN HYDROCHLORIDE
Motofen Tablets

DIFLORASONE DIACETATE
Florone Cream 0.05%
Florone E Emollient Cream 0.05%
Florone Ointment 0.05%
Maxiflor Cream
Maxiflor Ointment
Psorcon Cream 0.05%
Psorcon Ointment 0.05%
Diflucan Injection, Tablets, and Oral Suspension
   (ROERIG DIVISION)

DIFLUNISAL
Diflunisal Tablets, U.S.P.
Dolobid Tablets
Diflunisal Tablets, U.S.P. (WEST POINT PHARMA)
Digepepsin Pancreatin Enzyme Supplement
   (KENWOOD LABORATORIES)
Digibind (BURROUGHS WELLCOME CO.)

DIGITOXIN
Crystodigin Tablets

DIGOXIN
Digoxin Elixir
Digoxin Injection
Digoxin in Tubex
Lanoxicaps
Lanoxin Elixir Pediatric
Lanoxin Injection
Lanoxin Injection Pediatric
Lanoxin Tablets

UNDERLINE DENOTES GENERIC NAME

Digoxin Elixir (ROXANE LABORATORIES, INC.)
Digoxin Injection (ELKINS-SINN, INC.)
Digoxin in Tubex
 (WYETH-AYERST LABORATORIES)
DIGOXIN IMMUNE FAB (OVINE)
 Digibind
Dihistine DH Elixir (BARRE-NATIONAL INC.)
Dihistine Expectorant (BARRE-NATIONAL INC.)
DIHYDROCODEINE BITARTRATE
 DHCplus Capsules
 Synalgos-DC Capsules
DIHYDROERGOTAMINE MESYLATE
 D.H.E. 45 Injection
DIHYDROTACHYSTEROL
 DHT (Dihydrotachysterol) Tablets & Intensol
Dilacor XR Extended-release Capsules
 (RHONE-POULENC RORER PHARMACEUTICALS INC.)
Dilantin Infatabs (PARKE-DAVIS)
Dilantin Kapseals (PARKE-DAVIS)
Dilantin Parenteral (PARKE-DAVIS)
Dilantin-125 Suspension (PARKE-DAVIS)
Dilatrate-SR (REED & CARNRICK)
Dilaudid Cough Syrup
 (KNOLL PHARMACEUTICAL COMPANY)
Dilaudid Hydrochloride Ampules
 (KNOLL PHARMACEUTICAL COMPANY)
Dilaudid Injection
 (KNOLL PHARMACEUTICAL COMPANY)
Dilaudid Multiple Dose Vials (Sterile Solution)
 (KNOLL PHARMACEUTICAL COMPANY)
Dilaudid-5 Oral Liquid
 (KNOLL PHARMACEUTICAL COMPANY)
Dilaudid Powder
 (KNOLL PHARMACEUTICAL COMPANY)
Dilaudid Rectal Suppositories
 (KNOLL PHARMACEUTICAL COMPANY)
Dilaudid Tablets 2mg and 4mg
 (KNOLL PHARMACEUTICAL COMPANY)
Dilaudid Tablets - 8 mg
 (KNOLL PHARMACEUTICAL COMPANY)
Dilaudid-HP Injection
 (KNOLL PHARMACEUTICAL COMPANY)
Dilor Elixir (SAVAGE LABORATORIES)
Dilor Injectable (SAVAGE LABORATORIES)
Dilor-200 Tablets (SAVAGE LABORATORIES)
Dilor-400 Tablets (SAVAGE LABORATORIES)
Dilor-G Tablets & Liquid
 (SAVAGE LABORATORIES)
DILTIAZEM HYDROCHLORIDE
 Cardizem CD Capsules-120 mg, 180 mg, 240 mg
  and 300 mg
 Cardizem SR Capsules-60 mg, 90 mg and 120 mg
 Cardizem Injectable
 Cardizem Tablets-30 mg, 60 mg, 90 mg
  and 120 mg
 Dilacor XR Extended-release Capsules
 Diltiazem Hydrochloride Tablets
 Diltiazem Hydrochloride Tablets
Diltiazem Hydrochloride Tablets
 (LEDERLE STANDARD PRODUCTS)
Diltiazem Hydrochloride Tablets
 (MYLAN PHARMACEUTICALS INC.)
DIMENHYDRINATE
 DMH-Syrup
 Dimenhydrinate in Tubex
Dimenhydrinate in Tubex
 (WYETH-AYERST LABORATORIES)
Dimetane-DC Cough Syrup
 (A. H. ROBINS COMPANY, INC.)
Dimetane-DX Cough Syrup
 (A. H. ROBINS COMPANY, INC.)
DIMETHICONE
 Moisturel Cream

 Moisturel Lotion
 pH-Stabil Skin Protectant Cream
DIMETHYL SULFOXIDE
 Rimso-50
DINOPROSTONE
 Prepidil Gel
 Prostin E2 Suppository
Diocto Liquid and Syrup
 (BARRE-NATIONAL INC.)
Diocto-C Syrup
 (BARRE-NATIONAL INC.)
DIOXYBENZONE
 Solaquin Forte 4% Gel
 Solbar Plus 15 Cream
Dipentum Capsules
 (PHARMACIA ADRIA PHARMACIA INC.)
DIPHENHYDRAMINE
 DPH-Elixir, USP
DIPHENHYDRAMINE CITRATE
 Excedrin P.M. Analgesic/Sleeping Aid Tablets
  and Caplets
DIPHENHYDRAMINE HYDROCHLORIDE
 Actifed Allergy Daytime/Nighttime Caplets
 Actifed Sinus Daytime/Nighttime Caplets and
  Tablets
 Benadryl Allergy Liquid
 Benadryl Allergy/Sinus Headache Caplets
 Benadryl Capsules
 Benadryl Cold/Flu Tablets
 Benadryl Cream
 Benadryl Cream Maximum Strength
 Benadryl Decongestant Liquid
 Benadryl Decongestant Tablets
 Benadryl Dye-Free Allergy Liqui-Caps
 Benadryl Dye-Free Allergy Liquid
 Benadryl Itch Relief Stick
 Benadryl Kapseals
 Benadryl Kapseals
 Benadryl Parenteral
 Benadryl Spray Maximum Strength 2%
 Benadryl Spray Regular 1%
 Benadryl Steri-Vials, Ampoules, and
  Steri-Dose Syringe
 Benadryl Tablets
 Diphenhydramine Hydrochloride Elixir
 Diphenhydramine Hydrochloride Injection
 Diphenhydramine Hydrochloride in Tubex
 Dytuss
 TYLENOL Allergy Sinus NightTime Caplets
 TYLENOL Flu NightTime, Maximum
  Strength, Gelcaps
 TYLENOL Maximum Strength Allergy Sinus
  Nighttime Medicine
 TYLENOL Flu NightTime, Maximum Strength,
  Hot Medication
 TYLENOL PM, Extra Strength Pain
  Reliever/Sleep Aid Caplets, Gelcaps, Geltabs,
  Tablets
 Maximum Strength Unisom Sleepgels
 Unisom With Pain Relief-Nighttime Sleep Aid
  and Pain Reliever
Diphenhydramine Hydrochloride Elixir
 (ROXANE LABORATORIES, INC.)
Diphenhydramine Hydrochloride Injection
 (ELKINS-SINN, INC.)
Diphenhydramine Hydrochloride in Tubex
 (WYETH-AYERST LABORATORIES)
DIPHENIDOL
 Vontrol Tablets
DIPHENOXYLATE HYDROCHLORIDE
 Diphenoxylate Hydrochloride & Atropine Sulfate
  Tablets

 Diphenoxylate Hydrochloride & Atropine Sulfate
  Tablets & Oral Solution
 Lomotil Liquid
 Lomotil Tablets
**Diphenoxylate Hydrochloride & Atropine
 Sulfate Tablets**
 (MYLAN PHARMACEUTICALS INC.)
**Diphenoxylate Hydrochloride & Atropine Sulfate
 Tablets & Oral Solution**
 (ROXANE LABORATORIES, INC.)
DIPHTHERIA & TETANUS TOXOIDS AND
ACELLULAR PERTUSSIS VACCINE ADSORBED
 Tripedia
DIPHTHERIA & TETANUS TOXOIDS
ADSORBED, (FOR PEDIATRIC USE)
 Diphtheria & Tetanus Toxoids
  Adsorbed Purogenated
**Diphtheria & Tetanus Toxoids
 Adsorbed Purogenated**
 (LEDERLE LABORATORIES)
DIPHTHERIA & TETANUS TOXOIDS AND
PERTUSSIS VACCINE ADSORBED WITH
HEMOPHILUS B CONJUGATE VACCINE (D
 Tetramune
DIPHTHERIA & TETANUS TOXOIDS
COMBINED, PEDIATRIC, ALUMINUM
PHOSPHATE ADSORBED
 Diphtheria & Tetanus Toxoids Adsorbed
  (Pediatric) in Tubex
 Diphtheria & Tetanus Toxoids Adsorbed,
  Ultrafined, Pediatric
**Diphtheria & Tetanus Toxoids Adsorbed
 (Pediatric) in Tubex**
 (WYETH-AYERST LABORATORIES)
**Diphtheria & Tetanus Toxoids Adsorbed,
 Ultrafined, Pediatric**
 (WYETH-AYERST LABORATORIES)
DIPHTHERIA & TETANUS TOXOIDS W/ACEL-
LULAR PERTUSSIS VACCINE COMBINED,
ALUMINUM PHOSPHATE ADSORBED
 Acel-Imune Diphtheria and Tetanus Toxoids and
  Acellular Pertussis Vaccine Adsorbed
DIPHTHERIA & TETANUS TOXOIDS W/
PERTUSSIS VACCINE COMBINED, ALUMINUM
PHOSPHATE ADSORBED
 Diphtheria and Tetanus Toxoids and Pertussis
  Vaccine Adsorbed
 Tri-Immunol Adsorbed
DIPHTHERIA & TETANUS TOXOIDS
W/PERTUSSIS VACCINE COMBINED,
ALUMINUM POTASSIUM SULFATE ADSORBED
 Diphtheria and Tetanus Toxoids and Pertussis
  Vaccine Adsorbed USP (For Pediatric Use)
**Diphtheria and Tetanus Toxoids and
 Pertussis Vaccine Adsorbed**
 (SMITHKLINE BEECHAM PHARMACEUTICALS)
**Diphtheria and Tetanus Toxoids and Pertussis
 Vaccine Adsorbed USP (For Pediatric Use)**
 (CONNAUGHT LABORATORIES, INC.)
DIPOTASSIUM PHOSPHATE
 Uro-KP-Neutral
Diprivan Injection (STUART PHARMACEUTICALS)
Diprolene AF Cream (SCHERING CORPORATION)
Diprolene Gel 0.05% (SCHERING CORPORATION)
Diprolene Lotion 0.05%
 (SCHERING CORPORATION)
Diprolene Ointment 0.05%
 (SCHERING CORPORATION)

UNDERLINE DENOTES GENERIC NAME

DIPYRIDAMOLE
  Dipyridamole Tablets
  Persantine Tablets
Dipyridamole Tablets
  (LEDERLE STANDARD PRODUCTS)
Disalcid Capsules (3M PHARMACEUTICALS)
Disalcid Tablets (3M PHARMACEUTICALS)

DISODIUM PHOSPHATE
  Uro-KP-Neutral

DISOPYRAMIDE PHOSPHATE
  Disopyramide Phosphate Capsules
  Disopyramide Phosphate
    Extended-release Capsules
  Norpace Capsules
  Norpace CR Capsules
Disopyramide Phosphate Capsules
  (BIOCRAFT LABORATORIES, INC.)
**Disopyramide Phosphate Extended-release
  Capsules**
  (ETHEX CORPORATION)

DISULFIRAM
  Antabuse Tablets
Ditropan Syrup (MARION MERRELL DOW INC.)
Ditropan Tablets (MARION MERRELL DOW INC.)
Diucardin Tablets
  (WYETH-AYERST LABORATORIES)
Diupres Tablets (MERCK & CO., INC.)
Diuril Oral Suspension (MERCK & CO., INC.)
Diuril Sodium Intravenous
  (MERCK & CO., INC.)
Diuril Tablets (MERCK & CO., INC.)
Diutensen-R Tablets (WALLACE LABORATORIES)

DIVALPROEX SODIUM
  Depakote Sprinkle Capsules
  Depakote Tablets
Doan's Extra-Strength Analgesic
  (CIBA CONSUMER PHARMACEUTICALS)
Extra Strength Doan's P.M.
  (CIBA CONSUMER PHARMACEUTICALS)
Doan's Regular Strength Analgesic
  (CIBA CONSUMER PHARMACEUTICALS)
Doak Tar Distillate (DOAK DERMATOLOGICALS)
Doak Tar Lotion (DOAK DERMATOLOGICALS)
Doak Tar Oil (DOAK DERMATOLOGICALS)
Doak Tar Shampoo (DOAK DERMATOLOGICALS)

DOBUTAMINE HYDROCHLORIDE
  Dobutrex Solution Vials
Dobutrex Solution Vials
  (ELI LILLY AND COMPANY)

DOCUSATE SODIUM
  Dialose Tablets
  Dialose Plus Tablets
  Diocto Liquid and Syrup
  Docusate Sodium Syrup
  Docusate Sodium Capsules, USP (D-S-S)
  Docusate Sodium with Casanthranol Capsules
    (D-S-S Plus)
  Ferro-Sequels High Potency, Time-Release Iron
    Supplement
  Hemaspan Caplets
  Prenate 90 Tablets
  Senokot-S Tablets
Docusate Sodium Syrup
  (ROXANE LABORATORIES, INC.)
Docusate Sodium Capsules, USP (D-S-S)
  (WARNER CHILCOTT LABORATORIES)
**Docusate Sodium with Casanthranol Capsules
  (D-S-S Plus)**
  (WARNER CHILCOTT LABORATORIES)
Dolobid Tablets (MERCK & CO., INC.)
Dolophine Hydrochloride Ampoules & Vials
  (ELI LILLY AND COMPANY)

Dolophine Hydrochloride Tablets
  (ELI LILLY AND COMPANY)
**Domeboro Astringent Solution
  Effervescent Tablets**
  (MILES INC. CONSUMER HEALTHCARE PRODUCTS)
Domeboro Astringent Solution Powder Packets
  (MILES INC. CONSUMER HEALTHCARE PRODUCTS)
Donatussin DC Syrup (LASER, INC.)
Donatussin Drops (LASER, INC.)
Donnatal Capsules (A. H. ROBINS COMPANY, INC.)
Donnatal Elixir (A. H. ROBINS COMPANY, INC.)
Donnatal Extentabs (A. H. ROBINS COMPANY, INC.)
Donnatal Tablets (A. H. ROBINS COMPANY, INC.)
Donnazyme Tablets (A. H. ROBINS COMPANY, INC.)

DOPAMINE HYDROCHLORIDE
  Dopamine Hydrochloride Injection
  Dopamine Hydrochloride Injection, USP
Dopamine Hydrochloride Injection
  (ELKINS-SINN, INC.)
Dopamine Hydrochloride Injection, USP
  (ASTRA USA, INC.)
Dopar Capsules
  (ROBERTS PHARMACEUTICAL CORPORATION)
Dopram Injectable (A. H. ROBINS COMPANY, INC.)
Doral Tablets (WALLACE LABORATORIES)
Dorcol Children's Cough Syrup
  (SANDOZ PHARMACEUTICALS/ CONSUMER DIVISION)

DORNASE ALFA
  Pulmozyme Inhalation
Doryx Capsules (PARKE-DAVIS)
DOSAFLEX Liquid Laxative
  (RICHWOOD PHARMACEUTICAL COMPANY, INC.)
Dovonex Ointment 0.005%
  (WESTWOOD-SQUIBB PHARMACEUTICALS INC.)

DOXACURIUM CHLORIDE
  Nuromax Injection

DOXAPRAM HYDROCHLORIDE
  Dopram Injectable

DOXAZOSIN MESYLATE
  Cardura Tablets

DOXEPIN HYDROCHLORIDE
  Adapin Capsules
  Doxepin HCl Capsules
  Doxepin HCl Capsules
  Doxepin Hydrochloride Capsules
  Doxepin Oral Solution
  Sinequan Capsules
  Sinequan Oral Concentrate
  Zonalon Cream
Doxepin HCl Capsules
  (GENEVA PHARMACEUTICALS, INC.)
Doxepin HCl Capsules
  (PAR PHARMACEUTICAL, INC.)
Doxepin Hydrochloride Capsules
  (MYLAN PHARMACEUTICALS INC.)
Doxepin Oral Solution
  (WARNER CHILCOTT LABORATORIES)

DOXORUBICIN HYDROCHLORIDE
  Adriamycin PFS
  Adriamycin RDF
  Doxorubicin Hydrochloride for Injection, USP
  Doxorubicin Hydrochloride for Injection, USP
  Doxorubicin Hydrochloride Injection, USP
  Rubex
Doxorubicin Hydrochloride for Injection, USP
  (ASTRA USA, INC.)
Doxorubicin Hydrochloride for Injection, USP
  (CHIRON THERAPEUTICS)
Doxorubicin Hydrochloride Injection, USP
  (CHIRON THERAPEUTICS)

DOXYCYCLINE HYCLATE
  Bio-Tab Tablets

  Doryx Capsules
  Doxycycline Hyclate Capsules, Tablets
  Doxycycline Hyclate Capsules & Tablets
  Doxycycline Hyclate Capsules & Tablets, USP
  Doxycycline Hyclate for Injection
  Vibramycin Hyclate Capsules
  Vibramycin Hyclate Intravenous
  Vibra-Tabs Film Coated Tablets
Doxycycline Hyclate Capsules, Tablets
  (LEDERLE STANDARD PRODUCTS)
Doxycycline Hyclate Capsules & Tablets
  (MYLAN PHARMACEUTICALS INC.)
Doxycycline Hyclate Capsules & Tablets, USP
  (WARNER CHILCOTT LABORATORIES)
Doxycycline Hyclate for Injection
  (ELKINS-SINN, INC.)

DOXYCYCLINE MONOHYDRATE
  Monodox Capsules
  Vibramycin Monohydrate for Oral Suspension

DOXYLAMINE SUCCINATE
  Unisom Nighttime Sleep Aid

DRESSINGS, STERILE
  HydraSorb Sterile Dressings
  Pro-Clude Transparent Wound Dressing
  Water-Jel Sterile Burn Dressings
Drithocreme 0.1%, 0.25%, 0.5%, 1.0% (HP)
  (DERMIK LABORATORIES, INC.)
Dritho-Scalp 0.25%, 0.5%
  (DERMIK LABORATORIES, INC.)

DRONABINOL
  Marinol (Dronabinol) Capsules

DROPERIDOL
  Droperidol Injection, USP
  Fentanyl Citrate and Droperidol Injection
  Inapsine Injection
  Innovar Injection
Droperidol Injection, USP (ASTRA USA, INC.)
Drysol (PERSON & COVEY, INC.)
Duadacin Cold & Allergy Capsules
  (KENWOOD LABORATORIES)
Dulcolax Suppositories
  (CIBA CONSUMER PHARMACEUTICALS)
Dulcolax Tablets
  (CIBA CONSUMER PHARMACEUTICALS)
Duo-Medihaler Aerosol (3M PHARMACEUTICALS)
Durabolin (ORGANON INC.)
Duradrin Capsules
  (DURAMED PHARMACEUTICALS, INC.)
Duragesic Transdermal System
  (JANSSEN PHARMACEUTICA INC.)
Dura-Gest Capsules
  (DURA PHARMACEUTICALS, INC)
Duramorph (ELKINS-SINN, INC.)
Duranest Injections (ASTRA USA, INC.)
Dura-Tap/PD Capsules
  (DURA PHARMACEUTICALS, INC)
Duratex Capsules
  (DURAMED PHARMACEUTICALS, INC.)
Duratuss Tablets
  (WHITBY PHARMACEUTICALS, INC.)
Dura-Vent/A Capsules
  (DURA PHARMACEUTICALS, INC)
Dura-Vent/DA Tablets
  (DURA PHARMACEUTICALS, INC)
Duratuss HD Elixir
  (WHITBY PHARMACEUTICALS, INC.)
Dura-Vent Tablets
  (DURA PHARMACEUTICALS, INC)
Duricef (BRISTOL-MYERS SQUIBB COMPANY)
Dyazide Capsules
  (SMITHKLINE BEECHAM PHARMACEUTICALS)
Dyazide New Formulation
  (SMITHKLINE BEECHAM PHARMACEUTICALS)

UNDERLINE DENOTES GENERIC NAME

Dyclone 0.5% and 1% Topical Solutions, USP
  (ASTRA USA, INC.)

DYCLONINE HYDROCHLORIDE
  Dyclone 0.5% and 1% Topical Solutions, USP
Dynacin Capsules
  (MEDICIS DERMATOLOGICS, INC.)
DynaCirc Capsules
  (SANDOZ PHARMACEUTICALS CORPORATION)

DYPHYLLINE
  Dilor Elixir
  Dilor Injectable
  Dilor-200 Tablets
  Dilor-400 Tablets
  Dilor-G Tablets & Liquid
  Dyphylline GG Elixir
  Lufyllin Elixir
  Lufyllin Injection
  Lufyllin & Lufyllin-400 Tablets
  Lufyllin-GG Elixir & Tablets
Dyphylline GG Elixir (BARRE-NATIONAL INC.)
Dyrenium Capsules
  (SMITHKLINE BEECHAM PHARMACEUTICALS)
Dytuss (LUNSCO, INC.)

E

E.E.S. 400 Filmtab (ABBOTT LABORATORIES)
E.E.S. Granules (ABBOTT LABORATORIES)
E.E.S. 200 Liquid (ABBOTT LABORATORIES)
E.E.S. 400 Liquid (ABBOTT LABORATORIES)
E-Gems Soft Gels
  (J. R. CARLSON LABORATORIES, INC.)
E.N.T. Tablets (ION LABORATORIES, INC.)
E-Mycin Tablets (BOOTS LABORATORIES)

EPA (EICOSAPENTAENOIC ACID)
  Super Omega-3 Fatty Acids Soft Gels
**Ear Drops by Murine+13 (See Murine Ear Wax
  Removal System/Murine Ear Drops)**
  (ROSS PRODUCTS DIVISION)
Easprin (PARKE-DAVIS)

ECHOTHIOPHATE IODIDE
  Phospholine Iodide

ECONAZOLE NITRATE
  Spectazole (econazole nitrate 1%) Cream
**Ecotrin Enteric Coated Aspirin
  Low Strength Tablets**
  (SMITHKLINE BEECHAM CONSUMER HEALTHCARE, L.P.)
**Ecotrin Enteric Coated Aspirin Maximum
  Strength Tablets and Caplets**
  (SMITHKLINE BEECHAM CONSUMER HEALTHCARE, L.P.)
**Ecotrin Enteric Coated Aspirin Regular Strength
  Tablets and Caplets**
  (SMITHKLINE BEECHAM CONSUMER HEALTHCARE, L.P.)
Edecrin Sodium Intravenous (MERCK & CO., INC.)
Edecrin Tablets (MERCK & CO., INC.)

EDROPHONIUM CHLORIDE
  Enlon Injection
  Enlon-Plus Injection
  Reversol
  Tensilon Injectable
Effective Strength Cough Formula
  (BARRE-NATIONAL INC.)
**Effective Strength Cough Formula with
  Decongestant** (BARRE-NATIONAL INC.)
Effexor (WYETH-AYERST LABORATORIES)
Efudex Cream (ROCHE LABORATORIES)
Efudex Solutions (ROCHE LABORATORIES)
Elase Ointment (FUJISAWA USA, INC.)

Elase Vials (FUJISAWA USA, INC.)
Elase-Chloromycetin Ointment
  (FUJISAWA USA, INC.)
Elavil Injection (STUART PHARMACEUTICALS)
Elavil Tablets (STUART PHARMACEUTICALS)
Eldepryl Tablets
  (SOMERSET PHARMACEUTICALS, INC.)
Eldercaps (MAYRAND PHARMACEUTICALS, INC.)
Eldertonic (MAYRAND PHARMACEUTICALS, INC.)
Eldopaque Forte 4% Cream
  (ICN PHARMACEUTICALS, INC.)
Eldoquin Forte 4% Cream
  (ICN PHARMACEUTICALS, INC.)

ELECTROLYTE SOLUTION
  K+ Care Powder
  K+ Care ET
  K+ 10 Tablets
  Pedialyte Oral Electrolyte Maintenance Solution
  Rehydralyte Oral Electrolyte Rehydration
    Solution
Elimite (permethrin) 5% Cream
  (ALLERGAN HERBERT)
Elixophyllin Dye-Free Capsules
  (FOREST PHARMACEUTICALS, INC.)
Elixophyllin Elixir
  (FOREST PHARMACEUTICALS, INC.)
Elixophyllin-GG Oral Solution
  (FOREST PHARMACEUTICALS, INC.)
Elixophyllin-KI Elixir
  (FOREST PHARMACEUTICALS, INC.)
Elocon Cream 0.1% (SCHERING CORPORATION)
Elocon Lotion 0.1% (SCHERING CORPORATION)
Elocon Ointment 0.1% (SCHERING CORPORATION)
Elon Nail Conditioner, Formaldehyde Free
  (DARTMOUTH PHARMACEUTICALS, INC.)
Elspar (MERCK & CO., INC.)
Emcyt Capsules
  (PHARMACIA ADRIA PHARMACIA INC.)
Emecheck (SAVAGE LABORATORIES)
Emete-con Intramuscular/Intravenous
  (ROERIG DIVISION)
Emetrol Solution - Cherry
  (BOCK PHARMACAL COMPANY)
Emetrol Solution - Lemon-Mint
  (BOCK PHARMACAL COMPANY)
Emgel 2% Topical Gel (GLAXO DERMATOLOGY)
Eminase
  (SMITHKLINE BEECHAM PHARMACEUTICALS)
Emla Cream (ASTRA USA, INC.)
Empirin Tablets (WARNER WELLCOME)
Empirin with Codeine Tablets
  (BURROUGHS WELLCOME CO.)

ENALAPRIL MALEATE
  Vaseretic Tablets
  Vasotec Tablets

ENALAPRILAT
  Vasotec I.V.
Endal-HD (UAD LABORATORIES)
Endep Tablets (ROCHE PRODUCTS INC.)
Endorphenyl Capsules (d-Phenylalanine)
  (TYSON AND ASSOCIATES, INC.)
Enduron Tablets (ABBOTT LABORATORIES)
**Ener-B Vitamin B$_{12}$ Nasal Gel Dietary
  Supplement** (NATURE'S BOUNTY, INC.)

ENFLURANE
  Ethrane
Engerix-B Unit-Dose Vials
  (SMITHKLINE BEECHAM PHARMACEUTICALS)
Enlon Injection
  (OHMEDA PHARMACEUTICAL PRODUCTS DIVISION INC.)
Enlon-Plus Injection
  (OHMEDA PHARMACEUTICAL PRODUCTS DIVISION INC.)

ENOXACIN
  Penetrex Tablets

ENOXAPARIN
  Lovenox Injection
Ensure Complete Balanced Nutrition
  (ROSS PRODUCTS DIVISION)
**Ensure High Protein Complete Balanced
  Nutrition** (ROSS PRODUCTS DIVISION)
Ensure Plus High Calorie Complete Nutrition
  (ROSS PRODUCTS DIVISION)
Ensure With Fiber Complete, Balanced Nutrition
  (ROSS PRODUCTS DIVISION)
Entac Liquid (BARRE-NATIONAL INC.)
Enterogenic Concentrate and Tablets
  (TYLER ENCAPSULATIONS)
Entex Capsules
  (PROCTER & GAMBLE PHARMACEUTICALS, INC.)
Entex LA Tablets
  (PROCTER & GAMBLE PHARMACEUTICALS, INC.)
Entex Liquid
  (PROCTER & GAMBLE PHARMACEUTICALS, INC.)
Entex PSE Tablets
  (PROCTER & GAMBLE PHARMACEUTICALS, INC.)
Entozyme Tablets (A. H. ROBINS COMPANY, INC.)

ENTSUFON SODIUM
  pHisoHex
Enulose (BARRE-NATIONAL INC.)

ENZYMES, COLLAGENOLYTIC
  Collagenase Santyl Ointment

ENZYMES, DEBRIDEMENT
  Collagenase Santyl Ointment
  Panafil Ointment
  Panafil-White Ointment
  Travase Ointment

ENZYMES, DIGESTIVE
  Arco-Lase Plus Tablets
  Arco-Lase Tablets
  Digepepsin Pancreatin Enzyme Supplement
  Donnazyme Tablets
  Entozyme Tablets
  Kutrase Capsules
  Ku-Zyme Capsules
  Ku-Zyme HP Capsules
  Similase

ENZYMES, FIBRINOLYTIC
  Elase Ointment
  Elase Vials
  Elase-Chloromycetin Ointment

ENZYMES, PROTEOLYTIC
  Panafil Ointment
  Panafil-White Ointment
  Travase Ointment

EPHEDRINE HYDROCHLORIDE
  Broncholate Softgels
  Broncholate Syrup
  Mudrane Tablets
  Mudrane GG Elixir
  Mudrane GG Tablets
  Quadrinal Tablets

EPHEDRINE SULFATE
  Marax Tablets & DF Syrup

EPHEDRINE TANNATE
  Rynatuss Pediatric Suspension
  Rynatuss Tablets
Epifoam (REED & CARNRICK)
Epi-Lock Wound Dressing
  (CALGON VESTAL LABORATORIES, INC.)

EPINEPHRINE
  Epinephrine Injection
  Epinephrine Injection, USP
  Epinephrine in Tubex
  Epinephrine Mist
  EpiPen Jr.
  EpiPen–Epinephrine Auto-Injector

UNDERLINE DENOTES GENERIC NAME

Lidocaine Hydrochloride & Epinephrine Injection
Marcaine Hydrochloride with Epinephrine
  1:200,000
Sensorcaine with Epinephrine Injection
Sus-Phrine Injection
Xylocaine with Epinephrine Injections
Epinephrine Injection (ELKINS-SINN, INC.)
Epinephrine Injection, USP (ASTRA USA, INC.)
Epinephrine in Tubex
  (WYETH-AYERST LABORATORIES)
Epinephrine Mist (BARRE-NATIONAL INC.)

 EPINEPHRINE BITARTRATE
Sensorcaine-MPF with Epinephrine Injection

EPINEPHRINE HYDROCHLORIDE
Ana-Kit Anaphylaxis Emergency Treatment Kit
EpiPen Jr. (CENTER LABORATORIES)
EpiPen– Epinephrine Auto-Injector
  (CENTER LABORATORIES)

EPOETIN ALFA
Epogen for Injection
Procrit for Injection
Epogen for Injection (AMGEN INC.)
Equagesic Tablets (WYETH-AYERST LABORATORIES)
Equanil Tablets (WYETH-AYERST LABORATORIES)
Erex Tablets (ION LABORATORIES, INC.)
Ergamisol Tablets (JANSSEN PHARMACEUTICA INC.)

ERGOCALCIFEROL
Calciferol Drops
Calciferol in Oil Injection
Calciferol Tablets

ERGOLOID MESYLATES
Hydergine LC Liquid Capsules
Hydergine Liquid
Hydergine Oral Tablets
Hydergine Sublingual Tablets
Ergomar (LOTUS BIOCHEMICAL CORPORATION)
Ergostat (PARKE-DAVIS)

ERGOTAMINE TARTRATE
Bellergal-S Tablets
Cafergot Suppositories
Cafergot Tablets
Ergomar
Ergostat
Wigraine Tablets & Suppositories
ERYC (PARKE-DAVIS)
Erycette (erythromycin 2%) Topical Solution
  (ORTHO PHARMACEUTICAL CORPORATION DERMA-
  TOLOGICAL DIVISION)
Erygel Topical Gel (ALLERGAN HERBERT)
Erymax Topical Solution (ALLERGAN HERBERT)
EryPed Drops and Chewable Tablets
  (ABBOTT LABORATORIES)
EryPed 200 & EryPed 400 Granules
  (ABBOTT LABORATORIES)
Ery-Tab Tablets (ABBOTT LABORATORIES)
Erythra-Derm (formerly ETS-2%)
  (PADDOCK LABORATORIES, INC.)

ERYTHRITYL TETRANITRATE
Cardilate Oral/Sublingual Tablets
Erythrocin Stearate Filmtab
  (ABBOTT LABORATORIES)

ERYTHROMYCIN
A/T/S 2% Acne Topical Gel and Solution
Akne-mycin Ointment
Benzamycin Topical Gel
E-Mycin Tablets
Emgel 2% Topical Gel
ERYC
Erycette (erythromycin 2%) Topical Solution
Erygel Topical Gel
Erymax Topical Solution
Ery-Tab Tablets

Erythra-Derm (formerly ETS-2%)
Erythromycin Base Filmtab
Erythromycin Delayed-Release Capsules, USP
Erythromycin Topical Soln. USP 2%
Ilotycin Ophthalmic Ointment
PCE Dispertab Tablets
Pediazole
T-Stat 2.0% Topical Solution and Pads
Theramycin Z Topical Solution 2%
Erythromycin Base Filmtab
  (ABBOTT LABORATORIES)
Erythromycin Delayed-Release Capsules, USP
  (ABBOTT LABORATORIES)
Erythromycin Topical Soln. USP 2%
  (BARRE-NATIONAL INC.)

ERYTHROMYCIN ESTOLATE
Erythromycin Estolate Oral Susp. USP 125 mg/5 mL
Erythromycin Estolate Oral Susp. USP 250 mg/5 mL
Ilosone Liquid, Oral Suspensions
Ilosone Pulvules & Tablets
Erythromycin Estolate Oral Susp.
  USP 125 mg/5 mL (BARRE-NATIONAL INC.)
Erythromycin Estolate Oral Susp.
  USP 250 mg/5 mL (BARRE-NATIONAL INC.)

ERYTHROMYCIN ETHYLSUCCINATE
E.E.S. 400 Filmtab
E.E.S. Granules
E.E.S. 200 Liquid
E.E.S. 400 Liquid
EryPed Drops and Chewable Tablets
EryPed 200 & EryPed 400 Granules
Erythromycin Ethylsuccinate/ Sulfisoxazole
  Acetyl Oral Suspension
Erythromycin Ethylsuccinate Oral Susp. USP 200
  mg/5 mL
Erythromycin Ethylsuccinate Oral Susp. USP 400
  mg/5 mL
Erythromycin Ethylsuccinate Tablets
Eryzole Oral Suspension, USP
Pediazole
Erythromycin Ethylsuccinate/ Sulfisoxazole
  Acetyl Oral Suspension
  (LEDERLE STANDARD PRODUCTS)
Erythromycin Ethylsuccinate Oral Susp.
  USP 200 mg/5 mL (BARRE-NATIONAL INC.)
Erythromycin Ethylsuccinate Oral Susp.
  USP 400 mg/5 mL (BARRE-NATIONAL INC.)
Erythromycin Ethylsuccinate Tablets
  (MYLAN PHARMACEUTICALS, INC.)

ERYTHROMYCIN GLUCEPTATE
Ilotycin Gluceptate, IV, Vials

ERYTHROMYCIN LACTOBIONATE
Erythromycin Lactobionate for Injection
Sterile Erythromycin Lactobionate for Injection
Erythromycin Lactobionate for Injection
  (ELKINS-SINN, INC.)
Sterile Erythromycin Lactobionate for Injection
  (LEDERLE STANDARD PRODUCTS)

ERYTHROMYCIN STEARATE
Erythrocin Stearate Filmtab
Erythromycin Stearate Tablets
Erythromycin Stearate Tablets
  (MYLAN PHARMACEUTICALS, INC.)
Eryzole Oral Suspension, USP
  (ALRA LABORATORIES, INC.)
Esgic-Plus Tablets
  (FOREST PHARMACEUTICALS, INC.)
Esgic Tablets & Capsules
  (FOREST PHARMACEUTICALS, INC.)
Esidrix Tablets
  (CIBA PHARMACEUTICAL COMPANY)
Esimil Tablets
  (CIBA PHARMACEUTICAL COMPANY)

Eskalith Capsules
  (SMITHKLINE BEECHAM PHARMACEUTICALS)
Eskalith CR Controlled Release Tablets
  (SMITHKLINE BEECHAM PHARMACEUTICALS)

ESMOLOL HYDROCHLORIDE
Brevibloc Injection
Esophotrast Cream
  (RHONE-POULENC RORER PHARMACEUTICALS INC.)

ESTAZOLAM
ProSom Tablets
Estrace Cream and Tablets
  (BRISTOL-MYERS SQUIBB COMPANY)
Estraderm Transdermal System
  (CIBA PHARMACEUTICAL COMPANY)

ESTRADIOL
Emcyt Capsules
Estrace Cream and Tablets
Estraderm Transdermal System
Estradurin (WYETH-AYERST LABORATORIES)

ESTRAMUSTINE PHOSPHATE SODIUM
Emcyt Capsules
ESTRATAB Tablets (0.3, 0.625, 1.25, 2.5 mg)
  (SOLVAY PHARMACEUTICALS, INC.)
ESTRATEST Tablets
  (SOLVAY PHARMACEUTICALS, INC.)
ESTRATEST H.S. Tablets
  (SOLVAY PHARMACEUTICALS, INC.)

ESTROGENS, CONJUGATED
PMB 200 and PMB 400
Premarin Intravenous
Premarin with Methyltestosterone
Premarin Tablets
Premarin Vaginal Cream

ESTROGENS, ESTERIFIED
ESTRATAB Tablets (0.3, 0.625, 1.25, 2.5 mg)
ESTRATEST Tablets
ESTRATEST H.S. Tablets
Menest Tablets

ESTROPIPATE
Estropipate Tablets
Estropipate Tablets
Estropipate Tablets, USP
Ogen Tablets
Ogen Vaginal Cream
Ortho-Est .625 Tablets
Ortho-Est Tablets
Estropipate Tablets
  (DURAMED PHARMACEUTICALS, INC.)
Estropipate Tablets
  (WARNER CHILCOTT LABORATORIES)
Estropipate Tablets, USP
  (WATSON LABORATORIES, INC.)

ETHACRYNATE SODIUM
Edecrin Sodium Intravenous

ETHACRYNIC ACID
Edecrin Tablets

ETHAMBUTOL HYDROCHLORIDE
Myambutol Tablets
Ethamolin (REED & CARNRICK)

ETHANOLAMINE OLEATE
Ethamolin

ETHAVERINE HYDROCHLORIDE
Isovex Capsules

ETHCHLORVYNOL
Placidyl Capsules

ETHINYL ESTRADIOL
Brevicon 21-Day Tablets
Brevicon 28-Day Tablets
Demulen 1/35-21

Demulen 1/35-28
Demulen 1/50-21
Demulen 1/50-28
Desogen Tablets
Levlen 21 Tablets
Levlen 28 Tablets
Loestrin Fe 1/20
Loestrin Fe 1.5/30
Loestrin 21 1/20
Loestrin 21 1.5/30
Lo/Ovral Tablets
Lo/Ovral-28 Tablets
Modicon 21 Tablets
Modicon 28 Tablets
Nelova
Nordette-21 Tablets
Nordette-28 Tablets
Norinyl 1+35 21-Day Tablets
Norinyl 1+35 28-Day Tablets
Ortho-Cept Tablets
Ortho-Cyclen Tablets
Ortho-Novum 1/35 ☐ 21 Tablets
Ortho-Novum 1/35 ☐ 28 Tablets
Ortho-Novum 7/7/7 ☐ 21 Tablets
Ortho-Novum 7/7/7 ☐ 28 Tablets
Ortho-Novum 10/11 ☐ 21 Tablets
Ortho-Novum 10/11 ☐ 28 Tablets
Ortho Tri-Cyclen Tablets
Ovcon 35
Ovcon 50
Ovral Tablets
Ovral-28 Tablets
Tri-Levlen 21 Tablets
Tri-Levlen 28 Tablets
Tri-Norinyl 21-Day Tablets
Tri-Norinyl 28-Day Tablets
Triphasil-21 Tablets
Triphasil-28 Tablets
Ethiodol (SAVAGE LABORATORIES)

ETHIONAMIDE
Trecator-SC Tablets
Ethmozine Tablets
(ROBERTS PHARMACEUTICAL CORPORATION)

ETHOSUXIMIDE
Zarontin Capsules
Zarontin Syrup

ETHOTOIN
Peganone Tablets
Ethrane
(OHMEDA PHARMACEUTICAL PRODUCTS DIVISION INC.)

ETHYL ALCOHOL
Lavacol

ETHYL CHLORIDE
Ethyl Chloride, U.S.P.
Fluro-Ethyl
Ethyl Chloride, U.S.P. (GEBAUER COMPANY)

2-ETHYLHEXYL-P-METHOXYCINNAMATE
Eucerin Dry Skin Care Daily Facial Lotion
SPF 20

2-ETHYLHEXYL SALICYLATE
Eucerin Dry Skin Care Daily Facial Lotion
SPF 20

ETHYNODIOL DIACETATE
Demulen 1/35-21
Demulen 1/35-28
Demulen 1/50-21
Demulen 1/50-28

ETIDOCAINE HYDROCHLORIDE
Duranest Injections

ETIDRONATE DISODIUM (BIPHOSPHONATE)
Didronel I.V. Infusion

ETIDRONATE DISODIUM (DIPHOSPHONATE)
Didronel Tablets

ETODOLAC
Lodine Capsules and Tablets

ETOMIDATE
Amidate

ETOPOSIDE
VePesid Capsules and Injection
Etrafon-A Tablets (4-10)
(SCHERING CORPORATION)
Etrafon Forte Tablets (4-25)
(SCHERING CORPORATION)
Etrafon 2-10 Tablets (2-10)
(SCHERING CORPORATION)
Etrafon Tablets (2-25)
(SCHERING CORPORATION)

ETRETINATE
Tegison Capsules
Eucalyptamint 100% All Natural Ointment
(CIBA CONSUMER PHARMACEUTICALS)

EUCALYPTOL
Listerine Antiseptic
Cool Mint Listerine
Eucerin Dry Skin Care Cleansing Bar
(BEIERSDORF INC)
Eucerin Dry Skin Care Lotion
(BEIERSDORF INC)
**Eucerin Dry Skin Care Moisturizing Creme
(Unscented)** (BEIERSDORF INC)
Eucerin Dry Skin Care Daily Facial Lotion SPF 20
(BEIERSDORF INC)
Eucerin Plus Dry Skin Care Moisturizing Lotion
(BEIERSDORF INC)
Eucerin Plus Moisturizing Creme
(BEIERSDORF INC)

EUCERITE
Eucerin Dry Skin Care Cleansing Bar
Nephro-Derm Cream
Eulexin Capsules (SCHERING CORPORATION)
Eurax Cream & Lotion
(WESTWOOD-SQUIBB PHARMACEUTICALS INC.)
Evac-Q-Kwik (SAVAGE LABORATORIES)
Aspirin Free Excedrin Analgesic Caplets
(BRISTOL-MYERS PRODUCTS)
Excedrin Dual (BRISTOL-MYERS PRODUCTS)
**Excedrin Extra-Strength Analgesic Tablets &
Caplets** (BRISTOL-MYERS PRODUCTS)
**Excedrin P.M. Analgesic/Sleeping Aid Tablets
and Caplets** (BRISTOL-MYERS PRODUCTS)
**Sinus Excedrin Analgesic, Decongestant Tablets
& Caplets** (BRISTOL-MYERS PRODUCTS)
Exelderm Cream 1.0%
(WESTWOOD-SQUIBB PHARMACEUTICALS INC.)
Exelderm Solution 1.0%
(WESTWOOD-SQUIBB PHARMACEUTICALS INC.)
Exgest LA Tablets
(CARNRICK LABORATORIES, INC.)
Ex-Lax Chocolated Laxative Tablets
(SANDOZ PHARMACEUTICALS/ CONSUMER DIVISION)
Extra Gentle Ex-Lax Laxative Pills
(SANDOZ PHARMACEUTICALS/ CONSUMER DIVISION)
Ex-Lax Gentle Nature Laxative Tablets
(SANDOZ PHARMACEUTICALS/ CONSUMER DIVISION)
Maximum Relief Formula Ex-Lax Laxative Pills
(SANDOZ PHARMACEUTICALS/ CONSUMER DIVISION)
Regular Strength Ex-Lax Laxative Pills
(SANDOZ PHARMACEUTICALS/ CONSUMER DIVISION)
Ex-Lax Gentle Nature Laxative Pills
(SANDOZ PHARMACEUTICALS/ CONSUMER DIVISION)
Exna Tablets (A. H. ROBINS COMPANY, INC.)
Exosurf Neonatal for Intratracheal Suspension
(BURROUGHS WELLCOME CO.)
Exsel Shampoo/Lotion (ALLERGAN HERBERT)
Extendryl Chewable Tablets
(FLEMING & COMPANY)
Extendryl Sr. & Jr. T.D. Capsules
(FLEMING & COMPANY)
Extendryl Syrup (FLEMING & COMPANY)

Eye-Stream Eye Irrigating Solution
(ALCON LABORATORIES, INC.)

F

4-Way Cold Tablets (BRISTOL-MYERS PRODUCTS)
**4-Way Fast Acting Nasal Spray - Original
Formula (regular & mentholated) & Metered
Spray Pump (regular)**
(BRISTOL-MYERS PRODUCTS)
4-Way Long Lasting Nasal Spray
(BRISTOL-MYERS PRODUCTS)
FS Shampoo (HILL DERMACEUTICALS, INC.)

FACTOR VIII INHIBITOR BYPASSER
Feiba VH Immuno

FACTOR IX (HUMAN)
AlphaNine-SD Coagulation Factor IX (Human)
Mononine Coagulation Factor IX (Human)

FACTOR IX COMPLEX
Bebulin VH Immuno
Konȳne 80 Factor IX Complex
Proplex T, Factor IX Complex, Heat Treated

FACTOR IX COMPLEX (HUMAN)
Profilnine Heat-Treated Factor IX Complex
Factrel (WYETH-AYERST LABORATORIES)

FAMCICLOVIR
Famvir

FAMOTIDINE
Pepcid Injection
Pepcid Injection Premixed
Pepcid Oral Suspension
Pepcid Tablets
Famvir (SMITHKLINE BEECHAM
PHARMACEUTICALS)
Fansidar Tablets (ROCHE LABORATORIES)
Fastin Capsules
(SMITHKLINE BEECHAM PHARMACEUTICALS)

FATTY ACIDS
Super Omega-3 Fatty Acids Soft Gels
Fedahist Gyrocaps (SCHWARZ PHARMA)
Fedahist Timecaps (SCHWARZ PHARMA)
Feiba VH Immuno (IMMUNO-U.S., INC.)

FELBAMATE
Felbatol
Felbatol (WALLACE LABORATORIES)
Feldene Capsules
(PRATT PHARMACEUTICALS DIVISION)
**Feldene Capsules (see Pratt Pharmaceuticals
Division)** (PFIZER LABS DIVISION)

FELODIPINE
Plendil Extended-Release Tablets
Femcet Capsules (NORTHAMPTON MEDICAL, INC.)
Femstat Prefill Vaginal Cream 2%
(SYNTEX PUERTO RICO, INC.)
Femstat Vaginal Cream 2%
(SYNTEX PUERTO RICO, INC.)
Fenesin Tablets (DURA PHARMACEUTICALS, INC)
Fenesin DM (DURA PHARMACEUTICALS, INC)

FENFLURAMINE HYDROCHLORIDE
Pondimin Tablets

FENOPROFEN CALCIUM
Fenoprofen Calcium Tablets
Fenoprofen Calcium Tablets
Nalfon 200 Pulvules & Nalfon Tablets
Fenoprofen Calcium Tablets
(LEDERLE STANDARD PRODUCTS)
Fenoprofen Calcium Tablets
(MYLAN PHARMACEUTICALS INC.)

FENTANYL
  Duragesic Transdermal System

FENTANYL CITRATE
  Fentanyl Citrate Injection (Preservative-Free)
  Fentanyl Citrate and Droperidol Injection
  Fentanyl Oralet
  Innovar Injection
  Sublimaze Injection
Fentanyl Citrate Injection (Preservative-Free)
  (ELKINS-SINN, INC.)
Fentanyl Citrate and Droperidol Injection
  (ASTRA USA, INC.)
Fentanyl Oralet (ABBOTT LABORATORIES)
Feosol Capsules
  (SMITHKLINE BEECHAM CONSUMER HEALTHCARE, L.P.)
Feosol Elixir
  (SMITHKLINE BEECHAM CONSUMER HEALTHCARE, L.P.)
Feosol Tablets
  (SMITHKLINE BEECHAM CONSUMER HEALTHCARE, L.P.)
Fero-Folic-500 Filmtab
  (ABBOTT LABORATORIES)
Fero-Grad-500 Filmtab (ABBOTT LABORATORIES)
Fero-Gradumet Filmtab (ABBOTT LABORATORIES)
Fe-50 Caplets (NORTHAMPTON MEDICAL, INC.)
Ferro-Sequels High Potency, Time-Release Iron Supplement (LEDERLE LABORATORIES)

FERROUS FUMARATE
  Chromagen Capsules
  Ferro-Sequels High Potency, Time-Release Iron
    Supplement
  Fetrin Capsules
  Fumatinic Capsules
  Hemaspan Caplets
  Hemocyte Plus Tabules
  Hemocyte Tablets
  Hemocyte-C Tablets
  Hemocyte-F Tablets
  Ircon Tablets
  Ircon-FA Tablets
  Nephro-Fer Tablets
  Nephro-Fer Rx Tablets
  Nephro-Vite + Fe Tablets
  Pramilet FA
  Prenate 90 Tablets
  Trinsicon Capsules
  Vi-Daylin/F Multivitamin + Iron Chewable
    Tablets With Fluoride

FERROUS GLUCONATE
  Fosfree
  ILX B$_{12}$ Caplets Crystalline
  Iromin-G
  Megadose
  Mission Prenatal
  Mission Prenatal F.A.
  Mission Prenatal H.P.

FERROUS SULFATE
  Feosol Capsules
  Feosol Elixir
  Feosol Tablets
  Fero-Folic-500 Filmtab
  Fero-Grad-500 Filmtab
  Fero-Gradumet Filmtab
  Fe-50 Caplets
  Ferrous Sulfate Drops and Elixir
  Ferrous Sulfate Oral Solution & Tablets
  Iberet Filmtab
  Iberet-500 Filmtab
  Iberet-500 Liquid
  Iberet-Folic-500 Filmtab
  Iberet-Liquid
  Irospan Capsules
  Irospan Tablets
  Slow Fe Tablets
  Slow Fe with Folic Acid

  Vi-Daylin/F ADC Vitamins + Iron Drops With
    Fluoride
  Vi-Daylin/F Multivitamin + Iron Drops With
    Fluoride
Ferrous Sulfate Drops and Elixir
  (BARRE-NATIONAL INC.)
Ferrous Sulfate Oral Solution & Tablets
  (ROXANE LABORATORIES, INC.)
Fetrin Capsules (LUNSCO, INC.)
FEVERALL Children's Suppositories
  (UPSHER-SMITH LABORATORIES, INC.)
FEVERALL Infant's Suppositories
  (UPSHER-SMITH LABORATORIES, INC.)
FEVERALL Junior Strength Suppositories
  (UPSHER-SMITH LABORATORIES, INC.)
FEVERALL Sprinkle Caps Powder
  (UPSHER-SMITH LABORATORIES, INC.)

FIBER SUPPLEMENT
  Ensure With Fiber Complete, Balanced Nutrition
  Glucerna Specialized Nutrition with Fiber for
    Patients with Abnormal Glucose Tolerance
Fiberall Chewable Tablets, Lemon Creme Flavor
  (CIBA CONSUMER PHARMACEUTICALS)
Fiberall Fiber Wafers - Fruit & Nut
  (CIBA CONSUMER PHARMACEUTICALS)
Fiberall Fiber Wafers - Oatmeal Raisin
  (CIBA CONSUMER PHARMACEUTICALS)
Fiberall Powder, Natural Flavor
  (CIBA CONSUMER PHARMACEUTICALS)
Fiberall Powder, Orange Flavor
  (CIBA CONSUMER PHARMACEUTICALS)
FiberCon Tablets (LEDERLE LABORATORIES)

FIBRINOLYSIN
  Elase Ointment
  Elase Vials
  Elase-Chloromycetin Ointment

FILGRASTIM
  Neupogen for Injection

FINASTERIDE
  Proscar Tablets
Fioricet Tablets
  (SANDOZ PHARMACEUTICALS CORPORATION)
Fioricet with Codeine Capsules
  (SANDOZ PHARMACEUTICALS CORPORATION)
Fiorinal Capsules
  (SANDOZ PHARMACEUTICALS CORPORATION)
Fiorinal with Codeine Capsules
  (SANDOZ PHARMACEUTICALS CORPORATION)
Fiorinal Tablets
  (SANDOZ PHARMACEUTICALS CORPORATION)
Flagyl I.V. (SCS)
Flagyl I.V. RTU (SCS)
Flagyl Tablets (G.D. SEARLE & CO.)

FLAVOXATE HYDROCHLORIDE
  Urispas Tablets

FLECAINIDE ACETATE
  Tambocor Tablets
Fleet Babylax (C. B. FLEET CO., INC.)
Fleet Bisacodyl Enema (C. B. FLEET CO., INC.)
Fleet Children's Enema (C. B. FLEET CO., INC.)
Fleet Enema (C. B. FLEET CO., INC.)
Fleet Flavored Castor Oil Emulsion
  (C. B. FLEET CO., INC.)
Fleet Glycerin Laxative Rectal Applicators
  (C. B. FLEET CO., INC.)
Fleet Mineral Oil Enema (C. B. FLEET CO., INC.)
Fleet Phospho-Soda (C. B. FLEET CO., INC.)
Fleet Prep Kits (C. B. FLEET CO., INC.)
Flexeril Tablets (MERCK & CO., INC.)
Flintstones Children's Chewable Vitamins
  (MILES INC. CONSUMER HEALTHCARE PRODUCTS)

**Flintstones Children's Chewable Vitamins
  With Extra C**
  (MILES INC. CONSUMER HEALTHCARE PRODUCTS)
**Flintstones Children's Chewable Vitamins
  Plus Iron**
  (MILES INC. CONSUMER HEALTHCARE PRODUCTS)
**Flintstones Complete With Calcium, Iron &
  Minerals Children's Chewable Vitamins**
  (MILES INC. CONSUMER HEALTHCARE PRODUCTS)
Florinef Acetate Tablets (APOTHECON)
Florone Cream 0.05%
  (DERMIK LABORATORIES, INC.)
Florone E Emollient Cream 0.05%
  (DERMIK LABORATORIES, INC.)
Florone Ointment 0.05% (DERMIK LABORATORIES, INC.)
Floropryl Sterile Ophthalmic Ointment
  (MERCK & CO., INC.)
Florvite Chewable Tablets 0.5 mg & 1 mg
  (EVERETT LABORATORIES, INC.)
Florvite Drops 0.25 mg & 0.5 mg
  (EVERETT LABORATORIES, INC.)
**Florvite + Iron Chewable Tablets 0.5 mg and
  1 mg** (EVERETT LABORATORIES, INC.)
Florvite + Iron Drops 0.25 mg & 0.5 mg
  (EVERETT LABORATORIES, INC.)
Floxin I.V. (MCNEIL PHARMACEUTICAL)
Floxin Tablets (MCNEIL PHARMACEUTICAL)

FLOXURIDINE
  Sterile FUDR

FLUCONAZOLE
  Diflucan Injection, Tablets, and Oral Suspension

FLUCYTOSINE
  Ancobon Capsules
Fludara for Injection (BERLEX LABORATORIES)

FLUDARABINE PHOSPHATE
  Fludara for Injection

FLUDROCORTISONE ACETATE
  Florinef Acetate Tablets
Flumadine Tablets & Syrup
  (FOREST PHARMACEUTICALS, INC.)

FLUMAZENIL
  Romazicon

FLUNISOLIDE
  AeroBid Inhaler System
  Aerobid-M Inhaler System
  Nasalide Nasal Solution 0.025%

FLUOCINOLONE ACETONIDE
  Derma-Smoothe/FS Topical Oil
  FS Shampoo
  Fluocinolone Acetonide Cream USP 0.025%
  Fluocinolone Acetonide Cream USP 0.01%
  Fluonid Topical Solution
  Neo-Synalar Cream
  Synalar Creams 0.025%, 0.01%
  Synalar Ointment 0.025%
  Synalar Topical Solution 0.01%
  Synalar-HP Cream 0.2%
  Synemol Cream 0.025%
Fluocinolone Acetonide Cream USP 0.025%
  (BARRE-NATIONAL INC.)
Fluocinolone Acetonide Cream USP 0.01%
  (BARRE-NATIONAL INC.)
FLUOCINONIDE
  Dermacin Creme
  Fluocinonide Cream, USP 0.05%
  Fluocinonide Cream and Topical Solution, 0.05%
  Fluocinonide E Cream 0.05%
  Lidex Cream 0.05%
  Lidex Gel 0.05%
  Lidex Ointment 0.05%
  Lidex Topical Solution 0.05%
  Lidex-E Cream 0.05%

Fluocinonide Cream, USP 0.05%
(TARO PHARMACEUTICALS U.S.A., INC.)
Fluocinonide Cream and Topical Solution, 0.05%
(BARRE-NATIONAL INC.)
Fluocinonide E Cream 0.05%
(TARO PHARMACEUTICALS U.S.A., INC.)
Fluonid Topical Solution (ALLERGAN HERBERT)
Fluori-Methane (GEBAUER COMPANY)
Fluoroplex Topical Solution & Cream 1%
(ALLERGAN HERBERT)

FLUOROURACIL
Efudex Cream
Efudex Solutions
Fluoroplex Topical Solution & Cream 1%
Fluorouracil Injection
Fluorouracil Injection (ROCHE LABORATORIES)
Fluothane (WYETH-AYERST LABORATORIES)

FLUOXETINE HYDROCHLORIDE
Prozac Pulvules & Liquid, Oral Solution

FLUOXYMESTERONE
Halotestin Tablets

FLUPHENAZINE DECANOATE
Prolixin Decanoate

FLUPHENAZINE ENANTHATE
Prolixin Enanthate

FLUPHENAZINE HYDROCHLORIDE
Fluphenazine HCl Tablets
Fluphenazine HCl Tablets
Fluphenazine Hydrochloride Tablets
Prolixin Elixir
Prolixin Injection
Prolixin Oral Concentrate
Prolixin Tablets
Fluphenazine HCl Tablets
(GENEVA PHARMACEUTICALS, INC.)
Fluphenazine HCl Tablets
(PAR PHARMACEUTICAL, INC.)
Fluphenazine Hydrochloride Tablets
(MYLAN PHARMACEUTICALS INC.)

FLURANDRENOLIDE
Cordran Lotion
Cordran Ointment
Cordran SP Cream
Cordran Tape

FLURAZEPAM HYDROCHLORIDE
Dalmane Capsules
Flurazepam HCl Capsules
Flurazepam HCl Capsules
Flurazepam Hydrochloride Capsules
Flurazepam HCl Capsules
(PAR PHARMACEUTICAL, INC.)
Flurazepam HCl Capsules
(WARNER CHILCOTT LABORATORIES)
Flurazepam Hydrochloride Capsules
(MYLAN PHARMACEUTICALS INC.)

FLURBIPROFEN
Ansaid Tablets
Flurbiprofen Tablets
Flurbiprofen Tablets
(MYLAN PHARMACEUTICALS INC.)
Fluro-Ethyl (GEBAUER COMPANY)

FLUTAMIDE
Eulexin Capsules

FLUTICASONE PROPIONATE
Cutivate Cream
Cutivate Ointment

FLUVASTATIN SODIUM
Lescol Capsules
Fluzone (CONNAUGHT LABORATORIES, INC.)

FOLIC ACID
Cefol Filmtab
Eldercaps
Fero-Folic-500 Filmtab
Folvite Parenteral
Hemocyte-F Tablets
Iberet-Folic-500 Filmtab
Ircon-FA Tablets
Materna Tablets
May-Vita Elixir
Mega-B
Megadose
Mission Prenatal H.P.
Nephro-Fer Rx Tablets
Nephro-Vite + Fe Tablets
Nephro-Vite Rx Tablets
Niferex-150 Forte Capsules
Niferex Forte Elixir
Nu-Iron V Tablets
Nu-Iron Plus Elixir
Pramilet FA
Prenate 90 Tablets
Renal Multivitamin Formula Rx
Slow Fe with Folic Acid
Stuartnatal Plus Tablets
Trinsicon Capsules
Vitafol Caplets
Folvite Parenteral
(LEDERLE STANDARD PRODUCTS)
Forane
(OHMEDA PHARMACEUTICAL PRODUCTS DIVISION INC.)

FORMALDEHYDE
Formalyde-10 Spray
LazerFormalyde Solution
Formalyde-10 Spray (PEDINOL PHARMACAL INC.)
Fortaz (GLAXO PHARMACEUTICALS)

FOSCARNET SODIUM
Foscavir Injection
Foscavir Injection (ASTRA USA, INC.)
Fosfree (MISSION PHARMACAL COMPANY)

FOSINOPRIL SODIUM
Monopril Tablets
Fototar Cream (ICN PHARMACEUTICALS, INC.)

FRUCTOOLIGOSACCHARIDES
Enterogenic Concentrate and Tablets
Sterile FUDR (ROCHE LABORATORIES)
Fulvicin P/G Tablets (SCHERING CORPORATION)
Fulvicin P/G 165 & 330 Tablets
(SCHERING CORPORATION)
Fumatinic Capsules (LASER, INC.)
Fungizone Intravenous (APOTHECON)
Fungoid Creme (PEDINOL PHARMACAL INC.)
Fungoid & HC Cremes
(PEDINOL PHARMACAL INC.)
Fungoid Solution (PEDINOL PHARMACAL INC.)
Fungoid Tincture (PEDINOL PHARMACAL INC.)
Furacin Soluble Dressing
(ROBERTS PHARMACEUTICAL CORPORATION)
Furacin Topical Cream
(ROBERTS PHARMACEUTICAL CORPORATION)
Furacin Topical Solution 0.2%
(ROBERTS PHARMACEUTICAL CORPORATION)

FURAZOLIDONE
Furoxone Liquid
Furoxone Tablets

FUROSEMIDE
Furosemide Injection (Preservative-Free)
Furosemide Injection, USP
Furosemide Tablets
Furosemide Tablets
Furosemide Tablets
Furosemide Tablets & Oral Solution

Furosemide Tablets, USP
Lasix Injection, Oral Solution and Tablets
Furosemide Injection (Preservative-Free)
(ELKINS-SINN, INC.)
Furosemide Injection, USP (ASTRA USA, INC.)
Furosemide Tablets
(LEDERLE STANDARD PRODUCTS)
Furosemide Tablets
(MYLAN PHARMACEUTICALS INC.)
Furosemide Tablets
(WATSON LABORATORIES, INC.)
Furosemide Tablets & Oral Solution
(ROXANE LABORATORIES, INC.)
Furosemide Tablets, USP
(WARNER CHILCOTT LABORATORIES)
Furoxone Liquid
(ROBERTS PHARMACEUTICAL CORPORATION)
Furoxone Tablets
(ROBERTS PHARMACEUTICAL CORPORATION)

G

GABAPENTIN
Neurontin Capsules

GADODIAMIDE
Omniscan Injection
Gamimune N, 5% Immune Globulin Intravenous (Human), 5% (MILES INC. PHARMACEUTICAL
DIVISION BIOLOGICAL PRODUCTS)
Gamimune N, 10% Immune Globulin Intravenous (Human), 10%
(MILES INC. PHARMACEUTICAL DIVISION BIOLOGICAL PRODUCTS)

GAMMA GLOBULIN
Gammar, Immune Globulin (Human) U.S.P.
Gammar I.V., Immune Globulin Intravenous (Human), Lyophilized
HyperHep Hepatitis B Immune Globulin (Human)
Hyper-Tet Tetanus Immune Globulin (Human)
Gammagard, Immune Globulin, Intravenous (Human) (BAXTER HEALTHCARE CORPORATION)
Gammar, Immune Globulin (Human) U.S.P.
(ARMOUR PHARMACEUTICAL COMPANY)
Gammar I.V., Immune Globulin Intravenous (Human), Lyophilized
(ARMOUR PHARMACEUTICAL COMPANY)
Gamulin Rh, Rh$_0$(D) Immune Globulin (Human)
(ARMOUR PHARMACEUTICAL COMPANY)

GANCICLOVIR SODIUM
Cytovene Sterile Powder
Gantanol Tablets (ROCHE LABORATORIES)
Gantrisin Ophthalmic Solution
(ROCHE LABORATORIES)
Gantrisin Pediatric Suspension
(ROCHE LABORATORIES)
Gantrisin Syrup (ROCHE LABORATORIES)
Gantrisin Tablets (ROCHE LABORATORIES)
Garamycin Cream 0.1% (SCHERING CORPORATION)
Garamycin Injectable (SCHERING CORPORATION)
Garamycin Intrathecal Injection
(SCHERING CORPORATION)
Garamycin Ointment 0.1%
(SCHERING CORPORATION)
Garamycin Ophthalmic Ointment–Sterile
(SCHERING CORPORATION)
Garamycin Ophthalmic Solution–Sterile
(SCHERING CORPORATION)

UNDERLINE DENOTES GENERIC NAME

Garamycin Pediatric Injectable
  (SCHERING CORPORATION)
Gas-X Chewable Tablets
  (SANDOZ PHARMACEUTICALS/ CONSUMER DIVISION)
Extra Strength Gas-X Chewable Tablets
  (SANDOZ PHARMACEUTICALS/ CONSUMER DIVISION)
Gastrocrom Capsules
  (FISONS CORPORATION PRESCRIPTION PRODUCTS)
Gaviscon Antacid Tablets
  (SMITHKLINE BEECHAM CONSUMER HEALTHCARE, L.P.)
Gaviscon Extra Strength Relief Formula Antacid Tablets
  (SMITHKLINE BEECHAM CONSUMER HEALTHCARE, L.P.)
Gaviscon Extra Strength Relief Formula Antacid Liquid
  (SMITHKLINE BEECHAM CONSUMER HEALTHCARE, L.P.)
Gaviscon Liquid Antacid
  (SMITHKLINE BEECHAM CONSUMER HEALTHCARE, L.P.)

GELATIN PREPARATIONS
  Gelfoam Sterile Powder
  Gelfoam Sterile Sponge
Gelfoam Sterile Powder (THE UPJOHN COMPANY)
Gelfoam Sterile Sponge (THE UPJOHN COMPANY)
Gelpirin Tablets (ALRA LABORATORIES, INC.)
Gelpirin CCF Tablets (ALRA LABORATORIES, INC.)
Gelusil Liquid (WARNER WELLCOME)
Gelusil Tablets (WARNER WELLCOME)
Gemcor Tablets
  (UPSHER-SMITH LABORATORIES, INC.)

GEMFIBROZIL
  Gemcor Tablets
  Gemfibrozil Tablets
  Gemfibrozil Tablets
  Lopid Tablets
Gemfibrozil Tablets
  (LEDERLE STANDARD PRODUCTS)
Gemfibrozil Tablets
  (WARNER CHILCOTT LABORATORIES)

GENTAMICIN SULFATE
  Garamycin Cream 0.1%
  Garamycin Injectable
  Garamycin Intrathecal Injection
  Garamycin Ointment 0.1%
  Garamycin Ophthalmic Ointment–Sterile
  Garamycin Ophthalmic Solution–Sterile
  Garamycin Pediatric Injectable
  Gentamicin Sulfate Cream and Ointment, USP 0.1%
  Gentamicin Sulfate Injection
  G-myticin Creme and Ointment 0.1%
Gentamicin Sulfate Cream and Ointment, USP 0.1% (BARRE-NATIONAL INC.)
Gentamicin Sulfate Injection
  (ELKINS-SINN, INC.)
Gen-XENE Tablets (ALRA LABORATORIES, INC.)
Geocillin Tablets (ROERIG DIVISION)
Geref (sermorelin acetate for injection)
  (SERONO LABORATORIES, INC.)
Gerimed Tablets
  (THE FIELDING PHARMACEUTICAL COMPANY, INC.)
Geroton Forte (KENWOOD LABORATORIES)
Gevrabon Liquid (LEDERLE LABORATORIES)
Gevral T Tablets (LEDERLE LABORATORIES)
Glandosane Mouth Moisturizer
  (KENWOOD LABORATORIES)

GLIPIZIDE
  Glipizide Tablets
  Glucotrol Tablets
  Glucotrol XL Extended Release Tablets
Glipizide Tablets
  (MYLAN PHARMACEUTICALS INC.)

GLOBULIN, IMMUNE (HUMAN)
  Gamimune N, 5% Immune Globulin Intravenous (Human), 5%
  Gamimune N, 10% Immune Globulin Intravenous (Human), 10%
  Gammagard, Immune Globulin, Intravenous (Human)
  Gammar, Immune Globulin (Human) U.S.P.
  Gammar I.V., Immune Globulin Intravenous (Human), Lyophilized
  Hyper-Tet Tetanus Immune Globulin (Human)
  HypRho-D Full Dose Rho (D) Immune Globulin (Human)
  HypRho-D Mini-Dose Rho (D) Immune Globulin (Human)
  Iveegam
  MICRhoGAM Rh$_O$ (D) Immune Globulin (Human)
  Polygam S/D, Immune Globulin Intravenous (Human)
  RhoGAM Rh$_O$ (D) Immune Globulin (Human)
  Sandoglobulin I.V.
  Varicella-Zoster Immune Globulin (Human)
  Venoglobulin-I, Immune Globulin Intravenous (Human)
  Venoglobulin-S 5% Solution Solvent Detergent Treated, Immune Globulin Intravenous (Human)

GLUCAGON
  Glucagon for Injection Vials and Emergency Kit
Glucagon for Injection Vials and Emergency Kit
  (ELI LILLY AND COMPANY)
Glucerna Specialized Nutrition with Fiber for Patients with Abnormal Glucose Tolerance
  (ROSS PRODUCTS DIVISION)

GLUCONO-DELTA-LACTONE
  Renacidin Irrigation

GLUCOSAMINE
  Casamin
  Glusamin

GLUCOSE OXIDASE
  Tes-Tape

GLUCOSE POLYMERS
  Polycose Glucose Polymers
Glucotrol Tablets
  (PRATT PHARMACEUTICALS DIVISION)
Glucotrol XL Extended Release Tablets
  (PRATT PHARMACEUTICALS DIVISION)
Glusamin (VITALINE CORPORATION)

L-GLUTAMINE
  AlitraQ Specialized Elemental Nutrition With Glutamine

GLUTATHIONE
  Carotene Health Packs
  Glutathione Health Packs
  Glutathione-Forté Capsules
  Performance Packs
  Performance Packs-Light
Glutathione Health Packs
  (HEALTH MAINTENANCE PROGRAMS, INC.)
Glutathione-Forté Capsules
  (HEALTH MAINTENANCE PROGRAMS, INC.)
Glutofac Caplets (KENWOOD LABORATORIES)
Glutose 15, Glutose 45 (Oral Glucose Gel)
  (PADDOCK LABORATORIES, INC.)
Glutose Tablets
  (PADDOCK LABORATORIES, INC.)

GLYBURIDE
  DiaBeta Tablets
  Glynase PresTab Tablets
  Micronase Tablets

GLYCERIN
  Aquanil Lotion
  Auralgan Otic Solution
  DML Facial Moisturizer with Sunscreen
  DML Moisturizing Lotion
  Fleet Babylax
  Fleet Glycerin Laxative Rectal Applicators
  Glycerin USP
  Lubrin Vaginal Lubricating Inserts
  Nutraderm 30 Lotion
  Tucks Clear Gel
Glycerin USP
  (BARRE-NATIONAL INC.)

GLYCERYL STEARATE
  DHS Conditioning Rinse

GLYCOPYRROLATE
  Robinul Forte Tablets
  Robinul Injectable
  Robinul Tablets
Glynase PresTab Tablets
  (THE UPJOHN COMPANY)
Gly-Oxide Liquid (SMITHKLINE BEECHAM CONSUMER HEALTHCARE, L.P.)
G-myticin Creme and Ointment 0.1%
  (PEDINOL PHARMACAL INC.)

GOLD SODIUM THIOMALATE
  Myochrysine Injection
GoLYTELY (BRAINTREE LABORATORIES, INC.)

GONADORELIN ACETATE
  Lutrepulse for Injection
  Lutrepulse for Injection

GONADORELIN HYDROCHLORIDE
  Factrel
Gordochom Solution (GORDON LABORATORIES)

GOSERELIN ACETATE IMPLANT
  Zoladex

GRAMICIDIN
  Neosporin Ophthalmic Solution Sterile

GRANISETRON HYDROCHLORIDE
  Kytril
Granulex (DOW HICKAM PHARMACEUTICALS, INC.)
Green Soap (BARRE-NATIONAL INC.)
Grifulvin V (griseofulvin tablets) Microsize (griseofulvin oral suspension) Microsize
  (ORTHO PHARMACEUTICAL CORPORATION DERMATOLOGICAL DIVISION)
Grisactin Capsules
  (WYETH-AYERST LABORATORIES)
Grisactin Tablets
  (WYETH-AYERST LABORATORIES)
Grisactin Ultra Tablets
  (WYETH-AYERST LABORATORIES)

GRISEOFULVIN
  Fulvicin P/G Tablets
  Fulvicin P/G 165 & 330 Tablets
  Grifulvin V (griseofulvin tablets) Microsize (griseofulvin oral suspension) Microsize
  Grisactin Capsules
  Grisactin Tablets
  Grisactin Ultra Tablets
  Gris-PEG Tablets, 125 mg & 250 mg
Gris-PEG Tablets, 125 mg & 250 mg
  (ALLERGAN HERBERT)
Guaifed Capsules (Extended-Release)
  (MURO PHARMACEUTICAL, INC.)
Guaifed-PD Capsules (Extended-Release)
  (MURO PHARMACEUTICAL, INC.)
Guaifed Syrup (MURO PHARMACEUTICAL, INC.)

GUAIFENESIN
  Albatussin SR Caplets
  Anatuss DM Syrup

Anatuss DM Tablets
Anatuss LA Tablets
Asbron G Elixir
Asbron G Inlay-Tabs
Benylin Expectorant
Benylin Multi-Symptom
Broncholate Softgels
Broncholate Syrup
Brontex
Codiclear DH Syrup
Congess Jr. T.D. Capsules
Congess Sr. T.D. Capsules
Deconsal Sprinkle Capsules
Deconsal C Expectorant Syrup
Deconsal Pediatric Syrup
Deconsal II Tablets
D-FEDA II Tablets
Despec Caplets
Despec Liquid
Despec SF
Dilaudid Cough Syrup
Dilor-G Tablets & Liquid
Donatussin DC Syrup
Donatussin Drops
Dura-Gest Capsules
Duratex Capsules
Duratuss Tablets
Duratuss HD Elixir
Dura-Vent Tablets
Elixophyllin-GG Oral Solution
Entex Capsules
Entex LA Tablets
Entex Liquid
Entex PSE Tablets
Exgest LA Tablets
Fenesin Tablets
Fenesin DM
Gelpirin CCF Tablets
Guaifed Capsules (Extended-Release)
Guaifed-PD Capsules (Extended-Release)
Guaifenesin Syrup
Guaifenex Liquid
Guaifenex LA Extended-release Tablets
Guaifenex PSE 120 Extended-release Tablets
Guaimax-D Tablets
Guiatuss
Guiatuss AC Syrup
Guiatuss CF
Guiatuss DAC
Guiatuss DM
Guiatuss PE
Guiatuss Maximum Strength Cough Suppressant
Guiatuss Pediatric Cough & Cold
Guiatuss Pediatric Cough Suppressant
Humibid DM Sprinkle Capsules
Humibid DM Tablets
Humibid L.A. Tablets
Humibid Sprinkle Capsules
HycoClear Tuss Syrup
Isoclor Expectorant
Kwelcof Liquid
Liquibid Tablets
Liquibid-D Tablets
Lufyllin-GG Elixir & Tablets
Mudrane GG Elixir
Mudrane GG Tablets
Mudrane GG-2 Tablets
Nasabid Capsules
Nasatab LA Tablets
Norel
Novahistine Expectorant (+)
Nucofed Expectorant
Nucofed Pediatric Expectorant
Organidin NR Tablets and Liquid
P-V-TUSSIN Tablets

Phenylpropanolamine HCl and Guaifenesin Long
   Acting Tablets
Pneumomist Tablets
Pneumotussin HC Cough Syrup
Pseudoephedrine HCl and Guaifenesin Extended
   Release Tablets
Quibron Capsules
Quibron-300 Capsules
Rescon-GG Liquid
Respaire-SR Capsules 60, 120
Robitussin A-C Syrup
Robitussin-DAC Syrup
Ru-Tuss DE Tablets
Safe Tussin 30
Sinupan Capsules
Sinutab Non Drying Liquid Caps
SINUVENT Tablets
Slo-Phyllin GG Capsules
Slo-Phyllin GG Syrup
Sudafed Cold & Cough Liquid Caps
Sudafed Cough Syrup
Syn-Rx Tablets
Theolate Liquid
Touro DM Caplets
Touro EX Caplets
Touro LA Caplets
Triaminic Expectorant with Codeine
Triaminic Expectorant DH
Tussar-2
Tussar SF
Tussi-Organidin DM NR Liquid and DM-S NR
   Liquid
Tussi-Organidin NR Liquid and S NR Liquid
Vicodin Tuss Expectorant
Zephrex Tablets
Zephrex LA Tablets
Guaifenesin Syrup
   (ROXANE LABORATORIES, INC.)
Guaifenex Liquid (ETHEX CORPORATION)
Guaifenex LA Extended-release Tablets
   (ETHEX CORPORATION)
Guaifenex PSE 120 Extended-release Tablets
   (ETHEX CORPORATION)
Guaimax-D Tablets
   (CENTRAL PHARMACEUTICALS, INC.)
Guaitab Tablets (MURO PHARMACEUTICAL, INC.)

GUANABENZ ACETATE
   Guanabenz Acetate Tablets, USP
   Wytensin Tablets
Guanabenz Acetate Tablets, USP
   (WATSON LABORATORIES, INC.)

GUANADREL SULFATE
   Hylorel Tablets

GUANETHIDINE MONOSULFATE
   Esimil Tablets
   Ismelin Tablets

GUANFACINE HYDROCHLORIDE
   Tenex Tablets
Guiatuss (BARRE-NATIONAL INC.)
Guiatuss AC Syrup (BARRE-NATIONAL INC.)
Guiatuss CF (BARRE-NATIONAL INC.)
Guiatuss DAC (BARRE-NATIONAL INC.)
Guiatuss DM (BARRE-NATIONAL INC.)
Guiatuss PE (BARRE-NATIONAL INC.)
Guiatuss Maximum Strength Cough Suppressant
   (BARRE-NATIONAL INC.)
Guiatuss Pediatric Cough & Cold
   (BARRE-NATIONAL INC.)
Guiatuss Pediatric Cough Suppressant
   (BARRE-NATIONAL INC.)
Gynol II Extra Strength Contraceptive Jelly
   (ORTHO PHARMACEUTICAL CORPORATION)
Gynol II Original Formula Contraceptive Jelly
   (ORTHO PHARMACEUTICAL CORPORATION)

H

H-BIG
   (NABI (NORTH AMERICAN BIOLOGICALS, INC.))
HP Acthar Gel
   (RHONE-POULENC RORER PHARMACEUTICALS INC.)
Habitrol Nicotine Transdermal System
   (BASEL PHARMACEUTICALS)

HAEMOPHILUS B CONJUGATE VACCINE
   ActHIB
   HibTITER
   OmniHIB
   PedvaxHIB
   ProHIBiT Haemophilus b Conjugate Vaccine
      (Diphtheria Toxoid Conjugate)

HALCINONIDE
   Halog Cream, Ointment & Solution
   Halog-E Cream
Halcion Tablets (THE UPJOHN COMPANY)
Haldol Decanoate 50 (50 mg/mL) Injection
   (MCNEIL PHARMACEUTICAL)
Haldol Decanoate 100 (100 mg/mL) Injection
   (MCNEIL PHARMACEUTICAL)
Haldol Injection, Tablets and Concentrate
   (MCNEIL PHARMACEUTICAL)
Halfprin (KRAMER LABORATORIES INC.)

HALOBETASOL PROPIONATE
   Ultravate Cream 0.05%
   Ultravate Ointment 0.05%
Halog Cream, Ointment & Solution
   (WESTWOOD-SQUIBB PHARMACEUTICALS INC.)
Halog-E Cream
   (WESTWOOD-SQUIBB PHARMACEUTICALS INC.)

HALOPERIDOL
   Haldol Injection, Tablets and Concentrate
   Haloperidol Concentrate
   Haloperidol Oral Soln. USP 2 mg/mL
   Haloperidol Tablets
   Haloperidol Tablets
   Haloperidol Tablets
   Haloperidol Tablets
Haloperidol Concentrate
   (WARNER CHILCOTT LABORATORIES)
Haloperidol Oral Soln. USP 2 mg/mL
   (BARRE-NATIONAL INC.)
Haloperidol Tablets
   (GENEVA PHARMACEUTICALS, INC.)
Haloperidol Tablets
   (MYLAN PHARMACEUTICALS INC.)
Haloperidol Tablets
   (PAR PHARMACEUTICAL, INC.)
Haloperidol Tablets
   (ROXANE LABORATORIES, INC.)

HALOPERIDOL DECANOATE
   Haldol Decanoate 50 (50 mg/mL) Injection
   Haldol Decanoate 100 (100 mg/mL) Injection
Halotestin Tablets (THE UPJOHN COMPANY)

HALOTHANE
   Fluothane
Haltran Tablets
   (ROBERTS PHARMACEUTICAL CORPORATION)
Head & Shoulders Dandruff Shampoo
   (PROCTER & GAMBLE)
Head & Shoulders Dry Scalp Dandruff Shampoo
   (PROCTER & GAMBLE)
Head & Shoulders Intensive Treatment Dandruff
   and Seborrheic Dermatitis Shampoo
   (PROCTER & GAMBLE)
Hemaspan Caplets (BOCK PHARMACAL COMPANY)

UNDERLINE DENOTES GENERIC NAME

HEMIN FOR INJECTION
  Panhematin
Hemocyte Plus Tabules
  (U.S. PHARMACEUTICAL CORPORATION)
Hemocyte Tablets
  (U.S. PHARMACEUTICAL CORPORATION)
Hemocyte-C Tablets
  (U.S. PHARMACEUTICAL CORPORATION)
Hemocyte-F Tablets
  (U.S. PHARMACEUTICAL CORPORATION)
**Hemofil M, Antihemophilic Factor (Human),
  Method M, Monoclonal Purified**
  (BAXTER HEALTHCARE CORPORATION)
Hemorrhoidal HC Suppositories, 25 mg
  (BARRE-NATIONAL INC.)
Hepacolin (KENWOOD LABORATORIES)
Heparin Lock Flush Solution
  (WYETH-AYERST LABORATORIES)
Heparin Lock Flush Solution in Tubex
  (WYETH-AYERST LABORATORIES)

HEPARIN SODIUM
  Heparin Lock Flush Solution
  Heparin Lock Flush Solution in Tubex
  Heparin Flush Kits
  Heparin Sodium Injection
  Heparin Sodium Injection
  Heparin Sodium Injection, USP, Sterile Solution
  Heparin Sodium Vials
  Heparin Sodium in Tubex
  Hep-Lock (Heparin Lock Flush Solution)
  Hep-Lock (Preservative-Free Heparin Lock Flush
    Solution)
Heparin Flush Kits
  (WYETH-AYERST LABORATORIES)
Heparin Sodium Injection (ELKINS-SINN, INC.)
Heparin Sodium Injection
  (WYETH-AYERST LABORATORIES)
Heparin Sodium Injection, USP, Sterile Solution
  (THE UPJOHN COMPANY)
Heparin Sodium Vials (ELI LILLY AND COMPANY)
Heparin Sodium in Tubex
  (WYETH-AYERST LABORATORIES)

HEPATITIS B IMMUNE GLOBULIN (HUMAN)
  H-BIG
  Hep-B-Gammagee
  HyperHep Hepatitis B Immune Globulin
    (Human)

HEPATITIS B VACCINE
  Engerix-B Unit-Dose Vials
  Recombivax HB
Hep-B-Gammagee (MERCK & CO., INC.)
Hep-Forte Capsules (MARLYN HEALTH CARE)
Hep-Lock (Heparin Lock Flush Solution)
  (ELKINS-SINN, INC.)
**Hep-Lock (Preservative-Free Heparin Lock
  Flush Solution)** (ELKINS-SINN, INC.)
Hermal Bath Oil
  (HERMAL PHARMACEUTICAL LABORATORIES, INC.)
Herpecin-L Cold Sore Lip Balm Stick
  (CAMPBELL LABORATORIES INC.)
Hespan Injection (DUPONT PHARMA)

HESPERIDIN COMPLEX
  Peridin-C Tablets

HETASTARCH
  Hespan Injection

HEXACHLOROPHENE
  pHisoHex
Hexadrol Phosphate Injection (ORGANON INC.)
Hexadrol Tablets (ORGANON INC.)
Hexalen Capsules (U.S. BIOSCIENCE, INC.)
Helixate, Antihemophilic Factor (Recombinant)
  (ARMOUR PHARMACEUTICAL COMPANY)

Hibiclens Antimicrobial Skin Cleanser
  (STUART PHARMACEUTICALS)
Hibiclens Sponge/Brush with Nail Cleaner
  (STUART PHARMACEUTICALS)
Hibistat Germicidal Hand Rinse
  (STUART PHARMACEUTICALS)
Hibistat Towelette (STUART PHARMACEUTICALS)
HibTITER (LEDERLE LABORATORIES)
Hismanal Tablets
  (JANSSEN PHARMACEUTICA INC.)
HISTALET FORTE Tablets
  (SOLVAY PHARMACEUTICALS, INC.)

HISTAMINE PHOSPHATE
  Histatrol Vial
Histatrol Vial (CENTER LABORATORIES)

L-HISTIDINE
  Nephramine
  HISTINEX DM (ETHEX CORPORATION)
HISTINEX HC (ETHEX CORPORATION)
HISTINEX PV Syrup (ETHEX CORPORATION)

HISTRELIN ACETATE
  Supprelin Injection
Histussin HC (BOCK PHARMACAL COMPANY)
Hivid Tablets (ROCHE LABORATORIES)

HOMATROPINE METHYLBROMIDE
  Tussigon Tablets
**Humate-P, Antihemophilic Factor (Human),
  Pasteurized**
  (ARMOUR PHARMACEUTICAL COMPANY)
Humatrope Vials (ELI LILLY AND COMPANY)
Humibid DM Sprinkle Capsules
  (ADAMS LABORATORIES, INC.)
Humibid DM Tablets
  (ADAMS LABORATORIES, INC.)
Humibid L.A. Tablets
  (ADAMS LABORATORIES, INC.)
Humibid Sprinkle Capsules
  (ADAMS LABORATORIES, INC.)
Humorsol Sterile Ophthalmic Solution
  (MERCK & CO., INC.)
Humulin 50/50, 100 Units
  (ELI LILLY AND COMPANY)
Humulin 70/30, 100 Units
  (ELI LILLY AND COMPANY)
Humulin BR, 100 Units
  (ELI LILLY AND COMPANY)
Humulin L, 100 Units
  (ELI LILLY AND COMPANY)
Humulin N, 100 Units
  (ELI LILLY AND COMPANY)
Humulin R, 100 Units
  (ELI LILLY AND COMPANY)
Humulin U, 100 Units
  (ELI LILLY AND COMPANY)
**Hurricaine Topical Anesthetic Aerosol Spray,
  2 oz (wild cherry flavor)** (BEUTLICH L.P.)
Hurricaine Topical Anesthetic Spray Kit
  (BEUTLICH L.P.)
**Hurricaine Topical Anesthetic Gel, 1 oz Wild
  Cherry, Pina Colada, Watermelon, +101 oz
  Wild Cherry, Watermelon** (BEUTLICH L.P.)
**Hurricaine Topical Anesthetic Liquid, .25 gm,
  1 oz Wild Cherry and Pina Colada .25 ml Dry
  Handle Swab Wild Cherry, +101 oz Wild
  Cherry** (BEUTLICH L.P.)

HYALURONIC ACID
  DML Facial Moisturizer with Sunscreen

HYALURONIDASE
  Wydase, Lyophilized
HYATE:C Antihemophilic Factor (Porcine)
  (SPEYWOOD PHARMACEUTICALS, INC.)
HycoClear Tuss Syrup (ETHEX CORPORATION)

Hyco-Pap Capsules (LUNSCO, INC.)
Hycosin Expectorant (BARRE-NATIONAL INC.)
Hydeltrasol Injection, Sterile (MERCK & CO., INC.)
Hydeltra-T.B.A. Sterile Suspension
  (MERCK & CO., INC.)
Hydergine LC Liquid Capsules
  (SANDOZ PHARMACEUTICALS CORPORATION)
Hydergine Liquid
  (SANDOZ PHARMACEUTICALS CORPORATION)
Hydergine Oral Tablets
  (SANDOZ PHARMACEUTICALS CORPORATION)
Hydergine Sublingual Tablets
  (SANDOZ PHARMACEUTICALS CORPORATION)

HYDRALAZINE HYDROCHLORIDE
  Apresazide Capsules
  Apresoline Hydrochloride Tablets
  Hydralazine HCl Tablets
  Hydralazine HCl Tablets
  Hydra-Zide (Hydralazine HCl and
    Hydrochlorothiazide) Capsules
  Ser-Ap-Es Tablets
Hydralazine HCl Tablets
  (LEDERLE STANDARD PRODUCTS)
Hydralazine HCl Tablets
  (PAR PHARMACEUTICAL, INC.)
Hydramine Cough Syrup and Elixir
  (BARRE-NATIONAL INC.)
HydraSorb Sterile Dressings
  (CALGON VESTAL LABORATORIES, INC.)
**Hydra-Zide (Hydralazine HCl and
  Hydrochlorothiazide) Capsules**
  (PAR PHARMACEUTICAL, INC.)
Hydrea Capsules
  (BRISTOL-MYERS SQUIBB ONCOLOGY DIVISION)
Hydrisinol Creme & Lotion
  (PEDINOL PHARMACAL INC.)
Hydrocet Capsules
  (CARNRICK LABORATORIES, INC.)

HYDROCHLOROTHIAZIDE
  Aldactazide
  Aldoril Tablets
  Amiloride Hydrochloride and
    Hydrochlorothiazide Tablets
  Amiloride Hydrochloride and
    Hydrochlorothiazide Tablets
  Amiloride Hydrochloride and
    Hydrochlorothiazide Tablets, U.S.P.
  Amiloride HCl and Hydrochlorothiazide Tablets
  Apresazide Capsules
  Capozide
  Dyazide Capsules
  Dyazide New Formulation
  Esidrix Tablets
  Esimil Tablets
  Hydra-Zide (Hydralazine HCl and
    Hydrochlorothiazide) Capsules
  Hydrochlorothiazide Tablets
  Hydrochlorothiazide Tablets, U.S.P.
  HydroDIURIL Tablets
  Hydropres Tablets
  Inderide Tablets
  Inderide LA Long Acting Capsules
  Lopressor HCT Tablets
  Lotensin HCT
  Maxzide Tablets
  Maxzide-25 MG Tablets
  Methyldopa & Hydrochlorothiazide Tablets
  Methyldopa and Hydrochlorothiazide Tablets
  Methyldopa & Hydrochlorothiazide Tablets, USP
  Methyldopa & Hydrochlorothiazide Tablets
  Methyldopa and Hydrochlorothiazide Tablets
    USP
  Methyldopa and Hydrochlorothiazide Tablets,
    U.S.P.
  Moduretic Tablets

Oretic Tablets
Prinzide Tablets
Propranolol Hydrochloride &
    Hydrochlorothiazide Tablets
Ser-Ap-Es Tablets
Spironolactone & Hydrochlorothiazide Tablets
Timolide Tablets
Triamterene/Hydrochlorothiazide Tablets
Triamterene and Hydrochlorothiazide Tablets
Triamterene and Hydrochlorothiazide Tablets
Triamterene and HCTZ Tablets, USP
Vaseretic Tablets
Zestoretic
Ziac
Hydrochlorothiazide Tablets
    (LEDERLE STANDARD PRODUCTS)
Hydrochlorothiazide Tablets, U.S.P.
    (WEST POINT PHARMA)

HYDROCODONE BITARTRATE
    Anaplex HD Cough Syrup
    Anexsia 5/500 Tablets
    Anexsia 7.5/650 Tablets
    Azdone Tablets
    Bancap HC Capsules
    Codiclear DH Syrup
    Codimal DH Syrup
    Co-Gesic Tablets
    Damason-P
    Donatussin DC Syrup
    Duratuss HD Elixir
    Endal-HD
    HISTINEX HC
    HISTINEX PV Syrup
    Histussin HC
    HycoClear Tuss Syrup
    Hyco-Pap Capsules
    Hydrocet Capsules
    Hydrocodone Bitartrate and APAP Tablets
    Hydrocodone with APAP Tablets
    Kwelcof Liquid
    Lorcet Plus
    Lorcet-HD
    Lorcet 10/650
    Lortab ASA Tablets
    Lortab 2.5/500 Tablets
    Lortab 5/500 Tablets
    Lortab 7.5/500 Tablets
    Lortab Elixir
    P-V-TUSSIN Syrup
    P-V-TUSSIN Tablets
    Panacet 5/500 Tablets
    Panasal 5/500 Tablets
    Pneumotussin HC Cough Syrup
    Ru-Tuss with Hydrocodone
    Triaminic Expectorant DH
    Tussigon Tablets
    Vanex-HD Liquid
    Vicodin Tablets
    Vicodin ES Tablets
    Vicodin Tuss Expectorant
Hydrocodone Bitartrate and APAP Tablets
    (WATSON LABORATORIES, INC.)
Hydrocodone with APAP Tablets
    (WARNER CHILCOTT LABORATORIES)

HYDROCODONE POLISTIREX
    Tussionex Pennkinetic Extended-Release
        Suspension

HYDROCORTISONE
    Acetasol HC
    Aeroseb-HC Topical Aerosol Spray
    Anusol-HC Cream 2.5%
    Maximum Strength Bactine Hydrocortisone Anti-
        Itch Cream 1.0%

CORTENEMA
Cortic Ear Drops
Cortisporin Ointment
Cortisporin Ophthalmic Ointment Sterile
Cortisporin Ophthalmic Suspension Sterile
Cortisporin Otic Solution Sterile
Cortisporin Otic Suspension Sterile
Hemorrhoidal HC Suppositories, 25 mg
Hydrocortisone Cream 1/2% and 1%
Hydrocortisone Cream USP 0.5%
Hydrocortisone Cream USP 1% - OTC
Hydrocortisone Cream USP 1% - Rx
Hydrocortisone Cream USP 2.5%
Hydrocortisone Ointment 1/2% and 1%
Hydrocortisone 0.5% Ointment USP
Hydrocortisone Ointment USP 1% - OTC
Hydrocortisone Ointment USP 1% - Rx
Hydrocortone Tablets
Hytone Cream 1%, 2 1/2 %
Hytone Lotion 1%, 2 1/2 %
Hytone Ointment 1%, 2 1/2 %
Iodochlorhydroxyquin 3% w/Hydrocortisone
    1% Cream
LactiCare-HC Lotion, 1%
LactiCare-HC Lotion, 2 1/2%
LazerSporin-C Solution
Massengill Medicated Soft Cloth Towelettes
Nutracort Lotion
PediOtic Suspension Sterile
Penecort Cream 1%
Penecort Topical Solution 1%
ProctoCream-HC 2.5%
Synacort Creams 1%, 2.5%
VōSoLă Otic Solution
Vytone Cream 1%
Hydrocortisone Cream 1/2% and 1%
    (TARO PHARMACEUTICALS U.S.A., INC.)
Hydrocortisone Cream USP 0.5%
    (BARRE-NATIONAL INC.)
Hydrocortisone Cream USP 1% - OTC
    (BARRE-NATIONAL INC.)
Hydrocortisone Cream USP 1% - Rx
    (BARRE-NATIONAL INC.)
Hydrocortisone Cream USP 2.5%
    (BARRE-NATIONAL INC.)
Hydrocortisone Ointment 1/2% and 1%
    (TARO PHARMACEUTICALS U.S.A., INC.)
Hydrocortisone 0.5% Ointment USP
    (BARRE-NATIONAL INC.)
Hydrocortisone Ointment USP 1% - OTC
    (BARRE-NATIONAL INC.)
Hydrocortisone Ointment USP 1% - Rx
    (BARRE-NATIONAL INC.)

HYDROCORTISONE ACETATE
    Analpram-HC Rectal Cream 1% and 2.5%
    Anusol HC-1 Ointment
    Anusol-HC Suppositories
    Coly-Mycin S Otic w/Neomycin &
        Hydrocortisone
    Cortifoam
    Cortisporin Cream
    Epifoam
    Fungoid & HC Cremes
    Hydrocortisone Acetate 0.5% Cream w/Aloe
    Hydrocortone Acetate Sterile Suspension
    Mantadil Cream
    Pedinol's HC Creme
    Pramosone Cream, Lotion & Ointment
    ProctoCream-HC
    Proctofoam-HC
    Terra-Cortril Ophthalmic Suspension
    Zone-A Cream 1%
Hydrocortisone Acetate 0.5% Cream w/Aloe
    (BARRE-NATIONAL INC.)

HYDROCORTISONE BUTYRATE
    Locoid Cream, Ointment and Topical Solution
HYDROCORTISONE SODIUM PHOSPHATE
    Hydrocortone Phosphate Injection, Sterile
HYDROCORTISONE SODIUM SUCCINATE
    Solu-Cortef Sterile Powder
HYDROCORTISONE VALERATE
    Westcort Cream 0.2%
    Westcort Ointment 0.2%
Hydrocortone Acetate Sterile Suspension
    (MERCK & CO., INC.)
Hydrocortone Phosphate Injection, Sterile
    (MERCK & CO., INC.)
Hydrocortone Tablets (MERCK & CO., INC.)
HydroDIURIL Tablets (MERCK & CO., INC.)
HYDROFLUMETHIAZIDE
    Diucardin Tablets
Hydromet Syrup (BARRE-NATIONAL INC.)

HYDROGEN PEROXIDE
    Proxacol
HYDROMORPHONE HYDROCHLORIDE
    Dilaudid Cough Syrup
    Dilaudid Hydrochloride Ampules
    Dilaudid Injection
    Dilaudid Multiple Dose Vials (Sterile Solution)
    Dilaudid-5 Oral Liquid
    Dilaudid Powder
    Dilaudid Rectal Suppositories
    Dilaudid Tablets 2mg and 4mg
    Dilaudid Tablets - 8 mg
    Dilaudid-HP Injection
    Hydromorphone HCl Injection
    Hydromorphone Hydrochloride Injection
    Hydromorphone Hydrochloride in Tubex
    Hydromorphone Hydrochloride Tablets
    HydroStat IR Hydromorphone HCL Tablets
Hydromorphone HCl Injection (ASTRA USA, INC.)
Hydromorphone Hydrochloride Injection
    (ELKINS-SINN, INC.)
Hydromorphone Hydrochloride in Tubex
    (WYETH-AYERST LABORATORIES)
Hydromorphone Hydrochloride Tablets
    (ROXANE LABORATORIES, INC.)
Hydromox Tablets (LEDERLE LABORATORIES)
Hydropres Tablets (MERCK & CO., INC.)
HYDROQUINONE
    Eldopaque Forte 4% Cream
    Eldoquin Forte 4% Cream
    Melanex Topical Solution
    Solaquin Forte 4% Cream
    Solaquin Forte 4% Gel
HydroStat IR Hydromorphone HCL Tablets
    (RICHWOOD PHARMACEUTICAL COMPANY, INC.)
HYDROXYCHLOROQUINE SULFATE
    Plaquenil Sulfate Tablets
HYDROXYPROPYL CELLULOSE
    Lacrisert Sterile Ophthalmic Insert
HYDROXYPROPYL METHYLCELLULOSE
    Ocucoat
    Tears Naturale II Lubricant Eye Drops
    Tears Naturale Free
HYDROXYUREA
    Hydrea Capsules
HYDROXYZINE HYDROCHLORIDE
    Atarax Tablets & Syrup
    Hydroxyzine Syrup
    Hydroxyzine HCl Syrup USP 10 mg/5 mL
    Hydroxyzine Hydrochloride Injection
    Marax Tablets & DF Syrup
    Vistaril Intramuscular Solution

UNDERLINE DENOTES GENERIC NAME

Hydroxyzine Syrup
  (WARNER CHILCOTT LABORATORIES)
Hydroxyzine HCl Syrup USP 10 mg/5 mL
  (BARRE-NATIONAL INC.)
Hydroxyzine Hydrochloride Injection
  (ELKINS-SINN, INC.)

HYDROXYZINE PAMOATE
  Vistaril Capsules
  Vistaril Oral Suspension
Hygroton Tablets
  (RHONE-POULENC RORER PHARMACEUTICALS INC.)
Hylorel Tablets (FISONS CORPORATION)

HYOSCYAMINE
  Cystospaz Tablets
  Urised Tablets
  Urisedamine Tablets

HYOSCYAMINE SULFATE
  Anaspaz Tablets
  Arco-Lase Plus Tablets
  Atrohist Plus Tablets
  Bellatal Tablets
  Cystospaz-M Capsules
  Donnatal Capsules
  Donnatal Elixir
  Donnatal Extentabs
  Donnatal Tablets
  Kutrase Capsules
  Levsin Drops
  Levsin Elixir
  Levsin Injection
  Levsin Tablets
  Levsin/SL Tablets
  Levsinex Timecaps
  Rexatal Tablets
  Ru-Tuss Tablets
Hyperab Rabies Immune Globulin (Human)
  (MILES INC. PHARMACEUTICAL DIVISION
  BIOLOGICAL PRODUCTS)
**HyperHep Hepatitis B Immune Globulin
  (Human)** (MILES INC. PHARMACEUTICAL
  DIVISION BIOLOGICAL PRODUCTS)
Hyperstat I.V. Injection (SCHERING CORPORATION)
Hyper-Tet Tetanus Immune Globulin (Human)
  (MILES INC. PHARMACEUTICAL DIVISION
  BIOLOGICAL PRODUCTS)
**HypRho-D Full Dose Rho (D) Immune Globulin
  (Human)** (MILES INC. PHARMACEUTICAL
  DIVISION BIOLOGICAL PRODUCTS)
**HypRho-D Mini-Dose Rho (D) Immune Globulin
  (Human)** (MILES INC. PHARMACEUTICAL
  DIVISION BIOLOGICAL PRODUCTS)
Hyskon Hysteroscopy Fluid
  (MEDISAN PHARMACEUTICALS INC.)
Hytone Cream 1%, 2¹/₂%
  (DERMIK LABORATORIES, INC.)
Hytone Lotion 1%, 2¹/₂ %
  (DERMIK LABORATORIES, INC.)
Hytone Ointment 1%, 2¹/₂ %
  (DERMIK LABORATORIES, INC.)
Hytrin Tablets (ABBOTT LABORATORIES)

I

IBU Tablets (BOOTS LABORATORIES)
ILX B₁₂ Caplets Crystalline
  (KENWOOD LABORATORIES)
**ILX B₁₂ Elixir Crystalline and ILX B₁₂
  Sugar–Free Elixir**
  (KENWOOD LABORATORIES)

ILX Elixir (KENWOOD LABORATORIES)
Iberet Filmtab (ABBOTT LABORATORIES)
Iberet-500 Filmtab (ABBOTT LABORATORIES)
Iberet-500 Liquid (ABBOTT LABORATORIES)
Iberet-Folic-500 Filmtab (ABBOTT LABORATORIES)
Iberet-Liquid (ABBOTT LABORATORIES)

IBUPROFEN
  Children's Advil Suspension
  IBU Tablets
  Ibuprofen Tablets
  Ibuprofen Tablets
  Ibuprofen Tablets
  IBU-TAB OTC Tablets, Ibuprofen Tablets, USP
  IBU-TAB Rx Tablets, Ibuprofen Tablets, USP
  Children's Motrin Ibuprofen Suspension
  Motrin Tablets
  Nuprin Ibuprofen/Analgesic Tablets & Caplets
  Sine-Aid IB Caplets
Ibuprofen Tablets
  (MYLAN PHARMACEUTICALS INC.)
Ibuprofen Tablets (PAR PHARMACEUTICAL, INC.)
Ibuprofen Tablets
  (WARNER CHILCOTT LABORATORIES)
IBU-TAB OTC Tablets, Ibuprofen Tablets, USP
  (ALRA LABORATORIES, INC.)
IBU-TAB Rx Tablets, Ibuprofen Tablets, USP
  (ALRA LABORATORIES, INC.)

ICHTHAMMOL
  Ichthammol Ointment USP 10%
  Ichthammol Ointment USP 20%
Ichthammol Ointment USP 10%
  (BARRE-NATIONAL INC.)
Ichthammol Ointment USP 20%
  (BARRE-NATIONAL INC.)
Idamycin for Injection
  (PHARMACIA ADRIA PHARMACIA INC.)

IDARUBICIN HYDROCHLORIDE
  Idamycin for Injection
Identi-Dose (ELI LILLY AND COMPANY)
IFEX
  (BRISTOL-MYERS SQUIBB ONCOLOGY DIVISION)

IFOSFAMIDE
  IFEX
Iletin I, Lente (ELI LILLY AND COMPANY)
Iletin I, NPH (ELI LILLY AND COMPANY)
Iletin I, Regular (ELI LILLY AND COMPANY)
Iletin II, Pork Lente (ELI LILLY AND COMPANY)
Iletin II, Pork NPH (ELI LILLY AND COMPANY)
Iletin II, Pork Regular (ELI LILLY AND COMPANY)
Iletin II, Pork Regular (Concentrated), (ELI LILLY)
Ilopan-Choline Tablets
  (SAVAGE LABORATORIES)
Ilosone Liquid, Oral Suspensions
  (DISTA PRODUCTS COMPANY)
Ilosone Pulvules & Tablets
  (DISTA PRODUCTS COMPANY)
Ilotycin Gluceptate, IV, Vials
  (DISTA PRODUCTS COMPANY)
Ilotycin Ophthalmic Ointment
  (DISTA PRODUCTS COMPANY)
Imdur (KEY PHARMACEUTICALS, INC.)

IMIPENEM-CILASTATIN SODIUM
  Primaxin I.M.
  Primaxin I.V.

IMIPRAMINE HYDROCHLORIDE
  Imipramine Hydrochloride Tablets
  Imipramine HCl Tablets
  Imipramine HCl Tablets
  Imipramine Hydrochloride Tablets
  Tofranil Ampuls
  Tofranil Tablets
Imipramine Hydrochloride Tablets
  (BIOCRAFT LABORATORIES, INC.)

Imipramine HCl Tablets
  (GENEVA PHARMACEUTICALS, INC.)
Imipramine HCl Tablets
  (PAR PHARMACEUTICAL, INC.)
Imipramine Hydrochloride Tablets
  (ROXANE LABORATORIES, INC.)

IMIPRAMINE PAMOATE
  Tofranil-PM Capsules
Imitrex Injection (CERENEX)
Imodium A-D Caplets and Liquid
  (MCNEIL CONSUMER PRODUCTS COMPANY)
Imodium Capsules
  (JANSSEN PHARMACEUTICA INC.)
Imogam Rabies Immune Globulin (Human)
  (CONNAUGHT LABORATORIES, INC.)
Imovax Rabies I.D. Rabies Vaccine
  (CONNAUGHT LABORATORIES, INC.)
Imovax Rabies Vaccine
  (CONNAUGHT LABORATORIES, INC.)
Impregon Concentrate (FLEMING & COMPANY)
Imuran Injection (BURROUGHS WELLCOME CO.)
Imuran Tablets (BURROUGHS WELLCOME CO.)
Inapsine Injection (JANSSEN PHARMACEUTICA INC.)

INDAPAMIDE
  Lozol Tablets
Inderal Injectable
  (WYETH-AYERST LABORATORIES)
Inderal Tablets (WYETH-AYERST LABORATORIES)
Inderal LA Long Acting Capsules
  (WYETH-AYERST LABORATORIES)
Inderide Tablets
  (WYETH-AYERST LABORATORIES)
Inderide LA Long Acting Capsules
  (WYETH-AYERST LABORATORIES)
Indocin Capsules (MERCK & CO., INC.)
Indocin I.V. (MERCK & CO., INC.)
Indocin Oral Suspension (MERCK & CO., INC.)
Indocin SR Capsules (MERCK & CO., INC.)
Indocin Suppositories (MERCK & CO., INC.)

INDOMETHACIN
  Indocin Capsules
  Indocin Oral Suspension
  Indocin SR Capsules
  Indocin Suppositories
  Indomethacin Capsules
  Indomethacin Capsules
  Indomethacin Capsules 25 + 50
  Indomethacin Capsules
  Indomethacin Capsules and Extended-Release
    Capsules, USP
  Indomethacin Capsules, U.S.P.
  Indomethacin Extended-Release Capsules, U.S.P.
Indomethacin Capsules
  (LEDERLE STANDARD PRODUCTS)
Indomethacin Capsules
  (MYLAN PHARMACEUTICALS INC.)
Indomethacin Capsules 25 + 50
  (NOVOPHARM, USA INC.)
Indomethacin Capsules
  (PAR PHARMACEUTICAL, INC.)
**Indomethacin Capsules and Extended-Release
  Capsules, USP**
  (WARNER CHILCOTT LABORATORIES)
Indomethacin Capsules, U.S.P.
  (WEST POINT PHARMA)
Indomethacin Extended-Release Capsules, U.S.P.
  (WEST POINT PHARMA)

INDOMETHACIN SODIUM TRIHYDRATE
  Indocin I.V.
INFeD Iron Dextran Injection
  (SCHEIN PHARMACEUTICAL, INC.)

INFLUENZA VIRUS VACCINE
  Fluzone

UNDERLINE DENOTES GENERIC NAME

Influenza Virus Vaccine, Trivalent, Types A & B
(chromatographed and filter-purified subviron
antigen) FluShield
Influenza Virus Vaccine, Trivalent, Types A & B,
1994-95 Formula, in Tubex
**Influenza Virus Vaccine, Trivalent,
Types A & B (chromatographed and
filter-purified subviron antigen) FluShield**
(WYETH-AYERST LABORATORIES)
**Influenza Virus Vaccine, Trivalent,
Types A & B, 1994-95 Formula, in Tubex**
(WYETH-AYERST LABORATORIES)
**Infumorph 200 and Infumorph 500 Sterile
Solutions** (ELKINS-SINN, INC.)
Innovar Injection (JANSSEN PHARMACEUTICA INC.)
Inocor Lactate Injection
(SANOFI WINTHROP PHARMACEUTICALS)

INOSITOL
Amino-Cerv
Mega-B
Megadose
InspirEase (SCHERING CORPORATION)
INSTAT* Collagen Absorbable Hemostat
(JOHNSON & JOHNSON MEDICAL, INC.)
**INSTAT* MCH Microfibrillar Collagen
Hemostat** (JOHNSON & JOHNSON MEDICAL, INC.)

INSULIN, HUMAN ISOPHANE SUSPENSION
Novolin N

INSULIN, HUMAN NPH
Humulin N, 100 Units
Novolin N PenFill Cartridges
Novolin N Prefilled Syringe

INSULIN, HUMAN REGULAR
Humulin BR, 100 Units
Humulin R, 100 Units
Novolin R
Novolin R PenFill Cartridges
Novolin R Prefilled Syringe
NovoFine 30 Disposable Needle
NovolinPen
Velosulin Human

INSULIN, HUMAN REGULAR AND
HUMAN NPH MIXTURE
Humulin 50/50, 100 Units
Humulin 70/30, 100 Units
Novolin 70/30
Novolin 70/30 PenFill Cartridges
Novolin 70/30 Prefilled

INSULIN, HUMAN, ZINC SUSPENSION
Humulin L, 100 Units
Humulin U, 100 Units
Novolin L

INSULIN, NPH
NPH Insulin
NPH Purified Pork Isophane Insulin

INSULIN, REGULAR
Regular Insulin
Regular Purified Pork Insulin

INSULIN, ZINC CRYSTALS
INSULIN, ZINC SUSPENSION
Iletin I
Lente Insulin
Lente Purified Pork Insulin
Ultralente Insulin
Intal Capsules
(FISONS CORPORATION PRESCRIPTION PRODUCTS)
Intal Inhaler
(FISONS CORPORATION PRESCRIPTION PRODUCTS)
Intal Nebulizer Solution
(FISONS CORPORATION PRESCRIPTION PRODUCTS)
**INTERCEED* (TC7) Absorbable Adhesion
Barrier** (JOHNSON & JOHNSON MEDICAL, INC.)

INTERFERON ALFA-2A, RECOMBINANT
Roferon-A Injection

INTERFERON ALFA-2B, RECOMBINANT
Intron A

INTERFERON ALFA-N3 (HUMAN LEUKOCYTE
DERIVED)
Alferon N Injection

INTERFERON BETA-1B
Betaseron for SC Injection

INTERFERON GAMMA-1B
Actimmune

INTRINSIC FACTOR CONCENTRATE
Trinsicon Capsules
Intron A (SCHERING CORPORATION)
Inversine Tablets (MERCK & CO., INC.)

IODINE
Ethiodol
Pima Syrup
Prenate 90 Tablets

IODOCHLORHYDROXYQUIN
Iodochlorhydroxyquin 3% w/Hydrocortisone 1%
Cream
**Iodochlorhydroxyquin 3% w/Hydrocortisone 1%
Cream** (BARRE-NATIONAL INC.)

IODOQUINOL
Vytone Cream 1%
Yodoxin

IOHEXOL
Omnipaque
Ionamin Capsules
(FISONS CORPORATION PRESCRIPTION PRODUCTS)
Ionil Plus Shampoo
(GALDERMA LABORATORIES, INC.)
Ionil T Plus Shampoo
(GALDERMA LABORATORIES, INC.)
Iophen-C Liquid (BARRE-NATIONAL INC.)
Iophen DM (BARRE-NATIONAL INC.)
Iophen Elixir (BARRE-NATIONAL INC.)
Iophylline Elixir (BARRE-NATIONAL INC.)

IPECAC
Ipecac Syrup
Ipecac Syrup USP
Ipecac Syrup (ROXANE LABORATORIES, INC.)
Ipecac Syrup USP (BARRE-NATIONAL INC.)
IPOL Poliovirus Vaccine Inactivated
(CONNAUGHT LABORATORIES, INC.)

IPRATROPIUM BROMIDE
Atrovent Inhalation Aerosol
Atrovent Inhalation Solution
IPSATOL Cough Formula
(KENWOOD LABORATORIES)
Ircon Tablets (KENWOOD LABORATORIES)
Ircon-FA Tablets (KENWOOD LABORATORIES)
Iromin-G (MISSION PHARMACAL COMPANY)

IRON DEXTRAN
INFeD Iron Dextran Injection

IRON & AMMONIUM CITRATE
ILX B$_{12}$ Elixir Crystalline and ILX B$_{12}$
Sugar–Free Elixir
Irospan Capsules
(THE FIELDING PHARMACEUTICAL COMPANY, INC.)
Irospan Tablets
(THE FIELDING PHARMACEUTICAL COMPANY, INC.)
Ismelin Tablets (CIBA PHARMACEUTICAL COMPANY)
Ismo Tablets (WYETH-AYERST LABORATORIES)
Isoclor Expectorant
(FISONS CORPORATION PRESCRIPTION PRODUCTS)

ISOETHARINE
Bronkometer Aerosol

Bronkosol Solution
Isoetharine Inhalation Solution, USP, Arm-a-Med
Isoetharine Inhalation Solution
Isoetharine Inhalation Solution, Sulfite-Free, USP
Isoetharine Inhalation Solution, USP, Arm-a-Med
(ASTRA USA, INC.)
Isoetharine Inhalation Solution
(ROXANE LABORATORIES, INC.)
**Isoetharine Inhalation Solution, Sulfite-Free,
USP** (DEY LABORATORIES)

ISOFLURANE
Forane

ISOFLUROPHATE
Floropryl Sterile Ophthalmic Ointment

ISOMETHEPTENE MUCATE
Duradrin Capsules
Midrin Capsules
Migralam Capsules
Isomil DF Soy Formula For Diarrhea
(ROSS PRODUCTS DIVISION)
Isomil SF Sucrose Free Soy Formula
(ROSS PRODUCTS DIVISION)
Isomil Soy Formula with Iron
(ROSS PRODUCTS DIVISION)

ISONIAZID
Isoniazid Tablets
Nydrazid Injection
Rifamate Capsules
Rifater
Isoniazid Tablets
(DURAMED PHARMACEUTICALS, INC.)

ISOPROPYL ALCOHOL
Cetylcide Germicidal Concentrate

ISOPROTERENOL HYDROCHLORIDE
Duo-Medihaler Aerosol
Isoproterenol Hydrochloride Injection
Isuprel Hydrochloride Glossets
Isuprel Hydrochloride Injection 1:5000
Isuprel Hydrochloride Solution 1:200 & 1:100
Isuprel Mistometer
Isoproterenol Hydrochloride Injection
(ELKINS-SINN, INC.)

ISOPROTERENOL SULFATE
Medihaler-Iso Aerosol
Norisodrine with Calcium Iodide Syrup
Isoptin Ampules 5mg/2mL
(KNOLL PHARMACEUTICAL COMPANY)
Isoptin for Intravenous Injection 5mg/2mL
(KNOLL PHARMACEUTICAL COMPANY)
Isoptin Oral Tablets
(KNOLL PHARMACEUTICAL COMPANY)
Isoptin SR Tablets
(KNOLL PHARMACEUTICAL COMPANY)
Isordil Sublingual Tablets 2.5 mg, 5 mg & 10 mg
(WYETH-AYERST LABORATORIES)
Isordil Tembids Capsules (40 mg)
(WYETH-AYERST LABORATORIES)
Isordil Tembids Tablets (40 mg)
(WYETH-AYERST LABORATORIES)
Isordil 5 Titradose Tablets, 5 mg
(WYETH-AYERST LABORATORIES)
Isordil 10 Titradose Tablets, 10 mg
(WYETH-AYERST LABORATORIES)
Isordil 20 Titradose Tablets, 20 mg
(WYETH-AYERST LABORATORIES)
Isordil 30 Titradose Tablets, 30 mg
(WYETH-AYERST LABORATORIES)
Isordil 40 Titradose Tablets, 40 mg
(WYETH-AYERST LABORATORIES)

ISOSORBIDE DINITRATE
Dilatrate-SR
Isordil Sublingual Tablets 2.5 mg, 5 mg & 10 mg

UNDERLINE DENOTES GENERIC NAME

Isordil Tembids Capsules (40 mg)
Isordil Tembids Tablets (40 mg)
Isordil 5 Titradose Tablets, 5 mg
Isordil 10 Titradose Tablets, 10 mg
Isordil 20 Titradose Tablets, 20 mg
Isordil 30 Titradose Tablets, 30 mg
Isordil 40 Titradose Tablets, 40 mg
Isosorbide Dinitrate Tablets
Isosorbide Dinitrate Tablets
Sorbitrate Chewable Tablets
Sorbitrate Oral Tablets
Sorbitrate Sublingual Tablets
Isosorbide Dinitrate Tablets
   (GENEVA PHARMACEUTICALS, INC.)
Isosorbide Dinitrate Tablets
   (PAR PHARMACEUTICAL, INC.)

ISOSORBIDE MONONITRATE
   Imdur
   Ismo Tablets
   Monoket

ISOTRETINOIN
   Accutane Capsules
Isovex Capsules
   (U.S. PHARMACEUTICAL CORPORATION)

ISRADIPINE
   DynaCirc Capsules
Isuprel Hydrochloride Glossets
   (SANOFI WINTHROP PHARMACEUTICALS)
Isuprel Hydrochloride Injection 1:5000
   (SANOFI WINTHROP PHARMACEUTICALS)
Isuprel Hydrochloride Solution 1:200 & 1:100
   (SANOFI WINTHROP PHARMACEUTICALS)
Isuprel Mistometer
   (SANOFI WINTHROP PHARMACEUTICALS)
Itch-X Gel (B. F. ASCHER & COMPANY, INC.)

ITRACONAZOLE
   Sporanox Capsules
Iveegam (IMMUNO-U.S., INC.)

J

JAPANESE ENCEPHALITIS VACCINE

INACTIVATED
   JE-VAX
JE-VAX (CONNAUGHT LABORATORIES, INC.)
Jevity Isotonic Liquid Nutrition with Fiber
   (ROSS PRODUCTS DIVISION)

K

K+ 8 Tablets (ALRA LABORATORIES, INC.)
K+ Care Powder (ALRA LABORATORIES, INC.)
K+ Care ET (ALRA LABORATORIES, INC.)
K-Dur Microburst Release System (potassium chloride, USP) E.R. Tablets
   (KEY PHARMACEUTICALS, INC.)
K-Lor Powder Packets (ABBOTT LABORATORIES)
K-Lyte/Cl 50 Effervescent Tablets (APOTHECON)
K-Lyte/Cl Tablets (APOTHECON)
K-Lyte & K-Lyte DS Effervescent Tablets
   (APOTHECON)
K-Norm Extended-Release Capsules
   (FISONS CORPORATION PRESCRIPTION PRODUCTS)

K-Phos M.F. Tablets (BEACH PHARMACEUTICALS)
K-Phos Neutral Tablets
   (BEACH PHARMACEUTICALS)
K-Phos Original Formula "Sodium Free" Tablets
   (BEACH PHARMACEUTICALS)
K-Phos No. 2 Tablets (BEACH PHARMACEUTICALS)
K-Tab Filmtab (ABBOTT LABORATORIES)
K+ 10 Tablets (ALRA LABORATORIES, INC.)
Kabikinase (Streptokinase)
   (PHARMACIA ADRIA PHARMACIA INC.)
Kaltostat Wound Dressing
   (CALGON VESTAL LABORATORIES, INC.)
Kaochlor 10% Liquid (SAVAGE LABORATORIES)
Kaochlor S-F 10% Liquid (Sugar Free)
   (SAVAGE LABORATORIES)

KAOLIN
   Kaolin-Pectin Suspension
Kaolin-Pectin Suspension
   (ROXANE LABORATORIES, INC.)
Kaon CL 10 (SAVAGE LABORATORIES)
Kaon-CL 6.7 Meq Tablets SA
   (SAVAGE LABORATORIES)
Kaon-CL 20% Liquid (SAVAGE LABORATORIES)
Kaon Grape Elixir (SAVAGE LABORATORIES)
Kaopek (BARRE-NATIONAL INC.)
Kasof Capsules
   (ROBERTS PHARMACEUTICAL CORPORATION)
Kayexalate
   (SANOFI WINTHROP PHARMACEUTICALS)
Keflex Pulvules & Oral Suspension
   (DISTA PRODUCTS COMPANY)
Keftab Tablets (DISTA PRODUCTS COMPANY)
Kefurox Vials, Faspak & ADD-Vantage
   (ELI LILLY AND COMPANY)
Kefzol Vials, Faspak & ADD-Vantage
   (ELI LILLY AND COMPANY)
Kemadrin Tablets (BURROUGHS WELLCOME CO.)
Kenwood Therapeutic Liquid
   (KENWOOD LABORATORIES)
Keri Lotion - Original Formula
   (BRISTOL-MYERS PRODUCTS)
Keri Lotion - Silky Smooth Formula
   (BRISTOL-MYERS PRODUCTS)
Keri Lotion - Silky Smooth Fragrance-Free Formula (BRISTOL-MYERS PRODUCTS)
Kerlone Tablets (G.D. SEARLE & CO.)

KETOCONAZOLE
   Nizoral 2% Cream
   Nizoral 2% Shampoo
   Nizoral Tablets

KETOPROFEN
   Ketoprofen Capsules
   Ketoprofen Capsules
   Orudis Capsules
   Oruvail Capsules
Ketoprofen Capsules
   (BIOCRAFT LABORATORIES, INC.)
Ketoprofen Capsules
   (LEDERLE STANDARD PRODUCTS)

KETOROLAC TROMETHAMINE
   Acular
   Acular
   Toradol IM Injection
   Toradol Oral
Kionex (PADDOCK LABORATORIES, INC.)
Klonopin Tablets (ROCHE LABORATORIES)
Klor-Con/EF Tablets
   (UPSHER-SMITH LABORATORIES, INC.)
Klor-Con 8/Klor-Con 10 Tablets
   (UPSHER-SMITH LABORATORIES, INC.)
Klor-Con Powder
   (UPSHER-SMITH LABORATORIES, INC.)
Klor-Con/25 Powder
   (UPSHER-SMITH LABORATORIES, INC.)

Klorvess Effervescent Granules
   (SANDOZ PHARMACEUTICALS CORPORATION)
Klorvess Effervescent Tablets
   (SANDOZ PHARMACEUTICALS CORPORATION)
Klorvess 10% Liquid
   (SANDOZ PHARMACEUTICALS CORPORATION)
Klotrix Tablets (APOTHECON)
Koāte-HP Antihemophilic Factor (Human)
   (MILES INC. PHARMACEUTICAL DIVISION BIOLOGI-
   CAL PRODUCTS)
**KOGENATE Antihemophilic Factor
   (Recombinant)** (MILES INC. PHARMACEUTICAL
   DIVISION BIOLOGICAL PRODUCTS)
Kolyum Liquid
   (FISONS CORPORATION PRESCRIPTION PRODUCTS)
Konakion Injection (ROCHE LABORATORIES)
Konÿne 80 Factor IX Complex (MILES INC. PHAR-
   MACEUTICAL DIVISION BIOLOGICAL PRODUCTS)
Koro-Flex (GYNOPHARMA INC.)
Koromex (GYNOPHARMA INC.)
Kronofed-A Kronocaps
   (FERNDALE LABORATORIES, INC.)
Kronofed-A-Jr. Kronocaps
   (FERNDALE LABORATORIES, INC.)
Kutrase Capsules (SCHWARZ PHARMA)
Ku-Zyme Capsules (SCHWARZ PHARMA)
Ku-Zyme HP Capsules (SCHWARZ PHARMA)
Kwelcof Liquid (B. F. ASCHER & COMPANY, INC.)
Kwell Cream & Lotion (REED & CARNRICK)
Kwell Shampoo (REED & CARNRICK)
Kytril (SMITHKLINE BEECHAM PHARMACEUTICALS)

L

LABETALOL HYDROCHLORIDE
   Normodyne Injection
   Normodyne Tablets
   Trandate Injection
   Trandate Tablets
Lac-Hydrin 12% Lotion
   (WESTWOOD-SQUIBB PHARMACEUTICALS INC.)
Lacril Lubricant Ophthalmic Solution
   (ALLERGAN, INC.)
**Lacri-Lube S.O.P. Lubricant Ophthalmic
   Ointment** (ALLERGAN, INC.)
Lacrisert Sterile Ophthalmic Insert
   (MERCK & CO., INC.)
Lactaid Caplets (LACTAID, INC.)
Lactaid Drops (LACTAID, INC.)

LACTALBUMIN HYDROLYSATE
   Perative Specialized Liquid Nutrition

LACTASE (BETA-D-GALACTOSIDASE)
   Lactaid Caplets
   Lactaid Drops

LACTIC ACID
   Atrac-Tain, Moisturizing Cream
   Lactinol Lotion and Lactinol-E Creme
LactiCare-HC Lotion, 1%
   (STIEFEL LABORATORIES, INC.)
LactiCare-HC Lotion, 2^1/$_2$%
   (STIEFEL LABORATORIES, INC.)
Lactinol Lotion and Lactinol-E Creme
   (PEDINOL PHARMACAL INC.)
Lactocal-F Tablets (LASER, INC.)

LACTULOSE
   Cholac Lactulose Syrup
   Constilac Lactulose Syrup
   Constulose

UNDERLINE DENOTES GENERIC NAME

Enulose
Lactulose Solution
Lactulose Solution (ROXANE LABORATORIES, INC.)
Lamisil Cream 1%
  (SANDOZ PHARMACEUTICALS CORPORATION)
Lamprene Capsules (GEIGY PHARMACEUTICALS)

LANOLIN
  Eucerin Dry Skin Care Lotion
  Lanolin Hydrous USP
  Lanolin Modified USP
  pHisoHex
Lanolin Hydrous USP (BARRE-NATIONAL INC.)
Lanolin Modified USP (BARRE-NATIONAL INC.)

LANOLIN OIL
  Sween Cream
Lanoxicaps (BURROUGHS WELLCOME CO.)
Lanoxin Elixir Pediatric
  (BURROUGHS WELLCOME CO.)
Lanoxin Injection (BURROUGHS WELLCOME CO.)
Lanoxin Injection Pediatric
  (BURROUGHS WELLCOME CO.)
Lanoxin Tablets (BURROUGHS WELLCOME CO.)
Lariam Tablets (ROCHE LABORATORIES)
Larobec Tablets (ROCHE LABORATORIES)
Larodopa Tablets (ROCHE LABORATORIES)
Lasix Injection, Oral Solution and Tablets
  (HOECHST-ROUSSEL PHARMACEUTICALS INC.)
Lavacol (WARNER WELLCOME)
Lazer Creme (PEDINOL PHARMACAL INC.)
LazerFormalyde Solution
  (PEDINOL PHARMACAL INC.)
LazerSporin-C Solution
  (PEDINOL PHARMACAL INC.)

LECITHIN
  PhosChol Concentrate
  PhosChol Forte
  PhosChol 565 Softgels
  PhosChol 900 Softgels
  Pro-Hepatone Capsules
Ledercillin VK Oral Solution, Tablets
  (LEDERLE STANDARD PRODUCTS)
Lente Insulin
  (NOVO NORDISK PHARMACEUTICALS INC.)
Lente Purified Pork Insulin
  (NOVO NORDISK PHARMACEUTICALS INC.)
Lescol Capsules
  (SANDOZ PHARMACEUTICALS CORPORATION)

LEUCOVORIN CALCIUM
  Leucovorin Calcium for Injection,
    Wellcovorin Brand
  Leucovorin Calcium for Injection
  Leucovorin Calcium for Injection
    (Preservative-Free)
  Leucovorin Calcium for Injection
  Leucovorin Calcium Tablets, Wellcovorin Brand
  Leucovorin Calcium Tablets
Leucovorin Calcium for Injection, Wellcovorin Brand (BURROUGHS WELLCOME CO.)
Leucovorin Calcium for Injection
  (CHIRON THERAPEUTICS)
Leucovorin Calcium for Injection (Preservative-Free) (ELKINS-SINN, INC.)
Leucovorin Calcium for Injection
  (IMMUNEX CORPORATION)
Leucovorin Calcium Tablets, Wellcovorin Brand
  (BURROUGHS WELLCOME CO.)
Leucovorin Calcium Tablets
  (IMMUNEX CORPORATION)
Leukeran Tablets (BURROUGHS WELLCOME CO.)
Leukine for IV Infusion (IMMUNEX CORPORATION)
Leustatin (ORTHO BIOTECH INC.)

LEUPROLIDE ACETATE
  Lupron Depot 3.75 mg

Lupron Depot 7.5 mg
Lupron Depot-PED 7.5 mg, 11.25 mg and 15 mg
Lupron Injection

LEVAMISOLE HYDROCHLORIDE
  Ergamisol Tablets
Levatol (REED & CARNRICK)
Levlen 21 Tablets (BERLEX LABORATORIES)
Levlen 28 Tablets (BERLEX LABORATORIES)
Levo-Dromoran Injectable
  (ROCHE LABORATORIES)
Levo-Dromoran Tablets (ROCHE LABORATORIES)
LEVO-T Tablets (LEDERLE STANDARD PRODUCTS)

LEVOCARNITINE
  L-Carnitine Capsules
  L-Carnitine Capsules
  L-Carnitine 250mg and 500mg Tablets
  Carnitor Injection
  Carnitor Tablets and Solution

LEVODOPA
  Atamet
  Carbidopa and Levodopa Tablets, USP
  Dopar Capsules
  Larodopa Tablets
  Sinemet Tablets
  Sinemet CR Tablets

LEVONORGESTREL
  Levlen 21 Tablets
  Levlen 28 Tablets
  Nordette-21 Tablets
  Nordette-28 Tablets
  Norplant System
  Tri-Levlen 21 Tablets
  Tri-Levlen 28 Tablets
  Triphasil-21 Tablets
  Triphasil-28 Tablets
Levophed Bitartrate Injection
  (SANOFI WINTHROP PHARMACEUTICALS)
Levoprome (IMMUNEX CORPORATION)

LEVORPHANOL TARTRATE
  Levo-Dromoran Injectable
  Levo-Dromoran Tablets
  Levorphanol Tartrate Tablets
Levorphanol Tartrate Tablets
  (ROXANE LABORATORIES, INC.)
Levothroid Tablets
  (FOREST PHARMACEUTICALS, INC.)

LEVOTHYROXINE SODIUM
  Levothroid Tablets
  Levothyroxine Sodium Tablets
  Levothyroxine Sodium Tablets
  Levoxine Tablets
  Synthroid Injection
  Synthroid Tablets
  Thyrar Tablets
Levothyroxine Sodium Tablets
  (DURAMED PHARMACEUTICALS, INC.)
Levothyroxine Sodium Tablets
  (WARNER CHILCOTT LABORATORIES)
Levoxine Tablets
  (DANIELS PHARMACEUTICALS, INC.)
Levsin Drops (SCHWARZ PHARMA)
Levsin Elixir (SCHWARZ PHARMA)
Levsin Injection (SCHWARZ PHARMA)
Levsin Tablets (SCHWARZ PHARMA)
Levsin/SL Tablets (SCHWARZ PHARMA)
Levsinex Timecaps (SCHWARZ PHARMA)

LEVULOSE
  Emecheck
  Emetrol Solution - Cherry
  Emetrol Solution - Lemon-Mint
Librax Capsules (ROCHE PRODUCTS INC.)
Libritabs Tablets (ROCHE PRODUCTS INC.)

Librium Capsules (ROCHE PRODUCTS INC.)
Librium Injectable (ROCHE PRODUCTS INC.)
Lidex Cream 0.05% (SYNTEX PUERTO RICO, INC.)
Lidex Gel 0.05% (SYNTEX PUERTO RICO, INC.)
Lidex Ointment 0.05% (SYNTEX PUERTO RICO, INC.)
Lidex Topical Solution 0.05%
  (SYNTEX PUERTO RICO, INC.)
Lidex-E Cream 0.05% (SYNTEX PUERTO RICO, INC.)

LIDOCAINE
  Emla Cream
  Lidocaine Viscous 2%
  Neosporin Plus Maximum Strength Cream
  Neosporin Plus Maximum Strength Ointment
  Terramycin Intramuscular Solution
  Water-Jel Burn Jel
  Xylocaine 5% Ointment
  Xylocaine 10% Oral Spray

LIDOCAINE HYDROCHLORIDE
  Anestacon Jelly
  Decadron Phosphate with Xylocaine Injection,
    Sterile
  Lidocaine HCl Oral Topical Soln. USP 2%
  Lidocaine Hydrochloride Injection
  Lidocaine Hydrochloride Injection (Preservative-
    Free)
  Lidocaine Hydrochloride & Epinephrine Injection
  Xylocaine Injections
  Xylocaine with Epinephrine Injections
  Xylocaine Injections for Ventricular Arrhythmias
  Xylocaine 2% Jelly
  Xylocaine 1.5% Solution with Dextrose 7.5%
  Xylocaine 5% Solution with Glucose 7.5%
  4% Xylocaine-MPF Sterile Solution
  Xylocaine 4% Topical Solution
  Xylocaine 2% Viscous Solution
Lidocaine HCl Oral Topical Soln. USP 2%
  (BARRE-NATIONAL INC.)
Lidocaine Hydrochloride Injection
  (ELKINS-SINN, INC.)
Lidocaine Hydrochloride Injection (Preservative-Free) (ELKINS-SINN, INC.)
Lidocaine Hydrochloride & Epinephrine Injection (ELKINS-SINN, INC.)
Lidocaine Viscous 2%
  (ROXANE LABORATORIES, INC.)
Limbitrol DS Tablets (ROCHE PRODUCTS INC.)
Limbitrol Tablets (ROCHE PRODUCTS INC.)
Lindane Lotion USP 1% (BARRE-NATIONAL INC.)
Lindane Shampoo, USP 1%
  (BARRE-NATIONAL INC.)
Lincocin Capsules (THE UPJOHN COMPANY)
Lincocin Pediatric Capsules
  (THE UPJOHN COMPANY)
Lincocin Sterile Solution (THE UPJOHN COMPANY)

LINCOMYCIN HYDROCHLORIDE
  Lincocin Capsules
  Lincocin Pediatric Capsules
  Lincocin Sterile Solution

LINDANE
  Kwell Cream & Lotion
  Kwell Shampoo
  Lindane Lotion USP 1%
  Lindane Shampoo, USP 1%
Lioresal Intrathecal
  (MEDTRONIC, INC. NEUROLOGICAL DIVISION)
Lioresal Tablets (GEIGY PHARMACEUTICALS)

LIOTHYRONINE SODIUM
  Cytomel Tablets
  Thyrar Tablets
  Triostat Injection

LIOTRIX
  Thyrolar Tablets

LIPOLYTIC ENZYME
  Arco-Lase Tablets
  Cotazym
  Kutrase Capsules
  Ku-Zyme Capsules
  Ku-Zyme HP Capsules
Lippes Loop Intrauterine Double-S
  (ORTHO PHARMACEUTICAL CORPORATION)
Liquibid Tablets (ION LABORATORIES, INC.)
Liquibid-D Tablets (ION LABORATORIES, INC.)
Liquid Pred Syrup
  (MURO PHARMACEUTICAL, INC.)
Liquifilm Forte Lubricant Ophthalmic Solution
  (ALLERGAN, INC.)
Liquifilm Tears Lubricant Ophthalmic Solution
  (ALLERGAN, INC.)

LISINOPRIL
  Prinivil Tablets
  Prinzide Tablets
  Zestoretic
  Zestril Tablets
Listerex Scrub Golden (WARNER WELLCOME)
Listerex Scrub Herbal (WARNER WELLCOME)
Listerine Antiseptic (WARNER WELLCOME)
Cool Mint Listerine (WARNER WELLCOME)
Listermint with Fluoride (WARNER WELLCOME)

LITHIUM CARBONATE
  Eskalith Capsules
  Eskalith CR Controlled Release Tablets
  Lithium Carbonate Capsules & Tablets
  LITHONATE Capsules
  LITHOTABS Tablets
Lithium Carbonate Capsules & Tablets
  (ROXANE LABORATORIES, INC.)

LITHIUM CITRATE
  Lithium Citrate Syrup
Lithium Citrate Syrup
  (ROXANE LABORATORIES, INC.)
LITHONATE Capsules
  (SOLVAY PHARMACEUTICALS, INC.)
Lithostat (MISSION PHARMACAL COMPANY)
LITHOTABS Tablets
  (SOLVAY PHARMACEUTICALS, INC.)

LIVER PREPARATIONS
  Hep-Forte Capsules
  ILX B$_{12}$ Caplets Crystalline
  ILX B$_{12}$ Elixir Crystalline and ILX B$_{12}$
    Sugar–Free Elixir
  ILX Elixir
  Trinsicon Capsules
Locoid Cream, Ointment and Topical Solution
  (FERNDALE LABORATORIES, INC.)
Lodine Capsules and Tablets
  (WYETH-AYERST LABORATORIES)

LODOXAMIDE TROMETHAMINE
  Alomide
Lodrane LD Capsules (ECR PHARMACEUTICALS)
Lodrane Liquid (ECR PHARMACEUTICALS)
Loestrin Fe 1/20 (PARKE-DAVIS)
Loestrin Fe 1.5/30 (PARKE-DAVIS)
Loestrin 21 1/20 (PARKE-DAVIS)
Loestrin 21 1.5/30 (PARKE-DAVIS)

LOMEFLOXACIN HYDROCHLORIDE
  Maxaquin Tablets
Lomotil Liquid (G.D. SEARLE & CO.)
Lomotil Tablets (G.D. SEARLE & CO.)

LOMUSTINE (CCNU)
  CeeNU
Loniten Tablets (THE UPJOHN COMPANY)
Lo/Ovral Tablets (WYETH-AYERST LABORATORIES)
Lo/Ovral-28 Tablets
  (WYETH-AYERST LABORATORIES)

LOPERAMIDE HYDROCHLORIDE
  Imodium A-D Caplets and Liquid
  Imodium Capsules
  Loperamide HCl Oral Soln. 1 mg/5 mL
  Loperamide Hydrochloride Capsules
  Loperamide Hydrochloride Capsules USP
  Loperamide Hydrochloride Capsules and Oral
    Solution
  Loperamide Caplet, 2 mg
  Loperamide Capsules
  Loperamide Liquid
  Pepto Diarrhea Control
Loperamide HCl Oral Soln. 1 mg/5 mL
  (BARRE-NATIONAL INC.)
Loperamide Hydrochloride Capsules
  (MYLAN PHARMACEUTICALS INC.)
Loperamide Hydrochloride Capsules USP
  (NOVOPHARM, USA INC.)
Loperamide Hydrochloride Capsules and Oral
  Solution (ROXANE LABORATORIES, INC.)
Loperamide Caplet, 2 mg (NOVOPHARM, USA INC.)
Loperamide Capsules
  (GENEVA PHARMACEUTICALS, INC.)
Loperamide Liquid (NOVOPHARM, USA INC.)
Lopid Tablets (PARKE-DAVIS)
Lopressor Ampuls (GEIGY PHARMACEUTICALS)
Lopressor HCT Tablets
  (GEIGY PHARMACEUTICALS)
Lopressor Tablets (GEIGY PHARMACEUTICALS)
Loprox 1% Cream and Lotion
  (HOECHST-ROUSSEL PHARMACEUTICALS INC.)
Lorabid Suspension and Pulvules
  (ELI LILLY AND COMPANY)

LORACARBEF
  Lorabid Suspension and Pulvules

LORATADINE
  Claritin

LORAZEPAM
  Ativan Injection
  Ativan Tablets
  Ativan in Tubex
  Lorazepam Tablets
  Lorazepam Tablets
  Lorazepam Tablets, USP
Lorazepam Tablets (MYLAN PHARMACEUTICALS INC.)
Lorazepam Tablets
  (WARNER CHILCOTT LABORATORIES)
Lorazepam Tablets, USP
  (WATSON LABORATORIES, INC.)
Lorcet Plus (UAD LABORATORIES)
Lorcet-HD (UAD LABORATORIES)
Lorcet 10/650 (UAD LABORATORIES)
Lorelco Tablets (MARION MERRELL DOW INC.)
Lortab ASA Tablets
  (WHITBY PHARMACEUTICALS, INC.)
Lortab 2.5/500 Tablets
  (WHITBY PHARMACEUTICALS, INC.)
Lortab 5/500 Tablets
  (WHITBY PHARMACEUTICALS, INC.)
Lortab 7.5/500 Tablets
  (WHITBY PHARMACEUTICALS, INC.)
Lortab Elixir
  (WHITBY PHARMACEUTICALS, INC.)
Lotensin Tablets
  (CIBA PHARMACEUTICAL COMPANY)
Lotensin HCT (CIBA PHARMACEUTICAL COMPANY)
Lotrimin Cream 1% (SCHERING CORPORATION)
Lotrimin Lotion 1% (SCHERING CORPORATION)
Lotrimin Solution 1% (SCHERING CORPORATION)
Lotrisone Cream (SCHERING CORPORATION)

LOVASTATIN
  Mevacor Tablets
Lovenox Injection
  (RHONE-POULENC RORER PHARMACEUTICALS INC.)

LOXAPINE HYDROCHLORIDE
  Loxapine Capsules
  Loxitane C Oral Concentrate
  Loxitane IM
Loxapine Capsules
  (WARNER CHILCOTT LABORATORIES)

LOXAPINE SUCCINATE
  Loxapine Succinate Capsules
  Loxitane Capsules
Loxapine Succinate Capsules
  (WATSON LABORATORIES, INC.)
Loxitane C Oral Concentrate
  (LEDERLE LABORATORIES)
Loxitane Capsules (LEDERLE LABORATORIES)
Loxitane IM (LEDERLE LABORATORIES)
Lozol Tablets
  (RHONE-POULENC RORER PHARMACEUTICALS INC.)
Lubrin Vaginal Lubricating Inserts
  (KENWOOD LABORATORIES)
Ludiomil Tablets
  (CIBA PHARMACEUTICAL COMPANY)
Lufyllin Elixir (WALLACE LABORATORIES)
Lufyllin Injection (WALLACE LABORATORIES)
Lufyllin & Lufyllin-400 Tablets
  (WALLACE LABORATORIES)
Lufyllin-GG Elixir & Tablets
  (WALLACE LABORATORIES)
Lupron Depot 3.75 mg
  (TAP PHARMACEUTICALS INC.)
Lupron Depot 7.5 mg
  (TAP PHARMACEUTICALS INC.)
Lupron Depot-PED 7.5 mg, 11.25 mg and 15 mg
  (TAP PHARMACEUTICALS INC.)
Lupron Injection (TAP PHARMACEUTICALS INC.)
Luride Drops 50 ml
  (COLGATE ORAL PHARMACEUTICALS, INC.)
Luride Lozi-Tabs Tablets
  (COLGATE ORAL PHARMACEUTICALS, INC.)
Lurline PMS Tablets
  (THE FIELDING PHARMACEUTICAL COMPANY, INC.)
Lutrepulse for Injection
  (ORTHO PHARMACEUTICAL CORPORATION)
Lutrepulse for Injection
  (FERRING LABORATORIES, INC.)

LYMPHOCYTE IMMUNE GLOBULIN,

ANTITHYMOCYTE GLOBULIN (EQUINE)
  Atgam Sterile Solution

LYPRESSIN
  Diapid Nasal Spray

LYSINE HYDROCHLORIDE
  Klorvess Effervescent Granules
  Klorvess Effervescent Tablets
Lysodren
  (BRISTOL-MYERS SQUIBB ONCOLOGY DIVISION)

M

MB-TAB Meprobamate Tablets
  (ALRA LABORATORIES, INC.)
MDR Fitness Tabs for Men and Women
  (MDR FITNESS CORPORATION)
MICRhoGAM Rh+DN,o (D) Immune Globulin
  (Human) (ORTHO DIAGNOSTIC SYSTEMS INC.)
M-M-R$_{II}$ (MERCK & CO., INC.)
M-R-VAX$_{II}$ (MERCK & CO., INC.)
MS Contin Tablets
  (THE PURDUE FREDERICK COMPANY)
MSIR Oral Capsules
  (THE PURDUE FREDERICK COMPANY)

UNDERLINE DENOTES GENERIC NAME

MSIR Oral Solution
(THE PURDUE FREDERICK COMPANY)
MSIR Oral Solution Concentrate
(THE PURDUE FREDERICK COMPANY)
MSIR Tablets (THE PURDUE FREDERICK COMPANY)
MS/L Morphine Sulfate Liquid
(RICHWOOD PHARMACEUTICAL COMPANY, INC.)
MS/L Concentrate Morphine Sulfate Liquid
(RICHWOOD PHARMACEUTICAL COMPANY, INC.)
MS/S Suppositories Morphine Sulfate
(RICHWOOD PHARMACEUTICAL COMPANY, INC.)
M.V.I. Pediatric for Infusion
(ASTRA USA, INC.)
M.V.I.-12 Multi-Vitamin Infusion
(ASTRA USA, INC.)
Maalox Antacid Caplets
(RHONE-POULENC RORER PHARMACEUTICALS INC.)
Maalox Anti-Diarrheal
(RHONE-POULENC RORER PHARMACEUTICALS INC.)
Maalox Anti-Gas
(RHONE-POULENC RORER PHARMACEUTICALS INC.)
Maalox Daily Fiber Therapy
(RHONE-POULENC RORER PHARMACEUTICALS INC.)
Maalox Heartburn Relief Antacid Suspension
(RHONE-POULENC RORER PHARMACEUTICALS INC.)
Maalox Heartburn Relief Antacid Tablets
(RHONE-POULENC RORER PHARMACEUTICALS INC.)
Maalox Suspension
(RHONE-POULENC RORER PHARMACEUTICALS INC.)
Maalox Antacid Plus Anti-Gas
(RHONE-POULENC RORER PHARMACEUTICALS INC.)
Extra Strength Maalox Antacid Plus
Anti-Gas Suspension
(RHONE-POULENC RORER PHARMACEUTICALS INC.)
Maalox TC Suspension Antacid
(RHONE-POULENC RORER PHARMACEUTICALS INC.)
Extra Strength Maalox Antacid Plus
Anti-Gas Tablets
(RHONE-POULENC RORER PHARMACEUTICALS INC.)
Macrobid Capsules
(PROCTER & GAMBLE PHARMACEUTICALS, INC.)
Macrodantin Capsules
(PROCTER & GAMBLE PHARMACEUTICALS, INC.)

MAFENIDE ACETATE
Sulfamylon Cream
Magan (SAVAGE LABORATORIES)

MAGNESIUM CARBONATE
Mylanta Gelcaps Antacid
Renacidin Irrigation

MAGNESIUM CHLORIDE
Chlor-3 Condiment

MAGNESIUM GLUCONATE
Magonate Tablets and Liquid

MAGNESIUM HYDROXIDE
Aludrox Oral Suspension
Alumina and Magnesia Oral Suspension
Alumina, Magnesia, and Simethicone Oral
Suspension I
Arthritis Pain Ascriptin
Regular Strength Ascriptin Tablets
Gelusil Liquid
Gelusil Tablets
Maalox Antacid Plus Anti-Gas
Extra Strength Maalox Antacid Plus
Anti-Gas Suspension
Maalox TC Suspension Antacid
Extra Strength Maalox Antacid Plus
Anti-Gas Tablets
Milk of Magnesia & Milk of Magnesia-
Concentrated
Milk of Magnesia-Cascara Suspension
Concentrated

Milk of Magnesia-Mineral Oil Emulsion &
Emulsion (Flavored)
Mylanta Liquid
Mylanta Tablets
Mylanta Double Strength Liquid
Mylanta Double Strength Tablets

MAGNESIUM LACTATE
MagTab SR Caplets

MAGNESIUM OXIDE
Beelith Tablets
Caltrate PLUS
Mag-Ox 400
Uro-Mag

MAGNESIUM SALICYLATE
Magsal Tablets

MAGNESIUM SULFATE
Eldercaps
Eldertonic
Magnesium Sulfate Injection, USP
Magnesium Sulfate Injection, USP
(ASTRA USA, INC.)
Magonate Tablets and Liquid
(FLEMING & COMPANY)
Mag-Ox 400 (BLAINE COMPANY, INC.)
Magsal Tablets
(U.S. PHARMACEUTICAL CORPORATION)
MagTab SR Caplets
(NICHE PHARMACEUTICALS, INC.)
Maltsupex Liquid, Powder & Tablets
(WALLACE LABORATORIES)
Mandol Vials, Faspak & ADD-Vantage
(ELI LILLY AND COMPANY)

MANGANESE
May-Vita Elixir

MANGANESE SULFATE
Caltrate PLUS
Eldercaps
Eldertonic
Mann-Dino Chewable (VITALINE CORPORATION)

MANNITOL
Mannitol Injection, USP, 25%
Mannitol Injection, USP, 25%
(ASTRA USA, INC.)
Mantadil Cream (BURROUGHS WELLCOME CO.)

MAPROTILINE HYDROCHLORIDE
Ludiomil Tablets
Maprotiline Tablets
Maprotiline Hydrochloride Tablets
Maprotiline Hydrochloride Tablets, USP
Maprotiline Tablets
(WARNER CHILCOTT LABORATORIES)
Maprotiline Hydrochloride Tablets
(MYLAN PHARMACEUTICALS INC.)
Maprotiline Hydrochloride Tablets, USP
(WATSON LABORATORIES, INC.)
Marax Tablets & DF Syrup (ROERIG DIVISION)
Marblen Suspension Peach/Apricot
(FLEMING & COMPANY)
Marblen Tablets (FLEMING & COMPANY)
Marcaine Hydrochloride with
Epinephrine 1:200,000
(SANOFI WINTHROP PHARMACEUTICALS)
Marcaine Hydrochloride Injection
(SANOFI WINTHROP PHARMACEUTICALS)
Marcaine Spinal
(SANOFI WINTHROP PHARMACEUTICALS)
Marinol (Dronabinol) Capsules
(ROXANE LABORATORIES, INC.)
Marlyn Formula 50 Capsules
(MARLYN HEALTH CARE)

MASOPROCOL
Actinex Cream
Massengill Disposable Douche
(SMITHKLINE BEECHAM CONSUMER HEALTHCARE, L.P.)
Massengill Fragrance-Free Soft Cloth Towelette
& Baby Powder Scent
(SMITHKLINE BEECHAM CONSUMER HEALTHCARE, L.P.)
Massengill Liquid Concentrate
(SMITHKLINE BEECHAM CONSUMER HEALTHCARE, L.P.)
Massengill Medicated Disposable Douche
(SMITHKLINE BEECHAM CONSUMER HEALTHCARE, L.P.)
Massengill Medicated Liquid Concentrate
(SMITHKLINE BEECHAM CONSUMER HEALTHCARE, L.P.)
Massengill Medicated Soft Cloth Towelettes
(SMITHKLINE BEECHAM CONSUMER HEALTHCARE, L.P.)
Massengill Powder
(SMITHKLINE BEECHAM CONSUMER HEALTHCARE, L.P.)
Materna Tablets (LEDERLE LABORATORIES)
Matulane Capsules (ROCHE LABORATORIES)
Maxair Autohaler (3M PHARMACEUTICALS)
Maxair Inhaler (3M PHARMACEUTICALS)
Maxaquin Tablets (G.D. SEARLE & CO.)
Maxiflor Cream (ALLERGAN HERBERT)
Maxiflor Ointment (ALLERGAN HERBERT)
Maxzide Tablets (LEDERLE LABORATORIES)
Maxzide-25 MG Tablets (LEDERLE LABORATORIES)
May-Vita Elixir
(MAYRAND PHARMACEUTICALS, INC.)
Mazanor Tablets (WYETH-AYERST LABORATORIES)

MAZINDOL
Mazanor Tablets
Sanorex Tablets

MEASLES VIRUS VACCINE LIVE
Attenuvax

MEASLES & RUBELLA VIRUS VACCINE LIVE
M-R-VAX +DN,II

MEASLES, MUMPS & RUBELLA VIRUS
VACCINE LIVE
M-M-R$_{II}$
Mebaral Tablets
(SANOFI WINTHROP PHARMACEUTICALS)

MEBENDAZOLE
Vermox Chewable Tablets

MECAMYLAMINE HYDROCHLORIDE
Inversine Tablets

MECHLORETHAMINE HYDROCHLORIDE
Mustargen
Meclan (mecloycycline sulfosalicylate) Cream
(ORTHO PHARMACEUTICAL CORPORATION
DERMATOLOGICAL DIVISION)

MECLIZINE HYDROCHLORIDE
Antivert, Antivert/25 Tablets, & Antivert/50
Tablets
Bonine Tablets
Meclizine HCl Tablets
Meclizine HCl Tablets
Meclizine HCl Tablets
(GENEVA PHARMACEUTICALS, INC.)
Meclizine HCl Tablets
(PAR PHARMACEUTICAL, INC.)

MECLOCYCLINE SULFOSALICYLATE
Meclan (mecloycycline sulfosalicylate) Cream

MECLOFENAMATE SODIUM
Meclofenamate Sodium Capsules
Meclofenamate Sodium Capsules
(MYLAN PHARMACEUTICALS INC.)
Medicated Blue Shampoo (BARRE-NATIONAL INC.)
Medigesic Capsules
(U.S. PHARMACEUTICAL CORPORATION)
Medihaler-Iso Aerosol (3M PHARMACEUTICALS)

Mediplex (U.S. PHARMACEUTICAL CORPORATION)
Medrol Dosepak Unit of Use
　(THE UPJOHN COMPANY)
Medrol Tablets (THE UPJOHN COMPANY)

MEDROXYPROGESTERONE ACETATE
　Amen Tablets
　Cycrin Tablets
　Depo-Provera Contraceptive Injection
　Depo-Provera Sterile Aqueous Suspension
　Medroxyprogesterone Tablets
　Provera Tablets
Medroxyprogesterone Tablets
　(WARNER CHILCOTT LABORATORIES)

MEFENAMIC ACID
　Ponstel

MEFLOQUINE HYDROCHLORIDE
　Lariam Tablets
Mefoxin (MERCK & CO., INC.)
Mefoxin Premixed Intravenous Solution
　(MERCK & CO., INC.)
Mega-B (ARCO PHARMACEUTICALS, INC.)
Megace Oral Suspension
　(BRISTOL-MYERS SQUIBB ONCOLOGY DIVISION)
Megace Tablets
　(BRISTOL-MYERS SQUIBB ONCOLOGY DIVISION)
Megadose (ARCO PHARMACEUTICALS, INC.)

MEGESTROL ACETATE
　Megace Oral Suspension
　Megace Tablets
　Megestrol Acetate Tablets
Megestrol Acetate Tablets
　(PAR PHARMACEUTICAL, INC.)
Melanex Topical Solution
　(NEUTROGENA DERMATOLOGICS)
Mellaril Concentrate
　(SANDOZ PHARMACEUTICALS CORPORATION)
Mellaril Tablets
　(SANDOZ PHARMACEUTICALS CORPORATION)
Mellaril-S Suspension
　(SANDOZ PHARMACEUTICALS CORPORATION)

MELPHALAN
　Alkeran Tablets

MELPHALAN HYDROCHLORIDE
　Alkeran for Injection
Menest Tablets
　(SMITHKLINE BEECHAM PHARMACEUTICALS)

MENINGOCOCCAL POLYSACCHARIDE

VACCINE
　Menomune-A/C/Y/W-135
Menomune-A/C/Y/W-135
　(CONNAUGHT LABORATORIES, INC.)

MENOTROPINS
　Pergonal (menotropins for injection, USP)

MENTHOL
　Listerine Antiseptic
　Cool Mint Listerine
　Menthol Chest Rub
　Nephro-Derm Cream
　Panalgesic Gold Cream
　Panalgesic Gold Liniment
　PrameGel
　Thera-Gesic
　Therapeutic Mineral Ice, Pain Relieving Gel
Menthol Chest Rub (BARRE-NATIONAL INC.)
Mepergan Injection
　(WYETH-AYERST LABORATORIES)
Mepergan in Tubex
　(WYETH-AYERST LABORATORIES)

MEPERIDINE HYDROCHLORIDE
　Demerol Hydrochloride Carpuject

Demerol Hydrochloride Injection
Demerol Hydrochloride Syrup
Demerol Hydrochloride Tablets
Demerol Hydrochloride Uni-Amp
Mepergan Injection
Mepergan in Tubex
Meperidine Hydrochloride Injection
Meperidine Hydrochloride Injection
Meperidine Hydrochloride in Tubex
Meperidine Hydrochloride Injection
　(ASTRA USA, INC.)
Meperidine Hydrochloride Injection
　(ELKINS-SINN, INC.)
Meperidine Hydrochloride in Tubex
　(WYETH-AYERST LABORATORIES)

MEPHENYTOIN
　Mesantoin Tablets

MEPHOBARBITAL
　Mebaral Tablets
Mephyton Tablets (MERCK & CO., INC.)

MEPIVACAINE HYDROCHLORIDE
　Carbocaine Hydrochloride Injection
　Polocaine Injection, USP

MEPROBAMATE
　Equagesic Tablets
　Equanil Tablets
　MB-TAB Meprobamate Tablets
　Meprospan Capsules
　Miltown Tablets
　PMB 200 and PMB 400
Mepron Tablets (BURROUGHS WELLCOME CO.)
Meprospan Capsules (WALLACE LABORATORIES)

MERCAPTOPURINE
　Purinethol Tablets
Meruvax II (MERCK & CO., INC.)

MESALAMINE
　Asacol Delayed-Release Tablets
　Pentasa
　ROWASA Rectal Suppositories, 500 mg
　ROWASA Rectal Suspension Enema 4.0
　　grams/unit (60 mL)
Mesantoin Tablets
　(SANDOZ PHARMACEUTICALS CORPORATION)

MESNA
　Mesnex Injection
Mesnex Injection
　(BRISTOL-MYERS SQUIBB ONCOLOGY DIVISION)

MESORIDAZINE BESYLATE
　Serentil Ampuls
　Serentil Concentrate
　Serentil Tablets
Mestinon Injectable
　(ICN PHARMACEUTICALS, INC.)
Mestinon Syrup (ICN PHARMACEUTICALS, INC.)
Mestinon Tablets (ICN PHARMACEUTICALS, INC.)
Mestinon Timespan Tablets
　(ICN PHARMACEUTICALS, INC.)

MESTRANOL
　Nelova
　Norinyl 1+50 21-Day Tablets
　Norinyl 1+50 28-Day Tablets
　Ortho-Novum 1/50 □ 21 Tablets
　Ortho-Novum 1/50 □ 28 Tablets
Metamucil Effervescent Sugar Free, Lemon-Lime
　Flavor(PROCTER & GAMBLE)
Metamucil Effervescent Sugar Free, Orange
　Flavor (PROCTER & GAMBLE)
Metamucil Powder, Orange Flavor
　(PROCTER & GAMBLE)
Metamucil Original Texture Powder, Regular
　Flavor (PROCTER & GAMBLE)

Metamucil Smooth Texture, Citrus Flavor
　(PROCTER & GAMBLE)
Metamucil Smooth Texture, Sugar Free, Citrus
　Flavor (PROCTER & GAMBLE)
Metamucil Smooth Texture Powder,
　Orange Flavor (PROCTER & GAMBLE)
Metamucil Smooth Texture Powder, Sugar Free,
　Orange Flavor (PROCTER & GAMBLE)
Metamucil Smooth Texture, Sugar Free, Regular
　Flavor (PROCTER & GAMBLE)
Metamucil Wafers, Apple Crisp and Cinnamon
　Spice Flavors (PROCTER & GAMBLE)
Metaprel Inhalation Aerosol Bronchodilator
　(SANDOZ PHARMACEUTICALS CORPORATION)
Metaprel Inhalation Solution
　(SANDOZ PHARMACEUTICALS CORPORATION)
Metaprel Syrup
　(SANDOZ PHARMACEUTICALS CORPORATION)
Metaprel Tablets
　(SANDOZ PHARMACEUTICALS CORPORATION)

METAPROTERENOL SULFATE
　Alupent Inhalation Aerosol
　Alupent Inhalation Solution
　Alupent Syrup
　Alupent Tablets
　Metaprel Inhalation Aerosol Bronchodilator
　Metaprel Inhalation Solution
　Metaprel Syrup
　Metaprel Tablets
　Metaproterenol Sulfate Inhalation Solution, USP,
　　Arm-a-Med
　Metaproterenol Sulfate Inhalation Solution
　Metaproterenol Sulfate Inhalation Solution, USP
　Metaproterenol Sulfate Syrup
　Metaproterenol Sulfate Tablets
　Metaproterenol Sulfate Tablets
Metaproterenol Sulfate Inhalation Solution, USP,
　Arm-a-Med (ASTRA USA, INC.)
Metaproterenol Sulfate Inhalation Solution
　(PAR PHARMACEUTICAL, INC.)
Metaproterenol Sulfate Inhalation Solution, USP
　(DEY LABORATORIES)
Metaproterenol Sulfate Syrup
　(BIOCRAFT LABORATORIES, INC.)
Metaproterenol Sulfate Tablets
　(PAR PHARMACEUTICAL, INC.)
Metaproterenol Sulfate Tablets
　(BIOCRAFT LABORATORIES, INC.)

METARAMINOL BITARTRATE
　Aramine Injection
Metastron
　(MEDI-PHYSICS, INC., AMERSHAM HEALTHCARE)

METAXALONE
　Skelaxin Tablets

METHACHOLINE CHLORIDE
　Provocholine for Inhalation

METHADONE HYDROCHLORIDE
　Dolophine Hydrochloride Ampoules & Vials
　Dolophine Hydrochloride Tablets
　Methadone Hydrochloride Diskets
　Methadone Hydrochloride Oral Concentrate
　Methadone Hydrochloride Oral Solution &
　　Tablets
Methadone Hydrochloride Diskets
　(ELI LILLY AND COMPANY)
Methadone Hydrochloride Oral Concentrate
　(ROXANE LABORATORIES, INC.)
Methadone Hydrochloride Oral Solution &
　Tablets (ROXANE LABORATORIES, INC.)

METHAMPHETAMINE HYDROCHLORIDE
　Desoxyn Gradumet Tablets

METHANAMINE SULFOSALICYLATE
　Unguentum Bossi

METHAZOLAMIDE
　Methazolamide Tablets
　Methazolamide Tablets
　Neptazane Tablets
Methazolamide Tablets
　(GENEVA PHARMACEUTICALS, INC.)
Methazolamide Tablets
　(LEDERLE STANDARD PRODUCTS)

METHENAMINE
　Prosed/DS
　Urised Tablets
　Uro-Phosphate Tablets

METHENAMINE HIPPURATE
　Urex Tablets

METHENAMINE MANDELATE
　Methenamine Mandelate Oral Susp.
　　USP 500 mg/5 mL
　Urisedamine Tablets
　Uroqid-Acid No. 2 Tablets
**Methenamine Mandelate Oral Susp. USP 500
mg/5 mL** (BARRE-NATIONAL INC.)
Methergine Injection
　(SANDOZ PHARMACEUTICALS CORPORATION)
Methergine Tablets
　(SANDOZ PHARMACEUTICALS CORPORATION)

METHIMAZOLE
　Tapazole Tablets

METHIONINE
　Amino-Cerv

METHOCARBAMOL
　Methocarbamol Tablets
　Methocarbamol and Aspirin Tablets
　Robaxin Injectable
　Robaxin Tablets
　Robaxin-750 Tablets
　Robaxisal Tablets
Methocarbamol Tablets
　(LEDERLE STANDARD PRODUCTS)

METHOHEXITAL SODIUM
　Brevital Sodium Vials
Methocarbamol and Aspirin Tablets
　(PAR PHARMACEUTICAL, INC.)

METHOTREXATE SODIUM
　Methotrexate Sodium Tablets, for Injection and
　　LPF Injection
　Methotrexate Tablets
　Rheumatrex Methotrexate Dose Pack
**Methotrexate Sodium Tablets, for Injection and
LPF Injection** (IMMUNEX CORPORATION)
Methotrexate Tablets
　(MYLAN PHARMACEUTICALS INC.)

METHOTRIMEPRAZINE
　Levoprome

METHOXAMINE HYDROCHLORIDE
　Vasoxyl Injection

METHOXSALEN
　Oxsoralen Lotion 1%
　Oxsoralen-Ultra Capsule

METHSCOPOLAMINE BROMIDE
　Pamine Tablets

METHSCOPOLAMINE NITRATE
　AH-CHEW Chewable Tablets
　D.A. Chewable Tablets
　Dallergy Caplets, Syrup, Tablets
　Dura-Vent/DA Tablets
　Extendryl Chewable Tablets

　Extendryl Sr. & Jr. T.D. Capsules
　Extendryl Syrup
　OMNIHIST L.A. Tablets

METHSUXIMIDE
　Celontin Kapseals

METHYCLOTHIAZIDE
　Aquatensen Tablets
　Diutensen-R Tablets
　Enduron Tablets
　Methyclothiazide Tablets
Methyclothiazide Tablets
　(MYLAN PHARMACEUTICALS INC.)

METHYL SALICYLATE
　Listerine Antiseptic
　Cool Mint Listerine
　Panalgesic Gold Cream
　Panalgesic Gold Liniment
　Thera-Gesic

METHYLDOPA
　Aldoclor Tablets
　Aldomet Oral Suspension
　Aldomet Tablets
　Aldoril Tablets
　Methyldopa & Hydrochlorothiazide Tablets
　Methyldopa and Hydrochlorothiazide Tablets
　Methyldopa & Hydrochlorothiazide Tablets, USP
　Methyldopa Tablets
　Methyldopa Tablets
　Methyldopa Tablets USP, 200 + 500
　Methyldopa Tablets, U.S.P.
　Methyldopa & Hydrochlorothiazide Tablets
　Methyldopa and Hydrochlorothiazide
　　Tablets USP
　Methyldopa and Hydrochlorothiazide
　　Tablets, U.S.P.
Methyldopa & Hydrochlorothiazide Tablets
　(LEDERLE STANDARD PRODUCTS)
Methyldopa and Hydrochlorothiazide Tablets
　(PAR PHARMACEUTICAL, INC.)
Methyldopa & Hydrochlorothiazide Tablets, USP
　(WARNER CHILCOTT LABORATORIES)
Methyldopa Tablets
　(LEDERLE STANDARD PRODUCTS)
Methyldopa Tablets
　(MYLAN PHARMACEUTICALS INC.)
Methyldopa Tablets USP, 200 + 500
　(NOVOPHARM, USA INC.)
Methyldopa Tablets, U.S.P.
　(WEST POINT PHARMA)
Methyldopa & Hydrochlorothiazide Tablets
　(MYLAN PHARMACEUTICALS INC.)
**Methyldopa and Hydrochlorothiazide Tablets
USP** (NOVOPHARM, USA INC.)
**Methyldopa and Hydrochlorothiazide Tablets,
U.S.P.** (WEST POINT PHARMA)

METHYLDOPATE HYDROCHLORIDE
　Aldomet Ester HCl Injection
　Methyldopate Hydrochloride Injection
Methyldopate Hydrochloride Injection
　(ELKINS-SINN, INC.)

METHYLENE BLUE
　Prosed/DS
　Urised Tablets
　Urolene Blue

METHYLERGONOVINE MALEATE
　Methergine Injection
　Methergine Tablets

METHYLPHENIDATE HYDROCHLORIDE
　Ritalin Hydrochloride Tablets
　Ritalin-SR Tablets

METHYLPREDNISOLONE
　Medrol Dosepak Unit of Use
　Medrol Tablets
　Methylprednisolone Tablets
Methylprednisolone Tablets
　(DURAMED PHARMACEUTICALS, INC.)

METHYLPREDNISOLONE ACETATE
　Depo-Medrol Single-Dose Vial
　Depo-Medrol Sterile Aqueous Suspension

METHYLPREDNISOLONE SODIUM SUCCINATE
　Solu-Medrol Sterile Powder

METHYLTESTOSTERONE
　Android Capsules, 10 mg
　Android-10 Tablets
　Android-25 Tablets
　ESTRATEST Tablets
　ESTRATEST H.S. Tablets
　Oreton Methyl
　Premarin with Methyltestosterone
　Testred Capsules
　Virilon

METHYSERGIDE MALEATE
　Sansert Tablets

METOCLOPRAMIDE
　Metoclopramide Oral Solution
　Metoclopramide Oral Soln. USP 5 mg/5 mL
　Metoclopramide Tablets
　Metoclopramide Tablets
　Metoclopramide Tablets
Metoclopramide Oral Solution
　(BIOCRAFT LABORATORIES, INC.)
Metoclopramide Oral Soln. USP 5 mg/5 mL
　(BARRE-NATIONAL INC.)
Metoclopramide Tablets
　(BIOCRAFT LABORATORIES, INC.)
Metoclopramide Tablets
　(DURAMED PHARMACEUTICALS, INC.)
Metoclopramide Tablets
　(LEDERLE STANDARD PRODUCTS)

METOCLOPRAMIDE HYDROCHLORIDE
　Metoclopramide HCl Syrup and Tablets
　Metoclopramide Hydrochloride Tablets
　Reglan Injectable
　Reglan Syrup
　Reglan Tablets
Metoclopramide HCl Syrup and Tablets
　(WARNER CHILCOTT LABORATORIES)
Metoclopramide Hydrochloride Tablets
　(WATSON LABORATORIES, INC.)

METOCURINE IODIDE
　Metubine Iodide Vials

METOLAZONE
　Mykrox Tablets
　Zaroxolyn Tablets

METOPROLOL SUCCINATE
　Toprol-XL Tablets

METOPROLOL TARTRATE
　Lopressor Ampuls
　Lopressor HCT Tablets
　Lopressor Tablets
　Metoprolol Tartrate Tablets
　Metoprolol Tartrate Tablets
　Metoprolol Tartrate Tablets, USP
Metoprolol Tartrate Tablets
　(MYLAN PHARMACEUTICALS INC.)
Metoprolol Tartrate Tablets
　(WARNER CHILCOTT LABORATORIES)
Metoprolol Tartrate Tablets, USP
　(WATSON LABORATORIES, INC.)

Metrodin (urofollitropin for injection)
  (SERONO LABORATORIES, INC.)
MetroGel (GALDERMA LABORATORIES, INC.)
MetroGel-Vaginal (CURATEK PHARMACEUTICALS)

METRONIDAZOLE
  Flagyl I.V. RTU
  Flagyl Tablets
  MetroGel
  MetroGel-Vaginal
  Metronidazole Compressed Tablets
  Metronidazole Redi-Infusion (Preservative-Free)
  Protostat Tablets
Metronidazole Compressed Tablets
  (PAR PHARMACEUTICAL, INC.)
Metronidazole Redi-Infusion (Preservative-Free)
  (ELKINS-SINN, INC.)

METRONIDAZOLE HYDROCHLORIDE
  Flagyl I.V.
Metubine Iodide Vials (DISTA PRODUCTS COMPANY)

METYROSINE
  Demser Capsules
Mevacor Tablets (MERCK & CO., INC.)

MEXILETINE HYDROCHLORIDE
  Mexitil Capsules
Mexitil Capsules
  (BOEHRINGER INGELHEIM PHARMACEUTICALS)
Mezlin (MILES INC. PHARMACEUTICAL DIVISION)
Mezlin Pharmacy Bulk Package
  (MILES INC. PHARMACEUTICAL DIVISION)

MEZLOCILLIN SODIUM
  Mezlin
  Mezlin Pharmacy Bulk Package
Miacalcin Injection
  (SANDOZ PHARMACEUTICALS CORPORATION)

MICONAZOLE
  Monistat I.V.

MICONAZOLE NITRATE
  Breezee Mist Antifungal Foot Powder
  Fungoid Creme
  Fungoid Tincture
  Miconazole Nitrate Cream 2%
  Miconazole Nitrate 2% Cream
  Miconazole Nitrate Vaginal Suppositories, USP
    100mg, 200mg
  Monistat Dual-Pak
  Monistat 3 Vaginal Suppositories
  Monistat-Derm (miconazole nitrate 2%) Cream
  Ony-Clear Nail Spray
Miconazole Nitrate Cream 2%
  (BARRE-NATIONAL INC.)
Miconazole Nitrate 2% Cream
  (TARO PHARMACEUTICALS U.S.A., INC.)
Miconazole Nitrate Vaginal Suppositories, USP
  100mg, 200mg (BARRE-NATIONAL INC.)
Micro-K Extencaps (A. H. ROBINS COMPANY, INC.)
Micro-K 10 Extencaps (A. H. ROBINS COMPANY, INC.)
Micro-K LS Packets (A. H. ROBINS COMPANY, INC.)
Micronase Tablets (THE UPJOHN COMPANY)
Micronor Tablets
  (ORTHO PHARMACEUTICAL CORPORATION)
Midamor Tablets (MERCK & CO., INC.)

MIDAZOLAM HYDROCHLORIDE
  Versed Injection
Midrin Capsules (CARNRICK LABORATORIES, INC.)
Migralam Capsules (RICO PHARMACAL)
Miles Nervine Nighttime Sleep-Aid
  (MILES INC. CONSUMER HEALTHCARE PRODUCTS)
Milk of Magnesia & Milk of Magnesia-
  Concentrated (ROXANE LABORATORIES, INC.)
Milk of Magnesia-Cascara Suspension
  Concentrated (ROXANE LABORATORIES, INC.)

Milk of Magnesia-Mineral Oil Emulsion &
  Emulsion (Flavored)
  (ROXANE LABORATORIES, INC.)
Milontin Kapseals (PARKE-DAVIS)

MILRINONE LACTATE
  Primacor Injection
Miltown Tablets (WALLACE LABORATORIES)

MINERAL OIL
  Agoral Liquid
  Anusol Hemorrhoidal Ointment
  Aquaphor Healing Ointment
  Aquaphor Healing Ointment, Original Formula
  Eucerin Dry Skin Care Lotion
  Eucerin Dry Skin Care Moisturizing Creme
    (Unscented)
  Eucerin Plus Dry Skin Care Moisturizing Lotion
  Eucerin Plus Moisturizing Creme
  Fleet Mineral Oil Enema
  Milk of Magnesia-Mineral Oil Emulsion &
    Emulsion (Flavored)
  Mineral Oil, Topical Light
  Nutraderm Cream & Lotion
Mineral Oil, Topical Light
  (ROXANE LABORATORIES, INC.)

MINERAL WAX
  Aquaphor Healing Ointment, Original Formula
Mini-Gamulin Rh, Rh$_0$ (D) Immune
  Globulin (Human)
  (ARMOUR PHARMACEUTICAL COMPANY)
Minipress Capsules (PFIZER LABS DIVISION)
Minitran Transdermal Delivery System
  (3M PHARMACEUTICALS)
Minizide Capsules (PFIZER LABS DIVISION)
Minocin Intravenous (LEDERLE LABORATORIES)
Minocin Oral Suspension
  (LEDERLE LABORATORIES)
Minocin Pellet-Filled Capsules
  (LEDERLE LABORATORIES)

MINOCYCLINE HYDROCHLORIDE
  Dynacin Capsules
  Minocin Intravenous
  Minocin Oral Suspension
  Minocin Pellet-Filled Capsules
  Minocycline Hydrochloride Capsules
  Minocycline HCl Capsules
Minocycline Hydrochloride Capsules
  (BIOCRAFT LABORATORIES, INC.)
Minocycline HCl Capsules
  (WARNER CHILCOTT LABORATORIES)

MINOXIDIL
  Loniten Tablets
  Minoxidil Tablets
  Rogaine Topical Solution
Minoxidil Tablets (PAR PHARMACEUTICAL, INC.)
Mintezol Chewable Tablets (MERCK & CO., INC.)
Mintezol Suspension (MERCK & CO., INC.)
Mio-Rel Injectable
  (INTERNATIONAL ETHICAL LABS.)

MISOPROSTOL
  Cytotec
Mission Prenatal (MISSION PHARMACAL COMPANY)
Mission Prenatal F.A.
  (MISSION PHARMACAL COMPANY)
Mission Prenatal H.P.
  (MISSION PHARMACAL COMPANY)
Mission Prenatal RX
  (MISSION PHARMACAL COMPANY)
Mithracin
  (MILES INC. PHARMACEUTICAL DIVISION)

MITOMYCIN (MITOMYCIN-C)
  Mutamycin

MITOTANE
  Lysodren

MITOXANTRONE HYDROCHLORIDE
  Novantrone for Injection Concentrate
Mitraflex Wound Dressing
  (CALGON VESTAL LABORATORIES, INC.)
Mivacron Injection (BURROUGHS WELLCOME CO.)
Mivacron Premixed Infusion
  (BURROUGHS WELLCOME CO.)

MIVACURIUM CHLORIDE
  Mivacron Injection
  Mivacron Premixed Infusion
Moban Tablets and Concentrate
  (TEVA PHARMACEUTICALS)
Mobigesic Analgesic Tablets
  (B. F. ASCHER & COMPANY, INC.)
Mobisyl Analgesic Creme
  (B. F. ASCHER & COMPANY, INC.)
Modane Bulk Powder (SAVAGE LABORATORIES)
Modane Soft (SAVAGE LABORATORIES)
Modane Tablets (SAVAGE LABORATORIES)
Modane Plus Tablets (SAVAGE LABORATORIES)
Modicon 21 Tablets
  (ORTHO PHARMACEUTICAL CORPORATION)
Modicon 28 Tablets
  (ORTHO PHARMACEUTICAL CORPORATION)
Moduretic Tablets (MERCK & CO., INC.)
Moisturel Cream
  (WESTWOOD-SQUIBB PHARMACEUTICALS INC.)
Moisturel Lotion
  (WESTWOOD-SQUIBB PHARMACEUTICALS INC.)

MOLINDONE HYDROCHLORIDE
  Moban Tablets and Concentrate
Moxilin Capsules
  (INTERNATIONAL ETHICAL LABS.)
Moxilin O/S (INTERNATIONAL ETHICAL LABS.)

MOMETASONE FUROATE
  Elocon Cream 0.1%
  Elocon Lotion 0.1%
  Elocon Ointment 0.1%
Monistat Dual-Pak
  (ORTHO PHARMACEUTICAL CORPORATION)
Monistat I.V. (JANSSEN PHARMACEUTICA INC.)
Monistat 3 Vaginal Suppositories
  (ORTHO PHARMACEUTICAL CORPORATION)
Monistat-Derm (miconazole nitrate 2%) Cream
  (ORTHO PHARMACEUTICAL CORPORATION
  DERMATOLOGICAL DIVISION)

MONOBENZONE
  Benoquin Cream 20%
Monocid Injection
  (SMITHKLINE BEECHAM PHARMACEUTICALS)
Monoclate-P Factor VIII:C, Pasteurized,
  Monoclonal Antibody Purified Antihemophilic
  Factor (Human)
  (ARMOUR PHARMACEUTICAL COMPANY)
Monodox Capsules
  (OCLASSEN PHARMACEUTICALS, INC.)
Mono-Gesic Tablets
  (CENTRAL PHARMACEUTICALS, INC.)
Monoket (SCHWARZ PHARMA)
Mononine Coagulation Factor IX (Human)
  (ARMOUR PHARMACEUTICAL COMPANY)
Monopril Tablets
  (BRISTOL-MYERS SQUIBB COMPANY)

MORICIZINE HYDROCHLORIDE
  Ethmozine Tablets

MORPHINE SULFATE
  Astramorph/PF Injection, USP
    (Preservative-Free)
  Duramorph

Infumorph 200 and Infumorph 500
　　Sterile Solutions
MS Contin Tablets
MSIR Oral Capsules
MSIR Oral Solution
MSIR Oral Solution Concentrate
MSIR Tablets
MS/L Morphine Sulfate Liquid
MS/L Concentrate Morphine Sulfate Liquid
MS/S Suppositories Morphine Sulfate
Morphine Sulfate Injection
Morphine Sulfate Injection, USP
Morphine Sulfate Oral Solution & Tablets
Morphine Sulfate in Tubex
OMS Concentrate CII
Oramorph SR (Morphine Sulfate Sustained
　　Release Tablets)
RMS Suppositories CII
Rescudose (Morphine Sulfate Oral Solution)
Roxanol (Morphine Sulfate Concentrated
　　Oral Solution)
Roxanol 100 (Morphine Sulfate Concentrated
　　Oral Solution)
Roxanol Suppositories (Morphine Sulfate)
Roxanol UD Morphine Sulfate Oral Solution
Morphine Sulfate Injection (ELKINS-SINN, INC.)
Morphine Sulfate Injection, USP (ASTRA USA, INC.)
Morphine Sulfate Oral Solution & Tablets
　　(ROXANE LABORATORIES, INC.)
Morphine Sulfate in Tubex
　　(WYETH-AYERST LABORATORIES)

MORRHUATE SODIUM
Scleromate
Motofen Tablets
　　(CARNRICK LABORATORIES, INC.)
Children's Motrin Ibuprofen Suspension
　　(MCNEIL CONSUMER PRODUCTS COMPANY)
Motrin Tablets (THE UPJOHN COMPANY)
Mucosil Acetylcysteine Solution
　　(DEY LABORATORIES)
Mudrane Tablets (ECR PHARMACEUTICALS)
Mudrane GG Elixir (ECR PHARMACEUTICALS)
Mudrane GG Tablets (ECR PHARMACEUTICALS)
Mudrane GG-2 Tablets (ECR PHARMACEUTICALS)
Multi-antibiotic Cream (BARRE-NATIONAL INC.)
**Multitest CMI Skin Test Antigens for
　　Cellular Hypersensitivity**
　　(CONNAUGHT LABORATORIES, INC.)
Multi Vit Drops with Iron (BARRE-NATIONAL INC.)

MUMPS VIRUS VACCINE, LIVE
Mumpsvax
Mumpsvax (MERCK & CO., INC.)

MUPIROCIN
Bactroban Ointment
**Murine Ear Wax Removal System/Murine Ear
　　Drops** (ROSS PRODUCTS DIVISION)
Murine Lubricating Eye Drops
　　(ROSS PRODUCTS DIVISION)
**Murine Plus Lubricating Redness Reliever Eye
　　Drops** (ROSS PRODUCTS DIVISION)

MUROMONAB-CD3
Orthoclone OKT3 Sterile Solution
Mustargen (MERCK & CO., INC.)
Mutamycin
　　(BRISTOL-MYERS SQUIBB ONCOLOGY DIVISION)
Myambutol Tablets (LEDERLE LABORATORIES)
Mycelex OTC Cream Antifungal
　　(MILES INC. CONSUMER HEALTHCARE PRODUCTS)
Mycelex OTC Solution Antifungal
　　(MILES INC. CONSUMER HEALTHCARE PRODUCTS)
Mycelex Troches
　　(MILES INC. PHARMACEUTICAL DIVISION)
Mycelex-7 Vaginal Cream Antifungal
　　(MILES INC. CONSUMER HEALTHCARE PRODUCTS)

Mycelex-7 Vaginal Inserts Antifungal
　　(MILES INC. CONSUMER HEALTHCARE PRODUCTS)
Mycelex-G 500 mg Vaginal Tablets
　　(MILES INC. PHARMACEUTICAL DIVISION)
Mycobutin Capsules
　　(PHARMACIA ADRIA PHARMACIA INC.)
Mycostatin Cream and Topical Powder
　　(WESTWOOD-SQUIBB PHARMACEUTICALS INC.)
Mycostatin Pastilles
　　(BRISTOL-MYERS SQUIBB ONCOLOGY DIVISION)
Mykrox Tablets
　　(FISONS CORPORATION PRESCRIPTION PRODUCTS)
Mylanta Gas Tablets-40 mg
　　(JOHNSON & JOHNSON • MERCK CONSUMER
　　PHARMACEUTICALS CO.)
Mylanta Gas Tablets-80 mg
　　(JOHNSON & JOHNSON • MERCK CONSUMER
　　PHARMACEUTICALS CO.)
Maximum Strength Mylanta Gas Tablets-125 mg
　　(JOHNSON & JOHNSON • MERCK CONSUMER
　　PHARMACEUTICALS CO.)
Mylanta Gelcaps Antacid
　　(JOHNSON & JOHNSON • MERCK CONSUMER
　　PHARMACEUTICALS CO.)
Mylanta Liquid
　　(JOHNSON & JOHNSON • MERCK CONSUMER
　　PHARMACEUTICALS CO.)
Mylanta Natural Fiber Supplement
　　(JOHNSON & JOHNSON • MERCK CONSUMER
　　PHARMACEUTICALS CO.)
Mylanta Soothing Lozenges
　　(JOHNSON & JOHNSON • MERCK CONSUMER
　　PHARMACEUTICALS CO.)
Mylanta Tablets
　　(JOHNSON & JOHNSON • MERCK CONSUMER
　　PHARMACEUTICALS CO.)
Mylanta Double Strength Liquid
　　(JOHNSON & JOHNSON • MERCK CONSUMER
　　PHARMACEUTICALS CO.)
Mylanta Double Strength Tablets
　　(JOHNSON & JOHNSON • MERCK CONSUMER
　　PHARMACEUTICALS CO.)
Myleran Tablets (BURROUGHS WELLCOME CO.)
Mylicon Infants' Drops
　　(JOHNSON & JOHNSON • MERCK CONSUMER
　　PHARMACEUTICALS CO.)
Myochrysine Injection (MERCK & CO., INC.)
Myotonachol (GLENWOOD, INC.)
Mysoline Suspension
　　(WYETH-AYERST LABORATORIES)
Mysoline Tablets (WYETH-AYERST LABORATORIES)
Mytrex Cream & Ointment
　　(SAVAGE LABORATORIES)

N

NPH Insulin
　　(NOVO NORDISK PHARMACEUTICALS INC.)
NPH Purified Pork Isophane Insulin
　　(NOVO NORDISK PHARMACEUTICALS INC.)

NABUMETONE
Relafen Tablets

NADOLOL
Nadolol Tablets
Nadolol Tablets (MYLAN PHARMACEUTICALS INC.)

NAFARELIN ACETATE
Synarel Nasal Solution for Central Precocious
　　Puberty
Synarel Nasal Solution for Endometriosis

NAFCILLIN SODIUM
Unipen Capsules
Unipen Injection

NAFTIFINE HYDROCHLORIDE
Naftin Cream 1%
Naftin Gel 1%
Naftin Cream 1% (ALLERGAN HERBERT)
Naftin Gel 1% (ALLERGAN HERBERT)
Nail Scrub (PEDINOL PHARMACAL INC.)

NALBUPHINE HYDROCHLORIDE
Nalbuphine Hydrochloride Injection
Nubain Injection
Nalbuphine Hydrochloride Injection
　　(ASTRA USA, INC.)
Naldelate Pediatric Drops and Syrup
　　(BARRE-NATIONAL INC.)
Naldelate Syrup (BARRE-NATIONAL INC.)
Nalex-A Tablets (BLANSETT PHARMACAL)
Nalex Capsules (BLANSETT PHARMACAL)
Nalex DH Liquid (BLANSETT PHARMACAL)
Nalex JR Capsules (BLANSETT PHARMACAL)
Nalfon 200 Pulvules & Nalfon Tablets
　　(DISTA PRODUCTS COMPANY)

NALIDIXIC ACID
NegGram Caplets
NegGram Suspension

NALOXONE HYDROCHLORIDE
Naloxone Hydrochloride Injection, USP
Naloxone Hydrochloride Injection
Narcan Injection
Talwin Nx
Naloxone Hydrochloride Injection, USP
　　(ASTRA USA, INC.)
Naloxone Hydrochloride Injection
　　(ELKINS-SINN, INC.)

NALTREXONE HYDROCHLORIDE
Trexan Tablets

NANDROLONE DECANOATE
Deca-Durabolin

NANDROLONE PHENPROPIONATE
Durabolin

NAPHAZOLINE HYDROCHLORIDE
4-Way Fast Acting Nasal Spray - Original
　　Formula (regular & mentholated) & Metered
　　Spray Pump (regular)
Naphcon-A Ophthalmic Solution
Naphcon-A Ophthalmic Solution
　　(ALCON LABORATORIES, INC.)
Naprosyn Suspension (SYNTEX PUERTO RICO, INC.)
Naprosyn Tablets (SYNTEX PUERTO RICO, INC.)

NAPROXEN
Naprosyn Suspension
Naprosyn Tablets
Naproxen Tablets, 250 mg
Naproxen Tablets, 375 mg
Naproxen Tablets, 500 mg
Naproxen Tablets
Naproxen Tablets
Naproxen Tablets
Naproxen Tablets, 250 mg (NOVOPHARM, USA INC.)
Naproxen Tablets, 375 mg (NOVOPHARM, USA INC.)
Naproxen Tablets, 500 mg (NOVOPHARM, USA INC.)

NAPROXEN SODIUM
Aflaxen Tablets
Aleve
Anaprox and Anaprox DS Tablets
Naproxen Sodium Tablets, 275 mg, + 550 mg
Naproxen Sodium Tablets
Naproxen Sodium Tablets, 275 mg, + 550 mg
　　(NOVOPHARM, USA INC.)

Naproxen Sodium Tablets
(GENEVA PHARMACEUTICALS, INC.)
Naproxen Tablets
(GENEVA PHARMACEUTICALS, INC.)
Naproxen Tablets
(LEDERLE STANDARD PRODUCTS)
Naproxen Tablets
(MYLAN PHARMACEUTICALS INC.)
Narcan Injection
(ENDO LABORATORIES, L.L.C.)
Nardil (PARKE-DAVIS)
Nasabid Capsules
(ABANA PHARMACEUTICALS, INC.)
Nasacort Nasal Inhaler
(RHONE-POULENC RORER PHARMACEUTICALS INC.)
Nasalcrom Nasal Solution
(FISONS CORPORATION PRESCRIPTION PRODUCTS)
Nasalide Nasal Solution 0.025%
(SYNTEX PUERTO RICO, INC.)
Nasatab LA Tablets (ECR PHARMACEUTICALS)
Nature's Remedy Natural Vegetable
Laxative Tablets
(SMITHKLINE BEECHAM CONSUMER HEALTHCARE, L.P.)
Navane Capsules and Concentrate
(ROERIG DIVISION)
Navane Intramuscular (ROERIG DIVISION)
Nebcin Vials, Hyporets & ADD-Vantage
(ELI LILLY AND COMPANY)
NebuPent for Inhalation Solution
(FUJISAWA USA, INC.)

NEDOCROMIL SODIUM
　Tilade
NegGram Caplets
(SANOFI WINTHROP PHARMACEUTICALS)
NegGram Suspension
(SANOFI WINTHROP PHARMACEUTICALS)
Nelova (WARNER CHILCOTT LABORATORIES)
Nembutal Sodium Capsules
(ABBOTT LABORATORIES)
Nembutal Sodium Solution
(ABBOTT LABORATORIES)
Nembutal Sodium Suppositories
(ABBOTT LABORATORIES)
Neo-Calglucon Syrup
(SANDOZ PHARMACEUTICALS CORPORATION)
NeoDecadron Sterile Ophthalmic Ointment
(MERCK & CO., INC.)
NeoDecadron Sterile Ophthalmic Solution
(MERCK & CO., INC.)
NeoDecadron Topical Cream
(MERCK & CO., INC.)
Neoloid Emulsified Mint Castor Oil
(KENWOOD LABORATORIES)

NEOMYCIN
　Neosporin Original Ointment
　Neosporin Plus Maximum Strength Cream
　Neosporin Plus Maximum Strength Ointment

NEOMYCIN SULFATE
　Coly-Mycin S Otic w/Neomycin &
　　Hydrocortisone
　Cortisporin Cream
　Cortisporin Ointment
　Cortisporin Ophthalmic Ointment Sterile
　Cortisporin Ophthalmic Suspension Sterile
　Cortisporin Otic Solution Sterile
　Cortisporin Otic Suspension Sterile
　LazerSporin-C Solution
　NeoDecadron Sterile Ophthalmic Ointment
　NeoDecadron Sterile Ophthalmic Solution
　NeoDecadron Topical Cream
　Neomycin Sulfate Tablets
　Neomycin Sulfate Tablets
　Neosporin G.U. Irrigant Sterile
　Neosporin Ophthalmic Ointment Sterile

　Neosporin Ophthalmic Solution Sterile
　Neo-Synalar Cream
　PediOtic Suspension Sterile
Neomycin Sulfate Tablets
(BIOCRAFT LABORATORIES, INC.)
Neomycin Sulfate Tablets
(ROXANE LABORATORIES, INC.)
Neopap Suppositories
(POLYMEDICA PHARMACEUTICALS (U.S.A.), INC.)
NEOSAR Lyophilized/Neosar
(PHARMACIA ADRIA PHARMACIA INC.)
Neosporin G.U. Irrigant Sterile
(BURROUGHS WELLCOME CO.)
Neosporin Original Ointment
(WARNER WELLCOME)
Neosporin Plus Maximum Strength Cream
(WARNER WELLCOME)
Neosporin Plus Maximum Strength Ointment
(WARNER WELLCOME)
Neosporin Ophthalmic Ointment Sterile
(BURROUGHS WELLCOME CO.)
Neosporin Ophthalmic Solution Sterile
(BURROUGHS WELLCOME CO.)

NEOSTIGMINE BROMIDE
　Prostigmin Tablets

NEOSTIGMINE METHYLSULFATE
　Neostigmine Methylsulfate Injection
　Neostigmine Methylsulfate Injection
　Prostigmin Injectable
Neostigmine Methylsulfate Injection
(ASTRA USA, INC.)
Neostigmine Methylsulfate Injection
(ELKINS-SINN, INC.)
Neo-Synalar Cream
(SYNTEX PUERTO RICO, INC.)
Neo-Synephrine Hydrochloride 1% Carpuject
(SANOFI WINTHROP PHARMACEUTICALS)
Neo-Synephrine Hydrochloride 1% Injection
(SANOFI WINTHROP PHARMACEUTICALS)
Neo-Synephrine Hydrochloride (Ophthalmic)
(SANOFI WINTHROP PHARMACEUTICALS)
Nephramine (R&D LABORATORIES, INC.)
Nephro-Calci Tablets
(R&D LABORATORIES, INC.)
Nephrocaps (FLEMING & COMPANY)
Nephro-Derm Cream (R&D LABORATORIES, INC.)
Nephro-Fer Tablets (R&D LABORATORIES, INC.)
Nephro-Fer Rx Tablets (R&D LABORATORIES, INC.)
Nephro-Vite Tablets (R&D LABORATORIES, INC.)
Nephro-Vite + Fe Tablets
(R&D LABORATORIES, INC.)
Nephro-Vite Rx Tablets
(R&D LABORATORIES, INC.)
Nephrox Suspension (FLEMING & COMPANY)
Nepro Specialized Liquid Nutrition
(ROSS PRODUCTS DIVISION)
Neptazane Tablets (LEDERLE LABORATORIES)
Nesacaine Injections (ASTRA USA, INC.)
Nesacaine-MPF Injection (ASTRA USA, INC.)
Nestabs FA Tablets
(THE FIELDING PHARMACEUTICAL COMPANY, INC.)

NETILMICIN SULFATE
　Netromycin Injection 100 mg/ml
Netromycin Injection 100 mg/ml
(SCHERING CORPORATION)
Neurochol Dietary Supplement
(KENWOOD LABORATORIES)
Neupogen for Injection (AMGEN INC.)
Neuroforte-R Vial
(INTERNATIONAL ETHICAL LABS.)
Neuroforte-Six Monovial
(INTERNATIONAL ETHICAL LABS.)
Neurontin Capsules (PARKE-DAVIS)
Neutrexin (U.S. BIOSCIENCE, INC.)

NIACIN
　Niacinol
　Niacin-Time
　Nicobid
　Nicolar Tablets
　Slo-Niacin Tablets
Niacinol (TYLER ENCAPSULATIONS)
Niacin-Time (J. R. CARLSON LABORATORIES, INC.)

NIACINAMIDE
　Eldercaps
　Eldertonic
　Glutofac Caplets
　ILX B$_{12}$ Caplets Crystalline
　May-Vita Elixir
　Mega-B
　Prenate 90 Tablets

NICARDIPINE HYDROCHLORIDE
　Cardene Capsules
　Cardene I.V.
　Cardene SR Capsules
Niclocide Chewable Tablets
(MILES INC. PHARMACEUTICAL DIVISION)

NICLOSAMIDE
　Niclocide Chewable Tablets
Nicobid
(RHONE-POULENC RORER PHARMACEUTICALS)
Nicoderm Nicotine Transdermal System
(MARION MERRELL DOW INC.)
Nicolar Tablets
(RHONE-POULENC RORER PHARMACEUTICALS INC.)
Nicorette
(SMITHKLINE BEECHAM CONSUMER HEALTHCARE, L.P.)
Nicorette DS
(SMITHKLINE BEECHAM CONSUMER HEALTHCARE, L.P.)

NICOTINAMIDE
　ILX B$_{12}$ Elixir Crystalline and ILX B$_{12}$
　　Sugar–Free Elixir

NICOTINE
　Habitrol Nicotine Transdermal System
　Nicoderm Nicotine Transdermal System
　Nicotrol Nicotine Transdermal System
　Prostep (nicotine transdermal system)

NICOTINE POLACRILEX
　Nicorette
　Nicorette DS
Nicotinex Elixir (FLEMING & COMPANY)

NICOTINIC ACID
　(See also under NIACIN)
　Slo-Niacin Tablets
Nicotrol Nicotine Transdermal System
(MCNEIL CONSUMER PRODUCTS COMPANY)

NIFEDIPINE
　Adalat Capsules (10 mg and 20 mg)
　Adalat CC
　Nifedipine Capsules USP
　Nifedipine Capsules
　Procardia Capsules
　Procardia XL Extended Release Tablets
Nifedipine Capsules USP (NOVOPHARM, USA INC.)
Nifedipine Capsules
(WARNER CHILCOTT LABORATORIES)
Niferex-150 Capsules
(CENTRAL PHARMACEUTICALS, INC.)
Niferex Daily Tablets
(CENTRAL PHARMACEUTICALS, INC.)
Niferex Elixir
(CENTRAL PHARMACEUTICALS, INC.)
Niferex-150 Forte Capsules
(CENTRAL PHARMACEUTICALS, INC.)
Niferex Forte Elixir
(CENTRAL PHARMACEUTICALS, INC.)

UNDERLINE DENOTES GENERIC NAME

Niferex Tablets
(CENTRAL PHARMACEUTICALS, INC.)
Niferex w/Vitamin C Tablets
(CENTRAL PHARMACEUTICALS, INC.)
Niferex-PN Forte Tablets
(CENTRAL PHARMACEUTICALS, INC.)
Niferex-PN Tablets
(CENTRAL PHARMACEUTICALS, INC.)
Nilstat for Preparation of Oral Suspension
(LEDERLE STANDARD PRODUCTS)
Nilstat Oral Suspension
(LEDERLE STANDARD PRODUCTS)

NIMODIPINE
Nimotop Capsules
Nimotop Capsules
(MILES INC. PHARMACEUTICAL DIVISION)
Nite Time Cold Formula-Cherry Flavor and Original Flavor (BARRE-NATIONAL INC.)
Nite Time Cold Formula - Children's
(BARRE-NATIONAL INC.)
Nitro-Bid IV (MARION MERRELL DOW INC.)
Nitro-Bid Ointment (MARION MERRELL DOW INC.)
Nitrodisc
(ROBERTS PHARMACEUTICAL CORPORATION)
Nitro-Dur (nitroglycerin) Transdermal Infusion System (KEY PHARMACEUTICALS, INC.)

NITROFURANTOIN
Macrodantin Capsules
Nitrofurantoin Capsules
Nitrofurantoin Capsules
(WARNER CHILCOTT LABORATORIES)

NITROFURANTOIN MONOHYDRATE
Macrobid Capsules

NITROFURAZONE
Furacin Soluble Dressing
Furacin Topical Cream
Furacin Topical Solution 0.2%
Nitrogard Tablets
(FOREST PHARMACEUTICALS, INC.)

NITROGLYCERIN
Deponit NTG Transdermal Delivery System
Minitran Transdermal Delivery System
Nitro-Bid IV
Nitro-Bid Ointment
Nitrodisc
Nitro-Dur (nitroglycerin) Transdermal Infusion System
Nitrogard Tablets
Nitroglycerin Extended-release Capsules
Nitroglycerin Transdermal System Patches
Nitroglyn Extended+14 Release Capsules
Nitrolingual Spray
Nitrostat Tablets
Transdermal-NTG
Transderm-Nitro Transdermal Therapeutic System
Nitroglycerin Extended-release Capsules
(ETHEX CORPORATION)
Nitroglycerin Transdermal System Patches
(MYLAN PHARMACEUTICALS INC.)
Nitroglyn Extended+14 Release Capsules
(KENWOOD LABORATORIES)
Nitrol Ointment Appli-Kit (SAVAGE LABORATORIES)
Nitrolingual Spray
(RHONE-POULENC RORER PHARMACEUTICALS INC.)
Nitrostat Tablets (PARKE-DAVIS)
Nix Creme Rinse (WARNER WELLCOME)

NIZATIDINE
Axid Pulvules
Nizoral 2% Cream (JANSSEN PHARMACEUTICA INC.)
Nizoral 2% Shampoo
(JANSSEN PHARMACEUTICA INC.)

Nizoral Tablets (JANSSEN PHARMACEUTICA INC.)
No Doz Maximum Strength Caplets
(BRISTOL-MYERS PRODUCTS)
Nolahist Tablets (CARNRICK LABORATORIES, INC.)
Nolamine Timed-Release Tablets
(CARNRICK LABORATORIES, INC.)
Nolvadex Tablets (ZENECA PHARMACEUTICALS)
Norcuron (ORGANON INC.)
Nordette-21 Tablets
(WYETH-AYERST LABORATORIES)
Nordette-28 Tablets
(WYETH-AYERST LABORATORIES)
Norel (U.S. PHARMACEUTICAL CORPORATION)
Norel Plus (U.S. PHARMACEUTICAL CORPORATION)

NOREPINEPHRINE BITARTRATE
Levophed Bitartrate Injection

NORETHINDRONE
Brevicon 21-Day Tablets
Brevicon 28-Day Tablets
Micronor Tablets
Modicon 21 Tablets
Modicon 28 Tablets
Nelova
Norinyl 1+35 21-Day Tablets
Norinyl 1+35 28-Day Tablets
Norinyl 1+50 21-Day Tablets
Norinyl 1+50 28-Day Tablets
Nor-Q D Tablets
Ortho-Novum 1/35 □ 21 Tablets
Ortho-Novum 1/35 □ 28 Tablets
Ortho-Novum 1/50 □ 21 Tablets
Ortho-Novum 1/50 □ 28 Tablets
Ortho-Novum 7/7/7 □ 21 Tablets
Ortho-Novum 7/7/7 □ 28 Tablets
Ortho-Novum 10/11 □ 21 Tablets
Ortho-Novum 10/11 □ 28 Tablets
Ovcon 35
Ovcon 50
Tri-Norinyl 21-Day Tablets
Tri-Norinyl 28-Day Tablets

NORETHINDRONE ACETATE
Aygestin Tablets
Loestrin Fe 1/20
Loestrin Fe 1.5/30
Loestrin 21 1/20
Loestrin 21 1.5/30
Norflex Injection (3M PHARMACEUTICALS)
Norflex Sustained-Release Tablets
(3M PHARMACEUTICALS)

NORFLOXACIN
Chibroxin Sterile Ophthalmic Solution
Noroxin Tablets
Norgesic Forte Tablets (3M PHARMACEUTICALS)
Norgesic Tablets (3M PHARMACEUTICALS)

NORGESTIMATE
Ortho-Cyclen Tablets
Ortho Tri-Cyclen Tablets

NORGESTREL
Lo/Ovral Tablets
Lo/Ovral-28 Tablets
Ovral Tablets
Ovral-28 Tablets
Ovrette Tablets
Norinyl 1+35 21-Day Tablets
(SYNTEX PUERTO RICO, INC.)
Norinyl 1+35 28-Day Tablets
(SYNTEX PUERTO RICO, INC.)
Norinyl 1+50 21-Day Tablets
(SYNTEX PUERTO RICO, INC.)
Norinyl 1+50 28-Day Tablets
(SYNTEX PUERTO RICO, INC.)

Norisodrine with Calcium Iodide Syrup
(ABBOTT LABORATORIES)
Normodyne Injection (SCHERING CORPORATION)
Normodyne Tablets (SCHERING CORPORATION)
Noroxin Tablets (MERCK & CO., INC.)
Norpace Capsules (G.D. SEARLE & CO.)
Norpace CR Capsules (G.D. SEARLE & CO.)
Norplant System (WYETH-AYERST LABORATORIES)
Norpramin Tablets (MARION MERRELL DOW INC.)
Nor-Q D Tablets (SYNTEX PUERTO RICO, INC.)
Nortriptyline Capsules
(GENEVA PHARMACEUTICALS, INC.)

NORTRIPTYLINE HYDROCHLORIDE
Nortriptyline Capsules
Nortriptyline Hydrochloride Capsules
Pamelor Capsules
Pamelor Solution
Nortriptyline Hydrochloride Capsules
(MYLAN PHARMACEUTICALS INC.)
Norvasc Tablets (PFIZER LABS DIVISION)
Novacet Lotion (GENDERM CORPORATION)
Novahistine DH (+)
(SMITHKLINE BEECHAM CONSUMER HEALTHCARE, L.P.)
Novahistine DMX
(SMITHKLINE BEECHAM CONSUMER HEALTHCARE, L.P.)
Novahistine Elixir
(SMITHKLINE BEECHAM CONSUMER HEALTHCARE, L.P.)
Novahistine Expectorant (+)
(SMITHKLINE BEECHAM CONSUMER HEALTHCARE, L.P.)
Novantrone for Injection Concentrate
(IMMUNEX CORPORATION)
Novocain Hydrochloride for Spinal Anesthesia
(SANOFI WINTHROP PHARMACEUTICALS)
Novocain Hydrochloride Injection
(SANOFI WINTHROP PHARMACEUTICALS)
Novolin L (NOVO NORDISK PHARMACEUTICALS INC.)
Novolin N (NOVO NORDISK PHARMACEUTICALS INC.)
Novolin N PenFill Cartridges
(NOVO NORDISK PHARMACEUTICALS INC.)
Novolin N Prefilled Syringe
(NOVO NORDISK PHARMACEUTICALS INC.)
Novolin 70/30
(NOVO NORDISK PHARMACEUTICALS INC.)
Novolin 70/30 PenFill Cartridges
(NOVO NORDISK PHARMACEUTICALS INC.)
Novolin 70/30 Prefilled
(NOVO NORDISK PHARMACEUTICALS INC.)
Novolin R (NOVO NORDISK PHARMACEUTICALS INC.)
Novolin R PenFill Cartridges
(NOVO NORDISK PHARMACEUTICALS INC.)
Novolin R Prefilled Syringe
(NOVO NORDISK PHARMACEUTICALS INC.)
NovoFine 30 Disposable Needle
(NOVO NORDISK PHARMACEUTICALS INC.)
NovolinPen
(NOVO NORDISK PHARMACEUTICALS INC.)
Nubain Injection (ENDO LABORATORIES, L.L.C.)
Nucofed Expectorant
(ROBERTS PHARMACEUTICAL CORPORATION)
Nucofed Pediatric Expectorant
(ROBERTS PHARMACEUTICAL CORPORATION)
Nucofed Syrup and Capsules
(ROBERTS PHARMACEUTICAL CORPORATION)
Nucotuss Expectorant (BARRE-NATIONAL INC.)
Nucotuss Pediatric Expectorant
(BARRE-NATIONAL INC.)
Nu-Iron 150 Capsules
(MAYRAND PHARMACEUTICALS, INC.)
Nu-Iron V Tablets
(MAYRAND PHARMACEUTICALS, INC.)
Nu-Iron Elixir
(MAYRAND PHARMACEUTICALS, INC.)
Nu-Iron Plus Elixir
(MAYRAND PHARMACEUTICALS, INC.)
NuLYTELY (BRAINTREE LABORATORIES, INC.)

UNDERLINE DENOTES GENERIC NAME

Numorphan Injection (DUPONT PHARMA)
Numorphan Suppositories (DUPONT PHARMA)
Nupercainal Hemorrhoidal and Anesthetic Ointment (CIBA CONSUMER PHARMACEUTICALS)
Nupercainal Pain Relief Cream
(CIBA CONSUMER PHARMACEUTICALS)
Nupercainal Suppositories
(CIBA CONSUMER PHARMACEUTICALS)
Nuprin Ibuprofen/Analgesic Tablets & Caplets
(BRISTOL-MYERS PRODUCTS)
Nuromax Injection (BURROUGHS WELLCOME CO.)
Nursoy, Soy Protein Formula for Infants, Concentrated Liquid, Ready-to-Feed, and Powder (WYETH-AYERST LABORATORIES)
Nutracort Lotion (GALDERMA LABORATORIES, INC.)
Nutraderm Cream & Lotion
(GALDERMA LABORATORIES, INC.)
Nutraderm 30 Lotion
(GALDERMA LABORATORIES, INC.)
NutraVescent (NORTHAMPTON MEDICAL, INC.)
NUTRIENTS
Nutropin (GENENTECH, INC.)
Nydrazid Injection (APOTHECON)
NYSTATIN
Mycostatin Cream and Topical Powder
Mycostatin Pastilles
Mytrex Cream & Ointment
Nystatin Cream, USP
Nystatin Cream, Ointment, or Oral Suspension, USP
Nystatin Oral Suspension
Nystatin Oral Suspension, USP
Nystatin Oral Suspension
Nystatin Tablets
Nystatin & Triamcinolone Acetonide Ointment, USP
Nystatin, USP for Extemporaneous Preparation of Oral Suspension
Nystatin/Triamcinolone Acetonide Cream or Ointment
Nystatin and Triamcinolone Acetonide Cream, USP
Pedi-Dri Topical Powder
Nystatin Cream, USP
(TARO PHARMACEUTICALS U.S.A., INC.)
Nystatin Cream, Ointment, or Oral Suspension, USP (BARRE-NATIONAL INC.)
Nystatin Oral Suspension
(ROXANE LABORATORIES, INC.)
Nystatin Oral Suspension, USP
(WARNER CHILCOTT LABORATORIES)
Nystatin Oral Suspension
(BIOCRAFT LABORATORIES, INC.)
Nystatin Tablets (PAR PHARMACEUTICAL, INC.)
Nystatin & Triamcinolone Acetonide Ointment, USP (TARO PHARMACEUTICALS U.S.A., INC.)
Nystatin, USP for Extemporaneous Preparation of Oral Suspension
(PADDOCK LABORATORIES, INC.)
Nystatin/Triamcinolone Acetonide Cream or Ointment (BARRE-NATIONAL INC.)
Nystatin and Triamcinolone Acetonide Cream, USP (TARO PHARMACEUTICALS U.S.A., INC.)

O

OMS Concentrate CII
(UPSHER-SMITH LABORATORIES, INC.)
Obenix Capsules
(ABANA PHARMACEUTICALS, INC.)

Obetrol Tablets (REXAR PHARMACAL)
Oby-Cap Phentermine HCl Capsules
(RICHWOOD PHARMACEUTICAL COMPANY, INC.)
Oby-Trim Capsules (REXAR PHARMACAL)
Occlusal-HP (GENDERM CORPORATION)
Ocucoat (LEDERLE LABORATORIES)
Ocean Nasal Mist (FLEMING & COMPANY)
OCTOCRYLENE
Solbar PF Ultra Cream SPF 50 (PABA Free)
Solbar PF Ultra Liquid SPF 30
OCTREOTIDE ACETATE
Sandostatin Injection
OCTYL DIMETHYL PABA
Solaquin Forte 4% Cream
Solaquin Forte 4% Gel
Solbar Plus 15 Cream
OCTYL METHOXYCINNAMATE
DML Facial Moisturizer with Sunscreen
Solbar PF 15 Cream (PABA Free)
Solbar PF 15 Liquid (PABA Free)
Solbar PF Ultra Cream SPF 50 (PABA Free)
Solbar PF Ultra Liquid SPF 30
Ocuflox (ALLERGAN, INC.)
Ocuvite Vitamin and Mineral Supplement
(LEDERLE LABORATORIES)
OFLOXACIN
Floxin I.V.
Floxin Tablets
Ocuflox
Ogen Tablets (THE UPJOHN COMPANY)
Ogen Vaginal Cream (THE UPJOHN COMPANY)
Oil of Olay Daily UV Protectant SPF 15 Beauty Fluid-Regular and Fragrance Free (Olay Co. Inc.) (PROCTER & GAMBLE)
Oil of Olay Daily UV Protectant SPF 15 Moisture Replenishing Cream (PROCTER & GAMBLE)
OLSALAZINE SODIUM
Dipentum Capsules
OMEPRAZOLE
Prilosec Delayed-Release Capsules
OmniHIB
(SMITHKLINE BEECHAM PHARMACEUTICALS)
OMNIHIST L.A. Tablets
(WE PHARMACEUTICALS, INC.)
Omnipaque
(SANOFI WINTHROP PHARMACEUTICALS)
Omnipen Capsules (WYETH-AYERST LABORATORIES)
Omnipen for Oral Suspension
(WYETH-AYERST LABORATORIES)
Omnipen-N Injection
(WYETH-AYERST LABORATORIES)
Omniscan Injection
(SANOFI WINTHROP PHARMACEUTICALS)
Oncaspar
(RHONE-POULENC RORER PHARMACEUTICALS INC.)
Oncovin Solution Vials & Hyporets
(ELI LILLY AND COMPANY)
Oncovite (MISSION PHARMACAL COMPANY)
ONDANSETRON HYDROCHLORIDE
Zofran Injection
Zofran Tablets
One-A-Day Essential Vitamins
(MILES INC. CONSUMER HEALTHCARE PRODUCTS)
One-A-Day Extras Antioxidant
(MILES INC. CONSUMER HEALTHCARE PRODUCTS)
One-A-Day Extras Garlic
(MILES INC. CONSUMER HEALTHCARE PRODUCTS)
One-A-Day Extras Vitamin C
(MILES INC. CONSUMER HEALTHCARE PRODUCTS)
One-A-Day Extras Vitamin E
(MILES INC. CONSUMER HEALTHCARE PRODUCTS)

One-A-Day Maximum Formula Vitamins and Minerals
(MILES INC. CONSUMER HEALTHCARE PRODUCTS)
One-A-Day Men's
(MILES INC. CONSUMER HEALTHCARE PRODUCTS)
One-A-Day Women's Multivitamin with Calcium, Extra Iron and Zinc
(MILES INC. CONSUMER HEALTHCARE PRODUCTS)
One-A-Day 55 Plus
(MILES INC. CONSUMER HEALTHCARE PRODUCTS)
Ony-Clear Nail Spray (PEDINOL PHARMACAL INC.)
OPIUM ALKALOIDS
B & O No. 15A & No. 16A Supprettes
Oramorph SR (Morphine Sulfate Sustained Release Tablets) (ROXANE LABORATORIES, INC.)
Orap Tablets (TEVA PHARMACEUTICALS)
Oratrast
(RHONE-POULENC RORER PHARMACEUTICALS INC.)
Oretic Tablets (ABBOTT LABORATORIES)
Oreton Methyl (ICN PHARMACEUTICALS, INC.)
Organidin NR Tablets and Liquid
(WALLACE LABORATORIES)
Orimune (LEDERLE LABORATORIES)
Ornade Spansule Capsules
(SMITHKLINE BEECHAM PHARMACEUTICALS)
ORPHENADRINE CITRATE
Mio-Rel Injectable
Norflex Injection
Norflex Sustained-Release Tablets
Norgesic Forte Tablets
Norgesic Tablets
Ortho-Cept Tablets
(ORTHO PHARMACEUTICAL CORPORATION)
Ortho-Cyclen Tablets
(ORTHO PHARMACEUTICAL CORPORATION)
Ortho Diaphragm Kit/All-Flex Arcing Spring
(ORTHO PHARMACEUTICAL CORPORATION)
Ortho Diaphragm Kit-Coil Spring
(ORTHO PHARMACEUTICAL CORPORATION)
Ortho Dienestrol Cream
(ORTHO PHARMACEUTICAL CORPORATION)
Ortho-Est .625 Tablets
(ORTHO PHARMACEUTICAL CORPORATION)
Ortho-Est Tablets
(ORTHO PHARMACEUTICAL CORPORATION)
Ortho-Gynol Contraceptive Jelly
(ORTHO PHARMACEUTICAL CORPORATION)
Ortho-Novum 1/35 □ 21 Tablets
(ORTHO PHARMACEUTICAL CORPORATION)
Ortho-Novum 1/35 □ 28 Tablets
(ORTHO PHARMACEUTICAL CORPORATION)
Ortho-Novum 1/50 □ 21 Tablets
(ORTHO PHARMACEUTICAL CORPORATION)
Ortho-Novum 1/50 □ 28 Tablets
(ORTHO PHARMACEUTICAL CORPORATION)
Ortho-Novum 7/7/7 □ 21 Tablets
(ORTHO PHARMACEUTICAL CORPORATION)
Ortho-Novum 7/7/7 □ 28 Tablets
(ORTHO PHARMACEUTICAL CORPORATION)
Ortho-Novum 10/11 □ 21 Tablets
(ORTHO PHARMACEUTICAL CORPORATION)
Ortho-Novum 10/11 □ 28 Tablets
(ORTHO PHARMACEUTICAL CORPORATION)
Ortho Tri-Cyclen Tablets
(ORTHO PHARMACEUTICAL CORPORATION)
Ortho-White Diaphragm Kit-Flat Spring
(ORTHO PHARMACEUTICAL CORPORATION)
Orthoclone OKT3 Sterile Solution
(ORTHO BIOTECH INC.)
Orthoxicol Cough Syrup
(ROBERTS PHARMACEUTICAL CORPORATION)
Orudis Capsules (WYETH-AYERST LABORATORIES)
Oruvail Capsules (WYETH-AYERST LABORATORIES)
Os-Cal 250+D Tablets
(SMITHKLINE BEECHAM CONSUMER HEALTHCARE, L.P.)

UNDERLINE DENOTES GENERIC NAME

Os-Cal 500 Chewable Tablets
(SMITHKLINE BEECHAM CONSUMER HEALTHCARE, L.P.)
Os-Cal 500 Tablets
(SMITHKLINE BEECHAM CONSUMER HEALTHCARE, L.P.)
Os-Cal 500+D Tablets
(SMITHKLINE BEECHAM CONSUMER HEALTHCARE, L.P.)
Os-Cal Fortified Tablets
(SMITHKLINE BEECHAM CONSUMER HEALTHCARE, L.P.)
Osmolite Isotonic Liquid Nutrition
(ROSS PRODUCTS DIVISION)
**Osmolite HN High Nitrogen Isotonic Liquid
Nutrition** (ROSS PRODUCTS DIVISION)
Ostiderm (PEDINOL PHARMACAL INC.)
Ostiderm Roll On (PEDINOL PHARMACAL INC.)
Otic Domeboro Solution
(MILES INC. PHARMACEUTICAL DIVISION)
Otic Tridesilon Solution 0.05%
(MILES INC. PHARMACEUTICAL DIVISION)
Otocain (ABANA PHARMACEUTICALS, INC.)
Otrivin Nasal Drops
(CIBA CONSUMER PHARMACEUTICALS)
Otrivin Pediatric Nasal Drops
(CIBA CONSUMER PHARMACEUTICALS)
Ovcon 35 (BRISTOL-MYERS SQUIBB COMPANY)
Ovcon 50 (BRISTOL-MYERS SQUIBB COMPANY)
Ovral Tablets (WYETH-AYERST LABORATORIES)
Ovral-28 Tablets (WYETH-AYERST LABORATORIES)
Ovrette Tablets (WYETH-AYERST LABORATORIES)

OXACILLIN SODIUM
   Oxacillin Sodium Capsules
   Oxacillin Sodium for Oral Solution
Oxacillin Sodium Capsules
(BIOCRAFT LABORATORIES, INC.)
Oxacillin Sodium for Oral Solution
(BIOCRAFT LABORATORIES, INC.)

OXAPROZIN
   Daypro Caplets

OXAZEPAM
   Oxazepam Capsules
   Serax Capsules
   Serax Tablets
Oxazepam Capsules
(WARNER CHILCOTT LABORATORIES)

OXICONAZOLE NITRATE
   Oxistat Cream
   Oxistat Lotion
Oxistat Cream (GLAXO DERMATOLOGY)
Oxistat Lotion (GLAXO DERMATOLOGY)
Oxsoralen Lotion 1%
(ICN PHARMACEUTICALS, INC.)
Oxsoralen-Ultra Capsule
(ICN PHARMACEUTICALS, INC.)

OXTRIPHYLLINE
   Choledyl Tablets
   Choledyl SA Tablets
Oxy Medicated Cleanser
(SMITHKLINE BEECHAM CONSUMER HEALTHCARE, L.P.)
**Oxy Medicated Pads - Regular, Sensitive Skin
and Maximum Strength**
(SMITHKLINE BEECHAM CONSUMER HEALTHCARE, L.P.)
Oxy Medicated Soap
(SMITHKLINE BEECHAM CONSUMER HEALTHCARE, L.P.)
**Oxy Night Watch Nighttime Acne Medication -
Maximum Strength and Sensitive
Skin Formulas**
(SMITHKLINE BEECHAM CONSUMER HEALTHCARE, L.P.)
Oxy 10 Benzoyl Peroxide Wash
(SMITHKLINE BEECHAM CONSUMER HEALTHCARE, L.P.)
Oxy-5 and Oxy-10 Tinted and Vanishing
(SMITHKLINE BEECHAM CONSUMER HEALTHCARE, L.P.)

OXYBENZONE
   DML Facial Moisturizer with Sunscreen

   Solaquin Forte 4% Cream
   Solbar PF 15 Cream (PABA Free)
   Solbar PF 15 Liquid (PABA Free)
   Solbar PF Ultra Cream SPF 50 (PABA Free)
   Solbar PF Ultra Liquid SPF 30
   Solbar Plus 15 Cream

OXYBUTYNIN CHLORIDE
   Ditropan Syrup
   Ditropan Tablets

OXYCODONE HYDROCHLORIDE
   Percocet Tablets
   Percodan Tablets
   Roxicet 5/500 Caplets (Oxycodone &
     Acetaminophen)
   Roxicet Tablets & Oral Solution (Oxycodone &
     Acetaminophen)
   Roxicodone Tablets, Oral Solution & Intensol
     (Oxycodone)
   Roxiprin Tablets (Oxycodone & Aspirin)
   Tylox Capsules

OXYCODONE TEREPHTHALATE
   Percodan Tablets

OXYMETAZOLINE HYDROCHLORIDE
   4-Way Long Lasting Nasal Spray
   12 Hour Nasal Spray

OXYMETHOLONE
   Anadrol-50 Tablets

OXYMORPHONE HYDROCHLORIDE
   Numorphan Injection
   Numorphan Suppositories

OXYQUINOLINE SULFATE
   Aci-Jel Therapeutic Vaginal Jelly

OXYTETRACYCLINE
   Terramycin Intramuscular Solution

OXYTETRACYCLINE HYDROCHLORIDE
   Terra-Cortril Ophthalmic Suspension
   Terramycin with Polymyxin B Sulfate
     Ophthalmic Ointment
   Urobiotic-250 Capsules

OXYTOCIN
   Oxytocin Injection
   Oxytocin in Tubex
   Syntocinon Injection
   Syntocinon Nasal Spray
Oxytocin Injection
(WYETH-AYERST LABORATORIES)
Oxytocin in Tubex
(WYETH-AYERST LABORATORIES)

P

P-A-C (Revised Formula) Analgesic Tablets
(ROBERTS PHARMACEUTICAL CORPORATION)

PACLITAXEL
   Taxol

PAH (PARA-AMINO ANALOG OF HIPPURIC ACID)
   Aminohippurate Sodium Injection
PBZ Tablets (GEIGY PHARMACEUTICALS)
PBZ-SR Tablets (GEIGY PHARMACEUTICALS)
**PC-CAP Propoxyphene Hydrochloride
Compound, USP** (ALRA LABORATORIES, INC.)
PCE Dispertab Tablets (ABBOTT LABORATORIES)
pHisoDerm
(SANOFI WINTHROP PHARMACEUTICALS)
pHisoHex (SANOFI WINTHROP PHARMACEUTICALS)

PMB 200 and PMB 400
(WYETH-AYERST LABORATORIES)
**PP-CAP Propoxyphene Hydrochloride Capsules,
USP** (ALRA LABORATORIES, INC.)
PPD Tine Test (LEDERLE LABORATORIES)
P-V-TUSSIN Syrup
(SOLVAY PHARMACEUTICALS, INC.)
P-V-TUSSIN Tablets
(SOLVAY PHARMACEUTICALS, INC.)
Pacaps Capsules (LUNSCO, INC.)

PADIMATE O (OCTYL DIMETHYL PABA)
   Herpecin-L Cold Sore Lip Balm Stick
PALS Internal Deodorant
(PALISADES PHARMACEUTICALS, INC.)

PAMABROM
   Lurline PMS Tablets
Pamelor Capsules
(SANDOZ PHARMACEUTICALS CORPORATION)
Pamelor Solution
(SANDOZ PHARMACEUTICALS CORPORATION)

PAMIDRONATE DISODIUM
   Aredia for Injection
Pamine Tablets (KENWOOD LABORATORIES)
Panacet 5/500 Tablets (ECR PHARMACEUTICALS)
Panafil Ointment (RYSTAN COMPANY, INC.)
Panafil-White Ointment (RYSTAN COMPANY, INC.)
Panalgesic Gold Cream (ECR PHARMACEUTICALS)
Panalgesic Gold Liniment
(ECR PHARMACEUTICALS)
Panasal 5/500 Tablets (ECR PHARMACEUTICALS)
Pancrease Capsules (MCNEIL PHARMACEUTICAL)
Pancrease MT Capsules
(MCNEIL PHARMACEUTICAL)

PANCREATIN
   CREON 10 Capsules
   Donnazyme Tablets
   Entozyme Tablets

PANCRELIPASE
   Cotazym
   Cotazym-S
   CREON 20 Capsules
   Ku-Zyme HP Capsules
   Pancrease Capsules
   Pancrease MT Capsules
   Ultrase Capsules
   Viokase Powder
   Viokase Tablets
   Zymase Capsules

PANCURONIUM BROMIDE INJECTION
   Pancuronium Bromide Injection
   Pancuronium Bromide Injection
   Pavulon
Pancuronium Bromide Injection
(ASTRA USA, INC.)
Pancuronium Bromide Injection
(ELKINS-SINN, INC.)
Panhematin (ABBOTT LABORATORIES)
PanOxyl 5 Acne Gel
(STIEFEL LABORATORIES, INC.)
PanOxyl 10 Acne Gel
(STIEFEL LABORATORIES, INC.)
PanOxyl AQ 2$^{1}/_{2}$ Acne Gel
(STIEFEL LABORATORIES, INC.)
PanOxyl AQ 5 Acne Gel
(STIEFEL LABORATORIES, INC.)
PanOxyl AQ 10 Acne Gel
(STIEFEL LABORATORIES, INC.)

PAPAIN
   Panafil Ointment
   Panafil-White Ointment

PAPAVERINE HYDROCHLORIDE
   Papaverine Hydrochloride Vials and Ampoules

Papaverine Hydrochloride Vials and Ampoules
(ELI LILLY AND COMPANY)

PARA-AMINOBENZOATE, POTASSIUM
Potaba

PARA-AMINOBENZOIC ACID
Mega-B
Paradione Capsules (ABBOTT LABORATORIES)
Paraflex Caplets (MCNEIL PHARMACEUTICAL)
Parafon Forte DSC Caplets
(MCNEIL PHARMACEUTICAL)
**ParaGard T380A Intrauterine Copper
Contraceptive** (GYNOPHARMA INC.)

PARAMETHADIONE
Paradione Capsules
Paraplatin for Injection
(BRISTOL-MYERS SQUIBB ONCOLOGY DIVISION)
Parathar
(RHONE-POULENC RORER PHARMACEUTICALS)

PAREGORIC
Paregoric USP
Paregoric USP (BARRE-NATIONAL INC.)
Parepectolin Suspension
(RHONE-POULENC RORER PHARMACEUTICALS INC.)
Parlodel Capsules
(SANDOZ PHARMACEUTICALS CORPORATION)
Parlodel SnapTabs
(SANDOZ PHARMACEUTICALS CORPORATION)
Parnate Tablets
(SMITHKLINE BEECHAM PHARMACEUTICALS)

PAROXETINE HYDROCHLORIDE
Paxil Tablets
PASER Granules
(JACOBUS PHARMACEUTICAL CO., INC.)
Pathocil Capsules (WYETH-AYERST LABORATORIES)
Pathocil for Oral Suspension
(WYETH-AYERST LABORATORIES)
Pavulon (ORGANON INC.)
Paxil Tablets
(SMITHKLINE BEECHAM PHARMACEUTICALS)
Pazo Hemorrhoid Ointment & Suppositories
(BRISTOL-MYERS PRODUCTS)

PECTIN
Kaolin-Pectin Suspension
PediaCare Cold-Allergy Chewable Tablets
(MCNEIL CONSUMER PRODUCTS COMPANY)
PediaCare Cough-Cold Chewable Tablets
(MCNEIL CONSUMER PRODUCTS COMPANY)
PediaCare Cough-Cold Liquid
(MCNEIL CONSUMER PRODUCTS COMPANY)
PediaCare Infants' Decongestant Drops
(MCNEIL CONSUMER PRODUCTS COMPANY)
PediaCare NightRest Cough-Cold Liquid
(MCNEIL CONSUMER PRODUCTS COMPANY)
Pediacof Cough Syrup
(SANOFI WINTHROP PHARMACEUTICALS)
Pediaflor Drops (ROSS PRODUCTS DIVISION)
Pedialyte Oral Electrolyte Maintenance Solution
(ROSS PRODUCTS DIVISION)
Pediapred Oral Liquid
(FISONS CORPORATION PRESCRIPTION PRODUCTS)
PediaSure Complete Liquid Nutrition
(ROSS PRODUCTS DIVISION)
PediaSure With Fiber Complete Liquid Nutrition
(ROSS PRODUCTS DIVISION)
**Pediatric Vicks 44d Dry Hacking Cough & Head
Congestion** (PROCTER & GAMBLE)
**Pediatric Vicks 44e Chest Cough & Chest
Congestion** (PROCTER & GAMBLE)
Pediatric Vicks 44m Cough & Cold Relief
(PROCTER & GAMBLE)
Pediazole (ROSS PRODUCTS DIVISION)
Pedi-Boro Soak Paks (PEDINOL PHARMACAL INC.)

Pedi-Dri Topical Powder
(PEDINOL PHARMACAL INC.)
Pedi-Joy Chewable (VITALINE CORPORATION)
Pedinol's HC Creme (PEDINOL PHARMACAL INC.)
PediOtic Suspension Sterile
(BURROUGHS WELLCOME CO.)
Pedi-Pro Topical Powder
(PEDINOL PHARMACAL INC.)
PedvaxHIB (MERCK & CO., INC.)

PEGADEMASE BOVINE
Adagen (pegademase bovine) Injection

PEGASPARGASE
Oncaspar
Peganone Tablets (ABBOTT LABORATORIES)

PEMOLINE
Cylert Chewable Tablets
Cylert Tablets
Pen•Kera Creme (B. F. ASCHER & COMPANY, INC.)
Pen•Vee K for Oral Solution
(WYETH-AYERST LABORATORIES)
Pen•Vee K Tablets
(WYETH-AYERST LABORATORIES)

PENBUTOLOL SULFATE
Levatol
Penecort Cream 1% (ALLERGAN HERBERT)
Penecort Topical Solution 1%
(ALLERGAN HERBERT)
Penetrex Tablets
(RHONE-POULENC RORER PHARMACEUTICALS INC.)

PENICILLAMINE
Cuprimine Capsules
Depen Titratable Tablets

PENICILLIN G BENZATHINE
Bicillin C-R Injection
Bicillin C-R in Tubex
Bicillin C-R 900/300 Injection
Bicillin C-R 900/300 in Tubex
Bicillin L-A Injection
Bicillin L-A in Tubex

PENICILLIN G POTASSIUM
Pfizerpen for Injection

PENICILLIN G PROCAINE
Bicillin C-R Injection
Bicillin C-R in Tubex
Bicillin C-R 900/300 Injection
Bicillin C-R 900/300 in Tubex
Wycillin Injection

PENICILLIN V POTASSIUM
Ledercillin VK Oral Solution, Tablets
Pen•Vee K for Oral Solution
Pen•Vee K Tablets
Penicillin V Potassium for Oral Solution
Penicillin V Potassium Tablets
Penicillin V Postassium Tablets
Penicillin V Potassium Tablets, USP
Penicillin VK for Oral Solution, USP
Penicillin V Potassium for Oral Solution
(BIOCRAFT LABORATORIES, INC.)
Penicillin V Potassium Tablets
(BIOCRAFT LABORATORIES, INC.)
Penicillin V Postassium Tablets
(MYLAN PHARMACEUTICALS INC.)
Penicillin V Potassium Tablets, USP
(WARNER CHILCOTT LABORATORIES)
Penicillin VK for Oral Solution, USP
(WARNER CHILCOTT LABORATORIES)
PenNeedle Disposable Needle
(NOVO NORDISK PHARMACEUTICALS INC.)
Pentacarinat, Sterile Pentamidine Isethionate
(ARMOUR PHARMACEUTICAL COMPANY)

PENTAGASTRIN
Peptavlon
Pentam 300 Injection (FUJISAWA USA, INC.)

PENTAMIDINE ISETHIONATE
NebuPent for Inhalation Solution
Pentacarinat, Sterile Pentamidine Isethionate
Pentam 300 Injection
Pentaspan Injection (DUPONT PHARMA)
Pentasa (MARION MERRELL DOW INC.)

PENTASTARCH
Pentaspan Injection

PENTAZOCINE HYDROCHLORIDE
Talacen
Talwin Compound
Talwin Nx

PENTAZOCINE LACTATE
Talwin Ampuls
Talwin Carpuject
Talwin Injection

PENTOBARBITAL SODIUM
Nembutal Sodium Capsules
Nembutal Sodium Solution
Nembutal Sodium Suppositories
Pentobarbital Sodium in Tubex
Pentobarbital Sodium in Tubex
(WYETH-AYERST LABORATORIES)

PENTOXIFYLLINE
Trental Tablets
Pentrax Anti-dandruff Shampoo
(GENDERM CORPORATION)
Pepcid Injection (MERCK & CO., INC.)
Pepcid Injection Premixed (MERCK & CO., INC.)
Pepcid Oral Suspension (MERCK & CO., INC.)
Pepcid Tablets (MERCK & CO., INC.)
Peptavlon (WYETH-AYERST LABORATORIES)
Pepto-Bismol Liquid, Tablets and Caplets
(PROCTER & GAMBLE)
Maximum Strength Pepto-Bismol Liquid
(PROCTER & GAMBLE)
Pepto Diarrhea Control (PROCTER & GAMBLE)
Perative Specialized Liquid Nutrition
(ROSS PRODUCTS DIVISION)
Percocet Tablets (DUPONT PHARMA)
Percodan Tablets (DUPONT PHARMA)
Percogesic Analgesic Tablets (PROCTER & GAMBLE)
Perdiem Fiber Granules
(RHONE-POULENC RORER PHARMACEUTICALS INC.)
Perdiem Granules
(RHONE-POULENC RORER PHARMACEUTICALS INC.)
Performance Packs
(HEALTH MAINTENANCE PROGRAMS, INC.)
Performance Packs-Light
(HEALTH MAINTENANCE PROGRAMS, INC.)

PERGOLIDE MESYLATE
Permax Tablets
Pergonal (menotropins for injection, USP)
(SERONO LABORATORIES, INC.)
Periactin Syrup (MERCK & CO., INC.)
Periactin Tablets (MERCK & CO., INC.)
Peridex (PROCTER & GAMBLE)
Peridin-C Tablets (BEUTLICH L.P.)
Permax Tablets (ATHENA NEUROSCIENCES, INC.)

PERMETHRIN
Elimite (permethrin) 5% Cream
Nix Creme Rinse
Rid Lice Control Spray

PERPHENAZINE
Etrafon-A Tablets (4–10)
Etrafon Forte Tablets (4-25)
Etrafon 2-10 Tablets (2-10)
Etrafon Tablets (2-25)

UNDERLINE DENOTES GENERIC NAME

Perphenazine Tablets
Perphenazine & Amitriptyline Hydrochloride
   Tablets
Perphenazine/Amitriptyline HCl Tablets
Triavil Tablets
Trilafon Concentrate
Trilafon Injection
Trilafon Tablets
Perphenazine Tablets
   (GENEVA PHARMACEUTICALS, INC.)
Perphenazine & Amitriptyline Hydrochloride
   Tablets (MYLAN PHARMACEUTICALS, INC.)
Perphenazine/Amitriptyline HCl Tablets
   (GENEVA PHARMACEUTICALS, INC.)
Persa-Gel (benzoyl peroxide)
   (ORTHO PHARMACEUTICAL CORPORATION
   DERMATOLOGICAL DIVISION)
Persa-Gel W (benzoyl peroxide)
   (ORTHO PHARMACEUTICAL CORPORATION
   DERMATOLOGICAL DIVISION)
Persantine Tablets
   (BOEHRINGER INGELHEIM PHARMACEUTICALS, INC.)

PETROLATUM
   Aquaphor Healing Ointment
   Aquaphor Healing Ointment, Original Formula
   DML Facial Moisturizer with Sunscreen
   DML Forte Cream
   DML Moisturizing Lotion
   Eucerin Dry Skin Care Moisturizing Creme
     (Unscented)
   Moisturel Cream
   Nutraderm 30 Lotion

PETROLATUM, WHITE
   Borofax
   Prophyllin CCC Topical Emollient Ointment
   White Petrolatum USP
Petro-Phylic Soap (DOAK DERMATOLOGICALS)
Pfizerpen for Injection (ROERIG DIVISION)
Phazyme (REED & CARNRICK)

PHENACEMIDE
   Phenurone Tablets
Phenadex Children's Cough/Cold Syrup
   (BARRE-NATIONAL INC.)
Phenadex Pediatric Cough/Cold Drops
   (BARRE-NATIONAL INC.)
Phenadex Senior Cough/Cold Liquid
   (BARRE-NATIONAL INC.)
Phenaphen with Codeine Capsules
   (A. H. ROBINS COMPANY, INC.)

PHENAZOPYRIDINE HYDROCHLORIDE
   Azo Gantanol Tablets
   Azo Gantrisin Tablets
   Azo-Standard Tablets
   Prodium
   Pyridium
   Urobiotic-250 Capsules

PHENDIMETRAZINE TARTRATE
   Bontril PDM Tablets
   Bontril Slow-Release Capsules
   Plegine Tablets
   Prelu-2 Timed Release Capsules
   X-Trozine Capsules and Tablets
   X-Trozine L.A. Capsules

PHENELZINE SULFATE
   Nardil
Phenergan with Codeine
   (WYETH-AYERST LABORATORIES)
Phenergan with Dextromethorphan
   (WYETH-AYERST LABORATORIES)
Phenergan Injection
   (WYETH-AYERST LABORATORIES)

Phenergan Suppositories
   (WYETH-AYERST LABORATORIES)
Phenergan Syrup Fortis
   (WYETH-AYERST LABORATORIES)
Phenergan Syrup Plain
   (WYETH-AYERST LABORATORIES)
Phenergan Tablets (WYETH-AYERST LABORATORIES)
Phenergan in Tubex
   (WYETH-AYERST LABORATORIES)
Phenergan VC (WYETH-AYERST LABORATORIES)
Phenergan VC with Codeine
   (WYETH-AYERST LABORATORIES)

PHENINDAMINE TARTRATE
   Nolahist Tablets
   Nolamine Timed-Release Tablets
   P-V-TUSSIN Tablets

PHENIRAMINE MALEATE
   Naphcon-A Ophthalmic Solution
   Poly-Histine Elixir
   Poly-Histine-D Capsules
   Poly-Histine-D Elixir
   Poly-Histine-D Ped Caps
   Ru-Tuss with Hydrocodone
   Triaminic Expectorant DH
   Triaminic Oral Infant Drops

PHENOBARBITAL
   Antrocol Elixir
   Arco-Lase Plus Tablets
   Bellatal Tablets
   Bellergal-S Tablets
   Donnatal Capsules
   Donnatal Elixir
   Donnatal Extentabs
   Donnatal Tablets
   Mudrane Tablets
   Mudrane GG Elixir
   Mudrane GG Tablets
   Phenobarbital Elixir and Tablets
   Phenobarbital Elixir & Tablets
   Phenobarbital Elixir USP 20 mg/5 mL
   Phenobarbital Tablets, USP
   Quadrinal Tablets
   Rexatal Tablets
   Solfoton Tablets, Capsules
Phenobarbital Elixir and Tablets
   (ELI LILLY AND COMPANY)
Phenobarbital Elixir & Tablets
   (ROXANE LABORATORIES, INC.)
Phenobarbital Elixir USP 20 mg/5 mL
   (BARRE-NATIONAL INC.)
Phenobarbital Tablets, USP
   (WARNER CHILCOTT LABORATORIES)

PHENOBARBITAL SODIUM
   Phenobarbital Sodium Injection
   Phenobarbital Sodium in Tubex
Phenobarbital Sodium Injection
   (ELKINS-SINN, INC.)
Phenobarbital Sodium in Tubex
   (WYETH-AYERST LABORATORIES)

PHENOL
   Castellani Paint Modified
   Ostiderm
   Ostiderm Roll On

PHENOLPHTHALEIN
   Agoral Liquid
   Alophen Pills
   Dialose Plus Tablets

PHENOXYBENZAMINE HYDROCHLORIDE
   Dibenzyline Capsules

PHENSUXIMIDE
   Milontin Kapseals

PHENTERMINE HYDROCHLORIDE
   Adipex-P Tablets and Capsules
   Fastin Capsules
   Obenix Capsules
   Oby-Cap Phentermine HCl Capsules
   Oby-Trim Capsules
   Zantryl Capsules

PHENTERMINE RESIN
   Ionamin Capsules

PHENTOLAMINE MESYLATE
   Regitine
Phenurone Tablets (ABBOTT LABORATORIES)

PHENYL SALICYLATE
   Prosed/DS
   Urised Tablets

PHENYLALANINE
   Endorphenyl Capsules (d-Phenylalanine)

2-PHENYLBENZIMIDAZOLE-5-SULFONIC ACID
   Eucerin Dry Skin Care Daily Facial Lotion
     SPF 20

PHENYLEPHRINE BITARTRATE
   Duo-Medihaler Aerosol

PHENYLEPHRINE HYDROCHLORIDE
   AH-CHEW Chewable Tablets
   AH-CHEW D Chewable Tablets
   Albatussin SR Caplets
   Anaplex HD Cough Syrup
   Atrohist Plus Tablets
   Codimal DH Syrup
   Codimal DM Syrup
   Codimal PH Syrup
   Comhist LA Capsules
   D.A. Chewable Tablets
   Dallergy Caplets, Syrup, Tablets
   Deconsal Sprinkle Capsules
   Despec Liquid
   Despec SF
   Donatussin DC Syrup
   Donatussin Drops
   Dura-Gest Capsules
   Duratex Capsules
   Dura-Vent/DA Tablets
   Endal-HD
   Entex Capsules
   Entex Liquid
   Extendryl Chewable Tablets
   Extendryl Sr. & Jr. T.D. Capsules
   Extendryl Syrup
   4-Way Fast Acting Nasal Spray - Original
     Formula (regular & mentholated) & Metered
     Spray Pump (regular)
   Guaifenex Liquid
   HISTALET FORTE Tablets
   HISTINEX HC
   HISTINEX PV Syrup
   Histussin HC
   Liquibid-D Tablets
   Neo-Synephrine Hydrochloride 1% Carpuject
   Neo-Synephrine Hydrochloride 1% Injection
   Neo-Synephrine Hydrochloride (Ophthalmic)
   OMNIHIST L.A. Tablets
   Pediacof Cough Syrup
   Phenergan VC
   Phenergan VC with Codeine
   Phenylephrine HCl Nasal Soln. USP, 1%
   Phenylephrine Hydrochloride Injection
   Protid Tablets
   Rescon-GG Liquid
   Ru-Tuss with Hydrocodone
   Ru-Tuss Tablets
   Sinupan Capsules
   Tympagesic Ear Drops

UNDERLINE DENOTES GENERIC NAME

Vanex Forte Caplets
Vanex-HD Liquid
Phenylephrine HCl Nasal Soln. USP, 1%
(BARRE-NATIONAL INC.)
Phenylephrine Hydrochloride Injection
(ELKINS-SINN, INC.)

PHENYLEPHRINE TANNATE
Atrohist Pediatric Suspension
R-Tannate Tablets and Pediatric Suspension
Ricobid-D Pediatric Suspension
Ricobid Tablets and Pediatric Suspension
Rynatan Tablets
Rynatan-S Pediatric Suspension
Rynatuss Pediatric Suspension
Rynatuss Tablets
Triotann Pediatric Suspension
Triotann Tablets

PHENYLPROPANOLAMINE HYDROCHLORIDE
Atrohist Plus Tablets
Comtrex Maximum Strength Multi-Symptom
    Cold Reliever Tablets/Caplets/Liqui-
    Gels/Liquid
Despec Caplets
Despec Liquid
Despec SF
Dimetane-DC Cough Syrup
Duadacin Cold & Allergy Capsules
Dura-Gest Capsules
Duratex Capsules
Dura-Vent/A Capsules
Dura-Vent Tablets
E.N.T. Tablets
Entex Capsules
Entex LA Tablets
Entex Liquid
Exgest LA Tablets
Gelpirin CCF Tablets
Guaifenex Liquid
HISTALET FORTE Tablets
HISTINEX DM
Nolamine Timed-Release Tablets
Ornade Spansule Capsules
Phenylpropanolamine HCl and Guaifenesin
    Long Acting Tablets
Poly-Histine CS
Poly-Histine DM Syrup
Poly-Histine-D Capsules
Poly-Histine-D Elixir
Poly-Histine-D Ped Caps
Propagest Tablets
Rescon Liquid
Ru-Tuss with Hydrocodone
Ru-Tuss Tablets
Sinulin Tablets
SINUVENT Tablets
Triaminic Expectorant with Codeine
Triaminic Expectorant DH
Triaminic Oral Infant Drops
Vanex Forte Caplets
Phenylpropanolamine HCl and
    Guaifenesin Long Acting Tablets
    (DURAMED PHARMACEUTICALS, INC.)

PHENYLTOLOXAMINE CITRATE
Comhist LA Capsules
Kutrase Capsules
Poly-Histine Elixir
Poly-Histine-D Capsules
Poly-Histine-D Elixir
Poly-Histine-D Ped Caps

PHENYLTOLOXAMINE DIHYDROGEN CITRATE
Magsal Tablets

PHENYTOIN
Dilantin Infatabs
Dilantin-125 Suspension

PHENYTOIN SODIUM
Dilantin Kapseals
Dilantin Parenteral
Phenytoin Sodium Injection
Phenytoin Sodium Injection (ELKINS-SINN, INC.)
PhosChol Concentrate
(AMERICAN LECITHIN COMPANY)
PhosChol Forte (AMERICAN LECITHIN COMPANY)
PhosChol 565 Softgels
(AMERICAN LECITHIN COMPANY)
PhosChol 900 Softgels
(AMERICAN LECITHIN COMPANY)
PhosLo Tablets (BRAINTREE LABORATORIES, INC.)

PHOSPHATIDYLCHOLINE
PhosChol Concentrate
PhosChol Forte
PhosChol 565 Softgels
PhosChol 900 Softgels
Phospholine Iodide
(WYETH-AYERST LABORATORIES)

PHOSPHORIC ACID
Emecheck
Emetrol Solution - Cherry
Emetrol Solution - Lemon-Mint
Photoplex Broad Spectrum Sunscreen Lotion
(ALLERGAN HERBERT)
Phrenilin Forte Capsules
(CARNRICK LABORATORIES, INC.)
Phrenilin Tablets
(CARNRICK LABORATORIES, INC.)
pH-Stabil Skin Protectant Cream
(HERMAL PHARMACEUTICAL LABORATORIES, INC.)

PHYSOSTIGMINE SALICYLATE
Antilirium Injectable

PHYTONADIONE
AquaMEPHYTON Injection
Konakion Injection
Mephyton Tablets

PILOCARPINE HYDROCHLORIDE
Salagen Tablets
Pima Syrup (FLEMING & COMPANY)

PIMOZIDE
Orap Tablets

PINDOLOL
Pindolol Tablets
Pindolol Tablets
Pindolol Tablets
Pindolol Tablets, 5 mg
Pindolol Tablets, 10 mg
Pindolol Tablets
Visken Tablets
Pindolol Tablets (GENEVA PHARMACEUTICALS, INC.)
Pindolol Tablets (PAR PHARMACEUTICAL, INC.)
Pindolol Tablets (MYLAN PHARMACEUTICALS INC.)
Pindolol Tablets, 5 mg (NOVOPHARM, USA INC.)
Pindolol Tablets, 10 mg (NOVOPHARM, USA INC.)
Pindolol Tablets
(WARNER CHILCOTT LABORATORIES)

PIPECURONIUM BROMIDE
Arduan

PIPERACILLIN SODIUM
Pipracil
Zosyn
Zosyn Pharmacy Bulk Package

PIPERONYL BUTOXIDE
Rid Lice Killing Shampoo
Pipracil (LEDERLE LABORATORIES)

PIRBUTEROL ACETATE
Maxair Autohaler
Maxair Inhaler

PIROXICAM
Feldene Capsules
Piroxicam Capsules
Piroxicam Capsules
Piroxicam Capsules
Piroxicam Capsules, 10 mg
Piroxicam Capsules, 20 mg
Piroxicam Capsules
(LEDERLE STANDARD PRODUCTS)
Piroxicam Capsules
(MYLAN PHARMACEUTICALS INC.)
Piroxicam Capsules
(PAR PHARMACEUTICAL, INC.)
Piroxicam Capsules, 10 mg
(NOVOPHARM, USA INC.)
Piroxicam Capsules, 20 mg
(NOVOPHARM, USA INC.)
Placidyl Capsules (ABBOTT LABORATORIES)

PLAGUE VACCINE
Plague Vaccine
Plague Vaccine
(MILES INC. PHARMACEUTICAL DIVISION
BIOLOGICAL PRODUCTS)
Plaquenil Sulfate Tablets
(SANOFI WINTHROP PHARMACEUTICALS)

PLASMA FRACTIONS, HUMAN
Autoplex T, Anti-Inhibitor Coagulant Complex,
    Dried, Heat Treated
Buminate 5%, Albumin (Human),
    USP, 5% Solution
Buminate 25%, Albumin (Human),
    USP, 25% Solution
Hyperab Rabies Immune Globulin (Human)
HyperHep Hepatitis B Immune Globulin
    (Human)
Hyper-Tet Tetanus Immune Globulin (Human)
HypRho-D Full Dose Rho (D) Immune
    Globulin (Human)
HypRho-D Mini-Dose Rho (D) Immune
    Globulin (Human)
Profilate OSD Antihemophilic Factor (Human)
Protenate 5%, Plasma Protein Fraction (Human),
    USP, 5% Solution
Venoglobulin-I, Immune Globulin
    Intravenous (Human)
Plasma-Plex Plasma Protein Fraction (Human)
(ARMOUR PHARMACEUTICAL COMPANY)

PLASMA PROTEIN FRACTION (HUMAN)
Plasma-Plex Plasma Protein Fraction (Human)
Plasmatein 5% Plasma Protein Fraction (Human)
Plasmatein 5% Plasma Protein Fraction
(Human) (ALPHA THERAPEUTIC CORPORATION)
Platinol
(BRISTOL-MYERS SQUIBB ONCOLOGY DIVISION)
Platinol-AQ Injection
(BRISTOL-MYERS SQUIBB ONCOLOGY DIVISION)
Plegine Tablets (WYETH-AYERST LABORATORIES)
Plendil Extended-Release Tablets (ASTRA MERCK)

PLICAMYCIN
Mithracin

PNEUMOCOCCAL VACCINE, POLYVALENT
Pneumovax 23
Pnu-Imune 23
Pneumomist Tablets (ECR PHARMACEUTICALS)
Pneumotussin HC Cough Syrup
(ECR PHARMACEUTICALS)
Pneumovax 23 (MERCK & CO., INC.)
Pnu-Imune 23 (LEDERLE LABORATORIES)

UNDERLINE DENOTES GENERIC NAME

PODOFILOX
Condylox

POLIOVIRUS VACCINE INACTIVATED, TRIVALENT TYPES 1,2,3
IPOL Poliovirus Vaccine Inactivated

POLIOVIRUS VACCINE LIVE ORAL, TRIVALENT, TYPES 1,2,3 (SABIN)
Orimune
Polocaine Injection, USP (ASTRA USA, INC.)
Polycitra Syrup
(BAKER NORTON PHARMACEUTICALS, INC.)
Polycitra-K Crystals
(BAKER NORTON PHARMACEUTICALS, INC.)
Polycitra-K Oral Solution
(BAKER NORTON PHARMACEUTICALS, INC.)
Polycitra-LC
(BAKER NORTON PHARMACEUTICALS, INC.)
Polycose Glucose Polymers
(ROSS PRODUCTS DIVISION)

POLYESTRADIOL PHOSPHATE
Estradurin

POLYETHYLENE GLYCOL
Colyte and Colyte flavored
GoLYTELY
NuLYTELY
Polygam S/D, Immune Globulin Intravenous (Human) (AMERICAN RED CROSS)
Poly-Histine CS (BOCK PHARMACAL COMPANY)
Poly-Histine DM Syrup
(BOCK PHARMACAL COMPANY)
Poly-Histine Elixir (BOCK PHARMACAL COMPANY)
Poly-Histine-D Capsules
(BOCK PHARMACAL COMPANY)
Poly-Histine-D Elixir
(BOCK PHARMACAL COMPANY)
Poly-Histine-D Ped Caps
(BOCK PHARMACAL COMPANY)

POLYMYXIN B SULFATE
Cortisporin Cream
Cortisporin Ointment
Cortisporin Ophthalmic Ointment Sterile
Cortisporin Ophthalmic Suspension Sterile
Cortisporin Otic Solution Sterile
Cortisporin Otic Suspension Sterile
LazerSporin-C Solution
Neosporin G.U. Irrigant Sterile
Neosporin Original Ointment
Neosporin Plus Maximum Strength Cream
Neosporin Plus Maximum Strength Ointment
Neosporin Ophthalmic Ointment Sterile
Neosporin Ophthalmic Solution Sterile
PediOtic Suspension Sterile
Polymyxin B Sulfate, Aerosporin Brand Sterile Powder
Polysporin Ointment
Polysporin Ophthalmic Ointment Sterile
Polysporin Powder
Polytrim Ophthalmic Solution Sterile
Terramycin with Polymyxin B Sulfate Ophthalmic Ointment
Polymyxin B Sulfate, Aerosporin Brand Sterile Powder (BURROUGHS WELLCOME CO.)

POLYSACCHARIDE IRON COMPLEX
May-Vita Elixir
Niferex-150 Capsules
Niferex Daily Tablets
Niferex Elixir
Niferex-150 Forte Capsules
Niferex Forte Elixir
Niferex Tablets
Niferex w/Vitamin C Tablets
Niferex-PN Forte Tablets
Niferex-PN Tablets

Nu-Iron 150 Capsules
Nu-Iron V Tablets
Nu-Iron Elixir
Nu-Iron Plus Elixir
Polysporin Ointment (WARNER WELLCOME)
Polysporin Ophthalmic Ointment Sterile
(BURROUGHS WELLCOME CO.)
Polysporin Powder (WARNER WELLCOME)

POLYTHIAZIDE
Minizide Capsules
Polytrim Ophthalmic Solution Sterile
(ALLERGAN, INC.)

POLYURETHANE FILM
Mitraflex Wound Dressing

POLYURETHANE FOAM
Epi-Lock Wound Dressing
Poly-Vi-Flor Drops
(MEAD JOHNSON NUTRITIONALS)
Poly-Vi-Flor Tablets
(MEAD JOHNSON NUTRITIONALS)
Poly-Vi-Flor with Iron Drops
(MEAD JOHNSON NUTRITIONALS)
Poly-Vi-Flor with Iron Tablets
(MEAD JOHNSON NUTRITIONALS)
Pondimin Tablets (A. H. ROBINS COMPANY, INC.)
Ponstel (PARKE-DAVIS)
Pontocaine Hydrochloride for Spinal Anesthesia
(SANOFI WINTHROP PHARMACEUTICALS)
Potaba (GLENWOOD, INC.)

POTASSIUM ACID PHOSPHATE
K-Phos M.F. Tablets
K-Phos Original Formula "Sodium Free" Tablets
K-Phos No. 2 Tablets

POTASSIUM BICARBONATE
Alka-Seltzer Effervescent Antacid
K+ Care ET
K-Lyte/Cl 50 Effervescent Tablets
K-Lyte/Cl Tablets
K-Lyte & K-Lyte DS Effervescent Tablets
Klor-Con/EF Tablets
Klorvess Effervescent Granules
Klorvess Effervescent Tablets

POTASSIUM BITARTRATE
Ceo-Two Rectal Suppositories

POTASSIUM CHLORIDE
Chlor-3 Condiment
K+ 8 Tablets
K+ Care Powder
K-Dur Microburst Release System (potassium chloride, USP) E.R. Tablets
K-Lor Powder Packets
K-Lyte/Cl 50 Effervescent Tablets
K-Lyte/Cl Tablets
K-Norm Extended-Release Capsules
K-Tab Filmtab
K+ 10 Tablets
Kaon CL 10
Klor-Con 8/Klor-Con 10 Tablets
Klor-Con Powder
Klor-Con/25 Powder
Klorvess Effervescent Granules
Klorvess Effervescent Tablets
Klorvess 10% Liquid
Klotrix Tablets
Kolyum Liquid
Micro-K Extencaps
Micro-K 10 Extencaps
Micro-K LS Packets
NuLYTELY
Potassium Chloride Extended-release Capsules, USP
Potassium Chloride Extended-Release Tablets, USP

Potassium Chloride Oral Soln. USP, 10% Sugar-Free
Potassium Chloride Oral Soln. USP, 10% Yellow
Potassium Chloride Oral Soln. USP, 20% Sugar-Free
Rum-K Syrup
Slow-K Extended-Rlease Tablets
Ten-K Extended-Release Tablets
Potassium Chloride Extended-release Capsules, USP (ETHEX CORPORATION)
Potassium Chloride Extended-Release Tablets, USP (WARNER CHILCOTT LABORATORIES)
Potassium Chloride Oral Soln. USP, 10% Sugar-Free (BARRE-NATIONAL INC.)
Potassium Chloride Oral Soln. USP, 10% Yellow
(BARRE-NATIONAL INC.)
Potassium Chloride Oral Soln. USP, 20% Sugar-Free (BARRE-NATIONAL INC.)

POTASSIUM CITRATE
Citrolith Tablets
K-Lyte/Cl 50 Effervescent Tablets
K-Lyte/Cl Tablets
K-Lyte & K-Lyte DS Effervescent Tablets
Polycitra Syrup
Polycitra-K Crystals
Polycitra-K Oral Solution
Polycitra-LC
Urocit-K

POTASSIUM GLUCONATE
Kolyum Liquid
Potassium Gluconate Elixir USP
Potassium Gluconate Elixir USP
(BARRE-NATIONAL INC.)

POTASSIUM IODIDE
Elixophyllin-KI Elixir
Mudrane Tablets
Pediacof Cough Syrup
Pima Syrup
Quadrinal Tablets
SSKI Solution

POTASSIUM PHOSPHATE, MONOBASIC
K-Phos Neutral Tablets
K-Phos Original Formula "Sodium Free'" Tablets
Povidine Douche (BARRE-NATIONAL INC.)
Povidine Surgical Scrub (BARRE-NATIONAL INC.)
Povidine Topical Soln. 1% (BARRE-NATIONAL INC.)

POVIDONE IODINE
Betadine Disposable Medicated Douche
Betadine First Aid Cream
Betadine Medicated Douche
Betadine Medicated Gel
Betadine Medicated Vaginal Suppositories
Betadine Ointment
Betadine Pre-Mixed Medicated Disposable Douche
Betadine Skin Cleanser
Betadine Solution
Betadine Surgical Scrub
Massengill Medicated Disposable Douche
Massengill Medicated Liquid Concentrate
Povidone Iodine Ointment 10%
Povidone Iodine Ointment 10%
(BARRE-NATIONAL INC.)

PRALIDOXIME CHLORIDE
Protopam Chloride for Injection
PrameGel (GENDERM CORPORATION)
Pramilet FA (ROSS PRODUCTS DIVISION)
Pramosone Cream, Lotion & Ointment
(FERNDALE LABORATORIES, INC.)

PRAMOXINE HYDROCHLORIDE
Analpram-HC Rectal Cream 1% and 2.5%
Anusol Hemorrhoidal Ointment
Caladryl Clear Lotion

Caladryl Cream For Kids
Caladryl Lotion
Cortic Ear Drops
Epifoam
PrameGel
Pramosone Cream, Lotion & Ointment
Prax Cream & Lotion
ProctoCream-HC
Proctofoam-HC
Zone-A Cream 1%
Pravachol (BRISTOL-MYERS SQUIBB COMPANY)

PRAVASTATIN SODIUM
Pravachol
Prax Cream & Lotion
(FERNDALE LABORATORIES, INC.)

PRAZIQUANTEL
Biltricide Tablets

PRAZOSIN HYDROCHLORIDE
Minipress Capsules
Minizide Capsules
Prazosin HCl Capsules
Prazosin Hydrochloride Capsules
Prazosin Hydrochloride Capsules
Prazosin HCl Capsules
(LEDERLE STANDARD PRODUCTS)
Prazosin Hydrochloride Capsules
(MYLAN PHARMACEUTICALS INC.)
Prazosin Hydrochloride Capsules
(WARNER CHILCOTT LABORATORIES)
PreCare Caplets (NORTHAMPTON MEDICAL, INC.)

PREDNICARBATE
Dermatop Emollient Cream 0.1%
Prednicen-M 21-Pak
(CENTRAL PHARMACEUTICALS, INC.)

PREDNISOLONE
Prelone Syrup

PREDNISOLONE ACETATE
Blephamide Liquifilm Sterile Ophthalmic
Suspension

PREDNISOLONE SODIUM PHOSPHATE
Hydeltrasol Injection, Sterile
Pediapred Oral Liquid

PREDNISOLONE TEBUTATE
Hydeltra-T.B.A. Sterile Suspension

PREDNISONE
Deltasone Tablets
Liquid Pred Syrup
Prednicen-M 21-Pak
Prednisone Tablets, Oral Solution & Intensol
Sterapred DS Unipak
Sterapred DS 12 Day Unipak
Sterapred Unipak
Prednisone Tablets, Oral Solution & Intensol
(ROXANE LABORATORIES, INC.)
**Prefrin Liquifilm Vasoconstrictor and Lubricant
Eye Drops** (ALLERGAN, INC.)
Pregnyl (ORGANON, INC.)
Prelone Syrup (MURO PHARMACEUTICAL, INC.)
Prelu-2 Timed Release Capsules
(BOEHRINGER INGELHEIM PHARMACEUTICALS, INC.)
Premarin Intravenous
(WYETH-AYERST LABORATORIES)
Premarin with Methyltestosterone
(WYETH-AYERST LABORATORIES)
Premarin Tablets
(WYETH-AYERST LABORATORIES)
Premarin Vaginal Cream
(WYETH-AYERST LABORATORIES)
Prenatal Maternal (ETHEX CORPORATION)
Prenatal MR 90 Fe (ETHEX CORPORATION)
Prenatal Rx (ETHEX CORPORATION)

Prenatal Z (ETHEX CORPORATION)
Prenate 90 Tablets (BOCK PHARMACAL COMPANY)
Prepidil Gel (THE UPJOHN COMPANY)
PreSun 15, 25 and 46 Moisturizing Sunscreens
(BRISTOL-MYERS PRODUCTS)
PreSun Active 15 and 30 Clear Gel Sunscreens
(BRISTOL-MYERS PRODUCTS)
PreSun for Kids Lotion
(BRISTOL-MYERS PRODUCTS)
PreSun 23 and For Kids, Spray Mist Sunscreens
(BRISTOL-MYERS PRODUCTS)
PreSun 15 and 29 Sensitive Skin Sunscreens
(BRISTOL-MYERS PRODUCTS)

PRILOCAINE
Emla Cream
Prilosec Delayed-Release Capsules (ASTRA MERCK)
Primacor Injection
(SANOFI WINTHROP PHARMACEUTICALS)
Primaxin I.M. (MERCK & CO., INC.)
Primaxin I.V. (MERCK & CO., INC.)
Primer Unna Boot (GLENWOOD, INC.)

PRIMIDONE
Mysoline Suspension
Mysoline Tablets
Prinivil Tablets (MERCK & CO., INC.)
Prinzide Tablets (MERCK & CO., INC.)
Priscoline Hydrochloride Ampuls
(CIBA PHARMACEUTICAL COMPANY)
Privine Nasal Solution and Drops
(CIBA CONSUMER PHARMACEUTICALS)
Privine Nasal Spray
(CIBA CONSUMER PHARMACEUTICALS)
Pro-Banthine Tablets
(ROBERTS PHARMACEUTICAL CORPORATION)

PROBENECID
Ampicillin-Probenecid for Oral Suspension
Benemid Tablets
ColBENEMID Tablets
Probenecid Tablets
Probenecid Tablets
(MYLAN PHARMACEUTICALS INC.)

PROBUCOL
Lorelco Tablets

PROCAINAMIDE HYDROCHLORIDE
Procainamide Hydrochloride Injection
Procan SR Tablets
Procainamide Hydrochloride Injection
(ELKINS-SINN, INC.)

PROCAINE HYDROCHLORIDE
Novocain Hydrochloride for Spinal Anesthesia
Novocain Hydrochloride Injection
Procan SR Tablets (PARKE-DAVIS)

PROCARBAZINE HYDROCHLORIDE
Matulane Capsules
Procardia Capsules
(PRATT PHARMACEUTICALS DIVISION)
Procardia XL Extended Release Tablets
(PRATT PHARMACEUTICALS DIVISION)

PROCHLORPERAZINE
Compazine Injection
Compazine Multi-dose Vials
Compazine Prefilled Disposable Syringes
Compazine Spansule Capsules
Compazine Suppositories
Compazine Syrup
Compazine Tablets

PROCHLORPERAZINE EDISYLATE
Prochlorperazine Edisylate Injection
Prochlorperazine Edisylate in Tubex
Prochlorperazine Edisylate Injection
(ELKINS-SINN, INC.)

Prochlorperazine Edisylate in Tubex
(WYETH-AYERST LABORATORIES)
Pro-Clude Transparent Wound Dressing
(CALGON VESTAL LABORATORIES, INC.)
Procrit for Injection (ORTHO BIOTECH INC.)
ProctoCream-HC (REED & CARNRICK)
ProctoCream-HC 2.5% (REED & CARNRICK)
Proctofoam-HC (REED & CARNRICK)

PROCYCLIDINE HYDROCHLORIDE
Kemadrin Tablets
Prodium (BRECKENRIDGE PHARMACEUTICAL, INC.)
**Profasi (chorionic gonadotropin for injection,
USP)** (SERONO LABORATORIES, INC.)
Profilate OSD Antihemophilic Factor (Human)
(ALPHA THERAPEUTIC CORPORATION)
Profilnine Heat-Treated Factor IX Complex
(ALPHA THERAPEUTIC CORPORATION)
Progestasert System (ALZA PHARMACEUTICALS)

PROGESTERONE
Progestasert System
Proglycem Capsules
(BAKER NORTON PHARMACEUTICALS, INC.)
Proglycem Suspension
(BAKER NORTON PHARMACEUTICALS, INC.)
Prograf (FUJISAWA USA, INC.)
Pro-Hepatone Capsules (MARLYN HEALTH CARE)
**ProHIBiT Haemophilus b Conjugate Vaccine
(Diphtheria Toxoid Conjugate)**
(CONNAUGHT LABORATORIES, INC.)
Prohim (BAKER NORTON PHARMACEUTICALS, INC.)
**Prolastin Alpha+DN,1 -Proteinase Inhibitor
(Human)** (MILES INC. PHARMACEUTICAL
DIVISION BIOLOGICAL PRODUCTS)
Proleukin for Injection
(CHIRON THERAPEUTICS)
Prolixin Decanoate (APOTHECON)
Prolixin Elixir (APOTHECON)
Prolixin Enanthate (APOTHECON)
Prolixin Injection (APOTHECON)
Prolixin Oral Concentrate (APOTHECON)
Prolixin Tablets (APOTHECON)
Proloprim Tablets (BURROUGHS WELLCOME CO.)

PROMETHAZINE HYDROCHLORIDE
Mepergan Injection
Mepergan in Tubex
Phenergan with Codeine
Phenergan with Dextromethorphan
Phenergan Injection
Phenergan Suppositories
Phenergan Syrup Fortis
Phenergan Syrup Plain
Phenergan Tablets
Phenergan in Tubex
Phenergan VC
Phenergan VC with Codeine
Promethazine Hydrochloride Injection
Promethazine VC with Codeine
Prometh Syrup Plain
Prometh with Codeine Cough Syrup
Prometh VC Plain
Prometh VC with Codeine Cough Syrup
Prometh with Dextromethorphan Cough Syrup
Promethazine Hydrochloride Injection
(ELKINS-SINN, INC.)
Promethazine VC with Codeine
(WARNER CHILCOTT LABORATORIES)
Prometh Syrup Plain (BARRE-NATIONAL INC.)
Prometh with Codeine Cough Syrup
(BARRE-NATIONAL INC.)
Prometh VC Plain (BARRE-NATIONAL INC.)
Prometh VC with Codeine Cough Syrup
(BARRE-NATIONAL INC.)
Prometh with Dextromethorphan Cough Syrup
(BARRE-NATIONAL INC.)

UNDERLINE DENOTES GENERIC NAME

Promit (MEDISAN PHARMACEUTICALS INC.)
Promote High Protein Liquid Nutrition
(ROSS PRODUCTS DIVISION)
Promote With Fiber, High-Protein Liquid Nutrition (ROSS PRODUCTS DIVISION)

PROPAFENONE HYDROCHLORIDE
Rythmol Tablets–150mg, 225mg, 300mg
Propagest Tablets (CARNRICK LABORATORIES, INC.)

PROPANTHELINE BROMIDE
Pro-Banthine Tablets
Propantheline Bromide Tablets
Propantheline Bromide Tablets
Propantheline Bromide Tablets
(PAR PHARMACEUTICAL, INC.)
Propantheline Bromide Tablets
(ROXANE LABORATORIES, INC.)
Prophyllin CCC Topical Emollient Ointment
(RYSTAN COMPANY, INC.)
Proplex T, Factor IX Complex, Heat Treated
(BAXTER HEALTHCARE CORPORATION)

PROPOFOL
Diprivan Injection
Propoxyphene Compound Capsules
(MYLAN PHARMACEUTICALS INC.)

PROPOXYPHENE HYDROCHLORIDE
Darvon Compound-65 Pulvules
Darvon Pulvules
PC-CAP Propoxyphene Hydrochloride Compound, USP
PP-CAP Propoxyphene Hydrochloride Capsules, USP
Propoxyphene Compound Capsules
Propoxyphene Hydrochloride & Acetaminophen Tablets
Propoxyphene Hydrochloride Capsules
Wygesic Tablets
Propoxyphene Hydrochloride & Acetaminophen Tablets (MYLAN PHARMACEUTICALS INC.)
Propoxyphene Hydrochloride Capsules
(MYLAN PHARMACEUTICALS INC.)

PROPOXYPHENE NAPSYLATE
Darvocet-N 50 Tablets
Darvocet-N 100 Tablets
Darvon-N Suspension & Tablets
Propoxyphene Napsylate/Acetaminophen Tablets
Propoxyphene Napsylate & Acetaminophen Tablets
Propoxyphene Napsylate/Acetaminophen Tablets
(GENEVA PHARMACEUTICALS, INC.)
Propoxyphene Napsylate & Acetaminophen Tablets (MYLAN PHARMACEUTICALS INC.)

PROPRANOLOL HYDROCHLORIDE
Inderal Injectable
Inderal Tablets
Inderal LA Long Acting Capsules
Inderide Tablets
Inderide LA Long Acting Capsules
Propranolol HCl Tablets, USP
Propranolol Hydrochloride Intensol & Oral Solution
Propranolol Hydrochloride Tablets
Propranolol Hydrochloride Tablets
Propranolol Hydrochloride Tablets, USP
Propranolol Hydrochloride & Hydrochlorothiazide Tablets
Propranolol HCl Tablets, USP
(WARNER CHILCOTT LABORATORIES)
Propranolol Hydrochloride Intensol & Oral Solution (ROXANE LABORATORIES, INC.)
Propranolol Hydrochloride Tablets
(LEDERLE STANDARD PRODUCTS)
Propranolol Hydrochloride Tablets
(MYLAN PHARMACEUTICALS INC.)

Propranolol Hydrochloride Tablets, USP
(WATSON LABORATORIES, INC.)
Propranolol Hydrochloride & Hydrochlorothiazide Tablets
(MYLAN PHARMACEUTICALS INC.)
Propulsid (JANSSEN PHARMACEUTICA INC.)

PROPYLENE GLYCOL
Eucerin Dry Skin Care Lotion

PROPYLTHIOURACIL
Propylthiouracil Tablets
Propylthiouracil Tablets
(LEDERLE STANDARD PRODUCTS)
Proscar Tablets (MERCK & CO., INC.)
Prosed/DS (STAR PHARMACEUTICALS, INC.)
ProSom Tablets (ABBOTT LABORATORIES)
Prostep (nicotine transdermal system)
(LEDERLE LABORATORIES)
Prostigmin Injectable
(ICN PHARMACEUTICALS, INC.)
Prostigmin Tablets (ICN PHARMACEUTICALS, INC.)
Prostin E2 Suppository (THE UPJOHN COMPANY)
Prostin VR Pediatric Sterile Solution
(THE UPJOHN COMPANY)

PROTAMINE SULFATE
Protamine Sulfate Ampoules & Vials
Protamine Sulfate Injection (Preservative-Free)
Protamine Sulfate Ampoules & Vials
(ELI LILLY AND COMPANY)
Protamine Sulfate Injection (Preservative-Free)
(ELKINS-SINN, INC.)
Protegra Antioxidant Vitamin & Mineral Supplement (LEDERLE LABORATORIES)

PROTEIN HYDROLYSATE
Alimentum Protein Hydrolysate Formula With Iron

PROTEIN PREPARATIONS
Marlyn Formula 50 Capsules
Nepro Specialized Liquid Nutrition
Nursoy, Soy Protein Formula for Infants, Concentrated Liquid, Ready-to-Feed, and Powder
Plasmatein 5% Plasma Protein Fraction (Human)
Protenate 5%, Plasma Protein Fraction (Human), USP, 5% Solution
(BAXTER HEALTHCARE CORPORATION)

PROTEOLYTIC ENZYMES
Arco-Lase Tablets
Cotazym
Kutrase Capsules
Ku-Zyme Capsules
Ku-Zyme HP Capsules
Panafil Ointment
Panafil-White Ointment
Travase Ointment
Protid Tablets (LUNSCO, INC.)

PROTIRELIN
THYREL TRH
Protopam Chloride for Injection
(WYETH-AYERST LABORATORIES)
Protostat Tablets
(ORTHO PHARMACEUTICAL CORPORATION)

PROTRIPTYLINE HYDROCHLORIDE
Vivactil Tablets
Protropin (GENENTECH, INC.)
Proventil Inhalation Aerosol
(SCHERING CORPORATION)
Proventil Repetabs Tablets
(SCHERING CORPORATION)
Proventil Solution for Inhalation 0.5%
(SCHERING CORPORATION)
Proventil Inhalation Solution 0.083%
(SCHERING CORPORATION)

Proventil Syrup (SCHERING CORPORATION)
Proventil Tablets (SCHERING CORPORATION)
Provera Tablets (THE UPJOHN COMPANY)
Provocholine for Inhalation
(ROCHE LABORATORIES)
Proxacol (WARNER WELLCOME)
Prozac Pulvules & Liquid, Oral Solution
(DISTA PRODUCTS COMPANY)

PSEUDOEPHEDRINE HYDROCHLORIDE
Actifed Allergy Daytime/Nighttime Caplets
Actifed Plus Tablets and Caplets
Actifed with Codeine Cough Syrup
Actifed Sinus Daytime/Nighttime Caplets and Tablets
Actifed Syrup
Actifed Tablets
Anatuss DM Syrup
Anatuss DM Tablets
Anatuss LA Tablets
Atrohist Sprinkle Capsules
Benadryl Allergy/Sinus Headache Caplets
Benadryl Cold/Flu Tablets
Benadryl Decongestant Liquid
Benadryl Decongestant Tablets
Benylin Multi-Symptom
Brexin L.A. Capsules
Bromarest DX Cough Syrup
Bromfed Capsules (Extended-Release)
Bromfed Tablets
Bromfed-DM Cough Syrup
Bromfed-PD Capsules (Extended-Release)
Codimal-L.A. Capsules
Codimal-L.A. HALF Capsules
Allergy-Sinus Comtrex Multi-Symptom Allergy Sinus Formula Tablets & Caplets
Comtrex Maximum Strength Multi-Symptom Cold Reliever Tablets/Caplets/Liqui-Gels/Liquid
Non-Drowsy Comtrex Maximum Strength Caplets
Congess Jr. T.D. Capsules
Congess Sr. T.D. Capsules
Dallergy-JR Capsules
Decofed Liquid
Deconamine SR Capsules, Tablets, Syrup
Deconsal C Expectorant Syrup
Deconsal Pediatric Syrup
Deconsal II Tablets
D-FEDA II Tablets
Dimetane-DX Cough Syrup
Dura-Tap/PD Capsules
Duratuss Tablets
Duratuss HD Elixir
Entex PSE Tablets
Fedahist Gyrocaps
Fedahist Timecaps
Guaifed Capsules (Extended-Release)
Guaifed-PD Capsules (Extended-Release)
Guaifenex PSE 120 Extended-release Tablets
Guaimax-D Tablets
Isoclor Expectorant
Kronofed-A Kronocaps
Kronofed-A-Jr. Kronocaps
Lodrane LD Capsules
Lodrane Liquid
Nasabid Capsules
Nasatab LA Tablets
Novahistine DH (+)
Novahistine Expectorant (+)
Nucofed Expectorant
Nucofed Pediatric Expectorant
Nucofed Syrup and Capsules
P-V-TUSSIN Syrup
PediaCare Cold-Allergy Chewable Tablets
PediaCare Cough-Cold Chewable Tablets

UNDERLINE DENOTES GENERIC NAME

PediaCare Cough-Cold Liquid
PediaCare Infants' Decongestant Drops
PediaCare NightRest Cough-Cold Liquid
Pseudoephedrine Hydrochloride Tablets
Pseudoephedrine HCl and Guaifenesin Extended
  Release Tablets
Rescon Capsules
Rescon-DM Liquid
Rescon-ED Capsules
Rescon JR Capsules
Respaire-SR Capsules 60, 120
Robitussin-DAC Syrup
Rondec Oral Drops
Rondec Syrup
Rondec Tablet
Rondec-DM Oral Drops
Rondec-DM Syrup
Rondec-TR Tablet
Ru-Tuss DE Tablets
Seldane-D Extended-Release Tablets
Semprex-D Capsules
Semprex-D
Sine-Aid IB Caplets
Sine-Aid Maximum Strength Sinus Headache
  Gelcaps, Caplets and Tablets
Sinutab Non Drying Liquid Caps
Sinutab Maximum Strength Sinus Allergy Tablets
Sinutab Sinus Maximum Strength Without
  Drowsiness Tablet
Sinutab Regular Strength Without Drowsiness
  Tablet
Children's Sudafed Liquid
Sudafed Cold & Cough Liquid Caps
Sudafed Cough Syrup
Sudafed Plus Liquid
Sudafed Plus Tablets
Sudafed Severe Cold Formula Tablets
Sudafed Sinus Tablets & Caplets
Sudafed 60 mg Tablets
Sudafed 30 mg Tablets
Sudafed 12 Hour Caplets
Syn-Rx Tablets
Touro A&H Capsules
Touro LA Caplets
Tuss-DA RX
Tussafed Drops & Syrup
Tussar-2
Tussar DM
Tussar SF
TYLENOL Allergy Sinus NightTime Caplets
Children's TYLENOL Cold Multi-Symptom
  Liquid Formula and Chewable Tablets
Children's TYLENOL Cold Multi-Symptom Plus
  Cough Liquid Formula and Chewable Tablets
TYLENOL Flu NightTime, Maximum Strength,
  Gelcaps
TYLENOL Cold Hot Medication Packets
TYLENOL Cold Medication No Drowsiness
  Formula Gelcaps and Caplets
TYLENOL Maximum Strength Allergy Sinus
  Medication Gelcaps and Caplets
TYLENOL Maximum Strength Allergy Sinus
  Nighttime Medicine
TYLENOL Cough Multi-Symptom Medication
  with Decongestant
TYLENOL Flu Maximum Strength Gelcaps
TYLENOL Cold Multi-Symptom Formula
  Medication Tablets and Caplets
TYLENOL, Maximum Strength, Sinus
  Medication Geltabs, Gelcaps, Caplets and
  Tablets
TYLENOL Flu NightTime, Maximum Strength,
  Hot Medication
ULTRABROM Capsules
ULTRABROM PD Capsules
Zephrex Tablets

Zephrex LA Tablets
Pseudoephedrine Hydrochloride Tablets
  (ROXANE LABORATORIES, INC.)
Pseudoephedrine HCl and Guaifenesin
  Extended Release Tablets
  (DURAMED PHARMACEUTICALS, INC.)

PSEUDOEPHEDRINE SULFATE
  Trinalin Repetabs Tablets
Psorcon Cream 0.05%
  (DERMIK LABORATORIES, INC.)
Psorcon Ointment 0.05%
  (DERMIK LABORATORIES, INC.)

PSYLLIUM PREPARATIONS
  Alramucil Instant Mix, Orange
  Alramucil Instant Mix, Regular
  Metamucil Effervescent Sugar Free, Lemon-
    Lime Flavor
  Metamucil Effervescent Sugar Free,
    Orange Flavor
  Metamucil Powder, Orange Flavor
  Metamucil Original Texture Powder,
    Regular Flavor
  Metamucil Smooth Texture, Citrus Flavor
  Metamucil Smooth Texture, Sugar Free,
    Citrus Flavor
  Metamucil Smooth Texture Powder,
    Orange Flavor
  Metamucil Smooth Texture Powder, Sugar Free,
    Orange Flavor
  Metamucil Smooth Texture, Sugar Free,
    Regular Flavor
  Metamucil Wafers, Apple Crisp and Cinnamon
    Spice Flavors
  Mylanta Natural Fiber Supplement

PUMPKIN SEED POWDER
  Urokin
Pulmocare Specialized Nutrition for Pulmonary
  Patients (ROSS PRODUCTS DIVISION)
Pulmozyme Inhalation (GENENTECH, INC.)
Pure-E Capsules and Liquid
  (HEALTH MAINTENANCE PROGRAMS, INC.)
Purge Concentrate (FLEMING & COMPANY)
Puri-Clens, Wound Deodorizer and Cleanser
  (SWEEN CORPORATION)
Purinethol Tablets (BURROUGHS WELLCOME CO.)

PYRAZINAMIDE
  Pyrazinamide Tablets
  Rifater
Pyrazinamide Tablets
  (LEDERLE STANDARD PRODUCTS)

PYRETHRUM EXTRACT
  Rid Lice Killing Shampoo
Pyridium (PARKE-DAVIS)

PYRIDOSTIGMINE BROMIDE
  Mestinon Injectable
  Mestinon Syrup
  Mestinon Tablets
  Mestinon Timespan Tablets
  Regonol

PYRILAMINE MALEATE
  Codimal DH Syrup
  Codimal DM Syrup
  Codimal PH Syrup
  4-Way Fast Acting Nasal Spray - Original
    Formula (regular & mentholated) & Metered
    Spray Pump (regular)
  HISTALET FORTE Tablets
  Poly-Histine Elixir
  Poly-Histine-D Capsules
  Poly-Histine-D Elixir
  Poly-Histine-D Ped Caps
  Ru-Tuss with Hydrocodone

  Triaminic Expectorant DH
  Triaminic Oral Infant Drops
  Vanex Forte Caplets

PYRILAMINE TANNATE
  Atrohist Pediatric Suspension
  R-Tannate Tablets and Pediatric Suspension
  Rynatan Tablets
  Rynatan-S Pediatric Suspension
  Triotann Pediatric Suspension
  Triotann Tablets

PYRIMETHAMINE
  Daraprim Tablets
  Fansidar Tablets
Pyrinyl Lice Control Kit (BARRE-NATIONAL INC.)
Pyrinyl Shampoo (BARRE-NATIONAL INC.)

PYRITHIONE ZINC
  DHS Zinc Dandruff Shampoo
PYRROXATE CAPSULES
  (ROBERTS PHARMACEUTICAL CORPORATION)

Q

Quadrinal Tablets
  (KNOLL PHARMACEUTICAL COMPANY)
Quarzan Capsules (ROCHE PRODUCTS INC.)

QUAZEPAM
  Doral Tablets
Questran Light
  (BRISTOL-MYERS SQUIBB COMPANY)
Questran Powder
  (BRISTOL-MYERS SQUIBB COMPANY)
Questran Tablets
  (BRISTOL-MYERS SQUIBB COMPANY)
Quibron Capsules
  (ROBERTS PHARMACEUTICAL CORPORATION)
Quibron-300 Capsules
  (ROBERTS PHARMACEUTICAL CORPORATION)
Quibron-T Tablets
  (ROBERTS PHARMACEUTICAL CORPORATION)
Quibron-T/SR Tablets
  (ROBERTS PHARMACEUTICAL CORPORATION)

QUINACRINE HYDROCHLORIDE
  Atabrine Hydrochloride Tablets
Quinaglute Dura-Tabs Tablets
  (BERLEX LABORATORIES)
Quinamm Tablets (MARION MERRELL DOW INC.)

QUINAPRIL HYDROCHLORIDE
  Accupril Tablets

QUINETHAZONE
  Hydromox Tablets
Quinidex Extentabs (A. H. ROBINS COMPANY, INC.)

QUINIDINE GLUCONATE
  Quinaglute Dura-Tabs Tablets

QUINIDINE POLYGALACTURONATE
  Cardioquin Tablets

QUINIDINE SULFATE
  Quinidex Extentabs
  Quinidine Sulfate Tablets
  Quinidine Sulfate Tablets
Quinidine Sulfate Tablets
  (LEDERLE STANDARD PRODUCTS)
Quinidine Sulfate Tablets
  (ROXANE LABORATORIES, INC.)

QUININE SULFATE
  Quinamm Tablets

UNDERLINE DENOTES GENERIC NAME

Q-vel Muscle Relaxant Pain Reliever
(CIBA CONSUMER PHARMACEUTICALS)

R

RH_O (D) IMMUNE GLOBULIN (HUMAN)
Gamulin Rh, Rh_O (D) Immune Globulin (Human)
HypRho-D Full Dose Rho (D) Immune Globulin
(Human)
HypRho-D Mini-Dose Rho (D) Immune Globulin
(Human)
MICRhoGAM Rh_O (D) Immune Globulin
(Human)
Mini-Gamulin Rh, Rh_O (D) Immune Globulin
(Human)
RhoGAM Rh_O (D) Immune Globulin (Human)
RMS Suppositories CII
(UPSHER-SMITH LABORATORIES, INC.)
R-Tannate Tablets and Pediatric Suspension
(WARNER CHILCOTT LABORATORIES)

RABIES IMMUNE GLOBULIN (HUMAN)
Hyperab Rabies Immune Globulin (Human)
Imogam Rabies Immune Globulin (Human)
Rabies Immune Globulin (Human), Imogam
Rabies Vaccine
**Rabies Immune Globulin (Human), Imogam
Rabies Vaccine**
(CONNAUGHT LABORATORIES, INC.)

RABIES VACCINE
Imovax Rabies I.D. Rabies Vaccine
Imovax Rabies Vaccine
Rabies Vaccine Adsorbed
Rabies Vaccine, Imovax Rabies I.D.
Rabies Vaccine Adsorbed
(SMITHKLINE BEECHAM PHARMACEUTICALS)
Rabies Vaccine, Imovax Rabies I.D.
(CONNAUGHT LABORATORIES, INC.)

RAMIPRIL
Altace Capsules

RANITIDINE HYDROCHLORIDE
Zantac 150 GELdose Capsules
Zantac 300 GELdose Capsules
Zantac Injection and Zantac Injection Premixed
Zantac Syrup
Zantac 150 & 300 Tablets
Zantac 150 EFFERdose Tablets
Zantac 150 EFFERdose Granules
Recombinant (BAXTER HEALTHCARE CORPORATION)
Recombivax HB (MERCK & CO., INC.)
Redutemp (INTERNATIONAL ETHICAL LABS.)
Refresh Plus Cellufresh Formula
(ALLERGAN, INC.)
Refresh Lubricating Eye Drops (ALLERGAN, INC.)
Refresh P.M. Lubricating Eye Ointment
(ALLERGAN, INC.)
Regitine (CIBA PHARMACEUTICAL COMPANY)
Reglan Injectable (A. H. ROBINS COMPANY, INC.)
Reglan Syrup (A. H. ROBINS COMPANY, INC.)
Reglan Tablets (A. H. ROBINS COMPANY, INC.)
Regonol (ORGANON INC.)
Regroton Tablets
(RHONE-POULENC RORER PHARMACEUTICALS INC.)
Regular Insulin
(NOVO NORDISK PHARMACEUTICALS INC.)
Regular Purified Pork Insulin
(NOVO NORDISK PHARMACEUTICALS INC.)
**Rehydralyte Oral Electrolyte Rehydration
Solution** (ROSS PRODUCTS DIVISION)

Relafen Tablets
(SMITHKLINE BEECHAM PHARMACEUTICALS)
**Relief Vasoconstrictor and Lubricating Eye
Drops** (ALLERGAN, INC.)
Remular-S (INTERNATIONAL ETHICAL LABS.)
Renacidin Irrigation
(GUARDIAN LABORATORIES)
Renal Multivitamin Formula Rx
(VITALINE CORPORATION)
Repan Tablets and Capsules
(EVERETT LABORATORIES, INC.)
REPAN-CF Tablets
(EVERETT LABORATORIES, INC.)
Replens Vaginal Moisturizer
(WARNER WELLCOME)
Rescon Capsules (ION LABORATORIES, INC.)
Rescon Liquid (ION LABORATORIES, INC.)
Rescon-DM Liquid (ION LABORATORIES, INC.)
Rescon-ED Capsules (ION LABORATORIES, INC.)
Rescon-GG Liquid (ION LABORATORIES, INC.)
Rescon JR Capsules (ION LABORATORIES, INC.)
Rescudose (Morphine Sulfate Oral Solution)
(ROXANE LABORATORIES, INC.)

RESERPINE
Demi-Regroton Tablets
Diupres Tablets
Diutensen-R Tablets
Hydropres Tablets
Regroton Tablets
Reserpine & Chlorothiazide Tablets
Ser-Ap-Es Tablets
Reserpine & Chlorothiazide Tablets
(MYLAN PHARMACEUTICALS INC.)

RESORCINOL
Bensulfoid Cream
Respaire-SR Capsules 60, 120 (LASER, INC.)
Respbid Tablets
(BOEHRINGER INGELHEIM PHARMACEUTICALS, INC.)
Restoril Capsules
(SANDOZ PHARMACEUTICALS CORPORATION)
Retin-A (tretinoin) Cream/Gel/Liquid
(ORTHO PHARMACEUTICAL CORPORATION
DERMATOLOGICAL DIVISION)
Retrovir Capsules (BURROUGHS WELLCOME CO.)
Retrovir I.V. Infusion (BURROUGHS WELLCOME CO.)
Retrovir Syrup (BURROUGHS WELLCOME CO.)
Reverse-numbered Package
(ELI LILLY AND COMPANY)
Reversol (ORGANON INC.)
Rexatal Tablets (REXAR PHARMACAL)
Rheomacrodex (MEDISAN PHARMACEUTICALS INC.)
Rheumatrex Methotrexate Dose Pack
(LEDERLE LABORATORIES)
Rhinocort Nasal Inhaler (ASTRA USA, INC.)
RhoGAM Rh_O (D) Immune Globulin (Human)
(ORTHO DIAGNOSTIC SYSTEMS INC.)

RIBAVIRIN
Virazole
Ribo-2 Enteric Tablets (Riboflavin 5' Phosphate)
(TYSON AND ASSOCIATES, INC.)

RIBOFLAVIN 5' PHOSPHATE
Ribo-2 Enteric Tablets (Riboflavin 5' Phosphate)

RICINOLEIC ACID
Aci-Jel Therapeutic Vaginal Jelly
Ricobid-D Pediatric Suspension
(RICO PHARMACAL)
Ricobid Tablets and Pediatric Suspension
(RICO PHARMACAL)
Rid Lice Control Spray
(PFIZER CONSUMER HEALTH CARE)
Rid Lice Killing Shampoo
(PFIZER CONSUMER HEALTH CARE)
Ridaura Capsules
(SMITHKLINE BEECHAM PHARMACEUTICALS)

RIFABUTIN
Mycobutin Capsules
Rifadin Capsules (MARION MERRELL DOW INC.)
Rifadin I.V. (MARION MERRELL DOW INC.)
Rifamate Capsules (MARION MERRELL DOW INC.)

RIFAMPIN
Rifadin Capsules
Rifadin I.V.
Rifamate Capsules
Rifater
Rimactane Capsules
Rifater (MARION MERRELL DOW INC.)
Rimactane Capsules
(CIBA PHARMACEUTICAL COMPANY)

RIMANTADINE HYDROCHLORIDE
Flumadine Tablets & Syrup
Rimso-50 (RESEARCH INDUSTRIES CORPORATION)
Risperdal (JANSSEN PHARMACEUTICA INC.)

RISPERIDONE
Risperdal
Ritalin Hydrochloride Tablets
(CIBA PHARMACEUTICAL COMPANY)
Ritalin-SR Tablets
(CIBA PHARMACEUTICAL COMPANY)

RITODRINE HYDROCHLORIDE
Yutopar Intravenous Injection
Yutopar Tablets
Robaxin Injectable (A. H. ROBINS COMPANY, INC.)
Robaxin Tablets (A. H. ROBINS COMPANY, INC.)
Robaxin-750 Tablets (A. H. ROBINS COMPANY, INC.)
Robaxisal Tablets (A. H. ROBINS COMPANY, INC.)
Robinul Forte Tablets
(A. H. ROBINS COMPANY, INC.)
Robinul Injectable (A. H. ROBINS COMPANY, INC.)
Robinul Tablets (A. H. ROBINS COMPANY, INC.)
Robitussin A-C Syrup
(A. H. ROBINS COMPANY, INC.)
Robitussin-DAC Syrup
(A. H. ROBINS COMPANY, INC.)
Rocaltrol Capsules (ROCHE LABORATORIES)
Rocephin Injectable Vials, ADD-Vantage
(ROCHE LABORATORIES)

ROCURONIUM BROMIDE
Zemuron
Roferon-A Injection (ROCHE LABORATORIES)
Rogaine Topical Solution (THE UPJOHN COMPANY)
Romazicon (ROCHE LABORATORIES)
Rondec Oral Drops (ROSS PRODUCTS DIVISION)
Rondec Syrup (ROSS PRODUCTS DIVISION)
Rondec Tablet (ROSS PRODUCTS DIVISION)
Rondec-DM Oral Drops
(ROSS PRODUCTS DIVISION)
Rondec-DM Syrup (ROSS PRODUCTS DIVISION)
Rondec-TR Tablet (ROSS PRODUCTS DIVISION)
Ross Hospital Formula System
(ROSS PRODUCTS DIVISION)
Alimentum Protein Hydrolysate Formula
With Iron
Isomil 20 Soy Formula With Iron
Pedialyte
Similac 20 Low-Iron Infant Formula
Similac With Iron 20 Infant Formula
Similac 24 Low-Iron Infant Formula
Similac With Iron 24 Infant Formula
Similac 27 Low-Iron Infant Formula
Similac Natural Care Low-Iron Human
Milk Fortifier
Similac PM 60/40 Low-Iron Infant Formula
Similac Special Care 20 Low-Iron Premature
Infant Formula
Similac Special Care 24 Low-Iron Premature
Infant Formula

UNDERLINE DENOTES GENERIC NAME

Similac Special Care With Iron 24 Premature
    Infant Formula
Sterilized Water
5% Glucose Water
10% Glucose Water
Ross Metabolic Formula System
    (ROSS PRODUCTS DIVISION)
    Calcilo XD Low-Calcium/Vitamin D-Free Infant
        Formula With Iron
    Cyclinex-1
    Cyclinex-2
    Flavonex Flavored Energy Supplement
    Glutarex-1
    Glutarex-2
    Hominex-1
    Hominex-2
    I-Valex-1
    I-Valex-2
    Ketonex-1
    Ketonex-2
    Phenex-1
    Phenex-2
    Pro-Phree
    Propimex-1
    Propimex-2
    ProViMin Protein-Vitamin-Mineral Formula
        Component With Iron
    RCF Ross Carbohydrate Free Low-Iron Soy
        Formula Base
    Similac PM 60/40 Low-Iron Infant Formula
    Tyromex-1
    Tyrex-2
ROWASA Rectal Suppositories, 500 mg
    (SOLVAY PHARMACEUTICALS, INC.)
ROWASA Rectal Suspension Enema
    4.0 grams/unit (60 mL)
    (SOLVAY PHARMACEUTICALS, INC.)
Roxanol (Morphine Sulfate Concentrated
    Oral Solution) (ROXANE LABORATORIES, INC.)
Roxanol 100 (Morphine Sulfate Concentrated
    Oral Solution) (ROXANE LABORATORIES, INC.)
Roxanol Suppositories (Morphine Sulfate)
    (ROXANE LABORATORIES, INC.)
Roxanol UD Morphine Sulfate Oral Solution
    (ROXANE LABORATORIES, INC.)
Roxicet 5/500 Caplets (Oxycodone &
    Acetaminophen) (ROXANE LABORATORIES, INC.)
Roxicet Tablets & Oral Solution (Oxycodone &
    Acetaminophen) (ROXANE LABORATORIES, INC.)
Roxicodone Tablets, Oral Solution & Intensol
    (Oxycodone) (ROXANE LABORATORIES, INC.)
Roxiprin Tablets (Oxycodone & Aspirin)
    (ROXANE LABORATORIES, INC.)

RUBELLA VIRUS VACCINE LIVE
    Meruvax II

RUBELLA & MUMPS VIRUS VACCINE LIVE
    Biavax II
Rubex
    (BRISTOL-MYERS SQUIBB ONCOLOGY DIVISION)
Rum-K Syrup (FLEMING & COMPANY)
Ru-Tuss DE Tablets
    (BOOTS PHARMACEUTICALS, INC.)
Ru-Tuss with Hydrocodone
    (BOOTS PHARMACEUTICALS, INC.)
Ru-Tuss Tablets
    (BOOTS PHARMACEUTICALS, INC.)
Rxosine Capsules (Tyrosine)
    (TYSON AND ASSOCIATES, INC.)
Ryna Liquid (WALLACE LABORATORIES)
Ryna-C Liquid (WALLACE LABORATORIES)
Ryna-CX Liquid (WALLACE LABORATORIES)
Rynatan Tablets (WALLACE LABORATORIES)
Rynatan-S Pediatric Suspension
    (WALLACE LABORATORIES)

Rynatuss Pediatric Suspension
    (WALLACE LABORATORIES)
Rynatuss Tablets (WALLACE LABORATORIES)
Rythmol Tablets–150mg, 225mg, 300mg
    (KNOLL PHARMACEUTICAL COMPANY)

S

SD ALCOHOL
    Solbar PF Ultra Liquid SPF 30
SMA Iron Fortified Infant Formula,
    Concentrated, Ready-To-Feed and Powder
    (WYETH-AYERST LABORATORIES)
SMA Lo-Iron Infant Formula, Concentrated,
    Ready-To-Feed and Powder
    (WYETH-AYERST LABORATORIES)
S-P-T "Liquid" Capsules (FLEMING & COMPANY)
SSD Cream (BOOTS PHARMACEUTICALS, INC.)
SSD AF Cream (BOOTS PHARMACEUTICALS, INC.)
SSD RP Cream (BOOTS LABORATORIES)
SSKI Solution
    (UPSHER-SMITH LABORATORIES, INC.)
Safe Tussin 30 (KRAMER LABORATORIES INC.)
SalAc (GENDERM CORPORATION)
Sal-Acid Plaster (PEDINOL PHARMACAL INC.)
Salactic Film (PEDINOL PHARMACAL INC.)
Salagen Tablets (MGI PHARMA, INC.)
Salflex Tablets
    (CARNRICK LABORATORIES, INC.)

SALICYLIC ACID
    Ionil Plus Shampoo
    Listerex Scrub Golden
    Listerex Scrub Herbal
    Occlusal-HP
    SalAc
    Sal-Acid Plaster
    Salactic Film
    Sal-Plant Gel
    Trans-Ver-Sal Wart Remover Dermal Patch
        Delivery System

SALICYLSALICYLIC ACID
    Disalcid Capsules
    Disalcid Tablets
    Mono-Gesic Tablets
    Salflex Tablets
Salinex Nasal Mist and Drops
    (MURO PHARMACEUTICAL, INC.)

SALMETEROL XINAFOATE
    Serevent Inhalation Aerosol
Sal-Plant Gel (PEDINOL PHARMACAL INC.)

SALSALATE
    Disalcid Capsules
    Disalcid Tablets
    Mono-Gesic Tablets
    Salflex Tablets
    Salsalate Tablets
    Salsitab Tablets
Salsalate Tablets
    (DURAMED PHARMACEUTICALS, INC.)
Salsitab Tablets
    (UPSHER-SMITH LABORATORIES, INC.)
Sandimmune I.V. Ampuls for Infusion
    (SANDOZ PHARMACEUTICALS CORPORATION)
Sandimmune Oral Solution
    (SANDOZ PHARMACEUTICALS CORPORATION)
Sandimmune Soft Gelatin Capsules
    (SANDOZ PHARMACEUTICALS CORPORATION)
Sandoglobulin I.V.
    (SANDOZ PHARMACEUTICALS CORPORATION)

Sandostatin Injection
    (SANDOZ PHARMACEUTICALS CORPORATION)
Sanorex Tablets
    (SANDOZ PHARMACEUTICALS CORPORATION)
Sansert Tablets
    (SANDOZ PHARMACEUTICALS CORPORATION)

SARGRAMOSTIM
    Leukine for IV Infusion
Scleromate
    (PALISADES PHARMACEUTICALS, INC.)

SCOPOLAMINE
    Transderm Scōp Transdermal Therapeutic System

SCOPOLAMINE HYDROBROMIDE
    Atrohist Plus Tablets
    Bellatal Tablets
    Donnatal Capsules
    Donnatal Elixir
    Donnatal Extentabs
    Donnatal Tablets
    Rexatal Tablets
    Ru-Tuss Tablets
Sea-Clens, Wound Cleanser
    (SWEEN CORPORATION)

SECOBARBITAL SODIUM
    Secobarbital Sodium in Tubex
    Seconal Sodium Pulvules
Secobarbital Sodium in Tubex
    (WYETH-AYERST LABORATORIES)
Seconal Sodium Pulvules
    (ELI LILLY AND COMPANY)

SECRETIN
    Secretin-Ferring
Secretin-Ferring
    (FERRING LABORATORIES, INC.)
Sectral Capsules
    (WYETH-AYERST LABORATORIES)
Sedapap Tablets 50 mg/650 mg
    (MAYRAND PHARMACEUTICALS, INC.)
Seldane Tablets (MARION MERRELL DOW INC.)
Seldane-D Extended-Release Tablets
    (MARION MERRELL DOW INC.)

SELEGILINE HYDROCHLORIDE
    Eldepryl Tablets

SELENIUM
    ACES Antioxidant Soft Gels

SELENIUM SULFIDE
    Exsel Shampoo/Lotion
    Selenium Sulfide Lotion USP, 2.5%
    Selsun Rx 2.5% Selenium Sulfide Lotion, USP
Selenium Sulfide Lotion USP, 2.5%
    (BARRE-NATIONAL INC.)
Selsun Blue Dandruff Shampoo
    (ROSS PRODUCTS DIVISION)
Selsun Gold for Women Dandruff Shampoo
    (ROSS PRODUCTS DIVISION)
Selsun Rx 2.5% Selenium Sulfide Lotion, USP
    (ROSS PRODUCTS DIVISION)
Semprex-D Capsules
    (ADAMS LABORATORIES, INC.)
Semprex-D (BURROUGHS WELLCOME CO.)

SENNA CONCENTRATES
    DOSAFLEX Liquid Laxative
    Senna X-Prep Bowel Evacuant Liquid
    Senokot Granules
    Senokot Syrup
    Senokot Tablets
    SenokotXTRA Tablets
    Senokot-S Tablets
Senna X-Prep Bowel Evacuant Liquid
    (GRAY PHARMACEUTICAL CO.)

UNDERLINE DENOTES GENERIC NAME

Senokot Granules
(THE PURDUE FREDERICK COMPANY)
Senokot Syrup
(THE PURDUE FREDERICK COMPANY)
Senokot Tablets
(THE PURDUE FREDERICK COMPANY)
SenokotXTRA Tablets
(THE PURDUE FREDERICK COMPANY)
Senokot-S Tablets
(THE PURDUE FREDERICK COMPANY)
Sensorcaine with Epinephrine Injection
(ASTRA USA, INC.)
Sensorcaine Injection (ASTRA USA, INC.)
Sensorcaine-MPF with Epinephrine Injection
(ASTRA USA, INC.)
Sensorcaine-MPF Spinal (ASTRA USA, INC.)
Septra DS Tablets (BURROUGHS WELLCOME CO.)
Septra Grape Suspension
(BURROUGHS WELLCOME CO.)
Septra I.V. Infusion (BURROUGHS WELLCOME CO.)
Septra I.V. Infusion ADD-Vantage Vials
(BURROUGHS WELLCOME CO.)
Septra Suspension (BURROUGHS WELLCOME CO.)
Septra Tablets (BURROUGHS WELLCOME CO.)
Ser-Ap-Es Tablets
(CIBA PHARMACEUTICAL COMPANY)
Serax Capsules (WYETH-AYERST LABORATORIES)
Serax Tablets (WYETH-AYERST LABORATORIES)
Serentil Ampuls
(BOEHRINGER INGELHEIM PHARMACEUTICALS, INC.)
Serentil Concentrate
(BOEHRINGER INGELHEIM PHARMACEUTICALS, INC.)
Serentil Tablets
(BOEHRINGER INGELHEIM PHARMACEUTICALS, INC.)
Serevent Inhalation Aerosol
(ALLEN & HANBURYS)
SERMORELIN ACETATE
Geref (sermorelin acetate for injection)
Seromycin Pulvules (ELI LILLY AND COMPANY)
Serophene (clomiphene citrate tablets, USP)
(SERONO LABORATORIES, INC.)

SERTRALINE HYDROCHLORIDE
Zoloft Tablets
Sigtab Tablets
(ROBERTS PHARMACEUTICAL CORPORATION)
Silvadene Cream 1% (MARION MERRELL DOW INC.)

SILVER SULFADIAZINE
SSD Cream
SSD AF Cream
SSD RP Cream
Silvadene Cream 1%
Silver Sulfadiazine Cream
Silver Sulfadiazine Cream
(PAR PHARMACEUTICAL, INC.)

SIMETHICONE
Alumina, Magnesia, and Simethicone Oral
Suspension I
Gelusil Liquid
Gelusil Tablets
Maalox Antacid Plus Anti-Gas
Extra Strength Maalox Antacid Plus Anti-
Gas Suspension
Extra Strength Maalox Antacid Plus Anti-
Gas Tablets
Mylanta Gas Tablets-40 mg
Mylanta Gas Tablets-80 mg
Maximum Strength Mylanta Gas Tablets-125 mg
Mylanta Liquid
Mylanta Tablets
Mylanta Double Strength Liquid
Mylanta Double Strength Tablets
Mylicon Infants' Drops
**Similac Natural Care Low-Iron Human Milk
Fortifier** (ROSS PRODUCTS DIVISION)

Similac PM 60/40 Low-Iron Infant Formula
(ROSS PRODUCTS DIVISION)
**Similac Special Care 20 Low-Iron Premature
Infant Formula** (ROSS PRODUCTS DIVISION)
**Similac Special Care 24 Low-Iron Premature
Infant Formula** (ROSS PRODUCTS DIVISION)
**Similac Special Care With Iron 24 Premature
Infant Formula** (ROSS PRODUCTS DIVISION)
Similac 13 Low-Iron Infant Formula
(ROSS PRODUCTS DIVISION)
Similac 20 Low-Iron Infant Formula
(ROSS PRODUCTS DIVISION)
Similac 24 Low-Iron Infant Formula
(ROSS PRODUCTS DIVISION)
Similac 27 Low-Iron Infant Formula
(ROSS PRODUCTS DIVISION)
Similac With Iron 20 Infant Formula
(ROSS PRODUCTS DIVISION)
Similac With Iron 24 Infant Formula
(ROSS PRODUCTS DIVISION)
Similase (TYLER ENCAPSULATIONS)

SIMVASTATIN
Zocor Tablets
Sine-Aid IB Caplets
(MCNEIL CONSUMER PRODUCTS COMPANY)
**Sine-Aid Maximum Strength Sinus Headache
Gelcaps, Caplets and Tablets**
(MCNEIL CONSUMER PRODUCTS COMPANY)
**Sine-Off Maximum Strength Allergy/Sinus
Formula Caplets**
(SMITHKLINE BEECHAM CONSUMER HEALTHCARE, L.P.)
**Sine-Off Maximum Strength No Drowsiness
Formula Caplets**
(SMITHKLINE BEECHAM CONSUMER HEALTHCARE, L.P.)
Sine-Off Sinus Medicine Tablets-Aspirin Formula
(SMITHKLINE BEECHAM CONSUMER HEALTHCARE, L.P.)
Sinemet Tablets (DUPONT PHARMA)
Sinemet CR Tablets (DUPONT PHARMA)
Sinequan Capsules (ROERIG DIVISION)
Sinequan Oral Concentrate (ROERIG DIVISION)
Singlet Tablets
(SMITHKLINE BEECHAM CONSUMER HEALTHCARE, L.P.)
Sinulin Tablets
(CARNRICK LABORATORIES, INC.)
Sinupan Capsules (ION LABORATORIES, INC.)
Sinutab Non Drying Liquid Caps
(WARNER WELLCOME)
**Sinutab Maximum Strength Sinus Allergy
Tablets** (WARNER WELLCOME)
**Sinutab Sinus Maximum Strength Without
Drowsiness Tablet** (WARNER WELLCOME)
**Sinutab Regular Strength Without Drowsiness
Tablet** (WARNER WELLCOME)
SINUVENT Tablets (WE PHARMACEUTICALS, INC.)
Skelaxin Tablets (CARNRICK LABORATORIES, INC.)

SKIN TEST ANTIGENS
Multitest CMI Skin Test Antigens for Cellular
Hypersensitivity
Skin Test Antigens for Cellular Hypersensitivity,
Multitest CMI
**Skin Test Antigens for Cellular Hypersensitivity,
Multitest CMI**
(CONNAUGHT LABORATORIES, INC.)
Slo-bid Gyrocaps
(RHONE-POULENC RORER PHARMACEUTICALS INC.)
Slo-Niacin Tablets
(UPSHER-SMITH LABORATORIES, INC.)
Slo-Phyllin GG Capsules
(RHONE-POULENC RORER PHARMACEUTICALS INC.)
Slo-Phyllin GG Syrup
(RHONE-POULENC RORER PHARMACEUTICALS INC.)
Slo-Phyllin Gyrocaps
(RHONE-POULENC RORER PHARMACEUTICALS INC.)
Slo-Phyllin 80 Syrup
(RHONE-POULENC RORER PHARMACEUTICALS INC.)

Slo-Phyllin Tablets
(RHONE-POULENC RORER PHARMACEUTICALS INC.)
Slow Fe Tablets
(CIBA CONSUMER PHARMACEUTICALS)
Slow Fe with Folic Acid
(CIBA CONSUMER PHARMACEUTICALS)
Slow-K Extended-Release Tablets
(SUMMIT PHARMACEUTICALS)

SOAP
Green Soap

SODIUM ACID PHOSPHATE
K-Phos M.F. Tablets
K-Phos No. 2 Tablets
Uroqid-Acid No. 2 Tablets

SODIUM BICARBONATE
Alka-Seltzer Effervescent Antacid
Alka-Seltzer Effervescent Antacid and
Pain Reliever
Alka-Seltzer Extra Strength Effervescent Antacid
and Pain Reliever
Ceo-Two Rectal Suppositories
NuLYTELY
Sodium Bicarbonate Injection, USP
Sodium Bicarbonate Injection, USP
(ASTRA USA, INC.)

SODIUM BIPHOSPHATE
Uro-Phosphate Tablets

SODIUM CARBOXYMETHYLCELLULOSE
Glandosane Mouth Moisturizer

SODIUM CHLORIDE
Chlor-3 Condiment
Dey-Pak
Dey-Vial
Massengill Powder
NuLYTELY
Sea-Clens, Wound Cleanser
Sodium Chloride, Bacteriostatic in Tubex
Sodium Chloride and Sterile Water for Inhalation,
Arm-a-Vial
Sodium Chloride Inhalation Solution
Sodium Chloride Injection, Bacteriostatic
Sodium Chloride Injection (Preservative-Free)
Sodium Chloride Inhalation Solutions, USP
Sodium Chloride, Bacteriostatic in Tubex
(WYETH-AYERST LABORATORIES)
**Sodium Chloride and Sterile Water for
Inhalation, Arm-a-Vial** (ASTRA USA, INC.)
Sodium Chloride Inhalation Solution
(ROXANE LABORATORIES, INC.)
Sodium Chloride Injection, Bacteriostatic
(ELKINS-SINN, INC.)
Sodium Chloride Injection (Preservative-Free)
(ELKINS-SINN, INC.)
Sodium Chloride Inhalation Solutions, USP
(DEY LABORATORIES)

SODIUM CITRATE
Alka-Seltzer Lemon Lime Effervescent
Antacid and Pain Reliever
Bicitra
Citrolith Tablets
Polycitra Syrup
Polycitra-LC

SODIUM FLUORIDE
Apatate Liquid with Fluoride
Listermint with Fluoride
Luride Drops 50 ml
Luride Lozi-Tabs Tablets
Pediaflor Drops
Vi-Daylin/F ADC Vitamins Drops With Fluoride
Vi-Daylin/F ADC Vitamins + Iron Drops With
Fluoride
Vi-Daylin/F Multivitamin Drops With Fluoride

UNDERLINE DENOTES GENERIC NAME

Vi-Daylin/F Multivitamin + Iron Drops With
   Fluoride
Vi-Daylin/F Multivitamin Chewable Tablets With
   Fluoride
Vi-Daylin/F Multivitamin + Iron Chewable
   Tablets With Fluoride

SODIUM HYPOCHLORITE
   Nail Scrub

SODIUM LACTATE
   Eucerin Plus Dry Skin Care Moisturizing Lotion
   Eucerin Plus Moisturizing Creme

SODIUM MONOBASIC
   Uro-KP-Neutral

SODIUM NITROPRUSSIDE
   Sodium Nitroprusside, Sterile
   Sodium Nitroprusside, Sterile (ELKINS-SINN, INC.)

SODIUM OXYCHLOROSENE
   Clorpactin WCS-90

SODIUM PHOSPHATE DIBASIC
   Fleet Children's Enema
   Fleet Enema
   Fleet Phospho-Soda
   Fleet Prep Kits
   K-Phos Neutral Tablets

SODIUM PHOSPHATE MONOBASIC
   Fleet Children's Enema
   Fleet Enema
   Fleet Phospho-Soda
   Fleet Prep Kits
   K-Phos Neutral Tablets

SODIUM POLYSTYRENE SULFONATE
   Kayexalate
   Kionex
   Sodium Polystyrene Sulfonate Suspension
   Sodium Polystyrene Sulfonate Suspension
      (ROXANE LABORATORIES, INC.)

SODIUM PROPIONATE
   Amino-Cerv

SODIUM SACCHARIN
   Barotrast
   **Sodium Sulamyd Ophthalmic Ointment
   10%-Sterile** (SCHERING CORPORATION)
   **Sodium Sulamyd Ophthalmic Solution
   10%-Sterile** (SCHERING CORPORATION)
   **Sodium Sulamyd Ophthalmic Solution
   30%-Sterile** (SCHERING CORPORATION)

SODIUM SULFACETAMIDE
   Novacet Lotion
   Sulfacet-R Acne Lotion

SODIUM SULFATE
   GoLYTELY

SODIUM TETRADECYL SULFATE
   Sotradecol (Sodium Tetradecyl Sulfate Injection)

SODIUM THIOSALICYLATE
   Thiocyl Injectable Solution
Solaquin Forte 4% Cream
   (ICN PHARMACEUTICALS, INC.)
Solaquin Forte 4% Gel
   (ICN PHARMACEUTICALS, INC.)
Solatene Capsules (ROCHE LABORATORIES)
Solbar PF 15 Cream (PABA Free)
   (PERSÓN & COVEY, INC.)
Solbar PF 15 Liquid (PABA Free)
   (PERSÓN & COVEY, INC.)
Solbar PF Ultra Cream SPF 50 (PABA Free)
   (PERSÓN & COVEY, INC.)
Solbar PF Ultra Liquid SPF 30
   (PERSÓN & COVEY, INC.)

Solbar Plus 15 Cream
   (PERSÓN & COVEY, INC.)
Solfoton Tablets, Capsules
   (ECR PHARMACEUTICALS)
Solganal Suspension (SCHERING CORPORATION)
Solu-Cortef Sterile Powder
   (THE UPJOHN COMPANY)
Solu-Medrol Act-O-Vial & Vials
   (THE UPJOHN COMPANY)
Solu-Medrol Sterile Powder
   (THE UPJOHN COMPANY)
Soma Compound w/Codeine Tablets
   (WALLACE LABORATORIES)
Soma Compound Tablets
   (WALLACE LABORATORIES)
Soma Tablets (WALLACE LABORATORIES)

SOMATREM
   Protropin

SOMATROPIN
   Humatrope Vials
   Nutropin

SORBITOL
   Actidose with Sorbitol
   Glandosane Mouth Moisturizer
Sorbitrate Chewable Tablets
   (ZENECA PHARMACEUTICALS)
Sorbitrate Oral Tablets
   (ZENECA PHARMACEUTICALS)
Sorbitrate Sublingual Tablets
   (ZENECA PHARMACEUTICALS)

SOTALOL HYDROCHLORIDE
   Betapace Tablets
Sotradecol (Sodium Tetradecyl Sulfate Injection)
   (ELKINS-SINN, INC.)

SOY HYDROLYSATE
   AlitraQ Specialized Elemental Nutrition
      With Glutamine

SOYBEAN PREPARATIONS
   Hermal Bath Oil
   Isomil DF Soy Formula For Diarrhea
   Isomil SF Sucrose Free Soy Formula
   Isomil Soy Formula with Iron
Spectazole (econazole nitrate 1%) Cream
   (ORTHO PHARMACEUTICAL CORPORATION
   DERMATOLOGICAL DIVISION)

SPECTINOMYCIN HYDROCHLORIDE
   Trobicin Sterile Powder
Spectrobid Tablets (ROERIG DIVISION)

SPIRONOLACTONE
   Aldactazide
   Aldactone
   Spironolactone Tablets
   Spironolactone & Hydrochlorothiazide Tablets
Spironolactone Tablets
   (MYLAN PHARMACEUTICALS INC.)
Spironolactone & Hydrochlorothiazide Tablets
   (MYLAN PHARMACEUTICALS INC.)
Sporanox Capsules
   (JANSSEN PHARMACEUTICA INC.)
Stadol Injection (APOTHECON)
Stadol NS Nasal Spray
   (BRISTOL-MYERS SQUIBB COMPANY)

STANOZOLOL
   Winstrol Tablets

STARCH
   Anusol Suppositories

STAVUDINE
   Zerit Capsules
Stelazine Concentrate
   (SMITHKLINE BEECHAM PHARMACEUTICALS)

Stelazine Injection
   (SMITHKLINE BEECHAM PHARMACEUTICALS)
Stelazine Multi-dose Vials
   (SMITHKLINE BEECHAM PHARMACEUTICALS)
Stelazine Tablets
   (SMITHKLINE BEECHAM PHARMACEUTICALS)
Sterapred DS Unipak
   (MAYRAND PHARMACEUTICALS, INC.)
Sterapred DS 12 Day Unipak
   (MAYRAND PHARMACEUTICALS, INC.)
Sterapred Unipak
   (MAYRAND PHARMACEUTICALS, INC.)
Sterile Water for Inhalation, USP
   (DEY LABORATORIES)
Stilphostrol Tablets and Ampuls
   (MILES INC. PHARMACEUTICAL DIVISION)
**Stimate (desmopressin acetate) Nasal Spray,
   1.5 mg/mL**
   (ARMOUR PHARMACEUTICAL COMPANY)

STREPTOKINASE
   Kabikinase (Streptokinase)

STREPTOMYCIN SULFATE
   Streptomycin Sulfate Injection
Streptomycin Sulfate Injection
   (ROERIG DIVISION)

STREPTOZOCIN
   Zanosar Sterile Powder
Stresstabs, Advanced Formula
   (LEDERLE LABORATORIES)
Stresstabs + Iron, Advanced Formula
   (LEDERLE LABORATORIES)
Stresstabs + Zinc, Advanced Formula
   (LEDERLE LABORATORIES)

STRONTIUM CHLORIDE
   Metastron
Strovite Plus Caplets
   (EVERETT LABORATORIES, INC.)
Strovite Tablets
   (EVERETT LABORATORIES, INC.)
Stuart Prenatal Tablets
   (WYETH-AYERST LABORATORIES)
Stuartnatal Plus Tablets
   (WYETH-AYERST LABORATORIES)
Sublimaze Injection
   (JANSSEN PHARMACEUTICA INC.)

SUCCIMER
   CHEMET (succimer) Capsules

SUCCINYLCHOLINE CHLORIDE
   Anectine Flo-Pack
   Anectine Injection
   Succinylcholine Chloride
Succinylcholine Chloride (ORGANON INC.)

SUCRALFATE
   Carafate Suspension
   Carafate Tablets
Children's Sudafed Liquid (WARNER WELLCOME)
Sudafed Cold & Cough Liquid Caps
   (WARNER WELLCOME)
Sudafed Cough Syrup (WARNER WELLCOME)
Sudafed Plus Liquid (WARNER WELLCOME)
Sudafed Plus Tablets (WARNER WELLCOME)
Sudafed Severe Cold Formula Tablets
   (WARNER WELLCOME)
Sudafed Sinus Tablets & Caplets
   (WARNER WELLCOME)
Sudafed 60 mg Tablets (WARNER WELLCOME)
Sudafed 30 mg Tablets (WARNER WELLCOME)
Sudafed 12 Hour Caplets (WARNER WELLCOME)
Sufenta Injection
   (JANSSEN PHARMACEUTICA INC.)

SUFENTANIL CITRATE
   Sufenta Injection

UNDERLINE DENOTES GENERIC NAME

SULBACTAM SODIUM
  Unasyn

SULCONAZOLE NITRATE
  Exelderm Cream 1.0%
  Exelderm Solution 1.0%

SULFABENZAMIDE
  Sultrin Triple Sulfa Cream
  Sultrin Triple Sulfa Vaginal Tablets
  Trysul Vaginal Cream
Sulfacet-R Acne Lotion
  (DERMIK LABORATORIES, INC.)

SULFACETAMIDE
  Sultrin Triple Sulfa Cream
  Sultrin Triple Sulfa Vaginal Tablets
  Trysul Vaginal Cream

SULFACETAMIDE SODIUM
  Bleph-10 Ophthalmic Ointment 10%
  Bleph-10 Ophthalmic Solution 10%
  Blephamide Liquifilm Sterile Ophthalmic
    Suspension
  Sodium Sulamyd Ophthalmic Ointment 10%-
    Sterile
  Sodium Sulamyd Ophthalmic Solution 10%-
    Sterile
  Sodium Sulamyd Ophthalmic Solution 30%-
    Sterile

SULFADIAZINE
  Sulfadiazine Tablets
Sulfadiazine Tablets
  (EON LABS MANUFACTURING, INC.)

SULFADOXINE
  Fansidar Tablets

SULFAMETHIZOLE
  Thiosulfil Forte Tablets
  Urobiotic-250 Capsules

SULFAMETHOXAZOLE
  Azo Gantanol Tablets
  Bactrim DS Tablets
  Bactrim I.V. Infusion
  Bactrim Pediatric Suspension
  Bactrim Tablets
  Gantanol Tablets
  Septra DS Tablets
  Septra Grape Suspension
  Septra I.V. Infusion
  Septra I.V. Infusion ADD-Vantage Vials
  Septra Suspension
  Septra Tablets
  Sulfamethoxazole & Trimethoprim Concentrate
    for Injection
  Sulfamethoxazole and Trimethoprim
    Oral Suspension
  Sulfamethoxazole and Trimethoprim
    Oral Suspension
  Sulfamethoxazole & Trimethoprim Tablets
  Sulfamethoxazole and Trimethoprim Tablets
  Sulfamethoxazole and Trimethoprim Tablets
    (Regular and Double Strength)
  Sulfatrim Pediatric Suspension
  Sulfatrim Suspension
**Sulfamethoxazole & Trimethoprim
  Concentrate for Injection** (ELKINS-SINN, INC.)
**Sulfamethoxazole and Trimethoprim Oral
  Suspension** (WARNER CHILCOTT LABORATORIES)
**Sulfamethoxazole and Trimethoprim Oral
  Suspension** (BIOCRAFT LABORATORIES, INC.)
Sulfamethoxazole & Trimethoprim Tablets
  (LEDERLE STANDARD PRODUCTS)
Sulfamethoxazole and Trimethoprim Tablets
  (BIOCRAFT LABORATORIES, INC.)

**Sulfamethoxazole and Trimethoprim Tablets
  (Regular and Double Strength)**
  (ROXANE LABORATORIES, INC.)
Sulfamylon Cream
  (DOW HICKAM PHARMACEUTICALS, INC.)

SULFANILAMIDE
  AVC Cream
  AVC Suppositories

SULFASALAZINE
  Azulfidine Tablets and EN-tabs
  Sulfasalazine Tablets
Sulfasalazine Tablets
  (LEDERLE STANDARD PRODUCTS)

SULFATHIAZOLE
  Sultrin Triple Sulfa Cream
  Sultrin Triple Sulfa Vaginal Tablets
  Trysul Vaginal Cream
Sulfatrim Pediatric Suspension
  (BARRE-NATIONAL INC.)
Sulfatrim Suspension (BARRE-NATIONAL INC.)

SULFINPYRAZONE
  Anturane Capsules
  Anturane Tablets

SULFISOXAZOLE
  Azo Gantrisin Tablets
  Gantrisin Tablets
  Pediazole

SULFISOXAZOLE ACETYL
  Erythromycin Ethylsuccinate/ Sulfisoxazole
    Acetyl Oral Suspension
  Eryzole Oral Suspension, USP

SULFISOXAZOLE DIOLAMINE
  Gantrisin Ophthalmic Solution
Sulfoam Medicated Antidandruff Shampoo
  (DOAK DERMATOLOGICALS)
Sulfoxyl Lotion Regular
  (STIEFEL LABORATORIES, INC.)
Sulfoxyl Lotion Strong
  (STIEFEL LABORATORIES, INC.)

SULFUR
  Bensulfoid Cream
  Novacet Lotion
  Sulfacet-R Acne Lotion
  Sulfoam Medicated Antidandruff Shampoo
  Sulfoxyl Lotion Regular
  Sulfoxyl Lotion Strong
  Sulpho-Lac Acne Medication
  Sulpho-Lac Acne Medicated Soap

SULINDAC
  Clinoril Tablets
  Sulindac Tablets
  Sulindac Tablets
  Sulindac Tablets
  Sulindac Tablets, U.S.P.
  Sulindac Tablets
Sulindac Tablets
  (GENEVA PHARMACEUTICALS, INC.)
Sulindac Tablets
  (LEDERLE STANDARD PRODUCTS)
Sulindac Tablets
  (WARNER CHILCOTT LABORATORIES)
Sulindac Tablets, U.S.P.
  (WEST POINT PHARMA)
Sulindac Tablets
  (MYLAN PHARMACEUTICALS INC.)
Sulpho-Lac Acne Medication
  (DOAK DERMATOLOGICALS)
Sulpho-Lac Acne Medicated Soap
  (DOAK DERMATOLOGICALS)
Sultrin Triple Sulfa Cream
  (ORTHO PHARMACEUTICAL CORPORATION)

Sultrin Triple Sulfa Vaginal Tablets
  (ORTHO PHARMACEUTICAL CORPORATION)

SUMATRIPTAN SUCCINATE
  Imitrex Injection
**Sunkist Children's Chewable Multivitamins -
  Complete** (CIBA CONSUMER PHARMACEUTICALS)
**Sunkist Children's Chewable Multivitamins -
  Plus Extra C**
  (CIBA CONSUMER PHARMACEUTICALS)
**Sunkist Children's Chewable Multivitamins -
  Plus Iron** (CIBA CONSUMER PHARMACEUTICALS)
**Sunkist Children's Chewable Multivitamins -
  Regular** (CIBA CONSUMER PHARMACEUTICALS)
Sunkist Vitamin C - Chewable
  (CIBA CONSUMER PHARMACEUTICALS)
Sunkist Vitamin C - Easy to Swallow
  (CIBA CONSUMER PHARMACEUTICALS)
Super (VITALINE CORPORATION)
Super Omega-3 Fatty Acids Soft Gels
  (J. R. CARLSON LABORATORIES, INC.)

SUPEROXIDE DISMUTASE
  Catasod
  Super
Suplena Specialized Liquid Nutrition
  (ROSS PRODUCTS DIVISION)
Supprelin Injection
  (ROBERTS PHARMACEUTICAL CORPORATION)
Suprane
  (OHMEDA PHARMACEUTICAL PRODUCTS DIVISION INC.)
Suprax for Oral Suspension
  (LEDERLE LABORATORIES)
Suprax Tablets (LEDERLE LABORATORIES)
SURGICEL* Absorbable Hemostat
  (JOHNSON & JOHNSON MEDICAL, INC.)
SURGICEL* NU-KNIT Absorbable Hemostat
  (JOHNSON & JOHNSON MEDICAL, INC.)
Surmontil Capsules
  (WYETH-AYERST LABORATORIES)
Survanta Beractant Intratracheal Suspension
  (ROSS PRODUCTS DIVISION)
Sus-Phrine Injection
  (FOREST PHARMACEUTICALS, INC.)

SUTILAINS
  Travase Ointment
Sween Cream (SWEEN CORPORATION)
Syllact Powder (WALLACE LABORATORIES)
Synacort Creams 1%, 2.5%
  (SYNTEX PUERTO RICO, INC.)
Synalar Creams 0.025%, 0.01%
  (SYNTEX PUERTO RICO, INC.)
Synalar Ointment 0.025%
  (SYNTEX PUERTO RICO, INC.)
Synalar Topical Solution 0.01%
  (SYNTEX PUERTO RICO, INC.)
Synalar-HP Cream 0.2%
  (SYNTEX PUERTO RICO, INC.)
Synalgos-DC Capsules
  (WYETH-AYERST LABORATORIES)
**Synarel Nasal Solution for Central Precocious
  Puberty** (SYNTEX PUERTO RICO, INC.)
Synarel Nasal Solution for Endometriosis
  (SYNTEX PUERTO RICO, INC.)
Synemol Cream 0.025%
  (SYNTEX PUERTO RICO, INC.)
Syn-Rx Tablets (ADAMS LABORATORIES, INC.)
Synthroid Injection
  (BOOTS PHARMACEUTICALS, INC.)
Synthroid Tablets (BOOTS PHARMACEUTICALS, INC.)
Syntocinon Injection
  (SANDOZ PHARMACEUTICALS CORPORATION)
Syntocinon Nasal Spray
  (SANDOZ PHARMACEUTICALS CORPORATION)
Syprine Capsules (MERCK & CO., INC.)

UNDERLINE DENOTES GENERIC NAME

T

TACRINE HYDROCHLORIDE
Cognex Capsules

TACROLIMUS
Prograf

TEA-LAURYL SULFATE
DHS Shampoo
DHS Clear Shampoo
T-PHYL Tablets
(THE PURDUE FREDERICK COMPANY)
T-Stat 2.0% Topical Solution and Pads
(WESTWOOD-SQUIBB PHARMACEUTICALS INC.)
Tac-3 Suspension (ALLERGAN HERBERT)
Tagamet Injection
(SMITHKLINE BEECHAM PHARMACEUTICALS)
Tagamet Liquid
(SMITHKLINE BEECHAM PHARMACEUTICALS)
Tagamet Tablets
(SMITHKLINE BEECHAM PHARMACEUTICALS)
Talacen (SANOFI WINTHROP PHARMACEUTICALS)
Talwin Ampuls
(SANOFI WINTHROP PHARMACEUTICALS)
Talwin Carpuject
(SANOFI WINTHROP PHARMACEUTICALS)
Talwin Compound
(SANOFI WINTHROP PHARMACEUTICALS)
Talwin Injection
(SANOFI WINTHROP PHARMACEUTICALS)
Talwin Nx (SANOFI WINTHROP PHARMACEUTICALS)
Tambocor Tablets (3M PHARMACEUTICALS)

TAMOXIFEN CITRATE
Nolvadex Tablets
Tao Capsules (ROERIG DIVISION)
Tapazole Tablets (ELI LILLY AND COMPANY)
Tavist Syrup
(SANDOZ PHARMACEUTICALS CORPORATION)
Tavist Tablets
(SANDOZ PHARMACEUTICALS CORPORATION)
Tavist-1 12 Hour Relief Medicine
(SANDOZ PHARMACEUTICALS/ CONSUMER DIVISION)
Tavist-D 12 Hour Relief Medicine
(SANDOZ PHARMACEUTICALS/ CONSUMER DIVISION)
Taxol
(BRISTOL-MYERS SQUIBB ONCOLOGY DIVISION)
Tazicef for Injection
(SMITHKLINE BEECHAM PHARMACEUTICALS)
Tazidime Vials, Faspak & ADD-Vantage
(ELI LILLY AND COMPANY)

TAZOBACTAM SODIUM
Zosyn
Zosyn Pharmacy Bulk Package
TE Anatoxal Berna (BERNA PRODUCTS, CORP.)
Tears Naturale II Lubricant Eye Drops
(ALCON LABORATORIES, INC.)
Tears Naturale Free (ALCON LABORATORIES, INC.)
Tears Plus Lubricating Eye Drops (ALLERGAN, INC.)
Tegison Capsules (ROCHE LABORATORIES)
Tegretol Chewable Tablets
(BASEL PHARMACEUTICALS)
Tegretol Suspension (BASEL PHARMACEUTICALS)
Tegretol Tablets (BASEL PHARMACEUTICALS)
Tel-E-Dose, Tel-E-Ject (unit dose) Products:
(ROCHE LABORATORIES)

Bumex Tablets
Fansidar Tablets
Gantanol Tablets
Gantrisin Tablets
Klonopin Tablets
Lariam Tablets
Trimpex Tablets

Tel-E-Dose (unit dose) Products:
(ROCHE PRODUCTS INC.)
Librax Capsules
Librium Capsules
Limbitrol DS Tablets
Limbitrol Tablets
Valium Tablets
Temaril Tablets, Syrup and Spansule Extended-Release Capsules (ALLERGAN HERBERT)

TEMAZEPAM
Restoril Capsules
Temazepam Capsules
Temazepam Capsules
Temazepam Capsules
Temazepam Capsules
(MYLAN PHARMACEUTICALS INC.)
Temazepam Capsules
(PAR PHARMACEUTICAL, INC.)
Temazepam Capsules
(WARNER CHILCOTT LABORATORIES)
Temovate Cream (GLAXO DERMATOLOGY)
Temovate Emollient Cream
(GLAXO DERMATOLOGY)
Temovate Gel (GLAXO DERMATOLOGY)
Temovate Ointment (GLAXO DERMATOLOGY)
Temovate Scalp Application
(GLAXO DERMATOLOGY)
Tencon Capsules
(INTERNATIONAL ETHICAL LABS.)
Tenex Tablets (A. H. ROBINS COMPANY, INC.)
Ten-K Extended-Release Tablets
(SUMMIT PHARMACEUTICALS)

TENIPOSIDE
Vumon
Tenoretic Tablets (ZENECA PHARMACEUTICALS)
Tenormin Tablets and I.V. Injection
(ZENECA PHARMACEUTICALS)
Tensilon Injectable
(ICN PHARMACEUTICALS, INC.)
Terazol 3 Vaginal Cream
(ORTHO PHARMACEUTICAL CORPORATION)
Terazol 3 Vaginal Suppositories
(ORTHO PHARMACEUTICAL CORPORATION)
Terazol 7 Vaginal Cream
(ORTHO PHARMACEUTICAL CORPORATION)

TERAZOSIN HYDROCHLORIDE
Hytrin Tablets

TERBINAFINE HYROCHLORIDE
Lamisil Cream 1%

TERBUTALINE SULFATE
Brethaire Inhaler
Brethine Ampuls
Brethine Tablets
Bricanyl Injection
Bricanyl Tablets

TERCONAZOLE
Terazol 3 Vaginal Cream
Terazol 3 Vaginal Suppositories
Terazol 7 Vaginal Cream

TERFENADINE
Seldane Tablets
Seldane-D Extended-Release Tablets

TERIPARATIDE ACETATE
Parathar
Terra-Cortril Ophthalmic Suspension
(ROERIG DIVISION)
Terramycin Intramuscular Solution
(ROERIG DIVISION)
Terramycin with Polymyxin B Sulfate Ophthalmic Ointment (ROERIG DIVISION)
Teraseptic Antibacterial Cleansing Liquid
(DOAK DERMATOLOGICALS)

Teslac
(BRISTOL-MYERS SQUIBB ONCOLOGY DIVISION)
Tessalon Perles
(FOREST PHARMACEUTICALS, INC.)
Tes-Tape (ELI LILLY AND COMPANY)
Testoderm Testosterone Transdermal System
(ALZA PHARMACEUTICALS)

TESTOLACTONE
Teslac

TESTOSTERONE
Testoderm Testosterone Transdermal System

TESTOSTERONE CYPIONATE
DEPO-Testosterone Sterile Solution
Virilon IM

TESTOSTERONE ENANTHATE
Delatestryl Injection
Testred Capsules (ICN PHARMACEUTICALS, INC.)

TETANUS ANTITOXIN
Hyper-Tet Tetanus Immune Globulin (Human)

TETANUS & DIPHTHERIA TOXOIDS ADSORBED (FOR ADULT USE)
Tetanus & Diphtheria Toxoids Adsorbed For Adult Use USP

TETANUS & DIPHTHERIA TOXOIDS COMBINED, ALUMINUM PHOSPHATE ADSORBED (FOR ADULT USE)
Tetanus & Diphtheria Toxoids Adsorbed for Adult Use
Tetanus & Diphtheria Toxoids Adsorbed for Adult Use in Tubex
Tetanus & Diphtheria Toxoids Adsorbed Purogenated
Tetanus & Diphtheria Toxoids Adsorbed for Adult Use
(WYETH-AYERST LABORATORIES)
Tetanus & Diphtheria Toxoids Adsorbed for Adult Use USP
(CONNAUGHT LABORATORIES, INC.)
Tetanus & Diphtheria Toxoids Adsorbed for Adult Use in Tubex
(WYETH-AYERST LABORATORIES)
Tetanus & Diphtheria Toxoids Adsorbed Purogenated
(LEDERLE LABORATORIES)

TETANUS IMMUNE GLOBULIN (HUMAN)
Hyper-Tet Tetanus Immune Globulin (Human)

TETANUS TOXOID, ADSORBED
TE Anatoxal Berna
Tetanus Toxoid Adsorbed Purogenated
Tetanus Toxoid Adsorbed Purogenated
(LEDERLE LABORATORIES)

TETANUS TOXOID, ALUMINUM PHOSPHATE ADSORBED
Tetanus Toxoid Adsorbed, Aluminum Phosphate Adsorbed, Ultrafined
Tetanus Toxoid Adsorbed, Aluminum Phosphate Adsorbed, Ultrafined in Tubex
Tetanus Toxoid Adsorbed, Aluminum Phosphate Adsorbed, Ultrafined
(WYETH-AYERST LABORATORIES)
Tetanus Toxoid Adsorbed, Aluminum Phosphate Adsorbed, Ultrafined in Tubex
(WYETH-AYERST LABORATORIES)

TETANUS TOXOID, FLUID
Tetanus Toxoid Fluid, Purified, Ultrafined
Tetanus Toxoid Fluid, Purified, Ultrafined in Tubex
Tetanus Toxoid Fluid, Purified, Ultrafined
(WYETH-AYERST LABORATORIES)

UNDERLINE DENOTES GENERIC NAME

Tetanus Toxoid Fluid, Purified, Ultrafined in Tubex (WYETH-AYERST LABORATORIES)
Tetramune (LEDERLE LABORATORIES)

TETRACAINE HYDROCHLORIDE
Cetacaine Topical Anesthetic
Pontocaine Hydrochloride for Spinal Anesthesia

TETRACHLOROSALICYLANILIDE
Impregon Concentrate

TETRACYCLINE HYDROCHLORIDE
Achromycin V Capsules
Achromycin Ophthalmic Ointment 1% (See PDR For Ophthalmology)
Achromycin Ophthalmic Suspension 1% (See PDR For Ophthalmology)
Tetracycline HCl Capsules, USP
Tetracycline Hydrochloride Capsules
Topicycline for Topical Solution
Tetracycline HCl Capsules, USP
(WARNER CHILCOTT LABORATORIES)
Tetracycline Hydrochloride Capsules
(MYLAN PHARMACEUTICALS INC.)

TETRAHYDROZOLINE HYDROCHLORIDE
Tyzine Nasal Solution/Nasal Spray/Pediatric Nasal Drops
Thalitone (HORUS THERAPEUTICS, INC.)
Theo-24 Extended Release Capsules
(WHITBY PHARMACEUTICALS, INC.)
Theoclear L.A.-130 & -260 Capsules
(CENTRAL PHARMACEUTICALS, INC.)
Theoclear-80 Syrup
(CENTRAL PHARMACEUTICALS, INC.)
Theo-Dur Sprinkle Sustained Action Capsules
(KEY PHARMACEUTICALS, INC.)
Theo-Dur Extended-Release Tablets
(KEY PHARMACEUTICALS, INC.)
Theolair Liquid (3M PHARMACEUTICALS)
Theolair Tablets (3M PHARMACEUTICALS)
Theolair-SR Tablets (3M PHARMACEUTICALS)
Theolate Liquid (BARRE-NATIONAL INC.)
Theomax DF Syrup (BARRE-NATIONAL INC.)

THEOPHYLLINE
Marax Tablets & DF Syrup
Mudrane GG Elixir
Mudrane GG Tablets
Quibron Capsules
Quibron-300 Capsules
Quibron-T Tablets
Quibron-T/SR Tablets
Slo-Phyllin GG Capsules
Theolate Liquid
Theophylline Controlled-Release Tablets
Theophylline Elixir
Theophylline Elixir 80 mg/15 mL
Theophylline ER Capsules and Tablets
Theophylline Oral Solution
Theophylline Controlled-Release Tablets
(WARNER CHILCOTT LABORATORIES)
Theophylline Elixir
(WARNER CHILCOTT LABORATORIES)
Theophylline Elixir 80 mg/15 mL
(BARRE-NATIONAL INC.)
Theophylline ER Capsules and Tablets
(WARNER CHILCOTT LABORATORIES)
Theophylline Oral Solution
(ROXANE LABORATORIES, INC.)

THEOPHYLLINE ANHYDROUS
Aerolate Jr. T.D. Capsules
Aerolate Liquid
Aerolate Sr. T.D. Capsules
Aerolate III T.D. Capsules
Elixophyllin Dye-Free Capsules
Elixophyllin Elixir
Elixophyllin-GG Oral Solution

Elixophyllin-KI Elixir
Respbid Tablets
Slo-bid Gyrocaps
Slo-Phyllin GG Syrup
Slo-Phyllin Gyrocaps
Slo-Phyllin 80 Syrup
Slo-Phyllin Tablets
T-PHYL Tablets
Theo-24 Extended Release Capsules
Theoclear L.A.-130 & -260 Capsules
Theoclear-80 Syrup
Theo-Dur Sprinkle Sustained Action Capsules
Theo-Dur Extended-Release Tablets
Theolair Liquid
Theolair Tablets
Theolair-SR Tablets
Theo-X Extended-Release Tablets
Uniphyl 400 mg Tablets

THEOPHYLLINE CALCIUM SALICYLATE
Quadrinal Tablets

THEOPHYLLINE SODIUM GLYCINATE
Asbron G Elixir
Asbron G Inlay-Tabs
Theo-X Extended-Release Tablets
(CARNRICK LABORATORIES, INC.)
TheraCys BCG Live (Intravesical)
(CONNAUGHT LABORATORIES, INC.)
TheraFlu Flu and Cold Hot Liquid Medicine
(SANDOZ PHARMACEUTICALS/ CONSUMER DIVISION)
TheraFlu Flu Cold & Cough Hot Liquid Medicine
(SANDOZ PHARMACEUTICALS/ CONSUMER DIVISION)
TheraFlu Maximum Strength Nighttime Flu, Cold & Cough Hot Liquid Medicine
(SANDOZ PHARMACEUTICALS/ CONSUMER DIVISION)
TheraFlu Maximum Strength Non-Drowsy Flu, Cold & Cough Hot Liquid Medicine
(SANDOZ PHARMACEUTICALS/ CONSUMER DIVISION)
Theraflu Maximum Strength Non-Drowsy Flu, Cold & Cough Caplets
(SANDOZ PHARMACEUTICALS/ CONSUMER DIVISION)
Thera-Gesic (MISSION PHARMACAL COMPANY)
Theragran Liquid with Niacin and Vitamin C
(BRISTOL-MYERS PRODUCTS)
Theragran Stress Formula
(BRISTOL-MYERS PRODUCTS)
Theragran Tablets (BRISTOL-MYERS PRODUCTS)
Theragran-M Tablets with Beta Carotene
(BRISTOL-MYERS PRODUCTS)
Theramycin Z Topical Solution 2%
(MEDICIS DERMATOLOGICS, INC.)
Therapeutic Mineral Ice, Pain Relieving Gel
(BRISTOL-MYERS PRODUCTS)
Therapeutic Mineral Ice Exercise Formula, Pain Relieving Gel (BRISTOL-MYERS PRODUCTS)
Therapeutic Mineral Ice Plus Moisturizers
(BRISTOL-MYERS PRODUCTS)
Theravite Liquid (BARRE-NATIONAL INC.)

THIABENDAZOLE
Mintezol Chewable Tablets
Mintezol Suspension
Thiamilate Enteric Tablets (Thiamine Pyrophosphate) (TYSON AND ASSOCIATES, INC.)

THIAMINE HYDROCHLORIDE
Apatate Liquid/Tablets
Apatate Liquid with Fluoride
Eldertonic
ILX B$_{12}$ Caplets Crystalline
ILX B$_{12}$ Elixir Crystalline and ILX B$_{12}$ Sugar–Free Elixir
Thiamine Hydrochloride Injection
Thiamine Hydrochloride in Tubex
Thiamine Hydrochloride Injection
(ELKINS-SINN, INC.)

Thiamine Hydrochloride in Tubex
(WYETH-AYERST LABORATORIES)

THIAMINE MONONITRATE
Mega-B

THIETHYLPERAZINE MALATE
Torecan Injection

THIETHYLPERAZINE MALEATE
Torecan Tablets
Thiocyl Injectable Solution
(RICO PHARMACAL)

THIOGUANINE
Thioguanine Tablets, Tabloid Brand
Thioguanine Tablets, Tabloid Brand
(BURROUGHS WELLCOME CO.)
Thiola Tablets (MISSION PHARMACAL COMPANY)

THIORIDAZINE
Mellaril-S Suspension

THIORIDAZINE HYDROCHLORIDE
Mellaril Concentrate
Mellaril Tablets
Thioridazine HCl Oral Soln. USP 100 mg/mL
Thioridazine HCl Tablets
Thioridazine Hydrochloride Tablets
Thioridazine HCl Oral Soln. USP 100 mg/mL
(BARRE-NATIONAL INC.)
Thioridazine HCl Tablets
(GENEVA PHARMACEUTICALS, INC.)
Thioridazine Hydrochloride Tablets
(MYLAN PHARMACEUTICALS INC.)
Thiosulfil Forte Tablets
(WYETH-AYERST LABORATORIES)

THIOTEPA
Thiotepa For Injection
Thiotepa For Injection
(IMMUNEX CORPORATION)

THIOTHIXENE
Navane Capsules and Concentrate
Navane Intramuscular
Thiothixene Capsules
Thiothixene Capsules
THIOTHIXENE CAPSULES
(GENEVA PHARMACEUTICALS, INC.)
Thiothixene Capsules
(MYLAN PHARMACEUTICALS INC.)

THIOTHIXENE HYDROCHLORIDE
Thiothixine HCl Oral Soln. USP (Concentrate) 5 mg/mL
Thiothixine HCl Oral Soln. USP (Concentrate) 5 mg/mL (BARRE-NATIONAL INC.)
Thorazine Ampuls
(SMITHKLINE BEECHAM PHARMACEUTICALS)
Thorazine Concentrate
(SMITHKLINE BEECHAM PHARMACEUTICALS)
Thorazine Multi-dose Vials
(SMITHKLINE BEECHAM PHARMACEUTICALS)
Thorazine Spansule Capsules
(SMITHKLINE BEECHAM PHARMACEUTICALS)
Thorazine Suppositories
(SMITHKLINE BEECHAM PHARMACEUTICALS)
Thorazine Syrup
(SMITHKLINE BEECHAM PHARMACEUTICALS)
Thorazine Tablets
(SMITHKLINE BEECHAM PHARMACEUTICALS)
Threamine DM Syrup (BARRE-NATIONAL INC.)
Threamine Expectorant
(BARRE-NATIONAL INC.)

L-THREONINE
Threostat Capsules (Threonine)
Threostat Capsules (Threonine)
(TYSON AND ASSOCIATES, INC.)

Throat Discs Throat Lozenges
(SMITHKLINE BEECHAM CONSUMER HEALTHCARE, L.P.)
THROMBATE III Antithrombin III (Human)
(MILES INC. PHARMACEUTICAL DIVISION
BIOLOGICAL PRODUCTS)

THROMBIN
Thrombogen Topical Thrombin, USP with
Diluent and Transfer Needle
Thrombogen Topical Thrombin, USP,
Spray Kit
**Thrombogen Topical Thrombin, USP with
Diluent and Transfer Needle**
(JOHNSON & JOHNSON MEDICAL, INC.)
Thrombogen Topical Thrombin, USP, Spray Kit
(JOHNSON & JOHNSON MEDICAL, INC.)

THYMOL
Listerine Antiseptic
Cool Mint Listerine
Thyrar Tablets
(RHONE-POULENC RORER PHARMACEUTICALS INC.)
THYREL TRH (FERRING LABORATORIES, INC.)

THYROID
Armour Thyroid Tablets
S-P-T "Liquid" Capsules
THYROLAR TABLETS
(FOREST PHARMACEUTICALS, INC.)

THYROTROPIN
Thytropar
Thytropar
(RHONE-POULENC RORER PHARMACEUTICALS INC.)
Ticar for Injection
(SMITHKLINE BEECHAM PHARMACEUTICALS)

TICARCILLIN DISODIUM
Ticar for Injection
Timentin for Injection
Tice BCG, USP (ORGANON INC.)
Ticlid Tablets (SYNTEX PUERTO RICO, INC.)

TICLOPIDINE HYDROCHLORIDE
Ticlid Tablets
Tigan Capsules
(SMITHKLINE BEECHAM PHARMACEUTICALS)
Tigan Injectable
(SMITHKLINE BEECHAM PHARMACEUTICALS)
Tigan Suppositories
(SMITHKLINE BEECHAM PHARMACEUTICALS)
Tilade
(FISONS CORPORATION PRESCRIPTION PRODUCTS)
Timentin for Injection
(SMITHKLINE BEECHAM PHARMACEUTICALS)
Timolide Tablets (MERCK & CO., INC.)

TIMOLOL MALEATE
Blocadren Tablets
Timolide Tablets
Timolol Maleate Tablets
Timolol Maleate Tablets
Timolol Maleate Tablets, U.S.P.
Timoptic in Ocudose
Timoptic Sterile Ophthalmic Solution
Timoptic-XE
Timolol Maleate Tablets
(MYLAN PHARMACEUTICALS INC.)
Timolol Maleate Tablets
(NOVOPHARM, USA INC.)
Timolol Maleate Tablets, U.S.P.
(WEST POINT PHARMA)
Timoptic in Ocudose (MERCK & CO., INC.)
Timoptic Sterile Ophthalmic Solution
(MERCK & CO., INC.)
Timoptic-XE (MERCK & CO., INC.)

TIOCONAZOLE
Vagistat-1

TIOPRONIN
Thiola Tablets

TITANIUM DIOXIDE
Eucerin Dry Skin Care Daily Facial Lotion SPF 20
TobraDex Ophthalmic Suspension and Ointment
(ALCON LABORATORIES, INC.)

TOBRAMYCIN
TobraDex Ophthalmic Suspension and Ointment

TOBRAMYCIN SULFATE
Nebcin Vials, Hyporets & ADD-Vantage
Tobramycin Sulfate Injection
Tobramycin Sulfate Injection
Tobramycin Sulfate Injection (ELKINS-SINN, INC.)
Tobramycin Sulfate Injection
(LEDERLE STANDARD PRODUCTS)

TOCAINIDE HYDROCHLORIDE
Tonocard Tablets
Tofranil Ampuls (GEIGY PHARMACEUTICALS)
Tofranil Tablets (GEIGY PHARMACEUTICALS)
Tofranil-PM Capsules (GEIGY PHARMACEUTICALS)

TOLAZAMIDE
Tolazamide Tablets
Tolazamide Tablets
(MYLAN PHARMACEUTICALS INC.)

TOLAZOLINE HYDROCHLORIDE
Priscoline Hydrochloride Ampuls

TOLBUTAMIDE
Tolbutamide Tablets
Tolbutamide Tablets
(MYLAN PHARMACEUTICALS INC.)
Tolectin (200, 400 and 600 mg)
(MCNEIL PHARMACEUTICAL)

TOLMETIN SODIUM
Tolectin (200, 400 and 600 mg)
Tolmetin Sodium Capsules USP 400, Tabs 600
Tolmetin Sodium Capsules
Tolmetin Sodium Capsules USP 400, Tabs 600
(NOVOPHARM, USA INC.)
Tolmetin Sodium Capsules
(MYLAN PHARMACEUTICALS INC.)

TOLNAFTATE
Tolnaftate 1% Cream
Tolnaftate Cream or Solution, 1%
Tolnaftate 1% Cream
(TARO PHARMACEUTICALS U.S.A., INC.)
Tolnaftate Cream or Solution, 1%
(BARRE-NATIONAL INC.)
Tonocard Tablets (ASTRA MERCK)
Topicort Emollient Cream 0.25%
(HOECHST-ROUSSEL PHARMACEUTICALS INC.)
Topicort Gel 0.05%
(HOECHST-ROUSSEL PHARMACEUTICALS INC.)
Topicort LP Emollient Cream 0.05%
(HOECHST-ROUSSEL PHARMACEUTICALS INC.)
Topicort Ointment 0.25%
(HOECHST-ROUSSEL PHARMACEUTICALS INC.)
Topicycline for Topical Solution
(ROBERTS PHARMACEUTICAL CORPORATION)
Toprol-XL Tablets (ASTRA USA, INC.)
Toradol IM Injection (SYNTEX PUERTO RICO, INC.)
Toradol Oral (SYNTEX PUERTO RICO, INC.)
Torecan Injection (ROXANE LABORATORIES, INC.)
Torecan Tablets (ROXANE LABORATORIES, INC.)
Tornalate Inhalation Solution, 0.2%
(DURA PHARMACEUTICALS, INC)
Tornalate Metered Dose Inhaler
(DURA PHARMACEUTICALS, INC)

TORSEMIDE
Demadex Tablets and Injection
Touro A&H Capsules
(DARTMOUTH PHARMACEUTICALS, INC.)

Touro DM Caplets
(DARTMOUTH PHARMACEUTICALS, INC.)
Touro EX Caplets
(DARTMOUTH PHARMACEUTICALS, INC.)
Touro LA Caplets
(DARTMOUTH PHARMACEUTICALS, INC.)
Tracrium Injection (BURROUGHS WELLCOME CO.)
Trancopal Caplets
(SANOFI WINTHROP PHARMACEUTICALS)
Trandate Injection (ALLEN & HANBURYS)
Trandate Tablets (ALLEN & HANBURYS)

TRANEXAMIC ACID
Cyklokapron Tablets and Injection
**Transderm Scōp Transdermal Therapeutic
System** (CIBA CONSUMER PHARMACEUTICALS)
Transdermal-NTG
(WARNER CHILCOTT LABORATORIES)
**Transderm-Nitro Transdermal Therapeutic
System** (SUMMIT PHARMACEUTICALS)
**Trans-Ver-Sal Wart Remover Dermal Patch
Delivery System** (DOAK DERMATOLOGICALS)
Tranxene T-TAB Tablets (ABBOTT LABORATORIES)
Tranxene-SD Half Strength Tablets
(ABBOTT LABORATORIES)
Tranxene-SD Tablets (ABBOTT LABORATORIES)

TRANYLCYPROMINE SULFATE
Parnate Tablets
Travase Ointment (BOOTS PHARMACEUTICALS, INC.)

TRAZODONE HYDROCHLORIDE
Desyrel and Desyrel Dividose
Trazodone HCl Tablets
Trazodone HCl Tablets
Trazodone HCl Tablets
(GENEVA PHARMACEUTICALS, INC.)
Trazodone HCl Tablets
(WARNER CHILCOTT LABORATORIES)
Trecator-SC Tablets
(WYETH-AYERST LABORATORIES)
Trental Tablets
(HOECHST-ROUSSEL PHARMACEUTICALS INC.)

TRETINOIN
Retin-A (tretinoin) Cream/Gel/Liquid
Trexan Tablets (DUPONT PHARMA)
Triacin-C Cough Syrup (BARRE-NATIONAL INC.)
Triad, Hydrophilic Wound Dressing
(SWEEN CORPORATION)

TRIAMCINOLONE
Aristocort Tablets
Nystatin & Triamcinolone Acetonide
Ointment, USP

TRIAMCINOLONE ACETONIDE
Aristocort A Topical Cream
Aristocort A Topical Ointment
Azmacort Oral Inhaler
Mytrex Cream & Ointment
Nasacort Nasal Inhaler
Nystatin/Triamcinolone Acetonide Cream
or Ointment
Nystatin and Triamcinolone Acetonide
Cream, USP
Tac-3 Suspension
Triamcinolone Acetonide Cream USP 0.025%
Triamcinolone Acetonide Cream or Ointment,
USP 0.1%
Triamcinolone Acetonide Dental Paste,
USP 0.1%
Triamcinolone Acetonide Cream USP 0.025%
(BARRE-NATIONAL INC.)
**Triamcinolone Acetonide Cream or Ointment,
USP 0.1%** (BARRE-NATIONAL INC.)
Triamcinolone Acetonide Dental Paste, USP 0.1%
(TARO PHARMACEUTICALS U.S.A., INC.)

UNDERLINE DENOTES GENERIC NAME

TRIAMCINOLONE DIACETATE
  Aristocort Suspension (Forte Parenteral)
  Aristocort Suspension (Intralesional)

TRIAMCINOLONE HEXACETONIDE
  Aristospan Suspension (Intra-articular)
  Aristospan Suspension (Intralesional)
TRIAMINIC ALLERGY TABLETS
  (SANDOZ PHARMACEUTICALS/ CONSUMER DIVISION)
Triaminic Cold Tablets
  (SANDOZ PHARMACEUTICALS/ CONSUMER DIVISION)
Triaminic Expectorant
  (SANDOZ PHARMACEUTICALS/ CONSUMER DIVISION)
Triaminic Expectorant with Codeine
  (SANDOZ PHARMACEUTICALS/ CONSUMER DIVISION)
Triaminic Expectorant DH
  (SANDOZ PHARMACEUTICALS/ CONSUMER DIVISION)
Triaminic Nite Light Syrup
  (SANDOZ PHARMACEUTICALS/ CONSUMER DIVISION)
Triaminic Oral Infant Drops
  (SANDOZ PHARMACEUTICALS/ CONSUMER DIVISION)
Triaminic Sore Throat Formula
  (SANDOZ PHARMACEUTICALS/ CONSUMER DIVISION)
Triaminic Syrup
  (SANDOZ PHARMACEUTICALS/ CONSUMER DIVISION)
**Triaminic-12 Maximum Strength 12 Hour
  Relief Tablets**
  (SANDOZ PHARMACEUTICALS/ CONSUMER DIVISION)
Triaminic-DM Syrup
  (SANDOZ PHARMACEUTICALS/ CONSUMER DIVISION)
Triaminicin Cold, Allergy, Sinus Tablets
  (SANDOZ PHARMACEUTICALS/ CONSUMER DIVISION)
**Triaminicol Multi-Symptom Cold and
  Cough Tablets**
  (SANDOZ PHARMACEUTICALS/ CONSUMER DIVISION)
Triaminicol Multi-Symptom Relief Syrup
  (SANDOZ PHARMACEUTICALS/ CONSUMER DIVISION)

TRIAMTERENE
  Dyazide Capsules
  Dyazide New Formulation
  Dyrenium Capsules
  Maxzide Tablets
  Maxzide-25 MG Tablets
  Triamterene/Hydrochlorothiazide Tablets
  Triamterene and Hydrochlorothiazide Tablets
  Triamterene and Hydrochlorothiazide Tablets
  Triamterene and HCTZ Tablets, USP
Triamterene/Hydrochlorothiazide Tablets
  (GENEVA PHARMACEUTICALS, INC.)
Triamterene and Hydrochlorothiazide Tablets
  (WARNER CHILCOTT LABORATORIES)
Triamterene and Hydrochlorothiazide Tablets
  (PAR PHARMACEUTICAL, INC.)
Triamterene and HCTZ Tablets, USP
  (WATSON LABORATORIES, INC.)
Triavil Tablets (MERCK & CO., INC.)

TRIAZOLAM
  Halcion Tablets
  Triazolam Tablets .125 mg
  Triazolam Tablets .25 mg
Triazolam Tablets .125 mg
  (PAR PHARMACEUTICAL, INC.)
Triazolam Tablets .25 mg
  (PAR PHARMACEUTICAL, INC.)

TRICHLOROMONOFLUOROMETHANE
  Fluori-Methane
Tricosal Tablets
  (DURAMED PHARMACEUTICALS, INC.)
Tridesilon Cream 0.05%
  (MILES INC. PHARMACEUTICAL DIVISION)
Tridesilon Ointment 0.05%
  (MILES INC. PHARMACEUTICAL DIVISION)
Tridione Capsules (ABBOTT LABORATORIES)
Tridione Dulcet Tablets (ABBOTT LABORATORIES)

TRIENTINE HYDROCHLORIDE
  Syprine Capsules

TRIETHANOLAMINE POLYPEPTIDE OLEATE-
CONDENSATE
  Cerumenex Drops

TRIETHYLENETHIOPHOSPHORAMIDE
  Thiotepa For Injection

TRIFLUOPERAZINE HYDROCHLORIDE
  Stelazine Concentrate
  Stelazine Injection
  Stelazine Multi-dose Vials
  Stelazine Tablets
  Trifluoperazine HCl Tablets
Trifluoperazine HCl Tablets
  (GENEVA PHARMACEUTICALS, INC.)

TRIFLURIDINE
  Viroptic Ophthalmic Solution, 1% Sterile

TRIHEXYPHENIDYL HYDROCHLORIDE
  Artane Elixir
  Artane Sequels
  Artane Tablets
Tri-Immunol Adsorbed (LEDERLE LABORATORIES)
Trilafon Concentrate (SCHERING CORPORATION)
Trilafon Injection (SCHERING CORPORATION)
Trilafon Tablets (SCHERING CORPORATION)
Tri-Levlen 21 Tablets (BERLEX LABORATORIES)
Tri-Levlen 28 Tablets (BERLEX LABORATORIES)
Trilisate Liquid
  (THE PURDUE FREDERICK COMPANY)
Trilisate Tablets
  (THE PURDUE FREDERICK COMPANY)

TRIMEPRAZINE TARTRATE
  Temaril Tablets, Syrup and Spansule Extended-
    Release Capsules

TRIMETHADIONE
  Tridione Capsules
  Tridione Dulcet Tablets

TRIMETHAPHAN CAMSYLATE
  Arfonad Ampuls

TRIMETHOBENZAMIDE HYDROCHLORIDE
  Tigan Capsules
  Tigan Injectable
  Tigan Suppositories

TRIMETHOPRIM
  Bactrim DS Tablets
  Bactrim I.V. Infusion
  Bactrim Pediatric Suspension
  Bactrim Tablets
  Proloprim Tablets
  Septra DS Tablets
  Septra Grape Suspension
  Septra I.V. Infusion
  Septra I.V. Infusion ADD-Vantage Vials
  Septra Suspension
  Septra Tablets
  Sulfamethoxazole & Trimethoprim Concentrate
    for Injection
  Sulfamethoxazole and Trimethoprim Oral
    Suspension
  Sulfamethoxazole and Trimethoprim Oral
    Suspension
  Sulfamethoxazole & Trimethoprim Tablets
  Sulfamethoxazole and Trimethoprim Tablets
  Sulfamethoxazole and Trimethoprim Tablets
    (Regular and Double Strength)
  Sulfatrim Pediatric Suspension
  Sulfatrim Suspension
  Trimethoprim Tablets
  Trimpex Tablets
Trimethoprim Tablets
  (BIOCRAFT LABORATORIES, INC.)

TRIMETHOPRIM SULFATE
  Polytrim Ophthalmic Solution Sterile

TRIMETREXATE GLUCURONATE
  Neutrexin

TRIMIPRAMINE MALEATE
  Surmontil Capsules
Trimpex Tablets (ROCHE LABORATORIES)
Trinalin Repetabs Tablets
  (KEY PHARMACEUTICALS, INC.)
Tri-Norinyl 21-Day Tablets
  (SYNTEX PUERTO RICO, INC.)
Tri-Norinyl 28-Day Tablets
  (SYNTEX PUERTO RICO, INC.)
Trinsicon Capsules
  (WHITBY PHARMACEUTICALS, INC.)
Triofed Syrup (BARRE-NATIONAL INC.)
Triotann Pediatric Suspension
  (DURAMED PHARMACEUTICALS, INC.)
Triotann Tablets
  (DURAMED PHARMACEUTICALS, INC.)
Triotann-S Pediatric Suspension
  (DURAMED PHARMACEUTICALS, INC.)
Triostat Injection
  (SMITHKLINE BEECHAM PHARMACEUTICALS)

TRIOXSALEN
  Trisoralen Tablets
Tripalgen Cold Syrup (BARRE-NATIONAL INC.)
Tripedia (CONNAUGHT LABORATORIES, INC.)

TRIPELENNAMINE HYDROCHLORIDE
  PBZ Tablets
  PBZ-SR Tablets
Triphasil-21 Tablets
  (WYETH-AYERST LABORATORIES)
Triphasil-28 Tablets
  (WYETH-AYERST LABORATORIES)
Triple Antibiotic Ointment (BARRE-NATIONAL INC.)
Triple Antibiotic Ointment, Maximum Strength
  (BARRE-NATIONAL INC.)
**Triple Antibiotic Ointment, Plus, Maximum
  Strength** (BARRE-NATIONAL INC.)
Triple Sulfa Vaginal Cream
  (BARRE-NATIONAL INC.)

TRIPROLIDINE HYDROCHLORIDE
  Actifed Plus Tablets and Caplets
  Actifed with Codeine Cough Syrup
  Actifed Syrup
  Actifed Tablets
Tri-Vi-Flor Drops
  (MEAD JOHNSON NUTRITIONALS)
Tri-Vi-Flor Tablets (MEAD JOHNSON NUTRITIONALS)
Tri-Vi-Flor 0.25 mg with Iron Drops (MEAD JOHN-
  SON NUTRITIONALS)
Trisoralen Tablets
  (ICN PHARMACEUTICALS, INC.)
Tri Vit Drops w/Fluoride 0.25 mg
  (BARRE-NATIONAL INC.)
Tri Vit Drops w/Fluoride 0.5 mg
  (BARRE-NATIONAL INC.)
Trobicin Sterile Powder (THE UPJOHN COMPANY)

TROLEANDOMYCIN
  Tao Capsules
Tronolane Anesthetic Cream for Hemorrhoids
  (ROSS PRODUCTS DIVISION)
Tronolane Hemorrhoidal Suppositories
  (ROSS PRODUCTS DIVISION)

TRYPSIN
  Granulex
Trysul Vaginal Cream (SAVAGE LABORATORIES)

TUBERCULIN, OLD
  Tuberculin, Old, Tine Test
Tuberculin, Old, Tine Test
  (LEDERLE LABORATORIES)

UNDERLINE DENOTES GENERIC NAME

TUBERCULIN, PURIFIED PROTEIN DERIVATIVE
FOR MANTOUX TEST
  Tubersol

TUBERCULIN, PURIFIED PROTEIN
DERIVATIVE, MULTIPLE PUNCTURE DEVICE
  PPD Tine Test
Tubersol (CONNAUGHT LABORATORIES, INC.)
Tubex Closed Injection System Products
  (WYETH-AYERST LABORATORIES)
Tubex Injector (WYETH-AYERST LABORATORIES)
Tucks Clear Gel (WARNER WELLCOME)
Tucks Pads (WARNER WELLCOME)
Tucks Take Alongs (WARNER WELLCOME)
Tums Antacid Tablets
  (SMITHKLINE BEECHAM CONSUMER HEALTHCARE, L.P.)
Tums Anti-gas/Antacid Formula Tablets,
  Assorted Fruit
  (SMITHKLINE BEECHAM CONSUMER HEALTHCARE, L.P.)
Tums E-X Antacid Tablets
  (SMITHKLINE BEECHAM CONSUMER HEALTHCARE, L.P.)
Tuss-DA RX (INTERNATIONAL ETHICAL LABS.)
Tussafed Drops & Syrup
  (EVERETT LABORATORIES, INC.)
Tussar-2
  (RHONE-POULENC RORER PHARMACEUTICALS INC.)
Tussar DM
  (RHONE-POULENC RORER PHARMACEUTICALS INC.)
Tussar SF
  (RHONE-POULENC RORER PHARMACEUTICALS INC.)
Tussex Cough Syrup (BARRE-NATIONAL INC.)
Tussigon Tablets
  (DANIELS PHARMACEUTICALS, INC.)
Tussionex Pennkinetic Extended-Release
  Suspension
  (FISONS CORPORATION PRESCRIPTION PRODUCTS)
Tussi-Organidin DM NR Liquid and DM-S NR
  Liquid (WALLACE LABORATORIES)
Tussi-Organidin NR Liquid and S NR Liquid
  (WALLACE LABORATORIES)
12 Hour Nasal Spray (BARRE-NATIONAL INC.)
TYLENOL acetaminophen Children's Chewable
  Tablets & Elixir
  (MCNEIL CONSUMER PRODUCTS COMPANY)
TYLENOL acetaminophen Children's
  Suspension Liquid
  (MCNEIL CONSUMER PRODUCTS COMPANY)
TYLENOL Allergy Sinus NightTime Caplets
  (MCNEIL CONSUMER PRODUCTS COMPANY)
Tylenol with Codeine Elixir
  (MCNEIL PHARMACEUTICAL)
Tylenol with Codeine Phosphate Tablets
  (MCNEIL PHARMACEUTICAL)
Children's TYLENOL Cold Multi-Symptom
  Liquid Formula and Chewable Tablets
  (MCNEIL CONSUMER PRODUCTS COMPANY)
Children's TYLENOL Cold Multi-Symptom Plus
  Cough Liquid Formula and Chewable Tablets
  (MCNEIL CONSUMER PRODUCTS COMPANY)
TYLENOL Flu NightTime, Maximum Strength,
  Gelcaps
  (MCNEIL CONSUMER PRODUCTS COMPANY)
TYLENOL Cold Hot Medication Packets
  (MCNEIL CONSUMER PRODUCTS COMPANY)
TYLENOL Cold Medication No Drowsiness
  Formula Gelcaps and Caplets
  (MCNEIL CONSUMER PRODUCTS COMPANY)
TYLENOL Extended Relief Caplets
  (MCNEIL CONSUMER PRODUCTS COMPANY)
TYLENOL, Extra Strength, acetaminophen
  Adult Liquid Pain Reliever
  (MCNEIL CONSUMER PRODUCTS COMPANY)
TYLENOL, Extra Strength, acetaminophen
  Gelcaps, Geltabs, Caplets, Tablets
  (MCNEIL CONSUMER PRODUCTS COMPANY)

TYLENOL, Extra Strength, Headache Plus Pain
  Reliever with Antacid Caplets
  (MCNEIL CONSUMER PRODUCTS COMPANY)
TYLENOL, Infants' Drops and Infants'
  Suspension Drops
  (MCNEIL CONSUMER PRODUCTS COMPANY)
TYLENOL, Junior Strength, acetaminophen
  Coated Caplets, Grape and Fruit
  Chewable Tablets
  (MCNEIL CONSUMER PRODUCTS COMPANY)
TYLENOL Maximum Strength Allergy Sinus
  Medication Gelcaps and Caplets
  (MCNEIL CONSUMER PRODUCTS COMPANY)
TYLENOL Maximum Strength Allergy Sinus
  Nighttime Medicine
  (MCNEIL CONSUMER PRODUCTS COMPANY)
TYLENOL Cough Multi-Symptom Medication
  (MCNEIL CONSUMER PRODUCTS COMPANY)
TYLENOL Cough Multi-Symptom
  Medication with Decongestant
  (MCNEIL CONSUMER PRODUCTS COMPANY)
TYLENOL Flu Maximum Strength Gelcaps
  (MCNEIL CONSUMER PRODUCTS COMPANY)
TYLENOL Cold Multi-Symptom Formula
  Medication Tablets and Caplets
  (MCNEIL CONSUMER PRODUCTS COMPANY)
TYLENOL, Maximum Strength, Sinus
  Medication Geltabs, Gelcaps,
  Caplets and Tablets
  (MCNEIL CONSUMER PRODUCTS COMPANY)
TYLENOL Flu NightTime, Maximum
  Strength, Hot Medication
  (MCNEIL CONSUMER PRODUCTS COMPANY)
TYLENOL, Regular Strength, acetaminophen
  Caplets and Tablets
  (MCNEIL CONSUMER PRODUCTS COMPANY)
TYLENOL PM, Extra Strength Pain
  Reliever/Sleep Aid Caplets, Gelcaps, Geltabs,
  Tablets
  (MCNEIL CONSUMER PRODUCTS COMPANY)
Tylox Capsules (MCNEIL PHARMACEUTICAL)

TYLOXAPOL
  Exosurf Neonatal for Intratracheal Suspension
Tympagesic Ear Drops (SAVAGE LABORATORIES)

TYPHOID VACCINE
  Typhoid Vaccine

TYPHOID VACCINE LIVE ORAL TY21A
  Vivotif Berna
Typhoid Vaccine (WYETH-AYERST LABORATORIES)

L-TYROSINE
  Catemine Enteric Tablets (Tyrosine)
  Rxosine Capsules (Tyrosine)
Tyzine Nasal Solution/Nasal Spray/Pediatric
  Nasal Drops (KENWOOD LABORATORIES)

U

ULTRABROM Capsules
  (WE PHARMACEUTICALS, INC.)
ULTRABROM PD Capsules
  (WE PHARMACEUTICALS, INC.)
Ultralente Insulin
  (NOVO NORDISK PHARMACEUTICALS INC.)
Ultrase Capsules (SCANDIPHARM, INC.)
Ultravate Cream 0.05%
  (WESTWOOD-SQUIBB PHARMACEUTICALS INC.)
Ultravate Ointment 0.05%
  (WESTWOOD-SQUIBB PHARMACEUTICALS INC.)
Unasyn (ROERIG DIVISION)

UNDECYLENIC ACID
  Fungoid Solution
  Gordochom Solution
Unguentum Bossi (DOAK DERMATOLOGICALS)
Unibase (WARNER CHILCOTT LABORATORIES)
Unipen Capsules (WYETH-AYERST LABORATORIES)
Unipen Injection (WYETH-AYERST LABORATORIES)
Uniphyl 400 mg Tablets
  (THE PURDUE FREDERICK COMPANY)
Maximum Strength Unisom Sleepgels
  (PFIZER CONSUMER HEALTH CARE)
Unisom Nighttime Sleep Aid
  (PFIZER CONSUMER HEALTH CARE)
Unisom With Pain Relief-Nighttime
  Sleep Aid and Pain Reliever
  (PFIZER CONSUMER HEALTH CARE)

UREA
  Amino-Cerv
  Atrac-Tain, Moisturizing Cream
  Carmol 10
  Eucerin Plus Dry Skin Care Moisturizing Lotion
  Eucerin Plus Moisturizing Creme
  Panafil Ointment
  Panafil-White Ointment
  Ureacin Lotion & Creme
Ureacin Lotion & Creme
  (PEDINOL PHARMACAL INC.)
Urecholine Injection (MERCK & CO., INC.)
Urecholine Tablets (MERCK & CO., INC.)
Urex Tablets (3M PHARMACEUTICALS)
Urised Tablets
  (POLYMEDICA PHARMACEUTICALS (U.S.A.), INC.)
Urisedamine Tablets
  (POLYMEDICA PHARMACEUTICALS (U.S.A.), INC.)
Urispas Tablets
  (SMITHKLINE BEECHAM PHARMACEUTICALS)
Uro-KP-Neutral (STAR PHARMACEUTICALS, INC.)
Urobiotic-250 Capsules (ROERIG DIVISION)
Urocit-K (MISSION PHARMACAL COMPANY)

UROFOLLITROPIN
  Metrodin (urofollitropin for injection)
Urokin (VITALINE CORPORATION)

UROKINASE
  Abbokinase
  Abbokinase Open-Cath
Urolene Blue (STAR PHARMACEUTICALS, INC.)
Uro-Mag (BLAINE COMPANY, INC.)
Uro-Phosphate Tablets (ECR PHARMACEUTICALS)
Uroqid-Acid No. 2 Tablets
  (BEACH PHARMACEUTICALS)
Ursinus Inlay-Tabs
  (SANDOZ PHARMACEUTICALS/ CONSUMER DIVISION)

URSODIOL
  Actigall Capsules

V

Vagistat-1 (BRISTOL-MYERS SQUIBB COMPANY)
Valium Injectable (ROCHE PRODUCTS INC.)
Valium Tablets (ROCHE PRODUCTS INC.)
Valium Tel-E-Ject (ROCHE PRODUCTS INC.)

VALPROIC ACID
  Depakene Capsules
  Depakene Syrup
Valrelease Capsules (ROCHE LABORATORIES)
Vancenase AQ Nasal Spray 0.042%
  (SCHERING CORPORATION)

UNDERLINE DENOTES GENERIC NAME

Vancenase PocketHaler Nasal Inhaler
(SCHERING CORPORATION)
Vanceril Inhaler (SCHERING CORPORATION)
Vancocin HCl, Oral Solution & Pulvules
(ELI LILLY AND COMPANY)
Vancocin HCl, Vials & ADD-Vantage
(ELI LILLY AND COMPANY)
Vancoled (LEDERLE STANDARD PRODUCTS)

VANCOMYCIN HYDROCHLORIDE
    Vancocin HCl, Oral Solution & Pulvules
    Vancocin HCl, Vials & ADD-Vantage
    Vancoled
    Vancomycin Hydrochloride, Sterile
Vancomycin Hydrochloride, Sterile
(ELKINS-SINN, INC.)
Vanex Forte Caplets
(ABANA PHARMACEUTICALS, INC.)
Vanex-HD Liquid
(ABANA PHARMACEUTICALS, INC.)
Vanseb Cream and Lotion Dandruff Shampoos
(ALLERGAN HERBERT)
**Vanseb-T Cream and Lotion Tar Dandruff
    Shampoos** (ALLERGAN HERBERT)
Vantin for Oral Suspension and Vantin Tablets
(THE UPJOHN COMPANY)
Varicella-Zoster Immune Globulin (Human)
(MASSACHUSETTS PUBLIC HEALTH BIOLOGIC
LABORATORIES)
Vascor (200, 300 and 400 mg) Tablets
(MCNEIL PHARMACEUTICAL)
Vascor Tablets (See McNeil Pharmaceutical)
(WALLACE LABORATORIES)
Vaseretic Tablets (MERCK & CO., INC.)
Vasotec I.V. (MERCK & CO., INC.)
Vasotec Tablets (MERCK & CO., INC.)
Vasoxyl Injection (BURROUGHS WELLCOME CO.)

VECURONIUM BROMIDE
    Norcuron

VEGETABLE OIL, HYDROGENATED
    Hydrisinol Creme & Lotion
Velban Vials (ELI LILLY AND COMPANY)
Velosulin Human
(NOVO NORDISK PHARMACEUTICALS INC.)

VENLAFAXINE HYDROCHLORIDE
    Effexor
**Venoglobulin-I, Immune Globulin Intravenous
    (Human)** (ALPHA THERAPEUTIC CORPORATION)
**Venoglobulin-S 5% Solution Solvent Detergent
    Treated, Immune Globulin Intravenous
    (Human)** (ALPHA THERAPEUTIC CORPORATION)
Ventolin Inhalation Aerosol and Refill
(ALLEN & HANBURYS)
Ventolin Inhalation Solution
(ALLEN & HANBURYS)
Ventolin Nebules Inhalation Solution
(ALLEN & HANBURYS)
Ventolin Rotacaps for Inhalation
(ALLEN & HANBURYS)
Ventolin Syrup (ALLEN & HANBURYS)
Ventolin Tablets (ALLEN & HANBURYS)
VePesid Capsules and Injection
(BRISTOL-MYERS SQUIBB ONCOLOGY DIVISION)

VERAPAMIL HYDROCHLORIDE
    Calan SR Caplets
    Calan Tablets
    Isoptin Ampules 5mg/2mL
    Isoptin for Intravenous Injection 5mg/2mL
    Isoptin Oral Tablets
    Isoptin SR Tablets
    Verapamil Hydrochloride Tablets
    Verapamil Hydrochloride Tablets
    Verelan Capsules
    Verelan Capsules

Verapamil Hydrochloride Tablets
(MYLAN PHARMACEUTICALS INC.)
Verapamil Hydrochloride Tablets
(WATSON LABORATORIES, INC.)
Verelan Capsules (LEDERLE LABORATORIES)
Verelan Capsules (WYETH-AYERST LABORATORIES)
Vermox Chewable Tablets
(JANSSEN PHARMACEUTICA INC.)
Versed Injection (ROCHE LABORATORIES)

VERSENATE, CALCIUM DISODIUM
    Calcium Disodium Versenate Injection
Vibramycin Hyclate Capsules
(PFIZER LABS DIVISION)
Vibramycin Hyclate Intravenous
(ROERIG DIVISION)
Vibramycin Monohydrate for Oral Suspension
(PFIZER LABS DIVISION)
Vibra-Tabs Film Coated Tablets
(PFIZER LABS DIVISION)
**Vicks Chloraseptic Cough and Throat Drops:
    Cherry, Menthol & Honey Lemon Flavors**
(PROCTER & GAMBLE)
Vicks Chloraseptic Gargle & Mouth Rinse
(PROCTER & GAMBLE)
**Vicks Chloraseptic Sore Throat Spray: Menthol
    Flavor** (PROCTER & GAMBLE)
**Vicks Chloraseptic Sore Throat Lozenges:
    Cherry and Menthol Flavors**
(PROCTER & GAMBLE)
Vicks Cough Drops: Cherry and Menthol Flavors
(PROCTER & GAMBLE)
Vicks DayQuil Allergy Relief 4 Hour Tablets
(PROCTER & GAMBLE)
**Vicks DayQuil Allergy Relief 12-Hour Extended
    Release** (PROCTER & GAMBLE)
**Vicks DayQuil Liquid & LiquiCaps Multi-
    Symptom Cold/Flu Relief**
(PROCTER & GAMBLE)
**Vicks Dayquil SINUS Pressure & CONGES-
    TION Relief** (PROCTER & GAMBLE)
**Vicks Dayquil SINUS Pressure & PAIN Relief
    with IBUPROFEN** (PROCTER & GAMBLE)
Vicks 44 Liquicaps Cough, Cold & Flu Relief
(PROCTER & GAMBLE)
**Vicks 44 Liquicaps Non-Drowsy Cough and
    Cold Relief** (PROCTER & GAMBLE)
Vicks 44 Dry Hacking Cough (PROCTER & GAMBLE)
**Vicks 44D Dry Hacking Cough & Head
    Congestion** (PROCTER & GAMBLE)
Vicks 44E Chest Cough & Chest Congestion
(PROCTER & GAMBLE)
Vicks 44M Cough, Cold & Flu Relief
(PROCTER & GAMBLE)
Vicks Nyquil Hot Therapy (PROCTER & GAMBLE)
**Vicks NyQuil Multi-Symptom Cold/Flu Relief
    (Liquid)** (PROCTER & GAMBLE)
**Vicks NyQuil LiquiCaps Milti-Symptom
    Cold/Flu Relief** (PROCTER & GAMBLE)
**Vicks Sinex Nasal Spray and Ultra Fine Mist
    for Sinus Relief** (PROCTER & GAMBLE)
**Vicks Sinex 12 hour Nasal Spray and Ultra Fine
    Mist for Sinus Relief** (PROCTER & GAMBLE)
Vicks Vapor Inhaler (PROCTER & GAMBLE)
Vicks VapoRub (cream) (PROCTER & GAMBLE)
Vicks VapoRub (ointment) (PROCTER & GAMBLE)
Vicks VapoSteam (PROCTER & GAMBLE)
Vicodin Tablets
(KNOLL PHARMACEUTICAL COMPANY)
Vicodin ES Tablets
(KNOLL PHARMACEUTICAL COMPANY)
Vicodin Tuss Expectorant
(KNOLL PHARMACEUTICAL COMPANY)
Vicon Forte Capsules
(WHITBY PHARMACEUTICALS, INC.)
Vicon Plus Capsules
(WHITBY PHARMACEUTICALS, INC.)

Vicon-C Capsules
(WHITBY PHARMACEUTICALS, INC.)
Vi-Daylin ADC Vitamins Drops
(ROSS PRODUCTS DIVISION)
Vi-Daylin ADC Vitamins + Iron Drops
(ROSS PRODUCTS DIVISION)
Vi-Daylin Multivitamin Drops
(ROSS PRODUCTS DIVISION)
Vi-Daylin Multivitamin + Iron Drops
(ROSS PRODUCTS DIVISION)
Vi-Daylin/F ADC Vitamins Drops With Fluoride
(ROSS PRODUCTS DIVISION)
**Vi-Daylin/F ADC Vitamins + Iron Drops
    With Fluoride** (ROSS PRODUCTS DIVISION)
Vi-Daylin/F Multivitamin Drops With Fluoride
(ROSS PRODUCTS DIVISION)
**Vi-Daylin/F Multivitamin + Iron Drops
    With Fluoride** (ROSS PRODUCTS DIVISION)
Vi-Daylin Multivitamin Chewable Tablets
(ROSS PRODUCTS DIVISION)
Vi-Daylin Multivitamin + Iron Chewable Tablets
(ROSS PRODUCTS DIVISION)
**Vi-Daylin/F Multivitamin Chewable Tablets
    With Fluoride** (ROSS PRODUCTS DIVISION)
**Vi-Daylin/F Multivitamin + Iron Chewable
    Tablets With Fluoride**
(ROSS PRODUCTS DIVISION)
Vi-Daylin Multivitamin Liquid
(ROSS PRODUCTS DIVISION)
Vi-Daylin Multivitamin + Iron Liquid
(ROSS PRODUCTS DIVISION)
**Videx Tablets, Powder for Oral Solution, &
    Pediatric Powder for Oral Solution**
(BRISTOL-MYERS SQUIBB ONCOLOGY DIVISION)
Viminate (BARRE-NATIONAL INC.)

VINBLASTINE SULFATE
    Velban Vials

VINCRISTINE SULFATE
    Oncovin Solution Vials & Hyporets

VINEGAR
    Massengill Disposable Douche
Viokase Powder (A. H. ROBINS COMPANY, INC.)
Viokase Tablets (A. H. ROBINS COMPANY, INC.)
Virazole (ICN PHARMACEUTICALS, INC.)
Virilon (STAR PHARMACEUTICALS, INC.)
Virilon IM (STAR PHARMACEUTICALS, INC.)
Viroptic Ophthalmic Solution, 1% Sterile
(BURROUGHS WELLCOME CO.)
Visken Tablets
(SANDOZ PHARMACEUTICALS CORPORATION)
Vistaril Capsules (PFIZER LABS DIVISION)
Vistaril Intramuscular Solution
(ROERIG DIVISION)
Vistaril Oral Suspension
(PFIZER LABS DIVISION)
Vitafol Caplets (EVERETT LABORATORIES, INC.)
Vitafol Syrup (EVERETT LABORATORIES, INC.)
**Vital High Nitrogen Nutritionally Complete
    Partially Hydrolyzed Diet**
(ROSS PRODUCTS DIVISION)

VITAMIN A
    ACES Antioxidant Soft Gels
    Aquasol A Vitamin A Capsules, USP
    Aquasol A Parenteral, USP
    Eldercaps
    Lazer Creme
    Materna Tablets
    Megadose
    NutraVescent
    Prenate 90 Tablets
    Vi-Daylin ADC Vitamins + Iron Drops
    Vi-Daylin/F ADC Vitamins Drops With Fluoride
    Vi-Daylin/F ADC Vitamins + Iron Drops
        With Fluoride

UNDERLINE DENOTES GENERIC NAME

VITAMIN A & VITAMIN D
　Eldercaps
　Sween Cream
　Vi-Daylin ADC Vitamins Drops
　Vitamin A & Vitamin D Ointment
　Vitamin A & Vitamin D Ointment
　　(BARRE-NATIONAL INC.)

VITAMIN B COMPLEX
　Apatate Liquid/Tablets
　Apatate Liquid with Fluoride
　Eldertonic
　ILX B_{12} Elixir Crystalline and ILX B_{12}
　　Sugar–Free Elixir
　Materna Tablets
　Mega-B

VITAMIN B COMPLEX WITH VITAMIN C
　Berocca Plus Tablets
　Berocca Tablets
　Carotene Health Packs
　Cefol Filmtab
　Eldercaps
　Gerimed Tablets
　Glutathione Health Packs
　Glutofac Caplets
　Hemocyte Plus Tabules
　ILX B_{12} Caplets Crystalline
　Iberet Filmtab
　Iberet-500 Filmtab
　Iberet-500 Liquid
　Iberet-Folic-500 Filmtab
　Iberet-Liquid
　Megadose
　Nephro-Vite Tablets
　Nephro-Vite + Fe Tablets
　Nephro-Vite Rx Tablets
　Neuroforte-Six Monovial
　Performance Packs
　Performance Packs-Light
　Prenate 90 Tablets
　Renal Multivitamin Formula Rx

VITAMIN B_1
　Mega-B
　Thiamilate Enteric Tablets (Thiamine
　　Pyrophosphate)

VITAMIN B_2
　Mega-B

VITAMIN B_6
　Aminoxin Tablets (Coenzymatic B_6)
　Apatate Liquid/Tablets
　Beelith Tablets
　Lurline PMS Tablets
　Marlyn Formula 50 Capsules
　May-Vita Elixir
　Mega-B

VITAMIN B_{12}
　Apatate Liquid/Tablets
　Cyanocobalamin (Vit. B_{12}) Injection
　Ener-B Vitamin B_{12} Nasal Gel Dietary
　　Supplement
　Mega-B
　Neuroforte-R Vial
　Niferex Forte Elixir
　Nu-Iron Plus Elixir
　Trinsicon Capsules
　Vitamin B_{12} (Cyanocobalamin) in Tubex
　Vitamin B_{12} (Cyanocobalamin) in Tubex
　　(WYETH-AYERST LABORATORIES)

VITAMIN C
　ACES Antioxidant Soft Gels
　ANTIOX Capsules
　Centrum Singles Vitamin C
　Chromagen Capsules

Fero-Folic-500 Filmtab
Fero-Grad-500 Filmtab
Fetrin Capsules
Glutathione-Fort+342 Capsules
Hemaspan Caplets
Hemocyte-C Tablets
Irospan Capsules
Irospan Tablets
Materna Tablets
Niferex w/Vitamin C Tablets
Nu-Iron V Tablets
Peridin-C Tablets
Protegra Antioxidant Vitamin & Mineral
　Supplement
Trinsicon Capsules
Vi-Daylin ADC Vitamins Drops
Vi-Daylin ADC Vitamins + Iron Drops
Vi-Daylin/F ADC Vitamins Drops With Fluoride
Vi-Daylin/F ADC Vitamins + Iron Drops With
　Fluoride

VITAMIN D
　Calcet
　Caltrate PLUS
　Caltrate 600 + D
　Citracal Caplets+D
　Materna Tablets
　Megadose
　NutraVescent
　Prenate 90 Tablets
　Vi-Daylin ADC Vitamins + Iron Drops
　Vi-Daylin/F ADC Vitamins Drops With Fluoride
　Vi-Daylin/F ADC Vitamins + Iron Drops With
　　Fluoride

VITAMIN D_2
　Calciferol Drops
　Calciferol in Oil Injection
　Calciferol Tablets
　Eldercaps

VITAMIN D_3
　Calel-D
　Carotene Health Packs
　Casamin
　Dical-D Tablets & Wafers
　Glusamin
　Performance Packs
　Performance Packs-Light

VITAMIN E
　ACES Antioxidant Soft Gels
　ANTIOX Capsules
　Carotene-E Forté Capsules
　Carotene Health Packs
　Cefol Filmtab
　Centrum Singles Vitamin E
　E-Gems Soft Gels
　Eldercaps
　Glutathione Health Packs
　Glutofac Caplets
　Lazer Creme
　Materna Tablets
　Megadose
　Performance Packs
　Performance Packs-Light
　Prenate 90 Tablets
　Protegra Antioxidant Vitamin & Mineral
　　Supplement
　Pure-E Capsules and Liquid

VITAMIN K_1
　AquaMEPHYTON Injection
　Konakion Injection
　Mephyton Tablets

VITAMINS WITH FLUORIDE
　Adeflor M Tablets
　Apatate Liquid with Fluoride

Florvite Chewable Tablets 0.5 mg & 1 mg
Florvite Drops 0.25 mg & 0.5 mg
Florvite + Iron Chewable Tablets 0.5 mg
　and 1 mg
Florvite + Iron Drops 0.25 mg & 0.5 mg
Poly-Vi-Flor Drops
Poly-Vi-Flor Tablets
Poly-Vi-Flor with Iron Drops
Poly-Vi-Flor with Iron Tablets
Tri-Vi-Flor Drops
Tri-Vi-Flor Tablets
Tri-Vi-Flor 0.25 mg with Iron Drops
Vi-Daylin/F ADC Vitamins Drops With Fluoride
Vi-Daylin/F ADC Vitamins + Iron Drops
　With Fluoride
Vi-Daylin/F Multivitamin Drops With Fluoride
Vi-Daylin/F Multivitamin + Iron Drops
　With Fluoride
Vi-Daylin/F Multivitamin Chewable Tablets
　With Fluoride
Vi-Daylin/F Multivitamin + Iron Chewable
　Tablets With Fluoride

VITAMINS WITH IRON
　Florvite + Iron Chewable Tablets 0.5 mg
　　and 1 mg
　Florvite + Iron Drops 0.25 mg & 0.5 mg
　Hemaspan Caplets
　Hemocyte Plus Tabules
　ILX B_{12} Caplets Crystalline
　ILX B_{12} Elixir Crystalline and ILX B_{12}
　　Sugar–Free Elixir
　ILX Elixir
　Iberet Filmtab
　Iberet-500 Filmtab
　Iberet-500 Liquid
　Iberet-Folic-500 Filmtab
　Iberet-Liquid
　Materna Tablets
　Multi Vit Drops with Iron
　Nephro-Vite + Fe Tablets
　Niferex Daily Tablets
　Niferex-PN Forte Tablets
　Niferex-PN Tablets
　Poly-Vi-Flor with Iron Drops
　Prenate 90 Tablets
　Trinsicon Capsules
　Tri-Vi-Flor 0.25 mg with Iron Drops
　Vi-Daylin ADC Vitamins + Iron Drops
　Vi-Daylin Multivitamin + Iron Drops
　Vi-Daylin/F ADC Vitamins + Iron Drops With
　　Fluoride
　Vi-Daylin/F Multivitamin + Iron Drops With
　　Fluoride
　Vi-Daylin Multivitamin + Iron Chewable Tablets
　Vi-Daylin/F Multivitamin + Iron Chewable
　　Tablets With Fluoride
　Vi-Daylin Multivitamin + Iron Liquid

VITAMINS WITH MINERALS
　Adeflor M Tablets
　Apatate Forte Liquid
　Berocca Plus Tablets
　Calcet Plus
　Cefol Filmtab
　Eldercaps
　Eldertonic
　Ensure With Fiber Complete, Balanced Nutrition
　Florvite Chewable Tablets 0.5 mg & 1 mg
　Florvite Drops 0.25 mg & 0.5 mg
　Florvite + Iron Drops 0.25 mg & 0.5 mg
　Gerimed Tablets
　Geroton Forte
　Glutathione Health Packs
　Glutofac Caplets
　Hemocyte Plus Tabules
　Hep-Forte Capsules

UNDERLINE DENOTES GENERIC NAME

Kenwood Therapeutic Liquid
MDR Fitness Tabs for Men and Women
M.V.I. Pediatric for Infusion
M.V.I.-12 Multi-Vitamin Infusion
Materna Tablets
May-Vita Elixir
Mediplex
Megadose
Mission Prenatal
Mission Prenatal F.A.
Mission Prenatal H.P.
Mission Prenatal RX
Nestabs FA Tablets
Niferex Daily Tablets
Niferex-PN Forte Tablets
Niferex-PN Tablets
Performance Packs
Performance Packs-Light
Poly-Vi-Flor with Iron Tablets
Pramilet FA
PreCare Caplets
Prenatal Maternal
Prenatal MR 90 Fe
Prenatal Rx
Prenatal Z
Prenate 90 Tablets
Pro-Hepatone Capsules
Pulmocare Specialized Nutrition for Pulmonary
  Patients
Strovite Plus Caplets
Stuartnatal Plus Tablets
Vicon Forte Capsules
Vitafol Caplets
Vitafol Syrup
Vitamist Intra-Oral Spray Dietary Supplements
ZENATE Tablets
Zincvit Vitamin-Mineral Formula

VITAMINS, MULTIPLE

Gerimed Tablets
Larobec Tablets
M.V.I. Pediatric for Infusion
M.V.I.-12 Multi-Vitamin Infusion
Mann-Dino Chewable
Nephrocaps
Niferex Daily Tablets
Niferex-PN Forte Tablets
Niferex-PN Tablets
Oncovite
Pedi-Joy Chewable
Strovite Tablets
Vi-Daylin ADC Vitamins Drops
Vi-Daylin Multivitamin Drops
Vi-Daylin/F ADC Vitamins Drops With Fluoride
Vi-Daylin/F Multivitamin Drops With Fluoride
Vi-Daylin/F Multivitamin + Iron Drops
  With Fluoride
Vi-Daylin Multivitamin Chewable Tablets
Vi-Daylin/F Multivitamin Chewable Tablets
  With Fluoride
Vi-Daylin/F Multivitamin + Iron Chewable
  Tablets With Fluoride
Vi-Daylin Multivitamin Liquid
Zincvit Vitamin-Mineral Formula

VITAMINS, PRENATAL

Lactocal-F Tablets
Materna Tablets
PreCare Caplets
Prenatal Maternal
Prenatal MR 90 Fe
Prenatal Rx
Prenatal Z
Prenate 90 Tablets
ZENATE Tablets
Vitamist Intra-Oral Spray Dietary Supplements
  (MAYOR PHARMACEUTICAL)

Anti-Oxidant
Multiple Adult/Child
PMS
Revitalizer
Smoke-less
Slendermist
Stress
Vitamin A
Vitamin B-12
Vitamin C + Zinc
Vitamin E
Aerobic
Anti-chol
Circuflex
Menopausal
Pre-natal
Vivactil Tablets (MERCK & CO., INC.)
Vivotif Berna (BERNA PRODUCTS, CORP.)
Vi-Zac Capsules
  (WHITBY PHARMACEUTICALS, INC.)
Volmax Extended-Release Tablets
  (MURO PHARMACEUTICAL, INC.)
Voltaren Tablets (GEIGY PHARMACEUTICALS)
Vontrol Tablets
  (SMITHKLINE BEECHAM PHARMACEUTICALS)
VōSoLā Otic Solution
  (WALLACE LABORATORIES)
VōSoL Otic Solution (WALLACE LABORATORIES)
Vumon
  (BRISTOL-MYERS SQUIBB ONCOLOGY DIVISION)
Vytone Cream 1% (DERMIK LABORATORIES, INC.)

W

Wallette Pill Dispenser (SYNTEX PUERTO RICO, INC.)

WARFARIN SODIUM

Coumadin Tablets

WATER, BACTERIOSTATIC

Water For Injection, Bacteriostatic
Water For Injection, Bacteriostatic
  (ELKINS-SINN, INC.)

WATER, STERILE

Sterile Water for Inhalation, USP
Water for Injection, Sterile (Preservative-Free)
Water for Injection, Sterile (Preservative-Free)
  (ELKINS-SINN, INC.)
Water-Jel Burn Jel
  (WATER-JEL TECHNOLOGIES, INC.)
Water-Jel Sterile Burn Dressings
  (WATER-JEL TECHNOLOGIES, INC.)
Wellbutrin Tablets (BURROUGHS WELLCOME CO.)
Westcort Cream 0.2%
  (WESTWOOD-SQUIBB PHARMACEUTICALS INC.)
Westcort Ointment 0.2%
  (WESTWOOD-SQUIBB PHARMACEUTICALS INC.)
White Petrolatum USP (BARRE-NATIONAL INC.)
Wigraine Tablets & Suppositories (ORGANON INC.)
Winstrol Tablets
  (SANOFI WINTHROP PHARMACEUTICALS)

WITCH HAZEL

Tucks Clear Gel
Tucks Pads
Tucks Take Alongs

WOOL WAX ALCOHOL

Eucerin Dry Skin Care Moisturizing Creme
  (Unscented)
**Woun' dress, Natural Collagen Hydrogel Wound
Dressing** (SWEEN CORPORATION)

**Wyanoids Relief Factor Hemorrhoidal
  Suppositorie** (WYETH-AYERST LABORATORIES)
Wycillin Injection (WYETH-AYERST LABORATORIES)
Wydase, Lyophilized
  (WYETH-AYERST LABORATORIES)
Wygesic Tablets (WYETH-AYERST LABORATORIES)
Wymox Capsules (WYETH-AYERST LABORATORIES)
Wymox for Oral Suspension
  (WYETH-AYERST LABORATORIES)
Wytensin Tablets
  (WYETH-AYERST LABORATORIES)

X

X-Trozine Capsules and Tablets
  (REXAR PHARMACAL)
X-Trozine L.A. Capsules (REXAR PHARMACAL)
Xanax Tablets (THE UPJOHN COMPANY)
Xerac AC (PERSŌN & COVEY, INC.)
Xylocaine Injections (ASTRA USA, INC.)
Xylocaine with Epinephrine Injections
  (ASTRA USA, INC.)
Xylocaine Injections for Ventricular Arrhythmias
  (ASTRA USA, INC.)
Xylocaine 2% Jelly (ASTRA USA, INC.)
Xylocaine Ointment 2.5% (ASTRA USA, INC.)
Xylocaine 5% Ointment (ASTRA USA, INC.)
Xylocaine 10% Oral Spray (ASTRA USA, INC.)
Xylocaine 1.5% Solution with Dextrose 7.5%
  (ASTRA USA, INC.)
Xylocaine 5% Solution with Glucose 7.5%
  (ASTRA USA, INC.)
4% Xylocaine-MPF Sterile Solution
  (ASTRA USA, INC.)
Xylocaine 4% Topical Solution
  (ASTRA USA, INC.)
Xylocaine 2% Viscous Solution
  (ASTRA USA, INC.)

Y

YELLOW FEVER VACCINE

YF-Vax
YF-Vax (CONNAUGHT LABORATORIES, INC.)
Yocon (PALISADES PHARMACEUTICALS, INC.)
Yodoxin (GLENWOOD, INC.)

YOHIMBINE HYDROCHLORIDE

Aphrodyne
Erex Tablets
Prohim
Yocon
Yohimex Tablets
Yovital Tablets
Yohimex Tablets (KRAMER LABORATORIES INC.)
Yovital Tablets (KENWOOD LABORATORIES)
Yutopar Intravenous Injection (ASTRA USA, INC.)
Yutopar Tablets (ASTRA USA, INC.)

UNDERLINE DENOTES GENERIC NAME

Z

ZALCITABINE
Hivid Tablets
Zanosar Sterile Powder (THE UPJOHN COMPANY)
Zantac 150 GELdose Capsules
(GLAXO PHARMACEUTICALS)
Zantac 300 GELdose Capsules
(GLAXO PHARMACEUTICALS)
Zantac Injection and Zantac Injection Premixed
(GLAXO PHARMACEUTICALS)
Zantac Syrup (GLAXO PHARMACEUTICALS)
Zantac 150 & 300 Tablets
(GLAXO PHARMACEUTICALS)
Zantac 150 EFFERdose Tablets
(GLAXO PHARMACEUTICALS)
Zantac 150 EFFERdose Granules
(GLAXO PHARMACEUTICALS)
Zantryl Capsules (ION LABORATORIES, INC.)
Zarontin Capsules (PARKE-DAVIS)
Zarontin Syrup (PARKE-DAVIS)
Zaroxolyn Tablets
(FISONS CORPORATION PRESCRIPTION PRODUCTS)
Zebeta Tablets (LEDERLE LABORATORIES)
Zefazone I.V. Solution (THE UPJOHN COMPANY)
Zefazone Sterile Powder (THE UPJOHN COMPANY)
Zemuron (ORGANON INC.)
ZENATE Tablets
(SOLVAY PHARMACEUTICALS, INC.)
Zephiran Chloride Aqueous Solution
(SANOFI WINTHROP PHARMACEUTICALS)
Zephiran Chloride Concentrate Solution
(SANOFI WINTHROP PHARMACEUTICALS)
Zephiran Chloride Spray
(SANOFI WINTHROP PHARMACEUTICALS)
Zephiran Chloride Tinted Tincture
(SANOFI WINTHROP PHARMACEUTICALS)
Zephiran Towelettes
(SANOFI WINTHROP PHARMACEUTICALS)
Zephrex Tablets (BOCK PHARMACAL COMPANY)
Zephrex LA Tablets (BOCK PHARMACAL COMPANY)
Zerit Capsules
(BRISTOL-MYERS SQUIBB ONCOLOGY DIVISION)
Zestoretic (STUART PHARMACEUTICALS)
Zestril Tablets (STUART PHARMACEUTICALS)
Zetar Emulsion (DERMIK LABORATORIES, INC.)
Ziac (LEDERLE LABORATORIES)

ZIDOVUDINE
Retrovir Capsules
Retrovir I.V. Infusion
Retrovir Syrup
Zinacef (GLAXO PHARMACEUTICALS)

ZINC
May-Vita Elixir
Prenate 90 Tablets

ZINC ACETATE
Benadryl Cream
Benadryl Cream Maximum Strength
Benadryl Itch Relief Stick
Benadryl Spray Maximum Strength 2%
Benadryl Spray Regular 1%
Caladryl Clear Lotion
Renal Multivitamin Formula Rx

ZINC GLUCONATE
Megadose

ZINC OXIDE
Anusol Hemorrhoidal Ointment
Borofax
Caltrate PLUS
Critic-Aid, Antimicrobial Skin Paste

Ostiderm
Primer Unna Boot
Triad, Hydrophilic Wound Dressing
Zinc Oxide Ointment USP
Zinc Oxide Ointment USP
(BARRE-NATIONAL INC.)

ZINC SULFATE
Eldercaps
Eldertonic
Hemocyte Plus Tabules

ZINC UNDECYLENATE
Pedi-Pro Topical Powder
Zincon Dandruff Shampoo
(LEDERLE LABORATORIES)
Zincvit Vitamin-Mineral Formula
(KENWOOD LABORATORIES)
Zithromax Capsules (PFIZER LABS DIVISION)
Zocor Tablets (MERCK & CO., INC.)
Zofran Injection (CERENEX)
Zofran Tablets (CERENEX)
Zoladex (ZENECA PHARMACEUTICALS)
Zoloft Tablets (ROERIG DIVISION)

ZOLPIDEM TARTRATE
Ambien Tablets
Zonalon Cream (GENDERM CORPORATION)
Zone-A Cream 1%
(UAD LABORATORIES)
Zostrix (GENDERM CORPORATION)
Zostrix-HP Topical Analgesic Cream
(GENDERM CORPORATION)
Zosyn (LEDERLE LABORATORIES)
Zosyn Pharmacy Bulk Package
(LEDERLE LABORATORIES)
Zovirax Capsules (BURROUGHS WELLCOME CO.)
Zovirax Ointment 5%
(BURROUGHS WELLCOME CO.)
Zovirax Sterile Powder
(BURROUGHS WELLCOME CO.)
Zovirax Suspension (BURROUGHS WELLCOME CO.)
Zovirax Tablets (BURROUGHS WELLCOME CO.)
Zovirax Suspension
(WYETH-AYERST LABORATORIES)
Zyloprim Tablets (BURROUGHS WELLCOME CO.)
Zymacap Capsules
(ROBERTS PHARMACEUTICAL CORPORATION)
Zymase Capsules (ORGANON INC.)

UNDERLINE DENOTES GENERIC NAME

COMMON MEDICAL ABBREVIATIONS

α alpha; Bunsen's solubility coefficient; first in a series; specific rotation term

a (specific) absorption (coefficient) (USUALLY ITALIC); (total) acidity; area; (systemic) arterial (blood) (SUBSCRIPT); asymmetric; atto-

A absorbance

A adenosine (or adenylic acid) (in polynucleotides); alveolar gas (subscript); ampere

Å angstrom; Ångström unit

āā [G.] *ana* of each (USED IN PRESCRIPTIONS)

AA amino acid; aminoacyl

Ab antibody

ABG arterial blood gas

abl Abelson murine (mouse) leukemia virus

ABLB alternate binaural loudness balance (test)

ABR abortus-Bang-ring (test); auditory brainstem response (audiometry)

abs feb [L.] *absente febre*, when fever is absent

γ-Abu γ-aminobutyric acid

ABVD Adriamycin (doxorubicin), bleomycin, vinblastine, (and) dacarbazine

ac acetyl; [L.] *ante cibum*, before a meal

aC arabinosylcytosine

Ac acetyl; actinium

AC acetate; acromioclavicular; atriocarotid

AC/A accommodation convergence-accommodation (ratio)

ACEI angiotensin-converting enzyme inhibitor

ac-g accelerator globulin

AcG accelerator globulin

Ach acetylcholine

aCL anticardiolipin (antibody)

ACP acyl carrier protein

ACTH adrenocorticotropic hormone (corticotropin)

AD [L.] *auris dexter*, right ear

add. [L.] *adde*, (please) add

Ade adenine

ADH antidiuretic hormone

adhib [L.] *adhibendus*, to be administered

ADL activities (of) daily living

ad lib [L.] *ad libitum*, freely, as desired

admov [L.] *admove*, apply

Ado adenosine

ADP adenosine 5'-diphosphate

ad sat [L.] *ad saturatum*, *ad saturandum*, to saturation

adst feb [L.] *adstante febre*, when fever is present

ad us. ext [L.] *ad usum externum*, for external use

adv [L.] *adversum*, against

A-E above-the-elbow (amputation)

AFORMED alternating failure of response, mechanical, (to) electrical depolarization

AFP α-fetoprotein

Ag antigen; [L.] *argentum*, silver

agit. ante us. [L.] *agita ante usum*, shake before using

agit. bene [L.] *agita bene*, shake well

A/G R albumin-globulin ratio

AHF antihemophilic factor

AHG antihemophilic globulin

AID artificial insemination donor

AIDS acquired immunodeficiency syndrome

AIH artificial insemination by husband; artificial insemination, homologous

A-K above-the-knee (amputation)

Al aluminum

Ala alanine (or its mono- or diradical)

ALA δ-aminolevulinic acid

ALD adrenoleukodystrophy

ALL acute lymphocytic leukemia

ALS antilymphocyte serum

ALT alanine aminotransferase

alt hor [L.] *alternis horis*, every other hour

Am americium

AMP adenosine monophosphate (adenylic acid)

amu atomic mass unit

ANF antinuclear factor

ANUG acute necrotizing ulcerative gingivitis

APA antipernicious anemia (factor)

APC acetylsalicylic (acid), phenacetin, (and) caffeine (combined as an antipyretic and analgesic); antigen-presenting cell

A-P-C adenoidal-pharyngeal-conjunctival (virus)

aPS antiphospholipid antibody syndrome

APTT activated partial thromboplastin time

Ar argon

araC arabinosylcytosine (cytarabine)

ARC AIDS-related complex

ARDS adult respiratory distress syndrome

Arg arginine (or its mono- or diradical)

ARV AIDS-related virus

As arsenic

a.s. [L.] *auris sinistra*, left ear

Asn asparagine (or its mono- or diradical)

Asp aspartic (acid) (or its radical forms)

AST aspartate aminotransferase

At astatine

ATL adult T-cell leukemia; adult T-cell lymphoma

atm (standard) atmosphere

ATP adenosine 5'-triphosphate

ATPase adenosine triphosphatase

ATPD ambient temperature (and) pressure, dry

ATPS ambient temperature (and) pressure, saturated (with water vapor)

at. wt. atomic weight

Au [L.] *aurum*, gold

Au Ag Australia antigen

AU [L.] *auris uterque*, each ear, both ears

AV arteriovenous

A-V arteriovenous; atrioventricular (block, bundle, conduction, dissociation, extrasystole)

AVN atrioventricular nodal (extrasystole)

AVP antiviral protein

AW atomic weight

ax. axis

AZT azidothymidine (zidovudine)

b blood (SUBSCRIPT)

B barometric (pressure) (SUBSCRIPT); boron

Ba barium

BADL basic activities (of) daily life

BAER brainstem auditory evoked response

BAL British anti-Lewisite (dimercaprol); bronchoalveolar lavage

BALB binaural alternate loudness balance (test)

BBB blood-brain barrier

BCG bacille bilié de Calmette-Guérin (vaccine); ballistocardiograph

Be beryllium

B-E below-the-elbow (amputation)

Bi bismuth

bib. [L.] *bibe*, (please) drink

BIB. [L.] *bibe*, (please)

drink

b.i.d. [L.] *bis in die*, twice (in) a day

BID [L.] *bis in die*, twice (in) a day

BIDS brittle (hair), impaired (intelligence), decreased (fertility), (and) short (stature)

BIPAP bilevel positive airway pressure

Bk Berkelium

BMR basal metabolic rate

BP blood pressure; boiling point; *British Pharmacopoeia*

BPF bronchopleural fistula

Bq becquerel (SI unit of radionuclide activity)

Br bromine

BSA body surface area

BSER brainstem evoked response (audiometry)

BSP brom(o)sulfophthalein (liver function)

BT bleeding time

BTPS body temperature, (ambient) pressure, saturated (with water vapor)

BTU British thermal unit

BUN blood urea nitrogen

C calorie (large); carbon; Celsius; centigrade; clearance (rate, renal) (FOLLOWED BY A SUBSCRIPT); compliance; concentration; cylindrical (lens); cytidine

c calorie (small); capillary (blood) (SUBSCRIPT); centi-

ca [L.] *circa*, (about, approximately)

c-a cardioarterial

Ca calcium; cathodal; cathode

CA cancer; carcinoma; cardiac arrest; chronologic age; croup-associated (virus); cytosine arabinoside

cal calorie (small)

Cal calorie (large)

cAMP cyclic AMP (adenosine monophosphate)

CAP catabolite (gene) activator protein

CAT computerized axial tomography

CBC complete blood (cell) count

CBG corticosteroid-binding globulin

Cbz carbobenzoxy (chloride)

c.c. cubic centimeter

C.C. chief complaint

CCNU chloroethylcyclohexylnitrosourea (lomustine)

CCU coronary care unit; critical care unit

cd candela

Cd cadmium

CDC Centers (for) Disease Control

cDNA complementary DNA

CDP cytidine 5'-diphosphate

Ce cerium

CEA carcinoembryonic antigen

CELO chicken embryo lethal orphan (virus)

CEP congenital erythropoietic porphyria

Cf californium

CF coupling factor

CG chorionic gonadotropin

CGA catabolite gene activator

cgs centimeter-gram-second (system, unit)

CGS centimeter-gram-second (system, unit)

Ch¹ Christchurch (chromosome)

µCi microcurie

Ci curie

CI color index; *Colour Index*

CIB [L.] *cibus*, food

CIQ cognitive laterality quotient

Cl chlorine

CL cardiolipin

CLL chronic lymphocytic leukemia

cm centimeter

cM centimorgan

Cm curium

CMA Certified Medical Assistant

CMC carpometacarpal

CMI cell-mediated immunity

CML chronic myelogenous leukemia

CMP cytidine 5'-phosphate (or any cytidine monophosphate)

CMT Certified Medical Transcriptionist

CMV controlled mechanical ventilation; cytomegalovirus

CNM Certified Nurse Midwife

CNS central nervous system

Co cobalt

CoA coenzyme A

COG center of gravity

conA concanavalin A

cont. rem. [L.] *continuetur remedium*, let the medicine be continued

COPD chronic obstructive pulmonary disease

CPAP continuous (or; constant) positive airway pressure

CPM continuous passive motility

CPPB continuous (or; constant) positive-pressure breathing

CPPV continuous positive-pressure ventilation

CPR cardiopulmonary resuscitation

cps cycles per second

Cr chromium; creatinine

CR conditioned reflex; crown-rump (length)

CRD chronic respiratory disease

CRH corticotropin-releasing hormone

CRL crown-rump length

CRNA Certified Registered Nurse Anesthetist

CRP cross-reacting protein

CRST calcinosis (cutis), Raynaud's (phenomenon), sclerodactyly, (and)

telangiectasia (syndrome)

Cs cesium

CSF cerebrospinal fluid

CT computed tomography

CTP cytidine 5'-triphosphate

Cu [L.] *cuprum*, copper

CV cardiovascular

CVA cerebral vascular accident (older classical term for stroke)

CVP central venous pressure

Cyd cytidine

cyl cylinder; cylindrical (lens)

Cys cysteine

Cyt cytosine

δ delta

Δ delta

d deci-

d deuterium

d- dextrorotatory

D dead (space gas) (SUBSCRIPT); deciduous; deuterium; diffusing (capacity); dihydrouridine (in nucleic acids); diopter; [L.] *dexter*, right (opposite of left); vitamin D potency of cod liver oil

da deca-

dA deoxyadenosine

DA developmental age

dAdo deoxyadenosine

dAMP deoxyadenylic acid

DANS 1-dimethylaminonaphthalene-5-sulfonic acid

dB decibel

db decibel

DC Dental Corps; Doctor (of) Chiropractic

D & C dilation and curettage

DCG dacryocystography

DCI dichloroisoproterenol

dCMP deoxycytidylic acid

DDS Doctor (of) Dental Surgery

DDT dichlorodiphenyltrichloroethane (chlorophenothane)

D & E dilation and evacuation

def decayed, extracted, (or) filled (deciduous

"baby" teeth)

DEF decayed, extracted, (or) filled (permanent "adult" teeth)

deglut [L.] *degluttiatur*, (please) swallow

DES diethylstilbestrol

det [L.] *detur*, (please) give

DET diethyltryptamine

DEV duck embryo vaccine; duck embryo virus

df decayed (and) filled (deciduous "baby" teeth)

DF decayed (and) filled (permanent "adult" teeth)

dGMP deoxyguanosine monophosphate (deoxyguanylic acid)

DIC disseminated intravascular coagulation

dieb alt [L.] *diebus alternis*, every other day

dil [L.] *dilue*, (please) dilute

dim. [L.] *dimidius*, one-half

DIP desquamative interstitial pneumonia

dir. prop. [L.] *directione propria*, with proper direction

div in par aeq [L.] *divide in partes aequales*, (please) divide into equal parts

dk deca-, deka-

dM decimorgan

DMD Doctor (of) Dental Medicine

dmf decayed, missing, (or) filled (deciduous "baby" teeth)

DMF decayed, missing, (or) filled (permanent "adult" teeth)

DMSO dimethyl sulfoxide

DMT *N, N*-dimethyltryptamine

DN dibucaine number

DNA deoxyribonucleic acid

DNAase deoxyribonucleic acid nuclease

DNase deoxyribonuclease

DNAse deoxyribonuclease

DNP deoxyribonucleopro-

tein; 2,4-dinitrophenol

DNR do not resuscitate

DNS Director (of) Nursing Service(s); Doctor (of) Nursing Services

DO Doctor (of) Osteopathy

DOA dead on arrival

DOC deoxycholic acid

DOC deoxycorticosterone

DOM 2,5-dimethoxy-4-methylamphetamine

DP Doctor (of) Podiatry

2,3-DPG 2,3-diphospho-glycerate

DPH Doctor (of) Public Health; Doctor (of) Public Hygiene

DPI dry powder inhaler

DPM Doctor (of) Physical Medicine; Doctor (of) Podiatric Medicine

DPN diphosphopyridine nucleotide

DPT dipropyltryptamine

dr dram

DR degeneration reaction, reaction (of) degeneration (muscle fibers)

DRG diagnosis-related group

DrPH Doctor (of) Pubic Health; Doctor (of) Public Hygiene

DRVVT dilute Russell's viper venom test

D-S Doerfler-Stewart (test)

DSA digital subtraction angiography

dT deoxythymidine

DT delirium tremens; duration (of) tetany

dTDP deoxythymidine 5'-diphosphate

dThd thymidine

DTIC (dimethyltrizeno)imidazole carboxamide (dacarbazine)

dTMP deoxythymidylic acid

DTP diphtheria-tetanus (toxoids)-pertussis (vaccine); distal tingling (on) percussion (Tinel's sign)

DTPA diethylenetriamine pentaacetic acid

DTR deep tendon reflex

dTTP deoxythymidine 5'-triphosphate

dur dol [L.] *durante dolore*, while pain lasts

DVM Doctor (of) Veterinary Medicine

Dy dysprosium

ϵ epsilon; molar absorption coefficient

E exa-; extraction (ratio)

EB Epstein-Barr (virus)

EBV Epstein-Barr virus

ECF extracellular fluid

ECF-A eosinophilic chemotactic factor (of) anaphylaxis

ECG electrocardiogram

ECHO enterocytopathogenic human orphan (virus)

ECMO extracorporeal-membrane oxygenation (pronounced ek´mō)

ECS electrocerebral silence

ECT electroconvulsive therapy

ED effective dose

EDTA ethylenediaminetetraacetic acid (edathamil, edetic acid)

EEG electroencephalogram

EENT eye, ear, nose, (and) throat

EIA enzyme immunoassay

EKG [German] *Elektrokardiogramme* electrocardiogram

EKY electrokymogram

ELISA enzyme-linked immunoadsorbent assay

EMC encephalomyocarditis (virus)

EMF electromotive force

EMG electromyogram; exomphalos, macroglossia, (and) gigantism (syndrome)

emp [L.] *emplastrum*, plaster; [L.] *ex modo praescripto*, in the manner prescribed

ENG electronystagmography

ENT ear, nose, (and)

throat

EOG electro-oculography

EPAP expiratory positive airway pressure

Er erbium

ER endoplasmic reticulum

ERBF effective renal blood flow

ERCP endoscopic retrograde cholangiopancreatography

ERG electroretinogram

ERPF effective renal plasma flow

ERV expiratory reserve volume

Es einsteinium

ESEP extreme somatosensory evoked potential

ESP extrasensory perception

ESR electron spin resonance; erythrocyte sedimentation rate

Eu europium

ev electron-volt

eV electron-volt

f femto- (one-quadrillionth [10⁻¹⁵]); (respiratory) frequency

F Fahrenheit; faraday (constant); fertility (factor); field (of vision); filial (generation); fluorine; force; fractional (concentration); free (energy)

F1.2 (prothrombin) fragment 1.2

Fab fragment (of immunoglobulin G involved in) antigen binding

FAD flavin(e) adenine dinucleotide

FANA fluorescent antinuclear antibody (test)

FDA Food (and) Drug Administration

Fe [L.] *ferrum*, iron

FEF forced expiratory flow

FET forced expiratory time

FEV forced expiratory volume

FF filtration fraction

FFD focus-film distance

FIA fluorescent immunoassay
FIGLU formiminoglutamic (acid)
Fm fermium
FMN flavin(e) mononucleotide
fps foot-pound-second (system, unit)
FPS foot-pound-second (system, unit)
Fr francium; French (gauge, scale)
FRC functional residual capacity (of lungs)
FRF follicle-stimulating hormone-releasing factor
FRS first rank symptom
Fru fructose
FSH follicle-stimulating hormone
FSH-RF follicle-stimulating hormone-releasing factor
FSH-RH follicle-stimulating hormone-releasing hormone
ft [L.] *fiat*, let it be done, let there be made
FTA-ABS fluorescent treponemal antibody-absorption (test)
FUO fever (of) unknown origin
FVC forced vital capacity
Fw F wave (fibrillary wave, flutter wave)
γ gamma; Ostwald's solubility coefficient; the third in a series
μg microgram
g gram
G giga-; glucose (as in UDPG, uridine-diphosphoglucose); gravitation (newtonian constant of); guanosine (or guanylic acid) residues in polynucleotides, as in poly(G)
G 1 gap 1
G 2 gap 2
Ga gallium
GABA γ-aminobutyric acid
Gal galactose
Gd gadolinium

GDP mannose-1-phosphate guanylyltransferase
Ge germanium
GFR glomerular filtration rate
GH glenohumeral; growth hormone
GHRF growth hormone-releasing factor
GH-RF growth hormone-releasing factor
GHRH growth hormone-releasing hormone
GH-RH growth hormone-releasing hormone
GI Gingival Index; gastrointestinal
GIP gastric inhibitory polypeptide
GLC gas-liquid chromatography
Gln glutamine; glutaminyl
Glu glutamic acid; glutamyl
Gly glycine; glycyl
gm gram
GMP guanosine monophosphate (guanylic acid)
GnRH gonadotropin-releasing hormone
GOT glutamic-oxaloacetic transaminase (aspartate aminotransferase)
GPI Gingival-Periodontal Index
GPT glutamic-pyruvic transaminase
gr grain
grad. [L.] *gradatim*, gradually
GSH reduced glutathione
GSR galvanic skin response
GSSG oxidized glutathione
gt [L.] *gutta*, a drop
GTP guanosine 5'-triphosphate
gtt [L.] *guttae*, drops, (plural of the abbreviation gt)
GU genitourinary
Guo guanosine
guttat [L.] *guttatim*, drop by drop
Gy gray (unit of absorbed

dose of ionizing radiation)
GYN gynecology
h hecto-
h Planck's constant
α-h the right-handed helical form assumed by many proteins
H henry; hydrogen; hyperopia; hyperopic
¹H hydrogen-1 (protium, light hydrogen)
²H hydrogen-2 (deuterium, heavy hydrogen)
³H hydrogen-3 (tritium, radioactive hydrogen)
H⁺ hydrogen ion
Ha hahnium
HA hyaluronic acid
HAA hepatitis-associated antigen
HAV hepatitis A virus
Hb hemoglobin
HbA adult hemoglobin
HbA₁ major (component of) adult hemoglobin
HbA₂ minor (fraction of) adult hemoglobin
HbAS heterozygosity for hemoglobin A and hemoglobin S (sickle cell trait)
HB_cAg hepatitis B core antigen
HbCO carboxyhemoglobin
HBe hepatitis B early (antigen)
HB_eAb hepatitis B early antibody
HB_eAg hepatitis B early antigen
HbF fetal hemoglobin
HbO₂ oxyhemoglobin, oxygenated hemoglobin
HbS sickle-cell hemoglobin
HB_sAb hepatitis B surface antibody
HB_sAg hepatitis B surface antigen
HBV hepatitis B virus
HCG human chorionic gonadotropin
HCS human chorionic somatomammotropin (hormone) (human placental lactogen)

Hct hematocrit
hd [L.] *hora decubitus*, at bedtime
HDL high density lipoprotein
HDRV human diploid (cell strain) rabies vaccine
HDV human delta virus
He helium
HEMPAS hereditary erythroblastic multinuclearity (associated with) positive acidified serum
Hf hafnium
HFJV high-frequency jet ventilation
HFOV high-frequency oscillatory ventilation
HFPPV high-frequency positive pressure ventilation
HFV high-frequency ventilation
Hg [L.] *hydrargyrum*, water-silver, mercury
HGH human (pituitary) growth hormone
HHA hepatitis-associated antigen
HI hemagglutination inhibition (test, titer)
His histidine
His- histidyl
-His histidino
HIV human immunodeficiency virus
Hl hyperopia, latent
HLA human lymphocyte antigen
Hm hyperopia, manifest (hypermetropia)
HMG human menopausal gonadotropin
HMO Health Maintenance Organization
HMWK high molecular weight kininogen (Fletcher factor)
Ho holmium
hor decub [L.] *hora decubitus*, at bedtime
hor som [L.] *hora somni*, at bedtime
HPL human placental lactogen
HPV human papilloma

virus

HS [L.] *hora somni*, at bedtime

HSV herpes simplex virus

Ht hyperopia, total

5-HT 5-hydroxytrypta-mine (serotonin)

HTLV human T-cell lym-phocytotrophic virus; human T-cell lymphoma/leukemia virus

HTLV-III human T-cell lymphotropic virus (type) III

HVL half-value layer

Hz hertz

I inspired (gas) (SUBSCRIPT); iodine

¹²³I iodine-123 (radioiso-tope)

¹²⁵I iodine-125

¹³¹I iodine-131

IADL instrumental activi-ties (of) daily living

IAP intermittent acute por-phyria

ICD *International Classification of Diseases of the World Health Organization*

ICDA *International Classification of Diseases, Adapted for Use in the United States*

ICF intracellular fluid

ICP intracranial pressure

ICSH interstitial cell-stim-ulating hormone

ICU intensive care unit

ID infective dose

IDDM insulin-dependent diabetes mellitus

IDU idoxuridine

IF initiation factor; intrin-sic factor

IFN interferon

Ig immunoglobulin

IGF insulin-like growth factor

IH infectious hepatitis

IL interleukin

ILA insulin-like activity

Ile isoleucine (or its radi-cal, isoleucyl)

IM internal medicine; intramuscular (injection site, or) intramuscularly

IMP inosine monophos-phate (inosinic acid)

IMV intermittent manda-tory ventilation

in d [L.] *in dies*, daily

In indium

Ino inosine

INR international normal-ized ratio

int cib [L.] *inter cibos*, between meals

IOML infraorbitomeatal line

IP interphalangeal (joint, keratosis); intraperi-toneal, intraperitoneally

IPAP inspiratory positive airway pressure

IPPB intermittent positive-pressure breathing

IPPV intermittent posi-tive-pressure ventilation

IPV inactivated poliovirus vaccine

IQ intelligence quotient

Ir iridium

IRV inspiratory reserve volume

ISI International Sensitivity Index

ITP idiopathic thrombocy-topenic purpura; inosine 5'-triphosphate

IU International Unit

IUCD intrauterine contra-ceptive device

IUD intrauterine device

IV intravenous, intra-venously; intraventricular

J joule

J flux (density)

k kilo-

K [Modern L.] *kalium* potassium; kelvin (SI fundamental unit of tem-perature)

kat katal (enzyme unit of measurement)

kc kilocycle

kcal kilocalorie

KCT kaolin clotting time

kg kilogram

Kr krypton

17-KS 17-ketosteroid

kv kilovolt

kVp kilovolt peak

μl microliter

l liter

L inductance; left; [L.] *limes* a boundary, a limit; liter

La lanthanum

LA lupus anticoagulant

LATS long-acting thyroid stimulator

LAV lymphadenopathy-associated virus

LBT lupus band test

LCAT lecithin-cholesterol acyltransferase (deficien-cy)

LCM lymphocytic chori-omeningitis (virus)

LD lethal dose

LDH lactate dehydroge-nase

LDL low-density lipopro-tein

LE left eye; lupus erythe-matosus

LEEP loop electrosurgical excision procedure

LETS large external trans-formation-sensitive (fibronectin)

LFA left frontoanterior (fetal position)

LFP left frontoposterior (fetal position)

LFT left frontotransverse (fetal position)

LH luteinizing hormone

LH/FSH-RF luteinizing hormone/follicle-stimu-lating hormone-releasing factor

LH-RF luteinizing hor-mone-releasing factor

LH-RH luteinizing hor-mone-releasing hormone

Li lithium

LM Licentiate (in) Midwifery

LMA left mentoanterior (fetal position)

LMP left mentoposterior (fetal position)

LMT left mentotransverse (fetal position)

LNPF lymph node perme-ability factor

LOA left occipitoanterior (fetal position)

LOP left occipitoposterior

(fetal position)

LOT left occipitotrans-verse (fetal position)

LPH lipotropic pituitary hormone (lipotropin)

LPN Licensed Practical Nurse

Lr lawrencium

LRH luteinizing (hor-mone)-releasing hormone

LSA left sacroanterior (fetal position)

LSD lysergic acid diethy-lamide

LSP left sacroposterior (fetal position)

L/S R lecithin/sphin-gomyelin ratio

LST left sacrotransverse (fetal position)

LTH luteotropic hormone

LTM long-term memory

Lu lutetium

LUQ left upper quadrant (of abdomen)

LVET left ventricular ejection time

LVN Licensed Visiting Nurse; Licensed Vocational Nurse

Lw (FORMER SYMBOL FOR) lawrencium (now Lr)

Lys lysine (or its radicals in peptides)

μ mu; micro-

m mass; meter; milli-; minim; molar

m- meta-

M mega-, meg-; molar; moles (per liter); morgan; myopic; myopia

M molar; moles (per liter)

m moles (per liter)

μμ micromicro-

μm micrometer

mμ millimicron

mA milliampere

MA mental age

MAA macroaggregated albumin

M + Am compound myopic astigmatism

man. pr. [L.] *mane primo*, early morning, first thing in the morning

MAO monoamine oxidase

MAOI monoamine oxidase inhibitor

mA-s milliampere-second

Mb myoglobin

MBC maximum breathing capacity

MbCO carbon monoxided myoglobin

MbO₂ oxymyoglobin (myoglobin in its combination with O_2)

MC Medical Corps

MCH mean cell hemoglobin

MCHC mean cell hemoglobin concentration

mCi millicurie

MCP metacarpophalangeal

MCV mean cell volume

Md mendelevium

MD [L.] *Medicinae Doctor,* Doctor of Medicine

MDF myocardial depressant factor

MDI metered-dose inhaler

Me methyl

MEDLARS Medical Literature Analysis and Retrieval System

MEP maximal expiratory pressure

meq milliequivalent

mEq milliequivalent

Met methionine (or its radicals in peptides)

MET metabolic equivalent (of) task

met-Hb methemoglobin

met-Mb metmyoglobin

MEV million electron-volts (10^6 ev)

mg milligram

Mg magnesium

MHC major histocompatibility complex

mho siemens unit

mHz megahertz

MI myocardial infarction

MID minimal infecting dose

MIP maximum inspiratory pressure

MK menaquinone (vitamin K_2)

mks meter-kilogram-second (system, unit)

MKS meter-kilogram-second (system, unit)

ml milliliter

MLC mixed lymphocyte culture (test)

MLD minimal lethal dose

mm millimeter

mmol millimole

MMPI Minnesota Multiphasic Personality Inventory (test)

MMR measles-mumps-rubella (vaccine)

Mn manganese

Mo molybdenum

MO Medical Officer; mineral oil

mol mole

mol wt molecular weight

MOPP Mustargen (mechlorethamine hydrochloride), Oncovin (vincristine sulfate), procarbazine hydrochloride, and prednisone

mor dict [L.] *more dicto,* in the manner stated

mor sol [L.] *more solito,* as usual, as customary

MPD maximal permissible dose

MPS mononuclear phagocyte system

MR milk-ring (test)

M_r molecular (weight) ratio

mrd minimal reacting dose

MRD minimal reacting dose

MRI magnetic resonance imaging

mRNA messenger RNA

ms millisecond

MS multiple sclerosis

msec millisecond

MSG monosodium glutamate

MSH melanocyte-stimulating hormone

MTP metatarsophalangeal (joint)

Mu Mache unit

mV millivolt

Mv mendelevium

MVE Murray Valley encephalitis (virus)

MVV maximal voluntary ventilation

MW molecular weight

My myopia

ν nu; kinematic viscosity

n index of refraction; nano-

N newton; nitrogen; normal (concentration)

N normal (SMALL CAPS)

Na [Modern L.] *natrium,* sodium

NAD nicotinamide adenine dinucleotide

NAD⁺ nicotinamide adenine dinucleotide (oxidized form)

NADH nicotinamide adenine dinucleotide (reduced form)

NADP nicotinamide adenine dinucleotide phosphate

NADP+ nicotinamide adenine dinucleotide phosphate (oxidized form)

NADPH nicotinamide adenine dinucleotide phosphate (reduced form)

NAME nevi, atrial (myxoma), myxoid (neurofibromas, and) ephelides (syndrome)

NANB non-A, non-B (hepatitis)

Nb niobium

NBT nitroblue tetrazolium (test)

Nd neodymium

Ne neon

NEEP negative end-expiratory pressure

NF National Formulary

ng nanogram

NGF nerve growth factor (antigen)

Ni nickel

NIDDM non-insulin-dependent diabetes mellitus

NIH National Institutes (of) Health

NK natural killer (cell)

NLM National Library (of) Medicine

nm nanometer

NMN nicotinamide mononucleotide

NMR nuclear magnetic resonance (imaging)

No nobelium

noc maneq [L.] *nocte maneque,* at night and in the morning

Np neptunium

NPN nonprotein nitrogen

NREM non-rapid eye movement (sleep)

nRNA nuclear RNA

NSAID nonsteroidal anti-inflammatory drug

NUG necrotizing ulcerative gingivitis

Ω omega; ohm

O [L.] *oculus,* an eye; opening (in formulas for electrical reactions); oxygen

OAV oculoauriculovertebral (dysplasia, syndrome)

OB obstetrics

OB/GYN obstetrics (and) gynecology

OBS organic brain syndrome

OD Doctor (of) Optometry; [L.] *oculus dexter,* the right eye; overdose, overdosage

ODD oculodentodigital (dysplasia, syndrome)

Oe oersted (centimeter-gram-second unit of magnetic field strength)

OFD orofaciodigital (dysostosis, syndrome)

OKT Ortho-Kung T (cell)

OML orbitomeatal line

OMM ophthalmo-mandibulomelic (dysplasia, syndrome)

omn hor [L.] *omni horã,* at every hour

OMS organic mental syndrome

OPV oral (attenuated) poliovirus vaccine

ORD optical rotatory dispersion

Orn ornithine (or its radical)

Oro orotate; orotic acid

Os osmium

OS [L.] *oculus sinister*, the left eye

OSHA Occupational Safety (and) Health Administration

OT occupational therapy; (Koch's) old tuberculin

OTC over the counter (non-prescription drug)

OU [L.] *oculus uterque*, each eye (both eyes)

OXT oxytocin

oz ounce

p pico-; pupil

P partial (pressure); peta- one quadrillion (10^{15}); phosphorus, phosphoric (residue); plasma (con- centration); pressure

^{32}P phosphorus-32

P1 first parental (genera- tion)

Pa pascal; protactinium

PA Physician Assistant, Physician's Assistant

PABA *p*-aminobenzoic acid, *para*-aminobenzoic acid

PAF platelet-aggregating (or -activating) factor

PAH *p*-aminohippuric (acid), *para*-aminohip- puric (acid)

PaO$_2$ partial (pressure of) arterial oxygen

part. aeq. [L.] *partes aequales*, equal parts (amounts)

part. vic. [L.] *partitis vicibus*, in divided doses

PAS *p*-aminosalicylic (acid), *para*-aminosali- cylic (acid)

PASA *p*-aminosalicylic acid, *para*-aminosalicylic acid

Pb [L.] *plumbum*, lead

PBG porphobilinogen

PBI protein-bound iodine (test)

pc [L.] *post cibum*, after a meal

PCB polychlorinated biphenyl

Pco$_2$ partial pressure (ten- sion) of carbon dioxide

PCP phencyclidine

Pd palladium

PD prism diopter

PDLL poorly differentiat- ed lymphocytic lym- phoma

PEEP positive end-expira- tory pressure

PET positron emission tomography

PF$_4$ platelet factor 4

PFT pulmonary function test

pg picogram

PGA prostaglandin A

PGB prostaglandin B

PGE prostaglandin E

PGF prostaglandin F

pH hydrogen ion concen- tration; p (power) of [H+]$_{10}$

Ph phenyl

Ph^1 Philadelphia (chromo- some)

PHA phytohemagglutinin (antigen)

Pharm D [L.] *Pharmaciae Doctor*, Doctor of Pharmacy

PhD [L.] *Philosophiae Doctor*, Doctor of Philosophy

Phe phenylalanine (or its radical)

PhG Graduate (in) Pharmacy

PhG [L.] *Pharmacopoeia Germanica*, German Pharmacopeia

PID pelvic inflammatory disease

PIF prolactin-inhibiting factor

pK negative logarithm of the ionization constant (K$_a$) of an acid

PK pyruvate kinase

PKU phenylketonuria

pm picometer

Pm promethium

PMS premenstrual syn- drome

PNP platelet neutralization procedure

PNPB positive-negative pressure breathing

Po polonium

PO$_2$ partial pressure (ten-

sion) of oxygen

P$_{O2}$ partial pressure (ten- sion) of oxygen

POEMS polyneuropathy, organomegaly, endocrinopathy, mono- clonal (protein, and) skin (changes) (syndrome)

polio poliomyelitis (pō´ lē-ō)

POMP prednisone, Oncovin (vincristine sul- fate), methotrexate, and Purinethol (6-mercaptop- urine)

POR problem-oriented (medical) record

PP pyrophosphate

PPCA proserum pro- thrombin conversion accelerator

PPD (Siebert) purified protein derivative (of tuberculin)

PPLO pleuropneumonia- like organism

ppm parts per million

PPO 2,5-diphenyloxazole

PPPPP pain, pallor, pulse (loss), paresthesia, paral- ysis

PPPPPP pain, pallor, paraesthesia, pulseless- ness, paralysis, prostra- tion

PPV positive pressure ven- tilation

Pr praseodymium; presby- opia

PRA plasma renin activity

PRF prolactin-releasing factor

PRL prolactin

prn [L.] *pro re nata*, as needed, as required

PRN [L.] *pro re nata*, as needed, as required

pro rat. aet. [L.] *pro ratione aetatis*, according to (patient's) age

Pro proline (or its radicals)

PSP phenolsulfonph- thalein (phenol red)

PSV pressure supported ventilation

Pt platinum

PT physical therapy; pro-

thrombin time

PTA plasma thromboplas- tin antecedent

PTAH phosphotungstic acid hematoxylin

PTH parathyroid hormone

PTU propylthiouracil

Pu plutonium

PUO pyrexia (of) unknown (or uncertain or undetermined) origin

PUPPP pruritic urticarial papules (and) plaques (of) pregnancy

PUVA (oral administration of) psoralen (and subse- quent exposure to) ultra- violet light of A wave- length (uv-a)

PVC polyvinyl chloride

PVP polyvinylpyrrolidone (povidone)

Q volume of blood flow

Q coulomb

Qco$_2$ microliters of CO$_2$ given off per milligram of dry weight of tissue per hour

qd [L.] *quaque die*, every day, each day

qh [L.] *quaque hora*, every hour, each hour

qid [L.] *quater in die*, four times (in) a day

ql [L.] *quantum libet*, as much as desired

Qo oxygen consumption

Qo$_2$ oxygen consumption

qs [L.] *quantum satis*, as much as is enough; [L.] *quantum sufficiat*, as much as may suffice, quantity sufficient

r racemic; roentgen

R gas constant (8.315 joules); (organic) radical; Réaumur (scale); [L.] *recipe*, (please) take; resistance determinant (plasmid); resistance (electrical); resistance (unit) (in the cardiovascu- lar system); resolution; respiration; respiratory (exchange ratio); roentgen

Ra radium

rad radian

RAS reticular activating system

RAST radioallergosorbent test

RAV Rous-associated virus

RAW resistance, airway

Rb rubidium

rbc red blood cell; red blood (cell) count

RBC red blood cell; red blood (cell) count

RBF renal blood flow

RD reaction (of) degeneration; reaction (of) denervation; Registered Dietician

RDH Registered Dental Hygienist

Re rhenium

RE right ear; right eye

rem roentgen-equivalent-man

REM rapid eye movement (sleep); reticular erythematous mucinosis

rep roentgen-equivalent-physical

RES reticuloendothelial system

RF release factor; rheumatoid factor

RFA right frontanterior (fetal position)

RFLP restriction fragment length polymorphism

RFP right frontoposterior (fetal position)

RFT right frontotransverse (fetal position)

Rh Rhesus (RH blood group); rhodium

RH releasing hormone

Rib ribose

RLL right lower lobe (of lung)

RLQ right lower quadrant (of abdomen)

RMA right mentoanterior (fetal position)

RML right middle lobe (of lung)

RMP right mentoposterior (fetal position)

RMT right mentotransverse (fetal position)

Rn radon

RN Registered Nurse

RNA ribonucleic acid

RNase ribonuclease

RNP ribonucleoprotein

ROA right occipitoanterior (fetal position)

ROM range of motion

ROP right occipitoposterior (fetal position)

ROT right occipitotransverse (fetal position)

RPF renal plasma flow

RPh Registered Pharmacist

rpm revolutions per minute

RPR rapid plasma reagent (test)

RQ respiratory quotient

rRNA ribosomal RNA

Rs resolution

RS respiratory syncytial (virus)

RSA right sacroanterior (fetal position)

RSP right sacroposterior (fetal position)

RST right sacrotransverse (fetal position)

RSV Rous-sarcoma virus; respiratory syncytial virus

rTMP ribothymidylic acid

Ru ruthenium

RUL right upper lobe (of lung)

RUQ right upper quadrant (of the abdomen)

RV residual volume

℞ recipe; [L.] *recipe*, (the first word on a prescription), (please) take

σ sigma; reflection coefficient; standard deviation

s [L.] *semis*, half; steady state (SUBSCRIPT); [L.] *sinister*, left (opposite of "right", does not mean "remaining")

S [L.] *sinister*, left (opposite of "right", does not mean "remaining"); saturation of hemoglobin (percentage of) (FOLLOWED BY SUBSCRIPT O₂ OR CO₂); siemens; spherical; spherical (lens); sul-

fur; Svedberg (unit)

S-A sinoatrial (block)

SaO₂ oxygen saturation (of) arterial (oxyhemoglobin)

sat. saturated

sat. sol. saturated solution

Sb [L.] *stibium*, antimony

SBE subacute bacterial endocarditis

sc subcutaneous, subcutaneously

Sc scandium

SC sternoclavicular; subcutaneous, subcutaneously

SD standard deviation; streptodornase

SDA specific dynamic action

Se selenium

Sf Svedberg flotation (constant, unit)

SGOT serum glutamic-oxaloacetic transaminase (aspartate aminotransferase)

SGPT serum glutamic-pyruvic transaminase (alanine aminotransferase)

SH serum hepatitis

Si silicon

SI [French] Système International d'Unités International System of Units

SID source-to-image (-receptor) distance

SIDS sudden infant death syndrome

sig [L.] *signa*, (please) affix a seal to, (please) inscribe

SIMV spontaneous intermittent mandatory ventilation; synchronized intermittent mandatory ventilation

SIRD source-to-image-receptor distance

SISI small-increment (or short-increment) sensitivity index (test)

SK streptokinase

SLE systemic lupus erythematosus

Sm samarium

Sn [L.] *stannum*, tin

SOAP subjective (data), objective (data), assessment, (and) plan (problem-oriented record)

sol solution

soln solution

s.o.s. [L.] *si opus sit*, if needed

SPCA serum prothrombin conversion accelerator (factor VII)

SPECT single photon emission computed tomography

SPF sun protection (or protective) factor

sp gr specific gravity

sph spherical (lens)

spm suppression (and) mutation

spp species (WHEN PLURAL), (PLURAL OF THE ABBREVIATION SP)

SQ subcutaneous

Sr strontium

SRF somatotropin-releasing factor

SRF-A slow-reacting factor (of) anaphylaxis

SRIF somatotropin-release inhibiting factor

sRNA soluble RNA

SRS slow-reacting substance (of anaphylaxis)

SRS-A slow-reacting substance (of) anaphylaxis

ST scapulothoracic

stat [L.] *statim*, immediately, at once

STD sexually transmitted disease

STEL short-term exposure limit

STH somatotropic hormone

STM short-term memory

STPD standard temperature (0° C) (and) pressure (760 mm Hg absolute), dry

Sv sievert (unit)

SV sievert (unit)

t metric ton

t temperature (Celsius); tritium

α-T α-tocopherol

T temperature, absolute (Kelvin); tension (intraocular); tera-; tesla; tetanus (toxoid vaccine); tidal (volume) (SUBSCRIPT); tocopherol; transverse (tubule); tritium; tumor (antigen)

T absolute temperature (Kelvin)

T₃ 3,5,3'-triiodothyronine

T₄ tetraiodothyronine (thyroxine)

T- decreased tension (pressure)

T+ increased tension (pressure)

Ta tantalum

TAB typhoid, (paratyphoid) A, (and paratyphoid) B (vaccine)

TAD transient acantholytic dermatosis

TAF tumor angiogenesis factor

TAR thrombocytopenia (with) absent radii (syndrome)

TAT thematic apperception test

Tb terbium

TBP thyroxine-binding protein

TBV total blood volume

Tc technetium

⁹⁹ᵐTc technetium-99m

TCN talocalcaneonavicular (joint)

Td tetanus-diphtheria (toxoid adult type vaccine)

TDP ribothymidine 5'-diphosphate

Te tellurium

TEDD total end-diastolic diameter

TEN toxic epidermal necrolysis

TESD total end-systolic diameter

Th thorium

Thr threonine (or its radicals)

tᵢ/tₜₒₜ duty cycle

Ti titanium

TIA transient ischemic attack

t.i.d. [L.] *ter in die*, three times (in) a day

tinct tincture

TITh 3,5,3'-triiodothyronine

Tl thallium

TLC thin-layer chromatography; total lung capacity

TLV threshold-limit value

tₘ temperature midpoint (Celsius)

Tm thulium; tubular maximal (excretory capacity of kidneys)

Tₘ temperature midpoint (Kelvin)

TM transport maximum

TMJ temporomandibular joint (dysfunction)

TMP ribothymidine 5'-monophosphate

TMT tarsometatarsal

Tn (ocular) tension; (intraocular) tension, normal

TNM tumor, node, metastasis (tumor staging)

TORCH toxoplasmosis, other (infections), rubella, cytomegalorvirus (infection, and) herpes (simplex) (titer)

TPA tissue plasminogen activator

TPHA *Treponema pallidum* hemagglutination (test)

TPI *Treponema pallidum* immobilization (test)

TPN total parenteral nutrition

tr tincture

TRH thyrotropin-releasing hormone (stimulation test)

TRIC trachoma inclusion conjunctivitis (organism)

tRNA transfer RNA

Trp tryptophan (and its radicals)

TSH thyroid-stimulating hormone (stimulation test)

TSS toxic shock syndrome

TSTA tumor-specific transplantation antigen

TU toxic unit, toxin unit

Tyr tyrosine (and its radicals)

U unit; uranium; uridine (in polymers); urinary (concentration)

UDP uridine diphosphate

UGIS upper gastrointestinal series

UMP uridine monophosphate (uridylic acid)

ung [L.] *unguentum*, ointment

Urd uridine

USAN United States Adopted Names (Council)

USP *United States Pharmacopeia*

USPHS United States Public Health Service

UTP uridine triphosphate

v venous (blood); volt

V vanadium; vision; visual (acuity); volt; volume (FREQUENTLY WITH SUBSCRIPTS DENOTING LOCATION, CHEMICAL SPECIES, AND CONDITIONS)

V̇ ventilation; gas flow (FREQUENTLY WITH SUBSCRIPTS INDICATING LOCATION AND CHEMICAL SPECIES); ventilation;

V₁–V₆ the unipolar precordial electrocardiogram chest leads

VA viral antigen

V̇ₐ alveolar ventilation

V-A ventriculoatrial

Val valine (and its radicals)

V̇a/Q̇ ventilation/perfusion ratio

VATER vertebral (defects), (imperforate) anus, tracheoesophageal (fistula with) esophageal (atresia, and) radial and renal (dysplasia) (complex)

VC vision, color; vital capacity

VCE vagina, ectocervix, endocervix

V_D (physiologic) dead (space)

VDRL Venereal Disease Research Laboratory (test)

VHDL very-high-density lipoprotein

VIP vasoactive intestinal polypeptide

vipoma vasoactive intestinal polypeptide (+ G. *ōma*, a tumor), (vi- pō´mă)

VLDL very-low-density lipoprotein

VMA vanillylmandelic acid (test)

Vₘₐₓ maximal velocity

VP vasopressin

VR vocal resonance

VS volumetric solution

V_T tidal volume

W watt; [German] *Wolfram* tungsten

Wb weber

WBC white blood cell; white blood (cell) count

WDLL well differentiated lymphocytic (or lymphatic) lymphoma

WHO World Health Organization

WR Wassermann reaction

X xanthosine

Xao xanthosine

Xe xenon

¹³³Xe xenon-133

Y yttrium

Yb ytterbium

Z carbobenzoxy (chloride)

ZEEP zero end-expiratory pressure

Zn zinc

⁶⁵Zn zinc-65

Zr zirconium

ZSR zeta sedimentation ratio

WORDFINDER

The following pages--WF1-WF116--contain a list of subentry terms from the A to Z vocabulary arranged alphabetically letter by letter according to the first word(s) of the term. Use WordFinder when you want to find where in Stedman's a multi-word term is defined. Stedman's is organized in main entry-subentry format, which means that subentry terms are grouped under main, governing terms, and readers must know the organizing term in order to find where a definition is located.

Multi-word terms are in bold face; organizing terms are in light face. For example:

To find	Look under
Colorado tick fever	virus
lenticular progressive	degeneration
luteinizing hormone-releasing	factor

A

α: fetoprotein; granules; helix; hemolysin; thalassemia; thalassemia intermedia

α′: hemolysis

α-: keto acid dehydrogenase; streptococci

A: bands; bile; cells; chain; disks; fibers; wave

A₂: thalassemia

A-: DNA; esotropia; exotropia; strabismus

aaa: disease

Aaron's: sign

Aarskog-Scott: syndrome

abacterial thrombotic: endocarditis

Abadie's: sign of tabes dorsalis

abapical: pole

abarticular: gout

Abbe: flap; operation

Abbé's: condenser

Abbott's: artery; method; stain for spores; tube

ABC: leads

A.B.C.: process

abdominal: angina; aorta; apoplexy; ballottement; canal; cavity; dropsy; fibromatosis; fissure; fistula; guarding; hernia; hysterectomy; hysteropexy; hysterotomy; migraine; myomectomy; nephrectomy; ostium of uterine tube; pad; part of aorta; part of esophagus; part of thoracic duct; part of ureter; pool; pregnancy; pressure; pulse; reflexes; regions; respiration; ring; sac; salpingectomy; salpingo-oophorectomy; salpingotomy; section; typhoid; zones

abdominal aortic: plexus

abdominal external oblique: muscle

abdominal internal oblique: muscle

abdominal muscle deficiency: syndrome

abdominocardiac: reflex

abdominojugular: reflux

abdominopelvic: cavity

abdominopelvic splanchnic: nerves

abdominothoracic: arch

abdominovaginal: hysterectomy

abducens: eminence; nucleus

abducent: nerve

abductor: muscle of great toe; muscle of little finger; muscle of little toe

abductor digiti minimi: muscle of foot; muscle of hand

abductor hallucis: muscle

abductor pollicis brevis: muscle

abductor pollicis longus: muscle

Abegg's: rule

Abell-Kendall: method

Abel's: bacillus

Abelson murine leukemia: virus

Abernethy's: fascia

aberrant: artery; bundles; complex; ducts; ductules; ganglion; goiter; hemoglobin; regeneration

aberrant bile: ducts

aberrant obturator: artery

aberrant ventricular: conduction

abnormal: cleavage of cardiac valve; correspondence; occlusion

ABO: antigens; factors

ABO hemolytic: disease of the newborn

aborted: systole

aborted ectopic: pregnancy

abortion: rate

abortive: neurofibromatosis; transduction

abortus: bacillus

abraded: wound

Abrahams': sign

Abrams' heart: reflex

abrasive: strip

abscopal: effect

absence: seizure

absent: state

absolute: agraphia; alcohol; dehydration; glaucoma; hemianopia; humidity; hydration; hyperopia; leukocytosis; oils; pressure; scale; scotoma; system of units; temperature; threshold; unit; viscosity; zero

absolute cell: increase

absolute intensity threshold: acuity

absolute refractory: period

absolute terminal innervation: ratio

absorbable gelatin: film; sponge

absorbable surgical: suture

absorbancy: index

absorbed: dose

absorbent: cotton; points; system; vessels

absorption: band; cell; chromatography; coefficient; collapse; fever; lines; spectrum

absorptive: cells of intestine

abstinence: symptoms; syndrome

abstract: intelligence; thinking

acanthocytosis with: chorea

acapnial: alkalosis

acarine: dermatosis

accelerated: conduction; eruption; hypertension; reaction; rejection

accelerator: factor; fibers; globulin; nerves

acceptor: RNA; site

acceptor splicing: site

access: opening

accessory: adrenal; atrium; auricles; breast; canal; cartilage; chromosome; cramp; flocculus; gland; ligaments; molecules; nerve; organs; organs of the eye; pancreas; placenta; portion of spinal accessory nerve; process; sign; spleen; symptom; thyroid; tragus; tubercle

accessory cephalic: vein

accessory cuneate: nucleus

accessory flexor: muscle of foot

accessory hemiazygos: vein

accessory lacrimal: glands

accessory meningeal: branch of middle meningeal artery

accessory nasal: cartilages

accessory nerve: lymph nodes; trunk

accessory obturator: artery

accessory olivary: nuclei

accessory pancreatic: duct

accessory parotid: gland

accessory phrenic: nerves

accessory plantar: ligaments

accessory quadrate: cartilage

accessory saphenous: vein

accessory suprarenal: glands

accessory thyroid: gland

accessory vertebral: vein

accessory visual: apparatus

accessory volar: ligaments

accident: neurosis

accidental: abortion; host; hypothermia; image; murmur; symptom
acclimating: fever
accolé: forms
accommodation: phosphene; reflex
accommodative: asthenopia; convergence; strabismus
accommodative convergence-accommodation: ratio
accompanying: vein; vein of hypoglossal nerve
accordion: graft
accoucheur's: hand
accretion: lines
accretionary: growth
accumulation: analysis; disease
acentric: chromosome; fragment
acephalic: migraine
acetabular: artery; branch; fossa; labrum; lip; notch
acetate replacement: factor
acetic: fermentation; solution
acetone: body; chloroform; compound; fixative; test
acetone-insoluble: antigen
aceto-orcein: stain
acetosoluble: albumin
acetyl: value
acetyl-activating: enzyme
Achard: syndrome
Achard-Thiers: syndrome
Achenbach: syndrome
achievement: age; motive; quotient; test
Achilles: bursa; reflex; tendon
achlorhydric: anemia
acholuric: jaundice
achondroplastic: dwarfism
achrestic: anemia
achromatic: apparatus; lens; objective; threshold; vision
acid: agglutination; alcohol; carboxypeptidase; cell; deoxyribonuclease; dextran; dyspepsia; fuchsin; gland; indigestion; intoxication; maltase; oxide; phosphatase; radical; reaction; rigor; salt; seromucoid; stain; sulfate; tartrate; tide; wave
α₁-acid: glycoprotein
acid-ash: diet
acid-base: balance; equilibrium
acid etch cemented: splint
acid-etched: restoration
acidic: amino acid; dyes
acidified serum: test
acidophil: adenoma; cell; granule
acidophilic: leukocyte

acidophilus: milk
acid perfusion: test
acid phosphatase: test for semen
acid reflux: test
acinar: carcinoma; cell
acinar cell: tumor
acinic cell: adenocarcinoma; carcinoma
acinose: carcinoma
acinotubular: gland
acinous: cell; gland
ackee: poisoning
acne: bacillus; keloid
acneform: syphilid
acorn-tipped: catheter
Acosta's: disease
acoustic: agraphia; aphasia; area; cell; crest; enhancement; impedance; lemniscus; lens; meatus; nerve; neurilemoma; neurinoma; neuroma; papilla; pressure; radiation; schwannoma; shadow; spots; striae; tetanus; tolerance; tubercle; vesicle
acousticofacial: crest; ganglion
acousticopalpebral: reflex
acoustic reference: level
acoustic trauma: deafness
acquired: agammaglobulinemia; character; cuticle; drives; hyperlipoproteinemia; hypogammaglobulinemia; ichthyosis; immunity; leukoderma; leukopathia; megacolon; methemoglobinemia; nevus; pellicle; reflex; sensitivity; toxoplasmosis in adults; trichoepithelioma
acquired centric: relation
acquired eccentric: relation
acquired epileptic: aphasia
acquired hemolytic: anemia; icterus
acquired immunodeficiency: syndrome
acquired tufted: angioma
acral lentiginous: melanoma
Acrel's: ganglion
acrid: poison
acridine: dyes
acrocentric: chromosome
acrodynic: erythema
acrofacial: dysostosis; syndrome
acromegalic: gigantism
acromelic: dwarfism
acromial: angle; artery; branch of suprascapular artery; branch of thoracoacromial artery; end of clavicle; extremity of

clavicle; plexus; process; reflex
acromial arterial: network
acromial articular: facies of clavicle; surface of clavicle
acromioclavicular: disk; joint; ligament
acromion: presentation
acromiothoracic: artery
acroparesthesia: syndrome
acrosomal: cap; granule; vesicle
acrylic: resin
acrylic resin: base; tooth; tray
ACTH-producing: adenoma
ACTH stimulation: test
actin: filament
actinic: cheilitis; conjunctivitis; dermatitis; granuloma; keratitis; keratosis; porokeratosis; prurigo; ray; reticuloid
actinide: elements
actinium: emanation
actinomycotic: appendicitis
action: current; potential; tremor
activated: acetaldehyde; amino acid; atom; carboxylic acid; charcoal; choline; fatty acid; glucose; hydrogen; macrophage; resin; sludge; state
activated clotting: time
activated partial thromboplastin: time
activated sludge: method
activation: analysis
active: acetate; aldehyde; anaphylaxis; carbon dioxide; caries; center; congestion; electrode; formaldehyde; formate; formyl; glycoaldehyde; hyperemia; immunity; immunization; inflammation; labor; methionine; methyl; movement; mutant; placebo; principle; prophylaxis; psychoanalysis; pyruvate; repressor; site; splint; succinate; sulfate; transport; treatment; vasoconstriction; vasodilation
active chronic: hepatitis
active length-tension: curve
activities of daily living: scale
activity: coefficient
actual: cautery
acuminate papular: syphilid
acupuncture: anesthesia
acute: abdomen; abscess; alcoholism; angle;

appendicitis; ataxia; chalazion; cholecystitis; chorea; delirium; glaucoma; glomerulonephritis; goiter; inflammation; malaria; mania; nephritis; nephrosis; pyelonephritis; rejection; rhinitis; rickets; schizophrenia; trypanosomiasis; tuberculosis; urticaria
acute adrenocortical: insufficiency
acute African sleeping: sickness
acute anterior: poliomyelitis
acute ascending: paralysis
acute atrophic: paralysis
acute bacterial: endocarditis
acute brachial: radiculitis
acute bulbar: poliomyelitis
acute catarrhal: conjunctivitis
acute cellular: rejection
acute compression: triad
acute contagious: conjunctivitis
acute crescentic: glomerulonephritis
acute cutaneous: leishmaniasis
acute decubitus: ulcer
acute disseminated: encephalomyelitis; myositis
acute epidemic: conjunctivitis; leukoencephalitis
acute febrile neutrophilic: dermatosis
acute fibrinous: pericarditis
acute follicular: conjunctivitis
acute fulminating: meningococcemia
acute fulminating meningococcal: septicemia
acute hallucinatory: paranoia
acute hemorrhagic: conjunctivitis; encephalitis; glomerulonephritis; leukoencephalitis; pancreatitis
acute idiopathic: polyneuritis
acute inclusion body: encephalitis
acute infectious nonbacterial: gastroenteritis
acute inflammatory: polyneuropathy
acute intermittent: porphyria
acute interstitial: nephritis; pneumonia; pneumonitis
acute isolated: myocarditis

acute lobar: nephrosis
acute miliary: tuberculosis
acute necrotizing: encephalitis; myelitis
acute necrotizing hemorrhagic: encephalomyelitis; leukoencephalitis
acute necrotizing ulcerative: gingivitis
acute organic brain: syndrome
acute parenchymatous: hepatitis
acute phase: reactants; reaction
acute post-streptococcal: glomerulonephritis
acute primary hemorrhagic: meningoencephalitis
acute promyelocytic: leukemia
acute pulmonary: alveolitis
acute radiation: syndrome
acute recurrent: rhabdomyolysis
acute reflex bone: atrophy
acute respiratory: failure
acute rheumatic: arthritis
acute scalp: cellulitis
acute schizophrenic: episode
acute situational: reaction
acute splenic: tumor
acute stress: reaction
acute transverse: myelitis
acute vascular: purpura
acute viral: conjunctivitis
acute yellow: atrophy of the liver
acyclic: compound
acyl-activating: enzyme
acyl carrier: protein
acylmercaptan: bond
Adair-Koshland-Némethy-Filmer: model
adamantine: membrane
Adams-Stokes: disease; syncope; syndrome
adansonian: classification
adaptation: diseases; syndrome of Selye
adaptive: behavior; enzyme; hypertrophy
adaptive behavior: scales
adaptor: hypothesis
addictive: drug
Addis: count; test
Addison-Biermer: disease
addisonian: anemia; crisis; syndrome
Addison's: anemia; disease
Addison's clinical: planes
addition: compound; mutation
addition-deletion: mutation
additive: effect; model
addressing: ligands

adductor: canal; hiatus; muscle of great toe; muscle of thumb; reflex; tubercle
adductor brevis: muscle
adductor hallucis: muscle
adductor longus: muscle
adductor magnus: muscle
adductor minimus: muscle
adductor pollicis: muscle
Aden: fever; ulcer
adeno-associated: virus
adenoid: facies; tissue; tumor
adenoidal-pharyngeal-conjunctival: virus
adenoid cystic: carcinoma
adenoid squamous cell: carcinoma
adenomatoid: tumor
adenomatoid odontogenic: tumor
adenomatous: goiter; polyp
adenosatellite: virus
adenosquamous: carcinoma
adequal: cleavage
adequate: stimulus
adherence: syndrome
adherent: leukoma; pericardium; placenta
adhesion: dyspepsia; molecules; phenomenon; test
adhesive: arachnoiditis; atelectasis; bandage; capsulitis; inflammation; otitis; pericarditis; peritonitis; phlebitis; pleurisy; tape; vaginitis
adhesive absorbent: dressing
Adie: syndrome
adient: behavior
Adie's: pupil
adipodermal: graft
adipokinetic: hormone
adipose: capsule; cell; degeneration; folds of the pleura; fossae; infiltration; tissue; tumor
adiposogenital: degeneration; dystrophy; syndrome
adjacent: angle
adjustable: articulator
adjustable axis: face-bow
adjustable occlusal: pivot
adjustment: disorders
adjuvant: vaccine
adlerian: psychoanalysis; psychology
Adler's: test
admaxillary: gland
adnexal: adenoma; carcinoma
adolescent: albuminuria; crisis; medicine
adolescent round: back

adoptive: immunity; immunotherapy
ADP: ribosylation
adrenal: androgen; apoplexy; body; capsule; cortex; crisis; gland; hermaphroditism; hypertension; leukodystrophy; rest; virilism
adrenal androgen-stimulating: hormone
adrenal cortex: injection
adrenal cortical: carcinomas; syndrome
adrenaline: reversal
adrenal virilizing: syndrome
adrenal weight: factor
β-adrenergic: receptors
α-adrenergic: receptors
adrenergic: amine; blockade; fibers; neurotransmitter; receptors
adrenergic blocking: agent
β-adrenergic blocking: agent
α-adrenergic blocking: agent
adrenergic neuronal blocking: agent
β-adrenergic receptor blocking: agent
adrenocortical: adenoma; hormones; insufficiency
adrenocorticotropic: hormone; peptide
adrenocorticotropic releasing: factor
adrenogenital: syndrome
adrenomedullary: hormones
adrenomimetic: amine
β-adrenoreceptor: antagonist
adrenotropic: hormone
Adson: forceps; maneuver
Adson's: test
adsorption: chromatography; theory of narcosis
adult: hypophosphatasia; medulloepithelioma; rickets; tuberculosis
adult lactase: deficiency
adult-onset: diabetes
adult pseudohypertrophic muscular: dystrophy
adult respiratory distress: syndrome
adult T-cell: leukemia; lymphoma
advanced multiple-beam equalization: radiography
advancement: flap
adventitial: cell; neuritis
adventitious: albuminuria; bursa; cyst
adverse: reaction
adversive: movement
adynamic: ileus

A-E: amputation
Aeby's: muscle; plane
aerial: mycelium; sickness
aerobic: dehydrogenase; respiration
aerogenic: tuberculosis
aerosol: generator
aerospace: medicine
aestivoautumnal: fever
affect: displacement; hunger; memory; spasms
affective: disorders; psychosis; tone
affective personality: disorder
afferent: fibers; lymphatic; nerve; vessel
afferent glomerular: arteriole
afferent loop: syndrome
affinity: antibody; chromatography; column
afibrillar: cementum
AFORMED: phenomenon
African: histoplasmosis; trypanosomiasis
African endomyocardial: fibrosis
African furuncular: myiasis
African hemorrhagic: fever
African horse: sickness
African horse sickness: virus
African sleeping: sickness
African swine: fever
African swine fever: virus
African tick: fever
after-: contraction; current; discharge; effect; movement; nystagmus; pains; potential; sound; taste
afterloading: screw
afunctional: occlusion
A/G: ratio
Ag-AS: stain
agene: process
age-related macular: degeneration
age-specific: rate
agglutinating: antibody
agglutination: test
agglutinative: thrombus
aggregate: anaphylaxis; glands
aggregated lymphatic: follicles; follicles of vermiform appendix; nodules
aggressive: instinct
aggressive infantile: fibromatosis
agitated: depression
aglossia-adactylia: syndrome
agminate: glands
agnogenic myeloid: metaplasia

agonal: clot; infection; leukocytosis; rhythm; thrombus
agranular: cortex; leukocyte
agranular endoplasmic: reticulum
agranulocytic: angina
A-H: interval
A-H conduction: time
Ahumada-Del Castillo: syndrome
Aicardi's: syndrome
AIDS: dementia
AIDS dementia: complex
AIDS-related: complex; virus
air: bladder; bronchogram; cells; cells of auditory tube; conduction; dose; embolism; pollution; sac; sickness; splint; syringe; thermometer; tube; vesicles
air-bone: gap
airborne: infection
airbrasive: technique
air-conditioner: lung
air contrast: enema
air contrast barium: enema
air-gap: radiography; technique
airplane: splint
air-slaked: lime
airspace-filling: pattern
airway: pattern; resistance
A-K: amputation
Akabane: disease; virus
akamushi: disease
Åkerlund: deformity
akinetic: mutism; seizure
Akureyri: disease
ala central: lobule
alactic oxygen: debt
Alanson's: amputation
alar: artery of nose; chest; folds; lamina of neural tube; ligaments; part of nasalis muscle; plate of neural tube; process; spine
alarm: reaction
alaryngeal: speech
Albarran's: glands; test
Albarran y Dominguez': tubules
albedo: retinae
Albers-Schönberg: disease
Albert's: disease; stain; suture
Albini's: nodules
albino: rats
Albinus': muscle
Albrecht's: bone
Albright's: disease; syndrome
Albright's hereditary: osteodystrophy
albumin-globulin: ratio
albuminized: iron

albuminocytologic: dissociation
albuminoid: degeneration
albuminous: cell; gland; swelling
albuminuric: retinitis
alcelaphine: herpesvirus 1
Alcock's: canal
alcohol: addiction; diuresis
alcohol amnestic: syndrome
alcoholic: cardiomyopathy; cirrhosis; deterioration; extract; fermentation; hyalin; myocardiopathy; pneumonia; polyneuropathy; psychoses; tincture
alcoholic hyaline: bodies
alcoholic withdrawal: tremor
alcohol-soluble: eosin
alcohol withdrawal: delirium
aldehyde: fuchsin; reaction
Alder: bodies
Alder's: anomaly
aldol: condensation
aldosterone: antagonist
Aldrich: syndrome
alecithal: ovum
Aleppo: boil
aleukemic: leukemia; myelosis
Aleutian mink : disease
Aleutian mink disease: virus
Alexander's: deafness; disease
alexin: unit
Alezzandrini's: syndrome
algid: malaria; stage
algid pernicious: fever
algoid: cell
Alice in Wonderland: syndrome
alicyclic: compounds
alignment: curve; mark
alimentary: apparatus; canal; diabetes; glycosuria; hyperinsulinism; lipemia; osteopathy; pentosuria; system; tract
alimentary tract: smear
aliphatic: compound
alisphenoid: cartilage
alizarin: indicator
alkali: disease; metal; reserve; therapy
alkali denaturation: test
alkali earth: metal
alkaline: earths; phosphatase; reaction; RNase; tide; toluidine blue O; water; wave
alkaline-ash: diet
alkaline earth: elements
alkaline milk: drip
alkaline reflux: gastritis
alkylating: agent

allantoenteric: diverticulum
allantoic: bladder; cyst; diverticulum; fluid; sac; stalk; vesicle
allantoid: membrane
allantoidoangiopagous: twins
allelic: exclusion; gene
Allen-Doisy: test; unit
Allen-Masters: syndrome
Allen's: test
allergenic: extract
allergic: angiitis; conjunctivitis; coryza; eczema; extract; granulomatosis; inflammation; purpura; reaction; rhinitis
allergic contact: dermatitis
allergic granulomatous: angiitis
allied: reflexes
alligator: forceps; skin
Allis: forceps
Allis': sign
all or none: law
allogeneic: antigen; graft; inhibition
allograft: rejection
allomeric: function
allopathic: keratoplasty
allosteric: enzyme; site
allotropic: personality
allotypic: determinants; marker
alloxan: diabetes
Almeida's: disease
Almén's: test for blood
almond: nucleus
Alpers: disease
Alpha: tests
alpha: alcoholism; angle; blocking; cells of anterior lobe of hypophysis; cells of pancreas; error; fibers; granule; particle; radiation; ray; rhythm; substance
alpha: units; wave
alpha-: oxidation
alpha methyl: dopa
Alpine: scurvy
Alport's: syndrome
Alström's: syndrome
ALT:AST: ratio
alterative: inflammation
altercursive: intubation
alternate: hemianesthesia
alternate binaural loudness balance: test
alternate cover: test
alternate day: strabismus
alternating: current; hemiplegia; mydriasis; pulse; strabismus; tremor
alternating light: test
alternative: hypothesis; inheritance; medicine; tremor

altitude: chamber; disease; erythremia; sickness
altitudinal: hemianopia
Altmann-Gersh: method
Altmann's: fixative; granule; theory
Altmann's anilin-acid fuchsin: stain
Alu: sequences
alu: family
alu-equivalent: family
alum: whey
aluminum: penicillin
alveolar: abscess; adenocarcinoma; air; angle; arch of mandible; arch of maxilla; atrophy; body; bone; border; canals; cell; crest; duct; foramina; gas; gingiva; gland; index; macrophage; mucosa; osteitis; part of mandible; pattern; periosteum; point; process; ridge; sac; septum; ventilation; yoke
alveolar-arterial oxygen: difference
alveolar cell: carcinoma
alveolar dead: space
alveolar duct: emphysema
alveolar gas: equation
alveolar hydatid: cyst
alveolar soft part: sarcoma
alveolar supporting: bone
alveolobuccal: groove; sulcus
alveolocapillary: membrane
alveolo-capillary: block
alveolodental: canals; ligament; membrane
alveololabial: groove; sulcus
alveololingual: groove; sulcus
alveolonasal: line
Alzheimer's: dementia; disease; sclerosis
Alzheimer type I: astrocyte
Alzheimer type II: astrocyte
Am: antigens
amacrine: cell
Amadori: rearrangement
amalgam: carrier; matrix; strip; tattoo
amaranth: solution
amaurotic: mydriasis; nystagmus; pupil
amaurotic cat's: eye
Ambard's: constant; laws
amber: codon; mutant; mutation; suppressor
Amberg's lateral sinus: line
ambient: behavior; cistern
ambiguous: nucleus
ambiguous atrioventricular: connections
ambiguous external: genitalia
amboceptor: unit

Amboyna: button
Ambu: bag
ambulant: edema; erysipelas; plague
ambulatory: anesthesia; automatism; schizophrenia; surgery; typhoid
amebic: abscess; colitis; dysentery; granuloma; vaginitis
ameboid: cell; movement
amelanotic: melanoma
ameloblastic: fibroma; fibrosarcoma; layer; odontoma; sarcoma
ameloblastic adenomatoid: tumor
ameloblastomatous: craniopharyngioma
amelodental: junction
amenorrhea-galactorrhea: syndrome
American: leishmaniasis; tarantula; trypanosomiasis
American Law Institute: rule
Ames: assay; test
amide: oximes
amino: sugars; terminal
amino acid: activation; analysis; reagent
amino acid activating: enzyme
4-aminobutyrate: pathway
p-**aminohippurate:** clearance
δ-**aminolevulinate dehydratase:** porphyria
ammonia: assimilation; detoxication; fixation; rash
ammoniacal: urine
ammoniated: mercuric chloride; mercury; tincture
Ammon's: fissure; horn; prominence
amnemonic: agraphia
amnestic: aphasia; psychosis; syndrome
amniocardiac: vesicle
amnioembryonic: junction
amniogenic: cells
amnion: ring
amniotic: adhesions; amputation; bands; cavity; corpuscle; duct; ectoderm; fluid; fold; raphe; sac
amniotic fluid: embolism; syndrome
amorphous: fraction of adrenal cortex; hydroxyapatite; phosphorus
amorphous insulin zinc: suspension
Amoss': sign
AMPA: receptor
Ampère's: postulate
amphibolic: fistula
amphiprotic: solvent
amphophil: granule

amphoric: rale; resonance; respiration; voice
amphoric voice: sound
amphoteric: electrolyte; element; reaction
amphotropic: virus
amplifier: host
amplitude of: accommodation; convergence
ampullar: abortion; pregnancy
ampullary: aneurysm; crest; crura of semicircular ducts; folds of uterine tube; limbs of semicircular ducts; sulcus
amputating: ulcer
amputation: knife; neuroma
Amsler: test
Amsler's: chart
Amsterdam: syndrome
Amussat's: valve; valvula
amygdaloid: body; complex; fossa; nucleus; tubercle
amylaceous: corpuscle
amylase-creatinine clearance: ratio
amylic: fermentation
amylogenic: body
amyloid: angiopathy; bodies of the prostate; degeneration; kidney; nephrosis; protein; tumor
amyotrophic lateral: sclerosis
A-N: interval
anabiotic: cells
anabolic: steroid
anaclitic: depression; psychotherapy
anacrotic: limb; pulse
anaerobic: cellulitis; dehydrogenase; respiration
anagen: effluvium
anal: atresia; canal; cleft; columns; crypts; ducts; erotism; fascia; fissure; fistula; gland; membrane; orifice; pecten; phase; pit; plate; reflex; region; sac; sinuses; triangle; valves; verge
analeptic: enema
analgesic: cuirass; nephritis; nephropathy
anal skin: tag
analytic: chemistry; psychiatry; study; therapy
analytical: psychology; sensitivity; specificity
analyzing: rod
anamnestic: reaction; response
anancastic: personality
anaphase: lag

anaphylactic: antibody; intoxication; reaction; shock
anaphylactoid: crisis; purpura; shock
anaplastic: astrocytoma; carcinoma; cell; oligodendroglioma
anaplastic large cell: lymphoma
anaplerotic: reaction
anarthritic rheumatoid: disease
anastomosed: graft
anastomosing: fibers; vessel
anastomotic: branch; branch of middle meningeal artery to lacrimal artery; stricture; ulcer; veins
anatid: herpesvirus 1
anatomic: rigidity; teeth
anatomical: age; airway; crown; element; neck of humerus; pathology; position; root; sphincter; tubercle; wart
anatomical dead: space
anatrophic: nephrotomy
anchor: splint
anchorage: dependence
anchoring: villus
anconal: fossa
anconeus: muscle
ancylostoma: dermatitis
Andernach's: ossicles
Anders': disease
Andersch's: ganglion; nerve
Andersen's: disease
Anderson: splint
Anderson-Collip: test
Anderson and Goldberger: test
Anderson-Hynes: pyeloplasty
Andral's: decubitus
androgen: unit
androgen binding: protein
androgenic: alopecia; hormone; zone
androgen resistance: syndromes
android: pelvis
anechoic: chamber
Anel's: method
anemic: anoxia; halo; hypoxia; infarct; murmur
anergic: leishmaniasis
aneroid: manometer
anesthesia: machine; record
anesthetic: circuit; depth; ether; gas; index; leprosy; shock; vapor
anestrous: ovulation
aneurysm: needle
aneurysmal: bruit; cough; murmur; phthisis; sac; varix
aneurysmal bone: cyst

Angelman: syndrome
angel's: wing
Angelucci's: syndrome
Anger: camera
Anghelescu's: sign
anginose: scarlatina
angioblastic: cells; cyst
angiodysgenetic: myelomalacia
angiofollicular mediastinal lymph node: hyperplasia
angiogenesis: factor
angiography: catheter
angioimmunoblastic: lymphadenopathy with dysproteinemia
angiolithic: degeneration; sarcoma
angiolymphoid: hyperplasia with eosinophilia
angiomatoid: tumor
angioneurotic: edema
angio-osteohypertrophy: syndrome
angiopathic: neurasthenia
angiopathic hemolytic: anemia
angioplasty: balloon
angiotensin-converting: enzyme
angiotensin-converting enzyme: inhibitors
angle of: convergence
angle-closure: glaucoma
Angle's: classification of malocclusion
Ångström: scale; unit
Ångström's: law
angular: acceleration; aldehyde; aperture; artery; cheilitis; conjunctivitis; convolution; curvature; gyrus; methyl; notch; spine; stomatitis; vein
anhepatic: jaundice
anhepatogenous: jaundice
anhidrotic ectodermal: dysplasia
anhydrous: alcohol; chloral; lanolin
anicteric: hepatitis; leptospirosis
anicteric virus: hepatitis
aniline: fuchsin
animal: charcoal; dextran; force; graft; magnetism; model; pole; psychology; soap; starch; toxin; viruses; wax
animal protein: factor
anion: gap
anion-exchange: resin
anionic: detergents
anionic neutrophil activating: peptide
anisometropic: amblyopia
anisotropic: disks; lipid
Anitschkow: cell; myocyte

ankle: bone; clonus; jerk; joint; reflex; region
ankyloglossia superior: syndrome
ankylosed: tooth
ankylosing: hyperostosis; spondylitis
annealing: lamp; tray
annectent: gyrus
annihilation: radiation
annular: band; cartilage; cataract; ligament; ligament of the radius; ligament of the stapes; ligaments of the trachea; lipid; pancreas; part of fibrous digital sheath; placenta; plexus; pulley; scleritis; scotoma; sphincter; staphyloma; stricture; synechia; syphilid
annulate: lamellae
annuloaortic: ectasia
annuloplasty: ring
annulospiral: ending; organ
anococcygeal: body; ligament; nerves
anocutaneous: line
anodal: current
anodal closure: contraction; tetanus
anodal duration: tetanus
anodal opening: contraction; tetanus
anode: rays
anogenital: band; raphe
anomalous: complex; conduction; correspondence; trichromatism; uterus; viscosity
anomalous atrioventricular: excitation
anomalous mitral: arcade
anomeric: carbon
anomic: aphasia
anonymous: veins
anorectal: angle; flexure; junction; lymph nodes; spasm; syndrome
anosognosic: epilepsy; seizures
anospinal: center
anovular: menstruation
anovular ovarian: follicle
anovulational: menstruation
anovulatory: cycle
anoxemia: test
anoxic: anoxia
ANP: receptors
ANP clearance: receptors
Anrep: effect; phenomenon
anserine: bursa; bursitis
ansiform: lobule
antagonistic: muscles; reflexes
antalgic: gait
antebrachial: fascia

antebrachial flexor: retinaculum
antecedent: sign
antecubital: space
antegonial: notch
antegrade: cardioplegia; conduction; cystography; pyelography; urography
antemortem: clot; thrombus
antenatal: diagnosis
anterior: aphasia; arch of atlas; asynclitism; belly of digastric muscle; border; border of eyelids; border of fibula; border of lung; border of pancreas; border of radius; border of testis; border of tibia; border of ulna; branch; canaliculus of chorda tympani; cells; centriole; chamber of eye; choroiditis; column; column of medulla oblongata; commissure; component of force; crus of stapes; curvature; cusp of atrioventricular valve; embryotoxon; epithelium of cornea; extremity; extremity of caudate nucleus; fontanel; fovea; funiculus; guide; horn; layer of rectus abdominis sheath; ligament of head of fibula; ligament of Helmholtz; ligament of malleus; limb of internal capsule; limb of stapes; lip of uterine os; lobe of hypophysis; margin; mediastinotomy; mediastinum; megalophthalmos; naris; neuropore; notch of cerebellum; notch of ear; nuclei of thalamus; occlusion; part; part of anterior commissure of brain; part of diaphragmatic surface of liver; part of fornix of vagina; part of pons; pillar of fauces; pillar of fornix; pituitary; pole of eyeball; pole of lens; process of malleus; pyramid; recess; recess of tympanic membrane; region of arm; region of elbow; region of forearm; region of leg; region of neck; region of thigh; rhinoscopy; rhizotomy; root; scleritis; sclerotomy; segment; sinuses; staphyloma; surface; surface of arm; surface of cornea; surface of elbow; surface of

eyelids; surface of forearm; surface of iris; surface of kidney; surface of leg; surface of lens; surface of lower limb; surface of maxilla; surface of pancreas; surface of patella; surface of petrous part of temporal bone; surface of prostate; surface of radius; surface of suprarenal gland; surface of thigh; surface of ulna; symblepharon; synechia; teeth; triangle of neck; tubercle of atlas; tubercle of cervical vertebrae; tubercle of thalamus; urethra; urethritis; uveitis; vein of septum pellucidum; vitrectomy; wall of middle ear; wall of stomach; wall of tympanic cavity; wall of vagina
anterior ampullar: nerve
anterior antebrachial: nerve; region
anterior articular: surface of dens
anterior atlanto-occipital: membrane
anterior auricular: branches of superficial temporal artery; groove; muscle; nerves; vein
anterior axillary: fold; line
anterior basal: branch; segment
anterior brachial: region
anterior cardiac: veins
anterior cardinal: veins
anterior carpal: region
anterior cecal: artery
anterior central: convolution; gyrus
anterior cerebellar: notch
anterior cerebral: artery; vein
anterior cervical: lymph nodes
anterior cervical intertransversarii: muscles
anterior cervical intertransverse: muscles
anterior chamber: trabecula
anterior chamber cleavage: syndrome
anterior choroidal: artery
anterior ciliary: artery
anterior circumflex humeral: artery
anterior clear: space
anterior communicating: artery
anterior condyloid: canal of occipital bone; foramen
anterior conjunctival: artery

anterior coronary: plexus
anterior corticospinal: tract
anterior costotransverse: ligament
anterior cranial: base; fossa
anterior cruciate: ligament
anterior crural: nerve; region
anterior cubital: region
anterior cutaneous: branches of intercostal nerves; branch of iliohypogastric nerve; nerves of abdomen
anterior deep cervical: lymph nodes
anterior descending: artery
anterior elastic: layer
anterior ethmoidal: artery; nerve
anterior ethmoidal air: cells
anterior facial: height; vein
anterior femoral cutaneous: nerves
anterior focal: point
anterior gray: column
anterior ground: bundle
anterior group of axillary: lymph nodes
anterior horn: cell
anterior humeral circumflex: artery
anterior hypothalamic: region
anterior inferior: segment
anterior inferior cerebellar: artery
anterior inferior iliac: spine
anterior inferior segmental: artery of kidney
anterior intercondylar: area of tibia
anterior intercostal: arteries; veins
anterior intermediate: groove; sulcus
anterior interosseous: artery; nerve
anterior interventricular: artery; groove
anterior intestinal: portal
anterior intraoccipital: joint; synchondrosis
anterior jugular: lymph nodes; vein
anterior junction: line
anterior knee: region
anterior labial: arteries; commissure; nerves; veins
anterior lacrimal: crest
anterior lateral malleolar: artery
anterior limiting: layer of cornea; ring
anterior lingual: gland
anterior longitudinal: ligament
anterior lunate: lobule

anterior medial malleolar: artery

anterior median: fissure of medulla oblongata; fissure of spinal cord; line

anterior mediastinal: arteries; lymph nodes

anterior medullary: velum

anterior meningeal: artery

anterior meniscofemoral: ligament

anterior myocardial: infarction

anterior nasal: aperture; spine

anterior ocular: segment

anterior palatine: arch; foramen

anterior parietal: artery

anterior parolfactory: sulcus

anterior pelvic: exenteration

anterior perforated: substance

anterior peroneal: artery

anterior piriform: gyrus

anterior pituitary: gonadotropin

anterior pituitary-like: hormone

anterior pontomesencephalic: vein

anterior primary: division

anterior pyramidal: fasciculus; tract

anterior quadrigeminal: body

anterior rectus: muscle of head

anterior sacrococcygeal: ligament

anterior sacroiliac: ligaments

anterior sacrosciatic: ligament

anterior scalene: muscle

anterior scrotal: branch of external pudendal artery; nerves; veins

anterior semicircular: canals

anterior serratus: muscle

anterior spinal: artery

anterior spinocerebellar: tract

anterior spinothalamic: tract

anterior sternoclavicular: ligament

anterior superficial cervical: lymph nodes

anterior superior: segment

anterior superior alveolar: arteries; branches of infraorbital nerve

anterior superior dental: arteries

anterior superior iliac: spine

anterior superior segmental: artery of kidney

anterior supraclavicular: nerve

anterior talar articular: surface of calcaneus

anterior talofibular: ligament

anterior talotibial: ligament

anterior temporal: artery

anterior thalamic: radiations; tubercle

anterior tibial: artery; bursa; lymph node; muscle; nerve; node; veins

anterior tibial compartment: syndrome

anterior tibial recurrent: artery

anterior tibiofibular: ligament

anterior tibiotalar: ligament; part of deltoid ligament

anterior tympanic: artery

anterior urethral: valve

anterior vertebral: vein

anterior white: commissure

anterodorsal thalamic: nucleus

anterofacial: dysplasia

anterograde: amnesia; block; conduction; memory

anteroinferior myocardial: infarction

anterolateral: column of spinal cord; cordotomy; fontanel; groove; sulcus; surface of shaft of humerus; system; tractotomy

anterolateral central: arteries

anterolateral myocardial: infarction

anterolateral striate: arteries

anterolateral thalamostriate: arteries

anteromedial: surface of shaft of humerus

anteromedial central: arteries; branches

anteromedial thalamic: nucleus

anteromedial thalamostriate: arteries

anteromedian: groove

anteroposterior: diameter of the pelvic inlet; projection

anteroseptal myocardial: infarction

anteroventral thalamic: nucleus

anthracotic: tuberculosis

anthrax: pneumonia; septicemia; toxin

anthropoid: pelvis

anthroponotic cutaneous: leishmaniasis

antialopecia: factor

antianemic: factor; principle

antianxiety: agent

anti-basement membrane: antibody; glomerulonephritis; nephritis

antiberiberi: factor; vitamin

antibiotic: enterocolitis; sensitivity

antibiotic sensitivity: test

anti-black-tongue: factor

antibody: excess

antibody combining: site

antibody deficiency: disease; syndrome

antibody-dependent cell-mediated: cytotoxicity

anticardiolipin: antibodies

anticoagulant: therapy

anticoding: strand

anticomplementary: factor; serum

anti-D: immunoglobulin

antidermatitis: factor

antidiuretic: hormone

antiepithelial: serum

antifoaming: agents

anti-G: suit

antigen: excess; interferon; unit

antigen-antibody: complex; reaction

antigen-binding: site

antigenic: competition; complex; determinant; drift; shift

antigen-presenting: cells

antigen-responsive: cell

antigen-sensitive: cell

antiglobulin: test

antigravity: muscles

antihemophilic: factor A; factor B; globulin; globulin A; globulin B; plasma

antihemorrhagic: factor; vitamin

antihuman: globulin

antihuman globulin: test

anti-idiotype: antibody; autoantibody

anti-kidney serum: nephritis

antilymphocyte: globulin; serum

antimicrobial: spectrum

anti-Monson: curve

antineuritic: factor; vitamin

antinuclear: antibody; factor

antiparallel: strand

antipellagra: factor

antipernicious anemia: factor

antiphospholipid: antibodies

antipodal: cone

anti-Pr cold: autoagglutinin

antipsychotic: agent

antirabies: serum

antirachitic: vitamins

antireflection: coating

antireticular cytotoxic: serum

antiscorbutic: vitamin

antisense: DNA; RNA; strand; therapy

antiseptic: dressing

antiserum: anaphylaxis

antisocial: personality

antisocial personality: disorder

antisterility: factor; vitamin

antitermination: protein

antithrombin: test

antitoxic: serum

antitoxin: rash; unit

antitragicus: muscle

antitragohelicine: fissure

antitrypsin: deficiency

α-1 antitrypsin deficiency: panniculitis

antitryptic: index

antitumor: enzyme; protein

antivenene: unit

antiviral: immunity; protein

Antoni type A: neurilemoma

Antoni type B: neurilemoma

Anton's: syndrome

antral: pouch; sphincter

Antyllus': method

anvil: sound

anxiety: disorders; dream; hysteria; neurosis; reaction; syndrome

anxiety tension: state

anxious: delirium

aortic: aneurysm; arch; arches; area; atresia; bodies; bulb; dissection; dwarfism; facies; foramen; hiatus; incompetence; insufficiency; knob; knuckle; murmur; nerve; nipple; notch; opening; orifice; ostium; reflex; regurgitation; sac; sinus; spindle; stenosis; sulcus; valve; vestibule; window

aortic arch: syndrome

aortic body: tumor

aortic lymphatic: plexus

aortico-left ventricular: tunnel

aorticopulmonary: window

aorticorenal: ganglia

aortic-pulmonic: window

aortic septal: defect

aortic sinus: aneurysm

aortoannular: ectasia

aortocoronary: bypass

aortoiliac: bypass

aortoiliac occlusive: disease

aortopulmonary: septum; window

aortorenal: bypass

AP: projection

APACHE: score

apallic: state; syndrome

apathetic: thyrotoxicosis

apatite: calculus

A-pattern: strabismus

A-P-C: virus

APC: compound

ape: fissure; hand

aperiodic: biopolymer

aperiosteal: amputation

Apert's: hirsutism; syndrome

aperture: diaphragm

apex: beat; impulse; pneumonia

Apgar: score

aphakic: eye; glaucoma

aphonic: pectoriloquy

aphthous: stomatitis

apical: abscess; angle; area; branch; branch of inferior lobar branch of right pulmonary artery; cap; complex; dendrite; foramen of tooth; gland; granuloma; infection; ligament of dens; periodontitis; process; segment; space

apical-aortic: conduit

apical dental: foramen

apical ectodermal: ridge

apical group of axillary: lymph nodes

apical lordotic: projection

apical periodontal: abscess; cyst

apicoposterior: artery; branch of left superior pulmonary vein; segment

aplanatic: lens

aplastic: anemia; lymph

apneic: oxygenation; pause

apneustic: breathing

apochromatic: lens; objective

apocrine: adenoma; carcinoma; chromhidrosis; gland; metaplasia; miliaria

apocrine sweat: glands

apolar: bond; cell; interaction

aponeurotic: fibroma; reflex

apophysary: point

apophysial: fracture

apoplectic: cyst; retinitis

apothecaries': weight

apparent: leukonychia; viscosity

appendiceal: abscess

appendicular: artery; colic; lymph nodes; muscle; skeleton; vein

apperceptive: mass

appetite: juice

appetitive: behavior

applanation: tonometer

apple jelly: nodules

applied: anatomy; anthropology; chemistry

appliqué: forms

apposition: suture

appositional: growth

approach-approach: conflict

approach-avoidance: conflict

approximation: suture

Apt: test

aptitude: test

APUD: cells

apyretic: tetanus; typhoid

aquagenic: pruritus

aqueduct: veil

aqueductal: intubation

aqueous: chambers; flare; humor; phase; solution; vaccine; vein

aqueous influx: phenomenon

aquo-: ion

arachnoid: cyst; foramen; granulations; mater; membrane; trabecula; villi

arachnoidal: granulations

Aran-Duchenne: disease

Arantius': ligament; nodule; ventricle

arborescent: cataract

arborization: block

arc: perimeter

arc-flash: conjunctivitis

arch: bar; form; length; wire

archaic-paralogical: thinking

arched: crest

archenteric: canal

arch length: deficiency

arch-loop-whorl: system

arciform: arteries; veins of kidney

arcon: articulator

arcuate: arteries of kidney; artery; crest; crest of arytenoid cartilage; eminence; fasciculus; fibers; fibers of cerebrum; line; line of ilium; line of rectus sheath; nuclei; nucleus; nucleus of thalamus; scotoma; uterus; veins of kidney; zone

arcuate popliteal: ligament

arcuate pubic: ligament

ardent: fever; spirits

areolar: choroiditis; choroidopathy; glands; tissue

areolar venous: plexus

argentaffin: cells; granules

Argentinean hemorrhagic: fever

Argentine hemorrhagic fever: virus

arginine: oxytocin; vasopressin; vasotocin

Argonz-Del Castillo: syndrome

Argyll Robertson: pupil

argyrophilic: cells; fibers

Arias-Stella: effect; phenomenon; reaction

Arie-Pitanguy: mammaplasty; operation

aristotelian: method

Aristotle's: anomaly

arithmetic: mean

Arlt's: operation; sinus

arm: phenomenon

Armanni-Ebstein: change; kidney

armed: macrophage; rostellum

armor: heart

armored: heart

Army Alpha: tests

Army Beta: tests

Army General Classification: Test

Arndt-Gottron: syndrome

Arndt's: law

Arneth: classification; count; formula; index; stages

Arnold-Chiari: deformity; malformation; syndrome

Arnold's: bodies; bundle; canal; ganglion; nerve; tract

aromatase: inhibitors

aromatic: bitters; castor oil; compound; series; water

aromatic ammonia: spirit

arousal: function; reaction

arrector pili: muscles

arrested: tuberculosis

arrested dental: caries

arrhenic: medication

Arrhenius: doctrine; equation; law

Arrhenius-Madsen: theory

arrow: poison

arrow point: tracing

Arruga's: forceps

arsenic: pigmentation

arsenical: keratosis; polyneuropathy; tremor

arseniureted: hydrogen

arterial: arcades; arches of colon; arches of ileum; arches of jejunum; arch of lower eyelid; arch of upper eyelid; blood; bulb; canal; capillary; circle of cerebrum; cone; duct; flap; forceps; grooves; hyperemia; hypotension; ligament; line; murmur; nephrosclerosis; sclerosis; segments of kidney; spider; tension; transfusion; vein; wave

arterial switch: operation

arterial thoracic outlet: syndrome

arteriocapillary: sclerosis

arteriococcygeal: gland

arteriolar: nephrosclerosis; network; sclerosis

arteriolosclerotic: kidney

arteriolovenular: anastomosis; bridge

arteriosclerotic: aneurysm; gangrene; kidney; psychosis; retinopathy

arteriovenous: anastomosis; aneurysm; fistula; nicking; shunt

arteriovenous carbon dioxide: difference

arteriovenous oxygen: difference

arthritic: atrophy; calculus

arthritic general: pseudoparalysis

arthrodial: articulation; cartilage; joint

Arthus: phenomenon; reaction

articular: branches; capsule; cartilage; cavity; chondrocalcinosis; circumference of radius; circumference of ulna; corpuscles; crepitus; crescent; crests; disc; disc of acromioclavicular joint; disc of distal radioulnar joint; disc of sternoclavicular joint; disc of temporomandibular joint; disk; eminence of temporal bone; facet; fossa of temporal bone; fracture; gout; labrum; lamella; leprosy; lip; margin; meniscus; muscle; muscle of elbow; muscle of knee; nerve; network; pit of head of radius; process; rheumatism; sensibility; surface; surface of acromion; surface of arytenoid cartilage; surface of head of fibula; surface of head of rib; surface of patella; surface of temporal bone; surface of tubercle of rib; tubercle of temporal bone

articularis cubiti: muscle

articularis genu: muscle

articular vascular: circle; network; network of elbow; network of knee

articulated: skeleton

articulating: paper

artificial: anatomy; ankylosis; anus; crown; dentition; eye; fever; heart; insemination; intelligence; kidney; melanin; pacemaker; pneumothorax;

pupil; radioactivity; respiration; selection; sphincter; stone; tears; ventilation
artificial active: immunity
artificial Carlsbad: salt
artificial Kissingen: salt
artificial passive: immunity
artificial Vichy: salt
artistic: anatomy
arycorniculate: synchondrosis
aryepiglottic: fold; muscle
arylated: alkyl
arytenoid: cartilage; glands; swelling
arytenoidal articular: surface of cricoid
asbestos: bodies; corn; liner; wart
ascending: aorta; artery; branch; branch of the inferior mesenteric artery; cholangitis; colon; current; degeneration; myelitis; neuritis; paralysis; part of aorta; part of duodenum; process; pyelonephritis
ascending anterior: branch
ascending cervical: artery
ascending frontal: convolution; gyrus
ascending lumbar: vein
ascending palatine: artery
ascending parietal: convolution; gyrus
ascending pharyngeal: artery; plexus
ascending posterior: branch
Ascher's: syndrome
Ascher's aqueous influx: phenomenon
Aschheim-Zondek: test
Aschner-Dagnini: reflex
Aschner's: phenomenon; reflex
Aschoff: bodies; cell; nodules
ascitic: agar
Ascoli: reaction
Ascoli's: test
ascorbate-cyanide: test
Aselli's: gland; pancreas
aseptic: fever; necrosis; surgery
asexual: dwarfism; generation; reproduction
Ashby: method
ashen: tuber; tubercle; wing
Asherman's: syndrome
Ashman's: phenomenon
ashy: dermatosis
asialoglycoprotein: receptor
Asian: influenza
Asiatic: cholera; schistosomiasis
asiderotic: anemia
Askanazy: cell

Ask-Upmark: kidney
aspermatogenic: sterility
aspheric: lens
asphyxiating thoracic: chondrodystrophy; dysplasia
aspirating: needle
aspiration: biopsy; pneumonia
asplenia: syndrome
Assam: fever
assertive: conditioning; training
Assézat's: triangle
assident: sign; symptom
assimilation: pelvis; sacrum
assist-control: ventilation
assisted: circulation; respiration; ventilation
assisted cephalic: delivery
assisted reproductive: technology
assistive: movement
Assmann's tuberculous: infiltrate
associated: antagonist; macrophage; movements
association: areas; constant; cortex; fibers; mechanism; neurosis; system; test; time; tract
associative: aphasia; reaction; strength
assortative: mating; mating
astacoid: rash
asteroid: body; hyalosis
asthenic: personality
asthenic personality: disorder
asthma: crystals
asthmatic: bronchitis
asthmatoid: wheeze
astigmatic: dial; lens
astral: fibers
astroglia: cell
Astwood's: test
asymmetric: disulfide
asymmetrical: chondrodystrophy
asymmetric motor: neuropathy
asymptomatic: coccidioidomycosis; neurosyphilis
asynchronous pulse: generator
atactic: abasia; agraphia
atavistic: epiphysis
ataxia telangiectasia: syndrome
ataxic: aphasia; breathing; dysarthria; gait; paramyotonia; paraplegia; tremor
atelectatic: rale
ateliotic: dwarfism
atheroma: embolism

atheromatous: degeneration; plaque
atherosclerotic: aneurysm
athlete's: foot; heart
athletic: heart
atlantic: part of vertebral artery
atlantoaxial: joint
atlanto-occipital: articulation; joint; membrane
atmospheric: pressure
atomic: core; heat; number; theory; volume; weight
atomic absorption: spectrophotometry
atomic mass: unit
atomistic: psychology
atonic: bladder; dyspepsia; ectropion; entropion; epiphora; seizure; ulcer
atopic: allergy; asthma; cataract; dermatitis; eczema; keratoconjunctivitis; reagin
ATP: citrate (*pro-3S*)-lyase; cobalamin adenoxyltransferase
atrabiliary: capsule
atraumatic: needle; suture
atresic: teratosis
atretic: corpus luteum
atretic ovarian: follicle
atrial: appendage; arteries; auricle; auricula; bigeminy; branches; capture; complex; diastole; dissociation; echo; extrasystole; fibrillation; flutter; gallop; kick; myxoma; sound; standstill; systole; tachycardia
atrial capture: beat
atrial chaotic: tachycardia
atrial fusion: beat
atrial natriuretic: factor; peptide
atrial septal: defect
atrial synchronous pulse: generator
atrial transport: function
atrial triggered pulse: generator
atrial ventricular canal: defect
atrial-well: technique
atriocarotid: interval
atriosystolic: murmur
atrioventricular: band; block; bundle; canal; conduction; connections; dissociation; extrasystole; gradient; groove; interval; node; septum; sulcus; valves
atrioventricular canal: cushions

atrioventricular junctional: bigeminy; rhythm; tachycardia
atrioventricular nodal: branch; extrasystole
atrophic: arthritis; excavation; gastritis; glossitis; heterochromia; inflammation; kidney; pharyngitis; rhinitis; rhinitis of swine; thrombosis; vaginitis
atropine: test
attached: craniotomy; gingiva
attached cranial: section
attachment: apparatus
attack: rate
attending: physician; staff; surgeon
attention deficit: disorder
attention deficit hyperactivity: disorder
attenuated: tuberculosis; vaccine; virus
attenuation: compensation
attitudinal: reflexes
attraction: sphere
attributable: risk
atypical: achromatopsia; fibroxanthoma; gingivitis; lipoma; measles; mycobacteria; pneumonia; pseudocholinesterase
atypical absence: seizure
atypical facial: neuralgia
atypical melanocytic: hyperplasia
atypical trigeminal: neuralgia
atypical verrucous: endocarditis
Au: antigen
Aub-DuBois: table
Aubert's: phenomenon
audiogenic: seizure
auditory: agnosia; alternans; aphasia; area; canal; capsule; cortex; fatigue; field; ganglion; hairs; hallucination; hyperesthesia; lemniscus; localization; nerve; nucleus; organ; ossicles; pathway; pits; placodes; process; reflex; striae; strings; teeth; threshold; tract; tube; vertigo; vesicle
auditory brainstem response: audiometry
auditory oculogyric: reflex
auditory receptor: cells
Auenbrugger's: sign
Auer: bodies; rods
Auerbach's: ganglia; plexus
Aufrecht's: sign
Auger: electron

augmentation: graft; mammaplasty
augmented: lead
augmented histamine: test
augmentor: fibers; nerves
Aujeszky's: disease
Aujeszky's disease: virus
aural: myiasis; vertigo
auramine O fluorescent: stain
auricle of: atrium
auricular: appendage; appendectomy; appendix; arc; branch of occipital artery; branch of vagus nerve; canaliculus; cartilage; complex; extrasystole; fissure; ganglion; index; ligaments; notch; point; reflex; standstill; surface of ilium; surface of sacrum; systole; tachycardia; triangle; tubercle; veins
auriculo-infraorbital: plane
auriculopalpebral: reflex
auriculopressor: reflex
auriculotemporal: nerve
auriculotemporal nerve: syndrome
auriculoventricular: groove; interval
auropalpebral: reflex
Aus: antigen
auscultatory: alternans; gap; percussion; sound
aussage: test
Austin Flint: murmur; phenomenon
Australia: antigen
Australian Q: fever
Australian tick: typhus
Australian X: disease; encephalitis
Australian X disease: virus
autacoid: substance
authoritarian: personality
authority: figure
autistic: disorder; parasite
autochthonous: ideas; malaria; parasite
autocrine: hypothesis
autodermic: graft
autoerythrocyte: sensitization
autoerythrocyte sensitization: syndrome
autogeneic: graft
autogenous: control; keratoplasty; union; vaccine
autohemolysis: test
autoimmune: disease; thyroiditis
autoimmune hemolytic: anemia
autoimmune neonatal: thrombocytopenia

autokinetic: effect
autologous: graft; protein
autolytic: enzyme
automated differential leukocyte: counter
automatic: audiometer; audiometry; beat; condenser; contraction; epilepsy; plugger
autonomic: disorder; epilepsy; ganglia; imbalance; nerve; nuclei; part; plexuses
autonomic motor: neuron
autonomic nervous: system
autonomic neurogenic: bladder
autonomous: psychotherapy
autoparenchymatous: metaplasia
autophagic: vacuole
autoplastic: graft
autopolymer: resin
autoscopic: phenomenon
autoserum: therapy
autosomal: gene
autumn: fever
auxanographic: method
auxetic: growth
auxiliary: abutment
auxotrophic: mutant; strains
A-V: anastomosis; difference; interval; junction; valves
available arch: length
avalanche: conduction
avascular: necrosis
Avellis': syndrome
average flow: rate
average pulse: magnitude
aversion: therapy
aversive: behavior; conditioning; control; stimulus; training
avian: achondroplasia; diphtheria; erythroblastosis; herpesvirus 1; herpesvirus 2; influenza; leukosis; lymphomatosis; malaria; monocytosis; myeloblastosis; reticuloendotheliosis; sarcoma; spirochetosis; trichomoniasis
avian encephalomyelitis: virus
avian erythroblastosis: virus
avian infectious: encephalomyelitis; laryngotracheitis
avian infectious laryngotracheitis: virus
avian influenza: virus
avian leukosis-sarcoma: complex; virus
avian lymphomatosis: virus
avian myeloblastosis: virus

avian neurolymphomatosis: virus
avian pneumoencephalitis: virus
avian sarcoma: virus
avian viral arthritis: virus
aviation: medicine; otitis
aviator's: disease; ear
avidity: antibody
A-V junctional: rhythm; tachycardia
Avogadro's: constant; hypothesis; law; number; postulate
avoidance: conditioning; training
avoidance-avoidance: conflict
avoidant: disorder of adolescence; disorder of childhood; personality
avoidant personality: disorder
A-V strabismus: syndrome
avulsed: wound
avulsion: fracture
axial: ametropia; aneurysm; angle; cataract; current; filament; hyperopia; illumination; muscle; myopia; neuritis; plane; plate; point; projection; section; skeleton; surface; view; walls of the pulp chambers
axial pattern: flap
axilla: thermometer
axillary: anesthesia; arch; artery; cavity; fascia; fold; fossa; glands; hair; line; lymph nodes; nerve; plexus; region; sheath; space; thermometer; triangle; vein
axillary arch: muscle
axillary sweat: glands
axiolabiolingual: plane
axiomesiodistal: plane
axis: corpuscle; cylinder; deviation; ligament of malleus; shift; traction
axis-traction: forceps
axoaxonic: synapse
axodendritic: synapse
axon: degeneration; hillock; reflex; terminals
axonal: degeneration; polyneuropathy; process
axonal terminal: boutons
axon loss: polyneuropathy
axoplasmic: transport
axosomatic: synapse
Ayala's: index; quotient
Ayerza's: disease; syndrome
Ayre: brush
A.-Z.: test
azin: dyes
azo: dyes; itch

azocarmine: dyes
Azorean: disease
azotemic: retinitis
azotobacter: nuclease
Aztec: ear
azure: lunula of nails
azurophil: granule
azygoesophageal: recess
azygos: artery of vagina; fissure; lobe of lung; vein
azygos vein: principle

B

β: corynebacteriophage; hemolysin; hemolysis; phage; thalassemia
β_{1C}: globulin
β_{1E}: globulin
β_{1F}: globulin
β-δ: thalassemia
β-: microglobulin
β_2-: microglobulin
B: bile; cell; chain; fibers; lymphocyte; virus; wave
B19: virus
B_T: factor
B-: DNA
Babbitt: metal
Babcock: tube
Babès': nodes
Babès-Ernst: bodies
Babinski: reflex
Babinski's: phenomenon; sign; syndrome
baby: tooth
baby bottle: syndrome
Baccelli's: sign
Bachman: test
Bachmann's: bundle
Bachman-Pettit: test
bacillary: angiomatosis; dysentery; hemoglobinuria; layer
Bacillus anthracis: toxin
bacillus Calmette-Guérin: vaccine
back: cross; mutation; pressure; teeth
back-action: plugger
backboard: splint
back of foot: reflex
background: level; radiation
back vertex: power
backward: curvature
backward heart: failure
backwash: ileitis
Bacon's: anoscope
bacteria-free stage of
bacterial: endocarditis
bacterial: allergy; antagonism; capsule; cast; cystitis; encephalitis; endarteritis; endocarditis; growth; hemolysin; interference; peliosis; pericarditis; photosynthesis; plaque;

pneumonia; toxin; vaginosis; vegetations; virus
bacterial food: poisoning
bacteriocin: factors
bacteriocinogenic: plasmids
bacteriogenic: agglutination
bacteriolytic: serum
bacteriophage: immunity; plaque; resistance; typing
bacteriostatic: agent
bacteriotropic: substance
Baehr-Lohlein: lesion
Baelz': disease
Baer's: law; vesicle
Baeyer's: theory
bag of: waters
bag-gel: implant
Baggenstoss: change
Bagolini: test
Baillarger's: bands; lines
Bailliart's: ophthalmodynamometer
Bainbridge: reflex
baked: tongue
Baker's: cyst
baker's: eczema; itch
Baker's acid: hematein
Baker's pyridine: extraction
baking: soda
balance: theory
balanced: anesthesia; articulation; bite; diet; occlusion; polymorphism; translocation
balancing: contact; side
balancing occlusal: surface
balancing side: condyle
balanic: hypospadias
balanitic: epispadias
balantidial: dysentery
BALB: test
Balbani: ring
bald: tongue
Baldy's: operation
Balint's: syndrome
Balkan: beam; frame; nephropathy; splint
ball: thrombus; valve; variance
Ballance's: sign
ball-and-socket: joint
ballerina-foot: pattern
balloon: atrioseptostomy; catheter; cell; sickness
balloon cell: nevus
balloon counter: pulsation
ballooning: degeneration
balloon-tip: catheter
Ball's: operation
ball valve: action
ball-valve: thrombus
Baló's: disease
Baltic myoclonus: disease
Bamberger-Marie: disease; syndrome
Bamberger's: albuminuria; disease; sign

bamboo: hair; spine
bancroftian: filariasis
band: cell; centrifugation; neutrophil
bandage: sign
bandbox: resonance
Bandl's: ring
bandpass: filter
band-shaped: keratopathy
Bang's: bacillus; disease
Bannister's: disease
Bannwarth's: syndrome
Banti's: disease; syndrome
bar: clasp
Bárány's: sign
Bárány's caloric: test
Barbados: leg
barbed: broach
barber's: itch
barber's pilonidal: sinus
bar clasp: arm
Barclay-Baron: disease
bar clip: attachments
Barcoo: rot; vomit
Barcroft-Warburg: apparatus; technique
Bardet-Biedl: syndrome
Bardinet's: ligament
bare: area of liver; area of stomach
bare lymphocyte: syndrome
barium: enema
bar joint: denture
Barkan's: operation
Barkman's: reflex
Barkow's: ligaments
Barlow: syndrome
Barlow's: disease
Barnes': curve; dystrophy; zone
barometric: pressure
baroreceptor: nerve
Barraquer's: disease; method
Barr chromatin: body
barrel: chest
barrel-shaped: thorax
Barré's: sign
Barrett's: epithelium; esophagus; syndrome
barrier: contraceptive
bar-sleeve: attachments
Bartholin's: abscess; anus; cyst; cystectomy; duct; gland
Barth's: hernia
Bartonella: anemia
Barton's: bandage; forceps; fracture
Bart's: syndrome
Bartter's: syndrome
Baruch's: law
baryta: water
basal: age; anesthesia; body; bone; cell; cistern; corpuscle; diet; ganglia; gland; granule; lamina; lamina of choroid; lamina

of ciliary body; lamina of cochlear; lamina of neural tube; lamina of semicircular duct; layer; layer of choroid; layer of ciliary body; membrane of semicircular duct; metabolism; nuclei; nucleus of Ganser; part of occipital bone; part of pulmonary artery; plate of neural tube; ridge; rod; seat; sphincter; striations; surface; tuberculosis; vein of Rosenthal; veins
basal body: temperature
basal cell: adenoma; carcinoma; epithelioma; hyperplasia; layer; nevus; papilloma
basal cell nevus: syndrome
basal joint: reflex
basal metabolic: rate
basaloid: carcinoma; cell
basal seat: area
basal skull: fracture
basal squamous cell: carcinoma
basal tentorial: branch of internal carotid artery
Basan's: syndrome
base: composition; deficit; excess; hospital; line; material; metal; pair; plate; projection; units; view; view
baseball: finger
Basedow's: disease; goiter; pseudoparaplegia
baseline: tonus; variability of fetal heart rate
baseline fetal heart: rate
basement: lamina; membrane
baseplate: wax
basibregmatic: axis
basic: amino acid; diet; dyes; esotropia; exotropia; fuchsin; oxide; personality; proteins; reaction; salt; stain
basic electrical: rhythm
basic fuchsin-methylene blue: stain
basic personality: type
basicranial: axis; flexure
basifacial: axis
basilar: angle; apophysis; artery; bone; cartilage; cell; crest of cochlear duct; fibrocartilage; impression; index; invagination; lamina; leptomeningitis; membrane; meningitis; migraine; part of the occipital bone; part of pons; plexus; process; process of occipital bone;

prognathism; sinus; sulcus; vertebra
basilar pontine: sulcus
basilic: vein
basinasal: line
basioccipital: bone
basipharyngeal: canal
basisphenoid: bone
basivertebral: vein
basket: cell
basophil: adenoma; cell of anterior lobe of hypophysis; granule; substance
basophilic: degeneration; leukemia; leukocyte; leukocytosis; leukopenia; substance
basosquamous: carcinoma
Bassen-Kornzweig: syndrome
Bassini's: operation
Bassler's: sign
Bassora: gum
Bastedo's: sign
bat: ear
batch: culture
bath: itch; pruritus
bathing trunk: nevus
Batson's: plexus
Batten: disease
Batten-Mayou: disease
battered child: syndrome
battered spouse: syndrome
Battey: bacillus
battle: fatigue; neurosis
battledore: placenta
Battle's: sign
Baudelocque's: diameter; operation
Baudelocque's uterine: circle
Bauer's: syndrome
Bauer's chromic acid leucofuchsin: stain
Bauhin's: gland; valve
Baumé: scale
Baumès: symptom
Baumgarten's: glands; veins
bauxite: pneumoconiosis
bay: sore
Bayes: theorem
Bayesian: hypothesis
Bayle's: disease
Bayley: Scales of Infant Development
bayonet: forceps; hair
Bazett's: formula
Bazex's: syndrome
Bazin's: disease
B6 bronchus: sign
B cell antigen: receptors
B-cell differentiating: factor
B cell differentiation/growth: factors
B-cell stimulatory: factor 2
BCG: vaccine

B-E: amputation
Be^a: antigens
beaded: hair
beak: sign
beaked: pelvis
beaker: cell
Beale's: cell
bearing-down: pain
beat-to-beat: variability of fetal heart rate
Beau's: lines
Bechterew-Mendel: reflex
Bechterew's: band; disease; nucleus; sign
Becker: antigen
Becker's: disease; nevus; stain for spirochetes
Becker type muscular: dystrophy
Becker type tardive muscular: dystrophy
Beckmann's: apparatus
Beck's: method; triad
Beckwith-Wiedemann: syndrome
Béclard's: anastomosis; hernia; triangle
Becquerel: rays
bed: rest; sore
Bednar: tumor
Bednar's: aphthae
bedside: radiography
bee: toxin
beechwood: sugar
beer: heart
Beer-Lambert: law
Beer's: knife; law
beet: sugar
beet-: tongue
Beevor's: sign
Begbie's: disease
Begg light wire differential force: technique
Béguez César: disease
behavior: chain; disorder; modification; reflex; therapy
behavioral: epidemic; genetics; health; immunogen; manifestation; medicine; pathogen; psychology
behavioristic: psychology
Behçet's: disease; syndrome
Behring's: law
Behr's: disease; syndrome
BEI: test
Békésy: audiometer; audiometry
Belgian Congo: anemia
bell: sound; stage
belladonna: extract; tincture
bell clapper: deformity
Bellini's: ducts; ligament
Bell-Magendie: law
bellmetal: resonance
bellows: murmur

Bell's: law; muscle; palsy; phenomenon; spasm
bell-shaped: crown
Bell's respiratory: nerve
Belsey Mark IV: operation; procedure
Belsey Mark V: procedure
belt: test
Bence Jones: albumin; cylinders; myeloma; proteins; proteinuria; reaction
bench: testing
Bender gestalt: test
Bender Visual Motor Gestalt: test
bending: fracture
Benedek's: reflex
Benedict-Hopkins-Cole: reagent
Benedict-Roth: apparatus; calorimeter
Benedict's: solution; test for glucose
Benedikt's: syndrome
benign: albuminuria; cementoblastoma; dyskeratosis; glycosuria; hypertension; lymphadenosis; lymphocytoma cutis; lymphoma of the rectum; mesothelioma; mesothelioma of genital tract; nephrosclerosis; stupor; tetanus; tumor
benign bone: aneurysm
benign bovine: theileriosis
benign childhood: epilepsy with centrotemporal spikes
benign dry: pleurisy
benign essential: tremor
benign familial: chorea; icterus
benign familial chronic: pemphigus
benign giant lymph node: hyperplasia
benign inoculation: lymphoreticulosis; reticulosis
benign juvenile: melanoma
benign lymphoepithelial: lesion
benign migratory: glossitis
benign mucosal: pemphigoid
benign myalgic: encephalomyelitis
benign neonatal: convulsions
benign paroxysmal: peritonitis
benign paroxysmal postural: vertigo
benign positional: vertigo
benign prostatic: hypertrophy
benign tertian: malaria

Bennett: angle; movement
Bennett's: fracture
Bennhold's Congo red: stain
Bensley's specific: granules
bentiromide: test
bentonite flocculation: test
benzene: nucleus; ring
benzidine: test
benzoinated: lard
benzyl: penicillin
Beradinelli's: syndrome
Bérard's: aneurysm
Béraud's: valve
Berger: cells; rhythm
Berger's: disease; space
Berger's focal: glomerulonephritis
Bergmann's: cords; fibers
Bergmeister's: papilla
Berg's: stain
beriberi: heart
Berkefeld: filter
Berlin's: edema
berloque: dermatitis
Bernard-Cannon: homeostasis
Bernard-Horner: syndrome
Bernard's: canal; duct; puncture
Bernard-Sergent: syndrome
Bernard-Soulier: disease; syndrome
Bernays': sponge
Bernhardt-Roth: syndrome
Bernhardt's: disease; formula
Bernheim's: syndrome
Bernoulli: distribution; effect
Bernoulli's: law; principle; theorem
Bernstein: test
berry: aneurysm; cell
Berry's: ligaments
Berson: test
Berthelot: reaction
Berthollet's: law
Bertin's: bones; columns; ligament; ossicles
beryllium: granuloma
Besnier-Boeck-Schaumann: disease; syndrome
Besnier's: prurigo
Best's: disease
Best's carmine: stain
Beta: tests
beta: alcoholism; angle; cell of anterior lobe of hypophysis; cell of pancreas; error; fibers; granule; particle; radiation; ray; rhythm
beta: wave
beta-: oxidation
beta-oxidation-condensation: theory
betel: cancer
Bethesda: system; unit

Betke-Kleihauer: test
Bettendorff's: test
Betz: cells
Beuren: syndrome
Bevan-Lewis: cells
bevelled: anastomosis
Bezold-Jarisch: reflex
Bezold's: abscess; ganglion; mastoiditis; sign; symptom; triad
BH: interval
Bi: antigen
Bial's: test
Bianchi's: nodule; valve
biauricular: axis
biaxial: joint
bi-bi: reaction
bicameral: abscess
bicanalicular: sphincter
BICAP: cautery
biceps: muscle of arm; muscle of thigh; reflex
biceps brachii: muscle
biceps femoris: muscle; reflex
Bichat's: canal; fat-pad; fissure; foramen; fossa; ligament; membrane; protuberance; tunic
bicipital: aponeurosis; bursitis; fascia; groove; rib; ridges; tuberosity
bicipitoradial: bursa
Bickel's: ring
biclonal: gammopathy
biconcave: lens
bicondylar: articulation; joint
biconvex: lens
bicornate: uterus
bicoudate: catheter
bicuspid: tooth; valve
bidirectional: replication
bidirectional ventricular: tachycardia
bidiscoidal: placenta
Biebl: loop
Biederman's: sign
Bielschowsky's: disease; sign; stain
Biemond: syndrome
Biermer's: anemia; disease; sign
Biernacki's: sign
Bier's: amputation; hyperemia; method
Biesiadecki's: fossa
bifid: penis; rib; thumb; tongue; uterus; uvula
bifidus: factor
bifocal: lens; spectacles
biforate: uterus
bifoveal: fixation
bifurcate: ligament
bifurcated: ligament
bifurcation: lymph nodes
big: ACTH; head
Bigelow's: ligament; septum

bigeminal: bodies; pregnancy; pulse; rhythm
big liver: disease
bilaminar: blastoderm
bilateral: hermaphroditism; left-sidedness; lithotomy; pleurisy; synchrony
bilateral medial orbital: ecchymoses
bile: acids; alcohol; capillary; cyst; duct; gastritis; papilla; peritonitis; pigments; salts; thrombus
bile acid tolerance: test
bi-leaflet: valve
bile esculin: test
bile pigment: hemoglobin
Bile's: antigen
bile salt: agar
bile solubility: test
bilharzial: appendicitis; dysentery; granuloma
biliary: atresia; calculus; canaliculus; cirrhosis; colic; duct; ductules; dyskinesia; fever of dogs; fever of horses; fistula; steatorrhea; xanthomatosis
bilious: headache; pneumonia; typhoid of Griesinger; vomit
bilious remittent: fever; malaria
bilirubin: encephalopathy
billowing mitral valve: syndrome
Billroth I: anastomosis
Billroth II: anastomosis
Billroth's: cords; operation I; operation II; venae cavernosae
Bill's: maneuver
bilobed: flap
bilocular: joint; stomach
bilocular femoral: hernia
bimanual: palpation; percussion; version
bimaxillary: protrusion
bimaxillary dentoalveolar: protrusion
bimaxillary protrusive: occlusion
binangle: chisel
binary: combination; complex; digit; fission; nomenclature; process
binasal: hemianopia
binaural: stethoscope
binaural alternate loudness balance: test
binding: constant; energy
Binet: age; scale; test
Binet-Simon: scale
Bingham: flow; model; plastic
Bing's: reflex
Binn's: bacterium

binocular: fixation; heterochromia; loupe; microscope; ophthalmoscope; parallax; rivalry; vision
binomial: distribution
Binswanger's: disease; encephalopathy
Binz': test
biochemical: genetics; metastasis; pharmacology; profile
biochemical oxygen: demand
bioelectric: potential
biogenetic: law
biogenic: amines
biologic: evolution; hemolysis; time
biological: assay; chemistry; coefficient; control; half-life; immunotherapy; psychiatry; sampling; vector
biological standard: unit
biomedical: engineering; model
biometrical: school
Biondi-Heidenhain: stain
biophysical: profile
biopsy: needle
biopsychosocial: model
biorbital: angle
biotic: community; factors; potential
Biot's: breathing; respiration; respiration; sign
Biot's breathing: sign
biparietal: diameter
bipartite: uterus; vagina
bipedicle: flap
bipennate: muscle
biphasic: insulin; response
biplane: angiography
bipolar: cautery; cell; disorder; lead; neuron; psychosis; taxis; version
Birbeck's: granule
Birch-Hirschfeld: stain
bird: face; unit
bird-breeder's: disease; lung
Bird's: sign
birdseed: agar
bird shot: retinochoroiditis
bird's nest: filter
birth: amputation; canal; control; defect; fracture; palsy; rate; trauma; weight
Bischof's: myelotomy
biscuit: bite
bisferious: pulse
Bishop's: sphygmoscope
Biskra: boil; button
bismuth: line
bite: analysis; fork; gauge; plane; rim
bitemporal: hemianopia
bitewing: film; radiograph

biting: louse; pressure; strength
Bitot's: spots
bitter: almond oil; orange peel; orange peel, dried; orange peel, fresh; orange peel oil; peptides; principles; tonic; water
Bittner: agent; virus
Bittner's milk: factor
Bittorf's: reaction
biundulant: meningoencephalitis
biuret: reaction; reagent; test
bivalent: antibody; chromosome
bivalent gas gangrene: antitoxin
bivalve: speculum
biventer: lobule
biventral: lobule
Bixler type: hypertelorism
Bizzozero's: corpuscle
Bizzozero's red: cells
Bjerrum: screen
Bjerrum's: scotoma; sign
Bjork-Shiley: valve
Bjornstad's: syndrome
BK: virus
B-K: amputation
black: box; cataract; death; disease; eye; fever; heel; lead; line; lung; measles; mustard; piedra; plague; sickness; spore; tarantula; tongue; urine; vomit; water
black currant: rash
black-dot: ringworm
Black's: classification; formula
black-tongue: disease
blackwater: fever
bladder: calculi; compliance; reflex; schistosomiasis; stone
blade: bone
Blagden's: law
Blainville: ears
Blair-Brown: graft
Blalock: shunt
Blalock-Hanlon: operation
Blalock-Taussig: operation; shunt
bland: diet; embolism; infarct
Blandin's: gland
blanket: suture
Blasius': duct
blast: cell; crisis; injury
blastodermic: disk; ectoderm; layers; vesicle
blastomycetic: dermatitis
blastoporic: canal
Blatin's: syndrome
bleached: wax
bleaching: powder
blear: eye
bleary: eye

bleeding: polyp; time
blending: inheritance
blennorrheal: conjunctivitis
blighted: ovum
blind: boil; enema; fistula; foramen of frontal bone; foramen of the tongue; gut; headache; passage; spot; staggers; study; test
blinding: disease; glare
blind loop: syndrome
blind nasotracheal: intubation
blister: agent
blister beetle: poisoning
blistering: collodion
blistering distal: dactylitis
Bloch's: reaction
Bloch-Sulzberger: disease; syndrome
block: anesthesia; vertebrae
block design: test
blocked: aerogastria; reading frame
blocking: activity; agent; antibody
Blocq's: disease
blood: agar; albumin; blister; calculus; capillary; cast; cell; circulation; clot; corpuscle; count; crisis; crystals; cyst; disk; dyscrasia; gases; group; island; islet; lymph; mole; motes; pH; plasma; plastid; plate; poisoning; pressure; relationship; serum; spavin; spots; substitute; sugar; tumor; type; vessel
blood-air: barrier
blood-aqueous: barrier
blood-brain: barrier
blood-cerebrospinal fluid: barrier
blood gas: analysis
blood group: agglutinins; agglutinogens; antibodies; antigen; antiserums; substance; systems
blood group-specific: substances A and B
bloodless: amputation; decerebration; operation; phlebotomy
blood plasma: fractions
blood pool: imaging
blood urea: nitrogen
blood-vascular: system
blood volume: nomogram
Bloom's: syndrome
Blount-Barber: disease
Blount's: disease
blow-out: fracture
blowout: pipette
blubber: finger
blue: asphyxia; atrophy; baby; cataract; dextran; disease; edema; fever; line;

nevus; ointment; pus;
  sclera; spot; vision
blueberry muffin: baby
bluecomb: disease of
  chickens; disease of
  turkeys; virus
blue cone: monochromatism
blue dome: cyst
blue dot: sign
blue-green: algae; bacteria;
  bacterium
blue pus: bacillus
blue rubber-bleb: nevi
blue toe: syndrome
bluetongue: virus
Blumberg's: sign
Blumenau's: nucleus
Blumenbach's: clivus
Blumer's: shelf
blunt duct: adenosis
blunted: affect
blunt-end: ligation
blunt-ended: DNA
B-mode: echocardiography
boat: conformation; form
boat-shaped: abdomen
Bochdalek's: foramen;
  ganglion; gap; hernia;
  muscle; valve
Bockhart's: impetigo
Bock's: ganglion; nerve
Bodansky: unit
Bödecker: index
Bodian's copper-
  PROTARGOL: stain
body: cavity; image;
  language; mechanics;
  plethysmograph; schema;
  stalk
body dysmorphic: disorder
body mass: index
body righting: reflexes
body-weight: ratio
Boeck's: disease; sarcoid
Boehmer's: hematoxylin
Boerhaave's: glands;
  syndrome
bog: spavin
Bogros': space
Bogros' serous: membrane
Bohn's: nodules
Bohr: effect; magneton
Bohr's: atom; equation;
  theory
boilermaker's: deafness
boiling: point
Boley: gauge
Bolivian hemorrhagic: fever
Bolivian hemorrhagic fever:
  virus
Bollinger: bodies; granules
Boll's: cells
Bolognini's: symptom
bolster: finger
Bolton: plane
Bolton-Broadbent: plane
Bolton-nasion: line; plane
bolus: dressing

bomb: calorimeter
Bombay: phenomenon; trait
bone: abscess; ache; age;
  block; canaliculus; cell;
  charcoal; chips;
  conduction; corpuscle;
  cyst; flap; forceps; graft;
  infarct; island; marrow;
  matrix; phosphate; plate;
  reflex; resorption; salt;
  sclerosis; sensibility;
  spavin; tissue; wax
bone Gla: protein
bone marrow: dose;
  embolism; transplantation
Bonhoeffer's: sign
Bonnet's: capsule
Bonney: test
Bonnier's: syndrome
Bonwill: triangle
bony: ankylosis; crepitus;
  heart; labyrinth; palate;
  part of auditory tube; part
  of external acoustic
  meatus; part of nasal
  septum
bony nasal: septum
bony semicircular: canals
Böök: syndrome
booster: dose; response
Bordeau: theory
Bordeaux: mixture
border: cells; disease;
  molding; movements; seal
borderline: case;
  hypertension; leprosy;
  personality; tumor
borderline personality:
  disorder
border tissue: movements
Bordet and Gengou:
  reaction
Bordet-Gengou: bacillus;
  phenomenon
Bordet-Gengou potato
  blood: agar
Börjeson-Forssman-
  Lehmann: syndrome
Born: method of wax plate
  reconstruction
Borna: disease
Borna disease: virus
Bornholm: disease
Bornholm disease: virus
Borrel: bodies
Borrel's blue: stain
Borst-Jadassohn type
  intraepidermal:
  epithelioma
bosch: yaws
Bosin's: disease
Boston: exanthema; opium
Botallo's: duct; foramen;
  ligament
bothropic: antitoxin
Bothrops: antitoxin
botryoid: sarcoma
botryoid odontogenic: cyst

Böttcher's: canal; cells;
  crystals; ganglion; space
botulinum: antitoxin
botulinus: toxin
botulism: antitoxin
Bouchard's: disease
Bouchut's: tube
Bouffardi's black:
  mycetoma
Bouffardi's white:
  mycetoma
Bouillaud's: disease
Bouin's: fixative
bound: water
boundary: lamina
bouquet: fever
Bourdon: tube
Bourgery's: ligament
Bourneville-Pringle: disease
Bourneville's: disease
boutonneuse: fever
boutonnière: deformity
Bovero's: muscle
bovine: acetonemia;
  achondroplasia; antitoxin;
  babesiosis; borreliosis;
  brucellosis; colloid;
  hemoglobinuria;
  herpesvirus 1; herpesvirus
  2; hyperkeratosis; ketosis;
  leukemia; lymphosarcoma;
  mastitis; porphyria;
  rhinoviruses;
  trichomoniasis
bovine cancer: eye
bovine congenital: ataxia
bovine ephemeral: fever
bovine ephemeral fever:
  virus
bovine herpes: mammillitis
bovine immunodeficiency:
  virus
bovine leukemia: virus
bovine leukosis: virus
bovine papular: stomatitis
bovine papular stomatitis:
  virus
bovine petechial: fever
bovine respiratory
  syncytial: virus
bovine serum: albumin
bovine spongiform:
  encephalopathy
bovine sporadic:
  encephalomyelitis
bovine ulcerative:
  mammillitis
bovine vaccinia: mammillitis
bovine virus: diarrhea
bovine virus diarrhea: virus
bow-: leg
Bowditch: effect
Bowditch's: law
bowed: tendon
bowel: bypass; movement;
  sounds
bowel bypass: syndrome
Bowenoid: cells

bowenoid: papulosis
Bowen's: disease
Bowen's precancerous:
  dermatosis
Bowie's: stain
Bowles type: stethoscope
Bowman-Birk: inhibitor
Bowman's: capsule; disks;
  gland; membrane; muscle;
  probe; space; theory
boxer's: ear; fracture
boxing: wax
Boyd communicating
  perforation: veins
Boyden: meal
Boyden's: sphincter
Boyer's: bursa; cyst
Boyle's: law
Bozeman-Fritsch: catheter
Bozeman's: operation;
  position
Bozzolo's: sign
B-P: fistula
Braasch: catheter
brachial: anesthesia; artery;
  fascia; gland; lymph nodes;
  muscle; neuritis; plexitis;
  plexus; veins
brachial birth: palsy
brachialis: muscle
brachial plexus: neuropathy
brachiocephalic: arteritis;
  muscle; trunk; veins
brachioradial: muscle;
  reflex
brachioradialis: muscle
Bracht: maneuver
Bracht-Wachter: lesion
brachypellic: pelvis
bracken: poisoning; staggers
Bradford: frame
bradykinetic: analysis
bradykinin-potentiating:
  peptide
bradytachycardia:
  syndrome
Brailsford-Morquio: disease
brain: cicatrix; concussion;
  congestion; contusion;
  death; edema; laceration;
  lipid; mantle; murmur;
  potential; sand; stem;
  sugar; swelling; wave
brain-heart infusion: agar
Brain's: reflex
brainstem: glioma;
  hemorrhage
brainstem evoked response:
  audiometry
brain wave: complex; cycle
branch: migration
branched: calculus
branched chain:
  ketoaciduria; ketonuria
brancher deficiency:
  glycogenosis
brancher glycogen storage:
  disease

branchial: apparatus; arches; cartilages; clefts; cyst; fissure; fistula; groove; mesoderm; pouches
branchial cleft: cyst
branchial efferent: column
branching: enzyme; factor
branchiomeric: muscles
branchiomotor: nuclei
Brandt-Andrews: maneuver
brandy: nose
Branham's: sign
branny: desquamation; tetter
Brasdor's: method
brass founder's: ague; fever
brassy: body; cough
Braune's: canal; muscle; valve
Braun's: anastomosis
brawny: arm; edema; scleritis
Braxton Hicks: contraction; sign; version
Brazelton's Neonatal Behavioral Assessment: Scale
Brazil: wax
Brazilian: blastomycosis; pemphigus
Brazilian hemorrhagic: fever
Brazilian purpuric: fever
Brazilian spotted: fever
BrDu-: banding
bread: pill
bread-and-butter: pericardium
break: shock
breakbone: fever
breakoff: phenomenon
breast: bone; pang; pump
breath analysis: test
breath-holding: test
breathing: bag; reserve
Breda's: disease
breech: delivery; extraction; presentation
bregmatic: fontanel
bregmatolambdoid: arc
bregmocardiac: reflex
Brenner: tumor
brephoplastic: graft
Breschet's: bones; canals; hiatus; sinus; vein
Brescia-Cimino: fistula
Breslow's: thickness
Breus: mole
Brewer's: infarcts
brewers': yeast
brickdust: deposit
Bricker: operation
brickmaker's: anemia
bridge: corpuscle
bridging hepatic: necrosis
bridle: stricture; suture
brief: psychotherapy
Brigg's: test

brightness difference: threshold
Bright's: disease
brilliant green salt: agar
Brill's: disease
Brill-Symmers: disease
Brill-Zinsser: disease
Brimacombe: fragment
Brinell hardness: number
Briquet's: ataxia; disease; syndrome
brisket: disease
Brissaud-Marie: syndrome
Brissaud's: disease; infantilism; reflex
bristle: cell
British: gum
British thermal: unit
brittle: bones; diabetes
broad: fascia; ligament of the uterus; spectrum
Broadbent's: law; sign
broad beta: disease
broadest: muscle of back
broad spectrum: antibiotic
Broca's: angles; aphasia; area; center; field; fissure; formula; pouch
Broca's basilar: angle
Broca's diagonal: band
Broca's facial: angle
Broca's parolfactory: area
Broca's visual: plane
Brock: operation
Brockenbrough: sign
Brock's: syndrome
Brocq's: disease
Brödel's bloodless: line
Brodie: fluid
Brodie's: abscess; bursa; disease; knee; ligament
Brodmann's: areas
Broesike's: fossa
bromide: acne
bromine: water
bromphenol: test
Brompton: cocktail
bromsulphalein: test
bronchial: adenoma; arteries; arteriography; asthma; atresia; breathing; bud; calculus; fremitus; glands; pneumonia; polyp; respiration; tubes; veins; voice
bronchic: cells
bronchiolar: adenocarcinoma; carcinoma
bronchiolar exocrine: cell
bronchioloalveolar: adenocarcinoma
bronchiolo-alveolar: carcinoma
bronchitic: asthma
bronchobiliary: fistula
bronchocavitary: fistula

bronchocentric: granulomatosis
bronchoesophageal: fistula; muscle
bronchogenic: carcinoma; cyst
bronchomediastinal: trunk
bronchopleural: fistula
bronchopneumonic: aspergillosis
bronchopulmonary: aspergillosis; dysplasia; lymph nodes; segment; sequestration; spirochetosis
bronchoscopic: brush; smear; sponge
bronchovesicular: respiration
Brønsted: acid; base; theory
bronze: diabetes
bronzed: diabetes; disease; skin
brood: capsules; cell
Brooke: ileostomy
Brooke's: disease; tumor
brother: complex
brow: presentation
brown: atrophy; edema; fat; induration of the lung; layer; lung; pellicle; striae; tumor
brown adipose: tissue
Brown-Adson: forceps
Brown-Brenn: stain
brownian: motion; movement
brownian-Zsigmondy: movement
Browning's: vein
Brown's: syndrome
Brown-Séquard's: paralysis; syndrome
brucella strain 19: vaccine
Bruch's: glands; membrane
Brücke-Bartley: phenomenon
Brücke's: muscle; tunic
Bruck's: disease
Brudzinski's: sign
Brug's: filariasis
Brugsch's: syndrome
Brumpt's white: mycetoma
Brunn: reaction
Brunner's: glands
Brunn's: membrane; nests
Bruns: ataxia
Bruns': nystagmus
Brunschwig's: operation
brush: biopsy; border; burn; catheter
brush burn: abrasion
Brushfield's: spots
Brushfield-Wyatt: disease
brush heap: structure
Bryant's: sign; traction; triangle
BSP: test
bubble gum: dermatitis

bubbling: rale
bubonic: plague
buccal: angles; artery; branches of facial nerve; caries; cavity; curve; digestion; embrasure; fat-pad; flange; gingiva; glands; lymph node; nerve; occlusion; pit; region; smear; surface; tablet; vestibule
buccinator: crest; muscle; nerve; node
buccocervical: ridge
buccogingival: ridge
buccolingual: diameter; dimension; relation
bucconasal: membrane
bucconeural: duct
bucco-occlusal: angle
buccopharyngeal: fascia; membrane; part of superior pharyngeal constrictor
Büchner: extract; funnel
Buchwald's: atrophy
buck: tooth
bucked: shins
bucket-handle: incision; tear
buckled: aorta
Buck's: extension; fascia; traction
buckthorn: polyneuropathy
Bucky: diaphragm
bud: fission; stage
Budd-Chiari: syndrome
Budde: process
buddeized: milk
Budd's: cirrhosis; syndrome
Budge's: center
Budin's obstetrical: joint
Buerger's: disease
buffalo: hump; neck; type
buffer: capacity; index; pair; value; value of the blood
buffered crystalline: penicillin G
buffy: coat
bulbar: apoplexy; conjunctiva; myelitis; palsy; paralysis; pulse; ridge; septum
bulbocavernosus: muscle; reflex
bulboid: corpuscles
bulbomimic: reflex
bulbosacral: system
bulbourethral: gland
bulbous: bougie
bulboventricular: loop; ridge
bulging eye: disease
bulk: modulus
bull: neck
bulldog: calf; forceps; head
bullet: bubo; forceps
bullous: edema; edema vesicae; emphysema; fever; impetigo of newborn;

keratopathy; myringitis;
pemphigoid; syphilid
**bullous congenital
ichthyosiform:**
erythroderma
bull's-eye: maculopathy
Bumke's: pupil
bundle: bone
bundle-branch: block
Bunnell's: suture
Bunsen-Roscoe: law
Bunsen's solubility:
coefficient
Bunyamwera: fever; virus
bunyavirus: encephalitis
buoyant: density
bur: drill
Burchard-Liebermann:
reaction
Burdach's: column;
fasciculus; nucleus; tract
Burdwan: fever
Bürger-Grütz: disease;
syndrome
Burger's: triangle
Burgundy: pitch
buried: flap; penis; suture
Burkitt's: lymphoma
Burlew: disk; wheel
burner: syndrome
Burnett's: syndrome
burning drops: sign
burning foot: syndrome
burning vulva: syndrome
Burn and Rand: theory
Burns': ligament; space
Burns' falciform: process
burnt: alum
Burow's: operation; solution;
triangle; vein
burr: cell
burrowing: hairs
bursal: abscess; cyst;
synovitis
Burton's: line
Buruli: ulcer
Bury's: disease
Buschke-Löwenstein: tumor
Buschke-Ollendorf:
syndrome
Buschke's: disease
bush: sickness; yaws
Busquet's: disease
Buss: disease
Busse-Buschke: disease
butanol-extractable: iodine
butanol-extractable iodine:
test
butter: stools
butterfly: eruption;
fragment; lung; patch;
pattern; rash; vertebra
button: suture
buttonhole: iridectomy;
stenosis
buttress: foot; plate
buyo cheek: cancer
Buzzard's: maneuver

Bwamba: fever; virus
By: antigen
Byler: disease
by-product: material
Byzantine arch: palate

C

C: bile; cell; chain; factors;
fibers; gene; value; wave
C1: esterase
C3: proactivator; proactivator
convertase
C-: terminus
c: wave
CA: virus
CAAT: box
cabbage: goiter
cable: graft
Cabot-Locke: murmur
Cabot's ring: bodies
cacao: butter
cachectic: diarrhea; edema;
endocarditis; fever; pallor
cadaveric: rigidity; spasm
caddis: worm
cafe: coronary
Caffey-Kempe: syndrome
Caffey's: disease; syndrome
Caffey-Silverman: syndrome
Cagot: ear
Cain: complex
caisson: disease; sickness
Cajal's: cell
Cajal's astrocyte: stain
cake: alum; kidney
caked: breast
Calabar: swelling
calabash: curare
calcaneal: arteries; bone;
bursitis; gait; petechiae;
process of cuboid bone;
region; sulcus; tuber;
tubercle; tuberosity
calcaneal arterial: network
calcaneal articular: surface
of talus
calcanean: tendon
calcaneocuboid: joint;
ligament
calcaneofibular: ligament
calcaneonavicular: ligament
calcaneotibial: ligament
calcareous: conjunctivitis;
degeneration; infiltration;
metastasis; pancreatitis
calcarine: artery; branch of
medial occipital artery;
fasciculus; fissure; sulcus
calcic: water
calcific: pancreatitis
calcification: lines of Retzius
calcific nodular aortic:
stenosis
calcified: cartilage
**calcifying epithelial
odontogenic:** tumor

**calcifying and keratinizing
odontogenic:** cyst
calcifying odontogenic: cyst
calcined: magnesia
calcinuric: diabetes
calcitonin gene related:
peptide
calcium: antagonist; gout;
pump; rigor; sign; tungstate
calcium channel: blocker
calcium channel-blocking:
agent
**calcium pyrophosphate
deposition:** disease
calculated mean: organism
calculated serum: osmolality
Caldani's: ligament
Caldwell: projection; view
Caldwell-Luc: operation
Caldwell-Moloy:
classification
calf: bone; diphtheria; pump;
scours
caliciform: cell
California: encephalitis;
virus
**California psychological
inventory:** test
caliper: micrometer
Calkins': sign
Callahan's: method
Callander's: amputation
Call-Exner: bodies
Callison's: fluid
callosal: convolution; gyrus;
sulcus
callosomarginal: artery;
fissure; sulcus
Calmette: test
Calmette-Guérin: bacillus;
vaccine
calomel: electrode
caloric: nystagmus; test;
value
calorigenic: action
Calori's: bursa
Calot's: triangle
calvarial: hook
Calvé-Perthes: disease
calyciform: ending
cambium: layer
cameloid: anemia; cell
camelpox: virus
CAMP: test
CAMP: factor
camp: fever; hospital
Campbell: sound
Campbell's: ligament
Camper's: chiasm; fascia;
ligament; line; plane
camphorated: menthol;
phenol
cAMP receptor: protein
camptomelic: dwarfism;
syndrome
Canada: balsam; snakeroot;
turpentine

canalicular: adenoma; ducts;
sphincter
canarypox: virus
Canavan's: disease; sclerosis
**Canavan-Van Bogaert-
Bertrand:** disease
cancellous: bone; tissue
cancer: bodies; family; juice
cancer antigen 125: test
cane: sugar
canefield: fever
canicola: fever
canine: adenovirus 1;
amebiasis; babesiosis;
borreliosis; carcinoma 1;
distemper; dysautonomia;
ehrlichiosis; eminence;
fossa; herpesvirus;
herpetovirus; hysteria;
leishmaniasis; panosteitis;
parvovirus 2; prominence;
spasm; tooth; typhus
canine distemper: virus
canine hereditary: blindness
canine infectious cyclic:
thrombocytopenia
canine malignant:
lymphoma
canine oral: papilloma
canine parvovirus: disease
canine venereal: granuloma
canities: poliosis
canker: sores
Cannizzaro's: reaction
cannon: bone; sound; wave
cannonball: pulse
Cannon-Bard: theory
Cannon's: point; ring; theory
Cantelli's: sign
cantering: rhythm
canthal: hypertelorism
cantharidal: collodion
cantharis: camphor
canthomeatal: plane
cantilever: beam; bridge
Cantor: tube
caoutchouc: pelvis
cap: splint; stage
capeline: bandage
Capgras': phenomenon;
syndrome
capillary: angioma; arteriole;
attraction; bed; circulation;
drainage; fracture; fragility;
hemangioma; hemangioma
of infancy; lake; loops;
nevus; pericyte; pulse;
vein; vessel
capillary fragility: test
capillary permeability:
factor
capillary resistance: test
capillary zone:
electrophoresis
Capim: viruses
capital: operation
capitate: bone
capitular: joint

Caplan's: nodules; syndrome
capon: unit
capon-comb: unit
capon-comb-growth: test
capped: elbow; hock; knee; uterus
capping: proteins
Capps': reflex
caprine: herpesvirus; herpetovirus
caprine arthritis-: encephalomyelitis
caprine arthritis-encephalomyelitis: virus
capsular: advancement; antigen; branches of renal artery; cataract; cirrhosis of liver; glaucoma; ligament; space
capsular flap: pyeloplasty
capsular precipitation: reaction
capsule: cell; forceps
capsulolenticular: cataract
capture-recapture: method
Capuron's: points
caput: epididymis
car: sickness
Carabelli: tubercle
Caraparu: virus
carbacrylamine: resins
carbamino: compound
carbamylcholine: chloride
carbocyclic: compound
carbohydrate: loading; metabolism
carbohydrate-induced: hyperlipemia
carbohydrate utilization: test
carbol: fuchsin
carbol-fuchsin: paint
carbol-thionin: stain
carbon: autotrophy
carbonated: water
carbonate dehydratase: inhibitor
carbon dioxide: acidosis; content; cycle; electrode; elimination
carbon dioxide combining: power
carbon dioxide-free: water
carbon disulfide: poisoning
carbonic: anhydrase
carbonic acid: gas
carbonic anhydrase: inhibitor
carbonic anhydrase II deficiency: syndrome
carbon monoxide: hemoglobin; poisoning
carboxy: terminal
carboxylic acid: ester
carboxymethyl: cellulose
carcinoembryonic: antigen
carcinoid: flush; syndrome; tumor

carcinomatous: encephalomyelopathy; implants; myelopathy; myopathy; neuromyopathy; pericarditis
Carden's: amputation
cardiac: accident; albuminuria; alternation; aneurysm; arrest; arrhythmia; asthma; catheter; cirrhosis; competence; contractility; cycle; decompression; diuretic; dropsy; dyspnea; dysrhythmia; edema; failure; ganglia; gating; gland; glands of esophagus; hemoptysis; heterotaxia; histiocyte; hormone; impression of liver; impression of lung; impulse; incompetence; index; infarction; insufficiency; jelly; liver; lung; mapping; massage; monitor; murmur; muscle; neurosis; notch; notch of left lung; opening; orifice; output; part of stomach; plexus; polyp; prominence; reserve; segment; shock; skeleton; souffle; sound; standstill; symphysis; syncope; tamponade; telemetry; tube; veins
cardiac depressor: reflex
cardiac fibrous: skeleton
cardiac lymphatic: ring
cardiac muscle: tissue; wrap
cardiac valve: prosthesis
cardiac valvular: incompetence
cardinal: ligament; points; symptom; veins
cardinal ocular: movements
cardioarterial: interval
cardiodiaphragmatic: angle
cardioesophageal: junction; relaxation
cardiofacial: syndrome
cardiogenic: plate; shock
cardiohepatic: angle; triangle
cardioid: condenser
cardiophrenic: angle
cardioplegic: arrest
cardiopulmonary: arrest; bypass; murmur; resuscitation; transplantation
cardiopulmonary splanchnic: nerves
cardiorespiratory: murmur
cardiothoracic: ratio
cardiotoxic: myolysis
cardiovascular: radiology; syphilis; system
Carey Coombs: murmur

carinal: lymph nodes
carinate: abdomen
Carlen's: tube
Carman's: sign
Carmody-Batson: operation
carnassial: tooth
carnauba: wax
carneous: degeneration; mole
Carnett's: sign
Carnoy's: fixative
Caroli's: disease; syndrome
β-carotene cleavage: enzyme
caroticoclinoid: ligament
caroticotympanic: arteries; canaliculi; nerve
carotid: arteries; body; bruit; bulb; canal; duct; endarterectomy; foramen; ganglion; groove; pulse; sheath; shudder; sinus; sulcus; triangle; tubercle; wall of middle ear
carotid body: tumor
carotid-cavernous: fistula
carotid sinus: branch; nerve; reflex; syncope; syndrome; test
carp: mouth
carpal: arches; artery; articulation; bones; canal; groove; joints; tunnel
carpal articular: surface of radius
carpal tunnel: syndrome
Carpenter's: syndrome
Carpentier-Edwards: valve
carpometacarpal: joints; joint of thumb; ligaments
carpopedal: contraction; spasm
Carpue's: method
Carrel-Lindbergh: pump
Carrel's: treatment
carrier: cell; electrophoresis; screening; state; strain
Carrington's: disease
Carrión's: disease
Carr-Price: reaction; test
Carr-Purcell: experiment
carrying: angle
Carter's: fever
Carter's black: mycetoma
cartesian: nomogram
cartilage: bone; capsule; cell; knife; lacuna; matrix; space
cartilage-hair: hypoplasia
cartilaginous: articulation; joint; neurocranium; part of auditory tube; part of external acoustic meatus; part of skeletal system; septum; tissue; viscerocranium
Carus': circle; curve
Carvallo's: sign

Casal's: necklace
cascade: stomach
case control: study
case fatality: rate; ratio
caseous: abscess; degeneration; lymphadenitis; necrosis; osteitis; pneumonia; tubercle
Caslick's: operation
Casoni intradermal: test
Casoni skin: test
Casselberry: position
Casser's: fontanel
Casser's perforated: muscle
cassette: mutagenesis
cassia: cinnamon
Castellani-Low: sign
Castellani's: bronchitis; paint
Castile: soap
casting: flask; ring; wax
Castleman's: disease
Castle's intrinsic: factor
castration: anxiety; cells; complex
cat: unit
catabolite: repression
catabolite gene: activator
catabolite (gene) activator: protein
catacrotic: pulse
catadicrotic: pulse
catalatic: reaction
catalytic: antibody; center
cataract: lens; needle; spoon
cataract-oligophrenia: syndrome
catarrhal: asthma; fever; gastritis; inflammation; jaundice; ophthalmia
catastrophe: theory
catastrophic: reaction
catatonic: dementia; excitement; pupil; rigidity; schizophrenia; stupor
catatropic: image
cat-bite: disease; fever
catchment: area
cat distemper: virus
catechol: estrogen
categorical: trait
caterpillar: cell; dermatitis; flap; rash
caterpillar-hair: ophthalmia
catgut: suture
catheter: embolus; fever; gauge; guide
cathodal closure: contraction; tetanus
cathodal duration: tetanus
cathodal opening: clonus; contraction; tetanus
cathode: rays
cathode ray: oscilloscope; tube
cation-anion: difference
cation-exchange: resin

WordFinder

cationic: detergents
cat-scratch: disease; fever
cat's cry: syndrome
cat's-eye: pupil; syndrome
Cattell Infant Intelligence: Scale
cattle: plague; warts
cattle plague: virus
Catu: virus
cauda: epididymis
cauda equina: syndrome
caudal: anesthesia; canal; flexure; ligament; neuropore; retinaculum; sheath; vertebrae
caudal neurosecretory: system
caudal pancreatic: artery
caudal pharyngeal: complex
caudal transtentorial: herniation
caudal transverse: fissure
caudate: branches; lobe; nucleus; process
cauliflower: ear
causal: additivity; independence; treatment
caustic: alkali; potash; soda
cautery: conization; knife
caval: fold; valve
cavalry: bone
cave: sickness
cavernous: angioma; arteries; body of clitoris; body of penis; branch of internal carotid artery; groove; hemangioma; lymphangiectasis; nerves of clitoris; nerves of penis; part of internal carotid artery; plexus of clitoris; plexus of conchae; plexus of penis; rale; resonance; respiration; rhonchus; sinus; tissue; transfer of portal vein; veins of penis; voice
cavernous sinus: branch of internal carotid artery; syndrome
cavernous voice: sound
caviar: lesion
cavity: liner; margin; preparation; wall
cavity line: angle
cavity preparation: base; form
cavopulmonary: anastomosis; shunt
cavosurface: angle; bevel
Cazenave's: vitiligo
CB: lead
C-banding: stain
C carbohydrate: antigen
CDE: antigens
cDNA: clone; library
ceasmic: teratosis

cecal: arteries; folds; foramen of frontal bone; foramen of the tongue; hernia; recess; volvulus
cecil: urethroplasty
cecocentral: scotoma
Ceelen-Gellerstedt: syndrome
Celestin: tube
celiac: artery; axis; branches of vagus nerve; disease; ganglia; glands; lymph nodes; plexus; rickets; sprue; syndrome; trunk
celiac (lymphatic): plexus
celiac (nervous): plexus
celiac plexus: reflex
celiotomy: incision
cell: body; bridges; center; culture; cycle; determination; fusion; hybridization; inclusions; line; marker; matrix; membrane; nests; organelle; plate; sap; strain; transformation; wall
cell adhesion: molecule
cell-bound: antibody
cell-mediated: immunity; reaction
cell surface: marker
cellular: biology; biophysics; cartilage; embolism; immunodeficiency with abnormal immunoglobulin synthesis; infiltration; mosaicism; pathology; polyp; spill; tenacity; tumor
cellular blue: nevus
cellular immune: theory
cellular immunity deficiency: syndrome
cellulitic: phlegmasia
cellulocutaneous: flap
celluloid: strip
cellulose tape: technique
CELO: virus
celomic: bay; pouches
celomic metaplasia: theory of endometriosis
Celsius: scale
Celsus: kerion
Celsus': alopecia; area; papules; vitiligo
cement: base; corpuscle; line
cemental: caries
cementodentinal: junction
cementoenamel: junction
cementum: hyperplasia
centigrade: scale
centimeter-gram-second: system; unit
central: amputation; apnea; apparatus; artery; artery of retina; bearing; body; bone; bone of ankle; bradycardia; callus; canal; canals of

cochlea; canal of spinal cord; canal of the vitreous; cataract; chromatolysis; complex; deafness; dogma; ganglioneuroma; gyri; illumination; implantation; incisor; inhibition; lacteal; lobule; lobule of cerebellum; necrosis; neuritis; osteitis; paralysis; pit; placenta previa; pneumonia; scotoma; spindle; sulcus; tendon of diaphragm; tendon of perineum; vein of retina; veins of liver; vein of suprarenal gland; vision
central angiospastic: retinitis; retinopathy
central areolar choroidal: atrophy; sclerosis
central-bearing: device; point
central-bearing tracing: device
central cementifying: fibroma
central cord: syndrome
central core: disease
Central European tick-borne: fever
Central European tick-borne encephalitis: virus
central excitatory: state
central fibrous: body
central gray: substance
central group of axillary: lymph nodes
central lateral: nucleus of thalamus
central and lateral intermediate: substance
central limit: theorem
central mesenteric: lymph nodes
central nervous: system
central ossifying: fibroma
central palmar: space
central pontine: myelinolysis
central retinal: fovea
central serous: choroidopathy; retinopathy
central sulcal: artery
central tegmental: fasciculus; tract
central terminal: electrode
central thalamic: radiations
central transactional: core
central type: neurofibromatosis
central venous: catheter; pressure
centrencephalic: epilepsy
centri-acinar: emphysema
centric: contact; fusion; occlusion; position
centric jaw: relation

centrifugal: casting; current; nerve
centrifugal fast: analyzer
centrilobular: emphysema
centripetal: current; nerve
centroacinar: cell
centrofacial: lentiginosis
centrolecithal: egg; ovum
centromedian: nucleus
centromere banding: stain
centromeric: index
centronuclear: myopathy
cephalic: angle; flexure; index; pole; presentation; reflexes; tetanus; triangle; vein; version
cephalic arterial: rami
cephalocaudal: axis
cephalomedullary: angle
cephalometric: analysis; radiograph; tracing
cephalo-oculocutaneous: telangiectasia
cephalo-orbital: index
cephalopalpebral: reflex
cephalorrhachidian: index
cephalotrigeminal: angiomatosis
ceramide lactoside: lipidosis
ceramo-metal: casting
ceratocricoid: ligament; muscle
ceratopharyngeal: part of middle pharyngeal constrictor
cerebellar: arteries; astrocytoma; ataxia; atrophy; cortex; cyst; fissures; folia; fossa; frenulum; gait; hemisphere; nuclei; pyramid; rigidity; speech; sulci; syndrome; tonsil; veins
cerebellohypothalamic: fibers
cerebellomedullary: cistern
cerebellomedullary malformation: syndrome
cerebellopontile: angle
cerebellopontine: angle; cisternography; recess
cerebellopontine angle: syndrome; tumor
cerebellorubral: tract
cerebellospinal: fibers
cerebellothalamic: tract
cerebral: agraphia; angiography; anthrax; aqueduct; arteries; arteriography; calculus; cladosporiosis; compression; cortex; death; decompression; decortication; diataxia; dominance; dysplasia; edema; fissures; flexure; gigantism; hemisphere; hemorrhage; hernia; index;

lacuna; layer of retina; lipidosis; localization; malaria; palsy; part of arachnoid; part of dura mater; part of internal carotid artery; peduncle; porosis; rheumatism; sinuses; sphingolipidosis; sulci; surface; tetanus; thrombosis; trigone; tuberculosis; veins; ventricles; vesicle; vomiting

cerebral amyloid: angiopathy
cerebral arterial: circle
cerebrocortical: necrosis
cerebrohepatorenal: syndrome
cerebroretinal: angiomatosis
cerebroside: lipidosis; lipoidosis
cerebrospinal: axis; fever; fluid; index; meningitis; nematodiasis; pressure; system
cerebrospinal fluid: otorrhea; rhinorrhea
cerebrotendinous: cholesterinosis; xanthomatosis
cerebrovascular: accident; disease
Cerenkov: radiation
ceroid: lipofuscinosis
certified: milk
certified pasteurized: milk
certified registered: nurse anesthetist
cerulean: cataract
ceruleus: nucleus
ceruminous: glands
cervical: amputation; anchorage; anesthesia; auricle; branch of facial nerve; canal; cap; cyst; diverticulum; duct; dysplasia; enlargement; enlargement of spinal cord; fibrositis; flexure; glands; glands of uterus; hydrocele; hygroma; hyperesthesia; ligament of uterus; line; loop; margin; margin of tooth; myelogram; myositis; myospasm; nerves; nystagmus; part of esophagus; part of internal carotid artery; part of spinal cord; part of thoracic duct; patagium; pleura; plexus; pregnancy; rib; segments of spinal cord; sinus; smear; spondylosis; triangle; vein; vertebrae; vesicle; zone; zone of tooth
cervical aortic: knuckle

cervical axillary: canal
cervical compression: syndrome
cervical disc: syndrome
cervical fusion: syndrome
cervical iliocostal: muscle
cervical interspinal: muscle
cervical interspinales: muscles
cervical intraepithelial: neoplasia
cervical longissimus: muscle
cervical rib: syndrome
cervical rib and band: syndrome
cervical rotator: muscles
cervical splanchnic: nerves
cervical tension: syndrome
cervicoaxillary: canal
cervicolumbar: phenomenon
cervico-oculo-acoustic: syndrome
cervicothoracic: ganglion; transition
cervicovaginal: artery
cesarean: hysterectomy; operation; section
Cestan-Chenais: syndrome
C1 esterase: inhibitor
Ceylon: cinnamon; moss
CF: antibody; lead; test
C group: viruses
Chaddock: reflex; sign
Chadwick's: sign
Chagas': disease
Chagas-Cruz: disease
chagasic: myocardiopathy
Chagres: virus
chain: reaction; reflex
α chain: disease
chain-compensated: spirometer
chair: form
chalice: cell
challenge: diet
chalybeate: water
Chamberlain: procedure
Chamberlain's: line
Chamberlen: forceps
Champy's: fixative
Chance: fracture
chancriform: pyoderma; syndrome
chancroidal: bubo
chandelier: sign
Chandler: syndrome
Chantemesse: reaction
chaos: theory
chaotic: heart
character: analysis; disorder; neurosis
characteristic: curve; emission; radiation
characterizing: group
Charcot-Böttcher: crystalloids
Charcot-Bouchard: aneurysm

Charcot-Leyden: crystals
Charcot-Marie-Tooth: disease
Charcot-Neumann: crystals
Charcot-Robin: crystals
Charcot's: arteries; disease; gait; joint; syndrome; triad; vertigo
Charcot's intermittent: fever
Charcot-Weiss-Baker: syndrome
Chargaff's: rule
charge: nurse
charge transfer: complex; system
Charles: law
Charlouis': disease
Charnley hip: arthroplasty
Charrière: scale
Charters': method
Chassaignac's: space; tubercle
Chastek: paralysis
Chauffard's: syndrome
Chaussier's: areola; line; sign
Chauveau's: bacterium
Chayes: method
Cheadle's: disease
Cheatle: slit
check: ligaments of eyeball, medial and lateral; ligaments of odontoid
Chédiak-Higashi: disease
Chédiak-Steinbrinck-Higashi: anomaly; syndrome
cheek: bone; muscle; tooth
cheese: maggot
cheese worker's: lung
cheesy: abscess; pus
chemical: antidote; attraction; burn; cautery; ceptor; complexity; conjunctivitis; depilatory; dermatitis; diabetes; energy; equation; evolution; formula; kinetics; knife; modification; peeling; peritonitis; pneumonia; potential; prophylaxis; ray; repair; sampling; shift; solution; sympathectomy; taxonomy
"chemical": thyroidectomy
chemically cured: resin
chemical shift: artifact
chemiosmotic: theory
chemoreceptor: tumor
chemotherapeutic: index
Cheney: syndrome
cherry: angioma
cherry-red: spot
cherry-red spot myoclonus: syndrome
cherubic: facies

chessboard: grafts
chest: index; leads; radiology; wall
Chevalier-Jackson: dilator
chevron: incision
chewing: cycle; force
Cheyne-Stokes: psychosis; respiration
chi: sequence; structure
chi-: sequences
Chian: turpentine
Chiari-Budd: syndrome
Chiari-Frommel: syndrome
Chiari II: syndrome
Chiari's: disease; net; syndrome
chiasma: syndrome
chiasmatic: cistern; groove; sulcus
Chicago: disease
chicken: breast
chicken embryo lethal orphan: virus
chicken fat: clot
chickenpox: immunoglobulin; virus
chickenpox immune: globulin (human)
Chick-Martin: test
chick nutritional: dermatosis
chiclero: ulcer
chief: agglutinin; artery of thumb; cell; cell of corpus pineale; cell of parathyroid gland; cell of stomach; complaint
Chievitz': layer; organ
chikungunya: virus
Chilaiditi's: syndrome
chilblain: lupus; lupus erythematosus
CHILD: syndrome
child: abuse; psychology
childbearing: age
childbed: fever
childhood: epilepsy with occipital paroxysms; hypophosphatasia; schizophrenia; tuberculosis
childhood absence: epilepsy
childhood muscular: dystrophy
childhood type: tuberculosis
Chilean: saltpeter
chimeric: antibodies; molecule
chimney sweep's: cancer
chimpanzee coryza: agent
chin: cap; jerk; muscle; reflex
chinchilla: giardiasis
Chinese: cinnamon; ginger; wax
Chinese restaurant: syndrome
chip: graft; syringe
chiral: crystal
chi-square: distribution; test

chlamydial: arthritis
chloride: depletion; shift
chlorinated: lime; paraffin
chlorine: acne; water
chlorohemin: crystals
chloropercha: method
chlorophyll: unit
chloroprocaine: penicillin O
chlorotic: anemia
chlorotriazine: dyes
choanal: atresia; polyp
chocolate: agar; cyst; poisoning
Chodzko's: reflex
choked: disk
cholangiolitic: cirrhosis; hepatitis
cholangitic: abscess
cholecystoduodenal: fistula
choledoch: duct
choledochal: cyst; sphincter
choledochoduodenal: junction
cholemic: nephrosis
cholera: agar; bacillus; toxin; vaccine
choleraic: diarrhea
cholera-red: reaction
choleric: jaundice
cholestatic: hepatitis; jaundice
cholesterinized: antigen
cholesterol: cleft; embolism
cholesterol ester storage: disease
cholesterol ester transport: proteins
cholestyramine: resin
cholinergic: agent; blockade; fibers; neurotransmitter; receptors; urticaria
cholinesterase: inhibitor
chondrification: center
chondrin: ball
chondrodystrophic: dwarfism
chondroectodermal: dysplasia
chondroglossus: muscle
chondroid: syringoma; tissue
chondromyxoid: fibroma
chondropharyngeal: part of middle pharyngeal constrictor
chondroxiphoid: ligament
Chopart's: amputation; joint
chorda: saliva
choreic: abasia; movement
chorioallantoic: graft; membrane; placenta
chorioamnionic: placenta
choriocapillary: layer
chorionic: ectoderm; epithelioma; gonadotropin; plate; sac; villi
chorionic gonadotropic: hormone

chorionic gonadotropin: unit
chorionic "growth: hormone-prolactin"
chorionic villus: biopsy
chorioptic: mange
choriovitelline: placenta
choroid: branches; fissure; glomus; plexus; plexus of fourth ventricle; plexus of lateral ventricle; plexus of third ventricle; skein; tela of fourth ventricle; tela of third ventricle; vein; veins of eye
choroidal: fissure; ring
choroidal vascular: atrophy
Chotzen's: syndrome
Chr^a: antigens
Christchurch: chromosome
Christensen-Krabbe: disease
Christian's: disease; syndrome
Christison's: formula
Christmas: disease; factor
Christ-Siemens-Touraine: syndrome
chromaffin: body; cell; reaction; system; tissue; tumor
chromate: stain for lead
chromatic: aberration; apparatus; audition; fiber; granule; spectrum; vision
chromatin: body; network; nucleolus; particles
chromatography: paper
chromatophorotropic: hormone
chrome: alum; ulcer
chrome alum hematoxylin-phloxine: stain
chrome-cobalt: alloys
chromic: catgut
chromic phosphate P 32 colloidal: suspension
chromidial: apparatus; net; substance
chromophil: adenoma; granule; substance
chromophobe: adenoma; cells of anterior lobe of hypophysis; granules
chromosomal: deletion; gap; region; RNA; syndrome; trait
chromosomal instability: syndromes
chromosome: aberration; band; mosaicism; pair; satellite; walking
chronic: abscess; alcoholism; anaphylaxis; appendicitis; ataxia; bronchitis; cholecystitis; conjunctivitis; dysentery of cattle; eczema; glaucoma;

glomerulonephritis; hepatitis; inflammation; malaria; nephritis; pancreatitis; pleurisy; pneumonia; pyelonephritis; rejection; rheumatism; rhinitis; shock; soroche; tamponade; trypanosomiasis; ulcer; urticaria; vertigo
chronic absorptive: arthritis
chronic acholuric: jaundice
chronic active: inflammation
chronic active liver: disease
chronic adrenocortical: insufficiency
chronic African sleeping: sickness
chronic allograft: rejection
chronic anterior: poliomyelitis
chronic atrophic: polychondritis; thyroiditis; vulvitis
chronic bacillary: diarrhea
chronic bullous: dermatosis of childhood
chronic cicatrizing: enteritis
chronic constrictive: pericarditis
chronic cutaneous: leishmaniasis
chronic cystic: mastitis
chronic desquamative: gingivitis
chronic diffuse sclerosing: osteomyelitis
chronic discoid: lupus erythematosus
chronic endemic: fluorosis
chronic eosinophilic: pneumonia
chronic familial: icterus; jaundice; polyneuritis
chronic fibrosing: alveolitis; pancreatitis
chronic fibrous: thyroiditis
chronic focal sclerosing: osteomyelitis
chronic follicular: conjunctivitis
chronic granulomatous: disease
chronic hemorrhagic villous: synovitis
chronic hypertensive: disease
chronic hypertrophic: vulvitis
chronic hyperventilation: syndrome
chronic idiopathic: jaundice; xanthomatosis
chronic inflammatory demyelinating: polyneuropathy
chronic interstitial: hepatitis; salpingitis

chronic interstitial hypertrophic: neuropathy
chronic lymphadenoid: thyroiditis
chronic lymphocytic: thyroiditis
chronic mountain: sickness
chronic nonleukemic: myelosis
chronic obstructive pulmonary: disease
chronic persistent: hepatitis
chronic persisting: hepatitis
chronic progressive: chorea
chronic progressive external: ophthalmoplegia
chronic progressive syphilitic: meningoencephalitis
chronic relapsing: pancreatitis
chronic respiratory: disease
chronic subglottic: laryngitis
chronic ulcerative: proctitis
chronologic: age
Churg-Strauss: syndrome
Chvostek's: sign
chyle: cistern; corpuscle; cyst; peritonitis; vessel
chyliform: ascites
chylomicron retention: disease
chylous: arthritis; ascites; hydrothorax; urine
chymotropic: pigment
α-chymotrypsin-induced: glaucoma
Ciaccio's: glands; stain
cicatricial: alopecia; conjunctivitis; ectropion; entropion; horn; pemphigoid
cicatrization: atelectasis
cigarette: drain
cigarette-paper: scars
ciliary: blepharitis; body; border of iris; canals; cartilage; crown; disk; folds; ganglion; glands; ligament; margin of iris; movement; muscle; part of retina; poliosis; process; ring; staphyloma; veins; wreath; zone; zonule
ciliary ganglionic: plexus
ciliated: epithelium
ciliospinal: center; reflex
cinchona: bark
cincture: sensation
cinematic: amputation
cineplastic: amputation
cingulate: convolution; gyrus; herniation; sulcus
cingulum: rest
circadian: rhythm
Circe: effect
circinate: retinitis; retinopathy

circle absorption: anesthesia
circling: disease
circular: amputation; anastomosis; bandage; dichroism; fibers; folds; layer of muscular coat; layers of muscular tunics; layer of tympanic membrane; reaction; sinus; sulcus of insula; sulcus of Reil
circulation: time
circulatory: arrest; collapse; system
circumalveolar: fixation
circumanal: glands
circumduction: gait
circumferential: cartilage; clasp; fibrocartilage; implantation; lamella; wiring
circumferential clasp: arm
circumflex: branch of left coronary artery; nerve; veins
circumflex femoral: arteries
circumflex fibular: artery
circumflex humeral: arteries
circumflex iliac: arteries
circumflex scapular: artery
circummandibular: fixation
circumscribed: craniomalacia; myxedema; peritonitis; pyocephalus
circumvallate: papilla
circumventricular: organs
circumzygomatic: fixation
circus: movement; rhythm
cirsoid: aneurysm; varix
cis: configuration
cis: phase
13-*cis*-: retinoic acid
***cis*-acting:** locus
***cis*-acting:** protein
cisternal: puncture
***cis/trans*:** test
citrate: intoxication
citrate cleavage: enzyme
citrated: calcium carbimide
citric acid: cycle
citrovorum: factor
Civatte: bodies
Civatte's: disease
Civinini's: canal; ligament; process
CL: lead
Clado's: anastomosis; band; ligament; point
Clagett: procedure for empyema
Claisen: condensation
clamp: forceps
clang: association
Clapton's: line
Clara: cell
Clark: electrode
Clarke: cells
Clarke-Hadfield: syndrome

Clarke's: column; nucleus
Clark's: level
Clark's weight: rule
clasp: arm; bar; guideline
clasping: reflex
clasp-knife: effect; rigidity; spasticity
class: switching
class I: antigens
classic: migraine
classical: conditioning; genetics; hemophilia
classical cesarean: section
classic cervical rib: syndrome
classifiable: character
class II: antigens
class III: antigens
clastic: anatomy
clathrate: crystal
Clauberg: test; unit
Claude's: syndrome
Claudius': cells; fossa
claustral: layer
clavate: papillae
clavicular: branch of thoracoacromial artery; facet; head of pectoralis major muscle; notch of sternum; part of pectoralis major muscle; percussion
clavipectoral: fascia
claw: foot; hand
Claybrook's: sign
clay pigeon: poisoning
clay shoveler's: fracture
cleansing: cream
clear: cell; layer of epidermis
clear cell: acanthoma; adenocarcinoma; carcinoma of kidney; hidradenoma
clearing: factors; medium
clear liquid: diet
cleavage: cavity; cell; division; lines; product; site; spindle
cleaved: cell
Cleemann's: sign
cleft: hand; lip; nose; palate; spine; tongue
cleidocranial: dysostosis; dysplasia
Cleland: nomenclature
Cleland's: reagent
clenched fist: sign
clerical: spectacles
Clevenger's: fissure
click: syndrome
clicking: rale; tinnitus
client-centered: therapy
climacteric: psychosis; syndrome
climatic: bubo; keratopathy
climbing: fibers
clinical: anatomy; burden; chemistry; crown; diagnosis; epidemiology;

eruption; fitness; genetics; lethal; medicine; nurse specialist; nurse specialist; pathology; pharmacologist; pharmacology; pharmacy; psychology; recording; root; sensitivity; spectrometry; spectroscopy; thermometer; trial
clinoid: process
clip: forceps
clipped: speech
clitoral: recession
cloacal: exstrophy; membrane; plate; theory
clomiphene: test
clonal: aging; expansion
clonal deletion: theory
clonal selection: theory
clonic: convulsion; seizure; spasm
cloning: vector
clonogenic: assay; cell
Cloquet's: canal; hernia; septum; space
close: bite
closed: anesthesia; bite; circle; comedo; dislocation; drainage; fracture; hospital; laparoscopy; reading frame; reduction of fractures; surgery; system
closed-angle: glaucoma
closed chain: compound
closed chest: massage
closed circuit: method
closed head: injury
closed-loop: obstruction
closed skull: fracture
closing: contraction; membranes; snap; volume
clostridial: myonecrosis
closure: principle
clot retraction: time
clotting: factor; time
clouding of: consciousness
Cloudman: melanoma
cloudy: swelling; urine
clover: disease
cloverleaf: model; skull
cloverleaf skull: syndrome
club: foot; hair; hand; moss
clubbed: digits; fingers; penis
cluster: analysis; headache; sample
Clutton's: joints
CO₂: narcosis
coagulation: factor; necrosis; time; vitamin
coal tar: naphtha
coaptation: splint; suture
coarctate: retina
coarse: dispersion; tremor
coated: pit; tongue; vesicle
Coats': disease
Cobb: syndrome

cobbler's: suture
cobra: hemotoxin; toxin
cobra venom: cofactor; factor
cocarde: reaction
coccidioidal: granuloma
coccidioidin: test
coccygeal: body; bone; cornua; dimple; fistula; foveola; ganglion; gland; horn; joint; muscle; nerve; part of spinal cord; plexus; segments of spinal cord; sinus; vertebrae; whorl
coccygeus: muscle
Cochin China: diarrhea
cochlear: aqueduct; area; branch of labyrinthine artery; canal; canaliculus; duct; ganglion; implant; joint; labyrinth; nerve; nuclei; part of vestibulocochlear nerve; prosthesis; recess; root of vestibulocochlear nerve; root of VIII nerve; window
cochlear hair: cells
cochleariform: process
cochleo-orbicular: reflex
cochleopalpebral: reflex
cochleopupillary: reflex
cochleostapedial: reflex
Cockayne's: disease; syndrome
Cockett communicating perforating: veins
cockscomb: ulcer
cock's comb: test
coconut: sound
codeine: phosphate; sulfate
codfish: vertebrae
coding: sequence; strand
Codman's: sign; triangle; tumor
codominant: allele; gene; inheritance; trait
Coe: virus
coelomic: metaplasia
coenzyme: factor
coffee-ground: vomit
Coffey: suspension
coffin: joint
Coffin-Lowry: syndrome
Coffin-Siris: syndrome
Cogan-Reese: syndrome
Cogan's: syndrome
cognitive: development; dissonance; psychology; therapy
cognitive dissonance: theory
cognitive laterality: quotient
cogwheel: phenomenon; respiration; rigidity
cogwheel ocular: movements
cohesive: gold
Cohnheim's: area; field; theory
cohort: study

coil: gland
coiled: artery of the uterus
coin: lesion of lungs; test
coincidental: evolution
cointegrate: structure
Coiter's: muscle
cold: abscess; agglutination;
  agglutinin; allergy;
  antibody; autoagglutinin;
  autoantibody; cautery;
  chain; conization; cream;
  erythema; gangrene;
  hemolysin; light; nodule;
  pack; snare; sore; stage;
  ulcer; urticaria; virus
cold bend: test
cold-blooded: animal
cold cure: resin
cold hemagglutinin: disease
cold pressor: test
cold-reactive: antibody
cold-rigor: point
cold sensitive: enzyme
cold-sensitive: mutant
Cole-Cecil: murmur
coli: granuloma
colic: arteries; impression;
  intussusception; lymph
  nodes; sphincter; surface of
  spleen; teniae; veins
coliform: bacilli
collagen: diseases; fiber;
  fibrils; helix; injection
collagenous: colitis;
  pneumoconiosis
collapse: delirium; therapy
collapsing: pulse
collar: bone; incision
collar-button: abscess
collared: flagellate
collar-stud: chalazion
collateral: artery; branches
  of posterior intercostal
  arteries 3–11; circulation;
  eminence; fissure;
  hyperemia; inheritance;
  ligament; sulcus; trigone;
  vessel
collateral digital: artery
collecting: tubule
collective: unconscious
Colles': fascia; fracture;
  ligament; space
Collet-Sicard: syndrome
Collier's: sign; tract
collier's: lung
Collier's tucked lid: sign
colliquative: albuminuria;
  degeneration; diarrhea;
  necrosis; sweat
Collis: gastroplasty
Collis-Belsey: procedure
collision: tumor
collodion: baby
colloid: acne; adenoma; bath;
  bodies; cancer; carcinoma;
  corpuscle; cyst;

degeneration; goiter;
  system; theory of narcosis
colloidal: dispersion; gel;
  metal; silicon dioxide;
  silver iodide; solution
colloidal gold: reaction; test
colloidal radioactive: gold
colocutaneous: fistula
coloileal: fistula
colon: bacillus
colon cutoff: sign
colonic: diverticula; fistula;
  smear
colony-stimulating: factors
color: aberration; agnosia;
  blindness; constancy;
  hearing; radical; scotoma;
  sense; spectrum; taste
Colorado tick: fever
Colorado tick fever: virus
color-contrast: microscope
colored: vision
colorimetric: titration
colorimetric caries
  susceptibility: test
colostomy: bag
colostrum: corpuscle
colovaginal: fistula
colovesical: fistula
Columbia Mental Maturity:
  Scale
Columbia S. K.: virus
column: cells;
  chromatography
columnar: epithelium; layer
coma: aberration; cast; scale;
  vigil
combat: exhaustion; neurosis
comb-growth: test
combination: beat;
  restoration
combination oral:
  contraceptive
combined: glaucoma;
  immunodeficiency;
  pregnancy; sclerosis;
  version
combined fat- and
  carbohydrate-induced:
  hyperlipemia
combined
  immunodeficiency:
  syndrome
combined system: disease
combining: site; weight
comblike: septum
combustion: equivalent
Comby's: sign
comet: sign
comet tail: sign
comfort: zone
comitant: strabismus
comma: bacillus; bundle of
  Schultze; tract of Schultze
commando: operation;
  procedure
commemorative: sign
commensal: parasite

comminuted: fracture
comminuted skull: fracture
commissural: cell; cheilitis;
  fibers; myelotomy
commisural: pits
common: antigen; baldness;
  crus of semicircular ducts;
  limb of membranous
  semicircular ducts;
  migraine; opsonin; salt;
  wart
common basal: vein
common bile: duct
common cardinal: veins
common carotid: artery;
  plexus
common cold: virus
common facial: vein
common fibular: nerve
common flexor: sheath
common hepatic: artery;
  duct
common iliac: artery; lymph
  nodes; vein
common interosseous: artery
common palmar digital:
  artery; nerves
common peroneal: nerve
common peroneal tendon:
  sheath
common plantar digital:
  artery; nerves
common tendinous: ring
common variable:
  immunodeficiency
communicable: disease
communicating: artery;
  branch; branch of chorda
  tympani to lingual nerve;
  branches of
  auriculotemporal nerve to
  facial nerve; branches of
  lingual nerve to
  hypoglossal nerve;
  branches of spinal nerves;
  branches of sympathetic
  trunk; branch of facial
  nerve with
  glossopharyngeal nerve;
  branch of facial nerve with
  tympanic plexus; branch of
  glossopharyngeal nerve
  with auricular branch of
  vagus nerve; branch of
  lacrimal nerve with
  zygomatic nerve; branch of
  median nerve with ulnar
  nerve; branch of otic
  ganglion to
  auriculotemporal nerve;
  branch of otic ganglion to
  chorda tympani; branch of
  otic ganglion with medial
  pterygoid nerve; branch of
  otic ganglion with
  meningeal branch of
  mandibular nerve; branch
  of peroneal artery; branch

of superior laryngeal nerve
  with recurrent laryngeal
  nerve; hematoma;
  hydrocele; hydrocephalus;
  rami of spinal nerves; rami
  of sympathetic trunk
community: dentistry;
  medicine; nurse;
  psychiatry; psychology
community health: nurse
Comolli's: sign
compact: bone; substance
companion: artery to sciatic
  nerve; lymph nodes of
  accessory nerve; vein;
  veins
comparative: anatomy;
  medicine; pathology;
  physiology; psychology
comparator: microscope
compartmental: syndrome
compensated: acidosis;
  alkalosis; glaucoma
compensated metabolic:
  alkalosis
compensated respiratory:
  acidosis; alkalosis
compensating: curve;
  emphysema; ocular
compensation: neurosis
compensatory: atrophy;
  circulation; hypertrophy;
  hypertrophy of the heart;
  pause; polycythemia
competing: risk
competitive: antagonist;
  inhibition
competitive binding: assay
competitor: DNA
complement: factor I;
  fixation; system; unit
complemental: air
complementarity
  determining: regions
complementary: air; colors;
  DNA; hypertrophy; role;
  strand; structures
complement binding: assay
complement chemotactic:
  factor
complement-fixation:
  reaction; test
complement-fixing: antibody
complete: abortion;
  achromatopsia; antibody;
  antigen; ascertainment;
  blood count; carcinogen;
  cataract; cleavage; denture;
  disinfectant; fistula;
  hemianopia; hernia;
  iridoplegia; medium;
  metamorphosis; tetanus;
  transduction
complete atrioventricular:
  dissociation
complete A-V: block
complete denture:
  impression

complex: locus; odontoma
complex febrile: convulsion
complex learning: processes
complex partial: seizure
complex precipitated: epilepsy
complicated: cataract; fracture; migraine
composite: flap; graft; joint; resin
composite dental: cement
compound: aneurysm; articulation; caries; character; cyst; dislocation; eye; fracture; gland; heterozygote; joint; lens; lipids; microscope; nevus; odontoma; pregnancy; protein; restoration
compound granule: cell
compound hyperopic: astigmatism
compound myopic: astigmatism
compound skull: fracture
comprehensive medical: care
compressed: sponge; tablet; yeast
compressible cavernous: bodies
compression: anesthesia; cyanosis; molding; neuropathy; paralysis; plating; retinopathy; syndrome; thrombosis
compressive: myelopathy; nystagmus; strength
compressor: muscle of lips
Compton: effect; scatter
compulsive: idea; neurosis; personality
computed: perimetry; radiography; tomography
computer: model; simulation
computerized axial: tomography
Concato's: disease
concave: lens; mirror
concavoconcave: lens
concavoconvex: lens
concealed: conduction; hemorrhage; hernia; penis
concentrated human red blood: corpuscle
concentration: gradient
concentric: fibroma; hypertrophy; lamella
concept: formation
concerted: evolution; model
conchal: cartilage; crest; crest of maxilla; crest of palatine bone
conchoidal: bodies
concomitant: immunity; strabismus; symptom
concordance: rate

concordant: alternans; alternation
concordant atrioventricular: connections
concrete: oils; operations; seborrhea; thinking
concurrent: disinfection; validity
concussion: cataract; myelitis
condensation: compound
condensed: milk
condensing: enzyme; osteitis
conditional: probability
conditional-lethal: mutant
conditionally lethal: mutant
conditioned: avitaminosis; hemolysis; insomnia; reflex; response; stimulus
conditioning: therapy
conduct: disorder
conducting: airway; system of heart
conduction: analgesia; anesthesia; aphasia; block
conductive: deafness; heat
condylar: articulation; axis; canal; fossa; guidance; guide; joint; process
condylar emissary: vein
condylar guidance: inclination
condylar hinge: position
condyle: cord; path
condyloid: process
cone: cell of retina; degeneration; disks; dystrophy; fiber; granule; vision
confidence: interval
confluent: articulation; smallpox
confluent and reticulate: papillomatosis
confocal: microscope
conformational: map
confrontation: method
confusion: colors
congelation: urticaria
congenic: strain
congenital: afibrinogenemia; amputation; anemia; ankyloblepharon; aplasia of thymus; baldness; bronchiectasis; cataract; choreoathetosis; conus; dysphagocytosis; elephantiasis; epulis of newborn; fibrosis of the extraocular muscles; glaucoma; hydrocele; hydrocephalus; hypophosphatasia; hypothyroidism; lymphedema; megacolon; methemoglobinemia; myxedema; nevus; nystagmus; pancytopenia;

paramyotonia; pneumonia; stridor; syphilis; torticollis; toxoplasmosis; valve
congenital adrenal: hyperplasia
congenital aplastic: anemia
congenital atonic: pseudoparalysis
congenital cerebellar: atrophy
congenital cerebral: aneurysm
congenital diaphragmatic: hernia
congenital dyserythropoietic: anemia
congenital dysplastic: angiectasia; angiomatosis
congenital ectodermal: defect; dysplasia
congenital erythropoietic: porphyria
congenital facial: diplegia
congenital generalized: fibromatosis
congenital heart: block
congenital hemolytic: anemia; icterus; jaundice
congenital hypoplastic: anemia
congenital ichthyosiform: erythroderma
congenital lobar: emphysema
congenital nonregenerative: anemia
congenital pulmonary arteriovenous: fistula
congenital pyloric: stenosis
congenital rubella: syndrome
congenital sebaceous: hyperplasia
congenital selective glucose and galactose: malabsorption
congenital spastic: paraplegia
congenital sutural: alopecia
congenital total: lipodystrophy
congenital virilizing adrenal: hyperplasia
congestive: cardiomyopathy; cirrhosis; splenomegaly
congestive heart: failure
Congolian red: fever
congophilic: angiopathy
Congo red: paper
congruent: points
congruous: hemianopia
conic: papillae
conical: catheter; cornea; papillae
conjoined: anastomosis; tendon; twins
conjoined asymmetrical: twins

conjoined equal: twins
conjoined symmetrical: twins
conjoined unequal: twins
conjoint: tendon; therapy
conjugal: cancer
conjugate: acid; axis; deviation of the eyes; diameter of pelvic inlet; diameter of pelvic outlet; division; foci; foramen; gaze; ligament; movement of eyes; nystagmus; point
conjugate acid-base: pair
conjugated: antigen; bilirubin; compound; estrogen; hapten; protein
conjugated double: bonds
conjugative: plasmid
conjunctival: arteries; cul-de-sac; fornix; glands; layer of bulb; layer of eyelids; reflex; ring; sac; varix; veins
connecting: cartilage; stalk; tubule
connective: tissue; tumor
connective-tissue: diseases
connective tissue: cell; group
connector: bar
Connell's: suture
Conn's: syndrome
conoid: ligament; process; tubercle
Conradi-Drigalski: agar
Conradi's: disease; line
consecutive: amputation; aneurysm; angiitis; esotropia
consensual: reaction; validation
consensual light: reflex
conservative: replication; treatment
consistency: principle
consolidation: chemotherapy
consonating: rale
constancy: phenomenon
constant: coupling; region
constant field: equation
constant infusion: pump
constitutional: cause; formula; hirsutism; psychology; reaction; symptom; thrombopathy; ulcer
constitutional hepatic: dysfunction
constitutive: enzyme; heterochromatin
constriction: hyperemia; ring
constrictive: bronchiolitis; endocarditis; pericarditis
construct: validity
constructional: agraphia; apraxia
consulting: staff

consumption: coagulopathy
contact: allergy; area; catalysis; ceptor; cheilitis; dermatitis; hypersensitivity; illumination; inhibition; lens; point; splint; surface of tooth
contact-type: dermatitis
contagious: agalactia; disease; ecthyma
contagious bovine: pleuropneumonia; pyelonephritis
contagious caprine: pleuropneumonia
contagious ecthyma (pustular dermatitis): virus of sheep
contagious equine: metritis
contagious pustular: dermatitis
contagious pustular stomatitis: virus
content: analysis; validity
contig: map
contingency: table
continued: fever
continuous: arrhythmia; beam; capillary; clasp; culture; eruption; murmur; phase; spectrum; suture; tremor; variable; variation
continuous ambulatory peritoneal: dialysis
continuous bar: retainer
continuous epidural: anesthesia
continuous loop: wiring
continuous passive: motion
continuous positive airway: pressure
continuous positive pressure: breathing; ventilation
continuous random: variable
continuous spinal: anesthesia
contour: lines of Owen
contraceptive: device; sponge
contracted: foot; heel; kidney; pelvis; tendon
contractile: stricture; vacuole
contraction: band
contraction band: necrosis
contraction stress: test
contractual: psychiatry; psychotherapy
contractural: diathesis
contracture: deformity
contralateral: hemiplegia; reflex; sign
contrast: agent; bath; echocardiography; enema; enhancement; material; medium; sensitivity; stain
contrasuppressor: cells

contrecoup: injury of brain
control: animal; experiment; gene; group; syringe
controlled: respiration; substance; ventilation
controlled mechanical: ventilation
control release: suture
contusion: pneumonia
convalescent: carrier; serum
convective: heat
convenience: form
conventional: animal; signs; thoracoplasty; tomography
convergence: excess; insufficiency; nucleus of Perlia
convergence-retraction: nystagmus
convergent: evolution; squint; strabismus
converging: meniscus
conversion: disorder; electron; hysteria; neurosis; reaction
conversion hysteria: neurosis
conversive: heat
convex: lens; mirror
convexoconcave: lens
convexoconvex: lens
convoluted: bone; gland; part of kidney lobule; tubule of kidney
convoluted seminiferous: tubule
convulsant: threshold
convulsive: reflex; seizure; state; therapy; tic
cooing: murmur
Cooke's: speculum
cooled-knife: method
Cooley's: anemia
Coolidge: tube
coolie: itch
Coombs: murmur
Coombs': serum; test
coonhound: paralysis
cooperative: enzyme
cooperativity: model
Coopernail's: sign
Cooper's: fascia; hernia; herniotome; ligaments
coordinate: convulsion
coordinate covalent: bond
coordinated: reflex
Cope's: clamp
copia: elements
copolymer: resin
copper: cataract; colic; nose; protein
copper phosphate: cement
copper sulfate: method
Coppet's: law
copra: itch
coptic: lung
coracoacromial: arch; ligament

coracobrachial: bursa; muscle
coracobrachialis: muscle
coracoclavicular: ligament
coracohumeral: ligament
coracoid: process; tuberosity
coral: calculus
coralliform: cataract
cord: blood; hydrocele
cordate: pelvis
cordiform: uterus
cordy: pulse
core: particle; pneumonia
Cori: cycle; ester
Cori's: disease
corn: ergot; sugar
corneal: astigmatism; corpuscles; decompensation; dystrophy; ectasia; facet; graft; layer of epidermis; lens; margin; pannus; reflex; space; spot; staphyloma; transplantation; trepanation
corneal endothelial: polymorphism
Cornelia de Lange: syndrome
corneocyte: envelope
corneoscleral: part of trabecular reticulum
Corner-Allen: test; unit
Corner's: tampon
corniculate: cartilage; tubercle
corniculopharyngeal: ligament
cornified: layer of nail
cornmeal: agar; disease
cornoid: lamella
cornual: pregnancy
coronal: epispadias; hypospadias; plane; pulp; section; suture
coronary: angiography; arteriosclerosis; arteritis; artery; atherectomy; band; bypass; cataract; endarterectomy; failure; groove; insufficiency; ligament of knee; ligament of liver; node; occlusion; plexus; sinus; steal; sulcus; tendon; thrombosis; valve; vein
coronary artery: aneurysm
coronary care: unit
coronary nodal: rhythm
coronary ostial: stenosis
coronary perfusion: pressure
coronary-prone: behavior
coronary sinus: rhythm
coronoid: fossa of humerus; process
corpora lutea: cysts
corpus: epididymis

corpuscular: lymph; radiation
corpus luteum: hematoma; hormone
corpus luteum deficiency: syndrome
corpus luteum hormone: unit
corralin: yellow
corrected: dextrocardia; transposition of the great vessels
corrective emotional: experience
correlation: coefficient
correlational: method
correlative: differentiation
Correra's: line
corridor: disease
Corrigan's: disease; pulse; sign
corrosion: preparation
corrosive: sublimate; ulcer
corrugator: muscle
corrugator cutis: muscle of anus
corrugator supercilii: muscle
cortical: apraxia; arches of kidney; arteries; audiometry; blindness; bone; cataract; convexity; deafness; dysplasia; epilepsy; hormones; implantation; lobules of kidney; osteitis; part; part of middle cerebral artery; sensibility; substance
corticobulbar: fibers; tract
corticonuclear: fibers
corticopontine: fibers; tract
corticoreticular: fibers
corticorubral: fibers
corticospinal: fibers; tract
corticosteroid-binding: globulin; protein
corticosteroid-induced: glaucoma
corticothalamic: fibers
corticotropic: hormone
corticotropin-like intermediate-lobe: peptide
corticotropin releasing: factor; hormone
Corti's: arch; canal; cells; ganglion; membrane; organ; pillars; rods; tunnel
Corti's auditory: teeth
Corvisart's: facies
corymbose: syphilid
coryneform: bacteria
cosmetic: dermatitis; surgery
cosmic: rays
costal: angle; arch; cartilage; chondritis; facets; fringe; groove; groove for subclavian artery; notch; part of diaphragm; pit of

transverse process; pleura; pleurisy; process; respiration; surface; surface of lung; surface of scapula; tuberosity

costal arch: reflex

Costen's: syndrome

costoaxillary: vein

costocervical: artery; trunk

costochondral: joint; junction; syndrome

costoclavicular: ligament; line; syndrome

costocolic: ligament

costodiaphragmatic: recess

costomediastinal: recess; sinus

costopectoral: reflex

costophrenic: angle; sulcus

costophrenic septal: lines

costotransverse: foramen; joint; ligament

costovertebral: joints

costoxiphoid: ligament

cot: death

Cotard's: syndrome

Cotte's: operation

Cotton: effect

cotton-dust: asthma

cotton-fiber: embolism

cotton-mill: fever

cotton-root: bark

cotton-wool: patches; spots

Cotunnius: disease

Cotunnius': aqueduct; canal; liquid; space

cotyledonary: placenta

cotyloid: cavity; joint; ligament; notch

couching: needle

cough: fracture; reflex

Coumel's: tachycardia

Councilman: body

Councilman's: lesion

counseling: psychology

count: density

counter: transference

counter-: shock

counter-current: mechanism

countercurrent: distribution

coup: injury of brain

coupled: beats; pulse; rhythm

coupling: defect; factors; interval; phase

Cournand's: dip

Courvoisier's: gallbladder; law; sign

Couvelaire: uterus

covalent: modification

cove: plane

cover: glass; test

covert: sensitization

cover-uncover: test

cow: face; kidney

Cowden's: disease

Cowdry's type A inclusion: bodies

Cowdry's type B inclusion: bodies

CO_2-withdrawal seizure: test

cowl: muscle

Cowling's: rule

cow milk: anemia

Cowper's: cyst; gland; ligament

cowpox: virus

coxal: bone

coxitic: scoliosis

Coxsackie: encephalitis; virus

CR: lead

crab: hand; yaws

Crabtree: effect

crack: cocaine

cracked: heel

cracked-pot: resonance; sound

crackling: jaw; rale

cradle: cap

Crafoord: clamp

craft: palsy

Cramer wire: splint

Crampton: test

Crampton's: line; muscle

Crandall's: syndrome

cranial: arteritis; base; bones; capacity; cavity; flexure; fontanels; index; nerves; neuropore; root of accessory nerve; roots; sinuses; sutures; synchondroses; vault; vertebra

cranial epidural: space

craniocardiac: reflex

craniocarpotarsal: dysplasia; dystrophy

craniodiaphysial: dysplasia

craniofacial: angle; appliance; axis; dysostosis; fixation; notch; surgery

craniofacial dysjunction: fracture

craniofacial suspension: wiring

craniometaphysial: dysplasia

craniometric: points

craniopharyngeal: canal; duct

craniosacral: system

craniospinal: ganglia

craniospinalia: ganglia

crater: arc

cravat: bandage

crazy chick: disease

C-reactive: protein

cream of: tartar

crease: wound

creatine kinase: isoenzymes

creatinine: clearance; coefficient

creative: thinking

Credé's: maneuvers; methods

creep: recovery

creeping: eruption; myiasis; palsy; thrombosis; ulcer

cremaster: muscle

cremasteric: artery; fascia; reflex

creola: bodies

crepitant: rale

crescendo: angina; murmur; sleep

crescent: cell

crescent cell: anemia

crescentic: lobules of the cerebellum

CREST: syndrome

Creutzfeldt-Jakob: disease

crevicular: epithelium; fluid

crib: death

cribriform: area of the renal papilla; fascia; hymen; plate of ethmoid bone

cribrous: lamina

Crichton-Browne's: sign

cricoarytenoid: articulation; joint

cricoarytenoid articular: capsule

cricoesophageal: tendon

cricoid: cartilage

cricopharyngeal: ligament; myotomy; part of inferior pharyngeal constrictor

cricopharyngeus: muscle

cricosantorinian: ligament

cricothyroid: artery; articulation; joint; ligament; membrane; muscle

cricothyroid articular: capsule

cricotracheal: ligament; membrane

cricovocal: membrane

cri-du-chat: syndrome

Crigler-Najjar: disease; syndrome

Crile's: clamp

Crimean: fever

Crimean-Congo hemorrhagic: fever

Crimean-Congo hemorrhagic fever: virus

criminal: abortion; anthropology; hygiene; insanity; irresponsibility; psychology

crisis: intervention

crisscross: heart

criterion-related: validity

critical: angle; illumination; organ; period; pH; point; pressure; rate; temperature

critical care: unit

critical flicker fusion: frequency

critical illness: polyneuropathy

critical micelle: concentration

crocodile: tears

crocodile tears: syndrome

Crocq's: disease

Crohn's: disease

Cronkhite-Canada: syndrome

Crookes': glass

Crooke's: granules

Crookes-Hittorf: tube

Crooke's hyaline: change; degeneration

crop: gland; milk

Crosby: capsule

cross: agglutination; birth; circulation; flap; hybridization; infection; mating; reaction; section; tolerance

crossbite: teeth

cross-cultural: psychiatry

cross-cut: bur

crossed: anesthesia; aphasia; cylinders; diplopia; embolism; eyes; fixation; hemianesthesia; hemianopia; hemiplegia; immunoelectrophoresis; jerk; laterality; paralysis; reflex; reflex of pelvis

crossed adductor: jerk; reflex

crossed extension: reflex

crossed knee: jerk; reflex

crossed phrenic: phenomenon

crossed pyramidal: tract

crossed renal: ectopia

crossed spino-adductor: reflex

crossed testicular: ectopia

cross-linked: polymer; resin

cross-over: study

cross-reacting: agglutinin; antibody; material

cross-sectional: echocardiography; method; study

cross-table lateral: projection

crotalaria: poisoning

Crotalus: antitoxin; toxin

croup-associated: virus

croupous: bronchitis; laryngitis; lymph; membrane

Crouzon's: disease; syndrome

crowing: inspiration

crown: cavity; flask; glass; tubercle

crown-heel: length

crown-rump: length

crucial: bandage; ligament

cruciate: anastomosis; eminence; ligament of the atlas; ligament of leg; ligaments of knee; muscle

cruciform: eminence; ligament of atlas; loops; part of fibrous digital sheath; part of fibrous sheath; pulley

crude: calcium sulfide; death rate; drug; urine

crural: arch; fascia; fossa; hernia; ring; septum; sheath; triangle

crural interosseous: nerve

crush: kidney; syndrome

crusted: ringworm; tetter

crutch: palsy; paralysis

Cruveilhier-Baumgarten: disease; murmur; sign; syndrome

Cruveilhier's: disease; fascia; fossa; joint; ligaments; plexus

Cruz: trypanosomiasis

cry: reflex

crypt: abscesses

cryptogenic: cirrhosis; epilepsy; infection; pyemia; septicemia

cryptophthalmus: syndrome

cryptorchid: testis

crystal: rash; structure

crystalline: capsule; cataract; digitalin; interface; lens

crystalline insulin zinc: suspension

crystallized: trypsin

crystal violet: vaccine

Csillag's: disease

"C" sliding: osteotomy

CT: number; unit

Cuban: itch

cube: pessary

cubic: centimeter; niter

cubital: bone; fossa; joint; lymph nodes; nerve

cuboid: bone

cuboidal: epithelium

cuboidal articular: surface of calcaneus

cuboideonavicular: joint; ligaments

cuboidodigital: reflex

cuirass: respirator

cul-de-sac: smear

Cullen's: sign

Culp: pyeloplasty

cultivated: yeast

cultural: anthropology; shock

culture: medium

Culver's: root

Cummer's: classification; guideline

Cumulative: Index Medicus

cumulative: action; dose; effect

cumulative trauma: disorders

cuneate: fasciculus; funiculus; nucleus

cuneiform: bone; cartilage; cataract; lobe; tubercle

cuneocerebellar: tract

cuneocuboid: joint; ligaments

cuneometatarsal: joints

cuneonavicular: articulation; joint; ligaments

cup biopsy: forceps

cupping: glass

cupular: cecum of the cochlear duct; part of epitympanic recess

cupular blind: sac

cupuliform: cataract

curative: dose

curb: tenotomy

curby: hock

curd: soap

curdy: pus

curlicue: ureter

Curling's: ulcer

currant jelly: clot

current of: injury

Curschmann's: disease; spirals

curvature: aberration; hyperopia; myopia

Cushing: effect; phenomenon; response

Cushing's: basophilism; disease; suture; syndrome; syndrome medicamentosus

Cushing's pituitary: basophilism

cusp: angle; height

cuspal: interference

cuspid: tooth

cuspless: tooth

cutaneomeningospinal: angiomatosis

cutaneomucous: muscle

cutaneomucouveal: syndrome

cutaneous: absorption; albinism; ancylostomiasis; anthrax; apoplexy; blastomycosis; branch of obturator nerve; diphtheria; emphysema; gangrene; glands; habronemiasis; hemorrhoids; horn; larva migrans; layer of tympanic membrane; leishmaniasis; lupus erythematosus; meningioma; muscle; myiasis; nerve; reaction; reflex; schistosomiasis japonica; test; tuberculosis; ureterostomy; vasculitis; vein

cutaneous cervical: nerve

cutaneous focal: mucinosis

cutaneous graft versus host: reaction

cutaneous loop: ureterostomy

cutaneous pupil: reflex

cutaneous tuberculin: test

cutireaction: test

cutis: graft; plate

cutting: edge; forceps; needle; teeth

cuttlefish: disk

cuvette: oximeter

Cuvier's: ducts; veins

cyanide: poisoning

cyanide-nitroprusside: test

cyanobacterium-like: bodies

cyanogenic: glycoside

cyanose: tardive

cyanotic: asphyxia; atrophy; atrophy of the liver; induration

cyclic: adenylic acid; albuminuria; compound; esotropia; guanosine 3′,5′-monophosphate; hematopoiesis; neutropenia; nucleotide; peptide; phosphate; phosphoric acid; strabismus; uridine 3′,5′-monophosphate

cyclopian: eye

cyclothymic: disorder; personality

cyclothymic personality: disorder

cylinder: retinoscopy

cylindrical: bronchiectasis; epithelium; lens

cylindroid: aneurysm

cylindromatous: carcinoma

cynic: spasm

Cyon's: nerve

cysteine: hydrolases

cystic: acne; artery; bronchiectasis; carcinoma; diathesis; disease of the breast; disease of renal medulla; duct; fibrosis; goiter; hygroma; hyperplasia; hyperplasia of the breast; kidney; lymphangiectasis; lymph node; mole; node; polyp; vein

cystic adenomatoid: malformation

cystic duct: cholangiography

cysticercus: disease

cystic medial: necrosis

cystic papillomatous: craniopharyngioma

cystine: bridge; calculus; disease

cystine storage: disease

cystinotic: leukocyte

cystoduodenal: ligament

cystoid: maculopathy

cystoid macular: edema

cystoscopic: urography

cythemolytic: icterus

cytochrome: system

cytocrine: secretion

cytogenetic: map

cytogenic: reproduction

cytoid: bodies

cytokeratin: filaments

cytologic: examination; screening; smear; specimen

cytologic filter: preparation

cytomegalic: cells

cytomegalic inclusion: disease

cytomegalovirus: disease

cytopathic: effect

cytopathogenic: virus

cytophagic histiocytic: panniculitis

cytophil: group

cytophilic: antibody

cytoplasmic: bridges; inheritance; matrix

cytoplasmic inclusion: bodies

cytoreductive: therapy

cytotonic: enterotoxin

cytotoxic: cell; reaction

cytotrophoblastic: cells; shell

cytotropic: antibody

cytotropic antibody: test

Czapek-Dox: medium

Czapek's solution: agar

Czerny-Lembert: suture

Czerny's: suture

D

D: antigen; cell; enzyme; loop; wave

D-: 3-hydroxybutyric acid dehydrogenase; proline reductase

Daae's: disease

DaCosta's: syndrome

Da Fano's: stain

daily: dose

Dakin-Carrel: treatment

Dakin's: fluid; solution

Dale: reaction

Dale-Feldberg: law

Dalen-Fuchs: nodules

Dalrymple's: sign

Dalton-Henry: law

Dalton's: law

Dam: unit

Damus-Kaye-Stancel: procedure

Damus-Stancel-Kaye: anastomosis

Dana's: operation

Dance's: sign

dancing: chorea; spasm

Dandy: operation

dandy: fever

Dandy-Walker: syndrome

Dane: particles
Dane's: stain
Danforth's: sign
Danielssen-Boeck: disease
Danielssen's: disease
Danubian endemic familial: nephropathy
Danysz: phenomenon
DAPI: stain
DA pregnancy: test
dapsone: neuropathy
d'Arcet's: metal
Darier's: disease; sign
dark: adaptation; cells; reaction
dark-adapted: eye
dark-field: condenser; illumination; microscope
dark-ground: illumination
Darling's: disease
d'Arsonval: current; galvanometer
dartoic: tissue
dartos: fascia; muscle
Darwinian: evolution
darwinian: ear
darwinian: reflex; theory; tubercle
date: boil; fever
datum: plane
Datura: poisoning
Daubenton's: angle; line; plane
daughter: cell; colony; cyst; isotope; star
Davidoff's: cells
Davidson: syringe
Daviel's: operation; spoon
Davies': disease
Davis: grafts
Davis-Crowe mouth: gag
Davis interlocking: sound
Dawbarn's: sign
dawn: phenomenon
Dawson's: encephalitis
day: blindness; hospital; residue; sight
Day's: test
dazzling: glare
d-dimer: test
dead: fingers; nerve; pulp; space; tooth; tracts
dead-end: host
dead fetus: syndrome
deadly: agaric; nightshade
deamidizing: enzymes
deaminating: enzymes
Dean's fluorosis: index
death: instinct; rate; trance
Deaver's: incision
DeBakey: forceps
DeBakey's: classification
de Bordeau: theory
debrancher: deficiency
debranching: enzymes; factors
debranching deficiency limit: dextrinosis

Debré: phenomenon
Debré-Sémélaigne: syndrome
debulking: operation
decapacitation: factor
decarboxylated: dopa
decay: constant; theory
decentered: lens
decerebrate: rigidity; state
decidual: cast; cell; endometritis; fissure; reaction
deciduate: placenta
deciduous: dentition; membrane; skin; tooth
decision: analysis
declamping: phenomenon; shock
de Clerambault: syndrome
decomposition of: movement
decompression: chamber; disease; operations; sickness
decorticate: rigidity; state
decoy: cells
decremental: conduction
decubital: gangrene
decubitus: film; radiograph; ulcer
de-emetinized: ipecacuanha
deep: artery of clitoris; artery of penis; artery of thigh; artery of tongue; bite; branch; branch of the lateral plantar nerve; branch of the medial femoral circumflex artery; branch of the medial plantar artery; branch of the radial nerve; branch of the transverse cervical artery; branch of the ulnar nerve; cell; cortex; fascia; fascia of arm; fascia of forearm; fascia of leg; fascia of neck; fascia of penis; fascia of thigh; head of flexor pollicis brevis; lamina; layer; layer of levator palpebrae superioris muscle; layer of temporalis fascia; muscles of back; part of external anal sphincter; part of flexor retinaculum; part of masseter muscle; part of parotid gland; percussion; reflex; scleritis; sensibility; vein of penis; veins of clitoris
deep abdominal: reflexes
deep auricular: artery
deep brachial: artery
deep cardiac: plexus
deep cerebral: veins
deep cervical: artery; fascia; vein

deep circumflex iliac: artery; vein
deep crural: arch
deep dorsal: vein of clitoris; vein of penis
deep dorsal sacrococcygeal: ligament
deep epigastric: artery; vein
deep facial: vein
deep femoral: vein
deep fibular: nerve
deep flexor: muscle of fingers
deep gray: layer of superior colliculus
deep hypothermic: arrest
deep infrapatellar: bursa
deep inguinal: lymph nodes; ring
deep lingual: artery; vein
deep lymphatic: vessel
deep middle cerebral: vein
deep palmar: branch of ulnar artery
deep palmar (arterial): arch
deep palmar venous: arch
deep parotid: lymph nodes
deep perineal: pouch; space
deep peroneal: nerve
deep petrosal: nerve
deep plantar: branch of dorsalis pedis artery
deep posterior sacrococcygeal: ligament
deep punctate: keratitis
deep temporal: artery; nerves; veins
deep transitional: gyrus
deep transverse: muscle of perineum
deep transverse metacarpal: ligament
deep transverse metatarsal: ligament
deep transverse perineal: muscle
deep white: layer of superior colliculus
deer-fly: disease; fever
Deetjen's: bodies
def caries: index
defective: bacteriophage; organism; phage; probacteriophage; prophage; virus
defective interfering: particle
defense: mechanism; reflex
defensive: circle; medicine
deferent: canal; duct
deferential: artery; plexus
deferred: shock
defervescent: stage
deficiency: anemia; disease; mutant; symptom
definitive: callus; host; lysosomes; method; prosthesis

deflective occlusal: contact
degenerative: arthritis; chorea; index; inflammation; myopia
degenerative joint: disease
degloving: injury
deglutition: apnea; pneumonia; reflex
Degos': acanthoma; disease; syndrome
degree of: kindred
Dehio's: test
dehydrated: alcohol
dehydration: fever
dehydrocholate: test
deionized: water
deiterospinal: tract
Deiters': cells; nucleus
Deiters' terminal: frames
déjà vu: phenomenon
Dejerine-Klumpke: palsy; syndrome
Dejerine-Lichtheim: phenomenon
Dejerine-Roussy: syndrome
Dejerine's: disease; reflex; sign
Dejerine's hand: phenomenon
Dejerine-Sottas: disease
Delafield's: hematoxylin
de Lange: syndrome
delayed: allergy; coma after hypoxia; conduction; dentition; eruption; flap; graft; hypersensitivity; implantation; reaction; reflex; sensation; suture
delayed reaction: experiment
Delbet's: sign
Del Castillo: syndrome
DeLee's: maneuver
deletion: mutation
Delhi: sore
delimiting: keratotomy
delirious: shock
delphian: node
delta: agent; alcoholism; antigen; bilirubin; cell of anterior lobe of hypophysis; cell of pancreas; granule; hepatitis; rhythm; virus; wave
deltoid: branch; crest; eminence; impression; ligament; muscle; region; tuberosity
deltoideopectoral: triangle; trigone
deltopectoral: flap
delusional: disorder
demand: pacemaker
demand pulse: generator
demarcation: current; line of retina; potential
Demarquay's: symptom

dematiaceous: fungi
demigauntlet: bandage
demilune: body
demodectic: acariasis;
  blepharitis; mange
Demoivre's: formula
demonstration:
  ophthalmoscope
De Morgan's: spots
de Morsier's: syndrome
de Musset's: sign
demyelinated: myelitis
demyelinating: disease;
  encephalopathy;
  polyneuropathy
denaturation: temperature of
  DNA
denatured: alcohol; protein
dendriform: keratitis
dendritic: calculus; cataract;
  cells; depolarization;
  process; spines; thorns
dendritic corneal: ulcer
dengue: fever; virus
dengue hemorrhagic: fever
dengue shock: syndrome
Denis Browne: splint
Denis Browne's: pouch
Denman's spontaneous:
  evolution
Dennie's: line
Dennie's infraorbital: fold
Denonvilliers': aponeurosis;
  ligament
dense-deposit: disease
density: gradient
density gradient:
  centrifugation
dental: abscess; anatomy;
  anesthesia; ankylosis;
  apparatus; arch;
  articulation; biomechanics;
  biophysics; branches; bulb;
  calculus; canals; caps;
  caries; cast; cement; cord;
  crest; crypt; curing; cuticle;
  drill; dysfunction;
  engineering; fistula; floss;
  follicle; forceps; formula;
  furnace; geriatrics; germ;
  granuloma; groove;
  hygienist; impaction;
  implants; index;
  jurisprudence; lamina;
  ledge; lever; lymph;
  material; neck; nerve;
  orthopedics; osteoma;
  papilla; pathology; plaque;
  polyp; process;
  prophylaxis; prosthesis;
  prosthetics; pulp; pump;
  rami; ridge; sac; sealant;
  senescence; shelf; surgeon;
  syringe; tubercle; tubules;
  ulcer; wedge
dental lamina: cyst
dentary: center

dentate: fascia; fissure;
  fracture; gyrus; ligament of
  spinal cord; line; nucleus
  of cerebellum; suture
dentatorubral: fibers
dentatorubral cerebellar:
  atrophy with
  polymyoclonus
dentatothalamic: fibers;
  tract
denticulate: hymen; ligament
dentigerous: cyst
dentin: bridge; dysplasia;
  globule
dentinal: canals; fibers;
  fluid; papilla; sheath;
  tubules
dentinocemental: junction
dentinoenamel: junction
dentoalveolar: joint
dentogingival: lamina
denture: base; border; brush;
  characterization; edge;
  esthetics; flange; flask;
  foundation; hyperplasia;
  packing; prognosis;
  retention; space; stability
denture basal: surface
denture-bearing: area
denture foundation: area;
  surface
denture impression: surface
denture occlusal: surface
denture polished: surface
denture sore: mouth
denture-supporting: area;
  structures
Denucé's: ligament
denumerable: character
Denver: classification; shunt
Denver Developmental
  Screening: Test
Denys-Leclef: phenomenon
deodorized: opium
deoxy: sugar
dependent: beat; drainage;
  edema; personality;
  variable
dependent personality:
  disorder
depersonalization: disorder;
  syndrome
de Pezzer: catheter
depletion: response
depletional: hyponatremia
depolarizing: block; relaxant
depot: injection; reaction;
  therapy
depressed: fracture
depressed skull: fracture
depressive: neurosis;
  psychosis; reaction; stupor;
  syndrome
depressor: fibers; muscle of
  epiglottis; muscle of
  eyebrow; muscle of lower
  lip; muscle of septum;
  nerve of Ludwig; reflex

depressor anguli oris:
  muscle
depressor labii inferioris:
  muscle
depressor septi: muscle
depressor supercilii: muscle
deprivation: amblyopia
depth: compensation; dose;
  perception; psychology;
  recording
de Quervain's: disease;
  fracture; thyroiditis
derby hat: fracture
Dercum's: disease
derivative: chromosome
derived: protein
dermal: bone; graft;
  leishmanoid; papillae;
  sinus; system; tuberculosis
dermal duct: tumor
dermal-fat: graft
dermatan: sulfate
dermatitis-arthritis-
  tenosynovitis: syndrome
dermatogenic: torticollis
dermatologic: paste
dermatomal: distribution
dermatomic: area
dermatopathic:
  lymphadenitis;
  lymphadenopathy
dermoepidermal: interface
dermoid: cyst; cyst of ovary;
  tumor
dermolytic bullous:
  dermatosis
dermotuberculin: reaction
Derzsy's: disease
De Sanctis-Cacchione:
  syndrome
Desault's: bandage
Descartes': law
Descemet's: membrane
descending: aorta; artery of
  knee; branch; branch of
  hypoglossal nerve; branch
  of lateral circumflex
  femoral artery; branch of
  occipital artery; colon;
  current; degeneration;
  neuritis; nucleus of the
  trigeminus; part of aorta;
  part of duodenum; part of
  facial canal; tract of
  trigeminal nerve
descending anterior: branch
descending genicular: artery
descending palatine: artery
descending posterior:
  branch
descending scapular: artery
Deschamps: needle
descriptive: anatomy;
  myology; psychiatry;
  statistics
desensitizing: paste
desert: fever; sore
desiccated: liver; pituitary

design: denture
Desmarres': dacryoliths
desmoid: tumor
desmoplastic: fibroma;
  medulloblastoma;
  trichoepithelioma
desmoplastic cerebral:
  astrocytoma
desmoplastic malignant:
  melanoma
desmoteric: medicine
despeciated: antitoxin
D'Espine's: sign
desquamative: pneumonia
desquamative
  inflammatory: vaginitis
desquamative interstitial:
  pneumonia
destructive: distillation
detachable: balloon
detached: craniotomy; retina
detached cranial: section
detector: coil
determinant: group
determinate: cleavage
De Toni-Fanconi: syndrome
detrusor: areflexia;
  compliance; hyperreflexia;
  instability; muscle of
  urinary bladder; pressure;
  stability
detrusor sphincter:
  dyssynergia
Deutschländer's: disease
developmental: age;
  anatomy; anomaly;
  disability; grooves; lines;
  psychology
Deventer's: pelvis
deviational: nystagmus
Devic's: disease
devil's: grip
Devine: exclusion
devitalized: tooth
Devonshire: colic
dew: claw; itch; point
Dewar: flask
de Wecker's: scissors
dexamethasone
  suppression: test
df caries: index
Dharmendra: antigen
d'Herelle: phenomenon
dhobie: itch; mark
dhobie mark: dermatitis
D.I.: particle
Di: antigen
diabetic: acidosis;
  amyotrophy; arthropathy;
  cataract; coma;
  dermopathy; diet;
  fetopathy; gangrene;
  gingivitis;
  glomerulosclerosis;
  lipemia; myelopathy;
  neuropathy;
  polyneuropathy;
  polyradiculopathy;

puncture; retinitis;
retinopathy
diabetic neuropathic:
cachexia
diabetic thoracic:
radiculopathy
diabetogenic: factor
diachronic: study
diagnosis related: group
diagnostic: anesthesia;
audiometry; cast;
sensitivity; specificity;
ultrasound
diagnostic diphtheria: toxin
diagonal: conjugate; section
diagonal conjugate:
diameter
diagonalis: stria
dial: manometer
dialysis: dementia; shunt
dialysis disequilibrium:
syndrome
dialysis encephalopathy:
syndrome
diamond: disk; fuchsin; skin
Diamond-Blackfan: anemia;
syndrome
diamond cutting:
instruments
diamond-shaped: murmur
diamond skin: disease
Diana: complex
diaper: dermatitis; rash
diaphragm: pessary
diaphragmatic: flutter;
hernia; ligament of the
mesonephros; nodes;
pacemaker; peritonitis;
pleura; pleurisy; surface
diaphragmatic myocardial:
infarction
diaphysial: aclasis; center;
dysplasia
diarthrodial: cartilage; joint
diastasis: cordis
diastatic skull: fracture
diastolic: afterpotential;
murmur; pressure; shock;
thrill
diastrophic: dwarfism
diathermic: therapy
diatomaceous: earth
diazo: reaction; reagent; stain
for argentaffin granules
diazonium: salts
dibasic: acid; amino acid;
ammonium phosphate;
calcium phosphate;
potassium phosphate;
sodium phosphate
dicarboxylic acid: cycle
dicentric: chromosome
dichorial: twins
dichorionic diamniotic:
placenta
Dick: method; test
Dickens: shunt
Dick test: toxin

dicrotic: notch; pulse; wave
dicumarol: resistance
didactic: analysis
dideoxy: procedure;
sequencing
Dieffenbach's: method
Diels: hydrocarbon
diencephalic: epilepsy;
syndrome of infancy
dientamoeba: diarrhea
dietary: amenorrhea; fiber
Dieterle's: stain
dietetic: albuminuria;
treatment
diethenoid: fatty acid
O-**diethylaminoethyl:**
cellulose
Dietl's: crisis
Dieuaide: diagram
Dieulafoy's: erosion; theory
Di Ferrante: syndrome
differential: diagnosis;
growth; manometer; stain;
stethoscope; thermometer;
threshold
differential blood: pressure
differential gene: expression
differential renal function:
test
differential spinal:
anesthesia
**differential ureteral
catheterization:** test
differential white: blood
count
diffuse: abscess; aneurysm;
angiokeratoma; choroiditis;
emphysema; ganglion;
glomerulonephritis; goiter;
leishmaniasis;
mastocytosis;
panbronchiolitis;
peritonitis; phlegmon
diffuse arterial: ectasia
diffuse cutaneous:
leishmaniasis; mastocytosis
diffused: reflex
diffuse deep: keratitis
diffuse esophageal: spasm
diffuse idiopathic skeletal:
hyperostosis
diffuse infantile familial:
sclerosis
diffuse mesangial:
proliferation
diffuse obstructive:
emphysema
diffuse small cleaved cell:
lymphoma
diffuse waxy: spleen
diffusible: stimulant
diffusing: capacity; factor
diffusion: anoxia;
coefficient; constant;
hypoxia; method;
respiration; shell

digastric: branch of facial
nerve; fossa; groove;
muscle; notch; triangle
DiGeorge: syndrome
digestive: apparatus;
enzymes; fever; glycosuria;
leukocytosis; system; tract;
tube; vacuole
digital: crease; dilatation;
fossa; furrow; joints;
plethysmograph; pulp;
radiography; reflex; veins;
whorl
digital collateral: artery
digital flexion: crease
digital gray: scale
digitalis: tincture; unit
digital subtraction:
angiography
digitate: dermatosis;
impressions; wart
digitonin: reaction
Di Guglielmo's: disease;
syndrome
dihydric: alcohol
dihydrogen: phosphate
2,8-dihydroxyalanine:
lithiasis
dilantin: gingivitis
dilated: cardiomyopathy;
pore
dilation: thrombosis
dilator: muscle; muscle of
ileocecal sphincter; muscle
of pylorus
dilator pupillae: muscle
dilute: alcohol; phosphoric
acid
diluted: acetic acid;
hydrochloric acid
dilution: anemia
dimensional: stability
dimidiate: hermaphroditism
Dimmer's: keratitis
dimorphic: anemia
dimorphous: leprosy
dimple: sign
dinitrophenylhydrazine: test
dinner: pad
dinoflagellate: toxin
dinucleotide: domain; fold
Diogenes: cup
dioptric: aberration
diovular: twins
DIP: joints
dip: phenomenon
diphasic: complex
diphasic milk: fever
diphenylhydantoin:
gingivitis
diphenylmethane: dyes;
laxatives
diphtheria: antitoxin; toxin
diphtheria antitoxin: unit
**diphtheria toxoid, tetanus
toxoid, and pertussis:**
vaccine

diphtheritic: conjunctivitis;
enteritis; membrane;
neuropathy; paralysis; ulcer
diphyllobothrium: anemia
diploic: canals; vein
diploid: nucleus
dipolar: buffer; ions
dipole: moment; theory
direct: calorimetry; current;
diuretic; embolism; flap;
fracture; illumination;
image; laryngoscopy; lead;
method for making inlays;
ophthalmoscope;
ophthalmoscopy; oxidase;
percussion; rays; retainer;
retention; technique;
transfusion; vision;
zoonosis
direct acrylic: restoration
direct bone: impression
direct composite resin:
restoration
direct Coombs': test
direct filling: resin
direct fluorescent antibody:
test
direct inguinal: hernia
directional: atherectomy
directive: psychotherapy
direct lytic: factor of cobra
venom
direct nuclear: division
direct pulp: capping
direct pyramidal: tract
direct reacting: bilirubin
direct resin: restoration
direct vision: spectroscope
disappearing bone: disease
disc: electrophoresis
discharging: tubule
Dische: reaction; reagent
Dische-Schwarz: reagent
disciform: degeneration;
keratitis
disciform macular:
degeneration
disclosing: solution
discoid: lupus erythematosus
discoidal: cleavage
disconjugate: movement of
eyes
disconnection: syndrome
discontinuation: test
discontinuous: culture;
phase; sterilization
discordant: alternans;
alternation
discordant atrioventricular:
connections
discrete: character; smallpox;
variable
discrete random: variable
discriminant: analysis;
function; stimulus
disease: determinants
dish: face
dishpan: fracture

disintegration: constant
disjoined: pyeloplasty
disjunctive: absorption
disk: kidney; space;
  syndrome
disk sensitivity: method
disk-shaped: cataract
dislocation of: lens
dislocation: fracture
disodium: phosphate
disorganized: schizophrenia
disparity: angle
dispensing: tablet
disperse: placenta
dispersed: phase
dispersing: electrode
dispersion: colloid; medium;
  phase
displacement: analysis; loop;
  threshold
disproportionate: dwarfism
disproportionating: enzyme
disputed neurogenic
  thoracic outlet: syndrome
dissecting: aneurysm;
  cellulitis
dissection: tubercle
disseminate:
  coccidioidomycosis
disseminated: aspergillosis;
  choroiditis;
  lipogranulomatosis; lupus
  erythematosus; sclerosis;
  tuberculosis
disseminated cutaneous:
  gangrene; leishmaniasis
disseminated gonococcal:
  infection
disseminated intravascular:
  coagulation
disseminated recurrent:
  infundibulofolliculitis
Disse's: space
dissociated: anesthesia;
  nystagmus
dissociation: constant;
  constant of an acid;
  constant of a base; constant
  of water; sensibility
dissociative: anesthesia;
  disorders; hysteria; reaction
distal: caries; centriole; end;
  ileitis; myopathy;
  occlusion; part of anterior
  lobe of hypophysis; surface
  of tooth; tingling on
  percussion
distal interphalangeal:
  joints
distal radioulnar:
  articulation; joint
distal spiral: septum
distal splenorenal: shunt
distal tibiofibular: joint
distance: ceptor
distant: flap
distemper: virus
distention: cyst; ulcer

distilled: water
distortion: aberration
distraction: conus
distributed: effort
distributing: artery
distribution: coefficient;
  curve; leukocytosis;
  volume
distributive: analysis
disulfide: bond; bridge
disuse: atrophy
Dittrich's: plugs; stenosis
diurnal: enuresis;
  periodicity; rhythm
divergence: insufficiency
divergence excess: exotropia
divergence insufficiency:
  exotropia
divergent: evolution; squint;
  strabismus
diverging: meniscus
divers': spectacles
diver's: palsy; paralysis
diverticular: disease
divided: dose; spectacles
diving: goiter; reflex
dizygotic: twins
djenkol: poisoning
dmfs caries: index
DNA: gap; helix; homology;
  hybridization;
  polymorphism; virus
DNA-RNA: hybrid
d'Ocagne: nomogram
docking: protein
Döderlein's: bacillus
Doerfler-Stewart: test
dog: disease; ear; nose; unit
dog distemper: virus
Dogiel's: cells; corpuscle
dogmatic: school
Döhle: bodies; inclusions
dolichoectatic: artery
dolichopellic: pelvis
doll's eye: sign
dolorogenic: zone
dome: cell
dominance: hierarchy
dominant: character; eye;
  frequency; gene;
  hemisphere; idea;
  inheritance; trait
dominant lethal: trait
dominantly inherited
  Lévi's: disease
Donath-Landsteiner:
  phenomenon
Donath-Landsteiner cold:
  autoantibody
Donders': glaucoma; law;
  pressure; rings
Donnan: equilibrium
Donné's: corpuscle
Donohue's: disease;
  syndrome
donor: insemination
Donovan's: bodies
Doose: syndrome

dopa: reaction
Doppler: echocardiography;
  effect; phenomenon; shift;
  ultrasonography
Doppler color: flow
Dor: procedure
Dorello's: canal
Dorendorf's: sign
Dorfman-Chanarin:
  syndrome
Dorno: rays
dorsal: artery of clitoris;
  artery of foot; artery of
  nose; artery of penis;
  branch; branch of the
  lumbar artery; branch of
  the posterior intercostal
  arteries 3–11; branch of the
  posterior intercostal veins
  4–11; branch of the
  subcostal artery; branch of
  the superior intercostal
  artery; branch of the ulnar
  nerve; column of spinal
  cord; fascia of foot; fascia
  of hand; flexure; funiculus;
  hood; mesocardium;
  mesogastrium; muscles;
  nerve of clitoris; nerve of
  penis; nerve of scapula;
  nerves of toes; nucleus;
  nucleus of trapezoid body;
  nucleus of vagus; nucleus
  of vagus nerve; pancreas;
  part of pons; plate of
  neural tube; position;
  reflex; root; spine; surface;
  surface of digit; surface of
  sacrum; surface of scapula;
  thalamus; tubercle of
  radius; vein of corpus
  callosum; veins of clitoris;
  veins of penis; vertebrae
dorsal accessory olivary:
  nucleus
dorsal calcaneocuboid:
  ligament
dorsal callosal: vein
dorsal carpal: branch of
  radial artery; branch of
  ulnar artery; ligament;
  network
dorsal carpometacarpal:
  ligaments
dorsal column: stimulation
dorsal cuboideonavicular:
  ligament
dorsal cuneocuboid:
  ligament
dorsal cuneonavicular:
  ligaments
dorsal digital: artery; nerves;
  nerves of foot; nerves of
  hand; veins of foot; veins
  of toes
dorsal hypothalamic: region

dorsal interosseous: artery;
  muscles of foot; muscles of
  hand; nerve
dorsalis pedis: artery
dorsal lateral cutaneous:
  nerve
dorsal lingual: branches of
  lingual artery; vein
dorsal longitudinal:
  fasciculus
dorsal medial cutaneous:
  nerve
dorsal metacarpal: artery;
  ligaments; veins
dorsal metatarsal: artery;
  ligaments; veins
dorsal motor: nucleus of
  vagus
dorsal nasal: artery
dorsal pancreatic: artery
dorsal primary: ramus of
  spinal nerve
dorsal radiocarpal: ligament
dorsal root: ganglion
dorsal sacrococcygeal:
  muscle
dorsal sacrococcygeus:
  muscle
dorsal sacroiliac: ligaments
dorsal scapular: artery;
  nerve; vein
dorsal talonavicular: bone;
  ligament
dorsal tegmental:
  decussation
dorsal thoracic: artery
dorsal vagal: nucleus
dorsal venous: arch of foot;
  network of foot; network
  of hand
Dorset's culture egg:
  medium
dorsispinal: veins
dorsolateral: fasciculus;
  plate of neural tube; tract
dorsomedial: nucleus;
  nucleus of hypothalamus
dorsomedial hypothalamic:
  nucleus
dorsosacral: position
dorsum pedis: reflex
dose-response: curve;
  relationship
dotted: tongue
double: athetosis; bind;
  bond; chin; consciousness;
  enterostomy; fracture;
  helix; hemiplegia;
  immunodiffusion;
  intussusception; lip;
  membrane; pleurisy;
  pneumonia; product;
  protrusion; quartan;
  refraction; salt; stain;
  tachycardia; tertian; vision
double antibody:
  immunoassay; method;
  precipitation

double antibody sandwich: assay
double aortic: arch; stenosis
double back: cross
double blind: experiment; study
double bubble: sign
double-channel: catheter
double compartment: hydrocephalus
double concave: lens
double congenital: athetosis
double contrast: enema
double convex: lens
double displacement: mechanism
double flap: amputation
double (gel) diffusion precipitin: test in one dimension; test in two dimensions
double inlet atrioventricular: connections
double loop: hernia
double-masked: experiment
double minute: chromosomes
double-mouthed: uterus
double outlet right: ventricle
double pedicle: flap
double-point: threshold
double quotidian: fever
double-reciprocal: plot
double-shock: sound
double-strand: break
double tertian: malaria
double track: sign
doubly: heterozygous
doubly armed: suture
douche: bath
Douglas: abscess; bag; graft; mechanism
Douglas': cul-de-sac; fold; line; pouch
Douglas' spontaneous: evolution
dousing: bath
dowager's: hump
downbeat: nystagmus
downer: cow
Downey: cell
Downs': analysis
Down's: syndrome
downward: drainage
Doyère's: eminence
Doyle's: operation
Doyne's honeycomb: choroidopathy
Drabkin's: reagent
Dragendorff: reagent
Dragendorff's: test
Dräger: respirometer
drainage: tube
drain-trap: stomach
Draper's: law
drawer: sign; test

dream: associations; pain
dreamy: state
drepanocytic: anemia
dressing: forceps
Dressler: beat
Dressler's: syndrome
Dreulofoy's: lesion
Dreyer's: formula
dried: alum; ferrous sulfate; yeast
dried human: albumin; serum
dried human plasma protein: fraction
drift: movements
Drigalski-Conradi: agar
Drinker: respirator
drip: phleboclysis; transfusion
drip-suck: irrigation
driver's: thigh
drooping lily: sign
drop: attack; finger; foot; hand; heart
droplet: infection; nuclei
dropped: beat
drug: abuse; allergy; eruption; fever; pathogenesis; psychosis; rash; resistance; tetanus
drug-induced: disease; hepatitis; lupus
drum: membrane
Drummond's: sign
drumstick: appendage
dry: abscess; amputation; beriberi; bronchiectasis; cup; distillation; dressing; drowning; gangrene; hernia; labor; leprosy; nurse; pack; pericarditis; pleurisy; rale; socket; synovitis; tetter; vomiting; weight
dry cutaneous: leishmaniasis
dry eye: syndrome
D-S: test
dual: personality; relationships
dual-cure: resin
Duane's: syndrome
Dubin-Johnson: syndrome
DuBois': formula
Dubois': abscesses; disease
Du Bois-Reymond's: law
Duboscq's: colorimeter
Dubowitz: score
Dubreuil-Chambardel: syndrome
Duchenne: dystrophy
Duchenne-Aran: disease
Duchenne-Erb: paralysis
Duchenne's: disease; sign; syndrome
duck: plague
duckbill: speculum
duck embryo origin: vaccine

duck hepatitis: virus
duck influenza: virus
duck plague: virus
duck viral: enteritis; hepatitis
Duckworth's: phenomenon
Ducrey: test
Ducrey's: bacillus
duct: carcinoma; papilloma
ductal: aneurysm; hyperplasia
ductless: glands
ductus: nodes
Duddell's: membrane
Duffy: antigens
Dugas': test
Duhring's: disease
Dührssen's: incisions
Duke bleeding time: test
Dukes': classification; disease
Dulong-Petit: law
dumb: rabies
dumbbell: ganglioneuroma
Dumdum: fever
dummy: consultand
Dumontpallier's: pessary
dumping: syndrome
Duncan's: disease; folds; mechanism; ventricle
duodenal: ampulla; bulb; cap; digestion; diverticulum; fistula; fossae; glands; impression; smear; sphincter
duodenojejunal: angle; flexure; fold; fossa; hernia; junction; recess; sphincter
duodenomesocolic: fold
duodenorenal: ligament
duodoneal: branches of superior pancreaticoduodenal artery
Duplay's: disease
duplex: echocardiography; kidney; transmission; ultrasonography; uterus
duplex Doppler: scan
duplication: cyst
duplicity: theory of vision
Dupré's: muscle
Dupuy-Dutemps: operation
Dupuytren's: amputation; canal; contracture; disease of the foot; fascia; fracture; hydrocele; sign; suture; tourniquet
dural: sheath; sheath of optic nerve
dural venous: sinuses
Duran-Reynals permeability: factor
duration: tetany
Dürck's: nodes
Duret's: hemorrhage; lesion
Durham: rule
Durham's: tube

Duroziez': disease; murmur; sign
dust: asthma; ball; cell; corpuscles
Dutton's: disease
Dutton's relapsing: fever
Duverney's: fissures; foramen; gland; muscle
dwarf: pelvis
dwarfed: enamel
dyadic: psychotherapy; symbiosis
dye-dilution: curve
dye exclusion: test
Dyggve-Melchior-Clausen: syndrome
dynamic: aorta; compliance of lung; CT; demography; disease; equilibrium; force; friction; ileus; murmur; psychiatry; psychology; psychotherapy; refraction; relations; school; splint; viscosity
dynamic computed: tomography
dynamic platform: posturography
dynein: arm
dysconjugate: gaze
dyscrasic: fracture
dysembryoplastic neuroepithelial: tumor
dysenteric: diarrhea
dysenteric algid: malaria
dysentery: antitoxin; bacillus
dysfunctional uterine: bleeding
dysgranular: cortex
dysharmonious: correspondence
dyshemopoietic: anemia
dysjunctive: nystagmus
dysmenorrheal: membrane
dysmnesic: psychosis; syndrome
dysplastic: nevus
dysplastic nevus: syndrome
dysproteinemic: retinopathy
dysspermatogenic: sterility
dysthymic: disorder
dysthyroidal: infantilism
dystonic: reaction; torticollis
dystrophic: calcification; calcinosis

E

E: rosette
EAC: rosette
EAC rosette: assay
Eadie-Hofstee: plot
Eagle: syndrome
Eagle-Barrett: syndrome
Eagle's basal: medium
Eagle's minimum essential: medium
EAHF: complex

WordFinder

Eales': disease
ear: bones; crystals; lobe; mange; wax
Earle L: fibrosarcoma
Earle's: solution
ear lobe: crease
early: deceleration; reaction; seizure; syphilis
early diastolic: murmur
early infantile: autism
early latent: syphilis
early-phase: response
early posttraumatic: epilepsy
early receptor: potential
earth: wax
earthy: water
East African: trypanosomiasis
East African sleeping: sickness
East Coast: fever
eastern equine: encephalomyelitis
eastern equine encephalomyelitis: virus
eating: disorders; epilepsy
Eaton: agent
Eaton agent: pneumonia
Eaton-Lambert: syndrome
EB: virus
Ebbinghaus: test
Eberth's: bacillus; lines; perithelium
Ebner's: glands; reticulum
Ebola: virus
Ebola hemorrhagic: fever
Ebstein's: anomaly; disease; sign
ECBO: virus
eccentric: amputation; fixation; hypertrophy; implantation; occlusion; position; relation
ecchymotic: mask
eccrine: acrospiroma; gland; poroma; spiradenoma
ecdysial: glands
ECG: trigger
ecgonine: benzoate
echinococcus: cyst; disease
ECHO: virus
echo: beat; reaction; speech
echocardiographic: differentiation
Eck: fistula
Ecker's: fissure
eclamptic: retinopathy
eclipse: blindness; period; phase
ECMO: virus
ecological: chemistry; ectocrine; system
economic: coefficient
ecotropic: virus
ECSO: virus
ectatic: aneurysm; emphysema

ectatic marginal: degeneration of cornea
ecthymatous: syphilid
ectocervical: smear
ectodermal: cloaca; dysplasia
ectogenic: teratosis
ectopic: beat; decidua; eyelash; hormone; impulse; pacemaker; pinealoma; pregnancy; rhythm; schistosomiasis; tachycardia; teratosis; testis; ureter
ectopic ACTH: syndrome
ectoplacental: cavity
ectotrophoblastic: cavity
ectrodactyly-ectodermal dysplasia-clefting: syndrome
ectromelia: virus
eczematoid: seborrhea
eddy: sounds
edema: disease
Eder-Pustow: bougie
edge: enhancement
edge-to-edge: bite; occlusion
edgewise: appliance
Edinger-Westphal: nucleus
Edlefsen's: reagent
Edman: method
Edman's: reagent
Edridge-Green: lamp
educational: psychology
Edwards': syndrome
EEE: virus
EEG: activation
effective: conjugate; dose; half-life; temperature
effective osmotic: pressure
effective refractory: period
effective renal blood: flow
effective renal plasma: flow
effective temperature: index
effector: cell
efferent: duct; ductules of testis; fibers; lymphatic; nerve; vessel
efferent glomerular: arteriole
effervescent: lithium citrate; magnesium citrate; magnesium sulfate; potassium citrate; salts; sodium phosphate
effort: syndrome
effort-induced: thrombosis
egg: albumin; cell; membrane
egg drop: syndrome
Egger's: line
Eggleston: method
egg shell: nail
eggshell: calcification
egg-white: injury; syndrome
Eglis': glands
ego: analysis; ideal; identity; instincts

ego-dystonic: homosexuality
Egyptian: hematuria; ophthalmia; splenomegaly
Ehlers-Danlos: syndrome
Ehrenritter's: ganglion
Ehret's: phenomenon
Ehrlich: reaction
Ehrlich's: anemia; phenomenon; postulate; theory
Ehrlich's acid hematoxylin: stain
Ehrlich's aniline crystal violet: stain
Ehrlich's benzaldehyde: reaction
Ehrlich's diazo: reaction; reagent
Ehrlich's inner: body
Ehrlich's triacid: stain
Ehrlich's triple: stain
Ehrlich-Türk: line
Eichhorst's: corpuscles; neuritis
Eicken's: method
eidetic: image
eighth: nerve
eighth cranial: nerve
eighth nerve: tumor
Einarson's gallocyanin-chrome alum: stain
Einthoven's: equation; law; triangle
Einthoven's string: galvanometer
Eisenlohr's: syndrome
Eisenmenger's: complex; defect; disease; syndrome; tetralogy
ejaculatory: duct
ejection: click; fraction; murmur; period; sounds
Ejrup: maneuver
Ekbom: syndrome
EKG: trigger
elastic: artery; bandage; bougie; cartilage; cone; fibers; lamella; laminae of arteries; layers of arteries; layers of cornea; ligature; limit; membrane; skin; tissue
elastic band: fixation
elastoid: degeneration
elastotic: degeneration
Elaut's: triangle
elbow: bone; jerk; joint; reflex
elbowed: bougie; catheter
elder: abuse
elective: abortion; culture; mutism
Electra: complex
electric: anesthesia; bath; cataract; cautery; chorea; dermatome; irritability; retinopathy; shock; sleep

electrical: alternans; alternation of heart; axis; diastole; failure; formula; systole
electrical heart: position
electric cardiac: pacemaker
electrocardiographic: complex; wave
electrochemical: gradient
electroconvulsive: therapy
electrode: knife
electrode catheter: ablation
electrodermal: audiometry
electroencephalographic: dysrhythmia
electrographic: seizure
electrohydraulic shock wave: lithotripsy
electrolyte: metabolism
electromagnetic: flowmeter; induction; radiation; unit
electromechanical: dissociation; systole
electromotive: force
electromuscular: sensibility
electron: beam; capture; interferometer; interferometry; magneton; micrograph; microscope; microscopy; radiography
electronegative: element
electronic: number; pacemaker
electronic cell: counter
electronic fetal: monitor
electronic pacemaker: load
electron paramagnetic: resonance
electron resonance: absorption
electron spin: resonance
electron transfer: flavin
electron-transport: chain; system
electron transport: particles
electrophonic: effect
electrophrenic: respiration
electrophysiologic: audiometry
electropositive: element
electroshock: therapy
electrostatic: bond; unit
electrotherapeutic: sleep
electrotherapeutic sleep: therapy
electrotonic: current; junction; synapse
elementary: bodies; granule; particle
elephant: leg
elephant man's: disease
elephantoid: fever
elevator: disease; muscle of anus; muscle of prostate; muscle of rib; muscle of scapula; muscle of soft palate; muscle of thyroid gland; muscle of upper

eyelid; muscle of upper lip; muscle of upper lip and wing of nose

eleventh cranial: nerve

elfin: facies

elimination: diet

Ellik: evacuator

Elliot's: operation; position

Elliott's: law

ellipsoidal: joint

elliptical: amputation; anastomosis; recess

elliptocytary: anemia

elliptocytic: anemia

elliptocytotic: anemia

Ellis type 1: glomerulonephritis; nephritis

Ellis type 2: glomerulonephritis

Ellis-van Creveld: syndrome

Ellsworth-Howard: test

Eloesser: procedure

elongation: factor

Elschnig: pearls

Elschnig's: spots

El Tor: vibrio

elusive: ulcer

E-M: syndrome

EMB: agar

Embden: ester

Embden-Meyerhof pathway

Embden-Meyerhof-Parnas: pathway

embedding: agents

embolic: abscess; gangrene; infarct; pneumonia

emboliform: nucleus

embolomycotic: aneurysm

embryo: transfer

embryonal: adenoma; area; carcinoma; carcinosarcoma; inducer; leukemia; medulloepithelioma; rhabdomyosarcomas; tumor; tumor of ciliary body

embryonic: anideus; axis; blastoderm; cataract; cell; circulation; diapause; disk; hemoglobin; membrane; shield

embryopathic: cataract

EMC: virus

emergency: theory

emergent: evolution

emerging: viruses

emery: disks

Emery-Dreifuss muscular: dystrophy

emesis: basin

EMG: biofeedback; examination; syndrome

EMI: scan

emigration: theory

emissary: vein

emissary sphenoidal: foramen

emission: electron

Emmet's: needle; operation

emotional: age; amenorrhea; amnesia; attitudes; deprivation; disease; disorder; disturbance; leukocytosis; overlay

empathic: index

emphysematous: cholecystitis; cystitis; gangrene; phlegmon

empiric: risk; treatment

empirical: formula

empty: sella

empyema: tube

empyemic: scoliosis

emulsifying: wax

emulsion: colloid

enamel: cap; cell; cleavage; cleaver; crypt; cuticle; drop; dysplasia; epithelium; fibers; fissure; germ; hypocalcification; hypoplasia; lamella; layer; ledge; membrane; niche; nodule; organ; pearl; prisms; projection; pulp; rods; tuft; wall

enamel rod: inclination; sheath

enarthrodial: joint

encapsulated: delusion

encephalic: vesicle

encephalithogenic: protein

encephalitis: virus

encephaloclastic: microcephaly

encephalocraniocutaneous: lipomatosis

encephaloid: cancer

encephalomyelonic: axis

encephalomyocarditis: virus

encephalotrigeminal: angiomatosis

encephalotrigeminal vascular: syndrome

encounter: group

encu: method

encysted: calculus; pleurisy

end: artery; bud; bulb; cell; organ; oxidation; piece; plate; point; product; stage

endaural: incision

end-cutting: bur

end-diastolic: volume

endemic: deafmutism; disease; funiculitis; goiter; hematuria; hemoptysis; hypertrophy; index; influenza; neuritis; stability; syphilis; typhus

endemic nonbacterial infantile: gastroenteritis

endemic paralytic: vertigo

Endo: agar

endobronchial: tube

endocardial: cushions; fibroelastosis; fibrosis; murmur; sclerosis

endocardial cushion: defect

endocervical: smear

endocervical sinus: tumor

endochondral: bone; ossification

endocrine: exophthalmos; glands; hormones; ophthalmopathy; part of pancreas; system

endodermal: canal; cells; cloaca; pouches

endodermal sinus: tumor

endodontic: stabilizer; treatment

endogenic: toxicosis

endogenous: cycle; depression; fibers; hyperglyceridemia; infection; pyrogens

endogenous creatinine: clearance

endolymphatic: duct; hydrops; sac

endomembrane: system

endometrial: cyst; implants; smear

endometrial stromal: sarcoma

endometrioid: carcinoma; tumor

endomyocardial: fibrosis

end-on mattress: suture

endo-osseous: implant

endopelvic: fascia

endoplasmic: reticulum

endorectal pull-through: procedure

Endo's: medium

endoscopic: biopsy

endoscopic retrograde: cholangiopancreatography

Endo's fuchsin: agar

endosteal: implant

endoteric: bacterium

endothelial: cell; cyst; dystrophy of cornea; leukocyte; myeloma

endothelial-leukocyte adhesion: molecule

endothelial relaxing: factor

endotheliochorial: placenta

endothelio-endothelial: placenta

endothelium-derived relaxing: factor

endothoracic: fascia

endotoxin: shock

endotracheal: anesthesia; intubation; stylet; tube

endovaginal: ultrasonography

endovenous: septum

end-point: measurement; nystagmus

end product: inhibition; repression

endstage: lung

end-systolic: volume

end-tidal: sample

end-to-end: bite; occlusion

energy: metabolism

energy-rich: bond; phosphates

Engelmann's: disease

Engelmann's basal: knobs

engine: reamer

Englisch's: sinus

English: disease; position; rhinoplasty

English sweating: disease

enrichment: culture

ensheathing: callus

ensiform: cartilage; process

ensu: method

enteric: fever; plexus; tuberculosis; viruses

enteric coated: tablet

enteric cytopathogenic bovine orphan: virus

enteric cytopathogenic human orphan: virus

enteric cytopathogenic monkey orphan: virus

enteric cytopathogenic swine orphan: virus

entericoid: fever

enteric orphan: viruses

enterochromaffin: cells

enterocutaneous: fistula

enterocyte cobalamin: malabsorption

enteroendocrine: cells

enterogastric: reflex

enterogenous: cyanosis; cysts; methemoglobinemia

enterohemorrhagic *:* Escherichia coli

enterohepatic: circulation

enteroinvasive *:* Escherichia coli

enterokinetic: agent

enteropathic: arthritis

enteropathogenic *:* Escherichia coli

enterotoxigenic *:* Escherichia coli

enterovaginal: fistula

enterovesical: fistula

Entner-Douderoff: pathway

entodermal: cells

entoptic: pulse

entorhinal: area

entrance: block

entrapment: neuropathy; neuropathy

entry: zone

envelope: conformation; flap

environmental: psychology

enzootic: abortion of ewes; ataxia; balanoposthitis; encephalomyelitis;

hematuria; pneumonia; stability

enzootic bovine: leukosis

enzootic encephalomyelitis: virus

enzygotic: twins

enzymatic: synthesis

enzyme: analog; antagonist; immunoassay; interconversion; isomerization; kinetics; parameters; regulation; repression

enzyme-catalyzed: ligation

enzyme inhibition: theory of narcosis

enzyme-linked immunosorbent: assay

enzyme-multiplied: immunoassay technique

enzyme-substrate: complex

eosin-methylene blue: agar

eosinopenic: reaction

eosinophil: adenoma; granule

eosinophil chemotactic: factor of anaphylaxis

eosinophilia-myalgia: syndrome

eosinophilic: cellulitis; cystitis; fasciitis; gastritis; gastroenteritis; granuloma; leukemia; leukocyte; leukocytosis; leukopenia; meningitis; meningoencephalitis; pneumonia; pneumonopathy

eosinophilic endomyocardial: disease

eosinophilic pustular: folliculitis

epactal: bones; ossicles

epamniotic: cavity

eparterial: bronchus

ependymal: cell; cyst; layer; zone

ephemeral: fever; fever of cattle

ephemeral fever: virus

epibranchial: placodes

epicanthal: fold

epicranial: aponeurosis; muscle

epicranius: muscle

epicritic: sensibility

epidemic: curve; disease; dropsy; encephalitis; exanthema; hemoglobinuria; hepatitis; hiccup; hysteria; keratoconjunctivitis; myalgia; myositis; nausea; neuromyasthenia; parotiditis; pleurodynia; polyarthritis; roseola; stomatitis; tetany; tremor; typhus; vertigo; vomiting

epidemic benign dry: pleurisy

epidemic cerebrospinal: meningitis

epidemic diaphragmatic: pleurisy

epidemic gangrenous: proctitis

epidemic gastroenteritis: virus

epidemic hemorrhagic: fever

epidemic keratoconjunctivitis: virus

epidemic myalgia: virus

epidemic myalgic: encephalomyelitis; encephalomyelopathy

epidemic nonbacterial: gastroenteritis

epidemic parotitis: virus

epidemic pleurodynia: virus

epidemic transient diaphragmatic: spasm

epidemiological: distribution; genetics

epidermal: cyst; ridges

epidermal growth: factor

epidermal ridge: count

epidermic: cell; graft

epidermic-dermic: nevus

epidermoid: cancer; carcinoma; cyst

epidermolytic: hyperkeratosis

epidural: anesthesia; block; cavity; hematoma; meningitis; space

epifascicular: epineurium

epigastric: angle; fold; fossa; hernia; reflex; region; veins; voice

epiglottic: cartilage; folds; tubercle; vallecula

epihyal: bone; ligament

epikeratophakic: keratoplasty

epilation: dose

epilemmal: ending

epileptic: dementia; seizure

epileptiform: neuralgia

epileptogenic: zone

epimastical: fever

epimerase deficiency: galactosemia

epimyoepithelial: islands

epinephrine: reversal

epiotic: center

epipapillary: membrane

epipericardial: ridge

epiphrenic: diverticulum

epiphysial: arrest; cartilage; eye; fracture; line; plate

epiphysial aseptic: necrosis

epiploic: appendage; appendix; branches; foramen; tags

epipteric: bone

epiretinal: membrane

episcleral: artery; lamina; space; veins

episodic dyscontrol: syndrome

episternal: bone

epithelial: attachment; body; cancer; cast; cell; cyst; dysplasia; dystrophy; ectoderm; inlay; lamina; layers; migration; nest; pearl; plug; tissue

epithelial choroid: layer

epithelial myoepithelial: carcinoma

epithelial reticular: cell

epitheliochorial: placenta

epithelioid: cell

epithelioid cell: nevus

epithermal: chemistry; neutron

epitrichial: layer

epitrochlear: nodes

epituberculous: infiltration

epitympanic: recess; space

epizoic: commensalism

epizootic: cellulitis; lymphangitis

epizootic bovine: abortion

epizootic hemorrhagic: disease of deer

epizootic hemorrhagic disease of deer: virus

epoxy: resin

epsilon: alcoholism

Epsom: salts

Epstein-Barr: virus

Epstein's: disease; pearls; sign; symptom

equal: cleavage

equatorial: cleavage; division; plane; plate; staphyloma

equianalgesic: dose

equilibrium: constant; dialysis

equine: babesiosis; encephalitis; encephalomyelitis; encephalosis; gait; gonadotropin; herpesvirus 3; herpesvirus 4; influenza; rhinopneumonitis; rhinoviruses; syphilis; typhoid

equine abortion: virus

equine arteritis: virus

equine biliary: fever

equine coital: exanthema

equine coital exanthema: virus

equine encephalosis: virus

equine gonadotropin: unit

equine infectious: anemia

equine infectious anemia: virus

equine influenza: viruses

equine monocytic: ehrlichiosis

equine nonthrombocytopenic: purpura

equine rhinopneumonitis: virus

equine serum: hepatitis

equine spinal: ataxia

equine viral: arteritis

equine virus: abortion

equiphasic: complex

equivalence: point; zone

equivalent: dose; extract; power; temperature; weight

equivalent form: reliability

equivocal: symptom

Eranko's fluorescence: stain

Erb: atrophy; disease; palsy; paralysis; sign

Erb-Charcot: disease

Erb spinal: paralysis

Erb-Westphal: sign

Erdheim: disease; tumor

Erdmann's: reagent

erect: illumination

erectile: tissue

erector: muscles of hairs; muscle of spine

erector spinae: muscles

erector-spinal: reflex

erethistic: shock

ergot: alkaloids; poisoning

ergot alkaloid-associated heart: disease

Erichsen's: sign

Erlenmeyer: flask

Erlenmeyer flask: deformity

erogenous: zone

E-rosette: test

erosive: adenomatosis of nipple

erotic: zoophilism

erotomanic type of paranoid: disorder

erroneous: projection

error-prone: repair

eruption: cyst

eruptive: fever; phase; stage; xanthoma

erythema: dose; threshold

erythematous: syphilid

erythremic: myelosis

erythroblastic: anemia

erythrocyte: indices

erythrocyte adherence: phenomenon; test

erythrocyte fragility: test

erythrocyte maturation: factor

erythrocyte sedimentation: rate

erythrocytic: series

erythrodysesthesia: syndrome

erythrogenic: toxin

erythroid: cell

erythronormoblastic: anemia

erythrophore: reaction

erythropoietic: hormone; porphyria; protoporphyria

Esbach's: reagent

escape: beat; conditioning; contraction; impulse; interval; phenomenon; rhythm; training

escape-capture: bigeminy

escape ventricular: contraction

Escherichia coli: enterotoxin; RNase I

Escherich's: sign

Esmarch: bandage; tourniquet

esodic: nerve

esophageal: achalasia; arteries; atresia; branches; branches of the inferior thyroid artery; branches of the left gastric artery; branches of the recurrent laryngeal nerve; branches of the thoracic aorta; branches of the vagus nerve; cardiogram; constrictions; dysrhythmia; glands; hiatus; impression; lead; manometry; mucosa; opening; plexus; reflux; smear; spasm; speech; varices; veins; web

esophagogastric: junction; orifice; vestibule

esophagosalivary: reflex

essential: albuminuria; amino acids; anemia; anisocoria; bradycardia; dysmenorrhea; fatty acid; fever; fructosuria; hypertension; nutrients; oils; pentosuria; phthisis bulbi; pruritus; tachycardia; telangiectasia; thrombocytopenia; tremor

essential food: factors

essential progressive: atrophy of iris

Esser: graft; operation

Essick's cell: bands

Essig: splint

established cell: line

esterified: estrogens

Estes: operation

esthesiodic: system

esthetic: dentistry; surgery

Estlander: flap; operation

estradiol benzoate: unit

estrogenic: hormone

estrone: unit

estrous: cycle

ether: convulsion; test

ethereal: oil; solution; tincture

ethinyl: estradiol

ethmoid: angle; bone; infundibulum

ethmoid air: cells

ethmoidal: bulla; cells; crest; crest of maxilla; crest of palatine bone; foramen; groove; infundibulum; labyrinth; notch; process; sinuses; veins

ethmoidal-lacrimal: fistula

ethmoidolacrimal: suture

ethmoidomaxillary: suture

ethmovomerine: plate

ethyl: eosin

ethynyl: estradiol

"e"-type: cholinesterase

eucalyptus: gum

euglobulin clot lysis: time

eugnathic: anomaly

Eulenburg's: disease

eunuchoid: gigantism; state; voice

eupeptide: bond

euplastic: lymph

European: snakeroot; tarantula; typhus

euroxenous: parasite

eustachian: catheter; cushion; tonsil; tube; tuber; valve

eutectic: alloy; temperature

euthyroid: hypometabolism

euthyroid sick: syndrome

Evans: forceps

Evans': syndrome

evoked: potential; response

evoked response: audiometry

evolutionary: fitness

Ewart's: procedure; sign

Ewing's: sarcoma; sign; tumor

examining: table

exanthematous: disease; fever; typhus

excentric: amputation

excess: lactate

exchange: transfusion

excision: biopsy; repair

excitable: area; gap

excitation: spectrum; wave

excitatory junction: potential

excitatory postsynaptic: potential

excited: atom; catatonia; state

exciting: cause; electrode; eye

excitor: nerve

excitoreflex: nerve

exclamation point: hair

excretory: duct; duct of seminal vesicle; ducts of lacrimal gland; ductules of lacrimal gland; gland

exercise: bone; imaging; test

exercise-induced: amenorrhea

exercise radionuclide: angiocardiography

exertional: dyspnea; rhabdomyolysis

exfoliation: syndrome

exfoliative: cytology; dermatitis; gastritis

exhaustion: atrophy; psychosis

existential: psychiatry; psychology; psychotherapy

exit: block; dose

Exner's: plexus

exoccipital: bone

exocelomic: membrane

exocrine: gland; part of pancreas

exocrine pancreatic: insufficiency

exodic: nerve

exoerythrocytic: cycle; stage

exogenic: toxicosis

exogenous: cycle; depression; fibers; hemochromatosis; hyperglyceridemia; ochronosis; pigmentation; pyrogens

exogenous creatinine: clearance

exophthalmic: goiter; ophthalmoplegia

exophthalmos-producing: substance

exoteric: bacterium

expansion: arch

expansive: delusion

expectation: neurosis

experimental: error; group; medicine; method; neurosis; psychology

experimental allergic: encephalitis; encephalomyelitis

experimenter: effects

expiratory: center; dyspnea; resistance; stridor

expiratory reserve: volume

expired: gas

exploratory: drive

exploring: electrode; needle

explosive: decompression; speech

exponential: distribution; growth

exposed: pulp

exposure: dose; keratitis

expressed: mustard oil

expressed skull: fracture

expression: vector

expressive: aphasia

expulsive: pains

exsanguination: transfusion

exsiccated: alum; sodium sulfite

exsiccation: fever

extemporaneous: mixture

extended: clasp; family; pyelotomy

extended family: therapy

extended insulin zinc: suspension

extended radical: mastectomy

extension: bridge; form

extensor: aponeurosis; expansion; muscle of fingers; muscle of little finger; retinaculum

extensor carpi radialis brevis: muscle

extensor carpi radialis longus: muscle

extensor carpi ulnaris: muscle

extensor digital: expansion

extensor digiti minimi: muscle

extensor digitorum: muscle

extensor digitorum brevis: muscle; muscle of hand

extensor digitorum longus: muscle

extensor hallucis brevis: muscle

extensor hallucis longus: muscle

extensor indicis: muscle

extensor pollicis brevis: muscle

extensor pollicis longus: muscle

external: absorption; aperture of cochlear canaliculus; aperture of vestibular aqueduct; artery of nose; axis of eye; base of skull; branch of accessory nerve; branch of superior laryngeal nerve; canthus; capsule; conjugate; defibrillator; fistula; fixation; genitalia; hemorrhoid; hemorrhoids; hydrocephalus; lip of iliac crest; malleolus; matrix; medium; meningitis; naris; nose; opening of urethra; ophthalmopathy; ophthalmoplegia; os of uterus; pacemaker; phase; pyocephalus; respiration; secretion; sheath of optic nerve; sphincterotomy; squint; strabismus; surface; surface of frontal bone; surface of parietal bone; traction; urethrotomy; wall of cochlear duct

external acoustic: foramen; meatus; pore

external anal: sphincter

external arcuate: fibers

WordFinder

external auditory: foramen; meatus
external cardiac: massage
external carotid: artery; nerves; plexus
external cephalic: version
external collateral: ligament of wrist
external conjugate: diameter
external cuneate: nucleus
external dental: epithelium
external exudative: retinopathy
external female genital: organs
external iliac: artery; lymph nodes; plexus; vein
external inguinal: ring
external intercostal: membrane; muscles
external jugular: vein
external male genital: organs
external malleolar: sign
external mammary: artery
external maxillary: artery; plexus
external nasal: branches; veins
external nuclear: layer of retina
external oblique: muscle; reflex; ridge
external obturator: muscle
external occipital: crest; protuberance
external pillar: cells
external pin: fixation; fixation, biphase
external pterygoid: muscle
external pudendal: arteries; veins
external respiratory: nerve of Bell
external root: sheath
external salivary: gland
external saphenous: nerve
external semilunar: fibrocartilage
external spermatic: artery; fascia; nerve
external sphincter: muscle of anus
external spiral: sulcus
external urethral: orifice; sphincter
exterofective: system
extinction: coefficient
Exton: reagent
extra-: systole
extra-abdominal: desmoid
extraamniotic: pregnancy
extraanatomic: bypass
extracapsular: ankylosis; fracture; ligaments
extracardiac: murmur

extracellular: cholesterolosis; enzyme; fluid; toxin
extracellular fluid: volume
extrachorial: pregnancy
extrachromosomal: DNA; element; gene; inheritance
extracoronal: retainer
extracorporeal: circulation; dialysis; photophoresis
extracorporeal shock wave: lithotripsy
extracranial: arteritis; ganglia; pneumatocele; pneumocele
extracranial-intracranial: bypass
extracting: forceps
extraction: coefficient; ratio
extradural: anesthesia; hematorrhachis; hemorrhage
extraembryonic: blastoderm; celom; ectoderm; membrane; mesoderm
extraglomerular: mesangium
extramammary Paget: disease
extramembranous: pregnancy
extramural: practice
extranuclear: inheritance
extraocular: muscles
extraoral: anchorage
extraoral fracture: appliance
extraperitoneal: fascia
extrapineal: pinealoma
extrapleural: pneumothorax
extrapyramidal: disease; dyskinesias; syndrome
extrapyramidal cerebral: palsy
extrapyramidal motor: system
extrapyramidal motor system: disease
extrasaccular: hernia
extrasensory: perception
extrasensory thought: transference
extraskeletal: chondroma
extrathyroidal: hypermetabolism
extrauterine: pregnancy
extravaginal: torsion
extravasation: cyst
extravascular: fluid
extravital: ultraviolet
extreme: capsule
extrinsic: asthma; color; factor; motivation; muscles; proteins; sphincter
extrinsic allergic: alveolitis
extrinsic incubation: period
extruded: teeth

exudation: cell; corpuscle; cyst
exudative: bronchiolitis; choroiditis; glomerulonephritis; inflammation; retinitis; tuberculosis; vitreoretinopathy
exudative discoid and lichenoid: dermatitis
exudative retinal: detachment
eye: capsule; cup; drops; lens; ointment; reflex; socket; speculum; tooth
eyeball compression: reflex
eyeball-heart: reflex
eye-closure: reflex
eye-closure pupil: reaction
eye-ear: plane
eyelash: sign

F

F: duction; factor; genote; pili; pilus; plasmid; thalassemia; waves
F: agent
F-: actin
f: distribution
FA: virus
Fab: fragment; piece
Faber's: anemia; syndrome
Fabricius': ship
Fabry's: disease
face: form; peel; presentation; validity
face-bow: fork; record
facet: joints; rhizotomy
facial: angle; artery; axis; bones; canal; cleft; colliculus; diplegia; eczema; eminence; height; hemiatrophy; hemiatrophy of Romberg; hemiplegia; hillock; index; lymph nodes; muscles; myokymia; nerve; neuralgia; nucleus; palsy; paralysis; plane; plexus; profile; reflex; root; spasm; surface of tooth; tic; triangle; trophoneurosis; vein; vision
facialis: phenomenon
facial motor: nucleus
facilitated: diffusion; transport
faciodigitogenital: dysplasia
facioscapulohumeral: atrophy
facioscapulohumeral muscular: dystrophy
factitial: dermatitis
factitious: disorder; purpura; urticaria
factorial: experiments
facultative: anaerobe; heterochromatin;

hyperopia; parasite; saprophyte
Faden: suture
fading: time
Faget's: sign
Fahraeus-Lindqvist: effect
Fahrenheit: scale
Fahr's: disease
faith: healing
falciform: cartilage; crest; ligament; ligament of liver; lobe; margin; process
falciform retinal: fold
falciparum: fever; malaria
fallen: arches
falling: palate; sickness
falling of the: womb
fallopian: aqueduct; arch; canal; hiatus; ligament; neuritis; pregnancy; tube
Fallot's: tetrad; triad
false: agglutination; albuminuria; anemia; aneurysm; angina; ankylosis; blepharoptosis; branching; cast; conjugate; coxa vara; cyanosis; cyst; dextrocardia; diphtheria; diverticulum; dominance; glottis; hellebore; hematuria; hermaphroditism; hypertrophy; image; joint; knots; labor; macula; masturbation; membrane; mole; neuroma; nucleolus; pains; paracusis; pelvis; pregnancy; projection; ribs; ringbone; suture; thirst; vertebrae; waters
false-negative: reaction
false-positive: reaction
false vocal: cord
familial: aggregation; amyloidosis; cancer; dysautonomia; emphysema; glycinuria; goiter; hyperbetalipoproteinemia; hyperbetalipoproteinemia and hyperprebetalipoproteine-mia; hypercholesterolemia; hypercholesterolemia with hyperlipemia; hyperchylomicronemia; hyperchylomicronemia with hyperprebetalipoproteine-mia; hyperlipoproteinemia; hyperprebetalipoproteine-mia; hypertriglyceridemia; hypobetalipoproteinemia; hypoparathyroidism; lipodystrophy; nephrosis; screening; tremor
familial amyloid: neuropathy
familial aortic: ectasia

familial aortic ectasia: syndrome
familial bipolar mood: disorder
familial chylomicronemia: syndrome
familial combined: hyperlipemia
familial erythroblastic: anemia
familial fat-induced: hyperlipemia
familial high density lipoprotein: deficiency
familial hypercholesteremic: xanthomatosis
familial hypertrophic: cardiomyopathy
familial hypogonadotropic: hypogonadism
familial hypophosphatemic: rickets
familial hypoplastic: anemia
familial intestinal: polyposis
familial juvenile: nephrophthisis
familial lipoprotein lipase: inhibitor
familial Mediterranean: fever
familial microcytic: anemia
familial multiple endocrine: adenomatosis
familial nonhemolytic: jaundice
familial paroxysmal: polyserositis; rhabdomyolysis
familial periodic: paralysis
familial pseudoinflammatory: maculopathy
familial pseudoinflammatory macular: degeneration
familial pyridoxine-responsive: anemia
familial recurrent: polyserositis
familial spinal muscular: atrophy
familial splenic: anemia
familial white folded: dysplasia
family: medicine; physician; practice; therapy
famine: dropsy; fever
fan: sign
Fañanás: cell
Fanconi's: anemia; pancytopenia; syndrome
far: point; sight
Farabeuf's: amputation; triangle
Faraday's: constant; laws
far-and-near: suture
Farber's: disease; syndrome

Far East hemorrhagic: fever
Far East Russian: encephalitis
farmer's: lung; skin
Farnsworth-Munsell color: test
far point of: convergence
Farrant's mounting: fluid
Farre's: line
Farr's: law
fascia: graft
fascial: hernia; sheath of eyeball; sheaths of extraocular muscles
fascicular: block; degeneration; graft; keratitis; ophthalmoplegia; sarcoma; ulcer
fasciculata: cell
fasciolar: gyrus
fast: smear
fastidious: organism
fastigial: nucleus
fastigiobulbar: fibers; tract
fastigiospinal: fibers
fasting: hypoglycemia
fat: body of cheek; body of ischiorectal fossa; body of orbit; cell; embolism; graft; hernia; indigestion; metabolism; necrosis; pad; solvents; tide
fatality: rate
fate: map
father: complex
fatigue: fever; fracture; strength
fat-soluble: vitamins
fat-storing: cell
fatty: acid; alcohol; ascites; atrophy; cast; change; cirrhosis; degeneration; diarrhea; heart; hernia; infiltration; kidney; layer of superficial fascia; liver; metamorphosis; oil; phanerosis; series; stool; tissue
fatty acid binding: protein
fatty acid oxidation: cycle
fatty liver: syndrome
fatty renal: capsule
faucial: branches of lingual nerve; diphtheria; paralysis; reflex; tonsil
faulty: union
faun tail: nevus
Favre-Durand-Nicholas: disease
Favre-Racouchet's: disease
Favre-Racouchot: syndrome
Favre's: dystrophy
Fc: fragment; piece; receptor
featural: surgery
febrile: albuminuria; convulsion; crisis;

psychosis; seizure; urine; urticaria
fecal: abscess; fistula; impaction; incontinence; tumor; vomiting
Fechner-Weber: law
feedback: activation; inhibition; system
feed-forward: activation
feeding: center; tube
feeling: tone
Feer's: disease
Fehling's: reagent; solution
feigned: eruption
Feiss: line
feline: agranulocytosis; distemper; leukemia; pneumonitis; polioencephalomyelitis
feline immunodeficiency: virus
feline infectious: anemia; enteritis; peritonitis
feline leukemia: virus
feline leukemia-sarcoma virus: complex
feline panleukopenia: virus
feline rhinotracheitis: virus
feline urolithiasis: syndrome
feline urological: syndrome
feline viral: rhinotracheitis
Felty's: syndrome
female: catheter; gonad; hermaphroditism; homosexuality; prostate; pseudohermaphroditism; sterility; urethra
female pattern: alopecia
female urethral: syndrome
femininity: complex
femoral: arch; artery; branch of genitofemoral nerve; canal; fossa; hernia; muscle; nerve; opening; plexus; reflex; region; ring; septum; sheath; triangle; vein
femoroabdominal: reflex
femoropatellar: joint
femoropopliteal: bypass
femoropopliteal occlusive: disease
fenestrated: capillary; membrane; sheath
fenestration: operation
Fenn: effect
Fenton: reaction
Fenwick-Hunner: ulcer
Fenwick's: disease
Fergusson's: incision
fermentation *Lactobacillus casei*: factor
fermentative: dyspepsia
fern: test
Fernandez: reaction
Fernbach: flask
Ferrata's: cell

Ferrein's: canal; cords; foramen; ligament; pyramid; tube; vasa aberrantia
ferric: alum
ferric and ammonium acetate: solution
ferric chloride: reaction of epinephrine; test
ferruginous: bodies
Ferry-Porter: law
fertile: period
fertility: agent; factor; ratio; vitamin
fertilization: membrane
fertilized: ovum
fescue: foot; poisoning
festinating: gait
fetal: age; attitude; bradycardia; circulation; cotyledon; death; distress; dystocia; electrocardiography; erythroblastosis; fracture; gigantism; habitus; hemoglobin; hydrops; inclusion; medicine; membrane; movement; ovoid; placenta; souffle; tachycardia; zone
fetal adrenal: cortex
fetal alcohol: syndrome
fetal aspiration: syndrome
fetal death: rate
fetal face: syndrome
fetal heart: rate
fetal hydantoin: syndrome
fetal trimethadione: syndrome
fetal warfarin: syndrome
fetomaternal: transfusion
fetoplacental: anasarca
Feulgen: reaction; stain
fever: blister; therapy
feverish: urine
Fevold: test
FGT cytologic: smear
fiberoptic: gastroscope
fibrillar: baskets
fibrillary: astrocyte; astrocytoma; chorea; contractions; myoclonia; neuroma; waves
fibrillation: threshold
fibrillatory: waves
fibrin: calculus; thrombus
fibrin/fibrinogen degradation: products
fibrinogen-fibrin conversion: syndrome
fibrinoid: degeneration; necrosis
fibrinolytic: purpura
fibrinopurulent: inflammation
fibrinous: adhesion; bronchitis; cast;

inflammation; iritis; lymph; pericarditis; pleurisy; polyp

fibrin-stabilizing: factor

fibroblast: interferon

fibrocartilaginous: ring of tympanic membrane

fibrocaseous: peritonitis

fibrocystic: condition of the breast; disease of the pancreas

fibroelastic: membrane of larynx

fibroepithelial: polyp

fibrohyaline: tissue

fibroid: adenoma; cataract; inflammation; lung; tumor

fibrolamellar liver cell: carcinoma

fibromatosis: virus of rabbits

fibromuscular: dysplasia; hyperplasia

fibrosing: adenomatosis; adenosis; alveolitis; mediastinitis

fibrositic: headache

fibrotic: ophthalmoplegia

fibrous: adhesion; ankylosis; appendix of liver; capsule; capsule of kidney; capsule of liver; capsule of parotid gland; capsule of spleen; capsule of thyroid gland; cavernitis; degeneration; dysplasia of bone; dysplasia of jaws; goiter; hamartoma of infancy; histiocytoma; joint; layer; mediastinitis; membrane; pericarditis; pericardium; pneumonia; polyp; protein; ring; ring of heart; ring of intervertebral disc; sheaths; skeleton of heart; skeleton of the heart; tissue; trigones of heart; tubercle; tunic of corpus spongiosum; tunic of eye; union; xanthoma

fibrous articular: capsule

fibrous bacterial: viruses

fibrous cortical: defect

fibrous digital: sheaths of foot; sheaths of hand

fibrous tendon: sheath

fibular: artery; lymph node; margin of foot; node; notch; veins

fibular articular: surface of tibia

fibular collateral: ligament; ligament of ankle

Fick: method; principle

Fick's: laws of diffusion

Ficoll-Hypaque: technique

fictitious: feeding

Fiedler's: myocarditis

field: block; fever; gradient; lens; survey

field of: consciousness

field block: anesthesia

field emission: tube

Fielding's: membrane

Field's rapid: stain

Fiessinger-Leroy-Reiter: syndrome

fifth: disease; finger; ventricle

fifth cranial: nerve

fig: wart

fight or flight: reaction

Figueira's: syndrome

figure-of-8: abnormality; bandage; suture

filamentary: keratitis; keratopathy

filament-nonfilament: count

filamentous: bacteriophage; colony

filamentous bacterial: viruses

filament polymorphonuclear: leukocyte

filar: mass; micrometer; substance

filarial: arthritis; dermatosis; funiculitis; hydrocele; periodicity; synovitis

filariform: larva

Filatov: flap

Filatov Dukes': disease

Filatov-Gillies: flap

Filatov-Gillies tubed: pedicle

Filatov's: disease; operation; spots

filial: generation

filiform: bougie; nucleus; papillae; pulse; wart

filler: graft

fillet: layer

filling: defect

filter: paper

filtering: cicatrix; operation

filtrable: virus

filtrate: factor; nitrogen

filtration: angle; coefficient; fraction; slits; space

fimbriated: fold

fimbriodentate: sulcus

final: host; impression

Finckh: test

fine: structure; tremor

fine needle: biopsy

finger: agnosia; percussion; phenomenon

finger-nose: test

fingerprint: dystrophy

finger-thumb: reflex

finger-to-finger: test

finishing: bur

Fink-Heimer: stain

Finney: pyloroplasty

Finney's: operation

first: dentition; finger; messenger; molar

first arch: syndrome

first cranial: nerve

first cuneiform: bone

first degree: burn

first degree A-V: block

first duodenal: sphincter

first heart: sound

first-order: reaction

first parallel pelvic: plane

first rank: symptoms

first-set: rejection

first temporal: convolution

first visceral: cleft

Fischer: projection

Fischer projection formulas of: sugars

Fischer's: sign; symptom

Fischer's projection: formulas

fish: poison; skin; test

Fishberg concentration: test

Fisher's: syndrome

Fisher's exact: test

fish eye: disease

Fishman-Lerner: unit

fish-mouth: meatus

fish-mouth mitral: stenosis

fish tapeworm: anemia

fission: fungi; product

fissural: cyst

fissure: bur; caries; sealant; sign

fissured: fracture; tongue

fistula: knife; test

fistulous: withers

FIT: test

Fitzgerald: factor

Fitz-Hugh and Curtis: syndrome

five-day: fever

five year survival: rate

fixation: disparity; nystagmus; reaction

fixational ocular: movement

fixator: muscle

fixed: alkali; alkaloid; bridge; contracture; coupling; dressing; idea; macrophage; oil; pupil; torticollis; virus

fixed drug: eruption

fixed partial: denture

fixed-rate: pacemaker

fixed rate pulse: generator

fixing: eye

flaccid: ectropion; membrane; paralysis; part of tympanic membrane

Flack's: node

flag: flap; sign

flagellar: agglutinin; antigen

flagellate: diarrhea

flail: chest; joint

flame: arc; figure; photometer; spots

flame emission: spectrophotometry

flammable: anesthetic

flange: contour

flank: bone; incision; position

flap: amputation; operation

flapless: amputation

flapping: tremor

flash: blindness; burn; dispersal; keratoconjunctivitis; method; point

flashing pain: syndrome

flask: closure

flat: affect; bone; chest; condyloma; electroencephalogram; flap; hand; pelvis; plate; wart

Flatau's: law

Flatau-Schilder: disease

flat papular: syphilid

flat top: waves

flatulent: dyspepsia

flatus: enema

Flaujeac: factor

flavin: nucleotide

flax-dresser's: disease

flea-bitten: kidney

flea-borne: typhus

Flechsig's: areas; fasciculi; tract

Flechsig's ground: bundles

fleck: dystrophy of cornea; retina of Kandori

flecked: retina

flecked retina: syndrome

fleece: worm

Flegel's: disease

Fleisch: pneumotachograph

Fleischer's: ring; vortex

Fleischer-Strumpell: ring

Fleischmann's: bursa

Fleischner: lines

Fleitmann's: test

Flemming's: fixative

Flemming's triple: stain

Flesch: formula

fleshy: mole; polyp

Fletcher: factor

flexible: collodion

flexion: crease

Flexner's: bacillus

flexor: reflex; retinaculum; retinaculum of forearm; retinaculum of lower limb

flexor carpi radialis: muscle

flexor carpi ulnaris: muscle

flexor digiti minimi brevis: muscle of foot; muscle of hand

flexor digitorum brevis: muscle

flexor digitorum longus: muscle

flexor digitorum profundus: muscle

flexor digitorum superficialis: muscle

flexor hallucis brevis: muscle

flexor hallucis longus: muscle

flexor pollicis brevis: muscle

flexor pollicis longus: muscle

flexural: eczema

flick: movements

flicker: fusion; perimetry; photometer

flicker fusion frequency: technique

Flieringa's: ring

flight: blindness; nurse

flight of: ideas

flight or fight: response

flint: disease; glass

Flint's: arcade; murmur

flip: angle

flip-over: disease

flittering: scotoma

floating: cartilage; kidney; organ; patella; ribs; spleen; villus

floccular: fossa

flocculation: reaction; test

flocculonodular: lobe

flood: fever

Flood's: ligament

floor: cell; plate

floppy valve: syndrome

Florence: flask

Florence's: crystals

Florey: unit

florid oral: papillomatosis

florid osseous: dysplasia

floriform: cataract

Florschütz': formula

floss: silk

flotation: constant; method

Flourens': theory

floury: cornea

flow: cytometry; cytophotometry; void

Flower's: bone

Flower's dental: index

flower-spray: ending; organ of Ruffini

flowing: hyperostosis

flow-over: vaporizer

flow-volume: curve

fluent: aphasia

fluid: extract; retinopexy; wave

fluid mosaic: model

fluorescein: angiography

fluorescein instillation: test

fluorescein string: test

fluorescence: microscope; microscopy; quenching; spectrum

fluorescence plus Giemsa: stain

fluorescent: antibody; screen; stain

fluorescent antibody: technique

fluorescent antinuclear antibody: test

fluorescent treponemal antibody-absorption: test

fluoridated: teeth

Flury strain: vaccine

Flury strain rabies: virus

flush: technique

flutter-fibrillation: waves

flux: density; ratio

fluxionary: hyperemia

fly: agaric; blister

flying: blister

flying spot: microscope

Flynn: phenomenon

Flynn-Aird: syndrome

FMD: virus

foam: cells

foam stability: test

foamy: agents; viruses

focal: amyloidosis; appendicitis; depth; distance; epilepsy; glomerulonephritis; illumination; infection; interval; necrosis; nephritis; point; reaction; sclerosis; spot

focal condensing: osteitis

focal dermal: hypoplasia

focal embolic: glomerulonephritis

focal epithelial: hyperplasia

focal lymphocytic: thyroiditis

focal metastatic: disease

focal motor: seizure

focal sclerosing: glomerulopathy

focal segmental: glomerulosclerosis

focused: grid

Fogarty: catheter; clamp

fogging: retinoscopy

Foix-Alajouanine: myelitis; syndrome

Foix-Cavany-Marie: syndrome

fold-back: elements

folded-lung: syndrome

folding: fracture

Foley: catheter; operation

Foley Y-plasty: pyeloplasty

foliate: papillae; papillitis

folic acid: antagonists; conjugate

folic acid deficiency: anemia

Folin-Looney: test

Folin's: reaction; reagent; test

folk: medicine

follian: process

follicle-stimulating: hormone; principle

follicle-stimulating hormone-releasing: factor; hormone

follicular: abscess; adenoma; antrum; carcinomas; conjunctivitis; cyst; cystitis; gland; goiter; hormone; impetigo; iritis; lymphoma; mange; mucinosis; papule; stigma; syphilid; trachoma; urethritis; vulvitis

follicular epithelial: cell

follicular ovarian: cells

follicular predominantly large cell: lymphoma

follicular predominantly small cleaved cell: lymphoma

Folling's: disease

Folli's: process

following: bougie

follow-up: study

Foltz': valvule

Fonio's: solution

Fontan: operation; procedure

Fontana-Masson silver: stain

Fontana's: canal; spaces; stain

food: asthma; ball; fever; impaction; poisoning

foot: plate; plugger; process; rot; yaws

foot-and-mouth: disease

foot-and-mouth disease: virus

foot-and-mouth disease virus: vaccines

football: calf

foothill: abortion

footling: presentation

foot-pound-second: system; unit

Foot's reticulin impregnation: stain

foraminal: herniation; lymph node; node

Forbes': disease

Forbes-Albright: syndrome

forced: alimentation; beat; cycle; duction; feeding; respiration

forced expiratory: flow; time; volume

forced grasping: reflex

forced vital: capacity

forceps: delivery

force-velocity: curve

Forchheimer's: sign

Fordyce's: angiokeratoma; disease; granules; spots

forebrain: eminence; prominence; vesicle

foreign: body; protein; serum

foreign-body: appendicitis

foreign body: granuloma; salpingitis; tumorigenesis

foreign body giant: cell

foreign protein: therapy

Forel's: decussation

forensic: dentistry; medicine; odontology; psychiatry; psychology

forequarter: amputation

forest: yaws

Forestier's: disease

Formad's: kidney

formal: operations

formaldehyde: fixative

formalin: pigment

formative: cells

formed visual: hallucination

formol: titration

formol-calcium: fixative

formol-Müller: fixative

formol-saline: fixative

formol-Zenker: fixative

formyl-methionyl-: tRNA

fornicate: gyrus

Forssman: antibody; antigen; hapten; reaction

Forssman antigen-antibody: reaction

Förster's: uveitis

Fort Bragg: fever

fortification: figures; spectrum

fortified: milk

fortified vitamin D: milk

forward: conduction

forward heart: failure

Fosdick-Hansen-Epple: test

Foshay: test

Foster: frame

Foster Kennedy's: syndrome

Fothergill's: disease; neuralgia; operation; sign

Fouchet's: reagent; stain

founder: effect; principle

foundryman's: fever

fountain: decussation; syringe

Fourier: analysis; transfer

Fournier's: disease; gangrene

four-tailed: bandage

fourth: disease; finger; ventricle

fourth cranial: nerve

fourth heart: sound

fourth lumbar: nerve

fourth parallel pelvic: plane

fourth turbinated: bone

foveated: chest

foveolar: cells of stomach

Foville's: fasciculus; syndrome

fowl: cholera; diphtheria; erythroblastosis; leukosis; lymphomatosis; paralysis; pest; plague; typhoid

Fowler's: position

fowl erythroblastosis: virus

fowl lymphomatosis: virus

fowl myeloblastosis: virus

fowl neurolymphomatosis: virus

fowl plague: virus

fowlpox: virus
fox: encephalitis
fox encephalitis: virus
Fox-Fordyce: disease
fractional: distillation; dose; sterilization
fractional epidural: anesthesia
fractional spinal: anesthesia
fracture: bed; box; dislocation
Fraenkel's: pneumococcus
Fraenkel-Weichselbaum: pneumococcus
fragile: site
fragile X: chromosome; syndrome
fragility: test
fragment: reaction
fragmentation: myocarditis
Fraley: syndrome
frambesiform: syphilid
frame-shift: mutagen; mutation
Framingham Heart: study
Franceschetti-Jadassohn: syndrome
Franceschetti's: syndrome
Francke's: needle
frank breech: presentation
Frankenhäuser's: ganglion
Frankfort: plane
Frankfort horizontal: plane
Frankfort-mandibular incisor: angle
Franklin: spectacles
franklinic: taste
Franklin's: disease
Frank-Starling: curve
Fräntzel's: murmur
Fraser-Lendrum: stain for fibrin
Fraser's: syndrome
fraternal: twins
Fraunhofer's: lines
Frazier's: needle
Frazier-Spiller: operation
Fredet-Ramstedt: operation
free: association; border; border of nail; border of ovary; electrophoresis; energy; field; flap; gingiva; graft; macrophage; margin; margin of eyelids; radical; tenia; villus; water
free bone: flap
free-floating: anxiety
free-hand: knife
free induction: decay
free mandibular: movements
Freeman-Sheldon: syndrome
free nerve: endings
free thyroxine: index
free water: clearance
freeway: space
freeze: fracture

freezing: point
Frei: test
Freiberg's: disease
Frei-Hoffmann: reaction
Frejka pillow: splint
French: chalk; flap; polio; scale
French proof: agar
Frenkel's: symptom
Frenkel's anterior ocular traumatic: syndrome
frequency: curve; distribution; spectrum
Frerichs': theory
fresh frozen: plasma
Fresnel: lens; prism
freudian: fixation; psychoanalysis
Freud's: theory
Freund's: adjuvant; anomaly; operation
Freund's complete: adjuvant
Freund's incomplete: adjuvant
Frey's: hairs; syndrome
friction: murmur; rub; sound
frictional: attachment
Fridenberg's stigometric card: test
Friderichsen-Waterhouse: syndrome
Friedländer's: bacillus; pneumonia; stain for capsules
Friedländer's bacillus: pneumonia
Friedman: curve
Friedreich's: ataxia; phenomenon; sign
Friend: disease; virus
Friend leukemia: virus
fright: reaction
Froehde's: reagent
frog: face
frog-leg lateral: projection
Fröhlich's: dwarfism; syndrome
Frohn's: reagent
Froin's: syndrome
Froment's: sign
frontal: angle of parietal bone; area; artery; belly of occipitofrontalis muscle; bone; border; border of parietal bone; border of sphenoid bone; branch of superficial temporal artery; cortex; crest; eminence; fontanel; foramen; grooves; horn; lobe; lobe of cerebrum; margin; nerve; notch; part of corpus callosum; plane; plate; pole; pole of cerebrum; process of maxilla; process of zygomatic bone; region of head; section; sinus;

sinusitis; squama; suture; triangle; tuber; veins
frontalis: muscle
frontal lobe: epilepsy
frontal sinus: aperture
frontoanterior: position
frontoethmoidal: suture
frontolacrimal: suture
frontomaxillary: suture
frontonasal: duct; primordium; process; prominence; suture
fronto-occipital: fasciculus
fronto-orbital: area
frontopontine: tract
frontoposterior: position
frontosphenoidal: process
frontotemporal: tract
frontotransverse: position
frontozygomatic: suture
front-tap: contraction; reflex
Froriep's: ganglion; induration
Frost: suture
frost: itch
frosted: heart; liver
frozen: pelvis; section; shoulder
fructose: malabsorption
fruit: sugar
fruiting: body
frustration: tolerance
frustration-aggression: hypothesis
FTA-ABS: test
Fuchs': adenoma; coloboma; spur; stomas; syndrome; uveitis
Fuchs' black: spot
Fuchs' epithelial: dystrophy
Fuchs' heterochromic: cyclitis
fuchsin: agar; bodies
fuchsinophil: cell; granule; reaction
fugitive: swelling; wart
fugu: poison
fulcrum: line
fulgurating: migraine
full: denture
fuller's: earth
full liquid: diet
full-thickness: burn; flap; graft
fulminant: hepatitis; hyperpyrexia
fulminating: dysentery; smallpox
fuming: nitric acid; sulfuric acid
functional: albuminuria; anatomy; aphasia; apoplexy; asplenia; autonomy; blindness; castration; congestion; contracture; deafness; disease; disorder; dysmenorrhea; dyspepsia;

dyspnea; group; hypertrophy; illness; murmur; neurosurgery; occlusion; pathology; pleiotropy; psychosis; spasm; sphincter; splint; stricture; visual loss
functional cardiovascular: disease
functional chew-in: record
functional jaw: orthopedics
functional mandibular: movements
functional occlusal: harmony
functional orthodontic: therapy
functional prepubertal castration: syndrome
functional refractory: period
functional residual: air; capacity
functional terminal innervation: ratio
functional vocal: fatigue
fundamental: frequency; tone
fundiform: ligament of foot; ligament of penis
fundus: glands; reflex
fungating: sore
fungiform: papillae
fungous: foot
fungus: ball
funic: souffle
funicular: graft; hydrocele; myelitis; myelosis; process
funnel: breast
funnel-shaped: pelvis
furcal: nerve
furfurol: reaction
furious: rabies
furnacemen's: cataract
furred: tongue
fused: kidney; silver nitrate; teeth
fusel: oil
fusible: metal
fusiform: aneurysm; cataract; cells of cerebral cortex; gyrus; layer; muscle
fusing: point
fusion: area; beat; energy; temperature (wire method)
fusional: movement
fusion-inferred threshold: test
fusospirochetal: disease; gingivitis; stomatitis
Futcher's: line
futile: cycle
Fy: antigens

G

γ: hemolysis

G: antigen; cells; factor; force; proteins; syndrome; unit of streptomycin
G$_{M1}$: gangliosidosis
G$_{M2}$: gangliosidosis
G-: actin; protein
GABA: pathway
Gaboon: ulcer
Gaddum and Schild: test
Gaenslen's: sign
Gaffky: scale; table
gag: reflex
Gairdner's: disease
Gaisböck's: syndrome
gait: apraxia
GAL: virus
galactagogue: factor
galactokinase: deficiency
galactokinase deficiency: galactosemia
galactophorous: canals; ducts
galactopoietic: factor; hormone
galactose: cataract; diabetes
galactose tolerance: test
galactosylceramide: lipoidosis
Galant's: reflex
Galassi's pupillary: phenomenon
Galeati's: glands
Galeazzi's: fracture
Galen's: anastomosis; nerve
gall: bladder; duct
Gallavardin's: phenomenon
gallbladder: fossa
Gallego's differentiating: solution
Gallie's: transplant
gallop: rhythm; sound
Gall's: craniology
gallstone: colic; ileus
gallus adeno-like: virus
galoche: chin
galtonian: genetics; inheritance; trait
Galtonian-Fisher: genetics
Galton's: delta; law; whistle
Galton's system of classification of: fingerprints
galvanic: cautery; current; nystagmus; threshold
galvanic skin: reaction; reflex; response
galvanocaustic: snare
Gambian: fever; trypanosomiasis
game: theory
gamekeeper's: thumb
gametic: nucleus
gametokinetic: hormone
Gamgee: tissue
gamma: alcoholism; angle; camera; cell of pancreas; crystallin; efferent;

encephalography; fibers; loop; radiation; rays
gamma motor: neurons; system
gamma ray: knife
Gamna-Favre: bodies
Gamna-Gandy: bodies; nodules
Gamna's: disease
Gandy-Gamna: bodies
Gandy-Nanta: disease
gangliated: cord; nerve
ganglion: cell; cells of dorsal spinal root; cells of retina; ridge
ganglionic: blockade; branches of lingual nerve; branches of maxillary nerve; branch of internal carotid artery; crest; layer of cerebellar cortex; layer of cerebral cortex; layer of optic nerve; layer of retina; saliva
ganglionic blocking: agent
ganglionic motor: neuron
ganglioside: lipidosis
gangrenous: appendicitis; cellulitis; emphysema; pharyngitis; pneumonia; rhinitis; stomatitis
Ganser's: commissures; syndrome
Gant's: clamp
Gantzer's: muscle
Gantzer's accessory: bundle
Ganzfeld: stimulation
Gap$_1$: period; phase
Gap$_2$: period; phase
gap: arthroplasty; junction; phenomenon
garapata: disease
Gardner-Diamond: syndrome
Gardnerella: vaginitis
Gardner's: syndrome
gargantuan: mastitis
Gariel's: pessary
Garland's: triangle
Garré's: disease; osteomyelitis
Gartner's: canal; cyst; duct
Gärtner's: bacillus; method; tonometer
Gärtner's vein: phenomenon
gas: abscess; bacillus; cautery; chromatography; constant; cyst; embolism; gangrene; peritonitis; phlegmon; retinopexy; thermometer
gaseous: mediastinography; pulse
gas gangrene: antitoxin
Gaskell's: bridge; clamp
gas-liquid: chromatography
gasping: disease
gasserian: ganglion

gastral: mesoderm
gastrea: theory
gastric: analysis; area; arteries; branches of anterior vagal trunk; branches of posterior vagal trunk; bypass; calculus; canal; colic; crisis; diastole; digestion; feeding; fistula; folds; follicles; freezing; glands; hemorrhage; impression; indigestion; juice; mucin; mucosa; neurasthenia; pit; plexuses of autonomic system; smear; stapling; surface of spleen; tetany; ulcer; veins; vertigo; volvulus
gastric algid: malaria
gastric inhibitory: peptide; polypeptide
gastric lymphatic: follicles
gastrocardiac: syndrome
gastrocnemius: muscle
gastrocolic: fistula; ligament; omentum; reflex
gastrocutaneous: fistula
gastrodiaphragmatic: ligament
gastroduodenal: artery; fistula; lymph nodes; orifice
gastroenteritis: virus type A; virus type B
gastroepiploic: arteries; veins
gastroesophageal: hernia; vestibule
gastrogenous: diarrhea
gastrografin: swallow
gastrohepatic: omentum
gastroileac: reflex
gastrointestinal: fistula; hormone; tract
gastrojejunal loop obstruction: syndrome
gastrolienal: ligament
gastro-omental: arteries
gastropancreatic: folds
gastrophrenic: ligament
gastrosplenic: ligament; omentum
Gatch: bed
gate-control: hypothesis; theory
gated radionuclide: angiocardiography
gating: mechanism
Gaucher: cells; disorder
Gaucher's: disease
gauge: pressure
gauntlet: bandage
Gauss': sign
gaussian: curve; distribution
gauze: bandage
Gavard's: muscle
gay bowel: syndrome

Gay-Lussac's: equation; law
Gay's: glands
gaze paretic: nystagmus
G-banding: stain
GC: content
Ge: antigen
Geigel's: reflex
Geiger-Müller: counter; tube
gel: diffusion; electrophoresis; filtration; structure
gelastic: seizure
gelatin: sugar
gelatinous: ascites; infiltration; nucleus; polyp; scleritis; substance; tissue; varix
gel diffusion: reactions
gel diffusion precipitin: tests; tests in one dimension; tests in two dimensions
gel filtration: chromatography
Gélineau's: syndrome
Gell and Coombs: Classification; reactions
Gellé: test
Gély's: suture
geminated: teeth
gemistocytic: astrocyte; astrocytoma; cell; reaction
genal: glands
gender: identity; role
gender dysphoria: syndrome
gender identity: disorders
gene: activation; deletion; duplication; expression; flow; frequency; mosaicism; pool; regulation; therapy
gene dosage: compensation; effect
general: anatomy; anesthesia; anesthetic; bloodletting; hospital; immunity; paresis; peritonitis; physiology; practice; sensation; stimulant; transduction; tuberculosis
general adaptation: reaction; syndrome
general duty: nurse
general fertility: rate
generalized: anaphylaxis; chondromalacia; elastolysis; emphysema; epilepsy; gangliosidosis; glycogenosis; lentiginosis; myokymia; paralysis; seizures; tetanus; vaccinia; xanthelasma
generalized anxiety: disorder
generalized cortical: hyperostosis

generalized epidermolytic: hyperkeratosis

generalized eruptive: histiocytoma

generalized pustular: psoriasis of Zambusch

generalized Shwartzman: phenomenon

generalized tonic-clonic: epilepsy; seizure

general somatic afferent: column

general somatic efferent: column

general visceral afferent: column

general visceral efferent: column

generated occlusal: path

generation: effect

generative: empathy

generator: potential

genesial: cycle

genetic: amplification; association; burden; carrier; code; colonization; compound; counseling; death; determinant; disequilibrium; dominance; drift; engineering; equilibrium; female; fingerprint; fitness; fixation; heterogeneity; homeostasis; isolate; lethal; linkage; load; locus; marker; material; model; penetrance; polymorphism; psychology; recombination; testing

genetic human: male

Gengou: phenomenon

genial: tubercle

genicular: arteries

geniculate: body; ganglion; neuralgia; otalgia; zoster

geniculatus lateralis: nucleus

geniculocalcarine: radiation; tract

genioglossal: muscle

genioglossus: muscle

geniohyoid: muscle

genital: branch of genitofemoral nerve; branch of iliohypogastric nerve; cord; corpuscles; duct; eminence; fold; furrow; gland; ligament; organs; phase; primacy; ridge; stage; swellings; system; tract; tubercle; wart

genitocrural: nerve

genitofemoral: nerve

genitoinguinal: ligament

genitourinary: apparatus; fistula; system

Gennari's: band; stria

genomic: DNA; library

gentian aniline: water

genucubital: position

genupectoral: position

geographic: choroidopathy; keratitis; stippling of nails; tongue

geometric: isomer; isomerism; mean

geometrical: sense

Geraghty's: test

Gerbich: antigen

Gerbode: defect

Gerdy's: fibers; fontanel; ligament; tubercle

Gerdy's hyoid: fossa

Gerdy's interatrial: loop

Gerhardt-Mitchell: disease

Gerhardt's: disease; reaction; sign; test for acetoacetic acid; test for urobilin in the urine

Gerhardt-Semon: law

geriatric: medicine; therapy

Gerlach's: tonsil; valve; valvula

Gerlach's annular: tendon

Gerlier's: disease

germ: cell; layer; line; membrane; nucleus; theory; tube

German: measles

German measles: virus

germinal: aplasia; area; cell; center of Flemming; cords; disk; epithelium; localization; mosaicism; pole; rod; streak; vesicle

germinative: layer; layer of nail

Germiston: virus

germ layer: theory

germ tube: test

Gerota's: capsule; fascia; method

Gerstmann: syndrome

Gerstmann-Sträussler: syndrome

gestalt: phenomenon; psychology; theory; therapy

gestational: age; diabetes; edema; proteinuria; psychosis

Gey's: solution

ghatti: gum

Gheel: colony

Ghon's: complex; focus; tubercle

Ghon-Sachs: bacillus

Ghon's primary: lesion

ghost: cell; corpuscle; tooth

ghost cell: glaucoma

ghoul: hand

Giannuzzi's: crescents; demilunes

Gianotti-Crosti: syndrome

giant: cell; chromosome; colon; condyloma; drusen; fibroadenoma; hives; hypertrophy of gastric mucosa; melanosome; urticaria

giant axonal: neuropathy

giant cell: aortitis; arteritis; carcinoma; carcinoma of thyroid gland; epulis; fibroma; granuloma; hepatitis; myeloma; myocarditis; pneumonia; sarcoma; thyroiditis; tumor of bone; tumor of tendon sheath

giant cell hyaline: angiopathy

giant cell monstrocellular: sarcoma of Zülch

giant follicular: lymphoblastoma; thyroiditis

giant gastric: folds

giant osteoid: osteoma

giant pigmented: nevus

Gibbs: energy of activation

Gibbs': theorem

Gibbs-Donnan: equilibrium

Gibbs free: energy

Gibbs-Helmholtz: equation

Gibb's phase: rule

Gibney's: boot

Gibney's fixation: bandage

Gibson: murmur

Gibson's: bandage

Giemsa: stain

Giemsa chromosome banding: stain

Gierke: cells

Gierke's: disease

Gierke's respiratory: bundle

Gifford's: reflex

gigantiform: cementoma

gigantocellular: glioma; nucleus of medulla oblongata

Gigli's: operation; saw

Gilbert's: disease; syndrome

Gilchrist's: disease; mycosis

gill: clefts

gill arch: skeleton

Gilles de la Tourette's: disease; syndrome

Gillette's suspensory: ligament

Gilliam's: operation

Gillies': operation

Gillmore: needle

Gilmer: wiring

Gil-Vernet: operation

Gimbernat's: ligament

ginger: paralysis

gingival: abrasion; abscess; atrophy; clamp; cleft; contour; crest; crevice; curvature; cyst; elephantiasis; embrasure;

enlargement; epithelium; festoon; fibromatosis; fistula; flap; fluid; hyperplasia; margin; massage; mucosa; pocket; proliferation; recession; repositioning; resorption; retraction; septum; space; sulcus; tissues; trough; zone

gingivobuccal: groove; sulcus

gingivodental: ligament

gingivolabial: groove; sulcus

gingivolingual: groove; sulcus

ginglymoid: joint

Giordano-Giovannetti: diet

Giovannetti: diet

Girard's: reagent

girdle: anesthesia; pain; sensation

Girdlestone: procedure

gitter: cell

glabrous: skin

glacial: acetic acid; phosphoric acid

glairy: mucus

glancing: wound

glanders: bacillus

glandular: branches; branches of anterior/lateral/posterior branches of superior thyroid artery; branches of facial artery; branches of inferior thyroid artery; branches of submandibular ganglion; cancer; carcinoma; epithelium; fever; lobe of hypophysis; mastitis; plague; substance of prostate; system; tularemia

glandulopreputial: lamella

glanular: hypospadias

Glanzmann's: disease; thrombasthenia

glaserian: artery; fissure

Glasgow's: sign

glass: body; electrode; factor; rays

glass bead: sterilizer

Glasser's: disease

glass ionomer: cement

glassworker's: cataract

glassy: membrane

Glauber's: salt

glaucomatocyclitic: crisis

glaucomatous: cataract; cup; excavation; halo; ring

glaucomatous nerve-fiber bundle: scotoma

Gleason's: score

Gleason's tumor: grade

Glenn: shunt

Glenner-Lillie: stain for pituitary

Glenn's: operation
glenohumeral: articulation; ligaments
glenoid: cavity; fossa; labrum; ligament; surface
glenoidal: lip
Gley's: glands
glia: cells
glial limiting: membrane
gliding: joint; occlusion
Glisson's: capsule; cirrhosis; sphincter
glitter: cells
global: aphasia; paralysis
globe cell: anemia
globin: insulin
globin zinc: insulin
globoid: cell
globoid cell: leukodystrophy
globosus: nucleus
globular: heart; leukocyte; process; protein; sputum; thrombus
globulomaxillary: cyst
glomerular: capsule; crescent; cysts; layer of olfactory bulb; nephritis; sclerosis
glomerular filtration: rate
glomerulosa: cell
glomiform: glands
glomus: body; tumor
glomus jugulare: tumor
glossoepiglottic: ligament
glossolabiolaryngeal: paralysis
glossopalatine: arch; fold
glossopalatolabial: paralysis
glossopharyngeal: breathing; nerve; neuralgia; part of superior pharyngeal constrictor; tic
glossopharyngeolabial: paralysis
glossy: skin
glove: anesthesia
gloved-finger: sign
Glover: phenomenon
glover's: suture
glucagonoma: syndrome
glucose oxidase: method
glucose oxidase paper strip: test
glucose-6-phosphatase hepatorenal: glycogenosis
glucose-6-phosphate dehydrogenase: deficiency
glucosephosphate isomerase: deficiency
glucose tolerance: factor; test
glucose transport: maximum
glucosidase: inhibitors
β-*d*-glucuronidase: deficiency
glue: ear
Gluge's: corpuscles
γ-glutamyl: cycle

glutaraldehyde: fixative
glutathione synthetase: deficiency
gluteal: cleft; crest; fold; furrow; hernia; line; lymph nodes; reflex; region; ridge; surface of ilium; tuberosity; veins
gluten: enteropathy
gluten-free: diet
gluteofemoral: bursa
gluteus maximus: gait; muscle
gluteus medius: bursae; gait; muscle
gluteus minimus: bursa; muscle
glycerin: suppository
glycerinated: gelatin; tincture
glycerophosphate: shuttle
glycine-succinate: cycle
glycogen: cardiomegaly; granule
glycogenic: acanthosis; cardiomegaly
glycogen-storage: disease
glycol: ethers
glycolipid: lipidosis
glycosyl: compound
glycosylated: hemoglobin
glycotropic: factor
glycyl: chain
glyoxylic acid: cycle
Gm: allotypes; antigens
Gmelin's: test
gnathic: index
gnome's: calf
goatpox: virus
goat's milk: anemia
goblet: cell
Godélier's: law
Godman's: fascia
Godwin: tumor
Goeckerman: treatment
Goethe's: bone
Gofman: test
Goggia's: sign
gold: alloy; casting; equivalent; inlay; number
Goldblatt: hypertension; kidney; phenomenon
Goldblatt's: clamp
Goldenhar's: syndrome
Goldflam: disease
Goldman: equation
Goldman-Fox: knives
Goldman-Hodgkin-Katz: equation
Goldmann: perimeter
Goldmann's applanation: tonometer
gold-myokymia: syndrome
Goldscheider's: test
gold sol: test
Goldstein's toe: sign
Goldthwait's: sign
golfer's: skin

golf-hole ureteral: orifice
Golgi: apparatus; body; complex; corpuscle; zone
Golgi epithelial: cell
Golgi internal: reticulum
Golgi-Mazzoni: corpuscle
Golgi's: cells; stain
Golgi's osmiobichromate: fixative
Golgi tendon: organ
Golgi type I: neuron
Golgi type II: neuron
Goll's: column
Goltz: syndrome
Gombault's: triangle
Gomori-Jones periodic acid-methenamine-silver: stain
Gomori's aldehyde fuchsin: stain
Gomori's chrome alum hematoxylin-phloxine: stain
Gomori's methenamine-silver: stain
Gomori's nonspecific acid phosphatase: stain
Gomori's nonspecific alkaline phosphatase: stain
Gomori's one-step trichrome: stain
Gomori's silver impregnation: stain
Gompertz': hypothesis; law
gompholic: joint
gonad: dose; nucleus
gonadal: agenesis; aplasia; cords; dose; dysgenesis; hormones; ridge; streak
gonadal steroid-binding: globulin
gonadotrophic: cycle
gonadotropic: hormone
gonadotropin-producing: adenoma
gonadotropin-releasing: factor; hormone
gonococcal: arthritis; conjunctivitis; stomatitis
gonorrheal: conjunctivitis; ophthalmia; rheumatism; salpingitis; urethritis
Good: antigen
good: object
Goodell's: dilator; sign
Goodenough draw-a-man: test
Goodman's: syndrome
goodness of fit: test
Goodpasture's: stain; syndrome
Goormaghtigh's: cells
goose: flesh; parvovirus
goose viral: hepatitis
Gopalan's: syndrome
Gordon: reflex
Gordon's: sign; symptom

Gordon and Sweet: stain
Gorham's: disease
Goriaew's: rule
Gorlin: cyst; formula
Gorlin-Chaudhry-Moss: syndrome
Gorlin's: sign; syndrome
Gorman's: syndrome
Gosselin's: fracture
Gothic: arch; palate
Gothic arch: tracing
Göthlin's: test
Gougerot and Blum: disease
Gougerot-Carteaud: syndrome
Gougerot-Sjögren: disease
Gould's: suture
Gouley's: catheter
gout: diet
gouty: arthritis; diathesis; pearl; tophus; urine
government: hospital
Gowers: disease
Gowers': column; contraction; syndrome; tract
Gr: antigen
graafian: follicle
gracile: fasciculus; habitus; lobule; nucleus; tubercle
gracilis: muscle; syndrome
grade I: astrocytoma
grade II: astrocytoma
grade III: astrocytoma
grade IV: astrocytoma
Gradenigo's: syndrome
gradient: elution
graduate: nurse
graduated: compress; pipette; tenotomy
Graefe: forceps
Graefenberg: ring
Graefe's: knife; operation; sign; spots
Graffi's: virus
graft versus host: disease; reaction
Graham-Cole: test
Graham Little: syndrome
Graham's: law
Graham Steell's: murmur
grain: alcohol; itch
gram: calorie; equivalent
gram-: ion
gram-atomic: weight
gram-molecular: weight
Gram's: iodine; stain
grand: climacteric; mal; multipara
granddaughter: cyst
grandiose: delusion
grandiose type of paranoid: disorder
grand mal: epilepsy; seizure
Grandry's: corpuscles
Granger: projection
Granger's: line
Granit's: loop

granny: knot
granular: cast; conjunctivitis; cortex; degeneration; kidney; layer of cerebellar cortex; layer of cerebellum; layer of epidermis; layers of cerebral cortex; layers of retina; layer of a vesicular ovarian follicle; leukoblast; leukocyte; lids; ophthalmia; pits; pneumonocytes; trachoma; urethritis; vaginitis
granular cell: myoblastoma; tumor
granular endoplasmic: reticulum
granulated: opium
granulation: tissue
granule: cell of connective tissue; cells
granulocyte colony-stimulating: factor
granulocyte-macrophage colony-stimulating: factor
granulocytic: leukemia; sarcoma; series
granulomatous: arteritis; colitis; disease; encephalomyelitis; endophthalmitis; enteritis; inflammation; mastitis; meningoencephalomyelitis; nocardiosis; rosacea
granulosa: cell
granulosa cell: tumor
granulosa lutein: cells
granulovacuolar: degeneration
grape: endings; mole; sugar
graphic: aphasia; formula
graphomotor: aphasia
grasp: reflex
grasping: reflex
grass: bacillus; tetany
Grasset-Gaussel: phenomenon
Grasset's: law; phenomenon; sign
Gratiolet's: fibers; radiation
gratuitous: inducer
Gräupner's: method
grave: wax
Graves': disease; ophthalmopathy; orbitopathy
Graves' optic: neuropathy
gravid: uterus
gravidic: retinitis; retinopathy
gravitation: abscess
gravitational: ulcer; units
Grawitz': basophilia; tumor
gray: cataract; columns; degeneration; fibers; hepatization; induration; infiltration; layer of

superior colliculus; matter; rami communicantes; scale; substance; syndrome; tuber; tubercle; wing
gray collie: syndrome
gray-scale: ultrasonography
grease: heel
greaseless: cream
greasy pig: disease
great: foramen; toe; vein of Galen
great adductor: muscle
great alveolar: cells
great anastomotic: artery
great auricular: nerve
great cardiac: vein
great cerebral: vein; vein of Galen
greater: circulation; cul-de-sac; curvature of stomach; horn of hyoid bone; omentum; pelvis; ring of iris; trochanter; tubercle of humerus; tuberosity of humerus; wing of sphenoid bone
greater alar: cartilage
greater arterial: circle of iris
greater multangular: bone
greater occipital: nerve
greater palatine: artery; canal; foramen; groove; nerve
greater pectoral: muscle
greater peritoneal: cavity
greater petrosal: nerve
greater posterior rectus: muscle of head
greater psoas: muscle
greater rhomboid: muscle
greater sciatic: notch
greater splanchnic: nerve
greater superficial petrosal: nerve
greater supraclavicular: fossa
greater tympanic: spine
greater vestibular: gland
greater zygomatic: muscle
greatest: length
great horizontal: fissure
great longitudinal: fissure
great pancreatic: artery
great radicular: artery
great saphenous: vein
great sciatic: nerve
great superior pancreatic: artery
great-toe: reflex
green: cancer; hemoglobin; pus; sickness; soap; sputum; stain; tooth; vision
Greenfield: filter
Greenhow's: disease
green monkey: virus
green soap: tincture
greenstick: fracture

green tobacco: sickness
Greig's: syndrome
grenz: ray; zone
Greville: bath
Grey Turner's: sign
grid: ratio
Gridley's: stain; stain for fungi
Griesinger's: disease; sign; symptom
grinding: surface
Grisolle's: sign
Gritti's: operation
Gritti-Stokes: amputation
Grocco's: sign; triangle
grocer's: itch
Grocott-Gomori methenamine-silver: stain
Groenouw's corneal: dystrophy
groin: ulcer
Grönblad-Strandberg: syndrome
groove: sign
grooved: tongue
Gross': virus
gross: anatomy; hematuria; lesion
Gross' leukemia: virus
gross reproduction: rate
ground: bundles; itch; lamella; state; substance
ground-glass: cytoplasm; pattern
ground itch: anemia
group: agglutination; agglutinin; antigens; dynamics; hospital; immunity; practice; psychotherapy; reaction; test; transfer; translocation
group A: streptococci
group A streptococcal necrotizing: fasciitis
group B: streptococci
group I: mycobacteria
group II: mycobacteria
group III: mycobacteria
group IV: mycobacteria
Grover's: disease
growing: fracture; pains
growing ovarian: follicle
growth: curve; factors; hormone; hormone-releasing hormone; medium; phase; quotient; rate; rate of population; regulators
growth arrest: lines
growth hormone inhibiting: hormone
growth hormone-producing: adenoma
growth hormone-releasing: factor
growth-onset: diabetes
Gruber-Landzert: fossa

Gruber's: cul-de-sac; method; reaction
Gruber-Widal: reaction
Grunert's: spur
Grunstein-Hogness: assay
Grynfeltt's: triangle
gryposis: penis
GTP binding: proteins
guaiac: gum; test
Guama: virus
guanine: cell
guar: gum
Guarnieri: bodies
Guarnieri's gelatin: agar
Guaroa: virus
gubernacular: canal; cord
Gubler's: line; paralysis; syndrome; tumor
Gudden's: commissures; ganglion
Gudden's tegmental: nuclei
Guéneau de Mussy's: point
Guérin's: fold; fracture; glands; sinus; valve
guide: plane; wire
Guillain-Barré: reflex; syndrome
guillotine: amputation
guinea corn: yaws
Guldberg-Waage: law
Gulf War: syndrome
Gullstrand's: slitlamp
gum: contour; lancet; line; resection; resin
Gumboro: disease
gummatous: abscess; syphilid; ulcer
Gumprecht's: shadows
Gunn: phenomenon; pupil
Gunning: splint
Günning's: reaction
Gunn's: dots; sign; syndrome
Gunn's crossing: sign
gunshot: wound
gunstock: deformity
Günz': ligament
Günzberg's: reagent; test
gurgling: rale
Gussenbauer's: suture
gustatory: anesthesia; bud; cells; hallucination; hyperesthesia; hyperhidrosis; lemniscus; nucleus; organ; pore; rhinorrhea
gustatory-sudorific: reflex
gustatory sweating: syndrome
gut: glucagon
gut-associated lymphoid: tissue
Guthrie: test
Guthrie's: muscle
gutta-percha: cone; points; spreader
guttate: choroidopathy

gutter: dystrophy of cornea; fracture; wound
guttural: duct; pouch; pulse; rale
Gutzeit's: test
Guyon's: amputation; isthmus; sign
GVH: disease
gym: -diol
gynecoid: pelvis
gynecophoric: canal
gyrate: atrophy of choroid and retina
gyrochrome: cell
gyromagnetic: ratio

H

H: agglutinin; antigen; band; colony; disk; fields; gene; graft; rays; reflex; shunt; substance
H-2: antigens; complex
H-: meromyosin
HA1: virus
HA2: virus
haarscheibe: tumor
Haase's: rule
habenular: commissure; nucleus; sulcus; trigone
habenulointerpeduncular: tract
habenulopeduncular: tract
Haber's: syndrome
Haber-Weiss: reaction
habit: chorea; scoliosis; spasm; tic
habitual: abortion
HACEK: group
Haeckel's: law
Haeckel's gastrea: theory
Haemophilus influenzae **type B:** vaccine
Haenel's: symptom
Haff: disease
Haffkine's: vaccine
hafussi: bath
Hagedorn: needle
Hageman: factor
Haglund's: deformity; disease
Hahn's oxine: reagent
Haidinger's: brushes
Hailey-Hailey: disease
hair: ball; bulb; cast; cells; crosses; cycle; disk; follicle; papilla; root; shaft; streams; transplant; whorls
hairline: fracture
hairpin: loops
hairy: cells; heart; leukoplakia; mole; tongue
hairy cell: leukemia
hairy shaker: disease
Halberstaedter-Prowazek: bodies

Haldane: chamber; effect; relationship; transformation; tube
Haldane-Priestley: sample
Haldane's: apparatus
Hales': piesimeter
Hale's colloidal iron: stain
half: cystine; hapten
half-: life; time
half amplitude pulse: duration
half-axial: projection
half axial: view
half-chair: form
half-glass: spectacles
half and half: nail
half-value: layer
Haller: cell
Hallermann-Streiff: syndrome
Hallermann-Streiff-François: syndrome
Haller's: annulus; ansa; arches; circle; cones; habenula; insula; line; plexus; rete; tripod; tunica vasculosa; unguis; vas aberrans
Haller's vascular: tissue
Hallervorden: syndrome
Hallervorden-Spatz: disease; syndrome
Hallé's: point
Hallgren's: syndrome
Hallopeau's: disease
hallucinatory: neuralgia
halo: cast; effect; melanoma; nevus; sign; sign of hydrops; traction; vision
halogen: acne
halothane: hepatitis
halothane-ether: azeotrope
Halstead-Reitan: battery
Halsted's: law; operation; suture
hamate: bone
Hamburger's: law; phenomenon
Hamilton's: pseudophlegmon
Hamilton-Stewart: formula; method
Hamman-Rich: syndrome
Hamman's: disease; murmur; sign; syndrome
Hammarsten's: reagent
hammer: finger; nose; toe
Hammerschlag's: method
hammock: bandage; ligament
Hammond's: disease
Hampton: line; maneuver; technique
Hampton's: hump
Ham's: test
hamstring: muscles; tendon

hamular: notch; process of lacrimal bone; process of sphenoid bone
Hancock's: amputation
hand: eczema; ratio
hand-and-foot: syndrome
hand-foot-and-mouth: disease
hand-foot-and-mouth disease: virus
Hand-Schüller-Christian: disease
Hanes: plot
hanging: drop; septum
hanging-block: culture
hangman's: fracture
Hanhart's: syndrome
Hanks: dilators
Hanks': solution
Hannover's: canal
Hanot's: cirrhosis
Hansemann: macrophage
Hansen's: bacillus; disease
Hantaan: virus
haphazard: sampling
haploid: set
haploscopic: vision
happy puppet: syndrome
Hapsburg: jaw; lip
hapten: inhibition of precipitation
haptic: hallucination
Harada's: disease; syndrome
hard: cataract; chancre; corn; palate; papilloma; paraffin; pulse; rays; soap; sore; tissue; tubercle; ulcer; water
hardened: pelvis
Harden-Young: ester
Harder's: gland
Harding-Passey: melanoma
hardness: scale
hard pad: disease; virus
hardware: disease
Hardy-Rand-Ritter: test
Hardy-Weinberg: equilibrium; law
hare's: eye
harlequin: fetus; ichthyosis; reaction
harmonic: mean; suture
harmonious: correspondence
Harrington-Flocks: test
Harris: syndrome; test
Harris': hematoxylin; lines; migraine
Harrison's: groove
Harris and Ray: test
Hartel: technique
Hartmann's: curette; operation; pouch; solution
Hartman's: solution
Hartnup: disease; disorder; syndrome
harvester: ant
Häser's: formula

Hashimoto's: disease; struma; thyroiditis
Hasner's: fold; valve
Hassall-Henle: bodies
Hassall's: bodies
Hassall's concentric: corpuscle
Hasson: cannula; trocar
hatchet: excavator
Haudek's: niche
Haverhill: fever
Havers': glands
haversian: canals; lamella; spaces; system
Hawley: appliance; retainer
Haworth: projection
Haworth conformational formulas of cyclic: sugars
Haworth perspective and conformational: formulas
Haworth perspective formulas of cyclic: sugars
Hawthorne: effect
hay: asthma; bacillus; fever
Hayem's: hematoblast; solution
Hayem-Widal: syndrome
Hayflick's: limit
Haygarth's: nodes; nodosities
hazard: rate
H and D: curve
He: antigens
head: botflies; cap; cavity; fold; kidney; mirror; nurse; presentation; process; tetanus; tremors
head-bobbing doll: syndrome
head-dropping: test
Head's: areas; lines; zones
healed: tuberculosis; ulcer
health: behavior; care; indicator; promotion; psychology
health maintenance: organization
health status: index
healthy worker: effect
Heaney's: operation
hearing: level
heart: antigen; arrest; beat; block; failure; hormone; massage; position; rate; sac; sounds; stroke; tamponade; tones; transplantation
heart failure: cells
heart-lung: machine; preparation; transplantation
heart-shaped: pelvis; uterus
heart valve: prosthesis
heat: apoplexy; capacity; cramps; edema; exhaustion; hyperpyrexia; lamp; prostration; rash; rigor; stroke; treatment; urticaria
heat coagulation: test

heat-curing: resin
Heath-Edwards: grades
heat instability: test
heat-rigor: point
heat shock: proteins
heat-stable: enzyme
heavy: chain; hydrogen; metal; nitrogen; oxygen; water
μ-heavy-chain: disease
α-heavy-chain: disease
γ-heavy-chain: disease
heavy chain: disease
heavy liquid: petrolatum
heavy metal: neuropathy
hebephrenic: dementia; schizophrenia
Heberden's: angina; nodes; nodosities
Hebra's: disease; prurigo
Hecht's: pneumonia
Heck's: disease
hectic: flush
hederiform: ending
Hedström: file
heel: bone; fly; jar; tap; tendon
heel-tap: reaction; test
heel-to-knee-to-toe: test
heel-to-shin: test
Heerfordt's: disease
Hegar's: dilators; sign
Hegglin's: anomaly; syndrome
Hehner: number; value
Heidelberger: curve
Heidenhain: pouch
Heidenhain's: crescents; demilunes; law
Heidenhain's azan: stain
Heidenhain's iron hematoxylin: stain
height of: contour
height: vertigo
height-length: index
Heilbronner's: thigh
Heim-Kreysig: sign
Heimlich: maneuver
Heineke-Mikulicz: pyloroplasty
Heinz: bodies
Heinz body: anemia; test
Heinz-Ehrlich: body
Heister's: diverticulum; valve
HeLa: cells
Helbings': sign
Held's: bundle; decussation
helical: CT
helical computed: tomography
helicine: arteries of the penis
helicis major: muscle
helicis minor: muscle
helicoid: choroidopathy; ginglymus
helicopod: gait
Helie's: bundle

helium: speech
Heller: myotomy; operation
Heller's: plexus
Hellin's: law
HELLP: syndrome
Helly's: fixative
helmet: cell
Helmholtz: energy; theory of accommodation; theory of color vision; theory of hearing
Helmholtz' axis: ligament
Helmholtz-Gibbs: theory
helminthic: dysentery
helper: cell; virus
Helweg-Larssen: syndrome
Helweg's: bundle
hemadsorption: virus type 1; virus type 2
hemadsorption virus: test
hemagglutinating cold: autoantibody
hemagglutination: inhibition; test
hemal: arches; gland; node; spine
hemangiectatic: hypertrophy
hemangioma-thrombocytopenia: syndrome
hematinic: principle
hematogenetic: calculus
hematogenous: abscess; embolism; jaundice; metastasis; osteitis; pigment; theory of endometriosis
hematoidin: crystals
hematopoietic: gland; system
hematoxylin: bodies
hematoxylin and eosin: stain
hematoxylin-malachite green-basic fuchsin: stain
hematoxylin-phloxine B: stain
hematuric bilious: fever
hemianopic: scotoma; spectacles
hemiazygos: vein
hemic: calculus; distomiasis; murmur
hemilateral: chorea
hemiplegic: amyotrophy; gait; migraine
hemisulfur: mustard
hemithoracic: duct
hemizona: assay
hemoccult: test
hemochorial: placenta
hemoclastic: reaction
hemoendothelial: placenta
hemoglobin C: disease
hemoglobin H: disease
hemoglobinuric: fever; nephrosis
hemolymph: gland; node

hemolysin: unit
β-hemolytic: streptococci
hemolytic: anemia; anemia of newborn; chain; disease of newborn; gas; jaundice; splenomegaly; streptococci
hemolytic uremic: syndrome
hemophilic: arthritis; joint
hemopoietic: tissue
hemorrhagic: anemia; ascites; bronchitis; colitis; cyst; cystitis; dengue; diathesis; disease of deer; disease of the newborn; endovasculitis; enteritis; fever; fever with renal syndrome; gangrene; glaucoma; infarct; iritis; measles; nephritis; pachymeningitis; pericarditis; pian; plague; pleurisy; rickets; scurvy; septicemia; shock; smallpox
hemorrhagic exudative: erythema
hemorrhoidal: nerves; plexus; veins; zone
hemostatic: collodion; forceps
HEMPAS: cells
hen-cluck: stertor
Henderson-Hasselbalch: equation
Henke's: space
Henle's: ampulla; ansa; fissures; glands; layer; loop; membrane; reaction; sheath; spine; tubules; warts
Henle's fenestrated elastic: membrane
Henle's fiber: layer
Henle's nervous: layer
Hennebert's: sign
Henoch's: chorea; purpura
Henoch-Schönlein: purpura; syndrome
Henry-Gauer: response
Henry's: law
Hensen's: canal; cell; disk; duct; knot; line; node; stripe
Hensing's: ligament
heparin: complement; unit
hepatic: adenoma; amebiasis; arteries; branches of vagus nerve; capsulitis; colic; coma; cords; cysts; duct; encephalopathy; fistula; flexure; infantilism; insufficiency; laminae; lobule; lymph nodes; plexus; porphyria; prominence; segments; steatosis; triad; veins
hepatic intermittent: fever
hepatic portal: system; vein

hepatic venous: segments
hepatitis A: virus
hepatitis-associated: antigen
hepatitis B: vaccine; virus
hepatitis B core: antigen
hepatitis B e: antigen
hepatitis B surface: antigen
hepatitis C: virus
hepatitis delta: virus
hepatitis E: virus
hepatocellular: adenoma; carcinoma; jaundice
hepatocolic: ligament
hepatocystic: duct
hepatoduodenal: ligament
hepatoenteric: recess
hepatoerythropoietic: porphyria
hepatoesophageal: ligament
hepatogastric: ligament
hepatogenous: jaundice; pigment
hepatojugular: reflex; reflux
hepatolenticular: degeneration; disease
hepatopancreatic: ampulla; sphincter
hepatophosphorylase deficiency: glycogenosis
hepatopleural: fistula
hepatorenal: ligament; pouch; recess; syndrome
herald: patch
Herbst's: corpuscles
herd: immunity; instinct
hereditary: amyloidosis; angioedema; ataxia; chorea; clubbing; coproporphyria; hyperthyroidism; lymphedema; methemoglobinemia; myokymia; nephritis; photomyoclonus; pyropoikilocytosis; spherocytosis; syphilis
hereditary angioneurotic: edema
hereditary areflexic: dystasia
hereditary benign intraepithelial: dyskeratosis
hereditary cerebellar: ataxia
hereditary deforming: chondrodystrophy
hereditary folate: malabsorption
hereditary fructose: intolerance
hereditary hemorrhagic: telangiectasia; thrombasthenia
hereditary hypertrophic: neuropathy
hereditary hypophosphatemic: rickets

hereditary methemoglobinemic: cyanosis

hereditary multiple: exostoses; trichoepithelioma

hereditary opalescent: dentin

hereditary progressive: arthro-ophthalmopathy

hereditary renal: hypouricuria

hereditary sensory radicular: neuropathy

hereditary spinal: ataxia

heredofamilial: tremor

Hering-Breuer: reflex

Hering's: test; theory of color vision

Hering's sinus: nerve

Herlitz: syndrome

Hermann's: fixative

Hermansky-Pudlak: syndrome; syndrome type VI

hernia: knife

hernial: aneurysm; sac

herniated: disk

herpes: encephalitis; virus

herpes B: encephalomyelitis

herpes simplex: encephalitis; virus

herpes zoster: virus

herpetic: fever; keratitis; keratoconjunctivitis; meningoencephalitis; ulcer; whitlow

herpetiform: aphthae

Herring: bodies

herring-worm: disease

Herrmann's: syndrome

Hers': disease

Hershberg: test

Hertwig's: sheath

hertzian: experiments

Herxheimer's: reaction

herz: hormone

Heschl's: gyri

Hess: screen

Hess': law; test

Hesselbach's: fascia; hernia; ligament; triangle

heterochromic: cyclitis; uveitis

heterocyclic: compound

heterocytotropic: antibody

heterodetic: peptide

heterogametic: embryo

heterogeneic: antigen

heterogeneous: nucleation; radiation; system

heterogeneous nuclear: RNA

heterogenetic: antibody; antigen; parasite

heterogenic enterobacterial: antigen

heterogenous: keratoplasty; vaccine

heterologous: antiserum; desensitization; graft; insemination; protein; serotype; stimulus; tumor; twins

heteromeric: cell; peptide

heterometabolous: metamorphosis

heterometric: autoregulation

heteronomous: psychotherapy

heteronymous: diplopia; hemianopia; image; parallax

heterophil: antibody; antigen; hemolysin

heterophile: antibody; antigen

heteroplastic: graft

heteropolar: bond

heteropyknotic: chromatin

heterospecific: graft

heterotopic: bones; graft; pregnancy; stimulus

heterotrophic oral gastrointestinal: cyst

heterotype: mitosis

heterotypic: cortex

heterotypical: chromosome

heterovaccine: therapy

heteroxenous: parasite

Heubner's: arteritis

Heuser's: membrane

hexacanth: embryo

hexaxial reference: system

hexazonium: salts

hexokinase: method

hexon: antigen

hexone: bases

hexose monophosphate: pathway; shunt

Heyer-Pudenz: valve

Heyns' abdominal decompression: apparatus

Hey's: amputation; hernia

Hey's internal: derangement

HFR: strain

HG: factor

hiatal: hernia

hibernating: gland; myocardium; myocardium

hidden: part

hidden nail: skin

hidebound: disease

hidrotic ectodermal: dysplasia

high: convex; enema; lithotomy; wine

high altitude: chamber

high-calorie: diet

high dose: tolerance

high-egg-passage: vaccine

high endothelial postcapillary: venules

high energy: compounds; phosphates

high energy phosphate: bond

higher order: conditioning

highest: concha

highest intercostal: artery; vein

highest nuchal: line

highest thoracic: artery

highest turbinated: bone

high-fat: diet

high-fiber: diet

high forceps: delivery

high frequency: current; deafness; transduction

high-kV: technique

high lip: line

high molecular weight: kininogen

Highmore's: body

high osmolar contrast: agent; medium

high output: failure

high-pass: filter

high-performance liquid: chromatography

high quality filter: paper

high-resolution: banding

high resolution computed: tomography

high spinal: anesthesia

high steppage: gait

Higoumenakia: sign

hilar: dance; lymph nodes; shadow

hilar cell: tumor of ovary

Hill: coefficient; constant; operation; plot; reaction

Hillis-Müller: maneuver

Hill's: equation; phenomenon; sign

Hill-Sachs: lesion

Hilton's: law; method; sac

Hilton's white: line

hilus: cells

hind: kidney

hindbrain: vesicle

hindquarter: amputation

Hines-Brown: test

hinge: axis; joint; movement; position; region

hinged: flap

Hinman: syndrome

Hinton: test

hip: bone; dysplasia; joint; phenomenon

hip-flexion: phenomenon

hippocampal: commissure; convolution; fissure; gyrus; sclerosis; sulcus

hippocratic: face; facies; fingers; nails; school; succussion

hippocratic succussion: sound

Hirschberg's: method

Hirschfeld's: canals

Hirschowitz: syndrome

Hirsch-Peiffer: stain

Hirschsprung's: disease

His': band; bundle; copula; line; rule; spindle

His bundle: electrogram

His' perivascular: space

Hiss': stain

Histalog: test

histamine: flush; liberators; shock; test

histaminic: cephalalgia; headache

His-Tawara: system

histiocytic: lymphoma

histiocytic medullary: reticulosis

histocompatibility: antigen; complex; gene

histoid: leprosy; neoplasm; tumor

histologic: accommodation

histoplasmin-latex: test

histotoxic: anoxia

histrionic: personality; spasm

histrionic personality: disorder

hitchhiker: thumbs

Hitzig's: girdle

Hjärre's: disease

HL-A: antigens

HLA: complex; typing

HMG CoA reductase: inhibitors

Ho: antigen

Hoagland's: sign

hobnail: cells; liver; tongue

Hoboken's: gemmules; nodules; valves

Hoche's: bundle; tract

Hodgen: splint

Hodge's: pessary

Hodgkin-Key: murmur

Hodgkin's: disease; lymphoma

Hodgson's: disease

hoe: excavator; scaler

Hofbauer: cell

Hoffa's: operation

Hoffmann's: duct; phenomenon; reflex; sign

Hoffmann's muscular: atrophy

Hoffman's: violet

Hofmann's: bacillus

Hofmeister: gastrectomy; series

Hofmeister-Pólya: anastomosis

Hofmeister's: operation

hog: cholera

Hogben: number

hog cholera: vaccines; virus

Hogness: box

holandric: gene; inheritance

Holden's: line

holiday: syndrome

holiday heart: syndrome

holistic: medicine; psychology
Hollander: test
Hollenhorst: plaques
Holliday: junction; structure
hollow: back; bone; wall
Holl's: ligament
Holmes: heart
Holmes': stain
Holmes-Adie: pupil; syndrome
Holmes-Rahe: questionnaire
Holmgrén-Golgi: canals
Holmgren's wool: test
holoblastic: cleavage
holocrine: gland
holoendemic: disease
hologynic: inheritance
holometabolous: metamorphosis
holosystolic: murmur
Holter: monitor
Holthouse's: hernia
Holt-Oram: syndrome
Holzknecht: unit
Homans': sign
home health: nurse
homeometric: autoregulation
homeostatic: equilibrium; lag
homeotic: genes
Homer-Wright: rosettes
Home's: lobe
homigrade: scale
hominal: physiology
homing: value
homocyclic: compound
homocytotropic: antibody
homodetic: peptide
homogametic: embryo
homogeneous: immersion; nucleation; radiation; system
homogenous: keratoplasty
homograft: reaction
homolecithal: egg
homologous: antigen; antiserum; chromosomes; desensitization; graft; insemination; proteins; series; serotype; stimulus; tumor
homologous serum: jaundice
homomeric: peptide
homonymous: diplopia; hemianopia; images; parallax
homoplastic: graft
homosexual: panic
homotypic: cortex
homovanillic acid: test
homozygous: achondroplasia
honey: urine
honeycomb: lung; macula; pattern; ringworm; tetter
Hong Kong: foot; influenza; toe
hooded: prepuce

hoof-and-mouth: disease
hookean: behavior
hooked: bone; bundle of Russell; fasciculus
Hooker-Forbes: test
Hooke's: law
hook-shaped: cataract
hookworm: anemia; disease
Hoover's: signs
Hopmann's: papilloma; polyp
horizontal: atrophy; cell of Cajal; cells of retina; fissure of cerebellum; fissure of right lung; fracture; heart; osteotomy; overlap; part of duodenum; part of facial canal; plane; plate of palatine bone; resorption; transmission; vertigo
horizontal beam: film
horizontal growth: phase
hormonal: gingivitis
hormone replacement: therapy
horn: fly
Horner's: muscle; pupil; syndrome; teeth
Horner-Trantas: dots
horny: cell; layer of epidermis; layer of nail
horsepox: virus
horseradish: peroxidases
horseshoe: fistula; kidney; placenta
Horsley's bone: wax
Hortega: cells
Hortega's neuroglia: stain
Horton's: arteritis; cephalalgia; headache
hospital: fever; formulary; gangrene; nurse; record
hot: abscess; flash; flush; gangrene; nodule; pack; spot
hot salt: sterilizer
Hottentot: tea
hound-dog: facies
Hounsfield: number; unit
hourglass: contraction; head; murmur; pattern; stomach; vertebrae
house: staff; surgeon
housekeeping: genes
housemaid's: knee
Houssay: animal; phenomenon; syndrome
Houston's: folds; muscle; valves
Howard: test
Howell: unit
Howell-Jolly: bodies
Howship's: lacunae
Hoyer's: anastomoses; canals
H-R conduction: time
H-shape: vertebrae
H-type: fistula

H-type tracheoesophageal: fistula
Hu: antigens
Hubbard: tank
Hubrecht's protochordal: knot
Hückel's: rule
Hucker-Conn: stain
Hudson-Stähli: line
Hueck's: ligament
Hueter's: maneuver; sign
Hüfner's: equation
Huggins': operation
Hughes-Stovin: syndrome
Huguier's: canal; circle; sinus
Huhner: test
Hull's: triad
human: babesiosis; botfly; ecology; ehrlichiosis; fibrinogen; genetics; herpesvirus 1; herpesvirus 2; herpesvirus 3; herpesvirus 4; herpesvirus 5; herpesvirus 6; herpesvirus 7; insulin; serum; thrombin
human antihemophilic: factor; fraction
human botfly: myiasis
human chorionic: gonadotropin; somatomammotropin
human chorionic somatomammotropic: hormone
human diploid cell: vaccine
human diploid cell rabies: vaccine
human fibrin: foam
human gamma: globulin
human granulocytic: ehrlichiosis
human immunodeficiency: virus
humanistic: psychology
human leukemia-associated: antigens
human lymphocyte: antigens
human measles immune: serum
human menopausal: gonadotropin
human normal: immunoglobulin
human papilloma: virus
human pertussis immune: serum
human placental: lactogen
human plasma protein: fraction
human α_1-proteinase: inhibitor
human scarlet fever immune: serum
human serum: jaundice

human T-cell lymphoma/leukemia: virus
human T-cell lymphotropic: virus
human T lymphotrophic: virus
Humby: knife
humeral: artery; articulation; head
humeroradial: articulation; joint
humeroulnar: head of flexor digitorum superficialis muscle; joint
humid: tetter
Hummelsheim's: operation
humoral: doctrine; immunity; pathology; theory
Humphry's: ligament
hunger: contractions; pain; swelling
Hunner's: stricture; ulcer
Hunter and Driffield: curve
Hunter's: canal; glossitis; gubernaculum; ligament; line; membrane; operation; syndrome
Hunter-Schreger: bands; lines
hunting: phenomenon; reaction
Huntington's: chorea; disease
Hunt's: atrophy; neuralgia; syndrome
Hunt's paradoxical: phenomenon
Hurler's: disease; syndrome
Hurler-Scheie: syndrome
Hurst: bougies
Hürthle: cell
Hürthle cell: adenoma; carcinoma; tumor
Huschke's: cartilages; foramen; valve
Huschke's auditory: teeth
Hutchinson-Gilford: disease; syndrome
Hutchinson's: facies; freckle; mask; patch; pupil; teeth; triad
Hutchinson's crescentic: notch
Hutchison: syndrome
Huxley's: layer; membrane; sheath
Huygens': ocular; principle
H-V: interval
HVA: test
H-V conduction: time
H-Y: antigen
hyaline: bodies; bodies of pituitary; cartilage; cast; degeneration; leukocyte; membrane; thrombus; tubercle

hyaline membrane: disease of the newborn; syndrome
hyalocapsular: ligament
hyaloid: artery; body; canal; fossa; membrane
hyaloideoretinal: degeneration
hybrid: prosthesis
hydatid: cyst; disease; fremitus; polyp; pregnancy; rash; resonance; sand; thrill
hydatidiform: mole
Hyde's: disease
hydralazine: syndrome
hydrate: crystal
hydrated: alumina
hydrate microcrystal: theory of anesthesia
hydraulic: conductivity
hydremic: edema
hydride: ion
hydroalcoholic: extract; tincture
hydroelectric: bath
hydrogen: acceptor; bond; carrier; donor; electrode; ion; number; pump; transport
hydrolytic: cleavage
hydrolyzing: enzymes
hydronium: ion
hydrophil: colloid
hydrophilic: ointment; petrolatum
hydrophobic: bond; colloid; interaction; tetanus
hydropic: degeneration
hydrops: pericardii
hydrostatic: dilator; pressure
hydrous: wool fat
17-hydroxycorticosteroid: test
17-hydroxylase deficiency: syndrome
5-hydroxy tryptamine: antagonists
hygienic laboratory: coefficient
hygroscopic: expansion
hylic: tumor
hymenal: caruncula
Hynes: pharyngoplasty
hyobranchial: cleft
hyoepiglottic: ligament
hyoglossal: membrane; muscle
hyoglossus: muscle
hyoid: apparatus; arch; bone
hyomandibular: cleft
Hypaque: enema
hypaque: swallow
hyparterial: bronchi
hyperabduction: syndrome
hyperactive child: syndrome
hyperacute: rejection
hyperacute purulent: conjunctivitis

hyperbaric: anesthesia; chamber; medicine; oxygen; oxygenation
hyperbaric oxygen: therapy
hyperbaric spinal: anesthesia
hypercalcemic: sarcoidosis; uremia
hyperchloremic: acidosis
hyperchromatic: macrocythemia
hyperchromic: anemia; effect
hypercyanotic: angina
hyperendemic: disease
hypereosinophilic: syndrome
hyperergic: encephalitis
hyperextension-hyperflexion: injury
hyperfunctional: occlusion
hypergenic: teratosis
hyperglobulinemic: purpura
hyperglycemic-glycogenolytic: factor
hypergonadotropic: eunuchoidism; hypogonadism
hyperimmune: serum
hyperimmunoglobulin E: syndrome
hyperkalemic periodic: paralysis
hyperkinetic: dysarthria; syndrome
hyperkinetic heart: syndrome
hyperlucent: lung
hypermature: cataract
hypernatremic: encephalopathy
hyperopic: astigmatism
hyperornithinemia-hyperammonemia-hypercitrullinuria: syndrome
hyperosmolar (hyperglycemic) nonketotic: coma
hyperostotic: spondylosis
hyperplastic: arteriosclerosis; gingivitis; graft; inflammation; osteoarthritis; polyp; pulpitis
hyperprolactinemic: amenorrhea
hyperquantivalent: idea
hyperreactive malarious: splenomegaly
hyperreflexic: bladder
hypersecretion: glaucoma
hypersegmented: neutrophil
hypersensitive: dentin
hypersensitive xiphoid: syndrome
hypersensitivity: angiitis; pneumonitis; reaction; vasculitis

hypertensive: angiopathy; arteriopathy; arteriosclerosis; encephalopathy; retinopathy
hyperthyroid: heart
hypertonic: bladder
hypertrophic: arthritis; cardiomyopathy; dystrophy; gastritis; pulpitis; rhinitis; rosacea; scar
hypertrophic cervical: pachymeningitis
hypertrophic hypersecretory: gastropathy
hypertrophic interstitial: neuropathy
hypertrophic pulmonary: osteoarthropathy
hypertrophic pyloric: stenosis
hypervariable: regions
hyperventilation: syndrome; test; tetany
hyperviscosity: syndrome
hypnagogic: hallucination; image
hypnogenic: spot
hypnoid: state
hypnopompic: hallucination; image
hypnotic: psychotherapy; relationship; sleep; state
hypobaric spinal: anesthesia
hypobranchial: eminence
hypocalcemic: cataract
hypochondriac: region
hypochondriacal: melancholia; neurosis
hypochondrial: reflex
hypochromic: anemia; effect
hypochromic microcytic: anemia
hypocomplementemic: glomerulonephritis; vasculitis
hypocycloidal: tomography
hypodermic: injection; needle; syringe; tablet
hypoferric: anemia
hypogastric: artery; ganglia; nerve; reflex; vein
hypoglossal: canal; eminence; nerve; nucleus; trigone
hypoglycemic: coma
hypogonadotropic: eunuchoidism; hypogonadism
hypohidrotic ectodermal: dysplasia
hypokalemic: nephropathy
hypokalemic periodic: paralysis
hypokinetic: dysarthria

hypometabolic: state; syndrome
hypoparathyroid: tetany
hypoparathyroidism: syndrome
hypopharyngeal: diverticulum
hypophyseal: cachexia; pouch
hypophyseoportal: system
hypophysial: amenorrhea; cachexia; duct; dwarf; fossa; infantilism; syndrome
hypophysial portal: circulation; system
hypophysioportal: system
hypophysio-sphenoidal: syndrome
hypophysiotropic: hormone
hypoplastic: anemia; heart
hypoplastic fetal: chondrodystrophy
hypoplastic left heart: syndrome
hypopyon: ulcer
hyporeninemic: hypoaldosteronism
hypostatic: abscess; congestion; ectasia; pneumonia
hypotensive: anesthesia
hypothalamic: amenorrhea; infundibulum; obesity; obesity with hypogonadism; sulcus
hypothalamocerebellar: fibers
hypothalamohypophysial: tract
hypothalamohypophysial portal: circulation; system; system
hypothenar: eminence; prominence
hypothermic: anesthesia
hypothetical mean: organism; strain
hypothyroid: dwarf; dwarfism; infantilism
hypoventilation: coma
hypovolemic: shock
hypoxanthine guanine phosphoribosyltransferase: deficiency
hypoxemia: test
hypoxia warning: system
hypoxic: hypoxia; nephrosis
hypoxic-hypercarbic: encephalopathy
hypsiloid: angle; cartilage; ligament
Hyrtl's: anastomosis; foramen; loop; sphincter
Hyrtl's epitympanic: recess
hysterical: amblyopia; anesthesia; aphonia; ataxia; blindness; chorea;

convulsion; deafness; gait;
joint; neurosis; paralysis;
polydipsia; pregnancy;
psychosis; syncope;
torticollis; tremor; vertigo

I

I: antigens; band; cell; disk;
pili; region
iatrogenic: transmission
iatromathematical: school
Ibaraki: virus
IBR: virus
ICAO standard: atmosphere
Iceland: disease; moss
I-cell: disease
ichorous: pus
ichthyosiform: erythroderma
icing: heart; liver
iconic: signs
icteric: index
icterohemolytic: anemia
icterohemorrhagic: fever
icterus: index
ICU: psychosis
id: reaction
ideal alveolar: gas
ideational: apraxia
identical: twins
identity: crisis; disorder;
matrix
ideokinetic: apraxia
idiodynamic: control
idiographic: approach
idiojunctional: rhythm
idiomuscular: contraction
idionodal: rhythm
idiopathic: aldosteronism;
bradycardia;
cardiomyopathy; disease;
epilepsy; gout; hirsutism;
hypercalcemia of infants;
hyperlipemia;
hypertension; infantilism;
megacolon; myocarditis;
neuralgia; proctitis; roseola
idiopathic bilateral:
vestibulopathy
idiopathic bone: cavity
idiopathic fibrous:
mediastinitis;
retroperitonitis
idiopathic hypercalcemic:
sclerosis of infants
idiopathic hypertrophic:
osteoarthropathy
**idiopathic hypertrophic
subaortic:** stenosis
idiopathic interstitial:
fibrosis
idiopathic muscular:
atrophy
idiopathic orthostatic:
hypotension
idiopathic paroxysmal:
rhabdomyolysis

idiopathic pulmonary:
fibrosis; hemosiderosis
**idiopathic
thrombocytopenic:**
purpura
idiosyncratic: sensitivity
idiotype: antibody;
autoantibody
idiotypic antigenic:
determinant
idioventricular: kick;
rhythm
IgA: nephropathy
IgM: nephropathy
ileal: arteries; bladder;
conduit; intussusception;
sphincter; veins
ileoanal: pouch
ileocecal: eminence; fold;
intussusception; junction;
opening; orifice; valve
ileocecocolic: sphincter
ileocolic: artery;
intussusception; lymph
nodes; valve; vein
Ilhéus: encephalitis; fever;
virus
iliac: arteries; bone; branch
of iliolumbar artery; bursa;
colon; crest; fascia; fossa;
horn; muscle; plexus;
region; roll; spine; steal;
tubercle; tuberosity; veins
iliacosubfascial: fossa;
hernia
iliacus: muscle
iliacus minor: muscle
iliococcygeal: muscle
iliococcygeus: muscle
iliocostal: muscle
iliocostalis: muscle
iliocostalis cervicis: muscle
iliocostalis lumborum:
muscle
iliocostalis thoracis: muscle
iliofemoral: ligament;
triangle
iliohypogastric: nerve
ilioinguinal: nerve
iliolumbar: artery; ligament;
vein
iliopectineal: arch; bursa;
eminence; fascia; fossa;
ligament; line
iliopelvic: sphincter
iliopsoas: muscle
iliopubic: eminence; tract
iliosciatic: notch
iliotibial: band; tract
iliotrochanteric: ligament
illegal: abortion
Ilosvay: reagent
image: amplifier
imbrication: lines of von
Ebner
Imerslünd-Grasbeck:
syndrome
imitative: tetanus

Imlach's: fat-pad; ring
immature: cataract;
granulocyte; neutrophil
immediate: allergy;
amputation; auscultation;
contagion; denture; flap;
hypersensitivity;
percussion; reaction;
transfusion
immediate hypersensitivity:
reaction
immediate insertion:
denture
immediate posttraumatic:
automatism; convulsion
immersion: bath; foot; lens;
microscopy; objective
imminent: abortion
immobilized: enzyme
immobilizing: antibody
immotile cilia: syndrome
immovable: bandage; joint
immune: adherence;
adsorption; agglutination;
agglutinin; complex;
deficiency; deviation;
hemolysin; hemolysis;
inflammation; interferon;
opsonin; paralysis;
precipitation; protein;
reaction; response; serum;
suppression; surveillance;
system; thrombocytopenia
immune adherence:
phenomenon
immune adhesion: test
immune complex: disease;
disorder;
glomerulonephritis;
nephritis
immune electron:
microscopy
immune fetal: hydrops
immune response: genes
immune serum: globulin
immune thrombocytopenic:
purpura
immunity: deficiency
immunoblastic:
lymphadenopathy;
lymphoma; sarcoma
immunochemical: assay
immunodeficiency:
syndrome
immunofluorescence:
method; microscopy
immunofluorescent: stain
immunologic: tolerance
immunological: competence;
deficiency; enhancement;
mechanism; paralysis;
surveillance; tolerance
immunologically activated:
cell
**immunologically
competent:** cell
immunologically privileged:
sites

immunologic high dose:
tolerance
immunologic pregnancy:
test
immunoproliferative:
disorders
**immunoproliferative small
intestinal:** disease
immunoradiometric: assay
immunoreactive: insulin
impact: resistance
impacted: fetus; fracture;
tooth
impaired glucose: tolerance
impedance: angle; method;
plethysmography
imperative: conception
imperfect: fungus; stage;
state
imperforate: anus; hymen
impetiginous: cheilitis;
syphilid
implant: denture
implantation: cone; cyst;
graft; theory of the
production of
endometriosis
implant denture:
substructure; superstructure
implanted: suture
implosive: therapy
impression: area; compound;
material; tray
impressive: aphasia
impulse control: disorder
impulsive: obsession
impure: flutter
inactivated: serum
inactivated poliovirus:
vaccine
inactive: mutant; repressor;
tuberculosis
inadequate: personality;
stimulus
inanition: fever
inapparent: infection
inappropriate: affect;
hormone
inborn: errors of
metabolism; reflex
inborn error of: metabolism
inborn lysosomal: disease
incarcerated: hernia;
placenta
incarceration: symptom
incarial: bone
incasement: theory
inception: rate
incest: barrier
incidence: density; rate
incident: angle; point; ray
incidental: color; learning;
parasite
incipient: abortion; caries
incisal: edge; embrasure;
guidance; guide; margin;
path; point; rest; surface
incisal guide: angle

WordFinder

incised: wound
incision: biopsy
incisional: hernia
incisive: bone; canal; duct; foramen; fossa; papilla; suture
incisive canal: cyst
incisor: crest; foramen; tooth
inclusion: blennorrhea; bodies; cell; compound; conjunctivitis; cyst; dermoid
inclusion body: disease; encephalitis; rhinitis
inclusion cell: disease
inclusion conjunctivitis: viruses
incomitant: strabismus
incompatible blood transfusion: reaction
incompetent cervical: os
incomplete: abortion; achromatopsia; agglutinin; alexia; antibody; antigen; ascertainment; cleavage; disinfectant; fistula; fracture; hemianopia; metamorphosis; neurofibromatosis; tetanus
incomplete atrioventricular: block; dissociation
incomplete conjoined: twins
incomplete foot: presentation
incongruent: nystagmus
incongruous: hemianopia
increased markings: emphysema
incremental: lines; lines of von Ebner
incrusted: cystitis
incubation: period
incubative: stage
incubatory: carrier
incudal: fold; fossa
incudiform: uterus
incudomalleolar: articulation; joint
incudostapedial: articulation; joint
indentation: hardness
independent: assortment; variable
indeterminate: cleavage; leprosy
index: ametropia; case; finger; hypermetropia; myopia
index extensor: muscle
indexical: signs
India ink capsule: stain
Indian: flap; ginger; gum; method; operation; podophyllum; rhinoplasty; sickness
Indian podophyllum: resin
Indian tick: typhus
indicator: system; yellow
indicator dilution: method

indicator-dilution: curve
indifference to pain: syndrome
indifferent: cell; electrode; genitalia; gonad; oxide; tissue; water
indirect: agglutination; assay; calorimetry; diuretic; fracture; laryngoscopy; lead; method for making inlays; ophthalmoscope; ophthalmoscopy; oxidase; placentography; rays; retainer; retention; technique; test; transfusion; vision
indirect Coombs': test
indirect fluorescent antibody: test
indirect hemagglutination: test
indirect inguinal: hernia
indirect nuclear: division
indirect pulp: capping
indirect pupillary: reaction
indirect reacting: bilirubin
individual: differences; psychology; therapy; tolerance
individuation: field
indole: test
indolent: bubo; ulcer
indophenol: method
induced: abortion; apnea; enzyme; fever; fit; hypotension; malaria; mutation; phagocytosis; radioactivity; sensitivity; symptom; trance
induced fit: model
induced psychotic: disorder
inducer: cell
induction: chemotherapy; period
inductive: resistance
indurative: myocarditis
industrial: deafness; disease; hygiene; psychiatry; psychology
industrial methylated: spirit
indwelling: catheter
inert: gases
inertia: time
inevitable: abortion
infant: death
infantile: acropustulosis; autism; beriberi; cataract; colic; convulsion; diplegia; dwarfism; eczema; fibrosarcoma; gastroenteritis; hemiplegia; hernia; hypothyroidism; leishmaniasis; myofibromatosis; myxedema; osteomalacia; pellagra; scurvy; sexuality; spasm; tetany

infantile acute hemorrhagic: edema of the skin
infantile celiac: disease
infantile cortical: hyperostosis
infantile digital: fibromatosis
infantile G_{M2}: gangliosidosis
infantile gastroenteritis: virus
infantile, generalized G_{M1}: gangliosidosis
infantile muscular: atrophy
infantile neuroaxonal: dystrophy
infantile neuronal: degeneration
infantile progressive spinal muscular: atrophy
infantile purulent: conjunctivitis
infantile spastic: paraplegia
infantile spinal muscular: atrophy
infant mortality: rate
infected: abortion
infection: calculus; immunity
infection control: nurse
infection-exhaustion: psychosis
infectious: anemia; coryza; disease; endocarditis; enterohepatitis; granuloma; hepatitis; icterus; jaundice; mononucleosis; myositis; nucleic acid; ophthalmia; papilloma of cattle; plasmid; polyneuritis; serositis; sinusitis of turkeys; synovitis; warts
infectious arteritis: virus of horses
infectious avian: bronchitis
infectious bovine: keratitis; keratoconjunctivitis; rhinotracheitis
infectious bovine rhinotracheitis: virus
infectious bronchitis: virus
infectious bulbar: paralysis
infectious bursal: disease
infectious bursal disease: virus
infectious canine: hepatitis
infectious ectromelia: virus
infectious eczematoid: dermatitis
infectious hepatitis: virus
infectious necrotic: hepatitis of sheep
infectious papilloma: virus
infectious porcine: encephalomyelitis
infectious porcine encephalomyelitis: virus
infective: embolism; jaundice; thrombus

inferential: statistics
inferior: angle of scapula; belly of omohyoid muscle; border; border of liver; border of lung; border of pancreas; branch; branches of transverse cervical nerve; branch of oculomotor nerve; branch of pubic bone; branch of superior gluteal artery; bursa of biceps femoris; colliculus; extremity; fascia of pelvic diaphragm; fascia of urogenital diaphragm; flexure of duodenum; fovea; ganglion of glossopharyngeal nerve; ganglion of vagus nerve; horn; horn of falciform margin of saphenous opening; horn of lateral ventricle; horn of thyroid cartilage; laryngotomy; ligament of epididymis; limb; lobe of lung; margin; mediastinum; olive; part; part of duodenum; part of lingular branch of left pulmonary vein; part of vestibular ganglion; part of vestibulocochlear nerve; pole; pole of kidney; pole of testis; polioencephalitis; retinaculum of extensor muscles; root of ansa cervicalis; root of vestibulocochlear nerve; segment; surface of cerebellar hemisphere; surface of pancreas; surface of petrous part of temporal bone; surface of tongue; tarsus; trunk of brachial plexus; veins of cerebellar hemisphere; vein of vermis; vena cava; wall of orbit; wall of tympanic cavity
inferior aberrant: ductule
inferior accessory: fissure
inferior alveolar: artery; nerve
inferior anastomotic: vein
inferior articular: facet of atlas; pit of atlas; surface of tibia
inferior basal: vein
inferior calcaneonavicular: ligament
inferior cardiac: vein
inferior carotid: triangle
inferior cerebellar: peduncle
inferior cerebral: surface; veins
inferior cervical: ganglion

inferior cervical cardiac:
branches of vagus nerve;
nerve

inferior choroid: vein

inferior cluneal: nerves

inferior constrictor: muscle
of pharynx

inferior costal: facet; pit

inferior dental: arch; artery;
branches of inferior dental
plexus; canal; foramen;
nerve; plexus; rami

inferior duodenal: fold;
fossa; recess

inferior epigastric: artery;
lymph nodes; vein

inferior esophageal:
sphincter

inferior extensor:
retinaculum

inferior frontal:
convolution; gyrus; sulcus

inferior gemellus: muscle

inferior gingival: branches
of inferior dental plexus

inferior gluteal: artery;
nerve; veins

inferior hemorrhoidal:
artery; nerves; plexuses;
veins

inferior hypogastric: plexus

inferior hypophysial: artery

inferior ileocecal: recess

inferior internal parietal:
artery

inferiority: complex

inferior labial: artery;
branches of mental nerve;
vein

inferior laryngeal: artery;
cavity; nerve; vein

**inferior lateral brachial
cutaneous:** nerve

inferior lateral genicular:
artery

inferior lingual: muscle

inferior lingular: branch of
lingular branch of left
pulmonary artery; segment

inferior longitudinal:
fasciculus; muscle of
tongue; sinus

inferior macular: arteriole;
venule

inferior maxillary: nerve

inferior medial genicular:
artery

inferior medullary: velum

inferior mesenteric: artery;
ganglion; lymph nodes >;
plexus; vein

inferior myocardial:
infarction

inferior nasal: arteriole of
retina; colliculus; concha;
venule of retina

inferior nuchal: line

inferior oblique: muscle;
muscle of head

inferior occipital: gyrus;
triangle

inferior olivary: nucleus

inferior omental: recess

inferior ophthalmic: vein

inferior orbital: fissure

inferior palpebral: veins

inferior pancreatic: artery

**inferior
pancreaticoduodenal:**
artery

inferior parietal: gyrus;
lobule

inferior pelvic: aperture

inferior petrosal: groove;
sinus; sulcus

inferior phrenic: artery;
lymph nodes; vein

inferior posterior serratus:
muscle

inferior pubic: ligament

inferior quadrigeminal:
brachium

inferior radioulnar: joint

inferior rectal: artery;
nerves; plexuses; veins

inferior rectus: muscle

inferior sagittal: sinus

inferior salivary: nucleus

inferior salivatory: nucleus

inferior segmental: artery of
kidney

inferior semilunar: lobule

inferior suprarenal: artery

inferior tarsal: muscle

inferior temporal: arteriole
of retina; convolution;
gyrus; line; sulcus; venule
of retina

inferior thalamic: peduncle

inferior thalamostriate:
veins

inferior thoracic: aperture

inferior thyroid: artery;
notch; plexus; tubercle;
vein

inferior tibiofibular: joint

inferior tracheobronchial:
lymph nodes

**inferior transverse
scapular:** ligament

inferior triangle: sign

inferior turbinated: bone

inferior tympanic: artery

inferior ulnar collateral:
artery

inferior ventricular: vein

inferior vesical: artery;
nerves; plexus

inferior vestibular: area;
nucleus

inferolateral: margin;
surface of prostate

inferolateral myocardial:
infarction

inferomedial: margin

infertile male: syndrome

infiltrating: lipoma

infiltration: anesthesia

infinite: distance

inflamed: ulcer

inflammatory: carcinoma;
corpuscle; edema; lymph;
macrophage; polyp;
pseudotumor; rheumatism

inflammatory fibrous:
hyperplasia

inflammatory papillary:
hyperplasia

inflatable: implant; splint

influenza: bacillus; viruses

influenzal: pneumonia

influenzal virus: pneumonia

influenza virus: vaccines

information: system; theory

informational: RNA

**infra-auricular deep
parotid:** lymph nodes

**infra-auricular subfascial
parotid:** lymph nodes

infrabony: pocket

infracardiac: bursa

infraclavicular: fossa;
infiltrate; part of brachial
plexus; triangle

infraclinoid: aneurysm

infracostal: line

infraduodenal: fossa

infraglenoid: tubercle;
tuberosity

infraglottic: cavity; space

infragranular: layer

infrahyoid: branch of
superior thyroid artery;
bursa; muscles

infralobar: part of posterior
branch of right pulmonary
vein

inframammary: region

infranatant: fluid

infranodal: extrasystole

infraorbital: artery; canal;
foramen; groove; margin;
nerve; region; suture

infraorbitomeatal: plane

infrapalpebral: sulcus

infrapatellar: branch of
saphenous nerve; fat-pad

infrapatellar fat: body

infrapatellar synovial: fold

infrared: cataract; light;
microscope; ray;
spectroscopy; spectrum;
thermography

infrascapular: artery; region

infrasegmental: part; veins

infraspinatus: bursa; fascia;
muscle

infraspinous: fossa

infrasternal: angle

infratemporal: crest; fossa;
surface of maxilla

infratrochlear: nerve

infundibular: part; recess;
stalk; stem; stenosis

infundibuliform: fascia;
hymen; sheath

infundibulo-ovarian:
ligament

infundibulopelvic: ligament

infusion: graft

infusion-aspiration:
drainage

Ingrassia's: apophysis; wing

ingrowing: toenail

ingrown: hairs; nail

inguinal: branches of
external pudendal arteries;
canal; crest; fold; fossa;
glands; hernia; ligament;
ligament of the kidney;
plexus; region; triangle;
trigone

inguinal aponeurotic: fold

inguinocrural: hernia

inguinolabial: hernia

inguinoscrotal: hernia

inguinosuperficial: hernia

inhalation: analgesia;
anesthesia; anesthetic;
therapy

inherited: character

inherited albumin: variants

inhibiting: antibody

inhibition: factor

inhibitory: fibers; nerve;
obsession

inhibitory junction:
potential

inhibitory postsynaptic:
potential

initial: contact; dose; heat;
hematuria; rate; velocity

initiating: agent; codon

initiation: codon; factor;
tRNA

injection: flask; mass;
molding

injury: potential

inkblot: test

inlay: graft; wax

innate: heat; immunity;
reflex

inner: malleolus; membrane;
table of skull

inner cell: mass

inner dental: epithelium

innermost intercostal:
muscle

innervation: apraxia

innocent: murmur; tumor

innocent bystander: cell

innominate: artery; bone;
fossa; substance; veins

innominate cardiac: veins

inorganic: acid; catalyst;
chemistry; compound;
murmur; orthophosphate;
phosphate;
pyrophosphatase

inorganic dental: cement

inotropic: agents
inquiline: parasite
insect: viruses
insensible: perspiration; thirst
insertion: sequence
insertional: inactivation; mutagenesis
insight: learning
insoluble: soap
inspiratory: capacity; center; stridor
inspiratory reserve: volume
inspired: gas
instantaneous: vector
instantaneous electrical: axis
instructive: theory
instrumental: amusia; conditioning
insufflation: anesthesia
insular: area; arteries; cortex; gyri; hypothesis; part; part of middle cerebral artery; sclerosis; veins
insulin: antagonist; injection; lipoatrophy; lipodystrophy; resistance; shock; unit
insulin-antagonizing: factor
insulin coma: therapy; treatment
insulin-dependent: diabetes mellitus
insulin hypoglycemia: test
insulin-like: activity
insulin-like growth: factors
insulinopenic: diabetes
insulin shock: treatment
insulin zinc: suspension
integral: dose; proteins
integrated rate: expression
integumentary: system
intellectual: aura
intelligence: quotient; test
intensification: chemotherapy
intensifying: screen
intensive: care; psychotherapy
intensive care: unit
intention: spasm; tremor
intentional: replantation
interaction process: analysis
interalveolar: pores; septum; space
interannular: segment
interarch: distance
interarticular: fibrocartilage; joints
interarytenoid: notch
interatrial: foramen primum; foramen secundum; septum
interauricular: arc
intercalary: neuron; staphyloma
intercalated: disk; ducts; nucleus

intercapillary: cell; glomerulosclerosis
intercapital: ligament
intercapitular: veins
intercarotid: body; nerve
intercarpal: joints; ligaments
intercartilaginous: part of glottic opening; part of rima glottidis
intercavernous: sinuses
intercellular: bridges; canaliculus; cement; digestion; junctions; lymph
intercellular adhesion: molecule-1
interceptive occlusal: contact
interchondral: articulations; joints
interclavicular: ligament; notch
interclinoid: ligament
intercolumnar: fasciae; fibers; tubercle
intercondylar: eminence; fossa; line of femur; tubercle
intercondyloid: fossa; notch
intercornual: ligament
intercostal: anesthesia; arteries; ligaments; lymph nodes; membranes; nerves; neuralgia; space; veins
intercostobrachial: nerves
intercostohumeral: nerves
intercrural: fibers; ganglion
intercuneiform: joints; ligaments
intercurrent: disease
intercuspal: position
interdental: canals; caries; papilla; septum; splint
interdigital: folds
interectopic: interval
interfacial: canals
interfacial surface: tension
interfascial: space
interfascicular: fasciculus
interference: beat; dissociation; microscope
interfoveolar: ligament
interganglionic: rami
intergenic: complementation; suppression
interglobular: dentin; space; space of Owen
interiliac: lymph nodes
interilioabdominal: amputation
interim: denture
interjudge: reliability
interlaminar: jelly
interlobar: arteries of kidney; artery; duct; surfaces of lung; veins of kidney
interlobular: arteries; arteries of kidney; arteries

of liver; duct; ductules; emphysema; pleurisy; septum; veins of kidney; veins of liver
interlocal: additivity
interlocking: gyri
intermaxillary: anchorage; bone; elastic; fixation; relation; segment; suture; traction
intermediary: metabolism; movements; nerve; system
intermediate: abutment; amputation; body of Flemming; bronchus; carcinoma; disk; filaments; ganglia; heart; hemorrhage; host; junction; lamella; layer; line of iliac crest; mass; mesoderm; nerve; part; part of adenohypophysis; part of vestibular bulb; rays; trait; uveitis; variable; vein of forearm
intermediate antebrachial: vein
intermediate basilic: vein
intermediate cephalic: vein
intermediate cervical: septum
intermediate cubital: vein
intermediate cuneiform: bone
intermediate dorsal cutaneous: nerve
intermediate great: muscle
intermediate hypothalamic: region
intermediate lacunar: lymph node; node
intermediate laryngeal: cavity
intermediate layer of the transversospinalis: muscles
intermediate lumbar: lymph nodes
intermediate sacral: crests
intermediate supraclavicular: nerve
intermediate temporal: artery
intermediate vastus: muscle
intermediolateral: nucleus
intermediolateral cell: column of spinal cord
intermediomedial: nucleus
intermembrane: space
intermembranous: part of glottic opening; part of rima glottidis
intermenstrual: pain
intermesenteric: plexus
intermesenteric arterial: anastomosis
intermetacarpal: joints

intermetatarsal: articulations; joints
intermittent: albuminuria; arthralgia; claudication; cramp; hemoglobinuria; hydrarthrosis; hydrosalpinx; malaria; pulse; sterilization; tetanus; torticollis
intermittent acute: porphyria
intermittent explosive: disorder
intermittent malarial: fever
intermittent mandatory: ventilation
intermittent positive pressure: breathing; ventilation
intermittent self-: obturation
intermuscular: septum
intermuscular gluteal: bursa
internal: attachment; axis of eye; base of skull; branch of accessory nerve; branch of superior laryngeal nerve; canthus; capsule; conjugate; decompression; energy; fistula; fixation; hemorrhage; hemorrhoids; hernia; hydrocephalus; lip of iliac crest; malleolus; medicine; meningitis; naris; nostril; ophthalmopathy; ophthalmoplegia; phase; pyocephalus; ramus of accessory nerve; resorption; respiration; sheath of optic nerve; squint; strabismus; surface; surface of frontal bone; surface of parietal bone; traction; urethrotomy
internal acoustic: foramen; meatus; pore
internal adhesive: pericarditis
internal anal: sphincter
internal arcuate: fibers
internal auditory: artery; foramen; meatus; veins
internal capsule: syndrome
internal carotid: artery; nerve
internal carotid (nervous): plexus
internal carotid venous: plexus
internal cephalic: version
internal cerebral: veins
internal collateral: ligament of the wrist
internal conversion: electron
internal female genital: organs
internal iliac: artery; lymph nodes; vein
internal inguinal: ring

internal intercostal: membrane; muscle
internal jugular: vein
internal lacrimal: fistula
internal male genital: organs
internal mammary: artery; plexus
internal maxillary: artery; plexus
internal medullary: lamina
internal nasal: branches
internal nuclear: layer of retina
internal oblique: line; muscle
internal obturator: muscle
internal occipital: crest; protuberance
internal pillar: cells
internal pterygoid: muscle
internal pudendal: artery; vein
internal root: sheath
internal salivary: gland
internal saphenous: nerve
internal semilunar: fibrocartilage of knee joint
internal spermatic: artery; fascia
internal sphincter: muscle of anus
internal spiral: sulcus
internal thoracic: artery; plexus; vein
internal thoracic lymphatic: plexus
internal urethral: opening; orifice; sphincter
internasal: suture
International: System of Units
international: unit
International Labour Organization: Classification
International System of: Units
interneuromeric: clefts
internodal: segment
internuncial: neuron
interobserver: error
interocclusal: clearance; distance; gap; record
interocclusal rest: space
interofective: system
interosseous: border; border of fibula; border of radius; border of tibia; border of ulna; bursa of elbow; cartilage; crest; fascia; groove; groove of calcaneus; groove of talus; margin; membrane of forearm; membrane of leg; muscles; nerve of leg
interosseous cuneocuboid: ligament

interosseous cuneometatarsal: ligaments
interosseous metacarpal: ligaments; spaces
interosseous metatarsal: ligaments; spaces
interosseous sacroiliac: ligaments
interosseous talocalcaneal: ligament
interosseous tibiofibular: ligament
interpalpebral: zone
interpapillary: ridges
interparietal: bone; sulcus; suture
interpectoral: lymph nodes
interpeduncular: cistern; fossa; ganglion; nucleus
interpelviabdominal: amputation
interpersonal: conflict
interphalangeal: articulations; joints of foot; joints of hand
interpleural: space
interpolated: extrasystole; flap
interposition: arthroplasty
interpositus: nucleus
interproximal: papilla; space
interpubic: disc; disk
interpulmonary: septum
interradicular: alveoloplasty; septa; space
interrater: reliability
interrenal: bodies; glands
interridge: distance
interrupted: respiration; suture
interscalene: triangle
interscapular: gland; hibernoma; reflex
interscapulothoracic: amputation
intersegmental: fasciculi; part of pulmonary vein; veins
interseptovalvular: space
intersheath: spaces of optic nerve
intersigmoid: hernia; recess
interspecific: graft
interspinal: line; muscles; plane
interspinales: muscles
interspinous: ligament
interspongioplastic: substance
intersternebral: joints
interstitial: absorption; brachytherapy; cells; cystitis; deletion; disease; emphysema; fluid; gastritis; gland; growth; hernia; implantation; inflammation; keratitis;

lamella; mastitis; myositis; nephritis; neuritis; nucleus; nucleus of Cajal; pattern; pregnancy; therapy; tissue
interstitial cell: tumor of testis
interstitial cell-stimulating: hormone
interstitial giant cell: pneumonia
interstitial plasma cell: pneumonia
interstitial pulmonary: fibrosis
intertarsal: articulations; joints
intertendinous: connections
interthalamic: adhesion
intertragic: notch
intertransversarii: muscles
intertransverse: ligament; muscles
intertrochanteric: crest; line
intertropical: anemia; hyphemia
intertubercular: bursitis; groove; line; plane; sheath; sulcus
intertubular: zone
interureteric: fold
intervaginal: space of optic nerve
interval: gout; operation; scale
intervening: sequence; variable
intervenous: tubercle
interventional: angiography; radiology
interventricular: foramen; grooves; septum
intervertebral: cartilage; disc; disk; foramen; ganglion; notch; symphysis; vein
intervillous: lacuna; spaces
interzonal: mesenchyme
intestinal: anastomosis; angina; anthrax; arteries; atresia; calculus; capillariasis; digestion; emphysema; fistula; follicles; glands; intoxication; juice; lipodystrophy; lymphangiectasis; metaplasia; myiasis; rotation; sand; schistosomiasis; sepsis; stasis; steatorrhea; surface of uterus; trunks; villi
intestinal arterial: arcades
intra-alveolar: septa
intra-aortic: balloon
intra-aortic balloon: counterpulsation; pump

intra-articular: cartilage; fracture; ligament of costal head
intra-articular sternocostal: ligament
intra-atrial: block; conduction
intra-atrial conduction: time
intrabulbar: fossa
intracanalicular: fibroadenoma
intracanicular: part of optic nerve
intracapsular: ankylosis; fracture; ligaments
intracapsular temporomandibular joint: arthroplasty
intracardiac: catheter; lead
intracardiac pressure: curve
intracavernous: aneurysm; plexus
intracellular: canaliculus; digestion; enzyme; fluid; toxin
intracerebral: hemorrhage
intracoronal: retainer
intracranial: aneurysm; cavity; ganglion; hematoma; hemorrhage; hypotension; part of optic nerve; part of vertebral artery; pneumatocele; pneumocele; pressure
intracranial granulomatous: arteritis
intractable: epilepsy; pain
intracutaneous: reaction
intracystic: papilloma
intradermal: nevus
intraductal: carcinoma; papilloma
intraembryonic: mesoderm
intraepidermal: carcinoma
intraepiploic: hernia
intraepithelial: carcinoma; dyskeratosis; glands
intrafusal: fibers
intragenic: complementation; suppression
intraglandular deep parotid: lymph nodes
intraglandular parotid: lymph nodes
intragracile: sulcus
intrailiac: hernia
intrajugular: process
intralaminar: nuclei of thalamus; part of optic nerve
intralesional: therapy
intraligamentary: pregnancy
intralobar: part of the right superior pulmonary vein
intralobular: duct
intralocal: additivity

intramaxillary: anchorage
intramedullary: anesthesia; reamer; tractotomy
intramembranous: ossification
intramural: hematoma; practice; pregnancy
intranasal: anesthesia
intraobserver: error
intraocular: fluid; implant; neuritis; part of optic nerve; pressure
intraoral: anchorage; anesthesia; antrostomy
intraoral fracture: appliance
intraosseous: anesthesia; fixation
intrapapillary: drusen
intraparietal: sulcus; sulcus of Turner
intraparotid: plexus of facial nerve
intrapartum: hemorrhage; period
intrapelvic: hernia
intraperiosteal: fracture
intraperitoneal: pregnancy
intrapersonal: conflict
intrapyretic: amputation
intrarenal: reflux
intraretinal: space
intrasegmental: part; veins
intraspinal: anesthesia
intratendinous: bursa of elbow
intrathecal: injection
intrathyroid: cartilage
intratracheal: anesthesia; intubation; tube
intrauterine: amputation; contraceptive device; devices; fracture; pneumonia; transfusion
intravagal: glomus
intravaginal: torsion
intravascular: ligature; lymph
intravascular papillary endothelial: hyperplasia
intravenous: anesthesia; anesthetic; bolus; cholangiography; drip; narcosis; pyelography; urography
intravenous regional: anesthesia
intraventricular: block; conduction; hemorrhage; injection
intravital: stain; ultraviolet
intrinsic: asthma; color; deflection; dysmenorrhea; factor; fibers; motivation; muscles; muscles of foot; proteins; reflex; sphincter
intrinsicoid: deflection
intrinsic sympathomimetic: activity

intromittent: organ
introspective: method
intuitive: stage
intumescent: cataract
intussusceptive: growth
inulin: clearance
inundation: fever
InV: allotypes
invaginate: planula
invasive: aspergillosis; carcinoma; mole
inverse: anaphylaxis; symmetry; syntropy
inversed jaw-winking: syndrome
inverse ocular: bobbing
inverse square: law
inversion: recovery
invert: sugar
inverted: image; papilloma; pelvis; reflex
inverted cone: bur
inverted follicular: keratosis
inverted radial: reflex
investigatory: reflex
investing: cartilage; fascia; layer of deep cervical fascia; tissues
investment: cast
InV group: antigen
invisible: differentiation; light; spectrum
involuntary: guarding; muscles
involuntary nervous: system
involution: cyst; form
involutional: depression; melancholia; psychosis
iodate: reaction of epinephrine
iodide: acne
iodide transport: defect
iodinated: glycerol
iodinated ^{131}I human serum: albumin
iodinated ^{125}I serum: albumin
iodine: cysts; eruption; number; reaction of epinephrine; stain; test; value
iodine-induced: hyperthyroidism
iodized: collodion
iodophil: granule
iodotyrosine deiodinase: defect
ion: channel; pump
ion exchange: chromatography
ion-exchange: resin
ionic: medication; strength
ionization: chamber
ionized: atom
ionizing: radiation
ion-selective: electrodes
ipecac: syrup
ipomea: resin

ipsilateral: reflex
iridescent: virus
iridial: part of retina
iridocorneal: angle
iridocorneal endothelial: syndrome
iridocorneal mesodermal: dysgenesis
iridopupillary: lamina
IRI/G: ratio
iris: dehiscence; freckles; pits
Irish: moss
Irish moss: gelatin
iris-nevus: syndrome
iron: hematoxylin; index; lung; sulfate
iron-binding: capacity
iron deficiency: anemia
iron-dextran: complex
iron-storage: disease
iron-sulfur: proteins
irradiated vitamin D: milk
irreducible: hernia
irregular: astigmatism; bone; dentin; emphysema; nystagmus; pulse
irresistible: impulse
irreversible: colloid; hydrocolloid; pulpitis; reaction; shock
irritable: breast; colon; heart
irritant contact: dermatitis
irritation: cell; fibroma
Irvine-Gass: syndrome
Isaac's: syndrome
ischemia-modifying: factors
ischemic: contracture of the left ventricle; hypoxia; lumbago; necrosis; neuropathy
ischemic mitral: regurgitation
ischemic muscular: atrophy
ischemic optic: neuropathy
ischiadic: plexus; spine
ischial: bone; bursa; ramus; spine; tuberosity
ischiatic: hernia; notch
ischioanal: fossa
ischiocapsular: ligament
ischiocavernous: muscle
ischiofemoral: ligament
ischiopubic: ramus
ischiorectal: abscess; fat-pad; fossa
Ishihara: test
island: disease; fever; flap
islet: cell; tissue
islet cell: adenoma
isoallotypic: determinants
isobaric spinal: anesthesia
isochromic: anemia
isocyclic: compound
isodiphasic: complex
isodynamic: law

isoelectric: electroencephalogram; line; period; point; zone
isoenzyme: electrophoresis
isogeneic: graft
isogenic: strain
isogenous: chondrocytes; nest
isoimmune neonatal: thrombocytopenia
isoionic: point
isolated: abutment; dextrocardia; dyskeratosis follicularis; proteinuria
isolated explosive: disorder
isolated parietal: endocarditis
isolecithal: egg; ovum
isologous: graft
isomeric: function; transition
isometric: chart; contraction; exercise; period of cardiac cycle; relaxation; ruler; traction
isometric contraction: period
isometric relaxation: period
isomorphic: response
isomorphous: gliosis
isoniazid: neuropathy; polyneuropathy
isopeptide: bond
isoperistaltic: anastomosis
isophane: insulin
isoplastic: graft
isoprene: rule
isopropanol precipitation: test
isopycnic: zone
isorhythmic: dissociation
isosbestic: point
isoserum: treatment
isotonic: coefficient; contraction; exercise; traction
isotope: clearance
isotropic: disk; lipid
isovolume pressure-flow: curve
isovolumetric: relaxation
isovolumic: interval; relaxation
Itai-Itai: disease
Italian: flap; method; operation; rhinoplasty
ITO: method
Ito: cells
Ito-Reenstierna: test
Ito's: nevus
^{131}I uptake: test
Ivemark's: syndrome
ivory: exostosis; membrane; vertebra
Ivy bleeding time: test
Ivy loop: wiring

J

WordFinder

J: chain; point
Jaboulay: pyloroplasty
Jaboulay's: amputation
Jaccoud's: arthritis; arthropathy
jacket: crown
Jacksonian: seizure
jacksonian: epilepsy
Jackson's: law; membrane; rule; sign; veil
Jacobaeus: operation
Jacobson's: anastomosis; canal; cartilage; nerve; organ; plexus; reflex
Jacquart's facial: angle
Jacquemet's: recess
Jacquemin's: test
Jacques': plexus
Jacquet's: erythema
Jadassohn-Lewandowski: syndrome
Jadassohn-Pellizzari: anetoderma
Jadassohn's: nevus
Jadassohn-Tièche: nevus
Jaeger's: test types
Jaffe: reaction
Jaffe-Lichtenstein: disease
Jaffe's: test
Jahnke's: syndrome
jail: fever
jake: paralysis
Jakob-Creutzfeldt: disease
jalap: resin
Jamaican vomiting: sickness
James: fibers; tracts
James-Lange: theory
Jamestown Canyon: virus
Janet's: test
Janeway: lesion
Jansen's: operation
Jansky-Bielschowsky: disease
Jansky's: classification
Japan: wax
Japanese: dysentery
Japanese B: encephalitis
Japanese B encephalitis: virus
Japanese river: fever
jargon: aphasia
Jarisch-Herxheimer: reaction
Jarjavay's: ligament
Jarvik artificial: heart
Jatene: procedure
jaw: bone; jerk; joint; reflex; repositioning; separation; skeleton
Jaworski's: bodies
jaw-winking: phenomenon; syndrome
jaw-working: reflex
JC: virus
jealous type of paranoid: disorder
Jeanselme's: nodules
Jeghers-Peutz: syndrome

jejunal: arteries
jejunal and ileal: veins
jejunogastric: intussusception
jejunoileal: bypass; shunt
Jellinek: formula
Jembrana: disease
Jendrassik's: maneuver
Jenner-Kay: unit
Jenner's: stain
Jensen's: disease; sarcoma
jerk: finger
jerky: nystagmus; respiration
Jerne: technique
Jervell and Lange-Nielsen: syndrome
Jesuit: tea
jet: injection; injector; nebulizer
jet ejector: pump
Jeune's: syndrome
jeweller's: forceps
Jewett: sound
Jewett and Strong: staging
j-g: complex
JH: virus
Jk: antigens
Job: syndrome
Jobbins: antigen
Jobert de Lamballe's: fossa; suture
Jocasta: complex
jock: itch
Jod-Basedow: phenomenon
Joest: bodies
Joffroy's: reflex; sign
Johne's: bacillus; disease
Johnson's: method
joint: branches; capsule; effusion; evil; gamete; ill; oil; probability; sense
jojoba: oil
Jolles': test
Jolly: bodies
Jolly's: reaction
Jones': test
Jonnesco's: fossa
Jonston's: alopecia; area
Joseph: knife; rhinoplasty
Joseph's: clamp
Joubert's: syndrome
Joule's: equivalent
Js: antigen
J-sella: deformity
Judkins: technique
jugal: bone; ligament; point
jugular: bulb; duct; embryocardia; foramen; fossa; ganglion; gland; glomus; nerve; notch of occipital bone; notch of temporal bone; plexus; process; pulse; sinus; tubercle; veins; wall of middle ear
jugular foramen: syndrome
jugular lymphatic: trunk
jugular venous: arch

jugulo-digastric: lymph node
jugulodigastric: node
jugulo-omohyoid: lymph node; node
jump: flap
jumping: disease; gene
jumping the: bite
jumping Frenchmen of Maine: disease
junction: nevus
junctional: complex; cyst; epithelium; escape; extrasystole; rhythm; tachycardia
jungian: psychoanalysis
jungle: fever
jungle yellow: fever
Jüngling's: disease
Jung's: muscle
Junin: virus
junk: DNA
Junod's: boot
juvenile: angiofibroma; arrhythmia; arthritis; carcinoma; cataract; cell; chorea; cirrhosis; diabetes; elastoma; hemangiofibroma; kyphosis; neutrophil; osteoporosis; papillomatosis; pattern; pelvis; periodontitis; polyp; retinoschisis; xanthogranuloma
juvenile absence: epilepsy
juvenile cerebellar: astrocytoma
juvenile chronic: arthritis
juvenile epithelial corneal: dystrophy
juvenile hyalin: fibromatosis
juvenile muscular: atrophy
juvenile myoclonic: epilepsy
juvenile-onset: diabetes
juvenile palmo-plantar: fibromatosis
juvenile spinal muscular: atrophy
juxta-articular: nodules
juxtacortical: chondroma
juxtacortical osteogenic: sarcoma
juxta-esophageal pulmonary: lymph nodes
juxtaglomerular: apparatus; body; cells; complex; granules
juxta-intestinal: lymph nodes
juxtamedullary: glomerulus
juxtaphrenic: peak
juxtapupillary: choroiditis
juxtarestiform: body

K

K: antigens; capture; cells; complex; region; shell; virus
K-: radiation
K:A: ratio
kabure: itch
Kaffir: pox
kainate: receptor
Kaiserling's: fixative
kallikrein: system
Kallmann's: syndrome
kang: cancer
kangri burn: carcinoma
Kanner's: syndrome
Kaposi's: sarcoma
Kaposi's varicelliform: eruption
kappa: angle; granule; particles
karaya: gum
Karman: cannula
Karmen: unit
Karnofsky: scale
Kartagener's: syndrome; triad
karyochrome: cell
karyopyknotic: index
Kasabach-Merritt: syndrome
Kasai: operation
Kashin-Bek: disease
Kasten's fluorescent Feulgen: stain
Kasten's fluorescent PAS: stain
Kasten's fluorescent Schiff: reagents
Katayama: disease; fever; syndrome
Katayama's: test
Kawasaki's: disease; syndrome
Kayser-Fleischer: ring
Kazanjian's: operation
Kearns-Sayre: syndrome
Keating-Hart's: method
kedani: fever
keeled: chest
Keen's: operation; sign
Kegel's: exercises
Kehr's: sign
Keith and Flack: node
Keith's: bundle; node
Kelev strain rabies: virus
Keller: bunionectomy
Keller-Madlener: operation
Kelly: clamp
Kelly's: operation
Kelly's rectal: speculum
Kelvin: scale
Kempner: diet
Kendall's: compounds; substance
Kennedy: classification
Kennedy's: disease; syndrome
kennel: cough
Kenny's: treatment

Kent-His: bundle
Kent's: bundle
Kenya: fever
Kerandel's: symptom
keratic: precipitates
keratin: filaments; pearl
keratinized: cell
keratinous: cyst
keratogenous: membrane
keratohyalin: granules
keratoid: exanthema
keratophakic: keratoplasty
keratorefractive: surgery
keratosic: cones
Kerckring's: center; folds; ossicle; valves
Kerley A: lines
Kerley B: lines
Kerley C: lines
Kernig's: sign
Kernohan's: notch
kern-plasma relation: theory
Kestenbaum's: number; sign
α-keto acid: dehydrogenase
α-keto acid dehydrogenase: complex
ketogenic: diet
ketogenic-antiketogenic: ratio
ketogenic corticoids: test
17-ketogenic steroid assay: test
α-ketoglutarate dehydrogenase: complex
ketone: body
ketonimine: dyes
ketosis-prone: diabetes
ketosis-resistant: diabetes
ketotic: hyperglycemia; hyperglycinemia
Kety-Schmidt: method
Kew Gardens: fever
key: attachment; ridge; vein
Key-Gaskell: syndrome
keyhole: deformity; pupil
key-in-lock: maneuver
Key-Retzius: corpuscles
keyway: attachment
Ki-1+: lymphoma
kidney: carbuncle
Kiel: classification
Kienböck's: atrophy; disease; dislocation; unit
Kiernan's: space
Kiesselbach's: area
Kilham rat: virus
Kiliani-Fischer: reaction; synthesis
Kilian's: line
killer: cells
Killian's: bundle; operation; triangle
kilogram: calorie
Kimmelstiel-Wilson: disease; syndrome
Kimura's: disease

kinematic: face-bow; viscosity
kineplastic: amputation
kinesthesia: hallucination
kinesthetic: aura; sense
kinetic: analyzer; ataxia; energy; measurement; perimetry; strabismus; system; tremor
kinetochore: fibers
King: unit
King-Armstrong: unit
king's: evil
Kingsley: splint
kinked: aorta
Kinkiang: fever
kinky: hair
kinky-hair: disease; disorder
Kinyoun: stain
Kirby-Bauer: test
Kirkland: knife
Kirk's: amputation
Kirschner's: apparatus; wire
Kisch's: reflex
Kisenyi sheep disease: virus
Kitasato's: bacillus
Kjeldahl: apparatus; method
Kjelland's: forceps
Klapp's: method
Klebs-Loeffler: bacillus
Kleihauer's: stain
Kleine-Levin: syndrome
Klein-Gumprecht shadow: nuclei
Klein's: muscle
Klenow: fragment
Klestadt's: cyst
Klinefelter's: syndrome
Klinger-Ludwig acid-thionin: stain for sex chromatin
Klippel-Feil: syndrome
Klippel-Trenaunay-Weber: syndrome
Klumpke: palsy
Klumpke's: paralysis
Klüver-Barrera Luxol fast blue: stain
Klüver-Bucy: syndrome
Km: allotypes; antigen
Knapp's: streaks; striae
knee: jerk; joint; phenomenon; presentation; reflex
knee-chest: position
knee-elbow: position
knee-jerk: reflex
Kniest: syndrome
knife: needle
knife-rest: crystal
knock-out: drops
Knoll's: glands
Knoop hardness: number; test
Knoop's: theory
knuckle: pads
Kobelt's: tubules
Kober: test

Köbner's: phenomenon
Kocher: clamp
Kocher-Debré-Sémélaigne: syndrome
Kocher's: incision; sign
Koch's: bacillus; law; node; phenomenon; postulates; triangle
Koch's blue: bodies
Koch's old: tuberculin
Koch-Weeks: bacillus
Kock: ileostomy; pouch
Koenen's: tumor
Koenig's: syndrome
Koerber-Salus-Elschnig: syndrome
Koerte-Ballance: operation
Koettstorfer: number
Köhler: illumination
Köhler's: disease
Kohlmeier-Degos: syndrome
Kohlrausch's: muscle; valves
Kohn's: pores
Kohnstamm's: phenomenon
Kojewnikoff's: epilepsy
kokoi: venom
Kölliker's: layer; reticulum
Kollmann's: dilator
Kolmer: test
Kommerell's: diverticulum
Kondoleon: operation
Konno: procedure
Konno-Rastan: procedure
Koongol: viruses
Koplik's: spots
Korean hemorrhagic: fever
Korean hemorrhagic fever: virus
Korff's: fibers
Kornberg: enzyme
Korotkoff: sounds
Korotkoff's: test
Korsakoff's: psychosis; syndrome
Koshland-Némethy-Filmer: model
Kossa: stain
Kostmann: syndrome
Krabbe's: disease
Kraske's: operation
Krause: graft
Krause's: bone; glands; ligament; method; muscle; valve
Krause's end: bulbs
Krause's respiratory: bundle
Krause-Wolfe: graft
Krebs: cycle
Krebs-Henseleit: cycle
Krebs-Kornberg: cycle
Krebs-Ringer: solution
Kretschmann's: space
Kreysig's: sign
Krogh: spirometer
Kromayer's: lamp
Kronecker's: stain

Krönig's: isthmus; steps
Krönlein: operation
Krönlein's: hernia
Krueger: instrument stop
Krukenberg's: amputation; spindle; tumor; veins
Kruse's: brush
Kufs: disease
Kugelberg-Welander: disease
Kugel's anastomotic: artery
Kühne's: fiber; methylene blue; phenomenon; plate; spindle
Kuhnt-Junius: degeneration; disease
Kuhnt's: spaces
Kulchitsky: cells
Külz's: cylinder
Kümmell's: spondylitis
Küntscher: nail
Kupffer: cells
Kurloff's: bodies
Kürsteiner's: canals
Kurunegala: ulcers
Kurzrok-Ratner: test
Kuskokwim: syndrome
Kussmaul: respiration
Kussmaul-Kien: respiration
Kussmaul's: aphasia; coma; disease; pulse; sign; symptom
Kussmaul's paradoxical: pulse
Kveim: antigen; test
Kveim-Stilzbach: antigen; test
Kyasanur Forest: disease
Kyasanur Forest disease: virus
kyphoscoliotic: pelvis
kyphotic: pelvis
Kyrle's: disease

L

L: chain; doses; form; unit of streptomycin
L⁺: dose
L-: meromyosin; radiation
ʟ-: serine dehydratase
Laband's: syndrome
Labbé's: triangle; vein
Labbé's neurocirculatory: syndrome
labeled: atom; thyroxine
labial: arch; bar; commissure; embrasure; flange; gingiva; glands; hernia; occlusion; part of orbicularis oris muscle; splint; sulcus; surface; swelling; tubercle; veins; vestibule
labile: affect; current; elements; factor; hypertension; pulse
labiodental: sulcus

labiogingival: lamina
labiolingual: appliance; plane
labioscrotal: folds; swellings
labor: pains
laboratory: diagnosis
labored: respiration
Labrador: keratopathy
labyrinthine: angiospasm; apoplexy; artery; nystagmus; placenta; reflexes; torticollis; veins; vertigo; wall of middle ear
labyrinthine righting: reflexes
Lac: operon
lacerated: foramen
Lachman: test
laciniate: ligament
lacis: cell
lacrimal: apparatus; artery; bay; bone; border of maxilla; calculus; canaliculus; caruncle; conjunctivitis; fascia; fistula; fold; fossa; gland; groove; hamulus; lake; margin of maxilla; nerve; notch; opening; papilla; part of orbicularis oculi muscle; process; punctum; reflex; sac; vein
lacrimoconchal: suture
lacrimo-gustatory: reflex
lacrimomaxillary: suture
La Crosse: virus
lactacid oxygen: debt
β-lactamase: inhibitors
lactase: persistence; restriction
lactate dehydrogenase: virus
lactated Ringer's: injection; solution
lactating: adenoma
lactation: amenorrhea; hormone
lactational: mastitis
lacteal: cyst; fistula; vessel
lactic: acidosis
lactic acid: bacillus; fermentation
lactiferous: ampulla; ducts; gland; sinus
lacto-: vegetarian
lactobacillary: milk
Lactobacillus bulgaricus: factor
Lactobacillus casei: factor
lactogenic: factor; hormone
lacto-ovo-: vegetarian
lactose: intolerance
lactose-litmus: agar
lacunar: abscess; amnesia; ligament; state; tonsillitis
ladder: splint
Ladd-Franklin: theory
Ladd's: band; operation
Laënnec's: cirrhosis; pearls

Lafora: body
Lafora body: disease
Lafora's: disease
lag: phase
lagophthalmic: keratitis
Lahey: forceps
Lahore: sore
laimer: triangle
Laki-Lorand: factor
laky: blood
Lallemand's: bodies
Lallouette's: pyramid
lamarckian: theory
Lamaze: method
LAMB: syndrome
lamb: dysentery
Lambda: phage
lambdoid: border of occipital bone; margin of occipital bone; suture
Lambert-Eaton: syndrome; syndrome
Lambert's: law; syndrome
lambing: paralysis; sickness
Lambl's: excrescences
Lambrinudi: operation
lamellar: bone; cataract; granule; ichthyosis; keratoplasty
lamellated: corpuscles
lamina: propria; propria of semicircular duct
laminar: flow
laminar cortical: necrosis; sclerosis
laminated: clot; cortex; epithelium; thrombus
laminated epithelial: plug
laminin: receptor
lampbrush: chromosome
Lan: antigen
Lancefield: classification
Lancisi's: sign
land: scurvy
Landau-Kleffner: syndrome
Landolfi's: sign
Landolt's: bodies
Landouzy-Dejerine: dystrophy
Landouzy-Grasset: law
Landry: syndrome
Landry-Guillain-Barré: syndrome
Landry's: paralysis
Landschutz: tumor
Landsteiner-Donath: test
Landström's: muscle
Landzert's: fossa
Lane's: band; disease; kink; plates
Langenbeck's: triangle
Langendorff's: method
Langerhans': cells; granule; islands
Langer's: arch; lines; muscle
Lange's: solution; test
Langhans': cells; layer; stria
Langhans'-type giant: cells

Langley's: granules
Langmuir: trough
language: game; zone
Lannelongue's: foramina; ligaments
Lanterman's: incisures; segments
lanugo: hair
Lanz's: line
L-AP$_4$: receptor
laparoscopic: cannula; cholecystotomy; knot; surgery
laparoscopically assisted: surgery
laparoscopic-assisted vaginal: hysteroscopy
laparotomy: pad
Lapicque's: law
Laplace's: forceps; law
Laquer's: stain for alcoholic hyalin
larch: turpentine
lardaceous: liver; spleen
large: bowel; calorie; intestine; muscle of helix; pelvis; vein
large cell: carcinoma; lymphoma
large interarch: distance
large pudendal: lip
large saphenous: vein
Larmor: frequency
Laron type: dwarfism
Laroyenne's: operation
Larrey's: amputation; cleft
Larrey-Weil: disease
Larsen's: syndrome
larval: conjunctivitis; plague
laryngeal: aperture; atresia; bursa; chorea; crisis; diphtheria; epilepsy; glands; granuloma; mask; mucosa; papillomatosis; part of pharynx; pharynx; polyp; pouch; prominence; reflex; sinus; stenosis; stridor; syncope; tonsils; veins; ventricle; vertigo
laryngeal lymphatic: follicles
laryngopharyngeal: branches of superior cervical ganglion
laryngospastic: reflex
laryngotracheal: diphtheria; diverticulum; groove
Lasègue's: disease; sign; syndrome
laser: corepraxy; iridotomy; microscope; photocoagulator; trabeculoplasty
Lash's: operation
Lassa: fever; virus
Lassa hemorrhagic: fever
Latarget's: nerve; vein

late: cyanosis; deceleration; diastole; reaction; rickets; seizure; syphilis; systole
late apical systolic: murmur
late benign: syphilis
late diastolic: murmur
late latent: syphilis
late luteal phase dysphoric: disorder
latency: period; phase
latent: allergy; carcinoma; carrier; coccidioidomycosis; content; diabetes; empyema; energy; gout; heat; homosexuality; hyperopia; infection; learning; microbism; nystagmus; period; reflex; schizophrenia; stage; syphilis; tetany; typhoid; zone
latent adrenocortical: insufficiency
latent rat: virus
late-phase: response
lateral: aberration; angle of eye; angle of scapula; angle of uterus; aperture of the fourth ventricle; border; border of foot; border of forearm; border of humerus; border of kidney; border of nail; border of scapula; branches; canal; canthus; cartilage; cartilage of nose; column; column of spinal cord; condyle; condyle of femur; condyle of tibia; cord of brachial plexus; crus; crus of facial canal; crus of the greater alar cartilage of the nose; crus of horizontal part of the facial canal; crus of the superficial inguinal ring; curvature; epicondyle of femur; epicondyle of humerus; excursion; fillet; folds; fossa of brain; funiculus; funiculus of spinal cord; ginglymus; head; hermaphroditism; horn; illumination; incisor; lacunae; lakes; lamina of cartilaginous auditory tube; layer of cartilaginous auditory tube; lemniscus; ligament of elbow; ligament of knee; ligament of malleus; ligaments of the bladder; ligament of temporomandibular joint; ligament of wrist; limb; line; lip of linea aspera; lithotomy; malleolus; margin; mass of atlas; mass of ethmoid bone; meniscus;

mesoderm; movement; nucleus of medulla oblongata; nucleus of thalamus; occlusion; part of longitudinal arch of foot; part of middle lobar branch of right superior pulmonary vein; part of occipital bone; part of posterior cervical intertransversarii muscles; part of sacrum; part of vaginal fornix; plate; plate of pterygoid process; pole; process of calcaneal tuberosity; process of malleus; process of talus; projection; recess of fourth ventricle; region; region of neck; root of median nerve; root of optic tract; segment; sinus; surface; surface of arm; surface of fibula; surface of finger; surface of leg; surface of lower limb; surface of ovary; surface of testis; surface of tibia; surface of toe; surface of zygomatic bone; tubercle of posterior process of talus; vein of lateral ventricle; ventricle; vertigo; wall of middle ear; wall of orbit; wall of tympanic cavity

lateral aberrant thyroid: carcinoma
lateral alveolar: abscess
lateral ampullar: nerve
lateral antebrachial cutaneous: nerve
lateral anterior thoracic: nerve
lateral arcuate: ligament
lateral atlantoaxial: joint
lateral atlantoepistrophic: joint
lateral atrial: vein
lateral basal: branch; segment
lateral bicipital: groove
lateral calcaneal: branches of sural nerve
lateral cartilaginous: layer
lateral central palmar: space
lateral cerebral: fissure; fossa; sulcus
lateral cervical: nuclei
lateral circumflex: artery of thigh
lateral circumflex femoral: artery; veins
lateral collateral: ligament of ankle
lateral condylar: inclination
lateral corticospinal: tract

lateral costal: branch of internal thoracic artery
lateral costotransverse: ligament
lateral cricoarytenoid: muscle
lateral cuneate: nucleus
lateral cuneiform: bone
lateral cutaneous: branch; branches of intercostal nerves; branches of ventral primary ramus of thoracic spinal nerves; nerve of calf; nerve of forearm; nerve of thigh
lateral decubitus: radiograph
lateral deep cervical: lymph nodes
lateral direct: veins
lateral dorsal cutaneous: nerve
lateral epicondylar: crest; ridge
lateral femoral: tuberosity
lateral femoral circumflex: artery
lateral femoral cutaneous: nerve
lateral frontobasal: artery
lateral geniculate: body
lateral glossoepiglottic: fold
lateral great: muscle
lateral ground: bundle
lateral group of axillary: lymph nodes
lateral humeral: epicondylitis
lateral hypothalamic: area; region
lateral inferior genicular: artery
lateral inguinal: fossa
lateral jugular: lymph nodes
lateral lacunar: lymph node; node
lateral line: system
lateral line sense: organ
lateral lingual: swellings
lateral longitudinal: arch of foot; stria
lateral lumbar intertransversarii: muscles
lateral lumbar intertransverse: muscles
lateral lumbocostal: arch
lateral malleolar: arteries; ligament; network; surface of talus
lateral malleolar subcutaneous: bursa
lateral malleolus: bursa
lateral mammary: branches; branches of lateral cutaneous branches of intercostal nerves; branches of lateral cutaneous branches of thoracic spinal

nerves; branches of lateral thoracic artery
lateral medullary: lamina of corpus striatum; syndrome
lateral midpalmar: space
lateral myocardial: infarction
lateral nasal: artery; branches of anterior ethmoidal nerve; fold; primordium; process; prominence
lateral oblique: radiograph
lateral occipital: artery; sulcus
lateral occipitotemporal: gyrus
lateral orbitofrontal: branch
lateral palpebral: commissure; ligament; raphe
lateral patellar: retinaculum
lateral pectoral: nerve
lateral pericardiac: lymph nodes
lateral periodontal: abscess; cyst
lateral pharyngeal: space
lateral plantar: artery; nerve
lateral plate: mesoderm
lateral popliteal: nerve
lateral preoptic: nucleus
lateral proprius: bundle
lateral pterygoid: muscle; plate
lateral puboprostatic: ligament
lateral pyramidal: fasciculus; tract
lateral ramus: radiograph
lateral rectus: muscle; muscle of the head
lateral recumbent: position
lateral reticular: nucleus
lateral sacral: artery; crests; veins
lateral sacrococcygeal: ligament
lateral semicircular: canals
lateral skull: radiograph
lateral spinal: sclerosis
lateral spinothalamic: tract
lateral splanchnic: arteries
lateral striate: arteries
lateral superficial cervical: lymph nodes
lateral superior genicular: artery
lateral supraclavicular: nerve
lateral supracondylar: crest; ridge
lateral sural cutaneous: nerve
lateral talocalcaneal: ligament
lateral tarsal: artery

lateral temporomandibular: ligament
lateral thalamic: peduncle
lateral thoracic: artery; vein
lateral thyrohyoid: ligament
lateral tuberal: nuclei
lateral umbilical: fold; ligament
lateral vaginal wall: smear
lateral vastus: muscle
lateral venous: lacunae
lateral ventral: hernia
lateral vestibular: nucleus
late replicating: chromosome
latex agglutination: test
latex fixation: test
latissimus dorsi: muscle
latitude: film
lattice corneal: dystrophy
latticed: layer
Latzko's cesarean: section
laudable: pus
laughing: disease; gas; sickness
laughter: reflex
Laugier's: hernia; sign
Laumonier's: ganglion
Launois-Bensaude: syndrome
Launois-Cléret: syndrome
laurel: fever
Laurence-Moon-Biedl: syndrome
Laurer's: canal
Lauth's: canal; ligament
Lavdovsky's: nucleoid
Lawrence-Seip: syndrome
lazarine: leprosy
LCAT: deficiency
L-chain: disease; myeloma
LCM: virus
L-D: body
LDH: agent
LDL receptor: disorder
LE: body; cell; factors; phenomenon
Le: antigens
lead: anemia; colic; encephalitis; encephalopathy; gout; line; neuropathy; palsy; paralysis; poisoning; stomatitis
leader: sequences
lead hydroxide: stain
leading: ancestor; edge
lead-pipe: colon; rigidity
leak point: pressure
leapfrog: position
Lear: complex
learned: drive
learning: disability; set; theory
least diffusion: circle
least squares: estimator
leather-bottle: stomach
Le Bel-van't Hoff: rule

WordFinder

Leber's: plexus
Leber's hereditary optic: atrophy
Leber's idiopathic stellate: neuroretinitis; retinopathy
LE cell: test
Le Chatelier's: law; principle
lecheguilla: poisoning
lecithin/sphingomyelin: ratio
LeCompte: maneuver; operation
Lederer's: anemia
Ledermann: formula
Leede-Rumpel: phenomenon
Lee's: ganglion
Leeuwenhoek's: canals
leeway: space
Lee-White: method
Le Fort: osteotomy; sound
Le Fort I: fracture
Le Fort II: fracture
Le Fort III: fracture
Le Fort III craniofacial: dysjunction
Le Fort's: amputation
left: atrium of heart; crus of atrioventricular bundle; crus of diaphragm; duct of caudate lobe; heart; lobe; lobe of liver; ventricle
left atrioventricular: valve
left auricular: appendage
left axis: deviation
left colic: artery; flexure; lymph nodes; vein
left coronary: artery; vein
left fibrous: trigone
left gastric: artery; lymph nodes; vein
left gastroepiploic: artery; lymph nodes; vein
left gastroomental: vein
left gastro-omental: artery; nodes
left heart: bypass
left hepatic: artery; duct; veins
left inferior pulmonary: vein
left lumbar: lymph nodes
left main: bronchus
left ovarian: vein
left pulmonary: artery
left sagittal: fissure
left-sided: appendicitis
left-sided heart: failure
left superior intercostal: vein
left superior pulmonary: vein
left suprarenal: vein
left testicular: vein
left-to-right: shunt
left triangular: ligament
left umbilical: vein
left ventricular: failure; myomectomy

left-ventricular assist: device
left ventricular ejection: time
leg: phenomenon
legal: blindness; dentistry; medicine
Legal's: test
Legendre's: sign
Legg-Calvé-Perthes: disease
Legionnaire's: disease
Leichtenstern's: phenomenon; sign
Leigh's: disease
Leiner's: disease
Leishman-Donovan: body
leishmanin: test
Leishman's: stain
Leishman's chrome: cells
Leiter International Performance: Scale
Lejeune: syndrome
Lelystad: virus
Lembert: suture
lemniscal: trigone
Lendrum's phloxine-tartrazine: stain
Lenègre's: disease; syndrome
length-breadth: index
lengthening: reaction
length-height: index
Lenhossék's: processes
Lennert: classification
Lennert's: lesion; lymphoma
Lennox: syndrome
Lennox-Gastaut: syndrome
Lenoir's: facet
lens: capsule; pits; placodes; stars; sutures; vesicle
lens-induced: uveitis
lente: insulin
lenticular: ansa; apophysis; astigmatism; bone; capsule; colony; fasciculus; fossa; ganglion; knife; loop; nucleus; papillae; process of incus; syphilid; vesicle
lenticular progressive: degeneration
lenticulostriate: arteries
lentiform: bone
leonine: facies
LEOPARD: syndrome
leopard: fundus; retina
Leopold's: maneuvers
Lepehne-Pickworth: stain
Lepore: thalassemia
lepra: cells
lepromatous: leprosy
lepromin: reaction; test
leprosy: bacillus
leprous: neuropathy
leptomeningeal: carcinoma; carcinomatosis; cyst; fibrosis
leptospiral: jaundice

Leriche's: operation; syndrome
Leri's: pleonosteosis; sign
Leri-Weill: disease; syndrome
Lermoyez': syndrome
Lerner: homeostasis
Lesch-Nyhan: syndrome
Leser-Trélat: sign
lesser: circulation; cul-de-sac; curvature of stomach; horn of hyoid bone; omentum; pancreas; pelvis; ring of iris; trochanter; tubercle of humerus; tuberosity of humerus; wing of sphenoid bone
lesser alar: cartilages
lesser arterial: circle of iris
lesser internal cutaneous: nerve
lesser multangular: bone
lesser occipital: nerve
lesser palatine: artery; foramina; nerves
lesser peritoneal: cavity; sac
lesser petrosal: nerve
lesser rhomboid: muscle
Lesser's: triangle
lesser sciatic: notch
lesser splanchnic: nerve
lesser superficial petrosal: nerve
lesser supraclavicular: fossa
lesser tympanic: spine
lesser vestibular: glands
lesser zygomatic: muscle
Lesshaft's: triangle
let-down: reflex
lethal: coefficient; dose; dwarfism; equivalent; factor; gene; mutation
lethality: rate
lethal midline: granuloma
lethargic: hypnosis
letter: blindness
Letterer-Siwe: disease
leucine: hypoglycemia
leucine-induced: hypoglycemia
Leudet's: tinnitus
leukemic: leukemia; myelosis; reticuloendotheliosis; reticulosis; retinitis; retinopathy
leukemic hyperplastic: gingivitis
leukemoid: reaction
leukocyte: cream; inclusions; interferon
leukocyte adherence assay: test
leukocyte bactericidal assay: test
leukocyte common: antigen
leukocytic: pyrogens; sarcoma

leukocytoclastic: vasculitis
leukocytosis-promoting: factor
leukoerythroblastic: anemia
leukopenic: factor; index; leukemia; myelosis
leukoplakic: vulvitis
Levaditi: stain
levator: cushion; hernia; muscle of thyroid gland; swelling
levator anguli oris: muscle
levator ani: muscle
levatores costarum: muscles
levator labii superioris: muscle
levator labii superioris alaeque nasi: muscle
levator palati: muscle
levator palpebrae superioris: muscle
levator prostatae: muscle
levator scapulae: muscle
levator veli palatini: muscle
Levay: antigen
LeVeen: shunt
Levin: tube
levoatrio-cardinal: vein
Levret's: forceps
Lev's: disease; syndrome
Lewis: acid; base
Lewy: bodies
Leyden-Möbius muscular: dystrophy
Leyden's: ataxia; crystals; neuritis
Leydig cell: adenoma
Leydig's: cells
Lf: dose
Lhermitte's: sign
libido: theory
Libman-Sacks: endocarditis; syndrome
Liborius': method
licensed practical: nurse
licensed vocational: nurse
lichen: amyloidosis
lichenoid: amyloidosis; dermatosis; eczema; keratosis
lichen planus-like: keratosis
Lichtheim's: sign
lid: reflex
lid-closure: reaction
lid crutch: spectacles
Liddell-Sherrington: reflex
Lieberkühn's: crypts; follicles; glands
Liebermann-Burchard: reaction; test
Liebermeister's: rule
Liebig's: theory
lienal: artery
lienophrenic: ligament
lienorenal: ligament
lienteric: diarrhea
Liesegang: rings

Lieutaud's: body; triangle; trigone; uvula
life: cycle; instinct; stress; table
life-belt: cataract
life-span: development
Li-Fraumeni cancer: syndrome
ligand binding: site
ligand-gated: channel
ligature: wire
light: adaptation; bath; cells of thyroid; chain; difference; metal; micrograph; microscope; reflex; sense; sleep; treatment
light-activated: resin
light-adapted: eye
light chain-related: amyloidosis
light-cured: resin
light differential: threshold
lighthouse: lens
light liquid: petrolatum
light-near: dissociation
lightning: strip
light-touch: palpation
light wire: appliance
Lignac-Fanconi: syndrome
ligneous: conjunctivitis; struma; thyroiditis
Likert: scale
Lillie's allochrome connective tissue: stain
Lillie's azure-eosin: stain
Lillie's ferrous iron: stain
Lillie's sulfuric acid Nile blue: stain
lilliputian: hallucination
limb: bud; lead; myokymia
limb-girdle muscular: dystrophy
limbic: lobe; system
limb-kinetic: apraxia
lime: water
liminal: stimulus; trait
limit: dextrin; dextrinase
limited range: audiometer
limiting: angle; layers of cornea; membrane of retina; sulcus; sulcus of Reil; sulcus of rhomboid fossa
limulus lysate: test
Lindau's: disease; tumor
Lindner's: bodies
line: angle; pairs; test
linear: acceleration; accelerator; amputation; atrophy; craniectomy; fracture; phonocardiograph
linear absorption: coefficient
linear energy: transfer
linear epidermal: nevus
linear IgA bullous: disease in children

linear skull: fracture
lined: flap
line spread: function
Lineweaver-Burk: equation; plot
Ling's: method
lingual: aponeurosis; arch; artery; bar; bone; branches; branch of facial nerve; crypt; embrasure; flange; flap; follicles; frenulum; gingiva; goiter; gyrus; hemiatrophy; lobe; lymph nodes; mucosa; nerve; occlusion; papilla; plate; plexus; quinsy; rest; septum; splint; surface of tooth; tonsil; trophoneurosis; vein
lingual-facial-buccal: dyskinesia
lingual salivary gland: depression
lingular: branch
linguocervical: ridge
linguofacial: trunk
linguogingival: fissure; groove; ridge
linin: network
lining: cell
linkage: analysis; disequilibrium; group; map; marker
linker: DNA
linking: number
linnaean: system of nomenclature
lion-jaw bone-holding: forceps
lip: pits; reflex; sulcus
lipase: test
lipedematous: alopecia
lipemic: retinopathy
lipid: granulomatosis; histiocytosis; keratopathy; pneumonia
lipid-mobilizing: hormone
lip and leg: ulceration
lipoatrophic: diabetes
lipoblastic: lipoma
lipogenous: diabetes
lipoid: dermatoarthritis; granuloma; nephrosis; proteinosis; theory of narcosis
lipomatous: hypertrophy; infiltration; polyp
lipomelanic: reticulosis
lipophagic: granuloma
lipophagic intestinal: granulomatosis
lipoprotein: electrophoresis; polymorphism
lipoprotein(a): hyperlipoproteinemia
lipoprotein-associated coagulation: inhibitor
lipotropic: factor; hormone

Lipschütz: cell
Lipschütz': ulcer
liquefaction: degeneration
liquefactive: necrosis
liquefied: phenol
liquid: air; extract; glucose; paraffin; petroleum; pitch; scatter
liquid crystal: thermography
liquid human: serum
liquid-liquid: chromatography
Lisch: nodule
Lisfranc's: amputation; joints; ligaments; operation; tubercle
Lison-Dunn: stain
Lissauer's: bundle; column; fasciculus; tract
Lissauer's marginal: zone
listeria: meningitis
Lister's: dressing; method; tubercle
Listing's: law
Listing's reduced: eye
Liston's: knives; shears; splint
literal: agraphia
lithium: carmine
lithotomy: position
litigious: paranoia
little: ACTH; finger; fossa of the cochlear window; fossa of the vestibular window; head of humerus
Little Leaguer's: elbow
Little's: area; disease
littoral: cell
Littré's: glands; hernia
Litzmann: obliquity
live: vaccine
liveborn: infant
livedo: vasculitis
livedoid: dermatitis
live oral poliovirus: vaccine
liver of: sulfur
liver: acinus; breath; bud; flap; palm; spot; starch
liver cell: carcinoma
liver filtrate: factor
liver kidney: syndrome
liver *Lactobacillus casei***:** factor
liver-shod: clamp
living: anatomy
L-L: factor
Lloyd's: reagent
Lo: dose
loading: dose
lobar: bronchi; pneumonia; sclerosis
Lobo's: disease
Lobry de Bruyn-van Ekenstein: transformation
Lobstein's: ganglion
lobster-claw: deformity
lobular: carcinoma; carcinoma in situ;

glomerulonephritis; neoplasia
local: anaphylaxis; anemia; anesthesia; anesthetics; asphyxia; bloodletting; death; epilepsy; flap; glomerulonephritis; hormone; immunity; reaction; sign; stimulant; symptom; syncope; tetanus; tic
local anesthetic: reaction
local excitatory: state
localization: agnosia
localization related: epilepsy
localized: osteitis fibrosa; pemphigoid of Brunsting-Perry; peritonitis; scleroderma
localized nodular: tenosynovitis
localizing: electrode; symptom
lock: finger
lock-: jaw
lock-and-key: model
locked: bite; facets; knee
locked-in: syndrome
Locke-Ringer: solution
Locke's: solutions
Lockwood's: ligament
locomotor: ataxia
locoweed: disease
loculated: empyema
loculation: syndrome
locust: gum
lod: method
Loeb's: deciduoma
Loeffler's: bacillus; methylene blue; stain
Loeffler's blood culture: medium
Loeffler's caustic: stain
Loevit's: cell
Loewenthal's: bundle; reaction; tract
Löffler's: disease; endocarditis; syndrome
Loffler's parietal fibroplastic: endocarditis
Logan's: bow
logarithmic: phase; phonocardiograph
logistic: curve; model
logit: transformation
lognormal: distribution
Lohlein-Baehr: lesion
Lohmann: reaction
Lombard voice-reflex: test
Lon: protease
London: forces
long: axis; axis of body; bone; chain; crus of incus; gyrus of insula; head; muscle of head; muscle of neck; process of malleus; pulse; root of ciliary ganglion; sight; vinculum

long abductor: muscle of thumb
long-acting thyroid: stimulator
long adductor: muscle
long axis: view
long buccal: nerve
long central: artery
long ciliary: nerve
long cone: technique
long extensor: muscle of great toe; muscle of thumb; muscle of toes
long fibular: muscle
long flexor: muscle of great toe; muscle of thumb; muscle of toes
long incubation: hepatitis
long interspersed: elements
longissimus: muscle
longissimus capitis: muscle
longissimus cervicis: muscle
longissimus thoracis: muscle
longitudinal: aberration; arch of foot; arc of skull; bands of cruciform ligament; canals of modiolus; dissociation; duct of epoöphoron; fissure of cerebrum; fold of duodenum; fracture; layer of muscular coat; layers of muscular tunics; lie; ligament; method; relaxation; section; sinus; study; sulcus of heart
longitudinal oval: pelvis
longitudinal pontine: bundles; fasciculi
longitudinal vertebral venous: sinus
long-leg: arthropathy
long levatores costarum: muscles
Longmire's: operation
long palmar: muscle
long peroneal: muscle
long plantar: ligament
long posterior ciliary: artery
long radial extensor: muscle of wrist
Long's: coefficient; formula
long saphenous: nerve; vein
long subscapular: nerve
long-term: memory
long terminal repeat: sequences
long thoracic: artery; nerve; vein
longus capitis: muscle
longus colli: muscle
loop: diuretic; excision; resection; stoma
loop electrocautery excision: procedure
loose: associations; body; cartilage; skin
Looser's: lines; zones

lop: ear
Lorain-Lévi: dwarfism; infantilism; syndrome
Lorain's: disease
lordosis: reflex
lordotic: albuminuria; pelvis
Lorenz': sign
Loschmidt's: number
Lou Gehrig's: disease
Louis': angle; law
Louis-Bar: syndrome
louping: ill
louping-ill: virus
louse: flies
louse-borne: typhus
Lovén: reflex
Lovibond's: angle
Lovibond's profile: sign
low: convex; delirium; wine
low-calorie: diet
low-density lipoprotein: receptors
low-egg-passage: vaccine
Löwenberg's: canal; forceps; scala
Lowenstein-Jensen: medium
Lowenstein-Jensen culture: medium
lower: airway; extremity; eyelid; jaw; lid; limb; lip; lobe of lung
lower abdominal periosteal: reflex
lower alveolar: point
lower esophageal: sphincter
lower lateral cutaneous: nerve of arm
lower motor: neuron
lower motor neuron: dysarthria; lesion
lower nephron: nephrosis
lower nodal: extrasystole
lower respiratory tract: smear
lower ridge: slope
Lower's: ring; tubercle
lower uterine: segment
lower uterine segment cesarean: section
Lowe's: syndrome
lowest lumbar: arteries
lowest splanchnic: nerve
lowest thyroid: artery
Lowe-Terrey-MacLachlan: syndrome
low-fat: diet
low flow: principle
low forceps: delivery
low frequency: transduction
low grade: astrocytoma
low lip: line
low malignant potential: tumor
low molecular weight: kininogen
Lown-Ganong-Levine: syndrome
low output: failure

low-pass: filter
low purine: diet
low residue: diet
Lowry-Folin: assay
Lowry protein: assay
low salt: diet; syndrome
Lowsley: tractor
low spinal: anesthesia
low tension: glaucoma
low tone: deafness
L-phase: variants
Lr: dose
L/S: ratio
Lu: antigens
Lubarsch's: crystals
lubricating: cream
Lucas': groove
lucid: interval
Lucio's: leprosy
Lucio's leprosy: phenomenon
Lucké: carcinoma
Lucké's: adenocarcinoma; virus
Lücke's: test
Luc's: operation
Ludloff's: sign
Ludwig's: angina; angle; ganglion; labyrinth; nerve; stromuhr
Luer: syringe
Luer-Lok: syringe
luetic: mask
Luft's: disease
Luft's potassium permanganate: fixative
Lugol's iodine: solution
Lukes-Collins: classification
lumbar: appendicitis; artery; branch of iliolumbar artery; cistern; enlargement; enlargement of spinal cord; flexure; ganglia; hernia; lymph nodes; myelogram; nephrectomy; nerves; part; part of diaphragm; part of spinal cord; plexus; puncture; region; rheumatism; rib; segments of spinal cord; triangle; trunks; veins; vertebrae
lumbar iliocostal: muscle
lumbar interspinal: muscle
lumbar interspinales: muscles
lumbar puncture: needle
lumbar quadrate: muscle
lumbar rotator: muscles
lumbar splanchnic: nerves
lumberman's: itch
lumbocostal: ligament
lumbocostoabdominal: triangle
lumbodorsal: fascia
lumboinguinal: nerve
lumbosacral: angle; joint; plexus; trunk

lumbrical: muscle of foot; muscle of hand
luminous: flux; intensity; retinoscope
lumpy: jaw
lumpy skin: disease
lumpyskin disease: virus
Luna-Ishak: stain
lunar: periodicity
lunate: bone; fissure; sulcus; surface of acetabulum
lunate cerebral: sulcus
lung: bud; unit; window
lung fluke: disease
Lunyo: virus
lupoid: hepatitis; leishmaniasis; sycosis; ulcer
lupus: anticoagulant; nephritis
lupus band: test
lupus erythematosus: cell; panniculitis
lupus erythematosus cell: test
lupus-like: syndrome
Luschka's: bursa; cartilage; ducts; gland; joints; ligaments; sinus; tonsil
Luschka's cystic: glands
Luse: bodies
luteal: cell; phase
luteal phase: defect; deficiency
luteinizing: hormone; hormone-releasing hormone; principle
luteinizing hormone/follicle-stimulating hormone-releasing: factor
luteinizing hormone-releasing: factor
Lutembacher's: syndrome
luteoplacental: shift
luteotropic: hormone
luting: agent
Lutz-Splendore-Almeida: disease
Luys': body
Lyell's: disease; syndrome
Lyme: arthritis; borreliosis; disease
lymph: capillary; cell; circulation; cords; corpuscle; embolism; follicle; gland; node; nodule; sacs; scrotum; sinus; space; varix; vessels
lymphadenoid: goiter
lymphadenopathy-associated: virus
lymphatic: angina; duct; edema; fistula; follicles of larynx; follicles of rectum; leukemia; nodule; plexus; ring of cardiac part of stomach; sarcoma; sinus;

stroma; system; tissue; valvule; vessels
lymphatic dissemination: theory of endometriosis
lymphedematous: keratoderma
lymph node permeability: factor
lymphoblastic: leukemia; lymphoma
lymphocyte: transformation
lymphocyte function associated: antigen
lymphocyte-mediated: cytotoxicity
lymphocytic: adenohypophysitis; choriomeningitis; hypophysitis; leukemia; leukemoid reaction; leukocytosis; leukopenia; series; thyroiditis
lymphocytic choriomeningitis: virus
lymphocytic interstitial: pneumonia; pneumonitis
lymphocytotoxic: antibodies
lymphoepithelial: cyst
lymphogenous: metastasis
lymphogranuloma venereum: antigen; virus
lymphoid: cell; hemoblast of Pappenheim; hypophysitis; leukemia; polyp; ring
lymphoid interstitial: pneumonia; pneumonia
lymphomatoid: granulomatosis; papulosis
lymphopenic thymic: dysplasia
lymphostatic: verrucosis
Lyon: hypothesis
lyophilic: colloid
lyophobic: colloid
lyotropic: series
lysinuric protein: intolerance
lysogenic: bacterium; induction; strain
lysosomal: disease
Lyt: antigens

M

M: antigen; band; concentration; line; phase; protein
M₁: antigen
MAC: complex
Macchiavello's: stain
MacConkey: agar
Macewen's: sign; symptom; triangle
Mach: effect; line; number
Machado-Guerreiro: test
machinery: murmur
Mach's: band
Machupo: virus

Mackay-Marg: tonometer
Mackenrodt's: ligament
Mackenzie's: amputation; polygraph
Maclagan's: test
Maclagan's thymol turbidity: test
Macleod's: rheumatism; syndrome
MacNeal's tetrachrome blood: stain
macroaggregated: albumin
macrobiotic: diet
macrocytic: anemia; anemia of pregnancy; anemia tropical; hyperchromia
macrocytic achylic: anemia
macrofollicular: adenoma
macroglia: cell
macro-Kjeldahl: method
macromolecular: chemistry
macrophage-activating: factor
macrophage colony-stimulating: factor
macrophage inflammatory: protein
macrophage migration inhibition: test
macroscopic: anatomy; sphincter
macular: amyloidosis; area; arteries; atrophy; coloboma; degeneration; drusen; dystrophy; erythema; evasion; fasciculus; leprosy; retinopathy; syphilid
mad: itch
mad cow: disease
Maddox's: rod
Madelung's: deformity; disease; neck
Mad Hatter: syndrome
Madlener: operation
Madura: boil; foot
maedi: virus
Maffucci's: syndrome
Magendie-Hertwig: sign; syndrome
Magendie's: foramen; law; spaces
magenta: tongue
magical: thinking
Magnan's: sign
Magnan's trombone: movement
magnesia and alumina oral: suspension
magnet: reaction; reflex
magnetic: attraction; field; implant; inertia
magnetic field: gradient
magnetic resonance: angiography; imaging; spectroscopy
magnetogyric: ratio

magnification: angiography; radiography
Magnus': sign
Mahaim: fibers
Maier's: sinus
maintenance: dose
maintenance drug: therapy
Maissiat's: band
maize: factor
Majocchi: granulomas
Majocchi's: disease
major: agglutinin; amblyoscope; amputation; calices; connector; depression; epilepsy; fissure; forceps; groove; hippocampus; hypnosis; hysteria; operation; surgery; tranquilizer
major duodenal: papilla
major histocompatibility: complex
major mood: disorder
major motor: seizure
major salivary: glands
major sublingual: duct
Makeham's: hypothesis
Malabar: itch; leprosy
malabsorption: syndrome
Malacarne's: pyramid; space
malar: arch; bone; flush; fold; foramen; lymph node; node; point; process
malariae: malaria
malarial: cachexia; crescent; fever; hemoglobinuria; knobs; periodicity; pigment
malarial pigment: stain
Malassez' epithelial: rests
malate-aspartate: shuttle
malate-condensing: enzyme
Maldonado-San Jose: stain
male: breast; gonad; hermaphroditism; homosexuality; hypogonadism; pseudohermaphroditism; sterility; urethra
Malecot: catheter
male pattern: alopecia; baldness
Malgaigne's: amputation; fossa; hernia; luxation; triangle
Malherbe's calcifying: epithelioma
malic: enzyme
malignant: anemia; bubo; catarrh of cattle; dysentery; dyskeratosis; edema; endocarditis; exophthalmos; glaucoma; granuloma; hepatoma; histiocytosis; hyperphenylalaninemia; hyperpyrexia; hypertension; hyperthermia; jaundice;

lymphadenosis; lymphoma; malnutrition; melanoma; melanoma in situ; meningioma; myopia; nephrosclerosis; pustule; scleritis; smallpox; stupor; synovioma; tumor
malignant atrophic: papulosis
malignant carcinoid: syndrome
malignant catarrhal: fever
malignant catarrhal fever: virus
malignant ciliary: epithelioma
malignant fibrous: histiocytoma
malignant lentigo: melanoma
malignant midline: reticulosis
malignant mixed müllerian: tumor
malignant mole: syndrome
malignant ovine and caprine: theileriosis
malignant tertian: fever; malaria
malignant tertian malarial: parasite
mallear: fold; prominence; stripe
malleolar: sulcus
malleolar articular: surface of fibula; surface of tibia
mallet: finger
Mallory: bodies
Mallory's: stain for actinomyces; stain for hemofuchsin
Mallory's aniline blue: stain
Mallory's collagen: stain
Mallory's iodine: stain
Mallory's phloxine: stain
Mallory's phosphotungstic acid hematoxylin: stain
Mallory's trichrome: stain
Mallory's triple: stain
Mallory-Weiss: lesion; syndrome; tear
Mall's: formula; ridges
Maloney: bougies
Maloney leukemia: virus
malpighian: bodies; capsule; cell; corpuscles; glands; glomerulus; layer; nodules; pyramid; rete; stigmas; stratum; tubules; tuft; vesicles
malt: liquor; sugar
Malta: fever
malt-worker's: lung
mamillary: body; ducts; line; process; tubercle; tubercle of hypothalamus
mamillotegmental: fasciculus

mamillothalamic: fasciculus; tract

mammary: branches; calculus; ducts; dysplasia; fistula; fold; gland; line; neuralgia; plexus; region; ridge; souffle

mammary cancer: virus of mice

mammary duct: ectasia

mammary tumor: virus of mice

mammotropic: factor; hormone

managed: care

Manchester: operation; ovoid

Manchurian: fever; typhus

Manchurian hemorrhagic: fever

Mandelin's: reagent

mandibular: arch; axis; canal; cartilage; condyle; dentition; disk; foramen; fossa; glide; joint; lymph node; movement; nerve; nodes; notch; process; protraction; reflex; retraction; tongue; torus

mandibular guide: prosthesis

mandibular hinge: position

mandibuloacral: dysostosis

mandibulofacial: dysostosis; dysplasia

mandibulofacial dysotosis: syndrome

mandibulomaxillary: fixation

mandibulo-oculofacial: syndrome

mango: dermatitis

mangrove: fly

manic: episode; excitement; psychosis

manic-depressive: disorder; illness; psychosis

manifest: content; hyperopia; strabismus; tetany; vector

manifesting: carrier; heterozygote

manna: sugar

Mann-Bollman: fistula

Mannkopf's: sign

mannose-6-phosphate: receptors

Mann's methyl blue-eosin: stain

Mann-Williamson: operation; ulcer

Manson's: disease; pyosis; schistosomiasis

Manson's eye: worm

Mantel-Haenszel: test

mantle: layer; radiotherapy; sclerosis; zone

Mantoux: pit; test

manual: pelvimetry; ventilation

manubriosternal: joint; junction; symphysis

map-dot-fingerprint: dystrophy

maple: sugar

maple bark: disease

maple syrup: urine

maple syrup urine: disease

maplike: skull

Marañón's: sign; syndrome

marantic: atrophy; edema; endocarditis; thrombosis; thrombus

marasmic: kwashiorkor

marathon group: psychotherapy

marble: bones

marble bone: disease

marble cutters': phthisis

Marburg: disease; virus

Marburg virus: disease

Marcacci's: muscle

march: fracture; hemoglobinuria

Marchand's: adrenals; rest

Marchand's wandering: cell

Marchant's: zone

Marchiafava-Bignami: disease

Marchiafava-Micheli: anemia; syndrome

Marchi's: fixative; reaction; stain; tract

Marcille's: triangle

Marcus Gunn: phenomenon; pupil; syndrome

Marcus Gunn's: sign

Marek's: disease

Marek's disease: virus

Marey's: law

Marfan's: disease; law; syndrome

margarine: disease

marginal: artery of colon; blepharitis; crest; fasciculus; gingivitis; gyrus; integrity of amalgam; keratitis; layer; part of orbicularis oris muscle; rays; ridge; sinuses of placenta; sphincter; tubercle; tubercle of zygomatic bone; zone

marginal corneal: degeneration

marginal mandibular: branch of facial nerve

marginal ring: ulcer of cornea

marginal tentorial: branch of internal carotid artery

marian: lithotomy

Marie-Robinson: syndrome

Marie's: ataxia; disease

Marie-Strümpell: disease

marine: pharmacology; soap

Marinesco-Garland: syndrome

Marinesco's succulent: hand

Marion's: disease

Mariotte: bottle

Mariotte's: experiment; law

Mariotte's blind: spot

marital: counseling; therapy

Marjolin's: ulcer

marked fetal: bradycardia

marker: chromosome; enzyme; locus; trait

Markov: process

Marme's: reagent

marmoset: virus

Maroteaux-Lamy: syndrome

Marquis': reagent

marriage: therapy

marrow: canal; cell

marrow-lymph: gland

Marseilles: fever

marsh: fever; gas

Marshall: syndrome; test

Marshall-Marchetti: test

Marshall-Marchetti-Krantz: operation

Marshall's: method

Marshall's oblique: vein

Marshall's vestigial: fold

marsupial: notch

Martegiani's: area; funnel

Martin-Gruber: anastomosis

Martinotti's: cell

Martin's: bandage; disease; tube

Martorell's: syndrome

masculine: pelvis; uterus

masculinity-femininity: scale

Masini's: sign

masked: epilepsy; gout; hyperthyroidism; virus

masklike: face

Maslow's: hierarchy

masochistic: personality

Mason: operation

Mason-Pfizer: virus

mason's: lung

MASS: syndrome

mass: hysteria; infection; law; movement; number; peristalsis; reflex; screening; spectrograph

mass action: theory

mass-action: ratio

Masselon's: spectacles

masseter: muscle; reflex

masseteric: artery; fascia; nerve; tuberosity; veins

massive: collapse

massive bowel resection: syndrome

Masson-Fontana ammoniacal silver: stain

Masson's: pseudoangiosarcoma

Masson's argentaffin: stain

Masson's trichrome: stain

mast: cell; leukocyte

mast cell: leukemia

Master: test

master: cast; eye; gland

Master's two-step exercise: test

mastery: motive

masticating: cycles; surface

masticator: nerve

masticatory: apparatus; diplegia; force; nucleus; spasm; surface; system

masticatory silent: period

mastoid: abscess; angle of parietal bone; antrum; artery; bone; border of occipital bone; branches of posterior auricular artery; branch of occipital artery; canaliculus; cells; empyema; fontanel; foramen; fossa; groove; lymph nodes; margin of occipital bone; notch; part of the temporal bone; process; sinuses; wall of middle ear

mastoid air: cells

mastoid emissary: vein

Masugi's: nephritis

mat: burn; gold

Matas': operation

matched: groups

maternal: cotyledon; death; dystocia; immunity; inheritance; placenta

maternal death: rate

maternal deprivation: syndrome

maternity: hospital

mathematical: chaos; determinant; genetics; model

mating: isolate; season

matrix: band; calculus; retainer

matrix Gla: protein

mattress: suture

maturation: arrest; factor; index; value

mature: bacteriophage; cataract; neutrophil

mature cell: leukemia

mature ovarian: follicle

maturity-onset: diabetes

maturity onset: diabetes of youth

matutinal: epilepsy

Mauchart's: ligaments

Maurer's: clefts; dots

Mauriac's: syndrome

Mauriceau-Levret: maneuver

Mauriceau's: maneuver

Mauthner's: cell; sheath; test

maxillary: angle; antrum; artery; dentition; eminence;

gland; hiatus; nerve;
plexus; process;
protraction; sinus; surface
of greater wing of sphenoid
bone; surface of palatine
bone; tuberosity; vein
maxillary sinus: radiograph
maxillofacial: prosthetics
maxillomandibular:
fixation; record;
registration; relation;
traction
maximal: dose; stimulus
maximal Histalog: test
maximal permissible: dose
Maxim-Gilbert: sequencing
Maximow's: stain for bone
marrow
maximum: temperature;
velocity
maximum breathing:
capacity
maximum likelihood:
estimator
maximum occipital: point
maximum permissible: dose
maximum urea: clearance
maximum voluntary:
ventilation
May apple: root
Mayaro: virus
**Mayer-Rokitansky-Küster-
Hauser:** syndrome
Mayer's: pessary; reflex
Mayer's hemalum: stain
Mayer's mucicarmine: stain
Mayer's mucihematein:
stain
May-Grünwald: stain
May-Hegglin: anomaly
Mayo: bunionectomy
Mayo-Robson's: point;
position
Mayo's: operation; vein
May-White: syndrome
Mazzoni: corpuscle
Mazzotti: reaction; test
McArdle's: disease;
syndrome
McArdle-Schmid-Pearson:
disease
McBurney's: incision; point;
sign
McCarthy's: reflexes
McCrea: sound
McCune-Albright:
syndrome
McDonald's: maneuver
McGoon's: technique
McIndoe: operation
McKee's: line
McMurray: test
McNemar's: test
McPhail: test
McRoberts: maneuver
McVay's: operation
M:E: ratio
meadow: dermatitis

Meadows': syndrome
meal: worm
mean: calorie; temperature;
vector
mean corpuscular:
hemoglobin; volume
**mean corpuscular
hemoglobin:** concentration
mean electrical: axis
mean foundation: plane
mean manifest: vector
measles: immunoglobulin;
virus
measles convalescent: serum
measles immune: globulin
(human)
**measles, mumps, and
rubella:** vaccine
measles virus: vaccine
measured: intelligence
meatal: cartilage; spine
Mecca: balsam
mechanical: abrasion;
alternation of the heart;
antidote; corepraxy;
dysmenorrhea; heart; ileus;
intelligence; jaundice;
strabismus; vector;
ventilation; vertigo
mechanically balanced:
occlusion
mechanism-based: inhibitor
mechanistic: school
mechanobullous: disease
Meckel: scan; syndrome
Meckel-Gruber: syndrome
Meckel's: band; cartilage;
cavity; diverticulum;
ganglion; ligament; plane;
space
Mecke's: reagent
meconial: colic
meconium: aspiration; ileus;
peritonitis
meconium blockage:
syndrome
medi: virus
medial: angle of eye;
aperture of the fourth
ventricle; arteriole of
retina; arteriosclerosis;
border; border of foot;
border of forearm; border
of humerus; border of
kidney; border of scapula;
border of suprarenal gland;
border of tibia; branches;
canthus; condyle; condyle
of femur; condyle of tibia;
cord of brachial plexus;
crest of fibula; crus; crus of
facial canal; crus of greater
alar cartilage of nose; crus
of the horizontal part of the
facial canal; crus of the
superficial inguinal ring;
eminence; epicondyle of
femur; epicondyle of

humerus; fillet; head;
lamina of cartilaginous
auditory tube; layer of
cartilaginous auditory tube;
lemniscus; ligament;
ligament of knee; ligament
of talocrural joint; ligament
of wrist; limb; lip of linea
aspera; malleolus; margin;
meniscus; nucleus of
thalamus; part of
longitudinal arch of foot;
part of middle lobar branch
of right superior pulmonary
vein; part of posterior
cervical intertransversarii
muscles; plate of pterygoid
process; pole of ovary;
process of calcaneal
tuberosity; root of median
nerve; root of optic tract;
rotator; segment; sulcus of
crus cerebri; surface;
surface of arytenoid
cartilage; surface of
cerebral hemisphere;
surface of fibula; surface of
lung; surface of ovary;
surface of testis; surface of
tibia; surface of toes;
surface of ulna; tubercle of
posterior process of talus;
vein of lateral ventricle;
venule of retina; wall of
middle ear; wall of orbit;
wall of tympanic cavity
medial accessory olivary:
nucleus
**medial antebrachial
cutaneous:** nerve
medial anterior thoracic:
nerve
medial arcuate: ligament
medial atrial: vein
medial basal: branch of
pulmonary artery; segment
medial bicipital: groove
medial brachial cutaneous:
nerve
medial calcaneal: branches
of tibial nerve
medial cartilaginous: layer
medial central: nucleus of
thalamus
medial cerebral: surface
medial circumflex: artery of
thigh
medial circumflex femoral:
artery; veins
medial collateral: ligament
of elbow
medial crural cutaneous:
branches of saphenous
nerve
medial cuneiform: bone
medial cutaneous: branch;
nerve of arm; nerve of
forearm; nerve of leg

medial dorsal cutaneous:
nerve
medial epicondylar: crest;
ridge
medial femoral: tuberosity
medial femoral circumflex:
artery
medial forebrain: bundle
medial frontobasal: artery
medial geniculate: body
medial great: muscle
medial inferior genicular:
artery
medial inguinal: fossa
medial lacunar: lymph
node; node
medial longitudinal: arch of
foot; bundle; fasciculus;
stria
**medial lumbar
intertransversarii:**
muscles
**medial lumbar
intertransverse:** muscles
medial lumbocostal: arch
medial malleolar: arteries;
network; surface of talus
**medial malleolar
subcutaneous:** bursa
medial mammary: branches
medial medullary: lamina of
corpus striatum
medial midpalmar: space
medial nasal: branches of
anterior ethmoidal nerve;
fold; primordium; process;
prominence
medial occipital: artery
medial occipitotemporal:
gyrus
medial palpebral:
commissure; ligament
medial patellar: retinaculum
medial pectoral: nerve
medial plantar: artery; nerve
medial popliteal: nerve
medial preoptic: nucleus
medial pterygoid: muscle;
plate
medial puboprostatic:
ligament
medial rectus: muscle
medial striate: artery
medial superior genicular:
artery
medial supraclavicular:
nerve
medial supracondylar:
crest; ridge
medial sural cutaneous:
nerve
medial talocalcaneal:
ligament
medial tarsal: artery
medial umbilical: fold;
ligament
medial vastus: muscle
medial vestibular: nucleus

median: aperture of the fourth ventricle; artery; bar of Mercier; eminence; groove of tongue; laryngotomy; line; lithotomy; nerve; plane; rhinoscopy; section; sternotomy; strumectomy; sulcus of fourth ventricle; vein of forearm; vein of neck

median antebrachial: vein

median anterior maxillary: cyst

median arcuate: ligament

median atlantoaxial: joint

median basilic: vein

median cephalic: vein

median cubital: vein

median frontal: sulcus

median glossoepiglottic: fold

median longitudinal: raphe of tongue

median mandibular: point

median maxillary anterior alveolar: cleft

median palatal: cyst

median palatine: suture

median raphe: cyst of the penis

median retruded: relation

median rhomboid: glossitis

median sacral: artery; crest; vein

median thyrohyoid: ligament

median tongue: bud

median umbilical: fold; ligament

mediastinal: arteries; branches; branches of internal thoracic artery; branches of thoracic aorta; emphysema; fibrosis; lipomatosis; part of lung; pleura; pleurisy; space; surface of lung; veins; window

mediate: auscultation; contagion; percussion; transfusion

medical: anatomy; biophysics; care; chemistry; diathermy; ethics; examiner; genetics; jurisprudence; model; mycology; pathology; psychology; record; selection; treatment

medical record: linkage

medicinal: charcoal; chemistry; eruption; zinc peroxide

medicinal soft: soap

mediocolic: sphincter

mediodorsal: nucleus

mediopubic: reflex

mediotarsal: amputation

Mediterranean: fever; lymphoma; theileriosis

Mediterranean exanthematous: fever

medium: artery; vein

medullary: arteries of brain; bone; callus; carcinoma; cavity; center; chemoreceptor; cone; cords; folds; groove; laminae of thalamus; layers of thalamus; membrane; plate; pyramid; pyramidotomy; ray; sarcoma; sheath; space; striae of fourth ventricle; stria of thalamus; substance; teniae; tube

medullary spinal: arteries

medullary sponge: kidney

medullated nerve: fiber

Medusa: head

Meeh: formula

Meeh-Dubois: formula

Mees': lines; stripes

Meesman: dystrophy

megacystic: syndrome

megacystitis-megaureter: syndrome

megacystitis-microcolon-intestinal hypoperistalsis: syndrome

megakaryocytic: leukemia

megaloblastic: anemia

megalocytic: anemia

meibomian: blepharitis; conjunctivitis; cyst; glands; sty

Meige's: disease

Meigs': syndrome

Meinicke: test

meiotic: division; drive; phase

Meissner's: corpuscle; plexus

melamine: resin

melanocyte-stimulating: hormone

melanophore-expanding: principle

melanotic: carcinoma; freckle; medulloblastoma; pigment; progonoma; whitlow

melanotic neuroectodermal: tumor of infancy

melanotropin release-inhibiting: hormone

melanotropin-releasing: factor; hormone

Meleney's: gangrene; ulcer

Melkersson-Rosenthal: syndrome

Melnick-Needles: syndrome

melon-seed: body

melting: point; temperature; temperature of DNA

Meltzer-Lyon: test

Meltzer's: law

membrane: bone; enzyme; potential

membrane attack: complex

membrane-coating: granule

membrane expansion: theory

membranoproliferative: glomerulonephritis

membranous: ampulla; cataract; cochlea; conjunctivitis; dysmenorrhea; glomerulonephritis; labyrinth; lamina of cartilaginous auditory tube; laryngitis; layer; layer of superficial fascia; lipodystrophy; neurocranium; ossification; part of interventricular septum; part of male urethra; part of nasal septum; pharyngitis; septum; urethra; viscerocranium; wall of middle ear; wall of trachea

memory: loop; span; trace

Mendel-Bechterew: reflex

Mendeléeff's: law

mendelian: character; genetics; inheritance; ratio; trait

Mendel's first: law

Mendel's instep: reflex

Mendelson's: syndrome

Mendel's second: law

Ménétrier's: disease; syndrome

Menge's: pessary

Mengo: encephalitis; virus

Ménière's: disease; syndrome

meningeal: branches; branch of internal carotid artery; branch of mandibular nerve; branch of occipital artery; branch of ophthalmic nerve; branch of spinal nerves; branch of vagus nerve; carcinoma; carcinomatosis; hernia; layer of dura mater; leukemia; neurosyphilis; plexus; veins

meningitic: streak

meningocerebral: cicatrix

meningococcal: meningitis

meningotyphoid: fever

meningovascular: neurosyphilis; syphilis

meniscofemoral: ligaments

meniscus: lens

Menkes': syndrome

menopausal: syndrome

menstrual: age; colic; cycle; edema; leukorrhea; molimina; period; sclerosis

menstrual extraction: abortion

mental: aberration; age; agraphia; apparatus; artery; branches of mental nerve; canal; chronometry; deficiency; disease; disorder; foramen; health; hospital; hygiene; illness; image; impairment; impression; nerve; point; process; protuberance; region; retardation; scotoma; spine; symphysis; tubercle

mentalis: muscle

mentoanterior: position

mentolabial: furrow; sulcus

mentoposterior: position

mentotransverse: position

mercapturic acid: pathway

Mercier's: bar; sound; valve

mercurial: diuretics; line; manometer; stomatitis; tremor

mercury: arc; poisoning

mercury vapor: lamp

Merendino's: technique

meridional: aberration; cleavage; fibers

Merkel cell: tumor

Merkel's: corpuscle; filtrum ventriculi; fossa; muscle

Merkel's tactile: cell; disk

mermaid: deformity

meroblastic: cleavage

merocrine: gland

Merrifield: knife; synthesis

Méry's: gland

Merzbacher-Pelizaeus: disease

mesangial: cell; nephritis

mesangial proliferative: glomerulonephritis

mesangiocapillary: glomerulonephritis

mesatipellic: pelvis

mesencephalic: flexure; nucleus of trigeminal nerve; tegmentum; tract of trigeminal nerve; veins

mesenchymal: cells; epithelium; hyloma; tissue

mesenteric: glands; hernia; lymph nodes; portion of small intestine; veins

mesenteric artery: occlusion

mesentericoparietal: fossa; recess

mesethmoid: bone

mesh: graft

mesial: angle; caries; displacement; occlusion; surface of tooth

meso: compounds

mesoblastic: nephroma; segment; sensibility
mesocaval: shunt
mesocolic: lymph nodes; tenia
mesodermal: factor
mesoglial: cells
mesomelic: dwarfism
mesometanephric: carcinoma
mesometric: pregnancy
mesonephric: adenocarcinoma; duct; fold; rest; ridge; tissue; tubule
mesonephroid: tumor
mesopic: perimetry
mesothelial: cell; hyloma
mesovarian: border of ovary; margin of ovary
messenger: RNA
messenger-like: RNA
metabisulfite: test
metabolic: acidosis; alkalosis; calculus; coma; craniopathy; disease; encephalopathy; equivalent; indican; pool
metabolized vitamin D: milk
metabotropic: receptor
metacarpal: bone; index; veins
metacarpohypothenar: reflex
metacarpophalangeal: articulations; joints
metacarpothenar: reflex
metacentric: chromosome
metachromatic: bodies; granules; leukodystrophy; stain
metafacial: angle
metaherpetic: keratitis
metahypophysial: diabetes
metal: base; interface
metal fume: fever
metal insert: teeth
metallic: rale; tremor
metameric nervous: system
metanephric: blastema; bud; cap; diverticulum; duct; tubule
metanephrogenic: tissue
metaphysial: dysostosis; dysplasia
metaphysial fibrous cortical: defect
metaplastic: anemia; carcinoma; ossification; polyp
metastasizing: septicemia
metastatic: abscess; calcification; carcinoma; choroiditis; mumps; ophthalmia; pneumonia; retinitis

metastatic carcinoid: syndrome
metatarsal: artery; bone; reflex
metatarsophalangeal: articulations; joints
metatropic: dwarfism
metatypical: carcinoma
Metchnikoff's: theory
Metenier's: sign
meter: angle
meter-kilogram-second: system; unit
methacrylate: resin
methamphetamine: base
methanol: fixative
methionine-activating: enzyme
methionine malabsorption: syndrome
methionyl: dipeptidase
methonium: compounds
3-methoxy-4-hydroxymandelic acid: test
methyl: mercaptan
methylglucamine: iodipamide
methyl green-pyronin: stain
methylol: riboflavin
metopic: point; suture
metrial: gland
metric: system
metroperitoneal: fistula
metrotrophic: test
Meulengracht's: diet
Mexican: typhus
Mexican hat: cell; corpuscle
Mexican spotted: fever
Meyenburg-Altherr-Uehlinger: syndrome
Meyenburg's: complex; disease
Meyer-Archambault: loop
Meyer-Betz: disease; syndrome
Meyerhof oxidation: quotient
Meyer-Overton: rule; theory of narcosis
Meyer's: cartilages; line; reagent; sinus
Meynert's: cells; commissures; decussation; fasciculus; layer
Meynert's retroflex: bundle
MHA-TP: test
MHC: restriction
mianeh: disease; fever
miasma: theory
Mibelli's: angiokeratomas; disease
Michaelis: complex; constant
Michaelis-Gutmann: body
Michaelis-Menten: constant; equation; hypothesis
Michel's: spur

microangiopathic hemolytic: anemia
micro-Astrup: method
microbial: genetics; persistence; RNase II; vitamin
micrococcal: endonuclease; nuclease
microcrystalline: cellulose
microcystic: disease of renal medulla
microcystic epithelial: dystrophy
microcytic: anemia
microdrepanocytic: anemia
microelectric: waves
microetching: technique
microfilarial: sheath
microfollicular: adenoma; goiter
microglandular: adenosis
microglia: cells
microhemagglutination-Treponema pallidum: test
microinvasive: carcinoma
micro-Kjeldahl: method
microlecithal: egg
micromelic: dwarfism
micrometastatic: disease
micromyeloblastic: leukemia
microprecipitation: test
microscopic: anatomy; field; hematuria; section; sphincter
microscopically controlled: surgery
microsphere: method
microsporidian: keratoconjunctivitis
microtubule-associated: proteins
microtubule-organizing: center
microvascular: anastomosis
microwave: therapy
micturition: reflex; syncope
midaxillary: line
midbrain: tegmentum; vesicle
midcarpal: joint
midclavicular: line
middiastolic: murmur
middle: cells; finger; kidney; lobe of prostate; lobe of right lung; mediastinum; pain; piece; trunk of brachial plexus
middle atlantoepistrophic: joint
middle axillary: line
middle cardiac: vein
middle carpal: joint
middle cerebellar: peduncle
middle cerebral: artery
middle cervical: fascia; ganglion
middle cervical cardiac: nerve

middle cluneal: nerves
middle colic: artery; lymph nodes; vein
middle collateral: artery
middle constrictor: muscle of pharynx
middle costotransverse: ligament
middle cranial: fossa
middle cuneiform: bone
middle ethmoidal: sinuses
middle ethmoidal air: cells
middle frontal: convolution; gyrus; sulcus
middle genicular: artery
middle glossoepiglottic: fold
middle gray: layer of superior colliculus
middle group of mesenteric: lymph nodes
middle hemorrhoidal: artery; plexuses; veins
middle hepatic: veins
middle lobe: branch; syndrome
middle meningeal: artery; branch of maxillary nerve; nerve; veins
middle meningeal artery: groove
middle nasal: concha
middle palmar: space
middle radioulnar: joint
middle rectal: artery; lymph node; node; plexuses; veins
middle sacral: artery; plexus
middle scalene: muscle
middle superior alveolar: branch of infraorbital nerve
middle supraclavicular: nerve
middle suprarenal: artery
middle talar articular: surface of calcaneus
middle temporal: artery; convolution; gyrus; sulcus; vein
middle thyroid: vein
middle transverse rectal: fold
middle turbinated: bone
middle umbilical: fold; ligament
midforceps: delivery
midgastric transverse: sphincter
midget bipolar: cells
midlife: crisis
midline: incision; myelotomy
midline malignant reticulosis: granuloma
midnodal: extrasystole
midpalmar: space
midsagittal: plane; section
midsigmoid: sphincter
midtarsal: joint
Miescher's: elastoma; granuloma; tubes

mignon: lamp
migraine: headache
migrating: abscess; teeth
migration: theory
migration inhibition: test
migration-inhibitory: factor
migration inhibitory factor: test
migratory: cell; pneumonia
mika: operation
Mikulicz: clamp
Mikulicz': aphthae; cells; disease; drain; operation; syndrome
Mikulicz-Vladimiroff: amputation
mild: silver protein
mild fetal: bradycardia
Miles: resection
Miles': operation
Milian's: disease; erythema
miliary: abscess; aneurysm; embolism; fever; pattern; tuberculosis
miliary papular: syphilid
milieu: therapy
military: medicine; neurosis
milk: anemia; colic; corpuscle; crust; cyst; ducts; factor; fever; gland; leg; line; ridge; scall; sickness; spots; sugar; tetter; tooth
milk of: calcium
milk-alkali: syndrome
milk-ejection: reflex
milkers': nodes; nodules
milker's nodule: virus
milk let-down: reflex
Milkman's: syndrome
milk-ring: test
milky: ascites; urine
mill: fever
Millard-Gubler: syndrome
milled-in: curves; paths
Miller-Abbott: tube
miller's: asthma
Miller's chemicoparasitic: theory
Millner: needle
Millon: reaction
Millon clinical multiaxial: inventory
Millon Clinical Multiaxial Inventory: test
Millon-Nasse: test
Millon's: reagent
mill wheel: murmur
Milroy's: disease
Milton's: disease
MIM: number
mimetic: chorea; muscles; paralysis
mimic: convulsion; genes; spasm; tic
Minamata: disease
mind: blindness; pain
mineral: water; wax

miner's: asthma; cramps; disease; elbow; lung; nystagmus
Minerva: jacket
miniature: stomach
miniature scarlet: fever
minicore-multicore: myopathy
minimal: air; dose
minimal alveolar: concentration
minimal amplitude: nystagmus
minimal anesthetic: concentration
minimal brain: dysfunction
minimal-change: disease
minimal-change nephrotic: syndrome
minimal deviation: melanoma
minimal infecting: dose
minimal inhibitory: concentration
minimal lethal: dose
minimally invasive: surgery
minimal reacting: dose
minimum: light; temperature
minimum light: threshold
minimum protein: requirement
mink enteritis: virus
Minnesota Multiphasic Personality: Inventory
Minnesota multiphasic personality inventory: test
minor: agglutinin; amputation; calices; connector; fissure; forceps; groove; hippocampus; hypnosis; hysteria; operation; surgery; tranquilizer
minor duodenal: papilla
minor motor: seizure
minor salivary: glands
minor sublingual: ducts
Minot-Murphy: diet
minus: lens
minute: output; volume
miostagmin: reaction
Mirchamp's: sign
Mirizzi's: syndrome
mirror: haploscope; image; speech
mirror-image: cell
mirror image: dextrocardia
misdirection: phenomenon
mismatch: repair
missed: abortion; labor; period
missense: mutation
mist: bacillus
Mitchell's: disease; treatment
mite: typhus
mite-born: typhus

mitochondrial: chromosome; gene; matrix; membrane; myopathy; sheath
mitogenic: lectin
mitotic: cycle; division; figure; index; period; rate; spindle
mitral: area; cells; click; commissurotomy; facies; gradient; incompetence; insufficiency; murmur; orifice; regurgitation; stenosis; tap; valve; valvotomy
mitral valve: prolapse
mitral valve prolapse: syndrome
Mitrofanoff: principle
Mitsuda: antigen; reaction
Mitsuo's: phenomenon
mixed: agglutination; aphasia; astigmatism; beat; chancre; disulfide; esotropia; gland; glioma; glycerides; hyperlipemia; hyperlipidemia; hypoglycemia; infection; leukemia; nerve; paralysis; thrombus; tocopherols concentrate; tumor; tumor of salivary gland; tumor of skin
mixed agglutination: reaction; test
mixed connective-tissue: disease
mixed discrete-continuous random: variable
mixed expired: gas
mixed function: oxygenase
mixed hyperlipoproteinemia familial, type 5: hyperlipidemia
mixed lymphocyte: culture
mixed lymphocyte culture: reaction; test
mixed mesodermal: tumor
Mixter: clamp
Miyagawa: bodies
MLC: test
MM: virus
M'Naghten: rule
mnemic: hypothesis; theory
MNSs: antigens
mobile: part of nasal septum; spasm
Mobitz: block
Mobitz types of atrioventricular: block
Möbius': sign; syndrome
modal: alteration
model: game
modeling: composition; compound; plastic
moderate: hypothermia
moderator: band; variable
modern: genetics

modified: milk; smallpox
modified radical: hysterectomy; mastectomy
modified zinc oxide-eugenol: cement
modifier: gene
modulation transfer: function
Moeller's: glossitis
Moeller's grass: bacillus
Mogen: clamp
Mohr: pipette
Mohrenheim's: fossa; space
Mohr's: syndrome
Mohs: scale
Mohs': chemosurgery; surgery
Mohs' fresh tissue chemosurgery: technique
Mohs' micrographic: surgery
moist: gangrene; papule; rale; tetter; wart
Mokola: virus
molar: absorptivity; behavior; concentration; glands; mass; pregnancy; tooth
molar absorbancy: index
molar absorption: coefficient
molar extinction: coefficient
mold: guide
mole: fraction
molecular: behavior; biology; biophysics; disease; dispersion; distillation; formula; genetics; heat; layer; layer of cerebellar cortex; layer of cerebellum; layer of cerebral cortex; layer of retina; layers of olfactory bulb; mass; movement; pathology; rotation; sieve; weight
molecular dispersed: solution
molecular dissociation: theory
molecular weight: ratio
Molisch's: test
Mollaret's: meningitis
Moll's: glands
molluscum: body; conjunctivitis; corpuscle
molluscum contagiosum: virus
Moloney: test
Moloney's: virus
molybdenum: cofactor
molybdenum target: tube
Monakow's: bundle; nucleus; syndrome; tract
Mönckeberg's: arteriosclerosis; calcification; degeneration; sclerosis

Mönckeberg's medial: calcification
Monday morning: sickness
Mondini: deafness; dysplasia
Mondonesi's: reflex
Mondor's: disease
Monge's: disease
mongolian: fold; macula; spot
moniliasis: pneumonia
moniliform: hair
monkey: hand; malaria
monkey B: virus
monkeypox: virus
monoamine oxidase: inhibitor
monoamniotic: twins
monobasic: acid; ammonium phosphate; potassium phosphate
monobromated: camphor
monochorial: twins
monochorionic diamniotic: placenta
monochorionic monoamniotic: placenta
monochromatic: aberration; rays
monoclonal: antibody; gammopathy; immunoglobulin; protein
monocrotic: pulse
monocular: diplopia; heterochromia; strabismus
monocyte chemoattractant: protein-1
monocyte derived neutrophil chemotactic: factor
monocytic: angina; leukemia; leukemoid reaction; leukocytosis; leukopenia
monocytoid: cell
Monod-Wyman-Changeux: model
monohydric: alcohol
monoleptic: fever
monomolecular: reaction
monomorphic: adenoma
mononuclear phagocyte: system
monophasic: complex
monophyletic: theory
monopolar: cautery
monopotassium: phosphate
monorecidive: chancre
monosodium: phosphate
monostotic fibrous: dysplasia
monotonic: sequence
monovalent: antiserum
monovular: twins
monozygotic: twins
Monro-Kellie: doctrine
Monro-Richter: line
Monro's: doctrine; foramen; line; sulcus

Monsel: solution
Monsel's: solution
Monson: curve
montan: wax
Monteggia's: fracture
Montenegro: test
Montgomery's: follicles; glands; tubercles
mood: disorders
mood-congruent: hallucination
mood-incongruent: hallucination
moon: blindness; face; facies
Moon's: molars
moon shaped: face
Mooren's: ulcer
Moore's: method
Moore's lightning: streaks
Mooser: bodies
moral: ataxia; treatment
Morand's: foot; spur
Morax-Axenfeld: diplobacillus
Moraxella: conjunctivitis
morbid: impulse; obesity; thirst
morbidity: rate
morcellation: operation
Morel's: ear
Morgagni-Adams-Stokes: syndrome
morgagnian: cyst
Morgagni's: appendix; cartilage; caruncle; cataract; columns; concha; crypts; disease; foramen; fossa; fovea; frenum; globules; humor; hydatid; lacuna; liquor; nodule; prolapse; retinaculum; sinus; spheres; syndrome; tubercle; valves; ventricle
Morgan's: bacillus; fold
Morison's: pouch
Mörner's: test
morning: diarrhea; sickness; vomiting
morning glory: anomaly; syndrome
Moro: reflex
morphine injector's: septicemia
morphogenetic: movement
morphologic: element
Morquio's: disease; syndrome
Morquio-Ullrich: disease
mortality: rate
mortar: kidney
mortise: joint
Morton's: neuralgia; plane; syndrome; toe
Morvan's: chorea; disease
mosaic: fundus; inheritance; pattern; wart
Moschcowitz: test
Moschcowitz': disease

Mosenthal: test
Mosler's: diabetes; sign
mosquito: clamp; forceps
Moss: tube
moss: starch
Mossman: fever
Mosso's: ergograph; sphygmomanometer
mossy: cell; fibers; foot
Motais': operation
moth: patch
moth-eaten: alopecia
mother: cell; colony; cyst; liquor; star; surrogate; yaw
mother superior: complex
motile: leukocyte
motility: test
motility test: medium
motion: sickness
motor: abreaction; agraphia; amusia; aphasia; apraxia; area; ataxia; cell; cortex; decussation; endplate; fibers; image; impersistence; nerve; nerve of face; neuron; nuclei; nucleus of facial nerve; nucleus of trigeminal nerve; nucleus of trigeminus; paralysis; plate; point; root; root of ciliary ganglion; roots of submandibular ganglion; root of trigeminal nerve; unit; urgency; zone
motor dapsone: neuropathy
motor neuron: disease
motor speech: center
motor system: disease
mottled: enamel; tooth
Motulsky dye reduction: test
Mounier-Kuhn: syndrome
mountain: anemia; balm; disease; sickness
mounting: medium
mouse: cancer; encephalomyelitis; hepatitis; leprosy; poliomyelitis; unit
mouse antialopecia: factor
mouse encephalomyelitis: virus
mouse hepatitis: virus
mouse leukemia: viruses
mouse mammary tumor: virus
mouse parotid tumor: virus
mouse poliomyelitis: virus
mousepox: virus
mousetail: pulse
mouse thymic: virus
mouse-tooth: forceps
mouth: breathing; mirror; rehabilitation
mouth-to-mouth: respiration; resuscitation

movable: heart; joint; kidney; pulse; spleen; testis
Mowry's colloidal iron: stain
moyamoya: disease
Mozart: ear
MP: joints
MR: angiography
MS-1: agent; hepatitis
MS-2: agent
MSB trichrome: stain
Mu: antigen
Mucha-Habermann: disease; syndrome
Much's: bacillus
mucilaginous: gland
mucin clot: test
mucinogen: granules
mucinoid: degeneration
mucinous: carcinoma
muciparous: gland
Muckle-Wells: syndrome
mucoalbuminous: cells
mucobuccal: fold
mucocutaneous: junction; leishmaniasis; muscle
mucocutaneous lymph node: syndrome
mucoepidermoid: carcinoma; tumor
mucoepithelial: dysplasia
mucoid: adenocarcinoma; colony; degeneration
mucoid impaction of: bronchus
mucoid medial: degeneration
mucomembranous: enteritis
mucoperichondrial: flap
mucoperiosteal: flap
mucopolysaccharide keratin: dystrophy
mucopurulent: conjunctivitis
mucosa of: colon
mucosal: disease; folds of gallbladder; graft; tunics
mucosal disease: virus
mucosal relief: radiography
mucoserous: cells
mucous: cast; cell; colitis; cyst; diarrhea; gland; glands of auditory tube; membranes; membrane of tympanic cavity; patch; plaque; plug; polyp; rale; sheath of tendon
mucous connective: tissue
mucous neck: cell
mucus: impaction
mud: bed; fever
Muehrcke's: lines
Mueller electronic: tonometer
Mueller-Hinton: agar; medium
Muehrcke's: sign
muffle: furnace
Muir-Torre: syndrome

mulberry: calculus; molar; ovary; spots
Mulder's: test
Mules': operation
mule-spinner's: cancer
mulibrey: nanism
müllerian: adenosarcoma
müllerian inhibiting: factor; substance
müllerian regression: factor
Müller's: capsule; duct; fibers; fixative; law; maneuver; muscle; sign; trigone; tubercle
Müller's radial: cells
multangular: bone
multiaxial: classification; joint
multicentric: reticulohistiocytosis
multi-colony-stimulating: factor
multicore: disease
multicuspid: tooth
multidrug: resistance
multienzyme: complex
multifactorial: inheritance
multifidus: muscle
multifocal: choroiditis; lens; osteitis fibrosa
multiform: layer
multiformat: camera
multi-infarct: dementia
multilamellar: body
multilocal: genetics
multilocular: cyst; fat
multilocular adipose: tissue
multilocular hydatid: cyst
multimammate: mouse
multinodular: goiter
multinomial: distribution
multinuclear: leukocyte
multipennate: muscle
multiphasic: screening
multiple: alcohol; amputation; anchorage; embolism; exostosis; fission; fracture; myeloma; myelomatosis; myositis; neuritis; parasitism; personality; pregnancy; sclerosis; serositis; stain; sulfatase deficiency; vision
multiple chemical: sensitivity
multiple ego: states
multiple endocrine: adenomatosis; neoplasia, type 2
multiple endocrine deficiency: syndrome
multiple epiphysial: dysplasia
multiple glandular deficiency: syndrome
multiple hamartoma: syndrome

multiple idiopathic hemorrhagic: sarcoma
multiple intestinal: polyposis
multiple lentigines: syndrome
multiple mucosal neuroma: syndrome
multiple personality: disorder
multiple puncture tuberculin: test
multiple self-healing squamous: epithelioma
multiple sleep latency: test
multiple symmetric: lipomatosis
multiplicative: division; growth; model
multipolar: cell; mitosis; neuron
multistage: model
multivalent: vaccine
multivariate: studies
multivesicular: bodies
mummification: necrosis
mummified: pulp
mumps: meningoencephalitis; virus
mumps sensitivity: test
mumps skin test: antigen
mumps virus: vaccine
mumu: fever
Munchausen: syndrome; syndrome by proxy
Münchhausen: syndrome
mung bean: nuclease
municipal: hospital
Munro's: abscess; microabscess; point
Munson's: sign
mural: cell; endocarditis; pregnancy; thrombosis; thrombus
murine: hepatitis; leukemia; typhus
murine sarcoma: virus
Murphy: drip
Murphy's: button; percussion; sign
Murray Valley: encephalitis; rash
Murray Valley encephalitis: virus
Murutucu: virus
muscarinic: antagonist; receptors
muscle: bundle; curve; epithelium; fascicle; hemoglobin; plasma; plate; proteins; relaxant; repositioning; resection; serum; sound; spasm; spindle
muscle phosphorylase: deficiency
muscle-tendon: attachment; junction

muscular: artery; asthenopia; atrophy; branches; coat; coat of bronchi; coat of colon; coat of ductus deferens; coat of esophagus; coat of female urethra; coat of gallbladder; coat of pharynx; coat of rectum; coat of small intestine; coat of stomach; coat of trachea; coat of ureter; coat of urinary bladder; coat of uterine tube; coat of uterus; coat of vagina; dystrophy; fascia of extraocular muscle; fibril; hyperesthesia; incompetence; insufficiency; lacuna; layer of mucosa; movement; part of interventricular septum of heart; process of arytenoid cartilage; pulley; reflex; relaxant; rheumatism; sense; substance of prostate; system; tissue; triangle; trophoneurosis; tunic of gallbladder; tunics
muscular subaortic: stenosis
musculocutaneous: amputation; flap; nerve; nerve of leg
musculophrenic: artery; veins
musculospiral: groove; nerve; paralysis
musculotendinous: cuff
musculotubal: canal
mushroom: poisoning
mushroom-worker's: lung
music: blindness
musical: agraphia; alexia; murmur
musician's: cramp
muskeag: moss
Musset's: sign
Mustard: operation; procedure
mustard: gas
mutant: gene
mutation: rate
mutational: frequency
mutilating: keratoderma; leprosy
mutton-fat keratic: precipitates
mutual: resistance
mutualistic: symbiosis
MVE: virus
MWC: model
myasthenic: crisis; facies; reaction; syndrome
mycoplasma: pneumonia of pigs
mycoplasmal: pneumonia

mycotic: aneurysm; endocarditis; keratitis
myelin: body; figure; protein A1; sheath
myelinated: nerve
myelinated nerve: fiber
myelinic: degeneration
myeloblastic: leukemia; protein
myelocytic: crisis; leukemia; leukemoid reaction
myelogenic: sarcoma
myeloid: cell; metaplasia; sarcoma; series; tissue
myelomonocytic: leukemia
myelophthisic: anemia
myeloproliferative: syndromes
myenteric: plexus; reflex
mylohyoid: artery; fossa; groove; line; muscle; nerve; ridge
mylopharyngeal: part of superior pharyngeal constrictor
myocardial: bridge; infarction; infarction in dumbbell form; insufficiency; ischemia; rigor mortis
myocardial depressant: factor
myoclonic: seizure
myoclonic astatic: epilepsy
myoclonus: epilepsy
myocutaneous: flap
myodermal: flap
myoelastic: theory
myoepicardial: mantle
myoepithelial: cell
myofacial pain-dysfunction: syndrome
myofascial: syndrome
myofunctional: therapy
myogenic: paralysis; potential; theory; tonus
myoid: cells
myomatous: polyp
myometrial arcuate: arteries
myometrial radial: arteries
myoneural: blockade; junction
myopathic: atrophy; facies; scoliosis
myophosphorylase deficiency: glycogenosis
myopic: astigmatism; choroidopathy; conus; crescent; degeneration
myosin: filament
myotatic: contraction; irritability; reflex
myotonic: cataract; dystrophy
myotubular: myopathy
myovascular: sphincter
myovenous: sphincter
myxedema: heart; voice

myxedematous: infantilism
myxoid: cyst; degeneration
myxomatosis: virus
myxomembranous: colitis
myxopapillary:
ependymoma

N

N-: terminus
nabothian: cyst; follicle
nacreous: ichthyosis
Nadi: reaction
Naegeli: syndrome
Naegeli type of monocytic:
leukemia
Naffziger: operation;
syndrome
Nägele: obliquity
Nägele's: pelvis; rule
Nagel's: test
Nageotte: cells
nail: bed; extension; fold;
horn; matrix; pits; plate;
pulse
nail-patella: syndrome
Nairobi sheep: disease
Nairobi sheep disease: virus
Nakanishi's: stain
naked: virus
NAME: syndrome
NANB: hepatitis
NANBNC: hepatitis
NANC: neuron
nanoid: enamel
nanukayami: fever
nape: nevus
napkin: rash
narcissistic: personality
narcissistic personality:
disorder
narcoleptic: tetrad
narcotic: blockade; hunger;
reversal
narrow-angle: glaucoma
nasal: arch; atrium; bone;
border of frontal bone;
calculus; capsule; catarrh;
cavity; crest; duct; feeding;
foramen; ganglion; glands;
glioma; height;
hemorrhage; index; margin
of frontal bone; meatus;
mucosa; muscle; myiasis;
nerve; notch; part of frontal
bone; part of pharynx;
pharynx; pits; placodes;
point; polyp; process;
reflex; region; ridge; sacs;
septum; spine of frontal
bone; surface of maxilla;
surface of palatine bone;
valve; venules of retina
nasalis: muscle
nasal septal: cartilage
nasal venous: arch
Nasik: vibrio

nasion-pogonion:
measurement
nasion-postcondylar: plane
nasion soft: tissue
Nasmyth's: cuticle;
membrane
nasoalveolar: cyst
nasobasilar: line
nasobregmatic: arc
nasociliary: nerve; root
nasofrontal: vein
nasogastric: tube
nasojugal: fold
nasolabial: cyst; groove;
lymph node; node
nasolacrimal: canal; duct
nasomandibular: fixation
nasomaxillary: suture
nasomental: reflex
naso-occipital: arc
nasopalatine: groove; nerve
nasopalatine duct: cyst
nasopharyngeal: groove;
leishmaniasis; passage
nasotracheal: intubation;
tube
Nasse's: law
natal: cleft; tooth
Natal's: sore
natiform: skull
native: albumin; protein
natural: antibody; dentition;
dyes; focus of infection;
hemolysin; immunity;
mutation; pigment;
products; selection
natural killer: cells
natural killer cell
stimulating: factor
nature-nurture: issue
Nauheim: bath; treatment
Nauta's: stain
navel: ill
navicular: abdomen; bone;
bone of hand; disease;
fossa of urethra
navicular articular: surface
of talus
NBT: test
ND: virus
near: drowning; point;
reaction; reflex; sight
nearest neighbor: frequency
near point of: convergence
near-total: thyroidectomy
Nebraska calf scours: virus
nebulous: urine
necessary: cause
neck: reflexes; sign
neck-shaft: angle
necrobiotic:
xanthogranuloma
necrogenic: wart
necrolytic migratory:
erythema
necrosis: bacillus

necrotic: angina; cirrhosis;
cyst; inflammation; pulp;
rhinitis of pigs
necrotic infectious:
conjunctivitis
necrotizing: angiitis;
arteriolitis; cellulitis;
encephalitis;
encephalomyelopathy;
encephalopathy;
enterocolitis; fasciitis;
papillitis; scleritis;
sialometaplasia
necrotizing hemorrhage:
leukomyelitis
necrotizing ulcerative:
gingivitis
needle: bath; biopsy; culture;
forceps
needle point: tracing
Needles' split cast: method
Neethling: virus
Neftel's: disease
negative: accommodation;
afterimage; anergy;
catalyst; chronotropism;
control; convergence;
cooperativity; electrode;
electrotaxis; feedback;
image; meniscus; phase;
politzerization; pressure;
scotoma; stain; taxis;
thermotaxis; transference;
valence
negative base: excess
negative end-expiratory:
pressure
negatively: bathmotropic;
dromotropic; inotropic
negative strand: virus
Negishi: virus
Negri: bodies; corpuscles
Negro's: phenomenon
Neisser's: coccus; stain;
syringe
Nélaton's: fold
Nélaton's: catheter;
dislocation; fibers; line;
sphincter
Nelson: syndrome; tumor
nemaline: myopathy
neonatal: anemia; apoplexy;
arthritis of foals;
conjunctivitis; death;
diagnosis; hepatitis; herpes;
hyperbilirubinemia;
hypoglycemia;
isoerythrolysis; jaundice;
line; lupus; medicine; ring;
screening; tetanus; tetany;
tooth
neonatal calf diarrhea:
virus
neonatal mortality: rate
neoplastic: arachnoiditis;
meningitis
neotype: culture; strain
neovascular: glaucoma

nephric: blastema; duct
nephritic: calculus; factor;
syndrome
nephrogenic: adenoma; cord;
diabetes insipidus; tissue
nephronic: loop
nephrostomy: tube
nephrotic: edema; syndrome
nephrotomic: cavity
Neptune's: girdle
Néri's: sign
Nernst's: equation; theory
nerve: avulsion; block; cell;
conduction; deafness;
decompression; ending;
fascicle; fiber; field; force;
ganglion; graft;
implantation; pain; papilla;
plexus; root; stroma;
suture; tract; trunk
nerve block: anesthesia
nerve cell: body
nerve conduction: velocity
nerve growth: cone; factor
nerve growth factor:
antiserum
nervous: asthenopia; asthma;
dyspepsia; indigestion;
lobe; lobe of hypophysis;
part of retina; system;
tissue; tunic of eyeball
Nessler's: reagent
net: flux; knot
Netherton's: syndrome
nettle: rash
nettling: hairs
Neubauer's: artery
Neuberg: ester
Neufeld: reaction
Neufeld capsular: swelling
Neumann's: cells; disease;
law; sheath
neural: arch; axis; canal;
crest; cyst; factor; folds;
groove; layer of optic
retina; layer of retina; part
of hypophysis; plate;
segment; spine; tube
neural crest: syndrome
neuralgic: amyotrophy
neurasthenic: personality
neurenteric: canal; cysts
neurilemma: cells
neuritic: atrophy; plaque
neuroaxonal: dystrophy
neurobiotactic: movement
neurocentral: joint; suture;
synchondrosis
neurochronaxic: theory
neurocirculatory: asthenia
neurocranial
granulomatous: arteritis
neurocutaneous: melanosis;
syndrome
neuroectodermal: junction
neuroendocrine: cell
neuroendocrine transducer:
cell

WordFinder

neuroepithelial: body; cells; layer of retina
neurofibrillar: nerve
neurofibrillary: degeneration; tangle
neurogenic: atrophy; bladder; fracture; tonus
neuroglia: cells
neurohemal: organs
neurohumoral: secretion; transmission
neurolemma: cells
neuroleptic: agent
neuroleptic malignant: syndrome
neuromast: organ
neuromuscular: cell; junction; relaxant; spindle; system
neuromuscular blocking: agents
neuronal: ceroid lipofuscinosis; hyperplasia
neuronal intestinal: dysplasia
neuroparalytic: keratitis; keratopathy
neuropathic: albuminuria; arthritis; arthropathy; bladder; joint
neuropsychologic: disorder
neurosecretory: cells; substance
neurosomatic: junction
neurotendinous: organ; spindle
neurotic: excoriation; manifestation
neurotonic: reaction
neurotrophic: atrophy; keratitis; keratitis
neurotropic: attraction; virus
neurovascular: flap; sheath
Neusser's: granules
neutral: axis of straight beam; element; fat; mutation; occlusion; oxide; point; reaction; spirits; stain; zone
neutral buffered formalin: fixative
neutralization: plate; test
neutralizing: antibody
neutral lipid storage: disease
neutron: radiation
neutropenic: angina
neutrophil: granule
neutrophil activating: factor; protein
neutrophil chemotactant: factor
neutrophilic: leukemia; leukocyte; leukocytosis; leukopenia
nevoid: amentia; elephantiasis; hypertrichosis

nevus: cell; cell, A-type; cell, B-type; cell, C-type
new: combination; growth; methylene blue; mutation
Newcastle: disease
Newcastle disease: virus
Newcomer's: fixative
new duck: disease
New Hampshire: rule
Newtonian: constant of gravitation
newtonian: aberration
newtonian: flow; fluid; viscosity
Newton's: disk; law
New World: leishmaniasis
new yellow: enzyme
New York Heart Association: classification
Neyman-Pearson statistical: hypothesis
Nezelof: syndrome
Nezelof type of thymic: alymphoplasia
NGF: antiserum
niacin: test
nick: translation
nickel: dermatitis
Nickerson-Kveim: test
Nick's: procedure
Nicol: prism
Nicolas-Favre: disease
Nicolle's: stain for capsules
Nicolle's white: mycetoma
nicotine: stomatitis
nicotinic: receptors
nicotinic acid: maculopathy
nicotinic cholinergic: receptor
nictitating: membrane; spasm
Nieden's: syndrome
Niemann: disease
Niemann-Pick: cell; disease
Niemann's: splenomegaly
Niewenglowski: rays
night: blindness; hospital; myopia; pain; sight; sweats; vision
nihilistic: delusion
Nikiforoff's: method
Nikolsky's: sign
nil: disease
nine mile: fever
ninhydrin: reaction
ninhydrin-Schiff: stain for proteins
ninth cranial: nerve
ninth-day: erythema
nipple: line; shield
nirvana: principle
Nissen's: operation
Nissl: bodies; degeneration; granules; substance
Nissl's: stain
Nitabuch's: layer; membrane; stria
niter: paper

nitinol: filter
nitrate: respiration
nitritoid: reaction
nitro: dyes
nitroblue: tetrazolium
nitroblue tetrazolium: test
nitrofurantoin: polyneuropathy
nitrogen: autotrophy; balance; cycle; equivalent; fixation; mustards; narcosis
nitrogenous: equilibrium
nitroid: shock
nitroprusside: test
NK: cells
NMDA: receptor
Noack's: syndrome
noble: element; gases; metal
Noble-Collip: procedure
Noble's: position; stain
Nocardia: dacryoliths
nociceptive: reflex
nocifensor: reflex
nocturnal: amblyopia; diarrhea; dyspnea; enuresis; epilepsy; myoclonus; periodicity; vertigo
nodal: bigeminy; bradycardia; fever; plane; point; rhythm; tachycardia; tissue
nodding: spasm
nodose: ganglion; rheumatism
nodoventricular: fibers
nodular: amyloidosis; arteriosclerosis; body; disease; episcleritis; fasciitis; headache; hidradenoma; hyperplasia of prostate; iritis; leprosy; lymphoma; melanoma; mesoneuritis; opacity; panencephalitis; scleritis; sclerosis; syphilid; transformation of the liver; tuberculid; vasculitis
nodular histiocytic: lymphoma
nodular nonsuppurative: panniculitis
nodular non-X: histiocytosis
nodular regenerative: hyperplasia
nodular subepidermal: fibrosis
nodus sinuatrialis: echo
noetic: anxiety
noise: pollution
noise–induced: deafness
Nomarski: optics
Nomarski interference: microscopy
nomenclatural: type
nominal: aphasia
nomothetic: approach
nonabsorbable: ligature

nonabsorbable surgical: suture
nonaccommodative: esotropia
non-adrenergic, non-cholinergic: neuron
nonan: malaria
nonanatomic: teeth
non-A, non-B: hepatitis
non-A, non-B hepatitis: virus
non-A, non-B, non-C: hepatitis
non-arcon: articulator
nonbacterial thrombotic: endocarditis
nonbacterial verrucous: endocarditis
nonbullous congenital ichthyosiform: erythroderma
nonchromaffin: paraganglioma
nonclassical: phenylketonuria
nonclonogenic: cell
noncohesive: gold
noncommunicating: hydrocele; hydrocephalus
noncompetitive: inhibition
noncomplementary: role
nonconjugative: plasmid
nonconvulsive: seizure
noncovalent: bond
nondeciduous: placenta
nondepolarizing: block; relaxant
nondepolarizing neuromuscular blocking: agent
nondiabetic: glycosuria
nondirective: psychotherapy
nonepileptic: seizure
nonessential: amino acids
nonfenestrated: forceps
nonfilament polymorphonuclear: leukocyte
nonfluent: aphasia
nongonococcal: urethritis
nongranular: leukocyte
non-heme iron: protein
non-Hodgkin's: lymphoma
nonhomologous: chromosomes
nonhyperglycemic: glycosuria
nonimmune: agglutination; serum
nonimmune fetal: hydrops
noninfiltrating lobular: carcinoma
noninflammatory: edema
non-insulin-dependent: diabetes mellitus
nonionic: surfactant
nonisolated: proteinuria

nonketotic: hyperglycemia; hyperglycinemia
nonlamellar: bone
nonlipid: histiocytosis
nonmedullated: fibers
nonmotile: leukocyte
nonneurogenic neurogenic: bladder
non-newtonian: fluid
nonobstructive: jaundice
nonoccluded: virus
nonorganic: aphonia
nonossifying: fibroma
nonosteogenic: fibroma
nonovulational: menstruation
nonparticipant: observer
nonpedunculated: hydatid
nonpenetrant: trait
nonpenetrating: keratoplasty; wound
nonphasic sinus: arrhythmia
nonpitting: edema
non-PKU: hyperphenylalaninemia
nonplasmatic: compartment
nonpolar: amino acid; compound; solvents
nonprecipitable: antibody
nonprecipitating: antibody
nonprotein: nitrogen
nonrandom: mating
non-rapid eye: movement
nonreactive: depression
nonrebreathing: anesthesia; mask; valve
nonrefractive accommodative: esotropia
nonrenal: azotemia
nonresponder: tolerance
nonsecretory: myeloma
nonsense: codon; mutation; syndrome; triplet
nonseptate: mycelium
nonsexual: generation
nonspecific: anergy; cholinesterase; protein; system; therapy; urethritis; vaginitis
nonsteroidal anti-inflammatory: drugs
nonstress: test
nonsuppressible insulin-like: activity
nonthrombocytopenic: purpura
nontoxic: goiter
nontransmural myocardial: infarction
nontropical: sprue
nonvenereal: syphilis
nonvital: pulp; tooth
noogenic: neurosis
Noonan's: syndrome
NOR-: banding
Nordhausen: sulfuric acid
no reflow: phenomenon
norma: basilaris

normal: animal; antibody; antithrombin; antitoxin; bite; concentration; distribution; hearing; occlusion; opsonin; ovariotomy; phosphate; serum; solution; tartrate; toxin; values
normal cholesteremic: xanthomatosis
normal electrical: axis
normal horse: serum
normal human: plasma; serum
normal human serum: albumin
normally posed: tooth
normal pressure: hydrocephalus
normochromic: anemia
normocytic: anemia
normoglycemic: glycosuria
normokalemic periodic: paralysis
normospermatogenic: sterility
normotriglyceridemic: abetalipoproteinemia
Norrie's: disease
Norris': corpuscles
North American: blastomycosis
Northern blot: analysis
North Queensland tick: fever; typhus
Norton's: operation
Norwalk: agent; virus
Norway: itch
Norwegian: scabies
Norwood: procedure
Norwood's: operation
nose: drops
nose-bridge-lid: reflex
nose-eye: reflex
nosocomial: gangrene
notched: teeth
note: blindness
Nothnagel's: syndrome
no-threshold: concept
notifiable: disease
notochordal: canal; plate; process; sheath; vertebrate
notoedric: mange
Novy and MacNeal's blood: agar
NPH: insulin
nu: body
nuchal: fascia; ligament; plane; tubercle
Nuck's: diverticulum; hydrocele
nuclear: atom; bag; cataract; chemistry; energy; envelope; family; fusion; hyaloplasm; jaundice; lamina; layers of retina; magneton; matrix; medicine; membrane;

ophthalmoplegia; pacemaker; pore; reaction; RNA; sap; sclerosis; spindle; stain
nuclear bag: fiber
nuclear chain: fiber
nuclear-cytoplasmic: ratio
nuclear inclusion: bodies
nuclear magnetic: resonance
nuclear magnetic resonance: imaging; tomography
nuclear Overhauser: effect
nucleate: endonuclease
nucleic acid: base; hybridization; probe
nucleinic: base
nucleocortical: fibers
nucleolar: chromosome; organizer; zone
nucleolar-nuclear: ratio
nucleolus: organizer
nucleolus organizer: region
nucleoplasmic: index
nucleoside: pair; phosphorylases
nucleotide: deletion
nude: mouse
Nuel's: space
Nuhn's: gland
null: cells; hypothesis
null-cell: adenoma
numerical: aperture; hypertrophy; taxonomy
nummular: dermatitis; eczema; sputum; syphilid
nun's: murmur
nurse: cells
nursemaid's: elbow
nursing bottle: caries
Nussbaum's: bracelet; experiment
nutmeg: liver
nutrient: agar; arteries of humerus; artery; artery of femur; artery of fibula; artery of the tibia; canal; enema; foramen; medium; vessel
nutritional: amblyopia; anemia; cirrhosis; dropsy; edema; encephalomalacia of chicks; energy; hemosiderosis; marasmus; polyneuropathy
nutritional macrocytic: anemia
nutritional type cerebellar: atrophy
nutritive: equilibrium; ratio
nymphocaruncular: sulcus
nymphohymenal: sulcus
nystagmus: test
nystagmus blockage: syndrome
Nysten's: law

O

ω3: fatty acids
O: agglutinin; antigen; colony
oasthouse urine: disease
oat: cell
oat cell: carcinoma
oatmeal-tomato paste: agar
OAV: syndrome
O'Beirne's: sphincter; valve
Obermayer's: test
Obermeier's: spirillum
Obersteiner-Redlich: line; zone
obesity: index
object: blindness; constancy; glass; libido; relationship
objective: optometer; perimetry; probability; psychology; sensation; sign; symptom; synonyms
obligate: aerobe; anaerobe; parasite
oblique: amputation; bandage; bundle of pons; cord; diameter; fibers of stomach; fissure; fissure of lung; fracture; head; illumination; lie; ligament of elbow joint; line; line of mandible; line of thyroid cartilage; muscle of auricle; part of cricothyroid muscle; projection; ridge; ridge of trapezium; section; sinus of pericardium; vein of left atrium
oblique arytenoid: muscle
oblique auricular: muscle
oblique facial: cleft
oblique pericardial: sinus
oblique pontine: fasciculus
oblique popliteal: ligament
obliquus capitis inferior: muscle
obliquus capitis superior: muscle
obliterating: pericarditis
obliterative: arachnoiditis; bronchitis
oblong: fovea of arytenoid cartilage; pit of arytenoid cartilage
obsessional: neurosis
obsessive: behavior; personality
obsessive-compulsive: disorder; neurosis; neurosis; personality
obsessive-compulsive personality: disorder
obstacle: sense
obstetric: conjugate; conjugate of pelvic outlet; position; ultrasound

WordFinder

obstetrical: binder; forceps; hand; palsy; paralysis
obstetric conjugate: diameter
obstructive: apnea; appendicitis; dysmenorrhea; hydrocephalus; jaundice; murmur; pneumonia; thrombus; uropathy
obturating: embolism
obturator: appliance; artery; canal; crest; fascia; foramen; groove; hernia; lymph nodes; membrane; nerve; tubercle; vein
obturator externus: muscle
obturator internus: muscle
occipital: anchorage; angle of parietal bone; artery; belly of occipitofrontalis muscle; bone; border; border of parietal bone; border of temporal bone; branch; condyle; fontanel; groove; gyri; horn; lobe; lobe of cerebrum; lymph nodes; margin; neuralgia; neurectomy; neuritis; operculum; part of corpus callosum; plane; plexus; point; pole; pole of cerebrum; region of head; sinus; somite; squama; triangle; vein
occipital cerebral: veins
occipital emissary: vein
occipital horn: syndrome
occipitalis: muscle
occipital lobe: epilepsy
occipitoanterior: position
occipitoaxial: ligaments
occipitocollicular: tract
occipitofrontal: diameter; fasciculus; muscle
occipitofrontalis: muscle
occipitomastoid: suture
occipitomental: diameter; projection
occipitopontine: tract
occipitoposterior: position
occipitotectal: tract
occipitotemporal: sulcus
occipitothalamic: radiation
occipitotransverse: position
occluded: virus
occluding: frame; ligature; paper; relation
occluding centric relation: record
occlusal: adjustment; analysis; balance; caries; clearance; correction; curvature; disharmony; embrasure; force; form; harmony; imbalance; path; pattern; pivot; plane; position; pressure;

radiograph; rest; rim; scheme; surface; system; table; trauma; wear
occlusal rest: bar
occlusal vertical: dimension
occlusion: rim
occlusive: dressing; ileus; meningitis
occult: bleeding; blood; border of nail; carcinoma; fracture; hydrocephalus
occupational: deafness; disease; neurosis; spasm; therapy
Ochoa's: law
ochre: codon; mutation
ochronotic: arthritis
Ochsner: clamp
Ochsner's: method
ocular: albinism; bobbing; cone; crisis; cup; dysmetria; flutter; humor; hypertelorism; larva migrans; lens; lymphomatosis; micrometer; migraine; muscles; myiasis; myopathy; nystagmus; onchocerciasis; paralysis; pemphigoid; prosthesis; rigidity; scoliosis; sparganosis; tension; torticollis; vertigo; vesicle
ocular motor: apraxia
ocular-mucous membrane: syndrome
oculoauriculovertebral: dysplasia
oculobuccogenital: syndrome
oculocardiac: reflex
oculocephalic: reflex
oculocephalogyric: reflex
oculocerebrorenal: syndrome
oculocutaneous: albinism; syndrome
oculodentodigital: dysplasia
oculodermal: melanosis
oculoencephalic: angiomatosis
oculogravic: illusion
oculogyral: illusion
oculogyric: crises
oculomandibulofacial: syndrome
oculomotor: nerve; nucleus; response; root of ciliary ganglion; system
oculopharyngeal: dystrophy; syndrome
oculovagal: reflex
oculovertebral: dysplasia; syndrome
oculovestibulo-auditory: syndrome
odd: chromosome
Oddi's: sphincter

Odland: body
odontoblastic: layer; process
odontogenic: cyst; dysplasia; fibroma; keratocyst; myxoma
odontoid: ligament; process; process of epistropheus; vertebra
odorant binding: protein
odoriferous: gland
O'Dwyer's: tube
oedipal: neurosis; period; phase
Oedipus: complex
Oehler's: symptom
Oehl's: muscles
OFD: syndrome
official: formula
Ofuji's: disease
Ogilvie's: syndrome
Ogino-Knaus: rule
Ogston-Luc: operation
Ogston's: line
Oguchi's: disease
Ogura: operation
O'Hara: forceps
17-OH-corticoids: test
Ohm's: law
Ohngren's: line
oil: bath; cyst; embolism; glands; immersion; pneumonia; sugar; tumor; vaccine
oil of American: wormseed
oil retention: enema
oily: granuloma
ointment: base
Okazaki: fragment
OKT: cells
Old World: leishmaniasis
old yellow: enzyme
olecranon: bursitis; fossa; process; reflex
olfactory: angle; area; bulb; bundle; cells; cortex; epithelium; esthesioneuroblastoma; fila; foramen; glands; glomerulus; groove; hallucination; hyperesthesia; hypesthesia; membrane; mucosa; nerves; neuroblastoma; organ; peduncle; pits; placodes; pyramid; region of tunica mucosa of nose; roots; striae; sulcus; sulcus of nasal cavity; tract; trigone; tubercle
olfactory receptor: cells
oligemic: shock
oligoclonal: band
oligodendroglia: cells
olivary: body; eminence
olive-tipped: catheter
olivocerebellar: tract
olivocochlear: bundle; fibers; tract

olivopontocerebellar: atrophy; degeneration
olivospinal: tract
Ollier: graft
Ollier's: disease; method; theory
Ollier-Thiersch: graft
olympian: forehead
Ombrédanne: operation
omega-3: fatty acids
omega-: oxidation
omega-oxidation: theory
Omenn's: syndrome
omental: branches; bursa; enterocleisis; graft; sac; tenia; tuber
Ommaya: reservoir
omnifocal: lens
omoclavicular: triangle
omohyoid: muscle
omotracheal: triangle
omphaloangiopagous: twins
omphalomesenteric: artery; cord; cyst; duct
omphalomesenteric duct: cyst
Omsk hemorrhagic: fever
Omsk hemorrhagic fever: virus
oncocytic hepatocellular: tumor
oncofetal: antigens; marker
oncogenic: virus
oncoplastic: carcinoma
oncosphere: embryo
oncotic: pressure
Ondine's: curse
Ondiri: disease
one-carbon: fragment
one-horned: uterus
onion: bodies
onion bulb: neuropathy; neuropathy
onlay: graft
Onodi: cell
on-off: phenomenon
ontogenic: homeostasis
Onuf's: nucleus
O'nyong-nyong: virus
o'nyong-nyong: fever
oophoritic: cyst
opacifying: gallstones
opal: codon; mutation
opalescent: dentin
opaline: patch
Opalski: cell
opaque: microscope
open: biopsy; bite; comedo; cordotomy; dislocation; drainage; flap; fracture; hospital; laparoscopy; pneumothorax; reading frame; reduction of fractures; system; tuberculosis; wound
open-angle: glaucoma
open chain: compound
open chest: massage

open circuit: method
open drop: anesthesia
open head: injury
open heart: surgery
opening: axis; contraction; movement; snap
open skull: fracture
opera-glass: hand
operant: behavior; conditioning
operating: microscope; table
operative: dentistry; myxedema
operator: gene
opercular: fold; part
ophryospinal: angle
ophthalmic: artery; hyperthyroidism; nerve; ointment; plexus; solutions; veins; vesicle
ophthalmomandibulomelic: dysplasia
ophthalmoplegic: migraine
opiate: receptors
opioid: antagonists
opossum: encephalitis
Oppenheim's: disease; reflex; syndrome
opponens digiti minimi: muscle
opponens pollicis: muscle
opponent: color
opportunistic: pathogen
opposer: muscle of little finger; muscle of thumb
oppositional: disorder
opsonic: index
optic: agnosia; ataxia; axis; canal; capsule; chiasm; cup; decussation; disk; fissure; foramen; groove; layer; nerve; neuritis; papilla; part of retina; pit; placodes; radiation; recess; stalk; tract; vesicle
optical: aberration; activity; antipode; density; illusion; image; iridectomy; isomerism; keratoplasty; pachymeter; rotation
optical righting: reflexes
optical rotatory: dispersion
optic nerve: drusen; glioma; head; hypoplasia
optic nerve sheath: decompression; fenestration
opticokinetic: nystagmus
optimum: dose; pH; temperature
optokinetic: nystagmus
O-R: system
oral: biology; cavity; cavity proper; contraceptive; fissure; hygiene; membrane; mucosa; part of pharynx; pathology; pharynx; phase;

physiotherapy; plate; primacy; region; shields; smear; stereotypy; surgeon; surgery; teeth; vestibule
oral epithelial: nevus
oral (erosive): lichen planus
oral focal: mucinosis
oral lactose tolerance: test
oral poliovirus: vaccine
oral submucous: fibrosis
Orbeli: effect
orbicular: bone; ligament; ligament of radius; muscle; muscle of eye; muscle of mouth; process; zone
orbicularis: muscle; phenomenon
orbicularis oculi: muscle; reflex
orbicularis oris: muscle
orbicularis pupillary: reflex
orbital: abscess; artery; axis; branch of middle meningeal artery; branch of pterygopalatine ganglion; cavity; decompression; eminence of zygomatic bone; exenteration; fasciae; fat-pad; gyri; height; hernia; implant; index; lamina of ethmoid bone; layer of ethmoid bone; margin of eyelids; muscle; nerve; opening; ophthalmoplegia; part of frontal bone; part of lacrimal gland; part of optic nerve; part of orbicularis oculi muscle; plane; plate; plate of ethmoid bone; process; region; rim; septum; sulci; surface; syndrome; tubercle of zygomatic bone; width
orbitalis: muscle
orbitofrontal: artery; cortex
orbitomeatal: line; plane
orbitonasal: index
orcinol: test
ordered: mechanism
ordered on-random off: mechanism
ordinal: scale
orf: virus
organ: culture
organic: acid; catalyst; chemistry; compound; contracture; deafness; delusions; disease; evolution; hallucinosis; headache; murmur; pain; phosphate; principle; stricture; vertigo
organic brain: syndrome
organic dental: cement
organic mental: disorder; syndrome
organic mood: syndrome

organification: defect
organized: pneumonia
organoid: nevus; tumor
organ-specific: antigen
Oriboca: virus
Oriental: boil; button; ringworm; schistosomiasis; sore; ulcer
orienting: reflex; response
Ormond's: disease
Ornish prevention: diets
Ornish reversal: diet
ornithine: cycle
ornithosis: virus
oroantral: fistula
orodigitofacial: dysostosis
orofacial: fistula
orofaciodigital: syndrome
oronasal: fistula; membrane
oropharyngeal: membrane; passage
orotracheal: intubation; tube
Oroya: fever
orphan: disease; drugs; products; viruses
Orsi-Grocco: method
orthodontic: appliance; band; therapy
orthoglycemic: glycosuria
orthognathic: surgery
orthograde: conduction; degeneration
orthomolecular: psychiatry; therapy
orthopaedic: surgery
orthopnea: position
orthopneic: position
orthoscopic: lens; spectacles
orthostatic: albuminuria; hypopiesis; hypotension; proteinuria; tachycardia
orthotopic: graft
Orth's: fixative; stain
oscillating: vision
oscillatory: potential
Osgood-Schlatter: disease
Osler: node
Osler's: disease; sign
Osler-Vaquez: disease
osmic acid: fixative
osmolal: clearance
osmotic: diuresis; diuretics; fragility; nephrosis; pressure; shock
osseous: ampulla; cell; labyrinth; lacuna; part of skeletal system; polyp; tissue
osseous hydatid: cyst
osseous spiral: lamina
ossicular: chain
ossific: center
ossifying: cartilage
osteochondrogenic: cell
osteoclast activating: factor
osteocollagenous: fibers
osteogenetic: fibers; layer

osteogenic: cell; sarcoma; tissue
osteoid: osteoma; tissue
osteomalacic: pelvis
osteomyelofibrotic: syndrome
osteopathic: medicine; physician; scoliosis
osteoperiosteal: graft
osteoplastic: amputation; craniotomy; necrotomy
osteoporotic marrow: defect
osteoprogenitor: cell
osteosclerotic: anemia
ostial: sphincter
ostiomeatal: complex; unit
Ostrum-Furst: syndrome
Ostwald's solubility: coefficient
Ot: antigen
Ota's: nevus
Othello: syndrome
otic: abscess; barotrauma; capsule; ganglion; pits; placodes; vesicle
otitic: hydrocephalus; meningitis
otodectic: mange
otogenous: abscess
otolithic: membrane
otomandibular: dysostosis; syndrome
otopalatodigital: syndrome
otopharyngeal: tube
Otto: pelvis
Otto's: disease
Ottoson: potential
Ouchterlony: technique; test
outbreak: epidemic
outer: malleolus; membrane; table of skull
outlet forceps: delivery
outline: form
outpatient: anesthesia
oval: amputation; area of Flechsig; corpuscle; fasciculus; fossa; window
ovale: malaria
ovalocytic: anemia
ovarian: amenorrhea; artery; branch of uterine artery; bursa; colic; cycle; cyst; dysmenorrhea; fimbria; fossa; ligament; plexus; pregnancy; varicocele; veins
ovarian tubular: adenoma
ovarian vein: syndrome
ovarioabdominal: pregnancy
overanxious: disorder
overflow: incontinence; wave
overhanging: restoration
overlap: hybridization
overlay: denture
overproduction: theory
overriding: aorta
overripe: cataract
overt: homosexuality

overvalued: idea
ovine: acetonemia; mastitis
ovo-: vegetarian
ovular: membrane; transmigration
ovulation: inhibitor
ovulational: sclerosis
ovulocyclic: porphyria
Owen's: lines
own: controls
Owren's: disease
ox: bots; heart
oxalate: calculus
oxazin: dyes
Oxford: unit
oxidase: reaction; test
oxidation-reduction: electrode; indicator; potential; reaction; system
oxidative: deamination; decarboxylation; metabolism; phosphorylation
oxidized: cellulose; glutathione
oxonium: ion
oxygen: capacity; consumption; debt; deficit; effect; electrode; poisoning; tent; therapy; toxicity
oxygen affinity: anoxia; hypoxia
oxygenated: hemoglobin
oxygen deprivation: theory of narcosis
oxygen derived free: radicals
oxygen utilization: coefficient
oxyntic: cell; gland
oxyphil: adenoma; cells; chromatin; granule
oxyphilic: leukocyte

P

ψ: factor
π: helix
P: antigens; cell; elements; enzyme; factor; wave
P-A: interval
PA: projection
Paas': disease
pacchionian: bodies; corpuscles; depressions; glands; granulations
pacemaker: failure; output; potential; sensitivity; syndrome
Pacheco's: disease
Pacheco's parrot disease: virus
Pachon's: method; test
pachydermoperiostosis: syndrome
pacing: catheter
pacinian: corpuscles

packed cell: volume
packed human blood: cells
packing: process
P-A conduction: time
Padykula-Herman: stain for myosin ATPase
Pagenstecher's: circle
Paget-Eccleston: stain
pagetoid: cells; reticulosis
Paget's: cells; disease
Paget-von Schrötter: syndrome
Pahvant Valley: fever; plague
pain: reaction; threshold; tolerance
painful: anesthesia; heel; hematuria; paraplegia; point; toe
painful-bruising: syndrome
painless: hematuria; jaundice
pain-pleasure: principle
painter's: colic
paired: allosome; associates; beats; organelles
Pajot's: maneuver
Palade: granule
palatal: abscess; bar; index; myoclonus; nystagmus; papillomatosis; plate; reflex; seal; shelf; triangle
palate: hook; myograph
palatine: aponeurosis; bone; glands; groove; papilla; process; raphe; ridge; spines; surface of horizontal plate of palatine bone; tonsil; torus; uvula; vein
palatoethmoidal: suture
palatoglossal: arch
palatoglossus: muscle
palatomaxillary: index; suture
palatopharyngeal: arch; muscle; sphincter
palatopharyngeus: muscle
palatouvularis: muscle
palatovaginal: canal; groove
pale: globe; hypertension; infarct; thrombus
paleostriatal: syndrome
Palfyn's: sinus
palindromic: DNA; encephalopathy; sequence
palisade: layer
pallesthetic: sensibility
palliative: treatment
pallidal: syndrome
palm: grasp; oil; wax
palmar: aponeurosis; branch of median nerve; branch of ulnar nerve; crease; fascia; fibromatosis; flexion; ligaments; monticuli; reflex; surface of fingers; syphilid

palmar carpal: branch of radial artery; branch of ulnar artery; ligament
palmar carpometacarpal: ligaments
palmar digital: veins
palmar interosseous: artery; muscle
palmaris brevis: muscle
palmaris longus: muscle
palmar metacarpal: artery; ligaments; veins
palmar radiocarpal: ligament
palmar ulnocarpal: ligament
palmate: folds
palm-chin: reflex
Palmer acid: test for peptic ulcer
palmin: test
palmomental: reflex
palmoplantar: keratoderma
palpable: rale
palpatory: percussion
palpebral: arteries; branches of infratrochlear nerve; conjunctiva; fissure; glands; part of lacrimal gland; part of orbicularis oculi muscle; raphe; veins
palpebronasal: fold
paludal: fever
pampiniform: body; plexus
panacinar: emphysema
pancake: kidney
pancervical: smear
Pancoast: syndrome; tumor
Pancoast's: suture
pancreatic: abscess; branches; calculus; cholera; colic; cystoduodenostomy; deoxyribonuclease; diabetes; diarrhea; digestion; diverticula; dornase; duct; encephalopathy; infantilism; islands; islets; juice; lithiasis; lymph nodes; notch; plexus; polypeptide; RNase; sphincter; steatorrhea; veins
pancreatic hyperglycemic: hormone
pancreaticoduodenal: lymph nodes; transplantation; veins
pancreaticoduodenal arterial: arcades
pancreaticoenteric: recess
pancreaticosplenic: lymph nodes
pancreatogenous: diarrhea
pancreozymin-secretin: test
Pandy's: reaction; test
Paneth's granular: cells
panhypopituitary: dwarfism
panic: attack; disorder

panleukopenia: virus of cats
panlobular: emphysema
Panner's: disease
pannicular: hernia
panniculus carnosus: muscle
panoptic: stain
panoramic: radiograph
panoramic rotating: machine
panoramic x-ray: film
Pansch's: fissure
pansystolic: murmur
pantaloon: embolism; hernia
pantoate-activating: enzyme
pantoscopic: spectacles
pantropic: virus
Panum's: area
PAP: technique
Pap: smear
Pap: test
Papanicolaou: examination; smear; stain
Papanicolaou smear: test
paper: autoradiography; chromatography; plate
paper mill worker's: disease
Papez: circuit
papillary: adenocarcinoma; adenoma of large intestine; carcinoma; cystadenoma lymphomatosum; ducts; ectasia; foramina of kidney; hidradenoma; layer; muscle; process; stasis; tumor
papillary cystic: adenoma
papillary muscle: dysfunction; syndrome
papilloma: virus
Papillon-Léage and Psaume: syndrome
Papillon-Lefèvre: syndrome
pappataci: fever
pappataci fever: viruses
Pappenheimer: bodies
Pappenheim's: stain
papular: acrodermatitis of childhood; dermatitis of pregnancy; fever; mucinosis; scrofuloderma; syphilid; tuberculid; urticaria
papular stomatitis: virus of cattle
papulonecrotic: tuberculid
papulosquamous: syphilid
papyraceous: scars
para-aortic: bodies
parabasal: body; filament
parabiotic: flap
paraboloid: condenser
parabrachial: nuclei
paracarcinomatous: encephalomyelopathy; myelopathy
paracarmine: stain
paracellular: transport

paracelsian: method
paracentral: artery; fissure; lobule; nucleus of thalamus; scotoma
paracentric: inversion
paracervical block: anesthesia
parachordal: cartilage; plate
parachute: deformity; reflex
parachute mitral: valve
paracoccidioidal: granuloma
paracolic: gutters; recesses
paracolon: bacillus
paracyclic: ovulation
paracystic: pouch
paradoxical: contraction; embolism; incontinence; movement of eyelids; pulse; pupil; reflex; respiration; sleep
paradoxical diaphragm: phenomenon
paradoxical extensor: reflex
paradoxical flexor: reflex
paradoxical patellar: reflex
paradoxical pupillary: phenomenon; reflex
paradoxical triceps: reflex
paraduodenal: fold; fossa; hernia; recess
paradysentery: bacillus
paraesophageal: hernia
paraffin: cancer; tumor; wax
parafollicular: cells
parafrenal: abscess
paraganglionic: cells
paragenital: tubules
paraglenoid: groove; sulcus
Paraguay: tea
parahiatal: hernia
parahippocampal: gyrus
parainfluenza: viruses
parajejunal: fossa
parallax: method; test
parallel: attachment; rays
paraluteal: cell
paralutein: cell
paralytic: dementia; ectropion; ileus; miosis; mydriasis; myoglobinuria; rabies; scoliosis; strabismus
paralyzing: vertigo
paramammary: lymph nodes
paramastoid: process
paramedian: incision
paramesonephric: duct
parametric: abscess; test
paranasal: sinuses
paraneoplastic: acrokeratosis; encephalomyelopathy; syndrome
paranephric: abscess; body
paraneural: infiltration
paranoid: disorder; personality; schizophrenia

paranoid personality: disorder
paranuclear: body
paraperitoneal: hernia
parapharyngeal: space
paraphysial: body; cysts
pararectal: fossa; lymph nodes; pouch
parasaccular: hernia
parasagittal: plane; section
paraseptal: cartilage; emphysema
parasinoidal: sinuses
parasite-host: ecosystem
parasitic: chylocele; cyst; disease; granuloma; hemoptysis; leiomyoma; melanoderma; otitis; thyroiditis; twin
parasitophorous: vacuole
parasol: insertion
paraspinal: line
parasternal: hernia; line; lymph nodes
parastriate: area; cortex
parasympathetic: ganglia; nerve; part; root of ciliary ganglion
parasympathetic nervous: system
parasystolic: beat
parataxic: distortion
paratenic: host
paraterminal: body; gyrus
parathyroid: gland; hormone; insufficiency; osteosis; tetany
parathyroid hormonelike: protein
parathyroprival: tetany
paratracheal: lymph node
paratuberculous: lymphadenitis
paratyphoid: bacillus; fever
paraumbilical: veins
paraurethral: ducts; glands
parauterine: lymph nodes
paravaccinia: virus
paravaginal: hysterectomy; lymph nodes
paraventricular: nucleus
paravertebral: anesthesia; ganglia; gutter; line; triangle
paravesical: fossa; lymph nodes; pouch
paraxial: mesoderm; rays
parchment: heart; skin
parenchymal: atelectasis; cell
parenchymatous: cartilage; cell of corpus pineale; degeneration; goiter; hemorrhage; mastitis; neuritis
parent: artery; cell; cyst
parental: generation; rejection

parenteral: absorption; alimentation; hyperalimentation; therapy
parenteric: fever
Paré's: suture
paretic: impotence; neurosyphilis
parietal: angle; arteries; bone; border; border of frontal bone; border of sphenoid bone; border of temporal bone; branch; branch of medial occipital artery; branch of middle meningeal artery; branch of superficial temporal artery; cell; eminence; eye; fistula; foramen; hernia; layer; layer of leptomeninges; layer of serous pericardium; layer of tunica vaginalis; lobe; lobe of cerebrum; lymph nodes; margin; nodes; notch; peritoneum; plate; pleura; region; thrombus; tuber; veins; wall
parietal emissary: vein
parietal lobe: epilepsy
parietal pelvic: fascia
parietomastoid: suture
parieto-occipital: artery; fissure; sulcus
parietopontine: tract
Parinaud's: conjunctivitis; ophthalmoplegia; syndrome
Parinaud's oculoglandular: syndrome
Paris: line
Parker-Kerr: suture
Parkinson's: disease; facies
Park's: aneurysm
Park-Williams: bacillus; fixative
paroccipital: process
parolfactory: area
Parona's: space
paroophoritic: cyst
parosteal: fasciitis; osteosarcoma
parotid: abscess; bed; branches; bubo; duct; fascia; gland; notch; papilla; recess; sheath; space; veins
parotideomasseteric: fascia
paroxysmal: sleep; tachycardia
paroxysmal cerebral: dysrhythmia
paroxysmal cold: hemoglobinuria
paroxysmal nocturnal: dyspnea; hemoglobinuria
parrot: disease; fever; jaw; mouth; virus
parrot-beak: nail
Parrot's: disease

parry: fracture
Parry's: disease
Parsonage-Turner: syndrome
partial: agglutinin; anencephaly; aneuploidy; anodontia; antigen; cystectomy; denture; denture, distal extension; enterocele; epilepsy; lipoatrophy; pressure; sclerectasia; seizure; volume
partial adrenocortical: insufficiency
partial breech: extraction
partial denture: impression; retention
partial face-sparing: lipodystrophy
partial heart: block
partial ileal: bypass
partial-thickness: burn; flap; graft
partial thromboplastin: time
participant: observer
partition: chromatography; coefficient
parturient: canal; paralysis; paresis
parvilocular: cyst
PAS: stain
Pascal's: law
Pascheff's: conjunctivitis
Paschen: bodies
Passavant's: bar; cushion; pad; ridge
passional: attitudes
passive: agglutination; anaphylaxis; atelectasis; clot; congestion; diffusion; duction; eruption; hemagglutination; hyperemia; immunity; immunization; incontinence; learning; medium; movement; prophylaxis; transference; transport; tremor; vasoconstriction; vasodilation
passive-aggressive: behavior; personality
passive cutaneous: anaphylaxis
passive cutaneous anaphylactic: reaction
passive cutaneous anaphylaxis: test
passive length-tension: curve
Pasteur: pipette; vaccine
Pasteur's: effect
Pastia's: sign
pastoral: counseling
Patau's: syndrome
patch: clamp; test

patchy: atelectasis
Patein's: albumin
patellar: fossa of vitreous;
  ligament; network; reflex;
  retinaculum; surface of
  femur
patellar tendon: reflex
patello-adductor: reflex
patent: ductus arteriosus;
  medicine
Paterson-Brown-Kelly:
  syndrome
Paterson-Kelly: syndrome
path: analysis
pathematic: aphasia
pathetic: nerve
pathogenic: occlusion
pathognomonic: symptom
pathologic: absorption;
  amenorrhea; amputation;
  calcification; diagnosis;
  fracture; glycosuria;
  histology; myopia;
  physiology; rigidity;
  sphincter
pathological: anatomy;
  model; pathways
pathologic retraction: ring
pathologic startle:
  syndromes
patient controlled: analgesia
Patois: virus
Paton's: lines
Patrick's: test
patterned: alopecia
pattern sensitive: epilepsy
Paul-Bunnell: test
Pauling-Corey: helix
Pauling's: theory
Pauli's exclusion: principle
Paul's: reaction; test
Pautrier's: abscess;
  microabscess
Pauzat's: disease
pavement: epithelium
Pavlov: method; pouch;
  stomach
pavlovian: conditioning
Pavlov's: reflex
Pavy's: disease
Paxton's: disease
Payne: operation
Payr's: clamp; membrane;
  sign
PBI: test
peak: magnitude
peak expiratory: flow
peak flow: rate
pearl: cyst; moss; tumor
pearl-worker's: disease
pear-shaped: area
peat: moss
peccant: humors
pecking: order
Pecquet's: cistern; duct;
  reservoir
pecten: band
pectin: sugar

pectinate: fibers; ligaments
  of iridocorneal angle;
  ligaments of iris; line;
  muscles; zone
pectineal: ligament; line; line
  of pubis; muscle
pectineus: muscle
pectiniform: septum
pectoral: branch of
  thoracoacromial artery;
  fascia; girdle; glands;
  reflex; region; ridge; veins
**pectoral and abdominal
  anterior cutaneous:**
  branch of intercostal nerves
pectoral group of axillary:
  lymph nodes
pectoralis major: muscle
pectoralis minor: muscle
pectorodorsal: muscle
pectorodorsalis: muscle
pedal: system
Pedersen's: speculum
pediatric: dentistry;
  radiology
pedicle: flap; graft
pediculous: blepharitis
pedigree: analysis
peduncular: ansa; loop;
  veins
pedunculated: hydatid;
  polyp
pedunculomamillary:
  fasciculus
peg-and-socket: articulation;
  joint
pegged: tooth
Pel-Ebstein: disease; fever
Pelger-Huët nuclear:
  anomaly
peliosis: hepatitis
Pelizaeus-Merzbacher:
  disease
pellagra-preventing: factor
Pellegrini's: disease
Pellegrini-Stieda: disease
pellet: implantation
Pellizzi's: syndrome
pellucid: zone
pelvic: abscess; axis; brim;
  canal; cavity; cellulitis;
  diaphragm; exenteration;
  fascia; ganglia; girdle;
  hematocele; index; inlet;
  kidney; limb; outlet; part;
  part of ureter; peritonitis;
  plane of greatest
  dimensions; plane of inlet;
  plane of least dimensions;
  plane of outlet; plexus;
  pole; presentation;
  promontory; surface of
  sacrum; version
pelvic inflammatory:
  disease
pelvic splanchnic: nerves;
  nerves
pelvirectal: sphincter

pelvivertebral: angle
pelvofemoral muscular:
  dystrophy
pemphigoid: syphilid
pen: grasp
pencil: tenderness
Pendred's: syndrome
pendular: movement;
  nystagmus
pendulous: abdomen; heart;
  palate
pendulum: rhythm
penetrant: trait
penetrating: keratoplasty;
  ulcer; wound
penicillin G: potassium
penile: epispadias;
  fibromatosis; hypospadias;
  implant; raphe; urethra
penis: bone; envy; spines;
  thorns
pennate: muscle
penopubic: epispadias
penoscrotal: hypospadias;
  transposition
Penrose: drain
pension: neurosis
pentagastrin: test
pentavalent gas gangrene:
  antitoxin
penton: antigen
pentose monophosphate:
  shunt
pentose phosphate: cycle;
  pathway
pep: pills
Pepper: syndrome
pepper and salt: fundus
peptic: cell; digestion; gland;
  ulcer
peptide: bond
peptidyl: leukotrienes
peptonized: iron
perambulating: ulcer
percept: analysis
perceptive: deafness
perceptual: expansion
percussion: sound; wave
percutaneous: absorption;
  cholangiography;
  nephrostomy; stimulation
percutaneous endoscopic:
  gastrostomy
**percutaneous
  radiofrequency:**
  gangliolysis
percutaneous transluminal:
  angioplasty
**percutaneous transluminal
  coronary:** angioplasty
Perez: reflex
Perez': sign
perfect: fungus; stage; state
perforated: layer of sclera;
  space; ulcer
perforating: abscess;
  appendicitis; arteries;
  arteries of foot; arteries of

hand; arteries of internal
  mammary; branches;
  branches of internal
  thoracic artery; branches of
  palmar metacarpal arteries;
  branches of plantar
  metatarsal arteries; branch
  of peroneal artery; fibers;
  folliculitis; keratoplasty;
  ulcer of foot; veins; wound
perforating peroneal: artery
performance: test
performic acid: reaction
perfusion: cannula
perhydrase: milk
periaccretio: pericardii
perialveolar: wiring
perianal odoriferous: glands
periapical: abscess;
  curettage; cyst; granuloma;
  osteofibrosis; radiograph;
  tissue
periapical cemental:
  dysplasia
periappendiceal: abscess
periarterial: pad; plexus;
  plexus of maxillary artery;
  plexus of vertebral artery;
  sympathectomy
periarticular: abscess
pericallosal: artery
pericanalicular:
  fibroadenoma
pericapillary: cell
pericardiacophrenic: artery;
  veins
pericardial: branch of
  phrenic nerve; branch of
  thoracic aorta; cavity;
  decompression; effusion;
  fremitus; knock; murmur;
  reflex; rub; tap; veins; villi
pericardial friction: sound
pericardioperitoneal: canal
pericardiopleural:
  membrane
pericemental: abscess;
  attachment
pericentral: fibrosis;
  scotoma
pericentric: inversion
perichondral: bone
perichoroid: space
perichoroidal: space
periclaustral: lamina
pericolic membrane:
  syndrome
periconchal: sulcus
pericoronal: abscess; flap
pericorpuscular: synapse
pericytic: venules
peridental: ligament;
  membrane
peridural: anesthesia
perihypoglossal: nuclei
peri-infarction: block
perilimbal suction: cup
perilunar: dislocation

perilymphatic: duct; space
perimortem: delivery
perimuscular: fibrosis
perinatal: death; medicine; mortality; torsion
perinatal mortality: rate
perineal: artery; body; branches of posterior femoral cutaneous nerve; flexure of rectum; hernia; hypospadias; lithotomy; membrane; muscles; nerves; raphe; region; section; spaces; urethrostomy; urethrotomy
perineovaginal: fistula
perinephric: abscess
perineural: anesthesia; infiltration
perineuronal: satellite
perinuclear: cataract; space
periodic: arthralgia; biopolymer; catatonia; disease; edema; fever; filariasis; law; neutropenia; ophthalmia; paralysis; peritonitis; polyserositis; system
periodic acid-Schiff: stain
periodic migrainous: neuralgia
periodontal: abscess; anesthesia; atrophy; file; ligament; membrane; pocket; probe
periodontal ligament: fibers
perioplic: band
periorbital: membrane
periosteal: bone; bud; chondroma; elevator; ganglion; graft; implantation; layer of dura mater; osteosarcoma; reaction; reflex; sarcoma
periosteoplastic: amputation
periotic: bone; cartilage
peripartum: cardiomyopathy
peripharyngeal: space
peripheral: aneurysm; arteriosclerosis; cataract; chemoreceptor; dysostosis; glare; iridectomy; part; proteins; resistance; scotoma; seal; tabes; vision
peripheral anterior: synechia
peripheral facial: paralysis
peripheral nervous: system
peripheral ossifying: fibroma
peripolar: cell
periportal: cirrhosis; space of Mall
perirectal: abscess
perirenal: fascia; insufflation
periscopic: lens; meniscus
perisinusoidal: space
peristatic: hyperemia

peristernal: perichondritis
peristriate: area; cortex
peritarsal: network
perithelial: cell
peritoneal: button; cavity; dialysis; fossae; transfusion; villi
peritoneovenous: shunt
peritonsillar: abscess
peritracheal: glands
peritubular: dentin; zone
peritubular contractile: cells
perityphlitis: actinomycotica
periungual: fibroma
periureteral: abscess
periurethral: abscess
perivascular: cuffs
perivascular fibrous: capsule
periventricular: fibers
perivisceral: cavity
perivitelline: space
Perlia's: nucleus
Perls': test
Perls' Prussian blue: stain
permanent: callus; cartilage; restoration; stricture; tooth
permanent dominant: idea
permanent pedicle: flap
permeability: coefficient; constant; theory of narcosis; vitamin
permissible exposure: limit
permissive: cell
perna: disease
pernicious: anemia; malaria; vomiting
pernicious anemia type: metarubricyte; prorubricyte; rubriblast
peroneal: artery; bone; node; phenomenon; pulley; retinaculum; trochlea of calcaneus; veins
peroneal anastomotic: ramus
peroneal communicating: branch; nerve
peroneal muscular: atrophy
peroneus brevis: muscle
peroneus longus: muscle
peroneus tertius: muscle
peroral: endoscopy
peroxidase: reaction; stain
perpendicular: fasciculus; plate; plate of ethmoid bone; plate of palatine bone
perpetual: arrhythmia
perpetually growing: tooth
persecution: complex
persecutory type of paranoid: disorder
Persian Gulf: syndrome
Persian relapsing: fever
persistent: cloaca; tremor; truncus arteriosus

persistent anterior hyperplastic primary: vitreous
persistent atrioventricular: canal
persistent chronic: hepatitis
persistent ectopic: pregnancy
persistent generalized: lymphadenopathy
persistent müllerian duct: syndrome
persistent posterior hyperplastic primary: vitreous
personal: equation; motivation; probability; space
personal growth: laboratory
personality: disorder; formation; integration; inventory; profile; test
perspiratory: glands
Perthes: disease
Perthes': test
Pertik's: diverticulum
pertrochanteric: fracture
pertussis: immunoglobulin; syndrome; vaccine
pertussis immune: globulin
pertussis-like: syndrome
Peruvian: tarantula; wart
pervasive developmental: disorder
pervenous: pacemaker
pesco-: vegetarian
pessary: cell; corpuscle
peste des petits ruminants: virus
petechial: angiomas; fever; hemorrhage
Peters': anomaly; ovum
Petersen's: bag
petit: mal
petite: mutant
petit mal: epilepsy; seizure
Petit's: aponeurosis; canals; hernia; herniotomy; ligament; sinus
Petit's lumbar: triangle
Petri: dish
petro-occipital: fissure; joint
petrosal: bone; branch of middle meningeal artery; foramen; fossa; fossula; ganglion; impression of the pallium; sinus; vein
petrosphenoidal: syndrome
petrosquamous: fissure; suture
petrotympanic: fissure
petrous: bone; part of internal carotid artery; part of temporal bone; pyramid
Pette-Döring: disease
Peutz-Jeghers: syndrome
Peutz's: syndrome

Peyer's: glands; patches
Peyronie's: disease
Peyrot's: thorax
Pezzer: catheter
Pfannenstiel's: incision
Pfaundler-Hurler: syndrome
Pfeiffer's: bacillus; phenomenon; syndrome
Pfeiffer's blood: agar
Pflüger's: law
Pfuhl's: sign
pH: scale; value
phacoanaphylactic: uveitis
phacogenic: glaucoma; uveitis
phacolytic: glaucoma
phacomorphic: glaucoma
phaeomycotic: cyst
phagedenic: ulcer
phagocyte: dysfunction
phagocytic: index; pneumonocyte
phagocytic dysfunction: immunodeficiency
phagocytic dysfunction disorders: immunodeficiency
phakic: eye
phalangeal: cell; joints
phallic: phase; tubercle
phantom: aneurysm; corpuscle; limb; pregnancy; tumor
phantom limb: pain
pharmaceutical: biology; chemistry
pharmacologic: mediators of anaphylaxis
pharmacologic stress: imaging
pharmacopeial: gel
pharmacoresistent: epilepsy
pharyngeal: arches; branch of the artery of pterygoid canal; branch of the ascending pharyngeal artery; branch of descending palatine artery; branches; branch of glossopharyngeal nerve; branch of inferior thyroid artery; branch of pterygopalatine ganglion; branch of vagus nerve; bursa; calculus; canal; cartilages; fistula; flap; fornix; glands; grooves; hypophysis; isthmus; membranes; mucosa; opening of auditory tube; opening of eustachian tube; pituitary; plexus; pouches; raphe; recess; reflex; ridge; space; tonsil; tubercle; veins
pharyngeal pouch: syndrome
pharyngobasilar: fascia

pharyngobranchial: ducts
pharyngoconjunctival: fever
pharyngoconjunctival fever: virus
pharyngoepiglottic: fold
pharyngoesophageal: cushions; diverticulum; pads
pharyngomaxillary: space
pharyngonasal: cavity
pharyngopalatine: arch
pharyngotympanic: groove; tube
phase: image; microscope; rule; shift
phase I: block
phase II: block
phasic: reflex
phasic sinus: arrhythmia
P-H conduction: time
Phemister: graft
phenanthrene: nucleus
phenobarbital: elixir
phenol: coefficient
phenolsulfonphthalein: test
phenotypic: mixing; threshold; value
phentolamine: test
phenylalanyl: chain
phenylethanolamine *N*-: methyltransferase
phenylhydrazine: hemolysis
phenylpyruvate: oligophrenia
phenylpyruvic: amentia
phenylthiocarbamoyl: peptide; protein
pheochrome: cell
phi: phenomenon
Phialophore-type: conidiophore
Philadelphia: chromosome; cocktail
philanthropic: hospital
Philippe's: triangle
Philippine hemorrhagic: fever
Philip's: glands
Phillips': catheter
Phillipson's: reflex
philosopher's: stone
phlebotomus: fever
phlebotomus fever: viruses
phlegmonous: abscess; cellulitis; enteritis; erysipelas; gastritis; mastitis; ulcer
phlogiston: theory
phlorizin: diabetes; glycosuria
phlyctenular: conjunctivitis; keratitis; ophthalmia; pannus
PhNCS: protein
phocomelic: dwarfism
phonemic: regression
phonic: spasm
phosphatase: unit

phosphate: diabetes; tetany
phosphogluconate: pathway
phosphohexose isomerase: deficiency
phospholipid: syndrome
phosphor: plate
phosphoroclastic: cleavage; reaction
phosphorylase-rupturing: enzyme
phosphotungstic acid: hematoxylin; stain
phosphureted: hydrogen
photechic: effect
photic: driving; stimulation
photo: cell
photoallergic: sensitivity
photochromic: lens; spectacles
photodynamic: sensitization
photoelectric: absorption; effect
photogenic: epilepsy
photomultiplier: tube
photon: density
photo-patch: test
photopic: adaptation; eye; vision
photoradiation: therapy
photoreactivating: enzyme
photoreceptor: cells
photorefractive: keratectomy
photosensor: oculography
photostimulable: phosphor
photostress: test
phototoxic: sensitivity
phrenic: ampulla; ganglia; nerve; nucleus; pleura; plexus; veins
phrenicoabdominal: branch of phrenic nerve
phrenicocolic: ligament
phrenicocostal: sinus
phrenicolienal: ligament
phrenicomediastinal: recess
phrenicopleural: fascia
phrenicosplenic: ligament
phrenic pressure: test
phrenogastric: ligament
phrenopericardial: angle
phrenosplenic: ligament
phrygian: cap
phthalein: test
phthinoid: chest
phyllodes: tumor
physaliphorous: cell
physical: age; allergy; anthropology; diagnosis; elasticity of muscle; examination; fitness; half-life; map; medicine; sign; therapy
Physick's: pouches
physiologic: age; albuminuria; amenorrhea; anemia; anisocoria; antidote; congestion; cup;

dwarfism; elasticity of muscle; equilibrium; excavation; hypertrophy; icterus; incompatibility; jaundice; leukocytosis; occlusion; sclerosis; scotoma; tremor; unit; vertigo
physiological: anatomy; chemistry; drives; homeostasis; saline; sphincter
physiologically balanced: occlusion
physiologic dead: space
physiologic rest: position
physiologic retraction: ring
pial: funnel
pial-glial: membrane
pianist's: cramp
piano: percussion
Picchini's: syndrome
Pick: cell
picker's: nodules
Pick's: atrophy; bodies; bundle; disease; syndrome
Pick's tubular: adenoma
pickwickian: syndrome
pi cone: monochromatism
picrocarmine: stain
picroformol: fixative
picro-Mallory trichrome: stain
picronigrosin: stain
picture: element
picture frame: vertebra
piebald: eyelash; skin
Pierre Robin: syndrome
piezoelectric: effect; transducer
piezogenic pedal: papule
pig: skin
pigeon: breast; chest
pigeon's: milk
pigment: cell; cells of iris; cell of skin; cells of retina; cirrhosis; epitheliopathy; epithelium; epithelium of optic retina; induration of the lung
pigmentary: cirrhosis; glaucoma; retinopathy; syphilid
pigmented: ameloblastoma; dermatofibrosarcoma protuberans; epulis; layer of ciliary body; layer of iris; layer of retina; liver; part of retina
pigmented hair epidermal: nevus
pigmented keratic: precipitates
pigmented purpuric lichenoid: dermatosis
pigmented villonodular: synovitis
Pignet's: formula

pigtail: catheter
pilar: cyst; tumor of scalp
pileous: gland
piliferous: cyst
pillar: cells; cells of Corti
pill-rolling: tremor
piloid: gliosis
pilomotor: fibers; reflex
pilon: fracture
pilonidal: cyst; fistula; sinus
Piltz: sign
pilular: mass
pin: amalgam; implant
Pinard's: maneuver
pincer: nail
pinch: graft
Pindborg: tumor
pineal: body; cells; cyst; eye; gland; habenula; recess; stalk
Pinel's: system
ping-pong: bone; fracture; mechanism
pinhole: pupil
pink: disease; eye
pink bread: mold
Pinkus: tumor
pinocytotic: vesicle
Pins': sign; syndrome
pinta: fever
pinworm: vaginitis
PIP: joints
pipe: bone
Piper's: forceps
pipe-smoker's: cancer
pipe stem: cirrhosis
pipestem: arteries; fibrosis
piqûre: diabetes
Pirie's: bone
piriform: area; cortex; fossa; muscle; opening; recess; sinus
piriformis: muscle
piriform neuron: layer
Pirogoff's: amputation; angle; triangle
Pirquet's: index; reaction; test
pisciform: cataract
pisiform: bone
pisohamate: ligament
pisometacarpal: ligament
pisotriquetral: joint
pisounciform: ligament
pisouncinate: ligament
pistol-shot: sound
pistol-shot femoral: sound
piston: pulse
pit: caries
pitch: poisoning; wart
pitch-worker's: cancer
pit and fissure: caries
pithecoid: theory
Pitot: tube
Pitres': area; sign
pitted: keratolysis
pitting: edema
Pittsburgh: pneumonia

Pittsburgh pneumonia: agent
pituitary: adamantinoma; adenoma; ameloblastoma; apoplexy; cachexia; diverticulum; dwarf; dwarfism; fossa; gigantism; gland; infantilism; membrane; myxedema; stalk
pituitary gonadotropic: hormone
pituitary growth: hormone
pituitary stalk: section
pivot: joint
pivot shift: test
pizzle: rot
P-J: interval
P-K: antibodies; test
place: theory
placenta: gonadotropin; protein
placental: barrier; circulation; dysfunction; dystocia; lobes; membrane; plasmodium; polyp; presentation; septa; sign; souffle; thrombosis; transfusion
placental dysfunction: syndrome
placental growth: hormone
placental parasitic: twin
placental site trophoblastic: tumor
placental sulfatase: deficiency
Placido da Costa's: disk
plague: bacillus; pneumonia; septicemia; vaccine
plain: film
Planck's: constant; theory
plane: joint; suture; wart
planoconcave: lens
planoconvex: lens
plant: agglutinin; antitoxin; casein; dermatitis; indican; RNase; toxin; viruses
plantar: aponeurosis; arch; cushion; fascia; fibromatosis; flexion; ligaments; muscle; reflex; space; surface of toe; syphilid; wart
plantar arterial: arch
plantar calcaneocuboid: ligament
plantar calcaneonavicular: ligament
plantar cuboideonavicular: ligament
plantar cuneocuboid: ligament
plantar cuneonavicular: ligaments
plantar digital: veins
plantar interosseous: muscle
plantaris: muscle

plantar metatarsal: artery; ligaments; veins
plantar muscle: reflex
plantar quadrate: muscle
plantar tendon: sheath of peroneus longus muscle
plantar venous: arch; network
plasma: albumin; cell; factor X; fibronectin; layer; membrane; proteins; scalpel; stain; substitute; therapy
plasma accelerator: globulin
plasma cell: balanitis; gingivitis; hepatitis; leukemia; mastitis; myeloma
plasmacrit: test
plasma iodoprotein: disorder
plasmal: reaction
plasma labile: factor
plasma renin: activity
plasma thromboplastin: antecedent; component; factor; factor B
plasmatic: compartment
plasminogen: activator
plasmin prothrombins conversion: factor
plasmocytic: leukemoid reaction
plasmodial: trophoblast
plaster: bandage; splint
plaster of Paris: disease
plastic: anatomy; bronchitis; corpuscle; cyclitis; induration; iritis; lymph; motor; operation; pleurisy; surgery; teeth
plastic restoration: material
plastic section: stain
plate: thrombosis
plateau: iris; pulse
Plateau-Talbot: law
platelet: actomyosin; cofactor I; cofactor II; factor 3
platelet-activating: factor
platelet-aggregating: factor
platelet aggregation: test
platelet-derived growth: factor
platelet tissue: factor
platelike: atelectasis
platypellic: pelvis
platypelloid: pelvis
platysma: muscle
Plaut's: bacillus
play: therapy
Pleasure: curve
pleasure: principle
pledgetted: suture
pleiotropic: gene
pleomorphic: adenoma; lipoma; oligodendroglioma
plethysmographic: goggle

pleural: calculus; canal; cavity; cupula; effusion; fluid; fremitus; lines; plaque; poudrage; pressure; rale; reaction; recesses; rub; sinuses; space; stripe; villi
pleural friction: rub
pleuritic: pneumonia; rub
pleuroesophageal: line; muscle
pleuropericardial: canals; fold; hiatus; membrane; murmur
pleuroperitoneal: canal; cavity; fold; foramen; hiatus; membrane
pleuropneumonia-like: organisms
plexiform: layer; layer of cerebral cortex; layers of retina; neurofibroma; neuroma
plexogenic pulmonary: arteriopathy
Plimmer's: bodies
plocytic: astrocytoma
Plotz: bacillus
plugging: instrument
Plummer's: dilator; disease
Plummer-Vinson: syndrome
plural: pregnancy
pluripotent: cells
plus: lens
PMA: index
pneocardiac: reflex
pneopneic: reflex
pneumatic: bone; otoscopy; retinopexy; space; tonometer
pneumatic tire: injury
pneumatoenteric: recess
pneumococcal: empyema; pneumonia; polysaccharide; vaccine
pneumococcal/suppurative: keratitis
Pneumocystis carinii: pneumonia
pneumogastric: nerve
pneumogenic: osteoarthropathy
pneumonia: virus of mice
pneumonic: plague
P/O: quotient; ratio
pocketed: calculus
podalic: extraction; version
podiatric: medicine
Podophyllum: resin
podophyllum: resin
POEMS: syndrome
point: angle; deletion; epidemic; mutation
pointed: condyloma; wart
point system: test types
Poirier's: gland; line
Poiseuille's: law; space

Poiseuille's viscosity: coefficient
Poisson: distribution
Poisson-Pearson: formula
Poitou: colic
poker: back; spine
pokeweed: mitogen
Poland's: syndrome
polar: amino acid; anemia; body; cataract; cell; compound; fibers; globule; hypogenesis; plates; presentation; ring; solvents; star; zone
polarized: light
polarizing: microscope
pole: ligation
Polenské: number
poliomyelitis: immunoglobulin; vaccines; virus
poliomyelitis immune: globulin (human)
poliovirus: vaccines
polishing: brush
Politzer: bag; method
Politzer's luminous: cone
polka: fever
poll: evil
pollen: antigen; extract
Pólya: gastrectomy
polyacrylamide gel: electrophoresis
polyalveolar: lobe
polyamine-methylene: resin
Pólya's: operation
polyaxial: joint
polybasic: acid
polycarboxylate: cement
polychlorinated: biphenyl
polychromatic: cell
polychromatophil: cell
polychrome: methylene blue
polyclonal: activator; antibody; gammopathy
polycystic: disease of kidneys; kidney; liver; ovary
polycystic liver: disease
polycystic ovary: syndrome
polydystrophic: dwarfism
polyendocrine deficiency: syndrome
polyester: resin
polygenic: inheritance
polyhedral: body
polyleptic: fever
polymerase chain: reaction
polymer fume: fever
polymorphic: neuron; reticulosis
polymorphic genetic: markers
polymorphic superficial: keratitis
polymorphocytic: leukemia
polymorphonuclear: leukocyte

polymorphous: layer; perversion
polymorphous light: eruption
polyneuritic: psychosis
polyol: pathway
polyoma: virus
polyostotic fibrous: dysplasia
polyovular ovarian: follicle
polyoxyethylene: alcohols
polyphenic: gene
polyphyletic: theory
polypoid: adenoma
polypous: endocarditis; gastritis
polysaccharide: sulfate esters
polysplenia: syndrome
polytene: chromosome
polyuria: test
polyvalent: allergy; antiserum; serum; vaccine
polyzygotic: twins
pomade: acne
Pomeroy's: operation
Pompe's: disease
pond: fracture
ponderal: index
Ponfick's: shadow
pontine: angle; arteries; cistern; flexure; hemorrhage; nuclei; veins
pontine angle: tumor
pontine gray: matter
pontis nervi trigeminalis: nucleus
pontobulbar: body
pontocerebellar: recess
ponto-geniculo-occipital: spike
pontomedullary: groove
pooled: serum
Pool's: phenomenon
Pool-Schlesinger: sign
poorly compliant: bladder
poorly crystalline: hydroxyapatite
poorly differentiated lymphocytic: lymphoma
popliteal: arch; artery; fascia; fossa; groove; line; lymph nodes; muscle; notch; plane of femur; plexus; region; space; surface of femur; vein
popliteal communicating: nerve
popliteal entrapment: syndrome
popliteus: muscle
population: genetics; pyramid
porcelain: gallbladder; inlay
porcine: adenoviruses; amelia; enterovirus; graft; herpesvirus 1; herpesvirus 2; parakeratosis;

parvovirus; polioencephalomyelitis; valve
porcine epidemic: diarrhea
porcine epidemic diarrhea: virus
porcine hemagglutinating encephalomyelitis: virus
porcine sarcoma: virus
porcine stress: syndrome
porcine transmissible: gastroenteritis
porcupine: skin
Porges: method
Porges-Meier: test
porphobilinogen synthase: porphyria
Porro: hysterectomy; operation
portable: radiography
portacaval: anastomoses; shunt
portal: canals; circulation; cirrhosis; fissure; hypertension; lobule of liver; pyemia; system; triad; vein
portal hypophysial: circulation
portal-systemic: anastomoses; encephalopathy
portasystemic: shunt
Porter's: fascia
Porter-Silber: chromogens; reaction
Porter-Silber chromogens: test
Portuguese-Azorean: disease
port-wine: mark; stain
Posadas: disease
position: agnosia; effect; sense
positional: nystagmus; vertigo of Bárány
positive: accommodation; afterimage; afterpotential; anergy; catalyst; chronotropism; control; convergence; cooperativity; electrode; electron; electrotaxis; feedback; meniscus; phase; rays; scotoma; stain; taxis; thermotaxis; transference; valence
positive contrast: orbitography
positive end-expiratory: pressure
positively: bathmotropic; dromotropic; inotropic
positive-negative pressure: breathing
positron emission: tomography
post: dam; implant

postadrenalectomy: syndrome
postage stamp: grafts
postanal: gut
postarsphenamine: jaundice
postaxillary: line
postbasic: stare
postcapillary: venules
postcardiotomy: syndrome
postcaval: ureter
postcentral: area; artery; fissure; gyrus; sulcus
postcentral sulcal: artery
postcholecystectomy: syndrome
postcloacal: gut
postcommissurotomy: syndrome
postcommunical: part of anterior cerebral artery
postconcussion: neurosis; syndrome
postcostal: anastomosis
post dam: area
postdiphtheritic: paralysis
postdrive: depression
posterior: aphasia; arch of atlas; asynclitism; belly of digastric muscle; border of eyelids; border of fibula; border of petrous part of temporal bone; border of radius; border of testis; border of ulna; branches; branch of great auricular nerve; branch of inferior pancreaticoduodenal artery; branch of lateral cerebral sulcus; branch of obturator artery; branch of obturator nerve; branch of recurrent ulnar artery; branch of renal artery; branch of right branch of portal vein; branch of right hepatic duct; branch of right superior pulmonary vein; branch of spinal nerves; branch of superior thyroid artery; canaliculus of chorda tympani; cells; centriole; chamber of eye; choroiditis; column; column of spinal cord; cord of brachial plexus; crus of stapes; cusp of atrioventricular valve; embryotoxon; extremity; fontanel; funiculus; horn; layer of rectus abdominis sheath; ligament of head of fibula; ligament of incus; ligament of knee; limb of internal capsule; limb of stapes; lip of uterine os; lobe of hypophysis; mediastinum; naris; nephrectomy; neuropore;

notch of cerebellum; occlusion; part; part of the diaphragmatic surface of the liver; pillar of fauces; pillar of fornix; pituitary; pole of eyeball; pole of lens; probability; process of septal cartilage; process of talus; pyramid of the medulla; recess; recess of tympanic membrane; region of arm; region of elbow; region of forearm; region of leg; region of neck; region of thigh; rhinoscopy; rhizotomy; root; scleritis; sclerosis; sclerotomy; segment; segment of eyeball; staphyloma; surface; surface of arm; surface of arytenoid cartilage; surface of cornea; surface of elbow; surface of eyelids; surface of fibula; surface of forearm; surface of iris; surface of kidney; surface of leg; surface of lens; surface of lower limb; surface of pancreas; surface of petrous part of temporal bone; surface of prostate; surface of radius; surface of shaft of humerus; surface of suprarenal gland; surface of thigh; surface of tibia; surface of ulna; symblepharon; synechia; teeth; triangle of neck; tubercle of atlas; tubercle of cervical vertebrae; urethra; urethritis; uveitis; vaginismus; vein of left ventricle; vein of septum pellucidum; vitrectomy; wall of middle ear; wall of stomach; wall of tympanic cavity; wall of vagina
posterior alveolar: artery
posterior ampullar: nerve
posterior antebrachial: nerve; region
posterior antebrachial cutaneous: nerve
posterior anterior jugular: vein
posterior articular: surface of dens
posterior atlanto-occipital: membrane
posterior auricular: artery; groove; muscle; nerve; plexus; vein
posterior axillary: fold; line
posterior basal: branch; segment
posterior brachial: region

posterior brachial cutaneous: nerve
posterior cardinal: veins
posterior carpal: region
posterior cecal: artery
posterior central: convolution; gyrus
posterior cerebellar: notch
posterior cerebral: artery; commissure
posterior cervical intertransversarii: muscles
posterior cervical intertransverse: muscles
posterior choroidal: artery
posterior circumflex humeral: artery
posterior column: cordotomy
posterior communicating: artery
posterior condyloid: foramen
posterior conjunctival: artery
posterior coronary: plexus
posterior costotransverse: ligament
posterior cranial: fossa
posterior cricoarytenoid: ligament; muscle
posterior cruciate: ligament
posterior crural: region
posterior cubital: region
posterior cutaneous: nerve of arm; nerve of forearm; nerve of thigh
posterior dental: artery
posterior descending: artery
posterior elastic: layer
posterior ethmoidal: artery; nerve
posterior ethmoidal air: cells
posterior facial: vein
posterior femoral cutaneous: nerve
posterior focal: point
posterior group of axillary: lymph nodes
posterior humeral circumflex: artery
posterior hypothalamic: area; nucleus; region
posterior inferior cerebellar: artery
posterior inferior cerebellar artery: syndrome
posterior inferior iliac: spine
posterior inferior nasal: branches of greater palatine nerve
posterior intercondylar: area of tibia

posterior intercostal: arteries 1–2; arteries 3-11; veins
posterior intermediate: groove; sulcus
posterior interosseous: artery; nerve
posterior interventricular: artery; groove
posterior intestinal: portal
posterior intraoccipital: joint; synchondrosis
posterior junction: line
posterior knee: region
posterior labial: arteries; commissure; nerves; veins
posterior lacrimal: crest
posterior lateral nasal: arteries
posterior limiting: layer of cornea
posterior longitudinal: bundle; ligament
posterior lunate: lobule
posterior marginal: vein
posterior median: fissure of the medulla oblongata; fissure of spinal cord; line; sulcus of medulla oblongata; sulcus of spinal cord
posterior mediastinal: arteries; lymph nodes
posterior medullary: velum
posterior meningeal: artery
posterior meniscofemoral: ligament
posterior myocardial: infarction
posterior nasal: spine
posterior neck: region
posterior occipitoaxial: ligament
posterior palatal: seal
posterior palatal seal: area
posterior palatine: arch; foramina; spine
posterior pancreaticoduodenal: artery
posterior parietal: artery
posterior parolfactory: sulcus
posterior parotid: veins
posterior pelvic: exenteration
posterior perforated: substance
posterior pericallosal: vein
posterior periventricular: nucleus
posterior peroneal: arteries
posterior primary: division
posterior quadrigeminal: body
posterior sacroiliac: ligaments

posterior sacrosciatic: ligament
posterior sagittal: diameter
posterior scalene: muscle
posterior scapular: nerve
posterior scrotal: branch of internal pudendal artery; nerves; veins
posterior segmental: artery of kidney
posterior semicircular: canals
posterior septal: artery of nose
posterior spinal: artery; sclerosis
posterior spinocerebellar: tract
posterior sternoclavicular: ligament
posterior subcapsular: cataract
posterior superior alveolar: artery; branches of maxillary nerve
posterior superior iliac: spine
posterior superior lateral nasal: branches of pterygopalatine ganglion
posterior superior medial nasal: branches of pterygopalatine ganglion
posterior supraclavicular: nerve
posterior talar articular: surface of calcaneus
posterior talofibular: ligament
posterior talotibial: ligament
posterior temporal: artery
posterior thalamic: radiations
posterior thoracic: nerve
posterior tibial: artery; lymph node; muscle; node; veins
posterior tibial recurrent: artery
posterior tibiofibular: ligament
posterior tibiotalar: ligament; part of deltoid ligament
posterior tooth: form
posterior tympanic: artery
posterior urethral: valves
posterior vaginal: hernia
posteroanterior: projection
posterolateral: fissure; fontanel; groove; sulcus
posterolateral central: arteries
posteromedial central: arteries
posteruption: cuticle
postextrasystolic: pause
postextrasystolic T: wave

postganglionic: fibers
postganglionic motor: neuron
postgastrectomy: syndrome
postglenoid: foramen
posthemiplegic: athetosis; chorea
posthemorrhagic: anemia
posthepatitic: cirrhosis
posthippocampal: fissure
posthypnotic: amnesia; psychosis; suggestion
posthypoglycemic: hyperglycemia
posticus: palsy; paralysis
postinfarction ventricular septal: defect
postinfectious: bradycardia; myelitis; polyneuritis; psychosis
post-kala azar dermal: leishmanoid
postlaminar: part of optic nerve
postlingual: deafness; fissure
postlunate: fissure
post-marketing: surveillance
postmature: infant
postmaturity: syndrome
postmeiotic: phase
postmeningitic: hydrocephalus
postmenopausal: atrophy
postmitotic: phase
postmortem: clot; delivery; examination; hypostasis; livedo; lividity; pustule; rigidity; suggillation; thrombus; tubercle; wart
postmyocardial infarction: pericarditis; syndrome
postnasal: drip
postnatal: life; pit of the newborn
postnecrotic: cirrhosis
postnormal: occlusion
postoperative: bronchopneumonia; parotiditis; pneumonia; tetany
postoperative pressure: alopecia
postoral: arches
postpalatal: seal
postpalatal seal: area
postpartum: alopecia; amenorrhea; cardiomyopathy; estrus; hemorrhage; hypertension; psychosis; tetanus
postpartum pituitary necrosis: syndrome
postparturient: hemoglobinuria
postperfusion: lung
postpericardiotomy: pericarditis; syndrome
postpharyngeal: space

postphlebitic: syndrome
postprandial: lipemia; pain
postprimary: tuberculosis
postpyloric: sphincter
postpyramidal: fissure
postreduction: phase
postrenal: albuminuria
postrhinal: fissure
postrubella: syndrome
postsphenoid: bone
poststationary: phase
post-steady: state
post-stenotic: dilation
poststeroid: panniculitis
postsulcal: part of tongue
postsynaptic: membrane
post-term: infant
postthrombotic: syndrome
posttraumatic: delirium;
  dementia; epilepsy;
  hydrocephalus; neurosis;
  osteoporosis; pericarditis;
  psychosis; syndrome
posttraumatic arterial:
  thrombosis
**posttraumatic
  leptomeningeal:** cyst
posttraumatic neck:
  syndrome
posttraumatic stress:
  disorder; syndrome
posttussis suction: sound
posttussive: suction
postural: albuminuria;
  contraction; drainage;
  hypotension; ischemia;
  myoneuralgia; position;
  reflex; set; syncope;
  tremor; version; vertigo
posture: sense
postvaccinal: encephalitis;
  encephalomyelitis; myelitis
pot: curare
potable: water
Potain's: sign
potassium: inhibition
potassium nitrate: paper
potassium sparing: diuretics
potato: nose; tumor of neck
potato dextrose: agar
potential: energy
potentiometric: titration
Potomac horse: fever
Potter-Bucky: diaphragm
Potter's: disease; facies;
  syndrome; version
Potts': anastomosis; clamp;
  operation
Pott's: abscess; aneurysm;
  curvature; disease; fracture;
  gangrene; paralysis;
  paraplegia
Pott's puffy: tumor
poultry handler's: disease
poultryman's: itch
Poupart's: ligament; line
povidone: iodine
Powassan: encephalitis; virus

powdered: gold; ipecac;
  opium; stomach
power: failure; injector;
  point
Pozzi's: muscle
P-P: interval
P and P: test
p-p: factor
P-Q: interval
PR: enzyme
P-R: interval; segment
practical: anatomy; nurse;
  units
Prader-Willi: syndrome
Prague: maneuver; pelvis
prairie: conjunctivitis; itch
Pratt: dilators
Pratt's: symptom
Prausnitz-Küstner:
  antibody; reaction
pravastatin: sodium
preanesthetic: medication
preauricular: groove; point;
  sulcus
preauricular deep parotid:
  lymph nodes
preautomatic: pause
preaxillary: line
pre-B: lymphocyte
precancerous: lesion;
  melanosis of Dubreuilh
precapillary: anastomosis
prececal: lymph nodes
precentral: area; artery;
  gyrus; sulcus
precentral cerebellar: vein
precentral sulcal: artery
precervical: sinus
prechiasmatic: sulcus
prechordal: plate
precipitate: labor
precipitated: calcium
  carbonate; sulfur
precipitating: antibody;
  cause
precipitation: curve; test
precipitin: reaction; test
precision: attachment; rest
precocious: pseudopuberty;
  puberty
precollagenous: fibers
precommissural: bundle;
  septum
precommissural septal: area
precommunical: part of
  anterior cerebral artery
preconceptual: stage
precordial:
  electrocardiography; leads
precordial catch: syndrome
precorneal: film
precostal: anastomosis
precuneal: artery
precursory: cartilage
predictive: validity; value
predisposing: cause; factors
predorsal: bundle
preejection: period

preen: gland
preexcitation: syndrome
preextraction: record
preferred provider:
  organization
preformation: theory
prefrontal: area; cortex;
  leukotomy; lobotomy;
  veins
preganglionic: fibers
preganglionic motor: neuron
pregenital: organization;
  phase
pregnancy: cells; diabetes;
  disease of sheep; hormone;
  luteoma; toxemia of sheep;
  tumor
pregnant mare's serum:
  gonadotropin
pregranulosa: cells
prehyoid: gland
preinfarction: angina;
  syndrome
preinterparietal: bone
Preisz-Nocard: bacillus
prelaminar: part of optic
  nerve
prelaryngeal: lymph nodes
preliminary: impression
prelingual: deafness
prelogical: mind; thinking
premammary: abscess
premature: alopecia; beat;
  birth; contact; contraction;
  delivery; ejaculation; labor;
  systole
premature senility:
  syndrome
prematurity: myopia
premaxillary: bone; suture
premeiotic: phase
premenstrual: edema;
  syndrome; tension
premenstrual salivary:
  syndrome
premenstrual tension:
  syndrome
premitotic: phase
premolar: tooth
premotor: area; cortex;
  syndrome
prenatal: diagnosis; life;
  screening
prenodular: fissure
Prentice's: rule
preoccipital: notch
pre-oedipal: phase
preoperative: record
preoptic: area; region
preoral: gut
prepapillary: sphincter
prepared: chalk;
  ipecacuanha; suet
prepared mutton: tallow
prepatellar: bursa; bursitis
prepatent: period
prepericardiac: lymph nodes
prepiriform: gyrus

preprostate urethral:
  sphincter
preputial: calculus; glands;
  sac
prepyloric: sphincter; vein
prepyramidal: tract
prerectal: lithotomy
prereduction: phase
prerenal: albuminuria
pre-Rolandic: artery
prerubral: field; nucleus
presacral: anesthesia; nerve;
  neurectomy;
  sympathectomy
presenile: dementia
presenile spontaneous:
  gangrene
presenting: symptom
presomite: embryo
presphenoid: bone
presplenic: fold
pressor: amine; base; fibers;
  nerve; substance
pressoreceptive: mechanism
pressoreceptor: nerve;
  reflex; system
pressure: alopecia;
  amaurosis; anesthesia;
  atrophy; collapse; dressing;
  epiphysis; gangrene; palsy;
  paralysis; plethysmograph;
  pneumothorax; point;
  reversal; sense; sore; stasis;
  urticaria
pressure-controlled:
  respirator
pressure-volume: index
pre-steady: state
presternal: notch; region
prestriate: area
presulcal: part of tongue
presumed ocular:
  histoplasmosis
presumptive: region
presynaptic: membrane
presystolic: gallop; murmur;
  thrill
pretectal: area; nucleus;
  region
preterm: infant
pretibial: fever; myxedema
pretracheal: fascia; layer;
  lymph nodes
preventive: dentistry; dose;
  medicine; treatment
prevertebral: fascia; ganglia;
  layer; lymph nodes; part of
  vertebral artery
previllous: chorion; embryo
Pribnow: box
Price-Jones: curve
prickle: cell
prickle cell: layer
prickly: heat
primal: repression
primaquine: sensitivity
primary: adhesion;
  aerodontalgia; alcohol;

aldosteronism; amenorrhea; amputation; amyloidosis; anesthetic; atelectasis; bronchus; bubo; carcinoma; cardiomyopathy; caries; cementum; center of ossification; choana; coccidioidomycosis; color; complex; constriction; dementia; dentin; dentition; deviation; digestion; disease; drives; dysmenorrhea; fissure of cerebellum; gain; gout; hemochromatosis; hemorrhage; hydrocephalus; hyperoxaluria and oxalosis; hyperparathyroidism; hypertension; hyperthyroidism; hypogammaglobulinemia; hypogonadism; irritant; lymphedema; lysosomes; megaureter; mesoderm; metabolism; metabolite; methemoglobinemia; narcissism; neurasthenia; nodule; nondisjunction; oocyte; organizer; palate; pentosuria; point of ossification; process; proteose; pyoderma; radiation; rays; reaction; reinforcement; rejection; screw-worm; sensation; sequestrum; shock; sodium phosphate; spermatocyte; structure; syphilis; telangiectasia; tooth; tuberculosis; union; villus; vitreous

primary adrenocortical: insufficiency
primary amebic: meningoencephalitis
primary atypical: pneumonia
primary biliary: cirrhosis
primary brain: vesicle
primary dental: lamina
primary dried: yeast
primary egg: membrane
primary embryonic: cell
primary erythroblastic: anemia
primary extrapulmonary: coccidioidomycosis
primary generalized: epilepsy
primary herpetic: stomatitis
primary idiopathic macular: atrophy
primary immune: response
primary interatrial: foramen
primary irritant: dermatitis
primary labial: groove

primary lateral: sclerosis
primary macular: atrophy of skin
primary medical: care
primary myeloid: metaplasia
primary neuroendocrine: carcinoma of the skin
primary neuronal: degeneration
primary ovarian: follicle
primary pigmentary: degeneration of retina
primary progressive cerebellar: degeneration
primary pulmonary: lobule
primary refractory: anemia
primary renal: calculus
primary renal tubular: acidosis
primary sclerosing: cholangitis
primary senile: dementia
primary sex: characters
primary skin: graft
primary visual: area; cortex
primer: extension
primitive: aorta; chorion; furrow; groove; gut; knot; meninx; node; palate; pit; ridge; streak
primitive costal: arches
primitive neuroectodermal: tumor
primitive perivisceral: cavity
primitive reticular: cell
primordial: cartilage; cell; cyst; dwarfism; gigantism; kidney
primordial germ: cell
primordial ovarian: follicle
princeps cervicis: artery
princeps pollicis: artery
Princeteau's: tubercle
principal: artery of thumb; focus; islets; piece; plane; point
principal optic: axis
principal sensory: nucleus of trigeminal nerve; nucleus of the trigeminus
Pringle's: disease
Prinzmetal's: angina
prion: protein
prior: probability
prism: diopter
prism cover: test
prism vergence: test
prison fever: typhus
private: antigens; blood group; hospital; nurse
private duty: nurse
privet: cough
privileged: site
proacrosomal: granules
proactive: inhibition
probability: curve; sample

probe: gorget; patency; syringe
problem-oriented: record
procentriole: organizer
procerus: muscle
process: schizophrenia
prochordal: plate
procursive: chorea; epilepsy
prodromal: period; stage
prodromic: sign
product: inhibition
productive: inflammation; peritonitis; pleurisy
product-moment: correlation
Profeta's: law
profile: record
profound: hypothermia
profunda brachii: artery
profunda femoris: artery
progestational: hormone
progesterone: unit
progress: curve
progressive: cataract; cleavage; lipodystrophy; pneumonia; processes; staining; vaccinia
progressive bacterial synergistic: gangrene
progressive bulbar: palsy; paralysis
progressive cerebellar: tremor
progressive cerebral: poliodystrophy
progressive choroidal: atrophy
progressive circumscribed cerebral: atrophy
progressive emphysematous: necrosis
progressive familial: scleroderma
progressive hypertrophic: polyneuropathy
progressive infantile spinal muscular: atrophy
progressive multifocal: leukoencephalopathy
progressive muscular: atrophy; dystrophy
progressive pigmentary: dermatosis
progressive pneumonia: virus
progressive spinal: amyotrophy
progressive spinal muscular: atrophy
progressive subcortical: encephalopathy
progressive supranuclear: palsy
progressive tapetochoroidal: dystrophy
progressive torsion: spasm
projectile: vomiting

projection: fibers; perimeter; system
projective: test
prolactin: cell; unit
prolactin-inhibiting: factor; hormone
prolactin-producing: adenoma
prolactin-releasing: factor; hormone
proliferating: pleurisy
proliferating systematized: angioendotheliomatosis
proliferating tricholemmal: cyst
proliferation: cyst; therapy
proliferative: arthritis; bronchiolitis; choroiditis; dermatitis; fasciitis; gingivitis; glomerulonephritis; inflammation; intimitis; myositis; retinopathy
proligerous: disk; membrane
prolonged action: tablet
prometaphase: banding
prominent: heel
promontory common iliac: lymph nodes
promoting: agent
prompt insulin zinc: suspension
pronator: reflex; ridge
pronator quadratus: muscle
pronator teres: muscle
prone: position
pronephric: duct; tubule
proof: spirit
propagated: thrombus
proparathyroid: hormone
proper: fasciculi; ligament of ovary; substance
properdin: factor A; factor B; factor D; factor E; system
proper hepatic: artery
properitoneal inguinal: hernia
proper palmar digital: artery; nerves
proper plantar digital: artery; nerves
property: emergence
prophylactic: membrane; odontotomy; treatment
proportional: counter; limit
proportionate: infantilism
proprietary: hospital; medicine
proprioceptive: mechanism; reflexes; sensibility
proprioceptive-oculocephalic: reflex
prosecretion: granules
prosector's: tubercle; wart
proserum prothrombin conversion: accelerator
prospective: fate

prostate: gland
prostate-specific: antigen
prostatic: adenoma; calculus; catheter; ducts; ductules; fluid; massage; plexus; sheath; sinus; urethra; utricle
prostatic intraepithelial: neoplasia
prostaticovesical: plexus
prostatic venous: plexus
prosthetic: dentistry; group; valves
prostomial: mesoderm
protamine zinc: insulin
protection: test
protective: block; colloid; protein; spectacles; zone
protective laryngeal: reflex
protein: factor; fever; malnutrition; metabolism; quotient; shock; synthesis
α-1-proteinase: deficiency
protein-bound: iodine
protein-bound iodine: test
protein-losing: enteropathy
protein shock: therapy
Proteus: syndrome
prothoracic: glands
prothrombin: accelerator; test; time
prothrombin and proconvertin: test
protochordal: knot
protodiastolic: gallop
proton: pump
protopathic: sensibility
protoplasmic: astrocyte; astrocytoma; movement
prototrophic: strains
protozoan: cyst
protruded: disk
protruding: teeth
protrusive: excursion; occlusion; position; record; relation
protrusive jaw: relation
protuberant: abdomen
proud: flesh
Proust's: law; space
provisional: callus; cortex; denture; ligature; prosthesis
provocation: typhoid
provocative: test
provocative Wassermann: test
Prowazek: bodies
Prowazek-Greeff: bodies
proximal: border of nail; caries; centriole; contact
proximal femoral focal: deficiency
proximal interphalangeal: joints
proximal radioulnar: articulation; joint
proximal spiral: septum
proximal tibiofibular: joint

proximal urethral: sphincter
proximate: cause; principle
prozone: reaction
prune: belly
prune belly: syndrome
prune-juice: expectoration; sputum
pruritic urticarial: papules and plaques of pregnancy
Prussak's: fibers; pouch; space
Prussian blue: stain
psalterial: cord
psammoma: bodies
psammomatous: meningioma
pseudo: psychosis
pseudo-: hemianopia
pseudoachondroplastic spondyloepiphysial: dysplasia
pseudoanaphylactic: shock
pseudobulbar: paralysis
pseudocholinesterase: deficiency
pseudochylous: ascites
pseudocoarctation of the aorta
pseudocowpox: virus
pseudoepitheliomatous: hyperplasia
pseudoexfoliative capsular: glaucoma
pseudofusion: beat
pseudo-Gaucher: cell
pseudo-Graefe: sign
pseudo-Graefe's: phenomenon
pseudo-Hurler: disease; polydystrophy
pseudohypertrophic muscular: dystrophy
pseudolepromatous: leishmaniasis
pseudolymphocytic choriomeningitis: virus
pseudolysogenic: strain
pseudomembranous: bronchitis; colitis; conjunctivitis; enteritis; enterocolitis; gastritis; inflammation
pseudomucinous: cyst
pseudoneurogenic: bladder
pseudoneurotic: schizophrenia
pseudo-osteomalacic: pelvis
pseudoplastic: fluid
pseudorabies: virus
pseudosarcomatous: fasciitis
pseudostratified: epithelium
pseudotubercular: yersiniosis
pseudotubular: degeneration
pseudounipolar: cell; neuron
pseudoxanthoma: cell
psi: factor; phenomenon
psittacosis: virus

psittacosis inclusion: bodies
psoas: abscess; margin
psoas major: muscle
psoas minor: muscle
psoriatic: arthritis
psoroptic: acariasis; mange
psychedelic: drug; therapy
psychiatric: nosology
psychic: blindness; contagion; determinism; energy; force; impotence; inertia; overtone; seizure; tic; trauma
psychoanalytic: psychiatry; psychotherapy; situation; therapy
psychocardiac: reflex
psychodysleptic: drug
psychogalvanic: reaction; reflex; response
psychogenic: deafness; pain; polydipsia; purpura; seizure; torticollis; tremor; vomiting
psychogenic nocturnal: polydipsia
psychogenic nocturnal polydipsia: syndrome
psychogenic pain: disorder
psychological: tests
psycholytic: drug
psychomotor: epilepsy; retardation; seizure; tests
psychopathic: personality
psychophysiologic: manifestation
psychosensory: aphasia
psychosexual: development; dysfunction
psychosomatic: disorder; medicine
psychotic: manifestation
psychotomimetic: drug
psychotropic: agent; drug
psyllium: husk
PTA: stain
PTC: protein
pterygium: syndrome
pterygoid: branch of maxillary artery; canal; chest; depression; fissure; fossa; fovea; hamulus; laminae; nerve; notch; pit; plates; plexus; process; ridge of sphenoid bone; tubercle; tuberosity
pterygomandibular: ligament; raphe; space
pterygomaxillary: fissure; fossa; notch
pterygopalatine: canal; fossa; ganglion; groove; nerves
pterygopharyngeal: part of superior constrictor muscle of pharynx
pterygospinal: ligament

pterygospinous: ligament; process
ptotic: organ
pubic: angle; arch; arteries; baldness; body; bone; branch of inferior epigastric artery; branch of obturator artery; crest; rami; region; spine; symphysis; tubercle
public: antigens; health; hospital
public health: dentistry; nurse
pubocapsular: ligament
pubococcygeal: muscle
pubococcygeus: muscle
pubofemoral: ligament
puboprostatic: ligament; muscle
puborectal: muscle
puborectalis: muscle
pubourethral: triangle
pubovaginal: muscle; operation
pubovaginalis: muscle
pubovesical: ligament; muscle
pubovesicalis: muscle
Puchtler-Sweat: stain for basement membranes; stain for hemoglobin and hemosiderin
pudding: opium
puddle: sign
pudendal: anesthesia; canal; cleavage; cleft; hematocele; hernia; nerve; sac; slit; ulcer; veins
pudic: nerve
puerile: respiration
puerperal: convulsions; eclampsia; fever; hemoglobinemia; hemoglobinuria; mastitis; morbidity; period; phlebitis; psychosis; sepsis; septicemia; tetanus
Puestow: procedure
pullorum: disease
pulmonary: acariasis; acinus; adenomatosis; adenomatosis of sheep; alveolus; amebiasis; anthrax; arc; area; artery; aspergillosis; atresia; branch of autonomic nervous system; bulla; cavity; circulation; cirrhosis; collapse; cone; conus; distomiasis; edema; embolism; emphysema; encephalopathy; fistula; glomangiosis; glomus; hamartoma; heart; hemosiderosis; hypertension; hypostasis; incompetence;

insufficiency; ligament;
lymph nodes; murmur;
orifice; osteoarthropathy;
pleura; pleurisy; plexus;
pressure; ridges; salient;
schistosomiasis; siderosis;
sinuses; stenosis; sulcus;
surface of heart; talcosis;
toilet; transpiration; trunk;
tuberculosis; tularemia;
valve; veins; ventilation
pulmonary alveolar:
microlithiasis; proteinosis
pulmonary artery:
aneurysm; banding
pulmonary capillary wedge:
pressure
pulmonary dysmaturity:
syndrome
pulmonic: plague;
regurgitation; tularemia;
valve
pulmonocoronary: reflex
pulp: abscess; amputation;
atrophy; calcification;
calculus; canal; cavity;
chamber; horn; nodule;
polyp; pressure; stone; test
pulpal: wall
pulpar: cell
pulpit: spectacles
pulpless: tooth
pulpy kidney: disease
pulsatile: hematoma
pulsatility: index
pulsating: empyema;
metastases; neurasthenia
pulse: curve; deficit;
duration; generator;
granuloma; period;
pressure; rate; therapy;
wave
pulse-chase: experiment
pulsed dye: laser
pulsed-field gel:
electrophoresis
pulse-field gel:
electrophoresis
pulse height: analyzer
pulseless: disease
pulsion: diverticulum
pulvinar: nucleus
pumiced: foot
pump: failure; lung
punch: biopsy; grafts
punchdrunk: syndrome
punctate: basophilia;
cataract; hemorrhage;
hyalosis; keratitis;
keratoderma; parotiditis;
retinitis
punctuation: codon
puncture: diabetes; wound
pupillary: axis; border of
iris; distance; margin of
iris; membrane; reflex;
zone
pupillary block: glaucoma

pupillary light-near:
dissociation
pupillary-skin: reflex
pupillotonic: pseudotabes
pure: absence; aphasias;
color; culture; flutter
pure random: drift
pure red cell: anemia;
aplasia
pure tone: audiogram
pure-tone: audiometer;
audiometry
purified: cotton; ozokerite;
water
purified placental: protein
**purified protein derivative
of:** tuberculin
purine: base; bodies
purine-free: diet
purine-restricted: diet
Purkinje: conduction; effect;
images; shift; system
Purkinje's: cells; corpuscles;
fibers; figures; layer;
network; phenomenon
Purkinje-Sanson: images
Purmann's: method
pursed lips: breathing
purse-string: corepexy;
instrument; suture
Purtscher's: disease;
retinopathy
purulent: conjunctivitis;
cyclitis; encephalitis;
inflammation; ophthalmia;
pericarditis; pleurisy;
pneumonia; retinitis;
synovitis
pus: basin; cell; corpuscle;
tube
push-back: procedure
pustular: blepharitis;
miliaria; psoriasis; syphilid
Putnam-Dana: syndrome
putrescent: pulp
putrid: bronchitis
Putti-Platt: operation;
procedure
putty: kidney
PVM: virus
pyelonephritic: kidney
pyelotubular: reflux
pyelovenous: backflow
pyemic: abscess; embolism
pyloric: antrum; artery;
canal; cap; constriction;
glands; incompetence;
insufficiency; lymph nodes;
orifice; part of stomach;
sphincter; stenosis; valve;
vein
Pym's: fever
pyogenic: arthritis;
bacterium; fever;
granuloma; infection;
membrane;
pachymeningitis;
salpingitis

pyramid: sign
pyramidal: bone; cataract;
cells; decussation; disease;
eminence; fibers; fracture;
lobe of thyroid gland;
muscle; muscle of auricle;
process; radiation; tract;
tractotomy
pyramidal auricular:
muscle
pyramidal cell: layer
pyramidalis: muscle
pyridoxine: dependency with
seizure
pyriform: apparatus
pyriform aperture: wiring
pyrimidine: base; dimer
pyroligneous: alcohol; spirit;
vinegar
pyrrol: cell
pyrrole: nucleus
pyruvate dehydrogenase:
complex
pyruvate kinase: deficiency
pyruvate oxidation: factor

Q

Q: angle; bands; disks;
enzyme; fever; wave
Q-banding: stain
Q-R: interval
Q-RB: interval
QRS: complex; interval
Q-S$_2$: interval
Q-T: interval
Q tip: test
quack: medicine
quadrangular: cartilage;
lobule; membrane; space;
therapy
quadrantic: hemianopia;
scotoma
quadrate: ligament; lobe;
lobule; muscle; muscle of
loins; muscle of sole;
muscle of thigh; muscle of
upper lip; part of liver
quadrate pronator: muscle
quadratus: muscle
quadratus femoris: muscle
quadratus lumborum:
muscle
quadratus plantae: muscle
quadriceps: muscle of thigh;
reflex
quadriceps femoris: muscle
quadrigeminal: bodies;
lamina; plate; pulse;
rhythm
quadrilateral: space
quadripedal extensor: reflex
quadruple: amputation;
rhythm
quail bronchitis: virus
qualitative: alteration;
analysis; trait
quality: control; factor

quality control: chart
quantitative: alteration;
analysis; genetics;
hypertrophy; perimetry
Quant's: sign
quantum: efficiency; limit;
mottle; requirement;
theory; yield
Quaranfil: virus
quarantine: period
quartan: fever; malaria;
parasite
quarter: evil
quartz: glass
quaternary: structure;
syphilis
quaternary carbon: atom
Quatrefages': angle
Queckenstedt-Stookey: test
Queensland tick: typhus
quellung: phenomenon;
reaction; test
Quénu-Muret: sign
Quénu's hemorrhoidal:
plexus
quick cure: resin
Quick's: method; test
quick-stop: mutant
quiet: iritis; lung
quiet hip: disease
quilted: suture
**quinacrine chromosome
banding:** stain
Quincke's: disease; edema;
pulse; puncture; sign
quinhydrone: electrode
quinine carbacrylic: resin
quinine carbacrylic resin:
test
Quinlan's: test
quintan: fever
quisqualate: receptor
quotidian: fever; malaria

R

ρ**:** factor
R: antigen; enzyme; factors;
pili; plasmids; wave
R$_f$: value
rabbit: fever; fibroma;
plague; snuffles
rabbit fibroma: virus
rabbit hemorrhagic: disease
rabbit myxoma: virus
rabbitpox: virus
rabies: immunoglobulin;
vaccine; vaccine, Flury
strain egg-passage; virus;
virus, Flury strain; virus,
Kelev strain
rabies immune: globulin
(human)
raccoon: eyes
racemic: calcium
pantothenate
racemose: aneurysm; gland;
hemangioma

rachitic: diet; pelvis; rosary; scoliosis
racial: melanoderma
racket: amputation; nail
racquet: hypha
Radford: nomogram
radial: acceleration; artery; border of forearm; bursa; clubhand; eminence of wrist; fossa of humerus; head; immunodiffusion; keratotomy; nerve; notch; phenomenon; pulse; reflex; scar; tuberosity; veins
radial aplasia-thrombocytopenia: syndrome
radial collateral: artery; ligament; ligament of elbow; ligament of wrist
radial flexor: muscle of wrist
radial growth: phase
radial index: artery
radialis indicis: artery
radial recurrent: artery
radial sclerosing: lesion
radial styloid: tendovaginitis
radiant: energy; heat; intensity
radiate: crown; layer of tympanic membrane; ligament; ligament of head of rib; ligament of wrist
radiate sternocostal: ligaments
radiation: anemia; biology; biophysics; burn; caries; cataract; chemistry; chimera; dermatosis; myelitis; myelopathy; oncologist; oncology; physics; pneumonitis; poisoning; risks; sickness; therapy
radiation weighting: factor
radical: cystectomy; hysterectomy; mastectomy; mastoidectomy; operation for hernia; pericardiectomy
radicular: abscess; arteries; cyst; fila; pulp; syndrome
radioactive: atom; constant; cyanocobalamin; equilibrium; iodine; isotope; probe; thyroxine
radioactive iodide uptake: test
radioallergosorbent: test
radiobicipital: reflex
radiocarpal: articulation; joint
radiochemical: purity
radiofrequency: pulse
radiographic: pelvimetry
radiographic parallel line: shadows
radioimmunosorbent: test

radioiodinated serum: albumin
radioisotopic: purity
radiolabeled: thyroxine
radiological: anatomy; enteroclysis; sphincter
radionuclide: angiocardiography; angiography; cisternography; generator; ventriculography
radionuclidic: purity
radioperiosteal: reflex
radiopharmaceutical: chemistry; purity
radioreceptor: assay
radiotelemetering: capsule
radiotherapy: localization
radioulnar: disk; syndesmosis
radium: emanation
radium beam: therapy
Raeder's paratrigeminal: syndrome
ragpicker's: disease
rag-sorter's: disease
ragsorter's: disease
Rahe-Holmes social readjustment rating: scale
Rahn-Otis: sample
RAI: test
railroad: disease; nystagmus; sickness
rainbow: symptom
Rainey's: corpuscles
Raji: cell
Raji cell radioimmune: assay
Ramachandran: plot
Raman: effect; spectrum
Rambourg's chromic acid-phosphotungstic acid: stain
Rambourg's periodic acid-chromic methenamine-silver: stain
Ramsay Hunt's: syndrome
Ramsden's: ocular
Ramstedt: operation
Randall's: plaques
Randall stone: forceps
random: coil; mating; mechanism; sample; sampling; variable; waves
randomized controlled: trial
random mating: equilibrium
random pattern: flap
Raney: alloy; catalyst
range of: accommodation; convergence
Ranikhet: disease
ranine: artery; tumor
rank-difference: correlation
Ranke's: angle; formula
Rankine: scale
Rankin's: clamp
Ransohoff's: sign

Ranvier's: crosses; disks; node; plexus; segment
Raoult's: law
raphe: nuclei
raphespinal: fibers
rapid: canities; decompression; film changer
rapid eye: movements
rapid eye movement: sleep
rapidly progressive: glomerulonephritis
rapid plasma reagin: test
Rapoport: test
Rapoport-Luebering: shunt
Rappaport: classification
Rappaport's: acinus
rare: earths
rare-earth: screen
rare earth: elements; metal
Rasmussen's: aneurysm
raspberry: tongue
Rastelli's: operation; operation
rat: leprosy
rat-bite: disease; fever
rate: constants; equation; meter
Rathke's: bundles; diverticulum; pocket; pouch
Rathke's cleft: cyst
Rathke's pouch: tumor
ratio: scale
rational: formula; therapy
rat mite: dermatitis
rat sialodacryoadenitis: virus
Rauber's: layer
Rau's: process
Rauscher leukemia: virus
Rauscher's: virus
Raussly: disease
Ravius': process
raw: score
ray: fungus; therapeutics
Rayer's: disease
Rayleigh: equation; test
Raynaud's: disease; phenomenon; sign; syndrome
R-banding: stain
reaction: center; formation; time
reactive: astrocyte; cell; depression; hyperemia; schizophrenia
reactive attachment: disorder
reactive perforating: collagenosis
reading-frame-shift: mutation
reaginic: antibody
real: focus; image
reality: adaptation; principle
real-time: ultrasonography

Réaumur: scale
rebound: phenomenon; tenderness
rebreathing: anesthesia; technique
Rebuck skin window: technique
Récamier's: operation
recapitulation: theory
receiver operating: characteristic
receiver operating characteristic: curve
receptive: aphasia
receptor: protein; site
recessive: character; inheritance; trait
reciprocal: anchorage; arm; beat; bigeminy; forces; inhibition; innervation; rhythm; transfusion; translocation
reciprocating: rhythm
reciprocity: law
Recklinghausen's: disease of bone; disease type I; tumor
reclotting: phenomenon
recognition: factors; time
recoil: atom; wave
recombinant: DNA; strain; vector
recombination: fraction
recombinatorial: repair
recommended daily: allowance
reconstructive: mammaplasty; psychotherapy; surgery
record: base; linkage; rim
recovery: score
recreational: drug
recrudescent: typhus
recrudescent typhus: fever
recruiting: response
rectal: alimentation; ampulla; anesthesia; columns; folds; plexuses; reflex; shelf; sinuses; valves; valvotomy
rectal venous: plexus
rectangular: amputation
rectified: spirit; tar oil; turpentine oil
rectifier: tube
rectocardiac: reflex
rectococcygeal: muscle
rectococcygeus: muscle
rectolabial: fistula
rectolaryngeal: reflex
rectosigmoid: junction; sphincter
rectourethral: fistula; muscle
rectourethralis: muscle
rectouterine: fold; muscle; pouch
rectovaginal: fistula; septum
rectovaginouterine: pouch

rectovesical: fascia; fistula; fold; muscle; pouch; septum
rectovesicalis: muscle
rectovestibular: fistula
rectovulvar: fistula
rectus: muscle of abdomen; muscle of thigh; sheath
rectus abdominis: muscle
rectus capitis anterior: muscle
rectus capitis lateralis: muscle
rectus capitis posterior major: muscle
rectus capitis posterior minor: muscle
rectus femoris: muscle
recurrence: rate; risk
recurrent: albuminuria; appendicitis; artery; artery of Heubner; caries; encephalopathy; fever; hypopyon; nerve; polyserositis; stricture; tetany
recurrent aphthous: stomatitis; ulcers
recurrent central: retinitis
recurrent corneal: erosion
recurrent herpetic: stomatitis
recurrent interosseous: artery
recurrent laryngeal: nerve
recurrent meningeal: branch of spinal nerves; nerve
recurrent pyogenic: cholangitis
recurrent radial: artery
recurrent scarring: aphthae
recurrent ulcerative: stomatitis
recurrent ulnar: artery
recurring digital: fibromas of childhood
red: atrophy; corpuscle; degeneration; fever; fibers; gum; half-moon; hepatization; induration; infarct; lead; mange; muscle; neuralgia; nucleus; precipitate; pulp; reflex; sweat; test; thrombus; vision; wine
red blood: cell
red blood cell: cast
red bone: marrow
red cell: cast
red cell adherence: phenomenon; test
redox: electrode; indicator; potential; system
red oxide of: lead
red pulp: cords
red strawberry: tongue
reduced: eye; glutathione; hematin; hemoglobin

reduced enamel: epithelium
reduced interarch: distance
reducible: hernia
reducing: diet; enzyme; sugar; valve
reduction: deformity; division; mammaplasty; nucleus; phase
reduplicated: cataract
redwater: fever
Reed: cells
Reed-Frost: theory of epidemics
reed instrument: theory
Reed-Sternberg: cells
reedy: nail
reel: foot
re-entrant: mechanism
reentry: phenomenon; theory
Rees-Ecker: fluid
refeeding: gynecomastia
reference: electrode; method; values
referred: pain; sensation
Refetoff: syndrome
reflected: colors; light; ray
reflected inguinal: ligament
reflecting: retinoscope
reflection: coefficient
reflex: angina; arc; asthma; control; cough; dyspepsia; epilepsy; headache; incontinence; inhibition; iridoplegia; ligament; movement; otalgia; sensation; symptom; tachycardia; therapy
reflex detrusor: contraction
reflex neurogenic: bladder
reflexogenic: pressosensitivity; zone
reflex sympathetic: dystrophy
reflux: conjunctivitis; esophagitis; nephropathy; otitis media
refracted: light
refracting: angle of a prism
refractive: amblyopia; index; keratoplasty; keratotomy
refractive accommodative: esotropia
refractory: anemia; cast; flask; investment; period; period of electronic pacemaker; rickets; state
refrigeration: anesthesia
Refsum's: disease; syndrome
Regaud's: fixative
regenerative: polyp
regional: anatomy; anesthesia; enteritis; enterocolitis; hypothermia; lymphadenitis; perfusion
regional granulomatous: lymphadenitis
registered: nurse

regressing atypical: histiocytosis
regression of the: mean
regression: analysis
regressive: staining
regressive-reconstructive: approach
regular: astigmatism; insulin
regular insulin: injection
regulator: gene
regulatory: albuminuria; sequence
regurgitant: fraction; murmur
regurgitation: jaundice
Rehfuss: method
Rehfuss stomach: tube
Reichel-Pólya stomach: resection
Reichert-Meissl: number
Reichert's: cartilage
Reichert's cochlear: recess
Reichstein's: compound; substance
Reid's base: line
Reifenstein's: syndrome
Reil's: ansa; band; ribbon; triangle
Reinecke: salt
reinfection: tuberculosis
reinforced: anchorage
Reinke: crystalloids
Reinke's: space
Reinsch's: test
Reisseisen's: muscles
Reissner's: fiber; membrane
Reiter: test
Reiter's: disease; syndrome
relapsing: appendicitis; fever; malaria; perichondritis; polychondritis
relapsing febrile nodular nonsuppurative: panniculitis
relational: threshold
relative: accommodation; dehydration; humidity; immunity; incompetence; leukocytosis; polycythemia; risk; scotoma; sensitivity; specificity; viscosity
relative afferent: pupillary defect
relative afferent pupillary: defect
relative molecular: mass
relative refractory: period
relaxant: reversal
relaxation: factor; response; suture; time
release: phenomenon
released: substance
releasing: factors; hormone
reliability: coefficient
relief: area; chamber
REM: syndrome

Remak's: fibers; ganglia; plexus; reflex; sign
Remak's nuclear: division
REM behavior: disorder
reminiscent: aura
remittent: fever; malaria
remittent malarial: fever
remote: memory
removable: bridge
removable partial: denture
renal: adenocarcinoma; agenesis; amyloidosis; artery; ballottement; branch of lesser splanchnic nerve; branch of vagus nerve; calculus; capsulotomy; carcinosarcoma; cast; colic; collar; columns; corpuscle; cortex; diabetes; epistaxis; failure; fascia; ganglia; glycosuria; hematuria; hemorrhage; hypertension; hypoplasia; impression; infantilism; insufficiency; labyrinth; lobe; medulla; nanism; osteitis fibrosa; osteodystrophy; papilla; pelvis; plexus; pyramid; reflex; retinopathy; rickets; segments; sinus; surface of spleen; surface of suprarenal gland; surface of the suprarenal gland; threshold; transplantation; veins
renal cell: carcinoma
renal cortical: adenoma; lobule
renal fibrocystic: osteosis
renal papillary: necrosis
renal portal: system
renal-splanchnic: steal
renal-splenic venous: shunt
renal tubular: acidosis
Renaut: body
Rendu-Osler-Weber: syndrome
reniform: pelvis
renin-angiotensin: system
renin-angiotensin-aldosterone: system
renovascular: hypertension
Renpenning's: syndrome
Renshaw: cells
REO: virus
reovirus-like: agent
repair: enzyme
reparative: dentin
reparative giant cell: granuloma
reperfusion: injury
repetition: rate; time
repetition-compulsion: principle
repetitive: DNA
replacement: bone; fibrosis; therapy
replica: plating

replication: site
replicative: form; intermediate
reportable: disease
repressible: enzyme
repressor: gene
reproductive: assimilation; cycle; nucleus; system
required arch: length
resectoscope: sheath
reserve: air; force
reserve tooth: germ
reservoir: bag; host
resident: physician
residual: abscess; affinity; air; body; body of Regaud; capacity; cleft; cyst; error; inhibition; inhibitor; lumen; ridge; schizophrenia; urine; volume
residual ovary: syndrome
resin: cement
resistance: factors; form; plasmids; pyrometer; thermometer
resistance-inducing: factor
resistance-transfer: factor
resistance-transferring: episomes
resistant ovary: syndrome
resistive: movement
resolution: acuity
resolving: power
resonance: theory of hearing
resonant: frequency
resorcinol: test
resorption: atelectasis; lacunae
respirable: aerosols
respiration: rate
respirator: brain
respiratory: acidosis; airway; alkalosis; apparatus; arrhythmia; ataxia; bronchioles; burst; capacity; center; chain; coefficient; enzyme; epithelium; frequency; hippus; inhibitor; insufficiency; lobule; metabolism; metal; mucosa; murmur; pause; pigments; poison; pulse; quotient; region of tunica mucosa of nose; scleroma; sound; system; tract
respiratory dead: space
respiratory distress: syndrome of the newborn
respiratory enteric orphan: virus
respiratory exchange: ratio
respiratory minute: volume
respiratory syncytial: virus
respondent: behavior; conditioning
response: hierarchy
response-produced: cues

rest: area; bite; body; nitrogen; pain; position; relation; seat
restiform: body; eminence
resting: cell; length; saliva; stage; tremor
resting tidal: volume
resting wandering: cell
rest jaw: relation
restless: legs
restless legs: syndrome
restorative: dentistry
restorative dental: materials
restored: cycle
restrained: beam
restriction: endonuclease; enzyme; map; methylation; site
restriction fragment length: polymorphism
restriction length: polymorphism
restriction-site: polymorphism
restrictive: cardiomyopathy
restructured: cell
rest vertical: dimension
retained: menstruation; placenta
retarded: dentition
rete: cords; cyst of ovary; pegs; ridges
retention: area; cyst; form; groove; jaundice; point; polyp; suture; vomiting
retentive: arm
retentive circumferential clasp: arm
retentive fulcrum: line
reticular: cartilage; cell; degeneration; dystrophy of cornea; fibers; formation; lamina; layer of corium; membrane; nuclei of the brainstem; nucleus of thalamus; substance; tissue
reticular activating: system
reticular erythematous: mucinosis
reticularis: cell
reticulated: bone; corpuscle
reticuloendothelial: cell; system
reticulohistiocytic: granuloma
reticulonodular: pattern
reticulospinal: tract
reticulum cell: sarcoma
retinal: adaptation; blood vessels; camera; cones; detachment; disparity; dysplasia; embolism; fold; image
retinal anlage: tumor
retinol-binding: protein
retractile: testis
retraction: syndrome
retroactive: inhibition

retroadductor: space
retroauricular: lymph nodes
retrobulbar: abscess; anesthesia; neuritis
retrocaval: ureter
retrocecal: abscess; lymph nodes; recess
retrocedent: gout
retrocochlear: deafness
retrocollic: spasm
retrocuspid: papilla
retroduodenal: artery; fossa; recess
retroflex: fasciculus
retrogasserian: neurectomy; neurotomy
retrograde: amnesia; aortography; beat; block; cardioplegia; chromatolysis; conduction; degeneration; embolism; hernia; intussusception; memory; menstruation; metamorphosis; pyelography; urography
retrograde P: wave
retrohyoid: bursa
retroiliac: ureter
retroinguinal: space
retrolental: fibroplasia
retrolenticular: limb of internal capsule; part of internal capsule
retromammary: mastitis
retromandibular: fossa; process of parotid gland; vein
retromolar: fossa; pad
retromylohyoid: space
retroperitoneal: fibrosis; hernia; space
retropharyngeal: abscess; lymph nodes; space
retropubic: hernia; space
retropyloric: lymph nodes; nodes
retrospective: falsification
retrosternal: hernia; space
retrotarsal: fold
retroviral: vector
retrusive: excursion; occlusion
Rett's: syndrome
return: extrasystole
returning: cycle
Retzius': cavity; fibers; foramen; gyrus; ligament; space; striae; veins
Reuss': formula; test
Reuss' color: tables
reverberating: circuit
Reverdin: graft
Reverdin's: method
reverse: banding; bevel; curve; genetics; mutation; osmosis; transcriptase; transcription

reversed: anaphylaxis; coarctation; peristalsis; shunt
reversed paradoxical: pulse
reversed passive: anaphylaxis
reversed phase: chromatography
reversed Prausnitz-Küstner: reaction
reversed reciprocal: rhythm
reversed-three: sign
reverse Eck: fistula
reverse Kingsley: splint
reverse passive: hemagglutination
reverse Trendelenburg: position
reversible: calcinosis; colloid; decortication; hydrocolloid; pulpitis; reaction; shock
Revilliod's: sign
Reye's: syndrome
Reynolds: number; pentad
Rh: antigens; factor
rhabditiform: larva
rhagiocrine: cell
Rh blocking: test
$Rh_o(D)$: immunoglobulin
$RH_o(D)$ immune: globulin
rhegmatogenous retinal: detachment
Rheinberg: microscope
Rhese: projection
Rhesus: factor
rhesus: disease
rheumatic: arteritis; carditis; chorea; disease; endocarditis; fever; pericarditis; pneumonia; tetany; torticollis; valvulitis
rheumatic heart: disease
rheumatoid: arteritis; arthritis; disease; factors; nodules; spondylitis
rhinal: fissure; sulcus
Rh null: syndrome
rho: factor
Rhodesian: trypanosomiasis
Rhodesian malignant: theileriosis
rhombencephalic: isthmus; tegmentum
rhombencephalic gustatory: nucleus
rhombic: grooves; lip
rhomboid: fossa; impression; ligament
rhomboidal: sinus
rhomboideus major: muscle
rhomboid minor: muscle
rhonchal: fremitus
rhus: dermatitis
Rhus toxicodendron: antigen
Rhus venenata: antigen
rhythm: method

rhythmic: chorea
rib: spreader
Ribas-Torres: disease
Ribbert's: theory
ribbon: arch
ribbon arch: appliance
Ribes': ganglion
riboflavin: deficiency; unit
ribosomal: RNA
ribosome-lamella: complex
Riccò's: law
rice: body; diet; disease; itch
rice-field: fever
rice-Tween: agar
rice-water: stool
Richard's: fringes
Richards-Rundle: syndrome
Richter-Monro: line
Richter's: hernia; syndrome
rickettsia: vaccine,
   attenuated
Rickles: test
Rida: virus
Rideal-Walker: coefficient;
   method
Ridell's: operation
rider's: bone; bursa; leg;
   muscles
ridge: extension; relation;
   resorption
riding: embolism
Ridley's: circle; sinus
Riedel's: disease; lobe;
   struma; thyroiditis
Rieder: cells
Rieder cell: leukemia
Rieder's: lymphocyte
Riegel's: pulse
Rieger's: anomaly; syndrome
Riehl's: melanosis
Rift Valley: fever
Rift Valley fever: virus
Riga-Fede: disease
right: atrium of heart; border
   of heart; branch; branch of
   portal vein; branch of
   proper hepatic artery; crus
   of atrioventricular bundle;
   crus of diaphragm; duct of
   caudate lobe; heart; lobe;
   lobe of liver; margin of
   heart; part of
   diaphragmatic surface of
   liver; ventricle
right angle: clamp
right atrioventricular: valve
right auricular: appendage
right axis: deviation
right colic: artery; flexure;
   lymph nodes; vein
right coronary: artery
right fibrous: trigone
right gastric: artery; lymph
   nodes; vein
right gastroepiploic: artery;
   lymph nodes; vein
right gastroomental: vein

right gastro-omental: artery;
   lymph nodes
right heart: bypass
right hepatic: artery; duct;
   veins
right inferior pulmonary:
   vein
righting: reflexes
right or left lateral
   decubitus: film
right lumbar: lymph nodes
right lymphatic: duct
right main: bronchus
right ovarian: vein
right ovarian vein:
   syndrome
right parasternal: impulses
right pulmonary: artery
right sagittal: fissure
right splicing: junction
right superior intercostal:
   vein
right superior pulmonary:
   vein
right suprarenal: vein
right testicular: vein
right-to-left: shunt
right triangular: ligament
right ventricular: failure;
   hypoplasia
rigid: dysarthria
Riley-Day: syndrome
Rimini's: test
rinderpest: virus
Rindfleisch's: cells; folds
ring: abscess; chromosome;
   compound; enhancement;
   finger; ligament; pessary;
   scotoma; syringe; test;
   ulcer of cornea
ringed: hair
Ringer's: injection; solution
ring-like corneal: dystrophy
ring precipitin: test
ring-wall: lesion
ringworm: yaws
Rinne's: test
Riolan's: anastomosis; arc;
   arcades; bones; bouquet;
   muscle
Ripault's: sign
ripe: cataract
rise: time
risk: factor
Risley's rotary: prism
risorius: muscle
Ritgen's: maneuver
Rittenhouse-Manogian:
   procedure
Ritter-Rollet: phenomenon
Ritter's: law
Ritter's opening: tetanus
ritualistic: behavior
Riva-Rocci:
   sphygmomanometer
river: blindness
Rivero-Carvallo: effect
Rivers': cocktail

Rivière's: salt
Rivinus': canals; ducts;
   gland; incisure; membrane;
   notch
RNA: enzyme; virus
RNA tumor: viruses
Roach: clasp
Roaf's: syndrome
Roberts: syndrome
Robert's: pelvis
Robertshaw: tube
Robertson: pupil
robertsonian: translocation
Robinow: dwarfism
Robinow's: syndrome
Robin's: syndrome
Robinson: catheter; index
Robinson's: disease
Robison: ester
Robison-Embden: ester
Robison ester:
   dehydrogenase
ROC: curve
Rochelle: salt
Rocher's: sign
rocket:
   immunoelectrophoresis
Rocky Mountain spotted:
   fever
Rocky Mountain spotted
   fever: vaccine
rod: cell of retina; disks;
   fiber; granule;
   monochromatism;
   myopathy; vision
rodent: ulcer
rod nuclear: cell
roentgen: ray; unit
Roesler-Bressler: infarct
Roger-Anderson pin
   fixation: appliance
Rogers': sphygmomanometer
Roger's: bruit; disease;
   murmur; reflex
Röhrer's: index
Rohr's: stria
Rokitansky-Aschoff: sinuses
Rokitansky-Küster-Hauser:
   syndrome
Rokitansky's: disease;
   hernia; pelvis
Rolandic: artery
rolandic: epilepsy
Rolando's: angle; area; cells;
   column; tubercle
Rolando's gelatinous:
   substance
role: conflict
roll: sulfur; tube
roller: bandage
Roller's: nucleus
Rolleston's: rule
Rollet's: stroma
rolling: circle
roll-tube: culture
Roman: fever
Romaña's: sign
Romano-Ward: syndrome

Romanowsky's blood: stain
Romberg: test
Romberg-Howship:
   symptom
Romberg's: disease; sign;
   symptom; syndrome;
   trophoneurosis
Römer's: test
Rónne's nasal: step
R-on-T: phenomenon
roof: nucleus; plate
room: temperature
root: abscess; amputation;
   apex; avulsion; canal of
   tooth; caries; dehiscence;
   filaments; foramen;
   resection; resorption;
   sheath; tip
root canal: file; orifice;
   plugger; restoration;
   spreader; therapy;
   treatment
root caries: index
root end: cyst; granuloma
rooting: reflex
rope: burn; flap
Ropes: test
Rorschach: test
rosacea-like: tuberculid
Rosai-Dorman: disease
rosanilin: dyes
Roscoe-Bunsen: law
rose: cold; spots
rose bengal radioactive
   (^{131}I): test
Rose-Bradford: kidney
rose cephalic: tetanus
Rosenbach-Gmelin: test
Rosenbach's: disease; law;
   sign; test
Rosenmüller's: fossa; gland;
   node; recess; valve
Rosenthal: fiber
Rosenthaler-Turk: reagent
Rosenthal's: canal; vein
Roser-Nélaton: line
Rose's: position
Rose's cephalic: tetanus
rosette: test
rosette-forming: cells
Rose-Waaler: test
Ross: cycle
Ross-Jones: test
Rossolimo's: reflex; sign
Ross River: fever; virus
rostral: lamina; layer;
   neuropore
rostral transtentorial:
   herniation
rostrate: pelvis
rotary: joint
rotating: anode
rotating anode: tube
rotation: flap; therapy
rotational: axis; nystagmus
rotator: cuff of shoulder;
   muscles
rotatores: muscles

rotatores cervicis: muscles
rotatores lumborum: muscles
rotatores thoracis: muscles
rotatory: nystagmus; spasm; tic
Rotch's: sign
rote: learning
Roth-Bernhardt: disease
Rothera's nitroprusside: test
Rothmund's: syndrome
Rothmund-Thomson: syndrome
Roth's: disease; spots
Rotor's: syndrome
Rouget: cell
Rouget-Neumann: sheath
Rouget's: bulb; muscle
rough: colony; line
rough-surfaced endoplasmic: reticulum
Roughton-Scholander: apparatus; syringe
Rougnon-Heberden: disease
rouleaux: formation
round: atelectasis; bur; eminence; fasciculus; foramen; heart; ligament of elbow joint; ligament of femur; ligament of liver; ligament of uterus; pelvis; window
round cell: sarcoma
round heart: disease
round pronator: muscle
Rous: sarcoma; tumor
Rous-associated: virus
Rous sarcoma: virus
Roussy-Lévy: disease; syndrome
Roux: spatula
Roux-en-Y: anastomosis; operation
Roux's: method; stain
Rovsing's: sign
Rowntree and Geraghty: test
royal: touch
RPR: test
R-R: interval
Rs: virus
RST: segment
Rubarth's: disease
Rubarth's disease: virus
rubber: dam; pelvis; tissue
rubber-bulb: syringe
rubber dam: clamp
rubber dam clamp: forceps
rubber shod: clamp
rubbing: alcohol
rubella: cataract; retinopathy; virus
rubella HI: test
rubella virus: vaccine, live
rubeola: virus
Rubin: test
Rubinstein-Taybi: syndrome

Rubner's: laws of growth; test
rubrobulbar: tract
rubroreticular: fasciculi; tract
rubrospinal: decussation; tract
ruby: spots
Rud's: syndrome
Ruffini's: corpuscles
rufous: albinism
rugal: columns of vagina
rugger jersey: vertebra
Ruhemann's: purple
rum: nose
rumination: disorder
Rummel: tourniquet
Rumpel-Leede: phenomenon; sign; test
runaway: pacemaker
Runeberg's: formula
running: time
runt: disease
runting: syndrome
rupial: syphilid
ruptured: aneurysm; disk
rural cutaneous: leishmaniasis
Rushton: bodies
Russell: bodies; effect; traction
Russell's: sign; syndrome; viper
Russell's viper: venom
Russell's viper venom clotting: time
Russian: fly; influenza
Russian autumn: encephalitis
Russian autumn encephalitis: virus
Russian spring-summer: encephalitis (Eastern subtype); encephalitis (Western subtype)
Russian spring-summer encephalitis: virus
Russian tick-borne: encephalitis
Rust's: disease; phenomenon
rusty: sputum
Ruysch's: membrane; muscle; tube; veins
Rye: classification
Ryle's: tube

S

σ: factor
S: antigen; factor; peptide; phase; potential; protein; sign of Golden; unit of streptomycin; wave
S_7: gallop
S-A: node
saber: shin; tibia
saber-sheath: trachea
Sabin: vaccine

Sabin-Feldman dye: test
sabot: heart
Sabouraud-Noiré: instrument
Sabouraud's: agar; pastils
Sabouraud's dextrose: agar
saccadic: movement
sacciform: recess
saccular: aneurysm; bronchiectasis; gland; nerve; spot
sacculated: pleurisy
Sachs': bacillus
Sachs-Georgi: test
sacral: anesthesia; canal; cornua; crest; flexure; flexure of rectum; foramen; ganglia; hiatus; horns; index; lymph nodes; nerves; part of spinal cord; plexus; promontory; region; triangle; tuberosity; veins; vertebrae
sacral splanchnic: nerves
sacral venous: plexus
sacred: bone
sacroanterior: position
sacrococcygeal: disc; joint; junction; teratoma
sacrodural: ligament
sacrogenital: folds
sacroiliac: articulation; joint
sacropelvic: surface of ilium
sacroposterior: position
sacrosciatic: notch
sacrospinous: ligament
sacrotransverse: position
sacrotuberous: ligament
sacrouterine: fold
sacrovaginal: fold
sacrovesical: fold
saddle: anesthesia; back; embolism; head; joint; nose
saddle block: anesthesia
sadomasochistic: relationship
Saemisch's: section; ulcer
Saenger's: macula; operation; sign
Saethre-Chotzen: syndrome
safe: sex
safety: lens; spectacles
sagittal: axis; border of parietal bone; crest; fontanel; groove; line; plane; section; sulcus; suture; synostosis
sagittal split mandibular: osteotomy
sago: spleen
Saigon: cinnamon
sail: sound
sailor's: skin
Saint Anthony's: dance
Saint Ignatius': itch
Saint's: triad
Sakaguchi: reaction
Sakati-Nyhan: syndrome

Sakurai-Lisch: nodule
sakushu: fever
salaam: attack; convulsions; spasm
Salah's sternal puncture: needle
salicylic acid: collodion
saline: agglutinin; purgative; solution; water
Salinem: fever; infection
Salisbury common cold: viruses
saliva: ejector; pump
salivary: calculus; colic; corpuscle; digestion; duct; fistula; gland; virus
salivary gland: disease; hormone; virus
salivary gland virus: disease
Salk: vaccine
Salla: disease
salmon: disease; patch; poisoning
Salmonella food: poisoning
salpingopalatine: fold
salpingopharyngeal: fold; muscle
salpingopharyngeus: muscle
salt: action; bridge; depletion; dye; edema; fever; loading; poisoning; sensitivity; solution; wasting
saltatory: chorea; conduction; evolution; spasm
salt-depletion: crisis
salt depletion: syndrome
salted: plasma; serum
Salter-Harris: classification of epiphysial plate injuries
Salter's incremental: lines
salt-losing: defect; nephritis; syndrome
saltpeter: paper
salt water: boils; soap
salvage: chemotherapy; cystectomy; pathway
Salzmann's nodular corneal: degeneration
Samter's: syndrome
Sanarelli: phenomenon
Sanarelli-Shwartzman: phenomenon
Sanchez Salorio: syndrome
sand: bath; bodies; tumor
sandal: foot
sandal strap: dermatitis
sandfly: fever
sandfly fever: viruses
Sandhoff's: disease
Sandison-Clark: chamber
sandpaper: disks; gallbladder
Sandström's: bodies
sandworm: disease
Sanfilippo's: syndrome
Sanger: method

Sanger's: reagent
sanguineous: cyst
sanious: pus
San Joaquin: fever
San Joaquin Valley: disease; fever
San Miguel sea lion: virus
Sansom's: sign
Sanson's: images
Santini's booming: sound
Santorini's: canal; cartilage; concha; duct; fissures; incisures; labyrinth; muscle; plexus; tubercle; vein
Santorini's major: caruncle
Santorini's minor: caruncle
Sao Paulo: typhus
São Paulo: fever
saphenous: branch of descending genicular artery; hiatus; nerve; opening; veins
saponification: number
Sappey's: fibers; plexus; veins
sarcogenic: cell
sarcoidal: granuloma
sarcomatoid: carcinoma
sarcoplasmic: reticulum
sarcoptic: acariasis; mange
sartorius: bursae; muscle
satellite: abscess; cells; cell of skeletal muscle; DNA; metastasis
satellite-rich: heterochromatin
satiety: center
Sattler's: veil
Sattler's elastic: layer
saturated: color; fat; fatty acid; hydrocarbon; solution
saturation: analysis; index
saturnine: colic; encephalopathy; gout; tremor
saucer-shaped: cataract
Saundby's: test
sausage: fingers
Savage: syndrome
Savage's perineal: body
Savary: bougies
Sayre's: jacket
Sayre's suspension: apparatus; traction
S-BP: line
scabbard: trachea
scabby: mouth
scaffold-associated: regions
scalar: electrocardiogram
scalded skin: syndrome
scalene: hiatus; tubercle; tubercle of Lisfranc
scalenus anterior: muscle; syndrome
scalenus medius: muscle
scalenus minimus: muscle
scalenus posterior: muscle

scalp: contusion; hair; infection; laceration; muscle
scalpriform: incisors
scaly: leg; ringworm; tetter
scamping: speech
scanning: speech
scanning electron: microscope
scanning equalization: radiography
Scanzoni's: maneuver
Scanzoni's second: os
scaphoid: abdomen; bone; fossa; fossa of sphenoid bone; scapula; tuberosity
scapular: line; notch; reflex; region
scapulocostal: syndrome
scapulohumeral: atrophy; reflex
scapulohumeral muscular: dystrophy
scapuloperiosteal: reflex
scar: cancer; cancer of the lungs; carcinoma
Scardino vertical flap: pyeloplasty
scarf: bandage
scarification: test
scarlatinal: nephritis
scarlatiniform: erythema
scarlet: fever
scarlet fever: antitoxin
scarlet fever erythrogenic: toxin
Scarpa's: fascia; fluid; foramina; ganglion; habenula; hiatus; liquor; membrane; method; sheath; staphyloma; triangle
scarring: alopecia
Scatchard: plot
scattered: radiation
scavenger: cell
scent: glands
Schacher's: ganglion
Schaeffer-Fulton: stain
Schaer's: reagent
Schäfer's: method
Schaffer's: test
Schäffer's: reflex
Schamberg's: dermatitis
Schanz: syndrome
Schapiro's: sign
Schardinger: dextrins; enzyme; reaction
Schatzki's: ring
Schaudinn's: fixative
Schaumann: bodies
Schaumann's: lymphogranuloma; syndrome
Schauta vaginal: operation
Schede's: clot; method
scheduled: drug
Scheele's: green
Scheibe's: deafness

Scheibler's: reagent
Scheie's: syndrome
Scheiner's: experiment
Schellong: test
Schellong-Strisower: phenomenon
schematic: eye
Schenck's: disease
Scheuermann's: disease
Schick: method; test
Schick test: toxin
Schiff: base
Schiff's: reagent
Schiff-Sherrington: phenomenon
Schilder's: disease
Schiller's: test
Schilling: test
Schilling's: blood count; index
Schilling's band: cell
Schilling type of monocytic: leukemia
Schindler: disease
schindyletic: joint
Schiötz: tonometer
Schirmer: test
schistosomal: dermatitis
schistosome: granuloma
schizencephalic: microcephaly
schizo-affective: psychosis
schizoid: personality
schizophreniform: disorder
schizotypical: personality
Schlatter's: disease
Schlemm's: canal
Schlesinger's: sign
schlieren: optics
Schmidel's: anastomoses
Schmid-Fraccaro: syndrome
Schmidt: diet
Schmidt-Lanterman: clefts; incisures
Schmidt's: syndrome
Schmidt-Strassburger: diet
Schmidt-Thannhauser: method
Schmorl's: bacillus; jaundice; nodule
Schmorl's ferric-ferricyanide reduction: stain
Schmorl's picrothionin: stain
schneiderian: membrane
schneiderian first rank: symptoms
Schneider's: carmine
Schneider's first rank: symptoms
Scholander: apparatus
Scholz': disease
Schönbein's: operation; test
Schönlein-Henoch: syndrome
Schönlein's: disease; purpura
school: nurse; phobia

Schott: treatment
Schottmueller's: bacillus; disease
Schreger's: lines
Schridde's cancer: hairs
Schroeder's: operation
Schuchardt's: operation
Schüffner's: dots; granules
Schüller's: disease; ducts; phenomenon; syndrome
Schultz: reaction; stain
Schultz-Charlton: phenomenon; reaction
Schultz-Dale: reaction
Schultze's: cells; fold; mechanism; membrane; phantom; placenta; sign
Schütz: rule
Schütz': bundle; law
Schwabach: test
Schwalbe's: corpuscle; nucleus; ring; spaces
Schwann: cells
Schwann cell: unit
Schwann's white: substance
Schwartz: syndrome; tractotomy
Schweninger-Buzzi: anetoderma
Schweninger's: method
sciatic: foramen; hernia; nerve; neuralgia; neuritis; plexus; scoliosis; spine
scimitar: sign
scintigraphic: angiography
scintillating: scotoma
scintillation: camera; counter
scirrhous: carcinoma
scissor: gait
scleral: ectasia; resection; rigidity; ring; roll; spur; staphyloma; sulcus; veins
scleral buckling: operation
sclerocorneal: junction
sclerocystic: disease of the ovary
sclerosing: adenosis; agent; hemangioma; inflammation; keratitis; leukoencephalitis; mastoiditis; osteitis; therapy
sclerotic: bodies; coat; dentin; gastritis; kidney; stomach; teeth
sclerotic cemental: mass
scoliotic: pelvis
scombroid: poisoning
scorbutic: anemia
Scotch: cramp
scotopic: adaptation; eye; perimetry; vision
Scott: operation
Scott-Wilson: reagent
scout: film; radiograph
scratch: reflex in dogs; test
screen: defense; memory
screening: audiometry; test

WordFinder

screw: arteries; elevator; joint
screwdriver: teeth
Scribner: shunt
scrivener's: palsy
scrofulous: keratitis; rhinitis
scroll: bones; ear
scrotal: arteries; hernia; raphe; septum; swelling; tongue; veins
scrub: nurse; typhus
Scultetus': bandage; position
scurvy: rickets
sea: scurvy; sickness
sea-blue: histiocyte
sea-blue histiocyte: disease
sea gull: murmur
seal: fingers
sealed jar: technique
seal-fin: deformity
seamstress's: cramp
Seashore: test
seasonal affective: disorder
sea urchin: granuloma
sebaceous: adenoma; cyst; epithelioma; follicles; glands; horn; tubercle
Sebileau's: hollow; muscle
seborrheic: blepharitis; blepharoconjunctivitis; dermatitis; dermatosis; eczema; keratosis; verruca; wart
Seckel: dwarfism; syndrome
seclusion of: pupil
second: finger; incisor; law of thermodynamics; messenger; molar; sight; sound; tooth
secondarily generalized tonic-clonic: seizure
secondary: adhesion; aerodontalgia; agammaglobulinemia; alcohol; aldosteronism; amenorrhea; amputation; amyloidosis; anesthetic; atelectasis; axis; buffer; calcium phosphate; carcinoma; cardiomyopathy; caries; cataract; cementum; center of ossification; choana; coccidioidomycosis; constriction; degeneration; dementia; dentin; dentition; deviation; dextrocardia; digestion; disease; drives; drowning; dysmenorrhea; elaboration; encephalitis; failure; fissure of cerebellum; follicle; gain; glaucoma; gout; hemochromatosis; hemorrhage; host; hydrocephalus; hyperparathyroidism; hypertension;

hyperthyroidism; hypogammaglobulinemia; hypogonadism; hypothyroidism; immunodeficiency; infection; lysosomes; megaureter; mesoderm; metabolism; metabolite; methemoglobinemia; narcissism; nodule; nondisjunction; oocyte; palate; pellagra; point of ossification; process; proteose; pyoderma; radiation; rays; reinforcement; retinitis; saturation; screw-worm; spermatocyte; structure; suture; syphilid; syphilis; telangiectasia; thrombus; tuberculosis; union; villus; vitreous
secondary abdominal: pregnancy
secondary adrenocortical: insufficiency
secondary antibody: deficiency
secondary aortic: area
secondary egg: membrane
secondary generalized: epilepsy
secondary immune: response
secondary interatrial: foramen
secondary medical: care
secondary myeloid: metaplasia
secondary pulmonary: lobule
secondary refractory: anemia
secondary renal: calculus
secondary renal tubular: acidosis
secondary sensory: cortex; nuclei
secondary sex: characters
secondary spiral: lamina; plate
secondary tympanic: membrane
secondary visual: area; cortex
secondary X: zone
second cranial: nerve
second cuneiform: bone
second degree: burn
second degree A-V: block
second gas: effect
second heart: sound
second-look: operation
second-order: conditioning
second parallel pelvic: plane
second set: rejection
second signaling: system

second temporal: convolution
second tibial: muscle
Secrétan's: syndrome
secretin: test
secretomotor: nerve
secretor: factor
secretory: canaliculus; carcinoma; component; cyst; duct; granule; immunoglobulin; immunoglobulin A; nerve; otitis media
sectional: impression; radiography
sector: iridectomy; scan
secular: equilibrium
sedimentary: cataract
sedimentation: coefficient; constant; rate; velocity
seed: corn
seedy: toe
Seeligmüller's: sign
seesaw: murmur; nystagmus
Seessel's: pocket; pouch
segmental: anesthesia; arteries of kidney; atelectasis; bronchus; fracture; glomerulonephritis; neuritis; plate; sphincter; tubule; zone
segmental alveolar: osteotomy
segmental demyelinating: polyneuropathy
segmentation: cavity; nucleus
segmented: cell; leukocyte; neutrophil
segmenting: body
segregation: analysis; ratio
Seidel's: scotoma; sign
Seidlitz: mixture
Seignette's: salt
Seiler's: cartilage
Seldinger: technique
selection: coefficient; pressure
selective: angiography; grinding; hypoaldosteronism; immunoglobulin A deficiency; inattention; inhibition; injection; medium; memory; reduction; stain
selenium: poisoning
self: concept
self-curing: resin
self-limited: disease
self-registering: thermometer
self-retaining: catheter
Selivanoff's: test
Sellick's: maneuver
Selters: water
semantic: aphasia
semi-: vegetarian

semicircular: canals; ducts; line; line of Douglas
semi-closed: anesthesia; circle
semiconservative: replication
semidirect: leads
semihorizontal: heart
semilente: insulin
semilunar: bone; cartilage; cusp; fascia; fasciculus; fibrocartilage; fold; fold of colon; ganglion; hiatus; line; notch; nucleus of Flechsig; valve
semilunar conjunctival: fold
semimembranosus: muscle; reflex
seminal: capsule; colliculus; duct; fluid; gland; granule; hillock; lake; vesicle
seminal vesical: cyst
seminiferous: epithelium; tubule
seminiferous tubule: dysgenesis
semi-open: anesthesia
semioval: center
semipermeable: membrane
semipolar: bond
semiprone: position
semispinal: muscle; muscle of head; muscle of neck; muscle of thorax
semispinalis: muscle
semispinalis capitis: muscle
semispinalis cervicis: muscle
semispinalis thoracis: muscle
semisulfur: mustard
semitendinosus: muscle
semivertical: heart
Semon-Hering: theory
Semon's: law
Semple: vaccine
Sendai: virus
Senear-Usher: disease; syndrome
Seneca: snakeroot
senegal: gum
Sengstaken-Blakemore: tube
senile: amyloidosis; arteriosclerosis; atrophoderma; atrophy; cataract; chorea; degeneration; delirium; dementia; deterioration; dwarfism; ectasia; emphysema; fibroma; gangrene; halo; hemangioma; involution; keratoderma; keratoma; keratosis; lentigo; melanoderma; memory; nephrosclerosis; osteomalacia; plaque;

psychosis; retinoschisis; tremor; vaginitis; wart
senile dental: caries
senile hip: disease
senile lenticular: myopia
senile sebaceous: hyperplasia
senior: synonym
Sennetsu: fever
Senning: operation
sensation: time
sense: organs; strand
sense of: identity
sensible: heat; perspiration; temperature
sensitivity training: group
sensitized: antigen; cell; culture
sensitizing: dose; injection; substance
sensorial: areas
sensorimotor: area; theory
sensorineural: deafness
sensory: amblyopia; amusia; aphasia; ataxia; cell; cortex; crossway; decussation of medulla oblongata; deprivation; epilepsy; ganglion; image; inattention; nerve; neuron; neuronopathy; nuclei; paralysis; receptors; root of ciliary ganglion; root of pterygopalatine ganglion; root of trigeminal nerve; tract; urgency
sensory precipitated: epilepsy
sensory speech: center
sentinel: animal; gland; pile; tag
sentinel loop: sign
sentinel spinous process: fracture
separating: medium; wire
separation: anxiety
separation anxiety: disorder
septal: area; artery; bone; branches; cartilage; cell; cusp of tricuspid valve; gingiva; lines
septate: hymen; mycelium; uterus; vagina
septic: abortion; endocarditis; fever; infarct; intoxication; phlebitis; pneumonia; retinitis; shock; wound
septicemic: abscess; plague
septomarginal: fasciculus; trabecula; tract
septo-optic: dysplasia
sequence: hypothesis; pulse
sequence-tagged: sites
sequence-tagged site (STS): map
sequential: analysis
sequential multichannel: autoanalyzer
sequestration: cyst; dermoid

Sergent's white: line
serial: extraction; film changer; passage; radiography; section
serine: carboxypeptidase; hydrolases
serine protease: inhibitors
serofibrinous: inflammation; pleurisy
serologic: pipette
seromucous: cells; gland
serous: atrophy; cell; coat; cyst; demilunes; diarrhea; gland; hemorrhage; inflammation; iritis; layer of peritoneum; ligament; membrane; meningitis; otitis; pericardium; pleurisy; retinitis; synovitis; tunic
serpent: ulcer of cornea
serpentine: aneurysm
serpiginous: choroidopathy; keratitis; ulcer
serpiginous corneal: ulcer
serrate: suture
serratus anterior: muscle
serratus posterior inferior: muscle
serratus posterior superior: muscle
Serres': angle; glands
Sertoli cell: tumor
Sertoli-cell-only: syndrome
Sertoli's: cells; columns
serum: accelerator; accident; agar; agglutinin; albumin; disease; eruption; hepatitis; nephritis; proteins; rash; reaction; shock; sickness; therapy
serum accelerator: globulin
serumal: calculus
serum hepatitis: virus
serum prothrombin conversion: accelerator
Servetus': circulation
sesamoid: bone; cartilage of larynx; cartilages of nose
sessile: hydatid; polyp
set of: idiotopes
seton: operation; wound
setting: expansion
setting sun: sign
seven-day: fever
seventh: sense
seventh cranial: nerve
severe combined: immunodeficiency
severe postanoxic: encephalopathy
Severinghaus: electrode
sewer: gas
sewing: spasm
sex: cell; chromatin; chromosomes; cords; determination; factor;

hormones; linkage; object; ratio; reversal; role; skin
sex chromosome: imbalance
sex hormone-binding: globulin
sex-influenced: inheritance
sex-limited: inheritance
sex-linked: character; inheritance; locus
sex steroid-binding: globulin
sexual: abuse; deviation; dimorphism; dwarfism; generation; gland; infantilism; instinct; intercourse; life; neurasthenia; perversion; potency; reproduction; selection
sexually transmitted: disease
Sézary: cell; erythroderma; syndrome
shadow: cells; corpuscle; nucleus; test
Shaffer-Hartmann: method
shaggy: aorta; chorion; pericardium
shagreen: patch; skin
shake: culture; test
shaking: palsy
shallow: breathing
sham: feeding; rage
sham-movement: vertigo
shank: bone
shared psychotic: disorder
sharp: spoon
Sharpey's: fibers
shave: biopsy
Shaver's: disease
shaving: cramp
shawl: muscle
shear: flow; rate; stress; thinning
shearing: edge
sheath: ligaments; process of sphenoid bone; rot
sheathed: artery
Sheehan's: syndrome
sheep: bots
sheep-pox: virus
shelf: procedure
shell: nail; shock
shellac: base
Shemin: cycle
Shenton's: line
Shepherd's: fracture
Sherman: unit
Sherman-Bourquin: unit of vitamin B_2
Sherman-Munsell: unit
Sherrington: phenomenon
Sherrington's: law
sherry: wine
Shibley's: sign
shifting: dullness; pacemaker
Shiga: bacillus
Shiga-Kruse: bacillus
shilling: scars

shimamushi: disease
shin: bone
shin bone: fever
Shine-Dalgarno: sequence
ship: beriberi; fever
Shipley-Hartford: scale
shipping: fever
shipping fever: virus
Shirodkar: operation
shirt-stud: abscess
shock: antigen; index; lung; therapy; treatment
shocking: dose
shock wave: lithotripsy
shoddy: fever
shoe: boil
Shone's: anomaly; complex; syndrome
shop: typhus
Shope: fibroma; papilloma
Shope fibroma: virus
Shope papilloma: virus
short: bone; chain; crus of incus; gyri of insula; head; head of biceps brachii muscle; head of biceps femoris muscle; process of malleus; root of ciliary ganglion; sight; vinculum
short abductor: muscle of thumb
short adductor: muscle
short-bowel: syndrome
short central: artery
short ciliary: nerve
shortening: reaction
short extensor: muscle of great toe; muscle of thumb; muscle of toes
short fibular: muscle
short flexor: muscle of great toe; muscle of little finger; muscle of little toe; muscle of thumb; muscle of toes
short gastric: arteries; veins
short incubation: hepatitis
short interspersed: elements
short levatores costarum: muscles
short palmar: muscle
short peroneal: muscle
short posterior ciliary: artery
short radial extensor: muscle of wrist
short saphenous: nerve; vein
short-term: memory
short-term exposure: limit
short TI inversion: recovery
short wave: diathermy
shotgun: prescription
shot-silk: phenomenon; reflex; retina
shotted: suture
shoulder: bursitis; girdle; joint; presentation
shoulder-girdle: syndrome
shoulder-hand: syndrome

Shrapnell's: membrane
Shulman's: syndrome
shunt: cyanosis
shut-in: personality
shuttle: vector
Shwachman: syndrome
Shwartzman: phenomenon; reaction
Shy-Drager: syndrome
SI: units
Siamese: twins
Siberian tick: typhus
sibilant: rale
sibling: rivalry
Sibson's: aponeurosis; fascia; groove; muscle
Sibson's aortic: vestibule
sicca: complex; syndrome
sick: headache; role
sick building: syndrome
sick euthyroid: syndrome
sickle: cell; flap; form; scotoma
sickle cell: anemia; crisis; dactylitis; disease; hemoglobin; retinopathy; test; trait
sickle cell C: disease
sickle cell-thalassemia: disease
sick sinus: syndrome
side: chain
side-chain: theory
sideroblastic: anemia
sideropenic: dysphagia
siderotic: cataract; nodules
Siegert's: sign
Siegle's: otoscope
sieve: bone; graft; plate
Siggaard-Andersen: nomogram
sight: blindness
sigma: effect; factor; peptide
sigmoid: arteries; colon; flexure; fossa; groove; kidney; lymph nodes; notch; sinus; sulcus; veins; volvulus
sigmoidovesical: fistula
sign: blindness
signal: node; void
signal recognition: particle
signal-to-noise: ratio
signet: ring
signet ring: cells
signet-ring cell: carcinoma
Signorelli's: sign
silastic: band
silent: allele; area; electrode; gallstones; gap; ischemia; mutant; mutation; period
silent myocardial: infarction
silhouette: sign of Felson
silica: granuloma
silicate: cement; restorations
silicone: implant
silicotic: granuloma
silo-filler's: disease; lung

silver: cell; cone; point; poisoning; stain
silver-ammoniacal silver: stain
silver-fork: deformity; fracture
silverized: catgut
Silverman-Lilly: pneumotachograph
silver protein: stain
Silver-Russell: dwarfism; syndrome
Silverskiöld's: syndrome
silver-tin: alloy
Simbu: virus
simian: crease; fissure; hand; malaria; virus; virus 40
simian hemorrhagic: fever
simian hemorrhagic fever: virus
simian vacuolating: virus No. 40
Simmonds': disease
Simmons' citrate: medium
Simonart's: bands; ligaments; threads
Simons': disease
Simon's: position; sign
simple: absence; anchorage; anisocoria; beam; color; conjunctivitis; crus of semicircular duct; diplopia; dislocation; epithelium; fission; fracture; glaucoma; goiter; heterochromia; hypertrophy; joint; lipids; lobule; lymphangiectasis; mastectomy; microscope; myopia; necrosis; obesity; protein; retinitis; schizophrenia; ulcer; urethritis
simple bone: cyst
simple-central: anisocoria
simple hyperopic: astigmatism
simple membranous: limb of semicircular duct
simple myopic: astigmatism
simple partial: seizure
simple pulmonary: eosinophilia
simple skull: fracture
simple squamous: epithelium
Simpson's: forceps
Simpson uterine: sound
Sims': position
Sims uterine: sound
simulated: hypertrophy
simultaneous: contrast; perception
sincipital: presentation
Sindbis: fever; virus
singer's: nodes; nodules
single: ascertainment; bond; immunodiffusion; ventricle

single (gel) diffusion precipitin: test in one dimension; test in two dimensions
single photon emission computed: tomography
single-strand: break
single-stranded nucleate: endonuclease
singlet: oxygen; state
sinoatrial: block; node
sinoatrial conduction: time
sinoatrial nodal: artery
sinoatrial recovery: time
sinoauricular: block
sinoventricular: conduction
sinuatrial: chamber; node
sinuatrial nodal: branch of right coronary artery
sinuatrial node: artery
sinus: arrest; arrhythmia; barotrauma; bradycardia; histiocytosis with massive lymphadenopathy; nerve of Hering; node; pause; phlebitis; reflex; rhythm; septum; standstill; tachycardia; tubercle
sinus node: artery
sinusoidal: capillary
sinus venosus: syndrome
sinuvertebral: nerves
Sipple's: syndrome
sippy: diet
SISI: test
sister chromatid: exchange
Sister Joseph's: nodule
Sistrunk: operation
site-directed: mutagenesis
site specific: mutation; recombination
in situ: hybridization
situation: anxiety
situational: psychosis; test
in situ nucleic acid: hybridization
sitz: bath
sixth: disease; sense; ventricle
sixth cranial: nerve
sixth venereal: disease
sixth-year: molar
Sjögren-Larsson: syndrome
Sjögren's: disease; syndrome
Sjöqvist: tractotomy
skein: cell
skeletal: extension; muscle; survey; system; traction
skeletal muscle: fibers; tissue
skeleton: hand
Skene's: glands; tubules
skew: deviation; distribution; form
Skillern's: fracture
skim: milk
skin: botflies; dose; flap; furrows; graft; grooves;

pore; reaction; reflexes; ridges; stones; tag; test; traction
skinbound: disease
skin-muscle: reflexes
Skinner: box
skinnerian: conditioning
skin-puncture: test
skin-pupillary: reflex
skip: areas
skipped: generation
Sklowsky: symptom
skodaic: resonance
Skoda's: rale; sign; tympany
skull: fracture
slab-off: lens
slaframine: toxicosis
slaked: lime
slant: culture
slaty: anemia
sleep: apnea; dissociation; drunkenness; epilepsy; paralysis; spindle
sleep apnea: syndrome
sleep-induced: apnea
sleeping: sickness
sleep phase delay: syndrome
sleep terror: disorder
sleeve: graft
SLE-like: syndrome
slender: fasciculus; lobule; process of malleus
slew: rate
slide: micrometer
sliding: flap; hernia; hook
sliding esophageal hiatal: hernia
sliding filament: hypothesis
sliding hiatal: hernia
sliding oblique: osteotomy
slime: fever
sling: psychrometer
slipped: hernia; tendon
slipped tendon: disease
slipping: patella; rib
slipping rib: cartilage
slit: lamp; pores
slit ventricle: syndrome
slope: culture
slotted: attachment
sloughing: phagedena; ulcer
slow: combustion; fever; virus
slow channel-blocking: agent
slow-reacting: factor of anaphylaxis; substance
slow virus: disease
SLR: factor
Sluder's: neuralgia
sludged: blood
sluggish: layer
slurring: speech
Sly: syndrome
Sm: antigen
small: arteries; bowel; calorie; canal of chorda tympani; intestine;

pancreas; pelvis; trochanter; vein
small bowel: enema; series
small cardiac: vein
small cell: carcinoma
small cleaved: cell
small deep petrosal: nerve
smaller: muscle of helix
smaller pectoral: muscle
smaller posterior rectus: muscle of head
smaller psoas: muscle
smallest cardiac: veins
smallest scalene: muscle
smallest splanchnic: nerve
small increment sensitivity: index
small increment sensitivity index: test
small interarch: distance
small lymphocytic: lymphoma
small nuclear: RNA
small plaque: parapsoriasis
smallpox: vaccine; virus
small pudendal: lip
small saphenous: vein
small sciatic: nerve
smear: culture
Smellie's: scissors
smelling: salts
smelter's: chills; fever; shakes
Smith-Boyce: operation
Smith-Indian: operation
Smith-Lemli-Opitz: syndrome
Smith-Petersen: nail
Smith-Riley: syndrome
Smith-Robinson: operation
Smith's: fracture; operation
smoker's: patches; tongue
smooth: broach; chorion; colony; diet; leprosy; muscle
smooth muscle: relaxant; tissue
smooth muscular: sphincter
smooth surface: caries
smooth-surfaced endoplasmic: reticulum
smudge: cells
S-N: line
S-N-A: angle
snail: fever
snap: finger
snapping: hip; reflex
S-N-B: angle
Sneddon's: syndrome
Sneddon-Wilkinson: disease
sneezing: gas
Snellen's: sign; test types
Snell's: law
sniff: test
snout: reflex
Snow: procedure
snow: blindness; conjunctivitis

snowball: opacity; sampling
snowman: abnormality
snowshoe hare: virus
snub-nose: dwarfism
S1 nuclease: mapping
Snyder's: test
soapsuds: enema
Soave: operation
social: adaptation; control; diseases; instinct; intelligence; maladjustment; medicine; psychiatry; therapy
socialized: medicine
social network: therapy
sociometric: distance
socket: joint
soda: loading
sodium: chromate Cr 51; iodide iodine-131; methylprednisolone succinate; pertechnetate; pump
sodium-potassium: pump
sodium-responsive periodic: paralysis
Soemmerring's: ganglion; ligament; muscle; spot
soft: cataract; chancre; corn; diet; palate; papilloma; parts; pulse; rays; soap; sore; sulfur; tubercle; ulcer; wart; water
soft tissue: window
Sohval-Soffer: syndrome
solar: blindness; cheilitis; dermatitis; elastosis; energy; fever; ganglia; keratosis; lentigo; maculopathy; plexus; retinopathy; therapy; treatment; urticaria
soldier's: heart; patches
sole: nuclei; reflex
soleal: line
sole-plate: ending
sole tap: reflex
soleus: muscle
solid: edema
solid phase: immunoassay
solid-state: detector
solitary: bundle; fasciculus; follicles; foramen; glands; nodules of intestine; tract
solitary bone: cyst
solitary fibrous: tumor
solitary lymphatic: follicles
solitary osteocartilaginous: exostosis
solubility: test
soluble: antigen; ferric phosphate; glass; ligature; RNA; soap; starch; tartar
soluble gun: cotton
soluble specific: substance
solution: pressure
solvent: drag; ether; inhalation

somatic: agglutinin; antigen; arteries; cells; crossing-over; death; delusion; layer; mesoderm; mitosis; mutation; nerve; nucleus; reproduction; swallow; teniasis
somatic cell: genetics; hybridization
somatic motor: neuron; nuclei
somatic mutation: theory of cancer
somatic sensory: cortex
somatization: disorder
somatoform: disorder; pain
somatosensory evoked: potential
somatotropic: hormone
somatotropin release-inhibiting: factor; hormone
somatotropin-releasing: factor; hormone
somesthetic: area; system
somite: cavity
somitic: mesoderm
somnambulic: epilepsy
somnambulistic: trance
Somogyi: effect; method; phenomenon; unit
Sondermann's: canal
Songo: fever
sonic: waves
Sonne: bacillus; dysentery
sonomotor: response
sonorous: rale
soot: wart
sorbitol: pathway
sore: mouth; shins; throat
soremouth: virus
Sörensen: scale
Soret: band
Soret's: phenomenon
Sorsby's: syndrome
Sorsby's macular: degeneration
SOS: genes; repair
Sotos': syndrome
soul: pain
soundex: code
sound pressure: level
South African tick-bite: fever
South African type: porphyria
South American: blastomycosis; trypanosomiasis
Southern blot: analysis
Southey's: tubes
space: maintainer; medicine; myopia; nerve; retainer; sense; sickness
space adaptation: syndrome
spaced: teeth
spade: fingers; hand
Spallanzani's: law
spallation: product

Spanish: influenza
sparing: action; phenomenon
spasmodic: asthma; dysmenorrhea; laryngitis; stricture; tic; torticollis
spasmophilic: diathesis
spastic: abasia; anemia; aphonia; colon; diplegia; dysarthria; dysphonia; ectropion; entropion; gait; hemiplegia; ileus; miosis; mydriasis; paraplegia; speech; syndrome in cattle
spastic flat: foot
spastic spinal: paralysis
spatial: acuity; formula; localization; vector; vectorcardiography
spatula: needle
special: anatomy; hospital; nurse; sensation; sense
specialized: transduction
special somatic afferent: column
special visceral efferent: column; nuclei
special visceral motor: nuclei
species: tolerance
species-specific: antigen
specific: absorbance; action; activity; anergy; antigens; antiserum; bactericide; cause; cholinesterase; compliance; disease; epithet; extinction; gravity; heat; hemolysin; immunity; opsonin; parasite; reaction; serum; therapy; transduction; urethritis
specific absorption: coefficient
specific active: immunity
specific capsular: substance
specific dynamic: action
specific immune: globulin (human)
specificity: constant
specific optical: rotation
specific passive: immunity
specific soluble: polysaccharide; sugar
speck: finger
spectacle: eyes; plane
spectral: phonocardiograph; sensitivity
specular: glare; image
speculum: forceps
speech: audiogram; audiometer; audiometry; bulb; centers; pathology
Spens': syndrome
sperm: aster; cell; crystal; nucleus
spermacytic: seminoma
spermatic: cord; duct; filament; fistula; plexus; vein

sphagnum: moss
sphenoethmoidal: recess; suture; synchondrosis
sphenofrontal: suture
sphenoid: angle; bone; crest; process; process of palatine bone; process of septal cartilage
sphenoidal: angle of parietal bone; border of temporal bone; conchae; fissure; fontanel; herniation; part of middle cerebral artery; ridges; sinus; spine
sphenoidal sinus: aperture
sphenoidal turbinated: bones
sphenomandibular: ligament
sphenomaxillary: fissure; fossa; suture
spheno-occipital: joint; suture; synchondrosis
spheno-orbital: suture
sphenopalatine: artery; foramen; ganglion; neuralgia; notch
sphenoparietal: sinus; suture
sphenopetrosal: fissure; synchondrosis
sphenosquamous: suture
sphenotic: center; foramen
sphenovomerine: suture
sphenozygomatic: suture
spherical: aberration; amalgam; lens; nucleus; recess
spherical form of: occlusion
spherocylindrical: lens
spherocytic: anemia; jaundice
spheroid: articulation; colony; joint
sphincter: muscle; muscle of common bile duct; muscle of pancreatic duct; muscle of pupil; muscle of pylorus; muscle of urethra; muscle of urinary bladder
sphincter of Oddi: dysfunction
sphincteroid: tract of ileum
sphingomyelin: lipidosis
sphygmic: interval
spica: bandage
spider: angioma; cancer; cell; finger; hemangioma; mole; nevus; pelvis; telangiectasia
Spiegelberg's: criteria
Spiegler-Fendt: pseudolymphoma; sarcoid
Spielmeyer's acute: swelling
Spielmeyer-Sjögren: disease
Spielmeyer-Stock: disease
Spielmeyer-Vogt: disease
spigelian: hernia
Spigelius': line; lobe

spike: potential
spike and wave: complex
spin: density; echo
spinach: stools
spinal: analgesia; anesthesia; anesthetic; apoplexy; arteries; ataxia; block; canal; column; concussion; cord; curvature; decompression; fusion; ganglion; headache; induction; instability; lemniscus; length; marrow; muscle; muscle of head; muscle of neck; muscle of thorax; nerves; nucleus of accessory nerve; nucleus of the trigeminus; paralysis; part of accessory nerve; part of arachnoid; point; puncture; pyramidotomy; quotient; reflex; root of accessory nerve; shock; sign; stroke; tap; tract; tractotomy; tract of trigeminal nerve; veins
spinal accessory: nerve
spinal cord: concussion
spinalis: muscle
spinalis capitis: muscle
spinalis cervicis: muscle
spinalis thoracis: muscle
spinal trigeminal: nucleus
spindle: cataract; cell; fiber
spindle cell: carcinoma; lipoma; nevus; sarcoma
spindle-celled: layer
spindle-shaped: muscle
spine: cell; sign
Spinelli: operation
spin-lattice: relaxation
spinning disk: nebulizer
spino-adductor: reflex
spinocerebellar: ataxia; tracts
spinocervicothalamic: tract
spinoglenoid: ligament
spino-olivary: tract
spinoreticular: fibers; tract
spinotectal: tract
spinothalamic: cordotomy; tract; tractotomy
spinous: layer; process; process of tibia
spin-spin: relaxation
spiral: artery; bandage; canal of cochlea; canal of modiolus; crest; CT; fold of cystic duct; fracture; ganglion of cochlea; groove; hyphae; joint; ligament of cochlea; line; membrane; organ; plate; prominence; septum; suture; tubule; valve of cystic duct; vein of modiolus
spiral bulbar: septum

spiral cochlear: ganglion
spiral computed: tomography
spiral foraminous: tract
spiral tip: catheter
spirillar: dysentery
spirillum: fever
spirit: lamp; thermometer
spirituous: liquor
spiro-: index
spirochetal: jaundice
spironolactone: test
spiruroid: larva migrans
Spitz: nevus
Spitzer's: theory
Spitzka's: nucleus
Spitzka's marginal: tract; zone
Spix's: spine
splanchnesthetic: sensibility
splanchnic: anesthesia; cavity; ganglion; layer; mesoderm; nerve; wall
spleen: deoxyribonuclease; endonuclease; phosphodiesterases
Splendore-Hoeppli: phenomenon
splenial: gyrus
splenic: anemia; apoplexy; artery; branches of splenic artery; cells; cords; corpuscles; flexure; index; leukemia; lymph nodes; plexus; pulp; recess; sinus; vein
splenic flexure: syndrome
splenic lymph: follicles; nodules
splenic portal: venography
splenius: muscle of head; muscle of neck
splenius capitis: muscle
splenius cervicis: muscle
splenogonadal: fusion
splenorenal: ligament; shunt
splint: bone
splinted: abutment
splinter: hemorrhages
splintered: fracture
split: brain; fat; genes; hand; papules; pelvis; tolerance
split cast: method; mounting
split renal function: test
split-skin: graft
split-thickness: flap; graft
splitting: enzymes
splitting of heart: sounds
split-virus: vaccine
Spondweni: virus
spondyloepiphysial: dysplasia
spondylolisthetic: pelvis
sponge: biopsy; tent
spongiform: encephalopathy; pustule of Kogoj
spongy: body of penis; bone; degeneration of infancy;

part of the male urethra; spot; substance; urethra
spontaneous: abortion; agglutination; amputation; combustion; correction of placenta previa; evolution; fracture; gangrene of newborn; generation; mutation; phagocytosis; pneumothorax; recovery; remission; version
spontaneous breech: extraction
spontaneous cephalic: delivery
spontaneous intermittent mandatory: ventilation
spoon: nail
sporadic bovine: encephalomyelitis; leukosis
sporotrichositic: chancre
sports: medicine
spot: film; test for infectious mononucleosis
spot-film: radiography
spotted: fever; sickness
spouse: abuse
sprain: fracture
spreading: depression; factor
Sprengel's: deformity
spring: conjunctivitis; finger; lancet; ligament; ophthalmia
spurious: ankylosis; cast; meningocele; pregnancy; torticollis
sputum: smear
squamocolumnar: junction
squamomastoid: suture
squamoparietal: suture
squamotympanic: fissure
squamous: border; border of parietal bone; border of sphenoid bone; cell; margin; metaplasia; metaplasia of amnion; part of frontal bone; part of occipital bone; part of temporal bone; pearl; suture
squamous alveolar: cells
squamous cell: carcinoma; hyperplasia
squamous odontogenic: tumor
square: matrix
square wave: stimuli
squint: hook
squinting: eye
squirrel: porphyria
squirrel plague: conjunctivitis
ST: junction
S-T: segment
stab: cell; culture; drain; neutrophil; wound
stabilized: baseplate

stabilizing circumferential clasp: arm
stabilizing fulcrum: line
stable: colloid; equilibrium; factor; fracture; isotope
staccato: speech
Stader: splint
Staderini's: nucleus
staff: cell
Stafne bone: cyst
staghorn: calculus
stagnant: anoxia; hypoxia
stagnation: mastitis
Stahl's: ear
staircase: phenomenon
stalked: hydatid
standard: atmosphere; bicarbonate; cell; deviation; pressure; score; solution; substance; temperature; volume
standard error of: difference
standard error of the: mean
standardized mortality: ratio
standard limb: lead
standard serologic: tests for syphilis
standard urea: clearance
standby pulse: generator
standing: test
standing plasma: test
Stanford-Binet intelligence: scale
Stanley's cervical: ligaments
Stanley Way: procedure
Stannius: ligature
stapedial: artery; branch of stylomastoid artery; fold; membrane
stapedius: muscle
stapes: mobilization
stapes mobilization: operation
staphylococcal: enterotoxin; pneumonia
staphylococcal scalded skin: syndrome
staphylococcus: antitoxin; vaccine
Staphylococcus food: poisoning
staphylo-opsonic: index
starch: equivalent; glycerite; gum; sugar
starch-iodine: test
Stargardt's: disease
Starling's: curve; hypothesis; law; reflex
Starr-Edwards: valve
start: codon
starter: tRNA
starting: friction
startle: epilepsy; reaction; reflex
starvation: acidosis; diabetes

stasis: cirrhosis; dermatitis; eczema; ulcer
Stas-Otto: method
state: hospital
state-dependent: learning
static: arthropathy; ataxia; compliance; friction; gangrene; hysteresis; infantilism; perimetry; reflexes; refraction; relations; scoliosis; sense; system; tremor
static bone: cyst
station: test
stationary: anchorage; cataract; phase
statistical: genetics; model; power
statoacoustic: nerve
statoconial: membrane
statokinetic: reflex
statotonic: reflexes
Staub-Traugott: effect; phenomenon
Stauffer's: syndrome
steady: state
steady-state: rate; velocity
steady state: approximation
steal: phenomenon
steam-fitter's: asthma
Stearns alcoholic: amentia
Steele-Richardson-Olszewski: disease; syndrome
Steell's: murmur
Steenbock: unit
steeple: skull
steering wheel: injury
Steinberg thumb: sign
Steinert's: disease
Stein-Leventhal: syndrome
Steinmann: pin
Stein's: test
stellate: abscess; block; cataract; cells of cerebral cortex; cells of liver; fracture; ganglion; hair; ligament; neuroretinitis; reticulum; veins; venules
stellate skull: fracture
Stellwag's: sign
stem: bronchus; cell
stem cell: leukemia
Stender: dish
Stenger: test
stenopeic: disk; iridectomy; spectacles
stenosal: murmur
stenoxous: parasite
Stensen's: duct; experiment; foramen; plexus; veins
Stent: graft
Stenvers: projection; view
steppage: gait
stepping: reflex
stercoraceous: vomiting
stercoral: abscess; appendicitis; ulcer

sterculia: gum
stereochemical: formula; isomerism
stereoscopic: acuity; microscope; parallax; vision
stereotactic: cordotomy; instrument; surgery
stereotaxic: localization
sterile: abscess; cyst
sterile insect: technique
sternal: angle; arteries; bar; branches of internal thoracic artery; cartilage; end of clavicle; extremity of clavicle; joints; line; membrane; muscle; notch; part of diaphragm; plane; puncture; synchondroses
sternal articular: surface of clavicle
sternalis: muscle
Sternberg: cells
Sternberg-Reed: cells
Sternberg's: sign
sternobrachial: reflex
sternochondral: separation
sternochondroscapular: muscle
sternoclavicular: angle; disk; joint; ligament; muscle
sternocleidomastoid: branch of occipital artery; branch of superior thyroid artery; muscle; region; vein
sternocostal: articulations; head of pectoralis major muscle; joints; part of pectoralis major muscle; surface of heart; triangle
sternocostalis: muscle
sternohyoid: muscle
sternomanubrial: junction
sternomastoid: artery; muscle
sternopericardial: ligament
sternothyroid: muscle
Stern's: posture
steroid: acne; diabetes; fever; hormones; nucleus; ulcer
steroid metabolic clearance: rate
steroidogenic: diabetes
steroid production: rate
steroid secretory: rate
steroid withdrawal: syndrome
stertorous: breathing; respiration
stethoscopic: phonocardiograph
Stevens-Johnson: syndrome
Stewart-Hamilton: method; principle
Stewart-Holmes: sign
Stewart-Morel: syndrome

Stewart's: test
Stewart-Treves: syndrome
stichochrome: cell
Sticker's: disease
Stickler's: syndrome
sticky-ended: DNA
Stieda's: process
Stierlin's: sign
stiff: neck; toe
stiff heart: syndrome
stiff lamb: disease
stiff-man: syndrome
stifle: bone; joint
Stiles-Crawford: effect
still: layer
stillbirth: rate
stillborn: infant
Still-Chauffard: syndrome
Stilling color: tables
Stilling's: canal; column; nucleus; raphe
Stilling's gelatinous: substance
Still's: disease; murmur
stimulatory: protein 1
stimulus: control; generalization; substitution; threshold
stimulus sensitive: myoclonus
stippled: epiphysis; tongue
Stirling's modification of Gram's: stain
stitch: abscess
St. Louis encephalitis: virus
Stobo: antigen
stochastic: independence; process
stock: culture; strain; vaccine
Stocker's: line
Stockholm: syndrome
stocking: anesthesia
Stoerk's: blennorrhea
Stoffel's: operation
stoichiometric: number
stoker's: cramps
Stokes: amputation
Stokes': law
Stokes-Adams: disease; syndrome
stomach: ache; drops; pump; reefing; tooth; tube
stomal: ulcer
stomatognathic: system
stone: basket; heart
stone-mason's: disease
Stookey-Scarff: operation
stop: codon
stop-: needle; speculum
storage: disease; oscilloscope
storiform: neurofibroma
Stout's: wiring
strabismic: amblyopia
straddling: embolism
straight: gyrus; jacket; part of cricothyroid muscle; sinus; tubule; venules of kidney

WordFinder

straight back: syndrome
straight seminiferous: tubule
strain: fracture; gauge
strangulated: hernia
strap: cell; muscles
Strassburg's: test
Strassman's: phenomenon
stratified: epithelium; sample; thrombus
stratified ciliated columnar: epithelium
stratified squamous: epithelium
stratiform: fibrocartilage
stratographic: analysis
Straus: reaction
Straus': sign
straw: itch
strawberry: birthmark; gallbladder; hemangioma; mark; nevus; tongue
streak: culture; gonad; hyperostosis
streaming: movement
street: drug; virus
Streeter's: bands
strength-duration: curve
streptococcal: empyema; fibrinolysin; lymphadenitis; pneumonia
streptococcus erythrogenic: toxin
Streptococcus M: antigen
streptomycin: units
stress: echocardiography; fibers; fracture; immunity; inoculation; reaction; test; ulcers
stress-bearing: area
stress-strain: curve
stress urinary: incontinence
stretch: marks; receptors; reflex
striate: area; atrophy of skin; body; cortex; keratopathy; veins
striated: border; duct; membrane; muscle
striated muscular: sphincter
striatonigral: fibers
string: sign; test
stringed instrument: theory
stringent: factor; response
strionigral: fibers
stripped: atom
stripper's: asthma
stroboscopic: disk; microscope
Stroganoff's: method
stroke: output; volume
stroke work: index
stroma: plexus
stromal: hyperthecosis
strong: silver protein
strong silver: protein
Strong vocational interest: test

Stroud's pectinated: area
structural: color; formula; gene; interface; isomerism; pleiotropy
structure: proteins
structured: noise
Strümpell-Marie: disease
Strümpell's: disease; phenomenon; reflex
Strümpell-Westphal: disease
struvite: calculus
Stryker: frame; saw
Stryker-Halbeisen: syndrome
Stuart: factor
stuck: finger
student: nurse
Student's *t*: test
stump: cancer; hallucination; neuralgia
stunned: myocardium
stuporous: catatonia
Sturge-Kalischer-Weber: syndrome
Sturge-Weber: disease; syndrome
Sturmdorf's: operation
Sturm's: conoid; interval
stuttering: urination
Stuttgart: disease
styloauricular: muscle
styloglossus: muscle
stylohyoid: branch of facial nerve; ligament; muscle
styloid: cornu; process of fibula; process of radius; process of temporal bone; process of third metacarpal bone; process of ulna; prominence
stylomandibular: ligament
stylomastoid: artery; foramen; vein
stylomaxillary: ligament
stylopharyngeal: muscle
stylopharyngeus: muscle
styloradial: reflex
stylus: tracing
"s"-type: cholinesterase
styptic: collodion; colloid; cotton
Stypven time: test
subacromial: bursa; bursitis
subacute: glomerulonephritis; hepatitis; inflammation; nephritis; rheumatism
subacute bacterial: endocarditis
subacute combined: degeneration of the spinal cord
subacute granulomatous: thyroiditis
subacute inclusion body: encephalitis

subacute lymphocyte: thyroiditis
subacute migratory: panniculitis
subacute necrotizing: encephalomyelopathy; myelitis
subacute sclerosing: leukoencephalitis; panencephalitis
subacute spongiform: encephalopathy
subadventitial: fibrosis
subanconeus: muscle
subaortic: lymph nodes; stenosis
subapical: segment
subarachnoid: anesthesia; cavity; hemorrhage; space
subarachnoidal: cisterns
subarcuate: fossa
subareolar duct: papillomatosis
subastragalar: amputation
subcallosal: area; fasciculus; gyrus
subcapital: fracture
subcapsular: cataract
subcecal: fossa
subceruleus: nucleus
subchorial: lake; space
subclavian: artery; duct; groove; loop; muscle; nerve; plexus; steal; sulcus; triangle; vein
subclavian lymphatic: trunk
subclavian periarterial: plexus
subclavian steal: syndrome
subclavius: muscle
subclinical: diabetes; seizure
subcommissural: organ
subconscious: memory; mind
subcoracoid: bursa
subcoracoid-pectoralis minor tendon: syndrome
subcorneal pustular: dermatitis; dermatosis
subcoronal: hypospadias
subcortical arteriosclerotic: encephalopathy
subcostal: artery; groove; line; muscle; nerve; plane
subcrepitant: rale
subcrestal: pocket
subcrural: muscle
subcutaneous: bursa of the laryngeal prominence; bursa of lateral malleolus; bursa of medial malleolus; bursa of tibial tuberosity; emphysema; flap; implantation; mastectomy; myiasis; operation; part of external anal sphincter; phycomycosis; portion of external anal sphincter; ring; tenotomy; tissue;

transfusion; veins of abdomen; wound
subcutaneous acromial: bursa
subcutaneous calcaneal: bursa
subcutaneous fat: necrosis of newborn
subcutaneous infrapatellar: bursa
subcutaneous olecranon: bursa
subcuticular: suture
subdeltoid: bursa; bursitis
subdiaphragmatic: abscess; pyopneumothorax
subdigastric: node
subdural: cavity; cleavage; cleft; hematoma; hematorrhachis; hemorrhage; hygroma; space
subendocardial: layer
subendocardial myocardial: infarction
subendothelial: layer
subependymal giant cell: astrocytoma
subepidermal: abscess
subfalcial: herniation
subfascial prepatellar: bursa
subfornical: organ
subgaleal: emphysema; hemorrhage
subgerminal: cavity
subgingival: calculus; curettage; space
subhepatic: abscess; recess
subhyoid: bursa
subinguinal: fossa; triangle
subjective: fremitus; insomnia; probability; psychology; sensation; sign; symptom; synonyms; vision
sublenticular: limb of internal capsule; part of internal capsule
subleukemic: leukemia
sublimed: sulfur
subliminal: self; stimulus; thirst
sublingual: artery; bursa; caruncula; crescent; cyst; fold; fossa; ganglion; gland; medication; nerve; pit; tablet; vein
submammary: mastitis
submandibular: duct; fossa; ganglion; gland; lymph nodes; triangle
submaxillary: duct; fossa; ganglion; gland; triangle
submental: artery; lymph nodes; triangle; vein
submental vertex: projection; radiograph; radiograph

submentovertex: radiograph
submentovertical: projection
submerged: tonsil
submetacentric: chromosome
submitochondrial: particles
submucosal: implant; plexus
subnasal: point
subneural: apparatus
suboccipital: decompression; muscles; nerve; neuralgia; neuritis; part of vertebral artery; region; triangle
suboccipital venous: plexus
suboccipitobregmatic: diameter
suboccluding: ligature
subocclusal: surface
subpapillary: layer; network
subparietal: sulcus
subpellicular: fibril; microtubule
subperiodic: periodicity
subperiosteal: abscess; amputation; fracture; implant
subperitoneal: appendicitis; fascia
subphrenic: abscess; recesses
subplasmalemmal dense: zone
subpopliteal: recess
subpubic: angle
subpulmonic: effusion
subpyloric: lymph nodes; node
subquadricipital: muscle
subsartorial: canal; fascia
subscapular: artery; branches of axillary artery; bursa; fossa; muscle; nerves
subscapular group of axillary: lymph nodes
subscapularis: muscle
subsegmental: atelectasis
subseptate: uterus
subserous: layer; plexus
subsidiary atrial: pacemaker
subsistence: diet
substance: abuse; dependence
substance abuse: disorders
substance-induced organic mental: disorders
substantia: propria of cornea
substernal: angle; goiter
substituted: amide
substitution: product; therapy; transfusion
substitutive: therapy
substrate: cycle; inhibition; specificity
substrate-level: phosphorylation
subsuperior: segment
subsurface: cisterna

subtalar: joint
subtemporal: decompression
subtendinous: bursa of gastrocnemius muscle; bursa of the tibialis anterior muscle
subtendinous iliac: bursa
subtendinous prepatellar: bursa
subthalamic: fasciculus; nucleus
subthreshold: stimulus
subtotal: hysterectomy; thyroidectomy
subungual: abscess; exostosis; melanoma
subunit: vaccine
subvalvar: stenosis
subvalvular aortic: stenosis
subvocal: speech
succedaneous: dentition; tooth
succenturiate: placenta
successive: contrast
succinic acid: cycle
succussion: sound
sucking: cushion; louse; pad; wound
suckling: reflex
Sucquet-Hoyer: anastomoses; canals
Sucquet's: anastomoses; canals
sucrose hemolysis: test
suction: cup; drainage; ophthalmodynamometer; plate
sudanophobic: zone
sudden: death
sudden infant death: syndrome
Sudeck's: atrophy; syndrome
Sudeck's critical: point
sudomotor: fibers; nerves
sudoriferous: duct; glands
sudoriparous: abscess
sufficient: cause
suffocating: gas
suffocative: goiter
sugar: alcohol; cataract; ester; tumor
sugar-coated: spleen
sugar-icing: liver
suggestive: psychotherapy; therapeutics
Sugiura: procedure
suicide: gesture; substrate
suid: herpesvirus
sulcal: artery
sulcomarginal: tract
sulcular: epithelium; fluid
sulfate: respiration; water
sulfatide: lipidosis
sulfation: factor
sulfhydryl: reagent
sulfonium: ion
sulfosalicylic acid turbidity: test

sulfur: autotrophy; mustard; water
sulfurated: lime; potash
sulfureted: hydrogen
Sulkowitch's: reagent
Sulzberger-Garbe: disease; syndrome
summation: beat; gallop
summer: asthma; diarrhea; itch; prurigo; rash; sores
Sumner's: sign
sump: drain; syndrome
sun: stroke
sunflower: cataract
sun protection: factor
superciliary: arch; ridge
superconducting: magnet
superfatted: soap
superficial: angioma; branch; branch of the lateral plantar nerve; branch of the medial plantar artery; branch of the radial nerve; branch of the superior gluteal artery; branch of the transverse cervical artery; branch of the ulnar nerve; burn; cleavage; ectoderm; fascia; fascia of penis; fascia of perineum; head of flexor pollicis brevis muscle; implantation; lamina; layer; layer of deep cervical fascia; layer of the levator palpebrae superioris muscle; layer of temporalis fascia; part of duodenum; part of external anal sphincter; part of masseter muscle; part of parotid gland; reflex; vein
superficial back: muscles
superficial brachial: artery
superficial cardiac: plexus
superficial cerebral: veins
superficial cervical: artery; nerve
superficial circumflex iliac: artery; vein
superficial dorsal: veins of clitoris; veins of penis
superficial dorsal sacrococcygeal: ligament
superficial epigastric: artery; vein
superficial fibular: nerve
superficial flexor: muscle of fingers
superficial gray: layer of superior colliculus
superficial inguinal: lymph nodes; pouch; ring
superficial linear: keratitis
superficial lingual: muscle
superficial lymphatic: vessel
superficial middle cerebral: vein

superficial palmar: artery; branch of radial artery
superficial palmar (arterial): arch
superficial palmar venous: arch
superficial parotid: lymph nodes
superficial perineal: pouch; space
superficial peroneal: nerve
superficial posterior sacrococcygeal: ligament
superficial punctate: keratitis
superficial pustular: perifolliculitis
superficial spreading: melanoma
superficial temporal: artery; branch of auriculotemporal nerve; plexus; veins
superficial transverse: muscle of perineum
superficial transverse metacarpal: ligament
superficial transverse metatarsal: ligament
superficial transverse perineal: muscle
superficial volar: artery
superimposed: eclampsia; preeclampsia
superior: angle of scapula; belly of omohyoid muscle; border; border of pancreas; border of petrous part of temporal bone; border of scapula; border of spleen; border of suprarenal gland; branch; branch of the oculomotor nerve; branch of the pubic bone; branch of the right and left inferior pulmonary veins; branch of the superior gluteal artery; branch of the transverse cervical nerve; bursa of biceps femoris; cistern; colliculus; extremity; fascia of pelvic diaphragm; fascia of urogenital diaphragm; flexure of duodenum; fovea; ganglion of glossopharyngeal nerve; ganglion of vagus nerve; horn of falciform margin of saphenous opening; horn of thyroid cartilage; laryngotomy; ligament of epididymis; ligament of incus; ligament of malleus; limb; lobe of lung; mediastinum; olive; paraplegia; part of diaphragmatic surface of liver; part of duodenum; part of lingular branch of

WordFinder

left pulmonary vein; part of vestibular ganglion; part of vestibulocochlear nerve; pole of kidney; pole of testis; polioencephalitis; recess of lesser peritoneal sac; recess of tympanic membrane; retinaculum of extensor muscles; root of ansa cervicalis; root of vestibulocochlear nerve; segment; surface of cerebellar hemisphere; surface of talus; tarsus; trunk of brachial plexus; veins of cerebellar hemisphere; vein of vermis; vena cava; wall of orbit

superior aberrant: ductule
superior alveolar: nerves
superior anastomotic: vein
superior articular: facet of atlas; pit of atlas; process of sacrum; surface of tibia
superior auricular: muscle
superior azygoesophageal: recess
superior basal: vein
superior carotid: triangle
superior central tegmental: nucleus
superior cerebellar: artery; peduncle
superior cerebellar artery: syndrome
superior cerebral: veins
superior cervical: ganglion
superior cervical cardiac: branches of vagus nerve; nerve
superior choroid: vein
superior cluneal: nerves
superior constrictor: muscle of pharynx
superior costal: facet; pit
superior costotransverse: ligament
superior dental: arch; branches of superior dental plexus; nerves; plexus; rami
superior duodenal: fold; fossa; recess
superior epigastric: artery; veins
superior esophageal: sphincter
superior extensor: retinaculum
superior frontal: convolution; gyrus; sulcus
superior gastric: lymph nodes
superior gemellus: muscle
superior gingival: branches of superior dental plexus

superior gluteal: artery; nerve; veins
superior hemorrhagic: polioencephalitis
superior hemorrhoidal: artery; plexus; vein
superior hypogastric: plexus
superior hypophysial: artery
superior ileocecal: recess
superior intercostal: artery; vein
superior internal parietal: artery
superiority: complex
superior labial: artery; branches of infraorbital nerve; vein
superior laryngeal: artery; cavity; nerve; vein
superior lateral brachial cutaneous: nerve
superior lateral genicular: artery
superior limbic: keratoconjunctivitis
superior lingular: branch of lingular branch of superior lobar left pulmonary artery; segment
superior longitudinal: fasciculus; muscle of tongue; sinus; sulcus
superior macular: arteriole; venule
superior maxillary: nerve
superior medial genicular: artery
superior medullary: velum
superior mesenteric: artery; ganglion; lymph nodes; plexus; vein
superior mesenteric artery: syndrome
superior nasal: arteriole of retina; concha; venule of retina
superior nuchal: line
superior oblique: muscle; muscle of head
superior occipital: gyrus; sulcus
superior olivary: nucleus
superior omental: recess
superior ophthalmic: vein
superior orbital: fissure
superior palpebral: veins
superior pancreaticoduodenal: artery
superior parietal: gyrus; lobule
superior pelvic: aperture
superior petrosal: sinus; sulcus
superior phrenic: artery; lymph nodes; veins
superior posterior serratus: muscle

superior pubic: ligament; ramus
superior pulmonary sulcus: tumor
superior quadrigeminal: brachium
superior radioulnar: joint
superior rectal: artery; lymph nodes; plexus; vein
superior rectus: muscle
superior sagittal: sinus
superior salivary: nucleus
superior salivatory: nucleus
superior segmental: artery of kidney
superior semilunar: lobule
superior suprarenal: arteries
superior tarsal: muscle
superior temporal: arteriole of retina; convolution; fissure; gyrus; line; sulcus; venule of retina
superior thalamostriate: vein
superior thoracic: aperture; artery
superior thyroid: artery; notch; plexus; tubercle; vein
superior tibial: articulation
superior tibiofibular: joint
superior tracheobronchial: lymph nodes
superior transverse scapular: ligament
superior triangle: sign
superior turbinated: bone
superior tympanic: artery
superior ulnar collateral: artery
superior vena cava: syndrome
superior vesical: artery
superior vestibular: area; nucleus
supernatant: fluid
supernormal recovery: phase
supernumerary: breast; kidney; mamma; organs; placenta
superolateral: surface of cerebrum
superolateral cerebral: surface
superomedial: margin
supersaturated: solution
supersonic: rays; waves
supertraction: conus
supination: reflex
supinator: crest; jerk; muscle; reflex
supine: position
supine hypotensive: syndrome
supplemental: air; groove; lobe; ridge

supplementary: menstruation
supplementary motor: cortex
supplementary motor area: epilepsy
support: medium
supporting: area; cell; reactions; reflexes
supportive: psychotherapy
suppressed: menstruation
suppression: amblyopia
suppressor: cells; mutation; mutations; tRNA
suppressor-sensitive: mutant
suppurative: appendicitis; arthritis; cerebritis; choroiditis; encephalitis; gingivitis; hepatitis; hyalitis; inflammation; mastitis; necrosis; nephritis; periodontitis; pleurisy; pneumonia; pulpitis; synovitis
supra-acetabular: groove; sulcus
supra-arytenoid: cartilage
supra-auricular: point
supracallosal: gyrus
supracervical: hysterectomy
suprachoroid: lamina; layer
supraclavicular: lymph nodes; muscle; part of brachial plexus; triangle
supraclinoid: aneurysm
supracondylar: fracture; process
supracrestal: line; plane
supracristal: plane
supraduodenal: artery
supraepicondylar: process
supragingival: calculus
supraglenoid: tubercle
suprahepatic: spaces
suprahisian: block
suprahyoid: branch of lingual artery; gland; muscles
suprainterparietal: bone
supramarginal: convolution; gyrus
supramastoid: crest; fossa
supramaximal: stimulus
suprameatal: pit; spine; triangle
supranasal: point
supranormal: conduction; excitability
supranuclear: lesion; paralysis
supraoptic: commissures; nucleus; nucleus of hypothalamus
supraopticohypophysial: tract
supraorbital: arch; artery; foramen; margin; nerve;

neuralgia; notch; point; reflex; ridge; vein
supraorbitomeatal: plane
suprapatellar: bursa; reflex
supraperiosteal: implant
suprapineal: recess
suprapleural: membrane
suprapubic: cystotomy; lithotomy
suprapyloric: lymph node; node
suprarenal: body; capsule; cortex; gland; impression; medulla; plexus; veins
suprascapular: artery; ligament; nerve; notch; vein
suprasellar: cyst
supraspinalis: muscle
supraspinatus: muscle; syndrome
supraspinous: fossa; ligament; muscle
suprasternal: bone; notch; plane; pulsation; space
supratonsillar: fossa; recess
supratragic: tubercle
supratrochlear: artery; nerve; veins
supraumbilical: reflex
supravaginal: portion of cervix
supravalvar: stenosis
supravalvar aortic stenosis: syndrome
supravalvar aortic stenosis-infantile hypercalcemia: syndrome
supravalvular: stenosis
supraventricular: crest; extrasystole; tachycardia
supravesical: fossa
supravital: stain
supreme: concha
supreme intercostal: artery; vein
supreme nasal: concha
supreme turbinated: bone
sural: artery; nerve; region
surdocardiac: syndrome
surface: anatomy; catalysis; coil; epithelium; tension; thermometer
surface mucous: cells of stomach
surface tension: theory of narcosis
surface thalamic: veins
surgeon's: knot
surgical: abdomen; anatomy; anesthesia; appliance; diathermy; emphysema; eruption; erysipelas; ligation; maggot; microscope; neck of humerus; orthodontics; pathology; prosthesis; silk; splint; template

surgical ciliated: cyst
surging: faradism
surrogate: mother
survey: line
survival: analysis; time
susceptibility: testing
suspended: animation
suspension: colloid; laryngoscopy; stability
suspensory: bandage; ligament of axilla; ligament of clitoris; ligament of esophagus; ligament of eyeball; ligament of gonad; ligament of lens; ligament of ovary; ligament of penis; ligaments of breast; ligaments of Cooper; ligament of testis; ligament of thyroid gland; muscle of duodenum
sustained action: tablet
sustentacular: cell; fibers of retina
Sutton's: disease; nevus; ulcer
sutural: bones; cataract; ligament
suture: joint; ligature
Suzanne's: gland
SV40-adenovirus: hybrid
Svedberg: equation; unit
Sw^a: antigen
swallow: syncope
swallowing: reflex; threshold
swamp: fever; itch
swamp fever: virus
Swan-Ganz: catheter
Swann: antigens
swan-neck: deformity
sweat: duct; glands; pore; test
sweat gland: carcinoma
sweating: sickness; test
sweaty feet: syndrome
Swediauer's: disease
Swedish: gymnastics; movements
sweet: balm; itch; precipitate
sweet birch: oil
sweet clover: disease; poisoning
Sweet's: disease
Swift's: disease
swim: bladder
swimmer's: ear; itch
swimming: test
swimming pool: conjunctivitis; granuloma
swine: dysentery; erysipelas; fever; icteroanemia; influenza; pest; porphyria
swine encephalitis: virus
swine fever: virus
swineherd's: disease
swine influenza: viruses
swinepox: virus
swine vesicular: disease

swine vesicular disease: virus
swinging light: test
Swiss cheese: endometrium
Swiss mouse leukemia: virus
Swiss type: agammaglobulinemia
switching: site
swollen belly: disease; syndrome
swollen head: syndrome
swordfish: test
Swyer-James: syndrome
Swyer-James-MacLeod: syndrome
Sydenham's: chorea; disease
Sydney: crease; line
syllabic: speech
sylvatic: plague
Sylvest's: disease
Sylvian: cistern
sylvian: fissure; line; point; valve; ventricle
sylvian: angle; aqueduct
symbiotic fermentation: phenomenon
Syme's: amputation; operation
Symington's anococcygeal: body
Symmers' clay pipestem: fibrosis
symmetric: adenolipomatosis; asphyxia; disulfide
symmetrical: gangrene
symmetric distal: neuropathy
sympathetic: agent; amine; blockade; branch to submandibular ganglion; ganglia; heterochromia; hormone; hypertonia; imbalance; iridoplegia; iritis; nerve; ophthalmia; part; plexuses; root of ciliary ganglion; saliva; segment; symptom; trunk; uveitis
sympathetic formative: cell
sympathetic nervous: system
sympathetic reflex: dystrophy
sympathicotropic: cells
sympathizing: eye
sympathochromaffin: cell
sympathomimetic: amine
symphysial: surface of pubis
symphysic: teratosis
symptom: complex; formation; group; score; substitution
symptomatic: epilepsy; erythema; fever; headache; impotence; nanism; neuralgia; porphyria;

pruritus; reaction; tetany; torticollis; treatment; ulcer; varicocele
symptomatic myeloid: metaplasia
Syms: tractor
synaptic: boutons; cleft; conduction; endings; phase; resistance; terminals; trough; vesicles
synaptinemal: complex
synaptonemal: complex
synarthrodial: joint
synchondrodial: joint
synchronic: study
synchronized intermittent mandatory: ventilation
synchronous: reflex
synclonic: spasm
syncytial: bud; knot; sprout; trophoblast
syndesmochorial: placenta
syndesmodial: joint
synergic: control
synergistic: effect; muscles
syngeneic: graft
synovial: bursa; cell; chondromatosis; crypt; cyst; fluid; fold; frena; frenula; fringe; glands; hernia; joint; ligament; membrane; mesenchyme; osteochondromatosis; sarcoma; sheath; sheaths of digits of foot; sheaths of digits of hand; tufts; villi
synovial tendon: sheath
synovial trochlear: bursa
syntactical: aphasia
synthesis: period
synthetic: chemistry; dyes
syntonic: personality
syphilitic: abscess; aneurysm; aortitis; cirrhosis; fever; leukoderma; meningoencephalitis; nephritis; osteochondritis; roseola; teeth; ulcer
Syriac: ulcer
syringomyelic: dissociation; hemorrhage
systematic: anatomy; bacteriology; desensitization
systematized: delusion; nevus
systemic: anaphylaxis; anatomy; blastomycosis; chondromalacia; circulation; heart; hyalinosis; lupus erythematosus; mastocytosis; myelitis; poisoning; sclerosis
systemic autoimmune: diseases
systemic febrile: diseases

WordFinder

systemic vascular: resistance
systemic venous: hypertension
systolic: bruit; click; gallop; gradient; honk; murmur; pressure; shock; thrill; whoop
systolic/diastolic: ratio
systolic gallop: rhythm
systolic time: intervals

T

T: agglutinogen; antigens; cell; enzyme; fiber; group; lymphocyte; myelotomy; system; tube; tubule; wave
T-: bandage; binder
t: distribution; test
T.A.B.: vaccine
tabby cat: striation
tabetic: arthropathy; crisis; cuirass; dissociation; neurosyphilis
table: salt
tablet: triturate
Tac: antigen
Tacaribe: complex of viruses; virus
tachybradycardia: syndrome
tachycardia: window
tachycardia-bradycardia: syndrome
tactile: agnosia; anesthesia; cell; corpuscle; disk; elevations; fremitus; hair; hallucination; hyperesthesia; image; meniscus; organ; papilla; sense
Tactual Performance: Test
tadpole-shaped: pupil
Taenzer's: stain
tagged: atom
tagliacotian: operation
Tahyna: virus
tail: bone; bud; fold; sheath; vertebrae
tailor's: cramp; muscle; spasm
Tait's: law
Takahara's: disease
Takayama's: stain
Takayasu's: arteritis; disease; syndrome
talar: sulcus
talar articular: surface of calcaneus
talc: operation
Tallerman: treatment
tallow: soap
talocalcaneal: joint; ligament
talocalcaneonavicular: joint
talocrural: articulation; joint
talon: cusp
talonavicular: joint; ligament

tambour: sound
tamed: iodine
Tamm-Horsfall: mucoprotein; protein
tangent: screen
tangential: wound
Tangier: disease
tank: respirator
tanned red: cells
Tanner: stage
Tanner growth: chart
tanner's: ulcer
tannic acid: glycerite
tantalum: bronchography
tapered: bougie
tapetal light: reflex
tapetoretinal: degeneration
Tapia's: syndrome
tapir: mouth
Taq: polymerase
tar: acne; camphor; keratosis
Tardieu's: ecchymoses; petechiae; spots
tardive: cyanosis; dyskinesia
target: behavior; cell; gland; organ; patient; response
target cell: anemia
Tarin's: space; tenia; valve
Tarlov's: cyst
Tarnier's: forceps
tarry: cyst
tarsal: arch; bones; canal; cartilage; cyst; fold; glands; joints; ligaments; plates; sinus
tarsal tunnel: syndrome
tarsoepiphyseal: aclasis
tarsometatarsal: joints; ligaments
tarsophalangeal: reflex
tarsotibial: amputation
tart: cell
tartrated: antimony
taste: blindness; bud; bulb; cells; corpuscle; deficiency; hairs; pore; ridge
TATA: box
Taussig-Bing: disease; syndrome
tautomeric: fibers
Tawara's: node
Taylor's: apparatus; disease; splint
Taylor's back: brace
Tay-Sachs: disease
Tay's cherry-red: spot
^{99m}Tc: pyrophosphate
T cell antigen: receptors
T-cell growth: factor; factor-1; factor-2
T cell-rich, B cell: lymphoma
T cytotoxic: cells
T-dependent: antigen
TDTH: cells
T-E: fistula
teachers': nodes
teaching: hospital

TEAE-: cellulose
Teale's: amputation
tear: film; gas; sac; stone
technical: error
tectal: nucleus; stria
tectobulbar: tract
tectonic: keratoplasty
tectopontine: tract
tectorial: membrane; membrane of cochlear duct
tectospinal: decussation; tract
tegmental: decussations; fields of Forel; nuclei; syndrome; wall of middle ear
Teichmann's: crystals
telangiectatic: angioma; angiomatosis; cancer; fibroma; glioma; lipoma; wart
telangiectatic osteogenic: sarcoma
telencephalic: flexure; vesicle
telephone: theory
teleradium: therapy
telescopic: denture; spectacles
television: microscope
TeLinde: operation
telocentric: chromosome
telogen: effluvium
telolecithal: egg; ovum
telomeric R-banding: stain
temperate: bacteriophage; virus
temperature: coefficient; sense; spot
temperature-compensated: vaporizer
temperature-sensitive: mutant
template: RNA
temporal: aponeurosis; apophysis; arteritis; bone; branch of facial nerve; canal; cortex; dispersion; fascia; fossa; horn; line; lobe; muscle; plane; pole; pole of cerebrum; process; region of head; ridge; squama; surface; veins; venules of retina
temporalis: muscle
temporal lobe: epilepsy
temporary: base; callus; cartilage; denture; memory; parasite; restoration; stricture; tooth
temporofrontal: tract
temporomandibular: arthrosis; articulation; joint; ligament; nerve; syndrome
temporomandibular articular: disk
temporomandibular joint: dysfunction

temporomandibular joint pain-dysfunction: syndrome
temporomaxillary: vein
temporoparietal: muscle
temporoparietalis: muscle
temporopontine: tract
temporozygomatic: suture
tenaculum: forceps
tender: lines; points; zones
tendinous: arch; arch of levator ani muscle; arch of pelvic fascia; arch of soleus muscle; chiasm of the digital tendons; cords; inscription; intersection; opening; spot; synovitis; xanthoma
tendo Achillis: reflex
tendon: advancement; bundle; cells; graft; recession; reflex; sheath of abductor pollicis longus and extensor pollicis brevis muscles; sheath of extensor carpi radialis muscles; sheath of extensor carpi ulnaris muscle; sheath of extensor digiti minimi muscle; sheath of extensor digitorum and extensor indicis muscles; sheath of extensor digitorum longus muscle of foot; sheath of extensor hallucis longus muscle; sheath of extensor pollicis longus muscle; sheath of flexor carpi radialis muscle; sheath of flexor digitorum longus muscle of foot; sheath of flexor hallucis longus muscle; sheath of flexor pollicis longus muscle; sheath of superior oblique muscle; sheath of tibialis anterior muscle; sheath of tibialis posterior muscle; suture; transplantation
tendon sheath: syndrome
ten Horn's: sign
tennis: elbow; leg; thumb
Tenon's: capsule; space
tense: part of the tympanic membrane; pulse
tensile: strength; stress
tension: curve; headache; pneumothorax; suture
tensor: muscle of fascia lata; muscle of soft palate; muscle of tympanic membrane
tensor fasciae latae: muscle
tensor tarsi: muscle
tensor tympani: muscle
tensor veli palati: muscle
tenth cranial: nerve

tentorial: angle; nerve; notch; sinus; surface

teratoid: tumor

teratomatous: cyst

teres major: muscle

teres minor: muscle

term: infant

terminal: artery; bar; boutons; bronchiole; cisternae; crest; deletion; disinfection; endocarditis; filum; ganglion; hair; hematuria; ileus; infection; leukocytosis; line; nerves; notch of auricle; nuclei; oxidase; oxidation; part; plate; pneumonia; redundancy; sinus; stria; sulcus; thread; transferases; vein; ventricle; web

terminal addition: enzyme

terminal hinge: position

terminal jaw relation: record

terminal nerve: corpuscles

termination: codon; factor; sequence

termino-terminal: anastomosis

ternary: complex

Terrien's: valve

Terrien's marginal: degeneration

territorial: matrix

Terry's: nails; syndrome

Terson's: glands

tertian: fever; malaria; parasite

tertiary: alcohol; amputation; amyl alcohol; calcium phosphate; cortex; dentin; structure; syphilid; syphilis; villus; vitreous

tertiary egg: membrane

tertiary medical: care

Teschen: disease

Teschen disease: virus

Tesla: current

tessellated: fundus

Tessier: classification

test: cross; injection; meal; object; profile; solution; tube; type

test handle: instrument

testicular: appendage; artery; cord; duct; dysgenesis; feminization; implant; plexus; prosthesis; veins

testicular feminization: syndrome

testicular tubular: adenoma

testis: cords; ectopia

testis-determining: factor

testoid: hyperthecosis

testosterone-estrogen-binding: globulin

test-retest: reliability

test-tube: baby

tetanic: contraction; convulsion

tetanus: antitoxin; immunoglobulin; toxin; vaccine

tetanus antitoxin: unit

tetanus and gas gangrene: antitoxins

tetanus immune: globulin

tetanus-perfringens: antitoxin

tetany: cataract

Tete: viruses

tethered cord: syndrome

tetracyclic: antidepressant

tetracyclic steroid: nucleus

tetraethyl: poisoning

tetramethyl: acridine

tetrazonium: salts

Teutleben's: ligament

Texas: fever; snakeroot

text: blindness

Tg: cells

TGE: virus

Thal: procedure

thalamic: fasciculus; syndrome; tenia

thalamic gustatory: nucleus

thalamocortical: fibers

thalamostriate: veins

thallium: poisoning

thanatophoric: dwarfism

Thane's: method

Thayer-Martin: agar; medium

thebesian: circulation; foramina; valve; veins

theca: cells of stomach

theca cell: tumor

theca interna: cone

thecal: abscess; whitlow

theca lutein: cell

Theden's: method

Theiler's: disease; virus

Theiler's mouse encephalomyelitis: virus

Theiler's original: virus

Theile's: canal; glands; muscle

T helper: cells

thematic: paralogia; paraphasia

thematic apperception: test

thenar: eminence; prominence; space

Theobald Smith's: phenomenon

therapeutic: abortion; anesthesia; angiography; community; crisis; dose; electrode; fever; group; incompatibility; index; iridectomy; malaria; nihilism; optimism; pessimism; pneumothorax; range; ratio

thermal: anesthesia; burn; capacity; sense; spectrum

thermic: fever

thermo-: stromuhr

thermodynamic: potential; theory of narcosis

thermoelectric: pile

thermogenic: action

thermolabile: opsonin

thermoluminescence: dosimetry

thermoprecipitin: reaction

thermostable: enzyme; opsonin

thermostable opsonin: test

theta: antigen; rhythm; wave

Thezac-Porsmeur: method

thiamin chloride: unit

thiamin hydrochloride: unit

thiazide: diabetes

thiazin: dyes

Thiemann's: disease; syndrome

Thiersch: graft

Thiersch's: canaliculi; method; operation

Thiersch's graft: operation

thigh: bone; joint

thin: section

thin-layer: chromatography; electrophoresis; immunoassay

thiochrome: method

thioclastic: cleavage

thiocyanogen: number; value

thioflavine T: stain

thiol: enzyme; ester

third: corpuscle; disease; eyelid; finger; molar; ovary; sound; tonsil; trochanter; ventricle; ventriculostomy

third cranial: nerve

third cuneiform: bone

third degree: burn

third and fourth pharyngeal pouch: syndrome

third heart: sound

third occipital: nerve

third parallel pelvic: plane

third peroneal: muscle

third temporal: convolution

thirst: fever

Thiry's: fistula

Thiry-Vella: fistula

thixotropic: fluid

Thomas: splint

Thoma's: ampulla; fixative; laws

Thompson's: ligament; test

Thomsen's: disease

Thomson's: sign

thoracic: aorta; axis; cage; cavity; choke; compliance; duct; fistula; ganglia; girdle; glands; goiter; index; kidney; limb; nucleus; part of aorta; part of esophagus; part of spinal

cord; part of thoracic duct; respiration; spine; stomach; veins; vertebrae; wall

thoracic aortic: plexus

thoracic cardiac: branches of vagus nerve; nerves

thoracic interspinal: muscle

thoracic interspinales: muscles

thoracic intertransversarii: muscles

thoracic intertransverse: muscles

thoracic longissimus: muscle

thoracic outlet: syndrome

thoracic-pelvic-phalangeal: dystrophy

thoracic rotator: muscles

thoracic spinal: nerves

thoracic splanchnic: nerves

thoracoabdominal: nerves

thoracoacromial: artery; trunk; vein

thoracodorsal: artery; nerve

thoracoepigastric: vein

thoracolumbar: aponeurosis; fascia; system

thoracoscopic: surgery

thoracostomy: tube

thorium: emanation

Thormählen's: test

Thorn: test

thorn apple: crystals

Thorn's: syndrome

thought process: disorder

thready: pulse

threatened: abortion

3_{10}: helix

three-chambered: heart

three-cornered: bone

three-day: fever; measles

three-dimensional: record

three-glass: test

3.6_{13}: helix

thresher's: lung

threshold: body; differential; percussion; shift; stimulus; substance; trait

threshold limit: value

thrombin: time

thrombocytic: series

thrombocytopenia-absent radius: syndrome

thrombocytopenic: purpura

thromboembolic: meningoencephalitis

thrombopathic: syndrome

thrombopenic: purpura

thrombotic: gangrene; hydrocephalus; infarct; microangiopathy; phlegmasia

thrombotic thrombocytopenic: purpura

through: drainage

through-and-through myocardial: infarction
through transfer: imaging
thrush: fungus
thumb: forceps; lancet; reflex
Thygeson's: disease
thyme: camphor
thymic: abscesses; agenesis; alymphoplasia; arteries; branches of internal thoracic artery; corpuscle; hypoplasia; veins
thymic lymphopoietic: factor
thymine: dimer
thymol turbidity: test
thymus: gland; treatment
thymus-dependent: zone
thymus-independent: antigen
thyroarytenoid: muscle
thyrocardiac: disease
thyrocervical: trunk
thyroepiglottic: ligament; muscle
thyroglossal: duct
thyroglossal duct: cyst
thyrohyoid: membrane; muscle
thyrohypophysial: syndrome
thyroid: axis; body; bruit; cartilage; colloid; diverticulum; eminence; foramen; gland; insufficiency; lymph nodes; storm; therapy; toxicosis; veins
thyroidal articular: surface of cricoid
thyroid ima: artery
thyroid-stimulating: hormone; immunoglobulins
thyroid-stimulating hormone-releasing: factor
thyroid-stimulating hormone stimulation: test
thyroid suppression: test
thyrolingual: duct
thyropharyngeal: part of inferior pharyngeal constrictor muscle
thyrotoxic: coma; crisis; encephalopathy; myopathy; serum
thyrotoxic complement-fixation: factor
thyrotoxic heart: disease
thyrotropic: hormone
thyrotropin: resistance
thyrotropin-producing: adenoma
thyrotropin-releasing: factor; hormone
thyrotropin-releasing hormone stimulation: test
thyroxine-binding: globulin; prealbumin; protein

tibial: border of foot; crest; nerve; phenomenon; tuberosity
tibial collateral: ligament
tibial communicating: nerve
tibial intertendinous: bursa
tibialis anterior: muscle
tibialis posterior: muscle
tibiocalcaneal: ligament; part of deltoid ligament
tibiofemoral: index
tibiofibular: articulation; ligament; syndesmosis
tibionavicular: ligament; part of deltoid ligament
tick: fever; paralysis; pyemia; typhus
tick-borne: encephalitis (Central European subtype); encephalitis (Eastern subtype); fever; virus
tick-borne encephalitis: virus
tic-tac: rhythm; sounds
tidal: air; drainage; volume; wave
Tiedemann's: gland; nerve
tie-over: dressing
Tietze's: syndrome
tiger: heart
tight: junction
tigroid: bodies; fundus; retina; striation; substance
tilt: table; test
tilting disc: valve
tilting disc valve: prosthesis
time: constant; marker; sense
time-compensated: gain
time compensation: gain
time-gain: compensation
time-lapse: microscopy
time-varied: gain
time-varied gain: control
timothy-hay: bacillus
tine: test
Tinel's: sign
tinted: vision
tinted denture: base
Tiselius: apparatus
Tiselius electrophoresis: cell
Tissot: spirometer
tissue: basophil; culture; displaceability; displacement; factor; fluid; hormones; lymph; molding; registration; respiration; tension; valve
tissue-bearing: area
tissue culture infectious: dose
tissue plasminogen: activator
tissue-specific: antigen
tissue thromboplastin inhibition: time
tissue weighting: factor
titratable acidity: test

Tizzoni's: stain
Tj: antigen
Tm: cells
TNM: staging
TO: virus
toad: skin
to-and-fro: anesthesia; murmur; sound
toasted: shins
tobacco: heart
Tobia: fever
Tobruk: splint
Todaro's: tendon
Todd: unit
Todd's: paralysis
Todd's postepileptic: paralysis
Tod's: muscle
toe: clonus; itch; phenomenon
toilet: training
Toison's: stain
Tokelau: ringworm
tolbutamide: test
Toldt's: fascia; membrane
tolerance: dose
Tolosa-Hunt: syndrome
Tolu: balsam
Toma's: sign
Tomes': fibers; processes
Tomes' granular: layer
Tommaselli's: disease
tone: color
tone decay: test
tongue: bone; depressor; flap; phenomenon
tonic: contraction; control; convulsion; epilepsy; pupil; reflex; seizure; seizure; spasm
tonic-clonic: seizure
tonoclonic: spasm
tonsillar: branch of the facial artery; branch of glossopharyngeal nerve; calculus; crypt; fossa; fossulae; herniation; ring
tonsillolingual: sulcus
tooth: abrasion; avulsion; bud; cement; form; germ; ligation; plane; polyp; pulp; sac; socket; spasms; transplantation
tooth-and-nail: syndrome
tooth-borne: base
toothed: vertebra
toper's: nose
Töpfer's: test
tophaceous: gout
topical: anesthesia; anesthetic
Topinard's: line
Topinard's facial: angle
topographic: anatomy
Topolanski's: sign
toppling: gait
TORCH: syndrome
Torek: operation

toric: lens
Torkildsen: shunt
tornado: epilepsy
Tornwaldt's: abscess; cyst; disease; syndrome
Toronto: formula for pulmonary artery banding
Torre's: syndrome
torsion: disease of childhood; dystonia; fracture; neurosis; spasm
torsional: deformity
torsive: occlusion
Torsten Sjögren's: syndrome
torus: fracture
total: acidity; aphasia; ascertainment; cataract; cleavage; cystectomy; elasticity of muscle; energy; hematuria; hyperopia; keratoplasty; mastectomy; necrosis; placenta previa; sclerectasia; synechia; transfusion
total body: hypothermia; water
total breech: extraction
total catecholamine: test
total cell: count
total end-diastolic: diameter
total end-systolic: diameter
total joint: arthroplasty
total lung: capacity
total parenteral: nutrition
total or partial anomalous pulmonary venous: connections
total pelvic: exenteration
total peripheral: resistance
total push: therapy
total refractory: period
total spinal: anesthesia
totipotent: cell
totipotential: protoplasm
touch: cell; corpuscle
toughened: silver nitrate
Tourette: syndrome
Tourette's: disease
Tournay: sign
Tournay's: phenomenon
tourniquet: poditis; test
Tourtual's: membrane; sinus
Touton giant: cell
Tovell: tube
Towne: projection; view
Towne projection: radiograph
toxemic: jaundice; retinopathy of pregnancy
toxic: amaurosis; amblyopia; anemia; cataract; cirrhosis; cyanosis; delirium; dementia; equivalent; goiter; hemoglobinuria; hydrocephalus; megacolon; myocarditis; nephrosis;

neuritis; psychosis; retinopathy; shock; tetanus; unit
toxic epidermal: necrolysis
toxicogenic: conjunctivitis
toxic shock: syndrome
toxin: spectrum; unit
Toynbee's: corpuscles; muscle; tube
TPHA: test
TPI: test
Tr^a: antigen
trabecular: bone; carcinoma; meshwork; network; reticulum; zone
trabeculated: bladder
trace: conditioning; elements; nutrient
trace conditioned: reflex
tracheal: branches; cartilages; fenestration; fistula; glands; intubation; lymph nodes; mucosa; ring; triangle; tube; tug; ulceration; veins
trachealis: muscle
tracheal wall: stripe
trachelobregmatic: diameter
tracheloclavicular: muscle
tracheobronchial: diverticulum; dyskinesia; groove
tracheoesophageal: fistula; speech
tracheotomy: hook; tube
trachoma: bodies; glands; virus
trachomatous: conjunctivitis; keratitis; pannus
traction: alopecia; atrophy; diverticulum; epiphysis
tragicus: muscle
trained: reflex
training: analysis; group
train-of-four: stimulus
trainwheel: rhythm
tram: lines
trance: coma
trans: phase
transactional: analysis; psychotherapy
transaxial: plane
transcellular: fluids; transport; water
transcendental: anatomy
transcervical: fracture
transcondylar: fracture
transcortical: aphasia; apraxia
transcranial: radiograph
transducer: cell
transduodenal: sphincterotomy
transesophageal: echocardiography
transfer: coping; factor; genes; imaging; RNA

transferase deficiency: galactosemia
transference: neurosis
transferred: ophthalmia; sensation
transferring: enzymes
transfixion: suture
transformation: constant; zone
transformed: lymphocyte
transforming: agent; factor; gene
transforming growth: factor α; factor β; factors
transfusion: hepatitis; nephritis
trans-Golgi: reticulum
transhiatal: esophagectomy
transient: agammaglobulinemia; albuminuria; equilibrium; hypogammaglobulinemia of infancy; myopia; retinopathy
transient acantholytic: dermatosis
transient global: amnesia
transient ischemic: attack
transition: electron; mutation
transitional: cell; convolution; denture; epithelium; gyrus; leukocyte; zone
transitional cell: carcinoma; papilloma
transjugular intrahepatic portosystemic: shunt
translatory: movement
translocation: carrier; chromosome
translumbar: aortography
transmembrane: potential
transmethylation: factor
transmissible: dementia; enteritis; gastroenteritis of swine; plasmid
transmissible gastroenteritis: virus of swine
transmissible mink: encephalopathy
transmissible murine colonic: hyperplasia
transmissible turkey enteritis: virus
transmissible venereal: tumor
transmitted: light
transmural: pressure
transmural myocardial: infarction
transneuronal: atrophy
transnexus: channel
transorbital: leukotomy; lobotomy
transosseous: venography
transovarial: transmission

transparent: dentin; septum; ulcer of the cornea
transplantation: antigen; genetics
transplant lung: syndrome
transporionic: axis
transport: antibiotic; host; maximum; medium; number; tetany
transposable: element
transpulmonary: pressure
transpyloric: plane
transseptal: fibers; orchiopexy
transsexual: surgery
transstadial: transmission
transsynaptic: chromatolysis; degeneration
transtentorial: herniation
transthoracic: echocardiography; esophagectomy; pacemaker; pressure
transureteroureteral: anastomosis
transurethral: resection
transurethral resection: syndrome
transversalis: fascia
transversarial: part of vertebral artery
transverse: amputation; arch of foot; artery of neck; branches; colon; crest; crest of internal acoustic meatus; diameter; disk; ductules of epoöphoron; fasciculi; fissure of cerebellum; fissure of cerebrum; fissure of the lung; foramen; fornix; fracture; head; hermaphroditism; lie; ligament of acetabulum; ligament of the atlas; ligament of elbow; ligament of knee; ligament of leg; ligament of pelvis; ligament of perineum; lines of sacrum; muscle of abdomen; muscle of auricle; muscle of chin; muscle of nape; muscle of thorax; muscle of tongue; myelitis; myelitis; nerve of neck; part of left branch of portal vein; part of nasalis muscle; plane; presentation; process; relaxation; ridge; section; septum; sinus; sinus of pericardium; vein of face; vein of scapula; veins of neck; velum
transverse abdominal: incision

transverse anthelicine: groove
transverse arytenoid: muscle
transverse atlantal: ligament
transverse auricular: muscle
transverse carpal: ligament
transverse cervical: artery; nerve; veins
transverse costal: facet
transverse crural: ligament
transverse facial: artery; fracture; vein
transverse genicular: ligament
transverse horizontal: axis
transverse humeral: ligament
transverse metacarpal: ligament
transverse metatarsal: ligament
transverse nasal: groove
transverse occipital: sulcus
transverse oval: pelvis
transverse palatine: fold; ridge; suture
transverse pancreatic: artery
transverse pericardial: sinus
transverse perineal: ligament
transverse pontine: fibers
transverse rectal: folds
transverse rhombencephalic: flexure
transverse scapular: artery
transverse tarsal: articulation; joint
transverse temporal: convolutions; gyri; sulci
transverse tibiofibular: ligament
transverse vesical: fold
transversion: mutation
transversospinal: muscle
transversospinalis: muscle
transversovertical: index
transversus abdominis: muscle
transversus menti: muscle
transversus nuchae: muscle
transversus thoracis: muscle
Trantas': dots
trapezium: bone
trapezius: muscle
trapezoid: body; bone; ligament; line; ridge
Trapp-Häser: formula
Trapp's: formula
Traube-Hering: curves; waves
Traube's: bruit; corpuscle; dyspnea; plugs; sign
Traube's double: tone
Traube's semilunar: space

WordFinder

traumatic: alopecia;
amenorrhea; amnesia;
amputation; anemia;
anesthesia; aneurysm;
asphyxia; cataract;
dermatitis; encephalopathy;
fever; gastritis; herpes;
meningocele; neurasthenia;
neuritis; neuroma; neurosis;
occlusion; orchitis;
pneumonia; psychosis;
reticuloperitonitis;
retinopathy; tetanus
traumatic bone: cyst
traumatic cervical:
discopathy
traumatic progressive:
encephalopathy
traumatogenic: occlusion
Trautmann's triangular:
space
traveler's: diarrhea
Treacher Collins': syndrome
treatment: denture
trefoil: dermatitis;
polypeptide; tendon
Treitz': arch; hernia;
ligament; muscle
Treitz's: fascia; fossa
Trélat's: sign; stools
tremulous: iris
trench: fever; foot; hand;
lung; mouth; nephritis
Trendelenburg: radiograph
Trendelenburg's: operation;
position; sign; symptom;
test
trephine: biopsy
treponema-immobilizing:
antibody
treponemal: antibody
**Treponema pallidum
hemagglutination:** test
**Treponema pallidum
immobilization:** test
Treponema pallidum
immobilization: reaction
Tresilian's: sign
Treves': fold
Trevor's: disease
triadic: symbiosis
trial: base; case; denture;
frame; lenses
triangular: bandage; bone;
cartilage; crest; disk of
wrist; fascia; fold; fossa;
fovea of arytenoid
cartilage; lamella;
ligament; ligaments of
liver; muscle; nucleus;
part; pit of arytenoid
cartilage; recess; ridge;
uterus
triangularity of the: teeth
triaxial reference: system
triazolopyridine:
antidepressant

tribasic: calcium phosphate;
magnesium phosphate
tribasilar: synostosis
TRIC: agents
tricarboxylic acid: cycle
triceps: bursa; muscle of
arm; muscle of calf;
muscle of hip; reflex
triceps brachii: muscle
triceps coxae: muscle
triceps surae: muscle; reflex
trichilemmal: cyst
trichorhinophalangeal:
syndrome
trichrome: stain
tricuspid: area; atresia;
incompetence;
insufficiency; murmur;
orifice; stenosis; tooth;
valve
tricyclic: antidepressant
trident: hand
*O***-(triethylaminoethyl):**
cellulose
trifacial: nerve; neuralgia
trifid: stomach
trifocal: lens
trigeminal: cave; cavity;
crest; decompression;
ganglion; impression;
lemniscus; nerve;
neuralgia; pulse;
rhizotomy; rhythm;
tractotomy
trigeminofacial: reflex
trigeminothalamic: tract
trigger: area; finger; point;
zone
triggered: activity
trihydric: alcohol
triiodothyronine: toxicosis
triiodothyronine uptake:
test
triketohydrindene: reaction
trilaminar: blastoderm
trimalleolar: fracture
triphammer: pulse
triphenylmethane: dyes
triphyllomatous: teratoma
Tripier's: amputation
triplant: implant
triple: arthrodesis; bond;
helix; phosphate; point;
quartan; response; rhythm;
vision
triple symptom: complex
triplet: oxygen; state
triple X: syndrome
tripod: fracture
triquetral: bone
triquetrous: cartilage
trisodium: phosphate
trisomy 8: syndrome
trisomy 13: syndrome
trisomy 18: syndrome
trisomy 20: syndrome
trisomy 21: syndrome
trisomy C: syndrome

trisomy D: syndrome
trispiral: tomography
tritiated: thymidine
triticeal: cartilage
triton: tumor
trochanter: reflex
trochanteric: bursa; bursitis;
crest; fossa; syndrome
trochlear: fossa; fovea;
nerve; notch; nucleus; pit;
process; spine
trochlear synovial: bursa
trochoid: articulation; joint
Troisier's: ganglion; node
Trolard's: vein
Tröltsch's: corpuscles; fold;
pockets; recesses
Trömner's: reflex
trophic: changes; gangrene;
nucleus; ulcer; ulcer
trophoblastic: lacuna;
operculum
trophoneurotic: atrophy;
leprosy
trophotropic: zone of Hess
tropic: hormones
tropical: abscess; acne;
anemia; boil; bubo;
diarrhea; diseases; eczema;
eosinophilia; lichen; mask;
measles; medicine;
myositis; pyomyositis;
sore; splenomegaly; sprue;
theileriosis; typhus; ulcer
tropical canine:
pancytopenia
tropical splenomegaly:
syndrome
Trousseau-Lallemand:
bodies
Trousseau's: point; sign;
spot; syndrome
true: aneurysm; ankylosis;
cementoma; cholinesterase;
conjugate; diverticulum;
dwarfism; glottis;
hermaphroditism;
hypertrophy; knot; muscles
of back; pelvis; ribs; thirst;
vertebra
true vocal: cord
truncate: ascertainment
Trunecek's: sign
Trusler's: rule for
pulmonary artery banding
truth: serum
trypanosome: fever; stage
trypsin: inhibitor
α_1**-trypsin:** inhibitor
trypsin G-banding: stain
tsutsugamushi: disease;
fever
tubal: abortion; branch;
branch of the tympanic
plexus; branch of the
uterine artery; cartilage;
colic; dysmenorrhea;
extremity of ovary; folds of

uterine tubes; infantilism;
ligation; pregnancy;
prominence; tonsil
tubal air: cells
tube: cast; curare; teeth
tubed: flap
tubed pedicle: flap
tuberal: nuclei
tubercle: bacillus
tuberculin: test
tuberculin-type:
hypersensitivity
tuberculoid: leprosy; rosacea
tuberculo-opsonic: index
tuberculosis: lymphadenitis;
vaccine
tuberculous: abscess;
bronchopneumonia;
enteritis; lymphadenitis;
meningitis; nephritis;
pericarditis; peritonitis;
rheumatism; spondylitis;
wart
tuberoinfundibular: tract
tuberosity: reduction
tuberous: root; sclerosis
Tübinger: perimeter
tuboabdominal: pregnancy
tubo-ovarian: abscess;
pregnancy; varicocele
tuboreticular: structure
tubotympanic: canal; recess
tubouterine: pregnancy
tubular: adenoma;
aneurysm; carcinoma; cyst;
forceps; gland; maximum;
respiration; vision
tubular excretory: mass
tubuloacinar: gland
tubuloalveolar: gland
tubulointerstitial: nephritis
Tucker-McLean: forceps
tuffstone: body
tufted: cell; phalanx
tularemic: chancre;
conjunctivitis; pneumonia
Tullio's: phenomenon
Tulp's: valve
tumbu dermal: myiasis
tumor: antigens; embolism;
marker; stage; virus
tumoral: calcinosis
tumor angiogenic: factor
tumor-associated: antigen
tumor-infiltrating:
lymphocytes
tumor lysis: syndrome
tumor necrosis: factor;
factor-beta
**tumor-specific
transplantation:** antigens
tungsten arc: lamp
tuning: fork
tunnel: cells; disease; vision
Tuohy: needle
T$_3$ uptake: test
TUR: syndrome
turban: tumor

turbinal: varix
turbinated: body; bones; crest
Türck's: bundle; column; degeneration; tract
Turcot: syndrome
Türk: cell
turkey: rhinotracheitis
turkey gobbler: neck
turkey meningoencephalitis: virus
turkey rhinotracheitis: virus
Turkish: saddle
Türk's: leukocyte
Turlock: virus
Turner's: sulcus; syndrome; tooth
turnover: flap; number
turpentine: enema; poisoning
tussive: fremitus; syncope
Tuttle's: proctoscope
Tweed: triangle
Tweed edgewise: treatment
twelfth cranial: nerve
twelfth-year: molar
twenty-nail: dystrophy
twiddler's: syndrome
twilight: sleep; state; vision
twin: cone; crystal; helix; method; placenta; pregnancy
twin-twin: transfusion
twist: form
twisted: hairs
two-bellied: muscle
two-carbon: fragment
two-dimensional: chromatography; echocardiography; immunoelectrophoresis
two-glass: test
Twort: phenomenon
Twort-d'Herelle: phenomenon
two-step exercise: test
two-sympathin: theory
two-tail: test
2060: virus
two-way: catheter
tympanic: antrum; attic; body; bone; canal; canaliculus; cavity; cells; enlargement; ganglion; gland; groove; incisure; intumescence; labium of limbus of spiral lamina; lip of limbus of spiral lamina; membrane; nerve; notch; opening of auditory tube; opening of canaliculi for chorda tympani; opening of eustachian tube; part of temporal bone; plate of temporal bone; plexus; promontory; ring; scute;

sinus; veins; wall of cochlear duct
tympanic air: cells
tympanitic: resonance
tympanohyal: bone
tympanomastoid: fissure; suture
tympanosquamous: fissure
tympanostapedial: junction; syndesmosis
tympanostomy: tube
Tyndall: effect; phenomenon
type: culture; species; strain
type 1: dextrocardia; glycogenosis
type 2: dextrocardia; glycogenosis
type 3: dextrocardia; glycogenosis
type 4: dextrocardia; glycogenosis
type 5: glycogenosis
type 6: glycogenosis
type 7: glycogenosis
type A: behavior; personality
type B: behavior
Type 1 G$_{M1}$: gangliosidosis
type I: acrocephalosyndactyly; cells; collagen; diabetes; diabetes mellitus; dip; error
type I familial: hyperlipoproteinemia
type IH: mucopolysaccharidosis
type I H/S: mucopolysaccharidosis
type II: acrocephalosyndactyly; cells; collagen; diabetes; dip; error; mucopolysaccharidosis
type II familial: hyperlipoproteinemia
type III: acrocephalosyndactyly; collagen; mucopolysaccharidosis
type III familial: hyperlipoproteinemia
type III hypersensitivity: reaction
type IS: mucopolysaccharidosis
type IV: acrocephalosyndactyly; collagen
type IVA, B: mucopolysaccharidosis
type IV familial: hyperlipoproteinemia
type V: acrocephalosyndactyly; mucopolysaccharidosis
type V familial: hyperlipoproteinemia
type VI: mucopolysaccharidosis

type VII: mucopolysaccharidosis
type VIII: mucopolysaccharidosis
typhoid: bacillus; bacteriophage; cholera; fever; pleurisy; pneumonia; septicemia; vaccine
typhoid-paratyphoid A and B: vaccine
typhus: vaccine
typical: achromatopsia; pseudocholinesterase
typist's: cramp
Tyrode's: solution
Tyrrell's: fascia
Tyson's: glands
Tyzzer's: disease
Tzanck: cells; test

U

U: wave
Uffelmann's: reagent
Uhl: anomaly
Uhthoff: symptom; syndrome
Uhthoff's: sign
ulcerating: granuloma of pudenda
ulcerative: colitis; dermatosis; enteritis; pharyngitis; posthitis; stomatitis
ulceromembranous: gingivitis; pharyngitis
Ullmann's: line; syndrome
ulnar: artery; branch of medial antebrachial cutaneous nerve; bursa; clubhand; eminence of wrist; head; margin of forearm; nerve; notch; reflex; veins
ulnar collateral: ligament; ligament of elbow; ligament of wrist
ulnar communicating: branch of superficial radial nerve
ulnar extensor: muscle of wrist
ulnar flexor: muscle of wrist
ultimate: principle; strength
ultimobranchial: body; pouch
ultra-: microscope
ultradian: rhythm
ultrafiltration: coefficient; hemodialyzer
ultralente: insulin
ultrashortwave: diathermy
ultrasonic: cardiography; cephalometry; cleaning; lithotresis; microscope; nebulizer; rays; scaler; therapy; waves
ultrasonic egg: recovery

ultrasound: cardiography; transducer
ultrastructural: anatomy
ultraviolet: keratoconjunctivitis; lamp; microscope; rays; spectrum
ultropaque: method
Ulysses: syndrome
umber: codon; mutation
umbilical: artery; cord; cyst; duct; fissure; fistula; fossa; fungus; hernia; notch; part of left branch of portal vein; region; ring; souffle; vein; vesicle
umbilical prevesical: fascia
umbilicated: cataract
umbilicomammillary: triangle
umbilicovesical: fascia
Umbre: virus
unarmed: rostellum
unavoidable: hemorrhage
unbalanced: translocation
uncal: herniation
unciform: bone; fasciculus
uncinate: attack; bundle of Russell; epilepsy; fasciculus of Russell; fit; gyrus; pancreas; process of ethmoid bone; process of pancreas
uncompensated: acidosis; alkalosis
uncompetitive: inhibition
unconditioned: reflex; response; stimulus
unconjugated: bilirubin
unconscious: homosexuality
uncoupling: factors
uncovertebral: joints
uncrossed: diplopia
uncus: band of Giacomini
undercut: gauge
undermining: ulcer
Underwood's: disease
undescended: testis
undetermined: nitrogen
undifferentiated: cell
undifferentiated cell: adenoma
undifferentiated type: fevers
undulant: fever
undulating: fever; membrane; pulse
unequal: cleavage; pulse
unequal retinal: image
unerupted: tooth
unesterified free: fatty acid
uneven: crossing-over
unformed visual: hallucination
ungual: phalanx; tuberosity
uniaxial: joint
unicameral: cyst
unicameral bone: cyst
unicanalicular: sphincter
unicellular: gland; sclerosis

unicorn: uterus
unidentified: reading frame
unidirectional: block; flux;
  replication
unilateral: anesthesia;
  hemianopia;
  hermaphroditism
unilateral hyperlucent: lung
unilateral lobar: emphysema
unilocular: cyst; fat; joint
unilocular hydatid: cyst
unimolecular: reaction
uninducible: mutant
uninhibited neurogenic:
  bladder
uninterrupted: suture
uniovular: twins
unipennate: muscle
unipolar: cell;
  electrocardiogram; leads;
  neuron
unit: character; fibrils;
  membrane
unit of: convergence
uniting: canal; cartilage; duct
univalent: antibody
univentricular: connections;
  heart
universal: antidote;
  appliance; donor;
  infantilism; solvent
unmodified zinc oxide-
  eugenol: cement
unmyelinated: fibers; nerve
Unna-Pappenheim: stain
Unna's: disease; mark; stain
Unna-Taenzer: stain
unpaired: allosome;
  chromosome
unresolved: pneumonia
unroofed coronary sinus:
  syndrome
unsaturated: alcohols; fat;
  fatty acid
unsharp: masking
unstable: angina; bladder;
  colloid; equilibrium;
  fracture; hemoglobins
unstable hemoglobin
  hemolytic: anemia
unstrained jaw: relation
unstriated: muscle
unsystematized: delusion
ununited: fracture
Unverricht's: disease
unwinding: proteins
upbeat: nystagmus
upper: airway; extremity;
  extremity of fibula; eyelid;
  jaw; limb; lip; lobe of lung
upper abdominal
  periosteal: reflex
upper GI: series
upper jaw: bone
upper lateral cutaneous:
  nerve of arm
upper motor: neuron;
  neuron

upper motor neuron: lesion
upper nodal: extrasystole
upper subscapular: nerve
upper thoracic splanchnic:
  nerves
upper uterine: segment
up promoter: mutation
ur-: defenses
urachal: cyst; fistula; fold;
  ligament
uracil: mustard
uranium: nephritis
uranyl acetate: stain
urate crystals: stain
Urbach-Wiethe: disease
urban: typhus
urban cutaneous:
  leishmaniasis
Urban's: operation
urea: clearance; cycle; frost;
  nitrogen
urea clearance: test
urease: test
urecholine supersensitivity:
  test
uremic: breath; colitis;
  coma; lung; pericarditis;
  pneumonia; pneumonitis;
  polyneuropathy
ureteral: branches; colic;
  meatus; opening
ureteric: branches; branches
  of the ovarian artery;
  branches of the patent part
  of umbilical artery;
  branches of the renal
  artery; branches of the
  testicular artery; bud;
  dysmenorrhea; fold;
  orifice; pelvis; plexus
ureterocutaneous: fistula
uretero-ileal: anastomosis
ureteropelvic: junction;
  obstruction
ureteropelvic junction:
  obstruction
ureterorenal: reflux
ureterosigmoid: anastomosis
ureterotubal: anastomosis
ureteroureteral: anastomosis
ureterovaginal: fistula
ureterovesical: obstruction
urethral: artery; calculus;
  carina of vagina; caruncle;
  crest; crest of female; crest
  of male; dilation;
  diverticulum; fever; glands;
  groove; hematuria; lacuna;
  openings; papilla; plate;
  stricture; surface of penis;
  syndrome; valves
urethral pressure: profile
urethrovaginal: fistula
urge: incontinence
uric acid: infarct
uricolytic: index
urinary: apparatus; bladder;
  calculus; casts; cyst; fever;

fistula; nitrogen; organs;
  reflex; sand;
  schistosomiasis; smear;
  stuttering; system; tract
urinary concentration: test
urinary exertional:
  incontinence
urinary tract: infection
uriniferous: tubule
urogenital: apparatus; canal;
  cleft; diaphragm; fistula;
  membrane; mesentery;
  region; ridge; septum;
  sinus; system; triangle
uropoietic: system
uropygial: gland
urorectal: fold; membrane;
  septum
urticaria: pigmentosa
urticarial: fever; vasculitis
u-score: method
Usher's: syndrome
USP: unit
usual interstitial: pneumonia
  of Liebow
uterine: appendages; artery;
  calculus; cavity; colic;
  contraction; dysmenorrhea;
  extremity of ovary; glands;
  horn; inertia; insufficiency;
  milk; opening of uterine
  tubes; ostium of uterine
  tubes; part of uterine tube;
  pregnancy; sinus; sinusoid;
  souffle; tetanus; tube;
  tympanites; veins
uterine relaxing: factor
uterine venous: plexus
uteroabdominal: pregnancy
uteroepichorial: membrane
utero-ovarian: varicocele
uteroperitoneal: fistula
uteroplacental: apoplexy;
  sinuses
uterosacral: ligament
uterovaginal: canal; plexus
uterovesical: fold; ligament;
  pouch
utilization: time
utricular: cyst; nerve;
  reflexes; spot
utriculoampullar: nerve
utriculosaccular: duct
uveal: part of trabecular
  reticulum; staphyloma;
  tract
uveocutaneous: syndrome
uveo-encephalitic: syndrome
uveomeningitis: syndrome
uveoparotid: fever
uviol: lamp
uvulae: muscle
Uzbekistan hemorrhagic:
  fever

V

V: antigen; gene; lead; wave

V-2: carcinoma
V-: esotropia; exotropia
vaccine: bodies; lymph; virus
vaccinia: virus
vaccinoid: reaction
VACTERL: syndrome
vacuolar: degeneration;
  nephrosis
vacuolating: virus
vacuum: aspirator; casting;
  desiccator; extractor; flask;
  headache; investing; tube
vacuum disk: phenomenon
vagabond's: disease
vagal: attack; bradycardia;
  part; part of accessory
  nerve; trigone; trunk
vaginal: artery; atresia;
  celiotomy; columns;
  dysmenorrhea; fornix;
  gland; hysterectomy;
  hysterotomy; introitus;
  laceration; lithotomy;
  mucosa; myomectomy;
  nerves; opening; orifice;
  plug; pool; portion of
  cervix; process; process of
  peritoneum; process of
  sphenoid bone; process of
  testis; smear; synovitis
vaginal cornification: test
vaginal mucification: test
vaginal synovial: membrane
vaginal venous: plexus
vagovagal: reflex
vagrant's: disease
vagus: area; nerve; pulse
valence: electron
Valentine's: position; test
Valentin's: corpuscles;
  ganglion; nerve
vallate: papilla
vallecular: dysphagia
Valleix's: points
valley: fever
Valsalva: maneuver; test
Valsalva's: antrum;
  ligaments; muscle; sinus
valvotomy: knife
valvular: endocarditis;
  incompetence;
  insufficiency;
  pneumothorax; prolapse;
  regurgitation; sclerosis;
  thrombus
vampire: bat
Van Bogaert: encephalitis
van Buchem's: syndrome
van Buren: sound
van Buren's: disease
van Deen's: test
van den Bergh's: test
van der Hoeve's: syndrome
van der Kolk's: law
van der Velden's: test
van der Waals': forces
van Ermengen's: stain

van Gieson's: stain
van Helmont's: mirror
van Horne's: canal
vanillylmandelic acid: test
vanished testis: syndrome
vanishing: cream; lung
vanishing lung: syndrome
Van Slyke: apparatus
Van Slyke's: formula
van't Hoff's: equation; law; theory
vapor: density; pressure
Vaquez': disease
variable: coupling; deceleration; region
variance: ratio
variant: angina pectoris; hemoglobin
varicella: encephalitis
varicella-zoster: virus
varicose: aneurysm; eczema; ulcer; veins
variegate: porphyria
variola: virus
varioliform: syphilid
Varolius': sphincter
vascular: bud; cataract; circle; circle of optic nerve; cones; dementia; dentin; fold of the cecum; gland; headache; keratitis; lacuna; lamina of choroid; layer; layer of choroid coat of eye; leiomyoma; meninx; murmur; nerve; papillae; pedicle; plexus; polyp; ring; sclerosis; sheaths; spider; spur; stripe; system; tunic of eye; zone
vascularized: graft
vasculocardiac: syndrome of hyperserotonemia
vasculogenic: impotence
vasoactive: amine
vasoactive intestinal: peptide; polypeptide
vasodepressor: substance; syncope
vasoformative: cell
vasogenic: shock
vasomotor: angina; ataxia; center; epilepsy; fibers; imbalance; nerve; neurosis; paralysis; rhinitis; spasm
vasopressin-resistant: diabetes
vasopressor: reflex
vasovagal: attack; epilepsy; syncope; syndrome
vastoadductor: fascia
vastus intermedius: muscle
vastus lateralis: muscle
vastus medialis: muscle
VATER: complex
Vater-Pacini: corpuscles
Vater's: ampulla; corpuscles; fold
VCE: smear

VDRL: test
vector: cardiography; loop
VEE: virus
vegetable: alkali; base; calomel; charcoal; gelatin; sulfur; wax
vegetal: pole
vegetative: bacteriophage; endocarditis; life; reproduction; stage
vegetative nervous: system
veil: cell
veiled: cells; puff
veiling: glare
vein: stone
Vel: antigen
velamentous: insertion
veldt: disease; sore
Vella's: fistula
vellus: hair
velocity: coefficient; constants
velopharyngeal: closure; insufficiency; seal; sphincter
Velpeau's: bandage; canal; fossa; hernia
velvet: ant
Ven: antigen
vena cava: filter
vena caval: foramen
venereal: bubo; disease; lymphogranuloma; sore; ulcer; wart
Venezuelan equine: encephalomyelitis
Venezuelan equine encephalomyelitis: virus
Venice: turpentine
Venn: diagram
venocaval: filter
venom: hemolysis
veno-occlusive: disease of the liver
venorespiratory: reflex
venous: angioma; angle; artery; blood; capillary; circle of mammary gland; congestion; embolism; foramen; gangrene; grooves; heart; hum; hyperemia; insufficiency; lakes; ligament; murmur; plexus; plexus of bladder; plexus of foramen ovale; plexus of hypoglossal canal; pulse; segments of the kidney; segments of liver; sinuses; sinus of sclera; star; stasis; valve
venous occlusion: plethysmography
venous-stasis: retinopathy
ventilation: meter
ventilation-perfusion: scan
ventilation/perfusion: ratio
ventilatory: compliance

ventral: aortas; border; branch; decubitus; glands; hernia; horn; mesocardium; mesogastrium; mesogastrium; nucleus of thalamus; nucleus of trapezoid body; pancreas; part of pons; plate; plate of neural tube; root; surface of digit
ventral anterior: nucleus of thalamus
ventral intermediate: nucleus of thalamus
ventral lateral: nucleus of thalamus
ventral posterior: nucleus of thalamus
ventral posterior intermediate: nucleus of thalamus
ventral posterolateral: nucleus of thalamus
ventral posteromedial: nucleus of thalamus
ventral primary: rami of cervical spinal nerves; rami of lumbar spinal nerves; rami of sacral spinal nerves; ramus of spinal nerve
ventral sacrococcygeal: ligament; muscle
ventral sacrococcygeus: muscle
ventral sacroiliac: ligaments
ventral spinocerebellar: tract
ventral spinothalamic: tract
ventral splanchnic: arteries
ventral tegmental: decussation
ventral thalamic: peduncle
ventral tier thalamic: nuclei
ventral white: column
ventricular: aberration; afterload; aneurysm; arteries; band of larynx; bigeminy; bradycardia; capture; complex; conduction; diastole; diverticulum; escape; extrasystole; fibrillation; fluid; flutter; fold; gradient; layer; ligament; loop; plateau; preload; rhythm; septum; standstill; systole; tachycardia; trigone
ventricular assist: device
ventricular filling: pressure
ventricular fusion: beat
ventricular inhibited pulse: generator
ventricular pre-: excitation
ventricular septal: defect
ventricular synchronous pulse: generator

ventricular triggered pulse: generator
ventriculoatrial: conduction
ventriculoradial: dysplasia
ventrobasal: nucleus
ventromedial: nucleus of hypothalamus
Venturi: effect; meter; tube
verbal: agraphia; apraxia
Veress: needle
Verga's: ventricle
Verheyen's: stars
Verhoeff's elastic tissue: stain
vermian: fossa
vermicular: colic; movement; pulse
vermiform: appendage; appendix; process
vermilion: border; zone
verminous: abscess; aneurysm; appendicitis; bronchitis; ileus
vermis: folium
vernal: catarrh; conjunctivitis; encephalitis; keratoconjunctivitis
Verner-Morrison: syndrome
Vernet's: syndrome
Verneuil's: neuroma
Vernier: acuity
Verocay: bodies
verrucous: carcinoma; hemangioma; hyperplasia; nevus; scrofuloderma; vegetations; xanthoma
versive: seizure
vertebral: arch; artery; border of scapula; canal; column; foramen; formula; fusion; ganglion; groove; nerve; notch; part of the costal surface of the lungs; part of diaphragm; plexus; polyarthritis; pulp; region; ribs; vein; venography
vertebral-basilar: system
vertebral epidural: space
vertebral venous: plexus; system
vertebra prominens: reflex
vertebrate: hormones
vertebrated: catheter; probe
vertebroarterial: foramen
vertebrochondral: ribs
vertebrocostal: trigone
vertebropelvic: ligaments
vertebrosternal: ribs
vertex: presentation
vertical: axis; dimension; elastic; heart; hymen; illumination; index; muscle of tongue; nystagmus; opening; osteotomy; overlap; parallax; plate; strabismus; transmission; vertigo
vertical banded: gastroplasty

WordFinder

vertical growth: phase
vertical retraction: syndrome
verticosubmental: view
Vesalius': bone; foramen; vein
vesical: calculus; diverticulum; fistula; gland; hematuria; lithotomy; plexus; reflex; surface of uterus; triangle; veins
vesicalis: anus
vesicating: gas
vesicle: hernia
vesicocolic: fistula
vesicocutaneous: fistula
vesicointestinal: fistula
vesicoumbilical: ligament
vesicoureteral: reflux; valve
vesicourethral: canal
vesicouterine: fistula; ligament; pouch
vesicovaginal: fistula
vesicovaginorectal: fistula
vesicular: appendage; appendices of uterine tube; exanthema; keratitis; keratopathy; mole; murmur; rale; resonance; respiration; rickettsiosis; stomatitis; transport
vesicular exanthema of swine: virus
vesicular ovarian: follicle
vesicular stomatitis: virus
vesicular venous: plexus
vesiculocavernous: respiration
vesiculotympanitic: resonance
Vesling's: line
vestibular: anus; area; branches of labyrinthine artery; canal; cecum of the cochlear duct; crest; fissure of cochlea; fold; fossa; ganglion; glands; labium of limbus of spiral lamina; labyrinth; ligament; lip of limbus of spiral lamina; membrane; nerve; neuronitis; nucleus; nystagmus; organ; part of vestibulocochlear nerve; root; root of vestibulocochlear nerve; screen; surface of tooth; veins; wall of cochlear duct; window
vestibular blind: sac
vestibular hair: cells
vestibular ocular: reflex
vestibulocerebellar: ataxia
vestibulocochlear: nerve; nuclei; organ
vestibulo-equilibratory: control
vestibulospinal: reflex; tract

vestigial: fold; muscle; organ
Veterans Administration: hospital
veterinary: medicine
Vi: antibody; antigen
viable cell: count
vibrating: line
vibration: syndrome; tolerance
vibratory: massage; sensibility; urticaria
vibrionic: abortion
vicarious: hypertrophy; menstruation
Vicat: needle
vicious: cicatrix; circle; union
Vicq d'Azyr's: bundle; centrum semiovale; foramen
Victor-Michaelis-Menten: equation
Vidal's: disease
video: fluoroscopy
video-assisted thoracic: surgery
vidian: artery; canal; nerve; vein
Vierra's: sign
Vieussens': annulus; ansa; centrum; foramina; ganglia; isthmus; limbus; loop; ring; valve; veins; ventricle
view: box
villonodular pigmented: tenosynovitis
villous: adenoma; atrophy; carcinoma; papilloma; placenta; tenosynovitis; tumor
Vinca: alkaloids
Vincent's: angina; bacillus; disease; infection; spirillum; tonsillitis
Vincent's white: mycetoma
Vineberg: procedure
vinous: liquor
violinist's: cramp
Vipond's: sign
viral: cystitis; dysentery; encephalomyelitis; envelope; gastroenteritis; hemagglutination; hepatitis; hepatitis type A; hepatitis type B; hepatitis type C; hepatitis type D; hepatitis type E; neutralization; pericarditis; probe; strand; therapy; tropism; wart
viral hemorrhagic: fever
viral hemorrhagic fever: virus
Virchow-Hassall: bodies
Virchow-Holder: angle
Virchow-Robin: space
Virchow's: angle; cells; corpuscles; crystals;

disease; law; node; psammoma
virgin: generation; silk
virginal: membrane
Virginia: snakeroot
viridans: hemolysis
virile: member
virtual: focus; image
virulent: bacteriophage; bubo
virulent phage: mutant
virus: blockade; hepatitis; hepatitis of ducks; keratoconjunctivitis; pneumonia of pigs
virus A: hepatitis
virus-associated hemophagocytic: syndrome
virus B: hepatitis
virus C: hepatitis
virus-transformed: cell
virus X: disease
visceral: anesthesia; arches; brain; cavity; cleft; crises; disorder; epilepsy; inversion; larva migrans; layer; layer of serous pericardium; layer of tunica vaginalis of testis; leishmaniasis; leishmaniasis; lymph nodes; lymphomatosis; mesoderm; muscle; nerve; nodes; pericardium; peritoneum; plate; pleura; pleurisy; sense; skeleton; surface of liver; surface of the spleen; swallow
visceral disease: virus
visceral motor: neuron
visceral nervous: system
visceral pelvic: fascia
visceral traction: reflex
viscerogenic: reflex
visceromotor: reflex
visceropannicular: reflex
viscerosensory: reflex
viscerotrophic: reflex
viscoelastic: retardation
visibility: acuity
visible: spectrum
visiting: nurse
visna: virus
visual: acuity; agnosia; angle; aphasia; area; axis; blackout; cortex; cycle; efficiency; extinction; field; image; inattention; organ; pathway; pigments; projection; purple; threshold; violet; yellow
visual evoked: potential
visual orbicularis: reflex
visual receptor: cells
visual-spatial: agnosia
vita: glass

vital: capacity; center; force; index; knot; node; pulp; signs; spirits; stain; statistics; tooth; tripod; ultraviolet
vitality: test
vitamin A: unit
vitamin B_2: unit
vitamin B_{12}: neuropathy
vitamin B_6: unit
vitamin B_1 hydrochloride: unit
vitamin C: test; unit
vitamin D: milk; unit
vitamin D-binding: protein
vitamin D-resistant: rickets
vitamin E: unit
vitamin K: unit
vitelliform: degeneration
vitelline: artery; cord; duct; fistula; membrane; pole; reservoir; sac; vein; vessels
vitelliruptive: degeneration
vitellointestinal: cyst
vitiated: air
vitreoretinal choroidopathy: syndrome
vitreoretinal traction: syndrome
vitreo-tapetoretinal: dystrophy
vitreous: body; camera; cell; chamber of eye; detachment; hernia; humor; lamella; membrane; table
in vitro: fertilization
vivax: fever; malaria
in vivo: fertilization
Vladimiroff-Mikulicz: amputation
VMA: test
vocal: amusia; cord; fold; fremitus; ligament; muscle; process; process of arytenoid cartilage; resonance; shelf
vocal cord: nodules
vocalis: muscle
Vogel's: law
Voges-Proskauer: reaction
Vogt: syndrome
Vogt-Koyanagi: syndrome
Vogt's: angle
Vogt-Spielmeyer: disease
Vohwinkel: syndrome
voiding: cystogram
voiding flow: rate
Voigt's: lines
volar carpal: ligament
volar interosseous: artery; nerve
volatile: anesthetic; mustard oil; oil
volatile fatty acid: number
vole: bacillus
Volhard's: test
volitional: tremor

Volkmann's: canals; cheilitis; contracture; spoon
Vollmer: test
Volpe-Manhold: Index
voltage-gated: channel
voltaic: taste
Voltolini's: disease
volume: element; index; substitute; unit
volume-controlled: respirator
volume-displacement: plethysmograph
volumetric: analysis; flask; solution
voluntary: dehydration; guarding; hospital; muscle; mutism; nystagmus
volutin: granules
vomeral: groove; sulcus
vomerine: canal; cartilage
vomerobasilar: canal
vomeronasal: organ
vomerorostral: canal
vomerovaginal: canal; groove
vomiting: gas; reflex
von Economo's: disease
von Gierke's: disease
von Graefe's: sign
von Hippel-Lindau: syndrome
von Kossa: stain
von Langenbeck's bipedicle mucoperiosteal: flap
von Meyenburg's: disease
von Recklinghausen: disease
von Spee's: curve
von Willebrand: factor
von Willebrand's: disease
Voorhoeve's: disease
vortex: veins
vorticose: veins
Vossius' lenticular: ring
VS: virus
vulnerable: period; phase
vulnerable child: syndrome
Vulpian's: atrophy
vulsella: forceps
vulvar: dystrophy; slit
vulvovaginal: cystectomy; gland
Vw: antigen
V-Y: flap; plasty; procedure

W

W: chromosome; factor; procedure; rays
W-: arch
"w": hernia
Waardenburg: syndrome
Wachendorf's: membrane
Wachstein-Meissel: stain for calcium-magnesium-ATPase
Wada: test
waddingtonian: homeostasis

waddling: gait
Wagner's: disease; syndrome
Wagstaffe's: fracture
waiter's: cramp
Walcher: position
Waldenström's: macroglobulinemia; purpura; syndrome; test
Waldeyer's: fossae; glands; sheath; space; tract
Waldeyer's throat: ring
Waldeyer's zonal: layer
Walker: carcinoma; carcinosarcoma; tractotomy
Walker's: chart
walking: typhoid
walk-through: angina
Wallenberg's: syndrome
wallerian: degeneration; law
wallet: stomach
Walthard's cell: rest
Walther's: canals; dilator; ducts; ganglion; plexus
waltzed: flap
wandering: abscess; cell; erysipelas; goiter; kidney; liver; organ; pacemaker; pneumonia
Wangensteen: drainage; suction; tube
Wang's: test
war: neurosis
warble: botfly; fly
Warburg-Dickens-Horecker: shunt
Warburg-Lipmann-Dickens-Horecker: shunt
Warburg's: apparatus; theory
Warburg's old yellow: enzyme
Warburg's respiratory: enzyme
Ward-Romano: syndrome
Wardrop's: disease; method
Ward's: triangle
warehouseman's: itch
warm: agglutinins; autoantibody
warm-blooded: animal
warm-cold: hemolysin
Warren: shunt
Wartenberg's: symptom
Warthin-Finkeldey: cells
Warthin's: tumor
Warthin-Starry silver: stain
warty: dyskeratoma; horn
wash-: bottle
washed: sulfur
washed field: technique
washerman's: mark
washerwoman's: itch
washing: soda
washout: cannula; test
Wasmann's: glands
wasserhelle: cell

Wassermann: antibody; reaction; test
wasted: ventilation
wasting: disease; palsy; paralysis; syndrome
watchmaker's: cramp
water: aspirator; bath; bed; canker; depletion; diuresis; dressing; gas; glass; intoxication; itch; sore
water-clear: cell of parathyroid
water-drinking: test
water-hammer: pulse
Waterhouse-Friderichsen: syndrome
watering-can: perineum; scrotum
Waters': operation; projection; view
watershed: infarction
water-soluble: chlorophyll derivatives
Waterston: operation; shunt
Waters' view: radiograph
water-trap: stomach
water wheel: murmur
waterwheel: sound
water-whistle: sound
watery: eye
Watson-Crick: helix
Watson-Schwartz: test
wave: analyzer; form; number
wax: acid; alcohol; expansion; form; pattern
wax model: denture
wax-tipped: bougie
waxy: cast; degeneration; fingers; kidney; liver; spleen
WDHA: syndrome
wear-and-tear: pigment
weaver's: cough
weaving: syndrome
web: eye
Webb: antigen
webbed: fingers; neck; penis; toes
Weber-Christian: disease
Weber-Cockayne: syndrome
Weber-Fechner: law
Weber's: experiment; glands; law; organ; paradox; point; sign; syndrome; test for hearing; triangle
Webster's: operation; test
Wechsler-Bellevue: scale
Wechsler intelligence: scales
weddellite: calculus
Wedensky: effect; facilitation; inhibition
wedge: biopsy; bone; pressure; resection; spirometer
wedge-and-groove: joint; suture

wedge-shaped: fasciculus; tubercle
WEE: virus
weekend: hospital
Weeks': bacillus
weeping: eczema
Wegener's: granulomatosis
Wegner's: disease; line
Weibel-Palade: bodies
Weichselbaum's: coccus
Weidel's: reaction
Weigert-Gram: stain
Weigert's: law; stain for actinomyces; stain for elastin; stain for fibrin; stain for myelin; stain for neuroglia
Weigert's iodine: solution
Weigert's iron hematoxylin: stain
weight: sense
Weil-Felix: reaction; test
Weill-Marchesani: syndrome
Weil's: disease
Weil's basal: layer; zone
Weinberg's: reaction
Weingrow's: reflex
Weir Mitchell: treatment
Weir Mitchell's: disease
Weir's: operation
Weisbach's: angle
Weiss': sign
Weitbrecht's: cartilage; cord; fibers; foramen; ligament
Welch's: bacillus
Welcker's: angle
welder's: conjunctivitis; lung
well: counter
well-differentiated lymphocytic: lymphoma
Wells': syndrome
Wenckebach: block; period; phenomenon
Wenzel's: ventricle
Wepfer's: glands
Werdnig-Hoffmann: disease
Werdnig-Hoffmann muscular: atrophy
Werlhof's: disease
Wernekinck's: commissure; decussation
Werner's: syndrome; test
Wernicke-Korsakoff: encephalopathy; syndrome
Wernicke's: aphasia; area; center; disease; encephalopathy; field; radiation; reaction; region; sign; syndrome; zone
Wertheim's: operation
Werther's: disease
Wesselsbron: disease; fever
Wesselsbron disease: virus
West African: fever; trypanosomiasis

WordFinder

West African sleeping: sickness
Westberg's: space
Westergren: method
Westermark's: sign
Western blot: analysis
western equine: encephalomyelitis
western equine encephalomyelitis: virus
West Indian: smallpox
West Nile: fever; virus
West Nile encephalitis: virus
Westphal-Erb: sign
Westphal-Piltz: phenomenon
Westphal's: disease; phenomenon; pseudosclerosis; sign
Westphal's pupillary: reflex
Westphal-Strümpell: pseudosclerosis
West's: syndrome
wet: beriberi; compress; cup; dream; gangrene; lung; nurse; pack; pleurisy; shock; tetter
wet cutaneous: leishmaniasis
wet and dry bulb: thermometer
wettable: sulfur
Wetzel: grid
Wever-Bray: phenomenon
Weyers-Thier: syndrome
whale: fingers
Wharton's: duct; jelly
wheal-and-erythema: reaction
wheal-and-flare: reaction
wheat: germ; gum
wheat pasture: poisoning
Wheatstone's: bridge
Wheeler: method
Wheeler-Johnson: test
Wheelhouse's: operation
whetstone: crystals
whewellite: calculus
whey: alum; protein
whip: bougie
whiplash: injury
Whipple's: disease; operation
whispered: bronchophony; pectoriloquy
whistle-tip: catheter
whistling: deformity; rale
whistling face: syndrome
white: arsenic; beeswax; bile; commissure; corpuscle; diarrhea; fat; fiber; fingers; forelock; gangrene; graft; infarct; lead; leg; line; line of anal canal; line of Toldt; matter; muscle; mustard; petrolatum; piedra; pine; pitch; pulp; rami communicantes; reaction;

spot; substance; thrombus; turpentine; wax; yolk
white blood: cell
white blood cell: cast
white cell: cast
whitegraft: reaction
Whitehead: deformity
Whitehead's: operation
white mercuric: precipitate
white muscle: disease
white-out: syndrome
white pupillary: reflex
white soft: paraffin
white sponge: nevus
white spot: disease
Whitman's: frame
Whitmore's: bacillus; disease
Whitnall's: tubercle
whole: blood
whole-body: counter
whole-body titration: curve
whooping: cough
whooping-cough: vaccine
whorled: enamel
WI-38: cells
Wickham's: striae
Widal's: reaction; syndrome
wide: plane; spectrum
wide field: ocular
wide-latitude: film
Wigand: maneuver
wild: ginger; mandrake; tobacco; type; yeast
Wildermuth's: ear
Wilder's: diet; law of initial value; sign; stain for reticulum
Wildervanck: syndrome
Wilde's: cords; triangle
wildfire: rash
wild-type: strain
Wilhelmy: balance
Wilkie's: artery; disease
Willett's: forceps
Williams: factor; syndrome
Williams': stain; syndrome
Williams-Beurer: syndrome
Willis': centrum nervosum; cords; pancreas; paracusis; pouch
Williston's: law
Wilms': tumor
Wilson: block
Wilson-Mikity: syndrome
Wilson's: disease; lichen; method; muscle; syndrome
Windigo: psychosis
window: level; width
wine: spirit
wing: cell; plate
wing-beating: tumor
winged: catheter; scapula
Winiwarter-Buerger: disease
wink: reflex
winking: spasm
Winkler's: disease

Winslow's: foramen; ligament; pancreas; stars
winter: dysentery of cattle; eczema; itch; sleep
Winterbottom's: sign
Winternitz': sound
Wintersteiner: compound F; rosettes
wire: arch; splint
wire-loop: lesion
Wirsung's: canal; duct
wiry: pulse
wisdom: tooth
Wiskott-Aldrich: syndrome
Wissler's: syndrome
Wistar: rats
witch's: milk
withdrawal: reflex; symptoms; syndrome
wobble: base; hypothesis
Wohlfart-Kugelberg-Welander: disease
wolf: tooth
Wolfe: graft
Wolfe-Krause: graft
Wolfe's: method
Wolff-Chaikoff: block; effect
wolffian: body; cyst; duct; rest; ridge; tubules
wolffian duct: carcinoma
Wolff-Parkinson-White: syndrome
Wolff's: law
Wölfler's: gland
Wolf-Orton: bodies
Wolfring's: glands
Wollaston's: doublet; theory
Wolman's: disease; xanthomatosis
Wood: units
wood: charcoal; naphtha; spirit; sugar
wood: vinegar
woodcutter's: encephalitis
wooden: resonance; tongue of cattle
wooden-shoe: heart
Wood's: glass; lamp; light
wool: ball; fat; maggot; wax
Woolf-Lineweaver-Burk: plot
woolly: hair
woolly-hair: nevus
Woolner's: tip
wool-sorter's: pneumonia
woolsorter's: disease
word: deafness
Woringer-Kolopp: disease
working: bite; contacts; occlusion; side
working occlusal: surfaces
working side: condyle
worm: abscess; aneurysm
wormian: bones
Wormley's: test
Worth's: amblyoscope
Woulfe's: bottle

wound: botulism; clip; dehiscence; fever; myiasis
woven: bone
Wr^a: antigen
Wright: antigens; respirometer
Wright's: stain; syndrome; version
wrinkler: muscle of eyebrow
Wrisberg's: cartilage; ganglia; ligament; nerve; tubercle
wrist: clonus; joint; sign
wrist clonus: reflex
writer's: cramp
writhing: number
writing: hand
wrought: wire
wry: neck
Wurster's: reagent; test
Wyburn-Mason: syndrome

X

X: body; disease; disease of cattle; inactivation
X: zone
X-: strabismus
X-: esotropia; exotropia
x: wave
x^2: test
x-: ray
xanthene: dyes
xanthogranulomatous: cholecystitis; pyelonephritis
xanthoprotein: reaction
xenogeneic: graft
xenon-arc: photocoagulator
xenotropic: virus
xerotic: degeneration; keratitis
Xg: antigen
xiphisternal: joint
xiphisternal crunching: sound
xiphoid: cartilage; process
Xiphophorus: test
X-linked: gene; hypogammaglobulinemia; hypogammaglobulinemia with growth hormone deficiency; ichthyosis; inheritance; locus
XO: female; syndrome
x-ray: dosimetry; generator; microscope; therapy; tube
XX: male
XXX: female
XXY: male; syndrome
xylose: test
xylostyptic: ether
XYY: male; syndrome

Y

Y: body; cartilage
Y-: axis

y: wave
y-: angle
Yaba: tumor; virus
Yaba monkey: virus
Yangtze: edema
Yangtze Valley: fever
yeast: fungus; RNase
yeast artificial: chromosomes
yeast extract: agar
yellow: atrophy of the liver; body; cartilage; corallin; disease; enzyme; fever; fibers; hepatization; ligament; mercury iodide; nail; precipitate; skin; spot; vision; wax; yolk
yellow bone: marrow
yellow fever: vaccine; virus
yellow nail: syndrome
yellow soft: paraffin
yield: strength; stress
Y-linked: gene; inheritance; locus
yoke: bone
yolk: cells; cleavage; membrane; sac; stalk
yolk sac: carcinoma; tumor
Yorke's autolytic: reaction
Young: syndrome
Young-Helmholtz: theory of color vision
Young prostatic: tractor
Young's: modulus; rule
Y-shaped: ligament
Yt^a: antigen
Yvon's: test

Z

Z: band; disk; filament; gene; line; procedure
Z-: DNA; protein
Zaffaroni: system
Zaglas': ligament
Zahn's: infarct
Zambesi: ulcer
Zappert counting: chamber
zebra: body
Zeeman: effect
Zeis': glands
zeisian: sty
Zellweger: syndrome
Zenker's: degeneration; diverticulum; fixative; necrosis; paralysis
zero: gravity
zero degree: teeth
zero end-expiratory: pressure
zero-order: reaction
zero time-binding: DNA
zeta: potential
zeta sedimentation: ratio
Ziehen-Oppenheim: disease
Ziehl-Neelsen: stain
Ziehl's: stain
Ziemann's: dots; stippling
Zieve's: syndrome
Zika: fever; virus
Zimany's bilobed: flap
Zimmerlin's: atrophy
Zimmermann: reaction; test

Zimmermann's: corpuscle; granule
Zimmermann's elementary: particle
zinc: colic; finger; gelatin
zinc fume: fever
zinc phosphate: cement
zinc sulfate flotation centrifugation: method
Zinn's: artery; corona; ligament; membrane; ring; tendon; zonule
Zinn's vascular: circle
zirconium: granuloma
Zivert: syndrome
Zollinger-Ellison: syndrome; tumor
Zöllner's: lines
zonal: necrosis
zonary: placenta
Zondek-Aschheim: test
zone: centrifugation
zonular: band; cataract; fibers; layer; scotoma; spaces
zoo blot: analysis
zoonotic: infection; potential
zoonotic cutaneous: leishmaniasis
Zoon's: erythroplasia
zooplastic: graft
zoster: encephalomyelitis
zoster immune: globulin
Zsigmondy's: test
Z-tract: injection

Zubrod: scale
Zuckerkandl's: bodies; convolution; fascia
zwitter: hypothesis
zwitterionic: buffer; detergent; surfactant
zygal: fissure
zygapophyseal: joints
zygomatic: arch; bone; border of greater wing of sphenoid bone; branch of facial nerve; diameter; fossa; margin of greater wing of sphenoid bone; nerve; process of frontal bone; process of maxilla; process of temporal bone; region
zygomaticoauricular: index
zygomaticofacial: branch of zygomatic nerve; foramen
zygomaticomaxillary: suture
zygomatico-orbital: artery; foramen
zygomaticotemporal: branch of zygomatic nerve; foramen; suture
zygomaticus major: muscle
zygomaticus minor: muscle
zygomaxillary: point
zymogen: granule
zymogenic: cell
zymoplastic: substance
zymotic: papilloma
ZZ: genotype

ab

α 1. First letter of the Greek alphabet, alpha; used as a classifier in the nomenclature of many sciences. **2.** Symbol for Bunsen's solubility *coefficient*. **3.** In chemistry, denotes the first in a series, a position immediately adjacent to a carboxyl group, the first of a series of closely related compounds, an aromatic substituent on an aliphatic chain, or the direction of a chemical bond away from the viewer. **4.** Abbreviation for alpha *particle*. **5.** In chemistry, symbol for angle of optical *rotation*; degree of dissociation. For terms beginning with this prefix, see the specific term.

[α] Symbol for specific optical *rotation*.

α₁PI Symbol for human α_1-proteinase *inhibitor*.

A 1. Abbreviation for ampere; adenine; alanine; Helmholtz *energy*. **2.** As a subscript, refers to alveolar *gas*. **3.** Symbol (usually capitalized italic) for absorbance. **4.** Symbol for adenosine or adenylic acid in polynucleotides; alanine in polypeptides; first substrate in a multisubstrate enzyme=catalyzed reaction.

°A Symbol for degree absolute; replaced by K (kelvin).

Å Symbol for angstrom.

A⁻ Symbol for anion.

A. Symbol for absorbance.

a 1. Abbreviation for total *acidity*; ante; area; asymmetric; auris; artery; arteria [NA]. **2.** Symbol for atto-. **3.** As a subscript, refers to systemic arterial blood.

a Symbol for specific absorption *coefficient*. Abbreviation for absorptivity.

♲**a-, an-.** Not, without, -less; equivalent to L. *in-* and E. *un-*. [G. not, un-, usually *an-* before a vowel]

AA, aa Abbreviation for amino acid; aminoacyl.

aa. Abbreviation for arteriae [NA], arteries.

āā. Abbreviation for G. *ana*, of each; used in prescription writing following the name of two or more ingredients.

Aad Abbreviation for α-aminoadipic acid.

AAF Abbreviation for 2-acetylaminofluorene; 2-acetamidofluorene.

AAMC Abbreviation for Association of American Medical Colleges.

AAR Abbreviation for antigen-antibody *reaction*.

Aaron, Charles D., U.S. physician, 1866–1951. SEE A.'s *sign*.

Aarskog, Dagfinn J., Norwegian pediatrician, *1928. SEE A.-Scott *syndrome*.

AASH Abbreviation for adrenal androgen-stimulating *hormone*.

AAV Abbreviation for adeno-associated *virus*.

Ab Abbreviation for antibody.

♲**ab-, abs-.** **1.** From, away from, off. **2.** Prefix applied to electrical units in the CGS-electromagnetic system to distinguish them from units in the CGS-electrostatic system (prefix stat-) and those in the metric system or SI system (no prefix). [L. *ab*, from, usually *abs-* before c, q, and t; often *a-*before m, p, or v]

Abadie, Joseph Louis Irénée Jean, French neurosurgeon, 1873–1946. SEE A.'s *sign* of tabes dorsalis.

ab·am·pere (ab-am′pēr). Electromagnetic unit of current equal to 10 absolute amperes; a current that exerts a force of 2π dynes on a unit magnetic pole at the center of a circle of wire (1 cm in radius).

abap·i·cal (ă-bap′i-kăl). Opposite the apex.

abar·og·no·sis (ā-bar′og-nō′sis). Loss of ability to appreciate the weight of objects held in the hand, or to differentiate objects of different weights. When the primary senses are intact, caused by a lesion of the contralateral parietal lobe. [G. *a-* priv. + *baros*, weight, + *gnōsis*, knowledge]

aba·sia (ă-bā′zē-ă). Rarely used term for the inability to walk. SEE gait. [G. *a-* priv. + *basis*, step]

atactic a., ataxic a., difficulty in walking due to ataxia of the legs.

choreic a., a. related to choreiform movements of the legs.

spastic a., a. due to a spastic contraction of the muscles when an attempt is made to walk.

a. trep′idans, a. due to trembling of the lower limbs.

aba·si·a-asta·si·a. SEE astasia-abasia.

aba·sic (ă-bā′sik). **1.** Affected by, or associated with, abasia; also abatic (ă-bat′ik). **2.** Refers to loss of pyrimidine sites in DNA.

ab·ax·i·al, ab·ax·ile (ab-ak′sē-ăl, -ak′sīl). **1.** Lying outside the axis of any body or part. **2.** Situated at the opposite extremity of the axis of a part.

Abbe, Robert, U.S. surgeon, 1851–1928. SEE A. *flap, operation*.

Abbé, Ernst K., German physicist, 1840–1905. SEE A.'s *condenser*.

Abbott, Alexander C., U.S. bacteriologist, 1860–1935. SEE A.'s *stain* for spores.

Abbott, Edville G., U.S. orthopedic surgeon, 1871–1938. SEE A.'s *method*.

Abbott, W. Osler, U.S. physician, 1902–1943. SEE A.'s *tube;* Miller-A. *tube*.

Abbott's ar·tery. See under artery.

ab·cou·lomb (ab-kū-lom′). A unit of electrical charge equal to 10 coulombs. The charge that passes over a given surface in 1 second if a current of 1 abampere is flowing across the surface. [ab + coulomb]

ab·do·men (ab-dō′men, ab′dō-men) [NA]. The part of the trunk that lies between the thorax and the pelvis. The a. does not include the vertebral region posteriorly but is considered by some anatomists to include the pelvis (abdominopelvic cavity). It includes the greater part of the abdominal cavity (cavum abdominis [NA]), and is divided by arbitrary planes into nine regions. SEE ALSO abdominal *regions*, under *region*. SYN venter (1). [L. *abdomen*, etym. uncertain]

acute a., any serious acute intra-abdominal condition (such as appendicitis) attended by pain, tenderness, and muscular rigidity, and for which emergency surgery must be considered. SYN surgical a.

boat-shaped a., SYN scaphoid a.

carinate a., a sloping of the sides with prominence of the central line of the a.

navicular a., SYN scaphoid a.

a. obsti′pum, rarely used term for deformity of the a. due to congenitally short rectus muscles.

pendulous a., an a. with greatly relaxed walls that sag down over the pubic region.

protuberant a., unusual or prominent convexity of the a., due to excessive subcutaneous fat, poor muscle tone, or an increase in intra-abdominal content.

scaphoid a., a condition in which the anterior abdominal wall is sunken and presents a concave rather than a convex contour. SYN boat-shaped a., navicular a.

surgical a., SYN acute a.

ab·dom·i·nal (ab-dom′i-năl). Relating to the abdomen.

♲**abdomino-, abdomin-.** The abdomen, abdominal. [L. *abdomen, abdominis*]

♲ Combining forms	[NA] Nomina Anatomica
Word*Finder* **Multi-term entry finder** Preceding letter A	[MIM] Mendelian Inheritance in Man
A.D.A.M. Anatomy Plates Between letters L and M	☆ Official alternate term
Appendices: Following letter Z	☆[NA] Official alternate Nomina Anatomica term
SYN Synonym; Cf., compare	**High Profile Term**

ab·dom·i·no·cen·te·sis (ab-dom'i-nō-sen-tē'sis). Paracentesis of the abdomen. [abdomino- + G. *kentēsis,* puncture]

ab·dom·i·no·cy·e·sis (ab-dom'i-nō-sī-ē'sis). **1.** SYN abdominal *pregnancy.* **2.** SYN secondary abdominal *pregnancy.* [abdomino- + G. *kyēsis,* pregnancy]

ab·dom·i·no·cys·tic (ab-dom-i-nō-sis'tik). SYN abdominovesical. [abdomino- + G. *kystis,* bladder]

ab·dom·i·no·gen·i·tal (ab-dom'i-nō-gen'i-tăl). Relating to the abdomen and the genital organs.

ab·dom·i·no·hys·ter·ec·to·my (ab-dom'i-nō-his-ter-ek'tō-mē). SYN abdominal *hysterectomy.*

ab·dom·i·no·hys·ter·ot·o·my (ab-dom'i-nō-his-ter-ot'ō-mē). SYN abdominal *hysterotomy.*

ab·dom·i·no·pel·vic (ab-dom'i-nō-pel'vik). Relating to the abdomen and pelvis, especially the combined abdominal and pelvic cavities.

ab·dom·i·no·per·i·ne·al (ab-dom'i-nō-pār-i-nē'ăl). Relating to both abdomen and perineum, as in abdominoperineal resection of the rectum.

ab·dom·i·no·plas·ty (ab-dom'i-nō-plas-tē). An operation performed on the abdominal wall for esthetic purposes. [abdomino- + G. *plastos,* formed]

ab·dom·i·nos·co·py (ab-dom-i-nos'kŏ-pē). SYN peritoneoscopy. [abdomino- + G. *skopeō,* to examine]

ab·dom·i·no·scro·tal (ab-dom'i-nō-skrō'tăl). Relating to the abdomen and the scrotum.

ab·dom·i·no·tho·rac·ic (ab-dom'i-nō-thō-ras'ik). Relating to both abdomen and thorax.

ab·dom·i·no·vag·i·nal (ab-dom'i-nō-vag'i-năl). Relating to both abdomen and vagina.

ab·dom·i·no·ves·i·cal (ab-dom'i-nō-ves'i-kăl). Relating to the abdomen and urinary bladder, or to the abdomen and gallbladder. SYN abdominocystic.

ab·duce (ab-dūs'). SYN abduct.

ab·du·cens (ab-dū'senz). SYN abducent. [L.]

   a. oc'uli, SYN lateral rectus *muscle.*

ab·du·cent (ab-dū'sent). **1.** Abducting; drawing away, especially away from the median plane. **2.** SYN abducent *nerve.* SYN abducens. [L. *abducens*]

ab·duct (ab-dŭkt'). To move away from the median plane. SYN abduce.

ab·duc·tion (ab-dŭk'shŭn). **1.** Movement of a body part away from the median plane (of the body, in the case of limbs; of the hand or foot, in the case of digits). **2.** Monocular rotation (duction) of the eye toward the temple. **3.** A position resulting from such movement. Cf. adduction. [L. *abductio*]

ab·duc·tor (ab-dŭk'ter, -tōr). A muscle that draws a part away from the median plane; or, in the case of the digits, away from the normal axis of the middle finger or the second toe.

Abegg, Richard, Danish chemist, 1869–1910. SEE A.'s *rule.*

Abel, Rudolf, German bacteriologist, 1868–1942. SEE A.'s *bacillus.*

Abell-Kendall meth·od. See under method.

Abelson, Herbert T., U.S. pediatrician, *1941. SEE A. murine leukemia *virus.*

ab·em·bry·on·ic (ab'em-brē-on'ik). The area of the blastocyst opposite the region where the embryo is formed. [L. *ab,* from, + embryonic]

ab·en·ter·ic (ab-en-ter'ik). A rarely used term meaning away from the intestine, said of a morbid process occurring elsewhere that would normally occur in the intestine. [L. *ab,* from, + G. *enteron,* intestine]

Abernethy, John, British surgeon and anatomist, 1764–1831. SEE A.'s *fascia.*

ab·er·rant (ab-er'ant). **1.** Wandering off; said of certain ducts, vessels, or nerves deviating from the normal course or pattern. **2.** Differing from the normal; in botany or zoology, said of certain atypical individuals in a species. **3.** SYN ectopic (1). [L. *aberrans*]

ab·er·ra·tion (ab-er-ā'shŭn). **1.** Deviating from the normal

course or pattern. **2.** Deviant development or growth. SEE ALSO chromosome. [L. *aberratio*]

chromatic a., the difference in focus or magnification of an image arising because of a difference in the refraction of different wavelengths composing white light. SYN chromatism (2), color a., newtonian a.

chromosome a., any deviation from the normal number or morphology of chromosomes; also the phenotypic consequences thereof.

frequent numerical chromosome aberrations		
chromosome count (sex chromatin)		
autosomal trisomy G (Down syndrome)		
1 additional chromosome 21		
	a) regular kind of additional chromosome as mosaic	47 46/47
	b) translocation G/G additional chromosome, bound with a chromosome 21 or 22	46
	c) translocation D/G additional chromosome, bound with a chromosome of the D group	46
trisomy D (Paetau syndrome) 1 additional D$_1$ chromosome (no. 13)		47
trisomy E (Edward syndrome) 1 additional chromosome 18		47
sex chromosomes monosomy X-XO (Turner syndrome) 1 X-chromosome is missing, female phenotype		45 (∅)
trisomy XXX 1 additional X chromosome, female phenotype		47 (++)
trisomy XXY 1 additional X chromosome, male phenotype (Klinefelter syndrome)		47 (+)
1 additional Y chromosome, usually male phenotype		47 (∅)
tetrasomies (XXXY, XXYY) and pentasomies are rarely observed		

color a., SYN chromatic a.

coma a., (1) the distortion of image formation created when a bundle of light rays enters an optical system not parallel to the optic axis. **(2)** in botany, any tuft, as the hairs on a seed, or the greenery on a radish or a pineapple. SYN coma (3). [G. *komē,* hair, foliage]

curvature a., lack of spatial correspondence causing the image of a straight extended object to appear curved.

dioptric a., SYN spherical a.

distortion a., the faulty formation of an image arising because the magnification of the peripheral part of an object is different from that of the central part when viewed through a lens.

lateral a., in spherical a., the distance between paraxial focus of central rays on the optic axis.

longitudinal a., in spherical a., the distance separating the focus of paraxial and peripheral rays on the optic axis.

mental a., disturbed thought or behavior that connotes a psychological or psychiatric impairment. SEE delusion.

meridional a., an a. produced in the plane of a single meridian of a lens.

monochromatic a., a defect in an optical image arising because of the nature of lenses; the main types are spherical, coma, curvature, and distortion a., and astigmatism of oblique pencils.

newtonian a., SYN chromatic a.

optical a., failure of rays from a point source to form a perfect image after traversing an optical system.

spherical a., a monochromatic a. occurring in refraction at a spherical surface in which the paraxial and peripheral rays focus along the axis at different points. SYN dioptric a.

ventricular a., SYN aberrant ventricular *conduction*.

ab·er·rom·e·ter (ab-er-rom'ĕ-ter). An instrument for measuring optical aberration or any error in experimentation. [L. *aberratio*, aberration, + G. *metron*, measure]

abe·ta·lip·o·pro·tein·e·mia (ā-bā'tă-lip'ō-prō'tēn-ē'mē-ă) [MIM*200100]. A disorder characterized by an absence from plasma of low density lipoproteins that migrate electrophoretically as beta globules, presence of acanthocytes in blood, retinal pigmentary degeneration, malabsorption, engorgement of upper intestinal absorptive cells with dietary triglycerides, and neuromuscular abnormalities; autosomal recessive inheritance. SYN Bassen-Kornzweig syndrome. [G. *a-*, priv., + β, + lipoprotein + *-emia*, blood]

normotriglyceridemic a., a. with normal levels of triglycerides. This inherited disorder (possibly autosomal recessive) is probably due to the absence of apolipoprotein B-100.

abey·ance (ă-bā'ans). A state of temporary abolition of function. [fr. O. Fr.]

ab·far·ad (ab-far'ad). Electromagnetic unit of capacity equal to 10^9 farads.

ABG Abbreviation for arterial blood gas. SEE blood *gases*, under *gas*.

ab·hen·ry (ab-hen'rē). Electromagnetic unit of inductance equal to 10^{-9} henry.

ab·i·ent (ab'ē-ent). Having a tendency to move away from the source of a stimulus, as opposed to adient. [L. *abiens*, fr. *ab- eo*, to go from]

abil·i·ty (ă-bil'i-tē). The physical, mental, or legal competence to function. [L. *habilitas*, aptitude]

abi·ot·ic (ā-b-ī-ot'ik). **1.** Incompatible with life. **2.** Without life.

ab·i·ot·ro·phy (ab-ē-ot'rō-fē). An age-dependent manifestation of a trait that being genetically determined has been latent from the time of conception. [G. *a-* priv. + *bios*, life, + *trophē*, nourishment]

ab·ir·ri·tant (ab-ir'i-tănt). **1.** Obsolete term for soothing, or relieving irritation. **2.** Obsolete term for an agent possessing this property.

ab·ir·ri·ta·tion (ab-ir-i-ta'shŭn). Obsolete term for diminution or abolition of irritability in a part. [L. *ab*, from, + *irrito*, pp. *-atus*, to irritate]

ab·ir·ri·ta·tive (ab-ir'i-tā-tiv). Obsolete term for abirritant.

abl. An oncogene found in the Abelson strain of mouse leukemia virus and involved in the Philadelphia chromosome translocation in chronic granulocytic leukemia.

ab·lac·ta·tion (ab-lak-tā'shŭn). SYN weaning (1). [L. *ab*, from, + lactation]

ablas·te·mic (ā-blas-tem'ik). Not germinal or blastemic. [G. *a-* priv. + *blastēma*, sprout]

ablas·tin (ă-blas'tin). An antibody that seems to inhibit reproduction of trypanosomes; found in rats infected with *Trypanosoma lewisi*. [G. *a-* priv. + *blastos*, germ]

ab·late (ab-lāt'). To remove, or to destroy the function of. [L. *aufero*, pp. *ab- latus*, to take away]

ab·la·tion (ab-lā'shun). Removal of a body part or the destruction of its function, as by a surgical procedure, morbid process, or noxious substance. [L. see ablate]

electrode catheter a., a method of ablating the site of origin of arrhythmias whereby high energy elective shocks are delivered by intravascular catheters.

ab·la·tio pla·cen·tae (ab-lā'shē-ō pla-sen'tē). SYN abruptio placentae.

ableph·a·ria (ā-blef-ar'ē-ă) [MIM*200110]. Congenital absence, partial or complete, of the eyelids; recessive inheritance. SEE ALSO cryptophthalmus. [G. *a-* priv. + *blepharon*, eyelid]

ab·lu·ent (ab'lū-ent). **1.** Cleansing. **2.** Anything with cleansing properties. [L. *abluens*, fr. *ab-luo*, to wash off]

ab·lu·tion (ab-lū'shŭn). An act of washing or bathing. [L. *ablutio*, washing off, cleansing]

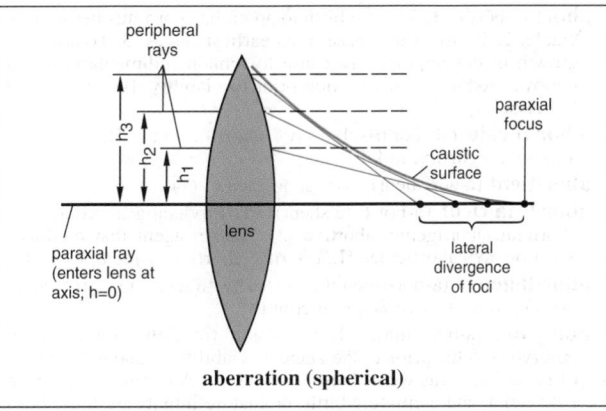

aberration (spherical)

ab·lu·to·ma·nia (ab-lū-tō-mā'nē-ă). Rarely used term for a morbid preoccupation with thoughts about cleanliness, exhibited by frequent washing, as seen in obsessive-compulsive disorder. [L. *ablutio*, washing, + G. *mania*, insanity]

ab·ner·val (ab-ner'văl). Away from a nerve; denoting specifically a current of electricity passing through a muscular fiber in a direction away from the point of entrance of the nerve fiber. SYN abneural (1).

ab·neu·ral (ab-nūr'ăl). **1.** SYN abnerval. **2.** Away from the neural axis. [L. *ab*, away from, + G. *neuron*, nerve]

ab·nor·mal (ab-nōr'măl). Not normal; differing in any way from the usual state, structure, condition, or rule.

ab·nor·mal·i·ty (ab-nōr-mal'i-tē). **1.** The state or quality of being abnormal. **2.** An anomaly, deformity, malformation, impairment, or dysfunction.

figure-of-8 a., a radiographic appearance associated with total anomalous drainage of the pulmonary venous circulation into enlarged right and anomalous left venae cavae, that produces a globular density above the heart; the silhouette suggests the figure 8. SEE snowman a. SYN snowman a.

snowman a., SYN figure-of-8 a.

ABO blood group. See Blood Groups appendix.

ABO blood group				
blood group	genotype	frequency in U.S. (%)	antigens of erythrocytes	antibodies in serum
A	AA or AO	32 pos 7 neg	A	anti-B (β)
B	BB or BO	9 pos 2 neg	B	anti-A (α)
AB	AB	3 pos 1 neg	A and B	none
O	OO	38 pos 8 neg	neither A nor B	α and β

ab·ohm (ab'ōm). Electromagnetic unit of resistance equal to 10^{-9} ohm.

aboi·e·ment (ah-bwah-mahn'). Rarely used term for the involuntary production of abnormal sounds, as seen in Gilles de la Tourette syndrome. [Fr. barking, yelping]

ab·o·ma·si·tis (ab'ō-mas-ī'tis). Inflammation of the abomasum.

ab·o·ma·sum (ab-ō-mā'sŭm). The fourth compartment and the glandular portion of the stomach of a ruminant. [L. *ab*, from, + *omasum*, bullock's tripe]

ab·o·rad, ab·o·ral (ab-ō'rad, -răl). In a direction away from the mouth; opposite of orad. [L. *ab*, from, + *os (or-)*, mouth]

abort (ă-bōrt'). **1.** To give birth to an embryo or fetus before it is viable. **2.** To arrest a disease in its earliest stages. **3.** To arrest in growth or development; to cause to remain rudimentary. **4.** To remove products of conception prior to viability. [L. *aborior,* to fail at onset]

a·bor·ti·cide (ah-bor'ti-sid). SYN abortifacient. [L. *abortus,,* abortion, + *caedo,,* to kill]

abor·tient (ă-bōr'shent). SYN abortifacient (1).

abor·ti·fa·cient (ă-bōr-ti-fā'shent). **1.** Producing abortion. SYN abortient, abortigenic, abortive (3). **2.** An agent that produces abortion. SYN aborticide. [L. *abortus,* abortion, + *facio,* to make]

abor·ti·gen·ic (ă-bōr-ti-jen'ik). SYN abortifacient (1). [L. *abortus,* abortion, + *genesis,* production]

abor·tion (ă-bōr'shŭn). **1.** Expulsion from the uterus of an embryo or fetus prior to the stage of viability at about 20 weeks of gestation (fetus weighs less than 500 g). A distinction is made between a. and premature birth: premature infants are those born after the stage of viability but prior to 37 weeks. A. may be either spontaneous (occurring from natural causes) or induced (artificial or therapeutic). **2.** The product of such nonviable birth. **3.** The arrest of any action or process before its normal completion.

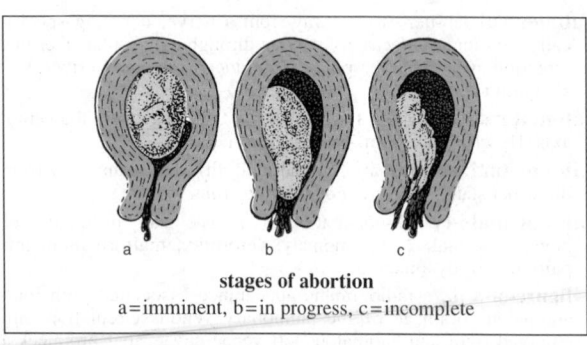

stages of abortion
a=imminent, b=in progress, c=incomplete

accidental a., a. due to a fall, blow, or other injury.

ampullar a., a. resulting from pregnancy in the ampulla of the fallopian tube.

complete a., (1) the complete expulsion or extraction from its mother of a fetus or embryo; **(2)** complete expulsion of any other product of gestation. (*e.g.,* hydatidiform mole).

criminal a., termination of pregnancy without legal justification. SYN illegal a.

elective a., an a. without medical justification but done in a legal way, as in the United States.

enzootic a. of ewes, a specific infectious a. of sheep caused by *Chlamydia psittaci.*

epizootic bovine a., an infectious disease of cattle transmitted by the tick *Ornithodoros coriaceus* and manifested as a. or weak calves at birth; occurs in the foothills of California, Nevada, and Oregon. SYN foothill a.

equine virus a., a highly contagious a. of mares, caused by equine rhinopneumonitis virus, a member of the family Herpesviridae.

foothill a., SYN epizootic bovine a.

habitual a., a condition in which a woman has had three or more consecutive, spontaneous a.'s.

illegal a., SYN criminal a.

imminent a., SYN incipient a.

incipient a., impending a. characterized by copious vaginal bleeding, uterine contractions, and cervical dilation. SYN imminent a.

incomplete a., a. in which part of the products of conception have been passed but part (usually the placenta) remains in the uterus.

induced a., a. brought on purposefully by drugs or mechanical means.

inevitable a., a. characterized by rupture of the membranes in the presence of cervical dilation in a previable pregnancy.

infected a., a septic complication of an a.

menstrual extraction a., a technique for aspiration of early products of conception from the uterus a few days after the first missed menstrual period.

missed a., a. in which the fetus dies *in utero* but the product of conception is retained *in utero* for two months or longer.

septic a., an infectious a. complicated by fever, endometritis, and parametritis.

spontaneous a., a. that has not been artificially induced.

therapeutic a., a. induced because of the mother's physical or mental health, or to prevent birth of a deformed child or a child resulting from rape.

threatened a., cramplike pains and slight show of blood that may or may not be followed by the expulsion of the fetus during the first 20 weeks of pregnancy.

tubal a., rupture of an oviduct, the seat of ectopic pregnancy, or extrusion of the product of conception through the fimbriated end of the oviduct; aborted ectopic pregnancy, the pregnancy having originated in the fallopian tubes. SYN aborted ectopic pregnancy.

vibrionic a., a. of cattle or sheep caused by *Campylobacter fetus.*

abor·tion·ist (ă-bōr'shŭn-ist). One who interrupts a pregnancy.

abor·tive (ă-bōr'tiv). **1.** Not reaching completion; *e.g.,* said of an attack of a disease subsiding before it has fully developed or completed its course. **2.** SYN rudimentary. **3.** SYN abortifacient (1). [L. *abortivus*]

abor·tus (ă-bōr'tŭs). Any product (or all products) of an abortion. [L.]

abou·lia (ă-bū'lē-ă). SYN abulia.

ABP Abbreviation for androgen binding *protein.*

ABPA Abbreviation for allergic bronchopulmonry aspergillosis.

ABR Abbreviation for auditory brainstem response. SEE auditory brainstem response *audiometry.*

abra·chia (ă-brā'kē-ă). Congenital absence of arms. SEE amelia. [G. *a-* priv. + *brachiōn,* arm]

abra·chi·o·ceph·a·ly, abra·chi·o·ce·pha·lia (ă-brā'kē-ō-sef'ă-lē, -se-fā'lē-ă). Congenital absence of arms and head. SYN acephalobrachia. [G. *a-* priv. + *brachiōn,* arm, + *kephalē,* head]

abrade (ă-brād'). **1.** To wear away by mechanical action. **2.** To scrape away the surface layer from a part. [L. *ab-rado,* pp. *-rasus,* to scrape off]

Abrahams, Robert, U.S. physician, 1861–1935. SEE A.'s *sign.*

Abrams, Albert, U.S. physician, 1863–1924. SEE A.'s heart *reflex.*

abra·sion (ă-brā'zhŭn). **1.** An excoriation, or circumscribed removal of the superficial layers of skin or mucous membrane. SYN abraded wound. **2.** A scraping away of a portion of the surface. **3.** In dentistry, the pathological grinding or wearing away of tooth substance by incorrect tooth-brushing methods, foreign objects, bruxism, or similar causes. SYN grinding. Cf. attrition. [see abrade]

brush burn a., SEE brush *burn.*

gingival a., a lesion of the gingiva resulting from mechanical removal of a portion of the surface epithelium.

mechanical a., SYN dermabrasion.

tooth a., loss or wearing away of tooth structure caused by the abrasive characteristics of substances other than foods.

abra·sive (a-brā'siv). **1.** Causing abrasion. **2.** Any material used to produce abrasions. **3.** A substance used in dentistry for abrading, grinding, or polishing.

abra·sive·ness (ă-brā'siv-nes). **1.** That property of a substance which causes surface wear by friction. **2.** The quality of being able to scratch or wear away another material.

ab·re·act (ab-rē-akt'). **1.** To show strong emotion while reliving a previous traumatic experience. **2.** To discharge or release repressed emotion.

ab·re·ac·tion (ab-rē-ak'shŭn). In freudian psychoanalysis, an episode of emotional release or catharsis associated with the bringing into conscious recollection previously repressed unpleasant experiences.

motor a., the release of an unconscious thought, idea, or impulse through motor or muscular expression.

abrin (ab′rin). A phytotoxin from jequirity seeds, the red seeds of *Abrus precatorius;* used in ophthalmology.

abrup·tion (ab-rŭp′shŭn). A tearing away, separation, or detachment.

ab·rup·tio pla·cen·tae (ab-rŭp′shē-ō pla-sen′tē). Premature detachment of a normally situated placenta. SYN ablatio placentae, amotio placentae.

Ab·rus (ā′brŭs). A genus of leguminous plants. The root of *A. precatorius,* Indian liquorice, is sometimes used as a substitute for liquorice; the seeds are toxic and may cause vomiting, diarrhea, convulsions, and death if chewed. [more correctly *Habrus,* from G. *habros,* graceful]

ABSCESS

ab·scess (ab′ses). **1.** A circumscribed collection of purulent exudate appearing in an acute or chronic localized infection, caused by tissue destruction and frequently associated with swelling and other signs of inflammation. **2.** A cavity formed by liquefactive necrosis within solid tissue. [L. *abscessus,* a going away]

acute a., a recently formed a. with little or no fibrosis in the wall of the cavity. SYN hot a.

alveolar a., an a. situated within the alveolar process of the jaws, most often caused by extension of infection from an adjacent nonvital tooth. SYN dental a., dentoalveolar a., root a.

amebic a., an area of liquefaction necrosis of the liver or other organ containing amebae, often following amebic dysentery. SYN tropical a.

apical a., **(1)** SYN periapical a. **(2)** an a. in the apex of the lung.

apical periodontal a., SYN periapical a.

appendiceal a., an intraperitoneal a., usually in the right iliac fossa, resulting from extension of infection in acute appendicitis, especially with perforation of the appendix. SYN periappendiceal a.

Bartholin's a., an a. of the vulvovaginal gland.

Bezold's a., an a. deep in the neck parapharyngeal space associated with suppuration in the mastoid tip cells.

bicameral a., an a. with two separate cavities or chambers.

bone a., suppuration within the medullary cavity (osteomyelitis), cortex, or periosteum of bone.

Brodie's a., a chronic a. of bone surrounded by dense fibrous tissue and sclerotic bone.

bursal a., suppuration within a bursa.

caseous a., an a. containing white solid or semisolid material of cheesy consistency; usually tuberculous. SEE ALSO cheesy a.

cheesy a., an a. that contains necrotic tissue with a cheese-like consistency; typically seen in tuberculosis.

cholangitic a. (kō-lan-ji′-tik), a focal area of pus formation in the liver resulting from infection arising in the biliary tract.

chronic a., a long-standing collection of pus surrounded by fibrous tissue.

cold a., **(1)** an a. without heat or other usual signs of inflammation; **(2)** SYN tuberculous a.

collar-button a., an a. consisting of two cavities connected by a narrow isthmus, usually formed by rupture of an a. through a fascial layer in the hand or foot. SYN shirt-stud a.

crypt a.'s, a.'s in crypts of Lieberkühn of the large intestinal mucosa; a characteristic feature of ulcerative colitis.

dental a., dentoalveolar a., SYN alveolar a.

diffuse a., a collection of pus not circumscribed by a well-defined capsule.

Douglas a., suppuration in Douglas pouch.

dry a., the remains of an a. after the pus is absorbed.

Dubois' a.'s, small cysts of the thymus containing polymorphonuclear leukocytes but lined by squamous epithelium; reported in congenital syphilis but also found in the absence of syphilis. SYN Dubois' disease, thymic a.'s.

embolic a., an a. arising at the point of arrest of a septic embolus.

fecal a., SYN stercoral a.

follicular a., an a. in a hair, tonsillar, or other follicle.

gas a., an a. containing gas caused by *Enterobacter aerogenes, Escherichia coli,* or other gas-forming microorganisms.

gingival a., an a. confined to the gingival soft tissue. SYN gumboil, parulis.

gravitation a., SYN perforating a.

gummatous a., an a. due to the softening and breaking down of a gumma, especially in bone. SYN syphilitic a.

hematogenous a., an a. caused by blood-borne organisms.

hot a., SYN acute a.

hypostatic a., SYN perforating a.

ischiorectal a., an a. involving the tissues in the ischiorectal fossa.

lacunar a., an a. involving the urethral lacunae.

lateral alveolar a., an alveolar a. located along the lateral root surface of a tooth. SYN pericemental a.

lateral periodontal a., an a. that forms at the depth of a periodontal pocket due to multiplication of pyogenic microorganisms or the presence of foreign material.

mastoid a., an a. of the mastoid air cells.

metastatic a., a secondary a. formed, at a distance from the primary focus, as a result of the transportation of pyogenic bacteria by the lymph or bloodstream.

migrating a., SYN perforating a.

miliary a., one of a number of minute collections of pus, widely disseminated throughout an area or the whole body.

Munro's a., SYN Munro's *microabscess.*

orbital a., a circumscribed collection of pus within the orbit; frequently an extension of purulent infection of the paranasal sinuses, usually the ethmoids. SYN retrobulbar a.

otic a., a cerebral a. usually involving the temporal lobe or cerebellar hemisphere, due to extension of suppuration of the middle ear. SYN otogenous a.

otogenous a., SYN otic a.

palatal a., **(1)** a lateral periodontal a. associated with the lingual surface of a maxillary tooth; **(2)** an alveolar a. that has eroded the cortical plate, allowing extension into the palatal soft tissues.

pancreatic a., an a. in the pancreatic or peripancreatic area usually related to pancreatitis.

parafrenal a., an a. that occurs on either side of the frenum of the penis.

parametric a., parametritic a., an a. in the connective tissue of the broad ligament of the uterus.

paranephric a., an a. in the region of the kidney, outside the renal fascia.

parotid a., rapidly progressive suppuration in the parotid gland; a complication of parotitis.

Pautrier's a., SYN Pautrier's *microabscess.*

pelvic a., an a. in the pelvic peritoneal cavity, developing as a complication of diffuse peritonitis or of localized peritonitis associated with abdominal or pelvic inflammatory disease, such as salpingitis; the pus frequently collects in the rectovesical or rectouterine pouch.

perforating a., an a. that breaks down tissue barriers to enter adjacent areas. SYN gravitation a., hypostatic a., migrating a., wandering a.

periapical a., an alveolar a. localized around the apex of a tooth root. SYN apical a. (1), apical periodontal a.

periappendiceal a., SYN appendiceal a.

periarticular a., an a. surrounding a joint, not necessarily involving it.

pericemental a., SYN lateral alveolar a.

pericoronal a., an a. developing in the inflamed dental follicular tissue overlaying the crown of a partially erupted tooth.

perinephric a., an a. within Gerota's fascia but outside the renal capsule.

periodontal a., an alveolar a. or a lateral periodontal a.

perirectal a., an a. in connective tissue adjacent to the rectum or anus.

peritonsillar a., extension of tonsillar infection beyond the capsule with abscess formation usually above and behind the tonsil.

periureteral a., an a. surrounding the ureter.

periurethral a., an a. involving the tissues around the urethra.

phlegmonous a., circumscribed suppuration characterized by intense surrounding inflammatory reaction which produces induration and thickening of the affected area.

Pott's a., tuberculous a. of the spine.

premammary a., an a. in the subcutaneous tissue covering the mammary gland.

psoas a., an a., usually tuberculous, originating in tuberculous spondylitis and extending through the iliopsoas muscle to the inguinal region.

pulp a., an a. involving the soft tissue within the pulp chamber of a tooth, usually a sequela of caries or less frequently of trauma.

pyemic a., a hematogenous a. resulting from pyemia, septicemia, or bacteremia. SYN septicemic a.

radicular a., alveolar a., an a. around a tooth root.

residual a., an a. recurring at the site of a former a. resulting from persistence of microbes and pus.

retrobulbar a., SYN orbital a.

retrocecal a., an a. located posterior to the cecum, usually resulting from perforation of a retrocecal appendix.

retropharyngeal a., an a. arising, usually, in retropharyngeal lymph nodes, most commonly in infants.

ring a., an acute purulent inflammation of the corneal periphery in which a necrotic area is surrounded by an annular girdle of leukocytic infiltration.

root a., SYN alveolar a.

satellite a., an a. closely associated with a primary a.

septicemic a., SYN pyemic a.

shirt-stud a., SYN collar-button a.

stellate a., a star-shaped necrotic area surrounded by histiocytes, seen within swollen inguinal lymph nodes in lymphogranuloma venereum.

stercoral a., a collection of pus and feces. SYN fecal a.

sterile a., an a. whose contents are not caused by pyogenic bacteria.

stitch a., an a. around a suture.

subdiaphragmatic a., SYN subphrenic a.

subepidermal a., a microscopic a. located in the dermis just beneath the epidermis.

subhepatic a., an a. located immediately beneath the liver.

subperiosteal a., an a. between the periosteum and cortical plate of the bone.

subphrenic a., an a. directly beneath the diaphragm. SYN subdiaphragmatic a.

subungual a., suppuration extending beneath a fingernail or toenail, usually from a parenychia.

sudoriparous a., a collection of pus in a sweat gland.

syphilitic a., SYN gummatous a.

thecal a., suppuration in a sheath or capsule.

thymic a.'s, SYN Dubois' a.'s.

Tornwaldt's a., chronic infection of the pharyngeal bursa. SEE ALSO Tornwaldt's *syndrome.*

tropical a., SYN amebic a.

tuberculous a., an a. caused by the tubercle bacillus. SYN cold a. (2).

tubo-ovarian a., a large a. involving a uterine tube and an adherent ovary, resulting from extension of purulent inflammation of the tube.

verminous a., SYN worm a.

wandering a., SYN perforating a.

worm a., a. due to parasitic worms or in which worms are found. SYN verminous a.

ab·scis·sa (ab-sis′ă). In a plane cartesian coordinate system, the

horizontal axis (*x*). Cf. ordinate. [L. *ab-scindo,* pp. *-scissus,* to cut away from]

ab·scis·sion (ab-si′shŭn). Cutting away. [L. *ab-scindo,* pp. *-scissus,* to cut away from]

ab·scon·sio (ab-skon′shē-ō). A recess, cavity, or depression; used especially in osteology to denote a bony cavity which accommodates the head of another bone. [Mod. L. fr. *abs-condo,* pp. *-conditus* or *-consus,* to hide]

ab·sco·pal (ab-skō′păl, -skop′ăl). Denoting the effect that irradiation of a tissue has on remote nonirradiated tissue. [ab- + G.*skopos,* target, + -al]

ab·sence (ab′sens). Paroxysmal attacks of impaired consciousness, occasionally accompanied by spasm or twitching of cephalic muscles, which usually can be brought on by hyperventilation; depending on the type and severity of the a., the EEG may show an abrupt onset of a 3/sec spike and wave pattern as in simple a., or in atypical cases, a 4/sec spike and wave or faster spike complexes. The clinical states accompanying these EEG abnormalities may be classified as: 1) a. with no overt manifestations, *e.g.,* simple a.; epileptic a.; subclinical a.; 2) a. with clonic movements, *e.g.,* myoclonic a.; 3) a. with atonic states, *e.g.,* atonic a.; 4) a. with tonic contractions, *e.g.,* hypertonic muscular contraction; 5) a. with automatisms, *e.g.,* various stereotyped movements, usually of the face or hands; 6) a. with atypical features, *e.g.,* bizarre motor activity. [L. *absentia*]

pure a., SYN simple a.

simple a., a brief clouding of consciousness accompanied by the abrupt onset of 3/sec spikes and waves on EEG. SYN pure a.

abs. feb. Abbreviation for L. *absente febre,* when fever is absent.

Ab·sid·ia (ab-sid′ē-ă). A genus of fungi (family Mucoraceae) commonly found in nature. Thermophilic species survive in compost piles at temperatures exceeding 45°C and may cause zygomycosis in humans.

ab·sinthe (ab′sinth). A liqueur consisting of an alcoholic extract of absinthium and other bitter herbs.

ab·sin·thin (ab′sin-thin). A bitter principle, $C_{30}H_{40}O_8$, obtained from absinthium.

ab·sin·thi·um (ab-sin′thē-ŭm). The dried leaves and tops of *Artemisia absinthium* (family Compositae). The infusion is now seldom used, but it has been used as a tonic; in large or frequently repeated doses it produces headache, trembling, and epileptiform convulsions. SYN wormwood. [L., fr. G. *apsinthion*]

ab·sin·thol (ab-sin′thawl). SYN thujone.

ab·so·lute (ab′sō-lūt). Unconditional; unlimited; uncombined; undiluted (as in case of alcohol); certain. [L. *absolutus,* complete, pp. of *ab-solvo,* to loosen from]

ab·sorb (ab-sōrb′). 1. To take in by absorption. 2. To reduce the intensity of transmitted light. [L. *ab-sorbeo,* pp. *-sorptus,* to suck in]

ab·sor·bance (A, A) (ab-sōr′bans). In spectrophotometry, equal to 2 minus the log of the percentage transmittance of light. SYN absorbancy, absorbency, extinction (2), optical density.

specific a., a. per unit of concentration. SEE specific absorption *coefficient.*

ab·sor·ban·cy (ab-sōr′ban-sē). SYN absorbance.

ab·sor·be·fa·cient (ab-sōr-bĕ-fā′shŭnt). 1. Causing absorption. 2. Any substance possessing such quality. [L. *ab-sorbeo,* to suck in, + *facio,* to make]

ab·sorb·en·cy (ab-sōrb′en-sē). SYN absorbance.

ab·sor·bent (ab-sōr′bent). 1. Having the power to absorb, soak up, or take into itself a gas, liquid, light rays, or heat. SYN absorptive, bibulous. 2. Any substance possessing such power. 3. Material (usually caustic) for removal of carbon dioxide from circuits in which rebreathing occurs; *e.g.,* anesthesia and basal metabolism equipment.

ab·sorb·er head (ab-sōr′ber hed). Portion of a rebreathing anesthesia circuit that contains carbon dioxide absorbent; often referred to as a canister.

ab·sorp·tion (ab-sōrp′shŭn). 1. The taking in, incorporation, or reception of gases, liquids, light, or heat. Cf. adsorption. 2. In radiology, the uptake of energy from radiation by the tissue or medium through which it passes. SEE half-value *layer.* 3. In radiation or medical physics, the number of disintegrations per second of a radionuclide. Radioactivity. Unit (SI): becquerel. [L. *absorptio*, fr. *absorbeo*, to swallow]

cutaneous a., SYN percutaneous a.

disjunctive a., a. of living tissue in immediate relation with a necrosed part, producing a line of demarcation.

electron resonance a., SEE electron spin *resonance*.

external a., the a. of substances through skin, mucocutaneous surfaces, or mucous membranes.

interstitial a., the removal of water or of substances in the interstitial fluid by the lymphatics.

parenteral a., a. by any route other than the alimentary tract.

pathologic a., parenteral a. of any excremental or pathologic material into the bloodstream, *e.g.*, pus, urine, bile, etc.

percutaneous a., the a. of drugs, allergens, and other substances through unbroken skin. SYN cutaneous a.

photoelectric a., interaction of an x-ray photon with matter in which the incident photon is completely absorbed, giving up all its energy by displacing an outer shell electron.

ab·sorp·tive (ab-sōrp′tiv). SYN absorbent (1).

ab·sorp·tiv·i·ty (*a*) (ab-sōrp-tiv′i-tē). **1.** SYN specific absorption *coefficient*. **2.** SYN molar absorption *coefficient*.

molar a., SYN molar absorption *coefficient*.

ab·sti·nence (ab′sti-nens). Refraining from the use of certain articles of diet, alcoholic beverages, illegal drugs, or from sexual intercourse. [L. *abs-tineo*, to hold back, fr. *teneo*, to hold]

ab·stract (ab′strakt). **1.** A preparation made by evaporating a fluid extract to a powder and triturating with milk sugar. **2.** A condensation or summary of a scientific or literary article or address. [L. *ab-straho*, pp. *-tractus*, to draw away]

ab·strac·tion (ab-strak′shŭn). **1.** Distillation or separation of the volatile constituents of a substance. **2.** Exclusive mental concentration. **3.** The making of an abstract from the crude drug. **4.** Malocclusion in which the teeth or associated structures are lower than their normal occlusal plane. SEE ALSO odontoptosis. **5.** The process of selecting a certain aspect of a concept from the whole. [L. *abs-traho*, pp. *-tractus*, to draw away]

ab·stric·tion (ab-strik′shŭn). In fungi, the formation of asexual spores by cutting off portions of the sporophore through the growth of dividing partitions. [L. *ab-*, from, + *strictura*, a contraction]

ab·ter·mi·nal (ab-ter′mi-năl). In a direction away from the end and toward the center; denoting the course of an electrical current in a muscle. [L. *ab*, from, + *terminus*, end]

ab·trop·fung (ab-trop′fŭng). A theory that nevus cells are epidermal cells (melanocytes) that proliferate and drop off (migrate) into the dermis. [Ger. *Abtropfung*, trickling down]

γ-Abu Abbreviation for γ-aminobutyric acid.

abu·lia (ă-bū′lē-ă). **1.** Loss or impairment of the ability to perform voluntary actions or to make decisions. **2.** Reduction in speech, movement, thought, and emotional reaction; a common result of bilateral frontal lobe disease. SYN aboulia. [G. *a-* priv. + *boulē*, will]

abu·lic (ă-bū′lik). Relating to, or suffering from, abulia.

a·bun·dance (a′bŭn-dans). The average number of types of macromolecules (*e.g.*, mRNAs) per cell.

abuse (ă-byūs′). **1.** Misuse, wrong use, especially excessive use, of anything. **2.** Injurious, harmful, or offensive treatment, as in child a. or sexual a.

child a., the psychological, emotional, and sexual a. of a child, typically by a parent, stepparent, or parent surrogate. SEE domestic *violence*.

drug a., habitual use of drugs not needed for therapeutic purposes, such as solely to alter one's mood, affect, or state of consciousness, or to affect a body function unnecessarily (as in laxative a.); non-medical use of drugs.

To qualify as drug dependant, a person must use a mood-altering substance daily, for a period of 2–3 weeks or longer. The drug-dependent person must also display certain characteristics, including psychological craving for the substance, symptoms of withdrawal indicating physi-

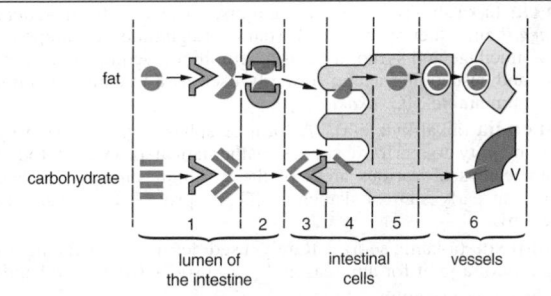

absorption (small intestine)
1) enzymatic division in the lumen; 2) forming of micelles with bile salts; 3) enzymatic division on the microvilli of the cells; 4) transport through the cuticular layer; 5) substance exchange in the enterocytes; 6) removal in blood (V) or lymph (L).

ological dependance, and tolerance (need for increased amounts of the drug to reproduce the initial level of response). Behaviorally, the dependent person manifests a reduced ability to function at work or home, and often will appear erratic, moody, or anxious. The use of virtually any drug may lead to dependance. Most commonly, drug dependance involves alcohol, nicotine, cocaine, and the opiates. In addition, some people use psychedelics, marijuana, caffeine, antihistamines, steroids, and solvents to a degree that qualifies as a substance use disorder. Treatment regimens vary in methodology and degree of success.

elder a., the physical or emotional a., including financial exploitation, of an elderly person, by one or more of the individual's children, nursing home caregivers, or others.

sexual a., SEE domestic *violence*.

spouse a., spousal a., SEE domestic *violence*.

substance a., maladaptive pattern of drug or alcohol use that may lead to social, occupational, psychological, or physical problems.

abut·ment (ă-bŭt′ment). In dentistry, a natural tooth or implanted tooth substitute, used for the support or anchorage of a fixed or removable prosthesis.

auxiliary a., a tooth other than the one supporting the direct retainer, assisting in the overall support of a removable partial denture.

intermediate a., a natural tooth, or an implanted tooth substitute, without other natural teeth in proximal contact, used along with the mesial and distal a.'s to support a prosthesis; often called a "pier."

isolated a., a lone-standing tooth, or root, used as an a. with edentulous areas mesial and distal to it.

splinted a., the joining of two or more teeth into a rigid unit by means of fixed restorations to form a single a. with multiple roots.

ABVD Abbreviation for a chemotherapy regimen of Adriamycin (doxorubicin), bleomycin, vinblastine, and dacarbazine; used to treat neoplastic diseases, such as Hodgkin's disease, shown to be resistant to MOPP therapy.

ab·volt (ab′vōlt). The CGS electromagnetic unit of difference of potential equal to 10^{-8} volt. The potential difference between two points such that 1 erg of work will be done when 1 abcoulomb of charge moves from point to point.

ab·zyme (ab′zīm). SYN catalytic *antibody*. [*ant*ibody + en*zyme*]

AC Abbreviation for alternating *current*.

Ac Symbol for actinium; acetyl.

aC Symbol for arabinosylcytosine.

a.c. Abbreviation for L. *ante cibum*, before a meal or *ante cibos*, before meals.

AC/A Abbreviation for accommodative convergence-accommodation *ratio*.

aca·cia (ă-kā′shē-ă). The dried gummy exudation from *Acacia senegal* and other species of *A.* (family Leguminosae), prepared as a mucilage and syrup; used as an emollient, demulcent excipient, and suspending agent; formerly used as a transfusion fluid. SYN gum arabic. [G. *akakia*]

acal·cu·lia (ā′kal-kyū′lē-a). A form of aphasia characterized by the inability to perform simple mathematical problems; found with lesions of various areas of the cerebral hemispheres, and often an early sign of dementia. [G. *a-* priv. + L. *calculo,* to reckon]

acamp·sia (ă-kamp′sē-ă). Rarely used term for stiffening or rigidity of a joint for any reason. [G. *a-* priv. + *kamptō,* to bend]

△**acanth-.** SEE acantho-.

acan·tha (ă-kan′thă). 1. A spine or spinous process. 2. The spinous process of a vertebra. [G. *akantha,* a thorn]

acan·tha·me·bi·a·sis (ă-kan′thă-mē-bī′ă-sis). Infection by free-living soil amebae of the genus *Acanthamoeba* that may result in a necrotizing dermal or tissue invasion, or a fulminating and usually fatal primary amebic meningoencephalitis.

Acan·tha·moe·ba (ă-kan-thă-mē′bă). A genus of free-living ameba (family Acanthamoebidae, order Amoebida) found in and characterized by the presence of acanthopodia. Human infection includes invasion of skin or colonization following injury, corneal invasion and colonization, and possibly lung or genitourinary tract colonization; a few cases of brain or CNS invasion have occurred, but not solely by the olfactory epithelium route of entry as with the more virulent infections caused by *Naegleria fowleri.* Species responsible are chiefly *A. culbertsoni,* but cases have been reported involving *A. castellanii, A. polyphaga,* and *A. astronyxis,* though most cases have been chronic rather than fulminating and rapidly fatal as with *Naegleria fowleri* infection. [G. *akantha,* thorn, spine, + Mod. L. *amoeba,* fr. G. *amoibē,* change]

ac·an·thel·la (ă-kan-thel′ă). An intermediate larva stage of Acanthocephala, formed within the arthropod host; a preinfective, nonencysted stage leading to the infective cystacanth. [G. *akantha,* thorn, spine]

acan·thes·the·sia (ă-kan-thes-thē′zē-ă). Paresthesia of a pinprick. [G. *akantha,* thorn, + *aisthēsis,* sensation]

Acan·thia lec·tu·lar·ia (ă-kan′thē-ă lek-tyū-lār′ē-ă). Early name for *Cimex lectularius.* [G. *akantha,* thorn, prickle; L. *lectus,* a bed]

acan·thi·on (ă-kan′thē-on). The tip of the anterior nasal spine. SYN akanthion. [G. *akantha,* thorn]

△**acantho-.** A spinous process; spiny, thorny. [G. *akantha,* a thorn, the backbone, the spine, fr. *akē,* a point, + *anthos,* a flower]

Acan·tho·ceph·a·la (ă-kan-thō-sef′ă-lă). The thorny-headed worms, a phylum (formerly considered a class) of obligatory parasites without an alimentary canal, characterized by an anterior introvertible spiny proboscis. They superficially resemble nematodes but are cestode-like in other traits, and hence are grouped as a distinctive phylum of helminths. In the adult stage they are parasites of vertebrate animals, mostly fish and amphibians; the larval stage is passed in invertebrates, chiefly crustaceans and insects. [acantho- + G. *kephalē,* head]

acan·tho·ceph·a·li·a·sis (ă-kan′thō-sef-ă-lī′ă-sis). An illness caused by infection with a species of Acanthocephala.

Acan·tho·chei·lo·ne·ma (ă-kan′thō-kī-lō-nē′mă). A genus of filarial worms parasitic in man, now considered part of the genus *Mansonella.* [acantho- + G. *cheilos,* lip, + *nēma,* thread]

acan·tho·cyte (ă-kan′thō-sīt). An erythrocyte characterized by multiple spiny cytoplasmic projections, as in acanthocytosis. SYN acanthrocyte. [acantho- + G. *kytos,* cell]

acan·tho·cy·to·sis (ă-kan′thō-sī-tō′sis). A rare condition in which the majority of erythrocytes are acanthocytes; a regular feature of abetalipoproteinemia. SYN acanthrocytosis.

acan·thoid (ă-kan′thoyd). Spine-shaped.

ac·an·thol·y·sis (ak-an-thol′i-sis). Separation of individual epidermal keratinocytes from their neighbor, as in conditions such as pemphigus vulgaris and Darier's disease. [acantho- + G. *lysis,* loosening]

ac·an·tho·ma (ak-an-thō′mă). A tumor formed by proliferation of epithelial squamous cells. SEE ALSO keratoacanthoma. [acantho- + G. *-oma,* tumor]

a. adenoi′des cys′ticum, SYN trichoepithelioma.

clear cell a., a sharply demarcated benign epidermal lesion of a leg or arm with acanthosis and accumulation of glycogen in keratinocytes having pale staining cytoplasm.

Degos' a., obsolete term for clear cell a.

a. fissura′tum, a fissure bordered by acanthosis developing at a site of friction by spectacle frames, usually behind the ears.

acan·tho·po·dia (ă-kan-thō-pō′dē-ă). Toothlike pseudopodia observed in some amebae, typically in members of the genus *Acanthamoeba.* [acantho- + G. *pous, podos,* foot]

acan·thor (ă-kan′thōr). The spindle-shaped embryo, with rostellar hooks and body spines, formed within the egg shell of Acanthocephala; this stage burrows into the body cavity of its first intermediate host, usually a crustacean in aquatic cycles, or insects in terrestrial cycles. [G. *akantha,* thorn or spine]

acan·thor·rhex·is (ă-kan-thō-rek′sĭs). Rupture of the intercellular bridges of the prickle cell layer of the epidermis, as in contact-type dermatitis. SEE spongiosis. [acantho + G. *rhexis,* rupture]

ac·an·tho·sis (ak-an-thō′sis). An increase in the thickness of the stratum spinosum of the epidermis. SYN hyperacanthosis. [acantho- + G. *-osis,* condition]

glycogenic a., elevated gray-white plaques of distal esophageal or vaginal mucosa, with epithelium thickened by proliferation of large glycogen-filled squamous cells.

a. ni′gricans, an eruption of velvety warty benign growths and hyperpigmentation occurring in the skin of the axillae, neck, anogenital area, and groins; in adults, may be associated with internal malignancy, endocrine disorders, or obesity; a benign (juvenile) type occurs in children. SEE ALSO pseudoacanthosis nigricans. SYN keratosis nigricans. [L. fr. *niger,* black]

ac·an·thot·ic (ak-an-thot′ik). Pertaining to or characteristic of acanthosis.

acan·thro·cyte (a-kan′thrō-sīt). SYN acanthocyte.

acan·thro·cy·to·sis (a-kan′thrō-sī-tō′sis). SYN acanthocytosis.

acap·nia (ă-kap′nē-ă). Absence of carbon dioxide in the blood; sometimes used erroneously for hypocapnia. [G. *a-* priv. + *kapnos,* smoke]

acar·bia (ă-kar′bē-ă). Obsolete term denoting pronounced reduction in bicarbonate of the blood (hypocarbia). [G. *a-* priv. + carbon]

acar·dia (ā-kar′dē-ă). Congenital absence of the heart; a condition sometimes occurring in monozygotic twins or in the smaller, parasitic member of conjoined twins when its partner monopolizes the placental blood supply. A. can also occur in triplet pregnancies. [G. *a-* priv. + *kardia,* heart]

acar·di·ac (ā-car′dē-ak). Without a heart.

acar·di·o·tro·phia (ă-kar′di-ō-trō′fē-ă). Obsolete term for atrophy of the myocardium. [G. *a-* priv. + *kardia,* heart, + *trophē,* nourishment]

acar·di·us (ă-kar′dē-ŭs). A twin without a heart, parasitic on, or utilizing the placental circulation of, its mate.

a. aceph′alus, acephalocardius; an acardiac fetus in which the head and thoracic organs are absent. Ribs and vertebrae may be present, and upper limbs are either absent or defective.

a. amor′phus, a shapeless mass covered by skin and hair.

a. an′ceps, an acardiac fetus with partly developed head and deformed face, trunk, and limbs. SEE hemiacardius.

ac·a·ri·a·sis (ak-ar-ī′ă-sis). Any disease caused by mites, usually a skin infestation. SEE mange. SYN acaridiasis, acarinosis.

demodectic a., SYN demodectic *mange.*

psoroptic a., infestation of mammalian skin with *Psoroptes* mites.

pulmonary a., infestation of the lungs of monkeys with the mite, *Pneumonyssus simicola.*

sarcoptic a., infestation of skin with *Sarcoptes scabiei.* SEE scabies (1).

acar·i·cide (ă-kar′i-sīd). An agent that kills acarines; commonly used to denote chemicals that kill ticks. [Mod. L. *acarus*, a mite, fr. G. *akari* + L. *caedo*, to cut, kill]

ac·a·rid (ak'ă-rid). A general term for a member of the family Acaridae or for a mite. SYN acaridan. [G. *akari*, mite]

Acar·i·dae (ă-kar'i-dē). A family of the order Acarina, a large group of exceptionally small mites, usually 0.5 mm or less, abundant in dried fruits and meats, grain, meal, and flour; frequently a cause of severe dermatitis among persons hypersensitized by frequent handling of infested products.

acar·i·dan (ă-kar'i-dan). SYN acarid.

ac·ar·i·di·a·sis (ak'ar-i-dī'ă-sis). SYN acariasis.

Ac·a·ri·na (ak-ă-rī'nă). An order of Arachnida that includes the mites and ticks. [G. *akari*, a mite]

ac·a·rine (ak'ă-rīn). A member of the order Acarina.

ac·ar·i·no·sis (ak'ă-ri-nō'sis, ă-kar'i-). SYN acariasis.

ac·a·ro·der·ma·ti·tis (ak'ă-rō-der-mă-tī'tis). A skin inflammation or eruption produced by a mite. [G. *akari*, mite, + *derma* (*dermat-*), skin]

  a. urticarioi'des, infestation with the grain itch mite, *Pyemotes ventricosus*.

ac·a·roid (ak'ă-royd). Resembling a mite. [G. *akari*, mite, + *eidos*, resemblance]

ac·a·rol·o·gy (ak-ă-rol'ō-jē). The study of acarine parasites, the ticks and mites, and the diseases they transmit. [G. *akari*, mite, + *logos*, study]

ac·a·ro·pho·bia (ak'ă-rō-fō'bē-ă). Morbid fear of small parasites, small particles, or of itching. [G. *akari*, mite, + *phobos*, fear]

Ac·a·rus (ak'ă-rŭs). A genus of mites of the family Acaridae. [G. *akari*, mite]

  A. bala'tus, a tropical species of mite that causes a particularly severe type of scabies-like irritation.

  A. folliculo'rum, SYN Demodex folliculorum.

  A. galli'nae, SYN Dermanyssus gallinae.

  A. horde'i, the barley mite, a species that penetrates beneath the skin.

  A. rhizoglyp'ticus hyacin'thi, a species that develops in spoiled onions and may cause dermatitis.

  A. scabie'i, former term for *Sarcoptes scabiei*.

acar·y·ote (ă-kar'ē-ōt). SYN akaryocyte.

acat·a·la·se·mia [MIM*115500]. SYN acatalasia.

acat·a·la·sia (ā-kat-ă-lā'zē-ă) [MIM*115500]. Absence or deficiency of catalase from blood and tissues, often manifested by recurrent infection or ulceration of the gums and related oral structures. Homozygotes may have complete absence (Japanese variety) or very low levels (Swiss variety) of catalase; heterozygotes have reduced catalase levels (hypocatalasia), which overlap with the normal range. SYN acatalasemia, Takahara's disease.

acat·a·ma·the·sia (ă-kat'ă-mă-thē'zē-ă). Obsolete term for the loss or impairment of understanding, especially speech comprehension. [G. *a-* priv. + *katamathēsis*, a thorough knowledge or understanding]

acat·a·pha·si·a (ă-kat-ă-fā'zē-ă). Inability to correctly formulate a statement. [G. *a-* priv. + *kataphasis*, affirmation]

ac·a·thec·tic (ak-ă-thek'tik). Rarely used term relating to acathexia.

ac·a·thex·ia (ak-ă-thek'sē-ă). Rarely used term for an abnormal release of secretions. [G. *a-* priv. + *kathexis*, retention]

ac·a·thex·is (ak-ă-thek'sis). Rarely used term for a mental disorder in which certain objects or ideas fail to arouse an emotional response in the individual. [G. *a-* priv. + *kathexis*, retention]

aca·thi·sia (ak-ă-thiz'ē-ă). SYN akathisia.

acau·dal, acau·date (ă-kaw'dăl, ă-kaw'dāt). Having no tail. [G. *a-* priv. + L. *cauda*, tail]

ACC Abbreviation for anodal closure *contraction*.

ac·cel·er·ans (ak-sel'er-anz). **1.** Accelerating. **2.** Obsolete term for an accelerator (sympathetic) nerve to the heart. [L. accelerator]

ac·cel·er·ant (ak-sel'er-ant). SYN accelerator.

ac·cel·er·a·tion (ak-sel-er-ā'shŭn). **1.** The act of accelerating. **2.**

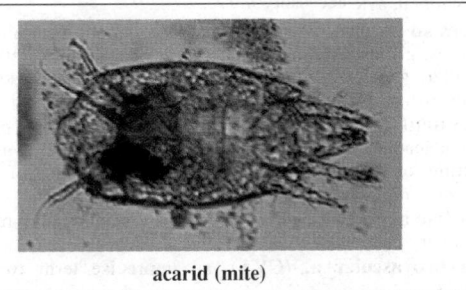

acarid (mite)

The rate of increase in velocity per unit of time; commonly expressed in *g* units; also expressed in centimeters or feet per second squared. **3.** The rate of increasing deviation from a rectilinear course. SEE radial a. [see accelerator]

  angular a., the rate of change of angular velocity; *e.g.,* when a centrifuge rotor is speeding up, or when there is a simultaneous change in velocity and direction, as in an aircraft in a tight spin.

  linear a., the rate of change of velocity without a change in direction; *e.g.,* when the speed of an aircraft increases while flying a straight pathway.

  radial a., the centripetal a. of a particle or vehicle moving along a curved path at a constant velocity; *e.g.,* turning a curve in an automobile, pulling out of a dive, or performing a loop maneuver in an aircraft. In aviation, a. varies directly with the square of the air speed and inversely with the radius of the turn ($a = {}^V/_r$, where V is air speed and r is radius of turn).

ac·cel·er·a·tor (ak-sel'er-ā-ter). **1.** Anything that increases rapidity of action or function. **2.** In physiology, a nerve, muscle, or substance that quickens movement or response. **3.** A catalytic agent used to hasten a chemical reaction. **4.** In nuclear physics, a device that accelerates charged particles (*e.g.,* protons) to high speed in order to produce nuclear reactions in a target, often for the production of radionuclides or for radiation therapy. SYN accelerant. [L. *accelerans*, pres. p. of *ac-celero*, to hasten, fr. *celer*, swift]

  linear a. (LINAC), a device imparting high velocity and energy to atomic and subatomic particles; an important device for radiation therapy.

  proserum prothrombin conversion a. (PPCA), SYN *factor* VIII.

  prothrombin a., SYN *factor* V.

  serum a., SYN *factor* VII.

  serum prothrombin conversion a. (SPCA), SYN *factor* VII.

ac·cel·er·in (ak-sel'er-in). Obsolete term for what was once considered an intermediary product of coagulation but is no longer thought to exist.

ac·cel·er·om·e·ter (ak-sel-er-om'ĕ-ter). An instrument for measuring the rate of change of velocity per unit of time.

ac·cen·tu·a·tor (ak-sent'yū-ā-ter). A substance, such as aniline, the presence of which allows a combination between a tissue or histologic element and a stain that might otherwise be impossible. [L. *accentus*, accent, fr. *cano*, to sing]

ac·cep·tor (ak-sep'ter). A compound that will take up a chemical group (*e.g.,* an amine group, a methyl group, a carbamoyl group) from another compound (the donor); under the action of alanine transaminase, L-glutamic acid is an amine donor while pyruvic acid is an amine a. [L. *ac-cipio,* pp. *-ceptus,* to accept]

  hydrogen a., SYN hydrogen *carrier*.

ac·cès per·ni·ci·eux (ak-sā' per-ni-syu'). A series of severe attacks of falciparum malaria, sometimes occurring in apparently mild cases; roughly classified as cerebral and algid. [Fr., pernicious attacks or symptoms]

ac·cess (ak'ses). A way or means of approach or admittance. In dentistry: **1.** The space required for visualization and for manipulation of instruments to remove decay and prepare a tooth for restoration. **2.** The opening in the crown of a tooth required to allow adequate admittance to the pulp space to clean, shape, and seal the root canal(s). SYN access opening. [L. *accessus*]

ac·ces·so·ri·us (ak-ses-ō'rē-ŭs). SYN accessory. [L.]

a. willis'ii, SYN accessory *nerve.*

ac·ces·so·ry (ak-ses′ō-rē). In anatomy, denoting certain muscles, nerves, glands, etc. that are auxiliary or supernumerary to some similar, generally more important thing. SYN accessorius. [L. *accessorius,* fr. *ac-cedo,* pp. *-cessus,* to move toward]

ac·ci·dent (ak′si-dent). An unanticipated but often predictable event leading to injury, *e.g.,* in traffic, industry, or a domestic setting, or such an event developing in the course of a disease. [L. *ac-cido,* to happen]

cardiac a., sudden cardiac catastrophe, such as may result from coronary occlusion.

cerebrovascular a. (CVA), an imprecise term for cerebral stroke.

serum a., anaphylactic shock resulting from injection of foreign serum for therapeutic purposes. SEE ALSO serum *sickness.*

ac·ci·dent-prone. **1.** Having a greater number of accidents than would be expected of the average person in similar circumstances. **2.** Having personality characteristics predisposing one to accidents.

ac·cli·ma·tion (ak-li-mā′shŭn). SYN acclimatization.

ac·cli·ma·ti·za·tion (ă-klī′mă-ti-zā′shŭn). Physiological adjustment of an individual to a different climate, especially to a change in environmental temperature or altitude. SYN acclimation.

ac·co·lé forms (ak-ōlā′). See under form.

ac·com·mo·da·tion (ă-kom′ŏ-dā′shŭn). **1.** The act or state of adjustment or adaptation. **2.** In sensorimotor theory, the alteration of schemata or cognitive expectations to conform with experience. [L. *ac-commodo,* pp. *-atus,* to adapt, fr. *modus,* a measure]

amplitude of a., the difference in refractivity of the eye at rest and when fully accommodated.

a. of eye, the increase in thickness and convexity of the eye's lens in order to focus the image of an external object upon the retina.

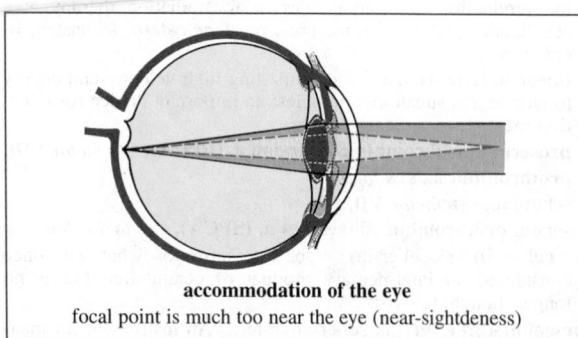

accommodation of the eye
focal point is much too near the eye (near-sightedness)

histologic a., change in shape of cells to meet altered physical conditions, as the flattening of cuboidal cells in cysts as a result of pressure. SYN pseudometaplasia.

negative a., the decrease of a. that occurs when shifting from near vision to distance vision.

a. of nerve, the property of a nerve by which it adjusts to a slowly increasing strength of stimulus, so that its threshold of excitation is greater than it would be were the stimulus strength to have risen more rapidly.

positive a., increased refractivity of the eye that occurs when shifting from the distance to a near object.

range of a., the distance between an object viewed with minimal refractivity of the eye and one viewed with maximal accommodation.

relative a., quantity of a. required for single binocular vision for any specified distance, or for any particular degree of convergence.

ac·com·mo·da·tive (ă-kom′ŏ-dā-tiv). Relating to accommodation.

ac·com·plice (ă-kom′plis). A bacterium which accompanies the main infecting agent in a mixed infection and which influences the virulence of the main organism. [M.E., fr. O.Fr., fr. L. *comples,* closely connected]

ac·couche·ment (a-kŭsh-mawn′). Childbirth, particularly parturition. SEE ALSO birth. [Fr. from *coucher,* to lie down]

a. forcé (fōr-sā′), forced, artificially hastened delivery, by means of forceps, version, etc.; originally applied to rapid dilation of the cervix with the hands, with version and forcible extraction of the fetus.

ac·cou·cheur (a-kū-sher′). Formerly used term for obstetrician.

ac·cre·men·ti·tion (ak′rē-men-tish′ŭn). **1.** Reproduction by budding or germination. **2.** SYN accretion (1). [L. *accresco,* pp. *-cretus,* to increase]

ac·cre·tio cor·dis (ă-krē′shē-ō kōr′dis). Adhesion of the pericardium to adjacent extracardiac structures.

ac·cre·tion (ă-krē′shŭn). **1.** Increase by addition to the periphery of material of the same nature as that already present; *e.g.,* the manner of growth of crystals. SYN accrementition (2). **2.** In dentistry, foreign material (usually plaque or calculus) collecting on the surface of a tooth or in a cavity. **3.** A growing together. [L. *accretio,* fr. *ad,* to, + *crescere,* to grow]

ac·cro·chage (ak-rō-shahj′). Intermittent synchronization of two different rhythms of the heart with one influencing the behavior of the other when neither is dominant; seen in cases of atrioventricular dissociation when an atrial beat falls shortly after a ventricular beat, the latter causing the atrial beat to occur sooner than expected. [Fr. hooking, hitching]

ac·cur·a·cy (ak′kyū-ră-sē). The degree to which a measurement, or an estimate based on measurements, represents the true value of the attribute that is being measured. In the laboratory a. of a test is determined when possible by comparing results from the test in question with results generated from an established reference method.

ACD Abbreviation for acid-citrate-dextrose.

ACE Abbreviation for angiotensin-converting *enzyme.*

ac·e·bu·to·lol (as-ĕ-byū′tō-lol). *N*-[3-Acetyl-4-[2-hydroxy-3-[(1-methylethyl)amino]propoxy]phenyl]butanamide; a β-adrenergic blocking agent.

acec·li·dine (a-sek′li-dēn). 3-Quinuclidinol acetate ester; a cholinergic drug used for topical therapy of glaucoma.

ac·e·dap·sone (as-ĕ-dap′sōn). Diacetyldiaminodiphenylsulfone; a derivative of dapsone with a longer duration of action; used to enhance the malaria chemoprophylaxis of quinine or of a combination of chloroquine-primaquine, and believed to act by interference with the utilization of folic acid.

ace·dia (ă-sē-dē′-ă). A mental syndrome, the chief features of which are listlessness, carelessness, apathy, and melancholia.

acef·yl·line pi·per·a·zine (ă-sef′i-lēn). Piperazine theophylline-7-acetate; a diuretic and smooth muscle relaxant.

ACEI Abbreviation for angiotensin-converting enzyme *inhibitors,* under *inhibitor.*

acel·lu·lar (ă-sel′yū-lăr). **1.** Devoid of cells. SYN noncellular (2). **2.** A term applied to unicellular organisms that do not become multicellular and are complete within a single cell unit; frequently applied to protozoans to emphasize their complete organization within a single cell. [G. *a-* priv. + L. *cellula,* a small chamber]

ace·lom (ā-sē′lom). Absence of a true celom or body cavity lined with mesothelium; typically found in Platyhelminthes (flatworms), which have a syncytial mass of parenchymal cells instead of a true body cavity. [G. *a-* priv. + *koilōma,* hollow (celom)]

ace·lo·mate, ace·lo·ma·tous (ā-sē′lō-māt, ā-sē-lō′mă-tŭs). Not having a celom or body cavity.

ace·nes·the·sia (ă-sē-nes-thē′zē-ă, ă-sen-es-). Absence of the normal sensation of physical existence, or of the consciousness of visceral functioning. [G. *a-* priv. + *koinos,* common, + *aisthēsis,* feeling]

acen·o·cou·ma·rin (ă-sē-nō-kū′mă-rin). SYN acenocoumarol.

acen·o·cou·ma·rol (ă-sē-nō-kū′mă-rol). 3-(α-acetonyl-*p*-nitrobenzyl)-4-hydroxycoumarin; an orally effective synthetic anticoagulant of the coumarin type, with similar actions. SYN acenocoumarin, nicoumalone.

acen·tric (ā-sen′trik). Lacking a center; in cytogenetics, denoting a chromosome fragment without a centromere. [G. *a-* priv. + *kentron*, center]

ace·pha·lia, aceph·a·lism (ă-se-fā′lē-ă, ă-sef′ă-lizm). SYN acephaly.

aceph·a·line (ă-sef′ă-līn). Denoting members of the protozoan suborder Acephalina (order Eugregarinida), characterized by simple noncompartmentalized bodies, that parasitize invertebrates.

aceph·a·lo·bra·chia (ă-sef′ă-lō-brā′kē-ă). SYN abrachiocephaly. [G. *a-* priv. + *kephalē*, head, + *brachiōn*, arm]

aceph·a·lo·car·dia (ă-sef′ă-lō-kar′dē-ă). Absence of head and heart in a parasitic twin. [G. *a-* priv. + *kephalē*, head, + *kardia*, heart]

aceph·a·lo·chei·ria, aceph·a·lo·chi·ria (ă-sef′ă-lō-kī′rē-ă). Congenital absence of head and hands. [G. *a-* priv. + *kephalē*, head, + *cheir*, hand]

aceph·a·lo·cyst (ă-sef′ă-lō-sist). A hydatid cyst with no daughter cyst; a sterile hydatid, so called because it fails to develop scoleces or tapeworm heads. [G. *a-* priv. + *kephalē*, head, + *kystis*, bladder]

aceph·a·lo·gas·ter·ia (ă-sef′ă-lō-gas-tēr′ē-ă). Congenital absence of head, thorax, and abdomen in a parasitic twin with pelvis and legs only.

aceph·a·lo·po·dia (ă-sef′ă-lō-pō′dē-ă). Congenital absence of head and feet. [G. *a-* priv. + *kephalē*, head, + *pous*, foot]

aceph·a·lor·rha·chia (ă-sef′ă-lō-rak′ē-ă). Congenital absence of head and vertebral column. [G. *a-* priv. + *kephalē*, head, + *rhachis*, spine]

aceph·a·lo·sto·mia (ă-sef′ă-lō-stō′mē-ă). Congenital absence of the greater part of the head with, however, the presence of a mouthlike opening. [G. *a-* priv. + *kephalē*, head, + *stoma*, mouth]

aceph·a·lo·tho·ra·cia (ă-sef′ă-lō-thōr-ā′sē-ă). Congenital absence of head and thorax. [G. *a-* priv. + *kephalē*, head, + *thorax*, chest]

aceph·a·lous (ă-sef′ă-lŭs). SYN acephalus.

aceph·a·lus (ă-sef′ă-lŭs). Headless. SYN acephalous. [G. *a-* priv. + *kephalē*, head]

a. acormus (ă-kōr′mŭs), condition in which a head without a body is attached to the placenta by an umbilical cord.

a. dibra′chius, a fetus lacking a head but having two recognizably developed upper limbs.

a. di′pus, a fetus lacking a head but showing two recognizably developed lower limbs.

a. monobra′chius, a fetus lacking a head and showing only one recognizable upper limb.

a. mon′opus, a fetus lacking a head and with fusion of the lower extremities so extreme that only a single foot is recognizable.

a. paraceph′alus, a malformed fetus with only partially developed skull and little or no brain.

a. sym′pus, an a. showing fusion of all of the lower limbs.

aceph·a·ly (ă-sef′ă-lē). Congenital absence of the head. SYN acephalia, acephalism. [G. *a-* priv. + *kephalē*, head]

ace·ro·la (ă-sĕ-rō′lă). Fruit of a bushy tree that grows in Central and South America and Puerto Rico. The berry is the richest known source of vitamin C (ascorbic acid).

acer·vu·line (ă-ser′vyū-līn). Occurring in clusters, aggregated. [Mod. L. *acervulus*, a little heap]

acer·vu·lus (ă-ser′vyū-lŭs). SYN *corpora* arenacea, under *corpus*. [Mod. L. dim. of L. *acervus*, a heap]

aces·to·ma (ă-ses-tō′mă). Exuberant granulations that form a cicatrix. [G. *akestos*, curable, + *-ōma*, tumor]

ace·sul·fame (ā-sē-sul-fām). A synthetic, noncaloric sweetener similar to saccharin.

◁acet-, aceto-. Combining forms denoting the two-carbon fragment of acetic acid.

ac·e·tab·u·la (as-ĕ-tab′yū-lă). Plural of acetabulum.

ac·e·tab·u·lar (as-ĕ-tab′yū-lăr). Relating to the acetabulum.

ac·e·tab·u·lec·to·my (as′ĕ-tab-yū-lek′tō-mē). Excision of the acetabulum. [acetabulum + G. *ektomē*, excision]

ac·e·tab·u·lo·plas·ty (as-ĕ-tab′yū-lō-plas-tē). Any operation aimed at restoring the acetabulum to as near a normal state as possible. [acetabulum + G. *plastos*, formed]

ac·e·tab·u·lum, pl. **ac·e·tab·u·la** (as-ĕ-tab′yū-lŭm, -lă) [NA]. A cup-shaped depression on the external surface of the hip bone, with which the head of the femur articulates. SYN cotyle (2), cotyloid cavity. [L. a shallow vinegar vessel or cup]

ac·e·tal (as′e-tal). Product of the addition of 2 moles of alcohol to one of an aldehyde, thus: $RCHO + 2R'OH \rightarrow RCH(OR')_2 + H_2O$; in mixed acetals (*e.g.*, glycosides), two different alcohols are bound to the original aldehyde group. SEE ALSO hemiacetal, hemiketal, ketal.

a. phosphatide, older trivial name for alk-1-enylglycerophospholipid.

ac·et·al·de·hyde (as-e-tal′dĕ-hīd). CH_3CHO; an intermediate in yeast fermentation of carbohydrate and in alcohol metabolism. It is a central agent for the toxic effects of ethanol. SYN acetic aldehyde, ethanal.

activated a., the activated form of acetaldehyde that is formed during the decarboxylation of active pyruvate. Formed in alcohol fermentation and in carbohydrate metabolism. SYN α-hydroxyethylthiamin pyrophosphate.

acet·a·mide (as-et-am′īd, ă-set′ă-mīd). CH_3CONH_2; Acetic amide; used in biomedical research. SYN acetic amide.

2-ac·et·am·i·do·flu·o·rene (AAF) (as′et-am′i-dō-flūr′ēn). SYN 2-acetylaminofluorene.

ac·et·a·min·o·phen (as-et-ă-mē′nō-fen). *N*-acetyl-*p*-aminophenol; *p*-acetamidophenol; an antipyretic and analgesic. SYN paracetamol.

ac·e·tam·in·o·sal·ol (as-ĕ-tam′in-ō-sal′ol). salicylic acid ester of acetyl-*p*-aminophenol; used as an analgesic, antipyretic, and intestinal antiseptic. SYN phenetsal.

ac·et·an·i·lid (as-ĕ-tan′i-lid). $C_6H_5NHCOCH_3$; *N*-Phenylacetamide; an analgesic and antipyretic; continued use causes cyanosis.

ac·et·ar·sol (as-ĕ-tar′sol). SYN acetarsone.

ac·et·ar·sone (as-ĕ-tar′sōn). acetylaminohydroxyphenylarsonic acid; *N*-acetyl-4-hydroxy-*m*-arsanilic acid; used in the treatment of amebiasis, and as a local application in Vincent's angina and in trichomoniasis vaginitis. The diethylamine salt is used as an antisyphilitic. SYN acetarsol.

ac·e·tate (as′e-tāt). CH_3COO^-; a salt or ester of acetic acid.

active a., SYN acetyl-CoA.

a. kinase [EC 2.7.2.1], a phosphotransferase forming acetyl phosphate and ADP from ATP and acetate. An important enzyme in the formation of "high-energy" phosphate in certain microorganisms. SYN acetokinase.

a. thiokinase, SYN *acetyl-CoA* ligase.

ac·e·tate-CoA ligase. SYN *acetyl-CoA* ligase.

acet·a·zol·a·mide (as′ĕ-tă-zol′ă-mīd). The heterocyclic sulfonamide, 5-acetylamido-1,3,4-thiadiazole-2-sulfonamide, which inhibits the action of carbonic anhydrase in the kidney, causing an increase in the urinary excretion of sodium, potassium, and bicarbonate, reduced excretion of ammonium, a rise in the pH of the urine, and a fall in the pH of the blood; used in respiratory acidosis for diuresis and control of fluid retention, in glaucoma to reduce intraocular pressure, and in epilepsy. A. sodium has the same actions and uses as a., but is more soluble and suitable for parenteral administration.

acet·e·nyl (a-sē′ten-il). SYN ethynyl.

ace·tic (a-sē′tik, -set′ik). **1.** Denoting the presence of the two-carbon fragment of acetic acid. **2.** Relating to vinegar; sour. [L. *acetum*, vinegar]

ace·tic ac·id. CH_3COOH; a product of the oxidation of ethanol and of the destructive distillation of wood; used locally as a counterirritant and occasionally internally, and also as a reagent. SYN ethanoic acid.

diluted a. a., contains 6% w/v of a. a.

glacial a. a., contains 99% absolute a. a.; a caustic for removal of corns and warts.

ace·tic al·de·hyde. SYN acetaldehyde.

ace·tic am·ide. SYN acetamide.

ace·ti·co·cep·tor (a-sē'ti-kō-sep'tōr). A side chain of molecules with a special affinity for the acetic acid radical. [L. *acetum,* vinegar, + *capio,* to take]

ace·tic phos·phor·ic an·hy·dride. SYN *acetyl* phosphate.

ace·ti·fy (ă-set'i-fī). To cause acetic fermentation; to make vinegar or become vinegar. [L. *acetum,* vinegar, + *facio,* to make; or *fieri,* to be made, to become]

ac·e·tim·e·ter (as-ĕ-tim'ĕ-ter). An apparatus for determining the content of acetic acid in vinegar or other fluid. SYN acetometer. [L. *acetum,* vinegar, + G. *metron,* measure]

⌂aceto-. SEE acet-.

ac·e·to·ac·e·tate (as'e-tō-as'e-tāt). A salt or ion of acetoacetic acid. A ketone body formed in ketogenesis. SYN diacetate (1).

a. decarboxylase [EC 4.1.1.4], a carboxy-lyase cleaving CO_2 from a. to form acetone.

ac·e·to·a·ce·tic ac·id (as'e-tō-a-sē'tik). CH_3COCH_2COOH; one of the ketone bodies, formed in excess and appearing in the urine in starvation or diabetes. SYN diacetic acid.

ac·e·to·a·ce·tyl-CoA (as'e-tō-a-sē'til). Intermediate in the oxidation of fatty acids and in the formation of ketone bodies; also formed from two molecules of acetyl-CoA; major role is condensation with acetyl-CoA to form the important β-hydroxy-β-methylglutaryl-CoA. SYN acetoacetyl-coenzyme A.

a.-CoA reductase [EC 1.1.1.36], an oxidoreductase catalyzing interconversion of a 3-oxoacyl-CoA and NADPH, and the corresponding D-3-hydroxyacyl-CoA, and $NADP^+$. A step in fatty acid synthesis.

a.-CoA thiolase, SYN *acetyl-CoA* acetyltransferase.

ac·e·to·a·ce·tyl-co·en·zyme A (as'e-tō-as'e-til-kō-en'zīm). SYN acetoacetyl-CoA.

ac·e·to·a·ce·tyl-suc·cin·ic thi·o·phor·ase (as'e-tō-as'e-til-sŭk-sin'ik). SYN 3-oxoacid-CoA transferase.

ac·e·to·hex·am·ide (as-ĕ-tō-heks'ă-mīd). 1-[(*p*-Acetylphenyl)-sulfonyl]-3-cyclohexylurea; an oral hypoglycemic agent that stimulates pancreatic insulin secretion; most useful therapeutically in mild cases of non-insulin dependent diabetes mellitus.

ac·e·to·hy·drox·a·mic ac·id (as'e-tō-hī-drok'să-mik). $C_2H_5NO_2$; *N*-Hydroxyacetamide; an inhibitor of urease, used as adjunctive therapy in chronic urea-splitting urinary infections.

acet·o·in (as-et'-ō-in). $CH_3CH(OH)COCH_3$; 3-Hydroxy-2-butanone; a condensation product of two molecules of acetaldehyde. SYN acetyl methylcarbinol.

ac·e·to·ki·nase (as'e-tō-kī'nās). SYN *acetate* kinase.

ac·e·tol (as'e-tol). Obsolete term for 1-hydroxy-2-propanone, or hydroxyacetone, $CH_2OH-CO-CH_3$; also used as a proprietary name for certain commercial items.

α-ac·e·to·lac·tic ac·id (as'e-tō-lak'tik). An intermediate in pyruvic acid catabolism and valine biosynthesis; $CH_3COC-(OH)(CH_3)-COOH$.

ac·e·tol·y·sis (as-e-tol'i-sis). Decomposition of an organic compound with the addition of the elements of acetic acid at the point of decomposition; analogous to hydrolysis and phosphorolysis.

ac·e·to·me·naph·thone (as'ĕ-tō-me-naf'thōn). SYN menadiol diacetate.

ac·e·tom·e·ter (as-ĕ-tom'ĕ-ter). SYN acetimeter.

ac·e·tone (as'e-tōn). CH_3COCH_3; a colorless, volatile, inflammable liquid; extremely small amounts are found in normal urine, but larger quantities occur in urine and blood of diabetic persons, sometimes imparting an ethereal odor to the urine and breath. It is one of the ketone bodies. The synthetic is used as a solvent in some pharmaceutical and commercial preparations. SYN dimethyl ketone.

ac·e·ton·e·mia (as'ĕ-tō-nē'mē-ă). The presence of acetone or acetone bodies in relatively large amounts in the blood, manifested at first by erethism, and later by a progressive depression. [acetone + G. *haima,* blood]

bovine a., SYN bovine *ketosis.*

ovine a., SYN pregnancy *toxemia* of sheep.

ac·e·to·ne·mic (as'ĕ-tō-nē'mik). Relating to or caused by acetonemia.

ac·e·to·ni·trile (as'e-tō-nī'tril). CH_3CN; Methyl cyanide; a colorless fluid of aromatic odor, soluble in water and alcohol.

ac·e·to·nu·ria (as'e-tō-nūr'ē-ă). Excretion in the urine of large amounts of acetone, an indication of incomplete oxidation of large amounts of lipids; commonly occurs in diabetic acidosis. [acetone + G. *ouron,* urine]

ac·e·to·phen·a·zine ma·le·ate (as-ĕ-tō-fē'nă-zēn mal'ē-āt). 2-Acetyl-10{3-[4-(2-hydroxyethyl)piperazinyl]-propyl}phenothiazine dimaleate; a phenothiazine tranquilizer.

ac·e·to·phe·net·i·din (as'ĕ-tō-fe-net'i-din). SYN phenacetin.

ac·e·to·sul·fone so·di·um (as'ĕ-tō-sŭl'fōn). 2-*N*-Acetyl-sulfamyl-4,4'-diaminodiphenylsulfone; a leprostatic administered orally.

ace·tous (as'e-tŭs). Relating to vinegar; sour-tasting.

ac·e·tri·zo·ate so·di·um (as-ĕ-trī-zō'āt). Salt of 3-acetamido-2,4,6-triiobenzoic acid, a formerly used water-soluble radiographic contrast medium.

ace·tum, pl. **ace·ta** (ă-sē'tŭm, -tă). SYN vinegar. [L. *vinum acetum,* soured wine, vinegar]

acet·u·rate (ă-set'yū-rāt). USAN-approved contraction for *N*-acetylglycinate, $CH_3CONHCH_2COO^-$.

ace·tyl (Ac) (as'e-til). $CH_3CO—$; the radical; an acetic acid molecule from which the hydroxyl group has been removed.

a. chloride, CH_3COCl; a colorless liquid used as a reagent; also corrosive, causing severe burns because of hydrolysis to HCl.

a. phosphate, $CH_3CO-OPO_3^{2-}$; a "high energy" phosphate that acts as an acetate donor in the metabolism of various bacteria. SYN acetic phosphoric anhydride.

a. transacylase, SYN ACP-acetyltransferase.

ace·tyl·ad·e·nyl·ate (as'e-til-ă-den'il-āt). Mixed anhydride between the carboxyl group of acetic acid and the phosphoric residue of adenosine 5'-monophosphoric acid; Ado(5')OP-(O_2H)—OCOCH_3.

2-ace·tylami·no·flu·o·rene (AAF) (as'e-til-am'i-nō-flūr'ēn). *N*-2-fluorenylacetamide; a potent carcinogenic compound. SYN 2-acetamidofluorene.

acet·y·lase (a-set'il-ās). Any enzyme catalyzing acetylation or deacetylation, as in the formation of *N*-acetylglutamate from glutamate plus acetyl-CoA, or the reverse; a.'s are usually called acetyltransferases.

***N*-ace·tyl·as·par·tate** (as'-ē-til-as-par'tāt). An acetylated derivative of aspartate found in the brain. Used as a marker in brain NMR and in neuroimaging.

acet·y·la·tion (a-set-i-lā'shŭn). Formation of an acetyl derivative.

ace·tyl·car·bro·mal (ă-sē'til-kar-brō'măl). *N*-acetyl-*N*'-(bromodiethylacetyl)urea; a sedative replaced by benzodiazepines and newer drugs.

***O*-ace·tyl·car·ni·tine** (as-e-til-kar'ni-ten). The acetyl derivative of carnitine formed by carnitine acetyltransferase. Facilitates acetyl transport into the mitochondria and is an important fuel source for sperm.

ace·tyl·cho·line (ACH, Ach) (as-e-til-kō'lēn). $CH_3CO-OCH_2CH_2N(CH_3)_3$; (2-acetoxyethyl)trimethylammonium ion; the acetic ester of choline, the neurotransmitter substance at cholinergic synapses, which causes cardiac inhibition, vasodilation, gastrointestinal peristalsis, and other parasympathetic effects. It is liberated from preganglionic and postganglionic endings of parasympathetic fibers and from preganglionic fibers of the sympathetic as a result of nerve injuries, whereupon it acts as a transmitter on the effector organ; it is hydrolyzed into choline and acetic acid by acetylcholinesterase before a second impulse may be transmitted.

a. chloride, a miotic, administered as an ophthalmic solution for parasympathomimetic effect; used in cataract surgery.

ace·tyl·cho·lin·es·ter·ase (as'e-til-kō-lin-es'ter-ās). The cholinesterases that hydrolyze acetylcholine to acetate and choline within the central nervous system and at peripheral neuroeffector junctions (*e.g.,* motor endplates and autonomic ganglia). SYN choline esterase I, "e"-type cholinesterase, specific cholinesterase, true cholinesterase.

ace·tyl-CoA. Condensation product of coenzyme A and acetic acid, symbolized as CoAS~COCH₃; intermediate in transfer of two-carbon fragment, notably in its entrance into the tricarboxylic acid cycle and in fatty acid synthesis. SYN acetyl-coenzyme A, active acetate.

a.-CoA acetyltransferase, an acetyltransferase forming acetoacetyl-CoA from two molecules of a.-CoA, releasing one CoA. A key step in ketogenesis and sterol synthesis. SYN acetoacetyl-CoA thiolase, a.-CoA thiolase, thiolase.

a.-CoA acylase, SYN a.-CoA hydrolase.

a.-CoA acyltransferase, an enzyme catalyzing the thioclastic cleavage by coenzyme A of β-ketoacyl-CoA, forming an acyl-CoA with a carbon chain shorter by two atoms, the missing two atoms appearing as a.-CoA. A step in fatty acid degradation. SEE ALSO a.-CoA acetyltransferase. SYN 3-ketoacyl-CoA thiolase, β-ketothiolase.

a.-CoA carboxylase, a ligase that catalyzes the reaction of a.-CoA, CO_2, H_2O, and ATP, with a divalent cation as catalyst and covalently bound biotin, to form malonyl-CoA, ADP, and P_i (or the reverse decarboxylase); N-carboxybiotin is an intermediate. A crucial enzyme in fatty acid synthesis.

a.-CoA deacylase, SYN a.-CoA hydrolase.

a.-CoA:α-glucosaminide acetyltransferase, an enzyme involved in the synthesis of certain carbohydrate moieties on proteins. A deficiency of this enzyme leads to mucopolysaccharidosis type III C.

a.-CoA hydrolase, a hydrolase that cleaves acetate and coenzyme A from a.-CoA. SYN a.-CoA acylase, a.-CoA deacylase.

a.-CoA ligase, a ligase that catalyzes the reaction of acetate and CoA and ATP to form AMP, pyrophosphate, and a.-CoA. A key step in the activation of acetate. SYN acetate thiokinase, acetate-CoA ligase, acetyl-activating enzyme, a.-CoA synthetase.

a.-CoA synthetase, SYN a.-CoA ligase.

a.-CoA thiolase, SYN a.-CoA acetyltransferase.

ace·tyl-co·en·zyme A (as′e-til-kō-en′zīm). SYN acetyl-CoA.

ace·tyl·cys·te·ine (as′ĕ-til-sis′tē-in). N-Acetyl-L-cysteine; a mucolytic agent that reduces the viscosity of mucous secretions; used to treat acetaminophen toxicity.

ace·tyl·dig·i·tox·in (ă-sē′til-dij-i-tok′sin). The α-acetyl ester of digitoxin derived from lanatoside A, having the same actions and uses as digitoxin, but more rapid onset and shorter duration of action.

ace·tyl·di·gox·in (ă-sē′til-dī-jok′sin). A digitalis glycoside with properties similar to those of digoxin; derived from digilanide C.

α-N-ace·tyl·ga·lac·to·sam·in·id·ase (as′ē-til-gal-ăk-tōs-a-min-i-dās). An enzyme that hydrolyzes 2-acetamido-2-deoxy-α-D-galactosides to the alcohol and free 2-acetamido-2-deoxy-D-galactose. A deficiency of this enzyme will result in Schindler disease.

N-ace·tyl·glu·co·sam·ine (as′ē-til-glu-cōs′a-mēn). An acetylated amino sugar that is an important moiety of glycoproteins.

α-N-ace·tyl·glu·co·sam·in·id·ase (as′ē-til-glu-cōs-a-min-i-dās). An enzyme that hydrolyzes glycosides of N-acetylglucosamine producing the alcohol and N-acetylglucosamine. A deficiency of this enzyme results in mucopolysaccharidosis III B.

N-ace·tyl·glu·ta·mate (NAG, AGA) (ă-sē′til-glū′tă-māt). The salt of N-acetylglutamic acid. An activator of carbamoyl phosphate synthetase I during urea synthesis; this amino acid causes a configurational change in the enzyme, increasing the activity of that enzyme. The inability to synthesize acetylglutamate results in a defect in urea biosynthesis.

ace·tyl·meth·a·dol (as′ē-til-meth-ă-dol). An opioid analgesic which exists in 4 different optical isomers. The l isomers are active and l-acetylmethadol (LAM) has a long duration of action and has been tried as a substitute for methadone in methadone maintenance programs and in programs where methadone is to be withdrawn, as in physical dependence of the morphine type.

ace·tyl meth·yl·car·bin·ol. SYN acetoin.

N-ace·tyl·neu·ra·min·ic ac·id (NeuAc) (as′ē-til-nur-a-min′ik-as′id). The most common form of sialic acid in mammals.

ace·tyl·or·ni·thin·ase (as′e-til-ōr′ni-thin-ās). SYN acetylornithine deacetylase.

ace·tyl·or·ni·thine de·a·cet·yl·ase (as′e-til-ōr′ni-thēn) [EC 3.5.1.16]. An enzyme catalyzing the hydrolysis of N^2-acetyl-L-ornithine to L-ornithine and acetate. SYN acetylornithinase.

3-ace·tyl·pyr·i·dine (as′e-til-pir′i-dēn). An antimetabolite of nicotinamide that produces symptoms of nicotinamide deficiency in mice.

ace·tyl·sal·i·cyl·ic ac·id (as′ĕ-til-sal-i-sil′ik). SYN aspirin.

N^1-ace·tyl·sul·fa·nil·a·mide. An antibacterial sulfa drug used topically and in the eye.

N^4-ace·tyl·sul·fa·nil·a·mide (as′e-til-sŭl-fă-nil′ă-mīd). An intermediate in the synthesis of sulfanilamide; formed in animal bodies by acetylation of sulfanilamide. SYN p-sulfamylacetanilide.

ace·tyl sul·fi·sox·a·zole. A derivative of sulfisoxazole with the same actions and uses; an antibacterial sulfa drug.

ace·tyl·tan·nic ac·id (as′ĕ-til-tan′ik). An astringent used for treatment of diarrhea. SYN diacetyltannic acid, tannylacetate.

ace·tyl·trans·fer·ase (as′e-til-trans′fer-ās). Any enzyme transferring acetyl groups from one compound to another. SEE ALSO *acetyl-CoA* acetyltransferase, *choline* acetyltransferase, dihydrolipoamide acetyltransferase. SYN transacetylase.

AcG, ac-g Abbreviation for accelerator *globulin*.

ACH, Ach Abbreviation for acetylcholine.

Ach. SEE ACH.

acha·la·sia (ak-ă-lā′zē-ă). Failure to relax; referring especially to visceral openings such as the pylorus, cardia, or any other sphincter muscles. [G. *a-* priv. + *chalasis,* a slackening]

esophageal a., an obstruction to the passage of food that develops in the terminal esophagus just proximal to the cardioesophageal junction caused by an autonomic nervous system abnormality; an associated dilation of the thoracic esophagus is commonly found. SYN cardiospasm, phrenospasm.

Achard, E. Charles, French physician, 1860–1941. SEE A. *syndrome;* A.-Thiers *syndrome.*

ache (āk). A dull, poorly localized pain, usually one of less than severe intensity.

bone a., a dull pain in the bones, often severe; an extreme variety occurs in dengue.

stomach a., pain in the abdomen, usually arising in the stomach or intestine. SYN gastralgia, gastrodynia.

achei·lia (ă-kī′lē-ă). Congenital absence of the lips. [G. *a-* priv. + *cheilos,* lip]

achei·lous, achi·lous (ă-kī′lŭs). Characterized by or relating to acheilia.

achei·ria (ă-kī′rē-ă). **1.** Congenital absence of one or both hands. **2.** Anesthesia in, with loss of the sense of possession of, one or both hands; a condition sometimes noted in hysteria. **3.** A form of dyscheiria in which the patient is unable to tell on which side of the body a stimulus has been applied. [G. *a-* priv. + *cheir,* hand]

achei·rop·o·dy, achi·rop·o·dy (ă-kī-rop′ō-dē, ă-kī-rop′ō-dē) [MIM*200500]. Congenital absence of the hands and feet; autosomal recessive inheritance. [G. *a-* priv. + *cheir,* hand, + *podos,* foot]

achei·rous, achi·rous (ă-kī′rŭs). Characterized by or relating to acheiria (1).

Achenbach, Walter, 20th century German internist. SEE A. *syndrome.*

Achilles, Mythical Greek warrior, vulnerable only in the heel. SEE A. *bursa, reflex, tendon.*

achil·lo·bur·si·tis (ă-kil′ō-ber-sī′tis). Inflammation of a bursa in proximity to the tendo calcaneus. SYN retrocalcaneobursitis.

achil·lo·dyn·ia (ă-kil-ō-din′ē-ă). Pain due to inflammation of the bursa between the calcaneus and the tendo calcaneus (achillobursitis). [Achilles (tendon) + G. *odynē,* pain]

ach·il·lor·rha·phy (ă-kil-ōr′ă-fē). Suture of the tendo calcaneus. [Achilles (tendon) + G. *rhaphē,* a sewing]

achil·lo·ten·o·my (ă-kil′ō-ten-ot′ō-mē). SYN achillotomy. [Achilles (tendon) + G. *tenōn,* tendon, + *tomē,* a cutting]

ach·il·lot·o·my (ă-kil-ot′ō-mē). Division of the tendo calcaneus. SYN achillotenotomy. [Achilles (tendon) + G. *tomē,* incision]

achi·ral (ā-kī'răl). Not chiral; denoting an absence of chirality. [G. *a*- priv. + *cheir,* hand]

achlor·hy·dria (ā-klōr-hī'drē-ă). Absence of hydrochloric acid from the gastric juice. [G. *a*- priv. + chlorhydric (acid)]

achlor·o·phyl·lous (ā-klōr-ō-fī'lŭs). Without chlorophyll, as in fungi.

Acho·le·plas·ma, pl. *Acho·le·plas·ma·ta* (ă-kō-lē-plas'mă, mah-tă). A genus of bacteria (order Mycoplasmatales) that have characteristics identical to those of the species in the genus *Mycoplasma,* with the exception that the acholeplasmas do not require sterol for growth; saprophytic and parasitic species occur. The type species is *A. laidlawii.*

A. axan'thum, a species originally found in a murine leukemia cell line; ecology not determined.

A. granula'rum, a species that occurs as a commensal in swine; pathogenicity not determined.

A. laidla'wii, a species that occurs as a saprophyte in sewage, manure, humus, and soil; type species of the genus *A.* SYN *Mycoplasma laidlawii.*

acho·lia (ă-kō'lē-ă). Suppressed or absent secretion of bile. [G. *a*- priv. + *cholē,* bile]

achol·ic (ă-kol'ik). Without bile, as in a. (pale) stools.

achol·u·ria (ā-kō-lū'rē-ă). Absence of bile pigments from the urine in certain cases of jaundice. [G. *a*- priv. + *cholē,* bile, + *ouron,* urine]

achol·u·ric (ā-kō-lū'rik). Without bile in the urine.

achon·dro·gen·e·sis (ă-kon-drō-jen'ĕ-sis) [MIM*200600 *200720]. Dwarfism accompanied by various bone aplasias of all four limbs, a normal or enlarged skull, and a short trunk with delayed ossification of the lower spine; autosomal recessive inheritance. A new dominant mutation of type II collagen has been reported. [G. *a*- priv., + *chondros,* cartilage, + *genesis,* origin]

achon·dro·pla·sia (ă-kon-drō-plā'zē-ă) [MIM*100800]. A type of chondrodystrophy characterized by an abnormality in conversion of cartilage into bone, predominantly affecting long bones, in which epiphysial growth is retarded and ceases early, resulting in dwarfism apparent at birth, with short extremities but normal trunk; the head may be enlarged, the effect being exaggerated by midfacial hypoplasia; stenosis at the foramen magnum and the spinal column commonly cause compression and neurological compromise; autosomal dominant inheritance. [G. *a*- priv. + *chondros,* cartilage, + *plasis,* a molding]

avian a., an autosomal dominant a. seen in several breeds of domestic chickens.

bovine a., SYN bulldog *calf.*

homozygous a., severe a. affecting progeny of two achondroplastic parents; usually fatal in the first year of life.

achon·dro·plas·tic (ă-kon-drō-plas'tik). Relating to or characterized by achondroplasia.

achor·date, achor·dal (ā-kōr'dāt, ā-kōr'dăl). Referring to animal forms below the Chordata that do not develop a notochord or chorda.

acho·re·sis (ă-kō-rē'sis). Permanent contraction of a hollow viscus, such as the stomach or bladder, whereby its capacity is reduced. [G. *a*- priv. + *chōreō,* to make room, fr. *chōros,* space]

Acho·ri·on (ă-kō'rē-on). Former name for *Trichophyton.* [G. *achōr,* dandruff]

achro·a·cyte (ă-krō'ă-sīt). A colorless cell. [G. *a*- priv. + *chroa,* color, + *kytos,* a hollow (cell)]

achro·a·cy·to·sis (ă-krō'ă-sī-tō'sis). Obsolete term for lymphocytosis.

ach·ro·dex·trin (ak-rō-deks'trin). SYN achroodextrin. [G. *a*- priv. + *chrōma,* color, + dextrin]

achro·ma·cyte (ă-krō'mă-sīt). SYN achromocyte.

ach·ro·ma·sia (ak-rō-mā'sē-ă). 1. Pallor associated with hippocratic facies, emaciation, and weakness, often heralding a moribund state. SYN cachectic pallor. 2. SYN achromia. [G. *achrōmos,* colorless]

achro·mat (ă-krō'măt). A person exhibiting achromatopsia. [G. *a*- priv. + *chrōma,* color]

ach·ro·mat·ic (ak-rō-mat'ik). 1. Colorless. 2. Not staining readily. 3. Refracting light without chromatic aberration. [G. *a*- priv. + *chrōma,* color]

achro·ma·tin (ă-krō'mă-tin). The weakly staining components of the nucleus, such as the nuclear sap and euchromatin.

achro·ma·tin·ic (ă-krō-mă-tin'ik). Relating to or containing achromatin.

achro·ma·tism (ă-krō'mă-tizm). 1. The quality of being achromatic. 2. The annulment of chromatic aberration by combining glasses of different refractive indexes and different dispersion.

achro·mat·o·cyte (ă-krō-mat'ō-sīt). SYN achromocyte.

achro·mat·ol·y·sis (ă-krō-mă-tol'i-sis). Dissolution of the achromatin of a cell or of its nucleus. SYN karyoplasmolysis.

achro·mat·o·phil (ă-krō-mat'ō-fil). 1. Not being colored by the histologic or bacteriologic stains. SYN achromophilic, achromophilous. 2. A cell or tissue that cannot be stained in the usual way. SYN achromophil. [G. *a*- priv. + *chrōma,* color, + *philos,* fond]

achro·mat·o·phil·ia (ă-krō'mat-ō-fil'ē-ă). A condition of being refractory to staining processes.

achro·ma·top·sia, achro·ma·top·sy (ă-krō-mă-top'sē-ă, ă-krō' mă-top-sē) [MIM*216900]. A severe congenital deficiency in color perception, often associated with nystagmus and reduced visual acuity. SYN achromatic vision, monochromasia, monochromasy, monochromatism (2). [G. *a*- priv. + *chrōma,* color, + *opsis,* vision]

atypical a., incomplete a. with normal visual acuity and no nystagmus. Cf. dyschromatopsia.

complete a., a. with absent color vision, nystagmus, reduced visual acuity, and light aversion. SYN rod monochromatism, typical a.

incomplete a., impaired, but not absent, color vision with less severely reduced visual acuity than in complete a.; inherited as an autosomal recessive [MIM*200930] or as an X-linked disorder [MIM*304020] (blue cone monochromism; pi cone monochromatism [MIM*303700]).

typical a., SYN complete a.

achro·ma·to·sis (ă-krō-mă-tō'sis). SYN achromia. [G. *a*- priv. + *chrōma,* color]

achro·ma·tous (ă-krō'mă-tŭs). Colorless.

achro·ma·tu·ria (ă-krō-mă-tū'rē-ă). The passage of colorless or very pale urine. [G. *a*- priv. + *chrōma,* color, + *ouron,* urine]

achro·mia (ă-krō'mē-ă). 1. Depigmentation; absence, or loss of natural pigmentation of the skin and iris; may be congenital or acquired. SEE ALSO depigmentation. 2. Lack of capacity to accept stains in cells or tissue. SYN achromasia (2), achromatosis. [G. *a*- priv. + *chrōma,* color]

a. parasit'ica, a phase of lessening or absence of pigmentation in cutaneous lesions, caused by the fungus *Malassezia furfur.* SEE ALSO *tinea* versicolor.

a. un'guium, SYN leukonychia.

achro·mic (ā-krō'mik). Colorless.

achro·mo·cyte (ă-krō'mō-sīt). A hypochromic, crescent-shaped erythrocyte, probably resulting from artifactual rupture of a red cell with loss of hemoglobin. SYN achromacyte, achromatocyte, ghost corpuscle, phantom corpuscle, Ponfick's shadow, shadow corpuscle, shadow (3), Traube's corpuscle. [G. *a*- priv. + *chrōma,* color, + *kytos,* hollow (cell)]

achro·mo·der·ma (ă-krō-mō-der'mă). SYN leukoderma.

achro·mo·phil (ă-krō'mō-fil). SYN achromatophil.

achro·mo·phil·ic, achro·moph·i·lous (ā-krō-mō-fil'ik, ā-krō-mof'i-lŭs). SYN achromatophil (1).

achro·mo·trich·ia (ă-krō-mō-trik'ē-ă). Absence or loss of pigment in the hair. SEE ALSO canities. [G. *a*- priv. + *chrōma,* color, + *thrix,* hair]

ach·ro·o·dex·trin (ak-rō'ō-deks'trin). Dextrin of low molecular weight, formed from starch in a stage of the digestion of the latter by amylase; it gives no color reaction with iodine. Cf. amylodextrin, erythrodextrin. SYN achrodextrin. [G. *achroos,* uncolored, + dextrin]

achy·lia (ă-kī′lē-ă). **1.** Absence of gastric juice or other digestive secretions. **2.** Absence of chyle. [G. *a-* priv. + *chylos,* juice]

a. gas′trica, diminished or abolished secretion of gastric juice associated with atrophy of the mucous membrane of the stomach.

a. pancreat′ica, deficiency or absence of pancreatic secretion, usually resulting in fatty stools, emaciation, and impaired nutrition.

achy·lous (ă-kī′lŭs). **1.** Lacking in gastric juice or other digestive secretions. **2.** Having no chyle. [G. *achylos,* without juice]

acic·u·lar (ă-sik′yū-lar). Needle-shaped or needle-pointed; applied particularly to leaves and crystals. [L. *acicular,* small pin]

ac·id (as′id). **1.** A compound yielding a hydrogen ion in a polar solvent (*e.g.,* in water); a.'s form salts by replacing all or part of the ionizable hydrogen with an electropositive element or radical. **2.** In popular language, any chemical compound that has a sour taste (given by the hydrogen ion). **3.** Sour; sharp to the taste. **4.** Relating to a.; giving an a. reaction. For individual acids, see specific names. [L. *acidus,* sour]

bile a.'s, steroid a.'s found in bile; *e.g.,* taurocholic and glycocholic a.'s, used when biliary secretion is inadequate and for biliary colic. Their physiological roles include fat emulsification. Their synthesis is reduced in disorders of the peroxisomes.

Brønsted a., an a. that is a proton donor.

conjugate a., the protonated compound of two compounds that differ in structure only by the presence of the labile proton.

dibasic a., an a. containing two ionizable atoms of hydrogen in the molecule. SEE acid (1).

fatty a., SEE fatty acid.

inorganic a., an a. made up of molecules not containing organic radicals; *e.g.,* HCl, H_2SO_4, H_3PO_4.

Lewis a., an a. that is an electron pair acceptor.

monobasic a., an a. containing one ionizable atom of hydrogen in the molecule. SEE acid (1).

organic a., an a. made up of molecules containing organic radicals; *e.g.,* acetic a., citric a., which contain the ionizable —COOH group.

polybasic a., an a. containing more than three ionizable atoms of hydrogen in the molecule. SEE acid (1).

ruberythric acid (rū-ber′ē-thrik), a glycoside of alizarin and a disaccharide containing D-xylose and D-glucose residues found in the roots of the madder plant.

wax a., a long-chain monocarboxylic a. with an even number of carbons, often found esterified in waxes (*e.g.,* lauric acid).

ac·id·am·i·nu·ria (as′id-am-i-nū′rē-ă). Obsolete term for aminoaciduria.

ac·id·-cit·rate-dex·trose (ACD). A citrate anticoagulant used for the collection and preservation of whole blood. It has largely been replaced by newer coagulants (CPD, Adsol) that allow for longer shelf life for blood and blood products.

ac·i·de·mia (as-i-dē′mē-ă). An increase in the H-ion concentration of the blood or a fall below normal in pH, notwithstanding alterations in bicarbonate concentration. Individual types of a. are listed by specific name, *e.g.,* isovalericacidemia, aminoacidemia, etc. [acid + G. *haima,* blood]

ac·id-fast (as′id-fast). Denoting bacteria that are not decolorized by acid-alcohol after having been stained with dyes such as basic fuchsin; *e.g.,* the mycobacteria and a few nocardiae.

acid·i·fy (a-sid′i-fī). **1.** To render acid. **2.** To become acid.

acid·i·ty (a-sid′i-tē). **1.** The state of being acid. **2.** The acid content of a fluid.

total a. (a), an obsolete expression of gastric a., the a. being determined by titration with sodium hydroxide, using phenolphthalein as indicator.

ac·i·do·cyte (ă-sid′ō-sīt). Obsolete term for eosinophilic *leukocyte.* [acid + G. *kytos,* cell]

ac·i·do·phil, ac·i·do·phile (ă-sid′ō-fil, ă-sid′ō-fīl). **1.** SYN acidophilic. **2.** One of the acid-staining cells of the anterior pituitary. **3.** A microorganism that grows well in a highly acid media. [acid + G. *philos,* fond]

ac·i·do·phil·ic (as′i-dō-fil′ik, ă-sid′ō-fil-ik). Having an affinity for acid dyes; denoting a cell or tissue element that stains with an acid dye, such as eosin. SYN acidophil (1), acidophile, oxychromatic.

ac·i·do·sis (as-i-dō′sis). A state characterized by actual or relative decrease of alkali in body fluids in relation to the acid content; depending on the degree of compensation for the a., the pH of body fluids may be normal or decreased; an accumulation of acid metabolites often is present, and tissue function may be disturbed (most importantly that of the central nervous system), if compensation is inadequate. [acid + G. *-ōsis,* condition]

carbon dioxide a., SYN respiratory a.

compensated a., an a. in which the pH of body fluids is normal; compensation is achieved by respiratory or renal mechanisms.

compensated respiratory a., retention of bicarbonate by the renal tubules to minimize the effect on the pH of the blood of retention of carbon dioxide by the lungs, such as occurs with hypoventilation.

diabetic a., decreased pH and bicarbonate concentration in the body fluids caused by accumulation of ketone bodies in diabetes mellitus.

hyperchloremic a., SYN renal tubular a.

lactic a., decreased pH and bicarbonate concentration in the body fluids caused by accumulation of lactic acid due to tissue hypoxia, drug reaction, or unknown etiology.

metabolic a., decreased pH and bicarbonate concentration in the body fluids caused either by the accumulation of acids or by abnormal losses of fixed base from the body, as in diarrhea or renal disease.

primary renal tubular a., a metabolic defect in the mechanism of urinary acidification that may be either the transient type, with onset in infancy, or the persistent type, with onset in childhood or adult years; both types are familial.

renal tubular a., a clinical syndrome characterized by decreased ability to acidify urine, and by low plasma bicarbonate and high plasma chloride concentrations, often with hypokalemia, often complicated by osteomalacia, nephrocalcinosis, or renal calculi. SEE ALSO primary renal tubular a., secondary renal tubular a. SYN hyperchloremic a.

respiratory a., a. caused by retention of carbon dioxide; due to inadequate pulmonary ventilation or hypoventilation, with decrease in blood pH unless compensated by renal retention of bicarbonate. SYN carbon dioxide a.

secondary renal tubular a., renal tubular a. that may occur as a complication of hypercalcemic states, hyperglobulinemic disorders, and in some other chronic renal conditions; a regular component of De Toni-Fanconi syndrome.

starvation a., ketoacidosis resulting from lack of food intake, leading to fat catabolism to provide energy, releasing acidic ketone bodies.

uncompensated a., an a. in which the pH of body fluids is subnormal, because restoration of normal acid-base balance is not possible or has not yet been achieved.

ac·i·dot·ic (as-i-dot′ik). Pertaining to or indicating acidosis.

ac·id red 87. SYN *eosin* y.

ac·id red 91. SYN *eosin* B.

acid·u·late (a-sid′yū-lāt). To render more acid or sour.

acid·u·lous (a-sid′yū-lŭs). Acid or sour.

ac·i·du·ria (as-i-dū′rē-ă). **1.** Excretion of an acid urine. **2.** Excretion of an abnormal amount of any specified acid. Individual types of a. are prefixed by the specific acid; *e.g.,* aminoaciduria, ketoaciduria. [acid + G. *ouron,* urine]

ac·i·du·ric (as-i-dū′rik). Pertaining to bacteria that tolerate an acid environment. [acid + L. *duro,* to endure]

ac·i·nar (as′i-nar). Pertaining to the acinus. SYN acinic.

Ac·i·ne·to·bac·ter (as-i-nē′tō-bak′ter). A genus of nonmotile, aerobic bacteria (family Neisseriaceae) containing Gram-negative or -variable coccoid or short rods, or cocci, often occurring in pairs. Spores are not produced. These bacteria grow on ordinary media without the addition of serum. They are oxidase-negative and catalase-positive; carbohydrates are oxidized or not attacked at all, and arginine dihydrolase is not produced. They are a frequent cause of nosocomial infections and can also cause severe primary infections in immunocompromised people. The type species is *A. calcoaceticus*. SYN *Lingelsheimia*.

A. calcoacet′icus, a species of bacteria originally found in a quinate enrichment; strains of this organism which were identified as *Bacterium anitratum* were found in the genitourinary tract; it is the type species of the genus *A*. SYN *Lingelsheimia anitrata*.

ac·i·ni (as′i-nī). Plural of acinus.

acin·ic (a-sin′ik). SYN acinar.

acin·i·form (a-sin′i-fŏrm). SYN acinous. [L. *acinus*, grape, + *forma*, shape]

ac·i·ni·tis (as-in-ī′tis). Inflammation of an acinus.

ac·i·nose (as′i-nōs). SYN acinous.

ac·i·nous (as′i-nŭs). Resembling an acinus or grape-shaped structure. SYN aciniform, acinose.

ac·i·nus, gen. and pl. **ac·i·ni** (as′i-nŭs, -nī) [NA]. One of the minute grape-shaped secretory portions of an acinous gland. Some authorities use the terms a. and alveolus interchangeably, whereas others differentiate them by the constricted openings of the a. into the excretory duct. [L. berry, grape]

liver a., the smallest functional unit of the liver, comprising all of the liver parenchyma supplied by a terminal branch of the portal vein and hepatic artery; typically involves segments of two lobules lying between two terminal hepatic venules. SYN Rappaport's a.

pulmonary a., that part of the airway consisting of a respiratory bronchiole and all of its branches. SYN primary pulmonary lobule, respiratory lobule.

Rappaport's a., SYN liver a.

a·clas·ia (ă-klā′zē-ă). SYN aclasis.

ac·la·sis (ak′lă-sis). A state of continuity between normal and abnormal tissue. SYN aclasia. [G. *a*- priv. + *klasis,* a breaking away, a fragment]

diaphysial a., SYN hereditary multiple *exostoses,* under *exostosis.*

tarsoepiphyseal a. (tăr′-sō-ep′ĭ-fiz′e- al), epiphysealis hemimelica, affects ankles and knees leading to limitation of motion. SYN Trevor's disease.

acleis·to·car·dia (ă-klīs-tō-kar′dē-ă). Obsolete term denoting patency of the foramen ovale of the heart. [G. *a*- priv. + *kleistos,* closed, + *kardia,* heart]

ac·me (ak′mē). The period of greatest intensity of any symptom, sign, or process. [G. *akmē,* the highest point]

ac·mes·the·sia (ak-mes-thē′zē-ă). **1.** Sensitivity to pinprick. **2.** A cutaneous sensation of a sharp point. [G. *acmē,* point, + *aisthēsis,* sensation]

ac·ne (ak′nē). An inflammatory follicular, papular, and pustular eruption involving the pilo sebaceous apparatus. [probably a corruption (or copyist's error) of G. *akmē,* point of efflorescence]

a. al′bida, a. caused by milia.

a. artificia′lis, a. produced by external irritants, such as tar (chloracne), or drugs internally administered, such as iodides or bromides. SYN a. venenata.

bromide a., follicular eruption on face, trunk, and extremities, due to bromide ingestion. SEE ALSO bromoderma.

a. cachectico′rum, a. occurring in persons who have a debilitating constitutional disease; characterized by large, soft, purulent, ulcerative, cystic, and scarred lesions.

chlorine a., SYN chloracne.

a. cilia′ris, follicular papules and pustules on the free edges of the eyelids.

colloid a., SYN colloid milium.

a. congloba′ta, severe cystic a., characterized by cystic lesion, abscesses, communicating sinuses, and thickened, nodular scars; usually sparing the face.

a. cosmet′ica, low-grade, non-inflammatory acne lesions from repeated application of comedogenic agents in cosmetics.

cystic a., severe a. in which the predominant lesions are follicular cysts which rupture and scar.

a. decal′vans, SYN *folliculitis* decalvans.

a. erythemato′sa, SYN rosacea.

a. fronta′lis, SYN a. varioliformis.

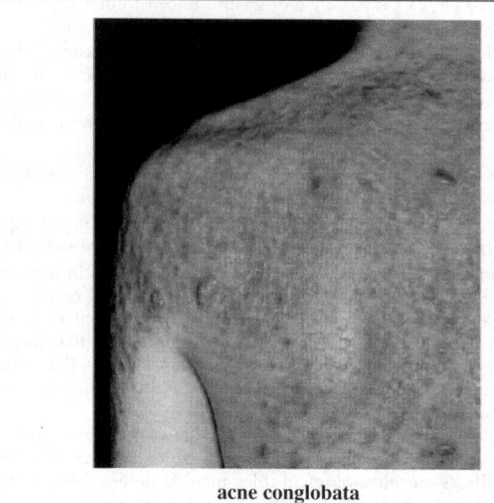

acne conglobata

a. fulminans (ak′nē ful′mi-nanz), severe scarring a. in teenaged males, which may be associated with fever, polyarthralgia, crusted ulcerative lesions, weight loss, and anemia. [*fulmen, fulminis,* thunder, lightning]

a. genera′lis, a. lesions involving the face, chest, and back.

halogen a., an acneform eruption caused by bromides or iodides.

a. hypertroph′ica, a. vulgaris in which the lesions, on healing, leave hypertrophic scars.

a. indura′ta, deeply seated a., with large papules and pustules, large scars, and hypertrophic scars.

iodide a., a follicular eruption on the face, trunk, and extremities, due to injection or ingestion of iodide in a hypersensitive individual. SEE ALSO iododerma.

a. kerato′sa, an eruption of papules consisting of horny plugs projecting from the hair follicles, accompanied by inflammation.

a. medicamento′sa, a. caused or exacerbated by drugs, *e.g.,* antiepileptic, halogens, steroids, tuberculostatic.

a. necrot′ica, SYN a. varioliformis.

a. neonato′rum, a condition in newborn infants, characterized by papules and comedones on forehead and cheeks.

a. papulo′sa, a. vulgaris in which the papular lesions predominate.

pomade a., a. commonly found on the forehead and temples of negro males after prolonged and repetitious application of hair creams.

a. puncta′ta, a. with black open comedones.

a. pustulo′sa, a. vulgaris in which pustular lesions predominate.

a. rosa′cea, SYN rosacea.

a. scrofulosorum, SYN *lichen* scrofulosorum.

a. sim′plex, simple a., SYN a. vulgaris.

steroid a., folliculitis similar to a. vulgaris, but resulting from topical or oral administration of steroids; comedones are rare.

a. syphilit′ica, SYN pustular *syphilid.*

tar a., SYN chloracne.

tropical a., a severe type of a. of the entire trunk, shoulders, upper arms, buttocks, and thighs; occurs in hot, humid climates.

a. urtica′ta, an eruption of acne-like lesions, beginning as urticarial papules and followed by slight scarring.

a. variolifor′mis, a pyogenic infection involving follicles occurring chiefly on the forehead and temples; involution of the umbilicated and crusting lesions is followed by scar formation. SYN a. frontalis, a. necrotica.

a. venena′ta, SYN a. artificialis.

a. vulga′ris, an eruption, predominantly of the face, upper back, and chest, composed of comedones, cysts, papules, and pustules on an inflammatory base; the condition occurs in a majority of people during puberty and adolescence, due to androgenic stimulation of sebum secretion, with plugging of follicles by keratinization, associated with proliferation of *Propionibacterium acnes.* SYN a. simplex, simple a.

ac·ne·form (ak′nē-fōrm). Resembling acne. SYN acneiform.

ac·ne·gen·ic (ak-nē-jen′ik). SYN comedogenic.

ac·ne·i·form (ak-nē′i-fōrm). SYN acneform.

ac·ne·mia, ak·ne·mia (ak-nē′mē-ă). **1.** Congenital absence of legs. **2.** Atrophy of the muscles of the calves of the legs. [G. *a-* priv. + *knēmē,* leg]

ac·o·kan·thera (ak-ō-kan′ther-ă). Juice from the leaves and stems of *Acokanthera ouabaio* (family Apocynaceae), a South African arrow poison containing ouabain. [G. *akōkē,* a point, + *anthēros,* blooming]

ac·o·la·sia (ak-ō-lā′sē-ă). Rarely used term for morbid intemperance or lust. [G. *akolasia,* licentiousness]

aco·lous (ak′ō-lŭs). Without limbs. [G. *a-* priv. + *kōlon,* limb]

aco·mia (ă-kō′mē-ă). SYN alopecia. [G. *a-* priv. + *komē,* hair of head]

acon·a·tive (ă-kon′ă-tiv). Without the desire or wish to act. [G. *a-* priv. + L. *conor,* to try]

acon·i·tase (ă-kon′i-tās). SYN aconitate hydratase.

acon·i·tate hy·dra·tase (ă-kon′i-tāt). An iron-containing enzyme catalyzing the dehydration of citric acid to *cis-*aconitic acid, a reaction of significance in the tricarboxylic acid cycle. SYN aconitase.

ac·o·nite (ak′ō-nīt). The dried root of *Aconitum napellus* (family Ranunculaceae), monkshood or wolfsbane; a powerful and rapid-acting poison formerly used as an antipyretic, diuretic, diaphoretic, anodyne, cardiac and respiratory depressant, and externally as an analgesic.

***cis*-ac·o·nit·ic ac·id** (ak-ō-nit′ik). Dehydration product of citric acid; an enzyme-bound intermediate in the tricarboxylic acid cycle.

acon·i·tine (a-kon′i-tēn). Acetylbenzoylaconine; the exceedingly poisonous active principle (diterpene alkaloid) of *Aconitum* sp. and *Delphinium* sp., formerly used as a cardiac sedative and applied externally for neuralgia.

aco·rea (ă-kō′rē-ă). Congenital absence of the pupil of the eye. [G. *a-* priv. + *korē,* pupil]

Acosta, Joseph (José) de, Spanish Jesuit missionary, 1539–1600. SEE A.'s *disease.*

acou·asm (ă-kū′ă-zm). SYN acousma.

acous·ma (ă-kūs′mă). Rarely used term for an auditory hallucination in which indefinite sounds, such as ringing or hissing, are heard. SYN acouasm. [G. *akousma,* something heard]

acous·ma·tam·ne·sia (ă-kūs′mă-tam-nē′zē-ă). Rarely used term for a loss of memory for sounds. [G. *akousma,* something heard, + *amnēsia,* forgetfulness]

acous·tic (ă-kūs′tik). Pertaining to hearing and the perception of sound, *e.g.,* acoustic meatus, acoustic nerve. [Gr. *akoustikos*]

acous·ti·co·pho·bia (ă-kūs′ti-kō-fō′bē-ă). Morbid fear of sounds. [G. *akoustikos,* acoustic, + *phobos,* fear]

acous·tics (ă-kūs′tiks). The science concerned with sounds and of their perception. [G. *akoustikos,* relating to hearing]

ACP Abbreviation for acyl carrier *protein.*

ACP-ace·tyl·trans·fer·ase. Enzyme transferring acetyl from acetyl-CoA to ACP and releasing CoA to begin fatty acid synthesis. SYN acetyl transacylase.

ACP-mal·o·nyl·trans·fer·ase. An enzyme transferring malonyl from malonyl-CoA to ACP and releasing free CoA; a key step in fatty acid synthesis. SYN malonyl transacylase.

ACPS Abbreviation for acrocephalosyndactyly.

ac·quired (ă-kwīrd′). Denoting a disease, predisposition, abnormality, etc. that is not inherited. [L. *ac-quiro* (*adq-*), to obtain, fr. *quaero,* to seek]

ac·qui·si·tion (ak-wi-zish′ŭn). In psychology, the empirical demonstration of an increase in the strength of the conditioned response in successive trials of pairing the conditioned and unconditioned stimulus.

ac·quis·i·tus (ă-kwiz′i-tŭs). Obsolete term for acquired.

ACR Abbreviation for American College of Radiology.

ac·ral (ak′răl). Relating to or affecting the peripheral parts, *e.g.,* limbs, fingers, ears, etc. [G. *akron,* extremity]

Acra·nia (ă-krā′nē-ă). A group of the phylum Chordata whose members possess a notochord, gill slits, and nerve cord but no vertebrae, ribs, or skull; *e.g., Amphioxus,* tunicates, and acorn worms. [G. *a-* priv. + *kranion,* skull]

acra·nia (ă-krā′nē-ă). Complete or partial absence of a skull; associated with anencephaly. [G. *a-* priv. + *kranion,* skull]

acra·ni·al (ă-krā′nē-ăl). Having no cranium; relating to acrania or an acranius.

acra·ni·us. A malformed fetus exhibiting acrania.

Acrel, Olof, Swedish surgeon, 1717–1806. SEE A.'s *ganglion.*

Ac·re·mo·ni·um (ak-rĕ-mō′nē-ŭm). A genus of fungi (family Moniliaceae, order Moniliales) that causes eumycotic mycetoma; three species, *A. falciforme, A. kiliense,* and *A. recifei,* produce whitish to yellow grains in the tissues. Produces keratomycosis and the antibiotic cephalosporin.

ac·ri·bom·e·ter (ak-ri-bom′ĕ-ter). An instrument for measuring very minute objects. [G. *akribēs,* exact, + *metron,* measure]

ac·rid (ak′rid). Sharp, pungent, biting, or irritating. [L. *acer* (*acr-*), pungent]

ac·ri·dine (ak′ri-dēn). 10-azaanthracene; a dye, dye intermediate, and antiseptic precursor (9-aminoacridine, acriflavine, proflavine hemisulfate) derived from coal tar and irritating to skin and mucous membranes. SYN dibenzopyridine.

tetramethyl a., SYN acridine orange.

ac·ri·dine or·ange [C.I. 46005]. 3,6-bis(dimethylamino)-acridine hydrochloride; a basic fluorescent dye useful as a metachromatic stain for nucleic acids; also used in screening cervical smears for abnormal and malignant cells, where unusual amounts of DNA and RNA occur during proliferation and in tumors (DNA fluoresces yellow to green; RNA fluoresces orange to red). SYN tetramethyl acridine.

ac·ri·dine yel·low. A faintly yellow solution with strong bluish-violet fluorescence; used as a topical antiseptic and as a fluorescent stain in histology. SYN 5-aminoacridine hydrochloride, 9-aminoacridine hydrochloride.

ac·ri·fla·vine (ak-ri-flā′vin) [C.I. 46000]. An acridine dye, a mixture of 3,6-diamino-10-methylacridinium chloride and 3,6-diaminoacridine; formerly used as a topical and urinary antiseptic, and used as one of Kasten's fluorescent Schiff reagents to reveal polysaccharides and DNA.

ac·ri·mo·nia (ak-ri-mō′nē-ă). In ancient humoral pathology, a sharp, pungent, disease-provoking humor. [L. pungency]

ac·ri·mo·ny (ak′rĭ-mō-nē). The quality of being intensely irritant, biting, or pungent. [L. *acrimonia,* pungency]

ac·ri·nol (ak′ri-nol). SYN ethacridine lactate.

ac·ri·sor·cin (ak-ri-sōr′sin). 9-Aminoacridine with 4-hexylresorcinol; a synthetic topical antifungal agent.

acrit·i·cal (ă-krit′i-kăl, ā-). Rarely used term for: **1.** Not critical; marked by no crisis; denoting diseases terminating by lysis. **2.** Indeterminate, especially concerning prognosis. [G. *a-* priv. + *kritikos,* critical]

acro-. Combining form meaning: **1.** Extremity, tip, end, peak, topmost. **2.** Extreme. [G. *akron,* highest point, extremity; *akros,* topmost, outermost, inmost, extreme, tip]

ac·ro·ag·no·sis (ak′rō-ag-nō′sis). Loss or impairment of the sensory recognition of a limb. Absence of acrognosis.

ac·ro·an·es·the·sia (ak′rō-an-es-thē′zē-ă). Anesthesia of one or more of the extremities. [acro- + G. *an-* priv. + *aisthēsis* sensation]

ac·ro·ar·thri·tis (ak-rō-arth-rī′tis). Inflammation of the joints of the hands or feet. [acro- + G. *arthron,* joint, + *-itis*]

ac·ro·as·phyx·ia (ak′rō-as-fik′sē-ă). Impaired digital circulation, possibly a mild form of Raynaud's disease, marked by a purplish or waxy white color of the fingers, with subnormal local temperature and paresthesia. SYN dead fingers, waxy fingers. [acro- + G. *asphyxia,* stoppage of the pulse]

ac·ro·a·tax·ia (ak′rō-ă-tak′sē-ă). Ataxia affecting the distal portion of the extremities, *i.e.,* hands and fingers, feet, and toes. Cf. proximoataxia. [acro- + ataxia]

ac·ro·blast (ak′rō-blast). Component of the developing spermatid composed of numerous Golgi elements; it contains the proacrosomal granules. [acro- + G. *blastos,* germ]

ac·ro·brach·y·ceph·a·ly (ak′rō-brak-i-sef′ă-lē). Type of craniosynostosis with premature closure of the coronal suture, resulting in abnormally short anteroposterior diameter of the skull. [acro- + G. *brachys,* short, + *kephalē,* head]

ac·ro·cen·tric (ak-rō-sen′trik). Having the centromere close to one end; said of a normal chromosome. [acro- + G. *kentron,* center]

ac·ro·ce·pha·lia (ak-rō-se-fā′lē-ă). SYN oxycephaly.

ac·ro·ce·phal·ic (ak-rō-se-fal′ik). SYN oxycephalic.

ac·ro·ceph·a·lo·pol·y·syn·dac·ty·ly (ak′rō-sef′ă-lō-pol′ē-sin-dak′ti-lē). Congenital malformation in which oxycephaly, brachysyndactyly of hand, and preaxial polydactyly of feet are associated with mental retardation; it is usually inherited as an autosomal recessive trait [MIM *200995, *201000] but there is also a dominant form [MIM*101120]. SYN Carpenter's syndrome (2), Goodman's syndrome, Noack's syndrome, Sakati-Nyhan syndrome.

ac·ro·ceph·a·lo·syn·dac·ty·ly (ACPS) (ak′rō-sef′ă-lō-sin-dak′ti-lē). A group of congenital syndromes characterized by peaking at the head, due to premature closure of skull sutures and fusion or webbing of digits. SYN acrodysplasia. [acrocephaly + G. *syn,* together, + *daktylos,* finger]

type I a., SYN Apert's syndrome.

type II a., SYN Vogt cephalodactyly.

type III a., an autosomal dominant syndrome with variable expression of brachycephaly, maxillary hypoplasia, prominent ear crus, syndactyly, facial asymmetry, shallow orbits, telecanthus, and nasal septal deviation; may show mental retardation. SYN Saethre-Chotzen syndrome.

type IV a. (ak′ro-sef′ă-lō-sin- dak′tĭ-lē), a. with pointed nose, hypertelorism, cleft palate, congenital heart disease and pseudohermaphroditism; contractures of elbows and knees; soft tissue syndactyly, absent first metatarsal and great toe. Autosomal recessive. SYN Waardenburg syndrome.

type V a., a. with broad short thumbs and great toes, often with duplication (polydactyly) of the great toes and variable syndactyly of other digits; autosomal dominant inheritance. SYN Pfeiffer's syndrome.

ac·ro·ceph·a·lous (ak-rō-sef′ă-lŭs). SYN oxycephalic.

ac·ro·ceph·a·ly (ak-rō-sef′ă-lē). SYN oxycephaly. [acro- + G. *kephalē,* head]

ac·ro·chor·don (ak-rō-kōr′don). SYN skin *tag.* [acro- + G. *chordē,* cord]

ac·ro·ci·ne·sia, ac·ro·ci·ne·sis (ak′rō-si-nē′zē-ă, -ē′sis). Excessive movement. SYN acrokinesia. [acro- + G. *kinēsis,* movement]

ac·ro·con·trac·ture (ak′rō-kon-trak′chŭr). Contracture of the joints of the hands or feet.

ac·ro·cy·a·no·sis (ak′rō-sī-ă-nō′sis). A circulatory disorder in which the hands, and less commonly the feet, are persistently cold and blue; some forms are related to Raynaud's phenomenon. SYN Crocq's disease, Raynaud's sign. [acro- + G. *kyanos,* blue, + *-osis,* condition]

ac·ro·cy·a·not·ic (ak′rō-sī-ă-not′ik). Characterized by acrocyanosis.

ac·ro·der·ma·ti·tis (ak′rō-der-mă-tī′tis). Inflammation of the skin of the extremities. [acro- + G. *derma,* skin, + *-itis,* inflammation]

a. chron′ica atroph′icans, a gradually progressive late skin manifestation of Lyme disease, appearing first on the feet, hands, elbows or knees, and comprised of indurated, erythematous plaques that become atrophic, giving a tissue-paper appearance of the involved sites. The disease is caused by *Borrelia* spirochetes, commonly transmitted by the *Ixodes ricinus* wood tick.

a. contin′ua, SYN *pustulosis* palmaris et plantaris.

a. enteropath′ica [MIM*201100], a progressive defect of zinc metabolism in young children (3 weeks to 18 months), often manifests first as a blistering, oozing, and crusting eruption on an extremity or around one of the orifices of the body, followed by loss of hair and diarrhea or other gastrointestinal disturbances;

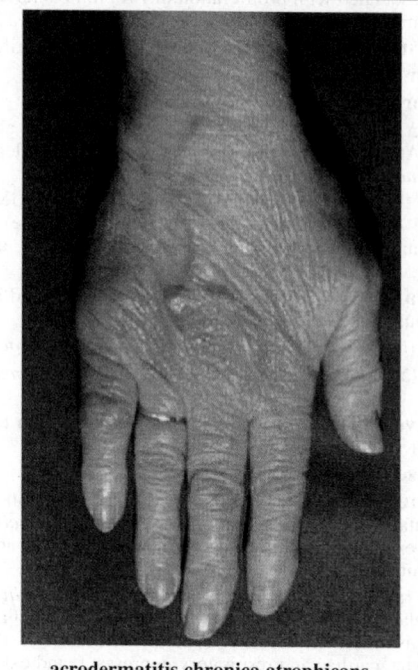

acrodermatitis chronica atrophicans

relieved by lifelong oral zinc supplementation; autosomal recessive trait.

a. hiema′lis, a. occurring chiefly in winter.

papular a. of childhood, SYN Gianotti-Crosti *syndrome.*

a. per′stans, SYN *pustulosis* palmaris et plantaris.

a. vesiculos′a trop′ica, a form occurring in hot climates in which the skin of the extremities is glossy and shows numerous small vesicles.

ac·ro·der·ma·to·sis (ak′rō-der-mă-tō′sis). Any cutaneous affection involving the more distal portions of the extremities. [acro- + G. *derma,* skin, + *-osis,* condition]

ac·ro·dont (ak′rō-dont). Tooth attachment in some lower vertebrates (mainly fish) in which the teeth rest on the edge of the jaw bone rather than in sockets or alveoli. [acro- + G. *odous,* tooth]

ac·ro·dyn·ia (ak-rō-din′ē-ă). 1. Pain in peripheral or acral parts of the body. 2. A syndrome caused almost exclusively by mercury poisoning: in children, characterized by erythema of the extremities, chest, and nose, polyneuritis, and gastrointestinal symptoms; in adults, by anorexia, photophobia, sweating, and tachycardia. SYN acrodynic erythema, dermatopolyneuritis, erythredema, Feer's disease, pink disease, Swift's disease. [acro- + G. *odynē,* pain]

ac·ro·dys·es·the·sia (ak′rō-dis-es-thē′zē-ă). Abnormal and unpleasant sensations in the peripheral portions of the extremities. [acro- + dysesthesia]

ac·ro·dys·os·to·sis (ak′rō-dis-os-tō′sis) [MIM*101800]. A disorder in which the hands and feet are short with stubby fingers and toes. Growth retardation is progressive. Mental retardation and marked nasal hypoplasia are also present; autosomal dominant inheritance. [acro- + dysostosis]

ac·ro·dys·pla·sia (ak′rō-dis-plā′zē-ă). SYN acrocephalosyndactyly. [acro- + dysplasia]

ac·ro·e·de·ma (ak′rō-ĕ-dē′mă). Edema of hand or foot, often permanent.

ac·ro·es·the·sia (ak′ro-es-thē′zē-ă). 1. An extreme degree of hyperesthesia. 2. Hyperesthesia of one or more of the extremities. [acro- + G. *aisthēsis,* sensation]

acrog·e·nous (ak-roj′ĕ-nŭs). Denoting conida of fungi produced by the conidiogenous cell at the tip of a conidiophore. [acro- + G. *genos,* birth]

ac·ro·ger·ia (ak-rō-jēr′ē-ă) [MIM*201200]. Congenital reduction or loss of subcutaneous fat and collagen of the hands and feet, giving the appearance of senility; the genetic evidence is ambiguous. [acro- + G. *gerōn,* old]

ac·rog·no·sis (ak-rog-nō′sis). Cenesthesia, or normal sensory perception, of the extremities. [acro- + G. *gnōsis,* knowledge]

ac·ro·hy·per·hi·dro·sis (ak′rō-hī′per-hī-drō′sis). Hyperhidrosis of the hands and feet.

ac·ro·ker·a·to·e·las·toi·do·sis (ak′rō-ker′ă-tō-ē-las-toy-dō′sis) [MIM*101850]. A developmental papular keratosis of the palms and soles, with disorganization of dermal elastic fibers; unrelated to sunlight and physical trauma. SEE ALSO keratoelastoidosis. [acro + G. *keras,* horn, + *elastos,* beaten, + *eidos,* resemblance, + *-ōsis,* condition]

ac·ro·ker·a·to·sis (ak′rō-ker-ă-tō′sis). Overgrowth of the horny layer of the skin, usually nodular configurations, of the dorsum of the fingers and toes, and occasionally on the rim of the ear and tip of the nose. [acro- + G. *keras,* horn, + *-osis,* condition]
paraneoplastic a., SYN Bazex's *syndrome.*

ac·ro·ker·a·to·sis ver·ru·ci·for·mis (ak′rō-ker-ă-tō′sis vĕ-rū-si-fōrm′is) [MIM*101900]. An outmoded dominant disorder characterized by warty papules of the hands and feet; autosomal dominant inheritance. [acro- + keratosis; L. *verruca,* a wart, + *forma,* form]

ac·ro·ki·ne·sia (ak′rō-ki-nē′zē-ă). SYN acrocinesia.

ac·ro·le·ic ac·ids (ak-rō′-lē-ik). SYN acrylic acids.

ac·ro·leu·kop·a·thy (ak′rō-lū-kop′ă-thē). Depigmentation of the extremities.

ac·ro·me·ga·lia (ak′rō-mĕ-gā′lē-ă). SYN acromegaly.

ac·ro·me·gal·ic (ak′rō-mĕ-gal′ik). Pertaining to or characterized by acromegaly.

ac·ro·meg·a·lo·gi·gan·tism (ak′rō-meg′ă-lō-jī′gan-tizm). Gigantism in which the facial features, disproportionate enlargement of the extremities, and other signs of acromegaly are prominent. [acro- + G. *megas,* great, + *gigas,* giant]

ac·ro·meg·a·loid·ism (ak-rō-meg′ă-loyd-izm). Rarely used term for a condition in which body proportions resemble those of acromegaly.

ac·ro·meg·a·ly (ak-rō-meg′ă-lē). A disorder marked by progressive enlargement of peripheral parts of the body, especially the head, face, hands, and feet, due to excessive secretion of somatotropin; organomegaly and metabolic disorders occur; diabetes mellitus may develop. SYN acromegalia. [acro- + G. *megas,* large]

ac·ro·mel·al·gia (ak-rō-mel-al′jē-ă). SEE erythromelalgia. [acro- + G. *melos,* limb, + *algos,* pain]

ac·ro·mel·ic (ak-rō-mel′ik). Affecting the terminal part of a limb. [acro- + G. *melos,* limb]

ac·ro·mes·o·me·lia (ak-rō-mē′lē-ă) [MIM*201250]. A form of dwarfism in which shortening is striking in the most distal segment of the limbs; autosomal recessive inheritance. SYN acromelic dwarfism. [acro- + G. *melos,* limb, + *ia,* condition]

ac·ro·met·a·gen·e·sis (ak′rō-met-ă-jen′ĕ-sis). Abnormal growth of the extremities resulting in deformity. [acro- + G. *meta,* beyond, + *genesis,* origin]

acro·mi·al (ă-krō′mē-ăl). Relating to the acromion.

ac·ro·mic·ria (ak-rō-mik′rē-ă, ak-rō-mī′krē-ă). The antithesis of acromegaly; a condition in which the bones of the face and extremities are small and delicate; possibly due to a deficiency of somatotropin. [acro- + G. *mikros,* small]

acro·mi·o·cla·vic·u·lar (ă-krō′mē-ō-kla-vik′yū-lăr). Relating to the acromion and the clavicle; denoting the articulation and ligaments between the clavicle and the acromion of the scapula. SYN scapuloclavicular (1).

acro·mi·o·cor·a·coid (ă-krō-mē-ō-kōr′ă-koyd). SYN coracoacromial.

acro·mi·o·hu·mer·al (ă-krō′mē-ō-hyū′mer-ăl). Relating to the acromion and the humerus.

acro·mi·on (ă-krō′mē-on) [NA]. The lateral end of the spine of the scapula which projects as a broad flattened process overhanging the glenoid fossa; it articulates with the clavicle and gives attachment to part of the deltoid and trapezius muscles. Its lateral border is a palpable landmark ("the point of the shoulder"). SYN acromial process. [G. *akrōmion,* fr. *akron,* tip, + *ōmos,* shoulder]

acro·mi·o·scap·u·lar (ă-krō′mē-ō-skap′yū-lăr). Relating to both the acromion and body of the scapula.

acro·mi·o·tho·rac·ic (ă-krō′mē-ō-thō-ras′ik). SYN thoracoacromial.

a·crom·pha·lus (ak-rom′fal-ŭs). Abnormal projection of the umbilicus. [acro- + G. *omphalos,* umbilicus]

ac·ro·my·o·to·nia (ak′rō-mī-ō-tō′nē-ă). Myotonia affecting the extremities only, resulting in spasmodic deformity of the hand or foot. SYN acromyotonus. [acro- + G. *mys,* muscle, + *tonos,* tension]

ac·ro·my·ot·o·nus (ak-rō-mī-ot′ō-nŭs). SYN acromyotonia.

ac·ro·nine (ak′rō-nēn). 3,12-Dihydro-6-methoxy-3,3,12-trimethyl-7*H*-pyrano[2,3-*c*]acridin-7-one; an antineoplastic agent.

ac·ro·os·te·ol·y·sis (ak′rō-os-tē-ol′i-sis) [MIM*102500]. Congenital condition manifested by palmar and plantar ulcerating lesions with osteolysis involving distal phalanges of the fingers and toes. Acquired a.-o. has been reported in workers exposed to vinyl chloride. There is an autosomal disorder, Cheney's syndrome [MIM*102500], in which this finding is combined with Wormian bones, hypolplasia of the mandibular rami and basilar osteoporosis. SEE ALSO Cheney *syndrome.* [acro- + G. *osteon,* bone, + *lysis,* loosening]

ac·ro·pachy (ak′rō-pak-ē, ă-krop′ă-kē). Thickening of peripheral tissues; seen most often in hypothyroidism and hypertrophic pulmonary osteoarthropathy. [acro- + G. *pachys,* thick]

ac·ro·pach·y·der·ma (ak′rō-pak-i-der′mă). SYN pachydermoperiostosis. [acro- + G. *pachys,* thick, + *derma,* skin]

ac·ro·par·es·the·sia (ak′rō-par-es-thēs′ē-a). **1.** Paresthesia of one or more of the extremities. **2.** Nocturnal paresthesia involving the hands, most often of middle-aged women; formerly attributed to a lesion in the thoracic outlet, but now known to be a classic symptom of carpal tunnel syndrome. [acro- + paresthesia]

acrop·a·thy (ă-krop′ă-thē) [MIM*119900]. SYN hereditary *clubbing.* [acro- + G. *pathos,* disease]

acrop·e·tal (ă-krop′ĕ-tăl). **1.** In a direction toward the summit. **2.** Produced successively toward the apex, with the youngest conidium formed at the tip and the oldest at the base of a chain of conidia; pertaining to asexual spore production in fungi by successive budding of the distal spore in a spore chain. [acro- + L. *peto,* to seek]

ac·ro·pho·bia (ak-rō-fō′bē-ă). Morbid fear of heights. [acro- + G. *phobos,* fear]

ac·ro·pig·men·ta·tion (ak′rō-pig-men-tā′shŭn). Hyperpigmentation of the dorsal surfaces of the fingers and toes beginning in early childhood and usually increasing with age; more common in persons of dark complexion.

ac·ro·pleu·rog·e·nous (ak′rō-plū-roj′ĕ-nŭs). Denoting spores developing at the tip and along the sides of fungal hyphae.

ac·ro·pus·tu·lo·sis (ak′rō-pŭs-tyū-lō′sis). Pustular eruptions of the hands and feet, often a form of psoriasis. [acro- + pustulosis]
infantile a., a cyclically recurrent papulopustular and crusting pruritic eruption, usually in black children, appearing soon after birth to 10 months; remission occurs at about 2 years of age.

ac·ro·scle·ro·der·ma (ak′rō-sklēr-ō-der′mă). SYN acrosclerosis. [acro- + G. *sklēros,* hard, + *derma,* skin]

ac·ro·scle·ro·sis (ak′rō-sklē-rō′sis). Stiffness and tightness of the skin of the fingers, with atrophy of the soft tissue and osteoporosis of the distal phalanges of the hands and feet; a limited form of progressive systemic sclerosis occurring with Raynaud's phenomenon. SEE CREST *syndrome.* SYN acroscleroderma, sclerodactyly, sclerodactylia.

ac·ro·sin (ak′rō-sin). A serine proteinase in spermatozoa similar in specificity to trypsin.

ac·ro·some (ak′rō-sōm). A cap-like organelle or saccule derived from the golgi. It surrounds the anterior two thirds of the nucleus of the sperm. Within this cap are enzymes that are thought to facilitate entry of the sperm into the ovum. [acro- + G. *soma,* body]

ac·ro·so·min (ak-rō-sō′min). A lipoglycoprotein complex present in the acrosomal cap.

ac·ro·spi·ro·ma (ak′rō-spī-rō′mă). A tumor of the distal dermal segment of a sweat gland. [scro- + G. *speira*, coil, + -oma, tumor]

    eccrine a., SYN clear cell *hidradenoma.*

ac·ros·te·al·gia (ak-ros-tē-al′jē-ă). Painful inflammation of the bones of the hands and feet. [acro- + G. *osteon*, bone, + *algos*, pain, + -ia]

ac·ro·ter·ic (ak-rō-ter′ik). Relating to the extreme peripheral or apical parts, such as the tips of fingers and toes, the end of the nose. [G. *akrōtērion*, the topmost point]

Ac·ro·the·ca (ak-rō-thē′kă). Former name for *Rhinocladiella.* [see acrotheca]

ac·ro·the·ca (ak-rō-thē′kă). In fungi, a type of spore formation characteristic of the genus *Fonsecaea*, in which conidia are formed along the ends and sides of irregular club-shaped conidiophores. [acro- + G. *thēkē*, box, case]

acrot·ic (ă-krot′ik). **1.** Marked by great weakness or absence of the pulse; pulseless. [G. *a-* priv. + *krotos*, a striking] **2.** Obsolete term relating to the surface of the body, especially the cutaneous glands. [G. *akrotēs*, extremity]

ac·ro·tism (ak′rō-tizm). Absence or imperceptibility of the pulse. [G. *a-* priv. + *krotos*, a striking]

ac·ro·troph·o·dyn·ia (ak′rō-trōf′ō-din′ē-a). Pain, paresthesia, sensory loss, and trophic changes affecting the distal extremities, usually the feet, that can follow prolonged exposure of the limbs to cold and moisture. [acro- + G. *trophē*, nourishment, + *odynē*, pain]

ac·ro·troph·o·neu·ro·sis (ak′rō-trof′ō-nū-rō′sis). Trophoneurosis of one or more of the extremities. [acro- + G. *trophē*, nourishment, + *neuron*, nerve, + *-osis*, condition]

a·cryl·ate (ă′kril-āt). A salt or ester of acrylic acid.

acryl·ic (ă-kril′ik). Denoting certain synthetic plastic resins derived from a. acid. SEE ALSO acrylic *resin.*

acryl·ic ac·ids. A series of unsaturated aliphatic acids of the general formula R=CH—COOH; the prototype, acrylic acid (R=CH$_2$) or 2-propenoic acid, is derived from propionic acid by reduction or from glycerol by dehydration. SYN acroleic acids.

ACT Abbreviation for activated clotting *time.*

ACTe Abbreviation for anodal closure *tetanus.*

ACTH Abbreviation for adrenocorticotropic *hormone.*

    big ACTH, a form of ACTH, produced by certain tumors, which is a larger and more acidic peptide molecule than little ACTH, but is not immunochemically distinguishable from it and does not exert any of the biological effects characteristic of ACTH; tryptic digestion of big ACTH yields hormonally active little ACTH.

    little ACTH, a term coined to denote the conventional ACTH molecule when contrasted with big ACTH.

ac·tin (ak′tin). One of the protein components into which actomyosin can be split; it can exist in a fibrous form (F-actin) or a globular form (G-actin).

    F-a., the association of G-a. subunits into a fibrous (F) protein caused by an increase in salt concentration; the conversion of G-a. to F-a. is catalyzed by small concentrations of magnesium ion, is reversible, and is accompanied by the conversion of the bound ATP molecule to ADP and the conversion of one reactive -thiol group to an unreactive form.

    G-a., the globular (G) subunits of the a. molecule, having a molecular weight 57,000 and containing one molecule of ATP; it is soluble in dilute salt, polymerizing to F-a. when the ionic strength is increased.

act·ing out. An overt act or set of actions that provides an emotional outlet for the expression of emotional conflicts (usually unconscious).

ac·tin·ic (ak-tin′ik). Relating to the chemically active rays of the electromagnetic spectrum. [G. *aktis* (*aktin*-), a ray]

ac·tin·i·des (ak′tin-ī-dēz). Those elements with atomic numbers 89 to 103, corresponding to the lanthanides in the Periodic Table. SYN actinide elements. [*actinium*, first element of the series]

α**-ac·tin·in** (ak-tin′in). An F-actin binding protein in vertebrate cells that cross-links actin filaments into regular parallel arrays.

ac·ti·nism (ak′tin-izm). Archaic term for the effect of radiant energy, such as light, on chemicals or tissue.

ac·tin·i·um (Ac) (ak-tin′ē-ŭm). An element, atomic no. 89, atomic wt. 227.05; it possesses no stable isotopes and exists in nature only as a disintegration product of uranium and thorium. [G. *aktis*, a ray]

△**actino-.** Combining form meaning a ray, as of light; applied to any form of radiation or to any structure with radiating parts. SEE ALSO radio-. [G. *aktis, aktinos*, a ray of light, a beam.]

ac·ti·no·bac·il·lo·sis (ak′tin-ō-bas-i-lō′sis). A disease of cattle and swine, occasionally reported in man, caused by *Actinobacillus lignieresii.* It affects the soft tissues, often the tongue and cervical lymph nodes, where granulomatous swellings are formed that eventually break down to form abscesses. SYN wooden tongue of cattle.

Ac·ti·no·ba·cil·lus (ak′tin-ō-bă-sil′lŭs). A genus of nonmotile, nonsporeforming, aerobic, facultatively anaerobic bacteria (family Brucellaceae) containing Gram-negative rods interspersed with coccal elements. The metabolism of these bacteria is fermentative. They are pathogenic to animals. The type species is *A. lignieresii.* [actino- + L. *bacillus*, a little rod]

    A. actinomycetemcom′itans, a species of doubtful taxonomic position; frequently associated with human periodontal disease as well as subacute and chronic endocarditis; occurs with actinomycetes in actinomycotic lesions. SYN *Haemophilus actinomycetemcomitans.*

    A. equu′li, a species causing suppurative lesions, particularly in the kidneys and joints in foals and piglets, and endocarditis in pigs.

    A. lignieres′ii, a species producing infections of the upper alimentary tract and mouth in cattle and swine (actinobacillosis) and suppurative lesions in the skin and lungs of sheep; it is the type species of its genus.

ac·ti·no·der·ma·ti·tis (ak′ti-nō-der-mă-tī′tis). **1.** SYN photodermatitis. **2.** Obsolete term for adverse reaction of skin to radiation therapy (ultraviolet, x-ray, or radium); more commonly, radiodermatitis. [actino- + G. *derma*, skin, + -*itis*, inflammation]

ac·tin·o·gram (ak-tin′ō-gram). Obsolete synonym for radiograph.

ac·ti·no·he·ma·tin (ak′ti-nō-hē′mă-tin). A red respiratory pigment found in certain forms of *Actinia* (sea anemones). [actino- + G. *haima*, blood]

ac·tin·o·lite (ak-tin′ō-līt). **1.** Any substance that undergoes a change when exposed to light. **2.** A greenish mineral, Ca(Mg, Fe)$_5$ Si$_8$O$_{22}$(OH, F)$_2$.

Ac·ti·no·mad·u·ra (ak′ti-nō-mad′yū-ră). A genus of aerobic, Gram-positive, non-acid-fast fungi where filaments fragment into spores. *A. pelletieri* is an agent of mycetoma. [actino- + *Madura*, India]

    A. africa′na, a species found in a case of mycetoma of the foot in South Africa.

    A. madurae, a member of the Eumycetes (true fungi); one of the etiologic agents of Madura foot and actiomycotic mycetoma.

ac·ti·no·my·ce·li·al (ak′ti-nō-mī-sē′lē-al). Relating to the mycelium-like filaments of the Actinomycetales.

Ac·ti·no·my·ces (ak′ti-nō-mī′sēz). A genus of slow-growing, nonmotile, nonsporeforming, anaerobic to facultatively anaerobic bacteria (family Actinomycetaceae) containing Gram-positive, irregularly staining filaments; diphtheroid cells are predominant. Has characteristic sulfur granules that exhibit true branching while forming mycelial type colonies. Most of the species produce a filamentous microcolony. The metabolism of these chemoheterotrophs is fermentative; the products of glucose fermentation include acetic, formic, lactic and succinic acids but not propionic acid. These organisms are pathogenic for man and/or other animals and can cause chronic suppurative infection in humans. The type species is *A. bovis.* [actino- + G. *mykēs*, fungus]

    A. bo′vis, a species of bacteria causing actinomycosis in cattle;

infection in man is not established; it is the type species of its genus.

A. israe′lii, a species of bacteria causing human actinomycosis and, occasionally, infections in cattle.

A. naeslun′dii, a species whose natural habitat is the oral cavity; human infections have been reported, and it produces periodontal destruction in some species of animals.

A. odontoly′ticus, a species whose normal habitat is the human oral cavity; it has been isolated from deep dental caries.

A. pyogenes, SYN *Corynebacterium pyogenes.*

A. visco′sus, a species that has been isolated from the oral cavity of humans and some species of other animals; it produces periodontal disease in animals and has been isolated from human dental calculus and root surface caries.

Ac·ti·no·my·ce·ta·ce·ae (ak′ti-nō-mī′sē-tā′sē-ē). A family of nonsporeforming, nonmotile, ordinarily facultatively anaerobic (some species are aerobic and others are anaerobic) bacteria (order Actinomycetales) containing Gram-positive, non-acid-fast, predominantly diphtheroid cells which tend to form branched filaments in tissue or in some stages of cultural development; the filaments readily fragment, producing diphtheroid or coccoid forms. The metabolism of these chemoheterotrophic bacteria is fermentative. This family contains the genera *Actinomyces* (type genus), *Arachnia, Bacterionema, Bifidobacterium,* and *Rothia.*

Ac·ti·no·my·ce·ta·les (ak′ti-nō-mī′sē-tā′lēz). An order of bacteria consisting of moldlike, rod-shaped, clubbed or filamentous forms with decided tendency to true branching, without endospores, but sometimes developing conidia; it includes the families Mycobacteriaceae, Actinomycetaceae, Streptomycetaceae, and Nocardiaceae.

ac·ti·no·my·cetes (ak′ti-nō-mī-sē′tēz). A term used to refer to members of the genus *Actinomyces;* sometimes improperly used to refer to any member of the family Actinomycetaceae or order Actinomycetales.

ac·ti·no·my·cin (ak′tin-ō-mī′sin). A group of peptide antibiotic agents, isolated from several species of *Streptomyces* (originally *Actinomyces*), that are active against Gram-positive bacteria, fungi, and neoplasms. A.'s are chromopeptides, most containing the chromophore actinocin, and are derivatives of phenoxazine that differ in their amino acids and their sequence in the peptide chains; they form complexes with DNA and therefore inhibit RNA synthesis, primarily the ribosomal type.

a. A, the first of the a.'s isolated in crystalline form.

a. C, SYN cactinomycin.

a. D, SYN dactinomycin.

a. F₁, KS4; produced by actinomycin C-elaborating strains of *Streptomyces chrysomallus;* used as an antineoplastic agent.

ac·ti·no·my·co·ma (ak′ti-nō-mī-kō′mă). A swelling caused by an actinomycete. SEE mycetoma. [actino- + G. *mykēs,* fungus, + *-oma,* tumor]

ac·ti·no·my·co·sis (ak′ti-nō-mī-kō′sis). A disease primarily of cattle and man caused by *Actinomyces bovis* in cattle and by *A. israelii* and *Arachnia propionica* in man. These actinomycetes are part of the normal bacterial flora of the mouth and pharynx, but when introduced into tissue they may produce chronic destructive abscesses or granulomas which eventually discharge a viscid pus containing minute yellowish granules (sulfur granules). In man, the disease commonly affects the cervicofacial area, abdomen, or thorax; in cattle, the lesion is commonly found in the mandible. SYN actinophytosis (1), lumpy jaw. [actino- + G. *mykēs,* fungus, + *-osis,* condition]

ac·ti·no·my·cot·ic (ak′ti-nō-mī-kot′ik). Relating to actinomycosis.

Ac·ti·no·myx·id·ia (ak′ti-nō-mik-sid′ē-ă). A sporozoan order having a double cellular envelope, three polar capsules, and eight spores; parasitic chiefly in segmented worms, such as the common earthworm. [actino- + G. *myxa,* mucus]

ac·ti·no·neu·ri·tis (ak′ti-nō-nū-rī′tis). Obsolete term for radioneuritis.

ac·tin·o·phage (ak-tin′ō-fāj). A virus specific for actinomycetes. [actino(myces) + G. *phagō,* to eat]

ac·ti·no·phy·to·sis (ak′ti-nō-fī-tō′sis). **1.** SYN actinomycosis. **2.** SYN botryomycosis.

Ac·ti·no·po·da (ak-ti-nop′ō-dă). A class of Sarcodina having slender pseudopodia with a central axial filament. [actino- + G. *pous,* foot]

ac·tin·o·sin (ak-tin′ō-sin). 2-Amino-4,6-dimethyl-3-oxo-3*H*-phenoxazine-1,9-dicarboxylic acid; a phenoxazone derivative that is the chromophore of the actinomycins.

ac·ti·no·ther·a·py (ak′ti-nō-thār′ă-pē). In dermatology, ultraviolet light therapy.

ac·tion (ak′shŭn). **1.** The performance of any of the vital functions, the manner of such performance, or the result of the same. **2.** The exertion of any force or power, physical, chemical, or mental. For the actions of some chemical substances, see under the substance. [L. *actio,* from *ago,* pp. *actus,* to do]

ball valve a., intermittent blockage of a tube or outlet of a cavity by some object or material that permits passage in one direction but not in the other.

calorigenic a., increase of heat production of the body, as by the thyroid hormone. SYN thermogenic a.

cumulative a., SYN cumulative *effect.*

salt a., any physicochemical effect produced by hypertonic concentrations of osmotically active electrolytes.

sparing a., the manner in which a nonessential nutritive component, by its presence in the diet, lowers the dietary requirement for an essential component; thus, nonessential L-cysteine spares essential L-methionine and nonessential L-tyrosine spares essential L-phenylalanine. SYN sparing phenomenon.

specific a., the a. of a drug or a method of treatment which has a direct and especially curative effect upon a disease, *e.g.,* the a. of vitamin B₁₂ in pernicious anemia.

specific dynamic a. (SDA), increase of heat production caused by the ingestion of food, especially of protein.

thermogenic a., SYN calorigenic a.

ac·ti·vate (ak′ti-vāt). **1.** To render active. **2.** To make radioactive.

ac·ti·va·tion (ak-ti-vā′shŭn). **1.** The act of rendering active. **2.** An increase in the energy content of an atom or molecule, through the raising of temperature, absorption of light photons, etc., which renders that atom or molecule more reactive. **3.** Techniques of stimulating the brain by light, sound, electricity, or chemical agents, in order to elicit abnormal activity in the electroencephalogram. **4.** Stimulation of peripheral nerve fibers to the point that action potentials are intiated. **5.** Stimulation of cell division in an ovum by fertilization or by artificial means. SEE cross-section. **6.** The act of making radioactive.

amino acid a., the formation of the amino acyl adenylate derivative (*e.g.,* during protein biosynthesis).

EEG a., the low voltage, fast pattern of attentive wakefulness.

feedback a., a. of an enzyme by an end product of a biochemical pathway in which that enzyme plays a part. For example, the activation of factors VIII and V by thrombin during blood clotting.

feed-forward a., the a. of an enzyme by a precursor of the substrate of that enzyme.

gene a., the process of a. of a gene so that it is expressed at a particular time. This process is crucial in growth and development.

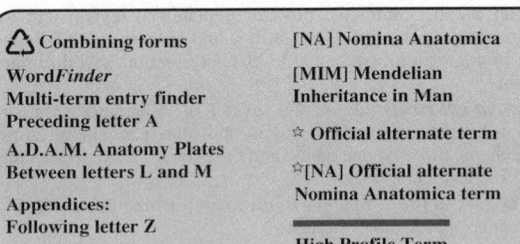

♻ **Combining forms**	**[NA] Nomina Anatomica**
Word*Finder*	**[MIM] Mendelian**
Multi-term entry finder	**Inheritance in Man**
Preceding letter A	
A.D.A.M. Anatomy Plates	☆ **Official alternate term**
Between letters L and M	
Appendices:	☆**[NA] Official alternate**
Following letter Z	**Nomina Anatomica term**
SYN Synonym; Cf., compare	**High Profile Term**

ac·ti·va·tor (ak′ti-vā-tōr). **1.** A substance that renders another substance, or catalyst, active, or that accelerates a process or reaction. **2.** The fragment, produced by chemical cleavage of a proactivator, that induces the enzymic activity of another substance. **3.** An apparatus for making substances radioactive; *e.g.,* neutron generator, cyclotron. **4.** A removable type of myofunctional orthodontic appliance that acts as a passive transmitter of force, produced by the function of the activated muscles, to the teeth and alveolar process that are in contact with it.

catabolite gene a. (CGA), SYN catabolite (gene) activator *protein.*

plasminogen a., a proteinase converting plasminogen to plasmin by cleavage of a single (usually Arg-Val) bond in the former. SYN urokinase.

polyclonal a. (pol-ē-klō′năl), a substance that will activate T cells, B cells, or both regardless of their specificities.

tissue plasminogen a. (TPA), thrombolytic serine protease catalyzing the enzymatic conversion of plasminogen to plasmin through the hypolysis of a single Arg-Val bond; a genetically engineered protein used as a thrombolytic agent in patients with thrombotic occlusion of a coronary artery.

ac·tiv·i·ty (ak-tiv′i-tē). **1.** In electroencephalography, the presence of neurogenic electrical energy. **2.** In physical chemistry, an ideal concentration for which the law of mass action will apply perfectly; the ratio of the a. to the true concentration is the a. coefficient (γ), which becomes 1.00 at infinite dilution. **3.** For enzymes, the amount of substrate consumed (or product formed) in a given time under given conditions; turnover *number.*

blocking a., repression or elimination of electrical activity in the brain by the arrival of a sensory stimulus.

insulin-like a. (ILA), a measure of substances, usually in plasma, that exert biologic effects similar to those of insulin in various bioassays; sometimes used as a measure of plasma insulin concentrations; always gives higher values than immunochemical techniques for the measurement of insulin.

intrinsic sympathomimetic a. (ISA), the property of a drug that causes activation of adrenergic receptors so as to produce effects similar to stimulation of the sympathetic nervous system.

nonsuppressible insulin-like a. (NSILA), plasma insulin-like a. not suppressed by antibodies to insulin and mostly present after pancreatectomy. Nonsuppressible insulin-like a. is mostly the action of polypeptide insulin-like growth factors IGF-I and IGF-II.

optical a., the ability of a compound in solution (one possessing no plane of symmetry, usually because of the presence of one or more asymmetric carbon atoms) to rotate the plane of polarized light either clockwise or counterclockwise.

plasma renin a. (PRA), estimation of renin in plasma by measuring the rate of formation of angiotensin I or II.

specific a., (1) radioactivity per unit mass of the stated element or compound; **(2)** for an enzyme, the amount of substrate consumed (or product formed) in a given time under given conditions per milligram of protein; **(3)** a. per unit mass of the stated radionuclide.

triggered a., one or a series of spontaneously generated heart beats originating from an action potential that produces an afterdepolarization which reaches activation threshold.

ac·to·my·o·sin (ak′-tō-mī′ō-sin). A protein complex composed of the actin and myosin; it is the essential contractile substance of muscle fiber, active with MgATP.

platelet a., the contractile protein of platelets, responsible for clot retraction, platelet aggregation, and release of ADP and other biologic amines essential to platelet function. SYN thrombosthenin.

Ac·u·a·ria spi·ra·lis (ak-ū-ā′rē-ă spī-rā′lis). A nematode parasite in the proventriculus and esophagus, and sometimes the intestine, of chickens, turkeys, pheasants, and other birds. [L. *acus,* needle; Mod. L. *spiralis,* spiral]

acu·i·ty (ă-kyū′i-tē). Sharpness, clearness, distinctness. [thr. Fr., fr. L. *acuo,* pp. *acutus,* sharpen]

absolute intensity threshold a., the minimal light that can be seen.

resolution a., detection of a target having two or more parts,

often measured by using the Snellen test types; indicated by two numbers: the first represents the distance at which an individual sees the test types (usually 6 meters or 20 feet), and the second, the distance at which the test types subtend an angle of 5 minutes; *e.g.,* vision of 6/9 indicates a test distance of 6 meters and recognition of symbols which subtend an angle of 5 minutes at a distance of 9 meters. SYN visual a.

spatial a., detection of the shape of a test object; *e.g.,* perceiving polygons of the same size but with different numbers of sides.

stereoscopic a., the detection of differences in distance by superimposition of slightly different retinal images into a single image to the brain.

Vernier a., detection of displacement of a portion of a line.

visibility a., recognition of an object on a background of different character.

visual a. (V), SYN resolution a.

acu·le·ate (ă-kyū′lē-āt). Pointed; covered with sharp spines. [L. *aculeatus,* pointed, fr. *acus,* needle]

acu·mi·nate (ă-kyū′mi-nāt). Pointed; tapering to a point. [L. *acumino,* pp. *-atus,* to sharpen]

ac·u·ol·o·gy (ak-yū-ol′ō-jē). The study of the use of needles for therapeutic purposes, as in acupuncture. [L. *acus,* needle, + G. *logos,* study]

a·cu·pres·sure. Application of pressure in sites used for acupuncture with therapeutic intent.

ac·u·punc·ture (ak-yū-punk′chūr). Puncture with long, fine needles: **1.** An ancient Oriental system of therapy. **2.** More recently, acupuncture *anesthesia* or analgesia. [L. *acus,* needle, + puncture]

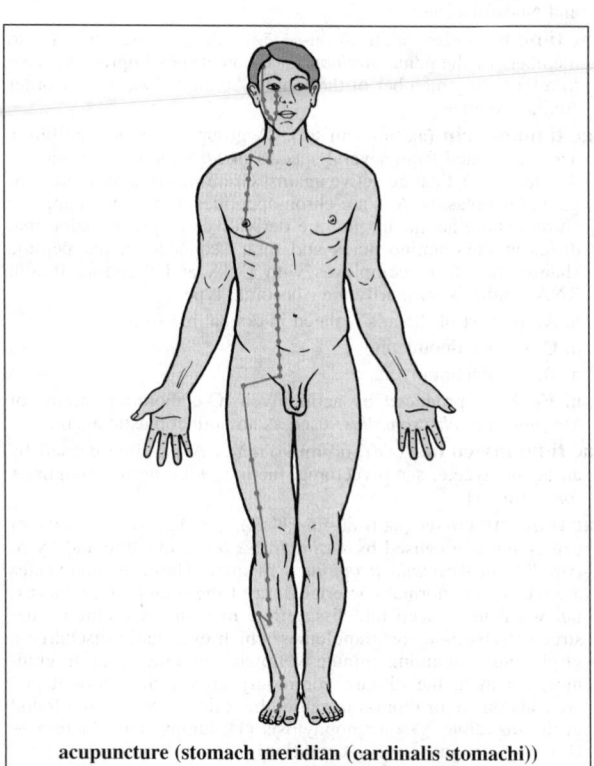

acupuncture (stomach meridian (cardinalis stomachi))

acus (ā′kŭs). Rarely used term for needle. [L.]

ac·u·sec·tion (ak′yū-sek-shŭn). Rarely used term for electrosurgery using a needle.

ac·u·sec·tor (ak′yū-sek-ter). Rarely used term for needle used for electrosurgery. [L. *acus,* needle, + *secare,* to cut]

acu·sis (ă-kyū′sis). The ability to perceive sound normally. SYN normal hearing. [G. *akousis,* hearing]

acute (ă-kyūt′). **1.** Referring to a health effect, brief; not chronic;

sometimes loosely used to mean severe. **2.** Referring to exposure, brief, intense, short-term; sometimes specifically referring to brief exposure of high intensity. [L. *acutus,* sharp]

acy·a·not·ic (ă-sī-ă-not′ik). Characterized by absence of cyanosis.

acy·clic (ā-si′klik). Not cyclic; denoting especially an a. compound.

acy·clo·guan·o·sine (ă-sī-klō-gwan′ō-sēn). SYN acyclovir.

acy·clo·vir (ā-sī′klō-vir). A synthetic acyclic purine nucleoside analogue used as an antiviral agent in the treatment of genital herpes; the sodium salt is used for parenteral therapy. SYN acycloguanosine.

ac·yl (as′il). An organic radical derived from an organic acid by the removal of the carboxylic hydroxyl group.

ac·yl-ACP de·hy·dro·gen·ase, ac·yl-ACP re·duc·tase. SYN enoyl-ACP reductase (NADPH).

ac·yl·ad·e·nyl·ate (as′il-ă-den′il-āt). A compound in which an acyl group is combined with AMP by elimination of H_2O between the OH's of a carboxyl group and of the phosphate residue of AMP, usually initially in the form of ATP and eliminating inorganic pyrophosphate in the condensation.

ac·yl·am·i·dase (as-il-am′i-dās). SYN amidase.

***n*-ac·yl·a·mi·no ac·id** (as-il-am′i-nō). RCO–NH–CHR–COOH; an amino acid to the N of which an acyl group is attached, as in hippuric acid (*N*-benzoylglycine) or phenaceturic acid.

ac·yl·a·tion (as-i-lā′shŭn). Introduction of an acyl radical into an organic compound or formation of such a radical within an organic compound.

acylcar·ni·tine (as′il-kar′ni-tēn). Condensation product of a carboxylic acid and carnitine. The transport form for a fatty acid crossing the mitochondrial membrane.

ac·yl-CoA. $RCH_2COSCoA$ or $RCH_2CO\text{~}SCoA$; condensation product of a carboxylic acid and coenzyme A, and metabolic intermediate of importance, notably in the oxidation and synthesis of fat. SYN acyl-coenzyme A.

a.-CoA dehydrogenase (NADPH⁺), enzyme catalyzing the reversible reduction of enoyl-CoA derivatives of chain length 4 to 16, with NADPH as the hydrogen donor, forming a.-CoA and $NADP^+$. SYN enoyl-CoA reductase.

a.-CoA synthetase, (1) general term for enzymes (EC 6.2.1) that form a.-CoA, now called ligases; **(2)** specifically, long-chain fatty acid–CoA ligase.

ac·yl-co·en·zyme A (as′il-kō-en′zīm). SYN acyl-CoA.

1-ac·yl·gly·ce·rol·-3-phos·phate ac·yl·trans·fer·ase. SEE *lysophosphatidic acid* acyltransferase.

ac·yl-mal·o·nyl-ACP syn·thase. SYN 3-oxoacyl-ACP synthase.

ac·yl·mer·cap·tan (as′il-mer-kap′tan). SYN thioester.

***N*-ac·yl·sphin·gol** (as-il-sfing′gol). Obsolete synonym for *N*-acylsphingosine.

***N*-ac·yl·sphin·go·sine** (as-il-sfing′gō-sēn). A condensation product of an organic acid with sphingosine at the amino group of the latter compound.

ac·yl·trans·fer·as·es (as-il-trans′fer-ā-sez) [EC class 2.3]. Enzymes catalyzing the transfer of an acyl group from an acyl-CoA to various acceptors. SYN transacylases.

acys·tia (ā-sis′tē-ă). Congenital absence of the urinary bladder. [G. *a-* priv. + *kystis,* bladder]

A.D. Abbreviation for *auris dexter* [L.], right ear.

△ad-. To, toward; increase; adherence; near; very.Prefix denoting increase, adherence, to, toward; increase; adherence; near; very. [L. *ad,* to, toward;]

△-ad. In anatomical nomenclature, -ward; toward or in the direction of the part indicated by the main portion of the word. [L. *ad,* to]

ADA Abbreviation for American Dental Association.

ad·a·cr·ya (dak′rē-ă). Absence of tears; tearlessness. [G. *a-* priv. + *dakryon,* tear, + -ia]

adac·ty·lous (ā-dak′tĭ-lŭs). Without fingers or toes.

adac·ty·ly (ā-dak′ti-lē). Congenital condition characterized by

the absence of digits (fingers or toes); autosomal recessive in Holstein cattle. [G. *a-* priv. + *daktylos,* digit]

Adair-Koshland-Némethy-Filmer mod·el (AKNF). See under model.

ad·a·man·tine (ad-ă-man′tēn). Exceedingly hard; formerly used in reference to the enamel of the teeth. [G. *adamantinos,* very hard]

ad·a·man·ti·no·ma (ad-ă-man-ti-nō′mă). Obsolete term for ameloblastoma.

a. of long bones, a rare tumor of limb bones, usually the tibia, that microscopically resembles an ameloblastoma; the histogenesis is uncertain.

pituitary a., SYN craniopharyngioma.

Adamkiewicz, Albert, Polish pathologist, 1850–1921. SEE *artery* of Adamkiewicz.

Adams, Robert, Irish physician, 1791–1875. SEE A.-Stokes *disease;* Stokes-A. *disease;* A.-Stokes *syncope, syndrome;* Stokes-A. *syndrome;* Morgagni-A.-Stokes *syndrome.*

Adams, Sir William, British surgeon, 1760–1829.

Adam's ap·ple. SYN laryngeal *prominence.*

ad·am·site (DM) (ad′ăm-sīt). A vomiting agent that has been used in military training and in riot control. [Roger *Adams,* Am. chemist]

Adanson, Michel, French naturalist, 1727–1806. SEE adansonian *classification.*

ad·ap·ta·tion (ad-ap-tā′shŭn). **1.** Preferential survival of members of a species because of a phenotype that give them an enhanced capacity to withstand the environment including the ecology. **2.** An advantageous change in function or constitution of an organ or tissue to meet new conditions. **3.** Adjustment of the sensitivity of the retina to light intensity. **4.** A property of certain sensory receptors that modifies the response to repeated or continued stimuli at constant intensity. **5.** The fitting, condensing, or contouring of a restorative material, foil, or shell to a tooth or cast so as to be in close contact. **6.** The dynamic process wherein the thoughts, feelings, behavior, and biophysiologic mechanisms of the individual continually change to adjust to a constantly changing environment. SYN adjustment (2). **7.** A homeostatic response. [L. *ad-apto,* pp. *-atus,* to adjust]

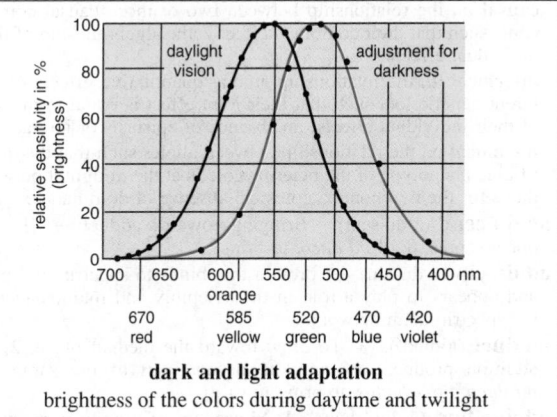

dark and light adaptation
brightness of the colors during daytime and twilight

dark a., the visual adjustment occurring under reduced illumination in which the retinal sensitivity to light is increased. SEE ALSO dark-adapted *eye.* SYN scotopic a.

light a., the visual adjustment occurring under increased illumination in which the retinal sensitivity to light is reduced. SEE ALSO light-adapted *eye.* SYN photopic a.

photopic a., SYN light a.

reality a., the ability to adjust to the world as it exists.

retinal a., adjustment to degree of illumination.

scotopic a., SYN dark a.

social a., adjustment to living in accordance with interpersonal, social, and cultural norms.

adapt·er, adap·tor (a-dap′ter, -tōr). **1.** A connecting part, joining two pieces of apparatus. **2.** A converter of electric current to a desired form.

ad·ap·tom·e·ter (ad-ap-tom′ĕ-ter). A device for determining the course of retinal dark adaptation and for measuring the minimum light threshold.

ad·ax·i·al (ad-ak′sē-ăl). Toward an axis, or on one or other side of an axis.

ADC Abbreviation for AIDS dementia *complex*.

ADCC Abbreviation for antibody-dependent cell-mediated *cytotoxicity*.

add. Abbreviation for L. *adde*, add; L. *addantur*, let them be added; *addendus*, to be added; and *addendo*, by adding.

ad·der. Common name for many members of the family Viperidae (the vipers), applied to several genera, although true a.'s are of the genus *Vipera*. [M.E. *naddre*, fr. O.E. *nǣdre*]

ad·dict (ad′ikt). A person who is habituated to a substance or practice, especially one considered harmful or illegal.

ad·dic·tion (ă-dik′shŭn). Habitual psychological and physiological dependence on a substance or practice that is beyond voluntary control. SYN alcohol a. [L. *ad-dico*, pp. *-dictus*, consent, fr. *ad-* + *dico*, to say]

　alcohol a., SYN addiction, alcoholism.

Addis, Thomas, U.S. internist, 1881–1949. SEE A. *count*.

Addison, Christopher, English anatomist, 1869–1951. SEE A.'s clinical *planes*, under *plane*.

Addison, Thomas, English physician, 1793–1860. SEE A.'s *anemia, disease;* addisonian *anemia;* addisonian *crisis;* A.-Biermer *disease.*

ad·di·so·ni·an (ad-i-sō′nē-an). Relating to or described by Thomas Addison; usually used in relation to pernicious *anemia*

ad·di·tive (ad′i-tiv). **1.** A substance not naturally a part of a material (*e.g.,* food) but deliberately added to fulfill some specific purpose (*e.g.,* preservation). **2.** Tending to add or be added; denoting addition. **3.** In metrical studies (*e.g.,* genetics, epidemiology, physiology, statistics), having the property that the total combined effect of two or more factors equals the sum of their individual effects in isolation. Cf. synergism.

ad·di·tiv·i·ty (ad-i-tiv′i-tē). The quality or state of being additive.

　causal a., the relationship between two or more causal components such that their combined effect is the algebraic sum of their individual effects.

　interlocal a., the relationship among quantitative effects of different genetic loci such that their joint effect is equal to the sum of their individual effects; an absence of epistasis or interaction.

　intralocal a., the relationship between alleles such that the quantifiable phenotype of the heterozygote is at the midpoint between those for the two homozygotes; an absence of dominance.

ad·du·cent (ă-dū′sent). Bringing toward; adducting. [L. *adducens*, pres. p. of *ad-duco*, to bring]

ad·du·cin (ă-dū′sen). A protein that binds to spectrin and actin and appears to play a role in the assembly and maintenance of the spectrin-actin network.

ad·duct (a-dŭkt′). **1.** To draw toward the median plane. **2.** An addition product, or complex, or one part of the same. [L. *ad-duco*, pp. *-ductus*, to bring toward]

ad·duc·tion (ă-dŭk′shŭn). **1.** Movement of a body part toward the median plane (of the body, in the case of limbs; of the hand or foot, in the case of digits). **2.** Monocular rotation (duction) of the eye toward the nose. **3.** A position resulting from such movement. Cf. abduction.

ad·duc·tor (ă-dŭk′ter, tōr). A muscle that draws a part toward the median plane; or, in the case of the digits, toward the normal axis of the middle finger or the second toe.

Ade Abbreviation for adenine.

ade·lo·mor·phous (ă-del-ō-mōr′fŭs). Of not clearly defined form. In the past this term was applied to certain cells of the gastric glands. [G. *adēlos,* uncertain, not clear, + *morphē,* shape]

△**aden-.** SEE adeno-.

ad·e·nal·gia (ad-ĕ-nal′jē-ă). Rarely used term for pain in a gland. [aden- + G. *algos,* pain]

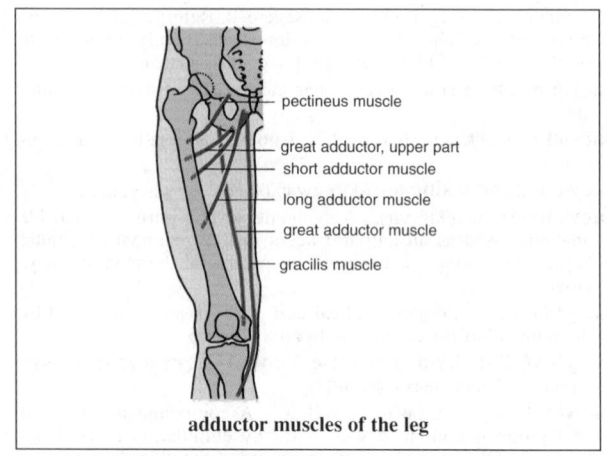
adductor muscles of the leg

pectineus muscle
great adductor, upper part
short adductor muscle
long adductor muscle
great adductor muscle
gracilis muscle

aden·dric (ā-den′drik). SYN adendritic.

aden·drit·ic (ā-den-drit′ik). Without dendrites. SYN adendric. [G., *a-* priv. + *dendron,* tree]

ad·e·nec·to·my (ad-ĕ-nek′tō-mē). Excision of a gland. [aden- + G. *ektomē,* excision]

ad·e·nec·to·pia (ad′ĕ-nek-tō′pē-ă). Presence of a gland other than in its normal anatomical position. [aden- + G. *ek,* out of, + *topos,* place]

ad·e·nem·phrax·is (ad′ĕ-nem-frak′sis). Rarely used term for an obstruction to the discharge of a glandular secretion. [aden- + G. *emphraxis,* stoppage]

aden·i·form (ă-den′i-fōrm). SYN adenoid (1).

ad·e·nine (A, Ade) (ad′ĕ-nēn). One of the two major purines (the other being guanine) found in both RNA and DNA, and also in various free nucleotides of importance to the body, such as AMP (adenylic acid), ATP, NAD$^+$ and NADP$^+$, and FAD; in all these smaller compounds, a. is condensed with ribose at the nitrogen-9, forming adenosine. For structure, see adenylic acid. SYN 6-aminopurine.

　a. arabinoside, misnomer for arabinosyladenine.

　a. deaminase, an enzyme that catalyzes the hydrolysis of a. to ammonia and hypoxanthine. A part of purine degradation.

　a. deoxyribonucleotide, SYN deoxyadenylic acid.

　a. nucleotide, SYN adenylic acid.

　a. phosphoribosyltransferase, an enzyme that catalyzes the reaction of a. with 5-phospho-α-D-ribose 1-diphosphate (PRPP) to form AMP and pyrophosphate. An important step in purine salvage. A deficiency of this enzyme can lead to 2,8-dihydroxyadenine lithiasis.

　a. sulfate, a. conjugated with sulfuric acid; used to stimulate leukocyte production in agranulocytosis.

ad·e·ni·tis (ad-ĕ-nī′tis). Inflammation of a lymph node or of a gland. [aden- + G. *-itis,* inflammation]

ad·e·ni·za·tion (ad-ĕ-nī-zā′shŭn). Conversion into glandlike structure.

△**adeno-, aden-.** A gland, glandular; corresponds to L. glandul-, glandi-.Combining forms denoting gland, glandular; corresponds to L. glandul-, glandi-. [G. *adēn, adenos* a gland]

ad·e·no·ac·an·tho·ma (ad′ĕ-nō-ak-an-thō′mă). A malignant neoplasm consisting chiefly of glandular epithelium (adenocarcinoma), usually well differentiated, with foci of metaplasia to squamous (or epidermoid) neoplastic cells. SYN adenoid squamous cell carcinoma.

ad·e·no·am·e·lo·blas·to·ma (ad′ĕ-nō-am′el-ō-blast-ō′mă). SYN adenomatoid odontogenic *tumor*.

ad·e·no·blast (ad′ĕ-nō-blast). A proliferating embryonic cell with the potential to form glandular parenchyma. [adeno- + G. *blastos,* germ]

ad·e·no·car·ci·no·ma (ad′ĕ-nō-ep-i-thē-lē-ō′mă). A malignant neoplasm of epithelial cells in glandular or glandlike pattern. SYN glandular cancer, glandular carcinoma.

ad

acinic cell a., an a. arising from secreting cells of a racemose gland, particularly the salivary glands. SYN acinar carcinoma, acinic cell carcinoma, acinose carcinoma, acinous carcinoma.

alveolar a., a. of the lung in which tumor cells form structures resembling alveoli.

a. in Barrett's esophagus, an a. arising in the lower third of the esophagus that has become columnar cell lined (Barrett's mucosa) due to gastroesophageal reflux.

bronchiolar a., SYN bronchiolar *carcinoma*.

bronchioloalveolar a., SYN bronchiolar *carcinoma*.

clear cell a., (1) a histologic type of renal a.; (2) a histologic type of a. occurring chiefly in the male and female genitourinary tracts which is characterized by distinctive hobnail cell growth of neoplastic cells in sheets, papillae, and coalescing glands.

Lucké's a., SYN Lucké *carcinoma*.

mesonephric a., SYN mesonephroma.

mucoid a., sometimes applied to mucinous carcinoma, or a. containing mucin secreting neoplastic cells.

papillary a., an a. containing finger-like processes of vascular connective tissue covered by neoplastic epithelium, projecting into cysts or the cavity of glands or follicles; occurs most frequently in the ovary and thyroid gland.

renal a., an a. arising in any part of the renal parenchyma, especially in middle-aged or older people of either sex (although more common in males). SYN clear cell carcinoma of kidney, hypernephroma, hypernephronia, renal cell carcinoma.

a. in si'tu, a noninvasive abnormal proliferation of glands believed to precede the appearance of invasive adenocarcinoma; reported in the endometrium, large intestine, cervix, and other sites.

ad·e·no·cel·lu·li·tis (ad′ĕ-nō-sel-yū-lī′tis). Inflammation of a gland, usually a lymph node, and of the adjacent connective tissue.

ad·e·no·chon·dro·ma (ad′ĕ-nō-kon-drō′mă). SYN pulmonary *hamartoma*. [adeno- + G. *chondros*, cartilage, + -*oma*, tumor]

ad·e·no·cys·to·ma (ad′ĕ-nō-sis-tō′mă). Adenoma in which the neoplastic glandular epithelium forms cysts.

ad·e·no·cyte (ad′ĕ-nō-sīt). A secretory cell of a gland. [adeno- + G. *kytos*, a hollow (cell)]

ad·e·no·di·as·ta·sis (ad′ĕ-nō-dī-as′tă-sis). Separation or ectopia of glands or glandular tissue from their usual anatomical sites, *e.g.,* pancreatic glands in the wall of the small intestine, gastric glands in the wall of the esophagus. [adeno- + G. *diastasis*, a separation]

ad·e·no·dyn·ia (ad′ĕ-nō-din′ē-ă). Rarely used term for adenalgia. [adeno- + G. *odynē*, pain]

ad·e·no·ep·i·the·li·o·ma. Obsolete term for an epithelioma containing glandular elements.

ad·e·no·fi·bro·ma (ad′ĕ-nō-fī-brō′mă). A benign neoplasm composed of glandular and fibrous tissues, with a relatively large proportion of glands.

ad·e·no·fi·bro·my·o·ma (ad′ĕ-nō-fī′brō-mī-ō′mă). SYN adenomatoid *tumor*.

ad·e·no·fi·bro·sis (ad′ĕ-nō-fī-brō′sis). SYN sclerosing *adenosis*.

ad·e·nog·en·ous (ad-ĕ-noj′en-ŭs). Having an origin from glandular tissue.

ad·e·no·hy·po·phy·si·al (ad′ĕ-nō-hī-pō-fiz′ē-ăl). Relating to the adenohypophysis.

ad·e·no·hy·poph·y·sis (ad′ĕ-nō-hī-pof′i-sis) [NA]. It consists of the distal part, intermediate part, and infundibular part. SEE ALSO hypophysis. SYN lobus anterior hypophyseos [NA], anterior lobe of hypophysis☆, glandular lobe of hypophysis, lobus glandularis hypophyseos.

ad·e·no·hy·poph·y·si·tis (ad′ĕ-nō-hī-pof-ĭ-sī′tis). Inflammatory reaction or sepsis affecting the anterior pituitary gland, often related to pregnancy.

lymphocytic a., a diffuse lymphocytic infiltration of the adenohypophysis, often related to pregnancy; probably a disturbance in the immune system.

ad·e·noid (ad′ĕ-noyd). **1.** Glandlike; of glandular appearance.

SYN adeniform, lymphoid (2). **2.** SEE adenoids. [adeno- + G. *eidos,* appearance]

ad·e·noid·ec·to·my (ad′ĕ-noy-dek′tō-mē). An operation for the removal of adenoid growths in the nasopharynx. [adenoid + G. *ektomē,* excision]

ad·e·noid·i·tis (ad′ĕ-noy-dī′tis). Inflammation of nasopharyngeal lymphoid tissue.

ad·e·noids (ad′ĕ-noydz). **1.** A normal collection of unencapsulated lymphoid tissue in the nasopharynx. Also called pharyngeal tonsils. **2.** Common terminology for the large (normal) pharyngeal tonsils of children. [G. *adēn,* gland, + -*eidos,* resemblance]

ad·e·no·lei·o·my·o·fi·bro·ma (ad′ĕ-nō-lī′ō-mī-ō-fī-brō′mă). SYN adenomatoid *tumor*. [adeno- + G. *leios,* smooth, + *mys,* muscle, + fibroma]

ad·e·no·li·po·ma (ad′ĕ-nō-li-pō′mă). A benign neoplasm composed of glandular and adipose tissues. [G. *adēn,* gland, + *lipos,* fat, + -*oma,* tumor]

ad·e·no·lip·o·ma·to·sis (ad′ĕ-nō-lip′ō-mă-tō′sis). A condition characterized by development of multiple adenolipomas.

symmetric a., SYN multiple symmetric *lipomatosis*.

ad·e·no·lym·pho·cele (ad′ĕ-nō-lim′fō-sēl). Cystic dilation of a lymph node following obstruction of the efferent lymphatic vessels. [adeno- + L. *lympha,* spring water, + G. *kēlē,* tumor]

ad·e·no·lym·pho·ma (ad′ĕ-nō-lim-fō′mă). A benign glandular tumor usually arising in the parotid gland and composed of two rows of eosinophilic epithelial cells, which are often cystic and papillary, together with a lymphoid stroma. SYN papillary cystadenoma lymphomatosum, Warthin's tumor.

ad·e·no·ma (ad-ĕ-nō′mă). An ordinarily benign neoplasm of epithelial tissue in which the tumor cells form glands or gland-like structures in the stroma; usually well circumscribed, tending to compress rather than infiltrate or invade adjacent tissue. [adeno- + G. -*oma,* tumor]

acidophil a., a tumor of the adenohypophysis in which cell cytoplasm stains with acid dyes; often growth hormone producing. SYN eosinophil a.

ACTH-producing a., a pituitary tumor composed of corticotrophs that produce ACTH, often a basophilic adenoma; may give rise to Cushing's disease or Nelson's syndrome.

adnexal a., an a. arising in, or forming structures resembling, skin appendages.

adrenocortical a., a benign tumor of adrenal cortical cells; small unencapsulated nodules of adrenal cortex are probably localized areas of hyperplasia rather than a.'s; true a.'s are rare and may be symptomless or associated with Cushing's syndrome or primary aldosteronism.

apocrine a., SYN papillary *hidradenoma*.

basal cell a., a benign tumor of major or minor salivary glands or other organs composed of small cells showing peripheral palisading.

basophil a., a tumor of the adenohypophysis in which the cell cytoplasm stains with basic dyes, often ACTH producing.

bronchial a., a slowly growing benign, or malignant but slowly progressing, polypoid epithelial tumor of bronchial mucosa, arising deep to the surface epithelium, possibly from mucous glands or their ducts; two histological types are recognized: carcinoid and cylindromatous.

canalicular a. (ca-na-nik′ū-lar), a variant of monomorphic a. composed of double rows of epithelial cells in long cords.

chromophil a., any a. composed of cells that stain readily.

chromophobe a., chromophobic a., a tumor of the adenohypophysis whose cells do not stain with either acid or basic dyes.

colloid a., a follicular a. of the thyroid, composed of large follicles containing colloid. SYN macrofollicular a.

embryonal a., a benign neoplasm in which the glandular epithelial elements are not fully differentiated, resembling immature tissue observed in embryonic development.

eosinophil a., SYN acidophil a.

fibroid a., a. fibro'sum, SYN fibroadenoma.

follicular a., an a. of the thyroid with a simple glandular pattern.

Fuchs' a., a benign epithelial tumor of the non-pigmented epithelium of the ciliary body, rarely exceeding 1 mm in diameter.

gonadotropin-producing a., a rare type of pituitary a. that produces FSH and LH; its cells can be identified only by immunochemical techniques.

growth hormone-producing a., an a. that produces the clinical picture of gigantism or acromegaly, although a third of the cells have no granules or are a mixture of acidophils and chromophobes; some tumors may secrete both growth hormone and prolactin; often an acidophil or eosinophil adenoma.

hepatic a., a benign tumor of the liver, usually occurring in women during the reproductive years in association with lengthy oral contraceptive use. The tumor is usually solitary, subcapsular and large, composed of cords of hepatocytes with postal triads. SYN hepatocellular a.

hepatocellular a., SYN hepatic a.

Hürthle cell a., an uncommon type of thyroid tumor characterized by abundant eosinophilic cytoplasm containing numerous mitochondria. Often malignant with widespread metastases; rarely takes up radioiodine. SEE ALSO Hürthle cell *tumor*.

islet cell a., a benign neoplasm of the pancreas composed of tissue similar in structure to that of the islets of Langerhans; it may contain functioning beta cells, and may cause hypoglycemia. SEE ALSO insulinoma. SYN nesidioblastoma.

lactating a., an uncommon a. of the breast composed of tubuloacinar structures with pronounced secretory changes such as seen in pregnancy and lactation.

Leydig cell a., small benign tumors of the testis that often produce testosterone, causing endocrine symptoms. SYN interstitial cell tumor of testis.

macrofollicular a., SYN colloid a.

microfollicular a., a fetal a. of the thyroid composed of very small follicles and solid alveolar groups of thyroid epithelial cells.

monomorphic a., a benign ductal neoplasm of the salivary glands, with a uniform epithelial pattern and lacking the chondromyxoid stroma of a pleomorphic a.

nephrogenic a., a benign tumor of the urinary bladder mucosa, composed of glandular structures resembling renal tubules.

a. of nipple, SYN subareolar duct *papillomatosis*.

null-cell a., an a. of the hypophysis composed of cells for which there is no overt evidence or hormone production, but which usually produces hypopituitarism and visual disturbances by compression of adjacent structures; approximately one third of these tumors have cells with abundant mitochondria (oncocytes) that are somewhat larger than the monocytic null cells. SYN undifferentiated cell a.

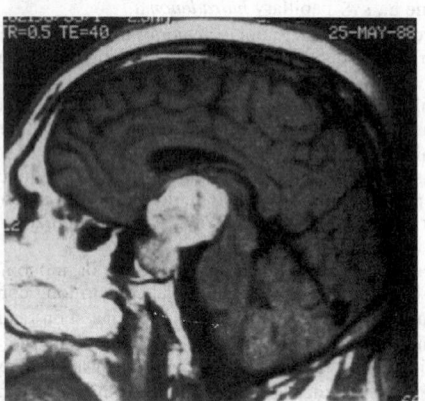

adenoma of the hypophysis
nuclear spin resonance tomography, after injection
of contrast medium

ovarian tubular a., SYN arrhenoblastoma.

oxyphil a., SYN oncocytoma.

papillary cystic a., an a. in which the lumens of the acini are

frequently distended by fluid, and the neoplastic epithelial elements tend to form irregular, fingerlike projections.

papillary a. of large intestine, SYN villous a.

Pick's tubular a., SYN androblastoma (1).

pituitary a., a benign neoplasm of the pituitary generally arising in the adenohypophysis.

pleomorphic a., SYN mixed *tumor* of salivary gland.

polypoid a., SYN adenomatous *polyp*.

prolactin-producing a., a pituitary adenoma composed of prolactin-producing cells; it gives rise to symptoms of nonpuerperal amenorrhea and galactorrhea (Forbes-Albright syndrome) in women and to impotence in men. SYN prolactinoma.

prostatic a., a term used for the growth in benign prostatic hyperplasia.

renal cortical a., one of the usually small a.'s sometimes found in the renal cortex and derived from renal tubular tissue.

sebaceous a., a benign neoplasm of sebaceous tissue, with a predominance of mature secretory sebaceous cells. Cf. a. sebaceum.

a. seba'ceum, archaic misnomer for a hamartoma occurring on the face, composed of fibrovascular tissue and appearing as an aggregation of red or yellow papules which may be associated with tuberous sclerosis; sebaceous glands may be present but are not increased. Cf. sebaceous a. SYN Pringle's disease.

testicular tubular a., SYN androblastoma (1).

thyrotropin-producing a., a rare pituitary adenoma usually associated with hypo- or hyperthyroidism.

tubular a., a benign neoplasm composed of epithelial tissue resembling a tubular gland.

undifferentiated cell a., SYN null-cell a.

villous a., appears as a solitary sessile, often large, tumor of colonic mucosa composed of mucinous epithelium covering delicate vascular projections; malignant change occurs frequently; hypersecretion occurs rarely. Also known as adenoma. SYN papillary a. of large intestine.

ad·e·no·ma·toid (ad-ĕ-nō′mă-toyd). Resembling an adenoma.

ad·e·no·ma·to·sis (ad′ĕ-nō-mă-tō′sis). A condition characterized by multiple glandular overgrowths.

erosive a. of nipple, SYN subareolar duct *papillomatosis*.

familial multiple endocrine a. [MIM*131100], presence of functioning tumors in more than one endocrine gland, commonly the pancreatic islets and parathyroid glands, which may be associated with Zollinger-Ellison syndrome; dominant inheritance. SYN multiple endocrine a.

fibrosing a., SYN sclerosing *adenosis*.

multiple endocrine a., SYN familial multiple endocrine a.

pulmonary a., a neoplastic disease in which the alveoli and distal bronchi are filled with mucus and mucus-secreting columnar epithelial cells; characterized by abundant, extremely tenacious sputum, chills, fever, cough, dyspnea, and pleuritic pain.

pulmonary a. of sheep, a chronic pulmonary disease of sheep of viral origin, caused by a member of Herpesviridae characterized by adenomatous proliferations in the alveoli and small bronchioles resembling neoplasia. SYN jaagsiekte.

ad·e·nom·a·tous (ad-ĕ-nō′mă-tŭs). Relating to an adenoma, and to some types of glandular hyperplasia.

ad·e·no·meg·a·ly (ad′ē-nō-meg′ă-lē). Enlargement of one or both adrenal glands. [adeno- + G. *megas*, large]

ad·e·no·mere (ad′ĕ-nō-mēr). Structural unit in the parenchyma of a developing gland which becomes the functional portion of the organ. [adeno- + G. *meros*, part]

ad·e·no·my·o·ma (ad′ĕ-nō-mī-ō′mă). A benign neoplasm of muscle (usually smooth muscle) with glandular elements; occurs most frequently in uterus and uterine ligaments. [G. *adēn*, gland, + *mys*, muscle, + *-oma*, tumor]

ad·e·no·my·o·sar·co·ma (ad′ĕ-nō-mī′ō-sar-kō′mă). SYN Wilms' *tumor*.

ad·e·no·my·o·sis (ad′ĕ-nō-mī-ō′sis). The ectopic occurrence or diffuse implantation of adenomatous tissue in muscle (usually smooth muscle). [G. *adēn*, gland, + *mys*, muscle, + *-osis* condition]

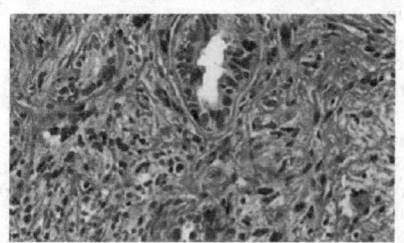
a. u′teri, a benign invasion of myometrium by endometrial tissue.

ad·e·no·neu·ral (ad′ĕ-nō-nū′răl).   Obsolete term relating to a gland and a nervous element. SEE neuroendocrine.

ad·e·nop·a·thy (ad-ĕ-nop′ă-thē).   Swelling or morbid enlargement of the lymph nodes. [adeno- + G. *pathos,* suffering]

ad·e·no·phleg·mon (ad′ĕ-nō-fleg′mon).   Acute inflammation of a gland and the adjacent connective tissue. [adeno- + G. *phlegmonē,* inflammation]

Ad·e·no·pho·ra·si·da (ad′ĕ-nō-fō-ras′i-dă).   A class of nematodes lacking lateral canals opening into the excretory system and phasmids, with few or no caudal papillae, eggs unsegmented, and with polar plugs or hatching *in utero.* It includes the genera *Trichuris, Capillaria,* and *Trichinella* among important parasites of man and domestic animals. SEE ALSO Secernentasida. SYN Adenophorea, Aphasmidia.   [G. *adēn,* gland, + *phōr,* thief]

Ad·e·no·pho·rea (ad′ĕ-nō-fō′rē-ă). SYN Adenophorasida.

ad·e·no·phy·ma (ad′ĕ-nō-fī′mă).   Obsolete term for any condition in which a gland or glandular organ is grossly enlarged as the result of inflammation. [adeno- + G. *phyma,* tumor]

ad·e·no·sal·pin·gi·tis (ad′ĕ-nō-sal-pin-jī′tis).   SYN *salpingitis* isthmica nodosa.

ad·e·no·sar·co·ma (ad′ĕ-nō-sar-kō′mă).   A malignant neoplasm arising simultaneously or consecutively in mesodermal tissue and glandular epithelium of the same part.

müllerian a., a tumor of the uterus or ovaries, of low grade malignancy, characterized by benign appearing glands and a sarcomatous stroma.

ad·e·nose (ad′ĕ-nōs).   Relating to a gland.

ad·e·no·sin·ase (ad-ĕ-nō′sin-ās).   SYN *adenosine* nucleosidase.

aden·o·sine (Ado) (ă-den′ō-sēn).   A condensation product of adenine and D-ribose; a nucleoside found among the hydrolysis products of all nucleic acids and of the various adenine nucleotides. A. accumulates in severe combined immunodeficiency disease. For structure, see adenylic acid. SYN 9-β-D-ribofuranosyladenine.

a. cyclic phosphate, SEE adenosine 3′,5′-cyclic monophosphate.

a. deaminase, an enzyme found in mammalian tissues, capable of catalyzing the deamination of adenosine, forming inosine and ammonia. A deficiency of a. can lead to one form of severe combined immunodeficiency disease.

a. diphosphate, SEE adenosine 5′-diphosphate.

a. kinase, enzyme catalyzing the transfer of a phosphate group from MgATP to adenosine, forming MgADP and AMP. An important step in nucleoside salvage.

a. monophosphate (AMP), specifically, adenosine-5′-monophosphate. SEE adenylic acid.

a. nucleosidase, an enzyme hydrolyzing adenosine to adenine and D-ribose. SYN adenosinase.

a. phosphate, specifically, adenosine 3′- or 5′-phosphate. SEE adenylic acid.

a. tetraphosphate, a condensation product of adenosine with tetraphosphoric acid at the 5′ position.

a. triphosphate, SYN adenosine 5′-triphosphate.

aden·o·sine 3′,5′-cy·clic monophos·phate (cAMP).   An activator of phosphorylase kinase and an effector of other enzymes, formed in muscle from ATP by adenylate cyclase and broken down to 5′-AMP by a phosphodiesterase; sometimes referred to as the "second messenger." A related compound (2′,3′) is also known. SYN cyclic adenylic acid, cyclic AMP, cyclic phosphate.

aden·o·sine 3′,5′-cy·clic phos·phate phos·pho·di·es·ter·-ase.   an enzyme that catalyzes the hydrolysis of adenosine 3′,5′-cyclic phosphate forming 5′-AMP. A crucial step in the regulation of cellular adenosine 3′,5′-cyclic phosphate levels. Inhibited by caffeine. SYN cAMP phosphodiesterase.

aden·o·sine 5′-di·phos·phate (ADP).   A condensation product of adenosine with pyrophosphoric acid, formed from ATP by the hydrolysis of the terminal phosphate group of the latter compound.

aden·o·sine 3′-phos·phate.   3′-Adenylic acid. SEE adenylic acid.

aden·o·sine 5′-phos·phate.   5′-Adenylic acid. SEE adenylic acid.

aden·o·sine 3′-phos·phate 5′-phos·pho·sul·fate (PAPS).   3′-phosphoadenosine 5′-phosphosulfate; an intermediate in the formation of urinary ethereal sulfates, notable for containing a "high energy" sulfate bond; the 3′-OH of adenosine is replaced by —OPO_3H_2, the 5′-OH by —$OP(O_2H)$–OSO_3H. SYN active sulfate.

aden·o·sine 5′-phos·pho·sul·fate (APS).   An intermediate in the formation of PAPS (active sulfate).

adenosine 5′-phosphosulfate kinase, the enzyme that catalyzes the formation of active sulfate from adenosine 5′-phosphosulfate and ATP.

ad·e·no·sine ·tri·phos·pha·tase (ATPase) (a-den′ō-sēn-trī-fos′fă-tās).   An enzyme in muscle (myosin) and elsewhere that catalyzes the release of the terminal phosphate group of adenosine 5′-triphosphate; visualized cytochemically in various cell membranes, mitochondria, and in the A band of striated muscle sarcomeres associated with myosin. SYN adenylpyrophosphatase, ATP-monophosphatase, triphosphatase.

aden·o·sine 5′-tri·phos·phate (ATP).   adenosine (5)pyrophosphate; adenosine with triphosphoric acid esterfied at its 5′ position; immediate precursors of adenine nucleotides in RNA. The primary energy currency of a cell. SYN adenosine triphosphate.

ad·e·no·sis (ad-ĕ-nō′sis).   A rarely used term for a more or less generalized glandular disease.

blunt duct a., a. of the breast in which the ducts are enlarged but not increased in number.

fibrosing a., SYN sclerosing a.

microglandular a., a. of the breast in which irregular clusters of small tubules are present in adipose or fibrous tissues, resembling tubular carcinoma but lacking stromal fibroblastic proliferation.

sclerosing a., a nodular, benign breast lesion occurring most frequently in relatively young women and consisting of hyperplastic distorted lobules of acinar tissue with increased collagenous stroma; the changes may be difficult to distinguish microscopically from carcinoma. Also, a benign nodular microscopic lesion of the prostate consisting of acimar tissue with increased stroma; the basal cell layer shows characteristic smooth muscle metaplasia. SYN adenofibrosis, fibrosing adenomatosis, fibrosing a.

aden·o·syl (a-den′ō-sil).   The radical of adenosine minus an H or OH from one of the ribosyl OH groups, usually the 5′, *e.g., S*-adenosyl-L-methionine.

ad·e·no·sylco·bal·a·min (a-den′ō-sil-kō-bal′ă-min).   A derivative of vitamin B_{12}. Its impaired biosynthesis can lead to methylmalonic acidemia.

S-aden·o·syl·-L-ho·mo·cys·te·ine (a-den′ō-sil-hō-mō-sis′te-ēn).   *S*-(5′-deoxy-5′-adenosyl)-L-homocysteine; the compound formed by the demethylation of *S*-adenosyl-L-methionine.

S-aden·o·syl·L-me·thi·o·nine (SAM, AdoMet) (a-den′ō-sil-me-thī′ō-nēn).   *S*-(5′-deoxy-5′-adenosyl)-L-methionine; condensation product of adenosine and L-methionine involving replacement of the —OPO_3H_2 of adenylic acid by —S^+(CH_3)-$CH_2CH_2CH(NH_3^+)CO_2$ of methionine; a sulfonium compound bearing a methyl group that is transferred in transmethylation

adenosarcoma (in the uterus)

reactions. SEE ALSO *methionine* adenosyltransferase. SYN active methionine.

ad·e·not·o·my (ad-ĕ-not'ō-mē). Incision of a gland. [adeno- + G. *tomē,* a cutting]

ad·e·no·ton·sil·lec·to·my (ad'ĕ-nō-ton-si-lek'tō-mē). Operative removal of tonsils and adenoids.

ad·e·nous (ad'ĕ-nŭs). Rarely used term for adenose.

Ad·e·no·vi·ri·dae (ad'ĕ-nō-vir'i-dē). A family of double-stranded DNA viruses, commonly known as adenoviruses, that develop in the nuclei of infected cells in mammals and birds. The virion is 70 to 90 nm in diameter, naked, and ether-resistant; the capsids are icosahedral and composed of 252 capsomeres. The family includes two genera, *Mastadenovirus* and *Aviadenovirus.*

ad·e·no·vi·rus (ad'ĕ-nō-vī'rŭs). Adenoidal-pharyngeal-conjunctival or A-P-C virus; any virus of the family Adenoviridae. More than 40 types are known to infect man causing upper respiratory symptoms, acute respiratory disease, conjunctivitis, gastroenteritis, hemorrhagic cystitis, and serous infections in neonates. SYN A-P-C virus, adenoidal-pharyngeal-conjunctival virus. [G. *adēn,* gland, + virus]

canine a. 1, a virus causing infectious canine hepatitis in dogs. SYN fox encephalitis virus, Rubarth's disease virus.

porcine a.'s, obsolete term for viruses of the genus *Mastadenovirus,* with four recognized serotypes, which can cause a mild upper respiratory tract disease in swine.

ad·e·nyl (ad'e-nil). The radical or ion of adenine; often used for adenylyl, as in adenylosuccinic acid.

aden·y·late (a-den'i-lāt). Salt or ester of adenylic acid.

a. cyclase, an enzyme acting on ATP to form 3',5'-cyclic AMP plus pyrophosphate. A crucial step in the regulation and formation of second messengers. SYN 3',5'-cyclic AMP synthetase.

a. kinase, adenylic acid kinase; a phosphotransferase that catalyzes the reversible phosphorylation of a molecule of ADP by MgADP, yielding MgATP and AMP. SYN adenylic acid kinase, myokinase.

ad·e·nyl cy·clase (ad'e-nil sī'klās). An enzyme that converts adenosine monophosphate to cyclic adenosine monophosphate, an intracellular second messenger of neural or hormonal activation.

ad·e·nyl·ic ac·id (ad-e-nil'ik). A condensation product of adenosine and phosphoric acid; a nucleotide found among the hydrolysis products of all nucleic acids. 3'-Adenylic acid (adenosine 3'-monophosphate) and 5'-adenylic acid (adenosine 5'-monophosphate [AMP]) differ in the place of attachment of the phosphoric acid to the D-ribose; deoxyadenylic acid differs in having H instead of OH at the 2' position of D-ribose. SEE ALSO AMP. SYN adenine nucleotide.

cyclic a. a., SYN adenosine 3',5'-cyclic monophosphate.

a. a. deaminase, SYN AMP deaminase.

a. a. kinase, SYN *adenylate* kinase.

ad·e·nyl·o·suc·ci·nase (ad'e-nil-ō-sŭk'sin-ās). SYN adenylosuccinate lyase.

ad·e·nyl·o·suc·ci·nate ly·ase (ad'e-nil-ō-sŭk'sin-āt). adenylylsuccinate lyase; an enzyme catalyzing the nonhydrolytic cleavage of adenylosuccinic acid producing AMP and fumarate and also of 4-(N-succinocarboxamido)-5-aminoimidazole nucleotide to yield fumarate and aminoimidazole carboxamide ribosyl-5-phosphate. Both are steps in purine nucleotide biosynthesis. SYN adenylosuccinase, adenylylsuccinate lyase.

ad·e·nyl·o·suc·ci·nate syn·thase. A ligase catalyzing the formation of adenylosuccinate, GDP, and P_i from inosinic acid, aspartate, and GTP. An important enzyme in purine nucleotide biosynthesis. SYN adenylylsuccinate synthase, IMP-aspartate ligase.

ad·e·nyl·o·suc·cin·ic ac·id (sAMP) (ad'e-nil-ō-sŭk'sin-ik). A condensation product of aspartic acid and inosine 5'-monophosphate; an intermediate in the biosynthesis of adenylic acid. Formally, it is adenylic acid with succinic acid replacing an H of the NH_2 group, forming a C–N. SYN adenylylosuccinic acid, N-succinyladenylic acid.

aden·yl·py·ro·phos·pha·tase. SYN adenosine triphosphatase.

aden·y·lyl (a-den'i-lil). The radical of adenylic acid minus an

OH from the phosphoric group; often shortened to adenyl in compound names, such as adenylosuccinic acid.

a. cyclase, former name for *adenylate* cyclase.

aden·y·lyl·o·suc·ci·nate ly·ase (a-den'i-lil-ō-sŭk'sin-āt). SYN adenylosuccinate lyase.

aden·y·lyl·o·suc·ci·nate syn·thase. SYN adenylosuccinate synthase.

aden·y·lyl·o·suc·cin·ic ac·id (a-den'i-lil-ō-sŭk'sin-ik). SYN adenylosuccinic acid.

aden·y·lyl·sul·fate ki·nase. SEE *adenosine 5'-phosphosulfate* kinase.

a·deps, gen. **adi·pis, adi·pes** (ad'eps, ad'i-pis, -pēz). **1.** Denoting fat or adipose tissue. **2.** The rendered fat of swine, lard, used in the preparation of ointments. SYN lard. SEE ALSO adeps lanae. [L. lard, fat]

a. re′nis, obsolete term for the layer of adipose tissue ("fatty capsule") surrounding the kidney (perirenal fat).

a·deps la·nae. The greasy substance obtained from the wool of the sheep *Ovis aries* (family Bovidae). Used as an emollient base for creams and ointments. SYN hydrous wool fat, lanolin, wool wax. [L. fat of wool]

ader·mia (ă-der'mē-ă). Congenital defect or absence of skin. [G. *a-* priv. + *derma,* skin]

ader·mo·gen·e·sis (ă-der-mō-jen'ĕ-sis). Failure or imperfection in the regeneration of the skin, especially the imperfect repair of a cutaneous defect. [G. *a-* priv. + *derma,* skin, + *genesis,* origin]

ADH Abbreviation for antidiuretic *hormone*; alcohol dehydrogenase.

ad·her·ence (ad-hēr'ens). **1.** The act or quality of sticking to something. SEE ALSO adhesion. **2.** The extent to which the patient continues the agreed-upon mode of treatment under limited supervision. Cf. compliance (2), maintenance. [L. *adhaereo,* to stick to]

immune a., the binding of antigen-antibody complexes or cells coated with antibodies or complement to cells bearing the appropriate complement or Fc receptors.

ad·he·sins (ad-hē'zins). Microbial surface antigens that frequently exist in the form of filamentous projections (pili or fimbriae) and bind to specific receptors on epithelial cell membranes; usually classified according to their ability to induce agglutination of erythrocytes from various species, their differential attachment to epithelial cells of various origins, or their susceptibility to reversal of such binding activities in the presence of mannose. [L. *ad-haereo,* pp. *ad-haesum,* to stick to, + -in]

ad·he·sio, pl. **ad·he·si·o·nes** (ad-hē'zē-ō, ad-hē-zē-ō'nēz) [NA]. SYN adhesion (1). [L.]

a. interthalam′ica [NA], SYN interthalamic *adhesion.*

ad·he·sion (ad-hē'zhŭn). **1.** The process of adhering or uniting of two surfaces or parts, especially the union of the opposing surfaces of a wound. SYN adhesio [NA], conglutination (1). **2.** In the plural, inflammatory bands that connect opposing serous surfaces. **3.** Physical attraction of unlike molecules for one another. **4.** Molecular attraction existing between the surfaces of bodies in contact. [L. *adhesio,* to stick to]

amniotic a.'s, SYN amniotic *bands,* under band.

fibrinous a., an a. that consists of fine threads of fibrin resulting from an exudate of plasma or lymph, or an extravasation of blood.

fibrous a., fibrous strands resulting from the organization of fibrinous a.'s.

interthalamic a., the variable connection between the two thalamic masses across the third ventricle; absent in about 20% of human brains. SYN adhesio interthalamica [NA], commissura cinerea, commissura grisea (1), intermediate mass, massa intermedia.

primary a., SYN *healing* by first intention.

secondary a., SYN *healing* by second intention.

ad·he·si·ot·o·my (ad-hē-sē-ot'ō-mē). Surgical section or lysis of adhesions.

ad·he·sive (ad-hē'siv). **1.** Relating to, or having the characteristics of, an adhesion. **2.** Any material that adheres to a surface or causes adherence between surfaces.

adhib. Abbreviation for L. *adhibendus*, to be administered.

ad·i·ad·o·cho·ci·ne·sia, ad·i·ad·o·cho·ci·ne·sis (ă-dī′ă-dō-kō-si-nē′sē-ă, -sis). SYN adiadochokinesis. [G. *a*-priv. + *diadochos*, successive, + *kinēsis*, movement]

ad·i·ad·o·cho·ki·ne·sis (ă-dī′ă-dō-kō-kin-ē′sis). Inability to perform rapid alternating movements. One of the clinical manifestations of cerebellar dysfunction. SEE ALSO dysdiadochokinesia. Cf. diadochokinesia. SYN adiadochocinesia, adiadochocinesis, dysdiadochokinesis. [G. *a*- priv. + *diadochos*, successive, + *kinēsis*, movement]

adi·a·pho·re·sis (ā′dī-ă-fō-rē′sis). SYN anhidrosis. [G. *a*- priv. + *diaphorēsis*, perspiration]

adi·a·pho·ret·ic (ā-dī′ă-fō-ret′ik). SYN anhidrotic.

adi·a·pho·ria (ă-dī-ă-fō′rē-ă). Failure to respond to stimulation after a series of previously applied stimuli. [G. *a*- priv. + *dia*, through, + *phoros*, bearing]

adi·a·spi·ro·my·co·sis (ā′dē-ă-spī′rō-mī-kō′sis). A rare pulmonary mycosis of humans and of rodents and other animals that dig in soil or are aquatic, caused by *Emmonsia parva*.

adi·a·spore (a′dē-ă-spōr). A fungus spore which, when produced in the lungs of an animal or incubated *in vitro* at elevated temperatures, increases greatly in size without eventual reproduction or replication. [G. *a*- priv. + *dia*, through, + *sporos*, seed]

adi·as·to·le (ă-dī-as′tō-lē). Absence or imperceptibility of the diastolic movement of the heart; diastolic ventricular functional abnormality. [G. *a*- priv. + *diastolē*, dilation]

adi·a·ther·man·cy (ă-dī-ă-ther′man-sē). Impermeability to heat. [G. *dia-thermainō*, to warm through, fr. *a*- priv. + *dia*, through, + *thermē*, heat]

Adie, William J., Australian physician, 1886–1935. SEE A.'s *pupil*; A. *syndrome*; Holmes-Adie *pupil*; Holmes-Adie *syndrome*.

ad·i·em·or·rhy·sis (ad′i-em-ōr′i-sis). Arrest of the capillary circulation. [G. *a*- priv. + *dia*, through, + *haima*, blood, + *rhysis*, a flowing]

ad·i·ent (ad′ē-ent). Having a tendency to move toward the source of a stimulus, as opposed to abient. [L. *adiens*, pr. p. of *adeo*, to go toward]

Adin·i·da (ă-din′i-dă). A suborder of dinoflagellates, in which the flagella are free and do not lie in furrows. [G. *a*- priv. + *dien*, a whirling]

△**adip-, adipo-.** Fat, fatty. Corresponds to G. lip-, lipo-. SEE ALSO lipo-. [L. *adeps, adipis*, soft animal fat, lard, grease; fatty tissue; obesity; akin to G. *aleipha*, unguent, anointing-oil, oil, fat, pitch, resin, *lipos*, animal fat, lard, tallow, vegetable oil]

ad·i·pec·to·my (ad-i-pek′tō-mē). Obsolete term for lipectomy. [L. *adeps*, fat, + G. *ektomē*, excision]

adiph·e·nine hy·dro·chlo·ride (ă-dif′ě-nen). α-Phenylbenzeneacetic acid 2-(diethylamino)ethyl ester hydrochloride; a spasmolytic agent used to decrease spasm of the biliary tract, gastrointestinal tract, uterus, and ureter.

adip·ic ac·id (ă-dip′ik). Hexanedioic acid; the dicarboxylic acid, HOOC(CH$_2$)$_4$COOH.

Ad·i·pi·o·done. SYN iodipamide.

△**adipo-.** SEE adip-.

ad·i·po·cel·lu·lar (ad′i-pō-sel′yū-lăr). Relating to both fatty and cellular tissues, or to connective tissue with many fat cells.

ad·i·po·cer·a·tous (ad-i-pō-ser′ă-tŭs). Relating to adipocere. SYN lipoceratous.

ad·i·po·cere (ad′i-pō-sēr). A fatty substance of waxy consistency into which dead animal tissues (as those of a corpse) are sometimes converted when kept from the air under certain favoring conditions of temperature. SYN grave wax, lipocere. [adipo- + L. *cera*, wax]

ad·i·po·cyte (ad′i-pō-sīt). SYN fat *cell*.

ad·i·po·gen·e·sis (ad′i-pō-jen′ě-sis). SYN lipogenesis.

ad·i·po·gen·ic, ad·i·pog·e·nous (ad′i-pō-jen′ik, ad′i-poj′ě-nŭs). SYN lipogenic.

ad·i·poid (ad′i-poyd). SYN lipoid. [adipo- + G. *eidos*, resemblance]

ad·i·po·ki·net·ic (ad′i-pō-ki-net′ik). Denoting a substance or factor that causes mobilization of stored lipid. [adipo- + G. *kinēsis*, movement]

ad·i·po·ki·nin (ad-i-pō-kī′nin). An anterior pituitary hormone that causes mobilization of fat from adipose tissue. SYN adipokinetic hormone.

ad·i·pom·e·ter (ad-i-pom′ě-ter). An instrument for determining the thickness of the skin. [adipo- + G. *metron*, measure]

ad·i·po·ne·cro·sis (ad′i-pō-ne-krō′sis). Rarely used term referring to necrosis of fat, as in hemorrhagic pancreatitis.

ad·i·po·sal·gia (ad′i-pō-sal′jē-ă). Condition in which painful areas of subcutaneous fat develop. [adipo- + G. *algos*, pain]

ad·i·pose (ad′i-pōs). Denoting fat.

ad·i·po·sis (ad-i-pō′sis). Excessive local or general accumulation of fat in the body. SYN lipomatosis, liposis (1), steatosis (1). [adipo- + G. *-osis*, condition]

a. cerebra′lis, obesity resulting from intracranial disease, most commonly of the hypothalamus, resulting in hyperphagia.

a. doloro′sa, a condition characterized by a deposit of symmetrical nodular or pendulous masses of fat in various regions of the body, with discomfort or pain. SYN Anders' disease, Dercum's disease, lipomatosis neurotica.

a. or′chica, SYN *dystrophia* adiposogenitalis.

a. tubero′sa sim′plex, a condition resembling a. dolorosa, in which the fat occurs in small, nodular masses, which are sensitive to touch and may be spontaneously painful, on the abdomen or on the extremities.

a. universa′lis, excessive deposition of fat throughout all parts of the body, including the viscera.

ad·i·pos·i·ty (ad-i-pos′i-tē). **1.** SYN obesity. **2.** Excessive accumulation of lipids in a site or organ.

ad·i·po·su·ria (ad′i-pō-sū′rē-ă). SYN lipuria. [adipo- + G. *ouron*, urine]

adip·sia, adip·sy (ă-dip′sē-ă, -dip′sē). Absence of thirst or the lack of desire to drink. [G. *a*- priv. + *dipsa*, thirst]

ad·i·tus, pl. **ad·i·tus** (ad′i-tŭs) [NA]. SYN aperture, inlet. [L. access, fr. *ad-eo*, pp. *-itus*, go to]

a. ad an′trum [NA], SYN *aperture* of mastoid antrum.

a. ad aqueduc′tum cer′ebri, SYN *anus* cerebri.

a. ad infundib′ulum, SYN infundibular *recess*.

a. ad sac′cum peritone′i mino′rem, SYN epiploic *foramen*.

a. glot′tidis infe′rior, SYN infraglottic *cavity*.

a. glot′tidis supe′rior, SYN intermediate laryngeal *cavity*.

a. laryn′gis [NA], SYN *inlet* of larynx.

a. or′bitae [NA], SYN orbital *opening*.

a. pel′vis, SYN superior pelvic *aperture*.

ad·just·ment (ă-jŭst′ment). **1.** In dentistry, any modification made upon a fixed or removable prosthesis during or after its insertion to perfect its adaptation and function. **2.** SYN adaptation (6). **3.** A summarizing procedure for a statistical measure in which the effects of differences in composition of the populations being compared have been minimized by statistical methods.

occlusal a., modification of the occluding and incising surfaces of teeth to develop harmonious relationships between these surfaces.

ad·ju·vant (ad′jū-vănt). **1.** A substance added to a drug product formulation which affects the action of the active ingredient in a predictable way. **2.** In immunology, a vehicle used to enhance antigenicity; *e.g.*, a suspension of minerals (alum, aluminum hydroxide or phosphate) on which antigen is adsorbed; or water-in-oil emulsion in which antigen solution is emulsified in mineral oil (Freund's incomplete a.), sometimes with the inclusion of killed mycobacteria (Freund's complete a.) to further enhance antigenicity. [L. *ad-juvo*, pres. p. *-juvans*, to give aid to]

Freund's a., SEE adjuvant.

Freund's complete a., water-in-oil emulsion of antigen, to which killed mycobacteria or tuberculosis bacteria are added.

Freund's incomplete a., water-in-oil emulsion of antigen, without mycobacteria.

ADL. Abbreviation for activities of daily living. SEE activities of daily living *scale*.

Adler, Alfred, Austrian psychiatrist, 1870–1937. SEE adlerian *psychology;* adlerian *psychoanalysis.*

Adler, Oscar, German physician, 1879–1932. SEE A.'s *test.*

ad·le·ri·an (ad-ler'ē-an). Relating to or described by Alfred Adler.

ad lib Abbreviation for L. *ad libitum,* freely, as desired.

adm. SEE admov.

ad·me·di·al, ad·me·di·an (ad-mē'dē-ăl, -dē-an). Toward or near the median plane.

ad·mi·nic·u·lum, pl. **ad·mi·nic·u·la** (ad-mi-nik'yū-lŭm, -yū-lă) [NA]. That which gives support to a part. [L. a hand-rest, prop, fr. *ad* + *manus,* hand]

  a. lin'eae al'bae [NA], a triangular fibrous expansion, sometimes containing a few muscular fibers, passing from the superior pubic ligament to the posterior surface of the linea alba.

admov. Abbreviation for L. *admove,* apply.

ad·ner·val (ad-ner'văl). SYN adneural.

ad·neu·ral (ad-nūr'ăl). **1.** Lying near a nerve. **2.** In the direction of a nerve; said of an electric current passing through muscular tissue toward the point of entrance of the nerve. SYN adnerval.

ad·nexa, sing. **ad·nex·um** (ad-nek'să, -sŭm). Parts accessory to the main organ or structure. SEE ALSO appendage. SYN annexa. [L. connected parts]

  a. o'culi, SYN accessory *organs* of the eye, under *organ.*

  a. u'teri, SYN uterine *appendages,* under *appendage.*

ad·nex·al (ad-nek'săl). Relating to the adnexa. SYN annexal.

ad·nex·ec·to·my (ad-nek-sek'tō-mē). **1.** Excision of any adnexa. **2.** In gynecology, excision of the fallopian tube and ovary if unilateral and excision of both tubes and ovaries (adnexa uteri) if bilateral. SYN annexectomy.

ad·nex·i·tis (ad-neks-ī'tis). Inflammation of the adnexa uteri. SYN annexitis. [L. *annexa,* adnexa, + *-itis,* inflammation]

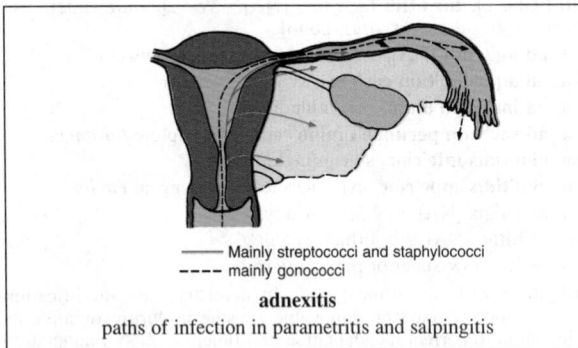

——— Mainly streptococci and staphylococci
- - - - mainly gonococci

adnexitis
paths of infection in parametritis and salpingitis

ad·nex·o·pexy (ad-neks'ō-pek-sē). Operation for suspension of the fallopian tube and ovary; usually, oophoropexy is accomplished without suspension of the tube. SYN annexopexy. [L. *annexa,* adnexa, + G. *pēxis,* fixation]

ad·nex·um (ad-nek'sŭm). Singular of adnexa.

Ado Symbol for adenosine.

ad·o·les·cence (ad-ō-les'ens). The period of life beginning with puberty and ending with completed growth and physical maturity. [L. *adolescentia*]

ad·o·les·cent (ad-ō-les'ent). **1.** Pertaining to adolescence. **2.** An individual in that stage of development.

AdoMet Abbreviation for *S*-adenosyl-L-methionine.

adon·is (a-don'is). Medicinal herb obtained from *Adonis vernalis* (family Ranunculaceae), grown in Eastern Europe and used there in the treatment of congestive heart failure. Contains strophanthidin and related cardiotonic glycosides. SYN false hellebore. [G. *Adōnis,* mythical figure, fr. Phoenicial *adon,* lord]

adon·i·tol (ă-don'i-tol). SYN ribitol.

ad·o·ral. Obsolete term for orad. [L. *ad,* to, + *os(or-),* mouth]

ADP Abbreviation for adenosine 5'-diphosphate.

ADPase. SYN apyrase.

⌂adren-. SEE adreno-.

ad·re·nal (ă-drē'năl). **1.** Near or upon the kidney; denoting the suprarenal (adrenal) gland. **2.** A suprarenal gland or separate tissue or product thereof. SEE ALSO suprarenal. [L. *ad,* to, + *ren,* kidney]

  accessory a., an island of cortical tissue separate from the adrenal gland, usually found in the retroperitoneal tissues, kidney, or genital organs. SYN adrenal rest.

  Marchand's a.'s, small collections of accessory a. tissue in the broad ligament of the uterus or in the testes. SYN Marchand's rest.

ad·re·nal·ec·to·my (ă-drē-năl-ek'tō-mē). Removal of one or both adrenal glands. [adrenal + G. *ektomē,* excision]

adren·a·line (ă-dren'ă-lin, -lēn). SYN epinephrine.

  a. oxidase, SYN *amine* oxidase (flavin-containing).

ad·re·nal·ism. SYN hypercorticoidism.

adre·nal·i·tis (ă-drē-năl-ī'tis). Inflammation of the adrenal gland.

adren·a·lone (ă-dren'ă-lōn). 3'4'-Dihydroxy-2-(methylamino)-acetophenone; 4-methylaminoacetopyrocatechol; precursor of epinephrine in some manufacturing processes; a topical adrenergic agent in ophthalmology.

adre·na·lop·a·thy (ă-drē-nă-lop'ă-thē). Any pathologic condition of the adrenal glands. SYN adrenopathy. [adrenal + G. *pathos,* suffering]

ad·ren·ar·che (ad'ren-ar-kē). **1.** Auxiliary and pubic hair growth during puberty induced by hyperactivity of the adrenal cortex. **2.** Physiologic change at puberty caused by adrenocortical secretion of androgenic hormones or precursors of them. [adren- + G. *archē,* beginning]

ad·re·ner·gic (ad-rĕ-ner'jik). **1.** Relating to nerve cells or fibers of the autonomic nervous system that employ norepinephrine as their neurotransmitter. Cf. cholinergic. **2.** Relating to drugs that mimic the actions of the sympathetic nervous system. SEE α-adrenergic *receptors,* under *receptor,* β-adrenergic *receptors,* under *receptor.* [adren- + G. *ergon,* work]

adren·ic (ă-drē'nik). Relating to the suprarenal gland.

⌂adreno-, adrenal-, adren-. Relating to the adrenal gland. [L. *ad,* to, near, + *renes,* the kidneys, + *-o-* + *-alis,* pertaining to]

adre·no·cep·tive (ă-dren-ō-sep'tiv). Referring to chemical sites in effectors with which the adrenergic mediator unites. Cf. cholinoceptive.

adre·no·cep·tor (ă-drē'sep'tor). SYN adrenergic *receptors,* under *receptor.*

adre·no·cor·ti·cal (ă-drē-nō-kōr'ti-kăl). Pertaining to suprarenal cortex.

adre·no·cor·ti·coid (ă-drē-nō-kor'ti-koid). SYN corticosteroid.

adre·no·cor·ti·co·mi·met·ic (ă-drē'nō-kōr'ti-kō-mi-met'ik). Mimicking or producing effects similar to adrenocortical function. [adrenal + cortex + G. *minētikos,* imitating]

adre·no·cor·ti·co·tro·pic, adre·no·cor·ti·co·tro·phic (ă-drē'nō-kōr'ti-kō-trō'pik, -trō'fik). Stimulating growth of the adrenal cortex or secretion of its hormones. SYN adrenotropic, adrenotrophic. [adrenal cortex + G. *trophē,* nurture; *tropē,* a turning]

adre·no·cor·ti·co·tro·pin (ă-drē'nō-kōr-ti-kō-trō'pin). SYN adrenocorticotropic *hormone.*

adre·no·gen·ic, adre·nog·e·nous (ă-drē-nō-jen'ik, a-drē-noj'e-nŭs). Of adrenal origin. [adreno- + G. *-gen,* producing]

adre·no·leu·ko·dys·tro·phy (ALD) (ă-drē'nō-lū-kō-dis'trō-fē) [MIM*300100]. An X-linked recessive disorder affecting young males, characterized by chronic adrenocortical insufficiency, skin hyperpigmentation, progressive dementia, spastic paralysis, and other intellectual and neurological disturbances; due to myelin degeneration in the white matter of the brain.

adre·no·lyt·ic (ă-dren-ō-lit'ik). Denoting antagonism to or inhibition or blockade of the action of epinephrine, norepinephrine, and related sympathomimetics. SEE ALSO adrenergic blocking *agent*. [adreno- + G. *lysis*, loosening, dissolution]

adre·no·meg·a·ly (ă-drē-nō-meg'ă-lē). Enlargement of the adrenal glands. [adreno- + G. *megas*, big]

adre·no·mi·met·ic (ă-drē'nō-mi-met'ik). Having an action similar to that of the compounds epinephrine and norepinephrine, which are liberated from the adrenal medulla and adrenergic nerves; term proposed to replace the less accurate term, sympathomimetic. Cf. adrenergic, cholinomimetic. [adreno- + G. *mimētikos*, imitative]

adre·no·my·e·lo·neu·rop·a·thy (ad-rē'nō-mī'e-lō-nū-rop'a-thē). A disorder of adult males, consisting of long standing adrenal insufficiency, hypogonadism, progressive myelopathy, peripheral neuropathy, and sphincter disturbances; considered a variant of adrenoleukodystrophy. [adreno- + G. *myelos*, medulla, + *neuron*, nerve, + *pathos*, suffering]

adre·nop·a·thy (ă-drē-nop'ă-thē). SYN adrenalopathy.

adre·no·pri·val (ă-drē-nō-prī'văl). Rarely used term indicating a loss of adrenal function, as a result of either disease or surgical excision. [adreno- + L. *privo*, to deprive]

adre·no·re·ac·tive (ă-drē'nō-rē-ak'tiv). Responding to the catecholamines.

adre·no·re·cep·tors (ă-drē'nō-rē-sep'terz). SYN adrenergic *receptors*, under *receptor*.

adre·nos·ter·one (a-drē-nos'ter-ōn). 4-androstene-3,11,17-trione; an androgen isolated from the adrenal cortex. SYN adrenosterone.

adre·no·tox·in (ă-drē-nō-tok'sin). A substance toxic for the adrenal glands. [adreno- + toxin]

adre·no·tro·pic, adre·no·tro·phic (ă-drē-nō-trō'pik, -trō'fik). SYN adrenocorticotropic.

adre·no·tro·pin (ă-drē-nō-trō'pin). SYN adrenocorticotropic *hormone*.

adri·a·my·cin (ā'drē-ă-mī'sin). SYN doxorubicin.

adro·mia (ă-drō'mē-ă). Failure of muscle innervation. [G. *a*-priv. + *dromos*, course]

ad sat Abbreviation for L. *ad saturatum*, to saturation.

Adson, Alfred W., U.S. neurosurgeon, 1887–1951. SEE A.'s *test;* A. *forceps, maneuver;* Brown-A. *forceps*.

ad·sorb (ad-sōrb'). To take up by adsorption. [L. *ad*, to, + *sorbeo*, to suck in]

ad·sorb·ate (ad-sōr'bāt). Any substance adsorbed.

ad·sorb·ent (ad-sōr'bent). **1.** A substance that adsorbs, *i.e.*, a solid substance endowed with the property of attaching other substances to its surface without any covalent bonding, *e.g.*, activated charcoal. **2.** An antigen or antibody used in immune adsorption.

ad·sorp·tion (ad-sōrp'shŭn). The property of a solid substance to attract and hold to its surface a gas, liquid, or a substance in solution or in suspension. For example, condensation of a gas onto a surface. Cf. absorption. [L. *ad*, to, + *sorbeo*, to suck up]
immune a., (1) removal of antibody (agglutinin or precipitin) from antiserum by use of specific antigen; after aggregation has occurred, the antigen-antibody complex is separated either by centrifugation or by filtration; (2) removal of antigen by specific antiserum in a similar manner.

ad·ster·nal (ad-ster'năl). Near or upon the sternum.

ADTe Abbreviation for anodal duration *tetanus*.

ad·ter·mi·nal (ad-ter'mi-năl). In a direction toward the nerve endings, muscular insertions, or the extremity of any structure.

adult (ă-dŭlt'). **1.** Fully grown and physically mature. **2.** A fully grown and mature individual. [L *adultus*, grown up fr. *adolesco*, to grow up]

adul·ter·ant (ă-dŭl'ter-ănt). An impurity; an additive that is considered to have an undesirable effect or to dilute the active material so as to reduce its therapeutic or monetary value.

adul·ter·a·tion (ă-dŭl-ter-ā'shŭn). The alteration of any substance by the deliberate addition of a component not ordinarily part of that substance; usually used to imply that the substance is debased as a result.

adul·to·mor·phism (ă-dŭl-tō-mōr'fizm). Interpretation of children's behavior in adult terms.

adv. Abbreviation for L. *adversum*, against.

ad·vance (ad-vans'). To move distally. [Fr. *avancer*, to set forward]

ad·vanced life sup·port. Definitive emergency medical care that includes defibrillation, airway management, and use of drugs and medications. Cf. basic life support.

ad·vance·ment (ad-vans'ment). Surgical procedure in which a ligamentous or partially tendinous insertion or a skin flap is partially severed or released from its attachment and sutured to a more distal point.
capsular a., surgical reattachment of the anterior portion of Tenon's capsule.
tendon a., excision of the tendon of an eye muscle and attachment of it to a more anterior location on the globe.

ad·ven·ti·tia (ad-ven-tish'ă). The outermost connective tissue covering of any organ, vessel, or other structure not covered by a serosa; instead, the covering is properly derived from without (*i.e.*, from the surrounding connective tissue) and does not form an integral part of such organ or structure. SYN tunica adventitia [NA], membrana adventitia (1). [L. *adventicius*, coming from abroad, foreign, fr. *ad*, to + *venio*, to come]

ad·ven·ti·tial (ad-ven-tish'ăl). Relating to the outer coat or adventitia of a blood vessel or other structure. SYN adventitious (3).

ad·ven·ti·tious (ad-ven-tish'ŭs). **1.** Arising from an external source or occurring in an unusual place or manner. SEE ALSO extrinsic. **2.** Occurring accidentally or spontaneously, as opposed to natural causes or hereditary. **3.** SYN adventitial.

ady·nam·ia (ā-dī-nam'ē-ă, ad-i-nă'mē-ă). **1.** SYN asthenia. **2.** Lack of motor activity or strength. [G. *a*- priv. + *dynamis*, power]
a. episodica hereditaria, hyperkalemic periodic *paralysis*, without myotonia.

ady·nam·ic (ă-dī-nam'ik). Relating to adynamia.

△**ae-.** For words so beginning and not found here, see under e-.

Aeby, Christopher T., Swiss anatomist, 1835–1885. SEE A.'s *muscle, plane*.

Aedes (ā-ē'dēz). A widespread genus of small mosquitoes frequently found in tropical and subtropical regions. [G. *aēdēs*, unpleasant, unfriendly]
A. aegyp'ti, the yellow fever mosquito, a species that is also the vector of the pathogen of dengue; characterized by white lyre-shaped markings on the thorax.
A. albopic'tus, species that is an important vector of dengue viruses widespread in the Pacific basin.
A. cabal'lus, species that is an important vector of Rift Valley fever in South Africa.
A. leucocelae'nus, species that transmits yellow fever in South America.
A. polynesien'sis, species that is an important vector of filariasis and dengue in the Polynesian region.
A. scapular'is, species that is a vector of myxomatosis of rabbits.
A. sollic'itans, a common salt-marsh mosquito species and vector of eastern equine encephalomyelitis on the Atlantic and Gulf coasts of the United States.
A. variegat'us, a species that is a vector of filarial parasites in the Pacific Islands (Gilbert and Ellice group).

ae·gyp·ti·a·nel·lo·sis (ē-jip'shē-a-nel-ō'sis). A tickborne disease of birds caused by rickettsiae of the genus *Aegyptianella* and characterized by punctiform hemorrhages of the serosa and anemia.

ae·lu·ro·pho·bia (ē-lū-rō-fō'bē-ă). SYN ailurophobia.

Aelu·ro·stron·gy·lus (ē'lūr-ō-stron'jī-lŭs). A common genus of lungworm in cats; land snails and slugs serve as intermediate hosts and snail-eating animals can serve as transport hosts. [G. *ailuros*, cat, + Mod. L., fr. G. *strongylus*, round]

ae·quo·rin (ē'kwō-rin). A luminescent protein isolated from the jellyfish *Aequorea* which emits blue light in the presence of even minute amounts of calcium ion; injected intracellularly, it is used to measure free calcium ion transients within cells. SEE ALSO fura-2, quin-2.

aer-, aero-. The air, a gas; aerial, gassy. [G. *aēr* (L. *aer*), air]

aer·ate (ār'āte). **1.** To supply (blood) with oxygen. **2.** To expose to the circulation of air for purification. **3.** To supply or charge (liquid) with a gas, especially carbon dioxide.

aer·en·do·car·dia (ār-en-dō-kar'dē-ă). Presence of undissolved air in the blood within the heart. [aer- + G. *endon,* within, + *kardia,* heart]

aero-. SEE aer-.

aer·o·at·el·ec·ta·sis (ār'ō-at-ē-lek'tă-sis). A partial, reversible, airless state of lung tissue most likely to occur in pilots exposed to high G forces, breathing 100% oxygen, and wearing an anti-G suit.

Aer·o·bac·ter (ār-ō-bak'ter). An officially rejected generic name of bacteria. The type species is *A. aerogenes.* Motile organisms previously placed in this species are now placed in *Enterobacter aerogenes;* the nonmotile organisms have been transferred to *Klebsiella pneumoniae.* The species *A. cloacae* is now known as *Enterobacter cloacae.* [aero- + G. *baktērion,* a small staff]

aer·obe (ār'ōb). **1.** An organism that can live and grow in the presence of oxygen. **2.** An organism that can use oxygen as a final electron acceptor in a respiratory chain. [aero- + G. *bios,* life]

obligate a., an organism which cannot live or grow in the absence of oxygen.

aer·o·bic (ār-ō'bik). **1.** Living in air. **2.** Relating to an aerobe. SYN aerophilous.

aer·o·bi·ol·o·gy (ār'ō-bī-ol'ō-jē). The study of atmospheric constituents, living and nonliving, of biological significance, *e.g.,* airborne spores, pathogenic bacteria, allergenic substances, pollutants.

aer·o·bi·o·scope (ār-ō-bī'ō-skōp). An apparatus for determining the bacterial content of the air. [aero- + G. *bios,* life, + *skopeō,* to view]

aer·o·bi·o·sis (ār-ō-bī-ō'sis). Existence in an atmosphere containing oxygen. [aero- + G. *biōsis,* mode of living]

aer·o·bi·ot·ic (ār-ō-bī-ot'ik). Relating to aerobiosis.

aer·o·cele (ār'ō-sēl). Distention of a small natural cavity with gas. [aero- + G. *kēlē,* tumor]

Aer·o·coc·cus (ār-ō-kok'ŭs). A genus of aerobic Gram-positive cocci that resemble enterococci but do not form chains. They are frequently isolated as airborne saphrophytes in hospitals and as a pathogen of lobsters; cause greening in blood agar and grow in the presence of 40% bile. In humans, they are found in endocarditis and in urinary tract infections. The type and only species is *A. viridans.* [aero- + G. *kokkos,* berry]

aer·o·col·pos (ār-ō-kol'pos). Distention of the vagina with gas. [aero- + G. *kolpos,* lap, hollow]

aer·o·der·mec·ta·sia (ār'ō-der-mek-tā'zē-ă). SYN subcutaneous *emphysema.* [aero- + G. *derma,* skin, + *ektasis,* a stretching out]

aer·o·don·tal·gia (ār'ō-don-tal'jē-ă). Dental pain caused by either increased or reduced atmospheric pressure. SYN aero-odontalgia, aero-odontodynia. [aero- + G. *odous,* tooth, + *algos,* pain]

primary a., dental pain associated with expansion of trapped gases within a tooth, as under a filling or in an infected pulp.

secondary a., pain referred to the dental area from an area of aerosinusitis.

aer·o·don·tia (ār-ō-don'shē-ă). The science of the effect of either increased or reduced atmospheric pressure on the teeth. [aero- + G. *odous,* tooth]

aer·o·dy·nam·ics (ār-ō-dī-nam'iks). The study of air and other gases in motion, the forces that set them in motion, and the results of such motion. [aero- + G. *dynamis,* force]

aer·o·dy·nam·ic size. In aerosols, the particle size with unit density that best represents the aerodynamic behavior of a particle.

aer·o·em·phy·se·ma (ār'ō-em-fi-sē'mă). Obsolete term for decompression *sickness.*

aer·o·gas·tria (ār-ō-gas'trē-ă). Distention of the stomach with gas.

blocked a., retention of gas in the stomach due to spasm of the sphincteric region of the lower esophagus which prevents belching.

aer·o·gen (ār'ō-jen). A gas-forming microorganism.

aer·o·gen·e·sis (ār-ō-jen'ē-sis). Production of gas, as by a microorganism. [aero- + G. *genesis,* origin]

aer·o·gen·ic, aer·og·e·nous (ār-ō-jen'ik, -oj'ē-nŭs). Gas-forming.

aer·o·hy·dro·ther·a·py (ār'ō-hī-drō-thār'ă-pē). Obsolete term for the treatment of disease by application, at different temperatures and by different methods, of both air and water. [aero- + G. *hydōr,* water, + *therapeia,* healing]

aer·o·med·i·cine (ār-ō-med'i-sin). SYN aviation *medicine.*

aer·o·mo·nad (ār-ō-mō'nad). A vernacular term used to refer to any member of the genus *Aeromonas.*

Aer·o·mo·nas (ār-ō-mō'nas). A genus of aerobic, facultatively anaerobic bacteria (family Vibrionaceae) containing gram-negative, rod-shaped to coccoid cells that occur singly or in pairs or in clumps of chains; motile cells ordinarily possess a single, polar flagellum; some species are nonmotile. The metabolism of these organisms is both respiratory and fermentative. These bacteria are found in water and sewage; some are pathogenic to fresh water and marine animals. The type species is *A. hydrophila.*

A. hydroph'ila, a species that causes cellulitis, wound infections, acute diarrhea (water-borne and shellfish-associated types), septicemia, and urinary tract infections in humans. Also causes red leg disease of frogs. The type species of *Aeromonas.*

aer·o·o·don·tal·gia (ār'ō-ō-don-tal'jē-ă). SYN aerodontalgia.

aer·o·o·don·to·dyn·ia (ār'ō-ō-don-tō-din'ē-ă). SYN aerodontalgia.

aer·op·a·thy (ār-op'ă-thē). Obsolete term for any morbid state induced by a pronounced change in atmospheric pressure; *e.g.,* altitude sickness, decompression sickness. [aero- + G. *pathos,* suffering]

aer·o·pause (ār'ō-pawz). An upper region of the atmosphere, between the stratosphere and outer space, in which gas particles are so sparse as to provide almost no support for man's physiologic requirements or for vehicles that require air for burning fuel.

aer·o·pha·gia, aer·oph·a·gy (ār-ō-fā'jē-ă, -of'ă-jē). An abnormal swallowing of air as seen in crib-biting and wind-sucking. SYN pneumophagia. [aero- + G. *phagō,* to eat]

aer·o·phil, aer·o·phile (ār'ō-fil, -fīl). **1.** Air-loving. **2.** An aerobic organism (aerobe), especially an obligate aerobe. [aero- + G. *philos,* fond]

aer·o·phil·ic, aer·oph·i·lous (ār-ō-fil'ik, ār-of'i-lŭs). SYN aerobic.

aer·o·pho·bia (ār-ō-fō'bē-ă). Morbid dread of fresh air or of air in motion. [aero- + G. *phobos,* fear]

aer·o·pi·e·so·ther·a·py (ār'ō-pī-ē'sō-thār'ă-pē). Treatment of disease by compressed (or rarified) air. [aero- + G. *piesis,* pressure, + *therapeia,* medical treatment]

aer·o·plank·ton (ār-ō-plank'tŏn). An organism or a substance carried by air, *e.g.,* bacterium, pollen grain. [aero- + G. *planktos,* ntr. *-on,* wandering]

aer·o·ple·thys·mo·graph (ār'ō-plē-thiz'mō-graf). Obsolete term for body *plethysmograph.* [aero- + G. *plēthysmos,* enlargement, + *graphō,* to write]

aer·o·si·al·oph·a·gy (ār'ō-sī-al-of'ă-jē). SYN sialoaerophagy.

aer·o·si·nus·i·tis (ār-ō-sī-nŭ-sī'tis). Inflammation of the paranasal sinuses caused by pressure difference within the sinus relative to ambient pressure, secondary to obstruction of the sinus orifice, sometimes due to high altitude flying or by descent from high altitude. SYN barosinusitis.

aer·o·sis (ār-ō'sis). Generation of gas in the tissues. [aero- + G. *-osis,* condition]

aer·o·sol (ār'ō-sol). **1.** Liquid or particulate matter dispersed in air in the form of a fine mist for therapeutic, insecticidal, or other purposes. **2.** A product that is packaged under pressure and contains therapeutically or chemically active ingredients intended for topical application, inhalation, or introduction into body orifices. [aero- + solution]

respirable a.'s, a.'s with an aerodynamic size under 10 μm.

aer·o·sol·i·za·tion (ār-ō-sol-i-zā′shŭn). Dispersion in air of a liquid material or a solution in the form of a fine mist, usually for therapeutic purposes, especially to the respiratory passages.

aer·o·ther·a·peu·tics, aer·o·ther·a·py (ār′ō-thār-ă-pyū′tiks, -thār′ă-pē). Treatment of disease by fresh air, by air of different degrees of pressure or rarity, or by air medicated in various ways.

aer·o·ti·tis me·dia (ār-ō-tī′tis mē′dē-ă). An acute or chronic inflammation of the middle ear caused by a reduction in pressure in the tympanic cavity relative to ambient pressure, secondary to eustachian tube obstruction; often occurs on descent from high altitude. SYN aviation otitis, aviator's ear, barotitis media. [aero- + G. *ous,* ear, + *-itis,* inflammation]

aer·o·ton·om·e·ter (ār′ō-ton-om′ĕ-ter). **1.** An instrument for estimating the tension or pressure of a gas. **2.** SYN tonometer (2). [aero- + G. *tonos,* tension, + *metron,* measure]

aes·cu·la·pi·an (es-kyū-lā′pē-an). Relating to Aesculapius, the art of medicine, or a medical practitioner. SYN esculapian. [L. *Aesculapius,* G. *Asklēpios,* the god of medicine]

aes·cu·lin (es′kyū-lin). SYN esculin.

aes·ti·val (es′ti-văl). SYN estival.

AFB Abbreviation for acid-fast bacillus. SEE acid-fast.

afe·brile (ā-feb′ril). SYN apyretic.

afe·tal (ă-fē′tăl). Without relation to a fetus or intrauterine life.

af·fect (af′fekt). The emotional feeling, tone, and mood attached to a thought, including its external manifestations. [L. *affectus,* state of mind, fr. *afficio,* to have influence on]

blunted a., a disturbance in mood seen in schizophrenic patients manifested by shallowness and a severe reduction in the expression of feeling.

flat a., absence of or diminution in the amount of emotional tone or outward emotional reaction typically shown by others or oneself under similar circumstances; a milder form is termed blunted a.

inappropriate a., emotional tone or outward emotional reaction out of harmony with the idea, object, or thought accompanying it.

labile a., rapid shifts in outward emotional expressions; often associated with organic brain syndromes such as intoxication.

af·fect dis·play. Facial expressions, postures, and gestures indicating emotional states.

af·fec·tion (ă-fek′shŭn). **1.** A moderate feeling of tenderness, caring, or love. **2.** An abnormal condition of body or mind. [L. *affectio,* fr. *af-ficio,* to affect, influence]

af·fec·tive (af-fek′tiv). Pertaining to mood, emotion, feeling, sensibility, or a mental state.

af·fec·tiv·i·ty (af-fek-tiv′i-tē). SYN feeling *tone.*

af·fec·to·mo·tor (af′fek-tō-mō′tor). Pertaining to muscular manifestations associated with affective tone.

af·fer·ent (af′er-ent). Inflowing; conducting toward a center, denoting certain arteries, veins, lymphatics, and nerves. Opposite of efferent. SYN centripetal (1), esodic. [L. *afferens,* fr. *af-fero,* to bring to]

af·fin·i·ty (ă-fin′i-tē). **1.** In chemistry, the force that impels certain atoms to bind to or unite with certain others to form complexes or compounds. **2.** Selective staining of a tissue by a dye or the selective uptake of a dye, chemical, or other substance by a tissue. [L. *affinis,* neighboring, fr. *ad,* to, + *finis,* end, boundary]

residual a., secondary forces that enable apparently saturated atoms, ions, or molecules to attract other atoms or groups, causing such phenomena as complex formation, hydration, adsorption, etc.

af·fi·nous (af′i-nŭs). Pertaining to a marriage in which the partners are related, not by consanguinity, but through another marriage. [L. *affinis,* related by marriage, fr. *ad,* to + *finis,* limit]

---

aerosol therapy (Relationship between particle size, target area, and mode of transport.)		
particle size	target area	mode of transport
< 1 μ	particles are exhaled	remain in gaseous state
1– 5 μ	peripheral bronchial passages	particles form a sediment
5 – 10 μ	upper respiratory passages and central bronchial passages	particles rebound
> 10 μ	upper respiratory passages	

af·fir·ma·tion (af-fer-mā′shŭn). The stage in autosuggestion in which one exhibits a positive reactive tendency. [L. *affirmatio,* fr. affirm, to make strong, fr *firmus,* strong]

af·flux, af·flux·ion (af′lŭks, af-lŭk′shŭn). A flowing toward; specifically, a flowing of blood toward any part. SEE congestion. [L. *af-fluo,* pp. *-fluxus,* to flow toward]

af·fu·sion (ă-fyū′zhŭn). Pouring of water upon the body or any of its parts for therapeutic purposes. [L. *af- fundo,* to pour into]

AFH Abbreviation for anterior facial *height.*

afi·bril·lar (ā-fī′bri-lăr). Denoting a biological structure that does not contain fibrils.

afi·brin·o·gen·e·mia (ā-fī′brin-ō-jĕ-nē′mē-ă). The absence of fibrinogen in the plasma. SEE ALSO hypofibrinogenemia.

congenital a. [MIM*202400], a rare disorder of blood coagulation in which little or no fibrinogen can be found in plasma because of a mutant form in one of the three fibrinogen loci. Leads to defective platelet aggregation; autosomal recessive inheritance.

Afipia felis. A cause of cat-scratch *disease.*

af·la·tox·i·co·sis (af′la-toks-ē-cō′sis). A disease caused by ingestion of aflatoxin.

af·la·tox·in (af′lă-tok′sin). Toxic metabolites of some strains of *Aspergillus flavus, Aspergillus parasitus, Aspergillus oryzae* as well as some *Penicillium* strains. They play a role in the etiology of primary cancer of the liver in humans and produce disease in animals eating peanut meal and other feed contaminated by these fungi.

AFORMED SEE AFORMED *phenomenon.*

AFP Abbreviation for α-*fetoproteins.* SEE fetoproteins.

af·ter·birth (af′ter-berth). The placenta and membranes that are extruded from the uterus after birth. SYN secundina, secundines.

af·ter·care (af′ter-kār). **1.** The care and treatment of a patient after an operation or during convalescence from an illness. **2.** Following psychiatric hospitalization, a continuing program of rehabilitation designed to reinforce the effects of the therapy; may include partial hospitalization, day hospital, or outpatient treatment.

af·ter·cat·a·ract (af′ter-kat′ă-rakt). SYN secondary *cataract* (2).

af·ter·chrom·ing (af′ter-krōm′ing). Additional treatment of a tissue specimen with chromate or a metal mordant to impart special staining properties. SYN postchroming.

af·ter·con·trac·tion (af′ter-kon-trak′shŭn). A muscular contraction persisting a noticeable time after the stimulus has ceased.

af·ter·cur·rent (af′ter-kŭr-ent). An electrical current induced in a muscle upon the termination of a constant current that has been passed through it.

af·ter·dis·charge (af-ter-dis′charj). Persistence of response of muscle or neural elements after cessation of stimulation.

af·ter·ef·fect (af′ter-ĕ-fekt′). A physical, physiologic, psychologic, or emotional effect that continues after removal of the stimulus. SEE flashback.

af·ter·gild·ing (af'ter-gild'ing). The treatment of a fixed and hardened histologic specimen of nervous tissue with gold salts.

af·ter·im·age (af'ter-im'ij). Persistence of a visual response after cessation of the stimulus. SYN accidental image, negative image.
  negative a., a. in which the lightness relationship is reversed; if chromatic, it appears in complementary color.
  positive a., a. in which the lightness relationship is the same as the original one; if chromatic, it appears in the same color.

af·ter·im·pres·sion (af'ter-im-presh'ŭn). SYN aftersensation.

af·ter·load (af'ter-lōd). **1.** The arrangement of a muscle so that, in shortening, it lifts a weight from an adjustable support or otherwise does work against a constant opposing force to which it is not exposed at rest. **2.** The load or force thus encountered in shortening.
  ventricular a., formerly, the arterial pressure or some other measure of the force that a ventricle must overcome while it contracts during ejection, contributed to by aortic or pulmonic artery impedance, peripheral vascular resistance, and mass and viscosity of blood; now, more rigorously expressed in terms of the wall stress, *i.e.,* the tension per unit cross-sectional area in the ventricular muscle fibers (calculated by an expansion of Laplace's law utilizing pressure, internal radius, and wall thickness) that is required to produce the intracavitary pressure required during ejection.

af·ter·move·ment (af'ter-moov'ment). Involuntary arm abduction that follows sustained isometric contraction of the deltoid and supraspinatus muscles (usually performed by pushing the upper extremity forcibly and against an immovable vertical surface while standing closely beside it). SYN Kohnstamm's phenomenon.

af·ter·pains (af'ter-pānz). Painful cramplike contractions of the uterus occurring after childbirth.

af·ter·per·cep·tion (af'ter-per-sep'shŭn). Subjective persistence of a stimulus after its cessation. Cf. palinopsia.

af·ter·po·ten·tial (af'ter-pō-ten'shǎl). The small change in electrical potential in a stimulated nerve that follows the main, or spike, potential; it consists of an initial negative deflection followed by a positive deflection in the oscillograph record.
  diastolic a., in the heart, a transmembrane potential change following repolarization, which may reach threshold magnitude and cause a rhythm disturbance; often recorded in poisoning, as by digitalis overdosage.
  positive a., a spontaneous or inducible increase in transmembrane potential of a cardiac or nerve cell following the completion of repolarization. In the heart, this usually corresponds to the electrocardiographic U wave.

af·ter·sen·sa·tion (af'ter-sen-sā'shŭn). Subjective persistence of sensation after cessation of stimulus. SYN afterimpression.

af·ter·sound (af'ter-sownd). Subjective persistence of an auditory stimulus after cessation of the stimulus.

af·ter·taste (af'ter-tāst). Subjective persistence of a gustatory stimulus after contact with the stimulating substance has ceased.

af·ter·touch (af'ter-tŭch). Persistence of tactile sensation after cessation of the stimulus.

af·to·sa (af-tō'sǎ). SYN foot-and-mouth *disease.* [Sp. *fiebre aftosa,* aphthous fever]

Ag 1. Symbol for silver (argentum). **2.** Abbreviation for antigen.

AGA Abbreviation for *N*-acetylglutamate.

ag·a·lac·tia (ă-gă-ak'shē-ă). Absence of milk in the breasts after childbirth. SYN agalactosis. [G. *a-* priv. + *gala* (*galakt-*), milk]
  contagious a., a generalized, debilitating disease of sheep and goats caused by *Mycoplasma agalactiae;* udder infection leads to a decrease in milk production.

aga·lac·tor·rhea (ā-ga-lak-tō-rē'ă). Absence of the secretion or flow of breast milk. [G. *a-* priv. + *gala,* milk, + *rhoia,* a flow]

ag·a·lac·to·sis (ă-gal-ak-tō'sis). SYN agalactia.

ag·a·lac·tous (ă-gal-ak'tŭs). Relating to agalactia, or to the diminution or absence of breast milk.

ag·a·mete (ā-gam'ēt, ag'a-mēt). A protozoan organism produced by asexual multiple fission. SEE ALSO schizogony. [G. *a-* priv. + *gametēs,* husband]

agam·ic (ā-gam'ik). Denoting nonsexual reproduction, as by fission, budding, etc. SYN agamous.

agam·ma·glob·u·lin·e·mia (ā-gam'ă-glob'yū-li-nē'mē-ă). Absence of, or extremely low levels of, the gamma fraction of serum globulin; sometimes used loosely to denote absence of immunoglobulins in general. SEE ALSO hypogammaglobulinemia.
  acquired a., SYN common variable *immunodeficiency.*
  secondary a., SYN secondary *immunodeficiency.*
  Swiss type a., SYN severe combined *immunodeficiency.*
  transient a., SYN transient *hypogammaglobulinemia* of infancy.

agam·o·cy·tog·e·ny (ā-gam'ō-sī-toj'ĕ-nē). SYN schizogony. [G. *agamos,* unmarried, + *kytos,* cell, + *genesis,* becoming]

Aga·mo·fi·lar·ia (ă-gam'ō-fī-lā'rē-ă). A name given to immature filarial forms, the genera of the adult forms being undetermined. [G. *agamos,* unmarried, + L. *filum,* thread]

ag·a·mo·gen·e·sis (ag'ă-mō-jen'ĕ-sis, ā-gam-ō-). SYN asexual *reproduction.* [G. *agamos,* unmarried, + *genesis,* production]

ag·a·mo·ge·net·ic (ag'ă-mō-jĕ-net'ik, -ā-gam-ō-). Indicating asexual reproduction.

ag·a·mog·o·ny (ag-ă-mog'ō-nē). SYN asexual *reproduction.* [G. *agamos,* unmarried, + *gonos,* offspring]

Ag·a·mo·mer·mis cu·li·cis (ag-ă-mō-mer'mis kyū'li-kis). A species of nematode parasitic in the mosquito; a few cases have been recorded in humans, usually larval worms found emerging from body openings, presumably after ingestion of infected insects or application of moist earth bearing free-living larval stages. [G. *agamos,* unmarried, + Mod. L., fr. G. *mermis,* cord; L. *culex,* gnat]

ag·a·mont (ag'ă-mont). SYN schizont. [G. *agamos,* unmarried, + *ōn* (*ont-*), being]

ag·a·mous (ag'ă-mŭs). SYN agamic. [G. *agamos,* unmarried]

agan·gli·on·ic (ā-gang-glē-on'ik). Without ganglia.

agan·gli·o·no·sis (ā-gang'glē-ō-nō'sis). The state of being without ganglia; *e.g.,* absence of ganglion cells from the myenteric plexus as a characteristic of congenital megacolon. [G. ā- priv. + ganglion + *-osis,* condition]

agap·ism (ah'gahp-izm). The doctrine that exalts nonsexual (brotherly) love. [G. *agapē,* brotherly love]

agar (ah'gar, ā'gar). A polysaccharide (a sulfated galactan) derived from seaweed (various red algae); used as a solidifying agent in culture media. [Bengalese]
  ascitic a., a form of serum a.
  bile salt a., an a. medium containing lactose, peptone, sodium taurocholate, and neutral red, for the growth and isolation of Gram-negative rods.
  birdseed a., media prepared from *Guizottia abyssinica* seeds used in culturing and in the presumptive diagnosis of *Cryptococcus neoformans.*
  blood a., a mixture of blood and nutrient a., used for the cultivation of many medically important microorganisms.
  Bordet-Gengou potato blood a., glycerine-potato a. with 25% of blood, used for the isolation of *Bordetella pertussis.*
  brain-heart infusion a., a medium used for the isolation of fastidious microorganisms, especially fungi.
  brilliant green salt a., a highly selective culture medium consisting of a. with peptone, lactose, sodium taurocholate, brilliant green, and picric acid solution used in the primary isolation of enteric pathogens such as *Salmonella* species.
  chocolate a., blood a. heated until the blood becomes brown or chocolate in color, used especially to isolate *Hemophilus* influenza or *Neisseria* species.
  cholera a., an alkaline a. medium for cultivating *Vibrio cholerae.*
  Conradi-Drigalski a., a selective, nutrient medium for isolation of *Salmonella typhi* and other intestinal pathogens from fecal specimens; it contains the dye crystal violet, which generally inhibits growth of Gram-positive, but not Gram-negative, bacteria. SYN Drigalski-Conradi a.
  cornmeal a., a culture medium that is low in nutrients, used

extensively in the study of yeastlike and filamentous fungi; it suppresses vegetative growth while stimulating sporulation of many species, and is widely used for producing the distinctive and rapidly diagnostic chlamydospores of *Candida albicans*.

Czapek's solution a., a culture medium used for the cultivation of fungus species and for identification of *Aspergillus* and *Penicillium* species. SYN Czapek-Dox medium.

Drigalski-Conradi a., SYN Conradi-Drigalski a.

EMB a., SYN eosin-methylene blue a.

Endo a., a medium containing peptone, lactose, dipotassium phosphate, a., sodium sulfite, basic fuchsin, and distilled water; originally developed for the isolation of *Salmonella typhi*, this medium is now most useful in the bacteriological examination of water; coliform organisms ferment the lactose, and their colonies become red and color the surrounding medium; non-lactose-fermenting organisms produce clear, colorless colonies against the faint pink background of the medium. SYN Endo's medium.

Endo's fuchsin a., nutrient a. containing lactose, alcoholic solution of fuchsin, sodium sulfite, and soda solution, used as a culture medium to differentiate *Salmonella typhi* from coliform bacteria. SYN fuchsin a.

eosin-methylene blue a., a. composed of peptone, lactose, and sucrose and containing eosin and methylene blue, used to distinguish between lactose-fermenting and non-lactose-fermenting Gram-negative bacteria. SYN EMB a.

French proof a., SYN Sabouraud's a.

fuchsin a., SYN Endo's fuchsin a.

Guarnieri's gelatin a., a type of a., similar to Stoddart's gelatin a., used for the cultivation of *Streptococcus pneumoniae*.

lactose-litmus a., a. made by adding 2% lactose and litmus to acid-free nutrient a.; formerly used in the identification of *Salmonella typhi*.

MacConkey a., medium containing peptone, lactose, bile salts, neutral red, and crystal violet used to identify Gram-negative bacilli and characterize them according to their status as lactose fermenters. Fermenters appear as red colonies while nonfermenters are colorless.

Mueller-Hinton a., medium containing beef infusion, peptone, and starch used primarily for the disk-agar diffusion method for antimicrobial susceptibility testing.

Novy and MacNeal's blood a., a nutrient a. containing two volumes of defibrinated rabbit's blood; suitable for the cultivation of a number of trypanosomes.

nutrient a., a simple solid medium containing beef extract, peptone, agar, and water; used for growing many common heterotrophic bacteria.

oatmeal-tomato paste a., a special culture medium for the production of ascospore formation in the dermatophytes.

Pfeiffer's blood a., solid a. with a few drops of human blood smeared on the surface.

potato dextrose a., a culture medium used extensively for the cultivation of fungi; especially good for development of conidia and other sporulating forms by which an organism is identified microscopically.

rice-Tween a., a useful medium for the development of the differential chlamydospores in *Candida albicans* and for preparation of slide cultures for other forms of sporulation in other fungal species.

Sabouraud's a., a culture medium for fungi containing neopeptone or polypeptone a. and glucose, with final pH 5.6; it is the standard, most universally used medium in mycology and is the international reference. Modified Sabouraud's a. (Emmons modification) with less glucose is better for pigment development in the colonies. SYN French proof a.

Sabouraud's dextrose a., a dextrose peptone media that supports the growth of most pathogenic fungi.

serum a., an enriched medium for cultivation of fastidious organisms; prepared by adding sterile serum to melted a.

Thayer-Martin a., a Mueller-Hinton a. with 5% chocolate sheep blood and antibiotics, used for transport and primary isolation of *Neisseria gonorrhoeae* and *Neisseria meningitides*. SYN Thayer-Martin medium.

yeast extract a., a medium used to induce sporulation and reduce vegetative growth in the cultivation of fungi.

agar·ic (ă-gar′ik). The dried fruit body of *Polyporus officinalis* (family Polyporaceae), occurring in the form of brownish or whitish light masses, which contains agaric acid. SYN amadou. [G. *agarikon,* a kind of fungus]

deadly a. a., SYN *Amanita phalloides*.

fly a. a., SYN *Amanita muscaria*.

agar·ic ac·id (ă-gar′ik). α-Hexadecylcitric acid; 2-hydroxy-1,2,3-nonadecanetricarboxylic acid; obtained from agaric and responsible for the anhidrotic action of the mushroom; used as an anhidrotic agent. SYN agaricic acid, agaricinic acid.

agar·ic·ic ac·id (ă-gă-ris′ik). SYN agaric acid.

agar·i·cin·ic ac·id (ă-gar-i-sin′ik). SYN agaric acid.

Agar·i·cus (ă-gar′i-kŭs). A large genus of mushrooms of which many are edible and others poisonous. [L. *agaricum,* fr. G. *agarikon,* a tree fungus]

agar·o·pec·tin (ag′ă-rō-pek′tin). A polysaccharide found in agar preparations consisting of D-galactose linked β1,3 glycosidically. Some of the galactosyl units are sulfated.

ag·a·rose (ag′ă-rōs). The neutral linear polysaccharide fraction found in agar preparations, generally comprised of D-galactose and altered 3,6-anhydrogalactose residues; used in chromatography.

agas·tric (ă-gas′trik). Without stomach or digestive tract. [G. *a-* priv. + *gastēr,* belly]

agas·tro·neu·ria (ă-gas-trō-nūr′ē-ă). Lessened nervous control of the stomach. [G. *a-* priv. + *gastēr,* belly, + *neuron,* nerve]

age (āj). **1.** The period that has elapsed since birth. **2.** One of the periods into which human life is divided, distinguished by physical evolution, equilibrium, and involution; *e.g.,* the seven a.'s of man are: infancy, childhood, adolescence, maturity, middle life, senescence, and senility. **3.** To grow old; to gradually develop changes in structure that are not due to preventable disease or trauma and that are associated with decreased functional capacity and an increased probability of death. **4.** To cause artificially the appearance characteristic of one who has lived long or of a thing that has existed for a long time. **5.** In dentistry, to heat an alloy for amalgam so as to make it set more slowly, increase strength, reduce flow, and have a stable shelf life; aging occurs by relieving internal strains. [F. *âge,* L. *aetas*]

achievement a., the relationship between the chronologic age and the age of achievement, as established by standard achievement tests.

anatomical a., a. in terms of structure rather than of function or of passage of time. SYN physical a.

basal a., highest mental a. level of the Stanford-Binet intelligence scale at which all items are passed.

Binet a., the a. of the normal child with whose intelligence (as measured by the Stanford-Binet scale) the intelligence of the abnormal child corresponds (the profoundly retarded individual functions like a child of 1 to 2 years; the moderately to severely retarded, 3 to 7 years; the borderline to mildly retarded, 8 to 12 years).

bone a., stage of development of bone as adjudged by radiography, in contrast to chronologic age.

childbearing a., the period in a woman's life between puberty and menopause.

chronologic a. (CA), a. expressed in years and months; used as a measurement against which to evaluate a child's mental a. in computing his Stanford-Binet intelligence quotient.

developmental a., (1) age estimated by anatomic development since implantation; SYN fetal a. (2) (DA), age of an individual estimated from the degree of anatomic, physiologic, mental, and emotional maturation.

emotional a., a measure of emotional maturity by comparison with average emotional development.

fetal a., SYN developmental a. (1).

gestational a., the a. of a fetus expressed in elapsed time since conception; usually measured from the first day of the last normal menstrual period.

menstrual a., a. of the conceptus computed from the start of the mother's last menstrual period.

mental a. (MA), a measure, expressed in years and months, of a child's measured intelligence relative to age norms as determined by testing with the Stanford-Binet intelligence scale.

physical a., SYN anatomical a.

physiologic a., a. estimated in terms of function.

agen·e·sis (ă-jen′ĕ-sis). Absence, failure of formation, or imperfect development of any part. [G. *a*- priv. + *genesis,* production]

gonadal a., SYN gonadal *aplasia.*

renal a., absence of one or both kidneys, most commonly unilateral with absence of the ipsilateral paramesonephric (müllerian) duct and its derivatives; renal function is normal as long as the remaining kidney is intact; bilateral or complete renal a. is associated with Potter's facies and neonatal death.

thymic a., absence of the thymus, which may be associated with parathyroid a. in DiGeorge syndrome.

agen·i·tal·ism (ă-jen′i-tal-izm). Congenital absence of genitalia.

agen·o·so·mia (ă-gen-ō-sō′mē-ă). Markedly defective formation or absence of the genitalia in a fetus; usually accompanied by protrusion of the abdominal viscera through an incomplete abdominal wall. [G. *a*- priv. + *genos,* sex, + *soma,* body]

agent (ā′jent). **1.** An active force or substance capable of producing an effect. For agents not listed here, see the specific name. **2.** Referring to disease, a factor such as a microorganism, chemical substance, or form of radiation whose presence, excessive presence, or relative absence (as in deficiency diseases) is essential for the occurrence of a disease. [L. *ago,* pres. p. *agens* (*agent*-), to perform]

adrenergic blocking a., a compound that selectively blocks or inhibits responses to sympathetic adrenergic nerve activity (sympatholytic a.) and to epinephrine, norepinephrine, and other adrenergic amines (adrenolytic a.); two distinct classes exist, alpha- and beta-adrenergic receptor blocking a.'s.

α-adrenergic blocking a., an agent that competitively blocks α-adrenergic receptors; used in the treatment of hypertension. SYN alpha-blocker.

β-adrenergic blocking a., a class of drugs that compete with β-adrenergic agonists for available receptor sites; some compete for both β_1 and β_2 receptors (*e.g.,* propranolol) while others are primarily either β_1 (*e.g.,* metoprolol) or β_2 blockers; used in the treatment of a variety of cardiovascular diseases where β-adrenergic blockade is desirable. SYN β-adrenergic receptor blocking a., β-adrenoreceptor antagonist, beta-blocker.

adrenergic neuronal blocking a., a drug that prevents the release of norepinephrine from sympathetic nerve terminals; it does not inhibit the responses of the adrenergic receptors to circulating epinephrine, norepinephrine, and other adrenergic amines.

β-adrenergic receptor blocking a., SYN β-adrenergic blocking a.

alkylating a., a drug or chemical that, via the formation of covalent bonds, forms a derivatized tissue constituent permanently containing part of the drug or chemical compound; frequently carcinogenic and mutagenic.

antianxiety a., a functional category of drugs useful in the treatment of anxiety and able to reduce anxiety at doses which do not cause excessive sedation (*e.g.,* diazepam). SYN anxiolytic (1), minor tranquilizer.

antifoaming a.'s, chemicals that lower surface tension (hence production of foam), used in laboratory evaporations, and also administered with oxygen to relieve the respiratory obstruction aggravated by the foam of edema fluid in pulmonary edema.

antipsychotic a., a functional category of neuroleptic drugs that are helpful in the treatment of psychosis and have a capacity to ameliorate thought disorders (*e.g.,* chlorpromazine, haloperidol). SEE ALSO neuroleptic (3). SYN antipsychotic (1), major tranquilizer.

bacteriostatic a., SYN bacteriostat.

Bittner a., SYN mammary tumor *virus* of mice.

blister a., SYN vesicant.

blocking a., a class of drugs that inhibit (block) a biologic

activity or process, such as axonal conduction or transmission, or ions across a cell membrane; frequently called "blockers."

calcium channel-blocking a., a class of drugs that have the ability to inhibit movement of calcium ions across the cell membrane; of particular value in the treatment of cardiovascular disorders because of pharmacologic effects such as depression of mechanical contraction of cardiac and smooth muscle and of both impulse formation and conduction velocity (*e.g.,* nifedipine). SYN calcium antagonist, slow channel-blocking a.

chimpanzee coryza a. (CCA), SYN respiratory syncytial *virus.*

cholinergic a., an a. that mimics the action of the parasympathetic nervous system (*e.g.,* methacholine).

contrast a., SYN contrast *medium.*

delta a., SYN hepatitis delta *virus.*

Eaton a., SYN *Mycoplasma pneumoniae.*

embedding a.'s, materials such as celloidin, paraffin, etc. in which specimens of tissue are set before being cut into sections for microscopic examination.

enterokinetic a., an a. used to relieve intestinal atony.

F a., SYN F *plasmid.*

fertility a., SYN F *plasmid.*

foamy a.'s, SYN foamy *viruses,* under *virus.*

ganglionic blocking a., an a. that impairs the passage of impulses in autonomic ganglia.

high osmolar contrast a. (HOCA), ionic water-soluble iodinated contrast media. SYN high osmolar contrast medium.

initiating a., SEE initiation.

inotropic a.'s, drugs that increase the force of contraction of cardiac muscle; examples include digitalis glycosides, amrinone, and epinephrine.

LDH a., SYN lactate dehydrogenase *virus.*

luting a., a fastening material or cement; *e.g.,* plaster or wax to hold casts to an articulator, or material to hold crowns to teeth.

MS-1 a., a strain of hepatitis A virus.

MS-2 a., a strain of hepatitis B virus.

neuroleptic a., any of a family of drugs producing sedation and tranquilization (*e.g.,* chlorpromazine, haloperidol). SEE ALSO antipsychotic a. SYN neuroleptic (1).

neuromuscular blocking a.'s, a group of drugs that prevent motor nerve endings from exciting skeletal muscle. They act either by competing for the neurotransmitter, acetylcholine, (like D-tubocurarine, mivacurium and pancuronium), or by first stimulating the postjunctional muscle membrane and subsequently desensitizing the muscle endplates to the acetylcholine (like succinylcholine or decamethonium); used in surgery to produce paralysis and facilitate manipulation of muscles.

nondepolarizing neuromuscular blocking a., a compound that paralyzes skeletal muscle primarily by inhibiting transmission of nerve impulses at the neuromuscular junction rather than by affecting the membrane potention of motor endplate or muscle fibers.

Norwalk a., a strain of epidemic gastroenteritis virus that appears to be related to the caliciviruses. [*Norwalk,* Ohio, where first implicated in disease]

Pittsburgh pneumonia a., SYN *Legionella micdadei.*

promoting a., SEE promotion.

psychotropic a., a chemical compound that influences the human psyche.

reovirus-like a., SYN rotavirus.

sclerosing a., a compound which acts by irritation of the veinous intimal epithelium; used in the treatment of varicose veins.

slow channel-blocking a., SYN calcium channel-blocking a.

sympathetic a., SEE sympathomimetic *amine.*

transforming a., SYN mitogen.

TRIC a.'s, strains of *Chlamydia trachomatis* that cause *tra*choma and *i*nclusion *c*onjunctivitis a.'s SEE *Chlamydia trachomatis.*

Agent Or·ange. An herbicide and defoliant, consisting of (2,4,5-trichlorophenoxy)acetic acid, (2,4-dichlorophenoxy)acetic acid, and dioxin, that was widely used in the Vietnam War; it has been shown to possess residual post-exposure carcinogenic and teratogenic properties in humans.

age·ra·sia (ă-jer-ā'zē-ă). An appearance of youth in old age. [G. *agērasia*, eternal youth, fr. *a-* priv. + *gēras*, old age]

ageu·sia (ă-gū'sē-ă). Loss of the sense of taste. SYN ageustia, gustatory anesthesia. [G. *a-* priv. + *geusis*, taste]

ageus·tia (ă-gūs'tē-ă). SYN ageusia.

ag·ger, pl. **ag·ger·es** (aj'er, -ēz; ag'er) [NA]. An eminence, projection, or shallow ridge. [L. mound]

a. na'si [NA], an elevation on the lateral wall of the nasal cavity lying between the atrium of the middle meatus and the olfactory sulcus; it is formed by the mucous membrane covering the base of the ethmoidal crest of the maxilla. SYN nasal ridge.

a. perpendicula'ris, SYN *eminence* of triangular fossa of auricle.

a. val'vae ve'nae, SYN *prominence* of venous valvular sinus.

ag·glom·er·ate, ag·glom·er·at·ed (ă-glom'er-āt). SYN aggregated. [L. *ag-glomero*, to wind into a ball; from *ad*, to, + *glomus*, a ball]

ag·glom·er·a·tion (ă-glom-er-ā'shŭn). SYN aggregation.

ag·glu·ti·nant (ă-glū'ti-nant). A substance that holds parts together or causes agglutination. [L. *ad*, to + *gluten*, glue]

ag·glu·ti·nate (ă-glū'ti-nāt). To accomplish, or be subjected to, agglutination.

ag·glu·ti·na·tion (ă-glū-ti-nā'shŭn). **1.** The process by which suspended bacteria, cells, or other particles of similar size are caused to adhere and form into clumps; similar to precipitation, but the particles are larger and are in suspension rather than being in solution. For specific a. reactions in the various blood groups, see Blood Groups appendix. **2.** Adhesion of the surfaces of a wound. [L. *ad*, to, + *gluten*, glue]

acid a., the clumping together of certain microorganisms at high hydrogen ion concentration.

bacteriogenic a., the clumping of erythrocytes as a result of effects of bacteria or their products.

cold a., a. of red blood cells by their own serum (see autoagglutination), or by any other serum when the blood is cooled below body temperature, but most pronounced below 25°C; the phenomenon results from cold agglutinins; may be seen occasionally in the blood of apparently normal persons or as a pathologic finding in patients with primary atypical pneumonia, infectious mononucleosis, and other viral diseases, certain protozoan infections, or lymphoproliferative neoplasms. SEE autoagglutination.

cross a., SYN group a.

false a., **(1)** SYN pseudoagglutination (1). **(2)** SYN rouleaux *formation*.

group a., a. by antibodies specific for minor (group) antigens common to several microorganisms, each of which possesses its own major specific antigen. SYN cross a.

immune a., a. caused by antibody (agglutinin) that is specific for the suspended microorganism, cell, or for an antigen that has been coated on a particle of suitable size.

indirect a., SYN passive a.

mixed a., SYN mixed agglutination *reaction*.

nonimmune a., **(1)** a. caused by a lectin having a degree of specificity, the mechanism of which is not understood; **(2)** a. that results from nonspecific factors, as in the case of acid a. or spontaneous a.

passive a., a. of particles that have been coated with soluble antigen, by antiserum specific for the adsorbed antigen. SYN indirect a.

spontaneous a., nonspecific clumping of organisms in saline related to lack of polar groups in electrolyte solution.

ag·glu·ti·na·tive (ă-glū'ti-nă-tiv). Causing, or able to cause, agglutination.

ag·glu·ti·nin (ă-glū'ti-nin). **1.** An antibody that causes clumping or agglutination of the bacteria or other cells which either stimulated the formation of the a., or contain immunologically similar, reactive antigen. SYN agglutinating antibody, immune a. **2.** A substance, other than a specific agglutinating antibody, that causes organic particles to agglutinate, commonly qualified, *e.g.*, plant a.

blood group a.'s, see Blood Groups appendix.

chief a., SYN major a.

cold a., an antibody which reacts more efficiently at temperatures below 37°C.

cross-reacting a., SYN group a.

flagellar a., SYN H a. (1).

group a., an immune a. specific for a group antigen. SYN cross-reacting a.

H a., **(1)** an a. that is formed as the result of stimulation by, and which reacts with, the thermolabile antigen(s) in the flagella of motile strains of microorganisms; SYN flagellar a. **(2)** see ABO blood group, Blood Groups appendix.

immune a., SYN agglutinin (1).

incomplete a. (ă-glū'ti-nin), antibody that binds to antigen but does not induce agglutination. These antibodies are usually of the IgG class and are referred to as incomplete antibody.

major a., immune a. present in greatest quantity in an antiserum and evoked by the most dominant of a mosaic of antigens. SYN chief a.

minor a., immune a. present in an antiserum in lesser concentration than the major a. SYN partial a.

O a., **(1)** an a. that is formed as the result of stimulation by, and that reacts with, the relatively thermostable antigen(s) in the cell bodies of microorganisms; SYN somatic a. **(2)** see ABO blood group, Blood Groups appendix.

partial a., SYN minor a.

plant a., a lectin.

saline a., an antibody which causes agglutination of erythrocytes when they are suspended either in saline or in a protein medium. SYN complete antibody.

serum a., an antibody which coats erythrocytes; the cells do not agglutinate when suspended in saline, but do agglutinate when suspended in serum or other protein media such as albumin. SYN incomplete antibody (2).

somatic a., SYN O a. (1).

warm a.'s, SEE autoantibody.

ag·glu·tin·o·gen (ă-glū-tin'ō-jen). An antigenic substance that stimulates the formation of specific agglutinin, which, under certain conditions, causes agglutination of cells that contain the antigen or particles coated with the antigen. SYN agglutogen. [agglutinin + G. *-gen*, production]

blood group a.'s, see Blood Groups appendix.

T a., an a. formed from a latent receptor on human red cells by the action of an enzyme in cultures of certain bacteria.

ag·glu·tin·o·gen·ic (ă-glū'tin-ō-jen'ik). Capable of causing the production of an agglutinin. SYN agglutogenic.

ag·glu·tin·o·phil·ic (ă-glū'tin-ō-fil'ik). Readily undergoing pronounced agglutination. [agglutination + G. *phileō*, to love]

ag·glu·tin·o·scope (ă-glū'tin-ō-skōp). Obsolete term for a magnifying glass or simple system of lenses used to observe agglutination *in vitro*. [agglutination + G. *skopeō*, to view]

ag·glu·to·gen (ă-glū'tō-jen). SYN agglutinogen.

ag·glu·to·gen·ic (ă-glū-tō-jen'ik). SYN agglutinogenic.

ag·gre·gate (ag'rĕ-gāt). **1.** To unite or come together in a mass or cluster. **2.** The total of individual units making up a mass or cluster. [L. *ag-grego*, pp. *-atus*, to add to, fr. *grex* (greg-), a flock]

ag·gre·gat·ed (ag'rĕ-gā-ted). Collected together, thereby forming a cluster, clump, or mass of individual units. SYN agglomerate, agglomerated, agminate, agminated.

ag·gre·ga·tion (ag-rĕ-gā'shŭn). A crowded mass of independent but similar units; a cluster. SYN agglomeration.

familial a., occurrence of a trait in more members of a family than can be readily accounted for by chance; presumptive but not cogent evidence of the operation of genetic factors.

ag·gre·gom·e·ter (ag-rē-gom'ĕ-ter). An instrument for measuring platelet adhesiveness.

ag·gres·sin (ă-gres'in). A substance postulated to inhibit the resistance mechanisms of the host. [L. *agressor*, an assailant, fr. *ad-gredio*, pp. *-gressus*, to attack]

ag·gres·sion (ă-gresh'ŭn). A domineering, forceful, or assaultive verbal or physical action toward another person as the motor component of the affects of anger, hostility, or rage. [L. *aggressio,* fr. *aggredior,* to accost, attack]

ag·gres·sive (ă-gres´iv). **1.** Denoting aggression. **2.** Denoting a competitive forcefulness or invasiveness, as of a behavioral pattern, a pathogenic organism, or a disease process.

ag·ing (ā´jing). **1.** The process of growing old, especially by failure of replacement of cells in sufficient number to maintain full functional capacity; particularly affects cells (*e.g.,* neurons) incapable of mitotic division. **2.** The gradual deterioration of a mature organism resulting from time-dependent, irreversible changes in structure that are intrinsic to the particular species, and that eventually lead to decreased ability to cope with the stresses of the environment, thereby increasing the probability of death. **3.** In the cardiovascular system, the progressive replacement of functional cell types by fibrous connective tissue. **4.** A demographic term, meaning an increase over time in the proportion of older persons in the population.

clonal a., the deterioration in successive generations of a clone; thus paramecia and other simple forms, if allowed to reproduce asexually for a number of generations, invariably undergo deterioration, the characters of each group of descendants progressively departing from those of the original sexually produced ancestor.

ag·i·to·graph·ia (aj´i-tō-graf´ē-ă). A condition in which one writes with great rapidity, leaving out words or parts of words. [L. *agito,* to hurry, + G. *graphō,* to write]

ag·i·to·la·lia (aj´i-tō-lā´lē-ă). SYN agitophasia.

ag·i·to·pha·sia (aj´i-tō-fā´zē-ă). Abnormally rapid speech in which words are imperfectly spoken or dropped out of a sentence. SYN agitolalia. [L. *agito,* to hurry, + G. *phasis,* speech]

ag·lo·bu·lia (ā-glō-byū´lē-ă). Obsolete term for anemia. [G. *a*- priv. + L. *globulus,* globule]

ag·lo·bu·li·o·sis (ā´glō-byū-lē-ō´sis). Obsolete term for a condition characterized by anemia.

aglob·u·lism (ā-glob´yū-lizm). Obsolete term for anemia.

aglo·mer·u·lar (ā-glō-mer´yū-lăr). Having no glomeruli; said especially of a kidney in which the glomeruli have been destroyed, or kidneys of certain fish, *e.g.,* toad fish, that possess tubules but no glomeruli.

aglos·sia (ă-glos´ē-ă). Congenital absence of the tongue. [G. *a*- priv. + *glōssa,* tongue]

aglos·so·sto·mia (ă-glos-ō-stō´mē-ă). Congenital absence of the tongue, with a malformed (usually closed) mouth. [G. *a*- priv. + *glōssa,* tongue, + *stoma,* mouth]

aglu·con (ā-glū´kon). The portion of a glucoside other than the glucose. [G. *a*- priv. + glucose + -on]

ag·lu·ti·tion (ā-glū-tish´ŭn). SYN dysphagia.

agly·ca, pl. **agly·con** (ā-glī´kon).

agly·con, a·gly·cone (ā-glī´kon). The noncarbohydrate portion of a glycoside (*e.g.,* digoxigenin). [G. *a*- priv. + *glykys,* sweet]

a·gly·cone. SEE aglycon.

agly·cos·u·ria (ā-glī-kō-sū´rē-ă). Absence of carbohydrate in the urine.

agly·cos·u·ric (ă-glī-kō-sū´rik). Relating to aglycosuria.

ag·men, pl. **ag·mina** (ag´men, ag´min-ă). Obsolete term for aggregation. [L. a multitude]

a. peyerian´um, SYN Peyer's *patches,* under *patch.*

ag·mi·nate, ag·mi·nat·ed (ag´mi-nāt, ag´mi-nā-ted). SYN aggregated. [L. *agmen,* a multitude]

ag·na·thia (ag-nā´thē-ă). Congenital absence of the lower jaw, usually accompanied by approximation of the ears. SEE ALSO otocephaly, synotia. [G. *a*- priv. + *gnathos,* jaw]

ag·na·thous (ag´nā-thŭs). Relating to agnathia.

ag·nea (ag-nē´ă). SYN agnosia. [G. *agnoia,* want of perception]

ag·no·gen·ic (ag-nō-jen´ik). SYN idiopathic. [G. *a*- priv. + *gnosis,* knowledge, + *genesis,* origin]

ag·no·sia (ag-nō´zē-ă). Impairment of ability to recognize, or comprehend the meaning of, various sensory stimuli, not attributable to disorders of the primary receptors or general intellect; a.'s are receptive defects caused by lesions in various portions of the cerebrum. SYN agnea. [G. ignorance; from *a*- priv. + *gnōsis,* knowledge]

auditory a., inability to recognize sounds, words, or music; caused by a lesion of the auditory cortex of the temporal lobe.

color a., inability to name or identify specific colors by sight; caused by lesions of the dominant occipital and temporal lobes.

finger a., inability to name or recognize individual fingers, of one's own or of other persons; most often caused by lesion of or near the angular gyrus of the dominant hemisphere.

localization a., inability to recognize the area where the skin is touched.

optic a., SYN visual a.

position a., failure to recognize the posture of an extremity.

tactile a., inability to recognize objects by touch, in the presence of intact cutaneous and proprioceptive hand sensation; caused by lesion in the contralateral parietal lobe. SYN astereognosis, stereoagnosis, stereoanesthesia.

visual a., inability to recognize objects by sight; usually caused by bilateral parieto-occipital lesions. SYN optic a.

visual-spatial a., inability to localize objects or to appreciate distance, motion, and spatial relationships; caused by lesion in the occipital lobe. Cf. simultanagnosia.

◬**-agogue, -agog.** Leading, promoting, stimulating; a promoter or stimulant of. [G. *agōgos,* leading forth, fr. *agō,* to lead.]

agom·phi·ous (ă-gom´-fē-us). SYN anodontia.

agom·pho·sis, agom·phi·a·sis (ag-om-fō´sis, fī´ă-sis). SYN anodontia. [G. *a*- priv. + *gomphos,* peg, bolt]

ago·nad·al (ă-gon´ă-dăl). Denoting the absence of gonads.

ag·o·nal (ag´on-ăl). Relating to the process of dying or the moment of death, so called because of the former erroneous notion that dying is a painful process.

ag·o·nist (ag´on-ist). **1.** Denoting a muscle in a state of contraction, with reference to its opposing muscle, or antagonist. **2.** A drug capable of combining with receptors to initiate drug actions; it possesses affinity and intrinsic activity. [G. *agōn,* a contest]

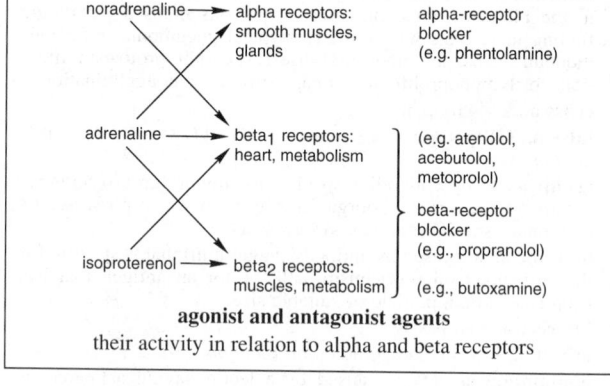

agonist and antagonist agents
their activity in relation to alpha and beta receptors

ag·o·ny (ag´ŏ-nē). Intense pain or anguish of body or mind. [G. *agōn,* a struggle, trial]

ag·o·ra·pho·bia (ag´ŏr-ă-fō´bē-ă). A mental disorder characterized by an irrational fear of leaving the familiar setting of home, or venturing into the open, so pervasive that a large number of external life situations are entered into reluctantly or are avoided; often associated with panic attacks. [G. *agora,* marketplace, + *phobos,* fear]

agor·a·pho·bic (ă-gōr-ă-fō´bik). Relating to or characteristic of agoraphobia.

agou·ti (ah-gu´tē). SYN *Dasyprocta.* [Fr., fr. native Indian]

◬**-agra.** Sudden onslaught of acute pain. [G. *agra,* a hunting, a catching, a trap]

agraffe (ă-graf´). An appliance for clamping together the edges of a wound, used in lieu of sutures. [Fr. *agrafe,* a hook, clasp]

ag·ram·mat·i·ca (ag-ră-mat´i-kă). SYN agrammatism.

agram·ma·tism (ā-gram´a-tizm). A form of aphasia characterized by an inability to construct a grammatical sentence, and the use of unintelligible or incorrect words; caused by a lesion in the dominant temporal lobe. SYN agrammatica, agrammatologia, jargon aphasia.

agram·ma·to·lo·gia (ă-gram′mă-tō-lō′jē-ă). SYN agrammatism.

agran·u·lo·cyte (ă-gran′yū-lō-sīt). A nongranular leukocyte. [G. *a-* priv. + L. *granulum,* granule, + G. *kytos,* cell]

agran·u·lo·cy·to·sis (ă-gran′yū-lō-sī-tō′sis). An acute condition characterized by pronounced leukopenia with great reduction in the number of polymorphonuclear leukocytes (frequently less than 500 granulocytes per mm³); infected ulcers are likely to develop in the throat, intestinal tract, and other mucous membranes, as well as in the skin. SYN agranulocytic angina, angina lymphomatosa, neutropenic angina.

feline a., SYN panleukopenia.

agran·u·lo·plas·tic (ă-gran′yū-lō-plas′tik). Capable of forming nongranular cells, and incapable of forming granular cells. [G. *a-* priv. + L. *granulum,* granule, + G. *plastikos,* formative]

agraph·ia (ă-graf′ē-ă). Inability to write properly in the absence of abnormalities of the limb; often accompanies aphasia and alexia; caused by lesions in various portions of the cerebrum, especially those in or near the angular gyrus. SYN anorthography, graphic aphasia, graphomotor aphasia, logagraphia. [G. *a-* priv. + *graphō,* to write]

absolute a., a. in which not even unconnected letters can be written. SYN atactic a., literal a.

acoustic a., inability to write from dictation.

amnemonic a., a. in which letters and words can be written, but not connected sentences.

atactic a., SYN absolute a.

cerebral a., the inability to express ideas in writing. SYN mental a.

constructional a., an a. in which letters and words can be written correctly, but not arranged appropriately on the writing surface.

literal a., SYN absolute a.

mental a., SYN cerebral a.

motor a., a. due to muscular incoordination.

musical a., an inability to write musical notation.

verbal a., a. in which single letters can be written, but not words.

agraph·ic (ă-graf′ik). Relating to or marked by agraphia.

agre·tope (ag-rē′tōp). That part of a processed antigen that binds to the major histocompatibility complex molecule; the agretope was derived from antigen restriction element. [antigen + *resric*tion + -tope]

ag·ri·o·thy·mia (ag′rē-ō-thī′mē-ă). Obsolete term for a wild, ferocious mania. [G. *agriothymos,* wild of temper, fr. *agrios,* wild, + *thymos,* spirit]

ag·ro·ma·nia (ag-rō-mā′nē-ă). Obsolete term for a morbid impulse to live in the open country or in solitude. [G. *agros,* field, + *mania,* frenzy]

agryp·nia (ă-grip′nē-ă). Rarely used term for insomnia. [G. sleeplessness, fr. *agreō,* to hunt after, + *hypnos,* sleep]

agryp·no·co·ma (ă-grip′nō-kō′mă). A wakeful, apathetic, or lethargic state. [G. *agrypnos,* sleepless, + *kōma,* coma]

ague (ā′gū). **1.** Archaic term for malarial fever. **2.** A chill. [Fr. *aigu,* acute]

brass founder's a., SYN brass founder's *fever.*

ag·yi·o·pho·bia (aj′ē-ō-fō′bē-ă). A form of agoraphobia characterized by a morbid fear of being in the street. [G. *agyia,* street, + *phobos,* fear]

agy·ria (ă-jī′rē-ă). Congenital lack or underdevelopment of the convolutional pattern of the cerebral cortex, owing to a defect of development. SYN lissencephalia, lissencephaly. [G. *a-* priv. + *gyros,* circle]

ahaus·tral (ă-haw′străl). Lacking haustra, smooth; describing the appearance of the colon on radiographs of a barium enema in ulcerative colitis. [G. *a-* priv. + haustra]

AHF Abbreviation for antihemophilic *factor* A.

AHG Abbreviation for antihemophilic *globulin.*

Ahumada, J.C., Argentinian physician. SEE A.-Del Castillo *syndrome.*

aHyl. Symbol for allohydroxylysine.

ahy·log·no·sia (ā-hī-log-nō′sē-ă). Inability to recognize differences of density, weight, and roughness. [G. *a-* priv. + *hylē,* matter, + *gnōsis,* recognition]

Aicardi, J. Dennis, 20th century French neurologist. SEE A.'s *syndrome.*

aich·mo·pho·bia (īk-mō-fō′bē-ă). Morbid fear of being touched by the finger or any slender pointed object. [G. *aichmē,* a point, + *phobos,* fear]

AID Abbreviation for donor of heterologous (artificial) insemination.

△**aidoi-, aidoio-.** (Archaic) the genitals; corresponds to L. pudend-. [G. *aidoia,* shameful things, the genitals]

⎯⎯⎯⎯

AIDS. A syndrome of the immune system characterized by opportunistic diseases, including candidiasis (both oropharyngeal and vulvovaginal), pneumocystis carinii pneumonia, oral hairy leukoplakia, herpes zoster, idiopathic thrombocytopenic purpura, cervical dysplasia and cervical carcinoma, Kaposi's sarcoma, pelvic inflammatory disease, toxoplasmosis, isosporiasis, cryptococcosis, non-Hodgkins lymphoma, and peripheral neuropathy. Tuberculosis may also be considered to be an opportunistic infection. The syndrome is caused by the human immunodeficiency virus (HIV-1, HIV-2), which is transmitted by exchange of body fluids (notably blood and semen) through sexual contact, sharing of contaminated neédles (by IV drug abusers), accidental needle sticks, contact with contaminated blood, or transfusion of contaminated blood/blood products. Hallmark of the immunodeficiency is depletion of T4⁺ helper/inducer lymphocytes, primarily the result of selective tropism of the virus for the lymphocytes. Persistent generalized lymphadenopathy, fever, weight loss, and diarrhea of long duration (lasting more than 1 month) are associated with early stages of the disease. SYN acquired immunodeficiency syndrome.

> As of 1994, the Centers for Disease Control put the number of HIV-infected people in the U.S. at 1 million, and those with full-blown AIDS at 339,250. Some 10 million people are estimated to be infected worldwide, with the highest suspected incidence in some Central and East African countries, where as much as a third of the adult population may be HIV-positive. Although in the U.S. the rise in new AIDS cases appears to have peaked among men, perhaps in part because of public education efforts, the number of new cases continues to rise rapidly among women and children (especially teens). Whereas female AIDS patients represented only 7% of total cases before 1985, they now account for an estimated 13%. Those groups showing the greatest rate of increase were Latino and black women who used IV drugs or had a partner who did. AIDS is the leading cause of death among men 25 to 44, and the fourth leading cause among women in the same age group. The speed with which researchers have identified and characterized the presumed causative agent of AIDS, the HIV virus, may be unparalleled in the history of medicine. However, therapies for halting or reversing the virally mediated collapse of immune function have yet to be devised, and work on vaccines has been stymied by the ability of HIV to mutate rapidly. See HIV.

⎯⎯⎯⎯

AIH Abbreviation for homologous (artificial) insemination.

AILD Abbreviation for angioimmunoblastic *lymphadenopathy* with dysproteinemia.

aIle. Abbreviation for alloisoleucine.

ai·lu·ro·pho·bia (ī′lū-rō-fō′bē-ă, ā′lu-). Morbid fear of or aversion to cats. SYN aelurophobia. [G. *ailouros,* cat, + *phobos,* fear]

ai·nhum (ī′yūm). An acquired slowly progressive painful fibrous constriction that develops in the digitoplantar fold, usually of the little toe, gradually resulting in spontaneous amputation of the toe; most commonly affects black males in the tropics. [fr. Af. (Lagos), to saw]

AIR Abbreviation for 5-aminoimidazole ribose 5′-phosphate and 5-aminoimidazole ribotide.

air (ār). **1.** A mixture of odorless gases found in the atmosphere

AIDS: Secondary Illnesses and Their Agents

Eyes:	Cytomegalovirus, *Toxoplasma gondii, Crytococcus neoformans* (chorioretinitis)
Skin and mucous membrane:	Herpes simplex virus (ulceration), varicella zoster virus (blistering), molluscum contagiosum virus, oral leukoplakia (Epstein-Barr virus?)
Bone marrow (depression):	*Mycobacteria* (*tuberculosis* and atypical), *Cryptococcus neoformans,* Histoplasma capsulatum, cytomegalovirus
Liver (hepatitis):	Hepatitis viruses, atypical *Mycobacteria,* cytomegalovirus, Epstein-Barr virus
Lungs (pneumonia):	*Pneumocystis carinii,* cytomegalovirus, *Cryptococcus neoformans, Mycobacteria* (*tuberculosis* and atypical)
Lymph nodes:	*Mycobacteria* (*tuberculosis* and atypical), cytomegalovirus, Epstein-Barr virus, human herpesvirus 6, *Cryptococcus neoformans,* lymphoid interstitial plasma cell pneumonia
Gastrointestinal tract:	
Esophagus:	*Candida albicans,* cytomegalovirus, Herpes simplex virus
Small and large intestines (diarrhea):	Cytomegalovirus (ulcers), *Cryptosporidia, Mycobacteria* (*tuberculosis* and atypical), *Isosporabelli, Giardia lamblia,* coccidiomycosis (in Central America), *Shigella, Salmonella,* herpes simplex virus
Fever (as yet undetermined):	*Mycobacteria* (atypical and *tuberculosis*), cytomegalovirus, *Toxoplasma gondii, Pneumocystis carinii*
Central nervous system (encephalitis, meningitis, dementia):	*Toxoplasma gondii, Cryptococcus neoformans,* papovavirus, cytomegalovirus, herpes simplex virus, *Mycobacteria* (atypical and *tuberculosis*), HIV

AIDS: CDC classification of adults

Group

I acute infections (HIV-positive)

II asymptomatic

III lymphadenopathic syndrome

IV

   A.   constitutional symptoms (fever, diarrhea, weight loss)

   B.   neurological conditions (HIV-associated)

   C.   1. opportunistic infections

         2. hairy leukoplakia, zoster (in several dermotomes), stomatitis candidiosa, nocardiosis, TB, salmonellosis (recrudescent), cryptococcosis, cryptosporidosis

   D.   Kaposi's sarcoma, non-Hodgkin's lymphoma, lymphoma of central nervous system

   E.   other HIV-associated symptoms not mentioned above

in the following approximate percentages by volume after water vapor has been removed: oxygen, 20.95; nitrogen, 78.08; argon 0.93; carbon dioxide, 0.03; other gases, 0.01. Formerly used to mean any respiratory gas, regardless of its composition. **2.** SYN ventilate. [G. *aēr;* L. *aer*]

alveolar a., SYN alveolar *gas.*

complemental a., SYN inspiratory reserve *volume.*

complementary a., SYN inspiratory *capacity.*

functional residual a., SYN functional residual *capacity.*

a. hunger, extremely deep ventilation such as occurs in patients with acidosis attempting to increase ventilation of alveoli and exhale more carbon dioxide. SEE ALSO Kussmaul *respiration.*

liquid a., a. that, by means of intense cold and pressure, has been liquefied.

minimal a., the volume of gas that remains in the lungs and cannot be expelled after they have been removed from the body, or after the chest has been opened.

reserve a., SYN expiratory reserve *volume.*

residual a., SYN residual *volume.*

supplemental a., SYN expiratory reserve *volume.*

tidal a., SYN tidal *volume.*

vitiated a., a. containing a reduced percentage of oxygen.

Aird, Robert B., U.S. neurologist, *1903. SEE Flynn-A. *syndrome.*

air·sac·cu·li·tis (ār'sak-yū-lī'tis). Inflammation of the mucous membrane of the air sacs of birds.

air·sick·ness. A condition resembling seasickness or other forms of motion sickness occurring in airplane or space flight as a result of erratic and continuous stimuli of the inner ear.

air·space (ār'spās). Pertaining to the portion of the lung distal to the conducting airways or bronchi; alveolar.

air·trap·ping (ār-trap'ing). Slow or incomplete emptying of air from all or part of a lung on expiration; implies obstruction of regional airways or emphysema.

air·way (ār'wā). **1.** Any part of the respiratory tract through which air passes during breathing. **2.** In anesthesia or resuscitation, a device for correcting obstruction to breathing, especially an oropharyngeal and nasopharyngeal a., endotracheal a., or tracheotomy tube.

anatomical a., SYN anatomical dead *space.*

conducting a., the a. from the nasal cavity to a terminal bronchiole.

lower a., the portion of the respiratory tract that extends from the subglottis to and including the terminal bronchioles.

respiratory a., that part of the a. where interchange of gases occurs; it includes respiratory bronchioles, alveolar ducts, sacs, and alveoli.

upper a., the portion of the respiratory tract that extends from the nares or mouth to and including the larynx.

Ajel·lo·my·ces cap·su·la·tum (ah-jĕ-lō-mī'sēz kap-sū-lā'tŭm). The ascomycetous (perfect, sexual, teleomorph) state of *Histoplasma capsulatum.* SYN Emmonsiella capsulata.

Ajel·lo·my·ces der·ma·tit·i·dis (ah-jĕ-lō-mī'sēz der-mă-tit'i-dis). The perfect (teleomorph) state of the fungus *Blastomyces dermatitidis;* the (+) and (-) mating types cause disease with equal frequency. This sexual state is placed in the family Gymnoascaceae.

aj·ma·line (aj′mă-lēn). An indole alkaloid from the roots of *Rauwolfia serpentina*, related to reserpine, serpentine, and yohimbine; has been used for treatment of hypertension and as a tranquilizer or sedative.

aj·o·wan oil (aj′ō-wan). A volatile oil distilled from the fruit of *Carum copticum*, one of the sources of thymol; a carminative, aromatic, and expectorant. SYN ptychotis oil.

akan·thi·on (ă-kan′thē-on). SYN acanthion.

akar·y·o·cyte (ā-kar′ē-ō-sīt). A cell without a nucleus (karyon), such as the erythrocyte. SYN acaryote, akaryote. [G. *a*- priv. + *karyon*, kernel, + *kytos*, a hollow (cell)]

akar·y·ote (ā-kar′ē-ōt). SYN akaryocyte. [G. *a*- priv. + *karyon*, kernel]

a·ka·thi·sia (ak-ă-thiz′ē-ă). A syndrome characterized by an inability to remain in a sitting posture, with motor restlessness and a feeling of muscular quivering; may appear as a side effect of antipsychotic and neuroleptic medication. SYN acathisia. [G. *a*- priv. + *kathisis*, a sitting]

akem·be (ă-kem′bē). SYN onyalai.

aker·a·to·sis (ă-ker-ă-tō′sis). Deficiency or absence of the horny layer of the epidermis.

Åkerlund, A. Olof, Swedish radiologist, 1885–1958. SEE A. *deformity.*

aki·ne·sia (ā-ki-nē′sē-ă, ā-kī-). **1.** Absence or loss of the power of voluntary movement, due to an extrapyramidal disorder. **2.** Obsolete term denoting the postsystolic interval of rest of the heart. **3.** A neurosis accompanied by paretic symptoms. SYN akinesis. [G. *a*- priv. + *kinēsis*, movement]

a. al′gera, a condition marked by severe generalized pain produced by any movement; often of psychogenic origin. [G. *algos*, pain]

a. amnes′tica, loss of muscular power from disuse.

aki·ne·sic (ā-ki-nē′sik, ā-kī-). SYN akinetic.

aki·ne·sis (ā-ki-nē′sis, ā-kī-). SYN akinesia.

akin·es·the·sia (ā-kin′es-thē′zē-ă). Inability to perceive movement or position. Absence of the sense of perception of movement or of the muscular sense. [G. *a*- priv. + *kinēsis*, motion, + *aisthēsis*, sensation]

aki·net·ic (ā-ki-net′ik, -kī-net′ik). Relating to or suffering from akinesia. SYN akinesic.

aki·ya·mi (ah-kē-yah′mē). SYN hasamiyami.

ak·lo·mide (ak′lō-mīd). 2-Chloro-4-nitrobenzamide; a coccidiostat used in veterinary practice.

ak·ne·mia. SEE acnemia.

AKNF. Abbreviation for Adair-Koshland-Némethy-Filmer *model.*

Al Symbol for aluminum.

ALA Abbreviation for δ-aminolevulinic acid. Cf. Ala.

Ala Symbol for alanine or its mono- or diradical.

ala, gen. and pl. **alae** (ā′lă, ā′lē). **1** [NA]. SYN **wing. 2.** Obsolete term for axilla. [L. wing]

a. au′ris, SYN auricle (1).

a. cerebel′li, SYN ala central *lobule.*

a. cine′rea, SYN vagal *trigone.*

a. cris′tae gal′li [NA], SYN *wing* of crista galli.

alae lin′gulae cerebel′li, SYN *vincula* lingulae cerebelli, under *vinculum.*

a. lob′uli centra′lis [NA], SYN ala central *lobule.*

a. ma′jor os′sis sphenoida′lis [NA], SYN greater *wing* of sphenoid bone.

a. mi′nor os′sis sphenoida′lis [NA], SYN lesser *wing* of sphenoid bone.

a. na′si [NA], SYN *wing* of nose.

a. orbitalis, SYN lesser *wing* of sphenoid bone.

a. os′sis il′ii [NA], SYN *wing* of ilium.

a. sacra′lis [NA], SYN *wing* of sacrum.

a. tempora′lis, SYN greater *wing* of sphenoid bone.

a. vespertilio′nis, obsolete term for broad *ligament* of the uterus. [L. bat's wing]

a. vo′meris [NA], SYN *wing* of vomer.

Alajouanine, Théophile, French neurologist, 1890–1980. SEE Foix-Alajouanine *myelitis;* Foix-Alajouanine *syndrome.*

ala·lia (ă-la′lē-ă). Mutism; inability to speak. SEE aphonia. [G. *a*- priv. + *lalia,* talking]

alal·ic (ă-lal′ik). Relating to alalia.

al·a·nine (A, Ala) (al′ă-nēn). $CH_3CH(NH_3)^+COO^-$; 2-aminopropionic acid; α-aminopropionic acid; the L-stereoisomer is one of the amino acids widely occurring in proteins.

β-al·a·nine. $^+NH_3CH_2CH_2 COO^-$; 3- or β-aminopropionic acid; a decarboxylation production of aspartic acid. Found in brain, in carnosine, and in coenzyme A.

al·a·nine ami·no·trans·fer·ase (ALT). An enzyme transferring amino groups from L-alanine to 2-ketoglutarate, or the reverse (from L-glutamate to pyruvate); there is a D-alanine transaminase that effects the same reaction, but with D-alanine and D-glutamate. Used in clinical diagnosis of viral hepatitis and myocardial infarction. SYN alanine transaminase, glutamic-pyruvic transaminase, serum glutamic-pyruvic transaminase.

al·a·nine-gly·ox·y·late ami·no·trans·fer·ase. An enzyme that reversibly catalyzes the transfer of an amino group of L-alanine to glyoxylate, thus producing pyruvate and glycine. An inherited disorder that results in an alteration of a.-g. a. activity is associated with primary hyperoxaluria type I.

al·a·nine-ox·o·mal·o·nate ami·no·trans·fer·ase. An enzyme that accomplishes the reversible transfer of the amino groups from L-alanine to oxomalonate, an action similar to that of alanine aminotransferase, producing pyruvate and aminomalonate.

β-ala·nine-py·ru·vate ami·no·trans·fer·ase. An enzyme that reversibly transfers the amino group of β-alanine to paruvate, thus producing L-alanine and malonate semialdehyde. A deficiency of this enzyme is believed to be the cause of hyper-β-alaninemia.

al·a·nine rac·e·mase. An enzyme, requiring pyridoxal phosphate as coenzyme, that catalyzes the reversible racemization of L-alanine to D-alanine; found in various microorganisms, where it plays a role in the biosynthesis of the D-amino acids present in the capsular proteins.

al·a·nine trans·am·i·nase. SYN alanine aminotransferase.

alan·o·sine (ă-lan′ō-sēn). An antibiotic substance produced by *Streptomyces alanosinicus;* possesses antineoplastic and antiviral activity.

Alanson, Edward, British surgeon, 1747–1823. SEE A.'s *amputation.*

alan·tin (ă-lan′tin). SYN inulin.

al·an·tol (al′an-tol). A yellowish liquid obtained by distillation from the root of *Inula helenium* or elecampane; used internally as an irritating tonic and externally as a mild rubefacient. SYN inulol.

al·ant starch (ă-lant′). SYN inulin.

al·a·nyl (al′ă-nil). The acyl radical of alanine.

alar (ā′lăr). **1.** Relating to a wing; winged. **2.** SYN axillary. **3.** Relating to the wings (ala) of such structures as the nose, sphenoid, sacrum, etc.

ALARA. Acronym for a philosophy of use of radiation based on

♻ **Combining forms**	**[NA] Nomina Anatomica**
Word*Finder*	**[MIM] Mendelian**
Multi-term entry finder	**Inheritance in Man**
Preceding letter A	
A.D.A.M. Anatomy Plates	☆ **Official alternate term**
Between letters L and M	
	☆**[NA] Official alternate**
Appendices:	**Nomina Anatomica term**
Following letter Z	
	━━━━━━━━
SYN Synonym; Cf., compare	**High Profile Term**

using dosages *as* low *as* reasonably *a*chievable to attain the desired diagnostic, therapeutic, or other goal.

alar·mone (ă-lar′mōn). A biochemical whose synthesis increases under certain stress conditions (for example, a nutritional deficiency affecting certain enzymes). [*alar*m + *-mone*]

alas·trim (ă-las′trim). A mild form of smallpox caused by a less virulent strain of the virus. SYN Cuban itch, Kaffir pox, milkpox, pseudosmallpox, pseudovariola, variola minor, West Indian smallpox, whitepox. [Pg. *alastrar,* to scatter over]

al·ba (al′bă). SYN white *matter.* [fem. of L. *albus,* white]

Albarran y Dominguez, Joaquin, Cuban urologist, 1860–1912. SEE Albarran's *glands,* under *gland;* Albarran's *test;* A.'s *tubules,* under *tubule.*

al·be·do (al-bē′dō). A white area of the retina due to edema or infarction. [L. whiteness]

Albers-Schönberg, Heinrich E., German radiologist, 1865–1921. SEE Albers-Schönberg *disease.*

Albert, Eduard, Austrian surgeon, 1841–1900. SEE A.'s *disease, suture.*

Albert, Henry, U.S. physician, 1878–1930. SEE A.'s *stain.*

al·bi·cans, pl. **al·bi·can·tia** (al′bi-kanz, -kan′tē-ă). **1.** SYN white. **2.** SYN *corpus* albicans. [L.]

al·bi·du·ria (al-bi-dū′rē-ă). The passing of pale or white urine of low specific gravity, as in chyluria. SYN albinuria. [L. *albidus,* whitish, + G. *ouron,* urine]

al·bi·dus (al′bi-dŭs). White, whitish. [L.]

Albini, Giuseppe, Italian physiologist, 1827–1911. SEE A.'s *nodules,* under *nodule.*

al·bi·nism (al′bi-nizm). A group of inherited (usually autosomal recessive) disorders with deficiency or absence of pigment in the skin, hair, and eyes, or eyes only, due to an abnormality in production of melanin. SEE ocular a., piebaldism. [albino + ism]

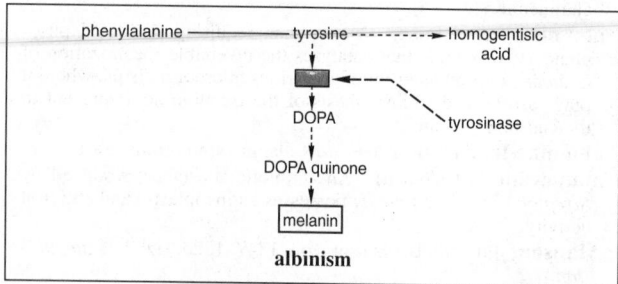

albinism

cutaneous a. [MIM*126070], an autosomal dominant condition characterized by patterned loss of skin pigment on extremities and ventral thorax; a white forelock is often present, but no ocular findings.

ocular a. [MIM*300650 & *300700], absence of pigment chiefly in the iris, choroid, and retinal pigment epithelium with deafness; X-linked inheritance.

oculocutaneous a., autosomal recessive deficiency of pigment in skin, hair, and eyes; in the *tyrosinase negative type* [MIM*203100], there is an absence of tyrosinase; in the *tyrosinase positive type* [MIM*203200], there is normal tyrosinase which cannot enter pigment cells; it is transmitted by an autosomal recessive inheritance. The compound heterozygote is normal so the two forms are not allelic. There are several types: type IA is characterized by absence of tyrosinase with life-long complete absence of melanin, marked photophobia, and nystagmus. Type IB, yellow a. with low or absent tyrosinase; improves with age. Type II, with normal tyrosinase activity is the most common; hair darkens and nevi and freckles develop. Type III is characterized by absent tyrosinase but pigmentation of the iris in the first decade. Type IV in Africans with normal tyrosinase. Type V with red hair. Type VI, Hermansky-Padlak syndrome, with hemorrhage due to platelet deficiency and low to absent tyrosinase. SYN Hermansky-Pudlak syndrome type VI.

rufous a., SYN xanthism.

al·bi·no (al-bī′nō). An individual with albinism. [Pg., little white one, fr. *albo,* white, fr. L. *albus* + *-ino,* dim. suffix]

al·bi·not·ic (al-bi-not′ik). Pertaining to albinism.

al·bi·nu·ria (al-bi-nū′rē-ă). SYN albiduria.

Albinus (Weiss), Bernhard S., German anatomist and surgeon, 1697–1770. SEE A.'s *muscle.*

al·bo·ci·ne·re·ous (al-bō-si-nē′rē-ŭs). Relating to both the white and the gray matter of the brain or spinal cord. [L. *albus,* white, + *cinereus,* ashen, fr. *cinis* (*ciner-*), ashes]

Albrecht, Karl M.P., German anatomist, 1851–1894. SEE A.'s *bone.*

Albright, Fuller, U.S. physician, 1900–1969. SEE A.'s *disease, syndrome,* hereditary *osteodystrophy;* Forbes-A. *syndrome;* McCune-A. *syndrome.*

al·bu·gin·ea (al-byū-jin′ē-ă). A white fibrous tissue layer, such as the tunica albuginea. SEE *tunica* albuginea, tunica albuginea of corpus spongiosum, *tunica* albuginea of corpora cavernosi, *tunica* albuginea oculi, *tunica* albuginea of testis. [L. *albugineus,* fr. *albugo,* white spot]

al·bu·gin·e·ot·o·my (al-byū-jin-ē-ot′ō-mē). Incision into any tunica albuginea. [albuginea + G. *tomē,* cutting]

al·bu·gin·e·ous (al-byū-jin′ē-ŭs). **1.** Resembling boiled white of egg. **2.** Relating to any tunica albuginea. [L. *albugineus,* fr. *albugo,* white spot]

al·bu·men (al-byū′men). SYN ovalbumin. [see albumin]

al·bu·min (al-byū′min). A type of simple protein, varieties of which are widely distributed throughout the tissues and fluids of plants and animals; a.'s are soluble in pure water, precipitable from solution by strong acids, and coagulable by heat in acid or neutral solution. [L. *albumen* (*-min-*), the white of egg]

a. A, the normal or common type of human serum a.

acetosoluble a., SYN Patein's a.

a. B, SEE inherited albumin *variants,* under *variant.*

Bence Jones a., SEE Bence Jones *proteins,* under *protein.*

blood a., SYN serum a.

bovine serum a. (BSA), a source of a. commonly used in *in vitro* biological studies.

dried human a., SYN normal human serum a.

egg a., SYN ovalbumin.

a. Ghent, SEE inherited albumin *variants,* under *variant.*

iodinated ^{131}**I human serum a.,** a sterile, buffered, isotonic solution prepared to contain not less than 10 mg of radioiodinated normal human serum a. per ml, and adjusted to provide not more than 1 mCi of radioactivity per ml; used as a diagnostic aid in the measurement of blood volume and cardiac output.

iodinated ^{125}**I serum a.,** a sterile, buffered, isotonic solution prepared to contain not less than 10 mg of radioiodinated normal human serum albumin per ml, and adjusted to provide not more than 1 mCi of radioactivity per ml; used as a diagnostic aid in determining blood volume and cardiac output. SYN radioiodinated serum a.

macroaggregated a. (MAA), conglomerates of human serum a. in a suspension; usually refers to particles 10 to 50 μm in size; used as a tagged agent for lung scanning.

a. Mexico, SEE inherited albumin *variants,* under *variant.*

a. Naskapi, SEE inherited albumin *variants,* under *variant.*

native a., a. existing in its natural state, the two principal forms being serum a. and egg a.; it is soluble in water and not precipitated by diluted acids.

normal human serum a., a sterile preparation of serum a. obtained by fractionating blood plasma proteins from healthy persons; used as a transfusion material and to treat edema due to hypoproteinemia. SYN dried human a.

Patein's a., a substance resembling serum a., but 'soluble in acetic acid. SYN acetosoluble a.

plasma a., SYN serum a.

radioiodinated serum a. (RISA), SYN iodinated ^{125}I serum a.

a. Reading, SEE inherited albumin *variants,* under *variant.*

serum a., the principal protein in plasma, present in blood plasma and in serous fluids. Participates in fatty acid transport and helps regulate the osmotic pressure of blood. SYN blood a., plasma a., seralbumin.

a. tannate, an astringent powder obtained by the action of tannic acid on a.; contains about 50% tannic acid; used as an astringent disinfectant in diarrhea and as a dusting powder.

al·bu·min·ate (al-byū′min-āt). The product of the reaction between native albumin and dilute acids or dilute bases, thereby resulting in acid a.'s or alkali a.'s; both types are characterized by solubility in dilute acid or alkali, and relative insolubility in water, dilute solutions of salts, and alcohol.

al·bu·mi·na·tu·ria (al-byū′mi-nă-tū′rē-ă). The presence of an abnormally large quantity of albuminates in the urine when voided. [albuminate + G. *ouron,* urine]

al·bu·min·if·er·ous (al-byū-min-if′er-ŭs). Producing albumin. [albumin + L. *fero,* to bear]

al·bu·min·ip·ar·ous (al-byū-min-ip′ăr-ŭs). Forming albumin. [albumin + L. *pario,* to bring forth]

al·bu·mi·no·cho·lia (al-byū′min-ō-kō′lē-ă). Obsolete term for albumin in the bile. [albumin + G. *cholē,* bile]

al·bu·min·og·e·nous (al-byū-min-oj′en-ŭs). Producing or forming albumin.

al·bu·mi·noid (al-byū′min-oyd). **1.** Resembling albumin. **2.** Any protein. **3.** A simple type of protein, insoluble in neutral solvents, present in horny and cartilaginous tissues and in the lens of the eye; *e.g.,* keratin, elastin, collagen. SYN glutinoid, scleroprotein.

al·bu·mi·nol·y·sis (al-byū-min-ol′i-sis). Proteolysis; often, specifically the proteolysis of albumins. [albumin + G. *lysis,* dissolution]

al·bu·mi·nop·ty·sis (al-byū-mi-nop′ti-sis). Albuminous expectoration. [albumin + G. *ptysis,* a spitting]

al·bu·mi·nor·rhea (al-byū-min-ō-rē′ă). SYN albuminuria. [albumin + G. *rhoia,* a flow]

al·bu·min·ous (al-byū′min-ŭs). Relating to, containing, or consisting of albumin.

al·bu·min·ur·ia (al-byū-mi-nū′rē-ă). Presence of protein in urine, chiefly albumin but also globulin; usually indicative of disease, but sometimes resulting from a temporary or transient dysfunction. SYN albuminorrhea, proteinuria (2). [albumin + G. *ouron,* urine]

adolescent a., functional a. occurring at about the time of puberty; it is usually cyclic or orthostatic a.

adventitious a., a. resulting from the presence of blood escaping somewhere in the urinary tract, of chyle, or of some other albuminous fluid, not caused by filtration of albumin from the blood through the kidneys. SYN false a.

a. of athletes, a form of functional a. following excessive muscular exertion.

Bamberger's a., obsolete term for hematogenous a. that is sometimes observed during the later phases of advanced anemia.

benign a., a collective term for types that are not the result of pathologic changes in the kidneys. SYN essential a.

cardiac a., a. caused by congestive heart failure.

colliquative a., an a. that is at first slight in degree, but unexpectedly becomes greatly increased during convalescence from highly febrile disease, *e.g.,* typhoid fever.

cyclic a., a functional a. sometimes observed intermittently in cycles of 12 to 36 hours' duration, chiefly in younger persons; the degree of a. is usually slight. SYN recurrent a.

dietetic a., the excretion of protein in the urine following the ingestion of certain foods.

essential a., SYN benign a.

false a., SYN adventitious a.

febrile a., a. associated with fever.

functional a., a collective term denoting types of benign a. that are associated with physical exertion or other conditions in which there are physiologic changes such as during pregnancy or adolescence. SYN physiologic a. (2).

intermittent a., functional a. occurring at intervals, such as cyclic a. or a. of athletes.

lordotic a., so-called on the theory that the a. results from pressure due to lordosis in the lumbar spine.

neuropathic a., a. associated with epilepsy or other convulsive disorders, trauma to the brain, and cerebral hemorrhage.

orthostatic a., the appearance of albumin in the urine when the patient is erect and its disappearance when recumbent. SYN orthostatic proteinuria, postural proteinuria, postural a.

physiologic a., (1) presence of slight traces of protein in otherwise normal urine; **(2)** SYN functional a.

postrenal a., a. caused by disease distal to the kidney.

postural a., SYN orthostatic a.

prerenal a., a. caused by disease other than disease of the kidney or genitourinary tract.

recurrent a., SYN cyclic a.

regulatory a., transitory a. occurring after unusual physical exertion.

transient a., a. of a temporary or short-lived nature.

al·bu·min·ur·ic (al-byū-mi-nū′rik). Relating to or characterized by albuminuria.

al·bu·ter·ol (al-byū′ter-ol). α′-[(*tert*-butylamino)methyl]-4-hydroxy-*m*-xylene-α,α′-diol; a sympathomimetic bronchodilator with relatively selective effects on β₂receptors, by inhalation. SYN salbutamol.

Al·ca·lig·e·nes (al-kā-lij′en-ēz). A genus of Gram-negative, rod-shaped, non-fermenting bacteria (family Achromobacteraceae) which are either motile and peritrichous or nonmotile. They are strictly aerobic; some strains are capable of anaerobic respiration in the presence of nitrate or nitrite. Their metabolism is respiratory, never fermentative. They do not utilize carbohydrates. They are found mostly in the intestinal canal, decaying materials, dairy products, water, and soil. They can be isolated from human respiratory and gastrointestinal tracts and wounds in hospitalized patients with compromised immune systems. Occasionally the cause of opportunistic infections, including nosocomial septicemia. The type species is *A. faecalis.* [alkali + G. *-gen,* producing]

al·cap·ton (al-kap′tŏn). SYN homogentisic acid.

al·cap·ton·u·ria, al·kap·ton·u·ria (al-kap-tō-nū′rē-ă). Excretion of homogentisic acid (alkapton) in the urine due to congenital lack of the enzyme homogentisate 1,2-dioxygenase, which mediates an essential step in the catabolism of phenylalanine and tyrosine; urine turns dark if allowed to stand or is alkalinized (a result of formation of polymerization products of homogentisic acid); frequently occurs throughout relatively long periods or may recur and subside at irregular intervals; arthritis and ochronosis are late complications; autosomal recessive inheritance. [alkapton + G. *ouron,* urine]

al·cap·ton·ur·ic, al·kap·to·nur·ic (al-kap-tō-nū-rik;). **1.** Relating to alcaptonuria. **2.** A person with alcaptonuria.

Al·ci·an blue (al′sē-an) [C.I. 74240]. A complex phthalocyanin dye used as a stain to distinguish sulfomucins from sialomucins and uronic acid mucins, to demonstrate sulfated polysaccharides, and to detect glycoproteins in electrophoresis; often used in combination with PAS or aldehyde fuchsin.

al·clo·fe·nac (al-klō′fē-nak). [4-(Allyloxy)-3-chlorophenyl]-acetic acid; an anti-inflammatory agent.

al·clo·met·a·sone (al-klō-met′ă-sōn). 7-Chloro-11,17,21-trihydroxy-16-methylpregna-1,4-diene-3,20-dione; a potent corticosteroid used as the 17,21-dipropionate in topical therapy for psoriasis and other deep-seated dermatoses.

Alcock, Benjamin, Irish anatomist, 1801–?. SEE A.'s *canal.*

al·co·gel (al′kō-jel). A hydrogel, with alcohol instead of water as the dispersion medium.

al·co·hol (al′kō-hol). **1.** One of a series of organic chemical compounds in which a hydrogen (H) attached to carbon is replaced by a hydroxyl (OH); a.'s react with acids to form esters and with alkali metals to form alcoholates. For individual a.'s not listed here, see specific name. **2.** CH_3CH_2OH; made from sugar, starch, and other carbohydrates by fermentation with yeast, and synthetically from ethylene or acetylene. It has been used in beverages and as a solvent, vehicle, and preservative; medicinally, it is used externally as a rubefacient, coolant, and disinfectant, and internally as an analgesic, stomachic, sedative, and antipyretic. SYN ethanol, ethyl alcohol, grain a., rectified spirit, wine spirit. **3.** The azeotropic mixture of CH_3CH_2OH and water

(92.3% by weight of ethanol at 15.56°C). [Ar. *al*, the, + *kohl*, fine antimonial powder, the term being applied first to a fine powder, then, to anything impalpable (spirit)]

absolute a., (1) 100% a., water having been removed; SYN anhydrous a. (2) a. with a minimum admixture of water, at most 1%. SYN dehydrated a.

acid a., ethyl a. (70%) containing 1% hydrochloric acid.

anhydrous a., SYN absolute a. (1).

bile a., one of a group of polyhydroxylated a.'s derived from cholestane.

dehydrated a., SYN absolute a. (2).

denatured a., ethyl a. rendered unfit for consumption as a beverage by the addition of one or several chemicals for commercial purposes (*e.g.,* sucrose octa-acetate). SYN industrial methylated spirit, methylated spirit.

dihydric a., a. containing two OH groups in its molecule; *e.g.,* ethylene glycol.

dilute a., an a. in water mixtures of various concentrations, *e.g.,* 90, 80, 70, 60, 50, 45, 25, and 20% v/v of C_2H_5OH.

fatty a., a long chain a., analogous to the fatty acids, of which the fatty a. may be viewed as a reduction product; *e.g.,* octadecanol from stearic acid. It is often found esterified in waxes. SYN wax a.

grain a., SYN alcohol (2).

monohydric a., an a. containing one OH group.

multiple a., an a. containing more than one OH group.

polyoxyethylene a.'s, used as emulsifying and wetting agents, antistats, solubilizers, defoamers, and other industrial applications. Laureth 9 as spermaticide; pharmaceutic aid (surfactant).

primary a., an a. characterized by the univalent radical, —CH₂OH.

pyroligneous a., SYN *methyl* alcohol.

rubbing a., an alcoholic mixture intended for external use; it usually contains 70% by volume of absolute a. or isopropyl a.; the remainder consists of water, denaturants (with and without coal tar colors), and perfume oils; used as a rubefacient for muscle and joint aches and pains.

secondary a., an a. characterized by the bivalent atom group,

$$\begin{matrix} R \\ \diagdown \\ & CHOH. \\ \diagup \\ R \end{matrix}$$

sugar a., SEE sugar alcohol.

tertiary a., an a. characterized by the trivalent atom group,

$$\begin{matrix} R \\ | \\ R—COH. \\ | \\ R \end{matrix}$$

trihydric a., an a. containing three OH groups; *e.g.,* glycerol.

unsaturated a.'s, those a.'s whose carbon chains contain one or more double or triple bonds.

wax a., SYN fatty a.

al·co·hol ac·ids. A group of compounds that contain both the carboxyl and hydroxy radicals; *e.g.,* glycolic acid.

al·co·hol·ate (al-kō-hol'āt). **1.** A tincture or other preparation containing alcohol. **2.** A chemical compound in which the hydrogen in the OH group of an alcohol is replaced by an alkali metal; *e.g.,* sodium methylate, CH₃ONa.

al·co·hol de·hy·dro·gen·ase (ADH). An oxidoreductase that reversibly converts an alcohol to an aldehyde (or ketone) with NAD⁺ as the H acceptor. For example, ethanol + NAD⁺ ↔ acetaldehyde + NADH. Plays an important role in alcoholism. SEE ALSO alcohol dehydrogenase (acceptor), alcohol dehydrogenase (NADP⁺).

al·co·hol de·hy·dro·gen·ase (ac·cep·tor). An oxidoreductase that reversibly converts primary alcohols to aldehydes with an H acceptor other than NADP⁺.

al·co·hol de·hy·dro·gen·ase (NADP⁺). An oxidoreductase reversibly converting alcohols to aldehydes (or ketones) with NAD(P)⁺ as H acceptor. SYN aldehyde reductase, DPNH → aldehyde transhydrogenase.

al·co·hol·ic (al-kō-hol'ik). **1.** Relating to, containing, or produced by alcohol. **2.** One who suffers from alcoholism. **3.** One who abuses or is dependent upon alcohol.

al·co·hol·ism (al'kō-hol-izm). Chronic alcohol abuse, dependence, or addiction; chronic excessive drinking of alcoholic beverages resulting in impairment of health and/or social or occupational functioning, and increasing adaptation to the effects of alcohol requiring increasing doses to achieve and sustain a desired effect; specific signs and symptoms of withdrawal usually are shown upon sudden cessation of such drinking.

acute a., a temporary deterioration in mental function, accompanied by muscular incoordination and paresis, induced by the rapid ingestion of alcoholic beverages. SYN intoxication (2).

alpha a., Jellinek's term for a still controllable and strictly psychological dependence on alcohol, as to relieve emotional or physical pain, with resulting interference with interpersonal relationships.

beta a., Jellinek's term for the physical complaints associated with excessive use of alcohol, such as polyneuropathy, gastritis, and liver cirrhosis.

chronic a., a pathologic condition, affecting chiefly the nervous and gastroenteric systems, associated with impairment in social and occupational functioning, caused by the habitual use of alcoholic beverages in toxic amounts. SEE ALSO gamma a.

delta a., Jellinek's term for an advanced form of gamma a. in which the individual has lost the ability to abstain from partaking of alcohol even for a brief period.

epsilon a., Jellinek's term for "spree-drinking," such as might occur during periods away from home.

gamma a., Jellinek's term for a severe stage of a. characterized by a progression from psychological to physiological dependence upon alcohol, including tissue dependence and withdrawal symptoms, with loss of control over alcohol intake and destructive effects on interpersonal relationships.

al·co·hol·i·za·tion (al'kō-hol-i-zā'shŭn). Permeation or saturation with alcohol.

al·co·hol·o·pho·bia (al'kō-hol-ō-fō'bē-ă). Morbid fear of alcohol, or of becoming an alcoholic. [alcohol + G. *phobos*, fear]

al·co·hol·y·sis (al-kō-hol'i-sis). Splitting of a chemical bond with the addition of the elements of alcohol at the point of splitting. [alcohol + G. *lysis*, dissolution]

al·cur·o·ni·um chlo·ride (al-kyūr-ō'nē-ŭm). *N,N'*-Diallylnortoxiferinium dichloride; a skeletal muscle relaxant active as a nondepolarizing neuromuscular blocking agent.

ALD Abbreviation for adrenoleukodystrophy.

al·da·di·ene (al-dă-dī'ēn). A metabolite of spironolactone that contains double bonds between C-4 and C-5 and between C-6 and C-7; formed upon removal of the 7α-acetylthiol side chain from spironolactone and as potent a diuretic as the parent compound.

al·dar·ic ac·id (al'dar-ik). One of a group of sugar acids characterized by the formula HOOC–(CHOH)ₙ–COOH; *e.g.,* saccharic acid.

al·de·hol (al'dĕ-hol). An oxidation product of kerosene; used for denaturing ethyl alcohol.

al·de·hyde (al'dĕ-hīd). A compound containing the radical —CH=O, reducible to an alcohol (CH₂OH), oxidizable to a carboxylic acid (COOH); *e.g.,* acetaldehyde.

activated glycol aldehyde, 2-(1,2-dihydroxyethyl)thiamin pyrophosphate; an intermediate in carbohydrate metabolism and in transketolization.

active a., any aldehyde derivative of thiamin pyrophosphate.

angular a., the a. group attached to carbon 13 (between rings C and D) of the steroid nucleus in aldosterone.

a. reductase, SYN alcohol dehydrogenase (NADP⁺).

al·de·hyde de·hy·dro·gen·ase (ac·yl·at·ing). An oxidoreductase converting an aldehyde and CoA to acyl-CoA with NAD⁺ as H acceptor.

al·de·hyde de·hy·dro·gen·ase (NAD⁺). An oxidoreductase reversibly converting aldehydes to acids with NADP⁺ as H acceptor.

al·de·hyde de·hy·dro·gen·ase (NAD(P)⁺). An oxidoreductase reversibly converting aldehydes to acids with NAD⁺ or NADP⁺ as H acceptor.

al·de·hyde→DPN trans·hy·dro·gen·ase. Aldehyde dehydrogenase (NAD⁺).

al·de·hyde-ly·as·es [EC sub-subgroup 4.1.2]. Enzymes catalyzing the reversal of an aldol condensation.

al·de·hyde→TPN trans·hy·dro·gen·ase. Aldehyde dehydrogenase (NADP⁺).

Alder, Albert von. SEE A.'s *anomaly; A. bodies*, under *body*.

al·dim·ine (al'dĕ-mēn). SYN Schiff *base*.

al·di·tol (al'di-tol). The polyalcohol derived by reduction of an aldose; *e.g.,* sorbitol. SEE ALSO *aldose* reductase.

al·do·bi·u·ron·ic ac·id (al'dō-bī-yū-ron'ik). Condensation products of an aldose and a uronic acid; such groupings occur among the components of various mucopolysaccharides, notably hyaluronic acid.

al·do·cor·tin (al'dō-kōr'tin). SYN aldosterone.

al·do·hex·ose (al-dō-heks'ōs). A 6-carbon sugar characterized by the (potential) presence of an aldehyde group in the molecule; *e.g.,* glucose, galactose.

al·do·ke·to·mu·tase (al'dō-kē-tō-myū'tās). SYN lactoylglutathione lyase.

al·dol (al'dōl). SEE aldol *condensation*.

al·dol·ase (al'dō-lās). **1.** Generic term for aldehyde-lyase. **2.** Name sometimes applied to fructose-bisphosphate aldolase.

al·don·ic ac·ids (al-don'ik). Monosaccharide derivatives in which the aldehyde group has been oxidized to a carboxyl group. They may form lactones (*e.g.,* galactonic acid). SYN glyconic acids.

al·do·pen·tose (al-dō-pen'tōs). A monosaccharide with five carbon atoms, of which one is a (potential) aldehyde group; *e.g.,* ribose.

al·dose (al'dōs). A monosaccharide potentially containing the characteristic group of the aldehydes, —CHO; a polyhydroxyaldehyde.

a. mutarotase, SYN aldose 1-epimerase.

a. reductase, polyol dehydrogenase (NADP⁺); an oxidoreductase that reversibly converts aldoses to alditols (*e.g.,* glucose to sorbitol) with NADPH as hydrogen donor. An important step in the metabolism of sorbitol and in the formation of diabetic cataracts. SEE ALSO D-sorbitol-6-phosphate dehydrogenase.

al·dose 1-ep·i·mer·ase. An enzyme catalyzing the reversible interconversion of α- and β-aldoses (*e.g.,* α- and β-D-glucose); also acts on L-arabinose, D-xylose, D-galactose, maltose, and lactose. SYN aldose mutarotase, mutarotase.

al·do·side (al'dō-sīd). A glucoside in which the sugar moiety is an aldose.

al·dos·ter·one (al-dos'ter-ōn). 11β,21-dihydroxy-3,20-dioxopregn-4-en-18-al(11→1 8 lactone); a mineralocorticoid hormone produced by the zona glomerulosa of the adrenal cortex; its major action is to facilitate potassium exchange for sodium in the distal renal tubule, causing sodium reabsorption and potassium and hydrogen loss; the principal mineralocorticoid. SYN aldocortin.

al·do·ste·ron·ism (al-dos'ter-on-izm). A disorder caused by excessive secretion of aldosterone. SYN hyperaldosteronism.

idiopathic a., SYN primary a.

primary a., an adrenocortical disorder caused by excessive secretion of aldosterone and characterized by headaches, nocturia, polyuria, fatigue, hypertension, potassium depletion, hypokalemic alkalosis, hypervolemia, and decreased plasma renin activity; may be associated with small benign adrenocortical adenomas. SYN Conn's syndrome, idiopathic a.

secondary a., a. resulting not from a defect intrinsic to the adrenal cortex but from a stimulation of hormonal secretion caused by extra-adrenal disorders; associated with increased plasma renin activity and occurs in heart failure, nephrotic syndrome, cirrhosis, and hypoproteinemia.

al·do·ste·ron·o·gen·e·sis (al-dos'ter-on-ō-jen'ĕ-sis). Formation of the hormone, aldosterone. [aldosterone + G. *genesis,* production]

al·do·tet·rose (al-dō-tet'rōs). A four-carbon aldose; *e.g.,* threose, erythrose.

al·do·tri·ose (al-dō-trī'os). A three-carbon aldose; *e.g.,* D- or L-glyceraldehyde.

al·dox·ime (al-doks'ēm). A compound derived by the reaction of an aldose with hydroxylamine, thus containing the a. group —HC=NOH.

Aldrich, Robert Anderson, U.S. pediatrician, *1917. SEE A. *syndrome;* Wiskott-Aldrich *syndrome.*

al·drin. A hexachlorohexahydrodimethanonaphthalene; a volatile chlorinated hydrocarbon used as an insecticide; if absorbed through the skin, it causes toxic symptoms consisting of irritability followed by depression.

alec·i·thal (ă-les'i-thal). Without yolk; denoting ova with little or no deutoplasm. [G. *a-* priv. + *lekithos,* yolk]

Alec·to·ro·bi·us ta·la·je (ă-lek-tōr-ō'bē-ŭs tă-lā'jē). An insect, commonly found in Mexico and South America, whose bites, like those of the bedbug, may suppurate.

alem·mal (ă-lem'ăl). Denoting a nerve fiber lacking a neurolemma. [G. *a-* priv. + *lemma,* husk]

ale·thia (ă-lēth'ē-ă). Rarely used term for an incapacity to forget past events. [G. *a-* priv. + *lēthē,* forgetfulness]

aleu·ke·mia (ă-lū-kē'mē-ă). **1.** Literally, a lack of leukocytes in the blood. The term is generally used to indicate varieties of leukemic disease in which the white blood cell count in circulating blood is normal or even less than normal (*i.e.,* no leukocytosis), but a few young leukocytes are observed; sometimes used more restrictedly for unusual instances of leukemia with no leukocytosis and no young forms in the blood. **2.** Leukemic changes in bone marrow associated with a subnormal number of leukocytes in the blood. SEE ALSO subleukemic *leukemia.* [G. *a-* priv. + *leukos,* white, + *haima,* blood]

aleu·ke·mic (ā-lū-kē'mik). Pertaining to aleukemia.

aleu·ke·moid (ā-lū-kē'moyd). Resembling aleukemia symptomatically.

aleu·kia (ā-lū'kē-ă). **1.** Absence or extremely decreased number of leukocytes in the circulating blood; sometimes also termed aleukemic myelosis. **2.** Obsolete name for thrombocytopenia. [G. *a-* priv. + *leukos,* white]

aleu·ko·cyt·ic (ā-lū-kō-sit'ik). Manifesting absence or extremely reduced numbers of leukocytes in blood or lesions.

aleu·ko·cy·to·sis (ā-lū-kō-sī-tō'sis). Absence or great reduction (relative or absolute) of the number of white blood cells in the circulating blood (*i.e.,* an advanced degree of leukopenia), or the lack of leukocytes in an anatomical lesion. [G. *a-* priv. + *leukos,* white, + *kytos,* a hollow (cell)]

aleu·ri·o·co·nid·i·um (ă-lū'rē-ō-kŏ-nid'ē-ŭm). A conidium developed from the blown out end of conidiogenous cells or hyphal branches, and released by rupture below the base of attachment. SYN aleuriospore. [G. *aleuron,* flour, + conidium]

aleu·ri·o·spore (ă-lū'rē-ō-spōr). SYN aleurioconidium.

al·eu·ron (al'ū-rōn). Protein granules in the endosperm of seeds, supposed to contain the vitamins of edible seeds and grains. [G. flour]

aleu·ro·nate (ă-lū'rō-nāt). Protein from the aleuron layer (endosperm) of cereal grains; used to make bread for diabetics.

aleu·ro·noid (ă-lū'rō-noyd). Resembling flour.

Alexander, Gustav, Austrian otolaryngologist, *1873. SEE A.'s *deafness.*

Alexander, W. Stewart, 20th century New Zealand pathologist. SEE A.'s *disease.*

alex·ia (ă-lek'sē-ă). An inability to comprehend the meaning of written or printed words and sentences, caused by a cerebral lesion. Also called **optical a., sensory a.,** or **visual a.,** in distinction to **motor a.** (anarthria), in which there is loss of the power to read aloud although the significance of what is written or printed is understood. SYN text blindness, word blindness, visual aphasia (1). [G. *a-* priv. + *lexis,* a word or phrase]

incomplete a., SYN dyslexia.

musical a., loss of the power to read musical notation. SYN music blindness, note blindness.

alex·ic (ă-lek'sik). Pertaining to alexia.

alex·in (ă-lek'sin). Obsolete term for the bactericidal substances of cell-free serum, the activity of which is destroyed by heating at 56°C; applied by Bordet to the heat-labile substance normally present in serum and distinct from the sensitizing substance (antibody) produced by infection or immunization. In this sense it is synonymous with complement. [G. *alexō,* to ward off]

alex·i·phar·mac (ă-lek-si-far'mak). **1.** SYN antidotal. **2.** An antidote. [G. *alexipharmakos,* preserving against poison]

alex·i·thy·mia (ă-lek-si-thī'mē-ă). Difficulty in recognizing and describing one's emotions, defining them in terms of somatic sensations or behavioral reactions. [G. *a-* priv. + *lexis,* word, + *-thymia,* feelings, passion]

aley·dig·ism (ă-lī'dig-izm). Aplasia of Leydig cells, seen in hypogonadotrophic hypogonadism.

Alezzandrini, Arturo Alberto, Argentinian ophthalmologist, *1932. SEE A.'s *syndrome.*

al·fa·cal·ci·dol (al-fă-kal'si-dol). 1-α-Hydroxycholecalciferol; a derivative of vitamin D used in the treatment of hypoparathyroidism, vitamin D dependent rickets, and rickets associated with malabsorption syndromes.

al·fen·ta·nil hy·dro·chlo·ride (al-fen'tă-nil). $C_{21}H_{32}N_6O_3 \cdot HCl \cdot H_2O$; a very potent, short acting narcotic agonist analgesic used as an anesthetic or as an adjunct in the maintenance of general anesthesia.

ALG Abbreviation for antilymphocyte *globulin.*

al·gae (al'jē). A division of eukaryotic, photosynthetic, nonflowering organisms that includes many seaweeds. [pl. of L. *alga,* seaweed]

blue-green a., former name for the blue-green bacteria, now classified as Cyanobacteria.

al·gal (al'găl). Resembling or pertaining to algae.

al·ga·ro·ba (al-gă-rō'bă). Ground meal of the fruit of *Ceratonia siliqua;* used as an adsorbent-demulcent in the treatment of diarrhea. SYN carob flour, locust gum.

⌂ **alge-, algesi-, algio-, algo-.** Pain; corresponds to L. dolor-. [G. *algos,* a pain]

al·ge·do·nic (al-jē-don'ik). Relating to a mixed sensation or emotion of pleasure and pain. [G. *algos,* pain, + *hēdonē,* pleasure]

al·ge·fa·cient (al-jē-fā'shent). An agent that has a cooling action. [L. *algeo,* to be cold, + *facio,* pr. pl. *-iens,* to make]

⌂ **algesi-.** SEE alge-.

al·ge·sia (al-jē'zē-ă). SYN algesthesia. [G. *algēsis,* a sense of pain]

al·ge·sic (al-jēz-ik). **1.** Painful; related to or causing pain. **2.** Relating to hypersensitivity to pain. SYN algetic.

al·ge·si·chro·nom·e·ter (al-jē'zē-krō-nom'ĕ-ter). An instrument for recording the time required for the perception of a painful stimulus. [G. *algēsis,* sense of pain, + *chronos,* time, + *metron,* measure]

al·ge·si·dys·tro·phy (al-jē-si-dis'trō-fē). SYN algodystrophy. [G. *algēsis,* sense of pain, + *dys-,* bad, + *trophē,* nourishment]

al·ge·sim·e·ter (al-jē-sim'ĕ-ter). SYN algesiometer.

al·ge·si·o·gen·ic (al-jē'zē-ō-jen'ik). Pain-producing. SYN algogenic. [G. *algēsis,* sense of pain, + *-gen,* production]

al·ge·si·om·e·ter (al-jē-zē-om'ĕ-ter). An instrument for measuring the degree of sensitivity to a painful stimulus. SYN algesimeter, algometer, odynometer. [G. *algēsis,* sense of pain, + *metron,* measure]

al·ges·the·sia (al-jes-thē'zē-ă). **1.** The appreciation of pain. **2.** Hypersensitivity to pain. SYN algesia, algesthesis. [G. *algos,* pain, + *aisthēsis,* sensation]

al·ges·the·sis (al-jes-thē'sis). SYN algesthesia.

al·ges·tone ac·e·to·phe·nide (al-jes'tōn ă-sē-tō-fē'nīd). 16α,17-dihydroxypregn-4-ene-3,20-dione cyclic acetal with acetophenone; a progestogen with contraceptive properties. SYN alphasone acetophenide.

al·get·ic (al-jet'ik). SYN algesic.

⌂ **-algia.** Pain, painful condition. [G. *algos,* a pain]

al·gi·cide (al'ji-sīd). An agent active against algae. [algae, + L. *caedo,* to kill]

al·gid (al'jid). Chilly, cold. [L. *algidus,* cold]

al·gin (al'jin). A carbohydrate product from a seaweed, *Macrocystis pyrifera;* used as a gel in pharmaceutical preparations. SYN sodium alginate.

al·gi·nate (al'ji-nāt). An irreversible hydrocolloid consisting of salts of alginic acid, a colloidal acid polysaccharide obtained from seaweed and composed of mannuronic acid residues; used in dental impression materials.

⌂ **algio-.** SEE alge-.

al·gi·o·mo·tor (al-jē-ō-mō'tōr). Causing painful muscular contractions. SYN algiomuscular. [algio- + L. *motor,* mover]

al·gi·o·mus·cu·lar (al'jē-ō-mŭs'kyū-lăr). SYN algiomotor.

al·gi·o·vas·cu·lar (al'jē-ō-vas'kyū-lăr). SYN algovascular.

⌂ **algo-.** SEE alge-.

al·go·dys·tro·phy (al-gō-dis'trō-fē). A painful local disturbance of growth, particularly due to focal aseptic necrosis of bone and cartilage. SYN algesidystrophy. [algo- + G. *dys-,* bad, + *trophē,* nourishment]

al·go·gen·e·sis, al·go·ge·ne·sia (al-gō-jen'ĕ-sis, -jĕ-nē'zē-ă). The production or origin of pain. [algo- + G. *genesis,* origin]

al·go·gen·ic (al-gō-jen'ik). SYN algesiogenic.

al·go·lag·nia (al-gō-lag'nē-ă). Form of sexual perversion in which the infliction or the experiencing of pain increases the pleasure of the sexual act or causes sexual pleasure independent of the act; includes both sadism (active a.) and masochism (passive a.). SYN algophilia (2). [algo- + G. *lagneia,* lust]

al·gol·o·gy (al-gōlō-jē). The study of pain. [G. *algos,* pain, + *-logy*]

al·gom·e·ter (al-gom'ĕ-ter). SYN algesiometer. [algo- + G. *metron,* measure]

al·gom·e·try (al-gom'ĕ-trē). The process of measuring pain.

al·go·phil·ia (al-gō-fil'ē-ă). **1.** Pleasure experienced in the thought of pain in others or in oneself. **2.** SYN algolagnia. [algo- + G. *phileō,* to love]

al·go·pho·bia (al-gō-fō'bē-ă). Abnormal fear of or sensitiveness to pain. [algo- + G. *phobos,* fear]

al·go·psy·cha·lia (al-go-si-ka'lǐ-ah). SYN psychalgia (1). [algo- + G. *psychē,* mind]

al·go·rithm (al'gō-rithm). A systematic process consisting of an ordered sequence of steps, each step depending on the outcome of the previous one. In clinical medicine, a step-by-step protocol for management of a health care problem; in computed tomography, the formulas used for calculation of the final image from the x-ray transmission data. [Mediev. L. *algorismus,* after Muhammad ibn-Musa *al-Khwarizmi,* Arbian mathematician, + G. *arithmos,* number]

al·gos·co·py (al-gos'kŏ-pē). SYN cryoscopy. [L. *algor,* cold, + G. *skopeō,* to view]

al·go·spasm (al'gō-spazm). Spasm produced by pain. [G. *algos,* pain, + *spasmos,* convulsion]

al·go·vas·cu·lar (al-gō-vas'kyū-lăr). Relating to changes in the lumen of the blood vessels occurring under the influence of pain. SYN algiovascular. [G. *algos,* pain]

al·i·ble (al'i-bl). SYN nutritive. [L. *alibilis,* nutritive, fr. *alo,* to nourish]

al·i·cy·clic (al-i-sik'lik). Denoting an alicyclic compound.

alien·a·tion (ā-lē-en-ā'shŭn). A condition characterized by lack of meaningful relationships to others, sometimes resulting in depersonalization and estrangement from others. [L. *alieno,* pp. *-atus,* to make strange]

ali·e·nia (ā-li-ē'nē-ă). Congenital absence of the spleen. [G. *a-* priv. + L. *lien,* spleen]

alien·ist (āl'yen-ist, ā-lē'en-ist). Obsolete term for one who treats mental diseases.

al·i·form (al'i-fōrm). Wing-shaped. [L. *ala,* + *forma,* shape]

align·ment (ă-līn'ment). **1.** The longitudinal position of a bone or limb. **2.** The act of bringing into line. **3.** In dentistry, the arrangement of the teeth in relation to the supporting structures and the adjacent and opposing dentitions. SYN alinement. [Fr. *aligner*, to line up, fr. L. *linea*, line]

al·i·ment (al′i-ment). **1.** SYN nourishment. **2.** In sensorimotor theory, that which is assimilated to a schema; analogous to a stimulus. [L. *alo*, to nourish]

al·i·men·ta·ry (al-i-men′ter-ē). Relating to food or nutrition. [L. *alimentarius*, fr. *alimentum*, nourishment]

al·i·men·ta·tion (al-i-men-tā′shŭm). Providing nourishment. SEE ALSO feeding.

forced a., SYN forced *feeding*.

parenteral a., providing nourishment intravenously.

rectal a., nourishment provided by retention enemas.

al·i·na·sal (al′i-nā′săl). Relating to the wings of the nose (alae nasi), or flaring portions of the nostrils. [L. *ala*, + *nasus*, nose]

aline·ment (ă-līn′ment). SYN alignment.

al·in·jec·tion (al′in-jek′shŭn). Injection of alcohol for hardening and preserving pathologic and histologic specimens.

al·i·phat·ic (al-i-fat′ik). Denoting the acyclic carbon compounds, most of which belong to the fatty acid series. [G. *aleiphar* (*aleiphat-*), fat, oil]

al·i·phat·ic ac·ids. The acids of nonaromatic hydrocarbons (*e.g.,* acetic, propionic, butyric acids); the so-called fatty acids of the formula R–COOH, where R is a nonaromatic (aliphatic) hydrocarbon.

ali·poid (ā-lip′oyd). Characterized by absence of lipoids. [G. *a*-priv. + *lipoidēs*, resembling fat]

alip·o·tro·pic (ā′lip-ō-trōp′ik). Having no effect upon fat metabolism, or upon the movement of fat to the liver. [G. *a*- priv. + *lipos*, fat, + *tropos*, a turning]

al·i·quant (al′ĭ-kwant). In chemistry and immunology, pertaining to a portion that results from dividing the whole in a manner that some is left after the a.'s (equal in volume or weight) have been apportioned.

al·i·quot (al′i-kwot). In chemistry and immunology, pertaining to a portion of the whole; loosely, any one of two or more samples of something, of the same volume or weight. [L. a few, several]

al·i·sphe·noid (al-i-sfē′noyd). Relating to the greater wing of the sphenoid bone. [L. *ala*, + *sphēn*, wedge]

aliz·a·rin (ă-liz′ă-rin) [C.I. 58000]. 1,2-Dihydroxyanthraquinone; a red dye that occurs in the root of madder (*Rubia tinctorum* and other *Rubiaceae*) in glucose combination (ruberythric acid) as orange needles, slightly soluble in water; used by the ancients as a dye. Now made synthetically from anthracene and used in the manufacture of dyes, *e.g.,* a. blue, a. orange, "Turkey red ". As an indicator, it changes from yellow to red at pH 5.5 to 6.8; other modified a.'s have other colors and change color at other pH values.

a. cyanin [C.I. 58610], disulfonate of hexahydroxyanthraquinone; an acid dye used as a nuclear stain after mordanting and as a fluorochrome in ultraviolet microscopy.

a. purpurin, SYN purpurin (2).

a. red S [C.I. 58005], sodium *a.* sulfonate; used as a stain for calcium in bone (calcium appears red-orange, magnesium, aluminum, and barium are varying shades of red), in the determination of fluorine; as a pH indicator it changes from yellow to purple between pH 3.7 and 5.2.

al·ka·di·ene (al-kă-dī′ēn). An acyclic hydrocarbon (alkane) containing two double bonds.

al·ka·le·mia (al-kă-lē′mē-ă). A decrease in H-ion concentration of the blood or a rise in pH, irrespective of alterations in the level of bicarbonate ion. [alkali + G. *haima*, blood]

al·ka·les·cence (al-ka-les′ens). **1.** A slight alkalinity. **2.** The process of becoming alkaline.

al·ka·les·cent (al-ka-les′ent). **1.** Slightly alkaline. **2.** Becoming alkaline.

al·ka·li, pl. **al·ka·lis, al·ka·lies** (al′kă-lī, -līz). **1.** A strongly basic substance yielding hydroxaide ions (OH·) in solution; *e.g.,* sodium hydroxide, potassium hydroxide. **2.** SYN base (3). **3.** SYN alkali *metal*. [Ar., *al*, the, + *qalīy*, soda ash]

caustic a., a highly ionized (in solution) alkali; *e.g.,* NaOH.

fixed a., any a. other than a weakly ionized one, like ammonia.

vegetable a., a mixture of potassium hydroxide and carbonate.

al·ka·line (al′kă-līn). Relating to or having the reaction of an alkali.

al·ka·lin·i·ty (al-kă-lin′i-tē). The state of being alkaline.

al·ka·lin·i·za·tion (al′kă-lin-i-zā′shŭn). SYN alkalization.

al·ka·li·nu·ria (al′kă-li-nū′rē-ă). The passage of alkaline urine. SYN alkaluria. [alkaline + G. *ouron*, urine]

al·ka·li·ther·a·py (al′kă-lī-thār′ă-pē). Therapeutic use of alkali for local or systemic effect.

al·ka·li·za·tion (al′kal-i-zā′shŭn). The process of rendering alkaline. SYN alkalinization.

al·ka·liz·er (al′kă-līz-er). An agent that neutralizes acids or renders a solution alkaline.

al·ka·loid (al′kă-loyd). Originally, any one of hundreds of plant products distinguished by alkaline (basic) reactions, but now restricted to heterocyclic nitrogen-containing and often complex structures possessing pharmacological activity; their trivial names usually end in -ine (*e.g.,* morphine, atropine, colchicine). A.'s are synthesized by plants and are found in the leaf, bark, seed, or other parts, usually constituting the active principle of the crude drug; they are a loosely defined group, but may be classified according to the chemical structure of their main nucleus. For medicinal purposes, due to improved water solubility, the salts of a.'s are usually used. See also individual a. or a. class. SYN vegetable base.

ergot a.'s (er′got), any of a large number of a.'s obtained from the ergot fungus *Claviceps purpurea* or semisynthetically derived; examples include ergotamine, ergonovine, dihydroergotamine, lysergic acid diethylamide (LSD), methysergide.

fixed a., a nonvolatile a.

Vinca a.'s, a.'s such as vincristine and vinblastine (antitumor agents) extracted from the periwinkle plant. SYN Catharanthus alkaloids.

al·ka·lo·sis (al-kă-lō′sis). A pathophysiological disorder characterized by H-ion loss or base excess in body fluids (metabolic a.), or caused by CO_2 loss due to hyperventilation (respiratory a.).

acapnial a., SYN respiratory a.

compensated a., a. in which there is a change in bicarbonate but the pH of body fluids approaches normal; respiratory a. may be compensated by increased production of metabolic acids or increased renal excretion of bicarbonate; metabolic a. is rarely compensated by hypoventilation.

compensated metabolic a., retention of acid, primarily carbon dioxide by the lung and acid ions by the renal tubules, to reduce the effect on the pH of the blood of excess alkali produced by ingestion or metabolism of alkali-producing substances.

compensated respiratory a., increased excretion of acid ions by the kidney to minimize the effect on the pH of the blood of excessive loss of carbon dioxide via the lungs, such as occurs with hyperventilation.

metabolic a., an a. associated with an increased arterial plasma bicarbonate concentration, possibly resulting from an excessive intake of alkaline materials or an excessive loss of acid in the urine or through persistent vomiting; the base excess and standard bicarbonate are both elevated. SEE ALSO compensated a.

respiratory a., a. resulting from abnormal loss of CO_2 produced by hyperventilation, either active or passive, with concomitant reduction in arterial plasma bicarbonate concentration. SEE ALSO compensated a. SYN acapnial a.

uncompensated a., a. in which the pH of body fluids is elevated because of lack of the compensatory mechanisms of compensated a.

al·ka·lot·ic (al-kă-lot′ik). Relating to alkalosis.

al·ka·lu·ria (al-kă-lū′rē-ă). SYN alkalinuria.

al·kane (al′kān). The general term for a saturated acyclic hydrocarbon; *e.g.,* propane, butane.

al·ka·net (al′kă-net) [C.I. 75530, 75520]. The root of a herb, *Alkanna*, or *Anchusa tinctoria* (family Boraginaceae), that yields red dyes alkannan and alkannin; used as a coloring agent; also used, combined with tannin, as an astringent.

al·kan·nan (al′kă-nan) [C.I. 75520]. A minor red dye component derived from alkanet.

al·kan·nin (al'kă-nin) [C.I. 75530]. (-)-5,8-dihydroxy-2-(1-hydroxy-4-methyl-3-pentenyl)-1,4-naphthoquinone; the major red dye derived from alkanet; used as an astringent, and in cosmetics and foods; can be used as an indicator: red at pH 6.8, changing to purple at pH 8.8 and blue at pH 10.0; also used as a fat stain. SYN anchusin.

al·kap·ton (al-kap'tŏn). SYN homogentisic acid. [Boedeker's coinage fr. alkali + L + G. *kaptein,* to suck up greedily]

al·ka·tri·ene (al-kă-trī'ēn). An acyclic hydrocarbon containing three double bonds; *e.g.,* 2,4,6-octatriene, CH_3—CH=CH—CH= CH—CH=CH— CH_3.

al·ka·ver·vir (al-kă-ver'vir). A mixture of alkaloids obtained by the selective extraction of *Veratrum viride* with various organic solvents; used orally or parenterally as a hypotensive agent.

al·kene (al'kēn). An acyclic hydrocarbon containing one or more double bonds; *e.g.,* ethylene, propene. SYN olefin.

al·ke·nyl (al'ken-il). The radical of an alkene.

alk-1-en·yl. The radical of an alkene in which the double bond indicated by "en(e)" is between carbons 1 and 2 (carbon 1 being the radical or "yl" carbon), *i.e.,* R—CH=CH—; sometimes expressed as alk-1-en-1-yl.

alk-1-en·yl·glyc·er·o·phos·pho·lip·id. A phosphatidate in which at least one of the radicals attached to the glycerol is an alk-1-enyl rather than the usual acyl radical (*i.e.,* is derived from an aldehyde rather than an acid, hence the older trivial names phosphatidal and acetal phosphatid(at)e); "plasmenic acid" has been proposed as a name for such phosphatidates.

al·kide (al'kīd). SYN alkyl (2).

al·kyl (al'kil). **1.** A hydrocarbon radical of the general formula C_nH_{2n+1}. **2.** A compound, such as tetraethyl lead, in which a metal is combined with alkyl radicals. SYN alkide.

arylated a., SYN aralkyl.

al·kyl·a·mine (al-kil'ă-mēn). An alkane containing an —NH_2 group in place of one H atom; *e.g.,* ethylamine.

al·kyl·at·ing agent. See under agent.

al·kyl·a·tion (al'ki-lā'shŭn). Substitution of an alkyl radical for a hydrogen atom; *e.g.,* introduction of a side chain into an aromatic compound.

ALL Abbreviation for acute lymphocytic leukemia.

al·la·ches·the·sia (al'ă-kes-thē'zē-ă). A condition in which a tactile sensation is referred to a point other than that to which the stimulus is applied. SEE ALSO allochiria. [G. *allaché,* elsewhere, + *aisthēsis,* sensation]

al·lan·ti·a·sis (al-an-tī'ă-sis). Obsolete term for sausage poisoning due to botulism. [G. *allas* (*allant*-), sausage]

⌂**allanto-, allant-.** Allantois; allantoid; sausage. [G. *allas, allantos,* sausage]

al·lan·to·ate de·im·i·nase. An enzyme that catalyzes the conversion of allantoic acid to ureidoglycine, NH_3, and CO_2.

al·lan·to·cho·ri·on (ă-lan-tō-kōr'ē-on). Extraembryonic membrane formed by the fusion of the allantois and chorion.

al·lan·to·gen·e·sis (ă-lan-tō-jen'ĕ-sis). Formation and development of the allantois. [allanto- + G. *genesis,* origin]

al·lan·to·ic (ă-lan-tō'ik). Relating to the allantois.

al·lan·to·ic ac·id (ă-lan-tō'ik as'id). diureidoacetic acid; a degradation product of allantoin.

al·lan·toid (ă-lan'toyd). **1.** Sausage-shaped. **2.** Relating to, or resembling, the allantois. [allanto- + G. *eidos,* appearance]

al·lan·toid·o·an·gi·op·a·gus (ă-lan-toyd'ō-an-jē-op'ă-gŭs). SYN omphaloangiopagus. SEE allantoidoangiopagous *twins,* under *twin.* [allantoid + G. *angeion,* vessel, + *pagos,* fastened]

al·lan·to·in (ă-lan'tō-in). 5-ureidohydantoin; a substance present in allantoic fluid, fetal urine, and elsewhere; also an oxidation product of uric acid and the end product of purine metabolism in animals other than humans and the other primates. SYN 3-ureidohydantoin, cordianine, glyoxyldiureide.

al·lan·to·in·ase (ă-lan-tō'i-nās). An enzyme (an amidohydrolase) that catalyzes the hydrolysis of allantoin to allantoic acid.

al·lan·to·in·u·ria (ă-lan'tō-in-yū'rē-ă). The urinary excretion of allantoin; normal in most mammals, abnormal in humans. [allantoin + G. *ouron,* urine]

al·lan·to·is (ă-lan'tō-is). A fetal membrane developing from the hindgut (or yolk sac, in humans). In humans it is vestigial; externally, in mammals, it contributes to the formation of the umbilical cord and placenta; in birds and reptiles it lies close beneath the porous shell and serves as an organ of respiration. SYN allantoid membrane. [allanto- + G. *eidos,* appearance]

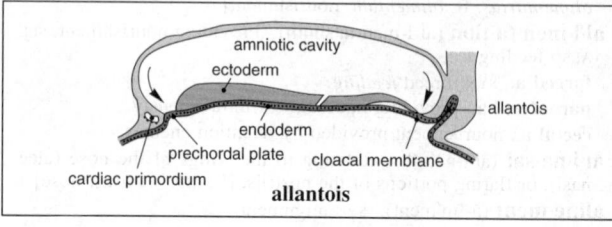

amniotic cavity
ectoderm
allantois
endoderm
prechordal plate — cloacal membrane
cardiac primordium
allantois

al·lax·is (ă-laks'is). SYN metamorphosis. [G. *allattein,* to alter]

al·lele (ă-lēl'). Any one of a series of two or more different genes that may occupy the same locus on a specific chromosome. As autosomal chromosomes are paired, each autosomal gene is represented twice in normal somatic cells. If the same a. occupies both units of the locus, the individual or cell is homozygous for this a. If the a.'s are different, the individual or cell is heterozygous for both a.'s. SEE DNA markers. SEE ALSO *dominance* of traits. SYN allelomorph. [G. *allēlōn,* reciprocally]

Dominant traits or conditions are caused by inheritance of a single allele from either parent; recessive ones by inheritance of a relevant allele from each parent. With the advent of DNA technology, the allele has become the focus of intense scrutiny, as molecular biologists attempt to track down genes responsible for physical and behavioral traits, and for the 3,500 human diseases that have been identified as chromosomally linked. Paired with radioisotopes or fluorescent dyes, alleles may serve as probes that allow for the identification of such genes.

codominant a., SEE codominant.
silent a., SYN amorph.

al·le·lic (ă-lē'lik). Relating to an allele. SYN allelomorphic.

al·lel·ism (al'ē-lizm). The state held in common by alleles. SYN allelomorphism.

al·le·lo·ca·tal·y·sis (ă-lē'lō-kă-tal'i-sis). Self-stimulation of growth in a bacterial culture by addition of similar cells. [G. *allēlōn,* mutually, reciprocally, + *catalytikos,* able to dissolve]

al·le·lo·cat·a·lyt·ic (ă-lē'lō-kat-ă-lit'ik). Mutually catalytic; denoting two substances each of which is decomposed in the presence of the other.

al·le·lo·chem·i·cals (ă-lē'lō-kem'i-kălz). Signal substances between individuals of different species. Cf. pheromones. [G. *allēlōn,* reciprocally, + chemical]

al·le·lo·morph (ă-lē'lō-mōrf). SYN allele. [G. *allēlōn,* reciprocally, + *morphē,* shape]

al·le·lo·mor·phic (ă-lē-lō-mōr'fik). SYN allelic.

al·le·lo·mor·phism (ă-lē-lō-mōr'fizm). SYN allelism.

al·le·lo·tax·is, al·le·lo·taxy (ă-lēl-ō-taks'is, -taks'ē). Development of an organ from a number of embryonal structures or tissues. [G. *allēlōn,* reciprocally, + *taxis,* an arranging]

Allen, Alfred Henry, U.S. chemist, 1846–1904. SEE A.'s *test.*

Allen, Edgar, U.S. endocrinologist, 1892–1943. SEE A.-Doisy *test, unit.*

Allen, Edgar Van Nuys, U.S. physician, 1900–1961. SEE A.'s *test.*

Allen, Willard Myron, U.S. gynecologist, *1904. SEE Corner-A. *test, unit;* A.-Masters *syndrome.*

al·ler·gen (al'er-jen). Term for an incitant of altered reactivity (allergy), an antigenic substance. [allergy + G. *-gen,* producing]

al·ler·gen·ic (al-er-jen'ik). SYN antigenic.

al·ler·gic (ă-ler'jik). Relating to any response stimulated by an allergen.

al·ler·gic sa·lute. A characteristic wiping or rubbing of the nose with a transverse or upward movement of the hand, as seen in children with allergic rhinitis.

al·ler·gin (al'er-jin). A seldom used term denoting the reactive substance in the passive transference of anaphylaxis.

al·ler·gist (al'er-jist). One who specializes in the treatment of allergies.

al·ler·gi·za·tion (al'er-ji-zā'shŭn). Active sensitization as a result of allergens being naturally or artificially brought into contact with susceptible tissues; the procedure of being allergized.

al·ler·gized (al'er-jīzd). Specifically altered in reactivity; rendered capable of exhibiting one or another aspect of allergy.

al·ler·go·sis (al'er-gō'sis). Any abnormal condition characterized by allergy. [allergy + G. -osis, condition]

al·ler·gy (al'er-jē). **1.** Hypersensitivity caused by exposure to a particular antigen (allergen) resulting in a marked increase in reactivity to that antigen upon subsequent exposure sometimes resulting in harmful immunologic consequences. SYN acquired sensitivity, induced sensitivity. SEE ALSO allergic *reaction,* anaphylaxis, immune. **2.** That branch of medicine concerned with the study, diagnosis, and treatment of allergic manifestations. **3.** An acquired hypersensitivity to certain drugs and biologic materials. [G. *allos,* other, + *ergon,* work]

atopic a., SEE atopy.

bacterial a., (1) the concept that the atopic kind of type I allergic reactions may be caused by bacterial allergens; **(2)** the delayed type of skin test, so-called because of its early association with bacterial antigens (*e.g.,* the tuberculin test).

cold a., physical symptoms produced by hypersensitivity to cold.

contact a., SYN allergic contact *dermatitis.*

delayed a., a type IV allergic reaction; so called because in a sensitized subject the reaction becomes evident hours after contact with the allergen (antigen), reaches its peak after 36 to 48 hours, then recedes slowly. Associated with cell-mediated responses. SEE ALSO delayed *reaction.* Cf. immediate a.

drug a., sensitivity (hypersensitivity) to a drug or other chemical.

immediate a., a type I allergic reaction; so called because in a sensitized subject the reaction becomes evident usually within minutes after contact with the allergen (antigen), reaches its peak within an hour or so, then rapidly recedes. SEE ALSO immediate *reaction,* anaphylaxis. Cf. delayed a.

latent a., a. that causes no signs or symptoms but can be revealed by means of certain immunologic tests with specific allergens.

physical a., excessive response to factors in the environment such as heat or cold.

polyvalent a., allergic response manifested simultaneously for several or numerous specific allergens.

Al·les·che·ria boy·dii (al-es-kē'rē-ă boy'dē-ī). SYN *Pseudallescheria boydii.*

al·les·the·sia (al-es-thē'zē-ă). SYN allochiria. [G. *allos,* other, + *aisthēsis,* sensation]

al·le·thrins (al'ĕ-thrinz). Allethrolone esters of chrysanthemum-monocarboxylic acids and synthetic analogs of pyrethrins, which are pyrethrolone esters of the same acids; viscous liquids, insoluble in water, that can be absorbed by lungs, skin, and mucous membranes and may cause liver and kidney injury, with lung congestion; used as an insecticide.

al·leth·ro·lone (ă-leth'rō-lōn). 2-Methyl-4-oxo-3-(2-propenyl)-2-cyclopentenol; an analog of pyrethrolone (2-propenyl replacing the 2,4-pentadienyl group) used in allethrins.

al·lied health pro·fes·sion·al. An individual trained to perform services in the care of patients other than a physician or registered nurse; includes a variety of therapy technicians (*e.g.,* pulmonary), radiology technicians, physical therapists, etc.

al·li·ga·tion (al-i-gā'shŭn). A rule of mixtures whereby 1) the cost of a mixture may be determined, given the proportions and prices of the several ingredients; or 2) in pharmacy, the relative amounts of solutions of different percentages which must be taken to form a mixture of a given strength. [L. *alligatio,* fr. *al-ligo (adl-),* pp. *-atus,* to bind to]

food allergies percentage distribution of foods implicated in 600 cases of food allergy	
food	%
cow's milk	42.0
hen's eggs	
egg white	14.5
egg yolk	9.0
white and yolk	9.7
fish	11.0
citrus fruit	4.5
legumes	2.5
horse meat	1.5
meat	1.3
vegetables	1.0
onions	1.0
other (nuts, chocolate)	2.0

Allis, Oscar Huntington, U.S. surgeon, 1836–1921. SEE A. *forceps;* A.'s *sign.*

al·lit·er·a·tion (ă-lit-er-ā'shŭn). In psychiatry, a speech disturbance in which words commencing with the same sounds, usually consonants, are notably frequent. [Fr. *alliteration,* fr. L. *ad,* to, + *littera,* letter of alphabet]

al·li·um (al'ē-ŭm). *Allium sativum* (family Liliaceae), whose bulb contains up to 0.9% of volatile irritating oil with antiseptic action; has been used as a diaphoretic, diuretic, and expectorant. SYN garlic. [L.]

all or none. SEE Bowditch's *law.*

allo-. **1.** Other; differing from the normal or usual. **2.** Chemical prefix formerly used with amino acids whenever their side chain contained an asymmetric carbon; for example, the alloisoleucines and allothreonines. [G. *allos,* other]

al·lo·al·bu·mi·ne·mia (al'ō-al-byū'mi-nē'mē-ă) [MIM*103600]. The autosomal dominant condition of having serum albumin of a variant type that differs in mobility on electrophoresis from the usual type A; individuals are heterozygous or homozygous for one of the genes for variant albumin types, a genetic polymorphism without known clinical significance. SEE ALSO inherited albumin *variants,* under *variant.* [allo- + albumin + G. *haima,* blood, + -ia]

al·lo·an·ti·body (al-ō-an'ti-bod-ē). An antibody specific for an alloantigen. Isoantibody is sometimes used in this sense.

al·lo·an·ti·gen (al-ō-an'ti-jen). An antigen that occurs in some, but not in other members of the same species. Isoantigen is sometimes used in this sense.

al·lo·bar·bi·tal (al-ō-bar'bi-tal). 5,5-Diallylbarbituric acid; a hypnotic with intermediate duration of action.

al·lo·cen·tric (al-ō-sen'trik). Characterized by or denoting interest centered in other persons rather than in one's self. Cf. egocentric. SYN heterocentric (2). [allo- + G. *kentron,* center]

al·lo·che·zia, al·lo·che·tia (al-ō-kē'zē-ă, -kē'shē-ă). Obsolete term for passage of feces through a fistula or other false passage. [allo- + G. *chezō,* to defecate]

al·lo·chi·ria, al·lo·chei·ria (al'-ō-kī'rē-ă, al-ō-kī'rē-ă). A form of allachesthesia in which the sensation of a stimulus in one limb is referred to the contralateral limb. SYN allesthesia, alloesthesia, Bamberger's sign (2). [allo- + G. *cheir,* hand]

al·lo·cho·lane (al-ō-kō'lān). Original term for 5α-cholane.

al·lo·cho·les·ter·ol (al-ō-kō-les'ter-ol). cholest-4-en-3β-ol; an isomer of cholesterol, differing in the position of the one double bond. SYN coprostenol.

al·lo·chro·ic (al-ō-krō'ik). Changed or changeable in color; relating to allochroism.

al·lo·chro·ism (al-ō-krō'izm). A change or changeableness in color. [allo- + G. *chrōa,* color]

al·lo·chro·ma·sia (al-ō-krō-mā'zē-ă). Change of color of the skin or hair. [allo- + G. *chrōma,* color]

al·lo·cor·tex (al'ō-kōr'teks). O. Vogt's term denoting several regions of the cerebral cortex, in particular the olfactory cortex and the hippocampus, characterized by fewer cell layers than the isocortex; SEE ALSO cerebral *cortex.* SYN heterotypic cortex. [allo- + L. *cortex,* bark (cortex)]

α-al·lo·cor·tol (al-ō-kōr'tol). 5α-Pregnane-3α,11β,17,20α,21-pentaol; the 5α enantiomer of α-cortol; a metabolite of hydroxycortisone found in the urine.

β-al·lo·cor·tol. 5α-Pregnane-3α,11β,17,20β,21-pentaol; the 20β isomer of α-allocortol and 5α enantiomer of β-cortol; a metabolite of hydrocortisone found in urine.

α-al·lo·cor·to·lone (al-ō-kōr'tō-lōn). 3α,17,20α,21-Tetrahydroxy-5α-pregnane-11-one; the 5α enantiomer of α-cortolone; a metabolite of hydrocortisone found in urine.

β-al·lo·cor·to·lone. 3α,17,20β,21-Tetrahydroxy-5α-pregnane-11-one; the 20β isomer of α-allocortolone and 5α enantiomer of β-cortolone; a metabolite of hydrocortisone found in urine.

al·lo·de·oxy·cho·lic ac·id (al-ō-dē-oks'e-ko'lik). 3α,12α-dihydroxy-5α-cholan-24-oic acid, one of the bile acids.

al·lo·dip·loid (al-ō-dip'loyd). SEE alloploid.

al·lo·dyn·ia (al-ō-din'ē-ă). Condition in which ordinarily nonpainful stimuli evoke pain. [allo- + G. *odynē,* pain]

al·lo·e·rot·ic (al'ō-ĕ-rot'ik). Pertaining to or characterized by alloerotism. SYN heteroerotic.

al·lo·e·rot·i·cism (al'ō-ĕ-rot'i-sizm). SYN alloerotism.

al·lo·er·o·tism (al-ō-ār'ō-tizm). Sexual attraction toward another person. Cf. autoerotism. SYN alloeroticism, heteroerotism. [allo- + G. *erōs,* love]

al·lo·es·the·sia (al-ō-es-thē'zē-ă). SYN allochiria.

al·log·a·my (al-og'ă-mē). Fertilization of the ova of one individual by the spermatozoa of another. Cf. autogamy. [allo- + G. *gamos,* marriage]

al·lo·gen·ic, al·lo·ge·ne·ic (al-ō-jen'ik, -jĕ-nē'ik). Used in transplantation biology. It pertains to different gene constitutions within the same species; antigenically distinct.

al·lo·go·tro·phia (al'ō-gō-trō'fē-ă). Growth or nourishment of one part or tissue at the expense of another part of the body. [allo- + G. *trophē,* nourishment]

al·lo·graft (al'ō-graft). A graft transplanted between genetically nonidentical individuals of the same species. SYN allogeneic graft, homologous graft, homoplastic graft.

al·lo·group (al'ō-grūp). A term formerly used to denote a haplotype composed of closely linked allotypic markers.

al·lo·hex·a·ploid (al-ō-heks'ă-ployd). SEE alloploid.

allohy·drox·y·ly·sine (aHyl) (ă-lō-hī-drok-sē-lī-sēn). 5-allohydroxylysine; a stereoisomer of 5-hydroxylysine; D-a is the diastereoisomer of D-5-hydroxylysine.

al·lo·i·so·leu·cine (aIle) (ă-lō-ī-sō-lū'sēn). A stereoisomer of isoleucine; D-a. is the diastereoisomer of D-isoleucine.

al·lo·i·so·mer (al-ō-ī'sŏm-er). A geometric isomer.

al·lo·ker·a·to·plas·ty (al-ō-ker'ă-tō-plas-tē). Replacement of opaque corneal tissue with a transparent prosthesis, usually plastic.

al·lo·ki·ne·sis (al-ō-ki-nē'sis, -kī-nē'sis). Passive or reflex movement; nonvoluntary movement. [allo- + G. *kinēsis,* movement]

al·lo·lac·tose (ă-lō-lăk'tōs). A sugar, isomeric with lactose, that is the true inducer of the *lac* operon.

al·lo·la·lia (al-ō-lā'lē-ă). Any speech defect, especially one caused by a cerebral disorder. [allo- + G. *lalia,* talking]

al·lo·ma·le·ic ac·id (al-ō-mal'ē-ik). SYN fumaric acid.

al·lom·er·ism (ă-lom'er-izm). The state of differing in chemical composition but having the same crystalline form. [allo- + G. *meros,* part]

al·lom·e·tron (al-ō-me'tron). An evolutionary change in form or proportion of organic beings. [allo- + G. *metron,* measure]

al·lo·mones (ă-lō-mōn). A pheromone that induces a behavioral or physiologic change in a member of another species that is of benefit to the producer. Cf. kairomones, pheromones. [G. *allos,* other, + -mone]

al·lo·mor·phism (al-ō-mōr'fizm). 1. Change of shape in cells due to mechanical causes, such as flattening from pressure, or to progressive metaplasia, such as the change of bile duct cells into liver cells. 2. The state of being similar in chemical composition but differing in form (especially crystalline). [allo- + G. *morphē,* form]

al·longe·ment (al-onzh'-maw). Rarely used term for lengthening of a structure during an operation by appropriate incisions. [Fr. elongation]

al·lon·o·mous (ă-lon'ō-mŭs). Governed by external stimuli. [allo- + G. *nomos,* law]

al·lo·path (al'ō-path). 1. One who is a practitioner of allopathy. 2. Erroneously, a traditional medical physician, as distinguished from eclectic or homeopathic practitioners. SYN allopathist.

al·lo·path·ic (al-ō-path'ik). Relating to allopathy.

al·lop·a·thist (al-op'ă-thist). SYN allopath.

al·lop·a·thy (al-op'ă-thē). A therapeutic system in which a disease is treated by producing a second condition that is incompatible with or antagonistic to the first. Cf. homeopathy. SYN heteropathy (2), substitutive therapy. [allo- + G. *pathos,* suffering]

al·lo·pen·ta·ploid (al-ō-pent'ă-ployd). SEE alloploid.

al·lo·phan·a·mide (al'ō-fan-am'id). SYN biuret.

al·lo·phan·ic ac·id (al-ō-fan'ik). NH₂CONHCOOH; urea carbonic acid; its amide is biuret (allophanamide). SYN carbamoylcarbamic acid, *N*-carboxyurea.

al·loph·a·sis (al-of'ă-sis). Speech that is incoherent, disordered. [allo- + G. *phasis,* speech]

al·lo·phe·nic (al-ō-fē'nik). Pertaining to an animal with different cellular phenotypes produced by combining dividing fertilized eggs (blastomeres) of different genotypes (*i.e.,* from different pairs of parents). SEE ALSO mosaic. [allo- + G. *phainō,* to appear, + -ic]

al·lo·phore (al'ō-fōr). SYN erythrophore.

al·loph·thal·mia (al-of-thal'mē-ă). SYN heterophthalmus.

al·lo·pla·sia (al-ō-plā'zē-ă). SYN heteroplasia. [allo- + G. *plasis,* a molding]

al·lo·plast (al'ō-plast). 1. A graft of an inert metal or plastic material. 2. A relatively inert foreign body used for implantation into tissues. [allo- + G. *plastos,* formed]

al·lo·plas·ty (al'ō-plas-tē). Repair of defects by allotransplantation.

al·lo·ploid (al'ō-ployd). Relating to a hybrid individual or cell with two or more sets of chromosomes derived from two different ancestral species; depending on the number of multiples of haploid sets, a.'s are referred to as allodiploids, allotriploids, allotetraploids, allopentaploids, allohexaploids, etc. SEE ALSO heterokaryon. [allo- + -ploid]

al·lo·ploi·dy (al-ō-ploy'dē). The condition of being alloploid.

al·lo·pol·y·ploid (al-ō-pol'i-ployd). An alloploid having three or more haploid sets of chromosomes. [allo- + polyploid]

al·lo·pol·y·ploi·dy (al-ō-pol'i-ploy-dē). The condition of being allopolyploid.

al·lo·preg·nane (al-ō-preg'nān). Original name for 5α-pregnane. SEE pregnane.

α-al·lo·preg·nane·di·ol (al'ō-preg-nān-dī'ol). 5α-Pregnane-3α,20α-diol; a metabolite of progesterone and adrenocortical hormones, found in urine.

β-al·lo·preg·nane·di·ol. The 5α-pregnane-3β,20α(and β)-diols; both are metabolites of progesterone and adrenocortical hormones; found in urine.

al·lo·psy·chic (al-ō-sī'kik). Denoting the mental processes in their relation to the outer world. [allo- + G. *psychē,* mind]

al·lo·pu·ri·nol (al-ō-pyū′ri-nol). 4-Hydroxypyrazolo-[3,4-*d*]-pyrimidine; inhibitor of xanthine oxidase to inhibit uric acid formation; used in the treatment of gout and to retard the rapid metabolic degradation of 6-mercaptopurine.

al·lo·rhyth·mia (al-ō-rith′mē-ă). An irregularity in the cardiac rhythm that repeats itself any number of times. [allo- + G. *rhythmos*, rhythm]

al·lo·rhyth·mic (al-ō-rith′mik). Relating to or characterized by allorhythmia.

al·lose (al′ōs). $C_6H_{12}O_6$; an aldohexose. D-A. is epimeric with D-glucose.

al·lo·sen·si·ti·za·tion (al′ō-sen′si-ti-zā-shun). Exposure to an alloantigen that induces immunological memory cells.

al·lo·some (al′ō-sōm). One of the chromosomes differing in appearance or behavior from the autosomes and sometimes unequally distributed among the germ cells. SYN heterochromosome, heterotypical chromosome. [allo- + G. *sōma*, body]

paired a., SYN diplosome.

unpaired a., SYN accessory *chromosome*.

al·lo·ste·ric (al-ō-stār′ik). Pertaining to or characterized by allosterism.

al·lo·ster·ism, al·lo·ste·ry (ă-los′ter-izm, -los′ter-ē). The influencing of an enzyme activity, or the binding of a ligand to a protein, by a change in the conformation of the protein, brought about by the binding of a substrate or other effector at a site (allosteric site) other than the active site of the protein. Cf. cooperativity, hysteresis.

al·lo·tet·ra·ploid (al-ō-tet′ră-ployd). SEE alloploid. [allo- + tetraploid]

al·lo·therm (al′ō-therm). SYN poikilotherm. [allo- + G. *thermē*, heat]

al·lo·thre·o·nines (al-o-thrē′ō-nēnz). Two of the four diastereoisomers of threonine, differing from the L- and D-threonines in the configuration of the hydroxyl group in the side chain.

al·lo·tope (al′ō-tōp). The antigenic determinant of an allotype. [allo- + -tope]

al·lo·to·pia (al-ō-tō′pē-ă). SYN dystopia. [allo- + G. *topos*, place]

al·lo·trans·plan·ta·tion (al′ō-tranz-plan-ta′shŭn). Transplantation of an allograft. SYN homotransplantation.

al·lo·trich·ia cir·cum·scrip·ta (al-ō-trik′ē-ă ser-kŭm-skrip′tă). SYN woolly-hair *nevus*. [allo- + G. *thrix*, hair, + L. *circumscriptio*, a boundary]

al·lot·ri·o·don·tia (al-ot′rē-ō-don′shē-ă). 1. Growth of a tooth in some abnormal location. 2. Transplantation of teeth. [G. *allotrios*, foreign, + *odous* (*odont-*), tooth]

al·lot·ri·o·geu·stia (al-ot′rē-ō-gū′stē-ă). Perverted taste for innutritious or unusual substances. [G. *allotrios*, foreign, + *geusis*, taste]

al·lot·ri·oph·a·gy (al-ot-rē-of′ă-jē). The habit of eating innutritious or unusual substances. SEE ALSO pica. [G. *allotrios*, foreign, + *phagō*, to eat]

al·lot·ri·os·mia (al-ot-rē-oz′mē-ă). Incorrect recognition of odors. SYN heterosmia. [G. *allotrios*, foreign, + *osmē*, smell]

al·lo·trip·loid (al-ō-trip′loyd). SEE alloploid. [allo + triploid]

al·lo·trope (al′ō-trōp). A substance in one of the allotropic forms that the element may assume. [allo- + G. *tropos*, a turning]

al·lo·tro·phic (al-o-trō′fik). Having an altered nutritive value. [allo- + G. *trophē*, nourishment]

al·lo·tro·pic (al-ō-trop′ik). 1. Relating to allotropism. 2. Denoting a type of personality characterized by a preoccupation with the reactions of others.

al·lot·ro·pism, al·lot·ro·py (ă-lot′rō-pizm, -lot′rō-pē). The existence of certain elements, in several forms differing in physical properties; *e.g.,* carbon black, graphite, and diamond are all pure carbon. [allo- + G. *tropos*, a turning]

al·lo·type (al′ō-tīp). Any one of the genetically determined antigenic differences within a given class of immunoglobulin that occur among members of the same species. SEE ALSO antibody. SYN allotypic marker. [allo- + G. *typos*, model]

Gm a.'s (ăl′lō-tīps), refers to human immunoglobulin gamma heavy chains that express different Gm allotypic determinants

(antigens). Each of the 25 different Gm a.'s is the product of genes within the constant regions of the human gamma heavy chain.

InV a.'s (ăl′lō-tīps), SYN Km a.'s.

Km a.'s (ăl′lō-tīp), refers to human kappa immunoglobulin light chains that express different Km allotypic determinants (antigens). SYN InV a.'s.

al·lo·typ·ic (al-ō-tip′ik). Pertaining to an allotype.

al·low·ance (a′lau-antz). 1. Permission. 2. A portion allotted.

recommended daily a. (RDA), the amount of daily nutrient intake judged to be adequate for the maintenance of good nutrition in an average adult.

al·lox·an (ă-loks′-an). An oxidation product of uric acid, 2,4,5,6-pyrimidinetetrone; administration to experimental animals causes hypoglycemia due to insulin liberation, followed by hyperglycemia due to destruction of the islets of Langerhans (alloxan diabetes).

al·lox·an·tin (ă-loks′an-tin). A condensation product of two molecules of alloxan, formed in the presence of reducing agents; a diabetogenic. SYN uroxin.

al·lox·a·zine (ă-loks′ă-zēn). Isomer of isoalloxazine.

al·lox·u·re·mia (al-oks-yū-rē′mē-ă, al-ok-sū-rē′mē-ă). The presence of purine bases in the blood. [alloxan + G. *haima*, blood]

al·lox·u·ria (al-oks-yū′rē-ă, al-ok-sū′rē-ă). The presence of purine bodies in the urine. [alloxan + G. *ouron*, urine]

al·loy (al′oy). A substance composed of a mixture of two or more metals.

chrome-cobalt a.'s, a.'s of cobalt and chromium containing molybdenum and/or tungsten plus trace elements; used in dentistry for denture bases and frameworks, and other structures.

eutectic a., an a., generally brittle and subject to tarnish and corrosion, with a fusion temperature lower than that of any of its components; used in dentistry mainly in solders.

gold a., an a. whose principal ingredient is gold, usually contains copper or platinum and silver; used in dentistry for restorations requiring considerable strength.

Raney a., an a. of Ni and Al in equal proportions, used in the preparation of Raney Nickel.

silver-tin a., any a. of silver and tin; commonly 3 parts Ag and 1 part Sn, forming Ag_3Sn, the chief intermetallic compound in dental amalgam.

all-*trans*-ret·i·nal. The orange retinaldehyde resulting from the action of light on the rhodopsin of the retina, which converts the 11-*cis*-retinal component of the rhodopsin to all-*trans*-retinal plus opsin. SYN *trans*-retinal, visual yellow.

all·spice oil (awl′spīs). SYN *pimenta* oil.

al·lu·lose (al′yū-lōs). Obsolete term for psicose.

al·lyl (al′il). 2-Propenyl; the monovalent radical, $CH_2=CHCH_2—$.

a. alcohol, $CH_2=CHCH_2OH$; 2-propenol; a colorless liquid of pungent odor used in making resins and plasticizers; highly irritating to mucous membranes and readily absorbed, causing depression and coma. SYN vinyl carbinol.

a. cyanide, $CH_2=CHCH_2CN$; 3-butenenitrile; found in some mustard oils.

a. isothiocyanate, $CH_2=CH–CH_2–NCS$; volatile mustard CH–allylisosulfocyanate; isothiocyanic allyl ester; obtained from *Brassica nigra* or produced synthetically; a vesicant, used in 10% solution in 50% alcohol as a counterirritant in neuralgia. Gives mustard its characteristics flavor and aroma. SEE ALSO mustard oil. SYN volatile mustard oil.

a. sulfide, $(CH_2=CHCH_2)S$; diallyl sulfide; thioallyl ether; "oil garlic"; a constituent of garlic oil used in the manufacture of flavors.

al·lyl·a·mine (al-il-am′ēn). $CH_2=CH–CH_2–NH_2$; 3-Aminopropylene; a colorless liquid derived from crude oil of mustard and used in the pharmaceutical industry, *e.g.,* in the manufacture of mercurial diuretics.

al·lyl·bar·bi·tal (al-il-bar′bi-tal). SYN butalbital.

al·lyl·es·tre·nol (al-il-es′trĕ-nol). 17-Allylestr-4-en-17β-ol; a progestational agent.

al·lyl·mer·cap·to·meth·yl·pen·i·cil·lin (al'il-mer-kap'tō-meth'-il-pen-i-sil'in). SYN *penicillin* O.

N-al·lyl·nor·mor·phine (al'il-nor-mor'fēn). SYN nalorphine.

al·ly·sines (al'i-sēnz). Two or more six-carbon α-amino acids connected by a carbon-carbon bond; constituents of connective tissue and other structural elements. SEE ALSO desmins.

Almeida, Floriano Paulo de, Brazilian physician, *1898. SEE A.'s *disease;* Lutz-Splendore-A. *disease.*

Almén, August Teodor, Swedish physiologist, 1833–1903. SEE A.'s *test* for blood.

al·mond oil (aw'mŭnd, awl'mŭnd). A fixed oil expressed from sweet almonds, the kernels of varieties of *Prunus amygdalus;* used in ointments.

bitter a. o., a volatile oil from the dried ripe kernels of bitter almonds and from other kernels containing amygdalin; it contains between 2 and 4% of hydrocyanic acid and 95% of benzaldehyde.

al·oe (al'ō). 1. The dried juice from the leaves of plants of the genus *Aloe* (family Liliaceae), from which are derived aloin, resin, emodin, and volatile oils. 2. The dried juice from the leaves of *Aloe perryi* (socotrine a.'s), of *A. barbadensis* (Barbados and Curaçao a.'s), or of *A. capensis* (Cape a.'s); used as a purgative; used topically in cosmetics where it has no demonstrated value.

al·oe-em·o·din (al'ō-em'ō-din). 1,8-dihydroxy-3-(hydroxymethyl)anthraquinone; 3-hydroxymethylchrysazin; the trimethyl ether of emodin; used as a laxative. SEE aloin, emodin. SYN rhabarberone.

al·o·e·tin (al-ō-ē'tin). SYN aloin.

alo·gia (ă-lō'jē-ă). 1. SYN aphasia. 2. Inability to speak due to mental deficiency or an episode of dementia. [G. *a-* priv. + *logos,* speech]

al·o·in (al'ō-in). 1,8-dihydroxy-3-hydroxymethyl-10-(6-hydroxymethyl-3,4,5-tr ihydroxy-2-pyranyl)anthrone; 10-(1',5'-anhydroglucosyl)-aloe-emodin-9- anthrone; a yellow crystalline principle made up of aloe-emodin and glucose, obtained from aloe; used as a laxative. SYN aloetin, barbaloin.

al·o·pe·cia (al-ō-pē'shē-ă). Loss of hair. SYN acomia, baldness, calvities, pelade. [G. *alōpekia,* a disease like fox mange, fr. *alōpēx,* a fox]

a. adnata, underdevelopment of the lashes. SEE ALSO a. congenitalis. SYN madarosis.

androgenic a., gradual decrease of scalp hair density in adults with transformation of terminal to vellus hairs which become lost as a result of familial increase susceptibility of hair follicles to androgen secretion following puberty. Two areas of the scalp are commonly affected in men; when it occurs in females it is associated with other evidence of excessive androgen activity, such as hirsutism. SEE female pattern a., male pattern a. SYN a. hereditaria, common baldness, patterned a.

a. area'ta [MIM*104000], a condition of undetermined etiology characterized by circumscribed, nonscarring, usually asymmetrical areas of baldness on the scalp, eyebrows, and bearded portion of the face. Hairy skin anywhere on the body may be affected; occasionally follows an autosomal dominant inheritance. Slow enlargement but eventual regrowth within one year is common, but relapse is frequent and progression to a. totalis may occur, especially with childhood onset.

a. cap'itis tota'lis, SYN a. totalis.

a. cel'si, obsolete term for a. areata.

Celsus' a., obsolete term for a. areata.

cicatricial a., SYN scarring a. [L. *cicatrix, cicatricis,* scar + suffix *-al,* characterized by]

a. cicatrisa'ta, SYN scarring a.

a. circumscrip'ta, obsolete term for a. areata.

a. congenita'lis [MIM*104130], absence of all hair at birth, associated with psychomotor epilepsy; autosomal dominant inheritance. SYN congenital baldness, hypotrichiasis (2).

congenital sutural a., SYN *dyscephalia* mandibulo-oculofacialis.

a. dissemina'ta, loss of hair from all parts of the body.

female pattern a., diffuse partial hair loss in the centroparietal

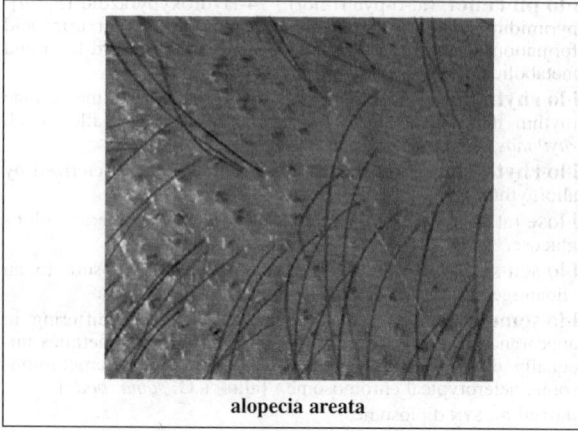
alopecia areata

area of the scalp, with preservation of the frontal and temporal hair lines; the most frequent type of androgenic a. in women.

a. follicula'ris, SYN *folliculitis* decalvans.

a. heredita'ria [MIM*109200], SYN androgenic a.

Jonston's a., obsolete term for a. areata.

a. leproti'ca, thinning or total loss of the lateral third of the eyebrows, eyelashes, and body hairs, seen in leprosy; loss of scalp hair is rare.

a. limina'ris fronta'lis, SYN a. marginalis.

lipedematous a., a. with itching, soreness, or tenderness of the scalp in adult negro women; the scalp is thickened and soft, subcutaneous fat is increased, and the hair is sparse and short.

male pattern a., the most common form of androgenic a., seen in men as receding frontal and bilateral triangular temple hair lines, and a balding patch on the vertex, which may progress to complete a. SYN male pattern baldness.

a. margina'lis, hair loss at the hair line, a condition most commonly seen in blacks; commonly transient and caused by chronic traction, although long-continued traction may cause permanent a. SYN a. liminaris frontalis.

a. medicamento'sa, diffuse hair loss, most notably of the scalp, caused by administration of various types of drugs.

moth-eaten a., patchy hair loss of parietal and occipital regions of the scalp, characteristic of secondary syphilis.

a. mucino'sa, follicular mucinosis with a. appearing in areas of erythema and edema in the bearded portion of the face or in the scalp.

a. neurot'ica, a. of trophoneurotic origin.

patterned a., SYN androgenic a.

a. pityro'des, a loss of hair, of the body as well as of the scalp, accompanied by an abundant branlike desquamation.

postoperative pressure a., loss of hair over a circumscribed area usually on the posterior scalp, resulting from continuous pressure on the occiput in a lengthy operative procedure, or unconsciousness following a drug overdose.

postpartum a., temporary diffuse telogen loss of scalp hair at the termination of pregnancy.

premature a., a. prematu'ra, male pattern baldness appearing at an unusually early age.

a. preseni'lis, ordinary or common baldness occurring in early or middle life without any apparent disease of the scalp.

pressure a., loss of hair over a circumscribed area usually on the posterior scalp, resulting from the continuous pressure on the occiput in a lengthy operative procedure, or unconsciousness following a drug overdose.

scarring a., a. in which hair follicles are irreversibly destroyed by scarring processes including trauma, burns, lupus erythematosus, lichen planopilaris, scleroderma, folliculitis decalvans, or of uncertain cause (pseudopelade). SYN a. cicatrisata, cicatricial a.

a. seni'lis, the normal loss of scalp hair in old age.

a. symptomat'ica, a. occurring in the course of various constitutional or local diseases, or following prolonged febrile illness.

a. syphilit′ica, moth-eaten a. of secondary syphilis.

a. tota′lis, total loss of hair of the scalp either within a very short period of time or from progression of localized a., especially a. areata. Cf. a. universalis. SYN a. capitis totalis.

a. tox′ica, hair loss attributed to febrile illness.

traction a., circumscribed or diffuse loss of hair resulting from repetitive traction on the hair by pulling or twisting; also occurs after excessive application of hair "softeners" such as permanent wave solutions or hot combs. A. marginalis is a form of traction a. SYN traumatic a.

traumatic a., SYN traction a.

a. triangularis (trī′ang-ū-la-ris), bilateral receding temporal hair lines in male pattern a.

a. triangula′ris congenita′lis, a congenital triangular patch of baldness on the frontal or temporal region of the scalp.

a. universa′lis, total loss of hair from all parts of the body. Cf. a. totalis.

al·o·pe·cic (al-ō-pē′sik). Relating to alopecia.

alox·i·prin (ă-lok′si-prin). A condensation product of aluminum oxide and aspirin, used as an analgesic.

Alpers, Bernard J., U.S. neurologist, 1900–1981. SEE A. *disease.*

al·pha (al′fă). First letter of the Greek alphabet, α.

al·pha am·y·lase. A starch-splitting enzyme obtained from a nonpathogenic bacterium of the *Bacillus subtilis* class, used in the treatment of inflammatory conditions and edema of soft tissues associated with traumatic injury; its therapeutic usefulness has not been fully established and its mode of action is not known.

al·pha-block·er (al′fă-blok′er). SYN α-adrenergic blocking *agent.*

al·pha·di·one (al-fă-dī′ōn). An intravenous anesthetic containing two steroids, alfaxalone, and alfadolone acetate, dissolved in 20% polyoxyethylated castor oil.

al·pha·pro·dine (al-fă-prō′dēn). α-1,3-Dimethyl-4-phenyl-4-piperidinyl propionate; a narcotic analgesic related to meperidine; physical and psychic dependence may develop.

al·pha·sone ac·e·to·phe·nide (al′fă-sōn). SYN algestone acetophenide.

Al·pha·vi·rus (al′fă-vī-rŭs). One of the genera of the family Togaviridae that was formerly classified as part of the "group A" arboviruses and includes the viruses that cause eastern equine, western equine, and Venezuelan encephalitis.

al·phos (al′fos). Obsolete term for psoriasis. [G. *alphos,* leprosy]

al·pi·dem (al-pī′dem). A benzodiazepine anxiolytic/sedative/hypnotic.

Alport, Arthur Cecil, South African physician, 1880–1959. SEE A.'s *syndrome.*

al·praz·o·lam (al-praz′ō-lam). A benzodiazepine minor tranquilizer used for management of anxiety disorders and panic attack; abuse may lead to habituation or addiction.

al·pren·o·lol hy·dro·chlo·ride (al-pren′ō-lol). The hydrochloride salt of 1-(*o*-allylphenoxy)-3-(isopropylamino)propan-2-ol; a β-receptor blocking agent, used for the treatment of cardiac arrhythmias.

al·pros·ta·dil (al-pros′tă-dil). 11,15-dihydroxy-9-oxoprost-13-en-1-oic acid; a vasodilator used for palliative therapy to temporarily maintain patency of the ductus arteriosus in neonates with congenital heart defects. SYN prostaglandin E_1.

ALS Abbreviation for amyotrophic lateral *sclerosis*; antilymphocyte *serum.*

al·ser·ox·y·lon (al′ser-ok′si-lon). A fat-soluble alkaloidal fraction extracted from the root of *Rauwolfia serpentina*, containing reserpine and other nonadrenolytic amorphous alkaloids; used as a sedative in psychoses, in mild hypertension, and as an adjunct to more potent hypotensive drugs.

Alström, Carl-Henry, Swedish geneticist, *1907. SEE A.'s *syndrome.*

ALT Abbreviation for alanine aminotransferase.

al·ter·a·tion (awl-ter-ā′shŭn). **1.** A change. **2.** A changing; a making different.

modal a., in electric irritability, a change in the mode of response of degenerated muscle to electric stimulation, the contraction being sluggish instead of quick.

qualitative a., in electric irritability, a change in which the muscle contracts as readily on application of the anode as on that of the cathode.

quantitative a., in electric irritability, a gradual loss of contractility in a muscle in response to static, faradic, and galvanic currents successively.

al·ter·e·go·ism (awl-ter-ē′gō-izm). Identification with people of similar personality to one's own.

al·ter·nans (awl-ter′nanz). Alternating; often used substantively for alternation of the heart, either electrical or mechanical. [L.]

auditory a., SYN auscultatory a.

auscultatory a., alternation in the intensity of heart sounds or murmurs in the presence of a regular cardiac rhythm as a result of alternation of the heart. SYN auditory a.

concordant a., simultaneous occurrence of right ventricular and pulmonary artery a. with left ventricular and peripheral pulsus a.

discordant a., presence of right ventricular and pulmonary artery a. with peripheral pulsus a., but with the strong beat of the right ventricle coinciding with the weak beat of the left and vice versa.

electrical a., electrical alternation of the heart.

Al·ter·nar·ia (al-ter-nā′rē-ă). A genus of fungi easily isolated from air and considered to be a common laboratory contaminant and an allergen; occasionally pathogenic in humans.

al·ter·na·tion (awl-ter-nā′shŭn). The occurrence of two things or phases in succession and recurrently; used interchangeably with alternans.

cardiac a., the occurrence of any cardiac phenomenon every other beat.

concordant a., a. in either the mechanical or electrical activity of the heart, occurring in both systemic and pulmonary circulations.

discordant a., a. in cardiac activities of either the systemic or the pulmonary circulations, but not of both, or in both but oppositely directed in each.

electrical a. of heart, a disorder in which the ventricular or atrial complexes or both are regular in time but of alternating pattern; detected by electrocardiography. The P, QRS, T, QRS-T, or P-QRST alternate singly or in combination.

a. of generations, a succession of generations of individuals like and unlike the original parents, or an a. of sexual and nonsexual generations.

mechanical a. of the heart, disorder in which contractions of the heart are regular but are alternately stronger and weaker.

al·ter·na·tor (awl′ter-nā-ter). Mechanical apparatus with movable transparent racks to which a large number of radiographs can be attached, to enable selection and viewing in front of a stationary bank of lights. [L. *alterno,* to do by turns, fr. *alter,* either of two]

al·ter·noc·u·lar (awl-ter-nok′yū-lăr). Denoting the use of each eye separately instead of binocularly. [L. *alternus,* by turns, + ocular]

al·te·ro·mo·nas. A Gram-negative bacteria that has curved rods and is motile by means of a single polar flagellum. It requires a seawater base for growth.

A. *putrefa′ciens,* a marine species implicated as a cause of fish spoilage but rarely as a human pathogen.

al·thea (al-thē′ă). Derived from *Althaea officinalis*, a perennial herb which is found wild in moist places in Europe. Contains a high proportion of starches, pectin, and sugars; used as a flavor and demulcent. SYN marshmallow root. [L., fr. G. *althaia,* marshmallow]

Altherr, Franz. SEE Meyenburg-A.-Uehlinger *syndrome.*

alt. hor. Abbreviation for L. *alternis horis,* every other hour.

al·ti·tu·di·nal (al-ti-tū′di-năl). Relating to vertical relationships; *e.g.,* a. hemianopsia.

Altmann, Richard, German histologist, 1852–1900. SEE A.'s *fixative, granule,* anilin-acid fuchsin *stain, theory;* A.-Gersh *method.*

al·tri·gen·drism (al-trī-jen′drizm). Natural, wholesome, nonerotic activity between the sexes. [L. *alter,* the other, + gender]

al·trose (al'trōs). An aldohexose isomeric with glucose, tallose, allose, etc. D-a. is epimeric with D-mannose.

al·um (al'ŭm). A double sulfate of aluminum and of an alkaline earth element or ammonium; chemically, an a. is any one of the markedly astringent double salts formed by a combination of a sulfate of aluminum, iron, manganese, chromium, or gallium with a sulfate of lithium, sodium, potassium, ammonium, cesium, or rubidium; used locally as styptics. [L. *alumen*]

burnt a., SYN dried a.

cake a., SYN *aluminum* sulfate octadecahydrate.

chrome a., the sulfate of chromium and potassium; used as a mordant in histologic staining.

dried a., a. deprived of its water of crystallization by heat; an astringent dusting powder. SYN burnt a.

exsiccated a., a. heated to complete dryness; a local astringent.

ferric a., SYN ferric ammonium sulfate.

whey a., an astringent and styptic preparation made by boiling a. (1 oz.) in milk (10 oz.).

al·um·he·ma·tox·y·lin (al'ŭm-hē-mă-tok'si-lin). A purple nuclear stain used in histology; a mixture of an aqueous solution of ammonium alum and an alcoholic solution of hematoxylin which is ripened or oxidized to hematein.

alu·mi·na (ă-lū'mi-nă). SYN *aluminum* oxide.

hydrated a., SYN *aluminum* hydroxide.

alu·mi·nat·ed (ă-lū'mi-nā-ted). Containing alum.

alu·mi·non (ă-lū'min-on). The ammonium salt of aurintricarboxylic acid, so-called because of its usefulness in the detection of aluminum in biologic material, foods, etc.

alu·mi·no·sis (ă-lū-min-ō'sis). A pneumoconiosis caused by inhalation of aluminum particles into the lungs.

alu·mi·num (Al) (ă-lū'min-ŭm). A white silvery metal of very light weight; atomic no. 13, atomic wt. 26.981539. Many salts and compounds are used in medicine and dentistry. [L. *alumen, alum*]

a. acetate, used as a disinfectant by embalmers; proposed as desiccant and deodorant powder for eczema and chronic skin ulcers.

a. acetotartrate, basic aluminum acetate (70%) and tartaric acid (30%); antiseptic.

a. acetylsalicylate, SYN a. aspirin.

a. ammonium sulfate, $AlNH_4(SO_4)_2$; an astringent.

a. aspirin, an analgesic and antipyretic. SYN a. acetylsalicylate.

a. bismuth oxide, SYN *bismuth* aluminate.

a. carbonate, basic, $Al_2O_3CO_2$; an a. hydroxide-carbonate complex consisting of white lumps, insoluble in water; aqueous suspensions bind phosphorus in the intestine and lower serum inorganic phosphorus resulting in an increase in reabsorption of phosphorus by renal tubules and reduction of urinary excretion of phosphorus; it reduces formation of phosphatic urinary calculi and gastric acidity.

a. chlorate nonahydrate, $Al(ClO_3)_3·9H_2O$; an antiseptic. SYN mallebrin.

a. chloride hexahydrate, $AlCl_3·6H_2O$; used as an astringent or antiseptic in solution.

a. diacetate, SYN a. subacetate.

a. hydrate, SYN a. hydroxide.

a. hydroxide, $Al(OH)_3$; an astringent dusting powder; also used internally as a mild astringent antacid. SYN a. hydrate, hydrated alumina.

a. hydroxide gel, a suspension containing Al_2O_3, mainly in the form of a. hydroxide, used as an antacid; a dried form, with the same use, is obtained by drying the product of interaction in aqueous solution of an a. salt with ammonium or sodium carbonate.

a. hydroxychloride, an antiperspirant.

a. magnesium silicate, SYN *magnesium* aluminum silicate.

a. monostearate, a compound of a. with a mixture of solid organic acids obtained from fats, and consisting chiefly of a. monostearate and a. monopalmitate; used as a suspending medium in pharmaceutical preparations.

a. nicotinate, tris(nicotinato)aluminum; a lipopenic agent with peripheral vasodilator action.

a. oleate, $Al(C_{18}H_{33}O_2)_3$; used as an ointment in certain cutaneous affections and in burns.

a. oxide, Al_2O_3; used as an abrasive, as a refractory, and in chromatography. SYN alumina.

a. penicillin, SEE aluminum *penicillin.*

a. phenolsulfonate, $Al(C_6H_4(OH)SO_3)_3$; antiseptic and astringent for local application, usually for cutaneous ulcers.

a. phosphate, $AlPO_4$; an infusible powder, insoluble in water but soluble in alkali hydroxides, used for dental cements with calcium sulfate and sodium silicate.

a. phosphate gel, an aqueous suspension of between 4.0 and 5.0% of a. phosphate; used as an antacid.

a. potassium sulfate, $AlK(SO_4)_2$; an astringent and styptic; also used in veterinary medicine for ulcerative stomatitis, leukorrhea, and conjunctivitis. SYN potassium alum.

a. salicylate, basic, used in the treatment of ozena and pharyngitis.

a. salicylate, basic, soluble, used in solution as a spray for diseases of the upper air passages.

a. silicate, SYN kaolin.

a. subacetate, $Al(CH_3CO_2)_2OH$; used in solution (as in Burow's solution) as an astringent, as an ingredient in mouthwashes, and in embalming fluids. SYN a. diacetate.

a. sulfate octadecahydrate, astringent detergent for skin ulcers. SYN cake alum.

alu·mi·num group. Aluminum, boron, gallium, indium, and thallium.

al·vei (al'vē-ī). Plural of alveus.

al·ve·o·al·gia (al'vē-ō-al'jē-ă). A postoperative complication of tooth extraction in which the blood clot in the socket disintegrates, resulting in focal osteomyelitis and severe pain. SYN alveolalgia, alveolar osteitis, dry socket. [alveolus + G. *algos,* pain]

al·ve·o·lal·gia (al'vē-ō-lal'jē-ă). SYN alveoalgia.

al·ve·o·lar (al-vē'ō-lăr). Relating to an alveolus.

al·ve·o·late (al-vē'ō-lāt). Pitted like a honeycomb. [L. *alveolus,* dim. of *alveus,* trough, hollow sac, cavity]

al·ve·o·lec·to·my (al'vē-ō-lek'tō-mē). Surgical excision of a portion of the dentoalveolar process, for recontouring of the alveolar ridge at the time of tooth removal to facilitate a dental prosthesis. [alveolus + G. *ektomē,* excision]

al·ve·o·li (al-vē'ō-lī). Plural of alveolus.

al·ve·o·lin·gual (al'vē-o-ling'gwăl). SYN alveololingual.

al·ve·o·li·tis (al'vē-ō-lī'tis). **1.** Inflammation of alveoli. **2.** Inflammation of a tooth socket.

acute pulmonary a., acute inflammation involving exudate into the pulmonary alveoli and impaired gas exchange; may result in necrosis with hemorrhage into the lungs; occurs in Goodpasture's syndrome, in association with a glomerulonephritis.

chronic fibrosing a., SYN idiopathic pulmonary *fibrosis.*

extrinsic allergic a., pneumoconiosis resulting from hypersensitivity due to repeated inhalation of organic dust, usually specified according to occupational exposure; in the acute form, respiratory symptoms and fever start several hours after exposure to the dust; in the chronic form, there is eventual diffuse pulmonary fibrosis after exposure over several years.

fibrosing a., SYN usual interstitial *pneumonia* of Liebow.

alveolo-. An alveolus, the alveolar process; alveolar. [L. *alveolus,* a concave vessel, a bowl, a basin, fr. *alveus,* a trough, + *-olus,* small, little; akin to *alvus,* the belly, the womb]

al·ve·o·lo·cla·sia (al-vē'ō-lō-klā'zē-ă). Destruction of the alveolus. [alveolo- + G. *klasis,* breaking]

al·ve·o·lo·den·tal (al-vē'ō-lō-den'tăl). Relating to the alveoli and the teeth.

al·ve·o·lo·la·bi·al (al-vē'ō-lō-lā'bē-ăl). Relating to the labial or vestibular (outer) surface of the alveolar processes of the upper or lower jaw.

al·ve·o·lo·la·bi·a·lis (al-vē'ō-lō-lā-bē-ā'lis). Relating to the alveololabial groove or region. [L.]

al·ve·o·lo·lin·gual (al-vē'ō-lō-ling'gwăl). Relating to the lingual (inner) surface of the alveolar process of the lower jaw. SYN alveolingual.

al·ve·o·lo·pal·a·tal (al-vē′ō-lō-pal′ă-tăl). Relating to the palatal surface of the alveolar process of the upper jaw.

al·ve·o·lo·plas·ty (al-vē′ō-lō-plas-tē). Surgical preparation of the alveolar ridges for the reception of dentures; shaping and smoothing of socket margins after extraction of teeth with subsequent suturing to insure optimal healing. SYN alveoplasty. [alveolo- + G. *plassō*, to form]

interradicular a., intraseptal a., removal of the interradicular bone and collapsing of the cortical plates to a more desirable alveolar contour.

al·ve·o·los·chi·sis (al-vē-ō-los′ki-sis). A cleft of the alveolar process. [alveolo- + G. *schisis,* cleaving]

al·ve·o·lot·o·my (al-vē-ō-lot′ō-mē). Surgical opening into a dental alveolus to allow drainage of pus from a periapical or other intraosseous abscess. [alveolo- + G. *tomē,* incision]

al·ve·o·lus, gen. and pl. **al·ve·o·li** (al-vē′ō-lŭs, -ō-lī) [NA]. A small cell, cavity, or socket. **1.** SYN pulmonary a. **2.** One of the terminal secretory portions of an alveolar or racemose gland. **3.** One of the honeycomb pits in the wall of the stomach. **4.** SYN tooth *socket.* [L. dim. of *alveus,* trough, hollow sac, cavity]

a. dentalis, pl. **alveoli dentales** [NA], SYN tooth *socket.*

pulmonary a., one of the thin-walled saclike terminal dilations of the respiratory bronchioles, alveolar ducts, and alveolar sacs across which gas exchange occurs between alveolar air and the pulmonary capillaries. SYN alveoli pulmonis [NA], alveolus (1) [NA], air cells (1), air vesicles, bronchic cells.

alveoli pulmo′nis [NA], SYN pulmonary a.

al·ve·o·plas·ty (al′vē-ō-plas-tē). SYN alveoloplasty.

al·ve·us, pl. **al·vei** (al′vē-ŭs, -vē-ī). A channel or trough. [L. tray, trough, cavity, fr. *alvus,* belly]

a. hippocam′pi [NA], SYN a. of hippocampus.

a. of hippocampus, a thin white band of fornix fibers covering the ventricular surface of the hippocampus. SYN a. hippocampi [NA].

a. urogenita′lis, obsolete term for prostatic *utricle.*

al·vin·o·lith (al-vin′ō-lith, al-vī′nō-lith). Obsolete term for coprolith. [L. *alvus,* belly, + G. *lithos,* stone]

A.L.W. Abbreviation for arch-loop-whorl *system.*

alym·phia (ă-lim′fē-ă). Absence or deficiency of lymph. [G. *a-* priv + lymph +-ia]

alym·pho·cy·to·sis (ă-lim′fō-sī-tō′sis). Absence or great reduction of lymphocytes.

alym·pho·pla·sia (ă-lim-fō-plā′zē-ă). Obsolete term for aplasia or hypoplasia of lymphoid tissue.

Nezelof type of thymic a., SYN cellular *immunodeficiency* with abnormal immunoglobulin synthesis.

thymic a., hypoplasia with absence of Hassall's corpuscles and deficiency of lymphocytes in the thymus and usually in lymph nodes, spleen, and gastrointestinal tract; there is peripheral lymphopenia and often hypogammaglobulinemia and absence of plasma cells; presents in early infancy with respiratory infections and leads to death within a few months. SEE ALSO *immunodeficiency* with hypoparathyroidism.

Alzheimer, Alois, German neurologist, 1864–1915. SEE A.'s *dementia, disease, sclerosis.*

Am Symbol for americium.

am Abbreviation for ammeter.

AMA. Abbreviation for American Medical Association.

am·a·crine (am′ă-krin). **1.** A cell or structure lacking a long, fibrous process. **2.** Denoting such a cell or structure. SEE ALSO amacrine *cell.* [G. *a-* priv. + *makros,* long, + *is* (*in-*), fiber]

am·a·dou (ahm′ah-dū). SYN agaric. [Fr.]

amal·gam (ă-mal′gam). An alloy of an element or a metal with mercury. In dentistry, primarily of two types: silver-tin alloy, containing small amounts of copper, zinc and perhaps other metals, and a second type containing more copper (12 to 30% by weight); they are used for restoring teeth and making dies. [G. *malagma,* a soft mass]

pin a., an a. restoration held in place largely by small metal rods protruding from holes drilled into tooth structure.

spherical a., an alloy for dental a. composed of spherical particles instead of filings.

amal·ga·mate (ă-mal′gă-māt). To make an amalgam.

amal·ga·ma·tion (ă-mal-gă-mā′shŭn). The process of combining mercury with a metal or an alloy to form a new alloy.

amal·ga·ma·tor (ă-mal′gă-mā-tŏr). A device for combining mercury with a metal or an alloy to form a new alloy.

Am·a·ni·ta (am-ă-nī′tă). A genus of fungi, many members of which are highly poisonous. [G. *amanitai,* fungi]

A. musca′ria, ha toxic species of mushroom with yellow to red pileus and white gills; it contains muscarine, which produces psychosis-like states and other symptoms. SYN fly agaric.

A. phalloi′des, a species containing poisonous principles, including phalloidin and amanitin, that cause gastroenteritis, hepatic necrosis, and renal necrosis. SYN deadly agaric.

α-am·a·ni·tin (am-ă-nī′tin). A highly toxic, heat-stable bicyclic oligopeptide in *Amanita phalloides*. It inhibits transcription by certain RNA polymerases.

aman·ta·dine hy·dro·chlo·ride (ă-man′tă-dēn). 1-Adamantanamine; an antiviral agent used for influenza; also used to treat parkinsonism where it increases dopamine release and reduces its reuptake into dopaminergic nerve terminals of substantia nigra neurons.

am·a·ra (ă-mah′ră). SYN bitters (2). [neut. pl. of L. *amarus,* bitter]

am·a·ranth, am·a·ran·thum (am′ă-ranth, am-ă-ran′thŭm) [C.I. 16185]. 1-(4-sulfo-1-naphthylazo)-2-naphthol-3,6-disulfonate (trisodium salt); an azo dye; a soluble reddish brown powder, the color turning to magenta red in solution; used as a food and cosmetic coloring agent, and occasionally in histology. [G. *amaranthon,* a never-fading flower]

am·a·rine (am′ă-rin). A name applied to various bitter principles derived from plants, especially to a poisonous substance, 2,4,5-triphenylimidazoline, obtained from oil of bitter almond. [L. *amarus,* bitter]

am·a·roid (am′ă-royd). A bitter extractive that does not belong to the class of glycosides, alkaloids, or any of the known proximate principles of plants. [L. *amarus,* bitter, + G. *eidos,* like]

am·a·roi·dal (am-ă-roy′dăl). Resembling bitters; having a slightly bitter taste.

ama·rum (ă-mah′rŭm). One of a class of vegetable drugs of bitter taste, such as gentian and quassia, used as appetizers and tonics. [neut. of L. *amarus,* bitter]

amas·tia (ă-mas′tē-ă). Absence of the breasts. SYN amazia. [G. *a-* priv. + *mastos,* breast]

amas·ti·gote (ă-mas′ti-gōt). SYN Leishman-Donovan *body.* [G. *a-* priv. + *mastix,* whip]

am·a·tho·pho·bia (ă-math-ō-fō′bē-ă). Morbid dread of dust or dirt. [G. *amathos,* dust, + *phobos,* fear]

am·a·tive·ness (ahm′ă-tiv-nes). Rarely used term for the propensity to love. [L. *amo,* pp. *amatus,* to love]

am·a·tox·in (am-a-tok′sin). One of a group of bicyclic octapeptides from *Amanita phalloides.*

am·au·ro·sis (am-aw-rō′sis). Blindness, especially that occurring without apparent change in the eye itself, as from a brain lesion. [G. *amauros,* dark, obscure, + *-osis,* condition]

a. congen′ita of Leber [MIM*204000 & MIM*204100], an autosomal recessive cone-rod abiotrophy causing blindness or severely reduced vision at birth.

a. fu′gax, a transient blindness that may result from a transient ischemia due to carotid artery insufficiency, retinal artery embolus, or to centrifugal force (visual blackout in flight).

pressure a., loss of vision occurring a few seconds after intraocular pressure exceeds systolic pressure of retinal arteries.

toxic a., blindness due to optic neuritis caused by methyl alcohol, lead, arsenic, quinine, or other poisons.

am·au·rot·ic (am-aw-rot′ik). Relating to or suffering from amaurosis.

amax·o·pho·bia (ă-mak-sō-fō′bē-ă). Rarely used term for morbid fear of, or of riding in, a vehicle. SYN hamaxophobia. [G. *amaxa, hamaxa,* a carriage, + *phobos,* fear]

ama·zia (ă-mā′zē-ă). SYN amastia.

am·ba·geu·sia (am-bă-gū′sē-ă). Loss of taste from both sides of the tongue. [L. *ambo,* both, + G. *a-* priv. + *geusis,* taste]

Ambard, Léon, French pharmacologist, 1876–1962. SEE A.'s *constant, laws,* under *law.*

am·be·no·ni·um chlo·ride (am-bē-nō′nē-ŭm). *N,N′*-Bis-2-[(2-chlorobenzyl)diethylammonium chloride]ethyloxamide; a cholinesterase inhibitor similar to neostigmine in actions; used chiefly in the management of myasthenia gravis and occasionally for intestinal and urinary tract obstruction.

AMBER (am′ber) Acronym for advanced multiple-beam equalization *radiography.*

am·ber (am′ber). **1.** A hard, dark yellow to tan, fossilized resin derived from pine trees. **2.** SEE amber *codon.* [Ar. *anbar*]

Amberg, Emil, U.S. otologist, 1868–1948. SEE A.'s lateral sinus *line.*

am·ber·gris (am′ber-gris). A grayish pathologic secretion from the intestine of the sperm whale that occurs as a flammable waxy mass (melting point about 60°C), insoluble in water; contains cholesterol and benzoic acid, and is used as a base for perfume. [Mod. L. *ambra grisea,* gray amber]

△**ambi-**. Around; on all (both) sides; both, double; corresponds to G. amphi-. SEE ALSO ambo-. [L., around, about, akin to *ambo,* both]

am·bi·dex·ter·i·ty (am-bi-deks-ter′i-tē). The ability to use both hands with equal ease. SYN ambidextrism.

am·bi·dex·trism (am-bi-deks′trizm). SYN ambidexterity.

am·bi·dex·trous (am-bi-deks′trŭs). Having equal facility in the use of both hands.

am·bi·ent (am′bē-ent). Surrounding, encompassing; pertaining to the environment in which an organism or apparatus functions. [L. *ambiens,* going around]

am·big·u·ous (am-big′yū-ŭs). **1.** Having more than one interpretation. **2.** In anatomy, wandering; having more than one direction. **3.** In neuroanatomy, applied to a nucleus (nucleus ambiguus) supplying special visceral efferent fibers to vagus and glossopharyngeal nerves. [L. *ambiguus,* fr. *ambigo,* to wander]

am·bi·lat·er·al (am-bi-lat′er-ăl). Relating to both sides. [ambi- + L. *latus,* side]

am·bi·le·vous (am-bi-lē′vŭs). Awkwardness in the use of both hands. SYN ambisinister, ambisinistrous. [ambi- + L. *laevus,* left]

am·bi·sex·u·al (am-bi-seks′yū-ăl). **1.** denoting sexual characteristics found in both sexes, *e.g.,* breast, pubic hair. **2.** Slang term for bisexual.

am·bi·sin·is·ter (am-bi-sin′is-ter). SYN ambilevous. [ambi- + L. *sinister,* left]

am·bi·si·nis·trous (am′bi-sin′is-trŭs). SYN ambilevous.

am·biv·a·lence (am-biv′ă-lens). The coexistence of antithetical attitudes or emotions toward a given person or thing, or idea, as in the simultaneous feeling and expression of love and hate toward the same person. [ambi- + L. *valentia,* strength]

am·biv·a·lent (am-biv′ă-lent). Relating to or characterized by ambivalence.

am·bi·vert (am′bi-vert). One who falls between the two extremes of introversion and extroversion, possessing some of the tendencies of each.

△**ambly-**. Dullness, dimness; blunt, dull, dim, dimmed. [G. *amblys,* blunt, dulled; faint, dim]

am·bly·a·phia (am-bli-ā′fē-ă). Diminution in tactile sensibility. [ambly- + G. *haphē,* touch]

am·bly·geus·tia (am-bli-gūs′tē-ă). A dimunition in the sense of taste. [ambly- + G. *geusis,* taste]

Am·bly·om·ma (am-blē-om′ă). A genus of ornate, hard ticks (family Ixodidae) characterized by having eyes, festoons, and deeply imbedded ventral plates near the festoons in males. [ambly- + G. *omma,* eye, vision]

A. america′num, the Lone-Star tick, a species that is an important pest and vector of Rocky Mountain spotted fever, found primarily in the southern United States and northern Mexico; it

occurs on dogs and many other hosts, including domestic animals, birds, and man; it bites man in larval, nymphal, and adult stages.

A. cajennen′se, the Cayenne tick, a species that is an important pest in southern Texas, Central and South America, and the larger Caribbean islands, and a vector of Rocky Mountain spotted fever in Mexico and Central and South America; all stages attack man and many species of domestic and wild animals.

A. hebrae′um, the South African bont tick, an important vector of heartwater in southern Africa.

A. macula′tum, the Gulf Coast tick, a species that is a pest of livestock in the southeastern United States.

A. variega′tum, the tropical bont tick, a serious pest of domestic livestock and an important vector of heartwater in Africa and the Caribbean; it is closely associated with the development of severe clinical dermatophilosis in cattle in the Caribbean.

am·bly·o·pia (am-blē-ō′pē-ă). This ancient word has meant "impaired vision" for many centuries. As knowledge increased, it became reserved for cases with poor vision in one eye without detectable cause. In most recent decades, as there came to be more discussion of "suppression amblyopia" in childhood, and as other causes of poor vision in one eye became evident, the word amblyopia has become almost synonymous with suppression amblyopia. [G. *amblyōpia,* dimness of vision, fr. *amblys* dull, + *ōps,* eye]

anisometropic a., a suppression of central vision due to an unequal refractive error (anisometropia) of at least two diopters. This induces a sufficient difference in image size (aniseikonia) that the two images cannot be fused. In order to avoid confusion, the blurrier image is suppressed. SYN refractive a.

deprivation a., SYN sensory a.

a. ex anop′sia, SYN suppression a.

hysterical a., functional visual loss.

nocturnal a., SYN nyctalopia.

nutritional a., a. resulting from lack of vitamin B-complex constituents.

refractive a., SYN anisometropic a.

sensory a., a suppression of central vision in one eye due to faulty image formation; for example, by a corneal scar, a cataract, or a droopy eyelid. SYN deprivation a.

strabismic a., a suppression of central vision due to the two eyes pointing in different directions. The two scenes cannot be fused into a single image, so, to avoid confusion, one of the images is suppressed.

suppression a., suppression of the central vision in one eye when the images from the two eyes are so different that they cannot be fused into one. This may be due to: 1) faulty image formation (sensory a.); 2) a large difference in refraction between the two eyes (anisometropic a.); or 3) the two eyes pointing in different directions (strabismic a.). Most suppression a. can be reversed if appropriately treated before age 6 years. SYN a. ex anopsia.

toxic a., SEE toxic *amaurosis.*

am·bly·o·pic (am-blē-ō′pik). Relating to, or suffering from, amblyopia.

am·bly·o·scope (am′blē-ō-skōp). A reflecting stereoscope used to evaluate or stimulate binocular vision. SEE ALSO haploscope. [amblyopia + G. *skopeō,* to view]

major a., an a. in which intensity of illumination as well as targets may be varied.

Worth's a., the original a.; a hand-held a. consisting of angled tubes that can be swiveled to any degree of convergence or divergence.

△**ambo-**. Around; on all (both) sides; corresponds to G. ampho-. SEE ALSO ambi-. [L. *ambo,* both]

am·bo·cep·tor (am′bō-sep-tŏr). Ehrlich's term for his concept, now obsolete, of the structure of complement-fixing antibody; now used chiefly to denote the anti-sheep erythrocyte antibody used in the hemolytic system of complement-fixation tests. [ambo- + L. *capio,* to take]

am·bo·mal·le·al (am-bō-mal′ē-ăl). SYN incudomallealear.

am·bos (am′bōs). Obsolete term for incus. [Ger.]

am·bro·sin (am-brō'sin). A principle in ragweed related to absinthin.

am·bu·cet·a·mide (am-byū-set'ă-mīd). α-Dibutylamino-α-(*p*-methoxyphenyl)acetamide; an intestinal antispasmodic.

am·bu·lance (am'byū-lans). A vehicle used to transport sick or injured persons to a treatment facility. [Fr., fr. *(hôpital) ambulant*, mobile hospital]

am·bu·la·to·ry, am·bu·lant (am'byū-lă-tōr-ē, am'byū-lant). Walking about or able to walk about; denoting a patient who is not confined to bed or hospital as a result of disease or surgery. [L. *ambulans*, walking]

am·bu·phyl·line (am-byū'fĭ-lin). A diuretic and bronchodilator. SYN theophylline aminoisobutanol.

am·bus·tion (am-bŭs'chŭn). Obsolete term for a burn or scald. [L. *amb-uro*, pp. *-ustus*, to burn around, scorch]

am·cin·o·nide (am-sin'ō-nid). A glucocorticoid used topically in the treatment of dermatoses.

am·di·no·cil·lin (am'di-nō-sil'in). $C_{15}H_{23}N_3O_3S$; a penicillin derivative of amidinopenicillamic acid which, unlike other penicillins, is very active against a wide range of Gram-negative bacteria. SYN mecillinam.

ame·ba, pl. **ame·bae, ame·bas** (ă-mē'bă, -bē, -băz). Common name for *Amoeba* and similar naked, lobose, sarcodine protozoa.

ame·ba·cide (ă-mē'bă-sīd). SYN amebicide.

ame·ba·ism (ă-mē'bă-izm). **1.** SYN ameboidism (1). **2.** SYN ameboididity.

am·e·bi·a·sis (ă-mē-bī'ă-sis). Infection with *Entamoeba histolytica* or other pathogenic amebas. [ameba + G. *-iasis*, condition]

canine a., infection of dogs with *Entamoeba histolytica* acquired from man; dogs are seldom cyst passers, and therefore are not a reservoir for human infection.

a. cu'tis, cutaneous a., appearing usually as an extension of underlying infection (*e.g.*, anus or colostomy site or over a liver abscess).

hepatic a., infection of the liver with *Entamoeba histolytica;* may occur with or without antecedent amebic dysentery.

pulmonary a., infection of the lung by amebae; usually indicates extension of *Entamoeba histolytica* infection from abscess of liver, penetrating through the diaphragm into the lung.

ame·bic (ă-mē'bik). Relating to, resembling, or caused by amebas.

ame·bi·ci·dal (ă-mē-bi-sī'dăl). Destructive to amebas.

ame·bi·cide (ă-mē'bi-sīd). Any agent that causes the destruction of amebas. SYN amebacide. [ameba + L. *caedo*, to kill]

ame·bi·form (ă-mē'bi-fōrm). Of the shape or appearance of an ameba. [ameba + L. *forma*, shape]

am·e·bi·o·sis (ă-mē-bī-ō'sis). Obsolete term for amebiasis.

ame·bism (ă-mē'bizm). Obsolete term for amebiasis.

ame·bo·cyte (ă-mē'bō-sīt). **1.** A wandering cell found in invertebrates. **2.** Obsolete term for leukocyte. **3.** An *in vitro* tissue culture leukocyte. [ameba, + *kytos*, cell]

ame·boid (ă-mē'boyd). **1.** Resembling an ameba in appearance or characteristics. **2.** Of irregular outline with peripheral projections; denoting the outline of a form of colony in plate culture. [ameba + G. *eidos*, appearance]

ame·boi·did·i·ty (ă-mē-boy-did'i-tē). The power of locomotion after the manner of an ameboid cell. SYN amebaism (2).

ame·boid·ism (ă-mē'boyd-izm). **1.** The performance of movements similar to those of an ameba. SYN amebaism (1). **2.** Denoting a condition sometimes seen in certain nerve cells.

am·e·bo·ma (ă-mē-bō'mă). A nodular, tumor-like focus of proliferative inflammation sometimes developing in chronic amebiasis, especially in the wall of the colon. SYN amebic granuloma. [ameba + G. *-oma*, tumor]

ame·bu·la, pl. **ame·bu·lae** (ă-mē'byū-lă, -lē). Term applied to the excysted young amebas of *Entamoeba* species that emerge from the cyst in the human or vertebrate gut and their immediate progeny, usually totalling eight, prior to their localization in the large intestine. [fr. G. *amoibē*, a change, alteration]

ame·bule (ă-mē'byūl). A minute ameba.

am·e·bu·ria (am-ē-byū'rē-ă). The presence of amebas in the urine. [ameba + G. *ouron*, urine]

amel·a·not·ic (ā-mel-ă-not'ik). Lacking in melanin. [G. *a-* priv. + *melas*, black]

ame·lia (ă-mē'lē-ă) [MIM104400]. Congenital absence of a limb or limbs. Mostly sporadic; any genetic factors are obscure. [G. *a-* priv. + *melos*, a limb]

porcine a., autosomal recessive a. in piglets.

ame·lio·ra·tion (ă-mēl-yō-rā'shŭn). Improvement; moderation in the severity of a disease or the intensity of its symptoms. [L. *ad*, to, + *melioro*, to make better]

am·e·lo·blast (ă-mel'ō-blast, am-ĕ-lō'blast). One of the columnar epithelial cells of the inner layer of the enamel organ of a developing tooth, concerned with the formation of enamel. SYN enamel cell, enameloblast, ganoblast. [Early E. *amel*, enamel, + G. *blastos*, germ]

am·e·lo·blas·to·ma (am'ĕ-lō-blas-tō'mă). A benign odontogenic epithelial neoplasm that histologically mimics the embryonal enamel organ but does not differentiate to the point of forming dental hard tissues; it behaves as a slowly growing expansile radiolucent tumor, occurs most commonly in the posterior regions of the mandible, and has a marked tendency to recur if inadequately excised. [ameloblast + G. *-oma*, tumor]

pigmented a., SYN melanotic neuroectodermal *tumor* of infancy.

pituitary a., SYN craniopharyngioma.

am·e·lo·den·tin·al (am'ĕ-lō-den'ti-năl). SYN dentinoenamel.

am·e·lo·gen·e·sis (am'ĕ-lō-jen'ĕ-sis). The deposition and maturation of enamel. SYN enamelogenesis.

a. imperfec'ta, a group of hereditary ectodermal disorders in which the enamel is defective in structure or deficient in quantity. Three major groups are recognized: hypoplastic types, with defective enamel matrix deposition but normal mineralization; hypomineralization types, with normal matrix but defective mineralization; and hypomaturation type, in which the enamel crystallites remain immature. The several types may be inherited as autosomal dominant [MIM*104500, 104510, 104550], recessive [MIM*205650, 204690, 204700] or X-linked [MIM*301100, 301200]. SYN enamel dysplasia, enamelogenesis imperfecta.

ame·nia (ă-mē'nē-ă). Rarely used term for amenorrhea. [G. *a-* priv. + *mēn*, month]

amen·or·rhea (ă-men-ō-rē'ă). Absence or abnormal cessation of the menses. [G. *a-* priv. + *mēn*, month, + *rhoia*, flow]

dietary a., loss of menstrual function due to severe weight loss or gain.

emotional a., a. caused by a strong emotional disturbance, *e.g.*, fright, grief.

exercise-induced a., temporary cessation of menstrual function due to strenuous, daily exercise, as in jogging; increased endorphins inhibiting hypothalamic function.

hyperprolactinemic a., a. associated with abnormally high levels of serum prolactin; often accompanied by unphysiological lactation.

hypophysial a., a. due to inadequate gonadotrophic secretions by the anterior lobe of the hypophysis.

hypothalamic a., secondary a. arising from defective hypothalamic stimulation of the anterior lobe of the hypophysis.

lactation a., physiological suppression of menses while nursing.

ovarian a., a. due to deficiency of estrogenic hormone.

pathologic a., a. due to organic disease, either uterine or other, *e.g.*, ovarian or pituitary failure, Simmonds' disease, inconstant and irrelevant debility.

physiologic a., a. of pregnancy or the menopause, not associated with an organic disorder.

postpartum a., permanent a. following childbirth, sometimes due to pituitary failure resulting from postpartum hemorrhage and consequent necrosis of the pituitary (Simmonds' *disease*).

primary a., a. in which the menses have never occurred.

secondary a., a. in which the menses appeared at puberty but subsequently ceased.

traumatic a., absence of menses because of endometrial scarring or cervical stenosis resulting from injury or disease.

amen·or·rhe·al, amen·or·rhe·ic (ă-men-ō-rē′ăl, -rē′ik). Relating to, accompanied by, or due to amenorrhea.

amen·tia (ă-men′shē-ă). **1.** SYN mental *retardation.* **2.** SYN dementia. [L. madness, fr. *ab*, from, + *mens*, mind]

nevoid a., SYN Brushfield-Wyatt *disease.*

phenylpyruvic a., a. accompanied by the appearance of phenylpyruvate in the urine.

Stearns alcoholic a., a temporary alcoholic mental disorder resembling delirium tremens but lasting for a longer time and showing a greater degree of amnesia and other mental defects.

amen·ti·al (ă-men′shē-al). Pertaining to amentia.

Amer·i·can Law In·sti·tute for·mu·la·tion. Used in certain jurisdictions to determine criminal responsibility in legal proceedings. SEE criminal *insanity.*

Amer·i·can Law In·sti·tute rule. See under rule.

Amer·i·can Red Cross. The national Red Cross society of the United States, established by Congress to assist in caring for the sick and wounded, serving as a communications link between members of the U.S. armed forces and their families, conducting disaster relief and prevention programs, and furnishing other humanitarian services, the largest of which is a network of regional blood centers providing blood and blood products.

am·er·i·ci·um (Am) (am′ĕ-ris′ē-ŭm). An element obtained by the bombardment of uranium with neutrons or β decay of plutoniums 241, 242, and 243; atomic no. 95; atomic weight 243.06. ^{241}Am (half-life of 432.2 years) has been used in the diagnosis of bone disorders. ^{243}Am has a half-life of 7370 years. [the Americas]

am·er·ism (am′er-izm). The condition or quality of not dividing into parts, segments, or merozoites. [G. *a-* priv. + *meros*, part]

am·er·is·tic (am-ĕ-ris′tik). Endowed with amerism; not dividing into parts or segments.

Ames, Bruce N., U.S. molecular geneticist, *1928. SEE A. *assay, test.*

am·e·thop·ter·in (ă-meth-ō-ter′in, am-ĕ-thop′tĕ-rin). SYN methotrexate.

ame·tria (ă-mē′trē-ă). Congenital absence of the uterus; the genetics is obscure. [G. *a-* priv. + *mētra*, uterus]

ame·tri·o·din·ic ac·id (ă′mĕ-trī-ō-din′ik). SYN iodamide.

am·e·tro·pia (am-ĕ-trō′pē-ă). The optical condition in which there is an error of refraction so that with the eye at rest the retina is not in conjugate focus with light rays from distant objects, *i.e.,* only objects located a finite distance from the eye are focused on the retina. [G. *ametros*, disproportionate, fr. *a-* priv. + *metron*, measure, + *ōps*, eye]

axial a., that resulting from a shortening or lengthening of the eyeball on the optic axis, causing hyperopia or myopia, respectively.

index a., that resulting from alteration in the refractive index of the lens of the eye.

am·e·tro·pic (am-ĕ-trō′pik). Relating to, or suffering from, ametropia.

am·i·an·ta·ceous (am′i-an-tā′shŭs). Asbestos-like; describing thin plates of inflammatory crusting of a cutaneous lesion. [G. *amiantus,* asbestos]

am·i·an·thoid (am-i-an′thoyd). Having a crystalline appearance like asbestos. SYN asbestoid. [G. *amianthus,* asbestos]

△**-amic.** Chemical suffix denoting the replacement of one COOH group of a dicarboxylic acid by a carboxamide group (—CONH₂); applied only to trivial names (*e.g.,* succinamic acid).

ami·cro·bic (ā-mī-krō′bik). Not microbic; not related to or caused by microorganisms.

ami·cro·scop·ic (ā′mī-krō-skop′ik). SYN submicroscopic.

am·i·dase (am′i-dās). An enzyme that catalyzes the hydrolysis of monocarboxylic amides to free acid plus NH₃; ω-a. acts on amides such as α-ketoglutaramic acid and α-ketosuccinamic acid. SYN acylamidase.

am·i·das·es. SYN amidohydrolases.

am·ide (am′īd, am′id). A substance formally derived from ammonia through the substitution of one or more of the hydrogen

atoms by acyl groups, R—CO—NH₂, or from a carboxylic acid by replacement of a carboxylic OH by NH₂. Replacement of one hydrogen atom constitutes a **primary a.**; that of two hydrogen atoms, a **secondary a.**; and that of three atoms, a **tertiary a.**.

substituted a., a secondary or tertiary a.; peptide linkages are substituted a.'s.

am·i·dine (am′i-din). The monovalent radical —C(NH)-NH₂.

am·i·di·no·hy·dro·las·es (am′i-din-ō-hī′drō-lās-ez) [EC subsubgroup 3.5.3]. Enzymes cleaving linear amidines; *e.g.,* arginase, creatinase.

am·i·din·o·trans·fer·as·es (am′i-din-ō-trans′fer-ās-ez) [EC subsubclass 2.1.4]. Enzymes catalyzing a transamidination reaction (*e.g.,* glycine amidinotransferase). SYN transamidinases.

△**amido-.** Prefix denoting the amide radical, R-CO-NH- or R-SO₂-NH-, etc. [am(monia) + -id(e) + -o-]

ami·do black 10B (am′i-dō) [C.I. 20470]. An acid diazo dye, C₁₂H₁₄N₆O₉S₂Na₂, used as a connective tissue stain, for staining protein in paper chromatography, and in electrophoresis.

ami·do·gen (am′i-dō-jen). Obsolete term for the amino group —(NH₂).

ami·do·hy·dro·las·es (am′i-dō-hī′drō-lā-sez) [EC class 3.5.1 and 3.5.2]. Enzymes hydrolyzing C-N bonds of amides and cyclic amides; *e.g.,* asparaginase, barbiturase, urease, amidase. SYN amidases, deamidases, deamidizing enzymes.

ami·do·naph·thol red (am′i-dō-naf′thol) [C.I. 18050]. An azo dye, C₁₈H₁₃N₃S₂Na₂, used in light and fluorescence microscopy as a real acid counterstain. SYN azophloxin.

ami·do·py·rine (am-i-dō-pī′rēn). SYN aminopyrine.

Am·i·dos·to·mum an·ser·is (am-i-dos′tō-mŭm an′ser-is). A species of bloodsucking nematodes, similar to those of the genus *Trichostrongylus,* that parasitizes the gizzard and sometimes also the proventriculus and esophagus of domestic and wild ducks and geese; it causes heavy mortality in young birds. [amido- + G. *stoma,* mouth, + L. *anser,* goose]

am·i·dox·imes (am-i-doks′īmz, -dok′sēmz). The oximes of amides with the general formula, R-C(NH₂)-NOH. SYN amide oximes.

am·i·dox·yl (am-i-dok′sil). The radical of an amide oxime (amidoxime), the terminal H (of the NOH) having been lost.

am·i·ka·cin sul·fate (am-i-kā′sin). An aminoglycoside antibiotic agent with antimicrobial activity similar to that of kanamycin; also effective against *Pseudomonas aeruginosa.*

amil·o·ride hy·dro·chlo·ride (ă-mil′ō-rīd). *N*-Amidino-3,5-diamino-6-chloropyrazinecarboxami de monohydrochloride dihydrate; a nonsteroidal compound exerting an effect similar to that of an aldosterone inhibitor, *i.e.,* urinary sodium excretion is enhanced and potassium excretion is reduced; a potassium sparing diuretic.

amim·ia (ā-mim′ē-a). **1.** Inability to express ideas by nonverbal communication, such as gestures or signs. **2.** Asymbolia; the inability to comprehend the meaning of gestures, signs, symbols, or pantomime. [G. *a-* priv. + *minos,* a mimic]

am·i·nac·rine hy·dro·chlo·ride (am′i-nak′rin). Bactericidal agent for external use. SEE ALSO acridine yellow. SYN 5-aminoacridine hydrochloride, 9-aminoacridine hydrochloride.

am·i·nate (am′i-nāt). To combine with ammonia.

am·i·na·tion (ă-me-nā′shŭn). The introduction of an amine moiety into a compound.

amine (ă-mēn′, am′in). A substance formally derived from ammonia by the replacement of one or more of the hydrogen atoms by hydrocarbon or other radicals. The substitution of one hydrogen atom constitutes a **primary a.**, *e.g.,* NH₂CH₃; that of two atoms, a **secondary a.**, *e.g.,* NH(CH₃)₂; that of three atoms, a **tertiary a.**, *e.g.,* N(CH₃)₃; and that of four atoms, a **quaternary ammonium ion,** *e.g.,* ⁺N(CH₃)₄, a positively charged ion isolated only in association with a negative ion. The a.'s form salts with acids.

adrenergic a., SYN sympathomimetic a.

adrenomimetic a., SYN sympathomimetic a.

biogenic a.'s, a class of compounds, each containing an a. group, produced by a living organism. This class normally does not include amino acids.

a. oxidase (copper-containing), an oxidoreductase containing copper, and perhaps pyridoxal phosphate, and carrying out the same reaction as a. oxidase (flavin-containing). SYN a. oxidase (pyridoxal-containing), diamine oxidase, diamino oxyhydrase, histaminase.

a. oxidase (flavin-containing), an oxidoreductase containing flavin and oxidizing amines with the aid of O_2 and water to aldehydes or ketones with the release of NH_3 and H_2O_2. Acted upon by antidepressants. SYN adrenaline oxidase, diamine oxidase, monoamine oxidase, tyraminase, tyramine oxidase.

a. oxidase (pyridoxal-containing), SYN a. oxidase (copper-containing).

pressor a., SYN pressor *base.*

sympathetic a., SYN sympathomimetic a.

sympathomimetic a., an agent that evokes responses similar to those produced by adrenergic nerve activity (*e.g.,* epinephrine, ephedrine, isoproterenol). SYN adrenergic a., adrenomimetic a., sympathetic a.

vasoactive a., a substance, such as histamine or serotonin, that contains amino groups and is pharmacologically characterized by its action on the blood vessels (altering vascular caliber or permeability).

am·in·er·gic (ă-mēn'er-gik). Relating to nerve cells or fibers.

△**amino-.** Prefix denoting a compound containing the radical, —NH_2. [an(monia) + in(e) + -o-]

ami·no·ace·tic ac·id (ă-mē'nō-a-sē'tik). SYN glycine.

ami·no ac·id (AA, aa) (ă-mē'nō). An organic acid in which one of the hydrogen atoms on a carbon atom has been replaced by NH_2. Usually refers to an aminocarboxylic acid. However, taurine is also an a. SEE ALSO α-amino acid.

acidic a. a., an a. a. with a second acid moiety, *e.g.,* glutamic acid, aspartic acid, cysteic acid.

activated a. a., SYN aminoacyl adenylate.

basic a. a., an a. a. containing a second basic group (usually an amino group); *e.g.,* lysine, arginine, ornithine. SYN dibasic a. a.

a. a. dehydrogenases, enzymes catalyzing the oxidative deamination of amino acids to the corresponding oxo (keto) acids; two relatively nonspecific varieties exist, L and D, for which L-amino acids and D-amino acids are the respective substrates; the products include NH_3 and a reduced hydrogen acceptor (NADH in the L case); a. a. dehydrogenases of greater specificity exist, (*e.g.,* glycine dehydrogenase). Cf. a. a. oxidases.

dibasic a. a., SYN basic a. a.

essential a. a.'s, α-amino acids nutritionally required by an organism and which must be supplied in its diet (*i.e.,* cannot be synthesized by the organism) either as free a. a. or in proteins.

nonessential a. a.'s, those a. a.'s that may be synthesized by an organism and are thus not required as such in its diet.

nonpolar a. a., an α-a. a. in which the functional group attached to the α-carbon (*i.e.,* R in $RCH(NH_2)COOH$) has hydrophobic properties; *e.g.,* valine, leucine, α-aminobutyrate.

a. a. oxidases, flavoenzymes oxidizing, with O_2 and H_2O, either L- or D-amino acids specifically, to the corresponding 2-keto acids, NH_3 and H_2O_2. Cf. a. a. dehydrogenases, yellow *enzyme.*

polar a. a., an α-a. a. in which the functional group attached to the α-carbon (*i.e.,* R in $RCH(NH_2)COOH$) has hydrophilic properties; *e.g.,* serine, cysteine, homocysteine.

α-**ami·no ac·id.** Typically, an amino acid of the general formula R-$CHNH_2$-$COOH$ (*i.e.,* the NH_2 in the α position); the L forms of these are the hydrolysis products of proteins. In rarer instances, this class of molecules also includes α-amino phosphoric acids and α-aminosulfonic acids.

ami·no·ac·i·de·mia (ă-mē'nō-as-i-dē'mē-ă, am'i-nō-). The presence of excessive amounts of specific amino acids in the blood. [amino acid + G. *haima,* blood]

ami·no·ac·id-tRNA li·gas·es. Recommended name for aminoacyl-tRNA synthetases (EC 6.1.1.1–EC 6.1.1.22); *e.g.,* tyrosine-tRNA ligase for tyrosyl-tRNA synthetase.

ami·no·ac·i·du·ria (am'i-nō-as-i-dū'rē-ă). Excretion of amino acids in the urine, especially in excessive amounts. SYN hyperaminoaciduria. [amino acid + G. *ouron,* urine]

hyperbasic aminoaciduria, An inherited disorder associated

α–amino acids			
alanine	(Ala;A)	leucine	(Leu;L)
arginine	(Arg;R)	lysine	(Lys;K)
asparagine	(Asn;N)	methionine	(Met;M)
aspartate	(Asp;D)	phenylalanine	(Phe;F)
cysteine	(Cys;C)	proline	(Pro;P)
glutamine	(Gln;Q)	serine	(Ser;S)
glutamate	(Glu;E)	threonine	(Thr;T)
glycine	(Gly;G)	tryptophan	(Trp;Try;W)
histidine	(His;H)	tyrosine	(Tyr;Y)
isoleucine	(Ile;I)	valine	(Val;V)

with a deficiency of a dibasic amino acid transport. Individuals do not display protein intolerance. Cf. lysinuric protein *intolerance.*

9-ami·no·ac·ri·dine (ă-mē-nō-ak'ri-dēn). 5-Aminoacridine; one of the acridine group of antiseptics (flavins); highly fluorescent in solution; used topically as an antiseptic.

5-ami·no·ac·ri·dine hy·dro·chlo·ride, 9-ami·no·ac·ri·dine hy·dro·chlo·ride. SYN acridine yellow, aminacrine hydrochloride.

ami·no·ac·yl (AA, aa) (ă-mē'nō-as'il). The radical formed from an amino acid by removal of OH from a COOH group.

ami·no·ac·yl a·den·y·late (ă-mē'nō-as-il-ă-den'i-lāt). The product formed by the condensation of the acyl radical of an amino acid and adenosine 5′-monophosphate (originally in the form of adenosine 5′-triphosphate, with elimination of a pyrophosphoric group). Formed in the first step of protein biosynthesis. SYN activated amino acid.

ami·no·ac·yl·ase (ă-mē'nō-as'i-lās). An enzyme catalyzing hydrolysis of a wide variety of *N*-acyl amino acids to the corresponding amino acid and an acid anion. SYN benzamide, dehydropeptidase II, hippuricase, histozyme.

α-**ami·no·ac·yl-pep·tide hy·dro·las·es.** SYN aminopeptidases.

ami·no·ac·yl-tRNA. Generic term for those compounds in which amino acids are esterfied through their COOH groups to the 3′ (or 2′) OH's of the terminal adenosine residues of transfer RNA's (*e.g.,* alanyl-tRNA, glycyl-tRNA); each compound involves one, or a small number, of tRNA's of specific chemical structure. Used in protein biosynthesis.

aminoacyl-tRNA ligases, SYN a.-tRNA synthetases.

a.-tRNA synthetases, enzymes catalyzing the formation of a specific a.-tRNA from an amino acid and adenosine 5′-triphosphate with the concomitant formation of adenosine 5′-monophosphate and pyrophosphate. SYN amino acid activating enzyme, aminoacyl-tRNA ligases.

ami·no·a·dip·ic δ-sem·i·al·de·hyde syn·thase. a bifunctional enzyme used in lysine degradation; it has a lysine:α-ketoglutarate reductase activity as well as a saccharopine dehydrogenase activity. A deficiency of this enzyme results in familial hyperlysinemia.

α-**ami·no·a·dip·ic ac·id (Aad)** (ă-mē'nō-ă-dip'ik). 2-amino-1,6-hexanedioic acid; an intermediate of lysine biosynthesis in higher fungi and bacteria, but not in algae and higher plants. Also in degradation of lysine in mammals.

ami·no·ben·zene (ă-mē'nō-ben'zēn). SYN aniline.

o-**ami·no·ben·zo·ic ac·id** (ă-mē'nō-ben-zō'ik). SYN anthranilic acid.

p-**ami·no·ben·zo·ic ac·id (PABA).** A factor in the vitamin B complex, a part of all folic acids and required for its formation; neutralizes the bacteriostatic effects of the sulfonamides since it furnishes an essential growth factor for bacteria, the utilization with which the sulfonamides interfere; used as an ultraviolet screen in lotions and creams. SYN paraamino benzoic acid, vitamin B_x.

D(-)-α-ami·no·ben·zyl·pen·i·cil·lin (ă-mē-nō-ben′zil-pen-i-sil′ in). SYN ampicillin.

γ-ami·no·bu·tyr·ic ac·id (GABA, γ-Abu) (ă-mē′nō-byū-tēr′ ik). $^+NH_3(CH_2)_3COO^-$; 4-aminobutyric acid; a constituent of the central nervous system; quantitatively the principal inhibitory neurotransmitter. Used in the treatment of a number of disorders (*e.g.,* epilepsy).

ami·no·ca·pro·ic ac·id (ă-mē′nō-că-prō′ik). ε-Aminocaproic acid; 6-aminohexanoic acid; an antifibrinolytic agent, used to prevent bleeding in hemophilia, and after heart and prostate surgery when plasminogen or urokinase may be activated.

am·i·no·car·bon·yl (am-i-nō-kar′bon-il). SYN carboxamide.

ami·no·car·box·yl·ic ac·id. SEE amino acid.

ami·no·cit·ric ac·id (ă-mē′no-sit′rik). $HOOCCH(NH_3^+)$ $C(COOH)(OH)CH_2CO$; OH; found in acid hydrolysates of ribonucleoprotein in human spleen.

2-ami·no·-2-de·oxy-D-ga·lac·tose. SEE galactosamine.

ami·no·eth·a·no·ic ac·id. SYN glycine.

2-ami·no·eth·a·nol. SEE ethanolamine.

α-ami·no·glu·tar·ic ac·id. SEE glutamic acid.

ami·no·glu·teth·i·mide (ă-mē′nō-glū-teth′i-mīd). 2-(*p*-Aminophenyl)-2-ethylglutarimide; an aromatase inhibitor used as an adjunct in the treatment of breast cancer; blocks the synthesis of estrogen; formerly tried as an anticonvulsant but no longer used for that purpose.

am·i·no·gly·co·side (am′i-nō-glī′kō-sīd). Any one of a group of bacteriocidal antibiotics derived from species of *Streptomyces* or *Micromonosporum* and characterized by two or more amino sugars joined by a glycoside linkage to a central hexose; a.'s act by causing misreading and inhibition of protein synthesis on bacterial ribosomes and are effective against aerobic Gram-negative bacilli and *Mycobacterium tuberculosis.* Some commonly used a.'s are streptomycin, neomycin, and gentamycin.

***p*-ami·no·hip·pu·ric ac·id (PAH)** (ă-mē′nō-hi-pyūr′ik). *N*-(4-Aminobenzoyl) glycine; used in renal function tests to measure renal plasma flow; actively secreted (and filtered) by the kidney.
p.-a. a. synthase, an enzyme in the liver that catalyzes the synthesis of *p*-aminohippuric acid from *p*-aminobenzoic acid (or the CoA-derivative) and glycine. It may be identical with glycine acyltransferase.

5-ami·no·im·id·az·ole ri·bose 5′-phos·phate (AIR) (ă-mē′ nō-im-id-az′ōl). 5-amino-1-β-D-ribofuranosylimidazole 5′-phosphate; an intermediate in the biosynthesis of purines. SYN 5-aminoimidazole ribotide.

5-a·mi·no·i·mid·a·zole ri·bo·tide (AIR). SYN 5-aminoimidazole ribose 5′-phosphate.

5-ami·no·im·id·a·zole-4-*N*-suc·ci·no·car·box·am·ide ri·bo·nu·cle·o·tide. An intermediate in purine biosynthesis.

β-ami·no·iso·bu·ty·rate:py·ru·vate ami·no·trans·fer·ase. β-aminoisobutyrate:pyruvate transaminase; an enzyme that catalyzes the reversible transfer of an amino group from β-aminoisobutyrate to pyruvate, producing L-alanine and methylmalonate semialdehyde. A step in valine degradation. A deficiency of β-aminoisobutyrate:pyruvate aminotransferase results in hyper-β-aminoisobutyric aciduria.

α-ami·no·iso·bu·tyr·ic ac·id (ă-mē′nō-ī-sō-byū-tēr′ik). 2-amino-2-methylpropionic acid; a synthetic amino acid useful in the study of amino acid transport across cell membranes and in the study of cytokine effects; it is not metabolized by the cell.

β-ami·no·i·so·bu·tyr·ic ac·id. 3-Amino-2-methylpropionic acid; an end product of thymine catabolism; high urinary levels (200-300 mg/day) have been noted in some individuals, either from some disease process or following a genetic pattern.

α-ami·no·-β-ke·to·a·dip·ic ac·id. 2-Amino-3-oxo-1,6-hexanedioic acid; an intermediate of porphobilinogen synthesis formed by δ-aminolevulinic acid synthase from succinyl-CoA and glycine; it rapidly decarboxylates to δ-aminolevulinic acid.

δ-ami·no·lev·u·li·nate de·hy·dra·tase (ă-mē′nō-lev-yū-lin′āt). SYN *porphobilinogen* synthase.

δ-ami·no·lev·u·lin·ic ac·id (ALA) (ă-mē′nō-lev-yū-lin′ik). $NH_2CH_2COCH_2CH_2COOH$; an acid formed by δ-aminolevulinate synthase from glycine and succinyl-coenzyme A; a precursor of porphobilinogen, hence an important intermediate in the biosynthesis of hematin. ALA levels are elevated in cases of lead poisoning.

δ-aminolevulinic acid synthase, an enzyme that catalyzes the reaction of succinyl-CoA with glycine to form δ-aminolevulinic acid, coenzyme A, and CO_2. The committed step in porphyrin biosynthesis.

am·i·nol·y·sis (am-i-nol′i-sis). Replacement of a halogen in an alkyl or aryl molecule by an amine radical, with elimination of hydrogen halide.

ami·no·met·ra·dine (ă-mē′nō-met′ră-dēn). SYN aminometramide.

ami·no·met·ra·mide (ă-mē′nō-met′ră-mīd). 1-allyl-6-amino-3-ethyluracil; synthetic uracil derivative; an orally effective diuretic that is believed to act by inhibiting the reabsorption of sodium by the renal tubules; used in the treatment of edema due to congestive heart failure, liver disease, pregnancy, and certain drugs. SYN aminometradine.

6-ami·no·pen·i·cil·lan·ic ac·id (6-APS) (ă-mē′nō-pen-i-sil-ăn′ ik). An important precursor in the synthesis of penicillin derivatives. By itself, it has no antibiotic activity. For structure, see under penicillin in which R = H. SYN penicin.

ami·no·pen·i·cil·lins (ă-mē′nō-pen-i-sil′inz). A class of penicillin-like antibiotics which chemically contain an amine group; this class includes ampicillin and amoxicillin; used in upper respiratory infections, urinary tract infections, meningitis, *salmonella* infections.

ami·no·pep·ti·dase(cy·to·sol). An enzyme of broad specificity, containing zinc, and catalyzing the hydrolysis of the N-terminal amino acid of a peptide (*i.e.,* an exopeptidase).

ami·no·pep·ti·dase(mi·cro·som·al). An aminopeptidase of broad specificity, but preferring alanine and discriminating against proline.

ami·no·pep·ti·das·es (ă-mē′nō-pep′ti-dās-ez) [EC sub-group 3.4.11]. Enzymes catalyzing the breakdown of a peptide, removing the amino acid at the amino end of the chain (*i.e.,* an exopeptidase); found in intestinal secretions. SYN α-aminoacyl-peptide hydrolases.

ami·no·phen·a·zone (ă-mē-nō-fen′ă-zōn). SYN aminopyrine.

am·i·noph·er·as·es (am-i-nof-er-ās-ez). SYN aminotransferases.

ami·no·phyl·line (ă-mē-nō-fil′in, am-i-nof′i-lin, -ēn) $(C_7H_8N_4O_2)$ $_2C_2H_4(NH_2)$ $_22H_2O$; a solubilized form of theophylline; a diuretic, vasodilator, and cardiac stimulant; also used as a bronchodilator in asthma and in veterinary medicine. SYN theophylline ethylenediamine.

ami·no·pro·ma·zine (ă-mē-nō-prō′mă-zēn). 10-[2,3-Bis-(dimethylamino)propyl]phenothiazine; an intestinal antispasmodic.

ami·no·pro·pi·on·ic ac·id (ă-mē′nō-prō-pē-on′ik). SEE alanine.

***p*-ami·no·pro·pi·o·phe·none (PAPP)** (ă-mē′nō-prō-pē-ō-fē′ nōn). 1-(4-Aminophenyl)-1-propanone; an antidote for cyanide poisoning.

am·i·nop·ter·in (am-i-nop′ter-in). 4-Aminopteroylglutamic acid; 4-aminofolic acid; a folic acid antagonist used in the treatment of acute leukemia and other neoplastic diseases.

6-ami·no·pu·rine (ă-mē′nō-pyūr′ēn). SYN adenine.

4-ami·no·pyr·i·dine (am-i-nō-pir′i-dēn). An antagonist of nondepolarizing neuromuscular blockade; devoid of muscarinic side-effects but associated with central nervous system stimulation.

ami·no·py·rine (am′i-nō-pī′rēn). dimethylaminoantipyrine 4-dimethylamino-2,3-dimethyl-1-phenyl-3-pyrazolin-5-one; used as an antipyretic and analgesic in rheumatism, neuritis, pulmonary tuberculosis, and common colds; may cause leukocytopenia; used to measure total body water. SYN amidopyrine, aminophenazone, dipyrine.

amin·o·rex (ă-min′ō-reks). 2-Amino-5-phenyl-2-oxazoline; a sympathomimetic appetite suppressant.

***p*-ami·no·sal·i·cyl·ic ac·id (PAS, PASA)** (am′i-nō-sal-i-sil′ ik). 4-Amino-2-hydroxybenzoic acid; a bacteriostatic agent against tubercle bacilli, used as an adjunct to streptomycin; the potassium, sodium, and calcium salts have the same use.

α-ami·no·suc·cin·ic ac·id (ă-mē′nō-sŭk-sin′ik). SYN aspartic acid.

ami·no-ter·mi·nal (ă-mē′nō-ter′min-ăl). The α-NH₂ group or the aminoacyl residue containing it at one end of a peptide or protein (usually at left as written). SYN NH₂-terminal.

ami·no-trans·fer·as·es (ă-mē′nō-trans′fer-ās-ez) [EC sub-group 2.6.1]. Enzymes transferring amino groups between an amino acid to (usually) a 2-keto acid; *e.g.*, ʟ-alanine and 2-ketoglutarate. Often, the amino acid is an α-amino acid. SYN aminopherases, transaminases.

ami·no-tri·a·zole (am′i-nō-trī′ă-zol). 3-amino-1*H*-1,2,4-triazole; an effective weed killer that also possesses some antithyroid activity. SYN amitrole.

ami·no·tri·pep·tid·ase (ă-mē′nō-trī-pep′tă-dās). An intestinal peptidase that acts on tripeptides, releasing an amino acid and a dipeptide.

am·i·nu·ria (am-i-nū′rē-ă). Excretion of amines in the urine. [amine + G. *ouron,* urine]

ami·o·da·rone hy·dro·chlo·ride (ă-mē′ō-dă-rōn). (2-Butyl-3-benzofuranyl)[4-[2-(diethylamino)ethoxyl]-3,5-d iiodophenyl]-methanone; a coronary vasodilator used in the control of ventricular and supraventricular arrhythmias, and in the management of angina pectoris. Causes significant and distinctive pulmonary toxicity.

am·i·thi·o·zone (am-i-thī′ō-zōn). 4′-formylacetanilide thiosemicarbazone; a leprostatic agent. SYN thiacetazone.

ami·to·sis (am-i-tō′sis). Direct division of the nucleus and cell, without the complicated changes in the nucleus that occur in the ordinary process of cell reproduction. SYN direct nuclear division, Remak's nuclear division. [G. *a-* priv. + mitosis]

ami·tot·ic (am-i-tot′ik). Relating to or marked by amitosis.

am·i·trip·ty·line hy·dro·chlo·ride (am-i-trip′ti-lēn). 10,11-Dihydro-*N,N*-dimethyl-5*H*-dibenzo[*a,d*]cycloheptene-Δ]-cycloheptene-Δ⁵,ᵞ-propylamine hydrochloride; chemically and pharmacologically related to imipramine hydrochloride; an antidepressant agent with mild tranquilizing properties, used in the treatment of mental depression and in the depressive phase of manic-depressive states; sometimes used in the treatment of sleep disorders.

am·i·trole (am′i-trōl). SYN aminotriazole.

am·lo·dip·ine (am-lō′dī-pēn). A calcium-blocking drug of the dihydropyridine series; belongs to the same class of agents as nifedipine.

am·me·ter (am) (am′mē-ter). An instrument for measuring strength of electric current in amperes.

Ammon, Friedrich von, German ophthalmologist and pathologist, 1799–1861. SEE A.'s *fissure, prominence.*

Ammon, Greek name of Egyptian god, Amun. SEE A.'s *horn.*

am·mo·ne·mia, am·mo·ni·e·mia (am-ō-nē′mē-ă). The presence of ammonia or some of its compounds in the blood, thought to be formed from the decomposition of urea; it usually results in subnormal temperature, weak pulse, gastroenteric symptoms, and coma. SYN hyperammonemia. [ammonia + G. *haima,* blood]

am·mo·nia (ă-mō′ne-ă). A colorless volatile gas, NH₃, very soluble in water, capable of forming the weak base, NH₄⁺OH⁻, which combines with acids to form ammonium compounds. [fr. L. *sal ammoniacus,* salt of Amen (G. *Ammōn*), obtained near a temple of Amen in Libya]

am·mo·ni·ac (ă-mō′ne-ak). A gum resin from a plant of western Asia, *Dorema ammoniacum* (family Umbelliferae); used internally as a stimulant and expectorant, and externally as a counter-irritant plaster.

am·mo·ni·a·cal (ă-mō-nī′ă-kl). Relating to ammonia.

am·mo·nia-ly·as·es. Enzymes removing ammonia or an amino compound nonhydrolytically (hence lyases, EC class 4), by rupture of a C—N bond leaving a double bond (EC subgroup 4.3); *e.g.,* aspartate ammonia-lyase (aspartase).

am·mo·ni·at·ed (ă-mō′nē-āt-ed). Containing or combined with ammonia.

△**ammonio-.** Combining form indicating an ammonium group; *e.g.,* trimethylammonioethanol (choline).

am·mo·ni·um (ă-mō′nē-ŭm). The ion, NH₄⁺, formed by combination of NH₃ and H⁺ (the pK_a value is 9.24); behaves as a univalent metal in forming ammonium compounds.

a. benzoate, C₆H₅COONH₄; a stimulant diuretic, urinary antiseptic, and antirheumatic.

a. bromide, NH₄Br; a sedative.

a. carbonate, (NH₄)₂CO₃; a cardiac and respiratory stimulant and carminative expectorant.

a. chloride, NH₄Cl; a stimulant expectorant and cholagogue; used to relieve alkalosis and to promote lead excretion; a urinary acidifier. SYN sal ammoniac.

dibasic a. phosphate, (NH₄)₂HPO₄; used for fireproofing, in baking powder, and as an antirheumatic.

a. ferric sulfate, SYN ferric ammonium sulfate.

a. ichthosulfonate, SYN ichthammol.

a. iodide, NH₄I; an expectorant.

a. mandelate, mandelic acid ammonium salt; a urinary antiseptic.

a. molybdate, H₂₄Mo₇N₆O₂₄; used in electron microscopy as a negative stain, and as a reagent for alkaloids and other substances.

monobasic a. phosphate, (NH₄)H₂PO₄; used in baking powder.

a. nitrate, NH₄NO₃; used in making nitrous oxide gas, in freezing mixtures, matches, and fertilizers; also used in veterinary medicine.

am·mo·ni·u·ria (ă-mō-nē-yū′rē-ă). Excretion of urine that contains an excessive amount of ammonia. SYN ammoniacal urine. [ammonia + G. *ouron,* urine]

am·mo·nol·y·sis (ă-mō-nol′i-sis). The breaking of a chemical bond with the addition of the elements of ammonia (NH₂ and H) at the point of breakage. [ammonia + G. *lysis,* dissolution]

am·mo·no·tel·ia (ă-mōn-ō-tēl′e-ă). The process or type of nitrogen excretion in which ammonia and ammonium ions are the primary form by which nitrogen is excreted from an organism. [ammonia + G. *telos,* end, outcome, + -ia]

am·mo·no·tel·ic (ă-mōn-ō-tēl′ik). Having the property of ammonotelism.

am·mo·no·tel·ism (ă-mōn-ō-tēl′izm). The excretion of ammonia and ammonium ions. Cf. ammonotelia.

am·ne·sia (am-nē′zē-ă). A disturbance in the memory of information stored in long-term memory, in contrast to short-term memory, manifested by total or partial inability to recall past experiences. [G. *amnēsia,* forgetfulness]

anterograde a., a. in reference to events occurring after the trauma or disease that caused the condition.

emotional a., a numbness of feeling and emotion whose etiology is psychological.

lacunar a., localized a., a. in reference to isolated events.

posthypnotic a., selective forgetting, after a hypnotic state, of events occurring during hypnosis or of information stored in long-term memory, such as one's name, address, and names of relatives.

retrograde a., a. in reference to events that occurred before the trauma or disease that caused the condition.

transient global a., a memory disorder seen in middle aged and

△ **Combining forms**	[NA] **Nomina Anatomica**
Word*Finder*	[MIM] **Mendelian**
Multi-term entry finder	**Inheritance in Man**
Preceding letter A	
A.D.A.M. Anatomy Plates	☆ **Official alternate term**
Between letters L and M	
Appendices:	☆[NA] **Official alternate**
Following letter Z	**Nomina Anatomica term**
SYN Synonym; Cf., compare	**High Profile Term**

elderly persons characterized by an episode of a. and bewilderment which persists for several hours; during the episode the patient has a memory defect for present and recent past events, but is fully alert, oriented, capable of high-level intellectual activity, and has a normal neurological examination. Typically, these amnesic episodes occur spontaneously, and most patients experience only one; of uncertain etiology—probably ischemic, but not due to atherosclerosis.

traumatic a., the loss or disturbance of memory following an insult or injury to the brain of the type that accompanies a head injury, or excessive use of alcohol, or following the cessation of alcohol ingestion or other psychoactive drugs; or loss or disturbance of memory of the type seen in hysteria and other forms of dissociative disorders.

am·ne·si·ac (am-nē′sē-ak). One suffering from amnesia.

am·ne·sic (am-nē′sik). Relating to or characterized by amnesia. SYN amnestic (1).

am·nes·tic (am-nes′tik). **1.** SYN amnesic. **2.** An agent causing amnesia. **3.** A disorder in which the essential feature is an impairment of the memory function.

△**amnio-.** The amnion. [G. *amnion*]

am·ni·o·cele (am′-nē-ō-sēl). SYN omphalocele.

am·ni·o·cen·te·sis (am′nē-ō-sen-tē′sis). Transabdominal aspiration of fluid from the amniotic sac. [amnio- + G. *kentēsis,* puncture]

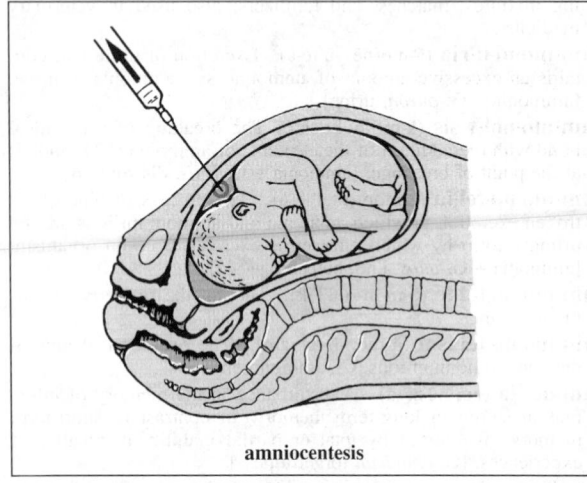
amniocentesis

am·ni·o·cho·ri·al, am·ni·o·cho·ri·on·ic (am′nē-ō-kōr′ē-ăl, -kōr-ē-on′ik). Relating to both amnion and chorion.

am·ni·o·gen·e·sis (am′nē-ō-jen′ĕ-sis). Formation of the amnion. [amnio- + G. *genesis,* production]

am·ni·og·ra·phy (am-nē-og′ră-fē). Radiography of the amniotic sac after the injection of radiopaque, water-soluble solution into the sac, which outlines the umbilical cord, the placenta, and the soft tissues of the fetal body; an obsolete technique. SEE ALSO fetography. [amnio- + G. *graphō,* to write]

am·ni·o·ma (am-nē-ō′mă). Broad flat tumor of the skin resulting from antenatal adhesion of the amnion. [amnio- + G. *-oma,* tumor]

am·ni·on (am′nē-on). Innermost of the extraembryonic membranes enveloping the embryo *in utero* and containing the amniotic fluid; it consists of an internal embryonic layer with its ectodermal component, and an external somatic mesodermal component; in the later stages of pregnancy the amnion expands to come in contact with and partially fuse to the inner wall of the chorionic vesicle; derived from the trophoblast cells. SYN amniotic sac. [G. the membrane around the fetus, fr. *amnios,* lamb]

a. nodo′sum, nodules in the a. that consist of typical stratified squamous epithelium. SYN squamous metaplasia of amnion.

am·ni·on·ic (am-nē-on′ik). Relating to the amnion. SYN amniotic.

am·ni·o·ni·tis (am′nē-ō-nī′tis). Inflammation resulting from infection of the amniotic sac, which, in turn, usually results from premature rupture of the membranes (a condition often associated with neonatal infection). [amnion + G. *-itis,* inflammation]

am·ni·or·rhea (am-nē-ō-rē′ă). Escape of amniotic fluid. [amnio- + G. *rhoia,* flow]

am·ni·or·rhex·is (am-nē-ō-rek′sis). Rupture of the amniotic membrane. [amnio- + G. *rhēxis,* rupture]

am·ni·o·scope (am′nē-ō-skōp). An endoscope for studying amniotic fluid through the intact amniotic sac.

am·ni·os·co·py (am-nē-os′kō-pē). Examination of the amniotic fluid in the lowest part of the amniotic sac by means of an endoscope introduced through the cervical canal. [amnio- + G. *skopeō,* to view]

Am·ni·o·ta (am′nē-ō′tă). A group of vertebrates whose embryos are enclosed in an amnion; it includes all the reptiles, birds, and mammals.

am·ni·ot·ic (am-nē-ot′ik). SYN amnionic.

am·ni·o·tome (am′nē-ō-tōm). An instrument for puncturing the fetal membranes. [amnio- + G. *tomē,* cutting]

am·ni·ot·o·my (am-nē-ot′ō-mē). Artificial rupture of the fetal membranes as a means of inducing or expediting labor.

am·o·bar·bi·tal (am-ō-bar′bi-tahl). 5-Ethyl-5-isoamylbarbituric acid; a central nervous system depressant with an intermediate duration of action; also used as the sodium salt.

A-mode. In diagnostic ultrasound, a one-dimensional presentation of a reflected sound wave in which echo amplitude (A) is displayed along the vertical axis and time of rebound (depth) along the horizontal axis; the echo information is presented from interfaces along a single line in the direction of the sound beam.

am·o·di·a·quine hy·dro·chlo·ride (am-ō-dī′ă-kwīn). 4-(7-Chloro-4-quinolylamino)-α-diethylamino-*o*-cresol dihydrochloride dihydrate; an antimalarial drug, also used in the treatment of amebic hepatitis; large doses may result in sialorrhea, nausea, vomiting, diarrhea, insomnia, palpitations, spasticity, and possibly convulsions.

△**amoeb-.** Ameba, *Amoeba.*

Amoe·ba (ă-mē′bă). A genus of naked, lobose, pseudopod-forming protozoa of the class Sarcodina (or Rhizopoda), that are abundant soil-dwellers, especially in rich organic debris, and are also commonly found as parasites. The typical amebic parasites of man are now placed in the genera *Entamoeba, Endolimax,* and *Iodamoeba.* SEE ALSO *Naegleria.* [Mod. L. fr. G. *amoibē*change]

A. bucca′lis, former name for *Entamoeba gingivalis.*

A. co′li, old, incorrect name *Entamoeba coli.*

A. denta′lis, former name for *Entamoeba gingivalis.*

A. dysenter′iae, old, incorrect name for *Entamoeba histolytica.*

A. histolyt′ica, old, incorrect name for *Entamoeba histolytica.*

A. meleag′ridis, SYN *Histomonas meleagridis.*

A. pro′teus, an abundant, nonparasitic species, remarkable for the number and varied shapes of its pseudopodia.

Amoe·bo·tae·nia (ă-mē′bō-tē′nē-ă). A genus of small intestinal tapeworms of birds, seldom possessing more than 30 segments. *A. cuneata* (*A. sphenoides*) is a species common in domestic fowl; its cysticercoid is developed in earthworms. [amoeb- + L. fr. G. *tainia,* band, tape, a tapeworm]

amok (ă-mok′). **1.** A culture-bound mental disorder originally observed in Malaya in which the subject becomes dangerously maniacal ("running amok"). **2.** Colloquialism denoting maniacal, wild, or uncontrolled behavior threatening injury to others. SYN amuck. [native word]

amorph (ā′mōrf). An allele that has no phenotypically recognizable product and therefore its existence can be inferred on molecular evidence only, depending on the subtlety of the means of detection available. SYN silent allele. [G. *a-* neg. + *morphē,* form, shape]

amor·phag·no·sia (ă-mōr-fag-nō′sē-ă). Inability to recognize the size and shape of objects. [G. *a-* priv. + *morphē,* shape, + *gnōsis,* recognition]

amor·phia, amor·phism (ă-mōr′fē-ă, -fizm). Condition of being amorphous (1). [G. *a-* priv. + *morphē,* form]

amor·pho·syn·the·sis (ă-mōr′fō-sin′thĕ-sis). Disorder of recognition of the right side of the body in spatial relationships, caused by a lesion of the left parietal lobe. [G. *a*- priv. + *morphē*, form, + synthesis]

amor·phous (ă-mōr'fŭs). **1.** Without definite shape or visible differentiation in structure. **2.** Not crystallized.

amor·phus (ă-mōr'fŭs). A malformed fetus with rudimentary head, limbs, and heart. [G. ā- priv. + *morphē*, form, shape]

Amoss, Harold L., U. S. physician, 1886–1956. SEE A.'s *sign.*

amo·tio pla·cen·tae (ă-mō'shē-ō plă-sen'tē). SYN abruptio placentae.

amox·a·pine (ă-mok'să-pēn). 2-Chloro-11-(1-piperazinyl)-dibenz[*b,f*][1,4]oxazepine; a tricyclic antidepressant/antipsychotic drug.

amox·i·cil·lin (ă-mok-si-sil'in). A semisynthetic penicillin antibiotic with an antimicrobial spectrum similar to that of ampicillin.

AMP Abbreviation for *adenosine* monophosphate; specifically, the 5'-monophosphate unless modified by a numerical prefix. SEE adenylic acid.

AMP de·am·i·nase. An enzyme hydrolyzing adenylic acid to inosinic acid and NH_3. A deficiency of AMP d. in muscles can lead to excess fatigue following exercise. SYN adenylic acid deaminase.

am·per·age (am'pēr-ij). Strength of electric current. SEE ampere.

Ampère, André-Marie, French physicist, 1775–1836. SEE ampere; statampere; A.'s *postulate.*

am·pere (A) (am-pēr'). The practical unit of electrical current; the absolute, practical a. originally was defined as having the value of 1/10 of the electromagnetic unit (see abampere and coulomb). Present definitions are: The practical unit of electrical current; the absolute, practical a. originally was defined as having the value of 1/10 of the electromagnetic unit (see abampere and coulomb). **2.** Legal definition: the current that, flowing for 1 second, will deposit 1.118 mg of silver from silver nitrate solution. **3.** Scientific (SI) definition: the current that, if maintained in two straight parallel conductors of infinite length and of negligible circular cross-sections and placed 1 m apart in a vacuum, produces between them a force of 2×10^{-7} N/m of length. [A. *Ampère*]

am·per·om·e·try (am-pĕ-rom'ĕ-trē). Determination of any analyte concentration by measurement of the current generated in a suitable chemical reaction.

amph-. SEE amphi-, ampho-.

am·phe·clex·is (am-fē-klek'sis). Reciprocal sexual selection, *i.e.,* by both male and female. [G. *amphi*, two-sided, + *eklexis*, selection]

am·phet·a·mine (am-fet'ă-mēn). $C_6H_5CH_2CH(NH_2)$ CH_3; α-Methylphenethylamine; 1-phenyl-2-aminopropane; (phenylisopropyl)amine; closely related in its structure and action to ephedrine and other sympathomimetic amines. A psychostimulant substance that can be abused.
a. (4-chlorophenoxy)acetate, same actions and uses as a. sulfate.
a. phosphate, same actions and uses as a. sulfate.
a. sulfate, exerts less vasopressor, cardiac, and bronchial effect than ephedrine, but has a greater central nervous stimulating effect, decreasing the sensation of fatigue; used in the treatment of narcolepsy and certain types of paralysis agitans, and to reduce appetite in obesity.

***d*-am·phet·a·mine phos·phate.** SYN dextroamphetamine phosphate.

***d*-am·phet·a·mine sul·fate.** SYN dextroamphetamine sulfate.

amphi-. On both sides, surrounding, double; corresponds to L. *ambi-*. [G. *amphi,*, *amphi-*, on both sides, about, around]

am·phi·ar·thro·di·al (am'fi-ar-thrō'dē-ăl). Relating to a symphysis (1) (amphiarthrosis).

am·phi·ar·thro·sis (am'fi-ar-thrō'sis). SYN symphysis (1). [amphi- + G. *arthrōsis*, joint]

am·phi·as·ter (am-fi-as'ter). The double-star figure formed by the two astrospheres and their connecting spindle fibers during mitosis. SYN diaster. [amphi- + G. *astēr*, star]

am·phi·bar·ic (am-fi-bar'ik). Denoting a pharmacologic material that may lower or elevate arterial blood pressure, depending on the dose. [amphi- + G. *baros*, pressure]

am·phi·bol·ic (am'fi-bol'ik). Referring to reactions or biological pathways that serve in both biosynthesis and degradation (*i.e.,* anabolism and catabolism). [amphi- + metabolic]

am·phi·ce·lous (am-fi-sē'lŭs). Concave at each end, as the body of a vertebra of a fish. [amphi- + G. *koilos*, hollow]

am·phi·cen·tric (am-fi-sen'trik). Centering at both ends, said of a rete mirabile that begins by the vessel breaking up into a number of branches and ends by the branches joining again to form the same vessel. [amphi- + G. *kentron*, center]

am·phi·chro·ic (am-fi-krō'ik). SYN amphichromatic.

am·phi·chro·mat·ic (am'fi-krō-mat'ik). Having the property of exhibiting either of two colors; *e.g.,* litmus, an a. pigment which is red in acids and blue in alkalis. SYN amphichroic. [amphi- + G. *chrōma*, color]

am·phi·cyte (am'fi-sīt). One of the cells located around the bodies of the cerebrospinal and sympathetic ganglionic neurons. SYN capsule cell. [amphi- + G. *kytos*, cell]

am·phi·dip·loid (am'fi-dip'loid). Having a complete diploid chromosome set from each parent strain. [*amphi* + diploid]

am·phi·kar·y·on (am'fē-kar'ē-on). A diploid nucleus containing two haploid sets of chromosomes. [amphi- + G. *karyon*, kernel]

am·phi·leu·ke·mic (am'fi-lū-kē'mik). Denoting a leukemic condition that corresponds in degree to the changes in the organ or tissue.

Am·phim·er·us (am-fim'er-ŭs). A genus of opisthorchid trematodes found in the bile ducts of mammals, birds, and reptiles; probably transmitted by fish. [amphi- + G. *meros*, segment]

am·phi·mi·crobe (am'fi-mī'krōb). A microorganism that is either aerobic or anaerobic, according to the environment.

am·phi·mic·tic (am'fi-mik'tik). The ability to freely interbreed and produce fertile offspring. [amphi + G. *miktos*, joined, mated, fr. *mignumi*, to mix, mae, + -ia]

am·phi·mix·is (am-fi-mik'sis). **1.** Union of the paternal and maternal chromatin after impregnation of the ovum. **2.** In psychoanalysis, a combination of genital and anal eroticism. [amphi- + G. *mixis*, mingling]

am·phi·nu·cle·o·lus (am'fi-nū-klē'ō-lŭs). A double nucleolus having both basophilic and oxyphilic components. [amphi- + L. *nucleolus*, dim. of *nucleus*, kernel]

am·phi·ons (am'fi-ons). SYN dipolar *ions*, under *ion.*

Am·phi·ox·us (am-fē-ok'sŭs). A genus of small, translucent, fishlike chordates found in warm marine waters. Members are structurally similar to vertebrates in having a notochord, gills, digestive tract, and nerve cord, but they lack paired fins, vertebrae, ribs, or a skull. [amphi- + G. *oxys*, sharp]

am·phi·path·ic (am-fē-path'ik). Denoting a molecule, such as comprises detergents or wetting agents, that contains groups with characteristically different properties, *e.g.,* both hydrophilic and hydrophobic properties. SYN amphiphilic, amphiphobic. [amphi- + G. *pathos*, feeling]

am·phi·phil·ic (am-fē-fil'ik). SYN amphipathic. [amphi- + G. *philos*, fond]

am·phi·pho·bic (am-fē-fōb'ik). SYN amphipathic. [amphi- + G. *phobos*, fear]

am·phis·tome (am-fis'tōm). A common name for any trematode of the genus *Paramphistomum*. [amphi- + G. *stoma*, mouth]

am·phi·thy·mia (am-fi-thī'mē-ă). Obsolete term for a mental condition marked by periods of depression and elation. [amphi- + G. *thymos*, soul]

am·phit·ri·chate, am·phit·ri·chous (am-fit'ri-kāt, am-fit'ri-kŭs). Having a flagellum or flagella at both extremities of a microbial cell; denoting certain microorganisms. [amphi- + G. *thrix*, hair]

am·phit·y·py (am-fit'i-pē). Exhibition of the properties characteristic of two types.

am·phix·en·o·sis (am-fiks-en-ō'sis). A zoonosis maintained in nature by man and lower animals, *e.g.,* certain staphylococcoses.

Cf. anthropozoonosis, zooanthroponosis. [amphi- + G. *xenos*, stranger, + G. *-osis*, condition]

⚠**ampho-.** On both sides, surrounding, double. [G. *amphō*, both]

am·pho·chro·mat·o·phil, am·pho·chro·mat·o·phile (am'fō-krō-mat'ō-fil, -ō-fīl). SYN amphophil.

am·pho·chro·mo·phil, am·pho·chro·mo·phile (am-fō-krō'mō-fil, -fīl). SYN amphophil. [ampho- + G. *chrōma*, color, + *philos*, fond]

am·pho·cyte (am'fō-sīt). SYN amphophil (2).

am·pho·dip·lo·pia (am'fō-di-plō'pē-ă). Obsolete term for double vision in each eye or bilateral monocular diplopia. SEE monocular *diplopia*. [ampho- + G. *diploos*, double, + *ōps*, vision]

am·pho·lyte (am'fō-līt). SYN amphoteric *electrolyte*.

am·pho·my·cin (am-fō-mī'sin). An antibiotic substance produced by *Streptomyces canus;* used topically for skin infections.

am·pho·phil, am·pho·phile (am'fō-fil, -fīl). **1.** Having an affinity both for acid and for basic dyes. SYN amphophilic, amphophilous. **2.** A cell that stains readily with either acid or basic dyes. SYN amphocyte. SYN amphochromatophil, amphochromatophile, amphochromophil, amphochromophile. [ampho- + G. *philos*, fond]

am·pho·phil·ic, am·phoph·i·lous (am-fō-fil'ik, am-fof'i-lŭs). SYN amphophil (1).

am·phor·ic (am-fōr'ik). Denoting the sound heard in percussion and auscultation, resembling the noise made by blowing across the mouth of a bottle. [G. *amphora*, a jar]

am·pho·ril·o·quy (am-fō-ril'ō-kwē). Presence of amphoric voice. [G. *amphora*, a jar, + *loquor*, to speak]

am·phor·oph·o·ny (am-fō-rof'ō-nē). SYN amphoric *voice*. [G. *amphora*, a jar, + *phōnē*, voice]

am·pho·ter·ic (am-fō-tār'ik). Having two opposite characteristics, especially having the capacity of reacting as either an acid or a base; *e.g.*, $Al(OH)_3 \equiv H_3AlO_3$ or an amino acid. [G. *amphoteroi* (pl.), both, fr. *amphō*, both]

am·pho·ter·i·cin, am·pho·ter·i·cin B (am-fō-tār'i-sin). $C_{46}H_{73}NO_{20}$; an amphoteric polyene antibiotic prepared from *Streptomyces nodosus* and available as the sodium deoxycholate complex; also a nephrotoxic antifungal agent used extensively in the treatment of systemic mycoses.

am·pho·to·nia, am·phot·o·ny (am-fō-tō'nē-ă, am-fot'ō-nē). Increased excitability of both the parasympathetic and sympathetic nervous systems. [ampho- + G. *tonos*, tension]

am·pi·cil·lin (am-pi-si'lin). D-(-)-α-Aminobenzylpenicillin; R– = $C_6H_5CH(NH_2)$–; an acid-stable semisynthetic penicillin derived from 6-aminopenicillanic acid; it has a broader spectrum of antimicrobial action than penicillin G, inhibits the growth of Gram-positive and Gram-negative bacteria, and is not resistant to penicillinase; also available as a. sodium and a. trihydrate. SYN D(-)-α-aminobenzylpenicillin.

ampl. Abbreviation for L. *amplus*, large.

am·plex·us (am-plek'sŭs). The pairing of male and female at the time that eggs and sperm are discharged simultaneously in those species, such as frogs, in which fertilization occurs externally. [L. an embrace, fr. *amplector*, pp. *-plexus*, to wind around]

am·pli·fi·ca·tion (am'pli-fi-kā'shŭn). The process of making larger, as in increasing an auditory or visual stimulus to enhance its perception. [L. *amplificatio*, an enlarging]

genetic a., a process for producing an increase in pertinent genetic material, particularly for increasing the proportion of plasmid DNA to that of bacterial DNA. Includes the production of extrachromosomal copies of the genes for RNA.

am·pli·fi·er. 1. A device that increases the magnification of a microscope. **2.** an electronic apparatus that increases the strength of input signals.

image amplifier, a device for converting a low light level fluoroscopic image to one that can be seen by the eye in a lighted environment; usually consists of an electronic light amplifier chained to a television tube. SYN image intensifier.

am·pli·tude (am'pli-tūd). Largeness; extent; breadth or range. [L. *amplitudo*, fr. *amplus*, large]

a. of pulse, SEE average pulse *magnitude*, peak *magnitude*.

am·poule (am'pul). SYN ampule.

am·pro·tro·pine phos·phate (am'prō-trō'pēn). 3-Diethylamino-2,2-dimethylpropyl tropate phosphate; an antispasmodic, similar in action to atropine.

am·pule, am·pul (am'pūl). A hermetically sealed container, usually made of glass, containing a sterile medicinal solution, or powder to be made up in solution, to be used for subcutaneous, intramuscular, or intravenous injection. SYN ampoule. [L. *ampulla*]

am·pul·la, gen. and pl. **am·pul·lae** (am-pul'lă, -ē) [NA]. A saccular dilation of a canal or duct. [L. a two-handled bottle]

a. canalic'uli lacrima'lis [NA], SYN a. of lacrimal canaliculus.

a. chy'li, SYN *cisterna* chyli.

a. duc'tus deferen'tis [NA], SYN a. of ductus deferens.

a. duc'tus lacrima'lis, incorrect term for a. of lacrimal canaliculus.

duodenal a., (1) the dilated portion of the superior part of the duodenum; SYN a. duodeni [NA]. SEE ALSO duodenal *cap*. **(2)** SYN hepatopancreatic a.

a. duode'ni [NA], SYN duodenal a. (1).

a. of gallbladder, SYN Hartmann's *pouch*.

Henle's a., SYN a. of ductus deferens.

hepatopancreatic a., the dilation within the major duodenal papilla that normally receives both the common bile duct and the main pancreatic duct. SYN a. hepatopancreatica [NA], duodenal a. (2), Vater's a.

a. hepat'opancreat'ica [NA], SYN hepatopancreatic a.

a. of lacrimal canaliculus, a slight dilation at the angle of the lacrimal canaliculus immediately beyond the lacrimal punctum. SYN a. canaliculi lacrimalis [NA].

a. lactif'era, SYN lactiferous *sinus*.

lactiferous a., SYN lactiferous *sinus*.

a. membrana'cea, pl. **ampullae membrana'ceae** [NA], SYN a. of the semicircular ducts.

membranous a., SYN a. of the semicircular ducts.

a. of milk duct, SYN lactiferous *sinus*.

a. os'sea, pl. **ampullae os'seae** [NA], SYN a. of the semicircular canals.

osseous a., SYN a. of the semicircular canals.

phrenic a., a physiologic localized dilatation of the distal esophagus, commonly demonstrated by esophagography.

rectal a., a dilated portion of the rectum just above the anal canal. SYN a. recti [NA], a. of rectum.

a. rec'ti [NA], SYN rectal a.

a. of rectum, SYN rectal a.

a. of the semicircular canals, a circumscribed dilation of one extremity of each of the three bony semicircular canals, anterior, posterior, and lateral; each contains an a. of the semicircular ducts. SYN a. ossea [NA], osseous a.

a. of the semicircular ducts, a nearly spherical enlargement of one end of each of the three semicircular ducts, anterior, posterior, and lateral, where they connect with the utricle. Each contains a neuroepithelial crista ampullaris. SYN a. membranacea [NA], membranous a.

Thoma's a., a dilation of the arterial capillary beyond the sheathed artery of the spleen.

a. tu'bae uteri'nae [NA], SYN a. of uterine tube.

a. of uterine tube, the wide portion of the uterine (fallopian) tube near the fimbriated extremity; it has a complexly folded mucosa with a columnar epithelium of mostly ciliated cells between which are secretory cells. SYN a. tubae uterinae [NA].

a. of ductus deferens, the dilation of the ductus deferens where it approaches its contralateral partner just before it is joined by the duct of the seminal vesicle. SYN a. ductus deferentis [NA], Henle's a.

Vater's a., SYN hepatopancreatic a.

am·pul·lar (am-pul'ăr). Relating in any sense to an ampulla.

am·pul·li·tis (am-pul-lī'tis). Inflammation of any ampulla, especially of the dilated extremity of the vas deferens or of the ampulla of Vater. [ampulla + G. *itis*, inflammation]

am·pul·lu·la (am-pul'ū-lă). A circumscribed dilation of any minute lymphatic or blood vessel or duct. [Mod. L. dim. of L. *ampulla*]

AMPUTATION

am·pu·ta·tion (am-pyū-tā′shŭn). **1.** The cutting off of a limb or part of a limb, the breast, or other projecting part. SYN congenital a. **2.** In dentistry, removal of the root of a tooth, or of the pulp, or of a nerve root or ganglion; a modifying adjective is therefore used (pulp a.; root a.). [L. *amputatio,* fr. *am-puto,* pp. *-atus,* to cut around, prune]

A-E a., acronym for *above-the-e*lbow a.

A-K a., acronym for *above-the-k*nee a.

Alanson's a., a circular a., the stump shaped like a cone.

amniotic a., SYN congenital a.

aperiosteal a., a. with removal of periosteum from bone at the site of a.

B-E a., acronym for *below-the-e*lbow a.

Bier's a., osteoplastic a. of tibia and fibula.

birth a., SYN congenital a.

B-K a., acronym for *below-the-k*nee a.

bloodless a., a. in which, by means of a tourniquet, the escape of blood from the cut surfaces is slight. SYN dry a.

Callander's a., tenontoplastic a. through the femur at the knee.

Carden's a., transcondylar a. of the leg, the femur is sawed through the condyles just above the articular surface.

central a., a. in which the flaps are so united that the cicatrix runs across the end of the stump.

cervical a., a. of the uterine cervix.

Chopart's a., a. through the midtarsal joint; *i.e.,* between the tarsal navicular and the calcaneocuboid joints. SYN mediotarsal a.

cinematic a., SYN cineplastic a.

cineplastic a., a method of a. of an extremity whereby the muscles and tendons are so arranged in the stump that they are able to execute independent movements and to communicate motion to a specially constructed prosthetic apparatus. SYN cinematic a., cineplastics, kineplastic a., kineplastics.

circular a., a. performed by a circular incision through the skin, the muscles being similarly divided higher up, and the bone higher still. SYN guillotine a., linear a.

congenital a. [MIM*217100], a. produced *in utero;* attributed to the pressure of constricting bands (amniotic); autosomal recessive inheritance. SYN amniotic a., amputation (1), birth a., intrauterine a., spontaneous a. (1).

consecutive a., a revision or secondary succeeding amputation of a limb.

a. in continuity, a. through a segment of a limb, not at a joint.

double flap a., a. in which a flap is cut from the soft parts on either side of the limb.

dry a., SYN bloodless a.

Dupuytren's a., a. of the arm at the shoulder joint.

eccentric a., a. with the scar of the stump off-center. SYN excentric a.

elliptical a., circular a. in which the sweep of the knife is not exactly vertical to the axis of the limb, the outline of the cut surface being therefore elliptical.

excentric a., SYN eccentric a.

Farabeuf's a., (1) a. of the leg, the flap being large and on the outer side; (2) a. of the foot; disarticulation of the foot through the subtalar joint and the talo-navicular joint.

flap a., an a. in which flaps of the muscular and cutaneous tissues are made to cover the end of the bone. SYN flap operation (1).

flapless a., an a. without any tissue to cover the stump

forequarter a., amputation of the arm with removal of the scapula and a portion of the clavicle. SYN interscapulothoracic a.

Gritti-Stokes a., supracondylar a. of the femur, the patella being

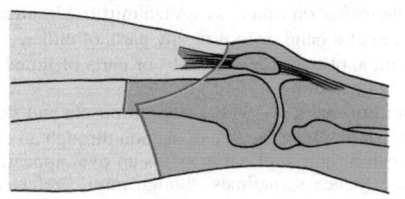

above-the-knee amputation
middle third (with flap amputation and circular incision through the muscles)

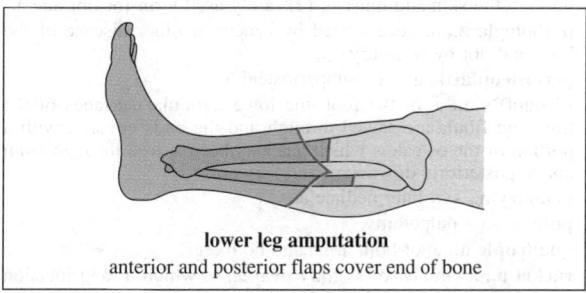

lower leg amputation
anterior and posterior flaps cover end of bone

preserved and applied to the end of the bone, its articular cartilage being removed so as to obtain union. SYN Gritti's operation.

guillotine a., SYN circular a.

Guyon's a., a. above the malleoli, a modification of Syme's a.

Hancock's a., a. of the foot through the astragalus.

Hey's a., a. of the foot in front of the tarsometatarsal joint.

hindquarter a., SYN hemipelvectomy.

immediate a., a. necessitated by irreparable injury to the limb, performed within twelve hours after the injury.

interilioabdominal a., SYN hemipelvectomy.

intermediate a., an a. formerly performed during the period between trauma or incipient gangrene and suppuration. SYN intrapyretic a., primary a.

interpelviabdominal a., SYN hemipelvectomy.

interscapulothoracic a., SYN forequarter a.

intrapyretic a., SYN intermediate a.

intrauterine a., SYN congenital a.

Jaboulay's a., SYN hemipelvectomy.

kineplastic a., SYN cineplastic a.

Kirk's a., a. at the lower end of the femur, using the tendon of the quadraceps extensor to cover the end of the bone.

Krukenberg's a., a cineplastic a. at the carpus with the distal end of the forearm used to create a fork-like stump; especially valuable in the blind because the stump has proprioception.

Larrey's a., a. at the shoulder joint.

Le Fort's a., a modification of Pirogoff's a.; the calcaneus is sawed through horizontally instead of vertically so that the patient steps on the same part of the heel as before.

linear a., SYN circular a.

Lisfranc's a., a. of the foot at the tarsometatarsal joint, the sole being preserved to make the flap. SYN Lisfranc's operation.

Mackenzie's a., a modification of Syme's a. at the ankle joint, the flap being taken from the inner side.

major a., a. of the lower or upper extremity above the ankle or the wrist, respectively.

Malgaigne's a., SYN subastragalar a.

mediotarsal a., SYN Chopart's a.

Mikulicz-Vladimiroff a., an osteoplastic resection of the foot in which the talus and calcaneus are excised, the anterior row of tarsal bones being united to the lower end of the tibia, the articular surfaces of both being removed; the lower end of the stump is therefore the anterior portion of the foot, the patient walking thereafter on tiptoe. SYN Vladimiroff-Mikulicz a.

minor a., a. of a hand or foot or any parts of either.

multiple a., a. of two or more limbs or parts of limbs performed at the same operation.

musculocutaneous a., a. with a flap of muscle and skin.

oblique a., a. in which the line of section through an extremity is at other than a right angle; this yields an oval appearance to the cut surface (hence sometimes, though rarely, referred to as an oval a.).

osteoplastic a., an a., *e.g.,* through the tarsus, in which the cut surface of another bone is brought in apposition with the one primarily divided so that the two unite, thus giving a better stump.

oval a., (1) a. in which the flaps are obained by oval incisions through the skin and muscle; **(2)** rarely used term for oblique a.

pathologic a., a. necessitated by cancer or other disease of the limb and not by an injury.

periosteoplastic a., SYN subperiosteal a.

Pirogoff's a., a. of the foot; the lower articular surfaces of the tibia and fibula are sawed through and the ends covered with a portion of the os calcis which has also been sawed through from above posteriorly downward and forward.

primary a., SYN intermediate a.

pulp a., SYN pulpotomy.

quadruple a., a. of both arms and both legs.

racket a., a circular or slightly oval a., in which a long incision is made in the axis of the limb.

rectangular a., a. in which the flaps are fashioned in the shape of a rectangle.

root a., surgical removal of one or more roots of a multirooted tooth, the remaining root canal(s) usually being treated endodontically. SYN radectomy, radiectomy, radisectomy.

secondary a., a. performed some time after a previous a. that has failed to heal satisfactorily.

spontaneous a., (1) SYN congenital a. **(2)** a. as the result of a pathologic process rather than external trauma.

Stokes a., a modification of the Gritti-Stokes a. in that the line of section of the femur is slightly higher.

subastragalar a., a. of the foot in which only the astragalus is retained. SYN Malgaigne's a.

subperiosteal a., a. in which the periosteum is stripped back from the bone and replaced afterward, forming a periosteal flap over the cut end. SYN periosteoplastic a.

Syme's a., a. of the foot at the ankle joint, the malleoli being sawed off, and a flap being made with the soft parts of the heel. SYN Syme's operation.

tarsotibial a., a. through the ankle joint.

Teale's a., (1) a. of the forearm in its lower half, or of the thigh, with a long posterior rectangular flap and a short anterior one; **(2)** a. of the leg, with a long anterior rectangular flap and a short posterior one.

tertiary a., an a. formerly performed after infection had been controlled.

a. by transfixion, a. performed by transfixing the soft parts with a long knife and cutting the flap or flaps from within outward.

transverse a., a. in which the line of section through the extremity is at right angles to the long axis.

traumatic a., a. resulting from accidental or nonsurgical injury; may be complete or incomplete.

Tripier's a., a modification of Chopart's a., in that a part of the calcaneus is also removed.

Vladimiroff-Mikulicz a., SYN Mikulicz-Vladimiroff a.

---

am·pu·tee (am′pyū-tē). A person with an amputated limb or part of limb.

am·ri·none lac·tate (am′ri-nōn). 5-Amino-(3,4′-bipyridin)-6(1*H*)-one; an inotropic agent with vasodilator activity, used in management of congestive heart failure.

Amsler, Marc, Swiss ophthalmologist, 1891–1968. SEE A.'s *chart;* A. *test.*

amu Abbreviation for atomic mass *unit.*

amuck (ă-mŭk′). SYN amok (2).

amu·sia (ă-myū′zē-ă). A form of aphasia characterized by an inability to produce or recognize music. [G. *a-* priv. + *mousa,* music]

instrumental a., loss of ability to play a musical instrument.

motor a., inability to produce music.

sensory a., inability to interpret or appreciate musical sounds.

vocal a., the inability to sing, although speech is intact.

Amussat, Jean Z., French surgeon, 1796–1856. SEE A.'s *valve, valvula.*

am·y·cho·pho·bia (am′ī-kō-fō′bē-ă). Morbid fear of being scratched. [G. *amychē,* a scratch, + *phobos,* fear]

Am·y·co·la·top·sis (Am-ē-kō-la-top′sis). A genus created in 1986. It can be isolated from soil, vegetable manner, and clinical specimens. The type species is *Amycolatopsis orientalis.*

Amycolatop′sis orienta′lis subsp. lu′rida, a species that produces ristocetin.

amyc·tic (ă-mik′tik). Obsolete term for itchy or irritating. [G. *amyssein,* to scratch, scarify]

amy·el·en·ce·pha·lia (ă-mī′el-en-sĕ-fā′lē-ă). Congenital absence of both brain and spinal cord. [G. *a-* priv. + *myelos,* marrow, + *enkephalos,* brain]

amy·el·en·ce·phal·ic, amy·el·en·ceph·a·lous (ă-mī′el-en-se-fal′ik, -sef′ă-lŭs). Denoting or characteristic of amyelencephalia.

amy·e·lia (ă-mī-ē′lē-ă). Congenital absence of the spinal cord, found in association with anencephaly. [G. *a-* priv. + *myelos,* marrow]

amy·el·ic (ă-mī-ē′lik). SYN amyelous.

amy·e·li·nat·ed (ă-mī′ĕ-li-nā′ted). SYN unmyelinated.

amy·e·li·na·tion (ă-mī′ĕ-li-nā′shŭn). Failure of formation of myelin sheath of a nerve.

amy·e·lin·ic (ă-mī′ĕ-lin′ik). SYN unmyelinated.

amy·e·lo·ic, amy·e·lon·ic (ă-mī-ĕ-lō′ik, ă-mī-ĕ-lon′ik). **1.** SYN amyelous. **2.** In hematology, sometimes used to indicate the absence of bone marrow or the lack of functional participation of bone marrow in hemopoiesis. [G. *a-* priv. + *myelos,* marrow]

amy·e·lous (ă-mī′ĕ-lŭs). Without spinal cord. SYN amyelic, amyeloic (1), amyelonic.

amyg·da·la, gen. and pl. **amyg·da·lae** (ă-mig′dă-lă, -lē). Denoting the cerebellar tonsil, as well as the lymphatic tonsils (pharyngeal, palatine, lingual, laryngeal, and tubal). [L. fr. G. *amygdalē,* almond; in Mediev. & Mod. L., a tonsil]

a. cerebel′li, SYN cerebellar *tonsil.*

amyg·da·lase (ă-mig′dă-lās). SYN β-D-glucosidase.

amyg·da·lin (ă-mig′dă-lin). mandelonitrile-β-gentiobioside; a cyanogenic glucoside present in almonds and seeds of other plants of the family Rosaceae; the principal component of laetrile. Emulsin splits a. into benzaldehyde, D-glucose, and hydrocyanic acid. SYN amygdaloside. [G. *amygdala,* almond, + -in]

amyg·da·line (ă-mig′dă-līn). **1.** Relating to an almond. **2.** Relating to a tonsil, or to the brain structure called amygdala or amygdaloid nuclear complex. **3.** SYN tonsillar.

amyg·da·loid (ă-mig′dă-loyd). Resembling an almond or a tonsil. [amygdala + G. *eidos,* appearance]

amyg·da·lo·side (ă-mig′dă-lō-sīd). SYN amygdalin.

am·yl (ā′mil). The radical formed from a pentane, C_5H_{12}, by removal of one H. Several isomeric forms exist, the more important being $CH_3CH_2CH_2CH_2CH_2$— (amyl or pentyl); $(CH_3)_2CHCH_2CH_2$— (isoamyl or isopentyl); $CH_3CH_2CH_2CH$-$(CH)_3$— and $(CH_3CH_2)_2CH$— (secondary amyl or pentyl); and $CH_3CH_2C(CH_3)_2$— (tertiary amyl or pentyl). SYN pentyl (1).

a. alcohol, 1-pentanol; used as a solvent for varnishes and oils; highly toxic, with irritating vapors. SEE ALSO fusel *oil.*

a. hydrate, SYN *amylene* hydrate.

a. nitrite, $C_5H_{11}NO_2$; a vasodilator used in angina pectoris and cyanide poisoning.

tertiary a. alcohol, SYN *amylene* hydrate.

a. valerate, isoamyl isovalerate; used as a sedative; formerly used in the treatment of gallstones because of its solvent action on cholesterol. SYN apple oil.

⚠**amyl-.** **1.** SEE amylo-. **2.** Pentyl- SEE amyl.

am·y·la·ceous (am′i-lā′shŭs). Starchy.

am·y·lase (am′il-ās). One of a group of amylolytic enzymes that cleave starch, glycogen, and related 1,4-α-glucans.

α-am·y·lase. A glucanohydrolase yielding α-glucose and maltose in a random manner from 1,4-α-glucans. An amylase that has been used clinically as a digestive aid. SYN glycogenase, ptyalin, Taka-diastase.

β-am·y·lase. A glucanohydrolase yielding β-maltose units from the nonreducing ends of 1,4-α-glucans. An exoamylase. SYN glycogenase, saccharogen amylase.

γ-am·y·lase. SYN exo-1,4-α-D-glucosidase.

am·y·la·su·ria (am-i-lā-sū′rē-ă). The excretion of amylase (sometimes termed diastase) in the urine, especially increased amounts likely in acute pancreatitis. SYN diastasuria.

am·y·le·mia (am-i-lē′mē-ă). The hypothetical presence of starch in the circulating blood. [amylo- + G. *haima*, blood]

am·yl·ene (am′i-lēn). $(CH_3)_2C$=$CHCH_3$; 2-methyl-2-butene; a flammable liquid hydrocarbon formed by the decomposition of amyl alcohol; has anesthetic properties but undesirable side actions. SYN trimethylethylene.

a. chloral, a hypnotic.

a. hydrate, *tert*-pentanol; an obsolete hypnotic used as a solvent for tribromoethanol. SYN amyl hydrate, tertiary amyl alcohol.

am·y·lin (am′i-lin). The cellulose of starch; the insoluble envelope of starch grains.

⚠**amylo-.** Starch, or polysaccharide nature or origin. [G. *amylon*, unmilled; starch, fr. *a-* + *mylē*, a mill]

am·y·lo·caine hy·dro·chlo·ride (am′i-lō-kān). 1-(Dimethylaminomethyl)-1-methylpropyl benzoate hydrochloride; benzoylethyldimethylaminopropanol hydrochloride; an early local anesthetic once widely used but eventually abandoned because of side effects.

am·y·lo·clast (am′i-lō-klast). Obsolete term for amylase. [amylo- + G. *klastos,* broken in pieces]

am·y·lo·dex·trin (am-i-lō-deks′trin). End product of hydrolysis of amylopectin by β-amylase; further hydrolysis requires amylo-1,6-glucosidase, which attacks the branch points. Identified by its color reaction with iodine (a. turns blue). Cf. achroodextrin, erythrodextrin.

am·y·lo·gen·e·sis (am-i-lō-jen′ě-sis). Biosynthesis of starch. [amylo- + G. *genesis,* production]

am·y·lo·gen·ic (am-i-lō-jen′ik). Relating to amylogenesis.

am·y·lo·-1,4:1,6-glu·can·trans·fer·ase. SYN 1,4-α-D-glucan branching enzyme.

am·y·lo·glu·co·si·dase (am-i-lō-glū′kō-si-dās). SYN exo-1,4-α-D-glucosidase.

am·y·lo·-1,6-glu·co·si·dase. An enzyme hydrolyzing α-D-1,6 links (branch points) in chains of 1,4-linked α-D-glucose residues, hence the term debranching enzyme or factor; deficiency causes type III glycogenosis. SYN dextrin 6-α-D-glucosidase.

am·y·loid (am′i-loyd). **1.** Any of a group of chemically diverse proteins that appears microscopically homogeneous, but is composed of linear nonbranching aggregated fibrils arranged in sheets when seen under the electron microscope; it stains dark brown with iodine, produces a characteristic green color in polarized light after staining with Congo red, is metachromatic with either methyl violet (pink-red) or crystal violet (purple-red), and fluoresces yellow after thioflavine T staining; a. occurs characteristically as pathologic extracellular deposits (amyloidosis), especially in association with reticuloendothelial tissue; the chemical nature of the proteinaceous fibrils is dependent upon the underlying disease process. **2.** Resembling or containing starch. [amylo- + G. *eidos,* resemblance]

am·y·loi·do·sis (am′i-loy-dō′sis). **1.** A disease characterized by extracellular accumulation of amyloid in various organs and tissues of the body; may be primary or secondary. **2.** The process of deposition of amyloid protein. [amyloid + G. *-osis,* condition]

a. of aging, characterized by deposition of Congo-red staining

material, derived from a variety of proteins, especially in nervous tissue, myocardium and pancreas. Associated with Alzheimer's syndrome; intractable congestive heart failure may result.

chronic amyloidosis, a. of long duration.

a. cu′tis, SYN lichenoid a.

familial a., SYN familial amyloid *neuropathy.*

focal a., SYN nodular a.

hereditary a., SYN familial amyloid *neuropathy.*

lichen a., SYN lichenoid a.

lichenoid a. (līk′en-oyd), localized cutaneous a. with pruritic brownish-red papules, most commonly on the lower legs, due to amyloid infiltration of the papillary dermis. SYN a. cutis, lichen a. [G. *leichēn,* lichen, a lichen-like eruption + *eidos,* resemblance]

light chain-related a., a form of primary a. in which the fibrillar amyloid deposits are derived from the amino terminal variable region of the light chains of immunoglobulin; seen in B-lymphocyte and plasma-cells dyscrasias.

macular a., a localized form of a. cutis characterized by pruritic symmetrical brown reticulated macules, especially on the upper back; microscopically, amyloid is deposited as small subepidermal globules.

a. of multiple myeloma, foci of a. in mesenchymal tissues of some persons with multiple myeloma; no direct relation between amyloid and Bence Jones protein is conclusively known.

nodular a., a localized form of a. in which amyloid occurs as masses or nodules beneath the skin or mucous membranes, *e.g.,* in the larynx. SYN amyloid tumor, focal a.

primary a., several forms of a. are known, following autosomal dominant [MIM *104750-*105230] recessive [MIM 204850-204900], and X-linked [MIM 301220] inheritance and not associated with other recognized disease. Tends to involve diffusely the arterial walls and mesenchymal tissues in the tongue, lungs, intestinal tract, skin, skeletal muscle, and myocardium; the amyloid frequently does not manifest the usual affinity for Congo red, and sometimes provokes a foreign-body type of inflammatory reaction in the adjacent tissue.

renal a., renal deposits of amyloid, especially in glomerular capillary walls, which may cause albuminuria and the nephrotic syndrome. SYN amyloid nephrosis (1).

secondary a., a. occurring in association with another chronic inflammatory disease; organs chiefly involved are the liver, spleen, and kidneys, and the adrenal glands less frequently.

senile a., a common form of a. in very old people, usually mild and limited to the heart. SEE ALSO a. of aging.

am·y·lol·y·sis (am-i-lol′i-sis). Hydrolysis of starch into soluble products. [amylo- + G. *lysis,* dissolution]

am·y·lo·lyt·ic (am-i-lō-lit′ik). Relating to amylolysis.

am·y·lo·malt·ase (am-i-lō-mal′tās). SYN 4-α-D-glucanotransferase.

am·y·lo·pec·tin (am-i-lō-pek′tin). A branched-chain polyglucose (glucan) in starch containing both 1,4 and 1,6 linkages. Cf. amylose.

am·y·lo·pec·tin 6-glu·can·o·hy·dro·lase. Former name for α-dextrin endo-1,6-α-glucosidase.

am·y·lo·pec·tin 1,6-glu·co·si·dase. Former name for an enzyme now known to be at least two enzymes, α-dextrin endoglucanohydrolase and isoamylase.

am·y·lo·pec·tin·o·sis (am′i-lō-pek-tin-ō′sis). SEE type 4 *glycogenosis.* [amylopectin + G. *-osis,* condition]

am·y·lo·pha·gia (am′i-lō-fā′jē-ă). A morbid craving for starch. SYN starch-eating. [amylo- + G. *phagō,* to eat]

am·y·lo·plast (am′i-lō-plast). A granule in the protoplasm of a plant cell that is the center of a starch-forming process. SYN amylogenic body. [amylo- + G. *plastos,* formed]

am·y·lo·psin (am-il-op′sin). The amylase of pancreatic juice.

am·y·lor·rhea (am′i-lō-rē′ă). Passage of undigested starch in the stools, implying a deficiency of amylase activity in the intestine. [amylo- + G. *rhoia,* flow]

am·y·lose (am′i-lōs). An unbranched polyglucose (glucan) in starch, similar to cellulose, containing $α(1→4)$ linkages. Cf. amylopectin.

am·y·lo·su·ria (am'i-lō-sū'rē-ă). Excretion of starch in the urine. SYN amyluria.

am·y·lo-(1,4→1,6)-trans·glu·co·si·dase, am·y·lo-(1,4→1,6)-trans·glu·co·syl·ase. SYN 1,4-α-D-glucan branching enzyme.

am·y·lum (am'i-lŭm). SYN starch.

am·y·lu·ria (am-i-lū'rē-ă). SYN amylosuria.

amy·o·car·dia (ă-mī-ō-kar'dē-ă). Obsolete term for weakness of the heart muscle. [G. *a*- priv. + *mys,* muscle, + *kardia,* heart]

amy·o·es·the·sia, amy·o·es·the·sis (ă-mī'ō-es-thē'zē-ă, -thē'sis). Absence of muscle sensation. [G. *a*- priv. + *mys,* muscle, + *aisthēsis,* perception]

amy·o·pla·sia (ă-mī-ō-plā'zē-ă). Deficient formation of muscle tissue and deficient muscle growth. [G. *a*- priv. + *mys,* muscle, + *plasis,* a molding]

    a. congen'ita, SYN *arthrogryposis* multiplex congenita.

amy·o·sta·sia (ă-mī-ō-stā'zē-ă). Difficulty in standing, due to muscular tremor or incoordination. [G. *a*- priv. + *mys,* muscle, + *stasis,* standing]

amy·o·stat·ic (ă-mī-ō-stat'ik). Showing muscular tremors.

amy·os·the·nia (ă-mī'os-thē'nē-ă). Muscular weakness. [G. *a*-priv. + *mys,* muscle, + *sthenos,* strength]

amy·os·then·ic (ă-mī-os-then'ik). Relating to or causing muscular weakness.

amy·o·taxy, amy·o·tax·ia (ă-mī'ō-tak-sē, ă-mī-ō-tak'sē-ă). Muscular ataxia. [G. *a*- priv. + *mys,* muscle, + *taxis,* order]

amy·o·to·nia (ă-mī-ō-tō'nē-ă). Generalized absence of muscle tone, usually associated with flabby musculature and an increased range of passive movement at joints. [G. *a*- priv. + *mys,* muscle, + *tonos,* tone]

    a. congen'ita, (1) atonic pseudoparalysis of congenital origin (neither familial nor hereditary), observed especially in infants and characterized by absences of muscular tone only in muscles innervated by the spinal nerves. SYN congenital atonic pseudoparalysis, myatonia congenita, Oppenheim's disease, Oppenheim's syndrome. **(2)** an indefinite term for a number of congenital neuromuscular disorders that cause generalized myotonia in young children, and that have a benign course (static or regressive).

amy·o·tro·phia (ă-mī-ō-trō'fē-ă). SYN amyotrophy.

amy·o·tro·phic (ă-mī-ō-trō'fik). Relating to muscular atrophy.

amy·ot·ro·phy (ă-mī-ot'rō-fē). Muscular wasting or atrophy. SYN amyotrophia. [G. *a*- priv. + *mys,* muscle, + *trophē,* nourishment]

    diabetic a., a type of diabetic neuropathy that primarily affects elderly patients with diabetes mellitus; clinically characterized by unilateral or bilateral anterior thigh pain, weakness, and atrophy; of abrupt or gradual onset and, when bilateral, of simultaneous or sequential onset, and usually asymmetrical; one type of diabetic polyradiculopathy. Sometimes referred to, erroneously, as diabetic femoral neuropathy.

    hemiplegic a., muscular atrophy seen in hemiplegic limbs.

    neuralgic a., a neurological disorder, of unknown cause, characterized by the sudden onset of severe pain, usually about the shoulder and often beginning at night, soon followed by weakness and wasting of various forequarter muscles, particularly shoulder girdle muscles; both sporadic and familial in occurrence with the former much more common; often preceded by some antecedent event, such as an upper respiratory infection, hospitalization, vaccination, or non-specific trauma; usually attributed to a brachial plexus lesion, because the nerve fibers involed are most often derived from the upper trunk, but actually multiple proximal mononeuropathies. SYN acute brachial radiculitis, brachial plexitis, brachial plexus neuropathy, Parsonage-Turner syndrome, shoulder-girdle syndrome.

    progressive spinal a., SYN amyotrophic lateral *sclerosis.*

am·y·ous (am'ē-ŭs). Lacking in muscular tissue, or in muscular strength. [G. *a*- priv. + *mys,* muscle]

amyx·or·rhea (ă-mik-sō-rē'ă). Absence of the normal secretion of mucus. [G. *a*- priv. + *myxa,* mucus, + *rhoia,* flow]

△**an-.** SEE a-.

ANA. Abbreviation for antinuclear *antibody;* American Nurses Association.

△**ana-.** Up, again, back; sometimes *an-* before a vowel; corresponds to L. *sursum-;* CAUTION: *an-* before a vowel usually stands for *a-* meaning not; sometimes *ana-* becomes *am-* before p, b, or ph. [G. *ana,* up]

An·a·bae·na (an-ă-bē'nă). A genus of Cyanobacteria causing odors in water supplies.

an·a·bi·o·sis (an'ă-bī-ō'sis). Resuscitation after apparent death. [G. a reviving, fr. *ana,* again, + *biōsis,* life]

an·a·bi·ot·ic (an'ă-bī-ot'ik). **1.** Resuscitating or restorative. **2.** A revivifying remedy; a powerful stimulant. [ana- + G. *bios,* life]

an·a·bol·ic (an-ă-bol'ik). Relating to or promoting anabolism.

anab·o·lism (ă-nab'ō-lizm). **1.** The building up in the body of complex chemical compounds from smaller simpler compounds (*e.g.,* proteins from amino acids), usually with the use of energy. Cf. catabolism, metabolism. **2.** The sum of synthetic metabolic reactions. [G. *anabolē,* a raising up]

anab·o·lite (ă-nab'ō-līt). Any substance formed as a result of anabolic processes.

an·a·bro·sis (an-ă-brō'sis). Archaic term for superficial erosion or ulceration. [G. fr. *ana,* up, + *bibrōskō,* to eat up]

an·a·brot·ic (an-ă-brot'ik). Obsolete term for a substance that produces ulceration or erosion of the skin surface.

an·a·camp·tom·e·ter (an-ă-kamp-tom'ĕ-ter). Instrument for measuring the intensity of the deep reflexes. [G. *anakampsis,* a bending back, reflection, + *metron,* measure]

an·a·car·di·ol (an-ă-kar'dē-ol). 3-Ethoxy-*N,N*-diethyl-4-hydroxybenzamide; an analeptic.

an·a·cat·es·the·sia (an'ă-kat'es-thē'zē-ă). A hovering sensation. [G. *ana,* up, + *kata,* down, + *aisthēsis,* sensation]

an·a·cid·i·ty (an-ă-sid'i-tē). Absence of acidity; used especially to denote absence of hydrochloric acid in the gastric juice.

anac·la·sis (ă-nak'lă-sis). **1.** Reflection of light or sound. **2.** Refraction of the ocular media. [G. a bending back, reflection]

an·a·clit·ic (an-ă-klit'ik). Leaning or depending upon; in psychoanalysis, relating to the dependence of the infant on the mother or mother substitute. SEE anaclitic *depression.* [G. *ana,* toward, + *klinō,* to lean]

an·ac·me·sis (an-ak'mē-sis). Obsolete spelling for anakmesis.

an·a·crot·ic (an-ă-krot'ik). Referring to the upstroke or ascending limb of the arterial pulse tracing; an abbreviated form for anadicrotic, twice beating on the upstroke. SYN anadicrotic.

anac·ro·tism (ă-nak'rō-tizm). Peculiarity of the pulse wave. SEE anacrotic *pulse.* SYN anadicrotism. [G. *ana,* up, + *krotos,* a beat]

an·a·cu·sis (an'ă-kū'sis). Total loss or absence of the ability to perceive sound as such. SYN anakusis. [G. *an-* priv. + *akousis,* hearing]

an·a·de·nia (an-ă-dē'nē-ă). Absence of glands or abeyance of glandular function. [G. *an-* priv. + *adēn,* gland]

    a. ventric'uli, absence of glands from the stomach.

an·a·di·crot·ic (an-ă-dī-krot'ik). SYN anacrotic.

an·a·di·cro·tism (an-ă-dik'rō-tizm). SYN anacrotism. [G. *ana,* up, + *di-krotos,* double beating]

an·a·did·y·mus (an-ă-did'i-mŭs). SYN *duplicitas* posterior. [G. *ana,* up, + *didymos,* twin]

an·a·dip·sia (an-ă-dip'sē-ă). Rarely used term for extreme thirst. SEE ALSO polydipsia. [G. *ana,* intensive, + *dipsa,* thirst]

an·ad·re·nal·ism (an-ă-drē'năl-izm). Complete lack of adrenal function.

an·aer·obe (an'ār-ōb, an-ār'ōb). A microorganism that can live and grow in the absence of oxygen. [G. *an-* priv. + *aēr,* air, + *bios,* life]

    facultative a., an a. that grows in the presence of air or under conditions of reduced oxygen tension.

    obligate a., an a. that will grow only in the absence of free oxygen.

an·aer·o·bic (an-ār-ō'bik). Relating to an anaerobe; living without oxygen.

an·aer·o·bi·o·sis (an-ār-ō-bī-ō'sis). Existence in an oxygen-free atmosphere. [G. *an-* priv. + *aēr,* air, + *biōsis,* way of living]

an·aer·o·gen·ic (an-ār-ō-jen'ik). Not producing gas. [G. *an-* priv. + *aēr,* air, + *-gen,* producing]

an·aer·o·phyte (an-ār'ō-fīt). 1. A plant that grows without air. 2. An anaerobic bacterium. [G. *an-* priv. + *aēr,* air, + *phyton,* plant]

an·aer·o·plas·ty (an-ār'ō-plas-tē). Treatment of wounds by exclusion of air. [G. *an-* not + *aēr,* air, + *plastos,* formed]

an·a·gen (an'ă-jen). Growth phase of the hair cycle, lasting about 3 to 6 years in human scalp hair. [G. *ana,* up, + *-gen,* producing]

an·a·gen·e·sis (an-ă-jen'ĕ-sis). 1. Repair of tissue. 2. Regeneration of lost parts. [G. *ana,* up, + *genesis,* production]

an·a·ge·net·ic (an'ă-jĕ-net'ik). Pertaining to anagenesis.

an·a·ges·tone ac·e·tate (an-ă-jes'tōn). 17-Hydroxy-6α-methyl-pregn-4-en-20-one acetate; a progestational agent.

Anagnostakis, Andrei, Cretan ophthalmologist, 1826–1897.

an·a·go·gy (an-ă-gō'jē). Psychic content of an idealistic or spiritual nature. [G. *anagōgē,* fr. *an-* *ago,* to lead up]

an·a·kat·a·did·y·mus, an·a·cat·a·did·y·mus (an'ă-kat-ă-did'i-mŭs). Conjoined twins united in the middle but separated above and below. SYN dicephalus dipygus. [G. *ana,* up, + *kata,* down, + *didymos,* twin]

an·á·khré (an-ah-krā'). SYN goundou. [Fr. fr. Af. native term meaning "big nose"]

an·ak·me·sis (an-ak'mē-sis). Arrest of maturation of leukocytes in their production centers, thereby resulting in greater numbers of young forms and progressively smaller proportions of mature granular cells in the bone marrow, as observed in agranulocytosis. [G. *an-* priv. + *akmēnos,* full grown, fr. *akmē,* highest point]

an·a·ku·sis (an-ă-kū'sis). SYN anacusis.

anal (ā'năl). Relating to the anus.

an·al·bu·mi·ne·mia (an'al-bū-mi-nē'mē-ă). Absence of albumin from the serum. [G. *an-* priv. + albumin + G. *haima,* blood]

an·a·lep·tic (an-ă-lep'tik). 1. Strengthening, stimulating, or invigorating. 2. A restorative remedy. 3. A central nervous system stimulant, particularly used to denote agents that reverse depressed central nervous system function. [G. *analēptikos,* restorative]

an·al·ge·sia (an-al-jē'zē-ă). A neurologic or pharmacologic state in which painful stimuli are so moderated that, though still perceived, they are no longer painful. Cf. anesthesia. [G. insensibility, fr. *an-* priv. + *algēsis,* sensation of pain]

a. al'gera, SYN a. dolorosa.

conduction a., SYN regional *anesthesia.*

a. doloro'sa, spontaneous pain in a body area that lacks sensation. SYN a. algera.

inhalation a., a. produced by inhalation of a central nervous system depressant gas (especially nitrous oxide) or vapor.

patient controlled a. (PCA), a method for control of pain based upon a pump for the constant intravenous or, less frequently, epidural infusion of a dilute narcotic solution that includes a mechanism for the self-administration at predetermined intervals of a predetermined amount of the narcotic solution should the infusion fail to relieve pain. SYN outpatient anesthesia (1).

spinal a., euphemism for spinal *anesthesia.*

an·al·ge·sic (an-ăl-jē'zik). 1. A compound capable of producing analgesia, *i.e.,* one that relieves pain by altering perception of nociceptive stimuli without producing anesthesia or loss of consciousness. SYN analgetic (1). 2. Characterized by reduced response to painful stimuli. SYN antalgic.

an·al·ge·sim·e·ter (an'ăl-jē-zim'i-ter). A device for eliciting painful stimuli in order to measure pain under experimental conditions. [analgesia + G. *metron,* measure]

an·al·get·ic (an-ăl-jet'ik). 1. SYN analgesic (1). 2. Associated with decreased pain perception.

anal·i·ty (ā-nal'i-tē). Referring to the psychic organization derived from, and characteristic of, the Freudian anal period of psychosexual development.

an·al·ler·gic (an-ă-ler'jik). Not allergic.

an·a·log (an'ă-log). 1. One of two organs or parts in different species of animals or plants which differ in structure or develop-

ment but are similar in function. 2. A compound that resembles another in structure but is not necessarily an isomer (*e.g.,* 5-fluorouracil is an analog of thymine); a.'s are often used to block enzymatic reactions by combining with enzymes (*e.g.,* isopropyl thiogalactoside vs. lactose). SYN analogue. [G. *analogos,* proportionate]

enzyme a., SYN synzyme.

anal·o·gous (ă-nal'ō-gŭs). Possessing a functional resemblance, but having a different origin or structure.

an·a·logue (an'ă-log). SYN analog.

an·al·pha·lip·o·pro·tein·e·mia (an-al'fă-lip'ō-prō'tēn-ē'mē-ă) [MIM*205400]. Familial high density lipoprotein deficiency; a heritable disorder of lipid metabolism characterized by almost complete absence from plasma of high density lipoproteins, and by storage of cholesterol esters in foam cells, tonsillar enlargement, an orange or yellow-gray color of the pharyngeal and rectal mucosa, hepatosplenomegaly, lymph node enlargement, corneal opacity, and peripheral neuropathy; autosomal recessive inheritance. SYN familial high density lipoprotein deficiency, Tangier disease. [G. *an-,* priv., + *alpha,* α, + lipoprotein + *-emia,* blood]

anal·y·sand (ă-nal'i-sand). In psychoanalysis, the person being analyzed. [analysis + L. *-andus,* gerundive ending]

anal·y·sis, pl. **anal·y·ses** (ă-nal'i-sis, -sēz). 1. The breaking up of a chemical compound or mixture into simpler elements; a process by which the composition of a substance is determined. 2. The examination and study of a whole in terms of the parts composing it. 3. SEE psychoanalysis. [G. a breaking up, fr. *ana,* up, + *lysis,* a loosening]

accumulation a., a technique in which an intermediate of a metabolic pathway accumulates due to selective inhibition of a particular step in that pathway or in a mutant that is deficient in a certain step. The intermediate is then isolated, analyzed, and identified.

activation a., the identification and quantification of unknown elements from their characteristic emissions and decay constants after they have been made radioactive by exposure to neutron or charged particle radiation.

amino acid a., (1) determination and identification of amino acid content of a macromolecule; **(2)** identification of a specific amino acid in macromolecules, often a mutated protein; **(3)** identification and quantitation of amino acid content in blood plasma or urine; a key diagnostic aid.

bite a., SYN occlusal a.

blood gas a., the direct electrode measurement of the partial pressure of oxygen and carbon dioxide in the blood.

bradykinetic a., the a. of a movement by means of slow cinematography.

cephalometric a., a study of the skeletal and dental relationships used in orthodontic case a.

character a., a. of the defenses and personality traits that characterize an individual.

cluster a., a set of statistical methods used to group variables or observations into strongly interrelated subgroups.

content a., any of a variety of techniques for classification and study of the verbal products of normal or of psychologically disabled individuals.

decision a., a derivative of operations research and game theory that involves identifying all available choices and the potential outcomes of each, in a series of decisions that have to be made about patient care—diagnostic procedures, therapeutic regimens, prognostic expectations; the range of choices can be plotted on a decision tree.

didactic a., SYN training a.

discriminant a., a statistical analytic technique used with discrete dependent variables, concerned with separating sets of observed values and allocating new values; an alternative to regression analysis.

displacement a., SYN competitive binding *assay.*

distributive a., the a. of information gained about the patient and its distribution by the physician, as indicated by the patient's complaint and symptoms.

Downs' a., a series of cephalometric criteria used as an aid in orthodontic diagnosis.

ego a., psychoanalytic study of the ways in which the ego deals with intrapsychic conflicts.

Fourier a., a mathematical approximation of a function as the sum of periodic functions (sine waves) of different frequencies; a method of converting a function of time or space into a function of frequency; used in reconstruction of images in computed tomography and magnetic resonance imaging in radiology and in analysis of any kind of signal for its frequency content. SYN Fourier transform.

gastric a., measurement of pH and acid output of stomach contents; basal acid output can be determined by collecting the overnight gastric secretion or by a 1-hr collection; maximal acid output is determined following injection of histamine; output is measured by titration with a strong base.

interaction process a., in psychology, a. of small group behavior in terms of 12 specific categories, *e.g.,* solidarity, tension release, agreement.

linkage a., the assessment of the linkage relationship between two loci by the examination of data in pedigrees. The classical concern is with estimating recombination fractions and (because of its elasticity, efficiency, and other optimal properties) the preferred method is maximum likelihood estimation. However, there are other more modern concerns, notably determining the order of loci, testing for additive and interactive properties in the mapping function, and reconciling the pedigree data with evidence from other methods (*e.g.,* cytogenetics, *in situ* hybridization studies, etc.).

Northern blot a., a procedure similar to the Southern blot a., used mostly to separate and identify RNA fragments; typically via transferring RNA fragments from an agarose gel to a nitrocellulose filter followed by detection with a suitable probe. [coined to distinguish it from eponymic Southern blot a.]

occlusal a., a study of the relations of the occlusal surfaces of opposing teeth and their effect upon related structures. SYN bite a.

path a., a mode of a. involving assumptions about the direction of causal relationships among linked sequences and configurations of variables.

pedigree a., the formal study of the pattern of a trait in a pedigree to determine such properties as its mode of inheritance, age of onset, and variability in phenotype.

percept a., psychologic survey of an individual's personality using Rorschach's series of inkblots.

qualitative a., determination of the nature, as opposed to the quantity, of each of the elements composing a substance.

quantitative a., determination of the amount, as well as the nature, of each of the elements composing a substance.

regression a., the statistical method of finding the "best" mathematical model to describe one variable as a function of another.

saturation a., SYN competitive binding *assay.*

segregation a., in genetics, the enumeration of progeny according to distinct and mutually exclusive phenotypes; used as a test of a putative pattern of inheritance, *e.g.,* mendelian, dominant autosomal, epistatic, age-dependent.

sequential a., a statistical method that allows an experiment to be ended as soon as a result of desired precision is obtained.

Southern blot a., a procedure to separate and identify DNA sequences; DNA fragments are separated by electrophoresis on an agarose gel, transferred (blotted) onto a nitrocellulose or nylon membrane, and hybridized with complementary (labeled) nucleic acid probes.

stratographic a., a former term for chromatography.

survival a., a class of statistical procedures for estimating survival rates and making inferences about effects of treatment, prognostic factors, etc.

training a., psychoanalytic treatment for the purpose of training of an analytic candidate carried out under the official auspices of a psychoanalytic training institute. SYN didactic a.

transactional a., a psychotherapy system, used in both individual and group treatment, involving a systematic understanding of the qualities of interpersonal interactions in the treatment sessions; includes four components: 1) structural analysis of intra-

psychic phenomena; 2) transactional a. proper, determination of the currently dominant ego state (parent, child, or adult) of each participant; 3) game analysis, identification of the games played in their interactions and of the gratifications provided; 4) script analysis, uncovering of the causes of the patient's emotional problems.

a. of variance (ANOVA), a statistical technique that isolates and assesses the contribution of categorical independent variables to variation in the mean of a continuous dependent variable.

volumetric a., quantitative a. by the addition of graduated amounts of a standard test solution to a solution of a known amount of the substance analyzed, until the reaction is just at an end; depends upon the stoichiometric nature of the reaction between the test solution and the unknown.

Western blot a., a procedure in which proteins separated by electrophoresis in polyacrylamide gels are transferred (blotted) onto nitrocellulose or nylon membranes and identified by specific complexing with antibodies that are either pre- or post-tagged with a labeled secondary protein. SEE ALSO immunoblot. SYN Western blot, Western blotting. [coined to distinguish it from eponymic Southern blot a.]

zoo blot a., a procedure using Southern blot a. to test the ability of a nucleic acid probe from one species to hybridize with the DNA fragment of another species.

an·a·lyst (an'ă-list). **1.** One who makes analytical determinations. **2.** Short term for psychoanalyst.

an·a·lyte (an'ă-līt). Any substance or chemical constituent of blood, urine, or other body fluid that is analyzed.

an·a·lyt·ic, an·a·lyt·i·cal (an-ă-lit'-ik, -i-kăl). **1.** Relating to analysis. **2.** Relating to psychoanalysis.

an·a·lyz·er, an·a·lyz·or (an'ă-līz-er, -ŏr). **1.** Any instrument that performs an analysis. **2.** The prism in a polariscope by means of which the polarized light is examined. **3.** The neural basis of the conditioned reflex; includes all of the sensory side of the reflex arc and its central connections. **4.** A device that electronically determines the frequency and amplitude of a particular channel of an electroencephalogram.

centrifugal fast a., an automatic spectrophotometer that uses centrifugal force to mix samples and reagents, and propels the reactants at high speed about a detector that makes multiple absorbance readings.

kinetic a., an instrument that measures the rate of change in a chemical substance; used mainly for enzyme measurement.

pulse height a., electronic circuitry that determines the energy of scintillations recorded by a detector, allowing use of a discriminator to select for photons of a specific type.

wave a., an apparatus that assesses a complex mixture of wave forms by separating out their component frequencies and displaying their distribution.

an·am·ne·sis (an-am-nē'sis). **1.** The act of remembering. **2.** The medical or developmental history of a patient. [G. *anamnēsis,* recollection]

an·am·nes·tic (an-am-nes'tik). **1.** Assisting the memory. SYN mnemonic. **2.** Relating to the medical history of a patient.

an·am·ni·on·ic, an·am·ni·ot·ic (an-am-nē-on'ik, -ot'ik). Without an amnion.

An·am·ni·o·ta (an-am-nē-ō'tă). A group of vertebrates whose embryos are not enclosed in an amnion; it includes the cyclostomes, fish, and amphibians.

ana·morph. A somatic or reproductive structure that originates without nuclear recombination (asexual reproduction); the imperfect part of the life cycle of fungi. [G. *ana,* up, + morphē, form]

an·a·mor·pho·sis (an'ă-mōr-fō'sis). **1.** In phylogeny, a progressive series of changes in the evolution of a group of animals or plants. **2.** In optics, the process of correcting a distorted image with a curved mirror. [G. *ana,* up, + morphē, form]

an·an·a·phy·lax·is (an'an-ă-fī-lak'sis). SYN desensitization (1).

an·an·a·sta·sia (an'an-ă-stā'zē-ă). Inability to stand up. [G. *a*-priv. + *anastasis,* stand up]

an·an·casm (an'an-kazm). Any form of repetitious stereotyped behavior which, if prevented, results in anxiety. [G. *anankasma,* compulsion]

an·an·cas·tia (an-an-kas′tē-ă). An obsession in which a person feels himself forced to act or think against his will. [G. *anankastos,* compelled]

an·an·cas·tic (an-an-kas′tik). Pertaining to anancasm or anancastia.

an·an·dria (an-an′drē-ă). Absence of masculinity. [G. want of manhood, fr. *an-* priv. + *anēr-* (*andr-*), man]

an·an·gi·o·pla·sia (an-an′jē-ō-pla′zē-ă). Imperfect vascularization of a part due to nonformation of vessels, or vessels with inadequate caliber. [G. *an-* priv. + *angeion,* vessel, + *plastos,* formed]

an·an·gi·o·plas·tic (an-an′jē-ō-plas′tik). Relating to, characterized by, or due to anangioplasia.

ANAP Abbreviation for anionic neutrophil activating *peptide.*

an·a·pei·rat·ic (an′ă-pī-rat′ik). Resulting from overuse; denoting certain occupational neuroses. [G. *ana-peiraomai,* to try again, fr. *peiraō,* to try]

an·a·phase (an′ă-fāz). The stage of mitosis or meiosis in which the chromosomes move from the equatorial plate toward the poles of the cell. In mitosis a full set of daughter chromosomes (46 in humans) moves toward each pole. In the first division of meiosis one member of each homologous pair (23 in humans), consisting of two chromatids united at the centromere, moves toward each pole. In the second division of meiosis the centromere divides, and the two chromatids separate with one moving to each pole. [G. *ana,* up, + *phasis,* appearance]

an·a·phia (an-ā′fē-ă, an-af′ē-ă). Absence of the sense of touch. SYN anhaphia. [G. *an-* priv. + *haphē,* touch]

an·a·pho·re·sis (an′ă-fō-rē′sis). Movement of negatively charged particles (anions) in a solution or suspension toward the anode in electrophoresis. Cf. cataphoresis. [G. *ana,* up + *phorēsis,* a being borne]

an·aph·o·ret·ic (an′ă-fō-ret′ik). Relating to anaphoresis (1).

an·aph·ro·di·sia (an′af-rō-diz′ē-ă). Rarely used term denoting absence of sexual feeling. [G. insensibility to love, from *an-* priv. + *Aphroditē,* the goddess of love]

an·aph·ro·di·si·ac (an′af-rō-diz′ē-ak). **1.** Relating to anaphrodisia. **2.** Repressing or destroying sexual desire. **3.** An agent that lessens or abolishes sexual desire. SYN antaphrodisiac, antaphroditic (1). [G. *an-* priv. + *aphrodisia,* sexual pleasure]

an·a·phy·lac·tic (an′ă-fī-lak′tik). Relating to anaphylaxis; manifesting extremely great sensitivity to foreign protein or other material.

an·a·phy·lac·to·gen (an′ă-fī-lak′tō-jen). A substance (antigen) capable of rendering an individual susceptible to anaphylaxis; a substance (antigen) that will cause an anaphylactic reaction in such a sensitized individual.

an·a·phy·lac·to·gen·e·sis (an′ă-fī-lak-tō-jen′ě-sis). The production of anaphylaxis.

an·a·phy·lac·to·gen·ic (an′ă-fī-lak-tō-jen′ik). Producing anaphylaxis; pertaining to substances (antigens) that result in an individual becoming susceptible to anaphylaxis.

an·a·phy·lac·toid (an′ă-fī-lak′toyd). Resembling anaphylaxis. SYN pseudoanaphylactic. [anaphylaxis + G. *eidos,* resemblance]

an·a·phyl·a·tox·in (an′ă-fil-ă-tok′sin). **1.** A substance postulated to be the immediate cause of anaphylactic shock and that is assumed to result from the *in vivo* combination of specific antibody and the specific sensitizing material, when the latter is injected as a shock dose in a sensitized animal. **2.** The small fragment (C3a) split from the third component (C3) of complement by C3 convertase and that releases histamine from rat peritoneal mast cells, causes pig ileum to contract, and produces a local wheal following intracutaneous injection in man; also used with reference to a small fragment (C5a) split from the fifth component (C5) of complement by the EAC1243 complex which has chemotactic properties as well. SYN anaphylotoxin. [anaphylaxis + toxin]

an·a·phyl·a·tox·in in·ac·ti·va·tor. An α-globulin (MW 300,000) which destroys the activity of the anaphylatoxic complement fragments. SEE anaphylatoxin (2).

an·a·phy·lax·is (an′ă-fī-lak′sis). A term coined by Portier and Richet to indicate a lessened resistance to a toxin which results

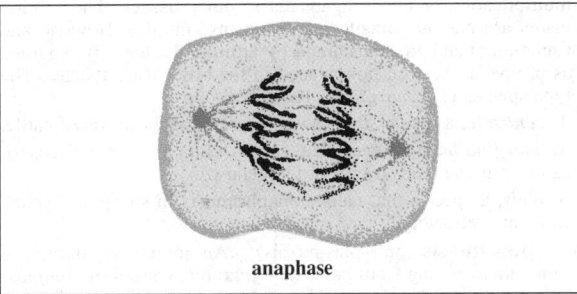
anaphase

from a previous inoculation of the same material, and in this sense was synonymous with hypersensitivity in its original usage of a postulated increased sensitivity to a toxin; shortly thereafter, a. was used by Arthus to indicate an induced sensitivity; at times a. is used for anaphylactic shock. The term is commonly used to denote the immediate, transient kind of immunologic (allergic) reaction characterized by contraction of smooth muscle and dilation of capillaries due to release of pharmacologically active substances (histamine, bradykinin, serotonin, and slow-reacting substance), classically initiated by the combination of antigen (allergen) with mast cell-fixed, cytophilic antibody (chiefly IgE); the reaction can be initiated, also, by relatively large quantities of serum aggregates (antigen-antibody complexes, and others) that seemingly activate complement leading to production of anaphylatoxin, a reaction sometimes termed "aggregate a." SYN anaphylactic reaction. [G. *ana,* away from, back from, + *phylaxis,* protection]

active a., reaction following inoculation of antigen in a subject previously sensitized to the specific antigen, in contrast to passive a.

aggregate a., SEE anaphylaxis.

antiserum a., SYN passive a.

chronic a., SYN *enteritis* anaphylactica.

generalized a., the immediate response, involving smooth muscles and capillaries throughout the body of a sensitized individual, that follows intravenous (and occasionally intracutaneous) injection of antigen (allergen). SEE ALSO anaphylactic *shock.* SYN systemic a.

inverse a., anaphylactic shock in an animal (*e.g.,* guinea pig) whose tissues contain Forssman antigen, resulting from an intravenous injection of serum that contains Forssman's antibody.

local a., the immediate, transient kind of response that follows the injection of antigen (allergen) into the skin of a sensitized individual and is limited to the area surrounding the site of inoculation. SEE ALSO skin *test.*

passive a., a reaction resulting from inoculation of antigen in an animal previously inoculated intravenously with specific antiserum from another animal, a latent period being required between the two inoculations. SYN antiserum a.

passive cutaneous a. (PCA), a reaction that occurs in the guinea pig when antiserum is injected into the skin and, 6 to 24 hours later, specific antigen and a dye such as Pontamine blue or Evans blue are inoculated intravenously; the size of the blue areas at the sites of the antibody injections is a measure of the degree of altered permeability to dye-bound albumin.

reversed a., SYN reversed passive a.

reversed passive a., an anaphylactic reaction induced in an animal injected with a specific antigen, which will bind to reactive tissue, and then, after a latent period, with serum from another animal previously sensitized to the identical antigen. SYN reversed a.

systemic a., SYN generalized a.

an·a·phyl·o·tox·in (an′ă-fil-ō-tok′sin). SYN anaphylatoxin.

an·a·pla·sia (an-ă-plā′sē-ă). Loss of structural differentiation, especially as seen in most, but not all, malignant neoplasms. SYN dedifferentiation (2). [G. *ana,* again, + *plasis,* a molding]

An·a·plas·ma (an-ă-plas′mă). A genus of bacteria (family Anaplasmataceae) that parasitize red blood cells, where they appear as spherical chromatic granules; there is no demonstrable multiplication of these organisms in other tissues. These organisms are natural parasites of ruminants (families Bovidae and Camelidae) and are transmitted by arthropods. Initially regarded as protozoa, they are now placed in the order Rickettsiales. The type species is *A. marginale.* [G. shape, copy]

A. centra'le, a species that causes benign anaplasmosis of cattle.

A. margina'le, a species that causes clinical anaplasmosis of cattle; it is the type species of the genus *A.*

A. o'vis, a species that causes anaplasmosis in sheep and goats; cattle are refractory.

an·a·plas·mo·sis (an'ă-plas-mō'sis). An infectious disease of ruminants, varying from peracute to chronic, caused by *Anaplasma* species and characterized by progressive anemia, and fever; it is transmitted by at least 20 species of ticks and mechanically by hematophagous insects including horseflies (*Tabanus*), stable flies (*Stomoxys*), deerflies (*Chrysops*), and mosquitoes.

an·a·plas·tic (an-ă-plas'tik). 1. Relating to anaplasty. 2. Characterized by or pertaining to anaplasia. 3. Growing without form or structure.

an·a·plas·ty (an'ă-plas-tē). Obsolete term for plastic *surgery.* [G. *ana,* again, + *plastos,* formed]

an·a·ple·ro·sis (an'ă-pler-ō'sis). The process of replenishment of depleted metabolic cycle or pathway intermediates; most commonly referring to the tricarboxylic acid cycle. [G. filling up, fr. *ana-,* up, + *plerosis,* filling, fr. *pleroō,* to fill]

an·a·ple·rot·ic (an'ă-pler-ŏ'tik). Referring to reactions or pathways that contribute to anaplerosis.

an·a·poph·y·sis (an-ă-pof'i-sis). An accessory spinal process of a vertebra, found especially in the thoracic or lumbar vertebrae. [G. *ana,* back, + *apophysis,* offshoot]

anap·tic (ă-nap'tik). Relating to anaphia.

an·a·rith·mia (an-ă-rith'mē-ă). Aphasia characterized by an inability to count or use numbers. [G. *an-* priv. + *arithmos,* number]

an·ar·thria (an-ar'thrē-a). Loss of the power of articulate speech. SEE ALSO aphasia, alexia, dysarthria. [G. fr. *an-anthos,* without joints; (of sound) inarticulate]

an·a·sar·ca (an-ă-sar'kă). A generalized infiltration of edema fluid into subcutaneous connective tissue. SYN hydrosarca. [G. *ana,* through, + *sarx* (*sark-*), flesh]

fetoplacental a., edema of fetus and placenta as found in fetal hydrops.

an·a·sar·cous (an-ă-sar'kŭs). Characterized by anasarca.

an·a·stig·mat·ic (an'as-tig-mat'ik). Not astigmatic.

an·as·tig·mats. 1. Lenses in which astigmatism is corrected. 2. Lenses in which both astigmatism and field curvature are corrected.

an·as·to·le (an-as'tō-lē). Obsolete term for the gaping of a wound. [G. *anastolē,* the laying bare of a wound]

anas·to·mose (ă-nas'tō-mōs). 1. To open one structure into another directly or by connecting channels, said of blood vessels, lymphatics, and hollow viscera; also incorrectly applied to nerves. 2. To unite by means of an anastomosis, or connection between formerly separate structures.

anas·to·mo·sis, pl. **anas·to·mo·ses** (ă-nas'tō-mō'sis, -sez). 1. A natural communication, direct or indirect, between two blood vessels or other tubular structures. Also incorrectly applied to nerves. SEE communication. 2. An operative union of two hollow or tubular structures. 3. An opening created by surgery, trauma, or disease between two or more normally separate spaces or organs. [G. *anastomōsis,* from *anastomoō,* to furnish with a mouth]

arteriolovenular a., SYN arteriovenous a.

a. arterioveno'sa [NA], SYN arteriovenous a.

arteriovenous a. (A-V a.), vessels through which blood is shunted from arterioles to venules without passing through the capillaries. SYN a. arteriovenosa [NA], arteriolovenular a.

A-V a., abbreviation for arteriovenous a.

Béclard's a., an a. between the right and the left end-branch of the deep lingual artery. SYN arcus raninus.

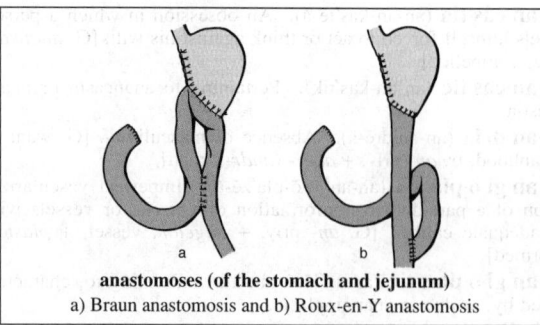
anastomoses (of the stomach and jejunum)
a) Braun anastomosis and b) Roux-en-Y anastomosis

bevelled a., a. performed after cutting each of the structures to be joined in an oblique fashion.

Billroth I a., SYN Billroth's *operation* I.

Billroth II a., SYN Billroth's *operation* II.

Braun's a., after gastroenterostomy, a. between afferent and efferent loops of jejunum.

cavopulmonary a., a means of palliating cyanotic heart disease by anastomosing the right pulmonary artery to the superior vena cava. SYN cavopulmonary shunt, Glenn shunt.

circular a., a. performed after cutting each structure to be joined in a plane vertical to the ultimate flow through the structures.

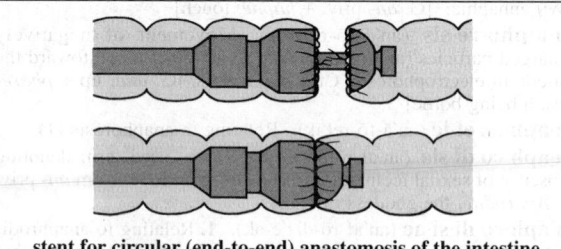
stent for circular (end-to-end) anastomosis of the intestine

Clado's a., a. in the right suspensory ligament of the ovary between the appendicular and ovarian arteries.

conjoined a., the joining together of two small blood vessels by side-to-side elliptical a. to create a single larger stoma for subsequent end-to-end a.

cruciate a., crucial a., a four-way a. between branches of the first perforating branch of the deep femoral, inferior gluteal and medial and lateral circumflex femoral arteries, located posterior to the upper part of the femur. Formerly described as commonly occurring; investigations show it rarely occurs in the four-way "cross" pattern.

Damus-Stancel-Kaye a., SYN Damus-Kaye-Stancel *procedure.*

elliptical a., a modification of direct a. whereby one or both tubular structures are spatulated beforehand, thus creating an ellipse of greater cross-sectional as well as circumferential dimension than would be possible with a bevelled or circular a.

Galen's a., SYN communicating *branch* of superior laryngeal nerve with recurrent laryngeal nerve.

Hofmeister-Pólya a., SEE Hofmeister's *operation,* Pólya's *operation.*

Hoyer's anastomoses, SYN Sucquet-Hoyer *canals,* under *canal.*

Hyrtl's a., SYN Hyrtl's *loop.*

intermesenteric arterial a., SYN intestinal arterial *arcades,* under *arcade.*

intestinal a., SYN enteroenterostomy.

isoperistaltic a., an a. allowing flow of contents in the same and normal direction.

Jacobson's a., a portion of the tympanic plexus.

Martin-Gruber a., a nerve anomaly in the forearm, consisting of a median to ulnar nerve communication; Also referred to a median–to–ulnar crossover.

microvascular a., a. of very small blood vessels performed under a surgical microscope.

portacaval anastomoses, SYN portal-systemic anastomoses.

portal-systemic anastomoses, (1) naturally-occurring venous communications between tributaries of the portal venous system and tributaries of the systemic venous system. The major portal-systemic anastomoses include: 1) esophageal branches of left gastric vein with esophageal veins, 2) superior rectal vein with middle and inferior rectal veins, 3) paraumbilical veins with subcutaneous veins of anterior abdominal wall, 4) retroperitoneal veins with venous branches of veins of the colon and bare area of the liver, and 5) a patent ductus venosus connecting left branch of portal vein to inferior vena cava (rare). These anastomoses are important clinically, providing collateral circulation during portal obstruction or hypertension, at which time they may become varicose; SEE *caput* medusae, esophageal *varices*, under *varix*, hemorrhoids. **(2)** surgically-created communications between the portal vein and the inferior vena cava or their tributaries, to relieve portal hypertension. SYN portacaval anastomoses.

postcostal a., longitudinal a. of intersegmental arteries giving rise to the vertebral artery.

Potts' a., SYN Potts' *operation.*

precapillary a., an a. between arterioles just before they become capillaries.

precostal a. (prē-kos-tal), longitudinal a. of intersegmental arteries in the embryo that gives rise to the thyrocervical and costocervical trunk.

Riolan's a., the specific portion of the marginal artery of the colon connecting the middle and left colic arteries. SYN Riolan's arc (3).

Roux-en-Y a., a. of the distal end of the divided jejunum to the stomach, bile duct, or another structure, with implantation of the proximal end into the side of the jejunum at a suitable distance below the first a., the bowel then forming a Y-shaped pattern.

Schmidel's anastomoses, abnormal channels of communication between the caval and portal venous systems.

Sucquet-Hoyer anastomoses, SYN Sucquet-Hoyer *canals,* under *canal.*

Sucquet's anastomoses, SYN Sucquet-Hoyer *canals,* under *canal.*

termino-terminal a., an operation by which the central end of an artery is connected with the peripheral end of the corresponding vein, and the peripheral end of the artery with the central end of the vein.

transureteroureteral a., SYN transureteroureterostomy.

uretero-ileal a., a. between the ureter and an isolated segment of ileum. SEE ALSO Bricker *operation.*

ureterosigmoid a., a. between the ureter and a segment of the sigmoid colon.

ureterotubal a., procedure for a. between the ureter and the fallopian tube.

ureteroureteral a., a. from one part of a ureter to another part of the same ureter.

anas·to·mot·ic (a-nas-tō-mot′ik). Pertaining to an anastomosis.

an·as·tral (an-as′trăl). Lacking an astrosphere.

an·a·tom·i·cal (an′ă-tom′i-kăl). **1.** Relating to anatomy. **2.** SYN structural. **3.** Denoting a strictly morphological feature distinct from its physiological or surgical considerations, *e.g.,* anatomical neck of humerus, anatomical dead space, anatomical lobulation of the liver.

an·a·tom·i·cal snuff·box (snŭf′boks). A hollow seen on the radial aspect of the wrist when the thumb is extended fully; it is bounded by the prominences of the tendon of the extensor pollicis longus posteriorly and of the tendons of the extensor pollicis brevis and abductor pollicis longus anteriorly. The radial artery crosses the floor which is formed by the scaphoid and the trapezium bones. SYN tabatière anatomique.

an·a·tom·i·co·med·i·cal (an-ă-tom′i-kō-med′i-kăl). Referring to both medicine and anatomy.

an·a·tom·i·co·path·o·log·i·cal (an-ă-tom′i-kō-path-ŏ-loj′i-kăl). Relating to anatomical pathology.

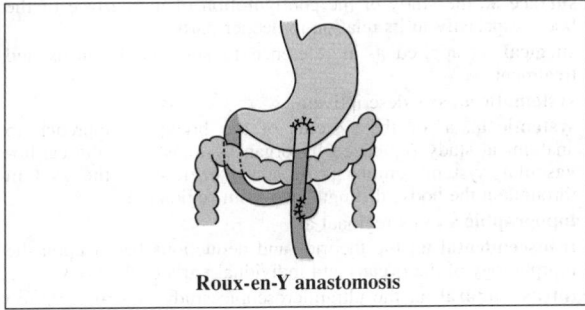

Roux-en-Y anastomosis

an·a·tom·i·co·sur·gi·cal (an-ă-tom′i-kō-ser′ji-kăl). Relating to surgical anatomy.

anat·o·mist (ă-nat′ŏ-mist). A specialist in the science of anatomy.

anat·o·my (ă-nat′ŏ-mē). **1.** The morphologic structure of an organism. **2.** The science of the morphology or structure of organisms. **3.** SYN dissection. **4.** A work describing the form and structure of an organism and its various parts. [G. *anatomē,* dissection, from *ana,* apart, + *tomē,* a cutting]

applied a., SYN clinical a.

artificial a., the manufacture of models of anatomic structures, or the study of a. from such models.

artistic a., the study of a. for artistic purposes, as applied to painting, drawing, or sculpture.

clastic a., the construction or study of models in layers which can be removed one after the other to show the structure of the organism and/or organ. SYN plastic a.

clinical a., the practical application of anatomical knowledge to diagnosis and treatment. SYN applied a.

comparative a., the comparative study of animal structure with regard to homologous organs or parts.

dental a., that branch of gross a. concerned with the morphology of teeth, their location, position, and relationships.

descriptive a., a description of, especially a treatise describing, physical structure, more particularly that of man. SYN systematic a.

developmental a., a. of the structural changes of an individual from fertilization to adulthood; includes embryology, fetology, and postnatal development.

functional a., a. studied in its relation to function. SYN morphophysiology, physiological a.

general a., the study of gross and microscopic structures as well as of the composition of the body, its tissues and fluids.

gross a., general a., so far as it can be studied without the use of the microscope; commonly used to denote the study of a. by dissection of a cadaver. SEE practical a. SYN macroscopic a.

living a., the study of a. in the living individual by inspection.

macroscopic a., SYN gross a.

medical a., a. in its bearing upon the diagnosis and treatment of diseases.

microscopic a., the branch of a. in which the structure of cells, tissues, and organs is studied with the light microscope. SEE histology.

pathological a., SYN anatomical *pathology.*

physiological a., SYN functional a.

plastic a., SYN clastic a.

practical a., a. studied by means of dissection. SEE gross a.

radiological a., the study of bodily sturcture using radiographs and other imaging methods.

regional a., an approach to anatomical study based on regions, parts, or divisions of the body (*e.g.,* the foot or the inguinal region), emphasizing the relationships of various systemic structures (*e.g.,* muscles, nerves, and arteries) within that area; distinguished from systemic a. SYN topographic a., topology (1).

special a., the a. of certain definite organs or groups of organs involved in the performance of special functions; descriptive a. dealing with the separate systems.

surface a., the study of the configuration of the surface of the body, especially in its relation to deeper parts.

surgical a., applied a. in reference to surgical diagnosis and treatment.

systematic a., SYN descriptive a.

systemic a., a. of the systems of the body; an approach to anatomical study organized by organ systems, *e.g.,* the cardiovascular system, emphasizing an overview of the system throughout the body; distinguished from regional a.

topographic a., SYN regional a.

transcendental a., the theories and deductions based upon the morphology of the organs and individual parts of the body.

ultrastructural a., the ultramicroscopic study of structures too small to be seen with a light microscope.

anat·o·pism (ă-nat′ō-pizm). Failure to conform to the cultural pattern. [G. *ana,* backward, + *topos,* place]

an·a·tox·ic (an-ă-tok′sik). Pertaining to the characteristic properties of anatoxin (toxoid).

an·a·tox·in (an-ă-tok′sin). SYN toxoid.

an·a·tri·crot·ic (an′ă-trī-krot′ik). Characterized by anatricrotism; denoting a sphygmographic tracing with three waves on the ascending limb.

an·a·tric·ro·tism (an′ă-trik′rō-tizm). A condition of the pulse manifested by a triple beat on the ascending limb of the sphygmographic tracing. [G. *ana,* up, + *tri-,* thrice, *krotos,* beating]

an·a·trip·sis (an-ă-trip′sis). Therapeutic use of rubbing or friction with or without simultaneous application of a medicament. [G. a rubbing, fr. *anatribō,* fr. *ana,* intensive, + *tribō,* to rub]

an·a·trip·tic (an-ă-trip′tik). **1.** Pertaining to anatripsis. **2.** A remedy to be applied by friction or rubbing.

an·ax·on, an·ax·one (an-aks′on, -aks′ōn). Having no axon; denoting certain nerve cells first described by S. Ramón y Cajal as amacrine cells in the retina, and later discovered in several brain regions. [G. *an-* priv. + *axōn,* axis]

an·a·zo·tu·ria (an′az-ō-tū′rē-ă). A deficiency or lack of nitrogenous metabolic products excreted in the urine; pertains especially to unusually small quantities of urea in the urine. [G. *an-* priv. + azoturia]

AnCC Abbreviation for anodal closure *contraction.*

an·ces·tor. A person in the direct line of descent from which a subject of interest is derived (parents, grandparents, etc.; but no collaterals or descendants).

leading ancestor, in genetic counseling given to a consultant unaffected by but possibly a carrier or a latent subject of the disease; the most recent ancestor in the direct line of descent known to have had the affected gene in question.

an·chor·age (ang′kōr-ij). **1.** Operative fixation of loose or prolapsed abdominal or pelvic organs. **2.** The part to which anything is fastened. In dentistry, a tooth or an implanted tooth substitute with which a fixed or removable partial denture, crown, or restoration is retained. **3.** The nature and degree of resistance to displacement offered by an anatomical unit when used for the purpose of effecting tooth movement. [L. *ancora,* fr. G. *ankyra,* anchor]

cervical a., a. in which the back of the neck is used for resistance by means of a cervical strap.

extraoral a., a. in which the resistance unit is outside the oral cavity; *e.g.,* cranial, occipital, or cervical a.

intermaxillary a., a. in which the units in one jaw are used to effect tooth movement in the other jaw.

intramaxillary a., a. in which the resistance units are all situated within the same jaw.

intraoral a., a. in which the resistance units are all located within the oral cavity.

multiple a., a. in which more than one type of resistance unit is utilized. SYN reinforced a.

occipital a., a. in which the top and back of the head are used for resistance by means of a headgear.

reciprocal a., a. in which the movement of one or more teeth is balanced against the movement of one or more opposing teeth.

reinforced a., SYN multiple a.

simple a., a. in which the resistance to the movement of one or more teeth comes solely from resistance to tipping movement of the a. unit.

stationary a., a. in which the resistance to the movement of one or more teeth comes from the resistance to bodily movement of the a. unit; a questionable concept since the selected teeth remain only relatively stable.

an·chor·in (ang′kōr-in). SYN ankyrin. [anchor + -in]

an·chu·sin (an′kū-sin). SYN alkannin.

an·cil·lary (an′si-lār-ē). Auxiliary, accessory, or secondary. [L. *ancillaris,* relating to a maid servant]

an·cip·i·tal, an·cip·i·tate, an·cip·i·tous (an-sip′i-tăl, -i-tāt, -i-tŭs). Two-headed; two-edged. [L. *anceps,* two- headed]

an·con (ang′kŏn). SYN elbow (1). [G. *ankon,* elbow]

an·co·nad (ang′kō-nad). Toward the elbow. [G. *ankōn,* elbow, + L. *ad,* to]

an·co·nal, an·co·ne·al (ang′kŏ-năl, ang-kō′nē-ăl). **1.** Relating to the elbow (ancon). **2.** Relating to the anconeus muscle.

an·co·ne·us (ang-kō′nē-ŭs). SYN anconeus *muscle.* [L.]

an·co·ni·tis (an-kō-nī′tis). Inflammation of the elbow joint. [G. *ankōn,* elbow, + *-itis,* inflammation]

an·co·noid (ang′kō-noyd). Resembling the elbow.

an·crod (an′krod). A fraction obtained from the venom of the pit viper, *Angkistrodon rhodostoma,* which contains a fibrinogen-splitting enzyme; produces hypofibrinogenemia and diminution of both whole blood and plasma viscosity for improvement of the rheologic properties of blood, and is used in treatment of chronic peripheral vascular disease.

△**ancylo-.** SEE ankylo-.

An·cy·los·to·ma (an-si-los′tō-mă, an-ki-). A genus of Nematoda, the Old World hookworm, the members of which are parasitic in the duodenum. They attach themselves to villi in the mucous membrane, suck blood, and may cause a state of anemia, especially in cases of malnutrition. The eggs are passed with the feces, and the larvae develop in moist soil to become infectious third-stage (filariform) larvae that enter the body of man through the skin and possibly in drinking water; they migrate by the bloodstream to lung alveoli, are carried to bronchi and trachea, swallowed, and passed to the intestine where they mature. SEE ALSO ancylostomiasis, *Necator.* SYN *Ankylostoma* (1). [G. *ankylos,* curved, hooked, + *stoma,* mouth]

A. brazilien′se, a species characterized by one pair of ventral buccal teeth, normally an intestinal parasite of dogs and cats but also found in man as a cause of human cutaneous larva migrans.

A. cani′num, a species possessing three pairs of ventral teeth in the oral cavity; common in dogs, but also occurring in human skin as a cause of cutaneous larva migrans.

A. ceylan′icum, species found in the civet cat of Ceylon; rarely reported from man as an intestinal parasite in Southeast Asia.

A. duodena′le, the Old World hookworm of man, a species widespread in temperate areas, in contrast to the more tropical distribution of the New World hookworm, *Necator americanus.* It is the only hookworm found in the U.S.

an·cy·lo·sto·mat·ic (an′si-lō-stō-mat′ik, an′ki-). Referring to hookworms of the genus *Ancylostoma.*

an·cy·lo·sto·mi·a·sis (an′si-lō-stō-mī′ă-sis, an′ki-). Hookworm disease caused by *Ancylostoma duodenale* and characterized by eosinophilia, anemia, emaciation, dyspepsia, and, in children with severe long-continued infections, swelling of the abdomen with mental and physical maldevelopment. SYN ankylostomiasis, intertropical hyphemia, tropical hyphemia, miner's disease (1), tunnel disease, uncinariasis.

cutaneous a., cutaneous larva migrans caused by larvae of hookworms. SYN ancylostoma dermatitis, a. cutis, coolie itch, dew itch, ground itch, swamp itch, swimmer's itch (1), toe itch, water itch (1), water sore.

a. cu′tis, SYN cutaneous a.

an·cy·roid (an′si-royd). Shaped like the fluke of an anchor; denoting the cornua of the lateral ventricles of the brain and the coracoid process of the scapula. SYN ankyroid. [G. *ankyra,* anchor, + *eidos,* resemblance]

Andernach, Johann W. (Guenther von Andernach), German physician, 1505–1574. SEE A.'s *ossicles,* under *ossicle.*

Anders, James Meschter, U.S. physician, 1854–1936. SEE A.'s *disease.*

Andersch, Carolus Samuel, German anatomist, 1732–1777. SEE A.'s *ganglion, nerve.*

Andersen, Dorothy Hansine, U.S. pediatrician, 1901–1963. SEE A.'s *disease.*

Anderson, Evelyn, U.S. physician, *1899. SEE A.-Collip *test.*

Anderson, James C., British urologist, *1899. SEE A.-Hynes *pyeloplasty.*

Anderson, Roger, U.S. surgeon, 1891–1971. SEE A. *splint.*

Anderson-Collip test. See under test.

an·di·ra (an-dī′ră). The bark of *Andira inermis,* a leguminous tree of tropical America, used as an emetic, purgative, and anthelmintic. SYN cabbage tree, worm bark. [West Indian native name]

an·di·rine (an-dī′rin). *N*-Methyltyrosine; an alkaloid derived from Andira that has negligible stimulating action.

Andral, Gabriel, French physician, 1797–1876. SEE A.'s *decubitus.*

an·dre·nos·ter·one (an-drĕ-nos′ter-ōn). SYN adrenosterone.

Andrews, C.J., U.S. surgeon. SEE Brandt-A. *maneuver.*

an·dri·at·rics, an·dri·a·try (an-dri-at′riks, -drī′ă-trē). Medical science relating to diseases of male genital organs and of men in general. [G. *anēr,* a man, + *iatreia,* medical treatment]

△**andro-.** Masculine. [G. *anēr, andros,* a male human being]

an·dro·blas·to·ma (an′drō-blas-tō′mă). **1.** A testicular tumor microscopically resembling fetal testis, with varying proportions of tubular and stromal elements; the tubules contain Sertoli cells, which may cause feminization. SYN Pick's tubular adenoma, Sertoli cell tumor, testicular tubular adenoma. **2.** SYN arrhenoblastoma. [G. *anēr (andre-),* man, + *blastos,* germ, + *-oma,* tumor]

an·dro·gen (an′drō-jen). Generic term for an agent, usually a hormone (*e.g.,* androsterone, testosterone), that stimulates activity of the accessory male sex organs, encourages development of male sex characteristics, or prevents changes in the latter that follow castration; natural a.'s are steroids, derivatives of androstane. SYN testoid (2).

  adrenal a., any androgenic hormone of adrenocortical origin; *e.g.,* dehydroepiandrosterone (and its sulfate), androstenedione, 11β-hydroxyandrostenedione.

an·dro·gen·e·sis (an-drō-jen′ĕ-sis). Egg development in the presence of paternal chromosomes only. [andro- + G. *genesis,* production]

an·dro·gen·ic (an-drō-jen′ik). Relating to an androgen; having a masculinizing effect. SYN testoid (1).

an·drog·e·nous (an-droj′ĕ-nŭs). Giving birth to males.

an·drog·y·nism (an-droj′i-nizm). SYN female *pseudohermaphroditism.*

an·drog·y·noid (an-droj′i-noyd). A male resembling a female, or possessing female features. [andro- + G. *gynē,* woman, + *eidos,* resemblance]

an·drog·y·nous (an-droj′i-nŭs). Pertaining to androgyny.

an·drog·y·ny (an-droj′i-nē). **1.** SYN female *pseudohermaphroditism.* **2.** Having both masculine and feminine characteristics, as in attitudes and behaviors that contain features of stereotyped, culturally sanctioned sexual roles of both male and female. [andro- + G. *gynē,* woman]

an·droid (an′droyd). SYN andromorphous. [andro- + G. *eidos,* resemblance]

an·drol·o·gy (an-drol′ō-jē). The branch of medicine concerned with diseases peculiar to the male sex, particularly infertility and sexual dysfunction. [andro- + G. *logos,* treatise]

an·dro·ma·nia (an-drō-mā′nē-ă). Obsolete term for nymphomania. [andro- + G. *mania,* frenzy]

an·drom·e·do·tox·in (an-drom′ĕ-dō-tok′sin). A strongly emetic active principle obtained from several species of *Andromeda* and *Rhododendron* (family Ericaceae); it is a cardiac poison, first stimulating and then paralyzing the vagus; it also paralyzes the motor nerve ends in striated muscle.

an·dro·mor·phous (an-drō-mōr′fŭs). Having a male form or habitus. SYN android. [andro- + G. *morphē,* form]

an·drop·a·thy (an-drop′ă-thē). Any disease, such as prostatitis, peculiar to the male sex. [andro- + G. *pathos,* suffering]

an·dro·pho·bia (an-drō-fō′bē-ă). Morbid fear of men, or of the male sex, resulting in avoidance of situations where men are present. [andro- + G. *phobos,* fear]

an·dro·stane (an′drō-stān). The parent hydrocarbon of the androgenic steroids. For structure, see steroids.

an·dro·stane·di·ol (an-drō-stān′dī-ol). 5α-Androstane-3β,17β-diol; a steroid metabolite, of which 5β isomers are also known.

an·dro·stane·di·one (an-drō-stān′dī-ōn). 5α-Androstane-3,17-dione; a steroid metabolite, of which the 5β isomer is also known.

an·dro·stene (an′drō-stēn). Androstane with an unsaturated (*i.e.,* —CH=CH—) bond in the molecule.

an·dro·stene·di·ol (an-drō-stēn′dī-ol). 5-Androsten-3β,17β-diol; a steroid metabolite differing from androstanediol by possessing a double bond between C-5 and C-6.

an·dro·stene·di·one (an-drō-stēn′dī-ōn). 4-Androstene-3,17-dione; androstanedione with a double bond between C-4 and C-5; an androgenic steroid of weaker biological potency than testosterone; secreted by the testis, ovary, and adrenal cortex.

an·dro·sten·o·lone (an-drō-stēn-ō-lōn). SYN dehydro-3-epiandrosterone.

an·dros·ter·one (an-dros′ter-ōn). *cis*-Androsterone; 3α-hydroxy-5α-androstan-17-one; (3α-hydroxyetioallocholan-17-one; 3-epihydroxyetioallocholan-17-one); a steroid metabolite, found in male urine, having weak androgenic potency. Formed in testes from progesterone.

AnDTe Abbreviation for anodal duration *tetanus.*

an·ec·dot·al (ă-nek′dō-tal). Report of clinical experiences based in individual cases, rather than an organized investigation with appropriate controls, etc. [G. *anekdota,* unpublished items, fr. *an-* priv + *ekdomi,* to publish]

an·e·cho·ic (an-ĕ-kō′ik). The property of appearing echo-free or without echoes on a sonographic image; a clear cyst appears anechoic. SEE transonic. SYN echo-free. [G. *an-* priv. + echo + ic]

an·ec·ta·sis (an-ek′tă-sis). SYN primary *atelectasis.* [G. *an-* priv. + *ektasis,* dilation]

Anel, Dominique, French surgeon, 1679–1725. SEE A.'s *method.*

an·e·lec·trode (an-ĕ-lek′trōd). SYN anode.

an·e·lec·tro·ton·ic (an-ē-lek-trō-ton′ik). Relating to anelectrotonus.

an·e·lec·trot·o·nus (an′ē-lek-trot′ō-nŭs). Changes in excitability and conductivity in a nerve or muscle cell in the neighborhood of the anode during the passage of a constant electric current. [anelectrode + G. *tonos,* tension]

ANEMIA

ane·mia (ă-nē′mē-ă). Any condition in which the number of red blood cells per cu mm, the amount of hemoglobin in 100 ml of blood, and the volume of packed red blood cells per 100 ml of blood are less than normal; clinically, generally pertaining to the concentration of oxygen-transporting material in a designated volume of blood, in contrast to total quantities as in oligocythemia, oligochromemia, and oligemia. A. is frequently manifested by pallor of the skin and mucous membranes, shortness of breath, palpitations of the heart, soft systolic murmurs, lethargy, and fatigability. [G. *anaimia,* fr. *an-* priv. + *haima,* blood]

  achlorhydric a., a form of chronic hypochromic microcytic a. associated with achlorhydria or achylia gastrica; observed most frequently in women in the third to fifth decades. SYN Faber's a., Faber's syndrome.

  achrestic a., a form of chronic progressive macrocytic a. that can

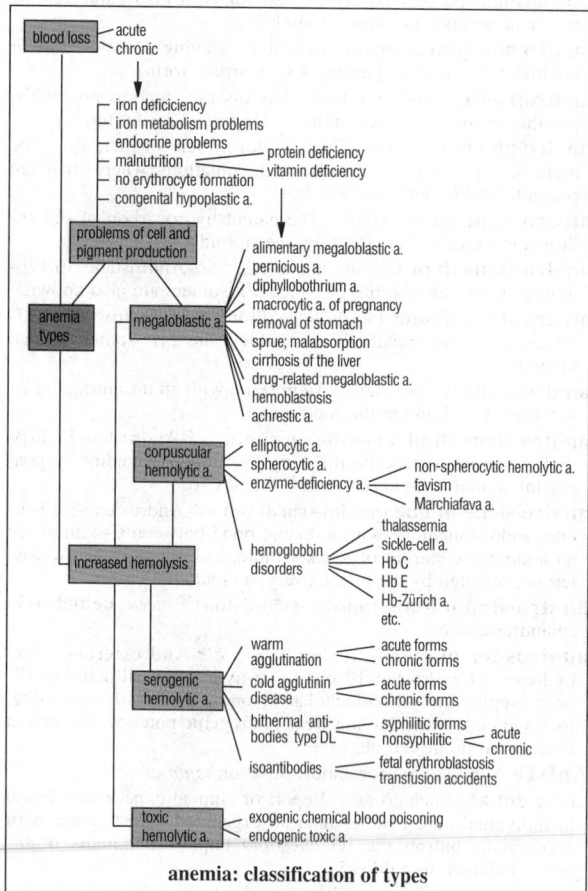

anemia: classification of types

high mortality. Occurs in central Andean mountains of northern South America; vector is phlebotomine sandfly, *Lutzomyia*.

Belgian Congo a., SYN kasai.

Biermer's a., SYN pernicious a.

brickmaker's a., a. associated with hookworm disease.

cameloid a., SYN elliptocytic a.

chlorotic a., SYN chlorosis.

congenital a., SYN *erythroblastosis* fetalis.

congenital aplastic a., SYN Fanconi's a.

congenital dyserythropoietic a., a group of autosomal recessive a.'s characterized by ineffective erythropoiesis, bone marrow erythroblastic multinuclearity, and secondary hemochromatosis. Three types are described: **type I** [MIM224100], macrocytic, megaloblastic a. with erythroblastic internuclear chromatin bridges; **type II**, [MIM*224100], normoblastic a. with multinucleated erythroblasts; **type III**, macrocytic a. with erythroblastic multinuclearity and gigantoblasts [MIM*105600].

congenital hemolytic a., accelerated destruction of red blood cells due to an inherited defect, such as in the membrane in hereditary spherocytosis.

congenital hypoplastic a. [MIM*205900], congenital nonregenerative, familial hypoplastic, or pure red cell a.; erythrogenesis imperfecta; Diamond-Blackfan syndrome; autosomal recessive normocytic normochromic a. resulting from congenital hypoplasia of the bone marrow, which is grossly deficient in erythroid precursors while other elements are normal; a. is progressive and severe, but leukocyte and platelet counts are normal or slightly reduced; survival of transfused erythrocytes is normal; minor congenital anomalies are found in some patients. SYN congenital nonregenerative a., Diamond-Blackfan a., Diamond-Blackfan syndrome, erythrogenesis imperfecta, familial hypoplastic a., pure red cell a.

congenital nonregenerative a., SYN congenital hypoplastic a.

Cooley's a., SYN *thalassemia* major.

cow milk a., a. occurring in infants fed cow milk without iron supplementation, attributed to digestive tract allergic reaction leading to blood loss and hence iron deficiency.

crescent cell a., SYN sickle cell a.

deficiency a., SYN nutritional a.

Diamond-Blackfan a., SYN congenital hypoplastic a.

dilution a., SYN hydremia.

dimorphic a., a. in which two distinct forms of red cells are circulating.

diphyllobothrium a., a rare form of macrocytic a. associated with *Diphyllobothrium latum* infection, especially in Finland. SYN fish tapeworm a.

drepanocytic a., SYN sickle cell a.

dyshemopoietic a., any a. resulting from defective function of the bone marrow.

Ehrlich's a., SYN aplastic a.

elliptocytary a. (ē-lip′tō-sī′tar-ē), a. with elliptocytosis; a heterogeneous group of inherited a.'s having in common elliptical red cells on blood smear. The defect may reside in dysfunction or deficiency of proteins of the red cell membrane skeleton. SYN elliptocytotic a.

elliptocytic a., a. characterized by elliptical erythrocytes (ovalocytes) resembling those observed normally in camels; 1 to 15% of erythrocytes in nonanemic persons may be oval, but greater proportions are observed in certain patients with microcytic a. SEE ALSO elliptocytosis. SYN cameloid a., ovalocytic a.

elliptocytotic a. (ē-lip′tō-sī-tot′ik), SYN elliptocytary a.

equine infectious a., a worldwide infectious disease of horses and other equids, caused by equine infectious a. virus and a member of the family Retroviridae, marked by general debility, remittent fever, staggering gait, progressive a., and loss of flesh; it is transmitted by bloodsucking insects and by contact, oral infection, or the use of unsterilized syringes and needles. SYN swamp fever (1).

erythroblastic a., SYN erythronormoblastic a.

erythronormoblastic a. (ĕ-rith′rō-nōr′mō-blast- ik), a. characterized by the presence of large numbers of nucleated red cells (normoblasts and erythroblasts) in the peripheral blood. Seen

be fatal in which the changes in bone marrow and circulating blood closely resemble those of pernicious a., but in which there is only transient or no response to therapy with vitamin B₁₂; glossitis, gastrointestinal disturbances, central nervous system disease, and pyrexia are not observed, and there is only little bleeding or hemolysis. [G. *a-* priv. + *chrēsis*, a using]

acquired hemolytic a., nonhereditary acute or chronic a. associated with or caused by extracorpuscular factors, *e.g.,* certain infectious agents, chemicals (including autoantibodies or therapeutic agents), burns, toxic materials from higher plant and animal forms (including snake venoms).

addisonian a., SYN pernicious a.

Addison's a., SYN pernicious a.

angiopathic hemolytic a., a rare postpartum a. of unknown etiology with uremia and nephrosclerosis; may be a rare complication following use of contraceptive steroids.

aplastic a., a. characterized by a greatly decreased formation of erythrocytes and hemoglobin, usually associated with pronounced granulocytopenia and thrombocytopenia, as a result of hypoplastic or aplastic bone marrow. SYN a. gravis, Ehrlich's a.

asiderotic a., SYN chlorosis.

autoimmune hemolytic a., **(1)** cold-antibody type, caused by hemagglutinating antibody (usually IgM class) maximally active at 4°C; and resulting from severe hemolysis in cold hemagglutinin disease; **(2)** warm-antibody type, acquired hemolytic a. due to serum autoantibodies (usually IgG class) maximally active at 37°C; that react with the patient's red blood cells; it varies in severity, occurs in all age groups of both sexes, and may be idiopathic or secondary to neoplastic, autoimmune, or other disease. The Coombs test is positive for IgG and complement, IgG alone, or complement alone.

Bartonella a., a. occurring in infection with *Bartonella bacilliformis* and characterized by an acute febrile a. of rapid onset and

especially in newborns with hemolytic a., such as that caused by Rh or ABO incompatibility. SYN erythroblastic a.

essential a., obsolete term for pernicious a.; also used formerly for any type of a. of unknown mechanism.

Faber's a., SYN achlorhydric a.

false a., SYN pseudoanaemia.

familial erythroblastic a., an outmoded term for thalassemia major.

familial hypoplastic a., SYN congenital hypoplastic a.

familial microcytic a. [MIM*206200], a rare type of autosomal recessive hypochromic microcytic a. associated with a defect of iron metabolism characterized by high serum iron, hepatic iron deposits, and absence of stainable bone marrow iron stores.

familial pyridoxine-responsive a. [MIM*206000], a rare autosomal recessive hereditary hypochromic a.; autosomal trait, responsive to pyridoxine.

familial splenic a., SYN Gaucher's *disease.*

Fanconi's a., a type of idiopathic refractory a. characterized by pancytopenia, hypoplasia of the bone marrow, and congenital anomalies, occurring in members of the same family (an autosomal recessive trait in at least two nonallelic types [MIM*227650 and 227660]); the a. is normocytic or slightly macrocytic, macrocytes and target cells may be found in the circulating blood, and the leukopenia usually is due to neutropenia; congenital anomalies include short stature, microcephaly, hypogenitalism, strabismus, anomalies of the thumbs, radii, and kidneys, mental retardation, and microphthalmia. SYN congenital aplastic a., congenital pancytopenia, Fanconi's syndrome (1).

feline infectious a. (FIA), an acute or chronic a. of domestic cats caused by the rickettsia *Haemobartonella felis.* SYN hemobartonellosis.

fish tapeworm a., SYN diphyllobothrium a.

folic acid deficiency a., a. due to deficiency of folic acid, characterized by large-sized red blood cells (macrocytosis) and presence of large nuclei in erythroid precursor cells (megaloblasts) in the bone marrow.

globe cell a., SYN hereditary *spherocytosis.*

goat's milk a., nutritional a. in infants maintained chiefly with goat's milk, which is relatively poor in iron content.

a. gra′vis, SYN aplastic a.

ground itch a., a. associated with hookworm disease.

Heinz body a., SEE unstable hemoglobin hemolytic a.

hemolytic a., any a. resulting from an increased rate of erythrocyte destruction.

hemolytic a. of newborn, (1) SYN *erythroblastosis* fetalis. **(2)** a disease similar to erythroblastosis fetalis, seen in foals, piglets, and puppies.

hemorrhagic a., a. resulting directly from loss of blood.

hookworm a., a. associated with heavy infestation by *Ancylostoma duodenale* or *Necator americanus.*

hyperchromic a., hyperchromatic a., a. characterized by a decrease in the ratio of the weight of hemoglobin to the volume of the erythrocyte, *i.e.,* the mean corpuscular hemoglobin concentration is less than normal; the individual cells contain less hemoglobin than they could under optimal conditions.

hypochromic a., a. characterized by a decrease in the ratio of the weight of hemoglobin to the volume of the erythrocyte, *i.e.,* the mean corpuscular hemoglobin concentration is less than normal; the individual cells contain less hemoglobin than they could have under optimal conditions.

hypochromic microcytic a., a. due to iron deficiency or thalassemia, and characterized by lower than normal mean corpuscular volume, mean corpuscular hemoglobin, and mean corpuscular hemoglobin concentration.

hypoferric a., SYN iron deficiency a.

hypoplastic a., progressive nonregenerative a. resulting from greatly depressed, inadequately functioning bone marrow; as the process persists, aplastic a. may occur.

icterohemolytic a., SYN hereditary *spherocytosis.*

infectious a., a. developing as a complication of infection; probably results from depressed formation and short survival of erythrocytes and abnormal iron metabolism.

intertropical a., an obsolete term for a. occurring in hookworm disease, chiefly necatoriasis.

iron deficiency a., hypochromic microcytic a. characterized by low serum iron, increased serum iron-binding capacity, decreased serum ferritin, and decreased marrow iron stores. SYN hypoferric a.

---

iron deficiency
the cause of chronic bleeding and posthemorrhagic anemia

in women:
1. hypermenorrhea (myomas of the uterus; i.u.d. or coil; retention of placenta; carcinomas; functional disorder)

in men and women:
2. – bleeding from the gastrointestinal tract: stomach or large intestine ulcers
   – carcinomas and benign stomach tumors
   – varices of the esophagus
   – hiatal hernias
   – hemorrhoids
   – colon-rectum carcinomas
   – polyps in colon or rectum
   – ulcerative colitis (proctitis), regional enteritis
   – diverticulosis coli (ancylostomiasis in the tropics, miner's disease)
   check stool for parasites

in rare cases:
3. – nose bleed
   – Osler syndrome
   – chronic hematuria of various causes
   – pulmonary hemosiderosis
   – excessive blood donation
   – loss of blood through suicide attempt

---

isochromic a., SYN normochromic a.

lead a., a. associated with poisoning from lead; thought to result from a defect in synthesis of hemoglobin based on the failure of iron being combined in the porphyrin ring.

Lederer's a., obsolete eponym for a form of acute acquired hemolytic a. associated with abnormal hemolysins and sometimes with hemoglobinuria.

leukoerythroblastic a., SYN leukoerythroblastosis.

local a., a. resulting from a decreased supply of blood to a part, as in the occlusion of a vessel.

macrocytic a., any a. in which the average size of circulating erythrocytes is greater than normal, *i.e.,* the mean corpuscular volume is 94 cu μm or more (normal range, 82 to 92 cu μm), including such syndromes as pernicious a., sprue, celiac disease, macrocytic a. of pregnancy, a. of diphyllobothriasis, and others. SYN megalocytic a.

macrocytic achylic a., SYN pernicious a.

macrocytic a. of pregnancy, an a. occurring in pregnancy, related to folate deficiency and characterized by a low level of hemoglobin and a reduced number of erythrocytes, which are larger than normal (macrocytes).

macrocytic a. tropical, the macrocytic, megaloblastic a. of tropical sprue.

malignant a., SYN pernicious a.

Marchiafava-Micheli a., SYN paroxysmal nocturnal *hemoglobinuria.*

megaloblastic a., any a. in which there is a predominant number of megaloblastic erythroblasts, and relatively few normoblasts, among the hyperplastic erythroid cells in the bone marrow (as in pernicious a.).

megalocytic a., SYN macrocytic a.

metaplastic a., pernicious a. in which the various formed elements in the blood are changed, *e.g.,* multisegmented, unusually large neutrophils (macropolycytes), immature myeloid cells, bizarre platelets.

microangiopathic hemolytic a., hemolysis due to narrowing or obstruction of small blood vessels usually due to inflammation, causing fragmentation and distortion in the shape of red blood cells.

microcytic a., any a. in which the average size of circulating erythrocytes is smaller than normal, *i.e.,* the mean corpuscular volume is 80 cu μm or less (normal range, 82 to 92 cu μm).

microdrepanocytic a., a., clinically resembling sickle cell a., in which individuals are compound heterozygous for the sickle cell gene and a thalassemia gene; about 60 to 80% of hemoglobin is Hb S, up to 20% Hb F, and the remainder Hb A. SYN sickle cell-thalassemia disease.

milk a., a type of hypochromic microcytic a., resulting from deficiency of iron, occurring in infants maintained on a milk diet for too long a time.

mountain a., term sometimes used for mountain sickness.

myelophthisic a., myelopathic a., SYN leukoerythroblastosis.

neonatal a., SYN *erythroblastosis* fetalis.

a. neonato´rum, SYN *erythroblastosis* fetalis.

normochromic a., any a. in which the concentration of hemoglobin in the erythrocytes is within the normal range, *i.e.,* the mean corpuscular hemoglobin concentration is from 32 to 36%. SYN isochromic a.

normocytic a., any a. in which the erythrocytes are normal in size, *i.e.,* the mean corpuscular volume ranges from 82 to 92 cu μm.

nutritional a., any a. resulting from a dietary deficiency of materials essential to red blood cell formation, *e.g.,* iron, vitamins (especially folic acid), protein. SYN deficiency a.

nutritional macrocytic a., macrocytic, megaloblastic anemia due to deficiency of either folate or vitamin B12.

osteosclerotic a., a. due to compromise of erythropoiesis due to osteosclerosis.

ovalocytic a., SYN elliptocytic a.

pernicious a. [MIM*361000], a chronic progressive a. of older adults (occurring more frequently during the fifth and later decades, rarely prior to 30 years of age), due to failure of absorption of Vitamin B$_{12}$, usually resulting from a defect of the stomach accompanied by mucosal atrophy and associated with lack of secretion of "intrinsic" factor; characterized by numbness and tingling, weakness, and a sore smooth tongue, as well as dyspnea after slight exertion, faintness, pallor of the skin and mucous membranes, anorexia, diarrhea, loss of weight, and fever; laboratory studies usually reveal greatly decreased red blood cell counts, low levels of hemoglobin, numerous characteristically oval shaped macrocytic erythrocytes (color index greater than normal, but not truly hyperchromic), and hypo- or achlorhydria, in association with a predominant number of megaloblasts and relatively few normoblasts in the bone marrow; the leukocyte count in peripheral blood may be less than normal, with relative lymphocytosis and hypersegmented neutrophils; a low level of vitamin B$_{12}$ is found in peripheral red blood cells; administration of vitamin B$_{12}$ results in a characteristic reticulocyte response, relief from symptoms, and an increase in erythrocytes, provided that pernicious a. is not complicated by another disease; the condition is not actually "pernicious," as it was prior to the availability of therapy with vitamin B$_{12}$. At least two autosomal recessive forms are known. In one there is a defect of intrinsic factor [MIM*26100] and in the other a defective absorption of vitamin B$_{12}$ from the intestine [MIM*261100]. SYN Addison's a., Addison-Biermer disease, addisonian a., Biermer's a., Biermer's disease, macrocytic achylic a., malignant a.

physiologic a., an obsolete term for apparent a. caused by increased fluid volume of the blood (overhydration).

polar a., a form of a. sometimes observed in natives of temperate climates when they migrate to the Arctic or Antarctic regions.

posthemorrhagic a., an acute a. caused by fairly sudden and rapid loss of blood, as by traumatic laceration of a relatively large vessel, erosion of an artery in a duodenal ulcer, hemorrhage in an ectopic pregnancy, or the result of such diseases as hemophilia and acute leukemia. SYN traumatic a.

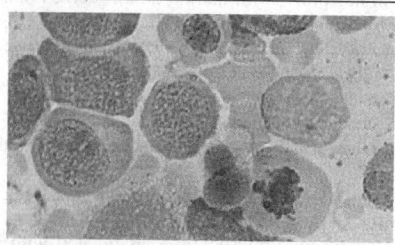

pernicious anemia (bone marrow smear)
note the typically loose chromatin structure of the megaloblasts

primary erythroblastic a., SYN *thalassemia* major.

primary refractory a., any of a group of anemic conditions in which there is persistent, frequently advanced a. that is not successfully treated by any means except blood transfusions, and that is not associated with another primary disease.

pure red cell a., SYN congenital hypoplastic a.

radiation a., hypoplastic a. sometimes occurring after high-level acute or low-level chronic exposure to ionizing radiation.

refractory a., (1) progressive a. unresponsive to therapy other than transfusion. SEE primary refractory a., secondary refractory a. SEE primary refractory a., secondary refractory a.

scorbutic a., a. occurring in patients with scurvy, usually due to coincident nutritional deficiency; *e.g.,* the "megaloblastic a. of scurvy" is due to concomitant folic acid deficiency.

secondary refractory a., any persistent a. that is successfully treated only by blood transfusions, and that is associated with another condition.

sickle cell a. [MIM*141900], an autosomal dominant a. [MIM141900] characterized by crescent- or sickle-shaped erythrocytes and by accelerated hemolysis, due to substitution of a single amino acid (valine for glutamic acid) in the sixth position of the beta chain of hemoglobin; affected homozygotes have 85-95% Hb S and severe anemia, while heterozygotes (said to have sickle cell trait) have 40-45% Hb S, the rest being normal Hb A; low oxygen tension causes polymerization of the abnormal beta chains, thus distorting the shape of the red blood cells to the sickle form. Homozygotes develop "crises" episodes of severe pain due to microvascular occlusions, bone infarcts, leg ulcers, and atrophy of the spleen associated with increased susceptibility to bacterial infections, especially streptococcal pneumonia. SYN crescent cell a., drepanocytic a., sickle cell disease.

sideroblastic a., sideroachrestic a., refractory a. characterized by the presence of sideroblasts in the bone marrow.

slaty a., an ash-gray pallor in poisoning from acetanelid or silver (argyria).

spastic a., local a. resulting from nontransitory contraction of the arterial vessels in the affected region.

spherocytic a., SYN hereditary *spherocytosis*.

splenic a., SYN Banti's *syndrome*.

target cell a., any a. with a conspicuous number of target cells in the peripheral blood; characteristic of the thalassemias and also found in several hemoglobinopathies.

toxic a., any a. resulting from the destructive effects of a chemical, metabolic poison, bacterial toxin, venom, and similar materials.

traumatic a., SYN posthemorrhagic a.

tropical a., various syndromes frequently observed in persons in tropical climates, usually resulting from nutritional deficiencies or hookworm or other parasitic diseases.

unstable hemoglobin hemolytic a., a congenital hemolytic a., due to autosomal inheritance of one of many unstable hemoglobins. The a. is of variable severity and characterized by the presence *in vivo* or *in vitro* of Heinz bodies.

ane·mic (ă-nē´mik). Pertaining to or manifesting the various features of anemia.

an·e·mom·e·ter (an-ĕ-mom′ĕ-ter). An instrument for measuring the velocity of air flow. [G. *anemos,* wind, + *metron,* measure]

a·nem·o·nol (ă-nem′ŏ-nol). A volatile oil, possessing markedly toxic properties, obtained from plants of the genus *Anemone.*

an·e·mo·pho·bia (an′ē-mō-fō′bē-ă). Morbid fear of wind. [G. *anemos,* wind, + *phobos,* fear]

an·e·mot·ro·phy (an-ĕ-mot′rō-fē). Lack of substances essential to the formation of blood, thereby resulting in hypoplastic anemia. [G. *an-* priv. + *haima,* blood, + *trophē,* nourishment]

an·en·ce·pha·lia (an′en-se-fā′lē-ă). SYN anencephaly.

an·en·ce·phal·ic (an-en-se-fal′ik). Relating to anencephaly. SYN anencephalous.

an·en·ceph·a·lous (an-en-sef′ă-lŭs). SYN anencephalic.

an·en·ceph·a·ly (an′en-sef′ă-lē). Congenital defective development of the brain, with absence of the bones of the cranial vault and absent or rudimentary cerebral and cerebellar hemispheres, brainstem, and basal ganglia. SYN anencephalia. [G. *an-* priv. + *enkephalos,* brain]

partial a., SYN hemicephalia.

an·en·ter·ous (an-en′ter-ŭs). Having no intestine; denoting certain parasites, such as tapeworms. [G. *an-* priv. + *entera,* intestines]

an·en·zy·mia (an-en-zī′mē-ă). Congenital absence of an enzyme.

aneph·ric (ă-nef′rik). Lacking kidneys. [*a-* priv. + G. *nephros,* kidney]

anep·ia (ă-nep′ē-ă). SYN aphasia. [G. *an-* priv. + *epos,* word]

an·ep·i·plo·ic (an-ep-i-plō′ik). Lacking an omentum (epiploon).

an·er·ga·sia (an-er-gā′zē-ă). Absence of psychic activity as the result of organic brain disease. [G. *an-* priv. + *ergasia,* work]

an·er·gas·tic (an-er-gas′tik). Pertaining to or characterized by anergasia.

an·er·gia (an-er′jē-ă). SYN anergy (2).

an·er·gic (an-er′jik). Relating to, or marked by, anergy.

an·er·gy (an′er-jē). **1.** Absence of ability to generate a sensitivity reaction in a subject to substances expected to be antigenic (immunogenic, allergenic) in that individual. **2.** Lack of energy. SYN anergia. [G. *an-* priv. + *energeia,* energy, from *ergon,* work]

negative a., a reduction of the normal or usual immunologic responses because of unrelated intervening disease. SYN nonspecific a.

nonspecific a., SYN negative a.

positive a., a reduction of the normal or usual immunologic response resulting from a reaction to a specific allergen. SYN specific a.

specific a., SYN positive a.

an·er·oid (an′er-oyd). Without fluid; denoting a form of barometer without mercury, in which the varying air pressure is indicated by a pointer governed by the movement of the elastic wall of an evacuated chamber. Also used to denote a mercury-free pressure gauge used with some sphygmomanometers. [G. *a-* priv. + *nēros,* wet, + *eidos,* form]

an·e·ryth·ro·pla·sia (an′ĕ-rith-rō-plā′zē-ă). A condition in which there is no formation of red blood cells. [G. *an-* priv. + erythro(cyte) + G. *plasis,* a molding]

an·e·ryth·ro·plas·tic (an′ĕ-rith-rō-plas′tik). Pertaining to or characterized by anerythroplasia.

an·e·ryth·ro·re·gen·er·a·tive (an-ĕ-rith′thrō-rē-jen′er-ă-tiv). Pertaining to or characterized by lack of regeneration of red blood cells.

an·es·the·ci·ne·sia (an-es′thē-si-nē′zē-ă). SYN anesthekinesia.

an·es·the·ki·ne·sia (an-es′thē-ki-nē′zē-ă). Combined sensory and motor paralysis. SYN anesthecinesia. [G. *an-* priv. + *aesthēsis,* sensation, + *kinēsis,* movement]

ANESTHESIA

an·es·the·sia (an′es-thē′zē-ă). **1.** Loss of sensation resulting from pharmacologic depression of nerve function or from neurological dysfunction. **2.** Broad term for anesthesiology as a clinical specialty. [G. *anaisthēsia,* fr. *an-* priv. + *aisthēsis,* sensation]

stages of anesthesia

acupuncture a., percutaneous insertion of, and stimulation by, needles placed in critical areas of the body to produce loss of sensation in another area.

ambulatory a., a. provided on an outpatient basis.

axillary a., loss of sensation in the distal two-thirds of the upper extremity following injection of a local anesthetic solution about the nerve trunks in the axilla.

balanced a., a technique of general a. based on the concept that administration of a mixture of small amounts of several neuronal depressants summates the advantages, but not the disadvantages of, the individual components of the mixture.

basal a., parenteral administration of one or more sedatives to produce a state of depressed consciousness short of a general a.

block a., SYN conduction a.

brachial a., anesthetization of an upper extremity by injection of local anesthetic solution about the brachial plexus.

caudal a., regional a. by injection of local anesthetic solution into the epidural space via the sacral hiatus.

cervical a., regional a. of the neck by injection of a local anesthetic solution about the cervical nerves or into the cervical epidural space.

circle absorption a., inhalation a. in which a circuit with carbon dioxide absorbent is used for complete (closed) or partial (semiclosed) rebreathing of exhaled gases.

closed a., inhalation a. in which there is total rebreathing of all exhaled gases, except carbon dioxide which is absorbed; gas flow into the anesthetic circuit consists only of oxygen, in amounts equal to the patient's metabolic consumption, plus small amounts of other gases (*e.g.,* nitrous oxide) which undergo continued uptake by and distribution in the patient.

compression a., SYN pressure a.

conduction a., regional a. in which local anesthetic solution is injected about nerves to inhibit nerve transmission; includes spinal, epidural, nerve block, and field block a., but not local or topical a. SYN block a.

continuous epidural a., insertion of a catheter into the lumbar or caudal epidural space for the repeated injection of local anesthetic solutions as a means of prolonging duration of anesthesia. SYN fractional epidural a.

continuous spinal a., insertion of a catheter into the spinal subarachnoid space and leaving it *in situ* to permit serial intermittent injection of local anesthetic solution for prolonged spinal a. SYN fractional spinal a.

crossed a., a. of one side of the head and the other side of the body due to a brainstem lesion.

dental a., general, conduction, local, or topical a. for operations upon the teeth, gingivae, or associated structures.

diagnostic a., a. induced for evaluation of the mechanism responsible for a painful condition.

differential spinal a., a form of diagnostic spinal a. producing blockade of different types of nerves in the subarachnoid space, based upon their differences in sensitivity to local anesthetics; also observed during surgical spinal a.

dissociated a., loss of some types of sensation with persistence of others; most often used in context of nerve blocks, wherein a loss of sensation for pain and temperature occurs without loss of tactile sense.

dissociative a., a form of general a., but not necessarily complete unconsciousness, characterized by catalepsy, catatonia, and amnesia, especially that produced by phenylcyclohexylamine compounds, including ketamine.

a. doloro′sa, severe spontaneous pain occurring in an anesthetic area. SYN painful a.

electric a., a., usually general a., produced by application of an electrical current.

endotracheal a., inhalation a. technique in which anesthetic and respiratory gases pass through a tube placed in the trachea via the mouth or nose. SYN intratracheal a.

epidural a., regional a. produced by injection of local anesthetic solution into the peridural space. SYN peridural a.

extradural a., anesthetization, by local anesthetics, of nerves near the spinal canal external to the dura mater; often refers to epidural a., but may include paravertebral a.

field block a., conduction a. in which small nerves are not anesthetized individually, as in nerve block a., but instead are blocked *en masse* by local anesthetic solution injected to form a barrier proximal to the operative site.

fractional epidural a., SYN continuous epidural a.

fractional spinal a., SYN continuous spinal a.

general a., loss of ability to perceive pain associated with loss of consciousness produced by intravenous or inhalation anesthetic agents.

girdle a., a. distributed as a band encircling the trunk.

glove a., loss of sensation in the distal upper extremity, *i.e.,* the hand and fingers.

gustatory a., SYN ageusia.

high spinal a., spinal a. in which the level of sensory denervation extends to the second or third thoracic dermatome.

hyperbaric a., inhalation of depressant gases or vapors at pressures greater than 1 atmosphere, especially as a means of producing general a. with agents too weak to produce a. at 1 atmosphere.

hyperbaric spinal a., spinal a. in which spread of local anesthetic solution in the subarachnoid space is controlled by adjusting the position of the patient when the density of local anesthetic is made greater than the density of cerebrospinal fluid (*i.e.,* hyperbaric) by the addition of glucose.

hypobaric spinal a., spinal a. in which spread of local anesthetic solution in the subarachnoid space is controlled by adjusting the position of the patient when the density of the local anesthetic solution is made less than the density of cerebrospinal fluid (*i.e.,* hypobaric) by the addition of distilled water.

hypotensive a., a. in which arterial hypotension is deliberately induced as a means of decreasing operative blood loss.

hypothermic a., general a. administered in conjunction with artificial lowering of body temperature.

hysterical a., a. as a manifestation of hysteria, usually involving half the body or isolated patches not conforming to neuroanatomical distribution.

infiltration a., a. produced by injection of local anesthetic solution directly into an area that is painful or about to be operated upon.

inhalation a., general a. resulting from breathing of anesthetic gases or vapors.

insufflation a., maintenance of inhalation a. by delivery of anesthetic gases or vapors directly to the airway of a spontaneously breathing patient.

intercostal a., regional a. produced by injection of local anesthetic solution about intercostal nerves.

intramedullary a., rarely used method of general a. by injection of intravenous anesthetic agent(s) into the medullary canal of long bones. SYN intraosseous a.

intranasal a., (1) insufflation a. in which an inhalation anesthetic is added to inhaled air passing through the nose or nasopharynx; (2) a. of nasal passages by infiltration and topical application of local anesthetic solution to nasal mucosa.

intraoral a., (1) insufflation a. in which an inhalation anesthetic is added to inhaled air passing through the mouth; (2) regional a. of the mouth and associated structures when local anesthetic solutions are used by topical application to oral mucosa, by local infiltration, or as nerve blocks.

intraosseous a., SYN intramedullary a.

intraspinal a., inaccurate synonym for spinal a.; local anesthetic solutions are not injected into the spinal cord.

intratracheal a., SYN endotracheal a.

intravenous a., general a. produced by injection of central nervous system depressants into the venous circulation.

intravenous regional a., regional a. by intravenous injection of local anesthetic solution distal to an occlusive tourniquet in an extremity previously exsanguinated by pressure or gravity. SYN Bier's method (1).

isobaric spinal a., spinal a. of same density as cerobrospinal fluid so that the level of a. is not influenced by a change in the position of the patient.

local a., a general term referring to topical, infiltration, field block, or nerve block a. but usually not to spinal or epidural a. SEE ALSO local *anesthetics,* under *anesthetic.*

low spinal a., spinal a. in which the level of sensory denervation extends to the tenth or eleventh thoracic dermatome.

nerve block a., conduction a. in which local anesthetic solution is injected about nerves, nerve trunks, or nerve plexuses.

nonrebreathing a., a technique for inhalation a. in which valves exhaust all exhaled air from the circuit.

open drop a., inhalation a. by vaporization of a liquid anesthetic placed drop by drop on a gauze mask covering the mouth and nose.

outpatient a., (1) SYN patient controlled *analgesia.*

painful a., SYN a. dolorosa.

paracervical block a., regional a. of the cervix uteri by injection of local anesthetic solution into tissues adjacent to the cervix.

paravertebral a., (1) a. by injection of local anesthetic solution about nerves as they exit from the vertebral canal; (2) combined presynaptic, postsynaptic, and ganglionic sympathetic block by injection of local anesthetic solution about paravertebral sympathetic chains.

patient controlled a. (PCA), a method for control of pain based upon a pump for the constant intravenous or, less frequently, epidural infusion of a dilute narcotic solution that includes a mechanism for the self-administration at predetermined intervals of a predetermined amount of the narcotic solution should the infusion fail to relieve pain. SYN outpatient a. (1).

peridural a., SYN epidural a.

perineural a., obsolete term for a. produced by injection of an anesthetic agent around a nerve.

periodontal a., a. of the periodontal ligament, produced by injection of a local anesthetic drug.

presacral a., injection of local anesthetic solution anterior to the sacrum, to block nerves as they exit from the sacral foramina.

pressure a., loss of sensation produced by pressure applied to a nerve. SYN compression a.

pudendal a., local a. produced by blocking the pudendal nerves near the spinal processes of the ischium; used in obstetrics.

rebreathing a., a technique for inhalation a. in which a portion or all of the gases that are exhaled are subsequently inhaled after carbon dioxide has been absorbed.

rectal a., general a. produced by instillation into the rectum of a solution containing a central nervous system depressant.

refrigeration a., SYN cryoanesthesia.

regional a., use of local anesthetic solution(s) to produce circumscribed areas of loss of sensation; a generic term including conduction, nerve block, spinal, epidural, field block, infiltration, and topical a. SYN conduction analgesia.

retrobulbar a., injection of a local anesthetic behind the eye to produce sensory denervation of the eye.

sacral a., regional a. limited to those areas innervated by sacral sensory nerves.

saddle a., SYN saddle block a.

saddle block a., a form of spinal a. limited in area to the buttocks, perineum, and inner surfaces of the thighs. SYN saddle a.

segmental a., loss of sensation limited to an area supplied by one or more spinal nerve roots.

semi-closed a., inhalation a. using a circuit in which a portion of the exhaled air is exhausted from the circuit and a portion is rebreathed following absorption of carbon dioxide.

semi-open a., inhalation a. in which a portion of inhaled gases is derived from an anesthesia circuit while the remainder consists of room air.

spinal a., (1) loss of sensation produced by injection of local anesthetic solution(s) into the spinal subarachnoid space; SYN subarachnoid a. **(2)** loss of sensation produced by disease of the spinal cord.

splanchnic a., loss of sensation in areas of the visceral peritoneum innervated by the splanchnic nerves. SYN visceral a.

stocking a., loss of sensation in the distal lower extremity, *i.e.,* the foot and toes.

subarachnoid a., SYN spinal a. (1).

surgical a., (1) any a. administered for the purpose of permitting performance of an operative procedure, as differentiated from obstetrical, diagnostic, and therapeutic a.; **(2)** loss of sensation with muscle relaxation adequate for an operative procedure.

tactile a., loss or impairment of the sense of touch.

therapeutic a., administration of an anesthetic as a means of treatment.

thermal a., thermic a., loss of temperature appreciation.

to-and-fro a., a. using of a valveless closed a. circuit in which respired gases pass back and forth through a carbon dioxide absorbent interposed between patient and respiratory reservoir bag.

topical a., superficial loss of sensation in conjunctiva, mucous membranes or skin, produced by direct application of local anesthetic solutions, ointments, or jellies.

total spinal a., spinal a. extensive enough to produce loss of sensation in all extracranial sensory roots.

traumatic a., loss of sensation resulting from nerve injury.

unilateral a., SYN hemianesthesia.

visceral a., SYN splanchnic a.

---

an·es·the·si·ol·o·gist (an′es-thē-zē-ol′ō-jist). **1.** A physician specializing solely in anesthesiology and related areas. **2.** An individual with a doctorate degree who is board-certified and legally qualified to administer anesthetics and related techniques. Cf. anesthetist.

an·es·the·si·ol·o·gy (an′es-thē-zē-ol′ō-jē). The medical specialty concerned with the pharmacological, physiological, and clinical basis of anesthesia and related fields, including resuscitation, intensive respiratory care, and acute and chronic pain. [anesthesia + G. *logos,* treatise]

an·es·thet·ic (an-es-thet′ik). **1.** A compound that reversibly depresses neuronal function, producing loss of ability to perceive pain and/or other sensations. **2.** Collective designation for anes-

thetizing agents administered to an individual at a particular time. **3.** Characterized by loss of sensation or capable of producing loss of sensation. **4.** Associated with or due to the state of anesthesia.

flammable a., an inhalation a. that supports combustion and forms explosive mixtures with oxidizing gases.

general a., a compound that produces loss of sensation associated with loss of consciousness.

inhalation a., a gas or a liquid with sufficient vapor pressure to produce general anesthesia when breathed.

intravenous a., a compound that produces anesthesia when injected intravenously.

local a.'s, drugs used for the interruption of the nerve transmission of pain sensations. They act at the site of application to prevent perception of pain; examples include procaine and lidocaine.

primary a., the compound that contributes most to loss of sensation when a mixture of anesthetics is administered.

secondary a., a compound that contributes to, but is not primarily responsible for, loss of sensation when two or more anesthetics are simultaneously administered.

spinal a., a local anesthetic agent producing loss of sensation when injected into the subarachnoid space.

topical a., a local a. preparation suitable for anesthetizing skin surfaces or mucous membranes. Can be used in the form of ointments, creams, jellies, sprays, or solutions.

volatile a., a liquid a. that at room temperature volatilizes to a vapor which when inhaled is capable of producing general anesthesia. SEE ALSO anesthetic *vapor.*

anes·the·tist (ă-nes′thĕ-tist). One who administers an anesthetic, whether an anesthesiologist, a physician who is not an anesthesiologist, a nurse a., or an anesthesia assistant.

anes·the·ti·za·tion (ă-nes′thĕ-ti-zā′shun). The act of producing loss of sensation.

anes·the·tize (ă-nes′thĕ-tīz). To produce loss of sensation.

an·es·trous (an-es′trŭs). Relating to the anestrus.

a·nes·trum (an-es′trŭm). The period between two estrus cycles [G. *an-* priv. + *oistros,* estrus]

an·es·trus (an-es′trŭs). The period of sexual quiescence between the estrus cycles of mammals; may be: 1) a prolonged period in monestrous animals (dogs) or seasonally polyestrous animals (sheep), or 2) a prolonged period of failure of estrus in mature nonpregnant, polyestrous animals. [G. *a-* priv. + *oistros,* a gadfly, mad desire (estrus)]

ane·tho·path (ă-nē′thō-path). A morally uninhibited person. [G. *an-* priv. + *ethos,* custom, + *pathos,* suffering]

an·e·to·der·ma (an-ĕ-tō-der′mă). Atrophoderma in which the skin becomes baglike and wrinkled. SYN atrophia maculosa varioliformis cutis, atrophoderma maculatum, macular atrophy, primary idiopathic macular atrophy, primary macular atrophy of skin. [G. *anetos,* relaxed, + *derma,* skin]

Jadassohn-Pellizzari a., cutaneous atrophy preceded by erythematous or urticarial lesions of the trunk and upper portions of the extremities, and enlarging to 2-3 cm before undergoing involution.

Schweninger-Buzzi a., sudden appearance of bluish-white balloon-like lesions, soft and readily indented, chiefly on the trunk and extremities of women.

⬙ **Combining forms**	[NA] **Nomina Anatomica**
Word*Finder* **Multi-term entry finder Preceding letter A**	[MIM] **Mendelian Inheritance in Man**
A.D.A.M. Anatomy Plates Between letters L and M	☆ **Official alternate term**
Appendices: Following letter Z	☆[NA] **Official alternate Nomina Anatomica term**
SYN Synonym; Cf., compare	**High Profile Term**

an·eu·ploid (an'yū-ployd). Having an abnormal number of chromosomes not an exact multiple of the haploid number, as contrasted with abnormal numbers of complete haploid sets of chromosomes, such as diploid, triploid, etc. [G. *an-* priv. + euploid]

an·eu·ploi·dy (an'yū-ploy-dē). State of being aneuploid.

partial a., a type of mosaicism in which some cells have a normal number of chromosomes and some have an abnormal number.

an·eu·rine (an'yū-rēn). SYN thiamin.

a. hydrochloride, SYN *thiamin* hydrochloride.

a. pyrophosphate, SYN *thiamin* pyrophosphate.

aneu·ro·lem·mic (ă-nū-rō-lem'ik). Without a neurolemma.

an·eu·rysm (an'yū-rizm). Circumscribed dilation of an artery connecting directly with the lumen of an artery or a cardiac chamber connecting directly with the lumen of an artery, usually due to an acquired or congenital weakness of the wall of the artery or chamber. [G. *aneurysma* (-*mat*-), a dilation, fr. *eurys*, wide]

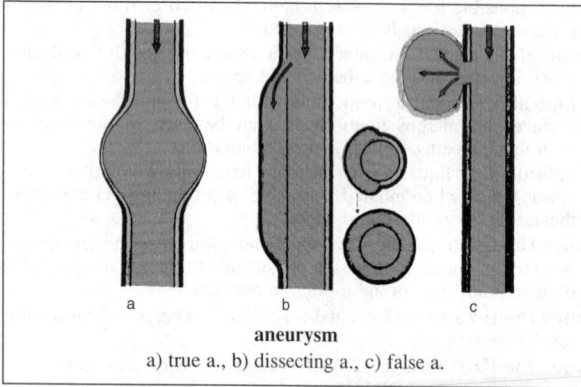

aneurysm
a) true a., b) dissecting a., c) false a.

ampullary a., SYN saccular a.

a. by anastomosis, a mass of dilated anastomosing vessels that produce a pulsating tumor usually in a superficial position.

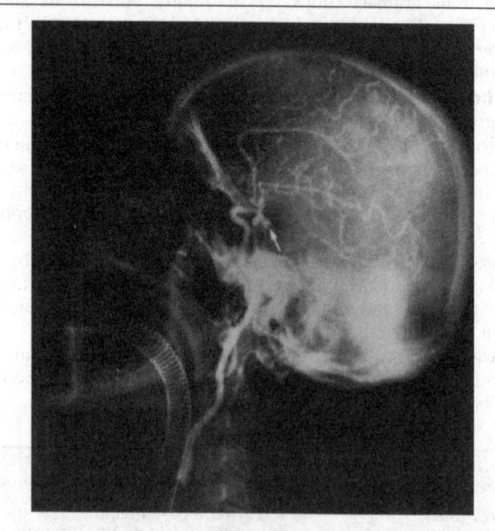

aneurysm
angiogram of an aneurysm in the posterior communicating artery (arrow)

aortic a., congenital absence of the aortic valve orifice. SEE ALSO dissecting a.

aortic sinus a., abnormal dilation of one or more of the three aortic sinuses situated behind the three aortic valve cusps.

arteriosclerotic a., the most common type of a., occurring in the abdominal aorta and other large arteries, primarily in the elderly. SYN atherosclerotic a.

arteriovenous a., (1) a dilated arteriovenous shunt. **(2)** communication between an artery and a vein, sometimes congenital.

atherosclerotic a., SYN arteriosclerotic a.

axial a., an a. involving the entire circumference of a blood vessel.

benign bone a., SYN aneurysmal bone *cyst*.

Bérard's a., an arteriovenous a. in the tissues outside the injured vein.

berry a., a small saccular a. of a cerebral artery that resembles a berry. Such a.'s frequently rupture causing a subarachnoid hemorrhage.

cardiac a., thinning, stretching, and bulging of a weakened ventricular wall, usually as a result of myocardial infarction; rarely postinflammatory or congenital. SYN mural aneurysm, ventricular a.

Charcot-Bouchard a., SYN miliary a.

cirsoid a., dilation of a group of blood vessels owing to congenital malformation with arteriovenous shunting. SYN cirsoid varix, racemose a., racemose hemangioma.

compound a., an a. in which some of the coats of the artery are ruptured, others intact.

congenital cerebral a., localized dilation of a cerebral vessel; usually a berry a.

consecutive a., SYN diffuse a.

coronary artery a., a. of the coronary artery, rarely congenital, usually due to atherosclerosis, inflammatory processes, or a coronary fistula.

cylindroid a., SYN tubular a.

diffuse a., an a. that has enlarged and spread to the surrounding tissues in consequence of rupture of its walls. SYN consecutive a.

dissecting a., splitting or dissection of an arterial wall by blood entering through an intimal tear or by interstitial hemorrhage; more common in the aorta, for example, with an intimal tear near the aortic valve (Type I) or subclavian artery and distal dissection of the media for a variable distance, frequently rupturing through the outer wall.

ductal a., of the patent ductus arteriosus, occurs either in infants or adults.

ectatic a., an a. in which all the coats of the artery, though stretched, are unruptured.

embolomycotic a., obsolete term for an a. caused by an embolism composed of an infected vegetation from a cardiac valve.

false a., (1) pulsating, encapsulated hematoma in communication with the lumen of a ruptured vessel; **(2)** ventricular pseudoaneurysm, a cardiac rupture contained and loculated by pericardium, which forms its external wall. **(3)** an a. whose walls consist of adventitia and periarterial fibrous tissue and hematoma.

fusiform a., an elongated spindle-shaped dilation of an artery.

hernial a., the protrusion of the stretched inner coats of an artery through a wound in the adventitia.

infraclinoid a., an intracranial a. occurring below the level of the anterior clinoid process of the sphenoid bone.

intracavernous a., an a. of the carotid artery within the cavernous sinus.

intracranial a., any a. located within the cranium. There are well authenticated autosomal dominant cases [MIM*105800].

miliary a., dilatation in the diameter of small arteries and arterioles secondary to lipohyalinosis from long-standing hypertension associated with intracerebral hematomas. SYN Charcot-Bouchard a.

mural aneurysm, SYN cardiac a.

mycotic a., an a. caused by the growth of fungi within the vascular wall, usually following impaction of a septic embolus; also used to refer to the growth of bacteria within the vascular wall of an a.; may result from impaction of septic embolus or from primary infection of the vessel wall.

Park's a., an arteriovenous a. in which the brachial artery communicates with the brachial and median basilic veins.

peripheral a., (1) a saclike a. springing from one side of an artery; (2) an a. of one of the smaller branches of an artery.

phantom a., a palpable throbbing aorta, mistaken by novices for an a.

Pott's a., SYN aneurysmal *varix*.

pulmonary artery a., a. of the pulmonary artery; rare in the absence of congenital heart disease.

racemose a., SYN cirsoid a.

Rasmussen's a., aneurysmal dilation of a branch of a pulmonary artery in a tuberculous cavity, rupture of which may cause serious hemoptysis.

a. of the right ventricle or right ventricular outflow patch, a. occurring after right ventriculostomy; the a. may either be a false or a true a.

ruptured a., an a. that is hemorrhaging into its wall or surrounding tissues.

saccular a., sacculated a., a saclike bulging on one side of an artery. SYN ampullary a.

serpentine a., dilation and tortuosity of an artery, sometimes affecting the temporal, splenic, or iliac arteries in the elderly.

a. of sinus of Valsalva, a congenital thin-walled tubular outpouching usually in the right or non-coronary sinus with an entirely intracardiac course that may rupture into the right or rarely the left heart chambers to form an aortocardiac fistula.

supraclinoid a., an intracranial a. located immediately above the anterior clinoid process of the sphenoid bone.

syphilitic a., an a., usually involving the thoracic aorta, resulting from tertiary syphilitic aortitis.

traumatic a., an a. resulting from physical damage to the wall of an artery; usually a false a. or arteriovenous a.

true a., localized dilation of an artery with an expanded lumen lined by stretched remnants of the arterial wall.

tubular a., the uniform dilation of an artery along a considerable distance. SYN cylindroid a.

varicose a., a blood-containing sac, communicating with both an artery and a vein.

ventricular a., SYN cardiac a.

a. of the ventricular portion of the membranous septum, an a. that bulges toward the right in systole, often consisting of the anterior leaflet of the tricuspid valve.

verminous a., an a. in horses caused by *Strongylus vulgaris* larvae; usually involving the mesenteric arteries. SYN worm a.

worm a., SYN verminous a.

an·eu·rys·mal, an·eu·rys·mat·ic (an-yū-riz′măl, -riz-mat′ik). Relating to an aneurysm.

an·eu·rys·mec·to·my (an-yū-riz-mek′tō-mē). Excision of an aneurysm. [aneurysm + G. *ektomē*, excision]

an·eu·rys·mo·gram. SYN aneurysmograph.

an·eu·rys·mo·graph (an′yū-riz′mŏg′răf). Demonstration of an aneurysm, usually by means of x-rays and a contrast medium. SYN aneurysmogram. [aneurysm + G. *graphō*, to write]

an·eu·rys·mo·plas·ty (an-yū-riz′mō-plas-tē). Repair of an aneurysm by opening the sac and suturing its walls to restore the normal dimension to the lumen of the artery. SEE ALSO aneurysmorrhaphy. SYN endoaneurysmoplasty, endoaneurysmorrhaphy. [aneurysm + G. *plastos*, formed]

an·eu·rys·mor·rha·phy (an′yū-riz-mōr′ă-fē). Closure by suture of the sac of an aneurysm to restore the normal lumen dimensions. [aneurysm + G. *rhaphē*, suture]

an·eu·rys·mot·o·my (an′yū-riz-mot′ō-mē). Incision into the sac of an aneurysm. [aneurysm + G. *tomē*, incision]

ANF Abbreviation for antinuclear *factor*; atrial natriuretic *factor*.

⌀angei-. SEE angio-.

an·gel·i·ca root (an-jel′i-kă). The root of *Angelica archangelica* (family Umbelliferae); a tonic and stimulant that may cause nausea; used as a carminative, diuretic, and externally as a counterirritant.

Angelucci, Arnaldo, Italian ophthalmologist, 1854–1934. SEE A.'s *syndrome*.

Anger, Hal, U.S. electrical engineer, *1920. SEE A. *camera*.

Anghelescu, Constantin, Roumanian surgeon, 1869–1948. SEE A.'s *sign*.

⌀angi-. SEE angio-.

an·gi·ec·ta·sia, an·gi·ec·ta·sis (an-jē-ek-tā′zē-ă, -ek′tă-sis). Dilation of a lymphatic or blood vessel. [angio- + G. *ektasis*, a stretching]

congenital dysplastic a., SYN Klippel-Trenaunay-Weber *syndrome*.

an·gi·ec·tat·ic (an-jē-ek-tat′ik). Marked by the presence of dilated blood vessels. [angio- + G. *ektatos*, capable of extension]

an·gi·ec·to·pia (an-jē-ek-tō′pē-ă). Abnormal location of a blood vessel. SYN angioplany. [angio- + G. *ektopos*, out of place]

an·gi·i·tis, an·gi·tis (an-jē-ī′tis, an-jī′tis). Inflammation of a blood vessel (arteritis, phlebitis) or of a lymphatic vessel (lymphangitis). SYN vasculitis. [angio- + G. *-itis*, inflammation]

allergic a., SYN cutaneous *vasculitis*.

allergic granulomatous a., SYN Churg-Strauss *syndrome*.

consecutive a., a. caused by extension of the inflammatory process from the surrounding tissues.

hypersensitivity a., an inflammatory reaction in a blood vessel, the result of a specific reaction to an antigenic (allergic) substance or other agents to which the individual expresses unusual vascular sensitization.

a. live′do reticula′ris, SYN *livedo* reticularis.

necrotizing a., inflammatory reaction of blood vessels resulting in fibrinoid necrosis of tissue, especially of the blood vessel wall.

an·gi·na (an′ji-nă, an-jī′nă). 1. A severe, often constricting pain, usually referring to a. pectoris. 2. Old term for a sore throat from any cause. [L. quinsy]

abdominal a., a. abdom′inis, intermittent abdominal pain, frequently occurring at a fixed time after eating, caused by inadequacy of the mesenteric circulation from arteriosclerosis or other arterial disease. SYN intestinal a.

agranulocytic a., SYN agranulocytosis.

crescendo a., a. pectoris that occurs with increasing frequency, intensity, or duration.

a. cru′ris, intermittent claudication of the leg.

a. decu′bitus, a. pectoris related to horizontal, usually supine, body position.

a. diphtherit′ica, obsolete term for diphtheria involving the pharynx or larynx.

a. of effort, a. pectoris precipitated by physical exertion.

false a., a.-like sensation(s) in absence of myocardial ischemia.

Heberden's a., SYN a. pectoris.

hypercyanotic a., anginal pain in cyanotic patients with congenital heart disease or chronic pulmonary disease, the pain developing with intensification of the cyanosis during activity.

intestinal a., SYN abdominal a.

a. inver′sa, SYN Prinzmetal's a.

Ludwig's a., cellulitis, usually of odontogenic origin, bilaterally involving the submaxillary, sublingual, and submental spaces, resulting in painful swelling of the floor of the mouth, elevation of the tongue, dysphasia, dysphonia, and (at times) compromise of the airway. [W.F. Ludwig]

lymphatic a., an affection resembling Vincent's disease marked by an increase in the number of lymphocytes in the blood.

a. lymphomato′sa, SYN agranulocytosis.

monocytic a., obsolete term for infectious mononucleosis.

necrotic a., obsolete term for a form of a. occurring usually as a complication of scarlet fever and more rarely of diphtheria, in which gangrenous patches are found in the mucous membrane of the air passages.

neutropenic a., SYN agranulocytosis.

a. no′tha, obsolete term for a. pectoris vasomotoria.

a. pec′toris, severe constricting pain in the chest, often radiating from the precordium to a shoulder (usually left) and down the arm, due to ischemia of the heart muscle usually caused by coronary disease. SYN breast pang, coronarism (2), heart stroke (2), Heberden's a., Rougnon-Heberden disease, stenocardia.

a. pec′toris decu′bitus, anginal pain developing while the subject is recumbent.

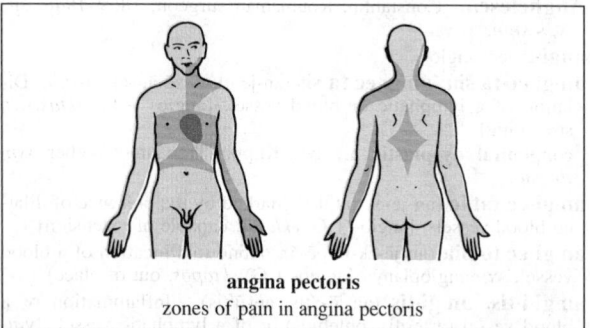

angina pectoris
zones of pain in angina pectoris

a. pec′toris si′ne dolor′e, SYN Gairdner's *disease*.

a. pec′toris vasomoto′ria, a. pectoris in which the breast pain is comparatively slight, but pallor followed by cyanosis, and coldness and numbness of the extremities, are marked. SYN a. spuria, a. vasomotoria, pseudangina, pseudoangina, reflex a., vasomotor a.

preinfarction a., obsolete term for unstable angina.

Prinzmetal's a., a form of a. pectoris, characterized by pain that is not precipitated by cardiac work, is of longer duration, is usually more severe, and is associated with unusual electrocardiographic manifestations including elevated ST segments in leads that are ordinarily depressed in typical a., and usually without reciprocal ST changes; occurring at night in bed. SYN a. inversa, variant a. pectoris.

reflex a., SYN a. pectoris vasomotoria.

a. scarlatino′sa, obsolete term for sore throat of scarlet fever.

a. si′ne do′lore, symptoms of coronary insufficiency occurring without pain.

a. spu′ria, SYN a. pectoris vasomotoria.

unstable a., (1) a. pectoris characterized by pain in the chest of coronary origin occurring in response to progressively less exercise or fewer other stimuli than ordinarily required to produce a.; often leading to myocardial infarction, if untreated, and caused by coronary artery spasm rather than increased myocardial oxygen and demand. **(2)** a. that has not achieved a constant or reproducible pattern in 30 or 60 days.

variant a. pectoris, SYN Prinzmetal's a.

vasomotor a., SYN a. pectoris vasomotoria.

a. vasomotor′ia, SYN a. pectoris vasomotoria.

Vincent's a., an ulcerative infection of the oral soft tissues including the tonsils and pharynx caused by fusiform and spirochetal organisms; it is usually associated with necrotizing ulcerative gingivitis and may progress to noma. Death from suffocation or sepsis may occur.

walk-through a., a circumstance in which despite continuing activity, such as walking, the pain of a. pectoris diminishes or disappears.

an·gi·nal (an′ji-năl, an-jī′). Relating to angina in any sense.

an·gi·ni·form (an-jin′i-fōrm). Resembling angina.

an·gi·noid (an′jin-oid). Rarely used term for resembling an angina, especially angina pectoris.

an·gin·o·pho·bia (an′ji-nō-fō′bē-ă). Extreme fear of an attack of angina pectoris. [angina + G. *phobos,* fear]

an·gi·nose, an·gi·nous (an′ji-nōs, -ji-nŭs). Rarely used term for relating to any angina.

⌂**angio-, angi-.** Blood or lymph vessels; a covering, an enclosure; corresponds to L. vas-,vaso-, vasculo-. [G. *angeion,* a vessel or cavity of the body, fr. *angos,* a vessel, vat, bucket, + *-eion,* small, little]

an·gi·o·ar·chi·tec·ture (an′jē-ō-ar′ki-tek-chūr). **1.** The arrangement and distribution of the blood vessels of any organ. **2.** The vascular framework of an organ or tissue.

an·gi·o·blast (an′jē-ō-blast). **1.** A cell taking part in blood vessel formation. SYN vasoformative cell. **2.** Primordial mesenchymal tissue from which embryonic blood cells and vascular endotheli-

um are differentiated. SYN angioderm. [angio- + G. *blastos,* germ]

an·gi·o·blas·to·ma (an′jē-ō-blas-tō′mă). SYN hemangioblastoma.

an·gi·o·car·di·og·ra·phy (an′jē-ō-kar-dē-og′ră-fē). X-ray imaging of the heart and great vessels made visible by injection of a radiopaque solution. SEE coronary *angiography.* SYN cardioangiography. [angio- + G. *kardia,* heart, + *graphō,* to write]

exercise radionuclide a., radionuclide a. while performing exercise, such as on a treadmill or bicycle.

gated radionuclide a., radionuclide a. using cardiac gating to combine images from several cardiac cycles to improve the quality of the images of separate phases (*e.g.,* systole and diastole).

radionuclide a., the display, by means of a stationary scintillation camera device, of the passage of a bolus of a rapidly injected radiopharmaceutical. SYN radionuclide ventriculography.

an·gi·o·car·di·o·ki·net·ic, an·gi·o·car·di·o·ci·net·ic (an′jē-ō-kar′dē-ō-ki-net′ik, -dē-ō-si-net′ik). Causing dilation or contraction in the heart and blood vessels. [angio- + G. *kardia,* heart, + *kinēsis,* movement]

an·gi·o·car·di·op·a·thy (an′jē-ō-kar-dē-op′ă-thē). Disease affecting both heart and blood vessels. [angio- + G. *kardia,* heart, + *pathos,* disease]

an·gi·o·cho·le·cys·ti·tis (an′jē-ō-kō′lē-sis-tī′tis). Rarely used term for inflammation of the bile vessels and gallbladder. [angio- + G. *cholē,* bile, + *kystis,* bladder, + *-itis,* inflammation]

an·gi·o·cho·li·tis (an′jē-ō-kō-lī′tis). SYN cholangitis.

an·gi·o·cyst (an′jē-ō-sist). A small vesicular aggregation of embryonic mesodermal cells that may give rise to vascular endothelium and blood cells.

an·gi·o·derm (an′jē-ō-derm). SYN angioblast (2).

an·gi·o·di·as·co·py (an′jē-ō-dī-as′kŏ-pē). Archaic term for examination of the vessels in a part by transillumination. [angio- + G. *dia,* through, + *skopeō,* to view]

an·gi·o·dys·pla·sia (an′jē-ō-dis-plā′zē-ă). Degenerative or congenital structural abnormality of the normally distributed vasculature.

an·gi·o·dys·tro·phy, an·gi·o·dys·tro·phia (an′jē-ō-dis′trō-fē, -dis-trō′fē-ă). Defective formation or growth associated with marked vascular changes. [angio- + G. *dys-,* bad, + *trophē,* nourishment]

an·gi·o·e·de·ma (an′jē-ō-ĕ-dē′mă). Recurrent large circumscribed areas of subcutaneous edema of sudden onset, usually disappearing within 24 hours; seen mainly in young women, frequently as an allergic reaction to foods or drugs. SYN angioneurotic edema, atrophedema, Bannister's disease, giant hives, giant urticaria, Milton's disease, periodic edema, Quincke's disease, Quincke's edema, urticaria tuberosa.

hereditary a., an inherited, autosomal dominant disease characterized by episodic appearance of brawny nonpitting edema, most often affecting the extremities but can involve any part of the body, including mucosal surfaces such as those of the intestine (causing abdominal pain) or respiratory tract (causing asphyxia, which can require intubation to avoid fatal outcome). Associated with deficiency of inhibitor of first component of complement pathway (C1). Emergency treatment with epinephrine, long-term treatment with a variety of agents is effective.

an·gi·o·el·e·phan·ti·a·sis (an′jē-ō-el′ĕ-fan-tī′ă-sis). Extensive increase in vascularity of the subcutaneous tissue, producing great thickening simulating large, diffuse angioma formation.

an·gi·o·en·do·the·li·o·ma·to·sis (an′jē-ō-en-dō-thē′lē-ō-mă-tō′sis). Proliferation of endothelial cells within blood vessels.

proliferating systematized a., a rare generalized cutaneous and visceral intracapillary proliferation of endothelial cells, with vascular thrombosis and obstruction. The condition has been divided into a benign reactive type and a rapidly fatal neoplastic type; however, most of the latter cases have been shown to be intravascular large-cell lymphomas.

an·gi·o·fi·bro·li·po·ma (an′jē-ō-fī′brō-li-pō′mă). A neoplasm composed of fibroblasts, capillaries, and adipose tissue. SYN angiolipofibroma.

an·gi·o·fi·bro·ma (an′jē-ō-fī-brō′mă). SYN telangiectatic *fibroma.*

juvenile a., a markedly vascular fibrous tumor occurring in the nasopharynx of males, usually in the second decade of life; epistaxis and local invasion may result, but spontaneous regression may occur after sexual maturity. SYN juvenile hemangiofibroma.

an·gi·o·fi·bro·sis (an'jē-ō-fī-brō'sis). Fibrosis of the walls of blood vessels.

an·gi·o·gen·e·sis (an'jē-ō-jen'ĕ-sis). Development of new blood vessels. [angio- + G. *genesis,* production]

an·gi·o·gen·ic (an'jē-ō-jen'ik). **1.** Relating to angiogenesis. **2.** Of vascular origin.

an·gi·o·gli·o·ma (an'jē-ō-glī-ō'mă). A mixed glioma and angioma.

an·gi·o·gli·o·ma·to·sis (an'jē-ō-glī'ō-mă-tō'sis). Occurrence of multiple areas of proliferating capillaries and neuroglia or a condition of multiple angiogliomas.

an·gi·o·gli·o·sis (an'jē-ō-glī-ō'sis). Glial scarring about a blood vessel or a condition of multiple angiogliomas.

an·gi·o·gram (an'jē-ō-gram). Radiograph obtained by angiography. [angio- + G. *gramma,* a writing]

an·gi·o·graph·ic (an-jē-ō-graf'ik). Relating to or utilizing angiography.

an·gi·og·ra·phy (an-jē-og'ră-fē). Radiography of vessels after the injection of a radiopaque contrast material; usually requires percutaneous insertion of a radiopaque catheter and positioning under fluoroscopic control. SEE ALSO arteriography, venography. [angio- + G. *graphō,* to write]

biplane a., synchronous a. in two planes at right angles to each other or in two orthogonal planes.

cerebral a., radiographic visualization of the blood vessels supplying the brain, including their extracranial portions; the injection of contrast media may be made percutaneously, by open exposure and puncture of the particular vessel, or by catheterization after introduction of the catheter at a distant site. SYN cerebral arteriography.

coronary a., imaging of the circulation of the myocardium by injection of contrast medium, usually by selective catheterization of each coronary artery, formerly by injection at the root of the aorta.

digital subtraction a. (DSA), computer-assisted roentgenographic a. permitting visualization of vascular structures without superimposed bone and soft tissue density; images made before and after contrast injection allow subtraction (separation and removal) of opacities not enhanced by the contrast medium. Other image-processing can be performed. Contrast material may be injected intravenously or in lower-than-usual amount intraarterially.

fluorescein a., photographic visualization of the passage of fluorescein through intraocular vessels after intravenous injection.

interventional a., SYN angioplasty.

magnetic resonance a., SYN MR a.

magnification a., enhanced imaging of small blood vessels using an increased distance from subject to film, as in magnification radiography.

MR a., imaging of blood vessels using special MR sequences which enhance the signal of flowing blood and suppress that from other tissues. SYN magnetic resonance a.

radionuclide a., scintillation camera imaging of tissue perfusion by intravascular injection of a radioactive pharmaceutical. SEE ALSO radionuclide *angiocardiography.* SYN scintigraphic a.

scintigraphic a., SYN radionuclide a.

selective a., a. in which visualization is improved by concentrating the contrast medium in the region to be studied by injection through a catheter positioned in a regional artery.

therapeutic a., use of angiographic catheters that have been modified to reduce or increase regional blood flow, or to deliver medicinal agents; interventional a. SEE angioplasty, balloon *catheter,* interventional a.

an·gi·o·hy·a·li·no·sis (an'jē-ō-hī'ă-li-nō'sis). Hyaline degeneration of the walls of the blood vessels. [angio- + G. *hyalos,* glass, + *-osis,* condition]

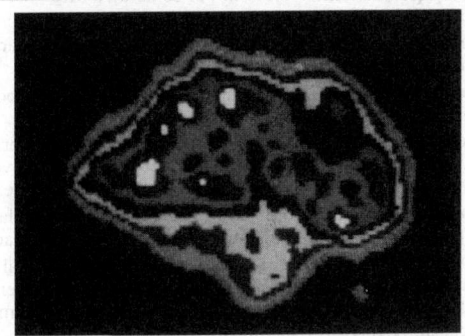

angiogram
in a right lateral projection after an injection of contrast medium into the right internal carotid artery; the large defect in the parietofrontal area is due to a large angioma

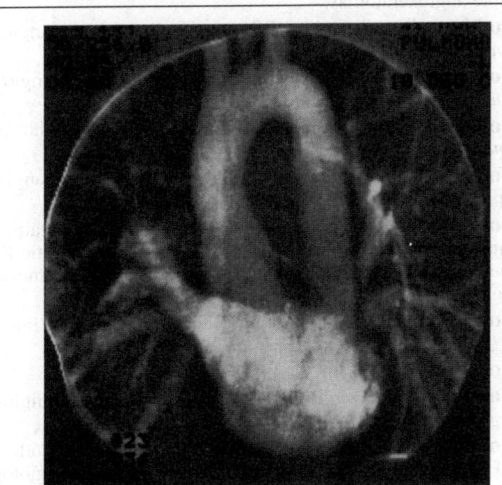

digital subtraction angiography of the heart

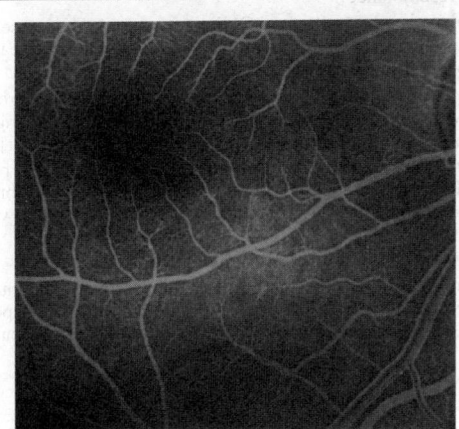

fluorescein angiography
fluorescein angiogram (early venous phase; the filling of the retinal capillary system is apparent)

an

an·gi·o·hy·per·to·nia (an′jē-ō-hī-per-tō′nē-ă). SYN vasospasm. [angio- + G. *hyper*, over, + *tonos*, tension]

an·gi·o·hy·po·to·nia (an′jē-ō-hī-pō-tō′nē-ă). SYN vasoparalysis. [angio- + G. *hypo*, under, + *tonos*, tension]

an·gi·oid (an′jē-oyd). Resembling blood vessels; an arborizing pattern. [angio- + G. *eidos*, resemblance]
a. streaks, breaks in Bruch's membrane visible in the peripapillary fundus oculi, and sometimes mistaken for choroidal vessels. SYN elastosis dystrophica, Knapp's streaks, Knapp's striae.

an·gi·o·in·va·sive (an′jē-ō-in-vā′siv). Denoting a neoplasm or other pathologic condition capable of entering the vascular bed.

an·gi·o·ker·a·to·ma (an′jē-ō-ker-ă-tō′mă). A superficial intradermal capillary acquired telangiectasis, over which there is a wartlike hyperkeratosis and acanthosis. SYN keratoangioma, telangiectasia verrucosa, telangiectatic wart. [angio- + G. *keras*, horn, + *-ōma*, tumor]
diffuse a., SYN Fabry's *disease*.
Fordyce's a., asymptomatic vascular papules of the scrotum, appearing in young adults; much less common in the vulva.
Mibelli's a.'s, telangiectatic small papules of the extremities, common in adolescent girls.

an·gi·o·ker·a·to·sis (an′jē-ō-ker-ă-tō′sis). The occurrence of multiple angiokeratomas.

an·gi·o·ki·ne·sis (an′jē-ō-ki-nē′sis). SYN vasomotion. [angio- + G. *kinēsis*, movement]

an·gi·o·ki·net·ic (an′jē-ō-ki-net′ik). SYN vasomotor. [angio- + G. *kinētikos*, pertaining to movement]

an·gi·o·lei·o·my·o·ma (an′jē-ō-lī′ō-mī-ō′mă). SYN vascular *leiomyoma*.

an·gi·o·lip·o·fi·bro·ma (an′jē-ō-lip′ō-fī-brō′mă). SYN angiofibrolipoma.

an·gi·o·li·po·ma (an′jē-ō-li-pō′mă). A lipoma that contains an unusually large number, or foci of proliferated, neoplastic-like, frequently dilated vascular channels. SYN lipoma cavernosum, telangiectatic lipoma.

an·gi·o·lith (an′jē-ō-lith). An arteriolith or a phlebolith. [angio- + G. *lithos*, stone]

an·gi·o·lith·ic (an′jē-ō-lith′ik). Relating to an angiolith.

an·gi·o·lo·gia (an′jē-ō-lō′jē-ă) [NA]. SYN angiology. [angio- + G. *logos*, treatise, discourse]

an·gi·ol·o·gy (an-jē-ol′ō-jē). The science concerned with the blood vessels and lymphatics in all their relations. SYN angiologia [NA]. [angio- + G. *logos*, treatise, discourse]

an·gi·o·lu·poid (an′jē-ō-lū′poyd). A sarcoid-like eruption of the skin in which the granulomatous telangiectatic papules are distributed over the nose and cheeks. [angio- + L. *lupus*, wolf, + G. *eidos*, resemblance]

an·gi·ol·y·sis (an-jē-ol′i-sis). Obliteration of a blood vessel, such as occurs in the newborn infant after tying of the umbilical cord. [angio- + G. *lysis*, destruction]

an·gi·o·ma (an-jē-ō′mă). A swelling or tumor due to proliferation, with or without dilation, of the blood vessels (hemangioma) or lymphatics (lymphangioma). [angio- + G. *-ōma*, tumor]
acquired tufted a., enlarging erythematous macules and plaques in children and adults, composed microscopically of lobules of capillaries and spindle cells that project into thin-walled venular dermal clefts.
capillary a., SYN capillary *hemangioma*.
cavernous a., vascular malformation composed of sinusoidal vessels without a large feeding artery; can be multiple, especially if inherited as an autosomal dominant trait. SYN nevus cavernosus.
cherry a., SYN senile *hemangioma*.
a. lymphat′icum, SYN lymphangioma.
petechial a.'s, multiple lesions resembling petechiae but due to dilation of capillary walls; they are obliterated by pressure.
a. serpigino′sum, the presence of rings of red dots on the skin, especially in female children, which tend to widen peripherally, due to dilatation of superficial capillaries. SYN essential telangiectasia (2), primary telangiectasia.
spider a., a telangiectatic arteriole in the skin with radiating

capillary branches simulating the legs of a a.; characteristic, but not pathognomonic of, parenchymatous liver disease; also seen in pregnancy, often disappearing after delivery, and at times in normal persons. SYN arterial spider, nevus arachnoideus, nevus araneus, spider hemangioma, spider mole, spider nevus, spider telangiectasia, spider (2), vascular spider.
superficial a., SYN capillary *hemangioma*.
telangiectatic a., a. composed of dilated vessels.
a. veno′sum racemo′sum, tortuous swelling caused by varicosities of superficial veins.
venous a., vascular anomaly composed of anomalous veins.

an·gi·o·ma·toid (an-jē-ō′mă-toyd). Resembling a tumor of vascular origin.

an·gi·o·ma·to·sis (an′jē-ō-mă-tō′sis). A condition characterized by multiple angiomas.
bacillary a., an infection of immunocompromised patients by a newly recognized Rickettsial species *Rochalimaea henselae*, characterized by fever and granulomatous cutaneous nodules, and peliosis hepatis in some cases. Skin biopsy shows vascular proliferation and infiltration of vessel walls by neutrophils and clumps of organisms seen with Warthin-Starry silver staining.
cephalotrigeminal a., SYN Sturge-Weber *syndrome*.
cerebroretinal a., SYN von Hippel-Lindau *syndrome*.
congenital dysplastic a. [MIM*185300 & MIM149000], autosomal dominant a. in which there is dysplasia of the underlying tissues, sometimes with overgrowth of bone (Klippel-Trenaunay-Weber syndrome), or encephalotrigeminal a. (Sturge-Weber syndrome) in which there is an angioma in the distribution of one or more branches of the trigeminal nerve, with vascular anomalies and calcification of the cerebral cortex.
cutaneomeningospinal a., SYN Cobb *syndrome*.
encephalotrigeminal a., SYN Sturge-Weber *syndrome*.
oculoencephalic a. [MIM*185300], an incomplete autosomal dominant form of Sturge-Weber syndrome, consisting of angiomas of the choroid and meninges only.
telangiectatic a., disseminated capillary and venous vascular malformations of the cerebral hemispheres and leptomeninges, occurring in Sturge-Weber syndrome.

an·gi·o·ma·tous (an-jē-ō′mă-tŭs). Relating to or resembling an angioma.

an·gi·o·meg·a·ly (an′jē-ō-meg′ă-lē). Enlargement of blood vessels or lymphatics. [angio- + G. *megas*, large]

an·gi·o·my·o·car·di·ac (an′jē-ō-mī′ō-kar′dē-ak). Relating to the blood vessels and the cardiac muscle. [angio- + G. *mys*, muscle, + *kardia*, heart]

an·gi·o·my·o·fi·bro·ma (an′jē-ō-mī′ō-fī-brō′mă). SYN vascular *leiomyoma*.

an·gi·o·my·o·li·po·ma (an′jē-ō-mī′ō-li-pō′mă). A benign neoplasm of adipose tissue (lipoma) in which muscle cells and vascular structures are fairly conspicuous; most commonly a renal tumor containing smooth muscle, often associated with tuberous sclerosis. [angio- + G. *mys*, muscle, + *lipos*, fat, + *-oma*, tumor]

an·gi·o·my·o·ma (an′jē-ō-mī-ō′mă). SYN vascular *leiomyoma*. [angio- + G. *mys*, muscle, + *-ōma*, tumor]

an·gi·o·my·o·neu·ro·ma (an′jē-ō-mī′ō-nū-rō′mă). Obsolete term for glomus *tumor*.

an·gi·o·my·op·a·thy (an′jē-ō-mī-op′ă-thē). Any disease of blood vessels involving the muscular layer. [angio- + G. *mys*, muscle, + *pathos*, suffering]

an·gi·o·my·o·sar·co·ma (an′jē-ō-mī′ō-sar-kō′mă). A myosarcoma that has an unusually large number of proliferated, frequently dilated, vascular channels.

an·gi·o·myx·o·ma (an′jē-ō-miks-ō′mă). A myxoma in which there is an unusually large number of vascular structures.

an·gi·o·neu·rec·to·my (an′jē-ō-nū-rek′tō-mē). **1.** Excision of the vessels and nerves of a part. [angio- + G. *neuron*, nerve, + *ektomē*, excision] **2.** Excision of a segment of the spermatic cord to produce sterility. [G. *neuron*, cord] [angio- + G. *neuron*, nerve, + *ektomē*, excision]

an·gi·o·neur·e·de·ma (an′jē-ō-nūr-ĕ-dē′mă). Obsolete term for angioneurotic *edema.* [angio- + G. *neuron,* nerve, + *oidēma,* a swelling]

an·gi·o·neu·ro·my·o·ma (an'jē-ō-nū'rō-mī-ō'mă). Obsolete term for glomus *tumor.*

an·gi·o·neu·rop·a·thy (an'jē-ō-nū-rop'ă- thē). A vascular disorder attributed to an abnormality of the autonomic nervous system fibers supplying the blood vessels (*i.e.,* the vasomotor system.

an·gi·o·neu·ro·ses (an'jē-ō-nū-rō'- sēz). A collective term for a number of conditions and symptoms, including Raynaud's disease, erythromelalgia, causalgia, and acroparesthesia, attributed to vasomotor system dysfunction. An obsolete concept.

an·gi·o·neu·ro·sis (an'jē-ō-nū-rō'sis). SYN vasomotor *neurosis.*

an·gi·o·neu·rot·ic (an'jē-ō-nū-rot'ik). Relating to angioneuroses.

an·gi·o·neu·rot·o·my (an'jē-ō-nū-rot'ō-mē). Division of both nerves and vessels of a part. [angio- + G. *neuron,* nerve, + *tomē,* a cutting]

an·gi·o·pa·ral·y·sis (an'jē-ō-pă-ral'i-sis). SYN vasoparalysis.

an·gi·o·pa·re·sis (an'jē-ō-pă-rē'sis, -par'ĕ-sis). SYN vasoparesis.

an·gi·o·path·ic (an'jē-ō-path'ik). Relating to angiopathy.

an·gi·op·a·thy (an-jē-op'ă-thē). Any disease of the blood vessels or lymphatics. SYN angiosis. [angio- + G. *pathos,* suffering]

amyloid a., deposition of acellular hyaline material in small arteries and arterioles of the leptomeninges and cerebral cortex in the elderly with resulting predilection for recurrent lobar intraparenchymal hematomas.

cerebral amyloid a., a pathological condition of small cerebral vessels characterized by deposits of amyloid in the vessel walls, which may lead to infarcts or hemorrhage; may also occur in Alzheimer's disease. SEE ALSO congophilic a.

congophilic a., a condition of blood vessels characterized by deposits in the vessel walls of a substance, usually amyloid, that take a Congo red stain. SEE ALSO cerebral amyloid a.

giant cell hyaline a., an inflammatory infiltrate containing foreign body giant cells and eosinophilic material. Fragments of foreign material resembling vegetable matter may be included. SYN pulse granuloma.

hypertensive a., a condition of turkeys of unknown etiology, associated with sudden death in rapidly growing male birds.

an·gi·o·phac·o·ma·to·sis, an·gi·o·phak·o·ma·to·sis (an'jē-ō-fak'ō-mă-tō'sis). The angiomatous phacomatoses: von Hippel-Lindau's disease and the Sturge-Weber syndrome.

an·gi·o·pla·ny (an'jē-ō-plā-nē). SYN angiectopia. [angio- + G. *planē,* a wandering]

an·gi·o·plas·ty (an'jē-ō-plas-tē). Reconstitution or recanalization of a blood vessel; may involve balloon dilation, mechanical stripping of intima, forceful injection of fibrinolytics, or placement of a stent. SYN interventional angiography. [angio- + G. *plastos,* formed, shaped]

percutaneous transluminal a. (PTA), an operation for enlarging a narrowed vascular lumen by inflating and withdrawing through the stenotic region a balloon on the tip of an angiographic catheter; may include positioning of an intravascular stent.

percutaneous transluminal coronary a. (PTCA), percutaneous transluminal a. of coronary artery or arteries.

an·gi·o·poi·e·sis (an'jē-ō-poy-ē'sis). Formation of blood or lymphatic vessels. SYN vasifaction, vasoformation. [angio- + G. *poiesis,* making]

an·gi·o·poi·et·ic (an'jē-ō-poy-et'ik). Relating to angiopoiesis. SYN vasifactive, vasofactive, vasoformative.

an·gi·or·rha·phy (an-jē-ōr'ă-fē). Suture repair of any vessel, especially of a blood vessel. [angio- + G. *rhaphē,* a seam]

an·gi·or·rhex·is (an'jē-ō-rek'sis). Obsolete term for rupture of any vessel, especially of a blood vessel. [angio- + G. *rhēxis,* rupture]

an·gi·o·sar·co·ma (an'jē-ō-sar-kō'mă). A rare malignant neoplasm occurring most often in the breast and skin, and believed to originate from the endothelial cells of blood vessels; microscopically composed of closely packed round or spindle-shaped cells, some of which line small spaces resembling vascular clefts.

an·gi·o·scope (an'jē-ō-skōp). A modified microscope for study-

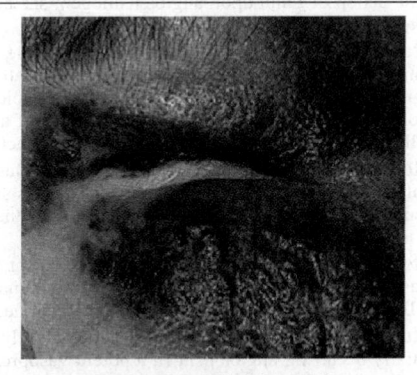

angiosarcoma (of the skin)

ing the capillary vessels and a scope used for viewing larger vessels. [angio- + G. *skopeō,* to view]

an·gi·os·co·py (an-jē-os'kō-pē). **1.** Visualization with a microscope of the passage of substances (*e.g.,* contrast media, radiopaque agents) through capillaries after intravenous injection. **2.** Visualization of the interior of blood vessels, especially the pulmonary arteries, using a fiberoptic catheter inserted through a peripheral artery. [angio- + G. *skopeō,* to view]

an·gi·o·sco·to·ma (an'jē-ō-skō-tō'mă). Ribbon-shaped defect of the visual fields caused by the retinal vessels overlying photoreceptors. [angio- + G. *skotōma,* dizziness, vertigo]

an·gi·o·sco·tom·e·try (an'jē-ō-skō-tom'ĕ-trē). The measurement or projection of the angioscotoma pattern.

an·gi·o·sis (an-jē-ō'sis). SYN angiopathy.

an·gi·o·spasm (an'jē-ō-spazm). SYN vasospasm.

labyrinthine a., SYN Lermoyez' *syndrome.*

an·gi·o·spas·tic (an'jē-ō-spas'tik). SYN vasospastic.

an·gi·o·ste·no·sis (an'jē-ō-stĕ-nō'sis). Narrowing of one or more blood vessels. [angio- + G. *stenōsis,* a narrowing]

an·gi·o·stron·gy·lo·sis (an'jē-ō-stron-ji-lō'sis). Infection of animals and man with nematodes of the genus *Angiostrongylus.* SYN eosinophilic meningitis.

An·gi·o·stron·gy·lus (an'jē-ō-stron'jĭ-lŭs). A genus of metastrongyle nematodes parasitic in respiratory or circulatory systems of rodents, carnivores, and marsupials. SYN *Parastrongylus.* [G. *angeion,* vessel, + *strongylos,* round]

A. cantonen'sis, lungworm of rodents, a species transmitted by infected mollusks ingested by rodents; larvae develop in the brain and migrate to lungs, where the adult worms are found; thought to cause eosinophilic encephalomeningitis in man in the Pacific basin; larvae have been removed from cerebrospinal fluid and the anterior chamber of the eye from persons in Thailand who had eaten raw snails.

A. costaricen'sis, a nematode parasite of rats and other rodents in Central America, recently found to infect humans, where they localize in the mesenteric arteries; infective third-stage larvae have been found in the slug, *Vaginulus plebeius.* SYN *Morerastrongylus costaricensis.*

A. malaysien'sis, species of *A.* found in Malaysia, a common rodent parasite similar to *A. cantonensis* and an actual or potential agent of eosinophilic meningitis in that region.

A. vaso'rum, a species occurring in the pulmonary artery and, rarely, in the right ventricle of the dog and fox; thrombi may occur in the lungs, and hypertrophy of the heart and liver may result in ascites; affected animals suffer from dyspnea and occasionally may die from cardiac insufficiency. SYN *Haemostrongylus vasorum.*

an·gi·o·te·lec·ta·sis, an·gi·o·tel·ec·ta·sia (an'jē-ō-tĕ-lek'tă-sis, -tel'ek-tā'sē-ă). Rarely used term for dilation of the terminal arterioles, venules, or capillaries. [angio- + G. *telos,* end, + *ektasis,* a stretching out]

an·gi·o·ten·sin (an-jē-ō-ten'sin). A family of peptides of known and similar sequence, with vasoconstrictive activity, produced by enzymatic action of renin upon angiotensinogen. SEE angiotensin I, angiotensin II, angiotensin III.

an·gi·o·ten·sin I. A decapeptide of slightly variable sequence, depending on the animal source, formed from the tetradecapeptide angiotensinogen by the removal of four amino acid residues, a reaction catalyzed by renin; a peptidase cleaves off a dipeptide (histidylleucine) to yield a. I II, the physiologically active form.

an·gi·o·ten·sin II. A vasoactive peptide that is produced by the action of a. II converting enzyme on a. II I; produces stimulation of vascular smooth muscle and stimulates sympathetic nerve centers in the brain.

an·gi·o·ten·sin III. A vasoactive protein less potent than a. III II on vascular smooth muscle but approximately equally potent with a. III II in promoting the secretion of aldosterone.

an·gi·o·ten·sin am·ide. A synthetic substance closely related to the naturally occurring angiotensin II; a potent vasopressor agent useful in the management of certain types of shock and circulatory collapse.

an·gi·o·ten·sin·ase (an-jē-ō-ten'sin-ās). Former name for the enzyme responsible for converting angiotensin I to II; now applied to the enzyme that degrades angiotensin II. It hydrolyses a peptide bond between a tyrosyl and an isoleucyl residue.

an·gi·o·ten·sin·o·gen (an'jē-ō-ten-sin'ō-jen). The substrate for renin whereupon through enzymatic action angiotensin I is liberated; an abundant α_2-globulin that circulates in the blood plasma. The precursor of angiotensin I. SYN angiotensin precursor.

an·gi·o·ten·sin·o·gen·ase (an'jē-ō-ten-sin'ō-jen-ās). SYN renin.

an·gi·o·ten·sin pre·cur·sor. SYN angiotensinogen.

an·gi·ot·o·my (an-jē-ot'ō-mē). Sectioning of a blood vessel, or the creation of an opening into a vessel prior to its repair. [angio- + G. *tomē*, cutting]

an·gi·o·to·nia (an'jē-ō-tō'nē-ă). SYN vasotonia.

an·gi·o·ton·ic (an'jē-ō-ton'ik). SYN vasotonic (1).

an·gi·o·to·nin (an'jē-ō-tō-nin). Former name for angiotensin.

an·gi·o·tro·phic (an'jē-ō-trof'ik). Rarely used term for vasotrophic. [angio- + G. *trophē*, nourishment]

Angle, Edward Hartley, U.S. orthodontist, 1855–1930. SEE A.'s *classification* of malocclusion.

ANGLE

an·gle (ang'gl). The meeting point of two lines or planes; the figure formed by the junction of two lines or planes; the space bounded on two sides by lines or planes that meet. For a.'s not listed below, see the descriptive term; *e.g.,* axioincisal, distobuccal, labiogingival, linguogingival (2), mesiogingival, proximobuccal, etc. SYN angulus [NA]. [L. *angulus*]

acromial a., the prominent angle at the junction of the posterior and lateral borders of the acromion. SYN angulus acromialis [NA].

acute a., any a. less than 90°.

adjacent a., an a. with a line in common with another a.

alpha a., (1) the a. between the visual and optic axes as they cross at the nodal point of the eye; (2) the a. between the visual line and the major axis of the corneal ellipse.

alveolar a., the a. between the horizontal plane and a line connecting the base of the nasal spine and the middle point of the projection of the alveolus of the maxilla.

a. of anomaly, an obsolete term for the degree of deviation from parallelism of the visual axes of the eyes.

anorectal a., (1) the a. formed by the junction of the rectum with the anus; may be important in maintenance of continence. (2) SYN perineal *flexure* of rectum.

a. of antetorsion, SYN a. of anteversion.

a. of anteversion, the a. formed by a line drawn through the center of the long axis of the neck of the femur meeting a line drawn in the transverse axis of the condyles, when the bone is viewed from above, looking straight down through the head of the femur; used to illustrate the normal degree of anteversion about 12° of the neck of the femur, which may be increased or decreased in some diseases. SYN a. of antetorsion.

a. of aperture, the a. formed by lines drawn from the ends of the diameter of a lens to its point of focus. SEE ALSO angular *aperture*.

apical a., the a. between two plane surfaces of a prism. SYN refracting a. of a prism.

axial a., an a. formed by two surfaces of a body, the line of union of which is parallel with its axis; the axial a.'s of a tooth are the distobuccal, distolabial, distolingual, mesiobuccal, mesiolabial, and mesiolingual.

basilar a., an a. formed by the intersection at the basion of lines coming from the nasal spine and the nasal point.

Bennett a., the a. formed by the sagittal plane and the path of the advancing condyle during lateral mandibular movement as viewed in the horizontal plane.

beta a., the a. formed by a line connecting the bregma and hormion meeting the radius fixus.

biorbital a., an a. formed by the meeting of the axes of the orbits.

Broca's a.'s, (1) SYN Broca's basilar a. **(2)** SYN Broca's facial a. **(3)** SYN occipital a. of parietal bone (1).

Broca's basilar a., the a. formed at the basion of lines drawn from the nasion and the alveolar point. SYN Broca's a.'s (1).

Broca's facial a., the a. formed by the intersection at the biauricular axis of lines drawn from the supraorbital point and the alveolar point. SYN Broca's a.'s (2).

buccal a.'s, a.'s formed by the buccal surface of a tooth joining the other surfaces.

bucco-occlusal a., the line of junction of the buccal and occlusal surfaces of a tooth.

cardiodiaphragmatic a., SYN cardiophrenic a.

cardiohepatic a., the a. formed by the upper border of the liver and the right border of the heart, especially as defined by percussion. SYN cardiohepatic triangle.

cardiophrenic a., the a. between the heart and the diaphragm at either lateral end of the cardiac projection on imaging (usually the chest x-ray film). The right cardiophrenic a. is normally indistinguishable from the cardiohepatic a. radiographically. SYN cardiodiaphragmatic a., phrenopericardial a.

carrying a., the a. made by the axes of the arm and the forearm, with the elbow in full extension.

cavity line a., in dentistry, the a. formed by two walls of a cavity, *e.g.,* a tooth cavity, meeting along a line.

cavosurface a., the a. formed by the junction of a cavity wall and the surface of the tooth.

cephalic a., one of several a.'s formed by the intersection of two lines passing through certain points of the face or cranium.

cephalomedullary a., the a. made by the junction of the cerebrum and the brain stem.

cerebellopontile a., SYN cerebellopontine a.

cerebellopontine a., the recess at the junction of the cerebellum, pons, and medulla. SYN cerebellopontile a., pontine a.

costal a., the rather abrupt change in curvature of the body of a rib posteriorly, such that the neck and head of the rib are directed upward. SYN angulus costae [NA].

costophrenic a., costophrenic sulcus as seen on chest radiograph.

craniofacial a., the a. formed by the basifacial and basicranial axes at the midpoint of the sphenoethmoidal suture.

critical a., the a. of incidence at which a ray of light, in passing between two media, changes from refraction to total reflection. SYN limiting a.

cusp a., (1) the a. made by the slopes of a cusp with the plane which passes through the tip of the cusp and which is perpendicular to a line bisecting the cusp, measured mesiodistally or buccolingually; (2) the a. made by the slopes of a cusp with a perpendicular line bisecting the cusp, measured mesiodistally or buccolingually; (3) one-half of the included a. between the buccal and lingual or mesial and distal cusp inclines.

Daubenton's a., an a. formed by the junction, at the opisthion, of lines coming from the basion and from the projection in the median plane of the lower border of the orbits. SEE ALSO Daubenton's *line*, Daubenton's *plane*. SYN angulus occipitalis ossis parietalis [NA], occipital a. of parietal bone (2).

a. of declination, obsolete term for a. of anteversion.

a. of depression, SYN a. of inclination.

a. of deviation, (1) in a prism, the sum of the a.'s of incidence and emergence minus the apical a. of a prism; **(2)** in optics, a. of refraction; **(3)** in strabismus, a. of anomaly.

disparity a., the difference in position of images on the retina, still permitting fusion.

duodenojejunal a., SYN duodenojejunal *flexure*.

a. of eccentricity, in strabismus, the a. between the line of fixation and the line of normal foveal fixation.

a. of emergence, the a. formed by a light ray emerging from the second surface of a prism and a line parallel to the incident ray. Cf. a. of deviation.

epigastric a., the a. formed by the xiphoid process with the body of the sternum.

ethmoid a., the a. made by the plane of the cribriform plate of the ethmoid bone extended to meet the basicranial axis.

facial a., (1) any of several variously named and variously defined anatomical a.'s that have been used to quantify facial protrusion; **(2)** in dentistry, the a. formed by the intersection of the orbitomeatal (Frankfort) plane with the nasion-pogonion line (inner lower a.), which establishes the anteroposterior relation of the mandible to the upper face at the orbitomeatal plane. SYN Frankfort-mandibular incisor a.

a. of femoral torsion, SYN a. of femoral torsion. SYN a. of femoral torsion.

filtration a., SYN iridocorneal a.

flip a., in a magnetic resonance imaging sequence, the rotation of the average axis of the protons induced by radiofrequency signals; low angles are used in rapid-imaging sequences and to show a signal from flowing blood.

Frankfort-mandibular incisor a., SYN facial a. (2).

frontal a. of parietal bone, the anterior superior angle of the parietal bone. SYN angulus frontalis ossis parietalis [NA].

a. of Fuchs, a crevice between the ciliary and pupillary zones of the iris formed by atrophy of superficial layers of the iris in the pupillary zone.

gamma a., the a. formed between a line joining the fixation point to the center of the eye and the optic axis.

hypsiloid a., SYN y-a.

impedance a., a term expressing the ratio of electric resistance to electric capacitance (ohms to microfarads) in the tissues of the body or any other substance.

a. of incidence, (1) the a. that a ray entering a refracting medium makes with a line drawn perpendicular to the surface of this medium; **(2)** the a. that a ray striking a reflecting surface makes with a line perpendicular to this surface. SYN incident a.

incident a., SYN a. of incidence.

incisal guide a., the a. formed with the horizontal plane by drawing a line in the sagittal plane between incisal edges of the maxillary and mandibular central incisors when the teeth are in centric occlusion.

a. of inclination, the a. formed by the meeting of a line drawn through the shaft of the femur with one passing through the long axis of the femoral neck; normally it is about 127°. SYN a. of depression, neck-shaft a.

inferior a. of scapula, the acute angle formed by junction of the medial and lateral borders of the scapula. SYN angulus inferior scapulae [NA].

infrasternal a., the angle between the lower borders of the costal cartilages of the two sides as they approach the sternum. SYN angulus infrasternalis [NA], substernal a.

iridocorneal a., the acute angle between the iris and the cornea at the periphery of the anterior chamber of the eye. SYN angulus iridocornealis [NA], a. of iris, angulus iridis, filtration a.

a. of iris, SYN iridocorneal a.

Jacquart's facial a., a facial a. with the intersection always at the nasal spine point; additional variation uses the supraorbital point instead of the glabella, and this latter version is also known as ophryospinal facial a. or Topinard's facial a.

a. of jaw, SYN a. of mandible.

kappa a., the a. between the pupillary axis and the visual axis; it is positive when the pupillary axis is nasal to the visual axis, and negative when the pupillary axis is temporal to the visual axis.

lateral a. of eye, the angle formed by the junction of the lateral parts of the upper and lower eyelids. SYN angulus oculi lateralis [NA], angulus oculi temporalis, external canthus, lateral canthus.

lateral a. of scapula, the blunt, concave head of the scapula forming the glenoid cavity at the junction of the superior and lateral borders of the bone. SYN angulus lateralis scapulae [NA].

lateral a. of uterus, the upper part of the side of the uterus at the point of its junction with the uterine tube.

limiting a., SYN critical a.

line a., in dentistry, the junction of two surfaces of the crown of a tooth, or of a tooth cavity (cavity line a.).

Louis' a., SYN sternal a.

Lovibond's a., the a. made at the meeting of the proximal nail fold and the nail plate when viewed from the radial aspect; normally, less than 180° but exceeding this in clubbing of the fingers. SYN Lovibond's profile sign.

Ludwig's a., SYN sternal a.

lumbosacral a., the angle between the long axis of the lumbar part of the vertebral column and that of the sacrum.

a. of mandible, the angle formed by the lower margin of the body and the posterior margin of the ramus of the mandible. SYN angulus mandibulae [NA], a. of jaw.

mastoid a. of parietal bone, the posteroinferior point of the parietal bone. SYN angulus mastoideus ossis parietalis [NA].

maxillary a., the a. formed by a line drawn from the ophryon and another from the point of the mandible and meeting at the contact between the upper and lower incisor teeth.

medial a. of eye, the angle formed by the union of the upper and lower eyelids medially. SYN angulus oculi medialis [NA], angulus oculi nasalis, internal canthus, medial canthus.

mesial a., the a. formed by the meeting of the mesial with the labial (or buccal) or lingual surface of a tooth.

metafacial a., the a. between the pterygoid processes and the base of the skull. SYN Serres' a.

meter a., the amount of convergence required to view binocularly an object 1 meter distant and exerting 1 diopter of accommodation. SYN unit of ocular convergence.

a. of mouth, the lateral limit of the oral fissure. SEE ALSO labial *commissure*. SYN angulus oris [NA].

neck-shaft a., SYN a. of inclination.

occipital a. of parietal bone, (1) the posterior superior angle of the parietal bone; SYN Broca's a.'s (3). **(2)** SYN Daubenton's a.

olfactory a., the a. formed by the plane of the lamina cribrosa and the basicranial axis.

ophryospinal a., SEE Jacquart's facial a.

parietal a., an a. formed by the meeting of the prolongation of two lines tangential to the most prominent part of the zygomatic arch and to the parietofrontal suture on each side; when the lines remain parallel the a. is zero; when they diverge it is negative. SYN Quatrefages' a.

pelvivertebral a., the a. made by the pelvis as defined by the plane of the superior pelvic aperture with the general axis of the trunk or vertebral column. SEE ALSO *inclination* of pelvis.

phrenopericardial a., SYN cardiophrenic a.

Pirogoff's a., SYN venous a. (1).

point a., the junction of three surfaces of the crown of a tooth, or of the walls of a cavity.

a. of polarization, the a. of incidence at which the reflected light is all polarized.

pontine a., SYN cerebellopontine a.

pubic a., SYN subpubic a.

Q a., the a. formed by lines representing the resultant pull of the quadriceps muscle and the axis of the patellar tendon.

Quatrefages' a., SYN parietal a.

Ranke's a., the a. formed by the horizontal plane of the head and a line passing from the center of the margin of the alveolar arch of the maxilla, below the nasal spine to the center of the fronto-nasal suture. [J. Ranke]

a. of reflection, the a. that a ray reflected from a surface makes with a line drawn perpendicular to this surface; it is equal to the a. of incidence (2).

refracting a. of a prism, SYN apical a.

a. of refraction, the a. that a ray leaving a refracting medium makes with a line drawn perpendicular to the surface of this medium.

Rolando's a., the a. which the fissure of Rolando (central sulcus) makes with the midplane.

Serres' a., SYN metafacial a.

S-N-A a., in cephalometrics, an a. measuring the anteroposterior relationship of the maxillary basal arch on the anterior cranial base; it shows the degree of maxillary prognathism. SEE ALSO subspinale. [sella-nasion-subspinale (or point *A*)]

S-N-B a., an a. showing the anterior limit of the mandibular basal arch in relation to the anterior cranial base. SEE ALSO supramentale. [sella-nasion-supramentale (or point *B*)]

sphenoid a., sphenoidal a., (1) a. formed by the intersection at the top of the sella turcica (dorsum sellae), of lines coming from the nasal point and from the tip of the rostrum of the sphenoid; **(2)** SYN sphenoidal a. of parietal bone.

sphenoidal a. of parietal bone, the anterior inferior angle of the parietal bone. SYN angulus sphenoidalis ossis parietalis [NA], sphenoid a. (2), sphenoidal a., Welcker's a.

sternal a., the angle between the manubrium and the body of the sternum at the manubriosternal junction. Marks the level of the second costal cartilage (rib) for counting ribs or intercostal spaces. Denotes level of aortic arch, bifurcation of trachea, and T4/T5 intervertebral disc. SYN angulus sterni [NA], Louis' a., Ludwig's a., manubriosternal junction.

sternoclavicular a., the a. formed by the junction of the clavicle with the sternum.

subpubic a., the a. formed between the inferior rami of the pubic bones. In the female, the angle approximates that a. between the widely extended thumb and index finger (90°); in the male, it approximates the a. between the widely abducted index and middle fingers (60°). SEE ALSO pubic *arch*. SYN angulus subpubicus [NA], pubic a.

substernal a., SYN infrasternal a.

superior a. of scapula, formerly named the medial angle, it lies at the junction of the superior and medial borders of the bone. SYN angulus superior scapulae [NA].

sylvian a., the a. formed by the sylvian line and a line perpendicular to the horizontal plane tangential to the highest point of the hemisphere.

tentorial a., the a. made by the plane of the tentorium and the basicranial axis.

Topinard's facial a., SEE Jacquart's facial a.

a. of torsion, the amount of rotation of a long bone along its axis or between two axes, measured in degrees.

venous a., (1) the junction of the internal jugular and subclavian veins, toward which converge the external and the anterior jugular and the vertebral veins, the thoracic duct in the left a. and the right lymphatic duct in the right a.; SYN Pirogoff's a. **(2)** in neuroradiology, the a. of union of the superior thalamostriate vein (vena terminalis) with the internal cerebral vein, usually closely behind the interventricular foramen of Monro.

Virchow-Holder a., SYN Virchow's a.

Virchow's a., an a. formed by the meeting of a line drawn from the middle of the nasofrontal suture to the base of the anterior nasal spine with a line drawn from this last point to the center of the external auditory meatus. SYN Virchow-Holder a.

visual a., the a. formed at the retina by the meeting of lines drawn from the periphery of the object seen.

Vogt's a., a craniometric a. formed by the nasobasilar and alveolonasal lines. [K. Vogt]

Weisbach's a., a craniometric a. formed by the junction, at the alveolar point, of lines passing from the basion and from the middle of the frontonasal suture.

Welcker's a., SYN sphenoidal a. of parietal bone.

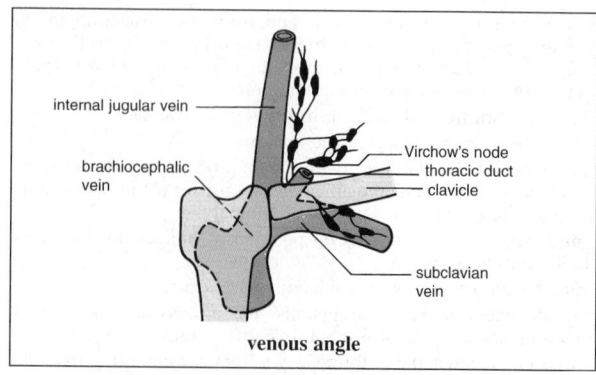

internal jugular vein

brachiocephalic vein

Virchow's node
thoracic duct
clavicle

subclavian vein

venous angle

y-a., in craniometry, the a. at the inion formed by lines drawn from the hormion and the lambda. SYN hypsiloid a.

an·gor (ang'gŏr). Rarely used term for extreme distress or mental anguish. [L. quinsy, anguish]

a. an'imi, the sense of being in the act of dying, differing from the fear of death or the desire for death; a symptom that may occur with angina pectoris and occasionally in diseases of the medulla. SYN a. pectoris (2).

a. pec'toris, (1) SYN Gairdner's *disease.* **(2)** SYN a. animi.

Ångström, Anders J., Swedish physicist, 1814–1874. SEE angstrom; A.'s *law;* A. *unit, scale.*

ang·strom (Å) (ang'strŏm). A unit of wavelength, 10^{-10} m, roughly the diameter of an atom; equivalent to 0.1 nm. [A.J. Ångström]

An·guil·lu·la (ang-gwil'lū-lă). Old name for a genus of free-living nematodes. SEE *Turbatrix.* [Mod. L. dim. of L. *anguilla,* eel]

an·gu·la·tion (ang'gū-lā'shŭn). Formation of an angle; an abnormal angle or bend in an organ.

an·gu·lus, gen. and pl. **an·gu·li** (ang'gyū-lŭs, -lī) [NA]. SYN angle. [L.]

a. acromia'lis [NA], SYN acromial *angle.*

a. cos'tae [NA], SYN costal *angle.*

a. fronta'lis os'sis parieta'lis [NA], SYN frontal *angle* of parietal bone.

a. infe'rior scap'ulae [NA], SYN inferior *angle* of scapula.

a. infrasterna'lis [NA], SYN infrasternal *angle.*

a. ir'idis, SYN iridocorneal *angle.*

a. iridocornea'lis [NA], SYN iridocorneal *angle.*

a. latera'lis scap'ulae [NA], SYN lateral *angle* of scapula.

a. mandib'ulae [NA], SYN *angle* of mandible.

a. mastoid'eus os'sis parieta'lis [NA], SYN mastoid *angle* of parietal bone.

a. occipita'lis os'sis parieta'lis [NA], SYN Daubenton's *angle.*

a. oc'uli latera'lis [NA], SYN lateral *angle* of eye.

a. oc'uli media'lis [NA], SYN medial *angle* of eye.

a. oc'uli nasa'lis, SYN medial *angle* of eye.

a. oc'uli temporalis, SYN lateral *angle* of eye.

a. o'ris [NA], SYN *angle* of mouth.

a. sphenoida'lis os'sis parieta'lis [NA], SYN sphenoidal *angle* of parietal bone.

a. ster'ni [NA], SYN sternal *angle.*

a. subpu'bicus [NA], SYN subpubic *angle.*

a. supe'rior scap'ulae [NA], SYN superior *angle* of scapula.

an·ha·line (an-hă'lin). SYN hordenine.

an·haph·ia (an-haf'ē-ă). SYN anaphia.

an·he·do·nia (an-hē-dō'nē-ă). Absence of pleasure from the performance of acts that would ordinarily be pleasurable. [G. *an*-priv. + *hedonē,* pleasure]

an·hi·dro·sis (an-hǐ-drō'sis). Inability to tolerate heat; absence of sweat glands. SYN adiaphoresis, anidrosis. [G. *an-* priv. + *hidrōs,* sweat]

an·hi·drot·ic (an-hī-drot'ik). **1.** Relating to, or characterized by, anhidrosis. **2.** SYN antiperspirant (2). **3.** Denoting a reduction or absence of sweat glands, characteristic of congenital ectodermal defect and anhidrotic ectodermal dysplasia. SYN adiaphoretic, anidrotic.

an·his·tic, an·his·tous (an-his'tik, -tŭs). Without apparent structure. [G. *an-* priv. + *histos,* web]

an·hy·drase (an-hī'drās). An enzyme that catalyzes the removal of water from a compound; most such enzymes are now known as hydrases, hydro-lyases, or dehydratases.

carbonic a., a zinc-containing enzyme that catalyzes the interconversion of CO_2 with HCO_3^- and H^+. There are at least seven human isozymes that appear predominantly in red blood cells, secretory tissues, muscle, etc. A deficiency of a. II can result in osteopetrosis and metabolic acidosis. The inhibition of a. IV and possibly a. II by sulfonamides is a current therapy in the treatment of glaucoma. SYN carbonate dehydratase, carbonate hydrolyase.

an·hy·dra·tion (an-hī-drā'shŭn). SYN dehydration (1).

an·hy·dride (an-hī'drīd). An oxide that can combine with water to form an acid or that is derived from an acid by the abstraction of water.

△**anhydro-.** Chemical prefix denoting the removal of water. Cf. pyro- (2). [G. *an-* priv., + *hydōr,* water]

3,6-an·hy·dro·ga·lac·tose (an-hī'drō-gă-lak'tōs). A galactose derivative found in a number of polysaccharides (*e.g.,* agarose).

an·hy·dro·gi·tal·in (an-hī'drō-jit'ă-lin). SYN gitoxin.

an·hy·dro·leu·cov·o·rin (an-hī'drō-lū-kō-vōr'in). An intermediate formed in the folic acid-catalyzed glycine-serine interconversion. SYN N^5,N^{10}-methenyltetrahydrofolic acid.

an·hy·dro·sug·ars (an-hī'drō-shug-ărz). Sugars from which one or more molecules of water, other than water of crystallization, have been eliminated. SYN dehydrosugars.

an·hy·drous (an-hī'drŭs). Containing no water, especially water of crystallization.

a·ni·a·cin·am·i·do·sis (ă-nī'ă-sin-am-i-dō'sis). Rarely used term for deficiency of niacinamide which may be associated with pellagra. [G. *a-* priv. + niacinamide + *-osis,* condition]

a·ni·a·cin·o·sis (ă-nī'ă-sin-ō'sis). Rarely used term for aniacinamidosis. [G> *a-* oruv. + niacin + *-osis* condition]

an·ic·ter·ic (an-ik-ter'ik). Not icteric.

an·id·e·an (an-id'ē-an). Shapeless; denoting a formless mass of tissue. SYN anidous. [see anideus]

an·id·e·us (an-id'ē-ŭs). A parasitic fetus consisting of a poorly differentiated mass of tissue with slight indications of parts. SEE ALSO *holoacardius* amorphus. [G. *an-* priv. + *eidos,* shape]

embryonic a., a blastoderm without axial organization.

an·i·dous (an-ī'dŭs). SYN anidean.

an·i·dro·sis (an-i-drō'sis). SYN anhidrosis.

an·i·drot·ic (an-i-drot'ik). SYN anhidrotic.

an·ile (ā'nīl, an'il). Obsolete term for senile or demented. [L. *anilis,* fr. *anus,* an old woman]

an·i·ler·i·dine (an-i-ler'i-dēn). Ethyl 1-(4-aminophenethyl)-4-phenylisonipecotate; related chemically and pharmacologically to meperidine hydrochloride; used for relief of moderate to severe pain; also mildly antihistaminic and spasmolytic; addiction liability is equivalent to that of morphine.

an·i·lide (an'i-lid). An *N*-acyl aniline; *e.g.,* acetanilide.

ani·linc·tion, ani·linc·tus (ā-ni-lingk'shŭn, -lingk'tŭs). SYN anilingus.

an·i·line (an'i-lin, -lēn). $C_6H_5(NH_2)$; an oily, colorless or brownish liquid, of aromatic odor and acrid taste, that is the parent substance of many synthetic dyes; formally derived from benzene by the substitution of the group —NH_2 for one of the hydrogen atoms. Aniline is highly toxic and may cause industrial poisoning. SYN aminobenzene, benzeneamine, phenylamine. [Ar. *an-nil,* indigo]

an·i·line blue [C.I. 42755]. A mixture of sulfonated triphenyl-

methane dyes used widely as a connective tissue stain and counterstain.

ani·lin·gus (ā-ni-ling'gŭs). Sexual stimulation by licking or kissing the anus; a type of oral-genital sexual activity. SYN anilinction, anilinctus. [L. *anus,* + *lingo,* to lick]

an·i·lin·ism (an'i-lin-izm). SYN anilism.

an·i·li·no·phil, an·i·li·no·phile (an-i-lin'ō-fil, -fīl). Denoting a cell or histologic structure that stains readily with an aniline dye. SYN anilinophilous. [aniline + G. *philos,* fond]

an·i·li·noph·i·lous (an-i-li-nof'ĭ-lŭs). SYN anilinophil.

an·il·ism (an'i-lizm). Chronic aniline poisoning characterized by gastric and cardiac weakness, vertigo, muscular depression, intermittent pulse, and cyanosis. SYN anilinism.

anil·i·ty (ă-nil'i-tē). SYN senility. [L. *anilitas,* fr. *anus,* an old woman]

an·i·ma (an'i-mă). **1.** The soul or spirit. SEE animus (4). **2.** In jungian psychology, the inner self, in contrast to persona; a female archtype in a man. Cf. animus (5). [L. breath, soul]

an·i·mal (an'i-măl). **1.** A living, sentient organism that has membranous cell walls, requires oxygen and organic foods, and is capable of voluntary movement, as distinguished from a plant or mineral. **2.** One of the lower a. organisms as distinguished from humans. [L.]

cold-blooded a., SYN poikilotherm.

control a., in research, an a. submitted to the same conditions as the others used for the experiment, but with the crucial factor (such as the injection of antitoxin, the administration of a drug, etc.) omitted. SEE ALSO control, control *experiment.*

conventional a., an a. colonized by the burden of resident microorganisms normally associated with its particular species.

Houssay a., an a. that has been pancreatectomized and hypophysectomized. Named after the discoverer of the principle that a.'s are more sensitive to insulin after removal of the pituitary, and that after this operation the intensity of diabetes in depancreatized a.'s is diminished.

normal a., in research, an experimental a. that has neither suffered an attack of a particular disease nor received an injection of a specific microorganism or its toxin.

sentinel a., an a. deliberately placed in a particular environment to detect the presence of an infectious agent, such as a virus.

warm-blooded a., SYN homeotherm.

an·i·mal black. SYN animal *charcoal.*

an·i·mal·cule (an-i-mal'kyūl). Term used by believers in the preformation theory to designate the supposed miniature body contained in a gamete. SEE homunculus. [Mod. L. *animalculum,* dim. of L. *animal,* a living being]

an·i·ma·tion (an-i-mā'shŭn). **1.** The state of being alive. **2.** Liveliness; high spirits. [L. *animo,* pp. *-atus,* to make alive; *anima,* breath, soul]

suspended a., a temporary state resembling death, with cessation of respiration; may also refer to certain forms of hibernation in animals or to endospore formation by some bacteria.

an·i·mat·ism (an'i-mă-tizm). Attribution of mental or spiritual qualities to both living beings and nonliving things. SEE ALSO animism.

an·i·mism (an'i-mizm). The view that all things in nature, both animate and inanimate, contain a spirit or soul; held by primitive peoples and young children. SEE ALSO animatism. [L. *anima,* soul]

an·i·mus (an'i-mŭs). **1.** An animating or energizing spirit. **2.** Intention to do something; disposition. **3.** In psychiatry, a spirit of active hostility or grudge. **4.** The ideal image toward which a person strives. **5.** In jungian psychology, a male archetype in a woman. Cf. anima (2). [L. *animus,* breath, rational soul in man, will]

an·i·on (A$^-$) (an'ī-on). An ion that carries a negative charge, going therefore to the positively charged anode; in salts, acid radicals are a.'s.

an·i·on ex·change. The process by which an anion in a mobile (liquid) phase exchanges with another anion previously bound to a solid, positively charged phase, the latter being an anion exchanger. It takes place when Cl$^-$ is exchanged for OH$^-$ in desalting. The reaction is Cl⁻ (in solution) + (OH⁻ on anion exchanger⁺) → (Cl⁻ on anion exchanger) + OH⁻ (in solution); combined with cation exchange, NaCl is removed from solution. Anion exchange may also be used chromatographically, to separate anions, and medicinally, to remove an anion (*e.g.*, Cl⁻) from gastric contents or bile acids in the intestine.

an·i·on ex·chang·er. An insoluble solid, usually a polystyrene or a polysaccharide, with cation groups (*e.g.*, —NR₃⁺ or —NR₂H⁺), which can attract and hold anions that pass by in a moving solution in exchange for anions previously held.

an·i·on·ic (an-ī-on′ik). Referring to a negatively charged ion.

an·i·on·ot·ro·py (an′-ī-on-ot′rō-pē). The migration of a negative ion in tautomeric changes.

an·i·rid·ia (an-i-rid′ē-ă) [MIM*106200]. Absence of the iris; when congenital, a rudimentary iris root is usually present. About 60 percent of cases are inherited as autosomal dominants, although somewhat irregularly manifested. Cf. irideremia. [G. *an-* priv. + irid- + -ia]

an·i·sa·ki·a·sis (an′i-să-kī′ă-sis). Infection of the intestinal wall by larvae of *Anisakis marina* and other genera of anisakid nematodes (*Contracaecum, Phocanema*), characterized by intestinal eosinophilic granuloma and symptoms like those of peptic ulcer or tumor. SYN herring-worm disease. [G. *anisos*, unequal, + *akis*, a point, + -*iasis*, condition]

an·i·sa·kid (an-i-sā′kid). Common name for nematodes of the family Anisakidae.

An·i·sa·ki·dae (an-i-sā′ki-dē). Family of large nematode worms (superfamily Heterocheilidae) found in the stomach and intestines of fish-eating birds and marine mammals, infection being acquired from marine fish; human cases of anisakiasis have been reported from Japan. SEE ALSO *Anisakis*.

An·i·sa·kis (an-i-sā′kis). Genus of nematodes (family Anisakidae) that includes many common parasites of marine fish-eating birds and marine mammals. [G. *anisos*, unequal, + *akis*, a point]

an·is·ate (an′ī-sāt). A salt of anisic acid, usually possessing antiseptic properties.

an·ise (an′is). The fruit of *Pimpinella anisum* (family Umbelliferae); an aromatic and carminative.

an·is·ei·ko·nia (an′ī-sī-kō′nē-ă). An ocular condition in which the image of an object in one eye differs in size or shape from the image of the same object in the fellow eye. SYN unequal retinal image. [G. *anisos*, unequal, + *eikōn*, an image]

anis·ic (an-is′ik). Relating to anise.

anis·ic ac·id (an-is′ik). A crystalline volatile acid obtained from anise; its compounds are the antiseptic anisates. SYN 4-methoxybenzoic acid.

an·i·sin·di·one (an′i-sin-dī′ōn). 2-*p*-Anisylindan-1,3-dione; an anticoagulant with pharmacologic actions similar to those of phenindione and bishydroxycoumarin.

△**aniso-.** Unequal, dissimilar, unlike. [G. *anisos*, unequal, fr. *an-*, not, + *isos*, equal]

an·i·so·ac·com·mo·da·tion (an-ī′sō-ă-kom-ō-dā′shŭn). Variation between the two eyes in accommodation capacity. [aniso- + L. *accommodo*, to adapt]

an·i·so·chro·ma·sia (an-ī′sō-krō-mā′zē-ă). The unequal distribution of hemoglobin in the red blood cells, such that the periphery is pigmented and the central region is virtually colorless, as observed in films of blood from persons with certain forms of anemia caused by deficiency of iron; normal red blood cells show mild a. because of their biconcave shape. [aniso- + G. *chrōma*, color]

an·i·so·chro·mat·ic (an-ī′sō-krō-mat′ik). Not uniformly of one color.

an·i·so·co·ria (an-ī-sō-kō′rē-ă). A condition in which the two pupils are not of equal size. [aniso- + G. *korē*, pupil]

essential a., SYN simple a.

physiologic a., SYN simple a.

simple a., a common (20% of normals) benign inequality of the pupils that may change from one hour to the next. SYN essential a., physiologic a., simple-central a.

simple-central a., SYN simple a.

an·i·so·cy·to·sis (an-ī′sō-sī-tō′sis). Considerable variation in the size of cells that are normally uniform, especially with reference to red blood cells. [aniso- + G. *kytos*, cell, + -*osis*, condition]

an·i·so·dac·ty·lous (an-ī′sō-dak′ti-lŭs). Relating to anisodactyly.

an·i·so·dac·ty·ly (an-ī′sō-dak′ti-lē). Unequal length in corresponding fingers. [aniso- + G. *daktylon*, finger]

an·i·sog·a·my (an′-i-sog′ă-mē). Fusion of two gametes unequal in size or form; fertilization as distinguished from isogamy or conjugation. [aniso- + G. *gamos*, marriage]

an·i·sog·na·thous (an-i-sog′nă-thŭs). Having jaws of unequal size, the upper being wider than the lower. [aniso- + G. *gnathos*, jaw]

an·i·so·kar·y·o·sis (an-ī′sō-kar-ē-ō′sis). Variation in size of nuclei, greater than the normal range for a tissue. [aniso- + G. *karyon*, nut (nucleus), + -*osis*, condition]

an·is·ole (an′i-sōl). C₆H₅OCH₃; Methoxybenzene; obtained from anisic acid; used in perfumery.

an·i·so·mas·tia (an-i-sō-mas′tē-ă). Breasts of unequal size. [aniso- + G. *mastos*, breast]

an·i·so·me·lia (an-i-sō-mē′lē-ă). A condition of inequality between two paired limbs. [aniso- + G. *melos*, limb]

an·i·so·me·tro·pia (an-ī′sō-me-trō′pē-ă). A difference in the refractive power of the two eyes. [aniso- + G. *metron*, measure, + *ōps*, sight]

an·i·so·me·tro·pic (an-ī′sō-me-trop′ik). 1. Relating to anisometropia. 2. Having eyes of unequal refractive power.

an·i·so·pi·e·sis (an-ī-sō-pī-ē′sis). Unequal arterial blood pressure on the two sides of the body. [aniso- + G. *piesis*, pressure]

an·i·sor·rhyth·mia (an-ī-sō-ridth′mē-ă). Irregular action of the heart, or absence of synchronism in the rate of atria and ventricles. [aniso- + G. *rhythmos*, rhythm]

an·i·so·sphyg·mia (an-ī-sō-sfig′mē-ă). Difference in volume, force, or time of the pulse in the corresponding arteries on two sides of the body, *e.g.*, the two radials, or femorals. [aniso- + G. *sphygmos*, pulse]

an·i·sos·then·ic (an-ī-sos-then′ik). Of unequal strength; denoting two muscles or groups of muscles that are either paired or are antagonists. [aniso- + G. *sthenos*, strength]

an·i·so·ton·ic (an-ī-sō-ton′ik). Not having equal tension; having unequal osmotic pressure. [aniso- + G. *tonus*, tension]

an·i·so·tro·pic (an-ī-sō-trop′ik). Not having properties that are the same in all directions. [aniso- + G. *tropos*, a turning]

an·i·so·tro·pine meth·yl·bro·mide (an′i-sō-trō′pēn). 8-Methyltropinium bromide 2-propylvalerate; an anticholinergic and intestinal antispasmodic.

Anitschkow, Nikolai, Russian pathologist, 1885–1964. SEE A. *cell, myocyte.*

an·kle (ang′kl). 1. SYN ankle *joint.* 2. The region of the a. joint. 3. SYN talus.

△**ankylo-.** Bent, crooked, stiff, fused, fixed, closed SEE ALSO ancylo-. [G. *ankylos*, bent, crooked; *ankylōsis*, stiffening of the joints, fr. *ankos*, a bend, a hollow]

an·ky·lo·bleph·a·ron (ang′ki-lō-blef′ă-ron). SYN blepharocoloboma. [ankylo- + G. *blepharon*, eyelid]

congenital a., congenital adhesion of the upper and lower eyelid by bands of tissue. SYN filiform adnatum.

an·ky·lo·col·pos (ang′ki-lō-kol′pos). SYN vaginal *atresia.* [ankylo- + G. *kolpos*, womb (vagina)]

an·ky·lo·dac·ty·ly, an·ky·lo·dac·tyl·ia (ang′ki-lō-dak′ti-lē, -dak-til′ē-ă). Adhesion between two or more fingers or toes. SEE ALSO syndactyly. [ankylo- + G. *daktylos*, finger]

an·ky·lo·glos·sia (ang′ki-lō-glos′ē-ă) [MIM 106280]. Partial or complete fusion of the tongue to the floor of the mouth; abnormal shortness of the frenulum linguae. SYN tongue-tie. [ankylo- + G. *glōssa*, tongue]

an·ky·lo·me·le (ang′ki-lō-mē′lē). A curved or bent probe. [ankylo- + G. *mēlē*, probe]

an·ky·lo·poi·et·ic (ang′ki-lō-poy-et′ik). Forming ankylosis.

an·ky·lo·proc·tia (ang′ki-lō-prok′shē-ă). Obsolete term for imperforation or stricture of the anus. [ankylo- + G. *prōktos*, anus]

an·ky·losed (ang'ki-lōsd). Stiffened; bound by adhesions; denoting a joint in a state of ankylosis.

an·ky·lo·sis (ang'ki-lō'sis). Stiffening or fixation of a joint as the result of a disease process, with fibrous or bony union across the joint. [G. *ankylōsis*, stiffening of a joint]

artificial a., SYN arthrodesis.

bony a., SYN synostosis.

dental a., bony union of the radicular surface of a tooth to the surrounding alveolar bone in an area of previous partial root resorption.

extracapsular a., stiffness of a joint due to induration or heterotopic ossification of the surrounding tissues. SYN spurious a.

false a., SYN fibrous a.

fibrous a., stiffening of a joint due to the presence of fibrous bands between and about the bones forming the joint. SYN false a., pseudankylosis.

intracapsular a., stiffness of a joint due to the presence of bony or fibrous adhesions between the articular surfaces of the joint.

spurious a., SYN extracapsular a.

true a., SYN synostosis.

An·ky·los·to·ma (ang-ki-los'tō-mă). **1.** SYN *Ancylostoma*. **2.** SYN trismus. [ankylo- + G. *stoma*, mouth]

an·ky·lo·sto·mi·a·sis (ang'ki-lō-stō-mī'ă-sis). SYN ancylostomiasis.

an·ky·lot·ic (ang-ki-lot'ik). Characterized by or pertaining to ankylosis.

an·ky·rin (ang'ki-rin). An erythrocyte membranal protein that binds spectrin. A deficiency in ankyrin may lead to a type of hereditary spherocytosis. SYN anchorin, syndein. [G. *ankyra*, anchor, + -in]

an·ky·roid (an'ki-royd). SYN ancyroid.

an·la·ge, pl. **an·la·gen** (ahn'lah-ge, -gen). **1.** SYN primordium. **2.** In psychoanalysis, genetic predisposition to a given trait or personality characteristic. [Ger. plan, outline]

an·neal (an-nēl'). **1.** To soften or temper a metal by controlled heating and cooling; the process makes a metal more easily adapted, bent, or swaged, and less brittle. **2.** In dentistry, to heat gold leaf preparatory to its insertion into a cavity, in order to remove adsorbed gases and other contaminants. **3.** The pairing of complementary single strands of DNA; or of DNA-RNA. **4.** The attachment of the ends of two macromolecules; *e.g.*, two microtubules annealing to form one longer microtubule. **5.** In molecular biology, annealing is a process in which short sections of single-stranded DNA from one source are bound to a filter and incubated with single-stranded, radioactively conjugated DNA from a second source. Where the two sets of DNA possess complementary sequences of nucleotides, bonding occurs. The degree of relatedness (homology) of the two sets of DNA is then estimated according to the radioactivity level of the filter. This technique plays a central role in the classification of bacteria and viruses. SYN nucleic acid hybridization. [A.S. *anaelan*, to burn]

an·nec·tent (a-nek'tent). Connected with; joined. [L. *an-necto*, pres. p. *-nectnes*, pp. *-nexus*, to join to]

An·nel·i·da (an'nĕ-lī'dă). A phylum that includes the segmented or true worms, such as the earthworm.

an·ne·lids (an'nĕ-lids). Common name for members of the phylum Annelida.

an·nel·lide (an'ĕ-līd). A conidiogenous cell that produces conidia in succession, each leaving a ringlike collar on the cell wall when released. [Fr. *annelide*, fr. L. *anellus*, a ring]

an·nel·lo·co·nid·i·um (an'ĕ-lō-kŏ-nid'ē-um). A conidium produced by an annellide.

an·nexa (a-nek'să). SYN adnexa.

an·nex·al (a-neks-ăl). SYN adnexal.

an·nex·ec·to·my (an-eks-ek'tō-mē). SYN adnexectomy.

an·nex·ins (a-nek'sinz). A family of Ca²⁺dependent phospholipid-binding proteins which may act as mediators of intracellular calcium signals.

an·nex·i·tis (an-eks-ī'tis). SYN adnexitis.

an·nex·o·pexy (an-eks'ō-pek-sē). SYN adnexopexy.

an·not·to (ă-not'ō). Coloring matter extracted from the seeds of *Bixa orellana;* contains bixin and several other yellow to orange-red pigments; used for coloring butter, margarine, cheese, and oils.

an·nu·lar (an'yū-lăr). Ring-shaped. SYN anular. [L. *anulus*, ring]

an·nu·lo·plasty (an'yū-lō-plas-tē). Reconstruction of the ring (or annulus) of an incompetent cardiac valve. [L. *anulus*, ring, + G. *plastos*, formed]

an·nu·lor·rha·phy (an-yū-lōr'ă-fē). Closure of a hernial ring by suture. [L. *anulus*, ring, + G. *rhaphē*, seam]

an·nu·lus (an'yū-lŭs) [NA]. SYN ring. SEE ALSO ring.

a. abdomina'lis, SYN deep inguinal *ring*.

a. cilia'ris, SYN ciliary *body*.

a. conjuncti'vae [NA], SYN conjunctival *ring*.

a. femora'lis [NA], SYN femoral *ring*.

a. fibrocartilagin'eus membranae tympani [NA], SYN fibrocartilaginous *ring* of tympanic membrane.

a. fibro'sus [NA], **(1)** SYN fibrous *ring* of heart. **(2)** SYN a. fibrosus of intervertebral disc.

a. fibrosus cordis [NA], SYN fibrous *ring* of heart.

a. fibrosus disci intervertebralis [NA], SYN a. fibrosus of intervertebral disc.

a. fibrosus of intervertebral disc, the ring of fibrocartilage and fibrous tissue forming the circumference of the intervertebral disc; surrounds the nucleus pulposus, which is prone to herniation when the a. fibrosus is compromised. SYN a. fibrosus disci intervertebralis [NA], a. fibrosus (2) [NA], fibrous ring of intervertebral disc, fibrous ring (2).

a. of fibrous sheath, SYN annular *part* of fibrous digital sheath.

Haller's a., SYN Haller's *insula*.

a. hemorrhoida'lis, SYN hemorrhoidal *zone*.

a. inguina'lis profun'dus [NA], SYN deep inguinal *ring*.

a. inguina'lis superficia'lis [NA], SYN superficial inguinal *ring*.

a. ir'idis, SYN *ring* of iris.

a. iridis major, SYN greater *ring* of iris.

a. iridis minor, SYN lesser *ring* of iris.

a. lymphat'icus car'diae [NA], SYN lymphatic *ring* of cardiac part of stomach.

a. ova'lis, SYN *limbus* fossae ovalis.

a. tendin'eus commu'nis [NA], SYN common tendinous *ring*.

a. tympan'icus [NA], SYN tympanic *ring*.

a. umbilica'lis [NA], SYN umbilical *ring*.

a. urethra'lis, SYN *sphincter* vesicae.

Vieussens' a., SYN *limbus* fossae ovalis.

AnOC Abbreviation for anodal opening *contraction*.

an·o·chle·sia (an'ō-klē'zē-ă). **1.** SYN catalepsy. **2.** Quietude. [G. *an-* priv. + *ochlēsis*, disturbance]

an·o·chro·ma·sia (an'ō-krō-mā'zē-ă). **1.** Failure of cells or other elements of tissue to be colored in the usual manner when treated with a stain (or stains). **2.** Accumulation of hemoglobin in the peripheral zone of erythrocytes, thereby resulting in a pale, virtually colorless central portion. [G. *anō*, upward, + *chrōma*, color]

ano·ci·as·so·ci·a·tion (ă-nō'sē-ă-sō-sē-ā'shŭn). Theory that afferent stimuli, especially pain, contribute to the development of surgical shock and, as a corollary, that conduction anesthesia at the surgical field and pre-surgical sedation protect against shock. [G. *a-* priv. + L. *noceo*, to injure, + association]

ano·coc·cyg·e·al (a-nō-kok-sij'ē-ăl). Relating to both anus and coccyx.

anod·al (an-ōd'ăl). Of, pertaining to, or emanating from an anode. SYN anodic.

an·ode (an'ōd). **1.** The positive pole of a galvanic battery or the electrode connected with it; an electrode toward which negatively charged ions (anions) migrate; a positively charged electrode. Cf. cathode. **2.** The portion, usually made of tungsten, of an x-ray tube from which x-rays are re leased by bombardment by cathode rays (electrons). SYN anelectrode, positive electrode. [G. *anodos*, a way up, fr. *ana*, up, + *hodos*, a way]

rotating a., in diagnostic radiography, modern x-ray tubes that have a mushroom-shaped anode that rotates rapidly to avoid local heat buildup from electron impact during x-ray generation.

an·o·derm (ā′nō-derm). Lining of the anal canal immediately inferior to the dentate line and extending for about 1.5 cm. to the anal verge; it is devoid of hair and sebaceous and sweat glands, and so is not true skin, although it is squamous epithelium; it is pale, smooth, thin, and delicate, and shiny when stretched; it is especially vulnerable to abrasion (as from rough toilet paper), chemical irritants (soaps), and is well-provided with tactile and nociceptive (pain, itch) endings innervated by the inferior rectal (pudendal) nerve.

an·od·ic (an-ōd′ik). SYN anodal.

an·o·don·tia (an-ō-don′shē-ă). Congenital absence of the teeth; developmental, not due to extraction or impaction. SYN agomphiasis, agomphious, agomphosis, agomphiasis. [G. *an-* priv. + *odous,* tooth]

partial a., SYN hypodontia.

an·o·dont·ism (an-ō-dont′izm). Congenital absence of tooth germ development.

an·o·dyne (an′ō-dīn). A compound less potent than an anesthetic or a narcotic but capable of relieving pain. [G. *an-* priv. + *odynē,* pain]

an·o·et·ic (an-ō-et′ik). Lacking the power of comprehension, as in severe and profound levels of mental retardation. [G. *anoēsia,* from *a-* priv. + *noos,* perception]

ano·gen·i·tal (ā′nō-jen′ĭ-tăl). Relating in any way to both the anal and the genital regions.

anom·a·lad (ă-nom′ă-lad). A malformation together with its subsequently derived structural changes. [see anomaly]

anom·a·lo·scope (ă-nom′ă-lō-skōp). An instrument used to diagnose abnormalities of color perception in which one-half of a field of color is matched by mixing two other colors. [G. *anōmalos,* irregular, + *skopeō,* to examine]

anom·a·ly (ă-nom′ă-lē). Deviation from the average or norm; anything that is structurally unusual or irregular or contrary to a general rule. Congenital defects are an example of the definition of anomaly. [G. *anōmalia,* irregularity]

Alder's a., coarse azurophilic granulation of leukocytes, especially granulocytes, which may be associated with gargoylism and Morquio's disease.

Aristotle's a., when a small object is held between the first and second fingers crossed in such a way that it touches or presses upon skin surfaces which ordinarily are not pressed upon simultaneously by a single object, it is perceived falsely as two.

Chédiak-Steinbrinck-Higashi a., SYN Chédiak-Steinbrinck-Higashi *syndrome.*

developmental a., an a. established during intrauterine life; a congenital a.

Ebstein's a., congenital downward displacement of the tricuspid valve into the right ventricle. SYN Ebstein's disease.

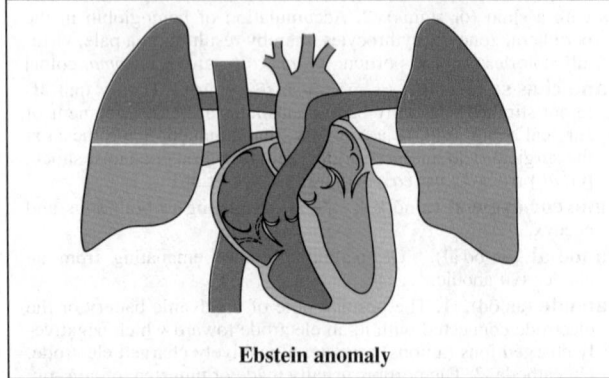

Ebstein anomaly

eugnathic a., SYN eugnathia.

Freund's a., a narrowing of the upper aperture of the thorax by shortening of the first rib and its cartilage; formerly believed to

predispose to tuberculosis because of defective expansion of the lung apex.

Hegglin's a., a disorder in which neutrophils and eosinophils contain basophilic structures known as Döhle or Amato bodies and in which there is faulty maturation of platelets, with thrombocytopenia; autosomal dominant inheritance. SYN May-Hegglin a.

May-Hegglin a., SYN Hegglin's a.

morning glory a., congenital a. of the optic disk in which the nerve head is funnel-shaped, with a dot of white tissue at the end of the excavation, and is surrounded by an elevated pigmented annulus; the retinal vessels seen are multiple narrow bands at the edge of the disk.

Pelger-Huët nuclear a. [MIM*169400], congenital inhibition of lobulation in the nuclei of neutrophilic leukocytes; most cells present band or bilobulate appearance, and only an occasional cell is trilobed; it is not associated with disease, but may be confused with leukocyte "shift to left"; autosomal dominant inheritance.

Peters' a., SYN anterior chamber cleavage *syndrome.*

Rieger's a., SYN iridocorneal mesodermal *dysgenesis.*

Shone's a., coarctation of the aorta, subaortic stenosis, and stenosing ring of the left atrium found in association with a parachute mitral valve.

Uhl a., right ventricular myocardial aplasia, causing a dilated, thin-walled right ventricle without murmurs; death results in early childhood.

an·o·mer (an′ō-mer). One of two sugar molecules that are epimeric at the hemiacetal or hemiketal carbon atom (carbon-1 in aldoses, carbon-2 in most ketoses); *e.g.,* α-D-glucose and β-D-glucose. SEE ALSO sugars. Cf. epimer.

ano·mia (ă-nō′mē-ă). SYN nominal *aphasia.* [G. *a-* priv. + *ōnoma,* name]

an·o·mie (an′ō-mē). **1.** Lawlessness; absence or weakening of social norms or values, with corresponding erosion of social cohesion. **2.** In psychiatry, absence or weakening of individual norms or values; characterized by anxiety, isolation, and personal disorientation. [Fr., fr. G. *anomia,* lawlessness]

an·o·nych·ia, an·o·ny·cho·sis (an-ō-nik′ē-ă, an-ō-nī-kō′sis). Absence of the nails. [G. *an-* priv. + *onyx* (*onych-*), nail]

anon·y·ma (ă-non′i-mă). Without name; a term formerly applied to the large vessels in the thorax (now called the brachiocephalic trunk and vein) and the hip bone. SYN innominate. [G. *an-* priv. + *onyma,* name]

Anoph·e·les (ă-nof′ě-lēz). A genus of mosquitoes (family Culicidae, subfamily Anophelinae). The sporogenous cycle of the malarial parasite is passed in the body cavity of female mosquitoes of certain species of this genus; a few selected vectors (from among over 90 species) are listed below. [G. *anōphelēs,* useless, harmful, fr. *an-* priv. + *ōpheleō,* to be of use]

A. albima′nus, a species having white hind feet, a common carrier of the malaria parasite in the West Indies and Central America.

A. albitar′sus, a South American species that transmits malaria.

A. balabacen′sis, a vector species in Southeast Asia, Burma, and India.

A. culicifa′cies, a species that is a common malaria vector in India and Sri Lanka, China, and elsewhere in the Orient.

A. darling′i, a South American species, an important carrier of the malarial parasite.

A. fluviatil′is, a species that is an important vector in India and Pakistan.

A. freebor′ni, a species that is a vector in the western U.S. (although endemic cases are no longer present).

A. funes′tus, an important African species that transmits malaria.

A. gam′biae, an African species that is a most important vector of malaria.

A. labranch′iae, a species that is an important vector in southern Europe and the Mediterranean basin.

A. macula′tus, a species that is a vector in Malaysia and Indonesia.

A. maculipen′nis, the type species of this genus; its wings are marked by spots formed of collections of scales; one of the most widely spread species active in the dissemination of malaria (formerly an important vector in continental Europe).

A. min'imus, a species that is an important vector throughout the Orient.

A. pseudopunctipen'nis, a South American vector species.

A. quadrimacula'tus, a species that was formerly an important carrier of malaria in the southern United States.

A. stephen'si, a widespread species that is an important vector of malaria in Asia.

A. sundai'cus, a species that is an important vector in the Orient and Southeast Asia.

A. superpic'tus, a species that is an important vector in the Mediterranean region, Middle East, and southern Asia.

anoph·e·li·cide (ă-nof′ĕ-li-sīd). An agent that destroys the *Anopheles* mosquito.

anoph·e·li·fuge (ă-nof′ĕ-li-fūj). An agent that drives away or prevents the bite of *Anopheles* mosquitoes.

Anoph·e·li·nae (an-of-ĕ-lī′nē). A subfamily of the mosquitoes (Culicidae) consisting of several genera, including *Anopheles*.

anoph·e·line (ă-nof′ĕ-līn). Referring to the *Anopheles* mosquito.

Anophe·li·ni (ă-nof-ĕ-lī′nī). The tribe of mosquitoes (family Culicidae) that includes the genus *Anopheles*. [G. *anōphelēs*, useless, troublesome]

anoph·e·lism (ă-nof′ĕ-lizm). The habitual presence in any region of *Anopheles* mosquitoes.

an·oph·thal·mia (an-of-thal′mē-ă). Congenital absence of all tissues of the eyes. [G. *an-* priv. + *ophthalmos*, eye]

ano·plas·ty (ā′nō-plas-tē). Plastic surgery of the anus. [L. *anus* + G. *plastos*, formed]

An·op·lo·ceph·a·la (an-op′lō-sef′ă-lă). A genus of large tapeworms (family Anoplocephalidae) with strong linear segmentation, numerous scattered testes, and eggs with a pyriform apparatus; they are parasitic in herbivores, with terrestrial mites serving as intermediate hosts. [G. *anoplos,* unarmed, + *kephalē,* head]

A. perfolia'ta, a cosmopolitan species of the horse, donkey, mule, and zebra; cysticercoid larvae are found in arthropods. SYN *Taenia equina, Taenia quadrilobata*.

An·o·plu·ra (an-ō-plū′ră). The order of insects that includes the bloodsucking lice of mammals, with some 450 species arranged in 6 families, of which 4 contain species of medical or veterinary importance: *Haematopinus, Linognathus,* and *Solenopotes* of domestic mammals, and the human sucking lice *Pediculus humanus*. [G. *anoplos,* unarmed, + *oura,* tail]

an·or·chia (an-ōr′kē-ă). SYN anorchism.

an·or·chism (an-ōr′kizm). Absence of the testes; may be congenital or acquired. SYN anorchia. [G. *an-* priv. + *orchis,* testis]

ano·rec·tal (ā′nō-rek′tăl). Relating to both anus and rectum.

an·o·rec·tic, an·o·ret·ic (an-ō-rek′tic, -ret′ik). **1.** Relating to, characteristic of, or suffering from anorexia, especially anorexia nervosa. **2.** An agent that causes anorexia. SYN anorexic.

an·o·rex·ia (an-ō-rek′sē-ă). Diminished appetite; aversion to food. [G. fr. *an-* priv. + *orexis,* appetite]

a. nervo'sa, a mental disorder manifested by extreme fear of becoming obese and an aversion to food, usually occurring in young women and often resulting in life-threatening weight loss, accompanied by a disturbance in body image, hyperactivity, and amenorrhea.

an·o·rex·i·ant (an-ō-rek′sē-ănt). A drug ("diet pills"), process, or event that leads to anorexia.

an·o·rex·ic (an-ō-rek′sik). SYN anorectic.

an·o·rex·i·gen·ic (an′ō-rek-si-jen′ik). Promoting or causing anorexia.

an·or·gas·my, an·or·gas·mia (an-ōr-gaz′mē, -gaz′mē-ă). Failure to experience an orgasm; may be biogenic (secondary to a physical disorder or medication), psychogenic (secondary to psychological or situational factors), or a combination of the two. [G. *an-* priv. + orgasm + *-ia*]

an·or·thog·ra·phy (an-ōr-thog′ră-fē). SYN agraphia. [G. *an-* priv. + *orthos,* straight, + *graphō,* to write]

ano·scope (ā′nō-skōp). A short speculum for examining the anal canal and lower rectum.

Bacon's a., an instrument resembling a rectal speculum, with a long slit on one side and an electric light opposite.

ano·sig·moid·os·co·py (ā′nō-sig-moy-dos′-kŏ-pē). Endoscopy of the anus, rectum and sigmoid colon.

an·os·mia (an-oz′mē-ă). Loss of the sense of smell. It may be: 1) essential or true, due to lesion of the olfactory nerve; 2) mechanical or respiratory, due to obstruction of the nasal fossae; 3) reflex, due to disease in some other part or organ; or 4) functional, without any apparent causal lesion. [G. *an-* priv. + *osmē,* sense of smell]

an·os·mic (an-oz′mik). Relating to anosmia.

ano·so·di·a·pho·ria (ă-nō′sō-dī-ă-fōr′ē-ă). Indifference, real or assumed, regarding the presence of disease, specifically of paralysis. [G. *a-* priv. + *nosos,* disease, + *diaphora,* difference]

ano·sog·no·sia (ă-nō′sog-nō′sē-ă). Ignorance of the presence of disease, specifically of paralysis. Most often seen in patients with non-dominant parietal lobe lesions, who deny their hemiparesis. [G. *a-* priv. + *nosos,* disease, + *gnōsis,* knowledge]

ano·sog·no·sic (ă-nō-sog-nō′sik). Relating to anosognosia.

ano·spi·nal (ā′nō-spī′năl). Relating to the anus and the spinal cord.

an·os·te·o·pla·sia (an-os′tē-ō-plā′zē-ă). Failure of bone formation. [G. *an-* priv. + *osteon,* bone, + *plassō,* to form]

an·os·to·sis (an-os-tō′sis). Failure of ossification. [G. *an-* priv. + *osteon,* bone]

an·o·tia (an-ō′shē-ă). Congenital absence of one or both auricles of the ears. [G. *an-* priv. + *ous,* ear]

ANOVA Acronym for *analysis* of variance.

ano·ves·i·cal (ā′nō-ves′i-kăl). Relating in any way to both anus and urinary bladder.

an·ov·u·lar (an-ov′yū-lăr). Absence of discharge of an ovum from the ovary during an ovarian cycle. SYN anovulatory.

an·ov·u·la·tion (an-ov-yū-lā′shŭn). Suspension or cessation of ovulation.

an·ov·u·la·to·ry (an-ov′yū-lă-tōr-ē). SYN anovular.

an·ox·e·mia (an-ok-sē′mē-ă). Absence of oxygen in arterial blood; formerly often used to include moderate decrease in oxygen now properly distinguished as hypoxemia. [G. *an-* priv. + oxygen + G. *haima,* blood]

an·ox·ia (an-ok′sē-ă). Absence or almost complete absence of oxygen from inspired gases, arterial blood, or tissues; to be differentiated from hypoxia. [G. *an-* priv. + oxygen]

anemic a., a term formerly considered synonymous with anemic hypoxia, but now reserved for extremely severe cases in which oxygen is almost completely lacking.

anoxic a., a term formerly considered synonymous with hypoxic hypoxia, but now reserved for extremely severe cases in which oxygen is almost completely lacking.

diffusion a., diffusion hypoxia severe enough to result in the absence of oxygen in alveolar gas.

histotoxic a., poisoning of the respiratory enzyme systems of the tissues, as in the inhibition of cytochrome oxidase by cyanides; owing to the inability of tissue cells to utilize oxygen, its tension in arterial and capillary blood is usually greater than normal.

a. neonator'um, any a. observed in newborn infants.

oxygen affinity a., a. due to inability of hemoglobin to release oxygen.

stagnant a., stagnant hypoxia severe enough to result in the absence of oxygen in tissues.

an·ox·ic (an-ok′sik). Denoting or characteristic of anoxia.

ANP Abbreviation for atrial natriuretic *peptide*.

Anrep, G.V., 20th century Lebanese physiologist in Britain. SEE A. *phenomenon*.

ANS Symbol for anterior nasal *spine*.

an·sa, gen. and pl. **an·sae** (an′să, -sē) [NA]. Any anatomical structure in the form of a loop or an arc. SEE ALSO loop. [L. loop, handle]

a. cervica'lis [NA], a loop in the cervical plexus consisting of

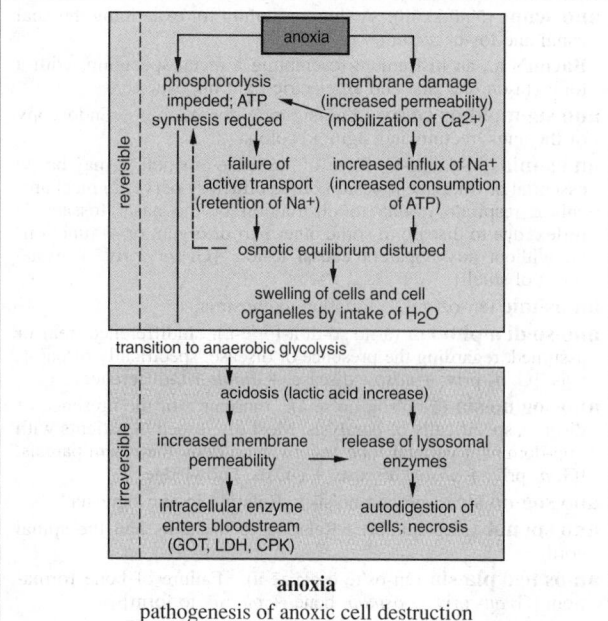

anoxia
pathogenesis of anoxic cell destruction

fibers from the first three cervical nerves. Fibers from a loop between the C-1 and C-2 spinal nerves accompany the hypoglossal nerve for a short distance, leaving it as the superior root of the a. cervicalis. Fibers from a loop between the C-2 and C-3 spinal nerves form the inferior root of the a. cervicalis. Most commonly, the roots merge, forming the a. cervicalis, which gives rise to branches innervating infrahyoid muscles. SYN cervical loop, loop of hypoglossal nerve.

Haller's a., SYN communicating *branch* of facial nerve with glossopharyngeal nerve.

Henle's a., SYN nephronic *loop.*

a. hypoglos'si, former name for a. cervicalis.

lenticular a., SYN lenticular *loop.*

a. lenticula'ris [NA], SYN lenticular *loop.*

ansae nervo'rum spina'lium, SYN *loops* of spinal nerves, under *loop.*

peduncular a., SYN a. peduncularis.

a. peduncula'ris [NA], a complex fiber bundle curving around the medial edge of the internal capsule and connecting the anterior or part of the temporal lobe (temporal cortex), amygdala, and olfactory cortex with the mediodorsal nucleus of the thalamus; it enters the thalamus as a component of the inferior thalamic peduncle which also contains a major part of the fibers connecting the mediodorsal nucleus to the orbitofrontal cortex. SYN peduncular a., peduncular loop, Reil's a.

Reil's a., SYN a. peduncularis.

a. sacra'lis, a nerve cord connecting one or both of the sympathetic nerve trunks with the ganglion impar.

a. subcla'via [NA], a nerve cord connecting the middle cervical and stellate sympathetic ganglia, forming a loop around the subclavian artery. SYN subclavian loop, Vieussens' a., Vieussens' loop.

Vieussens' a., SYN a. subclavia.

an·sate (an'sāt). SYN ansiform.

an·ser·ine. **1** (an'ser-īn). Resembling or characteristic of a goose. SEE *cutis* anserina, *pes* anserinus. **2** (an'ser-ēn). N^a-(β-alanyl)-π-methyl- L-histidine; present in muscle. SYN *N*-methylcarnosine. [L. *anserinus,* fr. *anser,* goose]

an·si·form (an'si-fōrm). In the shape of a loop or arc. SYN ansate. [L. *ansa,* handle, + *forma,* shape]

an·sot·o·my (an-sot'ō-mē). **1.** Surgical division of a loop, usually a constricting loop. **2.** Section of the ansa lenticularis for treatment of striatal syndromes. [L. *ansa,* handle + G. *tomē,* cutting]

△**ant-.** SEE anti-.

ant. One of the most numerous insects (order Hymenoptera), characterized by an extraordinary development of colonial dwelling and caste specialization.

harvester a., SYN *Pogonomyrmex.*

velvet a., a wingless mutilid wasp (family Mutilidae, order Hymenoptera) known for its venomous sting.

ant·ac·id (ant-as'id). **1.** Neutralizing an acid. **2.** Any agent that reduces or neutralizes acidity, as of the gastric juice or any other secretion. SYN antiacid.

an·tag·o·nism (an-tag'on-izm). **1.** Denoting mutual opposition in action between structures, agents, diseases, or physiologic processes. Cf. synergism. **2.** The situation in which the combined effect of two or more factors is smaller than the solitary effect of any one of the factors. SYN mutual resistance. [G. *antagōnisma,* from *anti,* against, + *agōnizomai,* to fight, fr. *agōn,* a contest]

bacterial a., the inhibition of one bacterium by products of another.

an·tag·o·nist (an-tag'ŏ-nist). Something opposing or resisting the action of another; certain structures, agents, diseases, or physiologic processes that tend to neutralize or impede the action or effect of others. Cf. synergist.

β-adrenoreceptor a., SYN β-adrenergic blocking *agent.*

aldosterone a., an agent that opposes the action of the adrenal hormone aldosterone on renal tubular mineralocorticoid retention; these agents, *e.g.,* spironolactone, are useful in treating the hypertension of primary hyperaldosteronism, or the sodium retention of secondary hyperaldosteronism.

associated a., one of two muscles or groups of muscles which pull in nearly opposite directions, but which, when acting together, move the part in a path between their diverging lines of action.

calcium a., SYN calcium channel-blocking *agent.*

competitive a., an antimetabolite.

enzyme a., an antimetabolite or inhibitor of enzyme action.

folic acid a.'s, modified pterins, such as aminopterin and amethopterin, that interfere with the action of folic acid and thus produce the symptoms of folic acid deficiency; have been used in cancer chemotherapy.

5-hydroxy tryptamine a.'s, agents which block serotonin receptors and hence interfere with the biological actions of serotonin (5-HT).

insulin a., substances in the β- and γ-globulin or $β_1$-lipoprotein fractions of serum which may induce a functional insulin deficiency; may include nonprecipitating antibodies against nonhuman insulin.

muscarinic a., drugs which bind with muscarinic cholinergic receptors but do not activate them, thus preventing access to acetylcholine; examples include atropine, scopolamine, propantheline, and pirenzepine.

opioid a.'s, agents such as naloxone and naltrexone which have high affinity for opiate receptors but do not activate these receptors. These drugs block the effects of exogenously administered opioids such as morphine, heroin, meperidine, and methadone, or of endogenously released endorphins and enkephalins.

ant·al·ge·sia (ant-al-jē'zē-ă). Rarely used term for lowering of a previous elevation in pain threshold. [anti- + G. *algēsis,* sense of pain]

ant·al·gic (ant-al'jik). SYN analgesic (2).

ant·al·ka·line (ant-al'kă-līn). Reducing or neutralizing alkalinity.

ant·aph·ro·di·si·ac (ant'af-rō-diz'ē-ak). SYN anaphrodisiac.

ant·aph·ro·dit·ic (ant'af-rō-dit'ik). **1.** SYN anaphrodisiac. **2.** SYN antivenereal.

ant·ar·thrit·ic (ant'ar-thrit'ik). Rarely used term for: **1.** Relieving arthritis. **2.** A remedy for arthritis. SYN antiarthritic.

ant·as·then·ic (ant-as-then'ik). **1.** Strengthening or invigorating. **2.** An agent possessing such qualities. [anti- + G. *astheneia,* weakness]

ant·asth·mat·ic (ant-az-mat'ik). **1.** Tending to relieve or prevent asthma. **2.** An agent that prevents or arrests an asthmatic attack. SYN antiasthmatic.

an·a·tro·phic (ant-ă-trof′ik). **1.** Preventing or curing atrophy. **2.** An agent that promotes the restoration of atrophied structures.

an·taz·o·line hy·dro·chlo·ride (an-taz′ō-lēn). 2-(*N*-benzylanilino- methyl)-2-imidazoline hydrochloride; a histamine-antagonizing agent used in treating allergy; also available as a. h. phosphate. SYN phenazoline hydrochloride.

△**ante-.** Before, in front of (in time or place or order). SEE ALSO pre-, pro- (1). [L. *ante*, before, in front of]

an·te·brach·i·al (an′te-brā′kē-ăl). Relating to the forearm.

an·te·bra·chi·um (an-te-brā′kē-ŭm) [NA]. SYN forearm. [ante- + L. *brachium*, arm]

an·te·car·di·um (an-te-kar′dē-ŭm). SYN precordia.

an·te·ced·ent (an-te-sē′dent). A precursor. [L. *antecedo*, to go before]

  plasma thromboplastin a. (PTA), SYN *factor* XI.

an·te ci·bum (an′tē sī′bŭm). Before a meal. The plural is ante cibos, before meals. [L.]

an·te·cu·bi·tal (an-te-kyū′bi-tăl). In front of the elbow. [ante- + L. *cubitum*, elbow]

an·te·fe·brile (an-te-feb′ril). Rarely used term for antepyretic. [ante- + L. *febris*, fever]

an·te·flex (an′te-fleks). To bend forward, or cause to bend forward. [ante- + L. *flecto*, pp. *flexus*, to bend]

an·te·flex·ion (an-te-flek′shŭn). A bending forward; a sharp forward curve or angulation; denoting especially the normal forward bend in the uterus at the junction of corpus and cervix uteri. **a. of iris,** rarely used term for an iris that is in part, folded forward after a severe iridodialysis so that the pigmented layer faces forward.

an·te·grade (an′tĕ-grād). In the direction of normal movement, as in blood flow or peristalsis. [ante- + L. *gradior*, to walk]

an·te·mor·tem (an′te-mōr-tem). Before death. Cf. postmortem. [ante- + L. acc. case of *mors* (*mort-*), death]

an·te·na·tal (an-te-nā′tăl). SYN prenatal. [ante- + L. *natus*, birth]

an·te·par·tum (an′te-par-tŭm). Before labor or childbirth. Cf. intrapartum, postpartum. [ante- + L. *pario*, pp. *partus*, to bring forth]

ant·eph·i·al·tic (ant′ef-i-al′tik). Alleviating nightmares or distressing dreams. [anti- + G. *ephialtēs*, nightmare]

an·te·po·si·tion (an′te-pō-si′shŭn). Forward or anterior position.

an·te·pros·tate (an-te-pros′tāt). Obsolete term for bulbourethral gland.

an·te·py·ret·ic (an′te-pī-ret′ik). Before the occurrence of fever; before the period of reaction following shock. [ante- + G. *pyretos*, fever]

an·te·ri·or (an-tēr′ē-ōr). **1** [NA]. In human anatomy, denoting the front surface of the body; often used to indicate the position of one structure relative to another, *i.e.*, situated nearer the front part of the body. SYN ventral (2). **2.** Near the head or rostral end of certain embryos. **3.** Undesirable and confusing substitute for *cranial* in quadrupeds. In veterinary anatomy, a. is restricted to parts of the eye and inner ear. **4.** Before, in relation to time or space. [L.]

△**antero-.** Anterior. [L. *anterior*, more before, earlier, fr. *ante*, before, + -r- -*ior*, more]

an·ter·o·ex·ter·nal (an′ter-ō-eks-ter′năl). In front and to the outer side.

an·ter·o·grade (an′ter-ō-grād). **1.** Moving forward. Cf. antegrade. **2.** Extending forward from a particular point in time; used in reference to amnesia. [L. *gradior*, pp. *gressus*, to step, go]

an·ter·o·in·fe·ri·or (an′ter-ō-in-fēr′ē-ōr). In front and below.

an·ter·o·in·ter·nal (an′ter-ō-in-ter′năl). In front and to the inner side.

an·ter·o·lat·er·al (an′ter-ō-lat′er-ăl). In front and away from the middle line.

an·ter·o·me·di·al (an′ter-ō-mē′dē-ăl). In front and toward the middle line.

an·ter·o·me·di·an (an′ter-ō-mē′dē-an). In front and in the central line.

an·ter·o·pos·te·ri·or (an′ter-ō-pos-tēr-ē-er). **1.** Relating to both

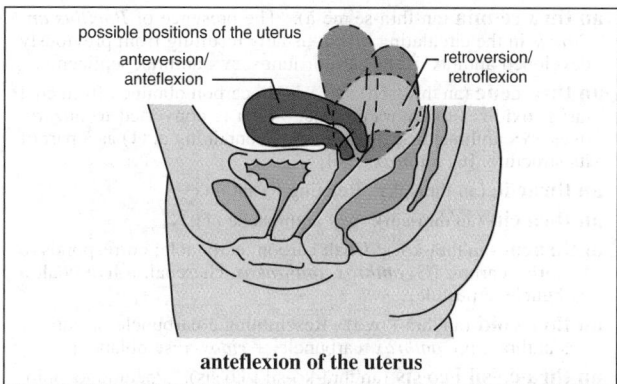

possible positions of the uterus
anteversion/anteflexion
retroversion/retroflexion

anteflexion of the uterus

front and rear. **2.** In x-ray imaging, describing the direction of the beam through the patient from anterior to posterior, *e.g.,* an A-P view of the abdomen.

an·ter·o·su·pe·ri·or (an′ter-ō-sū-pē′rē-er). In front and above.

ant·e·rot·ic (ant-er-ot′ik). Pertaining to an effort to avoid erotic feelings. [anti- + G. *erōtikos*, pertaining to love]

an·te·sys·to·le (an-te-sis′tō-lē). Premature activation of the ventricle responsible for the pre-excitation syndrome of the Wolff-Parkinson-White or Lown-Ganong-Levine types.

an·te·ver·sion (an-te-ver′shŭn). Turning forward, inclining forward as a whole without bending. [ante- + Mediev. L. *versio*, a turning]

an·te·vert·ed (an-te-vert′ed). Tilted forward; in a position of anteversion.

ant·he·lix (ant′hē-liks, an′thē-liks) [NA]. SYN antihelix. [anti- + G. *helix*, coil]

an·thel·min·thic (ant-hel-min′thik). SYN anthelmintic (1).

an·thel·min·tic (ant-hel-min′tik, an-thel-). **1.** An agent that destroys or expels intestinal worms. SYN anthelminthic, antihelminthic, helminthagogue, helminthic, helmintic, vermifuge. **2.** Having the power to destroy or expel intestinal worms. SYN vermifugal. [anti- + G. *helmins*, worm]

an·the·lone (an′thĕ-lōn). SYN urogastrone.

  a. E, SYN enterogastrone.

  a. U, SYN urogastrone.

ant·he·lot·ic (ant-hē-lot′ik). Obsolete term for a remedy for corns. [anti- + G. *hēlos*, nail, callus]

an·the·ma (an-thē′mă, an′thē). SYN exanthema. [G. *anthein*, to blossom]

an·ther·id·i·um (an′ther-id′ē-um). The male gametangium produced in the teleomorph part to the life cycle of fungi. [Mod. L. *anthera*, flower, fr. G *anthēros*, blooming, fr. *anthēo*, to bloom, + dim. suffix -*idium*, fr. G. -*idion*]

an·thi·o·li·mine (an-thī-ō′li-mēn). Lithium antimony thiomalate; used in the treatment of filariasis and schistosomiasis.

an·tho·cy·a·nins (an-thō-sī′ă-ninz). A group of floral pigments, existing as glycosides in combination with glucose or cellobiose molecules, that range from red to blue and are often pH dependent; soluble in water and alcohol but not in ether. A. are divided into derivatives of pelargonidin, cyanidins, and delphinidins. Some have been used as hematoxylin substitutes. [G. *anthos*, flower, + *kyanos*, a blue substance]

An·tho·my·ia (an-thō-mī′yă). A genus of muscoid flies similar in appearance to the common housefly. [G. *anthos*, flower, + *myia*, fly]

  A. canicula′ris, a small black horsefly, the larvae of which have been reported as accidental parasites in the intestine of humans, being hatched there from the ingested eggs; symptoms of gastro-enteric irritation may be caused by it; adults may transport eggs of the tropical warble fly or botfly to humans, *Dermatobia hominis,* a cause of myiasis.

an·tho·xan·thins (an-thō-zan′thinz). Compounds responsible for the yellow and ivory shades of flowers; usually divided into flavones and flavonols.

an·thra·ce·mia (an-thră-sē′mē-ă). The presence of *Bacillus anthracis* in the circulating blood, usually resulting from previously developed anthrax of the skin or lungs. SYN anthrax septicemia.

an·thra·cene (an′thră-sēn). **1.** A hydrocarbon obtained from coal tar; it oxidizes to anthraquinone, which is converted to alizarin dyes. SYN anthracin. **2.** A compound containing a. (1) as a part of its structure. [G. *anthrax,* coal]

an·thrac·ic (an-thras′ik). Relating to anthrax.

an·thra·cin (an′thră-sin). SYN anthracene (1).

△anthraco- (an′thră-kō-). Coal; carbon; carbuncle; corresponds to L. carb-, carbo-. [G. *anthrax, anthrakos,* charcoal, a live coal; a carbuncle, a pustule]

an·thra·coid (an′thră-koyd). Resembling a carbuncle or cutaneous anthrax. [G. *anthrax,* carbuncle, + *eidos,* resemblance]

an·thra·co·sil·i·co·sis (an′thră-kō-sil′i-kō′sis). Pneumonoconiosis from accumulation of carbon and silica in the lungs from inhaled coal dust; the silica content produces fibrous nodules. [anthraco- + silicosis]

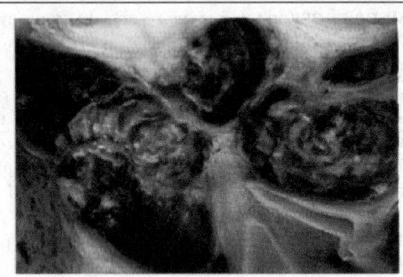

anthracosilicosis
cross-section of a lung

an·thra·co·sis (an-thră-kō′sis). Pneumonoconiosis from accumulation of carbon from inhaled smoke or coal dust in the lungs. SEE ALSO pneumomelanosis. SYN collier's lung, melanedema, miner's lung (1). [anthraco- + G. *-osis,* condition]

an·thra·cot·ic (an-thră-kot′ik). Characterized by anthracosis.

an·thra·lin (an′thră-lin). 1,8,9-anthracenetriol; 1,8,9-anthratriol; 1,8,9-dihydroxyanthranol; used as a substitute for chrysarobin in ointment for treatment of psoriasis and ringworm infestation. SYN dithranol.

an·thra·mu·cin (an-thră-myū′sin). A neutralizing material from the capsule of *Bacillus anthracis* that neutralizes serum and tissue antimicrobial action.

an·thra·nil·ic ac·id (an-thră-nil′ik). One of the products of tryptophan catabolism. SYN *o*-aminobenzoic acid.

an·thra·nil·o·yl (an-thră-nil′ō-il). The acyl radical of anthranilic acid.

an·thra·pur·pu·rin (an′thră-pūr′pū-rin). $C_{14}H_8O_5$; 1,2,7-Trihydroxyanthraquinone; a purple dye used in histology as a reagent for calcium, although the specificity has been questioned.

9,10-an·thra·qui·none (an′thră-kwi′nōn). **1.** 9,10-Dioxoanthracene; the basis of natural cathartic principles in plants; used as a reagent. **2.** A compound containing 9,10-anthraquinone (1) as a part of its structure; this class of compound comprises the largest group of naturally occurring quinones.

an·thrax (an′thraks). **1.** A disease in humans caused by infection by cutaneous anthrax (q.v.) followed by septicemia with *Bacillus anthracis* from infected animals through traumatized skin; marked by hemorrhage and serous effusions in various organs and body cavities and by symptoms of extreme prostration. Rarely, infection is airborne, with no cutaneous lesion. SYN carbuncle (2). **2.** An infectious disease of animals, especially herbivores, due to presence in the blood of *Bacillus anthracis.* SYN charbon. [G. *anthrax (anthrak-),* charcoal, coal, a carbuncle]

cerebral a., a form of a., associated with pulmonary or intestinal a., in which the specific bacilli invade the capillaries of the brain causing violent delirium; frequently associated with hemorrhagic meningitis.

cutaneous a., the skin of *B. anthracis* infection characteristic lesion that begins as a papule and soon becomes a vesicle and breaks, discharging a bloody serum; the seat of this vesicle, in about 36 hours, becomes a bluish black necrotic mass; constitutional symptoms of septicemia are severe: high fever, vomiting, profuse sweating, and extreme prostration; the infection is often fatal. SYN malignant pustule.

intestinal a., a usually fatal form of a. marked by chill, high fever, pain in the head, back, and extremities, vomiting, bloody diarrhea, cardiovascular collapse, and frequently hemorrhages from the mucous membranes and in the skin (petechiae). SEE ALSO *mycosis* intestinalis.

pulmonary a., a form of a. acquired by inhalation of dust containing *Bacillus anthracis;* there is an initial chill followed by pain in the back and legs, rapid respiration, dyspnea, cough, fever, rapid pulse, and extreme cardiovascular collapse. SYN anthrax pneumonia, ragpicker's disease, ragsorter's disease, ragsorter's disease, wool-sorter's pneumonia, woolsorter's disease, wool-sorter's disease.

an·throne (an′thrōn). 9,10-dihydro-9-oxoanthracene; a reagent used in the detection of carbohydrates.

△anthropo-. Human. [G. *anthrōpos,* a human being (of either sex)]

an·thro·po·bi·ol·o·gy (an′thrō-pō-bī-ol′ō-jē). The study of the biologic relationships of humans as a species.

an·thro·po·cen·tric (an′thrō-pō-sen′trik). With a human bias, under the assumption that man is the central fact of the universe. [anthropo- + G. *kentron,* center]

an·thro·po·gen·e·sis (an′thrō-pō-jen′ĕ-sis). SYN anthropogeny.

an·thro·po·gen·ic, an·thro·po·ge·net·ic (an′thrō-pō-jen′ik, -jĕ-net′ik). Relating to anthropogeny.

an·thro·pog·e·ny (an-thrō-poj′ĕ-nē). The origin and development of man, both individual and racial. SYN anthropogenesis, anthropogony. [anthropo- + G. *genesis,* origin]

an·thro·pog·o·ny (an-thrō-pog′ō-nē). SYN anthropogeny.

an·thro·pog·ra·phy (an-thrō-pog′ră-fē). The geographical distribution of the varieties of mankind. [anthropo- + G. *graphō,* to write]

an·thro·poid (an′thrō-poyd). **1.** Resembling man in structure and form. **2.** One of the monkeys resembling man; an ape. [G. *anthrōpo-eidēs,* man-like]

An·thro·poi·dea (an′thrō-pō-id′ē-ă). A suborder of Primates, including man and the monkeys.

an·thro·pol·o·gy (an-thrō-pol′ō-jē). The branch of science concerned with origin and development of humans in all their physical, social, and cultural relationships. [anthropo- + G. *logos,* treatise]

applied a., a fusion of modern cultural a. and some aspects of sociology in the study of literate peoples in their cultures and deriving applications therefrom.

criminal a., a. in relation to the physical and mental characteristics, heredity, and social relations of the criminal. SEE ALSO criminology.

cultural a., study of all aspects of culture resulting from human behavior, including, among others, speech and language, systems of thought, social systems, and the artifacts produced by a culture.

physical a., the study of the physical attributes of human beings.

an·thro·pom·e·ter (an-thrō-pom′ĕ-ter). An instrument for measuring various dimensions of the human body.

an·thro·po·met·ric (an-thrō-pō-met′rik). Relating to anthropometry.

an·thro·pom·e·try (an-thrō-pom′ĕ-trē). The branch of anthropology concerned with comparative measurements of the human body. [anthropo- + G. *metron,* measure]

an·thro·po·mor·phism (an′thrō-pō-mōr′fizm). Ascription of human shape or qualities to nonhuman creatures or inanimate objects. Cf. theriomorphism. [anthropo- + G. *morphē,* form]

an·thro·pon·o·my (an-thrō-pon′ō-mē). The study of the laws

an

governing the development of the human species and the relation to the environment. [anthropo- + G. *nomos,* law]

an·thro·pop·a·thy (an-thrō-pop′ă-thē). Attribution of human feelings to nonhumans, *e.g.,* to gods or lower animals. [anthropo- + G. *pathos,* suffering]

an·thro·po·phil·ic (an′thrō-pō-fil′ik). Human-seeking or human-preferring, especially with reference to: 1) bloodsucking arthropods, denoting the preference of a parasite for the human host as a source of blood or tissues over an animal host; and 2) dermatophytic fungi which grow preferentially on humans rather than other animals. [anthropo- + G. *phileō,* to love]

an·thro·po·pho·bia (an′thrō-pō-fō′bē-ă). Morbid aversion to or dread of human companionship. SYN phobanthropy. [anthropo- + G. *phobos,* fear]

an·thro·pos·co·py (an′thrō-pos′kŏ-pē). Judging body type and build by inspection. [anthropo- + G. *skopeō,* to view]

an·thro·po·so·ma·tol·o·gy (an′thrō-pō′sō-mă-tol′ō-jē). That part of anthropology concerned with the human body, *e.g.,* anatomy, physiology, or pathology. [anthropo- + G. *sōma,* body, + *logos,* study]

an·thro·po·zo·o·no·sis (an′thrō-pō-zō′ō-nō′sis). A zoonosis maintained in nature by animals and transmissible to man; *e.g.,* rabies, brucellosis. Cf. zooanthroponosis, amphixenosis. [anthropo- + G. *zōon,* animal, + *nosos,* disease]

△**anti-.** 1. Against, opposing, or, in relation to symptoms and diseases, curative. 2. Prefix denoting an antibody (immunoglobulin) specific for the thing indicated; *e.g.,* antitoxin (antibody specific for a toxin). [G. *anti,* against, opposite, instead of]

an·ti·ac·id (an-tē-as′id). SYN antacid.

an·ti·ad·ren·er·gic (an′tē-ad-rĕ-ner′jik). Antagonistic to the action of sympathetic or other adrenergic nerve fibers. SEE ALSO sympatholytic.

an·ti·ag·glu·ti·nin (an′tē-ă-glū′ti-nin). A specific antibody that inhibits or destroys the action of an agglutinin.

an·ti·a·lex·in (an′tē-ă-lek′sin). SYN anticomplement.

an·ti·al·ler·gic (an′tē-ă-ler′jik). Relating to any agent or measure that prevents, inhibits, or alleviates an allergic reaction.

an·ti·an·a·phy·lax·is (an′tē-an′ă-fī-lak′sis). SYN desensitization (1).

an·ti·an·dro·gen (an-tē-an′drō-jen). Any substance capable of preventing full expression of the biological effects of androgenic hormones on responsive tissues, either by producing antagonistic effects on the target tissue, as estrogens do, or by merely inhibiting androgenic effects, such as by competing for binding sites at the cell surface.

an·ti·a·ne·mic (an′tē-ă-nē′mik). Pertaining to factors or substances that prevent or correct anemic conditions.

an·ti·an·ti·body (an′tē-an′tē-bod-ē). Antibody specific for another antibody.

an·ti·an·ti·tox·in (an′tē-an-tē-tok′sin). An antiantibody that inhibits or counteracts the effects of an antitoxin.

an·ti·a·rach·nol·y·sin (an-tē-ar-ak-nol′i-sin). An antivenin counteracting the poison (lysin) of a spider. [anti- + G. *arachnē,* spider, + lysin]

an·ti·ar·rhyth·mic (an′tē-ă-rith′mik). Combating an arrhythmia. SYN antidysrhythmic.

an·ti·ar·thrit·ic (an′tē-ar-thrit′ik). SYN antarthritic.

an·ti·asth·mat·ic (an′tē-az-mat′ik). SYN antasthmatic.

an·ti·au·tol·y·sin (an′tē-aw-tol′i-sin). An antibody that inhibits or neutralizes the activity of an autolysin.

an·ti·bac·te·ri·al (an′tē-bak-tēr′ē-ăl). Destructive to or preventing the growth of bacteria.

an·ti·bech·ic (an-tē-bek′ik). SYN antitussive. [anti- + G. *bēx* (*bēch-*), cough]

an·ti·bi·o·gram (an-tē-bī′ō-gram). Obsolete term for a record of the resistance of microbes to various antibiotics.

an·ti·bi·ont (an-tē-bī′ont). A microorganism producing antimicrobial substance.

an·ti·bi·o·sis (an′tē-bī-ō′sis). 1. An association of two organisms which is detrimental to one of them, in contrast to probiosis. 2. Production of an antibiotic by bacteria or other organisms inhibi-

tory to other living things, especially among soil microbes. [anti- + G. *biōsis,* life]

an·ti·bi·ot·ic (an′tē-bī-ot′ik). 1. Relating to antibiosis. 2. Prejudicial to life. 3. A soluble substance derived from a mold or bacterium that inhibits the growth of other microorganisms. 4. Relating to such an action.

antibiotic groups
aminoglycosides (e.g., streptomycin, gentamicin, sisomicin, tobramycin, amicacin)
ansamycins (e.g., rifamycin)
antimycotics *polyenes* (e.g., nystatin, pimaricin, amphotericin B, pecilocin) *benzofuran derivatives* (griseofulvin)
β–lactam antibiotics *penicillins* (penicillin G. and its derivatives, oral penicillins, penicillinase-fixed penicillins, broad-spectrum penicillins, penicillins active against *Proteus* and *Pseudomonas*) *cephalosporins* (e.g., cephalothin, cephaloridine, cephalexin, cefazolin, cefotaxime)
chloramphenicol group (chloramphenicol, thiamphenicol, azidamphenicol)
linosamides (lincomycin, clindamycin)
macrolides (e.g., erythromycin, oleandomycin, spiramycin)
peptides, peptolides, polypeptides (e.g., polymyxin B. and E., bacitracin, tyrothrycin, capreomycin, vancomycin)
tetracyclines (e.g., tetracycline, oxytetracycline, minocycline, doxycycline)
other antibiotics (phosphomycin, fusidic acid)

broad spectrum a., an a. having a wide range of activity against both Gram-positive and Gram-negative organisms.

transport a., A substance that makes biomembranes permeable to certain ions.

an·ti·bi·ot·ic-re·sis·tant. Indicating microorganisms that continue to multiply although exposed to antibiotic agents.

an·ti·bi·o·tin (an-tē-bī′ō-tin). SYN avidin.

an·ti·blen·nor·rhag·ic (an′tē-blen-ō-raj′ik). Rarely used term for: 1. Preventive or curative of a mucous discharge (blennorrhagia). 2. A remedy possessing such properties.

an·ti·body (Ab) (an′tē-bod-i). An immunoglobulin molecule with a specific amino acid sequence evoked in man or other animals by an antigen, and characterized by reacting specifically with the antigen in some demonstrable way, antibody and antigen each being defined in terms of the other. It is believed that antibodies may also exist naturally, without being present as a result of the stimulus provided by the introduction of an antigen: 1) in the broad sense any body or substance, soluble or cellular, which is evoked by the stimulus provided by the introduction of antigen and which reacts specifically with antigen in some demonstrable way; 2) one of the classes of globulins (immunoglobulins) present in the blood serum or body fluids of an animal as a result of antigenic stimulus or occurring "naturally." Different genetically inherited determinants, Gm (found on IgG H chains), Am (found on IgA H chains), and Km (found on K-type L chains and formerly called InV), control the antigenicity of the antibody molecule; subclasses are denoted either alphabetically or numerically (*e.g.,* G3mb1 or G3m5). The various classes differ widely in their ability to react in different kinds of serologic tests. SEE ALSO immunoglobulin. SYN immune protein, protective protein, sensitizer (1).

affinity a., the measure of the interaction between molecules such as a receptor and its ligand. This interaction is reversible.

agglutinating a., SYN agglutinin (1).

anaphylactic a., SYN cytotropic a.

anti-basement membrane a., autoantibodies to renal glomerular basement membrane antigens.

anticardiolipin a.'s, a.'s directed against cardiolipid, a phosphorylated polysaccharide ester of fatty acids found in cell membranes. Associated with immune-mediated illnesses, syphilis, and stroke;s thought to be from a hypercoagulable state.

anti-idiotype a., an antiantibody, the activity of which is directed specifically against the idiotype of a particular immunoglobulin (antibody) molecule. SYN idiotype a.

antinuclear a. (ANA), an a. showing an affinity for cell nuclei, demonstrated by exposing a cell substrate to the serum to be tested, followed by exposure to an antihuman-globulin serum conjugated with fluorescein; development of specific nuclear fluorescence is a positive reaction; this a. is found in the serum of a high proportion of patients with systemic lupus erythematosus, rheumatoid arthritis, and certain collagen diseases, in some of their healthy relatives, and in about 1% of normal individuals.

antiphospholipid a.'s, a.'s directed against phosphorylated polysaccharide esters of fatty acids, includes lupus anticoagulant, VDRL, and anticardiolipin a.'s. Associated with immune-mediated illnesses, syphilis, and stroke; thought to be from a hypercoagulable disorder.

avidity a., the sum total of the functional binding strength between a polyvariant and its a. The total binding strength represents the sum strength of all the affinity bonds.

bivalent a., a. that causes a visible reaction with specific antigen as in agglutination, precipitation, and so on; so-called because according to the "lattice theory" aggregation occurs when the antibody molecule has two or more binding sites that can cross-link one antigen particle to another; probably a characteristic of the class of immunoglobulin.

blocking a., (1) a. which, in certain concentrations, does not cause precipitation after combining with specific antigen, and which, in this combined state, "blocks" activity of additional a. added to increase the concentration to a level at which precipitation would ordinarily occur; **(2)** the IgG class of immunoglobulin which combines specifically with an atopic allergen but does not elicit a type I allergic reaction, the combined IgG a. "blocking" available IgE class (reaginic) a. activity.

blood group a.'s, see Blood Groups appendix.

catalytic a., an a. that has been altered to give it a catalytic activity. SYN abzyme.

cell-bound a., a term used for a. on the surface of cells that may be bound either through antigen combining sites or other sites such as the Fc region.

CF a., SYN complement-fixing a.

chimeric a.'s, a. that may have the FAB fragment from one species fused with FC fragment from another.

cold a., SEE cold *agglutinin.*

cold-reactive a., SEE cold *agglutinin.*

complement-fixing a., a. that combines with and sensitizes antigen leading to the activation of complement, which may result in cell lysis. SYN CF a., sensitizing substance.

complete a., SYN saline *agglutinin.*

cross-reacting a., (1) a. specific for group antigens, *i.e.,* those with identical functional groups; **(2)** a. for antigens that have functional groups of closely similar, but not identical, chemical structure.

cytophilic a., SYN cytotropic a.

cytotropic a., a. that has an affinity for certain kinds of cells, in addition to and unrelated to its specific affinity for the antigen

that induced it, because of the properties of the Fc portion of the heavy chain. SEE ALSO heterocytotropic a., homocytotropic a., cytotropic antibody *test.* SYN anaphylactic a., cytophilic a.

fluorescent a., an immunoglobulin (antibody) to which a fluorescent dye has been attached.

Forssman a., a heterogenetic a. specific for the Forssman group of heterogenetic antigens. SYN heterophil a., heterophile a.

heterocytotropic a., a cytotropic a. (chiefly of the IgG class) similar in activity to homocytotropic a., but having an affinity for cells of a different species rather than for cells of the same or a closely related species.

heterogenetic a., an a. that reacts to a heterogenetic antigen.

heterophil a., SYN Forssman a.

heterophile a., SYN Forssman a.

homocytotropic a., a. of the IgE class which has an affinity for tissues (notably mast cells) of the same or a closely related species and that, upon combining with specific antigen, triggers the release of pharmacological mediators of anaphylaxis from the cells to which it is attached; the tropism seems to be dependent upon the Fc portion of the antibody molecule; the Prausnitz-Küstner a. (IgE class of immunoglobulins) is the prototype for this a., but in anaphylaxis in the guinea pig, the homocytotropic a. involved is of the γG class. SYN reaginic a.

idiotype a., SYN anti-idiotype a.

immobilizing a., SYN treponema-immobilizing a.

incomplete a., (1) SYN univalent a. **(2)** SYN serum *agglutinin.*

inhibiting a., SYN univalent a.

lymphocytotoxic a.'s, a.'s specific for histocompatibility antigens of lymphocytes and which, upon combining with the antigens, induce cellular damage or death.

———

monoclonal a. (MAB, MoAb), an a. produced by a clone or genetically homogenous population of hybrid cells *i.e.,* hybridoma; hybrid cells are cloned to establish cell lines producing a specific a. that is chemically and immunologically homogeneous.

> Invented in 1975 by molecular biologists Cesar Milstein and Georges Kohler, the technique for producing such antibodies has become a mainstay of immunological research and medical diagnosis. MoAbs serve as experimental probes in a number of fields, including cell biology, biochemistry, and parasitology; and are used in purification of biological substances and certain drugs (e.g., interferon). Because of their high specificity in binding to target antigens, they provide far more accurate assays than conventional antiserum. Yoked to radionuclides, they have been employed therapeutically to deliver radiation doses directly to cancerous tissues.

———

natural a., SYN normal a.

neutralizing a., a form of a. that reacts with an infectious agent (usually a virus) and destroys or inhibits its infectivity and virulence; may be demonstrated by means of mixing serum with the suspension of infectious agent, and then injecting the mixture into animals or cell cultures that are susceptible to the agent in question.

nonprecipitable a., SYN nonprecipitating a.

nonprecipitating a., a. that, under conditions normally employed in precipitin tests, is refractory to precipitation by specific a., demonstrable when antigen is added serially in small amounts; nonprecipitating a. will precipitate under special conditions such as addition of complement. SYN nonprecipitable a.

normal a., a. demonstrable in the serum or plasma of various persons or animals not known to have been stimulated by specific antigen, either artificially or as the result of naturally occurring contact. SYN natural a.

P-K a.'s, igE a.'s involved in the Prausnitz-Kustner reaction.

polyclonal a. (pol-ē-klō′năl), a. that is derived from different clones of plasma cells but reacts with a particular a.

Prausnitz-Küstner a., one of the IgE class of a.'s first demonstrated by Prausnitz and Küstner by passive transfer to the skin. SEE homocytotropic a. SYN atopic reagin.

precipitating a., SYN precipitin.

reaginic a., SYN homocytotropic a.

treponema-immobilizing a., a., evoked during syphilitic infections, possessing specific affinity for *Treponema pallidum*, and which in the presence of complement immobilizes the organism. SYN immobilizing a., treponemal a.

treponemal a., SYN treponema-immobilizing a.

univalent a., an "incomplete" form of a. that may coat antigen, but which according to the "lattice theory" does not have a second receptor for attachment to another molecule of antigen; in the case of Rh+ erythrocytes, such an anti-Rh antibody may coat the cells but not cause them to agglutinate in saline; however, agglutination does occur when such coated cells are suspended in serum or other protein media, such as albumin, therefore called serum agglutinin. SYN incomplete a. (1), inhibiting a.

Vi a., a form of a. that agglutinates highly virulent strains of *Salmonella typhi, i.e.,* cells with Vi antigen; such bacteria are not agglutinable with O antiserum until the Vi antigen is destroyed. SEE Vi *antigen.*

Wassermann a., a., evoked during syphilitic infections, that combines with cardiolipin in the presence of lecithin and cholesterol; it is distinct from the treponema-immobilizing a.

an·ti·bra·chi·al (an-tē-brā′kē-ăl). Incorrect spelling of antebrachial.

an·ti·bra·chi·um (an-tē-brā′kē-ŭm). Incorrect spelling of antebrachium.

an·ti·bro·mic (an-tē-brō′mik). **1.** Deodorizing. **2.** A deodorizer. [anti- + G. *brōmos,* smell]

an·ti·cal·cu·lous (an-tē-kal′kyū-lŭs). SYN antilithic.

an·ti·car·i·ous (an′tē-kār′ē-ŭs). Preventing or inhibiting caries.

an·ti·ca·thex·is (an′tē-kă-thek′sis). In psychoanalysis, the shifting of an emotional charge to an impulse or action of an opposite character; *e.g.,* unconscious hatred expressed as conscious love. SYN counterinvestment.

an·ti·ceph·a·lal·gic (an′tē-sef-ă-lal′jik). Headache-relieving or preventing.

an·ti·chol·a·gogue (an-tē-kol′ă-gog). Rarely used term for an agent or process that reduces or suspends the flow of bile.

an·ti·cho·lin·er·gic (an′tē-kol-i-ner′jik). Antagonistic to the action of parasympathetic or other cholinergic nerve fibers (*e.g.,* atropine).

an·ti·cho·lin·es·ter·ase (an′tē-kō-lin-es′ter-ās). One of the drugs that inhibit or inactivate acetylcholinesterase, either reversibly (*e.g.,* physostigmine) or irreversibly (*e.g.,* tetraethyl pyrophosphate.

α-₁-an·ti·chy·mo·tryp·sin (an′ti-kī′mō-trip-sin). An inhibiter protein of the digestive protease, chymotrypsin.

an·tic·i·pate (an-tis′i-pāt). To come before the appointed time; said of a periodic symptom or disease, such as a malarial paroxysm, when it recurs at progressively shorter intervals. [L. *anticipo,* pp. *-cipatus,* to anticipate, fr. *anti* (old form of *ante*), before, + *capio,* to take]

an·tic·i·pa·tion (an-tis-i-pā′shŭn). **1.** Appearance before the appointed time of a periodic symptom or sign, such as a malarial paroxysm. **2.** Progressively earlier age of manifestation of a hereditary disease in successive generations; may be factitious (because of heightened awareness to early signs of the disease or because they are more conspicuous in the young) or authentic (because of progressive loss of epistatic and modifier genes by recombination and segregation).

an·ti·cli·nal (an-tē-klī′năl). Inclined in opposite directions, as two sides of a pyramid. [anti- + G. *klinō,* to incline]

an·tic·ne·mi·on (an-tik-nē′mē-on). SYN anterior *border* of tibia. [G. *antiknēmion*]

an·ti·co·ag·u·lant (an′tē-kō-ag′yū-lant). **1.** Preventing coagulation. **2.** An agent having such action (*e.g.,* warfarin).

lupus a., antiphospholipid antibody causing elevation in partial thromboplastin time; associated with venous and arterial thrombosis.

an·ti·co·don (an-tē-kō′don). The trinucleotide sequence complementary to a codon found in one loop of a tRNA molecule; *e.g.,* if a codon is A-G-C, its anticodon is U (or T)-C-G. The complementarity principle arises from Watson-Crick base-pairing, in which A is complementary to U (or T) and G is complementary to C. Sometimes called "nodoc".

an·ti·com·ple·ment (an-tē-kom′plĕ-ment). A substance that combines with a complement and so neutralizes its action by preventing its union with the antibody. SYN antialexin.

an·ti·com·ple·men·ta·ry (an′tē-kom-plĕ-men′tă-rē). Denoting a substance possessing the power of diminishing or abolishing the action of a complement.

an·ti·con·ta·gious (an′tē-kon-tā′jŭs). Preventing contagion.

an·ti·con·vul·sant (an′tē-kon-vŭl′sant). **1.** Preventing or arrest-

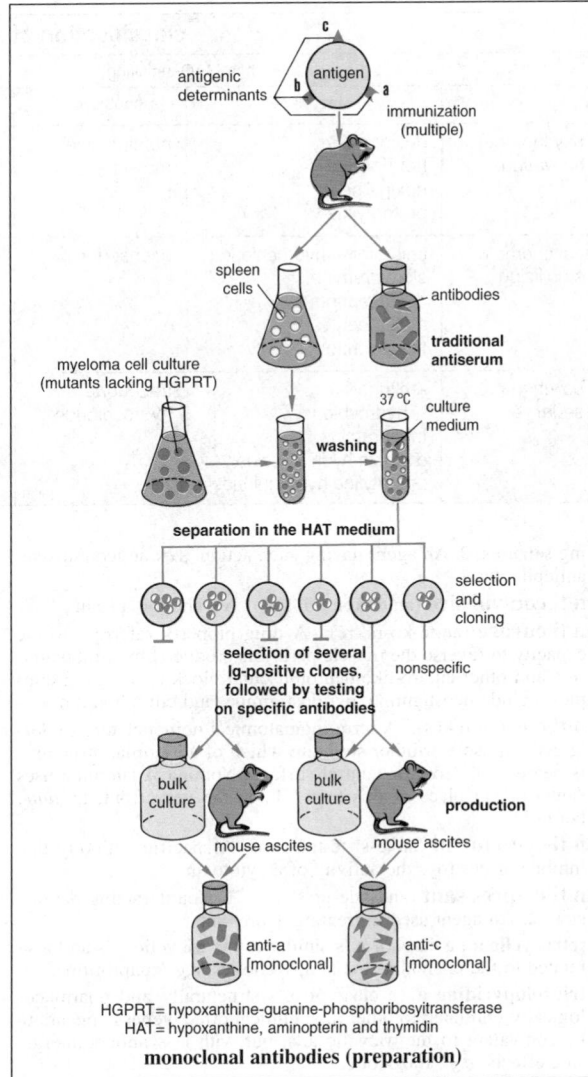

HGPRT = hypoxanthine-guanine-phosphoribosyitransferase
HAT = hypoxanthine, aminopterin and thymidin

monoclonal antibodies (preparation)

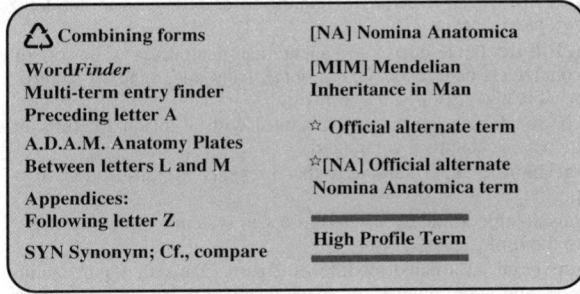

🔁 Combining forms	[NA] Nomina Anatomica
Word*Finder*	[MIM] Mendelian
Multi-term entry finder	Inheritance in Man
Preceding letter A	
A.D.A.M. Anatomy Plates	☆ Official alternate term
Between letters L and M	
	☆[NA] Official alternate
Appendices:	Nomina Anatomica term
Following letter Z	
	───────
SYN Synonym; Cf., compare	High Profile Term

classification of antidepressants				
non-MAO-inhibiting				MAO inhibiting
	tricyclic	nontricyclic	precursors	
psychomotor activating	desipramine nortriptyline noxiptiline protriptyline	nomifensine maleate		isocarboxazid iproclozid tranylcypromine
psychomotor stabilizing	imipramine hydrochloride clomipramine dibenzeprine melitracen dimetacrine	mianserine		
psychomotor sedative	amitriptyline hydrochloride trimipramine doxepin hydrochloride butriptyline hydrochloride	trazodone hydrochloride	L-tryptophan	

ing seizures. **2.** An agent having such action. SYN anticonvulsive, antiepileptic.

an·ti·con·vul·sive (an'tē-kon-vŭl'siv). SYN anticonvulsant.

an·ti·curare (an-tē-kō-rä'-rē). A drug property referring to the capacity to reverse the muscle paralysis produced by *d*-tubocurarine and other curare-like neuromuscular blocking drugs. Examples include neostigmine, pyridostigmine, and edrophonium.

an·ti·cus (an-tī'kŭs). A term in anatomical nomenclature to designate a muscle or other structure which of all similar structures is nearest the front or ventral surface. Nomina Anatomica uses "anterior" in place of this term. [L. in the very front, fr. *ante*, before]

an·ti·cy·to·tox·in (an'tē-sī-tō-tok'sin). A specific antibody that inhibits or destroys the activity of a cytotoxin.

an·ti·de·pres·sant (an'tē-dē-pres'ănt). **1.** Counteracting depression. **2.** An agent used in treating depression.

tetracyclic a., a class of a.'s similar to the tricyclic a.'s and also related to the phenothiazine antipsychotics; *e.g.,* maprotiline.

triazolopyridine a., a class of a.'s structurally and pharmacologically unrelated to other a.'s; clinical effectiveness appears to be equivalent to the tricyclic a.'s, but with less anticholinergic side effects; *e.g.,* trazodone.

tricyclic a., a chemical group of a. drugs that share a 3-ringed nucleus; *e.g.,* amitriptyline, imipramine, desipramine, and nortriptyline.

an·ti·di·a·bet·ic (an'tē-dī-ă-bet'ik). Counteracting diabetes; denoting an agent that lowers blood sugar.

an·ti·di·ar·rhe·al, an·ti·di·ar·rhet·ic (an'tē-dī-ă-re'ăl, -dī-ă-ret'ik). **1.** Having the property of opposing or correcting diarrhea. **2.** An agent having such action.

an·ti·di·u·re·sis (an'tē-dī-yū-re'sis). Reduction of urinary volume.

an·ti·di·u·ret·ic (an'tē-dī-yū-ret'ik). An agent that reduces the output of urine.

an·ti·di·u·re·tin (an'tē-dī-yū-ret'in). SYN vasopressin.

an·ti·dot·al (an-tē-dō'tăl). Relating to or acting as an antidote. SYN alexipharmac (1).

an·ti·dote (an'tē-dōt). An agent that neutralizes a poison or counteracts its effects. [G. *antidotos*, from *anti*, against, + *dotos*, what is given, fr. *didōmi*, to give]

chemical a., a substance that unites with a poison to form an innocuous chemical compound.

mechanical a., a substance that prevents the absorption of a poison.

physiologic a., an agent that produces systemic effects contrary to those of a given poison.

universal a., a dated mixture of 2 parts charcoal, 1 part tannic acid, and 1 part magnesium oxide intended to be administered to persons having consumed poison. The mixture is ineffective and no longer used; activated charcoal is useful.

an·ti·drom·ic (an-tē-drom'ik). Performing a nerve conduction study in such a manner that the nerve impulse is being propagated in a direction opposite to that in which the nerve fiber ordinarily conducts.

an·ti·dys·en·ter·ic (an'tē-dis-en-ter'ik). Relieving or preventing dysentery.

an·ti·dys·rhyth·mic (an'tē-dis-rith'mik). SYN antiarrhythmic.

an·ti·dys·u·ric (an'tē-dis-yū'rik). Preventing or relieving strangury or distress in urination.

an·ti·e·met·ic (an'tē-ĕ-met'ik). **1.** Preventing or arresting vomiting. **2.** A remedy that tends to control nausea and vomiting. [anti- + G. *emetikos*, emetic]

an·ti·e·ner·gic (an'tē-en-er'jik). Acting against or in opposition. [anti- + G. *energos*, active]

an·ti·en·zyme (an-tē-en'zīm). An agent or principle that retards, inhibits, or destroys the activity of an enzyme; may be an inhibitory enzyme or an antibody to an enzyme (*e.g.,* serum antitrypsin).

an·ti·ep·i·lep·tic (an'tē-ep-i-lep'tik). SYN anticonvulsant.

an·ti·es·tro·gen (an'tē-es'trō-jen). Any substance capable of preventing full expression of the biological effects of estrogenic hormones on responsive tissues, either by producing antagonistic effects on the target tissue, as androgens and progestogens do, or by competing with estrogens at estrogen receptors at the cellular level.

an·ti·fe·brile (an-tē-fē'brīl, -feb'ril). SYN antipyretic (1). [anti- + L. *febris*, fever]

an·ti·fibrillatory (an-tē-fī'bri-lă-tōr-ē). Any measure or medication that tends to suppress fibrillary arrhythmias (atrial fibrillation, ventricular fibrillation).

an·ti·fi·bri·nol·y·sin (an'tē-fī-bri-nol'i-sin). SYN antiplasmin.

an·ti·fi·bri·no·lyt·ic (an'tē-fī-brin-ō-lit'ik). Denoting a substance that decreases the breakdown of fibrin; *e.g.,* aminocaproic acid.

an·ti·fo·lic (an-tē-fō'lik). **1.** Antagonistic to the action of folic acid. **2.** Any agent with this effect. SEE ALSO folic acid *antagonists,* under *antagonist.*

an·ti·fun·gal (an-tē-fŭng'ăl). SYN antimycotic.

an·ti·G. In the strict sense, a term that means "antigravity" but, as commonly used, an adjectival term that implies protection against the effects of gravity (*e.g.,* anti-G *suit*).

an·ti·ga·lac·ta·gogue (an'tē-ga-lak'tă-gog). An agent for suppressing lactation.

an·ti·ga·lac·tic (an-tē-ga-lak'tik). Diminishing or arresting the secretion of milk. [anti- + G. *gala,* milk]

ANTIGEN

an·ti·gen (Ag) (an'ti-jen). Any substance that, as a result of coming in contact with appropriate cells, induces a state of sensitivity and/or immune responsiveness after a latent period (days to weeks) and which reacts in a demonstrable way with antibodies and/or immune cells of the sensitized subject *in vivo* or *in vitro*. Modern usage tends to retain the broad meaning of a., employing the terms "antigenic determinant" or "determinant group" for the particular chemical group of a molecule that confers antigenic specificity. SEE ALSO hapten. SYN immunogen. [anti(body) + G. *-gen,* producing]

ABO a.'s, see ABO blood group, Blood Groups appendix.

acetone-insoluble a., SYN cardiolipin.

allogeneic a. (al'ō-jĕ-ne'ik), genetic variations of the same a.'s within a given species.

Am a.'s, allotypic determinants (antigens) on human immunoglobulin alpha heavy chains.

Au a., (1) see Auberger blood group, Blood Groups appendix; (2) SYN Australia a.

Aus a., SYN Australia a.

Australia a., so-called because it was first recognized in an Australian aborigine, but now known to be an a. associated with hepatitis B virus surface antigen. SYN Au a. (2), Aus a.

Be^a a.'s, see low frequency blood groups, Blood Groups appendix. SYN Becker a.

Becker a., SYN Be^a a.'s.

Bi a., see low frequency blood groups, Blood Groups appendix. SYN Bile's a.

Bile's a., SYN Bi a.

blood group a., generic term for any inherited antigen found on the surface of erythrocytes that determines a blood grouping reaction with specific antiserum; a.'s of the ABO and Lewis blood groups may be found also in saliva and other body fluids; the genes controlling development of blood group a.'s vary in frequency in different population and ethnic groups. See also Blood Groups appendix. SYN blood group substance.

By a., see low frequency blood groups, Blood Groups appendix.

capsular a., that found only in the capsules of certain microorganisms; *e.g.,* the specific polysaccharides of various types of pneumococci.

carcinoembryonic a. (CEA), a glycoprotein constituent of the glycocalyx of embryonic endodermal epithelium, generally absent from adult cells with the exception of some carcinomas. It may also be detected in the serum of patients with colon cancer.

C carbohydrate a., an antigen found in the cell wall of *Streptococcus pneumoniae*. SEE β-hemolytic *streptococci,* under *streptococcus*.

CDE a.'s, see Rh blood group, Blood Groups appendix.

cholesterinized a., cardiolipin to which cholesterol has been added.

Chr^a a.'s, see low frequency blood groups, Blood Groups appendix.

class I a.'s, cell membrane bound glycoproteins that are coded by genes of the major histocompatibility complex.

class II a.'s, a cell membrane glycoprotein encoded by genes of the major histocompatibility complex. These antigens are distributed on a.-presenting cells such as macrophages, B cells, and dendritic cells.

class III a.'s, non-cell membrane molecules that are encoded by the S region of the major histocompatibility complex. These a.'s are not involved in determining histocompatibility and include the complement proteins.

common a., cross reacting antigen (epitope), a common antigen that occurs in 2 or more different molecules/organisms. SYN heterogenic enterobacterial a.

complete a., any a. capable of stimulating the formation of antibody with which it reacts *in vivo* or *in vitro,* as distinguished from incomplete a. (hapten).

conjugated a., SYN conjugated *hapten*.

D a., one of 6 antigens that compose the Rh locus. Antibody induced by D antigen is the most frequent cause of hemolytic disease of the newborn.

delta a., SYN hepatitis delta *virus*.

Dharmendra a., a chloroform-ether extracted suspension of *Mycobacterium leprae;* used to produce the Fernandez reaction in a lepromin test.

Di a., see Diego blood group, Blood Groups appendix.

Duffy a.'s, see Duffy blood group, Blood Groups appendix.

flagellar a., the heat-labile a.'s associated with bacterial flagella, in contrast to somatic a. SEE ALSO H a.

Forssman a., a type of heterogenetic a. found in dogs, horses, sheep, cats, turtles, eggs of some fish, in certain bacteria (*e.g.,* some strains of enteric organisms and pneumococci), and varieties of corn; usually found in the tissues and organs (not in blood), but is present in sheep erythrocytes, though not in this animal's tissues; with the exception of guinea pigs and hamsters, Forssman a. is not found in rodents, or in frogs, hogs, and most primates; the antibody that develops in infectious mononucleosis of man reacts specifically with the Forssman. a.

Fy a.'s, see Duffy blood group, Blood Groups appendix.

G a., an antigenic glycoprotein frequently associated with viral surfaces. [Ger. *gebundenes,* bound]

Ge a., see high frequency blood groups, Blood Groups appendix.

Gerbich a., glycophorin C. SEE glycophorins.

Gm a.'s, allotypic determinants (antigens) that are present on the heavy chain of immunoglobulin G. There are 25 different determinants present throughout the human population.

Good a., see low frequency blood groups, Blood Groups appendix.

Gr a., SYN Vw a. See Vw a. under MNSs blood group in Blood Groups Appendix.

group a.'s, a.'s that are shared by related genera of microorganisms.

H a., (1) the a. in the flagella of motile bacteria; so named because first identified in motile bacteria from a film (Ger. *Hauch*) of spreading growth on agar medium; SEE ALSO O a. (1). (2) the chemical precursor of a.'s of the ABO blood group locus.

H-2 a.'s, a.'s that are coded by the H-2 complex of genes in mice and are involved in self/nonself recognition.

He a.'s, see MNSs blood group, Blood Groups appendix. SYN Hu a.'s.

heart a., SYN cardiolipin.

hepatitis-associated a. (HAA), a term used for the surface a. of hepatitis B virus before its nature was established. SEE hepatitis B surface a.

hepatitis B core a. (HB_cAb, HB_cAg), the a. found in the core of the Dane particle (which is the complete virus) and also in hepatocyte nuclei in hepatitis B infections.

hepatitis B e a. (HB_eAb, HBe, HB_eAg), an a., or group of a.'s, associated with hepatitis B infection and distinct from the surface a. (HB_sAg) and the core a. (HB_cAg); it is associated with the viral nucleocapsid. Its presence indicates that the virus is replicating and the individual is potentially infectious.

hepatitis B surface a. (HB_sAb, HB_sAg), a. of the small (20 nm) spherical and filamentous forms of hepatitis B a., and a surface a. of the larger (42 nm) Dane particle (complete infectious hepatitis B virus). SEE ALSO hepatitis B core a., hepatitis B e a.

heterogeneic a., SEE heterophile a.

heterogenetic a., an a. which is possessed by a variety of different phylogenetically unrelated species; *e.g.,* the various organ- or tissue-specific a.'s, the alpha- and beta-crystalline protein of the lens of the eye, and Forssman a. SYN heterophil a.

heterogenic enterobacterial a., SYN common a.

heterophil a., SYN heterogenetic a.

heterophile a., an a. or antigenic determinant which is found in different tissues in more than one species.

hexon a., SEE hexon.

histocompatibility a., an a. on the surface of nucleated cells, particularly leucocytes and thrombocytes. SEE ALSO H-2 a.'s. SYN transplantation a.

HL-A a.'s, original designation for *h*uman *l*ymphocyte histo-compatibility a.'s determined by alleles at locus *A* (the first recognized); "HLA" is now the system designation, locus A being designated HLA-A. SEE human lymphocyte a.'s.

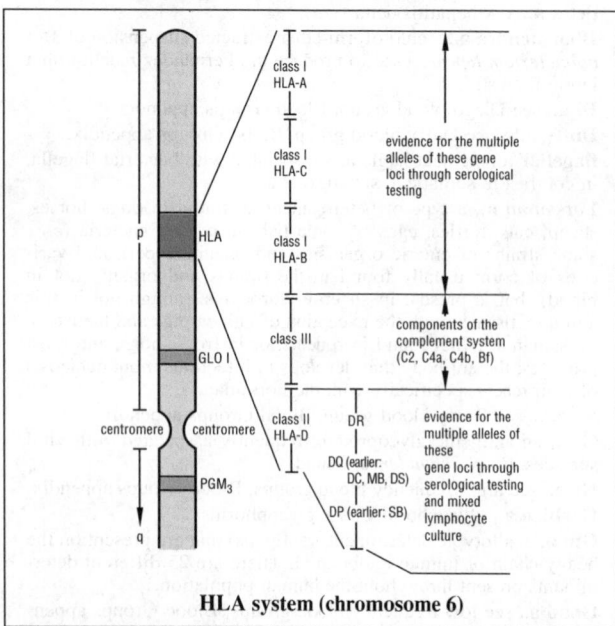

HLA system (chromosome 6)

Ho a., see low frequency blood groups, Blood Groups appendix.

homologous a. (hō′mō-log′us), the specific a. that generates the formation of an antibody that in turn can react with that antigen.

Hu a.'s, SYN He a.'s.

human leukemia-associated a.'s, a.'s on the surface of leuke-mic cells which seem not to be present on the surfaces of the same type of normal cells; the myeloblast a. of acute myeloge-nous leukemia found in chronic myelogenous leukemia is thought to be associated with a "blastic" transformation.

human lymphocyte a.'s (HLA) [MIM*142560], system desig-nation for the gene products of at least four linked loci (A, B, C, and D) and a member of subloci on the sixth human chromosome which have been shown to have a strong influence on human allotransplantation, transfusions in refractory patients, and cer-tain disease associations; more than 50 alleles are recognized, most of which are at loci HLA-A and HLA-B; autosomal domi-nant inheritance.

H-Y a., an a. factor, dependent on the Y chromosome, respon-sible for the differentiation of the human embryo into the male phenotype by inducing the initially bipotential embryonic gonad to develop into a testis; in the absence of this a., the indifferent gonad develops into an ovary. There are two loci involved, one that generates the a. [MIM*143170] and one that makes the receptor [MIM*143150], both are dominant.

I a.'s, see I blood group, Blood Groups appendix.

incomplete a., SYN hapten.

InV group a., SYN Km a.

Jk a.'s, see Kidd blood group, Blood Groups appendix.

Jobbins a., see low frequency blood groups, Blood Groups ap-pendix.

Js a., see Sutter Blood Group, Blood Groups Appendix.

K a.'s, see Kell blood group, Blood Groups appendix.

Km a., allotypic a.'s that are present on human kappa immuno-globulin light chains. SYN InV group a.

Kveim a., a saline suspension of human sarcoid tissue prepared from the spleen of an individual with active sarcoidosis; used in the Kveim test. SYN Kveim-Stilzbach a.

Kveim-Stilzbach a., SYN Kveim a.

Lan a., see high frequency blood groups, Blood Groups appen-dix.

Le a.'s, see Lewis blood group, Blood Groups appendix.

leukocyte common a. (lū′kō-sīt), family of glycoproteins found on most leukocytes and absent from other cell types. These cell surface a.'s can comprise up to 10% of the membrane proteins.

Levay a., see low frequency blood groups, Blood Groups appen-dix.

Lu a.'s, see Lutheran blood group, Blood Groups appendix.

lymphocyte function associated a. (LFA) (limf′ō-sit), a mem-ber of the integrin family that is expressed on all leukocytes and binds to ICAM-1 and ICAM-2 on a variety of cells.

lymphogranuloma venereum a., a sterile preparation of inacti-vated chlamydiae grown in the yolk sac of domestic fowl and used as an a. in the Frei *test*.

Lyt a.'s, a group of alloantigens that are present on either T or B murine lymphocytes, *e.g.,* Lyt 2,3 is equivalent to human CD8.

M a., an antigen found in the cell of *Streptococcus pyogenes;* associated with virulence. SEE β-hemolytic *streptococci,* under *streptococcus.*

M_1 a., M^g a., M^c a., M_2 a., see MNSs blood group, Blood Groups appendix.

Mitsuda a., an autoclaved suspension of human tissue naturally infected with *Mycobacterium leprae;* used to produce the Mitsuda reaction in a lepromin test.

MNSs a.'s, see MNSs blood group, Blood Groups appendix.

Mu a., see MNS blood group, Blood Groups appendix.

mumps skin test a., a sterile suspension of killed mumps virus in isotonic sodium chloride solution, used to determine suscepti-bility to mumps or to confirm previous exposure.

O a., (1) somatic a. of enteric gram-negative bacteria. External part of cell wall lipopolysaccharide; SEE ALSO H a. (1). (2) see ABO blood group, Blood Groups appendix.

oncofetal a.'s, tumor-associated a.'s present in fetal tissue but not in normal adult tissue, including α-fetoprotein and carcino-embryonic a.

organ-specific a., a heterogenetic antigen with organ specificity; *e.g.,* in addition to species-specific a., kidney of one species contains a. that is identical to that in kidney of other species. SYN tissue-specific a.

Ot a., see low frequency blood groups, Blood Groups appendix.

P a., see P blood group, Blood Groups appendix.

partial a., SYN hapten.

penton a., SEE penton.

pollen a., an extract of the antigenic protein from the pollen of plants; *i.e.,* pollen allergen, used in the diagnosis and prevention of hay fever.

private a.'s, see low frequency blood groups, Blood Groups appendix.

prostate-specific a. (PSA), a single chain 31 kilodalton glyco-protein with 240 amino acid residues and 4 carbohydrate side chains that is a kallikrein protease; found in normal seminal fluid and produced by the prostatic epithelial cells. Elevated levels of PSA in blood serum are associated with prostatic enlargement and prostatic adenocarcinoma, and this allows early detection of cancer in many cases.

> In about 70% of cases, the rise is owed to a cancerous condition. Thus, some studies have suggested that PSA testing may supplement an older test for prostatic acid phosphate (PAP), previously a fairly reliable gauge of metastatic prostate cancer. However, because no large-scale clinical studies have been completed, the medical and economic value of PSA testing remain uncertain.

public a.'s, see high frequency blood groups, Blood Groups appendix.

R a., SEE β-hemolytic *streptococci,* under *streptococcus.*

Rh a.'s, see Rh blood group, Blood Groups appendix.

Rhus toxicodendron a., an extract of fresh leaves of poison ivy, with 0.4% of procaine hydrochloride; used by intradermal injec-tion to determine sensitiveness to the poison of *Rhus toxicoden-dron.*

Rhus venenata a., an extract of fresh leaves of poison sumac;

used to determine sensitiveness to the plant or to relieve the dermatitis caused by contact with its leaves.

S a., SYN soluble a.

sensitized a., the complex formed when a. combines with specific antibody; so called because the a., by the mediation of antibody, is rendered sensitive to the action of complement.

shock a., an a. capable of producing anaphylactic shock in an animal that has been sensitized to it.

Sm a., see high frequency blood groups, Blood Groups appendix.

soluble a., viral a. that remains in solution after the particles of virus have been removed by means of centrifugation; in the case of the influenza viruses, it is the internal helical structure, free of the external envelope. SYN S a.

somatic a., an a. located in the cell wall of a bacterium in contrast to one in the flagella (flagellar a.) or in a capsule (capsular a.).

species-specific a., antigenic components in the tissues and fluids of members of a species of animal, by means of which various species may be immunologically distinguished; *e.g.,* serum albumin of horses is immunologically different from that of man, dogs, sheep, and so on.

specific a.'s, a.'s that characterize a single genus of microorganisms.

Stobo a., see low frequency blood groups, Blood Groups appendix.

Streptococcus M a., the somatic a. associated with virulence and type specificity of group A streptococci. SYN M protein (1).

Swᵃ a., see low frequency blood groups, Blood Groups appendix.

Swann a.'s, see low frequency blood groups, Blood Groups appendix.

T a.'s, tumor antigens associated wtih replication and transformation by certain DNA tumor viruses, including adenoviruses and papovaviruses. SEE ALSO β-hemolytic *streptococci,* under *streptococcus,* tumor a.'s.

Tac a., an antigenic determinant of the human interleukin 2 receptor that is identified by a murine monoclonal antibody, anti-Tac. Binding of this antigen prevents the proliferation of T cells, which is normally stimulated by binding interleukin-2.

T-dependent a., an a. that requires T helper cells in addition to appropriate B cells. Most a.'s are T-dependent.

theta a. (thā′tă), a surface glycoprotein that is present on thymocytes of mice and rats.

thymus-independent a., an a. that does not require T helper cell activation in order for the host's B cells to be stimulated. Repeating polymers such as polysaccharides are examples of T-independent a.'s.

tissue-specific a., SYN organ-specific a.

Tj a., see P blood group, Blood Groups appendix.

Trᵃ a., see low frequency blood groups, Blood Groups appendix.

transplantation a., SYN histocompatibility a.

tumor a.'s, (1) a.'s that may be frequently associated with tumors or may be specifically found on tumor cells of the same origin (tumor specific); **(2)** tumor antigens may also be associated with replication and transformation by certain DNA tumor viruses, including adenoviruses and papovaviruses. SYN neoantigens. SEE ALSO T a.'s.

tumor-associated a., a.'s that are highly correlated with certain tumor cells. They are not usually found, or are found to a lesser extent, on normal cells.

tumor-specific transplantation a.'s (TSTA), surface a.'s of DNA tumor virus-transformed cells, which elicit an immune rejection of the virus-free cells when transplanted into an animal that has been immunized against the specific cell-transforming virus.

V a., viral a. that is intimately associated with the virus particle, is protein in nature, has multiple antigenicities, and is strain-specific; antibody to such a. is demonstrable as protective or neutralizing antibody.

Vel a., see high frequency blood groups, Blood Groups appendix.

Ven a., see low frequency blood groups, Blood Groups appendix.

Vi a., "virulence a.," an external capsular a. of enterobacteria formerly thought to be related to increased virulence.

Vw a., see MNSs blood group, Blood Groups appendix. SYN Gr a.

Webb a., see low frequency blood groups, Blood Groups appendix.

Wrᵃ a., see low frequency blood groups, Blood Groups appendix.

Wright a.'s (Wrᵃ), see low frequency blood groups, Blood Groups appendix.

Xg a., see Xg blood group, Blood Groups appendix.

Ytᵃ a., see high frequency blood groups, Blood Groups appendix.

---

an·ti·ge·ne·mia (an′ti-jě-nē′mē-ă). Persistence of antigen in circulating blood; *e.g.,* HBₛ-antigenemia (presence of hepatitis B virus surface antigen in blood serum). [antigen + G. *haima,* blood]

an·ti·gen·ic (an-ti-jen′ik). Having the properties of an antigen (allergen). SYN allergenic, immunogenic.

an·ti·ge·nic·i·ty (an′ti-jě-nis′i-tē). The state or property of being antigenic. SYN immunogenicity.

an·ti·gon·or·rhe·ic (an′tē-gon-ō-rē′ik). Curative of gonorrhea.

an·ti·grav·i·ty (an-tē-grav′i-tē). SEE anti-G.

an·ti·HBc. Antibody to the hepatitis B core *antigen* (HBcAg).

an·ti·HBs. Antibody to the hepatitis B surface *antigen* (HBsAg).

an·ti·HB e. Antibody to the hepatitis B e *antigen* (HBeAg).

an·ti·he·lix (an-tē-hē′liks). An elevated ridge of cartilage anterior and roughly parallel to the posterior portion of the helix of the external ear. SYN anthelix [NA].

an·ti·helminthic (an′tē-hel-minth′ik). SYN anthelmintic (1).

an·ti·hem·ag·glu·ti·nin (an′tē-hē-mă-glū′ti-nin, an′tē-hem-ă-). A substance (including antibody) that inhibits or prevents hemagglutination.

an·ti·he·mo·ly·sin (an′tē-hē-mol′i-sin, an′tē-hem-ol′-). A substance (including antibody) that inhibits or prevents the effects of hemolysin.

an·ti·he·mo·lyt·ic (an′tē-hē-mō-lit′ik, an′tē-hem-ō-). Preventing hemolysis.

an·ti·hem·or·rhag·ic (an′tē-hem-ō-rāj′ik). Arresting hemorrhage. SYN hemostatic (2).

an·ti·hi·drot·ic (an′tē-hī-drot′ik, -hi-drot′ik). SYN antiperspirant.

an·ti·his·ta·mines (an-tē-his′tă-mēnz). Drugs having an action antagonistic to that of histamine; used in the treatment of allergy symptoms.

an·ti·his·ta·min·ic (an′tē-his-tă-min′ik). **1.** Tending to neutralize or antagonize the action of histamine or to inhibit its production in the body. **2.** An agent having such an effect, used to relieve the symptoms of allergy.

an·ti·hor·mones (an-tē-hōr′mōnz). Substances demonstrable in serum that inhibit or prevent the usual effects of certain hormones, *e.g.,* specific antibodies.

an·ti·hy·dri·ot·ic (an′tē-hī-drē-ot′ik). SYN antiperspirant.

an·ti·hy·drop·ic (an′tē-hī-drop′ik). **1.** Relieving edema (dropsy). **2.** An agent that mobilizes accumulated fluids.

an·ti·hy·per·ten·sive (an′tē-hī-per-ten′siv). Indicating a drug or mode of treatment that reduces the blood pressure of hypertensive individuals.

an·ti·hyp·not·ic (an′tē-hip-not′ik). **1.** Preventing or tending to prevent sleep. **2.** An arousing agent, or one antagonistic to sleep.

an·ti·hy·po·ten·sive (an′tē-hī′pō-ten′siv). Any measure or medication that tends to raise reduced blood pressure.

an·ti·ic·ter·ic (an′tē-ik-ter′ik). Rarely used term for preventing or curing icterus (jaundice).

an·ti·in·flam·ma·to·ry (an′tē-in-flam′ă-tō-rē). Reducing inflammation by acting on body mechanisms, without directly antagonizing the causative agent; denoting agents such as glucocorticoids and aspirin.

an·ti·-in·su·lin. A factor, usually an antibody, which antagonizes the action of insulin.

an·ti·ke·to·gen·e·sis (an′tē-kē-tō-jen′ĕ-sis). Prevention or reduction of ketosis either by decreased production or increased utilization of ketone bodies.

an·ti·ke·to·gen·ic (an′tē-kē-tō-jen′ik). Inhibiting the formation of ketone bodies, or accelerating their utilization.

an·ti·leu·koc·i·din (an′tē-lū-kos′i-din, lū-kō-sī′din). **1.** A substance that inhibits or prevents the effects of leukocidin. **2.** A leukocidin-specific antibody.

an·ti·leu·ko·tox·in (an′tē-lū-kō-tok′sin). A substance (including antibody) that inhibits or prevents the effects of leukocytoxin; frequently regarded as synonymous with antileukocidin.

an·ti·lew·is·ite (an-tē-lū′i-sīt). SYN dimercaprol.

an·ti·lip·o·tro·pic (an′tē-lip-ō-trop′ik). Pertaining to substances depressing choline synthesis (*e.g.*, by competing for methyl groups) and thus enhancing dietary fatty liver.

an·ti·lith·ic (an-tē-lith′ik). **1.** Preventing the formation of calculi or promoting their dissolution. **2.** An agent so acting. SYN anticalculous. [anti- + G. *lithos,* stone]

an·ti·lo·bi·um (an-tē-lō′bē-ŭm). SYN tragus (1). [L., fr. G. *antilobion*]

an·ti·lu·te·o·gen·ic (an′tē-lū-tē-ō-jen′ik). Inhibiting the growth or hastening involution of the corpus luteum.

an·ti·ly·sin (an-tē-lī′sin). An antibody that inhibits or prevents the effects of lysin.

an·ti·ma·lar·i·al (an′tē-mă-lā′rē-ăl). **1.** Preventing or curing malaria. **2.** A chemotherapeutic agent that inhibits or destroys malarial parasites.

an·ti·mer (an′ti-mer). SYN enantiomer.

an·ti·mere (an′ti-mēr). **1.** A segment of an animal body formed by planes cutting the axis of the body at right angles. **2.** One of the symmetrical parts of a bilateral organism. **3.** The right or left half of the body. [anti- + G. *meros,* a part]

an·ti·mes·en·ter·ic (an′tē-mez′en-ter′ik). Pertaining to the part of the intestine that lies opposite the mesenteric attachment.

an·ti·me·tab·o·lite (an′tē-me-tab′ō-līt). A substance that competes with, replaces, or antagonizes a particular metabolite; *e.g.*, ethionine is an a. of methionine.

an·ti·me·tro·pia (an′tē-me-trō′pē-ă). A form of anisometropia in which one eye is myopic and the other hypermetropic. [anti- + G. *metron,* measure, + *ōps,* eye]

an·ti·mi·cro·bi·al (an′tē-mī-krō′bē-ăl). Tending to destroy microbes, to prevent their multiplication or growth, or to prevent their pathogenic action.

an·ti·mi·tot·ic (an′tē-mī-tot′ik). **1.** Having an arresting action upon mitosis. **2.** A drug having such an effect; *e.g.*, a folic acid antagonist that is used in leukemia to inhibit the multiplication of white cells.

an·ti·mon·gol·oid (an-tē-mon′gō-loyd). The condition in which the lateral portion of the palpebral fissure is lower than the medial portion.

an·ti·mo·nid (an-tē-mō′nid). A chemical compound containing antimony in union with a more positive element; *e.g.*, sodium a., Na_3Sb.

an·ti·mo·nous ox·ide (an-ti-mō′nŭs). SYN *antimony* trioxide.

an·ti·mo·ny (Sb) (an′-ti-mō-nē). A metallic element, atomic no. 51, atomic wt. 121.757, valences 0, −3, +3, +5; used in alloys; toxic and irritating to the skin and mucous membranes. SYN stibium. [G. *anti* + *monos,* not found alone]

a. chloride, SYN a. trichloride.

a. dimercaptosuccinate, 2,3-dimercaptosuccinic acid cyclic thioantimonate; an antiparasitic effective against *Schistosoma mansoni* and *S. haematobium.* SYN stibocaptate.

a. oxide, SYN a. trioxide.

a. potassium tartrate, a compound used as an expectorant and in the treatment of schistosomiasis japonicum, although it is extremely toxic and must be administered very slowly intravenously; common toxic manifestations are phlebitis, tachycar-

dia, and hypotension; sudden deaths have been reported, chiefly from circulatory collapse. SYN potassium antimonyltartrate, tartar emetic, tartrated a.

a. sodium gluconate, SYN stibogluconate sodium (1).

a. sodium tartrate, $Na(SbO)C_4H_4O_6$; used in the treatment of schistosomiasis, and as an emetic. SYN sodium antimonyl tartrate.

a. sodium thioglycollate, a compound of a. trioxide and thioglycolic acid, used for tropical parasites.

tartrated a., SYN a. potassium tartrate.

a. thioglycollamide, $Sb(SCH_2CONH_2)_3$; the triamide of a. thioglycolic acid; used in the treatment of trypanosomiasis, kala azar, and filariasis.

a. trichloride, $SbCl_3$; combines with vitamin A to form a blue compound and with β-carotene to form a green one, as a method for assay of these substances; also used externally as a caustic. SYN a. chloride.

a. trioxide, Sb_2O_3; used technically in paints and flame-proofing; also used as an expectorant and emetic. SYN antimonous oxide, a. oxide, flowers of antimony.

an·ti·mo·nyl (an-tim′ō-nil). The univalent radical, SbO−, of antimony.

an·ti·mus·ca·rin·ic (an′tē-mŭs′kă-rin′ik). Inhibiting or preventing the actions of muscarine and muscarine-like agents, or the effects of parasympathetic stimulation at the neuroeffector junction (*e.g.*, atropine).

an·ti·mu·ta·gen (an-tē-myū′tă-jen). A factor that reduces or interferes with the mutagenic actions of effects of a substance.

an·ti·mu·ta·gen·ic (an′tē-myū-tă-jen′ik). Pertaining to or characteristic of an antimutagen.

an·ti·my·as·then·ic (an′tē-mī′as-then′ik). Tending toward the correction of the symptoms of myasthenia gravis, *e.g.,* as in the action of neostigmine.

an·ti·my·cot·ic (an′-tē-mī-kot′ik). Antagonistic to fungi. SYN antifungal. [anti- + G. *mykēs,* fungus]

an·ti·na·trif·er·ic (an′tē-nā-trif′er-ik). Tending to inhibit sodium transport.

an·ti·nau·se·ant (an-tē-naw′sē-ănt). Having an action to prevent nausea.

an·ti·ne·o·plas·tic (an′tē-nē-ō-plas′tik). Preventing the development, maturation, or spread of neoplastic cells.

an·ti·ne·phrit·ic (an′tē-nĕ-frit′ik). Rarely used term for preventing or relieving inflammation of the kidneys.

an·ti·neu·ral·gic (an′tē-nū-ral′jik). A rarely used term for an agent that relieves paroxysmal nerve pain.

an·ti·neu·rit·ic (an′tē-nū-rit′ik). A rarely used term for an agent that relieves nerve pain.

an·ti·neu·ro·tox·in (an′tē-nū-rō-tok′sin). An antibody to a neurotoxin.

an·tin·i·ad (an-tin′ē-ad). Toward the antinion.

an·tin·i·al (an-tin′ē-ăl). Relating to the antinion.

an·tin·i·on (an-tin′ē-on). The space between the eyebrows; the point on the skull opposite the inion. SEE ALSO glabella. [anti- + G. *inion,* nape of the neck]

an·tin·o·my (an-tin′ō-mē). A contradiction between two principles, each of which is considered true. [anti- + G. *nomos,* law]

an·ti·nu·cle·ar (an-tē-nū′klē-er). Having an affinity for or reacting with the cell nucleus.

an·ti·o·don·tal·gic (an′tē-ō-don-tăl-jik). **1.** Relieving toothache. **2.** A toothache remedy. [anti- + G. *odous,* tooth, + *algos,* pain]

an·ti·on·co·gene (an-tē-on′kō-jēn). A tumor-suppressing gene involved in controlling cellular growth; inactivation of this type of gene leads to deregulated cellular proliferation, as in cancer.

A number of antioncogenes have been identified. Their deletion, mutation, or inactivation opens the gateway for further cellular harm. Typically, the shut-off of an antioncogene results first in cell proliferation. In the presence of one or more oncogenes, this proliferation is accelerated and the cells become invasive.

an·ti·ox·i·dant (an-tē-oks′i-dănt). An agent that inhibits oxidation and thus prevents rancidity of oils or fats or the deterioration of other materials through oxidative processes (*e.g.*, ascorbic acid, vitamin E).

an·ti·pain (an′tē-pā-in). A peptide that inhibits the proteolytic enzymes, papain, trypsin, and plasmin. [*anti-* + pa*pain*]

an·ti·par·al·lel (an-tē-par′ă-lel). Denoting molecules that are parallel but point in opposite directions; *e.g.*, the two strands of a DNA double helix.

an·ti·par·a·sit·ic (an′tē-par-ă-sit′ik). Destructive to parasites.

an·ti·pa·ras·ta·ta (an′tē-pa-ras′tă-tă). Obsolete term for bulbourethral *gland*. [*anti-* + G. *parastatēs*, a testicle]

an·ti·pe·dic·u·lar (an′tē-pe-dik′yū-lăr). Destructive to lice.

an·ti·pe·dic·u·lot·ic (an′tē-pe-dik-yū-lot′ik). Effective in the treatment of pediculosis, especially denoting such an agent.

an·ti·pe·ri·od·ic (an′tē-pēr-ē-od′ik). Preventing the regular recurrence of a disease (*e.g.*, malaria) or a symptom.

an·ti·per·i·stal·sis (an′tē-per-i-stal′sis). SYN reversed *peristalsis*.

an·ti·per·i·stal·tic (an′tē-per-i-stal′tik). 1. Relating to antiperistalsis. 2. Impeding or arresting peristalsis.

an·ti·per·spi·rant (an-tē-per′spi-rant). 1. Having an inhibitory action upon the secretion of sweat. 2. An agent having such an action (*e.g.*, aluminum chloride). SYN anhidrotic (2). SYN antihidrotic, antihydriotic, antisudorific.

an·ti·phag·o·cyt·ic (an′tē-fag-ō-sit′-ik). Impeding or preventing the action of the phagocytes.

an·ti·phlo·gis·tic (an′tē-flō-jis′tik). 1. Older term denoting preventing or relieving inflammation. 2. An agent that reduces inflammation. SYN antipyrotic (1). [*anti-* + G. *phogistos*, burnt up]

an·ti·pho·bic (an-tē-fō′bik). A mechanism or drug designed to control phobias.

an·ti·plas·min (an-tē-plaz′min). A substance that inhibits or prevents the effects of plasmin; found in plasma and some tissues, especially the spleen and liver. SYN antifibrinolysin.

an·ti·plate·let (an-tē-plāt′let). A substance that manifests a lytic or agglutinative action on the blood platelets, thereby inhibiting or destroying the effects of the latter.

an·ti·pneu·mo·coc·cic (an′tē-nū-mō-kok′sik). Destructive to, or repressing the growth of, the pneumococcus (*e.g.*, penicillin).

an·tip·o·dal (an-tip′ŏ-dăl). Denoting opposite positions; positioned at opposite sides of a cell or other body.

an·ti·pode (an′ti-pōd). That which is diametrically opposite. [G. *antipous*, with the feet opposite]

    optical a., SYN enantiomer.

an·ti·port (an′tē-pōrt). The coupled transport of two different molecules or ions through a membrane in opposite directions by a common carrier mechanism (antiporter). Cf. symport, uniport. [*anti-* + L. *porto*, to carry]

an·ti·por·ter (an′tē-pōr-ter). A protein responsible for mediating the transport of two different molecules or ions simultaneously in opposite directions through a membrane.

an·ti·po·sic (an-tē-pō′sik). Rarely used term for: 1. Inhibitory to the drinking of water and other beverages. 2. An agent that has this effect. [*anti-* + G. *posis*, drinking, + *-ic*]

an·ti·pre·cip·i·tin (an′tē-prē-sip′i-tin). A specific antibody that inhibits or prevents the effects of a precipitin.

an·ti·pro·ges·tin (an′tē-prō-jes′tin). A substance that inhibits progesterone formation, that interferes with its carriage or stability in the blood, or that reduces its uptake by, or effects on, target organs (*e.g.*, RU-486).

an·ti·pros·tate (an-tē-pros′tāt). Obsolete term for bulbourethral *gland.*

an·ti·pro·throm·bin (an′tē-prō-throm′bin). An anticoagulant that inhibits or prevents the conversion of prothrombin into thrombin; examples are heparin, which is present in various tissues (especially in liver), and dicoumarin, which is isolated from partially decomposed sweet clover.

an·ti·pru·rit·ic (an′tē-prū-rit′ik). 1. Preventing or relieving itching. 2. An agent that relieves itching.

an·ti·pso·ric (an-tē-sō′rik). Obsolete term for curative of scabies, or of itching. [*anti-* + G. *psōra*, itch]

an·ti·psy·chot·ic (an′tē-sī-kot′ik). 1. SYN antipsychotic *agent*. 2. Denoting the actions of such an agent (*e.g.*, chlorpromazine).

an·ti·pu·rine (an′tē-pyūr′ēn). An analog of the purines and purine nucleotides that acts as an antimetabolite.

an·ti·py·o·gen·ic (an′tē-pī-ō-jen′ik). Preventing suppuration. [*anti-* + G. *pyon*, pus, + *-gen,* production]

an·ti·py·re·sis (an′tē-pī-rē′sis). Symptomatic treatment of fever rather than of the underlying disease.

an·ti·py·ret·ic (an′tē-pī-ret′ik). 1. Reducing fever. SYN antifebrile, febrifugal. 2. An agent that reduces fever (*e.g.*, acetaminophen, aspirin). SYN febrifuge. [*anti-* + G. *pyretos*, fever]

an·ti·py·rim·i·dine (an′tē-pir-im′i-dēn). An analog of the pyrimidines and pyrimidine nucleotides that acts as an antimetabolite.

an·ti·py·rine (an-tē-pī′rin, -pī′rēn). 2,3-Dimethyl-1-phenyl-3-pyrazoline-5-one; an obsolescent analgesic and antipyretic.
    a. acetylsalicylate, a compound of a. and aspirin; an antirheumatic and analgesic.
    a. salicylacetate, an analgesic, antirheumatic, and antipyretic.
    a. salicylate, an analgesic and antipyretic; used in dysmenorrhea, influenza, and acute rhinitis in the early stages.

an·ti·py·rot·ic (an′tē-pī-rot′ik). 1. SYN antiphlogistic. 2. Relieving the pain and promoting the healing of superficial burns. 3. A topical application for burns. [*anti-* + G. *pyrōtikos*, burning, inflaming]

an·ti·ra·chit·ic (an′tē-ră-kit′ik). Promoting the cure of rickets or preventing its development (*e.g.*, vitamin D preparations).

an·ti·rheu·mat·ic (an′tē-rū-mat′ik). 1. Denoting an agent which suppresses manifestations of rheumatic disease; usually applied to anti-inflammatory agents or agents that are capable of delaying progression of the basic disease process in inflammatory arthritis. 2. An agent possessing such properties (*e.g.*, gold compounds).

an·ti·ri·cin (an-tē-rī′sin). An antibody or antitoxin that inhibits or prevents the effects of ricin.

an·ti·ru·mi·nant (an-tē-rū′mi-nănt). Denoting a method to 1) control regurgitation of food or 2) break a compulsive trend of thought. [*anti-* + L. *rumino,* to chew the cud, fr. *rumen*, throat]

an·ti-S. See MNSs blood group, Blood Groups appendix.

an·ti·scor·bu·tic (an′tē-skōr-byū′tik). 1. Preventive or curative of scurvy (scorbutus). 2. A treatment for scurvy (*e.g.*, vitamin C).

an·ti·seb·or·rhe·ic (an′tē-seb-ō-rē′ik). 1. Preventing or relieving excessive secretion of sebum; preventing or relieving seborrheic dermatitis. 2. An agent having such actions.

an·ti·se·cre·to·ry (an′tē-sē-krē′tō-rī). Inhibitory to secretion, said of certain drugs that reduce or suppress gastric secretion (*e.g.*, ranitidine, omeprazole).

an·ti·sense (an′tē-sens). SEE antisense DNA, antisense RNA.

an·ti·sep·sis (an-tē-sep′sis). Prevention of infection by inhibiting the growth of infectious agents. SEE ALSO disinfection. [*anti-* + G. *sēpsis*, putrefaction]

an·ti·sep·tic (an-tē-sep′tik). 1. Relating to antisepsis. 2. An agent or substance capable of effecting antisepsis.

an·ti·se·rum (an-tē-sē′rŭm). Serum that contains demonstrable antibody or antibodies specific for one (monovalent or specific a.) or more (polyvalent a.) antigens; may be prepared from the blood of animals inoculated parenterally (under certain conditions) with an antigenic material or from the blood of animals and persons that have been stimulated by natural contact with an antigen (as in those who recover from an attack of disease). SYN immune serum.
    blood group a.'s, see Blood Groups appendix.
    heterologous a., an a. that reacts with (*e.g.*, agglutinates) certain microorganisms or other complexes of antigens, even though the a. was produced by means of stimulation with a different microorganism or antigenic material. SEE ALSO homologous a.
    homologous a., an a. in which there is complete correspondence between the content of antibodies and the antigenic material used for producing the a.
    monovalent a., SEE antiserum.
    nerve growth factor a., an a. containing antibodies against

nerve growth factor; when injected into newborn animals the majority of sympathetic ganglion cells are permanently destroyed, resulting in hypoinnervation of peripheral tissues. SYN NGF a.

NGF a., SYN nerve growth factor a.

polyvalent a., SEE antiserum.

specific a., SEE antiserum.

an·ti·shock gar·ment. SEE military antishock trousers, pneumatic antishock *garment.*

an·ti·si·al·a·gogue (an-tē-sī-al′ă-gog). An agent that diminishes or arrests the flow of saliva (*e.g.,* atropine). [anti- + G. *sialon,* saliva, + *agōgos,* drawing forth]

an·ti·si·der·ic (an-tē-sid′er-ik). Counteracting the physiological action of iron, probably by chelating or precipitation. [anti- + G. *sideros,* iron]

an·ti·so·cial (an-tē-sō′shŭl). Behaving in violation of the social or legal norms of society; *e.g.,* the antisocial personality, the psychopath. Cf. asocial.

an·ti·spas·mod·ic (an′tē-spaz-mod′ik). **1.** Preventing or alleviating muscle spasms (cramps). **2.** An agent that quiets spasm.

an·ti·staph·y·lo·coc·cic (an′tē-staf′i-lō-kok′sik). Antagonistic to staphylococci or their toxins.

an·ti·staph·y·lol·y·sin (an′tē-staf-i-lol′i-sin). A substance that antagonizes or neutralizes the action of staphylolysin.

an·ti·ste·ap·sin (an′tē-stē-ap′sin). An antibody counteracting the action of triacylglycerol lipase (steapsin).

an·ti·strep·to·coc·cic (an′tē-strep-tō-kok′sik). Destructive to streptococci or antagonistic to their toxins.

an·ti·strep·to·ki·nase (an′tē-strep-tō-kī′nās). An antibody that inhibits or prevents the dissolution of fibrin by streptokinase.

an·ti·strep·tol·y·sin (an′tē-strep-tol′i-sin). An antibody that inhibits or prevents the effects of streptolysin O elaborated by group A streptococci; the amount of a. in the serum is frequently increased during and after streptococcal disease, and comparative titers may be a diagnostic and prognostic aid.

an·ti·sub·stance (an-tē-sŭb′stans). Obsolete term for antibody.

an·ti·su·do·rif·ic (an′tē-sū-dōr-if′ic). SYN antiperspirant.

an·ti·-tac. Monoclonal antibody that recognizes a drain of the IL-2 receptor.

an·ti·te·tan·ic (an′tē-te-tan′ik). Preventing or alleviating muscular contraction.

an·ti·the·nar (an-tē-thē′nar). SYN hypothenar *eminence.*

an·ti·throm·bin (an-tē-throm′bin). Any substance that inhibits or prevents the effects of thrombin in such a manner that blood does not coagulate. A deficiency of a. results in impaired inhibition of coagulation factors IIa, IXa, and Xa in plasma, causing recurrent thrombosis.

a. III, an a. at present somewhat conjectural and biochemically not well characterized. Deficiency [MIM*107300] is commonly inherited as an autosomal dominant trait; one of the few known mendelizing disorders to which thrombotic disease occurs.

normal a., an a. naturally occurring in blood and certain tissues under normal conditions in contrast to abnormal states or a. from other sources.

an·ti·thy·roid (an-tē-thī′royd). Relating to an agent that suppresses thyroid function (*e.g.,* propylthiouracil).

an·ti·ton·ic (an-tē-ton′ik). Diminishing muscular or vascular tonus.

an·ti·tox·ic (an-tē-tok′sik). Neutralizing the action of a poison; specifically, relating to an antitoxin. SEE ALSO antidotal.

an·ti·tox·i·gen (an-tē-toks′i-jen). SYN antitoxinogen.

an·ti·tox·in (an-tē-tok′sin). Antibody formed in response to antigenic poisonous substances of biologic origin, such as bacterial exotoxins (*e.g.,* those elaborated by *Clostridium tetani* or *Corynebacterium diphtheriae*), phytotoxins, and zootoxins; in general usage, a. refers to whole, or globulin fraction, of serum from animals (usually horses) immunized by injections of the specific toxoid. A. neutralizes the pharmacologic effects of its specific toxin *in vitro,* and also *in vivo* if the toxin is not already fixed in the tissue cells. [anti- + G. *toxikon,* poison]

bivalent gas gangrene a., a. specific for the toxins of *Clostridium perfringens* and *C. septicum.*

bothropic a., a. specific for the venom of pit vipers of the genus *Bothrops* (*Bothrophora*) of the family Crotalidae. SYN Bothrops a.

Bothrops a., SYN bothropic a.

botulinum a., SYN botulism a.

botulism a., a. specific for a toxin of one or another strain of *Clostridium botulinum.* SYN botulinum a.

bovine a., a. prepared from cattle instead of horses, used in the treatment of persons who are sensitive to horse serum; the cattle are immunized against the toxin for which specific a. is desired.

Crotalus a., a. specific for venom of rattlesnakes (*Crotalus* species).

despeciated a., an antitoxic serum treated in an appropriate manner to alter the species-specific protein, so that a person sensitized to the animal protein is not likely to have a serious reaction when the a. is administered.

diphtheria a., a. specific for the toxin of *Corynebacterium diphtheriae.*

dysentery a., a. specific for the neurotoxin of *Shigella dysenteriae.*

gas gangrene a., a. specific for the toxin of one or more species of *Clostridium* that cause gaseous gangrene and associated toxemia, especially *C. perfringens C. novyi, C. histolyticum,* and commercially available preparations are usually polyvalent, *i.e.,* contain a. for two or more species. SYN pentavalent gas gangrene a.

normal a., serum that is capable of neutralizing an equivalent quantity of a normal toxin solution.

pentavalent gas gangrene a., SYN gas gangrene a.

plant a., a. specific for a phytotoxin.

scarlet fever a., a. specific for the erythrogenic toxin of strains of group A β-hemolytic streptococci.

staphylococcus a., a preparation from native serum containing antitoxic globulins or their derivatives that specifically neutralize the lethal, skin-necrosing, and hemolytic properties of the α-toxin of *Staphylococcus aureus.*

tetanus a., a. specific for the toxin of *Clostridium tetani.*

tetanus and gas gangrene a.'s, a mixture of antibodies obtained from animals immunized against the toxins of *Clostridium tetani, C. perfringens,* and *C. septicum.*

tetanus-perfringens a., an a. prepared from animals immunized against the toxins of *Clostridium tetani* and *C. perfringens* (*C. welchii*).

an·ti·tox·in·o·gen (an′tē-tok-sin′ō-jen). Any antigen that stimulates the formation of antitoxin in an animal or person, *i.e.,* a toxin or a toxoid. SYN antitoxigen. [antitoxin + G. *-gen,* producing]

an·ti·trag·i·cus (an′tē-traj′i-kŭs). SEE antitragicus *muscle.*

an·ti·tra·go·hel·i·cine (an′tē-trā′gō-hel′i-sēn). SEE antitragohelicine *fissure.*

an·ti·tra·gus (an-tē-trā′gŭs) [NA]. A projection of the cartilage of the auricle, in front of the tail of the helix, just above the lobule, and posterior to the tragus from which it is separated by the intertragic notch. [G. *anti-tragos,* the eminence of the external ear, fr. *anti,* opposite, + *tragos,* a goat, the tragus]

an·ti·trep·o·ne·mal (an′tē-trep-ō-nē′măl). SYN treponemicidal.

an·ti·tris·mus (an-tē-triz′mŭs). A condition of tonic muscular spasm that prevents closing.

an·ti·trope (an′ti-trōp). An organ or appendage that forms a symmetrically reversed pair with another of the same type, *e.g.,* the right and left legs of a vertebrate. [anti- + G. *tropē,* a turn]

an·ti·tro·pic (an-tē-trō′pik). Similar, bilaterally symmetrical, but in an opposite location (as in a mirror image), *e.g.,* the right thumb in relation to the left thumb.

an·ti·tryp·sic (an-tē-trip′sik). SYN antitryptic.

an·ti·tryp·sin (an-tē-trip′sin). A substance that inhibits or prevents the action of trypsin.

α_1-**an·ti·tryp·sin.** A glycoprotein that is the major protease inhibitor of human serum, is synthesized in the liver, and is genetically polymorphic due to the presence of over 20 alleles; individuals appropriately homozygous are deficient in α_1-trypsin and are predisposed to pulmonary emphysema and juvenile hepatic cirrhosis because of alterations in the amino acid and sialic acid components of the glycoprotein. α-a.'s also inhibits thrombin. SYN α_1-trypsin inhibitor, human α_1-proteinase inhibitor.

an·ti·tryp·tic (an-tē-trip'tik). Possessing properties of antitrypsin. SYN antitrypsic.

an·ti·tu·mor·i·gen·e·sis (an'tē-tū-mōr-i-jen'ĕ-sis). Inhibition of the development of a neoplasm.

an·ti·tus·sive (an-tē-tŭs'iv). **1.** Relieving cough. **2.** A cough remedy (*e.g.,* codeine). SYN antibechic. [anti- + L. *tussis,* cough]

an·ti·ty·phoid (an-tē-tī'foyd). Preventive or curative of typhoid fever.

an·ti·ve·nene (an-tē-vĕ-nēn'). SYN antivenin.

an·ti·ve·ne·al (an'tē-ve-nē'rē-ăl). Rarely used term for preventive or curative of venereal diseases. SYN antaphroditic (2).

an·ti·ven·in (an-tē-ven'in). An antitoxin specific for an animal or insect venom. SYN antivenene. [anti- + L. *venenum,* poison]

an·ti·vi·ral (an-tē-vī'răl). Opposing a virus; interfering with its replication; weakening or abolishing its action.

an·ti·vi·ta·min (an-tē-vī'tă-min). A substance that prevents a vitamin from exerting its typical biological effects. Most a.'s have chemical structures similar to vitamins (*e.g.,* pyridoxine and its a., deoxypyridoxine) and appear to function as competitive antagonists; some a.'s produce effects, in addition, that are unrelated to vitamin antagonism.

an·ti·viv·i·sec·tion (an'tē-viv-i-sek'shŭn). Opposition to the use of living animals for experimentation. SEE vivisection.

an·ti·xe·roph·thal·mic (an'tē-zē-rof-thal'mik). Denoting agents (vitamin A and retinoic acid) that inhibit pathologic drying of the conjunctiva (xerophthalmia). [anti- + G. *xēros,* dry, + *ophthalmos,* eye]

an·ti·xe·rot·ic (an'tē-zē-rot'ik). Preventing xerosis.

Anton, Gabriel, German neuropsychiatrist, 1858–1933. SEE A.'s *syndrome.*

Antoni, Nils, Swedish neurologist, 1887–1968. SEE A. type A *neurilemoma,* type B *neurilemoma.*

an·tra (an'tră). Plural of antrum.

an·tral (an'trăl). Relating to an antrum.

an·trec·to·my (an-trek'tō-mē). **1.** Removal of the walls of an antrum. **2.** Removal of the antrum (distal half) of the stomach; often combined with bilateral excision of portions of vagus nerve trunks (vagectomy) in treatment of peptic ulcer. [antrum + G. *ektomē,* excision]

⚠**antro-.** An antrum. [L. *antrum,* from G. *antron,* a cave]

an·tro·du·o·de·nec·to·my (an'trō-dū-ō-dĕ-nek'tō-mē). Surgical removal of the antrum of the stomach and the ulcer-bearing part of the duodenum.

an·tro·na·sal (an-trō-nā'săl). Relating to a maxillary sinus and the corresponding nasal cavity.

an·tro·phose (an'trō-fōz). A subjective sensation of light or color originating in the visual centers of the brain. SEE ALSO phosphene. [antro- + G. *phos,* light]

an·tro·py·lo·ric (an'trō-pī-lōr'ik). Related to or affecting the pyloric antrum.

an·tro·scope (an'trō-skōp). An instrument to aid in the visual examination of any cavity, particularly the antrum of Highmore maxillary sinus. [antro- + G. *skopeō,* to view]

an·tros·co·py (an-tros'cō-pē). Examination of any cavity, especially the antrum of Highmore, by means of an antroscope.

an·tros·to·my (an-tros'tō-mē). Formation of a permanent opening into any antrum (maxillary sinus). [antro- + G. *stoma,* mouth]

intraoral a., SYN Caldwell-Luc *operation.*

an·trot·o·my (an-trot'ō-mē). Incision through the wall of any antrum. [antro- + G. *tomē,* incision]

an·tro·to·nia (an-trō-tō'nē-ă). Tonus of the muscular walls of an antrum, such as that of the stomach.

an·tro·tym·pan·ic (an'trō-tim-pan'ik). Relating to the mastoid antrum and the tympanic cavity.

an·trum, gen. **an·tri,** pl. **an·tra** (an'trŭm, -trī, -tră). **1** [NA]. Any nearly closed cavity, particularly one with bony walls. **2.** SYN pyloric a. [L. fr. G. *antron,* a cave]

a. au'ris, SYN external acoustic *meatus.*

a. cardi'acum, a dilation that occasionally occurs in the esophagus near the stomach. SYN forestomach.

antra ethmoida'lia, SYN ethmoidal *sinuses,* under *sinus.*

follicular a., the cavity of an ovarian follicle filled with liquor folliculi.

a. of Highmore, SYN maxillary *sinus.*

mastoid a., a cavity in the petrous portion of the temporal bone, communicating posteriorly with the mastoid cells and anteriorly with the epitympanic recess of the middle ear via the aperture of the mastoid a. SYN a. mastoideum [NA], tympanic a., Valsalva's a.

a. mastoid'eum [NA], SYN mastoid a.

maxillary a., SYN maxillary *sinus.*

pyloric a., The initial portion of the pyloric part of the stomach, which may temporarily become partially or completely shut off from the remainder of the stomach during digestion by peristaltic contraction of the prepyloric "sphincter"; it is demarcated, sometimes, from the second part of the pyloric part of the stomach (pyloric canal) by a slight groove. SYN a. pyloricum [NA], antrum (2), lesser cul-de-sac.

a. pylor'icum [NA], SYN pyloric a.

tympanic a., SYN mastoid a.

Valsalva's a., SYN mastoid a.

ANTU Abbreviation for α-naphthylthiourea.

Antyllus, Greek physician, *ca.* 150 A.D. SEE A.'s *method.*

ANUG Abbreviation for acute necrotizing ulcerative *gingivitis.*

an·u·lar. SYN annular.

an·u·lus, pl. **an·u·li** (an'yū-lŭs, -lī) [NA]. ✫official alternate term for ring. [L.]

an·u·re·sis (an-yū-rē'sis). Obsolete term for inability to pass urine. [G. *an-* priv. + *ourēsis,* urination]

an·u·ret·ic (an-yū-ret'ik). Relating to anuresis.

an·u·ria (an-yū'rē-ă). Absence of urine formation.

an·u·ric (an-yūr'ik). Relating to anuria.

anus, gen. **ani,** pl. **anus** (ā'nŭs, -nī, -nŭs) [NA]. The lower opening of the digestive tract, lying in the cleft between the buttocks, through which fecal matter is extruded. SYN anal orifice. [L.]

artificial a., an opening into the bowel, usually in the right or left flank, as a result of a colostomy.

Bartholin's a., SYN a. cerebri.

a. cer'ebri, entrance to the cerebral aqueduct (of Sylvius) from the caudal part of the third ventricle. SYN aditus ad aqueductum cerebri, Bartholin's a., opening to cerebral aqueduct.

imperforate a., (1) SYN anal *atresia.* (2) SYN ectopic (1).

a. vesica'lis, rectal emptying into the urinary bladder.

vesicalis a. (ve-sĭ'kal-is), imperforate a. with urinary bladder opening into the a.

vestibular a., vulvovaginal a., a congenital malformation in which the a. is imperforate but the rectum opens into the vagina just above the vulva.

an·vil. SYN incus.

anx·i·e·ty (ang-zī'ĕ-tē). **1.** Apprehension of danger and dread accompanied by restlessness, tension, tachycardia, and dyspnea unattached to a clearly identifiable stimulus. **2.** In experimental psychology, a drive or motivational state learned from and thereafter associated with previously neutral cues. [L. *anxietas,* anxiety, fr. *anxius,* distressed, fr. *ango,* to press tight, to torment]

a. attack, an acute episode of anxiety.

castration a., SYN castration *complex.*

free-floating a., in psychoanalysis, a pervasive unrealistic expectation unattached to a clearly formulated concept or object of fear; observed particularly in a. neurosis and may be seen in some cases of latent schizophrenia.

noetic a., in existential psychotherapy, a. caused by confusion or loss of meaning in life.

separation a., a child's apprehension or fear associated with removal from or loss of a parent or significant other.

situation a., a. related to current life problems.

anx·i·o·lyt·ic (ang'zē-ō-lit'ik). **1.** SYN antianxiety *agent.* **2.** Denoting the actions of such an agent. [anxiety + G. *lysis,* a dissolution or loosening]

AOC Abbreviation for anodal opening *contraction.*

aor·ta, gen. and pl. **aor·tae** (ā-ōr'tă, ā-ōr'tē) [NA]. A large artery of the elastic type which is the main trunk of the systemic arterial system, arising from the base of the left ventricle and ending at the left side of the body of the fourth lumbar vertebra by dividing to form the right and left common iliac arteries. The a. is formed from: ascending a.; aortic arch; and descending a., which is divided into the thoracic a. and the abdominal a. SYN arteria aorta. [Mod. L. fr. G. *aortē,* from *aeirō,* to lift up]

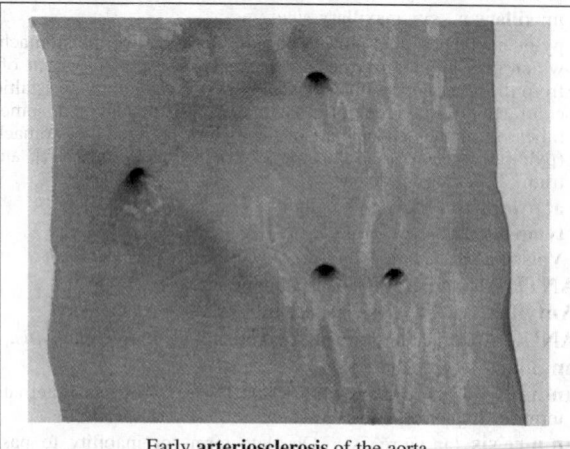

Early **arteriosclerosis** of the aorta.

abdominal a., the part of the descending a. that supplies structures below the diaphragm. SYN pars abdominalis aortae [NA], abdominal part of aorta, a. abdominalis.

a. abdomina′lis, SYN abdominal a.

a. angus′ta, congenital narrowness of a.

a. ascen′dens, SYN ascending a.

ascending a., the part of the a. prior to the aortic arch from which arise the coronary arteries. SYN a. ascendens, ascending part of aorta, pars ascendens aortae.

buckled a., SYN pseudocoarctation.

a. descen′dens, SYN descending a.

descending a., a part of the a., further divided into the thoracic a. and the abdominal a. SYN pars descendens aortae [NA], a. descendens, descending part of aorta.

dynamic a., abnormally marked pulsations of a.

kinked a., SYN pseudocoarctation.

overriding a., a congenitally malpositioned a. whose origin straddles the ventricular septum and so receives ejected blood from the right ventricle as well as from the left; it is found especially in tetralogy of Fallot.

primitive a., the paired aortic primordia in young embryos.

pseudocoarctation of the a., a rare abnormality of the arch of the a. that constricts that vessel but is not a true coarctation in that there is no significant encroachment on the lumen.

shaggy a., a colloquial but fitting description for severe arterial degeneration of the aorta, the surface of which is extremely friable and likely to cause atheroembolism.

thoracic a., the part of the descending a. that supplies structures as far down as the diaphragm. SYN pars thoracica aortae [NA], a. thoracica, thoracic part of aorta.

a. thorac′ica, SYN thoracic a.

ventral aortas, the paired vessels ventral to the pharynx, which give rise to the aortic arches.

aor·tal (ā-ōr'tăl). SYN aortic.

aor·tal·gia (ā-ōr-tal'jē-ă). Pain assumed to be due to aneurysm

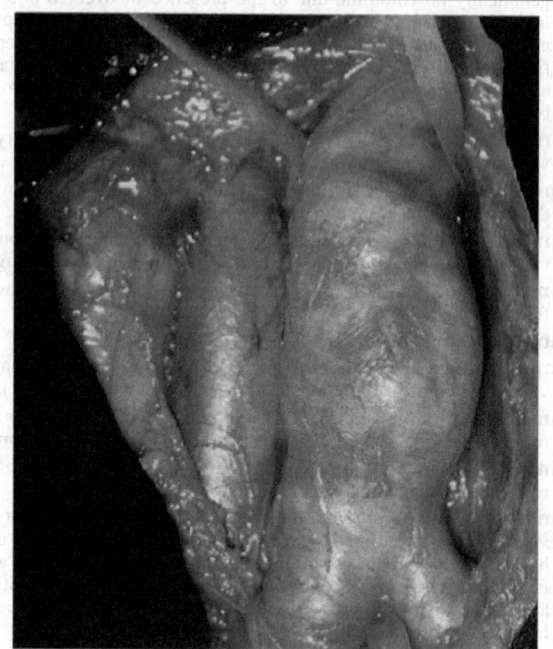

Aneurysm of the abdominal aorta (operative view); inferior vena cava at left.

or other pathologic conditions of the aorta. [aorta + G. *algos,* pain]

aor·tarc·tia (ā-ōr-tark'shē-ă). SYN aortostenosis. [aorta + L. *arcto,* properly *arto,* to narrow]

aor·tar·tia (ā-ōr-tar'shē-ă). SYN aortostenosis.

aor·tec·ta·sis, aor·tec·ta·sia (ā-ōr-tek'tă-sis, -tek-tā'zē-ă). Dilation of aorta. [aorta + G. *ektasis,* a stretching]

aor·tec·to·my (ā-ōr-tek'tō-mē). Excision of a portion of the aorta. [aorta + G. *ektomē,* excision]

aor·tic (ā-ōr'tik). Relating to the aorta or the a. orifice of the left ventricle of the heart. SYN aortal.

aor·tic cur·tain. an intertrigonal sheet of fibrous tissue between the aortic annulus and the anterior leaflet of the mitral valve.

aor·ti·co·re·nal (ā-ōr'ti-kō-rē'năl). Related to the aorta and kidney, specifically the ganglion aorticorenale.

aor·ti·tis (ā-ōr-tī'tis). Inflammation of the aorta.

giant cell a., giant cell arteritis involving the aorta.

syphilitic a., a common manifestation of tertiary syphilis, involving the thoracic aorta, where destruction of elastic tissue in the media results in dilation and aneurysm formation.

aor·to·cor·o·nary (ā-ōr'tō-kōr'ō-nār-ē). Relating to the aorta and the coronary arteries.

aor·to·gram (ā-ōr'tō-gram). The image or set of images resulting from aortography.

aor·tog·ra·phy (ā-ōr-tog'ră-fē). **1.** Radiographic imaging of the aorta and its branches, or a portion of the aorta, by injection of contrast medium. **2.** Imaging of the aorta by ultrasound or magnetic resonance. [aorta + G. *graphō,* to write]

retrograde a., a. by the injection of contrast medium into the aorta through one of its branches, *e.g.,* the brachial artery, in a direction against normal arterial blood flow.

translumbar a., early method of a. by injection into the abdominal aorta through a needle just below the twelfth rib and four fingerbreadths to the left of the spinal processes of the vertebrae.

aor·top·a·thy (ā-ōr-top'ă-thē). Disease affecting the aorta. [aorta + G. *pathos,* suffering]

aor·to·pex·y. A surgical procedure used to treat tracheomalacia or tracheal compression.

aor·to·plas·ty (ā-ōr′tō-plas′tē). A procedure for surgical repair of the aorta.

aor·top·to·sia, aor·top·to·sis (ā-ōr-top-tō′zē-ă, -top-tō′sis). A sinking down of the abdominal aorta in splanchnoptosia. [aorta + G. *ptōsis*, a failing]

aor·tor·rha·phy (ā-ōr-tōr′ă-fē). Suture of the aorta. [aorta + G. *rhaphē*, seam]

aor·to·scle·ro·sis (ā-ōr′tō-skler-ō′sis). Arteriosclerosis of the aorta.

aor·to·ste·no·sis (ā-ōr-tō-stě-nō′sis). Narrowing of the aorta. SYN aortarctia, aortartia. [aorta + G. *stenōsis*, a narrowing]

aor·tot·o·my (ā-ōr-tot′ō-mē). Incision of the aorta. [aorta + G. *tomē*, a cutting]

AP Abbreviation for *area postrema.*

APA Abbreviation for antipernicious anemia *factor.*

apall·es·the·sia (ă-pal-es-thē′zē-ă). SYN pallanesthesia. [G. *a*-priv. + *pallo*, to tremble, quiver, + *aisthēsis*, feeling]

apal·lic (ă-pal′ik). SYN apallic *state.* [G. *a*- priv. + L. *pallium*, brain mantle (cerebral cortex)]

apan·cre·at·ic (ă-pan-krē-at′ik). Without a pancreas.

apar·a·lyt·ic (ā-par′ă-lit′ik). Without paralysis; not causing paralysis.

apar·a·thy·re·o·sis (ă-par-ă-thī′rē-ō- sis). hypoparathyroidism, especially that caused by removal of the parathyroid glands. [G. *a*- priv. + parathyroid + *-osis*, condition]

apar·a·thy·roid·ism (ă-par-ă-thī′royd-izm). Congenital absence, deficiency, or surgical removal of the parathyroid glands, with an extreme degree of hypoparathyroidism.

apa·reu·nia (ă-par-yū′nē-ă). Absence or impossibility of coitus. [G. *a*- priv. + *para*, alongside, + *eunē*, bed]

ap·a·thet·ic (ap-ă-thet′ik). Exhibiting apathy; indifferent.

ap·a·thism (ap′ă-thizm). A sluggishness of reaction. Cf. erethism.

ap·a·thy (ap′ă-thē). Indifference; absence of interest in the environment. Often one of the earliest signs of cerebral disease. [G. *apatheia*, fr. *a*- priv. + *pathos*, suffering]

ap·a·tite (ap′ă-tīt). **1.** Generic name for a class of minerals with compositions that are variants of the formula D_5T_3M, where D is a divalent cation, T is a trivalent tetrahedral compound ion, and M is a monovalent anion; calcium phosphate a.'s are important mineral constituents of bones and teeth. SEE hydroxyapatite. **2.** $Ca_5(PO_4)_3(OH,F,Cl)$.

APC Acronym for *a*cetylsalicylic acid, *p*henacetin, and *c*affeine combined as an antipyretic and analgesic; antigen-presenting *cells*, under *cell*.

A-P-C. Abbreviation for adenoidal-pharyngeal-conjunctival.

ap·ei·do·sis (ap-ī-dō′sis). Rarely used term for departure from the normal histologic picture or the characteristic manifestations of a disease. [G. *apo*, away, + *eidos*, form]

apel·lous (ă-pel′ŭs). **1.** Without skin. **2.** Without foreskin; circumcised. [G. *a*- not + L. *pellis*, skin]

ap·en·ter·ic (ap-en-ter′ik). An obsolete term for abenteric. [G. *apo*, from, + *enteron*, intestine]

apep·sin·ia (ā-pep-sin′ē-ă). Rarely used term for lack of pepsin in the gastric juice.

ape·ri·od·ic (ā-pēr-ē-od′ik). Not occurring periodically.

aper·i·stal·sis (ā′per-i-stal′sis). Absence of peristalsis.

aper·i·tive (ā-per′i-tiv). Stimulating the appetite. [Fr. *apéritif*, from L. *aperio*, to open]

Apert, Eugène, French pediatrician, 1868–1940. SEE A.'s *hirsutism, syndrome.*

aper·to·gnath·ia (ă-per-tō-nath′ē-ă). An open bite deformity, a type of malocclusion characterized by premature posterior occlusion and absence of anterior occlusion. SYN open bite (2). [L. *apertus*, open, + G. *gnathos*, jaw]

ap·er·tom·e·ter (ap-er-tom′ě-ter). Instrument for measuring the angular aperture of a microscope objective.

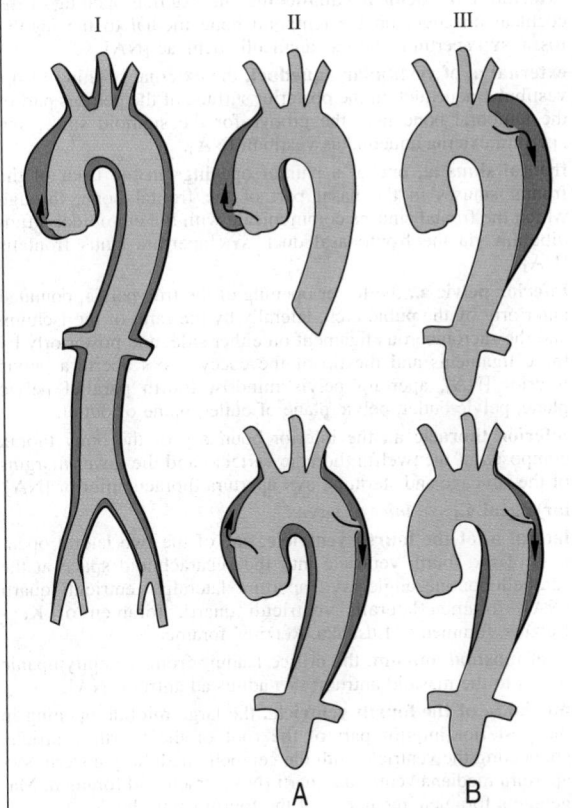

Classifications of acute dissecting **aneurysm** of the thoracic aorta: types I, II, and III (DeBakey); types A and B (Stanford).

ap·er·tu·ra, pl. **ap·er·tu·rae** (ap-er-tū′ră, -rē) [NA]. SYN aperture. [L. fr. *aperio*, pp. *apertus*, to open]

a. exter′na aqueduc′tus vestib′uli [NA], SYN external *aperture* of vestibular aqueduct.

a. exter′na canalic′uli coch′leae [NA], SYN external *aperture* of cochlear canaliculus.

a. latera′lis ventric′uli quar′ti [NA], SYN lateral *aperture* of the fourth ventricle.

a. media′na ventric′uli quar′ti [NA], SYN medial *aperture* of the fourth ventricle.

a. pel′vis infe′rior [NA], SYN inferior pelvic *aperture.*

a. pel′vis mino′ris, SYN inferior pelvic *aperture.*

a. pel′vis supe′rior [NA], SYN superior pelvic *aperture.*

a. pirifor′mis [NA], SYN anterior nasal *aperture.*

a. si′nus fronta′lis [NA], SYN frontal sinus *aperture.*

a. si′nus sphenoidal′is [NA], SYN *opening* of the sphenoidal sinus.

a. thora′cis infe′rior [NA], SYN inferior thoracic *aperture.*

a. thora′cis supe′rior [NA], SYN superior thoracic *aperture.*

a. tympan′ica canalic′uli chor′dae tym′pani [NA], SYN tympanic *opening* of canaliculi for chorda tympani.

ap·er·ture (ap′er-chŭr). **1.** An inlet or entrance to a cavity or channel. in anatomy, an open gap or hole. **2.** The diameter of the objective of a microscope. SYN aditus [NA], apertura [NA], opening. [L. *apertura*, an opening]

angular a., the angle, in air, of light that passes from the object to the ends of the diameter of the front lens of the microscope objective.

anterior nasal a., the anterior nasal opening in the skull. SYN apertura piriformis [NA], piriform opening.

external a. of cochlear canaliculus, the external opening of the cochlear aqueduct on the temporal bone medial to the jugular fossa. SYN apertura externa canaliculi cochleae [NA].

external a. of vestibular aqueduct, the external opening of the vestibular aqueduct on the posterior surface of the petrous part of the temporal bone near the groove for the sigmoid sinus. SYN apertura externa aqueductus vestibuli [NA].

frontal sinus a., one of a pair of openings in the floor of the frontal sinuses in the nasal part of the frontal bone, through which the frontal sinuses communicate with the ethmoidal infundibulum via the frontonasal duct. SYN apertura sinus frontalis [NA].

inferior pelvic a., the lower opening of the true pelvis, bounded anteriorly by the pubic arch, laterally by the rami of the ischium and the sacrotuberous ligament on either side, and posteriorly by these ligaments and the tip of the coccyx. SYN apertura pelvis inferior [NA], apertura pelvis minoris, fourth parallel pelvic plane, pelvic outlet, pelvic plane of outlet, plane of outlet.

inferior thoracic a., the inferior boundary of the bony thorax composed of the twelfth thoracic vertebra and the lower margins of the rib cage and sternum. SYN apertura thoracis inferior [NA].

laryngeal a., SYN *inlet* of larynx.

lateral a. of the fourth ventricle, one of the two lateral openings of the fourth ventricle into the subarachnoid space at the cerebellopontine angle. SYN apertura lateralis ventriculi quarti [NA], foramen lateralis ventriculi quarti, foramen of Key-Retzius, foramen of Luschka, Retzius' foramen.

a. of mastoid antrum, the orifice leading from the epitympanic recess to the mastoid antrum. SYN aditus ad antrum [NA].

medial a. of the fourth ventricle, the large midline opening in the posterior inferior part of the roof of the fourth ventricle, connecting the ventricle with the cerebellomedullary cistern. SYN apertura mediana ventriculi quarti [NA], arachnoid foramen, Magendie's foramen, median a. of the fourth ventricle.

median a. of the fourth ventricle, SYN medial a. of the fourth ventricle.

numerical a. (N.A.), defined by the formula n sine a, where n is the refractive index of the medium between the object and objective lens and a is the angle between the central and the marginal ray entering the objective.

a. of orbit, SYN orbital *opening*.

sphenoidal sinus a., SYN *opening* of the sphenoidal sinus.

superior pelvic a., the upper opening of the true pelvis, bounded anteriorly by the pubic symphysis and the pubic crest on either side, laterally by the iliopectineal lines, and posteriorly by the promontory of the sacrum. SYN apertura pelvis superior [NA], aditus pelvis, first parallel pelvic plane, pelvic brim, pelvic inlet, pelvic plane of inlet, plane of inlet.

superior thoracic a., the upper boundary of the bony thorax composed of the first thoracic vertebra and the upper margins of the first ribs and manubrium of the sternum. SYN apertura thoracis superior [NA].

apex, gen. **ap·i·cis,** pl. **ap·i·ces** (ā′peks, ap′i-sis, ap′i-sēs) [NA]. The extremity of a conical or pyramidal structure, such as the heart or the lung. [L. summit or tip]

a. of arytenoid cartilage, the pointed upper end of the cartilage which supports the corniculate cartilage and the aryepiglottic fold. SYN a. cartilaginis arytenoideae [NA].

a. auric′ulae [NA], SYN *tip* of auricle.

a. cap′itis fib′ulae [NA], SYN a. of head of fibula.

a. cartila′ginis arytenoi′deae [NA], SYN a. of arytenoid cartilage.

a. cor′dis [NA], SYN a. of heart.

a. cor′nus posterio′ris [NA], SYN a. of the posterior horn.

a. cus′pidis den′tis [NA], SYN a. of cusp of tooth.

a. of cusp of tooth, the tip of the peaklike projections from the crown of a tooth. SYN a. cuspidis dentis [NA].

a. of dens, the tip of the dens of the axis to which is attached the apical ligament of the dens. SYN a. dentis [NA].

a. den′tis [NA], SYN a. of dens.

a. of head of fibula, the pointed upper end of the fibular head to which is attached the arcuate popliteal ligament and part of the biceps femoris tendon. SYN a. capitis fibulae [NA], styloid process of fibula.

a. of heart, the blunt extremity of the heart formed by the left ventricle. SEE apex *beat*. SYN a. cordis [NA], vertex cordis.

a. lin′guae [NA], SYN *tip* of tongue.

a. of lung, the rounded, upper extremity of each lung that extends into the cupula of the pleura. SYN a. pulmonis [NA].

a. na′si [NA], SYN *tip* of nose.

a. of orbit, the posterior part of the orbit into which the optic canal opens; forms the tip of the pyramidal-shaped space.

a. os′sis sa′cri [NA], SYN a. of sacrum.

a. par′tis petro′sae ossis temporalis [NA], SYN a. of petrous part of temporal bone.

a. of patella, the pointed lower end of the patella from which the ligamentum patellae passes to insert on the tibial tuberosity. SYN a. patellae [NA].

a. patel′lae [NA], SYN a. of patella.

a. of petrous part of temporal bone, the irregular antero-medial extremity of the petrous part on which the anterior end of the carotid canal opens. SYN a. partis petrosae ossis temporalis [NA].

a. of the posterior horn, the pointed extremity of each posterior gray column or cornu of the spinal cord. SYN a. cornus posterioris [NA], caput cornus, tip of posterior horn.

a. pro′statae [NA], SYN a. of prostate.

a. of prostate, the lowermost part of the prostate, situated above the urogenital diaphragm. SYN a. prostatae [NA].

a. pulmo′nis [NA], SYN a. of lung.

a. rad′icis den′tis [NA], SYN *tip* of tooth root.

root a., SYN *tip* of tooth root.

a. of sacrum, the tapering lower end of the sacrum that articulates with the coccyx. SYN a. ossis sacri [NA].

a. sat′yri, SYN *tip* of auricle.

a. of urinary bladder, the junction of the superior and anteroinferior surfaces of the bladder, continuous above with the median umbilical ligament. SYN a. vesicae [NA].

a. vesi′cae [NA], SYN a. of urinary bladder.

apex·car·di·o·gram (ā-peks-kar′dē-ō-gram). Graphic recording of the movements of the chest wall produced by the apex beat of the heart.

apex·car·di·og·ra·phy (ā′peks-kar′dē-og-ră-fē). Noninvasive graphic recording of cardiac pulsations from the region of the apex, usually of the left ventricle, and resembling the ventricular pressure curve.

apex·i·fi·ca·tion (ā-pek′si-fi-kā′shŭn). Induced tooth root development or closure of the root apex by hard tissue deposition.

apex·i·graph (ā-pek′si-graf). A device for determining the size and position of the apex of a tooth root. [apex + G. *graphō*, to write]

APF Abbreviation for animal protein *factor*.

Apgar, Virginia, U.S. anesthesiologist, 1909–1974. SEE A. *score*.

apha·gia (ă-fā′jē-ă). Inability to eat. [G. *a-* priv. + *phagō*, to eat]

apha·kia (ă-fā′kē-ă). Absence of the lens of the eye. [G. *a-* priv. + *phakos*, lentil, anything shaped like a lentil]

apha·lan·gia (ă-fă-lan′jē-ă). Congenital absence of a digit, or more specifically, absence of one or more of the long bones (phalanges) of a finger or toe. [G. *a-* priv. + phalanx]

aphan·i·sis (ă-fan′i-sis). Loss of sexuality. [G. *aphaneia,* disappearance]

apha·sia (ă-fā′zē-ă). Impaired or absent comprehension or production of, or communication by, speech, writing, or signs, due to an acquired lesion of the dominant cerebral hemisphere. SYN alogia (1), anepia, logagnosia, logamnesia, logasthenia. [G. speechlessness, fr. *a-* priv. + *phasis,* speech]

acoustic a., SYN auditory a.

acquired epileptic a., SYN Landau-Kleffner *syndrome.*

amnestic a., amnesic a., SYN nominal a.

anomic a., SYN nominal a.

anterior a., SYN motor a.

associative a., SYN conduction a.

ataxic a., SYN motor a.

auditory a., an impairment in comprehension of the auditory forms of language and communication, including the ability to write from dictation in the presence of normal hearing. Spontaneous speech, reading, and writing are not affected. SYN acoustic a., word deafness.

Broca's a., SYN motor a.

conduction a., a form of a. in which the patient understands spoken and written words, is aware of his deficit, and can speak and write, but skips or repeats words, or substitutes one word for another (paraphasia);word repetition is severely impaired. The responsible lesion is in the associate tracks connecting the various language centers. SYN associative a.

crossed a., a. in a right-handed person due to a solely right cerebral lesion.

expressive a., SYN motor a.

fluent a., SYN sensory a.

functional a., nonorganic a. related to conversion hysteria.

global a., in which all aspects of speech and communication are severely impaired. At best, patients can understand or speak only a few words or phrases; they cannot read or write. SYN mixed a., total a.

graphic a., SYN agraphia.

graphomotor a., SYN agraphia.

impressive a., SYN sensory a.

jargon a., SYN agrammatism.

Kussmaul's a., mutism in psychosis; a misnomer; not actually an aphasia.

mixed a., SYN global a.

motor a., a type of a. in which there is a deficit in speech production or language output, often accompanied by a deficit in communicating by writing, signs, etc. The patient is aware of his impairment. SYN anterior a., ataxic a., Broca's a., expressive a., nonfluent a.

nominal a., an a. in which the principal deficit is difficulty in naming persons and objects seen, heard, or felt; due to lesions in various portions of the language area. SYN amnestic a., amnesic a., anomia, anomic a.

nonfluent a., SYN motor a.

pathematic a., mutism related to anger or strong emotions.

posterior a., SYN sensory a.

psychosensory a., SYN sensory a.

pure a.'s, rare a.'s affecting only one type of communication, *e.g.,* reading, while related communication forms such as writing, auditory comprehension, etc. remain intact.

receptive a., SYN sensory a.

semantic a., a. in which objects are correctly named; there is little disturbance in the articulation of words; individual words are understood, but the broader meaning of what is heard cannot be grasped.

sensory a., a. in which there is impairment in the comprehension of spoken and written words, associated with effortless, articulated, but paraphrasic, speech and writing; malformed words, substitute words, and enologisms are charcteristic. When severe, and speech is incomprehensible, it is called jargon a. The patient often appears unaware of his deficit. SYN fluent a., impressive a., posterior a., psychosensory a., receptive a., Wernicke's a.

syntactical a., a. in which the words are fairly well pronounced but are spoken in short phrases or poorly constructed sentences without articles, prepositions, or conjunctions.

total a., SYN global a.

transcortical a., an a. in which the unaffected motor and sensory language areas are isolated from the rest of the hemispheric

cortex. Subdivided into transcortical sensory and transcortical motor a.'s.

visual a., (1) SYN alexia. **(2)** improperly used as a synonym for anomia.

Wernicke's a., SYN sensory a.

apha·si·ac, apha·sic (ă-fā′zē-ak, ă-fā′sik). Relating to or suffering from aphasia.

apha·si·ol·o·gist (ă-fā′zē-ol′ŏ-gist). A specialist who deals with speech disorders caused by dysfunction of the language areas of the brain.

apha·si·ol·o·gy (ă-fā′zē-ol′ŏ-gē). The science of speech disorders caused by dysfunction of the cerebral language areas.

aphas·mid (ă-faz′mid). **1.** Lacking phasmids, as seen in nematodes of the class Adenophorasida (Aphasmidia). **2.** Common name for a member of the class Aphasmidia, now Adenophorasida.

Aphas·mid·ia (ă-faz-mid′ē-ă). SYN Adenophorasida.

aph·e·li·ot·ro·pism (ap-hē-lē-ot′rō-pizm). Negative heliotaxis. [G. *apo,* away, + *helios,* sun, + *tropein,* to turn]

aphe·mes·the·sia (ă-fē-mes-thē′zē-ă). Loss of the sense of articulate speech; inability to recognize what one is saying. [G. *a-* priv. + *phēmē,* speech, + *aisthēsis,* sensation]

aphe·mia (ă-fē′mē-ă). Obsolete term for a form of motor aphasia in which the ability to express ideas in spoken words is lost. [a- priv. + G. *phēmē,* voice]

aphe·mic (ă-fē′mik). Relating to aphemia.

aphe·pho·bia (a-fē-fō′bē-ă). SYN haphephobia.

apher·e·sis (ă-fer-ē′sis). Infusion of a patient's own blood from which certain cellular or fluid elements have been removed. [G. *aphairesis,* withdrawal]

aphil·op·o·ny (ă-fil-op′ō-nē). Obsolete term for an aversion, or lack of desire, to work. [G. *a-* priv. + *philō,* to like, + *ponos,* work]

apho·nia (ă-fō′nē-ă). Loss of the voice as a result of disease or injury to the larynx. [G. *a-* priv. + *phōnē,* voice]

hysterical a., loss of voice for psychogenic reasons, as in some varieties of hysteria. SYN nonorganic a.

nonorganic a., SYN hysterical a.

a. paralyt′ica, a. due to paralysis of the vocal cords.

spastic a., a. caused by spasmodic contraction of the laryngeal adductor muscles provoked by attempted phonation.

aphon·ic (ă-fon′ik). Relating to aphonia. SYN aphonous.

apho·no·ge·lia (ă-fon-ō-jē′lē-ă). Inability to laugh out loud. [G. *a-* priv. + *phonē,* sound, + *gelān,* to laugh]

aph·o·nous (af′ō-nŭs). SYN aphonic.

apho·tes·the·sia (ă-fō-tes-thē′zē-ă). Decreased sensitivity of the retina to light caused by excessive exposure to sunlight. [G. *a-* priv. + *phōs,* light, + *aisthēsis,* perception]

aphra·sia (ă-frā′zē-ă). Inability to speak, from any cause. [G. *a-* priv. + *phrasis,* speaking]

aph·ro·di·sia (af-rō-diz′ē-ă). Sexual desire, especially when excessive. [G. *aphrodisios,* relating to Aphrodite]

aph·ro·di·si·ac (af-rō-diz′ē-ak). **1.** Increasing sexual desire. **2.** Anything that arouses or increases sexual desire.

aph·ro·di·si·o·ma·nia (af-rō-diz′ē-ō-mā′nē-ă). Abnormal and excessive erotic interest. [G. *aphrodisia,* sexual pleasures, + *mania,* insanity]

aph·tha, pl. **aph·thae** (af′thă, af′thē). **1.** In the singular, a small ulcer(s) on a mucous membrane. **2.** In the plural, stomatitis charctized by intermittent episodes of painful oral ulcers of unknown etiology that are covered by gray exudate, are surrounded by an erythematous halo, and range from several millimeters to 2 cm in diameter; they are limited to oral mucous membranes that are not bound to periosteum, occur as solitary or multiple lesions, and heal spontaneously in one to two weeks. SYN aphthae minor, aphthous stomatitis, canker sores, recurrent aphthous stomatitis, recurrent aphthous ulcers, recurrent ulcerative stomatitis, ulcerative stomatitis. [G. *ulceration*]

Bednar's aphthae, traumatic ulcers located bilaterally on either side of the midpalatal raphe in infants.

herpetiform aphthae, a variant of oral aphthae, of unknown etiology, characterized by up to several dozen ulcers, 2-3 mm in diameter, organized in a clustered herpetiform distribution.

aphthae ma'jor, a severe form of aphthae characterized by unusually numerous, large, deep, and frequent ulcers; healing may take as long as six weeks and results in scarring. SYN Mikulicz' aphthae, periadenitis mucosa necrotica recurrens, recurrent scarring aphthae, Sutton's disease (2).

Mikulicz' aphthae, SYN aphthae major.

aphthae mi'nor, SYN aphtha (2).

recurrent scarring aphthae, SYN aphthae major.

aph·thoid (af'thoyd). Resembling aphthae.

aph·tho·sis (af-thō'sis). Any condition characterized by the presence of aphthae.

aph·thous (af'thŭs). Characterized by or relating to aphthae or aphthosis.

aphy·lac·tic (ā-fī-lak'tik). Rarely used term for pertaining to or characterized by aphylaxis.

aphy·lax·is (ā-fī-lak'sis). Rarely used term for lack of protection against disease. SYN nonimmunity. [G. *a-* priv. + *phylaxis,* a guarding]

ap·i·cal (ap'i-kăl). 1. Relating to the apex or tip of a pyramidal or pointed structure. 2. Situated nearer to the apex of a structure in relation to a specific reference point; opposite of basal. SYN apicalis [NA].

ap·i·ca·lis (ap-i-kā'lis) [NA]. SYN apical, apical. [L.]

ap·i·cec·to·my (ap-i-sek'tō-mē). 1. Opening and exenteration of air cells in the apex of the petrous part of the temporal bone. 2. In dental surgery, an obsolete synonym for apicoectomy. [L. *apex,* summit or tip, + G. *ektomē,* excision]

apic·e·ot·o·my (ă-pis-ē-ot'ō-mē). SYN apicotomy.

ap·i·ces (ap'i-sēs). Plural of apex.

ap·i·ci·tis (ap-i-sī'tis). Inflammation of the apex of a structure or organ.

⌂**apico-.** An apex; apical [L. *apex, apicis* a summit or a tip + -o-]

ap·i·co·ec·to·my (ap'ī-kō-ek'tō-mē). Surgical removal of a dental root apex. SYN root resection. [apico- + G. *ektomē,* excision]

ap·i·co·lo·ca·tor (ap'i-kō-lō'kă-tŏr). A device for locating the root apex of a tooth.

ap·i·col·y·sis (ap-i-kol'i-sis). Surgical collapse of the upper portion of the lung by the operative detachment of the parietal pleura allowing a medial displacement of the pulmonary apex. [apico- + G. *lysis,* destruction]

Api·com·plexa (ap-i-kom-plek'să). A phylum of the subkingdom Protozoa, which includes the class Sporozoea and the subclasses Coccidia and Piroplasmia, and is characterized by the presence of an apical complex. [L. *apex,* pl. *apicis,* tip, summit, + *complexus,* woven together]

ap·i·co·stome (ap'i-kō-stōm). The trocar and cannula used in apicostomy.

ap·i·cos·to·my (ap-i-kos'tō-mē). An operation in which the labial or buccal alveolar plate is perforated with a trocar and cannula; done to reach the root apex and to take bacterial cultures from this area. [apico- + G. *stoma,* mouth]

ap·i·cot·o·my (ap-i-kot'ō-mē). Incision into an apical structure. SYN apiceotomy. [apico- + G. *tomē,* a cutting]

apic·u·late (ă-pik'yū-lāt). Terminated abruptly by a small point. [L. *apiculus,* a tip or point]

apic·u·lus (ă-pik'yū-lŭs). A short, sharp projection on one end of a fungus spore at the point of attachment, or on the wall, of a hypha or condiophore. [L.]

ap·i·cu·ret·tage (ap-i-kyū'rĕ-tahzh). Apical curettage after removal of an infected tooth.

apin·e·al·ism (ă-pin'ē-al-izm). Acquired absence of the pineal gland.

api·pho·bia (ā-pi-fō'bē-ă). Morbid fear of bees. SYN melissophobia. [L. *apis,* bee, + G. *phobos,* fear]

api·tu·i·tar·ism (ā-pi-tū'i-tār-izm). Total lack of functional pituitary tissue; may be iatrogenic (*e.g.,* as a consequence of hypophysectomy) or the result of a spontaneous disease process.

apla·cen·tal (ā-pla-sen'tăl). Without a placenta; denoting the monotremes (which lay eggs and have no placenta) and the marsupials (which have a transitory simple yolk-sac placenta).

ap·la·nat·ic (ap-la-nat'ik). Pertaining to aplanatism, or to an aplanatic lens.

aplan·a·tism (ă-plan'ă-tizm). Freedom from spherical aberration; said of a lens. [G. *a-* priv. + *planētos,* wandering]

apla·sia (ă-plā'zē-ă). 1. Defective development or congenital absence of an organ or tissue. 2. In hematology, incomplete, retarded, or defective development, or cessation of the usual regenerative process. [G. *a-* priv. + *plasis,* a molding]

congenital a. of thymus, SYN DiGeorge *syndrome.*

a. cu'tis congen'ita [MIM*107600], congenital absence or deficiency of a localized area of skin, with the base of the defect covered by a thin translucent membrane; most often a single area near the vertex of the scalp, but may occur in other areas; underlying structures may also be affected; autosomal inheritance, either dominant or recessive.

germinal a., SYN seminiferous tubule *dysgenesis.*

gonadal a., congenital absence of essentially all gonadal tissue; the external genitalia and genital ducts are female, but if interstitial cells of Leydig are present, the external genitalia are commonly ambiguous and the genital ducts are female. SEE gonadal *dysgenesis.* Cf. Klinefelter's *syndrome,* Turner's *syndrome.* SYN gonadal agenesis.

pure red cell a., a transitory arrest of red blood cell production which may occur in the course of a hemolytic anemia, often preceded by infection, or as a complication of certain drugs; if the arrest persists anemia may result. SEE ALSO congenital hypoplastic *anemia.*

aplas·tic (ā-plas'tik, ă-). Pertaining to aplasia, or conditions characterized by defective regeneration, as in a. anemia.

apleu·ria (ă-plūr'ē-ă). Congenital absence of one or more ribs; usually associated with absent transverse process or processes. [*a-* priv. + G. *pleura,* rib]

ap·nea (ap'nē-ă). Absence of breathing. [G. *apnoia,* want of breath]

central a., a. as the result of medullary depression which inhibits respiratory movement.

deglutition a., inhibition of breathing during swallowing.

induced a., intentional respiratory arrest during general anesthesia produced by hypocapnia, a muscle relaxant drug, respiratory center depression, or sudden cessation of controlled respiration.

obstructive a., peripheral a., a. either as the result of obstruction of the air passages or inadequate respiratory muscle activity.

sleep a., central and/or peripheral a. during sleep, associated with frequent awakening and often with daytime sleepiness. Cf. sleep-induced a.

sleep-induced a., a. resulting from failure of the respiratory center to stimulate adequate respiration during sleep; divided into respiratory pause (cessation of air flow for less than 10 seconds) and apneic pause (cessation of air flow greater than 10 seconds).

ap·ne·ic (ap'nē-ik). Related to or suffering from apnea.

apneu·ma·to·sis (ap-nū-mă-tō'sis). Obsolete term for congenital atelectasis. [G. *a-* priv. + *pneumatoō,* to inflate, + *-osis,* condition]

ap·neu·mia (ap-nū'mē-ă). Congenital absence of the lungs. [G. *a-* priv. + *pneumōn,* lung]

ap·neu·sis (ap-nū'sis). An abnormal respiratory pattern consisting of a pause at full inspiration; a prolonged inspiratory cramp caused by a lesion at the mid or caudal pontine level of the brainstem. [G. *a-* priv. + *pneusis,* a breathing, fr. *pneō,* to breathe]

ap·neus·tic (ap-nū'stik). Obsolete term for apneusis.

apo Abbreviation for apoenzyme; apolipoprotein .

⌂**apo-.** Combining form meaning, usually, separated from or derived from. [G. *apo,* away from, off; *apo-* becomes *ap-,* especially before a vowel or h]

ap·o·bi·o·sis (ap-ō-bī-ō'sis). Death, especially local death of a part of the organism. [G. death, fr. *apo,* from, + *biōsis,* life]

ap·o·car·ter·e·sis (ap'ō-kar-ter-ē'sis). Suicide by starvation. [G. *apocartereō,* to starve oneself to death]

ap·o·clei·sis (ap-ō-klī′sis). Aversion to food. [G. *apo,* away, + *kleisis,* closure]

ap·o·crine (ap′ō-krin). Denoting a mechanism of glandular secretion in which the apical portion of secretory cells is shed and incorporated into the secretion. SEE ALSO apocrine *gland.* [G. *apo-krinō,* to separate]

ap·o·crus·tic (ap-ō-krŭs′tik). **1.** Astringent and repellent. **2.** An agent with such action. [G. *apokroustikos,* able to beat off, fr. *apo,* off, + *krouō,* to strike]

a·po·dal (ă-pō′dal). Relating to apodia. SYN apodous. [G. *a-* priv. + *pous,* foot]

ap·o·de·mi·al·gia (ap′ō-dē-mē-al′jē-ă). Wanderlust; longing to get away from home or to travel. Cf. nostalgia. [G. *apodēmia,* being away from home, + *algos,* pain]

apo·dia (ă-pō′dē-ă). Congenital absence of feet. SYN apody. [G. *a-* priv. + *pous,* foot]

ap·o·dous (ap′ō-dŭs). SYN apodal.

ap·o·dy (ap′ō-dē). SYN apodia.

ap·o·en·zyme (apo) (ap′ō-en-zīm). The protein portion of an enzyme as contrasted with the nonprotein portion, or coenzyme, or prosthetic portion (if present).

ap·o·fer·ri·tin (ap-ō-fer′i-tin). A protein in the intestinal wall that combines with a ferric hydroxide-phosphate compound to form ferritin, the first stage in the absorption of iron.

ap·o·gam·ia, apog·a·my (ap-ō-gam′ē-ă, ă-pog′ă-mē). SYN parthenogenesis. [G. *apo,* away, + *gameō,* to wed]

apo·gee. The peak of severity of the clinical manifestations of an illness. [Fr., fr. Mod. L. *apogaeum,* fr. G. *apogaios,* far from the earth, fr. *apo,* + gaia, earth]

ap·o·in·duc·er (ă′pō-in-dūs′er). A protein that binds to DNA to switch on transcription.

apo·lar (ă-pō′lăr). **1.** Without poles; denoting specifically embryonic nerve cells (neuroblasts) that have not yet begun to sprout processes. **2.** SYN hydrophobic (2).

ap·o·lip·o·pro·tein (apo) (ap′ō-lip-ō-prō′tēn). The protein component of lipoprotein complexes that is a normal constituent of plasma chylomicrons, HDL, LDL, and VLDL in man.

a. A-I, an a. found in HDL and chylomicrons. It is an activator of LCAT and a ligand for the HDL receptor. A deficiency of this a. has been associated with low HDL levels and with Tangier disease.

a. A-II, an a. found in HDL and chylomicrons.

a. A-IV, an a. secreted with chylomicrons.

a. B, a.'s found in LDL, VLDL, and IDL. Elevated in the plasma of individuals with familial hyperlipoproteinemia.

a. B-100, an a. found in LDL, VLDL, and IDL. The ligand for the LDL receptor; absent in certain types of abetalipoproteinemia.

a. B-48, an a. found in chylomicrons and chylomicron remnants. Retained in intestine of individuals with chylomicron retention disease.

a. C-I, an a. found in VLDL, HDL, and chylomicrons.

a. C-II, an a. found in VLDL, HDL, and chylomicrons; an activator of lipoprotein lipase; a deficiency will result in accumulation of chylomicrons and triacylglycerols.

a. C-III, an a. found in VLDL, HDL, and chylomicrons.

a. D, an a. found in HDL whose function is unclear.

a. E, an a. found in VLDL, HDL, chylomicrons, and chylomicron remnants. Elevated in individuals with type III hyperlipoproteinemia.

ap·o·mix·ia (ap-ō-mik′sē-ă). SYN parthenogenesis. [G. *apo,* from, + *mixis,* a mingling]

ap·o·mor·phine hy·dro·chlo·ride (ap-ō-mōr′fēn). $C_{17}H_{17}NO_2$- HC1; a derivative of morphine used as an emetic by the parenteral route of administration.

ap·o·neu·rec·to·my (ap′ō-nū-rek′tō-mē). Excision of an aponeurosis. [aponeurosis + G. *ektomē,* excision]

ap·o·neu·ror·rha·phy (ap′ō-nū-rōr′ă-fē). SYN fasciorrhaphy. [aponeurosis + G. *rhaphē,* suture]

ap·o·neu·ro·sis, pl. **ap·o·neu·ro·ses** (ap′ō-nū-rō′sis, -sēz) [NA]. A fibrous sheet or flat, expanded tendon, giving attachment to muscular fibers and serving as the means of origin or insertion of a flat muscle; it sometimes also performs the office of a fascia for other muscles. [G. the end of the muscle where it becomes tendon, fr. *apo,* from, + *neuron,* sinew]

bicipital a., a. bicipita′lis, radiating fibers from the tendon of insertion of the biceps which form a triangular band passing obliquely across the hollow of the elbow to the ulnar side and becoming merged into the deep fascia of the forearm. Formerly called "grace Dieu" fascia, it serves to protect the brachial artery and median nerve during phlebotomy of median cubital vein. SYN a. musculi bicipitis brachii [NA], bicipital fascia, lacertus fibrosus, semilunar fascia.

Denonvilliers' a., SYN rectovesical *septum.*

epicranial a., the aponeurosis or intermediate tendon connecting the frontalis and occipitalis muscles to form the epicranius. SYN a. epicranialis [NA], galea aponeurotica [NA], galea (2).

a. epicrania′lis [NA], SYN epicranial a.

extensor a., SYN extensor digital *expansion.*

a. of external abdominal oblique muscle, broad, flat tendinous portion of the external abdominal oblique muscle. The fleshy fibers of the muscle end in the a. along a line descending vertically from the costochondral joint of the ninth rib then turning laterally just below the level of the umbilicus toward the anterior superior iliac spine. The fibers of the aponeurosis run medially and inferiorly, contributing to the anterior wall of the sheath of the rectus abdominis muscle and decussating with those of the contralateral a. at the median linea alba. Inferomedially, the a. is attached to the upper border of the pubic symphysis, the pubic crest and pubic tubercle. Between the anterior superior iliac spine and the pubic tubercle, it is thickened and turned under, forming the inguinal ligaments. The portion of the a. attached to the pubic bone forms the superficial inguinal ring by splitting into medial and lateral crura. SEE ALSO external spermatic *fascia,* inguinal *ligament,* lacunar *ligament,* pectineal *ligament,* reflected inguinal *ligament,* superficial inguinal *ring,* rectus *sheath.*

a. of insertion, a tendinous sheet serving for the insertion of a broad muscle.

a. of internal abdominal oblique muscle, broad, flat tendinous portion of the internal abdominal oblique muscle. The fleshy fibers of the muscle end in the a. lateral to the semilunar line. The uppermost portion of the a. is attached to the outer surfaces and lower borders of the seventh to ninth costal cartilages. Of the portion extending between the costoxiphoid margin and the pubis, the upper two-thirds splits into anterior and posterior laminae at the lateral border of the rectus abdominis muscle to contribute to the anterior and posterior walls of the sheath of the rectus abdominis muscle as they extend to the midline linea alba. The lower third of the a. does not split but joins the aponeuroses of the external abdominal oblique and transversus abdominis muscles to form the anterior wall of the sheath of the rectus abdominis muscle. The fibers of the portion of the a. contributing to the rectus sheath decussate with those of the contralateral a. in the linea alba. The lowermost portion of the a. blends with the a. of the transversus abdominis muscle to form the conjoint tendon, attaching to the pubic crest and often the pecten pubis, thus forming the posterior wall of the inguinal canal at the superficial inguinal ring. SEE ALSO cremasteric *fascia,* conjoint *tendon,* rectus *sheath.*

a. of investment, a fibrous membrane covering and keeping in place a muscle or group of muscles.

a. lin′guae [NA], SYN lingual a.

lingual a., the thickened lamina propria of the tongue to which the lingual muscles attach. SYN a. linguae [NA].

a. mus′culi bicip′itis bra′chii [NA], SYN bicipital a.

a. of origin, a tendinous expansion serving as the attachment of origin of a broad muscle.

a. palati′na [NA], SYN palatine a.

palatine a., the expanded tendons of the tensor veli palatini muscles in the anterior two-thirds of the soft palate to which the other palatine muscles attach. SYN a. palatina [NA].

palmar a., the thickened, central portion of the fascia ensheathing the hand; it radiates toward the bases of the fingers from the tendon of the palmaris longus muscle. SYN a. palmaris [NA], Dupuytren's fascia, palmar fascia.

a. palma′ris [NA], SYN palmar a.

Petit's a., the posterior layer of the broad ligament of the uterus. [P. Petit]

a. pharyn′gea, SYN pharyngobasilar *fascia.*

plantar a., the very thick, central portion of the fascia investing the plantar muscles; it radiates toward the toes from the medial process of the calcaneal tuberosity and gives attachment to the short flexor muscle of the toes. SYN a. plantaris [NA], plantar fascia.

a. planta′ris [NA], SYN plantar a.

Sibson's a., SYN suprapleural *membrane.*

temporal a., SYN temporal *fascia.*

thoracolumbar a., SYN thoracolumbar *fascia.*

a. of vastus muscles, SEE patellar *retinaculum,* medial patellar *retinaculum,* lateral patellar *retinaculum.*

ap·o·neu·ro·si·tis (ap′ō-nū-rō-sī′tis). Inflammation of an aponeurosis.

ap·o·neu·rot·ic (ap′ō-nū-rot′ik). Relating to an aponeurosis.

ap·o·neu·ro·tome (ap-ō-nū′rō-tōm). Instrument for dividing an aponeurosis. [aponeurosis + G. *tomē,* a cutting]

ap·o·neu·rot·o·my (ap′ō-nū-rot′ō-mē). Incision of an aponeurosis.

ap·o·pa·thet·ic (ap′ō-pă-thet′ik). Denoting a form of behavior in which one conspicuously alters his conduct in the presence of other people. [G. *apo,* away, + *pathētikos,* relating to the feelings]

ap·o·phy·lax·is (ap′ō-fī-lak′sis). A diminution of the phylactic power of the body fluids, as sometimes observed in the negative phase of therapy with immunizing agents.

apoph·y·sary (ă-pof′i-sā-rē). SYN apophysial.

ap·o·phys·i·al, apoph·y·se·al (ă-pō-fiz′ē-ăl). Relating to or resembling an apophysis. SYN apophysary.

apoph·y·sis, pl. **apoph·y·ses** (ă-pof′i-sis, -sēz). An outgrowth or projection, especially one from a bone. A bony process or outgrowth that lacks an independent center of ossification. [G. an offshoot]

basilar a., SYN basilar *part* of the occipital bone.

a. con′chae, SYN *eminence* of concha.

a. hel′icis, SYN *spine* of helix.

Ingrassia's a., SYN lesser *wing* of sphenoid bone.

lenticular a., SYN lenticular *process* of incus.

temporal a., SYN mastoid *process.*

apoph·y·si·tis (ă-pof-i-sī′tis). Inflammation of any apophysis.

a. tibia′lis adolescen′tium, SYN Osgood-Schlatter *disease.*

ap·o·plas·mia (ap-ō-plaz′mē-ă). A decrease in the amount of blood plasma.

ap·o·plec·tic (ap-ŏ-plek′tik). Relating to, suffering from, or predisposed to apoplexy.

ap·o·plec·ti·form (ap-ŏ-plek′ti-fōrm). Resembling apoplexy.

ap·o·plexy (ap′ŏ-plek-sē) A classical but obsolete term for a cerebral stroke, most often due to intracerebral hemorrhage. [G. *apoplēxia*]

abdominal a., mesenteric hemorrhage, thrombosis, or embolus involving the mesenteric or abdominal blood vessels.

adrenal a., hemorrhage into the adrenal glands or thrombosis of the adrenal veins, followed by acute adrenal insufficiency, occurring in the Waterhouse-Friderichsen syndrome.

bulbar a., a. due to vascular lesion in the brainstem.

cutaneous a., archaic term for a sudden rush of blood to the skin and subcutaneous tissue.

functional a., a condition simulating a. without any cerebral lesion; a form of conversion hysteria.

heat a., (1) SYN heatstroke. **(2)** SYN ardent *fever.*

labyrinthine a., a clinical syndrome manifested as a single, abrupt attack of severe vertigo, nausea, and vomiting, with permanent loss of labyrinthine function on one side, but without associated hearing loss or tinnitus. Attributed to occlusion of the labyrinthine branch of the internal auditory artery.

neonatal a., intracranial hemorrhage in newborn children.

pituitary a., the sudden onset of visual loss, ophthalmoplegia, and meningeal pain due to infarction of a a. adenoma, producing compression of chiasm and cavernous sinus and some subarachnoid hemorrhage.

spinal a., stroke involving the spinal cord.

splenic a., peracute anthrax often seen in ruminants, in which death occurs very quickly after the appearance of the first signs of the disease; grossly enlarged spleen and capillary hemorrhages are often the only lesions.

uteroplacental a., SYN Couvelaire *uterus.*

ap·o·pro·tein (ap-ō-prō′tēn). A polypeptide chain (protein) not yet complexed with the prosthetic group that is necessary to form the active holoprotein.

ap·o·pto·sis (ap-ō-tō′sis, ap′op-tō′sis). Single deletion of scattered cells by fragmentation into membrane-bound particles which are phagocytosed by other cells; believed to be due to programmed cell death. [G. a falling or dropping off, fr. *apo,* off, + *ptosis,* a falling]

ap·o·re·pres·sor (ap′ō-rē-pres′er). SYN inactive *repressor.*

apo·ria (ă-pōr′ē-ă). Doubt, especially deriving from incompatible views on the same subject. [G. *aporia,* difficulty, doubt]

apo·ri·o·neu·ro·sis (ă-pōr′ē-ō-nū-rō′sis). Obsolete term for anxiety *neurosis.* [G. *aporia,* difficulty, doubt, + neurosis]

ap·o·some (ap′ō-sōm). A cytoplasmic inclusion produced by the cell itself. [G. *apo,* from, + *sōma,* body]

ap·o·stax·is (ap-ō-staks′is). Slight hemorrhage, or bleeding by drops. [G. a trickling down]

apos·thia (ă-pos′thē-ă). Congenital absence of the prepuce. [G. *a-* priv. + *posthē,* foreskin]

ap·o·stilb (ap′ō-stilb). A unit of brightness equal to 0.1 millilambert. [G. *apo,* from + *stilbē,* lamp]

ap·o·tha·na·sia (ap′-ō-thă-nā′zē-ă). Postponement of death; prolongation of life, as opposed to euthanasia. [G. *apo,* away, + *thanatos,* death]

apoth·e·car·y (ă-poth′ĕ-kār-ē). Obsolescent term for pharmacist or druggist. [G. *apothēkē,* a barn, storehouse, fr. *apo,* from, + *thēkē,* a box]

ap·o·them, ap·o·theme (ap′ō-them, ap′ō-thēm). A precipitate caused by long boiling of a vegetable infusion or by its exposure to air. [G. *apo,* from, + *thema,* something set down, fr. *tithēmi,* to place]

ap·ox·e·sis (ap-ok-sē′sis). SYN subgingival *curettage.* [G. *apo,* away, + *xeein,* to scrape]

ap·o·zem, apoz·e·ma (ap′ō-zem, ap-oz′ĕ-mă). SYN decoction. [apo- + G. *zema,* something boiled]

ap·pa·ra·tus, pl. **ap·pa·ra·tus** (ap-ă-rā′tŭs, -rat′ŭs). **1.** A collection of instruments adapted for a special purpose. **2.** An instrument made up of several parts. **3** [NA]. A group or system of glands, ducts, blood vessels, muscles, or other anatomical structures involved in the performance of some function. SEE ALSO system. [L. equipment. fr. *ap-paro,* pp. *-atus,* to prepare]

accessory visual a., SYN accessory *organs* of the eye, under *organ.*

achromatic a., the nonstaining asters and spindle fibers in a dividing cell.

alimentary a., SYN digestive *system.*

attachment a., the tissues that attach the tooth to the alveolar process: cementum, periodontal membrane, and alveolar bone.

Barcroft-Warburg a., SYN Warburg's a.

Beckmann's a., a. for the accurate measurement of melting points and boiling points in connection with molecular weight determinations.

Benedict-Roth a., a device employed to measure the amount of oxygen utilized in quiet breathing in the basal state for the estimation of the basal metabolic rate; the subject rebreathes oxygen through soda lime from a recording spirometer.

branchial a., the aggregate of the pharyngeal arches, pouches, clefts, and membranes seen in the developing embryo of vertebrates.

central a., the centrosome and centrosphere.

chromatic a., the deeply staining mass of chromosomes in a dividing cell.

chromidial a., the aggregate of extranuclear network, irregular strands, and masses of basophilic staining material permeating the protoplasm of the cell. SEE ALSO ribosome, endoplasmic *reticulum.*

dental a., SYN masticatory *system.*

digestive a., the digestive tract from the mouth to the anus with all its associated glands and organs. SYN a. digestorius [NA].

a. digesto′rius [NA], SYN digestive a.

genitourinary a., SYN urogenital *system.*

Golgi a., a membranous system of cisternae and vesicles located between the nucleus and the secretory pole or surface of a cell; concerned with the investment and intracellular transport of membrane-bounded secretory proteins. SYN dictyosome, Golgi body, Golgi complex, Golgi internal reticulum, Holmgrén-Golgi canals.

Haldane's a., a device used for the analysis of respiratory gases.

Heyns' abdominal decompression a., a vacuum chamber enclosing the abdomen of the pregnant woman, creating pressure during the first stage of labor.

hyoid a., veterinary anatomy term for hyoid bones, a modified portion of the ancestral branchial skeleton consisting of an articulated chain of bones extending from the mastoid region of the skull on each side to the base of the tongue; in humans, it is reduced to a single bone, os hyoideum; in a typical mammal (the dog), it consists of a tympanohyoid cartilage attached to the skull, followed by the stylohyoid, epihyoid, keratohyoid, basihyoid, and thyrohyoid bones. SYN a. hyoideus.

a. hyoi′deus, SYN hyoid a.

juxtaglomerular a., SYN juxtaglomerular *complex.*

Kirschner's a., SYN Kirschner's *wire.*

Kjeldahl a., an a. for distilling ammonia arising from acid decomposition of an organic compound; used in nitrogen analysis.

lacrimal a., consisting of the lacrimal gland, the lacrimal lake, the lacrimal canaliculi, the lacrimal sac, and the nasolacrimal duct. SYN a. lacrimalis [NA].

a. lacrima′lis [NA], SYN lacrimal a.

a. ligamento′sus col′li, SYN *ligamentum* nuchae.

a. ligamento′sus weitbrecht′i, SYN tectorial *membrane.*

masticatory a., (1) SYN masticatory *system.* **(2)** SYN stomatognathic *system.*

mental a., mental structure consisting of thoughts, feelings, cognitions, and memories; in psychoanalysis, the topographic structure of the mind.

pyriform a., a pear-shaped structure within the eggshell of certain tapeworms (family Anoplocephalidae), of uncertain function.

a. respirato′rius [NA], SYN respiratory *system.*

respiratory a., SYN respiratory *system.*

Roughton-Scholander a., a syringe-like device for analyzing the respiratory gases in a small sample of blood. SYN Roughton-Scholander syringe.

Sayre's suspension a., archaic term for Sayre's suspension *traction.*

Scholander a., a device used for determining the oxygen and carbon dioxide percentage in 0.5 ml of a respiratory gas.

subneural a., modified sarcoplasm in a motor end-plate.

a. suspenso′rius len′tis, SYN ciliary *zonule.*

Taylor's a., SYN Taylor's back *brace.*

Tiselius a., an a. for separating proteins in solution by electrophoresis and thus for determining the isoelectric point, molecular weight, and related physical properties; the direction and rate of migration of the protein and the characteristics of the boundary phase between the protein solution and the supernatant salt solution are recorded by photography of the changes in refractive index at the boundary.

urinary a., SYN urogenital *system.*

urogenital a., SYN urogenital *system.*

a. urogenita′lis [NA], SYN urogenital *system.*

Van Slyke a., an a. for determining the amounts of respiratory gases in the blood.

Warburg's a., an a. for measuring the oxygen consumption of

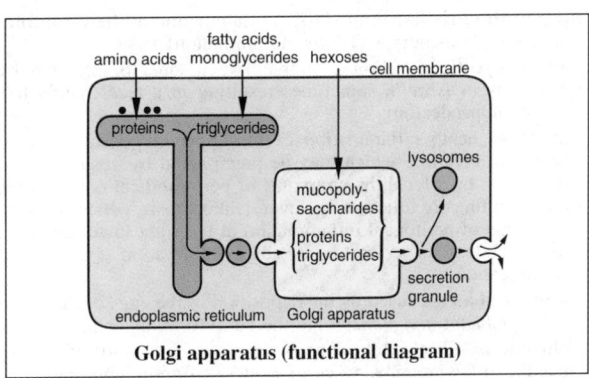

Golgi apparatus (functional diagram)

incubated tissue slices by manometric measurement of changes in gas pressure produced by oxygen absorption in an enclosed flask. SYN Barcroft-Warburg a.

ap·par·ent (ă-păr′ent). **1.** Manifest; obvious; evident; *e.g.,* a clinically a. infection. **2.** Frequently used (confusingly) to mean "seeming to be," ostensible, pseudo-. [L. *apparens,* visible, fr. *appareo,* to come in sight]

ap·pend·age (ă-pen′dij). Any part, subordinate in function or size, attached to a main structure. SEE ALSO adnexa. SYN appendix (1). [L. *appendix*]

atrial a., the small projection from each atrium hanging over like a small ear, more marked on the left, with a small cavity of its own.

auricular a., (1) SYN auricle of *atrium.* **(2)** a small congenital skin tag usually located anterior to the tragus of the ear, often called a skin tag; more often unilateral than bilateral.

drumstick a., an a. of the nucleus that represents the inactive heterochromatic X chromosome seen in 3% of the neutrophil leukocytes of human females. SEE sex *chromatin,* lyonization.

epiploic a., SYN *appendix* epiploica.

a.'s of eye, SYN accessory *organs* of the eye, under *organ.*

a.'s of the fetus, amnion, yolk sac, and the fetal (chorionic) part of the placenta together with the umbilical cord.

left auricular a., SYN *auricle* of left atrium.

right auricular a., SYN *auricle* of right atrium.

a.'s of skin, the hairs, nails, and sweat, sebaceous, and mammary glands.

testicular a., a vesicular nonpedunculated structure attached to the cephalic pole of the testis; a vestige of the cephalic end of the paramesonephric (müllerian) duct. SYN appendix testis [NA], appendix of the testis, nonpedunculated hydatid, ovarium masculinum, sessile hydatid.

uterine a.'s, the ovaries, uterine (fallopian) tubes, and associated ligaments. SYN adnexa uteri.

vermiform a., SYN vermiform *appendix.*

vesicular a., SYN vesicular *appendices* of uterine tube, under *appendix.*

ap·pen·dal·gia (ap-pen-dal′jē-ă). Obsolete term for pain in the right lower quadrant of the abdomen in the region of the vermiform appendix. [appendix + G. *algos,* pain]

ap·pen·dec·to·my (ap-pen-dek′tō-mē). Surgical removal of the vermiform appendix. SYN appendicectomy. [appendix + G. *ektomē,* excision]

auricular a., excision of the auricular appendix of an atrium, usually the left.

ap·pen·di·cal (ă-pen′di-kăl). SYN appendiceal.

ap·pen·dic·e·al (ă-pen-dis′ē-ăl). Relating to an appendix. SYN appendical.

ap·pen·di·cec·ta·sis (ap-pen-di-sek′tă-sis). Ectasia of the appendix.

ap·pen·di·cec·to·my (ap-pen-di-sek′tō-mē). SYN appendectomy.

ap·pen·di·cism (ă-pen′di-sizm). Rarely used term for any chronic disease of the vermiform appendix, or a symptomatic uneasiness in that area.

ap·pen·di·ci·tis (ă-pen-di-sī'tis). Inflammation of the vermiform appendix. [appendix + G. *-itis,* inflammation]

actinomycotic a., chronic suppurative a. due to infection by *Actinomyces israelii,* sometimes resulting in a fecal fistula following appendectomy.

acute a., acute inflammation of the appendix, usually due to bacterial infection, which may be precipitated by obstruction of the lumen by a fecalith; symptoms of periumbilical colicky pain and vomiting are followed by fever, leukocytosis, persistent pain, and signs of peritoneal inflammation in the right lower quadrant of the abdomen; perforation or abscess formation is a frequent complication.

bilharzial a., a. caused by the deposition of the eggs of the blood fluke, *Schistosoma mansoni,* in the vermiform appendix.

chronic a., fibrous adhesions, scarring, or deformity of the appendix following subsidence of acute a.; fibrous obliteration of the distal lumen is not abnormal in older persons; term frequently used to refer to repeated mild attacks of acute a.

focal a., acute a. involving only part of the appendix, sometimes at the site of, or distal to, an obstruction of the lumen.

foreign-body a., a. caused by obstruction of the lumen of the appendix by a foreign substance, such as a particulate foreign body.

gangrenous a., acute a. with necrosis of the wall of the appendix, most commonly developing in obstructive a. and frequently causing perforation and acute peritonitis.

left-sided a., a. occurring on the left side of the abdomen, usually the left-lower quadrant, due to abnormal rotation of the gut (such as situs inversus).

lumbar a., a retrodisplaced appendix in the lumbar region.

obstructive a., acute a. due to infection of retained secretion behind an obstruction of the lumen by a fecalith or some other cause, including carcinoma of the cecum.

perforating a., inflammation of the appendix leading to perforation of the wall of the appendix into the peritoneal cavity, resulting in peritonitis.

recurrent a., repeated episodes of right lower quadrant abdominal pain attributed to recurrence of inflammation of the appendix in an individual who did not have an appendectomy for prior episodes. SYN relapsing a.

relapsing a., SYN recurrent a.

stercoral a., a. following a lodgment of fecal material in the appendix.

subperitoneal a., a. of a subperitoneally displaced appendix.

suppurative a., acute a. with purulent exudate in the lumen and wall of the appendix.

verminous a., a. caused by obstruction or response to the presence of parasitic worms such as *Ascaris lumbricoides, Strongyloides stercoralis,* or the pinworm *Enterobius vermicularis.*

ap·pen·di·clau·sis (ă-pen-di-klaw'sis). Obsolete term for atrophy or obstruction of the appendix. [appendix + L. *clausus,* closed]

appendico-. An appendix, usually the vermiform appendix. [L. *appendix, appendicis* an appendage, fr. *appendo,* to hang something onto something, fr. *ad-, ap-,* to, onto, + *pendo,* to hang, + -o-]

ap·pen·di·co·cele (ă-pen'di-kō-sēl). The vermiform appendix in a hernial sac. [appendico- + G. *kēlē,* hernia]

ap·pen·di·co·en·ter·os·to·my (ă-pen'di-kō-en-ter-os'tō-mē). **1.** Formerly used term for the establishment of an artificial opening between the appendix and the small intestine. [appendico- + G. *enteron,* intestine, + *stoma,* mouth]

ap·pen·di·co·lith (ă-pen'dĭ-kō-lith). A calcified concretion in the appendix visible on an abdominal radiograph. [appendico- + G. *lithos,* stone]

ap·pen·di·co·li·thi·a·sis (ă-pen'di-kō-li-thī'ă-sis). The presence of concretions in the vermiform appendix. [appendico- + G. *lithos,* stone]

ap·pen·di·col·y·sis (ă-pen'di-kol'i-sis). An operation for freeing the appendix from adhesions. [appendico- + G. *lysis,* a loosening]

ap·pen·di·cos·to·my (ă-pen'di-kos'tō-mē). An operation for

opening into the intestine through the tip of the vermiform appendix, previously attached to the anterior abdominal wall. [appendico- + G. *stoma,* mouth]

ap·pen·di·co·ves·i·cos·to·my (ă-pen-di-ko'ves'ĭ-kos-tō-mē). Use of an isolated appendix on a vascularized pedicle as a catheterizable route of access to the bladder from the skin. SYN Mitrofanoff principle. [eppendico- + L. *vesica,* bladder, + G. *stoma,* mouth]

ap·pen·dic·u·lar (ap'en-dik'yū-lăr). **1.** Relating to an appendix or appendage. **2.** Relating to the limbs, as opposed to axial, which refers to the trunk and head.

ap·pen·dix, gen. **ap·pen·di·cis,** pl. **ap·pen·di·ces** (ă-pen'diks, -di-sis, -di-sēs). **1** [NA]. SYN appendage. **2.** Specifically, the vermiform appendix. [L. appendage, fr. *ap- pendo,* to hang something on]

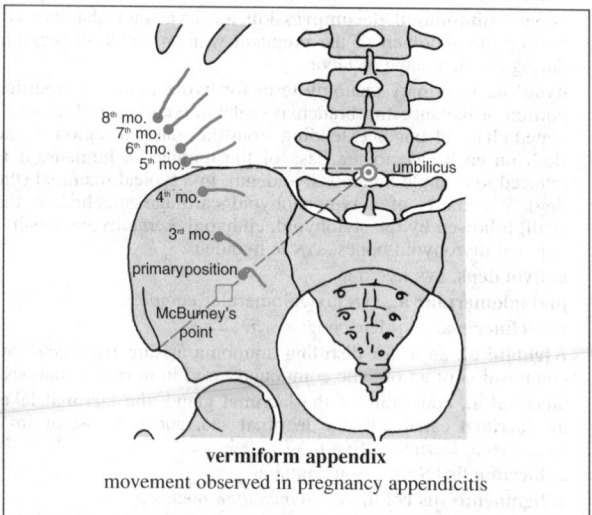

vermiform appendix
movement observed in pregnancy appendicitis

auricular a., SYN auricle of *atrium.*

a. ce'ci, SYN vermiform a.

a. epididym'idis [NA], SYN a. of epididymidis.

a. of epididymidis, a small pedunculated body often attached to the head of the epididymis which is a vestige of the embryonic mesonephric duct. SYN a. epididymidis [NA], pedunculated hydatid.

epiploic a., SYN a. epiploica.

a. epiplo'ica, pl. **appen'dices epiplo'icae** [NA], one of a number of little processes or sacs of peritoneum filled with adipose tissue and projecting from the serous coat of the large intestine, except the rectum; they are most evident on the transverse and sigmoid colon, being most numerous along the free tenia. SYN epiploic appendage, epiploic a., epiploic tags.

a. fibro'sa hep'atis [NA], SYN fibrous a. of liver.

fibrous a. of liver, a fibrous process, into which the tip of the left lobe of the liver may taper out, that passes with the left triangular ligament to be attached to the diaphragm. SYN a. fibrosa hepatis [NA].

Morgagni's a., SYN pyramidal *lobe* of thyroid gland.

a. tes'tis [NA], SYN testicular *appendage.*

a. of the testis, SYN testicular *appendage.*

a. ventric'uli laryn'gis, SYN *saccule* of larynx.

vermiform a., a wormlike intestinal diverticulum extending from the blind end of the cecum; it varies in length and ends in a blind extremity. SYN a. vermiformis [NA], a. ceci, processus vermiformis, vermiform appendage, vermiform process, vermix.

a. vermifor'mis [NA], SYN vermiform a.

vesicular appendices of uterine tube, a small fluid-filled cyst attached by a slender stalk to the fimbriated end of the uterine tube; a vestigial remnant of the embryonic mesonephric duct. SYN a. vesiculosa [NA], Morgagni's hydatid, morgagnian cyst, stalked hydatid, vesicular appendage.

a. vesiculo′sa, pl. **appen′dices vesiculo′sae** [NA], SYN vesicular appendices of uterine tube.

ap·per·cep·tion (ap-er-sep′shŭn). **1.** The final stage of attentive perception in which something is clearly apprehended and thus is relatively prominent in awareness; the full apprehension of any psychic content. **2.** The process of referring the perception of ideas to one's own personality. [L. *ad,* to, + *per- cipio,* pp. *-ceptus,* to take wholly, perceive]

ap·per·cep·tive (ap-er-sep′tiv). Relating to, involved in, or capable of apperception.

ap·per·son·a·tion, ap·per·son·i·fi·ca·tion (ă-per′sŏ-nā′shŭn, ap-er-son′i-fi-kā′shŭn). A delusion in which one assumes the character of another person.

ap·pe·stat (ap′e-stat). The mechanism in the brain (possibly in the hypothalamus) concerned with the appetite and control of food intake. [appetite + G. *statos,* standing]

ap·pe·tite (ap′ĕ-tīt). A desire or motive derived from a biologic or psychological need for food, water, sex, or affection; a desire or longing to satisfy any conscious physical or mental need. SYN orexia (2). [L. *ad-peto,* pp. *-petitus,* to seek after, desire]

ap·pe·ti·tion (ap-ĕ-tish′ŭn). Desire directed toward a definite goal or object. [L. *appetitio,* strong desire]

ap·pla·na·tion (ap′lan-ā′shŭn). In tonometry, the flattening of the cornea by pressure. Intraocular pressure is directly proportional to external pressure, and inversely proportional to the area flattened. SEE ALSO applanation *tonometer.* [L. *ad,* toward, + *planum,* plane]

ap·pla·nom·e·try (ap-lan-om′ĕ-trē). Use of an applanation tonometer.

ap·ple oil. SYN *amyl* valerate.

ap·pli·ance (ă-plī′ans). A device used to provide function to a part, or for therapeutic purposes. [fr, O. Fr. *aplier,* to apply, fr. L. *applico,* to fold together]

craniofacial a., a device used to immobilize and/or reduce mandibular or midfacial fractures. SEE ALSO fixation.

edgewise a., a fixed, multibanded orthodontic a. using an attachment bracket the slot of which receives a rectangular archwire horizontally, which gives precise control of tooth movement in all three planes of space.

extraoral fracture a., a device used for extraoral reduction and fixation of maxillary or mandibular fractures, in which pins, clamps, or screws interjoined with metal or acrylic connectors are used to align the fractured segments. SEE ALSO external pin *fixation.*

Hawley a., SYN Hawley *retainer.*

intraoral fracture a., a metal or acrylic device attached to the teeth with wire or cement; used to immobilize fractures of the maxilla and mandible.

labiolingual a., an orthodontic a. that consists of a maxillary labial arch wire and a mandibular lingual arch wire.

light wire a., an orthodontic a. utilizing small gauge labial wires with expansion and contraction loops formed into it and attached to bands fitted to individual teeth; sometimes called Begg light wire differential force technique.

obturator a., an a. used to obliterate congenital or acquired defects of the jaws and surrounding structures, usually made of acrylic or rubber.

orthodontic a., a mechanism for the application of pressure to the teeth and their supporting tissues to produce changes in the relationship of the teeth and/or the related osseous structures.

ribbon arch a., an a. consisting of a rectangular wire inserted into a specially designed bracket attached to the labial and buccal surfaces of the teeth.

Roger-Anderson pin fixation a., an a. used in extraoral fixation of mandibular fractures and prognathic corrections in which pins placed in the bone segments are joined by metal connecting rods. SEE ALSO external pin *fixation.*

surgical a., a metal or plastic a. constructed prior to surgery and used to immobilize or support mucosal, skin, bone, or bone marrow grafts during the postoperative phase.

universal a., a combination of the edgewise and ribbon arch a.

techniques, affording precise control of individual teeth in all planes of space.

applicand. Abbreviation for *applicandus,* to be applied. [L.]

ap·pli·ca·tor (ap′li-kā-tōr). A slender rod of wood, flexible metal, or synthetic material, at one end of which is attached a pledget of cotton or other substance for making local applications to any accessible surface. [L. *ap-plico,* to attach to]

ap·po·si·tion (ap-ō-zish′ŭn). **1.** The placing in contact of two substances. **2.** The condition of being placed or fitted together. **3.** The relationship of fracture fragments to one another. **4.** The process of thickening of the cell wall. [L. *ap-pono,* pp. *-positus,* to place at or to]

ap·proach (ă-prōch′). In psychiatry, a term used to describe how interpersonal relationships are negotiated. [M.E., fr. O. Fr., fr L.L. *appropio,* to come nearer, fr. *ad,* to + *propius,* nearer]

idiographic a., the comprehensive study of an individual as a basis for understanding human behavior in general.

nomothetic a., a frame of psychologic reference that attempts to provide norms and general principles of behavior by the study of groups.

regressive-reconstructive a., a form of psychotherapy in which regression, in order to resurrect some original psychic trauma, is an integral part of the treatment.

ap·prox·i·mate (ă-prok′si-māt). To bring close together. In dentistry: **1.** Proximate, denoting the contact surfaces, either mesial or distal, of two adjacent teeth. **2.** Close together; denoting the teeth in the human jaw, as distinguished from the separated teeth in certain of the lower animals. [L. *ad,* to, + *proximus,* nearest]

ap·prox·i·ma·tion (ă-prok-si-mā′shŭn). In surgery, bringing tissue edges into desired apposition for suturing.

steady state a., An assumption in the derivation of an enzyme rate expression in which the rate of change of the concentration of any enzyme species is zero or much smaller than d[P]/dt.

aprac·tag·no·sia (ā-prak-tag-nō′sē-ă). SYN constructional *apraxia.* [G. *a-* priv. + *praktea,* things to be done, + *gnōsis,* recognition]

aprac·tic (ă-prak′tik). SYN apraxic.

aprag·ma·tism (ă-prag′mă-tizm). An interest in theory or dogmatism rather than in practical results. [G. *a-* priv. + pragmatism]

aprax·ia (ă-prak′sē-ă). **1.** A disorder of voluntary movement, consisting of impairment in the performance of skilled or purposeful movements, notwithstanding the preservation of comprehension, muscular power, sensibility, and coordination in general; due to acquired cerebral disease. **2.** A psychomotor defect in which the proper use of an object can not be carried out although the object can be named and its uses described. SYN parectropia. [G. *a-* priv. + *prattō,* to do]

a. al′gera, a hysterical condition in which speaking, reading, writing, or consecutive thinking is impossible owing to the severe headache it causes.

constructional a., a. manifested as an impairment in activity such as building, assembling, and drawings; caused by parietal lobe lesions. SYN apractagnosia.

cortical a., SYN motor a.

gait a., a. for walking, accompanied by inability to make walking movements with the legs.

ideational a., ideatory a., obsolete term for the misuse of objects due to a disturbance of identification (agnosia).

ideokinetic a., ideomotor a., a form of a. in which simple acts are incapable of being performed, presumably because the connections between the cortical centers that control volition and the motor cortex are interrupted. SYN transcortical a.

innervation a., SYN motor a.

limb-kinetic a., SYN motor a.

motor a., an inability to make movements or to use objects for the purpose intended. SYN cortical a., innervation a., limb-kinetic a.

ocular motor a., a congenital inability to initiate horizontal saccades. Children with this condition often use head thrusts to move their eyes to the left and right.

transcortical a., SYN ideokinetic a.

verbal a., a speech disorder in which phonemic substitutions are constantly used for the desired syllable or word.

aprax·ic (ă-prak′sik). Marked by or pertaining to apraxia. SYN apractic.

ap·ri·cot ker·nel oil (ā′pri-kot). SEE persic oil.

ap·ro·bar·bi·tal (ap-rō-bar′bi-tawl). 5-Allyl-5-isopropylbarbituric acid; allylisopropylmalonylurea; a hypnotic and sedative with intermediate action; available as a. sodium, with the same uses.

aproc·tia (ă-prok′shē-ă). Congenital absence or imperforation of the anus. [G. *a*- priv. + *prōktos*, anus]

ap·ro·fen, ap·ro·fene, ap·ro·phen (ap′rō-fen, ap′rō-fēn, ap′rō-fen). 2-Diethylaminoethyl 2,2-diphenylpropionate; analgesic and antispasmodic.

ap·ro·pho·ria (ap′rō-fōr′ē-ă). Aphasia, including agraphia. [G. *a*- priv. + *prophora*, utterance]

apros·ex·ia (ap-rō-sek′sē-ă). Inattention, due to a sensorineural or mental defect. [G. *a*- priv. + *prosexis*, attention, fr. *pros-echō*, to hold to]

apros·o·dy (ă-pros′ō-dē). Absence, in speech, of the normal pitch, rhythm, and variations in stress. [G. *a*- priv. + *prosōdia*, voice modulation]

ap·ro·so·pia (ap-rō-sō′pē-ă). Congenital absence of the greater part or all of the face, usually associated with other malformations. [G. *a*- priv. + *prosōpon*, face]

apro·ti·nin (ā-prō′ti-nin). A protease and kallikrein inhibitor obtained from animal organs; a polypeptide with a molecular weight of about 6000. May be useful in the treatment of pancreatitis and in preventing bleeding after surgery involving cardiopulmonary bypass.

APS Abbreviation for adenosine 5′-phosphosulfate.

6-APS Abbreviation for 6-aminopenicillanic acid.

ap·tho·vi·rus. A genus in the family Picornaviridae associated with foot and mouth disease of cattle.

aPTT Abbreviation for activated partial thromboplastin *time*.

APUD. Proposed designation for a group of cells in different organs secreting polypeptide hormones. Cells in this group have certain biochemical characteristics in common, the first letters of which form the name: they contain amines, such as catecholamine and 5-hydroxytryptamine, take up precursors of these amines *in vivo*, and contain amino-acid decarboxylase. [*a*mine *p*recursor *u*ptake, *d*ecarboxylase]

apu·rin·ic ac·id (a-pyū-rin′ik). DNA from which the purine bases have been removed by mild acid treatment.

apyk·no·mor·phous (ă-pik-nō-mōr′fŭs). Denoting a cell or other structure that does not stain deeply because the stainable or chromophil material is not closely aggregated. [G. *a*- priv. + *pyknos*, thick, + *morphē*, shape, form]

ap·y·rase (ă-pī′rās). An enzyme catalyzing hydrolytic removal of two orthophosphate residues from adenosine 5′-triphosphate to yield adenosine 5′-monophosphate; *i.e.,* ATP + $2H_2O \rightarrow$ AMP + $2P_i$. SYN ADPase, ATP-diphosphatase.

apy·ret·ic (ā-pī-ret′ik). Without fever, denoting apyrexia; having a normal body temperature. SYN afebrile, apyrexial.

apy·rex·ia (ā-pī-rek′sē-ă). Absence of fever. [G. *a*- priv. + *pyrexis*, fever]

apy·rex·i·al (ā-pī-rek′sē-ăl). SYN apyretic.

apy·rim·i·din·ic ac·id (ă-pī′rim-i-din′ik). DNA from which the pyrimidine bases have been removed by chemical treatment (*e.g.,* exposure to hydrazine).

aq. Abbreviation for L. *aqua*, water.

aq. bull. Abbreviation for L. *aqua bulliens*, boiling water.

aq. dest. Abbreviation for L. *aqua destillata*, distilled water.

aq. ferv. Abbreviation for L. *aqua fervens*, hot water.

aq. frig. Abbreviation for L. *aqua frigida*, cold water.

aq·ua, gen. and pl. **aq·uae** (ak′wă, ah′kwah). H_2O. Pharmaceutical waters, aquae, are aqueous solutions of volatile substances. Pharmaceutical solutions, liquors, are aqueous solutions of nonvolatile substances. SEE water (3), solution (3). [L.]

a. re′gia, a. rega′lis, SYN nitrohydrochloric acid. [L. royal water, so called from its power to dissolve gold]

aq·ua·co·bal·a·min (ak′wă-kō-bal′ă-min). vitamin B_{12a} (tautomeric with B_{12b}); a cobalamin derivative in which the sixth coordinate bond of the cobaltic ion is attached to a water molecule. SEE ALSO *vitamin* B_{12}. SYN aquocobalamin.

aq·ua·pho·bia (ak-wă-fō′bē-ă). Morbid fear of water. [L. *aqua*, water, + G. *phobos*, fear]

aq·ua·punc·ture (ak-wă-pŭnk′chyūr). Rarely used term for a hypodermic injection of water. [L. *aqua*, water, + *punctura*, puncture]

Aq·ua·spi·ril·lum (ah-kwah-spī-ril′ŭm). A genus of motile, nonsporeforming, aerobic bacteria (family Spirillaceae) containing Gram-negative, rigid, helical or helically curved cells which are 0.2 to 1.5 μm in diameter. Motile cells contain fascicles of flagella at one or both poles. Some species can grow anaerobically with nitrate instead of oxygen as the terminal electron acceptor. These organisms are chemoorganotrophic, possessing a strictly respiratory metabolism. They do not ferment carbohydrates; a few species can oxidize a limited variety of carbohydrates. The habitat of these organisms is fresh water. The type species is *A. serpens*. [L. *aqua*, water, + *spirillum*, coil]

aquat·ic (ă-kwat′ik). **1.** Of or pertaining to water. **2.** Denoting an organism that lives in water.

aq·ue·duct (ak′we-dŭkt). A conduit or canal. SYN aqueductus [NA]. [L. *aquaeductus*]

cerebral a., an ependymal-lined canal in the mesencephalon about 20 mm long, connecting the third to the fourth ventricle. SYN aqueductus cerebri [NA], a. of cerebrum, aqueductus sylvii, iter a tertio ad quartum ventriculum, sylvian a.

a. of cerebrum, SYN cerebral a.

cochlear a., SYN perilymphatic *duct.*

Cotunnius' a., SYN a. of vestibule.

fallopian a., SYN facial *canal.*

sylvian a., SYN cerebral a.

a. of vestibule, a bony canal running from the vestibule and opening on the posterior surface of the petrous portion of the temporal bone, giving passage to the endolymphatic duct and a small vein. SYN aqueductus cotunnii, aqueductus vestibuli, Cotunnius' a., Cotunnius' canal.

aq·ue·duc·tus, pl. **aq·ue·duc·tus** (ak-we-dŭk′tŭs) [NA]. SYN aqueduct. [L. fr. *aqua*, water, + *ductus*, a leading, fr. *duco*, pp. *ductus*, to lead]

a. cer′ebri [NA], SYN cerebral *aqueduct.*

a. coch′leae, SYN perilymphatic *duct.*

a. cotun′nii, SYN *aqueduct* of vestibule.

a. fallo′pii, SYN facial *canal.*

a. syl′vii, SYN cerebral *aqueduct.*

a. vestib′uli, [NA] SYN *aqueduct* of vestibule.

aque·ous (ak′wē-ŭs, ā′kwē-ŭs). Watery; of, like, or containing water.

aquip·ar·ous (ă-kwip′er-ŭs). Secreting or excreting a watery fluid. [L. *aqua*, water, + *pario*, to bring forth]

aq·uo·co·bal·a·min (ak′wō-kō-bal′ă-min). SYN aquacobalamin.

aq·uo·i·on (ak′wō-ī′on). A hydrated ion; an ion containing one or more water molecules; *e.g.,* $Cu(H_2O)_4^{2+}$.

aquos·i·ty (ă-kwos′i-tē). **1.** The state of being watery. **2.** Moisture.

Ar Symbol for argon.

Ara Symbol for arabinose, or its mono- or diradical.

△ara-. Prefix for arabinose or arabinosyl.

△arab-. Gum arabic; similar gummy substances. [G. *Araps, Arabos*, an Arab]

ar·a·ban (a′ră-ban). A polysaccharide that yields arabinose on hydrolysis; a constituent of some pectins.

ar·a·bic (a′ră-bik). Relating to or derived from various species of *Acacia* having a gummy or resinous exudate.

ar·a·bic ac·id. SYN arabin.

ar·a·bin (a′ră-bin). A carbohydrate gum, hydrolyzing to D-arabinose and hexoses, found naturally in union with calcium, potassium, and magnesium ions, when it is called gum arabic. SYN arabic acid.

ar·a·bi·no·a·den·o·sine (a′ră-bin-ō-ah-den′ō-sēn). SYN arabinosyladenine.

ar·a·bi·no·cy·ti·dine (a′ră-bin-ō-sī′ti-dēn). SYN arabinosylcytosine.

ara·bin·o·fur·a·no·syl·ad·e·nine (a′ră-bin-ō-fūr′ă-nō-sil-ad′ĕ-nēn). An arabinoside that has antiviral activity.

ar·a·bi·no·fu·ra·no·syl·cy·to·sine (a′ră-bin-ō-fūr′ă-nō-sil-sī′tō-sēn). SYN arabinosylcytosine.

arab·i·nose (Ara) (ă-rab′i-nōs, a′ră-bin-ōs). A pentose whose D-isomer is widely distributed in plants, usually in complex polysaccharides; used in culture media. D-a. is an epimer of D-ribose. [arabin + -ose (1)]

a. 5-phosphate, a phosphorylated a. that is an intermediate in the pentose phosphate pathway.

a. 5-phosphate 2-epimerase, an enzyme in the pentose phosphate pathway that reversibly interconverts a. and ribose 5-phosphate.

ar·a·bi·no·sides (ă-rab′i-nō-sīdz). A ribonucleoside in which the sugar moiety is arabinose. It often has antibiotic activity.

arab·i·no·sis (ă-rab-i-nō′sis). Disordered metabolism of arabinose.

ar·a·bi·no·su·ria (ă-rab′i-nō-sū′rē-ă). Excretion of arabinose in the urine.

ar·a·bi·no·syl·ad·e·nine (a′ră-bin-ō-sil-ā′den-ēn). 9-β-D-arabinofuranosyladenine; used for herpes simplex corneae and vaccinial keratitis. SYN arabinoadenosine.

ar·a·bi·no·syl·cy·to·sine (aC, araC) (a′ră-bin-ō-sil-sī′tō-sēn). A compound of arabinose and cytosine, analogous to ribosylcytosine (cytidine), that inhibits the biosynthesis of DNA; used as a chemotherapeutic agent because of antiviral and tumor-growth inhibiting properties. SYN arabinocytidine, arabinofuranosylcytosine, cytarabine.

arab·i·tol (ă-rab′i-tol). $C_5H_{12}O_5$; 1,2,3,4,5-pentanepentol; a sugar alcohol obtained from the reduction of arabinose.

AraC. Abbreviation for *cytosine* arabinoside.

araC Symbol for arabinosylcytosine.

arach·ic ac·id (ă-rak′ik). SYN arachidic acid.

ar·a·chid·ic ac·id (a-ră-kid′ik). $CH_3(CH_2)_{18}COOH$; a fatty acid contained in peanut oil, butter, and other fats. SYN arachic acid, *n*-eicosanoic acid, *n*-icosanoic acid. [*Arachis,* fr. G. *arakis,* leguminous weed]

ar·a·chi·don·ic ac·id (ă-rak-i-don′ik). $CH_3(CH_2)_3(CH_2CH=CH)_4(CH_2)_3COOH$; 5,8,11,14-eicosatetraenoic (icosatetraenoic) acid; an unsaturated fatty acid, usually essential in nutrition; the biological precursor of the prostaglandins, the thromboxanes, and the leukotrienes collectively known as eicosanoids.

ar·a·chi·don·ic ac·id cas·cade. Eicosanoid synthetic pathway.

ar·a·chis oil (ar′ă-kis). SYN peanut oil.

arach·ne·pho·bia (ă-rak-nē-fō′bē-ă). Morbid fear of spiders. SYN arachnophobia. [G. *arachne,* spider, + *phobos,* fear]

Arach·nia (ă-rak′nē-ă). A genus of nonmotile, nonsporeforming, facultatively anaerobic bacteria (family Actinomycetaceae) containing Gram-positive, non-acid-fast, branched, diphtheroid rods (0.2 to 0.3 by 3.0 to 5.0 μm and longer). These organisms produce filamentous microcolonies. Their metabolism is fermentative. Primarily propionic and acetic acids are produced from glucose. Catalase is not produced. The cell wall contains diaminopimelic acid but not arabinose. These organisms are pathogenic for man, causing lacrimal canaliculitis and typical actinomycosis. The type species is *A. propionica.*

A. propio′nica, a species causing lacrimal canaliculitis and typical actinomycosis; it is the type species of the genus *A.* SYN *Propionibacterium propionicus.*

Arach·ni·da (ă-rak′ni-dă). A class of arthropods in the subphylum Chelicerata, consisting of spiders, scorpions, harvestmen, mites, ticks, and allies. [G. *arachnē,* spider]

arach·nid·ism (ă-rak′ni-dizm). Systemic poisoning following the bite of a spider (especially of the black widow spider).

arach·no·dac·ty·ly (ă-rak-nō-dak′ti-lē). A condition in which the hands and fingers, and often the feet and toes, are abnormally long and slender; a characteristic of Marfan's syndrome [MIM*154700], Achard syndrome [MIM*100700], the MASS syndrome [MIM*157700], and kindred hereditary disorders of connective tissue. SYN spider finger. [G. *arachnē,* spider, + *daktylos,* finger]

arach·noid (ă-rak′noyd). A delicate fibrous membrane forming the middle of the three coverings of the central nervous system. In life, its smooth external surface is closely applied (but not attached) to the internal surface of the dura mater, with only a potential space (subdural space) intervening. It is held against the dura by the pressure of the cerebrospinal fluid (CSF) which occupies the subarachnoid space which lies immediately deep to the a., intervening between it and the pia mater. Thus, in a spinal puncture, dura mater and a. are penetrated simultaneously as if a single layer. In the absence of CSF pressure in the cadaver, the a. falls away from the dura, the subdural space becoming an artifactual true space. The a. is named for the delicate, spider-web-like filaments that extend from its deep surface, through the CSF of the subarachnoid space, to the pia mater. SEE ALSO leptomeninges. SYN arachnoidea, arachnoides [NA], arachnoid a., arachnoid membrane, parietal layer of leptomeninges. [G. *arachnē,* spider, cobweb, + *eidos,* resemblance]

a. of brain, that portion of the a. which lies within the cranial cavity and surrounds the brain and the cranial portion of the subarachnoid space. In several sites it is relatively widely-separated from the pia mater, creating the cranial subarachnoid cisterns. SYN a. mater cranialis [NA], a. mater encephali✩, cerebral part of arachnoid.

arachnoid a., SYN arachnoid.

a. mater cranialis [NA], SYN a. of brain.

a. mater encephali, ✩official alternate term for a. of brain.

a.'s mater spinalis [NA], SYN a. of spinal cord.

a. of spinal cord, that portion of the a. which lies within the vertebral canal and surrounds the spinal cord and the vertebral portion of the subarachnoid space. It extends from the foramen magnum above to the S-2 vertebral level. Since the spinal cord ends at the L-2 vertebral level, a wide separation occurs between the a. and pia mater, the lumbar cistern, filled with cerebrospinal fluid in which the cauda equina is suspended. SYN a.'s mater spinalis [NA], spinal part of arachnoid.

ar·ach·noi·dal (ă-rak-noy′dăl). Relating to the arachnoid membrane, or arachnoidea.

ar·ach·noi·dea, ar·ach·noi·des (ă-rak-noyd′ē-ă, -dēz) [NA]. SYN arachnoid. [Mod. L. *arachnoideus* fr. G. *arachnē,* spider, + *eidos,* resemblance]

arach·noid·i·tis (ă-rak-noy-dī′tis). Inflammation of the arachnoid membrane often with involvement of the subjacent subarachnoid space. SEE ALSO leptomeningitis. [arachnoidea + -*itis*, inflammation]

adhesive a., thickening of the leptomeninges, sometimes with obliteration of the subarachnoid space; commonly related to acute or chronic leptomeningitis of bacterial or chemical origin. SEE ALSO leptomeningeal *fibrosis.* SYN obliterative a.

neoplastic a., SYN neoplastic *meningitis.*

obliterative a., SYN adhesive a.

arach·no·ly·sin (ă-rak-nol′i-sin). A hemolytic substance in the venom of certain spiders.

⟁ **Combining forms**	**[NA]** Nomina Anatomica
Word*Finder*	**[MIM]** Mendelian
Multi-term entry finder	**Inheritance in Man**
Preceding letter A	
	✩ **Official alternate term**
A.D.A.M. Anatomy Plates	
Between letters L and M	✩**[NA] Official alternate**
	Nomina Anatomica term
Appendices:	
Following letter Z	
	High Profile Term
SYN Synonym; Cf., compare	

arach·no·pho·bia (ă-rak-nō-fō'bē-ă). SYN arachnephobia.

ar·al·kyl (ă-ral'kil). A radical in which an aryl group is substituted for a hydrogen atom of an alkyl group; *e.g.,* C₆H₅CH₂–. SYN arylated alkyl.

Aran, François, French physician, 1817–1861. SEE A.-Duchenne *disease;* Duchenne-A. *disease.*

araneism. Rarely used term for arachnidism.

Arantius, (Aranzio), Giulio C., Italian anatomist and physician, 1530–1589. SEE A.'s *ligament, nodule, ventricle; corpus* arantii; *ductus* venosus arantii.

ara·phia (ă-rā'fē-ă). SYN holorachischisis. [G. *a-* priv. + *rhaphē,* a seam]

ar·bor, pl. **ar·bo·res** (ar'bŏr, ar-bō'rēz). In anatomy, a treelike structure with branchings. [L. tree]

a. vi'tae [NA], the arborescent appearance of gray and white matter in sagittal sections of the cerebellum.

a. vi'tae u'teri, SYN palmate *folds,* under *fold.*

ar·bo·res·cent (ar-bō-res'ent). SYN dendriform.

ar·bo·ri·za·tion (ar'bŏr-i-zā'shŭn). **1.** The terminal branching of nerve fibers or blood vessels in a branching treelike pattern. **2.** The branched pattern formed under certain conditions by a dried smear of cervical mucus.

ar·bo·rize (ar'bŏr-īz). To spread in a treelike branching pattern.

ar·bo·roid (ar'bŏr-oyd). Denoting a colony of protozoa, each of which remains attached to another cell or to the main stem at one point, forming a branching or dendritic figure. [L. *arbor,* tree, + G. *eidos,* resemblance]

ar·bor·vi·rus (ar'bŏr-vī'rŭs). SYN arbovirus.

classification of arboviruses		
families	genera	
	arboviruses	nonarboviruses
Togaviridae	alphavirus flavivirus (e.g., yellow fever)	rubivirus (rubella)
Bunyaviridae	bunyavirus, with over 145 species (at least 25 can infect humans)	
Rhabdoviridae	vesiculovirus (vesicular stomatitis)	Lyssa virus (rabies)
Reoviridae	orbivirus (e.g., Colorado tick fever)	reovirus rotavirus

ar·bo·vi·rus (ar'bō-vī'rŭs). A large, heterogenous group of RNA viruses, most ranging from 40 to 100 nm or more in diameter, and divisible into groups on the basis of characteristics of the virions. There are over 500 species, which are distributed among several families (Togaviridae, Flaviviridae, Bunyaviridae, Arenaviridae, Rhabdoviridae, Reoviridae) have been recovered from arthropods, bats, and rodents, and most, but not all, are arthropod-borne. These taxonomically diverse animal viruses are unified by an epidemiological concept, *i.e.,* transmission between vertebrate hosts by blood-feeding (hematophagous) arthropod vectors, such as mosquitoes, ticks, sandflies, and midges.. Although about 100 species can infect man, in most instances diseases produced by these viruses are of a very mild nature and difficult to distinguish from illnesses caused by viruses of other taxonomic groups. Apparent infections may be separated into several clinical syndromes: undifferentiated type fevers (systemic febrile disease), hepatitis, hemorrhagic fevers, and encephalitides. SYN arborvirus. [*ar,* arthropod, + *bo,* borne, + *virus*]

ARC Abbreviation for AIDS-related *complex.*

arc (ark). **1.** A curved line or segment of a circle. **2.** Continuous luminous passage of an electric current in a gas or vacuum between two or more separated carbon or other electrodes. [L. *arcus,* a bow]

auricular a., binauricular a., a line carried over the cranium from the center of one external auditory meatus to that of the other. SYN interauricular a.

bregmatolambdoid a., the line running along the sagittal suture from the bregma to the apex of the lambdoid suture.

crater a., an a. of a direct current that forms a pitlike excavation at the positive pole.

flame a., an a. between two impregnated electrodes that causes volatilization of the core with resultant flame.

interauricular a., SYN auricular a.

longitudinal a. of skull, the line carried over the skull in the midline from the nasion to the opisthion.

mercury a., an electric discharge through mercury vapor between electrodes, one of which is usually mercury; provides a rich source of therapeutic ultraviolet rays; the containing tube is usually quartz; may also be glass with a fluorite window.

nasobregmatic a., a line running through the midline of the forehead from the nasion to the bregma.

naso-occipital a., the a. in the midline from the root of the nose to the inferior limit of the external occipital protuberance.

pulmonary a., obsolete term for pulmonary *salient.*

reflex a., the route followed by nerve impulses in the production of a reflex act, from the peripheral receptor organ through the afferent nerve to the central nervous system synapse and then through the efferent nerve to the effector organ.

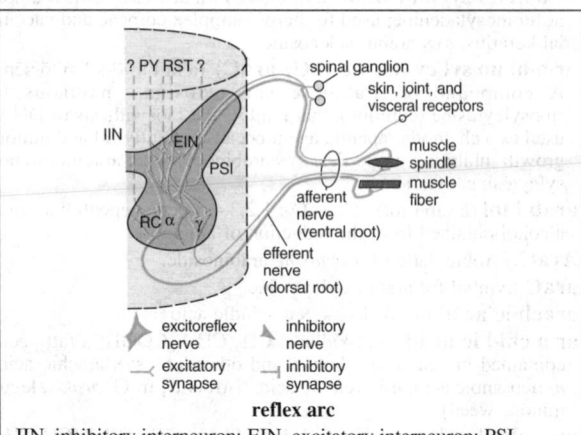

reflex arc
IIN, inhibitory interneuron; EIN, excitatory interneuron; PSI, presynaptic inhibition; RST, reticulospinal tract; PY, pyramidal tract; RC, Renshaw cell; α = α motorneuron; γ = motoneuron

Riolan's a., (1) SYN intestinal arterial *arcades,* under *arcade.* **(2)** SYN marginal *artery* of colon. **(3)** SYN Riolan's *anastomosis.*

ar·cade (ar-kād). An anatomical structure or structures (especially a blood vessel) taking the form of a series of arches. [L. *arcus,* arc, bow]

anomalous mitral a., short chordae tendineae extending from both papillary muscles to the central portion of the anterior leaflet of the mitral valve and resulting in stenosis or incompetence of the valve.

arterial a.'s, a series of anastomosing arterial arches, as the intestinal arterial a.'s between the branches of the jejunal and ileal arteries in the mesentery and the pancreaticoduodenal arteries on the head of the pancreas.

Flint's a., a series of vascular arches at the bases of the pyramids of the kidney.

intestinal arterial a.'s, the series of arterial arches formed in the mesentery by anastomoses between adjacent jejunal and ileal arteries and from which vasa recta arise. The arterial a.'s of the ileum are shorter and more complex than those of the jejunum. SEE ALSO arterial *arches* of ileum, under *arch,* arterial *arches* of jejunum, under *arch.* SYN intermesenteric arterial anastomosis, Riolan's arc (1), Riolan's a.'s.

pancreaticoduodenal arterial a.'s, anastomoses between the anterior and posterior pancreaticoduodenal arteries (from the gastroduodenal artery) and the anterior and posterior inferior pancreaticoduodenal arteries (from the superior mesenteric artery) on the anterior and posterior aspects of the head of the pancreas and the duodenum, supplying both structures.

Riolan's a.'s, SYN intestinal arterial a.'s. SEE ALSO Riolan's *anastomosis.*

Ar·can·o·bac·te·ri·um (ar-kā'nō-bac-tēr'ē-oom). A genus of nonmotile, facultatively anaerobic bacteria containing Gram-positive slender irregular rods, sometimes showing clubbed ends that may be in V formation with no filaments. These organisms are obligate parasites of the pharynx in farm animals and humans, occasionally causing lesions on the pharynx or skin. The type species is *A. haemolyticum.*

A. haemolyticum, a species that causes pharyngitis and chronic skin ulcers in humans as well as farm animals.

ar·cate (ar'kāt). SYN arcuate.

ARCH

arch. Any structure resembling a bent bow or an arch; an arc. In anatomy, any vaulted or archlike structure. SEE arcus. SYN arcus [NA]. [thru O. Fr. fr. L. *arcus,* bow]

abdominothoracic a., a bell-shaped line defined by the lower end of the sternum and the costal a.'s on each side, constituting a boundary line between the anterolateral portions of the thoracic and abdominal walls.

alveolar a. of mandible, the free margin of the alveolar process of the mandible. SYN arcus alveolaris mandibulae [NA], limbus alveolaris (1).

alveolar a. of maxilla, the free border of the alveolar process of the maxilla. SYN arcus alveolaris maxillae [NA], limbus alveolaris (2).

anterior a. of atlas, an arch that connects the lateral masses of the atlas anteriorly and articulates with the anterior articular facet of the dens of the axis. SYN arcus anterior atlantis [NA].

anterior palatine a., SYN palatoglossal a.

aortic a., (1) the curved portion between the ascending and descending parts of the aorta; it begins as a continuation of the ascending aorta posterior to the sternal angle, runs posteriorly and slightly to the left as it passes over the root of the left lung, and becomes the descending aorta as it reaches and begins to course along the vertebral column; it gives rise to the brachiocephalic trunk, the left common carotid and left subclavian arteries; SYN arch of the aorta. **(2)** any member of the several pairs of arterial channels encircling the embryonic pharynx in the mesenchyme of the brachial a.'s; there are potentially six pairs, but in mammals the fifth pair is poorly developed or absent. The first and second pairs are functional only in very young embryos; the third pair is involved in the formation of the carotids; the fourth a. on the left is incorporated in the a. of the aorta; the sixth pair forms the proximal part of the pulmonary arteries. SYN arcus aortae [NA].

aortic a.'s, a series of arterial channels encircling the embryonic pharynx in the mesenchyme of the branchial a.'s. There are potentially six pairs, but in mammals the fifth pair is poorly developed or absent. The first and second pairs are functional only in very young embryos; the third pair is involved in the formation of the carotids; the fourth a. on the left is incorporated in the a. of the aorta; the sixth pair forms the proximal part of the pulmonary arteries.

arterial a.'s of colon, anastomosing branches of the colic arteries that form a.'s in the mesocolon from which the walls of the colon are supplied. SEE marginal *artery* of colon.

arterial a.'s of ileum, a.'s formed in the mesentery by branches of the superior mesenteric artery from which vessels (*vasa* recta, under *vas*) arise to supply the wall of the ileum. SEE ALSO intestinal arterial *arcades,* under *arcade.*

arterial a.'s of jejunum, a.'s formed in the mesentery by

branches of the superior mesenteric artery from which vessels (*vasa recta,* under *vas*) arise to supply the walls of the jejunum. SEE ALSO intestinal arterial *arcades,* under *arcade.*

arterial a. of lower eyelid, formed by the medial palpebral artery which communicates with a branch of the lacrimal artery along the tarsal margin. SYN arcus palpebralis inferior [NA].

arterial a. of upper eyelid, formed by communicating branches of the medial and lateral palpebral arteries. Often two arches are present, one located near the free border of the tarsal plate, the other along the upper border of the tarsus. SYN arcus palpebralis superior [NA].

axillary a., SYN pectorodorsalis *muscle.*

branchial a.'s, typically, 6 a.'s in vertebrates; in the lower vertebrates, they bear gills; in the higher vertebrates, they appear transiently and give rise to specialized structures in the head and neck. SYN pharyngeal a.'s, visceral a.'s.

carpal a.'s, two anastomotic arterial twigs running transversely across the wrist: the *palmar* or *anterior* lies in front of the carpus, being formed by palmar carpal branches of the radial and ulnar arteries; the *dorsal* or *posterior* lies on the dorsal surface of the carpus, being formed by the dorsal carpal branches of the radial and ulnar arteries.

coracoacromial a., a protective a. formed by the smooth inferior aspect of the acromion and the coracoid process of the scapula with the coracoacromial ligament spanning between them. This osseoligamentous structure overlies the head of the humerus, preventing its upward displacement from the glenoid fossa.

cortical a.'s of kidney, the portions of renal substance (cortex) intervening between the bases of the pyramids and the capsule of the kidney.

Corti's a., the a. formed by the junction of the heads of Corti's inner and outer pillar cells.

costal a., that portion of the inferior aperture of the thorax formed by the articulated cartilages of the seventh to tenth (false) ribs. SYN arcus costalis [NA], arcus costarum.

a. of cricoid cartilage, the narrow part of the cartilage that encircles the air passage anterior to the lamina. SYN arcus cartilaginis cricoideae [NA].

crural a., SYN inguinal *ligament.*

deep crural a., SYN iliopubic *tract.*

deep palmar (arterial) a., the arterial arch located deep to the long flexor tendons in the hand. It is formed by the terminal part of the radial artery in conjunction with the deep palmar branch of the ulnar artery. The a. gives rise to palmar metacarpal and princeps pollicis arteries. SYN arcus palmaris profundus [NA], arcus volaris profundus.

deep palmar venous a., the venous arch that accompanies the deep palmar arterial arch; it usually consists of paired venae comitantes. SYN arcus venosus palmaris profundus [NA].

dental a., the curved composite structure of the natural dentition and the residual ridge, or the remains thereof after the loss of some or all of the natural teeth.

dorsal venous a. of foot, the arch in the subcutaneous tissue of the dorsum of the foot formed by the dorsal and digital veins; it unites medially with the dorsal vein of the great toe to form the great saphenous vein, and laterally with the dorsal vein of the little toe to form the small saphenous. SYN arcus venosus dorsalis pedis [NA].

double aortic a., congenital malformation of the aorta that splits and has a right and a left a. instead of a single a.

expansion a., an orthodontic appliance that moves the dental structures distally, bucally, or labially, creating increased molar to molar width and arch length.

fallen a.'s, a breaking down of the a.'s of the foot, either longitudinal, transverse, or both; the resulting deformity is flat or splay foot, or both.

fallopian a., SYN inguinal *ligament.*

femoral a., SYN inguinal *ligament.*

a.'s of the foot, SEE longitudinal a. of foot, plantar a.

glossopalatine a., SYN palatoglossal a.

Gothic a., SYN needle point *tracing.*

Haller's a.'s, SEE lateral arcuate *ligament,* medial arcuate *ligament.*

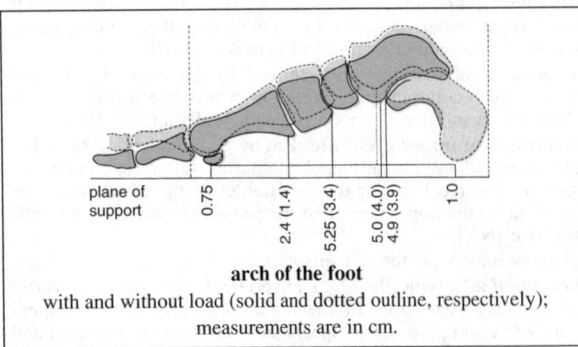

arch of the foot
with and without load (solid and dotted outline, respectively);
measurements are in cm.

plane of support   0.75   2.4 (1.4)   5.25 (3.4)   5.0 (4.0) 4.9 (3.9)   1.0

hemal a.'s, three or four V-shaped bones located ventral to the bodies of the third to sixth coccygeal vertebrae; they represent intercentra and usually enclose the ventral caudal artery and vein.

hyoid a., the second visceral, or branchial, a; the second postoral a. in the branchial a. series.

iliopectineal a., a thickened band of fused iliac and psoas fascia passing from the posterior aspect of the inguinal ligament anteriorly across the front of the femoral nerve to attach to the iliopectineal eminence of the hip bone posteriorly. The iliopectineal a. thus forms a septum which subdivides the space deep to the inguinal ligament into a lateral muscular lacunae and a medial vascular lacunae. When a psoas minor muscle is present, its tendon of insertion blends with the iliopectineal a. SYN arcus iliopectineus [NA], iliopectineal ligament, ligamentum iliopectineale.

inferior dental a., the teeth supported by the alveolar part of the mandible, whether the 10 deciduous teeth or the 16 permanent teeth. SYN arcus dentalis inferior [NA], mandibular dentition.

jugular venous a., a connecting vein between the two anterior jugular veins in the suprasternal space. SYN arcus venosus juguli [NA].

labial a., an orthodontic a. wire that approximates the labial surfaces of the teeth.

Langer's a., SYN axillary arch *muscle*.

lateral longitudinal a. of foot, formed by calcaneus, cuboid and two lateral metatarsals; the combined a. is supported normally by ligaments, intrinsic muscles, and the tendons of extrinsic muscles of the foot. SYN arcus pedis longitudinalis pars lateralis.

lateral lumbocostal a., SYN lateral arcuate *ligament*.

lingual a., an orthodontic a. wire that approximates the lingual surfaces of the teeth.

longitudinal a. of foot, SEE medial longitudinal a. of foot, lateral longitudinal a. of foot. SYN arcus pedis longitudinalis, lateral part of longitudinal arch of foot.

malar a., SYN zygomatic a.

mandibular a., the first postoral a. in the branchial a. series. SYN mandibular process.

medial longitudinal a. of foot, formed by the calcaneus, talus, navicular, three cuneiform bones, and the three medial metatarsals. SYN arcus pedis longitudinalis pars medialis.

medial lumbocostal a., SYN medial arcuate *ligament*.

nasal a., bridge of the nose, the upward arching roof of the piriform aperture formed by the nasal processes of the maxilla of each side and the nasal bones between them. Eyeglasses rest centrally on various portions of this a.

nasal venous a., an a. formed at the root of the nose by the two supratrochlear veins connected by a transverse vein.

neural a., SYN vertebral a.

a. of the palate, the vaulted roof of the mouth.

palatoglossal a., one of a pair of ridges or folds of mucous membrane passing from the soft palate to the side of the tongue; it encloses the palatoglossus muscle and forms anterior margin of the tonsillar fossa. Also demarcates oral cavity from isthmus of fauces. SYN arcus palatoglossus [NA], anterior palatine a., anterior pillar of fauces, arcus glossopalatinus, glossopalatine a., glossopalatine fold.

palatopharyngeal a., one of a pair of ridges or folds of mucous membrane which passes downward from the posterior margin of the soft palate to the lateral wall of the pharynx. It encloses the palatopharyngeus muscle and forms the posterior margin of the tonsillar fossa. It also demarcates the isthmus of fauces from oropharynx. SYN arcus palatopharyngeus [NA], pharyngopalatine a., posterior palatine a., posterior pillar of fauces.

pharyngeal a.'s, SYN branchial a.'s.

pharyngopalatine a., SYN palatopharyngeal a.

plantar a., (1) the arterial arch formed by the lateral plantar artery running across the bases of the metatarsal bones and anastomosing with the dorsal pedis artery; **(2)** either of two bony a.'s of the foot, longitudinal a. or transverse a. SEE ALSO medial longitudinal a. of foot, lateral longitudinal a. of foot, transverse a. of foot. SYN arcus plantaris [NA], plantar arterial a.

plantar arterial a., SYN plantar a.

plantar venous a., the arch formed by the plantar digital veins from the toes which accompanies the plantar arterial arch. SYN arcus venosus plantaris [NA].

popliteal a., SYN arcuate popliteal *ligament*.

posterior a. of atlas, the posterior arch of the atlas that connects the lateral masses of the atlas posteriorly, forming the posterior wall of the vertebral canal at this level. SYN arcus posterior atlantis [NA].

posterior palatine a., SYN palatopharyngeal a.

postoral a.'s, the series of branchial a.'s caudal to the mouth; the first is the mandibular, the second is the hyoid; caudal to the hyoid, the a.'s are unnamed, and designated only by their postoral number.

primitive costal a.'s, a.'s formed in the thoracic region of the vertebral column in the embryo from the costal processes or costal elements which give rise to the ribs.

pubic a., the arch formed by the symphysis, bodies and inferior rami of the pubic bones. SEE ALSO subpubic *angle*. SYN arcus pubis [NA].

ribbon a., a thin, ribbon-shaped, rectangular orthodontic a. wire applied to the dental a.'s so that its widest dimension is parallel to the labial or buccal surfaces of the teeth.

superciliary a., a fullness extending laterally from the glabella on either side, above the orbital margin of the frontal bone. SYN arcus superciliaris [NA], superciliary ridge.

superficial palmar (arterial) a., the arterial arch in the hand located superficial to the long flexor tendons approximately at the level of a line extrapolated across the palm from the distal side of the outstretched thumb. It is formed principally by the termination of the superficial ulnar artery and is usually completed by a communication with the superficial palmar branch of the radial artery. The a. gives rise to the common palmar digital arteries. SYN arcus palmaris superficialis [NA], arcus volaris superficialis.

superficial palmar venous a., the venous arch accompanying the superficial palmar arterial arch; it consists usually of paired venae comitantes and is drained by the superficial ulnar and radial veins. SYN arcus venosus palmaris superficialis [NA].

superior dental a., the teeth supported by the alveolar process of the two maxillae, whether the 10 deciduous teeth or the 16 permanent teeth. SYN arcus dentalis superior [NA], maxillary dentition.

supraorbital a., SYN supraorbital *margin*.

tarsal a., SEE arterial a. of lower eyelid, arterial a. of upper eyelid.

tendinous a., (1) a white, fibrous band attached to bone and/or muscle, arching over and thus protecting neurovascular elements passing beneath it from injurious compression; **(2)** a linear thickening of the deep fascia of a muscle which provides attachment for ligaments and/or muscle fibers. SYN arcus tendineus [NA].

tendinous a. of levator ani muscle, a thickened portion of the obturator fascia that extends in an arching line from the pubis posteriorly to the ischial spine and gives origin to part of the levator ani muscle. SYN arcus tendineus musculi levatoris ani [NA], arcus tendineus of obturator fascia.

tendinous a. of pelvic fascia, a linear thickening of the superior fascia of the pelvic diaphragm extending posteriorly from the body of the pubis alongside the bladder (and vagina in the female) and giving attachment to the supporting ligaments of the pelvic viscera. SYN arcus tendineus fasciae pelvis [NA].

tendinous a. of soleus muscle, a tendinous arch stretching over the popliteal vessels between the tibia and fibula, that gives origin to the central portion of the soleus muscle. SYN arcus tendineus musculi solei [NA].

a. of thoracic duct, SEE thoracic *duct.*

transverse a. of foot, the arch formed by the proximal parts of the metatarsal bones, the three cuneiform bones, and the cuboid. SYN arcus pedis transversalis.

Treitz' a., SYN paraduodenal *fold.*

vertebral a., the posterior projection from the body of a vertebra that encloses the vertebral foramen; it consists of paired pedicles and laminae; the spinous, transverse, and articular processes arise from the arch. In aggregate, the venous a.'s—and the ligamenta flava that unite them—form the posterior wall of the vertebral (spinal) canal. SYN arcus vertebrae [NA], neural a.

visceral a.'s, SYN branchial a.'s.

W-a., a fixed maxillary expansion device attached to the lingual part of the molars, with either bilateral or unilateral extension arms.

wire a., a wire conforming to the dental a.; used to restore the normal curve to the denture.

zygomatic a., the arch formed by the temporal process of the zygomatic bone that joins the zygomatic process of the temporal bone. SYN arcus zygomaticus [NA], cheek bone (2), malar a., zygoma (2).

---

arch-, arche-, archi-, archo-. Combining forms meaning primitive, or ancestral; also first, or chief. primitive, ancestral; first, chief, extreme. [G. *archē,* origin, beginning, + -o-]

ar·chae·o·cer·e·bel·lum (ar′kē-ō-ser′ĕ-bel′lŭm). SYN archicerebellum. [G. *archaios,* ancient, + cerebellum]

ar·chae·us (ar-kē′ŭs). Term first used by Valentine and later by Paracelsus and van Helmont to denote a spirit that presided over and governed bodily processes. SYN archeus. [L. fr. G. *archaios,* chief, leader]

ar·cha·ic (ar-kā′ik). Ancient; old; in jungian psychology, denoting the ancestral past of mental processes. [G. *archaikos,* ancient]

Archambault, LaSalle, U.S. neurologist, 1879–1940. SEE Meyer-A. *loop.*

arche-. SEE arch-.

arch·en·ter·on (ark-en′ter-on). SYN primitive *gut.* [G. *archē,* beginning, + *enteron,* intestine]

ar·che·o·cer·e·bel·lum. SYN vestibulocerebellum.

ar·che·o·ki·net·ic (ar-kē-ō-ki-net′ik). Denoting a low and primitive type of motor nerve mechanism, such as is found in the peripheral and the ganglionic nervous systems. Cf. neokinetic, paleokinetic. [G. *archaios,* ancient, + *kinētikos,* relating to movement]

ar·che·type (ar′kē-tīp). **1.** A primitive structural plan from which various modifications have evolved. **2.** In jungian psychology, structural manifestation of the collective unconscious. SYN imago (2). [G. *archetypos,* pattern, model, fr. *archē,* beginning, + *typtō,* to stamp out]

ar·che·us (ar-kē′ŭs). SYN archaeus.

archi-. SEE arch-.

ar·chi·cer·e·bel·lum (ar′ki-ser-ĕ-bel′ŭm) [NA]. The small, phylogenetically oldest portion of the cerebellum, also called vestibulocerebellum because its afferents arise from the vestibular ganglion and nuclei; in mammals, it is represented by four subdivisions of the cerebellum: nodulus, uvula vermis, flocculus, and lingula of cerebellum. SYN archaeocerebellum. [archi- + L. *cerebellum*]

ar·chi·cor·tex (ar′ki-kōr′teks). **1.** Typically, the phylogenetically older parts of the cerebral cortex. **2.** More specifically, the cortex forming the hippocampus. SEE ALSO allocortex, cerebral *cortex.* SYN archipallium. [archi- + L. *cortex*]

ar·chil (ar′kil) [old C.I. 1242]. A violet dye from the lichens

Rocella tinctoria and *R. fuciformis.* SYN orchella, orchil, roccellin.

ar·chin (ar′kin). SYN emodin.

ar·chi·pal·li·um (ar-ki-pal′ē-ŭm). SYN archicortex. [archi- + L. *pallium*]

ar·chi·tec·ton·ics (ar-ki-tek-ton′iks). SYN cytoarchitecture.

archo-. **1.** Variant of arch-. [G. *archē,* origin, beginning] **2.** OBSOLETE the rectum SEE procto-, recto-. [G. *archos,* rectum]

arch·wire (arch′wīr). A device consisting of a wire conforming to the alveolar or dental arch, used as an anchorage in correcting irregularities in the position of the teeth. SYN arch wire.

ar·ci·form (ar′ki-fōrm). SYN arcuate.

arc·ta·tion (ark-tā′shŭn). A narrowing, contraction, stricture, or coarctation. [L. *arto* (improp. *arcto*), pp. *-atus,* to tighten]

ar·cu·al (ar′kyū-ăl). Relating to an arch.

ar·cu·ate (ar′kyū-āt). Denoting a form that is arched or has the shape of a bow. SYN arcate, arciform. [L. *arcuatus,* bowed]

ar·cu·a·tion (ar-kyū-ā′shŭn). A bending or curvature.

ARCUS

---

ar·cus, gen. and pl. **ar·cus** (ar′kŭs) [NA]. SYN arch. [L. a bow]
a. adipo′sus, SYN a. cornealis.
a. alveola′ris mandib′ulae [NA], SYN alveolar *arch* of mandible.
a. alveola′ris maxil′lae [NA], SYN alveolar *arch* of maxilla.
a. ante′rior atlan′tis [NA], SYN anterior *arch* of atlas.
a. aor′tae [NA], SYN aortic *arch* (2).

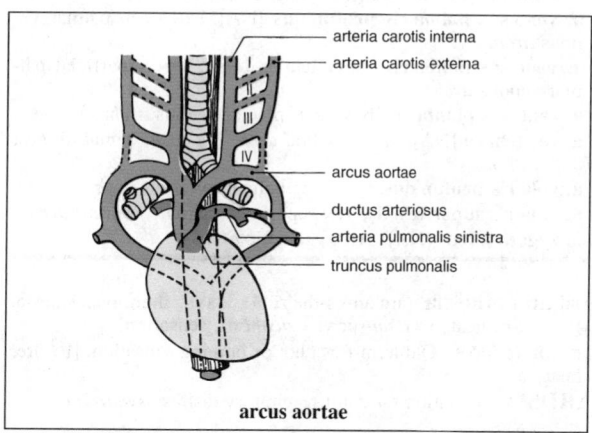

arteria carotis interna
arteria carotis externa

arcus aortae
ductus arteriosus
arteria pulmonalis sinistra
truncus pulmonalis

arcus aortae

a. cartila′ginis cricoi′deae [NA], SYN *arch* of cricoid cartilage.
a. cornea′lis, an opaque, grayish ring at the periphery of the cornea just within the sclerocorneal junction, of frequent occurrence in the aged; it results from a deposit of fatty granules in, or hyaline degeneration of, the lamellae and cells of the cornea. SYN anterior embryotoxon, a. adiposus, a. juvenilis, a. lipoides, a. senilis, gerontoxon, linea corneae senilis, lipoidosis corneae.
a. costa′lis [NA], SYN costal *arch.*
a. costa′rum, SYN costal *arch.*
a. denta′lis infe′rior [NA], SYN inferior dental *arch.*
a. denta′lis supe′rior [NA], SYN superior dental *arch.*
a. duc′tus thorac′ici [NA], SEE thoracic *duct.*
a. glossopalati′nus, SYN palatoglossal *arch.*
a. iliopectin′eus [NA], SYN iliopectineal *arch.*
a. inguina′lis [NA], ✗official alternate term for inguinal *ligament.*
a. juveni′lis, SYN a. cornealis.
a. lipoi′des, SYN a. cornealis.
a. lumbocosta′lis latera′lis, SYN lateral arcuate *ligament.*

a. lumbocosta′lis media′lis, SYN medial arcuate *ligament*.

a. palati′ni, SEE palatoglossal *arch*, palatopharyngeal *arch*.

a. palatoglos′sus [NA], SYN palatoglossal *arch*.

a. palatopharyn′geus [NA], SYN palatopharyngeal *arch*.

a. palma′ris profun′dus [NA], SYN deep palmar (arterial) *arch*.

a. palma′ris superficia′lis [NA], SYN superficial palmar (arterial) *arch*.

a. palpebra′lis infe′rior [NA], SYN arterial *arch* of lower eyelid.

a. palpebra′lis supe′rior [NA], SYN arterial *arch* of upper eyelid.

a. pe′dis longitudina′lis, SYN longitudinal *arch* of foot.

a. pe′dis transversa′lis, SYN transverse *arch* of foot.

a. planta′ris [NA], SYN plantar *arch*.

a. poste′rior atlan′tis [NA], SYN posterior *arch* of atlas.

a. pu′bis [NA], SYN pubic *arch*.

a. rani′nus, SYN Béclard's *anastomosis*.

a. seni′lis, SYN a. cornealis.

a. supercilia′ris [NA], SYN superciliary *arch*.

a. tar′seus, SEE arterial *arch* of lower eyelid, arterial *arch* of upper eyelid.

a. tendin′eus [NA], SYN tendinous *arch*.

a. tendin′eus fas′ciae pel′vis [NA], SYN tendinous *arch* of pelvic fascia.

a. tendin′eus mus′culi levato′ris ani [NA], SYN tendinous *arch* of levator ani muscle.

a. tendin′eus mus′culi so′lei [NA], SYN tendinous *arch* of soleus muscle.

a. tendineus of obturator fascia, SYN tendinous *arch* of levator ani muscle.

a. un′guium, SYN lunula (1).

a. veno′sus dorsa′lis pe′dis [NA], SYN dorsal venous *arch* of foot.

a. veno′sus jug′uli [NA], SYN jugular venous *arch*.

a. veno′sus palma′ris profun′dus [NA], SYN deep palmar venous *arch*.

a. veno′sus palma′ris superficia′lis [NA], SYN superficial palmar venous *arch*.

a. veno′sus planta′ris [NA], SYN plantar venous *arch*.

a. ver′tebrae [NA], SYN vertebral *arch*. SEE ALSO hemal *arches*, under *arch*.

a. vola′ris profun′dus, SYN deep palmar (arterial) *arch*.

a. vola′ris superficia′lis, SYN superficial palmar (arterial) *arch*.

a. zygomat′icus [NA], SYN zygomatic *arch*.

---

ard·an·es·the·sia (ard′an-es-thē′zē-ă). SYN thermoanesthesia. [L. *ardor,* heat, + G. *an-* priv. + *aisthēsis,* sensation]

ar·dor (ar′dŏr). Old term for a hot or burning sensation. [L. fire, heat]

ARDS Abbreviation for adult respiratory distress *syndrome*.

AREA

---

ar·ea (a), pl. **ar·e·ae** (ār′ē-ă, -ē). **1** [NA]. Any circumscribed surface or space. **2.** All of the part supplied by a given artery or nerve. **3.** A part of an organ having a special function, as the motor a. of the brain. SEE ALSO regio, region, space, spatium, zone. [L. a courtyard]

acoustic a., the floor of the lateral recess of the fourth ventricle, extending medially to the limiting sulcus and overlying the cochlear and vestibular nuclei of the rhombencephalon. SYN a. acustica.

a. acu′stica, SYN acoustic a.

anterior intercondylar a. of tibia, the broad depressed a. between the tibial condyles anteriorly to which attach the anterior ends of the menisci and the anterior cruciate ligament. SYN a. intercondylaris anterior tibiae [NA].

aortic a., the region of the chest wall over the second right costal cartilage, where sounds produced at the aortic orifice are often best heard.

apical a., the a. about the root end of a tooth.

association areas, SYN association *cortex*.

auditory a., SYN auditory *cortex*.

bare a. of liver, the a. on the posterior surface of the liver which is fused with the diaphragm and therefore not covered by peritoneum. SYN a. nuda hepatis [NA].

bare a. of stomach, the part of posterior surface of the fundus of the stomach between the two diverging layers of the gastrophrenic ligament, that is not covered by peritoneum.

basal seat a., that portion of the oral structures which is available to support a denture.

Broca's a., SYN Broca's *center*.

Broca's parolfactory a., SYN parolfactory a.

Brodmann's areas, a.'s of the cerebral cortex mapped out on the basis of the cortical cytoarchitectural patterns. SEE cerebral *cortex*.

a. of cardiac dullness, a triangular a. determined by percussion of the front of the chest; it corresponds to the part of the heart that is not covered by lung tissue.

catchment a., a term relating to community mental health center which delimits the geographic area surrounding each center, and thus the population of individuals who qualify for mental health services provided by each center.

Celsus' a., obsolete term for *alopecia* areata.

a. centra′lis, SYN *macula* retinae.

a. coch′leae [NA], SYN cochlear a.

cochlear a., the a. inferior to the transverse crest of the fundus of the internal acoustic meatus through which the filaments of the cochlear nerve pass to enter the cochlea; forms the base of the cone-shaped modiolus about which the cochlear canal spirals. SEE *base* of modiolus. SYN a. cochleae [NA].

Cohnheim's a., a polygonal mosaic-like figure formed by a group of myofibrils, as seen in the cross-section of a skeletal muscle fiber examined under the microscope; a shrinkage artifact of fixation. SYN Cohnheim's field.

contact a., that part of the proximal surface of a tooth which touches the adjacent tooth mesially or distally. SYN contact point, point of proximal contact.

cribriform a. of the renal papilla, the apex of a renal papilla pierced by 10 to 22 openings of the papillary ducts, the foramina papillaria. SYN a. cribrosa papillae renalis [NA].

a. cribro′sa papillae renalis [NA], SYN cribriform a. of the renal papilla.

denture-bearing a., SYN denture foundation a.

denture foundation a., that portion of the basal seat which supports the complete or partial denture base under occlusal load. SYN basal seat, denture-bearing a., denture-supporting a., stress-bearing a. (1), supporting a. (2), tissue-bearing a.

denture-supporting a., SYN denture foundation a.

dermatomic a., SYN dermatome (3).

embryonal a., embryonic a., the a. of the blastoderm on either side of, and immediately cephalic to, the primitive streak where the component cell layers have become thickened.

entorhinal a., Brodmann's a. 28, a cytoarchitecturally well-defined a. of multilaminate cerebral cortex on the medial aspect of the parahippocampal gyrus, immediately caudal to the olfactory cortex of the uncus; the a. is the origin of the major fiber system afferent to the hippocampus, the so-called perforant pathway.

excitable a., SYN motor *cortex*.

a. of facial nerve, the a. in the fundus of the internal acoustic meatus superior to the transverse crest through which the facial nerve passes to enter the facial canal. SYN a. nervi facialis [NA].

Flechsig's areas, three divisions (anterior, lateral, posterior) of each lateral half of the medulla as seen on transverse section, marked off by the root fibers of the hypoglossal and vagus nerves.

frontal a., SYN frontal *cortex*.

fronto-orbital a., SYN orbitofrontal *cortex*.

fusion a., SYN Panum's a.

gastric a., one of a number of small polygonal a.'s, 1–6 mm in diameter, separated by linear depressions on the surface of the mucous membrane of the stomach; they contain the gastric pits, with several gastric glands opening into each pit. SYN a. gastrica [NA].

a. gas′trica [NA], SYN gastric a.

germinal a., a. germinati′va, the place in the blastoderm where the embryo begins to be formed. SYN germinal *disk*.

Head's areas, a.'s of skin exhibiting reflex hyperesthesia and hyperalgesia due to visceral disease.

impression a., in dentistry, that surface which is recorded in an impression.

inferior vestibular a., the a. of the fundus of the internal acoustic meatus inferior to the transverse crest through which the interior portion of the vestibular (saccular) nerve passes. SYN a. vestibularis inferior [NA].

insular a., SYN insula (1).

a. intercondyla′ris ante′rior tibiae [NA], SYN anterior intercondylar a. of tibia.

a. intercondyla′ris poste′rior tibiae [NA], SYN posterior intercondylar a. of tibia.

Jonston's a., obsolete term for *alopecia* areata.

Kiesselbach's a., an a. on the anterior portion of the nasal septum rich in capillaries (Kiesselbach's plexus) and often the seat of epistaxis. SYN Little's a.

lateral hypothalamic a., SYN lateral hypothalamic *region*.

Little's a., SYN Kiesselbach's a.

macular a., SYN *macula* retinae.

Martegiani's a., SYN Martegiani's *funnel*.

mitral a., the region of the chest over the apex of the heart, where the sounds, normal or pathologic, produced at the mitral valves are usually heard most distinctly.

motor a., SYN motor *cortex*.

a. ner′vi facia′lis [NA], SYN a. of facial nerve.

a. nu′da hep′atis [NA], SYN bare a. of liver.

olfactory a., SYN anterior perforated *substance*.

a. opa′ca, the peripheral a. of the blastoderm of birds and reptiles which is opaque because of adherent yolk.

oval a. of Flechsig, SEE semilunar *fasciculus*.

Panum's a., the a. in and about the macula retinae in which stimulation of noncorresponding retinal points nevertheless results in stereoscopic vision. SYN fusion a.

parastriate a., SEE visual *cortex*.

a. parolfacto′ria [NA], SYN parolfactory a.

parolfactory a., a small region of cerebral cortex on the medial surface of the frontal lobe, formed by the junction of the straight gyrus with the cingulate gyrus, demarcated from the subcallosal gyrus by the posterior parolfactory sulcus. SYN a. parolfactoria [NA], Broca's parolfactory a.

pear-shaped a., SYN retromolar *pad*.

a. pellu′cida, the translucent central part of the blastoderm of birds and reptiles.

peristriate a., SEE visual *cortex*.

piriform a., SYN piriform *cortex*.

Pitres' a., prefrontal cortex of the cerebral hemisphere. SEE frontal *cortex*.

postcentral a., the cortex of the postcentral gyrus.

post dam a., SYN posterior palatal seal a.

posterior hypothalamic a., SYN posterior hypothalamic *region*.

posterior intercondylar a. of tibia, the deep notch between the tibial condyles posteriorly to which attaches the posterior cruciate ligament. SYN a. intercondylaris posterior tibiae [NA].

posterior palatal seal a., the soft tissues along the junction of the hard and soft palates on which pressure within the physiologic limits of the tissues can be applied by a denture to aid in the retention of the denture. SYN post dam a., postpalatal seal a.

postpalatal seal a., SYN posterior palatal seal a.

a. postre′ma (AP), a small, elevated a. in the lateral wall of the inferior recess of the fourth ventricle; one of the few loci in the brain where the blood-brain barrier is lacking; a chemoreceptor area associated with vomiting.

precentral a., the cortex of the precentral gyrus.

precommissural septal a., SYN subcallosal *gyrus*.

prefrontal a., SEE frontal *cortex*.

premotor a., SYN premotor *cortex*.

preoptic a., SYN preoptic *region*.

prestriate a., SEE visual *cortex*.

pretectal a., a narrow, transversally oriented rostral zone of the mesencephalic tectum, bounded caudally by the superior colliculus, rostrally by the habenular trigone, and laterally by the pulvinar thalami; the a. contains several nuclei that receive fibers from the optic tract; it has bilateral efferent connections with the Edinger-Westphal nucleus of the oculomotor nuclear complex by way of which it mediates the pupillary light reflex. SYN pretectal region, pretectum.

primary visual a., SEE visual *cortex*.

pulmonary a., the region of the chest at the second left intercostal space, where sounds produced at the pulmonary valve of the right ventricle are heard most distinctly.

relief a., in dentistry, the portion of the denture-bearing a. over which the denture base is altered to reduce functional pressure.

rest a., the portion of a tooth structure or of a restoration in a tooth that is prepared to receive the positive seating of the metallic occlusal, incisal, lingual, or cingulum rest of a removable prosthesis. SYN rest seat.

retention a., an a. of a tooth provided during its preparation for restoration that will aid in holding the restoration in place. SEE ALSO retention *groove*, retention *point*.

Rolando's a., SYN motor *cortex*.

secondary aortic a., region of the chest at the mid-left sternal bases where aortic diastolic murmurs are often best heard.

secondary visual a., SEE visual *cortex*.

sensorial areas, sensory areas, SEE cerebral *cortex*.

sensorimotor a., the precentral and postcentral gyri of the cerebral cortex.

septal a., the region of the cerebral hemisphere that stretches as a thin sheet of brain tissue between the fornix bundle and the ventral surface of the corpus callosum, forming the medial wall of the lateral ventricle's frontal horn; it extends ventrally through the narrow interval between the anterior commissure and the rostrum of corpus collosum as the precommissural septum or subcallosal gyrus, which is continuous caudally with the preoptic a. and hypothalamus, as well as more laterally with the innominate substance; its major functional connections are with the hippocampus and hypothalamus.

silent a., any a. of the cerebrum or cerebellum in which lesions cause no definite sensory or motor symptoms.

skip areas, subsidiary segments of diseased intestine or colon in regional enteritis or Crohn's colitis, separated from the region of major involvement.

somesthetic a., SYN somatic sensory *cortex*.

stress-bearing a., (1) SYN denture foundation a. **(2)** surfaces of oral structures that resist forces, strains, or pressures brought upon them during function.

striate a., SEE visual *cortex*.

Stroud's pectinated a., obsolete term for the a. of the anal canal lying just below the rectal columns.

a. subcallo′sa [NA], SYN subcallosal *gyrus*.

subcallosal a., SYN subcallosal *gyrus*.

superior vestibular a., the a. in the fundus of the internal acoustic meatus superior to the transverse crest through which the superior part of the vestibular nerve passes to reach the macula utriculus and the ampullae of the anterior and lateral semicircular ducts. SYN a. vestibularis superior [NA].

supporting a., (1) those areas of the maxillary and mandibular edentulous ridges which are considered best suited to carry the forces of mastication when the dentures are in function; **(2)** SYN denture foundation a.

tissue-bearing a., SYN denture foundation a.

tricuspid a., the region of the chest wall over the lower part of the body of the sternum, where the sounds produced at the tricuspid valve are heard most distinctly.

trigger a., SYN trigger *point*.

vagus a., a portion of the floor of the fourth ventricle overlying the vagoglossopharyngeal nuclei.

a. vasculo′sa, the part of the a. opaca of the embryonic blastoderm of the chick, where the first blood vessels appear.

vestibular a., SEE inferior vestibular a., superior vestibular a.

a. vestibula′ris infe′rior [NA], SYN inferior vestibular a.

a. vestibula′ris supe′rior [NA], SYN superior vestibular a.

visual a., SYN visual *cortex.*

Wernicke's a., SYN Wernicke's *center.*

---

ar·e·a·tus, ar·e·a·ta (ă-rē-ā′tŭs, -tă). Occurring in patches or circumscribed areas. [L.]

Are·ca (ar′ĕ-kă). A genus of palms of India and the Malay Archipelago. A species, *A. catechu,* furnishes a. nuts, or betel nuts, which contain arecoline and 15% red tannin, are chewed in the East Indies, and have an anthelmintic action. SEE ALSO betel nut. [Malay]

arec·ai·dine (ă-rek′ā-dēn). 1,2,5,6-tetrahydro-1-methylnicotinic acid; a crystalline alkaloid resembling betaine, derived from the betel nut. SYN arecaine.

are·caine (ar′e-kān). SYN arecaidine.

arec·o·line (ă-rek′ō-lēn). $C_8H_{13}NO_2$; a colorless oily alkaloid from the betel nut.

are·flex·ia (ā-rē-flek′sē-ă). Absence of reflexes.

detrusor a., a failure of the detrusor muscle to have a reflex contraction even though the bladder has reached or exceeded its capacity.

ar·e·na·ceous (ar-ĕ-nā′shŭs). Sandy; of sand-like consistency. [L. *arena,* sand]

Are·na·vi·ri·dae (ă-rē-nă-vir′i-dē). A family of at least 13 RNA viruses, many of which are natural parasites of rodents, that includes lymphocytic choriomeningitis virus, Lassa virus, and the Tacaribe virus complex. The virions are 50 to 300 nm (average 100 nm) in diameter, enveloped, ether-sensitive, and contain single-stranded, segmented RNA (molecular weight 3 to 5 × 10^6); they also contain electron-dense, RNA-containing granules (20 to 30 nm in diameter) that resemble ribosomes, with an electron-microscopic appearance of sandiness. [L. *arēna* (*harēna*), sand]

Are·na·vi·rus (ă-rē′nă-vī′rŭs). A genus in the family Arenaviridae that is associated with lymphocytic choriomeningitis and a number of hemorrhagic fevers.

are·o·la, pl. **are·o·lae** (ă-rē′ō-lă, -lē). **1** [NA]. Any small area. **2.** One of the spaces or interstices in areolar tissue. **3.** SYN a. of nipple. **4.** A pigmented, depigmented, or erythematous zone surrounding a papule, pustule, wheal, or cutaneous neoplasm. SYN halo (3). [L. dim. of *area*]

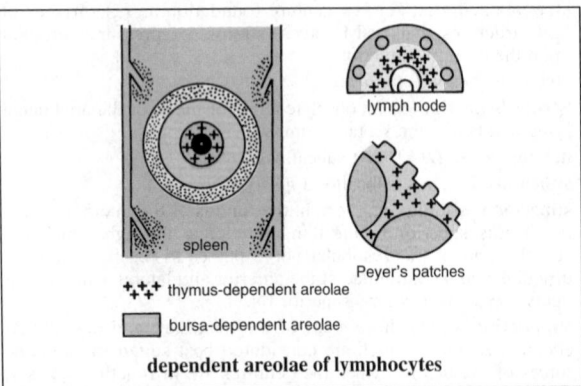

++++ thymus-dependent areolae

▨ bursa-dependent areolae

dependent areolae of lymphocytes

Chaussier's a., a ring of indurated tissue surrounding the lesion of cutaneous anthrax.

a. mam′mae [NA], SYN a. of nipple.

a. of nipple, a circular pigmented area surrounding the nipple or papilla mammae; its surface is dotted with little projections due

---

to the presence of Montgomery's glands beneath. SYN a. mammae [NA], a. papillaris, areola (3).

a. papilla′ris, SYN a. of nipple.

a. umbilicus, a pigmented ring around the umbilicus in the pregnant woman.

are·o·lar (ă-rē′ō-lăr). Relating to an areola.

ar·e·om·e·ter (ar-ē-om′ĕ-ter). SYN hydrometer. [G. *araios,* thin, + G. *metron,* measure]

ARF Abbreviation for acute respiratory *failure.*

Arg Symbol for arginine or its mono- or diradical.

Argas. A genus of soft ticks of the family Argasidae, some species of which usually infest birds but may attack man.

A. per′sicus, the abode, fowl, or Persian tick, a species that is a bloodsucking parasite of poultry; it transmits fowl spirochetosis.

A. reflex′us, the pigeon tick, a species that may cause a cutaneous inflammatory lesion in man.

ar·ga·sid (ar-gas′id). Common name for members of the family Argasidae.

Argas·i·dae (ar-gas′i-dē). Family of ticks (superfamily Ixodoidea, order Acarina), the soft ticks, so called because of their wrinkled, leathery, tuberculated appearance that fills out when the tick is engorged with blood. A dorsal shield (scutum) is not present; the mouthparts (capitulum) are subterminal or ventral in a depression (camerostome) that extends above the capitulum to form the anterior margin of the cephalothorax (hood). A. contains 4 genera: *Argas, Ornithodoros, Otobius,* and *Antricola;* argasid ticks, chiefly species of *Ornithodoros,* harbor and transmit spirochetes of the genus *Borrelia* that cause relapsing fever in birds and mammals.

ar·gen·taf·fin, ar·gen·taf·fine (ar-jen′tă-fin, -fēn). Pertaining to cells or tissue elements that reduce silver ions in solution, thereby becoming stained brown or black. [L. *argentum,* silver, + *affinitas,* affinity]

ar·gen·taf·fi·no·ma (ar′jen-tă-fi-nō′mă, -taf-i-nō′mă). SYN carcinoid *tumor.*

ar·gen·ta·tion (ar-jen-tā′shŭn). Impregnation with a silver salt. SEE ALSO argyria. [L. *argentum,* silver]

ar·gen·tic (ar-jen′tik). **1.** Relating to silver. SYN argyric (1). **2.** Denoting a chemical compound containing silver as the rare dication (Ag^{2+}).

ar·gen·tine (ar′jen-tēn). Relating to, resembling, or containing silver.

ar·gen·to·phil, ar·gen·to·phile (ar-jen′tō-fil, -fīl). SYN argyrophil.

ar·gen·tous (ar-jen′tŭs). Denoting a chemical compound containing silver as a singly charged (Ag^+) ion. The vast majority of silver compounds contain the a. ion; where the ionic state of silver is not specifically stated, as in silver nitrate, the a. state is assumed.

ar·gen·tum, gen. **ar·gen·ti** (ar-jen′tŭm, -jen′tī). SYN silver. [L.]

ar·gi·nase (ar′ji-nās). An enzyme of the liver that catalyzes the hydrolysis of L-arginine to L-ornithine and urea; a key enzyme of the urea cycle. A deficiency of a. leads to arginemia. SYN arginine amidase, canavanase.

ar·gi·nine (Arg) (ar′ji-nēn). 2-Amino-5-guanidinopentanoic acid; one of the amino acids occurring among the hydrolysis products of proteins, particularly abundant in the basic proteins such as histones and protamines. A dibasic amino acid.

a. amidase, SYN arginase.

a. deiminase, an enzyme catalyzing the hydrolytic deamination of L-a. to L-citrulline and ammonia. Cf. *nitric oxide* synthase. SYN a. dihydrolase, a. iminohydrolase.

a. dihydrolase, SYN a. deiminase.

a. glutamate, a compound composed of arginine and glutamic acid, given intravenously to detoxify ammonia; used in the treatment of ammoniemia resulting from liver dysfunction.

a. hydrochloride, a form of a. used for intravenous administration as an adjunct in the treatment of encephalopathies associated with liver diseases and ammoniacal azotemia.

a. iminohydrolase, SYN a. deiminase.

a. phosphate, SYN phosphoarginine.

ar·gi·ni·no·suc·ci·nase (ar'ji-ni-nō-sŭk'si-nās). SYN arginino-succinate lyase.

ar·gi·ni·no·suc·ci·nate ly·ase (ar'ji-ni-nō-sŭk'si-nāt). An enzyme cleaving L-argininosuccinate nonhydrolytically to L-arginine and fumarate; a deficiency of this enzyme leads to argininosuccinoaciduria; a key step in the urea cycle. SYN argininosuccinase.

ar·gi·ni·no·suc·cin·ic ac·id (ar'ji-ni-nō-sŭk-sin'ik). HOOC-CH₂CH(COOH)-NH-C(NH)-NH(CH₂)₃CHNH₂-COOH; formed as an intermediate in the conversion of L-citrulline to L-arginine in the urea cycle.

ar·gi·ni·no·suc·cin·ic·ac·i·du·ria (ar-ji-nin'ō-sŭk-sin'ik-as-i-dū'rē-ă) [MIM*207900]. An autosomal recessive disorder characterized by excessive urinary excretion of argininosuccinic acid, epilepsy, ataxia, mental retardation, liver disease, and friable, tufted hair; presumed to be the consequence of a deficiency of an enzyme responsible for splitting argininosuccinic acid to arginine and fumaric acid.

ar·gin·yl (ar'jin-il). The aminoacyl radical of arginine.

ar·gi·pres·sin (ar-ji-pres'in). SYN arginine *vasopressin.*

ar·gon (Ar) (ar'gon). A gaseous element, atomic no. 18, atomic wt. 39.948, present in the dry atmosphere in the proportion of about 0.94%; one of the noble gases. [G. ntr. of *argos,* lazy, inactive, fr. *a-* priv. + *ergon,* work]

Argonz, J., Argentinian physician. SEE A.-Del Castillo *syndrome.*

Argyll Robertson. SEE Robertson.

ar·gyr·ia (ar-jir'ē-ă, -jī'rē-ă). A slate-gray or bluish discoloration of the skin and deep tissues, due to the deposit of insoluble albuminate of silver, occurring after the medicinal administration for a long period of a soluble silver salt; formerly fairly common from use of proprietary preparations of silver-containing materials in the nose and sinuses. SYN argyriasis, argyrism, argyrosis, silver poisoning. [G. *argyros,* silver]

ar·gy·ri·a·sis (ar-ji-rī'ă-sis). SYN argyria.

ar·gyr·ic (ar-jir'ik). 1. SYN argentic (1). 2. Relating to argyria.

ar·gy·rism (ar'ji-rizm). SYN argyria.

ar·gy·rol. SYN mild *silver* protein.

ar·gyr·o·phil, ar·gyr·o·phile (ar-jī'rō-fil, -fīl). Pertaining to tissue elements that are capable of impregnation with silver ions and being made visible after an external reducing agent is used. SYN argentophil, argentophile. [G. *argyros,* silver, + *philos,* fond]

ar·gy·ro·sis (ar-ji-rō'sis). SYN argyria.

a·rhi·go·sis (ă-ri-gō'sis). Lack of perception of cold. [G. *a-* priv. + *rhigoō,* to shiver]

arhin·ia (ă-rin'ē-ă). Congenital absence of the nose. SYN arrhinia.

Arias-Stella, Javier, Peruvian pathologist, *1924. SEE Arias-Stella *effect;* Arias-Stella *phenomenon;* Arias-Stella *reaction.*

ari·bo·fla·vin·o·sis (ă-rī'bō-flā-vi-nō'sis). Properly hyporiboflavinosis: a nutritional condition produced by a deficiency of riboflavin in the diet, characterized by cheilosis and magenta tongue and usually associated with other manifestations of B vitamin deficiency.

Arie-Pi·tanguy mam·ma·plas·ty. See under mammaplasty.

Arie-Pi·tanguy op·er·a·tion. See under operation.

aris·to·loch·ic ac·id (ă-ris-tō-lō'kik). 8-Methoxy-6-nitrophenanthro[3,4-d]-1,3-dioxole-5-carboxylic acid; an aromatic bitter derived from plants of the genus *Aristolochia.*

ar·is·to·te·lian (ar'is-tō-tē'lē-ăn, ar'i-stŏ-tēl'yan). Attributed to or described by Aristotle.

Aristotle. Of Stagira, Greek philosopher and scientist, 384–322 B.C. SEE Aristotle's *anomaly,* aristotelian *method.*

arith·mo·ma·nia (ă-rith-mō-mā'nē-ă). A morbid impulse to count. [G. *arithmeō,* to count, fr. *arithmos,* number, + *mania,* madness]

A·ri·zo·na (ar'i-zō'nă). A genus of motile, peritrichous, non-sporeforming, aerobic to facultatively anaerobic bacteria (family Enterobacteriaceae) containing Gram-negative rods. These organisms do not produce urease and do not grow in media containing potassium cyanide. They decarboxylate lysine, arginine, and ornithine. Lactose is generally fermented. These organisms have been isolated from a wide variety of animals, including man; they may cause gastroenteritis in man and frequently are involved in localized lesions in man and lower animals. There is a single species, *A. hinshawii,* the type species.

A. hinshawii, former name for *Salmonella* subsp. *arizonae.*

Arlt, Carl Ferdinand von, Austrian ophthalmologist, 1812–1887. SEE A.'s *operation, sinus.*

arm. 1. Arm, specifically the segment of the upper limb between the shoulder and the elbow; commonly used to mean the whole superior limb. SYN brachium (1) [NA], brachio- (1). 2. An anatomical extension resembling an arm. 3. A specifically shaped and positioned extension of a removable partial denture framework. [L. *armus,* forequarter of an animal; G. *harmos,* a shoulder joint]

bar clasp a., a clasp a. which has its origin in the denture base or major connector; it consists of the a. which traverses but does not contact the gingival structures, and a terminal end which approaches its contact with the tooth in a gingivo-occlusal direction.

brawny a., a swollen arm caused by lymphedema, particularly after homolateral radical mastectomy.

circumferential clasp a., a clasp a. which has its origin in a minor connector and which follows the contour of the tooth approximately in a plane perpendicular to the path of insertion of the partial denture.

clasp a., a portion of a clasp of a removable partial denture which projects from the clasp body and helps retain the partial denture in position in the mouth. SEE clasp (2).

dynein a., a structure extending clockwise from one tubule of each of the 9 doublet microtubules toward the adjacent doublet seen in the axoneme of cilia or flagella (including human sperm tails); congenital absence of dynein, reflected structurally by absence of dynein a.'s, can account for symptoms seen in Kartagener's syndrome and in immotile cilia syndromes.

reciprocal a., a clasp a. or other extension used on a removable partial denture to oppose the action of some other part or parts of the appliance.

retentive a., retention a., a flexible segment of a removable partial denture that engages an undercut on an abutment and is designed to retain the denture.

retentive circumferential clasp a., an a. that is flexible and engages the infrabulge at the terminal end of the a.

stabilizing circumferential clasp a., an a. that is relatively rigid and embraces the height of contour of the tooth.

ar·ma·men·tar·i·um (ar'mă-men-tār'ē-ŭm). All the therapeutic means available to the health practitioner for the practice of his profession. [L. an arsenal, fr. *armamenta,* implements, tackle, fr. *arma,* armor, arms]

Armanni, Luciano, Italian pathologist, 1839–1903. SEE A.-Ebstein *kidney, change.*

ar·mar·i·um (ar-mar'ē-ŭm). Rarely used term for the physician's library, as part of his armamentarium. [L. a closet, chest, fr. *arma,* armor]

Ar·mil·li·fer (ar-mil'i-fer). A genus of Pentastomida (order Porocephalida, family Porocephalidae); adults are found in the lungs of reptiles and the young in many mammals, including man. [O. Fr. *armille,* fr. L. *armilla,* a bracelet]

A. armilla'tus, species occurring in the python, the larva or nymph being occasionally found in man. SYN *Porocephalus armillatus.*

arm·pit. SYN axilla.

Armstrong, Arthur Riley, Canadian physician, *1904. SEE King-A. *unit.*

Armstrong, Henry E., British physician.

Arndt, G., German physician, 1874—1929. SEE A.-Gottron *syndrome.*

Arndt, Rudolph, German psychiatrist, 1835–1900. SEE A.'s *law.*

Arneth, Joseph, German physician, 1873–1955. SEE A. *classification, count, formula, index, stages,* under *stage.*

ar·ni·ca (ar'ni-kă). The dried flower heads of *Arnica montana* (family Compositae); Obsolete cardiac sedative seldom given

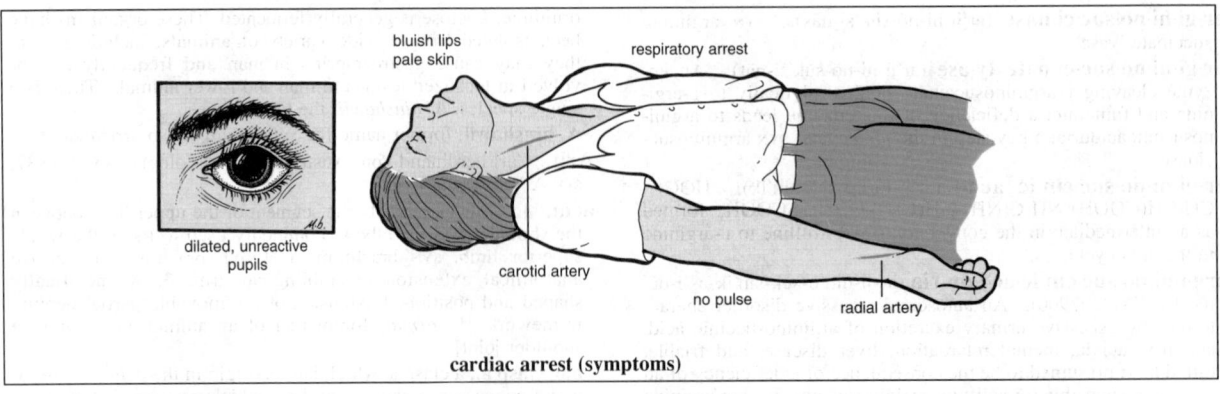

bluish lips
pale skin

respiratory arrest

dilated, unreactive
pupils

carotid artery

no pulse

radial artery

cardiac arrest (symptoms)

internally; used externally for sprains and bruises; formerly widely used as a counterirritant liniment. SYN leopard's bane. [Mod. L.]

Arnold, Friedrich, German anatomist, 1803–1890. SEE A.'s *bundle, canal, ganglion, nerve, tract; foramen* of A.

Arnold, Julius, German pathologist, 1835–1915. SEE A.'s *bodies,* under *body;* A.-Chiari *deformity, malformation, syndrome.*

ar·o·mat·ic (ar-ō-mat'ik). **1.** Having an agreeable, somewhat pungent, spicy odor. **2.** One of a group of vegetable drugs having a fragrant odor and slightly stimulant properties. **3.** SEE aromatic *compound.* [G. *arōmatikos,* fr. *arōma,* spice, sweet herb]

ar·o·mat·ic D-amino-ac·id de·car·box·yl·ase. An enzyme that catalyzes the decarboxylation of L-dopa to dopamine, of L-tryptophan to tryptamine, and of L-hydroxytryptophan to serotonin; important in the biosynthetic pathway of catecholamines and melanin. SYN dopa decarboxylase, hydroxytryptophan decarboxylase, tryptophan decarboxylase.

ar·o·yl (a'rō-il). The radical of an aromatic acid (*e.g.,* benzoyl); analogous to acyl, the more general term.

ar·rack (a-rak'). A strong alcoholic liquor distilled from dates, rice, sap of the coconut palm, and other substances. [Ar. sweet juice]

ar·rec·tor, pl. **ar·rec·to·res** (ă-rek'tōr, ă-rek-tō'rēz). SYN erector. [L. that which raises, fr. *ar-rigo,* pp. *-rectus,* to raise up]

arrecto'res pilo'rum, SYN arrector pili *muscles,* under *muscle.*

ar·rest (ă-rest'). **1.** To stop, check, or restrain. **2.** A stoppage; interference with, or checking of, the regular course of a disease, a symptom, or the performance of a function. **3.** Inhibition of a developmental process, usually at the ultimate stage of development; premature a. may lead to a congenital abnormality. [O. Fr. *arester,* fr. LL. *adresto,* to stop behind]

cardiac a. (CA), complete cessation of cardiac activity either electric, mechanical, or both; may be purposely induced for therapeutic reasons. SYN heart a.

cardioplegic a., stoppage of electrical and mechanical cardiac activity, used by surgeons when operating upon the heart.

cardiopulmonary a., an a. resulting in absence of cardiac and pulmonary activity.

circulatory a., cessation of the circulation of blood as a result of ventricular standstill or fibrillation.

deep hypothermic a., stoppage of electrical and mechanical cardiac activity that occurs when the heart is cooled.

epiphysial a., early and premature fusion between epiphysis and diaphysis.

heart a., SYN cardiac a.

maturation a., cessation of complete differentiation of cells at an immature stage; in spermatogenic maturation a., the seminiferous tubules contain spermatocytes, but no spermatozoa develop.

sinus a., cessation of sinus activity; the ventricles may continue to beat under ectopic atrial, A-V junctional, or idioventricular control. SEE ALSO sinus *standstill,* atrial *standstill.*

ar·rhaph·i·a. SYN *status* dysraphicus.

ar·rhen·ic (ă-ren'ik). Relating to arsenic. [G. *arrhenikon* (var.), arsenic]

Arrhenius, Svante, Swedish chemist and Nobel laureate, 1859–1927. SEE A. *doctrine, equation, law;* A.-Madsen *theory.*

ar·rhe·no·blas·to·ma (ă-rē'nō-blas-tō'mă). A rare ovarian tumor that produces masculinization and often contains tubules and luteinized cells. SYN androblastoma (2), gynandroblastoma (1), ovarian tubular adenoma. [G. *arrhēn,* male, + *blastos,* germ, + *-ōma,* tumor]

ar·rhin·en·ceph·a·ly, ar·rhin·en·ce·pha·lia, a·rhin·en·ceph·aly (ă-rin-en-sef'ă-lē, -se-fā'lē-ă). Congenital absence or rudimentary state of the rhinencephalon, or olfactory lobe of the brain, on one or both sides, with a corresponding lack of development of the external olfactory organs. [G. *a-* priv. + *rhis* (*rhin-*), nose, + *enkephalos,* brain]

ar·rhin·ia (ă-rin'ē-ă). SYN arhinia. [G. *a-* priv. + *rhis* (*rhin-*), nose]

ar·rhyth·mia (ă-ridh'mē-ă). Loss of rhythm; denoting especially an irregularity of the heartbeat. See also entries under rhythm. Cf. dysrhythmia. [G. *a-* priv. + *rhythmos,* rhythm]

cardiac a., SEE cardiac *dysrhythmia.*

continuous a., obsolete term for atrial *fibrillation.*

juvenile a., SYN sinus a.

nonphasic sinus a., sinus a. in which variations in rhythm are not related to the phases of respiration.

perpetual a., an obsolete term for atrial *fibrillation.*

phasic sinus a., sinus a. in which the irregularity is related to the phases of respiration, the rate being faster in inspiration and slower in expiration.

respiratory a., phasic sinus a. or any other rhythm fluctuation induced by respiratory fluctuation.

sinus a., rhythmic, repetitive irregularity of the heartbeat, the heart being under the control of its normal pacemaker, the sinoatrial node. SYN juvenile a.

ar·rhyth·mic (ă-ridh'mik, ā-). Marked by loss of rhythm; pertaining to arrhythmia.

ar·rhyth·mo·gen·ic (ă-ridh-mō-jen'ik). Capable of inducing cardiac arrhythmias. [G. *a-* priv. + *rhythmos,* rhythm, + *-gen,* production]

ar·row·root (ar'ō-rūt). The rhizome of *Maranta arundinacea,* a plant of tropical America, which is the source of a form of starch formerly used as a dietary supplement.

Arruga, Count Hermenegildo, Spanish ophthalmologist, 1886–1972. SEE A.'s *forceps.*

ar·sa·ce·tin (ar-să-sē'tin). *p*-Acetamidobenzenearsonic acid; formerly used as an antisyphilitic agent.

ar·sen·a·mide (ar-sen'ă-mīd). $H_2NCO-C_6H_4-As(SCH_2COOH)_2$; {[(*p*-Carbamoylphenyl)arsylene]dithio}diacetic acid; used in the treatment of filariasis.

ar·se·nate (ar'sĕ-nāt). A salt of arsenic acid.

ar·sen·i·a·sis (ar-sen-ī'ă-sis). Chronic arsenical poisoning. SYN arsenicalism.

ar·se·nic (As) (ar'sĕ-nik). A metallic element, atomic no. 33, atomic wt. 74.92159; forms a number of poisonous compounds, some of which are used in medicine. SYN arsenium, ratsbane. [L. *arsenicum*, G. *arsenikon*, fr. Pers. *zarnik*]

a. trihydride, SYN arsine.

a. trioxide, As_2O_3; dissolves in water to give arsenous acid, H_3AsO_3; used in the treatment of skin diseases and malaria, and as a tonic; also used externally as a caustic. SYN arsenous oxide, white a.

white a., SYN a. trioxide.

ar·se·nic (ar-sen'ik). Denoting the element arsenic or one of its compounds, especially arsenic acid.

ar·se·nic ac·id. $H_3AsO_4 \cdot \frac{1}{2}H_2O$; the hydrate of arsenic oxide or arsenic pentoxide which forms arsenates with certain bases.

ar·sen·i·cal (ar-sen'i-kăl). **1.** A drug or agent, the effect of which depends on its arsenic content. **2.** Denoting or containing arsenic.

ar·sen·i·cal·ism (ar-sen'i-kăl-izm). SYN arseniasis.

ar·se·nic-fast. Resistant to the poisonous action of arsenic; denoting especially spirochetes and other protozoan parasites, which acquire resistance after repeated administration of the drug.

ar·se·nide (ar'sĕ-nīd). A compound of arsenic with a metal or other positively charged atoms or groups in which the arsenic is not bound to any atoms of oxygen. SYN arseniuret.

ar·se·ni·ous (ar-sēn'ē-ŭs). Arsenic (adj.).

ar·se·ni·um (ar-sē'nē-ŭm). SYN arsenic.

ar·sen·iu·ret (ar-se'nyū-ret). SYN arsenide.

ar·sen·iu·ret·ed (ar-sē'nyū-ret-ed). Combined with arsenic so as to form an arsenide.

ar·se·no·ther·a·py (ar'sen-ō-thār'ă-pē). Therapeutic treatment with arsenic.

ar·se·nous (ar'-sen-ŭs). **1.** Denoting a compound of arsenic with a valence of +3. **2.** Arsenic (adj.).

ar·se·nous ac·id. SEE *arsenic* trioxide.

ar·se·nous hy·dride. SYN arsine.

ar·se·nous ox·ide. SYN *arsenic* trioxide.

ar·se·nox·i·des (ar-sĕ-nok'i-dēs). Oxidation products in the body of arsphenamines; believed to be the agents active against spirochetes.

ar·sine (ar'sēn). AsH_3; a cell and blood poison, many organic derivatives of which have been used in chemical warfare. SYN arsenic trihydride, arseniureted hydrogen, arsenous hydride.

ar·son·ic ac·id (ar-son'ik). A derivative of arsenic acid by replacement of a hydroxyl group by an organic radical.

ar·so·ni·um (ar-son'ē-ŭm). The positively charged ion, AsH_4^+; analogous to the ammonium ion, NH_4^+.

ars·phen·a·mine (ars-fen'ă-min). 3,3'-diamino-4,4'-dihydroxy-arsenobenzene dihydrochloride; formerly used in the treatment of syphilis, yaws, and some other diseases of protozoan origin, after neutralization with NaOH. The synthesis of a. in 1907 and the demonstration of its usefulness as a therapeutic agent by Paul Ehrlich and co-workers (1909) marked the beginning of chemotherapy. SYN phenarsenamine.

ars·thi·nol (ars'thī-nol). Cyclic (hydroxymethyl)ethylene ester of 3-acetamido-4-hydroxydithiobenzenearsonous acid; an amebicide.

ar·te·fact (ar'tĕ-fakt). SYN artifact.

ar·te·re·nol (ar'ter-ĕ-nol). The hydrochloride salt of norepinephrine. SEE norepinephrine.

△**arteri-.** SEE arterio-.

ARTERIA

ar·te·ri·a (a), gen. and pl. **ar·te·ri·ae (aa)** (ar-tēr'ē-ă, ar-tēr'ĭ-e) [NA]. SYN artery. SEE ALSO branch. [L. from G. *artēria*, the windpipe, later an artery as distinct from a vein]

a. acetab'uli, SYN acetabular *branch*.

a. alveola'ris infe'rior [NA], SYN inferior alveolar *artery*.

arteriae alveola'ris inferio'ris, SYN mylohyoid *artery*.

arteriae alveola'res supe'riores ante'riores [NA], SYN anterior superior alveolar *arteries*, under *artery*.

a. alveola'ris supe'rior poste'rior [NA], SYN posterior superior alveolar *artery*.

a. anastomot'ica auricula'ris mag'na, SYN Kugel's anastomotic *artery*.

a. anastomot'ica mag'na, (1) SYN inferior ulnar collateral *artery*. **(2)** SYN descending genicular *artery*.

a. angula'ris [NA], SYN angular *artery*.

a. aorta, SYN aorta.

a. appendicula'ris [NA], SYN appendicular *artery*.

a. arcua'ta [NA], SYN arcuate *artery*.

arte'riae arcua'tae renis [NA], SYN arcuate *arteries* of kidney, under *artery*. SYN arciform arteries.

a. articula'ris az'ygos, SYN middle genicular *artery*.

a. ascen'dens, (1) [NA], SYN ascending *artery*. **(2)** SYN ascending *branch* of the inferior mesenteric artery.

arteriae atria'les, SYN atrial *arteries*, under *artery*.

a. auditi'va inter'na, SYN labyrinthine *artery*.

a. auricula'ris poste'rior [NA], SYN posterior auricular *artery*.

a. auricula'ris profun'da [NA], SYN deep auricular *artery*.

a. axilla'ris [NA], SYN axillary *artery*.

a. basila'ris [NA], SYN basilar *artery*.

a. brachia'lis [NA], SYN brachial *artery*.

a. brachia'lis superficia'lis [NA], SYN superficial brachial *artery*.

a. bucca'lis [NA], SYN buccal *artery*.

a. bul'bi pe'nis [NA], SYN *artery* of bulb of penis.

a. bul'bi ure'thrae, SYN *artery* of bulb of penis.

a. bulbi vaginae, ☆official alternate term for *artery* of bulb of vestibule.

a. bul'bi vestib'uli [NA], SYN *artery* of bulb of vestibule.

a. calcari'na, SYN calcarine *branch* of medial occipital artery.

a. callo'somargina'lis [NA], SYN callosomarginal *artery*.

a. cana'lis pterygoid'ei [NA], SYN *artery* of pterygoid canal.

arte'riae carot'icotympan'icae arteriae carotidis internae [NA], SYN caroticotympanic *arteries*, under *artery*.

a. carot'is commu'nis [NA], SYN common carotid *artery*.

a. carot'is exter'na [NA], SYN external carotid *artery*.

a. carot'is inter'na [NA], SYN internal carotid *artery*. SEE pars.

a. cau'dae pancrea'tis [NA], SYN *artery* of the pancreatic tail.

a. ceca'lis ante'rior [NA], SYN anterior cecal *artery*.

a. ceca'lis poste'rior [NA], SYN posterior cecal *artery*.

a. celi'aca, SYN celiac *trunk*.

arte'riae centra'les anterolatera'les [NA], SYN lateral striate *arteries*, under *artery*.

arte'riae centra'les anteromedia'les [NA], SYN anteromedial central *arteries*, under *artery*.

arte'riae centra'les posterolatera'les [NA], SYN posterolateral central *arteries*, under *artery*.

arte'riae centra'les posteromedia'les [NA], SYN posteromedial central *arteries*, under *artery*.

a. centra'lis brev'is [NA], SYN short central *artery*.

a. centra'lis long'a [NA], SYN medial striate *artery*.

a. centra'lis ret'inae [NA], SYN central *artery* of retina.

a. cerebel'li infe'rior ante'rior [NA], SYN anterior inferior cerebellar *artery*.

a. cerebel'li infe'rior poste'rior [NA], SYN posterior inferior cerebellar *artery*.

a. cerebel'li supe'rior [NA], SYN superior cerebellar *artery*.

a. cer'ebri ante'rior [NA], SYN anterior cerebral *artery*.

a. cer'ebri me'dia [NA], SYN middle cerebral *artery*.

a. cer'ebri poste'rior [NA], SYN posterior cerebral *artery*.

a. cervica'lis ascen'dens [NA], SYN ascending cervical *artery*.

a. cervica'lis profun'da [NA], SYN deep cervical *artery*.

a. cervicalis superficialis, SYN superficial cervical *artery*. SEE ALSO superficial *branch* of the transverse cervical artery.

a. **cervicovagina′lis**, SYN cervicovaginal *artery*.

a. **choroi′dea ante′rior** [NA], SYN anterior choroidal *artery*.

a. **choroi′dea poste′rior,** SYN posterior choroidal *artery*.

a. **cilia′ris ante′rior** [NA], SYN anterior ciliary *artery*.

a. **cilia′ris poste′rior bre′vis** [NA], SYN short posterior ciliary *artery*.

a. **cilia′ris poste′rior lon′ga** [NA], SYN long posterior ciliary *artery*.

a. **circumflex′a fem′oris latera′lis** [NA], SYN lateral circumflex femoral *artery*.

a. **circumflex′a fem′oris media′lis** [NA], SYN medial circumflex femoral *artery*.

a. **circumflex′a hu′meri ante′rior** [NA], SYN anterior circumflex humeral *artery*.

a. **circumflex′a hu′meri poste′rior** [NA], SYN posterior circumflex humeral *artery*.

a. **circumflex′a ili′aca profun′da** [NA], SYN deep circumflex iliac *artery*.

a. **circumflex′a ili′aca superficia′lis** [NA], SYN superficial circumflex iliac *artery*.

a. **circumflex′a scap′ulae** [NA], SYN circumflex scapular *artery*.

a. **col′ica dex′tra** [NA], SYN right colic *artery*.

a. **col′ica me′dia** [NA], SYN middle colic *artery*.

a. **col′ica sinis′tra** [NA], SYN left colic *artery*.

a. **collatera′lis me′dia** [NA], SYN middle collateral *artery*.

a. **collatera′lis radia′lis** [NA], SYN radial collateral *artery*.

a. **collatera′lis ulna′ris infe′rior** [NA], SYN inferior ulnar collateral *artery*.

a. **collatera′lis ulna′ris supe′rior** [NA], SYN superior ulnar collateral *artery*.

a. **co′mes ner′vi phren′ici,** SYN pericardiacophrenic *artery*.

a. **com′itans ner′vi ischiad′ici** [NA], SYN *artery* to sciatic nerve.

a. **co′mitans ner′vi media′ni** [NA], SYN median *artery*.

a. **commu′nicans ante′rior** [NA], SYN anterior communicating *artery*.

a. **commu′nicans poste′rior** [NA], SYN posterior communicating *artery*.

a. **conjunctiva′lis ante′rior** [NA], SYN anterior conjunctival *artery*.

a. **conjunctiva′lis poste′rior** [NA], SYN posterior conjunctival *artery*.

a. **corona′ria dex′tra** [NA], SYN right coronary *artery*.

a. **corona′ria sinis′tra** [NA], SYN left coronary *artery*.

a. **cremaster′ica** [NA], SYN cremasteric *artery*.

a. **cys′tica** [NA], SYN cystic *artery*.

a. **deferentia′lis,** SYN *artery* of ductus deferens.

a. **digita′lis dorsa′lis** [NA], SYN dorsal digital *artery*.

a. **digita′lis palma′ris commu′nis** [NA], SYN common palmar digital *artery*.

a. **digita′lis palma′ris pro′pria** [NA], SYN proper palmar digital *artery*.

a. **digita′lis planta′ris commu′nis** [NA], SYN common plantar digital *artery*.

a. **digita′lis planta′ris pro′pria** [NA], SYN proper plantar digital *artery*.

a. **dorsa′lis clitor′idis** [NA], SYN dorsal *artery* of clitoris.

a. **dorsa′lis na′si** [NA], SYN dorsal nasal *artery*.

a. **dorsa′lis pe′dis** [NA], SYN dorsalis pedis *artery*.

a. **dorsa′lis pe′nis** [NA], SYN dorsal *artery* of penis.

a. **dorsa′lis scap′ulae** [NA], SYN dorsal scapular *artery*.

a. **duc′tus deferen′tis** [NA], SYN *artery* of ductus deferens.

a. **epigas′trica infe′rior** [NA], SYN inferior epigastric *artery*.

a. **epigas′trica superficia′lis** [NA], SYN superficial epigastric *artery*.

a. **epigas′trica supe′rior** [NA], SYN superior epigastric *artery*.

a. **episclera′lis** [NA], SYN episcleral *artery*.

a. **ethmoida′lis ante′rior** [NA], SYN anterior ethmoidal *artery*.

a. **ethmoida′lis poste′rior** [NA], SYN posterior ethmoidal *artery*.

a. **facia′lis** [NA], SYN facial *artery*.

a. **femora′lis** [NA], SYN femoral *artery*.

a. **fibula′ris** [NA], ⋆official alternate term for peroneal *artery*.

a. **fronta′lis,** SYN supratrochlear *artery*.

a. **frontobasa′lis latera′lis** [NA], SYN lateral frontobasal *artery*.

a. **frontobasa′lis media′lis** [NA], SYN medial frontobasal *artery*.

a. **gas′trica dex′tra** [NA], SYN right gastric *artery*.

arte′riae **gas′tricae bre′ves** [NA], SYN short gastric *arteries*, under *artery*.

a. **gas′trica sinis′tra** [NA], SYN left gastric *artery*.

a. **gastroduodena′lis** [NA], ⋆official alternate term for gastroduodenal *artery*.

a. **gastroepiplo′ica dex′tra,** ⋆official alternate term for right gastroepiploic *artery*.

a. **gastroepiplo′ica sinis′tra,** ⋆official alternate term for left gastroepiploic *artery*.

a. **gastro-omenta′lis dex′tra** [NA], SYN right gastroepiploic *artery*.

a. **gastro-omenta′lis sinis′tra** [NA], SYN left gastroepiploic *artery*.

a. **ge′nus descen′dens** [NA], SYN descending genicular *artery*.

a. **ge′nus infe′rior latera′lis** [NA], SYN inferior lateral genicular *artery*.

a. **ge′nus infe′rior media′lis** [NA], SYN inferior medial genicular *artery*.

a. **ge′nus me′dia** [NA], SYN middle genicular *artery*.

a. **ge′nus supe′rior latera′lis** [NA], SYN superior lateral genicular *artery*.

a. **ge′nus supe′rior media′lis** [NA], SYN superior medial genicular *artery*.

a. **glu′tea infe′rior** [NA], SYN inferior gluteal *artery*.

a. **glu′tea supe′rior** [NA], SYN superior gluteal *artery*.

a. **gy′ri angula′ris** [NA], SYN *artery* of angular gyrus.

arteriae **helici′nae penis** [NA], SYN helicine *arteries* of the penis, under *artery*.

a. **hepat′ica commu′nis** [NA], SYN common hepatic *artery*.

a. **hepat′ica pro′pria** [NA], SYN proper hepatic *artery*.

a. **hyaloi′dea** [NA], SYN hyaloid *artery*.

a. **hypogas′trica,** SYN internal iliac *artery*.

a. **hypophysia′lis infe′rior** [NA], SYN inferior hypophysial *artery*.

a. **hypophysia′lis supe′rior** [NA], SYN superior hypophysial *artery*.

arte′riae **ilea′les** [NA], SYN ileal *arteries*, under *artery*.

a. **ileocol′ica** [NA], SYN ileocolic *artery*.

a. **ili′aca commu′nis** [NA], SYN common iliac *artery*.

a. **ili′aca exter′na** [NA], SYN external iliac *artery*.

a. **ili′aca inter′na** [NA], SYN internal iliac *artery*.

a. **iliolumba′lis** [NA], SYN iliolumbar *artery*.

a. **infraorbita′lis** [NA], SYN infraorbital *artery*.

arte′riae **insula′res** [NA], SYN insular *arteries*, under *artery*.

arte′riae **intercosta′les posterio′res I et II** [NA], SYN posterior intercostal *arteries* 1–2, under *artery*.

arteriae **intercosta′les poste′riores III-XI** [NA], SYN posterior intercostal *arteries* 3-11, under *artery*.

a. **intercosta′lis supre′ma** [NA], SYN superior intercostal *artery*.

arte′riae **interloba′res re′nis** [NA], SYN interlobar *arteries* of kidney, under *artery*.

arteriae **interlobula′res** [NA], SYN interlobular *arteries*, under *artery*.

a. **interlobula′res (hepatis)** [NA], SYN interlobular *arteries* of liver, under *artery*.

a. **interlobula′res (renis)** [NA], SYN interlobular *arteries* of kidney, under *artery*.

a. **intermesenter′ica,** SYN ascending *branch* of the inferior mesenteric artery.

a. **interos′sea ante′rior** [NA], SYN anterior interosseous *artery*.

a. **interos′sea commu′nis** [NA], SYN common interosseous *artery*.

a. **interos′sea poste′rior** [NA], SYN posterior interosseous *artery*.

a. interos′sea recur′rens [NA], SYN recurrent interosseous *artery*.

a. interos′sea vola′ris, SYN anterior interosseous *artery*.

arte′riae intestina′les, SEE ileal *arteries*, under *artery*, jejunal *arteries*, under *artery*.

a. ischiad′ica, a. ischiat′ica, SYN inferior gluteal *artery*.

arteriae jejuna′les [NA], SYN jejunal *arteries*, under *artery*.

arte′riae labia′les anterio′res, SYN anterior labial *arteries*, under *artery*.

a. labia′lis infe′rior [NA], SYN inferior labial *artery*.

a. labia′lis supe′rior [NA], SYN superior labial *artery*.

a. labyrin′thi [NA], SYN labyrinthine *artery*.

a. lacrima′lis [NA], SYN lacrimal *artery*.

a. laryn′gea infe′rior [NA], SYN inferior laryngeal *artery*.

a. laryn′gea supe′rior [NA], SYN superior laryngeal *artery*.

a. liena′lis, ☆official alternate term for splenic *artery*.

a. ligamen′ti tere′tis u′teri [NA], SYN *artery* of round ligament of uterus.

a. lingua′lis [NA], SYN lingual *artery*.

a. lo′bi cauda′ti [NA], SYN *artery* of caudate lobe.

a. lumba′lis [NA], SYN lumbar *artery*.

arteriae lumba′les i′mae [NA], SYN lowest lumbar *arteries*, under *artery*.

a. luso′ria, an aberrant right subclavian artery arising from the descending aorta; it passes posterior to the esophagus, often producing dysphagia.

arte′riae malleola′res posterio′res latera′les, SYN lateral malleolar *arteries*, under *artery*.

arte′riae malleola′res posterio′res media′les, SYN medial malleolar *arteries*, under *artery*.

a. malleola′ris ante′rior latera′lis [NA], SYN anterior lateral malleolar *artery*.

a. malleola′ris ante′rior media′lis [NA], SYN anterior medial malleolar *artery*.

a. mamma′ria inter′na, SYN internal thoracic *artery*.

a. masseter′ica [NA], SYN masseteric *artery*.

a. maxilla′ris [NA], SYN maxillary *artery*.

a. maxilla′ris exter′na, SYN facial *artery*.

a. media′na, SYN median *artery*.

arte′riae mediastina′les ante′riores, SYN mediastinal *branches*, under *branch*.

a. menin′gea ante′rior [NA], SYN anterior meningeal *artery*.

a. menin′gea me′dia [NA], SYN middle meningeal *artery*.

a. menin′gea poste′rior [NA], SYN posterior meningeal *artery*.

a. menta′lis [NA], SYN mental *artery*.

a. mesenter′ica infe′rior [NA], SYN inferior mesenteric *artery*.

a. mesenter′ica supe′rior [NA], SYN superior mesenteric *artery*.

a. metacar′pea dorsa′lis [NA], SYN dorsal metacarpal *artery*.

a. metacar′pea palma′ris [NA], SYN palmar metacarpal *artery*.

a. metatar′sae [NA], SYN metatarsal *artery*.

a. metatar′sea dorsa′lis [NA], SYN dorsal metatarsal *artery*.

a. metatar′sea planta′ris [NA], SYN plantar metatarsal *artery*.

a. musculophren′ica [NA], SYN musculophrenic *artery*.

arte′riae nasa′les posterio′res latera′les [NA], SYN posterior lateral nasal *arteries*, under *artery*.

a. nasa′lis poste′rior sep′ti [NA], SYN posterior septal *artery* of nose.

a. na′si exter′na [NA], ☆official alternate term for dorsal nasal *artery*.

a. nervorum, arteries to nerves.

a. nutri′cia [NA], SYN nutrient *artery*.

arte′riae nutri′ciae hu′meri [NA], SYN nutrient *arteries* of humerus, under *artery*.

a. nu′triens fib′ulae [NA], SYN nutrient *artery* of fibula.

a. nu′triens tibia′lis [NA], SYN nutrient *artery* of the tibia.

a. obturato′ria [NA], SYN obturator *artery*.

a. obturato′ria accesso′ria [NA], SYN accessory obturator *artery*.

a. occipita′lis [NA], SYN occipital *artery*.

arte′riae occipita′lis [NA], SYN mastoid *artery*.

a. occipita′lis latera′lis [NA], SYN lateral occipital *artery*.

a. occipita′lis media′lis [NA], SYN medial occipital *artery*.

a. ophthal′mica [NA], SYN ophthalmic *artery*.

a. ova′rica [NA], SYN ovarian *artery*.

a. palati′na ascen′dens [NA], SYN ascending palatine *artery*.

a. palati′na descen′dens [NA], SYN descending palatine *artery*.

a. palati′na ma′jor [NA], SYN greater palatine *artery*.

a. palati′na mi′nor [NA], SYN lesser palatine *artery*.

arte′riae palpebra′les [NA], SYN palpebral *arteries*, under *artery*.

a. pancreat′ica dorsa′lis [NA], SYN dorsal pancreatic *artery*.

a. pancreat′ica infe′rior [NA], SYN inferior pancreatic *artery*.

a. pancreat′ica mag′na [NA], SYN great pancreatic *artery*.

a. pancreat′icoduodena′lis infe′rior [NA], SYN inferior pancreaticoduodenal *artery*.

a. pancreat′icoduodena′lis supe′rior [NA], SYN superior pancreaticoduodenal *artery*.

a. paracentra′lis [NA], SYN paracentral *artery*.

arte′riae parieta′les [NA], SYN parietal *arteries*, under *artery*.

a. parieta′les anterior, SYN anterior parietal *artery*.

a. parieta′les posterior, SYN posterior parietal *artery*.

a. pari′eto-occipita′lis [NA], SYN parieto-occipital *artery*.

arte′riae perforan′tes [NA], SYN perforating *arteries*, under *artery*.

a. pericallo′sa, ☆official alternate term for pericallosal *artery*.

a. pericardiacophren′ica [NA], SYN pericardiacophrenic *artery*.

a. perinea′lis [NA], SYN perineal *artery*.

a. peron′ea [NA], SYN peroneal *artery*.

a. pharyn′gea ascen′dens [NA], SYN ascending pharyngeal *artery*.

a. phren′ica infe′rior [NA], SYN inferior phrenic *artery*.

a. phren′ica supe′rior [NA], SYN superior phrenic *artery*.

a. planta′ris latera′lis [NA], SYN lateral plantar *artery*.

a. planta′ris media′lis [NA], SYN medial plantar *artery*.

arte′riae pon′tis [NA], SYN pontine *arteries*, under *artery*.

a. poplit′ea [NA], SYN popliteal *artery*.

a. precunea′lis [NA], SYN precuneal *artery*.

a. prin′ceps pol′licis [NA], SYN princeps pollicis *artery*.

a. profun′da bra′chii [NA], SYN profunda brachii *artery*.

a. profun′da clitor′idis [NA], SYN deep *artery* of clitoris.

a. profun′da fem′oris [NA], SYN profunda femoris *artery*.

a. profun′da lin′guae [NA], SYN deep lingual *artery*.

a. profun′da pe′nis [NA], SYN deep *artery* of penis.

arte′riae puden′dae exter′nae [NA], SYN external pudendal *arteries*, under *artery*.

a. puden′da inter′na [NA], SYN internal pudendal *artery*.

a. pulmona′lis, SYN pulmonary *trunk*.

a. pulmona′lis dex′tra [NA], SYN right pulmonary *artery*.

a. pulmona′lis sinis′tra [NA], SYN left pulmonary *artery*.

a. radia′lis [NA], SYN radial *artery*.

a. radia′lis in′dicis [NA], SYN radialis indicis *artery*.

a. radicula′ris mag′na, largest of the medullary arteries which supply the spinal cord by anastomosing with the anterior (longitudinal) spinal artery; it arises from a lower intercostal or upper lumbar artery (on the left side about 65% of the time) supplying most of the blood to the lower two-thirds of the anterior spinal artery. SEE medullary *arteries* of brain, under *artery*. SYN artery of Adamkiewicz, great anastomotic artery (3), great radicular artery.

a. rani′na, SYN deep lingual *artery*.

a. recta′lis infe′rior [NA], SYN inferior rectal *artery*.

a. recta′lis me′dia [NA], SYN middle rectal *artery*.

a. recta′lis supe′rior [NA], SYN superior rectal *artery*.

a. recur′rens [NA], SYN medial striate *artery*.

a. recur′rens radia′lis [NA], SYN radial recurrent *artery*.

a. recur′rens tibia′lis ante′rior [NA], SYN anterior tibial recurrent *artery*.

a. recur′rens tibia′lis poste′rior [NA], SYN posterior tibial recurrent *artery*.

a. recur′rens ulna′ris [NA], SYN recurrent ulnar *artery*.

a. rena′lis [NA], SYN renal *artery*.

arte′riae re′nis [NA], SYN segmental *arteries* of kidney, under *artery*.

a. ret′inae centra′lis, SYN central *artery* of retina.

a. retroduodena′lis [NA], SYN retroduodenal *artery*.

a. sacra′lis latera′lis [NA], SYN lateral sacral *artery*.

a. sacra′lis media′na [NA], SYN median sacral *artery*.

a. scapula′ris descen′dens, SYN dorsal scapular *artery*.

a. scapula′ris dorsa′lis [NA], ✩official alternate term for dorsal scapular *artery*.

a. segmen′ti anterio′ris inferio′ris re′nis [NA], SYN anterior inferior segmental *artery* of kidney. SEE ALSO segmental *arteries* of kidney, under *artery*.

a. segmen′ti anterio′ris superio′ris re′nis [NA], SYN anterior superior segmental *artery* of kidney. SEE ALSO segmental *arteries* of kidney, under *artery*.

a. segmen′ti inferio′ris re′nis [NA], SYN inferior segmental *artery* of kidney. SEE ALSO segmental *arteries* of kidney, under *artery*.

a. segmen′ti posterio′ris re′nis [NA], SYN posterior segmental *artery* of kidney. SEE ALSO segmental *arteries* of kidney, under *artery*.

a. segmen′ti superio′ris re′nis [NA], SYN superior segmental *artery* of kidney. SEE ALSO segmental *arteries* of kidney, under *artery*.

arte′riae sigmoi′deae [NA], SYN sigmoid *arteries*, under *artery*.

a. spermat′ica inter′na, SYN testicular *artery*.

a. sphe′nopalati′na [NA], SYN sphenopalatine *artery*.

a. spina′lis ante′rior [NA], SYN anterior spinal *artery*.

a. spina′lis poste′rior [NA], SYN posterior spinal *artery*.

a. sple′nica [NA], SYN splenic *artery*.

a. stylomastoi′dea [NA], SYN stylomastoid *artery*.

a. subcla′via [NA], SYN subclavian *artery*.

a. subcosta′lis [NA], SYN subcostal *artery*.

a. sublingua′lis [NA], SYN sublingual *artery*.

a. submenta′lis [NA], SYN submental *artery*.

a. subscapula′ris [NA], SYN subscapular *artery*.

a. sul′ci centra′lis [NA], SYN central sulcal *artery*.

a. sul′ci postcentra′lis [NA], SYN postcentral sulcal *artery*.

a. sul′ci precentra′lis [NA], SYN precentral sulcal *artery*.

a. supraduodena′lis [NA], SYN supraduodenal *artery*.

a. supraorbita′lis [NA], SYN supraorbital *artery*.

arteriae suprarena′les supe′riores [NA], SYN superior suprarenal *arteries*, under *artery*.

a. suprarena′lis infe′rior [NA], SYN inferior suprarenal *artery*.

a. suprarena′lis me′dia [NA], SYN middle suprarenal *artery*.

a. suprascapula′ris [NA], SYN suprascapular *artery*.

a. supratrochlea′ris [NA], SYN supratrochlear *artery*.

a. sura′lis [NA], SYN sural *artery*.

a. tar′sea latera′lis [NA], SYN lateral tarsal *artery*.

a. tar′sea media′lis [NA], SYN medial tarsal *artery*.

a. tempora′lis ante′rior [NA], SYN anterior temporal *artery*.

a. tempora′lis interme′dia [NA], SYN intermediate temporal *artery*.

a. tempora′lis media [NA], SYN middle temporal *artery*.

a. tempora′lis poste′rior [NA], SYN posterior temporal *artery*.

a. tempora′lis profun′da [NA], SYN deep temporal *artery*.

a. tempora′lis superficia′lis [NA], SYN superficial temporal *artery*.

a. testicula′ris [NA], SYN testicular *artery*.

arte′riae thalamostria′tae anterolatera′les, ✩official alternate term for lateral striate *arteries*, under *artery*.

arte′riae thalamostria′tae anteromedia′les [NA], ✩official alternate term for anteromedial central *arteries*, under *artery*.

a. thora′cica inter′na [NA], SYN internal thoracic *artery*.

a. thora′cica latera′lis [NA], SYN lateral thoracic *artery*.

a. thora′cica supe′rior [NA], SYN superior thoracic *artery*.

a. thoracoacromia′lis [NA], SYN thoracoacromial *artery*.

a. thoracodorsa′lis [NA], SYN thoracodorsal *artery*.

arte′riae thy′micae, SYN mediastinal *branches* of internal thoracic artery, under *branch*.

a. thyroi′dea i′ma [NA], SYN thyroid ima *artery*.

a. thyroi′dea infe′rior [NA], SYN inferior thyroid *artery*.

a. thyroi′dea supe′rior [NA], SYN superior thyroid *artery*.

a. tibia′lis ante′rior [NA], SYN anterior tibial *artery*.

a. tibia′lis poste′rior [NA], SYN posterior tibial *artery*.

a. transver′sa cer′vicis [NA], SYN transverse cervical *artery*.

a. transver′sa col′li [NA], ✩official alternate term for transverse cervical *artery*.

a. transver′sa facie′i [NA], SYN transverse facial *artery*.

a. tympan′ica ante′rior [NA], SYN anterior tympanic *artery*.

a. tympan′ica infe′rior [NA], SYN inferior tympanic *artery*.

a. tympan′ica poste′rior [NA], SYN posterior tympanic *artery*.

a. tympan′ica supe′rior [NA], SYN superior tympanic *artery*.

a. ulna′ris [NA], SYN ulnar *artery*.

a. umbilica′lis [NA], SYN umbilical *artery*.

a. urethra′lis [NA], SYN urethral *artery*.

a. uteri′na [NA], SYN uterine *artery*.

a. vagina′lis [NA], SYN vaginal *artery*.

arte′riae ventricula′res [NA], SYN ventricular *arteries*, under *artery*.

a. vertebra′lis [NA], SYN vertebral *artery*.

a. vesica′lis infe′rior [NA], SYN inferior vesical *artery*.

a. vesica′lis supe′rior [NA], SYN superior vesical *artery*.

a. vitelli′na, SYN vitelline *artery*.

a. vola′ris ind′icis radia′lis, SYN radialis indicis *artery*.

a. zygomat′ico-orbita′lis [NA], SYN zygomatico-orbital *artery*.

ar·te·ri·al (ar-tē′rē-ăl). Relating to one or more arteries or to the entire system of arteries.

ar·te·ri·al·i·za·tion (ar-tē′rē-ăl-ĭ-zā′shŭn). **1.** Making or becoming arterial. **2.** Aeration or oxygenation of the blood whereby it is changed in character from venous to arterial. **3.** SYN vascularization. **4.** Conversion of a venous structure to function as an artery.

ar·te·ri·arc·tia (ar-tēr-ē-ark′shē-ă). Obsolete term for vasoconstriction of the arteries. [L. *arteria*, artery, + *arcto*, to constrict]

ar·te·ri·ec·ta·sis, ar·te·ri·ec·ta·sia (ar-tēr-ē-ek′tă-sis, -ek-tā′zē-ă). Obsolete term for vasodilation of the arteries. [L. *arteria*, artery, + G. *ektasis*, distention]

ar·te·ri·ec·to·my (ar-tēr-ē-ek′tō-mē). Excision of part of an artery. [L. *arteria*, artery, + G. *ektomē*, excision]

△**arterio-, arteri-.** Artery. [L. *arteria*, fr. G. *artēria*, a windpipe, an artery]

ar·te·ri·o·at·o·ny (ar-tēr′ē-ō-at′ō-nē). An abnormally relaxed state of the arterial walls. [arterio- + G. *atonia*, atony]

ar·te·ri·o·cap·il·lary (ar-tēr′ē-ō-cap′i-lār-ē). Relating to both arteries and capillaries.

ar·te·ri·o·gram (ar-tēr′ē-ō-gram). Radiographic demonstration of an artery after injection of contrast medium into it. [arterio- + G. *gramma*, something written]

ar·te·ri·o·graph·ic (ar-tēr′ē-ō-graf′ik). Relating to or utilizing arteriography.

ar·te·ri·og·ra·phy (ar-tēr-ē-og′ră-fē). Visualization of an artery or arteries by x-ray imaging after injection of a radiopaque contrast medium. [arterio- + G. *graphō*, to write]

bronchial a., radiography of bronchial arteries by selective injection of the intercostal arteries from which they arise.

cerebral a., SYN cerebral *angiography*.

ar·te·ri·o·la, pl. **ar·te·ri·o·lae** (ar-tēr-ē-ō′lă, -ō′lē) [NA]. SYN arteriole. [Mod. L. dim. of *arteria*, artery]

a. glomerula′ris af′ferens [NA], SYN afferent glomerular *arteriole*.

a. glomerula′ris ef′ferens [NA], SYN efferent glomerular *arteriole*.

a. macula′ris infe′rior [NA], SYN inferior macular *arteriole*.

a. macula′ris supe′rior [NA], SYN superior macular *arteriole*.

a. media′lis ret′inae [NA], SYN medial *arteriole* of retina.

a. nasa′lis ret′inae infe′rior [NA], SYN inferior nasal *arteriole* of retina.

a. nasa′lis ret′inae supe′rior [NA], SYN superior nasal *arteriole* of retina.

arterio′lae rec′tae [NA], SYN *vasa* recta, under *vas*.

a. tempora′lis ret′inae infe′rior [NA], SYN inferior temporal *arteriole* of retina.

a. tempora′lis ret′inae supe′rior [NA], SYN superior temporal *arteriole* of retina.

ar·te·ri·o·lar (ar-ter-ē-ō′lăr). Of or pertaining to an arteriole or the arterioles collectively.

ar·te·ri·ole (ar-tēr′ē-ōl). A minute artery with a tunica media comprising only one or two layers of smooth muscle cells; a terminal artery continuous with the capillary network. SYN arteriola [NA].

afferent glomerular a., a branch of an interlobular artery of the kidney that conveys blood to the glomerulus. SYN arteriola glomerularis afferens [NA], vas afferens [NA], afferent vessel (2).

capillary a., a minute artery that terminates in a capillary.

efferent glomerular a., the vessel that carries blood from the glomerular capillary network to the capillary bed of the proximal convoluted tubule; collectively, these vessels constitute the renal portal system. SYN arteriola glomerularis efferens [NA], vas efferens (2) [NA], efferent vessel.

inferior macular a., *origin*, central artery of retina; *distribution*, inferior part of macula. SYN arteriola macularis inferior [NA].

inferior nasal a. of retina, the branch of the central artery of the retina that supplies the lower medial, or nasal, part of the retina. SYN arteriola nasalis retinae inferior [NA].

inferior temporal a. of retina, the branch of the central artery of the retina that passes laterally below the macula to supply the lower lateral or temporal part of the retina. SYN arteriola temporalis retinae inferior [NA].

medial a. of retina, an arteriole supplying the part of the retina between the optic disk and the macula. SYN arteriola medialis retinae [NA].

superior macular a., *origin*, central artery of retina; *distribution*, upper part of macula. SYN arteriola macularis superior [NA].

superior nasal a. of retina, the branch of the central artery of the retina that passes to the upper medial, or nasal, part of the retina. SYN arteriola nasalis retinae superior [NA].

superior temporal a. of retina, the branch of the central artery of the retina that passes laterally above the macula to supply the upper lateral or temporal part of the retina. SYN arteriola temporalis retinae superior [NA].

ar·te·ri·o·lith (ar-tēr′ē-ō-lith). A calcareous deposit in an arterial wall or thrombus. [L. *arteria*, artery, + G. *lithos*, a stone]

ar·ter·i·o·li·tis (ar-tēr′ē-ō-lī′tis). Inflammation of the wall of the arterioles. [L. *arteriola*, arteriole, + G. *-itis*, inflammation]

necrotizing a., necrosis in the media of arterioles, characteristic of malignant hypertension. SYN arteriolonecrosis.

⌂**arteriolo-.** The arterioles. [Modern L. *arteriola*, arteriole]

ar·te·ri·ol·o·gy (ar-tēr′ē-ol′ō-jē). The anatomy of the arteries: usually associated with the study of the other vessels under the name angiology. [L. *arteria*, artery, + G. *logos*, study]

ar·te·ri·o·lo·ne·cro·sis (ar-tēr-ē-ō′lō-ně-krō′sis). SYN necrotizing *arteriolitis*. [L. *arteriola*, arteriole, + G. *nekrōsis*, a killing]

ar·te·ri·o·lo·neph·ro·scle·ro·sis (ar-tēr-ē-ō′lō-nef′rō-skler-ō′sis). SYN arteriolar *nephrosclerosis*.

ar·te·ri·o·lo·scle·ro·sis (ar-tēr-ē-ō′lō-skler-ō′sis). Arteriosclerosis affecting mainly the arterioles, seen especially in chronic hypertension. SYN arteriolar sclerosis.

ar·te·ri·o·lo·ve·nous (ar-tēr-ē-ō′lō-vē′nŭs). Involving both the arterioles and veins. SYN arteriolovenular.

ar·te·ri·o·lo·ven·u·lar (ar-tēr-ē-ō′lō-vē′nyū-lăr). SYN arteriolovenous.

ar·te·ri·o·ma·la·cia (ar-tēr′ē-ō-mă-lā′shē-ă). Softening of the arteries. [arterio- + G. *malakia*, softness]

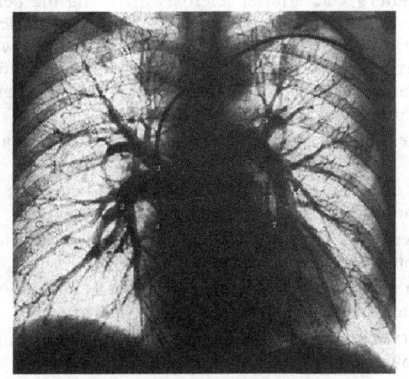

arteriography
normal finding for the pulmonary arteries

ar·te·ri·om·e·ter (ar-tēr-ē-om′ě-ter). An instrument for measuring the diameter of an artery, or its change in size during pulsation. [arterio- + G. *metron*, measure]

ar·te·ri·o·mo·tor (ar-tēr′ē-ō-mō′ter). Causing changes in the caliber of an artery; vasomotor with special reference to the arteries.

ar·te·ri·o·my·o·ma·to·sis (ar-tēr′ē-ō-mī′ō-mă-tō′sis). Thickening of the walls of an artery by an overgrowth of muscular fibers arranged irregularly, intersecting each other without any definite relation to the axis of the vessel. [arterio- + G. *mys*, muscle, + -*oma*, tumor, + -*osis*, condition]

ar·te·ri·o·neph·ro·scle·ro·sis (ar-tēr′ē-ō-nef′rō-skler-ō′sis). SYN arterial *nephrosclerosis*.

ar·te·ri·o·pal·mus (ar-tēr′ē-ō-pal′mŭs). Subjective sensation of throbbing of an artery. [arterio- + G. *palmos*, throbbing]

ar·te·ri·op·a·thy (ar-tēr-ē-op′ă-thē). Any disease of the arteries. [arterio- + G. *pathos*, suffering]

hypertensive a., arterial degeneration resulting from hypertension.

plexogenic pulmonary a., SYN Ayerza's *syndrome*.

ar·te·ri·o·pla·nia (ar-tēr′ē-ō-plā′nē-ă). Presence of an anomaly in the course of an artery. [arterio- + G. *plane*, a straying]

ar·te·ri·o·plas·ty (ar-tēr′ē-ō-plas-tē). Any operation for the reconstruction of the wall of an artery. [arterio- + G. *plastos*, formed]

ar·te·ri·o·pres·sor (ar-tēr′ē-ō-pres′ser). Causing increased arterial blood pressure.

ar·te·ri·or·rha·phy (ar-tēr-ē-ōr′ă-fē). Suture of an artery. [arterio- + G. *rhaphē*, seam]

ar·te·ri·or·rhex·is (ar-tēr′ē-ō-rek′sis). Rupture of an artery. [arterio- + G. *rhēxis*, rupture]

ar·te·ri·o·scle·ro·sis (ar-tēr′ē-ō-skler-ō′sis). Hardening of the arteries; types generally recognized are: atherosclerosis, Möncke-berg's a., and arteriolosclerosis. SYN arterial sclerosis, vascular sclerosis. [arterio- + G. *sklērōsis*, hardness]

coronary a., degenerative and metabolic changes of the walls of the coronary arteries usually beginning with atheroma of the intima and preceding to involve the media; also, calcified lesions known as Monckeberg's a.

hyperplastic a., hyperplasia of the intima and internal elastic layer and hypertrophy of the media independent of atheromatous lesions.

hypertensive a., progressive increase in muscle and elastic tissue of arterial walls, resulting from hypertension; in longstanding hypertension, elastic tissue forms numerous concentric layers in the intima and there is replacement of muscle by collagen fibers and hyaline thickening of the intima of arterioles; such changes can develop with increasing age in the absence of hypertension and may then be referred to as senile a.

medial a., SYN Mönckeberg's a.

Mönckeberg's a., arterial sclerosis involving the peripheral arteries, especially of the legs of older people, with deposition of calcium in the medial coat (pipestem arteries) but with little or no encroachment on the lumen. SYN medial a., Mönckeberg's calcification, Mönckeberg's degeneration, Mönckeberg's medial calcification, Mönckeberg's sclerosis.

nodular a., atheromas occurring in the arterial intima as discrete tumors.

a. oblit′erans, a. producing narrowing and occlusion of the arterial lumen.

peripheral a., a. in any of the vessels beyond the aorta; most often refers to the lower extremities.

senile a., a. similar to hypertensive a., but as a result of advanced age rather than hypertension.

ar·te·ri·o·scle·rot·ic (ar-tēr′ē-ō-skler-ot′ik). Relating to or affected by arteriosclerosis.

ar·te·ri·o·spasm (ar-tēr′ē-ō-spazm). Spasm of an artery or arteries.

ar·te·ri·o·ste·no·sis (ar-tēr′ē-ō-stĕ-nō′sis). Narrowing of the caliber of an artery, either temporary, through vasoconstriction, or permanent, through arteriosclerosis. [arterio- + G. *stenōsis,* a narrowing]

ar·te·ri·ot·o·my (ar-tēr-ē-ot′ō-mē). Any surgical incision into the lumen of an artery, *e.g.,* to remove an embolus. [arterio- + G. *tomē,* incision]

ar·te·ri·ot·o·ny (ar-tēr-ē-ot′ō-nē). SYN blood *pressure.* [arterio- + G. *tonos,* tension]

ar·te·ri·o·ve·nous (A-V) (ar-tēr′ē-ō-vē′nŭs). Relating to both an artery and a vein or to both arteries and veins in general; both arterial and venous, as an "arteriovenous (A-V) anastomosis."

ar·te·ri·tis (ar-ter-ī′tis). Inflammation involving an artery or arteries. [L. *arteria,* artery, + G. *-itis,* inflammation]

brachiocephalic a., giant-cell a. seen in older adults; characterized by inflammatory lesions in medium sized arteries, most commonly in the head, neck and/or shoulder girdle area; lesions include fragmented elastin, macrophages, and giant cells. Erythrocyte sedimentation rate is usually markedly elevated. Visual loss can occur.

coronary a., inflammation of any or all of the layers of coronary artery walls.

cranial a., SYN temporal a.

equine viral a., a highly contagious viral disease caused by equine arteritis virus, member of the family Togaviridae, and characterized by a high fever and respiratory and digestive tract signs; the essential lesions involve smaller arteries, with necrosis which may be followed by thrombosis, infarction, hemorrhages, and edema; abortion is a common result. SYN epizootic cellulitis, equine typhoid.

extracranial a., SYN temporal a.

giant cell a., SYN temporal a.

granulomatous a., SYN temporal a.

Heubner's a., inflammation of arteries within the circle of Willis secondary to chronic basal meningitis from tubercle bacillus or particular fungi such as *Cryptococcus, Histoplasma,* or *Coccidioides.*

Horton's a., SYN temporal a.

intracranial granulomatous a., a small vessel, giant cell a. that affects only intracranial blood vessels, of unknown etiology, and with diverse clinical manifestations, including those seen with an involving cerebral tumor, and with a low grade meningitis, leading to infarction of one portion of the cerebrum or cerebellum.

neurocranial granulomatous a., a small vessel giant cell a. which affects only intracranial blood vessels, of unknown etiology, and with diverse clinical manifestations, including those seen with an involving cerebral tumor, and with a lower grade meningitis, leading to infarction of one portion of the cerebrum or cerebellum.

a. nodo′sa, SYN *polyarteritis* nodosa.

a. oblit′erans, obliterating a., SYN *endarteritis* obliterans.

rheumatic a., a. due to rheumatic fever; Aschoff bodies are frequently found in the adventitia of small arteries, especially in the myocardium, and may lead to fibrosis and constriction of the lumens.

rheumatoid a., coronary a. associated with rheumatoid arthritis; aortitis with aortic valve incompetence accompanying ankylosing spondylitis may be related.

Takayasu's a., a progressive obliterative arteritis of unknown origin involving chronic inflammation of the aortic arch with fibrosis and marked luminal narrowing that affects the aorta and its branches, often with complete or near complete occlusion of segments of the aorta; most common in females. SEE ALSO aortic arch *syndrome.* SYN pulseless disease, Takayasu's disease, Takayasu's syndrome.

temporal a., a subacute, granulomatous a. involving the external carotid arteries, especially the temporal artery; occurs in elderly persons and may be manifested by constitutional symptoms, particularly severe headache, and sometimes sudden unilateral blindness. Shares many of the symptoms of *polymyalgia* rheumatica. SYN cranial a., extracranial a., giant cell a., granulomatous a., Horton's a.

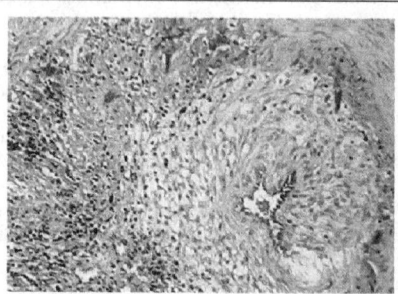

temporal arteritis (giant cell arteritis)

Arterivirus. A genus in the family Togaviridae which is associated with equine arteritis virus.

ARTERY

ar·tery (a) (ar′ter-ē). A relatively thick-walled, muscular, pulsating blood vessel conveying blood in a direction away from the heart. With the exception of the pulmonary and umbilical arteries, the arteries convey red or aerated blood. At the major arteries, the arterial branches are listed separately following the designation *branches.* SYN arteria [NA]. [L. *arteria,* fr. G. *artēria*]

Abbott's a., an anomalous a. arising from the posteromedial proximal descending aorta, important during coarctation repair.

aberrant a., a. having an unusual origin or course.

aberrant obturator a., SEE pubic *branch* of inferior epigastric artery.

accessory obturator a., term applied to the anastomosis of pubic branch of the inferior epigastric a. with the pubic branch of the obturator a. when it contributes a significant supply through the obturator canal. SYN arteria obturatoria accessoria [NA], ramus obturatorius arteriae epigastricae inferioris [NA].

acetabular a., SYN acetabular *branch.*

acromial a., SYN acromial *branch* of thoracoacromial artery.

acromiothoracic a., SYN thoracoacromial a.

a. of Adamkiewicz, SYN *arteria* radicularis magna.

alar a. of nose, a branch of the angular a. that supplies the ala of the nose.

angular a., (1) the terminal branch of the facial artery; *distribution,* muscles and skin of side of nose; *anastomoses,* lateral nasal, and dorsal artery of nose and palpebrals from the ophthalmic a., thereby providing an external-internal carotid arterial anastomosis; **(2)** SYN a. of angular gyrus. SYN arteria angularis [NA].

a. of angular gyrus, the last branch of the terminal part of the middle cerebral artery distributed to parts of the temporal parietal and occipital lobes. SYN arteria gyri angularis [NA], angular a. (2).

anterior cecal a., *origin,* ileocolic artery; *distribution,* anterior region of cecum. SYN arteria cecalis anterior [NA].

anterior cerebral a., one of the two terminal branches (with middle cerebral a.) of the internal carotid; it passes anterior, loops around the genu of the corpus callosum then posteriorly in the interhemispheric fissure along with its fellow of the opposite side, the two being joined by the anterior communicating artery; for descriptive purposes it is divided into two parts: the precommunical part (A_2 segment of clinical terminology), supplying branches to the thalamus and corpus striatum, and the postcommunical part, (A_2) or pericallosal a., supplying branches to the cortex of the medial parts of the frontal and parietal lobes. SYN arteria cerebri anterior [NA].

anterior choroidal a., *origin,* internal carotid or (rarely) middle cerebral artery; *distribution,* optic tract, crus cerebri, uncus, hippocampus, globus pallidus, posterior part of internal capsule, geniculate bodies of the thalamus, and choroid plexus in the inferior horn of the lateral ventricle. SYN arteria choroidea anterior [NA].

anterior ciliary a., one of several arteries derived from muscular branches of the ophthalmic which perforate the anterior part of the sclera and anastomose with posterior ciliary arteries. SYN arteria ciliaris anterior [NA].

anterior circumflex humeral a., *origin,* axillary; *distribution,* shoulder joint and biceps muscle; *anastomoses,* posterior circumflex humeral a. SYN arteria circumflexa humeri anterior [NA], anterior humeral circumflex a.

anterior communicating a., a short vessel joining the two anterior cerebral arteries and completing the cerebral arterial circle (circle of Willis) anteriorly. SYN arteria communicans anterior [NA].

anterior conjunctival a., one of a number of small branches of the anterior ciliary arteries that supplies the conjunctiva. SYN arteria conjunctivalis anterior [NA], conjunctival a.'s.

anterior descending a., SYN anterior interventricular a.

anterior ethmoidal a., *origin,* ophthalmic; *distribution,* cerebral membranes in anterior cranial fossa, anterior ethmoidal cells, frontal sinus, anterior upper part of nasal mucous membrane, skin of dorsum of nose. SYN arteria ethmoidalis anterior [NA].

anterior humeral circumflex a., SYN anterior circumflex humeral a.

anterior inferior cerebellar a., *origin,* basilar; *distribution,* lower surface of lateral lobes of cerebellum, choroid plexus in cerebellopontine angle; *anastomoses,* posterior inferior cerebellar; usual source of labyrinthine artery. SYN arteria cerebelli inferior anterior [NA].

anterior inferior segmental a. of kidney, *origin,* anterior branch of renal. SEE ALSO segmental a.'s of kidney. SYN arteria segmenti anterioris inferioris renis [NA], a. of anterior inferior segment of kidney.

a. of anterior inferior segment of kidney, SYN anterior inferior segmental a. of kidney.

anterior intercostal a.'s, one of the a.'s supplying the anterior portions of the intercostal spaces of the thoracic wall. Anterior intercostal a.'s 1–6 arise as branches of the internal thoracic a.; 7–11 arise as branches of the musculophrenic a. SYN rami intercostales anteriores [NA], rami intercostalis anteriores arteria thoracica interna.

anterior intercostal branches of internal thoracic artery, SEE anterior intercostal a.'s.

anterior interosseous a., *origin,* common interosseous; *distribution,* deep parts of the forearm anteriorly; *anastomoses,* posterior interosseous. SYN arteria interossea anterior [NA], arteria interossea volaris, volar interosseous a.

anterior interventricular a., anterior interventricular branch of left coronary artery. Terminal branch (with circumflex coronary a.) of left coronary a.; descends in anterior interventricular groove to apex, anastomosing with posterior interventricular a. Supplies most of sternal aspect of ventricles and anterior two-thirds of interventricular septum, including atrioventricular bundle of conducting tissue. SYN ramus interventricularis anterior arteriae coronariae sinistrae [NA], anterior descending a.

anterior labial a.'s, the anterior labial branches, branches of the external pudendal artery to the labium majus. SYN rami labiales anteriores arteriae pudendae externae [NA], arteriae labiales anteriores.

anterior lateral malleolar a., *origin,* anterior tibial; *distribution,* ankle joint; *anastomoses,* peroneal, lateral tarsal. SYN arteria malleolaris anterior lateralis [NA].

anterior medial malleolar a., *origin,* anterior tibial; *distribution,* ankle joint and neighboring integument; *anastomoses,* branches of posterior tibial. SYN arteria malleolaris anterior medialis [NA].

anterior mediastinal a.'s, SYN mediastinal *branches* of internal thoracic artery, under *branch.*

anterior meningeal a., *origin,* anterior ethmoidal; *distribution,* meninges in anterior cranial fossa; *anastomoses,* branches of middle meningeal and meningeal branches of internal carotid and lacrimal. SYN arteria meningea anterior [NA].

anterior parietal a., the branch distributed to the anterior part of the parietal lobe. SYN arteria parietales anterior.

anterior peroneal a., SEE perforating *branches,* under *branch.*

anterior spinal a., *origin,* intracranial part of vertebral; *distribution,* spinal cord and pia mater; *anastomoses,* spinal of intercostal and lumbar arteries. SYN arteria spinalis anterior [NA].

anterior superior alveolar a.'s, *origin,* infraorbital artery within intraorbital canal; *distribution,* via anterior alveolar canals to upper incisors and canine teeth, mucus membrane of maxillary sinus. SYN arteriae alveolares superiores anteriores [NA], anterior superior dental a.'s.

anterior superior dental a.'s, SYN anterior superior alveolar a.'s.

anterior superior segmental a. of kidney, *origin,* anterior branch of renal. SEE ALSO segmental a.'s of kidney. SYN arteria segmenti anterioris superioris renis [NA], a. of anterior superior segment of kidney.

a. of anterior superior segment of kidney, SYN anterior superior segmental a. of kidney.

anterior temporal a., a branch of the insular part of the middle cerebral artery distributed to the cortex of the anterior part of the temporal lobe. SYN arteria temporalis anterior [NA].

anterior tibial a., *origin,* popliteal; *branches,* posterior and anterior tibial recurrent, lateral and medial anterior malleolar, dorsalis pedis, lateral tarsal, medial tarsal, arcuate, dorsal metatarsal, and dorsal digital. SYN arteria tibialis anterior [NA].

anterior tibial recurrent a., a branch of the anterior tibial artery which ascends to supply the front and sides of the knee joint, thus contributing to the articular network of the knee. SYN arteria recurrens tibialis anterior [NA].

anterior tympanic a., *origin,* maxillary; *distribution,* middle ear; *anastomoses,* tympanic branches of internal carotid and ascending pharyngeal and stylomastoid. SYN arteria tympanica anterior [NA], glaserian a.

anterolateral central a.'s, SYN lateral striate a.'s.

anterolateral striate a.'s, SYN lateral striate a.'s.

anterolateral thalamostriate a.'s, SYN lateral striate a.'s.

anteromedial central a.'s, several small branches of the precommunical part of the anterior cerebral artery; they are distributed to the anteromedial part of the corpus striatum part of the thalamus. SYN arteriae centrales anteromediales [NA], arteriae thalamostriatae anteromediales ☆ [NA], anteromedial thalamostriate a.'s.

anteromedial thalamostriate a.'s, SYN anteromedial central a.'s.

apicoposterior a., a pulmonary a. branch to the apicoposterior segment of the upper lobe.

appendicular a., the branch of the ileocolic artery that descends posterior to the terminal ileum in the mesoappendix to supply the vermiform appendix. SYN arteria appendicularis [NA].

arciform a.'s, SYN *arteriae* arcuatae renis, under *arteria.*

arcuate a., *origin,* dorsalis pedis; *branches,* passes laterally dorsal to the bases of the metatarsals, giving rise to the 2nd, 3rd, and 4th dorsal metatarsal a.'s at the level of the medial cuneiform bone. SYN arteria arcuata [NA].

arcuate a.'s of kidney, curved a.'s at the corticomedullary border, arising from interlobar a.'s and giving rise to interlobular a.'s. SYN arteriae arcuatae renis [NA].

ascending a., the branch of the inferior branch of the ileocolic artery that passes superiorly up the ascending colon to communicate with a branch of the right colic artery and supplying the ascending colon. SYN arteria ascendens (1).

ascending cervical a., *origin,* usually a terminal branch of the thyrocervical trunk (along with interior thyroid a.); *distribution,* muscles of neck and spinal cord; *anastomoses,* branches of vertebral, occipital, ascending pharyngeal, and deep cervical. SYN arteria cervicalis ascendens [NA], cervicalis ascendens (2).

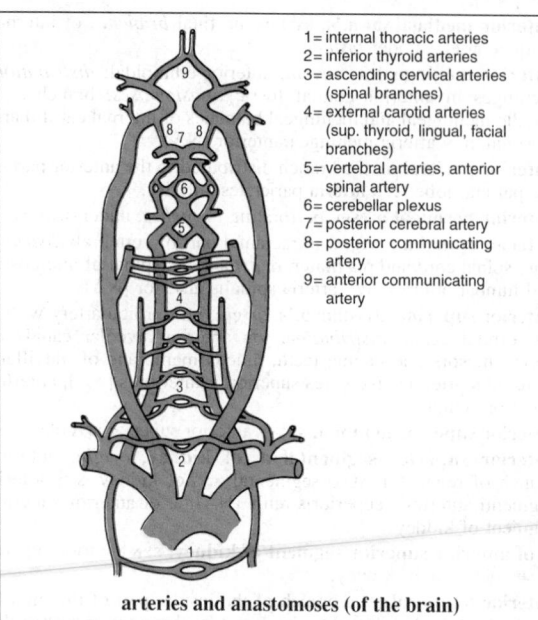

1 = internal thoracic arteries
2 = inferior thyroid arteries
3 = ascending cervical arteries (spinal branches)
4 = external carotid arteries (sup. thyroid, lingual, facial branches)
5 = vertebral arteries, anterior spinal artery
6 = cerebellar plexus
7 = posterior cerebral artery
8 = posterior communicating artery
9 = anterior communicating artery

arteries and anastomoses (of the brain)

ascending palatine a., *origin,* facial; *distribution,* lateral walls of pharynx, tonsils, auditory tubes, and soft palate; *anastomoses,* tonsillar branch of facial, dorsal lingual, and descending palatine. SYN arteria palatina ascendens [NA].

ascending pharyngeal a., *origin,* external carotid; *distribution,* wall of pharynx and soft palate, posterior cranial fossa. SYN arteria pharyngea ascendens [NA].

atrial a.'s, branches of the right and left coronary arteries distributed to the muscle of the atria. SYN arteriae atriales.

a. to atrioventricular node, the atrioventricular branches or the nodal branches, the small arteries supplying the atrioventricular node; they usually arise from the right coronary artery where it starts to descend the posterior interventricular sulcus. SYN ramus nodi atrioventricularis [NA], atrioventricular nodal branch, branch to atrioventricular node.

axillary a., the continuation of the subclavian a. after crossing the first rib to enter the axilla; becomes the brachial a. upon passing the inferior border of the teres major muscle. It is accompanied by the cords of the brachial plexus, and is enclosed with them and the axillary vein in the axillary sheath as it traverses the axilla. The parts of the axillary a. are described: proximal, posterior and distal to the pectoralis minor muscle. Branches: 1st part—superior thoracic a.; 2nd part—thoracoacromial arterial trunk, lateral thoracic a.; 3rd part—subscapular a., anterior and posterior humeral circumflex a.'s. SYN arteria axillaris [NA].

azygos a. of vagina, one of two a.'s that run longitudinally in the midline on the anterior and posterior aspects of the vagina; they take origin from the uterine a.

basilar a., formed by union of the intracranial portions of the two vertebral arteries; runs along the clivus in the pontine cistern of subarachnoid space from the lower to the upper border of the pons, where it bifurcates into the two posterior cerebral arteries; *branches,* anterior, inferior, cerebellar, labyrinthine, pontine, mesencephalic, and superior cerebellar. SYN arteria basilaris [NA].

brachial a., *origin,* is a continuation of the axillary beginning at the inferior border of the teres major muscle; *branches,* deep brachial, superior ulnar collateral, inferior ulnar collateral, muscular, and nutrient; terminates in the cubital fossa (elbow level) by bifurcating into radial and ulnar a.'s. SYN arteria brachialis [NA], humeral a.

bronchial a.'s, the bronchial branches or arteries, vessels or nerves distributed to the bronchi; the following have branches so named: 1) thoracic aorta; 2) internal thoracic artery; 3) vagus nerves. SYN rami bronchiales [NA].

buccal a., buccinator a., *origin,* maxillary; *distribution,* buccinator muscle, skin, and mucous membrane of cheek; *anastomoses,* buccal branch of facial. SYN arteria buccalis [NA].

a. of bulb of penis, a branch of the internal pudendal artery which supplies the bulb of the penis including the bulbar urethra. SYN arteria bulbi penis [NA], arteria bulbi urethrae.

a. of bulb of vestibule, the branch of the internal pudendal artery in the female that supplies the bulb of the vestibule. SYN arteria bulbi vestibuli [NA], arteria bulbi vaginae ✶.

calcaneal a.'s, the calcaneal branches or arteries, branches to the structures in the calcaneal region from 1) the posterior tibial artery and 2) the peroneal artery. SYN rami calcanei [NA].

calcarine a., SYN calcarine *branch* of medial occipital artery.

a. of calf, SYN sural a.

callosomarginal a., the second branch of the pericallosal artery running in the cingulate sulcus and sending branches to supply part of the medial and superolateral surfaces of the cerebral hemisphere. SYN arteria callosomarginalis [NA].

caroticotympanic a.'s, small branches from the petrous part of the internal carotid artery supplying the tympanic cavity; anastomose with the anterior tympanic and maxillary arteries. SYN arteriae caroticotympanicae arteriae carotidis internae [NA], rami caroticotympanici.

carotid a.'s, SEE common carotid a., external carotid a., internal carotid a.

carpal a., a.'s related to and supplying the wrist joint. SEE dorsal carpal *branch* of radial artery, dorsal carpal *branch* of ulnar artery, palmar carpal *branch* of radial artery, palmar carpal *branch* of ulnar artery.

caudal pancreatic a., SYN a. of the pancreatic tail.

a. of caudate lobe, *origin,* left branch of proper hepatic; *distribution,* caudate lobe of the liver. SYN arteria lobi caudati [NA].

cavernous a.'s, SYN cavernous sinus *branch* of internal carotid artery.

cecal a.'s, SEE anterior cecal a., posterior cecal a.

celiac a., SYN celiac *trunk.*

central a., SYN central sulcal a.

central a. of retina, a branch of the ophthalmic artery which penetrates the optic nerve 1 cm behind the eye to enter the eye at the optic papilla in the retina; it divides into superior and inferior temporal and nasal branches. SYN arteria centralis retinae [NA], arteria retinae centralis, Zinn's a.

central sulcal a., a branch of the terminal part of the middle cerebral artery distributed to the cortex on either side of the central sulcus. SYN arteria sulci centralis [NA], a. of central sulcus, central a., Rolandic a.

a. of central sulcus, SYN central sulcal a.

cerebellar a.'s, an artery related to and supplying the cerebellum. SEE anterior inferior cerebellar a., posterior inferior cerebellar a., superior cerebellar a.

cerebral a.'s, an artery related to and supplying the cerebral cortex. SEE anterior cerebral a., middle cerebral a., posterior cerebral a.

a.'s of cerebral hemorrhage, SYN lateral striate a.'s.

cervicovaginal a., an anastomotic communication between the uterine a. and the vaginal a.; it courses along the lateral aspect of the cervix and vagina. SYN arteria cervicovaginalis.

Charcot's a., SYN lenticulostriate a.'s (2).

chief a. of thumb, SYN princeps pollicis a.

circumflex femoral a.'s, SEE lateral circumflex femoral a., medial circumflex femoral a.

circumflex fibular a., the circumflex fibular branch, a branch of the posterior tibial artery which winds around the neck of the fibula and joins the anastomoses around the knee joint. SYN ramus circumflexus fibularis arteriae tibialis posterioris [NA].

circumflex humeral a.'s, SEE anterior circumflex humeral a., posterior circumflex humeral a.

circumflex iliac a.'s, SEE deep circumflex iliac a., superficial circumflex iliac a.

circumflex scapular a., *origin*, subscapular; *distribution*, muscles of shoulder and scapular region; *anastomoses*, branches of suprascapular and transverse cervical. SYN arteria circumflexa scapulae [NA].

coiled a. of the uterus, SYN spiral a.

colic a.'s, a.'s supplying the colon. SEE left colic a., middle colic a., right colic a.

collateral a., (**1**) one that runs parallel with a nerve or other structure; (**2**) one through which a collateral circulation is established. SEE articular vascular *network*.

collateral digital a., SYN proper palmar digital a.

common carotid a., *origin*, right from brachiocephalic, left from arch of aorta; runs upward in the neck and divides opposite upper border of thyroid cartilage (C-4 vertebral level) into *terminal branches*, external and internal carotid. SYN arteria carotis communis [NA].

common hepatic a., *origin*, celiac; *branches*, right gastric, gastroduodenal, and proper hepatic. SYN arteria hepatica communis [NA].

common iliac a., one of the two terminal branches of the abdominal aorta; opposite the lumbosacral joint, it bifurcates to form the internal iliac and the external iliac. SYN arteria iliaca communis [NA].

common interosseous a., *origin*, ulnar; *branches*, anterior and posterior interosseous. SYN arteria interossea communis [NA].

common palmar digital a., one of three arteries arising from the superficial palmar arch and running to the interdigital clefts where each divides into two proper palmar digital arteries. SYN arteria digitalis palmaris communis [NA].

common plantar digital a., one of four arteries arising from a superficial plantar arch, when present as a variation. They unite with the plantar metatarsal arteries. SYN arteria digitalis plantaris communis [NA].

communicating a., an a. that connects two larger a.'s. SEE anterior communicating a., posterior communicating a.

companion a. to sciatic nerve, SYN a. to sciatic nerve.

conjunctival a.'s, SYN anterior conjunctival a., posterior conjunctival a.

coronary a., (**1**) SEE right coronary a., left coronary a. (**2**) SYN left gastric a.

cortical a.'s, branches of the anterior, middle, and posterior cerebral a.'s that supply the cerebral cortex.

costocervical a., SYN costocervical *trunk*.

cremasteric a., *origin*, inferior epigastric; *distribution*, coverings of spermatic cord; *anastomoses*, external pudendal, spermatic, and perineal a. SYN arteria cremasterica [NA], external spermatic a.

cricothyroid a., a small branch of the superior thyroid artery that supplies the cricothyroid muscle. SYN ramus cricothyroideus [NA].

cystic a., *origin*, right branch of hepatic; *distribution*, gall bladder and visceral surface of the liver. SYN arteria cystica [NA].

deep auricular a., *origin*, first part of maxillary; *distribution*, articulation of jaw, parotid gland, and external acoustic meatus and external tympanic membrane; *anastomoses*, auricular branches of superficial temporal and posterior auricular. SYN arteria auricularis profunda [NA].

deep brachial a., SYN profunda brachii a.

deep cervical a., *origin*, terminal branch of costocervical trunk (along with superior intercostal artery); *distribution*, posterior deep muscles of neck; *anastomoses*, branches of occipital, as-

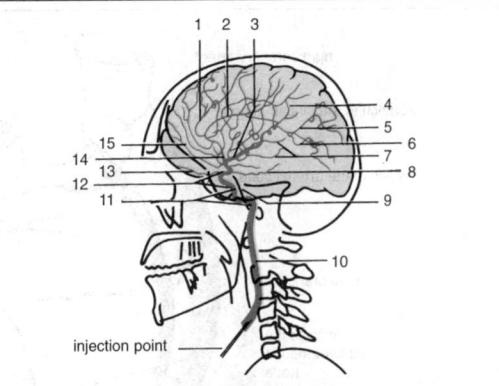

arteries (cerebral angiogram)

1) arteria callosomarginalis, 2) a. pericallosa, 3) a. cerebri media, 4) a. subcentralis, 5) a. supramarginalis, 6) a. gyri angularis, 7) aa. temporales, 8) a. choroidea anterior, 9) clivus (Blumenbachi), 10) a. carotis interna (pars cervicalis), 11) canalis caroticus (pars petrosa), 12) carotid siphon in sinus cavernosus (pars cavernosa), 13) a. opthalmica, 14) a. cerebri anterior, 15) a. frontopolaris

cending cervical, and vertebral. SYN arteria cervicalis profunda [NA].

deep circumflex iliac a., *origin*, external iliac; *distribution*, muscles and skin of lower abdomen, sartorius and tensor fasciae latae; *anastomoses*, lumbar, inferior epigastric, superior gluteal, iliolumbar, and superficial circumflex iliac. SYN arteria circumflexa iliaca profunda [NA].

deep a. of clitoris, the deep terminal branch of the internal pudendal artery in the female; it supplies the crus of the clitoris. SYN arteria profunda clitoridis [NA].

deep epigastric a., SYN inferior epigastric a.

deep lingual a., termination of lingual artery, *distribution*, muscles and mucous membrane of under surface of tongue. SYN arteria profunda linguae [NA], arteria ranina, deep a. of tongue, ranine a.

deep a. of penis, *origin*, terminal branch (with dorsal a. of penis) of the internal pudendal artery; *distribution*, corpus cavernosum of the penis via capillary beds and via helcine arteries and arteriovenous anastomoses to produce erection. SYN arteria profunda penis [NA].

deep temporal a., deep temporal artery, two in number, anterior and posterior; *origin*, maxillary; *distribution*, temporal muscle and periosteum, bone and diploe of temporal fossa; *anastomoses*, branches of superficial temporal, lacrimal, and middle meningeal. SYN arteria temporalis profunda [NA].

deep a. of thigh, SYN profunda femoris a.

deep a. of tongue, SYN deep lingual a.

deferential a., SYN a. of ductus deferens.

descending genicular a., *origin*, femoral, in adductor canal; *distribution*, penetrates vastoadductor fascia to supply knee joint and adjacent parts; *anastomoses*, medial superior genicular, medial inferior genicular, lateral superior genicular, lateral inferior genicular and anterior tibial recurrent a.'s, *i.e.*, articular network of knee. SYN arteria genus descendens [NA], arteria anastomotica magna (2), descending a. of knee, great anastomotic a. (2).

descending a. of knee, SYN descending genicular a.

descending palatine a., *origin*, maxillary; *distribution*, soft palate, gums, and bones and mucous membrane of hard palate; *anastomoses*, sphenopalatine, ascending palatine, ascending pharyngeal, and tonsillar branches of facial. SYN arteria palatina descendens [NA].

descending scapular a., SYN dorsal scapular a.

digital collateral a., SYN proper palmar digital a.

distributing a., SYN muscular a.

dolichoectatic a., a distorted, dilated, and elongated artery commonly compressing a neural structure.

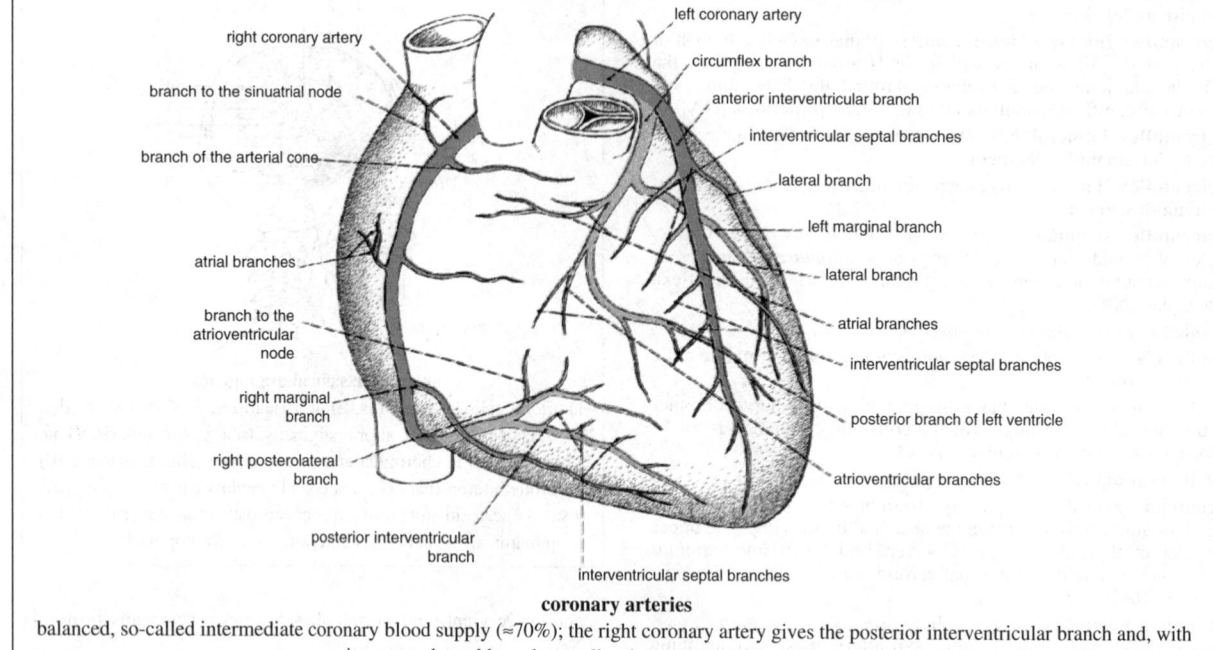

right coronary artery

branch to the sinuatrial node

branch of the arterial cone

atrial branches

branch to the atrioventricular node

right marginal branch

right posterolateral branch

posterior interventricular branch

left coronary artery

circumflex branch

anterior interventricular branch

interventricular septal branches

lateral branch

left marginal branch

lateral branch

atrial branches

interventricular septal branches

posterior branch of left ventricle

atrioventricular branches

interventricular septal branches

coronary arteries

balanced, so-called intermediate coronary blood supply (≈70%); the right coronary artery gives the posterior interventricular branch and, with its posterolateral branch, supplies the rear wall of the left ventricle

dorsal a. of clitoris, one of the two terminal branches of the internal pudendal artery in the female, the other being the deep a. of the clitoris. SYN arteria dorsalis clitoridis [NA].

dorsal digital a., one of the collateral digital branches of the dorsal metatarsal arteries in the foot, and/or of the dorsal metacarpal arteries in the hand. SYN arteria digitalis dorsalis [NA].

dorsal a. of foot, SYN dorsalis pedis a.

dorsal interosseous a., (1) SYN posterior interosseous a. **(2)** SYN dorsal metacarpal a.

dorsalis pedis a., continuation of anterior tibial artery after crossing ankle; *branches,* lateral tarsal, arcuate, dorsal metatarsal; a continuation of the anterior tibial; *anastomoses,* with the lateral plantar to form the plantar arch. SYN arteria dorsalis pedis [NA], dorsal a. of foot.

dorsal metacarpal a., one of four arteries taking origin from the dorsal carpal arch and running on the posterior aspect of the interosseous muscles of the hand. SYN arteria metacarpea dorsalis [NA], dorsal interosseous a. (2).

dorsal metatarsal a., one of four arteries arising from the dorsalis pedis (I) and arcuate (II–IV) arteries and running on the dorsum of the interosseous muscles of the foot. SYN arteria metatarsea dorsalis [NA].

dorsal nasal a., *origin,* ophthalmic; external artery of the nose; *distribution,* skin of side of root of nose; *anastomoses,* angular a. SYN arteria dorsalis nasi [NA], arteria nasi externa* [NA], dorsal a. of nose, external a. of nose.

dorsal a. of nose, SYN dorsal nasal a.

dorsal pancreatic a., *origin,* splenic; *distribution,* head and body of pancreas; *anastomoses,* superior pancreaticoduodenal. SYN arteria pancreatica dorsalis [NA], great superior pancreatic a.

dorsal a. of penis, the dorsal terminal branch of the internal pudendal artery in the male. SYN arteria dorsalis penis [NA].

dorsal scapular a., *origin,* subclavian or as the deep branch of the transverse cervical; *distribution,* passes deep to the rhomboid muscles, supplying them and other muscles and skin along the vertebral border of the scapula; *anastomoses,* suprascapular and scapular circumflex. SYN arteria dorsalis scapulae [NA], rami profundi arteriae transversae cervicis [NA], ramus profundus arteriae transversae colli [NA], arteria scapularis dorsalis* [NA], arteria scapularis descendens, deep branch of the transverse cervical artery, descending scapular a., ramus profundus arteria scapularis descendens.

dorsal thoracic a., SYN thoracodorsal a.

a. of Drummond, SYN marginal a. of colon.

a. of ductus deferens, *origin,* anterior division of internal iliac, or sometimes superior vesical; *distribution,* ductus deferens, seminal vesicles, testicle, ureter; *anastomoses,* testicular, cremasteric a.'s. SYN arteria ductus deferentis [NA], arteria deferentialis, deferential a.

elastic a., a large a., such as the aorta or pulmonary a., which has many elastic lamella in its tunica media.

end a., an a. with insufficient anastomoses to maintain viability of the tissue supplied if occlusion of the a. occurs. SYN terminal a.

episcleral a., one of many small branches of the anterior ciliary a.'s that arise as they perforate the sclera near the corneoscleral junction, and course on the sclera. SYN arteria episcleralis [NA].

esophageal a.'s, esophageal branches of the following: 1) inferior thyroid artery; 2) left gastric artery; 3) thoracic aorta.

external carotid a., *origin,* common carotid at C-4 vertebral level; *branches,* superior thyroid, lingual, facial, occipital, posterior auricular, ascending pharyngeal, and *terminal branches,* maxillary and superficial temporal at level of neck of mandible. SYN arteria carotis externa [NA].

external iliac a., *origin,* common iliac; *branches,* inferior epigastric, deep circumflex iliac; becomes the femoral at the inguinal ligament. SYN arteria iliaca externa [NA].

external mammary a., SYN lateral thoracic a.

external maxillary a., SYN facial a.

external a. of nose, SYN dorsal nasal a.

external pudendal a.'s, *origin,* femoral; *distribution,* skin over pubis, skin over penis and skin of scrotum or labium majus via anterior scrotal (labial) arteries; *anastomoses,* dorsal artery of penis or clitoris, posterior scrotal or labial arteries. SYN arteriae pudendae externae [NA].

external spermatic a., SYN cremasteric a.

facial a., *origin,* external carotid; *branches,* ascending palatine, tonsillar and glandular branches, submental, inferior labial, superior labial, masseteric, buccal, lateral nasal branches, and angular. SYN arteria facialis [NA], arteria maxillaris externa, external maxillary a.

femoral a., *origin,* continuation of external iliac, beginning at inguinal ligament; *branches,* external pudendal, superficial epigastric, superficial circumflex iliac, profunda femoris, descending genicular, terminating as the popliteal a. as it passes through the adductor hiatus to enter the popliteal space. SYN arteria femoralis [NA].

fibular a., SYN peroneal a.

frontal a., SYN supratrochlear a.

gastric a.'s, a.'s supplying the stomach along the lesser curvature. SEE left gastric a., right gastric a.

gastroduodenal a., *origin*, hepatic; terminal *branches*, right gastroepiploic, superior pancreaticoduodenal. SYN arteria gastroduodenalis ☆ [NA].

gastroepiploic a.'s, a.'s which supply the stomach and greater omentum as the course along the greater curvature of the stomach. SEE left gastroepiploic a., right gastroepiploic a. SYN gastroomental a.'s.

gastro-omental a.'s, SYN gastroepiploic a.'s.

genicular a.'s, a.'s contributing to the articular network of the knee. SEE descending genicular a., inferior lateral genicular a., inferior medial genicular a., middle genicular a., superior lateral genicular a., superior medial genicular a.

glaserian a., SYN anterior tympanic a.

great anastomotic a., (1) SYN inferior ulnar collateral a. **(2)** SYN descending genicular a. **(3)** SYN *arteria* radicularis magna.

greater palatine a., anterior branch of descending palatine artery, supplying the gums and mucous membrane of the hard palate. SYN arteria palatina major [NA].

great pancreatic a., *origin*, splenic; *distribution*, tail of pancreas; *anastomoses*, inferior pancreatic a. and a.'s of pancreatic tail. SYN arteria pancreatica magna [NA].

great radicular a., SYN *arteria* radicularis magna.

great superior pancreatic a., SYN dorsal pancreatic a.

helicine a.'s of the penis, the coiled terminal branches of the deep and dorsal a.'s of the penis. Parasympathetic stimulation causes them to uncoil, allowing blood at arterial pressure to fill the cavernous tissue causing erection. SYN arteriae helicinae penis [NA].

hepatic a.'s, a.'s involved in supplying blood to the liver. SEE common hepatic a., proper hepatic a., left hepatic a., right hepatic a.

a. of Heubner, SYN medial striate a.

highest intercostal a., SYN superior intercostal a.

highest thoracic a., SYN superior thoracic a.

humeral a., SYN brachial a.

hyaloid a., the terminal branch of the primitive ophthalmic artery, which forms in the embryo an extensive ramification in the primary vitreous and a vascular tunic around the lens; by 8½ months, these vessels have atrophied almost completely, but a few persistent remnants are evident entoptically as muscae volitantes. SYN arteria hyaloidea [NA].

hypogastric a., SYN internal iliac a.

ileal a.'s, *origin*, superior mesenteric; *distribution*, ileum; *anastomoses*, other branches of superior mesenteric. SYN arteriae ileales [NA].

ileocolic a., *origin*, superior mesenteric, often by a common trunk with the right colic; *distribution*, terminal part of ileum, cecum, vermiform appendix, and ascending colon; *anastomoses*, right colic and ileal. SYN arteria ileocolica [NA].

iliac a.'s, a.'s related to the ilium. SEE common iliac a., deep circumflex iliac a., external iliac a., internal iliac a., superficial circumflex iliac a.

iliolumbar a., *origin*, internal iliac; *distribution*, pelvic muscles and bones; *anastomoses*, deep circumflex iliac, lumbar. SYN arteria iliolumbalis [NA].

inferior alveolar a., *origin*, 1st part of maxillary artery; *distribution*, through mandibular foramen/canal to lower teeth and chin; *branches*, a. to mylohyoid, mental a., dental a.'s. SYN arteria alveolaris inferior [NA], inferior dental a.

inferior dental a., SYN inferior alveolar a.

inferior epigastric a., *origin*, external iliac; *branches*, cremasteric, muscular and pubic; *anastomoses*, superior epigastric, obturator. With overlying peritoneum, forms lateral umbilical ligament and forms a basis for distinguishing types of inguinal herni-

ae: direct hernias pass medial to the a.; indirect hernias pass laterally. SYN arteria epigastrica inferior [NA], deep epigastric a.

inferior gluteal a., *origin*, internal iliac; *distribution*, hip joint and gluteal region; *anastomoses*, branches of internal pudendal, lateral sacral, superior gluteal, obturator, medial and lateral circumflex femoral. SYN arteria glutea inferior [NA], arteria ischiadica, arteria ischiatica.

inferior hemorrhoidal a., SYN inferior rectal a.

inferior hypophysial a., a small branch of the cavernous part of the internal carotid to the hypophysis. SYN arteria hypophysialis inferior [NA].

inferior internal parietal a., SYN precuneal a.

inferior labial a., *origin*, facial; *distribution*, structures of lower lip; *anastomoses*, the artery from the opposite side, mental and sublabial. SYN arteria labialis inferior [NA].

inferior laryngeal a., *origin*, inferior thyroid; *distribution*, muscles and mucous membrane of larynx; *anastomoses*, superior laryngeal. SYN arteria laryngea inferior [NA].

inferior lateral genicular a., *origin*, popliteal; *distribution*, knee joint; *anastomoses*, lateral superior genicular and anterior tibial recurrent (and posterior); *i.e.*, articular vascular *network* of knee. SYN arteria genus inferior lateralis [NA], lateral inferior genicular a.

inferior medial genicular a., *origin*, popliteal; *distribution*, knee joint; *anastomoses*, anterior and posterior tibial recurrent and medial superior genicular, *i.e.*, articular vascular *network* of knee. SYN arteria genus inferior medialis [NA], medial inferior genicular a.

inferior mesenteric a., *origin*, abdominal aorta; *branches*, left colic, sigmoid, superior rectal; *anastomoses*, middle colic and middle rectal. SYN arteria mesenterica inferior [NA].

inferior pancreatic a., *origin*, dorsal pancreatic; *distribution*, body and tail of pancreas; *anastomoses*, great pancreatic a. SYN arteria pancreatica inferior [NA], transverse pancreatic a.

inferior pancreaticoduodenal a., *origin*, superior mesenteric; one of two arteries, anterior and posterior; *distribution*, head of pancreas, duodenum; *anastomoses*, superior pancreaticoduodenal. SYN arteria pancreaticoduodenalis inferior [NA].

inferior phrenic a., *origin*, the first paired branch from the abdominal aorta inferior to the diaphragm; *distribution*, diaphragm; *anastomoses*, superior phrenic, internal thoracic, and musculophrenic. SYN arteria phrenica inferior [NA].

inferior rectal a., *origin*, internal pudendal; *distribution*, anal canal, muscles and skin of the anal region, and skin of the buttock; *anastomoses*, middle rectal, perineal, and gluteal. SYN arteria rectalis inferior [NA], inferior hemorrhoidal a.

inferior segmental a. of kidney, *origin*, anterior branch of renal. SEE ALSO segmental a.'s of kidney. SYN arteria segmenti inferioris renis [NA], a. of inferior segment of kidney.

a. of inferior segment of kidney, SYN inferior segmental a. of kidney.

inferior suprarenal a., *origin*, renal; *distribution*, suprarenal gland. SYN arteria suprarenalis inferior [NA].

inferior thyroid a., *origin*, terminal branch of thyrocervical trunk (with ascending cervical artery); *branches*, inferior laryngeal, and muscular, esophageal, and tracheal. SYN arteria thyroidea inferior [NA].

inferior tympanic a., *origin*, ascending pharyngeal; *distribution*, middle ear; *anastomoses*, tympanic branches of other arteries. SYN arteria tympanica inferior [NA].

inferior ulnar collateral a., *origin*, brachial; *distribution*, arm muscles at back of elbow; *anastomoses*, anterior and posterior ulnar recurrent, superior ulnar collateral, profunda brachii, and recurrent interosseous, as part of the articular network of the elbow. SYN arteria collateralis ulnaris inferior [NA], arteria anastomotica magna (1), great anastomotic a. (1).

inferior vesical a., *origin*, internal iliac; *distribution*, base of bladder, ureter, and (in the male) seminal vesicles, ductus deferens, and prostate; *anastomoses*, middle rectal, and other vesical branches. SYN arteria vesicalis inferior [NA].

infraorbital a., *origin*, third part of maxillary; *distribution*, upper canine and incisor teeth, inferior rectus and inferior oblique muscles, lower eyelid, lacrimal sac, maxillary sinus, and upper lip; *anastomoses*, branches of ophthalmic, facial, superior labial, transverse facial, and buccal. SYN arteria infraorbitalis [NA].

infrascapular a., a small branch of the circumflex scapular a.

innominate a., Obsolete term for brachiocephalic *trunk*.

insular a.'s, branches from the insular part of the middle cerebral artery distributed to the cortex of the insula. SYN arteriae insulares [NA].

intercostal a.'s, a.'s which course in the thoracic wall between ribs. SEE anterior intercostal a.'s, posterior intercostal a.'s 1–2, posterior intercostal a.'s 3-11, superior intercostal a.

interlobar a., the descending right pulmonary a., which is contiguous with the right middle and lower lobes.

interlobar a.'s of kidney, the branches of the segmental arteries of the kidney; they run between the renal lobes and give rise to the arcuate arteries. SYN arteriae interlobares renis [NA].

interlobular a.'s, a.'s that pass between lobules of an organ. SEE interlobular a.'s of liver, interlobular a.'s of kidney. SYN arteriae interlobulares [NA].

interlobular a.'s of kidney, the branches of the interlobar a.'s of the kidney passing outward through the cortex and supplying the glomeruli. SYN arteria interlobulares (renis) [NA].

interlobular a.'s of liver, the many terminal branches of the hepatic a. passing between hepatic lobules. SYN arteria interlobulares (hepatis) [NA].

intermediate temporal a., a branch of the insular part of the middle cerebral artery supplying the cortex of the temporal lobe between the anterior and posterior temporal arteries. SYN arteria temporalis intermedia [NA].

internal auditory a., SYN labyrinthine a.

internal carotid a., arises from the common carotid opposite upper border of thyroid cartilage (C-4 vertebral level) and terminates in the middle cranial fossa by dividing into the anterior and middle cerebral arteries; for descriptive purposes it is divided into four parts: cervical, petrous, cavernous, and cerebral. SYN arteria carotis interna [NA].

internal iliac a., *origin*, common iliac; *branches*, iliolumbar, lateral sacral, obturator, superior gluteal, inferior gluteal, umbilical, superior vesical, inferior vesical, middle rectal, and internal pudendal. SYN arteria iliaca interna [NA], arteria hypogastrica, hypogastric a.

internal mammary a., SYN internal thoracic a.

internal maxillary a., SYN maxillary a.

internal pudendal a., *origin*, internal iliac; *branches*, inferior rectal, perineal, posterior scrotal (or labial), urethral, artery of bulb of penis (or of vestibule), deep artery of penis (or clitoris), dorsal artery of penis (or clitoris). SYN arteria pudenda interna [NA].

internal spermatic a., SYN testicular a.

internal thoracic a., *origin*, subclavian; *branches*, pericardiacophrenic, anterior intercostal, sternal, mediastinal, thymic, bronchial, muscular, and perforating branches, and bifurcates into the musculophrenic and superior epigastric. SYN arteria thoracica interna [NA], arteria mammaria interna, internal mammary a.

intestinal a.'s, SEE ileal a.'s, jejunal a.'s.

jejunal a.'s, *origin*, superior mesenteric; *distribution*, jejunum; *anastomoses*, by a series of arches with each other and with ileal arteries. SYN arteriae jejunales [NA].

a.'s of kidney, SYN segmental a.'s of kidney.

Kugel's anastomotic a., a vessel of variable origin, most commonly a branch of the circumflex a., coursing posteriorly through the base of the interatrial septum toward the crux of the heart, anastomosing with coronary a. branches supplying the atrioventricular node, the atrioventricular bundle (bundle of His), and the upper posterior walls of the left ventricle. SYN arteria anastomotica auricularis magna.

a. of labyrinth, SYN labyrinthine a.

labyrinthine a., internal acoustic meatal branch. a branch of the basilar artery that enters the labyrinth through the internal acoustic meatus. SYN arteria labyrinthi [NA], ramus meatus acustici interni ☆, arteria auditiva interna, a. of labyrinth, internal auditory a.

lacrimal a., *origin*, ophthalmic; *distribution*, lacrimal gland, lateral and superior rectus muscles, superior eyelid, forehead, and temporal fossa. SYN arteria lacrimalis [NA].

lateral circumflex femoral a., *origin*, profunda femoris; *distribution*, hip joint, thigh muscles; *anastomoses*, medial circumflex femoral, inferior gluteal, superior gluteal. SYN arteria circumflexa femoris lateralis [NA], lateral circumflex a. of thigh, lateral femoral circumflex a.

lateral circumflex a. of thigh, SYN lateral circumflex femoral a.

lateral femoral circumflex a., SYN lateral circumflex femoral a.

lateral frontobasal a., a branch of the insular part of the middle cerebral a. distributed to the cortex of the lateral, inferior part of the frontal lobe. SYN arteria frontobasalis lateralis [NA], ramus orbitofrontalis lateralis [NA], lateral orbitofrontal branch, orbitofrontal a.

lateral inferior genicular a., SYN inferior lateral genicular a.

lateral malleolar a.'s, lateral malleolar branches of peroneal artery. SYN rami malleolares laterales [NA], arteriae malleolares posteriores laterales, posterior peroneal a.'s.

lateral nasal a., a branch of the facial a. which supplies the dorsum and ala of the nose.

lateral occipital a., one of the terminal branches of the posterior cerebral artery; it supplies, by several named branches, the lateral portions of the temporal lobe. SYN arteria occipitalis lateralis [NA].

lateral plantar a., larger of the two terminal branches of the posterior tibial; *distribution*, forms the plantar arch and through it supplies the sole of the foot and plantar surfaces of the toes; *anastomoses*, medial plantar, dorsalis pedis. SYN arteria plantaris lateralis [NA].

lateral sacral a., usually one of two a.'s which arise from the internal iliac a. or its branches; they supply muscles and skin in the neighborhood and send branches into the sacral canal, supplying radicular and spinal a.'s, and continuing on to the skin and subcutaneous tissues overlying the sacrum. SYN arteria sacralis lateralis [NA].

lateral splanchnic a.'s, a.'s that arise in the embryo from the dorsal aorta to supply the mesonephros, testis or ovary, and adrenal gland.

lateral striate a.'s, numerous small branches from the sphenoidal part of the middle cerebral arteries supplying the lateral and anterior parts of the corpus striatum. SYN arteriae centrales anterolaterales [NA], arteriae thalamostriatae anterolaterales ☆, anterolateral central a.'s, anterolateral striate a.'s, anterolateral thalamostriate a.'s, a.'s of cerebral hemorrhage, lenticulostriate a.'s (1).

lateral superior genicular a., SYN superior lateral genicular a.

lateral tarsal a., *origin*, dorsalis pedis; *distribution*, tarsal joints and extensor digitorum brevis muscle; *anastomoses*, arcuate, peroneal, lateral plantar, anterior lateral malleolar. SYN arteria tarsea lateralis [NA].

lateral thoracic a., *origin*, axillary; *distribution*, muscles of chest and mammary gland. SYN arteria thoracica lateralis [NA], external mammary a., long thoracic a.

left colic a., *origin*, inferior mesenteric; *distribution*, descending colon and splenic flexure; *anastomoses*, middle colic, sigmoid. SYN arteria colica sinistra [NA].

left coronary a., *origin*, left aortic sinus; *distribution*, it divides into two major branches, an anterior interventricular which descends in the anterior interventricular sulcus, and a circumflex branch which passes to the diaphragmatic surface of the left ventricle; gives atrial, ventricular, and atrioventricular branches. SYN arteria coronaria sinistra [NA].

left gastric a., *origin*, celiac; *distribution*, cardia of stomach at lesser curvature, abdominal part of the esophagus, and, frequently, a portion of the left lobe of the liver via an aberrant left hepatic branch; *anastomoses*, esophageal, right gastric. SYN arteria gastrica sinistra [NA], coronary a. (2).

left gastroepiploic a., *origin*, splenic; *distribution*, greater curvature of stomach and greater omentum; *anastomoses*, right gastroepiploic and short gastric a.'s. SYN arteria gastro-omentalis sinistra [NA], arteria gastroepiploica sinistra[*], left gastro-omental a.

left gastro-omental a., SYN left gastroepiploic a.

left hepatic a., left branch of proper hepatic a.; terminal branch off proper hepatic a. supplying left lobe of the liver. SYN ramus sinister arteriae hepaticae propriae [NA].

left pulmonary a., the shorter of the two terminal branches of the pulmonary trunk, it pierces the pericardium to enter the hilum of the left lung. Its branches accompany the segmental and subsegmental bronchi. Branches to the superior lobe (rami lobi superioris [NA]) are apical (ramus apicalis [NA]), anterior ascending (ramus anterior ascendens [NA]), anterior descending (ramus anterior descendens [NA]), posterior (ramus posterior [NA]), and lingular (ramus lingularis [NA]), the last having inferior and superior branches (rami lingulares inferior et superior [NA]). Branches to the inferior lobe (rami lobi inferioris [NA]) are the superior branch of the inferior lobe (ramus superior lobi inferior [NA]) and the medial (medialis), anterior, lateral (lateralis) and posterior basal branches (rami basalis [NA]). SYN arteria pulmonalis sinistra [NA].

lenticulostriate a.'s, (1) SYN lateral striate a.'s. **(2)** any one of a variety of small a.'s entering the base of the brain through the anterior perforated substance and supplying the striatum, globus pallidus, and internal capsule; most of these perforating a.'s are branches of the M_1 segment (clinical terminology) of the middle cerebral and and (rarely) of the anterior choroidal a. SYN Charcot's a.

lesser palatine a., one of several posterior branches of the descending palatine in the greater palatine canal, distributed to the soft palate and tonsil. SYN arteria palatina minor [NA].

lienal a., SYN splenic a.

lingual a., *origin*, external carotid; *distribution*, runs along under surface of tongue, terminates as deep lingual a.; *branches*, suprahyoid and dorsal lingual branches and sublingual artery. SYN arteria lingualis [NA].

long central a., SYN medial striate a.

long posterior ciliary a., one of two branches of the ophthalmic running forward between the sclerotic and choroid coats to the iris, at the outer and inner margins of which they form by anastomosis two circles. SYN arteria ciliaris posterior longa [NA].

long thoracic a., SYN lateral thoracic a.

lowest lumbar a.'s, *origin*, middle sacral; *distribution*, sacrum and iliac muscle; *anastomosis*, deep circumflex iliac artery. SYN arteriae lumbales imae [NA].

lowest thyroid a., SYN thyroid ima a.

lumbar a., *origin*, abdominal aorta; one of four or five pairs; *distribution*, lumbar vertebrae, muscles of back, abdominal wall; *anastomoses*, intercostal, subcostal, superior and inferior epigastric, deep circumflex iliac, and iliolumbar. SYN arteria lumbalis [NA].

macular a.'s, SEE inferior macular *arteriole*, superior macular *arteriole*.

marginal a. of colon, a. formed by anastomoses between the right and left colic a.'s; it passes downward from the left colic flexure to the aboral end of the pelvic colon. SYN a. of Drummond, Riolan's arc (2).

masseteric a., *origin*, maxillary; *distribution*, deep surface of masseter muscle; *anastomoses*, branches of transverse facial and masseteric branches of facial. SYN arteria masseterica [NA].

mastoid a., mastoid branch of occipital artery, passing through the mastoid foramen; *distribution*, mastoid air cells; *anastomosis*,

middle meningeal a. SYN arteriae occipitalis [NA], ramus mastoideus arteriae occipitalis [NA], mastoid branch of occipital artery.

maxillary a., *origin*, external carotid; *branches*, deep auricular, anterior tympanic, middle meningeal, inferior alveolar, masseteric, deep temporal, buccal, posterior superior alveolar, infraorbital, descending palatine, artery of pterygoid canal, sphenopalatine. SYN arteria maxillaris [NA], internal maxillary a.

medial circumflex femoral a., *origin*, profunda femoris; *distribution*, hip joint, muscles of thigh; *anastomoses*, inferior gluteal, superior gluteal, lateral circumflex femoral. SYN arteria circumflexa femoris medialis [NA], medial circumflex a. of thigh, medial femoral circumflex a.

medial circumflex a. of thigh, SYN medial circumflex femoral a.

medial femoral circumflex a., SYN medial circumflex femoral a.

medial frontobasal a., the medial orbitofrontal branch, the first branch of the pericallosal artery; it supplies the medial half of the inferior surface of the frontal cortex. SYN arteria frontobasalis medialis [NA], ramus orbitofrontalis medialis [NA], orbital a.

medial inferior genicular a., SYN inferior medial genicular a.

medial malleolar a.'s, medial malleolar branches of posterior tibial artery. SYN rami malleolares mediales [NA], arteriae malleolares posteriores mediales.

medial occipital a., one of the terminal branches of the posterior cerebral artery; it is distributed, by several named branches, to the posterior corpus callosum and the medial and superolateral portions of the occipital lobe including the visual cortex. SYN arteria occipitalis medialis [NA].

medial plantar a., one of the terminal branches of the posterior tibial; *distribution*, medial side of the sole of the foot; *anastomoses*, dorsalis pedis, lateral plantar. SYN arteria plantaris medialis [NA].

medial striate a., arises at or just distal to the anterior communicating a.; *distribution*: anterior caudate and putamen and anterior limb of internal capsule. SYN arteria centralis longa [NA], arteria recurrens [NA], a. of Heubner, long central a., recurrent a. of Heubner, recurrent a. (2).

medial superior genicular a., SYN superior medial genicular a.

medial tarsal a., one of two small branches of the dorsalis pedis; *distribution*, to inner margin of foot. SYN arteria tarsea medialis [NA].

median a., *origin*, anterior interosseous; *distribution*, accompanies median nerve to palm; *anastomoses*, branches of superficial palmar arch. SYN arteria comitans nervi mediani [NA], arteria mediana.

median sacral a., *origin*, posterior aspect of abdominal aorta just above the bifurcation; *distribution*, lower lumbar vertebrae, sacrum, and coccyx; *anastomoses*, lateral sacral, superior and middle rectal. SYN arteria sacralis mediana [NA], middle sacral a.

mediastinal a.'s, SYN mediastinal *branches*, under *branch*.

medium a., SYN muscular a.

medullary a.'s of brain, branches of the cortical a.'s which penetrate to and supply the white matter of the cerebrum.

medullary spinal a.'s, a large caliber spinal or radicular a. which courses centrally along a dorsal or ventral root, perhaps supplying it and the surrounding meninges in the fashion of any spinal/radicular a., but which continues on to reach and anastomose with the anterior or posterior (longitudinal) spinal a. Only 4–9 of the spinal a.'s are medullary spinal a.'s, found mainly in the lower cervical, lower thoracic and upper lumbar levels, the largest of which is the great radicular a.

mental a., *distribution*, chin; the terminal branch of the inferior alveolar; *anastomoses*, inferior labial artery. SYN arteria mentalis [NA].

metatarsal a., one of four dorsal or four plantar a.'s coursing in relation to the metatarsal bones, each dividing distally into a medial and a lateral digital a., serving the dorsal or plantar aspects of adjacent sides of two toes. SEE dorsal metatarsal a., plantar metatarsal a. SYN arteria metatarsae [NA].

middle cerebral a., one of the two large terminal branches (with anterior cerebral a.) of the internal carotid artery; it passes laterally around the pole of the temporal lobe, then posteriorly in the depth of the lateral cerebral fissure; for descriptive purposes it is divided into three parts: 1) the sphenoidal part (M_1 segment of clinical terminology), supplying perforating branches to the internal capsule, thalamus, and striate body; 2) the insular part, supplying branches to the insula and adjacent cortical areas; and 3) the terminal part or cortical part, supplying a large part of the central cortical convexity (the latter two collectively forming M_2 segment). SYN arteria cerebri media [NA].

middle colic a., *origin*, superior mesenteric; *distribution*, transverse colon; *anastomoses*, right and left colic. SYN arteria colica media [NA].

middle collateral a., the posterior terminal branch of the profunda brachii, anastomosing with the arteries which form the articular network of the elbow. SYN arteria collateralis media [NA].

middle genicular a., *origin*, popliteal; *distribution*, synovial membrane and cruciate ligaments of knee joint. SYN arteria genus media [NA], arteria articularis azygos.

middle hemorrhoidal a., SYN middle rectal a.

middle meningeal a., *origin*, maxillary; *branches*, petrosal, superior tympanic, frontal and parietal; *distribution*, to parts mentioned and through terminal branches to anterior and middle cranial fossae; *anastomoses*, meningeal branches of occipital, ascending pharyngeal, ophthalmic and lacrimal, stylomastoid, accessory meningeal branch of maxillary, and deep temporal. SYN arteria meningea media [NA].

middle rectal a., *origin*, internal iliac; *distribution*, middle portion of rectum; *anastomoses*, inferior rectal and superior rectal. Because the latter is a tributary of the portal system, this is a portosystemic or portocaval anastomosis. SYN arteria rectalis media [NA], middle hemorrhoidal a.

middle sacral a., SYN median sacral a.

middle suprarenal a., *origin*, aorta; *distribution*, suprarenal gland. SYN arteria suprarenalis media [NA].

middle temporal a., *origin*, superficial temporal; *distribution*, temporal fascia and muscle; *anastomoses*, branches of maxillary. SEE ALSO intermediate temporal a., posterior temporal a. SYN arteria temporalis media [NA].

muscular a., an a. with a tunica media composed principally of circularly arranged smooth muscle. SYN distributing a., medium a.

musculophrenic a., *origin*, the lateral terminal branch of internal thoracic; *distribution*, diaphragm and intercostal muscles; *anastomoses*, branches of pericardiacophrenic, inferior phrenic, and posterior intercostal arteries. SYN arteria musculophrenica [NA].

mylohyoid a., branch of inferior alveolar artery to the mylohyoid muscle. SYN ramus mylohyoideus arteriae alveolaris inferioris [NA], arteriae alveolaris inferioris.

myometrial arcuate a.'s, branches of the uterine and ovarian a.'s.

myometrial radial a.'s, continuations of the myometrial arcuate a.'s.

Neubauer's a., SYN thyroid ima a.

nutrient a., an artery of variable origin that supplies the medullary cavity of a long bone. SYN arteria nutricia [NA], nutrient vessel.

nutrient a. of femur, one of two a.'s, superior and inferior, arising from the first and third perforating a.'s respectively (sometimes second and fourth).

nutrient a. of fibula, *origin*, peroneal (fibular); *distribution*, fibula. SYN arteria nutriens fibulae [NA].

nutrient a.'s of humerus, *origin*, deep brachial; *distribution*, the medullary cavity of the humerus. SYN arteriae nutriciae humeri [NA].

nutrient a. of the tibia, a. derived from the upper part of the posterior tibial a.; it enters through the nutrient foramen on the posterior surface of the tibia. SYN arteria nutriens tibialis [NA].

obturator a., *anastomoses*, iliolumbar, inferior epigastric, medial circumflex femoral; *origin*, anterior division of the internal iliac; *distribution*, ilium, pubis, obturator and adductor muscles; *branches*, pubic, acetabular, anterior, and posterior. SYN arteria obturatoria [NA].

occipital a., *origin*, external carotid; *branches*, sternocleidomastoid, meningeal, auricular, occipital, mastoid, and descending. SYN arteria occipitalis [NA].

omphalomesenteric a., obsolete term for vitelline a.

ophthalmic a., *origin*, internal carotid; *branches*, ciliary, central artery of retina, anterior meningeal, lacrimal, conjunctival, episcleral, supraorbital, ethmoidal, palpebral, dorsal nasal, and supratrochlear. SYN arteria ophthalmica [NA].

orbital a., SYN medial frontobasal a.

orbitofrontal a., SYN lateral frontobasal a.

ovarian a., *origin*, aorta; *distribution*, ureter, ovary, ovarian ligament and uterine tube; *anastomoses*, uterine. SYN arteria ovarica [NA].

palmar interosseous a., SYN palmar metacarpal a.

palmar metacarpal a., one of the three arteries springing from the deep palmar arch and running in the three medial interosseous spaces; they anastomose with the common palmar and dorsal metacarpal arteries. SYN arteria metacarpea palmaris [NA], palmar interosseous a.

palpebral a.'s, branches of the ophthalmic supplying the upper and lower eyelids, consisting of two sets, lateral and medial. SYN arteriae palpebrales [NA].

a. of the pancreatic tail, *origin*, splenic artery near the left gastroepiploic; *distribution*, the tail of the pancreas; *anastomoses*, with other pancreatic arteries. SYN arteria caudae pancreatis [NA], caudal pancreatic a.

paracentral a., the third branch of the pericallosal artery supplying the cerebral cortex of the paracentral lobule and both sides of the medial part of the central sulcus. SYN arteria paracentralis [NA].

parent a., the a. giving origin to a given a.; the a. of which a given a. is a branch.

parietal a.'s, branches of the terminal part of the middle cerebral a., divided into two branches: anterior parietal a. and posterior parietal a. SYN arteriae parietales [NA].

parieto-occipital a., the largest cortical branch of the pericallosal artery supplying the medial and superolateral surface of the parietal lobe posterior to the paracentral lobule; rarely does it extend to supply part of the occipital lobe. SYN arteria parieto-occipitalis [NA], superior internal parietal a.

a.'s of penis, SEE dorsal a. of penis, deep a. of penis.

perforating a.'s, *origin*, a. profunda femoris; *distribution*, as three or four vessels that pass through the aponeurosis of the adductor magnus to the posterior and anterior compartments of the thigh. SYN arteriae perforantes [NA].

perforating a.'s of foot, SYN perforating *branches* of plantar metatarsal arteries, under *branch*.

perforating a.'s of hand, SYN perforating *branches* of palmar metacarpal arteries, under *branch*.

perforating a.'s of internal mammary, SYN perforating *branches* of internal thoracic artery, under *branch*.

perforating peroneal a., SYN perforating *branches*, under *branch*.

pericallosal a., the continuation of the anterior cerebral artery after the anterior communicating artery; it supplies branches to the cerebral cortex as it passes along the corpus callosum. SYN pars postcommunicalis arteria cerebri anterior [NA], arteria pericallosa✩, postcommunical part of anterior cerebral artery.

pericardiacophrenic a., *origin*, internal thoracic; *distribution*, pericardium, diaphragm, and pleura; *anastomoses*, musculophrenic, inferior phrenic, mediastinal and pericardial branches of the internal thoracic. SYN arteria pericardiacophrenica [NA], arteria comes nervi phrenici.

perineal a., *origin*, internal pudendal; *distribution*, superficial structures of the perineum; *anastomoses*, external pudendal arteries. SYN arteria perinealis [NA].

peroneal a., *origin*, posterior tibial; *distribution*, soleus, tibialis posterior, flexor longus hallucis, peroneal muscles, inferior tibiofibular articulation, and ankle joint; *anastomoses*, anterior lateral malleolar, lateral tarsal, lateral plantar, dorsalis pedis. SYN arteria peronea [NA], arteria fibularis✩ [NA], fibular a.

pipestem a.'s, a.'s hardened by calcification as seen in Mönckeberg's arteriosclerosis; descriptive of the characteristic feeling to the finger of an examiner.

plantar metatarsal a., one of four branches of the plantar arterial arch that divide into plantar digital arteries to supply the toes. SYN arteria metatarsea plantaris [NA].

pontine a.'s, a.'s of pons, several small branches of the basilar artery distributed to the pons. SYN arteriae pontis [NA], rami ad pontem☆ [NA].

popliteal a., continuation of femoral a. in the popliteal space, bifurcating (at the lower border of the popliteus muscle as it passes deep to the arcus tendineus of the soleus muscle) into the anterior and posterior tibial a.'s; *branches*, lateral and medial superior genicular, middle genicular, lateral and medial inferior genicular, and sural arteries. SYN arteria poplitea [NA].

postcentral a., SYN postcentral sulcal a.

postcentral sulcal a., a branch of the terminal part of the middle cerebral artery distributing to the cortex on either side of the postcentral sulcus. SYN arteria sulci postcentralis [NA], a. of postcentral sulcus, postcentral a.

a. of postcentral sulcus, SYN postcentral sulcal a.

posterior alveolar a., SYN posterior superior alveolar a.

posterior auricular a., *origin*: posterior aspect of external carotid just above the digastric muscle; *course*: ascends first between parotid gland and styloid process then between cartilage of auricle and the mastoid process; *branches*: muscular (digastric, stylohyoid and sternocleidomastoid), glandular (parotid), stylomastoid a., occipital and auricular; *anastomoses*: anterior tympanic a. (via the stylomastoid a.) and occipital a. SYN arteria auricularis posterior [NA].

posterior cecal a., *origin*, ileocolic artery; *distribution*, posterior region of cecum. SYN arteria cecalis posterior [NA].

posterior cerebral a., formed by the bifurcation of the basilar artery; it passes around the cerebral peduncle to reach the medial aspect of the hemisphere; for descriptive purposes it is divided into three parts: 1) the precommunical part (P_1 segment of clinical terminology), the part before the junction with the posterior communicating artery, supplying parts of the thalamus, hypothalamus, and midbrain; 2) the postcommunical part (P_2), supplying the thalamus, cerebral peduncles, and the choroid plexuses of the lateral and third ventricles; and 3) the terminal or cortical part, supplying the cortex of the temporal (P_3) and occipital (P_4) lobes. SYN arteria cerebri posterior [NA].

posterior choroidal a., one of several choroid branches of the P_2 segment of the posterior cerebral artery that supply the choroid plexus of the body of the lateral ventricle and of the third ventricle. SYN arteria choroidea posterior.

posterior circumflex humeral a., *origin*, axillary; *distribution*, muscles and structures of shoulder joint; *anastomoses*, anterior circumflex humeral, suprascapular, thoracoacromial, and profunda brachii. SYN arteria circumflexa humeri posterior [NA], posterior humeral circumflex a.

posterior communicating a., *origin*, internal carotid; *distribution*, optic tract, crus cerebri, interpeduncular region, and hippocampal gyrus; *anastomoses*, with posterior cerebral to form the cerebral arterial circle (circle of Willis). SYN arteria communicans posterior [NA].

posterior conjunctival a., one of a series of branches from the arterial arches of the upper and lower eyelids that supplies the conjunctiva. SYN arteria conjunctivalis posterior [NA], conjunctival a.'s.

posterior dental a., SYN posterior superior alveolar a.

posterior descending a., SYN posterior interventricular a.

posterior ethmoidal a., *origin*, ophthalmic; *distribution*, posterior ethmoidal cells and upper posterior part of lateral wall of nasal cavity. SYN arteria ethmoidalis posterior [NA].

posterior humeral circumflex a., SYN posterior circumflex humeral a.

posterior inferior cerebellar a., *origin*, vertebral; *distribution*, lateral medulla, choroid plexus of fourth ventricle, and cerebellum; *anastomoses*, superior cerebellar and anterior inferior cerebellar. SYN arteria cerebelli inferior posterior [NA].

posterior intercostal a.'s 1–2, terminal branches of the superior intercostal a. (from costocervical trunk) supplying upper two intercostal spaces. SYN arteriae intercostales posteriores I et II [NA].

posterior intercostal a.'s 3-11, one of nine pairs of arteries arising from the thoracic aorta and distributed to the nine lower intercostal spaces, vertebral column, spinal cord, and muscles and integument of the back; they anastomose with branches of the musculophrenic, internal thoracic, superior epigastric, subcostal and lumbar. SYN arteriae intercostales posteriores III-XI [NA].

posterior interosseous a., *origin*, common interosseous artery; *distribution*, posterior compartment of forearm. SYN arteria interossea posterior [NA], dorsal interosseous a. (1).

posterior interventricular a., posterior interventricular branch of right coronary artery. Continuation of right coronary a. in posterior interventricular sulcus; descends to apex to anastomose with anterior interventricular a.; supplies most of diaphragmatic aspect of ventricles and posterior third of interventricular septum. SYN ramus interventricularis posterior arteriae coronariae dextrae [NA], posterior descending a.

posterior labial a.'s, the posterior labial branches, branches of the perineal artery to the labium majus. SYN rami labiales posteriores arteriae pudendae internae [NA].

posterior lateral nasal a.'s, branches of the sphenopalatine artery that supply the posterior parts of the conchae and lateral nasal wall. SYN arteriae nasales posteriores laterales [NA].

posterior mediastinal a.'s, SYN mediastinal *branches* of thoracic aorta, under *branch*.

posterior meningeal a., *origin*, ascending pharyngeal; *distribution*, dura mater of posterior cranial fossa; *anastomoses*, branches of middle meningeal and vertebral. SYN arteria meningea posterior [NA].

posterior pancreaticoduodenal a., SYN retroduodenal a.

posterior parietal a., the branch distributed to the posterior part of the parietal lobe. SYN arteria parietales posterior [NA].

posterior peroneal a.'s, SYN lateral malleolar a.'s.

posterior segmental a. of kidney, *origin*, continuation of the posterior branch of renal. SEE ALSO segmental a.'s of kidney. SYN arteria segmenti posterioris renis [NA], a. of posterior segment of kidney.

a. of posterior segment of kidney, SYN posterior segmental a. of kidney.

posterior septal a. of nose, a branch of the sphenopalatine artery that supplies the nasal septum and accompanies the nasopalatine nerve. SYN arteria nasalis posterior septi [NA].

posterior spinal a., *origin*, vertebral; *distribution*, medulla, spinal cord, and pia mater; *anastomoses*, spinal branches of intercostal arteries. SYN arteria spinalis posterior [NA].

posterior superior alveolar a., *origin*, 3rd part of maxillary a. within pterygopalatine fossa; *distribution*, molar and premolar teeth, gingiva and mucous membrane of maxillary sinus. SYN arteria alveolaris superior posterior [NA], posterior alveolar a., posterior dental a.

posterior temporal a., a branch of the insular part of the middle cerebral artery distributed to the cortex of the posterior part of the temporal lobe. SYN arteria temporalis posterior [NA].

posterior tibial a., the larger and more directly continuous of the two terminal branches of the popliteal; *branches*, peroneal, nutrient of fibula, lateral and medial posterior malleolar, nutrient of tibia, medial and lateral plantar. SYN arteria tibialis posterior [NA].

posterior tibial recurrent a., an inconstant branch of the posterior tibial artery which ascends anterior to the popliteus muscle, anastomoses with branches of the popliteal artery, and sends a twig to the tibiofibular joint. SYN arteria recurrens tibialis posterior [NA].

posterior tympanic a., *origin*, stylomastoid; *distribution*, middle ear; *anastomoses*, other tympanic arteries. SYN arteria tympanica posterior [NA].

posterolateral central a.'s, the circumflex mesencephalic branches, several small branches of the postcommunical part of the posterior cerebral artery distributed to the lateral posterior part of the midbrain. SYN arteriae centrales posterolaterales [NA].

posteromedial central a.'s, the interpeduncular perforating branches, several small branches from the precommunical part of the posterior cerebral artery supplying the posterior medial part of the midbrain. SYN arteriae centrales posteromediales [NA].

precentral a., SYN precentral sulcal a.

precentral sulcal a., a branch of the terminal part of the middle cerebral artery distributed to the cortex on either side of the precentral sulcus. SYN arteria sulci precentralis [NA], a. of precentral sulcus, pre-Rolandic a., precentral a.

a. of precentral sulcus, SYN precentral sulcal a.

precuneal a., the last cortical branch of the pericallosal artery; it supplies the inferior part of the precuneus. SYN arteria precunealis [NA], inferior internal parietal a.

pre-Rolandic a., SYN precentral sulcal a.

princeps cervicis a., SYN descending *branch* of occipital artery.

princeps pol'licis a., *origin*, radial (deep palmar (arterial) arch); *distribution*, palmar surface and sides of thumb; *anastomoses*, a.'s on dorsum of thumb. SYN arteria princeps pollicis [NA], chief a. of thumb, princeps pollicis, principal a. of thumb.

principal a. of thumb, SYN princeps pollicis a.

profunda brachii a., *origin*, brachial; *distribution*, humerus and muscles and integument of arm; *anastomoses*, posterior circumflex humeral, radial recurrent, recurrent interosseous, ulnar collateral, *i.e.*, articular vascular *network* of elbow. SYN arteria profunda brachii [NA], deep brachial a.

profunda fem'oris a., *origin*, femoral; *branches*, lateral circumflex femoral, medial circumflex femoral, terminating in three or four perforating a.'s. SYN arteria profunda femoris [NA], deep a. of thigh.

proper hepatic a., *origin*, common hepatic; *branches*, right and left hepatic. SYN arteria hepatica propria [NA].

proper palmar digital a., terminal branches of the common palmar digital a. that pass to the side of each finger. SYN arteria digitalis palmaris propria [NA], collateral digital a., digital collateral a.

proper plantar digital a., one of the digital branches of the plantar metatarsal arteries. SYN arteria digitalis plantaris propria [NA].

a. of pterygoid canal, *origin*: usually arises from the third part of the maxillary artery, but frequently from the greater palatine artery, within the pterygopalatine fossa. Passes posteriorly to run through the pterygoid canal with the corresponding nerve, supplying the contents and wall of the canal, the mucous membrane of the upper pharynx, the auditory tube and the tympanic cavity. SYN arteria canalis pterygoidei [NA], vidian a.

pubic a.'s, SEE pubic *branch* of inferior epigastric artery, pubic *branch* of obturator artery.

pulmonary a., SYN pulmonary *trunk*. SEE ALSO right pulmonary a., left pulmonary a.

a. of pulp, the first section of a penicillus of the spleen.

pyloric a., SYN right gastric a.

radial a., *origin*, brachial; *branches*, radial recurrent, dorsal metacarpal, dorsal digital, princeps pollicis, radial index, palmar metacarpal, and muscular, carpal, and perforating. SYN arteria radialis [NA].

radial collateral a., the anterior terminal branch of the profunda brachii, anastomosing with the radial recurrent, forming part of the articular network of the elbow. SYN arteria collateralis radialis [NA].

radial index a., SYN radialis indicis a.

radialis indicis a., *origin*, radial; *distribution*, radial side of index finger. SYN arteria radialis indicis [NA], arteria volaris indicis radialis, radial index a.

radial recurrent a., *origin*, radial; *distribution*, ascends around lateral side of elbow joint; *anastomoses*, radial collateral, interosseous recurrent. SYN arteria recurrens radialis [NA], recurrent radial a.

radicular a.'s, branches of spinal a.'s distributed to the dorsal and ventral roots of spinal nerves and their coverings. See entries under spinal a.'s..

ranine a., SYN deep lingual a.

recurrent a., (1) an a. which, upon or soon after originating, reflects or turns sharply to course in the general opposite direction to that of its parent a.; **(2)** SYN medial striate a.

recurrent a. of Heubner, SYN medial striate a.

recurrent interosseous a., *origin*, posterior interosseous; *distribution*, elbow joint; *anastomoses*, branches of profunda brachii

and inferior ulnar collateral, *i.e.*, articular vascular *network* of elbow. SYN arteria interossea recurrens [NA].

recurrent radial a., SYN radial recurrent a.

recurrent ulnar a., *origin*, ulnar artery; *distribution*, two branches, anterior and posterior, pass medially in front of and behind the elbow joint; *anastomoses*, superior and inferior ulnar collateral, *i.e.*, with articular vascular *network* of elbow. SYN arteria recurrens ulnaris [NA].

renal a., *origin*, aorta; *branches*, segmental, ureteral, and inferior suprarenal; *distribution*, kidney. SYN arteria renalis [NA].

retroduodenal a., *origin*, one of several small branches from the gastroduodenal artery posterior to the duodenum; *distribution*, first part of duodenum. SYN arteria retroduodenalis [NA], posterior pancreaticoduodenal a.

right colic a., *origin*, superior mesenteric, sometimes by a common trunk with the ileocolic; *distribution*, ascending colon; *anastomoses*, middle colic, ileocolic. SYN arteria colica dextra [NA].

right coronary a., *origin*, right aortic sinus; *distribution*, it passes around the right side of the heart in the coronary sulcus, giving branches to the right atrium and ventricle, including the atrioventricular branches and the posterior interventricular branch. SYN arteria coronaria dextra [NA].

right gastric a., *origin*, hepatic; *distribution*, pyloric portion of stomach on the lesser curvature; *anastomoses*, left gastric. SYN arteria gastrica dextra [NA], pyloric a.

right gastroepiploic a., *origin*, gastroduodenal; *distribution*, greater curvature and walls of stomach and greater omentum; *anastomoses*, frequently unites with left gastroepiploic, and branches from this arch anastomose with branches of right and left gastric. SYN arteria gastro-omentalis dextra [NA], arteria gastroepiploica dextra★, right gastro-omental a.

right gastro-omental a., SYN right gastroepiploic a.

right hepatic a., right branch of proper hepatic artery; terminal branch of proper hepatic a. supplying right lobe of liver; *branch*: cystic a. SYN ramus dexter arteriae hepaticae propriae [NA], right branch of proper hepatic artery.

right pulmonary a., the longer of the two terminal branches of the pulmonary trunk, it passes transversely across the mediastinum passing inferior to the aortic arch to enter the hilum of the right lung. Branches are distributed with the bronchi; frequent variations occurs. Typical branches to the superior lobe (rami lobi superioris [NA]) are apical (ramus apicalis [NA]), anterior ascending (rami anterior ascendens [NA]), anterior descending (ramus anterior descendens [NA]), posterior ascending (ramus posterior ascendens [NA]), and posterior descending (ramus posterior descendens [NA]); to the middle lobe (rami lobi medii [NA]) are medial (ramus medialis [NA]) and lateral (ramus lateralis [NA]); and to the inferior lobe (rami lobi inferioris [NA]) are superior (apical) branch of inferior lobe (ramus superior (apicalis) lobi inferioris [NA]), and the anterior, lateral (lateralis), medial (medialis) and posterior basal branches (rami basalis). SYN arteria pulmonalis dextra [NA].

Rolandic a., SYN central sulcal a.

a. of round ligament of uterus, *origin*, inferior epigastric; *distribution*, round ligament of uterus. SYN arteria ligamenti teretis uteri [NA].

a. to sciatic nerve, *origin*, inferior gluteal; *distribution*, sciatic nerve; *anastomoses*, branches of profunda femoris. SYN arteria comitans nervi ischiadici [NA], companion a. to sciatic nerve.

screw a.'s, coiled a.'s into the uterine mucosa or in the macular region of the retina.

scrotal a.'s, SEE anterior scrotal *branch* of external pudendal artery, under *branch*, posterior scrotal *branch* of internal pudendal artery, under *branch*.

segmental a.'s of kidney, the branches of the renal artery that supply the anatomical segments of kidney. Usually five in number, they are end a.'s and give off interlobar, arcuate and interlobular a.'s in sequence. The latter send afferent arterioles to the glomeruli as well as branches to the kidney capsule. The segmental a.'s of the kidney are identified as: (1) anterior inferior (arteriae segmenti anterioris inferioris renis [NA]); (2) anterior superior (arteriae segmenti anterioris superioris renis [NA]); (3)

inferior (arteriae segmenti inferioris renis [NA]); (4) posterior (arteriae segmenti posterioris renis [NA]); and (5) superior (arteriae segmenti superioris renis [NA]). SYN arteriae renis [NA], a.'s of kidney.

septal a., a branch of the superior labial a. that supplies the lower part of the nasal septum.

sheathed a., a subdivision of the penicillus of the spleen surrounded by macrophages and a reticular stroma.

short central a., a branch of the precommunical part of the anterior cerebral artery. SYN arteria centralis brevis [NA].

short gastric a.'s, four or five small arteries given off from the splenic, passing via the gastrosplenic ligament to the fundus of the stomach along the greater curvature, and anastomosing with the other arteries in that region. SYN arteriae gastricae breves [NA], vasa brevia.

short posterior ciliary a., one of approximately seven branches of the ophthalmic a. which pass around the optic nerve to supply the eyeball. Dividing into some 15–20 branches, they penetrate the sclera adjacent to the optic nerve, supplying the choroid and ciliary processes. *Anastomoses*: with central retinal a. and long and anterior ciliary arteries (at the ora serrata). SYN arteria ciliaris posterior brevis [NA].

sigmoid a.'s, *origin,* inferior mesenteric; *distribution,* descending colon and sigmoid flexure; *anastomoses,* left colic, superior rectal. SYN arteriae sigmoideae [NA].

sinoatrial nodal a., a branch usually of the right coronary a. SYN sinus node a.

a. to the sinuatrial (S-A) node, ascending atrial branch, usually (55%) arising from the anterior stem of the right coronary artery (but 35–45% arising from the circumflex branch of the left coronary artery), which runs around the base of the superior vena cava to reach the sinuatrial node. SYN ramus nodi sinuatrialis arteriae coronaria dextra [NA], branch to sinuatrial node, sinuatrial nodal branch of right coronary artery, sinuatrial node a.

sinuatrial node a., SYN a. to the sinuatrial (S-A) node.

sinus node a., SYN sinoatrial nodal a.

small a.'s, unnamed muscular a.'s, usually with fewer than six or seven layers of muscle.

somatic a.'s, a.'s that arise in the embryo from the dorsal aorta and supply the body wall; they persist almost unchanged as the posterior intercostal, subcostal, and lumbar a.'s.

sphenopalatine a., *origin,* third part of maxillary; *distribution,* posterior portion of lateral nasal wall and septum; *anastomoses,* branches of descending palatine, superior labial, and infraorbital. SYN arteria sphenopalatina [NA].

spinal a.'s, branches of the following arteries which supply the meninges, the roots of the spinal nerves, and in some cases, the spinal cord: 1) vertebral, 2) ascending cervical, 3) dorsal branch of posterior intercostal I to XI, 4) dorsal branch of subcostal, 5) dorsal branch of lumbar arteries, 6) lumbar branch of iliolumbar, 7) lateral sacral; all spinal a.'s give rise to radicular a.'s supplying dorsal and ventral roots of spinal nerves, but some (4–9), are large enough to reach and anastomose with the anterior and posterior spinal a.'s. SYN rami radiculares☆. SEE medullary spinal a.'s, *arteria* radicularis magna. SYN rami spinales (1) [NA].

spiral a., one of the corkscrew-like a.'s in premenstrual or progestational endometrium. SYN coiled a. of the uterus.

splenic a., *origin,* celiac trunk; *branches,* pancreatic, left gastroepiploic, short gastric, and (proper) splenic. SEE *arteria* radicularis magna. SYN arteria splenica [NA], arteria lienalis☆, lienal a.

stapedial a., a small a. in the embryo that passes through the ring of the stapes and is later obliterated; it is a second aortic arch derivative.

sternal a.'s, SYN sternal *branches* of internal thoracic artery, under *branch.*

sternomastoid a., SEE sternocleidomastoid *branch* of superior thyroid artery, sternocleidomastoid *branch* of occipital artery.

stylomastoid a., *origin,* posterior auricular; *distribution,* external acoustic meatus, mastoid cells, semicircular canals, stapedius muscle, and vestibule; *anastomoses,* tympanic branches of internal carotid and ascending pharyngeal, and labyrinthine a.'s. SYN arteria stylomastoidea [NA].

subclavian a., *origin,* right from brachiocephalic, left from arch of aorta; *branches,* vertebral, thyrocervical trunk, internal thoracic; costocervical trunk, descending scapular; it continues the axillary a. after crossing the first rib. SYN arteria subclavia [NA].

subcostal a., *origin,* thoracic aorta; *distribution,* inferior to twelfth rib in a manner similar to posterior intercostal arteries. SYN arteria subcostalis [NA].

sublingual a., *origin,* lingual; *distribution,* extrinsic muscles of tongue, sublingual gland, mucosa of region; *anastomoses,* the artery of opposite side and submental. SYN arteria sublingualis [NA].

submental a., *origin,* facial; *distribution,* mylohyoid muscle, submandibular and sublingual glands, and structures of lower lip; *anastomoses,* inferior labial, mental branch of inferior dental and sublingual. SYN arteria submentalis [NA].

subscapular a., *origin,* axillary; *branches,* circumflex scapular, thoracodorsal; *distribution,* muscles of shoulder and scapular region; *anastomoses,* branches of transverse cervical, suprascapular, lateral thoracic, and intercostals. SYN arteria subscapularis [NA].

sulcal a., a small branch of the anterior spinal a. running in the anterior median fissure of the spinal cord.

superficial brachial a., an occasional variation in which the brachial artery lies superficial to the median nerve in the arm. SYN arteria brachialis superficialis [NA].

superficial cervical a., *origin,* branch of thyrocervical trunk, running with spinal accessory nerve deep to trapezius muscle. SEE ALSO superficial *branch* of the transverse cervical artery. SYN arteria cervicalis superficialis.

superficial circumflex iliac a., *origin,* femoral; *distribution,* inguinal lymph nodes and integument of that region; sartorius, and tensor fasciae latae muscles; *anastomoses,* deep circumflex iliac. SYN arteria circumflexa iliaca superficialis [NA].

superficial epigastric a., *origin,* femoral; *distribution,* inguinal nodes and integument of lower abdomen; *anastomoses,* inferior epigastric, superficial circumflex iliac and external pudendal. SYN arteria epigastrica superficialis [NA].

superficial palmar a., SYN superficial palmar *branch* of radial artery.

superficial temporal a., *origin,* a terminal branch of the external carotid (with maxillary a.); *branches,* transverse facial, middle temporal, orbital, parotid, anterior auricular, frontal, and parietal. SYN arteria temporalis superficialis [NA].

superficial volar a., SYN superficial palmar *branch* of radial artery.

superior cerebellar a., *origin,* basilar; *distribution,* upper surface of cerebellum, colliculi, and most of the cerebellar nuclei; *anastomoses,* posterior inferior cerebellar. SYN arteria cerebelli superior [NA].

superior epigastric a., *origin,* the medial terminal branch of internal thoracic; *distribution,* abdominal muscles and integument, falciform ligament; *anastomoses,* inferior epigastric. SYN arteria epigastrica superior [NA].

superior gluteal a., *origin,* internal iliac; *distribution,* gluteal region; *anastomoses,* lateral sacral, inferior gluteal, internal pudendal, deep circumflex iliac, lateral circumflex femoral. SYN arteria glutea superior [NA].

superior hemorrhoidal a., SYN superior rectal a.

superior hypophysial a., a small branch of the cerebral part of the internal carotid artery supplying the hypophysis. SYN arteria hypophysialis superior [NA].

superior intercostal a., *origin,* costocervical trunk; *distribution,* structures of first and second intercostal spaces via its terminal branches, posterior intercostal a.'s 1 and 2; *anastomoses,* anterior intercostal branches of internal thoracic. SYN arteria intercostalis suprema [NA], highest intercostal a., supreme intercostal a.

superior internal parietal a., SYN parieto-occipital a.

superior labial a., *origin,* facial; *distribution,* structures of upper lip and, by a septal branch, the anterior and lower part of the nasal septum; *anastomoses,* the artery of the opposite side and the sphenopalatine. SYN arteria labialis superior [NA].

superior laryngeal a., *origin,* superior thyroid; *distribution,* muscles and mucous membrane of larynx; *anastomoses,* cricothyroid branch of superior thyroid and terminal branches of inferior laryngeal. SYN arteria laryngea superior [NA].

superior lateral genicular a., *origin,* popliteal; *distribution,* knee joint; *anastomoses,* lateral circumflex femoral, third perforating, anterior tibial recurrent, lateral inferior genicular, *i.e.,* the articular vascular network of the knee. SYN arteria genus superior lateralis [NA], lateral superior genicular a.

superior medial genicular a., *origin,* popliteal; *distribution,* knee joint; *anastomoses,* descending genicular, lateral superior genicular, *i.e.,* the articular vascular network of the knee. SYN arteria genus superior medialis [NA], medial superior genicular a.

superior mesenteric a., *origin,* abdominal aorta; *branches,* inferior pancreaticoduodenal, jejunal, ileal, ileocolic, appendicular, right colic, middle colic; *anastomoses,* superior pancreaticoduodenal and left colic. SYN arteria mesenterica superior [NA].

superior pancreaticoduodenal a., *origin,* gastroduodenal; one of two arteries, anterior and superior; *distribution,* head of pancreas, duodenum, common bile duct; *anastomoses,* inferior pancreaticoduodenal, splenic. SYN arteria pancreaticoduodenalis superior [NA].

superior phrenic a., one of a pair of small arteries given off from the thoracic aorta just superior to the diaphragm; *distribution,* diaphragm; *anastomoses,* musculophrenic, pericardiacophrenic, and inferior phrenic. SYN arteria phrenica superior [NA].

superior rectal a., *origin,* inferior mesenteric; *distribution,* upper part of rectum; *anastomoses,* middle and inferior rectal. As a tributary of the portal vein, its anastomosis with these a.'s forms a portosystemic or portocaval anastomosis. SYN arteria rectalis superior [NA], superior hemorrhoidal a.

superior segmental a. of kidney, *origin,* anterior branch of renal. SEE ALSO segmental a.'s of kidney. SYN arteria segmenti superioris renis [NA], a. of superior segment of kidney.

a. of superior segment of kidney, SYN superior segmental a. of kidney.

superior suprarenal a.'s, *origin,* inferior phrenic artery; *distribution,* suprarenal gland. SYN arteriae suprarenales superiores [NA].

superior thoracic a., *origin,* axillary; *distribution,* muscles of superior chest; *anastomoses,* branches of suprascapular, internal thoracic, and thoracoacromial. SYN arteria thoracica superior [NA], highest thoracic a.

superior thyroid a., *origin,* external carotid; *branches,* infrahyoid, superior laryngeal, sternocleidomastoid, cricothyroid, and two terminal branches. SYN arteria thyroidea superior [NA].

superior tympanic a., *origin,* middle meningeal; *distribution,* middle ear; *anastomoses,* other tympanic arteries. SYN arteria tympanica superior [NA].

superior ulnar collateral a., *origin,* brachial; *distribution,* elbow joint; *anastomoses,* posterior ulnar recurrent and inferior ulnar collateral, as part of the articular vascular network of the elbow. SYN arteria collateralis ulnaris superior [NA].

superior vesical a., *origin,* umbilical; *distribution,* bladder, urachus, ureter; *anastomoses,* other vesical branches. SYN arteria vesicalis superior [NA].

supraduodenal a., *origin,* gastroduodenal; *distribution,* first part of duodenum. SYN arteria supraduodenalis [NA].

supraorbital a., *origin,* ophthalmic; *distribution,* frontalis muscle and scalp; *anastomoses,* branches of the superficial temporal and supratrochlear. SYN arteria supraorbitalis [NA].

suprascapular a., *origin,* thyrocervical trunk; *distribution,* clavicle, scapula, muscles of shoulder, and shoulder joint; *anastomoses,* transverse cervical circumflex scapular. SYN arteria suprascapularis [NA], transverse scapular a.

supratrochlear a., *origin,* ophthalmic; *distribution,* anterior portion of scalp; *anastomoses,* branches of supraorbital. SYN arteria supratrochlearis [NA], arteria frontalis, frontal a.

supreme intercostal a., SYN superior intercostal a.

sural a., one of four or five arteries arising (sometimes by a common trunk) from the popliteal; *distribution,* muscles and integument of the calf; *anastomoses,* posterior tibial, medial, and lateral inferior genicular. SYN arteria suralis [NA], a. of calf.

terminal a., SYN end a.

testicular a., *origin,* aorta; *branches,* ureteral, cremasteric, epididymal; *distribution,* testicle and parts designated by names of branches; *anastomoses,* branches of renal, inferior epigastric, deferential. SYN arteria testicularis [NA], arteria spermatica interna, internal spermatic a.

thoracoacromial a., *origin,* axillary; *distribution,* muscles and skin of shoulder and upper chest; *anastomoses,* branches of superior thoracic, internal thoracic, lateral thoracic, posterior and anterior circumflex humeral, and suprascapular. SYN arteria thoracoacromialis [NA], acromiothoracic a., thoracic axis (1), thoracoacromial trunk.

thoracodorsal a., *origin,* subscapular; *distribution,* muscles of upper part of back; *anastomoses,* branches of lateral thoracic. SYN arteria thoracodorsalis [NA], dorsal thoracic a.

thymic a.'s, SYN mediastinal *branches* of internal thoracic artery, under *branch.*

thyroid ima a., an inconstant artery; *origin,* arch of aorta or brachiocephalic artery; *distribution,* thyroid gland. SYN arteria thyroidea ima [NA], lowest thyroid a., Neubauer's a.

transverse cervical a., *origin,* thyrocervical trunk; *branches,* superficial (superficial cervical) and deep (descending scapular). SYN arteria transversa cervicis [NA], arteria transversa colli☆ [NA], transverse a. of neck.

transverse facial a., *origin,* superficial temporal; *distribution,* parotid gland, parotid duct, masseter muscle, and overlying skin; *anastomoses,* infraorbital and buccal branches of maxillary, and buccal and masseteric branches of facial. SYN arteria transversa faciei [NA].

transverse a. of neck, SYN transverse cervical a.

transverse pancreatic a., SYN inferior pancreatic a.

transverse scapular a., SYN suprascapular a.

ulnar a., *origin,* brachial; *branches,* ulnar recurrent, common interosseous, dorsal and palmar carpal, deep palmar, and superficial palmar arch with its digital branches. SYN arteria ulnaris [NA].

umbilical a., before birth the a. is a continuation of the internal iliac; after birth it is obliterated between the bladder and umbilicus, forming the medial umbilical ligament, the remaining portion, between the internal iliac artery and bladder, being reduced in size and giving off the superior vesical arteries. SYN arteria umbilicalis [NA].

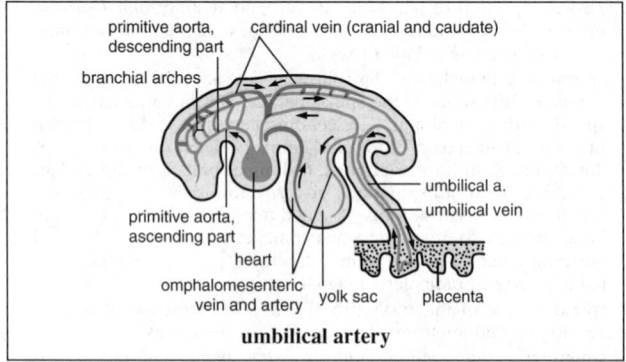

umbilical artery

urethral a., *origin,* perineal artery; *distribution,* membranous urethra. SYN arteria urethralis [NA].

uterine a., *origin,* internal iliac; *distribution,* uterus, upper part of vagina, round ligament, and medial part of uterine (fallopian) tube; *anastomoses,* ovarian, vaginal, inferior epigastric. Supplies maternal circulation to placenta during pregnancy. SYN arteria uterina [NA].

vaginal a., *origin,* internal iliac; *distribution,* vagina, base of bladder, rectum; *anastomoses,* uterine, internal pudendal. SYN arteria vaginalis [NA].

venous a., SYN pulmonary *trunk.*

ventral splanchnic a.'s, a.'s that arise on the embryo from the dorsal aorta and are distributed to the digestive tube.

ventricular a.'s, branches of the right and left coronary arteries distributed to the muscle of the ventricles. SYN arteriae ventriculares [NA].

vertebral a., the first branch of the subclavian artery; for descriptive purposes, divided into four parts: 1) prevertebral part, the portion before it enters the foramen of the transverse process of the sixth cervical vertebra; 2) transversarial part, the portion in the transverse foramina of the first six cervical vertebrae; 3) suboccipital (atlantic) part, the portion running along the posterior arch of the atlas; and 4) intracranial part, the portion within the cranial cavity to its union with the artery from the other side to form the basilar artery. SYN arteria vertebralis [NA].

vidian a., SYN a. of pterygoid canal.

vitelline a., an a. carrying blood to the yolk sac from the embryo. SYN arteria vitellina.

volar interosseous a., SYN anterior interosseous a.

Wilkie's a., the right colic a. when it occasionally crosses the duodenum.

Zinn's a., SYN central a. of retina.

zygomatico-orbital a., *origin,* superficial temporal, sometimes middle temporal; *distribution,* orbicularis oculi muscle and portions of the orbit; *anastomoses,* lacrimal and palpebral branches of ophthalmic. SYN arteria zygomatico-orbitalis [NA].

---

arthr-. SEE arthro-.

arth·rag·ra (arth-rag′ră). Obsolete term for articular *gout.* [G. *arthron,* joint, + *agra,* seizure]

ar·thral (ar′thrăl). SYN articular.

ar·thral·gia (ar-thral′jē-ă). Severe pain in a joint, especially one not inflammatory in character. SYN arthrodynia. [G. *arthron,* joint, + *algos,* pain]

  intermittent a., SYN periodic a.

  periodic a., a condition in which pain and swelling of one or more joints, most commonly the knee, occurs at regular intervals; there is sometimes abdominal pain, purpura, or edema. SYN intermittent a.

  a. saturni′na, severe pain, chiefly on flexion of the joints of the lower extremities, in lead poisoning.

ar·thral·gic (ar-thral′jik). Relating to or affected with arthralgia. SYN arthrodynic.

ar·threc·to·my (ar-threk′tō-mē). Excision of a joint. [G. *arthron,* joint, + *ektomē,* excision]

ar·thres·the·sia (ar-thres-thē′zē-ă). SYN articular *sensibility.* [G. *arthron,* joint, + *aisthesis,* sensation]

ar·thri·fuge (ar′thri-fūj). A gout remedy. [arthritis + L. *fugo,* to chase away]

ar·thrit·ic (ar-thrit′ik). Relating to arthritis.

ar·thri·tide (ar′thri-těd). Obsolete term for a skin eruption of assumed gouty or rheumatic origin. [Fr.]

ar·thrit·i·des (ar-thrit′i-dēz). Plural of arthritis.

ar·thri·tis, pl. **ar·thrit·i·des** (ar-thrī′tis, ar-thrit′i-dēz). Inflammation of a joint or a state characterized by inflammation of joints. SYN articular *rheumatism.* [G. fr. *arthron,* joint, + *-itis,* inflammation]

  acute rheumatic a., a. due to rheumatic fever.

  atrophic a., obsolete term for a. without new bone formation, now usually called rheumatoid a.

  chlamydial a., serous polyarthritis of cattle and sheep from chlamydial infection.

  chronic absorptive a., a. accompanied by pronounced resorption of bone with shortening and deformity, especially of the hands; when the deformity is extreme, the condition has also been termed a. mutilans.

  chylous a., a. with a high lymph content in synovial fluid, usually due to filariasis.

  a. defor′mans, SYN rheumatoid a.

  degenerative a., SYN osteoarthritis.

  enteropathic a., a form of a. sometimes resembling rheumatoid a. which may complicate the course of ulcerative colitis, Crohn's disease, or other intestinal disease.

filarial a., a. occurring in filariasis, probably due to extravasation of lipid-rich lymph resembling chyle into the joint space.

gonococcal a., joint space infection in humans caused by disseminated *Neisseria gonorrhoeae;* characteristically monarticular, but may be polyarticular. SYN gonorrheal arthritis.

gouty a., inflammation of the joints in gout.

hemophilic a., joint disease resulting from hemophilic bleeding into a joint.

hypertrophic a., SYN osteoarthritis.

Jaccoud's a., a rare form of chronic a., reported to occur after attacks of acute rheumatic fever, characterized by an unusual form of bone erosion of the metacarpal heads and by ulnar deviation of the fingers; it resembles rheumatoid a., but with less overt inflammation, and rheumatoid factor is absent. SYN Jaccoud's arthropathy.

juvenile a., juvenile rheumatoid a., chronic a. beginning in childhood, most cases of which are pauciarticular, *i.e.,* affecting few joints. Several patterns of illness have been identified: in one subset, primarily affecting girls, iritis is common and antinuclear antibody is usually present; another subset, primarily affecting boys, frequently includes spinal a. resembling ankylosing spondylitis; some cases are true rheumatoid a. beginning in childhood and characterized by the presence of rheumatoid factor and destructive deforming joint changes, often undergoing remission at puberty. SEE ALSO Still's *disease.* SYN juvenile chronic a.

juvenile chronic a., SYN juvenile a.

Lyme a., the arthritic manifestation of Lyme disease.

a. mu′tilans, a form of chronic rheumatoid a. in which osteolysis occurs with extensive destruction of the joint cartilages and bony surfaces with pronounced deformities, chiefly of the hands and feet; similar changes can occur in some cases of psoriatic a.

neonatal a. of foals, bacterial polyarthritis caused by umbilical infections by several bacterial species.

neuropathic a., SYN neuropathic *joint.*

a. nodo′sa, SYN rheumatoid a.

ochronotic a., osteoarthritis occurring as a complication of ochronosis.

proliferative a., rarely used term for rheumatoid a., based on the characteristic proliferation of the synovial membrane seen in joints affected by the disease.

psoriatic a., the concurrence of psoriasis and polyarthritis, resembling rheumatoid a. but thought to be a specific disease entity, seronegative for rheumatoid factor and often involving the digits. SEE ALSO a. mutilans. SYN arthropathia psoriatica.

pyogenic a., SYN suppurative a.

rheumatoid a., a systemic disease, occurring more often in women, which affects connective tissue; a. is the dominant clinical manifestation, involving many joints, especially those of the hands and feet, accompanied by thickening of articular soft tissue, with extension of synovial tissue over articular cartilages, which become eroded; the course is variable but often is chronic and progressive, leading to deformities and disability. SYN a. deformans, a. nodosa, nodose rheumatism (1).

suppurative a., acute inflammation of synovial membranes, with purulent effusion into a joint, due to bacterial infection; the usual route of infection is hemic to the synovial tissue, causing destruction of the articular cartilage, and may become chronic, with sinus formation, osteomyelitis, deformity, and disability. SYN purulent synovitis, pyarthrosis, pyogenic a., suppurative synovitis.

arthro-, arthr-. A joint, an articulation; corresponds to L. articul-. [G. *arthron,* a joint, fr. *arariskō,* to join, to fit together]

Arth·ro·bac·ter (ar-thrō-bak′ter). A genus of strictly aerobic, Gram-positive bacteria (family Corynebacteriaceae) whose cells undergo a change from a coccoid form to a rod shape following transfer to fresh complex growth medium. Although primarily found in soil, species identified as belonging to this genus have been found in the advancing front of lesions of dental caries. The type species is *A. globiformis.* [G. *arthron,* joint, + *baktron,* staff or rod]

ar·thro·cele (ar′thrō-sēl). **1.** Hernia of the synovial membrane through the capsule of a joint. **2.** Any swelling of a joint. [arthro- + G. *kēlē,* hernia, tumor]

ar·thro·cen·te·sis (ar′thrō-sen-tē′sis). Aspiration of fluid from a joint through a puncture needle. [arthro- + G. *kentēsis,* puncture]

ar·thro·chon·dri·tis (ar′thrō-kon-drī′tis). Inflammation of an articular cartilage. [arthro- + G. *chondros,* cartilage, + *-itis,* inflammation]

ar·thro·cla·sia (ar-thrō-klā′zē-ă). The forcible breaking up of the adhesions in ankylosis. [arthro- + G. *klasis,* a breaking]

ar·thro·co·nid·i·um (ar′thrō-kŏ-nid′ē-um). A conidium released by fragmentation or separation at the septum of cells of the hypha. SYN arthrospore. [G. *arthron,* joint, + conidium]

Arth·ro·der·ma (ar′thrō-der′mă). A genus of ascomycetous fungi comprised of the anamorph genera *Microsporium* and *Trichoderma* species.

ar·throd·e·sis (ar-throd′ĕ-sis, ar-thrō-dē′sis). The stiffening of a joint by operative means. SYN artificial ankylosis, syndesis. [arthro- + G. *desis,* a binding together]

triple a., surgical fusion of the talonavicular, talocalcaneal, and calcaneocuboid joints.

ar·thro·dia (ar-thrō′dē-ă). SYN plane *joint.* [G. *arthrōdia,* a gliding joint, fr. *arthron,* joint, + *eidos,* form]

ar·thro·di·al (ar-thrō′dē-ăl). Relating to arthrodia.

ar·thro·dyn·ia (ar-thrō-din′ē-ă). SYN arthralgia. [arthro- + G. *odynē,* pain]

ar·thro·dyn·ic (ar-thrō-din′ik). SYN arthralgic.

ar·thro·dys·pla·sia (ar′thrō-dis-plā′zē-ă). Hereditary congenital defect of joint development. [arthro- + G. *dys,* bad, + *plasis,* a molding]

ar·thro·en·dos·co·py (ar′thrō-en-dos′kŏ-pē). SYN arthroscopy.

ar·thro·e·rei·sis (ar-thrō-ĕ-rī′sis). SYN arthrorisis.

ar·throg·e·nous (ar-throj′ĕ-nŭs). **1.** Of articular origin; starting from a joint. **2.** Forming an articulation.

ar·thro·gram (ar′thrō-gram). Roentgenogram of a joint; usually implies the introduction of a contrast agent into the joint capsule. [arthro- + G. *gramma,* a writing]

ar·throg·ra·phy (ar-throg′ră-fē). Radiography of a joint after injecting one or more contrast media into the joint. [arthro- + G. *graphō,* to describe]

ar·thro·gry·po·sis (ar′thrō-gri-pō′sis). Congenital defect of the limbs characterized by contractures of joints. [arthro- + G. *gryphōsis,* a crooking]

a. mul′tiplex congen′ita, limitation of range of joint motion and contractures present at birth, usually involving multiple joints; a syndrome probably of diverse etiology that may result from changes in spinal cord, muscle, or connective tissue. Several forms exist, autosomal dominant [MIM*108110, 108120, 108130, 108140, 108145, 108200], recessive [MIM*208080, 208081, 208100, 208110, 208150, 208155, 208200], and X-linked [MIM*301820, 301830] SYN amyoplasia congenita.

ar·thro·ka·tad·y·sis (ar′thrō-kă-tad′i-sis). SYN Otto′s *disease.* [arthro- + G. *katadysis,* a dipping under, a setting, fr. *dyō,* to make sink]

ar·thro·lith (ar′thrō-lith). A loose body in a joint. [arthro- + G. *lithos,* stone]

ar·thro·li·thi·a·sis (ar′thrō-li-thī′ă-sis). Rarely used term for articular *gout.*

ar·thro·lo·gia (ar-thrō-lō′jē-ă) [NA]. SYN arthrology, arthrology.

ar·throl·o·gy (ar-throl′ō-jē). The branch of anatomy concerned with the joints. SYN arthrologia [NA], syndesmologia, syndesmology, synosteology. [arthro- + G. *logos,* study]

ar·throl·y·sis (ar-throl′i-sis). Restoration of mobility in stiff and ankylosed joints. [arthro- + G. *lysis,* a loosening]

ar·throm·e·ter (ar-throm′ĕ-ter). SYN goniometer (3).

ar·throm·e·try (ar-throm′ĕ-trē). Measurement of the range of movement in a joint. [arthro- + G. *metron,* measure]

ar·thro·no·sos (ar-thrō-nō′sos). Rarely used term for any disease of the joints. [arthro- + G. *nosos,* disease]

ar·thro·oph·thal·mop·a·thy (ar′thrō-of′thal-mop′ă-thē) [MIM*108300]. Disease affecting joints and eyes; autosomal dominant inheritance. [arthro- + ophthalmo- + G. *pathos,* suffering]

hereditary progressive a.-o. [MIM*108300], autosomal domi-

nant a.-o. associated with progressive multiple dysplasia of the epiphyses, overtubulation of long bones, cleft lip and palate, hypermobility of joints, flattened vertebral bodies, pelvic bone deformities, and deafness. SYN Stickler's syndrome.

ar·thro·path·ia (ar-thrō-path′ē-ă). SYN arthropathy. [L.]

a. psoriat′ica, SYN psoriatic *arthritis.*

ar·thro·pa·thol·o·gy (ar′thrō-pa-thol′ō-jē). The study of diseases of joints.

ar·throp·a·thy (ar-throp′ă-thē). Any disease affecting a joint. SYN arthropathia. [arthro- + G. *pathos,* suffering]

diabetic a., a neuropathic a. occurring in diabetes.

Jaccoud's a., SYN Jaccoud's *arthritis.*

long-leg a., a degenerative joint disease that develops, after many years, in the knee of the longer leg of a person with unequal leg lengths.

neuropathic a., SYN neuropathic *joint.*

static a., secondary involvement of a joint following disease in a joint of the same extremity; *e.g.,* knee or ankle involvement in hip disease.

tabetic a., a neuropathic a. that occurs with tabes dorsalis (tabetic neurosyphilis). SEE ALSO neuropathic *joint.* SYN Charcot's joint.

ar·thro·phy·ma (ar-thrō-fī′mă). An articular tumor or swelling. [arthro- + G. *phyma,* swelling, tumor]

ar·thro·plas·ty (ar′thrō-plas-tē). **1.** Creation of an artificial joint to correct ankylosis. **2.** An operation to restore as far as possible the integrity and functional power of a joint. [arthro- + G. *plastos,* formed]

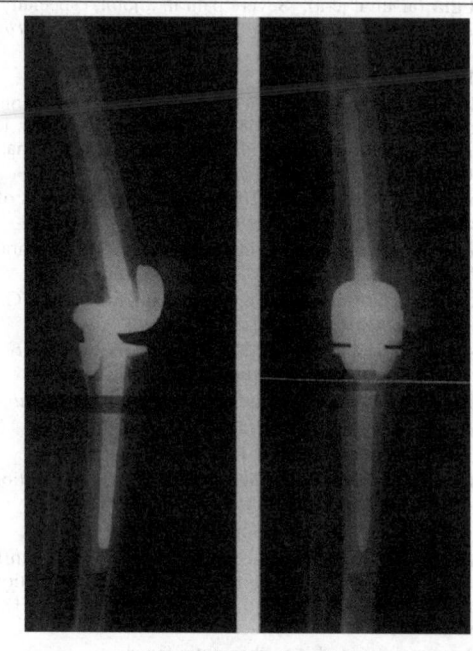

arthroplasty: joint prosthesis

Charnley hip a., a form of total hip replacement consisting of the application of an acetabular cup and a femoral head prosthesis.

gap a., the surgical correction of ankylosis by creating a space between the ankylosed part of a joint and the portion for which movement is desired.

interposition a., surgical correction of ankylosis by separation of the immobile part of a joint from the mobilized part and interposition of a substance (*e.g.,* fascia, cartilage, metal, or plastic) between them.

intracapsular temporomandibular joint a., operative recontouring of the articular surface of the mandibular condyle without the removal of the articular disk.

total joint a., a. in which both joint surfaces are replaced with artificial materials, usually metal and high-density plastic.

ar·thro·pneu·mo·ra·di·og·raph·y (ar′thrō-nū′mō-rā′ē-og′rǎ-fē). Radiographic examination of a joint after it has been injected with air. [arthro- + pneumo- + radiography]

ar·thro·pod (ar′thrō-pod). A member of the phylum Arthropoda. [arthro- + G. *pous,* foot]

Ar·throp·o·da (ar-throp′ŏ-dǎ). A phylum of the Metazoa that includes the classes Crustacea (crabs, shrimps, crayfish, lobsters), Insecta, Arachnida (spiders, scorpions, mites, ticks), Chilopoda (centipedes), Diplopoda (millipedes), Merostomata (horseshoe crabs), and various other extinct or lesser known groups. A. forms the largest assemblage of living organisms, 75% insects, of which over a million species are known. [arthro- + G. *pous,* foot]

ar·thro·po·di·a·sis (ar′thrō-pō-dī′ǎ-sis). Direct effects of arthropods upon vertebrates including acariasis, allergy, dermatosis, entomophobia, and actions of contact toxins.

ar·thro·po·dic, ar·throp·o·dous (ar-thrō-pō′dik, ar-throp′ŏ-dŭs). Pertaining to arthropods.

ar·thro·py·o·sis (ar′thrō-pī-ō′sis). Suppuration in a joint. [arthro- + G. *pyōsis,* suppuration]

ar·thro·ri·sis (ar′thrō-rī′sis). An operation for limiting motion in a joint in cases of undue mobility from paralysis, usually by means of a bone block. SYN arthroereisis. [arthro- + G. *ereisis,* a propping up]

ar·thro·scle·ro·sis (ar′thrō-skler-ō′sis). Stiffness of the joints, especially in the aged. [arthro- + G. *sklērōsis,* hardening]

ar·thro·scope (ar′thrō-skōp). An endoscope for examining joint interiors.

ar·thros·co·py (ar-thros′kŏ-pē). Endoscopic examination of the interior of a joint. SYN arthroendoscopy. [arthro- + G. *skopeō,* to view]

ar·thro·sis (ar-thrō′sis). **1.** SYN joint. [G. *arthrōsis,* a jointing] **2.** A degenerative affection of a joint. [arthro- + G. *-osis,* condition] **temporomandibular a.,** a noninfectious degenerative dysfunction of the temporomandibular joint characterized by pain, cracking, and limited mandibular opening. SEE ALSO myofacial pain-dysfunction *syndrome.*

ar·thro·spore (ar′thrō-spōr). SYN arthroconidium. [arthro- + G. *sporos,* seed]

ar·thros·te·i·tis (ar-thros-tē-ī′tis). Inflammation of the osseous structures of a joint. [arthro- + G. *osteon,* bone, + *-itis,* inflammation]

ar·thros·to·my (ar-thros′tō-mē). Establishment of a temporary opening into a joint cavity. [arthro- + G. *stoma,* mouth]

ar·thro·sy·no·vi·tis (ar′thrō-sin-ō-vī′tis). Inflammation of the synovial membrane of a joint.

ar·thro·tome (ar′thrō-tōm). A large, strong scalpel used in cutting cartilaginous and other tough joint structures.

ar·throt·o·my (ar-throt′ō-mē). Cutting into a joint. [arthro- + G. *tomē,* a cutting]

ar·thro·tro·pic (ar-thrō-trop′ik). Tending to affect joints. [arthro- + G. *tropos,* a turning]

ar·thro·ty·phoid (ar-thrō-tī′foyd). Obsolete term for typhoid fever with joint involvement due to metastatic infection.

ar·throx·e·sis (ar-throk′sĕ-sis). Removal of diseased tissue from a joint by means of the sharp spoon or other scraping instrument. [arthro- + G. *xesis,* a scraping]

Arthus, Nicolas Maurice, French bacteriologist, 1862–1945. SEE A. *phenomenon, reaction.*

ar·tic·u·lar (ar-tik′yū-lǎr). Relating to a joint. SYN arthral.

ar·tic·u·la·re (ar-tik-yū-lā′rē). In cephalometrics, the point of intersection of the external dorsal contour of the mandibular condyle and the temporal bone; the midpoint is used when a profile radiograph shows double projections of the rami.

ar·tic·u·late (ar-tik′yū-lit). **1.** SYN articulated. **2.** To join or connect together loosely to allow motion between the parts. **3.** Capable of distinct and connected speech. (ar-tik′yū-lāt). **4.** To speak distinctly and connectedly. [L. *articulo,* pp. *-atus,* to articulate]

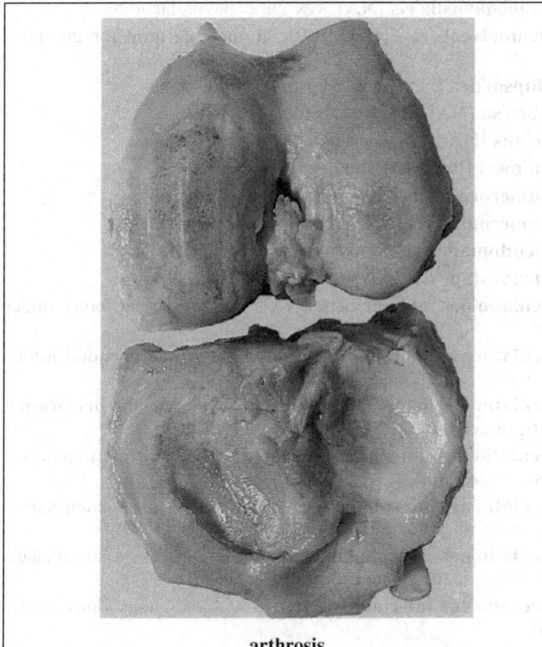

arthrosis
the cartilage of the knee is nearly destroyed

ar·tic·u·lat·ed (ar-tik′yū-lā-ted). Jointed. SYN articulate (1).

ARTICULATIO

ar·tic·u·la·tio, pl. **ar·tic·u·la·ti·o·nes** (ar-tik-yū-lā′shē-ō, -lā-shē-ō′nēz) [NA]. SYN joint. [L. a forming of vines]
a. acromioclavicula′ris [NA], SYN acromioclavicular *joint.*
a. atlantoaxia′lis latera′lis [NA], SYN lateral atlantoaxial *joint.*
a. atlantoaxia′lis media′na [NA], SYN median atlantoaxial *joint.*
a. atlan′to-occipita′lis [NA], SYN atlanto-occipital *joint.*
a. bicondyla′ris [NA], SYN bicondylar *joint.*
a. calca′neocuboi′dea [NA], SYN calcaneocuboid *joint.*
a. cap′itis cos′tae [NA], SYN *joint* of head of rib.
a. carpometacar′pea pol′licis [NA], SYN carpometacarpal *joint* of thumb.
articulatio′nes carpometacar′peae [NA], SYN carpometacarpal *joints,* under *joint.*
a. cartilag′inis [NA], SYN cartilaginous *joint.*
articulatio′nes cing′uli mem′bri inferio′ris [NA], SYN *joints* of pelvic girdle, under *joint.*
articulatio′nes cin′guli mem′bri superio′ris [NA], SYN *joints* of pectoral girdle, under *joint.*
a. complex′a [NA], SYN compound *joint.*
a. compos′ita [NA], SYN compound *joint.*
a. condyla′ris [NA], ★official alternate term for ellipsoidal *joint.*
a. costochondra′lis [NA], SYN costochondral *joint.*
a. cos′totransversa′ria [NA], SYN costotransverse *joint.*
articulatio′nes costovertebra′les [NA], SYN costovertebral *joints,* under *joint.*
a. cotyl′ica [NA], ★official alternate term for ball-and-socket *joint.*
a. cox′ae [NA], SYN hip *joint.*
a. cricoarytenoid′ea [NA], SYN cricoarytenoid *joint.*
a. cricothyroid′ea [NA], SYN cricothyroid *joint.*
a. cu′biti [NA], SYN elbow *joint.*

a. cuneonavicula′ris [NA], SYN cuneonavicular *joint*.

a. dentoalveola′ris [NA], ⭑official alternate term for gomphosis.

a. ellipsoi′dea [NA], SYN ellipsoidal *joint*.

a. fibro′sa [NA], SYN fibrous *joint*.

a. ge′nus [NA], SYN knee *joint*.

a. hu′meri [NA], SYN shoulder *joint*.

a. humeroradia′lis [NA], SYN humeroradial *joint*.

a. humeroulna′ris [NA], SYN humeroulnar *joint*.

a. incudomallea′ris [NA], SYN incudomalleolar *joint*.

a. incudostape′dia [NA], SYN incudostapedial *joint*.

articulatio′nes intercar′peae [NA], SYN intercarpal *joints*, under *joint*.

articulatio′nes interchondra′les [NA], SYN interchondral *joints*, under *joint*.

articulatio′nes intermetacar′peae [NA], SYN intermetacarpal *joints*, under *joint*.

articulatio′nes intermetatar′seae [NA], SYN intermetatarsal *joints*, under *joint*.

articulatio′nes interphalan′geae ma′nus [NA], SYN interphalangeal *joints* of hand, under *joint*.

articulatio′nes interphalan′geae pe′dis [NA], SYN interphalangeal *joints* of foot, under *joint*.

articulatio′nes intertar′seae [NA], SYN intertarsal *joints*, under *joint*.

a. lumbosacra′lis [NA], SYN lumbosacral *joint*.

a. mandibula′ris, SYN temporomandibular *joint*.

articulatio′nes ma′nus [NA], SYN *joints* of hand, under *joint*.

a. mediocar′pea [NA], SYN midcarpal *joint*.

articulatio′nes mem′bri inferio′ris li′beri [NA], SYN *joints* of free lower limb, under *joint*.

articulatio′nes mem′bri superio′ris li′beri [NA], SYN *joints* of free upper limb, under *joint*.

articulatio′nes metacarpophalan′geae [NA], SYN metacarpophalangeal *joints*, under *joint*.

articulatio′nes metatarsophalan′geae [NA], SYN metatarsophalangeal *joints*, under *joint*.

articulatio′nes ossiculo′rum audi′tus [NA], SYN *joints* of auditory ossicles, under *joint*.

a. os′sis pisifor′mis [NA], SYN pisotriquetral *joint*.

a. ovoida′lis, SYN saddle *joint*.

articulatio′nes pe′dis [NA], SYN *joints* of foot, under *joint*.

a. pla′na [NA], SYN plane *joint*.

a. radiocar′pea [NA], SYN wrist *joint*.

a. radioulna′ris dista′lis [NA], SYN distal radioulnar *joint*.

a. radioulna′ris proxima′lis [NA], SYN proximal radioulnar *joint*.

a. sacrococcyge′a [NA], SYN sacrococcygeal *joint*.

a. sacroili′aca [NA], SYN sacroiliac *joint*.

a. sellar′is [NA], SYN saddle *joint*.

a. sim′plex [NA], SYN simple *joint*.

a. spheroi′dea [NA], SYN ball-and-socket *joint*.

a. sternoclavicula′ris [NA], SYN sternoclavicular *joint*.

articulatio′nes sternocosta′les [NA], SYN sternocostal *joints*, under *joint*.

a. subtala′ris [NA], SYN subtalar *joint*.

a. synovia′lis [NA], SYN synovial *joint*.

a. tal′ocalca′neonavicula′ris [NA], SYN talocalcaneonavicular *joint*.

a. talocrural′is [NA], SYN ankle *joint*.

a. tar′si transver′sa [NA], SYN transverse tarsal *joint*.

articulatio′nes tarsometatar′seae [NA], SYN tarsometatarsal *joints*, under *joint*.

a. temporomandibula′ris [NA], SYN temporomandibular *joint*.

a. tibiofibula′ris [NA], SYN proximal tibiofibular *joint*.

a. trochoid′ea [NA], SYN pivot *joint*.

articulatio′nes zygapophysea′les [NA], SYN zygapophyseal *joints*, under *joint*.

ar·tic·u·la·tion (ar-tik-yū-lā′shŭn). **1.** SYN joint. **2.** A joining or connecting together loosely so as to allow motion between the parts. **3.** Distinct connected speech or enunciation. **4.** In dentistry, the contact relationship of the occlusal surfaces of the teeth during jaw movement. [see joint]

arthrodial a., SYN plane *joint*.

atlanto-occipital a., SYN atlanto-occipital *joint*.

balanced a., SYN balanced *occlusion*.

bicondylar a., SYN bicondylar *joint*.

carpal a., SYN wrist *joint*.

cartilaginous a., SYN cartilaginous *joint*.

compound a., SYN compound *joint*.

condylar a., SYN ellipsoidal *joint*.

confluent a., a tendency to run the syllables together in speech.

cricoarytenoid a., SYN cricoarytenoid *joint*.

cricothyroid a., SYN cricothyroid *joint*.

cuneonavicular a., SYN cuneonavicular *joint*.

dental a., the contact relationship of the occlusal surfaces of the upper and lower teeth when moving into and away from centric occlusion. SYN gliding occlusion.

distal radioulnar a., SYN distal radioulnar *joint*.

a.'s of foot, SYN *joints* of foot, under *joint*.

glenohumeral a., SYN shoulder *joint*.

a.'s of hand, SYN *joints* of hand, under *joint*.

humeral a., SYN shoulder *joint*.

humeroradial a., SYN humeroradial *joint*.

incudomalleolar a., SYN incudomalleolar *joint*.

incudostapedial a., SYN incudostapedial *joint*.

interchondral a.'s, SYN interchondral *joints*, under *joint*.

intermetatarsal a.'s, SYN intermetatarsal *joints*, under *joint*.

interphalangeal a.'s, SYN interphalangeal *joints* of hand, under *joint*.

intertarsal a.'s, SYN intertarsal *joints*, under *joint*.

metacarpophalangeal a.'s, SYN metacarpophalangeal *joints*, under *joint*.

metatarsophalangeal a.'s, SYN metatarsophalangeal *joints*, under *joint*.

peg-and-socket a., SYN gomphosis.

a. of pisiform bone, SYN pisotriquetral *joint*.

proximal radioulnar a., SYN proximal radioulnar *joint*.

radiocarpal a., SYN wrist *joint*.

sacroiliac a., SYN sacroiliac *joint*.

spheroid a., SYN ball-and-socket *joint*.

sternocostal a.'s, SYN sternocostal *joints*, under *joint*.

superior tibial a., SYN proximal tibiofibular *joint*.

talocrural a., SYN ankle *joint*.

temporomandibular a., SYN temporomandibular *joint*.

tibiofibular a., **(1)** SYN proximal tibiofibular *joint*. **(2)** SYN tibiofibular *syndesmosis*.

transverse tarsal a., SYN transverse tarsal *joint*.

trochoid a., SYN pivot *joint*.

ar·tic·u·la·tor (ar-tik′yū-lā-tŏr). A mechanical device which represents the temporomandibular joints and jaw members to which maxillary and mandibular casts may be attached. SYN occluding frame.

adjustable a., **(1)** an a. which may be adjusted to permit movement of the casts into recorded eccentric relationships; **(2)** an a. capable of adjustment to more than one eccentric position.

arcon a., **(1)** an a. with the equivalent condylar guides fixed to the upper member and the hinge axis to the lower member; **(2)** an instrument that maintains a constant relationship between the occlusal plane and the arcon guides at any position of the upper member, thereby making possible more accurate reproductions of mandibular movements.

non-arcon a., an a. with the equivalent condylar guides attached to the lower member and the hinge axis to the upper member.

ar·tic·u·la·to·ry (ar-tik′yū-lă-tō-rē). Relating to articulate speech.

ar·tic·u·lo·stat (ar-tik′yū-lō-stat). A research instrument that will position the dentition and the head of an x-ray machine in such a manner that films made at separate times may be accurately superimposed. [articulo- + G. *stasis*, a standing still]

ar·tic·u·lus (ar-tik′yū-lŭs). SYN joint. [L. joint]

ar·ti·fact (ar′ti-fakt). **1.** Anything, especially in a histologic specimen or a graphic record, that is caused by the technique used or is not a natural occurrence, but is merely incidental. **2.** A skin lesion produced or perpetuated by self-inflicted action, as in dermatitis artefacta. SYN artefact. [L. *ars*, art, + *facio*, pp. *factus*, to make]

chemical shift a., in magnetic resonance imaging, a dark band caused by a biochemical difference in resonant frequency of adjacent regions rather than a true anatomic separation.

ar·ti·fac·ti·tious (ar′ti-fak-tish′ŭs). SYN artifactual.

ar·ti·fac·tu·al (ar-ti-fak′chyū-ăl). Produced or caused by an artifact. SYN artifactitious.

Ar·ti·o·dac·ty·la (ar′ti-ō-dak′ti-lă). An order of even-toed ungulates having either two or four digits, with the axis between the third and fourth; *e.g.*, pig and hippopotamus with four; camel, deer, giraffe, antelope, and cow with two. [G. *artios*, even in number, + *daktylos*, finger]

ARV Abbreviation for AIDS-related *virus.*

ar·y·ep·i·glot·tic (ar′ē-ep-i-glot′ik). Relating to the arytenoid cartilage and the epiglottis; denoting a fold of mucous membrane (aryepiglottic fold) and a muscle contained in it (aryepiglottic muscle). SYN arytenoepiglottidean.

ar·yl (ar′il). An organic radical derived from an aromatic compound by removing a hydrogen atom.

a. acylamidase, an amidohydrolase cleaving the acyl group from an anilide by hydrolysis, producing aniline and an acid anion. SYN arylamidase.

ar·yl·am·i·dase (ar-il-am′i-dās). SYN *aryl* acylamidase.

ar·yl·ar·son·ic ac·id (ar′il-ar-son′ik). An arsonic acid containing an aryl radical; *e.g.*, arsenilic acid.

ar·yl·sul·fa·tase (ar-il-sŭl′fă-tās). An enzyme that cleaves phenol sulfates, including cerebroside sulfates (*i.e.*, a phenol sulfate + $H_2O \rightarrow$ a phenol + sulfate anion). Some a.'s are inhibited by sulfate (type II) and some are not (type I). SYN sulfatase (2).

ar·y·te·no·ep·i·glot·tid·e·an (a-rit′ĕ-nō-ep′i-glo-tid′ē-an). SYN aryepiglottic.

ar·y·te·noid (a-ri-tē′noyd). Denoting a cartilage (arytenoid cartilage) and muscles (oblique and transverse arytenoid muscles) of the larynx. [see arytenoideus]

ar·y·te·noi·dec·to·my (ar′ĭ-tē-noy-dek′tō-mē). Excision of an arytenoid cartilage, usually in bilateral vocal fold paralysis, to improve breathing. [arytenoid + G. *ektomē*, excision]

ar·y·te·noi·de·us (ar-ĭ-tē-noy′dē-ŭs). SYN oblique arytenoid *muscle*, transverse arytenoid *muscle*. [G. *arytainoeides*, ladle-shaped, applied to cartilage of the larynx, fr. *arytaina*, a ladle, + *eidos*, resemblance]

ar·yt·e·noi·di·tis (ă-rit′ĕ-noy-dī′tis). Inflammation of an arytenoid cartilage or its mucosal cover.

ar·y·te·noi·do·pexy (ar′ĭ-tĕ-noy′dō-pek′sē). Fixation by surgery of cartilages or muscles of arytenoids. [arytenoid + G. *pēxis*, fixation]

A.S. Abbreviation for *auris sinister* [L.], left ear.

As Symbol for arsenic.

as·a·fet·i·da (as-ă-fet′ĭ-dă). A gum resin, the inspissated exudate from the root of *Ferula foetida* (family Umbelliferae); used as a repellent against dogs, cats, and rabbits, and formerly used as an antispasmodic; in Asia, used as a condiment and flavoring agent. [Pers. *aza*, mastic, + L. *fetidus*, fetid]

Asa·rum (as′ar-ŭm). A genus of plants of the family Aristolochiaceae. [L., fr. G. *asaron*, hazelwort]

A. canaden′se, an aromatic stimulant and diaphoretic. SYN Canada snakeroot, Indian ginger, wild ginger.

A. europae′um, an emetic and cathartic. SYN European snakeroot, hazelwort.

as·bes·toid (as-bes′toyd). SYN amianthoid.

as·bes·tos (as-bes′tŏs). The commercial product, after mining and processing, obtained from a family of fibrous hydrated silicates divided mineralogically into amphiboles (amosite, anthrophyllite, and crocidolite) and serpentines (chrysotile); it is virtually insoluble and is used to provide tensile strength and moldability, thermal insulation, and resistance to fire, heat, and corrosion; inhalation of a. particles can cause asbestosis. [G. unquenchable; so called in the erroneous belief that when heated, it could not be quenched]

as·bes·to·sis (as-bes-tō′sis). Pneumoconiosis due to inhalation of asbestos fibers suspended in the ambient air; sometimes complicated by pleural mesothelioma or bronchogenic carcinoma; ferruginous bodies are the histologic hallmark of exposure to asbestos.

as·ca·ri·a·sis (as-kă-rī′ă-sis). Disease caused by infection with *Ascaris* or related ascarid nematodes. [G. *askaris*, an intestinal worm, + *-iasis*, condition]

as·ca·ri·cide (as-kar′i-sīd). **1.** Causing the death of ascarid nematodes. **2.** An agent having such properties. [ascarid + L. *caedo*, to kill]

as·ca·rid (as′kă-rid). **1.** A general name for any nematode of the family Ascarididae. **2.** Pertaining to such nematodes.

As·car·i·dae (as-kar′i-dē). Former spelling for Ascarididae.

As·car·i·da·ta (as-kă-rid′ă-tă). SYN Ascaridida.

As·ca·rid·i·a (as-kă-rid′i-ă). A genus of relatively large nematodes (family Heterakidae) that inhabit the intestine of birds and cause ascaridiasis. Their life cycle is direct, without an intermediate host; their appearance and habits are much like those of members of the family Ascarididae.

A. gal′li, a species abundant in the small intestine of chickens, turkeys, geese, guinea fowl, and many wild birds in most parts of the world.

as·car·i·di·a·sis (as′kă-ri-dī′ă-sis). Disease caused by infection with a species of *Ascaridia*, commonly occurring in the intestine of fowl.

As·ca·rid·i·da (as-kă-rid′i-dă). An order of nematode worms that includes many important human, domestic animal, and fowl parasites such as *Ascaris*, *Ascaridia*, *Subuluris*, *Heterakis*, and *Anisakis*. SYN Ascaridata, Ascarididea, Ascaridorida.

As·ca·rid·i·dae (as-kă-rid′i-dē). A family of large intestinal roundworms that includes the important nematode of man, *Ascaris lumbricoides*, the abundant roundworm of swine, *Ascaris suum*, and the common ascarids of dogs and cats, *Toxocara* and *Toxascaris* species. [G. *askaris*, an intestinal worm]

As·car·i·did·ea (as-kar-i-did′ē-ă). SYN Ascaridida.

As·car·i·doi·dea (as-kă-ri-doy′dē-ă). Superfamily of stout, 3-lipped intestinal roundworms that includes the family Ascarididae.

as·car·i·dole (as-kar′ĭ-dōl). 1,4-Peroxido-*p*-menth-2-ene; a major constituent of oil of chenopodium; an anthelmintic.

As·car·i·dor·i·da (as-kări-dōr′i-dă). SYN Ascaridida.

As·ca·ris (as′kă-ris). A genus of large, heavy-bodied roundworms parasitic in the small intestine; abundant in man and many other vertebrates. [G. *askaris*, an intestinal worm]

A. equo′rum, SYN *Parascaris equorum*.

A. lumbricoi′des, a large roundworm of man, one of the commonest human parasites (8 to 12 inches in length); various symptoms such as restlessness, fever, and sometimes diarrhea, are attributed to its presence, but usually it causes no definite symptoms; the similar species, *A. suum* (or *A. lumbricoides suum*) is very common in swine, but is not readily transmitted to man, and vice versa; the types are morphologically and immunologically similar but apparently are host-adapted types, considered distinct species or races.

As·ca·roi·dea (as-kă-roy′dē-ă). Former spelling for Ascaridoidea.

as·ca·ron (as-kă-ron). A toxic peptone present in helminths, especially the ascaridids; symptoms of a. poisoning are similar to those of anaphylactic shock. [G. *askaris*, an intestinal worm, + *hormōn*, pres. part. of *hormaō*, to excite]

As·ca·rops stron·gy·li·na (as′kă-rops stron-ji-lī′nă). A small

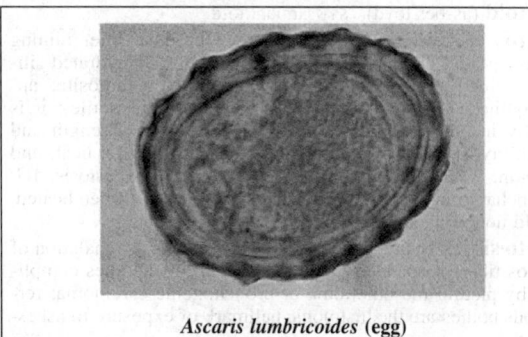

Ascaris lumbricoides (egg)

bloodsucking worm found in the stomach of pigs and wild boars in many parts of the world. Larvae of this species develop in coprophagous beetles; worms adhere to the gastric mucosa of the pig, and may cause inflammation and ulceration in heavy infections. [G. *askaris,* an intestinal worm; *strongylos,* round]

as·cen·dens (as-sen′denz). Ascending. Going upward, ascending, toward a higher position. [L.]

ascen·sus (ă-sen′sŭs). A moving upward; having an abnormally high position. [L. ascent]

as·cer·tain·ment (as-ser-tān′ment). In epidemiological and genetic research, the method by which a person, pedigree, or cluster is brought to the attention of an investigator; has a bearing on the interpretation of segregation ratios, concordance rates, linkage analysis, and other probability features.

  complete a., method by which all families with at least one affected individual in a population are certain or have an equal chance of being identified by survey or an appropriate random sampling technique.

  incomplete a., method of locating affected individuals in which probability of locating any specific patient has a known value between 0 and 1. SYN truncate a.

  single a., method of a. of locating affected individuals by hospital or clinic admission or another way in which probability of encountering the same family twice approaches zero; thus, the probability that a family will be ascertained is proportional to the number of affected members.

  total a., method by which all members of a population at risk of a trait are discerned or equally likely to be contained in a sample thereof.

  truncate a., SYN incomplete a.

Asc·hel·min·thes (ask-hel-min′thēz). A former phylum of the Metazoa which included the class Nematoda and a disparate assortment of other pseudocelomates, each now accorded separate phylum status; they are nonsegmented, bilaterally symmetric, and cylindric or filiform, with a pseudocele body cavity and rounded or pointed ends; they vary considerably in size, and the male is usually smaller than the female.

Ascher, Karl W., U.S. ophthalmologist, 1887–1971. SEE A.'s aqueous influx *phenomenon, syndrome.*

Aschheim, Selmar, German obstetrician and gynecologist, 1878–1965. SEE A.-Zondek *test.*

Aschner, Bernhard, Austrian gynecologist, 1883–1960. SEE A.'s *phenomenon, reflex;* A.-Dagnini *reflex.*

Aschoff, Karl Ludwig, German pathologist, 1866–1942. SEE A. *bodies,* under *body, nodules,* under *nodule; node* of A. and Tawara; Rokitansky-A. *sinuses,* under *sinus;* A. *cell.*

as·ci·tes (ă-sī′tēz). Accumulation of serous fluid in the peritoneal cavity. SYN abdominal dropsy, hydroperitoneum, hydroperitonia. [L. fr. G. *askos,* a bag, + *-ites*]

  a. adipo′sus, SYN chylous a.

  chyliform a., SYN chylous a.

  chylous a., a. chylo′sus, presence in the peritoneal cavity of a milky fluid containing suspended fat, ordinarily caused by an obstruction or injury of the thoracic duct or cisterna. SYN a. adiposus, chyliform a., chyloperitoneum, fatty a., milky a.

  fatty a., SYN chylous a.

gelatinous a., SYN *pseudomyxoma* peritonei.

hemorrhagic a., bloody or blood-stained serous fluid, frequently resulting from metastatic carcinoma, in the peritoneal cavity.

milky a., SYN chylous a.

pseudochylous a., presence in the peritoneum of an opalescent or cloudy fluid that does not contain fat.

ascit·ic (ă-sit′ik). Relating to ascites.

as·ci·tog·e·nous (as-i-toj′ĕ-nŭs). Producing ascites.

Asclepias (as-klē′pē-as). A genus of plants (family Asclepiadaceae), commonly called milkweeds; some species, *e.g., A. eriocarpa* and *A. galioides,* are toxic to herbivorous animals and fowl. [G. *Asklēpios,* Aesculapius]

as·co·carp (as′kō-karp). A fungus structure, of varying complexity, which bears asci and ascospores. [G. *askos,* bag, + *karpos,* fruit]

as·cog·e·nous (as-koj′ĕ-nŭs). Denoting ascus-bearing fungus hypha or cell.

as·co·go·ni·um (as-kō-gō′nē-ŭm). The female cell in an ascomycete that is fertilized by the male cell.

Ascoli, Alberto, Italian serologist, 1877–1957. SEE Ascoli *reaction;* Ascoli's *test.*

As·co·my·ce·tes (as′kō-mī-sē′tēz). A class of fungi characterized by the presence of asci and ascospores. Such fungi have generally two distinct reproductive phases, the sexual or perfect stage and the asexual or imperfect stage. *Ajellomyces capsulatum* and *Ajellomyces dermatitidis* are pathogenic members of this class. [G. *askos,* a bag, + *mykēs,* mushroom]

as·co·my·ce·tous (as′kō-mī′sē-tus). Fungi related to the Ascomycota.

As·co·my·co·ta (as′kō-mī-kō-tă). A phylum of fungi characterized by the presence of asci and ascospores. Some mycologists have moved the class Ascomycetes to the phylum or division level.

as·cor·base (as-kōr′bās). SYN *ascorbate* oxidase.

ascor·bate (as-kōr′bāt). A salt or ester of ascorbic acid.

  a. oxidase, a copper-containing enzyme that catalyzes the oxidation of L-ascorbic acid with O_2 to L-dehydroascorbic acid. Some forms of a. use $NADP^+$ as well. Used as an antitumor enzyme. SYN ascorbase.

ascor·bic ac·id (as-kōr′bik). 2,3-didehydro-L-*threo*-hexono-1,4-lactone; used in preventing scurvy, as a strong reducing agent, and as an antioxidant in foodstuffs. SYN antiscorbutic vitamin, cevitamic acid, vitamin C. [G. *a*- priv. + Mod.L. *scorbutus,* scurvy, fr. Germanic]

ascor·byl pal·mi·tate (as-kōr′bil pal′mi-tāt). L-Ascorbic acid-6-palmitate; used as a preservative in pharmaceutical preparations.

as·co·spore (as′kō-spōr). A spore formed within an ascus; the sexual spore of Ascomycetes. [G. *askos,* bag, + *sporos,* seed]

as·cus, pl. **as·ci** (as′kŭs, as′ī). The saclike cell of Ascomycetes in which ascospores develop following nuclear fusion and meiosis. [G. *askos,* bag]

-ase. A termination denoting an enzyme, suffixed to the name of the substance (substrate) upon which the enzyme acts; *e.g.,* phosphatase, lipase, proteinase. May also indicate the reaction catalyzed *e.g.,* decarboxylase, oxidase. Enzymes named before the convention was established generally have an -*in* ending; *e.g.,* pepsin, ptyalin, trypsin. [Fr. *(diast)ase,* an amylase that converts starch to maltose, fr. G. *diastasis,* separation, fr. *dia*-, through, apart, + *stasis,* a standing]

ase·cre·to·ry (ā-sē-krē′tō-rē). Without secretion.

Aselli (Asellius, Asellio), Gasparo, Italian anatomist at Cremona, 1581–1626. SEE A.'s *gland, pancreas.*

as·e·ma·sia, ase·mia (as-ĕ-mā′zē-ă, ă-sē′mē-ă). SYN asymbolia. [G. *a*- priv. + *sēmasia,* the giving of a signal, fr. *sēma,* sign]

asep·sis (ă-sep′sis, ā-). A condition in which living pathogenic organisms are absent; a state of sterility (2). [G. *a*- priv. + *sēpsis,* putrefaction]

asep·tate (ă-sep′tāt, ā-). In fungi, a term describing absence of cross walls in a hyphal filament or a spore. [G. *a*- priv. + L. *saeptum,* a partition]

asep·tic (ă-sep′tik, ā-). Marked by or relating to asepsis.

asep·ti·cism (ă-sep′ti-sizm, ā-). The practice of aseptic surgery.

ase·quence (ă-sē′kwens). Lack of normal sequence, specifically, between atrial and ventricular contractions.

asex·u·al (ā-seks′yū-ăl). **1.** Referring to reproduction without nuclear fusion in an organism. **2.** Having no sexual desire or interest. [G. *a-* priv. + sexual]

ASF Abbreviation for African swine *fever.*

Ashby, Winifred, 20th century hematologist. SEE Ashby *method.*

Asherman, Joseph G., Czechoslovakian gynecologist, *1889. SEE A.'s *syndrome.*

Ashman, R., 20th century U.S. physiologist. SEE A.'s *phenomenon.*

Ashman's phe·nom·e·non. See under phenomenon.

asi·a·lo·gly·co·pro·tein (ā-sī-al′ō-glī-kō-prō-tēn). A glycoprotein without a sialic acid moiety; such proteins are recognized by a. receptors and are targeted for degradation.

asit·ia (ă-sish′ē-ă). Disgust at the sight or thought of food. [G. *a-* priv. + *sitos,* food]

Askanazy, Max, German pathologist, 1865–1940. SEE A. *cell.*

Ask-Upmark, E., 20th century Swedish pathologist. SEE Ask-Upmark *kidney.*

Asn Symbol for asparagine or its mono- or diradical.

aso·cial (ā-sō′shŭl). Not social; withdrawn from society; indifferent to social rules or customs; *e.g.,* a recluse, a regressed schizophrenic person, a schizoid personality. Cf. antisocial.

aso·ma, pl. **aso·ma·ta** (ā-sō′mă, -sō′mă-tă). A fetus with only a rudimentary body. [G. *a-* priv. + *sōma,* body]

Asp Symbol for aspartic acid or its radical forms.

as·pal·a·so·ma (as-pal-ă-sō′mă). Obsolete term for a malformed fetus with eventration at the lower part of the abdomen, presenting separate openings for intestine, bladder, and sexual organs. [G. *aspalax,* a mole + *soma,* body]

as·par·a·gi·nase (as-par′ă-ji-nās). **1.** L-Asparaginase; an enzyme catalyzing the hydrolysis of L-asparagine to L-aspartic acid and ammonia. **2.** The enzyme from *Escherichia coli,* used in the treatment of acute leukemia and other neoplastic diseases.

as·par·a·gine (N, Asn) (as-par′ă-jin). $NH_2COCH_2CH(NH_3^+)$ COO^-; α-amino-β-succinamic acid; the β-amide of aspartic acid, the L-isomer is a nonessential amino acid occurring in proteins; a diuretic. SYN aspармide.

a. ligase, an acid:ammonia ligase (amide synthetase) forming L-asparagine and L-glutamate from L-aspartate and L-glutamine, with the concomitant cleavage of ATP to AMP and pyrophosphate. Under nonphysiological conditions, the mammalian enzyme can use ammonia as the nitrogen donor. A. also displays a glutaminase-like activity. SYN a. synthetase.

a. synthetase, SYN a. ligase.

as·par·a·gin·ic ac·id (as′par-ă-jin′ik). SYN aspartic acid.

as·pa·rag·i·nyl (as-par′ă-jin-il). The aminoacyl radical of asparagine.

As·par·a·gus (as-par′ă-gŭs). A genus of plants of the family Liliaceae. *A. officinalis* is an edible vegetable, the rhizome and roots of which, together with the young edible shoots, are used as a diuretic. [L. fr. G. *asparagos*]

as·par·mide (as′par-mīd). SYN asparagine.

as·par·tame (as′par-tām). N-L-α-Aspartyl-Lphenylalanine 1-methyl ester; a low-calorie sweetening agent about 200 times as sweet as sucrose.

as·par·tase (as-par′tās). SYN *aspartate* ammonia-lyase.

as·par·tate (as-par′tāt). A salt or ester of aspartic acid.

a. aminotransferase (AST), an enzyme catalyzing the reversible transfer of an amine group from L-glutamic acid to oxaloacetic acid, forming α-ketoglutaric acid and L-aspartic acid; a diagnostic aid in viral hepatitis and in myocardial infarctions. SYN a. transaminase, glutamic-aspartic transaminase, glutamic-oxaloacetic transaminase, serum glutamic-oxaloacetic transaminase.

a. ammonia-lyase, a nonmammalian enzyme catalyzing the conversion of L-aspartic acid to fumaric acid, splitting out ammonia. SYN aspartase, fumaric aminase.

a. carbamoyltransferase, an enzyme catalyzing formation of ureidosuccinate (*N*-carbamoyl-L-aspartate) and P_i by the transfer of a carbamoyl moiety from carbamoylphosphate to the amino group of L-aspartate; participates in pyrimidine biosynthesis.

a. kinase, an enzyme catalyzing the phosphorylation by ATP of L-aspartate to form 4-phospho-L-aspartate (β-aspartyl phosphate) and ADP.

a. transaminase, SYN a. aminotransferase.

as·par·tate 1-de·car·box·yl·ase. SYN *glutamate* decarboxylase.

as·par·tate 4-de·car·box·yl·ase. Aspartate β-decarboxylase; a carboxy-lyase converting L-aspartate to L-alanine (releasing CO_2); it decarboxylates aminomalonate and (in bacteria) removes SO_2 from cysteinesulfinate. SEE ALSO desulfinase.

as·par·tic ac·id (Asp) (as-par′tik). $HOOC–CH_2–CH(NH_2)–COOH$; the L-isomer is one of the amino acids occurring in proteins. SYN α-aminosuccinic acid, asparaginic acid.

as·par·tyl (as-par′til). The aminoacyl radical of aspartic acid.

β-as·par·tyl(ace·tyl·glu·cos·a·mine) (as-par′til-as′e-til-glū′kō-să-mēn). Misnomer for 1-(β-asparagino)-*N*-acetylglucosamine or 1-(β-aspartamido)-*N*-acetylglucosamine, or, formally, 1-(β-L-aspartamido)-*N*-2-acetamido-1,2-dideoxy-β-D-glucose; a compound of *N*-acetylglucosamine and asparagine, linked via the amide nitrogen of the latter and carbon-1 of the former. An important structural linkage in many glycoproteins.

as·par·tyl·gly·co·sa·mine (as-par′til-glī′kō-să-mēn). Generic term for compounds of asparagine and a 2-amino sugar; *e.g.,* β-aspartyl(acetylglucosamine).

as·par·tyl·gly·cos·a·mi·nid·ase (as-par′til-glī′kō-să-mi-ni-dās). A hydrolytic enzyme that cleaves off L-aspartate from aspartyl-glycosamines. A deficiency of a. can result in aspartylglycosaminuria.

as·par·tyl·gly·cos·a·mi·nu·ria (as-par′til-glī′kō-să-mi-nūr′ē-ă) [MIM*208400]. One of the disorders of glycoprotein catabolism resulting from the absence of aspartylglycosamine amidohydrolase, characterized by aspartylglycosamine in the urine and spinal fluid. Symptoms develop in the first months of life, with recurrent infections and diarrhea. Mental retardation, coarse facial features, and skeletal abnormalities are evident by adolescence.

as·pect (as′pekt). **1.** The manner of appearance; looks. **2.** The side of an object that is directed in any designated direction. [L. *aspectus,* fr. *a-spicio,* pp. *-spectus,* to look at]

as·per·gil·lic ac·id (as-per-jil′ik). 2-Hydroxy-3-isobutyl-6-(1-methylpropyl)pyrazine-1-oxide; produced by *Aspergillus flavus;* an antibiotic agent moderately active against Gram-positive and Gram-negative bacteria, but toxic to animal tissues.

as·per·gil·lin (as-per-jil′in). A black pigment obtained from various species of *Aspergillus;* improperly used to designate various antibiotics obtained from *Aspergillus.*

as·per·gil·lo·ma (as′per-ji-lō′mă). **1.** An infectious granuloma caused by *Aspergillus.* **2.** A variety of bronchopulmonary aspergillosis; a ball-like mass of *Aspergillis fumigatus* colonizing an existing cavity in the lung. [aspergillus + -oma, tumor]

as·per·gil·lo·my·co·sis (as′per-ji-lō′sis). SYN aspergillosis. [aspergillus + G. *mykēs,* fungus, + -osis, condition]

as·per·gil·lo·sis (as′per-ji-lō′sis). **1.** The presence of *Aspergillus* in the tissues or on a mucous surface of humans and animals, and the symptoms produced thereby. **2.** Infection of the lungs and air sacs of birds, especially chickens and turkeys, with *Aspergillus fumigatus,* frequently introduced in spoiled, moldy feed. SYN aspergillomycosis.

bronchopneumonic a. (brong′kō-nū-mon′ik), SYN bronchopulmonary a.

bronchopulmonary a., an inflammatory and destructive disease of the bronchi and lungs due to the presence and growth of *Aspergillus fumigatus.* There are four varieties: 1) a bronchial infection with allergic manifestations, in which the fungus grows in the mucus (evoked by the inflammation), which may be expectorated as yellow bronchial casts and may cause intermittent bronchial obstruction, with transient pulmonary shadows seen radiographically; asthma is often present, and bronchial wall

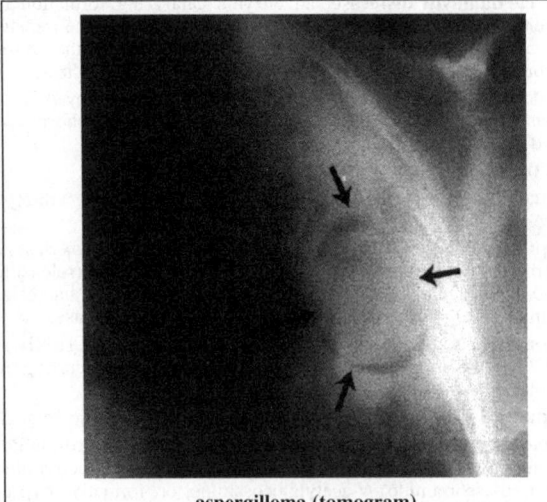

aspergilloma (tomogram)
fungal infection in a tuberculous lung cavern

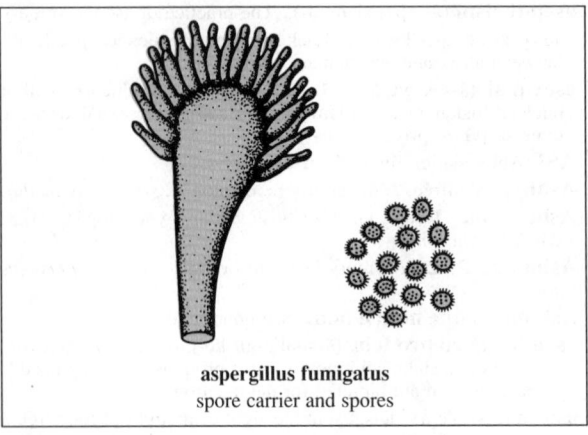

aspergillus fumigatus
spore carrier and spores

destruction may eventually result in a proximal form of bronchiectasis; 2) aspergilloma; 3) an infection with pulmonary necrosis as a pneumonic involvement of the lung in debilitated subjects; 4) disseminated a. SYN bronchopneumonic a., pulmonary a.

disseminated a., a variety of bronchopulmonary a., characterized by a generalized infection of the lung with *Aspergillus* occurring usually in subjects with defective immune response.

invasive a., so-called because of the peculiar predilection of *Aspergillus fumigatus* to invade blood vessels and cause tissue infarction; it is second only to candidiasis as a cause of opportunistic fungal infection in patients whose immune mechanisms have been suppressed by chemotherapy.

pulmonary a., SYN bronchopulmonary a.

As·per·gil·lus (as-per-jil′ŭs). A genus of fungi (class Ascomycetes) that contains many species, a number of them with black, brown, or green spores. A few species are pathogenic for man, other animals, and avians. There are about 300 species in this genus. [Med. L. a sprinkler, fr. L. *aspergo,* to sprinkle]

A. clava′tus, a species isolated from soil and feces; it yields a carcinogenic mycotoxin known as patulin.

A. fla′vus, a species with yellow-green conidia that is found growing on grains; may produce aflatoxin, which is the cause of aflatoxicosis in poultry and cattle, and is carcinogenic for rats and humans; occasionally causes aspergillosis in humans and animals.

A. fumiga′tus, a species that yields the antibiotics fumigacin and fumigatin, and is the common cause of aspergillosis in humans and birds.

A. nid′ulans, a species that causes one form of mycetoma, and occasionally causes aspergillosis in humans and other animals.

A. ni′ger, a pathogenic species with black spores, often present in the external auditory meatus but not necessarily pathogenic; used in the commercial manufacturing of citric and gluconic acids.

A. ter′reus, a species that produces the antibiotic citrinin; it has been isolated from otomycosis, especially in Japan and Taiwan, and occasionally causes aspergillosis in humans and animals.

asper·mat·o·gen·ic (ā-sper′mă-tō-jen′ik, ă-sper′). Failing in the production of spermatozoa. [G. *a-* priv. + *sperma,* seed, + *-gen,* production]

asper·mia (ā-sper′mē-ă, ă-sper′). Lack of secretion or expulsion of semen following ejaculation.

as·per·sion (as-per′zhŭn). A form of hydrotherapy in which water of a given temperature is sprinkled on the body. [L. *aspersio,* a sprinkling]

aspher·ic (ā-sfer′ik). Denoting a paraboloidal surface, especially of a lens or mirror, that eliminates spherical aberration. [G. *a-* priv. + *sphaira,* sphere]

as·phyg·mia (as-fig′mē-ă). Temporary absence of pulse. [G. *a-* priv. + *sphygmos,* pulse]

as·phyx·ia (as-fik′sē-ă). Impaired or absent exchange of oxygen and carbon dioxide on a ventilatory basis; combined hypercapnia and hypoxia or anoxia. [G. *a-* priv. + *sphyzō,* to throb]

blue a., SYN a. livida.

cyanotic a., a. to the point of sufficient destruction of hemoglobin to produce cyanosis.

a. liv′ida, a form of a. neonatorum in which the skin is cyanotic, but the heart is strong and the reflexes are preserved. SYN blue a.

local a., stagnation of the circulation, sometimes resulting in local gangrene, especially of the fingers; one of the symptoms usually associated with Raynaud's disease.

a. neonato′rum, a. occurring in the newborn.

a. pal′lida, a form of a. of the newborn, in which the skin is pale, the pulse weak and slow, and the reflexes absent.

symmetric a., SYN Raynaud's *syndrome.*

traumatic a., cyanotic a. due to trauma; the extravasation of blood into the skin and conjunctivae, produced by a sudden mechanical increase in venous pressure, analogous to the Rumpel-Leede test; it is common in those who have been hanged, and is seen occasionally in crush injuries. SYN pressure stasis.

as·phyx·i·al (as-fik′sē-ăl). Relating to asphyxia.

as·phyx·i·ant (as-fik′sē-ănt). **1.** Producing asphyxia. SYN asphyxiating. **2.** Anything, especially a gas, that produces asphyxia.

as·phyx·i·ate (as-fik′sē-āt). To induce asphyxia.

as·phyx·i·at·ing (as-fik′sē-āt-ing). SYN asphyxiant (1).

as·phyx·i·a·tion (as-fik-sē-ā′shŭn). The production of, or the state of, asphyxia.

As·pic·u·lu·ris tet·rap·tera (as-pik-yū-lū′ris tet-rap′ter-ă). The mouse pinworm, an abundant oxyurid nematode of the mouse cecum or large intestine, along with another common oxyurid pinworm of mice, *Syphacia obvelata;* it is also found in other rodents, including *Rattus.* [Pers. *espic,* fr. L. *spica,* ear, spike; *tetra-* + *pteron,* feather, wing]

as·pid·in (as-pid′in). A toxic active principle, $C_{25}H_{32}O_8$, contained in aspidium.

as·pid·i·nol (as-pid′i-nol). An alcohol, $C_{12}H_{16}O_4$, occurring in aspidium.

as·pid·i·um (as-pid′ē-ŭm). The rhizomes and stipes of *Dryopteris filix-mas* (European a. or male fern), or of *Dryopteris marginalis* (American a. or marginal fern) (family Polypodiaceae); used in the treatment of tapeworm infestation, usually in the form of the oleoresin or extract, but because of its potential toxicity, its use is restricted to patients who do not respond to treatment with safer drugs such as dichlorophen, niclosamide, or quinacrine. [G. *aspidion,* a little shield, dim. of *aspis,* shield]

as·pi·do·sam·ine (as'pi-dō-sam'ēn). A strong base, $C_{22}H_{28}N_2O_2$, derived from quebracho; a toxic irritant.

as·pi·do·sper·mine (as'pi-dō-sper'mēn). An alkaloid, $C_{22}H_{30}N_2O_2$, obtained from quebracho, an irritant.

as·pi·rate. 1 (as'pi-rāt). To remove by aspiration. **2** (as'pi-rit). The substance removed by aspiration. [L. *a-spiro*, pp. *-atus*, to breathe on, give the H sound]

as·pi·ra·tion (as-pi-rā'shŭn). **1.** Removal, by suction, of a gas or fluid from a body cavity, from unusual accumulations, or from a container. **2.** The inspiratory sucking into the airways of fluid or foreign body, as of vomitus. **3.** A surgical technique for cataract, requiring a small corneal incision, severance of the lens capsule, fragmentation of the lens material, and removal with a needle. [L. *aspiratio*, fr. *aspiro*, to breathe on]

meconium a., intrauterine a. by the fetus of amniotic fluid contaminated by meconium resulting from fetal hypoxic distress.

as·pi·ra·tor (as'pi-rā-ter, -tōr). An apparatus for removing fluid by aspiration from any of the body cavities; it consists usually of a hollow needle or trocar and cannula, connected by tubing with a container vacuumized by a syringe or reversed air (suction) pump.

vacuum a., an instrument for removing the products of conception by suction after cervical dilation.

water a., a jet ejector pump operated by water and commonly used as a laboratory suction pump.

as·pi·rin (as'pi-rin). $C_6H_4(OCOCH_3)COOH$; a widely used analgesic, antipyretic, and anti-inflammatory agent; also used as an antiplatelet agent. SYN acetylsalicylic acid.

asple·nia (ă-splē'nē-ă). Congenital absence of the spleen.

functional a., absence of splenic function due to spontaneous infarction of the spleen, as occurs in sickle cell *anemia.*

asplen·ic (ă-splen'ik). Having no spleen.

aspo·rog·e·nous (as-pō-roj'ĕ-nŭs). Not producing spores. [G. *a*-priv. + *sporos*, seed, + *-gen*, production]

aspo·rous (as-pōr'ŭs). Incapable of producing spores. [G. *a*-priv. + *sporos*, seed]

aspor·u·late (as-pōr'yū-lāt). Nonsporeforming.

as·sas·sin bug (ă-sas'in). An insect of the family Reduviidae (order Hemiptera) that inflicts irritating, painful bites in animals and man; related to the cone-nosed bugs (triatomines), a vector of American trypanosomiasis. [Fr., fr. It. *assassino*, fr. Ar. *hashshāshin*, those addicted to hashish]

as·say (as'sā, ă-sā'). **1.** Test of purity; trial. **2.** To examine; to subject to analysis. **3.** The quantitative or qualitative evaluation of a substance for impurities, toxicity, etc; the results of such an evaluation. [M.E>, fr. O>Fr. *essaier*, fr. L>L> *exagium*, a weighing]

Ames a., SYN Ames *test.*

biological a., SYN biotest.

clonogenic a., *in vitro* culturing of neoplastic cells to test their radiosensitivity or chemosensitivity, and probable clinical efficacy of a therapeutic agent.

competitive binding a., general term for an a. in which a binder competes for labeled versus unlabeled ligand; following separation of free and bound ligand, the ligand (the analyte assayed) is quantitated by relating bound and unbound ratios to known standards. SEE ALSO enzyme-linked immunosorbent a., radioreceptor a., immunoassay, enzyme-multiplied *immunoassay* technique, radioimmunoassay. SYN displacement analysis, saturation analysis.

complement binding a., a test for the detection of immune complexes.

double antibody sandwich a., for antigen; an application of the ELISA method in which material being tested for antigen is added to wells coated with known antibody; the presence of antigen fixed to the antibody coat can be determined either directly, by adding human antibody linked to the enzyme of the indicator system, or indirectly, by first adding unlabeled known antibody, the attachment of which to the antigen can be demonstrated by addition of immunoglobulin-specific antibody linked to the enzyme.

EAC rosette a. (ro-zet' as'sā), SEE EAC *rosette.*

enzyme-linked immunosorbent a. (ELISA), a sensitive method for serodiagnosis of specific infectious diseases; an *in vitro* competitive binding a. in which an enzyme and its substrate serve as the indicator system rather than a radioactive substance; in positive tests, the two yield a colored or other easily recognizable substance; tests are made in wells in polystyrene or other material to which immunoglobulins or antigenic (viral or other) preparations readily adsorb; the enzyme is linked to known immunoglobulin (or antigen) and in positive tests remains in the well as part of the antigen-antibody complex available to react with its substrate when added.

Grunstein-Hogness a., a procedure for identifying plasmid clones by colony hybridization.

hemizona a. (hem'ē-zō-nă), diagnostic test evaluating the binding capacity of sperm to the zona pellucida.

immunochemical a., SYN immunoassay.

immunoradiometric a., an a. that differs from conventional radioimmunoassay in that the compound to be measured combines directly with radioactively labeled antibodies.

indirect a., for antibody; an application of the ELISA method in which serum being tested for antibody is added to wells coated with known antigen; presence of antibody bound to the antigen coat can be determined by addition of immunoglobulin-specific antibody to which is linked the enzyme of the indicator system, followed by addition of substrate to the washed aggregate.

Lowry-Folin a., SYN Lowry protein a.

Lowry protein a., a method for determining protein concentrations using the Folin-Ciocalteu reagent. SYN Lowry-Folin a.

radioreceptor a., a competitive binding a. in which the binder is a membrane or tissue receptor rather than an antibody.

Raji cell radioimmune a., for immune complexes; a procedure by which immune complexes adsorbed from a test serum by a standard preparation of lymphoblastoid (Raji) cells are assayed by the capacity to bind ^{125}I-labeled antibody to immunoglobulin.

Assézat, Jules, French anthropologist, 1832–1876. SEE A.'s *triangle.*

as·sim·i·la·ble (ă-sim'i-lă-bl). Capable of undergoing assimilation. SEE assimilation.

as·sim·i·la·tion (ă-sim-i-lā'shŭn). **1.** Incorporation of digested materials from food into the tissues. **2.** Amalgamation and modification of newly perceived information and experiences into the existing cognitive structure. [L. *as-similo*, pp. *-atus*, to make alike]

ammonia a., the utilization of ammonia (or ammonium ions) in the net synthesis of nitrogen-containing molecules; *e.g.,* glutamine synthetase. SYN ammonia fixation.

reproductive a., in sensorimotor theory, an active cognitive process by which past experience is applied to novel situations.

Assmann, Herbert, German internist, 1882–1950. SEE A.'s tuberculous *infiltrate.*

as·so·ci·ate. 1 (ă-sō'shi-ăt). Any item or individual grouped with others by some common factor. **2** (ă-sō'shē-āt). To accomplish association.

paired a.'s, words, syllables, digits, or other items learned in pairs, so that when one is given, its a. is to be recalled.

as·so·ci·a·tion (ă-sō-sē-ā'shŭn). **1.** A connection of persons, things, or ideas by some common factor. **2.** A functional connection of two ideas, events, or psychological phenomena established through learning or experience. SEE ALSO conditioning. **3.** Statistical dependence between two or more events, characteristics, or other variables. [L. *as-socio*, pp. *-sociatus*, to join to; *ad + socius*, companion]

clang a., psychic a.'s resulting from sounds; often encountered in the manic phase of manic-depressive psychosis.

dream a.'s, the memories and emotions mentioned by a patient trying to understand a dream at the request of a psychoanalyst.

free a., an investigative psychoanalytic technique in which the patient verbalizes, without reservation or censor, the passing contents of his or her mind; the verbalized conflicts that emerge constitute resistances that are the basis of the psychoanalyst's interpretations.

genetic a., the occurrence together in a population, more often than can be readily explained by chance, of two or more traits of which at least one is known to be genetic.

loose a.'s, a manifestation of a thought disorder whereby the patient's responses do not relate to the interviewer's questions or one paragraph, sentence, or phrase is not logically connected to those that occur before or after.

as·so·ci·a·tion·ism (ă-sō-sē-ā′shŭn-izm). In psychology, the theory that man's understanding of the world occurs through ideas associated with sensory experience rather than through innate ideas.

as·sort·ment (ă-sōrt′ment). In genetics, the relationship between nonallelic genetic traits that are transmitted from parent to child more or less independently in accordance with the degree of linkage between the respective loci.

independent a., the pattern of transmission of unlinked loci.

as·sump·tion. Belief posited at the outset of an argument as a basis for deduction and inference. Commonly confused with a hypothesis, a conclusion at the end of the argument or an inference based on empirical data.

AST Abbreviation for *aspartate* aminotransferase.

asta·sia (ă-stā′zē-ă). Inability, through muscular incoordination, to stand. [G. unsteadiness, from *a*-priv. + *stasis*, standing]

asta·sia-aba·sia (ă-stā′zē-ă-ă-bā′zē-ă). The inability to either stand or walk in a normal manner; the gait is bizarre and is not suggestive of a specific organic lesion; often the patient sways wildly and nearly falls, but recovers at the last moment; a symptom of hysteria-conversion reaction. SYN Blocq's disease.

astat·ic (ā-stat′ik). Pertaining to astasia.

as·ta·tine (At) (as′tă-tēn). An artificial radioactive element of the halogen series; atomic no. 85, atomic wt. 211. [G. *astatos*, unstable]

aste·a·to·des (ă-stē-ă-tō′dēz). SYN asteatosis.

aste·a·to·sis (ă-stē-ă-tō′sis). Diminished or arrested secretion of the sebaceous glands. SYN asteatodes. [G. *a*- priv. + *stear* (*steat*-), fat]

a. cu′tis, dry, scaly integument with decrease in sebaceous secretion.

astem·i·zole. An H-1 type histamine-blocking drug with low sedating tendency.

as·ter (as′ter). SYN astrosphere. [Mod. L. fr. G. *astēr*, a star]

sperm a., SEE sperm-aster.

aster·e·og·no·sis (ă-stēr-og-nō′sis). SYN tactile *agnosia*. [G. *a*-priv. + *stereos*, solid + *gnōsis*, knowledge]

as·te·ri·on (ăs-tē′rē-on). A craniometric point in the region of the posterolateral, or mastoid, fontanel, at the junction of the lambdoid, occipitomastoid and parietomastoid sutures. [G. *asterios*, starry]

as·ter·i·o·sap·on·ins (ă-stēr′ē-ō-sap′ō-ninz). SYN asteriosaponins. SYN asteriosaponins.

as·ter·i·o·tox·ins (ă-stēr′ē-ō-tok′sinz). Toxic steroids produced by starfish (Asteroidea).

aster·ix·is (as-ter-ik′sis). Involuntary jerking movements, especially in the hands, best elicited by having the patient extend the arms, dorsiflex the wrists, and spread the fingers; due to arrhythmic lapses of sustained posture; seen primarily with various metabolic and toxic encephalopathies, especially hepatic encephalopathy. SYN flapping tremor. [G. *a*- priv. + *stērixis*, fixed position]

aster·nal (ā-ster′năl). **1.** Not related to or connected with the sternum, *e.g.,* a. rib. **2.** Without a sternum. [G. *a*- priv. + *sternon*, chest]

aster·nia (ă-ster′nē-ă). Congenital absence of the sternum.

As·ter·o·coc·cus. SYN *Mycoplasma*. [Mod. L. fr. G. *astēr*, a star, + *kokkos*, a berry]

as·ter·oid (as′tĕ-royd). Resembling a star. [G. *astēr*, star, + *eidos*, resemblance]

as·the·nia (as-thē′nē-ă). Weakness or debility. SYN adynamia (1). [G. *astheneia*, weakness, fr. *a*- priv. + *sthenos*, strength]

neurocirculatory a., an obsolete term for a type of anxiety neurosis formerly encountered often among military personnel during times of war, in which cardiorespiratory symptoms, such as palpitation, rapid pulse, and precordial pain, were prominent. SYN DaCosta's syndrome, effort syndrome.

as·then·ic (as-then′ik). **1.** Relating to asthenia. **2.** Denoting a thin, delicate body habitus.

as·the·no·pia (as-thĕ-nō′pē-ă). Subjective symptoms of ocular fatigue, discomfort, lacrimation, and headaches arising from use of the eyes. SYN eyestrain. [G. *astheneia*, weakness, + *ōps*, eye]

accommodative a., a. due to errors of refraction and excessive contraction of the ciliary muscle.

muscular a., a. due to imbalance of the extrinsic ocular muscles.

nervous a., a. due to functional or organic nervous disease.

as·the·nop·ic (as-thĕ-nop′ik). Relating to or suffering from asthenopia.

as·the·no·sper·mia (as-thē-nō-sper′mē-ă). Loss or reduction of motility of the spermatozoa, frequently associated with infertility. [G. *astheneia*, weakness, + *sperma*, seed, semen]

asth·ma (az′mă). Originally, a term used to mean "difficult breathing"; now used to denote bronchial a. [G.]

atopic a., bronchial a. due to atopy.

bronchial a., a condition of the lungs in which there is widespread narrowing of airways, varying over short periods of time either spontaneously or as a result of treatment, due in varying degrees to contraction (spasm) of smooth muscle, edema of the mucosa, and mucus in the lumen of the bronchi and bronchioles; these changes are caused by the local release of spasmogens and vasoactive substances (*e.g.,* histamine, or certain leukotrienes or prostaglandins) in the course of an allergic process.

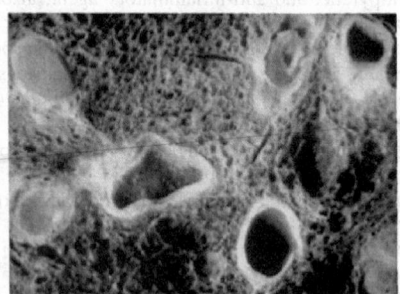

bronchial asthma (cross-section of lung)
mucus blocks the passages

bronchitic a., a. precipitated by bronchitis. SYN catarrhal a.

cardiac a., an asthmatic attack, the bronchoconstriction being secondary to the pulmonary congestion and edema of left ventricular failure.

catarrhal a., SYN bronchitic a.

cotton-dust a., SYN byssinosis.

dust a., a. aggravated by inhalation of dust, especially seen as occupational disease resulting from cotton dust.

extrinsic a., bronchial a. resulting from an allergic reaction to foreign substances, such as inhaled particles, vapors, or gases, or ingested foods, beverages, or drugs.

food a., a. caused by allergic reaction to a dietary item.

hay a., an asthmatic stage of hay fever.

intrinsic a., bronchial a. in which no extrinsic causes can be identified, and which is assumed to be due to an endogenous process, possibly allergic.

miller's a., a. caused by flour or grain allergens.

miner's a., the dyspnea of anthracosis or other pneumoconioses in miners.

nervous a., a. precipitated by psychic stress.

reflex a., a. occurring as a reflex in disease of the viscera, the nose, or other parts.

spasmodic a., a. due to spasm of the bronchioles.

steam-fitter's a., a. associated with asbestosis acquired by exposure to asbestos-insulated heating and plumbing components.

stripper's a., a. associated with byssinosis.

summer a., a. associated with hay fever or allergy to summer vegetation.

asth·mat·ic (az-mat′ik). Relating to or suffering from asthma.

asth·ma-weed. **1.** SYN lobelia. **2.** SYN *Euphorbia pilulifera.*

asth·mo·gen·ic (az′mō-jen′ik). Causing asthma.

as·tig·mat·ic (as′tig-mat′ik). Relating to or suffering from astigmatism.

astig·ma·tism (ă-stig′mă-tizm). **1.** A lens or optical system having different refractivity in different meridians. **2.** A condition of unequal curvatures along the different meridians in one or more of the refractive surfaces (cornea, anterior or posterior surface of the lens) of the eye, in consequence of which the rays from a luminous point are not focused at a single point on the retina. SYN astigmia. [G. *a-* priv. + *stigma* (*stig- mat-*), a point]
a. against the rule, a. when the greater curvature or refractive power is in the horizontal meridian.
compound hyperopic a., a. in which all meridians are hyperopic but to different degrees.
compound myopic a., a. in which all meridians are myopic but to different degrees.
corneal a., a. due to a defect in the curvature of the corneal surface.
hyperopic a., that form of a. in which one meridian is hyperopic and the one at right angle to it is without a refractive error. SYN simple hyperopic a.
irregular a., a. in which different parts of the same meridian have different degrees of curvature.
lenticular a., a. due to defect in the curvature, position, or index of refraction of the lens.
mixed a., a. in which one meridian is hyperopic while the one at right angle to it is myopic.
myopic a., that form of a. in which one meridian is myopic and the one at right angle to it is without refractive error. SYN simple myopic a.
a. of oblique pencils, an aberration occurring when a bundle of light rays strikes a refracting medium in some other direction than parallel to the axis of the lens.
regular a., a. in which the curvature in each meridian is equal throughout its course, and the meridians of greatest and least curvature are at right angles to each other.
simple hyperopic a., SYN hyperopic a.
simple myopic a., SYN myopic a.
a. with the rule, a. when the greater curvature or refractive power is in the vertical meridian.

astig·ma·tom·e·try, as·tig·mom·e·try (ă-stig-mă-tom′ĕ-trē, as-tig-mom′ĕ-trē). Determination of the form and measurement of the degree of astigmatism.

astig·mia (ă-stig′mē-ă). SYN astigmatism.

asto·ma·tous (ă-stō′mă-tŭs). Without a mouth. SYN astomous.

asto·mia (ă-stō′mē-ă). Congenital absence of a mouth. [G. *a-* priv. + *stoma,* mouth]

asto·mous (ă-stō′mŭs). SYN astomatous.

as·trag·a·lar (as-trag′ă-lar). Relating to the astragalus or talus.

as·trag·a·lec·to·my (as-trag-ă-lek′tō-mē). Removal of the astragalus, or talus. [astragalus, + G. *ektomē,* excision]

as·trag·a·lo·cal·ca·ne·an (as-trag′ă-lō-kal-kā′nē-an). Relating to both the talus (astragalus) and the calcaneus (os calcis).

as·trag·a·lo·fib·u·lar (as-trag′ă-lō-fib′yū-lar). Relating to both the talus (astragalus) and the fibula.

as·trag·a·lo·scaph·oid (as-trag′ă-lō-scaf′oyd). SYN talonavicular.

as·trag·a·lo·tib·i·al (as-trag′ă-lō-tib′ē-ăl). Relating to both the talus (astragalus) and the tibia.

As·trag·a·lus (as-trag′ă-lŭs). A genus of plants (family Leguminosae), notably *A. mollissimus* (locoweed) on the range lands of western North America, capable of taking selenium from the soil and causing poisoning in sheep, cattle, and horses. *A. gummifer* is a source of tragacanth.

as·tral (as′trăl). Relating to an astrosphere.

as·tra·po·pho·bia (as′tră-pō-fō′bē-ă). Morbid fear of lightning. [G. *astrapē,* lightning, + *phobos,* fear]

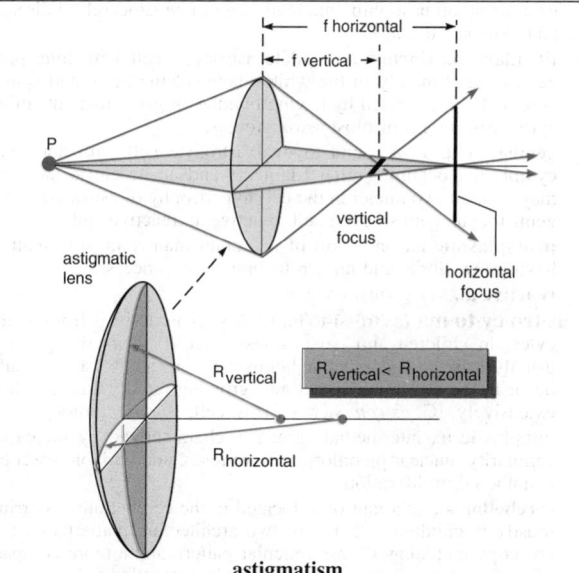

astigmatism
in an astigmatic lens, the curvatures (R) in the two meridians are unequal; thus the lens has two different focal distances and a point P appears as a line (horizontal and vertical focus); in the region between the two focal points, P appears as an ellipse

as·tric·tion (as-trik′shŭn). **1.** Astringent action. **2.** Compression to arrest hemorrhage.

as·trin·gent (as-trin′jent). **1.** Causing contraction of the tissues, arrest of secretion, or control of bleeding. **2.** An agent having these effects. [L. *astringens*]

as·tro·blast (as′trō-blast). A primitive cell developing into an astrocyte. [G. *astron,* star, + *blastos,* germ]

as·tro·blas·to·ma (as′trō-blas-tō′mă). A relatively poorly differentiated glioma composed of young, immature, neoplastic cells of the astrocytic series, frequently arranged radially with short fibrils terminating on small blood vessels. [astro- + G. *blastos,* germ, + *-oma,* tumor]

as·tro·cele (as′trō-sēl). SYN centrosphere. [G. *astron,* star, + *koilia,* hollow]

as·tro·cyte (as′trō-sīt). One of the large neuroglia cells of nervous tissue. SEE ALSO neuroglia. SYN astroglia cell, astroglia, Cajal's cell (2), Deiters' cells (2), macroglia cell, macroglia, spider cell (1). [G. *astron,* star, + *kytos,* hollow (cell)]

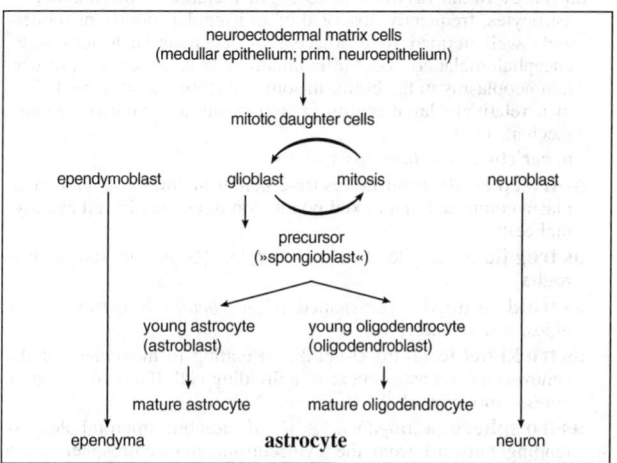

astrocyte

Alzheimer type I a., enlarged frequently multinucleated a.'s, seen in progressive multifocal leukoencephalopathy.

Alzheimer type II a., enlarged a.'s with vesicular nuclei and one or more small basophilic nucleoli, seen in hepatocerebral disease and Wilson's disease.

fibrillary a., fibrous a., stellate astrocytic cell with long processes found mainly in the white matter of the brain and spinal cord and characterized by having bundles of glial filaments in its cytoplasm; origin of most astrocytomas.

gemistocytic a., a round to oval astrocyte cell with abundant cytoplasm containing glial filaments and an eccentric nucleus; may contain two nuclei in the cell hypertrophy of astrocytes. SYN gemistocyte, gemistocytic cell, reactive a., reactive cell.

protoplasmic a., one form of a., found mainly in gray matter, having few fibrils and numerous branching processes.

reactive a., SYN gemistocytic a.

as·tro·cy·to·ma (as'trō-sī-tō'mă). A glioma derived from astrocytes; in children and persons less than 20 years of age, a.'s usually arise in a cerebellar hemisphere; in adults, a.'s usually occur in the cerebrum, sometimes growing rapidly and invading extensively. [G. *astron*, star, + *kytos*, cell, + *-oma*, tumor]

anaplastic a., intermediate grade a. characterized by increased cellularity, nuclear pleomorphism, mitoses, and variable vascular endothelial proliferation.

cerebellar a., a variant of a. located in the cerebellum occurring mostly in children, consists of two architectural patterns on microscopy including a loose reticular pattern and a more compact often spindled cell pattern. SYN juvenile cerebellar a.

desmoplastic cerebral a., a rare variant of a. most frequently occurring in infancy, the tumor has a spindled cell appearance.

fibrillary a., a. derived from fibrillary astrocytes.

gemistocytic a., an astrocytoma composed primarily of gemistocytic-type astrocytes. SYN gemistocytoma.

grade I a., solid or cystic a. of high differentiation or low grade.

grade II a., a. of intermediate grade.

grade III a., a. of intermediate grade. SEE ALSO glioblastoma multiforme.

grade IV a., SYN glioblastoma multiforme.

juvenile cerebellar a., SYN cerebellar a.

low grade a., a. characterized by an increased cellularity of uneven distribution and mild nuclear pleomorphism.

piloid astrocytoma, SYN plocytic a.

plocytic a., a slowing growing a. composed histologically of elongated fibrous astrocytes; often located in the optic chiasm or hypothalamus. SYN piloid astrocytoma.

protoplasmic a., a neoplasm composed primarily of protoplasmic-type astrocytes.

subependymal giant cell a., a rare a., frequently located in the wall of the lateral ventricle, comprised of large glial cells with abundant eosinophilic cytoplasm and intermixed elongated astrocytes, associated with tuberous sclerosis.

as·tro·cy·to·sis (as'trō-sī-tō'sis). An increase in the number of astrocytes, frequently observed in an irregular, poorly or moderately well defined zone adjacent to degenerative lesions (*e.g.,* encephalomalacia), focal inflammations (*e.g.,* abscesses), or certain neoplasms in the brain; in some instances, a. may be diffuse in a relatively large region; a. represents a reparative defense mechanism.

a. cer'ebri, SYN *gliomatosis* cerebri.

as·tro·ep·en·dy·mo·ma (as'trō-ē-pen'di-mō'mă). A glial neoplasm composed of a mixed population of astrocytic and ependymal cells.

as·trog·lia (as-trog'lē-ă). SYN astrocyte. [G. *astron*, star, + neuroglia]

as·troid (as'troyd). Star-shaped. [G. *astroeidēs*, fr. *astron*, star, + *eidos*, resemblance]

as·tro·ki·net·ic (as'trō-ki-net'ik). Relating to movement of the centrosome and astrosphere of a dividing cell. [G. *astron*, star, + *kinēsis*, movement]

as·tro·sphere (as'trō-sfēr). A set of radiating microtubules extending outward from the cytocentrum and centrosphere of a dividing cell. SYN aster, attraction sphere, Lavdovsky's nucleoid, paranuclear body. [G. *astron*, star, + *sphaira*, ball]

Astrup, Poul, Danish clinical chemist, *1915. SEE micro-A. method.

Astwood, Edwin B., U.S. endocrinologist, 1909–1976. SEE A.'s test.

as·ver·in (as'ver-in). 1-Methyl-3-piperidylidenedi(2-thienyl)-methane; an antitussive.

Asx. Symbol meaning Asp or Asn.

asyl·la·bia (ā-si-lā'bē-ă). Form of alexia in which one recognizes individual letters, but cannot comprehend them when arranged collectively in syllables or words. [G. *a-* priv. + *syllablē*, syllable]

asy·lum (ă-sī'lŭm). Old term for an institution for the housing and care of those who by reason of age or mental or bodily infirmities are unable to care for themselves. [L. fr. G. *asylon*, a sanctuary, fr. *a-* priv. + *sylē*, right of seizure]

asym·bo·lia (ă-sim-bō'lē-ă). A form of aphasia in which the significance of signs and symbols is not appreciated. SYN sight blindness. SYN asemasia, asemia. [G. *a-* priv. + *symbolon*, an outward sign]

asym·met·ric (a) (ā-sim-et'rik). Not symmetrical; denoting a lack of symmetry between two or more like parts.

asym·me·try (ā-sim'e-trē). 1. Lack of symmetry; disproportion between two normally alike parts; 2. Significant difference in amplitude or frequency of EEG activity recorded simultaneously from the two sides of the brain under identical conditions. SYN dissymmetry.

asymp·tom·at·ic (ā'simp-tō-mat'ik). Without symptoms, or producing no symptoms.

asymp·tot·ic (ā'simp-tot'ik). Pertaining to a limiting value, for example of a dependent variable, when the independent variable approaches zero or infinity.

asyn·cli·tism (ă-sin'kli-tizm). Absence of synclitism or parallelism between the axis of the presenting part of the child and the pelvic planes in childbirth. SYN obliquity. [G. *a-* priv. + *synklino*, to incline together]

anterior a., SYN Nägele *obliquity.*

posterior a., SYN Litzmann *obliquity.*

asyn·de·sis (ă-sin'dĕ-sis). 1. Rarely used term for a mental defect in which separate ideas or thoughts cannot be joined into a coherent concept. 2. A breaking up of the connecting links in language, said to be characteristic of the language disturbance of schizophrenics. [G. *a-* priv. + *syn*, together, + *desis*, binding]

asyn·ech·ia (ă-si-nek'ē-ă). Discontinuity of structure. [G. *a-* priv. + *synecheia*, continuity]

asy·ner·gia (ă-sin-er'jē-ă). SYN asynergy. [G. *a-* priv. + *syn*, with, + *ergon*, work]

asyn·er·gic (ā'sin-er'jik). Characterized by asynergia.

asyn·er·gy (ă-sin'er-jē). Lack of coordination among various muscle groups during the performance of complex movements, resulting in loss of skill and speed. When severe, results in decomposition of movement, wherein complex motor acts are performed in a series of isolated movements; caused by cerebellar disorders. SYN asynergia.

asy·ne·sia, asyn·e·sis (ă-si-nē'zē-ă, -nē'sis). Lack of easy comprehension and practical intelligence. [G. *a-* priv. + *synesis*, union, understanding]

asys·tem·at·ic (ā'sis-tĕ-mat'ik). Not systematic; not relating to one system or set of organs.

asys·to·le (ă-sis'tō-lē). Absence of contractions of the heart. SYN asystolia, cardiac standstill. [G. *a-* priv, + *systolē*, a contracting]

asys·to·lia (ă-sis-tō'lē-ă). SYN asystole.

asys·tol·ic (ă-sis-tol'ik). 1. Relating to asystole. 2. Not systolic.

AT Abbreviation for the adenine-thymine hydrogen-bonded base pair observed in double-stranded polynucleotides.

At Symbol for astatine.

ata Abbreviation for *atmosphere* absolute.

atac·til·ia (ā-tak-til'ē-ă). Loss of the sense of touch. [G. *a-* priv. + L. *tactilis*, relating to touch, fr. *tango*, pp. *tactus*, to touch]

at·a·rac·tic (at-ă-rak'tik). 1. Having a calming or tranquilizing effect. 2. A tranquilizer. SYN ataraxic. [G. *ataraktos*, calm]

at·a·rax·ia (at-ă-rak'sē-ă). Calmness and peace of mind; tranquility. [G. *a-* priv. + *taraktos*, disturbed, + *-ia*]

at·a·rax·ic (at-ă-rak′sik). SYN ataractic.

at·a·vism (at′ă-vizm). The appearance in an individual of characteristics presumed to have been present in some remote ancestor; reversion to an earlier biological type. [L. *atavus,* a remote ancestor]

at·a·vis·tic (at-ă-vis′tik). Relating to atavism.

atax·ia (ă-tak′sē-ă). An inability to coordinate muscle activity during voluntary movement, so that smooth movements occur. Most often due to disorders of the cerebellum or the posterior columns of the spinal cord; may involve the limbs, head, or trunk. SYN ataxy, incoordination. [G. *a-*prov. + *taxis,* order]

acute a., generalized a. of abrupt onset, most often caused by drug intoxications, poisonings, or vestibular neuronitis.

ataxia-telangiectasia, SEE a. telangiectasia.

bovine congenital a., an autosomal recessive a. seen in several European breeds of cattle.

Briquet's a., weakening of the muscle sense and increased sensibility of the skin, in hysteria. SYN hysterical a.

Bruns a., difficulty in initiation of movements of the feet when they are in contact with the ground; a condition related to a frontal lobe lesion.

a. of calves, a specific cerebellar a. in the Jersey breed, probably a recessive genetic trait.

cerebellar a., loss of muscle coordination caused by disorders of the cerebellum.

chronic a., persistent a., most often caused by hereditary cerebellar or metabolic disorders.

a. cor′dis, SYN atrial *fibrillation.*

enzootic a., a metabolic disease of lambs characterized clinically by progressive incoordination of the hind limbs and pathologically by disruption of neuron and myelin development in the central nervous system; caused by a deficiency of metabolizable copper in the ewe during the last half of her pregnancy. SYN swayback.

equine spinal a., a disease of young horses characterized by progressive weakness and incoordination, most evident in the hind legs; it is associated with lesions in the cervical region of the spinal cord and is the result of compression of the spinal cord by malformed cervical vertebrae.

Friedreich's a., SYN hereditary spinal a.

hereditary a., a simple autosomal recessive trait in fox terrier dogs that produces a progressive general a.

hereditary cerebellar a., (1) a disease of later childhood and early adult life, marked by ataxic gait, hesitating and explosive speech, nystagmus, and sometimes optic neuritis. It probably comprises several distinct conditions with diverse patterns of inheritance. **(2)** collective term for a number of hereditary disorders in which cerebellar signs are the most prominent finding.

hereditary spinal a. [MIM*229300], sclerosis of the posterior and lateral columns of the spinal cord, occurring in children and marked by a. in the lower extremities, extending to the upper, followed by paralysis and contractures; autosomal recessive inheritance. SEE ALSO spinocerebellar a. SYN Friedreich's a., heredotaxia.

hysterical a., SYN Briquet's a.

kinetic a., SYN motor a.

a. of lambs, myelination failure seen in ewes on a copper-deficient diet.

Leyden's a., SYN pseudotabes.

locomotor a., the severe gait ataxia seen with tabetic neurosyphilis. Patients walk with the feet wide apart, slapping them clumsily to the floor with each step, and depend on visual cues to maintain balance. SEE ALSO tabetic *neurosyphilis.*

Marie's a., obsolete term for a variety of non-Friedreich hereditary ataxias.

moral a., inconstancy of ideas and of conscious intent, as a manifestation of hysteria.

motor a., a. developing upon attempting to perform coordinated muscular movements. SYN kinetic a.

optic a., an inability to guide the hand toward an object using visual information; seen in Balint's *syndrome.*

respiratory a., SYN Biot's *respiration.*

sensory a., an a. due to impairment of position sense caused by lesions located at some point along the central or peripheral sensory pathways.

spinal a., a. due to spinal cord disease, as in tabes dorsalis.

spinocerebellar a., the most common hereditary a., with onset in middle to late childhood, manifested as limb a., nystagmus, kyphoscoliosis, and pes cavus; the major pathological changes are found in the posterior columns of the spinal cord; most often autosomal recessive inheritance.

static a., inability to preserve equilibrium while standing, due to loss of myesthesia; present during the resting state.

a. telangiectasia, ataxia-telangiectasia, a slowly progressive multisystem disorder with the following manifestations: a. appearing with the onset of walking; telangiectases of the conjunctiva and skin of the face, neck, and ears; athetosis and nystagmus; and recurrent infections of the respiratory system caused by immunoglobulin deficiencies. Due to an autosomal recessive trait, with major pathological changes involving the cerebellar cortex, posterior columns, spinocerebellar tracks, anterior horn cells, dorsal roots, and peripheral nerves. Approximately 70% of the patients have an IgA deficiency concomitant with decreased T helper cell function. There are numerous chromosome breaks and alpha-fetoprotein levels in the sera are usually elevated. SYN ataxia telangiectasia syndrome, Louis-Bar syndrome.

vasomotor a., a form of autonomic a. causing irregularity in the peripheral circulation, marked by alternations of pallor and suffusion, due to spasm of the smaller blood vessels.

vestibulocerebellar a., a. due to disease of the central vestibular system or its cerebellar components, manifested clinically by an unsteady gait, nystagmus, and incoordination of arm and leg movements.

atax·i·a·dy·nam·ia (ă-tak′sē-ă-dī-nam′ē-ă). Muscular weakness combined with incoordination.

atax·i·a·gram (ă-tak′sē-ă-gram). The recording made by an ataxiagraph.

atax·i·a·graph (ă-tak′sē-ă-graf). An instrument for measuring the degree and direction of the swaying of the body and head in static ataxia, with the individual's eyes closed. SYN ataxiameter.

atax·i·a·me·ter (ă-tak′sē-ă-mē′ter). SYN ataxiagraph.

atax·i·a·pha·sia (ă-tak′sē-ă-fā′zē-ă). Inability to form connected sentences, although single words may perhaps be used intelligibly. [G. *a-* priv. + *taxis,* order, + *phasis,* an affirmation, speech]

atax·ia-tel·an·gi·ec·ta·sia. See under ataxia.

atax·ic (ă-tak′sik). Relating to, marked by, or suffering from ataxia.

atax·i·o·phe·mia (ă-tak-sē-ō-fē′mē-ă). Incoordination of the muscles concerned in speech production. [G. *a-* priv. + *taxis,* order, + *phēmē,* voice, speech]

atax·i·o·pho·bia (ă-tak′sē-ō-fō′bē-ă). Morbid dread of disorder or untidiness. [G. *a-* priv. + *taxis,* order, + *phobos,* fear]

ataxy (ă-tak′sē). SYN ataxia.

♻**-ate.** Termination used as a replacement for "-ic acid" when the acid is neutralized (*e.g.,* sodium acetate) or esterfied (*e.g.,* ethyl acetate).

at·e·brine hy·dro·chlo·ride (ă′tē-brin). SYN quinacrine hydrochloride.

at·el·ec·ta·sis (at-ĕ-lek′tă-sis). Absence of gas from a part or the

♻ **Combining forms**	**[NA] Nomina Anatomica**
Word*Finder* **Multi-term entry finder** **Preceding letter A**	**[MIM] Mendelian** **Inheritance in Man**
A.D.A.M. Anatomy Plates **Between letters L and M**	☆ **Official alternate term**
Appendices: **Following letter Z**	☆**[NA] Official alternate** **Nomina Anatomica term**
SYN Synonym; Cf., compare	**High Profile Term**

whole of the lungs, due to failure of expansion or resorption of gas from the alveoli. SEE ALSO pulmonary *collapse*. [G. *atelēs,* incomplete, + *ektasis,* extension]

adhesive a., alveolar collapse in the presence of patent airways, especially when surfactant is inactivated or absent, especially in respiratory distress syndrome of the newborn, acute radiation pneumonitis, or viral pneumonia.

cicatrization a., the decrease in air per unit lung volume due to fibrosis, causing decreased lung compliance, and increased tissue.

parenchymal a., the collapse that occurs when pulmonary air is absorbed and not replaced, thus reducing lung volume.

passive a., the pulmonary collapse that occurs due to a space-occupying intrathoracic process such as pneumothorax or hydrothorax.

patchy a., decreased aeration and collapse of multiple small areas of lung.

platelike a., SYN subsegmental a.

primary a., nonexpansion of the lungs after birth, found in all stillborn infants and in liveborn infants who die before respiration is established. SYN anectasis.

resorption a., the slow partial collapse of a lobe that occurs when communication between alveoli and trachea is obstructed.

round a., SYN folded-lung *syndrome.*

secondary a., pulmonary collapse at any age, but particularly of infants, due to hyaline membrane disease or elastic recoil of the lungs while dying from other causes.

segmental a., partial collapse of one or more individual pulmonary segments.

subsegmental a., collapse of the portion of the lung distal to an obstructed subsegmental bronchus, manifested as a linear opacity on a chest radiograph. SEE Fleischner *lines,* under *line.* SYN platelike a.

at·e·lec·tat·ic (at-ĕ-lek-tat′ik). Relating to atelectasis.

ate·lia (ă-tē′lē-ă). SYN ateliosis.

atel·i·o·sis (ă-tē′lē-ō′sis). Incomplete development of the body or any of its parts, as in infantilism and dwarfism. SYN atelia. [G. *atelēs,* incomplete, + *-osis,* condition]

atel·i·ot·ic (ă-tē-lē-ot′ik). Marked by ateliosis.

atel·op·id·tox·in (ā-tel-op′id-tok′sin). A potent poison from the skin of the golden arrow frog (*Atelopus zeteki*) of Central and South America.

aten·o·lol (ă-ten′ō-lol). 4-[2-Hydroxy-3[(1-methylethyl)amino]-propoxy]benzeneacetami; a relatively cardioselective β-adrenergic blocking agent used primarily in the treatment of angina pectoris and hypertension; it possesses lower lipid solubility than other members of this class and hence apparently less central nervous system side effects.

athe·lia (ă-thē-lē-ă). Congenital absence of the nipples. [G. *a-* priv. + *thēlē,* nipple]

ath·er·ec·to·my (ath-e-rek′tō-mē). Any removal by surgery or specialized catheterization of an atheroma in the coronary or any other artery.

coronary a., instrumental removal, via catheter, of atheromas in coronary arteries.

directional a., removal of coronary atherometer with instrumented catheter.

ather·man·cy (ă-ther′man-sē). Impermeability to heat. [G. *athermantos,* not heated, fr. *a-* priv. + *thermaino,* to heat, fr. *thermē,* heat]

ather·ma·nous (ă-ther′mă-nŭs). Absorbing radiant heat; not permeable to heat rays.

ather·mo·sys·tal·tic (ă-ther′mō-sis-tal′tik). Not contracted or constricted by ordinary variations of temperature; said of certain tissues. [G. *a-* priv. + *thermos,* hot, + *systaltikos,* constringent]

⌂**athero-.** Gruel-like, soft, pasty materials; atheroma, atheromatous. [G. *athērē,* gruel, porridge]

ath·er·o·em·bo·lism (ath′er-ō-em′bō-lizm). Cholesterol embolism, with or without calcific matter, originating from an atheroma of the aorta or other diseased artery.

ath·er·o·gen·e·sis (ath′er-ō-jen′ĕ-sis). Formation of atheroma, important in the pathogenesis of arteriosclerosis.

ath·er·o·gen·ic (ath-er-ō-jen′ik). Having the capacity to initiate, increase, or accelerate the process of atherogenesis.

ath·er·o·ma (ath-er-ō′mă). The lipid deposits in the intima of arteries, producing a yellow swelling on the endothelial surface; a characteristic of atherosclerosis. SYN atherosis. [G. *athērē,* gruel, + *-ōma,* tumor]

ath·er·om·a·tous (ath-er-ō′mă-tŭs). Relating to or affected by atheroma.

ath·er·o·scle·ro·sis (ath′er-ō-skler-ō′sis). Arteriosclerosis characterized by irregularly distributed lipid deposits in the intima of large and medium-sized arteries; such deposits provoke fibrosis and calcification. In lower animals, a. of swine and fowl mostly resemble a. of man. SYN nodular sclerosis.

Atherosclerosis is a multistage process set in motion when cells lining the arteries are damaged as a result of high blood pressure, smoking, toxic substances in the environment, and other agents. Plaques develop when high density lipoproteins accumulate at the site of arterial damage and platelets act to form a fibrous cap over this fatty core. Deposits block, or eventually entirely shut off, blood flow. Because atherosclerosis greatly raises the risk of angina, stroke, or heart attack (the leading cause of death in the U.S.), a primary goal of American health officials since the 1970s has been to educate individuals concerning the dangers of cholesterol. Plaque buildups, particularly in the carotid arteries, can be spotted by arteriography and ultrasound. Balloon and laser angioplasty have proved effective at minimizing plaques and restoring blood flow. However, prevention appears to be the primary means of attacking atherosclerosis: through low-fat diets, regular vigorous exercise, control of high blood pressure or diabetes, and avoidance of tobacco. See free radicals, low-fat diets.

ath·er·o·scle·rot·ic (ath′er-ō-skler-ot′ik). Relating to or characterized by atherosclerosis.

ath·er·o·sis (ath-er-ō′sis). SYN atheroma.

ath·er·o·throm·bo·sis (ath′er-ō-throm-bō′sis). Thrombus formation in an atheromatous vessel.

ath·er·o·throm·bot·ic (ath′er-ō-throm-bot′ik). Denoting, characteristic of, or caused by atherothrombosis.

ath·e·toid (ath′ĕ-toyd). Resembling athetosis.

ath·e·to·sic, ath·e·tot·ic (ath-ĕ-tō′sik, -tot′ik). Pertaining to, or marked by, athetosis.

ath·e·to·sis (ath-ĕ-tō′sis). A condition in which there is a constant succession of slow, writhing, involuntary movements of flexion, extension, pronation, and supination of the fingers and hands, and sometimes of the toes and feet. Usually caused by an extrapyramidal lesions. SYN extrapyramidal cerebral palsy, Hammond's disease. [G. *athetos,* without position or place]

double a., a type of cerebral palsy manifested predominantly as bilateral involuntary movements, beginning at about the age of 2 years, and preceded by generalized hypotonia and delayed motor development. Due to various causes, including kernicterus and birth hypoxia. SYN congenital choreoathetosis, double congenital a., Vogt syndrome.

double congenital a., SYN double a.

posthemiplegic a., a unilateral athetosis involving hemiplegic limbs, usually seen in children. SYN posthemiplegic chorea.

aThr Abbreviation for allothreonine. SEE allothreonines.

athrep·sia, ath·rep·sy (ă-threp′sē-ă, ath′rep-sē). **1.** Obsolete term for marasmus. **2.** As used by Ehrlich, immunity to transplanted neoplastic cells due to a lack of nourishment in the sense of a deficiency of supposed substances required for the development of such cells. SYN atrepsy. [G. *a-* priv. + *threpsis,* nourishment]

ath·ro·cy·to·sis (ath′rō-sī-tō′sis). The capacity of cells to absorb and retain electronegative colloids, as shown by macrophages and at the apical surface of proximal convoluted tubule cells of the kidney. [G. *athrō*, gathered together, + *kytos*, cell, + *-osis*, condition]

athrom·bia (ă-throm'bē-ă) [MIM*209050]. A defect of blood clotting characterized by deficiency in formation of thrombin; autosomal recessive inheritance. [G. *a*- priv. + thrombin]

athy·mia (ă-thī'mē-ă). **1.** Absence of affect or emotivity; morbid impassivity. **2.** Congenital absence of the thymus gland, often with associated immunodeficiency. SYN athymism. [G. *a*-priv. + *thymos*, mind, also thymus]

athy·mism (ă-thī'mizm). SYN athymia (2).

athy·rea (ă-thī'rē-ă). **1.** SYN hypothyroidism. **2.** SYN athyroidism.

athy·roid·ism (ă-thī'royd-izm). Congenital absence of the thyroid gland or suppression or absence of its hormonal secretion. SEE hypothyroidism. SYN athyrea (2), athyrosis.

athy·ro·sis (ă-thī-rō'sis). SYN athyroidism.

athy·rot·ic (ă-thī-rot'ik). Relating to athyroidism.

ATL Abbreviation for adult T-cell *leukemia* or adult T-cell *lymphoma*.

at·lan·tad (at-lan'tad). In a direction toward the atlas.

at·lan·tal (at-lan'tăl). Relating to the atlas. SYN atloid.

⚠**atlanto-, atlo-.** The atlas (the bone that supports the head), as Atlas supported the sky. [G. *Atlas, Atlantos*, Atlas, the mythical Titan who supported the dome of the sky on his shoulders]

at·lan·to·ax·i·al (at-lan'tō-ak'sē-ăl). Pertaining to the atlas and the axis; denoting the joint between the first two cervical vertebrae. SYN atlantoepistrophic, atloaxoid.

at·lan·to·did·y·mus (at-lan'tō-did'ē-mŭs). Conjoined twins with two heads on one neck and a single body. SYN atlodidymus. [atlanto- + G. *didymos*, twin]

at·lan·to·ep·i·stroph·ic (at-lan'tō-ep'i-strof'ik). SYN atlantoaxial.

at·lan·to·oc·cip·i·tal (at-lan'tō-ok-sip'i-tăl). Relating to the atlas and the occipital bone. SYN atlo-occipital.

at·lan·to·odon·toid (at-lan'tō-ō-don'toyd). Relating to the atlas and the dens of the axis.

at·las (at'las) [NA]. First cervical vertebra, articulating with the occipital bone and rotating around the dens of the axis. [G. *Atlas*, in Greek mythology a Titan who supported the earth on his shoulders]

⚠**atlo-.** SEE atlanto-.

at·lo·ax·oid (at-lō-ak'soyd). SYN atlantoaxial.

at·lo·did·y·mus (at-lō-did'ē-mŭs). SYN atlantodidymus.

at·loid (at'loyd). SYN atlantal.

at·lo·oc·cip·i·tal (at'lō-ok-sip'i-tăl). SYN atlanto-occipital.

atm Symbol for standard *atmosphere*.

⚠**atmo-.** Prefix denoting steam or vapor; or derived by action of steam or vapor. [G. *atmos*, steam, vapor]

at·mol·y·sis (at-mol'i-sis). Separation of mixed gases by passing them through a porous diaphragm, the lighter gases diffusing through at a faster rate. [atmo- + G. *lysis*, dissolution]

at·mom·e·ter (at-mom'ĕ-ter). An instrument for measuring the rate of evaporation. [atmo- + G. *metron*, measure]

at·mos Obsolete abbreviation for a unit of pressure; replaced by atm. [abbreviation of atmosphere]

at·mo·sphere (at'mŏs-fēr). **1.** SYN ventilate. **2.** Any gas surrounding a given body; a gaseous medium. **3.** A unit of air pressure. SEE ALSO standard a., torr. [atmo- + G. *sphaira*, sphere]

a. absolute (ata), a unit of absolute pressure (also known as barometric pressure) expressed in atm.

ICAO standard a., the standard a. adopted by the International Civil Aviation Organization, used for calibrating altimeters and for expressing hypobaric chamber pressures in terms of equivalent altitude; it ignores many deviations found in nature.

standard a. (atm), (1) the pressure of the a. at mean sea level, equivalent to 1,013,250 dynes/cm^2 or 101,325 Pa (N/m^2 in the SI system); **(2)** a standardized expression of the relation of barometric pressure, temperature, and other atmospheric variables as a function of altitude above sea level.

at·mo·spher·i·za·tion (at'mŏ-sfēr-i-zā'shŭn). Conversion of venous into arterial blood.

At·mungs·fer·ment (aht'mungz-fer-ment). **1.** A system of cytochromes and their oxidases that participate in respiratory processes. **2.** Often, specifically, cytochrome oxidase. SYN Warburg's respiratory enzyme. [Ger.]

at·om (at'ŏm). The once ultimate particle of an element, believed to be as indivisible as its name indicates. Discovery of radioactivity demonstrated the existence of subatomic particles, notably protons, neutrons, and electrons, the first two comprising most of the mass of the atomic nucleus. We now know that subatomic particles are further divisible ino hadrons, leptons, and quarks. [G. *atomos*, indivisible, uncut]

activated a., an a. possessing more than normal energy as a result of input of energy. SEE ALSO excited *state*. SYN excited a.

Bohr's a., a concept or model of the a. in which the negatively charged electrons move in circular or elliptical orbits around the positively charged nucleus, energy being emitted or absorbed when electrons change from one orbit to another.

excited a., SYN activated a.

ionized a., an a. that possesses an electrostatic charge as a result of loss or gain of electrons; *e.g.*, H^+, Ca^{2+}, Cl^-, O^{2-}.

labeled a., a radioactive a., or a stable but rare one, which by its presence in a molecule helps localization or measurement of that molecule. SYN tagged a.

nuclear a., a concept or model of the a. characterized by the presence of a small, massive nucleus at its center.

quaternary carbon a., an a. of carbon to which four other carbon a.'s are attached.

radioactive a., an a. with an unstable nucleus, which emits particulate or electromagnetic radiation (radioactive emission) to achieve greater stability. SEE radionuclide, half-life, Becquerel.

recoil a., the remainder of an a. from which a nuclear particle has been emitted or ejected at high velocity; the remainder recoils with a velocity inversely proportional to its mass.

stripped a., an a. minus all its electrons; a nucleus.

tagged a., SYN labeled a.

atom·ic (ă-tom'ik). Relating to an atom.

at·om·ism (at'ŏm-izm). The approach to the study of a psychological phenomenon through analysis of the elementary parts of which it is assumed to be composed. Cf. holism.

at·om·is·tic (at-ŏm-is'tik). Pertaining to atomism or a. psychology.

at·om·i·za·tion (at-ŏm-i-zā'-shŭn). Spray production; reduction of a fluid to small droplets.

at·om·iz·er (at'ŏm-ī-zer). A device used to reduce liquid medication to fine particles in the form of a spray or aerosol; useful in delivering medication to the nose and throat. SEE ALSO nebulizer, vaporizer. [G. *atomos*, indivisible particle]

ato·nia (ā-tō'nē-ă). SYN atony. [G. languor]

aton·ic (ă-ton'ik). Relaxed; without normal tone or tension.

at·o·nic·i·ty (at-ō-nis'i-tē). SYN atony.

at·o·ny (at'ŏ-nē). Relaxation, flaccidity, or lack of tone or tension. SYN atonia, atonicity. [G. *atonia*, languor]

at·o·pen (at'ō-pen). The excitant causing any form of atopy.

atop·ic (ă-top'ik). Relating to or marked by atopy. [G. *atopos*, out of place; strange]

atop·og·no·sia, atop·og·no·sis (ă-top-og-nō'zē-ă, -og-nō'sis). Sensory inattention; inability to locate a sensation properly. Usually caused by a contralateral parietal lobe lesion. [G. *a*- priv. + *topos*, place, + *gnōsis*, knowledge]

at·o·py (at'ō-pē). A genetically determined state of hypersensitivity to environmental allergens. Type I allergic reaction is associated with the IgE antibody and a group of diseases, principally asthma, hay fever, and atopic dermatitis. [G. *atopia*, strangeness, fr. *a*- priv. + *topos*, a place]

atox·ic (ā-tok'sik). Not toxic.

ATP Abbreviation for adenosine 5'-triphosphate.

ATPase Abbreviation for adenosine triphosphatase.

ATP cit·rate ly·ase. SEE ATP *citrate* (*pro-3S*)-lyase.

ATPD Symbol indicating that a gas volume has been expressed as if it had been dried at the ambient temperature and pressure.

ATP-di·phos·pha·tase. SYN apyrase.

ATP-mon·o·phos·pha·tase. SYN adenosine triphosphatase.

ATPS Symbol indicating that a gas volume has been expressed as if it were saturated with water vapor at the ambient temperature and barometric pressure; the condition of an expired gas equilibrated in a spirometer.

ATP sul·fur·y·lase. SYN *sulfate* adenylyltransferase.

at·ra·bil·i·ary (at-ră-bil′ē-ār-ē). Obsolete term for depressed melancholic. [L. *atra bilis,* black bile]

atrac·to·syl·id·ic ac·id (ă-trak′tō-sil-id′ik). SYN atractyligenin.

atrac·tyl·ic ac·id (ă-trak′til-ik). A highly poisonous steroid glycoside from *Atractylis gummifera* L. (*Compositae*), having a strychnine-like action that produces convulsions of a hypoglycemic nature; the aglycon, atractyliginin, is combined with glucose and isovaleric acid, and is the toxic principle. A. a. interferes with oxidative reactions, the citric acid cycle, and nerve conduction.

atrac·tyl·i·gen·in (ă-trak′til-i-jen′in). The steroid aglycon and toxic principle of atractylic acid. SYN atractosylidic acid, atractylin.

atrac·tyl·in (ă-trak′til-in). SYN atractyligenin.

atra·cu·ri·um be·syl·ate (a-tră-kyūr′ē-ŭm). $C_{65}H_{82}N_2O_{18}S_2$; a non-depolarizing neuromuscular relaxant of intermediate duration of action; used as an adjunct to general anesthesia; a curare-like agent.

atrep·sy (ă-trep′sē). SYN athrepsia (2). [G. *a-* priv. + *trephō,* to nourish]

atre·sia (ă-trē′zē-ă). Absence of a normal opening or normally patent lumen. SYN clausura. [G. *a-* priv. + *trēsis,* a hole]

anal a., a. a′ni, congenital absence of an anal opening due to the presence of a membranous septum (persistence of the cloacal membrane) or to complete absence of the anal canal. SYN imperforate anus (1), proctatresia.

aortic a., congenital absence of the normal valvular orifice into the aorta.

biliary a., a. of the major bile ducts, causing cholestasis and jaundice, which does not become apparent until several days after birth; periportal fibrosis develops and leads to cirrhosis, with proliferation of small bile ducts unless these are also atretic; giant cell transformation of hepatic cells also occurs. Cf. neonatal *hepatitis.*

bronchial a., severe focal narrowing or obliteration of a segmental or lobar bronchus, usually associated with distal air trapping.

choanal a., congenital failure of one or both choanae to open owing to failure of the bucconasa membrane to rupture.

esophageal a., congenital failure of the full esophageal lumen to develop; commonly associated with tracheoesophageal fistula.

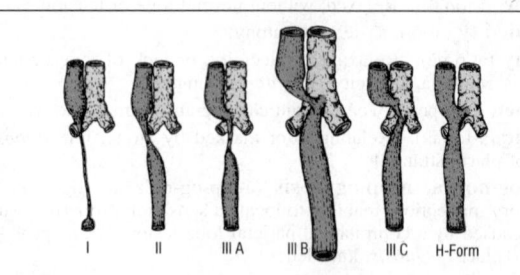

Vogt's classification
(of esophageal atresia [I–IIIC] and the so-called H type)

a. follic′uli, a normal process affecting the primordial ovarian follicles in which death of the ovum results in cystic degeneration followed by cicatricial closure.

intestinal a., an obliteration of the lumen of the small intestine, with the ileum involved in 50% of cases and the jejunum and duodenum next in frequency; most frequent cause of intestinal

obstruction in the newborn; etiology may be related to a failure of recanalization during early development or to some impairment of blood supply during intrauterine life.

a. i′ridis, congenital absence of the pupillary opening. SYN atretopsia.

laryngeal a., congenital failure of the laryngeal opening to develop, resulting in partial or total obstruction at or just above or below the glottis.

pulmonary a., congenital absence of the pulmonary valve orifice.

tricuspid a., congenital lack of the tricuspid orifice.

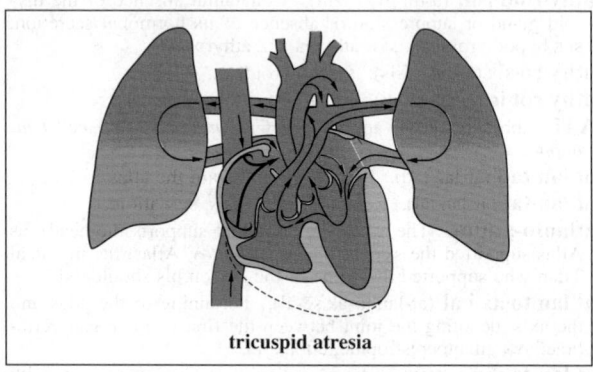

tricuspid atresia

vaginal a., congenital or acquired imperforation or occlusion of the vagina, or adhesion of the walls of the vagina. SYN ankylocolpos, colpatresia.

atre·sic (ă-trē′zik). SYN atretic.

atret·ic (ă-tret′ik). Relating to atresia. SYN atresic, imperforate.

atreto-. Lack of an opening. [G. *atrētos,* imperforate fr. *a-,* not + *trētos,* perforated, fr. *tetrainō, titrēmi,* to bore through, to pierce.]

atre·to·ble·pha·ria (ă-trē′tō-ble-fār′ē-ă). SYN symblepharon. [atreto- + G. *blepharon,* eyelid]

atre·to·cys·tia (ă-trē′tō-sis′tē-ă). Congenital or acquired absence of an opening of a bladder. [atreto- + G. *kystis,* bladder]

atre·to·gas·tria (ă-trē′tō-gas′trē-ă). Congenital absence of an opening of the stomach. [atreto- + G. *gastēr,* stomach]

atre·top·sia (ă-trē-top′sē-ă). SYN *atresia* iridis. [atreto- + G. *ōps,* eye]

atria (ā′trē-ă). Plural of atrium.

atri·al (ā′trē-ăl). Relating to an atrium.

atrich·ia (ă-trik′ē-ă). Absence of hair, congenital or acquired. SYN atrichosis. [G. *a-* priv. + *thrix* (trich-), hair]

atri·cho·sis (at-ri-kō′sis). SYN atrichia.

at·ri·chous (at′ri-kŭs). Without hair.

atrio-. The atrium; atrial. [L. *atrium,* an entrance hall]

atri·o·meg·a·ly (ā′trē-ō-meg′ă-lē). Enlargement of the atrium. [atrio- + G. *megas,* great]

atri·o·nec·tor (ā-trē-ō-nek′ter, -tōr). SYN sinuatrial *node.* [atrio- + L. *necto,* to join]

atri·o·pep·tin (ā′trē-ō-pep′tin). SYN atrial natriuretic *peptide.* [atrio- + peptide + suffix *-in,* material]

atri·o·sep·to·plas·ty (ā′trē-ō-sep′tō-plas-tē). Surgical repair of an atrial septal defect. [atrio- + L. *septum,* partition, + G. *plastos,* formed]

atri·o·sep·tos·to·my (ā′trē-ō-sep-tos′tō-mē). Establishment of a communication between the two atria of the heart. [atrio- + L. *septum,* partition, + G. *stoma,* mouth]

balloon a., tearing or enlarging the foramen ovale by pulling a balloon-bearing catheter across the atrial septum for the purpose of augmenting interatrial mixing of blood in the treatment of cyanotic congenital heart disease.

atri·ot·o·my (ā-trē-ot′ō-mē). Surgical opening of an atrium. [atrio- + G. *tomē,* incision]

atri·o·ven·tric·u·lar (A-V) (ā′trē-ō-ven-trik′yū-lar). Relating to both the atria and the ventricles of the heart, especially to the ordinary, orthograde transmission of conduction or bloodflow.

atrip·li·cism (ă-trip'li-sizm). An intoxication caused by the ingestion of certain species of *Atriplex*, eaten as greens in China; it is marked by pain and swelling of the fingers, spreading to the forearm; bullae and ulcers form, and the fingers may become gangrenous. [L. *atriplex* (*-plic-*), the orach, a vegetable]

atri·um, pl. **atria** (ā'trē-ŭm, ā'trē-ă). **1** [NA]. A chamber or cavity to which are connected several chambers or passageways. **2.** SYN a. of heart. **3.** That part of the tympanic cavity that lies immediately deep to the eardrum. **4.** SYN nasal a. **5.** In the lung, a subdivision of the alveolar duct from which alveolar sacs open. [L. entrance hall]

accessory a., SYN *cor* triatriatum.

auricle of a., a small conical ("ear-shaped") pouch projecting from the upper anterior portion of each atrium of the heart, increasing slightly the atrial volume. SEE *auricle* of left atrium, *auricle* of right atrium. SYN auricula atrialis [NA], atrial auricle, atrial auricula, auricle (2), auricula (2), auricular appendage (1), auricular appendix, skin tag.

a. cor'dis [NA], SYN a. of heart.

a. dex'trum cordis [NA], SYN right a. of heart.

a. glot'tidis, SYN *vestibule* of larynx.

a. of heart, the upper chamber of each half of the heart. SYN a. cordis [NA], atrium (2).

left a. of heart, a. of the left side of the heart which receives the blood from the pulmonary veins. SYN a. sinistrum cordis [NA], a. pulmonale.

a. mea'tus me'dii [NA], SYN nasal a.

nasal a., the anterior expanded portion of the middle meatus of the nose, just above the vestibule. SYN a. meatus medii [NA], atrium (4).

a. pulmona'le, SYN left a. of heart.

right a. of heart, right a., the a. of the right side of the heart which receives the blood from the venae cavae and coronary sinus. SYN a. dextrum cordis [NA].

a. sinis'trum cordis [NA], SYN left a. of heart.

At·ro·pa (at'rō-pă). A genus of plants (family Solanaceae) of which *A. belladonna* is typical. SEE belladonna. [G. *Atropos,* one of the Fates cutting the thread of life, because of the lethal effects of the plant]

atroph·e·de·ma (ă-trof'ĕ-dē'mă). SYN angioedema.

atro·phia (ă-trō'fē-ă). SYN atrophy. [G. fr. *a-* priv. + *trophē,* nourishment]

a. cu'tis, SYN atrophoderma.

a. maculo'sa varioliform'mis cu'tis, SYN anetoderma.

a. pilo'rum pro'pria, a general term that includes fragilitas crinium, trichorrhexis nodosa, monilethrix, and atrophy of the hair.

atroph·ic (ă-trof'ik). Denoting atrophy.

atro·phie blanche (ă'trō-fi blahnsh'). Small smooth ivory-white areas with hyperpigmented borders and telangiectasis, developing into atrophic stellate scars; seen especially on the legs and ankles of middle-aged women, and associated with livedo reticularis and dermal hyalinizing vasculitis. [Fr.]

at·ro·phied (at'rō-fēd). Characterized by atrophy.

at·ro·pho·der·ma (at'rō-fō-der'mă). Atrophy of the skin that may occur either in discrete localized areas or in widespread areas. SEE ALSO anetoderma. SYN atrophia cutis.

a. al'bidum, stocking-like type of atrophy affecting the extremities, probably congenital; first noted in early childhood on the lower limbs as a symmetric thinning that renders the parts sensitive.

a. biotrip'ticum, obsolete term for senile cutaneous atrophy.

a. diffu'sum, diffuse idiopathic cutaneous atrophy.

a. macula'tum, SYN anetoderma.

a. neurit'icum, SYN glossy *skin.*

a. of Pasini and Pierini, a form of slate-colored atrophy of the skin occurring in discrete, 2-cm or larger lesions, either singly or multiply, and occasionally confluent, increasing in number and size over a period of years and then remaining constant; thought by some to be of two types: one preceded by morphea, and the other appearing with no preceding identifiable pathology.

a. reticula'tum symmet'ricum facie'i, a rarely used term for *folliculitis* ulerythematosa reticulata.

senile a., a. seni'lis, the loss of collagen, with thinning and decreased elasticity of the skin associated with old age.

a. stria'tum, SYN *striae* cutis distensae, under *stria.*

a. vermicula'tum, SYN *folliculitis* ulerythematosa reticulata.

at·ro·pho·der·ma·to·sis (at'rō-fō-der-mă-tō'sis). Any cutaneous affection in which a prominent symptom is skin atrophy.

at·ro·phy (at'rō-fē). A wasting of tissues, organs, or the entire body, as from death and reabsorption of cells, diminished cellular proliferation, decreased cellular volume, pressure, ischemia, malnutrition, lessened function, or hormonal changes. SYN atrophia. [G. *atrophia,* fr. *a-* priv. + *trophē,* nourishment]

acute reflex bone a., SYN Sudeck's a.

acute yellow a. of the liver, a lesion in which there is extensive and rapid death of parenchymal cells of the liver, sometimes with fatty degeneration of the size of the organ; the necrosis may result from fulminant viral infection or chemical poisoning; associated with jaundice. SYN acute parenchymatous hepatitis, Rokitansky's disease (1).

alveolar a., diminution in size of the supportive tissues of the teeth due to lack of function, reduced blood supply, or unknown causes.

arthritic a., a. of muscles rendered inactive by a chronically inflamed or fixed joint.

blue a., depressed blue atrophic scars due to injections in the skin of impure substances, as seen in narcotics addicts.

brown a., a. of the heart wall, especially in the elderly, in which the muscle is dark reddish brown and reduced in volume; the muscle fibers become pigmented especially about the nuclei, by lipochrome granules.

Buchwald's a., a progressive form of cutaneous a.

central areolar choroidal a., SYN areolar *choroidopathy.*

cerebellar a., a degeneration of the cerebellum, particularly the Purkinje cells, as the result of abiotrophy or of toxic agents, as in alcoholism.

choroidal vascular a., a. affecting either all choroidal vessels or only the choriocapillaris, occurring either diffusely or confined to the posterior pole of the eye.

compensatory a., a. especially of an endocrine organ as a result of its function being assumed by a new source of hormone.

congenital cerebellar a., familial disorder that causes degeneration of various cells in the cerebellum. Two types are recognized, one in which the granular layer cells degenerate, the other in which the Purkinje cells degenerate.

cyanotic a., a. due to destruction of the parenchymatous cells of an organ as a consequence of chronic venous congestion. SYN red a.

cyanotic a. of the liver, a sequela of longstanding hepatic congestion due to high pressure in the right atrium as in chronic constrictive pericarditis and severe, protracted right ventricular failure.

dentatorubral cerebellar a. with polymyoclonus, SYN *dyssynergia* cerebellaris myoclonica.

disuse a., muscle wasting caused by immobilization, such as casting.

Erb a., SYN progressive muscular *dystrophy.*

essential progressive a. of iris, progressive a. of the iris without inflammatory signs, characterized by patchy loss of all layers of the iris with hole formation, migration of the pupil, degeneration of the corneal endothelium, peripheral anterior synechiae, and secondary glaucoma; usually unilateral, predominantly affecting women in their middle years.

exhaustion a., a., especially of glandular cells, believed to result from excessive functional activity or overstimulation.

facioscapulohumeral a., SYN facioscapulohumeral muscular *dystrophy.*

familial spinal muscular a., SYN infantile spinal muscular a.

fatty a., fatty infiltration secondary to an a. of the essential elements of an organ or tissue.

gingival a., SYN gingival *recession*.

gyrate a. of choroid and retina [MIM*258870], a slowly progressive a. of the choriocapillaris, pigmentary epithelium, and sensory retina, with irregular confluent atrophic areas and an associated ornithinuria; autosomal recessive inheritance; due to a deficiency of ornithine δ-aminotransferase.

Hoffmann's muscular a., SYN infantile spinal muscular a.

horizontal a., a progressive loss of alveolar and supporting bone surrounding the teeth, beginning at the most coronal level of the bone. SYN horizontal resorption.

Hunt's a., obsolete term for a. of the small muscles of the hand without sensory disturbances; two types are recognized: *thenar*, from compression of the thenar branch of the median nerve; *hypothenar*, from compression of the deep palmar branch of the ulnar nerve.

idiopathic muscular a., SYN progressive muscular *dystrophy*.

infantile muscular a., SYN infantile spinal muscular a.

infantile progressive spinal muscular a., SYN infantile spinal muscular a.

infantile spinal muscular a. [MIM*253300], transmitted as autosomal recessive on chromosome 5q. Progressive dysfunction of the anterior horn cells in the spinal cord and brainstem cranial nerves with profound weakness and bulbar dysfunction occurring in the first two years of life. Three groups, based on age of clinical onset, are recognized. SYN familial spinal muscular a., Hoffmann's muscular a., infantile muscular a., infantile progressive spinal muscular a., progressive infantile spinal muscular a., Werdnig-Hoffmann disease, Werdnig-Hoffmann muscular a.

ischemic muscular a., SEE Volkmann's *contracture*.

juvenile muscular a., SYN juvenile spinal muscular a.

juvenile spinal muscular a. [MIM*253600], slowly progressive proximal muscular weakness and wasting, beginning in childhood, caused by degeneration of motor neurons in the anterior horns of the spinal cord; onset usually between 2 and 17 years of age; usually autosomal recessive inheritance. SYN juvenile muscular a., Kugelberg-Welander disease, Wohlfart-Kugelberg-Welander disease.

Kienböck's a., acute a. of bone in an extremity following inflammation.

Leber's hereditary optic a. [MIM*308900], hereditary degeneration of the optic nerve and papillomacular bundle with resulting rapid loss of central vision, progressive for several weeks, then usually stationary with permanent central scotoma; age of onset is variable, most often in the third decade; more males than females are affected and transmission is cytoplasmic and strictly on the female side. Mutation on the mitochondrial chromosome involved, which presumably interacts with an X-linked mutant. This mechanism may explain the bizarre sex ratio, which differs significantly from one country to another.

linear a., SYN *striae* cutis distensae, under *stria*.

macular a., SYN anetoderma.

marantic a., SYN marasmus.

muscular a., wasting of muscular tissue. Cf. myopathic a. SYN myatrophy, myoatrophy.

myopathic a., muscular a. caused by a primary disorder of muscle.

neuritic a., SYN trophoneurotic a.

neurogenic a., SYN trophoneurotic a.

neurotrophic a., SYN trophoneurotic a.

nutritional type cerebellar a., a restricted type of cerebellar cortical degeneration, affecting particularly the Purkinje cells of the anterior and superior vermis; probably caused by thiamin deficiency; most frequently seen in chronic alcoholics and then called alcoholic cerebellar degeneration.

olivopontocerebellar a., a group of genetically distinct, mostly autosomal dominant progressive neurologic diseases characterized by loss of neurons in the cerebellar cortex, basis pontis, and inferior olivary nuclei; results in ataxia, tremor, involuntary movement, and dysarthria; five clinical types (four with dominant, one with recessive inheritance) have been described, each type characterized by additional findings, such as sensory loss, retinal degeneration, ophthalmoplegia, and extrapyramidal signs. Several loci are involved, autosomal dominant [MIM*164400 to *164600] and recessive [MIM*258200]. SYN olivopontocerebellar degeneration.

periodontal a., decrease in size and/or cellular elements of the periodontium after it has reached normal maturity.

peroneal muscular a. [MIM*118200 to 118220], a group of three familial peripheral neuromuscular disorders, sharing the common feature of marked wasting of the more distal extremities, particularly the peroneal muscle groups, resulting in "stork legs." Two of the three subtypes are hereditary sensorimotor polyneuropathies, one demyelinating in type and the other axon loss in type, while the third subgroup is an anterior horn cell disorder. It usually involves the legs before the arms; pes cavus is often the first sign; autosomal dominant, autosomal recessive, and X-linked recessive types exist [MIM*302800 to *302908], with severity related to genetic type. SYN Charcot-Marie-Tooth disease.

Pick's a., circumscribed a. of the cerebral cortex. SYN lobar sclerosis, progressive circumscribed cerebral a.

postmenopausal a., a. following menopause, as of the genital organs.

pressure a., the wasting of hard or soft tissue resulting from excessive pressure applied to tissue by a denture base.

primary idiopathic macular a., SYN anetoderma.

primary macular a. of skin, SYN anetoderma.

progressive choroidal a., SYN choroideremia.

progressive circumscribed cerebral a., SYN Pick's a.

progressive infantile spinal muscular a., SYN infantile spinal muscular a.

progressive muscular a., SYN amyotrophic lateral *sclerosis*.

progressive spinal muscular a., one of the subgroups of motor neuron disease; a progressive degenerative disorder of the motor neurons of the spinal cord, manifested as progressive, often symmetrical, weakness and wasting, typically beginning in the distal portions of the limbs, particularly in the upper extremities, and spreading proximally; fasciculation potentials are often present, but evidence of corticospinal tract disease (*e.g.,* increased deep tendon reflexes, Babinski sign) is not.

pulp a., diminution in size and/or cellular elements of the dental pulp due to interference with the blood supply.

red a., SYN cyanotic a.

scapulohumeral a., SYN Vulpian's a.

senile a., wasting of tissues and organs with advancing age from decreased catabolic or anabolic processes, at times due to endocrine changes, decreased use, or ischemia. SYN geromarasmus.

serous a., a degenerative change occurring in fat cells, the fat being absorbed and its place being taken by a serous fluid.

striate a. of skin, SYN *striae* cutis distensae, under *stria*.

Sudeck's a., a. of bones, commonly of the carpal or tarsal bones, following a slight injury such as a sprain. SEE ALSO causalgia, reflex sympathetic *dystrophy*. SYN acute reflex bone a., posttraumatic osteoporosis, Sudeck's syndrome. [L. English sweat]

traction a., SYN *striae* cutis distensae, under *stria*.

transneuronal a., SYN transsynaptic *degeneration*.

trophoneurotic a., abnormalities of the skin, hair, nails, subcutaneous tissues and bone, caused by peripheral nerve lesions. SYN neuritic a., neurogenic a., neurotrophic a., trophic changes.

villous a., abnormality of the small intestinal mucosa with crypt hyperplasia, resulting in flattening of the mucosa and the appearance of a. of villi; clinically seen in malabsorption syndromes such as sprue.

Vulpian's a., progressive spinal muscular a. beginning in the shoulder. SYN scapulohumeral a.

Werdnig-Hoffmann muscular a., SYN infantile spinal muscular a.

yellow a. of the liver, SEE acute yellow a. of the liver.

Zimmerlin's a., a variety of hereditary progressive muscular a. in which the a. begins in the upper half of the body.

at·ro·pine (at′rō-pēn). $C_{17}H_{23}NO_3$; *dl*-tropyl tropate; a racemic mixture of d- and l-hyoscyamine, alkaloids obtained from the leaves and roots of *Atropa belladonna*; an anticholinergic, with diverse effects (tachycardia, mydriasis, cycloplegia, constipation, urinary retention, antisudorific) attributable to reversible competitive blockade of acetylcholine at muscarinic type cholinergic receptors; used in the treatment of poisoning with organophosphate insecticides or nerve gases. The (–) form is by far the more active. SYN *dl*-hyoscyamine, tropine tropate.

a. methonitrate, the methylnitrate of a., with the same actions and uses as a., but less lipid soluble and hence fewer central nervous system effects; a quaternary compound.

a. methylbromide, SYN methylatropine bromide.

a. sulfate, an anticholinergic; a widely used soluble salt of atropine.

atrop·in·ic (at'rō-pin-ik). Term used to indicate a sharing of pharmacologic properties with atropine. This means blocking parasympathetic neuroeffector junctions leading to a constellation of effects including tachycardia, urinary retention, dry mouth, constipation, mydriasis, cycloplegia, and other anticholinergic effects.

at·ro·pin·ism (at'rō-pin-izm). Symptoms of poisoning by atropine or belladonna.

at·ro·pin·i·za·tion (at-rō'pin-i-zā'shŭn). Administration of atropine or belladonna to the point of achieving the pharmacologic effect.

atros·cine. *dl*-scopolamine. SEE scopolamine. [atropine + hyoscine]

at·ro·tox·in (at-rō-toks'in). A component of diamondback rattlesnake (*Crotalus atrox*) venom that specifically and reversibly increases voltage-dependent calcium ion currents in isolated myocytes.

at·tach·ment (ă-tach'ment). **1.** A connection of one part with another. **2.** In dentistry, a mechanical device for the fixation and stabilization of a dental prosthesis.

bar clip a.'s, SYN bar-sleeve a.'s.

bar-sleeve a.'s, fixed bar joints or rigid bar units used for splinting abutments with removable sleeves or clips within the partial denture for supporting and/or retaining the prosthesis. SYN bar clip a.'s.

epithelial a., SYN junctional *epithelium*.

frictional a., SYN precision a.

internal a., SYN precision a.

key a., SYN precision a.

keyway a., SYN precision a.

muscle-tendon a., the union of a muscle and tendon fiber in which sarcolemma intervenes between the two; the end of the muscle fiber may be rounded, conical, or tapered. SYN muscle-tendon junction.

parallel a., SYN precision a.

pericemental a., the tissues surrounding the cementum of the tooth, *i.e.,* the periodontal ligament and alveolar bone.

precision a., (1) a frictional or mechanically retained unit used in fixed or removable prosthodontics, consisting of closely fitting male and female parts; **(2)** an a. that may be rigid in function or may incorporate a movable stress control unit to reduce the torque on the abutment. SYN frictional a., internal a., key a., keyway a., parallel a., slotted a.

slotted a., SYN precision a.

at·tack (ă-tak'). The occurrence of some disorder or episode, ordinarily with dramatic and sudden onset, such as an a. of shingles or heart a.

drop a., an episode of sudden falling that occurs during standing or walking, without warning and without loss of consciousness, vertigo, or postictal behavior. The patients are usually elderly and have normal electroencephalograms; of unknown cause.

panic a., sudden onset of intense apprehension, fear, terror, or impending doom accompanied by increased autonomic nervous system activity and by various constitutional disturbances, depersonalization, and derealization.

salaam a., SYN nodding *spasm*.

transient ischemic a. (TIA), a sudden focal loss of neurological function with complete recovery usually within 24 hours; caused by a brief period of inadequate perfusion in a portion of the territory of the carotid or vertebral basilar arteries.

uncinate a., SYN uncinate *epilepsy*.

vagal a., SYN Gowers' *syndrome*. SYN vasovagal syndrome.

vasovagal a., SYN Gowers' *syndrome*.

at·tar of rose (at'ăr). SYN *rose* oil, *oil* of rose. [Pers. *attara,* to smell sweet]

at·tend·ing (ă-tend'ing). In psychology, an aroused readiness to percieve, as in listening or looking; focusing of sense organs is sometimes involved. [L. *attendo,* to bend to, notice]

at·ten·u·ant (ă-ten'yū-ănt). **1.** Denoting that which attenuates. **2.** An agent, means, or method that attenuates.

at·ten·u·ate (ă-ten'yū-āt). To dilute, thin, reduce, weaken, diminish. [L. *at-tenuo,* pp. *-tenuatus,* to make thin or weak, fr. *tenuis,* thin]

at·ten·u·a·tion (ă-ten-yū-ā'shŭn). **1.** The act of attenuating. **2.** Diminution of virulence in a strain of an organism, obtained through selection of variants which occur naturally or through experimental means. **3.** Loss of energy of a beam of radiant energy due to absorption, scattering, beam divergence, and other causes as the beam propagates through a medium. **4.** Regulation of termination of transcription; involved in control of gene expression in specific tissues.

at·ten·u·a·tor (ă-ten'yū-ā-tŏr, -tōr). **1.** An electrical system of resistors and capacitors used to reduce the strength of electrical signals as in ultrasonography. **2.** The terminator sequence in DNA at which attenuation occurs.

at·tic (at'ik). SYN epitympanic *recess*.

tympanic a., SYN epitympanic *recess*.

at·ti·co·mas·toid (at'i-kō-mas'toyd). Relating to the attic of the tympanic cavity and the mastoid antrum or cells.

at·ti·cot·o·my (at-i-kot'ō-mē). Operative opening into the tympanic attic. [attic + G. *tomē,* incision]

at·ti·tude (at'i-tūd). **1.** Position of the body and limbs. **2.** Manner of acting. **3.** In social or clinical psychology, a relatively stable and enduring predisposition or set to behave or react in a certain way toward persons, objects, institutions, or issues. [Mediev. L. *aptitudo,* fr. L. *aptus,* fit]

emotional a.'s, SYN passional a.'s.

fetal a., SYN fetal *habitus*.

passional a.'s, a.'s expressive of any of the great passions; *e.g.,* anger, lust. SYN emotional a.'s.

at·ti·tu·di·nal (at-i-tū'di-năl). Relating to a posture of the body; *e.g.,* a. (statotonic) reflex.

atto- (a). Prefix used in the SI and metric systems to signify one quintillionth (10^{-18}). [Danish *atten,* eighteen]

at·tol·lens (ă-tol'ens). Raising up; in anatomy, muscle action that lifts. [L. *at-* tollo, pres. p. *-tollens,* to lift up]

a. au'rem, a. auric'ulam, SYN superior auricular *muscle*.

a. oc'uli, SYN superior rectus *muscle*.

at·trac·tion (ă-trak'shŭn). The tendency of two bodies to approach each other. [L. *at-traho,* pp. *-tractus,* to draw toward]

capillary a., the force that causes fluids to rise up very fine tubes or through the pores of a loose material.

chemical a., the force impelling atoms of different elements or molecules to unite to form new substances or compounds.

magnetic a., the force that draws iron or steel toward a magnet.

neurotropic a., the pull of a regenerating axon toward the motor end-plate.

at·tra·hens (at'ră-henz). Drawing toward, denoting a muscle (attrahens aurem or auriculam) rudimentary in man, that tends to draw the pinna of the ear forward. SEE anterior auricular *muscle*. [see attraction]

at·tri·tion (ă-trish'ŭn). **1.** Wearing away by friction or rubbing. **2.** In dentistry, physiological loss of tooth structure caused by the abrasive character of food or from bruxism. Cf. abrasion. [L. *at-tero,* pp. *-tritus,* to rub against, rub away]

at wt Abbreviation for atomic *weight*.

atyp·ia (ā-tip'ē-ă). State of being not typical. SYN atypism.

atyp·i·cal (ā-tip'i-kal). Not typical; not corresponding to the normal form or type. [G. *a-* priv. + *typikos,* conformed to a type]

atyp·ism (ā-tip'izm). SYN atypia.

A.U. Abbreviation for *auris uterque* [L.], each ear or both ears.

Au Symbol for gold (aurum).

Aub, Joseph C., U.S. physician, 1890–1973. SEE A.-DuBois *table*.

Auberger blood group, Au blood group. See Blood Groups appendix.

Aubert, Hermann, German physiologist, 1826–1892. SEE A.'s *phenomenon*.

Auch·mer·o·my·ia (awk′mer-ō-mī′yă). A genus of bloodsucking botflies (family Calliphoridae, order Diptera). [G. *auchmeros*, without rain, hence unwashed, squalid, + *myia*, a fly]

A. _lute′ola_, the Congo floor maggot; the bloodsucking larva of this botfly species is found in Africa south of the Sahara, usually in or near human habitations; the resistant larvae or maggots crawl to sleeping humans and suck blood for 15 to 20 minutes, detach, and hide, repeating these nightly attacks during their developmental period; no disease transmission is known from this insect.

¹⁹⁸Au col·loid. SYN radiogold colloid.

au·dile (aw′dil). **1.** Relating to audition. **2.** Denoting the type of mental imagery in which one recalls most readily that which has been heard rather than seen or read. Cf. motile, visile. **3.** SYN auditive.

△**audio-.** The sense of hearing. [L. *audio*, to hear]

au·di·o·an·al·ge·sia (aw′dē-ō-an-ăl-jē′zē-ă). Use of music or sound delivered through earphones to mask pain during dental or surgical procedures.

au·di·o·gen·ic (awd′ē-ō-jen′ik). **1.** Caused by sound, especially a loud noise. **2.** Sound-producing. [audio- + G. *genesis*, production]

au·di·o·gram (aw′dē-ō-gram). The graphic record drawn from the results of hearing tests with the audiometer, charts the threshold of hearing at various frequencies against sound intensity in decibels. [audio- + G. *gramma*, a drawing]

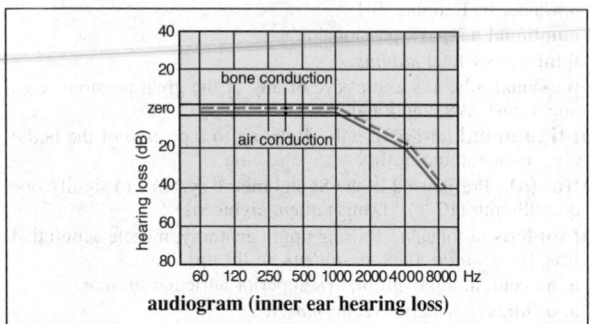

audiogram (inner ear hearing loss)

pure tone a., a chart of the threshold for hearing acuity at various frequencies usually expressed in decibels above normal threshold and usually covering frequencies from 128 to 8000 Hz.

speech a., the record of thresholds for spondaic word lists and scores for phonetically balanced word lists.

au·di·ol·o·gist (aw-dē-ol′ōjist). A specialist in evaluation and rehabilitation of those whose communication disorders center in whole or in part in the hearing function.

au·di·ol·o·gy (aw-dē-ol′ō-jē). The study of hearing disorders through the identification and measurement of hearing function loss as well as the rehabilitation of persons with hearing impairments.

au·di·om·e·ter (aw-dē-om′ĕ-ter). An electrical instrument for measuring the threshold of hearing for pure tones of frequencies generally varying from 128 to 8000 Hz (recorded in terms of decibels). [audio- + G. *metron*, measure]

automatic a., an a. that is operated by the patient, enabling him to control the intensity of the tone presented to him and thus track his own hearing thresholds.

Békésy a., an automatic a. in which the tone sweeps the audiometric scale while the patient controls intensity by pressing a button when he cannot hear the tone; may be operated either at a fixed frequency or at steadily changing frequencies.

limited range a., a pure-tone a. designed to test restricted ranges of frequency and sound pressure.

pure-tone a., an electroacoustical generator which produces pure tones of selected frequencies and calibrated output.

speech a., an a. that provides spoken material at controlled sound pressure levels to obtain speech reception thresholds, tolerance for loud speech, and discrimination ability, utilizing either a live voice with a microphone or a recorded voice played over a turntable or tape recorder.

au·di·o·met·ric (aw′dē-ō-met′rik). Related to measurement of hearing levels.

au·di·om·e·trist (aw-dē-om′ĕ-trist). A person trained in the use of the audiometer in testing hearing acuity.

au·di·om·e·try (aw-dē-om′ĕ-trē). Use of the audiometer.

auditory brainstem response a. (ABR), ABR a., an electrophysiologic measure of auditory function utilizing responses produced by the auditory nerve and the brainstem to repetitive acoustic stimuli.

automatic a., an audiometric technique using an automatic audiometer, which enables the patient to track his own hearing thresholds by controlling the intensity of the signal being presented to him, while the audiometer sweeps through the audible frequency range.

Békésy a., automatic a. utilizing the Békésy audiometer; the patient makes two threshold tracings, one in which the tone is rapidly turned on and off (interrupted tone) and one in which the tone is presented steadily (continuous tone); results may be suggestive of middle-ear, cochlear, or eighth nerve lesions.

brainstem evoked response a., BSER a., auditory brainstem response a.

cortical a., measurement of the potentials that arise in the auditory system above the level of the brainstem.

diagnostic a., measurement of hearing threshold levels to determine the nature and degree of hearing loss (*e.g.,* conductive, sensorineural, or mixed).

electrodermal a., a form of electrophysiologic a. used to determine hearing thresholds by measuring changes in skin resistance as a conditioned response to noise stimuli.

electrophysiologic a., measurement of a patient's response to a sound stimulus by using various types of objective audiometric equipment or techniques without necessarily having the patient's conscious cooperation.

evoked response a. (ERA), a type of electrophysiologic a. in which electrical potentials of neural impulses from the cochlear nerve and various levels in the brain in response to acoustic stimulation are used to localize the site of a lesion causing a hearing loss.

pure-tone a., a. utilizing tones of various frequencies and intensities as auditory stimuli to measure hearing, including comparisons of results from testing air conduction and bone conduction.

screening a., rapid measurement of the hearing of an individual or a group against a predetermined limit of normalcy; auditory responses to different frequencies presented at a constant intensity level are tested.

speech a., measurement of overall performance in hearing, understanding, and responding to speech for a general assessment of hearing and an estimate of degree of practical handicap.

au·di·o·vi·su·al (aw′dē-ō-vizh′yū-ăl). Pertaining to a communication or teaching technique that combines both audible and visible symbols.

au·dit. An examination or review that establishes the extent to which a condition, process, or performance conforms to predetermined standards or criteria. [L. *auditus*, a hearing, fr. *audio*, to hear]

au·di·tion (aw-dish′ŭn). SYN hearing. [L. *auditio*, a hearing, fr. *audeo*, to hear]

chromatic a., SYN color *hearing*.

au·di·tive (aw′di-tiv). One who recalls most readily that which has been heard. SYN audile (3).

au·di·to·ry (aw′di-tōr-ē). Pertaining to the sense of hearing or to the organs of hearing. [L. *audio*, pp. *auditus*, to hear]

Auenbrugger, Leopold, Austrian physician, 1722–1809. SEE A.'s *sign.*

Auer, John, U.S. physician, 1875–1948. SEE A. *bodies,* under *body, rods,* under *rod.*

Auerbach, Leopold, German anatomist, 1828–1897. SEE A.'s *ganglia,* under *ganglion, plexus.*

Aufrecht, Emanuel, German physician, 1844–1933. SEE A.'s *sign.*

Auger (aw′ger). Pierre-Victor, French physicist, *1899. SEE Auger *electron.*

aug·na·thus (awg-nā′thŭs). SYN dignathus. [G. *au,* again, + *gnathos,* jaw]

Aujeszky, Aládár, Hungarian pathologist, 1869–1933. SEE A.'s *disease,* disease *virus.*

aur. Abbreviation for auris.

au·ra, pl. **au·rae** (aw′ră, -rē). **1.** Subjective symptoms occurring at the onset of a partial epileptic seizure; often characteristic for the brain region involved in the seizure, *e.g.,* visual aura, occipital lobe auditory aura, temporal lobe. **2.** Subjective symptoms at the onset of a migraine headache. [L. breeze, odor, gleam of light]
   intellectual a., a dreamy, detached, or reminiscent a. SYN reminiscent a.
   kinesthetic a., an a. consisting of a subjective feeling of movement of a part of the body.
   reminiscent a., SYN intellectual a.

au·ral (aw′răl). **1.** Relating to the ear (auris). **2.** Relating to an aura.

au·ra·mine O (aw′ră-mēn) [C.I. 41000]. A yellow fluorescent dye, $C_{17}H_{22}N_3Cl$, used as a stain for the tubercle bacillus and as a stain for DNA in Kasten's fluorescent Feulgen stain.

au·ran·o·fin (aw-ran′ō-fin). $C_{20}H_{34}AuO_9PS$; an oral form of gold complex used in the treatment of rheumatoid arthritis. It is thought to arrest the progression of disease.

au·ran·ti·a·sis cu·tis (aw-ran-tī′ă-sis kyū′tis). Obsolete term for carotenosis cutis. [L. *aurantium,* orange, + G. *-iasis,* condition; *cutis,* skin]

au·re·o·lic ac·id (aw-rē-ō′lik). SYN mithramycin.

⚘**auri-.** Combining form denoting the ear. SEE ALSO ot-, oto-. [L. *auris,* an ear.]

au·ri·a·sis (aw-rī′ă-sis). SYN chrysiasis.

au·ric (aw′rik). Relating to gold (aurum).

au·ri·cle (aw′ri-kl). **1** [NA]. The projecting shell-like structure on the side of the head, constituting, with the external acoustic meatus, the external ear. SYN ala auris, auricula (1), pinna (1). **2.** SYN auricle of *atrium.*
   accessory a.'s, small, fleshy nodules or folds, sometimes with supporting cartilage, occasionally found along the margins of the embryonic branchial clefts.
   atrial a., SYN auricle of *atrium.* SEE ALSO left *atrium* of heart, right *atrium* of heart.
   cervical a., accessory a. on the neck.
   a. of left atrium, the small conical projection from the left atrium of the heart. SYN auricula sinistra [NA], left auricular appendage.
   a. of right atrium, the small conical projection from the right atrium of the heart. SYN auricula dextra [NA], right auricular appendage.

au·ric·u·la, pl. **au·ric·u·lae** (aw-rik′yū-lă, -lē). **1** [NA]. SYN auricle (1). **2.** SYN auricle of *atrium.* [L. the external ear, dim. of *auris,* ear]
   atrial a., SYN auricle of *atrium.* SEE ALSO left *atrium* of heart, right *atrium* of heart.
   a. a′tria′lis [NA], SYN auricle of *atrium.* SEE ALSO left *atrium* of heart, right *atrium* of heart.
   a. dex′tra [NA], SYN *auricle* of right atrium.
   a. sinis′tra [NA], SYN *auricle* of left atrium.

au·ric·u·lar (aw-rik′yū-lăr). Relating to the ear, or to an auricle in any sense.

au·ric·u·la·re, pl. **au·ric·u·lar·ia** (aw-rik-yū-lā′rē, -rē-ă). A craniometric point at the center of the opening of the external acoustic meatus; or, in certain cases, the middle of the upper edge of this opening. SYN auricular point. [L. *auricularis,* pertaining to the ear]

au·ric·u·lo·cra·ni·al (aw-rik′yū-lō-krā′nē-ăl). Relating to the auricle or pinna of the ear and the cranium.

au·ric·u·lo·tem·po·ral (aw-rik′yū-lō-tem′pō-răl). Relating to the auricle or pinna of the ear and the temporal region.

au·ric·u·lo·ven·tric·u·lar (aw-rik′yū-lō-ven-trik′yū-lăr). Obsolete synonym for atrioventricular.

au·rid, pl. **au·ri·des** (aw′rid, aw′ri-dēz). A skin lesion due to injection of gold salts. [L. *aurum,* gold, + *-id* (1)]

au·ri·form (aw′ri-fōrm). Ear-shaped.

au·rin (aw′rin) [C.I. 43800]. A triphenylmethane derivative used as an indicator (changes from yellow to red at pH 6.8 to 8.2) and as a dye intermediate; also used to help differentiate tubercle bacilli from other acid-fast microorganisms. SYN corallin, *p*-rosolic acid.

au·rin·tri·car·box·yl·ic ac·id (aw′rin-trī′kar-boks-il′ik). Tris(3-carboxy-4-hydroxyphenyl)methane; a chelating agent that has a special affinity for beryllium and certain other materials, and may therefore be of use in combating beryllium poisoning; the ammonium salt is known as aluminon.

au·ris (a, a, aur), pl. **au·res** (aw′ris, aw′rēz) [NA]. SYN ear. [L.]
   a. exte′rna [NA], SYN external *ear.* SEE ear. SEE ALSO auricle, external acoustic *meatus,* pinna.
   a. inter′na [NA], SYN internal *ear.* SEE ear. SEE ALSO labyrinth.
   a. me′dia [NA], SYN middle *ear.* SEE ear. SEE ALSO tympanic *cavity.*

au·ro·chro·mo·der·ma (aw′rō-krō-mō-der′mă). SYN chrysiasis. [L. *aurum,* gold, + *chrōma,* color, + derma, skin]

au·ro·mer·cap·to·ac·et·an·i·lid (aw′rō-mer-kap′tō-as-ĕ-tan′i-lid). $AuSCH_2CONH–C_6H_5$; {[(phenylcarbamoyl)methyl]-thio}gold; an organic gold compound, insoluble in water; used in the treatment of rheumatoid arthritis, and administered by intramuscular injection; more slowly absorbed than the water-soluble gold salts. SYN aurothioglycanide.

au·rone (aw′rōn). **1.** 2-benzylidene-3(2*H*)-benzofuranone; the parent compound of a series of plant pigments; they are substituted coumaranones, and may be formed from chalcones. They are often found as glycosides. **2.** A class of compounds based on a. (1). SYN benzalcoumaran-3-one.

au·ro·ther·a·py (aw-rō-thār′ă-pē). SYN chrysotherapy. [L. *aurum,* gold]

au·ro·thi·o·glu·cose (aw′rō-thī-ō-glū′kōs). Organic gold preparation with –SAu group in place of 1-OH group of glucose; used in treatment of rheumatoid arthritis and nondisseminated lupus erythematosus. SYN gold thioglucose.

au·ro·thi·o·gly·ca·nide (aw′-rō-thī-ō-glī′kă-nīd). SYN auromercaptoacetanilid.

au·rum (aw′rŭm). SYN gold. [L.]

aus·cul·tate, aus·cult (aws′kŭl-tāt, aws-kŭlt′). To perform auscultation.

aus·cul·ta·tion (aws-kŭl-tā′shŭn). Listening to the sounds made by the various body structures as a diagnostic method. [L. *ausculto,* pp. *-atus,* to listen to]
   immediate a., direct a., a. by application of the ear to the surface of the body.
   mediate a., a. performed with the use of a stethoscope.

aus·cul·ta·to·ry (aws-kŭl′tă-tō-rē). Relating to auscultation.

Austin Flint. SEE Flint. SEE Flint.

⚘**aut-.** SEE auto-.

au·ta·coid (aw-tă′-koyd). A substance, formed metabolically by one set of cells, which alters the function of other cells. (This term is sometimes used in place of the term hormone.) [aut- + G. *akos,* relief, resource]

au·te·cic, au·te·cious (aw-tē′sik, aw-tē′shŭs). Denoting a parasite that infects, throughout its entire existence, the same host. [G. *autos,* same, + *oikion,* house]

au·te·me·sia (aw-tĕ-mē′zē-ă). Rarely used term for: **1.** Idiopathic

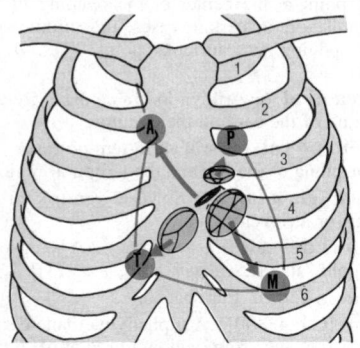

auscultation

projection of the heart valves, and the areas of relative cardiac dullness (red lines) on the pectus; the blue arrows show the direction of the valve sounds; red dots are points of auscultation (A = aortic valve; P = pulmonary valve; T = tricuspid valve; M = mitral valve)

or functional vomiting. **2.** Vomiting induced by provoking the gag reflex. [G. *autos,* self, + *emesis,* vomiting]

au·then·tic·i·ty (aw-then-tis′i-tē). **1.** The quality of being authentic, genuine, and valid. **2.** In psychological functioning and personality, applied to the conscious feelings, perceptions, and thoughts that one expresses and communicates honestly and genuinely. [G. *authentikos,* original, primary]

au·tism (aw′tizm). A tendency to morbid self-absorption at the expense of regulation by outward reality. SYN autistic disorder. [G. *autos,* self]

early infantile a., SYN infantile a.

infantile a., a severe emotional disturbance of childhood characterized by qualitative impairment in reciprocal social interaction and in communication, language, and social development. SYN autistic disorder, childhood schizophrenia, early infantile a., Kanner's syndrome.

au·tis·tic (aw-tis′tik). Pertaining to or characterized by autism.

⌂ **auto-, aut-.** Prefixes meaning self, same. [G. *autos,* self]

au·to·ac·ti·va·tion (aw′tō-ak-ti-vā′shŭn). SYN autocatalysis.

au·to·ag·glu·ti·na·tion (aw′to-ă-glū-ti-nā′shŭn). **1.** Nonspecific agglutination or clumping together of cells (*e.g.,* bacteria, erythrocytes) due to physical-chemical factors. **2.** The agglutination of an individual's red blood cells in his own serum, as a consequence of specific autoantibody.

au·to·ag·glu·ti·nin (aw′tō-ă-glū′ti-nin). An agglutinating autoantibody.

anti-Pr cold a., a cold a. specific for the Pr (protease-sensitive) antigen of erythrocytes.

cold a., a heterogeneous group of autoantibodies that react at temperatures below 37°C, often most actively at 4°C; most are the IgM class of immunoglobulins with affinity for the Ii system of erythrocyte antigens, but some are anti-Pr cold a.'s; cold a.'s may be associated with infection (*e.g.,* primary atypical pneumonia, infectious mononucleosis and other virus infections, certain protozoan infections) and in such instances usually are not active *in vivo.*

au·to·al·ler·gic (aw′tō-ă-ler′jik). Pertaining to autoallergy.

au·to·al·ler·gi·za·tion (aw′tō-al′er-ji-zā′shŭn). Induction of autoallergy.

au·to·al·ler·gy (aw-tō-al′er-jē). An altered reactivity in which antibodies (autoantibodies) are produced against an individual's own tissues, causing a destructive rather than a protective effect. SYN autoimmunity (2).

au·to·a·nal·y·sis (aw′tō-ă-nal′i-sis). Attempted analysis, or psychoanalysis, of one's self. SYN self-analysis.

au·to·an·a·lyz·er (aw-tō-an′ă-līz-er). An instrument capable of conducting analyses automatically; commonly used in chemical analyses.

sequential multichannel a. (SMA), an automated instrument capable of performing multiple (usually chemical) analyses simultaneously by propelling samples and reagents in continuous flow fashion along tubes to the detector mechanisms.

au·to·an·a·phy·lax·is (aw′tō-an′ă-fī-lak′sis). Old term for certain kinds of autoimmunity.

au·to·an·ti·body (aw-tō-an′ti-bod-ē). Antibody occurring in response to antigenic constituents of the host's tissue, and which reacts with the inciting tissue component.

autoantibodies	
antibody type	pathologies
antibodies and erythrocytes	
incomplete warm Ab warm hemolysin	idiopathic and symptomatic hemolytic anemia
incomplete cold Ab abnormal increase of complete cold agglutinin monothermal cold hemolysin	cold hemagglutinin disease
bithermal cold hemolysin	paroxysmal cold hemoglobinuria
antibodies and leukocytes	
leukocytagglutinin, leukocytolysin leukocyte nuclear Ab (?)	chronic leukopenia LE
antibodies and thrombocytes	
platelet agglutinin plateletolysin	idiopathic thrombocytopenia (thrombocytopenic purpura)

anti-idiotype a., an a., the specificity of which is directed against one of one's own idiotypes. SEE ALSO anti-idiotype *antibody.* SYN idiotype a.

cold a., an a. that reacts at temperatures below 37°c.

Donath-Landsteiner cold a., an a. of the IgG class responsible for paroxysmal cold hemoglobinuria; it is adsorbed to red cells only at temperatures of 20°C or lower, causing the red cells to lyse in the presence of complement at higher temperatures; it has only slight agglutinating properties in spite of its marked lytic activity, and has a specificity within the blood group P; it is also occasionally present for short periods of time following measles and other infections, and formerly was frequently associated with syphilis. SYN cold hemolysin.

hemagglutinating cold a., a cold autoagglutinin.

idiotype a., SYN anti-idiotype a.

warm a., an a. that reacts optimally at 37°C.

au·to·an·ti·com·ple·ment (aw′tō-an-ti-com′plĕ-ment). An anti-complement that is formed in the body of an animal and inhibits or destroys the complement of the same animal.

au·to·an·ti·gen (aw-to-an′ti-jen). A "self" antigen; any tissue constituent that evokes an immune response to the host's tissues.

au·to·as·say (aw′tō-as-ā). Detection or estimation of the amount of a substance produced in an organism by means of a test object in that organism, as, for example, use of the denervated heart *in situ* of a cat to assay for epinephrine or sympathin liberated into its bloodstream.

au·to·aug·men·ta·tion (aw′-tō-awg′men-tā-shŭn). Augmentation of the bladder by incision and excision of detrusor muscle leaving only bladder epithelium. SYN autocystoplasty, Snow procedure.

au·to·blast (aw′tō-blast). **1.** An independent cell. **2.** A single, independent microbe, protozoon, or single-celled (acellular) organism. [auto- + G. *blastos,* germ]

au·to·ca·tal·y·sis (aw′tō-kă-tal′i-sis). A reaction in which one or more of the products formed acts to catalyze the reaction; beginning slowly, the rate of such a reaction rapidly increases. Cf. chain *reaction*. SYN autoactivation.

au·to·cat·a·lyt·ic (aw′tō-kat-ă-lit′ik). Relating to autocatalysis.

au·to·cath·e·ter·i·za·tion, au·to·cath·e·ter·ism (aw′tō-kath-ĕ-ter-i-zā′shŭn, -kath′ĕ-ter-izm). Passage of a catheter by the patient.

au·toch·thon·ous (aw-tok′thon-ŭs). **1.** Native to the place inhabited; aboriginal. **2.** Originating in the place where found; said of a disease originating in the part of the body where found, or of a disease acquired in the place where the patient is. [auto- + G. *chthon,* land, ground, country]

au·toc·la·sis, au·to·cla·sia (aw-tok′lă-sis, aw-tō-klā′zē-ă). **1.** A breaking up or rupturing from intrinsic or internal causes. **2.** Progressive immunologically induced tissue destruction. [auto- + G. *klasis,* breaking]

au·to·clave (aw′tō-klāv). **1.** An apparatus for sterilization by steam under pressure; it consists of a strong closed boiler containing a small quantity of water and, in a wire basket, the articles to be sterilized. **2.** To sterilize in an autoclave. [auto- + L. *clavis,* a key, in the sense of self-locking]

au·to·coid (aw′tō-koyd). A chemical substance produced by one type of cell that affects the function of different types of cells in the same region, thus functioning as a local hormone or messenger. [G. *autos,* self, + *eidos,* form]

au·to·crine (aw′tō-krin). Denoting self-stimulation through cellular production of a factor and a specific receptor for it. [auto- + G. *krinō,* to separate]

au·to·cys·to·plas·ty (aw-tō-sis′tō-plas-tē). SYN autoaugmentation. [auto- + G. *kystis,* bladder, + *plastos,* formed]

au·to·cy·to·ly·sin (aw′tō-sī-tol′i-sin). SYN autolysin.

au·to·cy·tol·y·sis (aw′tō-sī-tol′i-sis). SYN autolysis.

au·to·cy·to·tox·in (aw′tō-sī-tō-toks′in). A cytotoxic autoantibody.

au·to·der·mic (aw-tō-der′mik). Relating to one's own skin; denoting especially an autodermic graft or dermatoautoplasty. [auto- + G. *derma,* skin]

au·to·di·ges·tion (aw′tō-dī-jes′chŭn). SYN autolysis.

au·to·dip·loid (aw-tō-dip′loyd). SEE autoploid.

au·to·drain·age (aw-tō-drān′ij). Drainage into contiguous tissues.

au·to·ech·o·la·lia (aw′tō-ek-ō-lā′lē-ă). A morbid repetition of another person's or one's own words. [auto- + echolalia]

au·to·e·rot·ic (aw′tō-ĕ-rot′ik). Pertaining to autoerotism.

au·to·e·rot·i·cism (aw′tō-ĕ-rot′i-sizm). SYN autoerotism.

au·to·e·ro·tism (aw-tō-ār′ō-tizm). **1.** Sexual arousal or gratification using one's own body, as in masturbation. **2.** Sexual self-love. SEE ALSO narcissism (1). Cf. alloerotism. SYN autoeroticism, autosexualism (1). [auto- + G. *erōtikos,* relating to love]

au·to·flu·o·ro·scope (aw-tō-flūr′ō-skōp). A type of scintillation camera consisting of a matrix of individual sodium iodide crystals, each with its separate light pipe and photomultiplier tube; used for radioisotope imaging procedures.

au·tog·a·mous (aw-tog′ă-mŭs). Relating to or characterized by autogamy.

au·tog·a·my (aw-tog′ă-mē). A form of self-fertilization in which fission of the cell nucleus occurs without division of the cell, the two pronuclei so formed reuniting to form the synkaryon; in other cases, the cell body also divides, but the two daughter cells immediately conjugate. SYN automixis. [auto- + G. *gamos,* marriage]

au·to·gen·e·sis (aw-tō-jen′ĕ-sis). **1.** The origin of living matter within the organism itself. **2.** In bacteriology, the process by which vaccine is made from bacteria obtained from the patient's own body. [auto- + G. *genesis,* production]

au·to·ge·net·ic, au·to·gen·ic (aw′tō-jĕ-net′ik, jen′ik). Relating to autogenesis. SYN autogenous (1).

au·tog·e·nous (aw-toj′ĕ-nŭs). **1.** SYN autogenetic. **2.** Originating within the body, applied to vaccines prepared from bacteria or other cells obtained from the affected person. Cf. endogenous. [G. *autogenēs,* self-produced]

au·tog·no·sis (aw-tog-nō′sis). Recognition of one's own charac-

ter, tendencies, and peculiarities. SYN self-knowledge. [auto- + G. *gnōsis,* knowledge]

au·to·graft (aw′tō-graft). A tissue or an organ transferred by grafting into a new position in the body of the same individual. SYN autogeneic graft, autologous graft, autoplast, autoplastic graft, autotransplant. [auto- + A.S. *graef*]

au·to·graft·ing (aw-tō-graft′ing). SYN autotransplantation.

au·to·gram (aw′tō-gram). A wheal-like lesion on the skin following pressure by a blunt instrument or by stroking. [auto- + G. *gramma,* something written]

au·tog·ra·phism (aw-tog′ră-fizm). SYN dermatographism.

au·to·hem·ag·glu·ti·na·tion (aw′tō-hē′mă-glū-ti-nā′shŭn). Autoagglutination of erythrocytes.

au·to·he·mo·ly·sin (aw′tō-hē-mol′i-sin). An autoantibody that in the presence of complement causes lysis of erythrocytes in the same individual in whose body the lysin is formed.

au·to·he·mol·y·sis (aw′tō-hē-mol′i-sis). Hemolysis occurring in certain diseases as a result of an autohemolysin.

au·to·he·mo·trans·fu·sion (aw′tō-hē-mō-tranz-fyū′zhŭn). SYN autotransfusion.

au·to·hex·a·ploid (aw-tō-heks′ă-ployd). SEE autoploid.

au·to·hyp·no·sis (aw′tō-hip-nō′sis). Self-induced hypnosis, accomplished by concentrating on self-absorbing thought or on the idea of being hypnotized. SYN autohypnotism, idiohypnotism, statuvolence.

au·to·hyp·not·ic (aw′tō-hip-not′ik). Relating to autohypnosis.

au·to·hyp·no·tism (aw-tō-hip′nō-tizm). SYN autohypnosis.

au·to·im·mune (aw-tō-i-myūn′). Arising from and directed against the individual's own tissues, as in autoimmune disease.

au·to·im·mu·ni·ty (aw′tō-i-myū′ni-tē). **1.** Literally, the condition in which "self" is exempt. **2.** In immunology, the condition in which one's own tissues are subject to deleterious effects of the immune system, as in autoallergy and in autoimmune disease; specific humoral or cell-mediated immune response against the body's own tissues. SYN autoallergy.

au·to·im·mu·ni·za·tion (aw′tō-im′yū-ni-zā′shŭn). Induction of autoimmunity.

au·to·im·mu·no·cy·to·pe·nia (aw-tō-im′yū-nō-sī-tō-pē′nē-ă). Anemia, thrombocytopenia, and leukopenia resulting from cytotoxic autoimmune reactions.

au·to·in·fec·tion (aw′tō-in-fek′shŭn). **1.** Reinfection by microbes or parasitic organisms on or within the body that have already passed through an infective cycle, such as a succession of boils, or a new infective cycle with production of a new generation of larvae and adults, as by the nematode *Strongyloides stercoralis* or the cestode *Hymenolepis nana*. **2.** Self-infection by direct contagion as with parasite eggs passed in the infectious state transmitted by fingernails (anal-oral route), as with the pinworm, *Enterobius vermicularis.* SYN autoreinfection, self-infection.

au·to·in·fu·sion (aw′tō-in-fyū′shŭn). Forcing the blood from the extremities or other areas such as the spleen, as by the application of a bandage or pressure device, to raise the blood pressure and fill the vessels in the vital centers; resorted to after excessive loss of blood or other body fluids. Cf. autotransfusion.

au·to·in·oc·u·la·ble (aw′tō-in-ok′yū-lă-bl). Susceptible to autoinoculation.

au·to·in·oc·u·la·tion (aw′tō-in-ok-yū-lā′shŭn). A secondary infection originating from a focus of infection already present in the body.

au·to·in·tox·i·cant (aw′tō-in-toks′i-kant). An endogenous toxic agent that causes autointoxication. SYN autotoxin.

au·to·in·tox·i·ca·tion (aw′tō-in-toks-i-kā′shŭn). A disorder resulting from absorption of the waste products of metabolism, decomposed matter from the intestine, or the products of dead and infected tissue as in gangrene. SYN autotoxicosis, endogenic toxicosis, enterotoxication, enterotoxism, intestinal intoxication, self-poisoning.

au·to·i·sol·y·sin (aw′tō-ī-sol′i-sin). An antibody that in the presence of complement causes lysis of cells in the individual in whose body the lysin is formed, as well as in others of the same species.

au·to·ker·a·to·plas·ty (aw-tō-ker′ă-tō-plas-tē). Grafting of corneal tissue from one eye of a patient to the fellow eye. [auto- + G. *keras,* horn, + *plastos,* formed]

au·to·ki·ne·sia, au·to·ki·ne·sis (aw-tō-ki-ne′sē-ă, aw-tō-ki-nē′sis). Voluntary movement. [auto- + G. *kinēsis,* movement]

au·to·ki·net·ic (aw-tō-kĭ-net′ik). Relating to autokinesis.

au·to·le·sion (aw-tō-lē′zhŭn). A self-inflicted injury.

au·tol·o·gous (aw-tol′ŏ-gŭs). 1. Occurring naturally and normally in a certain type of tissue or in a specific structure of the body. 2. Sometimes used to denote a neoplasm derived from cells that occur normally at that site, *e.g.,* a squamous cell carcinoma in the upper esophagus. 3. In transplantation, referring to a graft in which the donor and recipient areas are in the same individual. [auto- + G. *logos,* relation]

au·tol·y·sate (aw-tol′i-sāt). The mixture of substances resulting from autolysis.

au·to·lyse (aw′tō-līs). SYN autolyze.

au·tol·y·sin (aw-tol′i-sin). An antibody that in the presence of complement causes lysis of the cells and tissues in the body of the individual in whom the lysin is formed. SYN autocytolysin.

au·tol·y·sis (aw-tol′i-sis). 1. Enzymatic digestion of cells (especially dead or degenerate) by enzymes present within them (autogenous). 2. Destruction of cells as a result of a lysin formed in those cells or others in the same organism. SYN autocytolysis, autodigestion, isophagy. [auto- + G. *lysis,* dissolution]

au·to·lyt·ic (aw-tō-lit′ik). Pertaining to or causing autolysis.

au·to·lyze (aw′tō-līz). To undergo autolysis. SYN autolyse.

au·to·mal·let (aw′tō-mal-et). Obsolete term for automatic *plugger* or condenser.

au·tom·a·tism (aw-tom′ă-tizm). 1. The state of being independent of the will or of central innervation; applicable, for example, to the heart's action. 2. An epileptic attack consisting of stereotyped psychic, sensory, or motor phenomena carried out in a state of impaired consciousness and of which the individual usually has no knowledge. 3. A condition in which an individual is consciously or unconsciously, but involuntarily, compelled to the performance of certain motor or verbal acts, often purposeless and sometimes foolish or harmful. SYN telergy. [G. *automatos,* self-moving, + -in]

ambulatory a., a person's automatic performance of an action or series of actions without being consciously aware of the processes involved in the performance.

immediate posttraumatic a., a posttraumatic state in which the patient performs automatically without immediate or later memory of that behavior.

au·to·mat·o·graph (aw-tō-mat′ō-graf). An instrument for recording automatic movements.

au·to·mix·is (aw-tō-miks′is). SYN autogamy. [auto- + G. *mixis,* intercourse]

au·tom·ne·sia (aw-tom-nē′zē-ă). Spontaneous revival of memories of an earlier condition of life. [auto- + G. *mnēsis,* a remembering]

au·to·my·so·pho·bia (aw′tō-mis-ō-fō′bē-ă). Morbid dread of personal uncleanliness. [auto- + G. *mysos,* dirt, + *phobos,* fear]

au·to·nom·ic (aw-tō-nom′ik). 1. Relating to the autonomic nervous system. 2. Obsolete term for autonomous.

au·to·nom·o·tro·pic (aw′tō-nom-ō-trop′ik). Acting on the autonomic nervous system. [autonomic + G. *trepo,* to turn]

au·ton·o·mous (aw-ton′ŏ-mŭs). Having independence or freedom from control by external forces or, in a narrow sense, by the cerebrospinal nerve centers.

au·ton·o·my (aw-ton′ŏ-mē). The condition or state of being autonomous. [auto- + G. *nomos,* law]

functional a., in social psychology, the tendency of a developed motive system (*e.g.,* motive of acquisition) to become independent of the primary or innate drive from which it originated (*e.g.,* need for food).

au·to·ox·i·da·tion (aw′tō-oks-i-dā′shŭn). The direct combina-

tion of a substance with molecular oxygen at ordinary temperatures. SYN autoxidation.

au·to·ox·i·diz·a·ble (aw′tō-oks-i-dīz′ă-bl). Denoting substances that react directly with oxygen (*e.g.,* b hemochromogen in cytochrome) and do not require the action of dehydrogenases.

au·to·path·ic (aw-tō-path′ik). Rarely used synonym for idiopathic.

au·to·pen·ta·ploid (aw-tō-pen′tă-ployd). SEE autoploid.

au·to·pep·sia (aw-tō-pep′sē-ă). Rarely used term for self-digestion, said of ulceration of the gastric mucous membrane by its own secretion, or the digestion of the skin surrounding a gastrostomy or colostomy opening. [auto- + G. *pepsis,* digestion]

au·to·pha·gia (aw-tō-fā′jē-ă). 1. Biting one's own flesh; *e.g.,* as a symptom of Lesch-Nyhan syndrome. 2. Maintenance of the nutrition of the whole body by metabolic consumption of some of the body tissues. 3. SYN autophagy. [auto- + G. *phagō,* to eat]

au·to·pha·gic (aw-tō-fā′jik). Relating to or characterized by autophagia.

au·to·pha·go·ly·so·some (aw′tō-fā-gō-lī′sō-sōm). The digestive vacuole of autophagy that results from the fusion of a primary lysosome with an autophagic vacuole.

au·toph·a·gy (aw-tof′ă-jē). Segregation and disposal of damaged organelles within a cell. SYN autophagia (3). [auto- + G. *phagō,* to eat]

au·to·phil·ia (aw-tō-fil′ē-ă). SYN narcissism (1). [auto- + G. *phileō,* to love]

au·to·pho·bia (aw-tō-fō′bē-ă). Morbid fear of solitude or of self. [auto- + G. *phobos,* fear]

au·toph·o·ny (aw-tof′ŏ-nē). Increased resonance of one's own voice, breath sounds, arterial murmurs, etc., noted especially in disease of the middle ear or of the nasal fossae. SYN tympanophonia (2), tympanophony. [auto- + G. *phōnē,* sound]

au·to·plast (aw′tō-plast). SYN autograft. [auto- + G. *plastos,* formed]

au·to·plas·tic (aw′tō-plas-tik). Relating to autoplasty.

au·to·plas·ty (aw′tō-plas-tē). Repair of defects by autotransplantation.

au·to·ploid (aw′tō-ployd). Relating to an individual or cell with two or more copies of a single haploid set; depending on the number of multiples of the haploid set, a.'s are referred to as autodiploids, autotriploids, autotetraploids, autopentaploids, autohexaploids, etc. [auto- + -ploid]

au·to·ploi·dy (aw′tō-ploy-dē). The condition of being autoploid.

au·to·plug·ger (aw′tō-plŭg-er). Obsolete term for automatic *plugger.*

au·to·pod (aw′tō-pod). SYN autopodium.

au·to·po·di·um, pl. **au·to·po·dia** (aw′tō-pō′dē-ŭm, dē-ă). The distal major subdivision of a limb (hand or foot). SYN autopod. [auto- + G. *pous (pod-),* foot]

au·to·poi·son·ous (aw-tō-poy′zŭn-ŭs). SYN autotoxic.

au·to·pol·y·mer (aw-tō-pol′i-mer). SEE autopolymer *resin.*

au·to·po·lym·er·i·za·tion (aw-tō-pol′i-mer-i-zā′shŭn). Polymerization without the use of external heat, as a result of the addition of an activator and a catalyst.

au·to·pol·y·ploid (aw-tō-pol′i-ployd). An autoploid having two or more multiples of the haploid sets of chromosomes.

au·to·pol·y·ploi·dy (aw-tō-pol′i-ploy-dē). The condition of being allopolyploid.

au·top·sy (aw′top-sē). 1. An examination of the organs of a dead body to determine the cause of death or to study the pathologic changes present. SYN necropsy, thanatopsy. 2. In the terminology of the ancient Greek school of empirics, the intentional reproduction of an effect, event, or circumstance that occurred in the course of a disease and observation of its influence in ameliorating or aggravating the patient's symptoms. SYN postmortem examination. [G. *autopsia,* seeing with one's own eyes]

au·to·ra·di·o·gram (aw-tō-rā′dē-ō-gram). SYN autoradiograph. [auto- + radiogram]

au·to·ra·di·o·graph (aw-tō-rā′dē-ō-graf). Image of the distribution and concentration of radioactivity in a tissue or other substance made by placing a photographic emulsion on the surface of, or in close proximity to, the substance. SYN autoradiogram.

au·to·ra·di·og·ra·phy (aw′tō-rā-dē-og′ră-fē). The process of producing an autoradiograph. SYN radioautography.

paper a., a. in which compounds are separated by paper chromatography.

au·to·reg·u·la·tion (aw′tō-reg-yū-lā′shŭn). **1.** The tendency of the blood flow to an organ or part to remain at or return to the same level despite changes in the pressure in the artery which conveys blood to it. **2.** In general, any biologic system equipped with inhibitory feedback systems such that a given change tends to be largely or completely counteracted; *e.g.,* baroreceptor reflexes form a basis for autoregulation of the systemic arterial blood pressure.

heterometric a., intrinsic regulation of the strength of cardiac contraction as a function of diastolic fiber length (volume), independent of afterload, autonomic nerves and other extrinsic influences. Heterometric a. is also known as the length-tension relationship, the relationship of end diastolic volume to end diastolic pressure, Starling's law of the heart or the Frank-Starling mechanism.

homeometric a., intrinsic regulation of strength of cardiac contraction in response to influences that do not depend on change in fiber length, *i.e.,* the Frank-Starling mechanism, (*e.g.,* the Anrep effect in which strength increases in response to increased afterload, and the Bowditch staircase effect (treppe) in which strength increases in response to increased heart rate) and do not depend on extrinsic regulation (*e.g.,* in which strength increases in response to sympathetic nerve stimulation or norepinephrine).

au·to·re·in·fec·tion (aw′tō-rē-in-fek′shŭn). SYN autoinfection.

au·to·re·pro·duc·tion (aw′tō-rē-prō-duk′shŭn). The ability of a gene or virus, or nucleoprotein molecule generally, to bring about the synthesis of another molecule like itself from smaller molecules within the cell.

au·tor·rha·phy (aw-tōr′ă-fē). Wound closure using strands of fascia from the edges of the wound. [auto- + G. *rhaphē,* sewing]

au·to·sen·si·tize (aw-tō-sen′si-tīz). To sensitize against one's own body cells. SYN isosensitize.

au·to·sep·ti·ce·mia (aw′tō-sep-ti-sē′mē-ă). Septicemia apparently originating from microorganisms existing within the individual and not introduced from without. [auto- + G. *sēpsis,* decay, + *haima,* blood]

au·to·se·ro·ther·a·py (aw′tō-sē-rō-thār′ă-pē). The treatment of certain conditions, such as dermatoses, by injection of the patient's own blood serum. SYN autotherapy (3).

au·to·se·rum (aw-tō-sē′rŭm). Serum obtained from the patient's own blood and used in autoserotherapy.

au·to·sex·u·al·ism (aw-tō-sek′shū-ă-lizm). **1.** SYN autoerotism. **2.** SYN narcissism.

au·to·site (aw′tō-sīt). That member of abnormal, unequal conjoined twins that is able to live independently and nourish the other member (parasite) of the pair. [auto- + G. *sitos,* food]

au·tos·mia (aw-toz′mē-ă). The smelling of one's own body odor. [auto- + G. *osmē,* smell]

au·to·so·mal (aw-tō-sō′măl). Pertaining to an autosome.

au·to·so·ma·tog·no·sis (aw-tō-sō′mă-tog-nō′sis). The sensation that an amputated portion of the body is still present. SEE phantom *limb*. [auto- + G. *sōma,* body, + *gnōsis,* recognition]

au·to·so·ma·tog·nos·tic (aw-tō-sō′mă-tog-nos′tik). Pertaining to autosomatognosis.

au·to·some (aw′tō-sōm). Any chromosome other than a sex chromosome; a.'s normally occur in pairs in somatic cells and singly in gametes. SYN euchromosome. [auto- + G. *sōma,* body]

au·to·sug·gest·i·bil·i·ty (aw′tō-sŭg-jes-ti-bil′i-tē). A mental state in which autosuggestion (1) readily occurs.

au·to·sug·ges·tion (aw′tō-sŭg-jes′chŭn). **1.** Constant dwelling upon an idea or concept, thereby inducing some change in the mental or bodily functions. SEE ALSO autohypnosis. **2.** Reproduction in the brain of impressions previously received which become then the starting point of new acts or ideas.

au·to·syn·noia (aw′tō-sin-noy′ă). A mental disorder in which one never has a thought not connected with oneself. SYN self-centeredness. [auto- + G. *synnoia,* deep thought, fr. *syn,* with + *noeō,* to think]

au·to·syn·the·sis (aw-tō-sin′thĕ-sis). Self-reproduction or -replication.

au·to·te·lic (aw-tō-tel′ik). Denoting those traits closely associated with the central purposes of an individual. [auto- + G. *telos,* end, completeness, purpose]

au·to·tem·nous (aw-tō-tem′nŭs). Denoting a cell that propagates itself by fission without previous conjugation. [auto- + G. *temnō,* to cut]

au·to·tet·ra·ploid (aw-tō-tet′ră-ployd). SEE autoploid.

au·to·ther·a·py (aw-tō-thār′ă-pē). **1.** Self-treatment. **2.** Spontaneous cure. **3.** SYN autoserotherapy. **4.** An obsolete method of treating disease by the administration of the patient's own pathologic excretions.

au·tot·o·my (aw-tot′ŏ-mē). The act of casting off a body part as a means of escape; *e.g.,* the limb of a crab or the tail of a lizard. [auto- + G. *tomē,* a cutting]

au·to·top·ag·no·sia (aw′tō-top′ag-nō′zē-ă). Inability to recognize or to orient any part of one's own body; caused by a parietal lobe lesion. Cf. somatotopagnosis. [auto- + G. *topos,* place, + G. *a*- priv. + gnōsis]

au·to·tox·e·mia (aw′tō-tok-sē′mē-ă). Autointoxicants present in the blood, usually resulting in autointoxication.

au·to·tox·ic (aw-tō-toks′ik). Relating to autointoxication. SYN autopoisonous.

au·to·tox·i·co·sis (aw′tō-tok-si-kō′sis). SYN autointoxication.

au·to·tox·in (aw-tō-tok′sin). SYN autointoxicant.

au·to·trans·fu·sion (aw′tō-tranz-fyū′zhŭn). Withdrawal and reinjection/transfusion of the patient's own blood. Cf. autoinfusion. SYN autohemotransfusion.

au·to·trans·plant (aw-tō-tranz′plant). SYN autograft.

au·to·trans·plan·ta·tion (aw′tō-tranz-plan-tā′shŭn). The performance of an autograft. SYN autografting.

au·to·trip·loid (aw-tō-trip′loyd). SEE autoploid.

au·to·troph (aw′tō-trōf). A microorganism that uses only inorganic materials as its source of nutrients; carbon dioxide serves as the sole carbon source. [auto- + G. *trophē,* nourishment]

au·to·tro·phic (aw-tō-trof′ik). **1.** Self-nourishing. The ability of an organism to produce food from inorganic compounds. **2.** Pertaining to an autotroph.

au·to·tro·phy (aw′tō-trōf-ē;). The state of being self-sustaining and being able to produce food from inorganic compounds.

carbon autotrophy, ability to assimilate CO_2 from the air.

nitrogen autotrophy, ability to assimilate nitrate or to do nitrogen fixation.

sulfur autotrophy, ability to assimilate sulfate.

au·to·vac·ci·na·tion (aw′tō-vak-si-nā′shŭn). A second vaccination with virus from a vaccine sore on the same individual.

au·tox·i·da·tion (aw-tok-si-dā′shŭn). SYN auto-oxidation.

au·to·zy·gous (aw-tō-zī′gŭs). Denoting genes in a homozygote that are copies of the identical ancestral gene as a result of a consanguineous mating. [auto- + G. *zygōtos,* yoked]

⌂**auxano-, auxo-, aux-.** Increase, *e.g.,* in size, intensity, speed. [G. *auxanō,* to increase]

aux·an·o·gram (awk-san′ō-gram). A plate culture of bacteria in which variable conditions are provided in order to determine the effect of these conditions on the growth of the bacteria. [auxano- + G. *gramma,* something written]

aux·an·o·graph·ic (awk′san-ō-graf′ik). Pertaining to auxanogram or auxanography.

aux·a·nog·ra·phy (awk-să-nog′ră-fē). The study, using auxanograms, of the effects of different conditions on the growth of bacteria.

aux·an·ol·o·gy (awk-sa-nol′ō-jē). The study of growth. [auxano- + G. *logos,* study]

aux·e·sis (awk-sē′sis). Increase in size, especially as in hypertrophy. [G. increase]

aux·il·ia·ry (og-zil′yă-rē). **1.** Functioning in an augmenting capacity; supplementary. **2.** Functioning as a subordinate; secondary.

aux·il·i·o·mo·tor (awg-zil′ē-ō-mō-tŏr). Aiding motion.

aux·i·lyt·ic (awk′si-lit′ik). Increasing the destructive power of a lysin, or favoring lysis. [G. *auxō,* to increase, + *lysis,* dissolution]

△**auxo-.** SEE auxano-.

aux·o·car·dia (awk-sō-kar′dē-ă). **1.** Enlargement of the heart, either by hypertrophy or dilation. **2.** Diastole of the heart. [auxo- + G. *kardia,* heart]

aux·o·chrome (awk′sō-krōm). The chemical group within a dye molecule by which the dye is bound to reactive end groups in tissues. [auxo- + G. *chrōma,* color]

aux·o·drome (awk′sō-drōm). A course of growth as plotted on a Wetzel grid. [auxo- + G. *dromos,* course]

aux·o·flore (awk′sō-flōr). An atom or group of atoms that, by its presence in a molecule, shifts the latter's fluorescent radiation in the direction of the shorter wavelength, or increases the fluorescence. Cf. bathoflore.

aux·o·gluc (awk′sō-gluk). An atomic grouping that, when present in a molecule, intensifies its sweetness. [G. *auxanō,* to increase, + *glykys,* sweet]

aux·o·ton·ic (awk-sō-ton′ik). Denoting the condition in which a contracting muscle shortens against an increasing load. Cf. isometric (2), isotonic (3).

aux·o·tox (awk′sō-toks). An atomic grouping that, when present in a molecule, intensifies its poisonous characteristics. [G. *auxanō,* to increase, + *toxikon,* poison]

aux·o·troph (awk′sō-trōf). A mutant microorganism that requires some nutrient that is not required by the organism (prototroph) from which the mutant was derived. Cf. polyauxotroph, monoauxotroph. [auxo- + G. *trophē,* nourishment]

aux·o·tro·phic (awk-sō-trof′ik, -trō′fik). Pertaining to an auxotroph.

A-V Abbreviation for arteriovenous; atrioventricular.

aval·vu·lar (ā-val′vyū-lăr). Nonvalvular; without valves.

avas·cu·lar (ă-vas′kyū-ler, ā). Without blood or lymphatic vessels; may be a normal state as in certain forms of cartilage, or the result of disease. SYN nonvascular.

avas·cu·lar·i·za·tion (ă-vas′kyū-lar-ī-zā′shŭn, ā-). **1.** Expulsion of blood from a part, as by means of an Esmarch tourniquet or arterial compression. **2.** Loss of vascularity, as by scarring.

AVC Abbreviation for atrioventricular *conduction.*

AVD Abbreviation for atrioventricular *dissociation.*

AVE Abbreviation for atrioventricular *extrasystole.*

Avellis, Georg, German laryngologist, 1864–1916. SEE A.'s *syndrome.*

ave·nin (ă-vē′nin). A prolamine, about 25% L-glutamic acid residues, found in oats (*Avena*) and in various legumes; considered highly nutritious. SYN legumin, plant casein.

av·er·age. A value that represents or summarizes the relevant features of a set of values; it is usually computed by a mathematical manipulation of the individual values in a set. [M.E. *averays,* loss from damage to ship or cargo, fr. It. *avaris,* fr. Ar. *'awariya,* damaged goods, + damage]

aVF, aVL, aVR Abbreviation for augmented electrocardiographic leads from the foot (left), left arm, and right arm, respectively.

Avi·ad·e·no·vi·rus (ā′vē-ad′ĕ-nō-vī′rŭs). A genus of viruses (family Adenoviridae) that includes types (species) of viruses found in birds. [L. *avis,* bird, + G. *adēn,* gland, + virus]

avi·an (ā′vē-ăn). Pertaining to birds. [L. *avis,* bird]

av·i·din (av′i-din). A glycoprotein, obtained from egg whites, which possesses a high affinity for biotin. Labeled a. is allowed to bind to biotin-tagged antibodies in order to amplify antigen-antibody reactions that may be difficult to visualize. SYN antibiotin. [L. *avidus,* eager fr. *aveo,* to crave + -in]

avid·i·ty. The binding strength of an antibody for an antigen. [L. *avidus,* greedy, eager fr. *aveo,* to crave]

A·vi·pox·vi·rus (ā′vē-poks-vī′rŭs). The genus of viruses (family Poxviridae) that includes the poxviruses of birds, including canarypox and fowlpox viruses. [L. *avis,* bird, + pox + virus]

avir·u·lent (ā-vir′yū-lent). Not virulent.

avi·ta·min·o·sis (ā-vī′tă-min-ō′sis). Properly, hypovitaminosis. **conditioned a.,** a. caused by any number of pathologic states or dysfunctions in which the supply of a vitamin absorbed by the body is inadequate for the needs under particular circumstances; *e.g.,* the reduced bacterial synthesis of the vitamins in the alimentary canal produced by antibiotic agents.

avive·ment (ah-vēv-maw′). Obsolete term for the excision of the edges of a wound to assist the healing process. [Fr. *aviver,* to quicken, revive]

A-V node. Abbreviation for atrioventricular *node.*

Avogadro, Amadeo, Italian physicist, 1776–1856. SEE A.'s *constant, hypothesis, law, number, postulate.*

av·oir·du·pois (av′er-du-poyz′). A system of weights in which 16 ounces make a pound, equivalent of 453.59237 g. See Weights and Measures appendix. [Fr. to have weight, corrupted fr. O. Fr. *avoir,* property, + *de,* of, + *pois,* weight]

AVP Abbreviation for antiviral *protein*; arginine *vasopressin.*

A-V shunt Abbreviation for arteriovenous *shunt.*

avul·sion (ă-vŭl′shŭn). A tearing away or forcible separation. Cf. evulsion. [L. *a-vello,* pp. *-vulsus,* to tear away]
nerve a., the tearing away of a peripheral nerve at its point of origin from its parent nerve due to traction.
root a., the tearing away of the anterior and posterior primary nerve roots from the spinal cord, due to severe traction; most often the C5 through T1 roots are affected.
tooth a., the traumatic separation of a tooth from its alveolus.

AW Abbreviation for atomic *weight.*

ax Abbreviation for axis.

Axenfeld, K. Theodor P.P., German ophthalmologist, 1867–1930. SEE Morax-A. *diplobacillus.*

axen·ic (ā-zen′ik). Sterile, denoting especially a pure culture; *e.g.,* a protozoan culture free from bacteria. Also used to denote "germ-free" animals born and raised in a sterile environment. SEE ALSO gnotobiote. [G. *a-* priv. + *xenos,* foreign]

ax·er·oph·thol (ak′ser-of′thōl). SYN *vitamin* A. [antixerophthalmic + -ol]

ax·es (ak′sēz). Plural of axis.

ax·i·al (ak′sē-ăl). **1.** Relating to an axis. SYN axile. **2.** Relating to or situated in the central part of the body, in the head and trunk as distinguished from the limbs, *e.g.,* axial skeleton. **3.** In dentistry, relating to or parallel with the long axis of a tooth. **4.** In radiology, an axial image is one obtained by rotating around the axis of the body, producing a transverse planar image, *i.e.,* a section transverse to the axis.

ax·if·u·gal (ak-sif′yū-găl). Extending away from an axis or axon. SYN axofugal. [L. *axis* + *fugio,* to flee from]

ax·il (ak′sil). SYN axilla.

ax·ile (ak′sīl). SYN axial (1).

ax·il·la, gen. and pl. **ax·il·lae** (ak′sil′ă, ak-sil′ē). The space below the shoulder joint, bounded by the pectoralis major anteriorly, the latissimus dorsi posteriorly, the serratus anterior medially, and the humerus laterally; it has a superior opening between the clavicle, scapula, and first rib (cervicoaxillary canal), and an inferior opening covered by the axillary fascia; it contains the axillary artery and vein, the infraclavicular part of the brachial plexus, axillary lymph nodes and vessels, and areolar tissue. SYN fossa axillaris [NA], armpit, axil, axillary cavity, axillary fossa, axillary space, maschale. [L.]

ax·il·lary (ak′sil-ār-ē). Relating to the axilla. SYN alar (2).

△**axio-.** An axis. SEE ALSO axo-. [L. *axis*]

ax·i·o·buc·cal (ak′sē-ō-bŭk′ăl). Referring to the junction of the axial and buccal planes of a tooth, usually a line.

ax·i·o·buc·co·gin·gi·val (ak′sē-ō-bŭk-ō-jin′ji-văl). Referring to the junction of the axial, buccal and gingival planes of teeth; usually a point.

ax·i·o·in·ci·sal (ak′sē-ō-in-sī′săl). Referring to the line angle formed by the junction of the incisal edge and axial walls of a tooth.

ax·i·o·la·bi·al (ak′sē-ō-lā′bē-ăl). Referring to the line angle of a cavity formed by the junction of the axial and the labial walls of a tooth.

ax·i·o·la·bi·o·lin·gual (ak′sē-ō-lā′bē-ō-ling′gwăl). Referring to a section from labial to lingual along the longitudinal axis of a tooth.

ax·i·o·lin·gual (ak′sē-ō-ling′gwăl). Referring to the line angle of a cavity formed by the junction of an axial and a lingual wall of a tooth.

ax·i·o·lin·guo·cer·vi·cal (ak′sē-ō-ling′gwō-ser′vi-kăl). Referring to the point angle formed by the junction of an axial, lingual, and cervical (gingival) wall of a tooth cavity.

ax·i·o·lin·guo·clu·sal (ak′sē-ō-ling′gwō-klū′săl). Referring to the point angle formed by the junction of an axial, lingual, and occlusal wall of a tooth cavity.

ax·i·o·lin·guo·gin·gi·val (ak′sē-ō-ling′gwō-jin′ji-văl). Referring to the point angle formed by the junction of an axial, lingual, and gingival (cervical) wall of a tooth cavity.

ax·i·o·me·si·al (ak′sē-ō-mē′zē-ăl). Referring to the line angle of a tooth cavity formed by the junction of an axial and a mesial wall.

ax·i·o·me·si·o·cer·vi·cal (ak′sē-ō-mē′zē-ō-ser′vi-kăl). Referring to the point angle formed by the junction of an axial, mesial, and cervical (gingival) wall of a tooth cavity.

ax·i·o·me·si·o·dis·tal. SEE axiomesiodistal *plane*.

ax·i·o·me·si·o·gin·gi·val (ak′sē-ō-mē′zē-ō-jin′ji-văl). Referring to the point angle formed by the junction of an axial, mesial, and gingival (cervical) wall of a tooth cavity.

ax·i·o·me·si·o·in·ci·sal (ak′sē-ō-mē′zē-ō-in-sī′săl). Referring to the point angle formed by the junction of an axial, mesial, and incisal wall of a tooth cavity.

ax·i·on (ak′sē-on). The brain and spinal cord (cerebrospinal axis).

ax·io-oc·clu·sal (ak′sē-ō-ŏ-klū′săl). Pertaining to the line angle formed by the junction of the axial and occlusal walls of a tooth.

ax·i·o·plasm (ak′sē-ō-plazm). SYN axoplasm.

ax·i·o·po·di·um, pl. **ax·i·o·po·dia** (ak′sē-ō-pō′dē-ŭm, -dē-ă). SYN axopodium.

ax·i·o·pul·pal (ak′sē-ō-pŭl′păl). Referring to the line angle formed by the junction of an axial and pulpal wall of a tooth cavity.

ax·i·o·ver·sion (ak′sē-ō-ver′zhŭn). Abnormal inclination of the long axis of a tooth.

ax·ip·e·tal (ak-sip′ĕ-tăl). SYN centripetal (2). [L. *axis* + *peto*, to seek]

ax·i·ram·if·i·cate (ak′sē-ram-if′i-kāt). Denoting a nerve cell whose axon, usually short, breaks up into many branches, *e.g.*, Golgi's type II cells. [G. *axōn*, axis + *grapho*, to write]

ax·is (ax), pl. **ax·es** (ak′sis, ak′sēz). **1.** A straight line passing through a spherical body between its two poles, and about which the body may revolve. **2.** The central line of the body or any of its parts. **3.** The vertebral column. **4.** The central nervous system. **5** [NA]. The second cervical vertebra. SYN epistropheus, odontoid vertebra, toothed vertebra, vertebra dentata. **6.** An artery that divides, immediately upon its origin, into a number of branches, *e.g.*, celiac axis. SEE trunk. [L. axle, axis]

basibregmatic a., a line extending from the basion to the bregma.

basicranial a., a line drawn from the basion to the midpoint of the sphenoethmoidal suture.

basifacial a., a line drawn from the subnasal point to the midpoint of the sphenoethmoidal suture. SYN facial a.

biauricular a., a straight line joining the two auricles. Cf. auriculare.

a. bul′bi exter′nus [NA], SYN external a. of eye.

a. bul′bi inter′nus [NA], SYN internal a. of eye.

celiac a., SYN celiac *trunk*.

cephalocaudal a., SYN long a. of body.

cerebrospinal a., the central nervous system; the brain and spinal cord. SYN encephalomyelonic a., neural a.

condylar a., a line through the two mandibular condyles around which the mandible may rotate during a part of the opening movement. SYN condyle cord.

conjugate a., SYN *conjugate* of pelvic inlet.

craniofacial a., a straight line passing through the mesethmoid, presphenoid, basisphenoid, and basioccipital bones.

electrical a., the net direction of the electromotive forces developed in the heart during its activation, usually represented in the frontal plane. SEE triaxial reference *system.*

embryonic a., the cephalocaudal a. established in the embryo by the primitive streak.

encephalomyelonic a., SYN cerebrospinal a.

external a. of eye, that part of the optic a. from the midpoint of anterior surface of the cornea to the posterior surface of the posterior pole of the external surface of the sclera. SYN a. bulbi externus [NA].

facial a., SYN basifacial a.

hinge a., SYN transverse horizontal a.

instantaneous electrical a., the resultant a. of the electromotive forces developing in the heart at any given moment.

internal a. of eye, that part of the optic a. from the midpoint of the posterior surface of the cornea to the anterior surface of the retina opposite the posterior pole. SYN a. bulbi internus [NA].

a. of lens, a line connecting the anterior and posterior poles of the lens of the eye. SYN a. lentis [NA].

a. len′tis [NA], SYN a. of lens.

long a., a line extending through the center of an object lengthwise; in dentistry, the line extending inciso- (occluso-) cervically parallel to axial surfaces of a tooth.

long a. of body, SYN cephalocaudal a.

mandibular a., SYN transverse horizontal a.

mean electrical a., the average magnitude and direction of all the electromotive forces developed during the cardiac event under consideration; *e.g.*, atrial or ventricular depolarization, or ventricular repolarization. SEE ALSO axis *deviation.*

neural a., SYN cerebrospinal a.

neutral a. of straight beam, the a. perpendicular to the plane of loading of a beam at stresses within the proportional limit; it lies at the gravity a. of the cross-section of the beam.

normal electrical a., a mean electrical a. of the heart situated between -30° and +90°. SEE hexaxial reference *system.*

opening a., an imaginary line around which the mandibular condyles may rotate during opening and closing movements. Cf. fulcrum *line.*

optic a., the a. of the eye connecting the anterior and posterior poles; it usually diverges from the visual a. by five degrees or more. SYN a. opticus [NA].

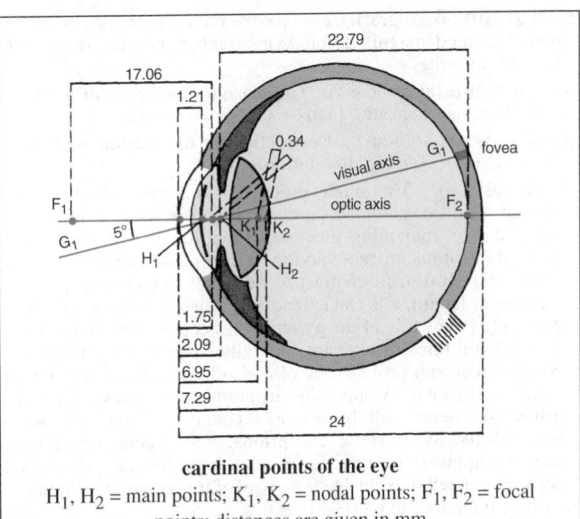

cardinal points of the eye
H_1, H_2 = main points; K_1, K_2 = nodal points; F_1, F_2 = focal points; distances are given in mm

a. op′ticus [NA], SYN optic a.

orbital a., the line from the center of the optic foramen (apex of orbit) extending anteriorly, laterally, and inferiorly to the middle of the orbital opening.

pelvic a., a hypothetical curved line joining the center point of each of the four planes of the pelvis, marking the center of the pelvic cavity at every level. SYN a. pelvis [NA], plane of pelvic canal.

a. pel'vis [NA], SYN pelvic a.

principal optic a., a line passing through the center of the lens of a refracting system at right angles to its surface.

pupillary a., a line perpendicular to the surface of the cornea, passing through the center of the pupil; the "direction of gaze."

rotational a., SYN fulcrum *line.*

sagittal a., in dentistry, the line in the frontal plane around which the working side condyle rotates during mandibular movement.

secondary a., any ray passing through the optical center of a lens.

a. of symmetry, an a. through a particle (*e.g.,* a virus) on such a plane that, if the particle is rotated on the a., there are two or more positions at which the particle appears identical.

thoracic a., (**1**) SYN thoracoacromial *artery.* (**2**) SYN thoracoacromial *vein.*

thyroid a., SYN thyrocervical *trunk.*

transporionic a., an imaginary line connecting the upper central points of the external auditory meatuses; used in radiographic cephalometry. SEE porion.

transverse horizontal a., an imaginary line around which the mandible may rotate through the horizontal plane. SYN hinge a., mandibular a.

vertical a., in dentistry, the line around which the working side condyle rotates in the horizontal plane during mandibular movement.

visual a., the straight line extending from the object seen, through the center of the pupil, to the macula lutea of the retina. SYN line of vision.

Y-a., a cephalometric indicator of the vertical and horizontal coordinates of mandibular growth expressed in degrees of the inferior facial angle formed by the intersection of the sella-gnathion plane with the Frankfort horizontal plane.

△**axo-.** Axis; axion. [G. *axōn,* axis]

ax·o·ax·on·ic (ak'sō-ak-son'ik). Relating to synaptic contact between the axon of one nerve cell and that of another. SEE synapse.

ax·o·den·drit·ic (ak'sō-den-drit'ik). Pertaining to the synaptic relationship of an axon with a dendrite of another neuron. SEE synapse.

ax·of·u·gal (ak-sof'yū-găl). SYN axifugal. [axo- + L. *fugio,* to flee]

ax·o·graph (ak'sō-graf). A device for recording scales or axes of predetermined magnitude on kymographic records. [axo- + G. *graphō,* to write]

ax·o·lem·ma (ak'sō-lem'ă). The plasma membrane of the axon. SYN Mauthner's sheath. [axo- + G. *lemma,* husk]

ax·ol·y·sis (ak-sol'i-sis). Destruction or dissolution of a nerve axon. [axo- + G. *lysis,* dissolution]

ax·on (ak'son). The single process of a nerve cell that under normal conditions conducts nervous impulses away from the cell body and its remaining processes (dendrites). It is a relatively even filamentous process varying in thickness from about 0.25 to more than 10 μm. In contrast to dendrites, which rarely exceed 1.5 mm in length, a.'s can extend great distances from the parent cell body (some a.'s of the pyramidal tract are 40 to 50 cm long). A.'s 0.5 μm thick or over are generally enveloped by a segmented myelin sheath provided by oligodendroglia cells (in brain and spinal cord) or Schwann cells (in peripheral nerves). Like dendrites and nerve cell bodies, a.'s contain a large number of neurofibrils. With some exceptions, nerve cells synaptically transmit impulses to other nerve cells or to effector cells (muscle cells, gland cells) exclusively by way of the synaptic terminals of their a. [G. *axōn,* axis]

ax·o·nal (ak'sō-năl). Pertaining to an axon.

ax·o·neme (ak'sō-nēm). **1.** The central thread running in the axis of the chromosome. **2.** SYN axial *filament.* **3.** The distinctive array of microtubules in the core of eukaryotic cilia and flagella

comprising a central pair surrounded by a sheaf of nine doublet microtubules. [axo- + G. *nēma,* a thread]

ax·on·og·ra·phy (ak-sŏ-nog'ră-fē). The recording of electrical changes in axons. SYN electroaxonography.

ax·o·nop·a·thy (aks'on-op'a-thē). A disorder affecting primarily the axons of peripheral nerve fibers, (although secondary demyelination occurs) in contrast to one that affects only myelin (myelinopathy).

ax·on·ot·me·sis (ak'son-ot-mē'sis). Interruption of the axons of a nerve followed by complete degeneration of the peripheral segment, without severance of the supporting structure of the nerve; such a lesion may result from pinching, crushing, or prolonged pressure. SEE ALSO neurapraxia, neurotmesis. [axon + G. *tmēsis,* a cutting]

ax·op·e·tal (ak-sop'ĕ-tăl). Extending in a direction toward an axon. [axo- + L. *peto,* to seek]

ax·o·plasm (ak'sō-plazm). Neuroplasm of the axon. SYN axioplasm.

ax·o·po·di·um, pl. **ax·o·po·dia** (ak-sō-pō'dē-ŭm, -ă). A permanent pseudopodium containing a stiff axial filament of differentiated protoplasm. SYN axiopodium. [Mod. L., fr. L. *axis* + G. *podion,* dim. of *pous* (*pod-*), foot]

ax·o·so·mat·ic (ak-sō-sō-mat'ik). Relating to the synaptic relationship of an axon with a nerve cell body. SEE synapse. [axo- + G. *sōma,* body]

ax·o·style (ak'sō-stīl). An elongate supporting rod or tubule that runs the length of certain flagellate protozoans, frequently projecting out of the posterior end. Single or multiple, filamentous or rigid, they vary with the species but serve as an endoskeletal framework and may function in locomotion as well. [axo- + G. *stylos,* pillar]

ax·ot·o·my (ak-sot'ō-mē). Incision or transection of an axon. [axo- + G. *tomē,* to cut]

ay·a·hua·sca (ī'ă-wa-skă). SYN caapi.

Ayala, G., Italian neurologist, 1878–1943. SEE A.'s *index, quotient.*

Ayerza, L., Argentinian physician, 1861–1918. SEE A.'s *disease, syndrome.*

Ayre, J. Ernest, U.S. gynecologist, *1910. SEE A. *brush.*

aza·crine (ā'ză-krēn). 2-Methoxy-6-chloro-9-(5'-diethylamino-2'-pentyl)amino-3-azoacridine; an antimalarial; an effective schizontocide in acute falciparum infection.

aza·cy·clo·nol hy·dro·chlo·ride (ā'ză-sī'klō-nol). γ-Pipradol hydrochloride; α,α-diphenyl-4-piperidine-methanol hydrochloride; a structural isomer of pipradol hydrochloride partially antagonistic to its actions, used with varying results in the treatment of hallucinations and confusion.

9-az·a·flu·o·rene (ā-ză-flūr'ēn). SYN carbazole.

8-aza·gua·nine (ā-ză-gwah'nēn). Guanine with N for C in position 8; a guanine antagonist that has been used in the treatment of acute leukemia. SYN guanazolo, triazologuanine.

aza·me·tho·ni·um bro·mide (ā'ză-me-thō'nē-ŭm). [(Methylimino)diethylene]bis-[ethyldimethylammonium bromide]; a ganglionic blocking agent.

aza·per·one (ā'za-per-ōn). 4'-Fluoro-4-[4-(2-pyridyl)-1-piperazinyl]butyrophenone; a tranquilizing agent.

azap·e·tine phos·phate (ā-zap'ĕ-tēn). 6-Allyl-6,7-dihydro-5*H*-dibenz[*c.e*]azepine phosphate; a potent adrenergic (α-receptor) blocking agent similar in action and uses to those of tolazoline; used in the treatment of peripheral vascular diseases.

azar·i·bine (ā-zar'i-bēn). 2',3',5'-Triacetyl derivative of 6-azauridine; an antipsoriatic agent no longer used because of a high incidence of severe adverse reactions.

aza·ser·ine (ā-ză-sēr'ēn). $N_2CH-CO-O-CH_2CH(NH_2)COOH$; *O*-diazoacetyl-L-serine; an antibiotic inhibitor of purine synthesis; a glutamine analog; mutagenic and antitumorogenic. SYN serine diazoacetate.

aza·spi·ro·dec·ane·di·one (ā-ză-spī'rō-dek-ān-dī'ōn). A class of antianxiety agents not chemically or pharmacologically related to other classes of sedative and anxiolytic drugs; *e.g.,* buspirone hydrochloride.

azat·a·dine ma·le·ate (ă-zat'ă-dēn). 6,11-Dihydro-11-(1-methyl-4-piperidylidene)-5H-benzo[5,6]cyclohepta[1,2-b]pyridine dimaleate; an antihistamine with anticholinergic and antiserotonin properties.

az·a·thi·o·prine (ā-ză-thī'ō-prēn). 6-(1-Methyl-4-nitro-5-imidazolyl)thiopurine; a derivative of 6-mercaptopurine, used as a cytotoxic and immunosuppressive agent in organ transplantation and in the treatment of autoimmune diseases such as hemolytic anemias, systemic lupus erythematosus, rheumatoid arthritis and leukemias.

6-aza·thy·mine (ā-ză-thī'mēn). Thymine with N for C in position 6; an antimetabolite of thymine.

6-az·au·ri·dine (AZUR) (az-aw'ri-dēn). Uridine with N for C in position 6; a triazine analogue of uridine and an antimetabolite with selectivity for human neoplastic leukocytes; produces partial remissions in certain acute leukemias of adults.

aze·o·trope (ā-zē'ō-trōp). A mixture of two or more liquids that boils without change in proportion of the liquids, either in the liquid or the vapor phase; *e.g.,* 95% ethanol (actually 94.9% by volume, the rest being water). [G. *a-* priv. + *zeein,* to boil, + *tropos,* a turning]

    halothane-ether a., an azeotropic mixture in the proportions halothane 68 to diethyl ether 32, by volume, that combines the advantages of each anesthetic yet is non-flammable.

aze·o·tro·pic (ā-zē-ō-trop'ik). Denoting or characteristic of an azeotrope.

az·ide (az'īd). A compound that contains the monovalent –N$_3$ group.

az·i·do·thy·mi·dine (AZT) (az'i-dō-thī'mi-dēn). SYN zidovudine.

az·lo·cil·lin so·di·um (az-lō-sil'in). Sodium (6R)-6-[D-2-(2-oxoimidazolidine-1-carboxamido)-2-phenylacetamido]-penicillanate; an extended spectrum penicillin used in treatment of infections caused by *Pseudomonas aeruginosa, Escherichia coli,* and *Haemophilus influenzae.*

△**azo-.** Prefix denoting the presence in a molecule of the group ≡C–N=N–C≡. Cf. diazo-. [Fr. *azote,* name for nitrogen proposed by A.L. Lavoisier (1743-1794)]

az·o·bil·i·ru·bin (az'ō-bil-i-rū'bin). The red-violet pigment formed by the condensation of diazotized sulfanilic acid with bilirubin in the van den Bergh reaction.

az·o·car·mine (ā'zō-kar'mīn). A series of azo dyes used in preparing tissue stains.

az·o·car·mine B, az·o·car·mine G (az-ō-kar'mīn) [C.I. 50090, C.I. 50085]. Red acid dyes, the former more soluble in water, useful in Heidenhain's azan stain.

azo·ic (ă-zō'ik, ā-). Containing no living things; without organic life. [G. *a-* priv. + *zōikos,* relating to an animal]

az·ole (az'ōl). SYN pyrrole.

az·o·lit·min (az-ō-lit'min) [old C.I. 1242]. A purplish red coloring matter obtained from natural litmus or synthesized by oxidizing orcinol in the presence of ammonia, lime, and potash; used as a broad indicator of pH (red at 4.5, blue at 8.3).

a·zo·o·sper·mia (ā-zō-ō-sper'mē-ă). Absence of living spermatozoa in the semen; failure of spermatogenesis. SEE ALSO aspermia. [G. *a-* priv. + *zōon,* animal, + *sperma,* seed]

az·o·phlox·in (az-ō-flok'sin). SYN amidonaphthol red.

az·o·pro·tein (az-ō-prō'tēn). Any of the modified proteins produced by treatment with diazonium derivatives of various aromatic amines; used to elicit antibody formation and demonstrate antibody specificity.

az·o·sul·fa·mide (az-ō-sŭl'fă-mīd). 2-(4′-Sulfamylphenylazo)-7-acetamido-1-hydroxynaphthalene-3,6-disulfonate; a reddish derivative, soluble in water, less toxic but less effective than sulfanilamide; it owes its antibacterial activity to the sulfanilamide released.

az·o·te·mia (az-ō-tē'mē-ă). SYN uremia. [azo- (azote) + G. *haima,* blood]

    nonrenal a., prerenal a., nitrogen retention resulting from something other than primary renal disease.

az·o·tem·ic (az-ō-tēm'ik). Relating to azotemia.

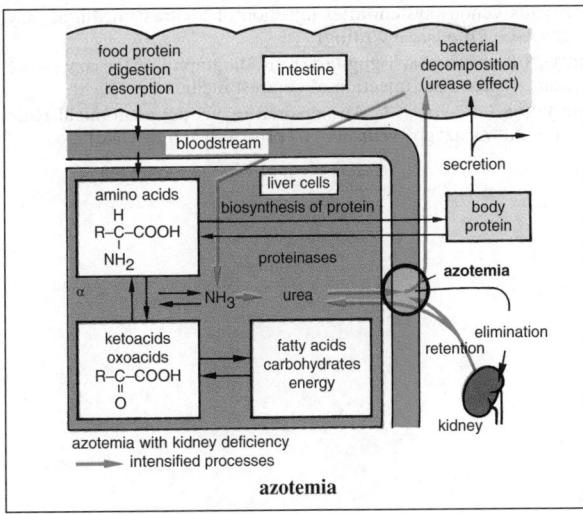

azotemia

az·o·ther·mia (az-ō-ther'mē-ă). Rarely used term for fever resulting from uremia. [azote + G. *thermē,* heat]

azo·tu·ria (az-ō-tūr'ē-ă). An increased elimination of urea in the urine. [azo- (azote) + G. *ouron,* urine]

    a. of horses, an afebrile disease of horses, characterized by massive muscle degeneration, a rapidly developing paralysis of the hind legs, and myoglobinuria; onset is sudden, usually appearing shortly after the horse has returned to work after a few days' rest. SYN black water, hemoglobinemia paralytica, Monday morning sickness, paralytic myoglobinuria.

az·o·van blue (az'ō-van). SYN Evans blue.

AZT Abbreviation for azidothymidine.

az·tre·o·nam (az-trē'ō-nam). 2-[[[1-(2-Amino-4-thiazolyl)-2-[2-methyl-4-oxo-1-sulf-3-az etidinyl)amino]-2-oxoethylidene]-amino]oxy]-2-methylpropan o ic acid; a synthetic bactericidal monolactam antibiotic with a wide spectrum of activity against Gram-negative aerobic pathogens.

az·ul (azh'yūl). SYN pinta. [Sp. blue]

AZUR Abbreviation for 6-azauridine.

az·ure (azh'yūr). A term for a group of basic blue methylthionine or phenothiazine dyes; used as biological stains, especially in blood and nuclear stains.

    a. A [C.I. 52005], C$_{14}$H$_{14}$N$_3$SCl; asymmetrical dimethylthionine chloride; a blue dye used as a component of MacNeal's tetrachrome blood stain and of Romanowsky-type blood stains; also used as a stain for mucins, nucleic acids, and mast cell granules; gives a metachromatic violet to red color to highly acidic substances in tissues.

    a. B [C.I. 52010], C$_{15}$H$_{16}$N$_3$SCl; trimethylthionine chloride; a blue dye used like a. A; also as a. B bromide to give metachromatic staining of RNA and DNA.

    a. C [C.I. 52002], C$_{13}$H$_{12}$N$_3$SCl; monomethylthione chloride; a blue-violet thiazin dye used in the metachromatic staining of mucins and cartilage.

    a. I, a mixture of a. A and B. SYN methylene azure.

    a. II, a mixture of a. I and methylene blue; the eosinate, a. II-eosin, is the principal ingredient of Giemsa stain.

az·u·res·in (azh'yū-res'in). A complex of azure A and carbacrylic resin; used as an indicator for the detection of gastric achlorhydria without intubation. SYN quinine carbacrylic resin.

az·u·ro·phil, az·u·ro·phile (azh'yū-rō-fil, -fīl). Staining readily with an azure dye, denoting especially the hyperchromatin and reddish purple granules of certain blood cells. [azure + G. *philos,* fond]

az·u·ro·phil·ia (az'yū-rō-fil'ē-ă). A condition in which the blood contains cells having azurophil granulations.

azy·go·gram (az'i-gō-gram). Radiographic demonstration of the azygos venous system after injection of contrast medium. [azygos + G. *gramma*, a writing]

azy·gog·ra·phy (az′i-gog′ră-fē). Radiography of the azygos venous system after injection of contrast medium.

az·y·gos (az′ĭ-gos). **1.** An unpaired (azygous) anatomical structure. **2.** SYN azygos *vein.* [G. *a*- priv. + *zygon,* a yoke]

a. continuation (of the inferior vena cava), a congenital anomaly in which the infrahepatic portion of the vena cava fails to form, and venous drainage of the lower body is maintained through a persistent right supracardinal vein, which becomes a large azygos vein.

az·y·gous (az′ĭ-gŭs, ă-zī′gŭs). Unpaired; single. [L. *azygos*] β. **1.** Second letter of the Greek alphabet, beta. **2.** In chemistry, denotes the second in a series, the second carbon from a functional (*e.g.,* carboxylic) group, or the direction of a chemical bond toward the viewer. For terms having this prefix, see the specific term.

β⁺. Symbol for positron.

B 1. Symbol for boron; for aspartic acid or asparagine when it is unclear which of the two amino acids is present; for bromouridine; second substrate in a multisubstrate enzyme-catalyzed reaction. **2.** As a subscript, refers to barometric *pressure.*

b. 1. As a subscript, refers to blood. **2.** Abbreviation for bis [L], twice.

Ba Symbol for barium.

Babbitt, Isaac, U.S. inventor, 1799–1862. SEE B. *metal.*

Babcock, Stephen M., U.S. chemist, 1843–1931. SEE B. *tube.*

Babès, Victor, Roumanian bacteriologist, 1854–1926. SEE *Babesia;* B.'s *nodes,* under *node;* B.-Ernst *bodies,* under *body.*

Ba·be·sia (bă-bē′zē-ă). The economically most important genus of the family Babesiidae; characterized by multiplication in host red blood cells to form pairs and tetrads; it causes babesiosis (piroplasmosis) in most types of domestic animals, and two species cause disease in splenectomized or normal people; vectors are ixodid or argasid ticks. [V. *Babès*]

B. argenti′na, SYN B. *bovis.*

B. ber′bera, SYN B. *bovis.*

B. bigem′ina, species that is a cause of bovine babesiosis, transmitted by *Boophilus* ticks.

B. bo′vis, a species that is a cause of bovine babesiosis; this parasite is smaller than B. *bigemina* and is transmitted by ticks of the genus *Boophilus.* SYN B. *argentina,* B. *berbera.*

B. cabal′li, species that is a cause of equine babesiosis in many parts of the world, including the southeastern U.S.; vector ticks are species of *Dermacentor, Hyalomma,* and *Rhipicephalus.*

B. ca′nis, species found in dogs, wolves, and jackals in many tropical and subtropical areas of the Americas, Europe, Asia, and Africa; it is most pathogenic in dogs, causing mild to severe canine babesiosis, the severest disease occurring in dogs imported into areas where the disease is enzootic; the most important vector is *Rhipicephalus sanguineus.*

B. diver′gens, commonest species of *Babesia* in western and central Europe, causing a disease of cattle similar to that produced by B. *bovis;* vector tick is *Ixodes ricinus;* it has caused human babesiosis in splenectomized individuals in France, Ireland, Scotland, Croatia, Georgia, a part of the former Soviet Union, and Sweden; also found in reindeer.

B. e′qui, species that occurs in horses, mules, donkeys, and zebras; it has a geographic distribution similar to that of B. *caballi,* but is smaller and more pathogenic, causing equine babesiosis.

B. fe′lis, species found in domestic and wild members of the cat family, chiefly in Africa and India, causing babesiosis less severe than that caused by B. *canis.*

B. gibso′ni, species that infects dogs, wolves, and jackals, chiefly in India, Sri Lanka, and China, and is smaller than B. *canis;* only slightly pathogenic for the natural host, the jackal, but highly pathogenic in the dog.

B. micro′ti, a malaria-like protozoan naturally parasitizing certain rodents (*Peromyscus* and *Microtus* spp.) in North America; a number of human cases have been reported from Nantucket and Martha's Vineyard islands and nearby coastal New England. The local tick vector is *Ixodes dammini,* whose numbers and infection levels have greatly increased in recent years with the increase in the deer population, which serves as an abundant blood source for *I. dammini.* SEE ALSO *Borrelia burgdorferi.*

B. mota′si, species that causes acute or chronic disease of sheep and goats in southern Europe, Africa, the Middle East, the area formerly known as the U.S.S.R., and other areas; transmitted by ticks of the genera *Rhipicephalus, Haemaphysalis,* and *Dermacentor.*

B. o′vis, species described from sheep and goats in many tropical and subtropical areas of the eastern hemisphere as a cause of icterohematuria; it is smaller and less pathogenic than B. *motasi,* and immunologically distinct.

B. trautman′ni, species that causes mild or fatal babesiosis in pigs in southern Europe, the area formerly known as the U.S.S.R., and Africa; the vector is *Rhipicephalus sanguineus.*

Ba·be·si·el·la (bă-bē-zē-el′ă). SEE *Babesia.*

Ba·be·si·i·dae (ba′bē-zī′i-dē, -zē′i-dē). A family of protozoan parasites (class Sporozoea, order Piroplasmida) occurring in the red blood cells of various mammals. The organisms are piriform, round, or oval in shape and reproduce by schizogony to form tetrads or by binary fission to form pairs in the red blood cells; transmission is effected by ticks. The family includes the genera *Babesia, Echinozoon,* and *Entopolypoides; Aegyptianella,* formerly included, is now thought to be a rickettsia. SEE ALSO Theileriidae.

ba·be·si·o·sis (bă-bē′zē-ō′sis). A disease caused by infection with a species of *Babesia,* the infection being transmitted by ticks. In animals, the disease is characterized by fever, malaise, listlessness, severe anemia, and hemoglobulinuria; the death rate frequently is higher in adult than in young animals. SYN piroplasmosis.

bovine b., an infectious disease of cattle caused by *Babesia* species and transmitted by ticks. SYN bovine hemoglobinuria, redwater fever (1), Texas fever, tick fever (3).

canine b., malignant fever in dogs caused by *Babesia* species.

equine b., a disease of horses caused by species of *Babesia* and characterized by high fever, icterus, and enlargement of the spleen and lymph nodes. SYN biliary fever of horses, equine biliary fever.

human b., a rare human disease caused by infection with *Babesia* species (most frequently B. *divergens* in Europe and B. *microti* in the U.S.) that has been fatal in some splenectomized individuals.

Babinski, Joseph F., French neurologist, 1857–1932. SEE B.'s *phenomenon, sign;* B. *reflex;* B.'s *syndrome.*

ba·by (bā′bē). An infant; a newborn child.

average birth measurements	
length	49–52 cm
suboccipitobregmatic diameter	9.5 cm
occipitofrontal diameter	12.0 cm
occipitomental diameter	13.5 cm
suboccipitobregmatic circumference	32.0 cm
occipitofrontal circumference	34.0 cm
occipitomental circumference	35.0 cm
shoulder width	12.0 cm
shoulder girth	35.0 cm
hip width	10–11 cm
hip girth	27.0 cm

blue b., a child born cyanotic because of a congenital cardiac or pulmonary defect causing incomplete oxygenation of the blood.

blueberry muffin b., jaundice and purpura, especially of the face in the newborn, which may result from intrauterine viral infection.

collodion b. [MIM*146600], a newborn child with lamellar ichthyosis; at birth, the skin is bright red, shiny, translucent, and drawn tight, giving a distorted appearance (as if having been painted with collodion) of immobilization of the face; contraction of the skin causes ectropion, a pressed down appearance of the nose, and a gaping of the mouth and the labia; autosomal dominant inheritance.

test-tube b., popular term for a b. born after uterine implantation of a maternal ovum fertilized *in vitro*.

bac·am·pi·cil·lin hy·dro·chlo·ride (bak'am-pi-sil'in). 1-(Ethoxycarbonyloxy)ethyl(6R)-6-(α-D-phenylglycylamino)penicillanate hydrochloride; a semisynthetic penicillin with the same activity and uses as ampicillin, but better absorbed on oral administration.

bac·cate (bak'āt). Berry-like. [L. *bacca*, berry]

Baccelli, Guido, Italian physician, 1832–1916. SEE B.'s *sign*.

bac·ci·form (bak'sĭ-fōrm). Berry-shaped. [L. *bacca*, berry]

Bachman, George W., U.S. parasitologist, *1890. SEE B.-Pettit *test.*

Bachmann, Jean George, U.S. physiologist, 1877–1959. SEE B.'s *bundle.*

Bachmann. SEE Rivinus.

Ba·cil·la·ce·ae (bă-si-lā'sē-ē). A family of aerobic or facultatively anaerobic, sporeforming, ordinarily motile bacteria (order Eubacteriales) containing Gram-positive rods. These organisms are chemoheterotrophic. Some species are pathogenic. Ordinarily two genera, *Bacillus* and *Clostridium*, are included. The type genus is *Bacillus*.

ba·cil·lar, bac·il·la·ry (bas'i-lar, bas'i-lā-rē). Shaped like a rod; consisting of rods or rodlike elements.

Ba·cil·le bi·lié de Calmette-Guérin (BCG), Ba·cil·le Calmette-Guérin (bah-sēl' bi-lē-ā). An attenuated strain of *Mycobacterium bovis* used in the preparation of BCG vaccine that is used for immunization against tuberculosis and in cancer chemotherapy. SYN Calmette-Guérin bacillus. [Fr.]

bac·il·le·mia (bas-i-lē'mē-ă). The presence of rod-shaped bacteria in the circulating blood. [bacillus + G. *haima*, blood]

ba·cil·li (bă-sil'ī). Plural of bacillus.

ba·cil·li·form (ba-sil'i-fōrm). Rod-shaped. [L. *bacillus*, a rod, + *forma*, form]

ba·cil·lin (ba-sil'in). An antibiotic substance produced by *Bacillus subtilis*.

ba·cil·lo·myx·in (ba-sil-ō-mik'sin). An antibiotic active against certain pathogenic fungi obtained from cultures of *Bacillus subtilis*. [*Bacillus* + G. *mykēs*, fungus, + -in]

bac·il·lo·sis (bas-i-lō'sis). A general infection with bacilli.

bac·il·lu·ria (bas-i-lū'rē-ă). The presence of bacilli in the urine. [bacillus + G. *ouron*, urine]

Ba·cil·lus (ba-sil'ŭs). A genus of aerobic or facultatively anaerobic, sporeforming, ordinarily motile bacteria (family Bacillaceae) containing Gram-positive rods. Motile cells are peritrichous. These organisms are chemoheterotrophic. They are found primarily in soil. A few species are animal pathogens; some species produce antibodies. The type species is *B. subtilis*. [L. dim. of *baculus*, rod, staff]

B. amyloliquefa'ciens, a highly amylolytic species of soil bacteria that produces subtilisin.

B. an'thracis, a species that causes anthrax in man, cattle, swine, sheep, rabbits, guinea pigs, and mice.

B. bre'vis, a species found in soil, air, dust, milk, and cheese; some strains produce the antibiotic gramicidin or tyrocidin.

B. ce'reus, a species that causes an emetic type and a diarrheal type of food poisoning in humans, and can cause infections in humans and other mammals.

B. hemoly'ticus, former name for *Clostridium haemolyticum*.

B. histoly'ticus, former name for *Clostridium histolyticum*.

B. megate'rium, a saprophytic species of experimental interest; strains produce bacteriocins (megacins).

B. piliformis, a species causing Tyzzer's disease in animals.

B. polymyx'a, a species found in soil, water, milk, feces, and decaying vegetables; some strains produce the antibiotic polymyxin.

B. sphae'ricus, a species that is an insect pathogen and that has

been associated with human and other mammalian infections, especially in compromised hosts.

B. subti'lis, a species found in soil and decomposing organic matter; some strains produce the antibiotic subtilin, subtenolin, or bacillomycin; it is the type species of the genus *B*. SYN grass bacillus, hay bacillus.

B. thuringien'sis, a species that is an insect pathogen and that has been implicated in human and mammalian infections.

ba·cil·lus, pl. **ba·cil·li** (ba-sil'ŭs, -ī). 1. A vernacular term used to refer to any member of the genus *Bacillus*. 2. Term formerly used to refer to any rod-shaped bacterium. [L. dim. of *baculus*, a rod, staff]

Abel's b., *Klebsiella pneumoniae subsp. ozaenae* SEE *Klebsiella ozaenae*.

abortus b., SYN *Brucella abortus*.

acne b., SYN *Propionibacterium acnes*.

Bang's b., SYN *Brucella abortus*.

Battey b., SYN *Mycobacterium intracellulare*. [Battey hospital in Rome, GA]

blue pus b., SYN *Pseudomonas aeruginosa*.

Bordet-Gengou b., SYN *Bordetella pertussis*.

Calmette-Guérin b., SYN Bacille bilié de Calmette-Guérin.

cholera b., SYN *Vibrio cholerae*.

coliform bacilli (kō'li-fōrm, kol'i-fōrm), common name for *Escherichia coli* that is used as an indicator of fecal contamination of water, measured in terms of coliform count. Occasionally used to refer to all lactose-fermenting enteric bacteria.

colon b., SYN *Escherichia coli*.

comma b., SYN *Vibrio cholerae*.

Döderlein's b., a large, Gram-positive bacterium occurring in normal vaginal secretions; although thought by some to be identical with *Lactobacillus acidophilus*, the identity of Döderlein's b. is still doubtful.

Ducrey's b., SYN *Haemophilus ducreyi*.

dysentery b., an organism of the genus *Shigella* which causes dysentery.

Eberth's b., SYN *Salmonella typhi*.

Flexner's b., SYN *Shigella flexneri*.

Friedländer's b., SYN *Klebsiella pneumoniae*.

Gärtner's b., SYN *Salmonella enteritidis*.

gas b., SYN *Clostridium perfringens*.

Ghon-Sachs b., SYN *Clostridium septicum*.

glanders b., SYN *Pseudomonas mallei*.

grass b., SYN *Bacillus subtilis*.

Hansen's b., SYN *Mycobacterium leprae*.

hay b., SYN *Bacillus subtilis*.

Hofmann's b., SYN *Corynebacterium pseudodiphtheriticum*.

influenza b., SYN *Haemophilus influenzae*.

Johne's b., SYN *Mycobacterium paratuberculosis*.

Kitasato's b., SYN *Yersinia pestis*.

Klebs-Loeffler b., SYN *Corynebacterium diphtheriae*.

Koch's b., (1) SYN *Mycobacterium tuberculosis*. (2) SYN *Vibrio cholerae*.

Koch-Weeks b., SYN *Haemophilus influenzae*.

lactic acid b., a member of the genus *Lactobacillus*.

leprosy b., SYN *Mycobacterium leprae*.

Loeffler's b., SYN *Corynebacterium diphtheriae*.

mist b., *Mycobacterium smegmatis* (formerly *M. lacticola*)

Moeller's grass b., SYN *Mycobacterium phlei*.

Morgan's b., SYN *Morganella morganii*.

Much's b., an alleged non-acid-fast granular form of the tubercle b.; not demonstrable by the Ziehl stain, but takes a modified Gram stain; it is said to be the form present in the tuberculous skin lesion.

necrosis b., SYN *Fusobacterium necrophorum*.

paracolon b., any one of a number of diverse enteric bacteria which fail to ferment lactose promptly.

paradysentery b., SYN *Shigella flexneri*.

paratyphoid b., one of the three organisms causing the three forms, A, B, and C, of paratyphoid fever. SEE ALSO paratyphoid *fever.*

Park-Williams b., a special strain of *Corynebacterium diphtheriae* used for toxin production.

Pfeiffer's b., SYN *Haemophilus influenzae.*

plague b., SYN *Yersinia pestis.*

Plaut's b., probably *Fusobacterium nucleatum,* differentiated by some from Vincent's b.; the former is motile and nonpathogenic, the latter is nonmotile and pathogenic.

Plotz b., a small, Gram-positive bacterium suggested as the pathogenic agent of typhus fever.

Preisz-Nocard b., SYN *Corynebacterium pseudotuberculosis.*

Sachs' b., SYN *Clostridium septicum.*

Schmorl's b., SYN *Fusobacterium necrophorum.*

Schottmueller's b., SYN *Salmonella schottmülleri.*

Shiga b., SYN *Shigella dysenteriae.*

Shiga-Kruse b., SYN *Shigella dysenteriae.*

Sonne b., SYN *Shigella sonnei.*

timothy hay b., SYN *Mycobacterium phlei.*

tubercle b., (1) SYN *Mycobacterium tuberculosis.* **(2)** SYN *Mycobacterium bovis.* **(3)** SYN *Mycobacterium avium.*

typhoid b., SYN *Salmonella typhi.*

Vincent's b., probably *Fusobacterium nucleatum.*

vole b., an acid-fast b. isolated from voles and used in the production of a vaccine against human and bovine tuberculosis.

Weeks' b., SYN *Haemophilus influenzae.*

Welch's b., SYN *Clostridium perfringens.*

Whitmore's b., SYN *Pseudomonas pseudomallei.*

bac·i·tra·cin (bas-i-trā′sin). An antibacterial antibiotic polypeptide of known chemical structure isolated from cultures of an aerobic, Gram-positive, spore-bearing bacillus (member of the *Bacillus subtilis* group); active against hemolytic streptococci, staphylococci, and several types of Gram-positive, aerobic, rod-shaped organisms; usually applied locally. Zinc b. is also available. [*Bacillus* + Margaret *Tracy,* source of orig. culture]

back (bak). **1.** Posterior aspect of trunk, below neck and above buttocks; **2.** Vertebral column with associated muscles (erector spinae and transversospinalis) and overlying integument. SEE dorsum.

adolescent round b., SYN Scheuermann's *disease.*

hollow b., SYN lordosis.

poker b., SYN *spondylitis* deformans.

saddle b., SYN lordosis.

back·ache (bak′āk). Nonspecific term used to describe back pain; generally refers to pain below the cervical level.

back·bone (bak′bōn). SYN vertebral *column.*

back·cross (bak′kros). **1.** Mating of an individual heterozygous at one or more loci to an individual homozygous at the same loci. **2.** SYN testcross.

back·flow. The reversal of the normal flow of a current. SEE ALSO regurgitation.

pyelovenous backflow, retrograde movement of fluid (urine or injected contrast materials) from renal pelvis into renal venous system. This occurs under conditions of distal obstruction or injection of solutions into renal collecting system.

back·ing (bak′ing). In dentistry, a metal support which serves to attach a facing to a prosthesis.

back·knee (bak′nē′). SYN *genu* recurvatum.

back·pro·jec·tion (bak′prō-jek′shŭn). In computed tomography or other imaging techniques requiring reconstruction from multiple projections, an algorithm for calculating the contribution of each voxel of the structure to the measured ray data, in order to generate an image; the oldest and simplest method of image reconstruction. SYN apical lordotic projection.

back·scat·ter (bak′skat-er). Induced radiation deflected more than 90° from the primary beam. SEE scattered *radiation.*

bac·lo·fen (bak′lō-fen). β-(Aminomethyl)-*p*-chlorohydrocinnamic acid; a muscle relaxant used in the symptomatic treatment of spinal cord injuries and multiple sclerosis; an agonist at GABA_b receptors.

Bacon, Harry E., U.S. proctologist, *1900. SEE B.'s *anoscope.*

bac·te·re·mia (bak-tēr-ē′mē-ă). The presence of viable bacteria in the circulating blood; may be transient following trauma such as dental or other iatrogenic manipulation or may be persistent or recurrent as a result of infection. SYN bacteriemia. [bacteria + G. *haima,* blood]

♻**bacteri-.** SEE bacterio-.

bac·te·ria (bak-tēr′ē-ă). Plural of bacterium.

blue-green bacteria, SEE Cyanobacteria.

coryneform bacteria, common name for nondiphtheria corynebacterium, usually a nonpathogenic component of skin and oropharyngeal flora in humans and animals can cause opportunistic infections in the immunocompromised host.

bac·te·ri·al (bak-tēr′ē-ăl). Relating to bacteria.

bac·te·ri·cho·lia (bak′tēr-i-kō′lē-ă). Bacteria in bile.

bac·te·ri·cid·al (bak-tēr′i-sī′dăl). Causing the death of bacteria. Cf. bacteriostatic. SYN bacteriocidal.

bac·te·ri·cide (bak-tēr′i-sīd). An agent that destroys bacteria. Cf. bacteriostat. SYN bacteriocide. [bacteria + L. *caedo,* to kill]

specific b., a bacteriolytic substance *i.e.,* immune serum destructive to one bacterial species or genus only.

bac·ter·id (bak′ter-id). **1.** A recurrent or persistent eruption of discrete sterile pustules of the palms and soles, thought to be an allergic response to infection at a remote site. **2.** A dissemination of a previously localized bacterial skin infection. [bacteria + -id (1)]

bac·te·ri·e·mia (bak-tēr-ē-ē′mē-ă). SYN bacteremia.

♻**bacterio-, bacteri-.** Bacteria. [see bacterium]

bac·te·ri·o·ag·glu·ti·nin (bak-tēr′ē-ō-ă-glū′ti-nin). An antibody that agglutinates bacteria.

bac·te·ri·o·chlo·rin (bak-tēr′-ē-ō-klōr′in). 7,8,17,18-Tetrahydroporphyrin; the basic structure of the bacteriochlorophylls.

bac·te·ri·o·chlo·ro·phyll (bak-tēr-ē-ō-klōr′ō-fil). Either of two forms of chlorophyll in photosynthetic bacteria: 1) α or a, $-CH=CH_2$ replaced by $-CO-CH_3$ in the chlorophyll α structure, two hydrogens also being added; 2) β or b, $-CH=CH_2$ replaced by $-CO-CH_3$ and $-CH_2-CH_3$ replaced by $-C\equiv CH$ in the chlorophyll β structure, two hydrogens also being added.

bac·te·ri·o·cid·al (bak-tēr′ē-ō-sī′dăl). SYN bactericidal.

bac·ter·i·o·cide (bak-tēr′ē-ō-sīd). SYN bactericide.

bac·te·ri·o·cid·in (bak-tēr′ē-ō-sī′din). Antibody having bactericidal activity.

bac·te·ri·o·cin·o·gens (bak-tēr′ē-ō-sin′ō-jenz). SYN bacteriocinogenic *plasmids,* under *plasmid.*

bac·te·ri·o·cins (bak-tēr′ē-ō-sinz). Proteins that are produced by certain bacteria possessing bacteriocinogenic plasmids and that exert a lethal effect on closely related bacteria; in general, b.'s have a narrower range of activity than antibiotics do and are more potent.

bac·te·ri·oc·la·sis (bak-tēr-ē-ok′lă-sis). Fragmentation of bacteria, as in the Twort phenomenon. [bacterio- + G. *klasis,* a breaking]

bac·te·ri·o·flu·o·res·cin (bak-tēr′ē-ō-flūr-es′in). A fluorescent material produced by bacteria.

bac·te·ri·o·gen·ic (bak-tēr′ē-ō-jen′ik). Caused by bacteria.

ba

bac·te·ri·og·e·nous (bak-tēr-ē-oj'e-nŭs). **1.** Producing bacteria. **2.** Of bacterial origin or causation.

bac·te·ri·oid (bak-tēr'ē-oyd). **1.** Resembling bacteria. **2.** Intracellular forms of Rhizobium spp. in the root nodules of leguminous plants. [bacterio- + G. *eidos*, resemblance]

bac·te·ri·o·log·ic, bac·te·ri·o·log·i·cal (bak'tēr-ē-ō-loj'ik, -i-kăl). Relating to bacteria or to bacteriology.

bac·te·ri·ol·o·gist (bak'ter-ē-ol'ŏ-jist). One who primarily studies or works with bacteria.

bac·te·ri·ol·o·gy (bak-tēr-ē-ol'ŏ-jē). The branch of science concerned with the study of bacteria. [bacterio- + G. *logos*, study]

systematic b., that branch of b. concerned with nomenclature and classification (taxonomy).

bac·te·ri·ol·y·sin (bak-tēr-ē-ol'i-sin). Specific antibody that combines with bacterial cells (*i.e.,* antigen) and, in the presence of complement, causes lysis or dissolution of the cells.

bac·te·ri·ol·y·sis (bak-tēr-ē-ol'i-sis). The dissolution of bacteria, *e.g.,* by means of hypotonic solutions or by specific antibody and complement. [bacterio- + G. *lysis,* dissolution]

bac·te·ri·o·lyt·ic (bak-tēr-ē-ō-lit'ik). Pertaining to lytic destruction of bacteria; manifesting the ability to cause dissolution of bacterial cells.

bac·te·ri·o·lyze (bak-tēr'ē-ō-līz). To cause the digestion or solution of bacterial cells.

bac·te·ri·o·pexy (bak-tēr'ē-ō-pek-sē). Immobilization of bacteria by phagocytic cells. [bacterio- + G. *pēxis,* fixation]

bac·te·ri·o·phage (bak-tēr'ē-ō-fāj). A virus with specific affinity for bacteria, and the active agent in d'Herelle's phenomenon. B.'s have been found in association with essentially all groups of bacteria, including the Cyanobacteria; like other viruses they contain either (but never both) RNA or DNA and vary in structure from the seemingly simple filamentous bacterial virus to relatively complex forms with contractile "tails"; their relationships to the host bacteria are rather specific and, as in the case of temperate b., may be genetically intimate. B.'s are named after the bacterial species, group, or strain for which they are specific, *e.g.,* corynebacteriophage, coliphage; a number of families are recognized and have been assigned provisional names: Corticoviridae, Cystoviridae, Inoviridae, Leviviridae, Microviridae, Myoviridae, Plasmaviridae, Podoviridae, Styloviridae, and Tectiviridae. SEE ALSO coliphage. SYN phage. [bacterio- + G. *phagō,* to eat]

defective b., a temperate b. mutant whose genome does not contain all of the normal components and cannot become fully infectious virus, yet can replicate indefinitely in the bacterial genome as defective probacteriophage; many defective b.'s are mediators of transduction. SYN defective phage.

filamentous b., a b. that is rod-shaped and elongated lacking the head-and-tail structure characteristic of many b.'s.

mature b., the complete, infective form of b.

temperate b., b. whose genome incorporates with, and replicates with, that of the host bacterium; dissociation (and resultant development of vegetative b.) occurs at a slow rate resulting occasionally in lysis of a bacterium and release of mature b., thus rendering the bacterial culture capable of inducing general lysis if transferred to a culture of a susceptible bacterial strain.

typhoid b., b. specific for *Salmonella typhi.*

vegetative b., the form of b. in which the b. nucleic acid (lacking its coat) multiplies freely within the host bacterium, independently of bacterial multiplication.

virulent b., a b. that regularly causes lysis of the bacteria that it infects; it may exist in one or the other of only two forms, vegetative or mature; it does not have a probacteriophage form (*i.e.,* its genome does not incorporate with that of the host bacterium), therefore it does not effect lysogenization.

bac·te·ri·o·pha·gia (bak-tēr-ē-ō-fā'jē-ă). SYN Twort-d'Herelle *phenomenon.*

bac·te·ri·o·pha·gol·o·gy (bak-tēr-ē-ō-fă-gol'ō-jē). The study of bacteriophages. SYN protobiology.

bac·te·ri·o·phe·o·phor·bide (bak-tēr'ē-ō-fē-ō-fōr'bīd). Bacteriophorbin with the side chains found in bacteriochlorophyll, but lacking the phytyl group.

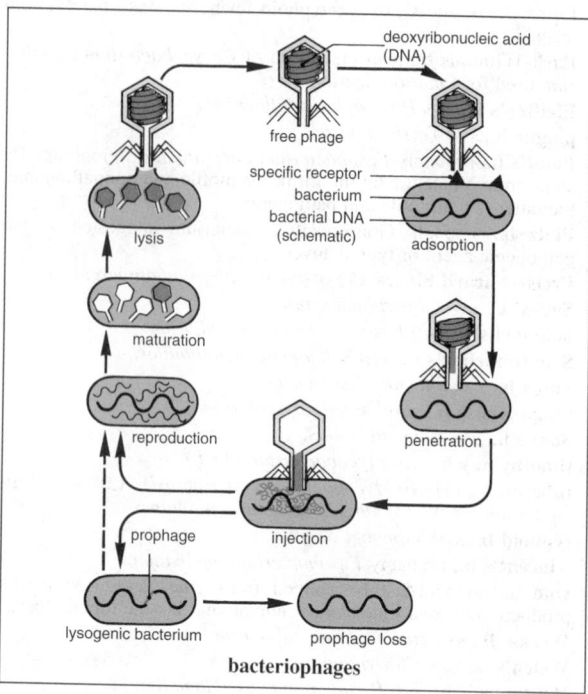

bacteriophages

bac·te·ri·o·phe·o·phor·bin (bak-tēr'ē-ō-fē-ō-fōr'bin). De-esterfied bacteriopheophorbide, derived from bacteriochlorin.

bac·te·ri·o·phe·o·phy·tin (bak-tēr'ē-ō-fē-ō-fī'tin). Bacteriopheophorbide with a phytyl ester on the C-17 propionic residue; bacteriochlorophyll less its magnesium residue.

bac·te·ri·o·phor·bin (bak-tēr'ē-ō-fōr'bin). Phorbin further saturated by addition of two hydrogens to C-7 and C-8.

bac·te·ri·o·phy·to·ma (bak-tēr'ē-ō-fī-tō'mă). A growth in plant tissues produced by bacteria. [bacterio- + G. *phytos,* plant, + *-oma,* growth]

bac·te·ri·o·pro·tein (bak-tēr'ē-ō-prō'tēn). One of the albuminous substances, or proteins, within the cells of bacteria; these substances vary in their character and properties.

bac·te·ri·op·so·nin (bak-tēr-ē-op'sō-nin). An opsonin acting upon bacteria, as distinguished from a hemopsonin which affects red blood corpuscles.

bac·te·ri·o·sis (bak-tēr-ē-ō'sis). A localized or generalized bacterial infection.

bac·te·ri·o·sper·mia (bak'ter-ē-ō-sper-mē-ă). Bacteria in the semen or ejaculate.

bac·te·ri·o·sta·sis (bak-tēr-ē-os'tă-sis). An arrest or retardation of growth of bacteria. [bacterio- + G. *stasis,* a standing still]

bac·te·ri·o·stat (bak-tēr'ē-ō-stat). Any agent that inhibits or retards bacterial growth. SYN bacteriostatic agent.

bac·te·ri·o·stat·ic (bak-tēr'ē-ō-stat'ik). Inhibiting or retarding the growth of bacteria.

bac·te·ri·o·tox·ic (bak-tēr'ē-ō-tok'sik). Poisonous or toxic to bacteria.

bac·te·ri·o·tro·pic (bak-tēr'ē-ō-trop'ik). Turning toward or moving in the direction of bacteria; having an affinity for bacteria. [bacterio- + G. *tropē,* a turning]

bac·te·ri·ot·ro·pin (bak-tēr-ē-ot'rō-pin). A constituent of the blood, usually a specific antibody, *i.e.,* opsonin, that combines with bacterial cells and renders them more susceptible to phagocytes.

bac·te·ri·o·tryp·sin (bak-tēr'ē-ō-trip'sin). A trypsin-like enzyme produced by bacteria, particularly *Vibrio cholerae.*

Bac·te·ri·um (bak-tēr'ē-ŭm). A bacterial generic name placed on the list of rejected names by the Judicial Commission and the International Committee on Systematic Bacteriology of the International Association of Microbiological Societies. As a consequence, *B.* is no longer used in bacteriology. Identifiable organisms formerly placed in the genus *B.* have all been transferred to other genera. Specifically, *B. anitratum* is now known as *Acinetobacter calcoaceticus; B. coli* is now called *Escherichia coli.* [Mod. L. fr. G. *baktērion,* dim. of *baktron,* a staff or club]

bac·te·ri·um, pl. **bac·te·ria** (bak-tēr'ē-ŭm, -ă). A unicellular prokaryotic microorganism that usually multiplies by cell division and has a cell wall that provides a constancy of form; they may be aerobic or anaerobic, motile or nonmotile, and freeliving, saprophytic, parasitic, or pathogenic. SEE ALSO Cyanobacteria. [Mod. L. fr. G. *baktērion,* dim. of *baktron,* a staff]

Binn's b., a type of the typhoid-paratyphoid subgroups of the nonlactose-fermenting bacteria.

blue-green b., SEE Cyanobacteria.

Chauveau's b., former name for *Clostridium chauvoei.*

endoteric b., a b. that forms an endotoxin.

exoteric b., a b. that secretes an exotoxin.

lysogenic b., (1) a b. in the symbiotic condition in which its genome includes the genome (probacteriophage) of a temperate bacteriophage; in occasional instances the probacteriophage dissociates from the bacterial genome, develops into vegetative bacteriophage, and then matures, causing lysis of the respective host b. and release into the culture medium of infective temperate bacteriophage; **(2)** formerly, a pseudolysogenic bacterial strain, *i.e.,* a "carrier" strain of bacteriophage of low infectivity.

pyogenic b., a b. that causes a pyogenic infection, such as the pyogenic cocci (staphylococci, streptococci, pneumococci, meningococci) and *Haemophilus influenzae.*

bac·te·ri·u·ria (bak-tēr-ē-ū'rē-ă). The presence of bacteria in the urine.

bac·te·roid (bak'ter-oyd). Resembling bacteria.

Bac·te·roi·da·ce·ae (bak'ter-oy-dā'sē-ē). A family of obligate anaerobic (microaerophilic species may occur), nonsporeforming bacteria (order Eubacteriales) containing Gram-negative rods which vary in size from minute, filterable forms to long, filamentous, branching forms; pronounced pleomorphism may occur. Motile and nonmotile species occur; motile cells are peritrichous. Body fluids are frequently required for growth. Carbohydrates are usually fermented with the production of acid; gas may be produced in glucose or peptone media. These organisms occur primarily in the intestinal tracts and mucous membranes of warm-blooded animals. They may be pathogenic. The type genus is *Bacteroides.*

Bac·te·roi·des (bak-ter-oy'dēz). A genus of obligate anaerobic, nonsporeforming bacteria (family Bacteroidaceae) containing Gram-negative rods. Both motile and nonmotile species occur; motile cells are peritrichous. Some species ferment carbohydrates and produce combinations of succinic, lactic, acetic, formic, or propionic acids, sometimes with short-chained alcohols; butyric acid is not a major product. Those species which do not ferment carbohydrates produce from peptone either trace to moderate amounts of succinic, formic, acetic, and lactic acids or major amounts of acetic and butyric acids with moderate amounts of alcohols and isovaleric, propionic, and isobutyric acids. They are part of the normal flora of the oral, respiratory, intestinal, and urogenital cavities of humans and animals; some species are pathogenic. The type species is *B. fragilis.* [G. *bacterion* + *eidos,* form]

B. bivius, a species usually isolated from urogenital and abdominal infections and linked to pelvic inflammatory disease.

B. capillo'sus, a species isolated from human cysts and wounds, the mouth, and feces, and from the intestinal tracts of some animals.

B. corro'dens, former name for *Eikenella corrodens.*

B. di'siens, a species isolated from abdominal and urogenital infections, and from the mouth. SYN *Prevotella disiens.*

B. frag'ilis, a species that is one of the predominant organisms in the lower intestinal tract of man and other animals; also found in specimens from appendicitis, peritonitis, rectal abscesses, pilonidal cysts, surgical wounds, and lesions of the urogenital tract; it is the type species of the genus *B.*

B. furco'sus, a species found in an infected appendix, in lung and abdominal abscesses, and in feces.

B. melaninogenicus, SYN *Prevotella melaninogenica.*

B. nodo'sus, a species involved in the causation of foot rot in sheep and goats. SYN *Dichelobacter nodosus.*

B. ora'lis, a species found in the gingival crevice area of man and in infections of the oral cavity and upper respiratory and genital tracts. SYN *Prevotella oralis.*

B. o'ris, a species isloated from the gingival crevice, systemic infections, face, neck, and chest abscesses, wound drainages, and blood and various bodily fluids. SYN *Prevotella oris.*

B. pneumosin'tes, a species found in the nasopharynx, gingival crevice and periodontal pockets, blood, respiratory tract, brain abscesses, and head and neck infections.

B. praeacu'tus, a species isolated from the intestinal tracts of infants and adults, gangrenous lesions, lung abscesses, and blood. SYN *Tissierella praeacuta.*

B. putredi'nis, a species isolated from feces, cases of acute appendicitis, and abdominal and rectal abscesses; also from foot rot of sheep and from farm soil.

B. thetaiotamicron, a species implicated in intra-abdominal infections.

B. ureolyt'icus, a species isolated from infections of the respiratory and intestinal tracts, and from the buccal cavity, intestinal tract, urogenital tract, and blood after a dental extraction.

bac·te·roi·do·sis (bak-ter-oy-dō'sis). Rarely used term for an infection with *Bacteroides.*

bac·u·li·form (bă-kyū'li-fōrm). Rod-shaped. [L. *baculum,* a rod, + *forma,* form]

Bac·u·lo·vi·ri·dae (bak-yū-lō-vir'i-dē). A family of viruses that multiply only in invertebrates; virions are rod-shaped and measure 40 to 70 nm by 250 to 400 nm; genomes are of double-stranded, supercoiled DNA (MW 80 to 100×10^6). Genera of viruses that multiply only in invertebrates are also included in other families: *Iridovirus* (Iridoviridae), *Entomopoxvirus* (Poxviridae), *Densovirus* (Parvoviridae), cytoplasmic polyhedral virus group (Reoviridae), and *Sigmavirus* (Rhabdoviridae). Baculovirus derived vectors are frequently used to express foreign genes in insect cells. [L. *baculum,* rod]

bac·u·lo·vi·rus (bak'ū-lō-vī-rŭs). A virus that infects insect cells; used extensively in expression systems for recombinant proteins that require eucaryotic processing systems. [L. *baculum,* rod, + virus]

bac·u·lum (bak'yū-lŭm). SYN *os* penis. [L. a rod]

Baehr, George, U.S. physician, 1887–1978. SEE B.-Lohlein *lesion.*

Baelz, Erwin, German physician in Tokyo, 1849–1913. SEE B.'s *disease.*

BAER Abbreviation for brainstem auditory evoked response. SEE evoked *response.*

Baer, Karl E. von, German-Russian embryologist, 1792–1876. SEE B.'s *law, vesicle.*

Baer's ves·i·cle. See under vesicle.

Baeyer, Johann F.W.A. von, German chemist and Nobel laureate, 1835–1917. SEE B.'s *theory.*

bag. A pouch, sac, or receptacle. [A.S. *baelg*]

Ambu b., proprietary name for a self-reinflating b. with nonrebreathing valves to provide positive pressure ventilation during resuscitation with oxygen or air.

breathing b., a collapsible reservoir from which gases are inhaled and into which gases may be exhaled during general anesthesia or artificial ventilation. SYN reservoir b.

colostomy b., a bag worn over an artifical anus to collect feces.

Douglas b., a large b. in which expired gas is collected for several minutes to determine oxygen consumption in humans under conditions of actual work. [C.G. Douglas]

nuclear b., the aggregation of nuclei occurring in the nonstriated center of an intrafusal muscle fiber of a neuromuscular spindle.

Petersen's b., an obsolete device consisting of a rubber b. introduced into the rectum and inflated to push up the bladder to facilitate suprapubic cystotomy.

Politzer b., a pear-shaped rubber b. used for forcing air through the eustachian tube by the Politzer method.

ba

classification of bacteria

kingdom:	prokaryotes (Prokaryotae)		
phylum I:	gracilicutes (mostly Gram-negative)		
class 1:	Spirochetes		
	order I: Spirochaetales	family I: Spirochaetaceae	genera: e.g., *Treponema, Borrelia*
		family II: Leptospiraceae	genus: *Leptospira*
class 2:	aerobic or microaerophilic, motile, spiral or bent Gram-negative bacteria		genera: e.g., *Spirillum, Campylobacter*
class 4:	Gram-negative aerobic bacilli and cocci		
		family I: Pseudomonadaceae	genus: e.g., *Pseudomonas*
		family VII: Legionellaceae	genus: *Legionella*
		family VIII: Neisseriaceae	genera: e.g., *Neisseria, Moraxella (Branhamella), Acinetobacter*
	other genera: e.g., *Alcaligenes, Brucella, Bordetella, Francisella*		
class 5:	Gram-negative facultative anaerobic bacilli		
		family I: Enterobacteriaceae	genera: *Escherichia, Shigella, Salmonella, Citrobacter, Klebsiella, Enterobacter, Erwinia, Serratia, Hafnia, Edwardsiella, Proteus, Providencia, Morganella, Yersinia*
		family II: Vibrionaceae	genera: e.g., *Vibrio, Aeromonas, Plesiomonas*
		family III: Pasteurellaceae	genera: *Pasteurella, Haemophilus, Actinobacillus*
	other genera: *Zymomonas, Chromobacterium, Cardiobacterium, Calymmatobacterium, Gardnerella, Eikenella, Streptobacillus*		
class 6:	Anaerobic Gram-negative straight, curved, and spiral-formed bacilli		
		family I: Bacteroidaceae	genera: e.g., *Bacteroides, Fusobacterium, Leptotrichia*
class 9:	Rickettsia		
	order I: Rickettsiales	family I: Rickettsiaceae	genera: e.g., *Rickettsia, Coxiella*
		family II: Bartonellaceae	genus: e.g., *Bartonella*
	order II: Chlamydiales	family I: Chlamydiaceae	genus: *Chlamydia*
phylum II:	firmicutes (mostly Gram-positive)		
class 12:	Gram-positive cocci		
		family: Micrococcaceae	genera: *Micrococcus, Stomatococcus, Planococcus, Staphylococcus*
		family: Deinococcaceae	genus: *Deinococcus*
	other organisms: e.g., streptococci		
class 13:	endospore-forming Gram-positive bacilli and cocci		genera: e.g., *Bacillus, Clostridium*
class 14:	regularly formed, asperogenous Gram-positive bacilli		genera: e.g., *Lactobacillus, Listeria, Erysipelothrix*
class 15:	irregularly formed, asperogenous Gram-positive bacilli		genera: e.g., *Corynebacterium, Gardnerella, Brevibacterium, Propionibacterium, Eubacterium, Actinomyces, Bifidobacterium*
class 16:	Mycobacteria	family: Mycobacteriaceae	genus: *Mycobacterium*
class 17:	Nocardioforms		genus: e.g., *Nocardia*
[class 18]	Mycoplasmids		
phylum III:	Tenericutes (without cell wall)	class I: Mollicutes	
	order I: Mycoplasmatales	family I: Mycoplasmataceae	genus: *Mycoplasma*
phylum IV:	Mendosicutes		
	class I: Archaeobacteria (cell wall without muramic acid)		methanogenous bacteria, extremely halophilic b., extremely thermophilic b.

reservoir b., SYN breathing b.

b. of waters, colloquialism for the amniotic sac and contained amniotic fluid.

bag·as·so·sis (bag-ă-sō′sis). Extrinsic allergic alveolitis following exposure to sugar cane fiber (bagasse); variously attributed to inhalation of spores of soil fungi and, particularly, thermophilic actinomycetes.

Baggenstoss, Archie H., U.S. pathologist, *1908. SEE B. change.

Bagolini, 20th century Italian ophthalmologist. SEE B. test.

bah·nung (bah′nŭng). Increased ease of transmission of a nerve impulse in a nerve tract as a result of prior stimulation. [Ger. Bahnung, the making of a pathway]

Baillarger, Jules G.F., French neurologist, 1809–1890. SEE B.'s bands, under band, lines, under line.

Bailliart, Paul, French ophthalmologist, 1877–1969. SEE B.'s ophthalmodynamometer.

Bainbridge, Francis A., English physiologist, 1874–1921. SEE B. reflex.

Baker, James Porter, U.S. physician, *1902. SEE Charcot-Weiss-B. syndrome.

Baker, John Randal, English zoologist, *1900. SEE B.'s pyridine extraction, acid hematein.

Baker, William M., English surgeon, 1839–1896. SEE B.'s cyst.

BAL Abbreviation for British anti-Lewisite.

⛛**balan-.** SEE balano-.

bal·ance (bal′ans). **1.** An apparatus for weighing; e.g., scales. **2.** The normal state of action and reaction between two or more parts or organs of the body. **3.** Quantities, concentrations, and proportionate amounts of bodily constituents. **4.** The difference between intake and utilization, storage, or excretion of a substance by the body. SEE ALSO equilibrium. [L. bi-, twice, + lanx, dish, scale]

acid-base b., the normal b. between acid and base in the blood plasma, expressed in the hydrogen ion concentration or pH, resulting from the relative amounts of acidic and basic materials ingested and produced by body metabolism, compared to the relative amounts of acidic and basic materials excreted from the body and consumed by body metabolism; the normal state of acid-base b. is not one of neutrality, with equal concentrations of hydrogen and hydroxyl ions, but a more alkaline state with a certain excess of hydroxyl ions. SYN acid-base equilibrium.

nitrogen b., the difference between the total nitrogen intake by an organism and its total nitrogen loss. A normal, healthy adult has a zero nitrogen b., $N_{in} > N_{out}$ (i.e., a positive nitrogen b.

occlusal b., a condition in which there are simultaneous contacts of the occluding units of the opposing dental arches in centric and eccentric positions within the functional range.

Wilhelmy b., a device for measuring surface tension in terms of the pull exerted on a thin plate of platinum or other material suspended vertically through the surface; used in a Langmuir trough to study pulmonary surfactant.

ba·lan·ic (ba-lan′ik). Relating to the glans penis or glans clitoridis. [G. balanos, acorn, glans]

Ba·la·ni·tes ae·gyp·ti·a·ca (bal-ă-nī′tēz ē-jip-tī′ā-kă). A genus of trees growing in the Near East, whose berries contain an active principle that is deadly to mollusks, miracidia, cercariae, tadpoles, and fish and that is used as a prophylactic against schistosomiasis by adding it to drinking water. [L. balanos, acorn]

bal·a·ni·tis (bal-ă-nī′tis). Inflammation of the glans penis or clitoris. [G. balanos, acorn, glans, + -itis, inflammation]

b. circumscripta plasmacellularis, SYN plasma cell b.

b. diabet′ica, glanular inflammation in diabetics related to urinary infection or concomitant posthitis.

plasma cell b., benign circumscribed b. characterized microscopically by subepithelial plasma cell infiltration and clinically by small erythematous papular lesions. SYN b. circumscripta plasmacellularis, b. of Zoon, Zoon's erythroplasia.

b. xerot′ica oblit′erans, lichen sclerosus et atrophicus of the glans penis, which may result in urethral stenosis.

b. of Zoon, SYN plasma cell b.

⛛**balano-, balan-.** Glans penis. [G. balanos, acorn, glans]

bal·a·no·plas·ty (bal′an-ō-plas-tē). Surgical reconstruction of the glans penis. [balano- + G. plastos, formed]

bal·a·no·pos·thi·tis (bal′an-ō-pos-thī′tis). Inflammation of the glans penis and overlying prepuce. [balano- + G. posthē, prepuce, + -itis, inflammation]

enzootic b., SYN ulcerative posthitis.

bal·an·ti·di·a·sis (bal′an-ti-dī′ă-sis). A disease caused by the presence of Balantidium coli in the large intestine; characterized by diarrhea, dysentery, and occasionally ulceration. SYN balantidosis.

Ba·lan·ti·di·um (bal-an-tid′ē-ŭm). A genus of ciliates (family Balantidiidae) found in the digestive tract of vertebrates and invertebrates. [G. balantidion, dim of ballantion, a bag]

B. co′li, a very large parasitic ciliate species, usually 50 to 80 μm in length, reaching up to 200 μm in pigs, found in the cecum or large intestine, swimming actively in the lumen; usually harmless in man but may invade and ulcerate the intestinal wall, producing a colitis resembling amebic dysentery.

B. su′is, a species originally considered distinct from the ciliate parasite of man, B. coli, but now considered synonymous with it; nonpathogenic in swine.

bal·an·ti·do·sis (bal′an-ti-dō′sis). SYN balantidiasis.

bal·a·nus (bal′ă-nŭs). SYN glans penis. [G. balanos, acorn, glans penis]

bald (bawld). Having no hair, or a decrease in the amount of hair of the scalp. [M.E. balled]

bald·ness (bawld′nes). SYN alopecia.

common b., SYN androgenic alopecia.

congenital b., SYN alopecia congenitalis.

male pattern b., SYN male pattern alopecia.

pubic b., loss of pubic hair. SYN pubomadesis.

Baldy, John M., U.S. gynecologist, 1860–1934. SEE B.'s operation.

Balint, Rudolph, Hungarian neurologist and psychiatrist, 1874–1929. SEE B.'s syndrome.

Ball, Sir Charles, Irish surgeon, 1851–1916. SEE B.'s operation.

ball. **1.** A round mass. SEE bezoar. **2.** In veterinary medicine, a large pill or bolus.

chondrin b., one of the globular masses formed by a group of cells enclosed in a capsule, in hyaline cartilage.

dust b., a mass sometimes found in the stomach or intestine of an animal fed on mill cleanings.

food b., SYN phytobezoar.

b. of the foot, the padded portion of the sole, at the anterior extremity of the heads of the metatarsals, upon which the weight rests when the heel is raised.

fungus b., a compact mass of fungal mycelium and cellular debris, 1 to 5 cm in diameter, residing within a lung cavity; such cavities may be produced by bacterial as well as mycotic infectious agents, but they are usually produced by Aspergillus fumigatus or, more rarely, by A. niger. SEE ALSO aspergilloma (2).

hair b., SYN trichobezoar.

wool b., a trichophytobezoar formed chiefly of wool and vegetable matter in the stomach of sheep.

Ballance, Sir Charles A., English surgeon, 1856–1936. SEE B.'s sign; Koerte-B. operation.

bal·ling gun, bal·ling iron. An instrument used for administering boluses or capsules to animals.

bal·lism (bal′izm). SYN ballismus.

bal·lis·mus (bal-iz′mŭs). A type of involuntary movement affecting the proximal limb musculature, manifested as jerking, flinging movements of the extremity; caused by a lesion of or near the contralateral subthalamic nucleus. Usually only one side of the body is involved, resulting in hemiballismus. SYN ballism. [G. ballismos, a jumping about]

bal·lis·to·car·di·o·gram (bal-is-tō-kar′dē-ō-gram). A record of the body's recoil caused by cardiac contraction, the ejection of blood into the aorta, and ventricular filling forces; has been used as a basis for calculating the cardiac output in man, but its lack of accuracy and reproducibility has caused it to be discarded. [G. *ballō*, to throw, + *kardia*, heart, + *gramma*, something written]

bal·lis·to·car·di·o·graph (BCG) (bal-is-tō-kar′dē-ō-graf). Instrument for taking a ballistocardiogram, consisting either of a moving table suspended from the ceiling, or of an apparatus that rests upon the patient's body, usually on the shins, together with a graphic recording system.

bal·lis·to·car·di·og·ra·phy (bal-is-tō-kar-dē-og′ră-fē). **1.** The graphic recording of movements of the body imparted by ballistic forces (cardiac contraction and ejection of blood, ventricular filling, acceleration, and deceleration of blood flow through the great vessels); these minute movements are amplified and recorded on moving chart paper after being translated into an electrical potential by a pickup device. **2.** The study and interpretation of ballistocardiograms.

bal·lis·to·pho·bia (bal-is-tō-fō′bē-ă). Morbid fear of a projectile or missile. [G. *ballista,* catapult, fr. G. *ballistēs* fr. *ballō,* + *phobos,* fear]

bal·loon (bă-lūn). **1.** An inflatable spherical or ovoid device used to retain tubes or catheters in, or provide support to, various body structures. **2.** A distensible device used to stretch or occlude a stenotic viscus or blood vessel. **3.** To distend a body cavity with a gas or fluid to facilitate its examination, dilate a structure, or occlude its lumen. [Fr. *ballon,* fr. It. *ballone,* fr. *balla,* ball, fr. Germanic]

angioplasty b., a b. near the tip of an angiographic catheter, designed to distend narrowed vessels. SEE balloon-tip *catheter.*

detachable b., a small b., attached to the tip of a catheter, which can be released to occlude a vessel.

intra-aortic b., an externally and intermittently inflatable balloon placed into the descending aorta and which, on activation during diastole, augments blood pressure and organ perfusion by its pulsatile thrust; then, on deflation, decreases the cardiac work with each systole—the so-called counterpulsation principle—by reducing cardiac afterload.

bal·loon·sep·tos·to·my (bă-lūn′sep-tos′tō-mē). Creation of an artificial interatrial septal defect by cardiac catheterization during which an inflated balloon is pulled across the interatrial septum through the foramen ovale; used in cases of transposition of the great vessels and tricuspid atresia.

bal·lot·ta·ble (bal-ot′ă-bl). Capable of exhibiting the phenomenon of ballottement.

bal·lotte·ment (bal-ot-maw′). **1.** Maneuver used in physical examination to estimate the size of an organ not near the surface, particularly when there is ascites, by a flicking motion of the hand or fingers similar to that of dribbling a basketball. **2.** An obsolete method of diagnosis of pregnancy: with the tip of the forefinger in the vagina, a sharp tap is made against the lower segment of the uterus; the fetus, if present, is tossed upward and (if the finger is retained in place) will be felt to strike against the wall of the uterus as it falls back. [Fr. *balloter,* to toss up]

abdominal b., examination of the abdomen by palpation to detect excessive amounts of fluid (ascites) by causing organs to bob up and down in the fluid milieu.

renal b., a maneuver in which the kidney is moved by pressure from behind, allowing it to be felt between the hands and its size, shape, and mobility determined.

balm (bawlm). **1.** SYN balsam. **2.** An ointment, especially a fragrant one. **3.** A soothing application. [L. *balsamum,* fr. G. *balsamon,* the balsam tree]

b. of Gilead, an oleoresin from *Commiphora opobalsamum* (family Burseraceae), probably the myrrh of the Bible; used in perfumery. SYN Mecca balsam, opobalsamum.

mountain b., SYN eriodictyon.

sweet b., SYN melissa.

bal·ne·o·ther·a·peu·tics, bal·ne·o·ther·a·py (bal′nē-ō-thār-ă-pyū′tiks, -thār′ă-pē). Immersion of part or all of the body in a mineral water bath as a form of therapy. [L. *balneum,* bath]

Baló, Jozsef, Hungarian physician, *1896. SEE B.'s *disease.*

bal·sam (bawl′sam). A fragrant, resinous or thick, oily exudate from various trees and plants. SYN balm (1), oleoresin (3). [G. *balsamon;* L. *balsamum*]

Canada b., a yellowish liquid resin from the b. fir, *Abies balsamea* (family Pinaceae); contains kinene and bornyl acetate; used for mounting histologic specimens and as a cement for lenses. SYN Canada turpentine.

b. of copaiba, SYN copaiba.

Mecca b., SYN *balm* of Gilead.

b. of Peru, a thick, dark brown liquid b. obtained from *Toluifera pereirae* (family Leguminosae), containing 60% cinnamein; used as a healing application to wounds.

Tolu b., a yellowish brown soft mass obtained from *Toluifera balsamum* (family Leguminosae), containing cinnamic and benzoic acids and esters; used as a stimulant expectorant.

bal·sam·ic (bawl-sam′ik). **1.** Relating to balsam. **2.** Fragrant.

Bamberger, Eugen, Austrian physician, 1858–1921. SEE B.-Marie *disease, syndrome.*

Bamberger, Heinrich von, Austrian physician, 1822–1888. SEE B.'s *albuminuria, disease, sign.*

ba·mif·yl·line hy·dro·chlo·ride (bă-mif′i-lin). 8-Benzyl-7-{2-[ethyl(2-hydroxyethyl)amino] ethyl}theophylline hydrochloride; a vasodilator and smooth muscle relaxant.

bam·i·pine (bam-i-pēn). 4-*N*-Benzylanilino-1-methylpiperidine; an antihistaminic.

ban·crof·ti·a·sis, ban·crof·to·sis (ban-krof-tī′ă-sis, -tō′sis). Infection with *Wuchereria bancrofti.*

band. 1. Any appliance or part of an apparatus that encircles or binds a part of the body. SEE ALSO zone. **2.** Any ribbon-shaped or cordlike anatomical structure that encircles or binds another structure or that connects two or more parts. SEE fascia, line, linea, stripe, stria, tenia. **3.** A narrow strip containing one or more macromolecules (on occasions, small molecules) detected in electrophoresis or certain types of chromatography.

A b.'s, the dark-staining anisotropic cross striations in the myofibrils of muscle fibers, comprising regions of overlapping thick (myosin) and thin (actin) filaments. SYN A disks, anisotropic disks, Q b.'s (1), Q disks.

absorption b., the range of wavelengths or frequencies in the electromagnetic spectrum where radiant energy is absorbed by passage through a gaseous, liquid, or dissolved substance; it is exploited for analytical purposes in colorimetry or spectrophotometry, and is usually described in terms of the wavelength where maximum absorbance occurs (*i.e.,* λ_{max}).

amniotic b.'s, strands of amniotic tissue adherent to the embryo or fetus; they may cause constriction of embryonic limbs. SEE ALSO congenital *amputation.* SYN amniotic adhesions, annular b., constriction ring (2), Simonart's b.'s (1), Simonart's ligaments, Simonart's threads, Streeter's b.'s.

annular b., SYN amniotic b.'s.

anogenital b., the first indication of the perineum in the embryo.

atrioventricular b., SYN atrioventricular *bundle.*

Baillarger's b.'s, SYN Baillarger's *lines,* under *line.*

b. bands, SYN Muehrcke's *sign.*

Bechterew's b., SYN b. of Kaes-Bechterew.

Broca's diagonal b., a white fiber bundle descending in the precommissural septum toward the base of the forebrain, immediately rostral to the lamina terminalis; at the base, the bundle turns in the caudolateral direction; traveling through a ventral stratum of the innominate substance alongside the optic tract, it fades before reaching the amygdala.

chromosome b., a region of darker or contrasting staining across the width of a chromosome; the pattern of b.'s is characteristic for most chromosomes. SEE banding.

Clado's b., the suspensory ligament of the ovary.

b.'s of colon, SYN *teniae* coli, under *tenia.*

contraction b., a microscopic change in myocardial cells in which excessive contraction, associated with elevated intracellular calcium and serum norepinephrine, causes the formation of transverse amorphous b. in the fibers which are then incapable of contracting again. SYN contraction band necrosis.

coronary b., a region of the pododerm; a prominent ridge of corium and underlying tela subcutanea at the top of the hoof from which most of the wall of the hoof grows. SYN corium coronae.

Essick's cell b.'s, groups of cells in the developing rhomben-cephalon which migrate in two b.'s, one of which eventually forms the inferior olivary nucleus and the arcuate nucleus, and the other the pontine nuclei.

Gennari's b., SYN *line* of Gennari.

b. of Giacomini, SYN uncus b. of Giacomini.

H b., the paler area in the center of the A b. of a striated muscle fiber, comprising the central portion of thick (myosin) filaments that are not overlapped by thin (actin) filaments. SYN H disk, Hensen's disk, Hensen's line.

His' b., SYN atrioventricular *bundle.*

Hunter-Schreger b.'s, alternating light and dark lines seen in dental enamel that begin at the dentoenamel junction and end before they reach the enamel surface; they represent areas of enamel rods cut in cross-sections dispersed between areas of rods cut longitudinally. SYN Hunter-Schreger lines, Schreger's lines.

I b., a light b. on each side of the Z line of striated muscle fibers, comprising a region of the sarcomere where thin (actin) filaments are not overlapped by thick (myosin) filaments. SYN I disk, isotropic disk.

iliotibial b., SYN iliotibial *tract.*

b. of Kaes-Bechterew, b. of horizontal myelinated fibers in the most superficial part of the third layer of the isocortex. SYN Bechterew's b., layer of Bechterew, line of Bechterew, line of Kaes.

Ladd's b., a peritoneal attachment of an incompletely rotated cecum, causing obstruction of the duodenum, found in malrotation of the intestine.

Lane's b., a congenital b. on the distal ileum causing stasis. SYN Lane's kink.

longitudinal b.'s of cruciform ligament, ligamentous slips forming the "upright" or vertical beam of the cruciform ligament. SYN fasciculi longitudinales ligamenti cruciformis atlantis [NA].

M b., SYN M *line.*

Mach's b., a relatively bright or dark b. perceived in a zone where the luminance increases or decreases rapidly.

Maissiat's b., SYN iliotibial *tract.*

matrix b., a metal or plastic b. secured around the crown of a tooth to confine restorative material to be adapted into a prepared cavity.

Meckel's b., the portion of the anterior ligament of the malleus that extends from the base of the anterior process through the petrotympanic fissure, to attach to the spine of the sphenoid. SEE anterior *ligament* of malleus. SYN Meckel's ligament.

moderator b., SYN septomarginal *trabecula.*

oligoclonal b., small discrete b.'s in the gamma globulin region of the spinal fluid electrophoresis, indicating local central nervous system production of IgG; b.'s are frequently seen in patients with multiple sclerosis but can also be found in other diseases of the central nervous system including syphilis, sarcoidosis, and chronic infection or inflammation.

orthodontic b., a thin strip of metal closely adapted to the crown of a tooth to which wires may be attached for tooth movement.

pecten b., a fibrous induration of the anal pecten resulting from passive congestion or a chronic form of inflammation in this region.

perioplic b., a narrow b. of corium and underlying tela subcutanea proximal to the coronary b. at the top of the hoof; the periople develops from it.

Q b.'s, (1) SYN A b.'s. **(2)** SEE Q-banding *stain.*

Reil's b., (1) SYN septomarginal *trabecula.* **(2)** SYN medial *lemniscus.*

silastic b. (si′lăs-tik), a small silastic ring placed around each fallopian tube to achieve permanent sterilization.

Simonart's b.'s, (1) SYN amniotic b.'s. **(2)** weblike band of tissue partially filling the gap between the medial and lateral portions of a cleft lip.

Soret b., the absorption b. of all porphyrins at about 400 nm.

Streeter's b.'s, SYN amniotic b.'s.

uncus b. of Giacomini, a slender whitish b., the attenuated anterior continuation of the dentate gyrus (fascia dentata), crossing transversely the surface of the recurved part of the uncus

gyri parahippocampalis. SYN b. of Giacomini, cauda fasciae dentatae, frenulum of Giacomini, tail of dentate gyrus.

ventricular b. of larynx, SYN vestibular *fold.*

Z b., SYN Z *line.*

zonular b., SYN *zona* orbicularis.

ban·dage (ban′dij). **1.** A piece of cloth or other material, of varying shape and size, applied to a body part to make compression, absorb drainage, prevent motion, retain surgical dressings. **2.** To cover a body part by application of a b.

adhesive b., a dressing of plain absorbent gauze affixed to plastic or fabric coated with a pressure-sensitive adhesive.

Barton's b., a figure-of-8 b. supporting the mandible below and anteriorly; used in mandibular fracture.

capeline b., a b. covering the head or an amputation stump like a cap. [L. *capella,* a cap]

circular b., one encircling an extremity, or a portion of it, or the trunk.

cravat b., a b. made by bringing the point of a triangular b. to the middle of the base and then folding lengthwise to the desired width.

crucial b., a b. in the shape of a cross; *e.g.,* a T-b..

demigauntlet b., a gauntlet b. that covers only the hand, leaving the fingers exposed.

Desault's b., a b. for fracture of the clavicle; the elbow is bound to the side, with a pad placed in the axilla.

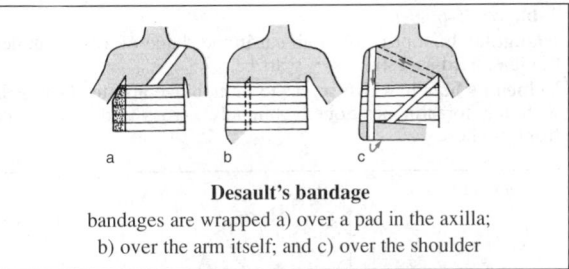

Desault's bandage
bandages are wrapped a) over a pad in the axilla;
b) over the arm itself; and c) over the shoulder

elastic b., a b. containing stretchable material; used to make local pressure.

Esmarch b., SYN Esmarch *tourniquet.*

figure-of-8 b., a b. applied alternately to two parts, usually two segments of a limb above and below the joint, in such a way that the turns describe the figure 8; used primarily for the treatment of fractures of the clavicle.

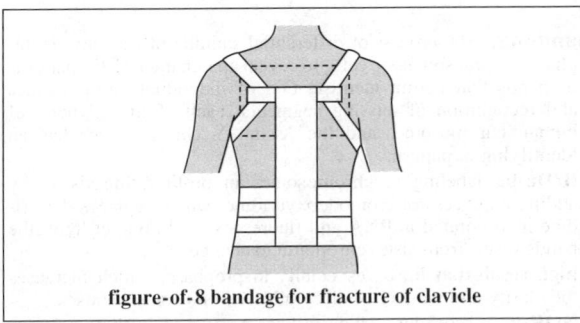

figure-of-8 bandage for fracture of clavicle

four-tailed b., a strip of cloth split in two except for a central portion placed under the chin, with four tails tied over the head; used to limit motion of the mandible.

gauntlet b., a figure-of-8 b. covering the hand and fingers.

gauze b., SEE gauze.

Gibney's fixation b., herring-bone strapping of the foot and leg for sprain of the ankle.

Gibson's b., a b., resembling Barton's b., for stabilizing a fracture of the mandible.

hammock b., a b. for retaining dressings on the head: the dressings are covered by a wide gauze strip, the ends of which are brought down over the ears and held while a narrow circular b. is passed around the head; the ends of the gauze strip are then turned up over the circular b. and other turns are made securing them firmly.

immovable b., a b. of cloth impregnated with plaster of Paris, liquid glass, or the like, which hardens soon after its application.

Martin's b., a roller b. of soft rubber used to make compression on a limb in the treatment of varicose veins or ulcers.

oblique b., a b. in which the successive turns proceed obliquely up or down the limb.

plaster b., a roller b. impregnated with plaster of Paris and applied moist; used to make a rigid dressing for a fracture or diseased joint.

roller b., a strip of material, of variable width, rolled into a compact cylinder to facilitate its application.

scarf b., SYN triangular b.

Scultetus' b., a large oblong cloth, the ends of which are cut into narrow strips, which is applied to the thorax or abdomen, the strips being tied or overlapped and pinned.

spica b., successive strips of material applied to the body and the first part of a limb, or to the hand and a finger, which overlap slightly in a V to resemble an ear of grain. [L. *spica,* ear of grain]

spiral b., an oblique b. encircling a limb, the successive turns overlapping those preceding.

suspensory b., a bag of expansile fabric for supporting the scrotum and its contents.

T-b., SYN T-*binder.*

triangular b., a piece of cloth cut in the shape of a right-angled triangle, used as a sling. SYN scarf b.

Velpeau's b., a b. which serves to immobilize arm to chest wall, with the forearm positioned obliquely across and upward on front of chest.

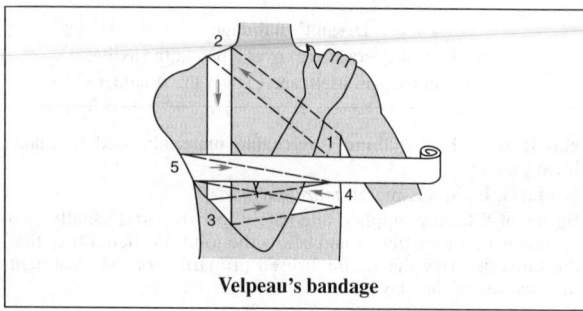

Velpeau's bandage

band·ing. The process of differential staining of (usually) metaphase chromosomes of cells to reveal the characteristic patterns of bands that permit identification of individual chromosomes and recognition of missing segments; each of the 22 pairs of human chromosomes and the X and Y chromosomes has an identifying b. pattern.

BrDu-b., labeling of chromosomes in proliferating tissue by adding an excess of bromodeoxyuridine, which replaces the uridine incorporated in RNA and fluoresces in ultraviolet light; the bands result from sister chromatid exchanges.

high-resolution b., b., especially in prophase, which increases the clarity and number of discernible chromosome bands.

NOR-b., a procedure which utilizes a silver stain that preferentially accumulates in the *n*ucleoli-*o*rganizing *r*egions, *i.e.,* the satellite regions of the acrocentric chromosomes.

prometaphase b., b. done in the stage of mitosis intermediate between prophase and metaphase.

pulmonary artery b., a surgical method of decreasing pulmonary blood flow and thereby volume overload of the left ventricle, alleviating CHF in certain congenital heart defects.

reverse b., SEE R-banding *stain.*

Bandl, Ludwig, German obstetrician, 1842–1892. SEE B.'s *ring.*

band·width. The range of frequency or wavelengths over which a device is intended to operate.

ban·dy-leg (ban'dē-leg). SYN *genu* varum.

bane (bān). A poison or blight. [O.E. *bana*]

Bang, Bernhard L.F., Danish veterinarian and physician, 1848–1932. SEE B.'s *bacillus, disease.*

ba·nis·te·rine (ba-nis'tĕ-rēn). SYN harmine.

Bannister, Henry M., U.S. physician, 1844–1920. SEE B.'s *disease.*

Banti, Guido, Italian physician, 1852–1925. SEE B.'s *disease, syndrome.*

bap·ti·tox·ine. SYN cytisine.

bar. **1.** A unit of pressure equal to 1 megadyne (10^6 dyne) per cm^2 in the CGS system, 0.9869233 atmosphere, or 10^5 Pa (N/m^2) in the SI system. **2.** One of the two convergent ridges on the ground surface of the hoof of a horse, united by the frog, and fused with the sole in front. SYN connector b. (1). **3.** A metal segment of greater length than width that serves to connect two or more parts of a removable partial denture. SEE ALSO major *connector.* **4.** A segment of tissue or bone that unites two or more similar structures.

arch b., any one of several types of wires, b., or splints conforming to the arch of the teeth, extending from one side of the arch to the other and located labially, or lingually; used for the treatment of jaw fractures and/or stabilization of injured teeth.

b. of bladder, SYN interureteric *fold.*

clasp b., SEE clasp.

connector b., **(1)** SYN bar (2). **(2)** SEE major *connector,* minor *connector.*

labial b., a major connector located labial to the dental arch joining two or more bilateral parts of a mandibular removable partial denture.

lingual b., a major connector located lingual to the dental arch joining two or more bilateral parts of a mandibular removable partial denture.

median b. of Mercier, a prominent band of fibromuscular tissue involving the interureteric ridge or neck of the urinary bladder, occasionally resulting in urinary obstruction.

Mercier's b., SYN interureteric *fold.*

occlusal rest b., a minor connector used to attach an occlusal rest to a major part of a removable partial denture.

palatal b., a major connector which crosses the palate and unites two or more parts of a maxillary removable partial denture.

Passavant's b., SYN Passavant's *cushion.*

sternal b., one of the transverse units of the developing sternum formed by the union of paired primordia.

terminal b., dark spots or b. (depending on the plane of section) in the lateral boundary between the apical ends of columnar epithelial cells; this region corresponds with the area of the junctional complex and the thin filaments that anchor on the zonula adherens.

bar·ag·no·sis (bar-ag-nō'sis). Loss of ability to appreciate the weight of objects held in the hand, or to differentiate objects of different weights. When the primary senses are intact, caused by a lesion of the contralateral parietal lobe. [G. *baros,* weight + *a-*priv., + *gnōsis,* a knowing]

Bárány, Robert, Austrian-Hungarian otologist and Nobel laureate, 1876–1936. SEE B.'s *sign,* caloric *test;* positional *vertigo* of B.

bar·ba (bar'bă). **1** [NA]. The beard. **2.** A hair of the beard. [L.]

barb·al·o·in (bar-bal'ō-in). SYN aloin.

Barber, Glenn, 20th century U.S. orthopedic surgeon. SEE Blount-Barber *disease.*

bar·bi·e·ro (bar-bē-ā'rō). Brazilian term for the bloodsucking hemipteran triatomid bug, *Panstrongylus megistus,* an important vector of Chagas' disease, caused by *Trypanosoma cruzi.* [Pg. the barber]

bar·bi·tal (bar'bi-tawl). A hypnotic and sedative; available as b. sodium (soluble b.), with the same uses; often used as a buffer. SYN 5,5-diethylbarbituric acid, barbitone, Veronal.

bar·bi·tone. SYN barbital.

bar·bi·tu·rate (bar-bich'yūr-āt). A derivative of barbituric acid, including phenobarbital and others, that act as CNS depressants and are used for their tranquilizing, hypnotic, and anti-seizure effects; most b.'s have the potential for abuse.

bar·bi·tu·ric ac·id (bar-bi-chyūr'ik). 2,4,6-trioxohexahydropyrimidine; 2,4,6-(1*H*,3*H*,5*H*)-pyrimidinetrione; a crystalline dibasic acid from which barbital and other barbiturates are derived; has no sedative action. SYN malonylurea.

bar·bi·tu·rism (bar'bi-chyūr-izm). Chronic poisoning by any of the derivatives of barbituric acid; symptoms, which are not very distinctive, include cutaneous eruption accompanied by chills, fever, and headache.

bar·bo·tage (bar-bō-tahzh'). A method of spinal anesthesia in which a portion of the anesthetic solution is injected into the cerebral spinal fluid, which is then aspirated back into the syringe and reinjected. [Fr. *barboter,* to dabble]

bar·bu·la hir·ci (bar'byū-lă hir'sī). The hairs growing from the tragus, antitragus, and incisura intertragica at the opening of the external acoustic meatus. [L. dim. of *barba,* beard, + gen. sing. of *hircus,* goat]

Barclay, Alfred E., English physician, 1877–1949. SEE B.-Baron *disease.*

Barcroft, Sir Joseph F., English physiologist, 1872–1947. SEE B.-Warburg *apparatus, technique.*

Bard, Philip, U.S. physiologist, 1898–1945. SEE Cannon-B. *theory.*

Bardet, Georges, French physician, *1885. SEE B.-Biedl *syndrome.*

Bardinet, Barthélemy A., French physician, 1809–1874. SEE B.'s *ligament.*

bar·es·the·sia (bar-es-thē'zē-ă). SYN pressure *sense.* [G. *baros,* weight, + *aisthēsis,* sensation]

bar·es·the·si·om·e·ter (bar'es-thē'zē-om'ĕ-ter). An instrument for measuring the pressure sense. [G. *baros,* weight, + *aisthēsis,* sensation, + *metron,* measure]

bar·i·at·ric (bar-ē-at'rik). Relating to bariatrics.

bar·i·at·rics (bar-ē-at'riks). That branch of medicine concerned with the management (prevention or control) of obesity and allied diseases. [G. *baros,* weight, + *iatreia,* medical treatment]

bar·ic (ba'rik). Relating to barometric pressure (as in isobar) or to weight generally.

ba·ric·i·ty (ba-ris'i-tē). The weight of one substance compared to the weight of an equal volume of another substance at the same temperature. [G. *baros,* weight]

ba·ril·la (ba-ril'ă). Commercial, usually impure, sodium carbonate and sulfate.

bar·i·to·sis (bar-i-tō'sis). A form of pneumoconiosis caused by barite or barium dust.

bar·i·um (Ba) (ba'rē-ŭm, bā'rē-ŭm). A metallic, alkaline, divalent earth element; atomic no. 56, atomic wt. 137.327. Salts are often used in diagnosis. [G. *barys,* heavy]

b. chloride, formerly used as a heart tonic and for varicose veins; extremely toxic.

b. hydroxide, Ba(OH)₂; a caustic compound combined with calcium hydroxide in a carbon dioxide absorbent; used in anesthetic circuits. SEE ALSO absorbent (3).

b. meal, oral administration of b. sulfate suspension for radiographic study of the upper gastrointestinal tract (British usage).

b. oxide, b. monoxide, BaO; it is caustic, forming the strong base, Ba(OH)₂, in water; used as a dehydrating agent. SYN baryta.

b. sulfate, BaSO₄; given as a suspension orally, rectally, or through a tube, for radiographic visualization of a part of the gastrointestinal tract. SEE enteroclysis, barium *enema.* SEE ALSO barium *enema.*

b. sulfide, a poisonous grayish yellow powder, used as a depilatory.

b. swallow, oral administration of b. sulfate suspension for radiographic investigation of the hypopharynx and esophagus.

bark. 1. The envelope or covering of the roots, trunk, and branches of plants. B. of pharmacological significance not listed below are alphabetized under specific names. 2. SYN cinchona.

cinchona b., SYN cinchona.

cotton-root b., dried root b. of *Gossypium herbaceum* and other

barbiturates		
no.	short name	effects*
1	allobarbital	i
2	amobarbital	i
3	aprobarbital	i
4	barbital	l
5	cyclobarbital	s
6	cyclopentobarbital	s
7	heptabarb	i
8	pentobarbital	s
9	phenobarbital	l
10	propallynonal	s
11	proxibarbal	i
12	(sec)butabarbital	i
13	secobarbital	s
14	vinylbital	i
thiobarbiturates		
15	thiopental (Na-salt)	us
16	thiobutabarbital (Na)	s
N-substituted barbiturate		
17	hexobarbital	us
18	methohexital	us
* for induction of anesthesia: s = short, i = intermediate, l = long, us = ultra short		

species of *Gossypium* (family Malvaceae). Has been used as an abortifacient and oxytocic.

Barkan, Otto, U.S. ophthalmologist, 1887–1958. SEE B.'s *operation.*

Barkman, Åke, 20th century Swedish internist. SEE B.'s *reflex.*

Barkow, Hans K.L., German anatomist, 1798–1873. SEE B.'s *ligaments,* under *ligament.*

Barlow, John, 20th century South African cardiologist. SEE B. *syndrome.*

Barlow, Sir Thomas, British physician, 1845–1945. SEE B.'s *disease.*

barn. A unit of area for effective cross-section of atomic nuclei with respect to atomic projectiles; equal to 10⁻²⁴ cm². [fr. "big as the side of a barn" by humorous comparison with much smaller areas]

Barnes, Robert, British obstetrician, 1817–1907. SEE B.'s *curve, zone.*

Barnes. Stanley, British physician, 1875–1955. SEE Barnes' *dystrophy.*

baro-. Weight, pressure. [G. *baros,* weight]

bar·o·cep·tor (bar'ō-sep-ter, -tōr). SYN baroreceptor.

bar·og·no·sis (bar'og-nō'sis). Ability to appreciate the weight of objects, or to differentiate objects of different weights. [G. *baros,* weight, + *gnōsis,* knowledge]

bar·o·graph (bar'ō-graf). A device that gives a continuous record of barometric pressure. SYN barometrograph.

bar·o·met·ro·graph (bar-ō-met'rō-graf). SYN barograph.

Baron. SEE Barclay-Baron *disease.*

bar·o·phil·ic (bar'ō-fil'ik). Thriving under high environmental pressure; applied to microorganisms. [G. *baros,* weight, + *phileō,* to love]

bar·o·re·cep·tor (bar'ō-rē-sep'ter, -tōr). 1. In general, any sensor of pressure changes. 2. Sensory nerve ending in the wall of the auricles of the heart, vena cava, aortic arch, and carotid sinus, sensitive to stretching of the wall resulting from increased pressure from within, and functioning as the receptor of central reflex mechanisms that tend to reduce that pressure. SYN baroceptor, pressoreceptor. [G. *baros,* weight, + receptor]

bar·o·re·flex (bar-ō-rē'fleks). A reflex triggered by stimulation of a baroreceptor.

bar·o·scope (bar'ō-skōp). An instrument measuring changes in atmospheric pressure.

bar·o·si·nus·i·tis (bar'ō-sī-nus-ī'tis). SYN aerosinusitis. [G. *baros,* weight, pressure, + sinusitis]

bar·o·stat (bar'ō-stat). A pressure-regulating device or structure, such as the baroreceptors of the carotid sinus and aortic arch, when connected to effectors providing negative feedback. [G., *baros,* weight, pressure, + *statos,* made to stand]

bar·o·tax·is (bar-ō-tak'sis). Reaction of living tissue to changes in pressure. SYN barotropism. [G. *baros,* weight, + *taxis,* order]

bar·o·ti·tis me·dia (bar-ō-tī'tis mē'dē-ă). SYN aerotitis media.

bar·o·trau·ma (băr'ō-traw'mă). A term once used to describe injury to the middle ear or paranasal sinuses, resulting from imbalance between ambient pressure and that within the affected cavity. Now mostly used to refer to lung injury that occurs when a patient is on a ventilator and is subjected to excessive airway pressure (pulmonary barotrauma). [G. *baros,* weight, + trauma]

otic b., injury caused to the ear by imbalance in pressure between ambient air and the air in the middle ear.

sinus b., injury to paranasal sinuses, resulting from imbalance in pressure between ambient air and air in the paranasal sinuses. SEE ALSO aerosinusitis.

bar·ot·ro·pism (bar-ot'rō-pizm). SYN barotaxis. [G. *baros,* weight, + *tropē,* a turning]

Barr, Murray L., Canadian microanatomist, *1908. SEE B. chromatin *body.*

Barr, Yvonne M., English virologist, *1932. SEE Epstein-B. *virus.*

Barraquer, HIgnacio, Spanish ophthalmologist, 1884–1965. SEE B.'s *method.*

Barraquer Roviralta, Luis, Spanish physician, 1855–1928. SEE Barraquer's *disease.*

Barré, Jean A., French neurologist, *1880. SEE B.'s *sign;* Guillain-B. *reflex, syndrome;* Landry-Guillain-B. *syndrome.*

bar·ren (bar'en). Unable to produce a pregnancy. [M.E. *bareyne*]

Barrett, Norman R., British physician, *1903. SEE *adenocarcinoma* in B.'s esophagus; B. *esophagus, epithelium, syndrome.*

bar·ri·er (bar'ē-er). **1.** An obstacle or impediment. **2.** In psychiatry, a conflictual agent that blocks behavior which could help resolve a personal struggle. [M.E., fr. O.Fr. *barriere,* fr. L.L. *barraria*]

blood-air b., the material intervening between alveolar air and the blood; it consists of a nonstructural film or surfactant, alveolar epithelium, basement lamina, and endothelium.

blood-aqueous b., a selectively permeable b. between the capillary bed in the processes of the ciliary body and the aqueous humor in the anterior chamber of the eye; consists of two layers of simple cuboidal epithelium joined at their apical surfaces with junctional complexes.

blood-brain b. (BBB), a selective mechanism opposing the passage of most ions and large-molecular weight compounds from the blood to brain tissue located in a continuous layer of endothelial cells connected by tight junctions; similar capillaries are found in the retina, iris, inner ear, and within the endoneurium of peripheral nerves.

blood-cerebrospinal fluid b., blood-CSF b., a b. located at the tight junctions which surround and connect the cuboidal epithelial cells on the surface of the choroid plexus; capillaries and connective tissue stroma of the choroid do not represent a b. to protein tracers or dyes.

incest b., in psychoanalysis, the learning or internalization of parental and social prohibitions against incest.

placental b., SYN placental *membrane.*

Bart, Bruce J., U.S. dermatologist, *1936. SEE B.'s *syndrome.*

Bart. Nickname of St. Bartholomew's Hospital in London, where *hemoglobin* Bart's was first isolated from a patient.

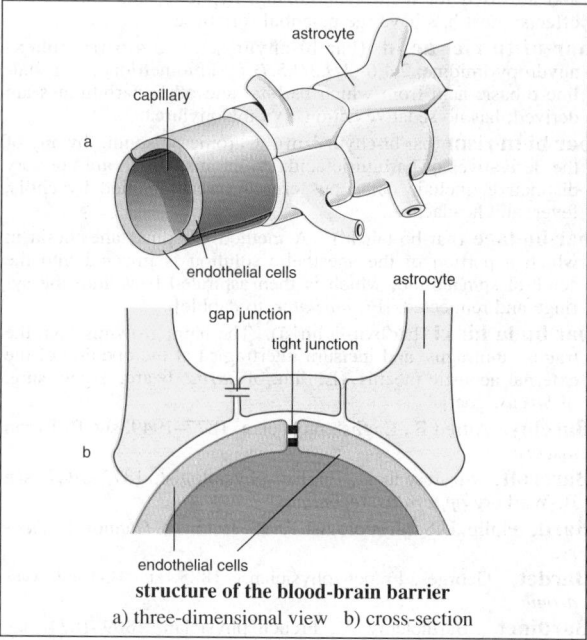

structure of the blood-brain barrier
a) three-dimensional view   b) cross-section

Bartels, Peter H., German scientist in U.S., specializing in optics and computer science, *1929.

Barth, Jean, Strasburg physician, 1806–1877. SEE B.'s *hernia.*

Bartholin, Casper, Danish anatomist, 1655–1738. SEE B.'s *abscess, cyst, cystectomy, duct, gland.*

Bartholin, Thomas, Danish anatomist, 1616–1680. SEE B.'s *anus.*

bar·tho·lin·i·tis (bar-tō-lin-ī'tis). Inflammation of a vulvovaginal (Bartholin's) gland.

Bartley, Samuel H., U.S. psychologist, *1901. SEE Brücke-B. *phenomenon.*

Barton, John Rhea, U.S. surgeon, 1794–1871. SEE B.'s *bandage, forceps, fracture.*

Bar·ton·el·la (bar-tō-nel'ă). A genus of bacteria (family Bartonellaceae) placed in the order Rickettsiales; these organisms multiply in fixed-tissue cells and in erythrocytes and reproduce by binary fission; they are found in man and in arthropod vectors. [A. L. *Barton*]

B. bacillifor'mis, a species found in the blood and epithelial cells of lymph nodes, spleen, and liver in Oroya fever (it is the cause of Oroya fever) and in blood and eruptive elements in verruga peruana; probably also found in sandflies (*Phlebotomus verrucarum*); known to be established only on the South American continent and perhaps in Central America; it is the type species of the genus *B.*

bar·ton·el·lo·sis (bar-tō-nel-ō'sis). A disease, endemic in certain valleys of the Andes in Peru, Chile, Ecuador, Bolivia, and Colombia, caused by *Bartonella bacilliformis* which is transmitted by the bite of the nocturnally biting sandfly, *Phlebotomus verrucarum;* occurs in three forms: 1) Oroya fever; 2) verruga peruana 3) a combination or sequence of these.

Bart's syn·drome. See under syndrome.

Bartter, Frederic C., U.S. physician, 1914–1983. SEE B.'s *syndrome.*

Baruch, Simon, U.S. physician, 1840–1921. SEE B.'s *law.*

bar·u·ria (bar-yū'rē-ă). Rarely used term for excretion of urine that has an unusually high specific gravity, *e.g.,* greater than 1.025 to 1.030. [G. *barys,* heavy, + *ouron,* urine]

△**bary-.** Heavy. [G. *barys*]

bar·ye (ba'rē). The CGS unit of pressure, equal to 1 dyne/cm² or 10^{-6} bar. SEE bar (1). [G. *barys,* heavy]

ba·ry·ta (ba-rī'tă). SYN *barium* oxide. [G. *barytēs,* weight]

⚲ **baryto-.** Prefix indicating the presence of barium in a mineral.

ba·sad (bā′sad). In a direction toward the base of any object or structure.

ba·sal (bā′săl). **1.** Situated nearer the base of a pyramid-shaped organ in relation to a specific reference point; opposite of apical. SYN basalis [NA]. **2.** In dentistry, denoting the floor of a cavity in the grinding surface of a tooth. **3.** Denoting a standard or reference state of a function, as a basis for comparison. More specifically, denoting the exact conditions for measurement of basal metabolic *rate* (*q.v.*); b. conditions do not always denote a minimum value, *e.g.*, metabolic rate in sleep is usually less than the b. rate, but is inconvenient for standard measurement.

ba·sal·i·o·ma (bā-sal-ē-ō′mă). Obsolete term for basal cell *carcinoma*.

ba·sa·lis (bā-sā′lis) [NA]. SYN basal (1). [L.]
  norma b. [NA], SYN external *base* of skull.

ba·sa·loid (bā′să-loyd). Resembling that which is basal, but not necessarily basal in origin or position.

ba·sa·lo·ma (bā-să-lō′mă). Obsolete term for basal cell *carcinoma*.

ba·sal ra·tion. Minimal diet containing only essential components.

Basan, Marianne, 20th century German physician. SEE Basan's *syndrome*.

Basan's syn·drome. See under syndrome.

base (bās). **1.** The lower part or bottom; the part of a pyramidal or cone-shaped structure opposite the apex; the foundation. SYN basis [NA], basement (1). **2.** In pharmacy, the chief ingredient of a mixture. **3.** In chemistry, an electropositive element (cation) that unites with an anion to form a salt; a compound ionizing to yield hydroxyl ion. SYN alkali (2). SEE ALSO Brønsted b., Lewis b. **4.** Nitrogen-containing organic compounds (*e.g.*, purines, pyrimidines, amines, alkaloids, ptomaines) that act as Brønsted b.'s. **5.** Cations, or substances forming cations. [L. and G. *basis*]

acrylic resin b., a form made of acrylic resin molded to conform to the tissues of the alveolar process and used to support the teeth of a prosthesis.

aldehyde base, obsolete term for an imide.

anterior cranial b., SYN anterior cranial *fossa*.

b. of arytenoid cartilage, the part of the arytenoid cartilage that articulates with the cricoid cartilage and from which the muscular process extends laterally and the vocal process projects anteriorly. SYN basis cartilaginis arytenoideae [NA].

b. of bladder, SYN *fundus* of urinary bladder.

b. of brain, the inferior surface of the brain visible when seen from below. SYN facies inferior cerebri [NA], basis cerebri, inferior cerebral surface.

Brønsted b., any molecule or ion that combines with a proton; *e.g.*, OH⁻, CN⁻, NH₃; this definition replaces the older and more limited concepts of base (3).

cavity preparation b., SYN cement b.

cement b., in dentistry, a layer of dental cement, sometimes medicated, that is placed in the deep portion of a cavity preparation to protect the pulp, reduce the bulk of a metallic restoration, or eliminate undercuts. SYN cavity preparation b.

b. of cochlea, the enlarged part of the cochlea that is directed posteriorly and medially and lies close to the internal acoustic meatus. SYN basis cochleae [NA].

cranial b., SYN b. of skull.

denture b., (**1**) that part of a denture which rests on the oral mucosa and to which teeth are attached; (**2**) that part of a complete or partial denture which rests upon the basal seat and to which teeth are attached. SYN saddle (2).

external b. of skull, external aspect of the b. of skull SYN norma basilaris [NA], basis cranii externa✶ [NA], norma inferior, norma ventralis.

b. of heart, that part of the heart that lies opposite the apex, formed mainly by the left atrium but to a small extent by the posterior part of the right atrium; it is directed backward and to the right and is separated from the vertebral column by the esophagus and aorta. SYN basis cordis [NA].

hexone b.'s, histone b.'s, the α-amino acids arginine, histidine, and lysine, which are basic by virtue of the presence in the side chains of a guanidine, imidazole, and amine group, respectively; the term "hexone" is a misnomer since histidine does not have six carbons.

b. of hyoid bone, SYN *body* of hyoid bone.

internal b. of skull, the interior aspect of the skull b. on which the brain rests; the floor of the cranial cavity. SEE ALSO b. of skull. SYN basis cranii interna [NA].

Lewis b., a b. that is an electron-pair donor.

b. of lung, the lower concave part of the lung that rests upon the convexity of the diaphragm. SYN basis pulmonis [NA].

b. of mandible, the rounded inferior border of the body of the mandible. SYN basis mandibulae [NA].

b. of metacarpal bone, the expanded proximal extremity of each metacarpal that articulates with one or more of the distal row of carpal bones. SYN basis ossis metacarpalis [NA].

metal b., a metallic portion of a denture b. forming a part of the wall of the basal surface of the denture; it serves as a b. for the attachment of the plastic (resin) part of the denture and the teeth.

b. of metatarsal bone, the expanded proximal extremity of each metatarsal bone; it articulates with one or more of the distal row of tarsal bones. SYN basis ossis metatarsalis [NA].

methamphetamine b., a form of methamphetamine that can be readily volatilized.

b. of modiolus, the part of the modiolus enclosed by the basal turn of the cochlea; it faces the lateral end of the internal acoustic meatus. SEE cochlear *area*. SYN basis modioli [NA].

nucleic acid b., a purine or pyrimidine; found in naturally occurring nucleic acids such as DNA.

nucleinic b., obsolete term for purine.

ointment b., the vehicle into which active ingredients may be incorporated. Petrolatum (which may be stiffened with wax) is the most widely used greasy ointment b. and is suitable for the incorporation of oleaginous materials. lin-containing b.'s will absorb water (and dissolved materials) and form water-in-oil type emulsions. Water soluble (washable) b.'s are often derived from polymers of ethylene glycol (PEGS); these will absorb water and ingredients dissolved in the water. Ointment b.'s are usually pharmacologically inert but may entrap water and serve to keep the skin from dying or to provide an emollient protective film.

b. of patella, the superior border of the patella to which the tendon of the rectus femoris attaches. SYN basis patellae [NA].

b. of phalanx, the expanded proximal end of each phalanx in the hand or foot that articulates with the head of the next proximal bone in the digit. SYN basis phalangis [NA].

pressor b., (**1**) one of several products of intestinal putrefaction believed to cause functional hypertension when absorbed; (**2**) any alkaline substance that raises blood pressure. SYN pressor amine, pressor substance.

b. of prostate, the broad upper surface of the prostate contiguous with the bladder wall. SYN basis prostatae [NA].

purine b., a purine.

pyrimidine b., a pyrimidine.

record b., SYN baseplate.

b. of renal pyramid, the outer broad part of a renal pyramid that lies next to the cortex. SYN basis pyramidis renis [NA].

b. of sacrum, the upper end of the sacrum that articulates with the body of the fifth lumbar vertebra in the midline and the alae on either side. SYN basis ossis sacri [NA].

Schiff b., R–CH=N–R′; condensation products of aldehydes and ketones with primary amine; the compounds are stable if there is at least one aryl group on the nitrogen or carbon. Cf. ketimine. SYN aldimine.

shellac b., a resinous wafer adapted to maxillary or mandibular casts to form baseplates.

b. of skull, the sloping floor of the cranial cavity. It comprises both the external b. of skull (external view) and the internal b. of skull (internal view). SEE ALSO internal b. of skull. SYN basis cranii, cranial b.

b. of stapes, the flat portion of the stapes that fits in the oval window. SYN basis stapedis [NA], footplate (1), foot-plate.

temporary b., SYN baseplate.

tinted denture b., a denture b. that simulates the coloring and shading of natural oral tissues.

b. of tongue, SYN *root* of tongue.

tooth-borne b., the denture b. restoring an edentulous area which has abutment teeth at each end for support; the tissue which it covers is not used for support.

trial b., SYN baseplate.

vegetable b., SYN alkaloid.

wobble b., the 3′ codon b. that is less strictly specified in the genetic code. SEE ALSO wobble, wobble *hypothesis*.

bas·e·doid (bahz′ĕ-doyd). Rarely used term denoting a condition resembling Graves' disease (Basedow's disease), but without toxic symptoms.

Basedow, Karl A. von, German physician, 1799–1854. SEE B.'s *disease, pseudoparaplegia;* Jod-B. *phenomenon;* B.'s *goiter.*

ba·se·dow·i·an (bahz′ĕ-dō′ē-an). Rarely used to denote terms described by or attributed to K. Basedow.

base·ment (bās′ment). **1.** SYN base (1). **2.** A cavity or space partly or completely separated from a larger space above it.

base·plate (bās′plāt). A temporary form representing the base of a denture; used for making maxillomandibular (jaw) relation records and for the arrangement of teeth. SYN record base, temporary base, trial base.

stabilized b., a b. lined with plastic material to improve its fit and stability.

base-stack·ing. A clustering of DNA or RNA bases in which the rings lie on top of each other.

bas-fond (bah-fawn′). SYN *fundus* of urinary bladder.

Basham's mix·ture. SYN ferric and ammonium acetate *solution.*

△**basi-, basio-, baso-.** Base; basis. [G. and L. *basis*]

ba·si·a·lis (bā-sē-ā′lis). Relating to a basis or the basion.

ba·si·al·ve·o·lar (bā′sē-al-vē′ō-lăr). Relating to both basion and alveolar points; denoting especially the b. length, or the shortest distance between these two points.

ba·sic (bā′sik). Relating to a base.

ba·sic·i·ty (bā-sis′i-tē). **1.** The valence or combining power of an acid, or the number of replaceable atoms of hydrogen in its molecule. **2.** The characteristic(s) of being a chemical base.

ba·sic life sup·port. Emergency cardiopulmonary resuscitation, control of bleeding, treatment of shock, acidosis, and poisoning, stabilization of injuries and wounds, and basic first aid.

ba·si·cra·ni·al (bā′si-krā′nē-ăl). Relating to the base of the skull.

Ba·sid·i·ob·o·lus (ba-sid′ē-ō-bō′lŭs). A genus of fungi belonging to the class Zygomycetes. *B. haptosporus* has been isolated from cases of zygomycosis (entomophthoramycosis basidiobolae) in humans, especially in Indonesia, tropical Africa, and Southeast Asia. [Mod. L. *basidium,* dim. of G. *basis,* base, + L. *bolus,* fr. G. *bolos,* lump or clod]

Ba·sid·i·o·my·ce·tes (ba-sid′ē-ō-mī-sēt′ez). One of the four major classes of fungi, characterized by a spore-bearing organ (basidium), usually a single clavate cell, which bears basidiospores after karyogamy and meiosis. The class comprises the smuts, rusts, mushrooms, and puffballs. Excluding mycotoxins, there is only one human pathogen, the basidiomycetous stage of *Cryptococcus neoformans.* [Mod. L. *basidium,* dim. of G. *basis,* base, + *mykēs* (*mykēt*), fungus]

Ba·sid·i·o·my·co·ta (bă-sid′ē-ō-mī-kō-tă). A phylum of fungi characterized by a spore-bearing organ, the basidium, that is usually a clavate cell that bears basidiospores after karyogamy and meiosis. Some mycologists have raised the class Basidiomycetes to the phylum or division level.

ba·sid·i·o·spore (ba-sid′ē-ō-spōr). A fungal spore borne on a basidium, characteristic of the class Basidiomycetes. [G. *basidon,* small base, + *sporos,* seed]

ba·sid·i·um, pl. **ba·sid·ia** (ba-sid′ē-ŭm, -ă). A cell or spore-bearing organ usually club-shaped that is characteristic of the Basidiomycota. It bears basidiospores externally after karyogamy and meiosis. It is composed of a swollen terminal cell situated on a slender stalk, and gives rise to slender filaments (sterig-

mata), usually four in number, from the ends of which the basidiospores are developed. [L., fr G. *basis,* base]

ba·si·fa·cial (bā′si-fā′shăl). Relating to the lower portion of the face.

ba·si·hy·al (bā′si-hī′ăl). SYN *body* of hyoid bone.

ba·si·hy·oid (bā-zē-hī′oyd). SYN *body* of hyoid bone.

bas·i·lar, bas·i·la·ris (bas′i-lăr, bas-i-lā′ris). Relating to the base of a pyramidal or broad structure.

ba·si·lat·er·al (bā′si-lat′er-ăl). Relating to the base and one or more sides of any part.

ba·si·lem·ma (bā-si-lem′ă). SYN basement *membrane.* [basi- + G. *lemma,* rind]

ba·sil·i·cus (ba-sil′i-kŭs). Denoting a prominent or important part or structure. [L. fr. G. *basilikos,* royal]

ba·sin (bā′sin). A receptacle for fluids.

emesis b., kidney b., a shallow b. of curved, kidney-shaped design, used to collect body fluids or as a container for various other liquids.

pus b., a receptacle curved so as to fit closely the surface to which it is applied, used to receive the pus from a wound during its cleansing and redressing.

ba·si·na·sal (bā′si-nā′săl). Relating to the basion and the nasion; denoting especially the b. length, or the shortest distance between the two points.

△**basio-.** SEE basi-.

ba·si·oc·cip·i·tal (bā′sē-ok-sip′i-tăl). Relating to the basilar process of the occipital bone.

ba·si·oc·ci·put (bā-zē-ok′sē-put). SYN basilar *part* of the occipital bone.

ba·si·o·glos·sus (bā-sē-ō-glos′ŭs). The portion of the hyoglossus muscle that originates from the body of the hyoid bone.

ba·si·on (bā′sē-on) [NA]. The middle point on the anterior margin of the foramen magnum, opposite the opisthion. [G. *basis,* a base]

ba·sip·e·tal (ba-sip′ĕ-tăl). **1.** In a direction toward the base. **2.** Pertaining to asexual conidial production in fungi, in which successive budding of the basal conidium forms in an unbranched chain with the youngest at the base. [basi- + L. *peto,* to seek]

bas·i·pho·bia (bās-i-fō′bē-ă). Morbid fear of walking. [G. *basis,* a stepping, + *phobos,* fear]

ba·sis (bā′sis) [NA]. SYN base (1). [L. and G.]

b. cartilag′inis arytenoi′deae [NA], SYN *base* of arytenoid cartilage.

b. cer′ebri, SYN *base* of brain.

b. coch′leae [NA], SYN *base* of cochlea.

b. cor′dis [NA], SYN *base* of heart.

b. cra′nii, SYN *base* of skull.

b. cra′nii exter′na [NA], ✲official alternate term for external *base* of skull.

b. cra′nii inter′na [NA], SYN internal *base* of skull.

b. mandib′ulae [NA], SYN *base* of mandible.

b. modi′oli [NA], SYN *base* of modiolus.

b. os′sis metacarpa′lis [NA], SYN *base* of metacarpal bone.

b. os′sis metatarsa′lis [NA], SYN *base* of metatarsal bone.

b. os′sis sa′cri [NA], SYN *base* of sacrum.

b. patel′lae [NA], SYN *base* of patella.

b. pedun′culi, the base of the midbrain consisting of the crus cerebri and substantia nigra. SEE ALSO cerebral *peduncle.*

b. phalan′gis [NA], SYN *base* of phalanx.

b. pro′statae [NA], SYN *base* of prostate.

b. pulmo′nis [NA], SYN *base* of lung.

b. pyram′idis re′nis [NA], SYN *base* of renal pyramid.

b. stape′dis [NA], SYN *base* of stapes.

ba·si·sphe·noid (bā′si-sfē′noyd). Relating to the base or body of the sphenoid bone; denoting the independent center of ossification in the embryo that forms the posterior portion of the body of the sphenoid bone.

ba·si·tem·po·ral (bā′si-tem′pŏ-răl). Relating to the lower part of the temporal region.

ba·si·ver·te·bral (bā'si-ver'tĕ-brăl). Relating to the body of a vertebra.

bas·ket. 1. A basket-like arborization of the axon of cells in the cerebellar cortex, surrounding the cell body of Purkinje cells. **2.** Any basket-like device or structure. [M.E., from Celtic]

fibrillar b.'s, the scleral end of neuroglia fibers of Müller that as fine, tapering, needlelike fibrillae ascend the proximal parts of rods and cones, giving them a fibrillar appearance.

stone b., an instrument passed through an endoscope to capture and extract urinary calculi.

Basle Nom·i·na An·a·tom·i·ca (BNA). The name adopted in 1895 in Basel, Switzerland (French spelling, Basle) by members of the German Anatomical Society which met to compile a Latin nomenclature of anatomical terms. Revisions of the resulting nomenclature were published at intervals until, in 1955 in Paris, France, the international membership of the Congress of Anatomists adopted a modification of the Basle Nomina Anatomica terminology. That modification dropped the reference to the original meeting place. SEE Nomina Anatomica.

baso-. SEE basi-.

ba·so·cyte (bā'sō-sīt). SYN basophilic *leukocyte*. [G. *basis,* base, + *kytos,* cell]

ba·so·cy·to·pe·nia (bā'sō-sī-tō-pē'nē-ă). SYN basophilic *leukopenia.*

ba·so·cy·to·sis (bā'sō-sī-to'sis). SYN basophilic *leukocytosis.*

ba·so·e·ryth·ro·cyte (bā'sō-e-rith'rō-sīt). A red blood cell that manifests changes of basophilic degeneration, such as basophilic stippling, punctate basophilia, or basophilic granules.

ba·so·e·ryth·ro·cy·to·sis (bā'sō-ĕ-rith'rō-sī-tō'sis). An increase of red blood cells with basophilic degenerative changes, frequently observed in diseases characterized by prolonged hypochromic anemia.

ba·so·graph (bā'sō-graf). An instrument that makes graphic records of abnormalities of gait. [baso- + G. *graphō,* to write]

ba·so·lat·er·al (bā-sō-lat'er-ăl). Basal and lateral; specifically used to refer to one of the two major cytological divisions of the amygdaloid complex. SEE amygdaloid *body.*

ba·so·met·a·chro·mo·phil, ba·so·met·a·chro·mo·phile (bā'sō-met-ă-krō'mō-fil, -fīl). Staining metachromatically with a basic dye. SEE metachromasia.

ba·so·pe·nia (bā-sō-pē'nē-ă). SYN basophilic *leukopenia.* [baso- + G. *penia,* poverty]

ba·so·phil, ba·so·phile (bā'sō-fil, -fīl). **1.** A cell with granules that stain specifically with basic dyes. **2.** SYN basophilic. **3.** A phagocytic leukocyte of the blood characterized by numerous basophilic granules containing heparin and histamine; except for its segmented nucleus, it is morphologically and physiologically similar to the mast cell though they originate from different stem cells in the bone marrow. [baso- + G. *phileō,* to love]

tissue b., SYN mast *cell.*

ba·so·phil·ia (bā-sō-fil'ē-ă). **1.** A condition in which there is more than the usual number of basophilic leukocytes in the circulating blood (basophilic leukocytosis) or an increase in the proportion of parenchymatous basophilic cells in an organ (in the bone marrow, basophilic hyperplasia). **2.** A condition in which basophilic erythrocytes are found in circulating blood, as in certain instances of leukemia, advanced anemia, malaria, and plumbism. SYN Grawitz' b. SYN basophilism.

Grawitz' b., SYN basophilia (2).

punctate b., SYN stippling (1).

ba·so·phil·ic (bā'sō-fil'ik). Denoting tissue components having an affinity for basic dyes under specific pH conditions. SYN basophil (2), basophile.

ba·soph·i·lism (bā-sof'i-lizm). SYN basophilia.

Cushing's b., pituitary b., SYN Cushing's *syndrome.*

Cushing's pituitary b., SYN Cushing's *disease.*

ba·so·phil·o·cyte (bā-sō-fil'ō-sīt). SYN basophilic *leukocyte.*

ba·so·plasm (bā'sō-plazm). That part of the cytoplasm that stains readily with basic dyes.

Bassen, Frank A., U.S. physician, *1903. SEE B.-Kornzweig *syndrome.*

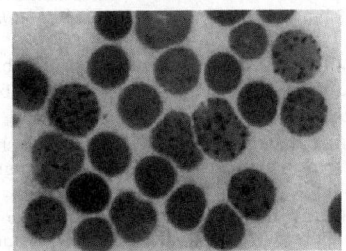

punctate basophilia (in chronic lead poisoning)

Bassini, Edoardo, Italian surgeon, 1844–1924. SEE B.'s *operation.*

Bassler, Anthony, U.S. physician, 1874–1959. SEE B.'s *sign.*

bas·sor·in (bas'ŏr-in). The insoluble portion (60 to 70%) of tragacanth that swells to form a gel; it contains complex methoxylated acids, particularly bassoric acid.

Bastedo, Walter A., U.S. physician, 1873–1952. SEE B.'s *sign.*

bat. A member of the mammalian order Chiroptera. [M.E. *bakke*]

vampire b., a member of the genus *Desmodus;* an important reservoir host of rabies virus in Central and South America.

bath. 1. Immersion of the body or any of its parts in water or any other yielding or fluid medium, or application of such medium in any form to the body or any of its parts. **2.** Apparatus used in giving a b. of any form, qualified according to the medium used, the temperature of the medium, the form in which the medium is applied, the medicament added to the medium, or according to the part bathed. **3.** Fluid used for maintenance of metabolic activities or growth of living organisms, *e.g.,* cells derived from body tissue. [A.S. *baeth*]

colloid b., prepared by adding soothing agents such as sodium bicarbonate or oatmeal to the b. water to relieve skin irritation and pruritus.

contrast b., a b. in which a part is immersed in hot water for a period of a few minutes and then in cold, the hot and cold periods alternated regularly at intervals, usually half-hours; used to increase the blood flow to the part.

douche b., the local application of water in the form of a large jet or stream.

dousing b., a luminous electric hot air b. given at a very high temperature.

electric b., electrotherapeutic b., (1) a b. in which the medium is charged with electricity; SYN hydroelectric b. **(2)** therapeutic application of static electricity, with the patient placed on an insulated platform.

Greville b., an obsolete treatment with nonluminous electric hot air given at a very high temperature.

hafussi b., a modification of the Nauheim treatment, with only the hands and feet of the patient being immersed in hot water through which carbon dioxide gas is made to pass. [Ger. *hand,* hand, + *fuss,* foot]

hydroelectric b., SYN electric b. (1).

immersion b., a therapeutic b. in which the whole person or a body part is totally immersed in the therapeutic substance.

light b., therapeutic exposure of the skin to radiant light.

Nauheim b., SYN Nauheim *treatment.*

needle b., a b. in which water is projected forcibly against the body in many very fine jets.

oil b., in chemistry, a vessel containing oil, in which a container holding a substance to be heated or evaporated can be immersed.

sand b., in chemistry, an arrangement whereby a substance to be treated is in a vessel protected from the direct action of fire by a layer of sand.

sitz b., immersion of only the perineum and buttocks, with the legs being outside of the tub. [Ger. *sitzen,* to sit]

water b., in chemistry, a vessel containing water, in which a container holding a substance to be heated or evaporated can be immersed.

ba

bath·mo·tro·pic (bath-mō-trō'pik). Influencing nervous and muscular irritability in response to stimuli. [G. *bathmos*, threshold, + *tropē*, a turning]

negatively b., lessening nervous or muscular irritability.

positively b., increasing nervous or muscular irritability.

⚠**batho-.** Depth. SEE ALSO bathy-. [G. *bathos*, depth]

bath·o·chro·mic (bath-ō-krō'mik). Denoting the shift of an absorption spectrum maximum to a longer wavelength. [batho- + G. *chrōma*, color]

bath·o·flore (bath'ō-flōr). An atom or group of atoms that, by its presence in a molecule, shifts the latter's fluorescent radiation in the direction of longer wavelength, or reduces the fluorescence. Cf. auxoflore.

bath·o·pho·bia (bath-ō-fō'bē-ă). Morbid fear of deep places or of looking into them. [G. *bathos*, depth, + *phobos*, fear]

⚠**bathy-.** Depth. SEE ALSO batho-. [G. *bathys*, deep]

bath·y·an·es·the·sia (bath'ē-an-es-thē'zē-ă). Loss of deep sensibility, *i.e.*, from muscles, ligaments, tendons, bones, and joints. [G. *bathys*, deep, + *an-* priv. + *aisthēsis*, sensation]

bath·y·car·dia (bath-ē-kar'dē-ă). A condition in which the heart occupies a lower position than normal but is fixed there, as distinguished from cardioptosia. [G. *bathys*, deep, + *kardia*, heart]

bath·y·es·the·sia (bath'ē-es-thē'zē-ă). General term for all sensation from the tissues beneath the skin, *i.e.*, muscles, ligaments, tendons, bones and joints. SEE ALSO myesthesia. SYN deep sensibility. [G. *bathys*, deep, + *aisthēsis*, sensation]

bath·y·gas·try (bath-ē-gas'trē). SYN gastroptosis. [G. *bathys*, deep, + *gastēr*, stomach]

bath·y·hy·per·es·the·sia (bath-ē-hī'per-es-thē'zē-ă). Exaggerated sensitiveness deep structures, *e.g.*, muscular tissue. [G. *bathys*, deep, + *hyper*, above, + *aisthēsis*, sensation]

bath·y·hyp·es·the·sia (bath-ē-hip'es-thē'zē-ă). Impairment of sensation in the structures beneath the skin, *e.g.*, muscle tissue. [G. *bathys*, deep, + *hypo*, under, + *aisthēsis*, sensation]

ba·trach·o·tox·in (ba-tra-kō-tok'sin). A neurotoxin from the Colombian arrow poison frog (*Phyllobates* sp.). It is nontoxic when ingested. If it is injected or if there are ulcers present, it will cause an irreversible increase in permeability of sodium ions in nerve membrane; produces paralysis; used in experimental pharmacological studies of neuromuscular transmission. [G. *batrachos*, frog, + toxin]

Batson, Oscar V., U.S. otolaryngologist, 1894–1979. SEE B.'s *plexus;* Carmody-B. *operation.*

Batten, Frederick E., British ophthalmologist, 1865–1918. SEE B.-Mayou *disease;* B. *disease.*

bat·tery (bat'er-ē). A group or series of tests administered for analytic or diagnostic purposes. [M.E. *batri*, beaten metal, fr. O.Fr. *batre*, to beat]

Halstead-Reitan b., a b. of neuropsychological tests (category test, tactual performance test, Seashore test, speech sounds perception test, finger oscillation test, trail-making test, dynamometer to measure strength of grip) used to study brain-behavior functions including determining the effects of brain damage on behavior. SYN Tactual Performance Test.

Battle, William H., English surgeon, 1855–1936. SEE B.'s *sign.*

Baudelocque, Jean L., French obstetrician, 1746–1810. SEE B.'s *diameter*, uterine *circle.*

Baudelocque, Louis A., French obstetrician, 1800–1864. SEE B.'s *operation.*

Bauer, Hans, 20th century German anatomist. SEE B.'s chromic acid leucofuchsin *stain.*

Bauer, Walter, U.S. internist, *1898. SEE B.'s *syndrome.*

Bauhin, Gaspard, Swiss anatomist, 1560–1624. SEE B.'s *gland, valve.*

Baumé, Antoine, French chemist and pharmacist, 1728–1805. SEE B. *scale.*

Baumès symp·tom. See under symptom.

Baumgarten, P. Clemens von, German pathologist, 1848–1928. SEE B.'s *veins*, under *vein;* Cruveilhier-B. *disease, murmur, sign, syndrome.*

bay (bā). **1.** In anatomy, a recess containing fluid. **2.** Especially, the lacrimal b.

celomic b., (1) medial and lateral recesses at either side of the urogenital mesentery of the embryo; **(2)** superior recess of the vestibule of the lesser peritoneal space; with the formation of the diaphragm, a portion of the right recess is cut off and becomes the infracardiac bursa; the portion below the diaphragm becomes the superior recess of the lesser peritoneal sac; the left recess is lost. SYN pneumatoenteric.

lacrimal b., SYN lacrimal *lake.*

bay·ber·ry bark (bā'ber-ē). SYN myrica.

Bayes, Thomas, British mathematician, 1702–1761. SEE B. *theorem.*

Bayle, Antoine L.J., French physician, 1799-1858. SEE B.'s *disease.*

Bayley, Nancy, U.S. psychologist, *1899. SEE B. *Scales* of Infant Development, under *scale.*

bay·lis·as·car·i·a·sis (bā-lē-sas'kar-ī-a-sis). The disease caused by nematode parasites of the genus *Baylisascaris;* migrating larvae of the raccoon parasite *B. procyonis* can cause a severe disease of the central nervous system in a variety of wild and domestic animal species and, rarely, in human beings; human disease has been manifested as either a fatal eosinophilic meningoencephalitis or a diffuse unilateral subacute neuroretinitis.

Bay·lis·as·ca·ris (Bāy-lis-as'kă-ris). A genus of ascarid nematodes found in the intestine of mammals.

B. procyonis, a large roundworm commonly found in raccoons; has been the cause of human visceral larva migrans and ocular larva migrans, following accidental ingestion of embryonated *B. procyonis* eggs in feces of infected raccoons. Central nervous system tissue following systemic migration by larvae of B. is thought to be due to cytotoxic eosinophil ungranule proteins released by the migration of these larvae. Can cause severe disease in a variety of wild and domestic animal species and in human beings. SEE ALSO visceral *larva migrans.*

bay·o·net (bā-ŏ-net'). An instrument having a blade or nib that is offset and parallel to the shaft. [Fr. *bayonette*, fr. *Bayonne*, France, where first made]

Bazett, Henry, English cardiologist, *1885. SEE Bazett's *formula.*

Bazett's for·mu·la. See under formula.

Bazex, A., 20th century French physician. SEE Bazex's *syndrome.*

Bazex's syn·drome. See under syndrome.

Bazin, Antoine P.E., French dermatologist, 1807–1878. SEE B.'s *disease.*

BBB Abbreviation for blood-brain *barrier.*

BBC. Abbreviation for bromobenzylcyanide.

BBOT Abbreviation for 2,5-bis(5-*t*-butylbenzoxazol-2-yl)thiophene, a liquid scintillator.

BCG Abbreviation for Bacille bilié de Calmette-Guérin; ballistocardiograph.

BCNU SYN carmustine.

bdel·lin (del'in). One of a group of protease inhibitors from the leech. [G. *bdella*, leech, + -in]

B.D.S. Abbreviation for Bachelor of Dental Surgery.

B.D.Sc. Abbreviation for Bachelor of Dental Science.

Be Symbol for beryllium.

bead·ed (bēd'ed). **1.** Marked by numerous small rounded projections, often arranged in a row like a string of beads. **2.** Applied to a series of noncontinuous bacterial colonies along the line of inoculation in a stab culture. **3.** Denoting stained bacteria in which more deeply stained granules occur at regular intervals in the organism.

bead·ing (bē'ding). **1.** Numerous small rounded projections, often in a row like a string of beads. **2.** The rounded elevation along the border of the tissue surface of the major connectors of a maxillary dental prosthesis. **3.** Protection of the formed borders of final impressions for a dental prosthesis done by placement of wax sticks or a plaster-pumice combination adjacent to the borders prior to forming the master cast.

b. of the ribs, SYN rachitic *rosary.*

beak (bēk). **1.** The nose of pliers used in dentistry for contouring and adjusting wrought or cast metal dental appliances. **2.** Sometimes used to describe a beak-shaped anatomical structure. SEE rostrum. [L. *beccus*]

beak·er (bē′ker). A thin glass vessel, with a lip (beak) for pouring, used as containers for liquids.

Beale, Lionel S., British physician, 1828–1906. SEE B.'s *cell.*

beam (bēm). **1.** Any bar whose curvature changes under load; in dentistry, frequently used instead of "bar." **2.** A collimated emission of light or other radiation, such as an x-ray b. [O.H.G. *Boum*]

Balkan b., SYN Balkan *frame.*

cantilever b., in dentistry, a b. that is supported by only one fixed support at only one of its ends.

continuous b., in dentistry, a b. that continues over three or more supports, those supports not at the b. ends being equally free supports.

electron b., a form of radiation used principally in superficial radiotherapy. SEE betatron.

restrained b., in dentistry, a b. that has two or more supports, at least one of which permits some freedom of rotation to the point of support but not as much as if the support were a free support.

simple b., in dentistry, a straight b. that has only two supports, one at either end.

bean (bēn). The flattened seed, contained in a pod, of various leguminous plants. B.'s of pharmacological significance are alphabetized by specific name. [O.E. *bean*]

bear·ing (bār′ing). A supporting point or surface.

central b., in dentistry, application of forces between the maxillae and mandible at a single point located as near as possible to the center of the supporting areas of the upper and lower jaws; used for the purpose of distributing closing forces evenly throughout the areas of the supporting structures during the recording of maxillomandibular (jaw) relations and during the correction of occlusal errors.

bear·ing down. Expulsive effort of a parturient woman in the second stage of labor.

beat (bēt). **1.** To strike; to throb or pulsate. **2.** A stroke, impulse, or pulsation, as of the heart or pulse. **3.** Activity of a cardiac chamber produced by catching a stimulus generated elsewhere in the heart. [A.S. *beatan*]

apex b., the visible and/or palpable pulsation made by the apex of the left ventricle as it strikes the chest wall in systole; normally in the fifth intercostal space, about 10 cm to the left of the median line.

atrial capture b., the cardiac cycle resulting when, after a period of A-V dissociation, the atria regain control of the ventricles; atrial depolarization due to retrograde transmission from a ventricular ectopic beat or an electronically paced ventricular impulse.

atrial fusion b., a b. that occurs when the atria are activated in part by the sinus impulse and in part by an ectopic or retrograde impulse from A-V junction or ventricle.

automatic b., in contrast to forced b., an ectopic b. that arises *de novo* and is not precipitated by the preceding b.; thus escaped and parasystolic b.'s are automatic. SYN automatic contraction.

combination b., SYN fusion b.

coupled b.'s, beats (usually premature) that recur at a fixed interval from a preceding (usually normal) beat.

dependent b., SYN forced b.

Dressler b., fusion b. interrupting a ventricular tachycardia and producing a normally narrow QRS complex as a result of the fusion of two impulses, one impulse from the ventricular tachycardia and the other from a supraventricular focus; Dressler b.'s strongly support the diagnosis of ventricular tachycardia by interruption of it.

dropped b., a heart b. that fails to appear.

echo b., extrasystole produced by the return of an impulse in the heart retrograde to a focus near its origin which then returns antegradely to produce a second depolarization.

ectopic b., a cardiac b. originating elsewhere than at the sinoatrial node.

escape b., escaped b., an automatic b., usually arising from the A-V junction or ventricle, occurring after the next expected normal b. has defaulted; it is therefore always a late b., terminating a longer cycle than the normal. SYN escape contraction.

forced b., (1) an extrasystole supposedly precipitated in some way by the preceding normal b. to which it is coupled; **(2)** an extrasystole caused by artificial stimulation of the heart. SYN dependent b.

fusion b., a b. triggered by more than a single electrical impulse, when the wave fronts coincide to act together on a single final pathway of activity; in the electrocardiogram, the atrial or ventricular complex when either atria or ventricles are activated jointly by two simultaneous or nearly simultaneous invading impulses. SYN combination b., mixed b., summation b.

heart b., a complete cardiac cycle, including spread of the electrical impulse and the consequent mechanical contraction. SYN ictus cordis.

interference b., ventricular capture in forms of A-V dissociation due to interference.

mixed b., SYN fusion b.

paired b.'s, SEE bigeminy.

parasystolic b., SYN parasystole.

premature b., SYN extrasystole.

pseudofusion b., an electrocardiographic representation of a cardiac depolarization produced by superimposition of an ineffectual electronic pacemaker spike upon a QRS-complex originating from a spontaneous focus within the heart; the pacemaker spike is ineffectual because the electronic discharge, which it represents graphically, occurred within the absolute refractory period of the spontaneous beat and is therefore not indicative of pacemaker malfunction.

reciprocal b., SEE reciprocal *rhythm.*

retrograde b., a b. occurring as an electrical activation of a portion of a heart chamber cephalad to the chamber of origin, *e.g.,* an atrial b. triggered by an impulse originating in the ventricle.

summation b., SYN fusion b.

ventricular fusion b., a fusion b. that occurs when the ventricles are activated partly by the descending sinus or A-V junctional impulse and partly by an ectopic ventricular impulse.

Beau, Joseph H.S., French physician, 1806–1865. SEE B.'s *lines,* under *line.*

Beau·var·ia (bō-vā′rē-ă). A genus of fungi (class Hyphomycetes). *B. bassiana* is pathogenic for insects, holds promise in the biologic control of insects, and has produced hyalohyphomycosis in humans.

be·can·thone hy·dro·chlo·ride (be-can′thŏn). 1-{[2- [Ethyl(2-hydroxy-2-methylpropyl)amino]ethyl]amino}- 4-methylthioxanthen-9-one; a schistosomicide.

Bechterew, Vladimir M. von, Russian neurologist, 1857–1927. SEE B.'s *band, disease; layer* of B.; B.'s *nucleus, sign; line* of B.; *band* of Kaes-B.; B.-Mendel *reflex;* Mendel-B. *reflex.*

Beck, Claude S., U.S. surgeon, 1894–1971. SEE B.'s *triad.*

Beck, Emil G., U.S. surgeon, 1866–1932. SEE B.'s *method.*

Beck, E.V.V., Russian physician. SEE Bek.

Becker, J.P. SEE B.'s *disease.*

Becker, Peter Emil, German geneticist, *1908. SEE B. type tardive muscular *dystrophy,* type muscular *dystrophy.*

Becker, Samuel W., U.S. dermatologist, 1894–1964. SEE B.'s *nevus.*

Becker's stain for spi·ro·chetes. See under stain.

Beckmann, Ernst O., German chemist, 1853–1923. SEE B.'s *apparatus.*

Beckwith, John Bruce, U.S. pathologist, *1933. SEE B.-Wiedemann *syndrome.*

Béclard, Pierre A., French anatomist, 1785–1825. SEE B.'s *anastomosis, hernia, triangle.*

be·clo·meth·a·sone di·pro·pi·o·nate (be-klō-meth′ă-sōn). Dipropionate salt of 9-chloro-11β,17,21-trihydroxy-16β-methylpregna-1,4-diene-3,20-dione; a topical anti-inflammatory agent; often used by inhalation in asthma.

Becquerel, Antoine H., French physicist and Nobel laureate, 1852–1908. SEE becquerel; B. *rays*, under *ray*.

bec·que·rel (Bq) (bek′rel). The SI unit of measurement of radioactivity, equal to 1 disintegration per second; 1 Bq = 0.027 × 10⁻⁹ Ci. SEE ALSO absorption. [A.H. *Becquerel*]

bed. 1. In anatomy, a base or structure that supports another structure. **2.** A piece of furniture used for rest, recuperation, or treatment.

b. of breast, structures against which the posterior surface of the breast lies; includes mainly the pectoralis major muscle, but also some serratus anterior and external abdominal oblique muscle; extends from second to sixth rib, and from parasternal to anterior axillary lines.

capillary b., the capillaries considered collectively and their volume capacity for blood.

fracture b., a narrow, extra-firm b. for treatment of fractures; usually incorporates an overhead frame for traction apparatus.

Gatch b., a b. with divided sections for independent elevation of a patient's head and knees.

mud b., a b. in which the mattress consists of semiliquid mud made from special clays, covered with a sheet of plastic material; used to widely distribute the pressure of the body weight over the dependent surface, for patients with burns or large anesthetic areas.

nail b., the area of the corium on which the nail rests; it is extremely sensitive and presents numerous longitudinal ridges on its surface. According to some anatomists, the nail bed is the portion covered by the body of the nail, the nail b. being only the part on which the root of the nail rests. SYN matrix unguis [NA], keratogenous membrane, nail matrix, onychostroma.

parotid b., the structures which surround and contact the parotid, forming the boundaries of the parotid space: anteriorly, the ramus of the mandible flanked by the masseter and medial pterygoid muscles; medially, the pharyngeal wall, carotid sheath and structures originating from the styloid process; posteriorly, the mastoid process, sternocleidomastoid muscle, and posterior belly of the digastric muscle; superiorly, the temporomandibular joint and the tympanic bone and cartilaginous portion of the external acoustic meatus.

b. of stomach, the structures against which the posteroinferior surface of the stomach lies, and from which it is separated, for the main part, by the omental bursa; includes diaphragm, left suprarenal gland, upper part of left kidney, splenic artery, anterior aspect of pancreatic body and tail, left colic flexure, and transverse mesocolon.

water b., a mattress in the form of a closed rubber bag filled with water; used to prevent or treat pressure sores by equalizing the distribution of the patient's weight against the support.

bed·bug. SYN *Cimex lectularius.*

bed·lam (bed′lăm). **1.** Pejorative colloquialism for a mental hospital or institution. **2.** A place or scene of wild or riotous behavior. **3.** A disturbing uproar. [corruption or contraction of St. Mary of *Bethlehem* Hospital in London]

bed·lam·ism (bed′lăm-izm). An obsolete term for acts associated with states of frenzy, excitement, wild tumult, and pandemonium.

Bednar, Alois, Austrian physician, 1816–1888. SEE B.'s *aphthae*, under *aphtha*.

Bednar, Blahoslav, 20th century Czech pathologist. SEE B. *tumor*.

bed·sore (bed′sōr). SYN decubitus *ulcer*.

bed·wet·ting. SYN nocturnal *enuresis.*

bee. An insect of the genus *Apis;* the honeybee, *A. mellifica,* is the source of honey and wax. [A.S. *beó, bī*]

beech oil. SYN beechwood tar.

beech·wood tar (bēch′wud). A thick, oily, dark brown liquid with the odor of creosote; largely used as a source of creosote. SYN beech oil.

Beer, August, German physicist, 1825–1863. SEE B.-Lambert *law;* B.'s *law.*

Beer, Georg J., Austrian ophthalmologist, 1763–1821. SEE B.'s *knife.*

bees·wax (bēz′waks). SYN wax (1).

white b., SYN white *wax.*

bee·tu·ria (bē-tū′rē-ă). Urinary excretion of betacyanin after ingestion of beets, found in most iron-deficient individuals and in some normal persons. SYN betacyaninuria.

Beevor, Charles E., English neurologist, 1854–1908. SEE B.'s *sign.*

Begbie, James, Scottish physician, 1798–1869. SEE B.'s *disease.*

Begg, P. Raymond, Australian orthodontist, *1898. SEE B. light wire differential force *technique.*

Béguez César, Antonio, Cuban pediatrician. SEE B.C. *disease.*

be·hav·ior (bē-hāv′yer). **1.** Any response emitted by or elicited from an organism. **2.** Any mental or motor act or activity. **3.** Specifically, parts of a total response pattern. [M.E., fr. O. Fr. *avoir,* to have]

adaptive b., any b. that enables an organism to adjust to a particular situation or environment.

adient b., SYN appetitive b.

ambient b., SYN aversive b.

appetitive b., movement of an organism toward a certain type of stimulus, such as food. Cf. aversive b. SYN adient b.

aversive b., movement of an organism away from a certain type of stimulus, such as electric shock. Cf. appetitive b. SYN ambient b.

coronary-prone b., b. that characterizes type A personality pattern.

health b., combination of knowledge, practices, and attitudes that together contribute to motivate the actions we take regarding health.

hookean b., the b. of a perfectly elastic body; *i.e.,* the strain is directly proportional to the stress. SEE ALSO Hooke's *law.*

molar b., in psychology, b. described in large response units rather than smaller ones. Cf. molecular b.

molecular b., in psychology, b. described in small response units rather than larger ones; a specific response. Cf. molar b.

obsessive b., the repetitive stylized b. seen in obsessive-compulsive neurosis.

operant b., b. whose continuation and frequency is determined by its consequences on the doer; central element of behavioral conditioning theory. SEE conditioning.

passive-aggressive b., apparently compliant b., with intrinsic obstructive or stubborn qualities, to cover deeply felt aggressive feelings that cannot be more directly expressed.

respondent b., b. in response to a specific stimulus; usually associated with classical conditioning. SEE conditioning.

ritualistic b., automatic b. of psychogenic or cultural origin.

target b., (1) SYN operant. **(2)** in b. modification therapy, the prescribed b.

type A b., a b. pattern characterized by aggressiveness, ambitiousness, restlessness, and a strong sense of time urgency; associated with increased risk for coronary heart disease.

type B b., a b. pattern characterized by the absence or obverse of type A b. characteristics.

be·hav·ior·al (bē-hāv′yer-ăl). Pertaining to behavior.

be·hav·ior·al sci·enc·es. A collective term for those disciplines or branches of science, such as psychology, sociology, and anthropology, and which derive their theories, concepts, and approaches from the observation and study of the behavior of living organisms.

be·hav·ior·ism (bē-hāv′yer-izm). A branch of psychology that formulates, through systematic observation and experimentation, the laws and principles which underlie the behavior of man and animals; its major contributions have been made in the areas of conditioning and learning. SYN behavioral psychology.

be·hav·ior·ist (bē-hāv′yer-ist). An adherent of behaviorism.

Behçet, Hulusi, Turkish dermatologist, 1889–1948. SEE B.'s *disease, syndrome.*

be·hen·ic ac·id (bĕ-hen′ik). CH₃(CH₂)₂₀COOH; a constituent of most fats and fish oils; large amounts are found in jamba, mustard seed, rapeseed oils, and cerebrosides. SYN *n*-docosanoic acid.

Behr, Carl, German ophthalmologist, 1874–1943. SEE B.'s *disease, syndrome.*

Behring, Emil A. von, German bacteriologist and Nobel laureate, 1854–1917. SEE B.'s *law.*

BEI Abbreviation for butanol-extractable *iodine.*

bej·el. Nonvenereal endemic syphilis now found chiefly among Arab children; apparently due to *Treponema pallidum.* SEE ALSO nonvenereal *syphilis.* [Ar. *bajlah*]

Bek (or Beck), E.V., Russian physician. SEE Kashin-B. *disease.*

Békésy, Georg von, Hungarian biophysicist in U.S. and Nobel laureate, 1899–1972. SEE B. *audiometer, audiometry.*

bel. Unit expressing the relative intensity of a sound. The intensity in bels is the logarithm (to the base 10) of the ratio of the power of the sound to that of a reference sound. Ordinarily, the reference sound is assumed to be one with a power of 10^{-16} watts per sq cm, approximately the threshold of a normal human ear at 1000 Hz. [A.G. *Bell,* Scottish-U.S. scientist, 1847–1922]

belch·ing. SYN eructation. [A.S. *baelcian*]

bel·em·noid (be-lem′noyd). Dart-shaped. [G. *belemnon,* a dart, + *eidos,* resemblance]

Bell, Sir Charles, Scottish surgeon, anatomist, and physiologist, 1774–1842. SEE B.'s *law;* B.-Magendie *law;* B.'s respiratory *nerve, palsy, spasm;* external respiratory *nerve* of B.

Bell, John, Scottish surgeon and anatomist, 1763–1820. SEE B.'s *muscle.*

bel·la·don·na (bel-ă-don′ă). *Atropa belladonna* (family Solanaceae); a perennial herb with dark purple flowers and shining purplish-black berries; the leaves (0.3% b. alkaloids) and root (0.5% b. alkaloids) orginally were source of atropine and related alkaloids, which are anticholinergic. B. is used as a powder (0.3% b. alkaloids, calculated as hyoscyamine) and tincture in asthma, colic, and hyperacidity. SYN deadly nightshade. [It. *bella,* beautiful, + *donna,* lady]

bel·la·don·nine (bel-ă-don′ēn). An artificial alkaloid derived from atropine by warming with hydrochloric acid.

bell-crowned (bel′krownd). Denoting a tooth the crown of which has a cross-sectional diameter much greater than that of the neck.

belle in·dif·fer·ence. SEE la belle indifférence.

Bellini, Lorenzo, Italian physician and anatomist, 1643–1704. SEE B.'s *ducts,* under *duct, ligament.*

bel·ly (bel′ē). **1.** The abdomen. **2.** The wide swelling part of a muscle. SYN venter (2). **3.** Popularly, the stomach or womb. [O.E. *belig,* bag]

anterior b. of digastric muscle, the portion of the digastric muscle which extends anteriorly from the intermediate tendon, and attaches to the posterior aspect of the mandible. SYN venter anterior musculi digastrici [NA].

b.'s of digastric muscle, SEE anterior b. of digastric muscle, posterior b. of digastric muscle.

frontal b. of occipitofrontalis muscle, the anterior belly of the occipitofrontalis muscle. SEE occipitofrontalis *muscle.* SYN venter frontalis musculi occipitofrontalis [NA], frontalis muscle.

inferior b. of omohyoid b., the inferior belly of the omohyoid muscle, attached to the superior border of the scapula. SYN venter inferior musculi omohyoidei [NA].

occipital b. of occipitofrontalis muscle, the posterior belly of the occipitofrontalis muscle. SEE occipitofrontalis *muscle.* SYN venter occipitalis musculi occipitofrontalis [NA], occipitalis muscle.

b.'s of omohyoid muscle, SEE inferior b. of omohyoid b., superior b. of omohyoid muscle.

posterior b. of digastric muscle, portion of digastric muscle posterior to the intermediate tendon, attaching to the digastric groove of the temporal bone. SYN venter posterior musculi digastrici [NA].

prune b., SEE abdominal muscle deficiency *syndrome.*

superior b. of omohyoid muscle, the superior belly of the omo-

hyoid muscle, attached to the hyoid bone. SYN venter superior musculi omohyoidei [NA].

bel·ly·ache (bel′ē-āk). Colloquialism·for abdominal pain, usually colicky.

bel·ly but·ton (bel′ē bŭt′ŏn). SYN umbilicus.

bel·o·ne·pho·bia (bel′ō-nē-fō′bē-ă). Morbid fear of needles, pins, and other sharp-pointed objects. [G. *belonē,* needle, + *phobos,* fear]

Belsey, Ronald, 20th century British surgeon. SEE B. Mark IV *operation,* Mark IV *procedure,* Mark V *procedure.*

bem·e·gride (bem′ĕ-grīd). 3-Ethyl-3-methylglutarimide; a central nervous system stimulant formerly used as an analeptic in intoxications due to barbiturates and other central nervous system depressant drugs.

ben Abbreviation for L. *bene,* well.

ben·ac·ty·zine hy·dro·chlo·ride (ben-ak′ti-zēn). 2-Diethylaminoethyl benzilate hydrochloride; an anticholinergic drug with the same actions but with approximately only one-fifth the activity of atropine; it is thought to raise the threshold of emotional reaction to external stimuli; now rarely used as a psychotherapeutic and tranquilizing agent.

Bence Jones, Henry, British physician, 1814–1873. SEE B. J. *albumin, cylinders,* under *cylinder, myeloma, proteins,* under *protein, reaction.*

ben·da·zac (ben′dă-zak). [(1-Benzyl-1*H*-indazol-3-yl)oxy]-acetic acid; a topical anti-inflammatory agent.

Bender, Lauretta, U.S. psychiatrist, 1897–1987. SEE B. gestalt *test,* Visual Motor Gestalt *test.*

ben·dro·flu·a·zide (ben-drō-flū′ă-zīd). SYN bendroflumethiazide.

ben·dro·flu·me·thi·a·zide (ben′drō-flū′mĕ-thī′ă-zīd). 3-benzyl-3,4-dihydro-6-(trifluoromethyl)-2*H*-1,2,4-benzothiadiazine-7-sulfonamide-1,1-dioxide; a thiazide diuretic and antihypertensive agent. SYN bendrofluazide.

bends (bendz). Colloquism for caisson *sickness;* decompression *sickness.* [fr. convulsive posture of those so afflicted]

ben·e·cep·tor (ben′ē-sep′ter, tōr). A nerve organ or mechanism (ceptor) for the appreciation and transmission of stimuli of a beneficial character. Cf. nociceptor. [L. *bene,* well, + *capio,* to take]

Benedek, Ladislaus (László), Austrian neurologist, 1887–1945. SEE B.'s *reflex.*

Benedict, Francis G., U.S. metabolist, 1870–1957. SEE B.-Roth *apparatus, calorimeter.*

Benedict, Stanley R., U.S. chemist, 1884–1936. SEE B.'s *solution, test* for glucose; B.-Hopkins-Cole *reagent.*

Benedikt, Moritz, Austrian physician, 1835–1920. SEE B.'s *syndrome.*

ben·e·fi·cence (be-nef′ĭ-sens). The ethical principle of doing good. [L. *beneficentia,* fr. *bene,* well, + *facio,* to do]

be·nign (bē-nīn′). Denoting the mild character of an illness or the nonmalignant character of a neoplasm. [thru O. Fr., fr. L. *benignus,* kind]

ben·ne oil (ben′nĕ). SYN *sesame* oil.

Bennett, Edward H., Irish surgeon, 1837–1907. SEE B.'s *fracture.*

Bennett, Norman G., British dentist, 1870–1947. SEE B. *angle, movement.*

Bennhold, H., German physician, *1893. SEE B.'s Congo red *stain.*

ben·ox·a·pro·fen (ben-oks-ă-prō′fen). (±)-2-(*p*-Chlorophenyl)-α-methyl-5- benzoxazoleacetic acid; a nonsteroidal anti-inflammatory and analgesic agent, no longer clinically used.

ben·per·i·dol (ben-per′i-dol). 1-{1-[3-(*p*-Fluorobenzoyl)propyl]-4-piperidyl}-2-benzimidazolin-one; a tranquilizer. SYN benzperidol.

ben·ser·a·zide (ben-ser′ă-zīd). An *l*-aromatic amino acid decarboxylase (dopa decarboxylase) inhibitor resembling carbidopa in action; given in combination with levodopa as an antiparkinsonian regimen. The benserazide prevents peripheral destruction of

be

levodopa and thus reduces cardiovascular side effects of treatment.

Bensley, Robert R., U.S.-Canadian anatomist, 1867–1956. SEE B.'s specific *granules*, under *granule*.

ben·tir·o·mide (ben-tir′ō-mīd). 4-[[(2-Benzoylamino)-3-(4-hydroxyphenyl)-1-oxopropyl]amino]benzoic acid; a peptide used as a screening test for exocrine pancreatic insufficiency and to monitor the adequacy of supplemental pancreatic therapy.

ben·ton·ite (ben′ton-īt). Native colloidal hydrated aluminum silicate; an absorbent clay found in the western U.S.; it is sometimes used in the treatment of diarrhea and skin disorders and was used as a suspending agent in lotions. [Fort *Benton*, Montana, + -ite]

△**benz-.** Combining form denoting association with benzene.

ben·zal·ac·e·to·phe·none (ben′zal-as-e-tō-fē′nōn). SYN chalcone.

ben·zal·cou·mar·an-3-one (ben-zal-kū′mar-an-thrē′ōn). SYN aurone.

benz·al·de·hyde (ben-zal′dĕ-hīd). C_6H_5CHO; an aldehyde produced artificially or obtained from oil of bitter almond, containing not less than 80% of b.; a flavoring agent used in orally administered medicines. SYN benzoic aldehyde.

ben·zal·ko·ni·um chlo·ride (ben-zal-kō′nē-ŭm). A mixture of alkylbenzyldimethylammonium chlorides in which the alkyls are long-chain compounds (C_8 to C_{18}); a surface-active germicide for many pathogenic nonsporulating bacteria and fungi. Aqueous solutions of this agent have a low surface tension, and possess detergent, keratolytic, and emulsifying properties that aid the penetration and wetting of tissue surfaces.

benz·am·ide (ben′ză-mīd). SYN aminoacylase.

benz[a]an·thra·cene (ben-zan′thră-sēn). 1,2-benzanthracene; a carcinogenic hydrocarbon. SYN benzanthrene.

ben·zan·threne (ben-zan′thrēn). SYN benz[a]anthracene.

ben·zene (ben′zēn). C_6H_6; the basic structure in most aromatic compounds; a highly toxic hydrocarbon from light coal tar oil; used as a solvent. SYN benzol, coal tar naphtha. [*benzoin*, + -ene]
b. bromide, a lacrimator or tear gas.

ben·zene·a·mine (ben-zēn′ă-mēn). SYN aniline.

o-**ben·zene·di·al·de·hyde.** SYN *o*-phthalaldehyde.

(γ)-**ben·zene hex·a·chlo·ride.** Incorrect name for 1,2,3,4,5,6-hexachlorocyclohexane (lindane).

ben·zes·trol (ben-zes′trol). 3-Ethyl-2,4-bis(*p*-hydroxyphenyl)-acetate; a synthetic estrogenic substance.

benz·e·tho·ni·um chlo·ride (benz-ĕ-thō′nē-ŭm). A synthetic quaternary ammonium compound, one of the cationic class of detergents; germicidal and bacteriostatic.

ben·zi·dine (ben′zi-dēn). $NH_2C_6H_4C_6$ H_4NH_2; *p*-Diaminodiphenyl; a colorless, crystalline compound used to detect sulfates in water analysis, for the identification of blood, and as a reagent in special stains; because it has been identified as a carcinogen, its current use is limited.

benz·im·id·az·ole (ben-zim-i-dā′zōl). A ring system comprised of a benzene ring fused with an imidazole ring; occurs in nature as part of the vitamin B_{12} molecule.

ben·zin, ben·zine (ben′zin, ben-zēn). SYN *petroleum* benzin.

ben·zin·da·mine hy·dro·chlo·ride (ben-zin′dă-mēn). SYN benzydamine hydrochloride.

ben·zi·o·da·rone (ben-zē′ō-dă-rōn). 2-Ethyl-3-benzofuranyl 4-hydroxy-3,5-diiodophenyl ketone; a coronary vasodilator.

ben·zo·ate (ben′zō-āt). A salt or ester of benzoic acid. The salts are often used as a food preservative. SYN benzoylecgonine.

ben·zo·at·ed (ben′zō-āt-ed). Containing benzoic acid or a benzoate, usually sodium benzoate.

ben·zo·caine (ben′zō-kān). $NH_2C_6H_4$–$COO(C_2H_5)$; the ethyl ester of *p*-aminobenzoic acid; a topical anesthetic agent. SYN ethyl aminobenzoate.

ben·zo·di·az·e·pine (ben′zō-dī-az′ĕ-pēn). Parent compound for the synthesis of a number of psychoactive compounds (*e.g.,* diazepam, chlordiazepoxide).

ben·zo·ic (ben-zō′ik). Relating to or derived from benzoin.

ben·zo·ic ac·id. C_6H_5COOH; occurs naturally in gum benzoin; it is used as a food preservative, locally as a fungistatic, and orally as an antiseptic, diuretic, and expectorant. It is excreted rapidly as hippuric acid. SYN benzoyl hydrate, flowers of benzoin.

ben·zo·ic al·de·hyde. SYN benzaldehyde.

ben·zo·in (ben′zō-in, ben′zoyn). A balsamic resin obtained from *Styrax benzoin* (family Styracaceae), used as a stimulant expectorant, but usually by inhalation in laryngitis and bronchitis; it retards rancidification of fats and is used for this purpose in the official benzoinated lard. SYN gum benjamin, gum benzoin. [It. *benzoino*, fr. Ar. *lubān jāwīy*, Javan incense]

ben·zol (ben′zol). SYN benzene.

ben·zo·mor·phan (ben-zō-mōr′fan). 6,7-Benzomorphan; 1,2,3,4,5,6-hexahydro-2,6-methano-3-benzazocine; the parent compound of a series of analgesics including pentazocine and phenazocine; it does not possess analgesic properties itself.

ben·zo·na·tate (ben-zō′nă-tāt). Nonaethyleneglycol monomethyl ether *p-n*-butylaminobenzoate; an antitussive agent related chemically to tetracaine; thought to act by depressing mechanoreceptors in the lungs.

ben·zo·pur·pu·rin 4B (ben-zō-per′pyū-rin) [C.I. 23500]. A red acid dye, $C_{34}H_{26}N_6O_6S_2Na_2$, formerly used as a plasma stain and as an indicator (changes from violet to red in the pH range 1.2 to 4.0).

1,4-ben·zo·qui·none (ben-zō-kwin′ōn). **1.** 2,5-cyclohexadiene-1,4-dione; an essential part of coenzyme Q and vitamin E, reducible to hydroquinone. SYN quinone (2). **2.** One of a class of benzoquinone derivatives.

ben·zo·qui·no·ni·um chlo·ride (ben′zō-kwī-nō′nē-ŭm). A skeletal muscle relaxant.

ben·zo·res·in·ol (ben-zō-res′i-nol). A resinous constituent of benzoin.

ben·zo·sul·fi·mide (ben-zō-sŭl′fi-mīd). SYN saccharin.

ben·zo·thi·a·di·a·zides (ben′zō-thī-ă-dī′ă-zīdz). A class of diuretics that increase the excretion of sodium and chloride and an accompanying volume of water, independent of alterations in acid-base balance; most of the compounds in this group are analogues of 1,2,4-benzothiadiazine-1,1-dioxide. SEE ALSO benzthiazide.

ben·zox·i·quine (ben-zoks′i-kwin). 8-quinolinol benzoate ester; a disinfectant. SYN benzoxyline.

ben·zox·y·line (ben-zoks′i-lēn). SYN benzoxiquine.

ben·zo·yl (ben′zō-il). The benzoic acid radical, C_6H_5CO—, forming benzoyl compounds.
b. chloride, C_6H_5COCl; a colorless liquid of pungent odor; a reagent for acylation reactions.
b. hydrate, SYN benzoic acid.
b. peroxide, C_6H_5CO–O–O–COC $_6H_5$; made by the interaction of sodium peroxide and b. chloride; used in oil as an application to ulcers and to burns and scalds, in promoting the polymerization of dental resins, and as a keratolytic in the treatment of acne.

ben·zo·yl·cho·lin·es·ter·ase (ben′zō-il-kō-lin-es′ter-ās). Obsolete term for cholinesterase.

benz·oy·lec·gon·ine (ben′zō-il-ek′gō-nēn). A metabolite of cocaine produced by hydrolysis; it can be found in the urine. SYN benzoate, ecgonine benzoate.

ben·zo·yl·pas cal·ci·um (ben-zō′il-pas). 4-Benzamidosalicylic acid calcium salt; an antituberculous agent.

benz·per·i·dol (benz-per′i-dol). SYN benperidol.

benz·phet·a·mine hy·dro·chlo·ride (benz-fet′ă-mēn). *N*-Benzyl-*N*,α-dimethylphenethylamine hydrochloride; a sympathomimetic agent used as an anorexiant.

benz·py·rene (benz-pī′rēn). An environmental carcinogen found in jet fuel exhaust, cigarette smoke, and charcoal broiled meats; a powerful enzyme inducer.

benz·pyr·in·i·um bro·mide (benz-pī-rin′ē-ŭm). 1-benzyl-3-hydroxypyridinium bromide diethylcarbamate; a cholinergic drug with action and uses similar to those of neostigmine. SYN benzstigminum bromidum.

benz·quin·a·mide (benz-kwin′ă-mīd). A benzoquinoline amide used as an antiemetic agent.

benz·stig·mi·num bro·mi·dum (benz-stig′mi-nŭm). SYN benzpyrinium bromide.

benz·thi·a·zide (benz-thī′ă-zīd). 3-[(Benzylthio)methyl]-6-chloro-2H-1,2,4-benzothiadiazine-7-sulfonamide 1,1-dioxide; a diuretic and antihypertensive agent.

benz·tro·pine mes·y·late (benz-trō′pēn). 3-Diphenylmethoxytropane methanesulfonate; a parasympatholytic agent with atropine-like and antihistaminic actions.

ben·zyd·a·mine hy·dro·chlo·ride (ben-zid′ă-mēn). 1-benzyl-3-[3-dimethylamino)propoxy]-1H-indazole; an analgesic and antipyretic. SYN benzindamine hydrochloride.

ben·zyl (ben′zil). The hydrocarbon radical, $C_6H_5CH_2$–.

b. alcohol, $C_6H_5CH_2OH$; possesses local anesthetic and bacteriostatic properties. SYN phenmethylol, phenylcarbinol.

b. benzoate, $C_6H_5CO–OCH_2C_6H_5$; an agent that reduces the contractility of unstriated muscular tissue, possessing marked antispasmodic properties; used now as a pediculicide and scabicide.

b. benzoate-chlorophenothane-ethyl aminobenzoate, a mixture of three components used in emulsions or ointments.

b. carbinol, SYN phenylethyl alcohol.

b. cinnamate, trans-cinnamic benzyl ester; a constituent of balsams of Peru, Tolu, and styrax. SYN cinnamein.

b. fumarate, $(C_6H_5CH_2)$ OOCCHCHCOO$(CH_2C_6H_5$; dibenzyl fumarate; used for the same purposes as b. benzoate.

b. mandelate, the b. ester of mandelic acid, having an antispasmodic action similar to that of b. benzoate.

b. succinate, $(C_6H_5CH_2)_2(CH_2CO_2)_2$; dibenzyl succinate; action and dosage are the same as those of b. benzoate.

ben·zyl·ic (ben-zil′ik). Relating to or containing benzyl.

ben·zyl·i·dene (ben-zil′i-dēn). The hydrocarbon radical, $C_6H_5CH=$.

benz·y·liso·quin·o·lines (ben′zil-ī-sō-kwin-ō-linz). A group of alkaloids found primarily in poppy plants (Papaveraceae). Curare alkaloids are bisbenzylisoquinolines.

ben·zyl·ox·y·car·bon·yl (Z, Cbz) (ben′zil-ok-sē-kar′bon-il). Amino-protecting radical used (as the chloride) in peptide synthesis, yielding PhCH₂OCO—NHR. SYN carbobenzoxy.

ben·zyl·pen·i·cil·lin (ben′zil-pen-i-sil′in). SYN penicillin G.

be·phen·i·um hy·drox·y·naph·tho·ate (be-fen′ē-ŭm hī-droks′ē-naf′thō-āt). Benzyldimethyl-(2-phenoxyethyl)ammonium 3-hydroxy-2-naphthoate; a drug used against Ancylostoma duodenale and Necator americanus (hookworms of man); now largely replaced by mebendazole.

BER Abbreviation for basic electrical rhythm.

Beradinelli, Waldemar, Argentinian physician, 1903–1956. SEE B.'s syndrome.

Bérard, Auguste, French surgeon, 1802–1846. SEE B.'s aneurysm.

Béraud, Bruno J., French surgeon, 1825–1865. SEE B.'s valve.

ber·ber·ine (ber′ber-ēn). $C_{20}H_{19}NO_5$; Umbellatine; an alkaloid from Hydrastis canadensis (family Berberidaceae); has been used as an antimalarial, antipyretic, and carminative, and externally for indolent ulcers.

be·reave·ment (bĕ-rēv-ment). An acute state of intense psychological sadness and suffering experienced after the tragic loss of a loved one or some priceless possession. [M.E., bireven, to deprive, + -ment]

Berger, Emil, Austrian ophthalmologist, 1855–1926. SEE B.'s space.

Berger, Hans, German neurologist, 1873–1941. SEE B. rhythm.

Berger, Jean, 20th century French nephrologist. SEE B.'s disease, focal glomerulonephritis.

Berger cells. See under cell.

Bergmann, Gottlieb H., German neurologist and anatomist, 1781–1861. SEE B.'s cords, under cord, fibers, under fiber.

Bergmeister, O., Austrian ophthalmologist, 1845–1918. SEE B.'s papilla.

Berg's stain. See under stain.

beri beri. SEE beriberi.

ber·i·beri, beri beri (ber′ē-ber′ē). A specific nutritional deficiency syndrome (a nutritional polyneuropathy), occurring in endemic form in eastern and southern Asia, sporadically in other parts of the world without reference to climate, and sometimes in alcoholics, resulting mainly from a dietary deficiency of thiamin; the "dry" form is characterized by painful polyneurites; sensory nerves are more likely to be affected than motor nerves, with symptoms beginning in the feet and working upward with the hands affected late in the course of the disease; the "wet" form is characterized by edema resulting from a high-output form of heart failure. SEE ALSO nutritional polyneuropathy. SYN endemic neuritis, kakké, panneuritis endemica. [Singhalese, extreme weakness]

dry b., paraplegic b., affecting chiefly the peripheral nerves; its clinical pattern is predominantly that of a polyneuropathy without associated congestive failure.

infantile b., b. appearing in a breast-fed infants whose mother has b. due to thiamin deficiency. It is mainly the "wet" form of b., characterized by heart failure with marked peripheral edema (which is otherwise unusual in heart failure in infancy). An often fatal disease, acute in onset, which was formerly common in the Far Eastern countries where rice is consumed; reversible with thiamin.

ship b., a form of thiamine deficiency seen among sailors.

wet b., edematous b., in which congestive heart failure occurs in addition to polyneuropthy.

berke·li·um (Bk) (berk′lē-um). An artificial transuranium radioactive element; atomic no. 97, atomic wt. 247.07. [Berkeley, Calif., city where first prepared]

Berlin, Rudolf, German ophthalmologist, 1833–1897. SEE B.'s edema.

Ber·lin blue [C.I. 77510]. $Fe_4(Fe(CN)_6)_3$; ferric ferrocyanide; a dye used to color injection masses for blood vessels and lymphatics, and in staining of siderocytes. SYN Prussian blue.

Bernard, Claude, French physiologist, 1813–1878. SEE B.'s canal, duct, puncture; B.-Cannon homeostasis; B.-Horner syndrome; B.-Sergent syndrome.

Bernard, Jean, French physician, *1907. SEE B.-Soulier disease, syndrome.

Bernays, Augustus C., U.S. surgeon, 1854–1907. SEE B.'s sponge.

Bernhardt, Martin, German neurologist, 1844–1915. SEE B.'s disease; Roth-B. disease; B.-Roth syndrome.

Bernhardt's for·mu·la. See under formula.

Bernheim, P., early 20th century French physician.

Bernheim's syn·drome. See under syndrome.

Bernoulli, Daniel, Swiss mathematician, 1700–1782. SEE B. effect; B.'s law, principle, theorem.

Bernoulli tri·al. A single random event for which there are two and only two possible outcomes that are mutually exclusive and have a priori fixed (and complementary) probabilities of resulting. The trial is the realization of this process. Conventionally one outcome is termed a success and is assigned the score 1, the other is a failure and has the score zero. Thus the outcome might be 0 (no heads, one tail) or 1 (1 head, no tails).

Bernstein, Lionel M., U.S. internist, *1923. SEE B. test.

Berry, Sir James, Canadian surgeon, 1860–1946. SEE B.'s ligaments, under ligament.

Berson, Solomon A., U.S. internist, 1918–1972.. SEE B. test.

Berthelot, Pierre Eugene Marcellin, French chemist, 1827–1907. SEE B. reaction.

Berthollet, Claude L., French chemist, 1748–1822. SEE B.'s law.

ber·ti·el·lo·sis (ber′tē-ĕ-lō′sis). Infection of primates including man with cestodes of the genus Bertiella.

Bertin, Exupère Joseph, French anatomist, 1712–1781. SEE B.'s bones, under bone, columns, under column, ligament, ossicles, under ossicle.

Bertrand, Ivan Georges, 20th century French neurologist. SEE Canavan-Van Bogaert-Bertrand disease.

be·ryl·li·o·sis (be-ril-ē-ō'sis). Beryllium poisoning characterized by the occurrence of granulomatous fibrosis, especially of the lungs, from chronic inhalation of beryllium.

be·ryl·li·um (Be) (be-ril'ē-ŭm). A white metal element belonging to the alkaline earths; atomic no. 4., atomic wt. 9.012182. [G. *beryllos, beryl*]

Besnier, Ernest, French dermatologist, 1831–1909. SEE B.'s *prurigo;* B.-Boeck-Schaumann *syndrome.*

Bes·noi·tia (bes-noy'tē-ă). A genus of protozoan parasites (family Besnoitiidae, class Sporozoea), closely related to *Toxoplasma,* that localize in subcutaneous, connective, serous, and other tissues and are surrounded by a heavy, nucleated wall of host tissue, forming a cyst; hosts include domestic ruminants, reindeer, caribou, rodents, opossums, and reptiles.

B. bennet'ti, species occurring in horses and asses in North America and Africa, and causing a chronic disease with scabbing, scarring, and thickening of the skin.

B. besno'iti, species causing besnoitiasis of cattle, goats, and larger antelopes in Europe, Africa, the Middle East, South America, and Asia; it primarily causes a chronic low-grade infection; mechanical transmission is by bloodsucking tabanid horseflies.

B. taran'di, a species occurring in reindeer and caribou, giving rise to a condition called "cornmeal disease" because of the granular nature of the lesions on the skin.

bes·noi·ti·a·sis (bes-noy-tē-ā'sis). A disease of cattle primarily caused by *Besnoitia besnoiti.* Cysts occur chiefly in the connective tissue of the skin, nasal mucous membranes, and serous membranes. Following a febrile stage, depilatory and seborrheic changes occur in the skin. SYN besnoitiosis.

Bes·noi·ti·i·dae (bes-noy'tē-i-dē). A family of protozoan parasites, similar to those of the family Toxoplasmatidae, to which the genus *Besnoitia* belong.

bes·noi·ti·o·sis (bes'noy-tē-ō'sis). SYN besnoitiasis.

Best, Franz, German pathologist, 1878–1920. SEE B.'s *disease,* carmine *stain.*

bes·ti·al·i·ty (bes-tē-al'i-tē). Sexual relations with an animal. SYN zooerastia. [L. *bestia,* beast]

be·syl·ate (bes'il-āt). USAN-approved contraction for benzenesulfonate.

be·ta (bā'tă). Second letter of the Greek alphabet, β (see entry at start of letter "B's". [G.]

be·ta-block·er (bā'tă-blok'er). SYN β-adrenergic blocking *agent.*

be·ta·cism (bā'tă-sizm). A defect in speech in which the sound of *b* is given to other consonants. [G. *bēta,* the second letter of the alphabet]

be·ta·cy·a·nin (bā'tă-sī-ă-nin). One of several red plant pigments; a betalain. An example is betanin. Elevated in urine of individuals with beeturia. [L. *beta,* beet, + G. *kyanos,* dark blue substance, + -in]

be·ta·cy·a·ni·nu·ria (bā-tă-sī'ă-ni-nū'rē-ă). SYN beeturia. [betacyanin + G. *ouron,* urine]

be·ta·his·tine hy·dro·chlo·ride (bā-tă-his'tēn). 2-[2-(Methylamino)ethyl]pyridine dihydrochloride; an inhibitor of diamine oxidase used as a histamine-like agent for treatment of Ménière's disease.

be·ta·ine (bē'tă-ēn). **1.** $(CH_3)_3N^+- CH_2COO^-$; an oxidation product of choline and a transmethylating intermediate in metabolism. **2.** A class of compounds related to b.(1) (*i.e.,* $R_3 N^=-CHR'-COO^-$). SYN glycine betaine, glycyl betaine, oxyneurine, trimethylglycine, trimethylglycocoll anhydride.

b. aldehyde, $(CH_3)_3N^+ -CH_2CHO$; an intermediate in the interconversion of betaine and choline.

b. hydrochloride, $C_5H_{12}ClNO_2$; trimethylglycine hydrochloride; an acidifying agent used in the treatment of achlorhydria and hypochlorhydria.

be·ta·ine-al·de·hyde de·hy·dro·gen·ase. An oxidizing enzyme that catalyzes the oxidation of betaine aldehyde with NAD^+ and water to betaine and NADH; part of the choline oxidase system and of choline metabolism.

bet·a·lains (bā'tă-lāns). A group of plant pigments found almost exclusively in the family Centrospermae, for example, betamin.

be·ta·meth·a·sone (bā-tă-meth'ă-sōn). Betadexamethasone 9-fluoro-11β,17,21-trihydroxy-16β-methyl-1,4-pre gnadiene-3,20-dione; 9α-fluoro-16β-methylprednisolone; a semisynthetic glucocorticoid with anti-inflammatory effects and toxicity similar to those of cortisol; not useful in the treatment of adrenal insufficiency because it causes little sodium retention. For systemic and topical therapy, its actions are similar to those of prednisone, but more potent. Also available as b. sodium phosphate, b. acetate, and b. valerate.

be·tan·i·dine sul·fate (be-tan'i-dēn). SYN bethanidine sulfate.

be·tan·in (bā'tă-nin). The red pigment in beets (*Beta vulgaris*); elevated in urine of individuals with beeturia. [fr. *betacyanin*]

be·ta sheets. a structure of proteins where the peptide is extended and stabilized by hydrogen bonding between NH and CO groups of different polypeptide chains or separate regions of the same chain.

be·ta·tron (bā'tă-tron). A circular electron accelerator that is a source of either high energy electrons or x-rays.

be·tax·o·lol hy·dro·chlo·ride (be-taks'ō-lol). 1-[4-[2-(cyclopropylmethoxy)ethyl]phenoxy]-3-isopropylaminopropan-2-ol hydrochloride; a β-adrenergic blocking agent used primarily in the treatment of ocular hypertension and chronic open-angle glaucoma.

be·ta·zole hy·dro·chlo·ride (bā'tă-zōl). An analogue of histamine that stimulates gastric secretion with less tendency to produce the side effects seen with histamine; used, in place of histamine, to measure the gastric secretory response.

be·tel (bē'tl). The dried leaves of *Piper betle* (family Piperaceae), a climbing East Indian plant; used as a stimulant and narcotic. [Pg. *betel, betle,* fr. Malayalam or Tamil *vetilla*]

be·tel nut. Areca nut, the nut of the areca palm, *Areca catechu* (family Palmae), of the East Indies, chewed by the natives; produces central nervous system stimulation; stains teeth and gums red.

be·tha·ne·chol chlo·ride (be-than'ĕ-kol). Carbamoylmethylcholine chloride; (2-hydroxypropyl)trimethylammonium chloride carbamate; a parasympathomimetic agent, used to relieve constipation, paralytic ileus, and urinary retention.

be·than·i·dine sul·fate (be-than'i-dēn). 1-benzyl-2,3-dimethylguanidine; an adrenergic blocking agent used for palliative treatment of hypertension. SYN betanidine sulfate.

Bethesda-Ballerup Group. A group of citrate-utilizing, slow lactose-fermenting bacteria (family Enterobacteriaceae) which share a similar series of antigens with the lactose-fermenting citrobacters; these organisms are now included in the genus *Citrobacter* without a distinction between prompt and slow lactose fermentation.

Betke-Kleihauer test. See under test.

Bettendorff, Anton J., German chemist, 1839–1902. SEE B.'s *test.*

bet·u·la. European white birch, bark and leaves of *Betula alba* (family Betulaceae); native to Europe, northern Asia, and North America, north of Pennsylvania. It contains betulin (betula camphor), betuloresinic acid, volatile oil, saponins, betulol (sesquiterpine alcohol), apigenin, dimethyl ether, betuloside, gaultherin, methyl salicylate, and ascorbic acid; has odor of wintergreen and is used as a pharmaceutic aid (flavor/aromatic).

bet·u·la oil (bet'yū-lă). See under oil.

Betz, Vladimir A., Russian anatomist, 1834–1894. SEE B. *cells,* under *cell.*

Beuren, Alois J. SEE Beuren *syndrome.*

Bevan-Lewis, William, English physician and physiologist, 1847–1929. SEE Bevan-Lewis *cells,* under *cell.*

bev·el (bev'ĕl). **1.** A surface having a sloped or slanting edge. **2.** The incline that one surface or line makes with another when not at right angles. **3.** The edge of a cutting instrument. **4.** To create a slanting edge on a body structure.

cavosurface b., the incline of the cavosurface angle of a prepared cavity wall in relation to the plane of the enamel wall.

reverse b., the sloping edge of a cutting instrument.

be·vo·ni·um meth·yl sul·fate (be-vō'nē-ŭm). 2-(hydroxymethyl)-1,1-dimethylpiperidinium methyl sulfate benzylate; an anticholinergic agent. SYN pyribenzyl methyl sulfate.

be·zoar (bē′zōr). A concretion formed in the alimentary canal of animals, and occasionally man; formerly considered to be a useful medicine with magical properties and apparently still used for this purpose in some places; according to the substance forming the ball, may be termed trichobezoar (hairball), trichophytobezoar (hair and vegetable fiber mixed), or phytobezoar (foodball). [Pers. *padzahr,* antidote]

Bezold, Albert von, German physiologist, 1836–1868. SEE B.'s *ganglion;* B.-Jarisch *reflex.*

Bezold, Friedrich, German otologist, 1842–1908. SEE B.'s *abscess, mastoiditis, sign, symptom, triad.*

BGP Abbreviation for bone Gla *protein.*

BHA Abbreviation for butylated hydroxyanisole.

bhang (bang). Name given in the East to powdered preparation of *Cannabis sativa* which is chewed or smoked by the local residents. SEE ALSO cannabis. [Hind.]

BHN Abbreviation for Brinell hardness *number.*

BHT Abbreviation for butylated hydroxytoluene.

Bi Symbol for bismuth.

⌂**bi-.** **1.** Prefix meaning twice or double, referring to double structures, dual actions, etc. **2.** In chemistry, used to denote a partially neutralized acid (an acid salt); *e.g.,* bisulfate. Cf. bis-, di-. [L.]

Bial, Manfred, German physician, 1869–1908. SEE B.'s *test.*

Bianchi, Giovanni, Italian anatomist, 1681–1761. SEE B.'s *nodule, valve.*

bi·ar·tic·u·lar (bī′ar-tik′yū-lăr). SYN diarthric.

bi·as (bī′-as). **1.** Systematic error between two laboratory procedures; may be constant or proportionate and if large may adversely affect test results. **2.** Deviation of results or inferences from the truth, or processes leading to such deviation; any trend in the collection, analysis, interpretation, publication, or review of data that can lead to conclusions that are systematically different from the truth. [Fr. *biais,* obliquity, perh. fr. L. *bifax,* two-faced]

bi·as·te·ri·on·ic (bī-as-ter-ē-on′ik). Relating to both asterions, especially the b. diameter, or b. width, the shortest distance from one asterion to the other.

bi·au·ric·u·lar (bī-aw-rik′yū-lăr). Relating to both auricles, in any sense.

bib. Abbreviation for L. *bibe,* drink.

bi·ba·sic (bī′bās-ik). SYN dibasic.

bib·li·o·ma·nia (bib′lē-ō-mā′nē-ă). Morbidly intense desire to collect and possess books, especially rare books. [G. *biblion,* book, + *mania,* frenzy]

bib·u·lous (bib′yū-lŭs). SYN absorbent (1). [L. *bibulus,* drinking freely, absorbent]

bi·cam·er·al (bī-kam′er-ăl). Having two chambers; denoting especially an abscess divided by a more or less complete septum. [bi- + L. *camera,* chamber]

bi·cap·su·lar (bī-kap′sū-lăr). Having a double capsule.

bi·car·bon·ate (bī-kar′bon-āt). HCO_3^-; the ion remaining after the first dissociation of carbonic acid; a central buffering agent in blood.

    standard b., the plasma b. concentration of a sample of whole blood that has been equilibrated at 37°C with a carbon dioxide pressure of 40 mm Hg and an oxygen pressure greater than 100 mm Hg; abnormally high or low values indicate metabolic alkalosis or acidosis, respectively.

bi·car·di·o·gram (bī-kar′dē-ō-gram). The composite curve of an electrocardiogram representing the combined effects of the right and left ventricles.

bi·cel·lu·lar (bī-sel′yū-lăr). Having two cells or subdivisions.

bi·ceph·a·lus (bī-sef′ă-lŭs). SYN dicephalus.

bi·ceps (bī′seps). A muscle with two origins or heads. Commonly used to refer to the biceps brachii *muscle.* [bi- + L. *caput,* head]

Bichat, Marie F.X., French anatomist, physician, and biologist,

1771–1802. SEE B.'s *canal, fat-pad, fissure, foramen, fossa, ligament, membrane, protuberance, tunic.*

bi·chlo·ride (bī-klōr′īd). SYN dichloride.

bi·cho (bē′cho). SYN epidemic gangrenous *proctitis.*

bi·chro·mate (bī-krō′māt). SYN dichromate.

bi·cil·i·ate (bī-sil′ē-āt). Having two cilia.

bi·cip·i·tal (bī-sip′i-tăl). **1.** Two-headed. **2.** Relating to a biceps muscle. [bi- + L. *caput,* head]

Bickel, Gustav, 19th century German physician. SEE B.'s *ring.*

bi·clo·nal (bī-klō′năl). Pertaining to or characterized by biclonality.

bi·clon·al·i·ty (bī-klōn-al′i-tē). A condition in which some cells have markers of one cell line and other cells have markers of another cell line, as in biclonal leukemias.

bi·clo·nal peak. Two narrow electrophoretic bands thought to represent immunoglobulin of two cell lines.

bi·con·cave (bī-kon′kāv). Concave on two sides; denoting especially a form of lens. SYN concavoconcave.

bi·con·vex (bī-kon′veks). Convex on two sides; denoting especially a form of lens. SYN convexoconvex.

bi·cor·nous, bi·cor·nu·ate, bi·cor·nate (bī-kōr′nŭs, -nū-āt, -nāt). Two-horned; having two processes or projections. [bi- + L. *cornu,* horn]

⌂**bicro-.** SYN pico- (2).

bi·cron (bī′kron). SYN picometer.

bi·cu·cul·line (bī′cū-cu-lēn). An alkaloid naturally occurring in the *d*-form; found in *Dicentra cucullaria* and *Adlumia fungosa* (family Fumariaceae) and several *Corydalis* species; a powerful convulsant that acts by antagonizing γ-aminobutyric acid, an inhibitory neurotransmitter.

bi·cus·pid (bī-kŭs′pid). **1.** Having two points, prongs, or cusps. **2.** Teeth having two cusps. Humans have eight: two in front of each group of molars. SEE bicuspid *tooth.* [bi- + L. *cuspis,* point]
    b. aortic valve, SEE familial aortic ectasia *syndrome.*

bi·cus·pi·di·za·tion (bī-kŭs′pi-di-zā′shŭn). Surgical change of a normally tricuspid valve into a functioning bicuspid valve; performed in correction of tricuspid valvar disease.

b.i.d. Abbreviation for L. *bis in die,* twice a day.

bi·dac·ty·ly (bī-dak′ti-lē). Abnormality in which the medial digits are lacking, with only the first and fifth represented. SEE ALSO lobster-claw *deformity,* ectrodactyly. [bi- + G. *daktylos,* finger]

bi·det (bē-dā′). A tub for a sitz bath, having also an attachment for giving vaginal or rectal infusions. [Fr. a small horse]

bi·dis·coi·dal (bī′dis-koy′dăl). Resembling, or consisting of, two disks.

BIDS [MIM*234050] Acronym for *b*rittle hair, *i*mpaired intelligence, *d*ecreased fertility, and *s*hort stature; usually manifested as an inherited deficiency of a high-sulfur protein.

bid·u·ous (bid′yū-ŭs). Rarely used term denoting of two days' duration. [L. *biduus,* lasting two days, fr. *bi-* + *dies,* day]

Biebl, M. SEE B. *loop.*

Biebrich scar·let red [C.I. 26905]. SYN scarlet red. [*Biebrich,* Germany]

Biederman, Joseph, U.S. physician, *1907. SEE B.'s *sign.*

Biedl, Artur, Austrian physician, 1869–1933. SEE Bardet-B. *syndrome.*

⌂ **Combining forms**   **[NA] Nomina Anatomica**

Word*Finder*
Multi-term entry finder
Preceding letter A   **[MIM] Mendelian Inheritance in Man**

A.D.A.M. Anatomy Plates
Between letters L and M   ☆ **Official alternate term**

Appendices:
Following letter Z   ☆**[NA] Official alternate Nomina Anatomica term**

SYN Synonym; Cf., compare   **High Profile Term**

Bielschowsky, Alfred, German ophthalmologist, 1871–1940. SEE B.'s *sign.*

Bielschowsky, Max, German neuropathologist, 1869–1940. SEE B.'s *disease, stain;* Jansky-B. *disease.*

Biemond, A., 20th century French neurologist. SEE B. *syndrome.*

Bier, August K.G., German surgeon, 1861–1949. SEE B.'s *amputation, hyperemia, method.*

Biermer, Anton, German physician, 1827–1892. SEE B.'s *anemia, disease, sign;* Addison-B. *disease.*

Biernacki, Edmund A., Polish pathologist, 1866–1912. SEE B.'s *sign.*

Biesiadecki, Alfred von, Polish physician, 1839–1888. SEE B.'s *fossa.*

bi·fas·cic·u·lar (bī'fă-sik'yū-lăr). Involving two of the presumed three major fascicles of the ventricular conduction system of the heart.

bi·fid (bī'fid). Split or cleft; separated into two parts. [L. *bifidus,* cleft in two parts]

Bi·fi·do·bac·te·ri·um (bī'fī-dō-bak-tēr'ē-ŭm). A genus of anaerobic bacteria (family Actinomycetaceae) containing Gram-positive rods of highly variable appearance; freshly isolated strains characteristically show bifurcated V and Y forms, uniform or branched, and club or spatulate forms. They frequently stain irregularly; two or more granules may stain with methylene blue, while the remainder of the cell is unstained. They are not acid-fast, are nonmotile, and do not produce spores; acetic and lactic acids are produced from glucose. Pathogenicity for man or other animals has not been reported, although they have been found in the feces and alimentary tract of infants, older people, and other animals. The type species is *B. bifidum.* [L. *bifidus,* cleft in two parts, + bacterium]

B. bi'fidum, type species of the genus *Bifidobacterium;* it is found in the feces and alimentary tract of breast- and bottle-fed infants and of older persons, rats, turkeys, and chickens; also found in the rumen of cattle; pathogenicity for man and other animals has not been reported. Associated with a growth factor belonging to a group of *N*-containing polysaccharides with a high hexosamine content and known as bifidus factor.

bi·fo·cal (bī-fō'kăl). Having two foci.

bi·fo·rate (bī-fō'rāt). Having two openings. [bi- + L. *foro,* pp. *-atus,* to bore, pierce]

bi·func·tion·al (bī-fŭnc'shŭn-ăl). Referring to a molecule containing two reactive functional groups; cross-linking reagents are bifunctional compounds.

bi·fur·cate, bi·fur·cat·ed (bī-fer'kāt, -kā-ted). Forked; two-pronged; having two branches. [bi- + L. *furca,* fork]

bi·fur·ca·tio (bī'fer-kā'shē-ō) [NA]. SYN bifurcation.

b. aor'tae [NA], SYN *bifurcation* of aorta.

b. tra'cheae [NA], SYN *bifurcation* of trachea.

b. trun'ci pulmona'lis [NA], SYN *bifurcation* of pulmonary trunk.

bi·fur·ca·tion (bī-fer-kā'shŭn). A forking; a division into two branches. SYN bifurcatio [NA].

b. of aorta, the division of the aorta into right and left common iliac arteries; it occurs at the level of the fourth and fifth lumbar vertebral body. SYN bifurcatio aortae [NA].

b. of pulmonary trunk, the division of the pulmonary trunk into right and left pulmonary arteries. SYN bifurcatio trunci pulmonalis [NA].

b. of trachea, the division of the trachea into the right and left main bronchi; it occurs at the level of the fifth or sixth thoracic vertebral body and is marked internally by the presence of a carina or keel-like ridge between the diverging bronchi. SYN bifurcatio tracheae [NA].

Bigelow, Henry J., U.S. surgeon, 1818–1890. SEE B.'s *ligament, septum.*

bi·gem·i·na (bī-jem'i-nă). SYN bigeminal *pulse.*

bi·gem·i·nal (bī-jem'i-năl). Paired; double; twin.

bi·gem·i·ni (bī-jem'i-nī). SYN bigeminy.

bi·gem·i·num (bī-jem'i-nŭm). One of the corpora bigemina. [L. ntr. of *bigeminus,* doubled]

bi·gem·i·ny (bī-jem'i-nē). Pairing; especially, the occurrence of heart beats in pairs. SYN bigemini. [bi- + L. *geminus,* twin]

atrial b., pairing of atrial beats, as when an atrial extrasystole is coupled to each sinus beat.

atrioventricular junctional b., paired beats, each pair consisting of an A-V nodal extrasystole coupled to a beat of the dominant, usually sinus, rhythm. SYN nodal b.

escape-capture b., paired beats, each couplet consisting of an escape beat followed by a conducted sinus beat.

nodal b., SYN atrioventricular junctional b.

reciprocal b., paired beats, each pair consisting of an A-V nodal beat followed by a reciprocal beat.

ventricular b., paired ventricular beats, the common form consisting of ventricular extrasystoles coupled to sinus beats.

bi·ger·min·al (bī-jer'min-ăl). Relating to two germs or ova.

big·head. 1. In horses, usually denotes osteodystrophia fibrosa. **2.** Gas gangrene infection of tissues of the head, caused by *Clostridium novyi* in sheep, usually young rams with head wounds. **3.** Photosensitization in sheep.

bi·git·a·lin (bī-jit'ă-lin). SYN gitoxin.

bi·gly·can (bī'glī-kan). A small interstitial proteoglycan that contains two glycosaminoglycan chains. SYN proteoglycan I.

Bignami, Amico, Italian physician, 1862–1929. SEE Marchiafava-B. *disease.*

bi·kun·in (bik'ū-nin). A plasma glycoprotein that is found in both the free state and covalently bound to the heavy chains of certain protease inhibitors.

bi·labe (bī'lāb). A forceps for seizing and removing urethral or small vesical calculi. [bi- + L. *labium,* lip]

bi·lat·er·al (bī-lat'er-ăl). Relating to, or having, two sides. [bi- + L. *latus,* side]

bi·lat·er·al·ism (bī-lat'er-ăl-izm). A condition in which the two sides are symmetrical.

bile (bīl). The yellowish brown or green fluid secreted by the liver and discharged into the duodenum where it aids in the emulsification of fats, increases peristalsis, and retards putrefaction; contains sodium glycocholate and sodium taurocholate, cholesterol, biliverdin and bilirubin, mucus, fat, lecithin, and cells and cellular debris. SYN gall (1). [L. *bilis*]

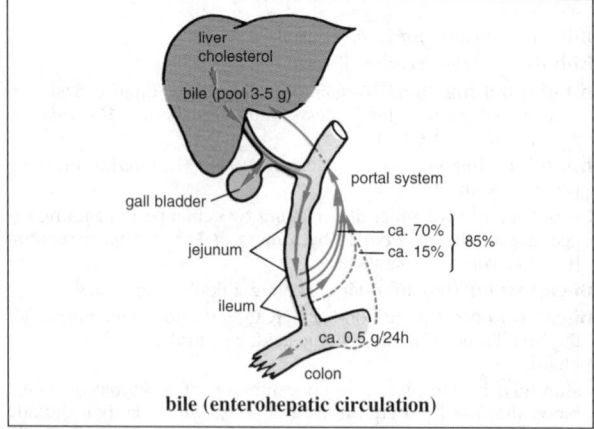

bile (enterohepatic circulation)

A b., b. from the common duct.

B b., b. from the gallbladder.

C b., b. from the hepatic duct.

white b., designating the relatively clear, almost colorless, clear viscid fluid that occurs in the gallbladder, intestines, or both as a result of obstruction of the b. ducts in various sites; actually the secretion of the mucous membrane, without the usual color resulting from b. pigments. SYN leukobilin.

Bil·har·zia (bil-har'zē-ă). An early name for *Schistosoma.* [T. *Bilharz*]

bil·har·zi·a·sis (bil-har-zī'ă-sis). SYN schistosomiasis.

bil·har·zi·o·ma (bil-har-zē-ō′mă). A tumor-like swelling of the skin, due to schistosomiasis.

bil·har·zi·o·sis (bil-har-zē-ō′sis). SYN schistosomiasis.

bili-. Bile. [L. *bilis*, bile]

bil·i·ary (bil′ē-ār-ē). Relating to bile or the biliary tract. SYN bilious (1).

bil·i·fac·tion, bil·i·fi·ca·tion (bil-i-fak′shŭn, -fi-kā′shŭn). Rarely used terms for bile formation. [bili- + L. *facio*, pp. *factus*, to make]

bil·if·er·ous (bil-if′er-ŭs). Rarely used term for containing or carrying bile.

bil·i·gen·e·sis (bil-i-jen′ĕ-sis). Bile production. [bili- + G. *genesis*, production]

bil·i·gen·ic (bil-i-jen′ik). Bile-producing.

bi·lin, bi·line (bī′lin). The chain of four pyrrole residues resulting from the cleavage of one bond of one of the four methylidene residues of the porphin part of a porphyrin; specifically, the unsubstituted tetrapyrrole; bilirubin and biliverdin are bilins.

bil·ious (bil′yŭs). 1. SYN biliary. 2. Relating to or characteristic of biliousness. 3. Formerly, denoting a temperament characterized by a quick, irritable temper. SYN choleric.

bil·ious·ness (bil′yŭs-nes). An imprecisely delineated congestive disturbance with anorexia, coated tongue, constipation, headache, dizziness, pasty complexion, and, rarely, slight jaundice; assumed to result from hepatic dysfunction.

bil·ip·ty·sis (bil-ip′ti-sis). Occurrence of bile in the sputum. [bili- + G. *pytalon*, saliva]

bil·i·ra·chia (bil-i-rā′kē-ă). Occurrence of bile pigments in the spinal fluid. [bili- + G. *rhachis*, spine]

bil·i·ru·bin (bil-i-rū′bin). A red bile pigment found as sodium bilirubinate (soluble), or as an insoluble calcium salt in gallstones, formed from hemoglobin during normal and abnormal destruction of erythrocytes by the reticuloendothelial system; a bilin with substituents on the 2, 3, 7, 8, 12, 13, 17, and 18 carbon atoms and with oxygens on carbons 1 and 19. Excess b. is associated with jaundice. [bili- + L. *ruber*, red]

conjugated b., SYN direct reacting b.

delta b., the fraction of b. covalently bound to albumin; in conventional methods it is measured as part of conjugated b. Because of its covalent bond during the recovery phase of hepatocellular *jaundice*, it may persist in the blood for a week or more after urine clears.

direct reacting b., the fraction of serum b. which has been conjugated with glucuronic acid in the liver cell to form b. diglucuronide; so called because it reacts directly with the Ehrlich diazo reagent; increased levels are found in hepatobiliary diseases, especially of the obstructive variety. SYN conjugated b.

indirect reacting b., the fraction of serum b. which has not been conjugated with glucuronic acid in the liver cell; so called because it reacts with the Ehrlich diazo reagent only when alcohol is added; increased levels are found in hepatic disease and hemolytic conditions. SYN unconjugated b.

b. UDPglucuronyltransferase (gloo-kū′ron-il-trans′fer-ās), an enzyme that catalyzes the reaction of UDPglucuronate and bilirubin forming UDP and bilirubin-glucuronoside; a deficiency of this enzyme is associated with Crigler-Najjar syndrome.

unconjugated b., SYN indirect reacting b.

bil·i·ru·bi·ne·mia (bil′i-rū-bin-ē′mē-ă). The presence of bilirubin in the blood, where it is normally present in relatively small amounts; the term is usually used in relation to increased concentrations observed in various pathologic conditions where there is excessive destruction of erythrocytes or interference with the mechanism of excretion in the bile. Determination of the quantity of bilirubin in the blood serum reveals two fractions, namely direct reacting (conjugated) and indirect reacting (nonconjugated) bilirubin; determination of conjugated and total bilirubin in serum is an important and frequently used clinical laboratory test. [bilirubin + G. *haima*, blood]

bil·i·ru·bin·glob·u·lin (bil-i-rū′bin-glob′yū-lin). A bilirubin-globulin complex; a transport form of bilirubin to the liver where bilirubin is converted to a diglucuronic acid derivative and passes into the bile.

bil·i·ru·bin-glu·cu·ron·o·side glu·cu·ron·o·syl·trans·fer-·ase. Bilirubin monoglucuronide transglucuronidase; a transferase that transfers a glucuronoside from one molecule of bilirubin glucuronoside to another, forming bilirubin bisglucuronoside and unconjugated bilirubin. A step in heme catabolism.

bil·i·ru·bin·oids (bil-i-rū′bin-oydz). Generic term denoting intermediates in the conversion of bilirubin to stercobilin by reductive enzymes in intestinal bacteria. Included are mesobilirubin, mesobilane mesobilene-b, urobilinogen, urobilin, reduction products of mesobilane (stercobilinogen) and mesobilene (stercobilin), and mesobiliviolin; most are found in normal urine and feces. Products related to these intermediates and found in pathological conditions (*e.g.*, jaundice, liver disease) are the structurally indefinite probilifuscins and propentdyopents found in gallstones.

bil·i·ru·bi·nu·ria (bil′i-rū-bi-nū′rē-ă). The presence of bilirubin in the urine. [bilirubin + G. *ouron*, urine]

bil·i·ther·a·py (bil-i-thār′ă-pē). Treatment with bile or bile salts.

bil·i·u·ria (bil-ē-yū′rē-ă). The presence of various bile salts, or bile, in the urine. SYN choleuria, choluria. [bili- + G. *ouron*, urine]

bil·i·ver·din, bil·i·ver·dine (bil-i-ver′din). A green bile pigment formed from the oxidation of bilirubin; a bilin with a structure almost identical to that of bilirubin. SYN choleverdin, dehydrobilirubin, verdine.

bil·i·ver·din·glo·bin (bil-i-ver′din-glō′bin). Obsolete term for choleglobin.

Bill, Arthur H., U.S. obstetrician, 1877–1961. SEE B.'s *maneuver*.

Billroth, C.A. Theodor, Austrian surgeon, 1829–1894. SEE B.'s *cords*, under *cord*, *operation* I, under *operation* II, *venae* cavernosae, under *vena*; B. I *anastomosis*, II *anastomosis*.

bi·lo·bate, bi·lobed (bī-lō′bāt, bī′lōbd). Having two lobes.

bi·lo·bec·to·my (bī′lōb-ek′tō-mē). Surgical excision of two lobes (of the lung).

bi·lob·u·lar (bī-lob′yū-lăr). Having two lobules.

bi·loc·u·lar, bi·loc·u·late (bī-lok′yū-lăr, -yū-lāt). Having two compartments or spaces. [bi- + L. *loculus*, dim. of *locus*, a place]

bi·loph·o·dont (bī-lof′ō-dont). Having two longitudinal ridges on the premolar and molar teeth; designating certain animals, such as the kangaroo. [bi- + G. *lophos*, ridge, + *odous*, tooth]

bi·man·u·al (bī-man′yū-ăl). Relating to, or performed by, both hands. [bi- + L. *manus*, hand]

bi·mas·toid (bī-mas′toyd). Relating to both mastoid processes.

bi·max·il·lary (bī-mak′si-lār-e). Relating to both the right and left maxillae; sometimes used when describing something affecting both halves of the upper jaw.

bi·mod·al (bī-mō′dăl). Denoting a frequency curve characterized by two peaks.

bi·mo·lec·u·lar (bī-mō-lek′yū-lăr). Involving two molecules, as in a b. reaction.

bin·an·gle (bin-ang′-ŭl). 1. The second angle given the shank of an angled instrument to bring its working end close to the axis of the handle in order to prevent it from turning about the axis. 2. A dental instrument possessing the above characteristics. [L. *bini*, pair, + *angulus*, angle]

bi·na·ry (bī′nār-ē). 1. Denoting or comprised of two components, elements, molecules, etc. 2. Denoting a choice of two mutually exclusive outcomes for one event (*e.g.*, male or female; heads or tails; affected or unaffected). [L. *binarius*, consisting of two, fr. *bini*, two at a time]

bin·au·ral (bin-aw′răl). Relating to both ears. SYN binotic. [L. *bini*, a pair, + *auris*, ear]

bind (bīnd). 1. To confine or encircle with a band or bandage. 2. To join together with a band or ligature. 3. To combine or unite molecules by means of reactive groups, either in the molecules *per se* or in a chemical added for that purpose; frequently used in relation to chemical bonds that may be fairly easily broken (*i.e.*, noncovalent), as in the binding of a toxin with antitoxin, or a heavy metal with a chelating agent, etc. 4. A close interpersonal relationship in which one person feels compelled to act in a certain way to obtain the approval of the other person. [A.S. *bindan*]

double b., a type of personal interaction in which one receives two mutually conflicting verbal or nonverbal instructions or demands from the same person or different individuals, resulting in a situation in which either compliance or noncompliance with either alternative threatens one of the needed relationships.

bind·er (bīnd′er). **1.** A broad bandage, especially one encircling the abdomen. **2.** Anything that binds. SEE bind (3).

obstetrical b., a supporting garment covering the abdomen from the ribs to the trochanters, tightly pinned at the back, affording support after childbirth or, rarely, during childbirth.

T-b., two strips of cloth at right angles; used for retaining dressing, as on the perineum. SYN T-bandage.

Binet, Alfred, French psychologist, 1857–1911. SEE B. *age*, *scale*, *test*; B.-Simon *scale*; Stanford-B. intelligence *scale*.

Bing, Paul Robert, German neurologist, 1878–1956. SEE B.'s *reflex*.

Bing, Richard J., U.S. physician, *1909. SEE Taussig-B. *disease*, *syndrome*.

Bingham, E.C., U.S. chemist, 1878–1945. SEE B. *flow*, *model*, *plastic*.

Binn's bac·te·ri·um. See under bacterium.

bin·oc·u·lar (bin-ok′yū-lăr). Adapted to the use of both eyes; said of an optical instrument. [L. *bini*, paired, + *oculus*, eye]

bi·no·mi·al (bī-nō′mē-ăl). A set of two terms or names; in the probabilistic or statistical sense it corresponds to a Bernoulli trial. SEE ALSO binary *combination*. [bi- + G. *nomos*, name]

bin·ot·ic (bin-ot′ik). SYN binaural. [L. *bini*, a pair, + G. *ous* (*ōt*-), ear]

Binswanger, Otto Ludwig, German neurologist, 1852–1929. SEE B.'s *disease*, *encephalopathy*.

bi·nu·cle·ar, bi·nu·cle·ate (bī-nū′klē-ăr, -klē-āt). Having two nuclei.

bi·nu·cle·o·late (bī-nū′klē-ō-lāt). Having two nucleoli.

Binz, Carl, German pharmacologist, 1832–1913. SEE B.'s *test*.

△**bio-.** Combining form denoting life. [G. *bios*, life]

bi·o·a·cous·tics (bī′ō-ă-kūs′tiks). The science dealing with the effects of sound fields or mechanical vibrations in living organisms.

bi·o·ac·tive (bī′ō-ăk′tiv). Referring to a substance that can be acted upon by a living organism or by an extract from a living organism.

bi·o·as·say (bī-ō-as′ā). Determination of the potency or concentration of a compound by its effect upon animals, isolated tissues, or microorganisms, as compared with an analysis of its chemical or physical properties.

bi·o·as·tro·nau·tics (bī′ō-as-trō-naw′tiks). The study of the effects of space travel and space habitation on living organisms.

bi·o·a·vail·a·bil·i·ty (bī′ō-ă-vāl′ă-bil′i-tē). The physiological availability of a given amount of a drug, as distinct from its chemical potency; proportion of the administered dose which is absorbed into the bloodstream.

bi·o·cat·a·lyst (bī′ō-kat-ă-list). A substance of biological origin that can catalyze a reaction; *e.g.*, an enzyme.

bi·o·ce·no·sis (bī-ō-se-nō′sis). An assemblage of species living in a particular biotope. SYN biotic community. [bio- + G. *koinos*, common]

bi·o·chem·i·cal (bī-ō-kem′i-kăl). Relating to biochemistry.

bi·o·chem·is·try (bī-ō-kem′is-trē). The chemistry of living organisms and of the chemical, molecular, and physical changes occurring therein. SYN biological chemistry, physiological chemistry.

bi·o·chem·or·phic (bī-ō-kem-ōr′fik). Denoting the relationship between biologic action and chemical structure, as in food and drugs.

bi·o·che·mor·phol·o·gy (bī′ō-kem-ōr-fol′ō-jē). **1.** The study of the relationship between biologic action and chemical structure. **2.** Macroscopic or gross morphology as revealed by biochemical techniques; *e.g.*, selective staining of enzymes, antibodies. [bio- + chemistry + G. *morphē*, shape, + *logos*, study]

bi·o·chrome (bī′ō-krōm). SYN natural *pigment*. [bio- + G. *chrōma*, color]

bi·o·cid·al (bī-ō-sī′dăl). Destructive of life; particularly pertaining to microorganisms. [bio- + L. *caedo*, to kill]

bi·o·cli·ma·tol·o·gy (bī′ō-klī-mă-tol′ō-jē). The science of the relationship of climatic factors to the distribution, numbers, and types of living organisms; an aspect of ecology.

bi·o·cy·ber·net·ics (bī′ō-sī-ber-net′iks). The science of communication and control within a living organism, particularly on a molecular basis.

bi·o·cy·tin (bī-ō-sī′tin). ε-*N*-biotinyl-L-lysine; biotin condensed through its carboxyl group with the ε-amino group of a lysyl residue in the apoenzymes to which biotin is the coenzyme; the predominant linkage in which biotin is found. SYN biotinyllysine.

bi·o·cy·tin·ase (bī-ō-sī′tin-ās). An enzyme in blood that catalyzes the hydrolysis of biocytin to biotin and lysine (or, lysyl residue if the lysine is in a protein); probably biotinidase.

bi·o·de·grad·a·ble (bī′ō-dē-grād′ă-bl). Denoting a substance that can be chemically degraded or decomposed by natural effectors (*e.g.*, weather, soil bacteria, plants, animals).

bi·o·de·gra·da·tion. SYN biotransformation.

bi·o·dy·nam·ic (bī′ō-dī-nam′ik). Relating to biodynamics.

bi·o·dy·nam·ics (bī′ō-dī-nam′iks). The science dealing with the force or energy of living matter. [bio- + G. *dynamis*, force]

bi·o·e·col·o·gy (bī-ō-ē-kol′ō-jē). SYN ecology.

bi·o·el·e·ment (bī′ō-el′ĕ-ment). An element required by a living organism.

bi·o·en·er·get·ics (bī′ō-en-er-jet′iks). **1.** The study of energy changes involved in the chemical reactions within living tissue. **2.** The study of energy exchanges between living organisms and their environments.

bi·o·en·gi·neer·ing (bī′ō-en-jin-ēr′ing). SEE biomedical *engineering*.

bi·o·feed·back (bī-ō-fēd′bak). A training technique that enables an individual to gain some element of voluntary control over autonomic body functions; based on the learning principle that a desired response is learned when received information such as a recorded increase in skin temperature (feedback) indicates that a specific thought complex or action has produced the desired physiological response.

EMG b., a form of b. that uses an electromyographic measure of muscle tension as the physical symptom to be deconditioned, such as tension in the frontalis muscle in the head which can cause headaches.

bi·o·fla·vo·noids (bī-ō-flāv′on-oydz). Naturally occurring flavone or coumarin derivatives having the activity of the so-called vitamin P, notably rutin and esculin.

bi·o·gen·e·sis (bī-ō-jen′ĕ-sis). **1.** Term given by Huxley to the principle that life originates from preexisting life only and never from nonliving material. SEE spontaneous *generation*, recapitulation *theory*. **2.** SYN biosynthesis. [bio- + G. *genesis*, origin]

bi·o·ge·net·ic (bī′ō-jĕ-net′ik). Relating to biogenesis.

bi·o·gen·ic (bī′ō-jen-ik). Produced by a living organism.

bi·o·geo·chem·is·try (bī′ō-jē-ō-kem′is-trē). The study of the influence of living organisms and life processes on the chemical structure and history of the earth.

bi·o·grav·ics (bī-ō-grav′iks). That field of study dealing with the effect on living organisms (particularly man) of abnormal gravitational effects produced, *e.g.*, by acceleration or by free fall; in the former case, heavier than normal weight is induced, and in the latter weightlessness. [bio- + L. *gravis*, weight]

Bi(OH)₃ Abbreviation for *bismuth* hydroxide.

bi·o·in·stru·ment (bī′ō-in′strū-ment). A sensor or device usually attached to or embedded in the human body or other living animal to record and to transmit physiologic data to a receiving and monitoring station.

bi·o·ki·net·ics (bī′ō-ki-net′iks). The study of the growth changes and movements that developing organisms undergo. [bio- + G. *kinēsis*, motion]

bi·o·log·ic, bi·o·log·i·cal (bī′ō-loj′ik, -loj′i-kăl). Relating to biology.

bi·ol·o·gist (bī-ol'ō-jist). A specialist or expert in biology.

bi·ol·o·gy (bī-ol'ō-jē). The science concerned with the phenomena of life and living organisms. [bio- + G. *logos,* study]

cellular b., SYN cytology.

molecular b., study of phenomena in terms of b. molecular (or chemical) interactions; it differs from biochemistry in that it historically has an emphasis on chemical interactions involved in the replication of DNA, its "transcription"; into RNA, and its "translation"; into or expression in protein, *i.e.,* in the chemical reactions connecting genotype and phenotype.

oral b., that aspect of b. devoted to the study of biological phenomena associated with the oral cavity in health and disease (*e.g.,* dental caries, mastication, periodontal disease).

pharmaceutical b., SYN pharmacognosy.

radiation b., field of science that studies the biological effects of ionizing radiation.

bi·o·lu·mi·nes·cence (bī'ō-lū-min-es'ens). 1. Light produced by certain organisms from the oxidation of luciferins through the action of luciferases and with negligible production of heat, chemical energy being converted directly into light energy. SYN cold light (1). 2. Any light produced by a living organism. [bio- + L. *lumen* (*-inis*), light]

bi·ol·y·sis (bī-ol'i-sis). Disintegration of organic matter through the chemical action of living organisms. [bio- + G. *lysis,* dissolution]

bi·o·lyt·ic (bī-ō-lit'ik). 1. Relating to biolysis. 2. Capable of destroying life.

bi·o·mac·ro·mol·e·cule (bī'ō-māk-rō-mol'ĕ-kyūl). A naturally occurring substance of large molecular weight (*e.g.,* protein, DNA).

bi·o·mass (bī'ō-mas). The total weight of all living things in a given area, biotic community, species population, or habitat; a measure of total biotic productivity.

bi·ome (bī'ōm). The total complex of biotic communities occupying and characterizing a particular geographic area or zone. [bio- + -ome]

bi·o·me·chan·ics (bī-ō-me-kan'iks). The science concerned with the action of forces, internal or external, on the living body.

dental b., SYN dental *biophysics.*

bi·o·med·i·cal (bī-ō-med'i-kăl). 1. Pertaining to those aspects of the natural sciences, especially the biologic and physiologic sciences, that relate to or underlie medicine. 2. Biological and medical, *i.e.,* encompassing both the science(s) and the art of medicine.

bi·o·mem·brane (bī-ō-mem'brān). A structure bounding a cell or cell organelle; it contains lipids, proteins, glycolipids, steroids, etc. SYN membrana [NA], membrane (2).

bi·om·e·ter (bī-om'ĕ-ter). A device for measuring carbon dioxide given off by organisms and, hence, for determining the quantity of living matter present. [bio- + G. *metron,* measure]

bi·o·me·tri·cian (bī-ō-me-trish'ăn). One who specializes in the science of biometry.

bi·om·e·try (bī-om'ĕ-trē). The application of statistical methods to the study of numerical data based on biological observations and phenomena. [bio- + G. *metron,* measure]

b. fetal, ultrasound measurement of fetal dimensions to evaluate gestational age of fetal size.

bi·o·mi·cro·scope (bī-ō-mī'krō-skōp). SYN slitlamp.

bi·o·mi·cros·co·py (bī'ō-mī-kros'kŏ-pē). 1. Microscopic examination of living tissue in the body. 2. Examination of the cornea, aqueous humor, lens, vitreous humor, and retina by use of a slitlamp combined with a binocular microscope.

Bi·om·pha·la·ria (bī-om-fă-lā'rē-ă). An important genus of freshwater snails (family Planorbidae, subfamily Planorbinae), several species of which serve as intermediate hosts of *Schistosoma mansoni* in Africa, Saudi Arabia and Yemen, South America, and the Caribbean. Host snails formerly were placed in the genera *Australorbis, Tropicorbis,* and *Taphius* but are no longer considered generically distinct.

bi·on (bī'on). A living thing. [G. pres. p. ntr. of *bioō,* to live]

Biondi, Aldolpho, Italian pathologist, 1846–1917. SEE B.-Heidenhain *stain.*

bi·o·ne·cro·sis (bī-ō-ne-krō'sis). SYN necrobiosis.

bi·on·ic (bī-on'ik). Relating to or developed from bionics.

bi·on·ics (bī-on'iks). 1. The science of biologic functions and mechanisms as applied to electronic chemistry; such as computers, employing various aspects of physics, mathematics, and chemistry; *e.g.,* improving cybernetic engineering by reference to the organization of the vertebrate nervous system. 2. The science of applying the knowledge gained by studying the characteristics of living organisms to the formulation of nonorganic devices and techniques. [bio- + electronics]

bi·o·nom·ics (bī-ō-nom'iks). 1. SYN bionomy. 2. SYN ecology.

bi·on·o·my (bī-on'ō-mē). The laws of life; the science concerned with the laws regulating the vital functions. SYN bionomics (1). [bio- + G. *nomos,* law]

bi·o·phage (bī'ō-fāj). An organism that derives the nourishment for its existence from another living organism.

bi·oph·a·gism (bī-of'ă-jizm). The deriving of nourishment from living organisms. SYN biophagy. [bio- + G. *phagō,* to eat]

bi·oph·a·gous (bī-of'ă-gŭs). Feeding on living organisms; denoting certain parasites.

bi·oph·a·gy (bī-of'ă-jē). SYN biophagism.

bi·o·phar·ma·ceu·tics (bī'ō-far-mă-sū'tiks). The study of the physical and chemical properties of a drug, and its dosage form, as related to the onset, duration, and intensity of drug action.

bi·o·phil·ia (bī-ō-fil'ē-ă). The instinct of self-preservation. [bio- + G. *philia,* love, fondness for]

bi·o·pho·tom·e·ter (bī-ō-fō-tom'ĕ-ter). An obsolete instrument once used for measuring the rate and degree of dark adaptation. Cf. adaptometer.

bi·o·phy·lac·tic (bī'ō-fī-lak'tik). Relating to biophylaxis.

bi·o·phy·lax·is (bī-ō-fī-lak'sis). Nonspecific defense reactions of the body, *e.g.,* phagocytosis, vascular and other reactions of inflammatory processes. [bio- + G. *phylaxis,* protection]

bi·o·phys·ics (bī-ō-phyz'iks). 1. The study of biological processes and materials by means of the theories and tools of physics. 2. The study of physical processes (*e.g.,* electricity, luminescence) occurring in organisms.

cellular b., b. concerned with cellular processes.

dental b., the relationship between the biologic behavior of oral structures and the physical influence of a dental restoration. SYN dental biomechanics.

medical b., b. related to diagnosis and therapy.

molecular b., b. concerned with membrane processes, conformational and configurational properties of macromolecules, bioelectrical phenomena, etc.

radiation b., the study of the effects of radiation on cells, tissues, biomolecules, and living organisms.

bi·o·plasm (bī'ō-plazm). Protoplasm, especially in its relation to living processes and development. [bio- + G. *plasma,* thing formed]

bi·o·plas·mic (bī-ō-plas'mik). Relating to bioplasm.

bi·o·pol·y·mer (bī'ō-pol'ē-mer). A naturally occurring compound that is a polymer of identical or similar subunits.

aperiodic b., a b. consisting of nonidentical subunits present in a nonperiodic sequence.

periodic b., a b. in which there are identical, repeating subunits.

bi·op·sy (bī'op-sē). 1. Process of removing tissue from living patients for diagnostic examination. 2. A specimen obtained by b. [bio- + G. *opsis,* vision]

aspiration b., SYN needle b.

brush b., b. obtained by passing a bristled catheter into the ureter or pyelocalyceal system to remove cells from suspected areas of disease by entrapping them in the bristles.

chorionic villus b., transcervical or transabdominal sampling of the chorionic villi for genetic analysis.

endoscopic b., b. obtained by instruments passed through an endoscope or obtained by a needle introduced under endoscopic guidance.

bi

excision b., excision of tissue for gross and microscopic examination in such a manner that the entire lesion is removed.

fine needle b., removal of tissue or suspensions of cells through a small needle.

incision b., removal of only a part of a lesion by incising into it.

needle b., any method in which the specimen for b. is removed by aspirating it through an appropriate needle or trocar that pierces the skin, or the external surface of an organ, and into the underlying tissue to be examined. SYN aspiration b.

open b., surgical incision or excision of the region from which the b. is taken.

punch b., any method that removes a small cylindrical specimen for b. by means of a special instrument that pierces the organ directly or through the skin or a small incision in the skin. SYN trephine b.

shave b., a b. technique performed with a surgical blade or a razor blade; used for lesions that are elevated above the skin level or confined to the epidermis and upper dermis, or to protrusions of lesions from internal sites.

sponge b., abrasion of a lesion with a suitable sponge.

trephine b., SYN punch b.

wedge b., excision of a cuneiform specimen.

bi·o·psy·chol·o·gy (bī'ō-sī-kol'ō-jē). An interdisciplinary area of study involving psychology, biology, physiology, biochemistry, the neural sciences, and related fields.

bi·o·psy·cho·social (bī-ō-sī'kō-sō- shăl). Involving interplay of biological, psychological and social influences.

bi·op·ter·in (bī-op'ter-in). 6-(1,2-Dihydroxypropyl)pterin; a pterin found in yeast, the fruit fly, and in normal human urine.

bi·op·tome (bī-op'tōm). A biopsy instrument passed through a catheter into the heart to obtain pieces of tissue for diagnosis. [biopsy + G. tomē, a cutting]

bi·o·py·o·cul·ture (bī-ō-pī'ō-kŭl-chŭr). A culture made from purulent exudate in which various cells, including the phagocytes, are still viable. [bio- + G. pyon, pus, + culture]

bi·or·bit·al (bī-ōr'bī-tăl). Relating to both orbits. [bi- + G. orbita, orbit]

bi·o·rhe·ol·o·gy (bī'ō-rē-ol'ō-jē). The science concerned with deformation and flow in biological systems. [bio- + G. rheō, to flow, + logos, study]

bi·o·rhythm (bī'ō-rith-m). A biologically inherent cyclic variation or recurrence of an event or state, such as the sleep cycle, circadian rhythms, or periodic diseases. [bio- + G. rhythmos, rhythm]

bi·o·roent·gen·og·ra·phy (bī'ō-rent-jen-og'ră-fē). Obsolete term for the making of x-ray pictures of subjects in motion. SEE cineradiography. SEE ALSO video fluoroscopy. [bio- + roentgenography]

bi·o·safe·ty (b-ī'ō-saf'tē). Safety measures applied to the handling of biological materials or organisms with a known potential to cause disease in humans. Current recommendations from the Centers for Disease Control are to follow universal precautions, that is to treat all human samples of blood and body fluid as though they were infectious.

bi·ose (bī'ōs). SYN glycolaldehyde.

bi·o·side (bī'ō-sīd). SYN disaccharide.

bi·o·sis (bī-ō'sis). Life, in a general sense. [G. biōsis, way of living]

bi·o·so·cial (bī-ō-sō'shŭl). Involving the interplay of biological and social influences.

bi·o·spec·trom·e·try (bī-ō-spek-trom'ĕ-trē). Spectroscopic determination of the types and amounts of various substances in living tissue or fluid from a living body. SYN clinical spectrometry. [bio- + L. spectrum, an image, + G. metron, measure]

bi·o·spec·tros·co·py (bī'ō-spek-tros'kō-pē). Spectroscopic examination of specimens of living tissue, including fluids removed therefrom. SYN clinical spectroscopy. [bio- + L. spectrum, image, + G. skopeō, to examine]

bi·o·spe·le·ol·o·gy (bī'ō-spē'lē-ol'ō-jē). The study of organisms whose natural habitat is wholly or partly subterranean. [bio- + G. spēliaion, cave]

bi·o·sphere (bī'ō-sfēr). All the regions in the world where living organisms are found. [bio- + G. sphaira, sphere]

bi·o·stat·ics (bī-ō-stat'iks). The science of the relation between structure and function in organisms. [bio- + G. statikos, causing to stand]

bi·o·sta·tis·tics (bī'ō-stă-tis'tiks). The science of statistics applied to biological or medical data.

bi·o·syn·the·sis (bī-ō-sin'thĕ-sis). Formation of a chemical compound by enzymes, either in the organism (in vivo) or by fragments or extracts of cells (in vitro). SYN biogenesis (2).

bi·o·syn·thet·ic (bī'ō-sin-thet'ik). Relating to or produced by biosynthesis.

bi·o·sys·tem (bī'ō-sis-tem). A living organism or any complete system of living things that can, directly or indirectly, interact with others.

Biot, Camille, 19th century French physician. SEE B.'s breathing, respiration, respiration, breathing sign, sign.

bi·o·ta (bī-ō'tă). The collective flora and fauna of a region. [Mod. L., fr. G. bios, life]

bi·o·tax·is (bī-ō-tak'sis). 1. The classification of living beings according to their anatomical characteristics. 2. SYN cytoclesis. [bio- + G. taxis, arrangement]

bi·o·tech·nol·ogy (bī'ō-tek-nol'ō-jē). 1. The field devoted to applying the techniques of biochemistry, cellular biology, biophysics, and molecular biology to addressing issues related to human beings and the environment. 2. The use of recombinant DNA or hybridoma technologies for production of useful molecules, or for the alteration of biological processes to enhance some desired property.

bi·o·te·lem·e·try (bī-ō-tel-em'ĕ-trē). The technique of monitoring vital processes and transmitting data without wires to a point remote from the subject.

bi·o·test (bī'ō-test). A method for assessing the effect of a compound, technique, or procedure on an organism. SYN biological assay.

bi·ot·ic (bī-ot'ik). Pertaining to life.

bi·ot·ics (bī-ot'iks). The science concerned with the functions of life, or vital activity and force. [G. biōtikos, relating to life]

bi·o·tin (bī'ō-tin). cis-hexahydro-2-oxo-1H-thieno[3,4-d]-imidazoline-4-valeric acid; the D-isomer component of the vitamin B_2 complex occurring in or required by most organisms and inactivated by avidin; participates in biological carboxylations. It is a small molecule with a high affinity for avidin that can be readily coupled to a previously labeled antibody in order to allow visualization by enzymatic or histochemical means. SEE ALSO avidin. SYN coenzyme R, vitamin H, W factor.

b. carboxylase, a subunit of a number of enzymes (e.g., acetyl-CoA carboxylase). It catalyzes the formation of carboxybiotin (on a biotin carrier protein), ADP, and P_i from ATP, CO_2 and biotin.

b. oxidase, an enzyme (probably nonspecific) catalyzing the beta-oxidation of the b. side chain.

bi·o·tin·i·dase (bī-ō-tin'i-dās). An enzyme catalyzing the hydrolysis of biotin amide (forming biotin and ammonia), biocytin (forming biotin and lysine), and other biotinides. A deficiency of b. can lead to organic acidemia.

bi·ot·i·nides (bī-ot'i-nīdz). Compounds of biotin; e.g., biocytin.

bi·o·tin·yl·ly·sine (bī'ō-tin-il-lī'sin). SYN biocytin.

bi·o·tope (bī'ō-tōp). The smallest geographical area providing uniform conditions for life; the physical part of an ecosystem. [G. bios, life, + topos, place]

bi·o·tox·i·col·o·gy (bī'ō-tok-si-kol'ō-jē). The study of poisons produced by living organisms.

bi·o·tox·in (bī-ō-tok'sin). Any toxic substance formed in an animal body, and demonstrable in its tissues or body fluids, or both.

bi·o·trans·for·ma·tion (bī'ō-trans-fōr-mā'shŭn). The conversion of molecules from one form to another within an organism, often associated with change in pharmacologic activity; refers especially to drugs and other xenobiotics. SYN biodegradation.

bi·o·tro·pism (bī-ō-trō'pizm). Obsolete term for a theory that a drug eruption may be due to activation of a latent allergy by the drug. [bio- + G. *trope*, a turning]

bi·o·type (bī′ō-tīp). **1.** A population or group of individuals composed of the same genotype. **2.** In bacteriology, former name for biovar. [bio- + G. *typos*, model]

bi·o·var (bī′ō-var). A group (infrasubspecific) of bacterial strains distinguishable from other strains of the same species on the basis of physiological characters. Formerly called biotype. [bio- + *variant*]

bi·o·vu·lar (bī′ov-yū-lar). SYN diovular.

bi·pal·a·ti·noid (bī-pal′ă-ti-noyd). A capsule with two compartments, used for making remedies in nascent form; the reaction between the two substances takes place as the capsule dissolves in the stomach, thus activating the remedy.

bi·par·a·sit·ism (bī-par′ă-sit-izm). SYN hyperparasitism.

bi·pa·ren·tal (bī-pa-ren′tăl). Having two parents, male and female.

bi·pa·ri·e·tal (bī-pa-rī′ĕ-tăl). Relating to both parietal bones of the skull. [bi- + L. *paries*, wall]

bip·a·rous (bip′ă-rŭs). Bearing two young. [bi- + L. *pario*, to give birth]

bi·par·tite (bī-par′tīt). Consisting of two parts or divisions.

bi·ped (bī′ped). **1.** Two-footed. **2.** Any animal with only two feet. [bi- + L. *pes*, foot]

bi·ped·al (bī′ped-ăl). **1.** Relating to a biped. **2.** Capable of locomotion on two feet; *e.g.*, an iguana and some other lizards have this capability.

bi·pen·nate, bi·pen·ni·form (bī-pen′āt, pen′i-fōrm). Pertaining to a muscle with a central tendon toward which the fibers converge on either side like the barbs of a feather. [bi- + L. *penna*, feather]

bi·per·fo·rate (bī-per′fō-rāt). Having two foramina or perforations.

bi·per·i·den (bī-per′i-den). α-5-Norbornen-2-yl-α-phenyl-1-piperidinepropanol; an anticholinergic agent with sedative and central effects on the basal ganglia; used in the symptomatic treatment of parkinsonism and drug-induced parkinsonism. Also available as b. hydrochloride.

bi·phen·a·mine hy·dro·chlo·ride (bī-fen′ă-mēn). Xenysalate hydrochloride; 2-diethylaminoethyl 2-hydroxy-3-phenylbenzoate hydrochloride; an antiseborrheic agent.

bi·phe·no·ty·pic (bī′fē-nō-tip′ik). Pertaining to or characterized by biphenotypy.

bi·phe·no·ty·py (bī-fē′nō-tī′pē). The expression of markers of more than one cell type by the same cell, as in certain leukemias.

bi·phen·yl (bī-fen′il). SYN diphenyl.

polychlorinated b. (PCB), b. in which some or all of the hydrogen atoms attached to ring carbons are replaced by chlorine atoms; a probable human carcingogen and teratogen.

bi·po·lar (bī-pō′ler). Having two poles, ends, or extremes.

bi·po·ten·ti·al·i·ty (bī′pō-ten-shē-al′i-tē). Capability of differentiating along two developmental pathways. An example is the capacity of the gonad to develop into either an ovary or a testis.

bi·ra·mous (bī-rā′mŭs). Having two branches. [bi- + L. *ramus*, branch]

Birbeck, Michael S., contemporary British cancer researcher. SEE B.'s *granule.*

Birch-Hirschfeld, Felix V., German pathologist, 1842–1899. SEE Birch-Hirschfeld *stain.*

birch tar (berch). SYN birch tar oil.

birch tar oil. Pyroligneous oil obtained by the dry distillation of the wood of *Betula alba* and rectified by steam distillation; used externally in the treatment of skin diseases. SYN birch tar.

Bird, Samuel D., Australian physician, 1833–1904. SEE B.'s *sign.*

bi·re·frin·gence (bī-rē-frin′jens). SYN double *refraction.*

bi·re·frin·gent (bī-rē-frin′-jent). Refracting twice; splitting a ray of light in two.

Bir·na·vi·ri·dae (bir′nă-vī′rā-dā). A family of icosahedral nonenveloped viruses, 60 nm in diameter whose genome consists of two segments of linear double-stranded RNA.

Bir·navi·rus (bir′nă-vī-rŭs). A virus in the family Birnaviridae that includes infectious bursal disease virus of chickens and infectious pancreatic necrosis virus of fish. [bi- + RNA + virus]

bi·ro·ta·tion (bī-rō-tā′shŭn). SYN mutarotation.

birth (berth). **1.** Passage of the offspring from the uterus to the outside world; the act of being born. **2.** Specifically, in the human, complete expulsion or extraction from its mother of a fetus, irrespective of gestational age, and regardless of whether or not the umbilical cord has been cut or whether or not the placenta is attached.

b. certificate, official, legal document recording details of a live b., usually comprising name, date, place, identity of parents, and sometimes additional information such as b. weight.

cross b., obsolete term for: obsolete term for transverse *lie*; transverse *presentation.*

premature b., b. of an infant after viability has been achieved with gestation of at least 20 weeks or birth weight of at least 500 gr, but before 37 weeks.

birth·mark (berth′mark). A persistent visible lesion, usually on the skin, identified at or near birth; commonly due to nevus or hemangioma. SEE nevus (1).

strawberry b., SYN strawberry *nevus.*

bis-. **1.** Prefix signifying two or twice. **2.** In chemistry, used to denote, the presence of two identical but separated complex groups in one molecule. Cf. bi-, di-. [L.]

bis·ac·o·dyl (bis-ak′ō-dil). 4,4′-(2-Pyridylmethylene)diphenol diacetate; bis(*p*-acetoxyphenyl)-2-pyridylmethane; a laxative used orally or rectally for constipation.

bis·a·cro·mi·al (bis′ă-krō′mē-ăl). Relating to both acromion processes.

bis·al·bu·mi·ne·mia (bis′al-byū′mi-nē′mē-ă). The concurrence of having two kinds of serum albumin that differ in mobility on electrophoresis: normal albumin (albumin A) and any one of several variant types that migrate at other speeds; individuals are heterozygous for the gene for albumin A and the gene for the variant albumin type. SEE ALSO inherited albumin *variants*, under *variant.*

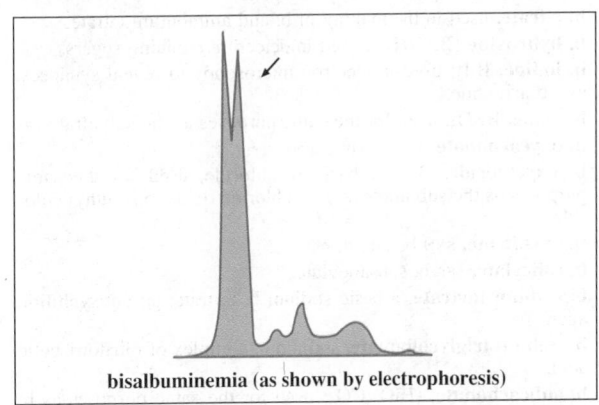

bisalbuminemia (as shown by electrophoresis)

bi·salt (bī′sawlt). SYN acid *salt.*

bis·ax·il·lary (bis-ak′si-lār-ē). Relating to both axillae.

bis·ben·zy·liso·quinoline al·ka·loids (bis-ben′zil-ī-sō-kwin′ō-lin ăl-ka-loids). A group of alkaloids whose base structure is two fused isoquinoline rings *e.g.*, curare alkaloids.

2,5-bis(5-*t*-bu·tyl·ben·zox·a·zol-2-yl)thi·o·phene (BBOT). A scintillator used in radioactivity measurements by scintillation counting.

Bischof, W., 20th century German neurosurgeon. SEE B.'s *myelotomy.*

bis·cuit (bis′kit). A term associated with the firing of porcelain, and applied to the fired article before glazing. May be any stage after the fluxes have flowed enough to provide rigidity to the structure up to the stage where shrinkage is complete. Referred to as low, medium or high b., depending on the completeness of vitrification, also as hard or soft b.

bis·cuit-bake. The initial bake(s) given fusing porcelain at lower than glazing temperature to control shrinkage during the process of building up the dental restoration. SYN biscuit-firing.

bis·cuit-fir·ing. SYN biscuit-bake.

bis·de·qua·lin·i·um chlo·ride (bis'de-kwă-lin'ē-ŭm). 1,1'-De-camethylene-4,4'-(1,10-decamethylenediimino)bis[quinaldinium chloride]; an antiseptic.

bis in die (bis in dē'ā). Twice a day. [L.]

bi·sex·u·al (bī-seks'yū-ăl). 1. Having gonads of both sexes. SEE ALSO hermaphroditism. 2. Denoting an individual who engages in both heterosexual and homosexual relations.

bis·fer·i·ent (bis-fer'ē-ent). SYN bisferious.

bis·fer·i·ous (bis-fēr'ē-ŭs). Striking twice; said of the pulse. SYN bisferient. [L. *bis*, twice, + *ferio*, to strike]

Bishop, Louis F., U.S. physician, 1864–1941. SEE B.'s *sphygmoscope*.

bis·hy·drox·y·cou·ma·rin (bis-hī-drox'ē-kū'mă-rin). SYN dicumarol.

bis·il·i·ac (bis-il'ē-ak). Relating to any two corresponding iliac parts or structures, as the iliac bones or iliac fossae.

Bismarck brown R [C.I. 21010]. A diazo dye similar to Bismarck brown Y.

Bismarck brown Y [C.I. 21000]. A diazo dye used for staining mucin and cartilage in histologic sections, in the Papanicolaou technique for vaginal smears, and as one of Kasten's Schiff-type reagents in the PAS and Feulgen stains. SYN vesuvin. [Ger. *bismarckbraun*, after Otto von *Bismarck*, Ger. chancellor]

bis·muth (Bi) (biz'mŭth). A trivalent metallic element; atomic no. 83, atomic wt. 20.98037. Several of its salts are used in medicine; some contain BiO^+, rather than Bi^{3+}, and are called subsalts. [Ger. *Wismut*, Weisse Masse, white mass]

b. aluminate, a gastric antacid. SYN aluminum bismuth oxide.

b. ammonium citrate, ammoniocitrate of b.; an intestinal astringent.

b. carbonate, SYN b. subcarbonate.

b. chloride oxide, SYN b. oxychloride.

b. citrate, used in the making of b. and ammonium citrate.

b. hydroxide (Bi(OH)₃), used in detecting reducing sugars.

b. iodide, BiI_3; used in electron microscopy to reveal synapses. SYN b. triiodide.

b. oxide, Bi_2O_3; used for the same purposes as the subnitrate.

b. oxycarbonate, SYN b. subcarbonate.

b. oxychloride, BiOCl; basic b. chloride, used for the same purposes as the subnitrate. SYN b. chloride oxide, bismuthyl chloride.

b. oxynitrate, SYN b. subnitrate.

b. salicylate, SEE b. subsalicylate.

b. sodium tartrate, a basic sodium b. tartrate; an antisyphilitic agent.

b. sodium triglycollamate, sodium b. complex of nitrilotriacetic acid.

b. subcarbonate, $(BiO)_2CO_3$; used for the same purposes as b. subnitrate, but has lower toxicity. SYN b. carbonate, b. oxycarbonate, bismuthyl carbonate.

b. subgallate, used internally in diarrhea and externally as an astringent and protective dusting powder.

b. subnitrate, a basic salt, the composition of which varies with the conditions of preparation; used internally as an intestinal astringent and externally as a mild astringent and antiseptic; the metal is used as an electron microscope stain for nucleic acids. SYN b. oxynitrate.

b. subsalicylate, used as an intestinal antiseptic.

b. tribromophenate, b. tribromophenol, used externally as an antiseptic.

b. trichloride, $BiCl_3$; addition of water results in formation of b. oxychloride. SYN butter of bismuth.

b. triiodide, SYN b. iodide.

bis·mu·tho·sis (bis-mŭ-thō'sis). Chronic bismuth poisoning.

bis·muth·yl (biz'mŭ-thil). The group, BiO^+, that behaves chemically as the ion of a univalent metal; its salts are subsalts of bismuth.

b. carbonate, SYN *bismuth* subcarbonate.

b. chloride, SYN *bismuth* oxychloride.

bis·ox·a·tin ac·e·tate (bis-ok'să-tin). 2,2-Bis(*p*-hydroxyphenyl)-2*H*-1,4-benzoxazin-3(4*H*)-one diacetate; a laxative.

1,4-bis(5-phen·yl·ox·a·zol-2-yl)ben·zene. A liquid scintillation agent used in radioisotope measurement.

bi·ste·phan·ic (bī'stĕ-fan'ik). Relating to both stephanions; denoting particularly the b. width of the cranium, or b. diameter, the shortest distance from one stephanion to the other.

bi·ste·roid (bī-stēr'oyd). A molecule composed of two molecules of a given steroid joined together by a carbon-to-carbon bond.

bis·tou·ry (bis'tū-rē). A long, narrow-bladed knife, with a straight or curved edge and sharp or blunt point (probe-point); used for opening or slitting cavities or hollow structures. [Fr. *bistouri*, fr. It. dialect *bistori*, perh. fr. *Pistoia*, Italy]

bi·stra·tal (bī-strā'tăl). Having two strata or layers.

bi·sul·fate (bī-sŭl'fāt). A salt containing HSO_4^-. SYN acid sulfate.

bi·sul·fide (bī-sŭl'fīd). A compound of the anion HS^-; an acid sulfide.

bi·sul·fite (bī-sŭl'fīt). A salt or ion of HSO_3^-.

bit. Acronym for binary *digit*.

bi·tar·trate (bī-tar'trāt). A salt or anion resulting from the neutralization of one of tartaric acid's two acid groups.

bitch. A female dog of breeding age. [O.E. *bicche*]

bite (bīt). 1. To incise or seize with the teeth. 2. The act of incision or seizure with the teeth. 3. A morsel of food held between the teeth. 4. Term used to denote the amount of pressure developed in closing the jaws. 5. Undesirable jargon for terms such as interocclusal record, maxillomandibular registration, denture space, and interarch distance. 6. A wound or puncture of the skin made by animal or insect. SEE bites. [A.S. *bītan*]

balanced b., SYN balanced *occlusion*.

biscuit b., SYN maxillomandibular *record*.

close b., SYN small interarch *distance*.

closed b., reduced vertical interarch distance with excessive vertical overlap of the anterior teeth.

deep b., an abnormally large vertical overlap of anterior teeth in centric occlusion.

edge-to-edge b., SYN edge-to-edge *occlusion*.

end-to-end b., SYN edge-to-edge *occlusion*.

jumping the b., an orthodontic technique for correcting a crossbite, usually anterior.

locked b., an occlusion in which the cusp arrangement restricts lateral excursions.

normal b., SYN normal *occlusion* (1).

open b., (1) SYN large interarch *distance*. (2) SYN apertognathia.

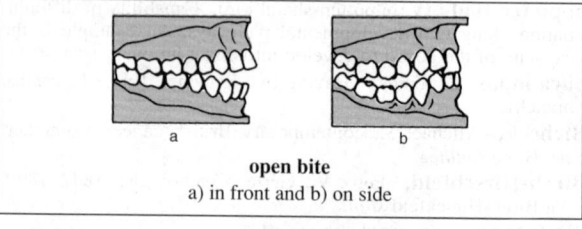

open bite
a) in front and b) on side

rest b., a misnomer for physiologic rest *position* of the mandible.

working b., SYN working *contacts*, under *contact*.

bi·tem·po·ral (bī-tem'pŏ-răl). Relating to both temples or temporal bones.

bite·plate, bite·plane (bīt'plāt, bīt'plān). A removable appliance that incorporates a plane of acrylic designed to occlude with the opposing teeth.

bites (bītz). Penetration of the skin (puncture or laceration) causing reactions that result from 1) mechanical injury; 2) injection of toxic material such as snake or scorpion venom; 3) injection of antigenic substance, especially by insect or arthropod bites, capable of inducing and eliciting allergic sensitization; 4) introduction of otherwise saprophytic flora such as *Staphylococcus pyogenes* in the instance of human bites; 5) invasion of the tissue as in myiasis; 6) transmission of disease such as typhus and rabies. Depending on the nature of the material propelled into the puncture of the skin and, in the case of antigenic material, on the previous exposure and immunity of the host, the local reaction will be immediate or delayed, accompanied by varying degrees of pain, itching and burning, and systemic manifestations specific for the offending agent. [see bite]

bite·wing (bīt′wing). SEE bitewing *radiograph.*

bi·thi·o·nol (bī-thī′ŏ-nol). 2,2′-Thiobis[4,6-dichlorophenol]; an antiparasitic agent used for treatment of the human lungworm, *Paragonimus westermani*, and the Oriental liver fluke, *Clonorchis sinensis;* also used as a bacteriostat in soaps and detergents; sodium bithionate is used as a topical bactericide and fungicide.

bi·tol·ter·ol mes·y·late (bī-tol′ter-ol). 4-[2-(*tert*-Butylamino)-1-hydroxyethyl]-o-phenylenedi(*p*-toluate)methanesulfonate; a sympathomimetic bronchodilator used in the prophylaxis and treatment of bronchial asthma and reversible bronchospasm.

Bitot, Pierre A., French physician, 1822–1888. SEE B.'s *spots*, under *spot.*

bi·tro·chan·ter·ic (bī-trō-kan-ter′ik). Relating to two trochanters, either to the two trochanters of one femur or to both great trochanters.

bi·tro·pic (bī-trop′ik). Having a dual affinity, as in tissues or organisms. [bi- + G. *tropē*, a turning]

bit·ter ap·ple. SYN colocynth.

bit·ters. 1. An alcoholic liquor in which bitter vegetable substances (*e.g.,* quinine, gentian) have been steeped. 2. Bitter vegetable drugs (*e.g.,* quassia, gentian, cinchona), usually used as tonics. SYN amara.

aromatic b., b. with a pleasant aromatic flavor.

Bittner, John J., U.S. oncologist, 1904–1961. SEE B. *agent;* B.'s milk *factor.*

Bittorf, Alexander, German physician, 1876–1949. SEE B.'s *reaction.*

bi·u·ret (bī-ū-ret′). NH(CONH₂)₂; a derivative of urea obtained by heating, eliminating one NH_3 between two ureas. Used in protein determinations. SYN allophanamide, carbamoylurea.

bi·va·lence, bi·va·len·cy (bī-vā′lens, bī-vā′len-sē). A combining power (valence) of 2. SYN divalence, divalency.

bi·va·lent (bī-vā′lent, biv′ă-lent). 1. Having a combining power (valence) of 2. SYN divalent. 2. In cytology, a structure consisting of two paired homologous chromosomes, each split into two sister chromatids, as seen during the pachytene stage of prophase in meiosis.

bi·ven·ter (bī-ven′ter). Two-bellied; denoting two-bellied muscles. [bi- + L. *venter,* belly]

b. cer′vicis, SYN spinalis capitis *muscle.*

b. mandib′ulae, SYN digastric *muscle.*

bi·ven·tral (bī-ven′tral). SYN digastric (1).

bi·ven·tric·u·lar (bī′ven-trik′ū-lar). Pertaining to both right and left ventricles.

bix·in (bik′sin). A monomethyl ester of a 24-carbon branched unsaturated dicarboxylic acid; a carotenoid (a carotene-dioic acid); the orange-red coloring matter from seeds of *Bixa orellana;* the ethyl ester is used as a food and drug colorant. SEE ALSO annotto.

bi·zy·go·mat·ic (bī′zī-gō-mat′ik). Relating to both zygomatic bones or arches.

Bizzozero, Giulio, Italian physician, 1846–1901. SEE B.'s *corpuscle.*

Bjerrum, Jannik P., Danish ophthalmologist, 1851–1926. SEE B.'s *scotoma;* B.'s *screen;* B.'s *sign.*

Bjork-Shiley valve. See under valve.

Bjornstad, R., 20th century Scandinavian dermatologist. SEE B.'s *syndrome.*

Bk Symbol for berkelium.

Black, Douglas A.K., Scottish physician, *1909. SEE B.'s *formula.*

Black, Greene V., U.S. dentist, 1836–1915. SEE B.'s *classification.*

Blackfan, Kenneth D., U.S. physician, 1883–1941. SEE Diamond-B. *anemia, syndrome.*

black·head (blak′hed). 1. SYN open *comedo.* 2. SYN histomoniasis.

black·leg (blak′leg). A highly fatal, specific, essentially gas-gangrenous infection caused by *Clostridium chavoei* and affecting the muscular upper parts of the legs of young cattle and sheep. SYN quarter evil.

black·out (blak′owt). 1. Temporary loss of consciousness due to decreased blood flow to the brain. 2. Momentary loss of consciousness as an absence. 3. Temporary loss of vision, without alteration of consciousness, due to positive (> normal) g (gravity) forces; caused by temporary decreased blood flow in the central retinal artery, and seen mostly in aviators. 4. A transient episode that occurs during a state of intense intoxication (alcoholic b.) for which the person has no recall, although not unconscious (as observed by others).

visual b., SEE *amaurosis* fugax.

blad·der (blad′er). A distensible musculomembranous organ serving as a receptacle for fluid, as the gallbladder. SEE detrusor. SYN vesica (1). [A.S. *blaedre*]

air b., a two-chambered gas-filled sac that is present in most fish and functions as a hydrostatic organ; it is located beneath the vertebral column, and is connected with the esophagus in some fish. SYN swim b.

allantoic b., a type of b. formed as an outgrowth of the cloaca.

atonic b., a large, dilated, and nonemptying b.; usually due to disturbance of innervation or to chronic obstruction.

autonomic neurogenic b., malfunctioning b., secondary to low spinal cord lesions.

gall b., SYN gallbladder.

hyperreflexic b., a b. exhibiting detrusor instability.

hypertonic b., a b. with poor compliance.

ileal b., SYN ileal *conduit.*

neurogenic b., SYN neuropathic b.

neuropathic b., any defective functioning of bladder due to impaired innervation, *e.g.,* cord b., neuropathic b. SYN neurogenic b.

nonneurogenic neurogenic b., detrusor-sphincter incoordination with urinary incontinence, constipation, UTI, upper tract changes. SYN Hinman syndrome, pseudoneurogenic b.

poorly compliant b., a b. that has high pressure at low volumes in the absence of detrusor activity.

pseudoneurogenic b., SYN nonneurogenic neurogenic b.

reflex neurogenic b., an abnormal condition of b. function whereby the b. is cut off from upper motor neuron control, but where the lower motor neuron arc is still intact.

swim b., SYN air b.

trabeculated b., characterized by thick wall and hypertrophied muscle bundles. Typically seen in instances of long-standing obstruction.

uninhibited neurogenic b., a condition, either congenital or acquired, of abnormal b. function whereby normal inhibitory control of detrusor function by the central nervous system is impaired or underdeveloped, resulting in precipitant or uncontrolled micturition and/or anuresis.

unstable b., characterized by uninhibited detrusor contractions.

urinary b., a musculomembranous elastic bag serving as a storage place for the urine. SYN vesica urinaria [NA], cystis urinaria, urocyst, urocystis.

blad·der cal·cu·li. See under calculus.

blad·der·worm (blad′er-werm). SYN *Cysticercus.*

blade·vent (blād′vent). A thin, wedge-shaped endo-osseous implant of metal that is inserted into a surgically prepared groove in the maxilla or mandible.

Blagden, Sir Charles, British physician, 1748–1820. SEE B.'s *law.*

blain (blān). Archaic term for a lesion on the skin. [A.S. *blegen*]

Blainville, Henri Marie Ducrotay de, French zoologist and anthropologist, 1777–1850. SEE B. ears, under *ear.*

Blair, Vilray P., U.S. surgeon, 1871–1955. SEE B.-Brown *graft.*

Blakemore, Arthur H., U.S. surgeon, 1897–1970. SEE Sengstaken-B. *tube.*

Blalock, Alfred, U.S. surgeon, 1899–1965. SEE B. *shunt;* B.-Hanlon *operation;* B.-Taussig *operation, shunt.*

Blandin, Philippe Frédéric, French anatomist and surgeon, 1798–1849. SEE B.'s *gland.*

blank. A solution consisting of all of the analytical components except the compound to be measured; this is used to establish a baseline of measurement intensity against which the compound of interest is compared. [M.E. white, fr. O.Fr. *blanc,* fr. Germanic]

blas. Term invented by van Helmont to denote a mystical spirit or vital force which presided over and governed the various processes of the body. Each bodily function was supposed to have its own special b.; b. appears to be the counterpart of the archaeus of Paracelsus. [a Middle E. variant of *blast*]

Blasius, Gerhard (Blaes), 17th century Dutch anatomist. SEE B.'s *duct.*

☖-blast. An immature precursor cell of the type indicated by the preceding word. [G. *blastos,* germ]

blas·te·ma (blas-tē′mă). **1.** The primordial cellular mass (precursor) from which an organ or part is formed. **2.** A cluster of cells competent to initiate the regeneration of a damaged or ablated structure. [G. a sprout]

metanephric b., SYN metanephric *cap.*

nephric b., the extension of nephrogenic cord tissue, caudal to the mesonephros, into which the ureteric buds grow to initiate development of the definitive mammalian kidney. SYN nephroblastema.

blas·tem·ic (blas-tem′ik). Relating to the blastema.

blas·tic (blas′tik). **1.** Describing the formation of a conidium by the blowing out process of a fertile hypha before being limited by a septum. **2.** Colloquial term for osteoblastic. [G. *blastos,* germ + -ic]

☖blasto-. Pertaining to the process of budding (and the formation of buds) by cells or tissue. [G. *blastos,* germ]

blas·to·cele (blas′tō-sēl). The cavity in the blastula of a developing embryo. SYN blastocoele, cleavage cavity, segmentation cavity. [blasto- + G. *koilos,* hollow]

blas·to·cel·ic (blas-tō-sē′lik). Relating to the blastocele. SYN blastocoelic.

blas·to·coele (blas′tō-sēl). SYN blastocele.

blas·to·coel·ic (blas′tō-sē′lik). SYN blastocelic.

Blas·to·co·nid·i·um (blas′tō-cŏ-nid′ē-ŭm). A holoblastic conidium that is produced singly or in chains, and detached at maturity leaving a bud scar, as in the budding of a yeast cell. SYN blastospore. [blasto- + conidium]

blas·to·cyst (blas′tō-sist). The modified blastula stage of mammalian embryos, consisting of the inner cell mass and a thin trophoblast layer enclosing the blastocele. SYN blastodermic vesicle. [blasto- + G. *kystis,* bladder]

Blas·to·cys·tis (blas′tō-sis′tis). A genus of yeastlike parasites in the digestive tract of mammals; generally considered nonpathogenic. Its relationship to fungi is now being questioned owing to protozoan characteristics, such as lack of cell walls, a membrane-bound central body, pseudopod activity, protozoan type of Golgi apparatus and mitochondria, and reproduction by sporulation or binary fission rather than by budding.

B. hominis, a species of B. widespread among humans, formerly considered harmless, now recognized as a cause of mild persistent diarrhea and other intestinal symptoms and eosinophilia when found in heavy infections.

blas·to·cyte (blas′tō-sīt). An undifferentiated blastomere of the morula or blastula stage of an embryo. [blasto- + G. *kytos,* cell]

blas·to·cy·to·ma (blas′tō-sī-tō′mă). SYN blastoma.

blas·to·derm, blas·to·der·ma (blas′tō-derm, -tō-der′ma). The thin, disk-shaped cell mass of a young embryo and its extraem-

bryonic extensions over the surface of the yolk; when fully formed, all three primary germ layers (ectoderm, endoderm, and mesoderm) are present. SYN germ membrane, germinal membrane, membrana germinativa. [blasto- + G. *derma,* skin]

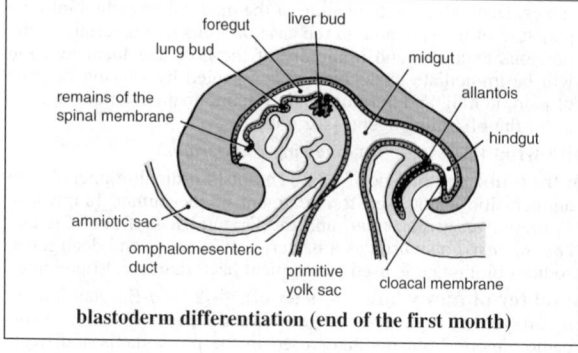

blastoderm differentiation (end of the first month)

bilaminar b., the b. of a young embryo when it consists of only two of the three primary germ layers it will ultimately have.

embryonic b., that part of the b. that takes part in the formation of the embryonic body.

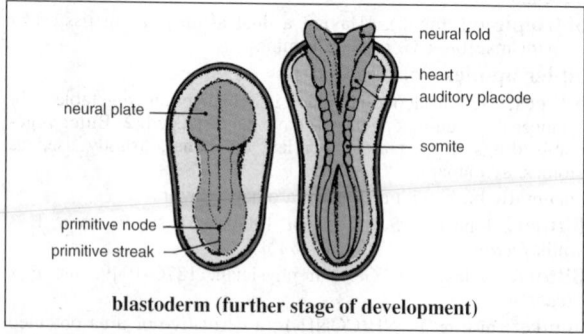

blastoderm (further stage of development)

extraembryonic b., that part of the b. which is not incorporated in the embryo but forms membranes concerned in its nourishment and protection.

trilaminar b., the b. after all three of the primary germ layers have been established.

blas·to·der·mal, blas·to·der·mic (blas-tō-der′măl, -der′mik). Relating to the blastoderm.

blas·to·disk (blas′tō-disk). **1.** The disk of active cytoplasm at the animal pole of a telolecithal egg. **2.** The blastoderm, especially in very young stages when its extent is small.

blas·to·gen·e·sis (blas-tō-jen′ĕ-sis). **1.** Reproduction of unicellular organisms by budding. **2.** Development of an embryo during cleavage and germ layer formation. **3.** Transformation of small lymphocytes of human peripheral blood in tissue culture into large, morphologically undifferentiated blast-like cells capable of undergoing mitosis; can be induced by a variety of agents including phytohemagglutinin, concanavalin A, certain antigens to which the cell donor has been previously immunized, and leukocytes from an unrelated individual. [blasto- + G. *genesis,* origin]

blas·to·ge·net·ic, blas·to·gen·ic (blas′tō-je-net′ik, -tō-jen′ik). Relating to blastogenesis.

blas·tol·y·sis (blas-tol′i-sis). Dissolution or destruction of the blastocyst or blast cells and subsequent death. [blasto- + G. *lysis,* loosening]

blas·to·lyt·ic (blas-tō-lit′ik). Relating to blastolysis.

blas·to·ma (blas-tō′mă). A neoplasm composed chiefly or entirely of immature undifferentiated cells (*i.e.,* blast forms), with little or virtually no stroma. SYN blastocytoma, embryonal carcinosarcoma. [blasto- + G. *-oma,* tumor]

blas·to·mere (blas′tō-mēr). One of the cells into which the egg divides after its fertilization. SYN cleavage cell, embryonic cell. [blasto- + G. *meros,* part]

blas·to·mer·ot·o·my (blas'tō-mēr-ot'ŏ-mē). SYN blastotomy. [blastomere + G. *tomē,* incision]

blas·to·mo·gen·ic (blas'tō-mō-jen'ik). Causing or producing a blastoma.

Blas·to·my·ces der·ma·tit·i·dis (blas-tō-mī'sēz der-mă-tit'i-dis). A dimorphic soil fungus that causes blastomycosis. It grows in mammalian tissues as budding cells and in culture as a white to buff-colored filamentous fungus bearing spherical or ovoid conidia on terminal or lateral short, slender conidiophores. In its perfect (teleomorph) state it is known as *Ajellomyces dermatitidis.* [blasto- + G. *mykēs,* fungus]

blas·to·my·cin (blas-tō-mī'sin). An antigen for intradermal testing prepared from sterile filtrates of cultures of the filamentous form of *Blastomyces dermatitidis.*

blas·to·my·co·sis (blas'tō-mī-kō'sis). A chronic granulomatous and suppurative disease caused by *Blastomyces dermatitidis;* originates as a respiratory infection and disseminates, usually with pulmonary, osseous, and/or cutaneous involvement predominating. Formerly called North American b., the disease now has been found in African states as well as in Canada and the U.S. SYN Gilchrist's disease.

Brazilian b., obsolete term for paracoccidioidomycosis.

cutaneous b., skin lesions seen with infection with *Blastomyces dermatitidis.*

North American b., SEE blastomycosis.

South American b., SYN paracoccidioidomycosis.

systemic b., infection with *Blastomyces dermatitidis* extending beyond the skin or the lung, the usual portals of entry; involvement of bone and genitourinary tract (esp. prostate and epididymis) are most frequent.

blas·to·neu·ro·pore (blas'tō-nū'rō-pōr). A temporary opening formed in some embryos by the union of the blastopore and neuropore. [blasto- + neuropore]

blas·to·phore (blas'tō-fōr). An early stage of division of a coccidial schizont in which spheroid or ellipsoid structures are formed with a single peripheral layer of nuclei; merozoites form at the surface of the b. over each nucleus, grow out radially, and separate from the residual body (remnant of the b.); in a first-generation schizont such as *Eimeria bovis,* about 120,000 merozoites are produced. [blasto- + G. *phorōs,* bearing]

blas·to·pore (blas'tō-pōr). The opening into the archenteron formed by invagination of the blastula to form a gastrula. SYN protostoma, protostome. [blasto- + G. *poros,* opening]

blas·to·spore (blas'tō-spōr). SYN Blastoconidium. [blasto- + G. *sporos,* seed]

blas·tot·o·my (blas-tot'ō-mē). Experimental destruction of one or more blastomeres. SYN blastomerotomy. [blasto- + G. *tomē,* incision]

blas·tu·la (blas'tyū-lă). An early stage of an embryo formed by the rearrangement of the blastomeres of the morula to form a hollow sphere. [G. *blastos,* germ]

blas·tu·lar (blas'tyū-lar). Pertaining to the blastula.

blas·tu·la·tion (blas-tyū-lā'shŭn). Formation of the blastula or blastocyst from the morula.

Blatin, Marc, French physician, *1878. SEE B.'s *syndrome.*

Blat·ta (blat'ă). A genus of insects (family Blattidae) that includes the abundant oriental cockroach, *B. orientalis.* The dried insect yields antihydropin, a diuretic principle. [L. cockroach]

Blat·tel·la (bla-tel'ă). A genus of cockroaches, (family Blattidae) that includes *B. germanica,* the German cockroach or croton bug, probably the most familiar and widespread of the cockroaches. [L. *blatta,* cockroach]

Blat·ti·dae (blat'i-dē). A family of insects (order Blattaria) consisting of over 4,000 species of cockroaches, largely tropical but worldwide in distribution, including a number of abundant pests of households, kitchens, and institutions or facilities, wherever food is present; noxious wherever found, yet not positively incriminated in natural transmission of pathogenic organisms to man. Common household pests include the German cockroach, *Blattella germanica,* the American cockroach, *Periplaneta amer-*

icana, and the oriental cockroach, *Blatta orientalis.* [L. *blatta,* cockroach]

bleb. A large flaccid vesicle.

bleed (blēd). To lose blood as a result of rupture or severance of blood vessels.

bleed·er (blēd'er). Colloquialism for one suffering from hemophilia, Christmas disease, Osler's disease, or other clotting disorders.

bleed·ing (blēd'ing). Losing blood as a result of the rupture or severance of blood vessels.

dysfunctional uterine b., uterine b. due to a benign endocrine abnormality rather than to any organic disease.

occult b., SEE occult *blood.*

blem·ish. 1. A small circumscribed alteration of the skin considered to be unesthetic but insignificant. **2.** To alter the skin, rendering an unesthetic appearance.

blen·nad·e·ni·tis (blen-ad-ĕ-nī'tis). Inflammation of the mucous glands. [G. *blennos,* mucus, + *adēn,* gland, + *-itis,* inflammation]

blen·ne·me·sis (blen-em'ĕ-sis). Rarely used term for vomiting of mucus. [G. *blennos,* mucus, + *emesis,* vomiting]

blenno-, blenn-. Mucus. [G. *blenna, blennos*]

blen·no·gen·ic (blen-ō-jen'ik). SYN muciparous. [blenno- + G. *-gen,* to produce]

blen·nog·e·nous (ble-noj'ĕ-nŭs). SYN muciparous.

blen·noid (blen'oyd). SYN muciform. [blenno- + G. *eidos,* resemblance]

blen·noph·thal·mia (blen-of-thal'mē-ă). **1.** SYN conjunctivitis. **2.** SYN gonorrheal *ophthalmia.*

blen·nor·rha·gia (blen-ō-rā'jē-ă). SYN blennorrhea. [blenno- + G. *rhēgnymi,* to burst forth]

blen·nor·rhag·ic (blen-ō-raj'ik). SYN blennorrheal.

blen·nor·rhea (blen-ō-rē'ă). **1.** Rarely used term for any mucous discharge, especially from the urethra or vagina. **2.** In ophthalmic usage, was synonymous with conjunctivitis, but is now obsolete. SYN blennorrhagia, myxorrhea. [blenno- + G. *rhoia,* a flow]

b. conjunctiva'lis, SYN gonorrheal *ophthalmia.*

inclusion b., a neonatal conjunctivitis caused by *Chlamydia trachomatis.*

b. neonato'rum, SYN *ophthalmia* neonatorum.

Stoerk's b., chronic, first purulent then dry, catarrh of the upper air passages with hypertrophy of the mucous membrane and submucosa, in many cases the same as scleroma.

blen·nor·rhe·al (blen-ō-rē'ăl). Rarely used term relating to blennorrhea. SYN blennorrhagic.

blen·nos·ta·sis (blen-os'tă-sis). Rarely used term for diminution or suppression of secretion from the mucous membranes. [blenno- + G. *stasis,* standing]

blen·no·stat·ic (blen-ō-stat'ik). Rarely used term for diminishing mucous secretion.

blen·nu·ria (ble-nū'rē-ă). The excretion of an excess of mucus in the urine. [blenno- + G. *ouron,* urine]

ble·o·my·cin sul·fate (blē-ō-mī'sin). An antineoplastic antibiotic obtained from *Streptomyces verticillus.*

blephar-. SEE blepharo-.

bleph·ar·ad·e·ni·tis (blef'ar-ad-ĕ-nī'tis). Inflammation of the meibomian glands or the marginal glands of Moll or Zeis. SYN blepharoadenitis. [blephar- + G. *adēn,* gland, + *-itis,* inflammation]

bleph·a·ral (blef'ă-răl). Referring to the eyelids.

bleph·a·rec·to·my (blef'a-rek'tō-mē). Excision of all or part of an eyelid. [blepharo- + G. *ektomē,* excision]

bleph·ar·e·de·ma (blef'ar-ĕ-dē'mă). Edema of the eyelids, causing swelling and often a baggy appearance.

bleph·a·ri·tis (blef'ă-rī'tis). Inflammation of the eyelids. [blepharo- + G. *-itis,* inflammation]

b. acar'ica, SYN demodectic b.

b. angula'ris, inflammation of the lid margins at the angles of the commissure.

ciliary b., SYN b. marginalis.

demodectic b., inflammation of the eyelid associated with *Demodex folliculorum.* SYN b. acarica.

b. follicula′ris, a deep-seated suppurative inflammation of ciliary follicles and the glands of Zeis and Moll of the eyelid. SYN pustular b.

marginal b., SYN b. marginalis.

b. margina′lis, inflammation of the margins of the eyelids. SYN ciliary b., marginal b.

meibomian b., inflammation of the eyelid margin and the meibomian glands.

b. oleo′sa, SYN seborrheic b.

b. parasit′ica, marginal b. due to the presence of lice. SYN b. phthiriatica, pediculous b.

pediculous b., SYN b. parasitica.

b. phthiriat′ica, SYN b. parasitica.

pustular b., SYN b. follicularis.

b. rosa′cea, inflammation of the margins of the eyelids in association with acne rosacea.

seborrheic b., a common type of chronic inflammation of the margins of the eyelids with erythema and white scales; often with an associated seborrheic dermatitis of scalp and face. SYN b. oleosa, b. squamosa.

b. sic′ca, inflammation of the margins of the eyelids in which the lashes are powdered with dry scales.

b. squamo′sa, SYN seborrheic b.

b. ulcero′sa, marginal b. with ulceration.

⌂**blepharo-, blephar-.** Eyelid. [G. *blepharon,* an eyelid]

bleph·a·ro·ad·e·ni·tis (blef′ă-rō-ad-ĕ-nī′tis). SYN blepharadenitis.

bleph·a·ro·ad·e·no·ma (blef′ă-rō-ad-ĕ-nō′mă). A tumor or adenoma of a gland of the eyelid. [blepharo- + G. *adēn,* gland, + *-oma,* tumor]

bleph·a·ro·chal·a·sis (blef′ă-rō-kal′ă-sis). A condition in which there is a redundancy of the skin of the upper eyelids so that a fold of skin hangs down, often concealing the tarsal margin when the eye is open. SYN ptosis adiposa. [blepharo- + G. *chalasis,* a slackening]

bleph·a·ro·chro·mi·dro·sis (blef′ă-rō-krō-mi-drō′sis). Chromidrosis of the eyelids. [blepharo- + G. *chrōma,* color, + *hidrōsis,* sweat]

bleph·a·ro·cloc·lo·nus (blef-ar-ok′lō-nŭs). Clonic spasm of the eyelids. [blepharo- + G. *klonos,* a tumult]

bleph·a·ro·col·o·bo·ma (blef′ă-rō-kol-ō-bō′mă). A defect of the eyelid; may be congenital or acquired. SYN ankyloblepharon. [blepharo- + coloboma]

bleph·a·ro·con·junc·ti·vi·tis (blef′ă-rō-kon-jŭnk-ti-vī′tis). Inflammation of the palpebral conjunctiva.

seborrheic b., SYN meibomian *conjunctivitis.*

bleph·a·ro·di·as·ta·sis (blef′ă-rō-dī-as′tă-sis). Abnormal separation or inability to completely close the eyelids. [blepharo- + G. *diastasis,* separation]

bleph·a·ro·ker·a·to·con·junc·ti·vi·tis (blef′ă-rō-ker′ă-tō-kon-jŭnk′ti-vī′tis). An inflammation involving the eyelids, cornea, and conjunctiva.

bleph·a·ron (blef′ă-ron). SYN eyelid. [G. *blepharon,* eyelid]

bleph·a·ro·phi·mo·sis (blef′ă-rō-fi-mō′sis). Decrease in the size of the palpebral aperture without fusion of lid margins. SYN blepharostenosis. [blepharo- + G. *phimōsis,* an obstruction]

bleph·a·ro·plast (blef′ă-rō-plast). SYN basal *body.* [blepharo- + G. *plastos,* formed]

bleph·a·ro·plas·tic (blef′ă-rō-plas′tik). Relating to blepharoplasty.

bleph·a·ro·plas·ty (blef′ă-ro-plast-tē). Any operation for the correction of a defect in the eyelids. [blepharo- + G. *plassō,* to form]

bleph·a·ro·ple·gia (blef′ă-rō-plē′jē-ă). Paralysis of an eyelid. [blepharo- + G. *plēgē,* stroke]

bleph·a·rop·to·sis, bleph·ar·op·to·sia (blef′ă-rop′tō-sis, -rop-tō′sē-ă). Drooping of the upper eyelid. SYN ptosis (2). [blepharo- + G. *ptōsis,* a falling]

b. adipo′sa, b. causing skin to hang over the free border of the eyelid.

false b., SYN pseudoptosis.

bleph·a·ro·spasm, bleph·a·ro·spas·mus (blef′ă-rō-spazm, -spaz′mŭs). Involuntary spasmodic contraction of the orbicularis oculi muscle; may occur in isolation or be associated with other dystonic contractions of facial, jaw, or neck muscles; usually initiated or aggravated by emotion, fatigue, or drugs.

bleph·a·ro·stat (blef′ă-rō-stat). SYN eye *speculum.* [blepharo- + G. *statos,* fixed]

bleph·a·ro·ste·no·sis (blef′ă-rō-ste-nō′sis). SYN blepharophimosis. [blepharo- + G. *stenōsis,* a narrowing]

bleph·a·ro·syn·ech·ia (blef′ă-rō-sin-ek′ē-ă). Adhesion of the eyelids to each other or to the eyeball. [blepharo- + G. *synecheia,* continuity, fr. *syn- echō,* to hold together]

bleph·a·rot·o·my (blef-ă-rot′ō-mē). A cutting operation on an eyelid. [blepharo- + G. *tomē,* incision]

blind (blīnd). Unable to see; without useful sight. SEE blindness.

blind·ness (blīnd′nes). **1.** Loss of the sense of sight; absolute b. connotes no light perception. SEE ALSO amblyopia, amaurosis. **2.** Loss of visual appreciation of objects although visual acuity is normal. **3.** Absence of the appreciation of sensation, *e.g.,* taste b. SYN typhlosis.

canine hereditary b., an autosomal dominant condition seen in dogs of the collie and several other breeds.

color b., misleading term for anomalous or deficient color vision; complete color b. is the absence of one of the primary cone pigments of the retina. SEE protanopia, deuteranopia, tritanopia.

cortical b., loss of sight due to an organic lesion in the visual cortex.

day b., SYN hemeralopia.

eclipse b., SYN solar *maculopathy.*

flash b., a temporary loss of vision produced when retinal light-sensitive pigments are bleached by light more intense than that to which the retina is physiologically adapted at that moment.

flight b., visual blackout in aviators. SEE ALSO *amaurosis* fugax.

functional b., apparent loss of vision related to suggestibility.

hysterical b., loss of vision or blurring of vision following a highly traumatic event such as seeing one's child killed by a truck.

legal b., generally, visual acuity of less than 6/60 or 20/200 using Snellen test types, or visual field restriction to 20° or less in the better eye; the criteria used to define legal b. vary among different groups.

letter b., visual agnosia for letters. The subject sees the letters but cannot identify them; caused by a lesion in the occipital cortex.

mind b., visual agnosia for objects. The subjet sees the object, but cannot identify it; due to a lesion in area 18 of the occipital cortex. SYN object b., psychanopsia, psychic b.

moon b., SYN periodic *ophthalmia.*

music b., SYN musical *alexia.*

night b., SYN nyctalopia.

note b., SYN musical *alexia.*

object b., SYN mind b.

psychic b., SYN mind b.

river b., SYN ocular *onchocerciasis.*

sight b., SYN asymbolia.

sign b., visual agnosia for signs.

snow b., severe photophobia secondary to ultraviolet keratoconjunctivitis.

solar b., SYN solar *maculopathy.*

taste b., inability to appreciate gustatory stimuli.

text b., word b., SYN alexia.

blis·ter. 1. A fluid-filled thin-walled structure under the epidermis or within the epidermis (subepidermal or intradermal). **2.** To form a b. with heat or some other vesiculating agent.

blood b., a b. containing blood; resulting from a pinch or crushing injury.

fever b., colloquialism for herpes simplex of the lips.

fly b., a cantharidal b. caused by discharge of a vesicating body fluid by certain beetles, particularly members of the family Meloidae which produce cantharidin, *e.g., Lytta (Cantharis) vesicatoria*, the notorious "Spanish fly;" non-cantharidin vesicating fluid is produced by other beetles, such as rove beetles (family Staphylinidae), especially the genus *Paederus*, whose fluid, on contact with the skin, produces an intensely painful b.

flying b., a misnomer for a vesicator agent applied successively to different skin areas and kept in one place just long enough to cause redness but not long enough to cause a b.

blis·ter·ing. SYN vesiculation (1).

bloat, bloat·ing (blōt, blōt′ing). **1.** Abdominal distention from swallowed air or intestinal gas from fermentation. **2.** Distention of the rumen of cattle, caused by the accumulation of gases of fermentation, particularly likely to occur when the animals are pastured on rich legume grasses; if unrelieved, the condition may quickly lead to death.

Bloch, Bruno, Swiss dermatologist, 1878–1933. SEE B.-Sulzberger *disease, syndrome.*

Bloch, Marcel, French physician, 1885–1925. SEE B.'s *reaction.*

block. 1. To obstruct; to arrest passage through. **2.** A condition in which the passage of an electrical impulse is arrested, wholly or in part, temporarily or permanently. **3.** SYN atrioventricular b. [Fr. *bloquer*]

alveolo-capillary b., the presence of material that impairs the diffusion of gases between the air in the alveolar spaces and the blood in alveolar capillaries; b. can be caused by edema, cellular infiltration, fibrosis, or tumor, and results in undersaturation of peripheral arterial blood with oxygen.

anterograde b., conduction b. of an impulse traveling anywhere in its ordinary direction, for example, from the sinoatrial node toward the ventricular myocardium.

arborization b., intraventricular b. supposedly due to widespread blockage in the Purkinje ramifications and manifested in the electrocardiogram by a pattern similar to bundle-branch b. but with complexes of low amplitude.

atrioventricular b., A-V b., partial or complete b. of electric impulses originating in the atrium or sinus node preventing them from reaching the atrioventricular node and ventricles. In first degree A-V b., there is prolongation of A-V conduction time (P-R interval); in second degree A-V b., some but not all atrial impulses fail to reach the ventricles, thus some ventricular beats are dropped; in complete A-V b., complete atrioventricular dissociation (2) occurs; no impulses can reach the ventricles despite even a slow ventricular rate (under 45 per minute); atria and ventricles beat independently. SYN block (3), heart b.

bone b., a surgical procedure in which the bone adjacent to the joint is modified to limit the motion of the joint mechanically; *e.g.,* at the ankle joint to correct foot-drop by preventing extension below 90°, but allowing flexion within 90°.

bundle-branch b., intraventricular b. due to interruption of conduction in one of the two main branches of the bundle of His and manifested in the electrocardiogram by marked prolongation of the QRS complex; b. of each branch has distinctive QRS morphology.

complete A-V b., SYN complete atrioventricular dissociation (2), complete A-V dissociation. SEE atrioventricular b.

conduction b., failure of impulse transmission at some point along a nerve, although conduction along the segments proximal and distal to it are unaffected. Clinically, most often caused by an area of focal demyelination; when caused by focal trauma, called neurapraxia.

congenital heart b., atrioventricular b. present *in utero* or at birth and usually of advanced or complete degree.

depolarizing b., skeletal muscle paralysis associated with loss of polarity of the motor endplate, as occurs following administration of succinylcholine.

entrance b., SYN protective b.

epidural b., an obstruction in the epidural space; used inaccurately to refer to epidural anesthesia.

exit b., inability of an impulse to leave its point of origin, the mechanism for which is conceived as an encircling zone of refractory tissue denying passage to the emerging impulse.

fascicular b., a condition based on the concept that the left branch of the bundle of His provides two of three major fascicles of a system of conduction, of which the right bundle branch constitutes the third, for the transmission of the cardiac impulse from the atrium above to the ventricles below the A-V node; block may occur in any or all fascicles, all three together producing complete A-V block. SEE ALSO hemiblock.

field b., regional anesthesia produced by infiltration of local anesthetic solution into tissues surrounding an operative field.

first degree A-V b., SEE atrioventricular b.

heart b., SYN atrioventricular b.

incomplete atrioventricular b., SYN partial heart b.

intra-atrial b., impaired conduction through the atria, manifested by widened and often notched P waves in the electrocardiogram.

intraventricular b. (IVB), I-V b., delayed conduction within the ventricular conducting system or myocardium, including bundle-branch, peri-infarction b.'s, the fascicular b.'s, excitation, and the W–P–W (pre-expectation) syndrome.

Mobitz b., second degree atrioventricular b. in which there is a ratio of two or more atrial deflections (P waves) to ventricular responses.

Mobitz types of atrioventricular b., type I, the dropped beat of the Wenckebach phenomenon; type II, a dropped cardiac cycle that occurs without alteration in the conduction of the preceding intervals.

nerve b., interruption of conduction of impulses in peripheral nerves or nerve trunks by injection of local anesthetic solution.

nondepolarizing b., skeletal mucle paralysis unaccompanied by changes in polarity of the motor endplate, as occurs following administration of tubocurarine.

partial heart b., impulses penetrate the atrioventricular junction in some relation to the ventricular rate. SYN incomplete atrioventricular b.

peri-infarction b., an electrocardiographic abnormality associated with an old myocardial infarct and caused by delayed activation of the myocardium in the region of the infarct; characterized by an initial vector directed away from the infarcted region with the terminal vector directed toward it.

phase I b., inhibition of nerve impulse transmission across the myoneural junction associated with depolarization of the motor endplate, as in the muscle paralysis produced by succinylcholine.

phase II b., inhibition of nerve impulse transmission across the myoneural junction unaccompanied by depolarization of the motor endplate, as in the muscle paralysis produced by tubocurarine.

protective b., an incompletely understood mechanism whereby a pacemaker is protected from being discharged by the impulse from another center; the mechanism, usually conceived as an encircling zone of unidirectionally refractory tissue permitting egress of impulses from the center but preventing access to the center, is seen in operation in ventricular parasystole where the parasystolic center is protected from discharge by the sinus pacemaker and so is able to maintain its intrinsic rhythm undisturbed. SYN entrance b., protection.

retrograde b., impaired conduction backward from the ventricles or A-V node into the atria.

second degree A-V b., SEE atrioventricular b.

sinoatrial b., S-A b., sinus b., blockade of the impulse leaving the sinus node before it can activate atrial muscle. SYN sinoauricular b.

sinoauricular b., SYN sinoatrial b.

spinal b., an obstruction to the flow of cerebrospinal fluid in the spinal subarachnoid space; used inaccurately to refer to spinal anesthesia.

stellate b., injection of local anesthetic solution in the vicinity of the stellate ganglion.

suprahisian b., atrioventricular conduction delay occurring above, or cephalad to, the bundle of His.

unidirectional b., b. that prevents passage of an impulse when it approaches from one direction but not from the other, as when b. in the A-V node prevents anterograde conduction to the ventricles while retrograde conduction to the atria remains intact.

Wenckebach b., a form of b. in any cardiac tissue (most often the atrioventricular junction) in which there is progressive lengthening of conduction until the beat is dropped.

Wilson b., the commonest form of right bundle-branch b., characterized in lead I by a tall slender R wave followed by a wider S wave of lower voltage.

Wolff-Chaikoff b., blocking of the organic binding of iodine and its incorporation into hormone caused by large doses of iodine; usually a transient effect, but in large doses in susceptible individuals it can be prolonged and cause iodine myxedema. SYN Wolff-Chaikoff effect.

block·ade (blok'ād). **1.** Intravenous injection of large amounts of colloidal dyes or other substances whereby the reaction of the reticuloendothelial cells to other influences (*e.g.,* by phagocytosis) is temporarily prevented. **2.** Arrest of peripheral nerve conduction or transmission at autonomic synaptic junctions, autonomic receptor sites, or myoneural junctions by a drug.

adrenergic b., selective inhibition by a drug of the responses of effector cells to adrenergic sympathetic nerve impulses (sympatholytic) and to epinephrine and related amines (adrenolytic).

cholinergic b., (**1**) inhibition by a drug of nerve impulse transmission at autonomic ganglionic synapses (ganglionic b.), at postganglionic parasympathetic effector cells (*e.g.,* by atropine), and at myoneural junctions (myoneural b.); (**2**) the inhibition of a cholinergic agent.

ganglionic b., inhibition of nerve impulse transmission at autonomic ganglionic synapses by drugs such as nicotine or hexamethonium.

myoneural b., inhibition of nerve impulse transmission at myoneural junctions by a drug such as curare.

narcotic b., the use of drugs to inhibit the effects of narcotic substances, as with naloxone.

sympathetic b., interruption of transmission in sympathetic ganglia or conduction of impulses in pre- or postganglionic sympathetic nerve fibers.

virus b., the interference of one virus by another, either attenuated or unrelated.

block·er (blok'er). **1.** An instrument used to obstruct a passage. **2.** SEE blocking *agent.*

calcium channel b., a class of drugs with the capacity to prevent calcium ions from passing through biologic membranes. These agents are used to treat hypertension, angina pectoris, and cardiac arrhythmias; examples include nifedipine, diltiazem, and verapamil.

block·ing (blok'ing). **1.** Obstructing; arresting of passage, conduction, or transmission. **2.** In psychoanalysis, a sudden break in free association occurring when a painful subject or repressed complex is touched. **3.** Sudden cessation of thoughts and speech, which may indicate the presence of a severe thought disorder or a psychosis.

alpha b., the attenuation of the occipital alpha rhythm (8–14 Hz brain waves as seen on an electroencephalogram), produced by opening the eyes or by intense mental concentration.

block·out (blok'owt). Elimination of undercuts by filling such areas with a medium such as wax or wet pumice.

Blocq, Paul O., French physician, 1860–1896. SEE B.'s *disease.*

blood (blŭd). The "circulating tissue" of the body; the fluid and its suspended formed elements that are circulated through the heart, arteries, capillaries, and veins; b. is the means by which 1) oxygen and nutritive materials are transported to the tissues, and 2) carbon dioxide and various metabolic products are removed for excretion. The b. consists of a pale yellow or gray-yellow fluid, plasma, in which are suspended red b. cells (erythrocytes), white b. cells (leukocytes), and platelets. SEE ALSO arterial b., venous b. [A.S. blōd]

arterial b., b. that is oxygenated in the lungs, found in the left chambers of the heart and in the arteries, and relatively bright red.

cord b., b. present in the umbilical vessels at the time of delivery.

laky b., b. that is undergoing or has undergone laking. SEE lake (2), laky.

occult b., b. in the feces in amounts too small to be seen but detectable by chemical tests.

sludged b., b. in which the corpuscles, as a result of some general abnormal state, *e.g.,* burns, traumatic shock, and similar stresses, become massed together in the capillaries, and thereby block the vessels or move slowly through them.

venous b., b. which has passed through the capillaries of various tissues, except the lungs, and is found in the veins, the right chambers of the heart, and the pulmonary arteries; it is usually dark red as a result of a lower content of oxygen.

whole b., b. drawn from a selected donor under rigid aseptic precautions; contains citrate ion or heparin as an anticoagulant; used as a b. replenisher.

blood bank. A place, usually a separate part or division of a hospital laboratory or a separate free-standing facility, in which blood is collected from donors, typed, separated into several components, stored, and/or prepared for transfusion to recipients.

blood count. Calculation of the number of red (RBC) or white (WBC) blood cells in a cubic millimeter of blood, by means of counting the cells in an accurate volume of diluted blood.

complete b. c. (CBC), a combination of the following determinations: red blood cell count, white blood cell count, erythrocyte indices, hematocrit, and differential blood count.

differential white b. c., an estimate of the percentage of white blood cell types which make up the total white blood cell count.

Schilling's b. c., a method of counting blood in which the polymorphonuclear neutrophils are separated into four groups according to the number and arrangement of the nuclear masses in these cells. SYN Schilling's index.

blood dust. SYN hemoconia.

blood group. A system of genetically determined antigens or agglutinogens located on the surface of the erythrocyte. Each b. g. is determined by closely linked loci. Because of the antigen differences existing between individuals, b. g.'s are significant in blood transfusions, maternal-fetal incompatibilities (erythroblastosis fetalis), tissue and organ transplantation, disputed paternity cases, and in genetic and anthropologic studies; certain b. g.'s have been supposed to be related to susceptibility or resistance to certain diseases. Often used as synonymous with blood type. See Blood Groups appendix for individual groups: ABO, Auberger, Diego, Duffy, I, Kell, Kidd, Lewis, Lutheran, MNSs, P, Rh, Sutter, Xg, and the low frequency and high frequency blood groups.

private b. g., a b. g. that is known to have occurred in only one family and is traceable to one single person.

blood group·ing. The classification of blood samples by means of laboratory tests of their agglutination reactions with respect to one or more blood groups. In general, a suspension of erythrocytes to be tested is exposed to a known specific antiserum; agglutination of the erythrocytes indicates that they possess the antigen for which the antiserum is specific. Certain antisera require special testing conditions.

blood·less (blŭd'les). Without blood.

blood·let·ting (blŭd'let-ing). Removing blood, usually from a vein (phlebotomy); formerly used as a general remedial measure, but used now in congestive heart failure and polycythemia.

general b., removing blood by arteriotomy or phlebotomy.

local b., removing blood from the smaller vessels, formerly by a cupping glass or by leeching.

blood puz·zles. Foreign bodies or deformed blood cells that may be misinterpreted as infectious agents (*e.g.,* bacteria, fungi) in stained films as a result of similarities in morphology and staining properties.

blood rel·a·tive. A relative of a person sharing some of the sources from which genes are derived. These will include many of the genes that operate in the blood and its constituents but no special importance attaches to the blood as a vehicle of inheritance. Spouses are not ordinarily blood relatives and when they are, the marriage is consanguineous and carries a higher risk than average of progeny homozygous by descent from ancestors in common. Such marriages are discouraged and within certain degrees of kindred may be illegal. [a folk metaphor of breeding]

blood·shot (blŭd'shot). Denoting locally congested smaller blood vessels of a part (*e.g.,* the conjunctiva) which are dilated and visible.

blood·stream (blŭd'strēm). The flowing blood as it is encountered in the circulatory system as distinguished from blood that has been removed from the circulatory system or sequestered in a part; thus, something added to the b. may be expected to become distributed to all parts of the body through which blood is flowing.

blood type. The specific reaction pattern of erythrocytes of an individual to the antisera of one blood group; *e.g.,* the ABO blood group consists of four major b. t.'s: O, A, B, and AB. This classification depends on the presence or absence of two major antigens: A or B. Type O occurs when neither is present and type AB when both are present. The b. t. is the genetic phenotype of the individual for one blood group system and may be determined using different antisera available for testing. See Blood Groups appendix.

blood ves·sel. A tube (artery, capillary, vein, or sinus) conveying blood.

retinal b. v.'s, the blood vasculature of the retina, including the branches and tributaries of the central retinal artery and vein, respectively, and the vascular circle of the optic nerve. SYN vasa sanguinea retinae [NA].

blood·worm (blŭd'werm). **1.** The filarial parasite of sheep, *Elaeophora schneideri.* **2.** Red aquatic larvae of certain dipterous gnats and midges. **3.** Marine annelids in the family Terebellidae with soft bodies and red blood. **4.** Blood-inhabiting worms, such as the blood flukes of man in the genus *Schistosoma.*

Bloom, David, U.S. dermatologist, *1892. SEE B.'s *syndrome.*

blot. SEE Northern blot *analysis,* Southern blot *analysis,* Western blot *analysis,* zoo blot *analysis.*

blotch. Commonly used term to denote a pigmented or erythematous lesion.

Blount, Walter P., U.S. orthopedic surgeon, *1900. SEE B.'s *disease;* B.-Barber *disease.*

blow·fly. SEE *Calliphora, Lucilia, Phormia regina.*

blow·fly strike. SYN cutaneous *myiasis.*

blue (blū). A color between green and violet on the spectrum. For individual blue dyes, see the specific name. SYN cerulean.

blue·bag. SYN ovine *mastitis.*

blue·tongue (blū'tŭng). An infectious disease of sheep caused by bluetongue virus, a member of the Reoviridae family and transmitted by bloodsucking midges of the genus *Culicoides;* manifested by catarrhal inflammation of the mucosae of the mouth, nose, and intestinal tract, accompanied frequently by foot involvement and lameness; infection or vaccination with attenuated virus during early pregnancy causes brain and heart anomalies in lambs; infection of cattle and goats is often inapparent, but disease can be severe in some wild ruminants such as deer. SYN soremuzzle.

Blum, Paul, French physician, 1878–1933. SEE Gougerot and B. *disease.*

Blumberg, Jacob M., German surgeon and gynecologist, 1873–1955. SEE B.'s *sign.*

Blumenau, Leonid W., Russian neurologist, 1862–1932. SEE B.'s *nucleus.*

Blumenbach, Johann F., German physiologist, 1752–1840. SEE B.'s *clivus.*

Blumer, George, U.S. physician, 1858–1940. SEE B.'s *shelf.*

blunt-end (blunt-ind). Refers to double-stranded DNA in which there are no unpaired bases at the end.

blush (blŭsh). **1.** A sudden and brief redness of the face and neck due to emotion. **2.** In angiography, used metaphorically to describe neovascularity or, in some cases, extravasation. [M.E., fr. O.E. *blyscan,*]

BLV Abbreviation for bovine leukemia *virus.*

B-mode. A two-dimensional diagnostic ultrasound presentation of echo-producing interfaces in a single plane; the intensity of the echo is represented by modulation of the brightness (B) of the spot, and the position of the echo is determined from the position of the transducer and the transit time of the acoustical pulse.

BMR Abbreviation for basal metabolic *rate.*

BNA Abbreviation for Basle Nomina Anatomica.

bob·bing. An up-and-down movement.

inverse ocular b., slow downward eye movement followed by delayed quick upward return.

ocular b., sudden conjugate downward deviation of the eyes with a slow return to the normal position; seen in some comatose patients who have bilateral hemisphere lesions.

bob·i·er·rite. The octahydrate of magnesium phosphate; $Mg_3(PO_4)_2 \cdot 8H_2O$; sometimes found in renal calculi. Cf. newberyite, struvite. [Pierre A. *Bobierre,* Fr. chemist, + -ite 4.]

BOC, *t*-BOC. Abbreviations formerly used for *t*-butoxycarbonyl; current usage is Boc.

Boc Abbreviation for *t*-butoxycarbonyl.

Bochdalek, Vincent A., Czechoslovakian anatomist, 1801–1883. SEE B.'s *foramen, ganglion, gap, hernia, muscle, valve;* flower basket of B.

Bock, August C., German anatomist, 1782–1833. SEE B.'s *ganglion.*

Bockhart, Max, German physician, 1883–1921. SEE B.'s *impetigo.*

BOD. Abbreviation for biochemical oxygen *demand.*

Bodansky, Aaron, U.S. biochemist, 1887–1961. SEE B. *unit.*

Bödecker, Charles F., U.S. oral histologist, embryologist, and pathologist, *1880. SEE B. *index.*

Bodian, David, U.S. anatomist, *1910. SEE B.'s copper-PROTARGOL *stain.*

Bo·do (bō'dō). A genus of free-living, ovoid or slightly pyriform protozoa with two flagella, one projecting anteriorly and the other posteriorly; may be ingested as encysted forms in food or drink, or possibly deposited in feces or urine after excretion; in either instance, cysts frequently develop into trophozoites if the specimen is permitted to remain at room temperature for a few hours prior to examination; the organisms are not pathogenic in man.

B. cauda'tus, a species that is found in specimens of human feces (especially in tropical regions); the organisms are frequently termed coprozoic flagellates.

B. sal'tans, a species of the intestinal tract sometimes observed in ulcers.

B. urina'rius, a species found occasionally in the urine.

BODY

body (bod'ē). **1.** The head, neck, trunk, and extremities. The human body, consisting of head (caput), neck (collum), trunk (truncus), and limbs (membra). **2.** The material part of a human, as distinguished from the mind and spirit. **3.** The principal mass of any structure. **4.** A thing; a substance. SEE ALSO corpus, soma. SYN corpus (1) [NA]. [A.S. *bodig*]

acetone b., SYN ketone b.

adrenal b., SYN suprarenal *gland.*

alcoholic hyaline b.'s, SYN Mallory b.'s.

Alder b.'s, granular inclusions in polymorphonuclear leukocytes; they take on a dark color with Giemsa-Wright stain and react metachromatically with toluidine blue. SEE ALSO Alder's *anomaly.*

alveolar b., SYN alveolar *process.*

amygdaloid b., a rounded mass of gray matter in the temporal lobe internal to the cortex of the uncus and immediately anterior to the inferior horn of the lateral ventricle; its major afferents are olfactory and its efferent connections are with the hypothalamus and mediodorsal nucleus of the thalamus and it is also reciprocally associated with the cortex of the temporal lobe; it is subdivided into two major nuclear groups; basolateral and corticomedial. SYN corpus amygdaloideum [NA], almond nucleus, amygdaloid complex, amygdaloid nucleus, nucleus amygdalae.

amylogenic b., SYN amyloplast.

amyloid b.'s of the prostate, obsolete term for small masses of colloid material often present in the tubules of the gland. SEE ALSO *corpus* amylaceum.

anococcygeal b., SYN anococcygeal *ligament.*

anterior quadrigeminal b., SYN superior *colliculus.*

aortic b.'s, SYN para-aortic b.'s.

Arnold's b.'s, small portions or minute fragments of erythrocytes (sometimes mistaken for blood platelets), or small "ghosts" of erythrocytes.

asbestos b.'s, ferruginous b.'s with asbestos fibers as a core; a histologic hallmark of exposure to asbestos.

Aschoff b.'s, a form of granulomatous inflammation characteristically observed in acute rheumatic carditis; fully developed Aschoff b.'s consist of fibrinoid change in connective tissue, lymphocytes, occasional plasma cells, and abnormal characteristic histiocytes. SYN Aschoff nodules.

asteroid b., (1) an eosinophilic inclusion resembling a star with delicate radiating lines, occurring in a vacuolated area of cytoplasm of a multinucleated giant cell; especially frequent in sarcoidosis, but occurs also in other granulomas; (2) a structure that is characteristic of sporotrichosis when found in the skin or secondary lesions of this mycosis; in tissue, it surrounds the 3- to 5-μm in diameter ovoid yeast of *Sporothrix schenkii.*

Auer b.'s, rod-shaped structures of uncertain nature in the cytoplasm of immature myeloid cells, especially myeloblasts, in acute myelocytic leukemia; may be an abnormal form of lysosomes; they contain peroxidase and acid phosphatase, and stain red by azure-eosin stains. SYN Auer rods.

Babès-Ernst b.'s, intracellular granules, present in many species of bacteria, which possess a strong affinity for nuclear stains.

Barr chromatin b., SYN sex *chromatin.*

basal b., an elongated centriolar structure situated at the base of each cilium at the apical margin of a cell. SYN basal corpuscle, basal granule, blepharoplast, kinetosome.

bigeminal b.'s, a bilateral single swelling of the roofplate of the embryonic midbrain that later in development becomes subdivided into a superior and an inferior colliculus. SEE quadrigeminal b.'s. SYN corpora bigemina.

Bollinger b.'s, relatively large, spheroid or ovoid, usually somewhat granular, acidophilic, intracytoplasmic inclusion b.'s observed in the infected tissues of birds with fowlpox; when b.'s are ruptured large numbers of fowlpox virus particles are released.

Borrel b.'s, particles of fowlpox virus; aggregates of Borrel b.'s in infected cells result in the formation of Bollinger b.'s.

brassy b., a dark-colored, usually shrunken erythrocyte in which there is a malarial parasite.

Cabot's ring b.'s, ring-shaped or figure-of-eight structures that stain red with Wright's stain, found in red blood cells in severe anemias, possibly a remnant of the nuclear membrane; a form of basophilic degenerative process.

Call-Exner b.'s, small fluid-filled spaces between granulosal cells in ovarian follicles and in ovarian tumors of granulosal origin; they may form a rosette-like structure.

cancer b.'s, discrete, acidophilic or amphophilic, hyaline b.'s of various shapes and sizes, occurring in the cytoplasm of some of the neoplastic cells and also extracellularly in the stroma of various carcinomas and sarcomas; formerly regarded by some observers as parasitic causal agents, but now thought to be products of cell necrosis (apoptosis).

carotid b., a small epithelioid structure located just above the bifurcation of the common carotid artery on each side. It consists of granular principal cells and nongranular supporting cells, a sinusoidal vascular bed, and a rich network of sensory fibers of the glossopharyngeal nerve. It serves as a chemoreceptor organ responsive to oxygen lack, carbon dioxide excess, and increased hydrogen ion concentration. SYN glomus caroticum [NA], intercarotid b., nodulus caroticus.

b. of caudate nucleus, the suprathalamic part of the caudate nucleus lying in the floor of the central part of the lateral ventricle. SYN corpus nuclei caudati [NA].

cavernous b. of clitoris, SYN *corpus* cavernosum clitoridis.

cavernous b. of penis, SYN *corpus* cavernosum penis.

cell b., the part of the cell containing the nucleus.

central b., SYN cytocentrum.

central fibrous b., the fibrous area where the leaflets of the aortic, mitral, and tricuspid valves meet in the heart.

chromaffin b., SYN paraganglion.

chromatin b., the genetic apparatus of bacteria. SEE nucleus (2).

ciliary b., a thickened portion of the vascular tunic of the eye between the choroid and the iris; it consists of three parts or zones; orbiculus ciliaris, corona ciliaris, and ciliary muscle. SYN corpus ciliare [NA], annulus ciliaris.

Civatte b.'s, eosinophilic hyaline spherical b.'s seen in or just beneath the epidermis, particularly in lichen planus, formed by necrosis of individual basal cells. SYN colloid b.'s.

b. of clavicle, the sinuous portion of the clavicle between the sternal and acromial extremities. SYN corpus claviculae [NA].

b. of clitoris, the shaft or pendulous portion of the clitoris, composed of two fused corpora cavernosa clitoridae, the distal end of which is the glans clitoris. SYN corpus clitoridis [NA].

coccygeal b., an arteriovenous (arteriolovenular) anastomosis supplied by the middle sacral artery and located on the pelvic surface of the coccyx. It was formerly called a gland (of Luschka) or a glomus and included with the paraganglia. SYN corpus coccygeum [NA], arteriococcygeal gland, coccygeal gland, glomus coccygeum.

colloid b.'s, SYN Civatte b.'s.

compressible cavernous b.'s, submucous venous plexuses found at the level of the pharyngoesophageal junction and anal canal, which assist in reducing or obliterating the lumen.

conchoidal b.'s, SYN Schaumann b.'s.

Councilman b., Councilman hyaline b., an eosinophilic globule, seen in the liver in yellow fever, derived from necrosis of a single hepatic cell. SYN Councilman's lesion.

Cowdry's type A inclusion b.'s, droplet-like masses of acidophilic material surrounded by clear halos within nuclei, with margination of chromatin on the nuclear membrane.

Cowdry's type B inclusion b.'s, droplet-like masses of acidophilic material surrounded by clear halos within nuclei, without other nuclear changes during early stages of development of the inclusion.

creola b.'s, large compact clusters of ciliated columnar cells found in the sputum of some asthmatic patients.

cyanobacterium-like b.'s, SYN *Cyclospora.*

cytoid b.'s, swollen retinal nerve fibers which look like cells when cut transversely; found in cotton-wool patches.

cytoplasmic inclusion b.'s, SEE inclusion b.'s.

Deetjen's b.'s, SYN platelet.

demilune b., a circular b. of extreme transparency except for a crescentic punctate substance on one edge which contains hemoglobin. The b. is much larger than a red blood cell, but is thought possibly to be a degenerated red blood cell swollen by imbibition; it has been found in malaria and in convalescence from typhoid fever; the transparent portion is called the glass b.

Döhle b.'s, discrete round or oval b.'s ranging in diameter from just visible to 2 μm, which stain sky blue to gray blue with Romanowsky stains, found in neutrophils of patients with infections, burns, trauma, pregnancy, or cancer. SYN Döhle inclusions, leukocyte inclusions.

Donovan's b.'s, clusters of blue or black staining, bipolar chromatin condensations in large mononuclear cells in granulation tissue infected with *Calymmatobacterium granulomatis.*

Ehrlich's inner b., a round oxyphil b. found in the red blood cell in case of hemocytolysis due to a specific blood poison. SYN Heinz-Ehrlich b.

elementary b.'s, (1) (E.B., EB), old term for virions, especially the largest virus particles, visible by light microscopy when stained; (2) SYN platelet.

b. of epididymis, the middle part that extends downward from the head to the tail of the epididymis on the posterior surface of the testis. SYN corpus epididymidis [NA].

epithelial b., SYN parathyroid *gland.*

fat b. of cheek, SYN buccal *fat-pad.*

fat b. of ischiorectal fossa, SYN ischiorectal *fat-pad.*

fat b. of orbit, SYN orbital *fat-pad*.

ferruginous b.'s, in the lungs, foreign inorganic or organic fibers coated by complexes of hemosiderin and glycoproteins, and believed to be formed by macrophages that have phagocytized the fibers. SEE ALSO asbestos b.'s.

foreign b., anything in the tissues or cavities of the b. that has been introduced there from without, and that is not rapidly absorbable.

b. of fornix, the middle part of the fornix situated ventral to the corpus callosum. SYN corpus fornicis [NA].

fruiting b., any fungal structure that bears spores.

fuchsin b.'s, (1) SYN Russell b.'s. **(2)** SYN hyaline b.'s.

b. of gallbladder, the main part of the gallbladder terminating in the rounded fundus below and continuing into the neck of the gallbladder above. SYN corpus vesicae biliaris [NA], corpus vesicae felleae [NA].

Gamna-Favre b.'s, characteristic, relatively large, intracytoplasmic basophilic inclusion b.'s observed in endothelial cells in lymphogranuloma venereum; probably composed of degenerated nuclear material. SEE ALSO Miyagawa b.'s.

Gamna-Gandy b.'s, small firm spheroidal or irregular foci that are yellow-brown, brown, or rustlike in color, occurring chiefly in the spleen in such conditions as congestive splenomegaly and sickle cell disease, and consisting of relatively dense fibrous tissue or collagenous fibers impregnated with iron pigment and calcium salts; probably result from organization and scarring of sites where small perivascular hemorrhages occurred. SYN Gamna-Gandy nodules, Gandy-Gamna b.'s, siderotic nodules.

Gandy-Gamna b.'s, SYN Gamna-Gandy b.'s.

geniculate b., SEE lateral geniculate b., medial geniculate b.

glass b., SEE demilune b.

glomus b., SYN glomus (2).

Golgi b., SYN Golgi *apparatus*.

Guarnieri b.'s, intracytoplasmic acidophilic inclusion b.'s observed in epithelial cells in variola (smallpox) and vaccinia infections, and which include aggregations of Paschen b.'s or virus particles.

Halberstaedter-Prowazek b.'s, SYN trachoma b.'s.

Hassall-Henle b.'s, hyaline b.'s on the posterior surface of Descemet's membrane at the periphery of the cornea. SYN Henle's warts.

Hassall's b.'s, SYN thymic *corpuscle*.

Heinz b.'s, intracellular inclusions usually attached to the red cell membrane, composed of denatured hemoglobin; they occur in thalassemia, enzymopathies, hemoglobinopathies, and after splenectomy. Visualization of these usually requires examination of red cells using supravital stains or by phase microscopy.

Heinz-Ehrlich b., SYN Ehrlich's inner b.

hematoxylin b.'s, hematoxyphil b.'s, poorly defined, homogeneous basophilic remnants of whole nuclei, an occasional finding in the fixed tissues of patients with systemic lupus erythematosus, but observed more frequently in the renal glomeruli and the walls of blood vessels, and probably related to the LE phenomenon; so named because of their affinity for hematoxylin stain.

Herring b.'s, accumulations of neurosecretory granules in dilated terminal endings of axons in the neurohypophysis.

Highmore's b., SYN *mediastinum* testis.

Howell-Jolly b.'s, spherical or ovoid eccentrically located granules, approximately 1 μm in diameter, occasionally observed in the stroma of circulating erythrocytes, especially in stained preparations (as compared with wet unstained films); probably represent nuclear remnants, inasmuch as they can be stained with dyes that are rather specific for chromatin; the significance of the b.'s is not exactly known; they occur most frequently after splenectomy or in megaloblastic or severe hemolytic anemia. SYN Jolly b.'s.

hyaline b.'s, homogeneous eosinophilic inclusions in the cytoplasm of epithelial cells; in renal tubules, hyaline b.'s represent droplets of protein reabsorbed from the lumen. SEE ALSO Mallory b.'s, drusen. SYN fuchsin b.'s (2).

hyaline b.'s of pituitary, accumulations of a gelatinous neurose-

cretory substance in the axons of the hypothalamohypophyseal tract in the posterior lobe of the hypophysis.

hyaloid b., SYN vitreous b.

b. of hyoid bone, the body of the hyoid bone, from which the greater and lesser horns extend. SYN corpus ossis hyoidei [NA], base of hyoid bone, basihyal, basihyoid.

b. of ilium, it forms the upper two-fifths of the acetabulum and joins the pubis and ischium in the acetabulum. It continues above into the ala or wing of the ilium. SYN corpus ossis ilii [NA].

inclusion b.'s, distinctive structures frequently formed in the nucleus or cytoplasm (occasionally in both locations) in cells infected with certain filtrable viruses, observed especially in nerve, epithelial, or endothelial cells; may be demonstrated by means of various stains, especially Mann's eosin methylene blue or Giemsa's techniques. Nuclear inclusion b.'s are usually acidophilic and are of two morphologic types: 1) granular, hyaline, or amorphous b.'s of various sizes, *i.e.,* Cowdry's type A inclusion b.'s, occurring in such diseases as herpes simplex infection or yellow fever; 2) more circumscribed b.'s, frequently with several in the same nucleus (and no reaction in adjacent tissue), *i.e.,* the type B b.'s, occurring in such diseases as Rift Valley fever and poliomyelitis. Cytoplasmic inclusion b.'s may be: 1) acidophilic, relatively large, spherical or ovoid, and somewhat granular, as in variola or vaccinia, rabies, and molluscum contagiosum; 2) basophilic, relatively large, complex combinations of viral and cellular material, as in trachoma, psittacosis, and lymphogranuloma venereum. In some instances, inclusion b.'s are known to be infective and probably represent aggregates of virus particles in combination with cellular material, whereas others are apparently not infective and may represent only abnormal products formed by the cell in response to injury. Inclusion b.'s that resemble some of those known to be related to viral infections are occasionally observed in degenerative diseases and in lead poisoning.

b. of incus, the main part of the incus that articulates with the malleus and from which the short and long limbs arise. SYN corpus incudis [NA].

infrapatellar fat b., SYN infrapatellar *fat-pad*.

intercarotid b., SYN carotid b.

intermediate b. of Flemming, SYN midbody.

interrenal b.'s, distinct paired or unpaired structures in all fishes, which lie in close proximity to the kidney, homologous to the cortical tissue of the mammalian adrenal gland. SYN interrenal glands.

b. of ischium, the entire ischium with the exception of the ramus. SYN corpus ossis ischii [NA].

Jaworski's b.'s, mucous shreds in the gastric contents in hyperchlorhydria.

Joest b.'s, intranuclear inclusion b.'s (Cowdry's type B) produced in certain nerve cells by Borna disease virus.

Jolly b.'s, SYN Howell-Jolly b.'s.

juxtaglomerular b., a collection of cells around the renal glomerular arterioles that contain cytoplasmic granules, probably composed of renin. SYN periarterial pad.

juxtarestiform b., a medial (smaller) subdivision of the inferior cerebellar peduncle (corpus restiforme) composed of fibers reciprocally connecting the vestibular nuclei with the cerebellum, in particular the latter's nodulus, flocculus, and uvula vermis. It also carries primary sensory fibers from the vestibular ganglia to the cerebellum, as well as cerebellar projections to the rhombencephalic reticular formation and vestibular nuclei.

ketone b., one of a group of ketones that includes acetoacetic acid, its reduction product, β-hydroxybutyric acid, and its decarboxylation product, acetone; high levels are found in tissues and body fluids in ketosis. SYN acetone b., acetone compound.

Koch's blue b.'s, schizonts of *Theileria parva,* the causative agent of East Coast fever; found principally within endothelial cells of the spleen and lymph nodes.

Kurloff's b.'s, palely basophilic, granular inclusions sometimes observed in the cytoplasm of the large mononuclear leukocytes (probably lymphocytes) of guinea pigs and certain other animals.

Lafora b. [MIM*254780], an intraneural intracytoplasmic inclusion b. composed of acid mucopolysaccharides, seen in familial myoclonus epilepsy; a recessive trait.

Lallemand's b.'s, (1) old term for small gelatinoid concretions sometimes observed in seminal fluid; **(2)** old term for Bence Jones *cylinders*, under *cylinder*. SYN Trousseau-Lallemand b.'s.

Landolt's b.'s, bipolar nerve cells lying between the retinal rods and cones in amphibia, reptiles, and birds.

lateral geniculate b., the lateral one of a pair of small oval masses that protrude slightly from the posteroinferior aspects of the thalamus; its main (dorsal) subdivision serves as a processing station in the major pathway from the retina to the cerebral cortex, receiving fibers from the optic tract and giving rise to the geniculocalcarine radiation to the visual cortex in the occipital lobe. SYN corpus geniculatum laterale [NA], corpus geniculatum externum.

L-D b., SYN Leishman-Donovan b.

LE b., the amorphous round b. in the cytoplasm of an LE cell.

Leishman-Donovan b., the intracytoplasmic, nonflagellated leishmanial form of certain intracellular parasites, such as species of *Leishmania* or the intracellular form of *Trypanosoma cruzi;* originally used for *Leishmania donovani* parasites in infected spleen or liver cells in kala azar. SYN amastigote, L-D b.

Lewy b.'s, intracytoplasmic inclusion b.'s especially noted in pigmented brainstem neurons and seen in Parkinson's disease.

Lieutaud's b., SYN *trigone* of bladder.

Lindner's b.'s, initial b.'s resembling inclusion b.'s found in scrapings of epithelial cells infected with trachoma.

loose b., a solid tissue fragment lying free in a body cavity, especially in a joint or the peritoneal cavity; *e.g.,* joint mice, melon-seed b., rice b.

Luse b.'s, collagen fibers with abnormally long spacing (exceeding 1000 Å) between electron-dense bands.

Luys' b., SYN subthalamic *nucleus.*

Mallory b.'s, large, poorly defined accumulations of eosinophilic material in the cytoplasm of damaged hepatic cells in certain forms of cirrhosis and marked fatty change especially due to alcoholism. SYN alcoholic hyalin, alcoholic hyaline b.'s.

malpighian b.'s, SYN splenic lymph *follicles,* under *follicle.*

mamillary b., a small, round, paired cell group that protrudes into the interpeduncular fossa from the inferior aspect of the hypothalamus. It receives hippocampal fibers through the fornix and projects fibers to the anterior thalamic nuclei and into the brainstem tegmentum. SYN corpus mamillare [NA], mamillary tubercle of hypothalamus.

b. of mammary gland, the principal part of the breast, consisting of glandular tissue and its supporting fibrous tissue. It forms a conical mass converging toward the nipple and is surrounded by adipose tissue. SYN corpus mammae [NA].

b. of mandible, the heavy, U-shaped, horizontal portion of the mandible extending posteriorly to the angle where it is continuous with the ramus; it supports the lower teeth. SYN corpus mandibulae [NA].

b. of maxilla, the central portion of the maxilla hollowed out by the maxillary sinus; it presents orbital, nasal, anterior, and infratemporal surfaces and supports four processes, frontal, zygomatic, palatine, and alveolar. SYN corpus maxillae [NA].

medial geniculate b., the medial one of a pair of prominent cell groups in the posteroinferior parts of the thalamus; it functions as the last of a series of processing stations along the auditory conduction pathway to the cerebral cortex, receiving the brachium of the inferior colliculus and giving rise to the auditory radiation to the auditory cortex in the superior temporal gyrus. SYN corpus geniculatum mediale [NA], corpus geniculatum internum.

melon-seed b., a small fibrous loose b. in the joints or tendon sheaths.

metachromatic b.'s, concentrated deposits consisting primarily of polymetaphosphate and occurring in many bacteria as well as in algae, fungi, and protozoa; m. b.'s differ in staining properties from the surrounding protoplasm. SEE metachromasia.

Michaelis-Gutmann b., a rounded homogenous or concentrically laminated b., 1 to 10 μ in diameter, containing calcium and iron; found within macrophages in the bladder wall in malakoplakia.

Miyagawa b.'s, a term previously used to refer to *Chlamydia trachomatis* (*Miyagawanella lymphogranulomatosis*), the elementary b.'s that develop in the intracytoplasmic microcolonies of lymphogranuloma venereum.

molluscum b., a distinctive intracellular spherical b. in the lesions of molluscum contagiosum caused by a member of the family Poxviridae; it consists of degenerated cytoplasm and the virus. SYN molluscum corpuscle.

Mooser b.'s, a term used to refer to the rickettsiae found in the exudate (and in tissue) from the tunica vaginalis in endemic typhus fever (caused by *Rickettsia typhi*).

multilamellar b., SYN cytosome (2).

multivesicular b.'s, membrane-bound b.'s, 0.5 to 1.0 μm wide, that occur in the cytoplasm of cells and contain a number of small vesicles; hydrolases (especially acid phosphatase) occur in the matrix.

myelin b., SYN myelin *figure.*

b. of nail, the exposed portion of the nail distal to its root. SYN corpus unguis [NA].

Negri b.'s, eosinophilic, sharply outlined, pathognomonic inclusion b.'s (2 to 10 μm in diameter) found in the cytoplasm of certain nerve cells containing the virus of rabies, especially in Ammon's horn of the hippocampus. SYN Negri corpuscles.

nerve cell b., the part of the neuron that includes the nucleus but excludes the processes.

neuroepithelial b., a corpuscular aggregate of nonciliated cells containing neurosecretory substance found in normal bronchial epithelium.

Nissl b.'s, SYN Nissl *substance.*

nodular b., in fungi, a compact, roughly spherical or squarish structure formed by coiling and twisting of the end of a hypha; considered to be abortive growths toward sexual reproduction.

nu b., SYN nucleosome.

nuclear inclusion b.'s, SEE inclusion b.'s.

Odland b., SYN keratinosome.

olivary b., SYN oliva.

onion b.'s, obsolete term for epithelial *nest.*

pacchionian b.'s, SYN arachnoid *granulations,* under *granulation.*

pampiniform b., SYN epoöphoron.

b. of pancreas, the part of the pancreas from the point where it crosses the portal vein to the point where it enters the lienorenal ligament. SYN corpus pancreatis [NA].

Pappenheimer b.'s, phagosomes, containing ferruginous granules, found in red blood cells in diseases such as sideroblastic anemia, hemolytic anemia, and sickle cell disease; may contribute to spurious platelet counts by electro-optical counters.

para-aortic b.'s, small masses of chromaffin tissue found near the sympathetic ganglia along the aorta; they are more prominent during fetal life. The chromaffin cells secrete noradrenalin; chemoreceptive endings monitor levels of blood gases. SYN corpora para-aortica [NA], aortic b.'s, corpus aorticum, glomera aortica, organs of Zuckerkandl, Zuckerkandl's b.'s.

parabasal b., a term formerly equivalent to the DNA kinetoplast, part of the giant mitochondrion of certain parasitic flagellates. The parabasal b. plus the basal b. were previously thought to comprise a kinetoplast, or locomotory apparatus, but kinetoplast is now restricted to part of the DNA giant mitochondrion and parabasal b. is a distinct structure near the nucleus, probably equivalent to the metazoan Golgi apparatus.

paranephric b., a mass of fat lying behind the renal fascia.

paranuclear b., SYN astrosphere.

paraphysial b., SYN paraphysis.

paraterminal b., SYN subcallosal *gyrus.*

Paschen b.'s, particles of virus observed in relatively large numbers in squamous cells of the skin (or the cornea of experimental animals) in variola (smallpox) or vaccinia.

b. of penis, the free pendulous portion of the penis, consisting of shaft and glans penis. SYN corpus penis [NA], scapus penis.

perineal b., SYN central *tendon* of perineum.

b. of phalanx, the shaft of each phalanx of the hand or foot. SYN corpus phalangis [NA].

Pick's b.'s, intracytoplasmic argentophilic inclusion b.'s seen in neurons in Pick's disease.

pineal b., a small, unpaired, flattened body, shaped somewhat like a pine cone, attached at its anterior pole to the region of the posterior and habenular commissures, and lying in the depression between the two superior colliculi below the splenium of the corpus callosum; it is a glandular structure, composed of follicles containing epithelioid cells and lime concretions called brain sand; despite its attachment to the brain, it appears to receive nerve fibers exclusively from the peripheral autonomic nervous system. It produces melatonin. SYN corpus pineale [NA], conarium, epiphysis cerebri, pineal gland, pinus.

Plimmer's b.'s, obsolete term for cancer b.'s

polar b., one of two small cells formed by the first and second meiotic division of oocytes; the first is usually released just prior to ovulation, the second not until discharge of the ovum from the ovary; in mammals, the second polar b. may fail to form unless the ovum has been penetrated by a sperm cell. SYN polar cell, polar globule, polocyte.

polyhedral b., an inclusion b. associated with replication of certain insect viruses.

pontobulbar b., a collection of nerve cells in the lower part of the medulla oblongata forming a ridge which crosses the restiform body obliquely. SYN corpus pontobulbare.

posterior quadrigeminal b., SYN inferior *colliculus*.

Prowazek b.'s, historic term for either of two types of inclusion b.'s associated with certain diseases: 1) trachoma b.'s; 2) tiny, ovoid, granular forms, frequently in pairs, observed in the cytoplasm and in Guarnieri b.'s in the cutaneous squamous cells of man and animals infected with variola (smallpox) or vaccinia virus; probably the same as Paschen b.'s.

Prowazek-Greeff b.'s, SYN trachoma b.'s.

psammoma b.'s, (1) mineralized b.'s occurring in the meninges, choroid plexus, and in certain meningiomas; composed usually of a central capillary surrounded by concentric whorls of meningocytes in various stages of hyaline change and mineralization; can also occur in benign and malignant epithelial tumors (often papillary) or with chronic inflammation; SYN sand b.'s. **(2)** SYN *corpora* arenacea, under *corpus*. **(3)** SYN calcospherite.

psittacosis inclusion b.'s, intracytoplasmic chlamydial microcolonies observed in bronchial epithelial cells infected with *Chlamydia psittaci.*

pubic b., b. of pubic bone, SYN b. of pubis.

b. of pubis, the flattened medial portion of the pubic bone entering into the pubic symphysis. From it extend the superior and inferior rami. SYN corpus ossis pubis [NA], pubic b., b. of pubic bone.

purine b.'s, any purine.

quadrigeminal b.'s, SEE inferior *colliculus*, superior *colliculus*. SYN corpora quadrigemina.

Renaut b., subperineurial structure comprised of loosely arranged and randomly oriented collagen fibers in a fine fibrillary material, seen in normal nerve as well as in certain pathologic states.

residual b., a cytoplasmic vacuole (lysosome) containing accumulated particulate products of metabolism, *e.g.,* lipofuscin.

residual b. of Regaud, the excess cytoplasm that separates from the spermatozoon during spermiogenesis.

rest b., a small mass of cytoplasm remaining after the nucleus and cytoplasm of the schizont of certain sporozoan protozoa have divided into asexual spores or merozoites.

restiform b., a lateral (larger) subdivision of the inferior cerebellar peduncle composed of a variety of fibers including, but not limited to, olivo-, reticulo-, cuneo-, trigemino-, and dorsal spinocerebellar. SEE ALSO inferior cerebellar *peduncle*. SYN corpus restiforme.

b. of rib, the shaft of a rib; the portion which extends laterally, anteriorly, and then medially from the tubercle. SYN corpus costae [NA].

rice b., one of the small, loose b.'s found in hygromas, tendon sheaths, and joints.

Rushton b., linear or curved hyaline bodies, presumably of hematogenous origin, found within the epithelial lining of odontogenic cysts.

Russell b.'s, small, discrete, variably sized, spherical, intracytoplasmic, acidophilic, hyaline b.'s that stain deeply with fuchsin; they occur frequently in plasma cells in chronic inflammation, where they are believed to consist of γ-globulin. SYN fuchsin b.'s (1).

sand b.'s, SYN psammoma b.'s (1).

Sandström's b.'s, SEE parathyroid *gland*.

Savage's perineal b., SYN central *tendon* of perineum.

Schaumann b.'s, concentrically laminated calcified b.'s found in granulomas, particularly in sarcoidosis. SYN conchoidal b.'s.

sclerotic b.'s, vegetative rounded muriform cells of dematiaceous fungi, characteristic of the causal agents of chromoblastomycosis in tissue. SYN copper pennies.

segmenting b., SYN schizont.

b. of sphenoid bone, the central portion of the sphenoid bone from which the greater and lesser wings and the pterygoid processes arise. The sphenoidal sinuses lie within it. SYN corpus ossis sphenoidalis [NA].

spongy b. of penis, SYN *corpus* spongiosum penis.

b. of sternum, the middle and largest portion of the sternum, lying between the manubrium superiorly and the xiphoid process inferiorly. SYN corpus sterni [NA], gladiolus, mesosternum, midsternum.

b. of stomach, the part of the stomach that lies between the fundus above and the pyloric antrum below; its boundaries are poorly defined. SYN corpus gastricum [ventriculi] [NA].

striate b., the caudate and lentiform (lenticular) nuclei; the striate appearance on section is caused by slender fascicles of myelinated fibers. Histologically, the striate b. can be subdivided into the generally small-celled striatum, consisting of the caudate nucleus and the outer segment of the lentiform nucleus (the putamen), and a large-celled globus pallidus composed of the two segments. SYN corpus striatum [NA].

suprarenal b., SYN suprarenal *gland*.

b. of sweat gland, the coiled tubular secretory portion of a sweat gland located in the subcutaneous tissue or deep in the corium and connected to the surface of the skin by a long duct. SYN corpus glandulae sudoriferae [NA].

Symington's anococcygeal b., SYN anococcygeal *ligament*.

b. of talus, the large posterior part of the talus forming the trochlea above for articulation with the tibia and fibula and articulating below with the calcaneus. SYN corpus tali [NA].

b. of thigh bone, SYN *shaft* of femur.

threshold b., SYN threshold *substance*.

thyroid b., SYN thyroid *gland*.

b. of tibia, SYN *shaft* of tibia.

tigroid b.'s, SYN Nissl *substance*.

b. of tongue, the oral part of the tongue anterior to the terminal sulcus. SYN corpus linguae [NA].

trachoma b.'s, distinctive, complex, intracytoplasmic forms found in the conjunctival epithelial cells of persons in the acute phase of trachoma, less frequently in later stages, varying from 1) discrete acidophilic granules (approximately 250 nm in diameter), to 2) irregular clumps of such material embedded in a basophilic matrix, to 3) relatively large basophilic b.'s (approximately 700 to 1000 nm in diameter), to 4) large basophilic b.'s that include discrete, tiny, acidophilic granules. SYN Halberstaedter-Prowazek b.'s, Prowazek-Greeff b.'s.

trapezoid b., a plate of transverse fibers running over the dorsal (deep) border of the pontine nuclei; it is formed by ascending auditory fibers that cross to the opposite side of the brainstem. SYN corpus trapezoideum [NA], trapezoid (4).

Trousseau-Lallemand b.'s, SYN Lallemand's b.'s.

tuffstone b., membrane-bound electron-dense granules, measuring about 0.5 μm in diameter, found primarily in Schwann cells of patients suffering from metachromatic leukodystrophy; the name alludes to their resemblance to volcanic limestone.

turbinated b., (1) a concha with its covering of mucous membrane and other soft parts; SYN turbinal. **(2)** SYN inferior nasal *concha*, middle nasal *concha*, superior nasal *concha*, supreme nasal *concha*.

tympanic b., SYN tympanic *gland*.

b. of ulna, SYN *shaft* of ulna. SYN corpus ulnae [NA].

ultimobranchial b., a diverticulum from the fourth pharyngeal pouch of an embryo, regarded by some as a rudimentary fifth pharyngeal pouch and by others as a lateral thyroid primordium; the ultimobranchial b.'s of lower vertebrates contain large amounts of calcitonin; in mammals, the ultimobranchial b.'s fuse with the thyroid gland and are thought to develop into the parafollicular cells. SEE ALSO ultimobranchial *pouch*.

b. of urinary bladder, the portion of the bladder between the apex and fundus. SYN corpus vesicae urinariae [NA].

b. of uterus, the part of the uterus above the isthmus, comprising about two thirds of the non-pregnant organ. SYN corpus uteri [NA].

vaccine b.'s, old term pertaining to intracellular b.'s that were erroneously thought to be forms in the life cycle of a protozoan organism, *Cytorrhyctes vaccinae,* postulated to be the causal agent of vaccinia.

Verocay b.'s, hyalinized acellular areas composed of reduplicated basement membrane outlined by opposing rows of prarallel nuclei; seen microscopically in neurilemomas.

b. of vertebra, the main portion of a vertebra anterior to the vertebral canal, as distinct from the arches. SYN corpus vertebrae [NA].

Virchow-Hassall b.'s, SYN thymic *corpuscle*.

vitreous b., a transparent jelly-like substance filling the interior of the eyeball behind the lens of the eye; it is composed of a delicate network (vitreous stroma) enclosing in its meshes a watery fluid (vitreous humor). SYN corpus vitreum [NA], hyaloid b., vitreous (2), vitreum.

Weibel-Palade b.'s, rod-shaped bundles of microtubules seen by electron microscopy in vascular endothelial cells.

wolffian b., SYN mesonephros.

Wolf-Orton b.'s, intranuclear inclusion b.'s seen in cells of malignant neoplasms, especially those of glial cell origin.

X b., obsolete term for Langerhans' *granule*.

Y b., a single fluorescent spot originating in the long arm of the Y chromosome and visible in somatic nuclei of buccal smears.

yellow b., SYN *corpus* luteum.

zebra b., metachromatically staining membrane-bound granules, measuring 0.5-1 μm in diameter and containing lamellae with a 5.8 nm spacing, reported in Schwann cells and macrophages of patients suffering from metachromatic leukodystrophy.

Zuckerkandl's b.'s, SYN para-aortic b.'s.

---

body bur·den. Activity of a radiopharmaceutical retained by the body at a specified time following administration.

Boeck, Caesar P.M., Norwegian dermatologist, 1845–1917. SEE B.'s *disease, sarcoid;* Besnier-B.-Schaumann *disease, syndrome.*

Boeck, Carl W., Norwegian physician, 1808–1875. SEE Danielssen-B. *disease.*

Boehmer, F. SEE B.'s *hematoxylin.*

Boerhaave, Hermann, Dutch physician, 1668–1738. SEE B.'s *glands,* under *gland, syndrome.*

bog·bean (bog'bēn). SYN buckbean.

Bogros, Antoine, 19th century French anatomist. SEE B.'s serous *membrane.*

Bogros, Jean-Annet, French anatomist, 1786–1823. SEE B.'s *space.*

Bohn, Heinrich, German physician, 1832–1888. SEE B.'s *nodules,* under *nodule.*

Bohr, Christian, Danish physiologist, 1855–1911. SEE B. *effect;* B.'s *equation.*

Bohr, Niels H.D., Danish physicist and Nobel laureate, 1885–1962. SEE B.'s *atom;* B. *magneton;* B.'s *theory.*

boil (boyl). SYN furuncle. [A.S. *byl,* a swelling]

  Aleppo b., Bagdad b., the lesion occurring in cutaneous leishmaniasis. SEE cutaneous *leishmaniasis.* SYN Biskra b.

Biskra b., SYN Aleppo b.

blind b., a furuncle that does not have a fluctuant central point; it appears as a dull red painful papule.

date b., Delhi b., Jericho b., the lesion occurring in cutaneous leishmaniasis.

Madura b., SYN mycetoma (1).

Oriental b., the lesion occurring in cutaneous leishmaniasis.

salt water b.'s, furuncles on hands and forearms of fishermen.

shoe b., olecranoid bursitis in the horse; so called because it may be caused by trauma from the shoe in the recumbent animal. SYN capped elbow.

tropical b., the lesion occurring in cutaneous leishmaniasis.

bol Abbreviation for bolus.

bol·de·none (bōl'dĕ-nōn). 17β-hydroxyandrosta-1,4-dien-3-one; an anabolic and androgenic agent used in veterinary medicine. SYN dehydrotestosterone.

bol·din (bol'din). A glycoside from boldus; a cholagogue and diuretic. SYN boldoglucin.

bol·dine (bol'dēn). A bitter alkaloid obtained from boldus.

boldine dimethyl ether. SYN glaucine.

bol·do (bol'dō). SYN boldus.

bol·do·glu·cin (bol-dō-glū'sin). SYN boldin.

bol·dus (bol'dŭs). The leaves of *Boldu boldus* or *Peumus boldus* (family Monimiaceae), an evergreen shrub of Chile; used in various disturbances of liver function. SYN boldo. [Chilean]

bol·et·ic ac·id (bol-et'ik). Obsolete term for fumaric acid.

Boley gauge. See under gauge.

Boll, Franz C., German histologist and physiologist, 1849–1879. SEE B.'s *cells,* under *cell.*

Bollinger, Otto, German pathologist, 1843–1909. SEE B. *bodies,* under *body, granules,* under *granule.*

Bollman, Jesse L., U.S. physiologist, *1896. SEE Mann-B. *fistula.*

Bolognini's symp·tom. See under symptom.

bo·lom·e·ter (bō-lom'ĕ-ter). 1. An instrument for determining minute degrees of radiant heat. 2. An obsolete instrument for measuring the force of the heartbeat as distinguished from the blood pressure. [G. *bolē,* a throw, a sunbeam, + *metron,* measure]

Bolton, Joseph S., English neurologist, 1867–1946. SEE B. *plane;* B.-Broadbent *plane;* B.-nasion *plane, line.*

bo·lus (bol) (bō'lŭs). 1. A single, relatively large quantity of a substance, usually one intended for therapeutic use, such as a b. dose of a drug. 2. A masticated morsel of food or another substance ready to be swallowed, such as a b. of barium for x-ray studies. 3. In high-energy radiation therapy, a quantity of tissue-equivalent material placed next to the irradiated region to increase the dose of secondary radiation to the superficial tissues. [L. fr. G. *bōlos,* lump, clod]

intravenous b., a relatively large volume of fluid or dose of a drug or test substance given intravenously and rapidly to hasten or magnify a response; in radiology, rapid injection of a large dose of contrast medium to increase opacification of blood vessels.

bom·bard. To expose a substance to particulate or electromagnetic radiations for the purpose of making it radioactive. [Mediev. L. *bombarda,* artillery assault, fr. *bombus,* a booming sound]

bom·be·sin (bomb'ĕ-sin). Pharmacologically active tetradecapeptide found in skins of European amphibians of the family Discoglossidae, principally *Bombina bombina* and *Bombina variegata variegata.* A potent stimulant of gastric and pancreatic secretions; a bombesin-like immunoreactive peptide is found in both brain and gut. Other actions include hypertensive, antidiuretic, and hyperglycemic activity. Has a strong effect on core temperature lowering in rats. High levels of intracellular bombesin have also been found in human small-cell lung carcinoma.

bond. In chemistry, the force holding two neighboring atoms in place and resisting their separation; a b. is electrovalent if it consists of the attraction between oppositely charged groups, or covalent if it results from the sharing of one, two, or three pairs of electrons by the bonded atoms.

acylmercaptan b., —CO—S—; a "high energy" b. formed by the condensation of a carboxyl group (—COOH) and a mercaptan (or thiol) group (—SH); widely formed in the course of intermediary metabolism, notably in the oxidation of fats, where the —SH is part of coenzyme A and the —COOH is part of the fatty acid being oxidized.

apolar b., SEE hydrophobic *interaction.*

conjugated double b.'s, two or more double b.'s separated by each single b.

coordinate covalent b., SYN semipolar b.

disulfide b., a single bond between two sulfurs; specifically, the —S—S— link binding two peptide chains (or different parts of one peptide chain); also occurs as part of the molecule of the amino acid, cystine, and is important as a structural determinant in many protein molecules, notably keratin, insulin, and oxytocin. A symmetric disulfide is R–S–S–R; R′–S–S–R is a mixed disulfide.

double b., a covalent b. resulting from the sharing of two pairs of electrons; *e.g.,* $H_2C=CH_2$ (ethylene).

electrostatic b., b. between atoms or groups carrying opposite charges (or, in some cases, partial charges). SYN heteropolar b., salt bridge.

energy-rich b., SEE high energy *compounds,* under *compound.*

eupeptide b., a peptide b. between the α-carboxyl group of one amino acid and the α-amino group of another amino acid. Cf. peptide b., isopeptide b.

heteropolar b., SYN electrostatic b.

high energy phosphate b., SEE high energy *phosphates,* under *phosphate.*

hydrogen b., a b. arising from the sharing of a hydrogen atom, covalently bound to an electronegative element (*e.g.,* N or O), with another electronegative element (*e.g.,* N, O, or a halogen). In substances of biological importance, the most common hydrogen b.'s are those in which H links N to O or N; such b.'s link purines on one strand to pyrimidines on the other strand of nucleic acids, thus maintaining double-stranded structures as in the Watson-Crick helix.

hydrophobic b., SEE hydrophobic *interaction.*

isopeptide b., an amide linkage between a carboxyl group of one amino acid and an amino group of another amino acid in which at least one of these groups is not on the α-carbon of one of the amino acids; for example, the bond between the glutamyl residue and the cysteinyl residue of glutathione. Cf. peptide b., eupeptide b.

noncovalent b., b. in which electrons are not shared between atoms; *e.g.,* electrostatic b., hydrogen b.

peptide b., the common link (—CO—NH—) between amino acids in proteins, actually a substituted amide, formed by elimination of H_2O between the —COOH of one amino acid and the H_2N— of another. Cf. eupeptide b., isopeptide b.

semipolar b., a b. in which the two electrons shared by a pair of atoms belonged originally to only one of the atoms; often represented by a small arrow pointing toward the electron receiver; *e.g.,* nitric acid, O(OH)N→O; phosphoric acid, $(OH)_3P$→O. SYN coordinate covalent b.

single b., a covalent b. resulting from the sharing of one pair of electrons; *e.g.,* H_3C—CH_3 (ethane).

triple b., a covalent b. resulting from the sharing of three pairs of electrons; *e.g.,* HC≡CH (acetylene).

BONE

---

bone (bōn). **1.** A hard connective tissue consisting of cells embedded in a matrix of mineralized ground substance and collagen fibers. The fibers are impregnated with a form of calcium phosphate similar to hydroxyapatite as well as with substantial quantities of carbonate, citrate sodium, and magnesium; by weight, b.

is composed of 75% inorganic material and 25% organic material; a portion of osseous tissue of definite shape and size, forming a part of the animal skeleton; in man there are 200 distinct ossa in the skeleton, not including the ossicula auditus of the tympanic cavity or the ossa sesamoidea other than the two patellae. Bone consists of a dense outer layer of compact substance or cortical substance covered by the periosteum, and an inner loose, spongy substance; the central portion of a long bone is filled with marrow. **2.** For definitions of bones as part of the animal skeleton, see os. For definitions of bones as part of the animal skelton, see Os. SYN os [NA]. [A.S. *bān*]

Albrecht's b., a small b. between the basioccipital and basisphenoid.

alveolar b., (1) SYN alveolar *process.* **(2)** in dentistry, the specialized bony structure which supports the teeth; it consists of the cortical b. that comprises the tooth socket into which the roots of the tooth fit, and is supported by the trabecular b. SYN alveolar supporting b.

alveolar supporting b., SYN alveolar b. (2).

ankle b., SYN talus.

basal b., the osseous tissue of the mandible and maxillae except the alveolar processes.

basilar b., the developmental basilar process of the occipital b. which unites with the condylar portions in about the fourth or fifth year, becoming the basilar *part* of the occipital bone. SYN basioccipital b., os basilare.

basioccipital b., SYN basilar b.

basisphenoid b., in comparative anatomy, the b. in the floor of the braincase in the region of the pituitary. SEE *body* of sphenoid bone.

Bertin's b.'s, SYN sphenoidal *conchae,* under *concha.*

blade b., SYN scapula.

breast b., SYN sternum.

Breschet's b.'s, SYN os suprasternale.

brittle b.'s, SYN *osteogenesis* imperfecta.

bundle b., immature b. containing thick bundles of collagen fibers arranged nearly parallel to one another with osteocytes in between; a similar type of b. is found in regions penetrated by fibers of Sharpey, as at ligament and tendon attachments.

calcaneal b., SYN calcaneus (1).

calf b., SYN fibula. [O.N. *kalfi,* fibula]

cancellous b., SYN *substantia* spongiosa.

cannon b., the middle metacarpal (or metatarsal b.) in the horse. SYN shank b. (1).

capitate b., SYN capitate (1).

carpal b.'s, eight bones arranged in two rows that articulate proximally with the radius and indirectly with the ulna, and distally with the five metacarpal bones; in domestic mammals, the bones of the proximal row are called radial, intermediate, ulnar, and accessory, while those of the distal row are termed first, second, third, and fourth carpal bones. SYN carpus (2) [NA], ossa carpi [NA].

cartilage b., SYN endochondral b.

cavalry b., SYN rider's b.

central b., SYN os centrale.

central b. of ankle, SYN navicular b.

cheek b., (1) SYN zygomatic b. **(2)** SYN zygomatic *arch.*

⌂ **Combining forms**

Word*Finder*
Multi-term entry finder
Preceding letter A

A.D.A.M. Anatomy Plates
Between letters L and M

Appendices:
Following letter Z

SYN Synonym; Cf., compare

[NA] Nomina Anatomica

[MIM] Mendelian
Inheritance in Man

☆ **Official alternate term**

☆**[NA] Official alternate**
Nomina Anatomica term

High Profile Term

bo

coccygeal b., SYN coccyx.

collar b., SYN clavicle.

compact b., the compact, noncancellous portion of bone that consists largely of concentric lamellar osteons and interstitial lamellae. SYN substantia compacta [NA], compact substance, substantia compacta ossium.

convoluted b., SEE inferior nasal *concha,* middle nasal *concha,* superior nasal *concha,* supreme nasal *concha.*

cortical b., the superficial thin layer of compact bone. SYN substantia corticalis [NA], cortical substance.

coxal b., SYN hip b.

cranial b.'s, SYN b.'s of skull.

cubital b., SYN triquetral b.

cuboid b., the lateral bone of the distal row of the tarsus, articulating with the calcaneus, lateral cuneiform, navicular (occasionally), and fourth and fifth metatarsal bones. SYN os cuboideum [NA].

cuneiform b., SEE triquetral b., intermediate cuneiform b., lateral cuneiform b., medial cuneiform b.

dermal b., a b. formed by ossification of the cutis.

b.'s of digits, the phalanges and sesamoid bones of the fingers and toes. SYN ossa digitorum [NA].

dorsal talonavicular b., an anomalous b. of the foot located near the head of the talus. SYN Pirie's b.

ear b.'s, SYN auditory *ossicles,* under *ossicle.*

elbow b., SYN olecranon.

endochondral b., a b. that develops in a cartilage environment after the latter is partially or entirely destroyed by calcification and subsequent resorption. SYN cartilage b., replacement b.

epactal b.'s, SYN sutural b.'s.

epihyal b., an ossified stylomastoid ligament.

epipteric b., a sutural b. occasionally present at the pterion or junction of the parietal, frontal, greater wing of the sphenoid, and squamous portion of the temporal b.'s. SYN Flower's b.

episternal b., SYN os suprasternale.

ethmoid b., an irregularly shaped bone lying between the orbital plates of the frontal and anterior to the sphenoid bone; it consists of two lateral masses of thin plates enclosing air cells, attached above to a perforated horizontal lamina, the cribriform plate, from which descends a median vertical or perpendicular plate in the interval between the two lateral masses; the bone articulates with the sphenoid, frontal, maxillary, lacrimal, and palatine bones, the inferior nasal concha, and the vomer; it enters into the formation of the anterior cranial fossa, the orbits, and the nasal cavity. SYN os ethmoidale [NA].

exercise b., SYN rider's b.

exoccipital b. (eks-ok-sip′i-tăl), SYN lateral *part* of occipital bone.

facial b.'s, the bones surrounding the mouth and nose and contributing to the orbits; they are the paired maxilla, zygomatic, nasal, lacrimal, palatine, inferior nasal concha; and the unpaired ethmoid, vomer, mandible, and hyoid. SYN ossa faciei [NA], b.'s of visceral cranium.

first cuneiform b., SYN medial cuneiform b.

flank b., SYN ilium.

flat b., a type of bone characterized by its thin, flattened shape, such as the scapula or certain of the cranial bones. SYN os planum [NA].

Flower's b., SYN epipteric b.

fourth turbinated b., SYN supreme nasal *concha.*

frontal b., the large single bone forming the forehead and the upper margin and roof of the orbit on either side; it articulates with the parietal, nasal, ethmoid, maxillary, and zygomatic bones, and with the lesser wings of the sphenoid. SYN os frontale [NA], coronale (1).

Goethe's b., SYN preinterparietal b.

greater multangular b., SYN trapezium.

hamate b., the bone on the medial (ulnar) side of the distal row of the carpus; it articulates with the fourth and fifth metacarpal, triquetral, lunate, and capitate. SYN os hamatum [NA], hamatum, hooked b., unciform b., unciforme, uncinatum.

heel b., SYN calcaneus (1).

heterotopic b.'s, b.'s that do not belong to the main skeleton but that regularly develop in certain organs, *e.g.,* the heart, penis, clitoris, and snout of some animals.

highest turbinated b., SYN supreme nasal *concha.*

hip b., a large flat bone formed by the fusion of the ilium, ischium, and pubis (in the adult), constituting the lateral half of the pelvis; it articulates with its fellow anteriorly, with the sacrum posteriorly, and with the femur laterally. SYN os coxae [NA], coxa (1), coxal b., innominate b., os innominatum.

hollow b., SYN pneumatic b.

hooked b., SYN hamate b.

hyoid b., (1) a U-shaped bone lying between the mandible and the larynx, suspended from the styloid processes by slender stylohyoid ligaments; (2) SEE hyoid *apparatus.* SYN os hyoideum [NA], lingual b., tongue b.

iliac b., SYN ilium.

incarial b., SYN *os* interparietale.

incisive b., SYN *os* incisivum.

b.'s of inferior limb, SYN b.'s of lower limb.

inferior turbinated b., SYN inferior nasal *concha.*

innominate b., SYN hip b.

intermaxillary b., SYN *os* incisivum.

intermediate cuneiform b., a bone of the distal row of the tarsus; it articulates with the medial and lateral cuneiform, navicular, and second metatarsal bones. SYN os cuneiforme intermedium [NA], mesocuneiform, middle cuneiform b., second cuneiform b., wedge b.

interparietal b., SYN *os* interparietale.

irregular b., one of a group of bones having peculiar or complex forms, *e.g.,* vertebrae, many of the skull bones. SYN os irregulare [NA].

ischial b., SYN ischium.

jaw b., SYN mandible.

jugal b., SYN zygomatic b.

Krause's b., small b. (secondary ossification center) in the triradiate cartilage between the ilium, the ischium, and the pubic b. in the growing acetabulum.

lacrimal b., an irregularly rectangular thin plate, forming part of the medial wall of the orbit behind the frontal process of the maxilla; it articulates with the inferior nasal concha, ethmoid, frontal, and maxillary bones. SYN os lacrimale [NA], os unguis.

lamellar b., the normal type of adult mammalian b., whether cancellous or compact, composed of parallel lamellae in the former and concentric lamellae in the latter; lamellar organization reflects a repeating pattern of collagen fibroarchitecture.

lateral cuneiform b., a bone of the distal row of the tarsus; it articulates with the intermediate cuneiform, cuboid, navicular, and second, third, and fourth metatarsal bones. SYN os cuneiforme laterale [NA], third cuneiform b., wedge b.

lenticular b., SYN lenticular *process* of incus.

lentiform b., SYN pisiform b.

lesser multangular b., SYN trapezoid b.

lingual b., SYN hyoid b.

long b., one of the elongated bones of the extremities, consisting of a tubular shaft (diaphysis) and two extremities (epiphysis) usually wider than the shaft; the shaft is composed of compact bone surrounding a central medullary cavity. Cf. short b. SYN os longum [NA], pipe b.

b.'s of lower limb, these include the inferior limb girdle (hip bone) and the skeleton of the free inferior limb (femur, tibia, fibula, patella, tarsus, metatarsus, and bones of the toes). SYN ossa membri inferioris [NA], b.'s of inferior limb.

lunate b., one of the proximal row in the carpus between the scaphoid and triquetral; it articulates with the radius, scaphoid, triquetral, hamate, and capitate. SYN os lunatum [NA], lunare, os intermedium.

malar b., SYN zygomatic b.

marble b.'s, SYN osteopetrosis.

mastoid b., SYN mastoid *process.*

medial cuneiform b., the largest of the three cuneiform bones, the medial bone of the distal row of the tarsus, articulating with the intermediate cuneiform, navicular, and first and second metatarsal bones. SYN os cuneiforme mediale [NA], first cuneiform b., wedge b.

medullary b., areas of b. formation present in the marrow spaces of the long b.'s of birds, which serve as a readily mobilized source of calcium for shell formation.

membrane b., a b. that develops embryologically within a membrane of vascularized primitive mesenchymal tissue without prior formation of cartilage.

mesethmoid b., in comparative anatomy, the b. present in some species as the most anterior b. of the floor of the braincase.

metacarpal b., one of the metacarpal bones, five long bones (numbered I to V, beginning with the bone on the radial or thumb side) forming the skeleton of the metacarpus or palm; they articulate with the bones of the distal row of the carpus and with the five proximal phalanges. SYN os metacarpale [NA].

metatarsal b., one of the metatarsal bones; the five long bones numbered I to V beginning with the bone on the medial side forming the skeleton of the anterior portion of the foot, articulating posteriorly with the three cuneiform and the cuboid bones, anteriorly with the five proximal phalanges. SYN os metatarsale [NA].

middle cuneiform b., SYN intermediate cuneiform b.

middle turbinated b., SYN middle nasal *concha.*

multangular b., SEE trapezium, trapezoid b.

nasal b., an elongated rectangular bone which, with its fellow, forms the bridge of the nose; it articulates with the frontal bone superiorly, the ethmoid and the frontal process of the maxilla posteriorly, and its fellow medially. SYN os nasale [NA].

navicular b., a bone of the tarsus on the medial side of the foot articulating with the head of the talus, the three cuneiform bones, and occasionally the cuboid. SYN os naviculare [NA], central b. of ankle, os centrale tarsi.

navicular b. of hand, SYN scaphoid b.

nonlamellar b., SYN woven b.

occipital b., a bone at the lower and posterior part of the skull, consisting of three parts (basilar, condylar, and squamous), enclosing a large oval hole, the foramen magnum; it articulates with the parietal and temporal bones on either side, the sphenoid anteriorly, and the atlas below. SYN os occipitale [NA].

orbicular b., SYN lenticular *process* of incus.

palatine b., an irregularly shaped bone posterior to the maxilla, which enters into the formation of the nasal cavity, the orbit, and the hard palate; it articulates with the maxilla, inferior nasal concha, sphenoid, and ethmoid bones, the vomer and its fellow of the opposite side. SYN os palatinum [NA].

parietal b., a flat, curved bone of irregular quadrangular shape, at either side of the vault of the cranium; it articulates, with its fellow medially, with the frontal anteriorly, the occipital posteriorly, and the temporal and sphenoid inferiorly. SYN os parietale [NA].

penis b., SYN *os* penis.

perichondral b., in the development of a long b. a collar or cuff of osseous tissue forms in the perichondrium of the cartilage model; the connective tissue membrane of this perichondral b. then becomes periosteum. SYN periosteal b.

periosteal b., SYN perichondral b.

periotic b., SYN petrous *part* of temporal bone.

peroneal b., SYN fibula.

petrosal b., SYN petrous *part* of temporal bone.

petrous b., SYN petrous *part* of internal carotid artery.

ping-pong b., the thin shell of osseous tissue at the periphery of a giant cell tumor in a b.

pipe b., SYN long b.

Pirie's b., SYN dorsal talonavicular b.

pisiform b., a small bone resembling a pea in size and shape, in the proximal row of the carpus, lying on the anterior surface of the triquetral with which alone it articulates; it gives insertion to the tendon of the flexor carpi ulnaris muscle. SYN os pisiforme [NA], lentiform b.

pneumatic b., a bone that is hollow or contains many air cells,

such as the mastoid process of the temporal bone. SYN os pneumaticum [NA], hollow b.

postsphenoid b., the posterior portion of the body of the sphenoid b.

preinterparietal b., a large sutural b. occasionally found detached from the anterior portion of the os interparietale. SYN Goethe's b.

premaxillary b., SYN *os* incisivum.

presphenoid b., in comparative anatomy, the b. in the floor of the braincase anterior to the basisphenoid b.

pubic b., SYN *mons* pubis.

pyramidal b., SYN triquetral b.

replacement b., SYN endochondral b.

reticulated b., SYN woven b.

rider's b., heterotopic bone ossification of the tendon of the adductor longus muscle from strain in horseback riding. SYN cavalry b., exercise b.

Riolan's b.'s, several small sutural b.'s sometimes present in the petro-occipital suture.

sacred b., SYN sacrum. [so called from belief in indestructibility of the bone as the basis for resurrection]

scaphoid b., the largest bone of the proximal row of the carpus on the lateral (radial) side, articulating with the radius, lunate, capitate, trapezium, and trapezoid. SYN os scaphoideum [NA], navicular b. of hand, os naviculare manus.

scroll b.'s, SEE inferior nasal *concha,* middle nasal *concha,* superior nasal *concha,* supreme nasal *concha.*

second cuneiform b., SYN intermediate cuneiform b.

semilunar b., obsolete term for lunate b.

septal b., SYN interalveolar *septum.*

sesamoid b., a bone formed in a tendon where it passes over a joint. SYN os sesamoideum [NA].

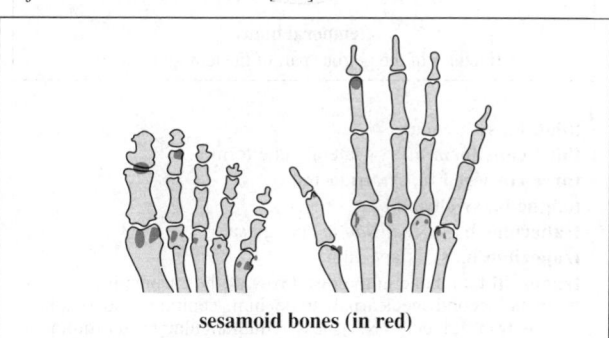

sesamoid bones (in red)

shank b., (1) SYN cannon b. (2) SYN tibia.

shin b., SYN tibia.

short b., one whose dimensions are approximately equal; it consists of a layer of cortical substance enclosing spongy substance and narrow. Cf. long b. SYN os breve [NA].

sieve b., SYN cribriform *plate* of ethmoid bone.

b.'s of skull, the paired inferior nasal concha, lacrimal, maxilla, nasal, palatine, parietal, temporal, and zygomatic; and the unpaired ethmoid, frontal, occipital, sphenoid, and vomer. SYN ossa cranii [NA], cranial b.'s.

sphenoid b., a bone of most irregular shape occupying the base of the skull; it is described as consisting of a central portion, or body, and six processes: two greater wings, two lesser wings and two pterygoid processes; it articulates with the occipital, frontal, ethmoid, and vomer, and with the paired temporal, parietal, zygomatic, palatine and sphenoidal concha bones. SYN os sphenoidale [NA], sphenoid (2).

sphenoidal turbinated b.'s, SYN sphenoidal *conchae,* under *concha.*

splint b., (1) the second or fourth, or internal or external small metacarpal b.'s in the horse; these are splinter-like in shape and lie on either side of the metacarpal or cannon b.; (2) SYN fibula.

spongy b., (1) SYN *substantia* spongiosa. (2) a turbinated bone.

stifle b., the patella of the stifle joint of a horse.

b.'s of superior limb, SYN b.'s of upper limb.

superior turbinated b., SYN superior nasal *concha.*

suprainterparietal b., a sutural b. at the posterior portion of the sagittal suture.

suprasternal b., SYN *os* suprasternale.

supreme turbinated b., SYN supreme nasal *concha.*

sutural b.'s, small irregular bones found along the sutures of the cranium, particularly related to the parietal bone. SYN ossa suturarum [NA], Andernach's ossicles, epactal b.'s, epactal ossicles, wormian b.'s.

tail b., SYN coccyx.

tarsal b.'s, the seven bones of the instep: talus, calcaneus, navicular, three cuneiform (wedge), and cuboid bones. SYN ossa tarsi [NA].

temporal b., a large irregular bone situated in the base and side of the skull; it consists of three parts, squamous, tympanic and petrous, which are distinct at birth; the petrous part contains the vestibulocochlear organ; the bone articulates with the sphenoid, parietal, occipital, and zygomatic bones, and by a synovial joint with the mandible. SYN os temporale [NA].

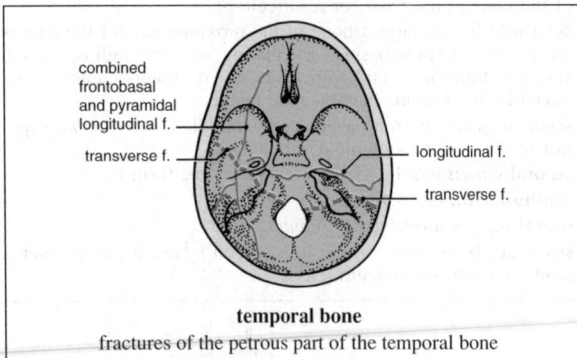

combined frontobasal and pyramidal longitudinal f.

transverse f.

longitudinal f.

transverse f.

temporal bone

fractures of the petrous part of the temporal bone

thigh b., SYN femur.

third cuneiform b., SYN lateral cuneiform b.

three-cornered b., SYN triquetral b.

tongue b., SYN hyoid b.

trabecular b., SYN *substantia* spongiosa.

trapezium b., SYN trapezium.

trapezoid b., a bone in the distal row of the carpus; it articulates with the second metacarpal, trapezium, capitate, and scaphoid. SYN os trapezoideum [NA], lesser multangular b., os multangulum minus, trapezoid (3).

triangular b., SYN *os* trigonum.

triquetral b., a bone on the medial (ulnar) side of the proximal row of the carpus, articulating with the lunate, pisiform, and hamate. SYN os triquetrum [NA], cubital b., os pyramidale, os triangulare (2), pyramidal b., pyramidale, three-cornered b., triquetrum.

turbinated b.'s, SEE inferior nasal *concha,* middle nasal *concha,* superior nasal *concha,* supreme nasal *concha.*

tympanic b., SYN tympanic *ring.*

tympanohyal b., a small nodule of b. forming the base of the cartilaginous styloid process of the temporal b. at birth.

unciform b., SYN hamate b.

upper jaw b., SYN maxilla.

b.'s of upper limb, these include the superior limb girdle (scapula and clavicle) and the skeleton of the free superior limb (humerus, radius, ulna, wrist bones, metacarpus, and bones of the fingers). SYN ossa membri superioris [NA], b.'s of superior limb.

Vesalius' b., SYN *os* vesalianum.

b.'s of visceral cranium, SYN facial b.'s.

wedge b., SYN intermediate cuneiform b., lateral cuneiform b., medial cuneiform b.

wormian b.'s, SYN sutural b.'s.

woven b., bony tissue characteristic of the embryonal skeleton, in which the collagen fibers of the matrix are arranged irregularly

in the form of interlacing networks. SYN nonlamellar b., reticulated b.

yoke b., SYN zygomatic b.

zygomatic b., a quadrilateral bone which forms the prominence of the cheek; it articulates with the frontal, sphenoid, temporal, and maxillary bone. SYN os zygomaticum [NA], cheek b. (1), jugal b., mala (2), malar b., os malare, yoke b., zygoma (1).

bone ar·chi·tec·ture. The pattern of trabeculae and associated structures. SEE ALSO Wolff's *law.*

bone ash. SYN tribasic *calcium* phosphate.

bone black. SYN animal *charcoal.*

bone·let (bōn′let). SYN ossicle.

bone-salt. The main chemical compound in bone, deposited as minute amorphous crystals in a netlike matrix of collagenous fibers containing collagen; it closely resembles the naturally occurring fluorapatite $3Ca_3(PO_4)_2 \cdot CaF_2$, but is probably a hydroxyapatite in which F is replaced by OH.

Bonhoeffer, Karl, German psychiatrist, 1868–1948. SEE B.'s *sign.*

Bonnet, Amédée, French surgeon, 1809–1858. SEE B.'s *capsule.*

Bonnevie, Kristine, German physician, 1872–1950.

Bonnier, Pierre, French clinician, 1861–1918. SEE B.'s *syndrome.*

Bonwill, William G.A., U.S. dentist, 1833–1899. SEE B. *triangle.*

Böök, Jan A., Swedish geneticist, *1915. SEE B. *syndrome.*

BOOP Abbreviation for *bronchiolitis* obliterans with organizing pneumonia, an idiopathic form of *bronchiolitis* obliterans.

Bo·oph·i·lus (bō-of′i-lŭs). A genus of hard ticks (family Ixodidae) infesting cattle; members are important vectors of bovine babesiosis and anaplasmosis in various parts of the world. Previously thought to be synonymous with *Margaropus,* but now considered distinct. [G. *bous,* ox, + *philos,* fond]

B. annula′tus, species that formerly was the vector of bovine babesiosis in the southern United States, but is still an important species in Mexico and northern African countries.

B. decolora′tus, species that is a vector of bovine babesiosis and anaplasmosis in sub-Saharan Africa.

B. mi′croplus, the tropical cattle tick, a species that is an important vector of bovine babesiosis and anaplasmosis in Mexico, Central and South America, the Caribbean Africa, Australia, the Orient and Micronesia, and of relapsing fever by *Borrelia theileri* in South Africa and Australia.

boost·er. SEE booster *dose.*

boot (būt). A boot-shaped appliance. [M. E. *bote,* fr. O. Fr.]

Gibney's b., adhesive tape treatment of a sprained ankle or similar condition, applied in a basket-weave fashion under the sole of the foot and around the back of the lower leg.

Junod's b., an airtight case into which the arm or leg is inserted and the air is then exhausted; used to divert a portion of the blood temporarily from the general circulation.

bo·rac·ic ac·id (bō-ras′ik). SYN boric acid.

bo·rate (bōr′āt). A salt of boric acid.

bo·rat·ed (bōr′āt-ed). Mixed or impregnated with borax or boric acid.

bo·rax (bō′raks). SYN *sodium* borate. [Pers. *būraq*]

bor·bo·ryg·mus, pl. **bor·bo·ryg·mi** (bōr-bō-rig′mŭs, -rig′mī). Rumbling or gurgling noises produced by movement of gas in the alimentary canal, and audible at a distance. [G. *borborygmos,* rumbling in the bowels]

Bordeau (Bordeu), Théophile de, French physician, 1722–1776. SEE B. *theory;* de B. *theory.*

bor·der (bōr′der). The part of a surface that forms its outer boundary. SEE ALSO edge, margin, border. SYN margo [NA].

alveolar b., (1) the most occlusal edge of the alveolar bone; **(2)** SYN alveolar *process.*

anterior b., the ventral or most forward margin of a structure. SYN anterior margin, ventral b.

anterior b. of eyelids, the anterior edge of the free margin of each eyelid, along close to which the eyelashes are embedded. SYN limbus palpebrales anteriores [NA].

anterior b. of fibula, a ridge on the shaft of the fibula to which is attached the anterior intermuscular septum of the leg. SYN margo anterior fibulae [NA].

anterior b. of lung, the thin anteromedial or sternal edge of the lung which overlaps the pericardial sac anteriorly and forms the boundary between the mediastinal and costal surfaces. SYN margo anterior pulmonis [NA].

anterior b. of pancreas, the sharp margin between the anterior and inferior surfaces of the pancreas. SYN margo anterior pancreatis [NA].

anterior b. of radius, the ridge on the shaft of the radius extending from the radial tuberosity to the anterior part of the styloid process. SYN margo anterior radii [NA].

anterior b. of testis, an imaginary convex line demarcating the lateral and medial surfaces. SYN margo anterior testis [NA].

anterior b. of tibia, the sharp subcutaneous ridge of the tibia that extends from the tuberosity to the anterior part of the medial malleolus. SYN margo anterior tibiae [NA], anticnemion, shin, tibial crest.

anterior b. of ulna, the ridge on the body of the ulna that extends from the tuberosity to the anterior part of the styloid process. SYN margo anterior ulnae [NA].

brush b., the apical epithelial surface bearing closely packed microvilli about 2 μm long, such as occur on the cells of the proximal tubule of the nephron. SYN limbus penicillatus.

ciliary b. of iris, the peripheral b. of the iris attached to the ciliary body. SYN margo ciliaris iridis [NA], ciliary margin of iris.

denture b., (**1**) the limit or boundary or circumferential margin of a denture base; (**2**) the margin of the denture base at the junction of the polished surface with the impression (tissue) surface; (**3**) the extreme edges of a denture base at the buccolabial, lingual, and posterior limits. SYN denture edge, periphery (2).

b.'s of eyelids, the anterior and posterior edges of the free margin of the upper and lower eyelids. SYN limbi palpebrales [NA].

free b., unattached edge of a sturcture, often opposite the attached edge. SEE free b. of nail, free b. of ovary. SYN margo liber [NA], free margin.

free b. of nail, the distal b. of the nail that overhangs the tip of the digit. SYN margo liber unguis [NA].

free b. of ovary, the unattached, posterior margin of the ovary. SYN margo liber ovarii [NA].

frontal b., edge of a bone which articulates with the frontal bone. SEE frontal b. of parietal bone, frontal b. of sphenoid bone. SYN margo frontalis [NA], frontal margin.

frontal b. of parietal bone, the margin of the parietal bone that articulates with the frontal bone. SYN margo frontalis ossis parietalis [NA].

frontal b. of sphenoid bone, the margin of the greater wing of the sphenoid bon that articulates with the frontal bone. SYN margo frontalis ossis sphenoidalis [NA].

inferior b., the caudal or lowermost margin of a structure. SYN inferior margin, margo inferior.

inferior b. of liver, the sharp border of the liver that separates the diaphragmatic and visceral surfaces. SYN margo inferior hepatis [NA].

inferior b. of lung, the sharp border of the lung that separates the diaphragmatic surface from the costal and mediastinal surfaces. SYN margo inferior pulmonis [NA].

inferior b. of pancreas, the border of the pancreas separating the inferior and posterior surfaces. SYN margo inferior pancreatis [NA], margo inferior splenis [NA].

interosseous b., edge of a bone to which a fibrous (interosseous) membrane is attached, by which the bone becomes attached to another bone. SEE interosseous b. of fibula, interosseous b. of radius, interosseous b. of tibia, interosseous b. of ulna. SYN margo interosseus [NA], interosseous crest, interosseous margin.

interosseous b. of fibula, the ridge along the medial b. of the fibula to which is attached the interosseous membrane. SYN margo interosseus fibulae [NA].

interosseous b. of radius, the ridge along the medial side of the radius to which is attached the interosseous membrane. SYN margo interosseus radii [NA].

interosseous b. of tibia, the ridge along the lateral b. of the tibia to which is attached the interosseous membrane. SYN margo interosseus tibiae [NA].

interosseous b. of ulna, the ridge along the lateral side of the body of the ulna to which is attached the interosseous membrane. SYN margo interosseus ulnae [NA].

lacrimal b. of maxilla, the margin of the nasal surface of the maxilla that articulates with the lacrimal bone. SYN margo lacrimalis maxillae [NA], lacrimal margin of maxilla.

lambdoid b. of occipital bone, the margin of the occipital squama that articulates with the parietal bones in the lambdoid suture. SYN margo lambdoideus squamae occipitalis [NA], lambdoid margin of occipital bone.

lateral b., the margin or edge of a structure which is farthest from the midline. SYN margo lateralis [NA], lateral margin.

lateral b. of foot, the border of the foot between the small toe and the heel. SYN margo lateralis pedis [NA], margo fibularis pedis*, fibular margin of foot.

lateral b. of forearm, an imaginary line running along the outermost extent of the forearm separating anterior and posterior surfaces laterally. SYN margo lateralis antebrachii [NA], margo radialis antebrachii*, radial b. of forearm.

lateral b. of humerus, the ridge on the humerus that extends from the greater tubercle to the lateral epicondyle. SYN margo lateralis humerii [NA].

lateral b. of kidney, the convex narrow edge separating the anterior and posterior surfaces. SYN margo lateralis renis [NA].

lateral b. of nail, the sides of the nail extending from the proximal to the free borders. SYN margo lateralis unguis [NA].

lateral b. of scapula, the edge of the scapula extending from the glenoid fossa to the inferior angle. SYN margo lateralis scapulae [NA].

mastoid b. of occipital bone, the margin of the occipital squama that articulates with the temporal bone. SYN margo mastoideus squamae occipitalis [NA], mastoid margin of occipital bone.

medial b., the b. of a structure closest to the medial plane. SYN margo medialis [NA], medial margin.

medial b. of foot, the inner b. of the foot extending from heel to the great toe. SYN margo medialis pedis [NA], margo tibialis pedis* [NA], tibial b. of foot.

medial b. of forearm, an imaginary line extrapolated from the medial epicondyle of the humerus to the styloid process of the ulna, forming a b. between the anterior and posterior surfaces. SYN margo medialis antebrachii [NA], margo ulnaris antebrachii* [NA], ulnar margin of forearm.

medial b. of humerus, the ridge on the humerus extending from the crest of the lesser tubercle to the medial epicondyle. SYN margo medialis humerii [NA].

medial b. of kidney, the concave b. of the kidney. SYN margo medialis renis [NA].

medial b. of scapula, the edge of the scapula closest to the vertebral column, extending from superior angle to inferior angle. SYN margo medialis scapulae, vertebral b. of scapula.

medial b. of suprarenal gland, the paravertebral edge of the suprarenal gland. SYN margo medialis glandulae suprarenalis [NA].

medial b. of tibia, the rounded b. of the tibia that separates the posterior and medial surfaces. SYN margo medialis tibiae [NA].

mesovarian b. of ovary, the border of the ovary to which the mesovarium is attached. SYN margo mesovaricus ovarii [NA], mesovarian margin of ovary.

nasal b. of frontal bone, the border of the frontal bone that articulates with the nasal bones. SYN margo nasalis ossis frontalis [NA], nasal margin of frontal bone.

occipital b., edge of a bone which articulates with the occipital bone. SEE occipital b. of parietal bone, occipital b. of temporal bone. SYN margo occipitalis [NA], occipital margin.

occipital b. of parietal bone, the posterior margin of the parietal bone that articulates with the occipital squama. SYN margo occipitalis ossis parietalis [NA].

occipital b. of temporal bone, that part of the temporal bone that articulates with the occipital squama. SYN margo occipitalis ossis temporalis [NA].

occult b. of nail, SYN proximal b. of nail.

parietal b., edge of a bone which articulates with the parietal bone. SEE parietal b. of frontal bone, parietal b. of sphenoid bone, parietal b. of temporal bone. SYN margo parietalis [NA], parietal margin.

parietal b. of frontal bone, the margin of the frontal bone that articulates with the parietal bone. SYN margo parietalis ossis frontalis [NA].

parietal b. of sphenoid bone, the margin of the greater wing of the sphenoid that articulates with the parietal bone. SYN margo parietalis ossis sphenoidalis [NA].

parietal b. of temporal bone, the b. of the squamous part of the temporal bone that articulates with the parietal bone. SYN margo parietalis ossis temporalis [NA].

posterior b. of eyelids, the posterior edge of the free margin of each eyelid, which is also the border of the conjunctiva.

posterior b. of fibula, the ridge on the posterior aspect of the fibula extending from the head to the medial aspect of the peroneal groove. SYN margo posterior fibulae [NA].

posterior b. of petrous part of temporal bone, the margin of the petrous part of the temporal bone that extends from the apex to the jugular notch; it articulates with the basal and jugular portions of the occipital bone. SYN margo posterior partis petrosae ossis temporalis [NA].

posterior b. of radius, the ridge on the radius that extends from the tuberosity to the tubercle on the posterior aspect of the distal extremity. SYN margo posterior radii [NA].

posterior b. of testis, the rounded posterior portion of the testis into which the vessels enter. SYN margo posterior testis [NA].

posterior b. of ulna, the sinuous palpable subcutaneous ridge on the posterior aspect of the ulna that extends from near the olecranon to the styloid process, demarcating "anterior" (flexor) from "posterior" (extensor) compartments of forearm. SYN margo posterior ulnae [NA].

proximal b. of nail, the proximal border of the nail entirely covered by the nail wall. SYN margo occultus unguis [NA], occult b. of nail.

pupillary b. of iris, the inner border of the iris that forms the edge of the pupil. SYN margo pupillaris iridis [NA], pupillary margin of iris.

radial b. of forearm, SYN lateral b. of forearm.

right b. of heart, the b. between the sternocostal and diaphragmatic surfaces of the heart; it is fairly well defined in fixed hearts but is rounded and indefinite in the living heart. SYN margo dexter cordis [NA], right margin of heart.

sagittal b. of parietal bone, the medial border of the parietal bone entering into the sagittal suture. SYN margo sagittalis ossis parietalis [NA].

sphenoidal b. of temporal bone, the part of the border of the squamous part of the temporal bone that articulates with the greater wing of the sphenoid. SYN margo sphenoidalis ossis temporalis [NA].

squamous b., edge of a bone which articulates with the squamous part of the temporal bone. SEE squamous b. of parietal bone, squamous b. of sphenoid bone. SYN margo squamosus [NA], squamous margin.

squamous b. of parietal bone, the lateral b. of the parietal bone that articulates with the squamous part of the temporal bone. SYN margo squamosus ossis parietalis [NA].

squamous b. of sphenoid bone, the margin of the greater wing of the sphenoid bone that articulates with the squamous part of the temporal bone. SYN margo squamosus ossis sphenoidalis [NA].

striated b., the free surface of the columnar absorptive cells of the intestine formed by closely packed microvilli about 1 μm long, giving the appearance of parallel striations. SYN limbus striatus.

superior b., the cranial or uppermost margin of a structure.

superior b. of pancreas, the uppermost border of the body of the pancreas that separates the anterior and posterior surfaces. SYN margo superior pancreatis [NA].

superior b. of petrous part of temporal bone, the margin that separates the anterior and posterior surfaces of the petrous part of the temporal bone and the lateral part of the middle cranial fossa from the posterior cranial fossa. SYN margo superior partis petrosae ossis temporalis [NA], crest of petrous part of temporal bone.

superior b. of scapula, the margin of the scapula that extends from the glenoid fossa to the superior angle. SYN margo superior scapulae [NA].

superior b. of spleen, the notched border of the spleen that separates the gastric and disphragmatic surfaces. SYN margo superior splenis [NA].

superior b. of suprarenal gland, the border of the suprarenal gland at the superior junction of the anterior and posterior surfaces. SYN margo superior glandulae suprarenalis [NA].

tibial b. of foot, SYN medial b. of foot.

b. of uterus, the right or left margin of the uterus along which the broad ligament is attached. The uterine tube and round ligament attach to the uterus at the upper part of the border. SYN margo uteri [NA].

ventral b., SYN anterior b.

vermilion b., the red margin of the upper and lower lip that commences at the exterior edge of the intraoral labial mucosa ("moist line") and extends outward, terminating at the extraoral labial cutaneous junction; a thinly keratinized type of stratified squamous epithelium deeply penetrated by well-vascularized dermal papillae which show through the translucent epidermis to impart the typical red appearance of the lips. SYN vermilion zone, vermilion transitional zone.

vertebral b. of scapula, SYN medial b. of scapula.

zygomatic b. of greater wing of sphenoid bone, the border of the greater wing of the sphenoid that articulates with the zygomatic bone. SYN margo zygomaticus alae majoris [NA], zygomatic margin of greater wing of sphenoid bone.

Bordet, Jules, Belgian bacteriologist and Nobel laureate, 1870–1961. SEE *Bordetella;* B.-Gengou potato blood *agar, bacillus, phenomenon;* B. and Gengou *reaction.*

Bor·de·tel·la (bōr-dĕ-tel′ă). A genus of strictly aerobic bacteria (family Brucellaceae) containing minute, Gram-negative coccobacilli. Motile and nonmotile species occur; motile cells are peritrichous. The metabolism of these organisms is respiratory. They require nicotinic acid, cysteine, and methionine; hemin (X factor) and coenzyme I (V factor) are not required. They are parasites and pathogens of the mammalian respiratory tract. The type species is *B. pertussis.* [J. *Bordet*]

B. bronchisep′tica, a species causing atrophic rhinitis of swine, bronchopneumonia in rodents, and bronchopneumonia secondary to distemper in dogs.

B. parapertus′sis, a species that causes a whooping cough-like disease.

B. pertus′sis, a species that causes whooping cough; it produces cell-destroying toxins and causes thick mucus to collect in the airway. The type species of the genus *B.* SYN Bordet-Gengou bacillus.

bo·ric ac·id (bō′rik). H_3BO_3; a very weak acid, used as an antiseptic dusting powder, in saturated solution as a collyrium, and with glycerin in aphthae and stomatitis. SYN boracic acid.

bor·ism (bōr′izm). Symptoms caused by the ingestion of borax or any compound of boron.

Börjeson, Mats, Swedish physician, *1922. SEE B.-Forssman-Lehmann *syndrome.*

Born, Gustav Jacob, German embryologist, 1851–1900. SEE B. *method* of wax plate reconstruction.

bor·nane (bōr′nān). 1,7,7-trimethylnorbornane; the monoterpene parent of borneols, camphene, and similar essential oils (terpenes).

bo·ro·glyc·er·in (bō-rō-glis′er-in). A soft mass obtained by heating glycerin and boric acid; an obsolete antiseptic, usually used mixed with equal parts of glycerin, constituting glycerite. SYN boroglycerol, glyceryl borate.

bo·ro·glyc·er·ol (bō-rō-glis′er-ol). SYN boroglycerin.

bo·ron (B) (bōr′on). A nonmetallic trivalent element, atomic no. 5, atomic wt. 10.811; occurs as a hard crystalline mass or as a brown powder, and forms borates and boric acid. A nutritional need has been reported with pregnant women. [Pers. *Burah*]

Borrel, Amédée, French bacteriologist, 1867–1936. SEE B. *bodies,* under *body;* B.'s blue *stain.*

Bor·rel·ia (bō-rē′lē-ă, bo-rel′ē-ă). A genus of bacteria (family Treponemataceae) containing cells 8 to 16 μm in length, with coarse, shallow, irregular spirals and tapered, finely filamented ends. These organisms are parasitic on many forms of animal life, are generally hematophytic, or are found on mucous membranes. Some borreliae are transmitted by the bites of arthropods. The type species is *B. anserina.* [A. *Borrell*]

B. anseri′na, a species that causes spirochetosis of fowls; found in the blood of infected geese, ducks, other fowls, and vector ticks; it is the type species of the genus *B.*

B. burgdor′feri, a species causing Lyme disease in humans and borreliosis in dogs, cattle, and possibly horses. The vector transmitting this spirochete to humans is the ixodid tick, *Ixodes dammini.*

B. cauca′sica, a species found as a cause of relapsing fever in the Caucasus; transmitted by *Ornithodoros verrucosus.*

B. crocidu′rae, a species that causes relapsing fever in Africa, the Near East, and central Asia, and is transmitted by the small variety of the tick *Ornithodoros erraticus.*

B. dutto′nii, a species causing Central and South African relapsing fever; transmitted by a tick, *Ornithodoros moubata.*

B. herm′sii, a species found as a cause of relapsing fever in British Columbia, California, Colorado, Idaho, Nevada, Oregon, and Washington; transmitted by a tick, *Ornithodoros hermsi.*

B. hispan′ica, a species causing relapsing fever in Spain, Portugal, and northwest Africa, transmitted by the large variety of the tick *Ornithodorus erratica.*

B. latysche′wii, a species that causes relapsing fever in Iran and central Asia; transmitted by the tick *Ornithodoros tartakovskyi* from rodents and reptiles.

B. mazzot′tii, a species that causes relapsing fever in Mexico and Central and South America; transmitted by the tick *Ornithodoros talajé.*

B. par′keri, a species found as a cause of relapsing fever in the western United States; transmitted by a tick, *Ornithodoros parkeri.*

B. per′sica, a species that causes relapsing fever in the Middle East and central Asia; the vector is the tick *Ornithodoros tholozani.*

B. recurren′tis, a species causing relapsing fever in South America, Europe, Africa, and Asia; transmitted by the bedbug, *Cimex lectularius,* and the louse, *Pediculus humanus* subsp. *humanus.* SYN Obermeier's spirillum, *Spirochaeta obermeieri.*

B. thei′leri, a species that causes borreliosis in cattle and other mammals in South Africa and Australia; transmitted by the ticks *Boophilus microplus* and *Rhipicephalus evertsi.*

B. turica′tae, a species found as a cause of relapsing fever in Mexico, New Mexico, Texas, Oklahoma, and Kansas; transmitted by *Ornithodoros turicata.*

B. venezuelen′sis, a species causing spirochetal relapsing fever in Central and South America; transmitted by *Ornithodoros rudis* and *O. venezuelensis.*

bor·re·li·o·sis (bō-rē-lē-ō′sis). Disease caused by bacteria of the genus *Borrelia.*

bovine b., a disease of cattle caused by *Borrelia burgdorferi* and characterized by laminitis, arthritis, and synovitis.

canine b., a disease of dogs caused by *Borrelia burgdorferi* and characterized by lameness due to a migratory, intermittent, oligoarticular arthritis.

Lyme b., SYN Lyme *disease.*

Borst, Maximilian, German pathologist, 1869–1946. SEE B.-Jadassohn type intraepidermal *epithelioma.*

Bosin's dis·ease. See under disease.

boss (baws). **1.** A protuberance; a circumscribed rounded swelling. **2.** The prominence of a kyphosis. [M. E. *boce,* fr. O. Fr.]

bos·se·lat·ed (baws′ĕ-lā-ted). Marked by numerous bosses or rounded protuberances. [Fr. *bosseler,* to emboss]

bos·se·la·tion (baws-ĕ-lā′shŭn). **1.** A boss. **2.** A condition in which one or more bosses, or rounded protuberances, are present.

Boston, Leonard N., U.S. physician, 1871–1931.

Botallo (Botallus), Leonardo, Italian physician in Paris, 1530–1600(?). SEE B.'s *duct, foramen, ligament.*

bot·fly (bot′flī). Robust, hairy fly of the order Diptera, often strikingly marked in black and yellow or gray, whose larvae produce a variety of myiasis conditions in man and various domestic animals, especially herbivores. SEE ALSO *Gasterophilus.*

head b.'s, flesh flies of the dipterous families Oestridae and Cuterebridae; robust, hairy, black, yellow, or gray flies that, while flying, deposit newly hatched larvae or, in some cases, eggs, on or near the nostrils of sheep, goats, deer, horses, camels, and, rarely, man.

human b., SYN *Dermatobia hominis.*

skin b.'s, SYN *Dermatobia hominis.* SEE ALSO *Cuterebra.*

warble b., SYN *Dermatobia hominis.* SEE ALSO *Hypoderma.*

both·ria (both′rē-ă). Plural of bothrium.

both·ri·o·ceph·a·li·a·sis (both′rē-ō-sef-ă-lī′ă-sis). SYN diphyllobothriasis.

Both·ri·o·ceph·a·lus (both′rē-ō-sef′ă-lŭs). A genus of pseudophyllid tapeworms with both plerocercoid and adult stages in fishes; sometimes historically confused with *Diphyllobothrium.* [G. *bothrion,* dim. of *bothros,* pit or trench, + *kephalē,* head]

B. corda′tus, a species common in dogs and man in Greenland.

B. la′tus, former name for *Diphyllobothrium latum.*

B. manso′ni, former name for *Spirometra mansoni.*

B. mansonoi′des, former name for *Spirometra mansonoides.*

both·ri·um, pl. **both·ria** (both′rē-ŭm, -rē-ă). One of the slitlike sucking grooves found on the scolex of pseudophyllidean tapeworms, such as the broad fish tapeworm of man, *Diphyllobothrium latum.* [G. *bothros,* pit or trench]

bot·ry·oid (bot′rē-oyd). Having numerous rounded protuberances resembling a bunch of grapes. SYN staphyline, uviform. [G. *botryoeidēs,* like a bunch of grapes (*botrys*)]

Bot·ry·o·my·ces (bot′rē-ō-mī′sēz). A generic name applied to a supposed fungus causing botryomycosis. Since this disease is now known to be caused by several kinds of bacteria, staphylococci most commonly, the name is invalid and rarely used. The name of the disease has been retained, nevertheless, to indicate a peculiar type of tissue reaction. [G. *botrys,* a bunch of grapes, + *mykēs,* fungus]

bot·ry·o·my·co·sis (bot′rē-ō-mī-kō′sis). A chronic granulomatous condition of horses, cattle, swine, and man, usually involving the skin but occasionally also the viscera, and characterized by granules in the pus, consisting of masses of bacteria, generally staphylococci but sometimes other types, surrounded by a hyaline capsule which sometimes exhibits clublike bodies around its periphery; the anatomic structure of the lesion resembles that of actinomycosis and mycetoma. SYN actinophytosis (2). [fr. *Botryomyces*]

bot·ry·o·my·cot·ic (bot′rē-ō-mī-kot′ik). Relating to or affected by botryomycosis.

bots. The larvae of several species of botflies. [Gael. *boiteag,* maggot]

ox b., cattle grub, the larvae of the warble flies, *Hypoderma bovis* and *H. lineatum.*

sheep b., *Oestrus ovis* larvae.

Böttcher, Arthur, Estonian anatomist, 1831–1889. SEE B.'s *canal, cells,* under *cell, crystals,* under *crystal, ganglion, space;* Charcot-B. *crystalloids,* under *crystalloid.*

bot·tle (bot′tl). A container for liquids.

Mariotte b., a stoppered b. with bottom outlet, used as a reservoir for constant infusions; air enters only by bubbling through a tube extending down through the stopper almost to the bottom; a partial vacuum thus supports the variable height of liquid above the air inlet, providing a constant gravity head for outflow.

wash-b., **(1)** a bottle with a tube passing to the bottom, through which gases are forced into water to purify them; **(2)** a stoppered bottle with two tubes, one ending above and the other below a fluid, so that air blowing through the short tube forces liquid in a small stream from the free end of the long one; used for washing chemical apparatus.

Woulfe's b., a b. with two or three necks, used in a series, connected with tubes, for working with gases (washing, drying, absorbing, etc.).

bot·u·lin (bot′yū-lin). SYN botulinus *toxin.*

bot·u·lin·o·gen·ic (bot′yū-lin-ō-jen′ik). SYN botulogenic.

bot·u·lism (bot′yū-lizm). Food poisioning caused by the ingestion of the neurotoxin *Clostridium botulinum* from improperly canned or preserved food; mainly affects man, chickens, water fowl, cattle, sheep, and horses, and is characterized by paralysis in all species; can be fatal; swine, dogs, and cats are somewhat resistant. SEE ALSO *Clostridium botulinum.* [L. *botulus,* sausage]

wound b., b. resulting from infection of a wound.

bot·u·lis·mo·tox·in (bot′yū-liz-mō-tok′sin). SYN botulinus *toxin.*

bot·u·lo·gen·ic (bot′yū-lō-jen′ik). Botulism-producing. SYN botulinogenic.

bou·bas (bū′bahs). SYN yaws. [native Brazilian]

Bouchard, Charles Jacques, French physician, 1837–1915. SEE B.'s *disease.*

bouche de ta·pir (būsh-dĕ-tā′pir). SYN tapir *mouth.* [Fr.]

Bouchut, Jean A.E., French physician, 1818–1891. SEE B.'s *tube.*

Bouffardi's my·ce·to·mas. SEE Bouffardi's white *mycetoma.*

bou·gie (bū-zhē′). A cylindrical instrument, usually somewhat flexible and yielding, used for calibrating or dilating constricted areas in tubular organs, such as the urethra or esophagus; sometimes containing a medication for local application. [Fr. candle]

b. à boule (bū-zhē′ă-būl′), a ball-tipped b.

bulbous b., a b. with a bulb-shaped tip, some of which are shaped like an acorn or an olive.

Eder-Pustow b., a metal olive-shaped b. with a flexible metal dilating system (for esophageal stricture).

elastic b., a b. made of rubber, latex, or other similarly flexible material.

elbowed b., a b. with a sharply angulated bend near its tip.

filiform b., a very slender b. usually used for gentle exploration of strictures or sinus tracts of small diameter where false passages can be encountered or created; the entering end can consist of either a straight or spiral tip, and the trailing end usually consists of a threaded cylinder into which the screw tip of a following b. can be inserted.

following b., a flexible tapered b. with a screw tip which is attached to the trailing end of a filiform b., to allow progressive dilation without danger of creating false passages.

Hurst b.'s, a series of mercury-filled tubes of graded diameter for dilating the cardioesophageal region.

Maloney b.'s, a series of b.'s similar to Hurst b.'s but having cone-shaped tips.

Savary b.'s, silastic tapered tip b.'s used over a guide wire in esophageal dilatation.

tapered b., a b. with gradually increasing caliber, used to dilate strictures.

wax-tipped b., a long slender flexible b. with a wax tip, used for endoscopic passage into the ureter to confirm the presence of a calculus by scratching the surface of the tip with the sharp edges of the stone.

whip b., a b. tapered to a threadlike tip at the end.

bou·gie·nage (bū-zhē-nahzh′). Examination or treatment of the interior of any canal by the passage of a bougie or cannula.

Bouillaud, Jean, French physician, 1796–1881. SEE B.'s *disease.*

bouil·lon (bū-yawn′). A clear beef tea. [Fr. broth, fr. *bouillir,* to boil]

Bouin, Paul, French histologist, 1870–1962. SEE B.'s *fixative.*

bou·lim·i·a (bū-lim′ē-ă). SYN bulimia *nervosa.*

bound (bownd). **1.** Limited, circumscribed; enclosed. **2.** Denoting a substance, such as iodine, phosphorus, calcium, morphine, or another drug, that is not in readily difusible form but exists in combination with a high molecular weight substance, especially protein. **3.** Fixed to a receptor, such as on a cell wall.

bou·quet (bū-ka′). A cluster or bunch of structures, especially of blood vessels, suggesting a b. [Fr.]

Riolan's b., the muscles and ligaments, "les fleurs rouges et les fleurs blanches" (the red and white flowers), arising from the styloid process.

Bourdon, Eugène, French engineer and inventor, 1808–1884. SEE B. *tube.*

Bourgery, Marc-Jean, French anatomist and surgeon, 1797–1849. SEE B.'s *ligament.*

Bourneville, Désiré-Magloire, French physician, 1840–1909. SEE B.'s *disease;* B.-Pringle *disease.*

Bourquin, Anne, U.S. chemist, *1897. SEE Sherman-B. *unit* of vitamin B$_2$.

bou·ton (bū-ton′). A button, pustule, or knob-like swelling. [Fr. button]

axonal terminal b.'s, SYN axon *terminals,* under *terminal.*

b. de Bagdad, b. d'Orient, the lesion occurring in cutaneous leishmaniasis. SYN bouton de Biskra.

b. en chemise, small abscess of the intestinal mucosa, occurring in amebic dysentery.

b.'s en passage, consecutive synapses along the course of an axon.

synaptic b.'s, SYN axon *terminals,* under *terminal.*

terminal b.'s, b. terminaux, SYN axon *terminals,* under *terminal.*

bou·ton·nière (bū-tŏn-nēr′, -når′). A traumatically produced slit or buttonhole-like opening. [Fr. buttonhole]

Bovero, Renaldo, 20th century Italian dermatologist. SEE Bovero's *muscle.*

Bo·vic·o·la (bō-vik′ō-lă). A genus of biting lice that is considered by some to be a subgenus of *Damalinia;* includes the species *B. bovis* (*Trichodectes scalaris*), the common red or biting ox louse of cattle; *B. caprae* (*Trichodectes climax*), found on sheep and goats; *B. equi* (*Trichodectes parumpilosus*), the common biting louse of horses; *B. ovis* (*Trichodectes sphaerocephalus*), the common biting louse of sheep. SEE ALSO *Trichodectes.*

Bovie. An instrument used for electrosurgical dissection and hemostasis. Frequently used as a verb, *i.e.,* to Bovie something is to dissect or cauterize it with the Bovie instrument.

bo·vine (bō′vīn, -vin). Relating to cattle. [L. *bos* (bov-), ox]

bow (bō). Any device bent in a simple curve or semicircle and possessing flexibility. [A.S. boga]

Logan's b., heavy stainless steel wire bent in an arc and taped to both cheeks to protect the incision and to relieve tension on a freshly repaired cleft lip.

Bowditch, Henry P., U.S. physiologist, 1840–1911. SEE B.'s *law;* B. *effect.*

bow·el. SYN intestinum (1). SEE small bowel *series.* [through the Fr. from L. *botulus,* sausage]

large b., the colon.

small b., proximal portion of the intestine distal to the stomach, comprising the duodenum, jejunum, and ileum.

Bowen, John T., U.S. dermatologist, 1857–1941. SEE B.'s *disease,* precancerous *dermatosis;* bowenoid *papulosis;* Bowenoid *cells,* under *cell.*

Bowie, Donald James, Canadian physician, *1887. SEE Bowie's *stain.*

Bowie's stain. See under stain.

bow·leg, bow-b. (bō′leg). SYN *genu* varum.

Bowles type steth·o·scope. See under stethoscope.

Bowman, Sir William, English ophthalmologist, anatomist, and physiologist, 1816–1892. SEE B.'s *capsule, disks,* under *disk, gland, membrane, muscle, probe, space, theory.*

box (boks). Container; receptacle. [L.L. *buxis,* fr. G. *puxis,* box tree]

black b., (1) (Jargon) descriptive of a method of reasoning or studying a problem, in which the methods and procedures, as such, are not described, explained, or perhaps even understood: conclusions relate solely to the empirical relationships observed; (2) in some contexts, the term can mean a piece of apparatus or

box 229 brachyesophagus

an experimental animal in which the pharmacologic or toxicologic pathway has not yet been worked out.

CAAT b., a sequence of nucleotides found in a conserved region of DNA located "upstream" (5′ direction) of the start points of eukaryotic transcription units; specific transcription factors appear to associate with it; found in many promoters at −75 bp with the consensus sequence: GG(T/C)CAATCT.

fracture b., an obsolete means of supporting a fractured leg, consisting of a container with only bottom and sides.

Hogness b., SEE homeobox.

homeobox, in molecular biology, a sequence of nucleotides rich in thymidylate (T) and deoxyadenylate (A) arranged in conventional 5′- to 3′- orientation which occurs in the promoter region of the DNA of many (if not all) genomes, just "upstream" (5′ direction) from the starting point of transcription by RNA polymerase. Sometimes called Hogness b. or Pribnow b. after the investigators who first noted the ubiquitous occurrence of the sequence in eukaryotes and prokaryotes, respectively. The b. contains a sequence of 180 base pairs, the homeodomain, which is very highly conserved. Several aberrant forms have been identified in individual disorders [MIM*142950-142993]. [*box,* fr. enclosure of nucleotide letters in a rectangle]

Pribnow b., SEE homeobox.

Skinner b., an experimental apparatus in which an animal presses a lever to obtain a reward or receive punishment.

TATA b., a highly conserved bacterial DNA sequence found about 25 bp upstream from the transcription start site of genes, usually flanked by GC rich sequences; binding site of transcription factors but not RNA polymerase. SEE homeobox.

view b., a light b. for display of radiographs or other photographic transparencies.

box·ing (boks′ing). In dentistry, the building up of vertical walls, usually in wax, around a dental impression after beading, to produce the desired size and form of the dental cast, and to preserve certain landmarks of the impression.

Boyce, William H., U.S. urologist, *1918. SEE Smith-B. *operation.*

Boyden, Edward A., U.S. anatomist, 1886–1977. SEE B. *meal;* B.'s *sphincter.*

Boyer, Baron Alexis, French surgeon, 1757–1833. SEE B.'s *bursa, cyst.*

Boyle, Hon. Robert, British physicist and chemist, 1627–1691. SEE B.'s *law.*

Bozeman, Nathan, U.S. surgeon, 1825–1905. SEE B.'s *operation, position;* B.-Fritsch *catheter.*

Bozzolo, Camillo, Italian physician, 1845–1920. SEE B.'s *sign.*

BP Abbreviation for blood *pressure;* British Pharmacopoeia.

b.p. Abbreviation for boiling *point.*

Bq. Abbreviation for becquerel.

Br Symbol for bromine.

Braasch, William F., U.S. urologist, 1878–1975. SEE B. *catheter.*

brace (brās). An orthosis or orthopedic appliance that supports or holds in correct position any movable part of the body and that allows motion of the part, in contrast to a splint, which prevents motion of the part. [M. E., fr. O. Fr., fr. L. *bracchium,* arm, fr. G. *brachion*]

Taylor's back b., a steel spinal support. SYN Taylor's apparatus, Taylor's splint.

brace·let (brās′let). An appliance for the wrist.

Nussbaum's b., an appliance designed for use with writer's cramp.

brac·es (brā′sez). Colloquialism for orthodontic appliances.

bra·chia (brā′kē-ă). Plural of brachium.

brach·i·al (brā′kē-ăl). Relating to the arm.

bra·chi·al·gia (brā-kē-al′jē-ă). Pain in the arm. [L. *brachium,* arm, + *algos,* pain]

b. stat′ica paresthet′ica, pain in the arm and transient paresthesia occurring only at night.

△**brachio-.** **1.** SYN arm (1). **2.** SYN radial. [L. *brachium*]

bra·chi·o·ce·phal·ic (brā′kē-ō-se-fal′ik). Relating to both arm and head.

bra·chi·o·cru·ral (brā′kē-ō-krū′răl). Relating to both arm and thigh.

bra·chi·o·cu·bi·tal (brā′kē-ō-kyū′bi-tăl). Relating to both arm and elbow or to both arm and forearm.

bra·chi·o·gram (brā′kē-ō-gram). Tracing of the brachial artery pulse.

bra·chi·um, pl. **bra·chia** (brā′kē-ŭm, brak′; -ă) [NA]. **1.** SYN arm (1). **2.** An anatomical structure resembling an arm. [L. arm, prob. akin to G. *brachiōn*]

b. collic′uli inferio′ris [NA], SYN b. of inferior colliculus.

b. collic′uli superio′ris [NA], SYN b. of superior colliculus.

b. conjuncti′vum cerebel′li, SYN superior cerebellar *peduncle.*

b. of inferior colliculus, a fiber bundle passing from the inferior colliculus on either side of the brainstem along the lateral border of the superior colliculus to the posterior part of the thalamus where it enters the medial geniculate body. It forms part of the major ascending auditory pathway. SYN b. colliculi inferioris [NA], b. quadrigeminum inferius, inferior quadrigeminal b.

inferior quadrigeminal b., SYN b. of inferior colliculus.

b. pon′tis, SYN middle cerebellar *peduncle.*

b. quadrigem′inum infe′rius, SYN b. of inferior colliculus.

b. quadrigem′inum supe′rius, SYN b. of superior colliculus.

b. of superior colliculus, a band of fibers of the optic tract bypassing the lateral geniculate body to terminate in the superior colliculus and pretectal region. SYN b. colliculi superioris [NA], b. quadrigeminum superius, superior quadrigeminal b.

superior quadrigeminal b., SYN b. of superior colliculus.

Bracht, E., 20th century German pathologist. SEE B.-Wachter *lesion.*

Bracht, Erich Franz, German obstetrician and gynecologist, *1882. SEE B. *maneuver.*

△**brachy-.** Short. [G. *brachys,* short]

brach·y·ba·sia (brak-ē-bā′sē-ă). The shuffling gait characteristic of pyramidal tract disease. [brachy- + G. *basis,* a stepping]

brach·y·ba·so·camp·to·dac·ty·ly (brak-ē-bā′sō-kamp-tō-dak′ti-lē). Combined disproportionate shortness and crookedness of the fingers. [brachy- + G. *basis,* base, + *campylos,* curved, + *daktylos,* finger]

brach·y·ba·so·pha·lan·gia (brak-ē-bā′sō-fă-lan′jē-ă). Abnormal shortness of the proximal phalanges. [brachy- + G. *basis,* base, + phalanx]

brach·y·car·dia (brak-ē-kar′dē-ă). SYN bradycardia.

brach·y·ce·pha·lia (brak-ē-sĕ-fā′lē-ă). SYN brachycephaly.

brach·y·ce·phal·ic (brak-ē-se-fal′ik). Relating to or characterized by brachycephaly. SYN brachycephalous.

brach·y·ceph·a·lism (brak-ē-sef′ă-lizm). SYN brachycephaly. [brachy- + G. *kephalē,* head]

brach·y·ceph·a·lous (brak-ē-sef′ă-lŭs). SYN brachycephalic.

brach·y·ceph·a·ly (brak-ē-sef′ă-lē). Disproportionate shortness of head, the skull having a cephalic index of over 80; among the brachycephalic races are the American Indians, Malayans, and Burmese. SYN brachycephalia, brachycephalism. [brachy- + G. *kephalē,* head]

brach·y·chei·lia, brach·y·chi·lia (brak′ē-kī′lē-ă). Abnormal shortness of the lips. [brachy- + G. *cheilos,* lip]

brach·y·cne·mic (brak-ē-nē′mik). Having short legs; specifically, relating to a tibiofemoral index of less than 82 with a shank disproportionately shorter than the thigh. [brachy- + G. *knēmē,* leg]

brach·y·cra·nic (brak-ē-krā′nik). Brachycephalic with a cephalic index of 80.0 to 84.9. [brachy- + G. *kranion,* skull]

brach·y·dac·tyl·ia (brak-ē-dak-til′ē-ă). SYN brachydactyly. [brachy- + G. *daktylos,* finger]

brach·y·dac·tyl·ic (brak-ē-dak-til′ik). Denoting brachydactyly.

brach·y·dac·ty·ly (brak-ē-dak′ti-lē). Abnormal shortness of the fingers. SYN brachydactylia. [brachy- + G. *daktylos,* finger]

brach·y·e·soph·a·gus (brak′ē-e-sof′ă-gŭs). An abnormally short esophagus. [brachy- + esophagus]

br

brach·y·fa·cial (brak-ē-fā'shăl). SYN brachyprosopic.

brach·y·glos·sal (brak-ē-glos'ăl). Denoting an abnormally short tongue. [brachy- + G. *glōssa*, tongue]

bra·chyg·na·thia (brak-ig-nā'thē-ă). Abnormal shortness or recession of the mandible. SEE ALSO micrognathia. SYN bird face. [brachy- + G. *gnathos*, jaw]

bra·chyg·na·thous (brak-ig'nā-thŭs). Having a receding underjaw.

brach·y·ker·kic (brak-ē-ker'kik). Relating to a radiohumeral index of less than 75, with a forearm relatively shorter than the upper arm. [brachy- + G. *kerkis*, radius]

brach·y·me·lia (brak-ē-mē'lē-ă). Disproportionate shortness of the limbs. [brachy- + G. *melos*, limb]

brach·y·me·so·pha·lan·gia (brak-ē-mes'ō-fă-lan'jē-ă). Abnormal shortness of the middle phalanges. [brachy- + G. *mesos*, middle, + phalanx]

brach·y·met·a·car·pa·lia, brach·y·met·a·car·pa·lism (brak'ē-met-ă-kar-pā'lē-ă, -met-ă-kar'pă-lizm). SYN brachymetacarpia.

brach·y·met·a·car·pia (brak'ē-met-ă-car'pē-ă). Abnormal shortness of the metacarpals, especially the fourth and fifth. SYN brachymetacarpalia, brachymetacarpalism.

brach·y·me·tap·o·dy (brak'ē-me-tap'ō-dē). Apparent shortness of toes or fingers resulting from shortness or hypoplasia of the metacarpals or metatarsals. [brachy- + G. *meta-* (tarsal) + *pous* (*pod*-), foot]

brach·y·met·a·tar·sia (brak'ē-met-ă-tar'sē-ă). Abnormal shortness of the metatarsals.

brach·y·mor·phic (brak'ē-mōr'fik). Having, or denoting, a shorter form than that of the usually accepted norm. [brachy- + G. *morphē*, form]

brach·y·o·dont (brak'ē-ō-dont). Having abnormally short teeth. [brachy- + G. *odous*, tooth]

brach·y·o·nych·ia (brak'ē-ō-nik'ē-ă). Short nails, in which the width of the nail plate and nail bed is greater than the length; may be congenital or result from nail biting, bone resorption in hyperparathyroidism, or psoriatic arthropathy. [G. *brachys*, short + *onyx*, *onychos*, nail, + suffix *-ia*, condition]

brach·y·pel·lic (brak-ē-pel'ik). Denoting a transverse oval pelvis. SEE brachypellic *pelvis*. SYN brachypelvic. [brachy- + pelvis]

brach·y·pel·vic (brak-ē-pel'vik). SYN brachypellic.

brach·y·pha·lan·gia (brak'ē-fă-lan'jē-ă). Abnormal shortness of the phalanges. [brachy- + phalanx]

bra·chyp·o·dous (bra-kip'ŏ-dŭs). Having abnormally short feet. [brachy- + G. *pous*, foot]

brach·y·pro·sop·ic (brak-ē-prō-sop'ik). Having a disproportionately short face. SYN brachyfacial. [brachy- + G. *prosōpikos*, facial]

brach·y·rhi·nia (brak-ē-rī'nē-ă). Abnormal shortness of the nose. [brachy- + G. *rhis*, nose]

brach·y·rhyn·chus (brak-ē-ring'kŭs). Abnormal shortness of the nose and maxilla, often associated with cyclopia. [brachy- + G. *rhynchos*, snout]

brach·y·skel·ic (brak-ē-skel'ik). Relating to abnormally short legs. [brachy- + G. *skelos*, leg]

brach·y·staph·y·line (brak-ē-staf'i-lin). Having a short palate; having a palatomaxillary index above 85. [brachy- + G. *staphylē*, uvula]

brach·y·syn·dac·ty·ly (brak'ē-sin-dak'ti-lē). Abnormal shortness of fingers or toes combined with a webbing between the adjacent digits. [brachy- + syndactyly]

brach·y·te·le·pha·lan·gia (brak-ē-tel'ē-fă-lan'jē-ă). Abnormal shortness of the distal phalanges. [brachy- + G. *telos*, end, + phalanx]

brach·y·ther·a·py (brak-ē-thār'ă-pē). Radiotherapy in which the source of irradiation is placed close to the surface of the body or within a body cavity; *e.g.*, application of radium to the cervix.
  interstitial b., radiotherapy by implantation of radioactive needles or other sources directly into and around the tissue to be irradiated.

brach·y·type (brak'ē-tīp). SYN endomorph.

brach·y·u·ran·ic (brak-ē-yū-ran'ik). Having a palatomaxillary index above 115. [brachy- + G. *ouranos*, the sky, roof of the mouth]

brac·ing (brās'ing). In dentistry, resistance to horizontal components of masticatory force. SEE *component* of force.

brack·et (brak'et). In dentistry, a small metal attachment that is soldered or welded to an orthodontic band or bonded directly to the teeth, serving to fasten the arch wire to the band or tooth.

Bradford, Edward H., U.S. orthopedist, 1848–1926. SEE B. *frame*.

△**brady-.** Slow. [G. *bradys*, slow]

bra·dy·ar·rhyth·mia (brad'ē-ă-rith'mē-ă). Any disturbance of the heart's rhythm resulting(by convention) in a rate under 60 beats per minute. [brady- + G. *a-* priv. + *rhythmos*, rhythm]

bra·dy·arth·ria (brad-ē-arth'rē-ă). A form of dysarthria characterized by an abnormal slowness or deliberation in speech. SYN bradyglossia (2), bradylalia, bradylogia. [brady- + G. *arthroō*, to utter distinctly, fr. *arthron*, a joint]

bra·dy·car·dia (brad-ē-kar'dē-ă). Slowness of the heartbeat, usually defined (by convention) as a rate under 60 beats per minute. SYN brachycardia, bradyrhythmia. [brady- + G. *kardia*, heart]
  central b., b. due to disease of the central nervous system, usually with increased intracranial pressure.
  essential b., a slow pulse for which no cause can be discovered. SYN idiopathic b.
  fetal b., a fetal heart rate of less than 100 beats per minute.
  idiopathic b., SYN essential b.
  marked fetal b., a fetal heart rate less than 100 beats per minute.
  mild fetal b., a fetal heart rate less than 120 beats per minute.
  nodal b., SYN atrioventricular junctional *rhythm*.
  postinfectious b., a toxic b. occurring during convalescence from various infectious diseases, such as influenza.
  sinus b., b. originating in the normal sinus pacemaker.
  vagal b., any excessive cardiac slowing due to stimulation of the vagus nerves.
  ventricular b., slowness of ventricular rate, usually implying the presence of atrioventricular block.

brad·y·car·di·ac (brad-ē-kar'dē-ak). Relating to or characterized by bradycardia. SYN bradycardic.

bra·dy·car·dic (brad-ē-kar'dik). SYN bradycardiac.

bra·dy·ci·ne·sia (brad-ē-si-nē'sē-ă). SYN bradykinesia.

bra·dy·crot·ic (brad-ē-krot'ik). Relating to or characterized by a slow pulse. [brady- + G. *krotos*, a striking]

bra·dy·di·as·to·le (brad-ē-dī-as'tō-lē). Prolongation of the diastole of the heart.

bra·dy·es·the·sia (brad-ē-es-thē'zē-ă). Slow sensory perception. [brady- + G. *aisthēsis*, sensation]

bra·dy·glos·sia (brad-ē-glos'ē-ă). **1.** Slow or difficult tongue movement. **2.** SYN bradyarthria. [brady- + G. *glōssa*, tongue]

bra·dy·ki·ne·sia (brad-ē-kin-ē'zē-ă). A decrease in spontaneity and movement. One of the features of extrapyramidal disorders, such as Parkinson's disease. SYN bradycinesia. [brady- + G. *kinēsis*, movement]

bra·dy·ki·net·ic (brad-ē-ki-net'ik). Characterized by or pertaining to slow movement.

bra·dy·ki·nin (brad-ē-kī'nin). The nonapeptide Arg-Pro-Pro-Gly-Phe-Ser-Pro-Phe-Arg, produced from the decapeptide kallidin (bradykininogen) that is produced from α_2-globulin by kallikrein, normally present in blood in an inactive form and similar to trypsin in action; b. is one of a number of the plasma kinins, is a potent vasodilator, and is one of the physiologic mediators of anaphylaxis released from cytotropic antibody-coated mast cells following reaction with antigen (allergen) specific for the antibody. SYN kallidin 9, kallidin I, kinin 9. [brady- + G. *kineō*, to move]

bra·dy·ki·nin·o·gen (brad'ē-ki-nin'ō-jen). SYN kallidin.

bra·dy·ki·nin po·ten·ti·a·tor B. Glp-Gly-Leu-Pro-Pro-Arg-Pro-Lys-Ile-Pro-Pro; the undecapeptide precursor of bradykinin and the angiotensins.

bra·dy·la·lia (brad-ē-lā'lē-ă). SYN bradyarthria. [brady- + G. *lalia*, speech]

bra·dy·lex·ia (brad-ē-lek'sē-ă). Abnormal slowness in reading. [brady- + G. *lexis,* word]

bra·dy·lo·gia (brad-ē-lō'jē-ă). SYN bradyarthria. [brady- + G. *logos,* word]

bra·dy·pep·sia (brad-ē-pep'sē-ă). Slowness of digestion. [brady- + G. *pepsis,* digestion]

bra·dy·pha·gia (brad-ē-fā'jē-ă). slowness in eating. [brady- + G. *phagō,* to eat]

bra·dy·pha·sia (brad-ē-fā'zē-ă). A form of aphasia characterized by abnormal slowness of speech. SYN bradyphemia. [brady- + G. *phasis,* speaking]

bra·dy·phe·mia (brad-ē-fē'mē-ă). SYN bradyphasia. [brady- + G. *phēmē,* speech]

bra·dyp·nea (brad-ip-nē'ă). Abnormal slowness of respiration, specifically a low respiratory frequency. [brady- + G. *pnoē,* breathing]

bra·dy·pra·gia (brad-ē-prā'jē-ă). Sluggish action; slow movement. [brady- + G. *prassō,* to do, act]

bra·dy·psy·chia (brad-ē-sī'kē-ă). Slowness of mental reactions. [brady- + G. *psychē,* soul]

bra·dy·rhyth·mia (brad-ē-rith'mē-ă). SYN bradycardia.

bra·dy·sper·ma·tism (brad-ē-sper'mă-tizm). Absence of ejaculatory force, so that the semen trickles away slowly. [brady, + G. *sperma (spermat-),* seed, + ism]

bra·dy·sphyg·mia (brad-ē-sfig'mē-ă). Slowness of the pulse; can occur without bradycardia, as in ventricular bigeminy when every alternate beat may fail to produce a peripheral pulse. [brady- + G. *sphygmos,* pulse]

bra·dy·stal·sis (brad-ē-stahl'sis). Slow bowel motion. [G. *bradys,* slow, + *(peri) stalsis,* contracting around]

bra·dy·tel·e·o·ci·ne·sia (brad'ē-tel-ē-ō-sin-ē'sē-ă). Sudden arrest of a movement just before its intended termination, then after a pause it is completed slowly or by jerks; a symptom of cerebellar disease. SYN bradyteleokinesis. [brady- + G. *teleos,* complete, + *kinēsis,* movement]

bra·dy·tel·e·o·ki·ne·sis (brad'ē-tel-ē-ō-ki-nē'sis). SYN bradyteleocinesia.

bra·dy·to·cia (brad-ē-tō'sē-ă). Tedious labor; slow delivery. [brady- + G. *tokos,* childbirth]

bra·dy·u·ria (brad-ē-yū'rē-ă). Slow micturition. [brady- + G. *ouron,* urine]

bra·dy·zo·ite (brad-ē-zō'īt). A slowly multiplying encysted form of sporozoan parasite typical of chronic infection with *Toxoplasma gondii.* It has also been called a merozoite or zoite; the complex of b.'s within an enclosing membrane has also been called a pseudocyst, though it is now regarded as a true cyst. [brady- + G. *zōē,* life]

braille (brāl). A system of writing and printing by means of raised dots corresponding to letters, numbers, and punctuation to enable the blind to read by touch. [Louis *Braille,* French teacher of blind, 1809–1852]

Brailsford, James Frederick, English radiologist, 1888–1961. SEE B.-Morquio *disease.*

Brain, W. Russell, Lord, English physician, 1895–1966. SEE B.'s *reflex.*

brain (brān). That part of the central nervous system contained within the cranium. SEE ALSO encephalon. Cf. cerebrum, cerebellum. [A.S. *braegen*]

   respirator b., a swollen and congested b. with necrotic and autolytic changes seen in patients who have been on a respirator.

   split b., a b. in which the corpus callosum and usually the anterior and posterior commissures have been sectioned; usually to treat certain refractory epilepsies.

   visceral b., SYN limbic *system.*

brain·case (brān'kās). SYN neurocranium.

brain·stem, brain stem (brān'stem). Originally, the entire unpaired subdivision of the brain, composed of (in anterior sequence) the rhombencephalon, mesencephalon, and diecephalon as distinguished from the brain's only paired subdivision, the

telencephalon. More recently, the term's connotation has undergone several arbitrary modifications: some use it to denote no more than rhombencephalon plus mesencephalon, distinguishing that complex from the prosencephalon (diencephalon plus telencephalon); others restrict it even further to refer exclusively to the rhombencephalon. From both developmental and architectural viewpoints, the original interpretation seems preferable.

brain·wash·ing (brān'wash'ing). Inducing a person to modify his attitudes and behavior in certain directions through various forms of psychological pressure or torture.

bran. A by-product of the milling of wheat, containing approximately 20% of indigestible cellulose; a bulk cathartic, usually taken in the form of cereal or special bran products.

branch. An offshoot; in anatomy, one of the primary divisions of a nerve or blood vessel. A branch. SEE ramus, artery, nerve, vein. SYN ramus (1) [NA].

   accessory meningeal b. of middle meningeal artery, a b. of either the middle meningeal or maxillary artery in the infratemporal fossa and passing superiorly through the foramen ovale to supply the trigeminal ganglion, dura mater and inner table of bone. SYN ramus meningeus accessorius arteriae meningeae mediae [NA].

   acetabular b., an arterial b. that supplies the acetabulum; two arteries, the obturator and the medial femoral circumflex, have such b.'s. SYN ramus acetabularis [NA], acetabular artery, arteria acetabuli.

   acromial b. of suprascapular artery, b. of suprascapular artery which pierces the origin of the trapezius muscle to run to the acromion; *anastomoses,* acromial b. of thoracoacromial artery. SYN ramus acromialis arteriae suprascapularis [NA].

   acromial b. of thoracoacromial artery, a b. of the thoracoacromial artery that runs over the coracoid process and under the deltoid muscle. SYN ramus acromialis arteriae thoracoacromialis [NA], acromial artery.

   anastomotic b., the anastomotic branch, a blood vessel that interconnects two neighboring vessels. It should not be used for the nervous system, because there is no analogy between a vascular anastomosing branch and a connection between nerves or their subdivisions. SYN ramus anastomoticus.

   anastomotic b. of middle meningeal artery to lacrimal artery, a b. of the middle meningeal artery arising in the cranial cavity which runs anteriorly through the superior orbital fissure to anastomose with the lacrimal artery. SEE orbital b. of middle meningeal artery. SYN ramus anastomoticus arteriae meningeae mediae cum lacrimali [NA].

   anterior b., the anterior branch of the following: 1) great auricular nerve; 2) lateral cerebral sulcus; 3) left and right superior pulmonary veins; 4) medial cutaneous nerve of the forearm; 5) obturator artery; 6) obturator nerve; 7) renal artery; 8) right branch of portal vein; 9) right hepatic duct; 10) superior thyroid artery; 11) ulnar recurrent artery. SYN ramus anterior [NA].

   anterior auricular b.'s of superficial temporal artery, *distribution,* auricle, earlobe and external acoustic meatus. SYN rami auriculares anteriores arteriae temporalis superficialis [NA].

   anterior basal b., anterior basal b. of (1) basal parts of the inferior lobar b.'s of the right and left pulmonary arteries, and (2) superior basal b.'s of the right and left inferior pulmonary veins. SYN ramus basalis anterior [NA].

   anterior cutaneous b. of iliohypogastric nerve, *distribution,* skin on pubis. SYN ramus cutaneus anterior nervi iliohypogastrici [NA], genital b. of iliohypogastric nerve.

   anterior cutaneous b.'s of intercostal nerves, medial mammary b.'s of anterior cutaneous b.'s of ventral primary rami of thoracic spinal nerves. SEE medial mammary b.'s.

   anterior scrotal b.'s of external pudendal artery, *distribution,* skin of anterior scrotum; *anastomoses,* posterior scrotal branches from internal pudendal artery. SYN rami scrotales anteriores arteriae pudendae externae [NA].

   anterior superior alveolar b.'s of infraorbital nerve, the b.'s of the superior alveolar nerve that supply the incisors, canines, premolars, and first molar by their contributions to the superior dental plexus. SYN rami alveolares superiores anteriores nervi infraorbitalis [NA].

anteromedial central b.'s, branches of the anterior communicating artery which supply part of the hypothalamus. SYN rami centrales anteromediales [NA].

apical b., the apical branch of the following: 1) superior lobar b.'s of left and right pulmonary arteries; 2) left superior pulmonary vein. SYN ramus superior (2) [NA]. SYN ramus apicalis [NA].

apical b. of inferior lobar branch of right pulmonary artery, b. (of the inferior lobar branch) of the right pulmonary artery serving the apical segment of the inferior lobe of the right lung. SYN ramus apicalis lobi inferioris arteriae pulmonalis dextrae [NA].

apicoposterior b. of left superior pulmonary vein, drains apicoposterior bronchopulmonary segment of superior lobe of left lung. SYN ramus apicoposterior venae pulmonalis sinistrae superioris [NA].

articular b.'s, b.'s distributed to joints. Almost any vessel related to a joint will supply articular rami. Most joints receive articular b.'s from the intramuscular b.'s of the motor nerves innervating the muscles crossing the joint (see Hilton's *law*). At this printing, Nomina Anatomica, however, specifically recognizes only the articular b.'s of the descending genicular artery, ramus articulares arteriae descendentis genicularis [NA]; supplying the knee joint. SYN rami articulares [NA], joint b.'s.

ascending b., a b. directed superiorly. Nomina Anatomica recognizes the ascending b. of the following: 1) deep circumflex iliac artery; 2) lateral cerebral sulcus; 3) lateral circumflex femoral artery. SYN ramus ascendens [NA].

ascending anterior b., the ascending anterior b. of the superior lobar b.'s of the left and right pulmonary arteries. SYN ramus anterior ascendens [NA].

ascending b. of the inferior mesenteric artery, b. of the left colic artery (from inferior mesenteric artery) that passes anteriorly to the left kidney into the transverse mesocolon, where it anastomoses with the middle colic artery. It thus forms an anastomosis between superior and inferior mesenteric arteries, and is a component of the marginal artery (Drummond) of the colon. SYN arteria ascendens (2), arteria intermesenterica.

ascending posterior b., the ascending posterior b. of the superior lobar branch of the right pulmonary artery. SYN ramus posterior ascendens [NA].

atrial b.'s, the atrial branches, the branches of the right coronary artery and the circumflex branch of the left coronary artery distributed to the right and left atrium, respectively. SYN rami atriales [NA].

atrioventricular nodal b., SYN *artery* to atrioventricular node.

b. to atrioventricular node, SYN *artery* to atrioventricular node.

auricular b. of occipital artery, *distribution,* posterior auricle; *anastomosis,* posterior auricular artery. SYN ramus auricularis arteriae occipitalis [NA].

auricular b. of vagus nerve, a b. of the superior ganglion of the vagus, supplying the back of the pinna and the external acoustic meatus. SYN ramus auricularis nervi vagi [NA], Arnold's nerve.

b. of auriculotemporal nerve to tympanic membrane, sensory b. of the auriculotemporal nerve supplying the external surface of the tympanic membrane. SYN ramus membranae tympani nervi auriculotemporalis [NA], nerve of tympanic membrane.

basal tentorial b. of internal carotid artery, a small b. from the cavernous part of the internal carotid artery to the base of the tentorium. SYN ramus basalis tentorii arteriae carotidis internae [NA].

buccal b.'s of facial nerve, motor b.'s of the facial nerve distributed to buccina or muscle and other muscles of facial expression below orbit and above chin. SYN rami buccales nervi facialis [NA].

calcarine b. of medial occipital artery, b. of medial occipital artery which runs in relationship to the calcarine sulcus. SYN ramus calcarinus arteriae occipitalis medialis [NA], arteria calcarina, calcarine artery.

capsular b.'s of renal artery, b.'s arising from the renal artery outside of the kidney that are distributed to the renal capsule. SYN rami capsulares arteriae renalis [NA].

carotid sinus b., SYN carotid sinus *nerve.*

caudate b.'s, b.'s of transverse part of left branch of portal vein

distributed to the caudate lobe before the vein enters the liver. SYN rami caudati [NA].

cavernous b. of internal carotid artery, a b. of the cavernous part of the internal carotid artery supplying the walls of the cavernous sinus.

cavernous sinus b. of internal carotid artery, a number of small b.'s of the cavernous part of the internal carotid artery. SEE ganglionic b. of internal carotid artery, cavernous sinus b. of internal carotid artery, basal tentorial b. of internal carotid artery, marginal tentorial b. of internal carotid artery. SYN ramus sinus cavernosi arteriae carotidis arteriae [NA], cavernous arteries.

celiac b.'s of vagus nerve, terminal b.'s of the posterior vagal trunk conveying presynaptic parasympathetic fibers to—and visceral afferent fibers from—the celiac plexus. SYN rami celiaci nervi vagi [NA].

cervical b. of facial nerve, the most inferior b. of the parotid plexus of the facial nerve, it descends to innervate the platysma muscle. SYN ramus colli nervi facialis [NA], ramus cervicalis nervi facialis ✫.

choroid b.'s, the choroid branches: *ramus* choroidei posteriores laterales [NA], lateral posterior choroid branches of posterior cerebral artery distributed to the choroid plexus of the lateral ventricle; *ramus* choroidei posteriores mediales [NA], medial posterior choroid branches of posterior cerebral artery distributed to the choroid plexus of the third ventricle; *ramus* choroidei ventriculi lateralis [NA], lateral ventricle choroid branch of anterior choroid artery distributed to the plexus of the lateral ventricle; *ramus* choroidei ventriculi tertii [NA], third ventricle choroid branch of anterior choroid artery to the third ventricle; *ramus* choroidei ventriculi quarti [NA], fourth ventricle choroid branch of posterior inferior cerebellar artery. SYN rami choroidei [NA].

circumflex b. of left coronary artery, terminal b. (with anterior interventricular artery) of left coronary artery which runs to left and then posteriorly in the coronary groove supplying atrial and ventricular b.'s. SYN ramus circumflexus arteriae coronariae sinistrae [NA].

clavicular b. of thoracoacromial artery, *distribution,* subclavius muscle and sternoclavicular joint. SYN ramus clavicularis arteriae thoracoacromialis [NA].

cochlear b. of labyrinthine artery, terminal b. (with vestibular b.) of labyrinthine artery; it divides into multiple fine b.'s which penetrate canals of modiolus to supply the plexus of the spiral lamina and basilar membrane. SYN ramus cochlearis arteriae labyrinthi [NA].

collateral b.'s of posterior intercostal arteries 3–11, b. arising near angle of rib and descending to run along superior border of rib below; *distribution:* lower half of intercostal spaces 3–11; *anastomoses:* collateral b.'s of anterior intercostal arteries. SYN ramus collateralis arteriarum intercostalium posteriorum III–XI [NA].

communicating b., a bundle of nerve fibers passing from one named nerve to join another. The term "communicating branch" is used in the nervous system to replace the inadequate "anastomosing branch" used for vascular systems. SYN ramus communicans [NA].

communicating b.'s of auriculotemporal nerve to facial nerve, b.'s conveying fibers from the auriculotemporal nerve to the facial nerve. SYN rami communicantes nervi auriculotemporalis cum nervo faciali [NA].

communicating b. of chorda tympani to lingual nerve, terminal b. of chorda tympani joining the lingual nerve in the infratemporal fossa; conveys sensory fibers for taste from anterior two-thirds of tongue and presynaptic parasympathetic fibers destined for submandibular ganglion for innervation of submandibular and sublingual salivary glands. SYN ramus communicans cum chorda tympani (1) [NA].

communicating b. of facial nerve with glossopharyngeal nerve, a small branch from the digastric branch of the facial nerve to the glossopharyngeal nerve. SYN ramus communicans cum nervo glossopharyngeo (1) [NA], Haller's ansa.

communicating b. of facial nerve with tympanic plexus, a fine b. of facial nerve joining the tympanic b. of the glossopharyngeal nerve. SYN ramus communicans nervi facialis cum plexu tympanico [NA].

communicating b. of glossopharyngeal nerve with auricular branch of vagus nerve, a small b. of the glossopharyngeal nerve which joins the auricular b. of the vagus, conveying tactile fibers. SYN ramus communicans cum nervo glossopharyngeo (2) [NA], ramus communicans nervi glossopharyngei cum ramo auriculari nervi vagalis.

communicating b. of lacrimal nerve with zygomatic nerve, nerve b. by which postsynaptic parasympathetic (secretomotor) fibers from the pterygopalatine ganglion are transferred from the zygomatic nerve to the lacrimal nerve (heretofore purely sensory) for distribution to the lacrimal gland. SYN ramus communicans nervi lacrimalis cum nervo zygomatico [NA].

communicating b.'s of lingual nerve to hypoglossal nerve, communicating b.'s between the lingual nerve (from mandibular nerve) and hypoglossal nerve forming a plexus on the hypoglossus muscle. SYN rami communicantes nervi lingualis cum nervo hypoglosso [NA].

communicating b. of median nerve with ulnar nerve, b. of median nerve joining the ulnar nerve in the hand; the anterior interosseous b. of the median nerve may also communicate with the ulnar nerve in the proximal forearm. SYN ramus communicans nervi mediani cum nervo ulnari [NA].

communicating b. of otic ganglion to auriculotemporal nerve, a b. of the otic ganglion joining the roots of the auriculotemporal nerve to convey postsynaptic parasympathetic fibers to the parotid gland. SYN ramus communicans ganglii otici cum nervo auriculotemporali [NA].

communicating b. of otic ganglion to chorda tympani, a small b. of the otic ganglion conveying sensory fibers to the chorda tympani. SYN ramus communicans cum chorda tympani (2) [NA].

communicating b. of otic ganglion with medial pterygoid nerve, b. of otic ganglion joining the nerve to the medial pterygoid muscle. SYN ramus communicans ganglii otici cum nervo pterygoideo mediali [NA].

communicating b. of otic ganglion with meningeal branch of mandibular nerve, a b. of otic ganglion to the meningeal branch of mandibular nerve conveying postsynaptic parasympathetic fibers which run back to the main stem of the mandibular nerve for distribution to the parotid gland via the auriculotemporal nerve. SYN ramus communicans ganglii otici cum ramo meningeo nervi mandibularis [NA].

communicating b. of peroneal artery, the communicating branch of the peroneal (fibular) artery. SYN ramus communicans arteriae fibularis [NA], ramus communicans arteriae peroneae.

communicating b.'s of spinal nerves, SYN white *rami* communicantes, under *ramus*.

communicating b. of superior laryngeal nerve with recurrent laryngeal nerve, b. of internal branch of superior laryngeal nerve communicating with the recurrent laryngeal nerve in the wall of the laryngopharynx supplying sensory fibers to the latter. SYN ramus communicans nervi laryngei recurrentis cum ramo laryngeo interno [NA], ramus communicans nervi laryngei superioris cum nervo laryngeo recurrenti [NA], Galen's anastomosis, Galen's nerve.

communicating b.'s of sympathetic trunk, SYN gray *rami* communicantes, under *ramus*.

cutaneous b. of obturator nerve, b. of the anterior branch of obturator nerve supplying skin of medial thigh above knee. SYN ramus cutaneus rami anterioris nervi obturatorii [NA].

deep b., b. which passes deeply, beneath, or farther from surface; usually in contrast to a superficial b. SYN ramus profundus [NA].

deep b. of the lateral plantar nerve, motor b. of lateral plantar nerve supplying lumbricals 2–4, plantar and dorsal interossei, and the adductor hallucis muscles. SYN ramus profundus nervi plantaris lateralis [NA].

deep b. of the medial femoral circumflex artery, distributed to posterior aspect of femoral head and neck. SYN ramus profundus arteriae circumflexae femoris medialis [NA].

deep b. of the medial plantar artery, b. running deep to abductor hallucis, supplying it and the flexor hallucis brevis muscle deep to the artery and the skin of the medial side of the distal foot. SYN rami profundi arteriae circumflexae femoris medialis [NA].

deep palmar b. of ulnar artery, b. of the ulnar artery which supplies the hypothenar muscles then passes deep into the palm to the flexor tendons and anastomoses with the deep palmar arch from the radial artery. SYN ramus palmaris profundus arteriae ulnaris [NA].

deep plantar b. of dorsalis pedis artery, deep plantar b. of arcuate artery or its first metatarsal artery b. which penetrates the foot between first and second metatarsal bones to anastomose with the termination of the plantar arterial arch. SYN ramus plantaris profundus arteriae dorsalis pedis [NA].

deep b. of the radial nerve, SYN posterior interosseous *nerve*.

deep b. of the transverse cervical artery, SYN dorsal scapular *artery*.

deep b. of the ulnar nerve, accompanies deep palmar b. of ulnar artery and deep palmar arch to supply wrist joint, lumbricals 3 & 4, palmar and dorsal interossei adductor pollicis and deep head of flexor pollicis brevis muscles. SYN ramus profundus nervi ulnaris [NA].

deltoid b., b.'s related to the deltoid muscle. Nomina Anatomica lists deltoid b.'s of the following: 1) thoracoacromial artery, ramus deltoideus arteriae thoracoacromialis [NA]; 2) profunda brachii artery, ramus deltoideus arteriae profundae brachii [NA]. SYN ramus deltoideus [NA].

dental b.'s, b.'s to the teeth. Nomina Anatomica lists dental b.'s of the following: 1) anterior superior alveolar artery, rami dentales arteriarum alveolarium superiorum anteriorum [NA]; 2) inferior alveolar artery, rami dentales arteriae alveolaris inferioris [NA]; 3) inferior dental plexus, rami dentales inferiores plexus dentalis inferioris [NA]; 4) posterior superior alveolar artery, rami dentales arteriae alveolaris superioris posterioris [NA]; 5) superior dental plexus, rami dentales superiores plexus dentalis superioris [NA]. SYN rami dentales [NA], dental rami.

descending b., b. of an artery or nerve passing inferiorly. Descending b.'s have been described for the following: (1) *descending b. of hypoglossal nerve,* superior root of ansa cervicalis; (2) *descending branch of lateral circumflex femoral artery;* (3) *descending b. of the occipital artery.* SYN ramus descendens [NA].

descending anterior b., the descending anterior b. of the superior lobar b.'s of the right and left pulmonry arteries. SYN ramus anterior descendens [NA].

descending b. of hypoglossal nerve, SYN superior *root* of ansa cervicalis.

descending b. of lateral circumflex femoral artery, a major b. of the lateral circumflex femoral artery accompanying the nerve to the vastus lateralis muscle along the anterior border of that muscle and deep to the rectus femoris muscle, supplying both muscles. *Anastomosis:* with lateral superior genicular artery, *i.e.,* it contributes to the articular network of the knee. SYN ramus descendens arteriae circumflexae femoris lateralis [NA].

descending b. of occipital artery, *origin:* occipital artery within occipital groove; *distribution:* posterior neck muscles and cervical trapezius muscle; *anastomoses:* superficial and deep cervical arteries, vertebral artery. SYN ramus descendens arteriae occipitalis [NA], princeps cervicis artery, princeps cervicis.

descending posterior b., the descending posterior b. of the superior lobar b. of the right pulmonary artery. SYN ramus posterior descendens [NA].

digastric b. of facial nerve, b. of the facial nerve innervating the posterior belly of the digastric muscle. SYN ramus digastricus nervi facialis [NA].

dorsal b., (1) SYN dorsal primary *ramus* of spinal nerve. (2) posteriorly-directed b.'s.

dorsal carpal b. of radial artery, a b. of the radial artery that passes to the back of the wrist to join the dorsal carpal network. SYN ramus carpalis dorsalis arteriae radialis, ramus carpeus dorsalis arteriae radialis.

dorsal carpal b. of ulnar artery, a b. of the ulnar artery that passes to the dorsal side of the carpus to enter the dorsal carpal network. SYN ramus carpeus dorsalis arteriae ulnaris [NA], ramus carpalis dorsalis arteriae ulnaris.

dorsal lingual b.'s of lingual artery, b.'s of the lingual artery to the posterior third or root of tongue. SYN rami dorsales linguae arteriae lingualis [NA].

dorsal b. of the lumbar artery, terminal b. (with ventral b.) of the 4–5 lumbar arteries, distributed to lumbar portion of back, posterior vertebral column, and spinal cord and environs. SYN ramus dorsalis arteriae lumbalium [NA].

dorsal b. of the posterior intercostal arteries 3–11, terminal b. (with ventral b.) of the 3rd through 11th posterior intercostal arteries, distributed to thoracic portion of posterior vertebral column, spinal cord and environs, and back. SYN ramus dorsalis arteriarum intercostalium posteriorum III–XI [NA].

dorsal b. of the posterior intercostal veins 4–11, major tributary of the 4th through 11th posterior intercostal veins; area drained is the same as that supplied by the dorsal b. of posterior intercostal arteries. SYN ramus dorsalis venarum intercostalium posteriorum IV–XI [NA].

dorsal b. of the subcostal artery, terminal b. (with ventral b.) of subcostal artery, distributed to posterior vertebral column, spinal cord and environs, and back at the T12–L1 vertebral level. SYN rami dorsales arteriae subcostalis [NA].

dorsal b. of the superior intercostal artery, b.'s of the 1st and 2nd posterior intercostal arteries which arise as b.'s of the supreme intercostal artery. The distribution is the same as for the dorsal b.'s of the other posterior intercostal arteries at the T1–T2 vertebral level. SYN rami dorsales arteriae intercostalis supremae [NA].

dorsal b. of the ulnar nerve, b. arising from the ulnar nerve proximal to the wrist for distribution to the medial side of the dorsum of the hand and proximal portion of the little finger and medial side of ring finger. SYN rami dorsales nervi ulnaris [NA].

duodeneal b.'s of superior pancreaticoduodenal artery, b.'s arising from both the anterior and posterior superior pancreaticoduodenal arteries for distribution to first and second parts of the duodenum. SYN rami duodenales arteriae pancreaticoduodenalis superioris [NA].

epiploic b.'s, b.'s to the greater omentum; epiploic b.'s arise from the left and right gastroepiploic arteries (rami omentales arteriae gastro-omentalis sinistrae et dextrae [NA]) opposite the gastric b.'s (rami gastrici [NA]) along the greater curvature of the stomach. SYN rami omentales [NA], omental b.'s, rami epiploicae.

esophageal b.'s, b.'s to the esophagus. SYN rami esophageales [NA], rami esophagei [NA].

esophageal b.'s of the inferior thyroid artery, *distribution:* upper one-quarter of esophagus; *anastomosis:* esophageal b.'s of thoracic aorta. SYN rami esophageales arteriae thyroideae inferioris [NA].

esophageal b.'s of the left gastric artery, ascends through esophageal hiatus of diaphragm to supply lowermost (cardiac) esophagus; *anastomosis:* esophageal b.'s of thoracic aorta. SYN rami esophageales arteriae gastricae sinistrae [NA].

esophageal b.'s of the recurrent laryngeal nerve, supply motor and sensory fibers to cervical esophagus on right side and to cervical and upper thoracic esophagus on left. SYN rami esophagei nervi laryngei recurrentis [NA].

esophageal b.'s of the thoracic aorta, b.'s arising directly from the anterior aspect of the portion of the thoracic aorta adjacent to the esophagus, by which most of the esophagus is supplied. SYN rami esophageales aortae thoracicae [NA].

esophageal b.'s of the vagus nerve, includes both b.'s passing directly from vagi and the b.'s from the recurrent laryngeal nerves that form the esophageal nerve plexus which surrounds esophagus, supplying it and adjacent portions of the pericardium. SYN rami esophagei nervi vagi [NA].

external b. of accessory nerve, portion of the accessory nerve trunk which exits independently from the jugular foramen, carrying fibers from the spinal root of the accessory nerve to the sternocleidomastoid and trapezius muscle.

external nasal b.'s, b.'s to external aspect of nose. The external nasal branches of 1) infraorbital nerve, rami nasales externi nervi infraorbitalis [NA], 2) nasociliary nerve, rami nasales externi nervi ethmoidalis anterioris [NA]. SYN rami nasales externi [NA].

external b. of superior laryngeal nerve, terminal b. of superior laryngeal nerve (with internal laryngeal nerve) supplying motor innervation to cricothyroid muscle. SYN ramus externus nervi laryngei superioris [NA].

faucial b.'s of lingual nerve, the faucial b.'s, b.'s to the isthmus of the fauces from the lingual nerve. SYN rami isthmi faucium nervi lingualis [NA], rami fauciales nervi lingualis⋆ [NA].

femoral b. of genitofemoral nerve, b. of genitofemoral nerve distributed to skin of uppermost part of anterior thigh. SYN ramus femoralis nervi genitofemoralis [NA].

frontal b. of superficial temporal artery, terminal b. of superficial temporal artery (with parietal b.) supplying anterolateral scalp and underlying musculature, periosteum, and outer table of cranium; *anastomosis:* across midline with contralateral partner; supratrochlear and supraorbital arteries. SYN ramus frontalis arteriae temporalis superficialis [NA].

ganglionic b. of internal carotid artery, b. to trigeminal ganglion; a small b. of the cavernous part of the internal carotid artery to the trigeminal ganglion. SYN ramus ganglii trigeminalis [NA].

ganglionic b. of lingual nerve, motor roots of submandibular ganglion; communicating b.'s between submandibular ganglion and lingual nerve. SYN rami communicantes ganglii submandibularis cum nervo linguali [NA], motor roots of submandibular ganglion.

ganglionic b.'s of maxillary nerve, the ganglionic branches, two short sensory branches of the maxillary nerve in the pterygopalatine fossa, the fibers of which pass through the pterygopalatine ganglion without synapse. SYN radix sensoria ganglii pterygopalatini [NA], rami ganglionici nervi maxillaris [NA], rami ganglionares⋆ [NA], nervi pterygopalatini, nervi sphenopalatini, pterygopalatine nerves, sensory root of pterygopalatine ganglion.

gastric b.'s of anterior vagal trunk, anterior gastric b.'s of the vagus; b.'s of the anterior vagal trunk to the anterior surface of the stomach. SYN rami gastrici anteriores nervi vagi [NA].

gastric b.'s of posterior vagal b., posterior gastric b.'s; b.'s of the posterior vagal trunk to the posterior surface of the stomach. SYN rami gastrici posteriores nervi vagi [NA].

genital b. of genitofemoral nerve, b. of genitofemoral nerve distributed to skin of anterior scrotum (male) or labia majora (female) and adjacent thigh and supplying a motor b. to the cremaster muscle. Usually passes through deep inguinal ring and canal. SYN ramus genitalis nervi genitofemoralis [NA], external spermatic nerve, nervus spermaticus externus.

genital b. of iliohypogastric nerve, SYN anterior cutaneous b. of iliohypogastric nerve.

glandular b.'s, b.'s distributed to glands. SYN rami glandulares [NA].

glandular b.'s of anterior/lateral/posterior branches of superior thyroid artery, b.'s of the branches of the superior thyroid artery to the thyroid gland. SYN ramus glandulares anterior/lateralis/posterior arteriae thyroideae superioris [NA].

glandular b.'s of facial artery, b.'s of facial artery to the submandibular gland. SYN rami glandulares arteriae facialis [NA].

glandular b.'s of inferior thyroid artery, b.'s of inferior thyroid artery to thyroid and parathyroid glands, anastomosing with b.'s of superior thyroid artery. SYN rami glandulares arteriae thyroideae inferioris [NA].

glandular b.'s of submandibular ganglion, b.'s of submandibular ganglion conveying postsynaptic parasympathetic fibers to the submandibular and sublingual glands. SYN rami glandulares ganglii submandibularis [NA].

b. of glossopharyngeal nerve to stylopharyngeus muscle, sole motor b. of the glossopharyngeal nerve to the stylopharyngeus muscle. SYN ramus musculi stylopharyngei nervi glossopharyngei [NA].

hepatic b.'s of vagus nerve, b.'s of the anterior and posterior vagal trunks distributed to the liver. SYN rami hepatici nervi vagi [NA].

iliac b. of iliolumbar artery, terminal b. of iliolumbar artery (with lumbar b.) distributed to iliac fossa to supply iliac muscle, ilium, and portions of muscles having attachment to the iliac crest. SYN ramus iliacus arteriae iliolumbalis [NA].

inferior b., a b. directed downward (caudally) or which is lowly-placed, usually in contrast with another b. (superior b.) which is directed upward (rostrally) or is highly-placed. SYN ramus inferior [NA].

inferior cervical cardiac b.'s of vagus nerve, the most inferior of the cervical b.'s of vagus nerve conducting presynaptic parasympathetic fibers to, and reflex afferent fibers from, the cardiac plexus; branching from the vagi at root of neck. SYN rami cardiaci cervicales inferiores nervi vagi [NA].

inferior dental b.'s of inferior dental plexus, b.'s passing from the inferior dental plexus to the roots of the teeth of the lower jaw. SYN rami dentales inferiores plexus dentalis inferioris [NA].

inferior gingival b.'s of inferior dental plexus, b.'s of inferior dental plexus to the gingiva of the lower jaw. SYN rami gingivales inferiores plexus dentalis inferioris [NA].

inferior labial b.'s of mental nerve, b.'s of mental nerve to lower lip. SYN rami labiales inferiores nervi mentalis [NA].

inferior lingular b. of lingular branch of left pulmonary artery, b. (of the lingular b.) of the left pulmonary artery serving the inferior lingular segment of the superior lobe of the left lung. SYN ramus lingularis inferior [NA].

inferior b. of oculomotor nerve, b. of oculomotor nerve providing motor b.'s to medial and inferior rectus and inferior oblique muscles and carrying presynaptic parasympathetic fibers which pass to the ciliary ganglion via the parasympathetic root. SYN ramus inferior nervi oculomotorii [NA].

inferior b. of pubic bone, SYN ramus inferior ossis pubis [NA]. SEE ischiopubic *ramus.*

inferior b. of superior gluteal artery, *distribution:* gluteus medius and minimus muscles; *anastomosis:* lateral circumflex femoral artery. SYN ramus inferior arteriae gluteae superioris [NA].

inferior b.'s of transverse cervical nerve, b. of transverse cervical nerve providing cutaneous innervation in lower part of anterior triangle of neck. SYN rami inferiores nervi transversi cervicalis [colli] [NA].

infrahyoid b. of superior thyroid artery, small b. from the initial part of the superior thyroid artery coursing along the hyoid bone deep to the thyrohyoid muscle to anastomose with its contralateral partner. SYN ramus infrahyoideus arteriae thyroidea superioris [NA].

infrapatellar b. of saphenous nerve, b. of saphenous nerve supplying skin over and below patella. SYN ramus infrapatellaris nervi sapheni [NA].

inguinal b.'s of external pudendal arteries, b.'s to the inguinal region which may arise as b.'s of external pudendal arteries or as direct b.'s of the femoral artery. Supply skin and subcutaneous tissues, including inguinal lymph nodes. SYN rami inguinales arteriae pudendae externae [NA].

internal b. of accessory nerve, b. of the accessory nerve trunk which carries fibers from the cranial root and which unites with the vagus nerve in the jugular foramen. SEE ALSO accessory *nerve.* SYN ramus internus nervi accessorii [NA], internal ramus of accessory nerve.

internal nasal b.'s, b.'s to nasal cavity. Internal nasal branches of 1) infraorbital nerve (rami nasales interni nervi infraorbitalis [NA]); 2) nasociliary nerve (rami nasales interni nervi ethmoidalis anterioris [NA]). SYN rami nasales interni [NA].

internal b. of superior laryngeal nerve, terminal b. of superior laryngeal nerve (with external b.) conveying sensory fibers to the supraglottic larynx. SYN ramus internus nervi laryngei superioris [NA].

joint b.'s, SYN articular b.'s.

laryngopharyngeal b.'s of superior cervical ganglion, b.'s conveying postganglionic sympathetic fibers from the superior cervical ganglion to the pharyngeal plexus. SYN rami laryngopharyngei ganglii cervicalis superioris [NA].

lateral b.'s, b.'s directed away from the midline, to the side. Nomina Anatomica lists lateral b.'s (ramus lasteralis/rami laterales) of the following: 1) anterior interventricular artery, ramus lateralis interventricularis anterioris arteriae coronariae sinistrae [NA]; 2) anterolateral central arteries, rami laterales arteriarum centralium anterolateralium [NA]; 3) dorsal primary rami of spinal nerves, rami laterales ramorum dorsalium nervorum cervicalium/thoracalium/lumbalium/sacralium; 4) left b. of portal vein, rami laterales rami sinistri venae portae hepatis [NA]; 5) left hepatic duct, ramus lateralis ductus hepatici sinistri [NA]; 6) middle lobe b. of right pulmonary artery, ramus lateralis ramorum lobarium medium arteriorum pulmonarium dextrum [NA]; 7) supraorbital nerve, ramus lateralis nervi supraorbitalis [NA]. SYN rami laterales [NA].

lateral basal b., lateral basal b. of the following: 1) basal part of inferior lobar b. of right pulmonary artery; 2) basal part of inferior lobar b. of left pulmonary artery. SYN ramus basalis lateralis [NA].

lateral calcaneal b.'s of sural nerve, b.'s of sural nerve providing cutaneous innervation to posterior aspect of distal leg and lateral aspect of proximal portion of foot. SYN rami calcanei laterales nervi suralis [NA].

lateral costal b. of internal thoracic artery, a variable b. of internal thoracic artery that runs lateral and parallel to the internal thoracic artery on the deep surface of the rib cage; *anastomosis:* posterior intercostal arteries. SYN ramus costalis lateralis arteriae thoracicae internae [NA].

lateral cutaneous b., lateral cutaneous b.'s of the following: 1) iliohypogastric nerve, ramus cutaneus lateralis nervi iliohypogastrici [NA]; 2) dorsal branch of thoracic nerves, ramus lateralis ramorum dorsalium nervorum thoracicorum [NA]; 3) dorsal branch of posterior intercostal arteries, ramus cutaneos lateralis ramorum posteriorum arterieae intercostalium [NA]. SYN ramus cutaneus lateralis [NA].

lateral cutaneous b.'s of intercostal nerves, SYN lateral cutaneous b.'s of ventral primary ramus of thoracic spinal nerves.

lateral cutaneous b.'s of ventral primary ramus of thoracic spinal nerves, b.'s arising in approximately the anterior axillary line at the level of the second through sixth intercostal spaces. SYN rami mammarii laterales nervorum intercostalium[☆], lateral cutaneous b.'s of intercostal nerves.

lateral mammary b.'s, b.'s primarily distributed to the lateral portion of the breast. SYN rami mammarii laterales [NA].

lateral mammary b.'s of lateral cutaneous branches of intercostal nerves, SYN lateral mammary b.'s of lateral cutaneous branches of thoracic spinal nerves.

lateral mammary b.'s of lateral cutaneous branches of thoracic spinal nerves, b.'s arising from the lateral cutaneous b.'s of the ventral primary rami of spinal nerves (intercostal nerves) T-3 to T-6 which run anteriorly to supply the lateral aspect of the breast. SYN rami mammarii laterales rami cutanei lateralis nervorum thoracicorum [NA], rami mammarii laterales rami cutanei lateralis nervorum intercostalium[☆], lateral mammary b.'s of lateral cutaneous branches of intercostal nerves.

lateral mammary b.'s of lateral thoracic artery, b.'s of the lateral thoracic artery which extend around the lateral borders of the pectoral muscles to supply the lateral aspect of the breast and mammary gland. SYN rami mammarii laterales arteriae thoracicae lateralis [NA].

lateral nasal b.'s of anterior ethmoidal nerve, b.'s of nasociliary nerve distributed to walls of nasal cavity. SYN rami nasales laterales nervi ethmoidalis anterioris [NA].

lateral orbitofrontal b., SYN lateral frontobasal *artery.*

lingual b.'s, b.'s to the tongue. Nomina Anatomica lists lingual b.'s of 1) hypoglossal nerve, rami linguales nervi hypoglossi [NA]; 2) lingual nerve, rami linguales nervi lingualis [NA]; 3) glossopharyngeal nerve, rami linguales nervi glossopharyngei [NA]. SYN rami linguales [NA].

lingual b. of facial nerve, lingual b. (inconstant) of the stylohyoid b. of the facial nerve. SYN ramus lingularis nervi facialis [NA].

lingular b., the lingular branch of 1) superior lobar b. of left pulmonary artery; 2) left superior pulmonary vein. SYN ramus lingularis [NA].

lumbar b. of iliolumbar artery, terminal b. of iliolumbar artery (with iliac b.) which ascends to supply psoas major and quadratus lumborum muscles; *anastomosis:* fourth lumbar artery. SYN ramus lumbalis arteriae iliolumbalis [NA].

mammary b.'s, SEE lateral mammary b.'s, medial mammary b.'s.

marginal mandibular b. of facial nerve, b. of facial nerve which parallels the mandibular margin innervating risorius muscle and muscles of lower lip and chin. SYN ramus marginalis mandibulae nervi facialis [NA].

marginal tentorial b. of internal carotid artery, a small b. from the cavernous part of the internal carotid artery to the free margin of the tentorium. SYN ramus marginalis tentorii arteriae carotidis internae [NA].

mastoid b. of occipital artery, SYN mastoid *artery*.

mastoid b.'s of posterior auricular artery, b.'s from stylomastoid b. of posterior auricular artery arising within the facial canal, distributed to the mastoid air cells. SYN rami mastoidei arteriae auricularis posterioris [NA].

medial b.'s, b.'s directed toward the midline, to the middle. Nomina Anatomica lists medial b.'s (ramus lateralis/rami mediales) of the following: 1) anterolateral central arteries, rami mediales arteriarum centralium anterolateralium [NA]; 2) dorsal primary rami of spinal nerves, rami medialis ramorum dorsalium nervorum cervicalium/thoracicalium/lumbalium/sacralium; 3) left b. of portal vein, rami mediales rami sinistri venae portae hepatis [NA]; 4) left hepatic duct, ramus medialis ductus hepatici sinistri [NA]; 5) middle lobar b. of right pulmonary artery, ramus medialis ramorum lobarium medium arteriorum pulmonarium dextrum [NA]; 6) supraorbital nerve, ramus medialis nervi supraorbitalis [NA]. SYN rami mediales [NA].

medial basal b. of pulmonary artery, a b. of the basal part of inferior lobar b.'s of the left and right pulmonary arteries. SYN ramus basalis medialis [NA].

medial calcaneal b.'s of tibial nerve, cutaneous b.'s of tibial nerve distributed to the inferior and medial heel. SYN rami calcanei mediales nervi tibialis [NA].

medial crural cutaneous b.'s of saphenous nerve, b.'s of saphenous nerve distributed to the skin of the medial side of the leg. SYN rami cutanei cruris mediales nervi sapheni [NA].

medial cutaneous b., Nomina Anatomica lists medial cutaneous b.'s of the following: 1) dorsal branch of thoracic nerves, ramus cutaneus medialis ramorum dorsalium nervorum thoracicorum [NA]; 2) dorsal branch of posterior intercostal arteries, ramus cutaneus medialis rami dorsalis arteriarum intercostalium posteriorum III–XI [NA]. SYN ramus cutaneus medialis [NA].

medial mammary b.'s, b.'s primarily distributed to the medial portion of the breast. Nomina Anatomica lists medial mammary b.'s (rami mammarii mediales...) of the following: 1) anterior cutaneous b.'s of ventral primary rami of thoracic spinal nerves (...rami cutanei anterioris ramorum ventralium nervorum thoracicorum [NA]; also known as anterior cutaneous b.'s of intercostal nerves (...rami cutanei anterioris nervorum intercostalium); nerve b.'s accompanying the perforating b.'s of internal thoracic artery. 2) perforating b.'s of internal thoracic artery (...rami perforantes arteriae thoracicae internae [NA]). SYN rami mammarii mediales [NA].

medial nasal b.'s of anterior ethmoidal nerve, b.'s of nasociliary nerve distributed to the nasal septum. SYN rami nasales mediales nervi ethmoidalis anterioris [NA].

mediastinal b.'s, b.'s distributed to the mediastinum. SYN rami mediastinales [NA], arteriae mediastinales anteriores, mediastinal arteries.

mediastinal b.'s of internal thoracic artery, small twigs supplying anterior mediastinal structures: mainly thymus and lymph nodes. SYN rami mediastinales arteriae thoracicae internae [NA], rami thymici [NA], anterior mediastinal arteries, arteriae thymicae, thymic arteries.

mediastinal b.'s of thoracic aorta, numerous small arteries supplying the pleura and lymph nodes of the posterior mediastinum. SYN rami mediastinales aortae thoracicae [NA], posterior mediastinal arteries.

meningeal b.'s, b.'s of vessels or nerves distributed to the coverings of the brain and spinal cord. SYN rami meningei.

meningeal b. of internal carotid artery, a b. from the cavernous part of the internal carotid artery to the meninges of the anterior cranial fossa. SYN ramus meningeus arteriae carotidis internae.

meningeal b. of mandibular nerve, a recurrent b. of the mandibular nerve that passes superiorly through foramen spinosum to be distributed with the posterior division of the middle meninge-

al artery to the meninges of the posterior portion of the middle cranial fossa. SYN rami meningeus nervi mandibularis [NA], ramus meningeus nervi mandibularis [NA], nervus spinosus.

meningeal b. of occipital artery, one of the variable b.'s of the occipital artery which may pass through the jugular or parietal foramina or condyloid canal to reach the dura mater and bone of the posterior cranial fossa, as well as the intracranial portions of the caudal four cranial neres. SYN ramus meningeus arteriae occipitalis [NA].

meningeal b. of ophthalmic nerve, SEE tentorial *nerve*.

meningeal b. of spinal nerves, a b. from the initial (mixed) part of each spinal nerve passing in a recurrent fashion back through the intervertebral foramen to supply spinal meninges, the posterior longitudinal ligament, posterolateral periphery of the intervertebral disc, and periosteum of the vertebrae. SYN ramus meningeus nervorum spinalium [NA], recurrent meningeal b. of spinal nerves, sinuvertebral nerves.

meningeal b. of vagus nerve, a b. of the superior ganglion of the vagus supplying the meninges of the posterior cranial fossa. SYN ramus meningeus nervi vagi [NA].

mental b.'s of mental nerve, mental branches of mental nerve. SYN rami mentales nervi mentalis [NA].

middle lobe b., middle lobe branch of 1) the right pulmonary artery (arteriae pulmonalis dextrae [NA]); 2) the right superior pulmonary vein (venae pulmonalis dextrae superior [NA]). SYN ramus lobi medii [NA].

middle meningeal b. of maxillary nerve, recurrent b. of maxillary nerve distributed with the anterior b. of the middle meningeal arteyr to the meninges of the anterior portion of the middle cranial fossa. SYN ramus meningeus medius nervi maxillaris [NA], middle meningeal nerve.

middle superior alveolar b. of infraorbital nerve, the middle superior alveolar branch, a branch of the superior alveolar nerve that contributes to the superior dental plexus. SYN ramus alveolaris superior medius nervi infraorbitalis [NA].

muscular b.'s, usually unnamed b.'s of nerves or vessels that supply the muscles. SYN rami musculares [NA].

occipital b., Nomina Anatomica lists occipital b.'s of 1) posterior auricular artery (rami occipitalis arteriae auricularis posterior [NA]; 2) posterior auricular nerve (rami occipitalis nervi auricularis posterioris [NA]; and 3) occipital artery, rami occipitales arteriae occipitis [NA]. SYN ramus occipitalis [NA].

omental b.'s, SYN epiploic b.'s.

orbital b. of middle meningeal artery, b. of middle meningeal artery traversing superior orbital fissure and running toward lacrimal gland. SEE anastomotic b. of middle meningeal artery to lacrimal artery. SYN ramus orbitalis arteriae meningeae mediae [NA].

orbital b.'s of pterygopalatine ganglion, b.'s of pterygopalatine ganglion traversing inferior orbital fissure, distributed in orbit to periorbita and mucosa of ethmoidal and sphenoidal sinuses. SYN ramus orbitalis ganglii pterygopalatini [NA].

ovarian b. of uterine artery, terminal b. of uterine artery (with tubal b.) which runs through mesovarium supplying ovary from medial aspect and anastomosing with ovarian b. of ovarian artery. SYN ramus ovaricus arteriae uterinae [NA].

palmar carpal b. of radial artery, a small b. of the radial artery that passes medially across the wrist to supply the carpal joints; it anastomoses with the anterior carpal branch of the ulnar artery. SYN ramus carpalis palmaris arteriae radialis, ramus carpeus palmaris arteriae radialis.

palmar carpal b. of ulnar artery, a b. of the ulnar artery that supplies the carpal joints and communicates with the anterior carpal branch of the radial artery. SYN ramus carpalis palmaris arteriae ulnaris, ramus carpeus palmaris arteriae ulnaris.

palmar b. of median nerve, b. of median nerve arising proximal to flexor retinaculum and running superficial to it to supply skin of proximal central palm and thenar eminence. Since it does not traverse carpal tunnel, it is not affected by carpal tunnel syndrome, even though it supplies skin distal to carpal tunnel. SYN ramus palmaris nervi mediani [NA].

palmar b. of ulnar nerve, b. of ulnar nerve arising in distal forearm and accompanying palmar artery into hand where it supplies skin of little finger and medial half of ring finger and adjacent parts of palm. SYN ramus palmaris nervi ulnaris [NA].

palpebral b.'s of infratrochlear nerve, b.'s of infratrochlear nerve supplying skin of medial aspects of upper and lower eyelids. SYN rami palpebrales nervi infratrochlearis [NA].

pancreatic b.'s, b.'s to the pancreas. Nomina Anatomica lists pancreatic b.'s of 1) splenic artery, rami pancreatici arteriae splenicae [NA]; 2) superior pancreaticoduodenal arteries, rami pancreatici arteriae pancreaticoduodenalis superioris [NA]. SYN rami pancreatici [NA].

parietal b., (1) b.'s coursing in relationship to and supplying the parietal bone or parietal lobe of cerebrum; **(2)** b.'s distributed to the body wall and limbs (the "parities") as opposed to visceral b.'s distributed to the body cavities. For example, the gray rami communicantes are the parietal b.'s of the sympathetic trunks (vs. the splanchnic nerves, which are visceral b.'s of the trunks). SYN rami parietales [NA].

parietal b. of medial occipital artery, an anterior b. of the medial occipital artery supplying the posterior section of the parietal lobe of the cerebrum. SYN ramus parietalis arteriae occipitalis medialis [NA].

parietal b. of middle meningeal artery, smaller terminal b. (with frontal b.) of middle meningeal artery supplying posterior portion of lateral and superior dura and cranium. SYN ramus parietalis arteriae meningeae mediae [NA].

parietal b. of superficial temporal artery, b.'s coursing in relationship to and/or supplying the parietal lobe of the brain. SYN ramus parietalis arteriae temporalis superficialis [NA].

parotid b.'s, b.'s to parotid gland; Nomina Anatomica lists parotid branches of 1) auriculotemporal nerve (rami parotidei nervi auriculotemporalis [NA]; 2) facial vein, rami parotidei venae facialis [NA]; 3) superficial temporal artery, ramus arteriae temporalis superficialis [NA]. SYN rami parotidei [NA].

pectoral and abdominal anterior cutaneous b. of intercostal nerves, SYN thoracoabdominal *nerves,* under *nerve.*

pectoral b.'s of thoracoacromial artery, pectoral branches of thoracoacromial artery. SYN rami pectorales arteriae thoracoacromialis [NA].

perforating b.'s, arterial b.'s which penetrate a wall or pass from the anterior to the posterior aspect or compartment of a structure such as the hand or foot to anastomose or be distributed. SYN ramus perforans [NA], perforating peroneal artery.

perforating b.'s of internal thoracic artery, small b.'s of the internal thoracic artery running between the costal cartilages to supply overlying skin and subcutaneous tissues. SYN ramus perforantes arteriae thoracicae internae [NA], perforating arteries of internal mammary.

perforating b.'s of palmar metacarpal arteries, the perforating b.'s of the palmar metacarpal arteries, three small arteries that pass dorsally through the second, third, and fourth interosseous spaces of the hand from the palmar metacarpal arteries. SYN ramus perforantes arteriarum metacarpalium palmarium [NA], perforating arteries of hand.

perforating b. of peroneal artery, the b. of the peroneal artery that perforates the interosseous membrane just above the anterior tibiofibular ligament. SYN ramus perforans arteriae fibularis [NA].

perforating b.'s of plantar metatarsal arteries, the perforating b.'s of the plantar metatarsal arteries, three small arteries that pass dorsally through the second, third, and fourth interosseous spaces of the foot from the plantar metatarsal arteries. SYN ramus perforantes arteriarum metatarsearum plantarium [NA], perforating arteries of foot.

pericardial b. of phrenic nerve, one of the b.'s of phrenic nerve distributed to the pericardium and adjacent mediastial parietal pleura. SYN ramus pericardiacus nervi phrenici [NA].

pericardial b.'s of thoracic aorta, small b.'s of thoracic aorta distributed to the pericardium, in the region of the oblique pericardial sinus, and to posterior mediastinal lymph nodes. SYN rami pericardiaci aortae thoracicae [NA].

perineal b.'s of posterior femoral cutaneous nerve, b.'s of posterior femoral cutaneous nerve which convey sensory fibers to the skin of the lateral-most perineum and adjacent portions of the upper medial thigh. SYN rami perineales nervi cutanei femoris posterioris [NA].

peroneal communicating b., the peroneal (fibular) communicating branch of the common peroneal (fibular) nerve; it arises from the common peroneal nerve in the popliteal space and passes over the lateral head of the gastrocnemius to the middle third of the leg, where it unites with the medial sural cutaneous nerve to form the sural nerve. SYN ramus communicans fibularis nervi fibularis communis [NA], ramus communicans peroneus nervi peronei communis ☆ [NA], nervus communicans fibularis, nervus communicans peroneus, peroneal anastomotic ramus, peroneal communicating nerve.

petrosal b. of middle meningeal artery, petrous b. of middle meningeal artery; first intracranial b. of middle meningeal artery; *anastomosis:* stylomastoid artery via hiatus of facial canal. SYN ramus petrosus arteriae meningeae mediae [NA].

pharyngeal b.'s, b.'s to the pharynx. SYN pharyngei [NA], rami pharyngeales [NA].

pharyngeal b. of the artery of pterygoid canal, distributed to uppermost nasopharynx (pharyngeal recesses). SYN ramus pharyngeus arteriae canalis pterygoidei [NA].

pharyngeal b. of the ascending pharyngeal artery, *distribution:* walls of oro- and nasopharynx. SYN rami pharyngeales arteriae pharyngeae ascendentis [NA].

pharyngeal b. of descending palatine artery, may arise as a separate b. or as a continuation of lesser palatine artery. SYN ramus pharyngeus arteriae palatini descendens [NA].

pharyngeal b. of glossopharyngeal nerve, conveys general sensory fibers to the mucosa of the oropharynx via the pharyngeal plexus. SYN rami pharyngei nervi glossopharyngei [NA].

pharyngeal b. of inferior thyroid artery, distributed to laryngopharynx. SYN rami pharyngeales arteriae thyroideae inferioris [NA].

pharyngeal b. of pterygopalatine ganglion, b. of pterygopalatine ganglion passing posteriorly through pharyngeal canal to supply postsynaptic parasympathetic fibers to mucus glands of nasopharynx. SYN ramus pharyngeus ganglii pterygopalatini [NA], Bock's nerve.

pharyngeal b. of vagus nerve, conveys motor fibers from the cranial root of the accessory nerve to the pharyngeal constrictor muscles, the intrinsic muscles of the soft palate and the levator palati muscle; may also bring some general sensory fibers to the pharyngeal plexus. SYN rami pharyngei nervi vagi [NA].

phrenicoabdominal b.'s of phrenic nerve, terminal b.'s of phrenic nerve providing motor innervation of diaphragm and sensory innervation to the diaphragm and the diaphragmatic pleura and peritoneum. SYN rami phrenicoabdominales nervi phrenici [NA].

posterior b.'s, b.'s directed dorsally or backward. SYN rami posteriores [NA].

posterior basal b., posterior basal b. of the basal part of the inferior lobar b. of the left and right pulmonary arteries. SYN ramus basalis posterior [NA].

posterior b. of great auricular nerve, provides general sensory fibers to skin of posterior auricle and over mastoid process. SYN ramus posterior nervi auricularis magni [NA].

posterior inferior nasal b.'s of greater palatine nerve, b. of greater palatine nerve to posterior inferior lateral wall of nasal cavity, including posterior aspect of mucosa over posterior portion of inferior nasal concha and meatus; may arise independently from pterygopalatine ganglion. SYN rami nasales posteriores inferiores nervi palatini majoris [NA].

posterior b. of inferior pancreaticoduodenal artery, the more dorsal of the two b.'s into which the inferior pancreaticoduodenal artery bifurcates; supplies uncinate process and head of pancreas, as well as the third and fourth parts of the duodenum; anastomoses with the posterior branch of the superior pancreaticuduodenal artery. SYN ramus posterior arteriae pancreaticoduodenalis inferioris [NA].

posterior b. of lateral cerebral sulcus, the long, posteriorly-directed continuation of the lateral cerebral sulcus which extends between the temporal lobe inferiorly and the parietal lobe superiorly, its termination surrounded by the supramarginal gyrus. SYN ramus posterior sulci lateralis cerebri [NA].

posterior b. of obturator artery, b. of obturator artery giving rise to acetabular b. and supplying muscles attached to ischium. SYN ramus posterior arteriae obturatoriae [NA].

posterior b. of obturator nerve, b. supplying obturator externus muscle; then passing posterior to adductor brevis, supplying it and the adductor portion of the adductor magnus muscle. SYN ramus posterior nervi obturatorii [NA].

posterior b. of recurrent ulnar artery, contributes to blood supply of flexor carpi ulnaris and to articular network of elbow. SYN ramus posterior arteriae recurrentis ulnaris [NA].

posterior b. of renal artery, terminal b. of renal artery (with anterior b.) becoming the posterior segmental artery of kidney. SYN ramus posterior arteriae renalis [NA].

posterior b. of right branch of portal vein, posterior segmental b. of portal vein; b. to posterior segments of right lobe of liver. SYN ramus posterior rami dextri venae portae hepatis [NA].

posterior b. of right hepatic duct, hepatic duct b. draining bile from posterior segments of right lobe of liver. SYN ramus posterior ductus hepatici dextri [NA].

posterior b. of right superior pulmonary vein, drains posterior portion of superior lobe of right lung. SYN ramus posterior venae pulmonalis dextrae superioris [NA].

posterior scrotal b.'s of internal pudendal artery, b.'s of perineal artery supplying skin of posterior scrotal sac. SYN rami scrotales posteriores arteriae pudendae internae [NA].

posterior b. of spinal nerves, SEE dorsal primary *ramus* of spinal nerve.

posterior superior alveolar b.'s of maxillary nerve, the b.'s of the superior alveolar nerves that supply the maxillary sinus and the molar tooth. SYN rami alveolares superiores posteriores nervi maxillaris [NA].

posterior superior lateral nasal b.'s of pterygopalatine ganglion, b.'s of pterygopalatine ganglion to upper posterior part of lateral wall of nasal cavity, including superior and middle nasal concha/meatuses, and posterior ethmoidal sinuses. SYN rami nasales posteriores superiores laterales ganglii pterygopalatini [NA].

posterior superior medial nasal b.'s of pterygopalatine ganglion, usually b.'s of the nasopalatine nerve to posterior superior nasal septum. SYN rami nasales posteriores superiores mediales ganglii pterygopalatini [NA].

posterior b. of superior thyroid artery, b. of superior thyroid artery which descends to supply the apical portion of the ipsilateral lobe of the thyroid, continuing along the posterior border of the gland to anastomose with the inferior thyroid artery. SYN ramus posterior arteriae thyroideae superioris [NA].

pterygoid b.'s of maxillary artery, pterygoid branches of middle meningeal artery. SYN rami pterygoidei arteriae maxillaris [NA].

pubic b. of inferior epigastric artery, b. arising from the inferior epigastric artery medial to the deep inguinal ring; runs medial to femoral ring onto posterior pubis; anastomosis, pubic b. of obturator artery. This anastomosis is frequently large, referred to as an "accessory obturator artery." In 20–30%, this anastomosis replaces the obturator artery, as an "aberrant" or "replaced" obturator artery. SYN ramus pubicus arteriae epigastricae inferioris [NA].

pubic b. of obturator artery, b. arising from the obturator artery just prior to its pasage through the obturator canal; the b. passes superiorly on the posterior aspect of the pubis. *Anastomosis:* with contralateral partner and pubic b. of inferior epigastric artery. SEE accessory obturator *artery*, pubic b. of inferior epigastric artery. SYN ramus pubicus arteriae obturatoriae [NA].

pulmonary b.'s of autonomic nervous system, pulmonary b.'s of cardiac plexuses and cardiaopulmonary splanchnic nerves. SYN rami pulmonales systematis autonomici [NA].

recurrent meningeal b. of spinal nerves, SYN meningeal b. of spinal nerves.

renal b. of lesser splanchnic b., b. of lesser splanchnic nerve to the aorticorenal plexus/ganglion. SYN ramus renalis nervi splanchnici minoris [NA].

renal b.'s of vagus nerve, b.'s of vagus nerve to kidney via the celiac plexus. SYN rami renales nervi vagi [NA].

right b., of a pair of b.'s, the b. passing to the right side of the body, to the right member of a bilateral pair of structures, or to the right portion of an unpaired structure; the other member of the pair being a left branch. SYN ramus dexter [NA].

right b. of portal vein, terminal b. of hepatic portal vein distributed to right lobe of liver tributary: cystic vein. SYN ramus dexter venae portae hepatis [NA].

right b. of proper hepatic artery, SYN right hepatic *artery.*

saphenous b. of descending genicular artery, b. of descending genicular artery supplying skin of the upper part of the medial aspect of the leg; *anastomosis:* medial inferior genicular artery (articular vascular *network* of knee). SYN ramus saphenus arteriae descendentis genicularis [NA].

b.'s of segmental bronchi, b.'s of segmental bronchi to the bronchopulmonary segments of the lungs. SYN rami bronchiales segmentorum [NA].

septal b.'s, the interventricular septal b.'s; b.'s of the anterior and posterior interventricular arteries distributed to the muscle of the interventricular septum. SYN rami interventriculares septales.

sinuatrial nodal b. of right coronary artery, SYN *artery* to the sinuatrial (S-A) node.

b. to sinuatrial node, SYN *artery* to the sinuatrial (S-A) node.

splenic b.'s of splenic artery, b.'s of proper splenic arteries; splenic artery entering spleen at hilum. SYN rami splenici arteriae splenicae [NA], rami lienales arteriae lienalis✴ [NA].

stapedial b. of stylomastoid artery, b. arising either directly from the stylomastoid artery or its b., the posterior tympanic artery; supplies stapedius muscle. SYN ramus stapedius arteriae stylomastoideae [NA].

sternal b.'s of internal thoracic artery, b.'s of internal thoracic artery which pass medially to supply the transversus thoracis muscle and posterior sternum. SYN rami sternales arteriae thoracicae internae [NA], sternal arteries.

sternocleidomastoid b. of occipital artery, b.'s of occipital artery to sternocleidomastoid muscle. One often hooks around hypoglossal nerve. It may arise as an independent b. of the external carotid, in which case it may be referred to as the sternomastoid *artery.* SYN rami sternocleidomastoidei arteriae occipitalis [NA].

sternocleidomastoid b. of superior thyroid artery, b. of superior thyroid artery to sternocleidomastoid muscle. SYN ramus sternocleidomastoideus arteriae thyroideae superioris [NA].

stylohyoid b. of facial nerve, b. of facial nerve to stylohyoid muscle. SYN ramus stylohyoideus nervi facialis [NA].

subscapular b.'s of axillary artery, b.'s of axillary artery passing directly to the subscapularis muscle. SYN rami subscapulares arteriae axillaris [NA].

superficial b., b. which passes above or closer to surface; usually in contrast to a deep b. SYN ramus superficialis [NA].

superficial b. of the lateral plantar nerve, mostly cutaneous b. to skin of small and lateral half of fourth toes and lateral side of sole of foot, but also supplies the flexor digiti minimi brevis muscle and the most lateral dorsal and plantar interosseous muscles. SYN ramus superficialis nervi plantaris lateralis [NA].

superficial b. of the medial plantar artery, gives rise to superficial digital arteries of medial three toes. SYN ramus superficialis arteriae plantaris medialis [NA].

superficial palmar b. of radial artery, the superficial palmar branch of the radial artery which supplies the thenar muscles then enters the palm to communicate with the superficial palmar arch from the ulnar artery. SYN ramus palmaris superficialis arteriae radialis [NA], superficial palmar artery, superficial volar artery, superficialis volae.

superficial b. of the radial nerve, cutaneous terminal b. (with deep b.) which runs under cover of brachioradialis muscle to wrist, then supplies skin of proximal portion of the dorsal aspects of thumb, index, middle and lateral half of ring fingers and the portion of the dorsum of the hand located proximally. SYN ramus superficialis nervi radialis [NA].

superficial b. of the superior gluteal artery, to upper gluteus maximus muscle. SYN ramus superficialis arteriae gluteae superioris [NA].

superficial temporal b.'s of auriculotemporal nerve, b.'s of auriculotemporal nerve to anterolateral scalp. SYN rami temporales superficiales nervi auriculotemporalis [NA].

superficial b. of the transverse cervical artery, b. of transverse cervical artery which accompanies the spinal accessory nerve on the deep surface of the trapezius muscle. Alternatively arises as a direct b. of the thyrocervical trunk, in which case it is called the superficial cervical artery.

superficial b. of the ulnar nerve, b. supplying skin of palmar aspect of little and medial half of ring fingers, the portion of the palm proximal to them and the palmaris brevis muscle. SYN ramus superficialis nervi ulnaris [NA].

superior b., b. which is directed upward or cranially or which is highly-placed, usually in contrast to an inferior b. SYN ramus superior [NA].

superior cervical cardiac b.'s of vagus nerve, uppermost of the b.'s of vagus nerve conducting presynaptic parasympathetic fibers to, and reflex afferent fibers from, the cardiac plexus; branching from the vagi close to the base of the skull. SYN rami cardiaci cervicales superiores nervi vagi [NA].

superior dental b.'s of superior dental plexus, b.'s passing from the superior dental plexus to the roots of the teeth of the upper jaw. SYN rami dentales superiores plexus dentalis superioris [NA].

superior gingival b.'s of superior dental plexus, b.'s of superior dental plexus to gingiva of upper jaw. SYN rami gingivales superiores plexus dentalis superioris [NA].

superior labial b.'s of infraorbital nerve, b.'s of infraorbital nerve to upper lip. SYN rami labiales superiores nervi infraorbitalis [NA].

superior lingular b. of lingular branch of superior lobar left pulmonary artery, b. (of the lingular b.) of the left pulmonary artery serving the superior lingular segment of the superior lobe of the left lung. SYN ramus lingularis superior [NA].

superior b. of the oculomotor nerve, b. of oculomotor nerve supplying the superior rectus and levator palpebrae superioris muscles. SYN ramus superior nervi oculomotorii [NA].

superior b. of the pubic bone, SYN superior pubic *ramus.*

superior b. of the right and left inferior pulmonary veins, tributaries of the right and left inferior pulmonary veins which receive oxygenated blood from the superior [S6] bronchopulmonary segments of the inferior lobes of the right and left lungs. SYN ramus superior venae pulmonalis dextrae/sinistrae inferioris [NA].

superior b. of the superior gluteal artery, runs between gluteus medius and minimus muscles, supplying both, and continuing to reach tensor fascia lata muscle. SYN ramus superior arteriae gluteae superioris [NA].

superior b. of the transverse cervical nerve, b. providing cutaneous innervation in upper part of anterior triangle of neck. SYN ramus superior nervi transversalis cervicalis (colli) [NA].

suprahyoid b. of lingual artery, b. of lingual artery which runs along hyoid bone; *anastomosis:* infrahyoid b. of superior thyroid artery and across midline with its contralateral partner. SYN ramus suprahyoideus arteriae lingualis [NA].

sympathetic b. to submandibular ganglion, b. to the submandibular ganglion composed of postsynaptic sympathetic fibers from the internal carotid plexus conveyed largely by a periarterial plexus of the facial artery. SYN ramus sympathicus [sympatheticus] ad ganglion submandibulare✻.

temporal b.'s of facial nerve, b.'s of facial nerve innervating the superior portion of the orbicularis oculi muscle and other muscles of facial expression above the eye. SYN rami temporales nervi facialis [NA].

thoracic cardiac b.'s of vagus nerve, b.'s of vagus nerve to the cardiac plexus which branch from the vagi at thoracic levels, conducting presynpatic parasympathetic fibers to, and reflex afferent fibers from, the cardiac plexus. SYN rami cardiaci thoracici nervi vagi [NA].

thymic b.'s of internal thoracic artery, SEE mediastinal b.'s of internal thoracic artery.

tonsillar b. of the facial artery, primary blood supply to palatine tonsil, with extensive anastomoses with other tonsillar arteries. SYN ramus tonsillaris arteriae facialis [NA].

tonsillar b.'s of glossopharyngeal nerve, b.'s of glossopharyngeal nerve conducting sensory fibers from the palatine tonsillar fossa. SYN rami tonsillares nervi glossopharyngei [NA].

tracheal b.'s, b.'s to the trachea. Nomina Anatomica lists tracheal branches of 1) inferior thyroid artery (rami tracheales arteriae thyroideae inferioris [NA]); and 2) recurrent laryngeal nerve (rami tracheales nervi laryngei recurrentis [NA]). SYN rami tracheales [NA].

transverse b.'s, b.'s which run transversly. Nomina Anatomica lists transverse b.'s of 1) lateral femoral circumflex artery (ramus transversus arteriae circumflexae femoris lateralis [NA]); and 2) medial femoral circumflex artery (ramus transversus arteriae circumflexae femoris medialis [NA]). SYN ramus transversus [NA].

b. to trigeminal ganglion, ganglionic b. of internal carotid artery.

tubal b., b. to a tubular structure. SYN ramus tubarius [NA].

tubal b. of the tympanic plexus, sensory b. of tympanic plexus (of glossopharyngeal nerve) to auditory tube. SYN ramus tubarius plexus tympanici [NA].

tubal b. of the uterine artery, terminal b. of uterine artery (with ovarian b.) supplying medial portion of uterine tube, anastomosing with tubal b. of ovarian artery. SYN ramus tubarius arteriae uterinae [NA].

ulnar communicating b. of superficial radial nerve, ulnar communicating b. of superficial b. of radial nerve, joining the dorsal b. of the ulnar nerve in the hand conveying sensation from the dorsal aspect of adjacent sides of the middle and ring fingers. SYN ramus communicans ulnaris nervi radialis [NA].

ulnar b. of medial antebrachial cutaneous nerve, b. of the medial antebrachial cutaneous nerve supplying the skin of the medial portion of the proximal two-thirds of the dorsal side of the forearm. SYN ramus ulnaris nervi cutanei antebrachii medialis [NA].

ureteral b.'s, SYN ureteric b.'s.

ureteric b.'s, b.'s distributed to the ureter. Although not listed by Nomina Anatomica, ureteric b.'s also rise regularly from the 1) abdominal aorta, 2) common iliac artery, and 3) internal iliac artery. Ureteric b.'s from the inferior vesical artery are constant in occurrence and supply the terminal portion of the ureter. SYN rami ureterici [NA], ureteral b.'s.

ureteric b.'s of the ovarian artery, b. of ovarian artery arising as it is crossed by the ureter in the female supplying mid portion of ureter. SYN rami ureterici arteriae ovaricae [NA].

ureteric b.'s of the patent part of umbilical artery, supplies pelvic portion of ureter. SYN rami ureterici partis patentis arteriae umbilicale [NA].

ureteric b.'s of the renal artery, supplies ureteric (renal) pelvis and superior portion of ureter. SYN rami ureterici arteriae renalis [NA].

ureteric b.'s of the testicular artery, b. of testicular artery arising as it is crossed by the ureter in the male; supplies mid portion of ureter. SYN rami ureterici arteriae testicularis [NA].

ventral b., SYN rami ventralis. SEE ventral primary *rami* of cervical spinal nerves, under *ramus,* ventral primary *rami* of lumbar spinal nerves, under *ramus,* ventral primary *rami* of sacral spinal nerves, under *ramus,* ventral primary *ramus* of spinal nerve.

vestibular b.'s of labyrinthine artery, b.'s of labyrinthine artery passing to the vestibule of the bony labyrinth to supply the membranous labyrinth.

zygomatic b.'s of facial nerve, b.'s of facial nerve crossing upper cheek to supply orbicularis oculi muscle. SYN rami zygomatici nervi facialis [NA].

zygomaticofacial b. of zygomatic nerve, penetrates zygomatic bone to supply skin of face over zygoma or cheekbone. SYN ramus zygomaticofacialis nervi zygomatici [NA].

zygomaticotemporal b. of zygomatic nerve, penetrates frontal process of zygomatic bone to supply skin of face lateral to orbit. SYN ramus zygomaticotemporalis nervi zygomatici [NA].

bran·chia, pl. **bran·chi·ae** (brang'kē-ă, -ē) [NA]. The gills, or organs of respiration, in water-living animals. [G. gill]

bran·chi·al (brang'kē-ăl). 1. Relating to branchiae or gills. 2. In embryology, denoting the various structures constituting the branchial *apparatus.*

branch·ing. Dividing into parts; sending out offshoots; bifurcating. SYN ramose, ramous. [Fr. *branche,* related to L. *branchium,* arm]

false b., in bacteriology, the appearance of b. produced when a cell is pushed out of the general line of growth and develops a new line of growth while the remaining cells continue to develop along the original line of growth.

bran·chi·o·gen·ic, bran·chi·og·en·ous (brang'kē-ō-jen'ik, -kē-oj'en-ŭs). Originating from the branchial arches. [G. *branchia,* gill, *-gen,* to produce]

bran·chi·o·ma (brang-kē-ō'mă). Obsolete term for a rare form of carcinoma that originates in remnants of epithelium in the branchial structures; most of the lesions occurring in this site are likely to be metastases from a primary neoplasm in another location. [G. *branchia,* gill + *-oma,* tumor]

bran·chi·o·mere (brang'kē-ō-mēr). An embryonic segment from which a branchial arch is developed. [G. *branchia,* gill, + *meros,* part]

bran·chi·om·er·ism (brang-kē-om'er-izm). Arrangement into branchiomeres.

bran·chi·o·mo·tor (brang'kē-ō-mō'tŏr). Relating to or controlling the movement of muscles derived from the branchial arches.

Brandt, M.L., U.S. obstetrician, *1894. SEE B.-Andrews *maneuver.*

bran·dy. An alcoholic liquid obtained by the distillation of the fermented juice of sound ripe grapes and usually containing 48 to 54% ethyl alcohol. [Du. *brandewijn,* burnt (distilled) wine]

Branham, H.H., 19th century U.S. surgeon. SEE B.'s *sign.*

Branham, Sara Elizabeth, U.S. bacteriologist, 1888–1962. SEE *Branhamella.*

Bran·ha·mel·la (bran-hă-mel'ă). A subgenus of aerobic, nonmotile, nonsporeforming bacteria (family Neisseriaceae) containing Gram-negative cocci that occur in pairs with adjacent sides flattened; these organisms differ from those of the genus *Moraxella* and of other genera in the family by their DNA base content and composition. They occur in the mucous membranes of the upper respiratory tract. The type species is *B. catarrhalis.* [Sara Branham]

B. catarrha'lis, SYN *Moraxella catarrhalis.*

bran·ny (bran'ē). Denoting desquamation of small husk-like scales. [M.E. *bran,* broken coat of cereal grain]

Brasdor, Pierre, French surgeon, 1721–1798. SEE B.'s *method.*

Braun, Christopher Heinrich, German surgeon, 1847–1911. SEE B.'s *anastomosis.*

Braune, Christian W., German anatomist, 1831–1892. SEE B.'s *canal, muscle, valve.*

brawny (brahw'nē). Thickened (lichenified) and dusky (a darkened hue), as of a swelling. [M.E. fleshy]

Braxton Hicks, John, British gynecologist, 1823–1897. SEE B.H. *contraction, sign, version.*

braxy (brak'sē). A fatal disease of sheep caused by *Clostridium septicum* and marked by inflammation of the abomasum and duodenum; symptoms preceding death in the less acute form are weakness, coma, and dyspnea. [Nor. *brad sot,* quick plague]

Bray, Charles William, U.S. otologist, *1904. SEE Wever-B. *phenomenon.*

Brazelton, T. Berry, U.S. pediatrician, *1918. SEE Brazelton's Neonatal Behavioral Assessment *Scale,* under *scale.*

bra·zil·ein (bră-zil'ē-in). $C_6H_{12}O_5$; a red oxidation product of brazilin.

braz·i·lin (bră-zil'in) [C.I. 75280]. A red natural dye, $C_{16}H_{14}O_5$, obtained from the bark of several species of tropical trees and oxidized to the active red dye brazilein; resembles hematoxylin in origin, chemistry, and usage; used as a nuclear stain and as an indicator (red in alkalies, yellow in acids).

braz·ing (brā'zing). In dentistry, soldering.

BrDu Abbreviation for bromodeoxyuridine.

break (brāk). To separate into parts. 2. A separation into parts.

double-strand b., a b. in double-stranded DNA in which both strands have been cleaved; however, the two strands have not separated from each other.

single-strand b., a b. in double-stranded DNA in which only one of the two strands has been cleaved; both strands have not separated from each other.

break·off (brāk'awf). A feeling of physical separation from the earth when piloting an aircraft at high altitude.

break·through (brāk'thrū). A sudden manifestation of new insights and more constructive attitudes following a period of resistance during psychotherapy.

breast (brest). 1. The pectoral surface of the thorax. 2. The organ of milk secretion; one of two hemispheric projections of variable size situated in the subcutaneous layer over the pectoralis major muscle on either side of the chest of the mature female; it is rudimentary in the male. SYN mamma [NA], teat (2). [A.S. *breōst*]

accessory b., SYN supernumerary b.

caked b., SYN stagnation *mastitis.*

chicken b., SYN *pectus* carinatum.

funnel b., SYN *pectus* excavatum.

irritable b., swelling and induration of the b., not due to a neoplasm, and usually of comparatively brief duration.

male b., one of the two, usually rudimentary, mammary glands in the male. SYN mamma masculina [NA], mamma virilis.

pigeon b., SYN *pectus* carinatum.

supernumerary b., a milk-secreting gland located elsewhere than at the normal place on the chest and existing in addition to the two usual mammae. SYN mamma accessoria [NA], accessory b., supernumerary mamma.

breath (breth). 1. The respired air. 2. An inspiration. [A.S. *braeth*]

liver b., SYN *fetor* hepaticus.

uremic b., characteristic odor of the b. in patients with chronic renal failure, variously described as "fishy," "ammoniacal," and "fetid," which is indicative of the systemic accumulation of volatile metabolites, usually excreted in the urine; dimethylamine and trimethylamine have been identified and correlated with the classic fishy odor.

breath-hold·ing (breth'hōld-ing). Voluntary or involuntary cessation of breathing; often seen in young children as a response to frustration.

breath·ing (brēdh'ing). Inhalation and exhalation of air or gaseous mixtures. SYN pneusis.

apneustic b., pauses in the respiratory cycle at full inspiration, caused by damage of the respiratory control centers in the more caudal pons.

ataxic b., SYN Biot's *respiration.*

Biot's b., SYN Biot's *respiration.*

bronchial b., breath sounds of a harsh or blowing quality, heard on auscultation of the chest, made by air moving in the large bronchi and barely, if at all, modified by the intervening lung; duration of the expiratory sound is as long as or longer than that of the inspiratory sound, and its pitch as high as or higher than that of the inspiratory sound; may be heard over a consolidated lung, above a pleural effusion due to an underlying compressed lung, and rarely over a pulmonary cavity; whispered pectoriloquy is another manifestation that usually can be elicited when bronchial b. is present.

continuous positive pressure b. (CPPB), SYN controlled mechanical *ventilation.*

glossopharyngeal b., respiration unaided by the usual primary muscles of respiration; the air is forced into the lungs by use of the tongue and muscles of the pharynx.

intermittent positive pressure b. (IPPB), SYN controlled mechanical *ventilation.*

mouth b., habitual respiration through the mouth instead of the nose, usually due to obstruction of the nasal airways.

positive-negative pressure b. (PNPB), inflation of the lungs with positive pressure and deflation with negative pressure by an automatic ventilator.

pursed lips b., a technique in which air is inhaled slowly through the nose and mouth and exhaled slowly through pursed lips; used by patients with chronic obstructive pulmonary disease to improve their breathing by increasing resistance to air flow, forcibly dilating small bronchi.

shallow b., a type of b. with abnormally low tidal volume.

stertorous b., SYN stertorous *respiration.*

Breda, Achille, Italian dermatologist, 1850–1933. SEE B.'s *disease.*

bre·douille·ment (brā-dwē-mahn′). Omission of parts of words related to extremely rapid speech. [Fr.]

breech (brēch). SYN buttocks. [A.S. *brēc*]

breed·ing (brēd′ing). Selected mating of individuals to produce a strain that is desirable or of scientific interest. SEE ALSO hybridization, linebreeding, inbreeding. [breed, fr. M.E. *breden,* fr. O.E. *brēdan,* + -ing]

breg·ma (breg′mă) [NA]. The point on the skull corresponding to the junction of the coronal and sagittal sutures. [G. the forepart of the head]

breg·mat·ic (breg-mat′ik). Relating to the bregma.

brei (brī). A fine mince or mush of tissue in which the cells are for the most part intact. Cf. homogenate. [Ger. pulp]

brems·strah·lung (bremz′strah-lŭng). Continuous spectrum radiation produced by the interaction of a beam of electrons and the nuclei that scatter them. [Ger. *Bremsstrahlung,* braking radiation]

Brenn, Lena, 20th century U.S. researcher. SEE Brown-B. *stain.*

Brenner, Fritz, German pathologist, *1877. SEE B. *tumor.*

⚠ **brepho-.** Rarely used prefix denoting a primitive stage of development. [G. *brephos,* embryo or newborn infant]

Breschet (Brechet), Gilbert, French anatomist, 1784–1845. SEE B.'s *bones,* under *bone, canals,* under *canal, hiatus, sinus, vein.*

Brescia, Michael J., U.S. nephrologist, *1933. SEE B.-Cimino *fistula.*

Breslow, Alexander, U.S. pathologist, 1928–1980. SEE B.'s *thickness.*

bre·tyl·i·um. An antihypertensive which on chronic oral dosing diminishes the release of norepinephrine from noradrenergic nerve endings.

bre·tyl·i·um tos·yl·ate (bre-til′ē-ŭm). (*o*-Bromobenzyl)-ethyldimethylammonium *p*-toluenesulfonate; a sympatholytic agent that prevents the release of norepinephrine from the nerve ending; used in the treatment of essential hypertension.

Breuer, Josef, Austrian internist, 1842–1925. SEE Hering-B. *reflex.*

Breus, Carl, Austrian obstetrician, 1852–1914. SEE B. *mole.*

brev·i·col·lis (brev-ē-kol′is). Abnormal shortness of the neck. [L. *brevis,* short, + *collum,* neck]

bre·vis (brev′is). Brief, short. [L. short]

bre·vo·tox·ins (BTX) (brev′ō-tok′sins). Structurally unique neurotoxins produced by the "red tide" dinoflagellate *Ptychodiscus brevis Davis* (*Gymnodinium breve Davis*). An algae responsible for large fish kills and mollusk and human food poisoning in the Gulf of Mexico and along the Florida coast. Unlike previously isolated dinoflagellate toxins, such as saxitoxin, which are water-soluble sodium channel blockers, the b. are lipid-soluble sodium channel activators. Used as tools in neurobiological research.

Brewer, George E., U.S. surgeon, 1861–1939. SEE B.'s *infarcts,* under *infarct.*

Bricker, Eugene M., U.S. urologist, *1908. SEE B. *operation.*

bridge (bridj). **1.** The upper part of the ridge of the nose formed by the nasal bones. **2.** One of the threads of protoplasm that appears to pass from one cell to another. **3.** SYN fixed partial *denture.*

arteriolovenular b., the largest capillary connecting arteriole to venule.

cantilever b., a fixed partial b. denture in which the pontic is retained only on one side by an abutment tooth. SYN extension b.

muscles used in breathing	
inspiration muscles	auxiliary muscles (inspiration)
diaphragm	sternocleidomastoid
external intercostal	scalene anterior, middle and posterior
internal intercostal, parasternal part (intercartilaginous)	greater pectoral
	lesser pectoral
	serratus posterior superior
	serratus anterior
expiration muscles	auxiliary muscles (expiration)
internal intercostal	rectus abdominis
transverse thoracic	transverse abdominis
subcostal	obliquus externus abdominis
	obliquus internus abdominis
	erector spinae
	quadratus lumborum
	serratus posterior inferior

cell b.'s, SYN intercellular b.'s.

cystine b., SYN disulfide b.

cytoplasmic b.'s, SYN intercellular b.'s.

dentin b., a deposit of reparative dentin or other calcific substances which forms across and reseals exposed tooth pulp tissue.

disulfide b., (1) a disulfide linkage between two cysteinyl residues in a poly- or oligopeptide or in a protein; (2) any disulfide linkage between any thiol-containing moieties of a larger molecule. SYN cystine b.

extension b., SYN cantilever b.

fixed b., SEE fixed partial *denture.*

Gaskell's b., SYN atrioventricular *bundle.*

intercellular b.'s, slender cytoplasmic strands connecting adjacent cells; in histological sections of the epidermis and other stratified squamous epithelia, the b.'s are processes attached by a desmosome and are shrinkage artifacts of fixation; true b.'s with cytoplasmic confluence exist between incompletely divided germ cells. SYN cell b.'s, cytoplasmic b.'s.

myocardial b., a b. of cardiac muscle fibers extending over the epicardial aspect of a coronary artery; this finding, in cases of sudden unexpected death, has led to speculation that cardiac contraction during exertion could constrict the coronary artery.

removable b., SYN removable partial *denture.*

salt b., SYN electrostatic *bond.*

Wheatstone's b., an apparatus for measuring electrical resistance; four resistors are connected to form the four sides or "arms" of a square; a voltage is applied to one diagonal pair of connections, while the voltage between the other diagonal pair is measured, *e.g.,* by a galvanometer; the bridge is "balanced" when the measured voltage is zero; then, the ratios of the two pairs of adjoining resistances must be identical.

⚠ **Combining forms**	**[NA]** Nomina Anatomica
Word*Finder*	**[MIM]** Mendelian
Multi-term entry finder	**Inheritance in Man**
Preceding letter A	
A.D.A.M. Anatomy Plates	☆ **Official alternate term**
Between letters L and M	
Appendices:	☆**[NA]** Official alternate
Following letter Z	**Nomina Anatomica term**
SYN Synonym; Cf., compare	**High Profile Term**

bridge·work (bridj′wŏrk). SYN partial *denture*.

bri·dle (brī′dl). **1.** SYN frenum. **2.** A band of fibrous material stretching across the surface of an ulcer or other lesion or forming adhesions between opposing serous or mucous surfaces. [M.E. *bridel*]

b. of clitoris, obsolete term for *frenulum* of clitoris.

Bright, Richard, English internist and pathologist, 1789–1858. SEE B.'s *disease*.

Brill, Nathan E., U.S. physician, 1860–1925. SEE B.'s *disease;* B.-Symmers *disease;* B.-Zinsser *disease*.

bril·liant cres·yl blue. SEE cresyl blue.

bril·liant green [C.I. 42040]. The sulfate of di-(*p*-diethylamino)-triphenyl carbinolanhydride. An indicator dye that changes from yellow to green at pH 0.0 to 2.6; also used as a topical antiseptic and as a selective bacteriostatic agent in culture media. SYN ethyl green.

bril·liant vi·tal red. SYN vital red.

bril·liant yel·low [C.I. 13085]. An indicator dye that changes from yellow to orange or red at pH 6.4 to 8.0.

brim. The upper edge or rim of a hollow structure.

pelvic b., SYN superior pelvic *aperture*.

brim·stone (brim′stōn). SYN sulfur. [A.S. *brinnan*, to burn]

brin·dle (brin′dl). A hair coat color in which there is a uniform mixture of gray or tawny hairs with others of white or black; a composite color. [diminutive of O.E. *brinded*]

Brinell, Johan A., Swedish metallurgist, 1849–1925. SEE B. hardness *number*.

Briquet, Paul, French physician, 1796–1881. SEE B.'s *ataxia, syndrome*.

brise·ment for·cé (briz-mon′fōr-sā′). Forcible manipulation, usually under anesthesia, in which the position of a deformed limb is corrected by tearing the soft tissue and crushing the bone, as in a once popular but no longer used correction for club foot deformities. [Fr. forcible breaking]

bris·ket. The part of a beef animal (sometimes used of other species) that constitutes the caudoventral part of the neck and lies cranially to and between the forelimbs of the animal. [O.E. *brusket*]

Brissaud, Edouard, French physician, 1852–1909. SEE B.'s *disease, infantilism, reflex;* B.-Marie *syndrome*.

Brit·ish an·ti-Lew·is·ite (BAL) (brit′ish an-tē-lū′is-īt). SYN dimercaprol.

Brit·ish Phar·ma·co·poe·ia (BP). SEE Pharmacopeia.

broach (brōch). A dental instrument for removing the pulp of a tooth or exploring the canal.

barbed b., a root canal instrument set with barbs; used for removing a dental pulp, pulp tissue remnants, or dentinal debris.

smooth b., an exploring instrument used in endodontic practice; a root canal tine.

Broadbent, Sir William H., British physician, 1835–1907. SEE B.'s *law, sign;* Bolton-B. *plane*.

broad-spec·trum. SEE spectrum.

Broca, Pierre P., French surgeon, neurologist, and anthropologist, 1824–1880. SEE B.'s *angles,* under *angle, aphasia,* basilar *angle,* facial *angle, area,* parolfactory *area,* diagonal *band, center, field, fissure, formula,* visual *plane, pouch*.

Brock, Sir Russell C., British surgeon, *1903. SEE B.'s *syndrome;* B. *operation*.

Brockenbrough, E.C., U.S. surgeon, *1930. SEE B. *sign*.

Brocq, Louis A.J., French dermatologist, 1856–1928. SEE B.'s *disease*.

bro·cre·sine (brō-krē′sēn). α-(Aminooxy)-6-bromo-*m*-cresol; a histidine decarboxylase inhibitor.

Brödel, Max, German medical artist in the U.S., 1870–1941. SEE B.'s bloodless *line*.

Brodie, Sir Benjamin C., British surgeon, 1783–1862. SEE B.'s *abscess, bursa, disease, knee*.

Brodie, Charles Gordon, Scottish anatomist and surgeon, 1860–1933. SEE B.'s *ligament*.

Brodie, Thomas Gregor, British physiologist, 1866–1916. SEE B. *fluid*.

Brodmann, Korbinian, German neurologist, 1868–1918. SEE B.'s *areas,* under *area*.

Broesike, Gustav, German anatomist, *1853. SEE B.'s *fossa*.

brom-, bromo-. Prefixes that most commonly indicate the presence of bromine in a compound. [G. *brōmos,* a stench]

bro·mate (brō′māt). Salt or anion of bromic acid.

bro·mat·ed (brō′māt-ĕd). Combined or saturated with bromine or any of its compounds. SYN brominated.

bro·ma·ze·pam (brō-mā′zĕ-pam). 7-Bromo-1,3-dihydro-5-(2-pyridinyl)-2*H*-1,4-benzodiazepin-2-one; an antianxiety agent.

bro·ma·zine hy·dro·chlo·ride (brō′mă-zēn). SYN bromodiphenhydramine hydrochloride.

brom·cre·sol green (brom-krē′sol). A substituted triphenylmethane dye (MW 698.021 g/mol, pK$_a$ 4.7), sparingly soluble in water but readily soluble in alcohol, diethyl ether, and ethyl acetate; used as an indicator of pH (yellow at pH 3.8, blue-green at pH 5.4).

brom·cre·sol pur·ple. A substituted triphenylmethane dye (MW 540.229 g/mol, pK$_a$ 6.3), practically insoluble in water but soluble in alcohol and dilute alkalies; used as an indicator of pH (yellow at pH 5.2, purple at pH 6.8).

bro·me·lain, bro·me·lin (brō′mĕ-lān, -lin). One of a group of peptide hydrolases, all thiol proteinases, obtained from pineapple stem; used in tenderizing meats and in producing hydrolysates of proteins; orally administered in the treatment of inflammation and edema of soft tissues associated with traumatic injury.

Bromelius, C., Swedish botanist, 1639–1705. SEE bromelain.

brom·hex·ine hy·dro·chlo·ride (brom-hek′sēn). 3,5-Dibromo-*N*^{α}-cyclohexyl-*N*^{α}-methyltoluene-α,2-diamine hydrochloride; an expectorant with mucolytic, antitussive, and bronchodilator properties.

brom·hi·dro·sis (brom-hi-drō′sis). SYN bromidrosis.

bro·mic (brō′mik). Relating to bromine; denoting especially bromic acid, HBrO$_3$.

bro·mide (brō′mīd). The anion Br$^-$; salt of hydrogen bromide (HBr); several salts formerly used as sedatives, hypnotics, and anticonvulsants.

bro·mi·dro·si·pho·bia (brō′mi-drō-si-fō′bē-ă). Morbid fear of giving forth a bad odor from the body, sometimes with the belief that such an odor is present. [bromidrosis + G. *phobos,* fear]

bro·mi·dro·sis (brōm-i-drō′sis). Fetid or foul smelling perspiration. SYN bromhidrosis, osmidrosis, ozochrotia. [G. *brōmos,* a stench, + *hidrōs,* perspiration]

bro·min·at·ed (brō′min-āt-ĕd). SYN bromated.

bro·min·di·one (brō-min-dī′ōn). 2-(*p*-Bromophenyl)-1,3-indandione; an oral anticoagulant.

bro·mine (Br) (brō′mēn, -min). A nonmetallic, reddish, volatile, liquid element; atomic no. 35, atomic wt. 79.904; valences 1 to 7, inclusive; it unites with hydrogen to form hydrobromic acid, and this reacts with many metals to form bromides, some of which are used in medicine. SYN bromum. [Fr. *brome,* bromine, fr. G. *bromos,* stench]

bro·mism, bro·min·ism (brō′mizm, -min-izm). Chronic bromide intoxication, characterized by headache, drowsiness, confusion and occasionally violent delirium, muscular weakness, cardiac depression, an acneform eruption, foul breath, anorexia, and gastric distress.

bromo-. SEE brom-.

bro·mo·ben·zyl·cy·an·ide (BBC) (brō′mō-benz-il-sī′a-nīd). A lacrimator used in tear gases in training and in riot control.

bro·mo·cre·sol green (brō-mō-krē′sol). Tetrabromo-m-cresol-sulfonphthalein; an indicator dye changing from yellow to blue at pH 4.7; used to track DNA in agarose electrophoresis, and in a dye-binding method for analysis of serum albumin.

bro·mo·crip·tine (brō-mō-krip′tēn). 2-Bromo-α-ergocryptine; an ergot derivative which slows dopamine turnover, inhibits prolactin secretion and release of prolactin by thyrotropin-releasing hormone, and retards tumor growth and hence is used in the treatment of hyperprolactinemia associated with various pituitary tumors; an agonist at dopamine receptors also used in Parkinson's disease.

bro·mo·de·ox·y·ur·i·dine (BrDu) (brō'mō-dē-ok'sē-yūr'i-dēn). A compound that competes with uridine for incorporation in RNA and fluoresces in ultraviolet light; used in BrDu-banding.

bro·mo·der·ma (brō-mō-der'mă). An acneform or granulomatous eruption due to hypersensitivity to bromide. [bromide + G. *derma,* skin]

bro·mo·di·phen·hy·dra·mine hy·dro·chlo·ride (brō'mō-dīfen-hī'dră-mēn). 2-(*p*-bromo-α-phenylbenzyloxy)-*N,N*-dimethylethylamine hydrochloride; an antihistamine that may cause drowsiness and xerostomia. SYN bromazine hydrochloride.

bro·mo·hy·per·hi·dro·sis, bro·mo·hy·per·i·dro·sis (brō'mō-hī'per-hi-drō'sis, -hī'per-i-drō'sis). Excessive secretion of sweat having a fetid odor. [G. *brōmos,* a stench, + *hyper,* over, + *hidrōsis,* sweating]

bro·mo·phe·nol blue (brō-mō-fē'nol). SYN bromphenol blue.

bro·mo·sul·fo·phtha·lein (brō'mō-sŭl'fō-thal'ē-in). SYN sulfobromophthalein sodium.

5-bro·mo·u·ra·cil (brō-mō-yū'ră-sil). Synthetic analogue (antimetabolite) of thymine, in which a bromine atom takes the place of the methyl group in thymine; a mutagen.

brom·phen·ir·a·mine ma·le·ate (brōm-fen-ir'ă-mēn). 2-[*p*-Bromo-α-(2-dimethylaminoethyl)benzyl]pyridine maleate; a potent antihistaminic agent.

brom·phe·nol blue (brom-fē-nol). A substituted triphenylmethane dye (MW 670, pK 4.0), used as an acid-base indicator (yellow at pH less than 3.1, blue at pH more than 4.7); also used for histochemical and electrophoretic demonstration of proteins. SYN bromophenol blue.

brom·sul·fo·phtha·lein (brom-sŭl'fō-thal'ē-in). SYN sulfobromophthalein sodium.

brom·thy·mol blue (brom-thī'mol). A substituted triphenylmethane dye (MW 624, pK 7.0), used primarily as a hydrogen ion indicator (yellow at pH 6.0, blue at pH 7.6); also a weak but toxic vital stain.

bro·mum (brō'mŭm). SYN bromine.

bron·ca·tar (bron'kă-tar). Camphoric acid compound (neutralized) with 2-amino-2-thiazoline (1:2); an antitussive and respiratory stimulant.

△**bronch-.** SEE broncho-.

bron·chi (brong'kī). Plural of bronchus.

△**bronchi-.** SEE broncho-.

bron·chia (brong'kē-ă). The smaller divisions of the bronchi. SEE ALSO bronchus, bronchiole. SYN bronchial tubes. [G. pl. of *bronchion,* dim. of *bronchos,* trachea]

bron·chi·al (brong'kē-ăl). Relating to the bronchi.

bron·chi·ec·ta·sia (brong'kē-ek-tā'zē-ă). SYN bronchiectasis.

b. sicca, SYN dry *bronchiectasis.*

bron·chi·ec·ta·sis (brong-kē-ek'tă-sis). Chronic dilation of bronchi or bronchioles as a sequel of inflammatory disease or obstruction. SYN bronchiectasia. [bronchi- + G. *ektasis,* a stretching]

congenital b., a rare form of b. due to developmental arrest in the tracheobronchial tree; may be unilateral or bilateral.

cylindrical b., b. resulting in dilated bronchi of cylindrical shape; *i.e.,* of uniform caliber.

cystic b., b. in which the bronchi end in blind sacs greater in diameter than the draining bronchi. SEE ALSO saccular b.

dry b., b. characterized by lack of productive cough and by occasional hemoptysis. SYN bronchiectasia sicca.

saccular b., b. resulting in dilated bronchi of saccular or irregular shape. SEE ALSO cystic b.

bron·chi·ec·tat·ic (brong-kē-ek-tat'ik). Relating to bronchiectasis.

bron·chil·o·quy (brong-kil'ō-kwē). Rarely used term for bronchophony [bronchi- + L. *loquor,* to speak]

bron·chi·o·gen·ic (brong-kē-ō-jen'ik). SYN bronchogenic.

bron·chi·ole (brong'kē-ōl). One of approximately six generations of increasingly finer subdivisions of the bronchi, all less than 1 mm in diameter, and having no cartilage in its wall, but

relatively abundant smooth muscle and elastic fibers. SYN bronchiolus [NA].

respiratory b.'s, the smallest bronchioles (0.5 mm in diameter) that connect the terminal bronchioles to alveolar ducts; alveoli rise from part of the wall. SYN bronchioli respiratorii [NA].

terminal b., the end of the nonrespiratory conducting airway; the lining is simple columnar or cuboidal epithelium without mucous goblet cells; most of the cells are ciliated, but a few nonciliated serous secreting cells occur. SYN bronchiolus terminalis.

bron·chi·o·lec·ta·sia (brong'kē-ō-lek-tā'zē-ă). SYN bronchiolectasis.

bron·chi·o·lec·ta·sis (brong'kē-ō-lek'tă-sis). Bronchiectasis involving the bronchioles. SYN bronchiolectasia. [bronchiole + G. *ektasis,* a stretching]

bron·chi·o·li (brong-kē'ō-lī). Plural of bronchiolus.

bron·chi·ol·i·tis (brong-kē-ō-lī'tis). Inflammation of the bronchioles, often associated with bronchopneumonia. [bronchiole + *-itis,* inflammation]

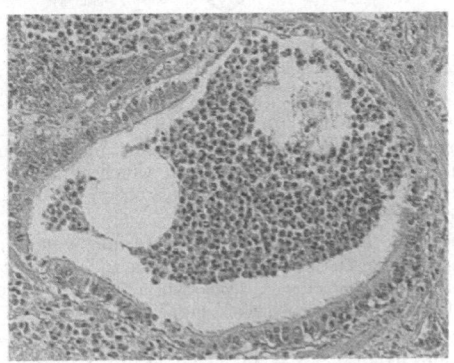

bronchiolitis
thick mass of granulocytes in a bronchiolar lumen

constrictive b., obliteration of bronchioles by scarring following b. obliterans. Cf. proliferative b.

exudative b., inflammation of the bronchioles, with fibrinous exudation.

b. fibro·sa oblit·erans, obstruction of bronchioles and alveolar ducts by fibrous granulation tissue induced by mucosal ulceration; the condition may follow inhalation of irritant gases (see silo-filler's *lung*) or may complicate pneumonia (see BOOP); associated with obstructive findings (see unilateral hyperlucent *lung,* Swyer-James *syndrome*). SYN b. obliterans.

b. oblit·erans, SYN b. fibrosa obliterans.

b. obliterans with organizing pneumonia (BOOP), b. fibrosa obliterans complicated by pneumonia with organization.

proliferative b., b. with obliteration of bronchiolar lumen and alveoli by epithelial proliferation, which may follow influenza and giant-cell pneumonia.

△**bronchiolo-.** Bronchiole. [L. *bronchiolus*]

bron·chi·o·lo·pul·mo·nary (brong'kē-ō-lō-pul'mō-nār-ē). Relating to the bronchioles and the lungs.

bron·chi·o·lus, pl. **bron·chi·o·li** (brong-kē'ō-lŭs, -ō-lī) [NA]. SYN bronchiole. [Mod. L. dim. of *bronchus*]

bronchi·oli respirato·rii [NA], SYN respiratory *bronchioles,* under *bronchiole.*

b. termina·lis, SYN terminal *bronchiole.*

bron·chi·o·ste·no·sis (brong'kē-ō-sten-ō'sis). Narrowing of the lumen of a bronchial tube.

bron·chit·ic (brong-kit'ik). Relating to bronchitis.

bron·chi·tis (brong-kī'tis). Inflammation of the mucous membrane of the bronchial tubes.

asthmatic b., b. that causes or aggravates bronchospasm.

Castellani's b., SYN hemorrhagic b.

chronic b., a condition of the bronchial tree characterized by

br

cough, hypersecretion of mucus, and expectoration of sputum over a long period of time, associated with frequent bronchial infection; usually due to inhalation, over a prolonged period, of air contaminated by dust or by noxious gases of combustion.

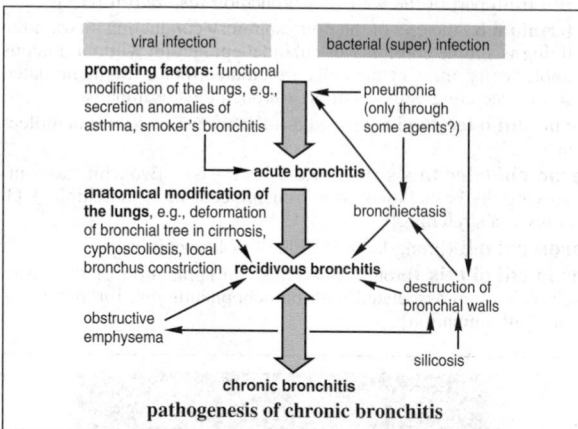

pathogenesis of chronic bronchitis

croupous b., obsolete term for fibrinous b.

fibrinous b., inflammation of the bronchial mucous membrane, accompanied by a fibrinous exudation, which often forms a cast of the bronchial tree with severe obstruction of air flow. SYN plastic b., pseudomembranous b.

hemorrhagic b., chronic b. due to infection with spirochetes (though other bacteria are usually present and contribute to the infection) and characterized by cough and bloody sputum. SYN bronchopulmonary spirochetosis, bronchospirochetosis, Castellani's b.

infectious avian b., a specific infectious disease of young birds, caused by infectious bronchitis virus, a member of Coronaviridae, and associated with blocking of respiratory passages by exudate; it is highly transmissible, and often causes heavy losses of young chicks and heavy production losses among older laying birds. SYN gasping disease.

obliterative b., b. oblit′erans, fibrinous b. in which the exudate is not expectorated but becomes organized, obliterating the affected portion of the bronchial tubes with consequent permanent collapse of affected portions of the lung.

plastic b., SYN fibrinous b.

pseudomembranous b., SYN fibrinous b.

putrid b., b. accompanied by an expectoration of foul-smelling sputum.

verminous b., b. and bronchopneumonia caused by invasion of the bronchi by lungworms; occurs commonly in cattle, swine, and sheep, but rarely in other species. SYN hoose, husk.

bron·chi·um (brong′kē-ŭm). SYN bronchus. [Mod. L. fr. G. *bronchion*]

♲**broncho-, bronch-, bronchi-.** Bronchus, and, in ancient usage, the trachea. [G. *bronchos,* windpipe]

bron·cho·al·ve·o·lar (brong′kō-al-vē′ō-lăr). SYN bronchovesicular.

bron·cho·cav·ern·ous (brong-kō-kav′er-nŭs). Relating to a bronchus or bronchial tube and a pulmonary pathologic cavity.

bron·cho·cele (brong′kō-sēl). A circumscribed dilation of a bronchus. [broncho- + G. *kēlē,* hernia]

bron·cho·con·stric·tion (brong-kō-kon-strik′shŭn). Reduction in the caliber of a bronchus or bronchi.

bron·cho·con·stric·tor (brong-kō-kon-strik′ter, -tōr). **1.** Causing a reduction in caliber of a bronchus or bronchial tube. **2.** An agent that possesses this action (*e.g.,* histamine).

bron·cho·di·la·ta·tion (brong′kō-dil-ă-tā′shŭn). Increase in caliber of the bronchi and bronchioles in response to pharmacologically active substances or autonomic nervous activity.

bron·cho·di·la·tion (brong′kō-dī-lā′shŭn). **1.** Alternative spelling for bronchodilatation. **2.** Rarely used term for bronchiectasis.

bron·cho·di·la·tor (brong-kō-dī-lā′ter, -tōr). **1.** Causing an increase in caliber of a bronchus or bronchial tube. **2.** An agent that possesses this power (*e.g.,* epinephrine).

bron·cho·e·de·ma (brong′kō-ĕ-dē′mă). Swelling of the mucosa of the bronchi.

bron·cho·e·soph·a·gol·o·gy (brong′kō-ē-sof-ă-gol′ō-jē). The specialty concerned with the diagnosis and treatment of diseases of the tracheobronchial tree and esophagus by endoscope and other means. [broncho- + G. *oisophagos,* esophagus, + *logos,* study]

bron·cho·e·soph·a·gos·co·py (brong′kō-ē-sof-ă-gos′kŏ-pē). Examination of the tracheobronchial tree or esophagus through appropriate endoscopes.

bron·cho·fi·ber·scope (brong-kō-fī′ber-skōp). A fiberoptic endoscope particularly adapted for visualization of the trachea and bronchi.

bron·cho·gen·ic (brong-kō-jen′ik). Of bronchial origin; emanating from the bronchi. SYN bronchiogenic.

bron·cho·gram (brong′kō-gram). A radiograph obtained by bronchography; radiographic visualization of a bronchus. [broncho- + G. *gramma,* a writing]

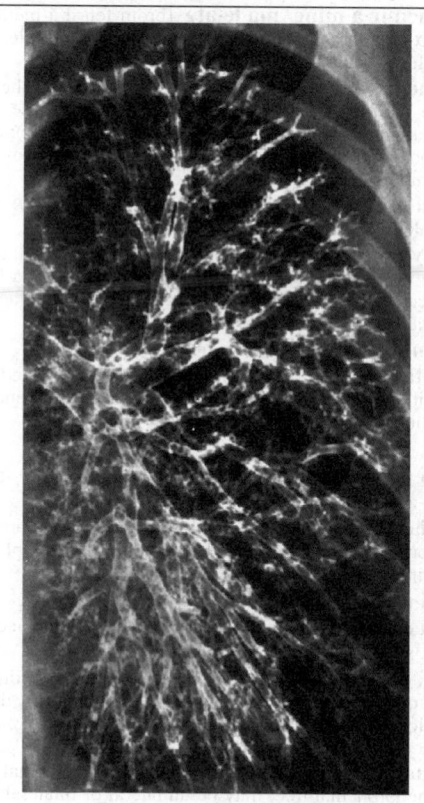

bronchogram (left lung)

air b., radiographic appearance of an air-filled bronchus surrounded by fluid-filled airspaces.

bron·chog·ra·phy (brong-kog′ră-fē). Radiographic examination of the tracheobronchial tree following introduction of a radiopaque material, usually an iodinated compound in a viscous suspension; rarely performed at this time, having been superseded by high resolution computed tomography. [broncho- + G. *graphē,* a drawing]

tantalum b., historically, b. using insufflated metallic tantalum powder.

bron·cho·lith (brong′kō-lith). A hard concretion in a bronchus or bronchial tube. SYN bronchial calculus. [broncho- + G. *lithos,* stone]

bron·cho·li·thi·a·sis (brong′kō-li-thī′ă-sis). Bronchial inflammation or obstruction caused by broncholiths.

bron·cho·ma·la·cia (brong′kō-mă-lā′shē-ă). Degeneration of elastic and connective tissue of bronchi and trachea. [broncho- + G. *malakia*, a softening]

bron·cho·mo·tor (brong-kō-mō′ter). **1.** Relating to a change in caliber, dilation, or contraction of a bronchus or bronchiole. **2.** An agent possessing this action. [broncho- + L. *motor*, mover]

bron·cho·my·co·sis (brong′kō-mī-kō′sis). Any fungus disease of the bronchial tubes or bronchi. [broncho- + G. *mykēs*, fungus]

bron·choph·o·ny (brong-kof′ō-nē). Increased intensity and clarity of voice sounds heard over a bronchus surrounded by consolidated lung tissue. SEE ALSO tracheophony. SYN bronchial voice. [broncho- + G. *phōnē*, voice]

whispered b., SYN whispered *pectoriloquy*.

bron·cho·plas·ty (brong′kō-plas-tē). Surgical alteration of the configuration of a bronchus. [broncho- + G. *plastos*, formed]

bron·cho·pneu·mo·nia (brong′ko-nu-mo′nĭ-ah). Acute inflammation of the walls of the smaller bronchial tubes, with varying amounts of pulmonary consolidation due to spread of the inflammation into peribronchiolar alveoli and the alveolar ducts; may become confluent or may be hemorrhagic. SYN bronchial pneumonia.

postoperative b., patchy pneumonia developing in a postoperative patient, usually following surgery to upper abdomen, with restricted diaphragmatic movement due to pain on inspiration, resulting in hypoventilation of the dependent portions of the lungs, with corresponding inadequate movement of secretions, allowing development of infection; likelihood minimized by early postoperative mobilization, deep breathing exercises.

tuberculous b., an acute form of pulmonary tuberculosis characterized by widespread patchy consolidations.

bron·cho·pul·mo·nary (brong-kō-pul′mō-nār-ē). Relating to the bronchi tubes and the lungs.

bron·chor·rha·phy (brong-kōr′ă-fē). Suture of a wound of the bronchus. [broncho- + G. *rhaphē*, a seam]

bron·chor·rhea (brong′kō-rē′ă). Excessive secretion of mucus from the bronchial mucous membrane. [broncho- + G. *rhoia*, a flow]

bron·cho·scope (brong′kō-skōp). An endoscope for inspecting the interior of the tracheobronchial tree, either for diagnostic purposes (including biopsy) or for the removal of foreign bodies. There are two types: flexible and rigid. [broncho- + G. *skopeō*, to view]

bron·chos·co·py (brong-kos′kŏ-pē). Inspection of the interior of the tracheobronchial tree through a bronchoscope.

bron·cho·spasm (brong′kō-spazm). Contraction of smooth muscle in the walls of the bronchi and bronchioles, causing narrowing of the lumen.

bron·cho·spas·mo·lyt·ic (brong′kō-spazm-mō-li-tik). Relieving a bronchospasm.

bron·cho·spi·ro·che·to·sis (brong′kō-spī′rō-kē-tō′sis). SYN hemorrhagic *bronchitis*.

bron·cho·spi·rog·ra·phy (brong′kō-spī-rog′ră-fē). Use of a single lumen endobronchial tube for measurement of ventilatory function of one lung. [broncho- + L. *spiro*, to breathe, + G. *graphō*, to write]

bron·cho·spi·rom·e·ter (brong′kō-spī-rom′ĕ-ter). A device for measurement of rates and volumes of air flow into each lung separately, using a double lumen endobronchial tube. [broncho- + L. *spiro*, to breathe, + G. *metron*, measure]

bron·cho·spi·rom·e·try (brong′kō-spī-rom′ĕ-trē). Use of a bronchospirometer to measure ventilatory function of each lung separately.

bron·cho·stax·is (brong′kō-stak′sis). Hemorrhage from the bronchi. [broncho- + G. *staxis*, a dripping]

bron·cho·ste·no·sis (brong-kō-sten-ō′sis). Chronic narrowing of a bronchus.

bron·chos·to·my (brong-kos′tō-mē). Surgical formation of a new opening into a bronchus. [broncho- + G. *stoma*, mouth]

bron·chot·o·my (brong-kot′ō-mē). Incision of a bronchus.

bron·cho·tra·che·al (brong-kō-trā′kē-ăl). Relating to the trachea and bronchi.

bron·cho·ve·sic·u·lar (brong′kō-vĕ-sik′yū-lăr). Relating to the bronchioles and alveoli in the lungs. SYN bronchoalveolar.

bron·chus, pl. **bron·chi** (brong′kŭs, brong′kī) [NA]. One of the two subdivisions of the trachea serving to convey air to and from the lungs. The trachea divides into right and left main bronchi, which in turn form lobar, segmental, and subsegmental bronchi. In structure, the intrapulmonary bronchi have a lining of pseudostratified ciliated columnar epithelium, and a lamina propria with abundant longitudinal networks of elastic fibers; there are spirally arranged bundles of smooth muscle, abundant mucoserous glands, and, in the outer part of the wall, irregular plates of hyaline cartilage. SYN bronchium. [Mod. L., fr. G. *bronchos*, windpipe]

eparterial b., right superior lobe b. which passes above the right pulmonary artery.

hyparterial bronchi, those bronchi which pass below the pulmonary arteries, *i.e.*, right middle and inferior lobar bronchi and left superior and inferior lobar bronchi.

intermediate b., b. intermedius, the portion of the right main b. between the upper lobe b. and the origin of the middle and inferior lobe bronchi. SYN b. intermedius.

left main b., it arises at the bifurcation of the trachea, passes in front of the esophagus and enters the hilum of the left lung where it divides into a superior lobe b. and an inferior lobe b. It is longer, of narrower caliber, and more nearly-horizontal than the right main b., hence, aspirated objects enter it less frequently. SYN b. principalis sinister [NA].

lobar bronchi, the divisions of the main bronchi that supply the lobes of the lungs; superior lobar b., b. lobaris superior [NA]; middle lobar b., b. lobaris medius [NA]; and inferior lobar b., b. lobaris inferior [NA] are the three lobar bronchi on the right; superior lobar b., b. lobaris superior [NA], and inferior lobar b., b. lobaris inferior [NA] are the two on the left. The lobar bronchi divide into segmental bronchi. SYN bronchi lobares [NA].

bronchi loba′res [NA], SYN lobar bronchi.

mucoid impaction of b., plugging of the lumen of bronchi due to thickened mucus, interfering with ventilation of corresponding lung segments and leading to characteristic clustered linear and grape-like radiologic densities and occasionally atelectasis and pneumonia; characteristically seen in cystic fibrosis but it can occur in a variety of disease states.

primary b., the main b. arising at the tracheal bifurcation and extending into the developing lung of the embryo.

b. principa′lis dex′ter [NA], SYN right main b.

b. principa′lis sinis′ter [NA], SYN left main b.

right main b., it arises at the bifurcation of the trachea and enters the hilum of the right lung, giving off the superior lobe b. and continuing downward to give off the middle and inferior lobe bronchi. It is shorter, of greater caliber, and more nearly-vertical than the left main b., thus, aspirated objects more frequently lodge on the right side. SYN b. principalis dexter [NA].

segmental b., one of the divisions of the lobar b. that supplies a bronchopulmonary segment. In the right lung there are commonly ten: *in the superior lobe,* the apical (B_1) segmental b., b. segmentalis apicalis [NA]; posterior (B_2) segmental b., b. segmentalis (BII) posterior [NA]; and anterior (B_3) segmental b., b. segmentalis (BIII) anterior [NA]; *in the middle lobe,* lateral (B_4) segmental b., b. segmentalis (BIV) lateralis [NA]; and medial (B_5) segmental b., b. segmentalis medialis (BV) [NA]; *in the inferior lobe,* superior (B_6) segmental b., b. segmentalis superior (BVI) [NA], medial basal (B_7) segmental b., b. segmentalis basalis medialis (BVII) [NA]; anterior basal (B_8) segmental b., b. segmentalis basalis anterior (BVIII) [NA]; lateral basal (B_9) segmental b., b. segmentalis basalis lateralis (BIX) [NA]; and posterior basal (B_{10}) segmental b., b. segmentalis basalis posterior (BX) [NA]. In the left lung there are commonly nine: *in the superior lobe,* the apicoposterior (B_{1+2}) segmental b., b. segmentalis apicoposterior (BI+I) [NA]; anterior (B_3) segmental b., b. segmentalis anterior (BIII) [NA]; superior lingular (B_4) segmental b., b. lingularis superior (BIV) [NA]; and inferior lingular (B_5) segmental b., b. lingularis inferior (BV) [NA]; *in the inferior lobe,* superior (B_6) segmental b., b. segmentalis superior

(BVI) [NA]; medial basal (B$_7$) segmental b., b. segmentalis basalis medialis (cardiacus) (BVII) [NA], anterior basal (B$_8$) segmental b., b. segmentalis basalis anterior (BVIII) [NA]; lateral basal (B$_9$) segmental b., b. segmentalis basalis lateralis (BIX) [NA]; and posterior basal (B$_{10}$) segmental b., b. segmentalis basalis posterior (BX) [NA]. SYN b. segmentalis [NA].

b. segmenta′lis [NA], SYN b. segmental b.

stem b., the main b. from which the branches of the bronchial tree arise.

Brǿnsted, Johannes N., Danish physical chemist, 1879–1947. SEE B. *acid, base, theory.*

bron·to·pho·bia (bront-ō-fō′bē-ǎ). Morbid fear of thunder. SYN tonitrophobia. [G. *brontē,* thunder, + *phobos,* fear]

brood (brūd). **1.** SYN litter (2). **2.** To ponder anxiously; to meditate morbidly.

Brooke, Bryan N., British surgeon, *1915. SEE B. *ileostomy.*

Brooke, Henry A.G., English dermatologist, 1854–1919. SEE B.'s *disease, tumor.*

bro·tiz·o·lam (brō′tiz-ō-lam). A triazolo-benzodiazepine derivative with a sulfur and bromine atom in the molecule. Used as a sedative and hypnotic.

brow. 1. The eyebrow. SEE eyebrow. **2.** SYN forehead. [A.S. *brū*]

brow·lift. Operation to elevate the eyebrows.

Brown, Harold W., U.S. ophthalmologist, *1898. SEE B.'s *syndrome.*

Brown, James, U.S. plastic surgeon, 1899–1971. SEE Blair-B. *graft;* B.-Adson *forceps.*

Brown, James H., U.S. microbiologist, *1884. SEE B.-Brenn *stain.*

Brown, Robert, English botanist, 1773–1858. SEE brownian *motion;* brownian *movement;* brownian-Zsigmondy *movement.*

Browne, Sir Denis John, British surgeon, *1892. SEE Denis B.'s *pouch;* Denis B. *splint.*

brown·i·an (brown′ē-ǎn). Relating to or described by Robert Brown.

Browning, William, U.S. anatomist and neurologist, 1855–1941. SEE B.'s *vein.*

Brown-Séquard, Charles E., French physiologist and neurologist, 1817–1894. SEE Brown-Séquard's *paralysis;* Brown-Séquard's *syndrome.*

Bruce, Sir David, British surgeon, 1855–1931. SEE *Brucella;* brucellosis.

Bru·cel′la (brū-sel′lǎ). A genus of encapsulated, nonmotile bacteria (family Brucellaceae) containing short, rod-shaped to coccoid, Gram-negative cells. These organisms do not produce gas from carbohydrates, are parasitic, invading all animal tissues and causing infection of the genital organs, the mammary gland, and the respiratory and intestinal tracts, and are pathogenic for man and various species of domestic animals. The type species is *B. melitensis.*

B. abor′tus, a species that causes abortion in cows (bovine brucellosis), mares, and sheep, undulant fever in man, and a wasting disease in chickens. SYN abortus bacillus, Bang's bacillus.

B. ca′nis, a species causing epididymitis, brucellosis, and abortion in dogs; occasionally causes mild human disease.

B. meliten′sis, a species that causes brucellosis in man, abortion in goats, and a wasting disease in chickens; it may infect cows and hogs and be excreted in their milk; it is the type species of the genus *B.*

B. su′is, a species causing abortion in swine, brucellosis in man, and a wasting disease in chickens; may also infect horses, dogs, cows, monkeys, goats, and laboratory animals.

Bru·cel·la·ce·ae (brū-sel-lā′sē-ē). A family of bacteria (order Eubacteriales) containing small, coccoid to rod-shaped, Gram-negative cells which occur singly, in pairs, in short chains, or in groups. The cells may or may not show bipolar staining. Motile and nonmotile species occur; motile cells are peritrichous. V (phosphopyridine nucleotide) and/or X (hemin) factors are sometimes required for growth. Blood serum may be required or may enhance growth. Increased carbon dioxide tension may also favor growth, especially on primary isolation. These organisms

are parasites and pathogens which affect warm-blooded animals, including man, rarely cold-blooded animals. It was formerly called Parvobacteriaceae. The type genus is *Brucella.*

bru·cel·ler·gin (brū-sel′er-jin). A fat-free nucleoprotein antigen derived from brucella; used in skin tests for brucellosis.

bru·cel·lin (brū-sel′in). A vaccine prepared from several species of *Brucella;* formerly thought to prevent or cure brucellosis.

bru·cel·lo·sis (brū-sel-ō′sis). An infectious disease caused by *Brucella,* characterized by fever, sweating, weakness, aches, and pains, and transmitted to man by direct contact with diseased animals or through ingestion of infected meat, milk, or cheese, and particularly hazardous to veterinarians, farmers, and slaughterhouse workers; although some crossing over by species may occur, *Brucella melitensis, B. abortus, B. canis,* and *B. suis* characteristically affect goats, cattle, dogs, and swine, respectively. SYN febris undulans, Malta fever, Mediterranean fever (1), undulant fever, undulating fever.

bovine b., a disease in cattle caused by *Brucella abortus;* in pregnant cows, characterized by abortion late in pregnancy, followed by retained placenta and metritis; in bulls, orchitis and epididymitis may occur; the organism may localize in the udder and thus appear in milk from infected cows. SYN Bang's disease.

Bruch, Carl W.L., German anatomist, 1819–1884. SEE B.'s *glands,* under gland, *membrane.*

bru·cine (brū-sēn, -in). 10,11-Dimethoxystrychnine; an alkaloid from *Strychnos nux-vomica* and *S. ignatii* (family Loganiaceae), that produces paralysis of sensory nerves and peripheral motor nerves; the convulsive action which is characteristic of strychnine is almost entirely absent; formerly used as a local anodyne and tonic. [fr. *Brucea* sp., a shrub, after James Bruce, Scottish explorer, †1794]

Bruck, Alfred, German physician, *1865. SEE B.'s *disease.*

Brücke, Ernst W. von, Austrian physiologist, 1819–1892. SEE B.'s *muscle, tunic;* B.-Bartley *phenomenon.*

Brudzinski, Josef von, Polish physician, 1874–1917. SEE B.'s *sign.*

Bru·gi·a (brū′jē-ǎ). A genus of filarial worms transmitted by mosquitoes to man, primates, felid carnivores, and a number of other mammals.

B. mala′yi, the Malayan filaria species, an important agent of human filariasis and elephantiasis in Southeast Asia and Indonesia, transmitted to man by species of *Mansonia* and *Anopheles* mosquitoes; adult parasites cause lymphangitis and lymphadenitis, but there is less involvement of the genital region and lower extremities, and a relatively greater incidence of disease in the upper extremities than with *Wuchereria bancrofti* infection. Formerly called *Wuchereria malayi.*

Brugsch's syn·drome. See under syndrome.

bruise (brūz). An injury producing a hematoma or diffuse extravasation of blood without rupture of the skin. [M.E. *bruisen,* fr. O.Fr., fr. Germanic]

bruisse·ment (brwēs-mawhn′). A purring auscultatory sound. [Fr.]

bru·it (brū-ē′). A harsh or musical intermittent auscultatory sound, especially an abnormal one. [Fr.]

aneurysmal b., blowing murmur heard over an aneurysm.

carotid b., a systolic murmur heard in the neck but not at the aortic area; any b. produced by blood flow in a carotid artery.

b. de canon, the loud first heart sound heard intermittently in complete atrioventricular block and in interference-dissociation when the ventricles happen to contract shortly after the atria. SYN cannon sound.

b. de claquement (brū-ē′ dě klak-maw′), the sound of cardiac clicks. SEE click.

b. de cuir neuf (brū-ē′ dě kwēr nuf), the sound of new leather (also bruit de craquement); a creaking pericardial friction sound heard mainly in chronic pericarditis.

b. de diable, SYN venous *hum.* [Fr. humming-top]

b. de frolement (brū-ē′ dě frōl′maw′), a rough, rustling sound made by a pleural or pericardial friction rub. [Fr. rustling]

b. de galop, SYN gallop. [Fr.]

b. de la roue de moulin, gurgling or splashing mill-wheel sounds heard when both fluid and air are present in the pericardial sac. [Fr. mill]

b. de lime, introduced by R. Laënnec to describe a rough rasping murmur. [Fr. file]

b. de rappel, applied by J. B. Bouillaud to describe the cadence of a split-second heart sound, or of the second sound followed by an opening snap or early third heart sound. SYN double-shock sound. [Fr. drum-beat]

b. de Roger, SYN Roger's *murmur.*

b. de scie (brū-ē' dĕ sē), a harsh heart murmur heard in systole and diastole that produces a sound resembling that of a saw. [Fr. *saw*]

b. de scie ou de rape, introduced by R. Laënnec to describe harsh, rasping murmurs. [Fr. saw, rasp]

b. de soufflet, introduced by R. Laënnec to describe a blowing murmur. [Fr. bellows]

b. de tabourka, a loud tambour-like or bell-like second heart sound heard at the aortic area in syphilitic aortitis. [Fr. tambour]

b. de tambour (brū-ē' dĕ tăm-bur'), reverberating, musical tone heard as the second heart sound over the aortic area, associated with syphilitic aortic valvular disease. SYN tambour sound. [Fr. sound of drum]

b. de triolet, introduced by L. Gallavardin to describe the triple cadence produced by a systolic click added to the first and second heart sounds. [Fr. a little trio]

Roger's b. (brū-ē'), SYN Roger's *murmur.*

systolic b., any abnormal sound or any murmur heard during systole.

thyroid b., vascular murmur heard over hyperactive thyroid gland, due to increased blood flow.

Traube's b., SYN gallop.

Brumpt, Emile, French parasitologist, 1877–1951. SEE B.'s white *mycetoma.*

Brunn, Albert von, German anatomist, 1849–1895. SEE B.'s *membrane, nests,* under *nest.*

Brunn, Fritz, 20th century Czechoslovakian physician. SEE B. *reaction.*

Brunner, Johann C., Swiss anatomist, 1653–1727. SEE B.'s *glands,* under *gland.*

brun·ner·o·ma (brŭn-er-ō'mă). An adenoma of Brunner's glands; a rare solitary tumor.

brun·ner·o·sis (brŭn-er-ō'sis). Benign nodular hyperplasia of Brunner's glands.

Bruns, Ludwig von, German neurologist, 1858–1916. SEE B. *ataxia;* B.'s *nystagmus.*

Brunschwig, Alexander, U.S. surgeon, 1901–1969. SEE B.'s *operation.*

brush (brŭsh). An instrument made of some flexible material, such as bristles, attached to a handle or to the tip of a catheter. [A.S. *byrst,* bristle]

Ayre b., a device, consisting of a long flexible tube with a b. at the distal end, for collecting gastric mucosal cells in cancer detection studies; after positioning in the stomach the b. is rotated and "sweeps" cells from the mucosa.

bronchoscopic b., a small b. for insertion through a bronchoscope to wipe off cells for microscopic identification in suspected bronchial carcinoma.

denture b., a b. used to clean removable dentures.

Haidinger's b.'s, the perception of two dark yellowish b. or sheaves radiating about 5 degrees from the point of fixation when an evenly illuminated surface, such as the blue sky, is viewed through a polarizing lens.

Kruse's b., a bunch of fine platinum wires attached to a holder; used in bacteriological work to spread material over the surface of a culture medium.

polishing b., a b. usually mounted in a rotating instrument, used to polish teeth or artificial replacements.

Brushfield, Thomas, British physician, 1858–1937. SEE B.'s *spots,* under *spot;* B.-Wyatt *disease.*

brush·ite (brŭsh'īt). CaHPO₄·2H₂O; a naturally occurring acid calcium phosphate occasionally found in dental calculus and renal calculi.

brux·ism (brŭk'sizm). A clenching of the teeth, associated with forceful lateral or protrusive jaw movements, resulting in rubbing, gritting, or grinding together of the teeth, usually during sleep; sometimes a pathologic condition. [G. *bruchō,* to grind the teeth]

Bryant, Sir Thomas, English surgeon, 1828–1914. SEE B.'s *sign, traction, triangle.*

BSA Abbreviation for bovine serum *albumin.*

BSE Abbreviation for bovine spongiform *encephalopathy.*

BSER Abbreviation for brainstem evoked response. SEE brainstem evoked response *audiometry.*

Bt₂cAMP. $N^6,O^{2'}$- dibutyryladenosine 3':5'-cyclic monophosphate, a dibutyryl derivative of cAMP.

BTPS Symbol indicating that a gas volume has been expressed as if it were saturated with water vapor at body temperature (37°C) and at the ambient barometric pressure; used for measurements of lung volumes.

BTU Abbreviation for British thermal *unit.*

BTX Abbreviation for brevotoxins.

bu·aki (bū-ak'ē). A nutritional (protein deficiency) disease observed in natives of the Congo and characterized by edema, skin lesions, and anemia; possibly related to kwashiorkor.

bu·ba mad·re (bū'bă mah'dre). SYN mother *yaw.*

bu·bas (bū'bahs). SYN yaws.

b. brazilia'na, SYN espundia.

bu·bo (bū'bō). Inflammatory swelling of one or more lymph nodes, usually in the groin; the confluent mass of nodes usually suppurates and drains pus. [G. *boubōn,* the groin, a swelling in the groin]

bullet b., a hard, painless swelling of a gland in the groin, accompanying a chancre.

chancroidal b., an ulcerating b., due to *Haemophilus ducreyi.* SYN virulent b.

climatic b., SYN venereal *lymphogranuloma.*

indolent b., an indurated enlargement of an inguinal node.

malignant b., the enlarged lymph node associated with bubonic plague.

parotid b., a swelling of the parotid gland due to secondary septic infection.

primary b., a b. occurring as the first sign of venereal infection.

tropical b., SYN venereal *lymphogranuloma.*

venereal b., an enlarged gland in the groin associated with any venereal disease, especially chancroid.

virulent b., SYN chancroidal b.

bu·bon·al·gia (bū'bon-al'jē-ă). Rarely used term for pain in the groin. [G. *boubōn,* groin, + *algos,* pain]

bu·bon·ic (bū-bon'ik). Relating in any way to a bubo.

bu·bon·u·lus (bū-bon'yū-lŭs). **1.** An abscess occurring along the course of a lymphatic vessel. **2.** One of a number of hard nodules, often breaking down into ulcers, which form along the course of acutely inflamed lymphatic vessels of the dorsum of the penis. [Mod. L. dim. of *bubo*]

bu·car·dia (byū-kar'dē-ă). SYN ox *heart.* [G. *bous,* ox, + *kardia,* heart]

buc·ca, gen. and pl. **buc·cae** (bŭk'ă, bŭk'ē) [NA]. SYN cheek. [L.]

buc·cal (bŭk'ăl). Pertaining to, adjacent to, or in the direction of the cheek.

buc·ci·na·tor. SEE buccinator *muscle.*

⌂ **bucco-.** Cheek. [L. *bucca*]

buc·co·ax·i·al (bŭk-ō-ak'sē-ăl). Referring to the line angle formed by the buccal and axial walls of a cavity.

buc·co·ax·i·o·cer·vi·cal (bŭk'ō-ak'sē-ō-ser'vi-kăl). Referring to the point angle formed by the junction of the buccal, axial, and cervical (gingival) walls of a cavity.

buc·co·ax·i·o·gin·gi·val (bŭk'ō-ak'sē-ō-jin'ji-văl). Referring to the point angle formed by the junction of a buccal, axial, and gingival (cervical) wall.

buc·co·cer·vi·cal (bŭk-ō-ser′vi-kăl). **1.** Relating to the cheek and the neck. **2.** In dental anatomy, referring to that portion of the buccal surface of a bicuspid or molar tooth adjacent to its cemento-enamel junction.

buc·co·clu·sal (bŭk-ō-klū′săl). Incorrect term referring to the line angle formed by the junction of a buccal and pulpal wall. SEE buccopulpal.

buc·co·dis·tal (buk-ō-dis′tăl). Referring to the line angle formed by the junction of a buccal and distal wall of a cavity.

buc·co·gin·gi·val (bŭk-ō-jin′ji-văl). Relating to the cheek and the gum.

buc·co·la·bi·al (bŭk-ō-lā′bē-ăl). **1.** Relating to both cheek and lip. **2.** In dentistry, referring to that aspect of the dental arch or those surfaces of the teeth in contact with the mucosa of lip and cheek.

buc·co·lin·gual (bŭk-ō-ling′wăl). **1.** Pertaining to the cheek and the tongue. **2.** In dentistry, referring to that aspect of the dental arch or those surfaces of the teeth in contact with the mucosa of the lip or cheek and the tongue.

buc·co·me·si·al (bŭk-ō-mē′zē-ăl). Referring to the line angle formed by the junction of a buccal and mesial wall of a cavity.

buc·co·pha·ryn·ge·al (bŭk′ō-fă-rin′jē-ăl). Relating to both cheek or mouth and pharynx.

buc·co·pul·pal (buk-ō-pŭl′păl). Referring to the line angle formed by the junction of a buccal and pulpal wall of a cavity.

buc·co·ver·sion (bŭk′ō-ver-zhŭn). Malposition of a posterior tooth from the normal line of occlusion toward the cheek.

buc·cu·la (bŭk′yū-lä). A fatty puffing under the chin. SYN double chin. [L. dim. of *bucca,* cheek]

Büchner, Eduard, German chemist and Nobel laureate, 1860–1917. SEE B. *extract, funnel.*

Büchner, Hans E.A., German bacteriologist, 1850–1902. SEE B. *extract.*

bu·chu (bū′kū). The dried leaves of *Barosma betulina, B. crenulata,* or *B. serratifolia* (family Rutaceae), a shrub growing in South Africa; used as a carminative, diuretic, and urinary antiseptic. SYN Hottentot tea. [native]

Buchwald, Hermann Edmund, German physician, *1903. SEE B.'s *atrophy.*

Buck, Gurdon, U.S. surgeon, 1807–1877. SEE B.'s *extension, fascia, traction.*

buck·bean. The leaves of *Menyanthes trifoliata* (family Gentianaceae); credited with emmenagogue, antiscorbutic, and simple bitter properties. SYN bogbean, menyanthes.

buck·thorn (bŭk′thōrn). SYN Rhamnus.

Bucky, Gustav, U.S. radiologist, 1880–1963. SEE B. *diaphragm.*

bu·cli·zine hy·dro·chlo·ride (bu′kli-zēn). 1-(*p-tert*-Butylbenzyl)-4-(*p*-phenylbenzyl)piperazine dihydrochloride; a mild sedative used for motion sickness, vertigo, and anxiety accompanying psychosomatic disorders.

buc·lo·sa·mide (buk-lō′să-mīd). *N*-Butyl-4-chlorosalicylamide; a topical antifungal agent.

bu·cry·late (byū′kri-lāt). Isobutyl 2-cyanoacrylate; a tissue adhesive used in surgery.

Bucy, Paul C., U.S. neurosurgeon, 1904–1992. SEE Klüver-B. *syndrome.*

bud (bŭd). **1.** An outgrowth that resembles the b. of a plant, usually pluripotential, and capable of differentiating and growing into a definitive structure. **2.** To give rise to such an outgrowth. SEE ALSO gemmation. **3.** a small outgrowth from a parent cell; a form of asexual reproduction.

bronchial b., one of the outgrowths from the primordial endodermal laryngotracheal tube giving rise to the primary bronchi. SEE laryngotracheal *diverticulum.*

end b., SYN tail b.

gustatory b., SYN taste b.

limb b., an ectodermally covered mesenchymal outgrowth on the embryonic flank giving rise to either the forelimb or hindlimb.

liver b., the primordial cellular diverticulum of the embryonic foregut endoderm that gives rise to the parenchyma of the liver.

lung b., SYN tracheobronchial *diverticulum.*

median tongue b., SYN *tuberculum* impar.

metanephric b., the primordial cellular outgrowth from the mesonephric duct that gives rise to the epithelial lining of the ureter, of the pelvis, and calyces of the kidney, and of the straight collecting tubules. SYN ureteric b.

periosteal b., a vascular connective tissue bud from the perichondrium that invades the ossification center of the cartilaginous model of a developing long bone.

syncytial b., SYN syncytial *knot.*

tail b., the rapidly proliferating mass of cells at the caudal extremity of the embryo; remnant of the primitive node. SYN end b.

taste b., one of a number of flask-shaped cell nests located in the epithelium of vallate, fungiform, and foliate papillae of the tongue and also in the soft palate, epiglottis, and posterior wall of the pharynx; it consists of sustentacular, gustatory, and basal cells between which the intragemmal sensory nerve fibers terminate. SYN caliculus gustatorius [NA], gustatory b., Schwalbe's corpuscle, taste bulb, taste corpuscle.

tooth b., the primordial structures from which a tooth is formed; the enamel organ, the dental papilla, and the dental sac enclosing them.

ureteric b., SYN metanephric b.

vascular b., an endothelial sprout arising from a blood vessel.

Budd, George, English physician, 1808–1882. SEE B.'s *cirrhosis, syndrome;* B.-Chiari *syndrome.*

Budde, E., Danish sanitary engineer, *1871. SEE B. *process.*

bud·ding (bŭd′ing). SYN gemmation.

Budge, Julius L., German physiologist, 1811–1888. SEE B.'s *center.*

bud·ge·ri·gar (buj-er′ē-gar). An Australian parakeet (*Melopsillacus undulatus*) commonly kept as a small pet bird.

bud·gie (buj′ē) Abbreviated form of budgerigar.

Budin, Pierre C., French gynecologist, 1846–1907. SEE B.'s obstetrical *joint.*

Buerger, Leo, Austrian-U.S. physician, 1879–1943. SEE Winiwarter-B. *disease;* B.'s *disease.*

⌂**bufa-, bufo-.** Combining forms denoting origin from toads; used in the systematic and trivial names of toxic substances (genins) isolated from plants and animals containing the bufanolide structure; prefixes denoting species origin are often attached. [L. *bufo,* toad]

bu·fa·di·en·o·lide (bū-fă-dī-en′ō-līd). SEE bufanolide.

bu·fa·gen·ins (bū′fă-jen-inz). SYN bufagins.

bu·fa·gins (bū′fă-jinz). A group of steroids (bufanolides) in the venom of a family of toads (Bufonidae) having a digitalis-like action upon the heart; cardiac glycosides having a six-membered lactone. SEE ALSO bufotoxins. SYN bufagenins, bufogenins.

bu·fan·o·lide (bū-fan′ō-līd). The fundamental steroid lactone of several vegetable (*e.g.,* squill) and animal (*e.g.,* toad) venoms or toxins; also found in the form of glycosides in plants (*e.g.,* digitalis). The steroid is essentially a 5β-androstane, with a 14β H. The lactone at C-17 is structurally related to the –CH(CH₃)-CH₂CH₂CH₃ radical attached to C-17 in the cholanes, and is in the same configuration as that of cholesterol (*i.e.,* 20*R*); in some species, b. is formed from cholesterol. Various b. derivatives having unsaturation in the lactone ring (20,22) or elsewhere (4) are known as **bufenolides** (one double bond), **bufadienolides** (two double bonds), **bufatrienolides** (three double bonds), etc; they have varying numbers of hydroxyl groups at positions 3, 5, 14, and 16, and these may be further substituted. For structure, see steroids.

bu·fa·tri·en·o·lide (bū-fă-trī-en′ō-līd). SEE bufanolide.

bu·fen·o·lide (bū-fen′ō-līd). SEE bufanolide.

buff·er (bŭf′er). **1.** A mixture of an acid and its conjugate base (salt), such as H_2CO_3/HCO_3^-; $H_2PO_4^-/HPO_4^{2-}$, that, when present in a solution, reduces any changes in pH that would otherwise occur in the solution when acid or alkali is added to it; thus, the pH of the blood and body fluids is maintained virtually constant (pH 7.45) although acid metabolites are continually being formed in the tissues and CO_2 (H_2CO_3) is lost in the lungs. SEE ALSO conjugate acid-base *pair.* **2.** To add a b. to a solution and thus give it the property of resisting a change in pH when it receives a limited amount of acid or alkali.

dipolar b., SYN zwitterionic b.

secondary b., SEE Hamburger's *law.*

zwitterionic b., b. whose structure can include opposite charges. SYN dipolar b.

⌂**bufo-.** SEE bufa-.

bu·fo·gen·ins (bū-fō-jen-inz). SYN bufagins.

Bu·fon·i·dae (bū-fon′ĭ-dē). A family of toads whose dermal glands secrete several kinds of pharmacologically active substances having a cardiac action similar to that of digitalis. [L. *bufo,* toad]

bu·for·min (bū-fōr′min). 1-Butylbiguanide; an oral hypoglycemic agent.

bu·fo·ten·ine (bū-fō-ten′ēn). 3-(2-dimethylaminoethyl)indol-5-ol; *N,N*-dimethylserotonin; a psychotomimetic agent isolated from the venom of certain toads (family Bufonidae) and also present in several plants and one of the active principles of cohoba; raises the blood pressure by a vasoconstrictor action and produces psychic effects including hallucinations. SYN mappine.

bu·fo·tox·ins (bū-fō-toks′inz). 1. A group of steroid lactones (conjugates of bufagins and suberylarginine at C-3) of digitalis present in the venoms of toads (family Bufonidae); their effects are similar to but weaker than those of the bufagins. 2. Specifically, the main toxin of the European toad (*Bufo vulgaris*).

bug. An insect belonging to the suborder Heteroptera. For organisms so called, see the specific term.

bug·gery (bŭg′ger-ē). SYN sodomy. [O.F. *bougre,* heretic, fr. Med. L. *Bulgaris,* a Bulgar (hence a heretic)]

bulb (bŭlb). 1. Any globular or fusiform structure. SYN bulbus [NA]. 2. A short vertical underground stem of plants, as of the onion and garlic. SYN bulbus [NA]. [L. *bulbus,* a bulbous root]

aortic b., the dilated first part of the aorta containing the aortic semilunar valves and the aortic sinuses. SYN bulbus aortae [NA], arterial b.

arterial b., SYN aortic b.

carotid b., SYN carotid *sinus.*

b. of corpus spongiosum, SYN b. of penis.

dental b., the papilla, derived from mesoderm, that forms the part of the primordium of a tooth that is situated within the cup-shaped enamel organ.

duodenal b., SYN duodenal *cap.*

end b., one of the oval or rounded bodies in which the sensory nerve fibers terminate in mucous membrane.

b. of eye, SYN eyeball.

hair b., SYN b. of hair.

b. of hair, hair bulb, the lower expanded extremity of the hair follicle that fits like a cap over the papilla pili. SYN bulbus pili [NA], hair b.

jugular b., SYN b. of jugular vein.

b. of jugular vein, one of two dilated parts of the internal jugular vein: (1) the superior bulb (Heister's diverticulum) is a dilation at the beginning of the internal jugular vein in the jugular fossa of the temporal bone; (2) the inferior bulb is a dilat ed portion of the vein just before it reaches the brachiocephalic vein. SYN jugular b. SYN bulbus venae jugularis [NA].

Krause's end b.'s, nerve terminals in skin, mouth, conjunctiva, and other parts, consisting of a laminated capsule of connective tissue enclosing the terminal, branched, convoluted ending of an afferent nerve fiber; generally believed to be sensitive to cold. SYN corpuscula bulboidea [NA], bulboid corpuscles.

b. of lateral ventricle, a rounded elevation in the dorsal part of the medial wall of the posterior horn of the lateral ventricle, produced by the major forceps.

olfactory b., the grayish expanded rostral extremity of the olfactory tract, lying on the cribriform plate of the ethmoid and receiving the olfactory filaments. SYN bulbus olfactorius [NA].

b. of penis, the expanded posterior part of the corpus spongiosum of the penis lying in the interval between the crura of the penis. SYN bulbus penis [NA], b. of corpus spongiosum, b. of urethra, bulbus urethrae.

b. of posterior horn of lateral ventricle of brain, SYN *bulbus* cornus posterioris.

Rouget's b., a venous plexus on the surface of the ovary.

speech b., a prosthetic speech aid; a restoration used to close a cleft or other opening in the hard or soft palate, or to replace absent tissue necessary for the production of good speech.

taste b., SYN taste *bud.*

b. of urethra, SYN b. of penis.

b. of vestibule, a mass of erectile tissue on either side of the vagina united anterior to the urethra by the commissura bulborum. SYN bulbus vestibuli vaginae [NA].

bul·bar (bŭl′bar). 1. Relating to a bulb. 2. Relating to the rhombencephalon (hindbrain). 3. Bulb-shaped; resembling a bulb.

bul·bi (bŭl′bī). Plural of bulbus.

bul·bi·tis (bŭl-bī′tis). Inflammation of the bulbous portion of the urethra.

⌂**bulbo-.** Bulb; bulbus [L. *bulbus*]

bul·bo·cap·nine (bul′bō-kap′nin). Drug derived from roots of *Corydalis cava* and *C. tuberosa* (family Fumariaceae) and *Dicentra canadensis* (family Papaveraceae); blocks the effects of dopamine on peripheral dopamine receptors.

bul·bo·cav·er·no·sus (bŭl′bō-kav-er-nō′sŭs). SEE *musculus* bulbocavernosus.

bul·boid (bŭl′boyd). Bulb-shaped. [bulbo- + G. *eidos,* resemblance]

bul·bo·nu·cle·ar (bŭl-bō-nū′klē-ar). Relating to the nuclei in the medulla oblongata.

bul·bo·pon·tine (bŭl-bō-pon′tēn). Relating to the rostral part of the rhombencephalon composed of the pons and overlying tegmentum.

bul·bo·sa·cral (bŭl′bō-sā′krăl). SEE bulbosacral *system.*

bul·bo·spi·nal (bŭl′bō-spī′năl). Relating to the medulla oblongata and spinal cord, particularly to nerve fibers interconnecting the two. SYN spinobulbar.

bul·bo·u·re·thral (bŭl′bō-yū-rē′thrăl). Relating to the bulbus penis and the urethra. SYN urethrobulbar.

bul·bus, gen. and pl. **bul·bi** (bŭl′bŭs, -bī) [NA]. SYN bulb (1), bulb. [L. a plant bulb]

b. aor′tae [NA], SYN aortic *bulb.*

b. cor′dis, a transitory dilation in the embryonic heart where the arterial trunk joins the ventral roots of the aortic arches.

b. cor′nus posterior′is [NA], bulb of posterior horn of lateral ventricle of the brain; a curved elevation on the inner wall of the posterior horn produced by the fibers of the forceps major of the corpus callosum as they bend backward into the occipital lobe. SYN bulb of posterior horn of lateral ventricle of brain.

b. oc′uli [NA], SYN eyeball.

b. olfacto′rius [NA], SYN olfactory *bulb.*

b. pe′nis [NA], SYN *bulb* of penis.

b. pi′li [NA], SYN *bulb* of hair.

b. ure′thrae, SYN *bulb* of penis.

b. ve′nae jugula′ris [NA], SYN *bulb* of jugular vein.

b. vestib′uli vaginae [NA], SYN *bulb* of vestibule.

bu·le·sis (bū-lē′sis). The will; a willing. [G. *boulēsis,* a willing]

bu·lim·ia (bū-lim′ē-ă). SYN b. nervosa. [G. *bous,* ox, + *limos,* hunger]

b. nervo′sa, a chronic morbid disorder involving repeated and secretive episodic bouts of eating characterized by uncontrolled rapid ingestion of large quantities of food over a short period of time (binge eating), followed by self-induced vomiting, use of laxatives or diuretics, fasting, or vigorous exercise in order to prevent weight gain; often accompanied by feelings of guilt, depression, or self-disgust. SYN boulimia, bulimia, hyperorexia.

bu·lim·ic (bū-lim′ik). Relating to, or suffering from, bulimia nervosa.

Bu·li·nus (byū-lī′nŭs). A genus and subgenus of freshwater snails in the family Planorbidae (subfamily Bulininae), which includes many species that are intermediate hosts of the human blood fluke, *Schistosoma haematobium,* in Africa and the Middle East; divided into two subgenera, *Physopsis* and *Bulinus,* the former being responsible for transmission of *S. haematobium* south of the Sahara, the latter responsible for transmission of this bladder blood fluke in north Africa and the Middle East. Important species include *B. truncatus* and *B. forskalii*, hosts for human and animal schistosomes and several domestic animal amphistome flukes.

bulk·age (bŭlk′ij). Anything, such as agar, that increases the bulk of material in the intestine, thereby stimulating peristalsis.

bull Abbreviation for L. *bulliens, bulliat,* or *bulliant,* boiling, let boil.

bul·la, gen. and pl. **bul·lae** (bul′ă, -ē). **1.** A large blister appearing as a circumscribed area of separation of the epidermis from the subepidermal structure (**subepidermal b.**) or as a circumscribed area of separation of epidermal cells (**intraepidermal b.**) caused by the presence of serum, or occasionally by an injected substance. **2** [NA]. A bubble-like structure. [L. bubble]

ethmoidal b., a bulging of the inner wall of the ethmoidal labyrinth in the middle meatus of the nose, just below the middle nasal concha; it is regarded as a rudimentary concha. SYN b. ethmoidalis [NA].

b. ethmoida′lis [NA], SYN ethmoidal b.

pulmonary b., (1) an air-filled blister on the surface of the lung; **(2)** a similar abnormality within the lung presenting as a thin-walled cavity.

b. tympan′ica, the bony capsule enclosing the middle ear of the cat and dog.

bul·lec·to·my (bul-ek′tō-mē). Resection of a bulla; helpful in treating some forms of bullous emphysema, in which giant bullae compress functioning lung tissue.

bull·nose (bul′nōz). SYN necrotic *rhinitis* of pigs.

bul·lous (bul′ŭs). Relating to, of the nature of, or marked by, bullae.

bu·met·a·nide (byū-met′ă-nīd). 3-Butylamino-4-phenoxy-5-sulfamoylbenzoic acid; a diuretic used in the treatment of edema associated with congestive heart failure, hepatic cirrhosis, and renal disease.

Bumke, Oswald C.E., German neurologist, 1877–1950. SEE B.'s *pupil.*

BUN Abbreviation for blood urea *nitrogen.*

bun·am·i·dine hy·dro·chlo·ride (bŭn-am′i-dēn). *N,N*-Dibutyl-4-hexyloxynaphthamidine monohydrochloride; an anthelmintic.

bun·dle (bŭn′dl). A structure composed of a group of fibers, muscular or nervous; a fasciculus.

aberrant b.'s, a group, or groups, of fibers from the corticobulbar or corticonuclear tract, directed to each of the motor nuclei of cranial nerves.

anterior ground b., SYN *fasciculus* anterior proprius. SEE *fasciculi* proprii, under *fasciculus.*

Arnold's b., SYN temporopontine *tract.*

atrioventricular b., the bundle of modified cardiac muscle fibers that begins at the atrioventricular node as the trunk of the atrioventricular bundle and passes through the right atrioventricular fibrous ring to the membranous part of the interventricular septum where the trunk divides into two branches, the right crus of the atrioventricular b. and the left crus of the atrioventricular b.; the two crura ramify in the subendocardium of their respective ventricles. SYN fasciculus atrioventricularis [NA], atrioventricular band, Gaskell's bridge, His' band, His' b., b. of His, Keith's b., Kent's b. (1), Kent-His b., ventriculonector.

Bachmann's b., division of the anterior internodal tract that continues into the left atrium providing a specialized path for interatrial conduction.

comma b. of Schultze, SYN semilunar *fasciculus.*

Flechsig's ground b.'s, fasciculus anterior proprius and fasciculus lateralis proprius. SEE *fasciculi* proprii, under *fasciculus.*

Gantzer's accessory b., SEE Gantzer's *muscle.*

Gierke's respiratory b., SYN solitary *tract.*

ground b.'s, SYN *fasciculi* proprii, under *fasciculus.*

Held's b., SYN tectospinal *tract.*

Helie's b., a vertically arched b. of fibers in the superficial layer of the myometrium.

Helweg's b., SYN olivospinal *tract.*

His' b., b. of His, SYN atrioventricular b.

Hoche's b., SEE semilunar *fasciculus.*

hooked b. of Russell, SYN uncinate b. of Russell.

Keith's b., SYN atrioventricular b.

Kent-His b., SYN atrioventricular b.

Kent's b., (1) SYN atrioventricular b. **(2)** a muscle fiber b. in the mammalian heart below the nodus atrioventricularis; may also occur in man.

Killian's b., SEE inferior constrictor *muscle* of pharynx.

Krause's respiratory b., SYN solitary *tract.*

lateral ground b., SYN lateral proprius b. SEE *fasciculi* proprii, under *fasciculus.*

lateral proprius b., SYN lateral ground b.

Lissauer's b., SYN dorsolateral *fasciculus.*

Loewenthal's b., SYN tectospinal *tract.*

longitudinal pontine b.'s, SYN longitudinal pontine *fasciculi,* under *fasciculus.*

medial forebrain b., a fiber system coursing longitudinally through the lateral zone of the hypothalamus, connecting the latter reciprocally with the midbrain tegmentum and with various components of the limbic system; it also carries fibers from norepinephrine-containing and serotonin-containing cell groups in the brainstem to the hypothalamus and cerebral cortex, as well as dopamine-carrying fibers from the substantia nigra to the caudate nucleus and putamen.

medial longitudinal b., SYN medial longitudinal *fasciculus.*

Meynert's retroflex b., SYN retroflex *fasciculus.*

Monakow's b., SYN rubrospinal *tract.*

muscle b., a group of muscle fibers ensheathed by connective tissue (perimysium).

oblique b. of pons, SYN oblique pontine *fasciculus.*

olfactory b., a fiber system, described by E. Zuckerkandl as "Reichbündel," descending from the transparent septum in front of the anterior commissure toward the base of the forebrain; it contains precommissural fibers of the fornix, fibers from the septum to the hypothalamus and innominate substance, as well as fibers ascending to the septum and hippocampus from the hypothalamus and midbrain; it bears no special relation to the sense of smell.

olivocochlear b., a b. of fibers that originates from the periolivary nuclei bilaterally, exits the brainstem on the vestibular nerve, joins the cochlear nerve in the inner ear, and terminates on outer hair cells. SYN b. of Rasmussen, olivocochlear fibers.

Pick's b., a b. of nerve fibers recurving rostralward from the pyramidal tract in the medulla oblongata, and believed to consist of corticonuclear fibers.

posterior longitudinal b., SYN medial longitudinal *fasciculus.*

precommissural b., SEE olfactory b.

predorsal b., SYN tectospinal *tract.*

b. of Rasmussen, SYN olivocochlear b.

Rathke's b.'s, SYN *trabeculae* carneae, under *trabecula.*

Schütz' b., SYN dorsal longitudinal *fasciculus.*

solitary b., SYN solitary *tract.*

tendon b., a group of tendon fibers surrounded by a sheath of irregular connective tissue (peritendineum).

Türck's b., SYN anterior pyramidal *tract.*

uncinate b. of Russell, fastigial efferent fibers that cross with the cerebellum and descend over the lateral surface of the superior cerebellar peduncle; these fibers largely terminate in the vestibular nuclei and the reticular formation of the pons and medulla. SYN hooked b. of Russell, uncinate fasciculus of Russell.

Vicq d'Azyr's b., SYN mamillothalamic *fasciculus.*

bun·gar·o·tox·ins (bung′gă-rō-tok′sinz). Constituent proteins of the venom of the South Asian banded krait *Bungarus multicinctus,* a snake of the Elapidae family. Used as pharmacologic tools in studying neuromuscular function.

bung·pag·ga (bŭng-pag′ă). SYN *myositis* purulenta tropica.

bun·ion (bŭn′yŭn). A localized swelling at either the medial or dorsal aspect of the first metatarsophalangeal joint, caused by an inflammatory bursa; a medial b. is usually associated with hallux valgus. [O.F. *buigne,* bump on the head]

bun·ion·ec·to·my (bŭn-yŭn-ek′tō-mē). Excision of a bunion.
Keller b., excision of the proximal portion of the proximal phalanx of the first toe.
Mayo b., excision of the head of the first metatarsal.

Bunnell, Sterling, U.S. surgeon, 1882–1957. SEE B.'s *suture;* Paul-B. *test.*

bu·no·dont (bū′nō-dont). Having molar teeth with rounded or low conical cusps, in contrast to lophodont. [G. *bounos,* mound, + *odous* (*odont-*), tooth]

bu·no·lol hy·dro·chlo·ride (byū′nō-lol). DL-5-[3-*tert*-(Butyl-amino)-2-hydroxypropoxy]-3,4-dihydro-1(2*H*)-naphthalenone hydrochloride; a β-adrenergic blocking agent for treatment of cardiac arrhythmias.

bu·no·loph·o·dont (bū-nō-lof′ō-dont). Having molar teeth with transverse ridges and rounded cusps on the occlusal surface. [G. bunos, mound, + *lophos,* ridge, + *odous,* tooth]

bu·no·se·le·no·dont (bū′nō-sĕ-len′ō-dont). Having molar teeth with crescentic ridges and rounded cusps on the occlusal surface. [*bunos,* + *selēnē,* moon, + *odous,* tooth]

Bu·nos·to·mum (byū-nō-stō′mŭm). A genus of hookworms (family Ancylostomatidae, subfamily Necatorinae) found in cattle and other herbivores; similar to *Necator.* [G. *bounos,* hill, mound, + *stoma,* mouth]
B. phlebot′omum, a species that occurs in cattle, sheep, and some wild ruminants in many parts of the world.
B. trigonoceph′alum, a cosmopolitan hookworm species in the small intestines of sheep and goats.

Bunsen, Robert W., German chemist and physicist, 1811–1899. SEE B. burner; B.'s solubility *coefficient;* B.-Roscoe *law.*

Bunsen burn·er. A gas lamp supplied with lateral openings admitting sufficient air so that the carbon is completely burned, thus giving a very hot but only slightly luminous flame. [R.W. Bunsen]

Bun·ya·vir·i·dae (bŭn-yă-vir′i-dē). A family of arboviruses composed of more than 200 virus serotypes and containing at least five genera: *Bunyavirus, Hantavirus, Phlebovirus, Nairovirus,* and *Uukuvirus.* Virions are 90–100 nm in diameter, sensitive to lipid solvents and detergents, and enveloped with glycopolypeptide surface projections; the nucleocapsid is of helical symmetry containing single-stranded segmented RNA (MW 7×10^6). [*Bunyamwere,* Uganda]

Bun·ya·vi·rus (bun′ya-vī-rus). A virus in the genus of the family Bunyaviridae that includes California encephalitis virus and LaCrosse encephalitis virus.

buph·thal·mia, buph·thal·mus, buph·thal·mos (būf-thal′mē-ă, -thal′mŭs, -thal′mos). An affection of infancy, marked by an increase of intraocular pressure with enlargement of the eyeball. SYN buphthalmos, congenital *glaucoma,* hydrophthalmia, hydrophthalmos, hydrophthalmus. [G. *bous,* ox, + *ophthalmos,* eye]

bu·piv·a·caine (byū-piv′ă-kān). *dl*-1-Butylpipecoloxylidide; a potent, long-acting local anesthetic used in regional anesthesia.

bu·pre·nor·phine hy·dro·chlo·ride (bū-pre-nōr′fēn). $C_{29}H_{41}NO_4 \cdot HCl$; a semisynthetic opioid analgesic used for relief of moderate to severe pain.

bu·pro·pi·on hy·dro·chlo·ride (bū-prō′pē-on). 1-Propanone,1-(3-chlorophenyl)-2-[1,1-dimethylethyl)amino]-hydrochloride; an antidepressant.

bur (bŭr). A rotary cutting instrument, used in dentistry, consisting of a small metal shaft and a head designed in various shapes; used at various rotational velocities for excavating decay, shaping cavity forms, and for reduction of tooth structure. SEE ALSO burr.
cross-cut b., a b. with blades located at right angles to its long axis.
end-cutting b., a b. with blades only on its end.
finishing b., a b. with numerous fine cutting blades placed close together; used to contour metallic restorations.
fissure b., a cylindrical or tapered rotary cutting tool intended for extending or widening fissures in a tooth, as for general surface reduction of tooth substance.
inverted cone b., a rotary cutting instrument in the shape of a

truncated cone with the smaller end attached to the shaft; generally used for entering carious pits or creating undercuts in cavity preparations.
round b., a dental b. with the cutting blades spherically arranged.

Burchard, H., 19th century German chemist. SEE B.-Liebermann *reaction;* Liebermann-B. *test.*

Burchard-Liebermann re·ac·tion. See under reaction.

Burdach, Karl F., German anatomist and physiologist, 1776–1847. SEE B.'s *column, fasciculus, nucleus, tract.*

bur·den (ber′den). SEE body burden.
clinical b., a b. that differs from genetic b. mainly in the added component of morbidity; a trait that is neither a clinical or a genetic lethal may be grossly disabling.
genetic b., the genetic debt due to harmful mutation but as yet undischarged. (In a large population of fixed size every mutation with diminished genetic fitness will eventually become extinct and depending on the details of inheritance and phenotype must be paid for by a fixed number of genetic deaths per mutation, the genetic debt.)

bu·ret, bu·rette (bū-ret′). A graduated glass tube with a tap as its lower end; used for measuring liquids in volumetric chemical analyses. [Fr.]

Bürger, Max, German physician, *1885. SEE B.-Grütz *syndrome, disease.*

Burger's tri·an·gle. See under triangle.

Burk, Dean, U.S. scientist, *1904. SEE Lineweaver-B. *equation, plot.*

Burkitt, Denis P., 20th century British physician in Uganda, died 1993. SEE B.'s *lymphoma.*

Burlew disk. See under disk.

Burlew wheel. See under wheel.

Burn, J.H. SEE B. and Rand *theory.*

burn (bern). **1.** To cause a lesion by heat or any other agent, similar to that caused by heat. **2.** To suffer pain caused by excessive heat, or similar pain from any cause. **3.** A lesion caused by heat or any cauterizing agent, including friction, electricity, and electromagnetic energy; types of b.'s resulting from different agents are relatively specific and diagnostic. The division of b.'s into three degrees (first degree, second degree, and third degree) is recognized for geographical designation. [A.S. *baernan*]

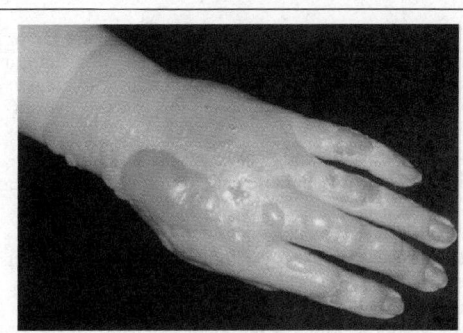

2nd degree burn (formation of blisters)

brush b., a b. caused by friction of a rapidly moving object against the skin or ground into the skin.
chemical b., a b. due to a caustic chemical.
first degree b., a b. involving only the epidermis and causing erythema and edema without vesiculation. SYN superficial b.
flash b., a b. due to very brief exposure to intense radiant heat; the typical b. produced by atomic explosion.
full-thickness b., SYN third degree b.
mat b., SEE brush b.
partial-thickness b., SYN second degree b.

radiation b., a b. caused by exposure to radium, x-rays, atomic energy in any form, ultraviolet rays, etc.

rope b., SEE brush b.

second degree b., a b. involving the epidermis and dermis and usually forming blisters that may be superficial, or by deep dermal necrosis, followed by epithelial regeneration extending from the skin appendages. SYN partial-thickness b.

superficial b., SYN first degree b.

thermal b., a b. caused by heat.

third degree b., a b. involving destruction of the entire skin; deep third-degree b.'s extend into subcutaneous fat, muscle, or bone and often cause much scarring. SYN full-thickness b.

burn·ers (bern′erz). Episodes of upper extremity burning pain. SEE ALSO burner *syndrome*. SYN stingers.

Burnett, Charles H., U.S. physician, 1901–1967. SEE B.'s *syndrome*.

bur·nish·er (bŭr′nish-er). An instrument for smoothing and polishing the surface or edge of a dental restoration. [O. F. *burnir,* to polish]

burn·out (bern′owt). **1.** In dentistry, the elimination, by heat, of an invested pattern from a set investment in order to prepare the mold to receive casting metal. **2.** A psychological state of physical and emotional exhaustion thought to be a stress reaction to a reduced ability to meet the demands of one's occupation; symptoms include fatigue, insomnia, impaired work performance, and an increased suscepibility to physical illness and substance abuse.

Burns, Allan, Scottish anatomist, 1781–1813. SEE B.'s *ligament,* falciform *process, space.*

Burow, Karl A. von, German surgeon, 1809–1874. SEE B.'s *operation, solution, triangle, vein.*

burr (bŭr). A drilling tool for enlarging a trephine hole in the cranium. SEE ALSO bur.

bur·row (ber′ō). **1.** A subcutaneous tunnel or tract made by a parasite, such as the itch mite. **2.** A sinus or fistula. **3.** To undermine or create a tunnel or tract through or beneath various tissue planes.

BURSA

bur·sa, pl. **bur·sae** (ber′să, ber′sē) [NA]. A closed sac or envelope lined with synovial membrane and containing fluid, usually found or formed in areas subject to friction; *e.g.,* over an exposed or prominent part or where a tendon passes over a bone. [Mediev. L., a purse]

Achil′les b., SYN b. of tendo calcaneus.

b. achil′lis [NA], ⋆official alternate term for b. of tendo calcaneus.

b. of acromion, SYN subcutaneous acromial b.

adventitious b., a b.-like cyst formed between two parts as a result of friction.

b. anseri′na [NA], SYN anserine b.

anserine b., the b. between the tibial collateral ligament of the knee joint and the tendons of the sartorius, gracilis, and semitendinosus muscles. SYN b. anserina [NA], tibial intertendinous b.

anterior tibial b., SYN subtendinous b. of the tibialis anterior muscle.

bicipitoradial b., the b. between the tendon of the biceps brachii muscle and the anterior part of the tuberosity of the radius. SYN b. bicipitoradialis [NA].

b. bicip′itoradia′lis [NA], SYN bicipitoradial b.

Boyer's b., SYN retrohyoid b.

Brodie's b., (1) medial subtendinous b. of gastrocnemius muscle; (2) SYN b. of semimembranosus muscle.

Calori's b., a b. between the arch of the aorta and the trachea.

coracobrachial b., a b. frequently present between the tendon of

the coracobrachialis and the subscapularis muscle. SYN b. musculi coracobrachialis [NA], subcoracoid b.

b. cubita′lis interos′sea [NA], SYN interosseous b. of elbow.

deep infrapatellar b., the b. between the upper part of the tibia and the patellar ligament. SYN b. infrapatellaris profunda [NA].

b. of extensor carpi radialis brevis muscle, the b. between the tendon of the extensor carpi radialis brevis and the base of the third metacarpal. SYN b. musculi extensoris carpi radialis brevis [NA].

b. fabric′ii, the b. of Fabricius in poultry, a blind saclike structure located on the posterodorsal wall of the cloaca; it performs a thymus-like function. SYN b. of Fabricius.

b. of Fabricius, SYN b. fabricii.

Fleischmann's b., SYN sublingual b.

b. of gastrocnemius, SYN subtendinous b. of gastrocnemius muscle.

gluteofemoral b., two or three small bursae between the tendon of the gluteus maximus and the linea aspera. SYN b. intermuscularis musculorum gluteorum [NA], intermuscular gluteal b.

gluteus medius bursae, the b. between the tendon of the gluteus medius and the greater trochanter and the b. between the piriformis and gluteus medius. SYN bursae trochantericae musculi glutei medii [NA].

gluteus minimus b., a fairly large b. usually located between the gluteus minimus and the greater trochanter. SYN b. trochanterica musculi glutei minimi [NA].

b. of great toe, the b. between the lateral side of the base of the first metatarsal bone and the medial side of the shaft of the second metatarsal.

b. of hyoid, SYN retrohyoid b.

iliac b., SYN subtendinous iliac b.

b. iliopecti′nea [NA], SYN iliopectineal b.

iliopectineal b., a large b. between the iliopsoas tendon and the iliopubic eminence. SYN b. iliopectinea [NA].

inferior b. of biceps fem′oris, the b. between the tendon of the biceps femoris and the fibular collateral ligament of the knee joint. SYN b. subtendinea musculi bicipitis femoris inferior [NA].

infracardiac b., a small serous sac sometimes present on the medial side of the base of the right lung in the embryo. SEE ALSO pneumatoenteric *recess,* celomic *bay.*

infrahyoid b., a b. sometimes found below the inferior margin of the body of the hyoid bone between the sternothyroid muscle and the median thyrohyoid membrane. SYN b. infrahyoidea [NA].

b. infrahyoi′dea [NA], SYN infrahyoid b.

b. infrapatella′ris profun′da [NA], SYN deep infrapatellar b.

infraspinatus b., the b. located between the tendon of the infraspinatus and the capsule of the shoulder joint. SYN b. subtendinea musculi infraspinati [NA].

intermuscular gluteal b., SYN gluteofemoral b.

b. intermuscula′ris mus′culorum gluteor′um [NA], SYN gluteofemoral b.

interosseous b. of elbow, an inconstant b. located between the tendon of the biceps and the ulna or the oblique cord. SYN b. cubitalis interossea [NA].

b. intratendin′ea olec′rani [NA], SYN intratendinous b. of elbow.

intratendinous b. of elbow, a b. sometimes present within the tendon of insertion of the triceps brachii. SYN b. intratendinea olecrani [NA], b. of Monro.

b. ischiad′ica mus′culi glu′tei max′imi [NA], SYN ischial b.

b. ischiad′ica mus′culi obturato′ris inter′ni [NA], SYN b. of obturator internus (1).

ischial b., the b. between the gluteus maximus muscle and the tuberosity of the ischium. SYN b. ischiadica musculi glutei maximi [NA].

laryngeal b., SYN subcutaneous b. of the laryngeal prominence.

lateral malleolar subcutaneous b., lateral malleolar b., the b. between the lateral malleolus and the skin. SYN b. subcutanea malleoli lateralis [NA], lateral malleolus b., subcutaneous b. of lateral malleolus.

lateral malleolus b., SYN lateral malleolar subcutaneous b.

b. of latiss′imus dor′si, a constant b. between the tendons of the teres major and the latissimus dorsi near their intersections. SYN b. subtendinea musculi latissimus dorsi [NA].

Luschka's b., SYN pharyngeal b.

medial malleolar subcutaneous b., the b. between the medial malleolus and the skin. SYN b. subcutanea malleoli medialis [NA], subcutaneous b. of medial malleolus.

b. of Monro, SYN intratendinous b. of elbow.

b. muco'sa, SYN synovial b.

b. mus'culi bicip'itis fem'oris supe'rior [NA], SYN superior b. of biceps femoris.

b. mus'culi coracobrachia'lis [NA], SYN coracobrachial b.

b. mus'culi extenso'ris car'pi radia'lis bre'vis [NA], SYN b. of extensor carpi radialis brevis muscle.

b. mus'culi pirifor'mis [NA], SYN b. of the piriformis muscle.

b. mus'culi semimembrano'si [NA], SYN b. of semimembranosus muscle.

b. mus'culi tenso'ris ve'li palati'ni [NA], SYN b. of tensor veli palatini muscle.

b. of ob'turator inter'nus, (1) the large, constant b. between the obturator internus tendon and the lesser sciatic notch; SYN b. ischiadica musculi obturatoris interni [NA]. **(2)** the b. between the tendon of the obturator internus muscle and the capsule of the hip joint. SYN b. subtendinea musculi obturatoris interni [NA].

b. of olecranon, SYN subcutaneous olecranon b.

omental b., an isolated portion of the peritoneal cavity lying dorsal to the stomach and extending craniad to the liver and diaphragm and caudad into the greater omentum; it opens into the general peritoneal cavity at the epiploic foramen. SYN b. omentalis [NA], lesser peritoneal cavity, lesser peritoneal sac, omental sac.

b. omenta'lis [NA], SYN omental b.

ovarian b., the peritoneal recess between the medial aspect of the ovary and the mesosalpinx. SYN b. ovarica.

b. ovar'ica, SYN ovarian b.

b. pharynge'a [NA], SYN pharyngeal b.

pharyngeal b., a cystic notochordal remnant found inconstantly in the posterior wall of the nasopharynx at the lower end of the pharyngeal tonsil. SYN b. pharyngea [NA], Luschka's b., Tornwaldt's cyst.

b. of the piriformis muscle, a small b. located between the tendons of the piriformis and superior gemellus and the femur. SYN b. musculi piriformis [NA].

b. of popliteus, SYN subpopliteal *recess.*

prepatellar b., a b. between the skin and the lower part of the patella. SYN b. subcutanea prepatellaris [NA].

b. quadra'ti fem'oris, between the anterior aspect of the quadratus femoris muscle and the lesser trochanter of the femur.

radial b., SYN tendon *sheath* of flexor pollicis longus muscle.

retrohyoid b., a b. between the posterior surface of the body of the hyoid bone and the thyrohyoid membrane. SYN b. retrohyoidea [NA], Boyer's b., b. of hyoid, subhyoid b.

b. retrohyoi'dea [NA], SYN retrohyoid b.

rider's b., an adventitious b. on the inner side of the knee caused by horseback riding.

sartorius bursae, bursae, sometimes separate from the anserine b., located between the tendons of the sartorius, semitendinosus, and gracilis muscles. SYN bursae subtendineae musculi sartorii [NA].

b. of semimembranosus muscle, it lies between the muscle, the head of the gastrocnemius, and the knee joint. SYN b. musculi semimembranosi [NA], Brodie's b. (2).

subacromial b., between the acromion and the capsule of the shoulder joint. SYN b. subacromialis [NA].

b. subacromia'lis [NA], SYN subacromial b.

subcoracoid b., SYN coracobrachial b.

b. subcuta'nea acromia'lis [NA], SYN subcutaneous acromial b.

b. subcuta'nea calca'nea [NA], SYN subcutaneous calcaneal b.

b. subcuta'nea infrapatella'ris [NA], SYN subcutaneous infrapatellar b.

b. subcuta'nea malle'oli latera'lis [NA], SYN lateral malleolar subcutaneous b.

b. subcuta'nea malle'oli media'lis [NA], SYN medial malleolar subcutaneous b.

b. subcuta'nea ole'crani [NA], SYN subcutaneous olecranon b.

b. subcuta'nea prepatella'ris [NA], SYN prepatellar b.

b. subcuta'nea prominen'tiae laryn'geae [NA], SYN subcutaneous b. of the laryngeal prominence.

b. subcuta'nea trochanter'ica [NA], SYN trochanteric b. (1).

b. subcuta'nea tuberosita'tis tib'iae [NA], SYN subcutaneous b. of tibial tuberosity.

subcutaneous acromial b., the b. between the acromion and the skin. SYN b. subcutanea acromialis [NA], b. of acromion.

subcutaneous calcaneal b., a b. between the skin and the posterior surface of the calcaneus. SYN b. subcutanea calcanea [NA].

subcutaneous infrapatellar b., a b. between the patellar ligament and the skin. SYN b. subcutanea infrapatellaris [NA].

subcutaneous b. of the laryngeal prominence, the b. located between the junction of the laminae of the thyroid cartilage and the skin. SYN b. subcutanea prominentiae laryngeae [NA], laryngeal b.

subcutaneous b. of lateral malleolus, SYN lateral malleolar subcutaneous b.

subcutaneous b. of medial malleolus, SYN medial malleolar subcutaneous b.

subcutaneous olecranon b., b. between the olecranon process of the ulna and the skin. SYN b. subcutanea olecrani [NA], b. of olecranon.

subcutaneous b. of tibial tuberosity, the b. located superficial to the tibial tuberosity, either subcutaneous or subfascial. SYN b. subcutanea tuberositatis tibiae [NA].

subdeltoid b., the b. between the deltoid muscle and the capsule of the shoulder joint. It may be combined with the subacromial b. SYN b. subdeltoidea [NA].

b. subdeltoid'ea [NA], SYN subdeltoid b.

b. subfascia'lis prepatella'ris [NA], SYN subfascial prepatellar b.

subfascial prepatellar b., a b. between the fascia lata and the quadriceps tendon anterior to the patella. SYN b. subfascialis prepatellaris [NA].

subhyoid b., SYN retrohyoid b.

sublingual b., an inconstant serous b. at the level of the frenulum linguae, between the surface of the genioglossus muscle and the mucous membrane of the floor of the mouth. SYN b. sublingualis, Fleischmann's b.

b. sublingua'lis, SYN sublingual b.

subscapular b., b. between the tendon of the subscapularis muscle and the neck of the scapula; it communicates with the shoulder joint. SYN b. subtendinea musculi subscapularis [NA].

b. subtendin'eae mus'culi gastrocne'mii [NA], SYN subtendinous b. of gastrocnemius muscle.

bursae subtendin'eae mus'culi sarto'rii [NA], SYN sartorius bursae.

b. subtendin'ea ili'aca [NA], SYN subtendinous iliac b.

b. subtendin'ea mus'culi bicip'itis fem'oris infe'rior [NA], SYN inferior b. of biceps femoris.

b. subtendin'ea mus'culi infraspinat'i [NA], SYN infraspinatus b.

b. subtendin'ea mus'culi latis'simus dor'si [NA], SYN b. of latissimus dorsi.

b. subtendin'ea mus'culi obturatoris inter'ni [NA], SYN b. of obturator internus (2).

b. subtendin'ea mus'culi subscapula'ris [NA], SYN subscapular b.

b. subtendin'ea mus'culi tere'tis majo'ris [NA], SYN b. of teres major.

b. subtendin'ea mus'culi tibia'lis anterio'ris [NA], SYN subtendinous b. of the tibialis anterior muscle.

b. subtendin'ea mus'culi trape'zii [NA], SYN b. of trapezius.

b. subtendin'ea mus'culi tricip'itus bra'chii [NA], SYN triceps b.

b. subtendin'ea prepatella'ris [NA], SYN subtendinous prepatellar b.

subtendinous b. of gastrocnemius muscle, consists of a lateral and a medial (Brodie's b. (1)) b. between the heads of the gastrocnemius and capsule of the knee joint. SYN b. subtendineae musculi gastrocnemii [NA], b. of gastrocnemius.

subtendinous iliac b., the b. at the attachment of the iliopsoas muscle into the lesser trochanter. SYN b. subtendinea iliaca [NA], iliac b.

subtendinous prepatellar b., a b. between the tendon of the quadriceps and the patella. SYN b. subtendinea prepatellaris [NA].

subtendinous b. of the tibialis anterior muscle, the small b. between the medial surface of the medial cuneiform bone and the tendon of the tibialis anterior. SYN b. subtendinea musculi tibialis anterioris [NA], anterior tibial b.

superior b. of biceps femoris, a b. frequently found between the tendon of the long head of the biceps femoris and the ischial tuberosity and the tendon of the semimembranosus. SYN b. musculi bicipitis femoris superior [NA].

suprapatellar b., a large b. between the lower part of the femur and the tendon of the quadriceps femoris muscle. It usually communicates with the cavity of the knee joint. SYN b. suprapatellaris [NA].

b. suprapatella′ris [NA], SYN suprapatellar b.

synovial b., a sac containing synovial fluid which occurs at sites of friction, as between a tendon and a bone over which it plays, or subcutaneously over a bony prominence. The NA lists the following types: subcutaneous synovial b., b. synovialis subcutanea [NA]; submuscular synovial b., b. synovialis submuscularis [NA]; subfascial synovial b., b. synovialis subfascialis [NA]; and subtendinous synovial b., b. synovialis subtendinea [NA]. SYN b. synovialis [NA], b. mucosa.

b. synovia′lis [NA], SYN synovial b.

synovial trochlear b., SYN tendon *sheath* of superior oblique muscle.

b. ten′dinis calca′nei [NA], SYN b. of tendo calcaneus.

b. of tendo calca′neus, b. between the tendo calcaneus and the upper part of the posterior surface of the calcaneum. SYN b. tendinis calcanei [NA], b. achillis* [NA], Achilles b.

b. of tensor veli palatini muscle, a small b. located where the tendon of the tensor passes around the pterygoid hamulus. SYN b. musculi tensoris veli palatini [NA].

b. of teres major, b. under the tendon of the teres major near its attachment. SYN b. subtendinea musculi teretis majoris [NA].

tibial intertendinous b., SYN anserine b.

b. of trapezius, a b. between the tendon of the trapezius muscle and the medial end of the scapular spine. SYN b. subtendinea musculi trapezii [NA].

triceps b., the b. located deep to the tendon of the triceps brachii near its insertion on the olecranon. SYN b. subtendinea musculi tricipitus brachii [NA].

trochanteric b., (1) the b. between the greater trochanter of the femur and the skin; SYN b. subcutanea trochanterica [NA]. **(2)** a multilocular b. between the gluteus maximus muscle and the greater trochanter of the femur. SYN b. trochanterica musculi glutei maximi [NA].

bur′sae trochanter′icae mus′culi glu′tei me′dii [NA], SYN gluteus medius bursae.

b. trochanter′ica mus′culi glu′tei max′imi [NA], SYN trochanteric b. (2).

b. trochanter′ica mus′culi glu′tei min′imi [NA], SYN gluteus minimus b.

trochlear synovial b., SYN tendon *sheath* of superior oblique muscle.

ulnar b., SYN common flexor *sheath*.

bur·sal (ber′săl). Relating to a bursa.

bur·sec·to·my (ber-sek′tō-mē). Surgical removal of a bursa. [bursa + G. *ektomē*, excision]

bur·si·tis (ber-sī′tis). Inflammation of a bursa. SYN bursal synovitis.

anserine b., inflammation of the anserine bursa lying between the pes anserinus and the upper medial surface of the tibia.

bicipital b., SYN intertubercular b.

calcaneal b., inflammation of one of the bursae related to the tuber calcanei, usually a result of trauma to the subcutaneous bursa; occurs most frequently in the horse. SYN capped hock.

intertubercular b., inflammation of the intertubercular bursa of the biceps brachii muscle of the shoulder of the horse, usually the result of trauma. SYN bicipital b., shoulder b.

olecranon b., inflammation of the olecranon bursa.

prepatellar b., SYN housemaid's *knee*.

shoulder b., SYN intertubercular b.

subacromial b., may be coalesced with subdeltoid b. SYN Duplay's disease.

subdeltoid b., may be coalesced with subacromial b.

trochanteric b., inflammation of one of the trochanteric bursae of the horse, and a common cause of hip lameness.

bur·so·lith (ber′sō-lith). A calculus formed in a bursa. [bursa + G. *lithos*, stone]

bur·sop·a·thy (ber-sop′ă-thē). Any disease of a bursa.

bur·sot·o·my (ber-sot′ō-mē). Incision through the wall of a bursa. [bursa + G. *tomē*, a cutting]

burst (berst). A sudden increase in activity.

respiratory b., the marked increase in metabolic activity that occurs in a phagocyte following ingestion of particles resulting in an increase in oxygen consumption, formation of superoxide anion, formation of hydrogen peroxide, and activation of the hexose monophosphate shunt.

b. size, the number of phages produced by an infected cell.

bur·su·la (ber′sū-lă). A small pouch or bag. [Mod. L. dim. of Mediev. L. *bursa*, purse]

b. tes′tium, archaic term for scrotum.

Burton, Henry, English physician, 1799–1849. SEE B.'s *line*.

Bury, Judson S., English dermatologist, 1852–1944. SEE B.'s *disease*.

Buschke, Abraham, German dermatologist, 1868–1943. SEE B.'s *disease;* Busse-B. *disease;* B.-Löwenstein *tumor;* B.-Ollendorf *syndrome*.

bu·spi·rone hy·dro·chlo·ride (byū-spī′rōn). *N*-[4-[4-(2-Pyrimidinyl)-1-piperazinyl]butyl]-hydrochloride; a non-benzodiazepine antianxiety agent used in the management of anxiety disorders or for short-term relief of the symptoms of anxiety.

Busquet, G. Paul, French physician, *1866. SEE B.'s *disease*.

Buss. Surname of the man on whose farm the disease was first diagnosed. SEE Buss *disease*.

Busse, Otto, German physician, 1867–1922. SEE B.-Buschke *disease*.

bu·sul·fan, bu·sul·phan (byū-sŭl′fan). CH_3O_2SO $(CH_2)_4OSO_2CH_3$; 1,4-Butanediol dimethanesulfonate; tetramethylene *bis*(methanesulfonate); an antineoplastic alkylating agent used in the treatment of chronic myelocytic leukemia; known to be teratogenic in humans.

bu·ta·bar·bi·tal (byū-tă-bar′bi-tawl). 5-*sec*-Butyl-5-ethylbarbituric acid; a sedative and hypnotic with intermediate duration of action; available as b. sodium, with same usages.

bu·ta·caine sul·fate (byū′tă-kān). 3-(Dibutylamino)-1-propanol *p*-aminobenzoate sulfate; a local anesthetic.

bu·tal·bi·tal (byū-tal′bi-tawl). 5-allyl-5-isobutylbarbituric acid; a barbiturate of intermediate duration of action; a sedative and hypnotic. SYN allylbarbital.

bu·tam·ben (byū-tam′ben). SYN *butyl* aminobenzoate.

bu·tane (byū′tān). C_4H_{10}; a gaseous hydrocarbon present in natural gas; two isomers are known, both of which are anesthetically active. *n*-Butane is $CH_3(CH_2)_2CH_3$ and isobutane is $CH_3CH(CH_3)CH_3$ (or 2-methylpropane).

bu·ta·no·ic ac·id (byū-tă-nō′ik). Systematic name for normal *n*-butyric acid.

bu·ta·nol (byū′tă-nol). Preferred chemical name for *n*-butyl alcohol.

bu·tan·o·yl (byū′tan-ō-il). $CH_3(CH_2)_2 COO^-$; the radical of butanoic acid. SYN butyryl.

bu·ta·per·a·zine (byū-tă-per′ă-zēn). 1-{10-[3-(4-Methyl-1-

piperazinyl)propyl]-phenothiazin-2-yl}-1-butanone; an antipsychotic.

bu·tav·er·ine (byū-tav′er-ēn). Butyl ester of β-phenyl-1-piperidinepropionic acid; an antispasmodic (as hydrochloride).

bu·te·thal (byū′tĕ-thawl). 5-Butyl-5-ethylbarbituric acid; a sedative and hypnotic.

bu·teth·a·mate (byū-teth′ă-māt). 2-Phenylbutyric acid 2-(diethylamino)ethyl ester; an intestinal antispasmodic agent.

bu·teth·a·mine hy·dro·chlo·ride (byū-teth′ă-mēn). 2-(Isobutylamino)ethyl-p-amino benzoate; a local anesthetic.

bu·thi·a·zide (byū-thī′ă-zīd). 6-chloro-3,4-dihydro-3-isobutyl-2H-1,2,4-benzothiadiazine-7-sulfonamide 1,1-dioxide; has diuretic and antihypertensive actions. SYN thiabutazide.

bu·to·con·a·zole   ni·trate (byū-tō-kō′nă-zōl). $C_{19}H_{17}Cl_3N_2S\cdot HNO_3$; an antifungal agent used primarily in the treatment of vulvovaginal candidiasis.

bu·to·py·ro·nox·yl (byū′tō-pī-rō-nok′sil). Butyl mesityl oxide oxalate; an insect repellent, effective against the biting stable fly (*Stomoxys calcitrans*)

bu·tor·pha·nol tar·trate (byū-tōr′fă-nōl). (-)-17-(Cyclobutylmethyl)morphinan-3,14-diol tartrate; a potent mixed agonist/antagonist narcotic analgesic agent.

bu·tox·a·mine hy·dro·chlo·ride (byū-tok′să-mēn). α-[1-(*tert*-Butylamino)ethyl]-2,5-dimethoxybenzyl alcohol hydrochloride; an antilipemic agent.

***t*-bu·tox·y·car·bon·yl (BOC, *t*-BOC, Boc)** (byū-toks-ē-kar′bŏn-il). $(CH_3)_3COCO$—; an amino-protecting group used in peptide synthesis. SYN *tert*-butyloxycarbonyl.

bu·trip·ty·line hy·dro·chlo·ride (byū-trip′tĭ-lēn). *dl*-10,11-Dihydro-N,N,β-trimethyl-5H-dibenzo[a,d]cycloheptene-5-propylamine; an antidepressant.

butt (bŭt). **1.** To bring any two square-ended surfaces in contact so as to form a joint. **2.** In dentistry, to place a restoration directly against the tissues covering the alveolar ridge.

but·ter (bŭt′er). **1.** A coherent mass of milk fat, obtained by churning or shaking cream until the separate fat globules run together, leaving a liquid residue, buttermilk. **2.** A soft solid having more or less the consistency of b. [L. *butyrum*, G. *boutyros*, prob. fr. *bous*, cow, + *tyros*, cheese]

b. of antimony, a concentrated acid solution of *antimony* trichloride.

b. of bismuth, SYN *bismuth* trichloride.

cacao b., cocoa b., SYN *theobroma* oil. SEE ALSO cacao.

b. of tin, stannic chloride pentahydrate, $SnCl_4\cdot 5H_2O$.

b. of zinc, SYN *zinc* chloride.

but·ter·fly (bŭt′er-flī). **1.** Any structure or apparatus resembling in shape a butterfly with outstretched wings. **2.** A scaling erythematous lesion on each cheek, joined by a narrow band across the nose; seen in lupus erythematosus and seborrheic dermatitis. SYN butterfly eruption, butterfly patch, butterfly rash.

but·ter·milk. The fluid containing casein and lactic acid, left after the process of making butter.

but·ter yel·low [C.I. 11160]. $C_6H_5N{:}NC_6H_4N(CH_3)_2$; a fat-soluble yellow dye (MW 225) that has hepatic carcinogenic action in experimental animals; used as an indicator of pH (red, at pH 2.9, yellow at pH 4.0). SYN dimethylaminoazobenzene, methyl yellow.

but·tocks (bŭt′oks). The buttocks; the prominence formed by the gluteal muscles on either side. SYN clunes [NA], nates [NA], breech.

but·ton (bŭt′ŏn). A structure, lesion, or device of knob shape. [M.E., fr. O.Fr. *bouton*, fr. *bouter*, to thrust, fr. Germanic]

Amboyna b., SYN yaws. [*Amboyna*, one of the Spice Islands in the Malay Archipelago]

Biskra b., the lesion occurring in cutaneous leishmaniasis.

Murphy's b., an obsolete appliance formerly used for intestinal anastomosis; it consists of two hollow cylinders, one of which is sutured into each open end of the intestine; the two are then joined and fasten automatically, maintaining the two ends of intestine in apposition by their serous surfaces; after firm union

has occurred the cylinders slough away and are passed in the stools.

Oriental b., the lesion occurring in cutaneous leishmaniasis.

peritoneal b., a device used to drain ascitic fluid to subcutaneous space.

but·ton·hole (bŭt′ŏn-hōl). **1.** A short straight cut made through the wall of a cavity or canal. **2.** The contraction of an orifice down to a narrow slit; *i.e.,* the so-called mitral b. in extreme mitral stenosis. SEE buttonhole *stenosis*.

bu·tyl (byū′til). $CH_3(CH_2)_3$—; a radical of *n*-butane.

b. alcohol, C_4H_9OH; several isomeric forms are known: **primary b. alcohol,** propylcarbinol, $CH_3CH_2CH_2CH_2OH$, the butyl alcohol of fermentation; isobutyl alcohol, isopropylcarbinol, 2-methyl-1-propanol, $(CH_3)_2CHCH_2OH$; narcotic in high concentrations; **secondary b. alcohol,** ethylmethylcarbinol, 2-butanol, $CH_3CH_2CH(CH_3)OH$; and **tertiary b. alcohol,** trimethylcarbinol, 2-methyl-2-propanol, $(CH_3)_3COH$, a denaturant for ethanol.

b. aminobenzoate, *n*-butyl *p*-aminobenzoate; a local anesthetic, very insoluble and only slightly absorbed. SYN butamben.

bu·tyl·at·ed hy·drox·y·an·is·ole (BHA) (bū-tĭ-lāt′ed hī′drok-sē-an′ĭ-sol). Exhibits antioxidant properties; often used with butylated hydroxytoluene propyl gallate, hydroquinone, methionine, lecithin, thiodipropionic acid, etc. Used as an antioxidant, especially in foods.

bu·tyl·at·ed hy·drox·y·tol·u·ene (BHT). Antioxidant for food, animal feed, petroleum products, synthetic rubbers, plastics, animal and vegetable oils, soap; also an antiskinning agent in paints and inks.

***tert*-bu·tyl·ox·y·car·bon·yl (tBoc)** (byū′til-oks′ē-kar′bŏn-il). SYN *t*-butoxycarbonyl.

bu·tyl·par·a·ben (byū-til-par′ă-ben). Butyl *p*-hydroxybenzoate; an antifungal preservative.

bu·ty·ra·ce·ous (byū-tir-ā′shĭ-us). Buttery in consistency.

bu·ty·rate (byū′ti-rāt). A salt or ester of butyric acid.

bu·ty·rate-CoA li·gase. Fatty acid thiokinase (medium chain), a ligase forming acyl-CoA's from medium-chain fatty acids and CoA with the conversion of ATP to AMP and PP_i. A key step in activation of fatty acids. SYN acyl-activating enzyme (2), butyryl-CoA synthetase, octanoyl-CoA synthetase.

bu·tyr·ic (byū-tir′ik). Relating to butter.

bu·tyr·ic ac·id (byū-tir′ik). An acid of unpleasant odor occurring in butter, cod liver oil, sweat, and many other substances. It exists in two forms: **normal b. a.** (also written as *n*-butyric acid), butanoic acid, $CH_3CH_2CH_2COOH$, which occurs in combination with glycerol in cow's butter; and isobutyric acid, 2-methyl-propanoic acid, $(CH_3)_2CHCOOH$, one of the intermediates in valine catabolism, found in combination with glycerol in croton oil and elsewhere.

γ-bu·tyr·o·be·taine (byū-tir′ō-be-tān). γ-(Trimethylammonium) butyric acid; a betaine of γ-aminobutyric acid; a precursor of carnitine by hydroxylation of the β-carbon.

bu·tyr·o·cho·lin·es·ter·ase (byū′tir-ō-kō-lin-es′ter-ās). SYN cholinesterase.

bu·ty·roid (byū′ti-royd). **1.** Buttery. **2.** Resembling butter.

bu·tyr·om·e·ter (byū-ti-rom′ĕ-ter). An instrument for determining the amount of butterfat in milk. [G. *boutyron*, butter, + *metron*, measure]

bu·ty·ro·phe·none (byū′tir-ō-fē′nōn). One of a group of derivatives of 4-phenylbutylamine that have neuroleptic activity; *e.g.,* haloperidol.

bu·tyr·ous (byū′ti-rŭs). Denoting a tissue or bacterial growth of butter-like consistency.

bu·tyr·yl (byū′ti-ril). SYN butanoyl.

bu·tyr·yl·cho·line es·ter·ase (byū′ti-ril-kō′lēn es′ter-ās). SYN cholinesterase.

bu·tyr·yl-CoA. $CH_3CH_2CH_2COSCoA$; condensation product of coenzyme A and *n*-butanoic acid; an intermediate in fatty acid degradation and in biosynthesis.

b.-C. synthetase, SYN butyrate-CoA ligase.

Buzzard, Thomas, English physician, 1831–1919. SEE B.'s *maneuver*.

Buzzi, Fausto, coworker of Ernst Schweninger. SEE Schwening-er-B. *anetoderma.*

Byler dis·ease. See under disease.

by·pass (bī´pas). **1.** A shunt or auxiliary flow. **2.** To create new flow from one structure to another through a diversionary channel. SEE ALSO shunt.

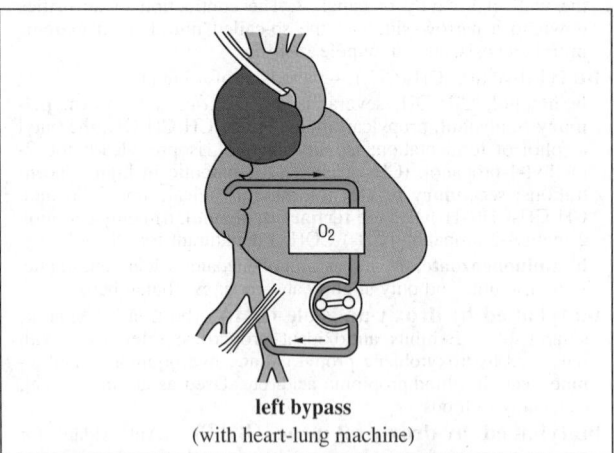

left bypass
(with heart-lung machine)

aortocoronary b., SYN coronary b.

aortoiliac b., an operation in which a vascular prosthesis is united with the aorta and iliac artery to relieve obstruction of the lower abdominal aorta, its bifurcation, and the proximal iliac branches.

aortorenal b., insertion of a graft of autogenous artery, saphenous vein, or synthetic material between the aorta and the distal renal artery, to circumvent an obstruction of the renal artery.

bowel b., SYN jejunoileal b.

cardiopulmonary b., diversion of the blood flow returning to the heart through a pump oxygenator (heart-lung machine) and then returning it to the arterial side of the circulation; used in operations upon the heart to maintain extracorporeal circulation.

coronary b., vein grafts or other conduits shunting blood from the aorta to branches of the coronary arteries, to increase the flow beyond the local obstruction. SYN aortocoronary b.

extraanatomic b., a vascular b. that does not conform to the preexisting anatomy.

extracranial-intracranial b., a vascular shunt created by the anastomosis of an extracranial vessel to an intracranial vessel, usually, the superficial temporal artery to a cortical branch of the middle cerebral artery.

femoropopliteal b., a vascular prosthesis that bypasses an obstruction in the femoral artery; may be synthetic material, autologous tissue, or heterologous tissue.

gastric b., high division of the stomach, anastomosis of the small upper pouch of the stomach to the jejunum, and closure of the distal part of the stomach that is retained; used for treatment of morbid obesity. SYN Mason operation.

jejunoileal b., anastomosis of the upper jejunum to the terminal ileum for treatment of morbid obesity. SYN bowel b., jejunoileal shunt.

left heart b., any procedure that shunts blood returning from the pulmonary circulation to the systemic circulation without passing through the left heart. This is utilized during some cardiac surgery and experimentally during severe left heart failure or cardiogenic shock.

partial ileal b., division of the small intestine approximately at the junction of the middle and lower one-third, closure of the distal end, and anastomosis of the proximal end to the cecum.

right heart b., introduction of a circuit shunting blood from the venae cavae around the right atrium and ventricle and directly into the pulmonary artery.

bys·si·no·sis (bis-i-nō´sis). Obstructive airway disease in people who work with unprocessed cotton, flax, or hemp; caused by reaction to material in the dust and thought to include endotoxin

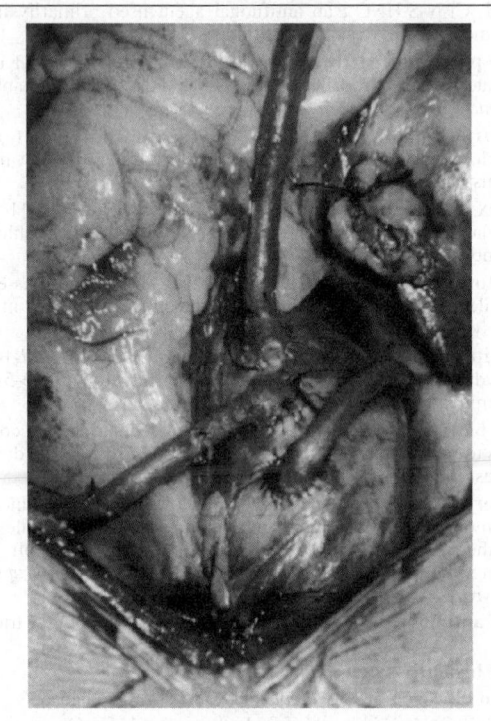

coronary bypass
aortal anastomosis (in a triple bypass)

from bacterial contamination. Sometimes called "monday morning asthma" since patients improve when away from work on the weekend. SYN cotton-dust asthma, cotton-mill fever, mill fever. [G. *byssos,* flax, + *-osis,* condition]

byte. A group of adjacent bits, commonly 4, 6 or 8, operating as a unit for the storage and manipulation of data in a computer.

C 1. Abbreviation or symbol for large *calorie*; carbon; cathodal; cathode; celsius; cervical vertebra (C1 to C7); closure (of an electrical circuit); congius (gallon); contraction; coulomb; curie; cylinder; cylindrical *lens*; cytidine; cysteine; cytosine; *component* of complement (C1 1/N C9); third substrate in a multisubstrate enzyme-catalyzed reaction. **2.** When followed by subscript letters, *e.g.*, C_{In}, indicates renal clearance of a substance (*e.g.*, inulin). When followed by subscript numbers, *e.g.*, C_{19}, indicates the number of carbon atoms in a molecule, *e.g.*, 19.

^{11}**C.** Symbol for carbon-11.

^{12}**C.** Symbol for carbon-12.

^{13}**C.** Symbol for carbon-13.

^{14}**C.** Symbol for carbon-14.

c 1. Abbreviation or symbol for centi-; small *calorie*; centum; concentration; speed of light in a vacuum; circumference. Abbreviation for curie. **2.** As a subscript, refers to blood *capillary*.

c̄ Abbreviation for L. *cum*, with.

CA Abbreviation for carcinoma; cardiac *arrest*; cancer; chronologic *age*; *cytosine* arabinoside.

CA-125. Abbreviation for cancer antigen 125 *test*.

CA125 Abbreviation for cancer antigen 125 *test*.

Ca 1. Abbreviation for cathode. **2.** Symbol for calcium.

^{45}**Ca.** Symbol for calcium-45.

^{47}**Ca** Abbreviation for calcium-47.

ca. Abbreviation for L. *circa* (about, approximately).

caa·pi (ka′pē). A hallucinogenic preparation obtained from *Banisteria caapi* (family Malpighaceae), a South American jungle vine; contains harmine and other psychotomimetic principles. SYN ayahuasca.

cab·bage tree (kab′ij trē). SYN andira.

Cabot, Richard, U.S. physician, 1868–1939. SEE C.'s ring *bodies*, under *body*; C.-Locke *murmur*.

Cabot-Locke mur·mur. See under murmur.

cac-. SEE caco-.

ca·cao (kă-ka′ō). Prepared c., or cocoa, a powder prepared from the roasted cured kernels of the ripe seed of *Theobroma cacao Linné* (family Sterculiaceae); the tree yields a fat, theobroma oil. SYN theobroma. [native Mexican origin]

c. oil, SYN *theobroma* oil.

CaCC Abbreviation for cathodal closure *contraction*.

Cacchione, Aldo, 20th century Italian psychiatrist. SEE De Sanctis-C. *syndrome*.

ca·ché (kah-shā′). An obsolete device consisting of a lead cone covered with several layers of paper, having a mica window at the bottom, used as an applicator in radiotherapy, the radium or other radioactive substance being at the apex of the cone and filters being placed below as required. [Fr. hidden, covered]

ca·chec·tic (kă-kek′tik). Relating to or suffering from cachexia.

cac·hec·tin (kak-hek′tin). A polypeptide hormone, produced by endotoxin-activated macrophages, which has the ability to modulate adipocyte metabolism, lyse tumor cells *in vitro*, and induce hemorrhagic necrosis of certain transplantable tumors *in vivo*. SYN tumor necrosis factor. [G. *kakos*, bad, + *hexis*, condition of body]

ca·chet (kă-shā′). A seal-shaped capsule or wafer for enclosing powders of disagreeable taste. [Fr. a seal]

ca·chex·ia (kă-kek′sē-ă). A general weight loss and wasting occurring in the course of a chronic disease or emotional disturbance. [G. *kakos*, bad, + *hexis*, condition of body]

c. aphtho′sa, SYN sprue (1).

c. aquo′sa, an edematous form of ancylostomiasis.

diabetic neuropathic c., a clinical syndrome seen almost exclusively in elderly diabetic males, consisting of the rather sudden onset of severe limb pain, marked weight loss, depression, and impotence. These patients appear to have a combination of a severe diabetic polyneuropathy, diffuse bilateral diabetic polyradiculopathy, and diabetic autonomic neuropathy.

hypophyseal c., SYN panhypopituitarism.

c. hypophys′eopri′va, a condition following total removal of the hypophysis cerebri resulting in panhypopituitarism marked by a fall of body temperature, electrolyte imbalance, and hypoglycemia, followed by coma and death.

hypophysial c., SYN Simmonds' *disease*, panhypopituitarism.

malarial c., SYN chronic *malaria*.

pituitary c., SYN Simmonds' *disease*.

c. strumipri′va, SYN c. thyropriva.

c. thyroid′ea, SYN c. thyropriva.

c. thyropri′va, signs and symptoms of hypothyroidism (with or without myxedema) resulting from the loss of thyroid tissue, either from surgery, radiotherapy, or disease. SYN c. strumipriva, c. thyroidea.

cach·in·na·tion (kak-i-nā′shŭn). Laughter without apparent cause, often observed in schizophrenia. [L. *cachinno*, to laugh immoderately and loudly]

caco-, caci-, cac-. Bad; ill. Cf. mal-. [G. *kakos*]

cac·o·de·mon·o·ma·nia (kak-ō-dē′mon-ō-mā′nē-ă). A mental condition in which the patient believes himself to be inhabited by or possessed by an evil spirit. [caco- + G. *daimōn*, spirit, + *mania*, frenzy]

cac·o·dyl (kak′ō-dil). $(CH_3)_2As$-$As(CH_3)_2$; an oil resulting from the distillation together of arsenous acid and potassium acetate. SYN dicacodyl, tetramethyldiarsine. [G. *kakōdēs*, foul-smelling]

cac·o·dyl·ate (kak′ō-dil-āt). A salt or ester of cacodylic acid. SEE cacodylic acid.

cac·o·dyl·ic (kak-ō-dil′ik). Relating to cacodyl; denoting especially c. acid.

cac·o·dyl·ic ac·id. $(CH_3)_2AsOOH$; prepared by treating cacodyl and cacodyl oxide with mercuric oxide, and forms cacodylates with various bases which were used in skin diseases, tuberculosis, malaria, and other affections in which arsenic was considered of value. SYN dimethylarsinic acid.

cac·o·geu·sia (kak-ō-gū′sē-ă). A bad taste. [caco- + G. *geusis*, taste]

cac·o·me·lia (kak-ō-mē′lē-ă). Congenital deformity of one or more limbs. [caco- + G. *melos*, limb]

cac·o·plas·tic (kak-ō-plas′tik). **1.** Relating to or causing abnormal growth. **2.** Incapable of normal or perfect formation. [caco- + G. *plastikos*, formed]

ca·cos·mia (kă-koz′mē-ă). A subjective perception of nonexistent disagreeable odors; a variety of parosmia. [G. *kakosmia*, a bad smell, fr. *kakos*, bad, + *osmē*, the sense of smell]

cac·ti·no·my·cin (kak′ti-nō-mī′sin). Produced by *Streptomyces chrysomallus*. A mixture of actinomycins C_1 (dactinomycin), C_2, and C_3 used as an antineoplastic, immunosuppressive agent. SEE ALSO actinomycin. SYN actinomycin C.

cac·u·men, pl. **cac·u·mi·na** (kak-yū′men, -mi-nă). The top or apex of a plant or an anatomical structure. [L. summit]

cac·u·mi·nal (kak-yū′mi-năl). Relating to a top or apex, particularly of a plant or anatomical structure.

ca·dav·er (kă-dav′er). A dead body. SYN corpse. [L. fr. *cado*, to fall]

ca·dav·er·ic (kă-dav′er-ik). Relating to a dead body.

ca·dav·er·ine (kă-dav′er-in). $H_2N(CH_2)_5NH_2$; 1,5-pentanediamine; 1,5-diaminopentane; a foul-smelling diamine formed by bacterial decarboxylation of lysine; poisonous and irritating to the skin.

ca·dav·er·ous (kă-dav′er-ŭs). Having the pallor and appearance resembling a corpse.

cade oil (kād). SYN *juniper* tar.

cad·her·ins. A family of integral-membrane glycoproteins that has a role in cell-cell adhesion and is important in morphogenesis and differentiation; E-c. is also known as uvomorulin and is

ca

concentrated in the belt desmosome in epithelial cells; N-c. is found in several cells, most notably in the nervous system and the neural ectoderm; N-c. helps maintain the integrity of neuronal aggregates; P-c. is expressed in many different types of cells. [cell + adhere + -in]

cad·mi·um (Cd) (kad′mē-ŭm). A metallic element, atomic no. 48, atomic wt. 112.411; its salts are poisonous and little used in medicine. Various compounds of c. are used commercially in metallurgy, photography, electrochemistry, etc.; a few have been used as ascaricides, antiseptics, and fungicides. [L. *cadmia,* fr. G. *kadmeia* or *kadmia,* an ore of zinc, calamine]

CaDTe Abbreviation for cathodal duration *tetanus.*

ca·du·ca (kă-dū′kă). SYN deciduous *membrane.* [L. fem. of *caducus,* fallen, falling]

ca·du·ce·us (kă-dū′sē-ŭs). A staff with two oppositely twined serpents and surmounted by two wings; emblem of the U.S. Army Medical Corps. For veterinary medicine the double serpent was changed in 1972 to its present form with a single serpent. SEE ALSO staff of Aesculapius. [L. the staff of Mercury; G. *kēryx* herald, the staff of Hermes]

CAE Abbreviation for caprine arthritis-*encephalomyelitis.*

⚫**cae-.** For words so beginning, see under ce-.

caf·fe·a·rine (kaf′ē-ă-rin). SYN trigonelline.

caf·feine (kaf′ēn). 1,3,7-trimethylxanthine; an alkaloid obtained from the dried leaves of *Thea sinensis,* tea, or the dried seeds of *Coffea arabica,* coffee; used as a central nervous system stimulant, diuretic, circulatory and respiratory stimulant, and as an adjunct in the treatment of headaches. SYN guaranine, thein.
c. citrate, citrated c., a mixture of equal parts of c. and citric acid.
c. hydrate, monohydrate of c., a central nervous system stimulant.
c. and sodium benzoate, a mixture of equal parts of sodium benzoate and c., used to meet the indication of c.
c. and sodium salicylate, a mixture of sodium salicylate and c. used for the relief of headache and neuralgia.

caf·fein·ism (kaf′ēn-izm). Caffeine intoxication characterized by restlessness, tremulousness, nervousness, excitement, insomnia, flushed face, diuresis, and gastrointestinal complaints, brought on by the ingestion of substances containing caffeine.

Caffey, John Patrick, U.S. physician, radiologist, and peditrician, the "the father of pediatric radiology", 1895–1978. SEE C.'s *disease, syndrome;* C.-Kempe *syndrome;* C.-Silverman *syndrome.*

cage (kāj). 1. An enclosure made partly or completely of open work and commonly used to house animals. 2. A structure resembling such an enclosure. [M.E., fr. O.Fr., fr. L. *cavea,* hollow, stall]
thoracic c., the skeleton of the thorax consisting of the thoracic vertebrae, ribs, costal cartilages, and sternum. SYN compages thoracis [NA], skeleton thoracicus✶.

Cajal (Ramón y Cajal), Santiago, Spanish histologist and Nobel laureate, 1852–1934. SEE C.'s *cell;* horizontal *cell* of C.; C.'s astrocyte *stain;* interstitial *nucleus* of C.

caj·e·put oil, caj·u·put oil (kaj′ĕ-pŭt, -yū-pŭt). A volatile oil distilled from the fresh leaves of *Cajuputi viridiflora,* a tree of tropical Asia and Australia; a stimulant, counterirritant, and expectorant.

caj·e·put·ol, caj·u·put·ol (kaj′ĕ-pyū-tol, -ŭ-pyū-tol). SYN cineole.

Cal Abbreviation for large *calorie.*

cal Abbreviation for small *calorie.*

Cal·a·bar bean (kal′ă-bar bēn). SYN physostigma.

cal·a·mine (kal′ă-mīn). Zinc oxide with a small amount of ferric oxide or basic zinc carbonate suitably colored with ferric oxide; used in dusting powders, lotions, and ointments, as a mild astringent and protective agent for skin disorders. [Mediev. L. *calamina,* fr. L. *cadmia,* fr. G. *kadmia,* Theban (earth), fr. *Kadmos,* founder of Thebes]

cal·a·mus (kal′ă-mŭs). 1. The dried, unpeeled rhizome of *Acorus calamus* (family Araceae), cultivated in Burma and Sri Lanka, a carminative and anthelminthic. 2. A reed-shaped structure. [L. reed, a pen]

c. scripto′rius, inferior part of the rhomboid fossa; the narrow lower end of the fourth ventricle between the two clavae. SYN Arantius' ventricle. [L. writing pen]

cal·ca·ne·al, cal·ca·ne·an (kal-kā′nē-al, kal-kā′nē-an). Relating to the calcaneus or heel bone.

⚫**calcaneo-.** The calcaneus. [L. *calcaneum,* heel]

cal·ca·ne·o·a·poph·y·si·tis (kal-kā′nē-ō-ă-pof-i-sī′tis). Inflammation at the posterior part of the os calcis, at the insertion of the Achilles tendon.

cal·ca·ne·o·as·trag·a·loid (kal-kā′nē-ō-as-trag′ă-loyd). Relating to the calcaneus, or os calcis, and the talus, or astragalus.

cal·ca·ne·o·cav·us (kal-ka′nē-ō-kā′vus). Combination of talipes calcaneus and talipes cavus.

cal·ca·ne·o·cu·boid (kal-kā′nē-ō-kyū′boyd). Relating to the calcaneus and the cuboid bone.

cal·can·e·o·dyn·ia (kal-kā′nē-ō-din′ē-ă). SYN painful *heel.* [calcaneo- + G. *odynē,* pain]

cal·ca·ne·o·na·vic·u·lar (kal-kā′nē-ō-na-vik′yū-lăr). Relating to the calcaneus and the navicular bone. SYN calcaneoscaphoid.

cal·ca·ne·o·scaph·oid (kal-kā′nē-ō-skaf′oyd). SYN calcaneonavicular.

cal·ca·ne·o·tib·i·al (kal-kā′nē-ō-tib′ē-ăl). Relating to the calcaneus and the tibia.

cal·ca·ne·o·val·go·cav·us (kal-ka′nē-ō-val′-go-kā′vus). Combination of talipes calcaneus, valgus, and cavus.

cal·ca·ne·o·val·gus (kal-kā′nē-ō-val′gŭs). SEE talipes calcaneovalgus.

cal·ca·ne·o·var·us (kal-kā′nē-ō-vā′rŭs). SEE talipes calcaneovarus.

cal·ca·ne·um (kal-kā′nē-ŭm). SYN calcaneus (1). [L. the heel]

cal·ca·ne·us, gen. and pl. **cal·ca·nei** (kal-kā′nē-ŭs, -kā′nē-ī). 1 [NA]. The largest of the tarsal bones; it forms the heel and articulates with the cuboid anteriorly and the talus above. SYN calcaneal bone, calcaneum, heel bone, os calcis. 2. SYN *talipes* calcaneus. [L. the heel (another form of *calcaneum*)]

cal·car (kal′kar). 1. A small projection from any structure; internal spurs (septa) at the level of division of arteries and confluence of veins when branches or roots form an acute angle. SEE ALSO vascular *spur.* 2. A dull spine or projection from a bone. 3. Archaic term for a horny outgrowth from the skin. SYN spur. [L. spur, cock's spur]
c. a′vis [NA], the lower of two elevations on the medial wall of the posterior horn of the lateral ventricle of the brain, caused by the depth of the calcarine sulcus. SYN Haller's unguis, hippocampus minor, minor hippocampus, Morand's spur, unguis avis.
c. femora′le, a bony spur springing from the underside of the neck of the femur above and anterior to the lesser trochanter, adding to the strength of this part of the bone. SYN Bigelow's septum.
c. pedis, SYN calx (2).

cal·car·e·ous (kal-kā′rē-ŭs). Chalky; relating to or containing lime or calcium, or calcific material. [L. *calcarius,* pertaining to lime, fr. *calx,* lime]

cal·ca·rine (kal′kă-rēn). 1. Relating to a calcar. 2. Spur-shaped.

cal·car·i·u·ria (kal-kar-ē-yū′rē-ă). Excretion of calcium (lime) salts in the urine. [L. *calcarius,* of lime, + G. *ouron,* urine]

cal·cer·gy (kal′ser-jē). Local calcification of soft tissue occurring at the site of injection of certain chemical compounds, such as lead acetate or cerium chloride; hydroxyapatite deposits are found in the calcified areas. [L. *calx,* chalk, calcium, + G. *ergon,* work, production]

cal·ces (kal′sēz). Plural of calx.

cal·cic (kal′sik). Relating to lime.

cal·ci·co·sis (kal-si-kō′sis). Pneumoconiosis from the inhalation of limestone dust.

cal·ci·di·ol (kal-sĭ-dī′ol). 25-hydroxycholecalciferol (a 3,25-diol); the first step in the biological conversion of vitamin D_3 to the more active form, calcitriol; it is more potent than vitamin D_3. SYN 25-hydroxycholecalciferol, calcifediol.
c. 1α-hydroxylase, 25-hydroxycholecalciferol 1α-hydroxylase, the monooxygenase that forms calcitriol from c.

using O_2 and NADPH; a deficiency in this enzyme can result in features of a vitamin D deficiency.

cal·ci·fe·di·ol (kal-sĭ-fĕ-dī′ol). SYN calcidiol.

cal·cif·er·ol (kal-sif′er-ol). SYN ergocalciferol.

cal·cif·er·ous (kal-sif′er-ŭs). **1.** Containing lime. **2.** Producing any of the salts of calcium. SYN calcophorous.

cal·cif·ic (kal-sif′ik). Forming or depositing calcium salts.

cal·ci·fi·ca·tion (kal′si-fi-kā′shŭn). **1.** Deposition of lime or other insoluble calcium salts. **2.** A process in which tissue or noncellular material in the body becomes hardened as the result of precipitates or larger deposits of insoluble salts of calcium (and also magnesium), especially calcium carbonate and phosphate (hydroxyapatite) normally occurring only in the formation of bone and teeth. SYN calcareous infiltration. [L. *calx*, lime, + *facio*, to make]

dystrophic c., c. occurring in degenerated or necrotic tissue, as in hyalinized scars, degenerated foci in leiomyomas, and caseous nodules.

eggshell c., a thin layer of c. around an intrathoracic lymph node, usually in silicosis, seen on a chest radiograph.

metastatic c., c. occurring in nonosseous, viable tissue (*i.e.,* tissue that is not degenerated or necrotic), as in the stomach, lungs, and kidneys (and rarely in other sites); the cells of these organs secrete acid materials, and, under certain conditions in instances of hypercalcemia, the alteration in pH seems to cause precipitation of calcium salts in these sites.

Mönckeberg's c., SYN Mönckeberg's *arteriosclerosis.*

Mönckeberg's medial c., SYN Mönckeberg's *arteriosclerosis.*

pathologic c., c. occurring in excretory or secretory passages as calculi, and in tissues other than bone and teeth.

pulp c., SYN endolith.

cal·ci·fy (kal′si-fī). To deposit or lay down calcium salts, as in the formation of bone.

cal·cig·er·ous (kal-sij′er-us). Producing or carrying calcium salts. [calcium + L. *gero*, to bear]

cal·ci·na·tion (kal-si-nā′shŭn). The process of calcining.

cal·cine (kal′sēn). To expel water and volatile matter by heat.

cal·ci·no·sis (kal-si-nō′sis). A condition characterized by the deposition of calcium salts in nodular foci in various tissues other than the parenchymatous viscera; the two well-known forms, c. circumscripta and c. universalis, are not associated with tissue damage or demonstrable metabolic disease; other forms are the result of abnormal calcium and/or phosphorous metabolism. [calcium + *-osis,* condition]

c. circumscrip′ta, localized deposits of calcium salts in the skin and subcutaneous tissues, usually surrounded by a zone of granulomatous inflammation; clinically, the lesions resemble the tophi of gout.

c. cu′tis, a deposit of calcium in the skin; usually occurs secondary to a preexisting inflammatory, degenerative, or neoplastic dermatosis, and is frequently seen in scleroderma. SYN dystrophic c., skin stones.

dystrophic c., SYN c. cutis.

c. intervertebra′lis, calcium deposit in vertebral disk.

reversible c., a form of c. sometimes observed in patients who constantly ingest large quantities of milk and alkaline medicines, as in the treatment of peptic ulcer.

tumoral c., calcification of collagen, chiefly at the site of large joints, in South African Negros; probably genetic.

c. universa′lis, diffuse deposits of calcium salts in the skin and subcutaneous tissues, connective tissue, and other sites; may be associated with dermatomyositis, occurs more frequently in young persons, and is often fatal; serum levels of calcium and phosphorus are generally within normal limits.

cal·ci·o·ki·ne·sis (kal′sē-ō-ki-nē′sis). Mobilization of stored calcium. [calcium + G. *kinēsis,* motion]

cal·ci·o·ki·net·ic (kal′sē-ō-ki-net′ik). Pertaining to or causing calciokinesis.

cal·ci·ol (kal′sē-ol). SYN cholecalciferol.

cal·ci·or·rha·chia (kal′sē-ō-ra′kē-ă). The presence of calcium in the cerebrospinal fluid. [calcium + G. *rhachis,* spine + -ia]

cal·ci·o·stat (kal′sē-ō-stat). Rarely used term denoting a postulated mechanism by which the parathyroid hormone production is increased when serum calcium is low and decreased when it is high. [calcium + G. *statos,* standing]

cal·ci·o·trau·mat·ic (kal′sē-ō-traw-mat′ik). Relating to the line of disturbed calcification that appears in the dentin of the incisor teeth of young rats placed on a rachitogenic diet: high in calcium and low in phosphorus, with no vitamin D.

cal·ci·pec·tic (kal-si-pek′tik). Pertaining to calcipexis.

cal·ci·pe·nia (kal-si-pē′nē-ă). A condition in which there is an insufficient amount of calcium in the tissues and fluids of the body. [calcium + G. *penia,* poverty]

cal·ci·pe·nic (kal-si-pē′nik). Pertaining to calcipenia.

cal·ci·pex·ic (kal-si-pek′sik). Related or pertaining to calcipexis.

cal·ci·pex·is, cal·ci·pexy (kal-si-pek′sis, kal′si-pek-sē). Fixation of calcium in the tissues, as an occasional cause of tetany in infants. [calcium + G. *pēxis,* a fixing]

cal·ci·phil·ia (cal-si-fil′ē-ă). A condition in which the tissues manifest an unusual affinity for, and fixation of, calcium salts circulating in the blood. [calcium + G. *phileō,* to love]

cal·ci·phy·lax·is (kal′si-fī-lak′sis). A condition of induced systemic hypersensitivity in which tissues respond to appropriate challenging agents with a sudden, but sometimes evanescent, local calcification.

cal·ci·priv·ia (kal-si-priv′ē-ă). Absence or deprivation of calcium in diet.

cal·ci·priv·ic (kal-si-priv′ik). Deprived of calcium.

cal·cite (kal′sīt). $CaCO_3$; a naturally occurring mineral found in several forms, *e.g.,* chalk, Iceland spar, limestone, marble. SEE ALSO *calcium* carbonate. SYN calcspar.

cal·ci·tet·rol (kal-si-tet′rol). The 1,24,25-triol (thus, a 1,3,24,24-tetrol) of cholecalciferol.

cal·ci·to·nin (kal-si-tō′nin). A peptide hormone, of which eight forms in five species are known; composed of 32 amino acids and produced by the parathyroid, thyroid, and thymus glands; its action is opposite to that of parathyroid hormone in that c. increases deposition of calcium and phosphate in bone and lowers the level of calcium in the blood; its level in the blood is increased by glucagon and by Ca^{2+}, and thus opposes postprandial hypercalcemia. SYN thyrocalcitonin. [calci- + G. *tonos,* stretching, + -in]

cal·ci·tri·ol (kal-si-trī′ol). 1α,25-Dihydroxycholecalciferol (thus, a 1,3,25-triol); formation of c. is the second step in the biological conversion of vitamin D_3 to its active form; it is more potent than calcidiol.

cal·ci·tro·ic ac·id (kal-si-trō′ik). Rarely used term for a metabolite of calcitriol, involving the loss of carbons 24, 25, 26, and 27 and the oxidation of carbon 23 to a carboxylic acid; its function is unknown.

CALCIUM

cal·ci·um (Ca), gen. **cal·′cii** (kal′sē-ŭm, -sē-ī). A metallic bivalent element; atomic no. 20, atomic wt. 40.078, density 1.55, melting point 842°C. The oxide of c. is an alkaline earth, CaO, quicklime, which on the addition of water becomes c. hydrate, $Ca(OH)_2$, slaked lime. For some organic c. salts not listed below, see the name of the organic acid portion. Many c. salts have crucial uses in metabolism and in medicine. C. salts are responsible for the radiopacity of bone, calcified cartilage, and arteriosclerotic plaques in arteries. Cathode electrons are fed from their source (battery or generator); in an x-ray or cathode ray tube, contains the filament from which electrons are accelerated toward the anode by the tube voltage. Cf. anode. [Mod. L. fr. L. *calx*, lime]

c. alginate, a topical hemostatic.

c. aminosalicylate, the c. salt of *p*-aminosalicylic acid, with the same uses.

c. benzoylpas, calcium 4-benzamidosalicylate; an antituberculous agent.

c. bromide, used to meet the same indications as potassium bromide.

c. carbide, CaC_2; blackish crystalline lumps which when in contact with water yield acetylene gas.

c. carbimide, Ca=N—C≡N; a fertilizer and weed seed killer that also exhibits antithyroid activity; like disulfiram, it impairs ethanol metabolism; workers in cyanamide-producing plants exhibit systemic symptoms ("Monday-morning illness") after ingestion of alcohol. SYN c. cyanamide.

c. carbonate, $CaCO_3$; an astringent and antacid. SEE ALSO calcite. SYN chalk, creta.

c. caseinate, the form of casein present in cow's milk; used in dietetic preparations; has been used for diarrhea in infants.

c. chloride, used to correct calcium deficiencies and in the treatment of magnesium intoxication and cardiac failure.

citrated c. carbimide, a mixture of two parts citric acid to one part c. carbimide; in the metabolism of ethanol, it slows the conversion of acetaldehyde to acetate; used in the treatment of alcoholism.

crude c. sulfide, used externally in the treatment of acne, scabies, and ringworm. SYN sulfurated lime.

c. cyanamide, SYN c. carbimide.

dibasic c. phosphate, $CaHPO_4 \cdot 2H_2O$; used as a c. and phosphorus dietary supplement. SYN c. monohydrogen phosphate, secondary c. phosphate.

c. folinate, SYN *leucovorin* calcium.

c. glubionate, calcium D-gluconate lactobionate monohydrate; a calcium replenisher.

c. gluceptate, used as a nutrient. SYN c. glucoheptonate.

c. glucoheptonate, SYN c. gluceptate.

c. gluconate, a salt of c. more palatable than the chloride, sometimes used as a calcium supplement.

c. glycerophosphate, a c. and phosphorus dietary supplement.

c. hippurate, said to be a solvent of uratic gravel and calculi.

c. hydroxide, $Ca(OH)_2$; used as a carbon dioxide absorbent.

c. hypophosphite, has been used for rickets and impaired nutrition.

c. iodate, used as a dusting powder and, in lotion and ointment, as an antiseptic and deodorant.

c. iodobehenate, a c. salt, $(C_{21}H_{42}ICOO)_2Ca$, formerly used to meet the indications of the ordinary iodides.

c. ipodate, calcium salt of 3-[(dimethylaminomethylene)amino]-2,4,6-triiodohydrocinnamic acid; a radiopaque medium used in cholangiography and cholecystography.

c. lactate, used as a calcium replenisher.

c. lactophosphate, a mixture of c. lactate, c. acid lactate, and c. acid phosphate; used as a c. and phosphorus dietary supplement.

c. leucovorin, SEE *leucovorin* calcium.

c. levulinate, a hydrated c. salt of levulinic acid; it has the usual effects of c. administered orally or intravenously.

c. mandelate, c. salt of mandelic acid; a urinary anti-infective agent.

milk of c., densely calcified fluid, most often found radiographically in the gallbladder in association with chronic obstruction.

c. monohydrogen phosphate, SYN dibasic c. phosphate.

c. oxalate, CaC_2O_4; found as sediment in the urine and in urinary calculi.

c. oxide, SYN lime (1).

c. pantothenate, the c. salt of pantothenic acid; a vitamin B filtrate factor.

precipitated c. carbonate, $CaCO_3$; used as an antacid in the management of peptic ulcers and other conditions of gastric hyperacidity.

c. propionate, the c. salt of propionic acid; an antifungal agent.

racemic c. pantothenate, a mixture of the c. salts of the dextrorotatory and levorotatory isomers of pantothenic acid; same uses as c. pantothenate.

c. saccharate, c. D-saccharate; used as an antacid in dyspepsia

and flatulence, as an antidote in carbolic acid poisoning, and as a stabilizer for c. gluconate solution for parenteral administration.

secondary c. phosphate, SYN dibasic c. phosphate.

c. stearate, used in the preparation of tablets as a lubricant for tablet machinery and to keep powder mixtures flowing.

c. sulfate, CaO_4S; used in exsiccated form to make plaster of Paris. SEE ALSO gypsum.

c. sulfite, used as an intestinal antiseptic, and locally in the treatment of parasitic skin diseases.

tertiary c. phosphate, SYN tribasic c. phosphate.

tribasic c. phosphate, $Ca_3(PO_4)_2$; used as an antacid. SYN bone ash, bone phosphate, tertiary c. phosphate, tricalcium phosphate, whitlockite.

c. trisodium pentetate, SYN pentetate trisodium calcium.

---

cal·ci·um-45 (⁴⁵Ca). Most easily available of the radioactive c.-45 isotopes; beta-emitter with a half-life of 162.7 days; used as a tracer.

cal·ci·um-47 (⁴⁷Ca). A radioisotope of calcium with a half-life of 4.54 days, used in the diagnosis of disorders of calcium metabolism.

cal·ci·um group. The metals of the alkaline earths: beryllium, magnesium, calcium, strontium, barium, and radium.

cal·ci·u·ria (kal-sē-yū'rē-ă). The urinary excretion of calcium; sometimes used as a synonym for hypercalciuria.

cal·co·dyn·ia (kal-kō-din'ē-ă). SYN painful *heel*. [L. *calx*, heel, + G. *odynē,* pain]

cal·coph·or·ous (kal-kof'er-ŭs). SYN calciferous. [L. *calx,* lime, + G. *phoros,* bearing]

cal·co·sphe·rite (kal-kō-sfēr'īt). A tiny, spheroidal, concentrically laminated body containing accretive deposits of calcium salts; found most frequently in papillary carcinoma of the thyroid and ovary, and in meningioma, probably as the result of degenerative changes in the fibrovascular stroma. SYN psammoma bodies (3). [L. *calx,* lime, + G. *sphaira,* sphere]

calc·spar (kalk'spar). SYN calcite.

cal·cu·li (kal'kyū-lī). Plural of calculus.

cal·cu·lo·sis (kal-kyū-lō'sis). The tendency or disposition to form calculi or stones. [L. *calculus,* small stone, + G. *-osis,* condition]

cal·cu·lus, gen. and pl. **cal·cu·li** (kal'kyū-lŭs, -lī). A concretion formed in any part of the body, most commonly in the passages of the biliary and urinary tracts; usually composed of salts of inorganic or organic acids, or of other material such as cholesterol. SYN stone (1). [L. a pebble, a calculus]

apatite c., a c. in which the crystalloid component consists of calcium fluorophosphate.

arthritic c., SYN gouty *tophus.*

biliary c., SYN gallstone.

bladder calculi, SYN bladder *stone,* under *stone.*

blood c., an angiolith or concretion of coagulated blood. SYN hemic c.

branched c., SYN staghorn c.

bronchial c., SYN broncholith.

cerebral c., SYN encephalolith.

coral c., SYN staghorn c.

cystine c., a c. composed of cystine, soft and faintly radiopaque.

dendritic c., SYN staghorn c.

dental c., (1) calcified deposits formed around the teeth; may appear as subgingival or supragingival c.; **(2)** SYN tartar (2).

encysted c., a urinary c. enclosed in a sac developed from the wall of the bladder. SYN pocketed c.

fibrin c., a urinary c. formed largely from fibrinogen in blood.

gastric c., SYN gastrolith.

hematogenetic c., SYN serumal c. (1).

hemic c., SYN blood c.

infection c., SYN secondary renal c.

intestinal c., a concretion in the bowel, either a coprolith or an enterolith.

lacrimal c., SYN dacryolith.

mammary c., a concretion in one of the ducts of the breast.

matrix c., a yellowish-white to light tan urinary c. containing calcium salts, with the consistency of putty; composed chiefly of an organic matrix consisting of a mucoprotein and a sulfated mucopolysaccharide, and usually associated with chronic infection.

metabolic c., a stone, usually a renal stone, caused by a metabolic abnormality resulting in increased excretion of a substance of low solubility in urine, such as urate or cystine.

mulberry c., a hard smooth urinary c. composed of calcium oxalate, so-called because of its resemblance to a mulberry.

nasal c., SYN rhinolith.

nephritic c., obsolete term for renal c.

oxalate c., a hard urinary c. of calcium oxalate; some are covered with minute sharp spines that can abrade the renal pelvic epithelium, whereas others are smooth.

pancreatic c., a concretion, usually multiple, in the pancreatic duct, associated with chronic pancreatitis. SYN pancreatolith, pancreolith.

pharyngeal c., SYN pharyngolith.

pleural c., SYN pleurolith.

pocketed c., SYN encysted c.

preputial c., a c. occurring beneath the foreskin. SYN postholith.

primary renal c., a c. formed in an apparently healthy urinary tract, usually composed of oxalates, urates, or cystine.

prostatic c., a concretion formed in the prostate gland, composed chiefly of calcium carbonate and phosphate (corpora amylacea). SYN prostatolith.

pulp c., SYN endolith.

renal c., a c. occurring within the kidney collecting system. SYN nephrolith.

salivary c., (1) a c. in a salivary duct or gland; (2) SYN supragingival c.

secondary renal c., a c. associated with infection and/or obstruction, usually composed of struvite (magnesium ammonium phosphate). SYN infection c.

serumal c., (1) a greenish or dark brown calcareous deposit on the tooth, usually apical to the gingival margin; SYN hematogenetic c. (2) SYN subgingival c.

staghorn c., a c. occurring in the renal pelvis, with branches extending into the infundibula and calices. SYN branched c., coral c., dendritic c.

struvite c., a c. in which the crystalloid component consists of magnesium ammonium phosphate.

subgingival c., calcareous deposit found on the tooth apical to the gingival margin. SYN serumal c. (2).

supragingival c., calcified plaques adherent to tooth surfaces coronal to the free gingival margin. SYN salivary c. (2).

tonsillar c., SYN tonsillolith.

urethral c., a stone impacted in urethra. May have formed proximally and gotten stuck there or may have formed in urethra; uncommon.

urinary c., a c. in the kidney, ureter, bladder, or urethra. SYN urolith.

uterine c., a calcified myoma of the uterus. SYN hysterolith, uterolith.

vesical c., a urinary c. formed or retained in the bladder. SYN cystolith.

weddellite c., a c. in which the crystalloid component consists of calcium oxalate dihydrate.

whewellite c., a c. in which the crystalloid component consists of calcium oxalate monohydrate.

Cal·cu·lus Sur·face In·dex (CSI). An index that measures only dental calculus, used for evaluating new calculus formation within a large group of test subjects.

Caldani, Leopoldo M.A., Italian anatomist, 1725–1813. SEE C.'s *ligament.*

cal·des·mon (kal-des′mon). An actin-binding protein that, at low or absent calcium levels, binds to tropomyosin and actin and prevents myosin binding. [calcium + G. *desmos*, bond, fr. *deō*, to bind]

Caldwell, Eugene W., U.S. radiologist, 1870–1918. SEE C. *projection, view.*

Caldwell, George W., U.S. physician, 1834–1918. SEE C.-Luc *operation.*

Caldwell, William E., U.S. obstetrician, 1880–1943. SEE C.-Moloy *classification.*

Caldwell pro·jec·tion. See under projection.

Caldwell view. See under view.

cal·e·fa·cient (kal-ĕ-fā′shent). **1.** Making warm or hot. **2.** An agent causing a sense of warmth in the part to which it is applied. [L. *calefacio,* fr. *caleo,* to be warm, + *facio,* to make]

calf, pl. **calves** (kaf, kavz). **1.** SYN sural *region.* **2.** A young bovine animal, male or female. [Gael. *kalpa*]

bulldog c., a c. with a short muzzle and brachycephalic skull, usually resulting from chondrodystrophy; associated with this condition are shortened limbs and anomalies of the vertebral centra; it often results in respiratory and feeding difficulties, and is sometimes fatal. SYN bovine achondroplasia.

football c., an obsolete term used to describe the doughy sensation elicited on palpation of the c. when muscle necrosis has developed as a consequence of acute ischemia produced by acute arterial embolism.

gnome's c., an obsolete term denoting the very full rounded c. occurring in pseudohypertrophic muscular dystrophy affecting the gastrocnemius muscles.

calf-bone. 1. SYN fibula. **2.** Bone from a calf (young cow) used in orthopaedic reconstruction.

cal·i·ber (kal′i-ber). The diameter of a hollow tubular structure. [Fr. *calibre,* of uncert. etym.]

cal·i·brate (kal′i-brāt). **1.** To graduate or standardize any measuring instrument. **2.** To measure the diameter of a tubular structure.

cal·i·bra·tion (kal-i-brā′shŭn). The act of standardizing or calibrating an instrument or laboratory procedure.

cal·i·bra·tor (kal′ĭ-brā-ter, -tōr). A standard or reference material or substance used to standardize or calibrate an instrument or laboratory procedure.

cal·i·ce·al (kal′i-se′al). Relating to the calix. SYN calyceal.

cal·i·cec·ta·sis (kal-i-sek′tă-sis). SYN caliectasis. [calix + G. *ektasis,* dilation]

cal·i·cec·to·my (kal-i-sek′tō-mē). SYN calicotomy. [calix, + G. *ektomē,* excision]

ca·li·ces (kal′i-sēz). Plural of calix.

ca·lic·i·form (kă-lis′i-fōrm). Shaped like a cup or goblet. SYN calyciform. [L. *calix* + *forma,* form]

cal·i·cine (kal′i-sēn). Of the nature of, or resembling a calix. SYN calycine.

Cal·i·ci·vi·ri·dae (kal′i-sē-vī′ră-dā). A family of naked icosahedral single-stranded positive sense RNA viruses 35–40 nm in diameter associated with epidemic viral gastroenteritis and certain forms of hepatitis in man.

Ca·lic·i·vi·rus (kă-lis′i-vī′rŭs). A genus in the family Caliciviridae that is associated with gastroenteritis. SEE Norwalk *agent.* [G. *kalyx,* cup, + virus]

ca·li·co·plas·ty (kă′lĭ-sō-plas-tē). SYN calioplasty. [calix, + G. *plastos,* formed]

ca

cal·i·cot·o·my (kal-ĭ-sot'ō-mē). Incision into a calix, usually for removal of a calculus. SYN calicectomy, caliotomy. [calix, + G. *tomē,* a cutting]

ca·lic·u·lus, pl. **ca·lic·u·li** (kă-lik'yū-lŭs, lī). A bud-shaped or cup-shaped structure, resembling the closed calyx of a flower. SYN calycle, calyculus. [L. dim. from G. *kalyx,* the cup of a flower]

c. gustato'rius [NA], SYN taste *bud.*

c. ophthal'micus, SYN optic *cup.*

ca·li·ec·ta·sis (kā-lē-ek'tă-sis). Dilation of the calices, usually due to obstruction or infection. SYN caliectasis, pyelocaliectasis.

cal·i·for·ni·um (Cf) (kal-i-fōr'nē-ŭm). An artificial transuranium element, symbol Cf, atomic no.˙98, atomic wt. 251.08 half-life of ^{251}Cf (the most stable known isotope) is 900 years. [*California,* state and university where first prepared]

ca·li·o·plas·ty (kā'lē-ō-plas-tē). Surgical reconstruction of a calix, usually designed to increase its lumen at the infundibulum. SYN calicoplasty.

ca·li·or·rha·phy (kā'lē-ōr-a-fē). **1.** Suturing of a calix. **2.** Plastic surgery of a dilated or obstructed calix to improve urinary drainage, often requiring combination of two or more calices or the massive movement of pelvic mucosa to rebuild the caliceal drainage system. [calix, + G. *rhaphē,* suture, seam]

ca·li·ot·o·my (kā-lē-ot'ō-mē). SYN calicotomy.

cal·i·pers (kal'i-perz). An instrument used for measuring diameters. [a corruption of *caliber*]

cal·is·then·ics (kal-is-then'iks). Systematic practice of various exercises with the object of preserving health and increasing physical strength. [G. *kalos,* beautiful, + *sthenos,* strength]

ca·lix, pl. **ca·li·ces** (kā'liks, kal'i-sēz) [NA]. A flower-shaped or funnel-shaped structure; specifically one of the branches or recesses of the pelvis of the kidney into which the orifices of the malpighian renal pyramids project. SYN calyx. [L. fr. G. *kalyx,* the cup of a flower]

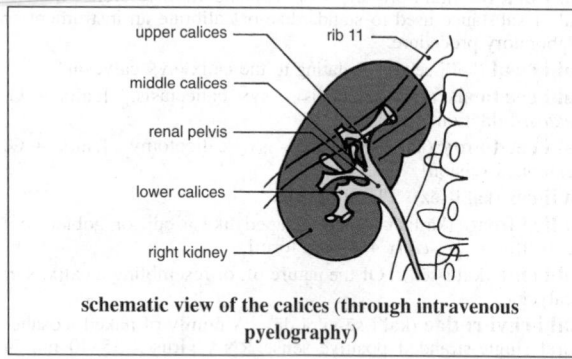

schematic view of the calices (through intravenous pyelography)

major calices, the primary subdivisions of the renal pelvis, usually two or three in number. SYN calices renales majores [NA].

minor calices, the subdivisions of the major calices, varying in number from 7 to 13, which receive the renal papillae. SYN calices renales minores [NA].

calices rena'les majo'res [NA], SYN major calices.

calices rena'les mino'res [NA], SYN minor calices.

Calkins, Leroy Adelbert, U.S. obstetrician-gynecologist, 1894–1960. SEE C.'s *sign.*

Call, Friedrich von, Austrian physician, 1844–1917. SEE C.-Exner *bodies,* under *body.*

Callahan, John R., U.S. endodontist, 1853–1918. SEE C.'s *method.*

Callander, Latimer, San Francisco surgeon, 1892–1947. SEE C.'s *amputation.*

Calleja (Calleja y Sanchez), Camilo, Spanish anatomist, †1913. SEE *islands* of C., under *island.*

Cal·liph·o·ra (kă-lif'ō-ră). A genus of blowflies (family Calliphoridae, order Diptera), the bluebottle flies, the larvae of which feed on dead flesh. *C. vomitoria* and *C. vicina* are common species in the U.S. [G. *kalli,* beauty, + *phoros,* bearing]

Callison, James S., U.S. physician, *1873. SEE C.'s *fluid.*

Cal·li·tro·ga (kal-i-trō'gă). Former name for *Cochliomyia.*

cal·lo·sal (ka-lō'săl). Relating to the corpus callosum.

cal·lose (kal'ōs). A 1,3-β-D-glucan formed by certain enzymes from UDP-glucose, differing from cellulose (a β-1,4-glucan formed from GDP-glucose) and starch amylose (an α-1,4-glucan formed from ADP-glucose).

cal·los·i·tas (ka-los'i-tas). SYN callosity.

cal·los·i·ty (ka-los'i-tē). A circumscribed thickening of the keratin layer of the epidermis as a result of repeated friction or intermittent pressure. SYN callositas, callus (1), keratoma (1), poroma (1), tyle, tyloma. [L. fr. *callosus,* thick-skinned]

cal·lo·so·mar·gin·al (ka-lō'sō-mar'jin-ăl). Relating to the corpus callosum and the cingulate gyrus; denoting the sulcus between them.

cal·lous (kal'ŭs). Relating to a callus or callosity.

cal·lus (kal'ŭs). **1.** SYN callosity. **2.** A composite mass of tissue that forms at a fracture site to establish continuity between the bone ends; it is composed initially of uncallused fibrous tissue and cartilage, and ultimately of bone. [L. hard skin]

central c., the c. within the medullary cavity of a fractured bone. SYN medullary c.

definitive c., the c. which has become converted into osseous tissue. SYN permanent c.

ensheathing c., the mass of c. around the outside of the fractured bone.

medullary c., SYN central c.

permanent c., SYN definitive c.

provisional c., the c. that develops to keep the ends of the fractured bone in apposition; it is absorbed after union is complete. SYN temporary c.

temporary c., SYN provisional c.

calm·a·tive (kahl'mă-tiv). Calming, quieting; allaying excitement; denoting such an agent.

Calmette, Leon A., French bacteriologist, 1863–1933. SEE Bacille bilié de C.-Guérin; bacillus C. *vaccine;* C. *test;* C.-Guérin *bacillus, vaccine.*

cal·mod·u·lin (kal-mod'yū-lin). A ubiquitous eukaryotic protein that binds calcium ions, thereby becoming the agent for many of the cellular effects long ascribed to calcium ions. This calcium-protein complex binds to the apoenzyme, to form the holoenzyme, of certain phosphodiesterases; through these, or other as yet unknown mechanisms, the complex regulates adenylate and guanylate cyclases, many kinases, phospholipase A_2 activity, and other basic cellular functions. [*calcium* + *modul*ate]

cal·o·mel (kal'ō-mel). HgCl; mild mercury chloride; mercury monochloride, protochloride, or subchloride; has been used as an intestinal antiseptic and laxative; replaced by safer agents. SYN mercurous chloride, sweet precipitate. [Mediev. L., fr. G. *kalos,* beutiful, + *melas,* black]

vegetable c., SYN podophyllum.

ca·lor (kā'lōr). Heat, as one of the four signs of inflammation (c., rubor, tumor, dolor) enunciated by Celsus. [L.]

Calori, Luigi, Italian anatomist, 1807–1896. SEE C.'s *bursa.*

ca·lor·ic (kă-lōr'ik). **1.** Relating to a calorie. **2.** Relating to heat. [L. *calor,* heat]

c. intake, the total number of calories in a daily diet allocation.

cal·o·rie (kal'ō-rē). A unit of heat content or energy. The amount of heat necessary to raise 1 g of water from 14.5°C to 15.5°C (small c.). Calorie is being replaced by joule, the SI unit equal to 0.239 calorie. SEE ALSO British thermal *unit.* SYN calory. [L. *calor,* heat]

gram c., SYN small c.

kilogram c. (kcal), SYN large c.

large c. (Cal, C), the quantity of energy required to raise the temperature of 1 kg of water 1°C, more precisely from 14.5° to 15.5°C; it is 1000 times the value of the small c.; used in measurements of the heat production of chemical reactions, including those involved in biology. SYN kilocalorie, kilogram c.

mean c., one hundredth of the energy required to raise the temperature of 1 g of water from 0°C to 100°C.

small c. (cal, c), the quantity of energy required to raise the temperature of 1 g of water 1°C, or from 14.5°C to 15.5°C in the case of normal or standard c. SYN gram c.

cal·o·rif·ic (cal-ŏ-rif′ik). Producing heat. [L. *calor,* heat]

ca·lor·i·gen·ic (kă-lōr-i-jen′ik). **1.** Capable of generating heat. **2.** Stimulating metabolic production of heat. SYN thermogenetic (2), thermogenic. [L. *calor,* heat, + G. *genesis,* production]

cal·o·rim·e·ter (kal-ō-rim′ĕ-ter). An apparatus for measuring the amount of heat liberated in a chemical reaction. [L. *calor,* heat, + G. *metron,* measure]

Benedict-Roth c., SEE Benedict-Roth *apparatus.*

bomb c., an instrument for determining the potential energy of organic substances, including those in foods. It consists of a hollow steel container, lined with platinum and filled with pure oxygen, into which a weighed quantity of substance is placed and ignited with an electric fuse; the heat produced is absorbed by water surrounding the bomb and, from the rise in temperature, the calories liberated are calculated.

cal·o·ri·met·ric (kă′lōr-i-met′rik). Relating to calorimetry.

cal·o·rim·e·try (kal-ō-rim′ĕ-trē). Measurement of the amount of heat given off by a reaction or group of reactions (as by an organism).

direct c., measurement of the heat produced by a reaction, as distinguished from indirect methods, which involve measurement of something other than heat production itself.

indirect c., determination of heat production of an oxidation reaction by measuring uptake of oxygen and/or liberation of carbon dioxide and nitrogen excretion, and then calculating the amount of heat produced.

ca·lor·i·tro·pic (kă-lōr′i-trop′ik). Relating to thermotropism.

cal·o·ry (kal′ō-rē). SYN calorie.

Calot, Jean-François, French surgeon, 1861–1944. SEE C.'s *triangle.*

cal·pains (kal′pāns). Calcium-dependent proteinases. [calcium + suffix *-pain,* protease, fr. *papain*]

cal·se·ques·trin (kal′sē-kwes′trin). A calcium-binding protein found in the interior of sarcoplasmic reticulum vesicles. [calcium + sequester + -in]

ca·lum·ba (kă-lŭm′bă). The dried root of *Jateorrhiza palmata* (family Menispermaceae), a tall climbing vine of east Africa; used as a bitter tonic.

ca·lum·bin (kal′ŭm-bin). $C_{21}H_{24}O_7$; an amaroid from calumba that accounts for the bitterness of the crude drug.

cal·u·ster·one (kal-yū′stĕ-rōn). 17β,17α-dimethyltestosterone; an antineoplastic agent.

cal·var·ia, pl. **cal·var·i·ae** (kal-vā′rē-ă, -vā′rē-ē) [NA]. The upper domelike portion of the skull. SYN roof of skull, skullcap. [L. a skull]

cal·var·i·al (kal-vār′ē-ăl). Relating to the skullcap.

cal·var·i·um (kal-vār′ē-ŭm). Incorrectly used for calvaria.

Calvé, Jacques, French orthopedic surgeon, 1875–1954. SEE C.-Perthes *disease;* Legg-C.-Perthes *disease.*

cal·vi·ti·es (kal-vish′e-ēz). SYN alopecia. [L. fr. *calvus,* bald]

calx, gen. **cal·cis,** pl. **cal·ces** (kalks, kal′sis, kal-sēs). **1.** SYN lime (1). [L. limestone] **2.** The posterior rounded extremity of the foot. SYN calcar pedis, heel (1). [L. heel]

cal·y·ce·al (kal′i-se′ăl). SYN caliceal.

ca·ly·ces (kal′i-sēz). Plural of calyx.

ca·lyc·i·form (kă-lis′i-fōrm). SYN caliciform.

ca·ly·cine (kal′i-sēn). SYN calicine.

ca·ly·cle, ca·lyc·u·lus (kal′i-kl, kă-lik′yū-lŭs). SYN caliculus.

Ca·lym·ma·to·bac·te·ri·um (kă-lim′mă-tō-bak-tēr′ē-ŭm). A genus of nonmotile bacteria (of uncertain taxonomic classification) containing Gram-negative, pleomorphic rods with single or bipolar condensations of chromatin; cells occur singly and in clusters. Outside of the human body, growth occurs only in the yolk sac or amniotic fluid of a developing chick embryo or in a medium containing embryonic yolk; the organisms are pathogenic only

for man. The type species is *C. granulomatis.* [G. *kalymma,* hood, veil, + *baktērion,* rod]

C. granulo′matis, a species causing granulomatous lesions (donovanosis) in man, particularly in the inguinal region (granuloma inguinale); the type species of the genus *C.*

ca·lyx, pl. **ca·ly·ces** (kā′liks, kal′i-sēz). SYN calix. [G. cup of a flower]

CAM Abbreviation for cell adhesion *molecule.*

cam·ben·da·zole (kam-ben′dah-zōl). Isopropyl 2-(4-triazolyl)-5-benzimidazolecarbamate; a anthelmintic.

cam·bi·um (kam′bē-ŭm). The inner layer of the periosteum in membranous ossification. [L. exchange]

cam·el·pox (kam′el-poks). A severe generalized disease of camels in northern Africa and southwestern Asia caused by the camelpox virus and characterized by extensive skin lesions.

cam·era, pl. **cam·er·ae, cam·er·as** (kam′er-ă, -ē). **1.** A closed box; especially one containing a lens, shutter, and light-sensitive film or plates for photography. **2** [NA]. In anatomy, any chamber or cavity, such as one of the chambers of the heart, or eye. [L. a vault]

Anger c., a scintigraphic imaging system or type of gamma camera; employing a single thin crystal and multiple photodetecting circuits, that views the entire field at once and is most effective in the 100- to 511-keV energy range.

c. ante′rior bul′bi [NA], SYN anterior *chamber* of eye.

gamma c., any one of several scintigraphic cameras that records simultaneously counts from the entire operative field of view. SYN scintillation c.

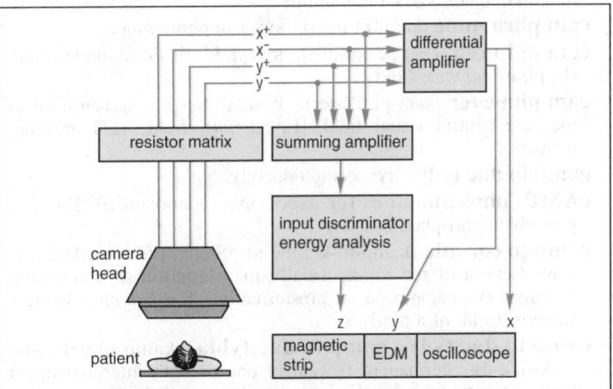

gamma camera (Anger camera) function
coordinate signals of only one photomultiplier are represented (EDM electronic data management)

multiformat c., photographic or laser printer for recording a variable number of video images on a sheet of film, as in computed tomography or ultrasound.

c. oc′uli ante′rior, SYN anterior *chamber* of eye.

c. oc′uli ma′jor, SYN anterior *chamber* of eye.

c. oc′uli mi′nor, SYN posterior *chamber* of eye.

c. oc′uli poste′rior, SYN posterior *chamber* of eye.

c. poste′rior bul′bi [NA], SYN posterior *chamber* of eye.

retinal c., an instrument for photographing the ocular fundus.

scintillation c., SYN gamma c.

c. vi′trea bul′bi [NA], SYN posterior *segment* of eyeball.

vitreous c., SYN posterior *segment* of eyeball.

cam·er·o·stome (kam′er-ō-stōm). Ventral depression of the anterior cephalothorax of soft ticks (family Argasidae) in which the mouthparts (capitulum) lie. [L. *camera,* a vault, + G. *stoma,* mouth]

cam·i·sole (kam′i-sōl). SYN straitjacket.

cam·o·mile (kam′ō-mil). SYN chamomile.

cAMP Abbreviation for adenosine 3′,5′-cyclic monophosphate (cyclic AMP).

Campbell, Meredith F., 20th century U.S. pediatric urologist. SEE C. *sound*.

Campbell, William F., U.S. surgeon, 1867–1926. SEE C.'s *ligament*.

Camper, Pieter, Dutch physician and anatomist, 1722–1789. SEE C.'s *chiasm, fascia, ligament, line, plane*.

cam·phene (kam'fēn). 2,2-Dimethyl-3-methylenenorbornane; a terpenoid occurring in many essential oils, *e.g.,* turpentine, camphor, citronella.

cam·phor (kam'fōr). 1,7,7-Trimethylbicyclo[2.2.1]heptan-2-one; a ketone distilled from the bark and wood of *Cinnamonum camphora,* an evergreen tree of Southeast Asia and the adjoining islands, and also prepared synthetically from oil of turpentine; used in a variety of commercial products and as a topical anti-infective and antipruritic agent. [mediev. L., fr. Ar. *kāfure*]

   cantharis c., SYN cantharidin.

   c. liniment, a mixture of camphor and cottonseed oil, or camphor and arachis oil; a mild counterirritant. SYN camphorated oil.

   monobromated c., obsolete term for an antispasmodic, soporific, and sedative.

   tar c., SYN naphthalene.

   thyme c., SYN thymol.

cam·pho·ra·ceous (kam-fō-rā'shŭs). Resembling camphor in appearance or odor.

cam·phor·at·ed (kam'fō-rā-ted). Containing camphor.

cam·phor·at·ed oil. SYN *camphor* liniment.

cam·pho·ta·mide (kam-fō'tă-mīd). 3-Diethylcarbamoyl-1-methylpyridinium camphorsulfonate; an analeptic and antianginal agent. SYN camphramine.

cam·phra·mine (kam'fră-mēn). SYN camphotamide.

cam·pi fo·re·li (kam'pē fōr-el'ē). SYN *fields* of Forel, under *field*. [L. pl. of *campus,* field]

cam·pim·e·ter (kam-pim'ĕ-ter). A small tangent screen used to measure central visual field. [L. *campus,* field, + G. *metron,* measure]

camp·lo·dac·ty·ly. SYN camptodactyly.

cAMP phos·pho·di·es·ter·ase. SYN adenosine 3',5'-cyclic phosphate phosphodiesterase.

camp·to·cor·mia (kamp-tō-kōr'mē-ă). Static, often marked forward flexion of the trunk; usually manifestation of conversion reaction. SYN camptospasm, prosternation. [G. *kamptos,* bent, + *kormos,* trunk of a tree]

camp·to·dac·ty·ly, camp·to·dac·tyl·ia (kamp-tō-dak'ti-lē, -dak-til'ē-ă). Permanent flexion of one or both interphalangeal joints of one or more fingers, usually the little finger; often congenital in origin. SYN camplodactyly, streblodactyly. [G. *kamptos,* bent, + *daktylos,* finger]

camp·to·me·lia (kamp-tō-mē'lē-ă). A skeletal dysplasia characterized by a bending of the long bones of the extremities, resulting in a permanent bowing or curvature of the affected part. [G. *kamptos,* bent, + *melos,* limb]

camp·to·mel·ic (kamp-tō-mel'ik). Denoting or characteristic of camptomelia. SEE camptomelic *syndrome*.

camp·to·spasm (kamp'tō-spazm). SYN camptocormia.

Cam·py·lo·bac·ter (kam'pi-lō-bak'ter). A genus of bacteria containing Gram-negative, nonspore-forming, spirally curved rods with a single polar flagellum at one or both ends of the cell; they are motile with a characteristic corkscrew-like motion. The type species is *C. fetus.* [G. *campylos,* curved, + *baktron,* staff or rod]

   C. fe'tus, a species that contains various subspecies which can cause human infections as well as abortion in sheep and cattle; it is the type species of the genus *C.*

   C. fetus subsp. *jejuni,* former name for *C. jejuni.*

   C. fetus subsp. venerealis, a subspecies causing a venereal disease of cattle characterized by infertility and early embryonic death.

   C. jejuni, a species that causes in man an acute gastroenteritis of sudden onset with constitutional symptoms (malaise, myalgia, arthralgia, and headache) and cramping abdominal pain; potential sources of human infection include poultry, cattle, sheep, pigs, and dogs. This species also causes abortion in sheep.

   C. pylori, SYN *Helicobacter pylori.*

   C. sputo'rum, a species found in the genital tract of sheep and cattle and in the gingival crevice of man.

cam·py·lo·bac·ter·i·o·sis (kam'pi-lō-bak'ter-ē-ō'sis). Infection caused by microaerophilic bacteria of the genus *Campylobacter.*

ca·myl·o·fine (kă-mil'ō-fin). *N*-[2-(diethylamino)ethyl]-2-phenylglycine isopentyl ester; an anticholinergic agent.

Canada, Wilma J., U.S. radiologist. SEE Cronkhite-C. *syndrome.*

can·a·dine (kan'ă-dēn). $C_{20}H_{21}NO_4$; tetrahydroberberine; an alkaloid present in *Hydrastis canadensis* (family Ranunculaceae) and in *Corydalis cava* (family Fumaraceae) with sedative and muscle relaxant properties. SYN xanthopuccine.

CANAL

---

ca·nal (kă-nal'). A duct or channel; a tubular structure. A canal or channel. SEE ALSO canal, duct. SYN canalis [NA]. [L. *canalis*]

abdominal c., SYN inguinal c.

accessory c., a channel leading from the root pulp laterally through the dentin to the periodontal tissue; may be found anywhere in the tooth root, but is more common in the apical third of the root. SYN lateral c.

adductor c., the space in middle third of the thigh between the vastus medialis and adductor muscles, converted into a canal by the overlying sartorius muscle. It gives passage to the femoral vessels and saphenous nerve, ending at the adductor hiatus. SYN canalis adductorius [NA], Hunter's c., subsartorial c.

Alcock's c., SYN pudendal c.

alimentary c., SYN digestive *tract.*

alveolar c.'s, canals in the body of the maxilla that transmit nerves and vessels from the alveolar foramina to the maxillary teeth. SYN canales alveolares [NA], alveolodental c.'s, dental c.'s.

alveolodental c.'s, SYN alveolar c.'s.

anal c., the terminal portion of the alimentary canal; it extends from the pelvic diaphragm to the anal orifice. SYN canalis analis [NA].

anterior condyloid c. of occipital bone, SYN hypoglossal c.

anterior semicircular c.'s, SEE bony semicircular c.'s.

archenteric c., invagination of the blastopore into the notochordal process to form a cavity. SEE neurenteric c. SYN notochordal c.

Arnold's c., SYN *hiatus* of canal of lesser petrosal nerve.

arterial c., SYN *ductus* arteriosus.

atrioventricular c., the c. in the embryonic heart leading from the common sinuatrial chamber to the ventricle.

auditory c., SYN external acoustic *meatus.*

basipharyngeal c., SYN vomerovaginal c.

Bernard's c., SYN accessory pancreatic *duct.*

Bichat's c., SYN *cistern* of great cerebral vein.

birth c., cavity of the uterus and vagina through which the fetus passes. SYN parturient c.

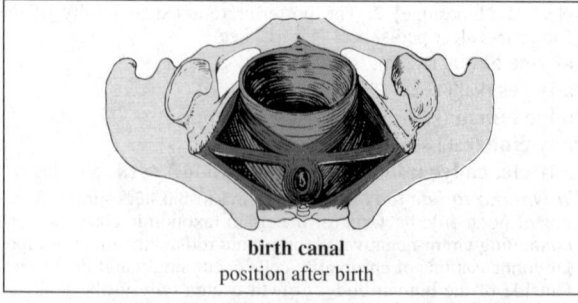

birth canal
position after birth

blastoporic c., obsolete term for primitive *pit.*

bony semicircular c.'s, the three bony tubes in the labyrinth of the ear within which the membranous semicircular ducts are located; they lie in planes at right angles to each other and are known as anterior semicircular canal, posterior semicircular canal, and lateral semicircular canal. SYN canales semicirculares ossei [NA].

Böttcher's c., SYN utriculosaccular *duct.*

Braune's c., the parturient c. formed by the uterine cavity, dilated cervix, vagina, and vulva.

Breschet's c.'s, SYN diploic c.'s.

carotid c., a passage through the petrous part of the temporal bone from its inferior surface upward, medially, and forward to the apex where it opens into the foramen lacerum. It transmits the internal carotid artery and plexuses of veins and autonomic nerves. SYN canalis caroticus [NA].

carpal c., (1) SYN carpal *tunnel.* **(2)** SYN carpal *groove.*

caudal c., the space occupied by the sacral extension of the epidural space.

central c., the ependyma-lined lumen (cavity) of the neural tube, the cerebral part of which remains patent to form the ventricles of the brain, while the spinal part in the adult often is reduced to a solid strand of modified ependyma. SYN canalis centralis medullae spinalis [NA], central c. of spinal cord, tubus medullaris. SYN syringocele (1).

central c.'s of cochlea, SYN longitudinal c.'s of modiolus.

central c. of spinal cord, SYN central c.

central c. of the vitreous, SYN hyaloid c.

cervical c., a fusiform canal extending from the isthmus of the uterus to the opening of the uterus into the vagina. SYN canalis cervicis uteri [NA].

cervical axillary c., c. through which the subclavian vessels and brachial vessels reach the upper extremities (or extremity).

cervicoaxillary c., superior opening to the axilla, bounded by clavicle anteriorly, scapula posteriorly and first rib medically. Axillary vessels and brachial plexus are transmitted.

ciliary c.'s, SYN *spaces* of iridocorneal angle, under *space.*

Civinini's c., SYN anterior *canaliculus* of chorda tympani.

Cloquet's c., SYN hyaloid c.

cochlear c., the winding tube of the bony labyrinth which makes two and a half turns about the modiolus of the cochlea; it is divided incompletely into two compartments by a winding shelf of bone, the bony spiral lamina. SYN canalis spiralis cochleae [NA], Rosenthal's c., spiral c. of cochlea.

condylar c., condyloid c., the inconstant opening through the occipital bone posterior to the condyle on each side that transmits the occipital emissary vein. SYN canalis condylaris [NA], posterior condyloid foramen.

Corti's c., SYN Corti's *tunnel.*

Cotunnius' c., SYN *aqueduct* of vestibule.

craniopharyngeal c., SYN pituitary *diverticulum.*

deferent c., SYN *ductus* deferens.

dental c.'s, SYN alveolar c.'s.

dentinal c.'s, SYN *canaliculi* dentales, under *canaliculus.*

diploic c.'s, channels in the diploë that accommodate the diploic veins. SYN canales diploici [NA], Breschet's c.'s.

Dorello's c., a bony c. sometimes found at the tip of the temporal bone enclosing the abducens nerve and inferior petrosal sinus as these two structures enter the cavernous sinus.

Dupuytren's c., SYN diploic *vein.*

endodermal c., SYN primitive *gut.*

facial c., the bony passage in the temporal bone through which the facial nerve passes; the facial c. commences at the internal auditory meatus with the horizontal part which passes at first anteriorly (medial crus of facial canal) then turns posteriorly at the geniculum of the facial c. to pass medial to the tympanic cavity (lateral crus of facial canal); finally, it turns downward (descending part of facial canal) to reach the stylomastoid foramen. SYN canalis nervi facialis [NA], aqueductus fallopii, fallopian aqueduct, fallopian c.

fallopian c., SYN facial c.

femoral c., the medial compartment of the femoral sheath. SYN canalis femoralis [NA].

Ferrein's c., SYN rivus lacrimalis.

Fontana's c., SYN *sinus* venosus sclerae.

galactophorous c.'s, SYN lactiferous *ducts,* under *duct.*

Gartner's c., SYN longitudinal *duct* of epoöphoron.

gastric c., furrow formed temporarily between longitudinal rugae of the gastric mucosa along the lesser curvature during swallowing; observed radiographically and endoscopically, it is formed because of the firm attachment of the gastric mucosa to the muscular layer, which is devoid of an oblique layer at this site; said to form a passageway favored by saliva and small quantities of masticated food and other fluids as they flow from cardia to gastroduodenal junction. SYN canalis gastricus [NA], canalis gastrici, magenstrasse.

greater palatine c., the c. formed between the maxilla and palatine bones; it transmits the descending palatine artery and the greater palatine nerve. SYN canalis palatinus major [NA], pterygopalatine c.

gubernacular c., a small c. located between the permanent tooth germ and the apex of the deciduous tooth, containing remnants of dental lamina and connective tissue.

c. of Guyon, passageway through the transverse carpal ligament by which the ulnar nerve and artery enter the palm; it is closely related to the pisiform and the hook of the hamate.

gynecophoric c., a ventral groove running the length of male schistosome flukes, into which the threadlike female worm fits.

Hannover's c., the potential space between the ciliary zonule and the vitreous body.

haversian c.'s, vascular c.'s that run longitudinally in the center of haversian systems of compact osseous tissue. SYN Leeuwenhoek's c.'s.

Hensen's c., SYN uniting *duct.*

c. of Hering, SYN cholangiole.

Hirschfeld's c.'s, SYN interdental c.'s.

Holmgrén-Golgi c.'s, SYN Golgi *apparatus.*

c. of Hovius, an anastomotic circle between the anterior twigs of the venae vorticosae in the eyes of some animals, but not in normal human eyes.

Hoyer's c.'s, SYN Sucquet-Hoyer c.'s.

Huguier's c., SYN anterior *canaliculus* of chorda tympani.

Hunter's c., SYN adductor c.

hyaloid c., a minute canal running through the vitreous from the discus nervi optici to the lens, containing in fetal life a prolongation of the central artery of the retina, the hyaloid artery. SEE vitreous, hyaloid *artery.* SYN canalis hyaloideus [NA], central c. of the vitreous, Cloquet's c., Stilling's c.

hypoglossal c., the canal through which the hypoglossal nerve emerges from the skull. SYN canalis hypoglossalis [NA], anterior condyloid c. of occipital bone, anterior condyloid foramen.

incisive c., incisor c., one of several bony canals leading from the floor of the nasal cavity into the incisive fossa on the palatal surface of the maxilla; they convey the nasopalatine nerves and branches of the greater palatine arteries which anastomose with the septal branch of the sphenopalatine artery. SYN canalis incisivus [NA].

inferior dental c., SYN mandibular c.

infraorbital c., a canal running beneath the orbital margin of the maxilla from the infraorbital groove, in the floor of the orbit, to the infraorbital foramen; it transmits the infraorbital artery and nerve. SYN canalis infraorbitalis [NA].

inguinal c., the obliquely directed passage through the layers of the lower abdominal wall that transmits the spermatic cord in the male and the round ligament in the female. SYN canalis inguinalis [NA], abdominal c., Velpeau's c.

interdental c.'s, c.'s that extend vertically through alveolar bone between roots of mandibular and maxillary incisor and maxillary bicuspid teeth. SYN Hirschfeld's c.'s.

interfacial c.'s, intercellular spaces occurring in relation to intercellular attachments by desmosomes in stratified squamous epithelium, generally resulting from shrinkage of an artifact of fixation.

Jacobson's c., SYN tympanic *canaliculus.*

Kürsteiner's c.'s, Küersteiner's c.'s, a fetal complex of vesicular, canalicular, and glandlike structures derived from parathyroid, thymus, or thymic cord; they are rudimentary and functionless unless persistent postnatally, when they may occur as cystic structures in the vicinity of parathyroid III and thymus III. Kürsteiner described three types, type II c.'s being associated with thyroaplasia.

lateral c., SYN accessory c.

lateral semicircular c.'s, SEE bony semicircular c.'s.

Laurer's c., a tube originating on the surface of the ootype of trematodes, directed dorsally to or near the surface; it may have originally served as a vagina or possibly as a reservoir of excess shell material.

Lauth's c., SYN *sinus* venosus sclerae.

Leeuwenhoek's c.'s, SYN haversian c.'s.

c.'s for lesser palatine nerves, c.'s located in the posterior part of the palatine bone. SYN canales palatini minores [NA].

longitudinal c.'s of modiolus, centrally placed channels that convey vessels and nerves to the apical turns of the cochlea. SYN canales longitudinales modioli [NA], central c.'s of cochlea.

Löwenberg's c., SYN cochlear *duct*.

mandibular c., the canal within the mandible that transmits the inferior alveolar nerve and vessels. Its posterior opening is the mandibular foramen. SYN canalis mandibulae [NA], inferior dental c.

marrow c., SYN root c. of tooth.

mental c., SYN mental *foramen*.

musculotubal c., a canal beginning at the anterior border of the petrous portion of the temporal bone near its junction with the squamous portion, and passing to the tympanic cavity; it is divided by the cochleariform process into two semicanals: one for the auditory (eustachian) tube, the other for the tensor tympani muscle. SYN canalis musculotubarius [NA].

nasolacrimal c., the bony canal formed by the maxilla, lacrimal bone, and inferior concha that transmits the nasolacrimal duct from the orbit to the inferior meatus of the nose. SYN canalis nasolacrimalis [NA].

neural c., the c. within the embryonic neural tube; the primordium of the central c.

neurenteric c., a transitory communication between the neural tube, notochordal canal, and gut endoderm in vertebrate embryos, including humans.

notochordal c., SYN archenteric c.

c. of Nuck, SEE *processus* vaginalis of peritoneum.

nutrient c., a canal in the shaft of a long bone or in other locations in irregular bones through which the nutrient artery enters a bone. SYN canalis nutricius [NA].

obturator c., the opening in the superior part of the obturator membrane through which the obturator nerve and vessels pass from the pelvic cavity into the thigh. SYN canalis obturatorius [NA].

optic c., the short canal through the lesser wing of the sphenoid bone at the apex of the orbit that gives passage to the optic nerve and the ophthalmic artery. SYN canalis opticus [NA], foramen opticum, optic foramen.

palatovaginal c., SYN pharyngeal c.

parturient c., SYN birth c.

pelvic c., the passage from the superior to the inferior aperture of the pelvis.

pericardioperitoneal c., the portion of the embryonic celom that joins the pericardial cavity to the peritoneal cavity, developing into the pleural cavities. SYN pleural c.

persistent atrioventricular c., a condition that is caused when the atrial and ventricular septa fail to meet, as in normal development, resulting in a low atrial and high ventricular septal defect or a common atrioventricular c. SYN endocardial cushion defect.

Petit's c.'s, SYN zonular *spaces*, under *space*.

pharyngeal c., on the undersurface of the vaginal process of the sphenoid bone, a furrow that is converted into a canal by the sphenoidal process of the palatine bone; it transmits the pharyngeal branch of the maxillary artery and the pharyngeal nerve from the pterygopalatine ganglion. SYN canalis palatovaginalis [NA], palatovaginal c.

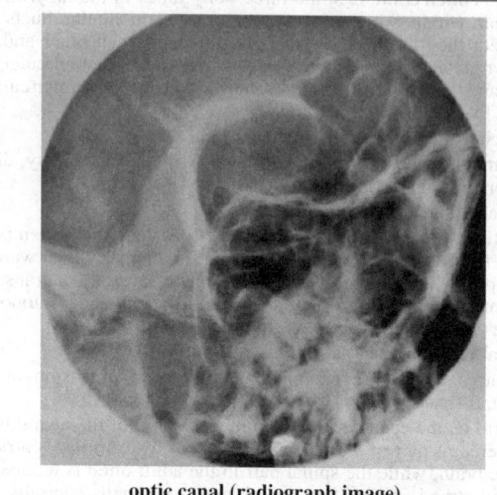

optic canal (radiograph image)

pleural c., SYN pericardioperitoneal c.

pleuropericardial c.'s, in the embryo, spaces or channels, one on each side, connecting the pericardial and pleural cavities.

pleuroperitoneal c., the communication between the embryonic pleural and peritoneal cavities.

portal c.'s, connective tissue spaces in the substance of the liver that are occupied by preterminal ramifications of the bile ducts, portal vein, and hepatic artery, as well as nerves and lymphatics.

posterior semicircular c.'s, SEE bony semicircular c.'s.

pterygoid c., an opening through the base of the medial pterygoid process of the sphenoid bone through which pass the artery, vein, and nerve of the pterygoid canal. SYN canalis pterygoideus [NA], vidian c.

pterygopalatine c., SYN greater palatine c.

pudendal c., the space within the obturator internis fascia lining the lateral wall of the ischiorectal fossa that transmits the pudendal vessels and nerves. SYN canalis pudendalis [NA], Alcock's c.

pulp c., SYN root c. of tooth.

pyloric c., the aboral segment (about 2 to 3 cm long) of the stomach; it succeeds the antrum and ends at the gastroduodenal junction. SYN canalis pyloricus [NA].

Rivinus' c.'s, SEE major sublingual *duct*, minor sublingual *ducts*, under *duct*.

root c. of tooth, the chamber of the dental pulp lying within the root portion of a tooth. SYN canalis radicis dentis [NA], marrow c., pulp c.

Rosenthal's c., SYN cochlear c.

sacral c., the continuation of the vertebral canal in the sacrum. SYN canalis sacralis [NA].

Santorini's c., SYN accessory pancreatic *duct*.

c.'s of Scarpa, separate c.'s for the nasopalatine nerves and vessels. These c.'s normally fuse to form the incisive c.

Schlemm's c., SYN *sinus* venosus sclerae.

semicircular c.'s, SEE bony semicircular c.'s.

small c. of chorda tympani, SYN posterior *canaliculus* of chorda tympani.

Sondermann's c., a blind outpouching of Schlemm's c., extending toward, but not communicating with, the anterior chamber of the eye.

spinal c., SYN vertebral c.

spiral c. of cochlea, SYN cochlear c.

spiral c. of modiolus, the space in the modiolus in which the spiral ganglion of the cochlear nerve lies. SYN canalis spiralis modioli [NA].

Stilling's c., SYN hyaloid c.

subsartorial c., SYN adductor c.

Sucquet-Hoyer c.'s, arteriovenous anastomoses controlling blood flow in the glomus bodies in the digits. SYN Hoyer's anastomoses, Hoyer's c.'s, Sucquet's anastomoses, Sucquet's c.'s, Sucquet-Hoyer anastomoses.

Sucquet's c.'s, SYN Sucquet-Hoyer c.'s.

tarsal c., SYN tarsal *sinus.*

temporal c., a c. in the zygomatic bone transmitting the zygomaticofacial and zygomaticotemporal nerves and vessels.

Theile's c., SYN transverse pericardial *sinus.*

tubotympanic c., SEE tubotympanic *recess.*

tympanic c., SYN tympanic *canaliculus.*

uniting c., SYN uniting *duct.*

urogenital c., SYN urethra.

uterovaginal c., a median tubular structure produced in the embryo from the fusion of the caudal parts of the paramesonephric ducts.

van Horne's c., SYN thoracic *duct.*

Velpeau's c., SYN inguinal c.

vertebral c., the canal that contains the spinal cord, spinal meninges, and related structures. It is formed by the vertebral foramina of successive vertebrae of the articulated vertebral column. SYN canalis vertebralis [NA], spinal c., tubus vertebralis.

vesicourethral c., the cranial portion of the primitive urogenital sinus from which develop the urinary bladder and part of the urethra.

vestibular c., SYN *scala* vestibuli.

vidian c., SYN pterygoid c.

Volkmann's c.'s, vascular c.'s in compact bone that, unlike those of the haversian system, are not surrounded by concentric lamellae of bone; they run for the most part transversely, perforating the lamellae of the haversian system, and communicate with the c.'s of that system.

vomerine c., SYN vomerovaginal c.

vomerobasilar c., SYN vomerorostral c.

vomerorostral c., a small canal between the superior border of the vomer and the rostrum of the sphenoidal bone. SYN canalis vomerorostralis [NA], vomerobasilar c.

vomerovaginal c., an opening between the vaginal process of the sphenoid and the ala of the vomer on either side. It conveys a branch of the sphenopalatine artery. SYN canalis vomerovaginalis [NA], basipharyngeal c., vomerine c.

Walther's c.'s, SYN minor sublingual *ducts,* under *duct.*

Wirsung's c., SYN pancreatic *duct.*

---

ca·na·les (kă-nā-lēz). Plural of canalis.

can·a·lic·u·lar (kan-ă-lik′yū-lăr). Relating to a canaliculus. [L. *canaliculus,* small channel, dim. fr. *canalis,* canal, + suffix -*ar,* pertaining to]

can·a·lic·u·li (kan-ă-lik′yū-lī). Plural of canaliculus.

can·a·lic·u·li·tis (kan′ă-lik-yū-lī′tis). Inflammation of the lacrimal canaliculus. [canaliculus + G. -*itis,* inflammation]

can·a·lic·u·li·za·tion (kan-ă-lik′yū-lī-zā′shŭn). The formation of canaliculi, or small canals, in any tissue.

can·a·lic·u·lus, pl. **can·a·lic·u·li** (kan-ă-lik′yū-lŭs, -lī) [NA]. A small canal or channel. SEE ALSO iter. [L. dim. fr. *canalis,* canal]

anterior c. of chorda tympani, a canal in the petrotympanic or glaserian fissure, near its posterior edge, through which the chorda tympani nerve issues from the skull. SYN Civinini's canal, Huguier's canal, iter chordae anterius.

auricular c., SYN mastoid c.

biliary c., one of the intercellular channels, about 1 μm or less in diameter, that occurs between liver cells forming the first portion of the bile system. SYN bile capillary.

bone c., the c. interconnecting bone lacunae with one another or with a haversian canal; contains the interconnecting cytoplasmic processes of osteocytes.

caroticotympanic canaliculi, small openings within the carotid canal that afford passage to the tympanic cavity of branches of the internal carotid artery and carotid sympathetic plexus. SYN canaliculi caroticotympanici [NA].

canaliculi caroticotympan′ici [NA], SYN caroticotympanic canaliculi.

c. chor′dae tym′pani [NA], SYN posterior c. of chorda tympani.

c. coch′leae [NA], SYN cochlear c.

cochlear c., a minute canal in the temporal bone that passes from the cochlea inferiorly to open in front of the medial side of the jugular fossa. It contains the perilymphatic duct. SYN c. cochleae [NA].

canalic′uli denta′les [NA], minute, wavy, branching tubes or canals in the dentin; they contain the long cytoplasmic processes of odontoblasts and extend radially from the pulp to the dentoenamel junction. SYN dental tubules, dentinal canals, dentinal tubules, tubuli dentales.

c. innomina′tus, SYN petrosal *foramen.*

intercellular c., one of the fine channels between adjoining secretory cells, such as those between serous cells in salivary glands.

intracellular c., a fine canal formed by invagination of the cell membrane into the cytoplasm of a cell, such as those of the parietal cells of the stomach.

lacrimal c., a curved canal beginning at the lacrimal punctum in the margin of each eyelid near the medial commissure and running transversely medially to empty with its fellow into the lacrimal sac. SYN c. lacrimalis [NA].

c. lacrima′lis [NA], SYN lacrimal c.

mastoid c., the canal that extends from the jugular fossa laterally through the mastoid process. It transmits the auricular branch of the vagus. SYN c. mastoideus [NA], auricular c.

c. mastoid′eus [NA], SYN mastoid c.

posterior c. of chorda tympani, a canal leading from the facial canal to the tympanic cavity through which the chorda tympani nerve enters this cavity. SYN c. chordae tympani [NA], iter chordae posterius, small canal of chorda tympani.

c. reu′niens, SYN uniting *duct.*

secretory c., SEE intercellular c., intracellular c.

Thiersch's canaliculi, minute channels in newly formed reparative tissue, permitting the circulation of nutritive fluids, precursors of new vascularization.

tympanic c., a minute canal passing from the inferior surface of the petrous portion of the temporal bone between the jugular fossa and carotid canal to the floor of the tympanic cavity. Located in the wedge of bone separating the jugular canal and carotid canal, it transmits the tympanic branch of the glossopharyngeal nerve. SYN c. tympanicus [NA], Jacobson's canal, tympanic canal.

c. tympan′icus [NA], SYN tympanic c.

ca·na·lis, pl. **ca·na·les** (ka-nā′lis, -lēz) [NA]. SYN canal. [L.]

c. adductor′ius [NA], SYN adductor *canal.*

cana′les alveola′res [NA], SYN alveolar *canals,* under *canal.*

c. ana′lis [NA], SYN anal *canal.*

c. carot′icus [NA], SYN carotid *canal.*

c. car′pi [NA], SYN carpal *tunnel.*

c. centra′lis medul′lae spina′lis [NA], SYN central *canal.*

c. cerv′icis u′teri [NA], SYN cervical *canal.*

c. condyla′ris [NA], SYN condylar *canal.*

cana′les diplo′ici [NA], SYN diploic *canals,* under *canal.*

c. femora′lis [NA], SYN femoral *canal.*

c. gastrici, SYN gastric *canal.*

c. gastricus [NA], SYN gastric *canal.*

c. hyaloid′eus [NA], SYN hyaloid *canal.*

c. hypoglossa′lis [NA], SYN hypoglossal *canal.*

c. incisi′vus [NA], SYN incisive *canal.*

c. infraorbita′lis [NA], SYN infraorbital *canal.*

c. inguina′lis [NA], SYN inguinal *canal.*

cana′les longitudina′les modi′oli [NA], SYN longitudinal *canals* of modiolus, under *canal.*

c. mandib′ulae [NA], SYN mandibular *canal.*

c. musculotuba′rius [NA], SYN musculotubal *canal.*

c. nasolacrima′lis [NA], SYN nasolacrimal *canal.*

c. ner′vi facia′lis [NA], SYN facial *canal.*

c. ner'vi petro'si superficial'is mino'ris, SYN *hiatus* of canal of lesser petrosal nerve.

c. nutri'cius [NA], SYN nutrient *canal.*

c. obturato'rius [NA], SYN obturator *canal.*

c. op'ticus [NA], SYN optic *canal.*

cana'les palati'ni mino'res [NA], SYN *canals* for lesser palatine nerves, under *canal.*

c. palati'nus ma'jor [NA], SYN greater palatine *canal.*

c. palatovagina'lis [NA], SYN pharyngeal *canal.*

c. pterygoi'deus [NA], SYN pterygoid *canal.*

c. pudenda'lis [NA], SYN pudendal *canal.*

c. pylor'icus [NA], SYN pyloric *canal.*

c. rad'icis den'tis [NA], SYN root *canal* of tooth.

c. reu'niens, SYN uniting *duct.*

c. sacra'lis [NA], SYN sacral *canal.*

canales semicirculares anterior, anterior semicurcular canal. SEE bony semicircular *canals,* under *canal.*

canales semicirculares lateralis, lateral semicircular canal. SEE bony semicircular *canals,* under *canal.*

cana'les semicircula'res os'sei [NA], SYN bony semicircular *canals,* under *canal.*

canales semicirculares posterior, posterior semicircular canal. SEE bony semicircular *canals,* under *canal.*

c. spira'lis coch'leae [NA], SYN cochlear *canal.*

c. spira'lis modi'oli [NA], SYN spiral *canal* of modiolus.

c. umbilica'lis, SYN umbilical *ring.*

c. vertebra'lis [NA], SYN vertebral *canal.*

c. vomerorostra'lis [NA], SYN vomerorostral *canal.*

c. vomerovagina'lis [NA], SYN vomerovaginal *canal.*

can·a·li·za·tion (kan-ăl-ĭ-zā'shŭn). The formation of canals or channels in a tissue.

Canavan, Myrtelle M., U.S. pathologist, 1879–1953. SEE C.'s *disease, sclerosis;* C.-Van Bogaert-Bertrand *disease.*

can·av·a·nase (kan-av'ă-nās). SYN arginase.

can·a·van·ine (kan-ă-van'ĭn). 2-amino-4-guanidinohydroxybutyric acid; $H_2NC(NH)NHO(CH_2)_2CH(NH_2)COOH$ H; an analog of arginine found in certain legumes; used in studies of arginine-dependent systems. [*Canavalia* + -ine]

can·cel·lat·ed (kan'sĕ-lā-ted). SYN cancellous. [L. *cancello,* to make a lattice work]

can·cel·lous (kan'sĕ-lŭs). Denoting bone that has a lattice-like or spongy structure. SYN cancellated.

can·cel·lus, pl. **can·cel·li** (kan-sel'ŭs, -lī). A lattice-like structure, as in spongy bone. [L. a grating, lattice]

can·cer (CA) (kan'ser). General term frequently used to indicate any of various types of malignant neoplasms, most of which invade surrounding tissues, may metastasize to several sites, and are likely to recur after attempted removal and to cause death of the patient unless adequately treated; especially, any such carcinoma or sarcoma, but, in ordinary usage, especially the former. [L. a crab, a cancer]

betel c., carcinoma of the mucous membrane of the cheek, observed in certain East Indian natives, probably as a result of irritation from chewing a preparation of betel nut and lime rolled within a betel leaf. SYN buyo cheek c.

buyo cheek c., SYN betel c. [Philippine *buyo,* betel]

chimney sweep's c., a squamous cell carcinoma of the skin of the scrotum, occurring as an occupational disease in chimney sweeps. The first reported form of occupational cancer (by Sir Percival Pott).

colloid c., SYN mucinous *carcinoma.*

conjugal c., c. à deux occurring in husband and wife.

c. à deux, carcinomas occurring at approximately the same time, or in fairly close succession, in two persons who live together. [Fr. *deux,* two]

encephaloid c., obsolete term for medullary *carcinoma.*

c. en cuirasse (on-kwē-rahs', Fr. breastplate), a carcinoma that involves a considerable portion of the skin of one or both sides of the thorax. [Fr. breastplate]

epidermoid c., SYN epidermoid *carcinoma.*

epithelial c., any malignant neoplasm originating from epithelium, *i.e.,* a carcinoma.

familial c., c. aggregating among blood relatives; exceptionally the mode of inheritance is clearly mendelian, either dominant, as in retinoblastoma, basal cell nevus syndrome, neurofibromatosis, and intestinal polyposis, or recessive, as in xeroderma pigmentosum. SEE ALSO cancer *family.*

glandular c., SYN adenocarcinoma.

green c., obsolete term for chloroma.

kang c., kangri c., a carcinoma of the skin of the thigh or abdomen in certain Indian or Chinese workers; thought to result from irritation by heat from a hot brick oven (kang) or fire basket (kangri). SYN kangri burn carcinoma.

mouse c., any of various types of malignant neoplasms that occur naturally in mice, especially in certain inbred "c. strains" used for research studies.

mule-spinner's c., carcinoma of the scrotum or adjacent skin exposed to oil, observed in some workers in cotton-spinning mills.

paraffin c., carcinoma of the skin occurring as an occupational disease in paraffin workers.

pipe-smoker's c., squamous cell carcinoma of the lips occurring in pipe smokers.

pitch-worker's c., carcinoma of the skin of the face or neck, arms and hands, or the scrotum, resulting from exposure to carcinogens in pitch, which occurs naturally as asphalt, or as a residue in the distillation of tar.

scar c., SYN scar *carcinoma.*

scar c. of the lungs, a pulmonary c. intimately related to a localized area of parenchymal fibrosis; the c. probably induces the fibrosis.

spider c., obsolete term for a malignant neoplasm with a rhizoid or filamentous edge of thin, threadlike, red lines that represent dilated vascular channels associated with the neoplasm; a form of telangiectatic c.

stump c., carcinoma of the stomach developing after gastroenterostomy or gastric resection for benign disease.

telangiectatic c., a c. with numerous dilated capillaries and "lakes" of blood within relatively large endothelium-lined channels.

can·cer·a·tion (kan-ser-ā'shŭn). Obsolete term for a change that results in properties and features usually associated with malignant neoplasms, *e.g.,* as in the development of a carcinoma in a site previously involved by a benign condition.

can·cer·i·ci·dal (kan'ser-i-sī'dăl). SYN carcinolytic. [cancer + L. *caedo,* to kill]

can·cer·i·gen·ic (kan'ser-i-jen'ik). SYN carcinogenic.

can·cer·o·ci·dal (kan'ser-ō-sī'dăl). SYN carcinolytic.

can·cer·o·pho·bia (kan'ser-ō-fō'bē-ă). A morbid fear of acquiring a malignant growth. SYN carcinophobia. [cancer + G. *phobos,* fear]

can·cer·ous (kan'ser-ŭs). Relating to or pertaining to a malignant neoplasm, or being afflicted with such a process.

can·cra (kang'kră). Plural of cancrum.

can·cri·form (kang'kri-fōrm). Resembling cancer. SYN cancroid (1).

can·croid (kang'kroyd). 1. SYN cancriform. 2. Obsolete term for a malignant neoplasm that manifests a lesser degree of malignancy than that frequently observed with carcinoma or sarcoma. [cancer + G. *eidos,* resemblance]

can·crum, pl. **can·cra** (kang'krŭm, -kră). A gangrenous, ulcerative, inflammatory lesion. [Mod. L., fr. L. *cancer,* crab]

c. na'si, gangrenous, necrotizing, and ulcerative rhinitis, especially in children.

c. o'ris, SYN noma.

can·de·la (cd) (kan'de-lă). The SI unit of luminous intensity, 1 lumen per m²; the luminous intensity, in a given direction, of a source that emits monochromatic radiation of frequency 540×10^{12} hertz and that has a radiant intensity in that direction of 1/683 watt per steradian (solid angle). SYN candle. [L.]

can·di·cans (kan'di-kanz). One of the corpora albicantia. [L. *candico,* pres. p. *-ans,* to be whitish]

can·di·ci·din (kan-di-sī'din). A fungistatic and fungicidal polyene antibiotic agent derived from a soil actinomycete similar to *Streptomyces griseus;* used in the treatment of vaginal candidiasis.

Can·di·da (kan'did-ă). A genus of yeastlike fungi commonly found in nature; a few species are isolated from the skin, feces, and vaginal and pharyngeal tissue, but the gastrointestinal tract is the source of the single most important species, *C. albicans.* [L. *candidus,* dazzling white]

C. al'bicans, a species ordinarily a part of humans' normal gastrointestinal flora, but which becomes pathogenic when there is a disturbance in the balance of flora or in debilitation of the host from other causes; resulting disease states may vary from limited to generalized cutaneous or mucocutaneous infections, to severe and fatal systemic disease including endocarditis, septicemia, and meningitis. SYN thrush fungus.

can·di·de·mia (kan-di-dē'mē-ă). Presence of cells of *Candida* species in the peripheral blood. [*Candida* + G. *haima,* blood]

can·di·di·a·sis (kan-di-dī'ă-sis). Infection with, or disease caused by, *Candida,* especially *C. albicans.* This disease usually results from debilitation (as in immunosuppression and especially AIDS), physiologic change, prolonged administration of antibiotics, and iatrogenic and barrier breakage. SYN candidosis, moniliasis.

can·di·do·sis (kan-di-dō'sis). SYN candidiasis.

can·dle (kan'dl). SYN candela.

can·dle-me·ter (kan'dl-mē'ter). SYN lux.

can·dle-pow·er (kan'dl-pow'er). SYN luminous *intensity.*

Can·i·dae (kan'i-dē). A family of the *Carnivora* including the dogs, coyotes, wolves, and foxes. [L. *canis,* dog]

ca·nine (kā'nīn). **1.** Relating to a dog. **2.** Relating to the c. teeth. **3.** SYN canine *tooth.* **4.** Referring to the cuspid tooth. [L. *caninus*]

ca·ni·ni·form (kă-nī'ni-fōrm). Resembling a canine tooth.

can·is·ter (kan'is-ter). A box or container; in anesthesiology, the container for carbon dioxide absorbent.

ca·ni·ti·es (kă-nish'ē-ēz). Graying of hair. SEE ALSO poliosis. [L., fr. *canus,* hoary, gray]

canities c., SYN ectopic *eyelash.*

c. circumscrip'ta, SYN piebald *eyelash.*

rapid c., whitening of hair overnight or over a few days; in the latter case, may be seen in alopecia areata, when surviving pigmented hairs are preferentially shed from gray hair.

c. un'guium, SYN leukonychia.

can·ker (kang'ker). **1.** In cats and dogs, acute inflammation of the external ear and auditory canal. SEE aphthae. **2.** In the horse, a process similar to but more advanced than thrush; the horny frog is generally under-run with a whitish, cheeselike exudate, and the entire sole and even the wall of the hoof may be undermined. **3.** In man, an outmoded term for aphthae. [L. *cancer*]

water c., SYN noma.

can·na·bi·di·ol (kan-ă-bi-dī'ol). $C_{21}H_{30}O_2$; a constituent of *Cannabis,* related to cannabinol.

can·nab·i·noids (ka-nab'i-noydz). Organic substances present in *Cannabis sativa,* having a variety of pharmacologic properties.

can·na·bi·nol (ka-nab'i-nol). 6,6,9-Trimethyl-3-pentyl-6*H*-dibenzo[*b,d*]-pyran-i-ol; a constituent of the resinous exudate of the pistillate flowers of *Cannabis sativa;* it has no psychotomimetic action as do the tetrahydro derivatives isolated from marijuana.

can·na·bis (kan'ă-bis). The dried flowering tops of the pistillate plants of *Cannabis sativa* (family Moraceae) containing isomeric tetrahydrocannabinols, cannabinol, and cannabidiol. Preparations of c. are smoked or ingested by members of various cultures and subcultures to induce psychotomimetic effects such as euphoria, hallucinations, drowsiness, and other mental changes. C. was formerly used as a sedative and analgesic; now available for restricted use in management of iatrogenic anorexia, especially that associated with oncologic chemotherapy and radiation therapy. Known by many colloquial or slang terms such as marijuana; marihuana; pot; grass; bhang; charas; ganja; hashish. [L., fr. G. *kannabis,* hemp]

can·na·bism (kan'ă-bizm). Poisoning by preparations of cannabis.

Cannizzaro, Stanislao, Italian chemist, 1826–1910. SEE C.'s *reaction.*

Cannon, Walter B., U.S. physiologist, 1871–1945. SEE C.'s *ring, theory;* C.-Bard *theory;* Bernard-C. *homeostasis.*

can·nu·la (kan'yū-lă). A tube which can be inserted into a cavity, usually by means of a trocar filling its lumen; after insertion of the c., the trocar is withdrawn and the c. remains as a channel for the transport of fluid. [L. dim. of *canna,* reed]

Hasson c., a laparoscopic instrument for open (rather than blind needle insufflation) placement of the initial port. The Hasson has a blunt-tipped oburator instead of a sharp trocar and a balloon on the distal portion of the sheath to hold it in place. SYN laparoscopic c.

Karman c., a flexible plastic c. used in performing early (menstrual extraction) abortion.

laparoscopic c., SYN Hasson c.

perfusion c., a double-barreled c. used for irrigation of a cavity, the wash fluid passing into the cavity through one tube and out through the other.

washout c., a c. that can be irrigated without removal from the artery.

can·nu·la·tion, can·nu·li·za·tion (kan-yū-lā'shŭn, -yū-lī-zā' shŭn). Insertion of a cannula.

Cantelli's sign. See under sign.

can·thal (kan'thăl). Relating to a canthus.

can·thar·i·dal (kan-thar'i-dăl). Relating to or containing cantharides.

can·thar·i·date (kan-thar'i-dāt). A salt of cantharidic acid.

can·thar·i·des (kan-thar'i-dēz). Plural of cantharis.

can·thar·i·dic ac·id (kan-thar'i-dik). $C_{10}H_{14}O_5$; an acid, derived from cantharis, that forms salts (cantharidates) with alkalis.

can·thar·i·din (kan-thar'i-din). $C_{10}H_{12}O_4$; hexahydro-3α,7α-dimethyl-4,7-epoxyisobenzofura n-1,3-dione; the active principle of cantharis; the anhydride of cantharic acid. SYN cantharis camphor.

can·tha·ris, gen. **can·thar·i·dis,** pl. **can·thar·i·des** (kan'tharis, kan-thar'i-dis, -dēz). A dried beetle, *Lytta (Cantharis) vesicatoria,* used as a counterirritant and vesicant. SYN Russian fly, Spanish fly. [L., fr. G. *kantharis,* a beetle]

can·thec·to·my (kan-thek'tō-mē). Excision of a palpebral canthus. [G. *kanthos,* canthus, + *ektomē,* excision]

can·thi (kan'thī). Plural of canthus.

can·thi·tis (kan-thī'tis). Inflammation of a canthus.

can·thol·y·sis (kan-thol'i-sis). SYN canthoplasty (1). [G. *kanthos,* canthus, + *lysis,* loosening]

can·tho·plas·ty (kan'thō-plas-tē). **1.** An operation for lengthening the palpebral fissure by incision through the lateral canthus. SYN cantholysis. **2.** An operation for restoration of the canthus. [G. *kanthos,* canthus, + *plassō,* to form]

can·thor·rha·phy (kan-thōr'ă-fē). Suture of the eyelids at either canthus. [G. *kanthos,* canthus, + *rhaphē,* suture]

can·thot·o·my (kan-thot'ō-mē). Slitting of the canthus. [G. *kanthos,* canthus, + *tomē,* incision]

can·thus, pl. **can·'thi** (kan'thŭs, -thī). The angle of the eye. [G. *kanthos,* corner of the eye]

external c., SYN lateral *angle* of eye.

internal c., SYN medial *angle* of eye.

lateral c., SYN lateral *angle* of eye.

medial c., SYN medial *angle* of eye.

Cantor, Meyer O., U.S. physician, *1907. SEE C. *tube.*

CaOC Abbreviation for cathodal opening *contraction.*

CaOCl Abbreviation for cathodal opening *clonus.*

CAP Abbreviation for catabolite (gene) activator *protein.*

cap (kap). **1.** Any anatomical structure that resembles a c. or cover. **2.** A protective covering for an incomplete tooth. **3.** Collo-

ca

quialism for restoration of the coronal part of a natural tooth by means of an artificial crown. **4.** The nucleotide structure found at the 5′ terminus of many eukaryotic messenger RNAs, consisting of a 7-methylguanosine connected, via its 5′-hydroxyl group, by a triphosphate group to the 5′-hydroxyl group of the first nucleoside encoded by the DNA; usually symbolized as $m^7G^{5'}ppp^{5'}N$, where N is nucleoside number 1 in the transcribed mRNA and is often itself methylated; the c. is added posttranscriptionally.

acrosomal c., a collapsed membranous vesicle that covers the anterior part of the nucleus of the spermatozoon, derived from the acrosomal granule; the carbohydrate-rich substance of the c. is associated with hydrolytic enzymes that aid in sperm penetration of the zona pellucida of the ovum. SYN head c.

c. of the ampullary crest, SYN *cupula* cristae ampullaris.

apical c., a curved shadow at the apex of one or both hemithoraces on chest x-ray; caused by pleural and pulmonary fibrosis.

cervical c., a contraceptive diaphragm that fits over the cervix uteri.

chin c., an extraoral appliance designed to exert an upward and backward force on the mandible by applying pressure to the chin, thereby preventing forward growth.

cradle c., colloquialism for seborrheic dermatitis of the scalp of the newborn.

dental c.'s, deciduous cheek teeth in the horse which remain attached to erupting permanent teeth.

duodenal c., the first portion of the duodenum, as seen in a roentgenogram or by fluoroscopy. SYN duodenal bulb.

enamel c., the enamel covering the crown of a tooth.

head c., SYN acrosomal c.

metanephric c., the concentrated mass of mesodermal cells about the metanephric bud in a young embryo; the cells of the cap form the uriniferous tubules of the permanent kidney. SYN metanephric blastema.

phrygian c., on cholecystography, an incomplete septum, or a fold in the gallbladder, whose shape suggests the liberty cap of the French Revolution.

pyloric c., archaic term for duodenal c.

ca·pac·i·tance (kă-pas′i-tans). The quantity of electric charge that may be stored upon a body per unit electric potential; expressed in farads, abfarads, or statfarads.

ca·pac·i·ta·tion (kă-pas′i-tā′shŭn). C. is a process whereby the glycoprotein coat and seminal proteins are removed from the surface of the sperm's acrosome. There are no morphological changes. C. can occur in *in vitro* fertilization. Once c. has occurred perforation of the acrosome can occur. [L. *capacitas,* fr. *capax,* capable of]

ca·pac·i·tor (kă-pas′i-ter, -tŏr). A device for holding a charge of electricity. SYN condenser (4).

ca·pac·i·ty (kă-pas′i-tē). **1.** The potential cubic contents of a cavity or receptacle. **2.** Power to do. SEE ALSO volume. [L. *capax,* able to contain; fr. *capio,* to take]

buffer c., the amount of hydrogen ion (or hydroxyl ion) required to bring about a specific pH change in a specified volume of a buffer. SEE ALSO buffer *value.*

cranial c., the cubic content of the skull obtained by determining the cubage of small shot, seeds, or beads required to fill the skull.

diffusing c. (symbol, D, followed by subscripts indicating location and chemical species), the amount of oxygen taken up by pulmonary capillary blood per minute per unit average oxygen pressure gradient between alveolar gas and pulmonary capillary blood; units are: ml/min/mm Hg; also applied to other gases such as carbon monoxide.

forced vital c. (FVC), vital c. measured with the subject exhaling as rapidly as possible; data relating volume, expiratory flow, and time form the basis for other pulmonary function tests, *e.g.,* flow-volume curve, forced expiratory volume, forced expiratory time, forced expiratory flow.

functional residual c. (FRC), the volume of gas remaining in the lungs at the end of a normal expiration; it is the sum of expiratory reserve volume and residual volume. SYN functional residual air.

heat c., the quantity of heat required to raise the temperature of a system 1°C. SYN thermal c.

inspiratory c., the volume of air that can be inspired after a normal expiration; it is the sum of the tidal volume and the inspiratory reserve volume. SYN complementary air.

iron-binding c. (IBC), the c. of iron-binding protein in serum (transferrin) to bind serum iron.

maximum breathing c. (MBC), SYN maximum voluntary *ventilation.*

oxygen c., the maximum quantity of oxygen that will combine chemically with the hemoglobin in a unit volume of blood; normally it amounts to 1.34 ml of O_2 per gm of Hb or 20 ml of O_2 per 100 ml of blood.

residual c., SYN residual *volume.*

respiratory c., SYN vital c.

thermal c., SYN heat c.

total lung c. (TLC), the inspiratory c. plus the functional residual c.; *i.e.,* the volume of air contained in the lungs at the end of a maximal inspiration; also equals vital c. plus residual volume.

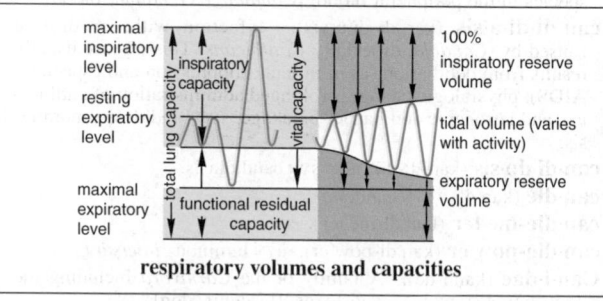

respiratory volumes and capacities

vital c. (VC), the greatest volume of air that can be exhaled from the lungs after a maximum inspiration. SYN respiratory c.

cap·ac·tins (kap-ak′tinz). A class of proteins capping the ends of actin filaments.

CAPD Abbreviation for continuous ambulatory peritoneal *dialysis.*

Capgras, Jean Marie Joseph, French psychiatrist, 1873–1950. SEE C.'s *phenomenon, syndrome.*

cap·il·lar·ec·ta·sia (kap′i-lar-ek-tā′zē-ă). Rarely used term for dilation of the capillary blood vessels. [capillary + G. *ektasis,* extension]

Ca·pil·la·ria (kap-i-lā′rē-ă). A genus of aphasmid nematode worms, characterized by threadlike appearance; related to *Trichuris.* [L. *capillaris,* fr. *capillus,* hair]

C. aeroph′ila, species occurring in the bronchi, bronchioles, and nasal sinuses of dogs, cats, and foxes; it causes rhinotracheitis, bronchitis, and nasal discharge in young animals.

C. bo′vis, species occurring in the small intestine of cattle, sheep, and goats.

C. brev′ipes, species found in the small intestine of cattle, sheep, and goats.

C. hepat′ica, species of threadworm that infects the liver in rodents; occasionally reported from man.

C. philippinen′sis, a species of threadworm that has been implicated as a cause of intestinal capillariasis among northern Philippine fishermen.

C. pli′ca, a fine threadworm species occurring in the urinary bladder and sometimes the renal pelvis of the dog and cat.

ca·pil·la·ri·a·sis (kap′i-lār-ī′ă-sis). A parasitic disease caused by infection with species of *Capillaria.*

intestinal c., a sprue-like diarrheal disease caused by infection with *Capillaria philippinensis,* large populations of which are built up by internal autoinfection in the intestinal mucosa; characterized by abdominal pain, edema, diarrhea, cachexia, hypoproteinemia, hypotension, cardiac failure, and hyporeflexia; severe infection is often manifested as a fulminating disorder that may be fatal.

cap·il·lar·i·o·mo·tor (kap-i-lār′ē-ō-mō′tŏr). Vasomotor, with special reference to the capillaries.

cap·il·lar·i·os·co·py (kap'i-lar-ē-os'kŏ-pē). Viewing the cutaneous capillaries at the base of the fingernail through the low power of the microscope. SYN capillaroscopy, microangioscopy.

cap·il·lar·i·tis (kap'i-lar-ī'tis). Inflammation of a capillary or capillaries.

cap·il·lar·i·ty (kap-i-lar'i-tē). The rise of liquids in narrow tubes or through the pores of a loose material, as a result of capillary action.

cap·il·la·ron (kap'i-lă-ron). An anatomical module composed of parenchymal cells together with their blood capillaries and extra-capillary fluid in a compliant capsule; functions as a hydraulic unit that provides a theoretical basis for proposing that blood flow is regulated at the capillary.

cap·il·la·rop·a·thy (kap'i-lă-rop'ă-thē). Any disease of the capillaries, often applied to vascular changes in diabetes mellitus. SYN microangiopathy. [capillary + G. *pathos,* disease]

cap·il·lar·os·co·py (kap'i-lar-os'kō-pē). SYN capillarioscopy.

cap·il·lary (kap'i-lār-ē). **1.** Resembling a hair; fine; minute. **2.** A capillary vessel; *e.g.,* blood c., lymph c. SYN vas capillare [NA], capillary vessel. **3.** Relating to a blood or lymphatic c. vessel. [L. *capillaris,* relating to hair]

arterial c., a c. opening from an arteriole or metarteriole.

bile c., SYN biliary *canaliculus.*

blood c. (symbol c, as a subscript), a vessel whose wall consists of endothelium and its basement membrane; its diameter, when the c. is open, is about 8 μm; with the electron microscope, fenestrated c.'s and continuous c.'s are distinguished.

continuous c., a c. in which small vesicles (caveolae) are numerous and pores are absent.

fenestrated c., a c., found in renal glomeruli, intestinal villi, and some glands, in which ultramicroscopic pores of variable size occur; usually these are closed by a delicate diaphragm, although diaphragms are lacking in at least some renal glomerular c.'s.

lymph c., the beginning of the lymphatic system of vessels; it is lined with a highly attenuated endothelium with poorly developed basement membrane and a lumen of variable caliber. SEE lacteal (2).

sinusoidal c., SYN sinusoid.

venous c., a c. opening into a venule.

ca·pil·lus, gen. and pl. **ca·pil·li** (ka-pil'ŭs, -lī) [NA]. SYN scalp *hair.* [L. hair]

cap·i·stra·tion (kap-i-strā'shŭn). Obsolete term for paraphimosis (1). [L. *capistrum,* muzzle]

ca·pi·ta (kap'i-tă). Plural of caput.

cap·i·tate (kap'i-tāt). **1.** The largest of the carpal bones; located in the distal row. SYN os capitatum [NA], capitate bone, magnum, os magnum. **2.** Head-shaped; having a rounded extremity. [L. *caput (capit-),* head]

cap·i·tel·lum (kap-i-tel'ŭm). **1.** SYN capitulum (1). **2.** SYN *capitulum* of humerus. [L. dim. of *caput,* head]

ca·pit·i·um (kă-pit'ē-ŭm). Obsolete term for bandage for the head. [L. *caput,* head]

cap·i·ton·nage (kap'i-tō-nahzh). Rarely used term for closure of a cyst cavity by use of sutures. [Fr. upholstering]

cap·i·to·ped·al (kap-i-tō-ped'ăl). Relating to the head and the feet. [L. *caput,* head, + *pes (ped-),* foot]

ca·pit·u·la (kă-pit'yū-lă). Plural of capitulum.

ca·pit·u·lar (kă-pit'yū-lăr). Relating to a capitulum.

ca·pit·u·lum, pl. **ca·pit·u·la** (kă-pit'yū-lŭm, -lă). **1** [NA]. A small head or rounded articular extremity of a bone. SYN capitellum (1). SEE ALSO caput. **2.** The bloodsucking, probing, sensing, and holdfast mouthparts of a tick, including the basal supporting structure; relative size and shape of mouthparts forming the c. are characteristic for the genera of hard ticks. [L. dim. of *caput,* head]

c. hu'meri [NA], SYN c. of humerus.

c. of humerus, the small rounded eminence on the lateral half of the distal end of the humerus for articulation with the radius. SYN c. humeri [NA], capitellum (2), little head of humerus.

Caplan, Anthony, British physician, 1907–1976. SEE C.'s *nodules,* under *nodule, syndrome.*

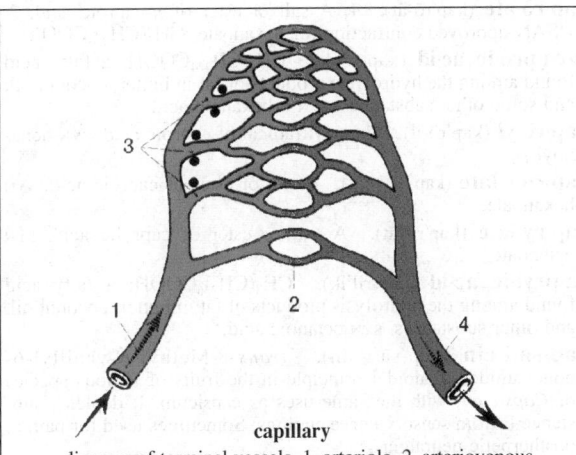

capillary
diagram of terminal vessels. 1. arteriole, 2. arteriovenous anastomosis, 3. capillaries, with precapillary sphincters, 4. venule

Cap·no·cy·to·pha·ga (kap'nō-sī-tō-fā'jē-ah). A genus of Gram-negative, fusiform-shaped, bacteria that requires carbon dioxide for growth and exhibits gliding motility; associated with human periodontal disease.

C. canimor'sus, a species linked to infections from dog bites (including bacteremia, endocarditis, and meningitis. Formerly designated DF-2 by the CDC. These infections usually occur in patients with impaired immune systems.

cap·no·gram (kap'nō-gram). A continuous record of the carbon dioxide content of expired air. [G. *kapnos,* smoke, + *gramma,* something written]

cap·no·graph (kap'nō-graf). Instrument by which a continuous graph of the carbon dioxide content of expired air is obtained.

cap·ping. Covering.

direct pulp c., a procedure for covering and protecting an exposed vital pulp.

indirect pulp c., the application of a suspension of calcium hydroxide to a thin layer of dentin overlying the pulp (near exposure) in order to stimulate secondary dentin formation and protect the pulp.

Capps, Joseph A., U.S. physician, 1872–1964. SEE C.'s *reflex.*

Cap·ra (kap'ră). A genus of ruminants (family Bovidae) that includes the goat, ibex, and related animals; *C. hircus* is the domestic goat. [L. a she-goat]

cap·rate (kap'rāt). A salt or ester of capric acid.

cap·re·o·my·cin sul·fate (kap'rē-ō-mī'sin). Sulfate salt of the cyclic peptide antibiotic obtained from *Streptomyces capreolus,* used in the treatment of tuberculosis.

n-cap·ric ac·id (kap'rik). $CH_3(CH_2)_8COOH$; a fatty acid found among the hydrolysis products of fat in goat's milk, cow's milk, and other substances. Cf. *n*-caproic acid, caprylic acid. SYN *n*-decanoic acid.

ca·pril·o·quism (kă-pril'ō-kwizm). SYN egophony. [L. *caper,* goat, + *loquor,* to speak]

cap·rin (kap'rin). tridecanoylglycerol; one of the substances found in butter upon which its flavor depends. SYN decanoin, glyceryl tricaprate.

cap·rine (kă'prīn). Relating to goats; goatlike. [L. *caprinus,* of goats]

cap·rine ar·thri·tis-en·ceph·a·lo·my·e·li·tis (CAE). See under encephalomyelitis.

Cap·ri·pox·vi·rus (kap'ri-poks-vī'rŭs). The genus of Poxviridae that includes the viruses of sheep-pox and goatpox. [L. *capra,* she-goat, + virus]

cap·ri·zant (kap'ri-zant). Bounding; leaping; denoting a form of pulse beat. [Fr., leaping, fr. L. *caper,* goat]

cap·ro·ate (kap′rō-āt). **1.** A salt or ester of *n*-caproic acid. **2.** USAN-approved contraction for hexanoate, $CH_3(CH_2)_4COO^-$.

***n*-ca·pro·ic ac·id** (kap-rō′ik). $CH_3(CH_2)_4COOH$; a fatty acid found among the hydrolysis products of fat in butter, coconut oil, and some other substances. SYN *n*-hexanoic acid.

cap·ro·yl (kap′rō-il). The acyl radical of caproic acid. SYN hexanoyl.

cap·ro·y·late (kap′rō-i-lāt). A salt or ester of caproic acid. SYN hexanoate.

cap·ry·late (kap′ri-lāt). A salt or ester of caprylic acid. SYN octanoate.

ca·pryl·ic ac·id (kap-ril′ik). $CH_3(CH_2)_6COOH$; a fatty acid found among the hydrolysis products of fat in butter, coconut oil, and other substances. SYN octanoic acid.

cap·sa·i·cin (cap-sā′i-sin). *trans*-8-Methyl-*N*-vanillyl-6-nonenamide; alkaloidal principle in the fruits of various species of *Capsicum*, with the same uses as capsicum. It depletes substance P from sensory nerve endings; Sometimes used for pain in postherpetic neuralgia.

cap·si·cin (kap′sī-sin). A yellowish red oleoresin containing the active principle of capsicum.

cap·si·cum (kap′si-kŭm). Cayenne, African, or red pepper, the dried ripe fruit of *Capsicum frutescens* (family Solanaceae); used as a carminative, gastrointestinal stimulant, and externally as a rubefacient.

cap·sid (kap′sid). SEE virion.

cap·so·mer, cap·so·mere (kap′sō-mēr). A subunit of the protein coat or capsid of a virus particle. SEE ALSO hexon, penton, virion.

cap·su·la, gen. and pl. **cap·su·lae** (kap′sū-lă, -lē) [NA]. **1.** A membranous structure, usually dense collagenous connective tissue, that envelops an organ, a joint, or any other part. **2.** An anatomical structure resembling a capsule or envelope. SYN capsule (1). [L. dim. of *capsa*, a chest or box]

c. adipo′sa re′nis [NA], SYN fatty renal *capsule*.

c. articula′ris [NA], SYN articular *capsule*.

c. articula′ris cricoarytenoi′dea [NA], SYN cricoarytenoid articular *capsule*.

c. articula′ris cricothyroi′dea [NA], SYN cricothyroid articular *capsule*.

c. bul′bi, SYN fascial *sheath* of eyeball.

c. cor′dis, SYN pericardium.

c. exter′na [NA], SYN external *capsule*.

c. extre′ma, SYN extreme *capsule*.

c. fibro′sa, SYN fibrous *capsule*.

c. fibro′sa glan′dulae thyroi′deae [NA], SYN fibrous *capsule* of thyroid gland.

c. fibro′sa per′ivascula′ris [NA], SYN fibrous *capsule* of liver (1).

c. fibro′sa re′nis [NA], SYN fibrous *capsule* of kidney.

c. glomer′uli [NA], SYN glomerular *capsule*.

c. inter′na [NA], SYN internal *capsule*.

c. len′tis [NA], SYN lens *capsule*.

c. li′enis, SYN fibrous *capsule* of spleen.

c. vasculo′sa len′tis, in the embryo, the vascular mesenchymal capsule that invests the lens of the eye; the vessels of the dorsal part of the capsule are branches of the hyaloid artery; those of the ventral part are derived from the anterior ciliary arteries; normally all the vessels are atrophied by the end of the eighth month of intrauterine life.

cap·su·lar (kap′sū-lăr). Relating to any capsule.

cap·su·la·tion (kap-sū-lā′shŭn). Enclosure in a capsule.

cap·sule (kap′sūl). **1.** SYN capsula. **2.** A fibrous tissue layer enveloping an organ or a tumor, especially if benign. **3.** A solid dosage form in which the drug is enclosed in either a hard or soft soluble container or "shell" of a suitable form of gelatin. **4.** A hyaline glycosaminoglycan sheath on the wall of a fungus cell, blastoconidium, or spore. [L. *capsula*, dim. of *capsa*, box]

adipose c., SYN fatty renal c.

adrenal c., SYN suprarenal *gland*.

articular c., a sac enclosing a joint, formed by an outer fibrous articular c. and an inner synovial membrane. SYN capsula articularis [NA], joint c.

atrabiliary c., SYN suprarenal *gland*.

auditory c., the cartilage that, in the embryo, surrounds the developing auditory vesicle and develops into the bony labyrinth of the inner ear.

bacterial c., a layer of slime of variable composition which covers the surface of some bacteria; capsulated cells of pathogenic bacteria are usually more virulent than cells without capsules because the former are more resistant to phagocytic action.

Bonnet's c., the anterior part of the vagina bulbi.

Bowman's c., SYN glomerular c.

brood c.'s, small hollow projections from the lining membrane of a hydatid cyst from which the scoleces arise.

cartilage c., the more intensely basophilic matrix in hyaline cartilage surrounding the lacunae in which the cartilage cells lie. SYN territorial matrix.

cricoarytenoid articular c., the capsule enclosing the joint between the arytenoid and cricoid cartilages. SYN capsula articularis cricoarytenoidea [NA].

cricothyroid articular c., the capsule enclosing the cricothyroid joint. SYN capsula articularis cricothyroidea [NA].

Crosby c., an attachment to the end of a flexible tube, used for peroral biopsy of the small intestine, by which a piece of mucosa is sucked into an opening in the c. and cut off.

crystalline c., SYN lens c.

external c., a thin lamina of white substance separating the claustrum from the putamen. It joins the internal c. at either extremity of the putamen, forming a c. of white matter external to the lenticular nucleus. SYN capsula externa [NA], periclaustral lamina.

extreme c., the layer of white matter separating the claustrum from the cortex of the insula, probably representing largely corticopetal and corticofugal fibers of the insular cortex. SYN capsula extrema.

eye c., SYN fascial *sheath* of eyeball.

fatty renal c., the perirenal fat. SYN capsula adiposa renis [NA], adipose c.

fibrous c., any fibrous envelope of a part. the fibrous capsule of an organ. SYN stratum fibrosum [NA], tunica fibrosa [NA], capsula fibrosa.

fibrous articular c., the outer fibrous part of the capsule of a synovial joint, which may in places be thickened to form capsular ligaments. SYN membrana fibrosa [NA], stratum fibrosum [NA], fibrous membrane.

fibrous c. of kidney, a fibrous membrane ensheathing the kidney. SYN capsula fibrosa renis [NA], tunica fibrosa renis.

fibrous c. of liver, (1) a layer of connective tissue ensheathing the hepatic artery, portal vein, and bile ducts as these ramify within the liver; SYN capsula fibrosa perivascularis [NA], perivascular fibrous c. **(2)** connective tissue c. surrounding the outer surface of the liver, but continuous with septae of some animals which divide parenchyme into lobule, and with the perivascular fibrous c. at the porta hepatis. SYN tunica fibrosa hepatis [NA], Glisson's c.

fibrous c. of parotid gland, SYN parotid *fascia*.

fibrous c. of spleen, the fibrous capsule of the spleen, containing collagen, elastic fibers, and smooth muscle. SYN tunica fibrosa splenis [NA], tunica fibrosa lienis ☆ [NA], capsula lienis, tunica propria lienis.

fibrous c. of thyroid gland, the fibrous sheath of the thyroid gland. SYN capsula fibrosa glandulae thyroideae [NA].

Gerota's c., SYN renal *fascia*.

Glisson's c., SYN fibrous c. of liver (2).

glomerular c., the expanded beginning of a nephron composed of an inner and outer layer: the visceral layer consists of podocytes which surround a tuft of capillaries (glomerulus); the parietal layer is simple squamous epithelium which becomes cuboidal at the tubular pole. SYN capsula glomeruli [NA], Bowman's c., malpighian c. (1), Müller's c.

internal c., a massive layer (8 to 10 mm thick) of white matter separating the caudate nucleus and thalamus (medial) from the more laterally situated lentiform nucleus (globus pallidus and putamen). It consists of 1) fibers ascending from the thalamus to the cerebral cortex that compose, among others, the visual, auditory, and somatic sensory radiations, and 2) fibers descending from the cerebral cortex to the thalamus, subthalamic region, midbrain, hindbrain, and spinal cord. The internal c. is the major route by which the cerebral cortex is connected with the brainstem and spinal cord. Laterally and superiorly it is continuous with the corona radiata which forms a major part of the cerebral hemisphere's white matter; caudally and medially it continues, much reduced in size, as the crus cerebri which contains, among others, the pyramidal tract. On horizontal section it appears in the form of a V opening out laterally; the V's obtuse angle is called genu (knee); its anterior and posterior limbs, respectively, the crus anterior and crus posterior. SYN capsula interna [NA].

joint c., SYN articular c.

lens c., the capsule enclosing the lens of the eye. SYN capsula lentis [NA], crystalline c., lenticular c., phacocyst.

lenticular c., SYN lens c.

malpighian c., (1) SYN glomerular c. **(2)** a thin fibrous membrane enveloping the spleen and continued over the vessels entering at the hilus.

Müller's c., SYN glomerular c.

nasal c., the cartilage around the developing nasal cavity of the embryo.

optic c., the concentrated zone of mesenchyme around the developing optic cup; the primordium of the sclera of the eye.

otic c., the cartilage c. surrounding the inner ear mechanism; in elasmobranchs, it remains cartilaginous in the adult; in the embryos of higher vertebrates, it is cartilaginous at first but later becomes bony (at approximately 23 weeks in humans).

perivascular fibrous c., SYN fibrous c. of liver (1).

radiotelemetering c., an instrument that transmits measurements by radio impulses, from within the body; *e.g.,* measurements of pressure from within the small bowel. SYN radiopill.

seminal c., SYN seminal *vesicle.*

suprarenal c., SYN suprarenal *gland.*

Tenon's c., SYN fascial *sheath* of eyeball.

cap·sul·ec·to·my. Removal of a capsule, as around a breast implant

cap·su·li·tis (kap'sū-lī'tis). Inflammation of the capsule of an organ or part, as of the liver or the lens of the eye.

adhesive c., a condition in which there is limitation of motion in a joint due to inflammatory thickening of the capsule, a common cause of stiffness in the shoulder. SYN frozen shoulder.

hepatic c., SYN perihepatitis.

cap·su·lo·len·tic·u·lar (kap'sū-lō-len-tik'yū-lăr). Referring to the lens of the eye and its capsule.

cap·su·lo·plas·ty (kap'sū-lō-plas-tē). Plastic surgery of a capsule; more specifically, the capsule of a joint. [L. *capsula,* capsule, + G. *plastos,* formed]

cap·su·lor·rha·phy (kap-sū-lōr'ă-fē). Suture of a tear in any capsule; specifically, suture of a joint capsule to prevent recurring dislocation of the articulation. [L. *capsula,* capsule, + *rhaphē,* suture]

cap·su·lo·tome (kap'sū-lō-tōm). SYN cystotome (2).

cap·su·lot·o·my (kap-sū-lot'ō-mē). **1.** Division of a capsule as around a breast implant. **2.** Creation of an opening through a capsule; *e.g.,* of a scar that might form around a foreign body. **3.** Specifically, incision of the capsule of the lens in the extracapsular cataract operation. [L. *capsula,* capsule, + G. *tomē,* a cutting]

renal c., incision of the capsule of the kidney.

cap·to·pril (kap'tō-pril). 1-(3-Mercapto-2-methyl-1-oxopropyl)-L-proline; an angiotensin converting enzyme inhibitor used in the treatment of hypertension and congestive heart failure.

cap·ture (kap'chūr). Catching and holding a particle or an electrical impulse originating elsewhere. [L. *capio,* pp. *-tus,* to take, seize]

atrial c., control of the atria for one or more beats after a period of independent beating, as in complete A-V block or in junctional or ventricular ectopic beats or tachycardias by a retrograde impulse.

electron c., a mode of radioactive disintegration, in which an orbital electron, usually from the K shell, is captured by the nucleus, converting a proton into a neutron with ejection of a neutrino and emission of a gamma ray, and emission of characteristic x-rays as the missing K-shell electron is replaced. SYN K c.

K c., SYN electron c.

ventricular c., capture of the ventricle(s) by an impulse arising in the atria or A-V junction.

Capuron, Joseph, French physician, 1767–1850. SEE C.'s *points,* under *point.*

ca·put, gen. **ca·pi·tis,** pl. **ca·pi·ta** (kap'ut, ka'put; kap'i-tis; kap'ĭ-tă). **1** [NA]. The upper or anterior extremity of the animal body, containing the brain and the organs of sight, hearing, taste, and smell. **2** [NA]. The upper, anterior, or larger extremity, expanded or rounded, of any body, organ, or other anatomical structure. **3.** The rounded extremity of a bone. **4.** That end of a muscle which is attached to the less movable part of the skeleton. SYN head. [L.]

c. angula're quadra'ti la'bii superio'ris, SYN levator labii superioris alaeque nasi *muscle.*

c. bre've [NA], SYN short *head.*

c. breve musculi bicipitis brachii [NA], SYN short *head* of biceps brachii muscle.

c. breve musculi bicipitis fem'oris, SYN short *head* of biceps femoris muscle.

c. cor'nus, SYN *apex* of the posterior horn.

c. cos'tae [NA], SYN *head* of rib.

c. epididymid'is [NA], SYN *head* of epididymis.

c. fem'oris, SYN *head* of femur.

c. fib'ulae [NA], SYN *head* of fibula.

c. gallinaginis (gal-i-naj'i-nis), SYN seminal *colliculus.* [Mod. L. snipe's head]

c. humera'le [NA], SYN humeral *head.*

c. humerale musculi flexoris carpi ulnaris [NA], humeral head of flexor carpi ulnaris muscle. SEE humeral *head.*

c. humerale musculi pronatoris teretis [NA], humeral head of pronator teres muscle. SEE humeral *head.*

c. hu'meri [NA], SYN *head* of humerus.

c. humeroulna're musculi flexoris digitorum superificialis [NA], SYN humeroulnar *head* of flexor digitorum superficialis muscle.

c. infraorbita'le quadra'ti la'bii superio'ris, SYN levator labii superioris *muscle.*

c. latera'le [NA], SYN lateral *head.*

c. laterale musculi gastrocnemii [NA], lateral head of gastrocnemius muscle. SEE lateral *head.*

c. laterale musculi tricipitis brachii [NA], lateral head of triceps brachii. SEE lateral *head.*

c. long'um [NA], SYN long *head.*

c. longum musculi bicipitis brachii [NA], long head of biceps brachii muscle. SEE long *head.*

c. longum musculi bicipitis fem'oris [NA], long head of biceps femoris muscle. SEE long *head.*

c. longum musculi tricipitis brachii [NA], long head of triceps brachii muscle. SEE long *head.*

c. mal'lei [NA], SYN *head* of malleus.

c. mandib'ulae [NA], SYN *head* of mandible.

c. media'le [NA], SYN medial *head.*

c. mediale musculi gastrocnemii [NA], medial head of gastrocnemius muscle. SEE medial *head.*

c. mediale musculi tricipitis brachii [NA], medial head of triceps brachii muscle. SEE medial *head.*

c. medu'sae, (1) varicose veins radiating from the umbilicus, seen in the Cruveilhier-Baumgarten syndrome; **(2)** dilated ciliary arteries girdling the corneoscleral limbus in rubeosis iridis. SYN Medusa head. [*Medusa,* G. myth. char.]

c. nu'clei cauda'ti [NA], SYN *head* of the caudate nucleus.

c. obli'quum [NA], SYN oblique *head.*

ca

c. obliquum musculi adductoris hallucis [NA], oblique head of adductor hallucis muscle. SEE oblique *head.*

c. obliquum musculi adductoris pollicis [NA], oblique head of adductor pollicis muscle. SEE oblique *head.*

c. os'sis fem'oris [NA], SYN *head* of femur.

c. os'sis metacarpa'lis [NA], SYN *head* of metacarpal bone.

c. os'sis metatarsa'lis [NA], SYN *head* of metatarsal bone.

c. pancrea'tis [NA], SYN *head* of pancreas.

c. phalan'gis [NA], SYN *head* of phalanx.

c. profun'dum musculi flexoris pollicis brevis [NA], SYN deep *head* of flexor pollicis brevis.

c. quadra'tum, a head of large size and square shape, owing to thickened parietal and frontal eminences, seen in rachitic children.

c. radia'le [NA], SYN radial *head.*

c. ra'dii [NA], SYN *head* of radius.

c. sta'pedis [NA], SYN *head* of stapes.

c. succeda'neum, an edematous swelling formed on the presenting portion of the scalp of an infant during birth; the effusion overlies the periosteum and consists of edema; contrasted with cephalhematoma, in which condition the effusion lies under the periosteum and consists of blood.

c. superficia'le musculi flexoris pollicis brevis [NA], SYN superficial *head* of flexor pollicis brevis muscle.

c. ta'li [NA], SYN *head* of talus.

c. transver'sum [NA], SYN transverse *head.*

c. transversum musculi adductoris hallucis [NA], transverse head of adductor hallucis muscle. SEE transverse *head.*

c. transversum musculi adductoris pollicis [NA], transverse head of adductor pollicis muscle. SEE transverse *head.*

c. ul'nae [NA], SYN *head* of ulna.

c. ulna're [NA], SYN ulnar *head.*

c. ulnare musculi flexoris carpi ulnaris [NA], ulnar head of flexor carpi ulnaris muscle. SEE ulnar *head.*

c. ulnare musculi pronatoris teretis [NA], ulnar head of pronator teres muscle. SEE ulnar *head.*

c. zygomat'icum quadra'ti la'bii superio'ris, SYN zygomaticus minor *muscle.*

Carabelli, Georg (Edler von Lunkaszprie), Austrian dentist, 1787–1842. SEE *cusp* of C.; C. *tubercle.*

car·a·mel (kar'ă-mel). Burnt sugar; a concentrated solution of the substance obtained by heating sugar with an alkali; a thick, dark brown liquid used as a coloring and flavoring agent in pharmaceutical preparations. [Sp., fr. L.L. *calamellus*, fr. L. *calamus*, reed]

ca·ram·i·phen eth·ane·di·sul·fo·nate (ka-ram'i-fen eth'ăn-dī-sŭl'fō-nāt). Diethylaminoethyl 1-phenylcyclopentanecarboxylate ethanedisulfonate; an antitussive.

ca·ram·i·phen hy·dro·chlo·ride. Diethylaminoethyl-1-phenylcyclopentane-1-carboxylate hydrochloride; a synthetic spasmolytic drug; used in the treatment of diseases of the basal ganglia, *e.g.,* parkinsonism and hepatolenticular degeneration.

ca·ra·te (kă-rah'tē). SYN pinta.

⌂carb-, carbo-. Prefixes indicating carbon, especially the attachment of a group containing a carbon atom. [L. *carbo,* charcoal]

car·ba·chol (kar'bă-kol). A parasympathetic stimulant used locally in the eye for the treatment of glaucoma.

car·ba·dox (kar'bă-doks). Methyl 3-(2-quinoxalinylmethylene)-carbazate N^1,N^4- dioxide; an antibacterial agent.

car·ba·mate (kar'bă-māt). **1.** A salt or ester of carbamic acid forming the basis of urethane hypnotics. **2.** A group of cholinesterase inhibiting insecticides resembling organophosphates; the most frequent c. is carbaril. SYN carbamoate, carbaril.

c. kinase, a phosphotransferase catalyzing the reaction of carbamoyl phosphate and ADP to form ATP, NH_3, and CO_2.

car·bam·az·e·pine (kar-bam-az'ĕ-pēn). 5-*H*-Dibenz[*b,f*]-azepine-5-carboxamide; an anticonvulsant; also useful in alleviating the pain of trigeminal neuralgia.

car·bam·ic ac·id (kar-bam'ik). A hypothetical acid, NH_2-COOH, forming carbamates; the acyl radical is carbamoyl.

car·bam·ide (kar'bă-mīd). Obsolete term for urea.

carb·a·mi·no·he·mo·glo·bin (kar-bam'i-nō-hē-mō-glō'bin). Carbon dioxide bound to hemoglobin by means of a reactive amino group on the latter, *i.e.,* Hb-NHCOOH; approximately 20% of the total content of carbon dioxide in blood is combined with hemoglobin in this manner. SYN carbhemoglobin, carbohemoglobin.

car·ba·moate. SYN carbamate.

car·bam·o·yl (kar'bă-mō-il). The acyl radical, NH_2-CO-, the transfer of which plays an important role in certain biochemical reactions; *e.g.,* in the urea cycle, via carbamoyl phosphate.

car·bam·o·yl·as·par·tate de·hy·drase (kar'bă-mō-il-as-par'tāt). SYN dihydro-orotase.

N-**car·bam·o·yl·as·par·tic** (kar'bă-mō-il-as-par'tik). SYN ureidosuccinic acid.

car·bam·o·yl·a·tion (kar-bă-mō-il-ā'shŭn). Transfer of the carbamoyl from a carbamoyl-containing molecule (*e.g.,* carbamoyl phosphate) to an acceptor moiety such as an amino group.

car·bam·o·yl·car·bam·ic ac·id (kar'bă-mō-il-kar-bam'ik). SYN allophanic acid.

N-**car·bam·o·yl·glu·tam·ic ac·id** (kar'bă-mō-il-glū-tam'ik). HOOC$(CH_2)_2$CH$(NHCONH_2)$COOH; an intermediate in the carbamoylation of ornithine to citrulline in the urea cycle; used in the treatment of individuals having a deficiency of the enzyme that synthesizes *N*-acetylglutamate.

car·bam·o·yl phos·phate. H_2NCO-OPO_3^{2-}; a reactive intermediate capable of transferring its carbamoyl group (H_2NCO-) to an acceptor molecule, forming citrulline from ornithine in the urea cycle, and ureidosuccinic acid from aspartic acid in pyrimidine ring formation.

c. p. synthetase, a phosphotransferase catalyzing the formation of c. p. There are two significant isozymes. c. p. synthetase I is a mitochondrial enzyme that catalyzes the reaction of 2ATP, NH_3, CO_2, and H_2O to c. p., 2ADP, and P_i. It is activated by *N*-acetylglutamate and participates in urea biosynthesis. A deficiency of c. p. synthetase I can result in hyperammonemia. c. p. synthetase II is a cytosolic enzyme that, under physiological conditions, uses L-glutamine as the nitrogen source (producing L-glutamate) instead of NH_3, is not activated by *N*-acetylglutamate, and is found in pyrimidine biosynthesis.

car·bam·o·yl·trans·fer·as·es (kar'bă-mō-il-trans'fer-ās-ĕz) [EC group 2.1.3]. Enzymes transferring carbamoyl groups from one compound to another (*e.g.,* aspartate carbamoyltransferase, ornithine carbamoyltransferase). SYN transcarbamoylases.

car·bam·o·yl·u·rea (kar'bă-mō-il-yū-rē'ă). SYN biuret.

car·ba·myl (kar'bă-mil). Former spelling of carbamoyl.

car·ba·myl·a·tion (kar'bă-mil-ā'shŭn). Former spelling of carbamoylation.

carb·an·i·on (karb-an'ī-on). An organic anion in which the negative charge is on a carbon atom; the specific names are formed by adding -ide, -diide, etc. to the name of the parent compound; *e.g.,* methanide, $(CH_3)^-$.

car·bar·il (car-bar-il'). SYN carbamate.

car·bar·sone (kar-bar'sōn). 4-Ureidobenzenearsonic acid; *N*-carbamoylarsanilic acid; an amebicide.

car·bar·yl (kar'bă-ril). A contact insecticide. A pediculicide and ectoparasiticide. Toxic to humans, causing nausea, vomiting, diarrhea, bronchoconstrictions, blurring vision, excessive salivation, muscle twitching, cyanosis, convulsions, coma, respiratory failure.

car·ba·zides (kar'bă-zīdz). 1,3-diaminoureas; rNH-NHCONH-NHR'. SYN carbohydrazides.

car·baz·o·chrome sa·lic·y·late (kar-baz'ō-krōm). Adrenochrome monosemicarbazone-sodium salicylate complex; an oxidation product of epinephrine used for the systemic control of capillary bleeding associated with increased capillary permeability.

car·ba·zole (kar'bă-zōl). Reacts with carbohydrates (including uronates and deoxypentoses) giving colors characteristic of the sugar type; used for assay and analysis of carbohydrates and formaldehyde, and as a dye intermediate; sensitive to ultraviolet light. SYN 9-azafluorene, diphenylenimine.

carb·a·zot·ic ac·id (kar-bă-zot'ik). SYN picric acid.

car·ben·i·cil·lin di·so·di·um (kar-ben-i-sil′in). Disodium salt of 6-(α-carboxy-α-phenylacetamido)penicillanic acid (α-carboxybenzylpenicillin); a semisynthetic extended spectrum penicillin active against a wide variety of Gram-positive and Gram-negative bacteria.

car·be·ni·um (kar-ben′ē-ŭm). SEE carbonium.

car·ben·ox·o·lone di·so·di·um (kar-ben-oks′ŏ-lōn dī-sō′dē-ŭm). 3β-Hydroxy-11-oxoolean-12-en-30-oic hydrogen succinate disodium salt; a glucocorticoid used as an anti-inflammatory agent for the treatment of peptic ulcer.

car·be·ta·pen·tane cit·rate (kar′be-tă-pen′tān). 2-(Diethylaminoethoxy)ethyl 1-phenylcyclopentyl-1-carboxylate citrate; it has atropine-like and local anesthetic actions and effectively suppresses acute cough due to common upper respiratory infections.

carb·he·mo·glo·bin (karb′hē-mō-glō′bin). SYN carbaminohemoglobin.

car·bide (kar′bīd). A compound of carbon with an element more electropositive than itself; *e.g.,* CaC_2, calcium carbide.

car·bi·do·pa (kar-bi-dō′pă). α-Methyldopahydrazine; (-)-L-α-hydrazino-3,4-dihydroxy-α-methylhydrocinnamic monohydrate; a dopa decarboxylase inhibitor which does not enter the brain used in conjunction with levodopa in the treatment of Parkinson's disease to reduce L-dopa doses and reduce side effects.

car·bi·ma·zole (kar-bī′mă-zōl). 1-Methyl-2-imidazolethiol ethyl carbonate; used in the treatment of hyperthyroidism.

car·bi·nol (kar′bi-nol). SYN *methyl* alcohol.

car·bi·nox·a·mine ma·le·ate (kar-bi-nok′să-mēn). Paracarbinoxamine maleate 2-[*p*-chloro-α-(2-dimethylaminoethoxy)benzyl]pyridine maleate; an antihistaminic agent.

car·bo. SYN charcoal. [L. coal]

carbo-. SEE carb-.

car·bo·ben·zoxy (Z, Cbz) (kar′bō-ben-zok′sē). SYN benzyloxycarbonyl.

car·bo·cat·i·on (kar-bō-kat′ī-on). SEE carbonium.

car·bo·he·mo·glo·bin (kar′bō-hē-mō-glō′bin). SYN carbaminohemoglobin.

car·bo·hy·drates (kar-bō-hī′drāts). Class name for the aldehydic or ketonic derivative of polyhydric alcohols, the name being derived from the fact that the most common examples of such compounds have formulas that may be written $C_n(H_2O)_n$ (*e.g.,* glucose, $C_6(H_2O)_6$; sucrose, $C_{12}(H_2O)_{11}$), although they are not true hydrates and the name is in that sense a misnomer. The group includes compounds with relatively small molecules, such as the simple sugars (monosaccharides, disaccharides, etc.), as well as macromolecular (polymeric) substances such as starch, glycogen, and cellulose polysaccharides. The c.'s most typical of the class contain carbon, hydrogen, and oxygen only, but carbohydrate metabolic intermediates in tissue contain phosphorus. SEE saccharides.

car·bo·hy·drat·u·ria (kar′bō-hī-dră-tū′rē-ă). General term denoting the excretion of one or more carbohydrates in the urine (*e.g.,* glucose, galactose, lactose, pentose), thus including such conditions as glycosuria (melituria), galactosuria, lactosuria, pentosuria, etc.

car·bo·hy·dra·zides (kar-bō-hī′dră-zīdz). SYN carbazides.

car·bo·late (kar′bō-lāt). 1. SYN phenate. 2. To carbolize.

car·bo·lat·ed (kar′bō-lā-ted). SYN phenolated.

car·bol-fuch·sin (kar′bol-fuk′sin). 1. SEE Ziehl's *stain.* 2. SEE carbol-fuchsin *paint.*

car·bol·ic ac·id (kar-bol′ik). SYN phenol.

car·bo·lize (kar′bō-līz). To mix with or add carbolic acid (phenol).

car·bo·lu·ria (kar-bō-lū′rē-ă). The presence of phenol (carbolic acid) in the urine. [carbolic acid + G. *ouron,* urine]

car·bo·mer (kar′bō-mer). A polymer of acrylic acid cross-linked with a polyfunctional compound, hence, a poly (acrylic acid) or polyacrylate; a suspending agent for pharmaceuticals.

car·bom·e·try (kar-bom′ě-trē). SYN carbonometry.

car·bo·my·cin (kar′bō-mī′sin). A macrolide antibiotic isolated

from *Streptomyces halstedii;* similar to erythromycin and used as an antibacterial and antimicrobial.

car·bon (C) (kar′bŏn). A nonmetallic tetravalent element, atomic no. 6, atomic wt. 12.011; the major bioelement. It has two natural isotopes, ^{12}C and ^{13}C (the former, set at 12.00000, being the standard for all molecular weights), and two artificial, radioactive isotopes of interest, ^{11}C and ^{14}C. The element occurs in three pure forms, diamond, graphite, and in the fullerines; in amorphous form in charcoal, coke, and soot; and in the atmosphere as CO_2. Its compounds are found in all living tissues, and the study of its vast number of compounds constitutes most of organic chemistry. [L. *carbo,* coal]

active c. dioxide, activated c. dioxide, a complex of *N*-carboxybiotin (biotin + CO_2) and an enzyme; the form in which c. dioxide is added to other molecules in carboxylations; *e.g.,* to methylcrotonyl-CoA to form β-methylglutaconyl in the catabolism of leucine, and to acetyl-CoA to form malonyl-CoA. SEE ALSO *acetyl-CoA* carboxylase.

anomeric c., the reducing c. of a sugar; C-1 of an aldose, C-2 of a 2-ketose.

c. bisulfide, SYN c. disulfide.

c. dichloride, SYN tetrachlorethylene.

c. dioxide, CO_2; the product of the combustion of c. with an excess of air; in concentrations not less than 99.0% by volume of CO_2, used as a respiratory stimulant. SYN carbonic acid gas, carbonic anhydride.

c. dioxide snow, solid c. dioxide used in the treatment of warts, lupus, nevi, and other skin affections, and as a refrigerant. SYN dry ice.

c. disulfide, CS_2; an extremely flammable (flashpoint -30°C), colorless, toxic liquid with a characteristic ethereal odor (fetid when impure); it is a parasiticide. SYN c. bisulfide.

c. monoxide (CO), a colorless, practically odorless, and poisonous gas formed by the incomplete combustion of c.; its toxic action is due to its strong affinity for hemoglobin, myoglobin, and the cytochromes, reducing oxygen transport and blocking oxygen utilization.

c. tetrachloride, CCl_4; a colorless, mobile liquid having a characteristic ethereal odor resembling that of chloroform; it is used as a cleansing fluid and as a fire extinguisher, and has been used as an anthelmintic, especially against hookworm. SYN tetrachloromethane.

car·bon-11 (^{11}C). A cyclotron-produced, positron-emitting radioisotope of carbon with a half-life of 20.3 minutes; used in positron-emitting tomography.

car·bon-12 (^{12}C). The standard of atomic mass, 98.90% of natural carbon.

car·bon-13 (^{13}C). A stable natural isotope, 1.1% of natural carbon.

car·bon-14 (^{14}C). A beta-emitter with a half-life of 5715 years, widely used as a tracer in studying various aspects of metabolism; naturally occurring ^{14}C, arising from cosmic ray bombardment, is used to date relics containing natural carbonaceous materials.

car·bon·ate (kar′bŏn-āt). 1. A salt of carbonic acid. 2. The ion $CO_3^=$.

c. dehydratase, SYN carbonic *anhydrase.*

c. hydro-lyase, SYN carbonic *anhydrase.*

car·bon·ic (kar-bon′ik). Relating to carbon. See also under carbonate.

car·bon·ic ac·id. H_2CO_3, formed from H_2O and CO_2.

car·bon·ic an·hy·drase. See under anhydrase.

car·bon·ic an·hy·dride. SYN *carbon* dioxide.

car·bo·ni·um (kar-bŏn′ē-ŭm). An organic cation in which the positive charge is on a carbon atom; *e.g.,* $(CH_3)^+$. It is now recommended that carbocation be used as the class name and carbenium be used for specific compound names.

car·bo·nom·e·ter (kar-bō-nom′ě-ter). An obsolete device used in carbonometry. [L. *carbo (carbon-),* coal, + G. *metron,* measure]

car·bo·nom·e·try (kar-bō-nom′ě-trē). An obsolete method for the determination of the presence and the proportion of carbon dioxide in the air or expired breath by the precipitation of calcium carbonate from lime water. SYN carbometry.

car·bo·nu·ria (kar-bo-nū′rē-ă). Rarely used term denoting the excretion of carbon dioxide or other carbon compounds in the urine.

car·bon·yl (kar′bŏn-il). The characteristic group, —CO—, of the ketones, aldehydes, and organic acids.

car·bo·plat·in (kar′bō-plă′tin). A platinum-containing anticancer agent much like cisplatin but more toxic to the myeloid elements of bone marrow while producing less nausea and neuro-, oto-, and nephrotoxicity; used in the chemotherapy of solid tumors.

car·bo·prost tro·meth·a·mine (kar′bō-prost trō-meth′ă-mēn). $C_{25}H_{38}O_5$; a prostaglandin used as an abortifacient and in the treatment of refractory postpartum bleeding.

car·box·am·ide (kar-boks′am-īd). A molecular configuration (–CONH₂) that, together with the related carboximides (iminocarbonyls) (–CONH–), is a constituent of many hypnotics, including barbiturates, hydantoins, and thiazines. SYN aminocarbonyl.

car·box·im·ide (kar-boks′im-īd). SEE carboxamide.

⌂**carboxy-.** Combining form indicating addition of CO or CO₂.

N-car·box·y·an·hy·drides (kar-bok′sē-an-hī′drīdz). Heterocyclic derivatives of amino acids from which polypeptides may be synthesized.

car·box·y·ca·thep·sin (kar-bok′sē-kă-thep′sin). SYN peptidyl dipeptidase A.

car·box·y·dis·mu·tase (kar-bok-sē-dis′mū-tās). SYN ribulose-1,5-bisphosphate carboxylase.

4-car·box·y·glu·tam·ic ac·id (Gla) (kar-bok′sē-glū-tam′ik). A carboxylated form of glutamic acid found in certain proteins (e.g., prothrombin, factors VII, IX, and X, osteocalcin). Its synthesis is vitamin K-dependent.

car·box·y·he·mo·glo·bin (HbCO) (kar-bok′sē-hē-mō-glō′bin). A fairly stable union of carbon monoxide with hemoglobin. The formation of c. prevents the normal transfer of carbon dioxide and oxygen during the circulation of blood; thus, increasing levels of c. result in various degrees of asphyxiation, including death. SYN carbon monoxide hemoglobin.

car·box·y·he·mo·glo·bi·ne·mia (kar-bok′sē-hē′mō-glō-bi-nē′mē-ă). Presence of carboxyhemoglobin in the blood, as in carbon monoxide poisoning.

car·box·yl (kar-bok′sil). The characterizing group (—COOH) of certain organic acids; e.g., HCOOH (formic acid), CH₃COOH (acetic acid), CH₃CH(NH₂)COOH (alanine), etc. Cf. carboxylic acid.

car·box·yl·ase (kar-bok′sil-ās). **1.** One of several carboxy-lyases, trivially named carboxylases or decarboxylases (EC subclass 4.1.1), catalyzing the addition of CO₂ to all or part of another molecule to create an additional —COOH group (e.g., ribulose-1,5-bisphosphate carboxylase). **2.** Obsolete name for *pyruvate* decarboxylase.

car·box·yl·a·tion (kar-bok-si-lā′shŭn). Addition of CO₂ to an organic acceptor, as in formation of malonyl-CoA or in photosynthesis, to yield a —COOH group; catalyzed by carboxylases.

car·box·yl·ic ac·id (kar-bok′sil-ik). An organic acid with a carboxyl group. Cf. carboxyl.

activated c. a., derivative of a carboxyl group that is more susceptible to nucleophilic attack than a free carboxyl group; e.g., acid anhydrides, thioesters.

car·box·yl·trans·fer·as·es (kar-bok-sil-trans′fer-ās-ez) [EC group 2.1.3]. Enzymes transferring carboxyl groups from one compound to another. SYN transcarboxylases.

car·box·y·meth·yl·cel·lu·lose (kar-bok-sē-meth′il-sel′yū-lōs). A cellulose derivative which forms a colloidal dispersion in water; indigestible and nonabsorbable systemically; absorbs water and is used as a bulk laxative. Can also be used as a suspending agent.

car·box·y·pep·ti·dase (kar-bok-sē-pep′ti-dās). A hydrolase that removes the amino acid at the free carboxyl end of a polypeptide chain; an exopeptidase.

acid c., SYN serine c.

serine c., a c. of broad specificity for terminal amino acid residues of peptides; the optimum pH is 4.5 to 6.0; sensitive to diisopropyl fluorophosphate; contains a serine at the active site. SYN acid c.

car·box·y·pep·ti·dase A. A hydrolase that releases C-terminal amino acids, with the exception of C-terminal arginyl, lysyl, and prolyl residues. A zinc-containing exopeptidase.

car·box·y·pep·ti·dase B. A hydrolase that releases C-terminal lysyl or arginyl residues preferentially. A zinc-containing exopeptidase. SYN protaminase.

car·box·y·pep·ti·dase C [EC 3.4.12.1]. SEE serine *carboxypeptidase*.

car·box·y·pep·ti·dase G. SYN γ-glutamyl hydrolase.

N-car·box·y·u·rea (kar-bok′sē-yū-rē′ă). SYN allophanic acid.

car·bro·mal (kar′brō-mal). Obsolete hypnotic agent which is a monoureide-containing bromine.

car·bun·cle (kar′bŭng-kl). **1.** Deep-seated pyogenic infection of the skin and subcutaneous tissues, usually arising in several contiguous hair follicles, with formation of connecting sinuses; often preceded or accompanied by fever, malaise, and prostration. **2.** SYN anthrax (1). [L. *carbunculus,* dim. of *carbo,* a live coal, a carbuncle]

kidney c., renal c., formerly used term for coalescent multiple intrarenal abscesses.

car·bun·cu·lar (kar-bŭng′kyū-lăr). Relating to a carbuncle.

car·bun·cu·lo·sis (kar-bŭng-kyū-lō′sis). A condition marked by the occurrence of several carbuncles simultaneously or within a short period of time.

car·bu·ret (kar′bū-ret). **1.** Archaic term for carbide. **2.** To combine with carbon. **3.** To enrich a gas with volatile hydrocarbons, as in a carburetor.

car·bu·ta·mide (kar-bū′tă-mīd). Aminophenurobutane; 1-butyl-3-sulfanilylurea; an oral hypoglycemic agent.

car·bu·te·rol hy·dro·chlo·ride (kar-bū′tĕ-rol). [5-[2-(*tert*-Butylamino)-1-hydroxyethyl]-2-hydro xyphenyl]urea monohydrochloride; a sympathomimetic drug with bronchodilatory activity.

car·cass (kar′kăs). The body of a dead animal; in reference to animals used for human food, the body after the hide, head, tail, extremities, and viscera have been removed. [F. *carcasse,* fr. It. *carcassa*]

⌂**carcino-, carcin-.** Cancer; crab. [G. *karkinos,* crab, cancer]

car·ci·no·em·bry·on·ic (kar′si-nō-em-brē-on′ik). Relating to a carcinoma-associated substance present in embryonic tissue, as a c. antigen.

car·cin·o·gen (kar-sin′ō-jen, kar′si-nō-jen). Any cancer-producing substance or organism, such as polycyclic aromatic hydrocarbons, or agents such as in certain types of irradiation. [carcino- + G, -gen, producing]

complete c., a chemical c. that is able to induce cancer without provocation by a tumor-promoting agent introduced during therapy.

car·ci·no·gen·e·sis (kar′si-nō-jen′ĕ-sis). The origin or production, or development of cancer, including carcinomas and other malignant neoplasms. [carcino- + G. *genesis,* generation]

car·ci·no·gen·ic (DAB) (kar′si-nō-jen′ik). Causing cancer. SYN cancerigenic.

car·ci·noid (kar′si-noyd). SEE carcinoid *tumor,* carcinoid *syndrome.*

car·ci·no·lyt·ic (kar′si-nō-lit′ik). Destructive to the cells of carcinoma. SYN cancericidal, cancerocidal. [carcino- + G. *lytikos,* causing a solution]

CARCINOMA

car·ci·no·ma (CA), pl. **car·ci·no·mas, car·ci·no·ma·ta** (kar-si-nō′mă, -măz, -nō′mă-tă). Any of the various types of malignant neoplasm derived from epithelial tissue in several sites, occurring more frequently in the skin and large intestine in both sexes, the lung and prostate gland in men, and the lung and breast in women. C.'s are identified histologically on the basis of invasiveness and the changes that indicate anaplasia, *i.e.,* loss of polarity of nuclei, loss of orderly maturation of cells (especially in squamous cell type), variation in the size and shape of cells, hyperchromatism of nuclei (with clumping of chromatin), and increase in the nuclear-cytoplasmic ratio. C.'s may be undifferentiated, or the neoplastic tissue may resemble (to varying degree) one of the types of normal epithelium. [G. *karkinōma,* fr. *karkinos,* cancer, + *-oma,* tumor]

Cancer of the breast or axillary nodes is second only to lung cancer as a cause of cancer death among U.S. women. There were an estimated 182,000 new cases and 46,000 deaths caused by it in 1994. Breast cancer has been the subject of a major public health effort since the 1980s. Various groups, including the American Cancer Society, have campaigned for increased federal funding for breast cancer research and health insurer coverage of diagnostic mammography. A controversial statistic, publicized by the American Cancer Society, indicates that breast cancer will afflict 1 in 9 American women. However, this is a cumulative probability figure calculated on the basis of a hypothetical 100 women between the ages of 30 and 110. A more accurate representation of the statistical model is that a woman between the ages of 30 and 55 has a 1 in 40 chance of breast cancer, and only a 1 in 180 chance of dying from it. Ninety percent of those with breast cancer report no breast cancer in their families. Risk appears slightly elevated for women who have no children, or undergo their first pregnancy after age 35; who experience an early menarche or late menopause; or who have more than two first-degree relatives who have had premenopausal or bilateral breast cancers. In 1993, 10–25% of new cancers seen were preinvasive ductal carcinoma in situ; a decade earlier, such pre- invasive tumors represented just 3% of cases. The increase is attributable to mammography. It is estimated that 20–50% of ductal carcinomas in situ go on to become invasive, with a latency period of 5–10 years. Because the milk ducts are distributed throughout the breast, radical mastectomy is the recommended treatment for this type of cancer. Meanwhile, breast conservation surgery has been shown to be highly effective for more compact tumors.

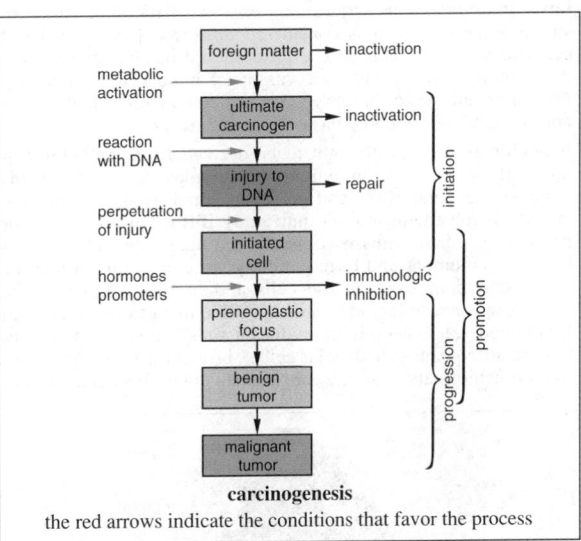

carcinogenesis
the red arrows indicate the conditions that favor the process

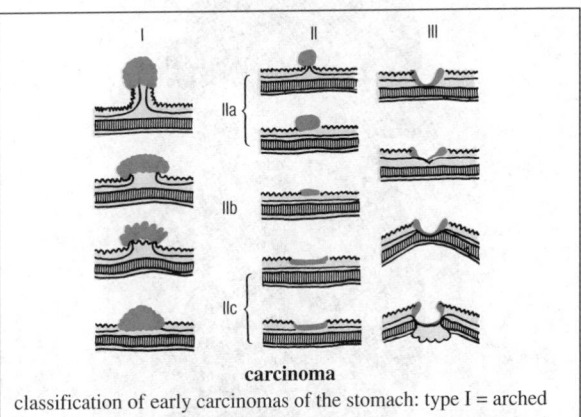

carcinoma
classification of early carcinomas of the stomach: type I = arched form; type II = superficial form (a = raised, b = level, c = sunken); type III = excavated form

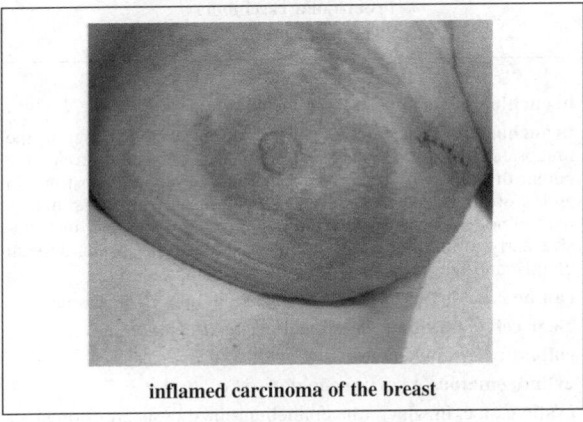

inflamed carcinoma of the breast

acinar c., SYN acinic cell *adenocarcinoma.*

acinic cell c., SYN acinic cell *adenocarcinoma.*

acinose c., acinous c., SYN acinic cell *adenocarcinoma.*

adenoid cystic c., a histologic type of c. characterized by large epithelial masses containing round, glandlike spaces or cysts which frequently contain mucus or collagen and are bordered by a few or many layers of epithelial cells without intervening stroma, forming a cribriform pattern like a slice of Swiss cheese; perineural invasion and hematogenous metastasis are common; occurs most commonly in salivary glands. SYN cylindromatous c.

adenoid squamous cell c., SYN adenoacanthoma.

adenosquamous c., a type of lung tumor exhibiting areas of clear cut glandular and squamous cell differentiation along with regions of the undifferentiated c.

adnexal c., a c. arising in, or forming structures resembling, skin appendages.

adrenal cortical carcinomas, large invasive and metastasizing tumors which may cause virilism or Cushing's syndrome.

alveolar cell c., SYN bronchiolar c.

anaplastic c., c. with absence of epithelial structural differentiation.

apocrine c., (1) a c. composed predominantly of cells with abundant eosinophilic granular cytoplasm, occurring in the breast; **(2)** a c. of the apocrine glands.

basal cell c., a slow-growing, invasive, but usually non-metastasizing neoplasm recapitulating normal basal cells of the epider-

mis or hair follicles, most commonly rising in sun-damaged skin of the elderly and fair-skinned. SYN basal cell epithelioma.

basaloid c., a poorly differentiated squamous cell c. of the anus that has some microscopic resemblance to basal cell c. of the skin, but which frequently metastasizes.

basal squamous cell c., SYN basosquamous c.

basosquamous c., basisquamous c., a c. of the skin which in structure and behavior is considered transitional between basal cell and squamous cell c. The term should not be used for the much more common keratotic variety of basal cell c., in which the tumor cells are of basal type but which contains small foci of abrupt keratinization. SYN basal squamous cell c.

bronchiolar c., a c., thought to be derived from epithelium of terminal bronchioles, in which the neoplastic tissue extends along the alveolar walls and grows in small masses within the alveoli; involvement may be uniformly diffuse and massive, or nodular, or lobular; microscopically, the neoplastic cells are cuboidal or columnar and form papillary structures; mucin may be demonstrated in some of the cells and in the material in the alveoli, which also includes denuded cells; metastases in regional lymph nodes, and even in more distant sites, are known to occur, but are infrequent. SYN alveolar cell c., bronchiolar adenocarcinoma, bronchiolo-alveolar c., bronchioloalveolar adenocarcinoma.

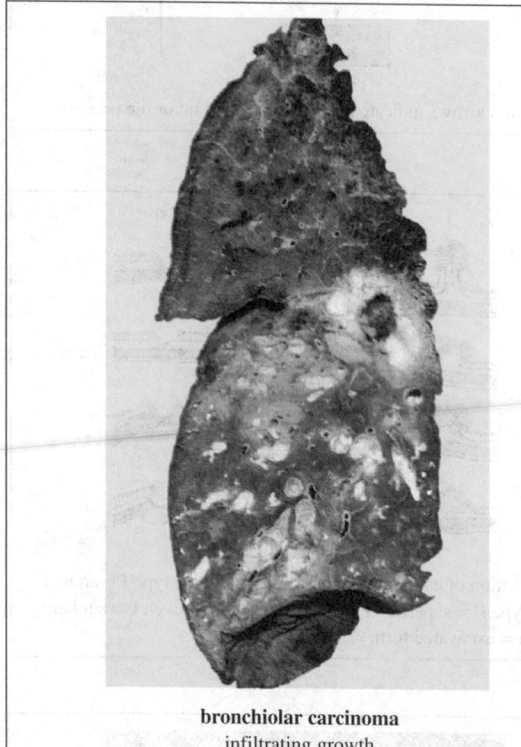

bronchiolar carcinoma
infiltrating growth

bronchiolo-alveolar c., SYN bronchiolar c.

bronchogenic c., squamous cell or oat cell c. that arises in the mucosa of the large bronchi and produces a persistent productive cough or hemoptysis; local growth causes bronchial obstruction and is observed radiologically as an enlarging lung mass; malignant tumor cells can be detected in the sputum, and they metastasize early to the thoracic lymph nodes and to the brain, adrenal glands, and other organs via the bloodstream.

canine c. 1, one of the few transplantable tumors of animals.

clear cell c. of kidney, SYN renal *adenocarcinoma*.

colloid c., SYN mucinous c.

cylindromatous c., SYN adenoid cystic c.

cystic c., a c. in which true epithelium-lined cysts are formed, or degenerative changes may result in cystlike spaces.

duct c., ductal c., a c. derived from epithelium of ducts, *e.g.,* in the breast or pancreas.

embryonal c., a malignant neoplasm of the testis, composed of large anaplastic cells with indistinct cellular borders, amphophilic cytoplasm, and ovoid, round, or bean-shaped nuclei that may have multiple large nuclei; in some instances, the neoplastic

bronchiolar carcinoma (TNM classification)		
T-classification	T_{IS}	preinvasive
	T_1	tumor < 3cm, is enclosed by lungs or visceral ribs; main bronchus is clear
	T_2	neither T_1 nor T_3
	T_3	neighboring tissues directly infiltrated (thoracic wall, diaphragm, etc.), or tumor is less than 2cm from the carina tracheae, or pleural effusion, or atelectasis, or obstructive pneumonia of entire lung
N-classification	N_0	regional lymph nodes not affected
	N_1	peribronchial hilus lymph nodes affected
	N_2	other mediastinal lymph nodes affected
M-classification	M_0	without sign of metastasis
	M_1	metastasis

cells may form tubular structures; embryonal c.'s may be malignant teratomas without differentiated elements.

endometrioid c., adenocarcinoma of the ovary or prostate resembling endometrial adenocarcinoma, possibly arising from ovarian foci of endometriosis.

epidermoid c., squamous cell c. of the skin. SYN epidermoid cancer.

epithelial myoepithelial c. (mī'yō-ep-i-thē'lē-al), a salivary gland malignancy composed of an inner layer of ductal cells surrounded by a layer of clear myoepithelial cells.

fibrolamellar liver cell c., primary hepatic c. in which malignant hepatocytes are intersected by fibrous lamellated bands. SYN oncocytic hepatocellular tumor.

follicular carcinomas, c.'s of the thyroid composed of well or poorly differentiated epithelial follicles without papillary formation, which are difficult to distinguish from adenomas; the criteria include blood vessel invasion and the finding of metastases of follicular thyroid tissue in other structures such as cervical lymph nodes and bone; follicular c.'s may take up radioactive iodine.

giant cell c., a malignant epithelial neoplasm characterized by unusually large anaplastic cells.

giant cell c. of thyroid gland, a rapidly progressive undifferentiated c. observed in the thyroid gland, characterized by numerous, unusually large, anaplastic cells derived from glandular epithelium of the thyroid gland.

glandular c., SYN adenocarcinoma.

hepatocellular c., SYN malignant *hepatoma.*

Hürthle cell c., SYN Hürthle cell *tumor.*

inflammatory c., c. of the breast presenting with edema, hyperemia, tenderness, and rapid enlargment of the breast; microscopically, there is extensive invasion of dermal lymphatics by the c.

intermediate c., obsolete term for basosquamous c.

intraductal c., a form of c. derived from the epithelial lining of ducts, especially in the breast, where most c.'s arise from ductal epithelium; the neoplastic cells proliferate in irregular papillary projections or masses, filling the lumens, that are solid, cribriform, or centrally necrotic; intraductal c. is a form of c. in situ as it is contained by the ductal basement membrane; when it invades surrounding stroma or metastasizes it is referred to as ductal c.

intraepidermal c., c. in situ of the skin; *e.g.,* Bowen's disease.

intraepithelial c., SYN c. in situ.

invasive c., a neoplasm in which collections of epithelial cells infiltrate or destroy the surrounding tissue.

juvenile c., SYN secretory c.

kangri burn c., SYN kang *cancer.*

large cell c., an anaplastic c., particularly bronchogenic, composed of cells which are much larger than those in oat cell c. of the lung.

latent c., an epithelial neoplasm showing microscopic features of malignancy believed to have remained localized and asymptomatic for a long period; *e.g.,* small c.'s of the prostate in old men, often found incidentally at autopsy.

lateral aberrant thyroid c., a cervical nodule of thyroid c. situated outside the thyroid gland, formerly thought to arise from ectopic thyroid tissue but now believed to be metastatic from an occult c. within the gland.

leptomeningeal c., SYN meningeal c.

liver cell c., SYN malignant *hepatoma.*

lobular c., a form of adenocarcinoma, especially of the breast, where lobular c. is less common than ductal c. and usually is composed of small cells.

lobular c. in situ, SYN noninfiltrating lobular c.

Lucké c., a herpesvirus-associated adenocarcinoma of the kidney in adult frogs. SYN Lucké's adenocarcinoma.

medullary c., a malignant neoplasm, comparatively soft and brainlike in consistency, that consists chiefly of neoplastic epithelial cells, with only a scant amount of fibrous stroma.

melanotic c., obsolete term for melanoma.

meningeal c., an infiltration of c. cells in the arachnoid and subarachnoid space; may be primary or secondary. SYN leptomeningeal c., leptomeningeal carcinomatosis, meningeal carcinomatosis.

mesometanephric c., SYN mesonephroma.

metaplastic c., a c. in which some of the tumor cells are spindle shaped, suggesting a sarcoma, or in which the stroma shows foci of bone or cartilage; such c.'s occur in the upper respiratory or alimentary tract or in the breast.

metastatic c., a c. that has appeared in a region remote from its site of origin, as in metastasis (2). SYN secondary c.

metatypical c., obsolete term for basosquamous c.

microinvasive c., a variety of c. seen most frequently in the uterine cervix, in which c. in situ of squamous epithelium, on the surface or replacing the lining of glands, is accompanied by small collections of abnormal epithelial cells that infiltrate a very short distance into the stroma; this may represent the earliest stage of invasion, in which the neoplastic cells are capable of intrusion but not of sustained growth in connective tissue.

mucinous c., a variety of adenocarcinoma in which the neoplastic cells secrete conspicuous quantities of mucin, and, as a result, the neoplasms are likely to be glistening, sticky, and gelatinoid in consistency. SYN colloid cancer, colloid c.

mucoepidermoid c., most commonly a salivary gland c. of low grade malignancy in children, but with variable malignancy in adults; composed of mucous, epidermoid, and intermediate cells, with mucous cells abundant only in low grade c.'s; recurrence is frequent, and high grade c.'s metastasize to cervical nodes. SYN mucoepidermoid tumor.

c. myxomato'des, obsolete term for a form of colloid cancer in which there is myxomatous metaplasia of the cellular fibrous stroma.

noninfiltrating lobular c., c. of the breast in which small tumor cells fill preexisting acini within lobules, without invading the surrounding stroma. SYN lobular c. in situ, lobular neoplasia.

oat cell c., an anaplastic, highly malignant, and usually bronchogenic c. composed of small ovoid cells with very scanty cytoplasm; this c. and small round cell c.'s comprise over one-third of c.'s of the lung. SYN small cell c. (2).

occult c., a small c., either asymptomatic or giving rise to metastases without symptoms due to the primary c.

oncoplastic c., obsolete term for an undifferentiated c. showing no evidence by light microscopy of origin from a specific epithelial tissue, *e.g.,* squamous or glandular epithelium.

papillary c., a malignant neoplasm characterized by the formation of numerous, irregular, finger-like projections of fibrous

stroma that is covered with a surface layer of neoplastic epithelial cells.

primary c., c. at the site of origin, with local invasion in that organ.

primary neuroendocrine c. of the skin, SYN Merkel cell *tumor.*

renal cell c., SYN renal *adenocarcinoma.*

sarcomatoid c., SYN spindle cell c.

scar c., c. of the lung, usually adenocarcinoma, arising from a peripheral lung scar or associated with interstitial fibrosis in a honeycomb lung. SYN scar cancer.

scirrhous c., a hard c., fibrous in nature, resulting from a desmoplastic reaction by the stromal tissue to the presence of the neoplastic epithelium. SYN fibrocarcinoma.

secondary c., SYN metastatic c.

secretory c., c. of the breast with pale-staining cells showing prominent secretory activity, as seen in pregnancy and lactation, but found mostly in children. SYN juvenile c.

signet-ring cell c., a poorly differentiated adenocarcinoma composed of cells with a cytoplasmic droplet of mucus that compresses the nucleus to one side along the cell membrane; arises most frequently in the stomach, occasionally in the large bowel or elsewhere.

c. sim'plex, obsolete term for any form of c. in which the relative proportions of stroma and neoplastic epithelial cells are not unusual, *i.e.,* stromal elements are not comparatively abundant, nor are they reduced in amount or lacking; an obsolete term for a c. lacking any identifiable microscopic pattern, such as glandular structure.

c. in si'tu (CIS), a lesion characterized by cytologic changes of the type associated with invasive c., but with the pathologic process limited to the lining epithelium and without histologic evidence of extension to adjacent structures; the distinctive changes are usually more apparent in the nucleus, *i.e.,* variation in size and shape, increase in chromatin, and numerous mitoses (including some that are atypical) in all layers of the epithelium, with loss of orderly maturation. The lesion is presumed to be the histologically recognizable precursor of invasive c., *i.e.,* a localized and curable phase of c. SYN intraepithelial c.

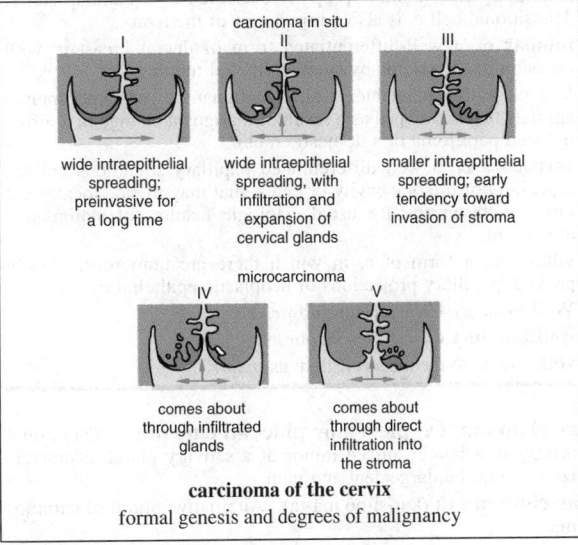

carcinoma in situ

I — wide intraepithelial spreading; preinvasive for a long time

II — wide intraepithelial spreading, with infiltration and expansion of cervical glands

III — smaller intraepithelial spreading; early tendency toward invasion of stroma

microcarcinoma

IV — comes about through infiltrated glands

V — comes about through direct infiltration into the stroma

carcinoma of the cervix
formal genesis and degrees of malignancy

small cell c., (1) an anaplastic c. composed of small cells; (2) SYN oat cell c.

spindle cell c., a c. composed of elongated cells, frequently a poorly differentiated squamous cell c. which may be difficult to distinguish from a sarcoma. SYN sarcomatoid c.

squamous cell c., a malignant neoplasm derived from stratified squamous epithelium, but which may also occur in sites, such as bronchial mucosa, where glandular or columnar epithelium is normally present; variable amounts of keratin are formed, in

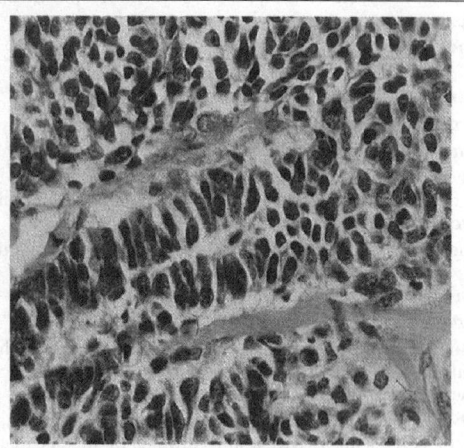

bronchiolar carcinoma (small-cell)

relation to the degree of differentiation, and, if the keratin is not on the surface, it accumulates in the neoplasm as a keratin pearl; in instances in which the cells are well differentiated, intercellular bridges may be observed between adjacent cells; a common example in lower animals is ocular squamous cell c. of Hereford cattle.

sweat gland c., usually a solitary tumor, nodular and fixed to the skin and underlying structure, having slow growth for long periods followed by rapid growth and dissemination.

trabecular c., SYN Merkel cell *tumor*.

transitional cell c., a malignant neoplasm derived from transitional epithelium, occurring chiefly in the urinary bladder, ureters, or renal pelves (especially if well differentiated); frequently papillary; these c.'s are graded 1 to 3 or 4 according to the degree of anaplasia, grade 1 appearing histologically benign but being liable to recurrence. So-called transitional cell c. of the upper respiratory tract is more properly classified as squamous cell c. Transitional cell c. is also a rare tumor of the ovary.

tubular c., a well-differentiated form of ductal breast c. with invasion of the stroma by small epithelial tubules.

V-2 c., a transplantable, highly malignant c. of experimental animals that developed as a result of malignant change in a virus-induced papilloma of a domestic rabbit.

verrucous c., a well differentiated papillary squamous cell c., especially of the oral cavity or penis, that may invade locally but rarely metastasizes; the usual cytologic features of malignancy are absent.

villous c., a form of c. in which there are numerous, closely packed, papillary projections of neoplastic epithelial tissue.

Walker c., SYN Walker *carcinosarcoma*.

wolffian duct c., SYN mesonephroma.

yolk sac c., SYN endocervical sinus *tumor*.

---

car·ci·no·ma ex ple·o·mor·phic ad·e·no·ma. Carcinoma arising in a benign mixed tumor of a salivary gland, characterized by rapid enlargement and pain.

car·ci·no·ma·ta (kar-si-nō′mă-tă). Alternative plural of carcinoma.

car·ci·no·ma·to·sis (kar′si-nō-mă-tō′sis). A condition resulting from widespread dissemination of carcinoma in multiple sites in various organs or tissues of the body; sometimes also used in relation to involvement of a relatively large region of the body. SYN carcinosis.

leptomeningeal c., SYN meningeal *carcinoma*.

meningeal c., SYN meningeal *carcinoma*.

car·ci·nom·a·tous (kar-si-nom′ă-tŭs). Pertaining to or manifesting the characteristic properties of carcinoma.

car·ci·no·pho·bia (kar′sin-ō-fō′bē-ă). SYN cancerophobia.

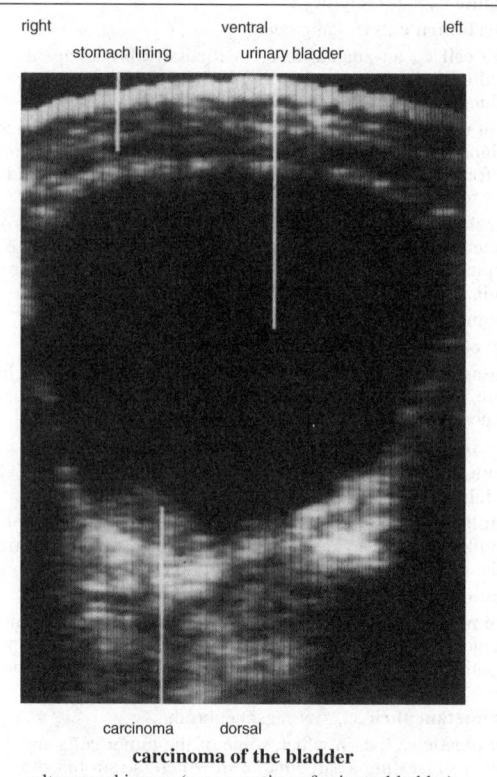

carcinoma of the bladder
ultrasound image (cross-section of urinary bladder)

car·ci·no·sar·co·ma (kar′si-nō-sar-kō′mă). A malignant neoplasm that contains elements of carcinoma and sarcoma so extensively intermixed as to indicate neoplasia of epithelial and mesenchymal tissue. SEE ALSO collision *tumor*.

embryonal c., SYN blastoma.

renal c., obsolete term for Wilms' *tumor*.

Walker c., a transplantable c. of the rat that originally appeared spontaneously in the mammary gland of a pregnant albino rat, and which now resembles a carcinoma in young transplants and a sarcoma in older transplants. SYN Walker carcinoma.

car·ci·no·sis (kar-si-nō′sis). SYN carcinomatosis.

car·ci·no·stat·ic (kar′si-nō-stat′ik). **1.** Pertaining to an arresting or inhibitory effect on the development or progression of a carcinoma. **2.** An agent that manifests such an effect.

car·co·ma (kar-kō′mă). Dark red-brown or mahogany-colored granular material that occurs in human feces in tropical regions; it yields a chemical reaction similar to that of urobilinogen and is composed of calcium oxide, iron, phosphoric and carbonic acids, urobilinogen, cholerythrogen, and other organic matter in varying proportions. [Sp. wood dust under the bark of a tree, caused by the wood louse]

car·da·mom (kar′dă-mom). Grains of paradise. Dried ripe seeds of *Elettaria cardamomum;* used for flavoring baked goods, confectionery, curry powder, and in the manufacture of *oil* of cardamom which is used for flavoring liqueurs. Pharmaceutical aid (flavor); adjuvant and carminative.

Carden, Henry D., British surgeon, †1872. SEE C.'s *amputation*.

car·den·o·lide (kar-den′ō-līd). A class of cardiac glycosides containing a five-membered lactone ring (*e.g.,* the *Digitalis* glycosides).

△**cardi-.** SEE cardio-.

car·dia (kar′dē-ă). SYN cardiac *part* of stomach. [G. *kardia,* heart]

car·di·ac (kar′dē-ak). **1.** Pertaining to the heart. **2.** Pertaining to the esophageal opening of the stomach. **3.** A remedy for heart disease. [L. *cardiacus*]

car·di·ac bal·let (kar′dē-ak bal-ā′). Short runs of cardiac dysrhythmia consisting of uniform sequences of repetitive multiform extrasystoles; so called from its undulating appearance, originally described by Bellet. SEE ALSO torsade de pointes.

car·di·ac gly·co·sides. Generic term for a large number of drugs with the capacity to increase the force of contraction of the failing heart. Examples include digitalis (foxglove) extracts as well as those obtained from other plant and animal sources.

car·di·al·gia (kar-dē-al′jē-ă). **1.** Obsolete term for pyrosis. **2.** SYN cardiodynia. [cardi- + G. *algos*, pain]

car·di·a·tax·ia (kar′dē-ă-tak′sē-ă). Extreme irregularity in the action of the heart. [cardi- + G. *ataxia*, disorder]

car·di·a·te·lia (kar′dē-ă-tē′lē-ă). Incomplete development of the heart. [cardi- + G. *atelēs*, incomplete]

car·di·ec·ta·sia (kar′dē-ek-tā′zē-ă). Dilation of the heart. [cardi- + G. *ektasis*, a stretching]

car·di·ec·to·my (kar-dē-ek′tō-mē). Excision of the cardiac part of the stomach. [cardi-(2) + G. *ektomē*, excision]

car·di·ec·to·pia (kar-dē-ek-tō′pē-ă). Abnormal placement of the heart. SEE *ectopia* cordis. [cardi- + G. *ektopos*, out of place]

car·di·nal (kar′di-năl). Chief or principal; in embryology, relating to the main venous drainage. [L. *cardinalis*, principal]

card·ing. The procedure of placing individual sets of anterior or posterior teeth in trays lined with a wax strip.

⌂**cardio-, cardi-.** **1.** The heart. **2.** The cardia (ostium cardiacum). [G. *kardia*, heart]

car·di·o·ac·cel·er·a·tor (kar′dē-ō-ak-sel′er-ā-ter). Accelerator of the heart beat.

car·di·o·ac·tive (kar′dē-ō-ak′tiv). Influencing the heart.

car·di·o·an·gi·og·ra·phy (kar′dē-ō-an-jē-og′ră-fē). SYN angiocardiography.

car·di·o·a·or·tic (kar′dē-ō-ā-ōr′tik). Relating to the heart and the aorta.

car·di·o·ar·te·ri·al (kar′dē-ō-ar-tēr′ē-ăl). Relating to the heart and the arteries.

Car·di·o·bac·te·ri·um. A genus of nonmotile, pleomorphic, gram negative, facultatively anaerobic, rod-shaped bacteria found in the nasal flora and associated with endocarditis in humans. The type species is *C. hominis*.

C. hom′inis, a species that causes endocarditis in humans. The type species of *Cardiobacterium*. SEE HACEK *group*.

car·di·o·cele (kar′dē-ō-sēl). A herniation or protrusion of the heart through an opening in the diaphragm, or through a wound. [cardio- + G. *kēlē*, hernia]

car·di·o·cha·la·sia (kar′dē-ō-kă-lā′zē-ă). Achalasia of the cardia.

car·di·o·di·o·sis (kar′dē-ō-dē-ō′sis). Rarely used term for maneuver to dilate the gastric cardia. [cardio- (2) + G. *diōsis*, a spreading open]

car·di·o·dy·nam·ics (kar′dē-ō-dī-nam′iks). The mechanics of the heart's action, including its movement and the forces generated thereby.

car·di·o·dyn·ia (kar′dē-ō-din′ē-ă). Pain in the heart. SYN cardialgia (2). [cardio- + G. *odynē*, pain]

car·di·o·e·soph·a·ge·al (kar′dē-ō-ē-sof-ă-jē′ăl). Denoting the area at the junction of the esophagus and cardiac part of the stomach.

car·di·o·gen·e·sis (kar-dē-ō-gen′ĕ-sis). Formation of the heart in the embryo. [cardio + G. *genesis*, origin]

car·di·o·gen·ic (kar′dē-ō-jen′ik). Of cardiac origin.

car·di·o·gram (kar′dē-ō-gram). **1.** The graphic tracing made by the stylet of a cardiograph. **2.** Generally used for any recording derived from the heart, with such prefixes as apex-, echo-, electro-, phono-, or vector- being understood. [cardio- + G. *gramma*, a diagram]

esophageal c., tracing of left atrial contractions made by recording displacements of the column of air in a sensor-equipped esophageal tube.

car·di·o·graph (kar′dē-ō-graf). An instrument for recording graphically the movements of the heart, constructed on the principle of the sphygmograph. [cardio- + G. *graphō*, to write]

car·di·og·ra·phy (kar-dē-og′ră-fē). The use of the cardiograph.

ultrasonic c., SYN echocardiography.

ultrasound c., SYN echocardiography.

vector c., the integration of scalar electrocardiographic recordings on two or three planes to produce a vector cardiogram consisting of loops divided by a timing mechanism for all the waves of the electrocardiogram.

car·di·o·he·mo·throm·bus (kar′dē-ō-hē-mō-throm′bŭs). SYN cardiothrombus.

car·di·o·he·pat·ic (kar′dē-ō-hĕ-pat′ik). Relating to the heart and the liver.

car·di·o·he·pa·to·meg·a·ly (kar′dē-ō-hep′ă-tō-meg′ă-lē). Enlargement of both heart and liver.

car·di·oid (kar′dē-oyd). Resembling a heart. [cardi- + G. *eidos*, resemblance]

car·di·o·in·hib·i·to·ry (kar′dē-ō-in-hib′ĭ-tō-rē). Arresting or slowing the action of the heart.

car·di·o·ki·net·ic (kar′dē-ō-kĭ-net′ik). Influencing the action of the heart. [cardio- + G. *kinēsis*, movement]

car·di·o·ky·mo·gram (kar′dē-ō-kī′mō-gram). Record made by a cardiokymograph.

car·di·o·ky·mo·graph (kar′dē-ō-kī′mō-graf). Noninvasive device, placed on the chest, capable of recording anterior left ventricle segmental wall motion; consists of a 5-cm diameter capacitive plate transducer as part of a high frequency, low-power oscillator with recording probe; changes in wall motion affect the magnetic field and thus the oscillatory frequency which is then recorded on a multichannel analog waveform polygraph.

car·di·o·ky·mog·ra·phy (kar′dē-ō-kī-mog′ră-fē). Use of a cardiokymograph.

car·di·o·lip·in (kar′dē-ō-lip′in). a 1,3-bis(phosphatidyl)glycerol found in many biomembranes with immunological properties; used in serological diagnosis of syphilis. When mixed with lecithin and cholesterol c. will combine with the Wassermann antibody but not with the treponema-immobilizing antibody. SYN acetone-insoluble antigen, heart antigen.

car·di·ol·o·gist (kar-dē-ol′ō-jist). Physician specializing in cardiology.

car·di·ol·o·gy (kar-dē-ol′ō-jē). The medical specialty concerned with the diagnosis and treatment of heart disease. [cardio- + G. *logos*, study]

car·di·ol·y·sis (kar-dē-ol′i-sis). An obsolete operation for breaking up the adhesions in chronic mediastinopericarditis; access is gained by resection of a portion of the sternum and the corresponding costal cartilages. [cardio- + G. *lysis*, loosening]

car·di·o·ma·la·cia (kar′dē-ō-mă-lā′shē-ă). Softening of the walls of the heart. [cardio- + G. *malakia*, softness]

car·di·o·meg·a·ly (kar-dē-ō-meg′ă-lē). Enlargement of the heart. SYN macrocardia, megacardia, megalocardia. [cardio- + G. *megas*, large]

glycogen c., a form of glycogenosis due to abnormal storage of glycogen within the heart muscle cells.

glycogenic c., enlargement of the heart due to glycogen storage disease; most often occurs in type II (lysosomal acid glucosidase deficiency), especially in infancy and childhood.

⌂ Combining forms	[NA] Nomina Anatomica
Word*Finder* Multi-term entry finder Preceding letter A	[MIM] Mendelian Inheritance in Man
A.D.A.M. Anatomy Plates Between letters L and M	☆ Official alternate term
Appendices: Following letter Z	☆[NA] Official alternate Nomina Anatomica term
SYN Synonym; Cf., compare	High Profile Term

car·di·om·e·try (kar-dē-om′ĕ-trē). Measurement of the dimensions of the heart or the force of its action. [cardio- + G. *metron*, measure]

car·di·o·mo·til·i·ty (kar′dē-ō-mō-til′ĭ-tē). Movements of the heart.

car·di·o·mus·cu·lar (kar′dē-ō-mŭs′kyū-lăr). Pertaining to the cardiac musculature.

car·di·o·my·o·li·po·sis (kar′dē-ō-mī′ō-li-pō′sis). Fatty degeneration of the myocardium. [cardio- + G. *mys*, muscle, + *lipos*, fat, + -*osis*, condition]

car·di·o·my·op·a·thy (kar′dē-ō-mī-op′ă-thē). Disease of the myocardium. As a disease classification, the term is used in several different senses, but is limited by the World Health Organization to: "Primary disease process of heart muscle in absence of a known underlying etiology" when referring to idiopathic cardiomyopathy. SYN myocardiopathy. [cardio- + G. *mys*, muscle, + *pathos*, disease]

---

classification of cardiomyopathies

primary cardiomyopathies

(dilated) congestive cardiomyopathy (CCM)

hypertrophic obstructive cardiomyopathy (HOCM)

hypertrophic nonobstructive cardiomyopathy (HNCM)

secondary cardiomyopathies

infectious heart muscle diseases

heart muscle diseases caused by nutritional or toxic injuries

heart muscle diseases from metabolic problems

heart muscle diseases in neuropathies and myopathies

infiltrative heart muscle diseases

physically conditioned heart muscle diseases

cardiomyopathy as a complication in pregnancy

---

alcoholic c., myocardial disease occurring in some chronic alcoholics; may result either from thiamin deficiency or be of unknown pathogenesis. SYN alcoholic myocardiopathy, beer heart.

congestive c., heart muscle disease of unknown or known origin involving cardiac muscle and not primarily involving any other structures, with systemic and pulmonary congestion through increased pressure and volume in the venous systems.

dilated c., decreased function of the left ventricle associated with its dilatation; most patients have global hypokinesia, although discrete regional wall movement abnormalities may occur; usually manifested by signs of overall cardiac failure, with congestive findings, as well as by fatigue indicative of a low output state.

familial hypertrophic c., familial occurrence of hypertrophic c. exhibiting an autosomal dominant pattern of inheritance. Familial c. of various kinds occurs with autosomal dominant inheritance [MIM*115200]. There is also an asymmetrical form affecting the ventricles and the interventricular septum [MIM*192600].

hypertrophic c., thickening of the ventricular septum and walls of the left ventricle with marked myofibril disarray; often associated with greater thickening of the septum than of the free wall resulting in narrowing of the left ventricular outflow tract and dynamic outflow gradient; diastolic compliance is greatly impaired.

idiopathic c., SYN primary c. (1).

peripartum c., cardiac failure due to heart muscle disease in the period before, during, or after delivery.

postpartum c., cardiomegaly and congestive heart failure developing in the puerperium in the absence of any of the known causes of heart disease.

primary c., (1) c. of unknown or obscure cause; SYN idiopathic c. **(2)** a disease that affects mainly the heart muscle, sparing other cardiac structures and usually resulting in fibrosis, hypertrophy, or both.

restrictive c., a diverse group of conditions characterized by restriction of diastolic filling; often confused with constrictive pericarditis and the infiltrative cardiomyopathies; left ventricular size and systolic function may be preserved but dyspnea results primarily from increase in left ventricular diastolic pressure; signs of right ventricular failure may be prominent.

secondary c., disease that affects the myocardium secondarily to systemic disease, infection, or metabolic disease.

car·di·o·my·o·plas·ty. an operation that uses stimulated latissimus dorsi muscle to assist cardiac function. The latissimus dorsi muscle is mobilized from the chest wall and moved into the thorax through the bed of the resected 2nd or 3rd rib. The muscle is then wrapped around the left and right ventricles and stimulated to contract during cardiac systole by means of an implanted burst-stimulator. SYN cardiac muscle wrap.

car·di·o·my·ot·o·my (kar′dē-ō-mī-ot′ō-mē). SYN esophagomyotomy. [cardio- (2) + G. *mys*, muscle, + *tomē*, cutting]

car·di·o·nat·rin. SYN atrial natriuretic *peptide*. [cardio- + Mod. L. *natrium*, sodium, + suffix -in, material]

car·di·o·ne·cro·sis (kar′dē-ō-nĕ-krō′sis). Necrosis of the myocardium.

car·di·o·nec·tor (kar′dē-ō-nek′tŏr, -tōr). Archaic term sometimes used for conducting *system* of heart. [cardio- + L. *necto*, to join]

car·di·o·neph·ric (kar′dē-ō-nef′rik). SYN cardiorenal.

car·di·o·neu·ral (kar′dē-ō-nūr′ăl). Relating to the nervous control of the heart. [cardio- + G. *neuron*, nerve]

car·di·o·neu·ro·sis (kar′dē-ō-nū-rō′sis). SYN cardiac *neurosis*.

car·di·o·o·men·to·pexy (kar′dē-ō-ō-men′tō-pek-sē). Operation for the attachment of omentum to the heart with the object of improving its blood supply. [cardio- + omentum, + G. *pēxis*, fixation]

car·di·o·pal·u·dism (kar′dē-ō-pal′ū-dizm). Irregularity in the heart's action due to malaria. [cardio- + paludism, malaria, fr. L. *palus*, marsh]

car·di·o·path (kar′dē-ō-path). A sufferer from heart disease.

car·di·o·path·ia nig·ra (kar-dē-ō-path′ē-ă nī′gra). SYN Ayerza's *syndrome*.

car·di·op·a·thy (kar-dē-op′ă-thē). Any disease of the heart. [cardio- + G. *pathos*, disease]

car·di·o·per·i·car·di·o·pexy (kar′dē-ō-pār-i-kar′dē-ō-pek-sē). An operation to increase the blood supply to the myocardium; sterile magnesium silicate (a form of talc) is spread within the pericardial sac or the sac is mechanically abraded to cause an adhesive pericarditis and an increase in blood supply to develop through the stimulation of interarterial coronary anastomoses and pericardial collaterals. [cardio- + pericardium, + G. *pēxis*, fixation]

car·di·o·pho·bia (kar′dē-ō-fō′bē-ă). Morbid fear of heart disease.

car·di·o·phone (kar′dē-ō-fōn). A stethoscope specially modified to aid in listening to the sounds of the heart. [cardio- + G. *phōnē*, sound]

car·di·oph·o·ny (kar′dē-of′ō-nē). A rarely used term for phonocardiography (1).

car·di·o·phre·nia (kar′dē-ō-frē′nē-ă). SYN phrenocardia.

car·di·o·plas·ty (kar′dē-ō-plas-tē). An operation on the cardia of the stomach. SYN esophagogastroplasty. [cardio- (2) + G. *plastos*, formed]

car·di·o·ple·gia (kar′dē-ō-plē′jē-ă). **1.** Paralysis of the heart. **2.** An elective stopping of cardiac activity temporarily by injection of chemicals, selective hypothermia, or electrical stimuli. [cardio- + G. *plēgē*, stroke]

antegrade c., c. effected by delivery of solutions through the coronary arteries.

retrograde c., c. effected by delivery of solutions via the coronary veins.

car·di·o·ple·gic (kar-dē-ō-plē′jik). Relating to cardioplegia.

car·di·op·to·sia (kar′dē-op-tō′sē-ă). A condition in which the heart is unduly movable and displaced downward, as distinguished from bathycardia. SEE ALSO *cor* mobile, *cor* pendulum. SYN drop heart. [cardio- + G. *ptōsis*, a falling]

car·di·o·pul·mo·nary (kar′dē-ō-pŭl′mo-nār-ē). Relating to the heart and lungs. SYN pneumocardial.

car·di·o·py·lo·ric (kar′dē-ō-pī-lōr′ik, -pi-lōr′ik). Relating to the cardiac and pyloric extremities of the stomach.

car·di·o·re·nal (kar′dē-ō-rē′năl). Relating to the heart and the kidney. SYN cardionephric, nephrocardiac, renicardiac.

car·di·or·rha·phy (kar-dē-ōr′ă-fē). Suture of the heart wall. [cardio- + G. *rhaphē*, suture]

car·di·or·rhex·is (kar-dē-ō-rek′sis). Rupture of the heart wall. [cardio- + G. *rhēxis*, rupture]

car·di·o·scope (kar′dē-ō-skōp). An instrument for inspecting the interior of the living heart. [cardio- + G. *skopeō*, to view]

car·di·o·se·lec·tive (kar′dē-ō-sĕ-lek′tiv). Denoting or having the properties of cardioselectivity.

car·di·o·se·lec·tiv·i·ty (kar′dē-ō-sĕ-lek-tiv′i-tē). The relatively predominant cardiovascular pharmacologic effect of a drug with multipharmacologic effects; used especially when describing beta-blocking agents.

car·di·o·spasm (kar′dē-ō-spazm). SYN esophageal *achalasia*.

car·di·o·sphyg·mo·graph (kar′dē-ō-sfig′mō-graf). An instrument for recording graphically the movements of the heart and the radial pulse. [cardio- + G. *sphygmos*, pulse, + *graphō*, to write]

car·di·o·ta·chom·e·ter (kar′dē-ō-tă-kom′ĕ-ter). An instrument for measuring the heart rate. [cardio- + G. *tachos*, rapidity, + *metron*, measure]

car·di·o·throm·bus (kar′dē-ō-throm′bŭs). A clot of blood within one of the heart's chambers. SYN cardiohemothrombus.

car·di·o·thy·ro·tox·i·co·sis (kar′dē-ō-thī-rō-tok-si-kō′sis). Hyperthyroidism with cardiac complications.

car·di·ot·o·my (kar-dē-ot′ō-mē). **1.** Incision of a heart wall. **2.** Incision of the cardiac part of the stomach. [cardio- + G. *tomē*, incision]

car·di·o·ton·ic (kar′dē-ō-ton′ik). Exerting a favorable, so-called tonic, effect upon the action of the heart; usually intended to indicate increased force of contraction. [cardio- + G. *tonos*, tension]

car·di·o·tox·ic (kar′dē-ō-tok′sik). Having a deleterious effect upon the action of the heart, due to poisoning of the cardiac muscle or of its conducting system. [cardio- + G. *toxikon*, poison]

car·di·o·tox·in (kar′dē-ō-tok′sin). **1.** A poisonous glycoside with specific cardiac effects. For example, causes irreversible depolarization of cell membranes. **2.** Specifically, one of the toxic principles from cobra venom. **3.** Any substance that can cause heart damage with toxic doses.

car·di·o·val·vu·li·tis (kar′dē-ō-val-vyū-lī′tis). Inflammation of the heart valves.

car·di·o·vas·cu·lar (CV) (kar′dē-ō-vas′kyū-lăr). Relating to the heart and the blood vessels or the circulation. SYN vasculocardiac. [cardio- + L. *vasculum*, vessel]

car·di·o·vas·cu·lo·re·nal (kar′dē-ō-vas′kyū-lō-rē′năl). Relating to the heart, arteries, and kidneys, especially as to function or disease.

car·di·o·ver·sion (kar′dē-ō-ver′zhŭn). Restoration of the heart's rhythm to normal by electrical countershock. [cardio- + con*version*]

car·di·o·vert (car′dē-ō-vert). The act of cardioversion.

car·di·o·ver·ter (kar′dē-ō-ver′ter). A machine used to perform cardioversion.

Car·di·o·vi·rus (kar′dē-ō-vī′rŭs). A genus of RNA viruses in the family Picornaviridae that are rarely associated with human disease and are recovered frequently from rodents.

car·di·tis (kar-dī′tis). Inflammation of the heart.
    rheumatic c., pancarditis occurring in rheumatic fever, characterized by formation of Aschoff bodies in the cardiac interstitial

tissue; may be associated with acute cardiac failure, endocarditis with small fibrin vegetations on the margins of closure of valve cusps (especially the mitral), and fibrinous pericarditis; it is frequently followed by scarring of the valves.

care (kār). In medicine and public health, a general term for the application of knowledge to the benefit of a community or individual.
    comprehensive medical c., a concept that includes not only the traditional c. of the acutely or chronically ill patient, but also the prevention and early detection of disease and the rehabilitation of the disabled.
    health c., services provided to individuals or communities by agents of the health services or professions for the purpose of promoting, maintaining, monitoring, or restoring health.
    intensive c., management and c. of critically ill patients. SEE ALSO intensive care *unit*.

    managed c., an arrangement whereby a third-party payer (*e.g.,* insurance company, federal government, or corporation) mediates between physicians and patients, negotiating fees for service and overseeing the types of treatment given.

> Managed care has virtually replaced unmanaged indemnity plans, where payment is automatic and oversight procedures are minimal. Whereas 96% of American workers had unmanaged indemnity in 1984, only 28% did in 1988. Typically, in managed care, the third-party payer requires second opinions and precertification review for patients requiring hospital admission. They obtain wholesale prices from doctors, and carry out cost-containment measures, including auditing hospitals and reviewing claims. Managed care has figured heavily in the national debate over health care.

    medical c., the portion of c. under a physician's direction.
    primary medical c., c. of a patient by a member of the health c. system who has initial contact with the patient.
    secondary medical c., medical c. by a physician who acts as a consultant at the request of the primary physician.
    tertiary medical c., specialized consultative c., usually on referral from primary or secondary medical c. personnel, by specialists working in a center that has personnel and facilities for special investigation and treatment.

Carey Coombs mur·mur. See under murmur.

ca·ri·bi (kă-rē′bē). SYN epidemic gangrenous *proctitis*.

car·i·ca (kar′i-kă). SYN papaya.

car·ies (kār′ēz). **1.** Microbial destruction or necrosis of teeth. **2.** Obsolete term for tuberculosis of bones or joints. [L. dry rot]

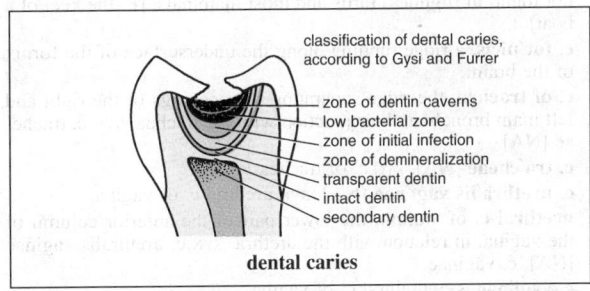

classification of dental caries, according to Gysi and Furrer
— zone of dentin caverns
— low bacterial zone
— zone of initial infection
— zone of demineralization
— transparent dentin
— intact dentin
— secondary dentin

dental caries

    active c., microbial-induced lesions of teeth that are increasing in size.
    arrested dental c., carious lesions that have become inactive and stopped progressing; they may exhibit changes in color and/or consistency.
    buccal c., c. beginning with decay on the buccal surface of a tooth.
    cemental c., c. of the cementum of a tooth.
    compound c., (**1**) c. involving more than one surface of a tooth; (**2**) two or more carious lesions joined to form one cavity.
    dental c., a localized, progressively destructive disease of the

ca

teeth which starts at the external surface (usually the enamel) with the apparent dissolution of the inorganic components by organic acids that are produced in immediate proximity to the tooth by the enzymatic action of masses of microorganisms (in the bacterial plaque) on carbohydrates; the initial demineralization is followed by an enzymatic destruction of the protein matrix with subsequent cavitation and direct bacterial invasion; in the dentin, demineralization of the walls of the tubules is followed by bacterial invasion and destruction of the organic matrix. SYN saprodontia.

distal c., loss of structure on the tooth surface that is directed away from the median plane of the dental arch.

fissure c., c. beginning in a fissure on the occlusal surfaces of posterior teeth.

incipient c., beginning c. or decay.

interdental c., c. between the teeth.

mesial c., c. on the tooth surface that is directed toward the median plane of the dental arch.

nursing bottle c., rampant c. of the primary dentition associated with the habitual use, after age 1, of a baby bottle as an aid for sleeping. SYN baby bottle syndrome.

occlusal c., c. starting from the occlusal surface of a tooth.

pit c., a carious lesion, usually small, beginning in a pit on the labial, buccal, lingual, or occlusal surface of a tooth.

pit and fissure c., c. initiated in the areas where developmental pits and fissures are located on the tooth surface.

primary c., initial lesions produced by direct extension from an external surface.

proximal c., c. occurring in the proximal surface, either distal or mesial, of a tooth.

radiation c., c. of the cervical regions of the teeth, incisal edges, and cusp tips secondary to xerostomia induced by radiation therapy to the head and neck.

recurrent c., c. recurring in an area due to inadequate removal of the initial decay, usually beneath a restoration or new decay at a site where caries has previously occurred.

root c., c. of the root surface of a tooth, usually appearing as a broad shallow defect in the area of the cemento-enamel junction.

secondary c., c. of enamel beginning at the dento-enamel junction due to a rapid lateral spread of decay from the original decay.

senile dental c., c. occurring in old age, usually interproximally and in the cementum.

smooth surface c., c. initiated on the smooth surfaces of teeth.

ca·ri·na, pl. **ca·ri·nae** (kă-rī′nă, -rī′nē). **1.** In man, a term applied or applicable to several anatomical structures forming a projecting central ridge. **2.** That portion of the sternum in a bird, bat, or mole that serves as the origin of the pectoral muscles; it is not found in flightless birds and most mammals. [L. the keel of a boat]

c. for′nicis, a ridge running along the undersurface of the fornix of the brain.

c. of trachea, the ridge separating the openings of the right and left main bronchi at their junction with the trachea. SYN c. tracheae [NA].

c. tra′cheae [NA], SYN c. of trachea.

c. urethra′lis vagi′nae [NA], SYN urethral c. of vagina.

urethral c. of vagina, the lower part of the anterior column of the vagina, in relation with the urethra. SYN c. urethralis vaginae [NA], c. vaginae.

c. vagi′nae, SYN urethral c. of vagina.

car·i·nate (kar′i-nāt). Shaped like a keel; relating to or resembling a carina.

cario-. Caries. [L. *caries*]

car·i·o·gen·e·sis (ka′rē-ō-jen′ĕ-sis). The process of producing caries; the mechanism of caries production.

car·i·o·gen·ic (ka′rē-ō-jen′ik). Producing caries; usually said of diets.

car·i·o·ge·nic·i·ty (ka′rē-ō-jĕ-nis′i-tē). Potential for caries production.

car·i·ol·o·gy (ka-rē-ol′ō-jē). The study of dental caries and cariogenesis.

car·i·o·stat·ic (kar-ē-ō-stat′ik). Exerting an inhibitory action upon the progress of dental caries.

car·i·ous (kār′ē-ŭs). Relating to or affected with caries.

car·i·so·pro·date (kar′i-sō-prō′dāt). SYN carisoprodol.

car·i·so·pro·dol (kar′i-so-prō′dol). isobamate; isopropyl meprobamate *N*-isopropyl-2-methyl-2-propyl-1,2-propanediol dicarbamate; a skeletal muscle relaxant, chemically related to meprobamate. SYN carisoprodate.

ca·ris·sin (ka-ris′sin). A glucoside obtained from *Carissa ovata stolonifera* of Australia; a powerful cardiac poison.

Carlen, Eric, 20th century Swedish otolaryngologist. SEE Carlen's *tube.*

Carlen's tube. See under tube.

carm·al·um (kar-mal′ŭm). A 1% solution of carmine in 10% alum water, used as a stain in histology.

Carman. Russell D., U.S. radiologist, 1875–1926. SEE Carman's *sign.*

car·mi·nate (kar′mi-nāt). A red salt of carminic acid.

car·min·a·tive (kar-min′ă-tiv). **1.** Preventing the formation or causing the expulsion of flatus. **2.** An agent that relieves flatulence. [L. *carmino,* pp. *-atus,* to card wool; special Mod. L. usage, to expel wind]

car·mine (kar′min, kar′mēn) [C.I. 75470]. Red coloring matter produced from coccinellin derived from cochineal; treatment of coccinellin with alum forms an aluminum lake of carminic acid, the essential constituent of c. [Mediev. L. *carminus,* contr. fr. *carmisinus,* fr. Ar. *qirmizē,* the cochineal insect]

lithium c., a vital stain for marophages.

Schneider's c., a stain consisting of a 10% solution of c. in 45% acetic acid, used for fresh chromosome preparations.

car·min·ic ac·id (kar-min′ik). A glucoside of an anthracenequinone carboxylic acid; the essential constituent of carmine.

car·min·o·phil, car·min·o·phile, car·mi·noph·i·lous (kar-min′ō-fil, -fil, kar-mi-nof′i-lŭs). Staining readily with carmine dyes. [G. *phileō,* to love]

Carmody, Thomas Edward, U.S. oral surgeon, *1875. SEE C.-Batson *operation.*

car·mus·tine (kar-mŭs′tēn). 1,3-Bis(2-chloroethyl)-1-nitrosourea; an antineoplastic agent. SYN BCNU.

car·nas·si·al (kar-nas′ē-ăl). Adapted for shearing flesh; denoting those teeth designed to cut flesh. [Fr. *carnassier,* carnivorous, fr. L. *caro,* flesh]

car·ne·ous (kar′nē-ŭs). Fleshy. [L. *carneus*]

car·nes (kar′nēz). Plural of caro. [L.]

Carnett, J. B., 20th century U.S. physician. SEE Carnett's *sign.*

Carnett's sign. See under sign.

car·ni·fi·ca·tion (kar′ni-fi-kā′shŭn). A change in tissues, whereby they become fleshy, resembling muscular tissue. [L. *caro (carn-),* flesh, + *facio,* to make]

car·ni·tine (kar′ni-tēn). L-3-hydroxy-4-(trimethylammonium)-butyrate; a trimethylammonium (betaine) derivative of γ-amino-β-hydroxybutyric acid, formed from $N^\epsilon, N^\epsilon, N^\epsilon$-trimethyllysine and from γ-butyrobetaine; the L-isomer is a thyroid inhibitor found in muscle, liver, and meat extracts; L-c. is an acyl carrier with respect to the mitochondrial membrane; it thus stimulates fatty acid oxidation. SYN B_T factor, vitamin B_T. [L. *caro carn-,* flesh + ine]

c. acetyltransferase, an enzyme found in mitochondria that catalyzes the reversible transfer of an acetyl group from acetyl-CoA to c., forming *O*-acetylcarnitine and coenzyme A. Acetylcarnitine is an important fuel source in sperm.

c. acylcarnitine translocase, a transport protein found in the inner mitochondrial membrane. Transports acylcarnitine derivatives into the mitochondria and transports c. out of the mitochondria. An important step in fatty acid oxidation.

c. palmitoyltransferase, (1) an enzyme that reversibly forms acylcarnitines and coenzyme A from carnitine and acylcoenzyme A (often, palmitoyl-CoA); important in fatty acid oxidation. Deficiency of isozyme I results in ketogenesis with hypoglycemia; deficiency of isozyme II affects primarily skeletal muscle.

Car·niv·o·ra (kar-niv′ō-ră). An order of chiefly flesh-eating mammals that includes the cats, dogs, bears, civets, minks, and hyenas, as well as the raccoon and panda; some species are omnivorous or herbivorous. [L. *carnivorus,* fr. *caro* (*carn-*), flesh, + *voro,* to devour]

car·ni·vore (kar'ni-vōr). One of the Carnivora.

car·niv·o·rous (kar-niv'ŏ-rŭs). Flesh-eating; subsisting on animals as food. SYN zoophagous.

car·nos·in·ase (kar'nō-si-nās). Mammalian enzyme that catalyzes the hydrolysis of carnosine, producing histidine and β-alanine; a deficiency of the serum enzyme leads to elevated carnosine levels.

car·no·sine (kar'nō-sēn). *N*-β-alanyl-L-histidine; the dominant nonprotein nitrogenous component of brain tissue, first found in relatively high amounts in muscle; chelates copper and activates myosin ATPase. SYN ignotine, inhibitine. [L. *carnosus,* fleshy, fr. *caro,* flesh, + -ia]

car·nos·ine·mia (kar'nō-si-nē'mē-ă). An autosomal recessive congenital disease, characterized by the presence of excess amounts of carnosine in the blood and urine and caused by a genetic deficiency of the enzyme carnosinase. Clinically characterized by progressive neurological damage, severe mental retardation, and myoclonic seizures. [carnosine + G. *haima,* blood + -ia]

car·nos·i·ty (kar-nos'i-tē). 1. Fleshiness. 2. A fleshy protuberance.

Carnoy, Jean Baptiste, French biologist, 1836–1899. SEE C.'s *fixative.*

ca·ro, gen. **car·nis,** pl. **car·nes** (kā'rō, kar'nis, -nes). The fleshy parts of the body; muscular and fatty tissues. [L.]

c. quadra′ta syl′vii, SYN quadratus plantae *muscle.*

car·ob flour (kar'ob). SYN algaroba.

Caroli, J., 20th century French physician. SEE C.'s *disease.*

car·o·ten·ase (kar'-ō-ten-ās). SYN β-carotene 15,15′-dioxygenase.

car·o·tene (kar'ō-tēn). A class of carotenoids, yellow-red pigments (lipochromes) widely distributed in plants and animals, notably in carrots, and closely related in structure to the xanthophylls and lycopenes and to the open-chain squalene; of particular interest in that they include precursors of the vitamins A (provitamin A carotenoids). Chemically, they consist of 8 isoprene units in a symmetrical chain with the 2 isoprenes at each end cyclized, forming either α-carotene or β-carotene (γ-carotene has only one end cyclized). The cyclic ends of β-carotene are identical β-ionine-like structures; thus, on oxidative fission, β-carotene yields 2 molecules of vitamin A. The cyclic ends of α-carotene differ: one is an α-ionone, the other a β-ionone; on fission, α-carotene, like γ-carotene, yields 1 molecule of vitamin A (a β-ionone derivative). SYN carotin.

c. oxidase, SYN lipoxygenase.

β-car·o·tene 15,15′-di·ox·y·gen·ase. An enzyme catalyzing the reaction of β-carotene plus O_2 producing two retinals. SYN β-carotene cleavage enzyme, carotenase, carotinase.

car·o·ten·e·mia (kar'ō-te-nē'mē-ă). Carotene in the blood, especially pertaining to increased quantities, which sometimes cause a pale yellow-red pigmentation of the skin that may resemble icterus. SYN carotinemia, xanthemia.

car·o·ten·o·der·ma (că-rot'en-ō-der-mă). SYN carotenosis cutis. [carotene + G. *derma,* skin]

ca·rot·e·noid (ka-rot'e-noyd). 1. Resembling carotene; having a yellow color. 2. One of the carotenoids. SYN carotinoid.

ca·rot·e·noids (ka-rot'e-noydz). Generic term for a class of carotenes and their oxygenated derivatives (xanthophylls) consisting of 8 isoprenoid units joined so that the orientation of these units is reversed at the center, placing the two central methyl groups in a 1,6 relationship in contrast to the 1,5 of others. All c. may be formally derived from the acyclic $C_{40}H_{56}$ structure (part I*A*, known as lycopene, of the accompanying group of structures) with its long central chain of conjugated double bonds by hydrogenation, dehydrogenation, oxidation, cyclization, or combinations of these. Included as c.'s are some compounds arising from certain rearrangements or degradations of the carbon skeleton (structure I*B*), but not retinol and related C_{20} com-

pounds. The nine-carbon end-groups may be acyclic with 1,2 and 5,6 double bonds (as in structure I*A*) or cyclohexanes with a single double bond at 5,6 or 5,4, or cyclopentanes or aryl groups; these are now designated by Greek letter prefixes (illustrated in part II of the accompanying group of structures) preceding "carotene" (α and δ, which are used in the trivial names α-carotene and δ-carotene, are not used for that reason). Suffixes (-oic acid, -oate, -al, -one, -ol) indicate certain oxygen-containing groups (acid, ester, aldehyde, ketone, alcohol); all other substitutions appear as prefixes (alkoxy-, epoxy-, hydro-, etc.). The configuration about all double bonds is *trans* unless *cis* and locant numbers appear. The prefix *retro-* is used to indicate a shift of one position of all single and double bonds; *apo-* indicates shortening of the molecule. Many c.'s have anticancer activities.

car·o·ten·o·pro·tein (ka-rot'en-ō-prō-tēn). A protein with a covalently-bound carotenoid.

car·o·te·no·sis cu·tis (kar-ō-te-nō'sis kyū'tis). A harmless reversible yellow coloration of the skin caused by an increase in carotene content. SYN carotenoderma, carotinosis cutis.

ca·rot·ic (kă-rot'ik). SYN stuporous. [G. *karōtikos,* stupefying]

ca·rot·i·co·tym·pan·ic (ka-rot'i-kō-tim-pan'ik). Relating to the carotid canal and the tympanum.

ca·rot·id (ka-rot'id). Pertaining to any c. structure. [G. *karōtides,* the carotid arteries, fr. *karoō,* to put to sleep (because compression of the c. artery results in unconsciousness)]

ca·rot·i·dyn·ia (kă-rot'i-din'ē-ă). SYN carotodynia.

car·o·tin (kar'ō-tin). SYN carotene.

car·o·ti·nase (kar'ō-ti-nās). SYN β-carotene 15,15′-dioxygenase.

car·o·tin·e·mia (kar'ō-ti-nē'mē-ă). SYN carotenemia.

car·o·ti·noid (ka-rot'i-noyd). SYN carotenoid.

car·o·ti·no·sis cu·tis (ka-rot-i-nō'sis kyū'tis). SYN carotenosis cutis.

ca·rot·o·dyn·ia (kă-rot'ō-din'ē-ă). Pain caused by pressure on the carotid artery. SYN carotidynia. [G. *odynē,* pain]

car·pal (kar'păl). Relating to the carpus.

car·pec·to·my (kar-pek'tō-mē). Excision of a portion or all of the carpus. [G. *karpos,* wrist, + *ektomē,* excision]

Carpenter, Charles J., U.S. immunologist, *1931. SEE C.'s *syndrome.*

Carpenter, George Alfred, British physician, 1859–1910. SEE C.'s *syndrome.*

Carpentier-Edwards valve. See under valve.

car·phen·a·zine ma·le·ate (kar-fen'ă-zēn). 1{10-(3-[4-(2-Hydroxyethyl)-1-piperazinyl]propyl)phenothia zine-2-yl}-1-propanone bis(hydrogen maleate); a phenothiazine tranquilizer of the piperazine group. Functionally classified as an antipsychotic agent, it is used in the treatment of chronic and acute schizophrenia; also possesses antiemetic, adrenolytic, anticholinergic, and dopamine-blocking actions.

car·pho·lo·gia, car·phol·o·gy (kar-fō-lō'jē-ă, -fol'ō-jē). SYN floccillation. [G. *karphologein*]

car·pi·tis (kar-pī'tis). Carpal arthritis in the horse and other animals.

car·po·car·pal (kar-pō-kar'păl). SYN midcarpal (2).

Car·po·glyp·tus (kar-pō-glip'tŭs). A genus of mites including *C. passularum,* the fruit mite, which causes a dermatitis among handlers of dried fruit. [G. *karpos,* fruit, + *glyphō,* , to carve]

car·po·met·a·car·pal (kar'pō-met-ă-kar'păl). Relating to both carpus and metacarpus.

car·po·ped·al (kar'pō-ped'ăl). Relating to the wrist and the foot, or the hands and feet; denoting especially c. spasm. [G. *karpos,* wrist, + L. *pes* (*ped-*), foot]

car·pop·to·sis, car·pop·to·sia (kar-pop-tō'sis, -tō'zē-ă). SYN *wrist*-drop. [G. *karpos,* wrist, + *ptōsis,* a falling]

Carpue, Joseph, British surgeon, 1764–1846. SEE C.'s *method.*

car·pus, gen. and pl. **car·pi** (kar'pŭs, kar'pī) [NA]. 1. SYN wrist. 2. SYN carpal *bones,* under *bone.* [Mod. L. fr. Gr. *karpos*]

c. cur′vus, SYN Madelung's *deformity.*

Carr, Francis H., British chemist, *1874. SEE C.-Price *reaction.*

car·ra·geen, car·ra·gheen (kar'ă-jēn, -gēn). **1.** SYN chondrus (2). **2.** SYN carrageenan.

car·ra·gee·nan, car·ra·gee·nin (kar-ă-gē'nan, -nin). A polysaccharide vegetable gum obtained from Irish moss; a galactosan sulfate resembling agar in molecular structure. SYN carrageen (2), carragheen. [*Carragheen,* Irish village]

car·re·four sen·si·tif (kar-fūr'son-sē-tēf'). A term given by Charcot to the posterior portion of the caudal limb of the internal capsule. [Fr. sensory crossroads]

Carrel, Alexis, French-U.S. surgeon and Nobel laureate, 1873–1944. SEE C.'s *treatment;* C.-Lindbergh *pump;* Dakin-C. *treatment.*

car·ri·er (ka'rē-er). **1.** A person or animal that harbors a specific infectious agent in the absence of discernible clinical disease and serves as a potential source of infection. **2.** Any chemical capable of accepting an atom, radical, or subatomic particle from one compound, then passing it to another; *e.g.,* cytochromes are electron c.'s; homocysteine is a methyl c. **3.** A substance which, by having chemical properties closely related to or indistinguishable from those of a radioactive tracer, is thus able to carry the tracer through a precipitation or similar chemical procedure; the best c.'s are the nonradioactive isotopes of the tracer in question. SEE ALSO label, tracer. **4.** A large immunogen which when coupled to a hapten will facilitate an immune response to the hapten.

amalgam c., an instrument used to transport triturated amalgam to a cavity preparation and to deposit it therein.

convalescent c., an individual who is clinically recovered from an infectious disease but is still capable of transmitting the infectious agent to others.

genetic c., (1) an unaffected heterozygote bearing a usually harmful recessive gene; (2) a c. that bears a dominant but latent age-dependent trait to have offspring with unbalanced karyotypes.

hydrogen c., a molecule that, in conjunction with a tissue enzyme system, carries hydrogen from one metabolite (oxidant) to another (reductant) or to molecular oxygen to form H_2O. SYN hydrogen acceptor.

incubatory c., an individual capable of transmitting an infectious agent to others during the incubation period of the disease.

latent c., a person, typically a prospective parent, bearing the appropriate genotype of a trait (homozygous for recessive, homozygous or heterozygous for dominant, hemizygous or homozygous for X-linked) that manifests the trait only under certain conditions, *e.g.,* age, an environmental insult, etc.

manifesting c., SYN manifesting *heterozygote.*

translocation c., a person with balanced translocation.

car·ri·er-free. A substance in which a radioactive or other tagged atom is found in every molecule; the highest possible specific activity.

Carrión, Daniel A., Peruvian medical student, 1859–1885, who inoculated himself with a disease later designated as Carrión's *disease,* and died thereof. SEE C.'s *disease.*

Carteaud, Alexandre, French physician, *1897. SEE Gougerot-C. *syndrome.*

Carter, Henry V., Anglo-Indian physician, 1831–1897. SEE C.'s *fever,* black *mycetoma.*

car·te·sian (kar-tē'zhŭn). Relating to Cartesius, Latinized form of Descartes.

car·tha·mus (kar'tha-mŭs). The dried florets of *Carthamus tinctorius* (family Compositae). SEE ALSO safflower oil. SYN safflower. [Ar. *qurtum,* fr. *qartama,* paint; the plant yields a dye]

CARTILAGE

car·ti·lage (kar'ti-lij). A connective tissue characterized by its nonvascularity and firm consistency; consists of cells (chondrocytes), an interstitial matrix of fibers (collagen), and a ground substance (proteoglycans). There are three kinds of c.: hyaline c., elastic c., and fibrocartilage. Nonvascular, resilient, flexible connective tissue found primarily in joints, the walls of the thorax, and tubular structures such as the larynx, air passages, and ears; comprises most of the skeleton in early fetal life, but is slowly replaced by bone. For gross anatomical description, see cartilage and its subentries. SYN cartilago [NA], chondrus (1), gristle. [L. *cartilago (cartilagin-),* gristle]

accessory c., a sesamoid c.

accessory nasal c.'s, variable small plates of cartilage located in the interval between the greater alar and lateral nasal cartilages. SYN cartilagines nasales accessoriae [NA], sesamoid c.'s of nose.

accessory quadrate c., SYN lesser alar c.'s.

c. of acoustic meatus, the cartilage that forms the wall of the lateral part of the external acoustic meatus. It is incomplete above and is firmly attached to the margins of the bony part of the external meatus. SYN cartilago meatus acustici [NA], meatal c.

alisphenoid c., the c. in the embryo from which the greater wing of the sphenoid bone is developed.

annular c., SYN cricoid c.

arthrodial c., SYN articular c.

articular c., the cartilage covering the articular surfaces of the bones participating in a synovial joint. SYN cartilago articularis [NA], arthrodial c., diarthrodial c., investing c.

arytenoid c., one of a pair of small triangular pyramidal laryngeal cartilages that articulate with the lamina of the cricoid cartilage. It gives attachment at its anteriorly-directed vocal process to the posterior part of the corresponding vocal ligament and to several muscles at its laterally-directed muscular process. The base of the cartilage is hyaline but the apex is elastic. SYN cartilago arytenoidea [NA], triquetrous c. (2).

c. of auditory tube, cartilage of auditory tube or of pharyngotympanic tube; tubal cartilage; the trough-shaped cartilage that forms the medial wall, roof, and part of the lateral wall of the auditory tube. SYN cartilago tubae auditivae [NA], c. of pharyngotympanic tube, tubal c.

auricular c., the cartilage of the auricle. SYN cartilago auriculae [NA], c. of ear, conchal c.

basilar c., the c. filling the foramen lacerum. SYN basilar fibrocartilage, fibrocartilago basalis.

branchial c.'s, c.'s developing within the vertebrate or embryonic branchial arches; they form the cartilaginous viscerocranium. SYN pharyngeal c.'s.

calcified c., c. in which calcium salts are deposited in the matrix; it occurs prior to replacement by osseous tissue and sometimes in aging c.

cellular c., an embryonic or immature stage of c. in which it consists chiefly of cells with very little matrix. SYN parenchymatous c.

ciliary c., incorrect term sometimes applied to the inferior tarsus and superior tarsus. SEE tarsus (2).

circumferential c., (1) SYN acetabular *labrum.* (2) SYN glenoid *labrum.*

conchal c., SYN auricular c.

connecting c., the c. in a cartilaginous joint such as the symphysis pubis. SYN interosseous c., uniting c.

corniculate c., a conical nodule of elastic cartilage surmounting the apex of each arytenoid cartilage. SYN cartilago corniculata [NA], corniculum laryngis, Santorini's c., supra-arytenoid c.

costal c., the cartilage forming the anterior continuation of a rib, providing the means by which it reaches and articulates with the sternum. SYN cartilago costalis [NA], costicartilage.

cricoid c., the lowermost of the laryngeal cartilages; it is shaped like a signet-ring, being expanded into a nearly quadrilateral plate (lamina) posteriorly; the anterior portion is called the arch (arcus). SYN cartilago cricoidea [NA], annular c.

cuneiform c., a small nonarticulating rod of elastic cartilage in the aryepiglottic fold anterolateral and somewhat superior to the corniculate cartilage. SYN cartilago cuneiformis [NA], Morgagni's c., Morgagni's tubercle, Wrisberg's c.

diarthrodial c., SYN articular c.

c. of ear, SYN auricular c.

elastic c., a c. in which the cells are surrounded by a territorial capsular matrix outside of which is an interterritorial matrix containing elastic fiber networks in addition to the collagen fibers and ground substance. SYN yellow c.

ensiform c., ensisternum c., obsolete term for xiphoid *process.*

epiglottic c., a thin lamina of elastic cartilage forming the central portion of the epiglottis. SYN cartilago epiglottica [NA].

epiphysial c., SYN epiphysial *plate.*

falciform c., SYN medial *meniscus.*

floating c., a loose piece of c. within a joint cavity, detached from the articular c. or from a meniscus. SYN loose c.

greater alar c., one of a pair of cartilages that form the tip of the nose. It consists of a medial crus that extends into the nasal septum with its fellow of the opposite side, and a lateral crus that forms the anterior part of the wing of the nose. SYN cartilago alaris major [NA].

Huschke's c.'s, two horizontal cartilaginous rods at the edge of the cartilaginous septum of the nose.

hyaline c., c. having a frosted glass appearance, with interstitial substance containing fine type II collagen fibers obscured by the ground substance; in adult c., the cells are present in isogenous groups.

hypsiloid c., SYN Y c.

interosseous c., SYN connecting c.

intervertebral c., SYN intervertebral *disc.*

intra-articular c., (1) SYN articular *disc.* **(2)** SYN articular *meniscus.*

intrathyroid c., a narrow slip of c. sometimes found joining the laminae of the thyroid c. of the larynx in infancy.

investing c., SYN articular c.

Jacobson's c., SYN *cartilago* vomeronasalis.

c.'s of larynx, SEE thyroid c., cricoid c., arytenoid c., cuneiform c., triticeal c., corniculate c., sesamoid c. of larynx, epiglottic c. SYN cartilagines laryngis [NA].

lateral c., cartilaginous plates that extend above the hoof from the caudal angles of the distal phalanx of the horse; they are readily palpated under the skin of the sides of the hoof and assist in distributing the animal's weight during locomotion.

lateral c. of nose, the cartilage located in the lateral wall of the nose above the alar cartilage. SYN cartilago nasi lateralis [NA].

lesser alar c.'s, the two to four cartilaginous plates of the wing of the nose posterior to the greater alar cartilage. SYN cartilagines alares minores [NA], accessory quadrate c.

loose c., SYN floating c.

Luschka's c., a small cartilaginous nodule sometimes found in the anterior portion of the vocal cord.

mandibular c., a c. bar in the mandibular arch that forms a temporary supporting structure in the embryonic mandible; the cartilagenous primordia of the malleus and incus develop from its proximal end, and it also gives rise to the sphenomandibular and anterior malleolar ligaments. SYN Meckel's c.

meatal c., SYN c. of acoustic meatus.

Meckel's c., SYN mandibular c.

Meyer's c.'s, the anterior sesamoid c.'s at the anterior attachments of the vocal ligaments.

Morgagni's c., SYN cuneiform c.

nasal septal c., a thin cartilaginous plate located between vomer, perpendicular plate of the ethmoid, and nasal bones, and completing the nasal septum anteriorly. SYN cartilago septi nasi [NA], c. of nasal septum, cartilaginous septum, pars cartilaginea septi nasi, quadrangular c., septal c.

c. of nasal septum, SYN nasal septal c.

c.'s of nose, SEE lateral c. of nose, greater alar c., nasal septal c., *cartilago* vomeronasalis, lesser alar c.'s, accessory nasal c.'s. SYN cartilagines nasi [NA].

ossifying c., SYN temporary c.

parachordal c., c. primordia adjacent on either side to the cephalic portion of the notochord in young embryos; they represent an initial step in the formation of the chondrocranium.

paraseptal c., SYN *cartilago* vomeronasalis.

parenchymatous c., SYN cellular c.

periotic c., a cartilaginous mass on either side of the chondrocranium surrounding the developing auditory vesicle in the fetus; the otic capsule in its early cartilaginous stage.

permanent c., c. that is not replaced by bone.

pharyngeal c.'s, SYN branchial c.'s.

c. of pharyngotympanic tube, SYN c. of auditory tube.

precursory c., SYN temporary c.

primordial c., c. in an early stage in its development.

quadrangular c., SYN nasal septal c.

Reichert's c., a c. in the mesenchyme of the second branchial arch in the embryo, from which develop the stapes, the styloid processes, the stylohyoid ligaments, and the lesser cornua of the hyoid bone.

reticular c., retiform c., rarely used terms for fibrocartilage.

Santorini's c., SYN corniculate c.

Seiler's c., a small rod of c. attached to the vocal process of the arytenoid c.

semilunar c., one of the articular menisci of the knee joint. SEE lateral *meniscus*, medial *meniscus.*

septal c., SYN nasal septal c.

sesamoid c. of larynx, a small nodule of elastic cartilage sometimes present on the lateral border of the arytenoid cartilage. SYN cartilago sesamoidea laryngis [NA].

sesamoid c.'s of nose, SYN accessory nasal c.'s.

slipping rib c., subluxation of rib c., at the costo-chondral junction, causing pain and audible click.

sternal c., a costal c. of one of the true ribs.

supra-arytenoid c., SYN corniculate c.

tarsal c., incorrect term sometimes applied to the inferior tarsus and superior tarsus. SEE tarsus (2).

temporary c., a c. that is normally replaced by bone, to form a part of the skeleton. SYN ossifying c., precursory c.

thyroid c., the largest of the cartilages of the larynx; it is formed of two approximately quadrilateral plates (*laminae*) joined anteriorly at an angle of from 90° to 120°, the prominence so formed constituting the laryngeal prominence (Adam's apple). SYN cartilago thyroidea [NA].

tracheal c.'s, the 16 to 20 incomplete rings of hyaline cartilage forming the skeleton of the trachea; the rings are deficient posteriorly for from one-fifth to one-third of their circumference. SYN cartilagines tracheales [NA], tracheal ring.

triangular c., SYN articular *disc* of distal radioulnar joint.

triquetrous c., (1) SYN articular *disc* of distal radioulnar joint. **(2)** SYN arytenoid c.

triticeal c., a rounded nodule of cartilage, the size of a grain of wheat, occasionally present in the posterior margin of the lateral thyrohyoid ligament. SYN cartilago triticea [NA], corpus triticeum, triticeum.

tubal c., SYN c. of auditory tube.

uniting c., SYN connecting c.

vomerine c., vomeronasal c., SYN *cartilago* vomeronasalis.

Weitbrecht's c., SYN articular *disc* of acromioclavicular joint.

Wrisberg's c., SYN cuneiform c.

xiphoid c., SYN xiphoid *process.*

Y c., Y-shaped c., the connecting c. for the ilium, ischium, and pubis; it extends through the acetabulum. SYN hypsiloid c.

yellow c., SYN elastic c.

---

car·ti·la·gi·nes (kar-ti-laj′i-nĕz). Plural of cartilago.

car·ti·lag·i·noid (kar-ti-laj′i-noyd). SYN chondroid (1).

car·ti·lag·i·nous (kar-ti-laj′i-nŭs). Relating to or consisting of cartilage. SYN chondral.

car·ti·la·go, pl. **car·ti·la·gi·nes** (kar-ti-lā′gō, -laj′i-nēs) [NA]. SYN cartilage. For histological description, see cartilage. [L. gristle]

cartila′gines ala′res mino′res [NA], SYN lesser alar *cartilages*, under *cartilage.*

c. ala′ris ma′jor [NA], SYN greater alar *cartilage.*

c. articula′ris [NA], SYN articular *cartilage.*

c. arytenoi′dea [NA], SYN arytenoid *cartilage.*

c. **auric′ulae** [NA], SYN auricular *cartilage*.

c. **cornicula′ta** [NA], SYN corniculate *cartilage*.

c. **costa′lis** [NA], SYN costal *cartilage*.

c. **cricoi′dea** [NA], SYN cricoid *cartilage*.

c. **cuneifor′mis** [NA], SYN cuneiform *cartilage*.

c. **epiglot′tica** [NA], SYN epiglottic *cartilage*.

c. **epiphysia′lis** [NA], SYN epiphysial *plate*.

cartila′gines laryn′gis [NA], SYN *cartilages* of larynx, under *cartilage*.

c. **mea′tus acus′tici** [NA], SYN *cartilage* of acoustic meatus.

cartila′gines nasa′les accessor′iae [NA], SYN accessory nasal *cartilages*, under *cartilage*.

cartila′gines na′si [NA], SYN *cartilages* of nose, under *cartilage*.

c. **na′si latera′lis** [NA], SYN lateral *cartilage* of nose.

c. **sep′ti na′si** [NA], SYN nasal septal *cartilage*.

c. **sesamoi′dea laryn′gis** [NA], SYN sesamoid *cartilage* of larynx.

c. **thyroid′ea** [NA], SYN thyroid *cartilage*.

cartila′gines trachea′les [NA], SYN tracheal *cartilages*, under *cartilage*.

c. **tritic′ea** [NA], SYN triticeal *cartilage*. [L. *triticum*, wheat]

c. **tu′bae auditi′vae** [NA], SYN *cartilage* of auditory tube.

c. **vomeronasa′lis** [NA], a narrow strip of cartilage located between the lower edge of the cartilage of the nasal septum and the vomer. SYN Jacobson's cartilage, paraseptal cartilage, vomer cartilagineus, vomerine cartilage, vomeronasal cartilage.

ca·ru·bin·ose (kă-rū′bin-ōs). Archaic word for mannose.

ca·run·cle (kar′ŭng-kl). SYN caruncula (1).

lacrimal c., a small reddish body at the medial angle of the eye, containing modified sebaceous and sweat glands. SYN caruncula lacrimalis [NA].

Morgagni's c., SYN middle *lobe* of prostate.

Santorini's major c., SYN major duodenal *papilla*.

Santorini's minor c., SYN minor duodenal *papilla*.

urethral c., a small, fleshy, sometimes painful protrusion of the mucous membrane at the meatus of the female urethra; it may be telangiectatic, papillomatous, or composed of granulation tissue.

ca·run·cu·la, pl. **ca·run·cu·lae** (kă-rŭng′kyū-lă, -lē). **1** [NA]. A small, fleshy protuberance, or any structure suggesting such a shape. SYN caruncle. **2.** In ungulates, one of about 200 specific disklike areas of the uterine endometrium that, in conjunction with the fetal cotyledon, forms a placentome of the placenta; as a site of fetal-maternal contact, the c. remains constant in position but enlarges greatly in size during pregnancy. [L. a small fleshy mass, fr. *caro*, flesh]

hymenal c., one of the numerous tabs or projections surrounding the orifice of the vagina. SYN c. hymenalis [NA], c. myrtiformis.

c. **hymena′lis**, pl. **carun′culae hymena′les** [NA], SYN hymenal c.

c. **lacrima′lis** [NA], SYN lacrimal *caruncle*.

c. **myrtifor′mis**, pl. **carun′culae myrtifor′mes**, SYN hymenal c.

c. **saliva′ris**, SYN sublingual c.

sublingual c., a papilla on each side of the frenulum of the tongue marking the opening of the submandibular duct. SYN c. sublingualis [NA], c. salivaris.

c. **sublingua′lis** [NA], SYN sublingual c.

Carus, Karl G., German anatomist and zoologist, 1789–1869. SEE C.'s *circle*, *curve*.

car·va·crol (kar′vă-krol). 2-*p*-Cymenol; an isomer of thymol that occurs in several volatile oils (marjoram, origanum, savory, and thyme), with properties and activity that closely resemble those of thymol; has antiseptic properties, but is used chiefly as a perfume.

Carvallo, SEE Rivero-Carvallo.

Carvallo's sign. See under sign.

car·ve·di·lol (kar′vē-dil-ol). An agent used as an antihypertensive, antianginal.

carv·er (kar′ver). A dental hand instrument, available in a wide variety of end shapes, used for forming and contouring wax, filling materials, etc.

△**caryo-.** Nucleus. SEE karyo-. [G. *karyon*, nut, kernel]

car·y·o·phyl·lus, car·y·o·phyl·lum (kar′ē-ō-fĭ′lŭs, -ŭm). Clove. [G. *karyophyllon*, clove tree, fr. *karyon*, nut, + *phyllon*, leaf]

car·y·o·the·ca (kar′ē-ō-thē′kă). SYN nuclear *envelope*. [caryo- + G. *thēkē*, sheath, box]

Casal, Gasper, Spanish physician, 1691–1759. SEE C.'s *necklace*.

cas·a·mi·no ac·ids (kās′ă-mē′nō). Trivial term for the mixture of amino acids derived by hydrolysis of casein; used in bacterial and similar growth media.

cas·cade (kas-kād′). **1.** A series of sequential interactions, as of a physiological process, which once initiated continues to the final one; each interaction is activated by the preceding one, sometimes with cumulative effect. **2.** To spill over, especially rapidly. [Fr., fr. It. *cascare*, to fall]

cas·cara (kas-kar′ă). SYN c. sagrada.

c. **amara**, the dried bark of a species of *Picramnia* (family Simarubaceae); used as a bitter tonic. SYN Honduras bark.

c. **sagrada**, the dried bark of *Rhamnus purshiana* (family Rhamnaceae); used as a laxative. SYN cascara.

case (kās). **1.** An instance of disease with its attendant circumstances. Cf. patient. **2.** A box or container. [L. *casus*, an occurrence]

borderline c., a patient, whose clinical findings are suggestive, but not fully convincing, of a specific diagnosis.

index c., SYN proband.

trial c., in refraction, a box containing lenses for testing.

ca·se·a·tion (kā-sē-ā′shŭn). A form of coagulation necrosis in which the necrotic tissue resembles cheese and contains a mixture of protein and fat that is absorbed very slowly; occurs particularly in tuberculosis. SEE ALSO caseous *necrosis*. SYN tyrosis (2). [L. *caseus*, cheese]

ca·sein (cā′sē-in, kā′sēn). The principal protein of cow's milk and the chief constituent of cheese. It is insoluble in water, soluble in dilute alkaline and salt solutions, forms a hard insoluble plastic with formaldehyde, and is used as a constituent of some glues; various components are designated α-, β-, and κ-caseins. β-c. is converted to γ-c. by milk proteases. There are several isoforms of α-c. κ-c. is not precipitated by calcium ions.

c. **iodine, iodinated c.**, a compound of c. with iodine formed by incubating the protein with the element, which becomes attached to tyrosine groups in the protein. SYN caseo-iodine.

plant c., SYN avenin.

ca·sein·ate (kā′sē-in-āt). A salt of casein.

ca·sein·o·gen (kā-sē-in′ō-jen). "Soluble" or κ-casein which, when acted upon by rennin, is converted into paracasein.

ca·seo·io·dine (kā′sē-ō-i′ō-dīn). SYN *casein* iodine.

ca·se·ose (kā′sē-ōs). Nondescript term for product resulting from the hydrolysis or digestion of casein.

ca·se·ous (kā′sē-ŭs). Pertaining to or manifesting the gross and microscopic features of tissue affected by caseation.

Caslick, Edward, 20th century U.S. veterinarian. SEE C.'s *operation*.

Casoni, Tommaro, Italian physician, 1880–1933. SEE C. intradermal *test*, skin *test*.

cas·sa·va starch (kă-sah′vah). SYN tapioca.

Casselberry, William E., U.S. laryngologist, 1858–1916. SEE C. *position*.

Casser (Casserio), Giulio, Italian anatomist, 1556–1616. SEE C.'s *fontanel*, perforated *muscle*.

cas·se·ri·an (ka-sē′rē-an). Relating to or described by Casser.

cas·sette (kă-set′). **1.** A plate, film, or tape holder for use in photography and radiography. **2.** A perforated holder in which tissue blocks are placed for paraffin embedding. [Fr., dim. of *casse*, box]

cas·sia bark (kash′yă). SYN cinnamon.

cas·sia fis·tu·la. The dried ripe fruit of *Cassia fistula*, used as a laxative. SYN purging cassia.

cas·sia oil. SYN cinnamon oil.

cast (kast). **1.** An object formed by the solidification of a liquid poured into a mold. **2.** Rigid encasement of a part, as with plaster or a plastic, for purposes of immobilization. **3.** An elongated or cylindrical mold formed in a tubular structure (*e.g.,* renal tubule, bronchiole) that may be observed in histologic sections or in material such as urine or sputum; results from inspissation of fluid material secreted or excreted in the tubular structures. **4.** Restraint of a large animal, usually a horse, with ropes and harnesses in a recumbent position. **5.** In dentistry, a positive reproduction of the form of the tissues of the upper or lower jaw, which is made by the solidification of plaster, metal, etc., poured into an impression, and over which denture bases or other dental restorations may be fabricated. [M.E. *kasten,* fr. O.Norse *kasta*]

bacterial c., a c. in the urine composed of bacteria.

blood c., a c. usually formed in renal tubules, but may occur in bronchioles; consists of inspissated material that includes various elements of blood (*i.e.,* erythrocytes, leukocytes, fibrin, and so on), resulting from bleeding into the glomerulus or tubule, or into the alveolus or bronchiole.

coma c., a renal c. of strongly refracting granules said to be indicative of imminent coma in diabetes. SYN Külz's cylinder.

decidual c., a mold of the interior of the uterus formed of the exfoliated mucous membrane in cases of extrauterine gestation.

dental c., a positive likeness of a part or parts of the oral cavity.

diagnostic c., a positive replica of the form of the teeth and tissues made from an impression.

epithelial c., a c. that contains epithelial cells and their remnants; occurs most frequently in renal tubules and urine as a marker for renal tubular necrosis.

false c., an elongated, ribbon-like mucous thread with poorly defined edges and pointed or split ends, often confused with a true urinary c. SYN cylindroid, mucous c., pseudocast, spurious c.

fatty c., a renal or urinary c. consisting largely of fat globules; those containing doubly refractile bodies (composed of cholesterol) are found in the nephrotic syndrome.

fibrinous c., a yellow c. that somewhat resembles a waxy c.; more likely to occur in the urine of certain patients with acute nephritis.

granular c., a relatively dark, dense urinary c. of coarsely or finely particulate cellular debris and other proteinaceous material, frequently seen in chronic renal disease but also in the recovery phase of acute renal failure. SEE ALSO waxy c.

hair c., a c. composed of parakeratotic scales attached to scalp hair but freely movable up and down the hair shaft; found in scaling dermatitis of the scalp, including dandruff, psoriasis, and seborrheic dermatitis. SYN pseudonit.

halo c., a c. applied to the shoulders in which metal bars are set that extend over the head to a halo, from which traction may be applied to the head by means of tongs or a halter.

hyaline c., a relatively transparent renal c. composed of proteinaceous material derived from disintegration of cells; seen in patients with renal disease or transiently with exercise, fever, congestive heart failure, and diuretic therapy.

investment c., SYN refractory c.

master c., a replica of the prepared tooth surfaces, residual ridge areas, and/or other parts of the dental arch as reproduced from an impression.

mucous c., SYN false c.

red blood cell c., a urinary c. composed of a matrix containing red cells in various stages of degeneration and visibility, characteristic of glomerular disease or renal parenchymal bleeding. SYN red cell c.

red cell c., SYN red blood cell c.

refractory c., a c. made of material that will withstand the high temperatures of metal casting or soldering without disintegrating. SYN investment c.

renal c., any type of c. formed in a renal tubule, and found in the urine consisting of various materials, *e.g.,* albumin, cells, blood. SYN tube c.

spurious c., SYN false c.

tube c., SYN renal c.

urinary c.'s, c.'s discharged in the urine.

waxy c., a form of urinary c. consisting of homogeneous proteinaceous material that has a high refractive index, in contrast to the low refractive index of hyaline c.'s; waxy c.'s probably represent

an advanced stage of the disintegrative process that results in coarsely and finely granular c.'s, and are usually indicative of oliguria or anuria.

white blood cell c., a urinary c. composed of polymorphonuclear leukocytes, characteristic of tubulointerstitial disease, especially pyelonephritis.

white cell c., a c. in the urine composed of white blood cells.

cast brace (kast brās). A specially designed plaster or plastic cast incorporating hinges and other brace components; used in the treatment of fractures to promote early activity and early joint motion.

Castellani, Sir Aldo, Italian physician, 1878–1971. SEE C.'s *bronchitis, paint;* C.-Low *sign.*

cast·ing (kas'ting). **1.** A metallic object formed in a mold. **2.** The act of forming a c. in a mold.

centrifugal c., c. molten metal into a mold by spinning the metal from a crucible at the end of a revolving arm.

ceramo-metal c., a c. made of alloys containing or excluding precious metals, to which dental porcelain can be fused.

gold c., a c. made of gold, usually formed to represent and replace lost tooth structure.

vacuum c., the c. of a metal in the presence of a vacuum.

Castle, William B., U.S. physician, *1897. SEE C.'s intrinsic *factor.*

Castleman, Benjamin, U.S. pathologist, 1906–1982. SEE C.'s *disease.*

cas·tor bean (kas'ter bēn). SYN Ricinus.

cas·tor oil. A fixed oil expressed from the seeds of *Ricinus communis* (family Euphorbiaceae); a purgative.

aromatic c. o., contains cinnamon oil 3, clove oil 1, vanillin 1, saccharin 0.5, alcohol 30, in c. o. to make 1000; a cathartic.

cas·trate (kas'trāt). To remove the testicles or the ovaries. [L. *castro,* pp. *-atus,* to deprive of generative power (male or female)]

cas·tra·tion (kas-trā'shŭn). **1.** Removal of the testicles or ovaries. SYN Huggins' *operation.* **2.** SEE castration *complex.* [see castrate]

functional c., gonadal atrophy produced by prolonged treatment with sex hormones.

ca·su·al·ty (kazh'ū-ăl-tē). An injury, or the victim of an accident.

CAT Abbreviation for computerized axial *tomography; chloramphenicol* acetyl transferase.

cata-. Down; opposite of ana-. SEE ALSO kata-. Cf. de-. [G. *kata,* down]

cat·a·ba·si·al (kat-ă-bā'sē-ăl). Denoting a skull in which the basion is lower than the opisthion. [cata- + Mod. L. *basion*]

cat·a·bi·ot·ic (kat'ă-bī-ot'ik). Used up in the carrying on of the vital processes other than growth, or in the performance of function, referring to the energy derived from food. [cata- + G. *biōtikos,* relating to life]

cat·a·bol·ic (kat-ă-bol'ik). Relating to or promoting catabolism.

ca·tab·o·lism (kă-tab'ō-lizm). **1.** The breaking down in the body of complex chemical compounds into simpler ones (*e.g.,* glycogen to CO_2 and H_2O), often accompanied by the liberation of energy. **2.** The sum of all degradative processes. SYN dissimilation (2). Cf. anabolism, metabolism. [G. *katabolē,* a casting down]

ca·tab·o·lite (kă-tab'ō-līt). Any product of catabolism.

cat·a·chron·o·bi·ol·o·gy (kat'ă-kron'ō-bī-ol'ō-jē). The study of the deleterious effects of time on a living system. [cata- + G. *chronos,* time, + biology]

cat·a·crot·ic (kat-ă-krot'ik). Denoting a pulse tracing in which the downstroke is interrupted by one or more upward waves.

ca·tac·ro·tism (kă-tak'rō-tizm). A condition of the pulse in which there are one or more secondary expansions of the artery following the main beat, producing secondary upward waves on the downstroke of the pulse tracing. [cata- + G. *krotos,* beat]

cat·a·di·crot·ic (kat'ă-dī-krot'ik). Denoting a pulse tracing in which there are two minor elevations interrupting the downstroke.

cat·a·di·cro·tism (kat-ă-dī'krō-tizm). A condition of the pulse

ca

marked by two minor expansions of the artery following the main beat, producing two secondary upward waves on the downstroke of the pulse tracing. [cata + G. *di-*, two, + *krotos,* beat]

cat·a·did·y·mus (kat-ă-did'i-mŭs). SYN *duplicitas* anterior. [cata- + G. *didymus,* twin]

cat·a·di·op·tric (kat-ă-dī-op'trik). Employing both reflecting and refractive optical systems.

cat·a·gen (kat'ă-jen). A regressing phase of the hair growth cycle during which cell proliferation ceases, the hair follicle shortens, and an anchored club hair is produced.

cat·a·gen·e·sis (kat-ă-jen'ĕ-sis). SYN involution. [cata- + G. *genesis,* origin]

cat·a·lase (kat'ă-lās). A hemoprotein catalyzing the decomposition of hydrogen peroxide to water and oxygen ($2H_2O_2 \rightarrow O_2 + 2H_2O$); a deficiency of c. is associated with acatalasemia.

cat·a·lep·sy (kat'ă-lep-sē). A morbid condition characterized by waxy rigidity of the limbs, which may be placed in various positions that are maintained for a time, lack of response to stimuli, mutism and inactivity; occurs with some psychosis, especially catatonic schizophrenia. SYN anochlesia (1). [G. *katalēpsis,* a seizing, catalepsy, fr. *kata,* down, + *lēpsis,* a seizure]

cat·a·lep·tic (kat-ă-lep'tik). Relating to, or suffering from, catalepsy.

cat·a·lep·toid (kat-ă-lep'toyd). Simulating or resembling catalepsy.

cat·a·lo·gia (kat'ă-lō'jē-a). SYN verbigeration.

ca·tal·y·sis (kă-tal'i-sis). The effect that a catalyst exerts upon a chemical reaction. [G. *katalysis,* dissolution]

contact c., a process wherein the catalyst is a solid and the catalyzed reaction is produced after the reactants (usually gases) have made contact with the solid.

surface c., c. at the surface of a solid particle or a macromolecule.

cat·a·lyst (kat'ă-list). A substance that accelerates a chemical reaction but is not consumed or changed permanently thereby. SYN catalyzer.

inorganic c., a c. such as a finely divided metal (Pt, Rh), carbon, etc.

negative c., a c. that retards a reaction.

organic c., (1) SYN enzyme, ribozyme. (2) a c. that is an organic molecule.

positive c., SEE catalyst.

Raney c., SYN Raney *Nickel.*

cat·a·lyt·ic (kat-ă-lit'ik). Relating to or effecting catalysis.

cat·a·lyze (kat'ă-līz). To act as a catalyst.

cat·a·lyz·er (kat'ă-līz-er). SYN catalyst.

cat·a·me·nia (kat-ă-mē'nē-ă). SYN menses. [G. the menses, ntr. pl. of *katamēnios,* monthly, fr. *mēn,* month]

cat·a·me·ni·al (kat-ă-mē'nē-ăl). SYN menstrual.

cat·a·men·o·gen·ic (kat'ă-men-ō-jen'ik). Causing menstruation.

cat·am·ne·sis (kat-am-nē'sis). The medical history of a patient after an illness; the follow-up history. [cata- + G *mnēmē,* memory]

cat·am·nes·tic (kat-am-nes'tik). Related to catamnesis.

cat·a·pasm (kat'ă-pazm). A dusting powder applied to raw surfaces or ulcers. [G. *katapasma,* a powder; *katapassō,* to sprinkle over]

cat·a·pha·sia (kat-ă-fā'zē-ă). SYN verbigeration. [cata- + G. *phasis,* a saying]

ca·taph·o·ra (kă-taf'ō-ră). Semicoma or somnolence interrupted by intervals of partial consciousness. [G. a falling down]

cat·a·pho·re·sis (kat'ă-fō-rē'sis). Movement of positively charged particles (cations) in a solution or suspension toward the cathode in electrophoresis. Cf. anaphoresis. [cata- + G. *phorēsis,* a being carried]

cat·a·pho·ret·ic (kat'ă-fō-ret'ik). Relating to cataphoresis.

cat·a·pla·sia, cat·a·pla·sis (kat-ă-plā'sē-ă, plā'sis). A degenerative change in cells or tissues that is the reverse of the constructive or developmental change; a return to an earlier or embryonic

stage. SYN retrograde metamorphosis (1), retrogression, retromorphosis. [cata- + G. *plasis,* a molding]

cat·a·plasm (kat'ă-plazm). SYN poultice. [G. *kataplasma,* poultice, fr. *kataplassō,* to spread over]

cat·a·plec·tic (kat-ă-plek'tik). **1.** Developing suddenly. **2.** Pertaining to cataplexy.

cat·a·plexy (kat'ă-plek-sē). A transient attack of extreme generalized muscular weakness, often precipitated by an emotional state such as laughing, surprise, fear, or anger. [cata- + G. *plēxis,* a blow, stroke]

CATARACT

cat·a·ract (kat'ă-rakt). Loss of transparency of the lens of the eye, or of its capsule. SYN cataracta. [L. *cataracta,* fr. G. *katarrhaktēs,* a downrushing, a waterfall, fr. *kata- rrhēgnymi,* to break down, rush down]

annular c., congenital c. in which a central white membrane replaces the nucleus. SYN disk-shaped c., life-belt c., umbilicated c.

arborescent c., obsolete term for dendritic c.

atopic c., a c. associated with atopic dermatitis.

axial c., a lenticular opacity in the visual axis of the lens.

black c., a c. in which the lens is hardened and of a dark brown color. In the 19th century, German black c. meant gutta severa (q.v.). SYN cataracta brunescens, cataracta nigra.

blue c., coronary c. of bluish color. SYN cataracta cerulea.

capsular c., a c. in which the opacity affects the capsule only.

capsulolenticular c., a c. in which both the lens and its capsule are involved. SEE ALSO membranous c.

central c., congenital c. limited to the embryonic nucleus.

cerulean c., a congenital c. with bluish coloring and radial lesions; appears to be at least sometimes autosomal dominant.

complete c., SYN mature c.

complicated c., SYN secondary c. (1).

concussion c., traumatic c. occurring with or without a hole in the lens capsule.

congenital c., c., usually bilateral, present at birth. It occurs as an autosomal recessive condition in calves of the Jersey breed. In humans approximately 25% of congenital c.'s are autosomal dominant [MIM*116200, *116700]; X-linked forms also exist [MIM*302200, *302300].

copper c., SYN *chalcosis* lentis.

coralliform c., congenital c. with round or elongated processes radiating from the center of the lens.

coronary c., peripheral cortical developmental c. occurring just after puberty; transmitted as a hereditary dominant characteristic.

cortical c., a c. in which the opacity affects the cortex of the lens. SYN peripheral c.

crystalline c., a hereditary c. with a coralliform or needle-shaped accumulation of crystals in the axial region of an otherwise clear lens.

cuneiform c., cortical c. in which the opacities radiate from the periphery like spokes of a wheel.

cupuliform c., a common form of senile c. often confined to a region just within the posterior capsule. SYN saucer-shaped c.

dendritic c., a congenital sutural c. with complicated branching.

diabetic c., c. occurring in insulin-dependent diabetes mellitus.

disk-shaped c., SYN annular c.

electric c., a c. caused by contact with a high-power electric current, or a lightning bolt. SYN cataracta electrica.

embryonic c. [MIM*115650], a congenital c. situated near the anterior Y suture of the fetal lens nucleus.

embryopathic c., congenital c. as a result of intrauterine infection, *e.g.,* rubella.

fibroid c., fibrinous c., a sclerotic hardening of the capsule of the lens, following exudative iridocyclitis.

floriform c., a congenital c. with opacities arranged like the petals of a flower.

furnacemen's c., SYN infrared c.

fusiform c., SYN spindle c.

galactose c., a neonatal c. associated with intralenticular accumulation of galactose alcohol. SEE galactosemia.

glassworker's c., SYN infrared c.

glaucomatous c., a nuclear opacity usually seen in absolute glaucoma.

gray c., a c. of gray color, usually seen in senile, mature, or cortical c.

hard c., SYN nuclear c.

hook-shaped c., congenital c. with hook-like figures between the fetal and embryonic nuclei.

hypermature c., a c. in which the lens cortex becomes liquid, with the nucleus gravitating within the capsule (Morgagni's c.). SYN overripe c.

hypocalcemic c., a c. occurring with low serum calcium.

immature c., a stage of partial lens opacification.

infantile c., a c. affecting a very young child.

infrared c., a c. secondary to absorption of heat by the lens, or by transmission from the adjacent iris. SYN furnacemen's c., glassworker's c.

intumescent c., a c. swollen because of fluid absorption.

juvenile c., a soft c. occurring in a child or young adult.

lamellar c., a c. in which the opacity is limited to the cortex. SYN zonular c.

life-belt c., SYN annular c.

mature c., a c. in which both the nucleus and cortex are opaque. SYN complete c., ripe c.

membranous c., a secondary c. composed of the remains of the thickened capsule and degenerated lens fibers.

Morgagni's c., a hypermature c. in which the nucleus gravitates within the capsule. SYN sedimentary c.

myotonic c., c. occurring in myotonic dystrophy.

nuclear c., a c. involving the nucleus. SYN hard c.

overripe c., SYN hypermature c.

perinuclear c., a lamellar c. in which the nucleus is clear but is surrounded by a ring of opacity.

peripheral c., SYN cortical c.

pisciform c., a hereditary c. with bilateral fish-shaped opacities in the axial region of the fetal nucleus.

polar c., a capsular c. limited to an area of the anterior or posterior pole of the lens.

posterior subcapsular c., a c. involving the cortex at the posterior pole of the lens.

progressive c., a c. in which the opacification process progresses to involve the entire lens.

punctate c., an incomplete c. in which there are opaque dots scattered through the lens.

pyramidal c., a cone-shaped, anterior polar c.

radiation c., a c. caused by excessive or prolonged exposure to ultraviolet rays, x-rays, radium, beta rays, gamma rays, heat, or radioactive isotopes.

reduplicated c., a type of congenital c. with opacities situated at various levels in the lens.

ripe c., SYN mature c.

rubella c., embryopathic c. secondary to intrauterine rubella infection.

saucer-shaped c., SYN cupuliform c.

secondary c., (1) a c. that accompanies or follows some other eye disease such as uveitis; SYN complicated c. **(2)** a c. occurring in the retained lens or capsule after a c. extraction. SYN aftercataract.

sedimentary c., SYN Morgagni's c.

senile c., a c. occurring spontaneously in the elderly; mainly a cuneiform c., nuclear c., or posterior subcapsular c., alone or in combination.

siderotic c., a c. resulting from deposition of iron from an iron-containing intraocular foreign body.

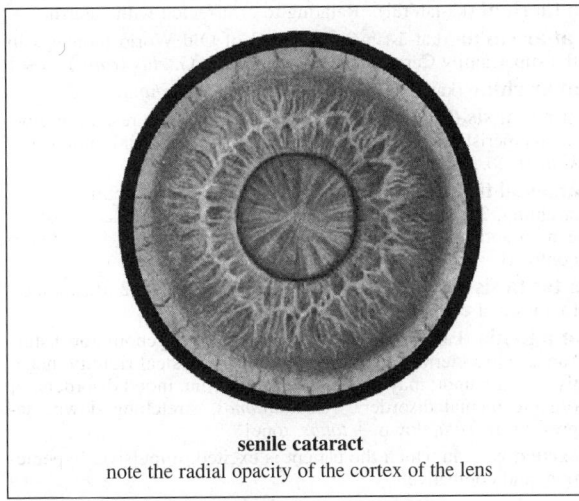

senile cataract
note the radial opacity of the cortex of the lens

soft c., an advanced or mature c. in which the nucleus is not well developed.

spindle c., a c. in which the opacity is fusiform, extending from one pole to the other. SYN fusiform c.

stationary c., a c. that does not progress.

stellate c., congenital c. with lens opacities radiating toward the periphery, with subcapsular and cortical changes.

subcapsular c., a c. in which the opacities are concentrated beneath the capsule.

sugar c., any c. associated with intralenticular accumulation of pentose or hexose alcohols.

sunflower c., SYN *chalcosis* lentis.

sutural c., a congenital type of c. with opacities along the Y sutures of the fetal lens nucleus; usually does not affect vision.

tetany c., a c. that develops in hypocalcemia.

total c., a c. involving the entire lens.

toxic c., a c. caused by drugs or chemicals.

traumatic c., a c. caused by contusion, rupture, or a foreign body.

umbilicated c., SYN annular c.

vascular c., congenital c. in which the degenerated lens is replaced with mesodermal tissue. SYN cataracta adiposa, cataracta fibrosa.

zonular c., SYN lamellar c.

cat·a·rac·ta (kat-ă-rak′tă). SYN cataract. [L.]

c. adipo′sa, SYN vascular *cataract.*

c. brunes′cens, SYN black *cataract.*

c. ceru′lea, SYN blue *cataract.*

c. elec′trica, SYN electric *cataract.*

c. fibro′sa, SYN vascular *cataract.*

c. ni′gra, SYN black *cataract.*

c. os′sea, an obsolete term for an ossified cataract.

cat·a·rac·to·gen·e·sis (kat′ă-rak-tō-jen′ĕ-sis). The process of cataract formation. [cataract + G. *genesis,* production]

cat·a·rac·to·gen·ic (kat′ă-rak-tō-jen′ik). Cataract-producing.

cat·a·rac·tous (kat-ă-rak′tŭs). Relating to a cataract.

ca·tar·ia (ka-tā′rē-ă). The dried flowering tops of *Nepeta cataria* (family Labiatae); an emmenagogue and antispasmodic; also reported to produce psychic effects. SYN catnep, catnip. [L. *cattus,* male cat (post-class)]

ca·tarrh (kă-tahr′). Inflammation of a mucous membrane with increased flow of mucus or exudate. [G. *katarrheō,* to flow down]

malignant c. of cattle, SYN malignant catarrhal *fever.*

nasal c., SYN rhinitis.

vernal c., SYN vernal *conjunctivitis.*

ca·tarrh·al (kă-tah′răl). Relating to or affected with catarrh.

Cat·ar·rhi·na (kat-ă-rī′nă). A genus of Old World monkeys in the superfamily Cercopithecoidea. [kata- + G. *rhis* (*rhin-*), nose]

cat·ar·rhine (kat′ă-rīn). Relating to the *Catarrhina.*

cat·a·stal·sis (kat-ă-stal′sis). A contraction wave resembling ordinary peristalsis but not preceded by a zone of inhibition. [G. *kata-stellō,* to put in order, check]

cat·a·stal·tic (kat-ă-stal′tik). **1.** Inhibitory, restricting, or restraining. **2.** An inhibitory or checking agent, such as an astringent or antispasmodic. [cata- + G. *staltos,* contracted, fr. *stellō,* to contract]

ca·tas·ta·sis (kă-tas′tă-sis). **1.** A condition or state. **2.** Restoration to a normal condition or a normal place. [G.]

cat·a·to·nia (kat-ă-tō′nē-ă). A syndrome of psychomotor disturbances characterized by periods of either physical rigidity, negativism, or stupor; may occur in schizophrenia, mood disorders, or organic mental disorders. [G. *katatonos,* stretching down, depressed, fr. *kata,* down, + *tonos,* tone]

excited c., c. in which the patient is excited, impulsive, hyperactive, and combative.

periodic c., regularly reappearing phases of catatonic excitement.

stuporous c., c. in which the patient is subdued, mute, and negativistic, accompanied by varying combinations of staring, rigidity, and cataplexy.

cat·a·ton·ic, cat·a·to·ni·ac (kat-ă-ton′ik, -tō′nē-ak). Relating to, or characterized by, catatonia.

cat·a·tri·chy (kat′ă-tri-kē) [MIM*116850]. Presence of a forelock of hair that is separate or different in appearance; may be inherited. SEE Waardenburg *syndrome.* [cata- + G. *thrix,* hair]

cat·a·tri·crot·ic (kat′ă-trī-krot′ik). Denoting a pulse tracing with three minor elevations interrupting the downstroke.

cat·a·tri·cro·tism (kat-ă-trī′krō-tizm). A condition of the pulse marked by three minor expansions of the artery following the main beat, producing three secondary upward waves on the downstroke of the pulse tracing. [cata- + G. *tri-,* three, + *krotos,* beat]

cat·e·chase (kat′ĕ-kās). SYN catechol 1,2-dioxygenase.

cat·e·chin (kat′ĕ-kin). 3,3′,4′,5,7-flavanpentol; derived from catechu, and used as an astringent in diarrhea and as a stain. SYN catechinic acid, catechuic acid, cyanidol.

cat·e·chin·ic ac·id (kat-ĕ-kin′ik). SYN catechin.

cat·e·chol (kat′ĕ-kol). **1.** SYN pyrocatechol. **2.** Term loosely used for catechin, which contains a pyrocatechol moiety, and as the root of catecholamines, which are pyrocatechol derivatives.

c.-*O*-methyltransferase, a transferase that catalyzes the methylation of the hydroxyl group at the 3 position of the aromatic ring of c.'s, including the catecholamines norepinephrine and epinephrine (thus, converting to normetanephrine and metanephrine, respectively), the methyl group coming from *S*-adenosyl-L-methionine. An important step in the catabolism of the catecholamines.

c. oxidase, an enzyme oxidizing c.'s to 1,2-benzoquinones, with O_2. SEE ALSO monophenol monooxygenase. SYN diphenol oxidase, *o*-diphenolase.

c. oxidase(dimerizing), an enzyme oxidizing a c., with O_2, to a diphenylenedioxide quinone (*e.g.,* 4 c. $+ 3O_2 \rightarrow 2$ dibenzo[1,4]-2,3-dione $+ 6H_2O$).

cat·e·chol·a·mines (kat-ĕ-kol′ă-mēnz). Pyrocatechols with an alkylamine side chain; examples of biochemical interest are epinephrine, norepinephrine, and L-dopa. C.'s are major elements in responses to stress.

cat·e·chol 1,2-di·ox·y·gen·ase. An oxidoreductase catalyzing oxidation of pyrocatechol, with O_2, to *cis-cis*-muconate. SYN catechase, pyrocatechase.

cat·e·chol 2,3-di·ox·y·gen·ase. An oxidoreductase oxidizing catechol, with O_2, to 2-hydroxymuconate semialdehyde. SYN metapyrocatechase.

cat·e·chu·ic ac·id (kat-ĕ-chū′ik, -kū′ik). SYN catechin.

cat·e·chu ni·grum. Black c. n., an extract of the heart wood of *Acacia catechu* (family Leguminosae), used as an astringent in diarrhea. SYN cutch.

cat·e·lec·trot·o·nus (kat′ē-lek-trot′ō-nŭs). The changes in excitability and conductivity in a nerve or muscle in the neighborhood of the cathode during the passage of a constant electric current. [cathode + electrotonus]

Ca·te·na·bac·te·ri·um (kat′ĕ-nă-bak-tēr′ē-ŭm). See entries under eubacterium lactobacillus. [L. *catena,* chain, + bacterium]
C. contor′tum, former name for *Eubacterium contortum.*

cat·en·ate (kat′e-nāt). To connect in a series of links like a chain; for example, two rings of mitochondrial DNA are often catenated. [L. *catenatus,* chained together, fr. *catena,* chain]

cat·e·nat·ing (kat′en-āt-ing). Occurring in a chain or series. [L. *catenatus,* chained]

cat·e·noid (kat′ĕ-noyd). **1.** Like a chain, such as a chain of fungus spores or a colony of protozoa in which the individuals are joined end to end. SYN catenulate. **2.** Surface of net zero curvature generated by the rotation of a catenary (curve of repose of a suspended chain); the interventricular septum of the heart in idiopathic hypertrophic subaortic stenosis resembles a c., which makes it ineffective in increasing intracavity pressure or in reducing its volume as defined in Laplace's law. [L. *catena,* chain, + G. *eidos,* resemblance]

ca·ten·u·late (ka-ten′yū-lāt). SYN catenoid (1).

cat·gut (kat′gŭt). An absorbable surgical suture material made from the collagenous fibers of the submucosa of certain animals; misnamed catgut (usually from sheep or cows). [probably from *kit,* a small violin, through confusion with kit, a small cat]

chromic c., c. impregnated with chromium salts to prolong its tensile strength and retard its absorption.

silverized c., c. prepared by immersion in a 2% solution of colloidal silver for 1 week and then in 95% alcohol for 15 to 30 minutes.

Catha ed·u·lis (kath′ă ed′yū-lis). A plant of Ethiopia and Arabia (family Celastraceae), cultivated for use as a stimulant; khat (the fresh leaves and twigs) is chewed or used in the preparation of a beverage; the active principle is pharmacologically related to the amphetamines, probably *d*-norisoephedrine. [Ar. *khat*]

Cath·ar·an·thus al·ka·loids (kath-ăr-ran′thus). SYN Vinca *alkaloids,* under *alkaloid.*

ca·thar·sis (kă-thar′sis). **1.** SYN purgation. **2.** The release or discharge of emotional tension or anxiety by psychoanalytically guided emotional reliving of past, especially repressed, events. SYN psychocatharsis. [G. *katharsis,* purification, fr. *katharos,* pure]

ca·thar·tic (kă-thar′tik). **1.** Relating to catharsis. **2.** An agent having purgative action.

ca·thec·tic (kă-thek′tik). Pertaining to cathexis.

ca·them·o·glo·bin (ka-thēm-ō-glō′bin). An artificial derivative of hemoglobin in which the globin is denatured and the iron oxidized.

ca·thep·sin (kă-thep′sin). One of a number of proteinases and peptidases (all endopeptidases) of animal tissues of varying specificities.

cath·e·ter (kath′ĕ-ter). **1.** A tubular instrument to allow passage of fluid from or into a body cavity. SEE ALSO line (4). **2.** Especially a c. designed to be passed through the urethra into the bladder to drain it of retained urine. [G. *kathetēr,* fr. *kathiēmi,* to send down]

acorn-tipped c., a c. used in ureteropyelography to occlude the ureteral orifice and prevent backflow from the ureter during and following the injection of an opaque medium.

angiography c., a thin-walled tube suitable for percutaneous puncture and powered injection of contrast media for radiography; c. diameter is measured on the French scale.

balloon c., a c. used in arterial embolectomy or to float into the pulmonary artery.

balloon-tip c., (1) a tube with a balloon at its tip that can be inflated or deflated without removal after installation; the balloon may be inflated to facilitate passage of the tube through a blood vessel (propelled by the bloodstream) or to occlude the vessel in which the tube alone would allow free flow; such c.'s are used to enter the pulmonary artery to facilitate hemodynamic measurements or to enter arteries and then remove them while inflated to withdraw clots (embolectomy catheter); SEE ALSO Swan-Ganz c. (2) SYN Fogarty c.

bicoudate c., c. bicoudé (bī-kū-dā′), an elbowed c. with a double bend. [bi + Fr. *coudé*, bent]

Bozeman-Fritsch c., a slightly curved double-channel uterine c. with several openings at the tip.

Braasch c., a bulb-tipped c. used for dilation and calibration.

brush c., a ureteral c. with a finely bristled brush tip that is endoscopically passed into the ureter or renal pelvis and by gentle to-and-fro movement brushes cells from the surface of suspected tumors.

cardiac c., SYN intracardiac c.

central venous c., a c. passed through a peripheral or central vein, ending in the thoracic vena cava or right atrium, for measurement of venous pressure or for infusion of concentrated solutions; the peripheral end may connect to a subcutaneous chamber for percutaneous injections given over periods of months or may exit from the skin at a distance from the vein.

conical c., a c. with a cone-shaped tip designed to dilate the ureter.

c. coudé (kū-da′), SYN elbowed c. [Fr. *coudé*, bent]

c. à demeure (ă-dem-ër′), an obsolete term for a c. that is retained for a considerable period in the urethra. [Fr. *demeurer*, to dwell]

de Pezzer c., a self-retaining c. with a bulbous extremity.

double-channel c., a c. with two lumens, allowing irrigation and aspiration. SYN two-way c.

elbowed c., a c. with an angular bend near the beak; used to rise over prostatic obstruction. SYN c. coudé, prostatic c.

eustachian c., a c. used for catheterization of the middle ear through the eustachian tube.

female c., a short, nearly straight c. for passage into the female bladder.

Fogarty c., a c. with an inflatable balloon near its tip; used to remove arterial emboli and thrombi from major veins (*e.g.,* iliofemoral) and to remove stones from the biliary ducts. SYN balloon-tip c. (2).

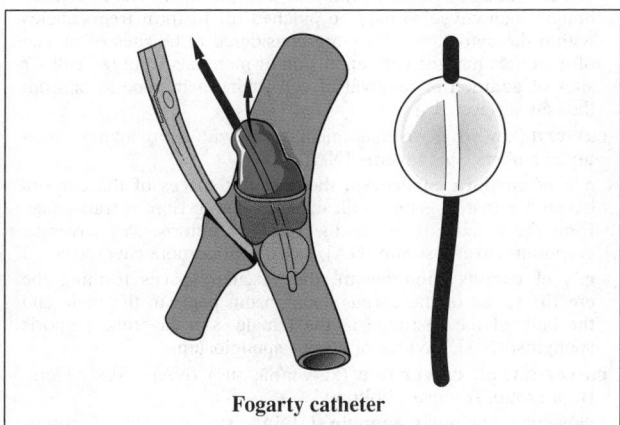

Fogarty catheter

Foley c., a c. with a retaining balloon.

Gouley's c., a solid curved steel instrument grooved on its inferior surface so that it can be passed over a guide through a urethral stricture.

indwelling c., a c. left in place in the bladder, usually a balloon c.

intracardiac c., a c. that can be passed into the heart through a vein or artery, to withdraw samples of blood, measure pressures within the heart's chambers or great vessels, and inject contrast media; used mainly in the diagnosis and evaluation of congenital, rheumatic, and coronary artery lesions and to evaluate systolic and diastolic cardiac function. SYN cardiac c.

Malecot c., a two- or four-winged c.

Nélaton's c., a flexible c. of red rubber.

olive-tipped c., a ureteral c. with an olive-shaped tip, used to dilate a constricted ureteral orifice; larger sizes are also used for dilating or calibrating urethral strictures.

pacing c., a cardiac c. with one or more electrodes at its tip which can be used to artificially pace the heart.

Pezzer c., SEE de Pezzer c.

Phillips' c., a c. with a filiform guide for the urethra.

pigtail c., an angiographic c. with a tightly curled end to reduce the impact of the injectant on the vessel wall.

prostatic c., SYN elbowed c.

Robinson c., a straight urethral c. with two to six holes to facilitate drainage, especially in the presence of blood clots which may occlude one or more openings.

self-retaining c., a c. so constructed that it remains in urethra and bladder until removed, *e.g.,* indwelling c.; Foley c.

spiral tip c., a c. with a helical filiform tip.

Swan-Ganz c., a thin (5 Fr), flexible, flow-directed c. using a balloon to carry it through the heart to a pulmonary artery; when it is positioned in a small arterial branch, pulmonary wedge pressure is measured in front of the temporarily inflated and wedged balloon.

two-way c., SYN double-channel c.

vertebrated c., a c. made of several segments moving on each other like the links of a chain.

whistle-tip c., a c. with an opening at the end and side.

winged c., a soft rubber c. with little flaps at each side of the beak to retain it in the bladder.

cath·e·ter·i·za·tion (kath′ĕ-ter-ī-zā′shŭn). Passage of a catheter.

cath·e·ter·ize (kath′ĕ-ter-īz). To pass a catheter.

cath·e·ter·o·stat (kath′ĕ-ter-ō-stat). A stand for holding catheters. [catheter + G. *statos*, standing]

ca·thex·is (kă-thek′sis). A conscious or unconscious attachment of psychic energy to an idea, object, or person. [G. *kathexis,* a holding in, retention]

cath·o·dal (C) (kath′ō-dăl). Of, pertaining to, or emanating from a cathode. SYN cathodic.

cath·ode (Ca, C) (kath′ōd). The negative pole of a galvanic battery or the electrode connected with it; the electrode toward which positively charged ions (cations) migrate and are reduced, and into which electrons are fed from their source (anode or generator). Cf. anode. SYN negative electrode. [G. *kathodos,* a way down, fr. *kata,* down, + *hodos,* a way]

ca·thod·ic (kă-thod′ik). SYN cathodal.

cath·ol·y·sis (kath-ol′ē-sis). Electrolysis with a cathode needle.

cat·i·on (kat′ī-on). An ion carrying a charge of positive electricity, therefore going to the negatively charged cathode. [G. *katiōn,* going down]

cat·i·on ex·change. The process by which a cation in a liquid phase exchanges with another cation present as the counter-ion of a negatively charged solid polymer (cation exchanger). A cation-exchange reaction in removal of the Na^+ of a sodium chloride solution is $RSO_3^-H^+ + Na^+ \rightarrow RSO_3^-Na^+ + H^+$ (R is the polymer, RSO_3^- is the cation exchanger); if this is combined with the anion-exchange reaction, NaCl is removed from the solution (desalting). Cation exchange may also be used chromatographically, to separate cations, and medicinally, to remove a cation; *e.g.,* H^+, from gastric contents, or Na^+ and K^+ in the intestine. SEE anion exchange.

cat·i·on ex·chang·er. An insoluble solid (usually a polystyrene or a polysaccharide) that has negatively charged radicals attached to it (*e.g.,* $-COO^-$, $-SO_3^-$), which can attract and hold cations that pass by in a moving solution if these are more attracted to the acid groups than the counter ion present.

cat·i·on·ic (kat-ī-on′ik). Referring to positively charged ions and their properties.

cat·i·on·o·gen (kat-ī-on′ō-jen). A substance that gives rise to positively charged ions.

cat·lin, cat·ling (kat′lin, -ling). A long, sharp-pointed, double-edged knife used in amputations.

cat·nep, cat·nip (kat′nep, kat′nip). SYN cataria.

cat·o·chus (kat'ō-kŭs). The trancelike phase of catalepsy in which the patient is conscious but cannot move or speak. [G. *katochē,* epilepsy (Galen), fr. *katechō,* to hold fast]

ca·top·tric (ka-top'trik). Relating to reflected light. [G. *katoptron,* mirror]

cau·da, pl. **cau·dae** (kaw'dă, kaw'dē) [NA]. SYN tail. [L. a tail]
c. epididym'idis [NA], SYN *tail* of epididymis.
c. equi'na [NA], the bundle of spinal nerve roots arising from the lumbosacral enlargement and medullary cone and running through the lumbar cistern (subarachnoid space) within the vertebral canal below the first lumbar vertebra; it comprises the roots of all the spinal nerves below the first lumbar. [L. horse tail]
c. fas'ciae denta'tae, SYN uncus *band* of Giacomini.
c. hel'icis [NA], SYN *tail* of helix.
c. nu'clei cauda'ti [NA], SYN *tail* of caudate nucleus.
c. pancre'atis [NA], SYN *tail* of pancreas.
c. stria'ti, SYN *tail* of caudate nucleus.

cau·dad (kaw'dad). **1.** In a direction toward the tail. **2.** Situated nearer the tail in relation to a specific reference point; opposite of craniad. SEE ALSO inferior.

cau·dal (kaw'dăl). Pertaining to the tail. SYN caudalis [NA]. [Mod. L. *caudalis*]

cau·da·lis (kaw-dā'lis) [NA]. SYN caudal, caudal.

cau·date (kaw'dāt). **1.** Tailed; possessing a tail. **2.** SYN caudate *nucleus.*

cau·da·to·len·tic·u·lar (kaw-dā'tō-len-tik'yū-lăr). Relating to the caudate nucleus and lenticularis. SYN caudolenticular.

cau·da·tum (kaw-dā'tŭm). SYN caudate *nucleus.*

cau·do·ceph·a·lad (kaw-dō-sef'ăl-ad). In a direction from the tail toward the head.

cau·do·len·tic·u·lar (kaw'dō-len-tik'yū-lăr). SYN caudatolenticular.

caul, cowl (kawl). **1.** The amnion, either as a piece of membrane capping the baby's head at birth or the whole membrane when delivered unruptured with the baby. SYN galea (4), veil (2), velum (2). **2.** SYN greater *omentum.* [Gaelic, *call,* a veil]

cau·mes·the·sia (kaw-mes-thē'zē-ă). Subjective heat sensation of uncomfortably high temperature; a type of thermal dysesthesia. [G. *kauma,* heat, + *aisthēsis,* sensation]

cau·sal·gia (kaw-zal'jē-ă). Persistent severe burning sensation, usually following partial injury of a peripheral nerve (especially median and tibial) or the brachial plexus, accompanied by trophic changes. [G. *kausis,* burning, + *algos,* pain]

cau·sal·i·ty (kawz'al-i-tē). The relating of causes to the effects they produce; the pathogenesis of disease, and epidemiology, are largely concerned with causality.

cause (kawz). That which produces an effect or condition; that by which a morbid change or disease is brought about. [L. *causa*]
constitutional c., a c. acting from within or through some systemic process or inborn error.
exciting c., the direct provoking c. of a condition. SYN procatarxis (1).
necessary c., an etiological factor without which a result in question will not occur; the occurrence of the result is proof that the factor is operating.
precipitating c., a factor that brings on the onset of manifestations of a disease process.
predisposing c., anything that produces a susceptibility or disposition to a condition without actually causing it.
proximate c., the immediate c. that precipitates a condition.
specific c., a c. the action of which definitely produces the condition in question.
sufficient c., an etiological factor that guarantees that a result in question will occur; non-occurrence of the result is proof that the factor is not operating.

caus·tic (kaws'tik). **1.** Exerting an effect resembling a burn. **2.** An agent producing this effect. **3.** Denoting a solution of a strong alkali; *e.g.,* caustic soda, NaOH. SYN pyrotic (2). [G. *kaustikos,* fr. *kaiō,* to burn]

cau·ter·ant (kaw'ter-ant). **1.** Cauterizing. **2.** A cauterizing agent.

cau·ter·i·za·tion (kaw-ter-ī-zā'shŭn). The act of cauterizing. SEE ALSO cautery.

cau·ter·ize (kaw'ter-īz). To apply a cautery; to burn with a cautery.

cau·tery (kaw'ter-ē). **1.** An agent or device used for scarring, burning, or cutting the skin or other tissues by means of heat, cold, electric current, or caustic chemicals. **2.** Use of a cautery. [G. *kautērion,* a branding iron]
actual c., a c., such as electrocautery, acting directly through heat and not by chemical means. SYN technocausis.
BICAP c., a form of bipolar electrocoagulation frequently used to arrest gastrointestinal bleeding.
bipolar c., electrocautery by high frequency electrical current passed through tissue from an active to a passive electrode; used for hemostasis.
chemical c., SYN chemocautery.
cold c., SYN cryocautery.
electric c., SYN electrocautery.
galvanic c., obsolete term for electrocautery.
gas c., c. by means of a measured amount of a lighted gas jet.
monopolar c., electrocautery by high frequency electrical current passed from a single electrode, where the cauterization occurs, the patient's body serving as a ground.

ca·va (kā'vă). SEE inferior *vena* cava, superior *vena* cava.

ca·va·gram (kā'vă-gram). SYN cavogram.

ca·val (kā'văl). Relating to a vena cava.

cav·a·scope (kav'ă-skōp). Obsolete term for celoscope. [L. *cavum,* hole, + G. *skopeō,* to view]

cave (kāv). A hollow or enclosed space or cavity. SEE cavity, cavitas, cavity, cavern, cavern.
trigeminal c., the cleft in the meningeal layer of dura of the middle cranial fossa near the tip of the petrous part of the temporal bone; it encloses the roots of the trigeminal nerve and the trigeminal ganglion. SYN cavum trigeminale [NA], Meckel's cavity, Meckel's space, trigeminal cavity.

cav·e·o·la, pl. **cav·e·o·lae** (kav-ē-ō'lă, -lē). A small pocket, vesicle, cave, or recess communicating with the outside of a cell and extending inward, indenting the cytoplasm and the cell membrane. Such caveolae may be pinched off to form free vesicles within the cytoplasm. They are considered to be sites of uptake of materials into the cell, expulsion of materials from the cell, or sites of addition or removal of cell (unit) membrane to or from the cell surface. [L.]

cav·ern (kav'ern). An anatomical cavity with many interconnecting chambers. SYN caverna [NA].
c.'s of corpora cavernosa, the vascular spaces of the corpora cavernosa that, together with the intervening fibrous trabeculae, form the erectile tissue of the penis or clitoris. SYN cavernae corporum cavernosorum [NA], cavities of corpora cavernosa.
c.'s of corpus spongiosum, the vascular spaces forming the erectile tissue of the corpus spongiosum penis in the male and the bulb of the vestibule in the female. SYN cavernae corporis spongiosi [NA], cavities of corpus spongiosum.

ca·ver·na, pl. **ca·ver·nae** (kă-ver'nă, -nē) [NA]. SYN cavern. [L. a grotto, fr. *cavus,* hollow]
cavernae cor'poris spongio'si [NA], SYN *caverns* of corpus spongiosum, under *cavern.*
cavernae cor'porum cavernoso'rum [NA], SYN *caverns* of corpora cavernosa, under *cavern.*

cav·er·nil·o·quy (kav-er-nil'ō-kwē). Low pitched resonant pectoriloquy heard over a lung cavity. [L. *caverna,* cavern, + *loquor,* to talk]

cav·er·ni·tis (kav-er-nī'tis). Inflammation of the corpus cavernosum penis. SYN cavernositis.
fibrous c., c. occasionally associated with Peyronie's disease.

cav·er·no·scope (kav'er-nō-skōp). Obsolete term for celoscope.

cav·er·nos·co·py (kav-er-nos'kŏ-pē). Obsolete term for celoscopy. [L. *caverna,* cavern, + G. *skopeō,* to view]

cav·er·no·si·tis (kav'er-nō-sī'tis). SYN cavernitis.

cav·er·nos·to·my (kav-er-nos'tō-mē). Obsolete term for opening of any cavity to establish drainage. [L. *caverna,* cavern, + G. *stoma,* mouth]

cav·ern·ous (kav′er-nŭs). Relating to a cavern or a cavity; containing many cavities.

Ca·via (kā′vē-ă). A genus of the family Caviidae that includes the guinea pigs. [Mod. L., fr. native Indian]

C. porcel′lus, a rodent with a very short tail that is not visible externally; native to South America, where it is raised for food; used widely as a laboratory animal in bacteriologic, pathologic, and pharmacologic research. SYN guinea pig.

cav·i·tary (kav′i-tā-rē). 1. Relating to a cavity or having a cavity or cavities. 2. Denoting any animal parasite that has an enteric canal or body cavity and that lives within the host's body.

cav·i·tas, pl. **cav·i·ta·tes** (kav′i-tas, -tā′tēs). SYN cavity. [Mod. L.]

c. abdomina′lis [NA], SYN abdominal *cavity.*

c. articula′ris [NA], SYN articular *cavity.*

c. corona′lis [NA], SYN crown *cavity.*

c. den′tis [NA], SYN pulp *cavity.*

c. glenoida′lis [NA], SYN mandibular *fossa.*

c. infraglot′ticum [NA], SYN infraglottic *cavity.*

c. laryn′gis [NA], SYN *cavity* of larynx.

c. medulla′ris [NA], SYN medullary *cavity.*

c. na′si [NA], SYN nasal *cavity.*

c. o′ris [NA], SYN oral *cavity.*

c. o′ris pro′pria, SYN oral *cavity* proper.

c. pel′vis [NA], SYN pelvic *cavity.*

c. pericardia′lis [NA], SYN pericardial *cavity.*

c. peritonea′lis [NA], SYN peritoneal *cavity.*

c. pharyn′gis [NA], SYN *cavity* of pharynx.

c. pleura′lis [NA], SYN pleural *cavity.*

c. thora′cis [NA], SYN thoracic *cavity.*

c. tympan′ica [NA], SYN tympanic *cavity.*

c. u′teri [NA], SYN uterine *cavity.*

cav·i·ta·tion (kav-i-tā′shŭn). 1. Formation of a cavity, as in the lung in tuberculosis. 2. The production of small vapor-containing bubbles or cavities in a liquid by ultrasound.

ca·vi·tis (kā-vī′tis). SYN celophlebitis.

cav·i·ty (kav′i-tē). 1. A hollow space. A hollow, hole, or cavity. SEE cave, cavity, cavitas, cavern, cavern. 2. Lay term for the loss of tooth structure due to dental caries. SYN cavum [NA], cavitas. [L. *cavus,* hollow]

abdominal c., the space bounded by the abdominal walls, the diaphragm, and the pelvis; it usually is arbitrarily separated from the pelvic cavity by a plane across the superior aperture of the pelvis; however, it may include the pelvis with the abdomen (see abdominopelvic c.); within the c. lie the greater part of the organs of digestion, the spleen, the kidneys, and the suprarenal glands. SYN cavitas abdominalis [NA], cavum abdominis, enterocele (2).

abdominopelvic c., abdominal c. plus pelvic c.

amniotic c., the fluid-filled c. inside the amnion which contains the developing embryo.

articular c., a joint cavity, the potential space bounded by the synovial membrane and articular cartilages of all synovial joints. Normally, the articular c. contains only sufficient synovial fluid to lubricate the internal surfaces. SYN cavitas articularis [NA], cavum articulare.

axillary c., SYN axilla.

body c., the collective visceral c. of the trunk (thoracic c. plus abdominopelvic c.), bounded by the superior thoracic aperture above, the pelvic floor below, and the body walls (parietes) in between. SYN celom (2), celoma, coelom.

buccal c., SYN oral *vestibule.*

cleavage c., SYN blastocele.

c. of concha, the space within the lower, larger portion of the concha below the crus helicis; it forms the vestibule leading into the external acoustic meatus. SYN cavum conchae [NA].

c.'s of corpora cavernosa, SYN *caverns* of corpora cavernosa, under *cavern.*

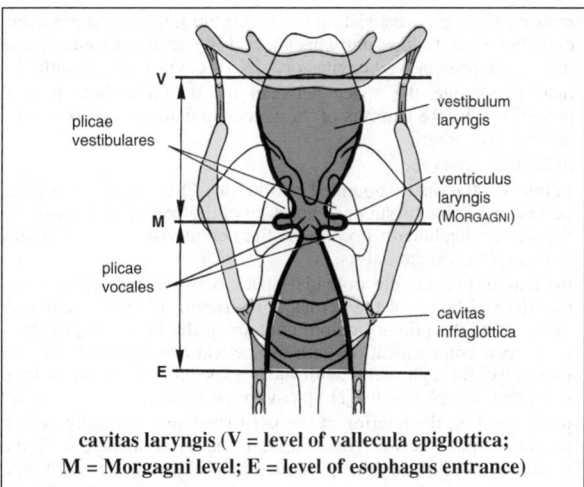

cavitas laryngis (V = level of vallecula epiglottica;
M = Morgagni level; E = level of esophagus entrance)

c.'s of corpus spongiosum, SYN *caverns* of corpus spongiosum, under *cavern.*

cotyloid c., SYN acetabulum.

cranial c., the space within the skull occupied by the brain, its coverings, and cerebrospinal fluid. SYN intracranial c.

crown c., the space within the crown of a tooth continuous with the root canal. SYN cavitas coronalis [NA], cavum coronale.

ectoplacental c., SYN epamniotic c.

ectotrophoblastic c., a developmental c. appearing between the trophoblast and the embryonic disk ectoderm in some mammals.

epamniotic c., a developmental c. that exists in some mammals and is derived by division of the proamniotic space; it is further removed from the embryo than the amniotic c. in some mammals. SYN ectoplacental c.

epidural c., the space between the walls of the vertebral canal and the dura mater of the spinal cord. SYN cavum epidurale [NA], epidural space.

glenoid c., SYN mandibular *fossa.*

greater peritoneal c., SYN peritoneal c.

head c., the cephalic region in the embryos of vertebrates containing the modified somites that give rise to the extrinsic eye muscles.

idiopathic bone c., SYN solitary bone *cyst.*

inferior laryngeal c., SYN infraglottic c.

infraglottic c., the part of the cavity of the larynx immediately below the glottis. SYN cavitas infraglotticum [NA], aditus glottidis inferior, cavum infraglotticum, inferior laryngeal c., infraglottic space.

intermediate laryngeal c., portion of the c. of the larynx between the vestibular and vocal folds, with which the ventricles communicate. SYN aditus glottidis superior.

intracranial c., SYN cranial c.

c. of larynx, a cavity that is continuous above with the pharynx at the level of the aryepiglottic folds and extends downward through the rima glottidis to the infraglottic space. SYN cavitas laryngis [NA], cavum laryngis.

lesser peritoneal c., SYN omental *bursa.*

Meckel's c., SYN trigeminal *cave.*

medullary c., the marrow cavity in the shaft of a long bone. SYN cavitas medullaris [NA], cavum medullare.

c. of middle ear, SYN tympanic c.

nasal c., the cavity on either side of the nasal septum, lined with ciliated respiratory mucosa, extending from the naris anteriorly to the choana posteriorly, and communicating with the paranasal sinuses through their orifices in the lateral wall, from which also project the three conchae; the cribriform plate, through which the olfactory nerves are transmitted, forms the roof; the floor is formed by the hard palate. SYN cavitas nasi [NA], cavum nasi.

nephrotomic c., SYN nephrocele (2).

oral c., the region consisting of the vestibulum oris, the narrow cleft between the lips and cheeks, and the teeth and gums, and the c. oris propria. SYN cavitas oris [NA], cavum oris, mouth (1).

oral c. proper, the space between the dental arches, limited posteriorly by the isthmus of the fauces (palatoglossal arch). SYN cavitas oris propria.

orbital c., SYN orbit.

pelvic c., the space bounded at the sides by the bones of the pelvis, above by the superior aperture of the pelvis, and below by the pelvic diaphragm; it contains the pelvic viscera. SYN cavitas pelvis [NA], cavum pelvis.

pericardial c., (1) the potential space between the parietal and the visceral layers of the serous pericardium; **(2)** in the embryo, that part of the primary celom containing the heart; originally it is in open communication with the pericardioperitoneal c.'s and indirectly, through them, with the peritoneal part of the celom. SYN cavitas pericardialis [NA], cavum pericardii.

peritoneal c., the interior of the peritoneal sac, normally only a potential space between the parietal and visceral layers of the peritoneum. SYN cavitas peritonealis [NA], cavum peritonei, greater peritoneal c.

perivisceral c., the space between the ectoderm and endoderm in the gastrula. SYN primitive perivisceral c.

pharyngonasal c., SYN nasopharynx.

c. of pharynx, it consists of a nasal part (nasopharynx) continuous anteriorly with the nasal cavity and receiving the openings of the auditory tubes, an oral part (oropharynx) opening through the fauces into the oral cavity, and a laryngeal part (laryngopharynx) leading into the vestibule of the larynx and to the esophagus. SYN cavitas pharyngis [NA], cavum pharyngis.

pleural c., the potential space between the parietal and visceral layers of the pleura. SYN cavitas pleuralis [NA], cavum pleurae, pleural space.

pleuroperitoneal c., that part of the embryonic celom later partitioned to give rise to the pleural and peritoneal c.'s.

primitive perivisceral c., SYN perivisceral c.

pulmonary c., the portion of the thoracic c. lying on either side of the mediastinum and occupied by a lung; the space existing when a lung is removed.

pulp c., the central hollow of a tooth consisting of the crown cavity and the root canal; it contains the fibrovascular dental pulp and is lined throughout by odontoblasts. SYN cavitas dentis [NA], c. of tooth, cavum dentis.

Retzius' c., SYN retropubic space. [A.A. Retzius]

segmentation c., SYN blastocele.

c. of septum pellucidum, a slitlike, fluid-filled space of variable width between the left and right transparent septum, which occurs in less than 10% of human brains and may communicate with the third ventricle. SYN cavum septi pellucidi [NA], Duncan's ventricle, fifth ventricle, pseudocele, pseudoventricle, sylvian ventricle, ventricle of Sylvius, ventriculus quintus, Vieussens' ventricle, Wenzel's ventricle.

somite c., SYN myocele (2).

splanchnic c., the celom or one of the body c.'s derived from it. SYN visceral c.

subarachnoid c., SYN subarachnoid space.

subdural c., SYN subdural space.

subgerminal c., SYN primitive gut.

superior laryngeal c., SYN vestibule of larynx.

thoracic c., the space within the thoracic walls, bounded below by the diaphragm and above by the neck. SYN cavitas thoracis [NA], cavum thoracis.

c. of tooth, SYN pulp c.

trigeminal c., SYN trigeminal cave.

tympanic c., an air chamber in the temporal bone containing the ossicles; it is lined with mucous membrane and is continuous with the auditory tube anteriorly and the tympanic antrum and mastoid air cells posteriorly. SYN cavitas tympanica [NA], c. of middle ear, cavum tympani, tympanum.

uterine c., c. of uterus, the space within the uterus extending from the cervical canal to the openings of the uterine tubes. SYN cavitas uteri [NA], cavum uteri.

visceral c., SYN splanchnic c.

ca·vo·gram (kā'vō-gram). An angiogram of a vena cava. SYN cavagram. [(vena) cava + G. gramma, a writing]

ca·vog·ra·phy (kā-vog'ră-fē). SYN venacavography.

ca·vo·sur·face (kā-vō-sŭr'făs). Relating to a cavity and the surface of a tooth.

ca·vum, pl. **ca·va** (ka'vŭm, -vă) [NA]. SYN cavity. [L. ntr. of adj. cavus, hollow]

c. abdom'inis, SYN abdominal cavity.

c. articula're, SYN articular cavity.

c. con'chae [NA], SYN cavity of concha.

c. corona'le, SYN crown cavity.

c. den'tis, SYN pulp cavity.

c. doug'lasi, SYN rectouterine pouch.

c. epidura'le [NA], SYN epidural cavity.

c. infraglot'ticum, SYN infraglottic cavity.

c. laryn'gis, SYN cavity of larynx.

c. mediastina'le, an inappropriate name sometimes applied to the mediastinum.

c. medulla're, SYN medullary cavity.

c. na'si, SYN nasal cavity.

c. o'ris, SYN oral cavity.

c. pel'vis, SYN pelvic cavity.

c. pericar'dii, SYN pericardial cavity.

c. peritone'i, SYN peritoneal cavity.

c. pharyn'gis, SYN cavity of pharynx.

c. pleu'rae, SYN pleural cavity.

c. psalte'rii, SYN Verga's ventricle.

c. ret'zii, SYN retropubic space. [A.A. Retzius]

c. sep'ti pellu'cidi [NA], SYN cavity of septum pellucidum.

c. subarachnoid'eum [NA], SYN subarachnoid space.

c. subdura'le, SYN subdural space.

c. thora'cis, SYN thoracic cavity.

c. trigemina'le [NA], SYN trigeminal cave.

c. tym'pani, SYN tympanic cavity.

c. u'teri, SYN uterine cavity.

c. ver'gae, SYN Verga's ventricle.

c. vesicouteri'num, SYN uterovesical pouch.

ca·vy (kā'vē). Common name for Cavia porcellus.

Cazenave, Pierre L. Alphée, French dermatologist, 1795–1877. SEE C.'s vitiligo.

Cb Symbol for columbium.

C-band·ing. SEE C-banding stain.

CBC Abbreviation for complete blood count.

CBF Abbreviation for cerebral or coronary blood flow.

CBG Abbreviation for corticosteroid-binding globulin.

Cbl Abbreviation for cobalamin.

CBPP Abbreviation for contagious bovine pleuropneumonia.

Cbz Abbreviation for carbobenzoxy (benzyloxycarbonyl).

C.C. Abbreviation for chief complaint, as recorded on a patient's medical history.

cc, c.c. Abbreviation for cubic centimeter.

CCA Abbreviation for chimpanzee coryza agent.

CCC Abbreviation for cathodal closure contraction.

CCDM Abbreviation for Control of Communicable Diseases in Man.

CCK Abbreviation for cholecystokinin.

CCNU SYN lomustine.

CCTe Abbreviation for cathodal closure tetanus.

CCU Abbreviation for coronary care unit; critical care unit.

CD Abbreviation for curative dose; circular dichroism; cluster of differentiation.

CD2 Abbreviation for cluster of differentiation 2.

CD3 Abbreviation for cluster of differentiation 3.

CD4 Abbreviation for cluster of differentiation 4.

CD8 Abbreviation for cluster of differentiation 8.

CD 54. SEE intercellular adhesion molecule-1.

CD^{50} Abbreviation for curative *dose*.

Cd Symbol for cadmium.

cd Symbol for candela.

CDC Abbreviation for Centers for Disease Control; previously known as the Communicable Disease Center.

CD4/CD8 count. The ratio of the number of helper-inducer T lymphocytes to cytotoxic-suppressor T lymphocytes, as measured by monoclonal antibodies to the CD4 surface antigen found on helper-inducer T cells, and the CD8 surface antigen found on cytotoxic-suppressor T cells. In healthy individuals, the H/S ratio ranges between 1.6 and 2.2.

> When the body mounts an immune response, as against a virus or a transplant, the ratio is almost always reduced because of a decrease in the number of circulating helper-inducer cells and an increase in suppressor cells. The CD4/CD8 count has been used to monitor for signs of organ rejection after transplants, and more recently has become a tool for assessing the relative condition of HIV patients. With the CD4 absolute count and the CD4 lymphocyte percentage, it provides a way of gauging the progression from HIV to AIDS.

CDE blood group. See Rh blood group, Blood Groups appendix.

cDNA Abbreviation for complementary DNA.

CDP Abbreviation for cytidine 5′-diphosphate.

CDP-cho·line Abbreviation for cytidine diphosphocholine.

CDP-glyc·er·ide Abbreviation for cytidine diphosphoglyceride.

CDP-sug·ar Abbreviation for cytidine diphosphosugar.

Ce Symbol for cerium.

CEA Abbreviation for carcinoembryonic *antigen*.

ce·bo·ceph·a·ly (sē-bō-sef′ă-lē). Malformation of the head in which the features are suggestive of a monkey; there is usually a tendency toward cyclopia, with defective or absent nose and closely set eyes. [G. *kēbos,* monkey, + *kephalē,* head]

⚠ **cec-.** SEE ceco-.

ce·ca (sē′kă). Plural of cecum.

ce·cal (sē′kăl). **1.** Relating to the cecum. **2.** Ending blindly or in a cul-de-sac.

ce·cec·to·my (sē-sek′tō-mē). Excision of the cecum. SYN typhlectomy. [ceco- + G. *ektomē,* excision]

Cecil, Arthur Bond, U.S. urologist, 1885–1967. SEE cecil *urethroplasty.*

ce·ci·tis (sē-sī′tis). Inflammation of the cecum. SYN typhlenteritis, typhlitis, typhloenteritis.

⚠ **ceco-, cec-.** The cecum. SEE ALSO typhlo- (1). Cf. typhlo-. [L. *caecum,* cecum, blind]

ce·co·co·los·to·my (sē′kō-kō-los′tō-mē). Formation of an anastomosis between cecum and colon.

ce·co·fix·a·tion (sē′kō-fik-sā′shŭn). SYN cecopexy.

ce·co·il·e·os·to·my (sē′kō-il-ē-os′tō-mē). SYN ileocecostomy.

ce·co·pexy (sē′kō-pek-sē). Operative anchoring of a movable cecum. SYN cecofixation, typhlopexy, typhlopexia. [ceco- + G. *pexis,* fixation]

ce·co·pli·ca·tion (sē′kō-pli-kā′shŭn). Operative reduction in size of a dilated cecum by the formation of folds or tucks in its wall. [ceco- + L. *plico,* pp. *-atus,* to fold]

ce·cor·rha·phy (sē-kōr′ă-fē). Suture of the cecum. SYN typhlorrhaphy. [ceco- + G. *rhaphē,* suture]

ce·co·sig·moid·os·to·my (sē′kō-sig-moy-dos′tō-mē). Formation of a communication between the cecum and the sigmoid colon.

ce·cos·to·my (sē-kos′tō-mē). Operative formation of a cecal fistula. SYN typhlostomy. [ceco- + G. *stoma,* mouth]

ce·cot·o·my (sē-kot′ō-mē). Incision into the cecum. SYN typhlotomy. [ceco- + G. *tomē,* incision]

ce·cum, pl. **ce·ca** (sē′kŭm, sē′kă) [NA]. **1.** The cul-de-sac, about 6 cm in depth, lying below the terminal ileum forming the first part of the large intestine. SYN blind gut, intestinum cecum,

typhlon. **2.** Any similar structure ending in a cul-de-sac. [L. ntr. of *caecus,* blind]

cupular c. of the cochlear duct, the upper blind extremity of the cochlear duct. SYN c. cupulare [NA], cupular blind sac, lagena (1).

c. cupula′re [NA], SYN cupular c. of the cochlear duct.

vestibular c. of the cochlear duct, the lower extremity of the cochlear duct, occupying the cochlear recess in the vestibule. SYN c. vestibulare [NA], vestibular blind sac.

c. vestibula′re [NA], SYN vestibular c. of the cochlear duct.

ce·dar leaf oil (sē′der). Oil obtained by steam distillation from the fresh leaves of *Thuja occidentalis;* used as an insect repellent and counterirritant, and in perfumery. SYN thuja oil.

ce·dar wood oil. Volatile oil obtained from the wood of *Juniperus virginiana* (family Pinaceae); used as an insect repellent, in perfumery, and as a clearing agent in microscopy.

Ceelen, Wilhelm, 1884–1964. SEE C.-Gellerstedt *syndrome.*

cef·a·clor (sef′ă-klōr). A semisynthetic broad spectrum antibiotic derived from cephalosporin C; used orally.

cef·a·drox·il (sef-ă-drok′sil). A semisynthetic broad spectrum antibiotic derived from cephalosporin C; used orally.

cef·a·man·dole nafate (sef-ă-man′dōl naf′āt). A semisynthetic broad spectrum antibiotic derived from cephalosporin C; used by injection.

ce·faz·o·lin (se-faz′ō-lin). A broad spectrum cephalosporin antibiotic used to treat a wide variety of serious infections; available as the sodium salt for intramuscular or intravenous administration.

ce·fon·i·cid di·so·di·um (se-fon′ĭ-sid). $C_{18}H_{16}N_6Na_2O_8S_3$; a broad spectrum long acting cephalosporin antibiotic structurally related to cefamandole.

ce·fo·per·a·zone so·di·um (se-fō-per′ă-zōn). $C_{25}H_{26}N_9NaO_8S_2$; a semisynthetic piperazine-cephalosporin antibiotic.

ce·for·a·nide (se-fōr′ă-nīd). $C_{20}H_{21}N_7O_6\ S_2$; a broad spectrum long-acting cephalosporin antibiotic.

ce·fo·tax·ime so·di·um (se-fō-taks′ēm). $C_{16}H_{16}N_5NaO_7S_2$; a broad spectrum cephalosporin antibiotic.

cef·o·te·tan di·so·di·um (sef′ō-te-tan). $C_{17}H_{15}N_7Na_2O_8S_4$; a broad spectrum cephalosporin antibiotic.

ce·fox·i·tin so·di·um (se-fok′si-tin). A semisynthetic antibiotic derived from cephamycin C but structurally and pharmacologically similar to the cephalosporins; used by injection.

cef·taz·i·dime so·di·um (sef-taz′i-dēm). $C_{22}H_{21}N_6NaO_7S_2$; a cephalosporin antibiotic especially effective against enterobacteria and species of *Pseudomonas.*

cef·ti·zox·ime so·di·um (sef-ti-zoks′ēm). $C_{13}H_{12}N_5NaO_5S_2$; a broad spectrum cephalosporin antibiotic similar to cefotaxime sodium.

cef·tri·ax·one di·so·di·um (sef-trī-aks′ōn). $C_{18}H_{16}N_8Na_2O_7S_3$; a semisynthetic parenteral cephalosporin antibiotic.

cel (sel). A unit of velocity; 1 cm per second. [L. *celer,* swift]

⚠ **-cele.** Swelling; hernia. [G. *kēlē,* tumor]

ce·lec·tome (sē′lek-tōm). Obsolete term for an instrument, such as the harpoon, for obtaining a bit of tissue from the interior of a tumor for examination. [G. *kēlē,* tumor, + *ektomē,* excision]

ce·len·ter·on (sē-len′ter-on). SYN primitive *gut.* [G. *koilos,* hollow, + *enteron,* intestine]

cel·ery seed (sel′er-ē). The dried ripe fruit of *Apium graveolens* (family Umbelliferae); has been used in dysmenorrhea and as a sedative.

Celestin, Felix, French physician, *1900. SEE C. *tube.*

ce·les·tine blue B (sě-les′tēn) [C.I. 51050]. A dye recommended as a substitute for hematoxylin when it is unavailable.

ce·li·ac (sē′lē-ak). Relating to the abdominal cavity. [G. *koilia,* belly]

ce·li·ag·ra (sē-lē-ag′ră). Rarely used term for sudden painful affection of the stomach or other abdominal organs. [G. *koilia,* belly, + *agra,* seizure]

ce·li·ec·to·my (sē-lē-ek′tō-mē). Obsolete term for excision of any abdominal organ, or part of one. [G. *koilia*, belly, + *ektomē*, excision]

△**celio-.** The abdomen. SEE ALSO celo- (3). [G. *koilia*, belly]

ce·li·o·cen·te·sis (sē′lē-ō-sen-tē′sis). Rarely used term for paracentesis of the abdomen. [celio- + G. *kentēsis*, puncture]

ce·li·o·en·ter·ot·o·my (sē′lē-ō-en-ter-ot′ō-mē). Obsolete term for opening into the intestine through an incision in the abdominal wall. [celio- + G. *enteron*, intestine, + *tomē*, incision]

ce·li·o·gas·tros·to·my (sē′lē-ō-gas-tros′tō-mē). Obsolete term for establishment of a gastric fistula through an incision in the abdominal wall. [celio- + G. *gastēr*, stomach, + *stoma*, mouth]

ce·li·o·gas·trot·o·my (sē′lē-ō-gas-trot′ō-mē). Obsolete term for abdominal section with incision of the stomach. [celio- + G. *gastēr*, stomach, + *tomē*, incision]

ce·li·o·hys·ter·ec·to·my (sē′lē-ō-his-ter-ek′tō-mē). SYN abdominal *hysterectomy*. [celio- + G. *hystera*, womb, + *ektomē*, excision]

ce·li·o·hys·ter·ot·o·my (sē′lē-ō-his-ter-ot′ō-mē). SYN abdominal *hysterotomy*. [celio- + G. *hystera*, womb, + *tomē*, incision]

ce·li·o·my·al·gia (sē′lē-ō-mī-al′jē-ă). Rarely used term for pain in the abdominal muscles. [celio- + G. *mys*, muscle, + *algos*, pain]

ce·li·o·my·o·mec·to·my (sē′lē-ō-mī-ō-mek′tō-mē). SYN abdominal *myomectomy*. [celio- + myoma, + G. *ektomē*, excision]

ce·li·o·my·o·mot·o·my (sē′lē-ō-mī-ō-mot′ō-mē). Obsolete term for incision into a myoma after abdominal incision. [celio- + myoma, + G. *tomē*, incision]

ce·li·o·my·o·si·tis (sē′lē-ō-mī-ō-sī′tis). Inflammation of the abdominal muscles. [celio- + G. *mys*, muscle, + *-itis*, inflammation]

ce·li·o·par·a·cen·te·sis (sē′lē-ō-par-ă-sen-tē′sis). Rarely used term for paracentesis of the abdomen. [celio- + G. *parakentēsis*, a puncture for dropsy]

ce·li·op·a·thy (sē-lē-op′ă-thē). Rarely used term for any abdominal disease. [celio- + G. *pathos*, disease]

ce·li·or·rha·phy (sē-lē-ōr′ă-fē). Suture of a wound in the abdominal wall. SYN laparorrhaphy. [celio- + G. *rhaphē*, seam]

ce·li·o·sal·pin·gec·to·my (sē′lē-ō-sal-pin-jek′tō-mē). SYN abdominal *salpingectomy*. [celio- + G. *salpinx*, trumpet + *ektomē*, excision]

ce·li·o·sal·pin·got·o·my (sē′lē-ō-sal-pin-got′ō-mē). SYN abdominal *salpingotomy*. [celio- + G. *salpinx*, trumpet, + *tomē*, incision]

ce·li·os·co·py (sē-lē-os′kŏ-pē). SYN peritoneoscopy. [celio- + G. *skopeō*, to view]

ce·li·ot·o·my (sē-lē-ot′ō-mē). Transabdominal incision into the peritoneal cavity. SYN abdominal section, laparotomy (2), ventrotomy. [celio- + G. *tomē*, incision]

vaginal c., opening the peritoneal cavity through the vagina. SYN culdotomy (2).

ce·li·tis (sē-lī′tis). Any inflammation of the abdomen. [G. *koilia*, belly, + *-itis*, inflammation]

CELL

---

cell (sel). **1.** The smallest unit of living structure capable of independent existence, composed of a membrane-enclosed mass of protoplasm and containing a nucleus or nucleoid. C.'s are highly variable and specialized in both structure and function, though all must at some stage replicate proteins and nucleic acids, utilize energy, and reproduce themselves. **2.** A small closed or partly closed cavity; a compartment or hollow receptacle. **3.** A container of glass, ceramic, or other solid material within which chemical reactions generating electricity take place. [L. *cella*, a storeroom, a chamber]

A c.'s, alpha c.'s of pancreas or of anterior lobe of hypophysis.

absorption c., a small glass chamber with parallel sides, in which absorption spectra of solutions can be obtained.

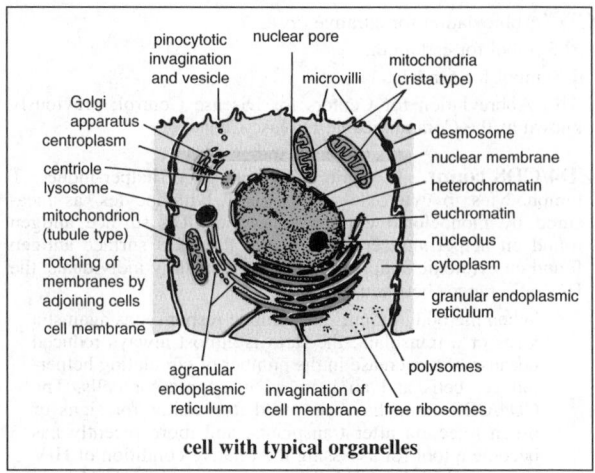

cell with typical organelles

absorptive c.'s of intestine, c.'s on the surface of villi of the small intestine and the luminal surface of the large intestine that are characterized by having microvilli on their free surface.

acid c., SYN parietal c.

acidophil c., a c. whose cytoplasm or its granules stain with acid dyes.

acinar c., any secreting c. lining an acinus, especially applied to the c.'s of the pancreas that furnish pancreatic juice and enzymes to distinguish them from the c.'s of ducts and the islets of Langerhans. SYN acinous c.

acinous c., SYN acinar c.

acoustic c., a hair c. of the organ of Corti.

adipose c., SYN fat c.

adventitial c., SYN pericyte.

air c.'s, (1) SYN pulmonary *alveolus*. **(2)** air-containing spaces in the skull.

air c.'s of auditory tube, SYN tubal air c.'s.

albuminous c., (1) SYN serous c. **(2)** SYN zymogenic c.

algoid c., a c. appearing like c.'s of algae, sometimes found in chronic diarrhea.

alpha c.'s of anterior lobe of hypophysis, acidophil c.'s that constitute about 35% of the c.'s of the anterior lobe. There are two varieties: one that elaborates somatotropin, another that elaborates prolactin.

alpha c.'s of pancreas, c.'s of the islets of Langerhans that secrete glucagon.

alveolar c., any of the c.'s lining the alveoli of the lung, including the squamous alveolar c.'s, the great alveolar c.'s, and the alveolar macrophages. SYN pneumocyte.

amacrine c., a nerve c. with short branching dendrites but believed to lack an axon; Cajal described and named such cells in the retina.

ameboid c., a c. such as a leukocyte, having ameboid movements, with a power of locomotion. SYN wandering c. SYN migratory c.

amniogenic c.'s, c.'s from which the amnion develops.

anabiotic c.'s, c.'s that are capable of resuscitation after apparent death; the existence of anabiotic tumor c.'s is postulated to explain the recurrence of a cancer after a very long symptomless period following operation.

anaplastic c., (1) a c. that has reverted to an embryonal state; **(2)** an undifferentiated c., characteristic of malignant neoplasms.

angioblastic c.'s, those c.'s in the early embryo from which primitive blood c.'s and endothelium develop.

Anitschkow c., SYN cardiac *histiocyte*.

anterior c.'s, SYN anterior ethmoidal air c.'s.

anterior ethmoidal air c.'s, the anterior group of air cells of the ethmoidal c.'s; each c. communicates with the middle meatus of the nasal cavity. SYN sinus ethmoidales anteriores [NA], anterior c.'s, anterior sinuses, cellulae anteriores.

anterior horn c., SYN motor *neuron*.

antigen-presenting c.'s (APC), c.'s that process protein antigens into peptides and present them on their surface in a form that can be recognized by lymphocytes. APCs include Langerhans c., dendritic c.'s, macrophages, B c.'s, and activated T c.'s.

antigen-responsive c., SYN antigen-sensitive c.

antigen-sensitive c., a small lymphocyte that, although not itself an immunologically activated c., responds to antigenic (immunogenic) stimulus by a process of division and differentiation that results in the production of immunologically activated cells. SYN antigen-responsive c.

apolar c., a neuron without processes.

APUD c.'s, SEE APUD.

argentaffin c.'s, c.'s that contain granules which precipitate silver from an ammoniacal silver nitrate solution. SEE ALSO enteroendocrine c.'s.

argyrophilic c.'s, c.'s that bind silver salts but that precipitate silver only in the presence of a reducing agent. SEE ALSO enteroendocrine c.'s.

Aschoff c., a large cell component of rheumatic nodules in the myocardium with a characteristic nucleus and relatively little cytoplasm.

Askanazy c., SYN Hürthle c.

astroglia c., SYN astrocyte.

auditory receptor c.'s, columnar c.'s in the epithelium of the organ of Corti, having hairs (stereocilia) on their apical ends. SEE Corti's c.'s.

B c., (1) beta c. of pancreas or of anterior lobe of hypophysis; (2) SYN B *lymphocyte*.

balloon c., (1) an unusually large degenerated c. with pale-staining vacuolated or reticulated cytoplasm, as in viral hepatitis or in degenerated epidermal c.'s in herpes zoster; (2) a large form of nevus c. with abundant nonstaining cytoplasm, formed by vacular degeneration of melanosomes.

band c., any c. of the granulocytic (leukocytic) series that has a nucleus that could be described as a curved or coiled band, no matter how marked the indentation, if it does not completely segment the nucleus into lobes connected by a filament. SYN band neutrophil, rod nuclear c., Schilling's band c., stab c., stab neutrophil, staff c.

basal c., a c. of the deepest layer of stratified epithelium. SYN basilar c.

basaloid c., a c., usually of the epidermis, resembling a basal c.

basilar c., SYN basal c.

basket c., (1) a neuron enmeshing the cell body of another neuron with its terminal axon ramifications; (2) SYN smudge c.'s. (3) a myoepithelial c. with branching processes that occurs basal to the secretory c.'s of certain salivary gland and lacrimal gland alveoli.

basophil c. of anterior lobe of hypophysis, SYN beta c. of anterior lobe of hypophysis.

beaker c., SYN goblet c.

Beale's c., a bipolar ganglion c. of the heart with one spiral and one straight prolongation.

Berger c.'s, SYN hilus c.'s.

berry c., a crenated red blood c. with surface spicules.

beta c. of anterior lobe of hypophysis, one of a population of functionally diverse c.'s that contain basophilic granules and secrete hormones such as ACTH, lipotropin, thyrotropin, and the gonadotropins. SYN basophil c. of anterior lobe of hypophysis.

beta c. of pancreas, the predominant c. of the islets of Langerhans that secretes insulin.

Betz c.'s, large pyramidal c.'s in the motor area of the precentral gyrus of the cerebral cortex. SYN Bevan-Lewis c.'s.

Bevan-Lewis c.'s, SYN Betz c.'s.

bipolar c., a neuron having two processes, such as those of the retina or the spiral and vestibular ganglia of the eighth nerve.

Bizzozero's red c.'s, nucleated red blood c.'s in human blood.

blast c., an immature precursor c.; *e.g.,* erythroblast, lymphoblast, neuroblast. SEE ALSO -blast.

blood c., one of the cells of the blood, a leukocyte or erythrocyte. SYN blood corpuscle.

Boll's c.'s, basal c.'s in the lacrimal gland.

bone c., SYN osteocyte.

border c.'s, c.'s forming the inner boundary of the organ of Corti.

Böttcher's c.'s, c.'s of the basilar membrane of the cochlea.

Bowenoid c.'s, c.'s characteristic of Bowen's disease; scattered large, round intraepidermal keratinocytes with a hyperchromatic nucleus and pole cytoplasm.

bristle c., hair c. of the inner ear.

bronchic c.'s, SYN pulmonary *alveolus*.

bronchiolar exocrine c., SYN Clara c.

brood c., SYN mother c.

burr c., a crenated red blood c.

C c., (1) a c. of the pancreatic islets of the guinea pig; SYN gamma c. of pancreas. (2) SYN parafollicular c.'s.

Cajal's c., (1) SYN horizontal c. of Cajal. (2) SYN astrocyte.

caliciform c., SYN goblet c.

cameloid c., SYN elliptocyte.

capsule c., SYN amphicyte.

carrier c., SYN phagocyte.

cartilage c., SYN chondrocyte.

castration c.'s, altered basophilic c.'s of the anterior lobe of the pituitary that develop following castration; the body of the c. is occupied by a large vacuole that displaces the nucleus to the periphery, giving the c. a resemblance to a signet ring. SYN signet ring c.'s.

caterpillar c., SYN cardiac *histiocyte*.

centroacinar c., a c. of the pancreatic ductule that occupies the lumen of an acinus; it secretes bicarbonate and water, providing an alkaline pH necessary for enzyme activity in the intestine.

chalice c., SYN goblet c.

chief c., the predominant cell type of a gland.

chief c. of corpus pineale, SYN pinealocyte.

chief c. of parathyroid gland, a round clear c. with a centrally located nucleus; secretes parathyroid hormone.

chief c. of stomach, SYN zymogenic c.

chromaffin c., a c. that stains with chromic salts, in adrenal medulla and paraganglia of the sympathetic nervous system.

chromophobe c.'s of anterior lobe of hypophysis, c.'s of the adenohypophysis that are devoid of specific acidophilic or basophilic granules when stained with common differential stains.

Clara c., a rounded, club-shaped, nonciliated c. protruding between ciliated c.'s in bronchiolar epithelium; believed to be secretory in function. SYN bronchiolar exocrine c.

Clarke c.'s, large multipolar c.'s characteristic of the thoracic nucleus (Clarke's nucleus in lamina VII) of the spinal cord.

Claudius' c.'s, columnar c.'s on the floor of the ductus cochlearis external to the organ of Corti.

clear c., (1) a c. in which the cytoplasm appears empty with the light microscope, as occurs in certain secretory c.'s of eccrine sweat glands and in the parathyroid glands when the glycogen is unstained; (2) any c., particularly a neoplastic one, containing abundant glycogen or other material that is not stained by hematoxylin or eosin, so that the c. cytoplasm is very pale in routinely stained sections.

cleavage c., SYN blastomere.

cleaved c., a c. with single or multiple clefts in the nuclear membrane.

clonogenic c., a c. that has the potential to proliferate and give rise to a colony of c.'s; some daughter c.'s from each generation retain this potential to proliferate.

cochlear hair c.'s, sensory c.'s in the organ of Corti in synaptic contact with sensory as well as efferent fibers of the cochlear (auditory) nerve; from the apical end of each c. about 100 stereocilia extend from the surface and make contact with the tectorial membrane. SYN Corti's c.'s.

column c.'s, neurons in the gray matter of the spinal cord whose axons are confined within the central nervous system.

commissural c., a neuron whose axon passes to the opposite side of the neuraxis. SYN heteromeric c.

compound granule c., SYN gitter c. SYN gitterzelle.

cone c. of retina, SYN cone (2).

connective tissue c., any of the c.'s of varied form occurring in connective tissue.

contrasuppressor c.'s (kon′tră-sŭ-pres′or), a subpopulation of T c.'s, distinct from T helper c.'s, which inhibit T suppressor c. function.

Corti's c.'s, SYN cochlear hair c.'s.

crescent c., SYN sickle c.

cytomegalic c.'s, c.'s containing large intranuclear and intra-cytoplasmic cytomegalic inclusion bodies caused by cytomegalo-virus; a member of the family Herpesviridae.

cytotoxic c., SYN suppressor c.'s.

cytotrophoblastic c.'s, stem c.'s that fuse to form the overlying syncytiotrophoblast of placental villi. SYN Langhans′ c.'s (2).

D c., SYN delta c. of pancreas.

dark c.'s, c.'s in eccrine sweat glands having many ribosomes and mucoid secretory granules.

daughter c., one of the two or more c.'s formed in the division of a parent c.

Davidoff's c.'s, SYN Paneth's granular c.'s.

decidual c., an enlarged, ovoid connective tissue c. appearing in the endometrium of pregnancy.

decoy c.'s, benign exfoliated epithelial c.'s with pyknotic nuclei seen in urinary infections; may be mistaken for malignant c.'s.

deep c., SYN mesangial c.

Deiters' c.'s, (1) SYN phalangeal c. (2) SYN astrocyte.

delta c. of anterior lobe of hypophysis, a variety of c. having basophilic granules.

delta c. of pancreas, a c. of the islets having fine granules and containing somatostatin. SYN D c.

dendritic c.'s, in embryonic ectoderm, c.'s of neural crest origin with extensive processes; they develop melanin early.

Dogiel's c.'s, the different cell types in cerebrospinal ganglia.

dome c., one of the rounded surface c.'s of the periderm layer of the fetal epidermis.

Downey c., the atypical lymphocyte of infectious mononucleo-sis.

dust c., SYN alveolar *macrophage*.

effector c., a terminally differentiated leukocyte that performs one or more specific functions. SEE ALSO effector.

egg c., the unfertilized ovum.

embryonic c., SYN blastomere.

enamel c., SYN ameloblast.

end c., a fully differentiated c., the mature c. of a lineage.

endodermal c.'s, embryonic c.'s forming the yolk sac and giving rise to the epithelium of the alimentary and respiratory tracts and to the parenchyma of associated glands. SYN entodermal c.'s.

endothelial c., one of the squamous c.'s forming the lining of blood and lymph vessels and the inner layer of the endocardium. SYN endotheliocyte.

enterochromaffin c.'s, SYN enteroendocrine c.'s.

enteroendocrine c.'s, c.'s with granules that may be either argentaffinic or argyrophilic; the c.'s, scattered throughout the digestive tract, are of several varieties and are believed to pro-duce at least 20 different gastrointestinal hormones and neuro-transmitters. SYN enterochromaffin c.'s, Kulchitsky c.'s.

entodermal c.'s, SYN endodermal c.'s.

ependymal c., a c. lining the central canal of the spinal cord (those of pyramidal shape) or one of the brain ventricles (those of cuboidal shape).

epidermic c., one of the c.'s of the epidermis.

epithelial c., one of the many varieties of c.'s that form epitheli-um.

epithelial reticular c., one of the many-branched epithelial c.'s that collectively form the supporting stroma for lymphocytes in the thymus; believed to produce thymosin and other factors that control thymic function.

epithelioid c., (1) a nonepithelial c. having certain characteristics of epithelium; (2) large mononuclear histiocytes having certain epithelial characteristics, particularly in tubercles where they are polygonal and have eosinophilic cytoplasm.

erythroid c., a c. of the erythrocytic series.

ethmoid air c.'s, the numerous small air-filled cells of the eth-moidal labyrinth. SEE anterior ethmoidal air c.'s, middle ethmoi-dal air c.'s, posterior ethmoidal air c.'s. SYN cellulae ethmoidales [NA], sinus ethmoidales [NA], ethmoidal c.'s.

ethmoidal c.'s, SYN ethmoid air c.'s.

external pillar c.'s, SEE pillar c.'s.

exudation c., SYN exudation *corpuscle*.

Fañanás c., a specialized astrocyte found in the cerebellar cor-tex.

fasciculata c., a c. of the zona fasciculata of the adrenal cortex that contains numerous lipid droplets due to the presence of corticosteroids.

fat c., a connective tissue c. distended with one or more fat globules, the cytoplasm usually being compressed into a thin envelope, with the nucleus at one point in the periphery. SYN adipocyte, adipose c.

fat-storing c., a multilocular fat-filled c. present in the perisinu-soidal space in the liver. SYN lipocyte.

Ferrata's c., SYN hemohistioblast.

floor c., an obsolete term for the cell body of pillar c.'s in the floor of the arch of Corti.

foam c.'s, c.'s with abundant, pale-staining, finely vacuolated cytoplasm, usually histiocytes that have ingested or accumulated material that dissolves during tissue preparation, especially lip-ids. SEE ALSO lipophage.

follicular epithelial c., a c. lining a follicle such as that of the thyroid gland.

follicular ovarian c.'s, c.'s of an ovarian follicle that surround the developing ovum; they form the stratum granulosum ovarii and cumulus oophorus.

foreign body giant c., a multinucleate "cell" or syncytium formed around particulate matter in chronic inflammatory reac-tions.

formative c.'s, inner cell mass c.'s of the blastocyst; collec-tively, these c.'s give rise to the embryo.

foveolar c.'s of stomach, theca c.'s of the foveolae of the stom-ach.

fuchsinophil c., a c. with a special affinity for fuchsin.

fusiform c.'s of cerebral cortex, spindle-shaped c.'s in the sixth layer of the cerebral cortex.

G c.'s, enteroendocrine c.'s that secrete gastrin, found primarily in the mucosa of the pyloric antrum of the stomach.

gamma c. of pancreas, SYN C c. (1).

ganglion c., originally, any nerve c. (neuron); in current usage, a neuron the c. body of which is located outside the limits of the brain and spinal cord, hence forming part of the peripheral ner-vous system; ganglion c.'s are either 1) the pseudounipolar c.'s of the sensory spinal and cranial nerves (sensory ganglia), or 2) the peripheral multipolar motor neurons innervating the viscera (visceral or autonomic ganglia). SYN gangliocyte.

ganglion c.'s of dorsal spinal root, pseudounipolar nerve c. bodies in the ganglia of the dorsal spinal nerve roots; the sensory spinal nerves are composed of the peripheral axon branches of these sensory ganglion c.'s, whereas the central axon branch of each such c. enters the spinal cord as a component of the dorsal root.

ganglion c.'s of retina, the nerve c.'s of the retina whose central processes (fibers) form the optic nerve; their peripheral processes synapse with the bipolar c.'s and through them with the rod and cone c.'s; these c. bodies are round or flask-shaped and vary considerably in size.

Gaucher c.'s, large, finely and uniformly vacuolated c.'s derived from the reticuloendothelial system, and found especially in the spleen, lymph nodes, liver, and bone marrow of patients with Gaucher's disease; Gaucher c.'s contain kerasin (a cerebroside), which accumulates as a result of a genetically determined ab-sence of the enzyme glucosylceramidase.

gemistocytic c., SYN gemistocytic *astrocyte*.

germ c., SYN sex c.

germinal c., a c. from which other c.'s proliferate.

ghost c., (1) a dead c. in which the outline remains visible, but without other cytoplasmic structures or stainable nucleus; **(2)** an erythrocyte after loss of its hemoglobin.

giant c., a c. of large size, often with many nuclei.

Gierke c.'s, small c.'s characteristic of the substantia gelatinosa (lamina II) of the dorsal horn of the spinal cord.

gitter c., a lipid-laden microglial phagocyte commonly seen at the edge of healing brain infarcts, a result of cellular phagocytosis of lipid from necrotic or degenerating brain c.'s. SYN compound granule c. [Ger. *Gitterzelle,* fr. *Gitter,* lattice, wire-net]

glia c.'s, SEE neuroglia.

glitter c.'s, polymorphonuclear leukocytes that stain pale blue with gentian violet and contain cytoplasmic granules that exhibit brownian movement; observed in urine sediment and characteristic of pyelonephritis.

globoid c., a large c. of mesodermal origin that is found clustered in the intracranial tissues in globoid cell leukodystrophy.

glomerulosa c., a c. of the zona glomerulosa of the adrenal cortex that is the source of aldosterone; the c.'s are arranged in spherical or oval groups.

goblet c., an epithelial c. that becomes distended with a large accumulation of mucous secretory granules at its apical end, giving it the appearance of a goblet. SYN beaker c., caliciform c., chalice c.

Golgi epithelial c., a glial cell found in the cerebellar cortex. SEE Bergmann's *fibers,* under *fiber.*

Golgi's c.'s, SEE Golgi type I *neuron,* Golgi type II *neuron.*

Goormaghtigh's c.'s, SYN juxtaglomerular c.'s.

granule c.'s, (1) small nerve cell bodies in the external and internal granular layers of the cerebral cortex; **(2)** small nerve cell bodies in the granular layer of the cerebellar cortex.

granule c. of connective tissue, SYN mast c.

granulosa c., a c. of the membrana granulosa lining the vesicular ovarian follicle that becomes a luteal c. of the corpus luteum after ovulation.

granulosa lutein c.'s, c.'s derived from the membrana granulosa of a mature ovarian follicle that secrete both estrogen and progesterone, and form the major component of the corpus luteum.

great alveolar c.'s, cuboidal c.'s connected with the squamous pulmonary alveolar c.'s and having in their cytoplasm lamellated bodies (cytosomes) that represent the source of the surfactant that coats the alveoli. SYN granular pneumonocytes, type II c.'s.

guanine c., a c. whose cytoplasm contains glistening crystals of guanine.

gustatory c.'s, SYN taste c.'s.

gyrochrome c., SEE gyrochrome.

hair c.'s, sensory epithelial c.'s present in the organ of Corti, in the maculae and cristae of the membranous labyrinth of the ear, and in taste buds; they are characterized by having long stereocilia or kinocilia (or both) which, with the light microscope, appear as fine hairs. SEE ALSO vestibular hair c.'s, cochlear hair c.'s, taste c.'s.

hairy c.'s, medium sized leukocytes that have features of reticuloendothelial c.'s and multiple cytoplasmic projections (hairs) on the c. surface, but which may be a variety of B lymphocyte; they are found in hairy cell leukemia.

Haller c., a variant of ethmoidal air cell developing into the floor of the orbit adjacent to the natural ostium of the maxillary sinus. A diseased Haller c. is capable of obstructing that ostium and producing a maxillary sinusitis.

heart failure c.'s, macrophages in the lung during left heart failure that often carry large amounts of hemosiderin. SEE ALSO siderophore.

HeLa c.'s, the first continuously cultured human malignant c.'s, derived from a cervical carcinoma of a patient, Henrietta Lacks; used in the cultivation of viruses.

helmet c., a schistocyte shaped like a military helmet.

helper c., a subset of T lymphocytes that acts in cooperation with B lymphocytes to permit antibody formation. SYN inducer c.

HEMPAS c.'s, the abnormal erythrocytes of type II congenital dyserythropoietic anemia. SEE HEMPAS.

Hensen's c., one of the supporting c.'s in the organ of Corti, immediately to the outer side of the c.'s of Deiters.

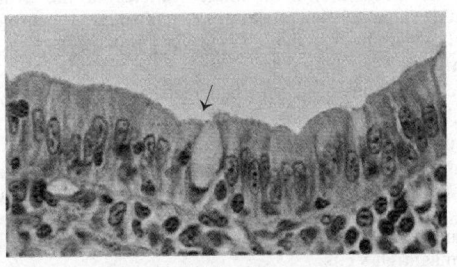

goblet cell

heteromeric c., SYN commissural c.

hilus c.'s, c.'s in the hilus of the ovary that produce androgens; they are thought to be the ovarian counterpart of the interstitial c.'s of the testis. SYN Berger c.'s.

hobnail c.'s, c.'s characteristic of a mesonephroma; a round expansion of clear cytoplasm projects into the lumen of neoplastic tubules, but the basal part of the c. containing the nucleus is narrow.

Hofbauer c., a large c. in the connective tissue of the chorionic villi; it appears to be a type of phagocyte.

horizontal c. of Cajal, a small fusiform c. found in the superficial layer of the cerebral cortex with its long axis placed horizontally. SYN Cajal's c. (1).

horizontal c.'s of retina, c.'s in the outer part of the inner nuclear layer of the retina that lie with their axes more or less parallel with the surface. They are thought to connect the rods of one part of the retina with cones of another part.

horny c., (1) SYN corneocyte.

Hortega c.'s, SYN microglia.

Hürthle c., a large, granular eosinophilic c. derived from thyroid follicular epithelium by accumulation of mitochondria, *e.g.,* in Hashimoto's disease. SYN Askanazy c.

I c., a cultured skin fibroblast containing membrane-bound inclusions; characteristic of mucolipidosis II. SEE ALSO immunocyte. SYN inclusion c.

immunologically activated c., an immunocyte that is in an elevated state of reactivity capable of carrying out an immune response, in contradistinction to an immunologically competent c.

immunologically competent c., a small lymphocyte capable of being immunologically activated by exposure to a substance that is antigenic (immunogenic) for the respective c.; activation involves either the capacity to produce antibody or the capacity to participate in cell-mediated immunity.

inclusion c., SYN I c.

indifferent c., an undifferentiated, nonspecialized c.

inducer c., SYN helper c.

innocent bystander c., the destruction of a c. by an immune process even though that c. was not directly targeted.

intercapillary c., SYN mesangial c.

internal pillar c.'s, SEE pillar c.'s.

interstitial c.'s, (1) c.'s between the seminiferous tubules of the testis that secrete testosterone; SYN Leydig's c.'s. **(2)** c.'s derived

⚠ **Combining forms**	**[NA] Nomina Anatomica**
WordFinder **Multi-term entry finder** **Preceding letter A**	**[MIM] Mendelian** **Inheritance in Man**
A.D.A.M. Anatomy Plates **Between letters L and M**	☆ **Official alternate term**
Appendices: **Following letter Z**	☆**[NA] Official alternate** **Nomina Anatomica term**
SYN **Synonym; Cf., compare**	**High Profile Term**

from the theca interna of atretic follicles of the ovary; they resemble luteal c.'s and are an important source of estrogens; **(3)** pineal c.'s similar to glial c.'s with long processes.

irritation c., SYN Türk c.

islet c., one of the c.'s of the pancreatic islets.

Ito c.'s, fat-containing c.'s lining hepatic sinusoids.

juvenile c., SYN metamyelocyte.

juxtaglomerular c.'s, c.'s, located at the vascular pole of the renal corpuscle that secrete renin and form a component of the juxtaglomerular complex; they are modified smooth muscle c.'s primarily of the afferent arteriole of the renal glomerulus. SYN Goormaghtigh's c.'s.

K c.'s, SYN killer c.'s.

karyochrome c., SEE karyochrome.

keratinized c., SYN corneocyte.

killer c.'s, cytotoxic c.'s involved in antibody-dependent c.-mediated immune responses; they appear to be T lymphocytes of the suppressor subset with receptors for the Fc portion of IgG molecules, and lyse or damage IgG coated target c.'s without mediation of complement. SEE antibody-dependent cell-mediated *cytotoxicity.* SYN K c.'s, null c.'s (1), T cytotoxic c.'s.

Kulchitsky c.'s, SYN enteroendocrine c.'s.

Kupffer c.'s, phagocytic c.'s of the mononuclear phagocyte series found on the luminal surface of the hepatic sinusoids. SYN stellate c.'s of liver.

lacis c. (lah-sē′), one of the c.'s of the juxtaglomerular apparatus found at the vascular pole of the renal corpuscle. [Fr. *lacis,* meshwork]

Langerhans' c.'s, dendritic clear c.'s in the epidermis, containing distinctive granules that appear rod- or racket-shaped in section, but lacking tonofilaments, melanosomes, and desmosomes; they carry surface receptors for immunoglobulin (Fc) and complement (C3), and are believed to be antigen fixing and processing c.'s of monocytic origin; active participants in cutaneous delayed hypersensitivity.

Langhans' c.'s, (1) multinucleated giant c.'s seen in tuberculosis and other granulomas; the nuclei are arranged in an arciform manner at the periphery of the c.'s; SYN Langhans'-type giant c.'s. **(2)** SYN cytotrophoblastic c.'s.

Langhans'-type giant c.'s, SYN Langhans' c.'s (1).

LE c., a polymorphonuclear leukocyte containing an amorphous round body that is a phagocytosed nucleus from another cell plus serum antinuclear globulin (IgG) and complement; formed *in vitro* in the blood of patients with systemic lupus erythematosus, or by the action of the patient's serum on normal leukocytes. SYN lupus erythematosus c.

Leishman's chrome c.'s, basophilic granular leukocytes (basophils) observed in the circulating blood of some persons with blackwater fever.

lepra c.'s, distinctive, large, mononuclear phagocytes (macrophages) with a foamlike cytoplasm, and also poorly staining saclike structures resulting from degeneration of such c.'s, observed characteristically in leprous inflammatory reactions; indistinct staining results from numerous, fairly closely packed leprosy bacilli, which are acid-fast and resistant to staining by ordinary methods but may be vividly demonstrated by acid-fast staining procedures.

Leydig's c.'s, SYN interstitial c.'s (1).

light c.'s of thyroid, SYN parafollicular c.'s.

lining c., SYN littoral c.

Lipschütz c., SYN centrocyte (1).

littoral c., the c.'s lining the lymphatic sinuses of lymph nodes and the blood sinuses of bone marrow. SYN lining c. [L. *littoralis,* the seashore]

Loevit's c., SYN erythroblast.

lupus erythematosus c., SYN LE c.

luteal c., lutein c., a c. of the corpus luteum of the ovary that is derived from the granulosa cells of the preovulatory follicle; it secretes progesterone and estrogen.

lymph c., SYN lymphocyte.

lymphoid c., a parenchymal c. of lymphatic tissue.

macroglia c., SYN astrocyte.

malpighian c., a c. of the stratum spinosum of the epidermis.

Marchand's wandering c., a c. of the mononuclear phagocyte system.

marrow c., any c. of bone marrow, especially hemopoietic c.'s.

Martinotti's c., a small multipolar nerve c. with short branching dendrites scattered through various layers of the cerebral cortex; its axon ascends toward the surface of the cortex.

mast c., a connective tissue c. that contains coarse, basophilic, metachromatic granules; the c. is believed to contain heparin and histamine. SYN granule c. of connective tissue, labrocyte, mastocyte, tissue basophil.

mastoid c.'s, SYN mastoid air c.'s.

mastoid air c.'s, numerous small intercommunicating cavities in the mastoid process of the temporal bone that empty into the mastoid or tympanic antrum. SYN cellulae mastoideae [NA], mastoid c.'s, mastoid sinuses.

Mauthner's c., a large neuron of the spinal cord with its c. body located in the metencephalon of fish and amphibia.

Merkel's tactile c., SYN tactile *meniscus.*

mesangial c., a phagocytic c. in the capillary tuft of the renal glomerulus, interposed between endothelial c.'s and the basement membrane in the central or stalk region of the tuft. SYN deep c., intercapillary c.

mesenchymal c.'s, fusiform or stellate c.'s found between the ectoderm and endoderm of young embryos; the shape of the c.'s in fixed material is indicative of the fact that in life they were moving from their place of origin to areas where they would become reaggregated and specialized; most mesenchymal c.'s are derived from established mesodermal layers, but in the cephalic region they also develop from neural crest or neural tube ectoderm; they are the most strikingly pluripotential c.'s in the embryonic body, developing at different locations into any of the types of connective or supporting tissues, to smooth muscle, to vascular endothelium, and to blood cells.

mesoglial c.'s, SYN mesoglia.

mesothelial c., one of the flat c.'s of mesenchymal origin that form the superficial layer of the serosal membranes lining the body cavities of the abdomen and thorax.

Mexican hat c., SYN target c. (1).

Meynert's c.'s, solitary pyramidal c.'s found in the cortex in the region of the calcarine fissure.

microglia c.'s, microglial c.'s, SYN microglia.

middle c.'s, SYN middle ethmoidal air c.'s.

middle ethmoidal air c.'s, the middle group of air cells of the ethmoidal c.'s; each c. communicates with the middle meatus of the nasal cavity. SYN sinus ethmoidales mediae [NA], cellulae mediae, middle c.'s, middle ethmoidal sinuses.

midget bipolar c.'s, bipolar c.'s in the inner nuclear layer of the retina that synapse with individual cone c.'s in the outer plexiform layer; other larger bipolar c.'s in the inner nuclear layer synapse with both rod and cone c.'s; the axons of both types synapse in the inner plexiform layer with the dendrites of the ganglion c.'s.

migratory c., SYN ameboid c.

Mikulicz' c.'s, foamy macrophages containing *Klebsiella rhinoscleromatis;* found in the mucosal nodules in rhinoscleroma.

mirror-image c., **(1)** a c. whose nuclei have identical features and are placed in the cytoplasm in similar fashion; **(2)** a binucleate form of Reed-Sternberg c. often found in Hodgkin's disease; the twin nuclei are disposed in relation to an imaginary plane between them like a single nucleus together with its image in a mirror.

mitral c.'s, large nerve c.'s in the olfactory lobe of the brain whose dendrites synapse (in glomeruli) with axons of the olfactory receptor c.'s of the nasal mucous membrane, and whose axons pass centrally in the olfactory tract to the olfactory cortex.

monocytoid c., a c. having morphological characteristics of a monocyte but which is nonphagocytic.

mossy c., one of the two types of neuroglia c.'s, consisting of a rather large body with numerous short branching processes.

mother c., a c. which, by division, gives rise to two or more daughter c.'s. SYN brood c., metrocyte, parent c.

motor c., a neuron whose axon innervates peripheral effector c.'s such as muscle fibers or gland c.'s.

mucoalbuminous c.'s, SYN mucoserous c.'s.

mucoserous c.'s, glandular c.'s intermediate in histologic characteristics between serous and mucous c.'s. SYN mucoalbuminous c.'s, seromucous c.'s.

mucous c., a c. secreting mucus; *e.g.,* a goblet c.

mucous neck c., one of the acidic mucin-secreting c.'s in the neck of a gastric gland.

Müller's radial c.'s, SYN Müller's *fibers* (2), under *fiber.*

multipolar c., a nerve c. with a number of dendrites arising from the c. body.

mural c., a nonendothelial c. enclosed within the basement membrane of retinal capillaries.

myeloid c., specifically, any young c. that develops into a mature granulocyte of blood, but frequently used as a synonym for marrow c.

myoepithelial c., a smooth muscle-like c. of ectodermal origin, found between the epithelium and basement membrane in a number of organs such as mammary, sweat, and lacrimal glands.

myoid c.'s, flattened smooth muscle-like c.'s of mesodermal origin that lie just outside the basal lamina of the seminiferous tubule. SYN peritubular contractile c.'s.

Nageotte c.'s, c.'s found in the cerebrospinal fluid, one or two per cubic millimeter in health, but in greater numbers in various diseases.

natural killer c.'s, large granular lymphocytes which do not express markers of either T or B c. lineage. These c.'s do possess Fc receptors for IgG and can kill target c.'s using antibody-dependent cell-mediated cytotoxicity. NK c.'s can also use perforin to kill c.'s in the absence of antibody. Killing may occur without previous sensitization. SYN NK c.'s.

nerve c., SYN neuron (1).

Neumann's c.'s, nucleated c.'s in the bone marrow developing into red blood c.'s.

neurilemma c.'s, SYN Schwann c.'s.

neuroendocrine c., (1) SEE neuroendocrine (2). (2) SYN paraneurone.

neuroendocrine transducer c., an endocrine c. that releases its hormonal product into the bloodstream only upon receipt of a nervous impulse.

neuroepithelial c.'s, SYN neuroepithelium.

neuroglia c.'s, SEE neuroglia.

neurolemma c.'s, SYN Schwann c.'s.

neuromuscular c., a c. of a lower metazoan organism that is both sensitive and contractile.

neurosecretory c.'s, nerve c.'s, such as those of the hypothalamus, that elaborate a chemical substance (such as a releasing factor, neuropeptide, or, more rarely, a true hormone) that influences the activity of another structure (*e.g.,* anterior lobe of the hypophysis). See also neurosecretion.

nevus c., the c. of a pigmented cutaneous nevus that differs from a normal melanocyte in that it lacks dendrites. SYN nevocyte.

nevus c., A-type, melanocytes in the epidermis in pigmented nevi, resembling epithelial c.'s and frequently containing melanin.

nevus c., B-type, small, usually non-pigmented melanocytes in the mid-dermis in pigmented nevi.

nevus c., C-type, non-pigmented spindle-shaped melanocytes in the lower dermis in pigmented nevi.

Niemann-Pick c., SYN Pick c.

NK c.'s, SYN natural killer c.'s.

nonclonogenic c., a c. that does not give rise to a colony of c.'s (large numbers of c.'s that are genetically identical); may undergo two or more c. divisions, but all daughter c.'s are destined to die or differentiate (losing all potential to divide).

null c.'s, (1) SYN killer c.'s. **(2)** large granular lymphocytes that lack surface markers/membrane associated proteins of either B or T lymphocytes.

nurse c.'s, SYN Sertoli's c.'s.

oat c., a short, bluntly spindle-shaped c. that contains a relatively large, hyperchromatic nucleus, frequently observed in some forms of undifferentiated bronchogenic carcinoma.

OKT c.'s, c.'s recognized by monoclonal antibodies to T lymphocyte antigens: OKT-3 c.'s are T lymphocytes as a class, since all share a common leukocyte differentiation antigen; OKT-4 c.'s are helper c.'s; OKT-8 c.'s are suppressor c.'s. OKT-4/OKT-8 expresses the ratio of helper to suppressor c.'s, sometimes used as a measure of the functional status of the immune system and thus a basis for clinical diagnosis and prognosis. Current usage favors using CD designations. [*Ortho-Kung T* cell]

olfactory c.'s, SYN olfactory receptor c.'s.

olfactory receptor c.'s, very slender nerve c.'s, with large nuclei and surmounted by six to eight long, sensitive cilia in the olfactory epithelium at the roof of the nose; they are the receptors for smell. SYN olfactory c.'s, Schultze's c.'s.

oligodendroglia c.'s, SEE oligodendroglia.

Onodi c., a variant of a posterior ethmoidal air c. in intimate relationship with the optic nerve just distal to the optic chiasm.

Opalski c., a characteristically altered glial c. in the basal ganglia and thalamus in hepatocerebral degeneration and Wilson's disease.

osseous c., SYN osteocyte.

osteochondrogenic c., one of the undifferentiated c.'s in the inner layer of the periosteum of an endochondrally developing bone capable of developing into an osteoblast or a chondroblast.

osteogenic c., one of the c.'s in the inner layer of the periosteum that forms osseous tissue.

osteoprogenitor c., a mesenchymal c. that differentiates into an osteoblast. SYN preosteoblast.

oxyntic c., SYN parietal c.

oxyphil c.'s, c.'s of the parathyroid gland that increase in number with age; the cytoplasm contains numerous mitochondria and stains with eosin. Similar c.'s, and tumors composed of them, are found in salivary glands and the thyroid; in the latter, also called Hürthle c.'s.

P c., a characteristic specialized c., with probable pacemaker function, found in the S-A node and A-V junction.

packed human blood c.'s, whole blood from which plasma has been removed; may be prepared any time during the dating period of the whole blood from which it is derived, but not later than six days after the blood has been drawn if separation of plasma and c.'s is achieved by centrifugation.

pagetoid c.'s, atypical melanocytes resembling Paget's c.'s, found in some cutaneous melanomas of the superficial spreading type.

Paget's c.'s, relatively large, neoplastic epithelial c.'s (carcinoma c.'s) with hyperchromatic nuclei and palely staining cytoplasm; in Paget's disease of the breast, such c.'s occur in neoplastic epithelium in the ducts and in the epidermis of the nipple, areola, and adjacent skin.

Paneth's granular c.'s, c.'s, located at the base of intestinal glands of the small intestine, which contain large acidophilic refractile granules and may produce lysozyme. SYN Davidoff's c.'s.

parafollicular c.'s, c.'s present between follicles or interspersed among follicular c.'s; they are rich in mitochondria and are believed to be the source of thyrocalcitonin. SYN C c. (2), light c.'s of thyroid.

paraganglionic c.'s, c.'s of the embryonic sympathetic nervous system that become chromaffin c.'s.

paraluteal c., SYN theca lutein c.

paralutein c. (par-ă-lū′tin), SYN theca lutein c.

parenchymal c., SEE parenchyma.

parenchymatous c. of corpus pineale, SYN pinealocyte.

parent c., SYN mother c.

parietal c., one of the c.'s of the gastric glands; it lies upon the basement membrane, covered by the chief c.'s, and secretes hydrochloric acid that reaches the lumen of the gland through fine intracellular and intercellular canals (canaliculi). SYN acid c., oxyntic c.

peptic c., SYN zymogenic c.

pericapillary c., SYN pericyte.

peripolar c., a granular c. located where the parietal and visceral capsules of the renal corpuscle meet; part of the c. faces the filtration space of Bowman.

perithelial c., SYN pericyte.

peritubular contractile c.'s, SYN myoid c.'s.

permissive c., a c. in which the late phase of viral infection follows the early phase and cell death is coupled with massive synthesis of virus; *e.g.,* monkey c.'s are permissive for SV40.

pessary c., a red blood c. in which the hemoglobin has disappeared from the center, leaving only the periphery visible.

phalangeal c., the supporting c.'s of the organ of Corti, attached to the basement membrane and receiving the hair c.'s between their free extremities. SEE ALSO phalanx (2). SYN Deiters' c.'s (1).

pheochrome c., (1) former term for enteroendocrine c.; **(2)** SYN pheochromocyte.

photo c., a light-detecting electronic device; the device that measures x-ray transmission through a patient for automatic termination of the exposure.

photoreceptor c.'s, rod and cone c.'s of the retina.

physaliphorous c., c.'s containing a bubbly or vacuolated cytoplasm, *e.g.,* as characteristically seen in chordoma.

Pick c., a relatively large, rounded or polygonal, mononuclear c., with indistinctly or palely staining, foamlike cytoplasm that contains numerous droplets of a phosphatide, sphingomyelin; such c.'s are widely distributed in the spleen and other tissues, especially those rich in reticuloendothelial components, in patients with Niemann-Pick disease. SYN Niemann-Pick c.

pigment c., a c. containing pigment granules.

pigment c.'s of iris, c.'s of the stromal layer of the iris; in dark eyes (but not in blue) they contain granules of pigment.

pigment c.'s of retina, c.'s in the outermost layer of the retina that contain pigment granules.

pigment c. of skin, SYN melanocyte.

pillar c.'s, c.'s forming the outer and inner walls of the tunnel in the organ of Corti. SYN Corti's pillars, Corti's rods, pillar c.'s of Corti, tunnel c.'s.

pillar c.'s of Corti, SYN pillar c.'s.

pineal c.'s, c.'s of the corpus pineale or pinealocyte.

plasma c., an ovoid c. with an eccentric nucleus having chromatin arranged like a clock face or spokes of a wheel; the cytoplasm is strongly basophilic because of the abundant RNA in its endoplasmic reticulum; plasma c.'s are derived from B type lymphocytes and are active in the formation of antibodies. SYN plasmacyte.

pluripotent c.'s, primordial c.'s that may still differentiate into various specialized types of tissue elements; *e.g.,* mesenchymal c.'s.

polar c., SYN polar *body.*

polychromatic c., a primitive erythrocyte in bone marrow, with basophilic material as well as hemoglobin (acidophilic) in the cytoplasm. SYN polychromatophil c.

polychromatophil c., SYN polychromatic c.

posterior c.'s, SYN posterior ethmoidal air c.'s.

posterior ethmoidal air c.'s, the posterior group of air cells of the ethmoidal c.'s; each c. communicates with the superior meatus of the nasal cavity. SYN sinus ethmoidales posteriores [NA], cellulae posteriores, posterior c.'s.

pregnancy c.'s, hypophysial chromophobe c.'s that increase in number and accumulate eosinophil granules during pregnancy.

pregranulosa c.'s, capsular c.'s surrounding the primordial ova in the embryonic ovary; they are derived from celomic epithelium.

prickle c., one of the c.'s of the stratum spinosum of the epidermis; so called because of typical shrinkage artifacts that occur in histological preparations, resulting in intercellular bridges at points of desmosomal adhesion. SYN spine c.

primary embryonic c., in a very young embryo, a c. still capable of differentiation.

primitive reticular c., a c. with processes making contact with those of other similar c.'s to form a cellular network; along with the network of reticular fibers, the reticular c.'s form the stroma of bone marrow and lymphatic tissues.

primordial c., a c. from a group that constitutes the primordium of an organ or part of the embryo.

primordial germ c., the most primitive undifferentiated sex cell, found initially outside the gonad. SYN gonocyte.

prolactin c., SYN mammotroph.

pseudo-Gaucher c., a plasma c., microscopically resembling a Gaucher c., found in the bone marrow in some cases of multiple myeloma.

pseudounipolar c., SYN unipolar *neuron.*

pseudoxanthoma c., relatively large phagocytic c.'s (macrophages) that contain numerous small lipid vacuoles or hemosiderin (or both), in organizing hemorrhagic or inflammatory lesions.

pulpar c., the specific macrophagic c. of the spleen substance.

Purkinje's c.'s, large nerve c.'s of the cerebellar cortex with a piriform cell body and dendrites arranged in a plane transverse to the folium. SYN Purkinje's corpuscles.

pus c., SYN pus *corpuscle.*

pyramidal c.'s, neurons of the cerebral cortex which, in sections perpendicular to the cortical surface, exhibit a triangular shape with a long apical dendrite directed toward the surface of the cortex; there are also lateral dendrites, and a basal axon that descends to deeper layers.

pyrrol c., pyrrhol c., a c. of the mononuclear macrophage system that has a special affinity for pyrrol blue, taking up the dye by a process of pinocytosis.

Raji c., a c. of a cultured line of lymphoblastoid c.'s derived from a Burkitt's lymphoma; it possesses numerous receptors for certain complement components and is thus suitable for use in detection of immune complexes. It expresses certain complement receptors as well as Fc receptors for immunoglobulin G.

reactive c., SYN gemistocytic *astrocyte.*

red blood c. (rbc, RBC), SYN erythrocyte.

Reed c.'s, SYN Reed-Sternberg c.'s.

Reed-Sternberg c.'s, large transformed lymphocytes generally regarded as pathognomonic of Hodgkin's disease; a typical c. has a pale-staining acidophilic cytoplasm and one or two large nuclei showing marginal clumping of chromatin and unusually conspicuous deeply acidophilic nucleoli; binucleate Reed-Sternberg c.'s frequently show a mirror-image form (mirror-image c.'s). SYN Reed c.'s, Sternberg c.'s, Sternberg-Reed c.'s.

Renshaw c.'s, inhibitory interneurons that are innervated by collaterals from motoneurons and in turn form synapses with the same and adjacent motoneurons to exert inhibition; identified physiologically and by intracellular injection technic.

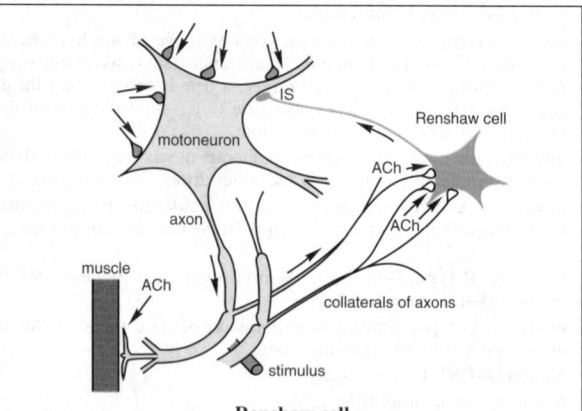

Renshaw cell

recurrent inhibition by Renshaw cell of spinal motoneuron (of cat); ACh, acetylcholine-releasing synapses; IS, inhibitory synapse

resting c., a quiescent c.; one not undergoing mitosis.

resting wandering c., SYN fixed *macrophage.*

restructured c., the viable c. produced by fusion of a karyoplast with a cytoplast.

reticular c., SEE primitive reticular c.

reticularis c., a c. of the zona reticularis of the innermost part of the adrenal cortex.

reticuloendothelial c., a c. of the reticuloendothelial system.

rhagiocrine c., SYN macrophage.

Rieder c.'s, abnormal myeloblasts (12 to 20 μm in diameter) in which the nucleus may be widely and deeply indented (*i.e.,* suggestive of lobulation), or may actually be a bi- or multi-lobate structure; such c.'s are frequently observed in acute leukemia, and probably represent a more rapid maturation of the nucleus than that of the cytoplasm.

Rindfleisch's c.'s, obsolete eponym for eosinophilic *leukocyte*.

rod nuclear c., SYN band c.

rod c. of retina, SYN rod (2).

Rolando's c.'s, the nerve c.'s in Rolando's gelatinous substance of the spinal cord.

rosette-forming c.'s, T lymphocytes with an affinity for sheep erythrocytes and which, when suspended in serum, bind the uncoated, nonsensitized erythrocytes in a rosette formation.

Rouget c., a c. with several slender processes that embraces the capillary wall in amphibia. SYN capillary pericyte.

sarcogenic c., SYN myoblast.

satellite c.'s, neuroglial c.'s surrounding the c. body of a ganglion c. in the spinal, cranial, and autonomic ganglia.

satellite c. of skeletal muscle, an elongated spindle-shaped c. occupying depressions in the sarcolemma and between it and the basal lamina; believed to play a role in muscle repair and regeneration by fusing with adjacent myofiber. SYN sarcoplast.

scavenger c., SYN phagocyte.

Schilling's band c., SYN band c.

Schultze's c.'s, SYN olfactory receptor c.'s.

Schwann c.'s, c.'s of ectodermal (neural crest) origin that compose a continuous envelope around each nerve fiber of peripheral nerves; such c.'s are comparable to the oligodendroglia c.'s of brain and spinal cord; like the latter, they may form membranous expansions that wind around axons and thus form the axon's myelin sheath. SYN neurilemma c.'s, neurolemma c.'s.

segmented c., a polymorphonuclear leukocyte matured beyond the band c. so that two or more lobes of the nucleus occur.

sensitized c., (1) a c., including a bacterial c., that has combined with specific antibody to form a complex capable of reacting with complement components; **(2)** a small, "committed," c. derived, by division and differentiation, from a transformed lymphocyte; **(3)** a c. that has been either exposed to antigen or opsonized with antibodies and/or complement.

sensory c., a c. in the peripheral nervous system that receives afferent (sensory) input; sensory receptor c.'s.

septal c., a round pale c. of the lungs in the septa between the pulmonary alveoli.

seromucous c.'s, SYN mucoserous c.'s.

serous c., a c., especially of the salivary gland, that secretes a watery or thin albuminous fluid, as opposed to a mucous c. SYN albuminous c. (1).

Sertoli's c.'s, elongated c.'s in the seminiferous tubules to which spermatids are attached during spermiogenesis; they secrete androgen-binding protein and establish the blood-testis barrier by forming tight junctions with adjacent Sertoli's c.'s. SYN nurse c.'s.

sex c., a spermatozoon or an ovum. SYN germ c.

Sézary c., an atypical T lymphocyte seen in the peripheral blood in the Sézary syndrome; it has a large convoluted nucleus and scanty cytoplasm containing PAS-positive vacuoles.

shadow c.'s, SYN smudge c.'s.

sickle c., an abnormal, crescentic erythrocyte that is characteristic of sickle c. anemia, resulting from an inherited abnormality of hemoglobin (hemoglobin S) causing decreased solubility at low oxygen tension. SYN crescent c., drepanocyte, meniscocyte.

signet ring c.'s, SYN castration c.'s.

silver c., one of a number of c.'s seen in plaques of multiple sclerosis, having round or oval nuclei, the body of the c. containing many yellow or light brown particles; the c.'s are characteristic of multiple sclerosis, but are found in other conditions, including syphilis.

skein c., SYN reticulocyte.

small cleaved c., a lymphoid c. of follicular center c. origin that has an irregularly shaped nucleus with clumped chromatin, absent nucleoli, and one or more clefts in the nuclear membrane.

smudge c.'s, immature leukocytes of any type that have undergone partial breakdown during preparation of a stained smear or tissue section, because of their greater fragility; smudge c.'s are seen in largest numbers in chronic lymphocytic leukemia. SYN basket c. (2), Gumprecht's shadows, shadow c.'s.

somatic c.'s, the c.'s of an organism, other than the germ c.'s.

sperm c., SYN spermatozoon.

spider c., (1) SYN astrocyte. **(2)** a c. in a rhabdomyoma of the heart, with central nucleus and cytoplasmic mass connected to the cell wall by strands of cytoplasm separated by clear glycogen-filled areas.

spindle c., a fusiform c., such as those in the deeper layers of the cerebral cortex.

spine c., SYN prickle c.

splenic c.'s, large round ameboid c.'s (macrophages) in the splenic pulp.

squamous c., a flat scale-like epithelial c.

squamous alveolar c.'s, highly attentuated squamous c.'s that form the gas-permeable epithelium lining the alveoli of the lungs. SYN type I c.'s.

stab c., SYN band c.

staff c., SYN band c.

standard c., an electrical c. having a definite known voltage; used to calibrate other electric c.'s.

stellate c.'s of cerebral cortex, small star-shaped c.'s in the second and fourth layers of the cortex, and large stellate c.'s in the deeper part of the third layer in the visual cortex.

stellate c.'s of liver, SYN Kupffer c.'s.

stem c., (1) any precursor cell; **(2)** a c. whose daughter c.'s may differentiate into other c. types.

Sternberg c.'s, SYN Reed-Sternberg c.'s.

Sternberg-Reed c.'s, SYN Reed-Sternberg c.'s.

stichochrome c., SEE stichochrome.

strap c., an elongated tumor c. of uniform width that may show cross-striations; found in rhabdomyosarcoma.

supporting c., SYN sustentacular c.

suppressor c.'s, cells of the immune system that inhibit or help to terminate an immune response, *e.g.,* suppressor macrophages and suppressor T cells. SYN cytotoxic c.

surface mucous c.'s of stomach, c.'s lining the gastric surface and foveolae; a glycoprotein product at the apical end of each c. is secreted and forms a mucous protective film. SYN theca c.'s of stomach.

sustentacular c., one of the ordinary elongated c.'s resting on the basement membrane that surround and serve as a support to the shorter specialized c.'s in certain organs, such as the labyrinth of the inner ear or olfactory epithelium. SYN supporting c.

sympathetic formative c., a neuroblast of the embryonic autonomic nervous system.

sympathicotropic c.'s, large epithelioid c.'s in the hilum of the ovary associated with unmyelinated nerve fibers.

sympathochromaffin c., the c. type in the embryonic suprarenal gland from which both sympathetic ganglion c.'s and chromaffin c.'s are developed.

synovial c., fibrotoplast-like c.'s that form 1–6 epithelioid layers in the synovial membrane of joints; believed to contribute proteoglycans and hyaluronate to the synovial fluid.

T c., SYN T *lymphocyte*.

tactile c., one of the epithelioid c.'s of a corpusculum tactus. SYN touch c.

tanned red c.'s, erythrocytes subjected to mild treatment with chemicals such as tannic acid so that they adsorb onto their surface soluble antigens; used in hemagglutination tests.

target c., (1) an erythrocyte in target c. anemia, with a dark center surrounded by a light band that again is encircled by a darker ring; it thus resembles a shooting target; such c.'s also appear after splenectomy; SYN Mexican hat c. **(2)** a c. lysed by cytotoxic T lymphocytes, as in graft rejection.

tart c., a monocyte with an engulfed nucleus in which the structure is still well preserved.

taste c.'s, darkly staining c.'s in a taste bud that appear to have extending into the gustatory pore long hair-like microvilli containing a number of closely packed microtubules; the taste c.'s stand in synaptic contact with sensory nerve fibers of the facial, glossopharyngeal, or vagus nerves. SYN gustatory c.'s.

T cytotoxic c.'s (Tc), SYN killer c.'s.

TDTH c.'s, a functional subset of T helper c.'s that are involved in delayed-type hypersensitivity reactions.

tendon c.'s, elongated fibroblastic c.'s arranged in rows between the collagenous tendon fibers.

Tg c.'s, a subset of T c.'s that have an Fc receptor for immunoglobulin G molecules.

theca lutein c., a steroid secretory c. of the corpus luteum that comes from the theca interna of the ovarian follicle at the time of ovulation. SYN paraluteal c., paralutein c.

theca c.'s of stomach, SYN surface mucous c.'s of stomach.

T helper c.'s (Th), a subset of lymphocytes that secrete various cytokines that regulate the immune response.

Tiselius electrophoresis c., the special container in a Tiselius apparatus containing the solution to be analyzed electrophoretically.

Tm c.'s, T helper c.'s that have an Fc receptor for immunoglobulin M molecules.

totipotent c., an undifferentiated c. capable of developing into any type of body c.

touch c., SYN tactile c.

Touton giant c., a xanthoma c. in which the multiple nuclei are grouped around a small island of nonfoamy cytoplasm.

transducer c., any c. responding to a mechanical, thermal, photic, or chemical stimulus by generating an electrical impulse synaptically transmitted to a sensory neuron in contact with the c.

transitional c., any c. thought to represent a phase of development from one form to another.

tubal air c.'s, occasional small air cells in the inferior wall of the auditory tube, near the tympanic orifice, communicating with the tympanic cavity. SYN cellulae pneumaticae tubae auditivae [NA], air c.'s of auditory tube.

tufted c., a particular type of c. in the olfactory bulb comparable to the bulb's mitral c. with respect to afferent and efferent relationships, but smaller and more superficially located.

tunnel c.'s, SYN pillar c.'s.

Türk c., a relatively large, immature c. with certain morphologic features resembling those of a plasma c., although the nuclear pattern is similar to that of a myeloblast; found in circulating blood only in pathologic conditions. SYN irritation c., Türk's leukocyte.

tympanic c.'s, SYN tympanic air c.'s.

tympanic air c.'s, numerous groovelike depressions in the walls of the tympanic cavity, communicating with the tubal air cells. SYN cellulae tympanicae [NA], tympanic c.'s.

type I c.'s, SYN squamous alveolar c.'s.

type II c.'s, SYN great alveolar c.'s.

Tzanck c.'s, acantholytic epithelial c.'s seen in the Tzanck test.

undifferentiated c., a primitive c. that has not assumed the morphologic and functional characteristics it will later acquire.

unipolar c., SYN unipolar *neuron*.

vasoformative c., SYN angioblast (1).

veil c., an antigen-presenting c. that has veil-like cytoplasmic processes and circulates in the blood and lymph. SYN veiled c.'s (1).

veiled c.'s, (1) SYN veil c. **(2)** SEE Langerhans' c.'s.

vestibular hair c.'s, c.'s in the sensory epithelium of the maculae and cristae of the membranous labyrinth of the inner ear; afferent and efferent nerve fibers of the vestibular nerve end synaptically upon them; from the apical end of each c. a bundle of stereocilia and a kinocilium extend into the statoconial membrane of the maculae and the cupula of the cristae.

Virchow's c.'s, (1) the lacunae in osseous tissue containing the bone c.'s; also the bone c.'s themselves; **(2)** SYN corneal *corpuscles*, under *corpuscle*.

virus-transformed c., a c. that has been genetically changed to a tumor c., the change being subsequently tramsmitted to all descendent c.'s; c.'s transformed by oncornaviruses continue to produce virus in high concentration without being killed; DNA tumor virus-transformed c.'s develop (along with other changes) tumor-associated antigens and rarely produce virus.

visual receptor c.'s, the rod and cone c.'s of the retina.

vitreous c., a c. occurring in the peripheral part of the vitreous body that may be responsible for production of hyaluronic acid and possibly of collagen. SYN hyalocyte.

wandering c., SYN ameboid c.

Warthin-Finkeldey c.'s, giant c.'s with multiple overlapping nuclei, found in lymphoid tissue in measles, especially during the prodromal stage.

wasserhelle c., SYN water-clear c. of parathyroid.

water-clear c. of parathyroid, a variety of chief c., so-called because the cytoplasm contains much glycogen that is not preserved or stained in the usual preparation. SYN wasserhelle c.

white blood c. (WBC), SYN leukocyte.

WI-38 c.'s, the first normal human cells, derived from fetal lung tissue, continuously cultivated. [*Wistar Institute*]

wing c., one of the polyhedral c.'s in the corneal epithelium beneath the surface layer.

yolk c.'s, primitive embryonic c.'s lying between the endoderm and mesoderm; they probably give rise to the endothelium of vitelline vessels.

zymogenic c., a c. that secretes an enzyme; specifically a chief c. of a gastric gland or an acinar c. of the pancreas. SYN albuminous c. (2), chief c. of stomach, peptic c.

---

cel·la, gen. and pl. **cel·lae** (sel'ă, sel'ē). A room or cell. [L. storeroom, or compartment]

c. me·dia, SYN *pars* centralis ventriculi lateralis.

cel·lic·o·lous (se-lik'ō-lŭs). Living within cells. [L. *cella*, cells, + *colo*, to abide in]

cel·lo·bi·ase (sel-ō-bī'ās). SYN β-D-glucosidase.

cel·lo·bi·ose (sel-ō-bī'ōs). A disaccharide obtained from cellulose and lichenin; a glucose-β(1 → 4)-glucoside, differing only from maltose in the nature of the glycoside bond. SYN cellose.

cel·lo·hex·ose (sel-ō-heks'ōs). SYN D-glucose.

cel·loi·din (se-loy'din). A solution of pyroxylin in ether and alcohol, used for embedding histologic specimens.

cel·lon (sel'on). SYN tetrachloroethane.

cel·lo·na (sel-ō'nă). A cellulose bandage impregnated with plaster of Paris.

cel·lose (sel'ōs). SYN cellobiose.

cel·lu·la, gen. and pl. **cel·lu·lae** (sel'yū-lă, -lē). **1** [NA]. In gross anatomy, a small but macroscopic compartment. SYN cellule. **2.** In histology, a cell. [L. a small chamber, dim. of *cella*]

cel′lulae anterio′res, SYN anterior ethmoidal air *cells*, under *cell*.

cel′lulae co′li, SYN *haustra* coli, under *haustrum*.

cel′lulae ethmoida′les [NA], SYN ethmoid air *cells*, under *cell*. SEE ALSO anterior ethmoidal air *cells*, under *cell*, middle ethmoidal air *cells*, under *cell*, posterior ethmoidal air *cells*, under *cell*.

cel′lulae mastoid′eae [NA], SYN mastoid air *cells*, under *cell*.

cel′lulae me′diae, SYN middle ethmoidal air *cells*, under *cell*.

cel′lulae pneumat′icae tu′bae auditi′vae [NA], SYN tubal air *cells*, under *cell*.

cel′lulae posterio′res, SYN posterior ethmoidal air *cells*, under *cell*.

cel′lulae tympan′icae [NA], SYN tympanic air *cells*, under *cell*.

cel·lu·lar (sel'yū-lăr). **1.** Relating to, derived from, or composed of cells. **2.** Having numerous compartments or interstices. [L. *cellula*, dim. of *cella*, storeroom]

cel·lu·lar·i·ty (sel-yū-lar'i-tē). The degree, quality, or condition of cells that are present.

cel·lu·lase (sel'yū-lās). Endo-1,4-β-glucase; an enzyme catalyzing the hydrolysis of 1,4-β-glucoside links in cellulose, lichenin, and other β-D-glucans; found in a variety of microorganisms in soil and in the digestive tracts of herbivores. Used to produce digestive tablets and in the removal of cellulose from foods for special diets.

cel·lule (sel′yūl). SYN cellula (1).

cel·lu·li·ci·dal (sel′yū-li-sī′dăl). Destructive to cells. [cellula + L. *caedo*, to kill]

cel·lu·lif·u·gal (sel-yū-lif′yū-găl). Moving from, or extending in a direction away from, a cell or cell body; denoting certain cells repelled by other cells, or processes extending from the body of a cell. [cellula + L. *fugio*, to flee]

cel·lu·lin (sel′yū-lin). SYN cellulose.

cel·lu·lip·e·tal (sel-yū-lip′ĕ-tăl). Moving toward, or extending in a direction toward, a cell or cell body. [cellula + L. *peto*, to seek]

cel·lu·lite (sel′yū-līt). **1.** Colloquial term for deposits of fat and fibrous tissue causing dimpling of the overlying skin. **2.** SYN lipoedema.

cel·lu·li·tis (sel-yū-lī′tis). Inflammation of cellular or connective tissue.

acute scalp c., deep inflammation of the scalp without suppuration.

anaerobic c., infection with subcutaneous soft tissues with any of a variety of anaerobic bacteria, usually a mixed culture including Bacteroides species, anaerobic cocci, and clostridia.

dissecting c., SYN *perifolliculitis* abscedens et suffodiens.

eosinophilic c., SYN Wells' *syndrome*.

epizootic c., SYN equine viral *arteritis*.

gangrenous c., infection of soft tissue with anaerobes, usually including clostridia, producing extensive tissue necrosis. SYN necrotizing c.

necrotizing c., SYN gangrenous c.

pelvic c., SYN parametritis.

phlegmonous c., obsolete term for diffuse *phlegmon.*

cel·lu·los·an (sel′yū-lō-san). SYN hemicellulose.

cel·lu·lose (sel′yū-lōs). A polysaccharide comprised of cellobiose residues, differing in this respect from starch, which is comprised of maltose residues; it forms the basis of vegetable fiber and is the most abundant organic compound. SYN cellulin. [L. *cellula*, cell, + -ose]

c. acetate, a polymer commonly used as a support medium for electrophoresis.

c. acetate phthalate, a reaction product of phthalic anhydride and a partial acetate ester of c.; used as a tablet-coating agent.

carboxymethyl c., c. in which some of the OH groups are modified to contain —CH_2—COOH groups; used in column chromatography. SYN CM-cellulose.

O-**diethylaminoethyl c.,** c. to which diethylaminoethyl groups have been attached; used in anion-exchange chromatography. SYN DEAE-cellulose.

microcrystalline c., purified, partially depolymerized c., prepared by treating α-cellulose, obtained as a pulp from fibrous plant material, with mineral acids; used as a tablet diluent.

oxidized c., (1) cellulosic acid in the form of an absorbable gauze; used as a hemostatic in operations where ligation is not feasible (capillary or venous bleeding from small vessels) because cellulosic acid has a pronounced affinity for hemoglobin and produces an artificial clot; **(2)** a sterile absorbable substance prepared by the oxidation of cotton containing not less than 16% and not more than 22% of carboxyl. SEE ALSO oxycellulose.

TEAE-c., c. to which triethylaminoethyl groups have been attached; used in ion-exchange chromatography. SYN *O*-(triethylaminoethyl) c.

O-**(triethylaminoethyl) c.,** SYN TEAE-c.

cel·lu·los·ic ac·id (sel-yū-los′ik). SEE oxidized *cellulose.*

△**celo-.** **1.** The celom. [G. *koilōma*, hollow (celom)] **2.** Hernia. [G. *kēlē*, hernia] **3.** The abdomen. SEE ALSO celio-. [G. *koilia*, belly]

ce·lom, ce·lo·ma (sē′lom, sē-lō′mă). **1.** The cavity between the splanchnic and somatic mesoderm in the embryo. **2.** SYN body cavity. [G. *koilōma*, a hollow]

extraembryonic c., that portion of the c. that extends beyond the confines of the embryonic body.

ce·lom·ic (sē-lom′ik). Relating to the body *cavity.*

ce·lo·nych·ia (sē-lō-nik′ē-ă). SYN koilonychia. [G. *koilos*, hollowed, + *onyx* (*onych*-), nail]

ce·lo·phle·bi·tis (sē-lō-flē-bī′tis). Inflammation of a vena cava. SYN cavitis. [G. *koilos*, hollow, + phlebitis]

ce·lo·scope (sē′lō-skōp). Rarely used term for an optical device for examining the interior of a body cavity. [G. *koilos*, hollow, + *skopeō*, to view]

ce·los·co·py (sē-los′kŏ-pē). Rarely used term for examination of any body cavity with an optical instrument.

ce·lo·so·mia (sē-lō-sō′mē-ă). Congenital protrusion of the abdominal or thoracic viscera, usually with a defect of the sternum and ribs as well as of the abdominal walls. SYN kelosomia. [G. *kēlē*, hernia, + *sōma*, body]

Ce·lo·vi·rus (sel′ō-vī-rŭs). An adenovirus found in chickens.

ce·lo·zo·ic (sē-lō-zō′ik). Inhabiting any of the cavities of the body; applied to certain parasitic protozoa, chiefly gregarines. [G. *koilos*, hollow, + *zoikos*, pertaining to animals]

Celsius, Anders, Swedish astronomer, 1701–1744. SEE Celsius *scale.*

cel·si·us (C). SEE Celsius *scale.*

Celsus, Aulus (Aurelius) Cornelius, Roman physician and medical writer, *ca.* 30 B.C.–45 A.D. SEE C.'s *alopecia, area;* C. *kerion;* C.'s *papules,* under *papule, vitiligo.*

ce·ment (se-ment′). **1.** SYN cementum. **2.** In dentistry, a nonmetallic material used for luting, filling, or permanent or temporary restorative purposes, made by mixing components into a plastic mass that sets, or as an adherent sealer in attaching various dental restorations in or on the tooth. [see cementum]

composite dental c., an organic dental c. modified by the inclusion of inorganic materials treated with a coupling agent to bond them to the polymers.

copper phosphate c., a dental preparation, the combination of a solution of orthophosphoric acid with a c. powder (usually zinc oxide) modified with varying proportions of copper oxide.

dental c., SEE cement (2).

glass ionomer c., a dental c. produced by mixing a powder prepared from a calcium aluminosilicate glass with an aqueous solution of polyacrylic acid. [ion + -mer (1)]

inorganic dental c., a dental c. consisting usually of metallic salts or oxides which, when mixed with a specific liquid, form a plastic mass that sets.

intercellular c., a hypothetical adhesive substance formerly believed to occur between some epithelial cells.

modified zinc oxide-eugenol c., dental c. obtained by mixing zinc oxide and eugenol with one or more additives.

organic dental c., a dental c. consisting mainly of synthetic polymers.

polycarboxylate c., a powder containing primarily zinc oxide mixed with a liquid containing polyacrylic acid which reacts to form a hard crystalline mass upon standing; when used to lute metal castings to teeth, it has the potential of bonding to the calcium contained in tooth structure as well as to any base metals contained in the casting.

resin c., a monomer or monomer/polymer system used as a dental luting agent; used in cementation of restorations or orthodontic brackets to the teeth.

silicate c., a dental filling material prepared by mixing a modified phosphoric acid solution with a powdered silica alumina fluoride glass.

tooth c., SYN cementum. SEE cement (2).

unmodified zinc oxide-eugenol c., a dental c. obtained by mixing zinc oxide and eugenol without modifiers.

zinc phosphate c., a powder, containing primarily zinc oxide mixed with a liquid containing orthophosphoric acid to form a hard crystalline mass on standing, used in dentistry as a luting agent for cast metal restorations and orthodontic bands, and as a temporary restorative material, or a base under restorations, particularly in deep cavities.

ce·men·ta·tion (sē-men-tā'shŭn). **1.** The process of attaching parts by means of a cement. **2.** In dentistry, attaching a restoration to natural teeth by means of a cement.

ce·ment·i·cle (se-men'ti-kl). A calcified spherical body, composed of cementum lying free within the periodontal membrane, attached to the cementum or imbedded within it.

ce·ment·i·fi·ca·tion (se-men'ti-fi-kā'shŭn). Metaplastic production of cementum or cementoid within a less differentiated connective tissue, *e.g.,* c. of a fibroma.

ce·ment·o·blast (se-men'tō-blast). One of the cells concerned with the formation of the layer of cementum on the roots of teeth. [L. *cementum*, cement, + G. *blastos*, germ]

ce·ment·o·blas·to·ma (se-men'tō-blas-tō'mă). A benign odontogenic tumor of functional cementoblasts; it appears as a mixed radiolucent-radiopaque lesion attached to a tooth root and may cause expansion of the bone cortex or be associated with pain. SYN benign c., true cementoma.

benign c., SYN cementoblastoma.

ce·ment·o·cla·sia (se-men-tō-klā'zē-ă). Destruction of cementum by cementoclasts. [L. *cementum*, cement, + G. *klasis*, fracture]

ce·ment·o·clast (se-men'tō-klast). One of the multinucleated giant cells, identical with osteoclasts, that are associated with the resorption of cementum. [L. *cementum*, cement, + G. *klastos*, broken]

ce·ment·o·cyte (se-men'tō-sīt). An osteocyte-like cell with numerous processes, trapped in a lacuna in the cementum of the tooth. [L. *cementum*, cement, + G. *kytos*, cell]

ce·ment·o·den·tin·al (se-men'tō-den'ti-năl). SYN dentinocemental.

ce·men·to·gen·e·sis (se-men'to-jen'ĕ-sis). The development of the cementum over the root dentin of a tooth. [cementum + G. *genesis*, production]

ce·men·to·ma (se-men-tō'mă). Nonspecific term referring to any benign cementum-producing tumor; four types are recognized: 1) periapical cemental dysplasia, 2) central ossifying fibroma, 3) cementoblastoma, 4) sclerotic cemental mass. When the type is not specified, c. usually refers to periapical cemental *dysplasia.* [L. *cementum*, cement, + G. *-ōma*, tumor]

gigantiform c., the familial occurrence of cemental masses in the jaws; inherited as an autosomal dominant characteristic. SEE ALSO sclerotic cemental *mass.*

true c., SYN cementoblastoma.

ce·men·tum (se-men'tŭm) [NA]. A layer of bone-like mineralized tissue covering the dentin of the root and neck of a tooth that blends with the fibers of the periodontal ligament. SYN cement (1), substantia ossea dentis, tooth cement. [L. *caementum*, rough quarry stone, fr. *caedo*, to cut]

afibrillar c., c. which, with the electron microscope, appears as laminated, electron-dense reticular material that sometimes overlies the enamel of the tooth.

primary c., c. that has no cementocytes; may cover the entire root of the tooth, but often is missing on the apical third of the root.

secondary c., c. that forms on the root surface after eruption; it contains cementocytes.

ce·nes·the·sia (sē-nes-thē'zē-ă). The general sense of bodily existence; the sensation caused by the functioning of the internal organs. SYN coenesthesia, sixth sense. [G. *koinos*, common, + *aisthēsis*, sensation]

ce·nes·the·sic, ce·nes·thet·ic (sē-nes-thē'zik, -sik; -thet'ik). Relating to cenesthesia.

ce·nes·thop·a·thy (sē-nes-thop'ă-thē). Rarely used term for a feeling or sense of general ill-being not related to any particular organ or part of the body. [G. *koinos*, common, + *aisthēsis*, sensation, + *pathos*, suffering]

⚠**ceno-.** **1.** Shared in common. [G. *koinos*, common] **2.** New, fresh. [G. *kainos*, new] **3.** Emptiness (rare). SEE ALSO coeno-. [G. *kenos*, empty]

ce·no·cyte (sē'nō-sīt). A multinucleate cell or hypha without cross walls, characteristic of the hyphae of zygomycetes. SEE

ALSO nonseptate *mycelium.* SYN coenocyte. [G. *koinos*, common, + *kytos*, cell]

ce·no·cyt·ic (sē-nō-sit'ik). Pertaining to or having characteristics of a cenocyte. SYN coenocytic.

cen·o·site (sē'nō-sīt). A facultative commensal organism; one that can sustain itself apart from its usual host. SYN coinosite. [G. *koinos*, common, + *sitos*, food]

ce·no·trope (sē'nō-trōp). A scientifically more accurate term than the earlier "instinct", denoting the behavior pattern shown by all members of a large group having the same biologic equipment and same experience. [G. *koinos*, common, + *tropē*, a turning]

cen·sor (sen'sōr). In psychoanalytic theory, the psychic barrier that prevents certain unconscious thoughts and wishes from coming to consciousness unless they are so cloaked or disguised as to be unrecognizable. [L. a judge, critic, fr. *censeo*, to value, judge]

cen·sus. An enumeration of a population, originally for taxation and military purposes, now with many other purposes; basic facts about all persons—age, sex, occupation, nature of residence, etc.— are recorded at the census, which often also includes some information about health status. [L., fr. *censeo*, to count]

cen·ter (sen'ter). **1.** The middle point of a body; loosely, the interior of a body. A center of any kind, especially an anatomical center. **2.** A group of nerve cells governing a specific function. SYN centrum [NA]. [L. *centrum;* G. *kentron*]

active c., the part of a macromolecule at which a substrate or ligand, upon binding, produces biological activity; for an enzyme, this is the catalytic c., the site on an enzyme that catalyzes the reaction.

anospinal c., the c. in the spinal cord that controls the contraction of the anal sphincter.

Broca's c., the posterior part of the inferior frontal gyrus of the left or dominant hemisphere, corresponding approximately to Brodmann's area 44; Broca identified this region as an essential component of the motor mechanisms governing articulated speech. SYN Broca's area, Broca's field, motor speech c.

Budge's c., SYN ciliospinal c.

catalytic c., SEE active c.

cell c., SYN cytocentrum.

chondrification c., a site of earliest cartilage formation in the body.

ciliospinal c., the preganglionic motor neurons in the first thoracic segment of the spinal cord which give rise to the sympathetic innervation of the dilator muscle of the eye's pupil. SYN Budge's c.

dentary c., a specific ossification c. of the mandible that gives rise to the lower border of its outer plate.

diaphysial c., primary c. of ossification in the shaft of a long bone.

epiotic c., the c. of ossification of the petrous part of the temporal bone that appears posterior to the posterior semicircular canal.

expiratory c., the region of the medulla oblongata that is electrically active during expiration and where electrical stimulation produces sustained expiration.

feeding c., a region of the lateral zone of the hypothalamus, electrical stimulation of which in the rat elicits uninterrupted eating; destruction of the region causes long-lasting anorexia.

germinal c. of Flemming, the lightly staining c. in a lymphatic nodule in which the predominant cells are large lymphocytes and macrophages. SYN reaction c.

inspiratory c., the region of the medulla oblongata that is electrically active during inspiration and where electrical stimulation produces sustained inspiration.

Kerckring's c., an occasional independent ossification c. in the occipital bone; it appears in the posterior margin of the foramen magnum at about the sixteenth week of gestation. SYN Kerckring's ossicle.

medullary c., SYN *centrum* semiovale.

microtubule-organizing c., a locus in interphase and mitotic cells from which most microtubules radiate; in the center of this c. is the centriole; this c. determines the polarity of cellular microtubules.

motor speech c., SYN Broca's c.

ossific c., SYN c. of ossification.

c. of ossification, the site of earliest bone formation via accumulation of osteoblasts within connective tissue (membranous ossification) or of earliest destruction of cartilage prior to onset of ossification (endochondral ossification). SYN punctum ossificationis [NA], ossific c., point of ossification.

primary c. of ossification, this is the first site where bone begins to form in the shaft of a long bone or in the body of an irregular bone. SYN punctum ossificationis primarium [NA], primary point of ossification.

reaction c., SYN germinal c. of Flemming.

respiratory c., the region in the medulla oblongata concerned with integrating afferent information to determine the signals to the respiratory muscles; the inspiratory and expiratory c.'s considered together.

c. of ridge, the buccolingual midline of the residual ridge.

c. of rotation, a point or line around which all other points in a body move. SEE axis.

satiety c., a term referring to the region of the ventromedial nucleus in the hypothalamus; destruction of this small region in the rat leads to continuous eating and extreme obesity.

secondary c. of ossification, this is the center of bone formation appearing later than the punctum ossificationis primarium, usually in epiphysis. SYN punctum ossificationis secundarium [NA], secondary point of ossification.

semioval c., SYN *centrum* semiovale.

sensory speech c., SYN Wernicke's c.

speech c.'s, areas of the cerebral cortex centrally involved in speech function; one is in the left inferior frontal gyrus, a second one in the supramarginal, angular, and first and second temporal gyri. SEE ALSO Broca's c., Wernicke's c.

sphenotic c., one of the paired c.'s of ossification of the sphenoid bone.

vasomotor c., diffuse area of the reticular formation in the lateral medulla containing neurons that control vascular tone; consists of separate vasodepressor and vasopressor areas.

vital c., c. essential to life; usually refers to the centers located in the medulla oblongata which are necessary for the maintenance of respiration and circulation.

Wernicke's c., the region of the cerebral cortex thought to be essential for understanding and formulating coherent, propositional speech; it encompasses a large region of the parietal and temporal lobes near the lateral sulcus of the left cerebral hemisphere; corresponding approximately to Brodmann's areas 40, 39, and 22. SYN sensory speech c., Wernicke's area, Wernicke's field, Wernicke's region, Wernicke's zone.

Cen·ters for Dis·ease Con·trol (CDC). The federal facility for disease eradication, epidemiology, and education headquartered in Atlanta, Georgia, which encompasses the Center for Infectious Diseases, Center for Environmental Health, Center for Health Promotion and Education, Center for Prevention Services, Center for Professional Development and Training, and Center for Occupational Safety and Health. Formerly named Center for Disease Control (1970), Communicable Disease Center (1946).

cen·te·sis (sen-tē'sis). Puncture, especially when used as a suffix, as in paracentesis. [G. *kentēsis*, puncture, fr. *kenteō*, to prick, pierce]

△**centi- (c).** Prefix used in the SI and metric systems to signify one hundredth (10^{-2}). [L. *centum*, one hundred]

cen·ti·bar (sen'ti-bar). One hundredth of a bar.

cen·ti·grade (C) (sen'ti-grād). 1. Basis of the former temperature scale in which 100 degrees separated the melting and boiling points of water. SEE Celsius *scale*. 2. One hundredth of a circle, equal to 3.6° of the astronomical circle. [L. *centum*, one hundred, + *gradus*, step, degree]

cen·ti·gram (sen'ti-gram). One hundredth of a gram; 0.15432358 grain.

cen·tile (sen'til). SYN quantile. [L. *centum*, one hundred, + *-ilis*, adj. suffix]

cen·ti·li·ter (sen'ti-lē-ter). 10 Milliliters; one hundredth of a liter; 162.3073 minims (U.S.).

cen·ti·me·ter (cm) (sen'ti-mē-ter). One hundredth of a meter; 0.3937008 inch.

cubic c. (cc, c.c.), one thousandth of a liter; 1 milliliter.

cen·ti·mor·gan (cM) (sen'ti-mōr-găn). SEE Morgan.

cen·ti·nor·mal (sen-ti-nōr'măl). One hundredth normal; denoting the concentration of a solution.

cen·ti·pede (sen'ti-pēd). A venomous predatory arthropod of the order Chilopoda, characterized by one pair of legs per leg-bearing segment. The venom is injected through the first pair of leg-like appendages, modified into piercing claws; the bites may be painful and locally necrotic, but seldom are dangerous, except to very young children. Genera found in the U.S. include *Scutigera*, *Lithobius*, *Scolopendra*, and *Geophilus*. [L. *centum*, hundred, + *pes* (*ped-*), foot]

cen·ti·poise (sen'ti-poyz). One hundredth of a poise.

cen·tra (sen'tră). Plural of centrum.

cen·trad (sen'trad). 1. Toward the center. 2. A unit of measurement of the refracting strength of a prism; it corresponds to the deviation of a ray of light, the arc of which is $^1/_{100}$ of the radius of the circle, or 0.57°.

cen·trage (sen'trāj). The condition in which the optical centers of all the reflecting and refracting surfaces of an optical system are on the same axis.

cen·tra·lis (sen-trā'lis) [NA]. Central; in the center. [L.]

cen·tre mé·di·an de Luys (sen'tr mă-dē-an). SYN centromedian *nucleus*. [Fr.]

cen·tren·ce·phal·ic (sen'tren-se-fal'ik). Relating to the center of the encephalon.

△**cen·tri-** (sen'trik). Combining form denoting center.

△**centric.** Having a center (of a specific kind or number) or having a specific thing as its center (of interest, focus, etc.). [G. *kentron*, center]

cen·tric·i·put (sen-tris'i-put). The central portion of the upper surface of the skull, between the occiput and the sinciput. [L. *centrum*, center, + *caput*, head]

cen·trif·u·gal (sen-trif'yū-găl). 1. Denoting the direction of the force pulling an object outward (away) from an axis of rotation. 2. Sometimes, by analogy, extended to describe any movement away from a center. Cf. eccentric (2). [L. *centrum*, center, + *fugio*, to flee]

cen·trif·u·gal·i·za·tion (sen-trif'yū-găl-i-zā'shŭn). SYN centrifugation.

cen·trif·u·gal·ize (sen-trif'yū-găl-īz). SYN centrifuge (2).

cen·trif·u·ga·tion (sen-trif-yū-gā'shŭn). Subjection to sedimentation, by means of a centrifuge, of solids suspended in a fluid. SYN centrifugalization.

band c., SYN density gradient c.

density gradient c., ultracentrifugation of substances in concentrated solutions of cesium salts or of sucrose; at equilibrium, the medium exhibits a concentration (hence density) gradient increasing in the direction of centrifugal force and the substances of interest collect in layers at the levels of their densities. SEE isopycnic *zone*. SYN band c., zone c.

zone c., SYN density gradient c.

cen·tri·fuge (sen'tri-fūj). 1. An apparatus by means of which particles in suspension in a fluid are separated by spinning the fluid, the centrifugal force throwing the particles to the periphery of the rotated vessel. 2. To submit to rapid rotary action, as in a c. SYN centrifugalize.

cen·tri·lob·u·lar (sen-tri-lob'yū-lăr). At or near the center of a lobule, *e.g.*, of the liver.

cen·tri·ole (sen'trē-ōl). Tubular structures, 150 nm by 300 to 500 nm, with a wall having 9 triple microtubules, usually seen as paired organelles lying in the cytocentrum; c.'s may be multiple and numerous in some cells, such as the giant cells of bone marrow. [G. *kentron*, a point, center]

anterior c., SYN proximal c.

distal c., the c. in the developing spermatozoon from which the flagellum develops. SYN posterior c.

posterior c., SYN distal c.

proximal c., the c. that lies in a depression in the wall of the posterior portion of the nucleus of the developing spermatozoon. SYN anterior c.

cen·trip·e·tal (sen-trip′ĕ-tăl). **1.** SYN afferent. **2.** Denoting the direction of the force pulling an object toward an axis of rotation. SYN axipetal. [L. *centrum,* center, + *peto,* to seek]

⌂**centro-.** Combining form denoting center. [G. *kentron*]

cen·tro·blast (sen′trō-blast). A lymphocyte with a large non-cleaved nucleus. [centro- + G. *blastos,* germ]

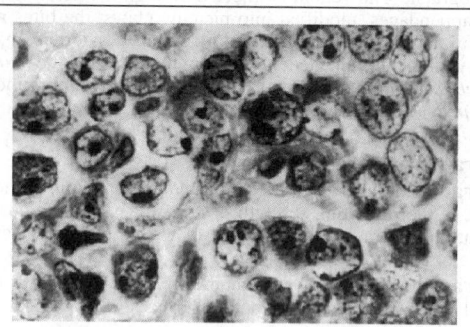

centroblasts
note relatively pale nuclei of c. in this lymphoma

Cen·tro·ces·tus (sen-trō-ses′tŭs). A genus of extremely small fish-borne flukes (family Heterophyidae) that may produce intestinal lesions similar to those caused by *Heterophyes heterophyes. C. formosana* has been reported from man in Taiwan. [G. *kentron,* point, center, + *kestos,* belt, both words fr. *kenteō,* to pierce]

cen·tro·cyte (sen′trō-sīt). **1.** A cell whose protoplasm contains single and double granules of varying size stainable with hematoxylin; seen in lesions of lichen planus. SYN Lipschütz cell. **2.** A lymphocyte with a small cleaved nuclei. [centro- + G. *kytos,* cell]

cen·tro·ki·ne·sia (sen′trō-ki-nē′sē-ă). Movement excited by a stimulus of central origin. [centro- + G. *kinēsis,* movement]

cen·tro·ki·net·ic (sen′trō-ki-net′ik). **1.** Relating to centrokinesia. **2.** SYN excitomotor.

cen·tro·lec·i·thal (sen-trō-les′i-thăl). Denoting an ovum in which the deutoplasm accumulates centrally. [centro- + G. *lekithos,* yolk]

cen·tro·mere (sen′trō-mēr). **1.** The nonstaining primary constriction of a chromosome which is the point of attachment of the spindle fiber; provides the mechanism of chromosome movement during cell division; the c. divides the chromosome into two arms, and its position is constant for a specific chromosome: near one end (acrocentric), near the center (metacentric), or between (submetacentric). [centro- + G. *meros,* part]

cen·tro·plasm (sen′trō-plazm). The substance of the cytocentrum. [centro- + G. *plasma,* thing formed]

cen·tro·some (sen′trō-sōm). SYN cytocentrum. [centro- + G. *sōma,* body]

cen·tro·sphere (sen′trō-sfēr). The specialized, often gelated cytoplasm of the cytocentrum. Contains the centrioles from which the astral fibers (microtubules) extend during mitosis. SYN astrocele, statosphere. [centro- + G. *sphaira,* a ball, sphere]

cen·tro·stal·tic (sen-trō-stal′tik). Relating to the center of motion. [centro- + G. *stallein,* set forth, fetch]

cen·trum, pl. **cen·tra** (sen′trŭm, sen′tră) [NA]. SYN center. [L. fr. G. *kentron*]

c. media′num, SYN centromedian *nucleus.*

c. medulla′re, SYN c. semiovale.

c. ova′le, SYN c. semiovale.

c. semiova′le, the great mass of white matter composing the interior of the cerebral hemisphere; the name refers to the general shape of this white core in horizontal sections of the hemisphere. SYN c. medullare, c. ovale, medullary center, semioval center, Vicq d'Azyr's c. semiovale, Vieussens' c.

c. tendin′eum diaphrag′matis [NA], SYN central *tendon* of diaphragm.

c. tendin′eum perine′i [NA], SYN central *tendon* of perineum.

c. of a vertebra, (1) the ossification center of the central mass of the body of a vertebra; **(2)** *body* of vertebra (as distinct from the arches).

Vicq d'Azyr's c. semiova′le, SYN c. semiovale.

Vieussens' c., SYN c. semiovale.

Willis' c. nervo′sum, SYN celiac *ganglia,* under *ganglion.*

Cen·tru·roi·des (sen-tru-roy′dēz). A genus of North American scorpions, the commonest species of which are *C. gracilis,* the margarite scorpion; *C. vittatus,* the stripe-back scorpion; and *C. sculpturatus,* the deadly sculptured scorpion. SEE ALSO Scorpionida.

cen·tum (c) (sen-tum). L. hundred [L. one hundred]

cen·u·ris, coe·nu·ris (se-nyū′ris). A tapeworm bladderworm with multiple inverted scoleces attached to the inner germinative layer; produced by taeniid cestodes of the genus *Multiceps,* typically found in the brain or tissues of herbivores and the adult worm in the intestine of wolves, dogs, or other canids; rare cases of c. infections in man have been reported. [G. *kenos,* empty, + G. *uris,* tail]

cen·u·ro·sis, ce·nu·ri·a·sis (sen-yū-rō′sis, sen-yū-rī′ă-sis). Disease produced by the presence of a cenuris cyst that, in sheep, causes a brain infection known as "gid" for the giddy gait induced in the infected animal; human c. has been reported but is extremely unusual, in contrast with hydatid disease. SYN coenurosis.

ce·pha·e·line (sef-a′ĕ-lēn). $C_{28}H_{38}N_2O_2$; Desmethylemetine; dihydropsychotrine; an alkaloid of ipecac; an emetic and amebicide.

Ceph·a·e·lis (sef-ă-ē′lis). SYN *Uragoga.* [G. *kephalē,* head, + *eilō,* to roll up, pack close]

⌂**cephal-.** SEE cephalo-.

ceph·a·lad (sef′ă-lad). In a direction toward the head. SEE ALSO cranial (1).

ceph·a·lal·gia (sef-al-al′jē-ă). SYN headache. [cephal- + G. *algos,* pain]

histaminic c., SYN cluster *headache.*

Horton's c., SYN cluster *headache.*

ceph·a·lea (sef-ă-lē′ă). SYN headache.

c. agita′ta, c. atton′ita, violent headache sometimes occurring in influenza and in the early stages of other infectious diseases.

ceph·al·e·de·ma (sef-al-ĕ-dē′mă). Edema of the head.

ceph·a·le·mia (sef-ă-lē′-mē-ă). Congestion, active or passive, of the brain. [cephal- + G. *haima,* blood]

ceph·a·lex·in (sef-ă-lek′sin). A broad spectrum antibiotic derived from cephalosporin C.

ceph·al·he·ma·to·cele (sef′ăl-hē-mat′ō-sēl). A cephalhematoma under the pericranium communicating with the dural sinuses. SYN cephalohematocele. [cephal- + G. *haima,* blood, + *kēlē,* tumor]

ceph·al·he·ma·to·ma (sef′ăl-hē-mă-tō′mă). A collection of blood due to an effusion of blood beneath the periosteum frequently in a newborn as a result of birth trauma; contrasted with caput succedaneum, in which the effusion overlies the periosteum and consists of serum. SYN cephalohematoma. [cephal- + G. *haima,* blood, + -*ōma,* tumor]

ceph·al·hy·dro·cele (sef-ăl-hī′drō-sēl). An accumulation of serous or watery fluid under the pencranium. [cephal- + G. *hydōr,* water, + *kēlē,* tumor]

ce·phal·ic (se-fal′ik). SYN cranial (1).

ceph·a·lin (sef′ă-lin). A term formerly applied to a group of phosphatidic esters resembling lecithin but containing either 2-ethanolamine or L-serine in the place of choline; these are now known as phosphatidylethanolamine and phosphatidylserine. They are widely distributed in the body, especially in the brain and spinal cord, and are used as local hemostatics and as reagents in liver function test. SYN kephalin.

ceph·a·line (sef′ă-līn). Denoting members of the protozoan suborder Cephalina (order Eugregarinida), characterized by bodies divided into chambers (anterior protomerite and posterior deutomerite, or anterior epimerite, protomerite, and terminal deutomerite); all are parasites of invertebrates.

ceph·a·li·tis (sef-ă-lī′tis). SYN encephalitis.

ceph·a·li·za·tion (sef′ăl-ĭ-zā′shŭn). **1.** Evolutionary tendency for important functions of the nervous system to move forward in the brain. **2.** Initiation and concentration of the growth tendency at the anterior end of the embryo.

◊**cephalo-, cephal-.** The head. [G. *kephalē*]

ceph·a·lo·cau·dal (sef′ă-lō-kaw′dăl). Relating to both head and tail, *i.e.,* to the long axis of the body. [cephalo- + L. *cauda,* tail]

ceph·a·lo·cele (sef′ă-lō-sēl). Protrusion of part of the cranial contents, *e.g.,* meningocele, encephalocele. SEE ALSO encephalocele.

ceph·a·lo·cen·te·sis (sef′ă-lō-sen-tē′sis). Passage of a hollow needle or trocar and cannula into the brain to drain or aspirate an abscess or the fluid of a hydrocephalus. [cephalo- + G. *kentēsis,* puncture]

ceph·a·lo·chord (sef′ă-lō-kōrd). Intracranial portion of the notochord in the embryo.

ceph·a·lo·did·y·mus (sef′ă-lō-did′i-mŭs). Conjoined twins fused except in the cephalic region; a variety of duplicitas posterior. SEE conjoined *twins,* under *twin.* [cephalo- + G. *didymos,* twin]

ceph·a·lo·di·pros·o·pus (sef′ă-lō-dī-pros′ō-pŭs). Asymmetrical conjoined twins with the head of the autosite carrying a reduced parasitic head. SEE conjoined *twins,* under *twin,* diprosopus. [cephalo- + G. *di-,* two, + *prosōpon,* face]

ceph·a·lo·dyn·ia (sef′ă-lō-din′ē-ă). Headache. [cephalo- + G. *odynē,* pain]

ceph·a·lo·gen·e·sis (sef′ă-lō-jen′ĕ-sis). Formation of the head in the embryonic period. [cephalo- + G. *genesis,* production]

ceph·a·lo·gly·cin (sef′ă-lō-glī′sin). A semisynthetic broad spectrum antibiotic produced from cephalosporin C.

ceph·a·lo·gram (sef′ă-lō-gram). SYN cephalometric *radiograph.*

ceph·a·lo·gy·ric (sef′ă-lō-jī′rik). Relating to rotation of the head. [cephalo- + G. *gyros,* a circle]

ceph·a·lo·he·ma·to·cele (sef′ă-lō-hē-mat′ō-sēl). SYN cephalhematocele.

ceph·a·lo·he·ma·to·ma (sef′ă-lō-hē-mă-tō′mă). SYN cephalhematoma.

ceph·a·lo·he·mom·e·ter (sef′ă-lō-hē-mom′ĕ-ter). An instrument showing the degree of intracranial blood pressure. [cephalo- + G. *haima,* blood, + *metron,* measure]

ceph·a·lo·meg·a·ly (sef′ă-lō-meg′ă-lē). Enlargement of the head. [cephalo- + G. *megas,* great]

ceph·a·lom·e·lus (sef-ă-lom′ĕ-lŭs). Malformed individual with an accessory limb, resembling a leg or arm, growing from the head. [cephalo- + G. *melos,* a limb]

ceph·a·lo·men·in·gi·tis (sef′ă-lō-men-in-jī′tis). Obsolete term for meningitis. [cephalo- + G. *mēninx* (*mēning-*), membrane]

ceph·a·lom·e·ter (sef-ă-lom′ĕ-ter). An instrument used to position the head to produce oriented, reproducible lateral and posterior-anterior headfilms. SYN cephalostat. [cephalo- + G. *metron,* measure]

ceph·a·lo·met·rics (sef-ă-lō-met′riks). In oral surgery and orthodontics: **1.** The scientific measurement of the bones of the cranium and face, utilizing a fixed, reproducible position for lateral radiographic exposure of skull and facial bones. **2.** A scientific study of the measurements of the head with relation to specific reference points; used for evaluation of facial growth and development, including soft tissue profile. [cephalo- + G. *metron,* measure]

ceph·a·lom·e·try (sef-ă-lom′ĕ-trē). Measurements on the living head, or head without removal of the soft parts. SEE ALSO cephalometrics. [cephalo- + G. *metron,* measure]

ultrasonic c., measurement of the fetal head by ultrasound.

ceph·a·lo·mo·tor (sef′ă-lō-mō′ter). Relating to movements of the head.

Ceph·a·lo·my·ia (sef′ă-lō-mī′yă). Former name for *Oestrus.* [cephalo- + G. *myia,* fly]

ceph·a·lont (sef′ă-lont). Adult stage of a cephaline gregarine, a sporozoan parasite commonly found in arthropods and other invertebrate hosts. The body is usually divided by a septum into an anterior epimerite and protomerite and a posterior deutomerite; acephaline gregarines lack a dividing septum. [cephalo- + G. *ōn* (*ont-*), being]

ceph·a·lop·a·gus (sef-ă-lop′ă-gŭs). Conjoined twins with heads fused but the remainder of the bodies separate. SEE conjoined *twins,* under *twin.* SEE ALSO craniopagus, *duplicitas* posterior. [cephalo- + G. *pagos,* something fixed]

ceph·a·lop·a·thy (sef-ă-lop′ă-thē). SYN encephalopathy. [cephalo- + G. *pathos,* suffering]

ceph·a·lo·pel·vic (sef′ă-lō-pel′vik). Pertaining to the size of the fetal head in relation to the maternal pelvis.

ceph·a·lo·pel·vim·e·try (sef′ă-lō-pel-vim′ĕ-trē). Roentgenographic measurement of the dimensions of the pelvis and the fetal head. SYN pelvicephalography, pelvocephalography. [cephalo- + pelvimetry]

ceph·a·lo·pha·ryn·ge·us (sef′ă-lō-fă-rin′jē-ŭs). SEE superior constrictor *muscle* of pharynx.

ceph·a·lor·i·dine (sef-ă-lōr′i-dēn). A broad spectrum antimicrobial derived from cephalosporin C.

ceph·a·lor·rha·chid·i·an (sef′ă-lō-ra-kid′ē-an). Relating to the head and the spine. [cephalo- + G. *rhachis,* spine]

ceph·a·lo·spor·an·ic ac·id (sef′ă-lō-spōr-an′ik). The basic chemical nucleus upon which cephalosporin antibiotic derivatives are based.

ceph·a·lo·spo·rin (sef′ă-lō-spōr′in). This is an antibiotic produced by a *Cephalosporium,* but since the antibiotic was discovered the name Cephalosporium has been removed and the new name is Acremonium.

c. C, an antibiotic whose activity is due to the 7-aminocephalosporanic acid portion of the cephalosporanic acid molecule; it is effective against Gram-positive and Gram-negative bacteria, but is less potent than c. N. Addition of side chains produced semisynthetic broad spectrum antibiotics with greater antibacterial activity than that of c. C; the antibiotic activity is due to interference with bacterial cell-wall synthesis.

c. N, D-4-amino-4-carboxybutyl penicillinic acid; an antibiotic active against Gram-positive and Gram-negative bacteria, but inactivated by penicillinase; on hydrolysis it yields penicillamine. SYN penicillin N, synnematin B.

c. P, a steroid antibiotic produced by *Cephalosporium,* chemically related to fusidic and helvolic acids, that is active only against Gram-positive bacteria.

ceph·a·lo·spor·i·nase (sef′ă-lō-spōr′i-nās). SYN β-lactamase.

Ceph·a·lo·spo·ri·um (sef′ă-lō-spō′rē-ŭm). Former name of *Acremonium.*

ceph·a·lo·stat (sef′ă-lō-stat). SYN cephalometer. [cephalo- + G. *statos,* stationary]

ceph·a·lo·thin (sef-ă-lō′thin). 7-(Thiophene-2-acetamido)-cephalosporanic acid; chemically modified cephalosporin C, a broad spectrum antibiotic.

ceph·a·lo·tho·rac·ic (sef′ă-lō-thō-ras′ik). Relating to the head and the chest.

ceph·a·lo·tho·ra·cop·a·gus (sef′ă-lō-thōr-ă-kop′ă-gŭs). Conjoined twins with the bodies fused in the cephalic and thoracic regions. SEE conjoined *twins,* under *twin.* [cephalo- + G. *thorax,* chest, + *pagos,* something fixed]

c. asym′metros, SYN c. monosymmetros.

c. disym′metros, a form of c. with the fused head showing equally developed faces directed laterally.

c. monosym′metros, a form of c. in which only one of the faces is well developed. SYN c. asymmetros.

ceph·a·lo·tome (sef′ă-lō-tōm). Instrument formerly used for cutting into the fetal head to permit its compression in cases of dystocia. [cephalo- + G. *tomē,* a cutting]

ceph·a·lot·o·my (sef-ă-lot′ō-mē). Formerly used operation of cutting into the head of the fetus.

ceph·a·lo·tox·in (sef′ă-lō-tok′sin). A poison, believed to be a protein, found in the salivary glands of cephalopods (octopus). SEE ALSO eledoisin.

ceph·a·lo·tribe (sef′ă-lō-trīb). Forceps-like instrument, with strong blades and a screw handle, formerly used to crush the fetal head in cases of dystocia. [G. *tribō*, to rub, bruise]

ceph·a·my·cins (sef'ă-mī'sin). A family of β-lactam antibiotics (similar to penicillin and cephalosporins) produced by various *Streptomyces* species.

ceph·a·pi·rin so·di·um (sef-ă-pī'rin). A semisynthetic broad spectrum antibiotic derived from cephalosporin C; it is used by injection.

ceph·ra·dine (sef'ră-dēn). A semisynthetic broad spectrum antibiotic derived from cephalosporin C; used orally and by injection.

cep·tor (sep'ter, tōr). SYN receptor (2). [L. *capio*, pp. *captus*, to take]

chemical c., c. that initiates chemical reactions in response to the appropriate stimuli.

contact c., a nerve c. in the surface layer of skin or mucous membrane by means of which impulses contributed by direct physical impact are received.

distance c., a nerve mechanism of one of the organs of special sense whereby the subject is brought into relation with his distant environment.

△-ceptor. Combining form denoting taker, receiver. [L. *capio*, pp. *captus*, to take]

ce·ra (sē'ră). SYN wax (1). [L.]

ce·ra·ceous (se-rā'shŭs). Waxen. [L. *cera*, wax]

cer·am·i·dase (ser-am'i-dās). An enzyme that hydrolyzes ceramides into sphingosine and a fatty acid. A deficiency of this enzyme is associated with Farber's disease.

cer·a·mide (ser'ă-mīd). Generic term for a class of sphingolipid, *N*-acyl (fatty acid) derivatives of a long chain base or sphingoid such as sphinganine or sphingosine; *e.g.,* $CH_3(CH_2)_{12}CH=CH-CHOH-CH(CH_2 OH)-NH-CO-R$, where *R* is the fatty-acid residue, attached in this example to 4-sphingenine (sphingosine) in amide linkage. C.'s accumulate in individuals with Farber's disease.

c. dihexoside, the accumulated glycolipid noted in glycolipid lipidosis.

c. lactosidase, a hydrolytic enzyme (a β-galactosidase) that acts on c. lactoside, producing glucosylceramide and galactose. A deficiency of this enzyme can result in c. lactoside liposis. Cf. cytolipin.

c. 1-phosphorylcholine, SYN sphingomyelins.

c. saccharide, SYN glycosphingolipid.

cer·a·sin (ser'ă-sin). SYN kerasin.

△cerat-. SEE kerat-.

ce·rate (sē'rāt). A rarely used unctuous solid preparation, harder than an ointment, containing sufficient wax to prevent it from melting when applied to the skin. [L. *cera*, wax]

cer·a·tin (ser'a-tin). SYN keratin.

△cerato-. SEE kerato-.

cer·a·to·cri·coid (ser'ă-tō-krī'koyd). Relating to the inferior cornua of the thyroid cartilage and to the cricoid cartilage, or the cricothyroid articulation. SYN keratocricoid.

cer·a·to·glos·sus (ser'ă-tō-glos'ŭs). SYN chondroglossus *muscle.* [L.]

cer·a·to·hy·al (ser'ă-tō-hī'ăl). Relating to one of the cornua of the hyoid bone. SYN keratohyal.

Cer·a·to·phyl·li·dae (ser'ă-tō-fil'i-dē). A family of mammal and bird fleas, many of which have a wide host range and serve as important vectors of plague, sustaining the infection among wild and domestic rodent hosts. Important genera include *Nosopsyllus* and *Ceratophyllus*. [G. *keras*, horn, + *phyllōdēs*, like leaves]

Cer·a·to·phyl·lus (ser-ă-tof'-ă-lŭs). A genus of fleas (family Ceratophyliidae) found in temperate climates; includes important fleas of poultry such as *C. niger*, the western chicken flea, and *C. gallinae*, the European chicken flea, though these fleas have a wide range of hosts, including man. [cerat- (kerat-) + G. *phyllon*, leaf]

C. punjaten'sis, a species abundant on wild and domestic rodents

in India; may serve as a liaison agent between wild rodents and man in the transmission of plague.

cer·car·ia, pl. **cer·car·i·ae** (ser-kā're-ă, -rē-ē). The free-swimming trematode larva that emerges from its host snail; it may penetrate the skin of a final host (as in *Schistosoma* of man), encyst on vegetation (as in *Fasciola*), in or on fish (as in *Clonorchis*), or penetrate and encyst in various arthropod hosts. Body and tail are greatly varied in form, and specialized function is adapted to the particular life cycle demands of each species. SEE ALSO sporocyst (1), redia. [G. *kerkos*, tail]

cer·ci (ser'sī). Plural of cercus.

cer·clage (sair-klazh'). **1.** Bringing into close opposition and binding together the ends of an obliquely fractured bone or the fragments of a broken patella by a ring or by an encircling, tightly drawn wire loop. **2.** Operation for retinal detachment in which the choroid and retinal pigment epithelium are brought in contact with the detached sensory retina by a band encircling the sclera posterior to the insertion of the ocular rectus muscles. **3.** The placing of a nonabsorbable suture around an incompetent cervical os. SYN tiring. [Fr. an encircling, hooping, banding]

cer·co·cys·tis (ser-kō-sis'tis). A specialized form of tapeworm cysticercoid larva that develops within the vertebrate host villus rather than in an invertebrate host; *e.g.,* the c. of *Hymenolepis nana* in its direct or egg-borne cycle in man. SEE ALSO cysticercus, cysticercoid. [G. *kerkos*, tail, + *kystis*, bladder]

cer·co·mer (ser'kō-mer). The caudal appendage of a larval cestode, the procercoid stage of pseudophyllid cestodes; it may also be found on the cysticercoid larvae of taenioid cestodes, as well as in many of the hymenolepidids (*e.g., Hymenolepis nana*). This appendage frequently bears the hooks originally used by the hexacanth in clawing its way into the intermediate host in which the procercoid or other larval stage develops. [G. *kerkos*, tail + *meros*, part]

cer·co·mo·nad (ser-kō-mō'nad). Common name for members of the genus *Cercomonas*.

Cer·co·mo·nas (ser-kō-mō'nas). A genus of freshwater and coprophilic protozoan flagellates in which members have one anterior and one posterior flagellum. Species have been described from the intestine or feces of man and several types of domestic livestock, but have usually proved to be other genera such as *Trichomonas* or *Chilomastix*. [G. *kerkos*, tail + *monas* (monad-), unit, monad]

Cer·co·pi·the·coi·dea (ser'kō-pith-ĕ-koy'dē-ă). One of the three superfamilies of the suborder Anthropoidea; includes apes, Old World monkeys, and man. [G. *kerkos*, tail, + *pithēkos*, monkey]

Cer·co·pi·the·cus (ser-kō-pith-ē'kŭs). A genus of the family Cercopithecidae, represented by guenons and common African monkeys.

cer·cus, gen. and pl. **cer·ci** (ser'kŭs, ker'kŭs; -sē, -kē). **1.** A stiff hairlike structure. **2.** A pair of specialized sensory appendages on the 11th abdominal segment of most insects. [Mod. L., fr. G. *kerkos*, tail]

ce·rea flex·i·bil·i·tas (sē'rē-ă flek-si-bil'i-tas). "Waxy flexibility," in which the limb remains where placed; often seen in catatonia. [L.]

cer·e·bel·lar (ser-e-bel'ar). Relating to the cerebellum.

cer·e·bel·lin (ser-ĕ-bel'in). A cerebellum-specific hexadecapeptide localized in the perikarya and dendrites of cerebellar Purkinje cells; used as a marker for Purkinje cell maturation studies of neural development.

cer·e·bel·li·tis (ser-ĕ-bel-ī'tis). Inflammation of the cerebellum.

△cerebello-. The cerebellum. [L. *cerebrum*, brain, + -*ellum*, dim. suff.]

cer·e·bel·lo·len·tal (ser-e-bel'ō-len'tăl). Relating to the cerebellum and the lens of the eye.

cer·e·bel·lo·med·ul·lary (ser-e-bel'ō-med'yū-lār-ē). Relating to the cerebellum and the medulla oblongata.

cer·e·bel·lo·ol·i·vary (ser-e-bel'ō-ol'i-vār-ē). Relating to the connections of the cerebellum with the inferior olive.

cer·e·bel·lo·pon·tine (ser-e-bel'ō-pon'tēn). Relating to the cerebellum and the pons; denoting especially the c. recess or angle between these two structures.

cer·e·bel·lo·ru·bral (ser-e-bel'ō-rū'brăl). Relating to the connections of the cerebellum with the red nucleus. [cerebello- + L. *ruber*, red]

cer·e·bel·lum, pl. **ce·re·bel·la** (ser-e-bel'ŭm, -bel'ă) [NA]. The large posterior brain mass lying dorsal to the pons and medulla and ventral to the posterior portion of the cerebrum; it consists of two lateral hemispheres united by a narrow middle portion, the vermis. [L. dim. of *cerebrum*, brain]

△**cerebr-.** SEE cerebro-.

ce·re·bra (sĕ-rē'bră). Plural of cerebrum.

ce·re·bral (ser'ĕ-brăl, sĕ-rē'brăl). Relating to the cerebrum.

cer·e·bral·gia (ser-ĕ-bral'jē-ă). SYN headache. [cerebrum + G. *algos*, pain]

cer·e·bra·tion (ser-ĕ-brā'shŭn). Activity of the mental processes; thinking. SEE ALSO mentation, cognition.

△**cerebri-.** SEE cerebro-.

cer·e·bri·form (se-rē'bri-fōrm). Resembling the external fissures and convolutions of the brain. [cerebri- + L. *forma*, shape, appearance, nature]

cer·e·bri·tis (ser-ĕ-brī'tis). Focal inflammatory infiltrates in the brain parenchyma.

    suppurative c., inflammation (phlegmon) of the brain with suppuration.

△**cerebro-, cerebr-, cerebri-.** The cerebrum. SEE ALSO encephalo-. [L. *cerebrum*, brain]

cer·e·bro·cu·pre·in (ser'ĕ-brō-kū'prē-in). SYN cytocuprein.

cer·e·bro·ga·lac·tose (ser'ĕ-brō-gă-lak'tōs). D-Galactose. SEE galactose.

cer·e·bro·ga·lac·to·side (ser'ĕ-brō-gă-lak'tō-sīd). SYN cerebroside.

cer·e·bro·ma. SYN encephaloma.

cer·e·bro·ma·la·cia (ser'ĕ-brō-mă-lā'shē-ă). SYN encephalomalacia.

cer·e·bro·men·in·gi·tis (ser'ĕ-brō-men-in-jī'tis). SYN meningoencephalitis.

cer·e·bron (ser'ĕ-bron). SYN phrenosin.

cer·e·bron·ic ac·id (ser-ĕ-bron'ik). 2-Hydroxylignoceric acid, 2-hydroxytetraeicosanoic acid; $CH_3\text{-}(CH_2)_{21}\text{-}CHOH\text{-}COOH$. a constituent of phrenosin (cerebron) and other glycolipids. SYN phrenosinic acid.

cer·e·bro·path·ia (ser'ĕ-brō-path'ē-ă). SYN encephalopathy.

cer·e·brop·a·thy (ser-ĕ-brop'ă-thē). SYN encephalopathy.

cer·e·bro·phys·i·ol·o·gy (ser'ĕ-brō-fiz-ē-ol'ō-jē). The physiology of the cerebrum.

cer·e·bro·scle·ro·sis (ser'ĕ-brō-sklēr-ō'sis). Encephalosclerosis, hardening of the cerebral hemispheres. [cerebro- + G. *sklērōsis*, hardening]

cer·e·brose (ser'ĕ-brōs). SYN galactose.

cer·e·bro·side (ser'ĕ-brō-sīd). A class of glycosphingolipid; specifically, a monoglycosylceramide (ceramide monosaccharide), the sugar being attached to the –CHOH– of the sphingoid. c's are found in the myelin sheath of nerve tissue; *e.g.*, kerasin, nervon, oxynervon, phrenosin, these names also being used for the fatty acid involved. C. is sometimes prefixed by gluco-, galacto-, etc., in place of the correct glucosylceramide, etc. The sulfate esters of c.'s are among the sulfatidates. SYN cerebrogalactoside.

    c.-sulfatase, c. sulfatidase, an enzyme that cleaves sulfate from a sulfated glycosphingolipid (such as a cerebroside 3-sulfate).

cer·e·bro·si·do·sis (ser'ĕ-brō-sī-dō'sis). A lipidosis as in Gaucher's *disease.*

cer·e·bro·spi·nal (ser'ĕ-brō-spī-năl, sĕ-rē'brō-). Relating to the brain and the spinal cord. SYN encephalorrhachidian, encephalospinal.

cer·e·bro·spi·nant (ser'ĕ-brō-spī'nant). Obsolete term for acting upon the cerebral nervous system, the brain and spinal cord and for an agent affecting the cerebrospinal system.

cer·e·bro·ste·rol (ser'ē-brō-stēr'ol). 24β-Hydroxycholesterol; a hydroxylated cholesterol found in the brain and spinal cord.

cer·e·brot·o·my (ser-ĕ-brot'ō-mē). Incision of the brain. [cerebro- + G. *tomē*, incision]

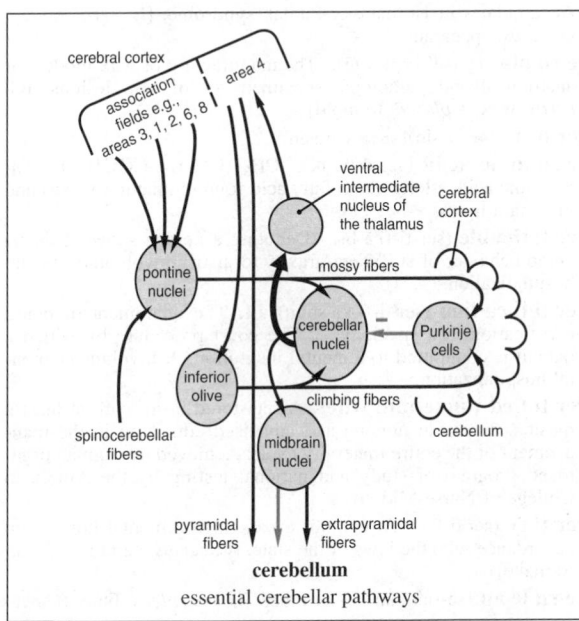

cerebellum
essential cerebellar pathways

cer·e·bro·to·nia (ser'ĕ-brō-tō'nē-ă). Rarely used term for a personality pattern proposed by William H. Sheldon associated with the relatively thin, ectomorphic bodily type and with predominance of intellectual processes; characterized by traits of inhibition, restraint, and concealment. [cerebro- + G. *tonos*, tone]

cer·e·bro·vas·cu·lar (ser'ĕ-brō-vas'kyū-lăr). Relating to the blood supply to the brain, particularly with reference to pathologic changes.

cer·e·brum, pl. **ce·re·bra**, **cer·e·brums** (ser'ĕ-brŭm, sĕ-rē'brŭm; -bră; -brŭmz) [NA]. Originally referred to the largest portion of the brain, including practically all parts within the skull except the medulla, pons, and cerebellum; it now usually refers only to the parts derived from the telencephalon and includes mainly the cerebral hemispheres (cerebral cortex and basal ganglia). [L., brain]

cere·cloth (sēr'kloth). Gauze or cheese cloth impregnated with wax containing an antiseptic; used in surgical dressings. [L. *cera*, wax]

Cerenkov, (Cherenkov) Pavel A., Russian physicist and Nobel laureate, *1904. SEE C. *radiation.*

cer·e·sin (ser'ĕ-sin). A natural mixture of hydrocarbons of high molecular weight; a substitute for beeswax, also used in dentistry for impressions. SYN cerin, cerosin, earth wax, mineral wax (2), purified ozokerite.

ce·rin (se'rin). SYN ceresin.

Cer·i·thid·ea (ser-i-thid'ē-ă). A genus of marine and brackish water operculate (prosobranch) snails that serve as first intermediate hosts of a number of trematodes. *C. cingulata* serves as host for *Heterophyes heterophyes* in Japan and Southeast Asia; *C. scalariformis* for cercariae that induce swimmer's itch in the southeastern U.S. from Florida to Texas.

ce·ri·um (Ce) (sēr'ē-ŭm). A metallic element, atomic no. 58, atomic wt. 140.115. [fr. *Ceres*, the planetoid]

    c. oxalate, a mixture of the oxalates of c., lanthanum, and other rare earths; has been used in the treatment of vomiting.

△**cero-.** Wax. [L. *cera*, wax]

ce·roid (sē'royd). A waxlike, golden or yellow-brown pigment first found in fibrotic livers of choline-deficient rats, and also known to be present in some of the cirrhotic livers (and certain other tissues) of human beings. C. is acid-fast, insoluble in fat solvents, and probably a type of lipofuscin, although differing from true lipofuscins by failing to stain with Schmorl's ferric-ferricyanide reduction stain; it also exhibits autofluorescence.

Accumulates in Hermansky-Pudlak syndrome. [L. *cera*, wax, + G. *eidos*, appearance]

ce·ro·plas·ty (sē'rō-plas-tē). The manufacture of wax models of anatomical and pathologic specimens or of skin lesions. [G. *kēros*, wax, + *plassō*, to mold]

cer·o·sin (ser'ō-sin). SYN ceresin.

ce·ro·tin·ic ac·id (ser-ō-tin'ik). $CH_3-(CH_2)_{24}-COOH$; *n*-hexacosanoic acid; a long-chain fatty acid found in natural waxes and in certain lipids.

cer·ti·fi·a·ble (ser-ti-fī'ă-bl). Denoting a person showing disordered behavior of sufficient gravity to justify involuntary mental hospitalization.

cer·ti·fi·ca·tion (ser'ti-fi-kā'shŭn). **1.** The attainment of board certification in a specialty. **2.** The court procedure by which a patient is committed to a mental institution. **3.** Involuntary mental hospitalization.

cer·ti·fied nurse-mid·wife. A registered n.-m. with at least a masters degree in nursing and advanced education in the management of the entire maternity cycle. Achieved through an organized program of study and national testing by the American College of Nurse-Midwives.

cer·ti·fy (ser'ti-fī). To commit a patient to a mental hospital in accordance with the laws of the state. [L. *certus*, certain, + *facio*, to make]

ce·ru·le·an (se-rū'lē-ăn). SYN blue. [L. *caeruleus*, blue, fr. *caelum*, sky]

ce·ru·le·in (se-rū'lē-in). A decapeptide with hypotensive activity; stimulates smooth muscle and increases digestive secretions; it is similar in structure to cholecystokinin and the gastrins, but much more potent as a stimulant to gallbladder contraction; also stimulates release of insulin. [fr. *Hyla caerulea*, from which isolated]

ce·ru·lo·plas·min (sĕ-rū'lō-plaz-min). A blue copper-containing α-globulin of blood plasma, with a molecular weight of about 140,000 and 8 atoms of copper per molecule; involved in copper transport and regulation, and can reduce O_2 directly without known intermediates; also has ferroxidase and polyamine oxidase properties of unknown significance. C. is absent in congenital Wilson's disease. [L. *caeruleus*, dark blue]

ce·ru·men (sĕ-rū'men). The soft, brownish yellow, waxy secretion (a modified sebum) of the ceruminous glands of the external auditory meatus. SYN ear wax, earwax. [L. *cera*, wax]

c. inspissa'tum, inspissated c., dried earwax plugging the external auditory canal.

ce·ru·mi·nal (se-rū'mi-năl). Relating to cerumen.

ce·ru·mi·no·lyt·ic (sĕ-rū'mi-nō-lit'ik). One of several substances instilled into the external auditory canal to soften wax. [cerumen, + G. *lysis*, a loosening]

ce·ru·mi·no·ma (sĕ-rū-mi-nō'mă). A usually benign adenomatous tumor of ceruminous glands of the external auditory canal.

ce·ru·mi·no·sis (se-rū-mi-nō'sis). Excessive formation of cerumen.

ce·ru·mi·nous (sĕ-rū'mi-nŭs). Relating to cerumen.

ce·ruse (sē'rūs). SYN lead carbonate. [L. *cerussa*]

cer·veau iso·lé (ser-vō' ē-sō-lā'). An animal with its mesencephalon transected; it breathes spontaneously but is unresponsive, with abnormal pupils (usually dilated) and a continuous sleep pattern in the electroencephalogram. Cf. encéphale isolé. [Fr. detached brain]

cer·vi·cal (ser'vĭ-kal). Relating to a neck, or cervix, in any sense. SYN cervicalis. [L. *cervix* (*cervic*-), neck]

cer·vi·ca·lis (ser-vi-kā'lis). SYN cervical.

c. ascen'dens, (1) SYN iliocostalis cervicis *muscle*. **(2)** SYN ascending cervical *artery*.

cer·vi·cec·to·my (ser-vi-sek'tō-mē). Excision of the cervix uteri. SYN trachelectomy. [cervix + G. *ektomē*, excision]

cer·vi·ces (ser'vi-sēz). Plural of cervix.

cer·vi·ci·tis (ser-vi-sī'tis). Inflammation of the mucous membrane, frequently involving also the deeper structures, of the cervix uteri. SYN trachelitis.

△cervico-. A cervix, or neck, in any sense. [L. *cervix*, neck]

cer·vi·co·brach·i·al (ser'vi-kō-brā'kē-ăl). Relating to the neck and the arm.

cer·vi·co·buc·cal (ser'vi-kō-bŭk'ăl). Relating to the buccal region of the neck of a premolar or molar tooth.

cer·vi·co·dyn·ia (ser'vi-kō-din'ē-ă). Neck pain. SYN trachelodynia. [cervico- + G. *odynē*, pain]

cer·vi·co·fa·cial (ser'vi-kō-fā'shăl). Relating to the neck and the face.

cer·vi·cog·ra·phy (ser-vi-kog'ră-fē). Technique, equivalent to colposcopy, for photographing part or all of the uterine cervix. [cervix + G. *graphō*, to write]

cer·vi·co·la·bi·al (ser'vi-kō-lā'bē-ăl). Relating to the labial region of the neck of an incisor or canine tooth.

cer·vi·co·lin·gual (ser'vi-kō-ling'gwăl). Relating to the lingual region of the cervix of a tooth.

cer·vi·co·lin·guo·ax·i·al (ser'vi-kō-ling'gwō-ak'sē-ăl). Referring to the point angle formed by the junction of the cervical (gingival), lingual, and axial walls of a cavity.

cer·vi·co·oc·cip·i·tal (ser'vi-kō-ok-sip'i-tăl). Relating to the neck and the occiput.

cer·vi·co·plas·ty (ser'vi-kō-plas-tē). Plastic surgery on the cervix uteri or on the neck.

cer·vi·co·tho·rac·ic (ser'vi-kō-thōr-as'ik). Relating to: **1.** The neck and thorax; **2.** The transition between the neck and thorax; **3.** The fusion of these vertebrae.

cer·vi·cot·o·my (ser-vi-kot'ō-mē). Incision into the cervix uteri. SYN trachelotomy. [cervico- + G. *tomē*, incision]

cer·vi·co·ves·i·cal (ser'vi-kō-ves'i-kăl). Relating to the cervix of the uterus and the bladder.

cer·vi·lax·in. SYN relaxin.

cer·vix, gen. **cer·vi·cis,** pl. **cer·vi·ces** (ser'viks, ser'vi-sis, -sēz) [NA]. **1.** SYN collum. **2.** Any necklike structure. **3.** SYN c. of uterus. [L. neck]

c. of the axon, the constricted portion of the axon just before the myelin sheath begins.

c. colum'nae posterio'ris, a slight constriction of the posterior gray column of the spinal cord, seen on cross-section just behind the gray commissure.

c. den'tis [NA], SYN *neck* of tooth.

c. u'teri [NA], SYN c. of uterus.

c. of uterus, the lower part of the uterus extending from the isthmus of the uterus into the vagina. It is divided into supravaginal and vaginal parts by its passage through the vaginal wall. SYN c. uteri [NA], cervix (3) [NA], neck of uterus, neck of womb.

c. vesi'cae urina'riae [NA], SYN *neck* of urinary bladder.

ce·ryl (sēr'il). The hydrocarbon radical, $C_{26}H_{53}-$, of ceryl alcohol (hexacosanol). SYN hexacosyl.

ce·sar·e·an (se-zā'rē-ăn). Denoting a c. section, which was included under *lex cesarea*, Roman law (715 B.C.); not because performed at the birth of Julius Caesar (100 B.C.).

ce·si·um (Cs) (sē'zē-ŭm). A metallic element, atomic no. 55, atomic wt. 132.90543; a member of the alkali metal group. [137]Cs (half-life equal to 30.1 years) is used in treatment of certain malignancies. [L. *caesius*, bluish gray]

Cestan, Raymond, French neurologist, 1872–1934. SEE C.-Chenais *syndrome*.

Ces·to·da (ses-tō'dă). A subclass of tapeworms (class Cestoidea), containing the typical members of this group, including the segmented tapeworms that parasitize man and domestic animals. SYN Eucestoda. [G. *kestos*, girdle]

Ces·to·dar·ia (ses-tō-dā'rē-ă). A subclass of the class Cestoidea, containing tapeworms that lack a scolex and are unsegmented (monozoic), in contrast to the typical tapeworms in the subclass Cestoda; larvae of c. (called lycophora) characteristically have 10 hooklets rather than six. C. are believed to be primitive tapeworms, parasitizing the intestine and celomic cavities of certain fish and a few reptiles.

ces·tode, ces·toid (ses'tōd, -toyd). Common name for tapeworms of the class Cestoidea or its subclasses, Cestoda and Cestodaria.

ces·to·di·a·sis (ses-tō-dī′ă-sis). Disease caused by infection with a cestode.

Ces·toi·dea (ses-toy′dē-ă). The tapeworms, a class of platyhelminth flatworms characterized by lack of an alimentary canal and, in typical forms (subclass Cestoda), by a segmented body with a scolex or holdfast organ at one end; adult worms are vertebrate parasites, usually found in the small intestine. [G. *kestos*, girdle, + *eidos*, form]

ce·ta·ce·um (sĕ-tā′shē-ŭm). SYN spermaceti. [G. *kētos*, a whale]

cet·al·ko·ni·um chlo·ride (set′al-kō′nē-ŭm). Benzylhexadecyldimethylammonium chloride; an antibacterial agent.

cet·hex·o·ni·um bro·mide (set-heks-ō′nē-ŭm). Hexadecyl(2-hydroxycyclohexyl)dimethylammonium bromide; an antiseptic.

ce·to·ste·a·ryl al·co·hol (se-tō-stē′ă-ril). A component of the hydrophilic ointment ingredient known as emulsifying wax; a mixture of solid aliphatic alcohols consisting chiefly of stearyl and cetyl alcohols.

ce·trar·ia (sē-trā′rē-ă). The dried plant, *Cetraria islandica* (family Parmeliaceae), a lichen, not a moss, used as a demulcent and as a folk remedy for bronchitis. SYN Iceland moss. [L. *caetra*, a short Spanish shield (from shape of the apothecia)]

ce·tri·mo·ni·um bro·mide (se-trī-mō′nē-ŭm). Hexadecyltrimethylammonium bromide; an antiseptic.

ce·tyl (sē′til). The univalent radical $C_{16}H_{33}$– of cetyl alcohol.

c. alcohol, the 16-carbon alcohol corresponding to palmitic acid, so called because it is isolated from among the hydrolysis products of spermaceti; it is used as an emulsifying aid and in the preparation of "washable" ointment bases. SYN 1-hexadecanol, palmityl alcohol.

c. palmitate, $C_{15}H_{31}CO–OC_{16}H_{31}$; a wax; the chief constituent of spermaceti.

ce·tyl·pyr·i·din·i·um chlo·ride (sē′til-pī-ri-din′ē-ŭm). The monohydrate of the quaternary salt of pyridine and cetyl chloride; a cationic detergent with antiseptic action against nonsporulating bacteria.

ce·tyl·tri·meth·yl·am·mo·ni·um bro·mide (sē′til-trī-me′thil-ă-mō′nē-ŭm). Cetrimide; a mixture of dodecyl-, tetradecyl-, and hexadecyltrimethylammonium bromides; an odorless surface-active agent, readily soluble in water; a disinfectant with a strong bacteriostatic action, used for the sterilization of instruments and utensils.

cev·a·dil·la (se-vă-dil′ă). SYN sabadilla. [Sp. dim. of *cebada*, barley]

cev·a·dine (sev′ă-dēn). $C_{32}H_{49}NO_9$; an alkaloid occurring in the seeds of *Schoenocaulon officinale* (*Sabadilla officinarum*), family Liliaceae; highly irritating to skin and mucous membranes. SEE ALSO veratrine.

ce·vi·tam·ic ac·id (sev-i-tam′ik). SYN ascorbic acid.

CF Abbreviation for citrovorum *factor*; coupling factor.

Cf Symbol for californium.

CFF Abbreviation for critical fusion frequency. SEE critical flicker fusion *frequency.*

CG Abbreviation for chorionic *gonadotropin*; phosgene.

CGA Abbreviation for catabolite gene *activator.*

cGMP Abbreviation for cyclic *guanosine* 3′,5′-monophosphate.

CGP Abbreviation for chorionic "growth *hormone*-prolactin".

CGRP Abbreviation for calcitonin gene related *peptide.*

CGS, cgs Abbreviation for centimeter-gram-second. SEE centimeter-gram-second *system*, centimeter-gram-second *unit.*

CH Abbreviation for crown-heel *length.*

Ch1 Abbreviation for Christchurch *chromosome.*

Cha·ber·tia (chă-ber′tē-ă). A genus of strongyle nematodes parasitic in animals. The species *C. ovina*, the bowel worm, is found in the digestive tract of sheep, goats, cattle, and some wild animals; it feeds on the mucosa of the gut, where in large numbers it can produce considerable damage.

Chaddock, Charles G., U.S. neurologist, 1861–1936. SEE C. *reflex, sign.*

Chadwick, James R., U.S. gynecologist, 1844–1905. SEE C.'s *sign.*

chae·ta (kē′tă). SYN seta. [Mod. L. fr. G. *chaitē*, stiff hair]

chafe (chāf). To cause irritation of the skin by friction. [Fr. *chauffer*, to heat, fr. L. *calefacio*, to make warm]

Chagas, Carlos, Brazilian physician, 1879–1934. SEE C.'s *disease;* C.-Cruz *disease.*

cha·go·ma (sha-gō′mă). The skin lesion in acute Chagas' disease.

chain (chān). **1.** In chemistry, a series of atoms held together by one or more covalent bonds. **2.** In bacteriology, a linear arrangement of living cells that have divided in one plane and remain attached to each other. [L. *catena*]

A c., **(1)** a polypeptide component of insulin containing 21 amino acyl residues, beginning with a glycyl residue (NH_2-terminus); insulin is formed by the linkage of an A c. to a B c. by two disulfide bonds; the amino-acid composition of the A c. is a function of species; SYN glycyl c. **(2)** in general, one of the polypeptides in a multiprotein complex.

B c., a polypeptide component of insulin containing 30 amino acyl residues, beginning with a phenylalanyl residue (NH_2-terminus); insulin is formed by the linkage of a B c. to an A c. by two disulfide bonds; the amino-acid composition of the B c. is a function of species. SYN phenylalanyl c.

behavior c., related behaviors in a series in which each response serves as a stimulus for the next response.

C c., SYN C-peptide.

cold c., a system of protection against high environmental temperatures for heat-labile vaccines, sera and other biological preparations.

electron-transport c., SYN respiratory c.

glycyl c., SYN A c. (1).

heavy c., a polypeptide c. of high molecular weight (about 400–500 residue), γ, α, μ, δ, or ε c.'s in immunoglobulin, determining the immunoglobulin class and subclass. SYN H chain.

hemolytic c., the hemolysis that occurs when complement is activated by the previously formed union of erythrocytes and specific antibody.

J c., a glycopeptide disulfide that is bonded to polymeric IgA and IgM; its function is to ensure correct polymerization of the subunits of IgA and IgM. [*joining*]

L c., SYN light c.

light c., a polypeptide c. with low molecular weight (about 200 residue), as the κ or λ c.'s in immunoglobulin. SYN L c.

long c., in bacteriology, a continuous line of more than eight cells.

ossicular c., SYN auditory *ossicles*, under *ossicle.*

phenylalanyl c., SYN B c.

respiratory c., a sequence of energy-liberating oxidation-reduction reactions whereby electrons are accepted from reduced compounds and eventually transferred to oxygen with the formation of water. SYN cytochrome system, electron-transport c., electron-transport system.

short c., in bacteriology, a string of two to eight cells.

side c., **(1)** a c. of noncyclic atoms linked to a benzene ring, or to any cyclic c. compound; **(2)** the atoms of an α-amino acid other than the α-carboxyl group, the α-amino group, the α-carbon, and the hydrogen attached to the α-carbon.

chain·ing (chān′ing). Learning related behaviors in a series in which each response serves as a stimulus for the next response.

cha·la·sia, cha·la·sis (kă-lā′zē-ă, -lā′sis). Inhibition and relaxation of any previously sustained contraction of muscle, usually of a synergic group of muscles. [G. *chalaō*, to loosen]

cha·la·za (kă-lā′ză). **1.** SYN chalazion. **2.** Suspensory ligament of the yolk in a bird's egg. [G. hail; a small tubercle, a sty (Galen)]

cha·la·zi·on, pl. **cha·la·zia** (ka-lā′zē-on, -zē-ă). A chronic inflammatory granuloma of a meibomian gland. SYN chalaza (1), meibomian cyst, tarsal cyst. [G. dim. of *chalaza*, a sty]

acute c., SYN *hordeolum* internum.

collar-stud c., a c. that extends through the tarsal plate anteriorly (c. externum) and toward the conjunctiva.

chal·cone (kal′kōn). $C_6H_5CH=CH-CO-C_6H_5$; 1,3-diphenyl-2-propen-1-one; the parent compound of a series of plant pigments.

All are flavonoids and typically are yellow to orange in color. SYN benzalacetophenone.

chal·co·sis (kal-kō'sis). Chronic copper poisoning. SYN chalkitis. [G. *chalkos,* copper, brass]

c. len'tis, a cataract caused by excessive intraocular copper. SYN copper cataract, sunflower cataract.

chal·i·co·sis (kal-i-kō'sis). Pneumoconiosis caused by the inhalation of dust incident to the occupation of stone cutting. SYN flint disease. [G. *chalix,* gravel]

chal·in·o·plas·ty (kal'in-ō-plas-tē). Obsolete term for the correction of defects of the mouth and lips, especially of the corners of the mouth. [G. *chalinos,* bridle, corner of the mouth, + *plastos,* formed]

chalk (chawk). SYN *calcium* carbonate. [L. *calx*]

French c., SYN talc.

prepared c., purified native calcium carbonate, usually molded into cones; used as a mild astringent and antacid.

chal·ki·tis (kal-kī'tis). SYN chalcosis. [G. *chalkos,* copper, brass]

cha·lone (kā'lōn). Originally, a hormone (*e.g.,* enterogastrone) that inhibits rather than stimulates; now, any one of a number of mitotic inhibitors (often glycoproteins) elaborated by a tissue and active only on that type of tissue, regardless of species; a reversible tissue-specific mitotic inhibitor. [G. + *chalaō,* to relax, + -one]

cha·ly·be·ate (kal-ib'ē-āt). Obsolete term for impregnated with or containing iron salts and for a therapeutic agent containing iron. [G. *chalyps* (*chalyb-*), steel]

cha·maz·u·lene (chǎ-maz'yū-lēn). 1,4-Dimethyl-7-ethylazulene; an anti-inflammatory agent.

cham·ber (chām'ber). A compartment or enclosed space. SEE ALSO camera. [L. *camera*]

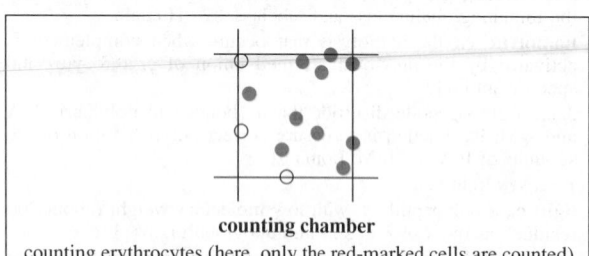

counting chamber
counting erythrocytes (here, only the red-marked cells are counted)

altitude c., a decompression c. for simulating a high altitude environment, particularly its low barometric pressure. SYN high altitude c.

anechoic c., a room designed to absorb all sound so as to eliminate all echoes; used for isolation and sound research on human subjects.

anterior c. of eye, the space between the cornea anteriorly and the iris/pupil posteriorly, filled with a watery fluid (aqueous humor) and communicating through the pupil with the posterior chamber. SYN camera anterior bulbi [NA], camera oculi anterior, camera oculi major.

aqueous c.'s, the combined anterior and posterior c.'s of the eye containing the aqueous humor. SEE anterior c. of eye, posterior c. of eye. SEE ALSO anterior *segment.*

decompression c., a c. for exposing organisms to pressures below that of the atmosphere.

Haldane c., an obsolete c. for metabolic studies on animals.

high altitude c., SYN altitude c.

hyperbaric c., a c. providing pressures greater than atmospheric, commonly used to treat decompression sickness and to provide hyperbaric oxygenation.

ionization c., a c. for detecting ionization of the enclosed gas; used for determining intensity of ionizing radiation.

posterior c. of eye, the ringlike space, filled with aqueous humor, between the iris/pupil anteriorly and the lens and ciliary body posteriorly. SYN camera posterior bulbi [NA], camera oculi minor, camera oculi posterior.

pulp c., that portion of the pulp cavity which is contained in the crown or body of the tooth.

relief c., a recess in the impression surface of a denture to reduce or eliminate pressure from that specific area of the mouth.

Sandison-Clark c., a c. that can be fitted over a hole punched in a rabbit's ear, so that tissue will grow to fill the defect between two transparent plates; if the distance between the plates is small, the living tissue can be studied microscopically.

sinuatrial c., the common c. formed by the single embryonic atrium and the right and left horns of the sinus venosus.

vitreous c. of eye, SYN posterior *segment* of eyeball.

Zappert counting c., a special, standardized glass slide used for counting cells (especially erythrocytes and leukocytes) and other particulate material in a measured volume of fluid; the central portion is precisely ground in such a manner that the uniformly flat surface is exactly 0.1 mm lower than that of two parallel ridges on which a special, uniformly flat coverslip may be placed; accurately etched lines on the flat central portion form the boundaries of groups of squares of known areas, thereby providing the basis for determining the volume of fluid in which the cells are counted. Glass slides of this type are frequently known as hemocytometers.

Chamberlain, W.E., U.S. radiologist, 1891–1947. SEE C.'s *line.*

Chamberlen, Peter, English obstetrician, 1560–1631. SEE C. *forceps.*

cham·e·ce·phal·ic (kam-ĕ-se-fal'ik). Having a flat head; denoting a skull with a vertical index of 70 or less; similar to tapinocephalic. SYN chamecephalous. [G. *chamai,* on the ground (low, stunted), + *kephalē,* head]

cham·e·ceph·a·lous (kam-ĕ-sef'ǎ-lus). SYN chamecephalic.

cham·e·pro·so·pic (kam'ĕ-prō-sop'ik). Having a broad face. [G. *chamai* (adv.), on the ground (low, spread out), + *prosōpikos,* facial]

cham·fer (sham'fer). A marginal finish on an extracoronal cavity preparation of a tooth which describes a curve from an axial wall to the cavosurface. [fr. O.Fr. *chanfrein(t),* beveled edge]

cham·o·mile (kam'ō-mīl). The flowering heads of *Anthemis nobilis* (family Compositae); a stomachic. SYN camomile. [G. *chamaimēlon,* chamomile, fr. *chamai,* on the ground, + *mēlon,* apple]

Champy, Christian, French physician, *1885. SEE C.'s *fixative.*

Chanarin, I., 20th century British hematologist. SEE Dorfman-C. *syndrome.*

Chance, G.Q., 20th century British radiologist. SEE C. *fracture.*

chan·cre (shang'ker). The primary lesion of syphilis, which begins at the site of infection after an interval of 10 to 30 days as a papule or area of infiltration, of dull red color, hard, and insensitive; the center usually becomes eroded or breaks down into an ulcer that heals slowly after 4 to 6 weeks. SYN hard c., hard sore, hard ulcer, syphilitic ulcer (1), ulcus venereum (1). [Fr. indirectly from L. *cancer*]

hard c., SYN chancre.

mixed c., a sore resulting from simultaneous inoculation of a site with syphilis and chancroid.

monorecidive c., a c. that recurs at the site of a previously healed lesion.

c. re'dux, a second c. occurring in a syphilitic subject, possibly an allergic reaction without the presence of the specific spirochete.

soft c., SYN chancroid.

sporotrichositic c., the initial lesion at the site of skin infection in sporotrichosis.

tularemic c., the primary lesion, usually of finger, thumb, or hand, in tularemia.

chan·cri·form (shang'kri-fōrm). Resembling chancre.

chan·croid (shang'kroyd). An infectious, painful, ragged venereal ulcer at the site of infection by *Haemophilus ducreyi,* beginning after an incubation period of 3 to 5 days; seen more commonly in men. SYN soft chancre, soft sore, soft ulcer, ulcus venereum (2), venereal sore, venereal ulcer. [chancre + G. *eidos,* resemblance]

chan·croi·dal (shang-kroy′dăl). Relating to or of the nature of chancroid.

chan·crous (shang′krŭs). Characterized by having a chancre.

Chandler, Paul A., U.S. ophthalmologist, *1896. SEE C. *syndrome.*

change (chanj). An alteration; in pathology, structural alteration of which the cause and significance is uncertain. SYN shift.

Armanni-Ebstein c., SYN Armanni-Ebstein *kidney.*

Baggenstoss c., distention of pancreatic acini by proteinaceous secretion, seen in dehydration.

Crooke's hyaline c., replacement of cytoplasmic granules of basophil cells of the anterior pituitary by homogenous hyaline material; a characteristic finding in Cushing's syndrome, but usually not present in the cells of a basophil adenoma. SYN Crooke's hyaline degeneration.

fatty c., SYN fatty *metamorphosis.*

c. of life, colloquialism for (1) menopause; (2) climacteric.

trophic c.'s, SYN trophoneurotic *atrophy.*

Changeux, Jean-Pierre, French 20th-century biochemist. SEE Monod-Wyman-Changeux *model.*

chan·nel (chan′ĕl). A furrow, gutter, or groovelike passageway. SEE ALSO canal. [L. *canalis*]

ion c., a specific macromolecular protein pathway, with an aqueous "pore," that traverses the lipid bilayer of a cell's plasma membrane and maintains or modulates the electrical potential across this barrier by allowing controlled influx or exit of small inorganic ions such as Na^+, K^+, Cl^-, and Ca^{2+}. It plays an important role in propagation of the action potential in neurons, but also may control transduction of extracellular signals and contraction in muscle cells. In general, ion c.'s are characterized by their selectivity for certain ions, their specific regulation or gating of these ions, and their specific sensitivity to toxins.

ligand-gated c., a class of ion c.'s whose ionic permeability is regulated by cell membrane receptors that respond to specific extracellular chemical signals.

transnexus c., a hexagonal 15-20Å hydrophilic c. capable of transporting small ions between cardiac muscle cells.

voltage-gated c., a class of ion c.'s that open and close in response to change in the electrical potential across the plasma membrane of the cell; voltage-gated Na^+ c.'s are important for conducting action potential along nerve cell processes.

Chantemesse, André, French bacteriologist, 1851–1919. SEE C. *reaction.*

cha·os. 1. State of such total disorganization that it has no constructive predicates. 2. A state in which no causal relationships are operating. [G., primeval formless void]

mathematical c., a dynamic system so sensitive to its precise current state (which in practice will never be known exactly) that its behavior, though deterministic, is indistinguishable from random.

cha·o·tro·pic (kā-ō-trōp′ik). Pertaining to chaotropism.

cha·o·tro·pism (kā-ō-trōp′izm). The property of certain substances, usually ions (*e.g.,* SCN^-, ClO_4^-, guanidinium), to disrupt the structure of water and thereby promote the solubility of nonpolar substances in polar solvents (*e.g.,* water), the unfolding of proteins, the elution from or movement through a chromatographic medium of an otherwise tightly bound substance, etc. [G. *chaos,* disorder, confusion, + *tropē,* a turning]

CHAP Acronym for cyclophosphamide, hexamethylmelamine, doxorubicin (Adriamycin), and cisplatin, a chemotherapy regimen used in the treatment of ovarian cancer.

cha·pe·rone (shap-ĕ-rōn). A protein required for the proper folding and/or assembly of another protein or protein complex. [Eng. escort, protector, fr. Fr. *chaperon,* hood, fr. *chape,* cape, fr. L.L. *cappa,* fr. L. *caput,* head]

chap·pa (chap′pă). A disease marked by subcutaneous nodules, the size of a pigeon's egg, which break down, release a fatty looking material, and form ulcers; the eruption is preceded by severe muscular and articular pains. [W. Af.]

chapped (chapt). Having or pertaining to skin, especially of the hands, that is dry, scaly, and fissured, owing to the action of cold

or to the excess rate of evaporation of moisture from the skin surface. [M.E. *chap,* to chop, split]

char·ac·ter (kar′ak-ter). An attribute in individuals that is amenable to formal and logical analysis and may be used as the basis of generalizations about classes and other statements that transcend individuality. SYN characteristic (1). [G. *kharakter,* stamp, mark, fr. *charassō,* to engrave]

acquired c., a c. developed in a plant or animal as a result of environmental influences during the individual's life.

classifiable c., a c. that allows individuals to be sorted into distinct but not quantitative classes, *e.g.,* blood types.

compound c., an inherited c. dependent upon two or more distinct genes.

denumerable c., classifiable c. that is also countable (*e.g.,* number of progeny, number of teeth). SYN discrete c.

discrete c., SYN denumerable c.

dominant c., an inherited c. determined by one kind of allele. SEE phenotype.

inherited c., a single attribute of an animal or plant that is transmitted at one locus from generation to generation in accordance with Mendel's law. SEE gene. SYN unit c.

mendelian c., an inherited c. under the control of a single locus (although perhaps modified by genes at other loci).

primary sex c.'s, the sex glands, testes or ovaries, and the accessory sex organs.

recessive c., an inherited c. determined by an allele in homozygous state only. SEE *dominance* of traits.

secondary sex c.'s, those c.'s peculiar to the male or female that develop at puberty, *e.g.,* the beard of men and the breasts of women.

sex-linked c., an inherited c. determined by a gene on a gonosome. SEE gene.

unit c., SYN inherited c.

char·ac·ter ar·mor. A habitual pattern of organized defenses against anxiety.

char·ac·ter·is·tic (kar′ak-ter-is′tik). 1. SYN character. 2. Typical or distinctive of a particular disorder.

receiver operating c. (ROC), a plot of the sensitivity of a diagnostic test as a function of nonspecificity (one minus the specificity). The ROC curve indicates the intrinsic properties of a test's diagnostic performance and can be used to compare the relative merits of competing procedures.

char·ac·ter·i·za·tion (kar′ak-ter-i-zā′shŭn). The discernment, description, or attributing of distinguishing traits.

denture c., modification of the form and color of the denture base and/or teeth to produce a more lifelike appearance.

cha·ras (char′as). A resin obtained from mature leaves of selected varieties of *Cannabis sativa;* used for smoking.

char·bon (shar-bawn′). SYN anthrax (2). [Fr. coal]

char·coal (char′kōl). Carbon obtained by heating or burning wood with restricted access of air. SYN carbo.

activated c., the residue from the destructive distillation of various organic materials, treated to increase its adsorptive power; used in diarrhea, as an antidote in various forms of poisoning, and in purification processes in industry and research. SYN medicinal c.

animal c., c. produced by incomplete combustion of animal tissues, especially bone. SYN animal black, bone black, bone c.

bone c., SYN animal c.

medicinal c., SYN activated c.

vegetable c., c. obtained by charring vegetable tissues, especially the wood of willow, beech, birch, or oak. SYN wood c.

wood c., SYN vegetable c.

Charcot, Jean M., French neurologist, 1825–1893. SEE C.'s *arteries, disease,* intermittent *fever, gait, joint, syndrome, triad, vertigo;* C.-Leyden *crystals,* under *crystal;* C.-Neumann *crystals,* under *crystal;* C.-Robin *crystals,* under *crystal;* C.-Böttcher *crystalloids,* under *crystalloid;* C.-Marie-Tooth *disease;* C.-Weiss-Baker *syndrome;* Erb-C. *disease.*

Chargaff, Erwin, Austrian-U.S. biochemist, *1905. SEE C.'s *rule.*

charge trans·fer. SEE charge transfer *complex.*

char·la·tan (shar'lă-tan). A mẹdical fraud claiming to cure disease by useless procedures, secret remedies, and worthless diagnostic and therapeutic machines. SYN quack. [Fr., fr. It. *ciarlare,* to prattle]

char·la·tan·ism (shar'lă-tan-izm). A fraudulent claim to medical knowledge; treating the sick without knowledge of medicine or authority to practice medicine. SYN quackery.

Charles, Jacques, French physicist, 1746–1823. SEE C. *law.*

char·ley horse (char'lē hōrs). Localized pain or muscle stiffness following a contusion of a muscle. [slang]

Charlouis, M., 19th century Dutch army surgeon in Java. SEE C.'s *disease.*

Charlton, Willy, German physician, *1889. SEE Schultz-C. *phenomenon, reaction.*

Charnley, Sir John, English surgeon, 1911–1988. SEE C. *hip arthroplasty.*

Charrière, Joseph F.B., French instrument maker, 1803–1876. SEE C. *scale.*

chart. **1.** A recording of clinical data relating to a patient's case. **2.** SYN curve (2). **3.** In optics, symbols of graduated size for measuring visual acuity, or test types for determining far or near vision. SEE Snellen's *test types.* [L. *charta,* sheet of papyrus]

Amsler's c., a 10-cm square divided into 5-mm squares upon which an individual may project a defect in the central visual field.

isometric c. (ī'sō-met-rik), a c. or graph that displays three dimensions on a plane surface.

quality control c., a c. illustrating the allowable limits of error in laboratory test performance, the limits being a defined deviation from the mean of a control serum, most commonly ±2 SD. SEE ALSO quality *control.*

Tanner growth c., a series of c.'s showing distribution of parameters of physical development, such as stature, growth curves, and skinfold thickness, for children by sex, age, and stages of puberty.

Walker's c., a system of plotting the relative fetal and placental sizes.

Charters, W.J., U.S. dentist. SEE C.'s *method.*

chart·ing. Making a record in tabular or graph form of the progress of a patient's condition. SYN clinical recording.

Chassaignac, Edouard P.M., French surgeon, 1804–1879. SEE C.'s *space, tubercle.*

Chastek. Surname of the owner of a farm on which the disease later known as Chastek *paralysis* was first reported. SEE Chastek *paralysis.*

Chaudhry, Anand P. SEE Gorlin-C.-Moss *syndrome.*

Chauffard, Anatole M.E., French physician, 1855–1932. SEE C.'s *syndrome;* Still-C. *syndrome.*

chaul·moo·gra oil (chawl-mū'gră). The fixed oil expressed from seeds of *Taraktogenos kurzii* and *Hydnocarpus wightiana* (family Flacourtiaceae); formerly used in the treatment of leprosy. SYN gynocardia oil, hydnocarpus oil.

Chaussier, François, French physician, 1746–1828. SEE C.'s *areola, line, sign.*

Chauveau, J.-B. Auguste, French veterinarian, physiologist, and microbiologist, 1827–1917. SEE C.'s *bacterium.*

Chayes, Herman E.S., U.S. prosthodontist, 1880–1933. SEE C.'s *method.*

Ch.B. Abbreviation for *Chirurgiae Baccalaureus,* Bachelor of Surgery.

Ch.D. Abbreviation for *Chirurgiae Doctor,* Doctor of Surgery.

Cheadle, Walter B., English pediatrician, 1835–1910. SEE C.'s *disease.*

Cheatle, Sir George L., British surgeon, 1865–1951. SEE C. *slit.*

Δ **check.** SYN delta check.

check·bite (chek'bīt). SYN interocclusal *record.*

check·er·ber·ry oil (chek'er-bār'ē). SYN methyl salicylate.

Chédiak, Moisés, 20th century Cuban physician. SEE C.-Higashi *disease;* C.-Steinbrinck-Higashi *anomaly, syndrome.*

cheek (chēk). The side of the face forming the lateral wall of the mouth. SYN bucca [NA], gena, mala (1). [A. S. *ceáce*]

△**cheil-.** SEE cheilo-.

chei·lal·gia, chi·lal·gia (kī-lal'jē-ă). Pain in the lip. [cheil- + G. *algos,* pain]

chei·lec·to·my, chi·lec·to·my (kī-lek'tō-mē). **1.** Excision of a portion of the lip. **2.** Chiseling away bony irregularities at osteochondral margin of a joint cavity that interfere with movements of the joint. [cheil- + G. *ektomē,* excision]

cheil·ec·tro·pi·on, chil·ec·tro·pi·on (kī-lek-trō'pē-on). Eversion of the lips or a lip. [cheil- + G. *ektropos,* a turning out]

chei·li·on (kī'lē-on). A cephalometric point located at the angle (corner) of the mouth. [G. *cheilos,* lips]

chei·li·tis, chi·li·tis (kī-lī'tis). Inflammation of the lips or of a lip. SEE ALSO cheilosis. [cheil- + G. *-itis,* inflammation]

actinic c., SYN solar c.

angular c., inflammation and fissuring radiating from the commissures of the mouth secondary to predisposing factors such as lost vertical dimension in denture wearers, nutritional deficiencies, atopic dermatitis, or *Candida albicans* infection. SYN angular stomatitis, commissural c., perlèche.

commissural c., SYN angular c.

contact c., inflammation of the lips resulting from contact with a primary irritant or specific allergen, including ingredients of lipsticks.

c. exfoliati'va, an exfoliative dermatitis; it may be related to atopic dermatitis or to contact sensitivity.

c. glandula'ris, an acquired disorder, of unknown etiology, of the lower lip characterized by swelling, ulceration, crusting, mucous gland hyperplasia, abscesses, and sinus tracts. SYN Baelz' disease, myxadenitis labialis, Volkmann's c.

c. granulomato'sa, chronic, diffuse, soft swelling of the lips, of unknown etiology, microscopically characterized by noncaseating granulomatous inflammation. SEE ALSO Melkersson-Rosenthal *syndrome.*

impetiginous c., pyoderma of the lips.

solar c., mucosal atrophy with drying, crusting, and fissuring of the vermillion border of the lower lip in older individuals, resulting from chronic exposure to sunlight; dysplastic (premalignant) changes are noted microscopically, analogous to solar keratosis. SYN actinic c.

c. venena'ta, allergic contact dermatitis of the lips, as in contact c.

Volkmann's c., SYN c. glandularis.

△**cheilo-, cheil-.** Lips. SEE ALSO chilo-, labio-. [G. *cheilos,* lip]

chei·lo·gnath·o·glos·sos·chi·sis (kī'lō-nath'ō-glos-os'ki-sis). Associated condition of cleft mandible and lower lip, and bifid tongue. [cheilo- + G. *gnathos,* jaw, + *glōssa,* tongue, + *schisis,* cleft]

chei·lo·gnath·o·pal·a·tos·chi·sis (kī'lō-nath'ō-pal-ă-tos'ki-sis). SYN cheilognathouranoschisis.

chei·lo·gnath·o·u·ra·nos·chi·sis (kī-lō-nath'ō-yū-ră-nos'ki-sis). Cleft lip with cleft upper jaw and palate. SYN cheilognathopalatoschisis. [cheilo- + G. *gnathos,* jaw, + *ouranos,* sky (roof of mouth), + *schisis,* cleft]

chei·lo·pha·gia, chi·lo·pha·gia (kī-lō-fā'jē-ă). Biting of the lips. [cheilo- + G. *phagō,* to eat]

chei·lo·plas·ty, chi·lo·plas·ty (kī'lō-plas-tē). Plastic surgery of the lips. SYN chiloplasty. [cheilo- + G. *plastos,* formed]

chei·lor·rha·phy, chi·lor·rha·phy (kī-lōr'ă-fē). Suturing of the lip. SYN chilorrhaphy. [cheilo- + G. *raphē,* suture]

chei·lo·sis, chi·lo·sis (kī-lō'sis). A condition characterized by dry scaling and fissuring of the lips, attributed by some to riboflavin and other nutritional deficiencies. SEE ALSO cheilitis. [cheil- + G. *-osis,* condition]

chei·lo·sto·ma·to·plas·ty, chi·lo·sto·ma·to·plas·ty (kī-lō-stō'mă-tō-plas-tē). Obsolete term for plastic surgery of the lips and mouth. [cheilo- + G. *stoma,* mouth, + *plastos,* formed]

chei·lot·o·my, chi·lot·o·my (kī-lot'ō-mē). Incision into the lip. SYN chilotomy. [cheilo- + G. *tomē,* incision]

△**cheir-.** SEE cheiro-.

chei·rar·thri·tis, chi·rar·thri·tis (kī′rar-thrī′tis). Obsolete term for inflammation of the joints of the hand. SYN chirarthritis. [cheir- + arthritis]

△**cheiro-, cheir-.** Hand. SEE ALSO chiro-. [G. *cheir*, a hand]

chei·ro·bra·chi·al·gia, chi·ro·bra·chi·al·gia (kī′rō-brā′kē-al′jē-ă). Obsolete term for pain and paresthesia in the hand and arm. SYN chirobrachialgia. [cheiro- + G. *brachiōn*, arm, + *algos*, pain]

chei·rog·nos·tic, chi·rog·nos·tic (kī′rog-nos′tik). Able to distinguish between right and left, as of the hands or of which side of the body is touched. SYN chirognostic. [cheiro- + G. *gnostikos*, perceptive]

chei·ro·kin·es·the·sia (kī′rō-kin-es-thē′zē-ă). The subjective sensation of movement of the hands. SYN chirokinesthesia. [cheiro- + G. *kinēsis*, movement, + *aisthēsis*, sensation]

chei·ro·kin·es·thet·ic (kī′rō-kin-es-thet′ik). Relating to cheirokinesthesia.

chei·rol·o·gy, chi·rol·o·gy (kī-rol′ō-jē). SYN dactylology. [cheiro- + G. *logos*, word]

chei·ro·meg·a·ly, chi·ro·meg·a·ly (kī′rō-meg′ă-lē). SYN macrocheiria. [cheiro- + G. *megas*, large]

chei·ro·plas·ty, chi·ro·plas·ty (kī′rō-plas-tē). Rarely used term for plastic surgery of the hand. SYN chiroplasty. [cheiro- + G. *plastos*, formed]

chei·ro·po·dal·gia, chi·ro·po·dal·gia (kī′rō-pō-dal′jē-ă). Pain in the hands and in the feet. SYN chiropodalgia. [cheiro- + G. *pous*, foot, + *algos*, pain]

chei·ro·pom·pho·lyx, chi·ro·pom·pho·lyx (kī-rō-pom′fō-liks). SYN dyshidrosis. [cheiro- + G. *pompholyx*, a bubble, fr. *pomphos*, a blister]

chei·ro·spasm, chi·ro·spasm (kī′rō-spazm). Spasm of the muscles of the hand, as in writers' cramp. SYN chirospasm. [cheiro- + G. *spasmos*, spasm]

che·late (kē′lāt). **1.** To effect chelation. **2.** Pertaining to chelation. **3.** A complex formed through chelation.

che·la·tion (kē-lā′shŭn). Complex formation involving a metal ion and two or more polar groupings of a single molecule; thus, in heme, the Fe^{2+} ion is chelated by the porphyrin ring. C. can be used to remove an ion from participation in biological reactions, as in the c. of Ca^{2+} of blood by EDTA, which thus acts as an anticoagulant. [G. *chēlē*, claw]

che·lic·era, pl. **che·lic·er·ae** (ke-lis′ĭ-ră, -ĭ-rē). One of the two anterior appendages of arachnids; in ticks and parasitic mites, the chelicerae are piercing and cutting structures, and constitute important feeding organs. [G. *chēlē*, claw, + *keras*, horn]

chel·i·don (kel′ĕ-don). SYN cubital *fossa*. [G. *chelidōn*, a swallow, because of fancied resemblance to the shape of a swallow's tail]

che·loid (kē′loyd). SYN keloid.

Che·lo·nia (kē-lō′nē-ă). An order of reptiles, embracing the turtles, tortoises, and terrapins, whose bodies are enclosed in a bony shell covered with epidermal scutes and formed dorsally by expanded ribs and ventrally by a sternal plastron. [G. *chelōnē*, a tortoise]

che·lo·ni·an (kē-lō′nē-an). Resembling or relating to a turtle, tortoise, or terrapin.

△**chem-.** SEE chemo-.

chem·ex·fo·li·a·tion (kem′eks-fō-lē-ā′shŭn). A chemosurgical technique designed to remove acne scars or treat chronic skin changes caused by exposure to sunlight. SYN chemical peeling.

chem·i·a·try (kem′i-ă-trē). SYN iatrochemistry.

chem·i·cal (kem′i-kăl). Relating to chemistry.

chem·i·co·cau·tery (kem′i-kō-kaw′ter-ē). SYN chemocautery.

chem·i·lu·mi·nes·cence (kem′ē-lū-min-es′ens). Light produced by chemical action usually at, or below, room temperature. SYN chemoluminescence.

chem·i·o·tax·is (kem′ē-ō-taks′is). SYN chemotaxis.

che·mise (shem-ēz′). A square of gauze fastened to a catheter passed through its center; used to retain a tampon packed around the catheter inserted into a wound, such as that resulting from a perineal section. [Fr. shirt]

chem·ist (kem′ist). **1.** A specialist or expert in chemistry. **2.** Pharmacist (British).

chem·is·try (kem′is-trē). **1.** The science concerned with the atomic composition of substances, the elements and their interreactions, and the formation, decomposition, and properties of molecules. **2.** The chemical properties of a substance. **3.** Chemical processes. [G. *chēmeia*, alchemy]

analytic c., the application of c. to the determination and detection of composition and identification of specific substances.

applied c., the application of the theories and principles of chemistry to practical purposes.

biological c., SYN biochemistry.

clinical c., **(1)** the c. of human health and disease; **(2)** c. in connection with the management of patients, as in a hospital laboratory.

ecological c., c. that concentrates on the effects of woman-made chemicals on the environment as well as the development of agents that are not harmful to the environment. **(2)** the study of the molecular interactions between species and between species and the environment.

epithermal c., so-called "hot atom" c.; the science concerned with the chemical reactions of recoil atoms and free radicals produced in low energy nuclear processes.

inorganic c., the science concerned with compounds not involving carbon-containing molecules.

macromolecular c., the c. of macromolecules (*e.g.,* proteins, nucleic acids) and polymers (nylon, polyethylene, etc.).

medical c., c. in its relation to pharmacy, physiology, or any science connected with medicine.

medicinal c., SYN pharmaceutical c.

nuclear c., the science concerned with the c. of nuclear reactions and processes.

organic c., that branch of c. concerned with covalently linked atoms, centering around carbon compounds of this type; originally, and still including, the c. of natural products.

pharmaceutical c., medicinal c. in its application to the analysis, development, preparation, and the manufacture of drugs. SYN medicinal c., pharmacochemistry.

physiological c., SYN biochemistry.

radiation c., the science concerned with the effects of ionizing or nuclear radiation on chemical reactions or materials.

radiopharmaceutical c., the science concerned with the labeling of pharmaceuticals with radionuclides.

synthetic c., the formation or building up of complex compounds by uniting the more simple ones.

△**chemo-, chem-.** Chemistry. [G. *chēmeia*, alchemy]

che·mo·au·to·troph (kem′ō-aw′tō-trōf, kē′mō). An organism that depends on chemicals for its energy and principally on carbon dioxide for its carbon. SYN chemolithotroph. [chemo- + G. *autos*, self, + *trophikos*, nourishing]

che·mo·au·to·tro·phic (kem′ō-aw-tō-trof′ik, kē′mo-). Pertaining to a chemoautotroph. SYN chemolithotrophic.

che·mo·bi·o·dy·nam·ics (kem′ō-bī-ō-dī-nam′iks, kē′mō-). Study devoted to elucidation of correlations between the chemical constitution of various materials and their ability to modify the function and morphology of biological systems. [chemo- + G. *bios*, life, + *dynamis*, power]

che·mo·cau·tery (kem′ō-kaw-ter-ē, kē′mō-). Any substance that destroys tissue upon application. SYN chemical cautery, chemicocautery.

che·mo·cep·tor (kem′ō-sep-tŏr, kē′mō-). SYN chemoreceptor.

che·mo·dec·to·ma (kem′ō-dek-tō′mă, kē′mō-). Aortic body, carotid body, chemoreceptor, or glomus jugulare tumor; nonchromaffin paraganglioma; receptoma; a relatively rare, usually benign neoplasm originating in the chemoreceptor tissue of the carotid body, glomus jugulare, and aortic bodies; consisting histologically of rounded or ovoid hyperchromatic cells that tend to be grouped in an alveolus-like pattern within a scant to moderate amount of fibrous stroma and a few large thin-walled vascular channels. Cf. paraganglioma. SYN aortic body tumor, carotid body tumor, chemoreceptor tumor, glomus jugulare tumor, non-

ch

chromaffin paraganglioma. [chemo- + G. *dektēs*, receiver, fr. *dechomai*, to receive, + *-oma*, tumor]

che·mo·dec·to·ma·to·sis (kem′ō-dek-tō-mă-to′sis, kē′mō-). Multiple tumors of perivascular tissue of carotid body or presumed chemoreceptor type, which have been reported in the lungs as minute neoplasms.

che·mo·dif·fer·en·ti·a·tion (kem′ō-dif-er-en-shē-ā′shŭn, kē′mō-). Differentiation of the cellular chemical constituents in the embryo prior to cytodifferentiation; sometimes recognizable histochemically. SYN invisible differentiation.

che·mo·het·er·o·troph (kem′ō-het′er-ō-trōf, kē′mō-). SYN chemoorganotroph. [chem- + G. *heteros*, other, + *trophē*, nourishment]

che·mo·het·er·o·troph·ic (kem′ō-het-er-ō-trof′ik, kē′mō-). SYN chemoorganotrophic.

che·mo·im·mu·nol·o·gy (kem′ō-im-yū-nol′ō-jē, kē′mō-). SYN immunochemistry.

che·mo·kines (kē′mō-kinz). A group of specific chemotactic polypeptides all of which have a 4-cysteine structure, *e.g.,* interleukin 8. [chemo- + G. *kineō,* to set in motion]

che·mo·ki·ne·sis (kem′ō-ki-nē′sis, kē′mō-). Stimulation of an organism by a chemical. [chemo- + G. *kinēsis,* movement]

che·mo·ki·net·ic (kem′-ō-ki-net′ik, kē′mo-). Referring to chemokinesis.

che·mo·lith·o·troph (kem′ō-lith′ō-trōf, kē′mō-). SYN chemoautotroph.

che·mo·lith·o·tro·phic (kem′ō-lith-ō-trof′ik, kē′mō-). SYN chemoautotrophic.

che·mo·lith·o·tro·phy (kem′ō-lith′ō-trōf-ē). The utilization of inorganic compounds or ions to obtain reducing equivalents and energy. [chemo- + G. *lithos,* stone, mineral, + *trophe,* nourishment]

che·mo·lu·mi·nes·cence (kem′ō-lū-min-es′ens, kē′mō-). SYN chemiluminescence.

chem·ol·y·sis (kem-ol′i-sis). Chemical decomposition. [chemo- + G. *lysis,* dissolution]

che·mo·nu·cle·ol·y·sis (kem′ō-nū-klē-ol′i-sis, kē′mō-). Injection of chymopapain into the nucleus pulposis of an intervertebral disc. A therapeutic option for the treatment of a herniated nucleus pulposis, *e.g.,* "slipped disc."

che·mo·or·ga·no·troph (kem′ō-ōr′gă-nō-trōf, kē′mō-). An organism that depends on organic chemicals for its energy and carbon. SYN chemoheterotroph. [chemo- + G. *organon,* organ, + *trophē,* nourishment]

che·mo·or·ga·no·tro·phic (kem′ō-ōr-gă-nō-trof′ik, kē′mō-). Pertaining to a chemoorganotroph. SYN chemoheterotrophic.

che·mo·pal·li·dec·to·my (kem′ō-pal-i-dek′tō-mē, kē′mō-). Destruction of the globus pallidus by injection of a chemical agent. SYN chemopallidotomy. [chemo- + globus pallidus + G. *ektomē,* excision]

che·mo·pal·li·do·thal·a·mec·to·my (kem′ō-pal′i-dō-thal-ă-mek′tō-mē, kē′mō-). Destruction of portions of the globus pallidus and thalamus by injection of a chemical substance. [chemo- + globus pallidus + thalamus + G. *ektomē,* excision]

che·mo·pal·li·dot·o·my (kēm′ō-pal-i-dot′ō-mē, kē′mō-). SYN chemopallidectomy. [chemo- + globus pallidus + G. *tomē,* incision]

che·mo·pro·phy·lax·is (kem′ō-pro′fi-lak′sis, kē′mō-). Prevention of disease by the use of chemicals or drugs.

che·mo·re·cep·tor (kem′ō-rē-sep′tŏr, kē′mō-). Any cell that is activated by a change in its chemical milieu and results in a nerve impulse. Such cells can be either 1) "transducer" cells innervated by sensory nerve fibers (*e.g.,* the gustatory receptor cells of the taste buds; cells in the carotid body sensitive to changes in the oxygen and carbon dioxide content of the blood); or 2) nerve cells proper, such as the olfactory receptor cells of the olfactory mucosa, and certain cells in the brainstem that are sensitive to changes in the composition of the blood or cerebrospinal fluid. SYN chemoceptor.

medullary c., the c.'s in or near the ventrolateral surface of the medulla that are stimulated by local acidity.

peripheral c., the c.'s in the carotid and aortic bodies that are

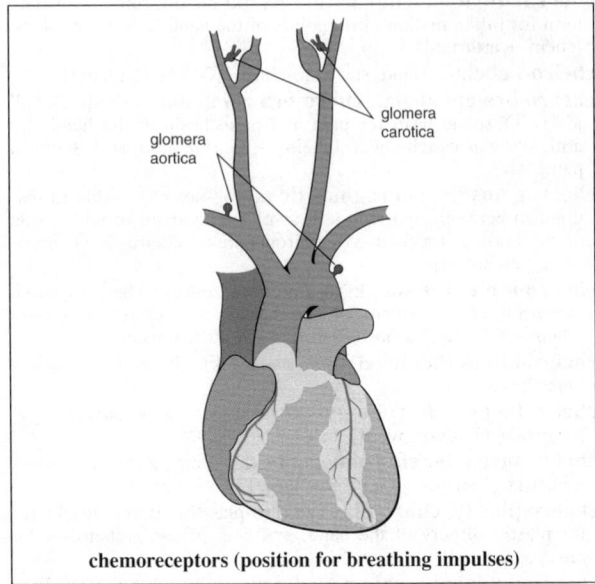

chemoreceptors (position for breathing impulses)

stimulated by chemical changes in the composition of the blood such as hypoxia.

che·mo·re·flex (kem-ō-rē′fleks, kē′mō-). A reflex initiated by the stimulation of chemoreceptors, *e.g.,* of a carotid body.

che·mo·re·sis·tance (kem′ō-rē-zis′tans, kē′mō-). The resistance of bacteria or malignant cells to the inhibiting action of certain chemical substances used in treatment.

che·mo·sen·si·tive (kem-ō-sen′si-tiv, kē′mō-). Capable of perceiving changes in the chemical composition of the environment, *e.g.,* changes in the oxygen and carbon dioxide content of the blood.

che·mo·se·ro·ther·a·py (kem′ō-sēr′ō-thār-ă-pē, kē′mō-). An obsolete treatment of disease with a combination of drugs and serum.

che·mo·sis (kē-mō′sis). Edema of the bulbar conjunctiva, forming a swelling around the cornea. [G. *chēmē,* a yawning, the cockle (from its gaping shell)]

chem·os·mo·sis (kem-os-mō′sis). Chemical reaction between substances initially separated by a membrane. [chem- + G. *ōsmos,* a thrusting, an impulsion]

che·mo·stat (kem′ō-stat). A fermenter for microbial growth in which the ratio of growth to synthesis of secondary products is controlled by the rate at which new medium is added to the culture.

che·mo·sur·gery (kem′ō-ser-jer-ē, kē′mō-). Excision of diseased tissue after it has been fixed *in situ* by chemical means.

Mohs' c., a technique for removal of skin tumors with a minimum of normal tissue, by prior necrosis with zinc chloride paste, mapping of the tumor site, and excision and microscopic examination of frozen section of thin horizontal layers of tissue, until all of the tumor is removed. More recently, the preliminary step of chemical necrosis has been omitted. SYN microscopically controlled surgery, Mohs' micrographic surgery, Mohs' surgery.

che·mo·syn·the·sis (kem′ō-sin′thĕ-sis). **1.** Chemical synthesis. **2.** Chemolithotrophy.

che·mo·tac·tic (kem-ō-tak′tik, kē′mō-). Relating to chemotaxis.

che·mo·tax·is (kem-ō-tak′sis, kē′mo-). Movement of cells or organisms in response to chemicals, whereby the cells are attracted (**positive c.**) or repelled (**negative c.**) by substances exhibiting chemical properties. SYN chemiotaxis, chemotropism. [chemo- + G. *taxis,* orderly arrangement]

che·mo·thal·a·mec·to·my (kem′ō-thal-ă-mek′tō-mē, kē′mō-). Chemical destruction of a part of the thalamus, usually for relief of pain or dyskinesia. SYN chemothalamotomy. [chemo- + thalamus, + G. *ektomē,* excision]

che·mo·thal·a·mot·o·my (kem′ō-thal-ă-mot′ō-mē, kē′mō-). SYN chemothalamectomy.

che·mo·ther·a·peu·tic (kem′ō-thār-ă-pyū′tik, kē′mō-). Relating to chemotherapy.

che·mo·ther·a·peu·tics (kem′ō-thār-ă-pyū′tiks, kē′mō). The branch of therapeutics concerned with chemotherapy.

che·mo·ther·a·py (kem′ō-thār-ă-pē, kē′mō-). Treatment of disease by means of chemical substances or drugs; usually used in reference to neoplastic disease. SEE ALSO pharmacotherapy.

consolidation c., repetitive cycles of treatment during the immediate post-remission period, used especially for leukemia. SYN intensification c.

induction c., use of c. as initial treatment before surgery or radiotherapy of a malignancy.

intensification c., SYN consolidation c.

salvage c., use of c. in a patient with recurrence of a malignancy following initial treatment, in hope of a cure or prolongation of life.

che·mot·ic (kē-mot′ic). Relating to chemosis.

che·mo·trans·mit·ter (kem-ō-trans′mit-er, kē-mō-). A chemical substance produced to diffuse and cause responses of neurons or effector cells.

che·mo·troph (kem-ō-trōf). An organism that obtains its energy by the oxidation of inorganic or organic nutrients.

che·mot·ro·pism (kem-ō-trōp′izm, kē-mō-). SYN chemotaxis. [chemo- + G. *tropos,* direction, turn]

Chenais, Louis J., French physician, 1872–1950. SEE Cestan-C. *syndrome.*

Cheney, William D., U.S. radiologist, *1918. SEE C. *syndrome.*

che·no·de·ox·y·cho·lic ac·id (kē′nō-dē-oks-ē-kō′lik). 3α,7α-dihydroxy-5β-cholan-24-oic acid; a major bile acid in many vertebrates, usually conjugated with glycine or taurine, which facilitates cholesterol excretion and fat absorption; administered to dissolve cholesterol gallstones. SYN chenodiol.

che·no·di·ol (kē-nō-dī′ol). SYN chenodeoxycholic acid.

che·no·po·di·um (kē-nō-pō′dē-ŭm). The dried ripe fruit of *Chenopodium ambrosoides* (family Chenopodiaceae), American wormwood, from which a volatile oil is distilled and used as an anthelmintic. SYN Jesuit tea, Mexican tea, wormseed (2). [G. *chēn,* goose, + *pous* (*pod-*), foot]

Cherenkov, SEE Cerenkov.

cher·ry juice (char′ē). The juice expressed from the fresh ripe fruit of *Prunus cerasus,* containing not less than 1.0% of malic acid; used as a flavoring agent, and as a vehicle for cough syrups and other preparations for oral administrations.

che·rub·ism (char′ŭb-izm) [MIM*118480]. Hereditary giant cell lesions of the jaws beginning in early childhood; multilocular radiolucencies and progressive symmetric painless swelling of the jaws; bilateral; occurs with no associated systemic manifestations. SYN fibrous dysplasia of jaws. [Hebr. *kerubh,* cherub]

chest. The anterior wall of the chest or thorax; the breast. SEE ALSO thorax. SYN pectus [NA], phthinoid. [A.S. *cest,* a box]

alar c., SYN flat c.

barrel c., a c. permanently resembling the shape of a barrel, *i.e.,* with increased anteroposterior diameter, roughly equaling the lateral diameter; usually with some degree of kyphosis; seen in cases of emphysema.

flail c., flapping chest wall; loss of stability of thoracic cage following fracture of sternum, ribs, or both.

flat c., a c. in which the anteroposterior diameter is shorter than the average. SYN alar c., pterygoid c.

foveated c., funnel c., SYN *pectus* excavatum.

keeled c., SYN *pectus* carinatum.

phthinoid c., a long narrow c., the lower ribs being more oblique than usual and sometimes reaching almost to the crest of the ilium, with the scapulae projecting backward, the manubrium sterni depressed, and Louis' angle sharper than normal; such a c. was once considered indicative of pulmonary tuberculosis.

pigeon c., SYN *pectus* carinatum.

pterygoid c., SYN flat c.

chest·nut (chest′nŭt). A small oval or round horny structure in the skin on the inner side of the legs of the horse. Since the architecture of c.'s varies in every individual, they may be used, like fingerprints of man, for positive identification of individuals.

Cheyne, John, Scottish physician, 1777–1836. SEE C.-Stokes *psychosis, respiration.*

chi (kī). **1.** The 22nd letter of the Greek alphabet, χ. **2.** In chemistry, denotes the 22nd in a series. **3.** Symbol for the dihedral angle between the α-carbon and the side-chains of amino acids in peptides and proteins.

Chiari, Hans, German pathologist, 1851–1916. SEE Arnold-C. *deformity, malformation, syndrome;* C.'s *disease, net, syndrome;* C. II *syndrome;* C.-Budd *syndrome;* Budd-C. *syndrome.*

Chiari, Johann B., German obstetrician, 1817–1854. SEE C.-Frommel *syndrome.*

chi·asm (kī′azm). **1.** The crossing of intertwined chromosomes during prophase. **2.** SYN chiasma. [G. *chiasma*]

Camper's c., SYN tendinous c. of the digital tendons.

optic c., a flattened quadrangular body in front of the tuber cinereum and infundibulum, the point of crossing or decussation of the fibers of the optic nerves; most of the fibers cross to the opposite side, some run directly forward on each side without crossing, some pass transversely on the posterior surface between the two optic tracts and others pass transversely on the anterior surface between the two optic nerves. SYN chiasma opticum [NA], optic decussation.

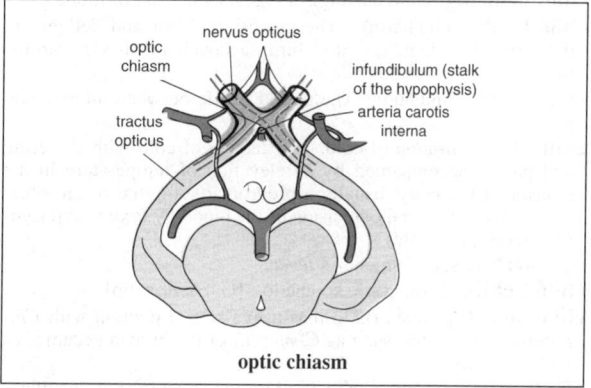

optic chiasm

tendinous c. of the digital tendons, crossing of the tendons, the passage of the tendons of the flexor digitorum profundus (flexor digitorum longus in the foot) through the interval left by the decussation of the fibers of the tendons of the flexor digitorum superficialis (flexor digitorum brevis in the foot). SYN chiasma tendinum [NA], Camper's c.

chi·as·ma, pl. **chi·as·ma·ta** (kī-az′mă, kī-az′mă-tă) [NA]. **1.** A decussation or crossing of two tracts, such as tendons or nerves; **2.** A site at which two homologous chromosomes appear to have exchanged material during meiosis. SYN chiasm (2). [G. *chiasma,* two crossing lines, fr. the letter *chi,* 3]

c. op′ticum [NA], SYN optic *chiasm.*

c. ten′dinum [NA], SYN tendinous *chiasm* of the digital tendons.

♻ Combining forms	[NA] Nomina Anatomica
Word*Finder*	[MIM] Mendelian
Multi-term entry finder	**Inheritance in Man**
Preceding letter A	
A.D.A.M. Anatomy Plates	☆ Official alternate term
Between letters L and M	
Appendices:	☆[NA] Official alternate
Following letter Z	**Nomina Anatomica term**
SYN Synonym; Cf., compare	High Profile Term

chi·as·ma·pexy (kī-as'mă-pek-sē). Surgical fixation of the optic chiasma. [G. *chiasma,* decussation, + *pēxis,* fixation]

chi·as·mat·ic (kī-az-mat'ik). Relating to a chiasm.

chick·en·pox (chik'en-poks). SYN varicella.

Chick-Martin test. See under test.

chi·cle (chik'el). The partially evaporated viscous, milky juice from *Manilkara zapotilla,* sapotaceae), which is native to the West Indies, Mexico, and Central America or a mixture of gutta with triterpene alcohols. Used in the manufacture of chewing gum. [Sp., from Nahuatl *chictli*]

Chievitz, Johan H., Danish anatomist, 1850–1901. SEE C.'s *layer, organ.*

chig·ger (chig'er). The six-legged larva of *Trombicula* species and other members of the family Trombiculidae; a bloodsucking stage of mites that includes the vectors of scrub typhus.

chig·oe (chig'ō). Common name for *Tunga penetrans.*

△**chil-.** SEE chilo-.

Chilaiditi, Demetrius, Austrian radiologist, *1883. SEE C.'s *syndrome.*

chil·blain (chil'blān). Erythema, itching, and burning, especially of the dorsa of the fingers and toes, and of the heels, nose, and ears caused by vascular constriction on exposure to extreme cold (usually associated with high humidity); lesions can be single or multiple, and can become blistered and ulcerated. SYN erythema pernio, perniosis. [chill + A.S. *blegen,* a blain]

CHILD SEE CHILD *syndrome.*

child·bear·ing (chīld'bār-ing). Pregnancy and parturition.

child·birth (chīld'berth). The process of labor and delivery in the birth of a child. SEE ALSO birth, accouchement. SYN parturition.

child·hood (chīld'hud). The period of life between infancy and puberty.

chill. 1. A sensation of cold. 2. A feeling of cold with shivering and pallor, accompanied by an elevation of temperature in the interior of the body; usually a prodromal symptom of an infectious disease due to the invasion of the blood by toxins. SYN rigor (2). [A.S. *cele,* cold]

smelter's c.'s, SYN smelter's *fever.*

△**chilo-, chil-.** Lips. SEE ALSO cheilo-. [G. *cheilos,* lip]

chi·lo·mas·ti·gi·a·sis (kī'lō-mas-ti-gī'ă-sis). Infection with *Chilomastix* flagellates, such as *C. mesnili* of the human cecum. SYN chilomastosis.

Chi·lo·mas·tix (kī-lō-mas'tiks). A genus of protozoan flagellates parasitic in the large intestine of man and other primates, and in many other mammals, birds, amphibia, and reptiles; it is ordinarily nonpathogenic, but one species, *C. mesnili,* may be an occasional cause of diarrhea in children. [chilo- + G. *mastix,* whip]

chi·lo·mas·to·sis (kī'lō-mas-tō'sis). SYN chilomastigiasis.

chi·lo·plas·ty (kī'lō-plas-tē). SYN cheiloplasty.

Chi·lo·po·da (kī-lop'ŏ-dă). A class of centipedes (phylum Arthropoda). [chilo- + G. *pous,* foot]

chi·lo·po·di·a·sis (kī'lō-pō-dī'ă-sis). Invasion of one of the cavities, especially the nasal cavity, by a species of Chilopoda.

chi·lor·rha·phy (kī-lōr'ă-fē). SYN cheilorrhaphy.

chi·lo·sto·ma·to·plas·ty (kī-lō-stō'ma-tō-plas-tē). Variant of cheilostomatoplasty.

chi·lot·o·my (kī-lot'ō-mē). SYN cheilotomy.

chi·me·ra (kī-mēr'ă, ki-). 1. In experimental embryology, the individual produced by grafting an embryonic part of one animal on to the embryo of another, either of the same or of another species. 2. An organism that has received a transplant of genetically and immunologically different tissue, such as bone marrow. 3. Dizygotic twins that retain each other as immunologically distinct types of erythrocytes. 4. Sometimes used as a synonym for mosaic. Chimeric antibodies may have the FAB fragment from one species fused with the Fc fragment from another. 5. A protein fusion in which two different proteins, usually from different species, are linked via peptide bonds; usually genetically engineered. 6. Any macromolecule fusion formed by two or more macromolecules from different species or from different

genes. [L. *Chimaera,* G. *Chimaira,* mythic monster, (lit. a she-goat)]

radiation c., an individual with mosaicism induced by exposure to ionizing radiation. SEE mosaic.

chi·mer·ic (kī-mēr'ik). 1. Relating to a chimera. Cf. chimera (5), chimeric *molecule.* 2. Composed of parts that are of different origin and are seemingly incompatible.

chi·me·rism (kī-mēr'izm). The state of being a chimera.

chim·pan·zee (chim-pan'zē, chim'pan-zē'). Generic name for *Pan panisus* and *P. troglodytes.* [African dial.]

chin. The prominence formed by the anterior projection of the mandible, or lower jaw. The chin. SYN mentum [NA]. [A.S. *cin*]

double c., SYN buccula.

galoche c. (ga-lōsh), an abnormally narrow, protruding c.

chin·ic ac·id (chin'ik). SYN quinic acid.

chi·ni·o·fon (kin'ē-ō-fon). A mixture of 7-iodo-8-hydroxyquinoline-5-sulfonic acid and sodium bicarbonate, used in the treatment of amebic dysentery.

chin·o·le·ine (chin'ō-lē-in). SYN quinoline (1).

chip. A small fragment resulting from breakage, cutting, or avulsion.

bone c.'s, small pieces of cancellous bone generally used to fill in bony defects and to promote reossification.

chip-blow·er. An instrument for blowing the debris out of, or drying, a tooth cavity that is being excavated for a filling; it consists of a rubber bulb with a metal nozzle.

chi·ral (kī'răl). Denoting an object, such as a molecule in a given configuration or conformation, that possesses chirality. A c. molecule has no plane, axis, or center of symmetry.

chi·ral·i·ty (kī-ral'i-tē). The property of nonidentity of an object with its mirror image; used in chemistry with respect to stereochemical isomers. [G. *cheir,* hand]

chi·rar·thri·tis (kī-rar-thrī'tis). SYN cheirarthritis.

△**chiro-, chir-.** The hand. SEE ALSO cheiro-. [G. *cheir,* hand]

chi·ro·bra·chi·al·gia (kī'rō-brā-kē-al'jē-ă). SYN cheirobrachialgia.

chi·rog·nos·tic (kī-rog-nos'tik). SYN cheirognostic.

chi·ro·kin·es·the·sia (kī-rō-kin-es-thē'zē-ă). SYN cheirokinesthesia.

chi·rol·o·gy (kī-rol'ō-jē). SYN dactylology.

chi·ro·meg·a·ly (kī-rō-meg'ă-lē). SYN macrocheiria.

chi·ro·plas·ty (kī'rō-plas-tē). SYN cheiroplasty.

chi·ro·po·dal·gia (kī'rō-pō-dal'jē-ă). SYN cheiropodalgia.

chi·rop·o·dist (kī-rop'ō-dist). SYN podiatrist. [chiro- + G. *pous,* foot]

chi·rop·o·dy (kī-rop'ō-dē). SYN podiatry.

chi·ro·pom·pho·lyx (kī-rō-pom'fō-liks). SYN dyshidrosis.

chi·ro·prac·tic (kī-rō-prak'tik). The system that in theory uses the recuperative powers of the body and the relationship between the musculoskeletal structures and functions of the body, particularly of the spinal column and the nervous system, in the restoration and maintenance of health. [chiro- + G. *praktikos,* efficient]

chi·ro·prac·tor (kī-rō-prak'tŏr). One who is licensed and certified to practice chiropractic.

Chi·rop·te·ra (kī-rop'ter-ă). The bats, an order of placental mammals of worldwide distribution, characterized by a modification of the forelimbs that enables them to fly. They are capable of emitting ultrasonic sounds that enable them to echolocate, find flying insect prey, and avoid objects in the dark. Though mostly insectivorous, some species feed on nectar, fruit, fish, and blood; the blood-feeding and insectivorous species are important reservoir hosts of rabies. [chiro- + G. *pteron,* wing]

chi·ro·scope (kī'rō-skōp). A haploscopic instrument used for coordinating hand and eye as the patient draws while looking through it. [chiro- + G. *skopeō,* to view]

chi·ro·spasm (kī'rō-spazm). SYN cheirospasm.

chirurg. Abbreviation for L. *chirurgicalis,* surgical.

chi·rur·geon (kī-rer'jon). Obsolete term for surgeon. [G. *cheirourgos,* fr. *cheir,* hand, + *ergon,* work]

chi·rur·gery (kī-rer′jer-ē). Obsolete term for surgery. [G. *cheirourgia*]

chi·rur·gi·cal (kī-rer′ji-kăl). Obsolete term for surgical. [L. surgical, fr. *chirurgia*, surgery, fr. G. *cheirourgia*, handicraft, fr. *cheir*, hand + *ergon*, work]

chis·el (chiz′l). A single beveled end-cutting blade with a straight or angled shank used with a thrust along the axis of the handle for cutting or splitting dentin and enamel.

binangle c., a c. with an angled shank to which a second angle is added in order to bring the cutting edge nearly in line with the axis of the handle so as to restore balance and to prevent it from turning about the axis; used when a c. must be angled for access.

chi-square (kī′ skwär). A statistical technique whereby variables are categorized to determine whether a distribution of scores is due to chance or experimental factors.

chi·tin (kī′tin). A polymer of *N*-acetyl-D-glucosamine, linked β(1→4), similar in structure to cellulose and the second most abundant polysaccharide in nature, comprising the horny substance in the exoskeleton of beetles, crabs, certain microorganisms, etc.

chi·ti·nase (kī′ti-nās). An enzyme catalyzing the random hydrolysis of β(1→4) linkages in chitin (ultimately releasing *N*-acetyl-D-glucosamine); some enzymes of this type display lysozyme activity. SYN chitodextrinase, poly-β-glucosaminidase.

chi·tin·ous (kī′tin-ŭs). Of or relating to chitin.

chi·to·bi·ose (kī-tō-bī′ōs). The disaccharide repeating unit in chitin; differs from cellobiose only in the presence of an *N*-acetylamino group on carbon-2 in place of the hydroxyl group.

chi·to·dex·tri·nase (kī-tō-deks′tri-nās). SYN chitinase.

chi·to·sa·mine (kī-tō′să-mēn). D-Glucosamine. SEE glucosamine.

chi·u·fa (chē-ū′fă). An acute gangrenous proctitis and colitis with high fever, seen in southern Africa and South America at high altitudes; in women, the vulva and vagina may be affected. SYN kanyemba.

CHL Abbreviation for crown-heel *length*.

Chla·myd·ia (kla-mid′ē-ă). The single genus of the family Chlamydiaceae, including all the agents of the psittacosis-lymphogranuloma-trachoma disease groups. Two species are recognized, *C. psittaci* and *C. trachomatis;* the latter is differentiated from the former by its intracytoplasmic production of glycogen and its susceptibility to sulfadiazine. The type species is *C. trachomatis.* Formerly called *Bedsonia.* SYN *Chlamydozoon.* [G. *chlamys*, cloak]

C. pneumo′niae, a species that causes pneumonia and upper and lower respiratory disease.

C. psi′ttaci, organisms that resemble *C. trachomatis*, but which form loosely bound intracytoplasmic microcolonies up to 12 μm in diameter, do not produce glycogen in sufficient quantity to be detected by iodine stains, and are not susceptible to sulfadiazine. Various strains of this species cause psittacosis in man and ornithosis in nonpsittacine birds; pneumonitis in cattle, sheep, swine, cats, goats, and horses; enzootic abortion of ewes; bovine sporadic encephalomyelitis; enteritis of calves; epizootic chlamydiosis of muskrats and hares; encephalitis of opossum; and conjunctivitis of cattle, sheep, and guinea pigs.

C. tracho′matis, spherical nonmotile organisms that form compact intracytoplasmic microcolonies up to 10 μm in diameter which (by division) give rise to infectious spherules 0.3 μm or more in diameter, accumulate glycogen for a limited period in sufficient quantity to be detected by iodine stain, and are susceptible to sulfadiazine and tetracycline; various strains of this species cause trachoma, inclusion and neonatal conjunctivitis, lymphogranuloma venereum, mouse pneumonitis, nonspecific urethritis, epididymitis, cervicitis, salpingitis, proctitis, and pneumonia; chief agent of bacterial sexually transmitted diseases in the U.S.; the type species of the genus *C.*

chla·myd·ia, pl. **chla·myd·i·ae** (kla-mid′ē-ă, -mid′ē-ē). A vernacular term used to refer to any member of the genus *Chlamydia.*

Chlam·y·di·a·ce·ae (kla-mid′ē-ā′sē-ē). A family of the order Chlamydiales (formerly included in the order Rickettsiales) that includes the agents of the psittacosis-lymphogranuloma-tracho-

ma group. The family contains small, coccoid, Gram-negative bacteria that resemble rickettsiae but which differ from them significantly by possessing a unique, obligately intracellular developmental cycle; intracytoplasmic microcolonies give rise to infectious forms by division. The classification of these organisms previously was in a state of flux, but they are now placed in a single genus, *Chlamydia*, the type genus of the family.

chla·myd·i·al (kla-mid′ē-ăl). Relating to or caused by any bacterium of the genus *Chlamydia.*

chla·myd·i·o·sis (klă-mid-ē-ō′sis). General term for diseases caused by *Chlamydia* species. SEE ALSO ornithosis, psittacosis.

chlam·y·do·co·nid·i·um (klam′i-dō-kŏ-nid′ē-um). A thallic conidium that is thick-walled and may be terminal or intercalary. Seen in a form of asexual reproduction. [G. *chlamys*, cloak, + conidium]

Chlam·y·do·phrys (kla-mid′ō-fris). A genus of shelled amebas, commonly found as fecal protozoans. [G. *chlamys*, cloak, + *ophrys*, brow]

Chlam·y·do·zo·on (klam′i-dō-zō′on). SYN *Chlamydia.*

chlo·as·ma (klō-az′mă). Melanoderma or melasma characterized by the occurrence of extensive brown patches of irregular shape and size on the skin of the face and elsewhere; the pigmented facial patches if confluent are also called the mask of pregnancy, and are associated most commonly with pregnancy and use of oral contraceptives. SYN moth patch. [G. *chloazō*, to become green]

c. bronzi′num, a bronze-colored pigmentation, probably produced by hormone imbalance, occurring in gradually increasing areas on the face, neck, and chest in persons exposed continuously to the tropical sun; similar to c. of the temperate zone, but intensified because of strong sunlight. SYN tropical mask.

chlo·phe·di·a·nol hy·dro·chlo·ride (klō-fĕ-dī′ă-nol). 2-Chloro-α-(2-dimethylaminoethyl)benzhydrol hydrochloride; an antitussive agent related chemically to the antihistamines.

△**chlor-, chloro-. 1.** Combining form denoting green. **2.** Combining form denoting association with chlorine. [G. *chloros*, green]

chlor·a·ce·tic ac·id (klōr-ă-sē′tik). SYN chloroacetic acid.

chlor·ac·ne (klōr-ak′nē). An occupational acne-like eruption due to prolonged contact with certain chlorinated compounds (naphthalenes and diphenyls); keratinous plugs (comedones) form in the pilosebaceous orifices, and variously sized small papules (2 to 4 mm) develop. SYN chlorine acne, tar acne.

chlo·ral (klōr′ăl). CCl₃-CHO; trichloroacetaldehyde; a thin oily liquid with a pungent odor, formed by the action of chlorine gas on alcohol. SYN anhydrous c.

anhydrous c., SYN chloral.

c. betaine, the adduct formed by chloral hydrate and betaine; it is slowly hydrolyzed in the alimentary tract to chloral hydrate; used as a hypnotic and sedative.

c. hydrate, $CCl_3CH(OH)_2$; a hypnotic, sedative, and anticonvulsant; it is also used externally as a rubefacient, anesthetic, and antiseptic.

m-**chlo·ral.** A polymer of chloral obtained by prolonged contact with sulfuric acid; it has properties similar to those of chloral hydrate. SYN metachloral, *p*-chloral, trichloral.

p-**chlo·ral.** SYN *m*-chloral.

chlo·ral al·co·hol·ate. A complex of chloral and ethanol. Prepared by refluxing trichloroacetaldehyde (chloral) or chloral hydrate with alcohol. Alleged to be an active constituent of a "Mickey Finn."

chlo·ral·ism (klōr′ăl-izm). Habitual use of chloral compounds as an intoxicant, or the symptoms caused thereby.

α-**chlor·a·lose** (klōr′ă-lōs). A conjugate of chloral and glucose used as an anesthetic in laboratory animals; it does not depress cardiovascular reflexes as much as most other anesthetic agents.

chlor·am·bu·cil (klōr-am′byū-sil). 4-{*p*-[bis(2-chloroethyl)-amino]phenyl}butyric acid; a nitrogen mustard derivative that depresses lymphocytic proliferation and maturation. SYN chloraminophene, chloroambucil.

chlo·ra·mine B (klōr′ă-mēn). Sodium *N*-chlorobenzenesulfonamide; a nontoxic antiseptic substance used in wound irrigation as a substitute for chloramine B T.

chlo·ra·mine T. sodium *N*-chloro-*p*-toluenesulfonamide; a nontoxic but strong antiseptic used in the irrigation of wounds and infected cavities. SYN chlorazene.

chlor·am·i·no·phene (klōr-am′i-nō-fēn). SYN chlorambucil.

chlor·am·i·phene (klōr-am′i-fēn). SYN clomiphene citrate.

chlor·am·phen·i·col (klōr-am-fen′i-kol). D-(-)-*threo*-2,2-Dichloro-*N*-[β-hydroxy-α-(hydroxymethyl)-*p*-nitrophenethyl]-acetamide; an antibiotic originally obtained from *Streptomyces Venezuelae*. It is effective against a number of pathogenic microorganisms including *Staphylococcus aureus*, *Brucella abortus*, Friedländer's bacillus, and the organisms of typhoid, typhus, and Rocky Mountain spotted fever; active by mouth. A serious reaction resulting in marrow damage with agranulocytosis or aplastic anemia may occur.

c. acetyl transferase (CAT), a bacterial enzyme often used as a marker for examining the control of eucaryotic gene expression.

c. palmitate, same action and use as c.

c. sodium succinate, chloramphenicol-α-(sodium succinate); the water-soluble sodium succinate derivative of c., suitable for parenteral administration; antibacterial activity, uses, and side effects are similar to those of the parent compound.

chlo·rate (klōr′āt). A salt of chloric acid.

chlo·raz·a·nil (klō-raz′ă-nil). 2-Amino-4-(*p*-chloroanilino)-*s*-triazine; a diuretic.

chlor·a·zene (klōr′ă-zēn). SYN chloramine T.

chlo·ra·zol black E (klor′ă-zol) [C.I. 30235]. An acid dye, $C_{34}H_{25}N_9O_7S_2Na_2$, used as a fat and general tissue stain, and to stain protozoa in fecal smears or in tissues.

chlor·ben·zox·a·mine (klōr-ben-zok′să-mēn). 1-[2-(*o*-chloro-α-phenylbenzyloxy)phenylbenzyloxy)ethyl]-4-*o*-methylbenzyl-piperazine; an anticholinergic agent. SYN chlorbenzoxyethamine.

chlor·ben·zox·y·eth·a·mine (klōr′ben-zok-sē-eth′ă-mēn). SYN chlorbenzoxamine.

chlor·bet·a·mide (klōr-bet′ă-mīd). 2,2-Dichloro-*N*-(2,4-dichlorobenzyl)-*N*-(2-hydroxyethyl)acetamide; an amebicide.

chlor·bu·tol (klōr-byū′tol). SYN chlorobutanol.

chlor·cy·cli·zine hy·dro·chlo·ride (klōr-sik′li-zēn). 1-(*p*-Chlorobenzhydryl)-4-methylpiperazine hydrochloride; an antihistaminic agent.

chlor·dane (klōr′dān). A chlorinated hydrocarbon used as an insecticide; it may be absorbed through the skin with resultant severe toxic effects: hyperexcitability of central nervous system, tremors, lack of muscular coordination, convulsions, and death; also causes damage to the liver, kidneys, and spleen. It is only mildly toxic to animals.

chlor·dan·to·in (klōr-dan′tō-in). 5-(1-Ethylpentyl)-3-(trichloromethylthio)hydantoin; a topical antifungal agent.

chlor·di·az·e·pox·ide hy·dro·chlo·ride (klōr′dī-az-ē-pok′sīd). The hydrochloride of 7-chloro-2-methylamino-5-phenyl-3*H*-1,4-benzodiazepine-4-oxide; an antianxiety agent.

chlor·e·mia (klō-rē′mē-ă). 1. SYN chlorosis. 2. SYN hyperchloremia.

chlor·eth·ene ho·mo·pol·y·mer (klōr′eth-ēn). SYN polyvinyl chloride.

chlor·gua·nide hy·dro·chlo·ride (klōr-gwah′nīd). SYN chloroguanide hydrochloride.

chlor·hex·i·dine hy·dro·chlo·ride (klōr-hek′si-dēn). 1,1′-Hexamethylenebis-[5-(*p*-chlorophenyl)biguanide]dihydrochloride; a topical antiseptic.

chlor·hy·dria (klōr-hī′drē-ă). SYN hyperchlorhydria.

chlo·ric ac·id (klōr′ik). An acid of pentavalent chlorine, $HClO_3$, existing only in solution and as chlorates.

chlo·ride (klōr′īd). A compound containing chlorine, at a valence of -1, as in the salts of hydrochloric acid.

carbamylcholine c., a cholinomimetic drug which reacts with and activates both muscarinic and nicotinic receptors. It is slowly hydrolyzed and thus its effects far outlast those of acetylcholine. Used medically to stimulate smooth muscle, as in paralytic ileus following surgery.

chlor·i·dim·e·try (klōr-ĭ-dim′ĕ-trē). The process of determining the amount of chlorides in the blood or urine, or in other fluids.

chlor·i·dom·e·ter (klōr-i-dom′ĕ-ter). An apparatus for determining the amount of chlorides in blood or urine, or other fluids.

chlor·i·du·ria (klōr-i-dū′rē-ă). SYN chloruresis.

chlo·rin (klōr′in). 2,3-Dihydroporphin(e); 2,3-dihydroporphyrin; one of the root structures of the chlorophylls (for structure, see porphyrin). Addition of the two-carbon bridge (see structure of chlorophyll) to c. yields phorbin(e); addition of side chains yields the phorbides, distinguished by a number of arbitrary prefixes (those found in the chlorophylls are pheo- and bacteriopheophorbide); esterification of the propionic group by phytyl yields the respective phytins, and the addition of magnesium yields the chlorophylls (magnesium phytinates). SEE porphyrins.

chlo·ri·nat·ed (klōr′in-āt-ĕd). Having been treated with chlorine.

chlo·ri·nat·ed lime. A mixture of varying proportions of complexes of chlorine with calcium oxide and calcium hydroxide. Contains 24–37% available chlorine. Decomposes in moist conditions to liberate chlorine. Strong irritant due to chlorine vapors. Used for disinfecting drinking water, sewage etc.; in the bleaching of wood pulp, linen, cotton, straw, oils, soaps, and laundry; as an oxidizer; in destroying caterpillars; and as a decontaminant for mustard gas and similar substances. SYN bleaching powder.

chlor·in·da·nol (klōr-in′dă-nol). 7-Chloro-4-indanol; a spermicide.

chlo·rine (Cl) (klōr′ēn). 1. A greenish, toxic, gaseous element; atomic no. 17, atomic wt. 35.4527; a halogen used as a disinfectant and bleaching agent in the form of hypochlorite or of c. water, because of its oxidizing power. One of the bioelements. 2. The molecular form of c. (1), Cl_2. [G. *chloros*, greenish yellow]

chlo·rine group. The halogens.

chlor·i·o·dized (klōr-ī′ō-dīzd). Containing both chlorine and iodine.

chlor·i·o·dized oil. Chlorinated and iodized peanut oil formed by the chemical addition of iodine monochloride; formerly used for radiography of sinus and bronchi. SYN iodochlorol.

chlor·i·o·do·quin (klōr′ē-ō-dō′kwin). SYN iodochlorhydroxyquin.

chlor·i·son·da·mine chlo·ride (klōr-i-son′dă-mēn). 4,5,6,7-Tetrachloro-2-(2-dimethylaminoethyl)-2-methylisoin dolinium chloride; a quaternary ammonium compound with ganglionic blocking action similar to, but more potent than, hexamethonium and pentolinium; used in the management of severe hypertension, including the malignant phase.

chlo·rite (klōr′īt). A salt of chlorous acid; the radical ClO_2^-.

chlor·mad·i·none ac·e·tate (klōr-mad′i-nōn). 6-chloro-17-hydroxy-4,6-pregnadiene-3,20-dione acetate; 6-chloro-6-dehydro-17α-acetoxyprogesterone; a progesterone derivative used in conjunction with estrogen as an oral contraceptive.

chlor·mer·od·rin (klōr-mer′od-rin). 1-[3-(Chloromercuri)-2-methoxypropyl]urea; a mercurial diuretic chemically related to meralluride.

chlor·mez·a·none (klōr-mez′ă-nōn). 2-(4-Chlorophenyl)-3-methyl-4-metathiazanone-1,1-dioxide; a muscle relaxant and tranquilizing agent with pharmacologic actions and uses similar to those of meprobamate.

△**chloro-.** SEE chlor-.

chlo·ro·a·ce·tic ac·id (klōr′ō-ă-sē′tik). An acetic acid in which one or more of the hydrogen atoms are replaced by chlorine. According to the number of atoms so displaced the acid is called monochloroacetic (chloroacetic; $ClCH_2COOH$), dichloroacetic ($Cl_2CHCOOH$), or trichloroacetic (Cl_3CCOOH). SYN chloracetic acid.

chlo·ro·ac·e·to·phe·none (klōr′ō-as′ĕ-tō-fē′nōn). $C_6H_5COCH_2Cl$; a lacrimatory gas; used in training and in riot control.

chlo·ro·am·bu·cil (klōr-ō-am′byū-sil). SYN chlorambucil.

chlo·ro·a·ne·mia (klōr-ō-ă-nē′mē-ă). SYN chlorosis.

chlo·ro·az·o·din (klōr-ō-az′ō-din). α,α′-Azo-bis(chloroformamidine); a bactericidal agent used as a surgical antiseptic.

o-**chlo·ro·benz·al·mal·o·no·ni·trile** (ōr′thō-klōr′ō-ben-zal-ma-lon′ō-nī-trīl). A strong lacrimator used in riot control.

chlo·ro·bu·ta·nol (klōr-ō-byū′tă-nol). $Cl_3CC(CH_3)_2OH$; trichloro-*tert*-butyl alcohol; a hypnotic sedative and local anesthetic; used chiefly in dermatologic preparations and as a preservative in multiple-dose vials for parenteral use. SYN acetone chloroform, chlorbutol.

chlo·ro·cre·sol (klōr-ō-krē′sol). *p*-Chloro-*m*-cresol; used as an antiseptic and disinfectant; it is more active in acid than in alkaline solutions.

chlo·ro·cru·o·rin (klōr-ō-krū′ōr-in). A greenish hemoglobin-like pigment found in certain worms; contains a porphyrin differing from protoporphyrin by a formyl group in place of the 2-vinyl group.

chlo·ro·eth·ane (klōr-ō-eth′ān). SYN *ethyl* chloride.

chlo·ro·eth·yl·ene (klōr-ō-eth′i-lēn). SYN *vinyl* chloride.

chlo·ro·form (klōr′ō-fōrm). CHCl₃; methylene trichloride; formerly used by inhalation to produce general anesthesia; also used as a solvent. SYN trichloromethane. [chlor(ine) + form(yl)]

acetone c., SYN chlorobutanol.

chlo·ro·form·ism (klōr′ō-fōrm-izm). Habitual chloroform inhalation, or the symptoms caused thereby.

chlo·ro·fu·cin (klōr-ō-fū′sin). SYN *chlorophyll c.* [chloro- + L. *fucus*, G. *phykos*, red lichen, + -in]

chlo·ro·gua·nide hy·dro·chlo·ride (klōr-ō-gwah′nīd). 1-(*p*-chlorophenyl)-5-isopropylbiguanide monohydrochloride; an antimalarial drug. SYN chlorguanide hydrochloride, proguanil hydrochloride.

chlo·ro·he·min (klōr-ō-hē′min). SYN hemin.

chlo·ro·leu·ke·mia (klōr-ō-lū-kē′mē-ă). SYN chloroma. [chloro- + G. *leukos*, white, + *haima*, blood]

chlo·ro·ma (klō-rō′mă). A condition characterized by the development of multiple localized green masses of abnormal cells (in most instances, myeloblasts), especially in relation to the periosteum of the skull, spine, and ribs; the clinical course is similar to that of acute myeloid leukemia, although the tumors may precede the findings in blood and bone marrow; observed more frequently in children and young adults. SEE ALSO granulocytic *sarcoma*. SYN chloroleukemia, chloromyeloma. [chloro- + G. -*ōma*, tumor]

***p*-chlo·ro·mer·cu·ri·ben·zo·ate (PCMB, *p*CMB, *p*-CMB)** (klōr′ō-mer′cyūr-ē-ben′zō-āt). Organic mercury compound (ClHgC₆H₄COO⁻, ClHgBzO⁻) that reacts with —SH groups of proteins; an inhibitor of action of those proteins (enzymes) that depend on —SH reactivity. SEE ALSO *p*-mercuribenzoate.

chlo·ro·meth·ane (klōr-ō-meth′ān). A refrigerant with anesthetic properties when inhaled; it hydrolyzes to methanol. SYN methyl chloride.

chlo·rom·e·try (klo-rom′ĕ-trē). The measurement of chlorine content, or the use of analytical techniques involving the release or titration of chlorine.

chlo·ro·my·e·lo·ma (klōr′ō-mī-ĕ-lō′mă). SYN chloroma. [chloro- + G. *myelos*, marrow, + -*ōma*, tumor]

chlo·ro·pe·nia (klōr-ō-pē′nē-ă). A deficiency in chloride. [chloro- + G. *penia*, poverty]

chlo·ro·per·cha (klōr-ō-per′chă). A solution of gutta-percha in chloroform, used in dentistry as an agent to lute gutta-percha filling material to the wall of a prepared root canal.

chlo·ro·phe·nol (klōr-ō-fē′nol). One of several substitution products obtained by the action of chlorine on phenol; used as antiseptics.

***o*-chlo·ro·phe·nol.** An antiseptic liquid, used in the treatment of lupus.

***p*-chlo·ro·phe·nol.** SYN parachlorophenol.

chlo·ro·phen·o·thane (klōr-ō-fen′ō-thān). SYN dichlorodiphenyltrichloroethane.

chlo·ro·phyll (klōr′ō-fil). The magnesium complex of the phorbin derivative found in photosynthetic organisms; light-absorbing green plant pigments that, in living plants, convert light energy into oxidizing and reducing power, thus fixing CO₂ and evolving O₂; the naturally occurring forms are c. *a*, *b*, *c*, and *d*. SEE ALSO phorbin.

c. *a*, magnesium(II) pheophytinate *a* [(pheophytina to *a*)magnesium(II)]; the major pigment found in all oxygen-evolving photosynthetic organisms (higher plants, and red and green algae).

c. *b*, (CH₃ at 7 replaced by CHO in the c. structure), magnesium-(II) pheophytinate *b* [(pheophytinato *b*) magnesium(II)]; the c. generally characteristic of higher plants (including the *Chlorophyta*, *Euglenaphyta*, and green algae). Absent in other types of algae.

c. *c*, the c. present in brown algae, diatoms, and flagellates. Two variants are known: *c*₁, in which two hydrogens are lost from C-17 and C-18, thus resembling phytoporphyrin, and the side chain at C-17 becomes an acrylic residue, —CH=CH₂COOH; *c*₂, in which the same changes are noted, but two more hydrogens are lost from the ethyl group at C-8, making this a vinyl residue like that at C-3. The two compounds can thus be named in terms of phytoporphyrin: magnesium $3^1,3^2,17^1,17^2$-tetradehydro-13^2-(methoxycarbonyl)phytoporphyrinate and magnesium $3^1,3^2,8^1,8^2,17^1,17^2$-hexadehydro-$13^2$-(methoxycarbonyl)-phytoporphyrinate. SYN chlorofucin.

c. *d*, —CH=CH₂ replaced by —CO—CH₃ in the *c.* structure; the c. found in red algae (*Rhodophyceae*), together with c. *a*.

c. esterase, SYN chlorophyllase.

water-soluble c. derivatives, the copper complex of sodium and/or potassium salts of saponified c., used topically for deodorization of chronic lesions and to promote wound repair.

chlo·ro·phyl·lase (klōr-ō-fil′-ās). A reversible hydrolyzing enzyme catalyzing the removal of the phytyl group from a chlorophyll, leaving a chlorophyllide. SYN chlorophyll esterase.

chlo·ro·phyl·lide, chlo·ro·phyl·lid (klōr′ō-fil-id). That which remains of a chlorophyll molecule when the phytyl group is removed.

chlo·ro·pic·rin (klōr-ō-pik′rin). CCl₃NO₂; trichloronitromethane; a toxic lung irritant and lacrimatory gas; it also causes vomiting, colic, and diarrhea, and therefore is called vomiting gas. SYN nitrochloroform.

chlo·ro·plast (klōr′ō-plast). A plant cell inclusion body containing chlorophyll; occurs in cells of leaves and young stems. Site of photosynthesis in higher plants. [chloro- + G. *plastos*, formed]

chlo·ro·pred·ni·sone (klōr-ō-pred′ni-sōn). 6α-Chloro-17,21-dihydroxypregna-1,4-diene-3,11,20-tr ione; a topical anti-inflammatory agent.

chlo·ro·pro·caine hy·dro·chlo·ride (klōr-ō-prō′kān). β-Diethylaminoethyl-2-chloro-4-aminobenzoate hydrochloride; a local anesthetic similar in action and use to procaine hydrochloride.

chlo·rop·sia (klo-rop′sē-ă). A condition in which objects appear to be colored green, as may occur in digitalis intoxication. SYN green vision. [chloro- + G. *opsis*, eyesight]

chlo·ro·pyr·a·mine (klōr-ō-pir′ă-mēn). 2-[*p*-Chlorobenzyl-(2-dimethylaminoethyl)amino]p yridine; an antihistaminic agent.

chlo·ro·quine (klōr′ō-kwīn). 7-chloro-4-(4-diethylamino-1-methylbutylamino)quinoline; an antimalarial agent used for the treatment and suppression of *Plasmodium vivax*, *P. malariae*, and *P. falciparum;* available as the phosphate and sulfate. It does not produce a radical cure because it has no effect on the exoerythrocytic stages; c.-resistant strains of *P. falciparum* have developed in Southeast Asia, Africa, and South America. It is also used for hepatic amebiasis and for certain skin diseases, *e.g.,* lupus erythematosus and lichen planus.

chlo·ro·sis (klōr-ō′sis). Rarely used term for a form of chronic hypochromic microcytic (iron deficiency) anemia, characterized by a great reduction in hemoglobin out of proportion to the decreased number of red blood cells; observed chiefly in females from puberty to the third decade and usually associated with diets deficient in iron and protein. SYN asiderotic anemia, chloremia (1), chloroanemia, chlorotic anemia, green sickness. [chloro- + G. -*osis,* condition]

chlo·ro·then cit·rate (klōr-ō-then). Chloromethapyrilene citrate; *N,N*-dimethyl-*N*′-(2-pyridyl)-*N*′-(5-chloro-2-thenyl)-ethylenediamine citrate; an antihistaminic agent.

chlo·ro·thi·a·zide (klōr-ō-thī′ă-zīd). 6-Chloro-7-sulfamyl-1,2,4-benzothiadiazine-1,1-dioxide; an orally effective diuretic inhibiting renal tubular reabsorption of sodium; used in the treatment of edema due to congestive heart failure, liver disease, pregnancy, premenstrual tension, and drugs; also used as an adjunct in the management of hypertension.

c. sodium, c. suitable for parenteral administration.

chlo·ro·thy·mol (klōr-ō-thī'mol). $C_{10}H_{13}OCl$; Monochlorothymol; an antibacterial for topical use. SYN chlorthymol.

chlo·rot·ic (klō-rot'ik). Pertaining to or having the characteristic features of chlorosis.

chlo·ro·tri·an·i·sene (klōr'ō-trī-an'i-sēn). Chlorotris(p-methoxyphenyl)ethylene; a synthetic estrogen derived from stilbene, active by mouth.

chlo·rous (klōr'ŭs). **1.** Relating to chlorine. **2.** Denoting compounds of chlorine in which its valence is +3; *e.g.,* c. acid.

chlo·rous ac·id. $HClO_2$; an acid forming chlorites with bases.

β-chlo·ro·vi·nyl·di·chlo·ro·ar·sine (klōr'ō-vī'nil-dī-klōr'ō-ar'sēn). SYN lewisite.

chlo·ro·zo·to·cin (klōr'ō-zō-tō-sin). A nitrogen mustard compound which is a chloroethylnitrosourea compound used in cancer chemotherapy; an antineoplastic.

chlor·phen·e·sin (klōr-fen'ĕ-sin). 3-(p-Chlorophenoxy)-1,2-propenediol; a topical antifungal agent.

c. carbamate, carbamic acid 3-(4-chlorophenoxy)-2-hydroxypropyl ester; a skeletal muscle relaxant.

chlor·phen·in·di·one (klōr-fen-in-dī'ōn). An anticoagulant related chemically to phenindione.

chlor·phen·ir·a·mine ma·le·ate (klōr-fen-ir'ă-mēn). (±)-2-[p-Chloro-α-[2-(dimethylamino)ethyl]benzyl]pyridine maleate; an antihistamine.

chlor·phe·nol red (klōr-fē'nol). An acid-base indicator (MW 423, pK 6.0): yellow at pH values below 5.1, red above 6.7.

chlor·phen·ox·a·mine (klōr-fen-ok'să-mēn). 2-(p-Chloro-α-methyl-α-phenylbenzyloxy)-N,N-dimethylethylamine hydrochloride; used in the management of idiopathic, arteriosclerotic, and postencephalitic parkinsonism, usually with concomitant administration of other anti-parkinsonian agents.

chlor·phen·ter·mine hy·dro·chlo·ride (klōr-fen'ter-mēn). 4-Chloro-α,α-dimethylphenethylamine hydrochloride; a sympathomimetic amine used as an anorexiant.

chlor·pro·eth·a·zine hy·dro·chlo·ride (klōr-prō-eth'ă-zēn). 2-Chloro-10-(3-diethylaminopropyl)phenothiazine; a skeletal muscle relaxant.

chlor·pro·guan·il hy·dro·chlo·ride (klōr-prō'gwah-nil). The 3,4-dichloro homologue of chloroguanide; used for causal prophylaxis and suppression of falciparum malaria.

chlor·prom·a·zine (klōr-prō'mă-zēn). 10-(3-Dimethylaminopropyl)-2-chlorophenothiazine; a phenothiazine antipsychotic agent with antiemetic, antiadrenergic, and anticholinergic actions. Although chemically related to promethazine, it has no antihistamine action, depresses conditioned reflexes and the hypothalamic centers, and has a hypotensive action of central origin.

c. hydrochloride, c. suitable for oral, intramuscular, and intravenous administration.

chlor·prop·a·mide (klōr-prō'pă-mīd). 1-(p-Chlorophenyl-sulfonyl)-3-propylurea; an orally effective hypoglycemic agent related chemically and pharmacologically to tolbutamide; used in controlling hyperglycemia in selected patients with adult onset (type II) diabetes mellitus.

chlor·pro·thix·ene (klōr-prō-thik'sēn). 2-Chloro-9-(3-dimethylaminopropylidene)thiaxanthene; an antipsychotic of the thioxanthene group; it also possesses antiemetic, adrenolytic, spasmolytic, and antihistaminic actions.

chlor·quin·al·dol (klōr-kwin'al-dol). 5,7-Dichloro-8-hydroxyquinaldine; a keratoplastic, antibacterial, and antifungal agent used in the treatment of cutaneous bacterial and mycotic infections.

chlor·tet·ra·cy·cline (klōr'tet-ră-sī'klēn). An antibiotic agent; a naphthacene derivative, obtained from *Streptomyces aureofaciens*; active against a wide range of pathogenic microorganisms including hemolytic streptococci, staphylococci, typhoid bacilli, and brucellae, as well as against certain viruses. Also available as c. calcium and c. hydrochloride.

chlor·thal·i·done (klōr-thal'i-dōn). 2-Chloro-5-(1-hydroxy-3-oxo-1-isoindolinyl)benzenesulfonamide; an orally effective diuretic and antihypertensive agent, used in the treatment of edema associated with congestive heart failure, renal disease, hepatic cirrhosis, pregnancy, and premenstrual tension; it produces an increase in the excretion of sodium, chloride, potassium, and water.

chlor·then·ox·a·zin (klōr-then-ok'să-zin). 2-(2-Chloroethyl)-2,3-dihydro-4H-1,3-benzoxazin-4-one; an antipyretic and analgesic.

chlor·thy·mol (klōr-thī'mol). SYN chlorothymol.

chlor·u·re·sis (klōr-yū-rē'sis). The excretion of chloride in the urine. SYN chloriduria, chloruria.

chlor·u·ret·ic (klōr-yū-ret'ik). Relating to an agent that increases the excretion of chloride in the urine, or to such an effect.

chlor·u·ria (klōr-yū'rē-ă). SYN chloruresis.

chlor·zox·a·zone (klōr-zok'să-zōn). 5-Chloro-2-benzoxazolol; a centrally acting skeletal muscle relaxant used in the treatment of painful muscle spasm due to musculoskeletal disorder.

cho·a·na, pl. **cho·a·nae** (kō'an-ă, kō-ā'nē) [NA]. The opening into the nasopharynx of the nasal cavity on either side. SYN isthmus pharyngonasalis, posterior naris, postnaris. [Mod. L. fr. G. *choanē*, a funnel]

primary c., primitive c., initial opening of the nasal pits and olfactory sac of the embryo into the rostral part of the primordial oronasal cavity, before the formation of the secondary palate.

secondary c., the definitive c. opening into the nasopharynx, after the nasal chambers have been lengthened by the formation of the secondary palate. SYN internal nostril.

cho·a·nal (kō'ă-năl). Pertaining to a choana.

cho·a·nate (kō'an-āt). Having a funnel, *i.e.,* with a ring or collar.

cho·a·no·flag·el·late (kō'an-ō-flaj'ĕ-lāt). SYN choanomastigote.

cho·a·noid (kō'ă-noyd). Funnel-shaped. SYN infundibuliform. [G. *choanē*, funnel, + *eidos*, resemblance]

cho·a·no·mas·ti·gote (kō'an-ō-mas'tī-gōt). A term, in the series used to describe developmental stages of the parasitic flagellates, denoting the "barleycorn" form of the flagellate in the genus *Crithidia* characterized by a collarlike extension surrounding the anterior and through which the single flagellum emerges. SEE ALSO amastigote, epimastigote, promastigote, trypomastigote. SYN choanoflagellate, collared flagellate. [G. *choanē*, a funnel, + *mastix*, whip]

Cho·a·no·tae·nia in·fun·dib·u·lum (kō-ā-nō-tē'nē-ă). An important species of cosmopolitan tapeworm of fowls, occurring in the small intestine and transmitted by houseflies and stableflies; related to *Dipylidium*, the double-pored dog tapeworm. [G. *choanē*, a funnel, + L., fr. G. *tainia*, tapeworm]

Chodzko's re·flex. See under reflex.

choke (chōk). **1.** To prevent respiration by compression or obstruction of the larynx or trachea. **2.** Any obstruction of the esophagus in herbivorous animals by a partly swallowed foreign body. [M.E. *choken*, fr. O.E. *āceōcian*]

thoracic c., obstruction by a foreign body in the thoracic portion of the esophagus of an animal.

chokes (chōks). A manifestation of decompression sickness or altitude sickness characterized by dyspnea, coughing, and choking.

△chol-. SEE chole-.

cho·la·gog·ic (kō-lă-goj'ik). SYN cholagogue (2).

cho·la·gogue (kō'lă-gog). **1.** An agent that promotes the flow of bile into the intestine, especially as a result of contraction of the gallbladder. **2.** Relating to such an agent or effect. SYN cholagogic. [chol- + G. *agōgos*, drawing forth]

cho·la·ic ac·id (kō-lā'ik). SYN taurocholic acid.

cho·lal·ic ac·id (kō-lal'ik). SYN cholic acid.

cho·lane, 5β-cho·lane (kō'lān). Parent hydrocarbon of the cholanic acids (cholic acids); androstane with a —CH(CH₃)-CH₂CH₂CH₃ group in the 17 position. 5α-Cholane is sometimes called allocholane. For structures, see steroids.

chol·a·ner·e·sis (kō-lă-ner'ĕ-sis). Increase in output of cholic acid or its conjugates. [cholane + G. *hairesis*, a taking]

cho·lan·ge·i·tis (kō'lan-jē-ī'tis). SYN cholangitis.

chol·an·gi·ec·ta·sis (kō-lan-jē-ek'tă-sis). Dilation of the bile ducts, usually as a sequel to obstruction. [chol- + G. *angeion,* vessel, + *ektasis,* a stretching]

chol·an·gi·o·car·ci·no·ma (kō-lan'jē-ō-kar-si-nō'mă). An adenocarcinoma, primarily in intrahepatic bile ducts, composed of ducts lined by cuboidal or columnar cells that do not contain bile, with abundant fibrous stroma; cirrhosis is usually absent.

chol·an·gi·o·en·ter·os·to·my (kō-lan'jē-ō-en-ter-os'tō-mē). Surgical anastomosis of bile duct to intestine.

chol·an·gi·o·fi·bro·sis (kō-lan'jē-ō-fī-brō'sis). Fibrosis of the bile ducts. [chol- + G. *angeion,* vessel, + fibrosis]

chol·an·gi·o·gas·tros·to·my (kō-lan'jē-ō-gas-tros'tō-mē). Formation of a communication between a bile duct and the stomach. [chol- + G. *angeion,* vessel, + *gastēr,* belly, + *stoma,* mouth]

chol·an·gi·o·gram (kō-lan'jē-ō-gram). The radiographic record of the bile ducts obtained by cholangiography.

chol·an·gi·og·ra·phy (kō-lan-jē-og'ră-fē). Radiographic examination of the bile ducts. [chol- + G. *angeion,* vessel, + *graphō,* to write]

cystic duct c., radiography of the biliary system after introduction of contrast medium through the cystic duct.

intravenous c., c. of bile ducts opacified by hepatic secretion of an intravenously injected contrast medium.

percutaneous c., radiography of the biliary system after introduction of contrast medium by introducing a needle through the skin inferior to the right costal margin, and inserting it into the substance of the liver or into the gallbladder.

chol·an·gi·ole (kō-lan'jē-ōl). A ductule occurring between a bile canaliculus and an interlobular bile duct. SYN canal of Hering. [chol- + G. *angeion,* vessel, + *-ole,* small]

chol·an·gi·o·li·tis (kō-lan'jē-ō-lī'tis). Inflammation of the small bile radicles or cholangioles.

chol·an·gi·o·ma (kō-lan'jē-ō'mă). A neoplasm of bile duct origin, especially within the liver; may be either benign or malignant (cholangiocarcinoma). [chol- + G. *angeion,* vessel, + *-oma,* tumor]

chol·an·gi·o·pan·cre·a·tog·ra·phy (kō-lan'jē-ō-pan-krē-ă-tog'ră-fē). Radiographic examination of the bile ducts and pancreas.

endoscopic retrograde c. (ERCP), a method of c. using an endoscope to inspect and cannulate the ampulla of Vater, with injection of contrast medium for radiographic examination of the pancreatic, hepatic, and common bile ducts.

chol·an·gi·os·co·py (kō-lan-jē-os'kŏ-pē). Visual examination of bile ducts utilizing a fiberoptic endoscope. [chol- + G. *angeion,* vessel, + *skopeō,* to examine]

chol·an·gi·os·to·my (kō-lan-jē-os'tō-mē). Formation of a fistula into a bile duct. [chol- + G. *angeion,* vessel, + *stoma,* mouth]

chol·an·gi·ot·o·my (ko-lan-jĭ-ot'o-mĭ). Incision into a bile duct. [chol- + G. *angeion,* vessel, + *tomē,* incision]

chol·an·gi·tis (kō-lan-jī'tis). Inflammation of a bile duct or the entire biliary tree. SYN angiocholitis, cholangeitis. [chol- + G. *angeion,* vessel, + *-itis,* inflammation]

ascending c., SYN c. lenta.

c. lenta (len-tă'), low-grade bacterial infection of the biliary tract; sometimes a cause of fever of unknown origin. SYN ascending c.

primary sclerosing c., recurrent or persistent obstructive jaundice, frequently with ulcerative colitis, due to extensive obliterative fibrosis of the extrahepatic or intrahepatic bile ducts; generally progresses to cirrhosis, portal hypertension, and liver failure; seen most commonly in young men.

recurrent pyogenic c., repeated attacks of c., commonly noted among Asians living in Asia, associated with the presence of multiple intrahepatic and extrahepatic bile duct stones and strictures.

cho·lan·ic ac·id (kō-lan'ik). SYN cholic acid.

cho·lan·o·poi·e·sis (kō'lan-ō-poy-ē'sis). Synthesis by the liver of cholic acid or its conjugates, or of natural bile salts. [chol- + G. *anō,* upward, + *poiēsis,* making]

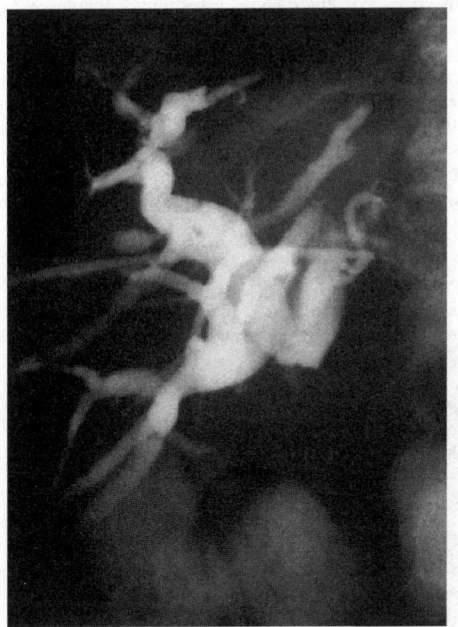

percutaneous transhepatic cholangiography
turmor-related obstruction in the area of the ductus hepaticus communis

cho·lan·o·poi·et·ic (kō'lan-ō-poy-et'ik). Pertaining to or promoting cholanopoiesis.

chol·an·threne (kō-lan'thrēn). A polycyclic, somewhat carcinogenic hydrocarbon, structural parent of the highly carcinogenic 3 (or 20)-methylcholanthrene.

cho·las·cos (kō-las'kos). Rarely used term for escape of bile into the free peritoneal cavity. [chol- + G. *askos,* bag]

cho·late (kō'lāt). A salt or ester of a cholic acid.

c. ligase, an enzyme that converts c., coenzyme A, and ATP, to choloyl-coenzyme A, AMP, and pyrophosphate. SYN cholyl-coenzyme A synthetase.

c. synthetase, c. thiokinase, cholate-CoA ligase.

⌂**chole-, chol-, cholo-.** Bile. Cf. bili-. [G. *cholē*]

cho·le·cal·cif·er·ol (kō'lē-kal-sif'er-ol). (5*Z*,7*E*)-(3*S*)-9,10-secocho lesta-5,7,10(19)-trien-3-ol; formed by breakage of 9,10 bond in 7-dehydrocholesterol by ultraviolet irradiation, yielding a double bond between C-10 and C-19; probably the vitamin D of animal origin found in the skin, fur, and feathers of animals and birds exposed to sunlight, and also in butter, brain, fish oils, and egg yolk. SYN vitamin D_3. SYN calciol.

cho·le·chro·mo·poi·e·sis (kō'lē-krō-mō-poy-ē'sis). Synthesis of bile pigments by the liver. [chole- + G. *chrōma,* color, + *poiesis,* making]

cho·le·cyst (kō'le-sist). SYN gallbladder.

cho·le·cys·ta·gog·ic (kō'lē-sis-tă-goj'ik). Stimulating activity of the gallbladder.

cho·le·cys·ta·gogue (kō-lē-sis'tă-gog). A substance that stimulates activity of the gallbladder. [chole- + G. *kystis,* bladder, + *agōgos,* leader]

cho·le·cys·tat·o·ny (kō'lē-sis-tat'ō-nē). Atonia, weakness, or failure of function of the gallbladder. [chole- + G. *kystis,* bladder, + *atonia,* atony]

cho·le·cys·tec·ta·sia (kō'lē-sis-tek-tā'zē-ă). Rarely used term for dilation of the gallbladder. [chole- + G. *kystis,* bladder, + *ektasis,* extension]

cho·le·cys·tec·to·my (kō'lē-sis-tek'tō-mē). Surgical removal of the gallbladder. [chole- + G. *kystis,* bladder, + *ektomē,* excision]

cho·le·cyst·en·ter·os·to·my (kō'lē-sist-en-ter-os'tō-mē). Formation of a direct communication between the gallbladder and the intestine. SYN enterocholecystostomy. [chole- + G. *kystis,* bladder, + *enteron,* intestine, + *stoma,* mouth]

cho·le·cyst·en·ter·ot·o·my (kō'lē-sist-en-ter-ot'ō-mē). Incision of both intestine and gallbladder. SYN enterocholecystotomy. [chole- + G. *kystis,* bladder, + *enteron,* intestine, + *tomē,* a cutting]

cho·le·cys·tic (kō-lē-sis'tik). Relating to the cholecyst, or gallbladder.

cho·le·cys·tis (kō-lē-sis'tis). SYN gallbladder. [chole- + G. *kystis,* bladder]

cho·le·cys·ti·tis (kō'lē-sis-tī'tis). Inflammation of the gallbladder. [chole- + G. *kystis,* bladder, + *-itis,* inflammation]

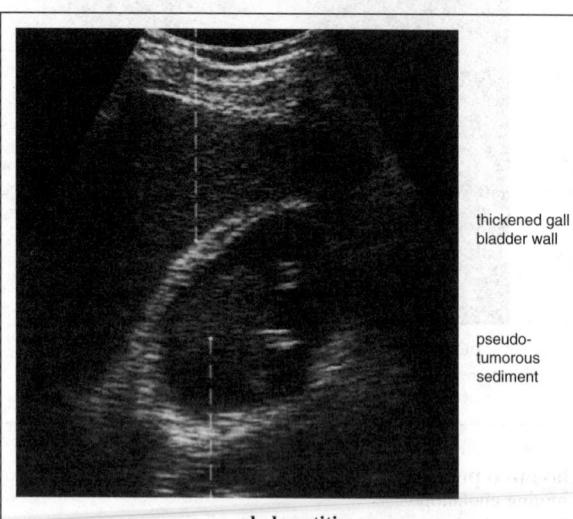

thickened gall bladder wall

pseudo-tumorous sediment

cholecystitis
thickened gall bladder wall in acute cholecystitis, with an inflamed mass of pseudotumorous sediment

acute c., inflammation and/or hemorrhagic necrosis, with variable infection, ulceration, and neutrophilic infiltration of the gallbladder wall; usually due to impaction of a stone in the cystic duct.

chronic c., chronic inflammation of the gallbladder, usually secondary to lithiasis, with lymphocytic infiltration and fibrosis that may produce marked thickening of the wall.

emphysematous c., c. due to infection with gas-producing bacteria, giving rise to gas in the gallbladder.

xanthogranulomatous c., chronic c. with conspicuous nodular infiltration by lipid macrophages; may be associated with biliary obstruction by calculi.

cho·le·cys·to·co·los·to·my (kō'lē-sis'tō-kō-los'tō-mē). Establishment of a communication between the gallbladder and the colon. SYN colocholecystostomy, cystocolostomy. [chole- + G. *kystis,* bladder, + *kōlon,* colon, + *stoma,* mouth]

cho·le·cys·to·du·o·de·nos·to·my (kō'lē-sis'tō-dū-ō-dē-nos'tō-mē). Establishment of a direct communication between the gallbladder and the duodenum. SYN duodenocholecystostomy, duodenocystostomy (1). [chole- + G. *kystis,* bladder, + L. *duodenum* + G. *stoma,* mouth]

cho·le·cys·to·gas·tros·to·my (kō-lē-sis'tō-gas-tros'tō-mē). Establishment of a communication between the gallbladder and the stomach. [chole- + G. *kystis,* bladder, + *gastēr,* stomach, + *stoma,* mouth]

cho·le·cys·to·gram (kō-lē-sis'tō-gram). The radiographic record of the gallbladder obtained by cholecystography.

cho·le·cys·tog·ra·phy (kō-lē-sis-tog'rǎ-fē). Radiographic study of the gallbladder after oral administration of a cholecystopaque; or scintigraphic imaging of the gallbladder and central bile ducts after administration of a radiopharmaceutical secreted by the liver. SYN Graham-Cole test. [chole- + G. *kystis,* bladder, + *grapho,* to write]

cho·le·cys·to·il·e·os·to·my (kō-lē-sis'tō-il-ē-os'tō-mē). Establishment of a communication between the gallbladder and the ileum. [chole- + G. *kystis,* bladder, + ileum + G. *stoma,* mouth]

cho·le·cys·to·je·ju·nos·to·my (kō-lē-sis'tō-jē-jū-nos'tō-mē). Establishment of a communication between the gallbladder and the jejunum. [chole- + G. *kystis,* bladder, + jejunum + G. *stoma,* mouth]

cho·le·cys·to·ki·nase (kō-lē-sis-tō-kī'nās). An enzyme catalyzing the hydrolysis of cholecystokinin.

cho·le·cys·to·ki·net·ic (kō'lē-sis'tō-ki-net'ik). Promoting emptying of the gallbladder.

cho·le·cys·to·ki·nin (CCK) (kō'lē-sis-tō-kī'nin). A polypeptide (of 33 residues) hormone liberated by the upper intestinal mucosa on contact with gastric contents; stimulates contraction of the gallbladder and secretion of pancreatic juice. SEE ALSO sincalide. SYN pancreozymin.

cho·le·cys·to·li·thi·a·sis (kō-lē-sis'tō-li-thī'ǎ-sis). Presence of one or more gallstones in the gallbladder. [chole- + G. *kystis,* bladder, + *lithos,* stone]

cho·le·cys·to·lith·o·trip·sy (kō-lē-sis'tō-lith'ō-trip-sē). Crushing or fragmentation of a gallstone by manipulation of the unopened gallbladder. [chole- + G. *kystis,* bladder, + *lithos,* stone, + *tripsis,* a rubbing]

cho·le·cys·to·my (kō-lē-sis'tō-mē). SYN cholecystotomy.

cho·le·cys·to·paque (kō-lē-sis'tō-pāk). A radiographic contrast medium that opacifies the gallbladder following oral administration, by virtue of hepatic secretion and gallbladder concentration; used in cholecystography.

cho·le·cys·top·a·thy (kō'lē-sis-top'ǎ-thē). Disease of the gallbladder.

cho·le·cys·to·pexy (kō-lē-sis'tō-pek-sē). Suture of the gallbladder to the abdominal wall. [chole- + G. *kystis,* bladder, + *pēxis,* fixation]

cho·le·cys·tor·rha·phy (kō'lē-sis-tōr'ǎ-fē). Suture of an incised or ruptured gallbladder. [chole- + G. *kystis,* bladder, + *rhaphē,* sewing]

cho·le·cys·to·so·nog·ra·phy (kō-lē-sis'tō-sō-nog'rǎ-fē). Ultrasonic examination of the gallbladder. [cholecysto- + sonography]

cho·le·cys·tos·to·my (kō'lē-sis-tos'tō-mē). Establishment of a fistula into the gallbladder. [chole- + G. *kystis,* bladder, + *stoma,* mouth]

cho·le·cys·tot·o·my (kō'lē-sis-tot'ō-mē). Incision into the gallbladder. SYN cholecystomy. [chole- + G. *kystis,* bladder, + *tomē,* incision]

laparoscopic c., minimally invasive surgical technique for removal of the gallbladder that uses a laparoscope for visualization of the gallbladder and placement of instruments into the abdominal cavity through trocars, therefore avoiding the traditional incision.

cho·le·doch (kō'lē-dok). SYN common bile *duct.* [G. *cholēdochos,* containing bile, fr. *cholē,* bile, + *dechomai,* to receive]

⌂choledoch-. SEE choledocho-.

cho·le·doch·al (kō-lē-dok'ǎl, kō-led'ō-kal). Relating to the common bile duct.

cho·led·o·chec·to·my (kō-led-ō-kek'tō-mē). Surgical removal of a portion of the common bile duct. [choledoch- + G. *ektomē,* excision]

cho·led·o·chen·dy·sis (kō'led-ō-ken'dī-sis). SYN choledochotomy. [choledoch- + G. *endysis,* an entering in]

cho·led·o·chi·arc·tia (kō'led-ō-ki-ark'tē-ǎ). Obsolete term for stenosis of the gall duct. [choledoch- + L. *artus* (improperly *arctus*), narrow]

cho·led·o·chi·tis (kō-led-ō-kī'tis). Inflammation of the common bile duct. [choledoch- + G. *-itis,* inflammation]

⌂choledocho-, choledoch-. The ductus choledochus (the common bile duct). [G. *cholēdochos,* containing bile, fr. *cholē,* bile, + *dechomai,* to receive]

cho·led·o·cho·cho·led·o·chos·to·my (kō-led'ō-kō-kō-led'ō-kos'tō-mē). Operative joining of divided portions of common bile duct. [choledocho- + choledocho- + G. *stoma*, mouth]

cho·led·o·cho·du·o·de·nos·to·my (kō-led'ō-kō-dū'ō-dē-nos'tō-mē). Formation of a communication, other than the natural one, between the common bile duct and the duodenum. [choledocho- + duodenum + G. *stoma*, mouth]

cho·led·o·cho·en·ter·os·tomy (kō-led'ō-kō-en-ter-os'tō-mē). Establishment of a communication, other than the natural one, between the common bile duct and any part of the intestine. [choledocho- + G. *enteron*, intestine, + *stoma*, mouth]

cho·led·o·chog·ra·phy (kō-led'ō-kog'ră-fē). Radiographic examination of the bile duct after the administration of a radiopaque substance. [choledocho- + G. *graphō*, to write]

cho·led·o·cho·je·ju·nos·to·my (kō-led'ō-kō-jĕ-jū-nos'tō-mē). Anastomosis between the common bile duct and the jejunum. [choledocho- + jejuno- + G. *stoma*, mouth]

cho·led·o·cho·lith (kō-led'ō-kō-lith). Stone in the common bile duct. [choledocho- + G. *lithos*, stone]

cho·led·o·cho·li·thi·a·sis (kō-led'ō-kō-lith-ī'ă-sis). Presence of a gallstone in the common bile duct.

cho·led·o·cho·li·thot·o·my (kō-led'ō-kō-li-thot'ō-mē). Incision of the common bile duct for the extraction of an impacted gallstone. [choledocho- + G. *lithos*, stone, + *tomē*, incision]

cho·led·o·cho·lith·o·trip·sy (kō-led'ō-kō-lith'ō-trip-sē). Crushing or fragmentation of a gallstone in the common bile duct by manipulation without opening of the duct. SYN choledocholithotrity. [choledocho- + G. *lithos*, stone, + *tripsis*, rubbing]

cho·led·o·cho·li·thot·ri·ty (kō-led'ō-kō-li-thot'ri-tē). SYN choledocholithotripsy.

cho·led·o·cho·plas·ty (kō-led'ō-kō-plas-tē). Plastic surgery of the common bile duct. [choledocho- + G. *plastos*, formed]

cho·led·o·chor·rha·phy (kō-led-ō-kōr'ră-fē). Suturing together the divided ends of the common bile duct. [choledocho- + G. *rhaphē*, suture]

cho·led·o·chos·to·my (kō-led-ō-kos'tō-mē). Establishment of a fistula into the common bile duct. [choledocho- + G. *stoma*, mouth]

cho·led·o·chot·o·my (kō-led-ō-kot'ō-mē). Incision into the common bile duct. SYN choledochendysis. [choledocho- + G. *tomē*, incision]

cho·led·o·chous (kō-led'ō-kŭs). Containing or conveying bile.

cho·led·o·chus (kō-led'ō-kŭs). SYN common bile *duct.* [see choledoch]

cho·le·glo·bin (kō-lē-glō'bin). A pigmented compound of globin and iron porphyrin (with an open ring due to cleavage of the α-methene bridge by α-methyl oxygenase); the first intermediate in the degradation of hemoglobin, further degraded successively to verdohemochrome, biliverdin, and bilirubin. SYN bile pigment hemoglobin, green hemoglobin, verdohemoglobin.

cho·le·he·ma·tin (kō-lē-hē'mă-tin). A red pigment in the bile of herbivorous animals; derived from chlorophyll and a product of hematin oxidation.

cho·le·he·mia (kō-lē-hē'mē-ă). SYN cholemia. [chole- + G. *haima*, blood]

cho·le·ic (kō-lē'ik). SYN cholic.

cho·le·ic ac·ids. Compounds of bile acids and sterols.

cho·le·lith (kō'lē-lith). SYN gallstone. [chole- + G. *lithos*, stone]

cho·le·li·thi·a·sis (kō'lē-li-thī'ă-sis). Presence of concretions in the gallbladder or bile ducts. SYN chololithiasis.

cho·le·li·thot·o·my (kō'lē-li-thot'ō-mē). Operative removal of a gallstone. [chole- + G. *lithos*, stone, + *tomē*, incision]

cho·le·lith·o·trip·sy (kō-lē-lith'ō-trip-sē). Rarely used term for the crushing of a gallstone. [chole- + G. *lithos*, stone, + *tripsis*, a rubbing]

cho·le·li·thot·ri·ty (kō-lē-li-thot'ri-tē). Rarely used term for the crushing of a gallstone. [chole- + G. *lithos*, stone, + L. *tero*, pp. *tritus*, to rub]

cho·lem·e·sis (kō-lem'ĕ-sis). Vomiting of bile. [chole- + G. *emesis*, vomiting]

cho·le·mia (kō-lē'mē-ă). The presence of bile salts in the circulating blood. SYN cholehemia. [chole- + G. *haima*, blood]

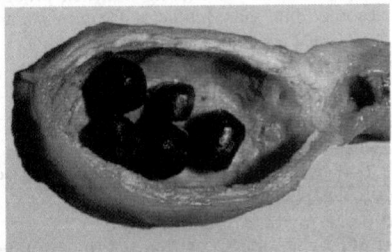

cholelithiasis
in chronic cholecystitis: note thickness of wall and roughness of mucous membrane

cho·lem·ic (kō-lē'mik). Relating to cholemia.

cho·le·path·ia (kō-lē-path'ē-ă). **1.** Disease of bile ducts. **2.** Irregularity in contractions of the bile ducts.

c. spas'tica, spastic contraction of the bile ducts.

cho·le·per·i·to·ne·um (kō'lē-pār-i-tō-nē'ŭm). Obsolete term for bile in the peritoneum, which may lead to bile peritonitis.

cho·le·per·i·to·ni·tis (kō'le-per-i-tō-nī'tis). SYN bile *peritonitis.*

cho·le·poi·e·sis (kō'lē-poy-ē'sis). Formation of bile. SYN cholopoiesis. [chole- + G. *poiēsis*, making]

cho·le·poi·et·ic (kō'lē-poy-et'ik). Relating to the formation of bile.

chol·era (kol'er-ă). **1.** Formerly, a nonspecific term for a variety of gastrointestinal disturbances. **2.** An acute epidemic infectious disease caused by the bacterium *Vibrio cholerae*, now occurring primarily in Asia. A soluble toxin elaborated in the intestinal tract by the bacterium activates the adenylate cylase of the mucosa, causing active secretion of an isotomic fluid resulting in profuse watery diarrhea, extreme loss of fluid and electrolytes, and dehydration and collapse, but no gross morphologic change in the intestinal mucosa. SYN Asiatic c. [L. a bilious disease, fr. G. *cholē*, bile]

Asiatic c., SYN cholera (2).

fowl c., a destructive disease of domestic fowls caused by *Pasteurella multocida.*

hog c., an acute, highly contagious, and fatal disease of swine caused by the hog cholera virus, a member of the Togaviridae, and characterized by a sudden onset, high fever, depression, diarrhea, cutaneous hemorrhages, and frequently encephalomyelitic symptoms; pigs may die of the virus infection alone, or from complications of secondary bacterial infections; transmission is by direct contact or ingestion of contaminated food, particularly garbage. SYN swine fever, swine pest.

c. infan'tum, old term for a disease of infants, characterized by vomiting, profuse watery diarrhea, fever, prostration, and collapse.

c. mor'bus, old term for acute severe gastroenteritis of unknown etiology, marked by severe colic, vomiting, and diarrhea with watery stools; formerly common during hot weather.

pancreatic c., SYN *diarrhea pancreatica.*

c. sic'ca, an old term for a malignant form of disease seen during epidemics of Asiatic c. in which death occurs without diarrhea.

typhoid c., old term for c. (2) with predominantly cerebral manifestations such as confusion or dementia.

chol·er·a·gen (kol'er-ă-jen). A term suggested for a factor(s) produced during growth *in vitro* of the cholera vibrio and causes diarrhea. [cholera + G. *-gen*, producing]

chol·er·a·ic (kol'er-ā'ik). Relating to cholera.

chol·er·a·phage (kol'er-ă-fāj). Bacteriophage of *Vibrio cholerae*. [cholera + G. *phagō*, to eat]

cho·le·re·sis (kō-ler-ē'sis). The secretion of bile as opposed to the expulsion of bile by the gallbladder. [chole- + G. *hairesis*, a taking]

cho·le·ret·ic (kol-er-et'ik). **1.** Relating to choleresis. **2.** An agent, usually a drug, that stimulates the liver to increase output of bile.

chol·e·rhe·ic (kol-ĕ-rē'ik). Denoting diarrhea produced secondary to unabsorbed bile salts. [chole- + G. *hairesis*, a taking]

chol·er·ic (kol'er-ik). SYN bilious (3).

chol·er·i·form (kol'er-i-fōrm). Resembling cholera. SYN choleroid.

chol·er·i·gen·ic, chol·er·ig·en·ous (kol'er-i-jen'ik, -ij'en-ŭs). Causing or engendering cholera.

chol·er·ine (kol'er-ēn). A mild form of diarrhea seen during epidemics of Asiatic cholera.

chol·er·oid (kol'er-oyd). SYN choleriform.

cho·ler·rha·gia (kō-lē-rā'jē-ă). Extensive flow of bile. [chole- + G. *rhegnymi*, to burst forth]

cho·ler·rha·gic (kō-lē-raj'ik). Referring to the flow of bile.

chol·e·scin·tig·ra·phy (kō-lē-sin-tig'ră-fē). Examination of the gall bladder and bile ducts by nuclear medicine scanning; radionuclide cholecystography. [chole- + scintigraphy]

cho·les·tane (kō'les-tān). The parent hydrocarbon of cholesterol. For structure, see steroids.

cho·les·ta·nol (kō-les'tan-ol). 5α-cholestan-3β-ol; 3β-hydroxycholestane; differing from cholesterol in the absence of the double bond.

cho·les·tan·one (kō-les'tan-ōn). An oxidation product of cholestanol, differing from it in the presence of a ketone oxygen in place of the 3-hydroxyl group; an isomer of coprostanone.

cho·le·sta·sia, cho·le·sta·sis (kō-les-tā'sē-ă, -les'tă-sis). An arrest in the flow of bile; c. due to obstruction of bile ducts is accompanied by formation of plugs of inspissated bile in the small ducts, canaliculi in the liver, and elevation of serum direct bilirubin and some enzymes. [chole- + G. *stasis*, a standing still]

cho·le·stat·ic (kō-les-tat'ik). Tending to diminish or stop the flow of bile.

cho·les·te·a·to·ma (kō-les-tē-ă-tō'mă). **1.** A mass of keratinizing squamous epithelium and cholesterol in the middle ear, usually resulting from chronic otitis media, with squamous metaplasia or extension of squamous epithelium inward to line an expanding cystic cavity that may involve the mastoid and erode surrounding bone. **2.** An epidermoid cyst arising in the central nervous system in man or animals. [cholesterol + G. *stear (steat)*, tallow, + *-ōma*, tumor]

cho·les·te·at·om·a·tous (kō-les-tē-ă-tō'mă-tŭs). Of or pertaining to cholesteatoma.

cho·les·ten·one (kō-les'ten-ōn). A dehydrocholestanone, differing from cholestanone by the presence of a double bond between carbons 4 and 5.

cho·les·ter·e·mia (kō-les-ter-ē'mē-ă). The presence of enhanced quantities of cholesterol in the blood. SYN cholesterinemia, cholesterolemia. [cholesterol + G. *haima*, blood]

cho·les·ter·ide (kō-les'ter-īd). Obsolete term for a cholesteryl ester of a fatty acid.

cho·les·ter·in (kō-les'ter-in). SYN cholesterol.

cho·les·ter·in·e·mia (kō-les'ter-in-ē'mē-ă). SYN cholesteremia.

cho·les·ter·in·o·sis (kō-les'ter-in-ō'sis). SYN cholesterolosis.
cerebrotendinous c., SYN cerebrotendinous *xanthomatosis*.

cho·les·ter·i·nu·ria (kō-les'ter-i-nū're-ă). SYN cholesteroluria. [cholesterin + G. *ouron*, urine]

cho·les·ter·o·der·ma (kō-les'ter-ō-der'mă). SYN xanthochromia.

cho·les·ter·ol (kō-les'ter-ol). 5-cholesten-3β-ol (cholestane with a 5,6 double bond and a 3β hydroxyl group); the most abundant steroid in animal tissues, especially in bile and gallstones, and present in food, especially that rich in animal fats; circulates in the plasma complexed to proteins of various densities and plays an important role in the pathogenesis of atheroma formation in arteries. SYN cholesterin.

cho·les·ter·ol·e·mia (kō-les'ter-ol-ē'mē-ă). SYN cholesteremia. [cholesterol + G. *haima*, blood]

cho·les·ter·ol·o·gen·e·sis (kō-les'ter-ol-ō-jen'ĕ-sis). The biosynthesis of cholesterol.

cho·les·ter·ol·o·sis (kō-les'ter-ol-ō'sis). **1.** A condition resulting from a disturbance in metabolism of lipids, characterized by deposits of cholesterol in tissue, as in Tangier disease. **2.** Choles-

terol crystals in the anterior chamber of the eye, as in aphakia with associated retinal separation. SYN cholesterinosis, cholesterosis.

extracellular c., obsolete term for erythema elevatum diutinum characterized by lipid deposits in vessel walls.

cho·les·ter·ol·u·ria (kō-les'ter-ol-ū'rē-ă). The excretion of cholesterol in the urine. SYN cholesterinuria.

cho·les·ter·o·sis (kō'les-ter-ō'sis). SYN cholesterolosis.
c. cu'tis, SYN xanthomatosis.

cho·le·styr·a·mine (kō-les'tēr-ă-mēn). An anion exchange resin used to bind dietary cholesterol and hence prevent its systemic absorption. Used to treat hypercholesteremia. Can bind many acidic drugs in the gastrointestinal tract and prevent their absorption.

cho·le·u·ria (kō-lē-yū'rē-ă). SYN biliuria.

cho·le·ver·din (kō-lē-ver'din). SYN biliverdin.

cho·lic (kō'lik). Relating to the bile. SYN choleic.

cho·lic ac·id. A family of steroids comprising the bile acids (or salts), generally in conjugated form (*e.g.,* glycocholic and taurocholic acids). Chemically, c. a.'s are cholan-24-oic (cholanic) acids (the terminal C_{24} of cholane becoming a —COOH group); biologically, c. a.'s are derived from cholesterol (a cholestane derivative) and display varying degrees of oxidation (OH groups) and orientation at positions 3, 7, and 12. It is these oxidations and orientations that distinguish the several c. a.'s; *e.g.,* c. a. is 3α,7α,12α-trihydroxy-5β-cholan-24-oic acid, deoxycholic acid is 3α,12α-dihydroxy-5β-cholanic acid. SYN cholalic acid, cholanic acid.

cho·li·cele (kō'li-sēl). Enlargement of the gallbladder due to retained fluids. [G. *cholē*, bile, + *kēlē*, tumor]

cho·line (kō'lēn). $HOCH_2CH_2N(CH_3)_3^+$; (2-hydroxyethyl)-trimethylammonium ion; found in most animal tissues either free or in combination as lecithin (phosphatidylcholine), acetate (acetylcholine), or cytidine diphosphate (cytidine diphosphocholine). It is included in the vitamin B complex; as acetylcholine (choline esterified with acetic acid), it is essential for synaptic transmission. Several salts of choline are used in medicine. SYN lipotropic factor, transmethylation factor.

c. acetylase, SYN c. acetyltransferase.

c. acetyltransferase, an enzyme catalyzing the condensation of choline and acetyl-coenzyme A, forming *O*-acetylcholine and coenzyme A. SYN c. acetylase.

activated c., SYN cytidine diphosphocholine.

c. chloride, a lipotropic agent.

c. dihydrogen citrate, (2-hydroxyethyl)trimethylammonium citrate; a lipotropic agent.

c. esterase I, SYN acetylcholinesterase.

c. esterase II, SYN cholinesterase.

c. kinase, an enzyme that catalyzes the formation of *O*-phosphocholine and ADP from choline and ATP. SYN c. phosphokinase.

c. phosphatase, SYN *phospholipase* D.

c. phosphate cytidylyltransferase, an enzyme that catalyzes a key step in lecithin biosynthesis: CTP + phosphocholine ↔ pyrophosphate + CDP-choline.

c. phosphokinase, SYN c. kinase.

c. salicylate, c. salt of salicyclic acid, an analgesic and antipyretic (because of the salicylate moiety).

c. theophyllinate, SYN oxtriphylline.

cho·line·phos·pho·trans·fer·ase (kō'lēn-fos-fō-trans'fer-ās). An enzyme catalyzing the reaction between CDP-choline and 1,2-diacylglycerol to form a phosphatidylcholine and CMP. The last step in lecithin biosynthesis.

cho·lin·er·gic (kol-in-er'jik). Relating to nerve cells or fibers that employ acetylcholine as their neurotransmitter. Cf. adrenergic. [choline + G. *ergon*, work]

cho·lin·es·ter (kō'lin-es-ter). An ester of choline; *e.g.,* acetylcholine.

cho·lin·es·ter·ase (kō-lin-es'ter-ās). One of a family of enzymes capable of catalyzing the hydrolysis of acylcholines and a few other compounds. Found in cobra venom. SEE ALSO acetylcholinesterase. SYN butyrocholinesterase, butyrylcholine esterase, choline esterase II, nonspecific c., pseudocholinesterase, "s"-type c.

"e"-type c., SYN acetylcholinesterase. ["e" in erythrocyte]

nonspecific c., SYN cholinesterase.

specific c., SYN acetylcholinesterase.

"s"-type c., SYN cholinesterase. ["s" in serum]

true c., SYN acetylcholinesterase.

cho·lin·es·ter·ase re·ac·ti·va·tor. A drug that reacts directly with the alkylphosphorylated enzyme to free the active unit; the drugs used therapeutically to reactivate phosphorylated forms of acetylcholinesterase are oximes, *e.g.,* diacetylmonoxime, monoisonitrosoacetone, 2-pralidoxime.

cho·lin·o·cep·tive (kō′lin-ō-sep′tiv). Referring to chemical sites in effector cells with which acetylcholine unites to exert its actions. Cf. adrenoceptive. [acetylcholine + L. *capio,* to take]

cho·li·no·lyt·ic (kō′lin-ō-lit′ik). Preventing the action of acetylcholine. [acetylcholine + G. *lysis,* loosening]

chol·i·no·mi·met·ic (kol′i-nō-mi-met′ik). Having an action similar to that of acetylcholine, the substance liberated by cholinergic nerves; term proposed to replace the less accurate term, parasympathomimetic. Cf. adrenomimetic. [acetylcholine + G. *mimētikos,* imitating]

cho·lin·o·re·ac·tive (kō′lin-ō-rē-ak′tiv). Responding to acetylcholine and related compounds.

chol·i·no·re·cep·tors (kol′i-nō-rē-sep′terz, -tōrz). SEE cholinergic *receptors,* under *receptor.*

cho·lis·tine sul·pho·meth·ate so·di·um (kō-lis′tēn sul-fō-meth′āt). SYN colistimethate sodium.

△cholo-. SEE chole-.

chol·o·lith (kol′ō-lith). Obsolete term for gallstone.

chol·o·li·thi·a·sis (kol-ō-li-thī′ă-sis). SYN cholelithiasis.

chol·o·lith·ic (kol-ō-lith′ik). Rarely used term relating in any way to gallstones.

chol·o·pla·nia (kol-ō-plā′nē-ă). The presence of bile salts in the blood or tissues. [cholo- + G. *planē,* a wandering]

chol·o·poi·e·sis (kō-lō-poy-ē′sis). SYN cholepoiesis.

chol·or·rhea (kol-ō-rē′ă). Obsolete term for an excessive secretion of bile. [cholo- + G. *rhoia,* a flow]

cho·los·co·py (kō-los′kŏ-pē). Rarely used term for cholangioscopy. [cholo- + G. *skopeō,* to view]

chol·o·tho·rax (kō-lō-thōr′aks). Bile in the pleural cavity.

cho·lo·yl (kō′lō-il). The radical of cholic acid or cholate.

chol·ur·ia (kō-lū′rē-ă). SYN biliuria. [G. *cholē,* bile, + *ouron,* urine]

cho·lyl-co·en·zyme A (kō′lil-kō-en′zīm). A condensation product of cholic acid and coenzyme A; an intermediate in the formation of bile salts from bile acids, as taurocholic acid from cholic acid.

c.-c. A synthetase, SYN *cholate* ligase.

chon·dral (kon′drăl). SYN cartilaginous. [G. *chondros,* cartilage]

chon·dral·gia (kon-dral′jē-ă). SYN chondrodynia. [G. *chondros,* cartilage, + *algos,* pain]

chon·dral·lo·pla·sia (kon′dral-ō-plā′zē-ă). Occurrence of cartilage in abnormal situations in the bony skeleton. [G. *chondros,* cartilage, + *allos,* other, + *plasia,* formed]

chon·drec·to·my (kon-drek′tō-mē). Excision of cartilage. [G. *chondros,* cartilage, + *ektomē,* excision]

Chon·drich·thyes (kon-drik′thi-ēz). Class of cartilaginous fishes, including the sharks, rays, and chimeras. [G. *chondros,* cartilage, + *ichthys,* a fish]

chon·dri·fi·ca·tion (kon′dri-fi-kā′shŭn). Conversion into cartilage. [G. *chondros,* cartilage, + L. *facio,* to make]

chon·dri·fy (kon′dri-fī). To become cartilaginous.

chon·drin (kon′drin). Obsolete term for a gelatin-like substance obtained from cartilage by boiling. SEE collagen.

△chondrio-. SEE chondro-.

chon·dri·o·some. Obsolete term for mitochondrion.

chon·dri·tis (kon-drī′tis). Inflammation of cartilage. [G. *chondros,* cartilage, + *-itis,* inflammation]

costal c., SYN costochondritis.

△chondro-, chondrio-. 1. Cartilage or cartilaginous. **2.** Granular or gritty substance. [G. *chondrion,* dim. of *chondros,* groats (coarsely ground grain), grit, gristle, cartilage]

chon·dro·blast (kon′drō-blast). A dividing cell of growing cartilage tissue. SYN chondroplast. [chondro- + G. *blastos,* germ]

chon·dro·blas·to·ma (kon′drō-blas-tō′mă). A benign tumor arising in the epiphyses of long bones, consisting of highly cellular tissue resembling fetal cartilage.

chon·dro·cal·cin (kon′drō-kal-sin). A 69,000 molecular weight protein believed to play a role in mineralization in hard tissue.

chon·dro·cal·ci·no·sis (kon′drō-kal-si-nō′sis). Calcification of cartilage. [chondro- + calcium + G. *-osis,* condition]

articular c. [MIM*118600], a disease characterized by deposits of calcium pyrophosphate crystals free of urate in synovial fluid, articular cartilage, and adjacent soft tissue; causes various forms of arthritis commonly characterized by goutlike attacks of pain, swelling of joints, and radiologic evidence of calcification in articular cartilage (pseudogout); sometimes inherited as an autosomal dominant trait and associated with certain diseases in others.

chon·dro·clast (kon′drō-klast). A multinucleated cell (giant cell) involved in the resorption of calcified cartilage; morphologically identical to osteoblasts. [chondro- + G. *klastos,* broken in pieces]

chon·dro·cos·tal (kon-drō-kos′tăl). SYN costochondral. [chondro- + L. *costa,* rib]

chon·dro·cra·ni·um (kon-drō-krā′nē-ŭm). A cartilaginous skull; the cartilaginous parts of the developing skull. [chondro- + G. *kranion,* skull]

chon·dro·cyte (kon′drō-sīt). A nondividing cartilage cell; occupies a lacuna within the cartilage matrix. SYN cartilage cell. [chondro- + G. *kytos,* a hollow (cell)]

isogenous c.'s, a clone of cartilage cells derived from one cell by division; occur in a cluster called an isogenous nest.

chon·dro·der·ma·ti·tis no·du·la·ris chron·i·ca he·li·cis (kon-drō-der-ma-tī′tis nod-yū-lar′is kron′i-kă hel′i-sis). A benign, chronic, small, painful nodule (or nodules) on the helix of the ear in elderly white males, which may occasionally become ulcerated. SYN Winkler's disease.

chon·dro·dyn·ia (kon-drō-din′ē-ă). Pain in cartilage. SYN chondralgia. [chondro- + G. *odynē,* pain]

chon·dro·dys·pla·sia (kon′drō-dis-plā′zē-ă). SYN chondrodystrophy. [chondro- + G. *dys,* bad, + *plasis,* a molding]

c. puncta′ta, SYN *dysplasia* epiphysialis punctata.

chon·dro·dys·tro·phia (kon′drō-dis-trō′fē-ă). SYN chondrodystrophy.

c. calcif′icans congen′ita, SYN *dysplasia* epiphysialis punctata.

c. congen′ita puncta′ta, SYN Conradi's *disease.*

chon·dro·dys·tro·phy (kon-drō-dis′trō-fē) [MIM*215150]. A disturbance in the development of the cartilage primordia of the long bones, especially the region of the epiphysial plates, resulting in arrested growth of the long bones and dwarfism in which the extremities are abnormally short, but the head and trunk are essentially normal; autosomal recessive inheritance. SYN chondrodysplasia, chondrodystrophia. [chondro- + G. *dys,* bad, + *trophē* nourishment]

asphyxiating thoracic c., SYN asphyxiating thoracic *dysplasia.*

asymmetrical c., SYN enchondromatosis.

hereditary deforming c., (1) SYN hereditary multiple *exostoses,* under *exostosis.* **(2)** SYN enchondromatosis.

hypoplastic fetal c., SYN *dysplasia* epiphysialis punctata.

chon·dro·ec·to·der·mal (kon′drō-ek-tō-der′măl). Relating to ectodermally derived cartilage; *e.g.,* branchial cartilages that may have developed from the neural crest.

chon·dro·fi·bro·ma (kon′drō-fī-brō′mă). SYN chondromyxoid *fibroma.*

chon·dro·gen·e·sis (kon-drō-jen′ē-sis). Formation of cartilage. SYN chondrosis (1). [chondro- + G. *genesis,* origin]

chon·dro·glos·sus (kon-drō-glos′ŭs). SEE chondroglossus *muscle.* [chondro- + G. *glossa,* tongue]

chon·droid (kon'droyd). **1.** Resembling cartilage. SYN cartilaginoid. **2.** Uncharacteristically developed cartilage, primarily cellular with a basophilic matrix and thin or nonexistent capsules. [chondro- + G. *eidos*, resemblance]

chon·dro·i·tin (kon-drō'i-tin). A (muco)polysaccharide (proteoglycan) composed of alternating residues of β-D-glucuronic acid and *N*-acetyl-D-galactosamine sulfate in alternating β(1-3) and β(1-4) linkages; present among the ground substance materials in the extracellular matrix of connective tissue.

c. sulfate A, c. with sulfuric residues esterifying the 4-hydroxyl groups of the galactosamine residues; found in connective tissue.

c. sulfate B, SYN dermatan *sulfate*.

c. sulfate C, c. with sulfuric residues esterifying the 6-hydroxyl groups of the galactosamine residues.

chon·drol·o·gy (kon-drol'ō-jē). The study of cartilage. [chondro- + G. *logos*, treatise]

chon·drol·y·sis (kon-drol'i-sis). Disappearance of articular cartilage as the result of disintegration or dissolution of the cartilage matrix and cells.

chon·dro·ma (kon-drō'mă). A benign neoplasm derived from mesodermal cells that form cartilage. [chondro- + G. *-ōma*, tumor]

extraskeletal c., a c. located in soft tissues, usually of the fingers, hands, and feet, not connected to underlying bone or periosteum.

juxtacortical c., SYN periosteal c.

periosteal c., a c. that develops from periosteum or periosteal connective tissue. SYN juxtacortical c.

chon·dro·ma·la·cia (kon'drō-mă-lā'shē-ă). Softening of any cartilage. [chondro- + G. *malakia*, softness]

c. feta'lis, an intrauterine form of c. in which the fetus is born dead with soft pliable limbs.

generalized c., SYN relapsing *polychondritis*.

c. of larynx, the presence of soft laryngeal cartilage, most often seen in epiglottis of young children. SYN laryngomalacia.

c. pate'llae, a softening of the articular cartilage of the patella; may cause patellalgia.

systemic c., SYN relapsing *polychondritis*.

chon·dro·ma·to·sis (kon'drō-mă-tō'sis). Presence of multiple tumor-like foci of cartilage.

synovial c., c. or osteocartilaginous nodules occurring in the synovial membrane of a joint. SYN synovial osteochondromatosis.

chon·dro·ma·tous (kon-drō'mă-tŭs). Pertaining to or manifesting the features of a chondroma.

chon·drome (kon'drōm). The genetic information contained in all of the mitochondria of a cell. [mitochondria + -ome]

chon·dro·mere (kon'drō-mēr). A cartilage unit of the fetal axial skeleton developing within a single metamere of the body; a primordial cartilaginous vertebra together with its costal component. [chondro- + G. *meros*, part]

chon·dro·mu·cin (kon-drō-myū'sin). SYN chondromucoid.

chon·dro·mu·coid (kon-drō-myū'koyd). Obsolete terms for a mucoprotein from cartilage; probably chondroitin sulfate, plus other materials. SYN chondromucin, chondroprotein.

chon·dro·myx·o·ma (kon'drō-mik-sō'mă). SYN chondromyxoid *fibroma*.

chon·dro·os·se·ous (kon-drō-os'ē-ŭs). Relating to cartilage and bone, either as a mixture of the two tissues or as a junction between the two, such as the union of a rib and its costal cartilage.

chon·dro·os·te·o·dys·tro·phy (kon'drō-os'tē-ō-dis'trō-fē). Term used for a group of disorders of bone and cartilage which includes Morquio syndrome and similar conditions. SYN osteochondrodystrophia deformans, osteochondrodystrophy.

chon·drop·a·thy (kon-drop'ă-thē). Any disease of cartilage. [chondro- + G. *pathos*, suffering]

chon·dro·pha·ryn·ge·us (kon'drō-făr-in-jē'ŭs). SEE middle constrictor *muscle* of pharynx.

chon·dro·phyte (kon'drō-fīt). An abnormal cartilaginous mass

that develops at the articular surface of a bone. [chondro- + G. *phytos*, a growth]

chon·dro·plast (kon'drō-plast). SYN chondroblast. [chondro- + G. *plastos*, formed]

chon·dro·plas·ty (kon'drō-plas-tē). Reparative or plastic surgery of cartilage. [chondro- + G. *plastos*, formed]

chon·dro·po·ro·sis (kon'drō-pōr-ō'sis). Condition of cartilage in which spaces appear, either normal (in the process of ossification) or pathologic. [chondro- + L. *porosus*, porous]

chon·dro·pro·tein (kon-drō-prō'tēn). SYN chondromucoid.

chon·dro·sar·co·ma (kon'drō-sar-kō'mă). A malignant neoplasm derived from cartilage cells, occurring most frequently in pelvic bones or near the ends of long bones, in middle-aged and old people; most c.'s arise *de novo*, but some may develop in a preexisting benign cartilaginous lesion.

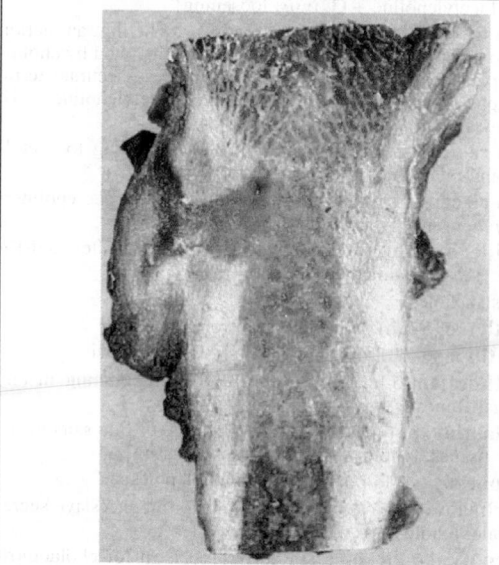

chondrosarcoma
on the proximal end of the femur

chon·dro·sin, chon·dro·sine (kon'drō-sin). A disaccharide composed of one molecule of D-glucuronic acid and one of D-galactosamine (chondrosamine); a component of the chondroitins.

chon·dro·sis (kon-drō'sis). **1.** SYN chondrogenesis. **2.** Obsolete term for a cartilaginous tumor.

chon·dro·skel·e·ton (kon'drō-skel'ĕ-tŏn). A skeleton formed of hyaline cartilage; *e.g.,* that of the human embryo or of certain adult fishes such as the shark or ray.

chon·dro·ster·nal (kon-drō-ster'năl). **1.** Relating to a sternal cartilage. **2.** Relating to the costal cartilages and the sternum.

chon·dro·ster·no·plas·ty (kon-drō-ster'nō-plas-tē). Surgical correction of malformations of the sternum.

chon·dro·tome (kon'drō-tōm). A very stiff scalpel-shaped knife used in cutting cartilage. SYN cartilage knife, ecchondrotome. [chondro- + G. *tomē*, cutting]

chon·drot·o·my (kon-drot'ō-mē). Division of cartilage. [chondro- + G. *tomē*, a cutting]

chon·dro·tro·phic (kon-drō-trof'ik). Influencing the nutrition and thereby the development and growth of cartilage. [chondro- + G. *trophē*, nourishment]

chon·dro·xi·phoid (kon-drō-zif'oyd). Relating to the xiphoid or ensiform cartilage. [chondro- + G. *xiphos*, sword, + *eidos*, appearance]

chon·drus (kon'drŭs). **1.** SYN cartilage. **2.** The plant *Chondrus crispus, Fucus crispus,* or *Gigartina mamillosa* (family Gigartinaceae); a demulcent in chronic and intestinal disorders. SYN carrageen (1), carragheen, Irish moss, pearl moss. [G. *chondros,* gristle]

cho·ne·chon·dro·ster·non (kō′nē-kon-drō-ster′non). SYN *pectus* excavatum. [G.*choanē* (*chonē*), funnel, + *chondros,* cartilage, + *sternon,* sternum]

CHOP Acronym for cyclophosphamide, doxorubicin, vincristine, and prednisone, a chemotherapy regimen for treatment of lymphomas.

Chopart, François, French surgeon, 1743–1795. SEE C.'s *amputation, joint.*

chord-. Cord. SEE ALSO cord-. [G. *chordē*]

chor·da, pl. **chor·dae** (kōr′dă, -dē) [NA]. A tendinous or a cord-like structure. SEE ALSO cord. [L., cord]

  c. chirurgica′lis, surgical catgut. [L.]

  c. dorsa′lis, SYN notochord (2).

  c. mag′na, SYN *tendo* calcaneus.

  c. obli′qua [NA], SYN oblique *ligament* of elbow joint.

  c. spermat′ica, SYN spermatic *cord.*

  c. spina′lis, SYN spinal *cord.*

  chor′dae tendin′eae [NA], the tendinous strands running from the papillary muscles to the atrioventricular valves (mitral and tricuspid). SYN tendinous cords.

  c. tym′pani [NA], a nerve given off from the facial nerve in the facial canal which passes through the posterior canaliculus of the c. tympani into the tympanic cavity, crosses over the tympanic membrane and handle of the malleus, and passes out through the anterior canaliculus of the c. tympani in the petrotympanic fissure to join the lingual branch of the mandibular nerve in the infratemporal fossa; it conveys taste sensation from the anterior two-thirds of the tongue and carries parasympathetic preganglionic fibers to the submandibular ganglion, for innervation of the submandibular and sublingual salivary glands. SYN cord of tympanum, tympanichord.

  c. umbilica′lis, SYN umbilical *cord.*

  c. vertebra′lis, obsolete term for notochord (2).

  c. voca′lis, pl. **chor′dae voca′les,** SYN vocal *fold.*

  chor′dae willis′ii, SYN Willis′ *cords,* under *cord.*

chord·al (kōr′dăl). Relating to any chorda or cord, especially to the notochord.

chor·da·me·so·derm (kor-dă-mes′ō-derm). That part of the protoderm of a young embryo which has the potentiality of forming notochord and mesoderm.

Chor·da·ta (kor-dā′tă). The phylum that includes the vertebrates, defined by possession of: 1) a single dorsal nerve cord (the brain and spinal cord of mammals); 2) a cartilaginous rod, the notochord, which forms dorsal to the primitive gut in the early embryo, and is surrounded and replaced by the vertebral column in the subphylum vertebrata; 3) by presence at some stage in development of gill slits in the pharynx or throat. [L. *chorda,* fr. G. *chordē,* a string]

chor·date (kōr′dāt). An animal of the phylum *Chordata.*

chor·dee (kōr-dē′). 1. Painful erection of the penis in gonorrhea or Peyronie's disease, with curvature resulting from lack of distensibility of the corpus cavernosum urethrae. SYN gryposis penis, penis lunatus. 2. Ventral curvature of the penis, most apparent on erection, as seen in hypospadias due to congenital shortness of the ventral skin and, on rare occasions, in patients with a normally situated meatus. [Fr. corded]

chor·di·tis (kōr-dī′tis). Inflammation of a cord; usually a vocal cord. [G. *chordē,* cord, + *-itis,* inflammation]

  c. voca′lis infe′rior, an inflammation limited mainly to the undersurface of the vocal cords and adjacent parts. SYN chronic subglottic laryngitis.

chor·do·ma (kōr-dō′mă). A rare solitary slowly growing neoplasm of skeletal tissue in adults, derived from persistent portions of the notochord; composed of cells arranged in lobules, with abundant quantities of extracellular mucus; some cells contain vacuoles of mucus that resemble soap bubbles (physaliphorous cells); most frequently in region clivus or lumbar-sacral cord. [(noto)chord + G. *-oma,* tumor]

chor·do·skel·e·ton (kōr-dō-skel′ĕ-tŏn). The part of the embryonic skeleton that develops in conjunction with the notochord.

chor·dot·o·my (kōr-dot′ō-mē). SYN cordotomy.

cho·rea (kōr-ē′ă). 1. Irregular, spasmodic, involuntary movements of the limbs or facial muscles, often accompanied by hypotonia. The location of the responsible cerebral lesion is not known. 2. SYN Sydenham's c. [L. fr. G. *choreia,* a choral dance, fr. *choros,* a dance]

  c.-acanthocytosis, a slowly progressive familial chorea with associated mental deterioration, diminished deep tendon reflexes, bilateral atrophy of the putamen and caudate nuclei and acanthocytosis (thorny appearance of blood erythrocytes); the disorder typically begins around late adolescence; inheritance is usually autosomal recessive. SYN acanthocytosis with c.

  acanthocytosis with c., SYN c.-acanthocytosis.

  acute c., SYN Sydenham's c.

  benign familial c., a rare, nonprogressive movement disorder characterized by c. and athetosis appearing in early childhood, most commonly manifested as gait ataxia and upper limb coordination. Intellect is unaffected. Probably autosomal-dominance inheritance with incomplete penetrance.

  chronic progressive c., SYN Huntington's c.

  c. cor′dis, cardiac irregularity related to c.

  dancing c., SYN procursive c.

  degenerative c., SYN Huntington's c.

  c. dimidia′ta, SYN hemichorea.

  electric c., (1) progressively fatal spasmodic disorder, possibly of malarial origin, occurring chiefly in Italy; **(2)** a severe form of Sydenham's c., in which the spasms are rapid and of a specially jerky character.

  fibrillary c., SYN myokymia.

  c. gravida′rum, sydenham's chorea occurring in pregnancy.

  habit c., SYN tic.

  hemilateral c., SYN hemichorea.

  Henoch's c., SYN spasmodic *tic.*

  hereditary c., SYN Huntington's c.

  Huntington's c., a progressive disorder usually beginning in young to middle age, consisting of a triad of choreoathetosis, dementia, and autosomal dominant inheritance with complete penetrance. Bilateral marked wasting of the putamen and the head of the caudate nucleus is characteristic. SYN chronic progressive c., degenerative c., hereditary c., Huntington's disease.

  hysterical c., conversion hysteria in which involuntary, quick, and purposeless (choreiform) movements constitute the chief feature.

  juvenile c., SYN Sydenham's c.

  laryngeal c., a spasmodic tic involving the muscles, resulting in an explosive manner of talking as in spasmotic dysphonia.

  c. ma′jor, a spasmodic attack occurring in patients with conversion hysteria.

  mimetic c., imitation of the c. movements of another person.

  c. mi′nor, SYN Sydenham's c.

  Morvan's c., SYN myokymia.

  posthemiplegic c., SYN posthemiplegic *athetosis.*

  procursive c., a form in which the patient whirls around, runs forward, or exercises a sort of rhythmic dancing movement. SYN dancing c.

  rheumatic c., SYN Sydenham's c.

  rhythmic c., patterned movement in conversion hysteria.

  saltatory c., rhythmic dancing movements, as in procursive c.

  senile c., a disorder resembling Sydenham's c., not associated with cardiac disease or dementia, occurring in the aged.

  Sydenham's c., a postinfectious c. appearing several months after a streptococcal infection with subsequent rheumatic fever. The c. typically involves the distal limbs and is associated with hypotonia and emotional lability. Improvement occurs over weeks or months and exacerbations occur without associated infection recurrence. SYN acute c., c. minor, chorea (2), juvenile c., rheumatic c., Sydenham's disease.

cho·re·al (kōr-ē′ăl). Relating to chorea.

cho·re·ic (kōr-ē′ik). Relating to or of the nature of chorea.

ch

cho·re·i·form (kōr-ē′i-fōrm). SYN choroid.

△**choreo-.** Chorea.

cho·re·o·ath·e·toid (kōr′ē-ō-ath′ĕ-toyd). Pertaining to or characterized by choreoathetosis.

cho·re·o·ath·e·to·sis (kōr′ē-ō-ath-ĕ-tō′sis). Abnormal movements of body of combined choreic and athetoid pattern. [choreo- + G. *athetos,* unfixed, + *-ōsis,* condition]
  congenital c., SYN double *athetosis.*

cho·re·oid (kōr′ē-oyd). Resembling chorea. SYN choreiform.

cho·re·o·phra·sia (kōr′ē-ō-frā′zē-ă). Continual repetition of meaningless phrases. [choreo- + G. *phrasis,* speaking]

△**chorio-.** Any membrane, especially that which encloses the fetus. [G. *chorion,* membrane]

cho·ri·o·ad·e·no·ma (kō′rē-ō-ad-ĕ-nō′mă). A benign neoplasm of chorion, especially with hydatidiform mole formation.
  c. destru′ens, hydatidiform mole in which there is an unusual degree of invasion of the myometrium or its blood vessels, causing hemorrhage, necrosis, and occasionally rupture of the uterus or embolism of molar tissue to the lungs; there is marked proliferation of the trophoblast, but avascular villi may also be found. SYN invasive mole.

cho·ri·o·al·lan·to·ic (kō′rē-ō-al-an-tō′ik). Pertaining to the chorioallantois.

cho·ri·o·al·lan·to·is (kō′rē-ō-ă-lan′tō-is). Extraembryonic membrane formed by the fusion of the allantois with the serosa or false chorion. In mammals it forms the fetal portion of the placenta; in avian embryos it is fused with the shell.

cho·ri·o·am·ni·o·ni·tis (kō′rē-ō-am′nē-ō-nī′tis). Infection involving the chorion, amnion, and amniotic fluid; usually the placental villi and decidua are also involved.

cho·ri·o·an·gi·o·ma (kō′rē-ō-an-jē-ō′mă). Benign tumor of placental blood vessels (hemangioma), usually of no clinical significance; large tumors may be associated with placental insufficiency and fetal hydrops; in some instances, the stroma is edematous and may resemble myxomatous tissue. SEE ALSO chorioangiosis. [chorion + angioma]

cho·ri·o·an·gi·o·ma·to·sis (kō′rē-ō-an′jē-ō-mă-tō′sis). SYN chorioangiosis.

cho·ri·o·an·gi·o·sis (kō′rē-ō-an-jē-ō′sis). An abnormal increase in the number of vascular channels in placental villi; severe c. is associated with a high incidence of neonatal death and major congenital malformations. SYN chorioangiomatosis. [chorio- + G. *angeion,* vessel, + *-osis,* condition]

cho·ri·o·cap·il·la·ris (kō′rē-ō-kap-i-lā′ris). SYN choriocapillary *layer.*

cho·ri·o·car·ci·no·ma (kō′rē-ō-kar-si-nō′mă). A highly malignant neoplasm derived from placental syncytial trophoblasts and cytotrophoblasts which forms irregular sheets and cords, which are surrounded by irregular "lakes" of blood; villi are not formed; neoplastic cells invade blood vessels. Hemorrhagic metastases develop relatively early in the course of the illness, and are frequently found in the lungs, liver, brain, and vagina and various other pelvic organs; c. may follow any type of pregnancy, especially hydatidiform mole, and occasionally originates in teratoid neoplasms of the ovaries or testes. SYN chorioepithelioma.

cho·ri·o·cele (kō′rē-ō-sēl). A hernia of the choroid coat of the eye through a defect in the sclera. [chorio- + G. *kēlē,* hernia]

cho·ri·o·ep·i·the·li·o·ma (kō′rē-ō-ep-i-thē-lē-ō′mă). SYN choriocarcinoma.

cho·ri·o·go·nad·o·tro·pin (kō′rē-ō-gon′ă-dō-trō-pin). SYN chorionic *gonadotropin.*

△**chorioid-, chorioido-.** For words beginning thus and not found here, see choroid-, choroido-.

cho·ri·o·ma (kō-rē-ō′mă). Rarely used term for a benign or malignant tumor of chorionic tissue.

cho·ri·o·mam·mo·tro·pin (kō′rē-ō-mam′ō-trō-pin). SYN human placental *lactogen.*

cho·ri·o·men·in·gi·tis (kō-rē-ō-men-in-jī′tis). A cerebral meningitis in which there is a more or less marked cellular infiltration

of the meninges, often with a lymphocytic infiltration of the choroid plexuses, particularly of the third and fourth ventricles.
  lymphocytic c., a form of viral meningitis that usually occurs in young adults during the fall and winter months. Caused by a virus carried by the common house mouse. SEE ALSO lymphocytic choriomeningitis *virus.*

cho·ri·on (kō′rē-on). The multilayered, outermost fetal membrane consisting of extraembryonic somatic mesoderm, trophoblast, and, on the maternal surface, villi bathed by maternal blood; as pregnancy progresses, part of the c. becomes the definitive fetal placenta. SYN chorionic sac, membrana serosa (1). [G. *chorion,* membrane enclosing the fetus]
  c. frondo′sum, the part of the c. where the villi persist, forming the fetal part of the placenta. SYN shaggy c.
  c. lae′ve, the portion of the c. from which the villi disappear in the later stages of pregnancy. SYN smooth c.
  previllous c., SYN primitive c.
  primitive c., the c. before its villi are well formed. SYN previllous c.
  shaggy c., SYN c. frondosum.
  smooth c., SYN c. laeve.

cho·ri·on·ic (kō-rē-on′ik). Relating to the chorion.

Cho·ri·op·tes (kō-rē-op′tēz). A genus of cosmopolitan and very common mange mites (family Psoroptidae) that cause chorioptic or symbiotic domestic animal mange, characterized by restriction of the mange to certain parts of the animal's body. Various species described, *i.e., C. equi* of horses, *C. caprae* of goats, *C. ovis* of sheep, *C. cuniculi* of rabbits, are now thought to be physiologic strains of one species, *C. bovis* of cattle. [G. *chorion,* membrane, + *optos,* visible]

cho·ri·o·ret·i·nal (kō-rē-ō-ret′i-năl). Relating to the choroid coat of the eye and the retina. SYN retinochoroid.

cho·ri·o·ret·i·ni·tis (kō′rē-ō-ret-i-nī′tis). SYN retinochoroiditis.
  c. sclopeta′ria, proliferation of fibrous tissue in the choroid and retina as the result of contusion of the sclera by a high velocity missile. [L. *sclopetum,* 14th century Italian handgun]

cho·ri·o·ret·i·nop·a·thy (kō′rē-ō-ret-i-nop′ă-thē). A primary abnormality of the choroid with extension to the retina. SEE ALSO choroidopathy.

cho·ris·ta (kō-ris′tă). A focus of tissue that is histologically normal per se, but is not normally found in the organ or structure in which it is located; *e.g.,* tissue displaced, during development, from its normal site. Cf. choristoma. [G. *chōristos,* separated]

cho·ris·to·blas·to·ma (kō-ris′tō-blas-tō′mă). An autonomous neoplasm composed of relatively undifferentiated cells of a choristoma. [choristoma + blastoma]

cho·ris·to·ma (kō-ris-tō′mă). A mass formed by maldevelopment of tissue of a type not normally found at that site. [G. *chōristos,* separated, + *-ōma*]

cho·roid (ko′royd). The middle vascular tunic of the eye lying between the retina and the sclera. SYN choroidea [NA]. [G. *choroeidēs,* a false reading for *chorioeidēs,* like a membrane)

cho·roi·dal (kō-roy′dăl). Relating to the choroid (choroidea).

cho·roi·dea (kō-royd′ē-ă) [NA]. SYN choroid. [see choroid]

cho·roi·der·e·mia (kō-roy-der-ē′mē-ă). Progressive degeneration of the choroid in males, occasionally in females, beginning with peripheral pigmentary retinopathy, followed by atrophy of the retinal pigment epithelium and of the choriocapillaris, night blindness, progressive constriction of visual fields, and finally complete blindness; X-linked inheritance; heterozygous females show a pigmentary retinopathy but without visual defect or peripheral progression. SYN progressive choroidal atrophy, progressive tapetochoroidal dystrophy. [choroid + G. *erēmia,* absence]

cho·roid·i·tis (kō-roy-dī′tis). Inflammation of the choroid. Cf. choroidopathy, chorioretinopathy. SYN posterior uveitis.
  anterior c., disseminated c. restricted to peripheral choroid.
  areolar c., inflammation of the choroid, with prominent pigment proliferation occurring first in the macular region and then more peripherally.
  diffuse c., a widespread exudative inflammation of the choroid, with progressive resolution of older lesions as new ones occur.

disseminated c., chronic inflammation of the choroid, with multiple isolated foci.

exudative c., a circumscribed inflammation of the choroid, often with multiple lesions.

juxtapupillary c., c. adjacent to the optic disk.

metastatic c., inflammation of the choroid arising from microbial emboli.

multifocal c., macular, peripapillary, and peripheral c., often designated presumed ocular histoplasmosis.

posterior c., disseminated c. restricted to the central choroid.

proliferative c., the dense scar tissue produced by severe choroiditis.

suppurative c., purulent inflammation of the choroid.

⌂choroido-. The choroid.

cho·roid·o·cy·cli·tis (kō-roy′dō-sī-klī′tis). Inflammation of the choroid coat and the ciliary body. [choroido- + G. *kyklos*, circle]

cho·roi·dop·a·thy (kō-roy-dop′ă-thē). Noninflammatory degeneration of the choroid.

areolar c., a slowly progressive pigmentary degeneration in young persons; characterized by black foci closely set together and coalescent at the posterior pole and macular region. SYN central areolar choroidal atrophy, central areolar choroidal sclerosis.

central serous c., detachment of the sensory retina induced by decreased adhesion between cells of the retinal pigment epithelium which permits plasma from the choriocapillaris to enter subretinal space. SYN central angiospastic retinopathy, central serous retinopathy.

Doyne's honeycomb c., obsolete term for macular *drusen.*

geographic c., bilateral acquired abnormality of retinal pigment epithelium and choroid in which irregular multiple progressive swelling is followed by atrophic scars in linear patterns. SYN helicoid c., serpiginous c.

guttate c., obsolete term for macular *drusen.*

helicoid c., SYN geographic c.

myopic c., chronic degeneration of the sclera and choroid with posterior staphyloma, accompanying high myopia.

serpiginous c., SYN geographic c.

cho·roid·o·ret·i·ni·tis (kō-roy′dō-ret-i-nī′tis). SYN retinochoroiditis.

cho·roi·do·sis (ko′-roy-dō′sis). Obsolete term for choroidopathy.

Chotzen, F., 20th century German physician. SEE C.'s *syndrome.*

Christ, J., German dermatologist, 1871–1948. SEE C.-Siemens-Touraine *syndrome.*

Christensen, Erna, Danish pathologist, 1906–1967. SEE C.-Krabbe *disease.*

Christian, Henry A., U.S. internist, 1876–1951. SEE C.'s *disease, syndrome;* Hand-Schüller-C. *disease;* Weber-C. *disease.*

Christison, Sir Robert, Scottish physician, 1797–1882. SEE C.'s *formula.*

Christmas. Surname of a child with the disease subsequently called Christmas *disease;* first case studied in detail. SEE ALSO Christmas *factor,* hemophilia B.

⌂chrom-, chromat-, chromato-, chromo-. Color. [G. *chrōma*]

chro·maf·fin (krō′maf-in). Giving a brownish yellow reaction with chromic salts; denoting certain cells in the medulla of the adrenal glands and in paraganglia. SYN chromaphil, chromatophil (3), chromophil (3), chromophile, pheochrome (1). [chrom- + L. *affinis,* affinity]

chro·maf·fin·o·ma (krō-maf-in-ō′mă). A neoplasm composed of chromaffin cells occurring in the medullae of adrenal glands, the organs of Zuckerkandl, or the paraganglia of the thoracolumbar sympathetic chain; some c.'s secrete catecholamines. SEE ALSO pheochromocytoma. SYN chromaffin tumor.

chro·maf·fin·op·a·thy (krō′maf-in-op′ă-thē). Any pathologic condition of chromaffin tissue, as in the medullae of adrenal glands or the organs of Zuckerkandl. [chromaffin + G. *pathos,* suffering]

chro·man, chro·mane (krō′man, -măn). 3,4-Dihydro-2*H*-1-benzopyran; fundamental unit of the tocopherols (vitamin E). SEE ALSO chromanol, chromene, chromenol.

chro·man·ol (krō′man-ol). 6-Hydroxychroman (6-chromanol) is the fundamental unit of the tocopherols (vitamin E), tocols, and tocotrienols, as well as of ubi-, toco-, and phyllochromanol. SEE ALSO chroman, chromene, chromenol. SYN hydroxychroman.

chro·ma·phil (krō′mă-fil). SYN chromaffin.

⌂chromat-. SEE chrom-.

chro·mate (krō′māt). A salt of chromic acid.

sodium c. Cr 51, anionic hexavalent radioactive chromium in the form of c. chromate ($Na_2{}^{51}CrO_4$) with a half-life of 27.8 days; used for the determination of circulating red cell volume and red cell survival time.

chro·mat·ic (krō-mat′ik). Of or pertaining to color or colors; produced by, or made in, a color or colors.

chro·ma·tid (krō′mă-tid). Each of the two strands formed by longitudinal duplication of a chromosome that becomes visible during prophase of mitosis or meiosis; the two c.'s are joined by the still undivided centromere; after the centromere has divided at metaphase and the two c.'s have separated, each c. becomes a chromosome. [G. *chrōma,* color, + -*id* (2),]

chro·ma·tin (krō′ma-tin). The genetic material of the nucleus, consisting of deoxyribonucleoprotein, which occurs in two forms during the phase between mitotic divisions: 1) as heterochromatin, seen as condensed, readily stainable clumps; 2) as euchromatin, dispersed lightly staining or nonstaining material. During mitotic division the c. condenses into chromosomes. [G. *chrōma,* color]

heteropyknotic c., SYN heterochromatin.

oxyphil c., SYN oxychromatin.

sex c., a small condensed mass of the inactivated X-chromosome usually located just inside the nuclear membrane of the interphase nucleus; the number of sex c. bodies per nucleus is one less than the number of X-chromosomes, hence normal males and females with Turner's syndrome (XO) have none (sex c. negative), normal females and males with Klinefelter's syndrome (XXY) have one, and (XXX) females have two c. masses. For technical reasons only about half the cells in a preparation show typical masses. SEE ALSO Lyon *hypothesis.* SYN Barr chromatin body.

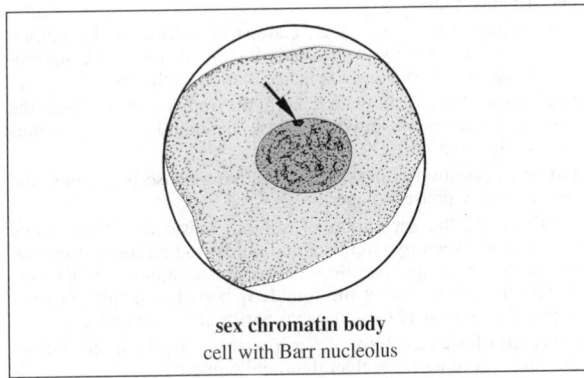

sex chromatin body
cell with Barr nucleolus

chro·ma·ti·nol·y·sis (krō′mă-ti-nol′i-sis). SYN chromatolysis.

chro·mat·i·nor·rhex·is (krō-mat′i-nō-rek′sis). Fragmentation of the chromatin. [chromatin + G. *rhēxis,* rupture]

chro·ma·tism (krō′mă-tizm). 1. Abnormal pigmentation. 2. SYN chromatic *aberration.* [G. *chrōma,* color]

⌂chromato-. SEE chrom-.

chro·ma·tog·e·nous (krō-mă-toj′ĕ-nŭs). Producing color; causing pigmentation. [chromato- + -*gen,* producing]

chro·mat·o·gram (krō-mat′ō-gram). The graphic record produced by chromatography.

chro·mat·o·graph (krō-mat′ō-graf). To perform chromatography.

chro·mat·o·graph·ic (krō′mat-ō-graf′ik). Pertaining to chromatography.

chro·ma·tog·ra·phy (krō-mă-tog′ră-fē). The separation of chemical substances and particles (originally plant pigments and other highly colored compounds) by differential movement through a two-phase system. The mixture of materials to be separated is percolated through a column or sheet of some suitable chosen absorbent (*e.g.,* an ion-exchange material); the substances least absorbed are least retarded and emerge the earliest; those more strongly absorbed emerge later. SYN absorption c. [chromato- + G. *graphō,* to write]

absorption c., SYN chromatography.

adsorption c., c. in which separation of substances is achieved by the difference in degree of adsorption of the compounds to a stationary phase.

affinity c., c. where the absorbent has a unique chemical affinity for a particular component of the passing solution. SYN affinity column.

column c., a form of partition, adsorption, ion exchange, or affinity c. in which one phase is liquid (aqueous) flowing down a column packed with the second phase, a solid; the dissolved substances form a partition between the solid and liquid phases depending on the chemical and physical conditions of each phase; the more strongly adsorbed solutes reach the bottom of the column later than the less strongly adsorbed ones.

gas c., a chromatographic procedure in which the mobile phase is a mixture of gases or vapors, which are separated in the process by their differential adsorption on a stationary phase.

gas-liquid c. (GLC), gas c., with the stationary phase being liquid rather than solid.

gel filtration c., SEE gel *filtration.*

high-performance liquid c. (HPLC), a chromatographic technology used to separate and quantitate mixtures of substances in solution. A sample is injected into a moving stream of solvent that flows through a column and detector. Separation during passage through the column occurs by absorption, partition, ion exchange, or size exclusion. The technique is commonly used in laboratories to measure organic compounds including steroid hormones, pesticides and poisons, toxic and carcinogenic compounds, and drugs. Also called high-pressure liquid c. SYN high-pressure liquid chromatography.

high-pressure liquid chromatography (HPLC), SYN high-performance liquid c.

ion exchange c., c. in which cations or anions in the mobile phase are separated by electrostatic interactions with the stationary phase. SEE ALSO anion exchange, cation exchange.

liquid-liquid c., c. in which both the moving phase and the stationary (or reverse-moving) phase are liquids, as in countercurrent distribution.

paper c., partition c. in which the moving phase is a liquid and the stationary phase is paper.

partition c., the separation of similar substances by repeated divisions between two immiscible liquids, so that the substances, in effect, cross the partition between the liquids in opposite directions; where one of the liquids is bound as a film on filter paper, the process is termed paper partition c. or paper c.

reversed phase c., a form of partitioning c. in which the stationary phase is more polar than the mobile phase.

thin-layer c. (TLC), c. through a thin layer of cellulose or similar inert material supported on a glass or plastic plate.

two-dimensional c., paper c. in which a spot, located originally in one corner of a sheet, is developed in one direction along one side of the sheet, after which the sheet is rotated 90° and developed, with another solvent, in the new direction; the resultant spots are thus spread over the entire paper, giving a "map" or "fingerprint." Also generalized to include c. followed by electrophoresis (or vice versa), column c. followed by paper c., etc.

chro·ma·toid (krō′mă-toyd). A refractile substance composed of chromatin, thought to be a non-glycogen food reserve contained within the cytoplasm of certain protozoa; seen in cysts of *Entamoeba histolytica* as rounded bars or chromatoidal bodies in contrast to the splintery form of c. bodies in cysts of *Entamoeba coli.* [chromato- + G. *eidos,* form]

chro·mat·o·ki·ne·sis (krō′mă-tō-ki-nē′sis). Rearrangement of the chromatin into various forms. [chromato- + G. *kinēsis,* movement]

chro·ma·tol·y·sis (krō-mă-tol′i-sis). The disintegration of the granules of chromophil substance (Nissl bodies) in a nerve cell body which may occur after exhaustion of the cell or damage to its peripheral process; other changes considered part of c. include swelling of the perikaryon and shifting of the nucleus from its central position to the periphery. SYN chromatinolysis, chromolysis, tigrolysis. [chromato- + G. *lysis,* dissolution]

central c., c. associated with significant axonal injury. SYN retrograde c.

retrograde c., SYN central c.

transsynaptic c., SYN transsynaptic *degeneration.*

chro·mat·o·lyt·ic (krō-mă-tō-lit′ik). Relating to chromatolysis.

chro·ma·tom·e·ter (krō-mă-tom′ĕ-ter). SYN colorimeter. [chromato- + G. *metron,* measure]

chro·mat·o·pec·tic (krō′mă-tō-pek′tik). Relating to or causing chromatopexis. SYN chromopectic.

chro·mat·o·pex·is (krō′mă-tō-pek′sis). The fixation of color or staining fluid. SYN chromopexis. [chromato- + G. *pēxis,* fixation]

chro·mat·o·phil (krō-mat′ō-fil). 1. SYN chromophilic. 2. SYN chromophil (2). 3. SYN chromaffin.

chro·mat·o·phil·ia (krō′mă-tō-fil′ĕ-ă). SYN chromophilia.

chro·mat·o·phil·ic, chro·ma·toph·i·lous (krō-mă-tō-fil′ik, -tof′i-lŭs). SYN chromophilic.

chro·mat·o·pho·bia (krō′mă-tō-fō′bē-ă). SYN chromophobia.

chro·mat·o·phore (krō-mat′ō-fōr). 1. A colored plastid, due to the presence of chlorophyll or other pigments, found in certain forms of protozoa. 2. Melanophage; a pigment-bearing phagocyte found chiefly in the skin, mucous membrane, and choroid coat of the eye, and also in melanomas. 3. SYN chromophore. 4. A colored plastid in plants; *e.g.,* chloroplasts, leukoplasts, etc. [chromato- + G. *phoros,* bearing]

chro·mat·o·pho·ro·tro·pic (krō′mă-tō-fōr′ō-trop′ik). Denoting the attraction of chromatophores to the skin or other organs. [chromatophore + G. *tropos,* a turning]

chro·mat·o·plasm (krō′mă-tō-plazm). The part of the cytoplasm containing pigment.

chro·ma·top·sia (krō-mă-top′sē-ă). A condition in which objects appear to be abnormally colored or tinged with color; designated according to the color seen: xanthopsia, yellow vision; erythropsia, red vision; chloropsia, green vision; cyanopsia, blue vision. SYN chromatic vision, colored vision, tinted vision. Cf. dyschromatopsia. [chromato- + G. *opsis,* vision]

chro·mat·o·some (krō-ma′tō-sōm). A nucleosome with one bound histone-1 protein.

chro·ma·tot·ro·pism (krō-mă-tot′rō-pizm). 1. A change of color. 2. The phenomenon of orientation in response to color. [chromato- + G. *tropē,* turn]

chro·ma·tu·ria (krō-mă-tū′rē-ă). Abnormal coloration of the urine. [chromato- + G. *ouron,* urine]

chrome (krōm). Chromium, especially as a source of pigment.

chro·mene (krō′mēn). 2*H*-1-Benzopyran; fundamental unit of the tocopherolquinones. SEE ALSO chroman, chromanol, chromenol.

chro·men·ol (krō′men-ol). 6-hydroxychromene (6-chromenol) is the fundamental unit of the tocopherolquinones (oxidized tocopherol) and plastochromenol-8. SEE ALSO chroman, chromanol, chromene. SYN hydroxychromene.

chrome red. Basic lead chromate, $PbCrO_4PbO$.

chro·mes·the·sia (krō-mes-thē′zē-ă). 1. The color sense. 2. A condition in which non-visual stimuli, such as taste or smell, cause the perception of color. [G. *chrōma,* color, + *aisthēsis,* sensation]

chrome yel·low [C.I. 77600]. A fine yellow powder used in paints and dyes. SYN lead chromate, Leipzig yellow, lemon yellow, Paris yellow.

chrom·hi·dro·sis (krōm-hī-drō′sis). A rare condition characterized by the excretion of sweat containing pigment. SYN chromidrosis. [chrom- + G. *hidros,* sweat]

apocrine c., excretion of colored sweat, usually black, from apocrine glands, due to an abnormal lipochrome content of the secretion, occurring on the face or the axillae in adult Negro males.

chro·mic ac·id (krō'mik). H_2CrO_4 or $H_2Cr_2O_7$; a strong oxidizing agent formed by dissolving chromium trioxide (CrO_3) in water. Has been used in solution as a topical antiseptic.

chro·mid·ia (krō-mid'ē-ă). Plural of chromidium.

chro·mid·i·a·tion (krō-mid-ē-ā'shŭn). SYN chromidiosis.

chro·mid·i·o·sis (krō-mid-ē-ō'sis). An outpouring of nuclear substance and chromatin into the cell protoplasm. SYN chromidiation.

chro·mid·i·um, pl. **chro·mid·ia** (krō-mid'ē-ŭm, -ē-ă). A basophilic particle or structure in the cell cytoplasm, rich in RNA, often found in specialized cells. [G. *chrōma*, color, + *-idion*, a diminutive termination]

chro·mi·dro·sis (krō-mi-drō'sis). SYN chromhidrosis.

chro·mi·um (Cr) (krō'mē-ŭm). A metallic element, atomic no. 24, atomic wt. 51.9961. A dietary essential bioelement. ^{51}Cr (half-life of 27.70 days) is used as a diagnostic aid in many disorders (*e.g.*, gastrointestinal protein loss). [G. *chroma*, color]

c. trioxide, CrO_3; chromic acid, used as a caustic in the removal of warts and other small growths from the skin and genitals; the hydrated acid, H_2CrO_4, forms variously colored salts with potassium, lead, and other bases.

△**chromo-**. SEE chrom-.

Chro·mo·bac·te·ri·um (krō-mō-bak-tēr'ē-ŭm). A genus of bacteria (family Rhizobiaceae) containing Gram-negative, motile rods. These microorganisms produce a violet pigment (violacein) and are occasionally pathogenic to man and other animals. The type species is *C. violaceum*.

C. viola'ceum, type species of the genus *C.*; it is found in soil and water.

chro·mo·blast (krō'mō-blast). An embryonic cell with the potentiality of developing into a pigment cell. [chromo- + G. *blastos*, germ]

chro·mo·blas·to·my·co·sis (krō'mō-blas'tō-mī-kō'sis). A localized chronic mycosis of the skin and subcutaneous tissues characterized by skin lesions so rough and irregular as to present a cauliflower-like appearance; caused by dematiaceous fungi such as *Phialophora verrucosa, P. dermatitidis, Fonsecaea pedrosoi, F. compacta,* and *Cladosporium carrionii*; fungal cells resembling copper pennies form rounded sclerotic bodies in tissue, with epidermal hyperplasia and intraepidermal microabscesses. SYN chromomycosis. [chromo- + G. *blastos*, germ, + *mykē*, fungus, + *-osis*, condition]

chro·mo·cen·ter (krō'mō-sen-ter). SYN karyosome.

chro·mo·cys·tos·co·py (krō'mō-sis-tos'kŏ-pē). SYN cystochromoscopy. [chromo- + G. *kystis*, bladder, + *skopeō*, to view]

chro·mo·cyte (krō'mō-sīt). Any pigmented cell, such as a red blood corpuscle. [chromo- + G. *kytos*, cell]

chro·mo·gen (krō'mō-jen). **1.** A substance, itself without definite color, that may be transformed into a pigment; denoting especially benzene and its homologues toluene, xylene, quinone, naphthalene, and anthracene, from which the aniline dyes are manufactured. **2.** A microorganism that produces pigment.

Porter-Silber c.'s, yellow phenylhydrazones formed by the reaction of 17,21-dihydroxy-20-oxosteroids with a phenylhydrazine-ethanol-sulfuric acid reagent; used chiefly to determine plasma cortisol concentrations and the urinary output of 17-hydroxycorticoids.

chro·mo·gen·e·sis (krō-mō-jen'ĕ-sis). Production of coloring matter or pigment. [chromo- + G. *genesis*, production]

chro·mo·gen·ic (krō-mō-jen'ik). **1.** Denoting a chromogen. **2.** Relating to chromogenesis.

chro·mo·gran·ins (krō'mō-gran-inz). Soluble proteins of chromaffin granules; c. A, an acidic glycoprotein, accounts for approximately half of the total protein of the granule matrix.

chro·mo·i·som·er·ism (krō'mō-ī-som'er-izm). Isomerism in which the isomers display different colors.

chro·mo·lip·id (krō-mō-lip'id). SYN lipochrome (1).

chro·mol·y·sis (krō-mol'i-sis). SYN chromatolysis.

chro·mo·mere (krō'mō-mēr). **1.** A condensed segment of a chromonema; densely staining bands visible in chromosomes under certain conditions. **2.** SYN granulomere. [chromo- + G. *meros*, a part]

chro·mom·e·ter (krō-mom'ĕ-ter). SYN colorimeter.

chro·mo·my·co·sis (krō'mō-mī-kō'sis). SYN chromoblastomycosis. [chromo- + G. *mykēs*, fungus, + *-osis,* condition]

chro·mo·nar hy·dro·chlo·ride (krō'mō-nar). [{3-[2-(diethylamino)ethyl]-4-methyl-2-oxo-2*H*-1-benzopyran-7-yl}oxy] acetic acid ethyl ester hydrochloride; used as a coronary vasodilator for treatment of angina pectoris.

chro·mone (krō'mōn). 4*H*-1-Benzopyran-4-one; fundamental unit of various plant pigments and other substances. SEE ALSO flavone, chromene, chroman.

chro·mo·ne·ma, pl. **chro·mo·ne·ma·ta** (krō-mō-nē'mă, -ma-tă). The coiled filament in which the genes are located, which extends the entire length of a chromosome and exhibits an intensely positive Feulgen test for DNA. SYN chromatic fiber. [chromo- + G. *nēma*, thread]

chro·mo·nych·ia (krō-mō-nik'ē-ă). Abnormality in the color of the nails. [chromo- + G. *onyx (onych-)*, nail]

chro·mo·pec·tic (krō-mō-pek'tik). SYN chromatopectic.

chro·mo·pex·is (krō-mō-pek'sis). SYN chromatopexis.

chro·mo·phage (krō'mō-fāj). A phagocyte that destroys pigment; an obsolete term applied by Metchnikoff to the cells believed by him to be active in the reduction of pigment of the hair. [chromo- + G. *phagein*, to eat]

chro·mo·phanes (krō'mō-phānz). The colored oil globules in the retinal cones of some animal species. [chromo- + G. *phaino*, to show]

chro·mo·phil, chro·mo·phile (krō'mō-fil, krō'mō-fīl). **1.** SYN chromophilic. **2.** A cell or any histologic element that stains readily. SYN chromatophil (2). **3.** SYN chromaffin. [chromo- + G. *phileō*, to love]

chro·mo·phil·ia (krō-mō-fil'ē-ă). The property possessed by most cells of staining readily with appropriate dyes. SYN chromatophilia. [chromo- + G. *phileō,* to love]

chro·mo·phil·ic, chro·moph·i·lous (krō-mō-fil'ik, -mof'i-lŭs). Staining readily; denoting certain cells and histologic structures. SYN chromatophil (1), chromatophilic, chromatophilous, chromophil (1), chromophile.

chro·mo·phobe (krō'mō-fōb). Resistant to stains, staining with difficulty or not at all; denoting certain degranulated cells in the anterior lobe of the pituitary gland. SYN chromophobic. [chromo- + G. *phobos*, fear]

chro·mo·pho·bia (krō-mō-fō'bē-ă). **1.** Resistance to stains on the part of cells and tissues. **2.** A morbid dislike of colors. SYN chromatophobia. [chromo- + G. *phobos*, fear]

chro·mo·pho·bic (krō-mō-fō'bik). SYN chromophobe. [chromo- + *phobos,* fear]

chro·mo·phore (krō'mō-fōr). The atomic grouping upon which the color of a substance depends. SYN chromatophore (3), color radical. [chromo- + G. *phoros*, bearing]

chro·mo·phor·ic, chro·moph·o·rous (krō-mō-fōr'ik, -mof'ŏr-ŭs). **1.** Relating to a chromophore. **2.** Producing or carrying color; denoting certain microorganisms.

chro·mo·pho·to·ther·a·py (krō'mō-phō'tō-thār'ă-pē). SYN chromotherapy. [chromo- + photo- + G. *therapeia*, medical treatment]

chro·mo·plast (krō'mō-plast). A chromophore filled with carotenoids.

chro·mo·plas·tid (krō-mō-plas'tid). A pigmented plastid, containing chlorophyll, formed in certain protozoans. [chromo- + G. *plastos*, formed, + *-id* (2)]

chro·mo·pro·tein (krō-mō-prō'tēn). One of a group of conjugated proteins, consisting of a combination of pigment (*i.e.*, a colored prosthetic group) with a protein; *e.g.*, hemoglobin.

chro·mo·som·al (krō-mō-sō'măl). Pertaining to chromosomes.

chro·mo·som·al map. A formal, stylized representation of the karyotype and of the positioning and ordering on it of those loci that have been localized by any of several mapping methods.

chro·mo·some (krō'mō-sōm). One of the bodies (normally 46 in humans) in the cell nucleus that is the bearer of genes, has the form of a delicate chromatin filament during interphase, contracts to form a compact cylinder segmented into two arms by the centromere during metaphase and anaphase stages of cell division, and is capable of reproducing its physical and chemical structure through successive cell divisons. In microbes, the c. is prokaryotic, not being enclosed within a nuclear membrane and not being subject to a mitotic mechanism. [chromo- + G. *sōma,* body]

---

chromosome set

n = haploid			
2n = diploid			
3n = triploid			
4n = tetraploid	anorthoploid	euploid or polyploid	
5n = pentaploid	orthoploid		heteroploid
6n = hexaploid			
n + 1	= simple disomal		
2n + 1	= simple trisomal	aneuploid or polysom	
2n + 2 (same)	= simple tetrasomal		
2n + 2 (diff.)	= double trisomal		

---

accessory c., a c. existing without its normal homologous c.; at the reduction division of gametogenesis an accessory c. is likely to be included in one daughter cell and not in the other, but may be lost completely by lagging behind on the equatorial plate. SYN monosome (1), odd c., unpaired allosome, unpaired c.

acentric c., a fragment of a c. lacking a centromere and unable to attach to the mitotic spindle, therefore unable to take part in the division of a nucleus and randomly distributed in daughter cells. SYN acentric fragment.

acrocentric c., a c. with the centromere placed very close to one end so that the short arm is very small, often with a satellite.

bivalent c., a pair of c.'s temporarily united.

Christchurch c. (Ch1), an abnormal small acrocentric c. (no. 21 or 22) with complete or almost complete deletion of the short arm; found in cultured leukocytes in some cases of chronic lymphocytic leukemia, also in some normal relatives of patients.

derivative c., an anomalous c. generated by translocation. SYN translocation c.

dicentric c., a c. with two centromeres that may result from reciprocal translocation.

double minute c.'s, paired, extrachromosomal elements lacking centromeres, often associated with a drug resistance gene.

fragile X c., an X c. with a fragile site near the end of the long arm, resulting in the appearance of an almost detached fragment; demonstrated only under special culture conditions; frequently associated with X-linked mental retardation. SEE Renpenning's *syndrome.*

giant c., (1) SYN polytene c. **(2)** SYN lampbrush c.

heterotypical c., SYN allosome.

homologous c.'s, members of a single pair of c.'s.

lampbrush c., lamp-brush c., (1) a large c. found in oocytes of certain animals characterized by many fine lateral projections giving the appearance of a test tube brush or lampbrush. **(2)** multiply looped chromosomal area of the chromatin of some species. SYN giant c. (2).

late replicating c., a c. (often anomalous) that is shown, *e.g.,* by incorporation of a labeled nucleotide, to undergo delayed duplication preliminary to mitosis; formerly used as a means of distinguishing members of a group of c.'s.

marker c., a c. with cytologically distinctive characteristics.

metacentric c., a c. with a centrally placed centromere that divides the c. into two arms of approximately equal length.

mitochondrial c., the DNA component of mitochondria, the chief function of which is synthesis of adenosine triphosphate and the management of cellular energy; the c. contains some 16,000 base pairs arranged in a circle. The inheritance is matrilineal, and the mutation rate is unusually high; since each cell contains thousands of copies a mutant form may assume an almost continuous gradation as in a galtonian process. Most of the mutations known have their impact on the respiratory chain.

nonhomologous c.'s, c.'s that are not members of the same pair.

nucleolar c., a c. regularly associated with a nucleolus.

odd c., SYN accessory c.

Philadelphia c. (Ph1), an abnormal minute c. formed by a rearrangement of c.'s 9 and 22; found in cultured leukocytes of many patients with chronic granulocytic leukemia.

polytene c., a stage of c. division that forms the giant c. found in the salivary gland of dipterous insects; the great width is the result of repeated divisions of the chromonema without subsequent lengthwise separation of the filaments. SYN giant c. (1).

c. puffs, expansions of particular c. regions; sites of RNA syntheses.

ring c., a c. with ends joined to form a circular structure. The ring form is abnormal in humans but the normal form of the c. in certain bacteria.

sex c.'s, the pair of c.'s responsible for sex determination. In humans and most animals, the sex c.'s are designated X and Y; females have two X c.'s, males have one X and one Y c. In certain birds, insects, and fishes the sex c.'s are designated Z and W; males have two Z c.'s, females may have one Z and one W c., or one Z and no W c. SYN gonosome.

submetacentric c., a c. with the centromere so placed that it divides the c. into two arms of strikingly unequal length.

telocentric c., a c. with a terminal centromere; such c.'s are unstable and arise by misdivision or breakage near the centromere and are usually eliminated within a few cell divisions.

translocation c., SYN derivative c.

unpaired c., SYN accessory c.

W c., X c., Y c., Z c., SEE sex c.'s.

yeast artificial c.'s (YAC), yeast DNA sequences that have incorporated into them very large foreign DNA fragments; the recombinant DNA is then introduced into the yeast by transformation; the use of yeast artificial c.'s permits the cloning of large genes with their flanking regulatory sequences.

chro·mo·some map. A systematic semiabstract representation of the physical location of loci on a karyotype. Cf. genetic map.

chro·mo·some map·ping. The process of determining the position of loci on specific chromosomes and constructing a diagram of each chromosome showing the relative positions of loci; techniques include family studies with linkage analysis, somatic cell hybridization, and chromosome deletion mapping.

chro·mo·some pair·ing. The process in synapsis whereby homologous c. p.'s align opposite each other before disjoining in the formation of the daughter cell; the apposition permits exchange of genetic material in crossing-over.

chro·mo·some walk·ing. A process of extending a genetic map by successive hybridization steps.

chro·mo·ther·a·py (krō-mō-thār'ă-pē). Treatment of disease by colored light. SYN chromophototherapy.

chro·mo·tox·ic (krō-mō-tok'sik). Caused by a toxic action on the hemoglobin, as in chromotoxic hyperchromemia, or resulting from the destruction of hemoglobin.

chro·mo·trich·ia (krō-mō-trik'ē-ă). Colored or pigmented hair. [chromo- + G. *thrix (trich-),* hair]

chro·mo·trich·i·al (krō-mō-trik'ē-ăl). Pertaining to the coloring of hair.

chro·mo·trope (krō'mō-trōp). Any of several dyes containing chromotropic acid and which have the property of changing from red to blue on afterchroming.

chro·mo·trope 2R [C.I. 16570]. A red acid dye, $C_{16}H_{10}N_2O_8S_2Na_2$, used as a counterstain and for staining red blood cells in sections.

chro·mo·tro·pic ac·id (krō'mō-trōp-ik). 4,5-Dihydroxynaphthalene-2,7-disulfonic acid; used as a reagent and in chromotropes.

chro·nax·ia (krō-nak'sē-ă). SYN chronaxie.

chro·nax·ie (krō′nak-sē). A measurement of excitability of nervous or muscular tissue; the shortest duration of an effective electrical stimulus having a strength equal to twice the minimum strength required for excitation. SYN chronaxia, chronaxis, chronaxy. [G. *chronos,* time, + *axia,* value]

chro·nax·im·e·ter (krō-nak-sim′ĕ-ter). An instrument for measuring chronaxie.

chro·nax·im·e·try (krō-nak-sim′ĕ-trē). The measurement of chronaxie. [G. *chronos,* time, + *axia,* value, + *metrein,* to measure]

chro·nax·is (krō-nak′sis). SYN chronaxie.

chro·naxy (krō′nak-sē). SYN chronaxie.

chron·ic. **1.** Referring to a health-related state, lasting a long time. **2.** Referring to exposure, prolonged or long-term, sometimes meaning also low-intensity. **3.** The U.S. National Center for Health Statistics defines a chronic condition as one of three months' duration or longer. [G. *chronos,* time]

chro·nic·i·ty (kron-is′i-tē). The state of being chronic.

△**chrono-.** Time. [G. *chronos*]

chro·no·bi·ol·o·gy (kron′ō-bī-ol′ŏ-jē). That aspect of biology concerned with the timing of biological events, especially repetitive or cyclic phenomena in individual organisms. [chrono- + G. *bios,* life, + *logos,* study]

chron·og·no·sis (kron-og-nō′sis). Perception of the passage of time. [chrono- + G. *gnōsis,* knowledge]

chro·no·graph (kron′ō-graf). An instrument for graphic measurement and recording brief periods of time. [chrono- + G. *graphō,* to record]

chro·nom·e·try (krō-nom′ĕ-trē). Measurement of intervals of time. [chrono- + G. *metron,* measure]

mental c., study of the duration of mental and behavorial processes.

chron·o·on·col·o·gy (kron′ō-on-kol′ō-jē). The study of the influence of biological rhythms on neoplastic growth; also used to describe anti-cancer treatment based on the timing of drug administration. [G. *chronos,* time, + oncology]

chro·no·phar·ma·col·o·gy (kron′ō-far-mă-kol′ō-jē). A branch of chronobiology concerned with the effects of drugs upon the timing of biological events and rhythms, and the relation of biological timing to the effects of drugs.

chro·no·pho·bia (kron′ō-fō′bē-ă). Morbid fear of the duration or immensity of time.

chro·no·pho·to·graph (kron-ō-fō′tō-graf). A photograph taken as one of a series for the purpose of showing successive phases of a motion.

chro·no·ta·rax·is (kron′ō-tă-rak′sis). Distortion or confusion of the sense of time. [chrono- + G. *taraxis,* confusion]

chro·no·tro·pic (kron′ō-trop′ik). Affecting the rate of rhythmic movements such as the heartbeat.

chro·not·ro·pism (kron-ot′rō-pizm). Modification of the rate of a periodic movement, *e.g.,* the heartbeat, through some external influence. [chrono- + G. *tropē,* turn, change]

negative c., retardation of movement, especially of the heart rate.

positive c., acceleration of movement, especially of the heart rate.

chro·o·coc·cals (krō-ō-kok-alz). A class of cyanobacteria in which the cells are solitary or colonial. [*Chroococcus* fr. G. *chrōs, chroos,* color, + *coccus*]

△**chrys-, chryso-.** Gold; corresponds to L. *auro-.* [G. *chrysos*]

chry·san·the·mum-car·box·yl·ic ac·ids (kri-san′thĕ-mŭm-kar-bok′si-lik). Cyclopropane carboxylic acids substituted in one position by two methyl groups, the other by 2-methyl-1-propenyl (chrysanthemum monocarboxylic acid) or by 3-methoxy-2-methyl-3-oxo-1-propenyl (chrysanthemum dicarboxylic acid methyl ester); these acids, esterified with allethrolone or pyrethrolone, are the allethrins and pyrethrins, respectively.

chrys·a·ro·bin (kris-ă-rō′bin). An extract of Goa powder; a complex mixture of reduction products of chrysophanic acid, emodin, and emodin monomethyl ether; used locally in ringworm, psoriasis, and eczema. [G. *chrysos,* gold, + Brazil Ind. *araroba,* bark]

chrys·a·zine (kris′ă-zin). SYN danthron.

chry·si·a·sis (kri-sī′ă-sis). A permanent slate-gray discoloration of the skin and sclera resulting from deposition of gold in the connective tissue of the skin and eye together with increased melanin formation after administration of gold. SYN auriasis, aurochromoderma, chrysoderma. [G. *chrysos,* gold]

chrys·o·cy·a·no·sis (kris′ō-sī-ă-nō′sis). Pigmentation of skin due to reaction to therapeutic use of gold salts.

chrys·o·der·ma (kris-ō-der′mă). SYN chrysiasis. [G. *chrysos,* gold, + *derma,* skin]

chrys·oi·din (kris′oy-din) [C.I. 11270]. 2,4-Diaminoazobenzene hydrochloride; a dye (MW 249) made from aniline, used in histology and as an indicator (changing from orange to yellow at pH 4.0 to 7.0); also employed as a substitute for Bismarck brown. C. citrate and c. thiocyanate are used as antiseptics.

Chrys·o·my·ia (kris-ō-mī′yă). A genus of myiasis-producing fleshflies (family Calliphoridae) with medium-sized metallic-colored adults; includes the Old World screw worm, *C. bezziana* (sometimes called *Cochliomyia bezziana*), which is a primary invader, comparable to *Cochliomyia hominivorax,* the New World screw worm fly, whereas *C. megacephala* is an Old World equivalent to *Cochliomyia macellaria,* both being secondary or saprophytic invaders. [G. *chrysos,* gold, + *myia,* fly]

Chrys·ops (kris′ops). The deerfly, a genus of biting flies with about 80 North American species, characterized by a splotched wing pattern; *C. discalis* is a vector of *Francisella tularensis* in the U.S.; *C. dimidiatus* and *C. silaceus* are the principal vectors of *Loa loa* in west Africa. [G. *chrysos,* gold, + *ōps,* eye]

Chrys·o·spo·ri·um par·vum (kris-ō-spōr′ē-ŭm par′vŭm). A species of soil fungus. The pathogenic organism that had this name has been changed to *Emmonsia parva* and does cause adiaspiromycosis.

chrys·o·ther·a·py (kris-ō-thār′ă-pē). Treatment of disease by the administration of gold salts. SYN aurotherapy. [G. *chrysos,* gold]

chthon·o·pha·gia, chthon·oph·a·gy (thon-ō-fā′jē-ă, -of′ă-jē). Rarely used terms for geophagia. [G. *chthōn,* earth, + *phagō,* to eat]

chunk·ing (chŭnk′ing). The process within short-term memory of combining disparate items of information so that they take up as little as possible of the limited space in short-term memory; *e.g.,* combining into one percept the three individual letters making up the word "cat".

Churg, Jacob, U.S. pathologist, *1910. SEE C.-Strauss *syndrome.*

chut·ta (chŭt′ă). Cancer of the roof of the mouth developing in Asians who smoke cigars with the lighted end inside the mouth. A similar association has been reported from South America and Sardinia.

Chvostek, Franz, Austrian surgeon, 1834–1884. SEE C.'s *sign.*

△**chyl-.** SEE chylo-.

chy·lan·gi·o·ma (kī-lan-jē-ō′mă). A mass of prominent, dilated lacteals and larger intestinal lymphatic vessels. [chyl- + G. *angeion,* vessel, + *-ōma,* tumor]

chy·la·que·ous (kī-lā′kwē-ŭs). Referring to watery chyle. [chyl- + L. *aqua,* water]

chyle (kīl). A turbid white or pale yellow fluid taken up by the lacteals from the intestine during digestion and carried by the lymphatic system via the thoracic duct into the circulation. The milky appearance is due to chylomicrons in the lymph. [G. *chylos,* juice]

chy·le·mia (kī-lē′mē-ă). The presence of chyle in the circulating blood. [chyl- + G. *haima,* blood]

chy·li·dro·sis (kī-li-drō′sis). Sweating of a milky fluid resembling chyle. [chyl- + G. *hidrōs,* sweat]

chy·li·fac·tion (kī-li-fak′shŭn). SYN chylopoiesis. [chyl- + L. *facio,* to make]

chy·li·fac·tive (kī-li-fak′tiv). SYN chylopoietic.

chy·lif·er·ous (kī-lif′er-ŭs). Conveying chyle. SYN chylophoric. [chyl- + L. *fero,* to carry]

chy·li·fi·ca·tion (kī′li-fi-kā′shŭn). SYN chylopoiesis.

chy·li·form (kī′li-fōrm). Resembling chyle.

ch

⌂**chylo-, chyl-.** Chyle. [G. *chylos*, juice.]

chy·lo·cele (kī′lō-sēl). A cystlike lesion resulting from the effusion of chyle into the tunica vaginalis propria and cavity of the tunica vaginalis testis. [chylo- + G. *kēlē*, tumor]

parasitic c., SYN *elephantiasis* scroti.

chy·lo·cyst (kī′lō-sist). SYN *cisterna* chyli. [chylo- + G. *kystis*, bladder]

chy·lo·der·ma (kī-lō-der′mă). SYN *elephantiasis* scroti. [chylo- + G. *derma*, skin]

chy·lo·me·di·as·ti·num (kī′lō-mē-dē-as-tī′nŭm). Abnormal presence of chyle in the mediastinum.

chy·lo·mi·cron, pl. **chy·lo·mi·cra, chy·lo·mi·crons** (kī-lō-mi′kron, -mī′kră, -mi′kronz). A lipid droplet (between 0.8 and 5 nm in diameter) of reprocessed lipid synthesized in epithelial cells of the small intestine and containing triacylglycerols, cholesterol esters, and several apolipoproteins (*e.g.,* A-I, B-48, C-I, C-II, C-III, E); the least dense (less than 0.95 g/mL) of the plasma lipoproteins which functions as a transport vehicle. [chylo- + G. *micros*, small]

chy·lo·mi·cro·ne·mia (kī′lō-mī-krō-nē′mē-ă). The presence of chylomicrons, especially an increased number, in the circulating blood, as in type I familial hyperlipoproteinemia. SEE ALSO familial chylomicronemia *syndrome.*

chy·lo·per·i·car·di·tis (kī′lō-pār-i-kar-dī′tis). SYN chylopericardium.

chy·lo·per·i·car·di·um (kī′lō-pār-i-kar′dē-ŭm). A milky pericardial effusion resulting from obstruction of the thoracic duct, from trauma, or of idiopathic origin. SYN chylopericarditis.

chy·lo·per·i·to·ne·um (kī′lō-pār-i-tō-nē′ŭm). SYN chylous *ascites.*

chy·lo·phor·ic (kī-lō-fōr′ik). SYN chyliferous. [chylo- + G. *phoros*, bearing]

chy·lo·pleu·ra (kī-lō-plūr′ă). SYN chylothorax.

chy·lo·pneu·mo·tho·rax (kī′lō-nū-mō-thōr′aks). Free chyle and air in the pleural space.

chy·lo·poi·e·sis (kī′lō-poy-ē′sis). Formation of chyle in the intestine. SYN chylifaction, chylification. [chylo- + G. *poiesis*, a making]

chy·lo·poi·et·ic (kī′lō-poy-et′ik). Relating to chylopoiesis. SYN chylifactive.

chy·lor·rhea (kī-lō-rē′ă). The flow or discharge of chyle. [chylo- + G. *rhoia*, flow]

chy·lo·sis (kī-lō′sis). The formation of chyle from the food in the intestine, its digestion and absorption by the intestinal mucosa, and its mixture with the blood and conveyance to the tissues.

chy·lo·tho·rax (kī-lō-thōr′aks). An accumulation of milky chylous fluid in the pleural space, usually on the left. SYN chylopleura, chylous hydrothorax.

chy·lous (kī′lŭs). Relating to chyle.

chy·lu·ria (kī-lū′rē-ă). The passage of chyle in the urine; a form of albiduria. [chyl- + G. *ouron*, urine]

chy·mase (kī′mās). SYN chymosin.

chyme (kīm). The semifluid mass of partly digested food passed from the stomach into the duodenum. SYN chymus, pulp (3). [G. *chymos*, juice]

chy·mi·fi·ca·tion (kī-mi-fi-kā′shŭn). SYN chymopoiesis. [G. *chymos*, juice, + L. *facio*, to make]

chy·mo·pa·pa·in (kī′mō-pap-ā′in). A cysteine proteinase similar to papain in specificity; rarely used to shrink slipped disks as an alternative to surgery, and as a meat tenderizer.

chy·mo·poi·e·sis (kī′mō-poy-ē′sis). The production of chyme; the physical state of food (semifluid) brought about by digestion in the stomach. SYN chymification. [G. *chymos*, juice, chyme, + *poiesis*, a making]

chy·mor·rhea (kī-mō-rē′ă). The flow of chyme. [G. *chymos*, juice, + *rhoia*, flow]

chy·mo·sin (kī′mō-sin). A proteinase structurally homologous with pepsin, formed from prochymosin; the milk-curdling enzyme obtained from the glandular layer of the stomach of the calf. Acts on a single peptide bond (–Phe–Met–) in κ-casein. SYN chymase, pexin, rennase, rennet, rennin.

chy·mo·sin·o·gen (kī-mō-sin′ō-jen). SYN prochymosin.

chy·mo·sta·tin (kī′mō-sta-tin). An oligopeptide that is known to inhibit chymotrypsin-like proteases (*e.g.,* cathepsin A, B, and D, and papain).

chy·mo·tryp·sin (kī-mō-trip′sin). C. A or B; a serine proteinase of the gastrointestinal tract that preferentially cleaves carboxyl links of hydrophobic amino acids, particularly at tyrosyl, tryptophanyl, phenylalanyl, and leucyl residues; synthesized in the pancreas as chymotrypsinogen, and subsequently converted to π-, δ-, and finally α-c. by successive trypsin-dependent cleavages; proposed for use in the treatment of inflammation and edema associated with trauma and to facilitate intracapsular cataract extraction. C. C is similar to c. but with broader specificity (*e.g.,* additionally acting on carboxyl links of methionyl, glutaminyl, and asparaginyl residues).

chy·mo·tryp·sin·o·gen (kī′mō-trip-sin′ō-jen). The precursor of chymotrypsin. Converted to π-chymotrypsin by the action of trypsin.

chy·mous (kī′mŭs). Relating to chyme.

chy·mus (kī′mŭs). SYN chyme.

Ci Abbreviation for curie.

Ciaccio, Carmelo, Italian pathologist, 1877–1956. SEE Ciaccio's *stain.*

Ciaccio, Giuseppe V., Italian anatomist, 1824–1901. SEE Ciaccio's *glands,* under *gland.*

cib. Abbreviation for L. *cibus*, food.

ci·bo·pho·bia (sī-bō-fō′bē-ă). Fear of eating, or loathing for, food. [L. *cibus*, food, + G. *phobos*, fear]

CIC Abbreviation for clean intermittent catheterization.

cic·a·trec·to·my (sik-ă-trek′tō-mē). Excision of a scar. [L. *cicatrix*, scar, + G. *ektomē*, excision]

cic·a·tri·ces (sik-ă-trī′sēz). Plural of cicatrix.

cic·a·tri·cial (sik-ă-trish′ăl). Relating to a scar.

cic·a·tri·cot·o·my, cic·a·tri·sot·o·my (sik′ă-trī-kot′ō-mē, -sot′ō-mē). Cutting a scar. [L. *cicatrix*, scar, + G. *tomē*, cutting]

cic·a·trix, pl. **cic·a·tri·ces** (sik′ă-triks, si-kā′triks; sik-ă-trī′sēz). A scar. [L.]

brain c., a scarring of the brain resulting from injury (reactive gliosis), characterized by proliferation of mesodermal (vascular) and ectodermal (glial) elements. SEE ALSO isomorphous *gliosis.*

filtering c., a c. through which fluid may seep; denoting especially a form of c. produced by an operation for glaucoma, through which there is subconjunctival drainage of aqueous humor.

meningocerebral c., scarring and adhesions involving contiguous brain and meninges; typically caused by head injury.

vicious c., a c. that by its contraction causes a deformity.

cic·a·tri·zant (sik-at′ri-zant). **1.** Causing or favoring cicatrization. **2.** An agent with such action.

cic·a·tri·za·tion (sik′ă-tri-zā′shŭn). **1.** The process of scar formation. **2.** The healing of a wound otherwise than by first intention.

ci·clo·pir·ox ol·a·mine (sī-klō-pir′oks ōl′ă-mēn). $C_{14}H_{24}N_2O_3$; a broad spectrum antifungal agent used to treat a variety of fungus and yeast skin infections.

cic·u·tox·in (sik-yū-tok′sin). (-)-Heptadeca-*trans*-8,10,12-triene-4,6-diyne-1,4-diol; a toxic principle present in water hemlock, *Cicuta virosa* (family Umbelliferae); pharmacologic action is similar to that of picrotoxin.

CIDP Abbreviation for chronic inflammatory demyelinating *polyneuropathy.*

ci·gua·te·ra (sēg-wah-tār′ă). Poisoning due to the ingestion of the flesh or viscera of various marine fish of the tropical Caribbean and Pacific, such as barracuda, grouper, red snapper, amberjack, and dolphin, which contain ciguatoxin acquired through their food chain and unaffected by preservation or preparation procedures; characterized by varying combinations of vomiting and diarrhea, myalgia, dysesthesia and paresthesia of the extremities and perioral region, pruritis, headache, weakness, and diaphoresis. [Sp., prob. *cigua*, sea snail]

ci·gua·tox·in (sēg-wă-tok′sin). A marine saponin of unknown structure but with the empirical formula $C_{35}H_{65}NO_8$; the toxic substance causing ciguatera.

ci·la·stat·in so·di·um (sī-lă-stat'in). $C_{16}H_{25}N_2NaO_5S$; an inhibitor of the renal dipeptidase, dehydropeptidase 1, used, in conjunction with antibiotics subject to metabolism in the kidneys, to increase therapeutic response to the antibiotic.

⌂**cili-.** SEE cilio-.

cil·ia (sil'ē-ă). Plural of cilium.

cil·i·ary (sil'ē-ar-ē). **1.** Relating to any cilia or hairlike processes, specifically, the eyelashes. **2.** Relating to certain of the structures of the eyeball. [Mod. L. *ciliaris*, relating to or resembling an eyelid, or eyelash, fr. L. *cilium*, eyelid]

cil·i·a·stat·ic (sil-ē-ă-stat'ik). Denoting a drug or condition that slows or stops the beating of cilia (generally used with reference to respiratory mucosal cilia).

Ci·li·a·ta (sil-ē-ā'tă). Formerly considered a class of Protozoa whose members bear cilia or structures derived from them, such as cirri or membranelles, but now placed within the phylum Ciliophora. Typical members, such as *Paramecium* or *Balantidium coli* (a parasite of man) possess two distinctive nuclei, a macronucleus and a micronucleus; only the latter bears the hereditary material exchanged in conjugation, a form of sexual reproduction found only in the C. [L. *cilium*, eyelid]

cil·i·at·ed (sil'ē-ā-ted). Having cilia.

cil·i·ates (sil'ē-āts). Common name for members of the Ciliata.

cil·i·ec·to·my (sil-ē-ek'tō-mē). SYN cyclectomy.

⌂**cilio-, cili-.** Cilia or meaning ciliary, in any sense; eyelashes. [L. *cilium*, eyelid (eyelash)]

cil·i·o·gen·e·sis (sil'ē-ō-jen'ĕ-sis). The formation of cilia.

Ci·li·oph·o·ra (sil'ē-of'ō-ră). A phylum of protozoa that includes the abundant free-living ciliates and the sessile suctorians; formerly classified as a subphylum of the phylum Protozoa. [cilio- + G. *phoros*, bearing]

cil·i·o·ret·i·nal (sil'ē-ō-ret'i-năl). Pertaining to the ciliary body and the retina.

cil·i·o·scle·ral (sil'ē-ō-sklē'răl). Relating to the ciliary body and the sclera.

cil·i·o·spi·nal (sil'ē-ō-spī'nal). Relating to the ciliary body and the spinal cord; denoting in particular the ciliospinal *center*.

cil·i·o·tox·ic·i·ty (sil'ē-ō-tok-sis'i-tē). The characteristic of a drug or condition which impairs ciliary activity (generally refers to respiratory mucosal cilia) (*e.g.*, tobacco smoke).

cil·i·um, pl. **cil·ia** (sil'ē-ŭm, -ă). **1** [NA]. SYN eyelash. **2.** A motile extension of a cell surface, *e.g.*, of certain epithelial cells, containing nine longitudinal double microtubules arranged in a peripheral ring, together with a central pair. [L. an eyelid]

cil·lo (sil'ō). SYN cillosis.

Cil·lo·bac·te·ri·um (sil'ō-bak-tēr'ē-ŭm). An obsolete genus of motile, anaerobic bacteria containing Gram-positive, straight or curved rods. Motile cells are peritrichous. These organisms may be pathogenic. The type species is *C. moniliforme*. This genus is no longer recognized, and most of its species have been transferred to *Eubacterium: C. combesi* is now *Eubacterium combesi*, *C. moniliforme* is now *Eubacterium moniliforme*, *C. multiforme* is now *Eubacterium multiforme*, and *C. tenue* is now *Eubacterium tenue*.

cil·lo·sis (sil-ō'sis). Obsolete term for spasmodic twitching of an eyelid. SYN cillo. [Mod. L., spelling influenced by Fr. *ciller*, to wink]

ci·met·i·dine (si-met'i-dēn). *N*-Cyano-*N*'-methyl-*N* ''-{2-[[(5-methyl-1*H*-imidazol-4-yl)methyl]thio]ethyl}guanidine; a histamine analogue and antagonist used to treat peptic ulcer and hypersecretory conditions by blocking histamine receptor (type 2) sites, thus inhibiting gastric acid secretion.

Ci·mex lec·tu·lar·i·us (sī'meks lek-tyū-lār-ē-ŭs). Member of the family Cimicidae, with a flat, reddish-brown wingless body, prominent lateral eyes, and a three-jointed beak; it produces a characteristic pungent odor from thoracic stink glands and is an abundant pest in human abodes, especially in the tropics under poor sanitary conditions. Although the bedbug's bite produces characteristic linear groups of pruritic wheals with a central hemorrhagic punctum, human disease has not been proved to be

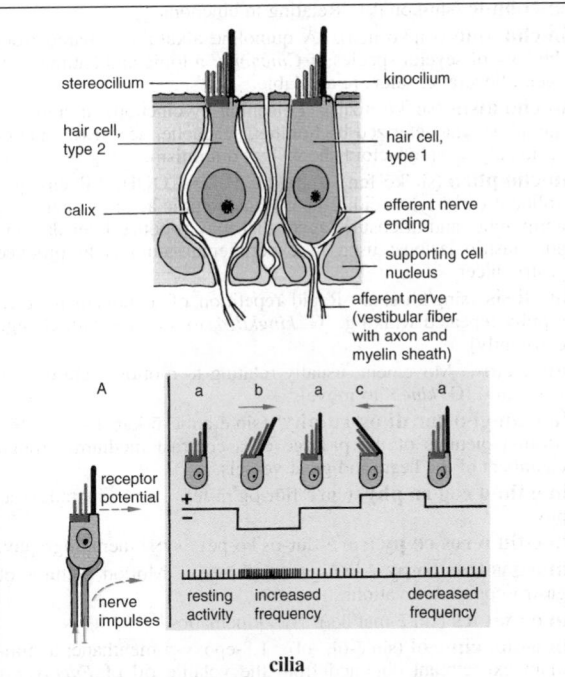

cilia

excitatory and inhibitory responses of stereocilia and kinocilia on hair cells (types I and II) of the vestibular apparatus to stimulation by movement in opposite directions. A) a) resting state; b) stimulation; c) inhibition.

transmitted by it, with the possible exception of hepatitis B. SYN bedbug. [L. *cimex*, bug, L. *lectulus*, a bed]

cim·i·co·sis (sim-i-kō'sis). Lesions produced by bedbug bites of *Cimex lectularius*.

Cimino, James E., U.S. nephrologist, *1928. SEE Brescia-C. *fistula*.

cIMP Abbreviation for cyclic inosine 3,5-monophosphate.

⌂**cin-.** SEE cine-.

cin·an·es·the·sia (sin'an-es-thē'zē-ă). SYN kinanesthesia.

ci·nan·ser·in hy·dro·chlo·ride (si-nan'ser-in). 2'-[[3-(Dimethylamino)propyl]thio]cinnamanilide monohydrochloride; a serotonin inhibitor.

cin·chol (sin'kol). SYN β-sitosterol.

cin·cho·na (sin-kō'nă). The dried bark of the root and stem of various species of *Cinchona*, a genus of evergreen trees (family Rubiaceae), native of South America but cultivated in various tropical regions. The cultivated bark contains 7 to 10% of total alkaloids; about 70% is quinine. C. contains more than 20 alkaloids, of which two pairs of isomers are most important: quinine and quinidine, and cinchonidine and cinchonine. SYN bark (2), cinchona bark, Jesuits' bark, Peruvian bark, quina, quinaquina, quinquina. [*Cinchona*, fr. Countess of *Chinch'on*]

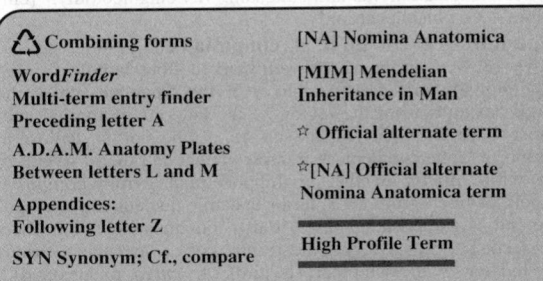

⌂ Combining forms	[NA] Nomina Anatomica
Word*Finder* **Multi-term entry finder Preceding letter A**	**[MIM] Mendelian Inheritance in Man**
A.D.A.M. Anatomy Plates Between letters L and M	☆ **Official alternate term**
Appendices: Following letter Z	☆**[NA] Official alternate Nomina Anatomica term**
SYN Synonym; Cf., compare	**High Profile Term**

cin·chon·ic (sin-kon′ik). Relating to cinchona.

cin·cho·nine (sin′kō-nēn). A quinoline alkaloid prepared from the bark of several species of *Cinchona;* a tonic and antimalarial agent. Several c. salts are available.

cin·cho·nism (sin′kō-nizm). Poisoning by cinchona, quinine, or quinidine; characterized by tinnitus, headache, deafness, and occasionally, anaphylactoid shock. SYN quininism.

cin·cho·phen (sin′kō-fen). $C_6H_5–(C_9H_5N)–COOH$; 2-Phenylquinoline-4-carboxylic acid; 2-phenylcinchoninic acid; an analgesic, antipyretic, and uricosuric agent that may produce liver damage and gastric lesions; used in experimental animals to produce gastric ulcer.

cin·cli·sis (sing′kli-sis). Rapid repetition of a movement, *e.g.,* rapidly repeated winking. [G. *kingklizō,* to wag the tail, change constantly]

⌂cine-, cin-. Movement, usually relating to motion pictures. SEE ALSO kin-. [G. *kineō,* to move]

cin·e·an·gi·o·car·di·og·ra·phy (sin′ē-an′jē-ō-kar-dē-og′rǎ-fē). Motion pictures of the passage of a contrast medium through chambers of the heart and great vessels.

cin·e·flu·o·rog·ra·phy (sin′ē-flūr-og′rǎ-fē). SYN cineradiography.

cin·e·flu·o·ros·co·py (sin′ē-flūr-os′kǒ-pē). SYN cineradiography.

cin·e·gas·tros·co·py (sin′ē-gas-tros′kǒ-pē). Motion pictures of gastroscopic observations.

cin·e·mat·ics (sin-ē-mat′iks). SYN kinematics.

cin·e·ole, cin·e·ol (sin′ē-ōl, -ol). 1,8-epoxy-*p*-menthane; a stimulant expectorant obtained from the volatile oil of *Eucalyptus globulus* and other species of *Eucalyptus.* SYN cajeputol, cajuputol, eucalyptol.

cin·e·pho·to·mi·crog·ra·phy (sin′ē-fō′tō-mī-krog′rǎ-fē). The making of a motion picture of microscopic objects; time lapse photography is often used.

cin·e·plas·tics (sin-ē-plas′tiks). SYN cineplastic *amputation.*

cin·e·ra·di·og·ra·phy (sin′ē-rā-dē-og′rǎ-fē). Radiography of an organ in motion, *e.g.,* the heart, the gastrointestinal tract. SYN cinefluorography, cinefluoroscopy, cineroentgenography.

ci·ne·rea (si-nē′rē-ǎ). 1. The gray matter of the brain and other parts of the nervous system. 2. Obsolete term for mantle *layer.* [L. fem. of *cinereus,* ashy, fr. *cinis,* ashes]

ci·ne·re·al (si-nē′rē-ǎl). Relating to the gray matter of the nervous system.

ci·ner·i·tious (si-ner-ish′ŭs). Ashen; denoting the gray matter of the brain, spinal cord, and ganglia.

cin·e·roent·gen·og·ra·phy (sin′ē-rent-gen-og′rǎ-fē). SYN cineradiography.

cin·e·seis·mog·ra·phy (sin′ē-sīz-mog′rǎ-fē). A technique for measuring movements of the body by continuous photographic recording of shaking or vibration.

ci·ne·to·plasm, ci·ne·to·plas·ma (sin-et′ō-plazm, sin-et-ō-plaz′mǎ). SYN kinetoplasm.

cin·gu·late (sing′gyū-lāt). Relating to a cingulum.

cin·gu·lec·to·my (sin-gyū-lek′tō-mē). SYN cingulotomy. [cingulum + G. *ektomē,* excision]

cin·gu·lot·o·my (sin-gyū-lot′ō-mē). Formerly, a unilateral or bilateral surgical excision of the anterior half of the cingulate gyrus, but now accomplished by electrolytic destruction of the anterior cingulate gyrus and callosum. SYN cingulectomy. [cingulum + G. *tomē,* a cutting]

cin·gu·lum, gen. **cin·′gu·li,** pl. **cin·gu·la** (sin′gyū-lŭm, -lē, -lǎ) [NA]. 1. SYN girdle. 2. A well-marked fiber bundle passing longitudinally in the white matter of the cingulate gyrus; the bundle extends from the region of the anterior perforated substance back over the dorsal surface of the corpus callosum; behind the latter's splenium it curves down and then forward in the white matter of the parahippocampal gyrus; composed largely of fibers from the anterior thalamic nucleus to the cingulate and parahippocampal gyri, it also contains association fibers connecting these gyri with the frontal cortex, and their various subdivisions with each other. [L. girdle, fr. *cingo,* to surround]

c. den′tis [NA], SYN c. of tooth.

c. mem′bri inferior′is [NA], SYN pelvic *girdle.*

c. mem′bri superior′is [NA], SYN shoulder *girdle.*

c. of tooth, a U- or W-shaped ridge at the base of the lingual surface of the crown of the upper incisors and cuspid teeth, the lateral limbs running for a short distance along the linguoproximal line angles, the central portion just above the gingiva. SYN c. dentis [NA], basal ridge (2), lingual lobe.

cin·na·mal·de·hyde (sin-ǎ-mal′de-hīd). 3-phenylpropenal; chief constituent of cinnamon oil. SYN cinnamic aldehyde.

cin·na·mate (sin′ǎ-māt). A salt or ester of cinnamic acid.

cin·nam·e·drine (sin-am′ē-drēn). α-[1-(Cinnamylmethylamino)ethyl]benzyl alcohol; a smooth muscle relaxant used in the treatment of menstrual cramping.

cin·nam·e·in (sin′am-ē-in). SYN *benzyl* cinnamate.

cin·na·mene (sin′ǎ-mēn). SYN styrene.

cin·nam·ic (si-nam′ik). Relating to cinnamon.

cin·nam·ic ac·id. $C_6H_5CH=CHCOOH$; 3-phenylpropenoic acid; obtained from cinnamon oil, Peruvian and tolu balsams, or storax. It has been used in lupus as paint and in infectious diseases to promote leukocytosis. SYN cinnamylic acid, phenylacrylic acid.

cin·nam·ic al·co·hol. SYN styrone.

cin·nam·ic al·de·hyde. SYN cinnamaldehyde.

cin·na·mon (sin′ǎ-mon). 1. The dried bark of *Cinnamomum loureirii* Nees (family Lauraceae), an aromatic bark used as a spice and, in medicine, as an adjuvant, carminative, and aromatic stomachic. SYN Saigon c. 2. The dried inner bark of the shoots of *Cinnamomum zeylanicum.* SYN Ceylon c. SYN cassia bark. [L. fr. G. *kinnamōmon,* cinnamon]

cassia c., *Cinnamomum cassia* Nees (family Lauraceae); the unofficial source of most of the cinnamon in the shops; the source of c. oil. SYN Chinese c.

Ceylon c., SYN cinnamon (2).

Chinese c., SYN cassia c.

Saigon c., SYN cinnamon (1).

cin·na·mon oil. The volatile oil distilled with steam from the leaves and twigs of *Cinnamomum cassia;* it contains not less than 80% by volume of the total aldehydes of cinnamon oil. SYN cassia oil.

cin·na·myl·ic ac·id (sin-ǎ-mil′ik). SYN cinnamic acid.

cin·nar·i·zine (si-nar′i-zēn). 1-cinnamyl-4-(diphenylmethyl)-piperazine; an antihistaminic. SYN cinnipirine.

cin·nip·i·rine (si-nip′i-rēn). SYN cinnarizine.

cin·o·cen·trum (sin-ō-sen′trŭm). SYN cytocentrum.

ci·nox·a·cin (si-noks′ǎ-sin). [1,3]Dioxolo[4,5-*g*]cinnoline-3-carboxylic acid, 1-ethyl-1,4-dihydro-4-oxo-; a synthetic organic acid, chemically related to nalidixic acid, used as an antibacterial to treat urinary tract infections.

ci·nox·ate (si-nok′sāt). 2-Ethoxyethyl *p*-methoxycinnamate; an ultraviolet screen for topical application on the skin.

ci·on (sī′on). Archaic term for uvula. [G. *kiōn,* pillar, the uvula]

cip·ro·flox·a·cin hy·dro·chlo·ride (sip-rō-floks′ǎ-sin). $C_{17}H_{18}FN_3O_3·HCl·H_2O$; a synthetic fluoroquinolone broad spectrum, antibacterial with activity against a wide range of Gram-negative and Gram-positive organisms.

cir·an·tin (sir-an′tin). SYN hesperidin.

cir·ca·di·an (ser-kā′dē-ǎn). Relating to biologic variations or rhythms with a cycle of about 24 hours. Cf. infradian, ultradian. [L. *circa,* about, + *dies,* day]

cir·cel·lus (sir-sel′ŭs). SYN circle. [L.]

c. veno′sus hypoglos′si, SYN venous *plexus* of hypoglossal canal.

cir·cho·ral (ser-kō′rǎl). Occurring cyclically about once an hour.

cir·ci·nate (ser′si-nāt). Circular; ring-shaped. [L. *circinatus,* made round, pp. of *circino,* to make round, fr. *circinus,* a pair of compasses]

cir·cle (ser′kl). 1. A ring-shaped structure or group of structures. 2. A line or process with every point equidistant from the center. SYN circellus. [L. *circulus*]

arterial c. of cerebrum, an anastomotic "circle" of arteries (roughly pentagonal in outline) at the base of the brain, formed, sequentially and in anterior to posterior direction, by the anterior communicating artery, the two anterior cerebral, the two internal carotid, the two posterior communicating, and the two posterior cerebral arteries. SYN circulus arteriosus cerebri [NA], c. of Willis.

articular vascular c., an anastomosis of vessels encircling a joint. SEE articular vascular *network*. SYN circulus articularis vasculosus [NA].

Baudelocque's uterine c., SYN pathologic retraction *ring*.

Carus' c., SYN Carus' *curve*.

cerebral arterial c., the roughly pentagonally shaped c. of vessels on the ventral aspect of the brain in the area of the optic chiasm, hypothalamus, and interpeduncular fossa. SEE c. of Willis.

closed c., a circuit for administration of an inhalation anesthetic in which there is complete rebreathing with carbon dioxide absorption.

defensive c., obsolete term for the addition of a secondary affection that limits or arrests the progress of the primary affection, as thought to occur when pneumothorax supervenes on pulmonary tuberculosis, the former having a therapeutic effect on the latter.

greater arterial c. of iris, an arterial circle at the ciliary border of the iris. SYN circulus arteriosus iridis major [NA].

Haller's c., (1) SYN vascular c. of optic nerve. **(2)** SYN areolar venous *plexus*.

Huguier's c., anastomosis around the isthmus of the uterus (junction of the cervix with the body) between the right and left uterine arteries.

least diffusion c., in the configuration of rays emerging from a spherocylindrical lens system, the place where diverging rays of the lens first forming a line image are balanced by converging rays of the second lens.

lesser arterial c. of iris, an arterial circle near the pupillary margin of the iris. SYN circulus arteriosus iridis minor [NA].

Pagenstecher's c., in the case of a freely movable abdominal tumor, the mass is moved throughout its entire range, its position at intervals being marked on the abdominal wall; when these points are joined, a c. is formed, the center of which marks the point of attachment of the tumor.

Ridley's c., SYN circular *sinus* (1).

rolling c., a mechanism for the replication of circular DNA.

semi-closed c., a circuit for administration of an inhalation anesthetic in which partial rebreathing with carbon dioxide absorption is combined with loss from the circuit of a portion of respired gases through valves.

vascular c., (1) the c. around the mouth formed by the inferior and superior labial arteries; **(2)** SYN areolar venous *plexus*.

vascular c. of optic nerve, a network of branches of the short ciliary arteries on the sclera around the point of entrance of the optic nerve. SYN circulus vasculosus nervi optici [NA], circulus arteriosus halleri, circulus zinnii, Haller's c. (1), Zinn's corona, Zinn's vascular c.

venous c. of mammary gland, SYN areolar venous *plexus*.

vicious c., (1) the mutually accelerating action of two independent diseases or phenomena, or of a primary and secondary affection; **(2)** the passage of food, after a gastroenterostomy, from the artificial opening through the intestinal loop by antiperistaltic action and back into the stomach again by the pyloric orifice, or the reverse.

c. of Willis, SYN arterial c. of cerebrum.

Zinn's vascular c., SYN vascular c. of optic nerve.

cir·cuit (ser'kit). The path or course of flow of cases or electric or other currents. [L. *circuitus,* a going round, fr. *circum,* around, + *eo,* pp. *itus,* to go]

anesthetic c., equipment used during inhalation anesthesia to regulate concentrations of inhaled gases; includes a reservoir bag and usually directional valves, breathing tubes, and a carbon dioxide absorber.

Papez c., a long circuitous conduction chain in the mammalian forebrain, leading from the hippocampus by way of the fornix to the mammillary body and thence returning to the hippocampus by way of, sequentially, the anterior thalamic nuclei, cingulate gyrus, and parahippocampal gyrus.

circadian rhythm and performance capacity

reverberating c., a theory of periodic conduction through the cerebral cortex of trains of impulses traveling in c.'s of neurons.

cir·cu·la·tion (ser-kyū-lā'shŭn). Movements in a circle, or through a circular course, or through a course which leads back to the same point; usually referring to blood c. unless otherwise specified. [L. *circulatio*]

assisted c., application of external devices to improve pressure, flow, or both in the heart or arteries.

blood c., the course of the blood from the heart through the arteries, capillaries, and veins back again to the heart.

capillary c., the course of the blood through the capillaries.

collateral c., c. maintained in small anastomosing vessels when the main vessel is obstructed.

compensatory c., c. established in dilated collateral vessels when the main vessel of the part is obstructed.

cross c., c. to an animal or one of its parts from the c. of another animal.

embryonic c., the basic plan of the c. of a young mammalian embryo, at first similar to that in aquatic forms, with an unpartitioned heart and conspicuous aortic arches in the branchial region; as gestation progresses, the arrangement of the major blood vessels gradually approaches that of an adult, but the routing of blood through the heart, characteristic of an adult, cannot be attained until lung breathing begins at birth.

enterohepatic c., c. of substances such as bile salts which are absorbed from the intestine and carried to the liver, where they are secreted into the bile and again enter the intestine.

extracorporeal c., the c. of blood outside of the body through a machine that temporarily assumes an organ's functions, *e.g.,* through a heart-lung machine or artificial kidney.

fetal c., the c. which serves the fetus *in utero*, with the placental circuit responsible for supplying oxygen and nutritive material and for eliminating CO_2 and nitrogenous wastes. SEE ALSO embryonic c.

greater c., SYN systemic c.

hypophysial portal c., SYN portal hypophysial c.

hypothalamohypophysial portal c., SYN portal hypophysial c.

lesser c., SYN pulmonary c.

lymph c., the slow passage of lymph through the lymphatic vessels and glands.

placental c., the c. of blood through the placenta during intrauterine life, serving the needs of the fetus for aeration, absorption, and excretion; also, maternal circulation through the intervillous space of the placenta.

portal c., (1) c. of blood to the liver from the small intestine, the right half of the colon, and the spleen via the portal vein; sometimes specified as the hepatic portal c.; **(2)** more generally, any part of the systemic circulation in which blood draining from the capillary bed of one structure flows through a larger vessel(s) to supply the capillary bed of another structure before returning to the heart; *e.g.,* the hypothalamohypophyseal portal system.

portal hypophysial c., a capillary network that carries hypophyseotropic hormones from the hypothalamus, where they are

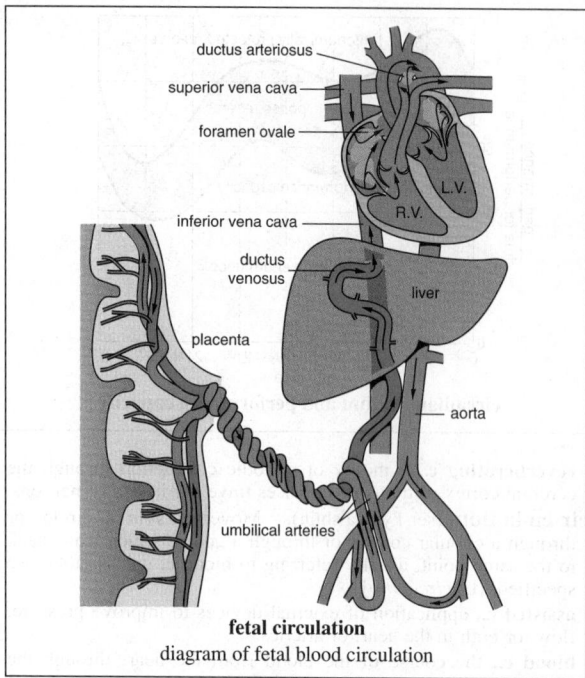

fetal circulation
diagram of fetal blood circulation

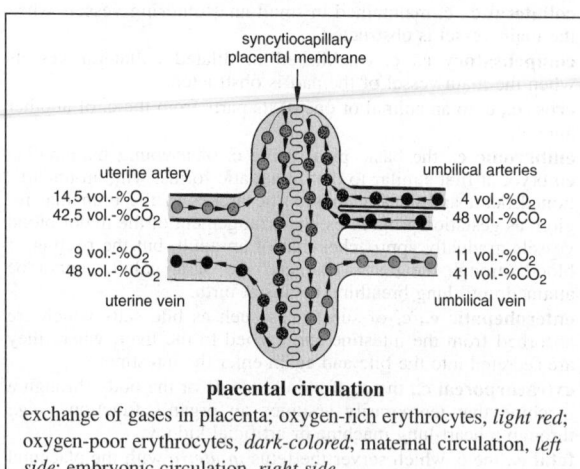

placental circulation
exchange of gases in placenta; oxygen-rich erythrocytes, *light red*; oxygen-poor erythrocytes, *dark-colored*; maternal circulation, *left side*; embryonic circulation, *right side*

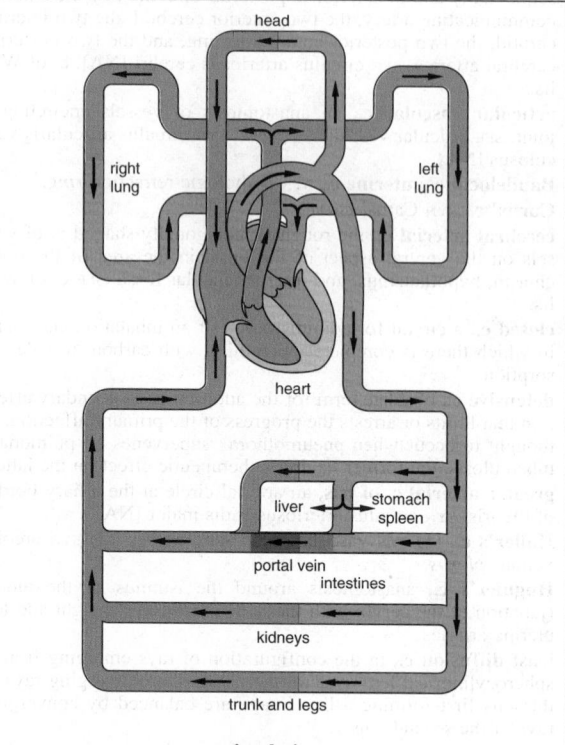

circulation
systemic circulation: through the body, from left ventricle to right atrium
pulmonary circulation: through the lungs, from the right ventricle to the left atrium

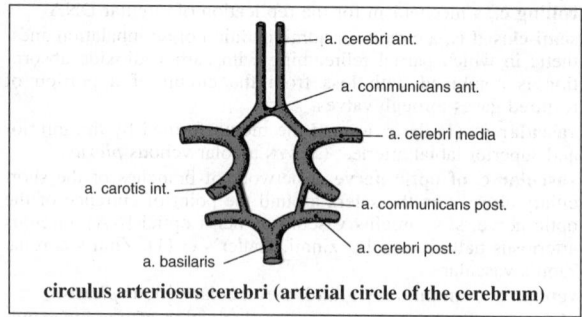

circulus arteriosus cerebri (arterial circle of the cerebrum)

secreted into blood, to their sites of action in the anterior hypophysis. SEE portal c., hypophysis, hypothalamus. SYN hypophyseoportal system, hypophysial portal c., hypophysial portal system, hypophysioportal system, hypothalamohypophysial portal c., hypothalamohypophysial portal system.

pulmonary c., the passage of blood from the right ventricle through the pulmonary artery to the lungs and back through the pulmonary veins to the left atrium. SYN lesser c.

Servetus' c., obsolete eponym for the pulmonary c.

systemic c., the c. of blood through the arteries, capillaries, and veins of the general system, from the left ventricle to the right atrium. SYN greater c.

thebesian c. (thē-bē′sē-an), the system of smaller veins in the myocardium.

cir·cu·la·to·ry (ser′kyū-lă-tō-rē). **1.** Relating to the circulation. **2.** SYN sanguiferous.

cir·cu·lus, gen. and pl. **cir·cu·li** (ser′kyū-lŭs, -lī). **1** [NA]. Any ringlike structure. **2.** A circle formed by connecting arteries, veins, or nerves. [L. dim. of *circus,* circle]

c. arterio′sus cer′ebri [NA], SYN arterial *circle* of cerebrum.

c. arterio′sus hal′leri, SYN vascular *circle* of optic nerve.

c. arterio′sus ir′idis ma′jor [NA], SYN greater arterial *circle* of iris.

c. arterio′sus ir′idis mi′nor [NA], SYN lesser arterial *circle* of iris.

c. articula′ris vasculo′sus [NA], SYN articular vascular *circle,* articular vascular *network.*

c. vasculo′sus ner′vi op′tici [NA], SYN vascular *circle* of optic nerve.

c. veno′sus hal′leri, SYN areolar venous *plexus.*

c. veno′sus rid′leyi, SYN circular *sinus* (1).

c. zin′nii, SYN vascular *circle* of optic nerve.

△**circum-.** A circular movement, or a position surrounding the part indicated by the word to which it is joined. SEE ALSO peri-. [L. around]

cir·cum·a·nal (ser-kŭm-ā'năl). Surrounding the anus. SYN perianal, periproctic.

cir·cum·ar·tic·u·lar (ser'kŭm-ar-tik'yū-lăr). Surrounding a joint. SYN periarthric, periarticular. [circum- + L. *articulus,* joint]

cir·cum·ax·il·lary (ser-kŭm-mak'si-lār-ē). Around the axilla. SYN periaxillary.

cir·cum·bul·bar (ser-kŭm-bŭl'bar). SYN peribulbar.

cir·cum·cise (ser'kŭm-sīz). To perform circumcision, especially of the prepuce.

cir·cum·ci·sion (ser-kŭm-sizh'ŭn). **1.** Operation to remove part or all of the prepuce. SYN peritomy (2). **2.** Cutting around an anatomical part (*e.g.,* the areola of the breast). SYN peritectomy (2). [L. *circumcido,* to cut around, fr. *circum,* around, + *caedo,* to cut]

cir·cum·cor·ne·al (ser-kŭm-kōr'nē-ăl). SYN pericorneal.

cir·cum·duc·tion (ser-kŭm-dŭk'shŭn). **1.** Movement of a part, *e.g.,* an extremity, in a circular direction. **2.** SYN cycloduction. [circum- + L. *duco,* pp. *ductus,* to draw]

cir·cum·fer·ence (c) (ser-kŭm'fer-ens). The outer boundary, especially of a circular area. SYN circumferentia [NA]. [L. *circumferentia, a bearing around*]

articular c. of radius, the portion of the head of the radius that articulates with the radial notch of the ulna. SYN circumferentia articularis radii [NA].

articular c. of ulna, the portion of the head of the ulna that articulates with the ulnar notch of the radius. SYN circumferentia articularis ulnae [NA].

cir·cum·fer·en·tia (ser-kŭm-fer-en'shē-ă) [NA]. SYN circumference, circumference. [L. a bearing around]

c. articula'ris ra'dii [NA], SYN articular *circumference* of radius.

c. articula'ris ul'nae [NA], SYN articular *circumference* of ulna.

cir·cum·flex (ser'kŭm-fleks). Describing an arc of a circle or that which winds around something; denotes several anatomical structures: arteries, veins, nerves, and muscles. [circum- + L. *flexus,* to bend]

cir·cum·gem·mal (ser-kŭm-jem'ăl). Surrounding a budlike or bulblike body; denoting a mode of nerve termination by fibrils surrounding an end bulb. SYN perigemmal. [circum- + L. *gemma,* a bud]

cir·cum·in·tes·ti·nal (ser'kŭm-in-tes'ti-năl). SYN perienteric.

cir·cum·len·tal (ser-kŭm-len'tăl). SYN perilenticular.

cir·cum·man·dib·u·lar (ser'kŭm-man-dib'yū-lăr). Around or about the mandible.

cir·cum·nu·cle·ar (ser-kŭm-nū'klē-ăr). SYN perinuclear.

cir·cum·oc·u·lar (ser-kŭm-ok'yū-lăr). Around the eye. SYN periocular, periophthalmic. [circum- + L. *oculus,* eye]

cir·cum·o·ral (ser-kŭm-ōr'ăl). SYN perioral. [circum- + L. *os (oris),* mouth]

cir·cum·or·bit·al (ser-kŭm-ōr'bi-tăl). Around the orbit. SYN periorbital (2).

cir·cum·re·nal (ser-kŭm-rē'năl). SYN perinephric. [circum- + L. *ren,* kidney]

cir·cum·scribed (ser'kŭm-skrībd). Bounded by a line; limited or confined. SYN circumscriptus. [circum- + L. *scribo,* to write]

cir·cum·scrip·tus (ser-kŭm-skrip'tŭs). SYN circumscribed. [L.]

cir·cum·stan·ti·al·i·ty (ser'kŭm-stan-shē-al'i-tē). A disturbance in the thought process, either voluntary or involuntary, in which one gives an excessive amount of detail (circumstances) that is often tangential, elaborate, and irrelevant, to avoid making a direct statement or answer to a question; observed in schizophrenia and in obsessional disorders. Cf. tangentiality. [L. *circum-sto,* pr. p. *-stans,* to stand around]

cir·cum·val·late (ser-kŭm-val'āt). Denoting a structure surrounded by a wall, as the c. (vallate) papillae of the tongue. [circum- + L. *vallum,* wall]

cir·cum·vas·cu·lar (ser-kŭm-vas'kyū-lăr). SYN perivascular. [circum- + L. *vasculum,* vessel]

cir·cum·ven·tric·u·lar (ser'kŭm-ven-trik'yū-lăr). Around or in the area of a ventricle, as the c. organs.

cir·cum·vo·lute (ser-kŭm-vol'ūt). Twisted around; rolled about. [L. *circum-volvo,* pp. *-volutus,* to roll around]

cir·rhog·e·nous, cir·rho·gen·ic (sir-roj'ĕ-nŭs, -rō-jen'ik). Rarely used term for tending to the development of cirrhosis. [G. *kirrhos,* yellow (liver), + *-gen,* producing]

cir·rhon·o·sus (sir-ron'ō-sŭs). A disease of the fetus marked anatomically by a yellow staining of the peritoneum and pleura. [G. *kirrhos,* yellow (liver), + *nosos,* disease]

cir·rho·sis (sir-rō'sis). Progressive disease of the liver characterized by diffuse damage to hepatic parenchymal cells, with nodular regeneration, fibrosis, and disturbance of normal architecture; associated with failure in the function of hepatic cells and interference with blood flow in the liver, frequently resulting in jaundice, portal hypertension, ascites, and ultimately hepatic failure. [G. *kirrhos,* yellow (liver), + *-osis,* condition]

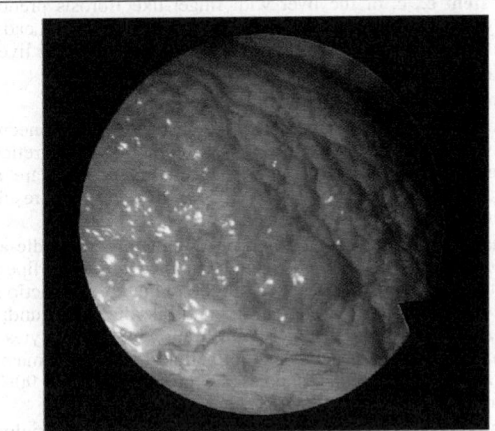

cirrhosis of the liver
small-node type (endoscopic view)

alcoholic c., c. that frequently develops in chronic alcoholism, characterized in an early stage by enlargement of the liver due to fatty change with mild fibrosis, and later by Laënnec's c. with contraction of the liver.

biliary c., c. due to biliary obstruction, which may be a primary intrahepatic disease or secondary to obstruction of extrahepatic bile ducts; the latter may lead to cholestasis and proliferation in small bile ducts with fibrosis, but marked disturbance of the lobular pattern is infrequent. SEE ALSO primary biliary c.

Budd's c., chronic enlargement of the liver without jaundice, formerly thought to be of intestinal origin.

capsular c. of liver, SYN Glisson's c.

cardiac c., an extensive fibrotic reaction within the liver as a result of chronic constrictive pericarditis or prolonged congestive heart failure; true c. with fibrous bridging of lobules is unusual. SYN cardiac liver, congestive c., pseudocirrhosis, stasis c.

cholangiolitic c., a form of c. in which there is diffuse inflammation of the cholangioles, with inflammation, fibrosis, and regeneration; characterized by chronicity, relapses, and febrile episodes.

congestive c., SYN cardiac c.

cryptogenic c., c. of unknown etiology, with no history of alcoholism or previous acute hepatitis.

fatty c., early nutritional c., especially in alcoholics, in which the liver is enlarged by fatty change, with mild fibrosis.

Glisson's c., chronic perihepatitis with thickening and subsequent contraction, resulting in atrophy and deformity of the liver. SYN capsular c. of liver.

Hanot's c., SYN primary biliary c.

juvenile c., SYN active chronic *hepatitis.*

Laënnec's c., c. in which normal liver lobules are replaced by small regeneration nodules, sometimes containing fat, separated by a fairly regular framework of fine fibrous tissue strands (hobnail liver); usually due to chronic alcoholism. Can progress to severe impairment of liver function, portal hypertension with ascites and esophageal varices, and life-threatening complications. SYN portal c.

necrotic c., SYN postnecrotic c.

nutritional c., c. occurring in persons or animals with general or specific dietary deficiencies; methionine and cystine deficiency may produce changes of c. in animals, but it is uncertain whether malnutrition in humans leads to c. or only to reversible fatty infiltration of the liver.

periportal c., c. of the liver with wide bands of fibrosis surrounding large segments of liver, with regenerative nodules.

pigment c., c. of the liver associated with dark brown discoloration seen in hemochromatosis.

pigmentary c., c. resulting from excessive deposits of iron in the liver, usually seen in hemochromatosis.

pipe stem c., c. of the liver with finger-like fibrosis predominantly around portal tracts, seen in schistosomiasis. Leads to portal hypertension but rarely to functional failure of the liver.

portal c., SYN Laënnec's c.

posthepatitic c., SYN active chronic *hepatitis.*

postnecrotic c., post-necrotic c., c. characterized by necrosis involving whole hepatic lobules, with collapse of the reticular framework to form large scars; regeneration nodules are also large; may follow viral or toxic necrosis, or develop as a result of ischemic necrosis. SYN necrotic c.

primary biliary c., a condition occurring mainly in middle-aged women, characterized by obstructive jaundice with hyperlipemia, pruritis, and hyperpigmentation of the skin; no obstruction of large bile ducts or proliferation of small bile ducts is found; the liver shows c. with marked portal infiltration by lymphocytes and plasma cells, and frequently by epithelioid cell granulomas; serum antimitochondrial antibodies are present in 85 to 90% of patients. SYN Hanot's c.

pulmonary c., fibrosis of the lungs; usually interstitial pulmonary fibrosis.

stasis c., SYN cardiac c.

syphilitic c., c. of the liver occurring as a result of tertiary or congenital syphilis.

toxic c., c. of the liver resulting from chronic poisoning, as by lead or carbon tetrachloride.

cir·rhot·ic (sir-rot'ik). Relating to or affected with cirrhosis or advanced fibrosis.

cir·ri (sir'ī). Plural of cirrus.

cir·rose, cir·rous (sir'ōs, sir'ŭs). Relating to or having cirri.

cir·rus, pl. **cir·ri** (sir'rŭs, -rī). A structure formed from a cluster or tuft of fused cilia, constituting one of the sensory or locomotor organs of certain ciliate protozoa. [L. a curl]

cir·sec·to·my (ser-sek'tō-mē). Obsolete term for excision of a section of a varicose vein. [G. *kirsos,* varix, + *ektomē,* excision]

cir·so·cele (ser'sō-sēl). SYN varicocele. [G. *kirsos,* varix, + *kēlē,* tumor]

cir·sod·e·sis (ser-sod'ĕ-sis). Obsolete term for ligation of varicose veins. [G. *kirsos,* varix, + *desis,* a binding, fr. *deō,* to bind]

cir·soid (ser'soyd). SYN variciform. [G. *kirsos,* varix, + *eidos,* appearance]

cir·som·pha·los (ser-som'fă-los). Rarely used term for *caput medusae* [G. *kirsos,* varix, + *omphalos,* umbilicus]

cir·soph·thal·mia (ser-sof-thal'mē-ă). Varicose dilation of the conjunctival blood vessels. [G. *kirsos,* varix, + *ophthalmos,* eye]

cir·so·tome (ser'sō-tōm). Obsolete term for cutting instrument used in operating upon varicose veins.

cir·sot·o·my (ser-sot'ō-mē). Obsolete term for treatment of varicose veins by multiple incisions. [G. *kirsos,* varix, + *tomē,* incision]

CIS Abbreviation for *carcinoma* in situ.

⚠**cis-. 1.** Prefix meaning on this side, on the near side; opposite of trans-. **2.** In genetics, a prefix denoting the location of two or more genes on the same chromosome of a homologous pair, in coupling. **3.** In organic chemistry, a form of geometric isomerism in which similar functional groups are attached on the same side

of the plane that includes two adjacent, fixed carbon atoms (*e.g.,* the 2- and 3-OH groups of ribofuranose) in a ring structure. SEE entgegen. **4.** In organic chemistry, a form of geometric isomerism with regards to carbon-carbon double bonds. Identical functional groups on the same side of the double bond are cis-. When the four moieties attached to the carbons of the double bond are all different, then the E/Z nomenclature has to be followed. SYN zusammen (1). SEE entgegen, zusammen. [L.]

cis·plat·in (sis'plă-tin). *cis*-Diamminedichloroplatinum; a chemotherapeutic agent with antitumor activity; c. binds DNA and interferes with DNA synthesis.

cis·sa (sis'ă). Craving for unusual or unwholesome foods during pregnancy. SEE ALSO pica, SYN citta, cittosis. [G. *kissa, kitta,* longing for strange food by pregnant women]

cis·tern (sis'tern). SYN cisterna. [L. *cisterna*]

ambient c., SYN c. of great cerebral vein.

basal c., SYN interpeduncular c.

cerebellomedullary c., the largest of the subarachnoid c.'s between the cerebellum and the medulla oblongata; may be divided into a dorsal c. located between the cerebellum and dorsal surface of the medulla (c. magna) and a lateral c. located between the cerebellum and the lateral aspect of the medulla. SYN cisterna cerebellomedullaris [NA], cisterna magna.

c. of chiasm, SYN chiasmatic c.

chiasmatic c., a dilation of the subarachnoid space below and anterior to the optic chiasm. SYN cisterna chiasmatis [NA], c. of chiasm.

chyle c., SYN *cisterna* chyli.

c. of cytoplasmic reticulum, SEE cisterna (2).

c. of great cerebral vein, an expansion of the subarachnoid space extending forward between the corpus callosum and the thalamus; it encloses the internal cerebral veins which caudally join to form the vena magna cerebri (Galen's vein). SYN ambient c., Bichat's canal, Bichat's foramen, c. of great vein of cerebrum, cisterna ambiens, cisterna superioris, cisterna venae magnae cerebri, superior c.

c. of great vein of cerebrum, SYN c. of great cerebral vein.

interpeduncular c., a dilation of the subarachnoid space in front of the pons, where the arachnoid membrane stretches across between the two temporal lobes over the base of the diencephalon. SEE interpeduncular *fossa.* SYN cisterna interpeduncularis [NA], basal c., cisterna basalis, cisterna cruralis, Tarin's space.

c. of lateral fossa of cerebrum, an elongated expansion of the subarachnoid space where the arachnoid bridges over the opening of the Sylvian fissure. SYN cisterna fossae lateralis cerebri [NA].

lumbar c., enlargement of subarachnoid space between inferior end of spinal cord (vertebral level L-2) and inferior end of subarachnoid space or dura mater (vertebral level S2); occupied by the dorsal and ventral roots of lumbosacral spinal nerves (which constitute the cauda equina), the filum terminal, and cerebrospinal fluid. Site for lumbar puncture and spinal anesthesia.

c. of nuclear envelope, SYN *cisterna* caryothecae.

Pecquet's c., SYN *cisterna* chyli.

pontine c., an upward continuation of the subarachnoid space of the spinal cord, continuous about the medulla with the cerebellomedullary c.l; may be divided into inferior (containing roots of C.N. 9–12) and superior (containing root of C.N. 5, 7, 8) parts. SYN cisterna pontis.

subarachnoidal c.'s, widening portions of the subarachnoid space within the cranium where the arachnoid bridges over a depression on the surface of the brain. SEE ALSO subarachnoid *space.* SYN cisternae subarachnoideales [NA].

superior c., SYN c. of great cerebral vein.

Sylvian c., the subarachnoid space associated with the lateral cerebral sulcus (Sylvian fissure); contains the M1 segment of the middle cerebral artery and the origin of lenticulostriate arteries, and proximal parts of the middle cerebral artery.

cis·ter·na, gen. and pl. **cis·ter·nae** (sis-ter'nă, -ter'nē). **1** [NA]. Any cavity or enclosed space serving as a reservoir, especially for chyle, lymph, or cerebrospinal fluid. **2.** An ultramicroscopic space occurring between the membranes of the flattened sacs of the endoplasmic reticulum, the Golgi complex, or the two membranes of the nuclear envelope. SYN cistern. [L. an underground cistern for water, fr. *cista,* a box]

c. am′biens, SYN *cistern* of great cerebral vein.

c. basa′lis, SYN interpeduncular *cistern.*

c. caryothe′cae, the space between the internal and external membranes of the nuclear envelope; may be continuous in places with cisterns of the endoplasmic reticulum. SYN cistern of nuclear envelope, perinuclear space.

c. cerebellomedulla′ris [NA], SYN cerebellomedullary *cistern.*

c. chias′matis [NA], SYN chiasmatic *cistern.*

c. chy′li [NA], a dilated sac at the lower end of the thoracic duct into which the intestinal trunk and two lumbar lymphatic trunks open; it occurs inconstantly and when present is located posterior to the aorta on the anterior aspect of the bodies of the first and second lumbar vertebrae. SYN ampulla chyli, chyle cistern, chylocyst, Pecquet's cistern, Pecquet's reservoir, receptaculum chyli, receptaculum pecqueti.

c. crura′lis, SYN interpeduncular *cistern.*

c. fos′sae latera′lis cer′ebri [NA], SYN *cistern* of lateral fossa of cerebrum.

c. interpeduncula′ris [NA], SYN interpeduncular *cistern.*

c. mag′na, SYN cerebellomedullary *cistern.*

c. perilymphat′ica, SYN perilymphatic *space.*

c. pon′tis, SYN pontine *cistern.*

cisternae subarachnoidea′les [NA], SYN subarachnoidal *cisterns,* under *cistern.*

subsurface c., a cistern of the endoplasmic reticulum that lies close to the plasma membrane; such cisternae occur especially in the cell bodies of neurons.

c. superior′is, SYN *cistern* of great cerebral vein.

terminal cisternae, pairs of transversely oriented tubules of the sarcoplasmic reticulum occurring at regular intervals in skeletal muscle fibers; together with an intermediate T tubule they make up a triad.

c. ve′nae mag′nae cer′ebri, SYN *cistern* of great cerebral vein.

cis·ter·nal (sis-ter′năl). Relating to a cisterna.

cis·tern·og·ra·phy (sis′tern-og′ră-fē). The radiographic study of the basal cisterns of the brain after the subarachnoid introduction of an opaque or other contrast medium, or a radiopharmaceutical with a suitable detector. [cisterna + G. *graphō,* to write]

cerebellopontine c., the radiographic study of the cerebellopontine angle and contiguous structures after the introduction of a radiopaque contrast medium into the subarachnoid space.

radionuclide c., scintigraphic imaging of the cisterns at the base of the brain following subarachnoid injection of a gamma-emitting radiopharmaceutical.

cis·tron (sis′tron). **1.** The smallest functional unit of heretability; a length of chromosomal DNA associated with a single biochemical function. Under classical concepts, a gene might consist of more than one c.; in modern molecular biology, the c. is essentially equivalent to the structural gene. **2.** The genetic unit defined by the *cis/trans* test. [*cis tr*-ans + -on]

cis·ves·tism, cis·ves·ti·tism (sis-ves′tizm, -ves′ti-tizm). The practice of dressing in clothes inappropriate to one's position or status. Cf. transvestism. [L. *cis,* on the near side of, + *vestio,* to dress]

Ci·tel·lus (si-tel′ŭs). A genus of ground squirrel. *C. beecheyi, C. grammurus, C. pygmaeus, C. townsendi,* and several other species act as an important reservoir of *Yersinia pestis.* [Mod. L.]

cito disp. Abbreviation for L. *cito dispensetur,* let it be dispensed quickly.

cit·ral (sit′răl). A monoterpene aldehyde consisting of both geometric isomers found in oils from lemon, orange, verbena, and lemon grass; c.-A is the trans-isomer and c.-B is the cis-isomer (neral).

cit·rase, cit·ra·tase (sit′rās, -ră-tās). SYN *citrate* lyase.

cit·rate (sit′rāt, sī′trāt). A salt or ester of citric acid; used as anticoagulants because they bind calcium ions.

c. aldolase, SYN c. lyase.

ATP c. (*pro-3S*)-lyase, an enzyme that catalyzes the reaction of ATP, citrate, and coenzyme A to form ADP, orthophosphate, oxaloacetate, and acetyl-CoA. An important step in fatty acid biosynthesis. SYN citrate cleavage enzyme.

c. lyase, *c. (pro-3S)*-lyase; an enzyme that catalyzes the cleavage of citrate to oxaloacetate and acetate, in the absence of coenzyme A. SYN citrase, citratase, c. aldolase, citridesmolase.

c. synthase, *c. (si)*-synthase; an enzyme catalyzing the condensation of oxaloacetate, water, and acetyl-CoA, forming citrate and coenzyme A; an important step in the tricarboxylic acid cycle. SYN citrogenase, condensing enzyme, oxaloacetate transacetase.

cit·rat·ed (sit′rā-ted). Containing a citrate; specifically denoting blood serum or milk to which has been added a solution of potassium or sodium citrate, or both.

cit·ric ac·id (sit′rik). 2-Hydroxypropane-1,2,3-tricarboxylic acid; the acid of citrus fruits, widely distributed in nature and a key intermediate in intermediary metabolism.

cit·ri·des·mo·lase (sit-ri-des′mō-lās). SYN *citrate* lyase.

cit·rin (sit′rin). SYN *vitamin P.*

Cit·ro·bac·ter (sit′rō-bak-ter). A genus of motile bacteria (family Enterobacteriaceae) containing Gram-negative rods which utilize citrate as a sole source of carbon; the motile cells are peritrichous. Fermentation of lactose by these organisms is delayed or absent; they produce trimethylene glycol from glycerol. The type species is *C. freundii.*

C. amalona′tica, a species found in feces, soil, water, and sewage; isolated from clinical specimens as an opportunistic pathogen. SYN *Levinea amalonatica.*

C. diver′sus, a species found in feces, soil, water, sewage, and food; isolated from urine, throat, nose, sputum, and wounds; reported in cases of neonatal meningitis. SYN *C. koseri, Levinea diversus, Levinea malonatica.*

C. freun′dii, a species found in water, feces, and urine; it appears to be an inhabitant of the normal intestine, but it may occur in alimentary infections and in infections of the urinary tract, gallbladder, middle ear, and meninges; it is the type species of the genus *C.*

C. ko′seri, SYN *C. diversus.*

ci·trog·en·ase (si-troj′en-ās). SYN *citrate* synthase.

cit·ro·nel·la (sit-rō-nel′ă). *Cymbopogon (Andropogon) nardus* (family Gramineae); a fragrant grass of Ceylon, from which is distilled a volatile oil (c. oil) used as a perfume and insect repellent.

cit·ro·nel·lal (sit′rōn-el′ăl). Principal volatile ingredient of lemon grass and citronella oil. Used in soap perfumes and as an insect repellent.

ci·trul·line (sit′rul-ēn). N^5-(Aminocarbonyl)-L-ornithine; α-amino-δ-ureidovaleric -ureidovaleric acid; 5-ureidonorvaline; an amino acid formed from L-ornithine in the course of the urea cycle as well as a product in nitric oxide biosynthesis; also found in watermelon (*Citrullus vulgaris*) and in casein. Elevated in individuals with a deficiency of argininosuccinate synthetase or argininosuccinate lyase.

cit·rul·li·ne·mia (sit′rul-i-nē′mē-ă) [MIM*215700]. A disease of amino acid metabolism (usually classed as a type of aminoaciduria) in which citrulline concentrations in blood, urine, and cerebrospinal fluid are elevated; manifested clinically by vomiting, ammonia intoxication, and mental retardation beginning in infancy; autosomal recessive inheritance.

cit·rul·li·nu·ria (sit′rŭl-i-nū′rē-ă). Enhanced urinary excretion of citrulline; a manifestation of citrullinemia.

cit·ta, cit·to·sis (si′tă, si-tō′sis). SYN cissa.

Civatte, Achille, French dermatologist, 1877-1956. SEE C. *bodies,* under *body;* C.'s *disease; poikiloderma* of C.

Civinini, Filippo, Italian anatomist, 1805–1844. SEE C.'s *canal, ligament, process.*

CJD Abbreviation for Creutzfeldt-Jakob *disease.*

CK Abbreviation for *creatine* kinase.

Cl Symbol for chlorine.

clad·i·o·sis (klad-ē-ō′sis). A dermatophytosis resembling sporotrichosis, characterized by verrucous lesions and ascending lymphangitis; caused by *Scopulariopsis blochii.* SEE *Scopulariopsis.* [G. *klados,* branch or root, + *-osis,* condition]

cl

Clado, Spiro, French gynecologist, 1856–1905. SEE C.'s *anastomosis, band, ligament, point.*

Cla·dor·chis wat·soni (kla-dōr′kis wat-sō′nī). Incorrect term for *Watsonius watsoni.*

clad·o·spo·ri·o·sis (klad′ō-spō-rē-ō′sis). Infection with a fungus of the genus *Cladosporium.*

cerebral c., cerebral chromoblastomycosis, a mycotic brain infection due to *Cladosporium trichoides* (*bantianum*); macroscopically infected tissue has a characteristic brown color.

Clad·o·spo·ri·um (klad-ō-spōr′i-ŭm). A genus of fungi having dematiaceous or dark-colored conidiophores with oval or round spores, commonly isolated in soil or plant residues. [G. *klados,* a branch, + *sporos,* seed]

C. bantia′num, a species that causes cerebral cladosporiosis.

C. carrion′ii, a species that is a cause of chromoblastomycosis in man.

C. cladosporioides (klad′ō-spor-ē-ō-ē-dēz), a species reported to cause local infection at the site of a skin test in an HIV-infected patient.

C. wernec′kii, SYN *Exophiala werneckii.*

clair·voy·ance (klār-voy′ans). Perception of objective events (past, present, or future) not ordinarily discernible by the senses; a type of extrasensory perception. [Fr.]

clam·ox·y·quin hy·dro·chlo·ride (klam-ok′si-kwin). 5-Chloro-7-{[(3-diethylaminopropyl) amino]methyl}8-quinolinol dihydrochloride; an amebicide.

clamp (klamp). An instrument for compression of a structure. Cf. forceps. [M.E., fr. Middle Dutch *klampe*]

Cope's c., a c. used in excision of colon and rectum.

Crafoord c., a c. used in heart, lung, and vascular operations.

Crile's c., a c. for temporary stoppage of blood flow.

Fogarty c., a c. with rubber-shod blades having serrated surfaces, to provide an atraumatic grip on tissues.

Gant's c., a right-angled c. used in hemorrhoidectomy.

Gaskell's c., an instrument for crushing the atrioventricular bundle in experimental animals and thus producing heart block.

gingival c., a springlike metal piece encircling or grasping the cervix of a tooth and shaped so as to retract the gingival tissue.

Goldblatt's c., a c. applied experimentally to the renal artery to damp pulse pressure and thereby produce chronic hypertension by activation of the renin-angiotensin system.

Joseph's c., a c. used after rhinoplasty to maintain or improve the alignment of the bony support of the nose.

Kelly c., a curved hemostat without teeth, introduced for gynecological surgery.

Kocher c., a heavy, straight hemostat with interlocking teeth on the tip.

liver-shod c., a c. with jaws covered by cloth to prevent injury to structures such as bowel when c. is closed.

Mikulicz c., a c. used to crush walls between proximal and distal colon in two-stage colectomy.

Mixter c., a right angle c.

Mogen c., a circumcision instrument. [Hebrew star]

mosquito c., a small hemostat, straight or curved, with or without teeth; used to hold delicate tissue or for hemostasis. SYN mosquito forceps.

Ochsner c., a straight hemostat with teeth.

patch c., SYN *patch* clamping.

Payr's c., a c. used in gastrectomy or enterectomy.

Potts' c., a fine-toothed, multiple-point, vascular fixation c. that imparts limited trauma to the vessel while securely holding it.

Rankin's c., a three-bladed c. used in resection of colon.

right angle c., a c. with a short 90° bend to its tip frequently used for dissection or passage of ligatures around vessels.

rubber dam c., a springlike metal piece encircling or grasping the cervix of a tooth and so shaped as to prevent a rubber dam from coming off the tooth.

rubber shod c., rubber-shod c., a small rubber-tipped c. that holds sutures in place during surgery.

clamp con·nec·tion. In fungi, a short hypha which bypasses a hyphal septum and is attached to the two cells adjacent to the septum; characteristic of most members of the phylum Basidiomycetes.

cla·po·tage, cla·pote·ment (kla-pō-tahz′, kla-pōt-mawn′). The splashing sound heard on succussion of a dilated stomach. [Fr.]

Clapton, Edward, English physician, 1830–1909. SEE C.'s *line.*

Clara, Max, Austrian anatomist, *1899. SEE C. *cell.*

cla·rif·i·cant (kla-rif′i-kant). An agent that makes a turbid liquid clear. [L. *clarus,* clear, + *facio,* to make]

clar·i·fi·ca·tion (klar′i-fi-kā′shŭn). The process of making a turbid liquid clear. SYN lucidification.

Clark, Alonzo, U.S pharmacologist, 1807–1887. SEE C.'s *weight rule.*

Clark, Eliot R., U.S. anatomist, 1881–1963. SEE Sandison-C. *chamber.*

Clark, Leland, Jr., U.S. biochemist, *1918. SEE C. *electrode.*

Clark, Wallace H., Jr., U.S. dermatopathologist, *1924. SEE C.'s *level.*

Clarke, Cecil. SEE C.-Hadfield *syndrome.*

Clarke, Jacob A.L., English anatomist, 1817–1880. SEE C.'s *column, nucleus.*

clas·mat·o·cyte (klaz-mat′ō-sīt). SYN macrophage. [G. *klasma,* a fragment, + *kytos,* a hollow (cell)]

clas·ma·to·sis (klaz-mă-tō′sis). The extension of pseudopodia-like processes in unicellular organisms and blood cells by plasmolysis rather than by a true formation of pseudopodia. [G. *klasma,* a fragment, + *-osis,* condition]

clasp. 1. A part of a removable partial denture that acts as a direct retainer and/or stabilizer for the denture by partially surrounding or contacting an abutment tooth. 2. A direct retainer of a removable partial denture, usually consisting of two arms joined by a body which connects with an occlusal rest; at least one arm of a clasp usually terminates in the infrabulge (gingival convergence) area of the tooth enclosed.

bar c., (1) a c. whose arms are bar-type extensions from major connectors or from within the denture base; the arms pass adjacent to the soft tissues and approach the point of contact on the tooth in a gingivo-occlusal direction; (2) a c. consisting of two or more separate arms located opposite to each other on the tooth; the bar arms arise from the framework or from a connector and may traverse the soft tissue; one arm (bar), the retentive arm, usually terminates in the infrabulge (gingival convergence) area of the tooth; the other, the reciprocal arm, usually terminates on the suprabulge (occlusal convergence) area. SYN Roach c.

circumferential c., (1) a c. that encircles more than 180° of a tooth, including opposite angles, and which usually contacts the tooth throughout the extent of the c., at least one terminal being in the infrabulge (gingival convergence) area; (2) a c. consisting of two circumferential c. arms, both of which originate from the same minor connector and are located on opposite surfaces of the abutment tooth.

continuous c., SYN continuous bar *retainer.*

extended c., a c. that extends from its minor connector along the lingual and/or facial surface of two or more teeth.

Roach c., SYN bar c.

class (klas). In biologic classification, the next division below the phylum (or subphylum) and above the order. [L. *classis,* a class, division]

clas·si·fi·ca·tion (klas′i-fi-kā′shŭn). A systematic arrangement into classes or groups based on perceived common characteristics; a means of giving order to a group of disconnected facts.

adansonian c., the c. of organisms based on giving equal weight to every character of the organism; this principle has its greatest application in numerical taxonomy. [M. *Adanson*]

Angle's c. of malocclusion, a c. of different types of malocclusion, based on the mesiodistal relationship of the permanent molars upon their eruption and locking, and comprised of three classes; *Class I:* normal relationship of the jaws, wherein the mesiobuccal cusp of the maxillary first molar occludes in the buccal groove of the mandibular first permanent molar; *Class II:* distal relationship of the mandible, wherein the distobuccal cusp of the maxillary first permanent molar occludes in the buccal groove of the mandibular first molar, and further classified as

Division 1, labioversion of maxillary incisor teeth, and Division 2, linguoversion of maxillary central incisors, both of which may be unilateral conditions; *Class III:* mesial relationship of the mandible, wherein the mesiobuccal cusp of the maxillary first molar occludes in the embrasure between the mandibular first and second permanent molars, further classified as a unilateral condition.

Arneth c., a c. of the polymorphonuclear neutrophils according to the number of their nuclear lobes. SEE Arneth *stages,* under *stage.*

Black's c., a c. of cavities of the teeth based upon the tooth surface(s) involved.

Caldwell-Moloy c., a c. of the variations in the female pelvis; namely gynecoid, android, anthropoid, and platypelloid pelvis, based on the type of the posterior and anterior segments of the inlet.

Cummer's c., a listing of several types of removable partial dentures in accordance with the distribution of direct retainers.

DeBakey's c., consists of three types: Type I extends into the transverse arch and distal aorta and type II is confined to the ascending aorta. Type III dissections begin in the descending aorta, with type IIIA extending toward the diaphragm and type IIIB extending below it.

Denver c., a system of nomenclature for human mitotic chromosomes, based on length and position of the centromere. [*Denver,,* Colorado, where agreed upon]

Dukes' c., a c. of the extent of operable adenocarcinoma of the colon or rectum commonly modified as follows: A (Duke's A), confined to the mucosa; B_1, into the muscularis mucosae; B_2, through the muscularis mucosae; C_1, limited to the bowel wall, with nodal metastases; C_2, through the bowel wall, with nodal metastases.

Gell and Coombs C. (gel koomz), a c. system that differentiates the 4 types of hypersensitivity reactions: Type I: anaphylactic reactions, Type II: cytotoxic reactions, Type III: immune complex reactions, and Type IV: cell-mediated reactions.

International Labour Organization C., ILO 1980 International Classification of Radiographs of the Pneumoconioses; a system for qualitative and semiquantitative description of the chest radiographic findings caused by pneumoconiosis, designed for epidemiologic studies; supersedes classifications of 1950, 1958, 1968, and 1971.

Jansky's c., the c. of human blood groups now designated O, A, B, and AB.

Kennedy c., a listing of several forms of partially edentulous jaws in accordance with the distribution of the missing teeth.

Kiel c., c. of non-Hodgkin's lymphoma into low-grade malignancy (lymphocytic, lymphoplasmacytoid, centrocytic, and centroblastic-centrocytic types) and high-grade malignancy (centroblastic, lymphoblastic of Burkitt's or convoluted cell, and immunoblastic types). SYN Lennert c.

Lancefield c., a serologic c. dividing hemolytic streptococci into groups (A to O) which bear a definite relationship to their sources, based upon precipitation tests depending upon group-specific substances that are carbohydrate in nature; *e.g., Group A* contains strains pathogenic for man; *B,* strains from mastitis in cows and from normal milk, including a few strains from the human throat and vagina; *C,* strains from various lower animals, including a number from cattle; *D,* strains from cheese; *E,* strains from certified milk; *F,* strains mainly from the human throat, associated with tonsillitis; *G,* strains from man, a few from monkeys and dogs; and *H, K,* and *O,* nonpathogenic strains from normal human respiratory tracts.

Lennert c., SYN Kiel c.

Lukes-Collins c., a c. of lymphomas according to the immunologic nature of the cell of origin, based on histologic and clinical data.

multiaxial c., a procedure used in DSM-III-R for diagnosing patients on five axes: 1) psychiatric syndrome present; 2) patient's history of personality and developmental disorders; 3) possible nonmental medical disorders; 4) severity of psychosocial stressors; 5) highest level of adaptive functioning in the past year.

Angle's classification of malocclusion

classes	anomalies
I	normal relationship of the jaws; neutroclusion
II	distal relationship of mandible; distoclusion
II div. 1	labioversion of maxillary incisors
div. 2	linguoversion of maxillary incisors
	– "pure class II": distoclusion without anomalies of teeth
	– class II "right" or "left": anomalies of teeth on right or left sides
III	mesial relationship of the mandible; mesioclusion

Denver classification

group	chromosome number	morphology
A	1–3	large chromosomes with nearly medial centromere, distinguished by its size and position
B	4–5	large chromosomes with sub-medial centromeres, 4 is longer than 5
C	6–12 plus an X	medium-large chromosomes; 6,7,8, and 11 have a more medial centromere; 9,10, and 12 have an extremely submedial centromere; X, though longer, is difficult to distinguish from 6
D	13–15	medium-large chromosomes with centromere nearly at end; 13 has a very distinct, 14 a small satellite on the short arm
E	16–18	very short chromosomes with nearly medial or submedial centromeres
F	19–20	short chromosomes with almost medial centromeres
G	21–22 plus a Y	very short chromosomes with centromere nearly at end, 21 has satellites on the short arm, Y is usually larger, with minimal divergence between the long arms

New York Heart Association c., a functional c. to assess cardiovascular disability. Class I: patients with cardiac disease without limitation of physical activity. Ordinary activity does not cause symptoms. Class II: patients with cardiac disease with slight limitation of activity; comfortable at rest. Ordinary physical activity results in fatigue, palpitation, dyspnea or angina. Class III: patients with cardiac disease producing marked limitation of activity: comfortable at rest. Less than ordinary physical activity causes symptoms. Class IV: patients with cardiac disease resulting in inability to carry on any physical activity without discomfort. Symptoms may be present even at rest.

Rappaport c., a histologic c. of lymphomas in use before the availability of recent methods for identification of B- and T-type lymphocytes.

Rye c., c. of Hodgkin's disease according to lymphocyte pre-

Lancefield classification		
group	type	pathogenic for:
A	Streptococcus pyogenes	+ humans
B	S. agalactiae	+ animals; rarely humans
C	S. equi, zooepidemicus, equisimilis, galactiae, pyogenes haemolyticus animalis	+ animals
D	S. faecalis, durans, liquefaciens, bovis	− or (+) humans
E	S. uberis, infrequens	−
F	S. minutus	(+) humans
G	S. anginosus	+ humans
H	S. sanguis, dysgalactiae	− humans
K-M	not further specified	− humans (K); animals (L,M)
N	S. lactis, cremoris	(+) humans
O-S	not further specified	− humans

dominance, nodular sclerosing, mixed cellularity, and lymphocyte depletion types. [*Rye, NY*, 1965]

Salter-Harris c. of epiphysial plate injuries, the c. of epiphysial plate injuries into five groups (I to V), according to the pattern of damage to epiphysis, physis, and/or metaphysis; the c. correlates with different prognoses regarding the effects of the injury on subsequent growth and subsequent deformity of the epiphysis.

Tessier c., an anatomical c. of facial, craniofacial, and laterofacial clefts that utilizes the orbit as the primary structure for reference. Fifteen locations for clefts are differentiated.

class switch. Change in the isotype of antibody produced after a B cell has encountered an antigen.

clas·tic (klas′tik). Breaking up into pieces, or exhibiting a tendency so to break or divide. [G. *klastos*, broken]

clas·to·gen (klas′tō-jen). An agent (*e.g.*, certain chemicals, x-rays, ultraviolet light) that causes breaks in chromosomes. [G. *klastos*, broken, + *genos*, birth]

clas·to·gen·ic (klas-tō-jen′ik). Relating to the action of a clastogen.

clas·to·thrix (klas′tō-thriks). SYN *trichorrhexis* nodosa. [G. *klastos*, broken, + *thrix*, hair]

clath·rate (klath′rāt). A type of inclusion compound in which small molecules are trapped in the cage-like lattice of macromolecules. [L. *clathrare*, pp. -*atus*, to furnish with a lattice]

clath·rin (klath′rin). The principal constituent of a polyhedral protein lattice that coats eukaryotic cell membranes (vesicles) and appears to be involved in protein secretion. [L. *clathri*, lattice]

Clauberg, Karl W., German bacteriologist, *1893. SEE C. *test*, *unit*.

Claude, Henri, French psychiatrist, 1869–1945. SEE C.'s *syndrome*.

clau·di·ca·tion (klaw-di-kā′shŭn). Limping, usually referring to intermittent c. [L. *claudicatio*, fr. *claudico*, to limp]

intermittent c., a condition caused by ischemia of the muscles; characterized by attacks of lameness and pain, brought on by walking, chiefly in the calf muscles; however, the condition may occur in other muscle groups. SYN Charcot's syndrome, myasthenia angiosclerotica.

clau·di·ca·tory (klaw′di-kă-tōr-ē). Relating to claudication, especially intermittent claudication.

Claudius, Friedrich M., German anatomist, 1822–1869. SEE C.'s *cells*, under *cell*, *fossa*.

Clausen. SEE Dyggve-Melchior-Clausen *syndrome*.

claus·tra (klaws′tră). Plural of claustrum.

claus·tral (klaws′trăl). Relating to the claustrum.

claus·tro·pho·bia (klaw-strō-fō′bē-ă). A morbid fear of being in a confined place. [L. *claustrum*, an enclosed space, + G. *phobos*, fear]

claus·tro·pho·bic (klaw-strō-fō′bik). Relating to or suffering from claustrophobia.

claus·trum, pl. **claus·tra** (klaws′trŭm, klaws′tră). **1.** One of several anatomical structures bearing a resemblance to a barrier. **2** [NA]. A thin, vertically placed lamina of gray matter lying close to the putamen, from which it is separated by the external capsule. C. consists of two parts: 1) an insular part and 2) a temporal part between putamen and the temporal lobe. Cells of the c. have reciprocal connections with sensory areas of the cerebral cortex. [L. barrier]

c. gut′turis, c. o′ris, obsolete term for soft *palate*.

c. virgina′le, an obsolete term for hymen.

clau·su·ra (klaw-sū′ră). SYN atresia. [L. a lock, bolt, fr. *claudo*, to close]

cla·va (klā′vă). SYN *tubercle* of gracile nucleus. [L. a club]

cla·val (klā′văl). Relating to the clava.

cla·vate (klā′vāt). Club-shaped. [L. *clava*, a club]

cla·vi (klā′vī). Plural of clavus.

Clav·i·ceps pur·pu·rea (klav′i-seps pū-pū′rē-ă). SEE ergot. [L. *clava*, club, + *caput*, head]

clav·i·cle (klav′i-kl). A doubly curved long bone that forms part of the shoulder girdle. Its medial end articulates with the manubrium sterni at the sternoclavicular joint, its lateral end with the acromion of the scapula at the acromioclavicular joint. SYN clavicula [NA], collar bone.

cla·vic·u·la, pl. **cla·vic·′u·lae** (klă-vik′yū-lă) [NA]. SYN clavicle. [L. *clavicula*, a small key, fr. *clavis*, key]

cla·vic·u·lar (kla-vik′yū-lăr). Relating to the clavicle.

cla·vic·u·lus, pl. **cla·vic·u·li** (kla-vik′yū-lŭs, -lī). One of the perforating collagen fibers of bone. [Mod. L. dim. of L. *clavus*, a nail]

clav·u·lan·ic ac·id (klav-yū-lan′ik). 3-(2-Hydroxyethylidene)-7-oxo-4-oxa-1-azabicyclo[3.2.0]heptane-2-carboxylic acid; a beta-lactam antibiotic structurally related to the penicillins that inactivate β-lactamase enzymes in penicillin-resistant organisms; usually used in combination with penicillins to enhance and broaden the spectrum of the penicillins.

cla·vus, pl. **cla·vi** (klā′vŭs, -vī). **1.** A small conical callosity caused by pressure over a bony prominence, usually on a toe. SYN corn (1), heloma. **2.** Obsolete term for a condition resulting from healing of a granuloma of the foot in yaws, in which a core falls out, leaving an erosion. [L. a nail, wart, corn]

cla·vus hys·ter·i·cus (klā′vŭs his-ter′ĕ-kŭs). Severe head pain, sharply defined, and typically described as feeling like a nail being driven into the head; usually regarded as a conversion symptom. [L. *clavus*, nail]

claw (klaw). A sharp, slender, usually curved nail on the paw of an animal. [L. *clavus*, a nail]

dew c., a rudimentary digit, not reaching the ground, on the feet of many quadrupeds.

claw·foot (klaw′fut). A condition of the foot characterized by hyperextension at the metatarsophalangeal joint and flexion at the interphalangeal joints, as a fixed contracture.

claw·hand (klaw′hand). Atrophy of the interosseous muscles of the hand with hyperextension of the metacarpophalangeal joints and flexion of the interphalangeal joints. SYN main en griffe.

Claybrook, Edwin B., U.S. surgeon, 1871–1931. SEE C.'s *sign*.

clean·ing (klēn′ing). In dentistry, a procedure whereby accretions are removed from the teeth or from a dental prosthesis. SEE ALSO dental *prophylaxis*.

ultrasonic c., in dentistry, the use of a high-frequency vibrating point to remove deposits from tooth structure; also the process of cleaning dentures by placing them in a special liquid in a container that generates high-frequency vibrations.

clear·ance (klēr′ans). **1** (*C* with a subscript indicating the substance removed). Removal of a substance from the blood, *e.g.,* by renal excretion, expressed in terms of the volume flow of arterial blood or plasma that would contain the amount of substance removed per unit time; measured in ml/min. Renal c. of any substance except urea or free water is calculated as the urine flow in ml/min multiplied by the urinary concentration of the substance divided by the arterial plasma concentration of the substance; normal human values are commonly expressed per 1.73 m² body surface area. **2.** A condition in which bodies may pass each other without hindrance, or the distance between bodies. **3.** Removal of something from some place; *e.g.,* "esophageal acid c." refers to removal from the esophagus of some acid that has refluxed into it from the stomach, evaluated by the time taken for restoration of a normal pH in the esophagus.

***p*-aminohippurate c.,** a good measure of renal plasma flow, which it slightly underestimates; when a low plasma concentration of *p*-aminohippurate (PAH) is maintained by intravenous infusion, the kidney extracts and excretes almost all of the PAH from the plasma before it reaches the renal vein.

creatinine c., measurement of the clearance of endogenous creatinine, used for evaluating the glomerular filtration rate (GFR).

endogenous creatinine c., a term distinguishing measurements based on the creatinine normally present in plasma; since no infusion is necessary, an average value may be obtained by collecting urine for a long period, *e.g.,* 24 hours.

exogenous creatinine c., a term distinguishing measurements based on infusing creatinine intravenously to raise its plasma concentration and facilitate its accurate chemical determination.

free water c., the amount of water excreted in the urine beyond that which would accompany the excreted solutes if the urine were isosmotic with plasma; it represents the loss of body water in excess of solute tending to raise body osmolality and making urine hyposmotic. Unlike other c.'s, it is calculated by subtracting the osmolal c. from the actual volume of urine excreted per minute. A negative value for free water c. represents the amount of water that the body has reclaimed from isosmotic tubule fluid to make the urine hyperosmotic and to lower body osmolality.

interocclusal c., SYN freeway *space.*

inulin c., an accurate measure of the rate of filtration through the renal glomeruli, because inulin filters freely with water and is neither excreted nor reabsorbed through tubule walls. Inulin is not a normal constituent of plasma and must be infused continously to maintain a steady plasma concentration and a steady rate of urinary excretion during the measurement. Inulin c. in a normal adult person is about 120 ml/min (range 100–150) per 1.73 m² body surface area.

isotope c., the rate at which an isotope is removed (usually by blood flow) from a tissue or organ such as the brain.

maximum urea c., the urea c. when the urine flow exceeds 2 ml/min; normal value is about 75 ml blood/min per 1.73 m² body surface area.

occlusal c., a condition in which the opposing occlusal surfaces may glide over one another without any interfering projection.

osmolal c., the volume of urine that would be excreted per minute if the urinary solutes were accompanied by just enough water to make the urine isosmotic with plasma, *i.e.,* so that the solute excretion did not change the osmolality of body fluids. To calculate it, the volume of urine excreted per minute is multiplied by the urinary osmolality (usually measured by freezing point depression) and divided by the plasma osmolality. Osmolal c. is less than actual urine flow when urine is hyposmotic and exceeds it when urine is hyperosmotic.

standard urea c., the value obtained when the square root of the urine flow (when below 2 ml/min) is multiplied by the urine urea concentration and divided by the whole blood urea concentration; represents an old empirical adjustment for the effect of low urine flow on urea excretion; sometimes corrected for body size by dividing by some function of body weight or surface area. Later, plasma concentration was substituted for blood concentra-

tion in the calculation. The normal value is about 54 ml/min per 1.73 m² in an adult person. SYN Van Slyke's formula.

urea c., the volume of plasma (or blood) that would be completely cleared of urea by one minute's excretion of urine; originally calculated as urine flow multiplied by urine urea concentration divided by concentration of urea in whole blood rather than plasma, representing blood urea c. rather than plasma urea c.

clear·er (klēr′er). An agent, used in histological preparations, which is miscible in both the dehydrating or fixing fluid and the embedding substance.

cleav·age (klēv′ij). **1.** Series of mitotic cell divisions occurring in the ovum immediately following its fertilization. SYN segmentation (2). SEE ALSO cleavage *division.* **2.** Splitting of a complex molecule into two or more simpler molecules. SYN scission (2). **3.** Linear clefts in the skin indicating the direction of the fibers in the dermis. SEE ALSO cleavage *lines,* under *line.* **4.** Midline depression or furrow between mature female breasts (common).

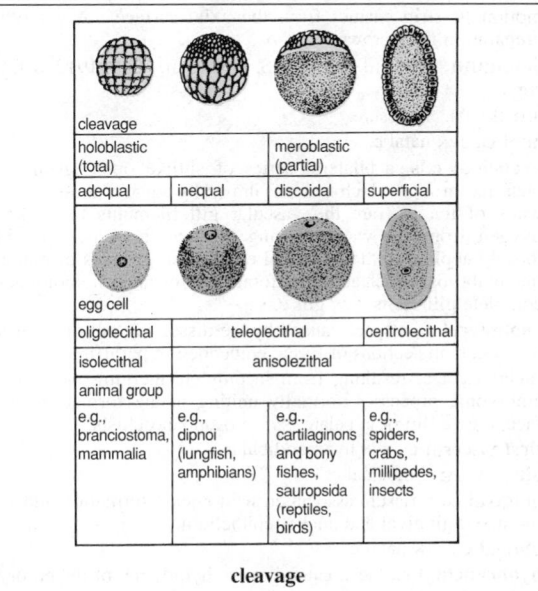

cleavage			
holoblastic (total)		meroblastic (partial)	
adequal	inequal	discoidal	superficial

egg cell			
oligolecithal	teleolecithal		centrolecithal
isolecithal	anisolezithal		
animal group			
e.g., branciostoma, mammalia	e.g., dipnoi (lungfish, amphibians)	e.g., cartilaginons and bony fishes, sauropsida (reptiles, birds)	e.g., spiders, crabs, millipedes, insects

cleavage

abnormal c. of cardiac valve, congenital malformation of a valve leaflet with a defect extending from the free margin.

adequal c., c. resulting in the formation of blastomeres of approximately equal size.

complete c., SYN holoblastic c.

determinate c., c. resulting in blastomeres each capable of developing only into a particular embryonic structure.

discoidal c., meroblastic c. limited to the small cap (animal pole) of protoplasm of large-yolked eggs, such as the telolecithal eggs of birds.

enamel c., the splitting of enamel in a plane parallel to the direction of the enamel rods.

equal c., c. producing blastomeres of like size.

equatorial c., c. in which the plane of cytoplasmic division is at right angles to the axis of the ovum.

holoblastic c., c. in which the blastomeres are completely separated; the entire egg participates in cell division. SYN complete c., total c.

hydrolytic c., SYN hydrolysis.

incomplete c., SYN meroblastic c.

indeterminate c., c. resulting in blastomeres of similar developmental potencies, each capable, when isolated, of producing an entire embryonic body.

meridional c., c. in a plane through the axis of the zygote.

meroblastic c., incomplete separation of the blastomeres, with the divisions being limited to the nonyolked portion of the egg. SYN incomplete c.

phosphoroclastic c., SYN phosphorolysis.

progressive c., in fungi, a type of sporulation in which c. planes in the cytoplasm first produce protospores and then sporangiospores in a sporangium.

pudendal c., SYN pudendal *cleft.*

subdural c., SYN subdural *space.*

superficial c., meroblastic c. with the divisions limited to the peripheral (surface) cytoplasm of a centrolecithal egg.

thioclastic c., the splitting of a bond in fashion analogous to hydrolysis or phosphorolysis except that the elements of a substituted hydrogen sulfide (usually coenzyme A) are added across the break.

total c., SYN holoblastic c.

unequal c., c. producing blastomeres of different sizes at the two poles.

yolk c., segmentation of the vitellus.

cleav·er (klē′ver). A heavy knife for cutting or chopping.

enamel c., an instrument with a heavy shank and a very short blade at about 90° to the axis of the handle; used with a hoeing motion to strip enamel from the axial surfaces of a tooth in preparation for a crown.

Cleemann, Richard Alsop, U.S. physician, 1840–1912. SEE C.'s *sign.*

cleft (kleft). A fissure.

anal c., SYN natal c.

branchial c.'s, a bilateral series of slitlike openings into the pharynx through which water is drawn by aquatic animals; in the walls of the c.'s are the vascular gill filaments that take up oxygen from the water passing through the c.'s; sometimes loosely applied to the branchial ectodermal grooves of mammalian embryos, which are imperforate, rudimentary homologues of complete gill clefts. SYN gill c.'s.

cholesterol c., a space caused by the dissolving out of cholesterol crystals in sections of tissue embedded in paraffin.

facial c., a c. resulting from incomplete merging or fusion of embryonic processes normally uniting in the formation of the face, *e.g.,* c. lip or c. palate. SYN prosopoanoschisis.

first visceral c., SYN hyomandibular c.

gill c.'s, SYN branchial c.'s.

gingival c., a fissure associated with pocket formation and lined by mixed gingival and pocket epithelium.

gluteal c., SYN natal c.

hyobranchial c., the c. caudal to the hyoid arch of the embryo.

hyomandibular c., the c. between the hyoid and mandibular arches of the embryo; the external auditory meatus is developed from its dorsal portion. SYN first visceral c.

interneuromeric c.'s, c.'s between the neuromeric or segmental elevations in the primitive rhombencephalon.

Larrey's c., SYN *trigonum* sternocostale.

Maurer's c.'s, SYN Maurer's *dots,* under *dot.*

median maxillary anterior alveolar c., an asymptomatic midline defect of the maxillary anterior ridge; the result of a failure of fusion or development of the lateral halves of the palate.

natal c., the sulcus between the buttocks (nates). SYN crena ani [NA], anal c., crena clunium, gluteal c.

oblique facial c., SYN prosoposchisis.

pudendal c., the cleft between the labia majora. SYN rima pudendi [NA], fissura pudendi, pudendal cleavage, pudendal slit, rima vulvae, urogenital c., vulvar slit.

residual c., the remnants of the pituitary diverticulum that occur between the pars distalis and pars intermedia; a distinct lumen is present in some animals, but, in humans, is present only during prenatal development and sometimes in young children. SYN residual lumen.

Schmidt-Lanterman c.'s, SYN Schmidt-Lanterman *incisures,* under *incisure.*

subdural c., SYN subdural *space.*

synaptic c., the space about 20 nm wide between the axolemma and the postsynaptic surface. SEE ALSO synapse.

urogenital c., SYN pudendal c.

visceral c., any c. between two branchial (visceral) arches in the embryo.

⌂**cleid-.** SEE cleido-.

clei·dag·ra, cli·dag·ra (klī-dag′ră). Rarely used term for a sudden severe pain in the clavicle, resembling gout. [cleid- + G. *agra,* seizure]

clei·dal (klī′dăl). Relating to the clavicle. SYN clidal.

⌂**cleido-, cleid-.** The clavicle; also spelled clido-, clid-. [G. *kleis,* bar, bolt]

clei·do·cos·tal (klī-dō-kos′tăl). Relating to the clavicle and a rib. SYN clidocostal. [cleido- + L. *costa,* rib]

clei·do·cra·ni·al (klī′dō-krā′nē-ăl). Relating to the clavicle and the cranium. SYN clidocranial. [G. *kleis,* clavicle, + *kranion,* cranium]

⌂**-cleisis.** Closure. [G. *kleisis,* a closing]

cleis·to·the·ci·um (klīs-tō-thē′sē-ŭm). In fungi, an ascocarp that is closed, with randomly dispersed asci. [G. *kleistos,* enclosed, + *thēkē,* box]

Cleland, W. Wallace, U.S. biochemist, *1930. SEE C.'s *reagent.*

clem·as·tine (klem′as-tēn). D-2-[2-[(*p*-chloro-α-methyl-α-phenylbenzyl)oxy]ethyl]-1-methylpyrrolidine; an antihistaminic. SYN meclastine.

clem·i·zole (klem′i-zōl). 1-Chlorobenzyl-2-(1-pyrrolidinylmethyl)benzimidazole; an antihistaminic.

cle·oid (klē′oyd). A dental instrument with a pointed elliptical cutting end, used in excavating cavities or carving fillings and waxes. [A. S. *cle,* claw + G. *eidos,* resemblance]

clep·to·par·a·site (klep-tō-par′ă-sīt). A parasite that develops on the prey of the parasite's host. [G. *kleptō,* to steal, + parasite]

Cléret, M., 20th century French physician. SEE Launois-C. *syndrome.*

Clevenger, Shobal V., U.S. neurologist, 1843–1920. SEE C.'s *fissure.*

click (klik). A slight sharp sound.

ejection c., a clicking ejection sound. SEE sound.

mitral c., the opening snap of the mitral valve.

systolic c., a sharp, clicking sound heard during cardiac systole; when heard in early systole it is usually an ejection sound; in late systole the c. usually signifies mitral insufficiency, as in the dysfunction of the mitral valvular apparatus when it prolapses into the left atrium during systole (see Barlow syndrome); rarely may also be due to pleuropericardial adhesions or other extracardiac mechanisms.

click·ing (klik′ing). A snapping, crepitant noise noted on excursions of the temporomandibular articulation, due to an asynchronous movement of the disk and condyle.

⌂**clid-.** SEE clido-.

cli·dal (klī′dăl). SYN cleidal.

cli·din·i·um bro·mide (klī-din′ē-ŭm). 3-Hydroxy-1-methylquinuclidinium bromide benzilate; an anticholinergic.

⌂**clido-, clid-.** The clavicle. SEE ALSO cleido-. [G. *kleis,* bar, bolt]

cli·do·cos·tal (klī-dō-kos′tăl). SYN cleidocostal.

cli·do·cra·ni·al (klī-dō-krā′nē-ăl). SYN cleidocranial.

cli·do·ic (klī-dō′ik). Cleidoic.

cli·ma·co·pho·bia (klī′mă-kō-fō′bē-ă). Morbid fear of stairs or of climbing. [G. *klimax,* ladder, + *phobos,* fear]

cli·mac·ter·ic (klī-mak′ter-ik, klī-mak-ter′ik). **1.** The period of endocrinal, somatic, and transitory psychologic changes occurring in the transition to menopause. **2.** A critical period of life. SYN climacterium. [G. *klimaktēr,* the rung of a ladder]

grand c., the sixty-third year; the ninth of the seven-year periods, each of which from the third (twenty-first year) was formerly regarded as a critical time of life.

cli·mac·ter·i·um (klī-mak-tēr′ē-ŭm). SYN climacteric.

cli·ma·tol·o·gy (klī-mă-tol′ō-jē). The study of climate and its relation to disease.

cli·ma·to·ther·a·py (klī′mă-tō-thār′ă-pē). Treatment of disease by removal of the patient to a region having a climate more favorable for recovery.

cli·max (klī′maks). **1.** The height or acme of a disease; its stage of greatest severity. **2.** SYN orgasm. [G. *klimax,* staircase]

cli·mo·graph (klī′mō-graf). A diagram showing the effect of climate on health. [G. *klima,* climate, + *graphō,* to record]

clin·da·my·cin (klin-dă-mī′sin). 7(*S*)-Chloro-7-deoxylincomycin; an antibacterial and antibiotic.

cline (klīn). A systematic relation between location and the frequencies of alleles; lines connecting points of equal frequency are termed isoclines, and the direction of the c. at any point is at right angles to an isocline. [G. *klinō*, to slope]

clin·ic (klin′ik). **1.** An institution, building, or part of a building where ambulatory patients are cared for. **2.** An institution, building, or part of a building in which medical instruction is given to students by means of demonstrations in the presence of the sick. **3.** A lecture or symposium on a subject relating to disease. [G. *klinē*, bed]

clin·i·cal (klin′i-kl). **1.** Relating to the bedside of a patient or to the course of his disease. **2.** Denoting the symptoms and course of a disease, as distinguished from the laboratory findings of anatomical changes. **3.** Relating to a clinic.

cli·ni·cian (klin-ish′ŭn). A health professional engaged in the care of patients, as distinguished from one working in other areas.

clin·i·co·path·o·log·ic (klin′i-kō-path-ō-loj′ik). Pertaining to the signs and symptoms manifested by a patient, and also the results of laboratory studies, as they relate to the findings in the gross and histologic examination of tissue by means of biopsy or autopsy, or both.

clino-. A slope (inclination or declination) or bend. [G. *klinō*, to slope, incline, or bend]

cli·no·ce·phal·ic, cli·no·ceph·a·lous (klī-nō-se-fal′ik, -sef′ă-lŭs). Relating to clinocephaly.

cli·no·ceph·a·ly (klī′nō-sef′ă-lē). Craniosynostosis in which the upper surface of the skull is concave, presenting a saddle-shaped appearance in profile. SYN saddle head. [clino- + G. *kephalē*, head]

cli·no·dac·ty·ly (klī′nō-dak′ti-lē). Permanent deflection of one or more fingers. [clino- + G. *daktylos*, finger]

cli·nog·ra·phy (klin-og′ră-fē). Graphic representation of the signs and symptoms exhibited by a patient. [G. *klinē*, bed, + *graphō*, to write]

cli·noid (klī′noyd). **1.** Resembling a four-poster bed. **2.** SYN clinoid *process*. [G. *klinē*, bed, + *eidos*, resemblance]

cli·no·scope (klī′nō-skōp). An obsolete instrument for measuring cyclophoria. [clino- + G. *skopeō*, to view]

cli·o·quin·ol (klī-ō-kwin′ol). SYN iodochlorhydroxyquin.

cli·ox·a·nide (klī-ok′să-nīd). 4′-Chloro-3,5-diiodosalicylanilide acetate; an anthelmintic.

CLIP Abbreviation for corticotropin-like intermediate-lobe *peptide*.

clip (klip′). A fastener used to hold a part or thing together with another.

  wound c., a metal clasp or device for surgical approximation of skin incisions.

clith·ro·pho·bia (klīth-rō-fō′bē-ă). Morbid fear of being locked in. [G. *kleithron*, a bolt, + *phobos*, fear]

clit·i·on (klit′ē-on). A craniometric point in the middle of the highest part of the clivus on the sphenoid bone. [G. *klitos*, a declivity]

clit·o·rid·e·an (klit′o-ri-dē′an). Relating to the clitoris.

clit·o·ri·dec·to·my (klit′ō-ri-dek′tō-mē). Removal of the clitoris. [clitoris + G. *ektomē*, excision]

clit·o·ri·di·tis (klit′ō-ri-dī′tis). Inflammation of the clitoris. SYN clitoritis. [clitoris + G. *-itis*, inflammation]

clit·o·ris, pl. **cli·to·ri·des** (klit′ō-ris, -tōr′i-dēz; klī′tō-ris) [NA]. A cylindric, erectile body, rarely exceeding 2 cm in length, situated at the most anterior portion of the vulva and projecting between the branched limbs or laminae of the labia minora, which form its prepuce and frenulum. It consists of a glans, a corpus, and two crura, and is the homologue of the penis in the male, except that it is not perforated by the urethra and does not possess a corpus spongiosum. [G. *kleitoris*]

clit·o·rism (klit′ō-rizm). Prolonged and usually painful erection of the clitoris; the analogue of priapism.

clit·o·ri·tis (klit-ō-rī′tis). SYN clitoriditis.

clit·or·o·meg·a·ly (klit′ōr-ō-meg′ă-lē). An enlarged clitoris. [clitoris + G. *megas*, great]

clit·or·o·plas·ty (klit′ō-rō-plas′tē). Any plastic procedure on the clitoris. [clitoris + G. *plastos*, formed]

cli·val (klī′văl). Pertaining to the clivus.

cli·vus, pl. **cli·vi** (klī′vŭs, -vē). **1.** A downward sloping surface. **2.** [NA]. The sloping surface from the dorsum sellae to the foramen magnum composed of part of the body of the sphenoid and part of the basal part of the occipital bone. SYN Blumenbach's c. [L. slope]

  Blumenbach's c., SYN clivus (2).

  c. ocula′ris, the sloping walls of the fovea leading to the foveola.

clo·a·ca (klō-ā′kă). **1.** In early embryos, the endodermally lined chamber into which the hindgut and allantois empty. **2.** In birds and monotremes, the common chamber into which open the hindgut, bladder, and genital ducts. [L. sewer]

  ectodermal c., the proctodeum of the embryo.

  endodermal c., terminal portion of the hindgut internal to the cloacal membrane of the embryo.

  persistent c., a condition in which the urorectal fold has failed to divide the c. of the embryo into rectal and urogenital portions. SYN sinus urogenitalis, urogenital sinus (2).

clo·a·cal (klō-ā′kăl). Pertaining to the cloaca.

clo·a·ci·tis (klō-ă-sī′tis). An inflammation of the cloacal mucosa of fowls, with ulceration and chronic discharge.

clo·ba·zam (klō-bă-zam). A novel benzodiazepine psychotherapeutic agent in which the nitrogens in the heterocyclic ring are in the 1,5- rather than in the more usual 1,4- positions; an anxiolytic.

clo·be·ta·sol pro·pi·o·nate (klō-bā′tă-sōl). Pregna-1,4-diene-3,20-dione,21-chloro-9-fluoro-11-hyroxy-16-methyl-17-(1-oxopropoxy)-,(11β,16β)-; an anti-inflammatory corticosteroid usually used in topical preparations.

clo·cor·to·lone (klō-kōr′tō-lōn). 9-Chloro-6α-fluoro-11β,21-dihydroxy-16α-methylpregna-1,4-diene-3,20-dione; an anti-inflammatory corticosteroid usually used in topical preparations; available as the acetate and the pivalate.

clo·faz·i·mine (klō-faz′ĭ-mēn). 3-(*p*-Chloroanilino)-10-(*p*-chlorophenyl)-2,10-dihydro-2-(isopropylimino)phenazine; a tuberculostatic and leprostatic agent.

clo·fen·a·mide (klō-fen′ă-mid). 4-chloro-*m*-benzenedisulfonamide; a diuretic. SYN monochlorphenamide.

clo·fi·brate (klō′fi-brāt). Ethyl chlorophenoxyisobutyrate; an antilipemic agent that reduces plasma levels of cholesterol, triglycerides, and uric acid; used in the treatment of hypercholesterolemia and atherosclerosis.

clo·ges·tone ac·e·tate (klō-jes′tōn). 6-Chloro-3β,17-dihydroxypregna-4,6-dien-20-one diacetate; a progestational agent.

clo·ma·cran phos·phate (klō′mă-kran). 2-Chloro-9-[3-(dimethylamino)propyl]acridan phosphate; a tranquilizer.

clo·me·ges·tone ac·e·tate (klō-me-jes′tōn). 6-Chloro-17-hydroxy-16α-methylpregna-4,6-diene-3,20-dione acetate; a progestational drug.

clo·mi·phene cit·rate (klō′mi-fēn). 2-[*p*-(2-chloro-1,2-diphenylvinyl)phenoxy]triethylamine dihydrogen citrate; an analog of the nonsteroid estrogen, chlorotrianisene; a pituitary gonadotropin stimulant used therapeutically to induce ovulation; it competes with estrogen at the hypothalamic level, interrupting the negative feedback system and resulting in increased gonadotropin secretion. SYN chloramiphene.

clo·mip·ra·mine hy·dro·chlo·ride (klō-mip′ră-mēn). Chlorimipramine hydrochloride; 3-chloro-5-[3-(dimethylamino)-propyl]-10,11-dihydro-5*H*-dibenz[*b,f*]azepine monohydrochloride; an antidepressant.

clo·nal (klō′năl). Pertaining to a clone.

clo·na·ze·pam (klō-nā′zē-pam). 5-(*o*-Chlorophenyl)-1,3-dihydro-7-nitro-2*H*-1,4-benzodiazepin-2-one; an anticonvulsant drug in the benzodiazepine class.

clone (klōn). **1.** A colony or group of organisms (or an individual organism), or a colony of cells derived from a single organism or cell by asexual reproduction, all having identical genetic constitutions. **2.** To produce such a colony or individual. **3.** A short section of DNA which has been copied by means of gene cloning. SEE cloning. [G. *klōn*, slip, cutting used for propagation]

cDNA c., a duplex DNA, representing an mRNA, carried in a cloning vector.

clo·nic (klon'ik). Relating to or characterized by clonus.

clon·ic·i·ty (klon-is'i-tē). The state of being clonic.

clon·i·co·ton·ic (klon'i-kō-ton'ik). Both clonic and tonic; said of certain forms of muscular spasm.

clo·ni·dine hy·dro·chlo·ride (klō'ni-dēn). 2-(2,6-Dichloroanilino)-2-imidazoline hydrochloride; an antihypertensive agent with central and peripheral actions; it stimulates adrenergic receptors in the brain leading to reduced sympathetic nervous system output.

---

clon·ing (klōn'ing). **1.** Growing a colony of genetically identical cells or organisms in vitro. **2.** Transplantation of a nucleus from a somatic cell to an ovum, which then develops into an embryo; many identical embryos can thus be generated by asexual reproduction. **3.** With blastocysts, dividing a cluster of cells through microsurgery and transferring one half the cells to a zona pellucida that has been emptied of its contents. The resulting embryos, genetically identical, may be implanted in an animal for gestation. **4.** A recombinant DNA technique used to produce millions of copies of a DNA fragment. The fragment is spliced into a cloning vehicle (*i.e.,* plasmid, bacteriophage, or animal virus). The cloning vehicle penetrates a bacterial cell or yeast (the host), which is then grown in vitro or in an animal host. In some cases, as in the production of genetically engineered drugs, the inserted DNA becomes activated and alters the chemical functioning of the host cell.

---

clo·nism (klon'izm). A long continued state of clonic spasms.

clo·no·gen·ic (klō-nō-jen'ik). Arising from or consisting of a clone.

clon·o·graph (klon'ō-graf). An instrument for registering the movements in clonic spasm. [G. *klonos*, tumult, + *graphō,* to write]

clo·nor·chi·a·sis (klō-nōr-kī'ă-sis). A disease caused by the fluke *Clonorchis sinensis,* affecting the distal bile ducts of man and other fish-eating animals after ingestion of raw, smoked, or undercooked fish or raw crayfish; initial infection may be benign, but repeated or chronic infection induces an intense proliferative and granulomatous condition. SYN clonorchiosis.

clo·nor·chi·o·sis (klō-nōr-kē-ō'sis). SYN clonorchiasis.

Clo·nor·chis si·nen·sis (klō-nōr'kis sī-nen'sis). The Oriental Chinese liver fluke, a species of trematodes (family Opisthorchiidae) that in the Far East infects the bile passages of man and other fish-eating animals; cyprinoid fish serve as chief second intermediate hosts, and various operculate snails serve as the first intermediate hosts. SYN *Opisthorchis sinensis.*

clon·o·spasm (klon'ō-spazm). SYN clonus.

clo·nus (klō'nŭs). A form of movement marked by contractions and relaxations of a muscle, occurring in rapid succession seen with, among other conditions, spasticity and some seizure disorders. SEE ALSO contraction. SYN clonospasm. [G. *klonos,* a tumult]

ankle c., a rhythmical contraction of the calf muscles following a sudden passive dorsiflexion of the foot, the leg being semiflexed.

cathodal opening c. (CaOCl, COCl), obsolete term for a c. produced near a cathode when the flow of current is stopped.

toe c., alternating movements of flexion and extension of the great toe following forcible extension at the metatarsophalangeal joint.

wrist c., rhythmical contractions and relaxations of the muscles of the forearm excited by a forcible passive extension of the hand.

clo·pam·ide (klō-pam'īd). 1-(4-Chloro-3-sulfamoylbenzamido)-2,6-dimethylpiperidine; a diuretic and antihypertensive agent.

Cloquet, Hippolyte, French anatomist, 1787–1840. SEE C.'s *space.*

Cloquet, Jules G., French anatomist, 1790–1883. SEE C.'s *canal, hernia, septum; node* of C.

clor·az·e·pate (klōr-az'ĕ-pāt). 7-Chloro-2,3-dihydro-2-oxo-5-phenyl-1*H*-1,4-benzodiazepine-3-carboxylate; the mono- or dipotassium salt is used as an anti-anxiety agent; a benzodiazepine prodrug for nordiazepam.

clor·pren·a·line hy·dro·chlo·ride (klōr-pren'ă-lēn). *o*-chloro-α-(isopropylaminomethyl)benzyl alcohol hydrochloride; a bronchodilator. SYN isoprophenamine hydrochloride.

clo·sir·a·mine acet·u·rate (klō-sir'ă-mēn). 8-Chloro-11-[2-(dimethylamino)ethyl]-6,11-dihydro-5*H*-benzo[5,6]-cyclohepta[1,2-*b*]pyridine compound with *N*-acetylglycine; an antihistaminic.

clos·trid·ia (klos-trid'ē-ă). Plural of clostridium.

clos·trid·i·al (klos-trid'ē-ăl). Relating to any bacterium of the genus *Clostridium.*

clos·trid·i·o·pep·ti·dase A (klos-trid'ē-ō-pep'ti-dās). SYN *Clostridium histolyticum* collagenase.

clos·trid·i·o·pep·ti·dase B. SYN clostripain.

CLOSTRIDIUM

Clos·trid·i·um (klos-trid'ē-ŭm). A genus of anaerobic (or anaerobic, aerotolerant), sporeforming, motile (occasionally nonmotile) bacteria (family Bacillaceae) containing Gram-positive rods; motile cells are peritrichous. Many of the species are saccharolytic and fermentative, producing various acids and gases and variable amounts of neutral products; other species are proteolytic, some attacking proteins with putrefaction or more complete proteolysis. Some species fix free nitrogen. Exotoxins are sometimes produced by these organisms. They may cause disease in man and other animals. They are generally found in soil and in the intestinal tract of man and other animals. The type species is *C. butyricum.* [G. *klōstēr,* a spindle]

C. bifermen'tans, a species found in putrid meat and gaseous gangrene; also commonly found in soil, feces, and sewage. Its pathogenicity varies from strain to strain.

C. botuli'num, a species that occurs widely in nature and is a frequent cause of food poisoning (botulism) from preserved meats, fruits, or vegetables which have not been properly sterilized before canning. The main types, A to F, are characterized by antigenically distinct, but pharmacologically similar, very potent neurotoxins, each of which can be neutralized only by the specific antitoxin; group C toxin contains at least two components; the recorded cases of human botulism have been due mainly to types A, B, E, and F; type Cα causes botulism in domestic and wild water fowl; Cβ and D are associated with intoxications in cattle.

C. butyr'icum, a species which occurs in naturally soured milk, in naturally fermented starchy plant substances, and in soil; it is not pathogenic. It is the type species of the genus *C.*

C. cadav'eris, a species found in a human cadaver and in the peritoneum of a rabbit; it is not pathogenic for guinea pigs or rabbits.

C. car'nis, a species found in a rabbit inoculated with soil; it is pathogenic for laboratory animals, in which an exotoxin produces edema, necrosis, and death.

C. chauvoe'i, a species which causes blackleg, black quarter, or symptomatic anthrax in cattle and other animals and which produces an exotoxin.

C. cochlear'ium, a species found in human war wounds and septic infections; it is not pathogenic for guinea pigs.

C. coli'num, a species causing ulcerative enteritis in quail and chickens.

C. diffi'cile (di-fi-sēl'), a species found in the feces of newborn infants; pathogenic for human beings, guinea pigs, and rabbits; frequent cause of colitis and diarrhea following antibiotic usage.

Found to be a cause of pseudomembranous colitis and associated with a number of intestinal diseases that are linked to antibiotic therapy. It is also the chief cause of nosocomial diarrhea. [L. difficult]

C. fal'lax, a species found in war wounds, appendicitis, and black leg of sheep; it produces a weak exotoxin.

C. haemoly'ticum, a species found in cattle dying of icterohemoglobinuria; it is pathogenic and toxic for guinea pigs and rabbits and produces an unstable, hemolytic toxin.

C. histoly'ticum, a species found in war wounds, where it induces necrosis of tissue; it produces a cytolytic exotoxin that causes local necrosis and sloughing on injection; it is not toxic on feeding; it is pathogenic for small laboratory animals.

C. innomina'tum, a species found in septic and gangrenous war wounds.

C. micro'sporum, a species found in the abdominal contents of a fatal case of peritonitis.

C. multifermen'tans, a species found in a human muscle infected with gas gangrene; also found in fermented olives and spoiled chocolate candy.

C. nigri'ficans, former name for *Desulfotomaculum nigrificans.*

C. no'vyi, a species consisting of three types, A, B, and C; type A, from a case of gaseous gangrene and from human necrotic hepatitis, produces γ-toxin (a hemolytic lecithinase); B, from black disease (infectious necrotic hepatitis) of sheep, produces β-toxin (a hemolytic lecithinase); and C, found in bacillary osteomyelitis of water buffaloes, does not produce toxin. SYN *C. oedematiens.*

C. oedema'tiens, SYN *C. novyi.*

C. parabotuli'num, a species containing organisms formerly referred to as *C. botulinum* types A and B; the types are identified by protection tests with known type antitoxin; it produces a powerful exotoxin and is pathogenic for man and other animals.

C. paraputri'ficum, a species found in feces, especially those of infants, gaseous gangrene, and postmortem fluid and tissue cultures; it is not pathogenic for rabbits or guinea pigs.

C. perfrin'gens, a species which is the chief causative agent of gas gangrene in man and a cause of gas gangrene in other animals, especially sheep; it may also be involved in causing enteritis, appendicitis, and puerperal fever; it is one of the most common causes of food poisoning in the U. S. This organism is found in soil, water, milk, dust, sewage, and the intestinal tract of man and other animals. SYN *C. welchii,* gas bacillus, Welch's bacillus.

C. ramo'sum, a species found in the natural cavities of man and other animals as well as in sea water; it is also found in association with mastoiditis, otitis, pulmonary gangrene, putrid pleurisy, appendicitis, intestinal infections, balanitis, liver abscess, osteomyelitis, septicemia, and urinary infections, as well as in the vagina and in feces. It was formerly the type species of the obsolete genus *Ramibacterium.*

C. sep'ticum, a species found in malignant edema of animals, in human war wounds, and in cases of appendicitis; it is pathogenic for guinea pigs, rabbits, mice, and pigeons and produces an exotoxin that is lethal and hemolytic. SYN Ghon-Sachs bacillus, Sachs' bacillus, *vibrion septique.*

C. sordel'li, a species causing big head in rams.

C. sphenoi'des, a species found in gangrenous war wounds; it is not pathogenic for guinea pigs or rabbits.

C. sporo'genes, a species found in intestinal contents, gaseous gangrene, and soil; it is not pathogenic for guinea pigs or rabbits, but does produce a slight, temporary, local tumefaction.

C. ta'le, a species found in a case of acute appendicitis and in canned fish; pathogenicity for laboratory animals is variable.

C. ter'tium, a species found in wounds, but that is nonpathogenic for laboratory animals.

C. tet'ani, the species that causes tetanus; it produces a potent exotoxin (neurotoxin) that is intensely toxic for man and other animals when formed in tissues or injected, but not when ingested.

C. tetanoi'des, a species found in war wounds, postmortem blood cultures, and garden soil.

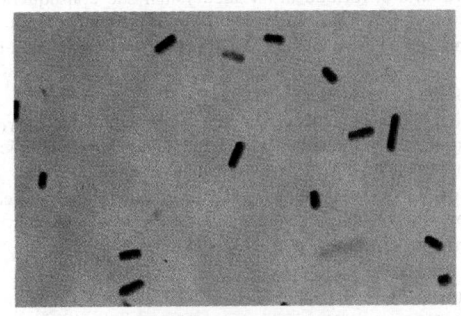

Clostridium perfringens
microscopic preparation: plump, Gram-positive bacilli

C. tetanomor'phum, a species found in war wounds and soil; it is not pathogenic for rabbits or guinea pigs.

C. thermosaccharoly'ticum, a species of thermophilic bacteria found in "hard swell" of canned goods; it is not pathogenic to laboratory animals.

C. welch'ii, SYN *C. perfringens.*

clos·trid·i·um, pl. **clos·trid·ia** (klos-trid′ē-ŭm, -ă). A vernacular term used to refer to any member of the genus *Clostridium.*

Clos·trid·i·um his·to·lyt·i·cum col·la·gen·ase. An enzyme that catalyzes the hydrolysis of collagen, preferentially at peptide bonds on the amino side of a glycylprolyl sequence. SYN clostridiopeptidase A, collagenase A, collagenase I.

Clos·trid·i·um his·to·lyt·i·cum pro·tein·ase B. SYN clostripain.

clos·tri·pain (klos′tri-pān). A cysteine proteinase cleaving preferentially at the carboxyl side of arginyl and lysyl residues. It also has an esterase activity. SYN clostridiopeptidase B, *Clostridium histolyticum* proteinase B.

clo·sure (klō′zhŭr). **1.** The completion of a reflex pathway. **2.** The place of coupling between stimuli in the establishment of conditioned learning. **3.** To achieve or experience a sense of completion in a mental task.

flask c., in dentistry, the procedure of bringing the two halves or parts of a flask together; trial flask c.'s are preliminary c.'s made to eliminate excess denture-base material and to ensure that the mold is completely filled; the final flask c. is the last c. of a flask before curing, following trial packing of the mold with denture-base material.

velopharyngeal c., the apposition of the palate to the upper posterior pharyngeal wall as in deglutition and in some speech sounds.

clo·sy·late (klō′si-lāt). USAN-approved contraction for *p-*chlorobenzenesulfonate.

clot (klot). **1.** To coagulate, said especially of blood. **2.** A soft, nonrigid, insoluble mass formed when a liquid (*e.g.,* blood or lymph) gels. [O.E. *klott,* lump]

agonal c., intravascular thrombosis ascribed to the process of dying.

antemortem c., a blood c., found at autopsy, formed in any of the heart cavities or the great vessels before death.

blood c., the coagulated phase of blood; the soft, coherent, jelly-like red mass resulting from the conversion of fibrinogen to fibrin, thereby entrapping the red blood cells (and other formed elements) within the coagulated plasma.

chicken fat c., c. formed *in vitro* or postmortem from leukocytes and plasma of sedimented blood.

currant jelly c., a jelly-like mass of red blood cells and fibrin formed by the *in vitro* or postmortem clotting of whole or sedimented blood.

laminated c., a c. formed in a succession of layers such as occurs in the natural course of an aneurysm.

passive c., a c. formed in an aneurysmal sac consequent to the cessation or slowing of circulation through the aneurysm.

postmortem c., a c. formed in the heart or great vessels after death.

Schede's c., SEE Schede's *method.*

clo·trim·a·zole (klō-trim′ă-zōl). 1-(*o*-Chloro-α,α-diphenylbenzyl)imidazole; an antifungal agent used topically to treat a variety of fungal and yeast infections.

clot·tage (klot′ij). Rarely used term for blocking of any canal or duct by a blood clot.

Cloudman, Arthur M., U.S. zoologist and pathologist, *1901. SEE C. *melanoma.*

clove oil (klōv). SYN *oil* of clove.

clox·a·cil·lin so·di·um (klok-să-sil′in). [5-Methyl-3-(*o*-chlorophenyl)-4-isoxazolyl]penicillin sodium; a penicillinase-resistant penicillin.

clo·za·pine (klō′ză-pēn). 8-Chloro-11-(4-methyl-1-piperazinyl)-5*H*-dibenzo[*b,e*][1,4]diazepine; a sedative and antipsychotic tricyclic dibenzodiazepine regarded as atypical because of low central antidopaminergic activity.

CLQ Abbreviation for cognitive laterality *quotient.*

club·bing (klŭb′ing). A condition affecting the fingers and toes in which proliferation of distal tissues, especially the nail-beds, results in thickening and widening of the extremities of the digits; the nails are abnormally curved and shiny.

hereditary c., Simple hereditary c. of the digits without associated pulmonary or other progressive disease, often more severe in males; most common in black patients; autosomal dominant inheritance. SYN acropathy.

club·foot (klŭb′fut). SYN *talipes* equinovarus.

club·hand (klŭb′hand). Congenital or acquired angulation deformity of the hand associated with partial or complete absence of radius or ulna; usually with intrinsic deformities in the hand in congenital variants.

radial c., c. with angular deviation towards radial side of limb. SEE *manus* valga.

ulnar c., c. with angular deviation toward ulnar side of limb. SEE *manus* vara.

clump (klŭmp). To form into clusters, small aggregations, or groups. [A.S. *clympre,* a lump]

clump·ing (klŭmp-ing). The massing together of bacteria or other cells suspended in a fluid.

clu·ne·al (klū′nē-ăl). Pertaining to the clunes.

clu·nes (klū′nēz) [NA]. SYN buttocks. [pl. of L. *clunis,* buttock]

clu·pan·o·don·ic ac·id (klū-pan′ō-don′ik). all-cis-7,10,13,16,19-docosapentaenoic acid; an ω-3 fatty acid with 22 carbons and five double bonds; found in fish oils and phospholipids in brain.

clus·ter of dif·fer·en·ti·a·tion (CD). Cell membrane molecules that are used to classify leukocytes into subsets. CD molecules are classified by monoclonal antibodies.

c. of d. 2 (CD2), a glycoprotein that is expressed on all peripheral T cells, large granular lymphocytes and most, but not all, thymocytes. CD2 is involved in signal transduction and cell adhesion.

c. of d. 3 (CD3), a complex of 5 polypeptides associated with the T cell receptor and is involved in signal transduction.

c. of d. 4 (CD4), a glycoprotein found on various subsets of T cells, *i.e.,* usually no helper and some T cytotoxic cells.

c. of d. 8 (CD8), membrane glycoprotein found on subsets of T lymphocytes. CD8 is expressed on T cytotoxic cells and T suppressor cells.

clut·ter·ing (klŭt′er-ing). A speech disorder usually occurring in childhood characterized by abnormally rapid rate, disturbed fluency, and erratic rhythm that makes it difficult to understand the speaker.

Clutton, Henry H., British surgeon, 1850–1909. SEE C.'s *joints,* under *joint.*

cly·sis (klī′sis). 1. An infusion of fluid, usually subcutaneously, for therapeutic purposes. 2. Formerly, a fluid enema; later, the

washing out of material from any body space or cavity by fluids. [G. *klysis,* a drenching by a clyster]

△-clysis. Combining form referring to injection or enema. [G. *klysis,* a drenching by a clyster]

clys·ter (klis′ter). An old term for enema. [G. *klystēr,* fr. *klyzō,* fut. *klysō,* to wash out]

C.M. Abbreviation for *Chirurgiae Magister,* Master in Surgery.

△CM- Symbol for carboxymethyl radical.

Cm Symbol for curium.

cM Abbreviation for centimorgan.

cm Abbreviation for centimeter; cm^2 for square centimeter; cm^3 for cubic *centimeter.*

CMA Abbreviation for Certified Medical Assistant.

p-CMB Abbreviation for *p*-chloromercuribenzoate.

cmc Abbreviation for critical micelle *concentration.*

CM-cel·lu·lose. SYN carboxymethyl *cellulose.*

CMG Abbreviation for cystometrogram.

CMI Abbreviation for cell-mediated *immunity.*

CML Abbreviation for cell-mediated lymphocytotoxicity.

CMO Abbreviation for calculated mean *organism.*

CMP Symbol for cytidine 5′-monophosphate (secondarily, for any cytidine monophosphate).

CMT Abbreviation for Certified Medical Transcriptionist. SEE medical transcriptionist.

CMV 1. Abbreviation for controlled mechanical *ventilation;* cytomegalovirus. 2. A cancer drug combination treatment consisting of cisplatin, methotrexate, and vinblastine, used in the treatment of bladder and other malignancies.

cne·mi·al (ne′mē-ăl). Relating to the leg, especially to the shin. [G. *knēmē,* leg]

cne·mis (nē′mis). The shin. [G. *knēmis* (*knēmid-*), a legging]

cni·da, pl. cni·dae (nī′dă, nī′dē). SYN nematocyst. [G. *knidē,* nettle]

cni·do·cyst (nī′dō-sist). SYN nematocyst.

cni·do·sis (nī-dō′sis). Obsolete term for urticaria. [G. *knidōsis,* nettle-rash, fr. *knidē,* a nettle]

Cnid·o·spora (nī-dō-spōr′ă). SYN Microspora. [G. *knidē,* nettle, sea nettle, + *sporos,* seed]

Cni·do·spo·rid·ia (nī′dō-spō-rid′ēă). SYN Microsporida. [G. *knidē,* nettle, sea nettle, + Mod. L., fr. G. *sporos,* seed]

C.N.M. Abbreviation for Certified Nurse Midwife.

CNS 1. Abbreviation for central nervous *system.* 2. Symbol for the thiocyanate radical, CNS⁻ or —CNS.

CO Symbol for *carbon* monoxide.

Co Symbol for cobalt; coccygeal.

^{57}Co. Symbol for cobalt-57.

^{58}Co. Symbol for cobalt-58.

^{60}Co. Symbol for cobalt-60.

△co-. SEE con-.

CoA Abbreviation for coenzyme A.

co·ac·er·vate (kō-as′er-vāt). An aggregate of colloidal particles separated out of an emulsion (coacervation) by the addition of some third component (coacervating agent). [L. *coacervare,* pp. *-atus,* to collect in a mass]

co·ac·er·va·tion (kō-as-er-vā′shŭn). Formation of a coacervate.

co·ad·ap·ta·tion (kō′ad-ap-ta′shŭn). The operation of selection jointly on two or more loci.

co·ag·glu·ti·nin (kō-ă-glū′ti-nin). A substance that per se does not agglutinate an antigen, but does result in agglutination of antigen that is appropriately coated with univalent antibody. SEE ALSO conglutination.

co·ag·u·la (kō-ag′yū-lă). Plural of coagulum.

co·ag·u·la·ble (kō-ag′yū-lă-bl). Capable of being coagulated or clotted.

co·ag·u·lant (kō-ag′yū-lant). 1. An agent that causes, stimulates, or accelerates coagulation, especially with reference to blood. 2. SYN coagulative.

co·ag·u·late (kō-ag′yū-lāt). 1. To convert a fluid or a substance in solution into a solid or gel. **2.** To clot; to curdle; to change from a liquid to a solid or gel. [L. *coagulo,* pp. *-atus,* to curdle]

co·ag·u·la·tion (kō-ag-yū-lā′shŭn). **1.** Clotting; the process of changing from a liquid to a solid, said especially of blood (*i.e.,* blood c.). In vertebrates, blood c. is a result of cascade regulation from fibrin. **2.** A clot or coagulum. **3.** Transformation of a sol into a gel or semisolid mass; *e.g.,* the c. of the white of an egg by means of boiling. In any colloidal suspension, the dispersion of the disperse phase from the continuous phase is greatly reduced, thereby leading to a complete or partial separation of the latter; usually an irreversible phenomenon unless the basic nature of the substance is chemically altered.

disseminated intravascular c. (DIC), a hemorrhagic syndrome which occurs following the uncontrolled activation of clotting factors and fibrinolytic enzymes throughout small blood vessels; fibrin is deposited, platelets and clotting factors are consumed, and fibrin degradation products inhibit fibrin polymerization, resulting in tissue necrosis and bleeding. SEE ALSO consumption *coagulopathy.*

co·ag·u·la·tive (kō-ag′yū-lă-tiv). Causing coagulation. SYN coagulant (2).

co·ag·u·lop·a·thy (kō-ag-yū-lop′ă-thē). A disease affecting the coagulability of the blood.

consumption c., a disorder in which marked reductions develop in blood concentrations of platelets with exhaustion of the coagulation factors in the peripheral blood as a result of disseminated intravascular coagulation.

co·ag·u·lum, pl. **co·ag·u·la** (kō-ag′yū-lŭm, -lă). A clot or a curd; a soft, nonrigid, insoluble mass formed when a sol undergoes coagulation. [L. a means of coagulating, rennet]

co·a·les·cence (kō-ă-les′ens). Fusion of originally separate parts. SYN concrescence (1).

coal oil (kōl). SYN petroleum.

coal tar. A by-product obtained during the destructive distillation of bituminous coal; a very dark semisolid of characteristic naphthalene-like odor and a sharp, burning taste; used in the treatment of skin diseases.

co·apt (kō′apt). To join or fit together.

co·ap·ta·tion (kō-ap-tā′shŭn). Joining or fitting together of two surfaces; *e.g.,* the lips of a wound or the ends of a broken bone. [L. *co-apto,* pp. *-aptatus,* to fit together]

co·arct (kō-arkt′). To restrict or press together. SYN coarctate (1). [L. *co-arcto,* pp. *-arctatus,* to press together]

co·arc·tate (kō-ark′tāt). **1.** SYN coarct. **2.** Pressed together.

co·arc·ta·tion (kō-ark-tā′shŭn). A constriction, stricture, or stenosis, usually of the aorta.

reversed c., aortic arch syndrome in which blood pressure in the arms is lower than in the legs.

co·arc·tec·to·my (kō′ark-tek′tō-mē). Excision of a coarctation (of the aorta).

co·arc·tot·o·my (kō-ark-tot′ō-mē). Division of a stricture. [coarct + G. *tomē,* cutting]

△**CoAS-, CoASH.** Symbols for the coenzyme A radical and reduced coenzyme A, respectively.

coat (kōt). **1.** The outer covering or envelope of an organ or part. **2.** One of the layers of membranous or other tissues forming the wall of a canal or hollow organ. SEE tunic.

buffy c., the upper, lighter portion of the blood clot (coagulated plasma and white blood cells), occurring when coagulation is delayed so that the red blood cells have had time to settle; the portion of centrifuged, anticoagulated blood which contains leukocytes and platelets. SYN crusta inflammatoria, crusta phlogistica, leukocyte cream.

muscular c., the muscular, usually middle, layer of a tubular structure; for most of the gastrointestinal tract, it consists of an outer longitudinal layer of muscle and an inner circular layer. SYN tunica muscularis [NA].

muscular c. of bronchi, muscular layer of the bronchial wall. SYN tunica muscularis bronchiorum [NA].

muscular c. of colon, muscular layer of the wall of the colon. SYN tunica muscularis coli [NA].

muscular c. of ductus deferens, muscular layer of the wall of

the ductus deferens. SYN tunica muscularis ductus deferentis [NA].

muscular c. of esophagus, muscular layer of the esophageal wall. SYN tunica muscularis esophagi [NA].

muscular c. of female urethra, muscular layer of the wall of the female urethra. SYN tunica muscularis urethrae femininae [NA].

muscular c. of gallbladder, muscular layer of the wall of the gallbladder. SYN tunica muscularis vesicae biliaris [NA], tunica muscularis vesicae felleae ☆ [NA].

muscular c. of pharynx, muscular layer of the pharyngeal wall. In contrast with the muscular coats of the rest of the gastrointestinal tract (except anal canal), that of the pharynx has an outer circular layer and an inner longitudinal layer. SYN tunica muscularis pharyngis [NA].

muscular c. of rectum, muscular layer of the wall of the rectum. SYN tunica muscularis recti [NA].

muscular c. of small intestine, muscular layer of the wall of the small intestine. SYN tunica muscularis intestini tenuis [NA].

muscular c. of stomach, muscular tunic of the stomach, consisting of smooth muscles arranged in three fairly well defined layers: an *outer longitudinal layer,* continuous with that of the esophagus but dividing at the cardia into two bands which run

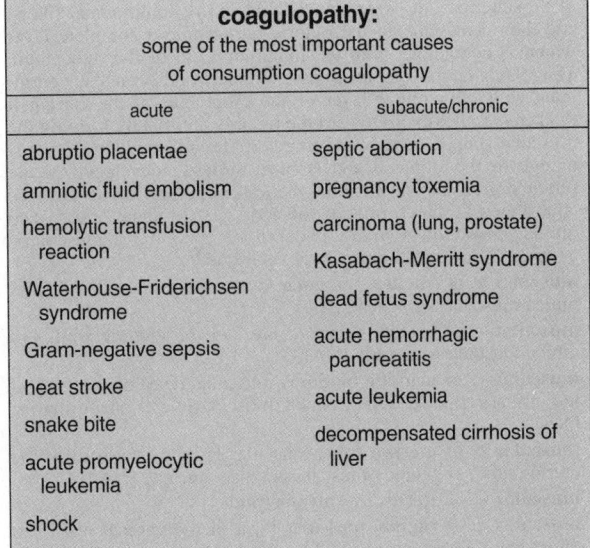

coagulopathy:
some of the most important causes
of consumption coagulopathy

acute	subacute/chronic
abruptio placentae	septic abortion
amniotic fluid embolism	pregnancy toxemia
hemolytic transfusion reaction	carcinoma (lung, prostate)
	Kasabach-Merritt syndrome
Waterhouse-Friderichsen syndrome	dead fetus syndrome
Gram-negative sepsis	acute hemorrhagic pancreatitis
heat stroke	acute leukemia
snake bite	decompensated cirrhosis of liver
acute promyelocytic leukemia	
shock	
purpura fulminans	

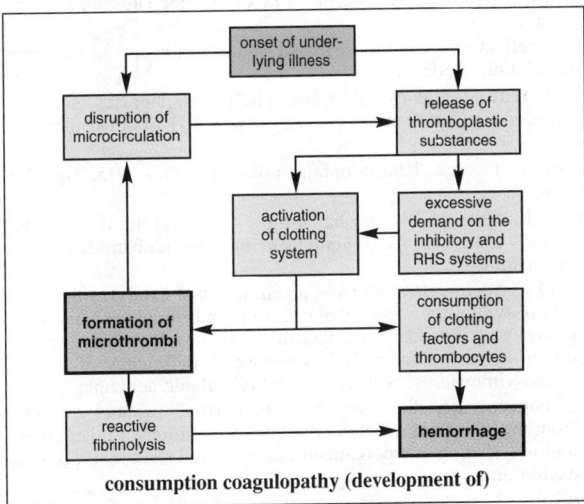

consumption coagulopathy (development of)

along the greater and lesser curvatures, leaving the middle areas of the anterior and posterior walls devoid of longitudinal fibers, and then coalescing in the pyloric region into a complete layer which is continuous with the longitudinal c. of the duodenum. The *middle circular layer* is most complete and strongest, continuous with the circular layer of the esophagus at the cardia; it thickens progressively toward the pylorus, ultimately forming the muscular ring of the pyloric sphincter. The *inner, oblique layer* is unique to the stomach and is most strongly developed in the fundic region and absent along the lesser curvature. This absence contributes to the formation of the "gastric canal." SEE ALSO oblique *fibers* of stomach, under *fiber*. SYN tunica muscularis gastrica [NA], tunica muscularis ventriculi ⋆.

muscular c. of trachea, muscular layer of the tracheal wall. SYN tunica muscularis tracheae [NA].

muscular c. of ureter, muscular layer of the ureteric wall. SYN tunica muscularis ureteris [NA].

muscular c. of urinary bladder, muscular layer of the wall of the urinary bladder. SYN tunica muscularis vesicae urinariae [NA].

muscular c. of uterine tube, muscular layer of the wall of the uterine tube. SYN tunica muscularis tubae uterinae [NA].

muscular c. of uterus, SYN myometrium.

muscular c. of vagina, muscular layer of the vaginal wall. SYN tunica muscularis vaginae [NA].

sclerotic c., SYN sclera.

serous c., SYN serosa.

coat·ing (kōt′ing). A covering; a layer of some substance spread over a surface.

antireflection c., a film of magnesium fluoride spread on a lens to minimize reflections.

CoA trans·fer·as·es [EC Class 2.8.3]. thiaphorases; enzymes transferring CoA from acetyl-CoA or succinyl-CoA to other acyl radicals.

Coats, George, British ophthalmologist, 1876–1915. SEE C.'s *disease*.

co·bal·a·min (Cbl) (kō-bal′ă-min). General term for compounds containing the dimethylbenzimidazolylcobamide nucleus of vitamin B$_{12}$.

ATP c. adenoxyltransferase, an enzyme that catalyzes the reaction of ATP, water, and cobalamin to form orthophosphate, pyrophosphate, and adenoxylcobalamin. Adenosylcobalamin is required by methylmalonyl-CoA mutase. A deficiency of ATP c. adenosyltransferase will lead to methylmalonic acidemia.

c. concentrate, the dried, partially purified product resulting from the growth of selected *Streptomyces* cultures or other cobalamin-producing microorganisms; contains at least 500 μg of c. in each gram.

co·balt (Co) (kō′bawlt). A steel-gray metallic element, atomic no. 27, atomic wt. 58.93320; a bioelement and a constituent of vitamin B$_{12}$; certain of its compounds are pigments, *e.g.,* c. blue. [Ger. *kobalt,* goblin or evil spirit]

co·balt-57 (^{57}Co). Half-life, 271.8 days; decays by electron capture with emission of a medium energy (122.06 keV) gamma ray. Used as a diagnostic aid with some metabolic disorders.

co·balt-58 (^{58}Co). Positron emitter with half-life of 70.88 days.

co·balt-60 (^{60}Co). Half-life, 5.271 years; emits beta particles and energetic gamma rays, for which reason it is used in radiation therapy and diagnostics in place of radium (radon) or x-rays. It is also used as a diagnostic aid in vitamin B$_{12}$-related problems.

co·bal·tous chlo·ride (kō-bawl′tŭs). CoCl$_2$·6H$_2$0; used in the treatment of various types of refractory anemia to improve the hematocrit, hemoglobin, and erythrocyte count.

Cobb, Stanley, U.S. neuropathologist, *1887. SEE C. *syndrome*.

co·bra (kō′bră). Members of the highly venomous snake genus, *Naja* (family Elapidae); six species are recognized, all African except for the Asiatic c.; typical behavior includes spreading of the neck (hood), rearing one-third of the body off of the ground, and, in some species, the spitting of venom, which is primarily neurotoxic. [Port. snake, from L. *coluber,* snake]

co·bro·tox·in (kō′brō-tok-sin). A polypeptide of 62 residues; action on cells is similar to that of melittin in that it promotes disruption of membranes; used as an investigational antirheumatic agent. SYN cobra toxin, direct lytic factor of cobra venom.

co·byr·ic ac·id (kō-bir′ik). The hexa-amide of cobyrinic acid; a part of the vitamin B$_{12}$ structure. SYN cobyrinamide, cobyrinic hexa-amide, factor V$_{1a}$.

co·byr·in·a·mide (kō-bir-in′ă-mīd). SYN cobyric acid.

co·byr·in·ic ac·id (kō-bir-in′ik). Corrin with 8 methyl groups at positions 1, 2, 5, 7, 12 (2), 15, 17; —CH$_2$COOH groups at positions 2, 7, 18; —CH$_2$CH$_2$COOH groups at positions 3, 8, 13, 17; and divalent cobalt centered among the four nitrogens. The acid side-chains are designated, in numerical order, *a, b, c, d, e, f, g.* It is a part of the vitamin B$_{12}$ structure.

co·byr·in·ic hex·a·am·ide. SYN cobyric acid.

COC Abbreviation for cathodal opening *contraction*.

co·ca (kō′kă). The dried leaves of *Erythroxylon coca,* yielding not less than 0.5% of ether-soluble alkaloids; the source of cocaine and several other alkaloids. [S. Am.]

co·caine (kō-kān′). Benzoylmethylecgonine; an alkaloid obtained from the leaves of *Erythroxylon coca* (family Erythroxylaceae) and other species of *Erythroxylon,* or by synthesis from ecgonine or its derivatives; it has moderate vasoconstrictor activity and pronounced psychotropic effects; its salts are used as a topical anesthetic.

crack c., a highly potent, smokable form of c. SEE street *drug*.

Within 10 seconds of being smoked, it provides a dramatic high lasting 3–5 minutes, and afterwards an intense craving for the drug arises in the user. Dependency can develop in less than 2 weeks. This ready-to-smoke freebase is manufactured from powdered cocaine, which is heated with water in a glass tube. Once the mixture cools, baking soda and cold water are added, and the resulting product hardened and broken into pieces. It is sometimes called "rock" or "ready rock" (although normally, rock is a hydrochloride product which is snorted). It is also sold in ridged lengths called "french fries" or "teeth." Like snorted or injected cocaine, it has both acute and chronic complications, including heart and nasopharyngeal damage, seizures, and sudden death, and fosters an assortment of mental problems, including cocaine psychosis. Street use of crack exploded upon its introduction in the 1980s, and accounted for rises in emergency room admissions for cocaine overdose and in births of cocaine dependant babies.

co·cain·i·za·tion (kō′kān-i-zā′shŭn). Production of topical anesthesia of mucous membranes by the application of cocaine.

co·car·box·yl·ase (kō-kar-boks′i-lās). SYN *thiamin* pyrophosphate.

co·car·cin·o·gen (kō-kar′si-nō-jen). A substance that works symbiotically with a carcinogen in the production of cancer.

Coc·ca·ce·ae (kok-kā′sē-ē). An obsolete term for a family of Eubacteriales which included all the spherical cells dividing in one (*Streptococcus*), two (*Micrococcus*), or three (*Sarcina*) planes, then forming cells, pairs, tetrads, cubes or larger packets, or chains. [G. *kokkos,* a berry]

coc·cal (kok′ăl). Relating to cocci.

coc·ci (kok′sī). Plural of coccus.

Coc·cid·ia (kok-sid′ē-ă). A subclass of important protozoa (class Sporozoea, phylum Apicomplexa) in which the mature trophozoites are small and typically intracellular; schizogony and sporogony can occur in the same host, in contrast to the gregarines (subclass Gregarinia of class Sporozoea), which have large extracellular trophozoites in various invertebrates and do not reproduce by schizogony. SYN Coccidiasina. [Mod. L., fr. G. *kokkos,* berry]

coccidia of cattle, SYN *Eimeria* of cattle.

coccidia of chickens, SYN *Eimeria* of chickens.

coccidia of geese, SYN *Eimeria* of geese.

coccidia of pheasants, SYN *Eimeria* of pheasants.

coccidia of rabbits, SYN *Eimeria* of rabbits.

coccidia of sheep and goats, SYN *Eimeria* of sheep and goats.

coccidia of swine, SYN *Eimeria* of swine.

coccidia of turkeys, SYN *Eimeria* of turkeys.

coc·cid·ia (kok-sid′ē-ă). Plural of coccidium.

coc·cid·i·al (kok-sid′ē-ăl). Relating to coccidia.

Coc·ci·di·as·i·na (kok-sid′ē-ā-sī′nă). SYN Coccidia.

coc·cid·i·oi·dal (kok-sid-ē-oy′dăl). Referring to the disease or to the infecting organism of coccidioidomycosis.

Coc·cid·i·oi·des (kok-sid-ē-oy′dēz). A genus of fungi found in the soil of the semi-arid areas of the Southwestern U.S. and smaller areas throughout Central and South America, but has not been found elsewhere. The only pathogenic species, *C. immitis,* causes coccidioidomycosis. [coccidium + G. *eidos,* resemblance]

coc·cid·i·oi·din (kok-sid-ē-oy′din). A sterile solution containing the by-products of growth of *Coccidioides immitis;* used as an intracutaneous skin test, diagnostically more valuable in non-endemic areas.

coc·cid·i·oi·do·ma (kok-sid′ē-oy-dō′mă). A benign localized residual granulomatous lesion or scar in a lung following primary coccidioidomycosis.

coc·cid·i·oi·do·my·co·sis (kok-sid-ē-oy′dō-mī-kō′sis). A variable, benign, severe, or fatal systemic mycosis due to inhalation of dust particles containing arthroconidia of *Coccidioides immitis.* In benign forms of the infection, the lesions are limited to the upper respiratory tract and lungs; in a low percentage of cases, the disease disseminates to other visceral organs, bones, joints, and skin and subcutaneous tissues. SYN Posadas disease. [coccidioides + G. *mykēs,* fungus, + *-osis,* condition]

asymptomatic c., SYN latent c.

disseminate c., a severe, chronic, and progressive form of c. resulting from rapid dissemination of endospores from the primary site of infection, or from reinfection in a previously sensitized patient, with widespread involvement of the central nervous system, bones, skin, and viscera.

latent c., a form of c. not differentiated clinically from upper respiratory infections of viral or bacterial etiology; positive skin tests are useful in demonstrating past and present infections; tests for circulating serum antibodies are prognostic as well as diagnostic in some cases. SYN asymptomatic c.

primary c., a disease common in the San Joaquin Valley of California and certain additional areas in the southwestern U.S. as well as the Chaco region of Argentina, caused by inhalation of the arthroconidia of *Coccidioides immitis;* acute onset of symptoms resemble pneumonia or pulmonary tuberculosis, productive of sputum usually containing spores of the fungus, and accompanied by aches, malaise, severe headache, and occasionally an early erythematous or papular eruption; erythema multiforme or erythema nodosum may appear; the coccidioidin test is positive. SYN desert fever, San Joaquin fever, San Joaquin Valley disease, San Joaquin Valley fever, valley fever.

primary extrapulmonary c., a rare form of c. presenting near the site of local trauma with painless firm nodules occurring at one to two weeks, accompanied by regional adenopathy, with spontaneous healing in a few weeks.

secondary c., progressive or disseminated extrapulmonary granulomatous lesions following primary c. SYN coccidioidal granuloma.

coc·cid·i·o·sis (kok-sid-ē-ō′sis). Group name for diseases due to any species of coccidia; a common and serious protozoan disease of many species of domestic animals and birds and many wild animals kept in captivity; both intestinal and pulmonary c. have been reported in human individuals with AIDS.

coc·cid·i·o·stat (kok-sid′ē-ō-stat). A chemical agent generally added to animal feed to partially inhibit or delay the development of coccidiosis.

coc·cid·i·um, pl. **coc·cid·ia** (kok-sid′ē-ŭm, -ē-ă). Common name given to protozoan parasites (order Eucoccidiida) in which schizogony occurs within epithelial cells, generally in the intestine, but in some species in the bile ducts and kidney; the final product of sexual fusion and differentiation that occurs within the host, the oocyst, generally passes to the soil in the feces, undergoes sporulation, and then acts as the infective form for

another host. Coccidia are parasitic in most domestic and wild birds and mammals, occasionally in man, and are highly host-specific; the majority are nonpathogenic, but certain species rank among the most serious and economically important pathogens, causing coccidiosis in birds and mammals. SEE *Eimeria, Isospora.* [Mod. L. dim. of G. *kokkos,* berry]

coc·ci·nel·la (kok-sin-el′ă). SYN cochineal.

coc·ci·nel·lin (kok-si-nel′in). The coloring principle derived from cochineal.

coc·co·bac·il·lary (kok′ō-bas′i-lār-ē). Relating to a coccobacillus.

coc·co·ba·cil·lus (kok′ō-bă-sil′ŭs). A short, thick bacterial rod of the shape of an oval or slightly elongated coccus. [G. *kokkos,* berry]

coc·coid (kok′oyd). Resembling a coccus. [G. *kokkos,* berry, + *eidos,* resemblance]

coc·cu·lin (kok′yū-lin). SYN picrotoxin.

coc·cus, pl. **coc·ci** (kok′ŭs, kok′sī). **1.** A bacterium of round, spheroidal, or ovoid form. **2.** SYN cochineal. [G. *kokkos,* berry]

Neisser's c., SYN *Neisseria gonorrhoeae.*

Weichselbaum's c., SYN *Neisseria meningitidis.*

coc·cy·al·gia (kok-sē-al′jē-ă). SYN coccygodynia. [coccyx + G. *algos,* pain]

coc·cy·ceph·a·ly (kok′si-sef′ă-lē). A malformation in which the cephalic profile suggests a beak. [G. *kokkyx,* cuckoo, + kephalē, head]

coc·cy·dyn·ia (kok-sē-din′ē-ă). SYN coccygodynia. [coccyx + G. *ōdyne, pain*]

coc·cy·gal·gia (kok-sē-gal′jē-ă). SYN coccygodynia. [coccyx + G. *algos,* pain]

coc·cyg·e·al (Co) (kok-sij′ē-ăl). Relating to the coccyx.

coc·cy·gec·to·my (kok-sē-jek′tō-mē). Removal of the coccyx. [coccyx + G. *ektomē,* excision]

coc·cyg·e·us. SEE coccygeus *muscle.*

coc·cy·go·dyn·ia (kok′si-gō-din′ē-ă). Coccyodynia pain in the coccygeal region. SYN coccyalgia, coccydynia, coccygalgia, coccyodynia. [coccyx + G. *odynē,* pain]

coc·cy·got·o·my (kok-sē-got′ō-mē). Operation for freeing the coccyx from its attachments. [coccyx + G. *tomē,* a cutting]

coc·cy·o·dyn·ia (kok′sē-ō-din′ē-ă). SYN coccygodynia.

coc·cyx, gen. **coc·cy·gis,** pl. **coc·cy·ges** (kok′siks, -si-jis, -si-jēs). The small bone at the end of the vertebral column in man, formed by the fusion of four rudimentary vertebrae; it articulates above with the sacrum. SYN os coccygis [NA], coccygeal bone, tail bone. [G. *kokkyx,* a cuckoo, the coccyx]

coch·i·neal (kotch′i-nēl) [C.I. 75470]. The dried female insects, *Coccus cacti,* enclosing the young larvae, or the dried female insect, *Dactylopius coccus,* containing eggs and larvae, from which coccinellin is obtained; used as a red coloring agent and a stain. SEE carmine. SYN coccinella, coccus (2). [O.Sp. *cochinilla,* wood louse, fr. G. *kokkinos,* berry]

co·chlea, pl. **co·chle·ae** (kok′lē-ă, lē-ē) [NA]. A cone-shaped cavity in the petrous portion of the temporal bone, forming one of the divisions of the labyrinth or internal ear. It consists of a spiral canal making two and a half turns around a central core of spongy bone, the modiolus; this spiral canal of the cochlea contains the membranous cochlea, or cochlear duct, in which is the spiral organ (Corti). [L. snail shell]

membranous c., SYN cochlear *duct.*

co·chle·ar (kok′lē-ăr). Relating to the cochlea.

co·chle·a·re (kō-klē′ă, kok-lē-ā′rē). A spoon. [L.]

c. am′plum, a tablespoonful. [L.]

c. mag′num, a tablespoonful. [L.]

c. me′dium, a dessertspoonful. [L.]

c. mod′icum, a dessertspoonful. [L.]

c. par′vum, a teaspoonful. [L.]

co·chle·ar·i·form (kok-lē-ar′i-fōrm). Spoon-shaped. [L. *cochleare,* spoon, + *forma,* form]

co·chle·ate (kok′lē-āt). **1.** Resembling a snail shell. **2.** Denoting the appearance of a form of plate culture. [L. *cochlea*, a snail shell]

co·chle·o·sac·cu·lot·o·my (kok'lē-ō-sac-yū-lot'ō-mē). An operation for Ménière's disease performed through the round window to create a shunt between the cochlear duct and the saccule.

co·chle·o·ves·tib·u·lar (kok'lē-ō-ves-tib'yū-lăr). Relating to the cochlea and the vestibule of the ear.

Co·chli·o·my·ia (kok'lē-ō-mī'yă). A genus of fleshflies (family Calliphoridae) whose larvae develop in decaying flesh or carrion or in wounds or sores.

C. american'a, incorrect name for *C. hominivorax*.

C. homini'vorax, the screw-worm fly, a species that is a serious pest of livestock from Mexico to Argentina and is the primary cause of myiasis in the western hemisphere; attracted by fresh blood, it deposits eggs on wounds, tick bites, or intact moist areas of the body, and the larvae invade living tissues, causing severe myiasis and often death; it is known to attack man, especially in the nose, although wounds, eyes, and other body openings have also been attacked.

C. macella'ria, the secondary screw-worm fly, a species attracted to decaying flesh (formerly used as surgical maggots); primarily a scavenger, but not implicated in primary myiasis as is *C. hominivorax*, though it may be a secondary wound invader in domestic animals in the Americas.

co·cil·la·na (ko'sĕ-lah'nă). The dried bark of *Guarea rusbyi*, a Bolivia tree, used as an expectorant in bronchitis.

Cockayne, Edward A., British physician, 1880–1956. SEE C.'s *disease, syndrome*; Weber-C. *syndrome*.

cock·tail (kok'tāl). A mixture that includes several ingredients or drugs.

Brompton c., a c. of morphine and cocaine usually used for analgesia in terminal cancer patients; the formulations vary, but typically it contains 15 mg of morphine hydrochloride and 10 mg of cocaine hydrochloride per 10 ml of the c. [*Brompton* Chest Hospital, London, England, where developed]

Philadelphia c., SYN Rivers' c.

Rivers' c., an intravenous slow injection of from 1000 to 2000 ml of 10% dextrose in isotonic saline to which thiamine hydrochloride and 25 units of insulin are added; used in acute alcoholism. SYN Philadelphia c.

COCl Abbreviation for cathodal opening *clonus*.

co·coa (kō'kō). A powder prepared from the roasted kernels of *Theobroma cacao* (family Sterculiaceae); used in the preparation of c. syrup, a flavoring agent. SEE ALSO cacao.

co·con·scious·ness (kō-kon'shŭs-nes). A splitting of consciousness into two streams.

co·con·ver·sion (kō'kon-ver'shŭn). The simultaneous correction of two sites on DNA during gene conversion.

cocto-. Prefix indicating boiled or modified by heat. [L. *coctus*, cooked]

coc·to·la·bile (kok-tō-lā'bil, -bīl). Subject to alteration or destruction when exposed to the temperature of boiling water.

coc·to·sta·bile, coc·to·sta·ble (kok-tō-stā'bil, -bīl; -stā'bl). Resisting the temperature of boiling water without alteration or destruction.

cod (kod). **1.** The fat-filled scrotum of a castrated bovine animal. **2.** A common marine fish (family Gadidae) related to the haddock and pollack.

code (kōd). **1.** A set of rules, principles, or ethics. **2.** Any system devised to convey information or facilitate communication. **3.** Term used in hospitals to describe an emergency requiring situation trained members of the staff, such as a cardiopulmonary resuscitation team, or the signal to summon such a team. **4.** A numerical system for ordering and classifying information, *e.g.*, about diagnostic categories. [L. *codex*, book]

genetic c., the genetic information carried by the specific DNA molecules of the chromosomes; specifically, the system whereby particular combinations of three consecutive nucleotides in a DNA molecule control the insertion of one particular amino acid in equivalent places in a protein molecule. The genetic c. is almost universal throughout the prokaryotic, plant, and animal kingdoms. There are two known exceptions. In ciliated protozo-

ans, the triplets AGA and AGG are read as termination signals instead of as L-arginine. This is also true of the mitochondrial c., which, in addition, uses AUA as a code for L-methionine (instead of isoleucine) and UGA for L-tryptophan (instead of a termination signal).

genetic code					
1. Position	2. Position				3. Position
	U(A)	C(G)	A(T)	G(C)	
U(A)	Phe	Ser	Tyr	Cys	U(A)
	Phe	Ser	Tyr	Cys	C(G)
	Leu	Ser	End	End	A(T)
	Leu	Ser	End	Trp	G(C)
C(G)	Leu	Pro	His	Arg	U(A)
	Leu	Pro	His	Arg	C(G)
	Leu	Pro	Gln	Arg	A(T)
	Leu	Pro	Gln	Arg	G(C)
A(T)	Ile	Thr	Asn	Ser	U(A)
	Ile	Thr	Asn	Ser	C(G)
	Ile	Thr	Lys	Arg	A(T)
	Met	Thr	Lys	Arg	G(C)
G(C)	Val	Ala	Asp	Gly	U(A)
	Val	Ala	Asp	Gly	C(G)
	Val	Ala	Glu	Gly	A(T)
	Val	Ala	Glu	Gly	G(C)

The so-called "code lexicon": it shows the relationship of mRNA codons (in parentheses after the DNA) to the coded amino acids. The triplets are arranged according to nucleic acid bases (A=adenine; C=cytosine; G=guanine; T=thymine; U=uracil; "end" indicates the termination of the codon). The three shadings indicate whether the amino acids are hydrophobic (green), hydrophilic (blue), or ambiphilic (pink).

soundex c., a sequence of letters used for recording names phonetically, especially in record linkage.

co·de·car·box·yl·ase (kō'dē-kar-boks'i-lās). SYN *pyridoxal 5'-phosphate*.

co·de·hy·dro·gen·ase I, co·de·hy·dro·gen·ase II (kō'dē-hī-droj'ĕ-nās). Obsolete names for nicotinamide adenine dinucleotide and nicotinamide adenine dinucleotide phosphate, respectively.

co·deine (kō'dēn). morphine monomethyl morphine 3-methyl ether; obtained from opium, which contains 0.7 to 2.5%, but usually made from morphine. Used as an analgesic and antitussive; drug dependence (physical and psychic) may develop, but c. is less liable to produce addiction than is morphine. SYN methylmorphine. [G. *kōdeia*, head, poppy head]

Co·dex med·i·ca·men·tar·i·us (kō'deks med'i-kă-men-tār'ē-ŭs). The official title of the French Pharmacopeia. [L. a book pertaining to drugs]

cod·ing. Translation of information, *e.g.*, diagnoses, questionnaire responses, into numbered categories for entry into a data processing system.

cod liv·er oil. The partially destearinated fixed oil extracted from the fresh livers of *Gadus morrhuae* and other species of the family Gadidae, containing vitamins A and D; used as a supplementary source of vitamins A and D.

Codman, Ernest Amory, U.S. surgeon, 1869–1940. SEE C.'s *sign, triangle, tumor.*

co·do·gen·ic (kō-dō-jen-ik). Formed by a code; specifically, the genetic code.

co·dom·i·nant (kō-dom′i-nant). In genetics, denoting an equal degree of dominance of two genes, both being expressed in the phenotype of the individual; *e.g.,* genes A and B of the ABO blood group are codominant; individuals with both are type AB.

co·don (kō′don). A set of three consecutive nucleotides in a strand of DNA or RNA that provides the genetic information to code for a specific amino acid which will be incorporated into a protein chain or serve as a termination signal. SYN triplet (3). [code + -on]

amber c., the termination codon UAG.

initiating c., the trinucleotide AUG (or sometimes GUG) that codes for the first amino acid in protein sequences, formylmethionine; the latter is often removed post-transcriptionally. SYN start c.

initiation c., a specific mRNA sequence (usually AUG, but sometimes GUG) that is the signal for the addition of fMet-tRNA and the beginning of translation.

nonsense c., SYN termination c.

ochre c., the termination c. UAA.

opal c., SYN umber c.

punctuation c., SYN termination c.

start c., SYN initiating c.

stop c., SYN termination c.

termination c., trinucleotide sequence (UAA, UGA, or UAG) that specifies the end of translation or transcription. Cf. amber c., ochre c., umber c. SYN nonsense c., punctuation c., stop c., termination sequence.

umber c., the termination c. UGA. SYN opal c.

△**coe-.** For words so beginning, and not found here, see ce-.

co·ef·fi·cient (kō-ě-fish′ěnt). **1.** The expression of the amount or degree of any quality possessed by a substance, or of the degree of physical or chemical change normally occurring in that substance under stated conditions. **2.** The ratio or factor that relates a quantity observed under one set of conditions to that observed under standard conditions, usually when all variables are either 1 or a simple power of 10. [L. *co-* + *efficio* (*exfacio*), to accomplish]

absorption c., (1) the milliliters of a gas at standard temperature and pressure that will saturate 100 ml of liquid; (2) the amount of light absorbed in passing through 1 cm of a 1 molar solution of a given substance, expressed as a constant in Beer-Lambert law; Cf. specific absorption c. (3) in x-ray, a measure of the rate of decrease of intensity of a beam in its passage through a substance, resulting from a combination of scattering and conversion to other forms of energy.

activity c. (γ), SEE activity (2).

biological c., rarely used term denoting the energy expended by the body at rest.

Bunsen's solubility c. (α), the milliliters of gas STPD dissolved per milliliter of liquid and per atmosphere (760 mm Hg) partial pressure of the gas at any given temperature.

c. of consanguinity, SYN c. of inbreeding.

correlation c., a measure of association that indicates the degree to which two variables have a linear relationship; this c., represented by the letter r, can vary between +1 and −1; when r = +1, there is a perfect positive linear relationship in which one variable relates directly with the other; when r = −1, there is a perfect negative linear relationship between the variables.

creatinine c., the number of milligrams of creatinine excreted daily per kilogram of body weight.

diffusion c., the mass of material diffusing across a unit area in unit time under a concentration gradient of unity. SYN diffusion constant.

distribution c., the ratio of concentrations of a substance in two immiscible phases at equilibrium; the basis of many chromatographic separation procedures. SYN partition c.

economic c., in growth and cultivation of microorganisms, the ratio of the mass produced to the substrate consumed.

extinction c. (ε), SYN specific absorption c.

extraction c., the percentage of a substance removed from the blood or plasma in a single passage through a tissue; *e.g.,* the extraction c. for *p*-aminohippuric acid (PAH) in the kidney is the difference between arterial and renal venous plasma PAH concentrations, divided by the arterial plasma PAH concentration.

filtration c., a measure of a membrane's permeability to water; specifically, the volume of fluid filtered in unit time through a unit area of membrane per unit pressure difference, taking into account both hydraulic and osmotic pressures.

Hill c., the slope of the line in a Hill plot; a measure of the degree of cooperativity. SYN Hill constant.

hygienic laboratory c., SYN Rideal-Walker c.

c. of inbreeding, the probability that the individual concerned is homozygous by descent at an autosomal locus picked at random; equal to the c. of kinship of the parents. SYN c. of consanguinity.

isotonic c., the amount of salts in the blood plasma, or the amount that should be added to distilled water in order to prepare an isotonic solution.

c. of kinship, the probability that two genes at the same locus, picked at random from each of two individuals, are identical by descent.

lethal c., that concentration of disinfectant that kills bacteria at 20–25°C in the shortest period of time.

linear absorption c., that fraction of ionizing radiation absorbed in a unit thickness of a substance or tissue. SEE ALSO absorption c. (3).

Long's c., SYN Long's *formula.*

molar absorption c. (ε), absorbance (of light) per unit path length (usually the centimeter) and per unit of concentration (moles per liter); a fundamental unit in spectrophotometry. SYN absorbancy index (2), absorptivity (2), molar absorbancy index, molar absorptivity, molar extinction c.

molar extinction c., SYN molar absorption c.

Ostwald's solubility c. (Λ), the milliliters of gas dissolved per milliliter of liquid and per atmosphere (760 mm of Hg) partial pressure of the gas at any given temperature. This differs from Bunsen's solubility c. (α) in that the amount of dissolved gas is expressed in terms of its volume at the temperature of the experiment, instead of STPD. Thus, λ = α (1 + 0.00367t), where t = temperature in degrees Celsius.

oxygen utilization c., the extraction c. for oxygen in any given tissue.

partition c., SYN distribution c.

permeability c., a c. associated with simple diffusion through a membrane that is proportional to the partition coefficient and the diffusion coefficient and inversely proportional to membrane thickness.

phenol c., SYN Rideal-Walker c.

Poiseuille's viscosity c., an expression of the viscosity as determined by the capillary tube method; the coefficient η = $(\pi P r^4/8vl)$, where P is the pressure difference between the inlet and outlet of the tube, r the radius of the tube, l its length, and v the volume of liquid delivered in the time t. If volume is in cm³, time is in seconds, and l and r are in cm, then n will be in poise.

reflection c. (σ), a measure of the relative permeability of a

---

△ **Combining forms**   [NA] Nomina Anatomica

Word*Finder*   [MIM] Mendelian Inheritance in Man
Multi-term entry finder
Preceding letter A
A.D.A.M. Anatomy Plates   ☆ Official alternate term
Between letters L and M
   ☆[NA] Official alternate
Appendices: Nomina Anatomica term
Following letter Z

SYN Synonym; Cf., compare   **High Profile Term**

particular membrane to a particular solute; calculated as the ratio of observed osmotic pressure to that calculated from van't Hoff's law; also equal to 1 minus the ratio of the effective pore areas available to solute and to solvent.

c. of relationship, the probability that a gene present in one mate is also present in the other and is derived from the same source.

reliability c., an index of the consistency of measurement often based on the correlation between scores obtained on the initial test and a retest (test-retest reliability) or between scores on two similar forms of the same test (equivalent-form reliability).

respiratory c., SYN respiratory *quotient.*

Rideal-Walker c., a figure expressing the disinfecting power of any substance; it is obtained by dividing the figure indicating the degree of dilution of the disinfectant that kills a microorganism in a given time by that indicating the degree of dilution of phenol which kills the organism in the same space of time under similar conditions. SYN hygienic laboratory c., phenol c.

sedimentation c. (s), SYN sedimentation *constant.*

selection c. (s), the proportion of progeny or potential progeny not surviving to sexual maturity; usually defined artificially by expressing the fitness of a phenotype as a fraction of the mean or optimal fitness to give the relative fitness, and subtracting this fraction from unity. If the mean size of family in the population is 3.2 and that for a particular genotype is 2.4 then the fitness of the phenotype is $2.4/3.2 = 0.75$ and the selection coefficient $= 1 - 0.75 = .25 = 5$

specific absorption c. (a), absorbance (of light) per unit path length (usually the centimeter) and per unit of mass concentration. Cf. molar absorption c. SYN absorbancy index (1), absorptivity (1), extinction c., specific extinction.

temperature c., the fractional change in any physical property per degree rise in temperature.

ultrafiltration c., the filtration c. of a semipermeable membrane.

c. of variation (CV), the ratio of the standard deviation to the mean.

velocity c., the rate of transformation of a unit mass of substance in a chemical reaction.

c. of viscosity, the value of the force per unit area required to maintain a unit relative velocity between two parallel planes a unit distance apart.

Coe·len·ter·a·ta (sē-len-tĕ-rā'tă). One of the major phyla of invertebrates, to which such forms as jellyfish belong.

coe·len·ter·ate (sē-len'ter-at). Common name for members of the Coelenterata.

coe·lom (sē'lom). SYN body *cavity.*

coe·nes·the·sia (kō-en-es-thē'zē-ă). SYN cenesthesia.

♻ **coeno-.** Shared in common. SEE ALSO ceno-. [G. *koinos,* common]

coe·no·cyte (sē'nō-sīt). SYN cenocyte.

coe·no·cyt·ic (sē-nō-sit'ik). SYN cenocytic.

coe·nu·ro·sis (sē-nū-rō'sis). SYN cenurosis.

Coe·nu·rus (sē-nū'rŭs). Former generic name, now used to designate larval forms of taenioid cestodes in which a bladder is formed with a number of invaginated scoleces developing within; distinguished from a hydatid cyst by the absence of free-floating daughter cyst colonies budded off within the bladder; C. larvae are found in members of the genus *Multiceps.* [G. *koinos,* common, + *oura,* tail]

C. cerebra'lis, the coenurus larvae of the tapeworm *Multiceps multiceps,* found in the brain and spinal cord of sheep, goats, and other ruminants (a few have been recorded in man); adults are found in the intestine of dogs, foxes, coyotes, and jackals.

C. seria'lis, the coenurus larvae of the tapeworm *Multiceps serialis,* found in subcutaneous and intramuscular tissues of rabbits and hares (a few have been recorded in man); adult worms are found in the intestine of dogs, foxes, and jackals.

co·en·zyme (kō-en'zīm). A substance (excluding solo metal ions) that enhances or is necessary for the action of enzymes; c.'s are of smaller molecular size than the enzymes themselves, are dialyzable and relatively heat-stable, and are usually easily dissociable from the protein portion of the enzyme; several vitamins are c. precursors. SYN cofactor (1).

co·en·zyme I, co·en·zyme II. Obsolete names for nicotinamide adenine dinucleotide and nicotinamide adenine dinucleotide phosphate respectively.

co·en·zyme A (CoA). A coenzyme containing pantothenic acid, adenosine 3'-phosphate 5'-pyrophosphate, and cysteamine; involved in the transfer of acyl groups, notably in transacetylations.

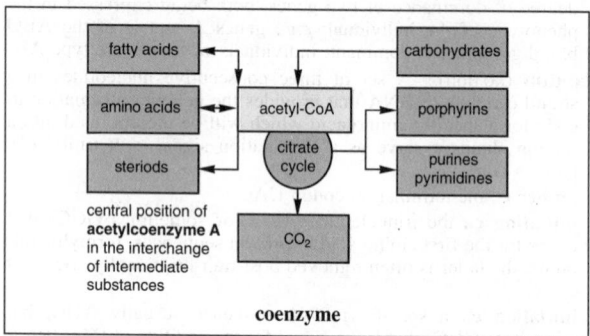

central position of **acetylcoenzyme A** in the interchange of intermediate substances

coenzyme

co·en·zyme F (kō-en'zīm). SYN tetrahydrofolic acid.

co·en·zyme Q (CoQ, Q). Quinones with isoprenoid side chains (specifically, ubiquinones) that mediate electron transfer between cytochrome *b* and cytochrome *c;* chemically similar to vitamins E and K, and to other tocopherols, quinones, and tocols.

co·en·zyme R. SYN biotin.

coeur (kūr). SYN heart. [Fr.]

c. en sabot (awn sah-bo'), the radiographic configuration of the heart in the tetralogy of Fallot; the elevated apex gives a silhouette like that of a wooden shoe. SYN sabot heart, wooden-shoe heart.

co·ev·o·lu·tion (kō-ev-ō-lū'shŭn). The process whereby genes or gene fragments are changing together and not diverging.

co·fac·tor (kō'fak'ter, tōr). **1.** SYN coenzyme. **2.** An atom or molecule essential for the action of a large molecule; *e.g.,* heme in hemoglobin, magnesium in chlorophyll. Solo metal ions are regarded as c.'s for proteins, but not as coenzymes.

cobra venom c., SYN properdin *factor* B.

molybdenum c. (mō-lib'dĕ-nŭm), a complex of molybdenum and molybdopterin required for a number of enzymes. A deficiency of this c. will result in lower activities of sulfite oxidase, xanthine dehydrogenase, and aldehyde oxidase causing elevated levels of sulfite, thiosulfite, xanthine, etc.

platelet c. I, SYN *factor* VIII.

platelet c. II, SYN *factor* IX.

co·fer·ment (kō'fer-ment). Obsolete term for coenzyme.

Coffey, Robert, U.S. surgeon, 1869–1933. SEE C. *suspension.*

Coffin, Grange S., U.S. pediatrician, *1923. SEE C.-Lowry *syndrome;* C.-Siris *syndrome.*

Cogan, David G., U.S. ophthalmologist, 1908–1993. SEE C.'s *syndrome;* C.-Reese *syndrome.*

cog·ni·tion (kog-ni'shŭn). **1.** Generic term embracing the mental activities associated with thinking, learning, and memory. **2.** Any process whereby one acquires knowledge. [L. *cognitio*]

cog·ni·tive (kog'ni-tiv). Pertaining to cognition.

co·he·sion (kō-hē'zhŭn). The attraction between molecules or masses that holds them together. [L. *co-haereo,* pp. -haesus, to stick together]

Cohnheim, Julius F., German histologist, pathologist, and physiologist, 1839–1884. SEE C.'s *area, field, theory.*

co·ho·ba (kō-hō'bă). A psychotomimetic hallucinogenic substance obtained from *Acacia niopo* (family Leguminosae), a Central American plant, *Piptadenia peregrina,* and other plants; among its constituents are bufotenine and dimethyltryptamine; used in native localities as snuff or enema.

co·hort (kō'hort). **1.** Component of the population born during a particular period and identified by period of birth so that its characteristics can be ascertained as it enters successive time and age periods. **2.** Any designated group followed or traced over a period, as in an epidemiological cohort study. [L. *cohors,* retinue, military unit]

coil (kōil). **1.** A spiral or series of loops. **2.** An object made of wire wound in a spiral configuration, used in electronic applications, or a loop of wire used as an antenna.

detector c., a c. used in magnetic resonance imaging as an antenna to record radiofrequency emissions of stimulated nuclei, *e.g.,* body coil, head coil.

random c., a structure of a macromolecule (typically, a biopolymer) which changes with time.

surface c., a detector c. applied directly to a body part for high resolution imaging; often a single loop of metal.

coin-count·ing (koyn′kownt′ing). A sliding movement of the tips of the thumb and index finger, occurring in paralysis agitans.

coin·o·site (koyn′ō-sīt). SYN cenosite.

co·in·te·grate. A structure resulting from replicative transposition where the transposon is duplicated.

co·i·tal (ko′i-tăl). Pertaining to coitus.

Coiter (Koyter), Volcher, Dutch surgeon and anatomist, 1534–1600. SEE C.'s *muscle.*

co·i·tion (kō-ish′ŭn). SYN coitus. [L. *co-eo,* pp. *-itus,* to come together]

co·i·to·pho·bia (kō′i-tō-fō′bē-ă). Morbid fear of sexual intercourse. [L. *coitus,* sexual intercourse, + G. *phobos,* fear]

co·i·tus (kō′i-tŭs). Sexual union between male and female. SYN coition, copulation (1), pareunia, sexual intercourse. [L.]

c. interrup′tus, sexual intercourse that is interrupted before the man ejaculates.

c. reserva′tus, c. in which ejaculation is postponed or suppressed.

col (kol). A crater-like area of the interproximal oral mucosa joining the lingual and buccal interdental papillae.

col-. SEE con-.

co·la (kō′lă). **1.** SYN kola. **2.** [L.], Strain (imperative form).

col·chi·cine (kol′chi-sin) [USP]. $C_{22}H_{25}NO_6$; an alkaloid obtained from *Colchicum autumnale* (family Liliaceae); used for gout.

Col·chi·cum corm (kŏl′chĭ-kum). Dried corm of *Colchicum autumnale,* the botanical source for colchicine, an alkaloidal drug used for the treatment of gout.

cold (kōld). **1.** A low temperature; the sensation produced by a temperature notably below an accustomed norm or a comfortable level. **2.** A virus infection involving the upper respiratory tract and characterized by congestion of the mucosa, watery nasal discharge, and general malaise, with a duration of 3 to 5 days. SEE ALSO rhinitis. SYN frigid (1).

c. in the head, SYN acute *rhinitis.*

rose c., allergic rhinitis occurring in the spring and early summer.

cold-blood·ed (kōld-blŭd′ed). SYN poikilothermic.

Cole, Laurent, French pathologist, *1903. SEE Benedict-Hopkins-C. *reagent.*

Cole, Rufus Ivory, U.S. physician, *1872.

Cole. Warren Henry, surgeon, *1898. Co-developer with E. A. Graham of cholecystography, first described in 1924. SEE Graham-Cole *test.*

Cole-Cecil mur·mur. See under murmur.

co·lec·ta·sia (kō-lek-tā′zē-ă). Distention of the colon. [G. *kolon,* colon, + *ektasis,* a stretching]

col·ec·to·my (kō-lek′tō-mē). Excision of a segment or all of the colon. [G. *kolon,* colon, + *ektomē,* excision]

coleo-. Sheath, specifically, the vagina. [G. *koleos,* sheath]

co·le·o·cele (kol′ē-ō-sēl). SYN colpocele (1). [G. *koleos,* sheath, + *kēlē,* tumor]

Co·le·op·te·ra (kō-lē-op′ter-ă). An order of insects, the beetles, characterized by the possession of a pair of hard, horny wing covers overlying a pair of delicate membranous flying wings; it is the largest of the insect orders with the largest number of

species of any animal or plant order. [G. *koleos,* sheath + *pteron,* wing]

co·le·op·to·sis (kō-lē-op′tō-sis). SYN coloptosis.

co·le·ot·o·my (kol-ē-ot′ō-mē). **1.** SYN pericardiotomy. **2.** SYN vaginotomy. [G. *koleos,* sheath, + *tomē,* incision]

co·les·ti·pol (kō-les′ti-pol). Tetraethylenepentamine polymer with 1-chloro-2,3-epoxypropane; an antilipemic drug.

colet. Abbreviation for L. *coletur,* let it be strained.

co·li·bac·il·lo·sis (kō′li-bas-i-lō′sis). Diarrheal disease caused by the bacterium *Escherichia coli.* Often called enteric c.

co·li·ba·cil·lus, pl. **co·li·ba·cil·li** (kō′li-bă-sil′ŭs). SYN *Escherichia coli.*

col·ic (kol′ik). **1.** Relating to the colon. **2.** Spasmodic pains in the abdomen. **3.** In young infants, paroxysms of gastrointestinal pain, with crying and irritability, due to a variety of causes, such as swallowing of air, emotional upset, or overfeeding. [G. *kōlikos,* relating to the colon]

appendicular c., colicky pain occurring early in acute appendicitis. SYN vermicular c.

biliary c., intense spasmodic pain felt in the right upper quadrant of the abdomen from impaction of a gallstone in the cystic duct. SYN gallstone c., hepatic c.

copper c., an affection similar to lead c. occurring in chronic poisoning by copper.

Devonshire c., SYN lead c.

gallstone c., SYN biliary c.

gastric c., colicky pain associated with gastritis or peptic ulcer.

hepatic c., SYN biliary c.

infantile c., episodes of abdominal pain due to abnormal muscular contraction of the intestine in infants.

lead c., severe colicky abdominal pain, with constipation, symptomatic of lead poisoning. SYN Devonshire c., painter's c., Poitou c., saturnine c.

meconial c., abdominal pain of newborn infants.

menstrual c., intermittent cramp-like lower abdominal pains associated with menstruation.

milk c., SYN enterotoxemia.

ovarian c., lower abdominal pain due to torsion or twisting of an ovary, as with an ovarian cyst.

painter's c., SYN lead c.

pancreatic c., severe colicky abdominal pain, resembling that of biliary c., caused by the passage of a pancreatic calculus.

Poitou c., SYN lead c.

renal c., severe colicky pain caused by the impaction or passage of a calculus in the ureter or renal pelvis.

salivary c., periodic attacks of pain in the region of a salivary duct or gland, accompanied by an acute swelling of the gland, occurring in cases of salivary calculus.

saturnine c., SYN lead c.

tubal c., lower abdominal pain due to spasmodic contraction of the oviduct excited by a blood clot, other irritant, or the injection of gas or oil.

ureteral c., paroxysm of pain due to abrupt obstruction of ureter from a calculus or blood clot in most instances.

uterine c., painful cramps of the uterine muscle sometimes occurring at the menstrual period, or in association with uterine disease.

vermicular c., SYN appendicular c.

zinc c., c. resulting from chronic zinc poisoning.

col·i·ca (kol′i-kă). A colic artery. SEE artery.

col·i·cin (kol′i-sin). Bacteriocin produced by strains of *Escherichia coli* and by other enterobacteria (*Shigella* and *Salmonella*) that carry the necessary plasmids. Many are toxic to related bacterial strains and bind to specific cellular receptors interfering with normal function. [(*Escherichia*) *coli* + bacteriocin]

col·i·ci·nog·e·ny (kol′i-si-noj′ĕ-nē). The bacterial property of producing a colicin.

col·icky (kol′i-kē). Denoting or resembling the pain of colic.

col·i·co·ple·gia (kol′i-kō-plē′jē-ă). Lead poisoning marked by both colic and palsy. [G. *kolikos,* suffering from colic, + *plēgē,* stroke]

CO

co·li·my·cin (kō-li-mī'sin). SYN colistin.

co·li·pase (kō'lip-ās). A small protein in pancreatic juice that is essential for the efficient action of pancreatic lipase. [co- + lipase]

co·li·phage (kō'li-fāj, kol'i-). A bacteriophage with an affinity for one or another strain of *Escherichia coli*. In general, c.'s, like other bacteriophages, are known by symbols that have significance only as a means of laboratory identification; additional notations, however, specifically identify variant characteristics, *e.g.,* λdgal denotes the deficient prophage (coliphage) λ, which carries the bacterial gene *gal* (galactose). [*(Escherichia) coli* + bacteriophage]

co·li·pli·ca·tion (kō'li-pli-kā'shŭn). SYN coloplication.

co·li·punc·ture (kō'li-pŭnk-chūr). SYN colocentesis.

co·lis·ti·meth·ate so·di·um (kō-lis-ti-meth'āte). Pentasodium colistinmethanesulfonate; contains the pentasodium salt of the penta(methanesulfonic acid) derivative of colistin A as the major component, with a small proportion of the pentasodium salt of the same derivative of colistin B; an effective antibiotic against most Gram-negative bacilli (except *Proteus*), given intramuscularly. SEE ALSO *colistin* sulfate, polymyxin. SYN cholistine sulphomethate sodium, colistin sulfomethate sodium.

co·lis·tin (kō-lis'tin). A mixture of cyclic polypeptide antibiotics from a strain of *Bacillus polymyxa;* separable into polymyxins. SYN colimycin.
c. sulfate, the sulfate salt of an antibacterial substance produced by the growth of a strain of *Bacillus polymyxa,* consisting primarily of colistin A with small amounts of colistin B; it is effective against most Gram-negative bacteria (except *Proteus*); given orally for intestinal antibacterial action. SEE ALSO colistimethate sodium, polymyxin.
c. sulfomethate sodium, SYN colistimethate sodium.

co·li·tis (kō-lī'tis). Inflammation of the colon. [G. *kōlon,* colon, + *-itis,* inflammation]
amebic c., inflammation of the colon in amebiasis.
collagenous c., c. occurring mostly in middle-aged women and characterized by persistent watery diarrhea and a deposit of a band of collagen beneath the basement membrane of colon surface epithelium.
c. cys'tica profun'da, intramural mucus-containing cysts of the large bowel; the condition may be mistaken for mucinous carcinoma but is not neoplastic.
c. cys'tica superficia'lis, a form of c. in which there is superficial cyst formation in the colon.
granulomatous c., changes, identical to those of regional enteritis, involving the colon.
c. gra'vis, obsolete term for ulcerative c.
hemorrhagic c., abdominal cramps and bloody diarrhea, without fever, attributed to a self-limited infection by a strain of *Escherichia coli.*
mucous c., an affection of the mucous membrane of the colon characterized by colicky pain, constipation or diarrhea (sometimes alternating), and passage of mucous or slimy pseudomembranous shreds and patches. SYN mucocolitis, myxomembranous c.
myxomembranous c., SYN mucous c.
pseudomembranous c., SYN pseudomembranous *enterocolitis.*
ulcerative c., a chronic disease of unknown cause characterized by ulceration of the colon and rectum, with rectal bleeding, mucosal crypt abscesses, inflammatory pseudopolyps, abdominal pain, and diarrhea; frequently causes anemia, hypoproteinemia, and electrolyte imbalance, and is less frequently complicated by peritonitis, toxic megacolon, or carcinoma of the colon.
uremic c., c. characterized by hemorrhages in the mucosa, occurring in renal failure, possibly owing to the irritant effect of ammonia formed by breakdown of increased urea in the intestinal secretions.

col·i·tose (kol'ĭ-tōs). A polysaccharide somatic antigen of *Salmonella* species.

col·la (kol'ă). Plural of collum.

col·la·cin (kol'ă-sin). Degenerated collagen. SYN collastin.

col·la·gen (kol'lă-jen). The major protein (comprising over half

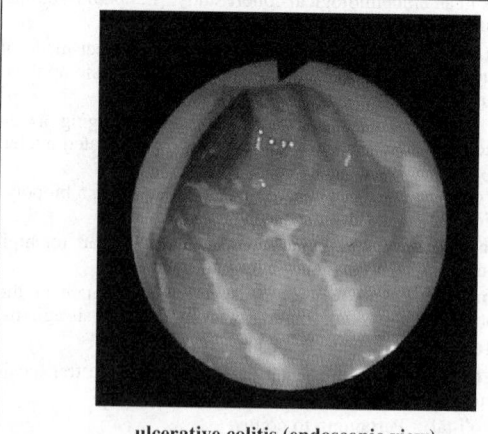
ulcerative colitis (endoscopic view)

of that in mammals) of the white fibers of connective tissue, cartilage, and bone, that is insoluble in water but can be altered to easily digestible, soluble gelatins by boiling in water, dilute acids, or alkalies. It is high in glycine, L-alanine, L-proline, and L-4-hydroxyproline, but is low in sulfur and has no L-tryptophan. C. comprises a family of genetically distinct molecules all of which have a unique triple helix configuration of three polypeptide subunits known as α-chains; 11 types of c. have been identified, each with a different polypeptide chain. SEE ALSO collagen *fiber.* SYN ossein, osseine, ostein, osteine. [G *koila,* glue, + *-gen,* producing]
type I c., the most abundant c., which forms large well-organized fibrils having high tensile strength.
type II c., c. unique to cartilage, nucleus pulposis, notochord, and vitreous body; it forms as thin highly glycosylated fibrils.
type III c., c. characteristic of reticular fibers.
type IV c., a less distinctly fibrillar form of c. characteristic of basement membranes.

col·la·gen·ase (kol-ă'jĕ-nās). A proteolytic enzyme that acts on one or more of the collagens.

col·la·gen·ase A, col·la·gen·ase I. SYN *Clostridium histolyticum* collagenase.

col·la·ge·na·tion (kol'ă-jĕ-nā'shŭn). SYN collagenization.

col·la·gen·ic (kol'ă-jen'ik). SYN collagenous.

col·lag·e·ni·za·tion (ko-laj'ĕ-ni-zā'shŭn). **1.** Replacement of tissues or fibrin by collagen. **2.** Synthesis of collagen by fibroblasts. SYN collagenation.

col·lag·e·no·lyt·ic (ko-laj'ĕ-nō-lit'ik). Causing the lysis of collagen, gelatin, and other proteins containing proline. [collagen + G. *lysis,* dissolving]

col·lag·e·no·sis (ko-laj-i-nō'sis). SEE collagen *diseases,* under *disease.*
reactive perforating c., a rare skin disorder characterized by extrusion of collagen fibers through the epidermis; usually begins in infancy or childhood and appears clinically as recurrent umbilicated papules that resolve spontaneously. The condition may be inherited or acquired, the latter differing from Kyrle's disease because follicular involvement is absent.

col·lag·e·nous (ko-laj'ĕ-nŭs). Producing or containing collagen. SYN collagenic.

col·lapse (kō-laps'). **1.** A condition of extreme prostration, similar to hypovolemic shock and due to the same causes. **2.** A state of profound physical depression. **3.** A falling together of the walls of a structure or the failure of a physiological system. [L. *col-labor,* pp. *-lapsus,* to fall together]
absorption c., pulmonary c. due to rapid complete obstruction of a large bronchus.
circulatory c., failure of the circulation, either cardiac or peripheral.
c. of dental arch, movement of teeth to fill a space which would

normally be filled by another, missing tooth, creating a malpositioning of adjacent and opposing teeth.

massive c., relatively sudden atelectasis of an entire lung or of a lobe.

pressure c., pulmonary c. due to external compression of the lung, as by a pleural effusion or pneumothorax.

pulmonary c., secondary atelectasis due to bronchial obstruction, pleural effusion or pneumothorax, cardiac hypertrophy, or enlargement of other structures adjacent to the lungs.

col·lar (kol′ăr). A band, usually denoting one encircling the neck.

renal c., in the embryo, a ring of veins around the aorta below the origin of the superior mesenteric artery.

c. of Venus, obsolete term for syphilitic *leukoderma* involving the anterior neck and chest.

col·lar·ette (kol′er-et′). The sinuous, scalloped line in the iris that divides the central pupillary zone from the peripheral ciliary zone and marks the embryonic site of the atrophied minor vascular circle of the iris. SYN iris frill.

col·las·tin (kol-as′tin). SYN collacin.

col·lat·er·al (ko-lat′er-ăl). 1. Indirect, subsidiary, or accessory to the main thing; side by side. 2. A side branch of a nerve axon or blood vessel.

col·lec·tins. A family of molecules that recognize and opsonize microbes during the preimmune response of a host.

Colles, Abraham, Irish surgeon, 1773–1843. SEE C.'s *fascia, fracture, ligament, space.*

Collet, Frédric-Justin, French otolaryngologist, *1870.

col·lic·u·lec·to·my (ko-lik-yū-lek′tō-mē). Excision of the colliculus seminalis.

col·lic·u·li·tis (ko-lik-yū-lī′tis). Inflammation of the urethra in the region of the colliculus seminalis. SYN verumontanitis.

col·lic·u·lus, pl. **col·lic·u·li** (ko-lic′yū-lŭs, -lī) [NA]. A small elevation above the surrounding parts. [L. mound, dim. of *collis,* hill]

c. of arytenoid cartilage, the elevation on the anterolateral surface of the arytenoid cartilage above the triangular fovea. SYN c. cartilaginis arytenoideae [NA].

c. cartila′ginis arytenoi′deae [NA], SYN c. of arytenoid cartilage.

facial c., prominent portion of the medial eminence, just rostral to the medullary striae in the rhomboidal fossa; it is formed by the internal genu of the facial nerve and the abducens nucleus around which the facial fibers curve. SYN c. facialis [NA], abducens eminence, eminentia abducentis, eminentia facialis, facial eminence, facial hillock.

c. facia′lis [NA], SYN facial c.

c. infe′rior [NA], SYN inferior c.

inferior c., the ovoid, paired, inferior eminence of the laminae of mesencephalic tectum; it receives the lateral lemniscus and projects by way of the brachium of inferior colliculus to the medial geniculate body of the thalamus, and is thus an essential way-station in the central auditory pathway. SYN c. inferior [NA], corpus quadrigeminum posterius, inferior nasal c., posterior quadrigeminal body.

inferior nasal c., SYN inferior c.

seminal c., an elevated portion of the urethral crest upon which open the two ejaculatory ducts and the prostatic utricle. SYN c. seminalis [NA], caput gallinaginis, c. urethralis, seminal hillock, verumontanum.

c. semina′lis [NA], SYN seminal c.

superior c., the paired, larger, rounded anterior eminence of the laminae of mesencephalic tectum; major afferent connections of the superficial layers are the retina and striate cortex; input to deep layers of the c. are polymodal. Its efferent connections are with the lower brainstem and spinal cord (tectobulbar tract and tectospinal tract) and with the pulvinar and other cell groups in the caudal part of the thalamus; participates in extrageniculate visual pathway. SYN c. superior [NA], anterior quadrigeminal body, corpus quadrigeminum anterius.

c. supe′rior [NA], SYN superior c.

c. urethra′lis, SYN seminal c.

Collier, James S., English physician, 1870–1935. SEE C.'s *tract, sign.*

col·li·ga·tion (kol-i-gā′shŭn). 1. A combination in which the components are distinguishable from one another. 2. The bringing of isolated events into a unified experience. [L. *cum,* together, + *ligo,* to bind]

col·li·ga·tive (ko-lig′ă-tiv). 1. Depending on numbers of particles. 2. Referring to properties of solutions that depend only on the concentration of dissolved substances and not on their nature (*e.g.,* osmotic pressure, elevation of boiling point, vapor pressure lowering, freezing point depression).

col·li·ma·tion (kol-i-mā′shŭn). The process, in x-ray, of restricting and confining the x-ray beam to a given area and, in nuclear medicine, of restricting the detection of emitted radiations from a given area of interest. [L. *collineo,* to direct in a straight line]

col·li·ma·tor (kol′i-mā-ter). A device of high absorption coefficient material used in collimation.

col·lin·e·ar·i·ty (kol′in-ē-ar′i-tē). The phenomena that the orderings of the corresponding elements of DNA, the RNA transcribed from it, and the amino acid translated from the RNA are identical. [L. *collineo,* to direct in a straight line]

Collins, Edward Treacher, English ophthalmologist, 1862–1919. SEE Treacher C.'s *syndrome.*

Col·lins. SEE Lukes-Collins *classification.*

col·li·ot·o·my (kol-ē-ot′ō-mē). Obsolete term for adhesiotomy. [G. *kolla,* glue, + G. *tomē,* incision]

Collip, James B., Canadian endocrinologist, 1892–1965. SEE Noble-C. *procedure;* Anderson-C. *test.*

col·li·qua·tion (kol-i-kwā′shŭn). 1. Excessive discharge of fluid. 2. Liquidification in the process of necrosis. [L. *col-,* together, + *liquo,* pp. *liquatus,* to cause to melt]

col·liq·ua·tive (ko-lik′wă-tiv). Denoting or characteristic of colliquation.

Collis, John Leighton, British thoracic surgeon, *1911. SEE C. *gastroplasty.*

col·lo·di·on (ko-lō′dē-on). A liquid made by dissolving pyroxylin or gun cotton in ether and alcohol; on evaporation it leaves a glossy contractile film; used as a protective for cuts or as a vehicle for the local application of medicinal substances. SYN collodium. [Mod. L. *collodium,* fr. G. *kolla,* glue]

blistering c., SYN cantharidal c.

cantharidal c., a powdered chloroform extract of cantharides in flexible c.; a vesicant. SYN blistering c., c. vesicans.

flexible c., a mixture of camphor, castor oil, and c., or a mixture of castor oil, Canada turpentine, and c., used for the same purposes as c., but its film possesses the advantage, for certain conditions, of not contracting.

hemostatic c., SYN styptic c.

iodized c., a 5% solution of iodine in flexible c.; a counterirritant.

salicylic acid c., a keratolytic agent used in the treatment of corns and verrucae.

styptic c., tannic acid in flexible c.; an astringent and local hemostatic. SYN hemostatic c., styptic colloid, xylostyptic ether.

c. vesicans, SYN cantharidal c.

col·lo·di·um (ko-lō′dē-ŭm). SYN collodion. [G. *kolla,* glue, + *eidos,* appearance]

col·loid (kol′oyd). 1. Aggregates of atoms or molecules in a finely divided state (submicroscopic), dispersed in a gaseous, liquid, or solid medium, and resisting sedimentation, diffusion, and filtration, thus differing from precipitates. SEE ALSO hydrocolloid. 2. Gluelike. 3. A translucent, yellowish, homogeneous material of the consistency of glue, less fluid than mucoid or mucinoid, found in the cells and tissues in a state of c. degeneration. SYN colloidin. 4. The stored secretion within follicles of the thyroid gland. For individual c.'s not listed below, see the specific name. [G. *kolla,* glue, + *eidos,* appearance]

bovine c., SYN conglutinin.

dispersion c., SYN dispersoid.

emulsion c., SYN emulsoid.

hydrophil c., hydrophilic c., SYN emulsoid.

hydrophobic c., SYN suspensoid.

irreversible c., a c. that is not again soluble in water after having been dried at ordinary temperature. SYN unstable c.

lyophilic c., SYN emulsoid.

lyophobic c., SYN suspensoid.

protective c., a c. that has the power of preventing the precipitation of suspensoids under the influence of an electrolyte.

c. pseudomilium, SYN colloid milium.

reversible c., a c. that is again soluble in water after having been dried at ordinary temperature. SYN stable c.

stable c., SYN reversible c.

styptic c., SYN styptic *collodion*.

suspension c., SYN suspensoid.

thyroid c., the semifluid material that occupies the lumen of thyroid follicles; it contains thyroglobulin mainly.

unstable c., SYN irreversible c.

col·loi·dal (ko-loyd′ăl). Denoting or characteristic of a colloid.

col·loi·din (ko-loy′din). SYN colloid (3).

col·loid mil·i·um (kol′loyd mil′ē-ŭm). Yellow papules developing in sun-damaged skin of the head and backs of the hands, composed of colloid material in the dermis resembling amyloid but with a different ultrastructure. SYN colloid acne, colloid pseudomilium, elastosis colloidalis conglomerata. [L. *milium,* millet]

col·loi·do·cla·sia, col·loi·do·cla·sis (ko-loy-dō-klā′sē-ă, -sis). Obsolete term for a rupture of the colloid equilibrium in the body. [colloid + G. *klasis,* fracture]

col·loi·do·clas·tic (ko-loy-dō-klas′tik). Obsolete term denoting colloidoclasia.

col·loi·do·gen (ko-loy′dō-jen). A substance capable of giving rise to a colloidal solution or suspension.

col·lox·y·lin (ko-lok′si-lin). SYN pyroxylin. [G. *kolla,* glue, + *xylinos,* woody, fr. *xylon,* wood]

col·lum, pl. **col·la** (kol′ŭm, kol′ă). **1** [NA]. The part between the shoulders or thorax and the head. **2.** A constricted or necklike portion of any organ or other anatomical structure. SYN cervix (1) [NA]. [L.]

c. anatom′icum hu′meri [NA], SYN anatomical *neck* of humerus.

c. chirur′gicum hu′meri [NA], SYN surgical *neck* of humerus.

c. cos′tae [NA], SYN *neck* of rib.

c. den′tis, SYN *neck* of tooth.

c. distor′tum, SYN torticollis.

c. fem′oris, SYN *neck* of femur.

c. fib′ulae [NA], SYN *neck* of fibula.

c. folli′culi pi′li, SYN *neck* of hair follicle.

c. glan′dis pe′nis [NA], SYN *neck* of glans penis.

c. hu′meri, SEE anatomical *neck* of humerus, surgical *neck* of humerus.

c. mal′lei [NA], SYN *neck* of malleus.

c. mandib′ulae [NA], SYN *neck* of mandible.

c. os′sis fem′oris [NA], SYN *neck* of femur.

c. ra′dii [NA], SYN *neck* of radius.

c. scap′ulae [NA], SYN *neck* of scapula.

c. ta′li [NA], SYN *neck* of talus.

c. vesi′cae biliar′is [NA], SYN *neck* of gallbladder.

c. vesi′cae fel′leae, ☆official alternate term for *neck* of gallbladder.

col·lu·to·ri·um (kol-yū-tō′rē-ŭm). SYN mouthwash. [Mod. L. fr. *col-luo,* pp. *-lutus,* to wash thoroughly]

col·lu·tory (kol′yū-tōr-ē). SYN mouthwash. [L. *colluere,* to rinse]

Col·lyr·i·clum (kol-ē-rik′lŭm). A genus of trematodes. *C. faba* causes the formation of subcutaneous cysts (cutaneous monostomiasis) in chickens, turkeys, and other birds.

col·lyr·i·um (ko-lir′ē-ŭm). Originally, any preparation for the eye; now, an eyewash. [G. *kollyrion,* poultice, eye salve]

⟁**colo-.** The colon. [G. *kolon,*]

col·o·bo·ma (kol-ō-bō′mă). Any defect, congenital, pathologic, or artificial, especially of the eye. [G. *kolobōma,* lit., the part taken away in mutilation, fr. *koloboō,* to dock, mutilate]

c. of choroid, a congenital defect of the choroid and retinal pigment epithelium exposing the sclera; the defect is usually situated below the optic disk in the region of fetal fissure.

Fuchs′ c., a congenital inferior crescent on the choroid at the edge of the optic disk; not associated with myopia. SYN congenital conus.

c. i′ridis, (1) retention of the choroid fissure causing a congenital cleft of the iris, often associated with c. of the choroid, viable in the inferior ocular fundus; (2) obsolete term for the iris defect resulting from a large surgical iridectomy.

c. len′tis, a segment of the lens equator devoid of zonular fibers, giving the appearance of a notch.

c. lo′buli, congenital fissure of the lobule of the ear.

macular c., a defect of the central retina as a result of arrested development or intrauterine retinal inflammation.

c. of optic nerve, a congenital notch in the formation of the optic nerve, appearing as a craterlike excavation at the optic disk.

c. palpebra′le, a congenital notch in the eyelid margin.

c. of vitreous, a congenital indentation of the vitreous body by mesoderm; associated with severe myopia.

co·lo·cen·te·sis (kō′lō-sen-tē′sis). Puncture of the colon with a trochar or scalpel to relieve distention. SYN colipuncture, colopuncture. [colo- + G. *kentēsis,* a puncture]

co·lo·cho·le·cys·tos·to·my (kō′lō-kō-lē-sis-tos′tō-mē). SYN cholecystocolostomy.

co·lo·col·ic (kō-lō-kol′ik). From colon to colon; said of a spontaneous or induced anastomosis between two parts of the colon.

co·lo·co·los·to·my (kō′lō-kō-los′tō-mē). Establishment of a communication between two noncontinuous segments of the colon. [colo- + colo- + G. *stoma,* mouth]

col·o·cynth (kol′ō-sinth). The peeled dried fruit of *Citrullus colcynthis* (family Cucurbitaceae), an herb of the sandy shores of the Mediterranean, resembling somewhat the watermelon plant; formerly widely used as a cathartic and laxative. SYN bitter apple. [G. *kolokynthē,* the round gourd or pumpkin]

co·lo·cys·to·plas·ty (kō-lō-sis′tō-plas-tē). Enlargement of the urinary bladder by attaching a segment of colon to it.

co·lo·en·ter·i·tis (kō′lō-en-ter-ī′tis). SYN enterocolitis.

co·lo·hep·a·to·pexy (kō-lō-hep′ă-tō-pek′sē). Attachment of the colon to the liver by adhesions. [colo- + G. *hēpar* (*hēpat-*), liver, + *pēxis,* fixation]

col·ol·y·sis (kō-lol′i-sis). Procedure of freeing the colon from adhesions. [colo- + G. *lysis,* loosening]

col·o·min·ic ac·id (kol-ō-min′ik). Polymer of α(1,5)-*N*-acetylneuraminic acid; found in *Escherichia coli.*

co·lon (kō′lon) [NA]. The division of the large intestine extending from the cecum to the rectum. [G. *kolon*]

c. ascen′dens [NA], SYN ascending c.

ascending c., the portion of the c. between the ileocecal orifice and the right colic flexure. SYN c. ascendens [NA].

c. descen′dens [NA], SYN descending c.

descending c., the part of the c. extending from the left colic flexure to the pelvic brim. SYN c. descendens [NA].

giant c., SYN megacolon.

iliac c., that portion of the descending c. which occupies the left iliac fossa, between the crest of the left ilium and the pelvic brim.

irritable c., tendency to colonic hyperperistalsis, sometimes with colicky pains and diarrhea.

lead-pipe c., the scarred rigid c. of advanced ulcerative colitis.

mucosa of c., the lining coat of the colon. SYN tunica mucosa coli [NA].

c. pelvi′num, SYN sigmoid c.

sigmoid c., the part of the c. describing an S-shaped curve between the pelvic brim and the third sacral segment; it is continuous with the rectum. SYN c. sigmoideum [NA], c. pelvinum, flexura sigmoidea, sigmoid flexure.

c. sigmoi′deum [NA], SYN sigmoid c.

spastic c., nonspecific term used to describe symptoms such as abdominal pain, flatulence, and alternating diarrhea with constipation thought to reflect increased muscular function of the colon.

transverse c., the part of the c. between the right and left colic flexures. It may extend somewhat transversely across the abdomen, but more often sags centally, frequently to subumbilical levels. SYN c. transversum [NA].

c. transver′sum [NA], SYN transverse c.

co·lon·al·gia (ko-lon-al′jē-ă). Rarely used term for pain in the colon. [colon + G. *algos,* pain]

co·lon·ic (ko-lon′ik). Relating to the colon.

col·o·ni·za·tion (kol′on-i-zā′shŭn). **1.** SYN innidiation. **2.** The formation of compact population groups of the same type of microorganism, as the colonies that develop when a bacterial cell begins reproducing. **3.** The care of certain persons, *e.g.,* lepers, mental patients, in community groups.

genetic c., propagation of a gene by a host into which the gene has been introduced, naturally or artificially.

co·lon·o·gram (ko-lon′ō-gram). Graphic recording of movements of the colon.

co·lo·nom·e·ter (kō′lō-nom′ĕ-ter). A device for counting bacterial colonies.

co·lon·op·a·thy (kō-lŏ-nop′ă-thē). Rarely used term for any disordered condition of the colon. SYN colopathy.

co·lon·or·rha·gia (kō-lon-ō-rā′jē-ă). Rarely used term for colorrhagia.

co·lon·or·rhea (kō′lon-ō-rē′ă). SYN colorrhea.

co·lon·o·scope (kō-lon′ō-skōp). An elongated endoscope, usually fiberoptic.

co·lon·os·co·py (kō-lon-os′kŏ-pē). Visual examination of the inner surface of the colon by means of a colonoscope. SYN coloscopy. [colon + G. *skopeō,* to view]

col·o·ny (kol′ŏ-nē). **1.** A group of cells growing on a solid nutrient surface, each arising from the multiplication of an individual cell; a clone. **2.** A group of people with similar interests, living in a particular location or area. [L. *colonia,* a colony]

daughter c., a secondary c. growing on the surface of an older c.; it is smaller and may have characteristics different from those of the mother c.

filamentous c., in bacteriology, a c. composed of long, interwoven, irregularly disposed threads.

Gheel c., a c. in Gheel, Belgium, originating in the 13th century, for the informal communal care, in private homes, of severely mentally disordered persons.

H c., a c. of motile organisms forming a thin film of growth. Cf. O c. [Ger. *Hauch,* breath]

lenticular c., a bacterial c. shaped like a lentil or a double-convex lens.

mother c., a c. which gives rise to a secondary c. (a daughter c.), the latter growing on the surface of the former; the mother c. is larger than the daughter c., and the characteristics of the c.'s may differ.

mucoid c., a c. showing viscous or sticky growth typical of an organism producing large quantities of a carbohydrate capsule.

O c., growth of a nonmotile bacterium in discrete, compact c.'s in contrast to a film of growth produced by some motile bacteria. Cf. H c. [Ger. *ohne Hauch,* without breath]

rough c., a bacterial c. with a granular, flattened surface; this type of c. is usually associated with loss of virulence with respect to that of smooth c.'s.

smooth c., a bacterial c. with a glistening, rounded surface; this type of c. is usually associated with increased virulence with respect to that of rough c.'s.

spheroid c., a c. of protozoa in which the individual cells are held together in a coherent spherical mass by a gelatinoid material.

co·lop·a·thy (kō-lop′ă-thē). SYN colonopathy.

co·lo·pex·os·to·my (kō′lō-peks-os′tō-mē). Rarely used term for establishment of an artificial anus by creation of an opening into the colon after its fixation to the abdominal wall. [colo- + G. *pēxis,* fixation, + *stoma,* mouth]

co·lo·pex·ot·o·my (kō′lō-pek-sot′ō-mē). Rarely used term for incision into the colon after its fixation to the abdominal wall. [colo- + G. *pēxis,* fixation, + *tomē,* incision]

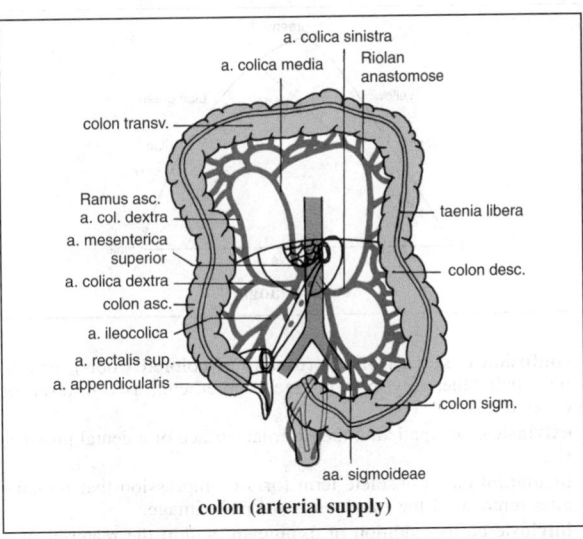

colon (arterial supply)

Labels: a. colica sinistra; Riolan anastomose; a. colica media; colon transv.; Ramus asc.; a. col. dextra; a. mesenterica superior; a. colica dextra; colon asc.; a. ileocolica; a. rectalis sup.; a. appendicularis; taenia libera; colon desc.; colon sigm.; aa. sigmoideae

colonies	
morphology of colonies	morphology of the single cell
1. S-form (smooth) with smooth surface	B-form (bacterial): bacilli
2. R-form (rough) with rough surface	F-form (filamental): chains of bacilli, or longer threads; arise from B-form colonies
3. M-form (mycoid) mucosal development	mycosis of the cell-wall
4. G-form (gonidial form) slowly growing, and thus smaller than the S- and R-forms; grow in moist nutritive base without causing visible change	C-form (coccoid); grow in coccal or granular form

col·o·pexy (kol′ō-pek-sē). Attachment of a portion of the colon to the abdominal wall. [colo- + G. *pēxis,* fixation]

co·lo·pho·ny (kō-lof′ō-nē). SYN rosin. [*Colophōn,* Summit, a town in Ionia]

co·lo·pli·ca·tion (kō′lō-pli-kā′shŭn). Reduction of the lumen of a dilated colon by making folds or tucks in its walls. SYN coliplication. [colo- + Mod. L. *plica,* fold]

co·lo·proc·tia (kō-lō-prok′shē-ă). Obsolete term for colostomy.

co·lo·proc·ti·tis (kō-lō-prok-tī′tis). Inflammation of both colon and rectum. SYN colorectitis, proctocolitis, rectocolitis. [colo- + G. *prōktos,* anus (rectum), + *-itis,* inflammation]

co·lo·proc·tos·to·my (kō′lō-prok-tos′tō-mē). Establishment of a communication between the rectum and a discontinuous segment of the colon. SYN colorectostomy. [colo- + G. *prōktos,* anus (rectum), + *stoma,* mouth]

co·lop·to·sis, co·lop·to·sia (kō-lop-tō′sis, -tō′sē-ă). Downward displacement, or prolapse, of the colon, especially of the transverse portion. SYN coleoptosis. [colo- + G. *ptōsis,* a falling]

co·lo·punc·ture (kō-lō-pŭnk′chūr). SYN colocentesis.

col·or (kŭl′ŏr). **1.** That aspect of the appearance of objects and light sources that may be specified as to hue, lightness (brightness), and saturation. **2.** That portion of the visible (370-760 nm) electromagnetic spectrum specified as to wavelength, luminosity, and purity. [L.]

complementary c.'s, pairs of different colors of light that produce white light when combined.

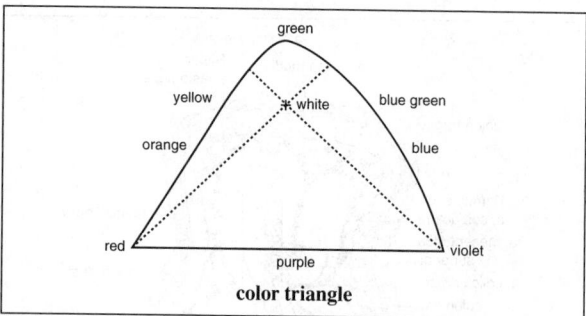

color triangle

confusion c.'s, a set of c.'s (usually of colored wools), cream, buff, pale blue, gray, brown, green, violet, etc., used in tests for c. blindness.

extrinsic c., c. applied to the external surface of a dental prosthesis.

incidental c., an obsolete term for a c. impression that remains after removal of the source. SEE ALSO afterimage.

intrinsic c., the addition of c. pigment within the material of a dental prosthesis.

opponent c., pairs of c. that share c. channels in the retina (red-green, blue-yellow, black-white).

primary c., the three c.'s of the retinal cone pigments (red, green, blue) that may be combined to match any hue. SYN simple c.

pure c., a visual sensation produced by light of a specific wavelength.

reflected c.'s, those c.'s seen in light falling upon a pigmented surface.

saturated c., a c. containing a minimum amount of whiteness.

simple c., SYN primary c.

structural c., a c. created by an optical effect (*e.g.,* via interference, refraction, or diffraction). Many naturally occurring blues fall in this class. Cf. natural *pigment.* SYN schemochromes.

tone c., SYN timbre.

co·lo·rec·tal (kol'ō-rek'tăl). Relating to the colon and rectum, or to the entire large bowel.

co·lo·rec·ti·tis (kō'lō-rek-tī'tis). SYN coloproctitis.

co·lo·rec·tos·to·my (kō'lō-rek-tos'tō-mē). SYN coloproctostomy.

col·or·im·e·ter (kŏl-er-im'ĕ-ter). An optical device for determining the color and/or intensity of the color of a liquid. SYN chromatometer, chrommeter.

Duboscq's c., an apparatus for measuring the depth of tint in a fluid by comparing it with a standard fluid; glass cylinders are immersed in each of two cups one containing standard fluid, the other the fluid to be tested; on looking through the cylinders, the tints are equalized by raising or lowering the cylinder in one cup, and the extent of this raising or lowering is indicated on a scale and gives the exact difference in tint.

col·or·i·met·ric (kŏl-er-i-met'rik). Relating to colorimetry.

col·or·im·e·try (kol-er-im'ĕ-trē). A procedure for quantitative chemical analysis, based on comparison of the color developed in a solution of the test material with that in a standard solution; the two solutions are observed simultaneously in a colorimeter, and quantitated on the basis of the absorption of light.

col·or match. The result of adjusting color mixtures until all visually apparent differences are minimal.

co·lor·rha·gia (kō-lō-rā'jē-ă). An abnormal discharge from the colon. [colo- + G. *rhēgnymi,* to burst forth]

co·lor·rha·phy (kō-lōr'ă-fē). Suture of the colon. [colo- + G. *rhaphē,* suture]

co·lor·rhea (kō-lō-rē'ă). Rarely used term for diarrhea thought to originate from a condition confined to or affecting chiefly the colon. SYN colonorrhea. [colo- + G. *rhoia,* a flow]

col·or sol·id. A schematic arrangement of color in space, the attributes of hue, saturation, and brightness being represented by cylindrical coordinates.

col·or tri·an·gle. A graph on which chromaticity coordinates are plotted.

co·los·co·py (kō-los'kŏ-pē). SYN colonoscopy. [colo- + G. *skopeō,* to view]

co·lo·sig·moi·dos·to·my (kō'lō-sig-moy-dos'tŏ-mē). Establishment of an anastomosis between any other part of the colon and the sigmoid colon.

co·los·to·my (kō-los'tō-mē). Establishment of an artificial cutaneous opening into the colon. [colo- + G. *stoma,* mouth]

co·los·tra·tion (kō-los-trā'shŭn). Infantile diarrhea attributed to the action of the colostrum.

co·los·tric (kō-los'trik). Relating to the colostrum.

co·los·tror·rhea (kō-los-trōr-rē'ă). Abnormally profuse secretion of colostrum. [colostrum, + G. *rhoia,* flow]

co·los·trous (kō-los'trŭs). Containing colostrum.

co·los·trum (kō-los'trŭm). A thin white opalescent fluid, the first milk secreted at the termination of pregnancy; it differs from the milk secreted later by containing more lactalbumin and lactoprotein; c. is also rich in antibodies which confer passive immunity to the newborn. SYN foremilk. [L.]

co·lot·o·my (kō-lot'ō-mē). Incision into the colon. [colo- + G. *tomē,* incision]

Col·our In·dex. A publication concerned with the chemistry of dyes, with each listed dye identified by a five-digit C.I. number, *e.g.,* methylene blue is C.I. 52015.

♻**colp-.** SEE colpo-.

col·pa·tre·sia (kol-pa-trē'zē-ă). SYN vaginal *atresia.* [colp- + G. *atrētos,* imperforate]

col·pec·ta·sis, col·pec·ta·sia (kol-pek'tă-sis, -pek-tā'si-ă). Distention of the vagina. [colp- + G. *aktasis,* stretching]

col·pec·to·my (kol-pek'tō-mē). SYN vaginectomy. [colp- + G. *ektomē,* excision]

♻**colpo-, colp-.** The vagina. SEE ALSO vagino-. [G. *kolpos,* fold or hollow]

col·po·cele (kol'pō-sēl). **1.** A hernia projecting into the vagina. SYN coleocele, vaginocele. **2.** SYN colpoptosis. [colpo- + G. *kēlē,* hernia]

col·po·clei·sis (kol-pō-klī'sis). Operation for obliterating the lumen of the vagina. [colpo- + G. *kleisis,* closure]

col·po·cys·ti·tis (kol'pō-sis-tī'tis). Obsolete term for inflammation of both vagina and bladder. [colpo- + G. *kystis,* bladder, + *-itis,* inflammation]

col·po·cys·to·cele (kol-pō-sis'tō-sēl). SYN cystocele. [colpo- + G. *kystis,* bladder, + *kēlē,* hernia]

col·po·cys·to·plas·ty (kol-pō-sis'tō-plas-tē). Plastic surgery to repair the vesicovaginal wall. [colpo- + G. *kystis,* bladder, + *plastos,* formed]

col·po·cys·tot·o·my (kol'pō-sis-tot'ō-mē). Incision into the bladder through the vagina. [colpo- + G. *kystis,* bladder, + *tomē,* incision]

col·po·cys·to·u·re·ter·ot·o·my (kol'pō-sis'tō-yū-rē-ter-ot'ō-mē). Incision into the ureter by way of the vagina and the bladder. [colpo- + G. *kystis,* bladder, + *ourēter,* ureter, + *tomē,* incision]

col·po·dyn·ia (kol-pō-din'ē-ă). SYN vaginodynia. [colpo- + G. *odynē,* pain]

col·po·hys·ter·ec·to·my (kol'pō-his-ter-ek'tō-mē). SYN vaginal *hysterectomy.* [colpo- + G. *hystera,* uterus, + *ektomē,* excision]

col·po·hys·ter·o·pexy (kol-pō-his'ter-ō-pek-sē). Operation for fixation of the uterus performed through the vagina. [colpo- + G. *hystera,* uterus, + *pēxis,* fixation]

col·po·hys·ter·ot·o·my (kol'pō-his-ter-ot'ō-mē). SYN vaginal *hysterotomy.* [colpo- + G. *hystera,* uterus, + *tomē,* incision]

col·po·mi·cro·scope (kol-pō-mī'krō-skōp). Special microscope for direct visual examination of the cervical tissue.

col·po·mi·cros·co·py (kol'pō-mī-kros'kŏ-pē). Direct observation and study of cells in the vagina and cervix magnified *in vivo,* in the undisturbed tissue, by means of a colpomicroscope.

col·po·my·co·sis (kol'pō-mī-kō'sis). SYN vaginomycosis.

col·po·my·o·mec·to·my (kol'pō-mī-ō-mek'tō-mē). SYN vaginal *myomectomy.* [colpo- + myoma + G. *ektomē,* excision]

col·pop·a·thy (kol-pop′ă-thē). SYN vaginopathy. [colpo- + G. *pathos*, suffering]

col·po·per·i·ne·o·plas·ty (kol′pō-pār-i-nē′ō-plas-tē). SYN vaginoperineoplasty. [colpo- + perineum, + G. *plastos*, formed]

col·po·per·i·ne·or·rha·phy (kol′pō-pār-i-nē-ōr′ă-fē). SYN vaginoperineorrhaphy. [colpo- + perineum, + G. *rhaphē*, sewing]

col·po·pexy (kol′pō-pek-sē). SYN vaginofixation. [colpo- + G. *pēxis*, fixation]

col·po·plas·ty (kol′pō-plas-tē). SYN vaginoplasty. [colpo- + G. *plastos*, formed]

col·po·poi·e·sis (kol′pō-poy-ē′sis). Surgical construction of a vagina. [colpo- + G. *poiēsis*, a making]

col·po·pto·sis, col·po·pto·sia (kol-pō-tō′sis, -tō′sē-ă; kol-pop-tō′sis). Prolapse of the vaginal walls. SYN colpocele (2). [colpo- + G. *ptōsis*, a falling]

col·po·rec·to·pexy (kol-pō-rek′tō-pek-sē). Repair of a prolapsed rectum by suturing it to the wall of the vagina. [colpo- + rectum + G. *pēxis*, fixation]

col·por·rha·gia (kol-pō-rā′jē-ă). A vaginal hemorrhage. [colpo- + G. *rhēgnymi*, to burst forth]

col·por·rha·phy (kol-pōr′ă-fē). Repair of a rupture of the vagina by excision and suturing of the edges of the tear. [colpo- + G. *rhaphē*, suture]

col·por·rhex·is (kol-pō-rek′sis). Tearing of the vaginal wall. SYN vaginal laceration. [colpo- + G. *rhēxis*, rupture]

col·po·scope (kol′pō-skōp). Endoscopic instrument that magnifies cells of the vagina and cervix *in vivo* to allow direct observation and study of these tissues.

col·pos·co·py (kol-pos′kŏ-pē). Examination of vagina and cervix by means of an endoscope. [colpo- + G. *skopeō*, to view]

The magnification afforded, between 5 and 50×, allows for visual inspection of dysplastic areas. Colposcopy generally takes place after an abnormal Pap smear, and it may aid in office procedures for removing dysplastic cells, such as cauterization or loop excision.

col·po·spasm (kol′pō-spazm). Spasmodic contraction of the vagina.

col·po·stat (kol′pō-stat). Appliance for use in the vagina, such as a radium applicator, for treatment of cancer of the cervix. [colpo- + G. *statos*, standing]

col·po·ste·no·sis (kol′pō-sten-ō′sis). Narrowing of the lumen of the vagina. [colpo- + G. *stenōsis*, narrowing]

col·po·ste·not·o·my (kol′pō-sten-ot′ō-mē). Surgical correction of a colpostenosis. [colpo- + G. *stenōsis*, narrowing, + *tomē*, incision]

col·pot·o·my (kol-pot′ō-mē). SYN vaginotomy. [colpo- + G. *tomē*, incision]

col·po·u·re·ter·ot·o·my (kol′pō-yū-rē-ter-ot′ō-mē). Incision into a ureter through the vagina. [colpo- + G. *tomē*, incision]

col·po·xe·ro·sis (kol-pō-zē-rō′sis). Abnormal dryness of the vaginal mucous membrane. [colpo- + G. *xērōsis*, dryness]

Co·lu·bri·dae (kol-yū′bri-dē). A family of largely nonpoisonous or mildly poisonous snakes comprising over 1000 species, found in North and South America, Asia, and Africa. [L. *coluber*, serpent]

co·lum·bi·um (Cb) (kol-ŭm′bē-ŭm). Former name for niobium. [*Columbia*, name for America]

col·u·mel·la, pl. **col·u·mel·lae** (kol-ū-mel′ă, -mel′ē). **1.** A column, or a small column. SYN columnella. **2.** In fungi, a sterile invagination of a sporangium, as in Zygomycetes. [L. dim. of *columna*, column]

c. au′ris, the middle ear ossicle of amphibians, reptiles, and birds; homologous with the stapes of mammals.

c. coch′leae, SYN *modiolus* labii.

c. na′si, the fleshy lower margin (termination) of the nasal septum.

col·umn (kol′ŭm). **1.** An anatomical part or structure in the form of a pillar or cylindric funiculus. SEE ALSO fascicle. **2.** A vertical object (usually cylindrical), mass, or formation. SYN columna [NA]. [L. *columna*]

affinity c., SYN affinity *chromatography*.

anal c.'s, a number of vertical ridges in the mucous membrane of the upper half of the anal canal formed as the caliber of the canal is sharply reduced from that of the rectal ampulla. SYN columnae anales [NA], Morgagni's c.'s, rectal c.'s.

anterior c., the pronounced, ventrally oriented ridge of gray matter in each half of the spinal cord; it corresponds to the anterior or ventral horn appearing in transverse sections of the cord, and contains the motor neurons innervating the skeletal musculature of the trunk, neck, and extremities. SEE ALSO gray c.'s. SYN columna anterior [NA].

anterior gray c., SYN central and lateral intermediate *substance*.

anterior c. of medulla oblongata, SYN *pyramid* of medulla oblongata.

anterolateral c. of spinal cord, SYN lateral *funiculus*.

Bertin's c.'s, SYN renal c.'s.

branchial efferent c., a c. of gray matter in the brainstem of the embryo, represented in the adult by the nucleus ambiguus and the motor nuclei of the trigeminal and facial nerves.

Burdach's c., SYN cuneate *fasciculus*.

Clarke's c., SYN thoracic *nucleus*.

dorsal c. of spinal cord, SYN posterior c.

c. of fornix, that part of the fornix that curves down in front of the thalamus and the interventricular foramen of Monro, then continues through the hypothalamus to the mamillary body; consisting primarily of fibers originating in the hippocampus and subiculum, the c. of fornix is the direct continuation of the body of the fornix. SYN columna fornicis [NA], anterior pillar of fornix.

general somatic afferent c., in the embryo, a c. of gray matter in the hindbrain and spinal cord, represented in the adult by the sensory nuclei of the trigeminal nerve and relay cells in the dorsal horn.

general somatic efferent c., a c. of gray matter in the embryo, represented in the adult by the nuclei of the oculomotor, trochlear, abducens, and hypoglossal nerves and by motor neurons of the ventral horn of the spinal cord.

general visceral afferent c., a c. of gray matter in the hindbrain and spinal cord of the embryo, developing into the nucleus of the solitary tract and relay cells of the spinal cord.

general visceral efferent c., a c. of gray matter in the hindbrain and spinal cord of the embryo, represented in the adult by the dorsal nucleus of the vagus, the superior and inferior salivatory and Edinger-Westphal nuclei and the visceral motor neurons of the spinal cord.

Goll's c., SYN *fasciculus* gracilis.

Gowers' c., SYN anterior spinocerebellar *tract*.

gray c.'s, the three somewhat ridge-shaped masses of gray matter (anterior, posterior, and lateral c.'s) that extend longitudinally through the center of each lateral half of the spinal cord; in transverse sections these c.'s appear as gray horns and are therefore commonly called ventral or anterior, dorsal or posterior, and lateral horn, respectively. SYN columnae griseae [NA].

intermediolateral cell c. of spinal cord, SYN intermediolateral *nucleus*.

lateral c., a slight protrusion of the gray matter of the spinal cord into the lateral funiculus of either side, especially marked in the thoracic region where it encloses preganglionic motor neurons of the sympathetic division of the autonomic nervous system; it corresponds to the lateral horn appearing in transverse sections of the spinal cord. SEE ALSO gray c.'s. SYN columna lateralis [NA], lateral c. of spinal cord.

lateral c. of spinal cord, SYN lateral c.

Lissauer's c., SYN dorsolateral *fasciculus*.

Morgagni's c.'s, SYN anal c.'s.

posterior c., the pronounced, dorsolaterally oriented ridge of gray matter in each lateral half of the spinal cord, corresponding to the posterior or dorsal horn appearing in transverse sections of the cord. SYN columna posterior [NA], dorsal c. of spinal cord, posterior c. of spinal cord (1).

posterior c. of spinal cord, (1) SYN posterior c. **(2)** in clinical parlance, the term often refers to the posterior funiculus of the spinal cord.

rectal c.'s, SYN anal c.'s.

renal c.'s, the prolongations of cortical substance separating the pyramids of the kidney. SYN columnae renales [NA], Bertin's c.'s.

Rolando's c., a slight ridge on either side of the medulla oblongata related to the descending trigeminal tract and nucleus.

rugal c.'s of vagina, two slight longitudinal ridges, anterior and posterior, in the vaginal mucous membrane, each marked by a number of transverse mucosal folds. SYN columnae rugarum [NA], vaginal c.'s.

Sertoli's c.'s, SEE Sertoli's *cells,* under *cell.*

special somatic afferent c., a c. of gray matter in the hindbrain of the embryo, represented in the adult by the nuclei of the auditory and vestibular nerves.

special visceral efferent c., a c. of gray matter in the hindbrain of the embryo, represented in the adult by the trigeminal and facial nuclei and the nucleus ambiguus.

spinal c., SYN vertebral c.

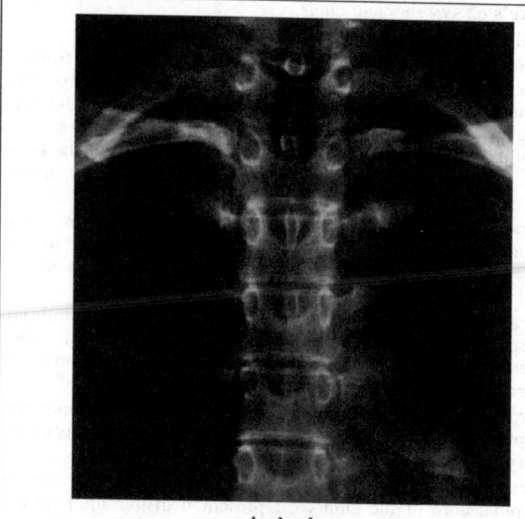

spinal column
x-ray view of T1–T5

c. of Spitzka-Lissauer, SEE dorsolateral *fasciculus.*

Stilling's c., SYN thoracic *nucleus.*

Türck's c., SYN anterior pyramidal *tract.*

vaginal c.'s, SYN rugal c.'s of vagina.

ventral white c., SYN white *commissure.*

vertebral c., the series of vertebrae that extend from the cranium to the coccyx, providing support and forming a flexible bony case for the spinal cord. SYN columna vertebralis [NA], backbone, dorsal spine, rachis, spina dorsalis, spina (2), spina (1), spinal c., spine (2), vertebrarium.

co·lum·na, gen. and pl. **co·lum·nae** (ko-lŭm′nă, -ne) [NA]. SYN column, column. [L.]

colum′nae ana′les [NA], SYN anal *columns,* under *column.*

c. ante′rior [NA], SYN anterior *column.*

colum′nae car′neae, SYN *trabeculae* carneae, under *trabecula.*

c. for′nicis [NA], SYN *column* of fornix.

colum′nae gris′eae [NA], SYN gray *columns,* under *column.*

c. latera′lis [NA], SYN lateral *column.*

c. poste′rior [NA], SYN posterior *column.*

colum′nae rena′les [NA], SYN renal *columns,* under *column.*

colum′nae ruga′rum [NA], SYN rugal *columns* of vagina, under *column.*

c. vertebra′lis [NA], SYN vertebral *column.*

co·lum·nel·la, pl. **col·um·nel·lae** (ko-lŭm-nel′ă, -nel′e). SYN columella (1). [L. dim. of *columna,* a column; another form of *columella*]

co·ly·pep·tic (ko-le-pep′tik). Rarely used term for retarding digestion. [G. *kolyo,* to hinder, + *pepsis,* digestion]

△**com-.** SEE con-.

co·ma (ko′mă). **1.** A state of profound unconsciousness from which one cannot be roused; may be due to the action of an ingested toxic substance or of one formed in the body, to trauma, or to disease. **2.** An aberration of spherical lenses; occurring in cases of oblique incidence (*e.g.,* the image of a point becomes comet-shaped). [G. *kome,* hair] **3.** SYN coma *aberration.* [G. *koma,* deep sleep, trance]

c. carcinomato′sum, c. occurring in the final stage of cancerous cachexia.

delayed c. after hypoxia, c. that develops a few days to 3 weeks after an acute hypoxic insult; the latter was usually severe enough to cause an initial bout of coma, which cleared, and was followed by a transient interval of apparent normality. SYN severe postanoxic encephalopathy.

diabetic c., c. that develops in severe and inadequately treated cases of diabetes mellitus and is commonly fatal, unless appropriate therapy is instituted promptly; results from reduced oxidative metabolism of the central nervous system that, in turn, stems from severe ketoacidosis and possibly also from the histotoxic action of the ketone bodies and disturbances in water and electrolyte balance. SYN Kussmaul's c.

hepatic c., c. that occurs with advanced hepatic insufficiency and portal-systemic shunts, caused by elevated blood ammonia levels; characteristic findings include asterixis in the precoma stage and paroxysms of bilaterally synchronous triphasic waves on EEG examination.

hyperosmolar (hyperglycemic) nonketotic c. (hi′per-os-mo′lăr), a complication seen in *diabetes* mellitus in which very marked hyperglycemia occurs (such as levels over 800 mg/dL) causing osmotic shifts in water in brain cells and resulting in coma. It can be fatal or lead to permanent neurologic damage. Ketoacidosis does not occur in these cases.

hypoglycemic c., a metabolic encephalopathy caused by hypoglycemia; usually seen in diabetics, and due to exogenous insulin excess.

hypoventilation c., coma seen with advanced lung failure and resultant hypoventilation. SYN CO_2 narcosis, hypoxic-hypercarbic encephalopathy, pulmonary encephalopathy.

Kussmaul's c., SYN diabetic c.

metabolic c., coma resulting from diffuse failure of neuronal metabolism, caused by such abnormalities as intrinsic disorders of neuron or glial cell metabolism, or extracerebral disorders that produce intoxication or electrolyte imbalances.

thyrotoxic c., c. preceding death in severe hyperthyroidism, as in thyroid storm or thyrotoxic crisis.

trance c., SYN lethargic *hypnosis.*

uremic c., a metabolic encephalopathy caused by renal failure.

co·ma·tose (ko′mă-tos). In a state of coma.

com·bi·na·tion (kom-bi-nā′shŭn). **1.** The act of combining (*i.e.,* by joining, uniting, or otherwise bringing into close association) separate entities. **2.** The state of being so combined.

binary c., the name of a species of bacteria consisting of two parts: a generic name and a specific epithet.

new c., the new name that results from the transfer of a microorganism from one genus to another; the generic name changes but, in most cases, the specific epithet remains the same.

com·bi·na·to·ri·al (kom′bin-ă-tor′e-ăl). Any system using a random assortment of components at any positions in the linear arrangement of atoms, *i.e.,* a combinatorial library of mutations could contain positions where all four bases have been randomly inserted.

com·bus·ti·ble (kom-bus′ti-bl). Capable of combustion.

com·bus·tion (kom-bŭs′chŭn). Burning, the rapid oxidation of any substance accompanied by the production of heat and light. [L. *comburo,* pp. *-bustus,* to burn up]

slow c., SEE decay.

spontaneous c., the ignition of a mass of material by heat developed within it by the oxidation of the substances composing it without external ignition.

Comby, Jules, French pediatrician, 1853–1947. SEE C.'s *sign.*

com·e·do, pl. **com·e·dos, com·e·do·nes** (kom′ē-dō, kō-mē′dō; kom′ē-dōz; kom-ē-dō′nēz). A dilated hair follicle infundibulum filled with keratin squamae, bacteria, particularly *Propionibacterium acnes,* and sebum; the primary lesion of acne vulgaris. [L. a glutton, fr. *com-edo,* to eat up]

closed c., a c. with a narrow or obstructed opening on the skin surface; closed c.'s may rupture, producing a low-grade dermal inflammatory reaction. SYN whitehead (2).

open c., a c. with a wide opening on the skin surface capped with a melanin-containing blackened mass of epithelial debris. SYN blackhead (1).

com·e·do·car·ci·no·ma (kō-mē′dō-kar-si-nō′mă). Form of carcinoma of the breast or other organ in which plugs of necrotic malignant cells may be expressed from the ducts.

com·e·do·gen·ic (kom′ē-dō-jen′ik). Tending to promote the formation of comedones. SYN acnegenic. [comedo + G. *genesis,* production]

com·e·do·ne·cro·sis (kom′ē-dō-nek-rō′sis). A type of necrosis occurring with glands in which there is central luminal inflammation with devitalized cells, usually occurring in the breast in intraductal carcinoma. [comedo + necrosis]

co·mes, pl. **com·i·tes** (kō′mēz, kom′i-tēz). A blood vessel accompanying another vessel or a nerve; the veins accompanying an artery, often two in number, are called venae comitantes or venae comites. [L. a companion, fr. *com-,* together, + *eo,* pp. *itus,* to go]

com·i·tance (kom′ē-tans). A characteristic of strabismus in which the misalignment of the eyes is maintained in all directions of gaze.

com·i·tant (komitant). having comitance; in a c. strabismus the same angle of misalignment of the eyes is maintained in all directions of gaze. SYN concomitant.

com·men·sal (kŏ-men′săl). **1.** Pertaining to or characterized by commensalism. **2.** An organism participating in commensalism.

com·men·sal·ism (kŏ-men′săl-izm). A symbiotic relationship in which one species derives benefit and the other is unharmed; *e.g., Entamoeba coli* in the human large intestine. Cf. metabiosis, mutualism, parasitism. [L. *con-,* with, together, + *mensa,* table]

epizoic c., SYN phoresis (2).

com·mi·nut·ed (kom′i-nū-ted). Broken into several pieces; denoting especially a fractured bone. [L. *com-minuo,* pp. *-minutus,* to make smaller, break into pieces, fr. *minor,* less]

com·mi·nu·tion (kom-i-nū′shŭn). A breaking into several pieces.

com·mis·su·ra, gen. and pl. **com·mis·sur·ae** (kom-i-syūr′ă, -syūr′ē) [NA]. SYN commissure. [L. a joining together, seam, fr. *com- mitto,* to send together, combine]

c. al′ba [NA], SYN white *commissure.*

c. ante′rior [NA], SYN anterior *commissure.*

c. ante′rior gris′ea, SEE *substantia* intermedia centralis et lateralis.

c. bulbor′um, ☆official alternate term for *commissure* of vestibular bulb.

c. cine′rea, SYN interthalamic *adhesion.*

c. colliculo′rum inferi′orum, SEE *commissure* of inferior colliculi.

c. colliculo′rum superio′rum, SEE *commissure* of superior colliculus.

c. for′nicis [NA], the triangular subcallosal plate of commissural fibers resulting from the converging of the right and left fornix bundles which exchange numerous fibers and which curve back in the contralateral fornix to end in the hippocampus of the opposite side. SYN c. hippocampi, commissure of fornix, delta fornicis, hippocampal commissure, psalterium (1), transverse fornix.

c. gris′ea, (1) SYN interthalamic *adhesion.* (2) SEE *substantia* intermedia centralis et lateralis.

c. habenula′rum [NA], the connection between the right and left

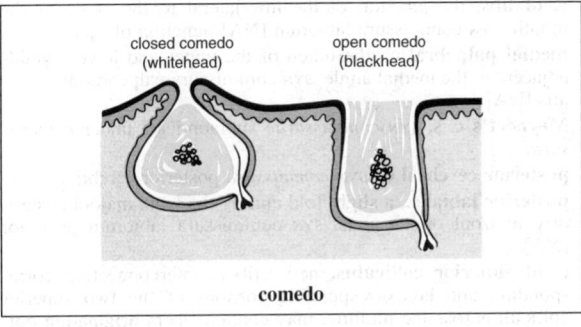

closed comedo (whitehead)   open comedo (blackhead)

comedo

habenular nuclei; the decussation of fibers of the two striae medullares, forming the dorsal portion of the peduncle of the pineal body. SYN commissure of habenulae, habenular commissure.

c. hippocam′pi, SYN c. fornicis.

c. labio′rum [NA], SYN *commissure* of lips.

c. labio′rum ante′rior [NA], SYN anterior labial *commissure.*

c. labio′rum poste′rior [NA], SYN posterior labial *commissure.*

c. palpebra′rum latera′lis [NA], SYN lateral palpebral *commissure.*

c. palpebra′rum media′lis [NA], SYN medial palpebral *commissure.*

c. poste′rior cer′ebri [NA], a thin band of white matter, crossing from side to side beneath the habenula of the pineal body and over the aditus ad aqueductum cerebri; it is largely composed of fibers interconnecting the left and right pretectal region and related cell groups of the midbrain; dorsally, it marks the junction of the diencephalon and mesencephalon. SYN posterior cerebral commissure.

c. poste′rior gris′ea, SEE *substantia* intermedia centralis et lateralis.

commissu′rae supraop′ticae [NA], the commissural fibers that lie above and behind the optic chiasm. SYN Ganser's commissures, Gudden's commissures, Meynert's commissures, supraoptic commissures.

c. ventra′lis al′ba, SYN white *commissure.*

com·mis·sur·al (kom-i-syūr′ăl). Relating to a commissure.

com·mis·sure (kom′i-syūr). **1.** Angle or corner of the eye, lips, or labia. **2.** A bundle of nerve fibers passing from one side to the other in the brain or spinal cord. SYN commissura [NA].

anterior c., a round bundle of nerve fibers that crosses the midline of the brain near the anterior limit of the third ventricle. It consists of a smaller anterior part, the fibers of which pass in part to the olfactory bulbs, and a larger posterior part, which interconnects the left and right temporal lobes. SYN commissura anterior [NA].

anterior labial c., the junction of the labia majora anteriorly at the mons pubis. SYN commissura labiorum anterior [NA].

anterior white c., SYN white c.

c. of cerebral hemispheres, SYN *corpus* callosum.

c. of fornix, SYN commissura fornicis.

Ganser's c.'s, SYN *commissurae* supraopticae, under *commissura.*

Gudden's c.'s, SYN *commissurae* supraopticae, under *commissura.*

c. of habenulae, SYN *commissura* habenularum.

habenular c., SYN *commissura* habenularum.

hippocampal c., SYN *commissura* fornicis.

c. of inferior colliculi, nerve fibers on the midline between the two inferior colliculi connecting the colliculi and containing some fibers originating from nontectal nuclei.

labial c., junction of upper and lower lip which occurs at corner of mouth. SEE ALSO *angle* of mouth.

lateral palpebral c., the union of the upper and lower eyelids adjacent to the lateral angle. SYN commissura palpebrarum lateralis [NA].

CO

c. of lips, the junction of the lips lateral to the angle of the mouth. SYN commissura labiorum [NA], junction of lips.

medial palpebral c., the union of the upper and lower eyelids adjacent to the medial angle. SYN commissura palpebrarum medialis [NA].

Meynert's c.'s, SYN *commissurae* supraopticae, under *commissura.*

posterior cerebral c., SYN *commissura* posterior cerebri.

posterior labial c., a slight fold uniting the labia majora posteriorly in front of the anus. SYN commissura labiorum posterior [NA].

c. of superior colliculus, nerve fibers interconnecting corresponding and noncorresponding portions of the two superior colliculi across the midline; may contain fibers originating outside the tectum.

supraoptic c.'s, SYN *commissurae* supraopticae, under *commissura.*

c. of vestibular bulb, a narrow median band that connects the two masses of erectile tissue (the bulbus vestibuli) on either side of the vaginal orifice. SYN pars intermedia commissura bulborum [NA], commissura bulborum★, intermediate part of vestibular bulb, pars intermedia bulborum.

Wernekinck's c., the decussation of the brachia conjunctiva before their entrance into the red nucleus of the tegmentum.

white c., a narrow band of white substance bordering on the anterior median fissure of the spinal cord in front of the anterior gray commissure, and consisting of nerve fibers crossing over from one half of the spinal cord to the other. SYN commissura alba [NA], anterior white c., commissura ventralis alba, ventral white column.

com·mis·sur·ot·o·my (kom'ĭ-syūr-ot'ō-mē). **1.** Surgical division of any commissure, fibrous band, or ring via surgery or a balloon catheter technique. **2.** SYN midline *myelotomy.*

mitral c., opening the narrowed mitral orifice for the relief of mitral stenosis.

com·mit·ment (kŏ-mit'ment). Legal consignment, by certification, or voluntarily, of an individual to a mental hospital or institution. [L. *com-mitto,* to deliver, consign]

com·mon ve·hi·cle spread. spread of disease agent from a source that is common to those who acquire the disease, *e.g.,* water, milk, air, syringe contaminated by infectious or noxious agents.

com·mo·tio (kō-mō'shē-ō). SYN concussion (2). [L. a moving, commotion, fr. *com-moveo,* pp. *-motus,* to set in motion, agitate]

c. cer'ebri, SYN brain concussion.

c. re'tinae, concussion of the retina that may produce a milky edema in the posterior pole that clears up after a few days.

com·mu·ni·ca·ble (kŏ-myūn'ĭ-kă-bl). Capable of being communicated or transmitted; said especially of disease.

com·mu·ni·cans, pl. **com·mu·ni·can·tes** (kŏ-myū'ni-kans, kŏ-myū-ni-kan'tēz). Communicating; connecting or joining. [L. pres. p. of *communico,* pp. *-atus,* to share with someone, make common]

com·mu·ni·ca·tion (kŏ-myū-ni-kā'shŭn). **1.** An opening or connecting passage between two structures. **2.** In anatomy, a joining or connecting, said of fibrous, solid structures, *e.g.,* tendons and nerves. Anastomosis is incorrectly used as a synonym. [L. *communicatio*]

com·mu·ni·ty (kŏ-myū'ni-tē). A given segment of a society or a population.

biotic c., SYN biocenosis.

therapeutic c., a specially structured mental hospital or community health center milieu that provides an effective environment for behavioral changes in patients through resocialization and rehabilitation.

com·mu·ni·ty men·tal health cen·ter. A mental health treatment center located in a neighborhood catchment area close to the homes of patients, introduced in the 1960's via new federal legislation designed to replace the large state hospitals, which usually were located in remote rural areas; features include offering a series of comprehensive services by one or more members of the four mental health professions, provision of continuity of care, participation of consumers in the centers, community location to provide accessibility, a combination of indirect or preventive and direct services, the use of program-centered as well as case-centered consultation, a requirement for program evaluation, and various linkages to a variety of health and human services.

Comolli, Antonio, Italian pathologist, *1879. SEE C.'s *sign.*

co·mor·bid·i·ty (kō-mōr-bid'i-tē). A concomitant but unrelated pathologic or disease process; usually used in epidemiology to indicate the coexistence of two or more disease processes. [co- + L. *morbidus,* diseased]

com·pac·ta (kom-pak'tă). SYN *stratum* compactum.

com·pa·ges tho·ra·cis (kom-pā'jēz thō-rā'sis) [NA]. SYN thoracic *cage.*

com·par·a·scope (kom-par'ă-skōp). A microscope accessory by means of which an observer may directly compare simultaneously the findings in two microscopic preparations. [L. *comparo,* to compare, + G. *skopeō,* to view]

com·part·ment (kom-part'ment). A separate division; specifically, a structural or biochemical portion of a cell that is separated from the rest of the cell.

nonplasmatic c., c. surrounded by a single biomembrane (*e.g.,* vacuoles, lysosomes).

plasmatic c., c. surrounded by a double biomembrane and containing polynucleotides (*e.g.,* mitochondria).

com·part·men·ta·tion (kom-part'ment-ā'shŭn). The division of a cell into different regions, either structurally or biochemically.

com·pat·i·bil·i·ty (kom-pat-ĭ-bil'i-tē). The condition of being compatible.

com·pat·i·ble (kom-pat'ĭ-bl). **1.** Capable of being mixed without undergoing destructive chemical change or exhibiting mutual antagonism; said of the elements in a properly constructed pharmaceutical mixture. **2.** Denoting the ability of two biologic entities to exist together without nullification of, or deleterious effects on, the function of either; *e.g.,* blood, tissues, or organs that cause no reaction when transfused or no rejection when transplanted. **3.** Denoting satisfactory relationships between two or more people as in work or in marriage or in sexual activities. [L. *con-,* with, + *patior,* to suffer]

com·pen·sa·tion (kom-pen-sā'shŭn). **1.** A process in which a tendency for a change in a given direction is counteracted by another change so that the original change is not evident. **2.** An unconscious mechanism by which one tries to make up for fancied or real deficiencies. [L. *com-penso,* pp. *-atus,* to weigh together, counterbalance]

attenuation c., SYN time-gain c.

depth c., SYN time-gain c.

gene dosage c., the putative mechanism that adjusts the X-linked phenotypes of males and females to compensate for the haploid state in males and the diploid state in females. It is now largely ascribed to lyonization which compensates the mean of the dose but not its variance, which is greater in females.

time-gain c. (TGC), in ultrasonography, an increase in receiver gain with time to compensate for loss in echo amplitude with depth, usually due to attenuation. SYN attenuation c., depth c., time compensation gain, time-compensated gain, time-varied gain control, time-varied gain.

com·pen·sa·to·ry (kom-pen'să-tōr-ē). Providing compensation; making up for a deficiency or loss.

com·pe·tence (kom'pĕ-tens). **1.** The quality of being competent or capable of performing an allotted function. **2.** The normal tight closure of a cardiac valve. **3.** The ability of a group of embryonic cells to respond to an organizer. **4.** The ability of a (bacterial) cell to take up free DNA, which may lead to transformation. **5.** In psychiatry, the mental ability to distinguish right from wrong and to manage one's own affairs, or to assist one's counsel in his or her defense in a legal proceeding. [Fr. *competence,* fr. L.L. *competentia,* congruity]

cardiac c., ability of the ventricles to pump the blood returning to the atria, so that atrial pressure does not rise abnormally.

immunological c., SYN immunocompetence.

com·pe·ti·tion (kom-pĕ-tish'ŭn). The process by which the activity or presence of one substance interferes with, or suppresses, the activity of another substance with similar affinities.

antigenic c., c. that occurs when two different antigens, each of which can evoke an immunological response when inoculated alone, are mixed in equal quantities and inoculated together; the response may be to only one, that to the other being largely or entirely suppressed.

com·plaint (kom-plānt'). A disorder, disease, or symptom, or the description of it. [O. Fr. *complainte*, fr. L. *complango*, to lament]

chief c., the primary symptom that a patient states as the reason for seeking medical care.

com·ple·ment (kom'plĕ-ment). Ehrlich's term for the thermolabile substance, normally present in serum, that is destructive to certain bacteria and other cells sensitized by a specific complement-fixing antibody. C. is a serum protein complex comprising at least 20 distinct proteins, the activity of which is affected by a series of interactions resulting in enzymatic cleavages and which can follow one or the other of at least two pathways. In the case of immune hemolysis (classical pathway), the complex comprises nine components (designated C1 through C9) which react in a definite sequence and the activation of which is effected by the antigen-antibody complex; only the first seven components are involved in chemotaxis, and only the first four are involved in immune adherence or phagocytosis or are fixed by conglutinins. An alternative pathway (see properdin *system*) is activated by factors other than antigen-antibody complexes and involves components other than C1, C4, and C2 in the activation of C3. SEE ALSO *component* of complement. [L. *complementum*, that which completes, fr. *com-pleo*, to fill up]

heparin c., the protein component of heparin in blood.

com·ple·men·tar·i·ty (kom-plĕ-men-tār'i-tē). **1.** The degree of base-pairing (A opposite U or T, G opposite C) between two sequences of DNA and/or RNA molecules. **2.** The degree of affinity, or fit, of antigen and antibody combining sites.

com·ple·men·ta·tion (kom'plĕ-men-tā'shŭn). **1.** Functional interaction between two defective viruses permitting replication under conditions inhibitory to the single virus. **2.** Interaction between two genetic units, one or both of which are defective, permitting the organism containing these units to function normally, whereas it could not do so if either unit were absent.

intergenic c., c. between pieces of genetic material that regulate the same function, such as a multienzyme pathway, but have defects in regions of separate genetic function; such c. permits synthesis of a normal end-product.

intragenic c., c. between pieces of genetic material, each of which has a different defect within the same locus; the resultant product of each is defective and nonfunctional, but the defective products may associate to produce a product which has some activity.

com·plex (kom'pleks). **1.** An organized constellation of feelings, thoughts, perceptions, and memories that may be in part unconscious and may strongly influence associations and attitudes. **2.** In chemistry, the relatively stable combination of two or more compounds into a larger molecule without covalent binding. **3.** A composite of chemical or immunological structures. **4.** A structural anatomical entity made up of three or more interrelated parts. **5.** An informal term used to denote a group of individual structures known or believed to be anatomically, embryologically, or physiologically related. [L. *complexus,* woven together]

aberrant c., an anomalous electrocardiographic c., more specifically an abnormal ventricular c. caused by abnormal intraventricular conduction of a supraventricular impulse.

AIDS dementia c. (ADC), a subacute or chronic HIV-1 encephalitis, the most common neurological complication in the later stages of HIV infection; manifested clinically as a progressive dementia, accompanied by motor abnormalities. SYN AIDS dementia, HIV encephalopathy.

AIDS-related c. (ARC), early manifestations of AIDS in individuals who have not yet developed deficient immune function, characterized by fever with generalized lymphadenopathy, diarrhea, and weight loss.

α-keto acid dehydrogenase c., SEE α-keto acid dehydrogenase.

amygdaloid c., SYN amygdaloid *body.*

anomalous c., a c. in the electrocardiogram differing significantly from the physiologic type in the same lead.

antigen-antibody c., SEE immune c.

antigenic c., a composite of different antigenic structures, such as a cell or a bacterium, or, by extension, a molecule containing two or more determinant groups of different antigenic specificities.

apical c., a set of anterior structures that characterize one or several developmental stages of members of the protozoan phylum Apicomplexa; includes the following structures, visible by electron microscopy: polar ring, conoid, rhoptries, micronemes, and subpellicular tubules.

atrial c., p wave in the electrocardiogram. SYN auricular c.

auricular c., SYN atrial c.

avian leukosis-sarcoma c., avian leukemia-sarcoma c., (1) a term applied to a group of transmissible virus-induced diseases of chickens causing sarcoma, myeloblastosis, erythroblastosis, leukosis, osteopetrosis, and lymphomatosis. These agents are closely related viruses (avian leukosis-sarcoma virus) causing prolferation of immature erythroid, myeloid, or lymphoid cells; **(2)** a division of the RNA tumor viruses (subfamily Oncovirinae) causing the avian leukosis-sarcoma c. of diseases; the viruses are subgrouped according to antigenic characteristics and growth in defined types of tissue culture cells. SYN avian erythroblastosis virus, avian leukosis-sarcoma virus, avian lymphomatosis virus (1), avian myeloblastosis virus, avian sarcoma virus, fowl erythroblastosis virus, fowl lymphomatosis virus, fowl myeloblastosis virus.

binary c., a noncovalent c. of two molecules; often referring to the enzyme-substrate c. in an enzyme-catalyzed reaction. Cf. central c., Michaelis c. SYN enzyme-substrate c.

brain wave c., a specific combination of fast and slow electroencephalographic activity that recurs frequently enough to be identified as a discrete phenomenon.

brother c., SYN Cain c.

Cain c., extreme envy or jealousy of a brother, leading to hatred. SYN brother c. [*Cain,* biblical personage]

castration c., (1) a child's fear of injury to the genitals by the parent of the same sex as punishment for unconcious guilt over oedipal feelings; **(2)** fantasied loss of the penis by a female or fear of its actual loss by a male; **(3)** unconscious fear of injury from those in authority. SYN castration anxiety.

caudal pharyngeal c., the ultimobranchial body associated with the embryonic fourth and transitory fifth pharyngeal pouches.

central c., in an enzyme-catalyzed reaction, the structural complex of the enzyme and all of the enzyme's substrates (or the enzyme with all of the enzyme's products) equivalent to the binary c. for a one-substrate enzyme. Cf. binary c., Michaelis c.

charge transfer c., (1) a c. between two organic molecules in which an electron from one (the donor) is transferred to the other (the acceptor), becoming generally distributed throughout the latter; subsequent transfer of a hydrogen atom completes the reduction of the acceptor; such c.'s are generally highly colored and may be so observed; **(2)** a network of hydrogen bridges at the catalytic center of certain proteases. SYN charge transfer system.

Diana c., ideas leading to the adoption of masculine traits and behavior in a female. [*Diana,* L. myth. char.]

diphasic c., a c. consisting of both positive and negative deflections.

EAHF c., a combination of allergies consisting of *eczema, a*sthma and *hay* fever.

Eisenmenger's c., the combination of ventricular septal defect with pulmonary hypertension and consequent right-to-left shunt through the defect, with or without an associated overriding aorta. SYN Eisenmenger's defect, Eisenmenger's disease, Eisenmenger's tetralogy.

Electra c., female counterpart of the Oedipus c. in the male; a term used to describe unresolved conflicts during childhood development toward the father which subsequently influence a woman's relationships with men. SYN father c. [*Electra,* daughter of Agamemnon]

electrocardiographic c., a deflection or group of deflections in the electrocardiogram.

enzyme-substrate c., SYN binary c.

equiphasic c., SYN isodiphasic c.

father c., SYN Electra c.

feline leukemia-sarcoma virus c., viruses from cats that induce transmissible leukemia or transmissible fibrosarcoma in kittens.

femininity c., in psychoanalysis, the unconscious fear, in boys and men, of castration at the hands of the mother with resultant identification with the aggressor and envious desire for breasts and vagina.

Ghon's c., SYN Ghon's *tubercle.*

Golgi c., SYN Golgi *apparatus.*

H-2 c., term that denotes genes of the major histocompatibility c.

histocompatibility c., a family of fifty or more genes on the sixth human chromosome that code for cell surface proteins and play a role in the immune response.

> Histocompatibility genes control the production of proteins on the outer membranes of tissue and blood cells, especially lymphocytes, and are vital elements in cell-cell recognition. The proteins also determine the level and type of immune response, and may serve other biochemical or immunologic functions. In the case of allografts, it is necessary to determine whether donor and recipient possess compatible sets of proteins (histocompatibility antigens), to minimize the likelihood of rejection. Histocompatibility testing (HLA tissue typing) provides this information.

HLA c., the major histocompatibility c. in humans. SEE ALSO human lymphocyte *antigens,* under *antigen.*

immune c., antigen combined with specific antibody, to which complement may also be fixed, and which may precipitate or remain in solution. Frequently associated with autoimmune disease.

inferiority c., a sense of inadequacy which is expressed in extreme shyness, diffidence, or timidity, or as a compensatory reaction in exhibitionism or aggressiveness.

iron-dextran c., a colloidal solution of ferric hydroxide in c. with partially hydrolyzed dextran; used in the treatment of iron deficiency anemias by intramuscular injection.

isodiphasic c., a diphasic c. whose positive and negative deflections are approximately equal. SYN equiphasic c.

j-g c., SYN juxtaglomerular c.

Jocasta c., a mother's libidinous fixation on a son. [*Jocasta,* mother and wife of Oedipus]

junctional c., the attachment zone between epithelial cells, typically consisting of the zonula occludens, the zonula adherens, and the macula adherens (desmosome).

juxtaglomerular c., a c. consisting of the juxtaglomerular cells, which are modified smooth muscle cells in the wall of the afferent glomerular arteriole and sometimes also the efferent arteriole; extraglomerular mesangium lacis cells, which are located in the angle between the afferent and efferent glomerular arterioles; the macula densa of the distal convoluted tubule; and granular epithelial peripolar cells located at the angle of reflection of the parietal to the visceral capsule of the renal corpuscle; believed to provide some feedback control of extracellular fluid volume and glomerular filtration rate. SYN j-g c., juxtaglomerular apparatus.

K c., high amplitude, diphasic frontocental slow waves in the electroencephalogram related to arousal from sleep by a sound; characteristic of sleep stages 2, 3, and 4.

α-ketoglutarate dehydrogenase c., SYN α-*ketoglutarate* dehydrogenase.

Lear c., a father's libidinous fixation on a daughter. [*Lear,* Shakespearean character]

MAC c., SYN membrane attack c.

major histocompatibility c. (MHC), a group of linked loci, collectively termed H-2 c. in the mouse and HLA c. in humans, that codes for cell-surface histocompatibility antigens and is the

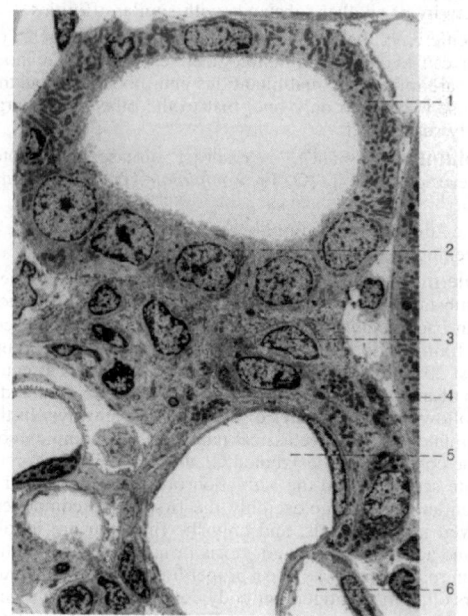

juxtaglomerular complex

1 = epithelium of the right part of the distal tubule; 2 = macula densa; 3 = extraglomerular mesangium; 4 = granular cells in the afferent glomerular arteriole; 5 = a.g. arteriole; 6 = visceral capsule

principal determinant of tissue type and transplant compatibility. SEE ALSO human lymphocyte *antigens,* under *antigen.*

membrane attack c. (MAC), a c. of complement components (C5–C9) that, when activate, bind to the membrane of a target cell, penetrating it with a hydrophobic residue exteriorly and a hydrophilic residue in the interior of the cell; this allows passage of ions and water, swelling of the cell and its eventual rupture. SYN MAC c.

Meyenburg's c., clusters of small bile ducts occurring in polycystic livers, separate from the portal areas.

Michaelis c., binary c. of an enzyme.

monophasic c., a c. in the electrocardiogram that is entirely negative or entirely positive.

mother superior c., the tendency of a psychotherapist to play a mothering role to the detriment of the therapeutic process.

multienzyme c., a structurally distinct and ordered collection of enzymes, often catalyzing successive steps in a metabolic pathway (*e.g.,* pyruvate dehydrogenase c.).

Oedipus c., a developmentally distinct group of associated ideas, aims, instinctual drives, and fears generally observed in male children 3 to 6 years old: coinciding with the peak of the phallic phase of psychosexual development, the child's sexual interest is attached primarily to the parent of the opposite sex and is accompanied by aggressive feelings toward the parent of the same sex; in psychoanalytic theory, it is replaced by the castration c. [*Oedipus,* G. myth. char.]

ostiomeatal c., point where the frontal and maxillary sinuses normally drain into the nasal cavity; obstruction produces inflammation of affected sinus cavities. SYN ostiomeatal unit.

persecution c., a feeling that others have evil designs against one's well-being.

primary c., the typical lesions of primary pulmonary tuberculosis, consisting of a small peripheral focus of infection, with hilar or paratracheal lymph node involvement.

pyruvate dehydrogenase c., SEE *pyruvate* dehydrogenase.

QRS c., portion of electrocardiogram corresponding to the depolarization of cardiac cells.

ribosome-lamella c., a cylindrical cytoplasmic inclusion composed of concentrically arranged sheets of membranes alternating with rows of ribosomes; characteristic of the hairy cell in leukemic reticuloendotheliosis.

Shone's c., an obstructive lesion of the mitral valve c. with left ventricular outflow obstruction and coarctation of the aorta.

sicca c., dryness of the mucous membranes, as of the eyes and mouth, in the absence of a connective tissue disease such as rheumatoid arthritis.

spike and wave c., a generalized, synchronous pattern seen on the electroencephalogram, consisting of a sharply contoured fast wave followed by a slow wave; particularly found in patients with generalized epilepsies. Spike and wave complexes are often characterized by their frequency, *e.g.,* s low spike and wave, fast spike and wave.

superiority c., term sometimes given to the compensatory behavior, *e.g.,* aggressiveness, self-assertion, associated with inferiority c.

symptom c., (1) SEE syndrome. **(2)** SEE complex (1).

synaptinemal c., a submicroscopic structure interposed between the homologous chromosome pairs during synapsis. SYN synaptonemal c.

synaptonemal c., SYN synaptinemal c.

Tacaribe c. of viruses, a group of arenaviruses that includes the antigenically interrelated arboviruses Amapari, Junin, Latino, Machupo, Parana, Pichinde, Tacaribe, and Tamiami.

ternary c., term used to describe the tripartite combination of, for example, enzyme-cofactor-substrate or enzyme-substrate$_1$-substrate$_2$ for a multisubstrate enzyme, the active form involved in many enzyme-catalyzed reactions.

triple symptom c., SYN Behçet's *syndrome.*

VATER c., a constellation of *v*ertebral defects, *a*nal atresia, *t*racheoesophageal fistula with *e*sophageal atresia, and *r*enal and *r*adial anomalies; associated with Fanconi's anemia.

ventricular c., the continuous QRST waves of each beat in the electrocardiogram.

com·plex·ion (kom-plek'shŭn). The color, texture, and general appearance of the skin of the face. [L. *complexio,* a combination, (later) physical condition]

com·plex·i·ty (kom-pleks'i-tē). The state of consisting of many interrelated parts.

chemical c., the level measured, via a chemical assay, of a DNA component.

com·plex·us (kom-plek'sŭs). Obsolete term for semispinalis capitis *muscle.* [L. an embracing, encircling]

com·pli·ance (kom-plī'ans). **1.** A measure of the distensibility of a chamber expressed as a change in volume per unit change in pressure. **2.** The consistency and accuracy with which a patient follows the regimen prescribed by a physician or other health professional. Cf. adherence (2), maintenance. **3.** A measure of the ease with which a structure or substance may be deformed. In medicine and physiology, usually a measure of the ease with which a hollow viscus (*e.g.,* lung, urinary bladder, gallbladder) may be distended, *i.e.,* the volume change resulting from the application of a unit pressure differential between the inside and outside of the viscus; the reciprocal of elastance. [M.E. fr. O. Fr., fr. L. *compleo,* to fulfill]

bladder c., relationship of volume to pressure; can be calculated from a cytometrogram's pressure volume curve. SYN c. of bladder.

c. of bladder, SYN bladder c.

detrusor c., change in volume of bladder for a given change in pressure.

dynamic c. of lung, the value obtained when lung c. is estimated during breathing by dividing the tidal volume by the difference in instantaneous transpulmonary pressures at the ends of the respiratory excursions, when flow in the airway is momentarily zero; this value deviates markedly from static c. in patients in whom resistances and compliances are not uniform throughout the lung (*i.e.,* uneven time constants).

c. of heart, the reciprocal of passive or diastolic stiffness of the ventricle of the heart, most commonly of the left ventricle; one may distinguish between c. of the muscle and c. of the supportive structures, although ordinarily both are considered together

(chamber c.); a hypertrophied or scarred heart will manifest a stiff wall, *i.e.,* decreased c.

specific c., (1) the c. of a structure divided by its initial volume; **(2)** more specifically for the lungs, the c. divided by the functional residual capacity.

static c., the value obtained when c. is measured at true equilibrium, *i.e.,* in the absence of any motion.

thoracic c., that portion of total ventilatory c. ascribable to c. of the thoracic cage.

ventilatory c., the sum of dynamic c. of the lung and thoracic c.

com·pli·cat·ed (kom'pli-kā-ted). Made complex; denoting a disease upon which a morbid process or event has been superimposed, altering symptoms and modifying its course for the worse. [L. *com-plico,* pp. *-atus,* to fold together]

com·pli·ca·tion (kom-pli-kā'shŭn). A morbid process or event occurring during a disease that is not an essential part of the disease, although it may result from it or from independent causes.

com·po·nent (kom-pō'nent). An element forming a part of the whole. [L. *com-pono,* pp. *-positus,* to place together]

anterior c. of force, a force operating to move teeth anteriorly.

c. of complement (C), any one of the nine distinct protein units (designated C1 through C9 and distributed in the α, β, and γ electrophoretic partitions of normal serum) that effect the immunological activities long associated with complement. C1 is a complex of three subunits: C1q, C1r, and C1s. C1$\bar{q}$ (overbar indicates "active form") activates proenzyme C1r to C1r̄ which activates C1s to C1s̄ (also known as C1 esterase), which converts proenzyme C2 to C2b and produces C4b from C4. C2b combines with C4b to form "classical-complement-pathway C3/C5 convertase" (also known as C3 convertase, C5 convertase, and C4̄2̄). This enzyme cleaves C3 to C3a and C3b, and C5 to yield C5a and C5b, as does "alternative-complement-pathway C3/C5 convertase" (also known as proenzyme factor B, properdin factor B, C3 proactivator, and heat-labile factor). Complement factor I (also known as C3b or C3b/C4b inactivator) inactivates C3b and C4b by a different proteolytic cleavage. Several autosomal recessive disorders have been identified in which one or more of the complement components have been deficient or completely absent.

c. of force, (1) one of the factors from which a resultant force may be compounded or into which it may be resolved; **(2)** one of the vectors into which a force may be resolved.

c.'s of mastication, the various jaw movements that are made during the act of mastication, as determined by the neuromuscular system, the temporomandibular articulations, the teeth, and the food being chewed; divided, for purposes of analysis or description, into opening, closing, left lateral, right lateral, and anteroposterior c.'s.

c.'s of occlusion, the various factors involved in occlusion, such as the temporomandibular joint, the associated neuromusculature, the teeth, and the denture-supporting structures.

plasma thromboplastin c. (PTC), SYN *factor* IX.

secretory c., a polypeptide chain found in external secretions (*e.g.,* tears, saliva, colostrum) associated with the immunoglobulins IgA and IgM. It also may occur in free form. The secretory piece is derived by proteolytic cleavage of the immunoglobulin receptor on epithelial cells.

com·pos·ite. A colloquial term for resin materials used in restorative dentistry. [L. *compositus,* put together, fr. *compono,* to put together]

com·po·si·tion (kom-pō-zish'ŭn). In chemistry, the kinds and numbers of atoms constituting a molecule. [L. *compono,* to arrange]

base c., the proportions of the four bases (adenine, cytosine, guanine, and thymine (or uracil) present in DNA or RNA; usually expressed as the percentage (mol %) of G plus C.

modeling c., SYN modeling *plastic.*

com·pos men·tis (kom'pos men'tis). Of sound mind; usually used in its opposite form, *non compos mentis.* [L. possessed of one's mind; *compos,* having control, + *mens(ment-),* mind]

com·pound (kom'pownd). **1.** In chemistry, a substance formed by the covalent or electrostatic union of two or more elements,

CO

generally differing entirely in physical characteristics from any of its components. **2.** In pharmacy, denoting a preparation containing several ingredients. For c.'s not listed here, see the specific chemical or pharmaceutical names. [thru O. Fr., fr. L. *compono*]

acetone c., SYN ketone *body*.

acyclic c., an organic c. in which the chain does not form a ring. SYN aliphatic c., open chain c.

addition c., (1) strictly, a complex of two or more complete molecules in which each preserves its fundamental structure and no covalent bonds are made or broken (*e.g.,* hydrates of salts, adducts); **(2)** loosely, association of acids with basic organic c.'s (*e.g.,* amines with HCl); **(3)** more loosely, addition of two molecules without loss of any atom, but forming new covalent bonds (*e.g.,* $CH_2=CH_2 + Br_2 \rightarrow BrCH_2—CH_2Br$).

alicyclic c.'s, SEE cyclic c.

aliphatic c., SYN acyclic c.

APC c., an analgesic tablet drug combination containing aspirin, phenacetin and caffeine. Very widely used in the 1940's through 1960's; original constituents of popular over-the-counter pain remedies. Use currently much diminished due to concerns about potential renal injury due to the phenacetin.

aromatic c., SEE cyclic c.

carbamino c., any carbamic acid derivative formed by the combination of carbon dioxide with a free amino group to form an *N*-carboxy group, -NH-COOH, as in hemoglobin forming carbaminohemoglobin.

carbocyclic c., SEE cyclic c.

closed chain c., SYN cyclic c.

condensation c., a c. resulting from the combination of two or more simple substances, with the splitting off of some other substance, such as alcohol or water; *e.g.,* a peptide. Cf. conjugated c.

conjugated c., a c. formed by the union of two c.'s (as by the elimination of water between an alcohol and an organic acid to form an ester) and easily converted to the original c.'s (hydrolysis). SEE ALSO conjugation (4). Cf. condensation c.

cyclic c., any c. in which the constituent atoms, or any part of them, form a ring. Used mainly in organic chemistry where: 1) numerous c.'s contain rings of carbon atoms (carbocyclic c.'s) or carbon atoms plus one or more atoms of other types (heterocyclic c.'s), usually nitrogen, oxygen, or sulfur; 2) where the atoms in the ring are all of the same element (homocyclic or isocyclic c.); 3) where the ring is saturated or contains nonconjugated double bonds (alicyclic c.), the c. is similar in properties to the corresponding acyclic c. (*e.g.,* cyclohexane resembles hexane); 4) where the ring contains conjugated double bonds in a closed loop in which there are $4n + 2$ (where n is an integer) delocalized π electrons (Hückel's rule) (aromatic c.; *e.g.,* benzene, pyridine), it is more stable than the corresponding saturated ring and exhibits unusual chemical properties characteristic of itself and not of other types of rings or of acyclic c.'s. These aromatic c.'s have the ability to sustain an induced ring current. SYN closed chain c., ring c.

genetic c., SYN compound *heterozygote*.

glycosyl c., the c. formed between a sugar and another organic substance in which the OH of the reducing (hemiacetal) group of the former is removed; *e.g.,* the natural nucleosides, in which a heterocyclic N becomes linked directly to the C-1 of ribose (or deoxyribose) to yield ribosyl compounds. Cf. glycoside.

heterocyclic c., SEE cyclic c.

high energy c.'s, classically, a group of phosphoric esters whose hydrolysis takes place with a standard free energy change of −5 to −15 kcal/mol (or, −20 to −63 kJ/mol) (in contrast to −1 to −4 kcal/mol or, −4 to −17 kJ/mol) for simple phosphoric esters like glucose 6-phosphate or α-glycerophosphates), thus being capable of driving energy-consuming reactions in living cells or reconstituted cell-free systems; adenosine 5′-triphosphate, with respect to the β- and γ-phosphates, is the best known and is regarded as the immediate energy source for most metabolic syntheses. The general types are acid anhydrides, phosphoric esters of enols, phosphamic acid ($R—NH—PO_3H_2$) derivatives, acyl thioesters (*e.g.,* of coenzyme A), sulfonium c.'s ($R_3—S^+$), and aminoacyl esters

of ribosyl moieties. SEE ALSO high energy *phosphates*, under *phosphate*.

homocyclic c., SEE cyclic c.

impression c., SYN modeling *plastic*.

inclusion c., the mechanical trapping of small molecules within spaces between other molecules; *e.g.,* the inclusion of iodine molecules by starch molecules to form the well-known red-to-black "addition c."

inorganic c., a c. in which the atoms or radicals consist of elements other than carbon and are typically held together by electrostatic forces rather than by covalent bonds; often are capable of dissociation into ions in polar solvents (*e.g.,* H_2O). Cf. organic c.

isocyclic c., SEE cyclic c.

Kendall's c.'s, a group of corticosteroids. Kendall's compound A (11-dehydrocorticosterone); Kendall's compound B (corticosterone); Kendall's compound E (cortisone); Kendall's compound F (cortisol). SYN Kendall's substance.

meso c.'s, c.'s containing more than one asymmetric carbon atom, with configurations about them so balanced that the molecule as a whole possesses a plane of symmetry, although the individual carbon atoms do not; such compounds are not optically active; *e.g.,* ribitol, mucic acid, *meso*-inositol, *meso*-cystine.

methonium c.'s, agents that block impulses in ganglia (*e.g.,* hexamethonium) and are used in arterial hypertension; also used for neuromusclar paralysis in surgery (*e.g.,* decamethonium).

modeling c., SYN modeling *plastic*.

nonpolar c., a c. composed of molecules that possess a symmetrical distribution of charge, so that no positive or negative poles exist, and that are not ionizable in solution; *e.g.,* hydrocarbons. SEE ALSO organic c.

open chain c., SYN acyclic c.

organic c., a c. composed of atoms (some of which are carbon) held together by covalent (shared electron) bonds. Cf. inorganic c.

polar c., a c. in which the electric charge is not symmetrically distributed, so that there is a separation of charge or partial charge and formation of definite positive and negative poles; *e.g.,* H_2O. See also inorganic c.

Reichstein's c., SYN Reichstein's *substance*.

ring c., SYN cyclic c.

Wintersteiner c. F, SYN cortisone.

com·pre·hen·sion (kom-prē-hen′shŭn). Knowledge or understanding of an object, situation, event, or verbal statement.

com·press (kom′pres). A pad of gauze or other material applied for local pressure. [L. *com-primo,* pp. *-pressus,* to press together]

graduated c., layers of cloth thickest in the center, becoming thinner toward the periphery.

wet c., gauze moistened with saline or antiseptic solution.

com·pres·sion (kom-presh′ŭn). A squeezing together; the exertion of pressure on a body in such a way as to tend to increase its density; the decrease in a dimension of a body under the action of two external forces directed toward one another in the same straight line.

c. of brain, SYN cerebral c.

cerebral c., pressure upon the intracranial tissues by an effusion of blood or cerebrospinal fluid, an abscess, a neoplasm, a depressed fracture of the skull, or an edema of the brain. SYN c. of brain.

c. of tissue, SYN tissue *displaceability*.

com·pres·sor (kom-pres′er, -ōr). **1.** A muscle, contraction of which causes compression of any structure. **2.** An instrument for making pressure on a part, especially on an artery to prevent loss of blood. SYN compressorium.

c. ve′nae dorsa′lis pe′nis, a variation of the bulbospongiosus muscle in which some fibers pass dorsal to the dorsal vein of the penis; thought at one time to be an important component in the mechanism of erection. SYN Houston's muscle.

com·pres·sor·i·um (kom-pres-ōr′ē-ŭm). SYN compressor (2).

Compton, Arthur H., U.S. physicist and Nobel laureate, 1892–1962. SEE C. *effect*.

Compton scat·ter·ing. SYN Compton *effect*.

com·pul·sion (kom-pŭl′shŭn). Uncontrollable thoughts or impulses to perform an act, often repetitively, as an unconscious mechanism to avoid unacceptable ideas and desires which, by themselves, arouse anxiety; the anxiety becomes fully manifest if performance of the compulsive act is prevented; may be associated with obsessive thoughts. [L. *com-pello* pp. *-pulsus,* to drive together, compel]

com·pul·sive (kom-pŭl′siv). Influenced by compulsion; of a compelling and irresistible nature.

com·put·er. A programmable electronic device that can be used to store and manipulate data in order to carry out designated functions; the two fundamental components are hardware, *i.e.,* the actual electronic device, and software, *i.e.,* the instructions or program used to carry out the function.

♻**con-.** With, together, in association; appears as com- before p, b, or m, as col- before l, and as co- before a vowel; corresponds to G. *syn-.* [L. *cum,* with, together]

conA, con A Abbreviation for concanavalin A.

con·al·bu·min (kon-al-byū′min). A glycoprotein containing D-mannose and D-galactose, constituting about 14% of egg white. SYN ovotransferrin.

con·a·nine (kon′ă-nēn). A steroid alkaloid; pregnane with a methylimino group bridging C-18 and C-20 (in α-configuration). SEE ALSO conessine.

co·nar·i·um (kō-nā′rē-ŭm). SYN pineal *body.* [G. *kōnarion* (dim. of *kōnos,* cone), the pineal body]

co·na·tion (kō-nā′shŭn). The conscious tendency to act, usually an aspect of mental process; historically aligned with cognition and affection, but more recently used in the wider sense of impulse, desire, purposeful striving. [L. *conātio,* an undertaking, effort]

co·na·tive (kon′ă-tiv). Pertaining to, or characterized by, conation.

co·na·tus (kō-nah′tŭs, -nā′tŭs). A striving toward self-preservation and self-affirmation. [L. attempt]

con·cam·er·a·tion (kon-kam-er-ā′shŭn). A system of interconnecting cavities. [L. *concameratio,* a vault; fr. *concamero,* pp. *-atus,* to vault over, fr. *camera,* a vault]

con·ca·nav·a·lin A (conA, con A) (kon-kă-nav′ă-lin). A phytomitogen, extracted from the jack bean (*Canavalia ensiformis*) that agglutinates the blood of mammals and reacts with glucosans; like other phytohemagglutinins, con A stimulates T lymphocytes more vigorously than it does B lymphocytes.

con·ca·ta·mer (kon-kāt-ă-mer). A linear repeat of restriction fragments. [*concate*nate + -mer]

con·cat·e·nate (kon-kat′ĕ-nāt). Denoting the arrangement of a number of structures, *e.g.,* enlarged lymph glands, in a row like the links of a chain. [L. *con-cateno,* pp. *-atus,* to link together, fr. *catena,* a chain]

Concato, Luigi M., Italian physician, 1825–1882. SEE C.'s *disease.*

con·cave (kon′kāv). Having a depressed or hollowed surface. [L. *concavus,* arched or vaulted]

con·cav·i·ty (kon-kav′i-tē). A hollow or depression, with more or less evenly curved sides, on any surface.

con·ca·vo·con·cave (kon-kā′vō-kon′kāv). SYN biconcave.

con·ca·vo·con·vex (kon-kā′vō-kon′veks). Concave on one surface and convex on the opposite surface.

con·cen·tra·tion (c) (kon-sen-trā′shŭn). **1.** A preparation made by extracting a crude drug, precipitating from the solution, and drying. **2.** Increasing the amount of solute in a given volume of solution by evaporation of the solvent. **3.** The quantity of a substance per unit volume or weight. In renal physiology, symbol U for urinary c., P for plasma c.; in respiratory physiology, symbol C for amount per unit volume in blood, F for fractional c. (mole fraction or volume per volume) in dried gas; subscripts indicate location and chemical species. [L. *con-,* together, + *centrum,* center]

critical micelle c. (cmc), the c. at which an amphipathic molecule (*e.g.,* a phospholipid) will form a micelle.

M c., the maximum number of bacterial cells which can be produced in a unit volume of growth medium.

mean corpuscular hemoglobin c. (MCHC), Hgb/Hct; the average hemoglobin c. in a given volume of packed red cells, calculated from the hemoglobin therein and the hematocrit, in erythrocyte indices.

minimal alveolar c., the end-alveolar c. of an inhalation anesthetic which prevents somatic response to a painful stimulus in 50% of individuals; an index of relative potency of inhalation anesthetics. SYN minimal anesthetic c.

minimal alveolar concentration (MAC) values of inhalation anesthetics, in order of increasing effectiveness		
	MAC values (% atm)	
	100% O_2	with 70% N_2O
methoxyflurane	0.16	0.07
halothane	0.75	0.29
isoflurane	1.15	0.50
enflurane	1.68	0.57
N_2O	110	—

minimal anesthetic c. (MAC), SYN minimal alveolar c.

minimal inhibitory c. (MIC), the lowest concentration of antibiotic sufficient to inhibit bacterial growth when tested *in vitro.*

molar c., SEE molar (4).

normal c. (N), SEE normal (3).

con·cen·tric (kon-sen′trik). Having a common center, such that two or more spheres, circles, or segments of circles are within one another.

con·cept (kon′sept). **1.** An abstract idea or notion. **2.** An explanatory variable or principle in a scientific system. SYN conception (1). [L. *conceptum,* something understood, pp. ntr. of *concipio,* to receive, apprehend]

no-threshold c., that the biologic effect of radiation is proportional to dose, even for minutely small doses.

self c., an individual's sense of self, including self definition in the various social roles he or she enacts, including assessment of his or her status on a single trait or on many human dimensions using societal or personal norms as criteria.

con·cep·ti (kon-sep′tī). Plural of conceptus.

con·cep·tion (kon-sep′shŭn). **1.** SYN concept. **2.** Act of forming a general idea or notion. **3.** Act of conceiving, or becoming pregnant; fertilization of the oocyte (ovum) by a spermatozoon to form a viable zygote. [L. *conceptio;* see concept]

imperative c., a concept that does not arise from association but appears spontaneously and refuses to be banished.

con·cep·tu·al (kon-sep′chŭ-ăl). Relating to the formation of ideas, usually higher order abstractions, to mental conceptions.

con·cep·tus, pl. **con·cep·ti** (kon-sep′tŭs, -sep′tī). The product of conception, *i.e.,* embryo and membranes.

con·cha, pl. **con·chae** (kon′kă, kon′kē) [NA]. In anatomy, a structure comparable to a shell in shape, as the auricle or pinna of the ear or a turbinated bone in the nose. [L. a shell]

c. auric′ulae [NA], SYN c. of ear.

c. bullosa, abnormal pneumatization of the middle turbinate which may interfere with normal ventilation of sinus ostia and can result in recurrent sinusitis.

c. of ear, the large hollow, or floor of the auricle, between the anterior portion of the helix and the antihelix; it is divided by the crus of the helix into the cymba above and the cavum below. SYN c. auriculae [NA].

highest c., SYN supreme nasal c.

inferior nasal c., (1) a thin, spongy, bony plate with curved margins, on the lateral wall of the nasal cavity, separating the middle from the inferior meatus; it articulates with the ethmoid, lacrimal, maxilla, and palate bones; **(2)** the above bony plate and its thick mucoperiosteum containing an extensive cavernous vas-

co

cular bed for heat exchange. SYN c. nasalis inferior [NA], inferior turbinated bone, turbinated body (2).

middle nasal c., (1) the middle thin, spongy, bony plate with curved margins, part of the ethmoidal labyrinth, projecting from the lateral wall of the nasal cavity and separating the superior meatus from the middle meatus; (2) the above bony plate and its thick mucoperiosteum containing a cavernous vascular bed for heat exchange. SYN c. nasalis media [NA], middle turbinated bone, turbinated body (2).

Morgagni's c., SYN superior nasal c.

c. nasa′lis infe′rior [NA], SYN inferior nasal c.

c. nasa′lis me′dia [NA], SYN middle nasal c.

c. nasa′lis supe′rior [NA], SYN superior nasal c.

c. nasa′lis supre′ma [NA], SYN supreme nasal c.

Santorini's c., c. santori′ni, SYN supreme nasal c.

sphenoidal conchae, paired ossicles of pyramidal shape, the spines of which are in contact with the medial pterygoid lamina, the bases forming the roof of the nasal cavity. SYN conchae sphenoidales [NA], Bertin's bones, Bertin's ossicles, sphenoidal turbinated bones.

con′chae sphenoida′les [NA], SYN sphenoidal conchae.

superior nasal c., (1) the upper thin, spongy, bony plate with curved margins, part of the ethmoidal labyrinth, projecting from the lateral wall of the nasal cavity and separating the superior meatus from the sphenoethmoidal recess; (2) the above bony plate and its thick mucoperiosteum, which is less vascular than that of the middle and inferior conchae. SYN c. nasalis superior [NA], Morgagni's c., superior turbinated bone, turbinated body (2).

supreme c., SYN supreme nasal c.

supreme nasal c., a small c. frequently present on the posterosuperior part of the lateral nasal wall; it overlies the supreme nasal meatus. SYN c. nasalis suprema [NA], fourth turbinated bone, highest c., highest turbinated bone, Santorini's c., c. santorini, supraturbinal, supreme c., supreme turbinated bone, turbinated body (2).

con·choi·dal (kon-koy′dăl). Shaped like a shell; having alternate convexities and concavities on the surface. [concha + G. *eidos,* appearance]

con·com·i·tance (kon-kom′i-tăns). In esotropia, one eye accompanying the other in all excursions, as in concomitant strabismus. [con- + L. *comito-,* pp. *-atus,* to accompany]

con·com·i·tant. SYN comitant.

con·cor·dance (kon-kŏr′dans). Agreement in the types of data that occur in natural pairs. For example, in a trait like schizophrenia, a pair of identical twins is concordant if both are affected or both are unaffected; it is discordant if one of them only is affected. Likewise, the pairs might be non-identical twins, or sibs, or husband and wife, etc. [L. *concordia,* agreeing, harmony]

con·cor·dant (kon-kŏr′dant). Denoting or exhibiting concordance.

con·cre·ment (kon′krĕ-ment). A concretion; a deposit of calcareous material in a part. [L. *con- cresco,* to grow together]

con·cres·cence (kon-kres′ens). 1. SYN coalescence. 2. In dentistry, the union of the roots of two adjacent teeth by cementum. [see concrement]

con·cre·tio cor·dis (kon-krē′shē-ō kŏr′dis). Extensive adhesion between parietal and visceral layers of the pericardium with partial or complete obliteration of the pericardial cavity. SYN internal adhesive pericarditis, synechia pericardii.

con·cre·tion (kon-krē′shŭn). The aggregation or formation of solid material. [L. *cum,* together, + *crescere,* to grow]

con·cret·i·za·tion (kon′krĕt-i-zā′shŭn). Inability to abstract with an overemphasis on specific details; seen in mental disorders, such as dementia and schizophrenia, and also normally in children. [L. *con-cresco,* pp. *-cretus,* to grow together, harden]

con·cus·sion (kon-kŭsh′ŭn). 1. A violent shaking or jarring. 2. An injury of a soft structure, as the brain, resulting from a blow or violent shaking. SYN commotio. [L. *concussio,* fr. *con- cutio,* pp. *-cussus,* to shake violently]

brain c., a clinical syndrome due to mechanical, usually traumatic, forces; characterized by immediate and transient impairment

of neural function, such as alteration of consciousness, disturbance of vision and equilibrium, etc. SYN commotio cerebri.

spinal c., SYN spinal cord c.

spinal cord c., injury to the spinal cord due to a blow to the vertebral column with transient or prolonged dysfunction below the level of the lesion. SYN spinal c.

con·cus·sor (kon-kŭs-er, -sōr). A hammer-like instrument for tapping the parts as a form of massage.

con·den·sa·tion (kon-den-sā′shŭn). 1. Making more solid or dense. 2. The change of a gas to a liquid, or of a liquid to a solid. 3. In psychoanalysis, an unconscious mental process in which one symbol stands for a number of others. 4. In dentistry, the process of packing a filling material into a cavity, using such force and direction that no voids result. [L. *con- denso,* pp. *-atus,* to make thick, condense]

aldol c., formation of an aldol (a β-hydroxy carbonyl compound) from two carbonyl compounds; the reverse reaction is an aldol cleavage; fructose 1,6-bisphosphate aldolase catalyzes such a reaction.

Claisen c., the formation of a β-keto ester from two esters, one of which has an α-hydrogen atom; malate synthase, citrate synthase, and ATP citrate lyase all catalyze such reactions.

con·dense (kon-dens′). To pack; to increase the density of; applied particularly to insertion of gold foil or silver amalgam in a cavity prepared in a tooth.

con·dens·er (kon-den′ser). 1. An apparatus for cooling a gas to a liquid, or a liquid to a solid. 2. In dentistry, a manual or powered instrument used for packing a plastic or unset material into a cavity of a tooth; variation in sizes and shapes allows conformation of the mass to the cavity outline. 3. The simple or compound lens on a microscope that is used to supply the illumination necessary for visibility of the specimen under observation. 4. SYN capacitor.

Abbé's c., a system of two or three wide-angle, achromatic, convex and planoconvex lenses that may be moved upward or downward beneath the stage of a microscope, thereby regulating the concentration of light (directly from a bulb or reflected from a mirror) that passes through the material to be examined on the stage.

automatic c., SYN automatic *plugger.*

cardioid c., a type of dark-field c.

dark-field c., an apparatus for throwing reflected light through the microscope field, so that only the object to be examined is illuminated, the field itself being dark.

paraboloid c., a type of dark-field c.

con·di·tion (kon-dish′ŭn). 1. To train; to undergo conditioning. 2. A certain response elicited by a specifiable stimulus or emitted in the presence of certain stimuli with reward of the response during prior occurrence. 3. Referring to several classes of learning in the behavioristic branch of psychology. [L. *conditio,* fr. *condico,* to agree]

con·di·tion·ing (kon-dish′ŭn-ing). The process of acquiring, developing, educating, establishing, learning, or training new responses in an individual. Used to describe both respondent and operant behavior; in both usages, refers to a change in the frequency or form of behavior as a result of the influence of the environment.

assertive c., SYN assertive *training.*

aversive c., SYN aversive *training.*

avoidance c., the technique whereby an organism learns to avoid unpleasant or punishing stimuli by learning the appropriate anticipatory response to protect it from further such stimuli. Cf. escape c. SYN avoidance training.

classical c., a form of learning, as in Pavlov's experiments, in which a previously neutral stimulus becomes a conditioned stimulus when presented together with an unconditioned stimulus. Also called stimulus substitution because the new stimulus evokes the response in question. SEE ALSO respondent c. SYN stimulus substitution.

escape c., the technique whereby an organism learns to terminate unpleasant or punishing stimuli by making the appropriate new response which ceases the delivery of such stimuli. Cf. avoidance c. SYN escape training.

higher order c., the use of a previously conditioned stimulus to condition further responses, in much the same way unconditioned stimuli are used.

instrumental c., c. in which the response is a prerequisite to achieving some goal; often used as a synonym for operant c., but some psychologists make distinctions in the usages of these two terms.

operant c., a type of c. developed by Skinner in which an experimenter waits for the target response (head scratching) to be conditioned to occur (emitted) spontaneously, immediately after which the organism is given a reinforcer reward; after this procedure is repeated many times, the frequency of emission of the targeted response will have significantly increased over its pre-experiment base rate. SEE ALSO *schedules* of reinforcement, under *schedule.* SYN skinnerian c.

pavlovian c., SYN respondent c.

respondent c., a type of c., first studied by I. P. Pavlov, in which a previously neutral stimulus (bell sound) elicits a response (salivation) as a result of pairing it (associating it contiguously in time) a number of times with an unconditioned or natural stimulus for that response (food shown to a hungry dog). SYN pavlovian c.

second-order c., the use of a previously successfully conditioned stimulus as the unconditioned stimulus for further c.

skinnerian c., SYN operant c.

trace c., c. when there is no temporal overlap between the c. stimulus and the unconditioned stimulus.

con·dom (kon′dom). Sheath or cover for the penis, or vagina for use in the prevention of conception or infection during coitus.

con·duc·tance (kon-dŭk′tans). **1.** A measure of conductivity; the ratio of the current flowing through a conductor to the difference in potential between the ends of the conductor; the c. of a circuit is the reciprocal of its resistance. **2.** The ease with which a fluid or gas enters and flows through a conduit, air passage, or respiratory tract; the flow per unit pressure difference.

con·duc·tion (kon-dŭk′shŭn). **1.** The act of transmitting or conveying certain forms of energy, such as heat, sound, or electricity, from one point to another, without evident movement in the conducting body. **2.** The transmission of stimuli of various sorts by living protoplasm. [L. *con- duco,* pp. *ductus,* to lead, conduct]

aberrant ventricular c., abnormal intraventricular c. of a supraventricular beat, especially where surrounding beats are normally conducted. SYN ventricular aberration.

accelerated c., any pathologically increased speed of c.; usually occurs between the atrium and ventricles as in the Wolff-Parkinson-White and Lown-Ganong-Levine syndromes; such accelerated pathways provide the bases for particular forms of reentry tachycardia.

air c., in relation to hearing, the transmission of sound to the inner ear through the external auditory canal and the structures of the middle ear.

anomalous c., c. of cardiac electrical impulses through any abnormal pathway.

antegrade c., SYN anterograde c.

anterograde c., c. in the expected normal direction between any cardiac structures. SYN antegrade c., forward c., orthograde c.

atrioventricular c. (AVC), A-V c., forward c. of the cardiac impulse from atria to ventricles via the A-V node or any bypass tract, represented in the electrocardiogram by the P-R interval. P-H c. time is from the onset of the P wave to the first high frequency component of the His bundle electrogram (normally 119 ± 38 msec); A-H c. time is from the onset of the first high frequency component of the atrial electrogram to the first high frequency component of the His bundle electrogram (normally 92 ± 38 msec); P-A conduction time is from the onset of the P wave to the onset of the atrial electrogram (normally 27 ± 18 msec).

avalanche c., the discharge of an impulse from a neuron into a large number of neurons of the same physiologic system, thus producing the liberation of a very large amount of nervous energy by a given stimulus.

bone c., in relation to hearing, the transmission of sound to the

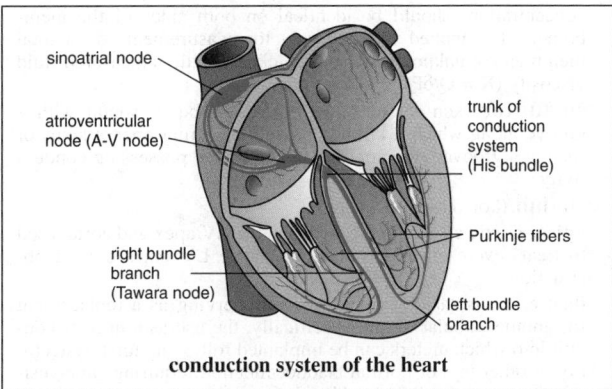

conduction system of the heart

inner ear through vibrations applied to the bones of the skull. SYN osteophony.

concealed c., c. of an impulse through a part of the heart without direct evidence of its presence in the electrocardiogram; c. is inferred only because of its influence on the subsequent cardiac cycle.

decremental c., impaired c. in a portion of a fiber because of progressively lessening response of the unexcited portion of the fiber to the action potential coming toward it; it is manifested by decreasing speed of c., amplitude of action potential, and extent of spread of the impulse.

delayed c., first-degree A-V block. SEE atrioventricular *block,* intraventricular *block,* bundle-branch *block.*

forward c., SYN anterograde c.

intra-atrial c., c. of the cardiac impulse through the atrial myocardium, represented by the P wave in the electrocardiogram.

intraventricular c., c. of the cardiac impulse through the ventricular myocardium, represented by the QRS complex in the electrocardiogram. H-R c. time is from the onset of the first high frequency component of the His bundle electrogram to the onset of the QRS complex of the surface electrocardiogram (normally 43 ± 12 msec); H-V c. time is from the onset of the first high frequency component of the His bundle electrogram to the onset of the ventricular electrogram (normally approximates the H-R interval but may be a little shorter). SYN ventricular c.

nerve c., the transmission of an impulse along a nerve fiber.

orthograde c., SYN anterograde c.

Purkinje c., c. of the cardiac impulse through the Purkinje system.

retrograde c., c. backward from the ventricles or from the A-V node into and through the atria. SYN retroconduction, ventriculoatrial c., V-A c.

saltatory c., c. in which the nerve impulse jumps from one node of Ranvier to the next.

sinoventricular c. (sī′nō-ven-trik′ū-lăr), a rare form of c. of the sinus impulse during paralysis of the atrial muscle by hyperkalemia. The impulse leaves the sinus node and enters the internodal tracts rapidly achieving the junctional tissues but without inscribing a P wave due to the inactivation of the atrial muscle cells.

supranormal c., transmission of an impulse during the brief period of the cardiac cycle when it would be expected to fail if it occurred outside this time interval. Cf. supranormal *excitability.*

synaptic c., the c. of a nerve impulse across a synapse.

ventricular c., SYN intraventricular c.

ventriculoatrial c. (VAC), V-A c., SYN retrograde c.

con·duc·tiv·i·ty (kon-dŭk-tiv′i-tē). **1.** The power of transmission or conveyance of certain forms of energy, as heat, sound, and electricity, without perceptible motion in the conducting body. **2.** The property, inherent in living protoplasm, of transmitting a state of excitation; *e.g.,* in muscle or nerve.

hydraulic c., ease of pressure filtration of a liquid through a membrane; specifically, $Kf = \eta(\dot{Q}/A) (\delta x/\delta P)$, where Kf = hydraulic c., η = viscosity of the liquid being filtered, $\dot{Q}/A$ = volume of liquid filtered per unit time and unit area, and $\delta x/\delta P$ = reciprocal of the pressure gradient through the membrane; solute concentrations should be identical on both sides of the membrane. Also applied more loosely to measurements on a total membrane of unknown area and thickness with unmeasured fluid viscosity ($K = \dot{Q}/\delta P$).

con·duc·tor (kon-dŭk'ter, -tōr). **1.** A probe or sound with a groove along which a knife is passed in slitting open a sinus or fistula; a grooved director. **2.** Any substance possessing conductivity.

con·duit (kon'dū-it). A channel.

apical-aortic c., a valved c. between the LV apex and aorta, used to treat severe otherwise unapproachable LV outflow tract obstruction.

ileal c., an isolated segment of ileum serving as a replacement for another tubular organ; specifically, the use as a urinary conduit into which ureters can be implanted following total cystectomy or other loss of normal bladder function requiring supravesical diversion. SYN ileal bladder.

con·du·pli·cate (kon-dū'pli-kāt). Folded upon itself lengthwise. [L. con-, with, + duplico, pp. -atus]

con·du·pli·ca·to cor·pore (kon-dū-pli-kā'tō kōr'pōr-ē). Condition in which the fetus is doubled up on itself in shoulder presentation.

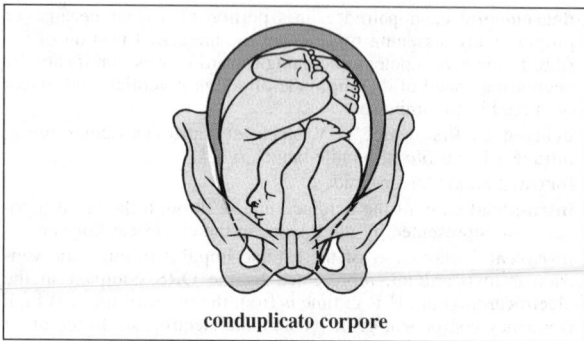

conduplicato corpore

con·du·ran·go (kon-dū-rang'gō). The bark of *Gonolobus condurango, Marsdenia condurango* (family Asclepiadaceae), a shrub of Ecuador and Peru; an aromatic bitter and astringent. [Peruv.]

con·dy·lar (kon'di-lăr). Relating to a condyle.

con·dy·lar·thro·sis (kon'di-lar-thrō'sis). A joint, like that of the knee, formed by condylar surfaces. [G. *kondylos*, condyle, + *arthrōsis*, a jointing]

con·dyle (kon'dīl). A rounded articular surface at the extremity of a bone. SYN condylus [NA].

balancing side c., in dentistry, the mandibular c. on the side away from which the mandible moves in a lateral excursion.

c. of humerus, the distal end of the humerus, including the trochlea, capitulum and the olecranon, coronoid and radial fossae. SYN condylus humeri [NA].

lateral c., c. farthest from the midline. SYN condylus lateralis [NA].

lateral c. of femur, the lateral c. is longer than the medial c. SYN condylus lateralis femoris.

lateral c. of tibia, the lateral c. is longer than the medial c. SYN condylus lateralis tibiae.

mandibular c., SYN condylar *process.*

medial c., c. closest to midline. SYN condylus medialis [NA].

medial c. of femur, the shorter c. closest to the midline. SYN condylus medialis femoris.

medial c. of tibia, the shorter c. closest to the midline. SYN condylus medialis tibiae.

occipital c., one of two elongated oval facets on the undersurface of the occipital bone, one on each side of the foramen magnum, which articulate with the atlas. SYN condylus occipitalis [NA].

working side c., in dentistry, the mandibular c. on the side toward which the mandible moves in a lateral excursion.

con·dy·lec·to·my (kon-di-lek'tō-mē). Excision of a condyle. [G. *kondylos*, condyle, + *ektomē*, excision]

con·dyl·i·on (kon-dil'ē-on). A point on the lateral outer or medial inner surface of the condyle of the mandible. [G. *kondylion*, dim. of *kondylos*, condyle]

con·dy·loid (kon'di-loyd). Relating to or resembling a condyle. [G. *kondylōdēs*, like a knuckle, fr. *kondylos*, condyle, + *eidos*, resemblance]

con·dy·lo·ma, pl. **con·dy·lo·ma·ta** (kon-di-lō'mă, -mah'tă). A wartlike excrescence at the anus or vulva, or on the glans penis. SYN verruca mollusciformis. [G. *kondylōma*, a knob]

c. acumina'tum, a contagious projecting warty growth on the external genitals or at the anus, consisting of fibrous overgrowths covered by thickened epithelium showing koilocytosis, due to sexual contact with infection by human papilloma virus; it is usually benign, although malignant change has been reported, associated with particular types of the virus. SYN genital wart, venereal wart.

flat c., (1) SYN c. latum. (2) a c. of the uterine cervix or other site caused by human papilloma virus infection and characterized histologically by koilocytosis without papillomatosis.

giant c., a large type of c. acuminatum found in the anus, vulva, or preputial sac of the penis of middle-aged, uncircumcised men; it tends to extend deeply and recur. SYN Buschke-Löwenstein tumor.

c. la'tum, a secondary syphilitic eruption of flat-topped papules, occurring in groups covered by a necrotic layer of epithelial detritus, and secreting a seropurulent fluid; they are found at the anus and wherever contiguous folds of skin produce heat and moisture. SYN flat c. (1), moist papule, mucous papule.

pointed c., obsolete term for c. acuminatum.

con·dy·lom·a·tous (kon-di-lō'mă-tŭs). Relating to a condyloma.

con·dy·lot·o·my (kon-di-lot'ō-mē). Division, without removal, of a condyle. [G. *kondylos*, condyle, + *tomē*, incision]

con·dy·lus (kon'di-lŭs) [NA]. SYN condyle. [L. fr. G. *kondylos*, knuckle, the knuckle of any joint]

c. hu'meri [NA], SYN *condyle* of humerus.

c. latera'lis [NA], SYN lateral *condyle.*

c. latera'lis fem'oris, SYN lateral *condyle* of femur.

c. latera'lis tib'iae, SYN lateral *condyle* of tibia.

c. media'lis [NA], SYN medial *condyle.*

c. media'lis fem'oris, SYN medial *condyle* of femur.

c. media'lis tibiae, SYN medial *condyle* of tibia.

c. occipita'lis [NA], SYN occipital *condyle.*

cone (kōn). **1.** A figure having a circular base with sides inclined so as to meet at a point above. **2.** The photosensitive, outward-directed, conical process of a c. cell essential for sharp vision and color vision; c.'s are the only photoreceptor in the fovea centralis and become interspersed with increasing numbers of rods toward the periphery of the retina. SYN cone cell of retina. **3.** Metallic cylinder or c. used to confine a beam of x-rays. SYN conus (1). [G. *kōnos*, cone]

antipodal c., the set of astral rays of a dividing cell extending from the centriole in a direction opposite to the equatorial plate.

arterial c., SYN *conus* arteriosus. SYN infundibulum (4).

c. down, to narrow a beam of x-rays to a region of interest using a collimator or c. (3); colloq., to delimit one's attention or activities.

elastic c., SYN *conus* elasticus (1).

gutta-percha c., a c.-shaped, semirigid root canal filling material composed of gutta-percha and zinc oxide.

Haller's c.'s, SYN *lobules* of epididymis, under *lobule.*

implantation c., SYN axon *hillock.*

keratosic c.'s, obsolete term for horny pointed or rounded elevations on the hands and feet, occasionally observed in cases of gonorrheal rheumatism.

c. of light, SYN *pyramid* of light.

medullary c., the tapering lower extremity of the spinal cord. SYN conus medullaris [NA].

nerve growth c., a highly motile structure at the leading edge of an elongating axon.

ocular c., the c. of light in the interior of the eyeball with the base formed by the rays entering through the pupil and the apex focused on the retina.

Politzer's luminous c., SYN *pyramid* of light.

pulmonary c., SYN *conus* arteriosus.

retinal c.'s, SEE cone (2).

silver c., pure silver c. with standard conical shape, used with cement to obturate dental root canals.

theca interna c., the conical thickening of thecal cells of an ovarian follicle with its apex pointed toward the surface.

twin c., two retinal c.'s fused together.

vascular c.'s, SYN *lobules* of epididymis, under *lobule.*

⌂**-cone.** The cusp of a tooth in the upper jaw.

co·nes·si (ko-nes′e). The bark of *Holarrhena antidysenterica* (family Apocynaceae), an Indian tree; used as an astringent and in the treatment of dysentery and amebiasis. SYN kurchi bark. [E. Ind.]

co·nes·sine (kon′ĕ-sēn). roquessine; 3β-(dimethylamino)con-5-enine; 3β-dimethylamino-18α:20α-methylimino-5-pregnene; a steroid alkaloid derived from *Holarrhena antidysenterica* (conessi); a yellow astringent, used in the treatment of amebic dysentery and vaginal trichomoniasis. SYN neriine, wrightine.

co·nex·us, pl. **co·nex·us** (ko-nek′sŭs) [NA]. ☆official alternate term for connection, connection. [L.]

c. intertendin′eus [NA], ☆official alternate term for intertendinous *connections,* under connection.

con·fab·u·la·tion (kon′fab-yū-lā′shŭn). The making of bizarre and incorrect responses, and a readiness to give a fluent but tangential answer, with no regard whatever to facts, to any question put; seen in amnesia, presbyophrenia, and Wernicke-Korsakoff syndrome. [L. *con-fabulor,* pp. *-fabulatus,* to talk together, fr. *fabula,* narrative]

con·fec·tio, gen. **con·fec·ti·o·nis,** pl. **con·fec·ti·o·nes** (kon-fek′shē-ō, -ō′nis, -ō′nēz). SYN confection. [L. fr. *conficio,* pp. *-fectus,* to make ready, prepare]

con·fec·tion (kon-fek′shŭn). A pharmaceutical preparation consisting of a drug mixed with honey or syrup; a soft solid, sometimes used as an excipient for pill masses. SYN confectio, conserve, electuary. [L. *confectio*]

con·fer·tus (kon-fer′tŭs). Arranged closely together; coalescing. [L. *confercio,* pp. *-fertus,* to cram together, fr. *farcio,* to fill full, cram]

con·fi·den·ti·al·i·ty (kon′fi-den-shē-al′i-tē). The statutorily protected right afforded specifically designated health professionals to nondisclosure of information discerned during consultation with a patient. [L. *con-fido,* to trust, be assured]

con·fig·u·ra·tion (kon-fig-yū-rā′shŭn). **1.** The general form of a body and its parts. **2.** In chemistry, the spatial arrangement of atoms in a molecule. The c. of a compound (*e.g.,* a sugar) is the unique spatial arrangement of its atoms such that no other arrangement of these atoms is superimposable thereon with complete correspondence, regardless of changes in conformation (*i.e.,* twisting or rotation about single bonds); change of c. requires breaking and rejoining of bonds, as in going from D to L c.'s of sugars. Cf. conformation.

cis c., (1) SEE cis- (4). **(2)** the property of two or more sites on the same molecule of DNA.

con·fine·ment (kon-fīn′ment). Lying-in; giving birth to a child. [L. *confine* (ntr.), a boundary, confine, fr. *con-* + *finis,* boundary]

con·flict (kon′flikt). Tension or stress experienced by an organism when satisfaction of a need, drive, motive, or wish is thwarted by the presence of other attractive or unattractive needs, drives, or motives.

approach-approach c., a situation of indecision and vacillation when an individual is confronted with two equally attractive alternatives.

approach-avoidance c., a situation of indecision and vacillation when the individual is confronted with a single object or event which has both attractive and unattractive qualities.

avoidance-avoidance c., a situation of indecision and vacillation when the individual is confronted with two equally unattractive alternatives.

c. of interest, a c. between the professional or personal interests

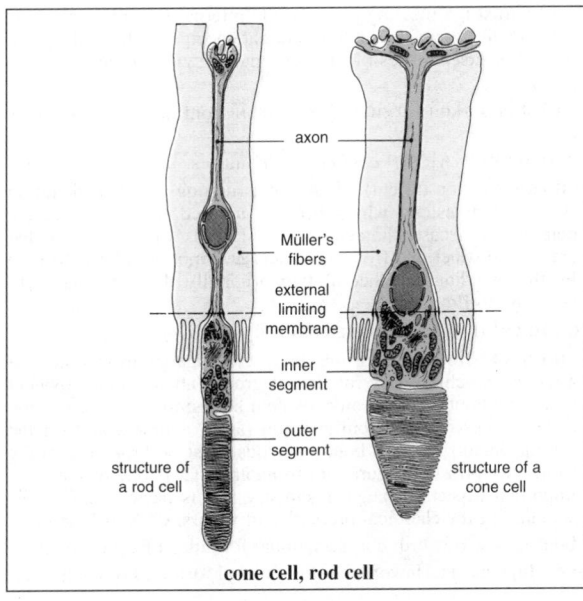

cone cell, rod cell

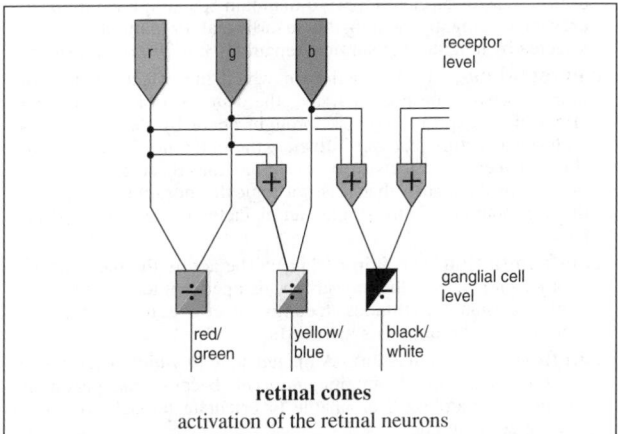

retinal cones
activation of the retinal neurons

and needs of a health provider and his or her professional responsibilities toward a patient or other consumer.

interpersonal c., relating to a conflict in the relations and social exchanges between persons. Cf. intrapersonal c.

intrapersonal c., a conflict that occurs solely in the psychological dynamics of the individual's own mind. SEE intrapsychic.

role c., the dilemma an individual experiences when required to play two different parts (*e.g.,* spouse and aggressive business competitor) that cannot be easily harmonized.

con·flu·ence (kon′flū-ĕns). A flowing together; a joining of two or more streams. SYN confluens [NA]. [L. *confluens*]

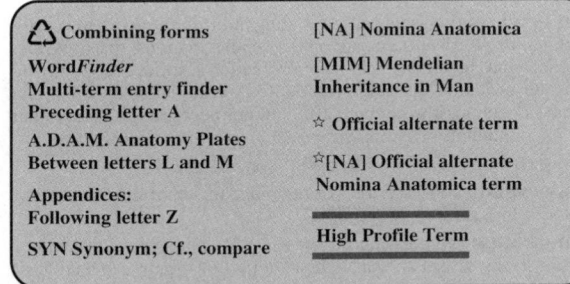

⌂ **Combining forms**	**[NA]** Nomina Anatomica
Word*Finder*	**[MIM]** Mendelian
Multi-term entry finder	**Inheritance in Man**
Preceding letter A	
A.D.A.M. Anatomy Plates	☆ **Official alternate term**
Between letters L and M	
Appendices:	☆**[NA] Official alternate**
Following letter Z	**Nomina Anatomica term**
SYN Synonym; Cf., compare	**High Profile Term**

c. of sinuses, a meeting place, at the internal occipital protuberance, of the superior sagittal, straight, occipital, drained by the two transverse sinuses of the dura mater. SYN confluens sinuum [NA].

con·flu·ens (kon-flū′enz) [NA]. SYN confluence, confluence. [L.]

c. si′nuum [NA], SYN *confluence* of sinuses.

con·flu·ent (kon′flū-ent). **1.** Joining; running together; denoting certain skin lesions which become merged, forming a patch; denoting a disease characterized by lesions which are not discrete, or distinct one from the other. **2.** Denoting a bone formed by the blending together of two originally distinct bones. [L. *con-fluo,* to flow together]

con·fo·cal (kon-fō′kal). SEE confocal *microscope.*

con·for·ma·tion (kon-fōr-mā′shŭn). The spatial arrangement of a molecule achieved by rotation of groups about single covalent bonds, without breaking any covalent bonds; the latter restriction differentiates c. from configuration (as in anomers and related stereoisomers) where a bond or bonds must be broken in going from one form (configuration) to another. C. is one of the most important aspects of sugar chemistry and is basic to an understanding of the chemical properties of sugars. Cf. configuration.

boat c., SEE Haworth conformational formulas of cyclic *sugars.*

envelope c., SEE Haworth conformational formulas of cyclic *sugars.*

con·form·er (kon-fōr′mer). A mold, usually of plastic material, used in plastic surgical repair to maintain space in a cavity or to prevent closing by healing of an artificial or natural opening affected by neighboring surgical repair. [L. *conformo,* to fashion]

con·found·ing. 1. A situation in which the effects of two or more processes are not separated; the distortion of the apparent effect of an exposure on risk, brought about by the association with other factors that can influence the outcome. **2.** A relationship between the effects of two or more causal factors observed in a set of data, such that it is not logically possible to separate the contribution of any single causal factor to the observed effects.

con·fron·ta·tion (kon-frŏn-tā′shŭn). The act by the therapist, or another patient in a therapy group, of openly interpreting a patient's resistances, attitudes, feelings, or effects upon either the therapist, the group, or its member(s).

con·fu·sion (kon-fyū′zhŭn). A mental state in which reactions to environmental stimuli are inappropriate because the person is bewildered, perplexed, or unable to orientate himself. [L. *con-fusio,* a confounding]

con·fu·sion·al (kon-fyū′zhŭn-ăl). Characterized by, or pertaining to, confusion.

con·ge·la·tion (kon-jĕ-lā′shŭn). **1.** SYN freezing. **2.** Obsolete term for frostbite. [L. *con-gelo,* pp. *-atus,* to freeze]

con·ge·ner (kon′jē-ner). **1.** One of two or more things of the same kind, as of animal or plant with respect to classification. **2.** One of two or more muscles with the same function. [L. *con-,* with, + *genus,* race]

con·ge·ner·ous (kon-jen′er-ŭs). **1.** Having the same function; denoting certain muscles that are synergistic. **2.** Derived from the same source, or of a similar nature. [see congener]

con·gen·ic (kon-jen′ik). Relating to an inbred strain of animals produced by repeated crossing of one gene line onto another inbred (isogenic) line. [con- + G. *genos,* birth, + -ic]

con·gen·i·tal (kon-jen′i-tăl). Existing at birth, referring to certain mental or physical traits, anomalies, malformations, diseases, etc. which may be either hereditary or due to an influence occurring during gestation up to the moment of birth. To establish that a trait is genetic, it is neither sufficient nor necessaary to show that it is congenital. SYN congenitus. [L. *congenitus,* born with]

con·gen·i·tus (kon-jen′i-tŭs). SYN congenital. [L.]

con·gest·ed (kon-jes′ted). Containing an abnormal amount of blood; in a state of congestion.

con·ges·tion (kon-jes′chŭn). Presence of an abnormal amount of fluid in the vessels or passages of a part or organ; especially, of blood due either to increased influx or to an obstruction to the return flow. SEE ALSO hyperemia. [L. *congestio,* a bringing together, a heap, fr. *con-gero,* pp. *-gestus,* to bring together]

active c., c. due to an increased flow of arterial blood to a part.

brain c., increased volume of the intravascular compartment of the brain; often associated with brain swelling. SYN encephalemia.

functional c., hyperemia occurring during functional activity of an organ. SYN physiologic c.

hypostatic c., c. due to pooling of venous blood in a dependent part. SYN hypostasis (2).

passive c., c. caused by obstruction or slowing of the venous drainage, resulting in partial stagnation of blood in the capillaries and venules.

physiologic c., SYN functional c.

venous c., overfilling and distention of the veins with blood as a result of mechanical obstruction or right ventricular failure.

con·ges·tive (kon-jes′tiv). Relating to congestion.

con·glo·bate (kon-glō′bāt). Formed in a single rounded mass. [L. *con-globo,* pp. *-atus,* to gather into a *globus,* ball]

con·glo·ba·tion (kon-glō-bā′shŭn). An aggregation of numerous particles into one rounded mass.

con·glom·er·ate (kon-glom′ĕ-rāt). Composed of several parts aggregated into one mass. [L. *con- glomero,* pp. *-atus,* to roll together, fr. *glomus,* a ball]

con·glu·ti·nant (kon-glū′ti-nant). Adhesive, promoting the union of a wound. [L. *con-glutino,* pp. *-atus,* to glue together, fr. *gluten,* glue]

con·glu·ti·na·tion (kon-glū-ti-nā′shŭn). **1.** SYN adhesion (1). **2.** Agglutination of antigen(erythrocyte)-antibody-complement complex by normal bovine serum (and certain other colloidal materials); the procedure provides a means of detecting the presence of nonagglutinating antibody.

con·glu·ti·nin (kon-glū′ti-nin). Bovine serum protein that, when absorbed by erythrocyte-antibody-complement complexes, causes them to agglutinate; it is comparatively thermostable and apparently dissociates when diluted with physiologic saline solution. SYN bovine colloid.

con·go·phil·ic (kon-gō-fil′ik). Denoting any substance that takes a Congo red stain.

Con·go red (kong′gō) [C.I. 22120]. An acid direct cotton dye, sodium diphenyldiazo-bis-α-naphthylaminesulfonate; used as an indicator (pH 3.0, blue-violet, to pH 5.0, red) in testing for free hydrochloric acid in gastric contents; the dye is absorbed by amyloid and induces green fluorescence to amyloid in polarized light; used as a laboratory aid in the diagnosis of amyloidosis and as a histologic stain. SEE Bennhold's Congo red *stain.*

co·ni (kō′nī). Plural of conus.

con·ic, con·i·cal (kon′ik, kon′i-kăl). Resembling a cone.

⌂**-conid.** The cusp of a tooth in the lower jaw.

co·nid·ia (ko-nid′ē-ă). Plural of conidium.

co·nid·i·al (ko-nid′ē-ăl). Relating to a conidium.

Co·nid·i·o·bo·lus (ko-nid′ē-ō-bō′lŭs). A genus of fungi containing two species, *C. coronatus* and *C. incongruus,* both of which cause zygomycosis (entomophthoramycosis).

co·nid·i·og·e·nous (ko-nid-ē-oj′ĕ-nŭs). Denoting a cell that gives rise to a conidium, *e.g.,* a phialide.

co·nid·i·o·phore (ko-nid′ē-ō-fōr). A specialized hypha which bears conidia in fungi. [conidium + G. *phoros,* bearing]

Phialophore-type c., a type of spore formation, characteristic of the genus *Phialophora,* in which conidia are formed endogenously in flask-like c.'s called phialids.

co·nid·i·um, pl. **co·nid·ia** (ko-nid′ē-ŭm, -ē-ă). An asexual spore of fungi borne externally in various ways. [Mod. L. dim. fr. G. *konis,* dust]

co·ni·ine (kō′nē-ēn). Cicutine; conicine; 2-propylpiperidine; the toxic active alkaloid of conium (hemlock); hydrobromide and hydrochloride salts have been used as an antispasmodic; principal toxin of poison hemlock (*Conium maculatum*).

co·ni·o·fi·bro·sis (kō′nē-ō-fī-brō′sis). Fibrosis produced by dust, especially of the lungs by inhaled dust. [G. *konis,* dust, + fibrosis]

co·ni·o·lymph·sta·sis (kŏ′nē-ō-limf′stă-sis). Stasis of lymph caused by dust, presumably through the intervention of fibrosis. [G. *konis*, dust, + lymph + G. *stasis*, a standing]

co·ni·om·e·ter (kō-nē-om′ĕ-ter). A device for estimating the amount of dust in the air. [G. *konis*, dust, + *metron*, measure]

co·ni·o·phage (kŏ′nē-ō-fāj). SYN alveolar *macrophage*. [G. *konis*, dust, + *phagein*, to eat]

co·ni·o·sis (kŏ-nē-ō′sis). Any disease or morbid condition caused by dust. [G. *konis*, dust]

co·ni·ot·o·my (kō-nē-ot′ō-mē). SYN cricothyrotomy.

co·ni·um (kō-nē′ŭm). The dried unripe fruit of *Conium maculatum* (family Umbelliferae), also known as spotted cowbane or spotted parsley; it has been used as a sedative, antispasmodic, and anodyne. SYN hemlock. [L. fr. G. *kōneion*, hemlock]

con·i·za·tion (kō-nī-zā′shŭn). Excision of a cone of tissue, *e.g.,* mucosa of the cervix uteri.

   cautery c., removal of a cone shape of endocervical tissue with electrocautery.

   cold c., obtaining a cone of endocervical tissue with a cold knife blade so as to preserve histological characteristics and avoid desiccating tissue.

con·ju·gant (kon′jū-gant). A member of a mating pair of organisms or gametes undergoing conjugation. SEE ALSO exconjugant. [L. *con-jugo,* to join]

con·ju·gase (kon′jū-gās). SYN γ-glutamyl hydrolase.

con·ju·ga·ta (kon-jū-gā′tă) [NA]. Conjugate diameters of the pelvis. SEE conjugate. [L. fem. of *conjugatus,* pp. of *con-jugo,* to join together]

   c. diagonal′is, SYN diagonal *conjugate*.

   c. vera, SYN *conjugate* of pelvic inlet.

con·ju·gate (kon′jū-gāt). **1.** Joined or paired. SYN conjugated. **2.** Conjugate diameters of the pelvis. The distance between any two specified points on the periphery of the pelvic canal. [L. *conjugatus,* joined together. See conjugata]

   diagonal c., the anteroposterior dimension of the inlet that measures the clinical distance from the promontory of the sacrum to the lower margin of the symphysis pubica. SYN conjugata diagonalis, diagonal conjugate diameter, false c. (1).

   effective c., the internal c. measured from the nearest lumbar vertebra to the symphysis, in spondylolisthesis. SYN false c. (2).

   external c., the distance in a straight line between the depression under the last spinous process of the lumbar vertebrae and the upper edge of the pubic symphysis. SYN Baudelocque's diameter, external conjugate diameter.

   false c., (1) SYN diagonal c. **(2)** SYN effective c.

   folic acid c., a folate with three molecules of glutamic acid (pteropterin) instead of one, or with seven (pteroylheptaglutamic acid or vitamin B$_c$ conjugate).

   internal c., SYN c. of pelvic inlet.

   obstetric c., the diameter that represents the shortest diameter through which the head must pass in descending into the superior strait and measures, by means of x-ray, the distance from the promontory of the sacrum to a point on the inner surface of the symphysis a few millimeters below its upper margin. SYN obstetric conjugate diameter.

   obstetric c. of pelvic outlet, the c. of the pelvic outlet lengthened by the posterior displacement of the coccyx.

   c. of pelvic inlet, distance from the promontory of the sacrum to the upper posterior edge of the pubic symphysis. SYN anteroposterior diameter of the pelvic inlet, conjugata vera, conjugate axis, conjugate diameter of pelvic inlet, diameter mediana, internal c., true c.

   c. of pelvic outlet, the distance from the tip of the coccyx to the lower edge of the pubic symphysis. SEE ALSO obstetric c. of pelvic outlet. SYN conjugate diameter of pelvic outlet.

   true c., SYN c. of pelvic inlet.

con·ju·gat·ed (kon′jū-gāt-ed). SYN conjugate (1).

con·ju·ga·tion (kon-jŭ-gā′shŭn). **1.** The union of two unicellular organisms or of the male and female gametes of multicellular forms followed by partition of the chromatin and the production of two new cells. **2.** Bacterial c., effected by simple contact,

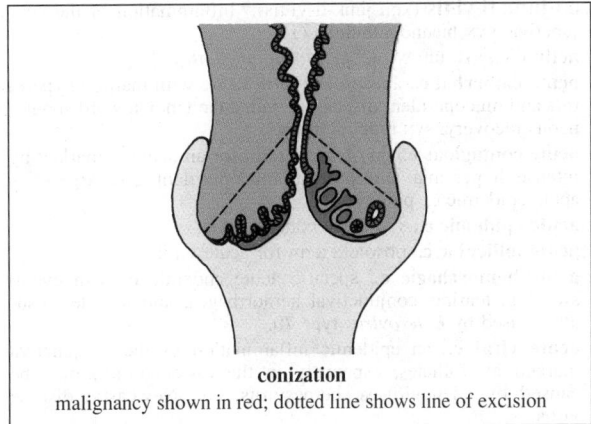

conization
malignancy shown in red; dotted line shows line of excision

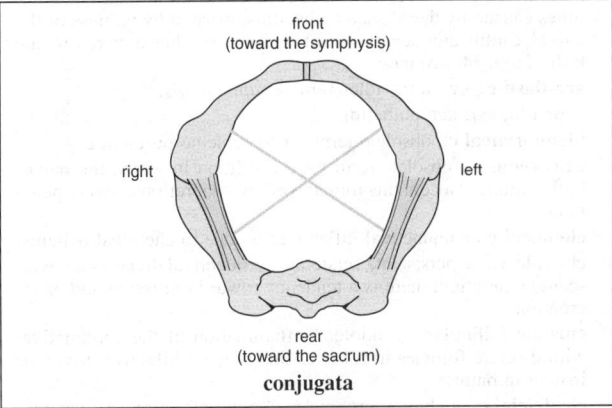

front
(toward the symphysis)

right   left

rear
(toward the sacrum)
conjugata

usually by means of specialized pili through which transfer genes and other genes of the plasmid are transferred to recipient bacteria. **3.** Sexual reproduction among protozoan ciliates, during which two individuals of appropriate mating types fuse along part of their lengths; their macronuclei degenerate and the micronuclei in each macronucleus divide several times (including a meiotic division); one of the resulting haploid pronuclei passes from each conjugant into the other and fuses with the remaining haploid nucleus in each conjugant; the organisms then separate (becoming exconjugants), undergo nuclear reorganization, and subsequently divide by asexual mitosis. **4.** The combination, especially in the liver, of certain toxic substances formed in the intestine, drugs, or steroid hormones with glucuronic or sulfuric acid; a means by which the biological activity of certain chemical substances is terminated and the substances made ready for excretion. **5.** The formation of glycyl or tauryl derivatives of the bile acids. [L. *con-jugo,* pp. *-jugatus,* to join together]

con·junc·ti·va, pl. **con·junc·ti·vae** (kon-jŭnk-tī′vă, -vē). The mucous membrane investing the anterior surface of the eyeball and the posterior surface of the lids. SYN tunica conjunctiva [NA]. [L. fem. of *conjunctivus,* from *conjungo,* pp. *-junctus,* to bind together]

   bulbar c., the part of the conjunctiva covering the anterior surface of the sclera and the surface epithelium of the cornea. SYN tunica conjunctiva bulbi [NA], conjunctival layer of bulb.

   palpebral c., the part of the conjunctiva lining the posterior surface of the eyelids and continuous with the bulbar conjunctiva at the conjunctival fornices. SYN tunica conjunctiva palpebrarum [NA], conjunctival layer of eyelids.

con·junc·ti·val (kon-jŭnk-tī′văl). Relating to the conjunctiva.

con·junc·tive (kon-jŭnk′tiv). Joining; connecting; connective.

con·junc·ti·vi·plas·ty (kon-jŭnk-tī′vi-plas-tē). SYN conjunctivoplasty.

con·junc·ti·vi·tis (kon-jŭnk-ti-vī′tis). Inflammation of the conjunctiva. SYN blennophthalmia (1).

actinic c., SYN ultraviolet *keratoconjunctivitis.*

acute catarrhal c., an obsolete term for c. with marked hyperemia and mucopurulent discharge, with a tendency toward spontaneous recovery. SYN mucopurulent c.

acute contagious c., an obsolete term for an acute c. marked by intense hyperemia and profuse mucopurulent discharge. SYN acute epidemic c., pinkeye (1).

acute epidemic c., SYN acute contagious c.

acute follicular c., obsolete term for acute viral c.

acute hemorrhagic c., specific acute endemic c. with eyelid swelling, tearing, conjunctival hemorrhages, and follicles; usually caused by *Enterovirus* type 70.

acute viral c., an epidemic inflammation of the conjunctiva marked by follicles, especially in the lower fornix; may be caused by adenoviruses, herpesvirus, and Newcastle disease virus.

allergic c., SYN vernal c.

angular c., a subacute bilateral conjunctival inflammation sometimes caused by the Moraxella bacillus, marked by redness of the lateral canthi and scanty, stringy discharge that adheres to the lashes. SYN Moraxella c.

arc-flash c., SYN ultraviolet *keratoconjunctivitis.*

c. ar′ida, SYN xerophthalmia.

blennorrheal c., obsolete term for hyperacute purulent c.

calcareous c., obsolete term for a condition in which the palpebral conjunctiva contains minute yellow concretions. SYN c. petrificans.

chemical c., conjunctival inflammation due to chemical irritants.

chronic c., a persistent, bilateral, conjunctival hyperemia with scanty exudation; there is a tendency toward remission and exacerbation.

chronic follicular c., indolent inflammation of the conjunctiva, with discrete follicles in fornices that may be infective, toxic, or irritant in nature.

cicatricial c., a chronic progressive ocular affection that produces scarring of the conjunctiva primarily and of the cornea sequentially.

diphtheritic c., a severe conjunctival inflammation caused by *Corynebacterium diphtheriae* and characterized by an infiltrating membrane which on removal leaves a raw surface. SYN membranous c.

follicular c., c. associated with hypertrophic lymphoid tissue in the conjunctival fornices.

gonococcal c., a type of hyperacute, purulent c.

gonorrheal c., SYN gonorrheal *ophthalmia.*

granular c., SYN trachomatous c.

hyperacute purulent c., c. caused by *Neisseria gonorrhea* and marked by swollen congested conjunctiva, edematous eyelids, and a purulent discharge.

inclusion c., a follicular c. caused by *Chlamydia trachomatis.*

infantile purulent c., SYN *ophthalmia* neonatorum.

lacrimal c., obsolete term for a secondary c. due to canaliculitis or dacryocystitis. SYN reflux c.

larval c., c. due to imbedding of larvae in the eye. SEE ophthalmomyiasis.

ligneous c., c. characterized typically by woody induration of the upper tarsal conjunctiva, whitish pseudomembrane, and, in severe cases, corneal opacity; usually bilateral.

c. medicamento′sa, a c. caused by medicine or toxin instilled into the conjunctival sac. SYN toxicogenic c.

meibomian c., an obsolete term for a c. associated with chronic inflammation of the meibomian glands, with swollen tarsal plates and frothy seborrheic secretion. SYN seborrheic blepharoconjunctivitis.

membranous c., SYN diphtheritic c.

molluscum c., c. associated with lesions of molluscum contagiosum of the eyelid.

Moraxella c., SYN angular c.

mucopurulent c., SYN acute catarrhal c.

necrotic infectious c., a unilateral, suppurative, necrotic inflammation of the conjunctiva characterized by scattered, elevated white spots in the fornices and palpebral conjunctiva, and ipsilateral swelling of preauricular, parotid, and submaxillary lymph glands. SYN Pascheff's c.

neonatal c., SYN *ophthalmia* neonatorum.

Parinaud's c., a chronic necrotic inflammation of the conjunctiva characterized by large, irregular, reddish follicles and regional lymphadenopathy.

Pascheff's c., SYN necrotic infectious c.

c. petrif′icans, SYN calcareous c.

phlyctenular c., a circumscribed c. accompanied by the formation of small red nodules of lymphoid tissue (phlyctenulae) on the conjunctiva. SYN phlyctenular ophthalmia.

prairie c., obsolete term for a chronic c., characterized by the presence of small white spots on the palpebral conjunctiva, especially of the lower lid.

pseudomembranous c., a nonspecific inflammatory reaction characterized by the appearance on the conjunctiva of a coagulated fibrinous plaque that may be peeled off from intact epithelium.

purulent c., a violently acute inflammation of the conjunctiva, with copious pus and a marked tendency for corneal involvement.

reflux c., SYN lacrimal c.

simple c., acute viral c., self-limited and of short duration.

snow c., SYN ultraviolet *keratoconjunctivitis.*

spring c., SYN vernal c.

squirrel plague c., one of the causes of Parinaud's c. SYN tularemic c., c. tularensis.

swimming pool c., a non-specific red-eye that can be caused by pool chlorination, adenovirus, and rarely, *Chlamydia.*

toxicogenic c., SYN c. medicamentosa.

trachomatous c., a chronic infection of the conjunctiva due to *Chlamydia trachomatis,* characterized by conjunctival follicles and subsequent cicatrization. SEE ALSO trachoma. SYN granular c.

tularemic c., c. tularen′sis, SYN squirrel plague c.

vernal c., a chronic, bilateral conjunctival inflammation with photophobia and intense itching that recurs seasonally during warm weather; characterized in the palpebral form by cobblestone papillae in the upper palpebral conjunctiva and in the bulbar form by gelatinous nodules adjacent to the corneoscleral limbus. SYN allergic c., spring c., spring ophthalmia, vernal catarrh, vernal keratoconjunctivitis.

welder's c., SYN ultraviolet *keratoconjunctivitis.*

con·junc·ti·vo·dac·ry·o·cys·to·rhi·nos·to·my (kon-jŭnk′ti-vō-dak′rē-ō-sis′tō-rī-nos′tō-mē). A procedure for providing lacrimal drainage when the canaliculi are closed; plastic tubes are inserted that extend from the conjunctival sac to the nose. [conjunctiva + G. *dakryon,* tear, + *kystis,* cyst, + *ris* (rhin-), nose, + *stoma,* mouth]

con·junc·ti·vo·dac·ry·o·cys·tos·to·my (kon-jŭnk′ti-vō-dak′rē-ō-sis-tos′tō-mē). **1.** A surgical procedure through the conjunctiva, which provides an opening into the lacrimal sac. **2.** The opening so produced. [conjunctiva + G. *dakryon,* tear, + *kystis,* sac, + *stoma,* mouth]

con·junc·ti·vo·plas·ty (kon-jŭnk-tī′vō-plas-tē, kon-jŭngk′ti-vō-). Plastic surgery on the conjunctiva. SYN conjunctiviplasty.

con·junc·ti·vo·rhi·nos·to·my (kon-jŭnk′ti-vō-rī-nos′tō-mē). **1.** A surgical procedure to construct a passageway through the conjunctiva into the nasal cavity. **2.** The opening so produced. [conjunctiva + G. *ris* (rhin), nose, + *stoma,* mouth]

Conn, Harold J., U.S. microbiologist, 1886–1975. SEE Hucker-C. *stain.*

Conn, Jerome, U.S. physician, *1907. SEE C.'s *syndrome.*

con·nec·tins (kon-nek′tinz). Collective term for the protein components of the cytoskeleton (connective tissue); originally described in muscle, but later observed in erythrocyte and other cell membranes.

con·nec·tion (kŏ-nek′shŭn). A union of elements or things; a connecting structure. SYN connexus [NA], conexus [NA].

ambiguous atrioventricular c.'s, c.'s in which half the atrioventricular junction is connected concordantly and the other half is discordantly connected.

atrioventricular c.'s, the five distinct and discrete ways in which the atrial chambers may be connected to the ventricles are concordant, discordant, ambiguous, double inlet, and univentricular.

concordant atrioventricular c.'s, c.'s in which the atrial chambers connect to the morphologically appropriate ventricles.

discordant atrioventricular c.'s, c.'s in which each atrium is connected with a morphologically inappropriate ventricle.

double inlet atrioventricular c.'s, c.'s in which both atrial chambers connect to the same ventricle.

intertendinous c.'s, fibrous bands passing obliquely between the diverging tendons of the extensor digitorum on the dorsum of the hand. SYN connexus intertendineus [NA], conexus intertendineus☆ [NA], juncturae tendinum.

total or partial anomalous pulmonary venous c.'s, c.'s in which some or all of the pulmonary veins connect to the right atrium or one of its tributaries.

univentricular c.'s, c.'s in which one of the atrial chambers is connected to a ventricle, but the other has no connection with the ventricular mass at all.

con·nec·tor (kŏ-nek'tŏr, -tōr). In dentistry, a part of a partial denture which unites its components.

major c., a plate or bar (lingual bar, palatal bar) used for the purpose of uniting partial denture bases.

minor c., the connecting link (tang) between the major c. or base of a partial denture and other units of the prosthesis, such as clasps, indirect retainers, and occlusal rests.

Connell, F. Gregory, U.S. surgeon, 1875–1968. SEE C.'s *suture.*

con·nex·ins, con·nex·ons (kon-neks'inz, -onz). Complex protein assemblies that traverse the lipid bilayer of the plasma membrane and forms a continuous channel with a pore diameter of approximately 1.5 nm; a pair of c.'s from two adjacent cells join to form a gap junction that bridges the 2–4-nm gap between the cells, resulting in both electrical and metabolic couplings; one type of c. makes up the gap junction in heart and may coordinate the beating of all muscle cells in one section of the heart.

con·nex·us (ko-nek'sŭs) [NA]. SYN connection. [L.]

c. intertendin′eus [NA], SYN intertendinous *connections,* under *connection.*

co·noid (kō'noyd). **1.** A cone-shaped structure. **2.** Part of the apical complex characteristic of the protozoan subphylum, Apicomplexa; seen in sporozoites, merozoites, or other developmental stages of sporozoans, less well developed in the piroplasms (families Babesiidae and Theileriidae). The function of the c. is unknown, but it is thought to be an organelle of penetration into the host cell, possibly aided by a protrusible form of the c. [G. *kōnoeidēs,* cone-shaped]

Sturm's c., in optics, the pattern of rays formed after passage through a spherocylindrical combination.

co·no·my·oi·din (kō-nō-mī'oy-din). Contractile protoplasm at the inner end of the inner segment of retinal cones; motility is most evident in fishes and amphibians, and slight or absent in mammals. [G. *kōnos,* cone, + *mys,* muscle, + *eidos,* resemblance]

con·qui·nine (kon'kwi-nēn). SYN quinidine.

Conradi, Andrew, Norwegian physician, 1809–1869. SEE C.'s *line.*

Conradi, Erich, 20th century German physician. SEE C.'s *disease.*

Conradi, Heinrich, German bacteriologist, *1876. SEE C.-Drigalski *agar;* Drigalski-Conradi *agar.*

con·san·guin·e·ous (kon-sang-gwin'ē-ŭs). Denoting consanguinity. [L. *cum,* with, + *sanguis,* blood: *consanguineus*]

con·san·guin·i·ty (kon-sang-gwin'i-tē). Kinship because of common ancestry. SYN blood relationship. [L. *consanguinitas,* blood relationship]

con·scious (con'shŭs). **1.** Aware; having present knowledge or perception of oneself, one's acts and surroundings. **2.** Denoting something occurring with the perceptive attention of the individual, as a c. act or idea, distinguished from automatic or instinctive. [L. *conscius,* knowing]

con·scious·ness (con'shŭs-nes). The state of being aware, or perceiving physical facts or mental concepts; a state of general wakefulness and responsiveness to environment; a functioning sensorium. [L. *con-scio,* to know, to be aware of]

clouding of c., a state in which the patient's mental state is clouded and thus not fully in contact with the environment.

double c., a condition in which one lives in two seemingly unrelated mental states, being, while in one, unaware of the other or of the acts performed in the other. SEE ALSO dual *personality.*

field of c., the content of awareness at any given moment.

con·sen·su·al (kon-sen'shū-ăl). Denoting what something is by the fact of agreement between the perceiving of several persons. SYN reflex (3). [L. *con-,* with, + *sensus,* sensation]

con·ser·va·tion (kon-ser-vā'shŭn). **1.** Preservation from loss, injury, or decay. **2.** In sensorimotor theory, the mental operation by which an individual retains the idea of an object after its removal in time or space. [L. *conservatio,* a preserving, keeping]

c. of energy, the principle that the total amount of energy in a closed system remains always the same, none being lost or created in any chemical or physical process or in the conversion of one kind of energy into another, within that system.

con·ser·va·tive (kon-ser'vă-tiv). Denoting treatment by gradual, limited, or well-established procedures, as opposed to radical.

con·serve (kon'serv). SYN confection.

con·sol·i·dant (kon-sol'i-dant). A substance that promotes healing or union.

con·sol·i·da·tion (kon-sol-i-dā'shŭn). Solidification into a firm dense mass; applied especially to inflammatory induration of a normally aerated lung due to the presence of cellular exudate in the pulmonary alveoli. [L. *consolido,* to make thick, condense, fr. *solidus,* solid]

con·spe·cif·ic (kon-spe-sif'ik). Of the same species. [L. *con-,* with, + specific]

con·spi·cu·i·ty (kon-spi-kyū'i-tē). The visibility of a structure of interest on a radiograph, a function of the inherent contrast of the structure and the complexity (noise) of the surrounding image.

con·stan·cy (kon'stan-sē). The quality of being constant. [L. *constantia,* fr. *consto,* to stand still]

color c., unchanging perception of the color of an object despite changes in lighting or viewing conditions.

object c., the tendency for objects to be perceived as unchanging despite variations in the positions and conditions under which the objects are observed; *e.g.,* a book's shape is always perceived as a rectangle regardless of the visual angle from which it is viewed.

con·stant (kon'stănt). A quantity that, under stated conditions, does not vary with changes in the environment.

Ambard's c., SEE Ambard's *laws,* under *law.*

association c., (1) in experimental immunology, a mathematical expression of hapten-antibody interaction: average association c., $K = $ [hapten-bound antibody]/[free antibody][free hapten]; **(2)** (K_a), the equilibrium c. involved in the association of two or more compounds or ions into a new compound; the reciprocal of the dissociation c. SYN binding c.

Avogadro's c., SYN Avogadro's *number.*

binding c., SYN association c.

decay c., the fractional change in the number of atoms of a radionuclide which occurs in unit time; the constant l in the equation for the fraction (DN/N) of the number of atoms (N) of a radionuclide disintegrating in time Dt, $DN/N = -lDt$. SYN disintegration c., radioactive c., transformation c.

diffusion c., SYN diffusion *coefficient.*

disintegration c., SYN decay c.

dissociation c. (K_d, K), the equilibrium c. involved in the dissociation of a compound into two or more compounds or ions. The reciprocal of the association c. (2).

dissociation c. of an acid (K_d, K_a), expressed by general equation $[H^+][A^-]/[HA] = K_a$, where HA is the undissociated acid.

dissociation c. of a base (K_b), expressed by the general equation $[B^+][OH^-]/[BOH] = K_b$, where BOH is the undissociated base.

dissociation c. of water (K_w), expressed by the equation $[H^+][OH^-] = K_w = 10^{-14}$ at 25°C.

CO

equilibrium c. (K_{eq}), in the reaction $A + B \leftrightarrow C + D$ at equilibrium (*i.e.*, no net change in concentrations of A, B, C, or D), the concentrations of the four components are related by the equation $K_{eq} = [C][D]/[A][B]$; K_{eq} is the equilibrium c. If any component in the reaction has a multiplier (*e.g.*, $H_2 \leftrightarrow 2H$), that multiplier appears as an exponent in the calculation of K (*e.g.*, $K_{eq} = [H]^2/[H_2]$). When this equation is applied to the ionization of a substance in solution, K_{eq} is called the dissociation c. (K_d) and its negative logarithm (base 10) is the pK_d. SEE ALSO Henderson-Hasselbalch *equation*, mass-action *ratio*.

Faraday's c. (F), SEE faraday.

flotation c. (S_f), characteristic sedimentation behavior of a lipoprotein fraction of plasma in a centrifugal field in a medium of appropriate density, achieved by adding a salt or D_2O to the plasma. SYN negative S, Svedberg of flotation.

gas c. (R), R (symbol for the constant) = 8.314×10^7 ergs per degree Celsius per mole = 8.314 J K^{-1} mol^{-1} (joules per kelvin mole).

Hill c., SYN Hill *coefficient*.

Michaelis c., (1) the true dissociation constant for the enzyme-substrate binary complex in a single-substrate rapid equilibrium enzyme-catalyzed reaction (usually symbolized by K_s); (2) the concentration of the substrate at which half the true maximum velocity of an enzyme-catalyzed reaction is achieved (when velocities are measured under initial rate and steady state conditions); the ratio of rate constants $(k_2 + k_3)/k_1$ in the single-substrate enzyme-catalyzed reaction: $E + S \leftrightarrow ES \leftrightarrow E + $ products where E represents the free enzyme, S is the substrate, and ES is the central binary complex. The expression for the Michaelis c. will be more complex for multisubstrate reactions. An apparent Michaelis c. is a c. determined either under conditions that are not strictly steady state and initial rate or one that varies with the concentration of one or more cosubstrates. SEE Michaelis-Menten *equation*. SYN Michaelis-Menten c.

Michaelis-Menten c. (K_m), SYN Michaelis c.

Newtonian c. of gravitation (G), a universal c. relating the gravitational force, f, attracting two masses, m_1 and m_2, toward each other when they are separated by a distance, r, in the equation: $f = G(m_1 m_2/r^2)$; it has the value of 6.67259×10^{-8} dyne cm^2 $g^{-2} = 6.67259 \times 10^{-11}$ m^3 kg^{-1} s^{-2} in SI units.

permeability c. (P with a subscript for the ion, P), a measure of the ease with which an ion can cross a unit area of membrane driven by a 1.0 M difference in concentration; usually expressed in centimeters per second. Cf. permeability *coefficient*.

Planck's c. (h), a c., $6.6260755 \times 10^{-34}$ J · s (joule-seconds) or $6.6260755 \times 10^{-27}$ erg-seconds = $6.6260755 \times 10^{-34}$ J Hz^{-1} (joule per hertz).

radioactive c. (Λ), SYN decay c.

rate c.'s (k), proportionality c.'s equal to the initial rate of a reaction divided by the concentration of the reactant(s); *e.g.*, in the reaction $A \rightarrow B + C$, the rate of the reaction equals $-d[A]/dt = k_1[A]$. The rate c. k_1 is a unimolecular rate c. since there is only one molecular species reacting and has units of reciprocal time (*e.g.*, sec^{-1}). For the reverse reaction, $B + C \rightarrow A$, the rate equals $-d[B]/dt = d[A]/dt = k_2[B][C]$. The rate c. k_2 is a bimolecular rate c. and has units of reciprocal concentration-time (*e.g.*, M^{-1} sec^{-1}). SYN velocity c.'s.

sedimentation c., the c. s in Svedberg's equation for estimating the molecular weight of a protein from the rate of movement in a centrifugal field:

$$M = s \frac{RT}{D(1 - \bar{V}\rho)}$$

where M is the molecular weight, R the gas constant, T the absolute temperature, D the diffusion constant (in square centimeters per second), $\bar{V}$ the partial specific volume of the protein, ρ the density of the solvent. The constant s, with dimensions of time per unit of field force ($s = \frac{d_{r_b}/dt}{\omega^2 r_b}$ where r_b is the position at time t, r_0 is the position at time 0, and ω is the angular velocity) is usually between 1×10^{-13} and 200×10^{-13} second. The Svedberg unit (S) is arbitrarily set at 1×10^{-13} second and is very often used to describe the sedimentation rate of macromolecules; *e.g.*, 4 S RNA. SYN sedimentation coefficient.

specificity c., ratio of the maximum velocity (V_{max}) or k_{cat} to the

true K_m value for a specific substrate in an enzyme-catalyzed reaction.

time c., that part of a circuit that determines the time interval over which the rate of electrical events will be averaged; in pulmonary physiology, the factors determining rate of flow in the airways.

transformation c., SYN decay c.

velocity c.'s (k), SYN rate c.'s.

con·stel·la·tion (kon-stel-ā'shŭn). In psychiatry, all the factors that determine a particular action. [L.L. *constellatio*, fr. *cum*, together, + *stella*, star]

con·sti·pate (kon'sti-pāt). To cause constipation.

con·sti·pat·ed (kon'sti-pāt-ed). Suffering from constipation.

con·sti·pa·tion (kon-sti-pā'shŭn). A condition in which bowel movements are infrequent or incomplete. SYN costiveness. [L. *con-stipo*, pp. *-atus*, to press together]

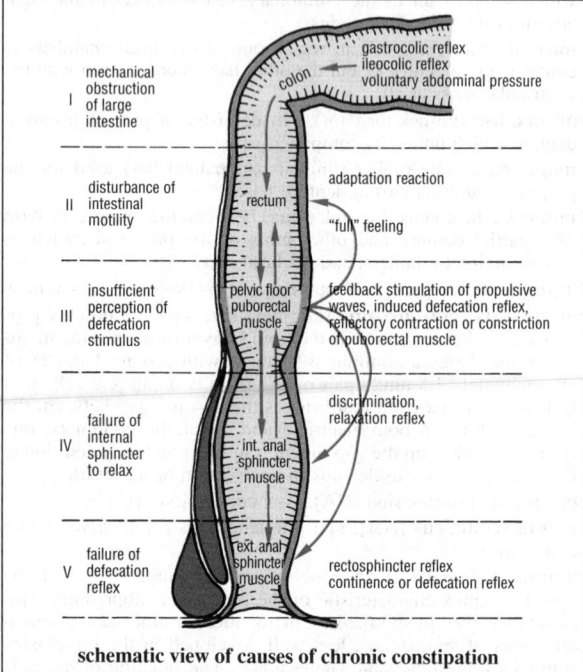

schematic view of causes of chronic constipation

con·sti·tu·tion (kon-sti-tū'shŭn). **1.** The physical makeup of a body, including the mode of performance of its functions, the activity of its metabolic processes, the manner and degree of its reactions to stimuli, and its power of resistance to the attack of pathogenic organisms. **2.** In chemistry, the number and kind of atoms in the molecule and the relation they bear to each other. [L. *constitutio*, constitution, disposition, fr. *constituo*, pp. *-stitutus*, to establish, fr. *statuo*, to set up]

con·sti·tu·tion·al (kon-sti-tū'shŭn-ăl). **1.** Relating to a body's constitution. **2.** General; relating to the system as a whole; not local.

con·sti·tu·tive (kon-sti'tū-tiv). **1.** SEE constitutive *enzyme*. **2.** In genetics, descriptive of a gene that is controlled by constantly active promoter.

con·stric·tion (kon-strik'shŭn). **1.** A normally or pathologically constricted or narrowed portion of a luminal structure. SEE ALSO stricture, stenosis. **2.** The act or process of binding or contracting, becoming narrowed; the condition of being constricted, squeezed. **3.** A subjective sensation of pressure or tightness, as if the body or any part were tightly bound or squeezed. [L. *con-str-ingo*, pp. *-strictus*, to draw together]

esophageal c.'s, three narrowings of the esophagus normally demonstrated radiographically following a barium swallow: the upper or pharyngeal esophageal constriction, at the beginning of the esophagus, is caused by the cricopharyngeus muscle, often referred to as the superior esophageal sphincter; the middle or aortic constriction is a left-sided narrowing due to the esophagus passing the aortic arch; the inferior or diaphragmatic esophageal c. corresponds to the passage of the esophagus through the esophageal hiatus of the diaphragm. SYN impressions of esophagus.

primary c., the narrowing between the two arms of the chromosome represented by the centromere.

pyloric c., a prominent fold of mucous membrane at the gastroduodenal junction overlying the pyloric sphincter. SYN pyloric valve, valvula pylori, valvulae pylori.

secondary c., a subsidiary narrowing of the chromosome associated in some cases with satellites.

c.'s of ureter, normal physiological narrowings of the ureter observable in a pyelogram; the uppermost occurs at the origin of the ureter from the renal pelvis; a second occurs as the ureter crosses the iliac vessels and pelvic brim; the inferiormost occurs as the ureter penetrates the wall of the urinary bladder.

con·stric·tor (kon-strik′ter, -tōr). **1.** Anything that binds or squeezes a part. **2.** A muscle, the action of which is to narrow a canal; a sphincter. [L. fr. *constringo,* to draw together]

con·struct. (noun) The combination of a bone graft, metal instrumentation, prosthetic devices and/or bone cement applied to a specific level of the spinal column in the setting of segmental spinal instability.

con·sul·tand (kon-sŭl′tand). A person about whose future offspring the genetic counselor is to make predictions; not to be confused with proband. [consult (for counsel) + L. *-andus,* gerundive suffix]

dummy c., a person in the line of descent from the leading ancestor to the c. proper; for logical simplicity, the dummy c. is analyzed as if the c. proper.

con·sul·tant (kon-sŭl′tant). **1.** A physician or surgeon who does not take full responsibility for a patient, but acts in an advisory capacity, deliberating with and counseling the attending physician or surgeon. **2.** A member of a hospital staff who has no active service but stands ready to advise in any case, at the request of the attending physician or surgeon. [L. *consulto,* pp. *-atus,* to deliberate, ask advice]

con·sul·ta·tion (kon-sŭl-tā′shŭn). Meeting of two or more physicians or surgeons to evaluate the nature and progress of disease in a particular patient and to establish diagnosis, prognosis, and/or therapy.

con·sump·tion (kon-sŭmp′shŭn). **1.** The using up of something, especially the rate at which it is used. **2.** Obsolete term for a wasting of the tissues of the body, usually tuberculous. [L. *con-sumo,* pp. *-sumptus,* to take up wholly, use up, waste]

oxygen c. ($\dot{V}_{O_2}$), (1) (Qo or Qo₂), the rate at which oxygen is used by a tissue; units: microliters of oxygen STPD used per milligram of tissue per hour; **(2)** ($\dot{V}_{O_2}$), the rate at which oxygen enters the blood from alveolar gas, equal in the steady state to the consumption of oxygen by tissue metabolism throughout the body; units: milliliters of oxygen STPD used per minute or mmol/min.

con·sump·tive (kon-sŭmp′tiv). Relating to, or suffering from, consumption.

con·tact (kon′takt). **1.** The touching or apposition of two bodies. **2.** A person who has been exposed to a contagious disease. [L. *con- tingo,* pp. *-tactus,* to touch, seize, fr. *tango,* to touch]

balancing c., (1) the c.'s between upper and lower dentures on the balancing or mediotrusive side for the purpose of stabilizing the dentures; **(2)** the c.'s between upper and lower dentures at the opposite side from the working or laterotrusive side (anteroposteriorly or laterally) for the purpose of stabilizing the dentures; **(3)** the c.'s between upper and lower natural or artificial teeth at the opposite side from the working or laterotrusive side. SYN balancing occlusal surface.

centric c., SYN centric *occlusion.*

deflective occlusal c., a condition of tooth c.'s which diverts the mandible from a normal path of closure to centric jaw relation. SYN cuspal interference, interceptive occlusal c., premature c.

initial c., (1) the first meeting of opposing teeth upon elevation

of the mandible toward the maxillae; **(2)** the initial occlusal c. of opposing teeth when the jaw is closed.

interceptive occlusal c., SYN deflective occlusal c.

premature c., SYN deflective occlusal c.

proximal c., proximate c., the area where the surfaces of two adjacent teeth in the same arch touch.

c. with reality, correctly interpreting external phenomena in relation to the norms of one's social or cultural milieu.

working c.'s, working or occlusion; c.'s of teeth made on the side of the occlusion toward which the mandible has been moved. SYN working bite, working occlusion.

con·tac·tant (kon-tak′tănt). Any of a heterogeneous group of allergens that elicit manifestations of induced sensitivity (hypersensitivity) by direct contact with skin or mucosa.

con·ta·gion (kon-tā′jŭn). **1.** SYN contagium. **2.** Transmission of infection by direct contact, droplet spread, or contaminated fomites. The term originated long before development of modern ideas of infectious disease and has since lost much of its significance, being included under the more inclusive term "communicable disease." **3.** Production via suggestion or imitation of a neurosis or psychosis in several or more members of a group. [L. *contagio;* fr. *contingo,* to touch closely]

immediate c., direct c. occurring as the result of actual contact with the sick.

mediate c., indirect c. effected through the medium of persons or objects that have been in contact with the sick.

psychic c., communication of a nervous disorder or lesser psychological symtoms by imitation, as in mass hysteria.

con·ta·gious (kon-tā′jŭs). Relating to contagion; communicable or transmissible by contact with the sick or their fresh secretions or excretions.

con·ta·gious·ness (kon-tā′jŭs-nes). The quality of being contagious.

con·ta·gium (kon-tā′jē-ŭm). The agent of an infectious disease. SYN contagion (1). [L. a touching]

con·tain·ment. The concept of regional or global eradication of communicable disease, proposed by Fred Lowe Soper (1893-1977) in 1949 for the eradication of smallpox.

con·tam·i·nant (kon-tam′i-nant). An impurity; any material of an extraneous nature associated with a chemical, a pharmaceutical preparation, a physiologic principle, or an infectious agent.

con·tam·i·nate (kon-tam′i-nāt). To cause or result in contamination. [L. *con-tamino,* to mingle, corrupt]

con·tam·i·na·tion (kon-tam-i-nā′shŭn). **1.** The presence of an infectious agent on a body surface; also on or in clothes, bedding, toys, surgical instruments or dressings, or other inanimate articles or substances including water, milk and food or that infectious agent itself. **2.** In epidemiology, the situation that exists when a population being studied for one condition or factor also possesses other conditions or factors that modify results of the study. **3.** Freudian term for a fusion and condensation of words. [L. *contamino,* pp. *-atus,* to stain, defile]

con·tent (kon′tent). **1.** That which is contained within something else, usually in this sense in the plural form, contents. **2.** In psychology, the form of a dream as presented to consciousness. **3.** Ambiguous usage for concentration (3); *e.g.,* blood hemoglobin c. could mean either its concentration or the product of its concentration and the blood volume. [L. *contentus,* fr. *con- tineo,* pp. *-tentus,* to hold together, contain]

carbon dioxide c., the total carbon dioxide available from serum or plasma following addition of acid; measured routinely in hospital laboratories as a component of electrolyte profiles.

GC c., the amount of guanine and cytosine in a polynucleic acid usually expressed in mole fraction (or percentage) of total bases; the melting temperature of such biopolymers varies with the GC c.

latent c., the hidden, unconscious meaning of thoughts or actions, especially in dreams or fantasies.

manifest c., those elements of fantasy and dreams which are consciously available and reportable.

con·tig. SEE contig *map.*

con·ti·gu·i·ty (kon-ti-gyū′i-tē). **1.** Contact without actual continuity, *e.g.*, the contact of the bones entering into the formation of a cranial suture. Cf. continuity. **2.** Occurrence of two or more objects, events, or mental impressions together in space (**spatial c.**) or time (**temporal c.**). [L. *contiguus*, touching, fr. *contingo*, to touch]

con·tig·u·ous (kon-tig′ū-ŭs). Adjacent or in actual contact.

con·ti·nence (kon′ti-nens). **1.** Moderation, temperance, or self-restraint in respect to the appetites, especially to sexual intercourse. **2.** The ability to retain urine and/or feces until a proper time for their discharge. [L. *continentia*, fr. *con- tineo*, to hold back]

con·ti·nent (kon′ti-nent). Denoting continence.

con·tin·ued (kon-tin′yūd). Continuous; without intermission; said especially of protracted fever without apyretic intervals, such as typhoid fever, compared with the paroxysms of fever in malaria. [L. *continuo*, to join together, make continuous]

con·ti·nu·i·ty (kon-ti-nu′i-tē). Absence of interruption, a succession of parts intimately united, *e.g.*, the unbroken conjunction of cells and structures that make up a single bone of the skull. Cf. contiguity. [L. *continuus*, continued]

con·tour (kon′tūr). **1.** The outline of a part; the surface configuration. **2.** In dentistry, to restore the normal outlines of a broken or otherwise misshapen tooth, or to create the external shape or form of a prosthesis. [L. *con-* (intens.), + *torno*, to turn (in a lathe), fr. *tornus*, a lathe]

   flange c., the design of the flange of a denture.

   gingival c., the shape or form of the gingiva, either natural or artificial, around the necks of the teeth. SYN gum c.

   gum c., SYN gingival c.

   height of c., SEE *height* of contour.

⌂**contra-.** Opposed, against. SEE ALSO counter-. Cf. anti-. [L.]

con·tra·an·gle (kon′tră-ang′gl). **1.** One of the double or triple angles in the shank of an instrument by means of which the cutting edge or point is brought into the axis of the handle. **2.** An extension piece added to the end of a dental handpiece which, through a set of bevel gears, changes the angle of the axis of rotation of the bur in relation to the axis of the handpiece.

con·tra·ap·er·ture (kon′tră-ap′er-chŭr). SYN counteropening.

con·tra·bev·el (kon′tră-bev′ĕl). A bevel located on the side opposite the customary side.

con·tra·cep·tion (kon-tră-sep′shŭn). Prevention of conception or impregnation.

con·tra·cep·tive (kon-tră-sep′tiv). **1.** An agent for the prevention of conception. **2.** Relating to any measure or agent designed to prevent conception. [L. *contra*, against, + conceptive]

   barrier c., a mechanical device designed to prevent spermatozoa from penetrating the cervical os; usually used in combination with a spermicidal agent, *i.e.*, vaginal diaphragm.

   combination oral c., a mixture of a steroid having progestational activity and an estrogen.

   intrauterine c. device, SEE intrauterine contraceptive *devices*.

   oral c., any orally effective preparation designed to prevent conception.

con·tract. **1** (kon-trakt′). To shorten; to become reduced in size; in the case of muscle, either to shorten or to undergo an increase in tension. **2** (kon-trakt′). To acquire by contagion or infection. **3** (kon′trakt). An explicit bilateral commitment by psychotherapist and patient to a defined course of action to attain the goal of the psychotherapy. [L. *con-traho*, pp. *-tractus*, to draw together]

con·trac·tile (kon-trak′tīl). Having the property of contracting.

con·trac·til·i·ty (kon-trak-til′i-tē). The ability or property of a substance, especially of muscle, of shortening, or becoming reduced in size, or developing increased tension.

   cardiac c., a measure of cardiac pump performance, the degree to which muscle fibers can shorten when activated by a stimulus independent of preload and afterload.

con·trac·tion (C) (kon-trak′shŭn). **1.** A shortening or increase in tension; denoting the normal function of muscular tissue. **2.** A shrinkage or reduction in size. **3.** Heart beat, as in premature c. See also entries under beat. [L. *contractio*, to draw together]

   after-c., SEE aftercontraction.

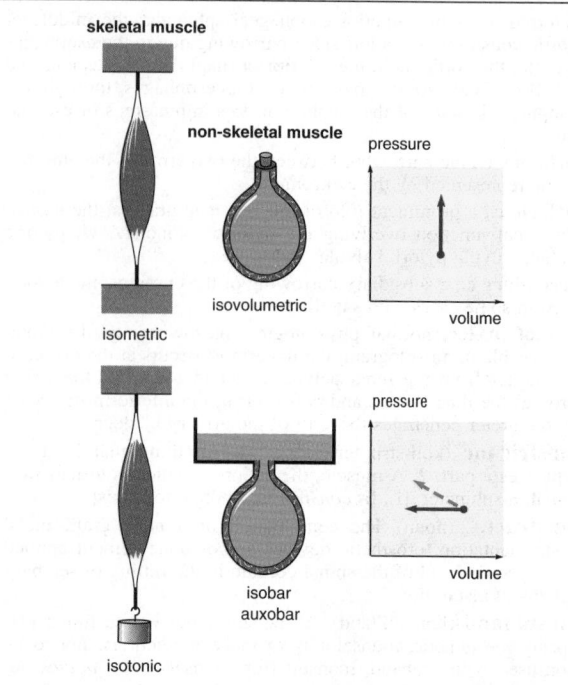

muscle contraction
contraction of skeletal muscle compared with that of nonskeletal muscle (such as heart muscle); during systole, the heart contracts isovolumetrically; during diastole, pressure increases and contraction is correctly designated as "auxobar"

   anodal closure c. (ACC, AnCC), obsolete term for the momentary c. of a muscle under the influence of the positive pole when the electrical circuit is established.

   anodal opening c. (AnOC, AOC), obsolete term for the momentary c. of a muscle under the influence of the positive pole when the circuit is broken.

   automatic c., SYN automatic *beat*.

   Braxton Hicks c., rhythmic myometrial activity occurring during the course of a pregnancy which causes no pain for the patient.

   carpopedal c., SYN carpopedal *spasm*.

   cathodal closure c. (CaCC, CCC), obsolete term for the momentary c. of a muscle under the influence of the negative pole when an electrical circuit is established.

   cathodal opening c. (CaOC, COC), obsolete term for the momentary c. of a muscle under the influence of the negative pole when the circuit is broken.

   closing c., c. produced at the time of closing of the circuit when using direct current to stimulate the muscle.

   escape c., SYN escape *beat*.

   escape ventricular c., an escape beat arising in the ventricle.

   fibrillary c.'s, c.'s occurring spontaneously in individual muscle fibers; they are seen commonly a few days after damage to the motor nerves supplying the muscle, and this type of activity is distinguished from fasciculation, which is related to activation of motor units.

   front-tap c., c. of the calf muscles when the anterior surface of the leg is struck. SYN Gowers' c.

   Gowers' c., SYN front-tap c.

   hourglass c., constriction of the middle portion of a hollow organ, such as the stomach or the gravid uterus.

   hunger c.'s, strong c.'s of the stomach associated with hunger pains.

   idiomuscular c., SYN myoedema.

   isometric c., force development at constant length. Cf. isotonic c.

isotonic c., shortening at constant force development. Cf. isometric c. SYN isotonic exercise.

myotatic c., a reflex c. of a skeletal muscle that occurs as a result of stimulation of the stretch receptors in the muscle, *i.e.,* as part of a myotatic reflex.

opening c., a c. produced at the time of opening the circuit when using direct current to stimulate the muscle or a motor nerve.

paradoxical c., a tonic c. of the anterior tibial muscles when a sudden passive dorsal flexion of the foot is made.

postural c., maintenance of muscular tension (usually isometric) sufficient to maintain posture.

premature c., SEE extrasystole.

reflex detrusor c., normal coordinated function of the bladder with sustained contractions of the bladder matched by simultaneous relaxation of the sphincteric outlet mechanisms to empty the bladder.

tetanic c., SEE tetanus (2).

tonic c., sustained contraction of a muscle, as employed in the maintenance of posture.

uterine c., rhythmic activity of the myometrium associated with menstruation, pregnancy, or labor.

con·trac·ture (kon-trak′chūr). Static muscle shortening due to tonic spasm or fibrosis, or to loss of muscular balance, the antagonists being paralyzed. [L. *contractura,* fr. *con-traho,* to draw together]

Dupuytren's c., a disease of the palmar fascia resulting in thickening and shortening of fibrous bands on the palmar surface of the hand and fingers.

fixed c., SYN organic c.

functional c., muscular shortening that ceases during sleep or general anesthesia, caused by prolonged active muscle contraction.

ischemic c. of the left ventricle, irreversible contraction of the left ventricle of the heart as a complication seen in the early period of cardiopulmonary bypass and now avoided by appropriate cardioplegic solutions. SYN myocardial rigor mortis, stone heart.

organic c., c., usually due to fibrosis within the muscle that persists whether the subject is conscious or unconscious. SYN fixed c.

Volkmann's c., ischemic c. resulting from irreversible necrosis of muscle tissue, produced by a compartment syndrome; classically involves the forearm flexor muscles.

con·tra·fis·sura (kon′tră-fi-shūr′ă). Fracture of a bone, as in the skull, at a point opposite that where the blow was received. [L. *contra,* against, counter, + *fissura,* fissure]

con·tra·in·di·cant (kon-tră-in′di-kant). Indicating the contrary, *i.e.,* showing that a method of treatment that would otherwise be proper is inadvisable by special circumstances in the individual case.

con·tra·in·di·ca·tion (kon-tră-in-di-kā′shun). Any special symptom or circumstance that renders the use of a remedy or the carrying out of a procedure inadvisable, usually because of risk.

con·tra·lat·er·al (kon-tră-lat′er-ăl). Relating to the opposite side, as when pain is felt or paralysis occurs on the side opposite to that of the lesion. SYN heterolateral. [L. *contra,* opposite, + *latus,* side]

c. partner, the corresponding structure on the opposite side.

con·trast (kon′trast). **1.** A comparison in which differences are demonstrated or enhanced. **2.** In radiology, the difference between the image densities of two areas is the c. between them; this is a function of the number of x-ray photons transmitted or the strength of the signals emitted by the two regions and the response of the recording medium. [L. *contra,* against, + *sto,* pp. *status,* to stand]

simultaneous c., the enhancement of the visual sensation of white when a white object is viewed adjacent to a black object; the black object also appears blacker as a result of the contiguity of white. Adjacent complementary colors also appear brighter; *e.g.,* green appears a brighter green and red a brighter red if these two colors are viewed side by side.

successive c., the visual effect caused by viewing a brightly

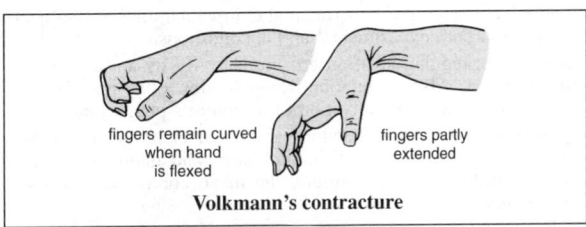

fingers remain curved when hand is flexed   fingers partly extended

Volkmann's contracture

colored object and then a gray surface; the latter appears tinged with the complementary color of the object. Viewing a surface colored in the complementary color of the object rather than in gray enhances the color intensity of the surface.

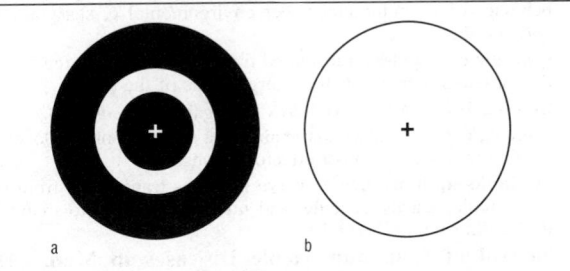

a   *b*

successive contrast

stare at white cross in *a* for about 30 secs. and then look at black cross in *b*; the image of *a* reappearing in the white field of *b* is a successive contrast

con·tra·stim·u·lant (kon-tră-stim′yū-lant). **1.** Annulling the effect of a stimulant. **2.** An agent whose action opposes that of a stimulant.

con·tre·coup (kawn-tr-kū′). Denoting the manner of a contrafissura, as in the skull, at a point opposite that at which the blow was received. SEE ALSO contrecoup *injury* of brain. [Fr. counterblow]

con·trec·ta·tion (kon-trek-tā′shun). **1.** Sexual foreplay prior to coition. **2.** The impulse to caress or embrace one of the opposite sex. [L. *con- trecto,* pp. *-trectatus,* to handle]

cont. rem. Abbreviation for L. *continuenter remedia,* continue the medicines.

con·trol (kon-trōl′). **1.** (v.) To regulate, restrain, correct, restore to normal. **2.** (n. or adj.) Ongoing operations or programs aimed at reducing or eliminating a disease. **3.** (n.) Person(s) in a comparison group that differs in disease experience or allocation to a regimen from the subjects of a study. **4.** (v). In statistics, to adjust or take into account extraneous influences. [Mediev. L. *contrarotulum,* a counterroll for checking accounts, fr. L. *rotula,* dim. of *rota,* a wheel]

autogenous c., regulation by the action of a gene product on the gene that codes for that product.

aversive c., control of the behavior of another individual by use of psychologically noxious means; *e.g.,* attempting to force better study habits by withholding a child's allowance, or withholding sexual contact unless the partner complies with a request.

biological c., c. of living organisms, including vectors and reservoirs of disease, by using their natural enemies (predators, parasites, competitors).

birth c., (1) restriction of the number of offspring by means of contraceptive measures; (2) projects, programs, or methods to control reproduction, by either improving or diminishing fertility.

idiodynamic c., nervous impulses from the medulla that preserve the normal trophic condition of the muscles.

negative c., regulation of an enzyme activity by an inhibitor of that enzyme or regulation of a protein by repression of transcription.

own c.'s, a method of experimental c. in which the same subjects are used in both experimental and c. conditions.

positive c., regulation of an enzyme activity by an activator of that enzyme. Also, regulation via induction of a specific protein's biosynthesis or activation of a protein's processing.

quality c., the c. of laboratory analytical error by monitoring analytical performance with control sera and maintaining error within established limits around the mean control values, most commonly ±2 SD.

reflex c., nerve impulses transmitted to the muscles to maintain normal reflex action.

social c., the influence on the behavior of a person exerted by other persons or by society as a whole; *e.g.,* through appropriate social norms, ostracism, or the criminal law.

stimulus c., the use of conditioning techniques to bring the target behavior of an individual under environmental c. SEE classical *conditioning*.

synergic c., impulses transmitted from the cerebellum regulating the muscular activity of the synergic units of the body.

time-varied gain c. (TGC), SYN time-gain *compensation*.

tonic c., nerve impulses that maintain a normal tonus or level of activity in muscle or other effector organs.

vestibulo-equilibratory c., nerve impulses transmitted from the semicircular canals, saccule, and utricle that serve to maintain the equilibrium of the body.

Con·trol of Com·mun·i·ca·ble Dis·eases in Man. The internationally recognized authoritative manual now in the 15th (1990) edition, published by the American Public Health Association.

con·tu·sion (kon-tū′shŭn). Any mechanical injury (usually caused by a blow) resulting in hemorrhage beneath unbroken skin. SEE ALSO bruise. [L. *contusio,* a bruising]

brain c., a bruising, usually of the surface, of the brain with extravasation of blood but without rupture of the pia-arachnoid; healing results in a superficial depressed sclerotic area, possibly with incorporated meninges. SEE ALSO brain *cicatrix*.

scalp c., intracutaneous or subcutaneous extravasation of blood without gross disruption of skin.

con·u·lar (kon′yū-lăr). Cone-shaped.

Co·nus (kō′nŭs). A genus of shellfish that inhabits the shores of some South Pacific islands. Several species, *C. geographus, C. textilis, C. aulicus, C. tulipa,* and *C. marmoreus* are poisonous, their sting or spine causing acute pain, edema, numbness, spreading paralysis, and sometimes coma and death.

co·nus, pl. **co·ni** (kō′nŭs, -nī). **1** [NA]. SYN cone. **2.** Posterior staphyloma in myopic choroidopathy. [L. fr. G. *kōnos,* cone]

c. arterio′sus [NA], the left or anterosuperior, smooth-walled portion of the cavity of the right ventricle of the heart, which begins at the supraventricular crest and terminates in the pulmonary trunk. SYN arterial cone, pulmonary cone, pulmonary c.

congenital c., SYN Fuchs' *coloboma*.

distraction c., a c. in which the optic nerve passes through the scleral canal in a markedly oblique direction.

c. elas′ticus [NA], **(1)** thicker lower portion of the elastic membrane of the larynx, extending between the cricoid cartilage and the vocal ligaments, the latter actually being a thickening of the free, superior margin of the c. elasticus; SYN cricovocal membrane, elastic cone. **(2)** SYN cricothyroid *ligament*.

co′ni epididym′idis [NA], ⋆official alternate term for *lobules* of epididymis, under *lobule*, *lobules* of epididymis, under *lobule*.

c. medulla′ris [NA], SYN medullary *cone*.

myopic c., SYN myopic *crescent*.

pulmonary c., SYN c. arteriosus.

supertraction c., a reddish yellow c. or ring at the nasal margin of the optic disk, produced by displacement of the retinal pigment epithelium and lamina vitrea of the choroid; occurs in high myopia.

co′ni vasculo′si, SYN *lobules* of epididymis, under *lobule*.

con·va·les·cence (kon-vă-les′ens). A period between the end of a disease and the patient's restoration to complete health. [L. *con-valesco,* to grow strong, fr. *valeo,* to be strong]

con·va·les·cent (kon-vă-les′ent). **1.** Getting well or one who is getting well. **2.** Denoting the period of convalescence.

con·val·lar·ia (kon-va-lăr′ē-ă). The flower, rhizome, and roots of *Convallaria majalis* (family Liliaceae), lily of the valley; they contain glycosides with digitalis-like action (*e.g.,* convallatoxin). [L. *convallis,* an enclosed valley]

con·vec·tion (kon-vek′shŭn). Conveyance of heat in liquids or gases by movement of the heated particles, as when the layer of water at the bottom of a heated pot rises or the warm air of a room ascends to the ceiling. [L. *con-veho,* pp. *-vectus,* to carry or bring together]

con·ver·gence (kon-ver′jens). **1.** The tending of two or more objects toward a common point. **2.** The direction of the visual lines to a near point. [L. *con-vergere,* to incline together]

accommodative c., the meter angle of c. expressed in diopters; equal to the product of the meter angles of c. times the interpupillary distance measured in centimeters.

amplitude of c., the distance between the near point and far point of c. SYN range of c.

angle of c., the angle that the visual axis makes with the median line when a near object is viewed.

far point of c., the point to which the visual lines are directed when c. is at rest.

near point of c., the point to which the visual lines are directed when c. is at its maximum.

negative c., the slight divergence of the visual axes when c. is at rest, as when observing the far point or during sleep.

positive c., inward deviation of the visual axes even when c. is at rest, as in cases of convergent squint.

range of c., SYN amplitude of c.

unit of c., SEE meter *angle*.

con·ver·gent (kon-ver′jent). Tending toward a common point.

con·ver·sion (kon-ver′zhŭn). **1.** SYN transmutation. **2.** An unconscious defense mechanism by which the anxiety which stems from an unconscious conflict is converted and expressed symbolically as a physical symptom; transformation of an emotion into a physical manifestation, as in c. hysteria. SEE conversion *hysteria*. **3.** In virology, the acquisition by bacteria of a new property associated with presence of a prophage. SEE ALSO lysogeny. [L. *con-verto,* pp. *-versus,* to turn around, to change]

con·ver·tase (kon′ver-tās). Proteases of complement that convert one component into another. SEE *component* of complement.

con·ver·tin (kon-ver′tin). Active form of factor VII designated VIIa.

con·vex (kon′veks, kŏn-veks′). Applied to a surface that is evenly curved outward, the segment of a sphere. [L. *convexus,* vaulted, arched, convex, fr. *con-veho,* to bring together]

high c., the segment of a sphere of short radius.

low c., the segment of a sphere of long radius.

con·vex·i·ty (kon-veks′i-tē). **1.** The state of being convex. **2.** A convex structure.

cortical c., SYN superolateral *surface* of cerebrum.

con·vex·o·ba·sia (kon-vek-sō-bā′sē-ă). Forward bending of the occipital bone. [L. *convexus,* outwardly curved, + *basis,* foundation]

con·vex·o·con·cave (kon-vek′sō-kon′kāv). Convex on one surface and concave on the opposite surface.

con·vex·o·con·vex (kon-vek′sō-kon′veks). SYN biconvex.

con·vo·lute (kon′vō-lūt). Rolled together with one part over the other; in the shape of a roll or scroll. SYN convoluted. [L. *con-volvo,* pp. *-volutus,* to roll together]

con·vo·lut·ed (kon′vō-lū-ted). SYN convolute.

con·vo·lu·tion (kon-vō-lū′shŭn). **1.** A coiling or rolling of an organ. **2.** Specifically, a gyrus of the cerebral or cerebellar cortex. [L. *convolutio*]

angular c., SYN angular *gyrus*.

anterior central c., SYN precentral *gyrus*.

ascending frontal c., SYN precentral *gyrus*.

ascending parietal c., SYN postcentral *gyrus*.

callosal c., SYN cingulate *gyrus*.

cingulate c., SYN cingulate *gyrus*.

first temporal c., SYN superior temporal *gyrus.*

hippocampal c., SYN parahippocampal *gyrus.*

inferior frontal c., SYN inferior frontal *gyrus.*

inferior temporal c., SYN inferior temporal *gyrus.*

middle frontal c., SYN middle frontal *gyrus.*

middle temporal c., SYN middle temporal *gyrus.*

posterior central c., SYN postcentral *gyrus.*

second temporal c., SYN middle temporal *gyrus.*

superior frontal c., SYN superior frontal *gyrus.*

superior temporal c., SYN superior temporal *gyrus.*

supramarginal c., SYN supramarginal *gyrus.*

third temporal c., SYN inferior temporal *gyrus.*

transitional c., SYN transitional *gyrus.*

transverse temporal c.'s, SYN transverse temporal *gyri,* under *gyrus.*

Zuckerkandl's c., SYN subcallosal *gyrus.*

con·vul·sant (kon-vŭl′sant). A substance that produces convulsions. SEE ALSO eclamptogenic, epileptogenic.

con·vul·sion (kon-vŭl′shŭn). **1.** A violent spasm or series of jerkings of the face, trunk, or extremities. **2.** SYN seizure (2). [L. *convulsio,* fr. *con-vello,* pp. *-vulsus,* to tear up]

benign neonatal c.'s, a familial, self-limited epilepsy, beginning at two or three days of age and resolving spontaneously by six months of age; autosomal dominant inheritance.

clonic c., a c. in which the contractions are intermittent, the muscles alternately contracting and relaxing.

complex febrile c., a febrile c. that is prolonged (greater than 15 minutes' duration) or is associated with focal neurological deficits.

coordinate c., a clonic c. in which the movements are seemingly purposeful, being exaggerations of those that may occur naturally.

ether c., a c. occasionally associated with divinyl and diethyl ether anesthesia.

febrile c., a brief seizure, lasting less than 15 minutes, seen in a neurologically normal infant or young child, associated with fever. SYN febrile seizure.

hysterical c., hysteroid c., SEE hysteria.

immediate posttraumatic c., a c. beginning very soon after injury.

infantile c., any c. occurring in infancy (0 to 2 years of age).

mimic c., SYN facial *tic.*

puerperal c.'s, SYN puerperal *eclampsia.*

salaam c.'s, SYN infantile *spasm.*

tetanic c., SYN tonic c.

tonic c., a c. in which muscle contraction is sustained. SYN tetanic c.

con·vul·sive (kon-vŭl′siv). Relating to convulsions; marked by or producing convulsions.

Cooke, A. Bennett, U.S. physician, *1869. SEE C.'s *speculum.*

Cooley, Thomas B., U.S. pediatrician, 1871–1945. SEE C.'s *anemia.*

Coolidge, William D., U.S. physicist, 1873–1974. SEE C. *tube.*

Coomassie bril·liant blue R-250 [C.I. 42660]. A general protein stain used in electrophoresis because of its unusual sensitivity. [originally, a proprietary name of Imperial Chemical; Coomassie (Kumasi), Ghana]

Coombs, Carey F., English physician, 1879–1932. SEE C. *murmur.*

Coombs, Robin R.A., English veterinarian and immunologist, *1921. SEE Gell and C. *reactions,* under *reaction;* C.'s *serum, test;* direct C. *test;* indirect C. *test.*

Cooper, Sir Astley Paston, English anatomist and surgeon, 1768–1841. SEE C.'s *fascia, hernia, herniotome, ligaments,* under *ligament;* suspensory *ligaments* of C., under *ligament.*

co·op·er·a·tiv·i·ty. A property of certain proteins (often enzymes) in which the bind curves or saturation curves or, in the case of enzyme, a plot of initial rates as a function of initial substrate concentration, are nonhyperbolic; suggests that the binding of a ligand has a different affinity at different ligand concentrations. Both allosterism and hysteresis are models that will display c. Cf. allosterism, hysteresis.

negative c., c. in which successive ligand molecules appear to bind with decreasing affinity.

positive c., c. in which successive ligand molecules appear to bind with increasing affinity.

Coo·pe·ria (kū-pē′rē-ă). A genus of small, slender nematodes (family Trichostrongylidae) inhabiting the small intestine, rarely the abomasum, of ruminants; when fresh they are a bright pink color; they produce serious effects only when present in large numbers. In partly immune animals, these worms become enclosed in nodules in the wall of the intestine; they are less pathogenic in sheep and goats than the trichostrongyles *Haemonchus, Ostertagia,* and *Trichostrongylus.*

C. biso′nis, species that occurs in cattle, sheep, bison, and pronghorn antelopes.

C. curti′cei, species that occurs in sheep, goats, and wild deer in Europe, although cosmopolitan in distribution.

C. fiel′dingi, SYN *C. punctata.*

C. oncoph′ora, species that occurs in cattle and domestic and wild sheep, but rarely in the horse; although worldwide in distribution, it is most common in the northern U.S. and Canada. SYN *Strongylus radiatus, Strongylus ventricosus.*

C. pectina′ta, species that occurs in cattle, sheep, water buffalo, dromedary camels, and various wild ruminants; it is common in the southern U.S.

C. puncta′ta, species that occurs mainly in cattle, less commonly in sheep, water buffalo, and several wild ruminants; although worldwide in distribution, it is especially widespread in North America and common in Hawaii. SYN *C. fieldingi.*

C. spatula′ta, a species that occurs in cattle and sheep in the southern U.S., Kenya, Australia, and Malaysia.

Coopernail, George P., U.S. surgeon, *1876. SEE C.'s *sign.*

co·or·di·nate. 1 (kō-ōr′di-nit). Any of the scales or magnitudes that serve to define the position of a point. **2** (kō-ōr′di-nāt). To perform the act of coordination. [see coordination]

co·or·di·na·tion (kō-ōr′di-nā′shun). The harmonious working together, especially of several muscles or muscle groups in the execution of complicated movements. [L. *co-,* together, + *ordino,* pp. *-atus,* to arrange, fr. *ordo* (*ordin-*), arrangement, order]

co·os·si·fi·ca·tion (kō-os′i-fi-kā′shŭn). State of being joined by bone formation.

co·os·si·fy (kō-os′i-fī). To unite into one bone. [L. *co-,* together, + *os,* bone, + *facio,* to make]

co·pai·ba (kō-pī′bă). The oleoresin of *Copaifera officinalis* and other species of *Copaifera* (family Leguminosae), a South American plant; c. oil is used as an expectorant, diuretic, and stimulant. SYN balsam of copaiba. [Sp.]

co·par·af·fi·nate (kō-par′af-i-nāt). A mixture of water-insoluble isoparaffinic acids partially neutralized with isooctyl hydroxybenzyldialkyl amines; used as an antifungal agent for external application.

COPD Abbreviation for chronic obstructive pulmonary *disease.*

Cope, Sir Vincent Z., English surgeon, 1881–1974. SEE C.'s *clamp.*

cope (kōp). **1.** The upper half of a flask in the casting art; hence applicable to the upper or cavity side of a denture flask. **2.** An act that enables one to adjust to the environmental circumstances.

co·pe·pod (kō′pē-pod). Any member of the order Copepoda.

Co·pep·o·da (kō-pep′ō-dă). An order of abundant, free-living, freshwater and marine crustaceans of basic importance in the aquatic food chain in both the marine and freshwater environments; some species are commonly called water fleas. Some are ectoparasites of both cold-blooded and warm-blooded aquatic vertebrates; the parasitic copepods of fish and whales are often highly modified for deep penetration of the skin or for adherence by suckers and hooks (*e.g.,* the fish lice, *Argulus*). Certain copepods (*Cyclops, Diaptomus*) are important as intermediate hosts of the tapeworm *Diphyllobothrium latum* and of the nematode *Dracunculus medinensis.* [G. *kōpē,* an oar, + *pous* (*pod-*), a foot]

cop·ing (kōp′ing). **1.** A thin metal covering or cap. **2.** An adaptive or otherwise successful method of dealing with individual or environmental situations that involve psychologic or physiologic stress or threat.

transfer c., in dentistry, a metallic, acrylic resin or other covering or cap used to position a die in an impression.

co·pol·y·mer (kō'pol-i-mer). A polymer in which two or more monomers or base units are combined.

cop·per (Cu) (kop'er). A metallic element, atomic no. 29, atomic wt. 63.546; several of its salts are used in medicine. A bioelement found in a number of proteins. [L. *cuprum*, orig. *Cyprium*, *Cyprus*, where it was mined]

c. arsenite, SYN cupric arsenite.

c. bichloride, SYN cupric chloride.

c. chloride, SYN cupric chloride.

c. citrate, SYN cupric citrate.

c. dichloride, SYN cupric chloride.

c. sulfate, c. sulphate, SYN cupric sulfate.

cop·per-64 (^{64}Cu). Beta and positron emitter with a half-life of 12.82 hr. Used in the study of Wilson's disease and in brain scans for tumors.

cop·per-67 (^{67}Cu). Beta and gamma emitter with a half-life of 2.580 days.

cop·per·as (kop'er-as). The impure commercial variety of ferrous sulfate.

cop·per·head (kop'er-hed). A poisonous snake of the genus *Denisonia* in Australia and *Agkistrodon* in the U.S.

cop·per pen·nies. SYN sclerotic *bodies,* under *body.*

Coppet, Louis de, French physicist, 1841–1911. SEE C.'s *law.*

co·pre·cip·i·ta·tion (kō'prē-sip-i-tā'shŭn). Precipitation of unbound antigen along with an antigen-antibody complex; may occur particularly when a soluble complex is precipitated by a second antibody specific for the Fc fragment of the immunoglobulin of the complex.

cop·rem·e·sis (kop-rem'ē-sis). SYN fecal *vomiting.* [G. *kopros,* dung, + emesis]

copro-. Filth, dung, usually used in referring to feces. SEE ALSO scato-, sterco-. [G. *kopros,* dung]

cop·ro·an·ti·bod·ies (kop'rō-an'ti-bod-ēz). Antibodies found in the intestine and in feces; they probably are formed by plasma cells in the intestinal mucosa and consist chiefly of the IgA class.

cop·ro·lag·nia (kop-rō-lag'nē-ă). A form of sexual perversion in which the thought or sight of excrement causes pleasurable sensation. [copro- + G. *lagneia,* lust]

cop·ro·la·lia (kop-rō-lā'lē-ă). Involuntary utterances of vulgar or obscene words; seen in Gilles de la Tourette's syndrome. SYN coprophrasia. [copro- + G. *lalia,* talk]

cop·ro·lith (kop'rō-lith). A hard mass consisting of inspissated feces. SYN fecalith, stercolith. [copro- + G. *lithos,* stone]

co·prol·o·gy (kop-rol'ō-jē). SYN scatology (1). [copro- + G. *logos,* study]

cop·ro·ma (kop-rō'mă). An accumulation of inspissated feces in the colon or rectum giving the appearance of an abdominal tumor. SYN fecal tumor, fecaloma, scatoma, stercoroma. [copro- + G. *-ōma,* tumor]

cop·ro·pha·gia. The eating of excrement. SYN coprophagy, rhypophagy, scatophagy.

co·proph·a·gous (kō-prof'ă-gŭs). Feeding on excrement.

co·proph·a·gy (kŏ-prof'ă-jē). SYN coprophagia. [copro- + G. *phagō,* to eat]

cop·ro·phil, cop·ro·phil·ic (kop'rō-fil, -fil'ik). **1.** Denoting microorganisms occurring in fecal matter. **2.** Relating to coprophilia. [see coprophilia]

cop·ro·phile (kop'rō-fīl). An organism that ingests fecal material from others organisms.

cop·ro·phil·ia (kop-rō-fil'ē-ă). **1.** Attraction of microorganisms to fecal matter. **2.** In psychiatry, a morbid attraction to, and interest in (with a sexual element), fecal matter. [copro- + G. *philos,* fond]

cop·ro·pho·bia (kop-rō-fō'bē-ă). Morbid fear of defecation and feces. [copro- + G. *phobos,* fear]

cop·ro·phra·sia (kop-rō-frā'zē-ă). SYN coprolalia.

cop·ro·plan·e·sia (kop-rō-plan-ē'zē-ă). Rarely used term for passage of feces through a fistula or artificial anus. [copro- + G. *planēsis,* a wandering]

cop·ro·por·phyr·ia (kop'rō-pōr-fir'ē-ă). Presence of coproporphyrins in the urine, as in variegate porphyria.

hereditary c., an inherited (autosomal dominant) disorder of a deficiency of coproporphyrinogen oxidase, resulting in overproduction of porphyrin precursors leading to neurological disturbances and photosensitivity.

cop·ro·por·phy·rin (kop-rō-pōr'fi-rin). One of two porphyrin compounds found normally in feces as a decomposition product of bilirubin (hence, from hemoglobin); certain c.'s are elevated in certain porphyrias. SEE ALSO porphyrinogens.

cop·ro·por·phy·rin·o·gen (kop'rō-pōr-fi-rin'ō-jen). SEE porphyrinogens.

c. oxidase, an enzyme that catalyzes a step in porphyrin biosynthesis, reacting coproporphyrinogen-III and O_2 to form protoporphyrinogen-IX and $2CO_2$. A deficiency of this enzyme will result in hereditary coproporphyria.

cop·ro·stane (kop-ros'tān). The parent hydrocarbon of coprosterol.

3β-co·pros·ta·nol (kop-ros'tan-ol). SYN coprosterol.

*epi-*co·pros·ta·nol. 5β-Cholestan-3α-ol. For structure of cholestane, see steroids. SYN *epi*-coprosterol.

cop·ros·tan·one (kop-ros'tan-ōn). 5β-Cholestan-3-one, an oxidation product of coprosterol.

cop·ro·sta·sis (kop-rō-stā'sis). Rarely used term for fecal impaction. [copro- + G. *stasis,* a standing]

cop·ros·ten·ol (kop-ros'ten-ol). SYN allocholesterol.

cop·ros·ter·in (kop-ros'ter-in). SYN coprosterol.

co·pros·ter·ol (kop-ros'ter-ol). 5β-cholastan-3β-ol; the main sterol of the feces produced by the reduction of cholesterol by intestinal bacteria. For structure of coprostane and cholestane, see steroids. SYN 3β-coprostanol, coprosterin, stercorin.

*epi-*co·pros·ter·ol. SYN *epi*-coprostanol.

cop·ro·stig·mas·tane (kop-rō-stig-mas'tān). The 5β isomer of stigmastane.

cop·ro·zoa (kop-rō-zō'ă). Protozoa that can be cultivated in fecal matter, although not necessarily living in feces within the intestine. [copro- + G. *zōon,* animal]

cop·ro·zo·ic (kop-rō-zō'ik). Relating to coprozoa.

cop·to·sis (kop-tō'sis). A state of perpetual fatigue. [G. *kopto,* to tire, + *osis,* condition]

cop·u·la (kop'yū-lă). **1.** In anatomy, a narrow part connecting two structures, *e.g.,* the body of the hyoid bone. **2.** A swelling that is formed during the early development of the tongue by the medial portion of the second branchial arch; it is overgrown by the hypobranchial eminence and is not present in the adult tongue. **3.** Obsolete term for zygote. [L. a bond, tie]

His' c., SYN hypobranchial *eminence.*

c. lin'guae, SYN hypobranchial *eminence.*

cop·u·la·tion (kop-yū-lā'shŭn). **1.** SYN coitus. **2.** In protozoology, conjugation between two cells that do not fuse but separate after mutual fertilization; observed in the ciliophora, as in *Paramecium.* [L. *copulatio,* a joining]

CoQ Abbreviation for coenzyme Q.

co·quille (kō-kēl'). A spherical curved lens of uniform thickness. [Fr.]

cor, gen. **cor·dis** (kōr, kōr'dis) [NA]. SYN heart. [L.]

c. adipo'sum, SYN fatty *heart* (2).

c. bilocula're, a heart in which the interatrial and interventricular septa are absent or incomplete.

c. bovi'num (kōr bō'vī-nŭm), SYN ox *heart.*

c. mo'bile, a heart that moves unduly on change of bodily position. SYN movable heart.

c. pen'dulum, an extreme form of c. mobile in which the heart appears to be suspended by the great vessels. SYN pendulous heart.

c. pulmona'le, chronic c. is characterized by hypertrophy of the right ventricle resulting from disease of the lungs, except for lung changes in diseases that primarily affect the left side of the heart and excluding congenital heart disease; acute c. p. is characterized by dilation and failure of the right side of the heart due to pulmonary embolism. In both types, characteristic electrocardiogram changes occur, and in later stages there is usually right-sided cardiac failure.

c. triatria′tum, a heart with three atrial chambers, the left atrium being subdivided by a transverse septum with a single small opening which separates the openings of the pulmonary veins from the mitral valve. SYN accessory atrium.

c. trilocula′re, three-chambered heart due to absence of the interatrial or the interventricular septum.

c. trilocula′re biatria′tum, absence of the interventricular septum.

c. trilocula′re biventriculare, absence of the interatrial septum.

cor·a·cid·i·um (kō-ră-sid′ē-ŭm). The ciliated first-stage aquatic embryo of pseudophyllid and other cestodes with aquatic cycles; within the ciliated embryophore is a hooked larva, the hexacanth, that develops in the intermediate host, usually an aquatic crustacean, into the next larval stage, the procercoid.

cor·a·co·a·cro·mi·al (kōr′ă-kō-ă-krō′mē-ăl). Relating to the coracoid and acromial processes. SYN acromiocoracoid.

cor·a·co·bra·chi·a·lis (kōr′ă-kō-brā-kē-ā′lis). Relating to the coracoid process of the scapula and the arm. SEE ALSO coracobrachialis *muscle,* coracobrachial *bursa.*

cor·a·co·cla·vic·u·lar (kōr′ă-kō-kla-vik′yū-lăr). Relating to the coracoid process and the clavicle. SYN scapuloclavicular (2).

cor·a·co·hu·mer·al (kōr′ă-kō-hyū′mer-ăl). Relating to the coracoid process and the humerus.

cor·a·coid (kōr′ă-koyd). Shaped like a crow's beak; denoting a process of the scapula. [G. *korakōdēs,* like a crow's beak, fr. *korax,* raven, + *eidos,* appearance]

cor·al·lin (kōr′ă-lin). SYN aurin.

yellow c., a sodium salt of aurin.

cord (kōrd). **1.** In anatomy, any long ropelike structure. A small, cordlike structure composed of several to many longitudinally oriented fibers, vessels, ducts, or combinations thereof. SEE ALSO chorda. **2.** In histopathology, a line of tumor cells only one cell in width. SYN funiculus [NA], funicle. [L. *chorda,* a string]

Bergmann's c.'s, SYN medullary *striae* of fourth ventricle, under *stria.*

Billroth's c.'s, SYN splenic c.'s.

condyle c., SYN condylar *axis.*

dental c., an aggregation of epithelial cells forming the rudimentary enamel organ.

false vocal c., SYN vestibular *fold.*

Ferrein's c.'s, SEE vocal *fold.*

gangliated c., SYN sympathetic *trunk.*

genital c., one of a pair of mesenchymal ridges bulging into the caudal part of the celom of a young embryo and containing the mesonephric and paramesonephric duct.

germinal c.'s, the gonadal c.'s of the embryonic ovary or testis. SYN sex c.'s.

gonadal c.'s, columns of germinal and follicle cells penetrating centripetally into the embryonic ovarian or testicular cortex.

gubernacular c., the content of the gubernacular canal, usually composed of remnants of dental lamina and connective tissue.

hepatic c.'s, liver laminae as seen in sections.

lateral c. of brachial plexus, in the brachial plexus, the bundle of nerve fibers formed by the anterior divisions of the superior and middle trunks which is located lateral to the axillary artery. This cord gives off the lateral pectoral nerve and terminates by dividing into the musculocutaneous nerve and the lateral root of the median nerve. SYN fasciculus lateralis plexus brachialis [NA].

lymph c.'s, SYN medullary c.'s (1).

medial c. of brachial plexus, in the brachial plexus, the bundle of nerve fibers formed by the anterior division of the inferior trunk which lies medial to the axillary artery; it gives off the medial pectoral nerve, the medial brachial cutaneous, and medial antebrachial cutaneous, nerves and end by dividing into the medial root of the median nerves and the ulnar nerve. SYN fasciculus medialis plexus brachialis [NA].

medullary c.'s, (1) c.'s of dense lymphoid tissue between the sinuses in the medulla of a lymph node; SYN lymph c.'s. **(2)** SYN rete c.'s.

nephrogenic c., a longitudinal dorsolateral tract of mesoderm derived from intermediate mesoderm; the primordium for both mesonephric and metanephric tubules.

oblique c., SYN oblique *ligament* of elbow joint.

omphalomesenteric c., SYN vitelline c.

posterior c. of brachial plexus, in the brachial plexus, the bundle of nerve fibers formed by the posterior divisions of the upper, middle and lower trunks which lies posterior to the axillary artery; it gives rise to the upper and lower subscapular and thoracodorsal nerves, terminates by dividing into the axillary, and radial nerves. SYN fasciculus posterior plexus brachialis [NA].

psalterial c., SYN *stria* vascularis of cochlea.

red pulp c.'s, SYN splenic c.'s.

rete c.'s, primordial cell c.'s (medullary c.'s and sex c.'s) in the embryonic gonads that connect with some of the mesonephric tubules and from which the rete testis of the male and the rete ovarii of the female develop. SYN medullary c.'s (2).

sex c.'s, SYN germinal c.'s.

spermatic c., the cord formed by the ductus deferens and its associated structures extending from the deep inguinal ring through the inguinal canal into the scrotum. SEE ALSO *coverings* of spermatic cord, under *covering.* SYN funiculus spermaticus [NA], chorda spermatica, testicular c., torsion testis.

spinal c., the elongated cylindrical portion of the cerebrospinal axis, or central nervous system, which is contained in the spinal or vertebral canal. SYN medulla spinalis [NA], chorda spinalis, spinal marrow.

splenic c.'s, the tissue occurring between the venous sinuses in the spleen. SYN Billroth's c.'s, red pulp c.'s.

tendinous c.'s, SYN *chordae* tendineae, under *chorda.*

testicular c., SYN spermatic c.

testis c.'s, the germinal c.'s of the embryonic testis.

true vocal c., SYN vocal *fold.*

c. of tympanum, SYN *chorda* tympani.

umbilical c., the definitive connecting stalk between the embryo or fetus and the placenta; at birth it is primarily composed of Wharton's jelly in which the umbilical vessels are embedded. SYN funiculus umbilicalis [NA], chorda umbilicalis, funis (1).

vitelline c., a persistent yolk stalk in the form of a solid cord of tissue connecting ileum to umbilicus. SYN omphalomesenteric c.

vocal c., SYN vocal *fold.*

Weitbrecht's c., SYN oblique *ligament* of elbow joint.

Wilde's c.'s, transverse markings on the corpus callosum.

Willis' c.'s, several fibrous c.'s crossing the superior sagittal sinus. SYN chordae willisii.

⌂ **cord-.** SEE chord-.

cor·date (kōr′dāt). Heart-shaped.

cor·dec·to·my (kōr-dek′tō-mē). Excision of a part or whole of a cord. [G. *chordē,* cord, + *ektomē,* excision]

cor·dial (kōr′jŭl). A sweet aromatic liquor. [Mediev. L. *cordialis,* fr. *cor* (cord-), heart]

cor·di·a·nine (kor-dī′ă-nēn). SYN allantoin.

cor·di·form (kōr′di-fōrm). Heart-shaped. [L. *cor* (cord-), heart, + *forma,* shape]

cor·dis (kōr′dis). Of the heart. [gen. of L. *cor,* heart]

diastasis c. (dī-as′tă-sis), any period of mechanical inactivity of the heart and particularly of the ventricles, usually appearing normally during slow heart rates when the ventricles complete their filling early and appear to be inactive.

cor·do·cen·te·sis (cor-dō-cen-tē′sis). Transabdominal blood sampling of the fetal umbilical cord, performed under ultrasound guidance. SYN funipuncture. [cord + G. *kentēsis,* puncture]

cor·don san·i·taire (kor-don′ san-i-tayr′). The barrier erected around a focus of infection. [Fr., sanitary barrier]

cor·do·pexy (kōr′dō-pek-sē). **1.** Operative fixation of any displaced anatomical cord. **2.** Lateral fixation of one or both vocal

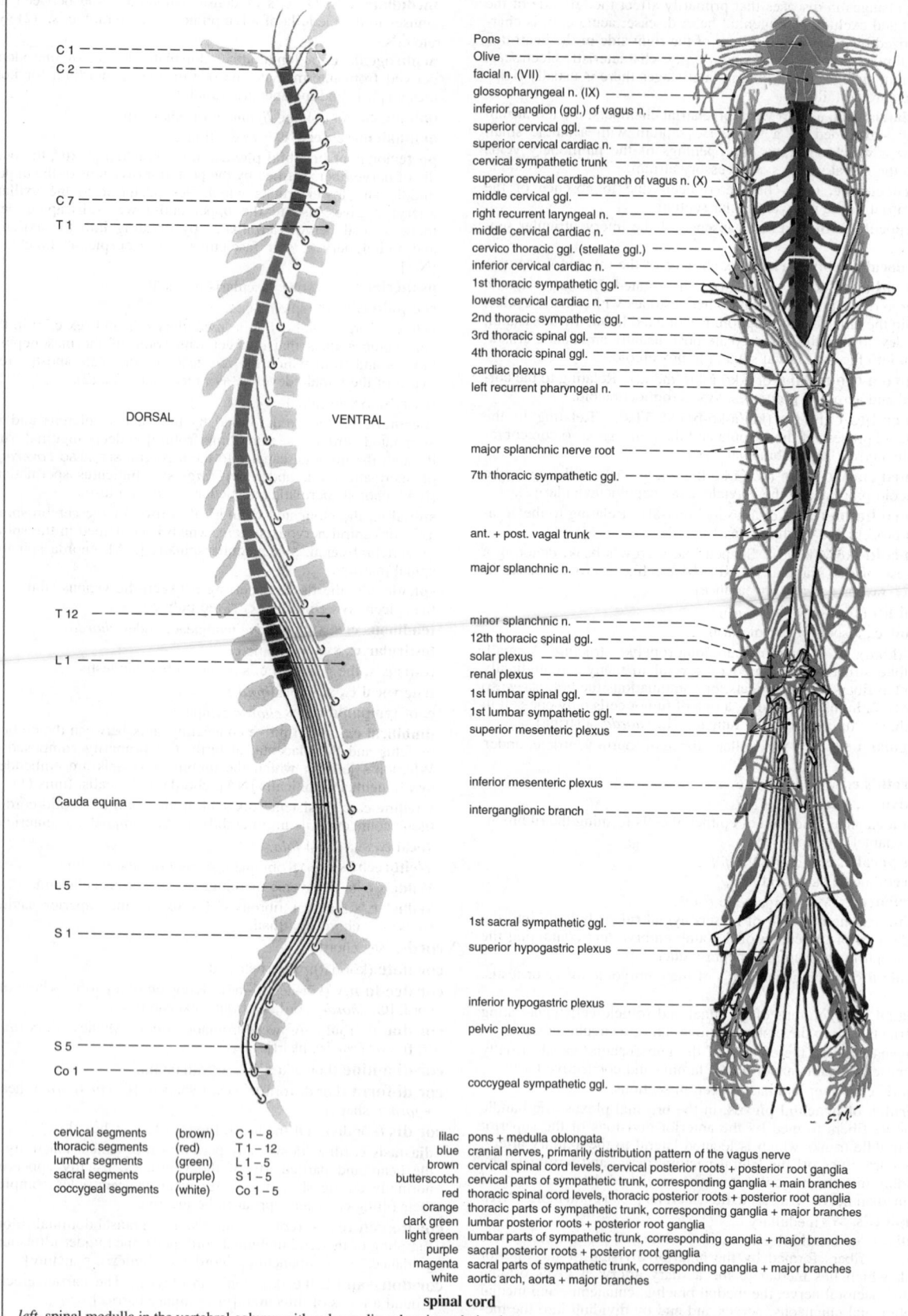

C 1
C 2
C 7
T 1
DORSAL
VENTRAL
T 12
L 1
Cauda equina
L 5
S 1
S 5
Co 1

Pons
Olive
facial n. (VII)
glossopharyngeal n. (IX)
inferior ganglion (ggl.) of vagus n.
superior cervical ggl.
superior cervical cardiac n.
cervical sympathetic trunk
superior cervical cardiac branch of vagus n. (X)
middle cervical ggl.
right recurrent laryngeal n.
middle cervical cardiac n.
cervico thoracic ggl. (stellate ggl.)
inferior cervical cardiac n.
1st thoracic sympathetic ggl.
lowest cervical cardiac n.
2nd thoracic sympathetic ggl.
3rd thoracic spinal ggl.
4th thoracic spinal ggl.
cardiac plexus
left recurrent pharyngeal n.

major splanchnic nerve root
7th thoracic sympathetic ggl.

ant. + post. vagal trunk

major splanchnic n.

minor splanchnic n.
12th thoracic spinal ggl.
solar plexus
renal plexus
1st lumbar spinal ggl.
1st lumbar sympathetic ggl.
superior mesenteric plexus

inferior mesenteric plexus
interganglionic branch

1st sacral sympathetic ggl.
superior hypogastric plexus

inferior hypogastric plexus
pelvic plexus

coccygeal sympathetic ggl.

cervical segments	(brown)	C 1 – 8		
thoracic segments	(red)	T 1 – 12	lilac	pons + medulla oblongata
lumbar segments	(green)	L 1 – 5	blue	cranial nerves, primarily distribution pattern of the vagus nerve
sacral segments	(purple)	S 1 – 5	brown	cervical spinal cord levels, cervical posterior roots + posterior root ganglia
coccygeal segments	(white)	Co 1 – 5	butterscotch	cervical parts of sympathetic trunk, corresponding ganglia + main branches
			red	thoracic spinal cord levels, thoracic posterior roots + posterior root ganglia
			orange	thoracic parts of sympathetic trunk, corresponding ganglia + major branches
			dark green	lumbar posterior roots + posterior root ganglia
			light green	lumbar parts of sympathetic trunk, corresponding ganglia + major branches
			purple	sacral posterior roots + posterior root ganglia
			magenta	sacral parts of sympathetic trunk, corresponding ganglia + major branches
			white	aortic arch, aorta + major branches

spinal cord

left, spinal medulla in the vertebral column with color coding showing relation between neural segments and vertebrae; *right*, color coding shows relation of sympathetic trunk to spinal nerves and branches cords to correct glottic stenosis. [G. *chordē*, cord, + *pēxis*, fixation]

cor·dot·o·my (kŏr-dot'ō-mē). **1.** Any operation on the spinal cord. **2.** Division of tracts of the spinal cord, which may be performed percutaneously (stereotactic c.) or after laminectomy (open c.) by various techniques such as incision or radio frequency coagulation. **3.** Incision through the membranous vocal fold to widen the posterior glottis in bilateral vocal paralysis. SYN chordotomy. [G. *chordē*, cord, + *tomē*, a cutting]

anterolateral c., division of the anterolateral quadrant of the spinal cord to section the spinothalamic tract. SYN anterolateral tractotomy, spinal tractotomy, spinothalamic c.

open c., SEE cordotomy (2).

posterior column c., division of the posterior column of the spinal cord.

spinothalamic c., SYN anterolateral c.

stereotactic c., SEE cordotomy (2).

Cor·dy·lo·bia (kŏr-di-lō'bē-ă). A genus of calliphorid fleshflies. [G. *kordylē*, a cudgel, swelling, or tumor]

C. anthropoph'aga, tumbu fly of Africa south of the Sahara; a species that causes a boil-like furuncular myiasis; many animals besides man are attacked, especially domestic dogs, though rats are probably the chief reservoir of human infection.

cor·dy·lo·bi·a·sis (kŏr-di-lō-bī'ă-sis). Infection of man and animals with larvae of flies of the genus *Cordylobia*. SYN African furuncular myiasis, tumbu dermal myiasis.

core (kŏr). **1.** The central mass of necrotic tissue in a boil. **2.** A metal casting, usually with a post in the canal of a tooth root, designed to retain an artificial crown. **3.** A sectional record, usually of plaster of Paris or one of its derivatives, of the relationships of parts, such as teeth, metallic restorations, or copings. [L. *cor,* heart]

atomic c., the nucleus plus the nonvalence electrons.

central transactional c., the reticular activating system of the brain.

⌂**core-, coreo-, coro-.** The pupil (of the eye). [G. *korē*, pupil]

cor·ec·to·pia (kŏr-ek-tō'pē-ă). Eccentric location of the pupil so that it is not in the center of the iris. [G. *korē*, pupil, + *ektopos*, out of place]

co·rel·y·sis (kō-rē-lī'sis). A rarely used term for freeing of adhesions between lens capsule and the iris. [G. *korē*, pupil, + *lysis*, a loosening]

co·re·mi·um (kō-rē'mē-ŭm). A sheaf-like tuft of conidiophores. [G. *korēma*, filth, refuse]

⌂**coreo-.** SEE core-.

cor·e·o·plas·ty (kŏr'ē-ō-plas-tē). The procedure to correct a misshapen, miotic, or occluded pupil. [G. *korē*, pupil, + *plassō*, to form]

cor·e·pexy. A suturing of the iris to modify the shape or size of the pupil.

purse-string c., a "pajama-string suture" threaded along the pupillary margin and tied down to make a large pupil small.

cor·e·praxy (kŏr-e-prak'sē). A procedure designed to widen a small pupil. [G. *korē*, pupil, + *praxis*, action]

laser c., the iris stroma is heated with a laser and the resultant contracture of iris tissue widens the pupil.

mechanical c., a procedure that lodges the pupillary margin in the groove of a device which, when widened, stretches the pupillary edge to make the pupil larger.

co·re·pres·sor (kō-rē-pres'ŏr). A molecule, usually a product of a specific metabolic pathway, that combines with and activates a repressor produced by a regulator gene. The repressor then attaches to an operator gene site and inhibits activity of the structural genes. This homeostatic mechanism regulates enzyme production in repressible enzyme systems.

Corey, R.B., U.S. chemist, 1897–1971. SEE Pauling-C. *helix.*

Cori, Carl F., Czech-U.S. biochemist and Nobel laureate, 1896–1984. SEE C. *cycle, ester.*

Cori, Gerty Theresa, Czech-U.S. biochemist and Nobel laureate, 1896–1957. SEE C.'s *disease.*

co·ria (kō'rē-ă). Plural of corium.

co·ri·an·der (kō-rē-an'der). The dried ripe fruit of *Coriandrum sativum* (family Umbelliferae); a mild stimulant aromatic and a flavoring agent.

co·ri·um, pl. **co·ria** (kō'rē-ŭm, -rē-ă) [NA]. SYN dermis. [L. skin, hide, leather]

c. coro'nae, SYN coronary *band.*

c. lim'bi, SYN periople.

c. pari'etis, the wall of the pododerm.

c. so'leae, the sole of the pododerm.

c. un'gulae, SYN pododerm.

corn (kŏrn). **1.** SYN clavus (1). **2.** A small inflammatory focus under the sole of the hoof of the horse; forefeet are most often affected, usually between the bar and the wall; sometimes seen in other hoofed animals. [L. *cornu*, horn, hoof]

asbestos c., a granulomatous or hyperkeratotic lesion of the skin at the site of deposit of asbestos particles. SYN asbestos wart.

hard c., the usual form of c. over a toe joint. SYN heloma durum.

seed c., a papilloma or wart on the sole of the foot.

soft c., a c. formed by pressure between two toes, the surface being macerated and yellowish in color. SYN heloma molle.

cor·nea (kŏr'nē-ă) [NA]. The transparent tissue constituting the anterior sixth of the outer wall of the eye, with a 7.7 mm radius of curvature as contrasted with the 13.5 mm of the sclera; it consists of stratified squamous epithelium continuous with that of the conjunctiva, a substantia propria, substantially regularly arranged collagen imbedded in mucopolysaccharide, and an inner layer of endothelium. It is the chief refractory structure of the eye. [L. fem. of *corneus*, horny]

conical c., SYN keratoconus.

c. farina'ta, bilateral speckling of the posterior part of the corneal stroma. SYN floury c.

floury c., SYN c. farinata.

c. uri'ca, bilateral deposition of crystalline deposits of urea and sodium urate within corneal stroma.

c. verticilla'ta, congenital whorl-like opacities in the c. SYN Fleischer's vortex.

cor·ne·al (kŏr'nē-ăl). Relating to the cornea.

cor·ne·o·bleph·a·ron (kŏr'nē-ō-blef'ă-ron). Adhesion of the eyelid margin to the cornea. [cornea + G. *blepharon*, eyelid]

cor·ne·o·cyte (kŏr'nē-ō-sīt). The dead keratin-filled squamous cell of the stratum corneum. SYN horny cell (1), keratinized cell. [*cornea*, L. fem. of *corneus*, horny, + G. *kytos*, cell]

cor·ne·o·sclera (kŏr'nē-ō-sklēr'ă). The combined cornea and sclera when considered as forming the external coat of the eyeball.

cor·ne·o·scler·al (kŏr'nē-ō-sklēr'ăl). Pertaining to the cornea and sclera.

cor·ne·ous (kŏr'nē-ŭs). SYN horny. [L. corneus, fr. *cornu*, horn]

Corner, Edred M., English surgeon, 1873–1950. SEE C.'s *tampon.*

Corner, George W., U.S. anatomist, 1889–1981. SEE C.-Allen *test, unit.*

cor·ne·um (kŏr'nē-ŭm). SEE *stratum* corneum epidermidis, *stratum* corneum unguis. [L., ntr. of *corneus,* horny, fr. *cornu,* horn]

cor·nic·u·late (kŏr-nik'yū-lāt). **1.** Resembling a horn. **2.** Having horns or horn-shaped appendages. [L. *corniculatus,* horned]

cor·nic·u·lum (kŏr-nik'yū-lŭm). A cornu of small size. [L. dim. of *cornu,* horn]

c. laryn'gis, SYN corniculate *cartilage.*

cor·ni·fi·ca·tion (kŏr-ni-fi-kā'shŭn). SYN keratinization. [L. *cornu,* horn, + *facio,* to make]

cor·ni·fied (kŏr'ni-fīd). SYN keratinized.

corn oil. The refined fixed oil expressed from the embryo of *Zea mays* (family Gramineae); a solvent. SYN maise oil.

corn·silk (kŏrn'silk). SYN zea.

corn smut (kŏrn'smŭt). SYN *Ustilago maydis.*

cor·nu, gen. **cor·nus,** pl. **cor·nua** (kŏr'nū, -nŭs, -nū-ă). **1** [NA]. SYN horn. **2.** Any structure composed of horny substance. **3.** One of the coronal extensions of the dental pulp underlying a cusp or lobe. **4.** The major subdivisions of the lateral ventricle in the

CO

cerebral hemisphere (the frontal horn, occipital horn, and temporal horn). SEE ALSO lateral *ventricle.* [L. horn]

c. ammo′nis, SYN Ammon's *horn.*

c. ante′rius [NA], SYN anterior *horn.*

coccygeal cornua, two processes that project upward from the dorsum of the base of the coccyx to articulate with the sacral c. SYN cornua coccygealia [NA], coccygeal horn.

cornua coccygea′lia [NA], SYN coccygeal cornua.

c. cuta′neum, SYN cutaneous *horn.*

cornua of falciform margin of saphenous opening, SEE inferior *horn* of falciform margin of saphenous opening, superior *horn* of falciform margin of saphenous opening.

cornua of hyoid bone, SEE greater *horn* of hyoid bone, lesser *horn* of hyoid bone.

c. infe′rius [NA], SYN inferior *horn.*

c. infe′rius cartila′ginis thyroi′deae [NA], SYN inferior *horn* of thyroid cartilage.

c. infe′rius margina′lis falcifor′mis hia′tus saphe′ni [NA], SYN inferior *horn* of falciform margin of saphenous opening.

c. infe′rius ventric′uli latera′lis [NA], SYN inferior *horn* of lateral ventricle.

c. latera′le [NA], SYN lateral *horn.*

cornua of lateral ventricle, SEE anterior *horn* (1), inferior *horn* of lateral ventricle, c. posterius ventriculi lateralis.

c. ma′jus os′sis hyoi′dei [NA], SYN greater *horn* of hyoid bone.

c. mi′nus os′sis hyoi′dei [NA], SYN lesser *horn* of hyoid bone.

c. posterius, SYN posterior *horn.*

c. poste′rius ventric′uli latera′lis [NA], SYN posterior *horn.*

sacral cornua, the most caudal parts of the intermediate sacral crest. On each side they form the lateral margin of the sacral hiatus and articulate with the coccygeal cornua. SYN cornua sacralia [NA], sacral horns.

cornua sacra′lia [NA], SYN sacral cornua.

cornua of spinal cord, SYN posterior *horn.* SEE anterior *horn* (2), lateral *horn.*

styloid c., SYN lesser *horn* of hyoid bone.

c. supe′rius cartila′ginis thyroi′deae [NA], SYN superior *horn* of thyroid cartilage.

c. supe′rius margin′alis falcifor′mis [NA], SYN superior *horn* of falciform margin of saphenous opening.

cornua of thyroid cartilage, SEE inferior *horn* of thyroid cartilage, superior *horn* of thyroid cartilage.

c. u′teri [NA], the portion of the uterus to which the intramural section of the uterine tube enters on either the right or left. SYN uterine horn, horn of uterus.

cor·nua (kōr′nū-ă). Plural of cornu.

cor·nu·al (kōr′nū-ăl). Relating to a cornu.

△**coro-.** SEE core-.

co·ro·na, pl. **co·ro·nae** (kō-rō′nă, -nē) [NA]. SYN crown. [L. garland, crown, fr. G. *korōnē*]

c. cap′itis, the topmost part of the head. SYN crown of head.

c. cilia′ris [NA], the circular figure on the inner surface of the ciliary body, formed by the processes and folds (plicae) taken together. SYN ciliary crown, ciliary wreath.

c. clin′ica [NA], SYN clinical *crown.*

c. den′tis [NA], SYN *crown* of tooth.

c. glan′dis [NA], SYN c. of glans penis.

c. of glans penis, the prominent posterior border of the glans penis. SYN c. glandis [NA].

c. radia′ta, (1) [NA], a fan-shaped fiber mass on the white matter of the cerebral cortex, composed of the widely radiating fibers of the internal capsule; **(2)** a single layer of columnar cells derived from the cumulus oophorus, which anchor on the pellucid zone of the oocyte in a secondary follicle. SYN radiate crown.

c. seborrhe′ica, a red band at the hair line along the upper border of the forehead and temples occasionally observed in seborrheic dermatitis of the scalp.

c. vene′ris, papular syphilitic lesions (secondary eruption) along the anterior margin of the scalp or on the back of the neck. SEE ALSO *crown* of Venus.

Zinn's c., SYN vascular *circle* of optic nerve.

cor·o·nad (kōr′ō-nad). In a direction toward any corona.

cor·o·nal (kōr′ō-năl). Relating to a corona or the coronal plane. SYN coronalis [NA].

cor·o·na·le (kōr-ō-nā′lē). **1.** SYN frontal *bone.* **2.** One of the two most widely separated points on the coronal suture at the poles of the greatest frontal diameter. [L. neuter of *coronalis,* pertaining to a *corona,* crown]

cor·o·na·lis (kōr-ō-nā′lis) [NA]. SYN coronal, coronal.

cor·o·na·ria (kōr-ō-nā′rē-ă). A coronary artery, of the heart.

cor·o·nar·ism (kōr′ō-nār-izm). **1.** SYN coronary *insufficiency.* **2.** SYN *angina* pectoris. [coronary (artery) + -ism]

cor·o·na·ri·tis (kōr′ō-nă-rī′tis). Inflammation of coronary artery or arteries.

cor·o·nary (kōr′o-nār-ē). **1.** Relating to or resembling a crown. **2.** Encircling; denoting various anatomical structures, *e.g.,* nerves, blood vessels, ligaments. **3.** Specifically, denoting the c. blood vessels of the heart and, colloquially, c. thrombosis. [L. *coronarius;* fr. *corona,* a crown]

cafe c., sudden collapse while eating that results from food impaction closing the glottis; often erroneously thought to stem from coronary artery disease.

Co·ro·na·vir·i·dae (kō-rō′nă-vir′i-dē). A family of single-stranded RNA-containing viruses of medium size, and made up of 4 antigenic groups; some of which cause upper respiratory tract infections in man similar to the "common cold"; others cause animal infections (infectious avian bronchitis, swine encephalitis, mouse hepatitis, neonatal calf diarrhea, and others). The viruses resemble myxoviruses except for the petal-shaped projections which give an impression of the solar corona. Virions are 80 to 130 nm in diameter, enveloped, and ether-sensitive. Nucleocapsids are thought to be of helical symmetry; they develop in cytoplasm and are enveloped by budding into cytoplasmic vesicles. *Coronavirus* is the only recognized genus. [L. *corona,* garland, crown]

Co·ro·na·vi·rus (kō-rō′nă-vī′rŭs). A genus in the family Coronaviridae that is associated with upper respiratory tract infections and possibly gastroenteritis in man.

co·ro·na·vi·rus (kō-rō′nă-vī′rŭs). Any virus of the family Coronaviridae.

cor·o·ner (kōr′on-er). An official whose duty it is to investigate sudden, suspicious, or violent death to determine the cause; in some communities, the office has been replaced by that of medical examiner. [L. *corona,* a crown]

cor·o·net (kōr′ō-net). The line of junction between the skin and the hoof or claw. [Fr. *coronette;* L. *corona,* crown]

co·ro·ni·on (kŏ-rō′nē-on). The tip of the coronoid process of the mandible; a craniometric point. SYN koronion. [G. *korōnē,* crow]

cor·o·ni·tis (kōr-ō-nī′tis). Inflammation of the coronary band of the horse's hoof, resulting in imperfect horn formation.

cor·o·noid (kōr′ō-noyd). Shaped like a crow's beak; denoting certain processes and other parts of bones. [G. *korōnē,* a crow, + *eidos,* resembling]

cor·o·noi·dec·to·my (kōr′ō-noy-dek′tō-mē). Surgical removal of the coronoid process of the mandible. [coronoid + G. *ektomē,* excision]

cor·po·ra (kōr′pōr-ă). Plural of corpus.

cor·po·re·al (kōr-pō′rē-ăl). Pertaining to the body, or to a corpus.

cor·po·rin (kōr′pŏ-rin). Obsolete term for corpus luteum *hormone.*

corpse (kōrps). SYN cadaver. [L. *corpus,* body]

corps ronds (kōr-ron′). Dyskeratotic round cells occurring in the epidermis, with a central round basophilic mass surrounded by a clear halo; characteristically found in keratosis follicularis. [Fr. round bodies]

cor·pu·lence, cor·pu·len·cy (kōr′pyū-lens, -len-sē). SYN obesity. [L. *corpulentia,* magnification of *corpus,* body]

cor·pu·lent (kōr′pyū-lent). SYN obese.

CORPUS

cor·pus, gen. **cor·po·ris**, pl. **cor·po·ra** (kōr′pŭs, -pōr-is, -pōr-ă) [NA]. **1.** SYN body. **2.** Any body or mass. **3.** The main part of an organ or other anatomical structure, as distinguished from the head or tail. SEE ALSO body, shaft, soma. [L. body]

c. adipo′sum [NA], SYN fat-pad.

c. adipo′sum buc′cae [NA], SYN buccal *fat-pad*.

c. adipo′sum fos′sae ischiorecta′lis [NA], SYN ischiorectal *fat-pad*.

c. adipo′sum infrapatella′re [NA], SYN infrapatellar *fat-pad*.

c. adipo′sum or′bitae [NA], SYN orbital *fat-pad*.

c. al′bicans [NA], a retrogressed c. luteum characterized by increasing cicatrization and shrinkage of the cicatricial core with an amorphous, convoluted, completely hyalinized lutein zone surrounding the central plug of scar tissue. SYN albicans (2), atretic c. luteum, c. candicans.

cor′pora alla′ta, a pair of juvenile hormone-producing endocrine glands located near the brain in insects; action of the juvenile hormone is interrelated with that of brain hormone and ecdysone; a high concentration of the hormone at the time of molting will cause production of an additional larval instar; removal at an early larval stage causes precocious pupation, resulting in the formation of a midget adult; implantation at late larval stages can cause development of an oversized adult.

c. amygdaloi′deum [NA], SYN amygdaloid *body*.

c. amyla′ceum, pl. **cor′pora amyla′cea**, one of a number of small ovoid or rounded, sometimes laminated, bodies resembling a grain of starch and found in nervous tissue, in the prostate, and in pulmonary alveoli; of little pathological significance, and apparently derived from degenerated cells or proteinaceous secretions. SYN amniotic corpuscle, amylaceous corpuscle, amyloid corpuscle, colloid corpuscle.

c. aor′ticum, SYN para-aortic *bodies*, under *body*.

c. aran′tii, SYN *nodule* of semilunar valve.

cor′pora arena′cea, small calcareous concretions in the stroma of the pineal and other central nervous system tissues. SYN acervulus, brain sand, psammoma bodies (2).

atretic c. luteum, SYN c. albicans.

c. atret′icum, SYN atretic ovarian *follicle*.

cor′pora bigem′ina, SYN bigeminal *bodies*, under *body*.

c. callo′sum [NA], the great commissural plate of nerve fibers interconnecting the cortical hemispheres (with the exception of most of the temporal lobes which are interconnected by the anterior commissure). Lying at the floor of the longitudinal fissure, and covered on each side by the cingulate gyrus, it is arched from behind forward and is thick at each extremity (splenium and genu) but thinner in its long central portion (truncus); it curves back underneath itself at the genu to form the rostrum of the c. callosum. SYN commissure of cerebral hemispheres.

c. can′dicans, SYN c. albicans.

c. caverno′sum clitor′idis [NA], one of the two parallel columns of erectile tissue forming the body of the clitoris; they diverge at the root to form the crura of the clitoris. SYN cavernous body of clitoris.

c. caverno′sum con′chae, SYN cavernous *plexus* of conchae.

c. caverno′sum pe′nis [NA], one of two parallel columns of erectile tissue forming the dorsal part of the body of the penis; they are separated posteriorly, forming the crura of the penis. SYN cavernous body of penis.

c. caverno′sum ure′thrae, SYN c. spongiosum penis.

c. cilia′re [NA], SYN ciliary *body*.

c. clavic′ulae [NA], SYN *body* of clavicle.

c. clitor′idis [NA], SYN *body* of clitoris.

c. coccy′geum [NA], SYN coccygeal *body*.

c. cos′tae [NA], SYN *body* of rib.

c. denta′tum, SYN dentate *nucleus* of cerebellum.

c. epididym′idis [NA], SYN *body* of epididymis.

c. fem′oris, SYN *shaft* of femur.

c. fibro′sum, the small fibrous cicatricial mass in the ovary formed following the atresia of an ovarian follicle; similar to a corpus albicans but smaller.

c. fib′ulae [NA], SYN *shaft* of fibula.

c. fimbria′tum, **(1)** SYN *fimbria* hippocampi. **(2)** the outer, ovarian extremity of the oviduct.

c. for′nicis [NA], SYN *body* of fornix.

c. gas′tricum [ventric′uli] [NA], SYN *body* of stomach.

c. genicula′tum exter′num, SYN lateral geniculate *body*.

c. genicula′tum inter′num, SYN medial geniculate *body*.

c. genicula′tum latera′le [NA], SYN lateral geniculate *body*.

c. genicula′tum media′le [NA], SYN medial geniculate *body*.

c. glan′dulae sudorif′erae [NA], SYN *body* of sweat gland.

c. hemorrhag′icum, a hematoma with a lining formed by the thinned-out bright yellow lutein zone; gradual resorption of the blood elements leaves a cavity filled with a clear fluid, *i.e.,* a c. luteum cyst. SYN corpus luteum hematoma.

c. high′mori, c. highmoria′num, SYN *mediastinum* testis.

c. hu′meri [NA], SYN *shaft* of humerus.

c. incu′dis [NA], SYN *body* of incus.

c. lin′guae [NA], SYN *body* of tongue.

c. lu′teum [NA], the yellow endocrine body, 1 to 1.5 cm in diameter, formed in the ovary at the site of a ruptured ovarian follicle immediately after ovulation; there is an early stage of proliferation and vascularization before full maturity; later, there is a festooned and bright yellowish lutein zone traversed by trabeculae of theca interna containing numerous blood vessels; the c. luteum secretes estrogen, as did the follicle, and also secretes progesterone. If pregnancy does not occur, it is called a **c. luteum spurium**, which undergoes progressive retrogression to a c. albicans. If pregnancy does occur, it is called a **c. luteum verum**, which increases in size, persisting to the fifth or sixth month of pregnancy before retrogression. SYN yellow body.

c. luy′si, SYN subthalamic *nucleus*.

c. mamilla′re [NA], SYN mamillary *body*.

c. mam′mae [NA], SYN *body* of mammary gland.

c. mandib′ulae [NA], SYN *body* of mandible.

c. maxil′lae [NA], SYN *body* of maxilla.

c. medulla′re cerebel′li [NA], the interior white substance of the cerebellum.

c. nu′clei cauda′ti [NA], SYN *body* of caudate nucleus.

c. oliva′re, SYN oliva.

c. os′sis fem′oris [NA], SYN *shaft* of femur.

c. os′sis hyoi′dei [NA], SYN *body* of hyoid bone.

c. os′sis il′ii [NA], SYN *body* of ilium.

c. os′sis isch′ii [NA], SYN *body* of ischium.

c. os′sis metacarpa′lis [NA], the shaft of one of the metacarpal bones.

c. os′sis pu′bis [NA], SYN *body* of pubis.

c. os′sis sphenoida′lis [NA], SYN *body* of sphenoid bone.

c. pampinifor′me, SYN epoöphoron.

c. pancrea′tis [NA], SYN *body* of pancreas.

c. papilla′re, SYN *stratum* papillare corii.

cor′pora para-aor′tica [NA], SYN para-aortic *bodies*, under *body*.

c. paratermina′le, SYN subcallosal *gyrus*.

c. pe′nis [NA], SYN *body* of penis.

c. phalan′gis [NA], SYN *body* of phalanx.

c. pine′ale [NA], SYN pineal *body*.

c. pon′tobulba′re, SYN pontobulbar *body*.

cor′pora quadrigem′ina, SYN quadrigeminal *bodies*, under *body*. SEE inferior *colliculus*, superior *colliculus*.

c. quadrigem′inum ante′rius, SYN superior *colliculus*.

c. quadrigem′inum poste′rius, SYN inferior *colliculus*.

c. ra′dii [NA], SYN *shaft* of radius.

c. restifor′me, SYN restiform *body*.

c. spongio′sum pe′nis [NA], the median column of erectile tissue located between and ventral to the two corpora cavernosa penis; posteriorly it expands into the bulbus penis and anteriorly it terminates as the enlarged glans penis; it is traversed by the urethra. SYN c. cavernosum urethrae, spongy body of penis.

c. spongio′sum ure′thrae mulie′bris, the submucous coat of the female urethra, containing a venous network that insinuates itself between the muscular layers, giving to them an erectile nature.

c. ster′ni [NA], SYN *body* of sternum.

c. stria′tum [NA], SYN striate *body.*

c. ta′li [NA], SYN *body* of talus.

c. tib′iae [NA], SYN *shaft* of tibia.

c. trapezoid′eum [NA], SYN trapezoid *body.*

c. triti′ceum, SYN triticeal *cartilage.*

c. ul′nae [NA], SYN *body* of ulna.

c. un′guis [NA], SYN *body* of nail.

c. u′teri [NA], SYN *body* of uterus.

c. ver′tebrae [NA], SYN *body* of vertebra.

c. vesi′cae bilia′ris [NA], SYN *body* of gallbladder.

c. vesi′cae fell′eae [NA], SYN *body* of gallbladder.

c. vesi′cae urina′riae [NA], SYN *body* of urinary bladder.

c. vit′reum [NA], SYN vitreous *body.* SEE ALSO vitreous.

---

cor·pus·cle (kōr′pŭs-l). **1.** A small mass or body. **2.** A blood cell. SYN corpusculum [NA]. [L. *corpusculum,* dim. of *corpus,* body]

amniotic c., SYN *corpus* amylaceum.

amylaceous c., amyloid c., SYN *corpus* amylaceum.

articular c.'s, encapsulated nerve terminations within joint capsules. SYN corpuscula articularia [NA].

axis c., axile c., the central portion of a tactile c.

basal c., SYN basal *body.*

Bizzozero's c., SYN platelet.

blood c., SYN blood *cell.*

bone c., SYN osteocyte.

bridge c., SYN desmosome.

bulboid c.'s, SYN Krause's end *bulbs,* under *bulb.*

cement c., a cementocyte contained within a lacuna or crypt of the cementum of a tooth; an entrapped cementoblast.

chyle c., a cell of the same appearance as a leukocyte, present in chyle.

colloid c., SYN *corpus* amylaceum.

colostrum c., one of numerous bodies present in the colostrum, supposed to be modified leukocytes containing fat droplets. SYN Donné's c., galactoblast.

concentrated human red blood c., c. prepared from one or more preparations of whole human blood which are not more than 14 days old and each of which has already been directly matched with the blood of the intended recipient.

corneal c.'s, connective tissue cells found between the laminae of fibrous tissue in the cornea. SYN Toynbee's c.'s, Virchow's cells (2), Virchow's c.'s.

Dogiel's c., an encapsulated sensory nerve ending.

Donné's c., SYN colostrum c.

dust c.'s, SYN hemoconia.

Eichhorst's c.'s, the globular forms sometimes occurring in the poikilocytosis of pernicious anemia.

exudation c., a cell present in an exudate that assists in the organization of new tissue. SYN exudation cell, inflammatory c., plastic c.

genital c.'s, special encapsulated nerve endings found in the skin of the genitalia and nipple. SYN corpuscula genitalia [NA].

ghost c., SYN achromocyte.

Gluge's c.'s, large pus cells containing fat droplets.

Golgi c., SEE Golgi-Mazzoni c.

Golgi-Mazzoni c., an encapsulated sensory nerve ending similar to a pacinian c. but simpler in structure.

Grandry's c.'s, general sensory endings in the beak, mouth, and tongue of birds; similar to Merkel's c.'s.

Hassall's concentric c.'s, SYN thymic c.

Herbst's c.'s, tactile c.'s, resembling pacinian c.'s, but much smaller; found in birds.

inflammatory c., SYN exudation c.

Key-Retzius c.'s, tactile c.'s, resembling pacinian c.'s, found in the beak of certain aquatic birds.

lamellated c.'s, small oval bodies in the skin of the fingers, in the mesentery, tendons, and elsewhere, formed of concentric layers of connective tissue with a soft core in which the axon of a nerve fiber runs, splitting up into a number of fibrils that terminate in bulbous enlargements; they are sensitive to pressure. SYN corpuscula lamellosa [NA], pacinian c.'s, Vater's c.'s, Vater-Pacini c.'s.

lymph c., lymphatic c., lymphoid c., a mononuclear type of leukocyte formed in lymph nodes and other lymphoid tissue, and also in the blood.

malpighian c.'s, (1) SYN renal c. **(2)** SYN splenic lymph *follicles,* under *follicle.*

Mazzoni c., a tactile c. apparently identical with Krause's end bulb. SEE ALSO Golgi-Mazzoni c.

Meissner's c., SYN tactile c.

Merkel's c., SYN tactile *meniscus.*

Mexican hat c., SEE target cell *anemia.*

milk c., one of the fat droplets in milk.

molluscum c., SYN molluscum *body.*

Negri c.'s, SYN Negri *bodies,* under *body.*

Norris' c.'s, decolorized red blood cells that are invisible or almost invisible in the blood plasma, unless they are appropriately stained.

oval c., SYN tactile c.

pacchionian c.'s, SYN arachnoid *granulations,* under *granulation.*

pacinian c.'s, SYN lamellated c.'s.

pessary c., an elongated red blood cell with hemoglobin concentrated in the peripheral portion.

phantom c., SYN achromocyte.

plastic c., SYN exudation c.

Purkinje's c.'s, SYN Purkinje's *cells,* under *cell.*

pus c., one of the polymorphonuclear leukocytes that comprise the chief portion of the formed elements in pus. SYN pus cell, pyocyte.

Rainey's c.'s, rounded, ovoidal, or sickle-shaped spores or bradyzoites, 12 to 16 by 4 to 9 μm, found within the elongated cysts (Miescher's tubes) of the protozoan *Sarcocystis.*

red c., SYN erythrocyte.

renal c., the tuft of glomerular capillaries and the capsula glomeruli that encloses it. SYN corpusculum renis [NA], malpighian c.'s (1).

reticulated c., SYN reticulocyte.

Ruffini's c.'s, sensory end-structures in the subcutaneous connective tissues of the fingers, consisting of an ovoid capsule within which the sensory fiber ends with numerous collateral knobs.

salivary c., one of the leukocytes present in saliva.

Schwalbe's c., SYN taste *bud.*

shadow c., SYN achromocyte.

splenic c.'s, SYN splenic lymph *follicles,* under *follicle.*

tactile c., one of numerous oval bodies found in the papillae of the skin, especially those of the fingers and toes; they consist of a connective tissue capsule in which the axon fibrils terminate around and between a pile of wedge-shaped epithelioid cells. SYN corpusculum tactus [NA], Meissner's c., oval c., touch c.

taste c., SYN taste *bud.*

terminal nerve c.'s, generic term denoting specialized encapsulated nerve endings such as the articular, bulboid, genital, lamellated, and tactile c.'s, and the tactile meniscus. SYN corpuscula nervosa terminalia [NA].

third c., SYN platelet.

thymic c., small spherical bodies of keratinized and usually squamous epithelial cells arranged in a concentric pattern around clusters of degenerating lymphocytes, eosinophils, and macrophages; found in the medulla of the lobules of the thymus. SYN Hassall's bodies, Hassall's concentric c.'s, Virchow-Hassall bodies.

touch c., SYN tactile c.

Toynbee's c.'s, SYN corneal c.'s.

Traube's c., SYN achromocyte.

Tröltsch's c.'s, minute spaces, resembling c.'s, between the radial fibers of the drum membrane of the ear.

Valentin's c.'s, small bodies, probably amyloid, found occasionally in nerve tissue.

Vater's c.'s, SYN lamellated c.'s.

Vater-Pacini c.'s, SYN lamellated c.'s.

Virchow's c.'s, SYN corneal c.'s.

white c., any type of leukocyte.

Zimmermann's c., SYN platelet.

cor·pus·cu·la (kōr-pŭs′kyū-lă). Plural of corpusculum.

cor·pus·cu·lar (kōr-pŭs′kyū-lăr). Relating to a corpuscle.

cor·pus·cu·lum, pl. **cor·pus·cu·la** (kōr-pŭs′kyū-lŭm, -kyū-lă) [NA]. SYN corpuscle.

corpus′cula articula′ria [NA], SYN articular *corpuscles,* under *corpuscle.*

corpus′cula bulboi′dea [NA], SYN Krause's end *bulbs,* under *bulb.*

corpus′cula genita′lia [NA], SYN genital *corpuscles,* under *corpuscle.*

corpus′cula lamello′sa [NA], SYN lamellated *corpuscles,* under *corpuscle.*

corpus′cula nervo′sa termina′lia [NA], SYN terminal nerve *corpuscles,* under *corpuscle.*

c. re′nis, pl. **corpus′cula re′nis** [NA], SYN renal *corpuscle.*

c. tac′tus, pl. **corpus′cula tac′tus** [NA], SYN tactile *corpuscle.*

cor·rec·tion (kō-rek′shŭn). The act of reducing a fault; the elimination of an unfavorable quality.

occlusal c., (1) the c. of malocclusion, by whatever means is employed; (2) elimination of disharmony of occlusal contacts.

spontaneous c. of placenta previa, the upward "migration" of the placenta away from the internal os by the differential growth rates of upper and lower uterine segments.

cor·rec·tive (kō-rek′tiv). **1.** Counteracting, modifying, or changing what is injurious. **2.** A drug that modifies or corrects an undesirable or injurious effect of another drug. SYN corrigent. [L. *cor-rigo* (conr-), pp. *-rectus,* to set right, fr. *rego,* to keep straight]

cor·re·la·tion (kōr-ĕ-lā′shŭn). **1.** The mutual or reciprocal relation of two or more items or parts. **2.** The act of bringing into such a relation. **3.** The degree to which variables change together.

product-moment c., a statistical procedure which yields the correlation coefficient referred to as r (-1.00 to +1.00) and involves the actual values, rather than the ranks (rank order) of the measurements.

rank-difference c., the relationship between paired series of measurements, each ranked according to magnitude, which yields a coefficient known as *rho;* the value of *rho* varies from zero (no relationship) to +1.00 (perfect relationship).

Correra's line. See under line.

cor·re·spon·dence (kōr-ĕ-spon′dens). In optics, those points on each retina that have the same visual direction.

abnormal c., SYN anomalous c.

anomalous c., abnormal c., a condition, frequent in strabismus, in which corresponding retinal points do not have the same visual direction; the fovea of one eye corresponds to an extrafoveal area of the fellow eye. SYN abnormal c.

dysharmonious c., a type of anomalous retinal c. in which the angle of the visual direction of the two retinas is different than the objective angle of the strabismus.

harmonious c., a type of anomalous retinal c. in which the angle of the visual direction of the two retinas is equal to the objective angle of strabismus.

Corrigan, Sir Dominic J., Irish pathologist and clinician, 1802–1880. SEE C.'s *disease, pulse, sign.*

cor·ri·gent (kōr′i-jent). SYN corrective.

cor·rin (kōr′in). The cyclic system of four pyrrole rings forming corrinoids, which are the central structure of the vitamins B_{12} and related compounds, differing from porphin (porphyrin) in that two of the pyrrole rings are directly linked (C-19 to C-1). [fr. *core* (of vitamin B_{12} molecule)]

cor·rin·oid (kōr′rin-oid). A compound containing a corrin ring.

cor·rode (kŏ-rōd′). To cause, or to be affected by, corrosion.

cor·ro·sion (kŏ-rō′shŭn). **1.** Gradual deterioration or consummation of a substance by another, especially by biochemical or chemical reaction. Cf. erosion. **2.** The product of corroding, such as rust. [L. *cor-rodo* (conr-), pp. *-rosus,* to gnaw]

cor·ro·sive (kŏ-rō′siv). **1.** Causing corrosion. **2.** An agent that produces corrosion; *e.g.,* a strong acid or alkali.

cor·ru·ga·tor (kōr′ŭ-gā-ter, -tōr). A muscle that draws together the skin, causing it to wrinkle. [L. *cor-rugo* (conr-), pp. *-atus,* to wrinkle, fr. *ruga,* a wrinkle]

CORTEX

cor·tex, gen. **cor·ti·cis,** pl. **cor·ti·ces** (kōr′teks, -ti-sis, -ti-sēz) [NA]. The outer portion of an organ, such as the kidney, as distinguished from the inner, or medullary, portion. [L. bark]

adrenal c., SYN suprarenal c.

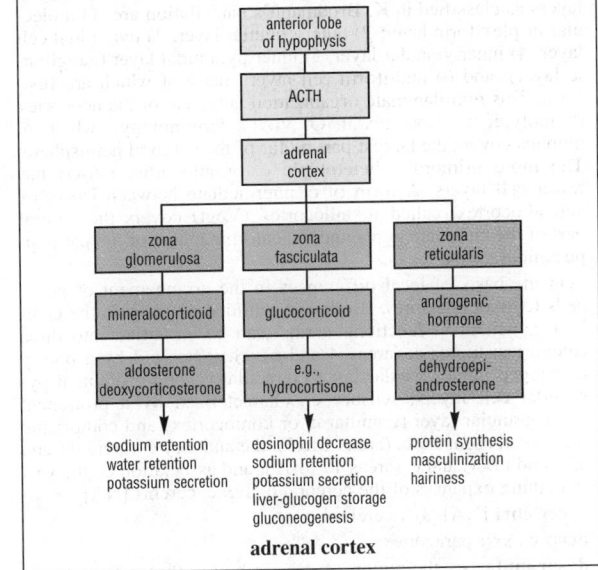

adrenal cortex

agranular c., SEE cerebral c.

association c., generic term denoting the large expanses of the cerebral c. that are not sensory or motor in the customary sense, but are involved in advanced stages of sensory information processing, multisensory integration, or sensorimotor integration. SEE ALSO cerebral c. SYN association areas.

auditory c., the region of the cerebral c. that receives the auditory radiation from the medial geniculate body, a thalamic cell group receiving auditory input from the cochlear nuclei in the rhombencephalon; it corresponds approximately to Brodmann's areas 41 and 42 and is tonotopically organized. SYN auditory area.

cerebellar c., the thin gray surface layer of the cerebellum, consisting of an outer molecular layer or stratum moleculare, a single layer of Purkinje cells (the ganglionic layer), and an inner granular layer or stratum granulosum. SYN c. cerebelli [NA].

c. cerebel′li [NA], SYN cerebellar c.

cerebral c., the gray cellular mantle (1 to 4 mm thick) covering the entire surface of the cerebral hemisphere of mammals; characterized by a laminar organization of cellular and fibrous components such that its nerve cells are stacked in defined layers

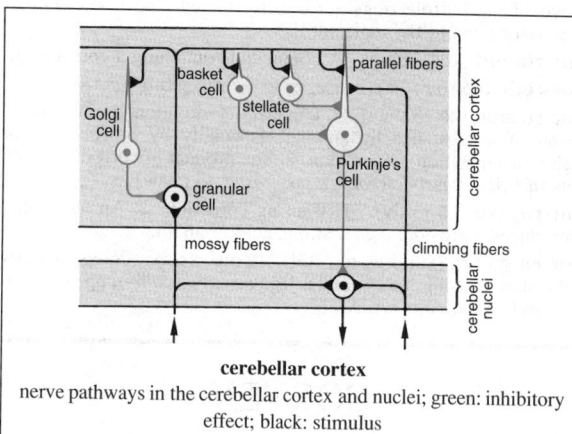

cerebellar cortex
nerve pathways in the cerebellar cortex and nuclei; green: inhibitory effect; black: stimulus

varying in number from one, as in the archicortex of the hippocampus, to five or six in the larger neocortex; the outermost (molecular or plexiform) layer contains very few cell bodies and is composed largely of the distal ramifications of the long apical dendrites issued perpendicularly to the surface by pyramidal and fusiform cells in deeper layers. From the surface inward, the layers as classified in K. Brodmann's parcellation are: 1) molecular or plexiform layer; 2) outer granular layer; 3) pyramidal cell layer; 4) inner granular layer; 5) inner pyramidal layer (ganglionic layer); and 6) multiform cell layer, many of which are fusiform. This multilaminate organization is typical of the neocortex (homotypic c.; isocortex in O. Vogt's terminology), which in humans covers the largest part by far of the cerebral hemisphere. The more primordial heterotypic c. or allocortex (Vogt) has fewer cell layers. A form of c. intermediate between isocortex and allocortex, called juxtallocortex (Vogt) covers the ventral part of the cingulate gyrus and the entorhinal area of the parahippocampal gyrus.

On the basis of local differences in the arrangement of nerve cells (cytoarchitecture), Brodmann outlined 47 areas in the cerebral c. which, in functional terms, can be classified into three categories: motor c. (areas 4 and 6), characterized by a poorly developed inner granular layer (agranular c.) and prominent pyramidal cell layers; sensory c., characterized by a prominent inner granular layer (granular c. or koniocortex) and comprising the somatic sensory c. (areas 1 to 3), the auditory c. (areas 41 and 42), and the visual c. (areas 17 to 19); and association c., the vast remaining expanses of the cerebral c. SYN c. cerebri [NA].

c. cer'ebri [NA], SYN cerebral c.

deep c., SYN paracortex.

dysgranular c., the region of the cerebral c. that is transitional between the agranular c. of the precentral gyrus and the granular frontal cortex (Brodmann's area 8).

fetal adrenal c., an extensive area of the adrenal gland present in primates during fetal life and for a short period after birth; located between the definitive cortex and the medulla, it contains large steroid-secreting cells arranged in a reticular pattern; involution of this zone in humans is largely completed by three months after birth. SYN androgenic zone (2), fetal reticularis (1), fetal zone, provisional c.

frontal c., c. of the frontal lobe of the cerebral hemisphere; **(1)** originally, the entire cortical expanse anterior to the central sulcus, including the agranular motor and premotor c. (Brodmann's areas 4 and 6), the dysgranular c. (area 8), and the granular frontal (prefrontal) c. anterior to the latter; **(2)** now more often refers to the granular frontal (prefrontal) c. SYN frontal area.

c. glan'dulae suprarena'lis [NA], SYN suprarenal c.

granular c., SEE cerebral c.

c. of hair shaft, the principal structural component of the hair shaft, composed of closely packed fusiform keratinized cells and invested by the cuticula pili.

heterotypic c., SYN allocortex.

homotypic c., SYN isocortex.

insular c., SYN insula (1).

laminated c., neocortex and allocortex.

c. of lens, the softer, more superficial part of the lens of the eye that encloses the central part or nucleus; its refractive power is less than that of the nucleus. SYN c. lentis [NA].

c. len'tis [NA], SYN c. of lens.

c. of lymph node, the outer portion of the lymph node underneath its capsule, consisting of fibrous trabeculae separating densely packed masses of lymphocytes arranged in nodules and separated from the trabeculae and capsule by lymph sinuses. SYN c. nodi lymphatici [NA].

motor c., the region of the cerebral c. most nearly immediately influencing movements of the face, neck and trunk, and arm and leg; it corresponds approximately to Brodmann's areas 4 and 6 of the precentral gyrus; its effects upon the motor neurons innervating the skeletal musculature are mediated by the pyramidal tract and are particularly essential for the human capacity to perform finely graded movements of arm and leg. SYN excitable area, motor area, Rolando's area.

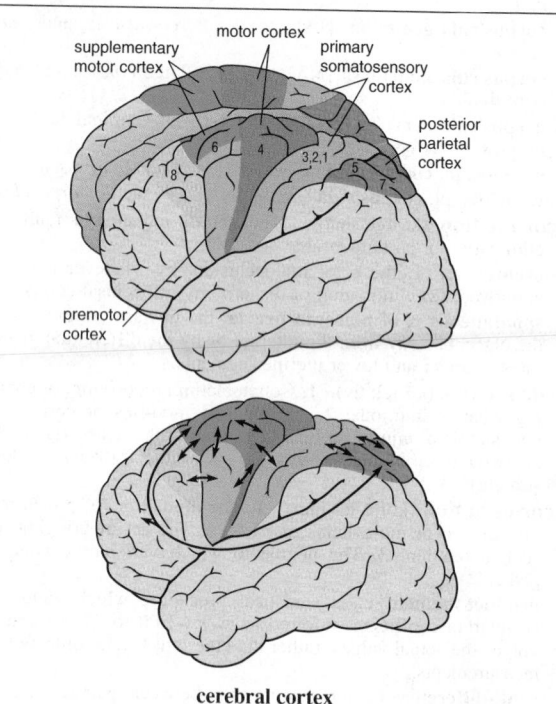

cerebral cortex
the essential regions of the cerebral cortex, which participate in voluntary motor functions; *above:* the areas (Brodmann's numbering) that take part in the strategy and accomplishment of movements lie near the motor cortex; *below:* corticocortical projections connect these regions; all connections are bidirectional

c. no'di lymphat'ici [NA], SYN c. of lymph node.

olfactory c., SYN piriform c.

orbitofrontal c., the cerebral c. covering the basal surface of the frontal lobes. SYN fronto-orbital area.

c. ova'rii [NA], SYN c. of ovary.

c. of ovary, the layer of the ovarian stroma lying immediately beneath the tunica albuginea, composed of connective tissue cells and fibers, among which are scattered primary and secondary (antral) follicles in various stages of development; the c. varies in thickness according to the age of the individual, becoming thinner with advancing years. SYN c. ovarii [NA].

parastriate c., SEE visual c.

peristriate c., SEE visual c.

piriform c., the olfactory c., corresponding to the rostral half of the uncus; receiving its major afferents from the olfactory bulb, it is classified as allocortex. SEE ALSO cerebral c. SYN olfactory c., piriform area.

prefrontal c., SEE frontal c.

premotor c., a somewhat ill-defined term usually referring to the agranular cortex of Brodmann's area 6. SYN premotor area.

primary visual c., SEE visual c.

provisional c., SYN fetal adrenal c.

renal c., the part of the kidney consisting of renal lobules in the outer zone beneath the capsule and also the lobules of the renal columns that are extensions inward between the pyramids; contains the renal corpuscles and the proximal and distal convoluted tubules. SYN c. renis [NA].

c. re′nis [NA], SYN renal c.

secondary sensory c., a cortical region occupying the parietal operculum (upper lip of the lateral sulcus) closely posterior to the foot of the postcentral gyrus; like the primary somatic-sensory c. of the postcentral gyrus, this region receives sensory impulses originating in face, trunk, and limbs; projections to the s.s.c. are from the ventral basal complex (ventral posteromedial and posterolateral thalamic nuclei) and from the primary somesthetic cortex.

secondary visual c., SEE visual c.

sensory c., formerly denoting specifically the somatic sensory c., but now used to refer collectively to the somatic sensory, auditory, visual, and olfactory regions of the cerebral c.

somatic sensory c., somatosensory c., the region of the cerebral c. receiving the somatic sensory radiation from the ventrobasal nucleus of the thalamus; it represents the primary cortical processing mechanism for sensory information originating at the body surfaces (touch) and in deeper tissues such as muscle, tendons, and joint capsules (position sense); it corresponds approximately to Brodmann's areas 1, 2, 3 on the postcentral gyrus. SYN somesthetic area.

striate c., SEE visual c.

supplementary motor c., a region from which, by electrical stimulation, the musculature of all bodily parts can be activated, as it also can by stimulation of the motor c. of the precentral gyrus; the region corresponds approximately to the expansion of Brodmann's area 6 over the medial surface of the cerebral hemisphere; this area has largely a bilateral representation and is concerned primarily with tonic and postural motor activities.

suprarenal c., the outer part of the adrenal gland, consisting of three zones from without inward: zona glomerulosa, zona fasciculata, and zona reticularis; this part of the adrenal c. yields steroid hormones such as corticosterone, deoxycorticosterone, and estrone. SYN c. glandulae suprarenalis [NA], adrenal c.

temporal c., SYN temporal *lobe.*

tertiary c., SYN paracortex.

c. of thymus, the outer part of a lobule of the thymus; it surrounds the medulla and is composed of masses of closely packed lymphocytes.

visual c., the region of the cerebral c. occupying the entire surface of the occipital lobe, and composed of Brodmann's areas 17 to 19. Area 17 (which is also called striate c. or area because the line of Gennari is grossly visible on its surface) is the primary visual c., receiving the visual radiation from the lateral geniculate body of the thalamus. The surrounding areas 18 (parastriate c. or area) and 19 (peristriate c. or area) are probably involved in subsequent steps of visual information processing; area 18 is referred to as the secondary visual c. SYN visual area.

---

cor·tex·o·lone (kōr-teks′ō-lōn). 17α,21-dihydroxy-pregn-4-ene-4,20-dione; a mineralocorticoid hormone from the adrenal cortex.

cor·tex·one (kōr-teks′ōn). SYN deoxycorticosterone.

Corti, Marquis Alfonso, Italian anatomist, 1822–1888. SEE C.'s *arch, canal, cells,* under *cell, ganglion, membrane, organ, pillars,* under *pillar, rods,* under *rod,* auditory *teeth,* under *tooth, tunnel;* pillar *cells* of C., under *cell.*

cor·ti·cal (kōr′ti-kăl). Relating to a cortex.

cor·ti·cal·i·za·tion (kōr′ti-kăl-i-zā′shŭn). In phylogenesis, the migration of function from subcortical centers to the cortex. SYN encephalization, telencephalization.

cor·ti·cal·os·te·ot·o·my (kōr′ti-kăl-os-tē-ot′ō-mē). An osteotomy through the cortex at the base of the dentoalveolar segment, which serves to weaken the resistance of the bone to the application of orthodontic forces.

cor·ti·cec·to·my (kōr-ti-sek′tō-mē). Removal of a specific portion of the cerebral cortex. [cortic- + G. *ektomē,* excision]

cor·ti·ces (kōr′ti-sēz). Plural of cortex.

cor·ti·cif·u·gal (kōr-ti-sif′yū-găl). Passing in a direction away from the outer surface; denoting especially nerve fibers conveying impulses away from the cerebral cortex. SYN corticoefferent, corticofugal. [L. *cortex,* rind, bark, + *fugio,* to flee]

cor·ti·cip·e·tal (kōr-ti-sip′e-tăl). Passing in a direction toward the outer surface; denoting nerve fibers conveying impulses toward the cerebral cortex. SYN corticoafferent. [L. *cortex,* rind, bark, + *peto,* to seek]

cor·ti·co·af·fer·ent (kōr′ti-kō-af′er-ent). SYN corticipetal.

cor·ti·co·bul·bar (kōr′ti-kō-bŭl′bar). Corticofugal fibers projecting to the rhombencephalon that terminate 1) directly on some motor cranial nerve nuclei, 2) in the reticular formation, and 3) on sensory relay nuclei, such as the cuneate nucleus and gracile nucleus and the spinal trigeminal nucleus.

cor·ti·co·cer·e·bel·lum (kor′ti-kō-ser-ĕ-bel′ŭm). SYN neocerebellum.

cor·ti·co·ef·fer·ent (kōr′ti-kō-ef′er-ent). SYN corticifugal.

cor·ti·cof·u·gal (kōr′ti-kō-fyū′găl). SYN corticifugal.

cor·ti·coid (kōr′ti-koyd). **1.** Having an action similar to that of a hormone of the adrenal cortex. **2.** Any substance exhibiting this action. **3.** SYN corticosteroid.

cor·ti·co·lib·er·in (kōr′ti-kō-lib′er-in). SYN corticotropin releasing *hormone.* SYN corticotropin releasing factor (1). [corticosteroid + L. *libero,* to free, + -in]

cor·ti·co·me·di·al (kōr′ti-kō-mē′dē-ăl). Cortical and medial; specifically used to refer to one of the two major cytological divisions of the amygdaloid complex. SEE *corpus* amygdaloideum.

cor·ti·co·ste·roid (kōr′ti-kō-stēr′oyd). A steroid produced by the adrenal cortex (*i.e.,* adrenal corticoid); a corticoid containing a steroid. SYN adrenocorticoid, corticoid (3), cortin.

cor·ti·cos·ter·one (kōr-ti-kos′ter-ōn). 11β,21-Dihydroxy-4-pregnene-3,20-dione; a corticosteroid that induces some deposition of glycogen in the liver, sodium conservation, and potassium excretion; the principal glucocortoid in the rat.

cor·ti·co·tha·lam·ic (kōr′ti-kō-thal′ă-mik). Pertaining to cortex and thalamus; the term is applied to fibers projecting from the cerebral cortex to the thalamus.

cor·ti·co·troph (kōr′ti-kō-trof). A cell of the adenohypophysis that produces adrenocorticotropic hormone (ACTH).

cor·ti·co·tro·pin (kōr′ti-kō-trō′pin). **1.** SYN adrenocorticotropic *hormone.* **2.** SYN β-corticotropin. [G. *tropē,* a turning]

c.-zinc hydroxide, purified c. absorbed on zinc hydroxide; same uses as c. but with a prolonged duration of action.

β-cor·ti·co·tro·pin. Acid- or pepsin-degraded β-corticotropin. SYN corticotropin (2).

Cor·ti·co·vir·i·dae (kōr′ti-kō-vir′i-dē). Provisional name for a family of nonenveloped, ether-sensitive bacterial viruses of me-

---

dium size, with a lipid-containing capsid and genome of cyclic, double-stranded DNA (MW 5×10^6), which accounts for about 12% of virion weight.

cor·tin (kōr′tin). SYN corticosteroid.

cor·ti·sol (kōr′ti-sol). SYN hydrocortisone.

c. acetate, SYN *hydrocortisone* acetate.

cor·ti·sone (kōr′ti-sōn). 17α,21-Dihydroxy-4-pregnene-3,11,20-trione; 17α-hydroxy-11-dehydrocorticosterone; a glucocorticoid not normally secreted in significant quantities by the human adrenal cortex. Endogenously, it is probably a metabolite of hydrocortisone but exhibits no biological activity until converted to hydrocortisone (cortisol); it acts upon carbohydrate metabolism and influences the nutrition and growth of connective (collagenous) tissues. SYN Wintersteiner compound F. [former acronym for corticosterone]

α-cor·tol (kōr′tol). 5β-Pregnane-3α,11β,17,20α,21-pentaol; the 5β enantiomer of α-allocortol; a reduction product of cortisone, present in the urine, differing from cortisone in that the three keto groups are reduced to hydroxyls.

β-cor·tol. α-Cortol with a 20β–OH group; the 5β enantiomer of β-allocortol, found in urine.

α-cor·to·lone (kōr′tŏ-lōn). 3α,17α,20α,21-Tetrahydroxy-5β-pregnane-11-one; the 5β enantiomer of α-allocortolone; a reduction product of cortisone, present in the urine, differing from cortisone in that two of the keto groups (at positions 3 and 20) are reduced to hydroxyls.

β-cor·to·lone. α-Cortolone with a 20β–OH group; the 5β enantiomer of β-allocortolone, found in urine.

co·run·dum (ko-rŭn′dŭm). Native crystalline aluminum oxide. [Hind. *kurand*]

cor·us·ca·tion (kōr-ŭs-kā′shŭn). Rarely used psychiatric term for a subjective sensation of a flash of light before the eyes. [L. *corusco,* to flash]

Corvisart des Marets, Baron Jean N., French clinician, 1755–1821. SEE Corvisart′s *facies.*

cor·yl·o·phy·line (kōr-il-ō-fī′lēn). SYN *glucose* oxidase.

co·rym·bi·form (kŏ-rim′bi-fōrm). Denoting the flower-like clustering configuration of skin lesions in granulomatous diseases (*e.g.,* syphilis, tuberculosis). [L. *corymbus,* cluster, garland]

cor·y·ne·bac·te·ria (kŏ-rī′nē-bak-tēr′ē-ă). Plural of corynebacterium.

cor·y·ne·bac·te·ri·o·phage (kŏ-rī′nē-bak-tēr′ē-ō-fāj). Any one of the bacteriophages specific for corynebacteria.

β c., a DNA-containing bacteriophage that induces toxigenicity in strains of *Corynebacterium diphtheriae* that are lysogenic for its prophage. SYN β phage.

Cor·y·ne·bac·te·ri·um (kŏ-rī′nē-bak-tēr′ē-ŭm). A genus of nonmotile (except for some plant pathogens), aerobic to anaerobic bacteria (family Corynebacteriaceae) containing irregularly staining, Gram-positive, straight to slightly curved, often club-shaped rods which, as a result of snapping division, show a picket fence arrangement. These organisms are widely distributed in nature. The best known species are parasites and pathogens of humans and domestic animals. The type species is *C. diphtheriae.* [G. *coryne,* a club, + *bacterium,* a small rod]

C. ac′nes, former name for *Propionibacterium acnes.*

C. bo′vis, a nonpathogenic species of bacteria found in freshly drawn cow′s milk.

C. diphthe′riae, a species that causes diphtheria and produces a powerful exotoxin causing degeneration of various tissues, notably myocardium, in man and experimental animals and catalyzes the ADP-ribosylation of elongation factor II; virulent strains of this organism are lysogenic; it is commonly found in membranes in the pharynx, larynx, trachea, and nose in cases of diphtheria; it is also found in apparently healthy pharynx and nose in carriers, and is occasionally found in the conjunctiva and in superficial wounds; it occasionally infects the nasal passages and wounds of horses; it is the type species of the genus *C.* SYN Klebs-Loeffler bacillus, Loeffler′s bacillus.

C. enzy′micum, a species found in human lungs, blood, and joints; pathogenic for laboratory animals.

C. e′qui, SYN *Rhodococcus equi.*

C. haemoly′ticum, former name for *Arcanobacterium haemolyticum.*

C. hofman′nii, former name for *C. pseudodiphtheriticum.*

C. kut′scheri, a species pathogenic to mice.

C. minutis′simum, a species that causes erythrasma in humans.

C. murisep′ticum, a species which causes septicemia in mice.

C. o′vis, former name for *C. pseudotuberculosis.*

C. par′vum, former name for *Propionibacterium acnes.*

C. pho′cae, a species found in an erysipelas occurring in the transition between the corium and the blubber of seals.

C. pseudodiphtherit′icum, a nonpathogenic species found in normal throats. SYN Hofmann′s bacillus.

C. pseudotuberculo′sis, a species found in necrotic areas in sheep kidney, in caseous lymphadenitis in sheep, and in ulcerative lesions in horses, cattle, and other warm-blooded animals. SYN Preisz-Nocard bacillus.

C. pyog′enes, a species which is probably the most frequently occurring pyogenic organism in cattle, swine, and sheep but which is not pathogenic for man; it produces a toxin and a heat-labile hemolysin and is frequently found alone, or with other bacteria, in a great variety of suppurative processes. SYN *Actinomyces pyogenes.*

C. rena′le, a species of bacteria which occurs in purulent infections of the urinary tract in cattle, sheep, horses, and dogs; is pathogenic to laboratory animals; causes ulcerative posthitis in sheep and goats.

C. stria′tum, a species found in nasal mucus and in the throat; also found in udders of cows with mastitis; pathogenic to laboratory animals.

C. xero′sis, a species found in normal and diseased conjunctiva; there is no evidence that this organism is pathogenic.

cor·y·ne·bac·te·ri·um, pl. **cor·y·ne·bac·te·ria** (kŏ-rī′nē-bak-tēr′ē-ŭm, -ă). A vernacular term used to refer to any member of the genus *Corynebacterium.*

co·ry·za (kŏ-rī′ză). SYN acute *rhinitis.* [G.]

allergic c., a rhinitis in an allergic individual due to the presence of an agent to which he is hypersensitive.

infectious c., an acute respiratory disease of chickens caused by the bacterium *Haemophilus paragallinarum* and characterized by nasal discharge, sneezing, and swelling of the face under the eyes; also occurs in pheasants, guinea fowl, and turkeys.

Co·ry·za·vi·rus (kŏ-rī′ză-vī′rŭs). Former name for *Rhinovirus.*

cos·me·sis (koz-mē′sis). A concern in therapeutics, especially in surgical operations, for the appearance of the patient; *i.e.,* a resort to an operation which will improve the appearance. [G. *kosmēsis,* an adorning, fr. *kosmeō,* to order, arrange, adorn, fr. *kosmos,* order]

cos·met·ic (koz-met′ik). **1.** Relating to cosmesis. **2.** Relating to the use of cosmetics.

cos·met·ics (koz-met′iks). Composite term for a variety of camouflages applied to the skin, lips, hair, and nails for purposes of beautifying in accordance with cultural dictates.

cos·mid (koz′mid). A recombinantly engineered plasmid, a circular DNA containing in order: a plasmid origin of replication and a drug-resistance marker, the *cos* (cohesive end) site from bacteriophage λ, and a fragment of eukaryotic DNA to be cloned; c.′s are constructed to permit cloning of fragments of up to about 40,000 base pairs in length, with one or more unique restriction sites being necessary to facilitate cloning.

cos·mo·pol·i·tan (koz-mō-pol′i-tan). In the biological sciences, a term denoting worldwide distribution. [G. *kosmos,* universe, + *polis,* city-state]

cos·ta, gen. and pl. **cos·tae** (kos′tă, -tē). **1** [NA]. SYN Rib. **2.** A rodlike internal supporting organelle that runs along the base of the undulating membrane of certain flagellate parasites such as *Trichomonas.* SYN basal rod. [L.]

c. cervica′lis [NA], SYN cervical *rib.*

cos′tae fluctuan′tes, SYN floating *ribs,* under *rib.*

cos′tae fluitan′tes [NA], SYN floating *ribs,* under *rib.*

cos′tae spu′riae [NA], SYN false *ribs,* under *rib.*

cos·tae ve′rae [NA], SYN true *ribs*, under *rib*.

cos·tal (kos′tăl). Relating to a rib.

cos·tal·gia (kos-tal′jē-ă). SYN pleurodynia. [L. *costa,* rib, + G. *algos,* pain]

cos·tec·to·my (kos-tek′tō-mē). Excision of a rib. [L. *costa,* rib, + G. *ektomē,* excision]

Costen, James B., U.S. otolaryngologist, 1895–1962. SEE C.'s *syndrome.*

cos·ti·car·ti·lage (kos-ti-kar′ti-lij). SYN costal *cartilage.*

cos·ti·form (kos′ti-fōrm). Rib-shaped. [L. *costa,* rib, + *forma,* form]

cos·tive (kos′tiv). Pertaining to or causing constipation. [contraction from L. *constipo,* to press together]

cos·tive·ness (kos′tiv-ness). SYN constipation.

△**costo-.** The ribs. [L. *costa,* rib]

cos·to·cen·tral (kos-tō-sen′trăl). SYN costovertebral.

cos·to·chon·dral (kos-tō-kon′drăl). Relating to the costal cartilages. SYN chondrocostal.

cos·to·chon·dri·tis (kos′tō-kon-drī′tis). Inflammation of one or more costal cartilages, characterized by local tenderness and pain of the anterior chest wall that may radiate, but without the local swelling typical of Tietze's syndrome. SYN costal chondritis. [costo- + G. *chondros,* cartilage, + *-itis,* inflammation]

cos·to·cla·vic·u·lar (kos-tō-klă-vik′yū-lăr). Relating to the ribs and the clavicle.

cos·to·cor·a·coid (kos-tō-kōr′ă-koyd). Relating to the ribs and the coracoid process of the scapula.

cos·to·gen·ic (kos-tō-jen′ik). Arising from a rib.

cos·to·in·fe·ri·or (kos-tō-in-fēr′ē-ōr). Relating to the lower ribs.

cos·to·scap·u·lar (kos-tō-skap′yū-lăr). Relating to the ribs and the scapula.

cos·to·sca·pu·la·ris (kos-tō-skap-yū-lā′ris). SYN serratus anterior *muscle.*

cos·to·ster·nal (kos-tō-ster′năl). Pertaining to the ribs and the sternum.

cos·to·ster·no·plas·ty (kos-tō-ster′nō-plas-tē). Operation to correct a malformation of the anterior chest wall. [costo- + G. *sternon,* chest, + *plastos,* formed]

cos·to·su·pe·ri·or (kos-tō-sū-pēr′ē-ōr). Relating to the upper ribs.

cos·to·tome (kos′tō-tōm). An instrument, knife or shears, designed for cutting through a rib.

cos·tot·o·my (kos-tot′ō-mē). Division of a rib. [costo- + G. *tomē,* a cutting]

cos·to·trans·verse (kos-tō-trans-vers′). Relating to the ribs and the transverse processes of the vertebrae articulating with them. SYN transversocostal.

cos·to·trans·ver·sec·to·my (kos′tō-tranz-ver-sek′tō-mē). Excision of a proximal portion of a rib and the articulating transverse process.

cos·to·ver·te·bral (kos-tō-ver′tĕ-brăl). Relating to the ribs and the bodies of the thoracic vertebrae with which they articulate. SYN costocentral, vertebrocostal (1).

cos·to·xi·phoid (kos-tō-zī′foyd). Relating to the ribs and the xiphoid cartilage of the sternum.

co·sub·strate (kō-sŭb′strāt). The second or other substrate of a multisubstrate enzyme; often, specifically refers to the coenzyme.

co·syn·tro·pin (kō-sin-trō′pin). α^{ACTH}; ^{24}- or β^{1-24}-corticotropin; tetracosactrin; a synthetic corticotrophic agent, comprising the first 24 amino acid residues of human ACTH, which sequence is found in several other species and which retains the full biologic activity of the complete ACTH; the remaining 15 residues differ among species and confer specific immunologic properties. SYN tetracosactide, tetracosactin.

Cotard, Jules, French neurologist, 1840–1887. SEE C.'s *syndrome.*

co·tar·nine (kō-tar′nēn). An alkaloidal principle, $C_{12}H_{15}NO_4$, derived from narcotine by oxidation; an astringent. [anagram of *narcotine*]

COTe Abbreviation of cathodal opening tetanus.

co·ti·nine (kō′ti-nēn). 1-Methyl-5-(3-pyridyl)-2-pyrrolidinone; one of the major detoxication products of nicotine; eliminated rapidly and completely by the kidneys. [anagram of *nicotine*]

co·trans·la·tion·al (kō′tranz-lā′shun-ăl). Any process involving the maturation or delivery of a protein that occurs during the process of translation.

co·trans·port (kō-trans′pōrt). The transport of one substance across a membrane, coupled with the simultaneous transport of another substance across the same membrane in the same direction.

Cotte, Gaston, French surgeon, 1879–1951. SEE C.'s *operation.*

Cotton, Frank A., U.S. chemist, *1930. SEE C. *effect.*

cot·ton (kot′ŭn). The white, fluffy, fibrous covering of the seeds of a plant of the genus *Gossypium* (family Malvaceae); used extensively in surgical dressings. [Ar. *qútun*]

absorbent c., c. from which all fatty matter has been extracted, so that it readily takes up fluids.

purified c., absorbent c. in which the hairs of the seed of varieties of *Gossypium* and other allied species are freed from adhering impurities, deprived of fatty matter, bleached, and sterilized; used for tampons, etc.

soluble gun c., SYN pyroxylin.

styptic c., absorbent c. wet with a dilute solution of ferric chloride, and then dried; applied locally as a hemostatic.

cot·ton·pox (kot′ŭn-poks). Obsolete name for *variola* minor.

cot·ton·seed oil (kot′ŭn-sēd). The refined fixed oil obtained from the seed of cultivated plants of various varieties of *Gossypium hirsutum* or of other species of *Gossypium* (family Malvaceae); a solvent.

Cotunnius (Cotugno), Domenico, Italian anatomist, 1736–1822. SEE C.'s *aqueduct, canal;* C. *disease;* C.'s *liquid, space; aqueductus* cotunnii; *liquor* cotunnii.

cot·y·le (kot′i-lē). 1. Any cup-shaped structure. 2. SYN acetabulum. [G. *kotylē,* anything hollow, the cup or socket of a joint]

cot·y·le·don (kot-i-lē′don). 1. SEE maternal c., fetal c. 2. In plants, a seed leaf, the first leaf to grow from a seed. 3. A placental unit. SEE maternal c. [G. *kotylēdon,* any cup-shaped hollow]

fetal c., a unit of the fetal placenta supplied by the vessels of a stem villus; several such c.'s may occur between two placental septa; traditionally called embryologists' c.

maternal c., a unit of the placenta made up of trophoblastic cells, fibrous tissue, and abundant blood vessels, which is visible grossly on the maternal surface as an irregularly shaped lobe circumscribed by a deep cleft and made up of a stem villus with numerous branching free villi and anchoring villi; placental vessels in the chorionic plate supply the stem villus and its branches, allowing gas and metabolite exchange across the trophoblastic layer with maternal blood in the intervillous space; traditionally called clinicians' c.

Cot·y·lo·gon·i·mus (kot-i-lō-gon′i-mŭs). A group of heterophyid flukes, now properly included in the genus *Heterophyes.* [G. *kotylē,* cup, + *gonimos,* productive]

cot·y·loid (kot′i-loyd). 1. Cup-shaped; cuplike. 2. Relating to the cotyloid cavity or acetabulum. [G. *kotylē,* a small cup, + *eidos,* appearance]

couch·ing (kowch′ing). An obsolete operation for cataract, consisting of displacement of the lens into the vitreous cavity out of the line of vision. [Fr. *coucher,* to lay down, to put to bed]

cough (kawf). 1. A sudden explosive forcing of air through the glottis, occurring immediately on opening the previously closed glottis, and excited by mechanical or chemical irritation of the trachea or bronchi, or by pressure from adjacent structures. 2. To force air through the glottis by a series of expiratory efforts. [echoic]

aneurysmal c., c. due to impingement of an aortic aneurysm on the recurrent laryngeal nerve or other nearby structures.

brassy c., loud metallic barking c. caused by subglottic edema.

kennel c., an imprecise term which has been used for a number of diseases in dogs which are characterized by bronchitis and caused by a variety of infectious agents.

CO

privet c., an allergic c., occurring in China during May and June, supposed to be caused by inhalation of the pollen of a species of privet (*Lingustrum*); it is analogous to the laurel fever seen in New England.

reflex c., a c. excited reflexly by irritation in some distant part, as the ear or the stomach.

weaver's c., obsolete term for c., dyspnea, and sense of constriction of the chest, caused in persons working with mildewed yarns.

whooping c., SYN pertussis.

cou·lomb (C, Q) (kū-lom'). The unit of electrical charge, equal to 3×10^9 electrostatic units; the quantity of electricity delivered by a current of 1 ampere in 1 second; equal to 1/96,485 faraday. [C. A. de *Coulomb*, Fr. physicist, 1736–1806]

cou·mar·a·none (kū-mar'ă-nōn). 3(2*H*)-Benzofuranone; the basis of many plant products; *e.g.,* aurone.

cou·ma·ric an·hy·dride (kū-mā'rik). SYN coumarin.

cou·ma·rin (kū'mă-rin). *ortho*-oxycinnamic anhydride; 2*H*-1-benzopyran-2-one; a fragrant neutral principle obtained from the Tonka bean, *Dypterix odorata,* and made synthetically from salicylic aldehyde; it is used to disguise unpleasant odors. SYN coumaric anhydride, cumarin. [*coumarou,* native name of Tonka bean]

cou·met·a·rol (kū-met'ă-rol). 3,3'-(2-methoxyethylidene)bis(4-hydroxycoumarin); an oral anticoagulant. SYN cumetharol, cumethoxaethane.

Councilman, William T., U.S. pathologist, 1854–1933. SEE C. *body;* C.'s *lesion.*

Coun·cil·ma·nia (kown-sil-man'ē-ă). Obsolete generic term for a group of amebas now recognized as *Entamoeba.* [W. Councilman]

coun·sel·ing (kown'sel-ing). A professional relationship and activity in which one person endeavors to help another to understand and to solve his or her adjustment problems; the giving of advice, opinion, and instruction to direct the judgment or conduct of another. SEE psychotherapy. [L. *consilium,* deliberation]

genetic c., the process whereby an expert in hereditary disorders provides information about risk and clinical burden of a disorder or disorders to patients or relatives in families with genetic disorders as an aid to making informed and responsible decisions about marriage, children, early diagnosis, and handling disability.

marital c., the process whereby a trained counselor assists married couples to resolve problems that arise and trouble them in their relationship; husband and wife are seen by the same counselor in separate and joint c. sessions focusing on immediate family problems.

pastoral c., the use of psychotherapeutic methods by members of the clergy, members of a religious community, and/or lay therapists for parishioners seeking help with personal problems.

count (kownt). 1. A reckoning, enumeration, or accounting. 2. To enumerate or score.

Addis c., a quantitative enumeration of the red blood c., white blood c., and casts in a 12-hr urine specimen; used to follow the progress of known renal disease.

Arneth c., the percentage distribution of polymorphonuclear neutrophils, based on the number of lobes in the nuclei (from 1 to 5). SEE ALSO Arneth *index.*

blood c., SEE blood count.

epidermal ridge c., an index of the frequency of sweat pores on the fingertips by enumeration along a set of arbitrarily defined lines; a classic example of a galtonian trait determined almost exclusively by genetic factors.

filament-nonfilament c., a differential c. of the number of neutrophils showing nuclear division and those showing no such division.

total cell c., number of cells in a given area or volume.

viable cell c., number of cells in a given area or volume that are thriving.

count·er (kown'ter). A device that counts.

automated differential leukocyte c., an instrument using digital imaging or cytochemical techniques to differentiate leukocytes.

electronic cell c., an automatic blood cell c. in which cells passing through an aperture alter resistance and are counted as voltage pulses, or in which cells passing through a flow cell deflect light; some types of c. are capable of multiple simultaneous measurements on each blood sample; *e.g.,* leukocyte count, red cell count, hemoglobin, hematocrit, and red cell indices.

Geiger-Müller c., an instrument for measuring radioactivity by counting the emission of radioactive particles; it consists of a metallic cylinder, negatively charged, in a tube containing a fine, positively charged wire at its center; radiations produce ionization of the gas molecules between the cylinder and the wire and result in an electrical discharge independent of the energy of the impinging particle or ray.

proportional c., a Geiger-Müller c. operating in the voltage range and under conditions in which pulse height is proportional to the energy of the particles or rays being counted, thus making discrimination between particles or rays of different energies possible.

scintillation c., an instrument used for the detection of radioactivity; the radiation is absorbed by a scintillator (a crystal or a compound, such as POPOP, in solution) which results in minute flashes of light that are detected by a photocathode. The resultant electron emission is amplified by a photomultiplier and an amplifier. SYN scintillometer, spinthariscope.

well c., a scintillation crystal shaped with a central hole to receive a small sample, plus associated detector and electronics.

whole-body c., shielding and instrumentation, usually involving more than one detector, designed to evaluate the total-body burden of various gamma-emitting nuclides.

⟳counter-. Opposite, opposed, against. SEE ALSO contra-. [L. *contra,* against]

count·er·bal·anc·ing (kown-ter-bal'ăn-sing). A procedure in behavioral research for distributing unwanted but unavoidable influences equally among the different experimental conditions or subjects.

count·er·con·di·tion·ing (kown'ter-kon-dish'ŭn-ing). Any of a group of specific behavior therapy techniques in which a second conditioned response (*e.g.,* approaching or even touching a snake) is introduced for the express purpose of counteracting or nullifying a previously conditioned or learned response (fear and avoidance of snakes).

count·er·cur·rent (kown'ter-ker'ent). 1. Flowing in an opposite direction. 2. A current flowing in a direction opposite to another current.

count·er·cur·rent ex·chang·er. A system in which heat or chemicals passively diffuse across a membrane separating two c. e. streams so that at each end the fluid leaving along one side of the membrane nearly resembles, in temperature or composition, the fluid entering the other; *e.g.,* the venae comites in the arms serve as a c. e. exchanger, the arterial blood serving to rewarm the cooler venous blood.

count·er·cur·rent mul·ti·pli·er. A system in which energy is used to transport material across a membrane separating two c. m. tubes connected at one end to form a hairpin shape; by this means a concentration can be achieved in the fluid in the hairpin bend, relative to the inflow and outflow fluids, that is much greater than the transport mechanism could produce between the two sides of the membrane at any point; *e.g.,* the nephronic loops in the renal medulla act as c. m.'s.

count·er·die (kown'ter-dī). The reverse image of a die, usually made of a softer and lower fusing metal than the die.

count·er·ex·ten·sion (kown'ter-eks-ten'shŭn). SYN countertraction.

count·er·im·mu·no·e·lec·tro·pho·re·sis (kown'ter-im'yū-nō-ē-lek'trō-fō-rē'sis). A modification of immunoelectrophoresis in which antigen (*e.g.,* serum containing hepatitis B virus) is placed in wells cut in the sheet of agar gel toward the cathode, and antiserum is placed in wells toward the anode; antigen and antibody, moving in opposite directions, form precipitates in the area between the cells where they meet in concentrations of optimal proportions.

count·er·in·ci·sion (kown'ter-in-sizh'ŭn). A second incision adjacent to a primary incision.

count·er·in·vest·ment (kown′ter-in-vest′ment). SYN anticathexis.

count·er·ir·ri·tant (kown-ter-ir′i-tant). **1.** An agent that causes irritation or a mild inflammation of the skin in order to relieve symptoms of a deep-seated inflammatory process. **2.** Relating to or producing counterirritation.

count·er·ir·ri·ta·tion (kown′ter-ir-i-tā′shŭn). Irritation or mild inflammation (redness, vesication, or pustulation) of the skin excited for the purpose of relieving symptoms of an inflammation of the deeper structures. SYN revulsion (1).

count·er·o·pen·ing (kown′ter-ō-pen-ing). A second opening made at the dependent part of an abscess or other cavity containing fluid, which is not draining satisfactorily through an opening previously made. SYN contra-aperture, counterpuncture.

count·er·pho·bic (kown-ter-fō′bik). **1.** Denoting a state of actual preference, on the part of a phobic person, for the very situation of which he is afraid. **2.** Opposed to the phobic impulse, as in c. mastery of a feared action by repeated engagement in the action.

count·er·pul·sa·tion (kown′ter-pŭl-sā′shŭn). A means of assisting the failing heart by automatically removing arterial blood just before and during ventricular ejection and returning it to the circulation during diastole; a balloon catheter is inserted into the aorta and activated by an automatic mechanism triggered by the ECG.

intra-aortic balloon c., rhythmic inflation and deflation of a catheter-borne balloon placed in the aorta distal to the aortic valve to facilitate ejection during systole and to limit regurgitation during diastole by the appropriate application of pressures. Usually an emergency treatment for cardiogenic shock or for intractable angina.

count·er·punc·ture (kown′ter-pŭnk-chūr). SYN counteropening.

count·er·shock (kown′ter-shok). An electric shock applied to the heart to terminate a disturbance of its rhythm.

count·er·stain (kown′ter-stān). A second stain of different color, having affinity for tissues, cells, or parts of cells other than those taking the primary stain, used to render more distinct the parts taking the first stain.

count·er·trac·tion (kown-ter-trak′shŭn). The resistance, or back-pull, made to traction or pulling on a limb; *e.g.,* in the case of traction made on the leg, c. may be effected by raising the foot of the bed so that the weight of the body pulls against the weight attached to the limb. SYN counterextension.

count·er·trans·fer·ence (kown′ter-trans-fer′ens). In psychoanalysis, the analyst's transference (often unconscious) toward the patient of his emotional needs and feelings, with personal involvement to the detriment of the desired objective analyst-patient relationship.

count·er·trans·port (kown-ter-tranz′pōrt). The transport of one substance across a membrane, coupled with the simultaneous transport of another substance across the same membrane in the opposite direction.

coup de sa·bre (kū-dĕ-sahb′). Linear scleroderma found over the scalp with scarring alopecia, face, or forehead. [Fr. stroke of a sword]

cou·ple (kŭ′pl). To copulate; to perform coitus; said especially of the lower animals.

cou·pling (kŭp′ling). **1.** Usually the result of the repeated pairing of a normal sinus beat with a ventricular extrasystole. **2.** SEE coupling *phase.* **3.** A condition in which one or more products of a reaction are the subsequent reactants (or substrates) of a second reaction.

constant c., SYN fixed c.

fixed c., where several premature beats are seen, the interval between each of them and the preceding normal beat is constant. SYN constant c.

variable c., where several extrasystoles are seen, the interval between each of them and the preceding sinus beat varies.

Courvoisier, Ludwig G., French surgeon, 1843–1918. SEE C.'s *law, sign, gallbladder.*

cou·vade (kū-vahd′). A primitive custom in certain cultures in which a man develops labor pains while his wife is in labor and then submits to the same postpartum purification rites and taboos. [Fr. *couver,* to hatch]

Couvelaire, Alexandre, French obstetrician, 1873–1948. SEE C. *uterus.*

cou·ver·cle (kū-ver′kl). Rarely used term for an external coagulum, especially a blood clot formed extravascularly. [Fr. cover, lid]

co·va·lent (kō-vāl′ent). Denoting an interatomic bond characterized by the sharing of 2, 4, or 6 electrons.

cov·er·age. A measure of the extent to which the services rendered cover the potential need for these services in a community; applied specifically to such services as immunization in developing countries.

cov·er·ing (kov′er-ing). A surrounding layer; something that covers or encloses, forming an outer layer. SEE ALSO tunica.

c.'s of spermatic cord, c.'s of the spermatic cord, including external and internal spermatic fasciae, and cremasteric muscle and fascia. SYN tunicae funiculi spermatici [NA].

cov·er·slip (kŭv′er-slip). SYN cover *glass.*

cow (kow). **1.** A generator for short-lived isotopes based upon successively eluting or otherwise separating ("milking") a short-lived radioactive daughter from a longer-lived parent; *e.g.,* ^{99m}Tc from ^{99}Mo, ^{113m}In from ^{113}Sn. **2.** The mature female of domestic cattle (genus *Bos*); also the mature female of certain other animals such as buffalo, elephant, and whale.

downer c., a recumbent c. that has failed to respond to treatment for its disease.

Cowden. Surname of the family from which the condition subsequently known as Cowden's *disease* was first reported.

Cow·dria ru·mi·nan·ti·um (kow′drē-ă rū-mi-nan′tē-ŭm). The rickettsial species causing heartwater in cattle, sheep, and goats in Sub-Saharan Africa and several islands in the Indian and Atlantic Oceans and in the Caribbean, transmitted by ticks of the genus *Amblyomma.* [E.V. *Cowdry*]

cow·dri·o·sis (kow-drē-ō′sis). SYN heartwater.

Cowdry, Edmund Vincent, U.S. cytologist, 1888–1975. SEE C.'s type A inclusion *bodies,* under *body,* type B inclusion *bodies,* under *body.*

cowl. SEE caul.

Cowling's rule. See under rule.

Cowper, William, English anatomist, 1666–1709. SEE cowperitis; C.'s *cyst, gland, ligament.*

cow·per·i·an (kow-pēr′ē-an). Relating to or described by Cowper.

cow·per·i·tis (kow-per-ī′tis). Inflammation of Cowper's gland.

cow·pox (kow′poks). A disease of milk cows, usually confined to the udder and teats, caused by the cowpox virus, a member of the family Poxviridae, but clinically indistinguishable from bovine vaccinia mammillitis caused by the vaccinia virus.

coxa, gen. and pl. **cox·ae** (kok′să, -sē). **1.** SYN hip *bone.* **2.** SYN hip *joint.* [L]

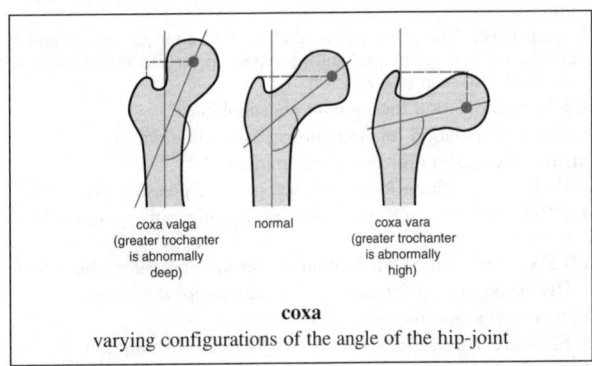

coxa valga (greater trochanter is abnormally deep)   normal   coxa vara (greater trochanter is abnormally high)

coxa
varying configurations of the angle of the hip-joint

c. adduc′ta, SYN c. vara.

false c. va′ra, approximation of the head of the femur to the shaft, due not to deformity of the neck of the femur, but to curvature of the shaft.

c. mag′na, enlargement and often deformation of femoral head; usually refers to a sequela of Legg-Calvé-Perthes disease or osteoarthritis.

c. pla′na, SYN Legg-Calvé-Perthes *disease*.

c. val′ga, alteration of the angle made by the axis of the femoral neck to the axis of the femoral shaft, so that the angle exceeds 135°; the femoral neck is in more of a straight-line relationship to the shaft of the femur.

c. va′ra, alteration of the angle made by the axis of the femoral neck to the axis of the femoral shaft so that the angle is less than 135°; the femoral neck becomes more horizontal. SYN c. adducta.

c. va′ra lux′ans, c. vara with dislocation of the femoral head.

cox·al·gia (koks-al′jē-ă). SYN coxodynia. [L. *coxa,* hip, + G. *algos,* pain]

Cox·i·el·la (kok-sē-el′ă). A genus of filterable bacteria (order Rickettsiales) containing small, pleomorphic, rod-shaped or coccoid, Gram-negative cells which occur intracellularly in the cytoplasm of infected cells and possibly extracellularly in infected ticks. These organisms have not been cultivated in cell-free media; they are parasitic on man and other animals. The type species is *C. burnetii.* [H. R. *Cox,* U.S. bacteriologist, *1907]

C. burnet′ii, a species that causes Q fever in man; it is more resistant than other rickettsiae and may be passed via aerosols as well as living vectors. Acute pneumonia and chronic endocarditis are also associated with this species. The type species of the genus *Coxiella.*

cox·i·tis (koks-ī′tis). Inflammation of the hip.

cox·o·dyn·ia (koks-ō-din′ē-ă). Pain in the hip joint. SYN coxalgia. [L. *coxa,* hip, + G. *odynē,* pain]

cox·o·fem·o·ral (kok-sō-fem′ŏ-răl). Relating to the hip bone and the femur.

cox·ot·o·my (koks-ot′ŏ-mē). Obsolete term for incision into the hip joint. [L. *coxa,* hip, + G. *tomē,* cutting]

cox·o·tu·ber·cu·lo·sis (koks′ō-tū-ber-kyū-lō′sis). Tuberculous hip-joint disease.

Cox·sack·ie·vi·rus (kok-sax′ē-vī′rŭs). A group of picornaviruses, included in the genus *Enterovirus,* of spherical shape and about 28 nm in diameter, causing myositis, paralysis, and death in young mice, and responsible for a variety of diseases in man, although inapparent infections are common. They are divided antigenically into two groups, A and B, each of which includes a number of serological types, *e.g., Enterovirus* coxsackie A1 to 24 and *Enterovirus* coxsackie B1 to 6. Type A viruses cause human herpangina and hand-foot-and-mouth disease; type B viruses cause epidemic pleurodynia; both type viruses may cause aseptic meningitis, myocarditis and pericarditis, and acute onset juvenile diabetes. [*Coxsackie,* N.Y., where first isolated]

co·zy·mase (kō-zī′mās). Former name for nicotinamide adenine dinucleotide.

c.p. Abbreviation for chemically pure.

CPAP Abbreviation for continuous positive airway *pressure.*

CPEO Acronym for chronic progressive external *ophthalmoplegia.*

C-pep·tide. The 30 amino-acid chain that connects the A and B chains of insulin in proinsulin; removed in the conversion of proinsulin to insulin. SYN C chain.

CPK Abbreviation for *creatine* phosphokinase.

CPM Abbreviation for continuous passive *motion.*

cpm Abbreviation for counts per minute.

CPPB Abbreviation for continuous positive pressure *breathing.*

CPPD Abbreviation for calcium pyrophosphate deposition *disease.*

CPPV Abbreviation for continuous positive pressure *ventilation.*

CPR Abbreviation for cardiopulmonary *resuscitation.*

cps Abbreviation for cycles per second.

CR Abbreviation for conditioned *reflex;* crown-rump *length.*

Cr 1. Symbol for chromium. **2.** Abbreviation for creatinine.

crab (krab). **1.** A crustacean, many varieties of which are edible. **2.** An insect, the crab louse, *Pthirus pubis.*

Crabtree, Herbert G., 20th century English physician and biochemist. SEE C. *effect.*

crack. A derivative of cocaine, usually smoked, resulting in a brief, intense high. C. is relatively inexpensive and extremely addictive. [slang]

crac·kle (krak′l). Short, sharp, or rough sounds heard with a stethoscope over the chest. Most often heard in pleurisy with fibrinous exudate. [echoic]

cra·dle (krā′dl). A frame used to keep bedclothes from coming in contact with an injured patient. [M.E. *cradel*]

Crafoord, Clarence, Swedish surgeon, *1899. SEE C. *clamp.*

Craig·ia (krā′gē-ă). Obsolete generic term for a group of amebas now recognized as *Entamoeba.* [C. *Craig*]

Cramer, Friedrich, German surgeon, 1847–1903. SEE C. wire *splint.*

cramp (kramp). **1.** A painful muscle spasm caused by prolonged tetanic contraction. **2.** A localized muscle spasm related to occupational use, qualified according to the occupation of the sufferer; *e.g.,* seamstress's c., writer's c. [M.E. *crampe,* fr. O. Fr., fr. Germanic]

accessory c., SYN torticollis.

heat c.'s, muscle spasms induced by severe exertion in intense heat, accompanied by considerable pain; sometimes related to salt deficiency, hyperventilation, or overindulgence in alcohol. SYN myalgia thermica.

intermittent c., (1) SYN tetany. (2) SYN benign *tetanus.*

miner's c.'s, c.'s caused by excessive salt loss through perspiration. SYN stoker's c.'s.

musician's c., an occupational dystonia, affecting those who play on musical instruments, and named usually according to the instrument played upon.

pianist's c., piano-player's c., an occupational dystonia affecting the muscles of the fingers and forearms in piano players.

Scotch c., SYN recurrent *tetany.*

seamstress's c., an occupational dystonia occurring in the fingers of women who sew. SYN sewing spasm.

shaving c., an occupational dystonia affecting the hands and fingers of barbers. SYN keirospasm, xyrospasm.

stoker's c.'s, SYN miner's c.'s.

tailor's c., an occupational dystonia affecting the forearms and hands of tailors. SYN tailor's spasm.

typist's c., an occupational dystonia affecting chiefly the long flexor muscles of the hands of typists.

violinist's c., a occupational dystonia affecting the digits of the fingering hand, or sometimes the bowing arm, in violin players.

waiter's c., an occupational dystonia characterized by spasm of the muscles of the back and dominant arm in persons who wait tables.

watchmaker's c., an occupational dystonia characterized by spasm of the orbicularis palpebrarum muscle from holding the lens to the eye and spasm of the muscles of the hand from performing the delicate movements of watch repairing.

writer's c., an occupation dystonia affecting chiefly the muscles of the thumb and two adjoining fingers of the writing hand, induced by excessive use of a writing instrument. SYN dysgraphia (2), graphospasm, mogigraphia, scrivener's palsy.

Crampton, Charles Ward, U.S. physician, *1877. SEE C. *test.*

Crampton, Sir Philip, Irish surgeon, 1777–1858. SEE C.'s *line, muscle.*

Crandall's syn·drome. See under syndrome.

crani-. SEE cranio-.

cra·nia (krā′nē-ă). Plural of cranium.

cra·ni·ad (krā′nē-ad). Situated nearer the head in relation to a specific reference point; opposite of caudad. SEE ALSO superior.

cra·ni·al (krā′nē-ăl). **1.** Relating to the cranium or head. SYN cranialis [NA], cephalic. SEE ALSO cephalad. **2.** SYN superior (2).

cra·ni·a·lis (krā-nē-ā′lis) [NA]. SYN cranial (1).

cra·ni·am·phit·o·my (krā-nē-am-fit′ō-mē). A decompression operation in which the entire circumference of the calvarium is divided. [G. *kranion*, skull, + *amphi*, around, + *tomē*, cutting]

Cra·ni·a·ta (krā-nē-ā'tă). SYN Vertebrata. [Mediev. L. *cranium*, fr. G. *kranion*, skull]

cra·ni·ec·to·my (krā-nē-ek'tō-mē). Excision of a portion of the skull, without replacement of the bone, *e.g.*, subtemporal or suboccipital. [G. *kranion*, skull, + *ektomē*, excision]

linear c., production of an artificial cranial suture.

△**cranio-, crani-.** The cranium. Cf. cerebro-. [G. *kranion*, skull]

cra·ni·o·au·ral (krā'nē-ō-aw'răl). Relating to the skull and the ear.

cra·ni·o·cele (krā'nē-ō-sēl). SYN encephalocele. [cranio- + G. *kēlē*, hernia]

cra·ni·o·ce·re·bral (krā'nē-ō-ser'ē-brăl). Relating to the skull and the brain.

cra·ni·o·cla·sia, cra·ni·o·cla·sis (krā-nē-ō-klā'sē-ă, krā-nē-ok'lă-sis). Formerly used operation for crushing of the fetal skull in cases of dystocia. [cranio- + G. *klasis*, a breaking]

cra·ni·o·clast (krā'nē-ō-klast). Instrument like a strong forceps formerly used for crushing and extracting the fetal head after perforation. [cranio- + G. *klaō*, to break in pieces]

cra·ni·o·clei·do·dys·os·to·sis (krā'nē-ō-klī'dō-dis-os-tō'sis). SYN cleidocranial *dysostosis*. [cranio- + G. *kleis*, clavicle, + dysostosis]

cra·ni·o·did·y·mus (krā'nē-ō-did'i-mŭs). Conjoined twins with fused bodies but with two heads. SEE conjoined *twins*, under *twin*. [cranio- + G. *didymos*, twin]

cra·ni·o·fa·cial (krā'nē-ō-fā'shăl). Relating to both the face and the cranium.

cra·ni·o·fe·nes·tria (krā'nē-ō-fe-nes'trē-ă). SYN craniolacunia. [cranio- + L. *fenestra*, window]

cra·ni·og·no·my (krā-nē-og'nō-mē). SYN phrenology. [cranio- + G. *gnōme*, judgment]

cra·ni·o·graph (krā'nē-ō-graf). An instrument for making drawings to scale of the diameters and general configuration of the skull.

cra·ni·og·ra·phy (krā-nē-og'ră-fē). The art of representing, by drawings made from measurements, the configuration of the skull and the relations of its angles and craniometric points. [cranio- + G. *graphō*, to write]

cra·ni·o·la·cu·nia (krā'nē-ō-lă-kū'nē-ă). Incomplete formation of the bones of the vault of the fetal skull so that there are nonossified areas in the calvaria. SYN craniofenestria. [cranio- + L. *lacuna*, cleft]

cra·ni·ol·o·gy (krā-nē-ol'ō-jē). The science concerned with variations in size, shape, and proportion of the cranium, especially with the variations characterizing the different races of humans. [cranio- + G. *logos*, study]

Gall's c., SYN phrenology.

cra·ni·o·ma·la·cia (krā'nē-ō-mă-lā'shē-ă). Softening of the bones of the skull. [cranio- + G. *malakia*, softness]

circumscribed c., SYN craniotabes.

cra·ni·o·me·nin·go·cele (krā'nē-ō-mě-ning'gō-sēl). Protrusion of the meninges through a defect in the skull. [cranio- + G. *mēninx*, membrane, + *kēlē*, hernia]

cra·ni·om·e·ter (krā-nē-om'ě-ter). An instrument for measuring the diameters of the skull.

cra·ni·o·met·ric (krā-nē-ō-met'rik). Relating to craniometry.

cra·ni·om·e·try (krā-nē-om'ě-trē). Measurement of the dry skull after removal of the soft parts, and study of its topography. [cranio- + G. *metron*, measure]

cra·ni·op·a·gus (krā-nē-op'ă-gŭs). Conjoined twins with fused skulls. SEE conjoined *twins*, under *twin*. SEE ALSO janiceps, syncephalus. [cranio- + G. *pagos*, something fixed]

c. occipita'lis, conjoined twins united at the occipital region of the skull. SYN iniopagus.

c. parasit'icus, a variety of c. in which one fetus is rudimentary in form and parasitic on the other. SEE ALSO epicomus.

cra·ni·op·a·thy (krā-nē-op'ă-thē). Any pathological condition of the cranial bones. [cranio- + G. *pathos*, suffering]

metabolic c., SYN Morgagni's *syndrome*.

cra·ni·o·pha·ryn·ge·al (krā'nē-ō-fă-rin'jē-ăl). Relating to the skull and to the pharynx.

cra·ni·o·pha·ryn·gi·o·ma (krā'nē-ō-fă-rin-jē-ō'mă). A suprasellar neoplasm, usually cystic, that develops from the nests of epithelium derived from Rathke's pouch; the histologic pattern, similar to that observed in adamantinomas, consists of nesting of squamous epithelium bordered by radially arranged cells; frequently accompanied by calcium deposition. SYN Erdheim tumor, pituitary adamantinoma, pituitary ameloblastoma, Rathke's pouch tumor, suprasellar cyst. [cranio- + pharyngio- + -oma]

ameloblastomatous c., a form of c. resembling an ameloblastoma.

cystic papillomatous c., a form of c. characterized by large cysts within which are fungating, irregular outgrowths of stratified squamous epithelium.

cra·ni·o·phore (krā'nē-ō-fōr). An apparatus for holding a skull while its angles and diameters are measured. [cranio- + G. *phoros*, bearing]

cra·ni·o·plas·ty (krā'nē-ō-plas-tē). Plastic surgery of the skull; a surgical correction of a skull defect. [cranio- + G. *plastos*, formed]

cra·ni·o·punc·ture (krā'nē-ō-pŭnk'chūr). Puncture of the brain for exploratory purposes.

cra·ni·or·rha·chid·i·an (krā'nē-ō-ră-kid'ē-an). SYN craniospinal. [cranio- + G. *rhachis*, spine]

cra·ni·or·rha·chis·chi·sis (krā'nē-ō-ră-kis'ki-sis). Severe congenital malformation in which there is incomplete closure of the skull and spinal column. [cranio- + G. *rhachis*, spine, + *schisis*, a cleaving]

cra·ni·o·sa·cral (krā'nē-ō-sā'krăl). Denoting the cranial and sacral origins of the parasympathetic division of the autonomic nervous system.

cra·ni·os·chi·sis (krā-nē-os'ki-sis). Congenital malformation in which there is incomplete closure of the skull. Usually accompanied by grossly defective development of the brain. [cranio- + G. *schisis*, a cleavage]

cra·ni·o·scle·ro·sis (krā'nē-ō-skler-ō'sis). Thickening of the skull. [cranio- + G. *sklēros*, hard, + -*osis*, condition]

cra·ni·os·co·py (krā-nē-os'kŏ-pē). Examination of the skull in the living subject for craniometric or diagnostic purposes. [cranio- + G. *skopeō*, to view]

cra·ni·o·spi·nal (krā'nē-ō-spī'năl). Relating to the cranium and spinal column. SYN craniorrhachidian.

cra·ni·o·ste·no·sis (krā'nē-ō-sten-ō'sis). Premature closure of cranial sutures resulting in malformation of the skull. [cranio- + G. *stenōsis*, a narrowing]

cra·ni·os·to·sis (krā'nē-os-tō'sis). SYN craniosynostosis. [cranio- + G. *osteon*, a bone, + -*osis*, condition]

cra·ni·o·syn·os·to·sis (krā'nē-ō-sin'os-tō'sis). Premature ossification of the skull and obliteration of the sutures. The particular sutures involved determine the resultant shape of the malformed head. SYN craniostosis.

cra·ni·o·tabes (krā'nē-ō-tā'bēz). A disease marked by the presence of areas of thinning and softening in the bones of the skull and widening of the sutures and fontanelles. Usually of syphilitic or rachitic origin. SYN circumscribed craniomalacia. [cranio- + L. *tabes*, a wasting]

cra·ni·o·tome (krā'nē-ō-tōm). Instrument formerly used for perforation and crushing of the fetal skull.

cra·ni·ot·o·my (krā-nē-ot'ō-mē). **1.** Opening into the skull, either by attached or detached c. or by trephination. **2.** Formerly used operation for perforation of the head of the fetus, removal of the contents, and compression of the empty skull, when delivery by natural means is impossible. [cranio- + G. *tomē*, incision]

attached c., c. with a segment of the calvaria and attached soft tissues turned as a flap to expose the cranial cavity. SYN attached cranial section, osteoplastic c.

detached c., c. with section of cranium separated from its soft tissue attachments. SYN detached cranial section.

osteoplastic c., SYN attached c.

cra·ni·o·to·nos·co·py (krā'nē-ō-tō-nos'kŏ-pē). Auscultatory

cr

percussion of the cranium. [cranio- + G. *tonos,* tone, + *skopeō,* to examine]

cra·ni·o·try·pe·sis (krā′nē-ō-tri-pē′sis). Trephining of the skull. [cranio- + G. *trypēsis,* a boring]

cra·ni·o·tym·pan·ic (krā′nē-ō-tim-pan′ik). Relating to the skull and the middle ear.

cra·ni·um, pl. **cra·nia** (krā′nē-ŭm, -ă) [NA]. SYN skull. [Mediev. L. fr. G. *kranion*]

c. bif′idum, bifid c., SYN encephalocele.

c. cerebra′le, cerebral c., SYN neurocranium.

c. viscera′le, visceral c., SYN viscerocranium.

crap·u·lent, crap·u·lous (krap′yū-lent, -lŭs). Rarely used term for drunken; due to alcoholic intoxication. [L. *crapula,* drunkenness]

crash cart. A movable collection of emergency equipment and supplies meant to be readily available for resuscitative effort. It includes medication as well as the equipment for defibrillation, intubation, intravenous medication, and passage of central lines.

cras·sa·men·tum (kras-ă-men′tŭm). **1.** Old term for blood *clot.* **2.** Old term for coagulum. [L. thickness, fr. *crassus,* thick]

cra·ter (krā′ter). The most depressed, usually central portion of an ulcer.

cra·ter·i·form (krā-ter′i-fōrm). Hollowed like a bowl or a saucer. [L. *crater,* bowl, + *forma,* shape]

cra·ter·i·za·tion (krā-ter-ī-zā′shŭn). SYN saucerization.

craw-craw (kraw′kraw). A term applied in west Africa to a pruritic papular skin eruption, which may lead to ulceration; some cases are caused by *Onchocerca.* SYN kra-kra.

Crawford, Brian H., British physicist, *1906. SEE Stiles-C. effect.

craz·ing (krā′zing). In dentistry, the appearance of minute cracks on the surface of plastic restorations such as filling materials, denture teeth, or denture bases.

CRD Abbreviation for chronic respiratory *disease.*

cream (krēm). **1.** The upper fatty layer which forms in milk on standing or which is separated from it by centrifugalization; it contains about the same amount of sugar and protein as milk, but from 12 to 40% more fat. **2.** Any whitish viscid fluid resembling c. **3.** A semisolid emulsion of either the oil-in-water or the water-in-oil type, ordinarily intended for topical use. [L. *cremor,* thick juice, broth]

cleansing c., a form of cold c. used to remove grime and cosmetics from the skin.

cold c., a water-in-oil emulsion of various oils, waxes, and water; the standard formula, rose water ointment, contains expressed almond oil, rose water, spermaceti, white paraffin wax, and sodium borate; used as a cleansing or lubricating c.

greaseless c., SYN vanishing c.

leukocyte c., SYN buffy *coat.*

lubricating c., a form of cold c. used as a massage c. or night c.; it contains lanolin or its derivatives.

vanishing c., an oil-in-water emulsion containing potassium, ammonium, or sodium stearate with water and holding in emulsified form more or less free stearic acid; it also contains a hygroscopic ingredient such as glycerol, and a small amount of a fatty ingredient; it leaves a protective, invisible film of stearic acid on the skin. SYN greaseless c.

crease (krēs). A line or linear depression as produced by a fold. SEE ALSO fold, groove, line.

digital c., one of the grooves on the palmar surface of a finger, at the level of an interphalangeal joint. SYN digital flexion c., digital furrow.

digital flexion c., SYN digital c.

ear lobe c., a diagonal c. found on one or both earlobes with a possible connection to coronary heart disease in males.

flexion c., a permanent c. in the skin on the flexor aspect of a movable joint.

palmar c., any of the several flexion c.'s normally found on the palm of the hand, occurring proximal to, but as a consequence of flexion at, the metacarpophalangeal joints.

simian c., a single transverse palmar c. formed by fusion of the distal and proximal palmar c.'s, so called because of its similarity to the transverse flexion crease seen in some monkeys; a common but not pathognomonic feature of Down's syndrome.

Sydney c., a variation of the proximal transverse palmar flexion c. that reaches the ulnar side of the palm; associated with acute lymphocytic anemia in early childhood, rubella embryopathy, and Down's syndrome. SYN Sydney line.

cre·a·ti·nase (krē′ă-tĭ-nās). An enzyme catalyzing the hydrolysis of creatine to sarcosine and urea.

cre·a·tine (krē′ă-tēn, -tin). H_2N-C(NH)-N(CH_3)-CH_2-COOH; *N*-(Aminoiminomethyl)-*N*-methylglycine; occurs in urine, sometimes as such, but generally as creatinine, and in muscle, generally as phosphocreatine. Elevated in urine in individuals with muscular dystrophy.

c. kinase (CK), an enzyme catalyzing the reversible transfer of phosphate from phosphocreatine to ADP, forming creatine and ATP; of importance in muscle contraction. Certain isozymes are elevated in plasma following myocardial infarctions. SYN c. phosphokinase.

c. phosphate, SYN phosphocreatine.

c. phosphokinase (CPK), SYN c. kinase.

cre·a·ti·ne·mia (krē′ă-ti-nē′mē-ă). The presence of abnormal concentrations of creatine in peripheral blood. [creatine + G. *haima,* blood]

cre·at·i·nin·ase (krē-at′i-nin-ās). An amidohydrolase catalyzing the conversion of creatine to creatinine.

cre·at·i·nine (Cr) (krē-at′i-nēn, -nin). A component of urine and the final product of creatine catabolism; formed by the nonenzymatic dephosphorylative cyclization of phosphocreatine to form the internal anhydride of creatine.

cre·a·tin·u·ria (krē′ă-ti-nū′rē-ă). The urinary excretion of increased amounts of creatine. [creatine + G. *ouron,* urine]

Credé, Karl S.F., German obstetrician and gynecologist, 1819–1892. SEE C.'s *methods,* under *method.*

creep (krēp). Any time-dependent strain developing in a material or an object in response to the application of a force or stress.

cre·mas·ter (krē-mas′ter). SEE cremasteric *fascia,* cremaster *muscle.* [G. *kremastēr,* a suspender, in pl. the muscles by which the testicles are retracted, fr. *kremannymi,* to hang]

crem·as·ter·ic (krē-mas-ter′ik). Relating to the cremaster.

crem·no·cele (krem′nō-sēl). A protrusion of intestine into the labium majus. [G. *krēmnos,* overhanging cliff, labium pudendi, + *kēlē,* hernia]

crem·no·pho·bia (krem-nō-fō′bē-ă). Morbid fear of precipices or steep places. [G. *krēmnos,* precipice, + *phobos,* fear]

cre·na, pl. **cre·nae** (krē′nă, krē′nē). A V-shaped cut or the space created by such a cut; one of the notches into which the opposing projections fit in the cranial sutures. [L. a notch]

c. a′ni [NA], SYN natal *cleft.*

c. clu′nium, SYN natal *cleft.*

c. cor′dis, (1) SYN anterior interventricular *groove.* **(2)** SYN posterior interventricular *groove.*

cre·nate, cre·nat·ed (krē′nāt, -nā-ted). Indented; denoting the outline of a shriveled red blood cell, as observed in a hypertonic solution. [L. *crena,* a notch]

cre·na·tion (krē-nā′shŭn). The process of becoming, or state of being, crenated.

cre·no·cyte (krē′nō-sīt). A red blood cell with serrated, notched edges. [L. *crena,* a notch, + G. *kytos,* a hollow (cell)]

cre·no·cy·to·sis (krē′nō-sī-tō′sis). The presence of crenocytes in the blood. [crenocyte + G. *-osis,* condition]

Cren·o·so·ma vul·pis (krē′nō-sō-mă vŭl′pis). A metastrongyle lungworm species of the fox, wolf, dog, raccoon, and other small carnivores in Europe, Asia, and North America; it occurs in the bronchi, causing bronchitis. [G. *krēnē,* a (mineral) spring, + *sōma,* body; L. *vulpes,* fox]

cre·oph·a·gy, cre·oph·a·gism (krē-of′ă-jē, krē-of′ă-jizm). Carnivorousness; flesh-eating. [G. *kreas,* flesh, + *phagō,* to eat]

cre·o·sol (krē′ō-sol). 2-Methoxy-*p*-cresol; a slightly yellowish aromatic liquid distilled from guaiac or from beechwood tar; a constituent of creosote. Cf. cresol.

cre·o·sote (krē′ō-sōt). A mixture of phenols (chiefly methyl guaiacol, guaiacol, and creosol) obtained during the distillation of wood-tar, preferably that derived from beechwood; used as a disinfectant and wood preservative. [G. *kreas,* flesh, + *sōtēr,* preserver]

crep·i·tant (krep′i-tant). 1. Relating to or characterized by crepitation. 2. Denoting a fine bubbling noise (rale) produced by air entering fluid in lung tissue; heard in pneumonia and in certain other conditions. 3. The sensation imparted to the palpating finger by gas or air in the subcutaneous tissues.

crep·i·ta·tion (krep-i-tā′shŭn). 1. Crackling; the quality of a fine bubbling sound (rale) that resembles noise heard on rubbing hair between the fingers. 2. The sensation felt on placing the hand over the seat of a fracture when the broken ends of the bone are moved, or over tissue, in which gas gangrene is present. SYN bony crepitus. 3. Noise or vibration produced by rubbing bone or irregular cartilage surfaces together as by movement of patella against femoral condyles in arthritis and other conditions. SYN crepitus (1). [see crepitus]

crep·i·tus (krep′i-tŭs). 1. SYN crepitation. 2. A noisy discharge of gas from the intestine. [L. fr. *crepo,* to rattle]

articular c., the grating of a joint.

bony c., SYN crepitation (2).

cre·pus·cu·lar (kre-pŭs′kyŭ-lăr). Pertaining to a twilight state of consciousness. [L. *crepusculum,* twilight]

cres·cent (kres′ent). 1. Any figure of the shape of the moon in its first quarter. 2. The figure made by the gray columns or cornua on cross-section of the spinal cord. 3. SYN malarial c. [L. *cresco,* pp. *cretus,* to grow]

articular c., SYN articular *meniscus.*

Giannuzzi's c.'s, SYN serous *demilunes,* under *demilune.*

glomerular c., proliferated epithelial cells partly encircling a renal glomerulus; it occurs in glomerulonephritis.

Heidenhain's c.'s, SYN serous *demilunes,* under *demilune.*

malarial c., the male or female gametocyte(s) of *Plasmodium falciparum,* whose presence in human red blood cells is diagnostic of falciparum malaria. SYN crescent (3), sickle form.

myopic c., a white or grayish white crescentic area in the fundus of the eye located on the temporal side of the optic disk; caused by atrophy of the choroid, permitting the sclera to become visible. SYN myopic conus.

sublingual c., the crescent-shaped area on the floor of the mouth formed by the lingual wall of the mandible and the adjacent part of the floor of the mouth.

cres·cen·tic (kres-sen′tik). Shaped like a crescent.

cres·co·graph (kres′kō-graf). A device for recording the degree and rate of growth. [L. *cresco,* to grow, + G. *graphō,* to draw or write]

cre·sol (krē′sol). HO–C₆H₄–CH₃; hydroxytoluene; methylphenol; a mixture of the three isomeric cresols, *o-, m-,* and *p*-cresol, obtained from coal tar. Its properties are similar to those of phenol, but it is less poisonous; used as an antiseptic and disinfectant. SYN tricresol.

m-cre·sol. A local antiseptic with a higher germicidal power than phenol and less toxicity to tissues; used in disinfectants and fumigants; its acetate derivative is used as a topical antiseptic and fungicide. SYN metacresol.

cre·so·lase (krē′sō-lās). SYN monophenol monooxygenase (1).

cre·sol red. An acid-base indicator with a pK value of 8.3; yellow at pH values below 7.4, red above 9.0.

CREST Acronym for *c*alcinosis, *R*eynaud's phenomenon, *e*sophageal motility disorders, *s*clerodactyly, and *t*elangiectasia. A ridge, crest, or elevated line projecting from a level or evenly rounded surface. SEE CREST *syndrome.*

CREST

crest (krest). 1. A ridge, especially a bony ridge. SEE ALSO crista.

2. The ridge of the neck of a male animal, especially of a stallion or bull. 3. Feathers on the top of a bird's head, or fin rays on the top of a fish's head. SYN crista [NA]. [L. *crista*]

acoustic c., SYN ampullary c.

acousticofacial c., the part of the neural c. from which the ganglia of the seventh and eighth cranial nerves develop.

alveolar c., (1) the portion of the alveolar bone extending beyond the periphery of the socket, lying interproximally; (2) the top of the residual alveolar bone.

c. of alveolar ridge, the top of the alveolar ridge or residual ridge; the highest continuous surface of the ridge, but not necessarily the center of the ridge.

ampullary c., an elevation on the inner surface of the ampulla of each semicircular duct; filaments of the vestibular nerve pass through the c. to reach hair cells on its surface; the hair cells are capped by the cupula, a gelatinous protein-polysaccharide mass. SYN crista ampullaris [NA], acoustic c., transverse septum (1).

anterior lacrimal c., a vertical ridge on the lateral surface of the frontal process of the maxilla that forms part of the medial rim of the orbit. SYN crista lacrimalis anterior [NA].

arched c., SYN arcuate c. of arytenoid cartilage.

arcuate c., SYN arcuate c. of arytenoid cartilage.

arcuate c. of arytenoid cartilage, the ridge on the anterior surface of the arytenoid cartilage that separates the triangular from the oblong fovea. SYN crista arcuata cartilaginis arytenoideae [NA], arched c., arcuate c.

articular c.'s, SYN intermediate sacral c.'s.

basilar c. of cochlear duct, an inward projection of the spiral ligament of the cochlea to which is attached the basilar membrane forming the floor of the cochlear duct. SYN crista basilaris ductus cochlearis [NA].

buccinator c., a ridge passing from the base of the coronoid process of the mandible to the region of the last molar tooth; it gives attachment to the mandibular part of the buccinator muscle. SYN crista buccinatoria.

c. of cochlear opening, SYN c. of fenestrae cochleae.

conchal c., bony ridge which articulates with, or provides attachment for, the inferior nasal concha. SEE conchal c. of maxilla, conchal c. of palatine bone. SYN crista conchalis [NA], turbinated c.

conchal c. of maxilla, ridge of the nasal surface of the body of the maxilla that articulates with the inferior nasal concha. SYN crista conchalis maxillae.

conchal c. of palatine bone, the ridge on the nasal surface of the perpendicular part of the palatine bone to which the inferior nasal concha attaches. SYN crista conchalis ossis palatini.

deltoid c., SYN deltoid *tuberosity.*

dental c., the maxillary ridge on the aleveolar processes of the maxillary bones in the fetus. SYN crista dentalis.

ethmoidal c., bony ridge which articulates with, or provides attachment for, any part of the ethmoid bone, especially the middle nasal concha. SEE ethmoidal c. of maxilla, ethmoidal c. of palatine bone. SYN crista ethmoidalis [NA].

ethmoidal c. of maxilla, a ridge on the upper part of the nasal surface of the frontal process of the maxilla that gives attachment to the anterior portion of the middle nasal concha. SYN crista ethmoidalis maxillae.

ethmoidal c. of palatine bone, a ridge on the medial surface of the perpendicular part of the palatine bone to which the middle nasal concha attaches posteriorly. SYN crista ethmoidalis ossis palatini.

external occipital c., a ridge extending from the external occipital protuberance to the border of the foramen magnum. SYN crista occipitalis externa [NA], linea nuchae mediana.

falciform c., SYN transverse c. of internal acoustic meatus.

c. of fenestrae cochleae, the edge of the opening of the cochlear window to which the secondary tympanic membrane is attached. SYN crista fenestrae cochleae [NA], c. of cochlear opening.

frontal c., a ridge arising at the termination of the sagittal sulcus on the cerebral surface of the frontal bone and ending at the foramen caecum. SYN crista frontalis [NA].

ganglionic c., SYN neural c.

gingival c., SYN gingival *margin.*

gluteal c., SYN gluteal *tuberosity.*

c. of greater tubercle, the ridge below the greater tubercle of the humerus into which the pectoralis major muscle inserts. SYN crista tuberculi majoris [NA], bicipital ridges, pectoral ridge.

c. of head of rib, the ridge that separates the superior and inferior articular surfaces of the head of a rib. SYN crista capitis costae [NA].

iliac c., the long, curved upper border of the wing of the ilium. SYN crista iliaca [NA].

incisor c., the front part of the nasal c. of the palatine process of the maxilla.

infratemporal c., a rough ridge marking the angle of union of the temporal and infratemporal surfaces of the greater wing of the sphenoid bone. SYN crista infratemporalis [NA], pterygoid ridge of sphenoid bone.

inguinal c., an elevation in the body wall of the embryo at the internal opening of the inguinal canal; part of the gubernaculum testis develops within it.

intermediate sacral c.'s, c.'s formed by the fusion of articular processes of all the sacral vertebrae. SYN articular c.'s, cristae sacrales intermediae.

internal occipital c., a ridge running from the internal occipital protuberance to the posterior margin of the foramen magnum, giving attachment to the falx cerebelli. SYN crista occipitalis interna [NA].

interosseous c., SYN interosseous *border.*

intertrochanteric c., the rounded ridge that connects the greater and lesser trochanters of the femur posteriorly and marks the junction of the neck and shaft of the bone. SYN crista intertrochanterica [NA], trochanteric c.

lateral epicondylar c., SYN lateral supracondylar *ridge.*

lateral sacral c.'s, c.'s which are rough ridges lying lateral to the sacral foramina; they represent the fused transverse processes of sacral vertebrae. SYN cristae sacrales laterales.

lateral supracondylar c., SYN lateral supracondylar *ridge.*

c. of lesser tubercle, the ridge below the lesser tubercle of the humerus into which the teres major muscle inserts. SYN crista tuberculi minoris [NA], bicipital ridges.

marginal c., the rounded borders which form the mesial and distal margins of the occlusal surface of a tooth. SYN crista marginalis [NA], marginal ridge.

medial epicondylar c., SYN medial supracondylar *ridge.*

medial c. of fibula, a ridge of bone, on the posterior surface of the fibula, separating the attachment of the posterior tibial muscle from that of the flexor hallucis longus and soleus muscles. SYN crista medialis fibulae [NA].

medial supracondylar c., SYN medial supracondylar *ridge.*

median sacral c., an unpaired c. formed by the fused spinous processes of the upper four sacral vertebrae. SYN crista sacralis mediana.

c.'s of nail bed, the numerous longitudinal ridges of the nail bed distal to the lunula. SYN cristae matricis unguis [NA].

nasal c., the midline ridge in the floor of the nasal cavity, formed by the union of the paired maxillae and palatine bones; the vomer attaches to the crest. SYN crista nasalis [NA], semicrista incisiva.

c. of neck of rib, the sharp upper margin of the neck of a rib. SYN crista colli costae [NA].

neural c., a band of neuroectodermal cells along either side of the line of closure of the embryonic neural groove; with the formation of the neural tube, these bands come to lie dorsolateral to the developing spinal cord and lateral to the brainstem, where they separate into clusters of cells that develop into, for example, dorsal-root ganglion cells, autonomic ganglion cells, the chromaffin cells of the adrenal medulla, Schwann cells, sensory ganglia of cranial nerves, 5, 7, 8, 9, and 10, part of the meninges, or integumentary pigment cells. SYN ganglion ridge, ganglionic c.

obturator c., a ridge that extends from the pubic tubercle to the acetabular notch, giving attachment to the pubofemoral ligament of the hip joint. SYN crista obturatoria [NA].

c. of palatine bone, palatine c., a transverse ridge near the posterior border of the bony palate, located on the inferior surface of the horizontal plate of the palatine bone. SYN crista palatina [NA].

c. of petrous part of temporal bone, SYN superior *border* of petrous part of temporal bone.

posterior lacrimal c., a vertical ridge on the orbital surface of the lacrimal bone which, together with the anterior lacrimal crest, bounds the fossa for the lacrimal sac. SYN crista lacrimalis posterior [NA].

pubic c., the rough anterior border of the body of the pubis, continuous laterally with the pubic tubercle. SYN crista pubica [NA].

sacral c., one of three rough irregular ridges on the posterior surface of the sacrum; median sacral c.; lateral sacral c.'s. SYN crista sacralis [NA].

sagittal c., a prominent ridge along the sagittal suture of the skull, present in some animals as a result of temporal muscle development.

c. of scapular spine, the posterior subcutaneous border of the spine of the scapula that expands in its medial part into a smooth triangular area.

sphenoid c., a vertical ridge in the midline of the anterior surface of the sphenoid bone that articulates with the perpendicular plate of the ethmoid bone. SYN crista sphenoidalis [NA].

spiral c., SYN spiral *ligament* of cochlea.

supinator c., c. of supinator muscle, the proximal part of the interosseous border of the ulna from which a portion of the supinator muscle takes origin. SYN crista musculi supinatoris [NA].

supramastoid c., the ridge that forms the posterior root of the zygomatic process of the temporal bone. SYN crista supramastoidea [NA].

supraventricular c., the internal muscular ridge that separates the conus arteriosus from the remaining part of the cavity of the right ventricle of the heart. SYN crista supraventricularis [NA].

terminal c., SYN *crista* terminalis.

tibial c., SYN anterior *border* of tibia.

transverse c., (1) SYN transverse c. of internal acoustic meatus. (2) SYN *crista* transversalis.

transverse c. of internal acoustic meatus, a horizontal ridge that divides the fundus of the internal acoustic meatus into a superior and an inferior area. In the former are the introitus of the facial canal and openings for the branches of the vestibular nerve to the utricle and to the ampullae of the anterior and lateral semicircular canals. In the latter are openings for the cochlear nerve, and for branches of the vestibular nerve to the saccule and to the ampulla of the posterior semicircular canal. SYN crista transversa [NA], falciform c., transverse c. (1).

triangular c., SYN *crista* triangularis.

trigeminal c., that part of the cranial neural c. from which the ganglion of the fifth cranial nerve develops.

trochanteric c., SYN intertrochanteric c.

turbinated c., SYN conchal c.

urethral c., longitudinal mucosal fold in the dorsal wall of the urethra. SEE urethral c. of female, urethral c. of male. SYN crista urethralis [NA].

urethral c. of female, a conspicuous longitudinal fold of mucosa on the posterior wall of the urethra. SYN crista urethralis femininae.

urethral c. of male, a longitudinal fold on the posterior wall of the urethra extending from the uvula of the bladder through the prostatic urethra; prominent in its midportion is the seminal colliculus. SYN crista phallica, crista urethralis masculinae.

vestibular c., c. of vestibule, an oblique ridge on the inner wall of the vestibule of the labyrinth, bounding the spherical recess above and posteriorly. SYN crista vestibuli [NA].

---

cres·ta (kres′tă). A small membranous organelle characteristic of certain flagellate protozoa, located near the pelta and seen in the living organism as an independently moving structure. [L. *crispus,* trembling]

cres·yl·ate (kres′i-lāt). A salt of cresylic acid, or cresol.

cres·yl blue, cres·yl blue bril·liant (kres′il) [C.I. 51010]. $C_{17}H_{20}N_3OCl$; Aminodimethylaminoethyldiphenazonium chloride; a basic oxazin dye used for staining the reticulum in young erythrocytes (reticulocytes); also used in vital staining and as a selective stain for gastric surface epithelial mucin and other acid mucopolysaccharides.

cres·yl echt, cres·yl fast vi·o·let. A metachromatic basic oxazin dye, $C_{19}H_{18}N_3O$-Cl, closely related to cresyl violet acetate and used for the same purposes.

cres·yl vi·o·let ac·e·tate. A metachromatic basic oxazin dye, $C_{18}H_{15}N_3O_3$, used as a stain for nuclei and Nissl substance; related to German derived dye known as cresyl echt violet or cresyl fast violet.

cre·ta (krē′tă). SYN *calcium* carbonate. [L. orig. adj. fr. *Creta*, Crete, *i.e.* Cretan earth, chalk]

cre·tin (krē′tin). An individual exhibiting cretinism. [Fr. *crétin*]

cre·tin·ism (krē′tin-izm). Obsolete term for congenital *hypothyroidism*. SEE infantile *hypothyroidism*.

cre·tin·is·tic (krē′tin-is-tik). SYN cretinous.

cre·tin·oid (krē′tin-oyd). Resembling a cretin; presenting symptoms similar to those of cretinism.

cre·tin·ous (krē′tin-ŭs). Relating to cretinism or a cretin; affected with cretinism. SYN cretinistic.

Creutzfeldt, Hans Gerhard, German neuropsychiatrist, 1885–1964. SEE C.-Jakob *disease;* Jakob-C. *disease.*

crev·ice (krev′is). A crack or small fissure, especially in a solid substance. [Fr. *crevasse*]

gingival c., SYN gingival *sulcus.*

cre·vic·u·lar (krĕ-vik′yū-lăr). 1. Relating to any crevice. 2. In dentistry, relating especially to the gingival crevice or sulcus.

CRF Abbreviation for corticotropin releasing *factor.*

CRH Abbreviation for corticotropin releasing *hormone.*

crib·ber (krib′er). A horse suffering from crib-biting.

crib·bit·ing (krib-bīt′ing). A behavior disorder of horses in which the animal grasps the edge of a convenient fixture and presses down, raising the floor of its mouth, forcing the soft palate open, and sometimes swallowing air. SEE aerophagia.

cri·bra (krī′bră, krib′ră). Plural of cribrum.

crib·rate (krib′rāt). SYN cribriform.

cri·bra·tion (kri-brā′shŭn). 1. Sifting; passing through a sieve. 2. The condition of being cribrate or numerously pitted or punctured.

crib·ri·form (krib′ri-fōrm). Sievelike; containing many perforations. SYN cribrate, polyporous. [L. *cribrum,* a sieve, + *forma,* form]

cri·brum, pl. **cri·bra** (krī′brŭm, krib′rŭm; -bră, -ra). SYN cribriform *plate* of ethmoid bone. [L. a sieve]

Cri·cet·i·nae (krī-sē′ti-nē). A subfamily of rodents (family Muridae) that includes the hamsters and the native American rats.

Cri·ce·tu·lus (kri-sē′tyū-lŭs). One of four genera of hamsters; *C. griseus,* the striped hamster native to Europe and Asia, is a reservoir for visceral leishmaniasis.

Cri·ce·tus (kri-sē′tŭs). One of four genera of hamsters; *C. cricetus* is used extensively as a research animal.

Crichton-Browne, Sir James, English physician, 1840–1938. SEE Crichton-Browne's *sign.*

Crick, Francis H.C., British biochemist and Nobel laureate, *1916. SEE Watson-C. *helix.*

cri·co·ar·y·te·noid (krī′kō-ar-i-tē′noyd). Relating to the cricoid and arytenoid cartilages.

cri·co·ar·y·te·noi·de·us (krī′kō-ar-i-te-noy′dē-ŭs). SEE lateral cricoarytenoid *muscle,* posterior cricoarytenoid *muscle.*

cri·coid (krī′koyd). Ring-shaped; denoting the cricoid cartilage. [L. *cricoideus,* fr. G. *krikos,* a ring, + *eidos,* form]

cri·coi·dyn·ia (krī′koy-din′ē-ă). Pain in the cricoid. [cricoid + G. *odynē,* pain]

cri·co·pha·ryn·ge·al (krī′kō-fă-rin′jē-ăl). Relating to the cricoid cartilage and the pharynx; a part of the inferior constrictor muscle of the pharynx. SEE inferior constrictor *muscle* of pharynx.

cri·co·thy·roid (krī-kō-thī′royd). Relating to the cricoid and thyroid cartilages.

cri·co·thy·roi·de·us (krī′kō-thī-roy′dē-ŭs). SEE cricothyroid *muscle.*

cri·co·thy·roi·dot·o·my (krī′kō-thī-roy-dot′ō-mē). SYN cricothyrotomy.

cri·co·thy·rot·o·my (krī′kō-thī-rot′ō-mē). Incision through the skin and cricothyroid membrane for relief of respiratory obstruction; used prior to or in place of tracheotomy in certain emergency respiratory obstructions. SYN coniotomy, cricothyroidotomy, inferior laryngotomy, intercricothyrotomy. [cricoid + thyroid + G. *tomē,* incision]

cri·cot·o·my (krī-kot′ō-mē). Division of the cricoid cartilage, as in cricoid split, to enlarge the subglottic airway. [cricoid + G. *tomē,* incision]

Crigler, John F., U.S. physician, *1919. SEE C.-Najjar *disease, syndrome.*

Crile, George W., U.S. surgeon, 1864–1943. SEE C.'s *clamp.*

crim·i·nol·o·gy (krim-i-nol′ō-jē). The branch of science concerned with the physical and mental characteristics and behavior of criminals. [L. *crimen,* crime, + G. *logos,* study]

crin·in (krin′in). Old term for a substance that will stimulate the production of secretions by specific glands. [G. *krinō,* to secrete, + -in]

cri·nis, pl. **cri·nes** (krī′nis, -nēz). SYN pilus (1). [L.]

crin·o·gen·ic (krin-ō-jen′ik). Causing secretion; stimulating a gland to increased function. [G. *krinō,* to separate, + *-gen,* to produce]

crin·oph·a·gy (krin-of′ă-jē). Disposal of excess secretory granules by lysosomes.

crip·pled (krip′ld). Denoting a person who, owing to a physical defect or injury, is partially or completely disabled. [A.S. *creopan,* to creep]

cri·sis, pl. **cri·ses** (krī′sis, -sēz). 1. A sudden change, usually for the better, in the course of an acute disease, in contrast to the gradual improvement by lysis. 2. A paroxysmal pain in an organ or circumscribed region of the body occurring in the course of tabetic neurosyphilis. SYN tabetic c. 3. A convulsive attack. [G. *krisis,* a separation, crisis]

addisonian c., SYN acute adrenocortical *insufficiency.*

adolescent c., the emotional turmoil often accompanying adolescence.

adrenal c., SYN acute adrenocortical *insufficiency.*

anaphylactoid c., (1) SYN anaphylactoid *shock.* (2) SYN pseudoanaphylaxis.

blast c., a sudden alteration in the status of a patient with leukemia in which the peripheral blood cells are almost exclusively blast cells of the type characteristic of leukemia; usually accompanied by a decrease in numbers of other formed elements of the blood, fever, and rapid clinical deterioration.

blood c., (1) the appearance of a large number of nucleated red blood cells in the peripheral blood, accompanied by reticulocytosis and occurring in "exhausted" bone marrow in pernicious anemia and in hemolytic icterus; (2) a suddenly appearing leukocytosis, indicating a change for the better in the course of a grave blood disease.

Dietl's c., intermittent pain, sometimes with nausea and emesis, caused by intermittent proximal obstruction of ureter. Originally believed due to a mobile kidney that caused ureter to kink with positional changes. SYN incarceration symptom.

febrile c., the stage in a febrile disease when spontaneous defervescence occurs.

gastric c., an attack, usually lasting several days, with severe pain in the abdomen or around the waist, accompanied by nausea and vomiting and occasionally diarrhea; occurs in tabetic neurosyphilis.

glaucomatocyclitic c., a form of monocular secondary open-angle glaucoma due to recurrent mild cyclitis.

identity c., a disorientation concerning one's sense of self, values, and role in society, often of acute onset and related to a particular and significant event in one's life.

laryngeal c., an attack of paralysis of the abductor, or spasm of the adductor, muscles of the larynx with dyspnea and noisy respiration, occurring in tabetic neurosyphilis.

midlife c., a point in a sequence of events during the middle years of life at which certain trends of prior and subsequent events in one's life are pondered, generally involving an aggregate of personal, career, or sexual dissatisfactions.

myasthenic c., severe, life-threatening exacerbation of the manifestations of *myasthenia* gravis requiring intensive treatment.

myelocytic c., a temporary but conspicuous and sudden increase in cells of the myelocytic series in the circulating blood.

ocular c., sudden and severe pain in the eyes.

oculogyric crises, incapacitating attacks of upward eye rolling seen in encephalitis lethargica and with phenothiazine drugs.

salt-depletion c., severe illness resulting from loss of sodium chloride, usually in urine (*i.e.,* salt-losing nephritis), in sweat following severe exercise in hot weather, or in intestinal secretions, as in cholera. Can occur as result of Addison's disease or Addisonian crisis; characterized by hypovolemia, hypotension.

sickle cell c., SEE sickle cell *anemia.*

tabetic c., SYN crisis (2).

therapeutic c., a turning point leading to positive or negative change in psychiatric treatment.

thyrotoxic c., thyroid c., the exacerbation of symptoms that occurs in severe thyrotoxicosis; can follow shock or injury or thyroidectomy; marked by rapid pulse (140 to 170 per minute), nausea, diarrhea, fever, loss of weight, extreme nervousness, and a sudden rise in the metabolic rate; coma and death may occur; occasionally the entire clinical picture is that of profound prostration, weakness, and collapse, without the phase of muscular overactivity and tachycardia. SYN thyroid storm.

visceral crises, attacks of severe, spreading epigastric pain that occur in patients with tabetic neurosyphilis.

cris·pa·tion (kris-pā′shŭn). **1.** A "creepy" sensation due to slight, fibrillary muscular contractions. **2.** Retraction of a divided artery or of muscular fibers or other tissues when cut across. [L. *crispo,* pp. *-atus,* to curl]

CRISTA

cris·ta, pl. **cris·tae** (kris′tă, -tē) [NA]. SYN crest. [L. crest]

c. ampulla′ris [NA], SYN ampullary *crest.*

c. arcua′ta cartila′ginis arytenoi′deae [NA], SYN arcuate *crest* of arytenoid cartilage.

c. basila′ris duc′tus cochlea′ris [NA], SYN basilar *crest* of cochlear duct.

c. buccinator′ia, SYN buccinator *crest.*

c. cap′itis cos′tae [NA], SYN *crest* of head of rib.

c. col′li cos′tae [NA], SYN *crest* of neck of rib.

c. concha′lis [NA], SYN conchal *crest.*

c. concha′lis max′illae, SYN conchal *crest* of maxilla.

c. concha′lis os′sis palati′ni, SYN conchal *crest* of palatine bone.

cris′tae cu′tis [NA], SYN epidermal *ridges,* under *ridge.*

c. denta′lis, SYN dental *crest.*

c. div′idens, the lower free edge of the septum secundum, forming the upper margin of the fetal foramen ovale; the limbus of the foramen ovale.

c. ethmoida′lis [NA], SYN ethmoidal *crest.*

c. ethmoida′lis max′illae, SYN ethmoidal *crest* of maxilla.

c. ethmoida′lis os′sis palati′ni, SYN ethmoidal *crest* of palatine bone.

c. fenes′trae coch′leae [NA], SYN *crest* of fenestrae cochleae.

c. fronta′lis [NA], SYN frontal *crest.*

c. gal′li [NA], the triangular midline process of the ethmoid bone extending superiorly from the cribriform plate; it gives anterior attachment to the falx cerebri.

c. glu′tea, SYN gluteal *tuberosity.*

c. hel′icis, SYN *crus* of helix.

c. ili′aca [NA], SYN iliac *crest.*

c. infratempora′lis [NA], SYN infratemporal *crest.*

c. intertrochanter′ica [NA], SYN intertrochanteric *crest.*

c. lacrima′lis ante′rior [NA], SYN anterior lacrimal *crest.*

c. lacrima′lis poste′rior [NA], SYN posterior lacrimal *crest.*

c. margina′lis [NA], SYN marginal *crest.*

cris′tae ma′tricis un′guis [NA], SYN *crests* of nail bed, under *crest.*

c. media′lis fi′bulae [NA], SYN medial *crest* of fibula.

cristae of mitochondria, cris′tae mitochondria′les, shelflike infoldings of the inner membrane of a mitochondrion.

c. mus′culi supinato′ris [NA], SYN supinator *crest.*

c. nasa′lis [NA], SYN nasal *crest.*

c. obturato′ria [NA], SYN obturator *crest.*

c. occipita′lis exter′na [NA], SYN external occipital *crest.*

c. occipita′lis inter′na [NA], SYN internal occipital *crest.*

c. palati′na [NA], SYN *crest* of palatine bone.

c. phal′lica, SYN urethral *crest* of male.

c. pu′bica [NA], SYN pubic *crest.*

c. quar′ta, a ridge that projects into the posterior end of the lateral semicircular duct of the labyrinth.

cris′tae sacra′les interme′diae, SYN intermediate sacral *crests,* under *crest.*

cris′tae sacra′les latera′les, SYN lateral sacral *crests,* under *crest.*

c. sacra′lis [NA], SYN sacral *crest.*

c. sacra′lis median′a, SYN median sacral *crest.*

c. sphenoida′lis [NA], SYN sphenoid *crest.*

c. spira′lis [NA], SYN spiral *ligament* of cochlea.

c. supracondyla′ris latera′lis [NA], SYN lateral supracondylar *ridge.*

c. supracondyla′ris media′lis [NA], SYN medial supracondylar *ridge.*

c. supramastoi′dea [NA], SYN supramastoid *crest.*

c. supraventricula′ris [NA], SYN supraventricular *crest.*

c. termina′lis [NA], a vertical crest on the interior wall of the right atrium that lies to the right of the sinus of the vena cava and separates this from the remainder of the right atrium. SYN tenia terminalis, terminal crest.

c. transver′sa [NA], SYN transverse *crest* of internal acoustic meatus.

c. transversa′lis [NA], a crest or ridge on the occlusal surface of a tooth formed by the union of two triangular crests. SYN transverse crest (2), transverse ridge.

c. triangula′ris [NA], a crest or ridge which extends from the apex of a cusp of a premolar or molar tooth toward the central part of the occlusal surface. SYN triangular crest, triangular ridge.

c. tuber′culi majo′ris [NA], SYN *crest* of greater tubercle.

c. tuber′culi mino′ris [NA], SYN *crest* of lesser tubercle.

c. urethra′lis [NA], SYN urethral *crest.*

c. urethra′lis femini′nae, SYN urethral *crest* of female.

c. urethra′lis masculi′nae, SYN urethral *crest* of male.

c. vestib′uli [NA], SYN vestibular *crest.*

cri·te·ri·on, pl. **cri·te·ria** (krī-tēr′ē-on, -ē-ă). **1.** A standard or rule for judging; usually plural (criteria) denoting a set of standards or rules. **2.** In psychology, a standard such as school grades against which test scores on intelligence tests or other measured behaviors are validated. **3.** A list of manifestations of a disease or disorder, a certain number of which must be present to warrant diagnosis in a given patient. [G. *kritērion,* a standard]

Spiegelberg's criteria (for diagnosis of ovarian pregnancy), 1) the oviduct on the affected side must be intact; 2) the amnionic sac must occupy the position of the ovary; 3) the amnionic sac must be connected to the uterus by the ovarian ligament; and 4) ovarian tissue must be present in the wall of the amnionic sac.

Cri·thid·ia (kri-thid′ē-ă). A genus of asexual, monogenetic, insect-parasitizing flagellates in the family Trypanosomatidae. [Mod. L., fr. G. *krithidion,* dim. of *krithē,* barley]

cri·thid·ia (kri-thid′ē-ă). Former term for epimastigote. [Mod. L. fr. G. *krithidion,* dim. of *krithē,* barley]

crit·i·cal (krit-ĭ-kăl). **1.** Denoting or of the nature of a crisis. **2.** Denoting a morbid condition in which death is possible. **3.** In sufficient quantity as to constitute a turning point.

CRL Abbreviation for crown-rump *length.*

CRM Abbreviation for cross-reacting *material.*

C.R.N.A. Abbreviation for certified registered *nurse* anesthetist.

cRNA. Abbreviation for complementary ribonucleic acid.

CRO Abbreviation for cathode ray *oscilloscope.*

croc·i·dis·mus (krok-i-dis'mŭs). SYN floccillation. [G. *krokē,* tuft of wool]

Crocq, Jean, Belgian physician, 1868–1925. SEE C.'s *disease.*

cro·cus (krō'kŭs). The dried stigmas of *Crocus sativus* (C. *of ficinalis*) (family Iridaceae), formerly used occasionally in flatulent dyspepsia; also formerly used as an antispasmodic in asthma and dysmenorrhea and as a coloring and flavoring agent. SYN saffron. [L. fr. G. *krokos,* the crocus, saffron (made from its stigmas)]

Crohn, Burrill, B., U.S. gastroenterologist, 1884–1983. SEE C.'s *disease.*

cro·mo·lyn so·di·um (krō'mō-lin). disodium 5,5'-[(2-hydroxytrimethylene)dioxy]bis[4-oxo-4*H*-1-benzopyran-2-carboxylate]; used for the prevention of asthmatic attack. SYN sodium cromoglycate.

Cronkhite, Leonard W., Jr., U.S. physician, *1919. SEE C.-Canada *syndrome.*

Crooke, Arthur, English pathologist, *1905. SEE C.'s *granules,* under *granule,* hyaline *change,* hyaline *degeneration.*

Crookes, Sir William, British physicist and chemist, 1832–1919; winner of the Nobel Prize in chemistry in 1907. SEE C.'s *glass;* C.-Hittorf *tube.*

Crosby, William Holmes, Jr., U.S. physician, *1914. SEE C. *capsule.*

cross (kros). **1.** Any figure in the shape of a c. formed by two intersecting lines. SYN crux. **2.** SYN *crux* of heart. **3.** A method of hybridization or the hybrid so produced. [F. *croix,* L. *crux*]

back c., the mating between an animal that is homozygous at a locus of interest and an animal that is heterozygous, commonly from the same ancestral stock.

double back c., a mating that is a back c. at each of two loci of interest; of special value and importance in linkage analysis.

hair c.'s, SYN *cruces* pilorum, under *crux.*

Ranvier's c.'s, black or brown figures in the shape of a c., marking Ranvier's nodes in the longitudinal section of a nerve stained with silver nitrate.

test c., in experimental genetics, a deliberate mating designed to test claims about the pattern of inheritance of one or more traits.

cross·bite (kros'bīt). An abnormal relation of one or more teeth of one arch to the opposing tooth or teeth of the other arch due to labial, buccal, or lingual deviation of tooth position, or to abnormal jaw position.

cross·breed (kros'brēd). **1.** SYN hybrid. **2.** To breed a hybrid.

cross·breed·ing (kros'brēd-ing). SYN hybridization.

cross-dress·ing. Clothing oneself in the clothes of the opposite sex. SEE transvestism.

cross-eye (kros'ī). Alternative spelling for crossed *eyes,* under *eye.*

cross·ing-over, cross·over (kros-ing-ō'ver, kros'ō-ver). Reciprocal exchange of material between two paired chromosomes during meiosis, resulting in the transfer of a block of genes from each chromosome to its homologue. In contrast to genetic recombination (2), which is a phenotypic phenomenon, c.-o. is genotypic. Any even number of c.-o. between two loci will cancel out phenotypically and no recombination will occur.

somatic c.-o., c.-o. that occurs during the mitosis of somatic cells, in contrast to that which occurs in meiosis.

uneven c.-o., unequal c.-o., c.-o. that happens when the breaks do not occur at precisely homologous points in two chromatid strands, and hence results in localized duplication of genetic material in one chromatid and complementary deletion in the other.

cross-link (kros-lingk). A covalent linkage between two polymers or between two different regions of the same polymer.

cross-match·ing (kros'match-ing). **1.** A test for incompatibility between donor and recipient blood, carried out prior to transfusion to avoid potentially lethal hemolytic reactions between the donor's red blood cells and antibodies in the recipient's plasma, or the reverse; performed by mixing a sample of red blood cells of the donor with plasma of the recipient (*major crossmatch*) and the red blood cells of the recipient with the plasma of the donor (*minor crossmatch*). Incompatibility is indicated by clumping of red blood cells and contraindicates use of the donor's blood. **2.** In allotransplantation of solid organs (*e.g.,* kidney), a test for identification of antibody in the serum of potential allograft recipients which reacts directly with the lymphocytes or other cells of a potential allograft donor; presence of these antibodies usually, if not always, contraindicates the performance of the transplantation because virtually all such grafts will be subject to a hyperacute type of rejection.

cross-sec·tion. **1.** A transverse section through a structure. **2.** The probability of an activation (5) by a nuclear reaction when a material is bombarded by neutrons, as in the production of radionuclides in a pile; unit: barn (10–24 cm^2/atom).

cross-sec·tion·al. SEE synchronic.

cross·way (kros'wā). The crossing of two nerve paths.

sensory c., the postlenticular portion of the posterior limb of the internal capsule of the brain.

Crosti, A., 20th century Italian dermatologist. SEE Gianotti-C. *syndrome.*

cro·ta·lid (krō'tă-lid). Any member of the snake family Crotalidae.

Cro·tal·i·dae (krō-tal'i-dē). A family of New World vipers characterized by the presence of a heat-sensitive loreal pit between each eye and nostril, and folding, caniculated, long anterior fangs.

cro·ta·lin (krot'ă-lin). A protein in rattlesnake venom. [*Crotalus,* a genus of rattlesnakes]

cro·ta·line (krot'ă-lēn). SYN monocrotaline.

cro·tal·ism (krō'tal-izm). SYN crotalaria *poisoning.*

Cro·ta·lus (krot'ă-lŭs). A genus of rattlesnakes (family Crotalidae) native to North America, having large fangs that are replaced periodically throughout life and a venom that is both neurotoxic and hemolytic. The largest species are the diamondbacks of the southern states (C. *adamanteus*) and western states (C. *atrox*); the smallest are the pigmy rattlers. [G. *krotalon,* a rattle, fr. *krotos,* a rattling noise]

cro·tam·i·ton (krō-tam'i-ton). *N*-Ethyl-*o*-crotonotoluide; a sarcopticide for topical use in scabies.

cro·taph·i·on (krō-taf'ē-on). The tip of the greater wing of the sphenoid bone; a point in craniometry. [G. *krotaphos,* the temple of the head]

cro·ton·ase (krō'ton-ās). SYN enoyl-CoA hydratase.

cro·ton oil (krō'ton). A fixed oil expressed from the seeds of *Croton tiglium* (family Euphorbiaceae), an East Indian shrub; used as an irritant purgative, and externally as a counterirritant and vesicant.

cro·to·nyl-ACP re·duc·tase (krō'ton-il). SYN enoyl-ACP reductase.

cro·tox·in (krō-tok'sin). The toxin from the venom of the North American rattlesnake. [*Crotalus* + toxin]

crot·tle. SYN cudbear.

croup (krūp). **1.** Laryngotracheobronchitis in infants and young children caused by parainfluenza viruses 1 and 2. **2.** Any affection of the larynx in children, characterized by difficult and noisy respiration and a hoarse cough. [Scots, probably from A.S. *kropan,* to cry aloud]

croup·ous (krū'pŭs). Relating to croup; marked by a fibrinous exudation.

croupy (krū'pē). Having the characteristics of croup, as a c. cough.

Crouzon, Octave, French physician, 1874–1938. SEE C.'s *disease, syndrome.*

crowd·ing (krowd′ing). A condition in which the teeth are crowded, assuming altered positions such as bunching, overlapping, displacement in various directions, torsiversion, etc.

Crowe, Samuel J., U.S. physician, 1883–1955. SEE Davis-C. mouth *gag.*

crown (krown). **1.** Any structure, normal or pathologic, resembling or suggesting a crown or a wreath. **2.** In dentistry, that part of a tooth that is covered with enamel, or an artificial substitute for that part. SYN corona [NA]. [L. *corona*]

anatomical c., SYN c. of tooth.

artificial c., a fixed restoration of the major part of the entire coronal part of a natural tooth; usually of gold, porcelain, or acrylic resin.

bell-shaped c., a c. of a tooth with an exaggerated occlusogingival contour; human deciduous molars typify the bell-shaped c.

ciliary c., SYN *corona* ciliaris.

clinical c., that part of the crown of a tooth visible in the oral cavity. SYN corona clinica [NA].

c. of head, SYN *corona* capitis.

jacket c., a hollow c. of acrylic resin, fused porcelain or cast gold, combinations of gold and acrylic or gold and porcelain; it fits over the prepared stump of the natural c.

radiate c., SYN *corona* radiata.

c. of tooth, the portion of a tooth covered with enamel. SYN corona dentis [NA], anatomical c.

c. of Venus, papular lesions of secondary syphilis on the forehead near the hair margin. SEE ALSO *collar* of Venus.

crown·ing (krown′ing). **1.** Preparation of the natural crown of a tooth and covering the prepared crown with a veneer of suitable dental material (gold or non-precious metal casting, porcelain, plastic, or combinations). **2.** That stage of childbirth when the fetal head has negotiated the pelvic outlet and the largest diameter of the head is encircled by the vulvar ring.

CRP Abbreviation for cAMP receptor *protein*; C-reactive *protein.*

CRT Abbreviation for cathode ray *tube.*

cru·ces (krū′sēz). Plural of crux.

cru·ci·ate (krū′shē-āt). Shaped like, or resembling, a cross. [L. *cruciatus*]

cru·ci·ble (krū′si-bl). A vessel used as a container for reactions or meltings at high temperature. [Mediev. L. *crucibulum*, a night lamp, later, a melting pot]

cru·fo·mate (krū′fō-māt). 4-*tert*-Butyl-2-chlorophenyl methyl methylphosphoramide; a veterinary anthelmintic.

cruor (krū′ōr). Coagulated blood. [L. blood (that flows from a wound)]

cru·ra (krū′ră). Plural of crus.

cru·ral (krū′răl). Relating to the leg or thigh, or to any crus.

cru·ra·lis pos·te·ri·or. SYN posterior *surface* of leg.

cru·re·us (krū-rē′ŭs). SYN vastus intermedius *muscle.* [Mod. L.]

crus, gen. **cru·ris,** pl. **cru·ra** (krūs, krū′ris, -ră) [NA]. **1.** SYN leg. **2.** Any anatomical structure resembling a leg; usually (in the plural) a pair of diverging bands or elongated masses. SEE ALSO limb. [L.]

ampullary crura of semicircular ducts, the dilated ends of the three semicircular ducts, each of which contains a specialized thickening of the epithelium known as the ampullary crest. SYN crura membranacea ampullaria ductus semicircularis [NA], ampullary limbs of semicircular ducts.

anterior c. of stapes, the anterior of the two delicate curving limbs of the stapes that pass from the head of the bone to the base or footplate. SYN c. anterius stapedis [NA], anterior limb of stapes.

c. ante′rius cap′sulae inter′nae [NA], SYN anterior *limb* of internal capsule.

c. ante′rius stape′dis [NA], SYN anterior c. of stapes.

c. anthel′icis [NA], SYN c. of antihelix.

c. of antihelix, one of two ridges, inferior and superior, bounding the fossa triangularis, by which the antihelix begins at the upper part of the auricle. SYN c. anthelicis [NA], leg of antihelix.

crura of bony semicircular canals, the extremities of the bony semicircular canals in which the corresponding membranous limbs of the semicircular ducts are located; they are the common bony c., simple bony c., and ampullary bony c. SYN crura ossea canalium semicircularium [NA], limbs of bony semicircular canals.

c. bre′ve incu′dis [NA], SYN short c. of incus.

c. cer′ebri [NA], specifically, the massive bundle of corticofugal nerve fibers passing longitudinally on the ventral surface of the midbrain on each side of the midline; it consists of fibers descending from the cortex to the tegmentum of the brainstem, pontine gray matter, and spinal cord. SEE ALSO cerebral *peduncle*, *basis* pedunculi.

c. clitor′idis [NA], SYN c. of clitoris.

c. of clitoris, the continuation on each side of the corpus cavernosum of the clitoris which diverges from the body posteriorly and is attached to the pubic arch. SYN c. clitoridis [NA].

common c. of semicircular ducts, the united, nonampullary ends of the superior and posterior semicircular ducts. SYN c. membranaceum commune ductus semicircularis [NA], common limb of membranous semicircular ducts.

c. cor′poris caverno′si pe′nis, SYN c. of penis.

c. dex′trum diaphrag′matis [NA], SYN right c. of diaphragm.

c. dex′trum fasci′culi atrioventricula′ris [NA], SYN right c. of atrioventricular bundle. SEE ALSO atrioventricular *bundle.*

c. for′nicis [NA], that part of the fornix that rises in a forward curve behind the thalamus to continue forward as the body for fornix ventral to the corpus callosum. SYN c. of fornix, posterior pillar of fornix.

c. of fornix, SYN c. fornicis.

c. hel′icis [NA], SYN c. of helix.

c. of helix, a transverse ridge continuing backward from the helix of the auricle, dividing the concha into an upper portion (cymba) and a lower portion (cavity of concha). SYN c. helicis [NA], crista helicis, limb of helix.

lateral c., limb or leg-like portion of a structure, farthest from midline. SYN c. laterale [NA], lateral limb.

c. latera′le [NA], SYN lateral c.

c. latera′le an′uli inguina′lis superficia′lis, SYN lateral c. of the superficial inguinal ring.

c. latera′le cartila′ginis ala′ris major′is, SYN lateral c. of the greater alar cartilage of the nose.

lateral c. of facial canal, laterally-placed, posteriorly-directed second portion of the horizontal part of the facial canal. SEE horizontal *part* of facial canal. SYN lateral c. of horizontal part of the facial canal.

lateral c. of the greater alar cartilage of the nose, portion of cartilage extending laterally and posteriorly in a wing-like fashion, supporting the wing of the nose and keeping the nostril patent. SYN c. laterale cartilaginis alaris majoris.

lateral c. of horizontal part of the facial canal, SYN lateral c. of facial canal. SEE horizontal *part* of facial canal.

lateral c. of the superficial inguinal ring, portion of the external oblique aponeurosis which passes lateral to the superficial inguinal ring blending into the inguinal ligament and forming the lateral boundary of the ring. SYN c. laterale anuli inguinalis superficialis.

left c. of atrioventricular bundle, the left leg or branch of the atrioventricular bundle which separates from the atrioventricular bundle just below the membranous portion of the interventricular septum to descend the septal wall of the left ventricle and begins to ramify subendocardially. SYN c. sinistrum fasciculi atrioventricularis [NA].

left c. of diaphragm, the muscular origin of the diaphragm from the upper two or three lumbar vertebrae that ascends to the left of the aorta to reach the central tendon. SYN c. sinistrum diaphragmatis [NA].

long c. of incus, the process of the incus that articulates with the stapes. SYN c. longum incudis [NA].

c. lon′gum incu′dis [NA], SYN long c. of incus.

medial c., limb or leg-like portion of a structure closest to the midline. SYN c. mediale [NA], medial limb.

c. media′le [NA], SYN medial c.

c. media′le ann′uli inguina′lis superficia′lis, SYN medial c. of the superficial inguinal ring.

c. media′le cartila′ginis ala′ris major′is, SYN medial c. of greater alar cartilage of nose.

medial c. of facial canal, medially-placed, anteriorly-directed first portion of the horizontal part of the facial canal. SEE horizontal *part* of facial canal. SYN medial c. of the horizontal part of the facial canal.

medial c. of greater alar cartilage of nose, portion of cartilage that forms the anterioinferior portion of the cartilaginous septum between nostrils. SYN c. mediale cartilaginis alaris majoris.

medial c. of the horizontal part of the facial canal, SYN medial c. of facial canal. SEE horizontal *part* of facial canal.

medial c. of the superficial inguinal ring, portion of the external oblique aponeurosis which passes medial to the superficial inguinal ring forming the medial boundary of the ring. SYN c. mediale annuli inguinalis superficialis.

cru′ra membrana′cea ampulla′ria duc′tus semicircula′ris [NA], SYN ampullary crura of semicircular ducts.

c. membrana′ceum commu′ne duc′tus semicircula′ris [NA], SYN common c. of semicircular ducts.

c. membrana′ceum sim′plex duc′tus semicircula′ris [NA], SYN simple c. of semicircular duct.

cru′ra os′sea cana′lium semicircula′rium [NA], SYN crura of bony semicircular canals.

c. pe′nis [NA], SYN c. of penis.

c. of penis, the posterior, tapering portion of the corpus cavernosum penis which diverges from its contralateral partner to be attached to the ischiopubic ramus. SYN c. penis [NA], c. corporis cavernosi penis.

posterior c. of stapes, the posterior of the two delicate limbs of the stapes that connect the head and base or footplate of the bone. SYN c. posterius stapedis [NA], posterior limb of stapes.

c. poste′rius cap′sulae inter′nae [NA], SYN posterior *limb* of internal capsule.

c. poste′rius stape′dis [NA], SYN posterior c. of stapes.

right c. of atrioventricular bundle, the right leg or branch of the atrioventricular bundle which diverges from the left c. just below the membranous portion of the interventricular septum to descend the septal wall of the right ventricle and ramify beneath the endocardium. SYN c. dextrum fasciculi atrioventricularis [NA].

right c. of diaphragm, the muscular origin of the diaphragm from the bodies of the upper three or four lumbar vertebrae that passes upward to the right of the aorta toward the central tendon; the esophageal hiatus is a parting of the fibers of the right c. to allow passage of the esophagus. SYN c. dextrum diaphragmatis [NA].

short c. of incus, the short c. of incus; the process of the incus that fits into a depression (fossa incudis) in the epitympanic recess. SYN c. breve incudis [NA].

simple c. of semicircular duct, the non-ampullary end of the lateral semicircular duct that opens independently into the utricle. SYN c. membranaceum simplex ductus semicircularis [NA], simple membranous limb of semicircular duct.

c. sinis′trum diaphrag′matis [NA], SYN left c. of diaphragm.

c. sinis′trum fasci′culi atrioventricula′ris [NA], SYN left c. of atrioventricular bundle. SEE ALSO atrioventricular *bundle.*

crus I (krūs). SYN superior semilunar *lobule.*

crus II (krūs). SYN inferior semilunar *lobule.*

crush (krŭsh). **1.** To squeeze injuriously between two hard bodies. **2.** A bruise or contusion from pressure between two solid bodies. [O. Fr. *cruisir*]

crus·ot·o·my (krŭs-ot′ō-mē). A mesencephalic pyramidal tractotomy. [L. *crus,* leg, + G. *tomē,* incision]

crust (krŭst). **1.** A hard outer layer or covering; cutaneous crusts are often formed by dried serum or pus on the surface of a ruptured blister or pustule. **2.** A scab. SYN crusta. [L. *crusta*]

milk c., SYN crusta lactea.

crus·ta, pl. **crus·tae** (krŭs′tă, -tē). SYN crust. [L.]

c. inflammato′ria, SYN buffy *coat.*

c. lac′tea, seborrhea of the scalp in an infant. SYN milk crust, milk scall.

c. phlogis′tica, SYN buffy *coat.*

Crus·ta·cea (krŭs-tā′shē-ă). A very large class of aquatic animals (phylum Arthropoda) with a chitinous exoskeleton and jointed appendages; *e.g.,* the crab, lobster, crayfish, shrimp, isopods, ostracods, and amphipods. Some, such as certain copepods, are parasitic; others serve as intermediate hosts for parasitic worms which cause disease in man and various vertebrates. SEE ALSO Copepoda. [L. *crusta,* a crust]

crutch (krŭtch). A device used singly or in pairs to assist in walking when the act is impaired by a lower extremity (or trunk) disability; it transfers all or part of weight-bearing to the upper extremity. [A. S. *cryce*]

Cruveilhier, Jean, French pathologist and anatomist, 1791–1874. SEE C.'s *disease, fascia, fossa; fossa* navicularis Cruveilhier; C.'s *joint, ligaments,* under *ligament, plexus;* C.-Baumgarten *disease, murmur, sign, syndrome.*

crux, pl. **cru·ces** (krŭks, krū′sēz). A junction or crossing. SYN cross (1). [L.]

c. of heart, the zone of junction of the septa and walls of the four chambers of the heart. SYN cross (2).

cru′ces pilo′rum [NA], crosslike figures formed by hairs growing from two directions that meet and then separate in a direction perpendicular to the original orientation. SYN hair crosses.

Cruz, Oswaldo, Brazilian physician, 1872–1917. SEE Chagas-C. *disease;* C. *trypanosomiasis.*

△**cry-.** SEE cryo-.

cry·al·ge·sia (krī-al-jē′zē-ă). Pain caused by cold. SYN crymodynia. [G. *kryos,* cold, + *algos,* pain]

cry·an·es·the·sia (krī′an-es-thē′zē-ă). Inability to perceive cold. [G. *kryos,* cold, + *an-* priv. + *aisthēsis,* sensation]

cry·es·the·sia (krī-es-thē′zē-ă). **1.** A subjective sensation of cold. **2.** Sensitiveness to cold. [G. *kryos,* cold, + *aisthēsis,* sensation]

cry for help. Telephone calls, notes left in conspicuous places, and other behaviors which communicate extreme distress and potential suicide.

△**crymo-.** Cold. SEE ALSO cryo-, psychro-. [G. *krymos,*]

cry·mo·dyn·ia (krī-mō-din′ē-ă). SYN cryalgesia. [crymo- + G. *odynē,* pain]

cry·mo·phil·ic (krī-mō-fil′ik). Preferring cold; denoting microorganisms which thrive best at low temperatures. SYN cryophilic. [crymo- + G. *philos,* fond]

cry·mo·phy·lac·tic (krī′mō-fi-lak′tik). Resistant to cold, said of certain microorganisms which are not destroyed even by freezing temperatures. SYN cryophylactic. [crymo- + G. *phylaxis,* a guarding against]

△**cryo-, cry-.** Cold. SEE ALSO crymo-, psychro-. [G. *kryos,*]

cry·o·an·es·the·sia (krī′ō-an-es-thē′zē-ă). Localized application of cold as a means of producing regional anesthesia. SYN refrigeration anesthesia.

cry·o·bi·ol·o·gy (krī′ō-bī-ol′ō-jē). The study of the effects of low temperatures on living organisms.

cry·o·cau·tery (krī′ō-kaw′ter-ē). Any substance, such as liquid air or carbon dioxide snow, or a low temperature instrument, the application of which causes destruction of tissue by freezing. SYN cold cautery.

cry·o·con·i·za·tion (krī′ō-kon-ī-zā′shŭn). Freezing of a cone of endocervical tissue *in vivo* with a cryoprobe.

cry·o·ex·trac·tion (krī′ō-ek-strak′shŭn). Removal of cataracts by the adhesion of a freezing probe to the lens; now rarely done.

cry·o·ex·trac·tor (krī′ō-ek-strak′tŏr, -tōr). An instrument, artificially cooled, for extraction of the lens by freezing contact.

cry·o·fi·brin·o·gen (krī′ō-fī-brin′ō-jen). An abnormal type of fibrinogen very rarely found in human plasma; it is precipitated upon cooling, but redissolves when warmed to room temperature.

cry·o·fi·brin·o·gen·e·mia (krī′ō-fī-brin′ō-je-nē′mē-ă). The presence in the blood of cryofibrinogens.

cry·o·flu·o·rane (krī-ō-flūr′ān). 1,2-Dichloro-1,1,2,2-tetrafluoroethane; used as a refrigerant and aerosol propellant; may be irritating to the respiratory tract and mildly narcotic.

cry·o·gen (krī'ō-jen). A freezing substance used to produce very low temperatures.

cry·o·gen·ic (krī-ō-jen'ik). **1.** Denoting or characteristic of a cryogen. **2.** Relating to cryogenics.

cry·o·gen·ics (krī-ō-jen'iks). The science concerned with the production and effects of very low temperatures, particularly temperatures in the range of liquid helium (<4.25 K). [cryo- + G. *-gen,* producing]

cry·o·glob·u·lin·e·mia (krī'ō-glob'yū-li-nē'mē-ă). The presence of abnormal quantities of cryoglobulin in the blood plasma.

cry·o·glob·u·lins (krī-ō-glob'yū-linz). Abnormal plasma proteins (paraproteins), now grouped with gamma globulins, characterized by precipitating, gelling, or crystallizing when serum or solutions of them are cooled; distinguished from Bence Jones proteins by their larger molecular weight (approximately 200,000 compared with 35,000 to 50,000); they may appear in patients with multiple myeloma.

cry·o·hy·drate (krī-ō-hī'drāt). A eutectic system of a salt and water.

cry·o·hy·poph·y·sec·to·my (krī'ō-hī-pof'i-sek'tō-mē). Destruction of hypophysis by the application of extreme cold. [cryo- + hypophysis + G. *ektomē,* excision]

cry·ol·y·sis (krī-ol'i-sis). Destruction by cold. [cryo- + G. *lysis,* dissolution]

cry·om·e·ter (krī-om'ĕ-ter). A device for measuring very low temperatures. [cryo- + G. *metron,* measure]

cry·o·pal·li·dec·to·my (krī'ō-pal-i-dek'tō-mē). Destruction of the globus pallidus by the application of extreme cold. [cryo- + globus pallidus + G. *ektomē,* excision]

cry·op·a·thy (krī-op'ă-thē). A morbid condition in which exposure to cold is an important factor. SYN frigorism. [cryo- + G. *pathos,* suffering]

cry·o·pexy (krī'ō-pek-sē). In retinal detachment surgery, sealing the sensory retina to the pigment epithelium and choroid by a freezing probe applied to the sclera. [cryo- + G. *pēxis,* a fixing in place]

cry·o·phil·ic (krī-ō-fil'ik). SYN crymophilic. [cryo- + G. *philos,* fond]

cry·o·phy·lac·tic (krī'ō-fī-lak'tik). SYN crymophylactic.

cry·o·pre·cip·i·tate (krī'ō-prē-sip'i-tāt). Precipitate which forms when soluble material is cooled, especially with reference to the precipitate that forms in normal blood plasma which has been subjected to cold precipitation and which is rich in factor VIII.

cry·o·pre·cip·i·ta·tion (krī'ō-prē-sip-i-tā'shŭn). The process of forming a cryoprecipitate from solution.

cry·o·pres·er·va·tion (krī'ō-pres-er-vā'shŭn). Maintenance of the viability of excised tissues or organs at extremely low temperatures.

cry·o·probe (krī'ō-prōb). An instrument used in cryosurgery to apply extreme cold to a selected area. [cryo- + L. *probo,* to test]

cry·o·pros·ta·tec·to·my (krī'ō-pros-tă-tek'tō-mē). Destruction of the prostate gland by freezing, utilizing a specially designed cryoprobe. [cryo- + L. *prostata,* prostate, + G. *ektomē,* excision]

cry·o·pro·tein (krī-ō-prō'tēn). A protein that precipitates from solution when cooled and redissolves upon warming.

cry·o·pul·vi·nec·to·my (krī'ō-pŭl-vi-nek'tō-mē). Destruction of the pulvinar by the application of extreme cold. [cryo- + pulvinar + G. *ektomē,* excision]

cry·o·scope (krī'ō-skōp). An instrument for measuring the freezing point.

cry·os·co·py (krī-os'kŏ-pē). The determination of the freezing point of a fluid, usually blood or urine, compared with that of distilled water. SYN algoscopy. [cryo- + G. *skopeō,* to examine]

cry·o·spasm (krī'ō-spazm). Spasm produced by cold. [cryo- + G. *spasmos,* convulsion]

cry·o·stat (krī'ō-stat). A freezing chamber. [cryo- + G. *statos,* standing]

cry·o·sur·gery (krī-ō-ser'jer-ē). An operation using freezing temperature (achieved by liquid nitrogen or carbon dioxide) to destroy tissue.

cry·o·thal·a·mec·to·my (krī'ō-thal-ă-mek'tō-mē). Destruction of the thalamus by the application of extreme cold. [cryo- + thalamus + G. *ektomē,* excision]

cry·o·ther·a·py (krī'ō-thār'ă-pē). The use of cold in the treatment of disease.

cry·o·tol·er·ant (krī-ō-tol'er-ant). Tolerant of very low temperatures.

crypt (kript). A pitlike depression or tubular recess. SYN crypta [NA].

anal c.'s, SYN anal *sinuses,* under *sinus.*

dental c., the space filled by the dental follicle.

enamel c., the narrow, mesenchyme-filled space between the dental ledge and an enamel organ. SYN enamel niche.

c.'s of Henle, infoldings of conjunctiva.

c.'s of iris, **(1)** pits near the pupillary margin of the anterior surface of the iris. **(2)** spaces in the anterior iris stroma through which the aqueous washes with every pupillary movement.

Lieberkühn's c.'s, SYN intestinal *glands,* under *gland.*

lingual c., a pit lined with epithelium in the lingual tonsil.

Morgagni's c.'s, SYN anal *sinuses,* under *sinus.*

synovial c., a diverticulum of the synovial membrane of a joint.

tonsillar c., one of the variable number of deep recesses that extend into the palatine and pharyngeal tonsils from the free surface where they open at the tonsillar fossa. SYN crypta tonsillaris [NA].

crypt-. SEE crypto-.

cryp·ta, pl. **cryp·tae** (krip'tă, -tē) [NA]. SYN crypt. [L. fr. G. *kryptos,* hidden]

c. tonsilla'ris, pl. **cryp'tae tonsilla'res** [NA], SYN tonsillar *crypt.*

cryp·tec·to·my (krip-tek'tō-mē). Excision of a tonsillar or other crypt. [crypt + G. *ektomē,* excision]

cryp·ten·a·mine ac·e·tates, cryp·ten·a·mine tan·nates (krip-ten'ă-mēn). Acetate or tannate salts of alkaloids from a nonaqueous extract of *Veratrum viride,* containing the hypotensive alkaloids protoveratrines A and B, germitrine, neogermetrine, germerine, germidine, jervine, rubijervine, isorubijervine, and germubide; used as an antihypertensive agent. SEE ALSO protoveratrine A and B.

cryp·tic (krip'tik). Hidden; occult; larvate. [G. *kryptikos*]

cryp·ti·tis (krip-tī'tis). Inflammation of a follicle or glandular tubule, particularly in the rectum.

crypto-, crypt-. Hidden, obscure; without apparent cause. [G. *kryptos,* hidden, concealed]

cryp·to·coc·co·ma (krip'tō-kok-ō'mă). An infectious granuloma, typically in the brain, but also found in the lung and elsewhere, caused by *Cryptococcus neoformans.* SYN toruloma. [*Cryptococcus* (genus name) + -oma]

cryp·to·coc·co·sis (krip'tō-kok-ō'sis). An acute, subacute, or chronic infection by *Cryptococcus neoformans,* causing a pulmonary, disseminated, or meningeal mycosis. The pulmonary form is usually transitory, mild, and unrecognized; cutaneous, skeletal, and visceral lesions may occur during dissemination; the most familiar and readily recognized form involves the central nervous system, with subacute or chronic meningitis. SYN Busse-Buschke disease.

Cryp·to·coc·cus (krip-tō-kok'ŭs). A genus of yeastlike fungi that reproduce by budding. [crypto- + G. *kokkos,* berry]

C. neofor'mans, a species that causes cryptococcosis in humans and other mammalians and parasitizes cats in some areas, although strains vary in virulence; the cells are spherical and may bud at any point on the surface or simultaneously at several points; a prominent feature is a mucoid polysaccharide capsule which may vary in width from very thin to several times the radius of the parent cell and buds combined. Once thought to be widespread in nature, its true niche appears to be narrowing to a saprobic association with the manure and nests of pigeons; it is therefore essentially global in distribution.

cryp·to·crys·tal·line (krip-tō-kris'tă-lēn). Having very minute crystals.

Cryp·to·cys·tis trich·o·dec·tis (krip-tō-sis'tis trī-kō-dek'tis). Name formerly applied to the larval form of the dog tapeworm, *Dipylidium caninum*, named for the cysticercoids found in the dog louse, *Trichodectes*. [crypto- + G. *kystis*, bladder; tricho- + G. *dektēs*, a beggar]

cryp·to·did·y·mus (krip'tō-did'i-mŭs). Conjoined twins, with the poorly developed parasitic twin concealed within the larger autosite. SEE conjoined *twins*, under *twin*. [crypto- + G. *didymos*, twin]

Cryp·to·gam·ia (krip-tō-gam'ē-ă). A montaxonomic division of the plant kingdom containing all forms of plant life that do not reproduce by means of seeds; included are the algae, bacteria, fungi, lichens, mosses, liverworts, ferns, horsetails, and club mosses. [crypto- + G. *gamos*, marriage]

cryp·to·gen·ic (krip-tō-jen'ik). Of obscure, indeterminate etiology or origin, in contrast to phanerogenic. [crypto- + G. *genesis*, origin]

cryp·to·lith (krip'tō-lith). A concretion in a gland follicle. [crypto- + G. *lithos*, stone]

cryp·to·men·or·rhea (krip'tō-men-ō-rē'ă). Occurrence each month of the general symptoms of the menses without any flow of blood, as in cases of imperforate hymen. [crypto- + G. *mēn*, month, + *rhoia*, flow]

cryp·toph·thal·mus, cryp·toph·thal·mia (krip-tof-thal'mŭs, -thal'mē-ă). Congenital absence of eyelids, with the skin passing continuously from the forehead onto the cheek over a rudimentary eye. [crypto- + G. *ophthalmos*, eye]

cryp·to·po·dia (krip-tō-pō'dē-ă). A swelling of the lower part of the leg and the foot, in such a manner that there is great distortion and the sole seems to be a flattened pad. [crypto- + G. *pous*, foot]

cryp·to·pyr·role (krip-tō-pir'ōl). 3-Ethyl-2,4-dimethylpyrrole; one of the pyrrole derivatives obtained by the drastic reduction of heme.

cryp·tor·chid (krip-tōr'kid). Relating to or characterized by cryptorchism. [crypto- + G. *orchis*, testis]

cryp·tor·chi·dism (krip-tōr'ki-dizm). SYN cryptorchism.

cryp·tor·chi·do·pexy (krip-tōr'ki-dō-pek'sē). SYN orchiopexy. [crypto- + G. *orchis*, testis, + *pēxis*, fixation]

cryp·tor·chism (krip-tōr'kizm). Failure of one or both of the testes to descend. SYN cryptorchidism.

cryp·to·scope (krip'tō-skōp). Early term for a simple x-ray fluoroscope. [G. *kryptos*, something hidden, + *skopeō*, to examine]

cryp·to·spo·rid·i·o·sis (krip'tō-spō-rid-ē-ō'sis). An enteric disease caused by waterborne protozoan parasites of the genus *Cryptosporidium;* characterized pathologically by villous atrophy and fusion and clinically by diarrhea in man, calves, lambs, and other animal species; disease in immunocompetent persons is manifest as a self-limiting diarrhea, whereas in immunocompromised persons it is manifest as a prolonged severe diarrhea that can be fatal.

Cryp·to·spo·rid·i·um (krip'tō-spō-rid'ē-ŭm). A genus of coccidian sporozoans (family Cryptosporiidae, suborder Eimeriina) that are important pathogens of calves and other domestic animals, and common opportunistic parasites of humans that flourish under conditions of compromised immune function.

Cryp·to·stro·ma cor·ti·ca·le (krip-tō-strō'mă kōr-ti-kā'lē). A species of fungus that is a common allergen, growing profusely under the bark of stacked maple logs; handlers who inhale the massive number of spores may develop pneumonitic as well as allergic reactions, including maple bark disease. [crypto- + G. *stroma*, bed]

cryp·to·tia (krip-tō'shē-ă). A deformity, usually congenital, in which the superior portion of the auricle is hidden under the scalp. [crypto- + G. *ōtos*, ear]

cryp·to·xan·thin (krip-tō-zan'thin). (3*R*)-β,β-Caroten-3-ol; β-caroten-3-ol; carotenoid (specifically, a xanthophyll) yielding 1 mole of vitamin A per mole. Found in many fruits and berries.

cryp·to·zo·ite (krip'tō-zō'īt). The exoerythrocyte stage of the malarial organism that develops directly from the sporozoite inoculated by the infected mosquito; development of the first generation of merozoites in vertebrate host tissues occurs in the liver parenchyma. [crypto- + G. *zōē*, life]

cryp·to·zy·gous (krip-toz'i-gŭs, -tō-zī'gŭs). Having a narrow face as compared with the width of the cranium, so that, when the skull is viewed from above, the zygomatic arches are not visible. [crypto- + G. *zygon*, yoke]

crys·tal (kris'tăl). A solid of regular shape and, for a given compound, characteristic angles, formed when an element or compound solidifies slowly enough, as a result either of freezing from the liquid form or of precipitating out of solution, to allow the individual molecules to take up regular positions with respect to one another. [G. *krystallos*, clear ice, crystal]

asthma c.'s, SYN Charcot-Leyden c.'s.

blood c.'s, SYN hematoidin.

Böttcher's c.'s, small c.'s observed microscopically in prostatic fluid that is treated with a drop or two of 1% solution of ammonium phosphate.

Charcot-Leyden c.'s, c.'s in the shape of elongated double pyramids, formed from eosinophils, found in the sputum in bronchial asthma and in other exudates or transudates containing eosinophils. SYN asthma c.'s, Charcot-Neumann c.'s, Charcot-Robin c.'s, Leyden's c.'s.

Charcot-Neumann c.'s, SYN Charcot-Leyden c.'s.

Charcot-Robin c.'s, SYN Charcot-Leyden c.'s.

chiral c., an enantiomorphic, dyssymmetric, optically active c.

chlorohemin c.'s, SYN Teichmann's c.'s.

clathrate c., lattice-like arrangement of molecules of one substance surrounding molecules of another substance.

ear c.'s, SYN statoliths.

Florence's c.'s, brown rhombic c.'s formed at the interface between a drop of Lugol's solution and a drop of fluid that contains semen; not a specific test for the latter.

hematoidin c.'s, SYN hematoidin.

hydrate c., one of several possible microstructural arrangements of water molecules based on intermolecular forces; suggested as being involved in the mode of action of inhalation anesthetics.

knife-rest c., a c. of ammoniomagnesium phosphate found in alkaline urine.

Leyden's c.'s, SYN Charcot-Leyden c.'s.

Lubarsch's c.'s, intracellular c.'s in the testis resembling sperm c.'s.

sperm c., spermin c., a c. of spermin phosphate found in the semen; possibly identical to Böttcher's c.'s.

Teichmann's c.'s, rhombic c.'s of hemin; used in microscopic detection of blood. SEE hemin. SYN chlorohemin c.'s.

thorn apple c.'s, ammonium urate c.'s in the shape of rounded bodies with many projecting points.

twin c., two c.'s that have grown together along a common face.

Virchow's c.'s, yellow-brown, amber, or burnt orange c.'s of hematoidin, frequently observed in extravasated blood in tissues.

whetstone c.'s, xanthine c.'s occasionally observed in urine.

crys·tal·lin (kris'tă-lin). A type of protein found in the lens of the eye; alpha (an embryonic single protein), beta, and gamma varieties (based on precipitibility) are known. Reptiles and birds have a δ-c. as well.

gamma c., the least rapidly mobile form of c. on electrophoresis.

crys·tal·line (kris'tă-lēn). 1. Clear; transparent. 2. Relating to a crystal or crystals.

crys·tal·li·za·tion (kris'tăl-i-zā'shŭn). Assumption of a crystalline form when a vapor or liquid becomes solidified, or a solute precipitates from solution.

crys·tal·lo·gram (kris'tă-lō-gram). A photograph produced when x-rays are diffracted by a crystal. [G. *krystallos*, crystal, + *gramma*, something written]

crys·tal·log·ra·phy (kris-tăl-log'ră-fē). The study of the shape and atomic structure of crystals.

crys·tal·loid (kris'tăl-oyd). 1. Resembling a crystal, or being such. 2. A body that in solution can pass through a semipermeable membrane, as distinguished from a colloid, which cannot do so.

cr

Charcot-Böttcher c.'s, spindle-shaped c.'s 10 to 25 μm long, found in human Sertoli cells.

Reinke c.'s, rod-shaped crystal-like structures with pointed or rounded ends present in the interstitial cells of the testis (Leydig cells) and ovary.

crys·tal·lo·pho·bia (kris'tăl-ō-fō'bē-ă). SYN hyalophobia. [G. *krystallon,* crystal, + *phobos,* fear]

crys·tal·lu·ria (kris-tă-lū'rē-ă). The excretion of crystalline materials in the urine.

crys·tal vi·o·let (kris'tăl) [C.I. 42555]. hexamethylpararosanilin chloride; a compound that has been used in the external treatment of burns, wounds, and fungal infections of skin and mucous membranes, and internally for pinworm and certain fluke infections; used also as a stain for chromatin, amyloid, platelets in blood, fibrin, and neuroglia, and to differentiate among bacteria. SYN methylrosaniline chloride.

cry·to·te·ta·ny (krī'tō). SYN latent *tetany*.

Cs Symbol for cesium.

C-sec·tion. SEE cesarean *section*.

CSF Abbreviation for cerebrospinal *fluid*; colony-stimulating *factors,* under *factor*.

CSI. Abbreviation for Calculus Surface Index.

Csillag, J. SEE C.'s *disease*.

CT Abbreviation for computed *tomography*.

dynamic CT, SYN dynamic computed *tomography*.

helical CT, SYN spiral computed *tomography*.

spiral CT, SYN spiral computed *tomography*.

CTD Abbreviation for cumulative trauma *disorders,* under *disorder*.

Cteno·ce·phal·i·des (tē-nō-se-fal'i-dēz). A genus of fleas. *C. canis* (dog flea) and *C. felis* (cat flea) are nearly universal ectoparasites of household pets; will attack man when starving owing to absence of pets. [G. *ktenōdēs,* like a cockle, + *kephalē,* head]

CTL Abbreviation for cytotoxic T lymphocytes.

CTP Abbreviation for cytidine 5′-triphosphate.

Cu Symbol for copper.

⁶⁴Cu. Symbol for copper-64.

⁶⁷Cu. Symbol for copper-67.

cu·beb (kyū'beb). The dried unripe, nearly full-grown fruit of *Piper cubeba* (family Piperaceae), a climbing plant of the West Indies, used as stimulant, carminative, and local irritant; c. oil has been used as a mild urinary antiseptic. [Ar. and Hindu, *kababa*]

cu·bi·tal (kyū'bi-tăl). Relating to the elbow or to the ulna.

cu·bi·tus, gen. and pl. **cu·bi·ti** (kyū'bi-tŭs, -tī) [NA]. **1.** SYN elbow (1). **2.** SYN ulna. [L. elbow]

c. val'gus, deviation of the extended forearm to the outer (radial) side of the axis of the limb.

c. va'rus, deviation of the extended forearm to the inward (ulnar) side of the axis of the limb.

cu·boid, cu·boi·dal (kyū'boyd, kyū-boy'dăl). **1.** Resembling a cube in shape. **2.** Relating to the os cuboideum. [G. *kybos,* cube, + *eidos,* resemblance]

cud·bear (kŭd'bār). Purple-red coloring agent derived from the lichen *Ochrolechia tartarea* (family Lecanoraceae) and for the coloring principles from Roccellaceae used for coloring liquid pharmaceutical preparations. SYN crottle.

cue (kyū). In conditioning and learning theory, a pattern of stimuli to which an individual has learned or is learning to respond.

response-produced c.'s, successive stimulus c.'s in a behavior chain, each response serving as a reinforcer for the previous response and as a stimulus, or c., for the next response. SEE higher order *conditioning,* behavior *chain*.

cuff (kŭf). Any structure shaped like a c.

musculotendinous c., SYN rotator c. of shoulder.

perivascular c.'s, SEE cuffing.

rotator c. of shoulder, the upper half of the capsule of the shoulder joint reinforced by the tendons of insertion of the supra-

1 corpus humeri
2 epicondylus medialis [humeri]
3 epicondylus lateralis [humeri]
4 capitulum humeri
5 trochlea humeri
6 caput radii (radiale)
7 collum radii
8 corpus radii
9 tuberositas radii
10 tuberositas ulnae

11 processus coronoideus [ulnae]
12 corpus ulnae
13 capsula articularis
14 articulatio radio-ulnaris proximalis
15 lig. collaterale radiale
16 lig. collaterale ulnare
17 lig. anulare radii
18 capsula articularis
19 membrana interossea antebrachii
20 fossa radialis
21 fossa coronoidea
22 chorda obliqua
23 foramina nutrientia

cubitus
the right elbow, frontal view; the joint capsule is exposed

spinatus, infraspinatus, teres minor, and subscapularis muscles. SYN musculotendinous c.

cuff·ing (kŭf'ing). A perivascular accumulation of various leukocytes seen in infectious, inflammatory, or autoimmune diseases. **2.** To surround a structure with fluid or cells, as with a cuff; in chest radiography, thickening of bronchial walls on the image. [M.E. *cuffe,* mitten]

cui·rass (kwē-ras'). The anterior surface of the thorax in relation to symptoms or disease changes. [Fr. *cuirasse,* a breastplate]

analgesic c., SYN tabetic c.

tabetic c., an analgesic or hypalgesic zone in the proximal thoracic region, found in tabetic neurosyphilis. SYN analgesic c., Hitzig's girdle.

cul-de-sac, pl. **culs-de-sac** (kŭl-de-sak'). **1.** A blind pouch or tubular cavity closed at one end; *e.g.,* diverticulum; cecum. **2.** SYN rectouterine *pouch*. [Fr. bottom of a sack]

conjunctival cul-de-sac, SYN conjunctival *fornix*.

Douglas' cul-de-sac, SYN rectouterine *pouch*.

greater cul-de-sac, SYN *fundus* of stomach.

Gruber's cul-de-sac, a lateral diverticulum in the suprasternal space beside the medial extremity of the clavicle behind the sternal attachment of the sternocleidomastoid muscle.

lesser cul-de-sac, SYN pyloric *antrum*.

cul·do·cen·te·sis (kŭl'dō-sen-tē'sis). Aspiration of fluid from the cul-de-sac (rectouterine excavation) by puncture of the vaginal vault near the midline between the uterosacral ligaments. [cul-de-sac + G. *kentēsis,* puncture]

cul·do·plas·ty (kŭl'dō-plas-tē). Plastic surgery to remedy relaxation of the posterior fornix of the vagina. [cul-de-sac + G. *plastos,* formed]

cul·do·scope (kŭl'dō-skōp). Endoscopic instrument used in culdoscopy.

cul·dos·co·py (kŭl-dos'kŏ-pē). Introduction of an endoscope through the posterior vaginal wall for viewing the rectovaginal pouch and pelvic viscera. [cul-de-sac + G. *skopeō,* to view]

cul·dot·o·my (kŭl-dot′ō-mē). **1.** Cutting into the cul-de-sac of Douglas. **2.** SYN vaginal *celiotomy.* [cul-de-sac + G. *tomē,* incision]

Cu·lex (kyū′leks). A genus of mosquitoes (family Culicidae) including over 2,000 species. Largely tropical but worldwide in distribution; they are vectors for a number of diseases of man and of domestic and wild animals and birds. [L. gnat]

C. pi′piens, a subspecies complex of the abundant polytypic species, the brown house mosquito or rainbarrel mosquito of temperate climates, which breeds commonly in standing water, especially in artificial containers, and has a 5- to 6-day cycle under optimal conditions; closely related forms are found in tropical areas.

C. tarsa′lis, a species that is an important vector of St. Louis and western equine encephalomyelitis viruses in horses, birds, and man.

Cu·lic·i·dae (kyū-lis′i-dē). A family of insects (order Diptera) that includes the true mosquitoes, which are all included in the subfamily Culicinae.

cu·li·ci·dal (kyū-li-sī′dăl). Destructive to mosquitoes. [L. *culex,* gnat, + *caedo,* to kill]

cu·li·cide (kyū′li-sīd). An agent that destroys mosquitoes.

cu·lic·i·fuge (kyū-lis′i-fūj). **1.** Driving away gnats and mosquitoes. **2.** An agent that keeps mosquitoes from biting. [L. *culex,* gnat + *fugo,* to drive away]

Cu·li·coi·des (kyū-li-koy′dēz). A genus of minute biting gnats or midges, vectors of several nonpathogenic human filariae (*Mansonella, Dipetalonema*), of *Onchocerca* in horses and cattle, and of several viral agents of domestic sheep and fowl. [L. *culex,* gnat]

C. aus′teni, species that is an intermediate host of the filarial worm, *Mansonella perstans,* chiefly in equatorial Africa.

C. fu′rens, species that is a vector of *Mansonella ozzardi,* in the West Indies.

C. mil′nei, a species that is one of the vectors of *Mansonella perstans* in West Africa.

C. variipen′nis, a species that is the primary vector of bluetongue virus in the U.S.

cu·li·co·sis (kyū′li-kō′sis). Dermatitis caused by *Culex* mosquitoes.

Cu·li·se·ta melanura (kū-li-sē′tă mel-ă-nū′ră). A species of mosquito that is the principal endemic vector of eastern equine encephalomyelitis virus; since this species feeds primarily on birds, other mosquitoes (*Aedes* spp.) transmit the virus from birds to humans and horses.

Cullen, Thomas S., U.S. gynecologist, 1868–1953. SEE C.'s *sign.*

cul·men, pl. **cul·′mi·na** (kul′men) [NA]. The anterior prominent portion of the monticulus of the vermis of the cerebellum; vermal lobule rostral to the primary fissure. SYN lobulus culminis. [L. summit]

Culp, Ormond S., U.S. urologist, 1910–1977. SEE C. *pyeloplasty.*

cult (kŭlt). A system of beliefs and rituals based on dogma or religious teachings and characterized by devoted adherents who display a readiness to obey, an unrealistic idealization of the leader, an abandonment of personal ambition and goals, and an eschewing of traditional societal values. [L. *cultus,* an honoring, adoration]

cul·ti·va·tion (kŭl-ti-vā′shŭn). SYN culture. [Mediev. L. *cultivo,* pp. *-atus,* fr. L. *colo,* pp. *cultus,* to till]

cul·tur·al di·ver·si·ty. The inevitable variety in customs, attitudes, practices, and behavior that exists among groups of individuals from different ethnic, racial, or national backgrounds who come into contact.

cul·ture (kŭl′chŭr). **1.** The propagation of microorganisms on or in media of various kinds. **2.** A mass of microorganisms on or in a medium. **3.** The propagation of mammalian cells, *i.e.,* cell culture. SEE cell c. SYN cultivation. [L. *cultura,* tillage, fr. *colo,* pp. *cultus,* to till]

batch c., a technique for large-scale production of microbes or microbial products in which, at a given point in time, the fermenter is stopped and the c. is worked up.

cell c., the maintenance or growth of dispersed cells after removal from the body, commonly on a glass surface immersed in nutrient fluid.

continuous c., a technique for production of microbes or microbial products in which nutrients are continuously supplied to the fermenter.

discontinuous c., a technique for production of microbes or microbial products in which the organisms are grown in a closed system until one nutrient factor becomes rate-limiting.

elective c., a method of isolating microorganisms capable of utilizing a specific substrate by incubating an inoculum in a medium containing the substrate; the medium usually contains substances or has characteristics that inhibit the growth of unwanted microorganisms. SYN enrichment c.

enrichment c., SYN elective c.

hanging-block c., the propagation of microorganisms on a cube of solidified agar medium which is inoculated, attached to a cover glass, and inverted over a moist chamber or hollowed slide.

mixed lymphocyte c., SEE mixed lymphocyte culture *test.*

needle c., SYN stab c.

neotype c., SYN neotype *strain.*

organ c., the maintenance or growth of tissues, organ primordia, or the parts or whole of an organ *in vitro* in such a way as to allow differentiation or preservation of the architecture or function.

pure c., in the ordinary bacteriologic sense, a c. consisting of the descendants of a single cell.

roll-tube c., a c. in a tube of medium which has been melted and allowed to solidify while the tube is being spun; the inside of the tube is thereby coated with a thin layer of solidified medium.

sensitized c., a live c. of an organism to which a specific antiserum is added; after the mixture is incubated for several minutes (during which the antibody in the serum combines with the organisms), the excess serum is removed by means of centrifugation, washing in physiologic saline solution, and recentrifugation; the sensitized organisms may then be resuspended in physiologic saline solution.

shake c., a c. made by inoculating a liquefied gelatin or agar medium, distributing the inoculum thoroughly by agitation, and then allowing the medium to solidify in the tube in an upright position.

slant c., a c. made on the slanting surface of a medium which has been solidified in a test tube inclined from the perpendicular so as to give a greater area than that of the lumen of the tube. SYN slope c.

slope c., SYN slant c.

smear c., a c. obtained by spreading material presumed to be infected on the surface of a solidified medium.

stab c., a c. produced by inserting an inoculating needle with inoculum down the center of a solid medium contained in a test tube. SYN needle c.

stock c., a c. of a microorganism maintained solely for the purpose of keeping the microorganism in a viable condition by subculture, as necessary, into fresh medium.

streak c., a c. produced by lightly stroking an inoculating needle or loop with inoculum over the surface of a solid medium.

tissue c., the maintenance of live tissue after removal from the body, by placing in a vessel with a sterile nutritive medium.

type c., a type strain of microorganism preserved in a c. collection as the standard.

cum (kum). With [L.]

cu·ma·rin (kyū′mă-rin). SYN coumarin.

cu·meth·a·rol (kyū-meth′ă-rol). SYN coumetarol.

cu·me·thox·a·eth·ane (kyū-me-thoks′ă-eth-ān). SYN coumetarol.

Cummer, William E., Canadian dentist, 1879–1942. SEE C.'s *classification, guideline.*

cUMP Abbreviation for cyclic *uridine* 3′,5′-monophosphate.

cu·mu·la·tive (kyū′myū-lă-tiv). Tending to accumulate or pile up, as with certain drugs that may have a c. effect.

cu·mu·lus, pl. **cu·mu·li** (kyū′myū-lŭs, -lī). A collection or heap of cells. [L. a heap]

c. oöph′orus, a mass of epithelial cells surrounding the ovum in the ovarian follicle. SYN discus proligerus, ovigerus, proligerous disk, proligerous membrane. [NA]

c. ova′ricus, rarely used term for c. oöphorus.

cu·ne·ate (kyū′nē-āt). Wedge-shaped. [L. cuneus, wedge]

cu·ne·i·form (kyū′nē-i-fōrm). Wedge-shaped. SEE intermediate cuneiform bone, lateral cuneiform bone, medial cuneiform bone.

cu·ne·o·cu·boid (kyū′nē-ō-kyū′boyd). Relating to the lateral cuneiform and the cuboid bones.

cu·ne·o·na·vic·u·lar (kyū-nē-ō-na-vik′yū-lăr). Relating to the cuneiform and the navicular bones. SYN cuneoscaphoid.

cu·ne·o·scaph·oid (kyū-nē-ō-skaf′oyd). SYN cuneonavicular.

cu·ne·us, pl. **cu·nei** (kyū′nē-ŭs, kū′nē-ī) [NA]. That region of the medial aspect of the occipital lobe of each cerebral hemisphere bounded by the parietooccipital fissure and the calcarine fissure. [L. wedge]

cu·nic·u·lus, pl. **cu·nic·u·li** (kyū-nik′yū-lŭs -lī). The burrow of the scabies mite in the epidermis. [L. a rabbit; an underground passage]

cun·ni·linc·tion, cun·ni·linc·tus (kŭn-i-lingk′shŭn, -lingk′tŭs). SYN cunnilingus.

cun·ni·lin·gus (kŭn-i-ling′gŭs). Oral stimulation of the vulva or clitoris; a type of oral-genital sexual activity; contrasted with fellatio, which is the oral stimulation of the penis. SYN cunnilinction, cunnilinctus. [L. cunnus, pudendum, + lingo, to lick]

Cun·ning·ham·el·la el·e·gans (kŭn-ing-ha-mel′ă el′ĕ-ganz). One of several species of fungi that can cause disseminated zygomycosis in man, and possibly abortion in cattle, swine, and other animals.

cun·nus (kŭn′ŭs). SYN vulva. [L.]

cup (kŭp). **1.** An excavated or cup-shaped structure, either anatomical or pathologic. SYN poculum. **2.** SYN cupping glass. [A.S. cuppe]

Diogenes c., SYN c. of palm.

dry c., a cupping glass formerly applied to the unbroken skin to draw blood to the area but without removing it.

eye c., a small oval receptacle used to apply a liquid to the external eye.

glaucomatous c., a deep depression of the optic disk combined with optic atrophy; caused by glaucoma. SYN glaucomatous excavation.

ocular c., SYN optic c.

optic c., the double-walled c. formed by the invagination of the embryonic optic vesicle; its inner component becomes the sensory layer of the retina, its outer layer, the pigment layer. SYN caliculus ophthalmicus, ocular c.

c. of palm, the palm of the hand when contracted and deepened by the action of the muscles on either side. SYN Diogenes c., poculum diogenis.

perilimbal suction c., a device for increasing intraocular pressure by impeding circulation and aqueous humor flow from the eye.

physiologic c., SYN excavation of optic disc.

suction c., one of the cupping glasses of various shapes, formerly used to produce local hyperemia according to Bier's method.

wet c., a cupping glass formerly applied to a part previously scarified or incised to draw and remove blood.

cu·po·la (kū′pŏ-lă, kyū′). SYN cupula.

cupped (kŭpt). Hollowed; made cup-shaped.

cup·ping (kŭp′ing). **1.** Formation of a hollow, or cup-shaped excavation. **2.** Application of a c. glass. SEE ALSO cup.

cu·pric (kū′prik, kyū-). Pertaining to copper, particularly to copper in the form of a doubly charged positive ion.

cu·pric ac·e·tate, cu·pric ac·e·tate nor·mal. Cu $(CH_3COOH)_2 \cdot H_2O$; a stimulating local caustic to ulcers.

cu·pric ar·se·nite. $CuHAsO_3$; a poisonous green crystalline powder, obsolete as a medicinal agent; now used as an insecticide and pigment. SYN copper arsenite, Scheele's green.

cu·pric chlo·ride. $CuCl_2 \cdot 2H_2O$; has been used as an antiseptic in the treatment of water supplies, ponds, and pools. SYN copper bichloride, copper chloride, copper dichloride.

cu·pric cit·rate. A salt of copper used as an astringent and antiseptic. SYN copper citrate.

cu·pric sul·fate. $CuSo_4 \cdot 5H_2O$; it is highly poisonous to algae, is a prompt and active emetic, and is used as an irritant, astringent, and fungicide. SYN copper sulfate, copper sulphate.

cu·pri·u·re·sis (kū′pri-yū-rē′sis, kyū′-). The urinary excretion of copper. [L. cuprum, copper, + G. ourēsis, a urinating]

cu·pu·la, pl. **cu·pu·lae** (kū′pū-lă, -lē; kyū′pyū-lă) [NA]. A cup-shaped or domelike structure. SYN cupola. [L. dim. of cupa, a tub]

c. of cochlea, the domelike apex of the cochlea. SYN c. cochleae [NA].

c. coch′leae [NA], SYN c. of cochlea.

c. cris′tae ampulla′ris [NA], a gelatinous mass that overlies the hair cells of the ampullary crests of the semicircular ducts; movement of endolymphatic fluid causes the c. to move across the hair cells of the ampullary crest. SYN cap of the ampullary crest.

c. pleu′rae [NA], SYN pleural c.

pleural c., the dome-shaped roof of the pleural cavity extending up through the superior aperture of the thorax. SYN c. pleurae [NA], cervical pleura.

cu·pu·lar (kū′pū-lăr, kyū′pyū-lăr). **1.** Relating to a cupula. **2.** Dome-shaped. SYN cupulate, cupuliform.

cu·pu·late (kū′pū-lāt, kyū′pyū-). SYN cupular (2).

cu·pu·li·form (kū′pŭ-lĭ-fōrm, kyū′pyū-). SYN cupular (2).

cu·pu·lo·gram (kū′pū-lō-gram). A graphic representation of vestibular function relative to normal performance.

cu·pu·lo·lith·i·a·sis (kū′pū-lō-li-thī′a-sis). SYN benign paroxysmal postural vertigo.

cu·rage (kyū′rij, kū-rahzh′). Curettage by means of the finger rather than the curet. [Fr. a cleansing]

cu·ra·re (koo-rah′rē). An extract of various plants, especially Strychnos toxifera, S. castelnaei, S. crevauxii, and Chondodendron tomentosum, that produces nondepolarizing paralysis of skeletal muscle after intravenous injection by blocking transmission at the myoneuronal junction; used clinically (e.g., as d-tubocurarine chloride, metocurine iodide) to provide muscle relaxation during surgical operations. Often classified by the vessels with which South American Indians stored c. SYN arrow poison (1). [S. Am.]

calabash c., (packed by Indians in hollow gourds), c. from Strychnos sp.; extremely poisonous; contains yohimbine, indole, and strychnine type alkaloids.

pot c., (c. stored in clay pots), c. from Chondodendron sp.; not highly poisonous.

tube c., (c. stored in bamboo tubes), c. from Chondodendron sp.; not highly poisonous; contains the alkaloid tubocurarine.

cu·ra·ri·form (kū-rar′i-fōrm). Denoting a drug having an action like curare.

cu·rar·i·mi·met·ic (kū-rar′i-mī-met′ik). Having a curare-like action.

cu·ra·rine (kyū′ră-rēn). $C_{40}H_{44}N_4O^{++}$; C-Curarine I; the alkaloid principle of calabash curare.

cu·ra·ri·za·tion (kyū-rah-ri-zā′shŭn). Induction of muscular relaxation or paralysis by the administration of curare or related compounds that have the ability to block nerve impulse transmission at the myoneural junction.

cur·a·tive (kyūr′ă-tiv). **1.** That which heals or cures. **2.** Tending to heal or cure.

curb (kerb). A hard, painful, inflammatory swelling on the back part of the hock of the horse; it occurs in the plantar ligament near its insertion, is characterized by swelling and heat in the part and generally by lameness, and is believed to be caused by straining the ligament in falling, jumping, or pulling. SYN curby hock.

cur·cum·in (kur'kū-min) A yellow pigment from roots and pods of *Curcuma longa;* used in liver and bile ailments; found in curry powder; used as an indicator. SYN tumeric yellow.

curd (kerd). The coagulum of milk.

cure (kyūr). **1.** To heal; to make well. **2.** A restoration to health. **3.** A special method or course of treatment. SEE dental *curing*. [L. *curo,* to care for]

cu·ret. SEE curette.

cu·ret·ment (kyū-ret'ment, kū-). SYN curettage.

cu·ret·tage (kyū-rĕ-tahzh', kū-). A scraping, usually of the interior of a cavity or tract, for the removal of new growths or other abnormal tissues, or to obtain material for tissue diagnosis. SYN curetment, curettement.

   periapical c., (1) removal of a cyst or granuloma from its pathologic bony crypt, utilizing a curette; (2) the removal of tooth fragments and debris from sockets at the time of extraction or of bone sequestra subsequently.

   subgingival c., removal of subgingival calculus, ulcerated epithelial and granulation tissues found in periodontal pockets. SYN apoxesis.

cu·rette, cu·ret (kyū-ret', kū-). Instrument in the form of a loop, ring, or scoop with sharpened edges attached to a rod-shaped handle, used for curettage. [Fr.]

   Hartmann's c., a c., cutting on the side, for the removal of adenoids.

cu·rette·ment (kyū-ret'ment, kū-). SYN curettage.

cu·rie (C, c, Ci) (kyū'rē). A unit of measurement of radioactivity, 3.70×10^{10} disintegrations per second; formerly defined as the radioactivity of the amount of radon in equilibrium with 1 gm. of radium; superseded by the S.I. unit, the becquerel (1 disintegration per second). [Marie (1867–1934) and Pierre (1859–1906) *Curie,* French chemists and physicists and Nobel laureates]

cur·ing (kyūr'ing). **1.** The act of accomplishing a cure. **2.** A process by which something is prepared for use, as by heating, aging, etc.

   dental c., the process by which plastic materials become rigid to form a denture base, filling, impression tray, or other appliance.

cu·ri·um (Cm) (kyū'rē-ŭm). An element, atomic no. 96, atomic wt. 247.07, not occurring naturally on earth, but first formed artificially in 1944 by bombarding ^{239}Pu with alpha particles; the most stable of the c. isotopes is ^{247}Cm, with a half-life of 15.6 million years. [see curie]

Curling, Thomas B., English surgeon, 1811–1888. SEE C.'s *ulcer.*

cur·rent (ker'rĕnt). A stream or flow of fluid, air, or electricity. [L. *currens,* pres. p. of *curro,* to run]

   action c., an electrical c. induced in muscle fibers when they are effectively stimulated; normally it is followed by contraction.

   after-c., SEE aftercurrent.

   alternating c. (AC), a c. that flows first in one direction then in the other; *e.g.,* 60-cycle c.

   anodal c., a c. produced in tissues under the anode when the circuit is closed.

   ascending c., the direction of c. flow in a nerve when the anode is placed peripheral to the cathode, in contrast to descending c.; the convention used is that c. flows from positive to negative. SYN centripetal c.

   axial c., the central rapidly moving portion of the bloodstream in an artery.

   centrifugal c., SYN descending c.

   centripetal c., SYN ascending c.

   d'Arsonval c., SYN high frequency c.

   demarcation c., SYN c. of injury.

   descending c., the direction of c. flow in a nerve when the cathode is placed peripheral to the anode, in contrast to ascending c. SYN centrifugal c.

   direct c. (DC), a c. that flows only in one direction; *e.g.,* that derived from a battery; sometimes referred to as galvanic c. SEE ALSO galvanism.

   electrotonic c., SEE electrotonus.

   galvanic c., SEE direct c., galvanism (1).

   high frequency c., an alternating electric c. having a frequency of 10,000 or more per second; it produces no muscular contractions and does not affect the sensory nerves. SYN d'Arsonval c., Tesla c.

   c. of injury, the c. set up when an injured part of a nerve, muscle, or other excitable tissue is connected through a conductor with the uninjured region; the injured tissue is negative to the uninjured. SYN demarcation c.

   labile c., an electrical c. applied to the body by means of electrodes that are constantly shifted about.

   Tesla c., SYN high frequency c.

Curschmann, Heinrich, German physician, 1846–1910. SEE C.'s *disease*, *spirals*, under *spiral*.

curse (kers). An affliction thought to be invoked by a malevolent spirit.

   Ondine's c., idiopathic central alveolar hypoventilation in which involuntary control of respiration is depressed, but voluntary control of ventilation is not impaired. [*Ondine,* char. in play by J. Giraudoux, based on Undine, Ger. myth. char.]

Curtis, Arthur H., U.S. gynecologist, 1881–1955. SEE Fitz-Hugh and C. *syndrome*.

cur·va·tu·ra, pl. **cur·va·tu·rae** (ker'vă-tū'ră, -tū'rē) [NA]. SYN curvature. [L.]

   c. ventric'uli ma'jor [NA], SYN greater *curvature* of stomach.

   c. ventric'uli mi'nor [NA], SYN lesser *curvature* of stomach.

cur·va·ture (ker'vă-chūr). A bending or flexure. SEE angulation. SYN curvatura [NA]. [L. *curvatura,* fr. *curvo,* pp. *-atus,* to bend, curve]

   angular c., a gibbous deformity, *i.e.,* a sharp angulation of the spine, occurring in Pott's disease. SYN Pott's c.

   anterior c., c. in which a more distal or cephalad part is deviated anteriorly with respect to the coronal anatomic plane.

   backward c., c. in which a more distal or cephalad part is deviated posteriorly with respect to the coronal anatomic plane.

   gingival c., the rounding of the gum along its line of attachment to the neck of a tooth.

   greater c. of stomach, the border of the stomach to which the greater omentum is attached. SYN curvatura ventriculi major [NA].

   lateral c., c. in which a more distal part is deviated away from the anatomic sagittal plane.

   lesser c. of stomach, the right border of the stomach to which the lesser omentum is attached. SYN curvatura ventriculi minor [NA].

   occlusal c., SYN *curve* of occlusion.

   Pott's c., SYN angular c.

   spinal c., SEE kyphosis, lordosis, scoliosis.

curve (kerv). **1.** A nonangular continuous bend or line. **2.** A chart or graphic representation, by means of a continuous line connecting individual observations, of the course of a physiological activity, of the number of cases of a disease in a given period, or of any entity that might be otherwise presented by a table of figures. SYN chart (2). [L. *curvo,* to bend]

   active length-tension c., the relationship between active isometric tension and preload (rest length) for a contracting muscle.

   alignment c., the line passing through the center of the teeth laterally in the direction of the c. of the dental arch.

cu

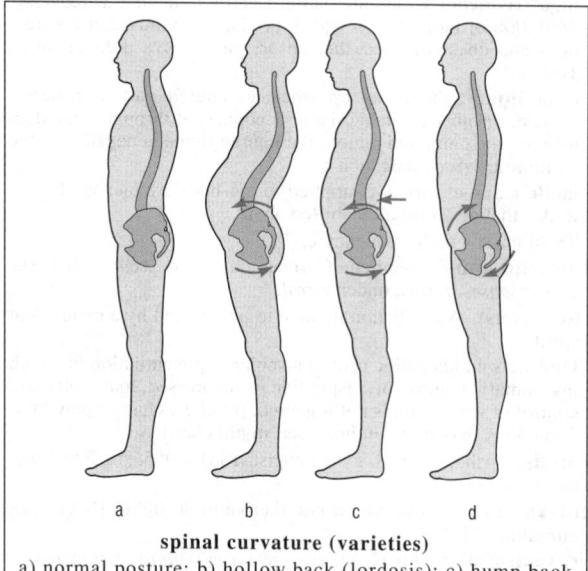

spinal curvature (varieties)
a) normal posture; b) hollow back (lordosis); c) hump back
(juvenile kyphosis); d) flat back

anti-Monson c., SYN reverse c.

Barnes' c., a c. corresponding in general with Carus' c., being the segment of a circle whose center is the promontory of the sacrum.

buccal c., the line of the dental arch from the canine, or cuspid tooth to the third molar.

Carus' c., an imaginary curved line obtained from a mathematical formula, supposed to indicate the outlet of the pelvic canal. SYN Carus' circle.

characteristic c., sensitometric c. of radiographic film, a plot of the film density versus the logarithm of the relative exposure. SYN H and D c., Hunter and Driffield c.

compensating c., the anteroposterior and lateral curvature in the alignment of the occluding surfaces and incisal edges of artificial teeth; used to develop balanced occlusion.

distribution c., a systematic grouping of data into classes or categories according to the frequency of occurrence of each successive value or ranges of such values, resulting in a graph of a frequency distribution. SYN frequency c.

dose-response c., a graph showing the relationship between the dose of a drug, infectious agent, etc. and the biological response.

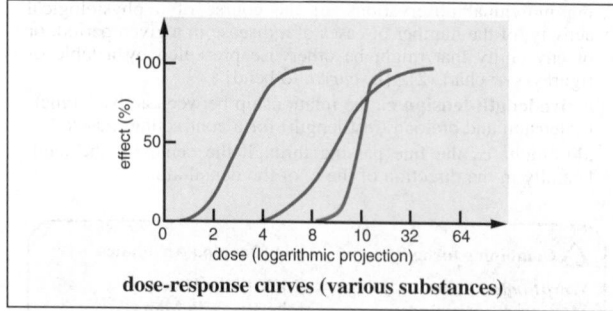

dose-response curves (various substances)

dye-dilution c., graph of the serial concentrations (dilutions) of a dye, *e.g.,* Evans blue, following its intravascular or intracardiac injection; useful in the diagnosis of congenital cardiac shunts, measurement of cardiac output, and detection of cardiovalvular incompetence. SYN indicator-dilution c.

epidemic c., a graph in which the number of new cases of a disease is plotted against an interval of time to describe a specific epidemic or outbreak.

flow-volume c., the graph produced by plotting the instantaneous flow of respiratory gas against the simultaneous lung volume, usually during maximal forced expiration.

force-velocity c., the relationship between isotonic velocity of shortening and afterload for a contracting muscle.

Frank-Starling c., SYN Starling's c.

frequency c., SYN distribution c.

Friedman c., a graph on which hours of labor are plotted against cervical dilation in centimeters.

gaussian c., SYN normal *distribution.*

growth c., a graphic representation of the change in size of an individual or a population over a period of time.

H and D c., SYN characteristic c.

Heidelberger c., SYN precipitation c.

Hunter and Driffield c., SYN characteristic c.

indicator-dilution c., SYN dye-dilution c.

intracardiac pressure c., c. of pressure recorded within the atrium or ventricle (intra-atrial and intraventricular pressure c.'s).

isovolume pressure-flow c., the relationship between transpulmonary pressure and respiratory air flow, expressed as a function of lung volume.

logistic c., an S-shaped c. which depicts the growth of a population in an area of fixed limits.

milled-in c.'s, SYN milled-in *paths,* under *path.*

Monson c., the c. of occlusion in which each cusp and incisal edge touches or conforms to a segment of the surface of a sphere 8 inches in diameter with its center in the region of the glabella.

muscle c., SYN myogram.

c. of occlusion, (1) a curved surface which makes simultaneous contact with the major portion of the incisal and occlusal prominences of the existing teeth; **(2)** the c. of a dentition on which the occlusal surfaces lie. SYN occlusal curvature.

passive length-tension c., the relationship between passive tension and preload (rest length) for a muscle at rest.

Pleasure c., a c. of occlusion which when viewed in sagittal section conforms to a line that is convex upward except for the last molars.

precipitation c., a graph of the quantity of precipitate formed as a function of the quantity of antigen added during the titration of an antibody with an antigen. SYN Heidelberger c.

Price-Jones c., a distribution c. of the measured diameters of red blood cells; it is to the right of the normal c. (*i.e.,* indicating larger diameters) in instances of pernicious anemia and other forms in which macrocytes are present, and to the left (*i.e.,* indicating smaller diameters) in iron deficiency and other forms of microcytic anemia.

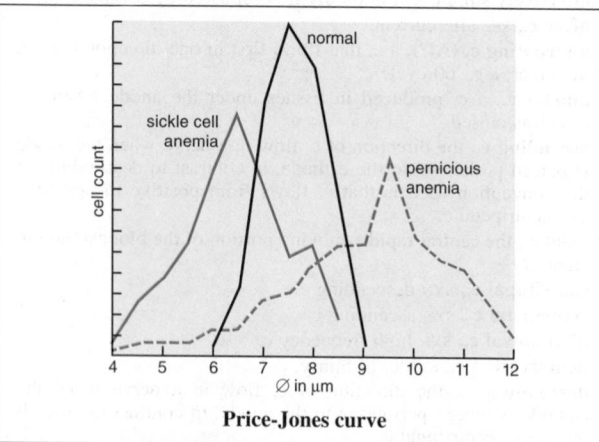

Price-Jones curve

probability c., a graph of the gaussian (normal) distribution representing relative probabilities.

progress c., a graphical representation of a chemical or enzyme-catalyzed reaction in which the product concentration or the substrate concentration or the ES binary complex are plotted against time.

pulse c., SYN sphygmogram.

receiver operating characteristic c., (1) a plot of true positive versus false positive results, usually in a trial of a diagnostic test. **(2)** a graphical means of assessing the ability of a screening test to discriminate between healthy and diseased persons. SYN ROC c.

reverse c., in dentistry, a c. of occlusion which is convex upward. SYN anti-Monson c.

ROC c., SYN receiver operating characteristic c.

c. of Spee, the anatomic curvature of the mandibular occlusal plane beginning at the tip of the lower cuspid and following the buccal cusps of the posterior teeth, continuing to the terminal molar. SYN von Spee's c.

Starling's c., a graph in which cardiac output or stroke volume is plotted against mean atrial or ventricular end-diastolic pressure; with increasing venous return and atrial pressure the output proportionately increases until further increments overload the heart and the output falls. SYN Frank-Starling c.

strength-duration c., a graph relating the intensity of an electrical stimulus to the length of time it must flow to be effective. SEE chronaxie, rheobase.

stress-strain c., a c. showing the ratio of deformation to load during the testing of a material in tension.

tension c., the direction of the trabeculae in cancellous bone tissue adapted to resist stress.

Traube-Hering c.'s, slow oscillations in blood pressure usually extending over several respiratory cycles; related to variations in vasomotor tone; rhythmical variations in blood pressure. SYN Traube-Hering waves.

von Spee's c., SYN c. of Spee.

whole-body titration c., a graphic representation of the *in vivo* changes in hydrogen ion, Pa_{CO_2}, and bicarbonate which occur in arterial blood in response to primary acid-base disturbances.

Cur·vu·la·ria (ker-vyū-lā′rē-ă). A genus of dark-colored fungi that grow rapidly on culture media. Generally regarded as contaminants, two species, *C. lunata* and *C. geniculata*, are among the true species of fungi capable of producing mycetoma in humans, keratomycosis, sinusitis, and pheohyphomycosis.

Cushing, Harvey W., U.S. neurosurgeon, 1869–1939. SEE C.'s *basophilism*, *disease*, *syndrome*, *syndrome* medicamentosus; C. *effect*, *phenomenon*, *response*; C.'s pituitary *basophilism*.

Cushing, Hayward W., U.S. surgeon, 1854–1934. SEE C.'s *suture*.

cush·ing·oid (kush′ing-oyd). Resembling the signs and symptoms of Cushing's disease or syndrome: buffalo hump obesity, striations, adiposity, diabetes, hypertension, and osteoporosis, usually due to exogenous corticosteroids.

cush·ion (kush′ŭn). In anatomy, any structure resembling a pad or c.

atrioventricular canal c.'s, a pair of mounds of embryonic connective tissue covered by endothelium, bulging into the embryonic atrioventricular canal; located one dorsally and one ventrally, they grow together and fuse with each other and with the lower edge of the septum primum, dividing the originally single canal into right and left atrioventricular orifices. SYN endocardial c.'s.

endocardial c.'s, SYN atrioventricular canal c.'s.

c. of epiglottis, SYN epiglottic *tubercle*.

eustachian c., SYN *torus* tubarius.

levator c., the bulge in the lateral wall of the nasopharynx, below the opening of the auditory tube, produced by the levator veli palatini muscle. SYN torus levatorius [NA], levator swelling.

Passavant's c., a prominence on the posterior wall of the nasopharynx formed by contraction of the superior constrictor of the pharynx during swallowing. SYN Passavant's bar, Passavant's pad, Passavant's ridge.

pharyngoesophageal c.'s, venous plexuses on the anterior and posterior walls of the pharyngoesophageal junction. SYN pharyngoesophageal pads.

plantar c., a dense mass of fibrofatty tissue overlying the frog in

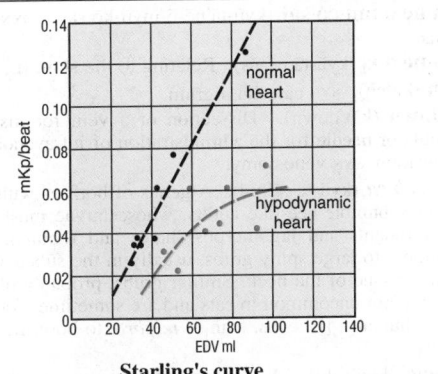

Starling's curve
pressure-volume-work, in relation to end diastolic volume (EDV)

the foot of the horse; serves an important shock-absorbing function.

sucking c., SYN buccal *fat-pad*.

cusp (kŭsp). **1.** In dentistry, a conical elevation arising on the surface of a tooth from an independent calcification center. SEE ALSO dental *tubercle*. **2.** A leaflet of one of the heart's valves. SYN cuspis [NA]. [L. *cuspis*, point]

anterior c. of atrioventricular valve, the anterior leaflet or valvule of either the tricuspid or mitral valves. SYN cuspis anterior valvae atrioventricularis dextrae/sinistrae [NA].

c. of Carabelli, a fifth c. found on the maxillary first molars, usually located lingual to the mesiolingual c.

posterior c. of atrioventricular valve, the posterior leaflet of either the tricuspid or mitral valves. SYN cuspis posterior valvae atrioventricularis dextrae/sinistrae [NA].

semilunar c., one of the three semilunar segments serving as the three c.'s of a valve preventing regurgitation at the beginning of the aorta; a similar valve guards the entrance of the pulmonary trunk; the segments are named, respectively, anterior, right, and left in the pulmonary valve, and posterior, right, and left in the aortic valve.

septal c. of tricuspid valve, the leaflet of the tricuspid valve located adjacent to the interventricular septum. SYN cuspis septalis valvae atrioventricularis dextrae [NA].

talon c., an anomalous c. that projects lingually from the cingulum of permanent incisors. [Eng. claw, heel, fr. O. Fr., fr. L. *talus*, ankle]

c. of tooth, an elevation or mound on the crown of a tooth making up a part of the occlusal surface. SYN cuspis dentis [NA], cuspis coronae☆ [NA].

cus·pad (kŭs′păd). In a direction toward the cusp of a tooth. [L. *ad*, to]

cus·pal (kŭs′păl). Pertaining to a cusp.

cus·pid (kŭs′pid). **1.** Having but one cusp. SYN cuspidate. **2.** SYN canine *tooth*. [L. *cuspis*, point]

cus·pi·date (kŭs′pi-dāt). SYN cuspid (1).

cus·pis, pl. **cus·pi·des** (kŭs′pis, kŭs′pi-dēz) [NA]. SYN cusp. [L. a point]

c. ante′rior val′vae atrioventricula′ris dex′trae/sinis′trae [NA], SYN anterior *cusp* of atrioventricular valve.

c. coro′nae [NA], ☆official alternate term for *cusp* of tooth, *cusp* of tooth.

c. den′tis [NA], SYN *cusp* of tooth.

c. poste′rior val′vae atrioventricula′ris dex′trae/sinis′trae [NA], SYN posterior *cusp* of atrioventricular valve.

c. septa′lis val′vae atrioventricula′ris dex′trae [NA], SYN septal *cusp* of tricuspid valve.

cu·sum (kū′sum). Acronym for cumulative sum of a series of measurements; used primarily in Great Britain.

cut (kŭt). In molecular biology, a hydrolytic cleavage of two opposing phosphodiester bonds in a double-stranded nucleic acid. Cf. nick.

cu·ta·ne·o·mu·co·sal (kyū-tā′nē-ō-myū-kō′săl). SYN mucocutaneous.

cu·ta·ne·ous (kyū-tā′nē-ŭs). Relating to the skin. [L. *cutis,* skin]

cutch (kŭtch). SYN catechu nigrum.

cut·down (kŭt′down). Dissection of a vein for insertion of a cannula or needle for the administration of intravenous fluids or medication. SYN venostomy.

Cu·te·reb·ra (kyū-te-rē′bră). A genus of botflies with large blue or black bumble-bee-like adults, whose larvae most commonly infest rodents and lagomorphs (hares and rabbits); the larvae develop into large spiny grubs, usually in the subcutaneous connective tissue of the neck. Similar grubs, probably of other species, are not uncommon in cats and are sometimes found in dogs and in humans. [L. *cutis,* skin, + *terebro,* to bore, fr. *terebra,* an auger]

cu·ti·cle (kyū′ti-kl). **1.** An outer thin layer, usually horny in nature. SYN cuticula (1). **2.** The layer, chitinous in some invertebrates, which occurs on the surface of epithelial cells. **3.** SYN epidermis. [L. *cuticula,* dim. of *cutis,* skin]

acquired c., acquired enamel c., SYN acquired *pellicle.*

dental c., SYN enamel c.

enamel c., the primary enamel cuticle, consisting of two extremely thin layers (the inner one clear and structureless, the outer one cellular), covering the entire crown of newly erupted teeth and subsequently abraded by mastication; it is evident microscopically as an amorphous material between the attachment epithelium and the tooth. SYN cuticula dentis [NA], adamantine membrane, dental c., membrana adamantina, Nasmyth's c., Nasmyth's membrane, skin of teeth.

c. of hair, SYN *cuticula* pili.

c. of nail, the exposed distal prolongation of the corneal layer of the deep surface of the proximal nail fold (eponychium (2)), seen as a thin "skin" overlapping and adherent to the body of the nail at its proximal portion (the area of the lunula). It is formed as a remnant of the eponychium (1) which otherwise degenerates by the eighth month of pregnancy.

Nasmyth's c., SYN enamel c.

posteruption c., SYN acquired *pellicle.*

c. of root sheath, SYN *cuticula* vaginae folliculi pili.

cu·tic·u·la, pl. **cu·tic·u·lae** (kyū-tik′yū-lă, -lē) **1** [NA]. SYN cuticle (1). **2.** SYN epidermis. [L. cuticle]

c. den′tis [NA], SYN enamel *cuticle.*

c. pi′li, a layer of overlapping shingle-like cells that invest the hair cortex and serve to lock the hair shaft in its follicle. SYN cuticle of hair.

c. vagi′nae follic′uli pi′li, cuticle of overlapping shingle-like cells lining the follicle of the hair. SYN cuticle of root sheath.

cu·tic·u·lar·i·za·tion (kyū-tik′yū-lar-ĭ-zā′shŭn). Obs. Covering an abraded area with epidermis.

cu·tin (kyū′tin). A specially prepared, thin, animal membrane used as a protective covering for wounded surfaces. [L. *cutis,* skin]

cu·ti·re·ac·tion (kyū′ti-rē-ak′shŭn). The inflammatory reaction in the case of a skin test in a sensitive (allergic) subject. SYN cutaneous reaction. [L. *cutis,* skin, + reaction]

cu·tis (kyū′tis) [NA]. SYN skin. [L.]

c. anseri′na, contraction of the arrectores pilorum produced by cold, fear, or other stimulus, causing the follicular orifices to become prominent. SYN goose flesh, gooseflesh.

c. lax′a [MIM*123700], a congenital or acquired condition characterized by deficient elastic fibers of the skin hanging in folds; vascular anomalies may be present; inheritance is either dominant or recessive, the latter sometimes in association with pulmonary emphysema and diverticula of the alimentary tract or bladder. SYN dermalaxia, dermatochalasis, generalized elastolysis, loose skin, pachydermatocele (1).

c. marmora′ta, a normal, physiologic, pink, marble-like mottling of the skin in infants, persisting abnormally in some children on exposure to cold.

c. rhomboida′lis nu′chae, geometric furrowed configurations of the skin of the back of the neck as a result of prolonged exposure to sunlight with solar elastosis.

c. unctuo′sa, SYN *seborrhea* oleosa.

c. ve′ra, SYN dermis.

c. ver′ticis gyra′ta, a congenital condition in which the skin of the scalp is hypertrophied and thrown into folds forming anterior to posterior furrows; it may be a component of pachydermoperiostosis.

cu·ti·sec·tor (kyū′ti-sek′tōr). **1.** Rarely used term for instrument for cutting small pieces of skin for grafting. **2.** Rarely used term for instrument used to remove a section of skin for microscopic examination. [L. *cutis,* skin, + *sector,* a cutter]

cu·ti·za·tion (kyū-ti-zā′shŭn). The transition from mucous membrane to skin at the mucocutaneous margins.

cu·vet, cu·vette (kū-vet′). A small container or cup in which solutions are placed for photometric analysis.

Cuvier, Baron Georges L.C.F.D. de la, French scientist, 1769–1832. SEE C.'s *ducts,* under duct, veins, under vein.

CV Abbreviation for *coefficient* of variation; cardiovascular; closing *volume.*

CVA Abbreviation for cerebrovascular *accident.*

CVP Abbreviation for central venous *pressure.*

CX Abbreviation for *phosgene* oxime.

cy·a·mem·a·zine (sī-ă-mem′ă-zēn). 10-(3-Dimethylamino-2-methylpropyl)-phenothiazine-2-carbonitrile; a sedative with antihistaminic and antispasmodic properties.

⌂**cyan-.** SEE cyano-.

cy·an·al·co·hols (sī-an-al′kō-holz). SYN cyanohydrins.

cy·an·a·mide (sī-an′i-mīd). An irritating and caustic water-soluble substance, H_2NCN or $HN=C=NH$; often used in referring to calcium cyanamide.

cy·a·nate (sī′an-āt). The radical $-O-C\equiv N$ or ion $(CNO)^-$.

cy·a·ne·mia (sī-a-ne′mē-ă). Obsolete term for cyanosis. [cyan- + G. *haima,* blood]

cy·a·nide (sī′an-īd). **1.** The radical $-CN$ or ion $(CN)^-$. The ion is extremely poisonous, forming hydrocyanic acid in water; inhibits respiratory proteins. **2.** A salt of HCN or a cyano-containing molecule.

c. methemoglobin, SYN cyanmethemoglobin.

cy·a·nid·e·non (sī-ă-nid′ĕ-non). SYN luteolin.

cy·an·i·dol (sī′an-i-dol). SYN catechin.

cy·an·met·he·mo·glo·bin (sī′an-met-hē′mō-glō-bin). A relatively nontoxic compound of cyanide with methemoglobin, which is formed when methylene blue is administered in cases of cyanide poisoning. SYN cyanide methemoglobin.

⌂**cyano-, cyan-.** **1.** Combining form meaning blue. **2.** Chemical prefix frequently used in naming compounds that contain the cyanide group, CN. [G. *kyanos,* a dark blue substance]

Cy·a·no·bac·te·ria (sī′ă-nō-bak-tēr′ē-ă). A division of the kingdom Prokaryotae consisting of unicellular or filamentous bacteria that are either nonmotile or possess a gliding motility, reproduce by binary fission, and perform photosynthesis with the production of oxygen. These blue-green bacteria were formerly referred to as blue-green algae. SYN Cyanophyceae.

cy·a·no·chro·ic, cy·an·och·rous (sī-an-ō-krō′ik, sī-an-ok′rŭs). SYN cyanotic. [cyano- + G. *chroia,* color]

cy·a·no·co·bal·a·min (sī′an-ō-kō-bal′ă-min). A complex of cyanide and cobalamin, as in vitamin B_{12}.

radioactive c., cyano[^{57}Co]cobalamin, cyano[^{58}Co]cobalamin, or cyano[^{60}Co]cobalamin produced by the growth of certain microorganisms on a medium containing cobalt-57, cobalt-58, or cobalt-60; used in the investigation of the absorption and metabolism of cyanocobalamin (vitamin B_{12}).

cy·an·o·gen (sī-an′ō-jen). A compound of two cyano radicals, NC-CN; its highly toxic compounds (general formula X-CN, where X is a halogen) are used in chemical syntheses and as tissue preservatives. SYN ethanedinitrile.

c. chloride, CNCl; a highly volatile liquid; a systemic poison used as a warning agent in fumigation with hydrogen cyanide.

cy·a·no·gen·ic (sī′an-ō-jen′ik). Capable of producing hydrocyanic acid; said of plants such as sorghum, Johnson grass, arrowgrass, and wild cherry which may cause cyanide poisoning in herbivorous animals.

cy·a·no·hy·drins (sī'an-ō-hī'drinz). R-CHOH-CN; addition compounds of HCN and aldehydes. SYN cyanalcohols.

cy·an·o·phil, cy·an·o·phile (sī'an-ō-fil, -fīl). A cell or element that is differentially colored blue by a staining procedure. [cyano- + G. *philos,* fond]

cy·a·noph·i·lous (sī-ă-nof'i-lŭs). Readily stainable with a blue dye.

Cy·a·no·phy·ce·ae (sī'ă-nō-fī'sē-ē). SYN Cyanobacteria. [cyano- + G. *phykos,* seaweed]

cy·a·no·pia (sī-ă-nō'pē-ă). SYN cyanopsia.

cy·a·nop·sia (sī-ă-nop'sē-ă). A condition in which all objects appear blue; may temporarily follow cataract extraction. SYN blue vision, cyanopia. [cyano- + G. *opsis,* vision]

cy·a·nosed (sī'ă-nōsd). SYN cyanotic.

cy·a·no·sis (sī-ă-nō'sis). A dark bluish or purplish coloration of the skin and mucous membrane due to deficient oxygenation of the blood, evident when reduced hemoglobin in the blood exceeds 5 g per 100 ml. [G. dark blue color, fr. *kyanos,* blue substance]

compression c., c. accompanied by edema and petechial hemorrhages over the head, neck, and upper part of the chest, as a venous reflex resulting from severe compression of the thorax or abdomen; the conjunctiva and retinas are similarly affected.

enterogenous c., apparent c. caused by the absorption of nitrites or other toxic materials from the intestine with the formation of methemoglobin or sulfhemoglobin; the skin color change is due to the chocolate color of methemoglobin.

false c., c. due to the presence of an abnormal pigment, such as methemoglobin, in the blood, and not resulting from a deficiency of oxygen.

hereditary methemoglobinemic c., SYN congenital *methemoglobinemia.*

late c., SYN cyanose *tardive.*

c. ret'inae, venous congestion of the retina.

shunt c., any blue color of the entire skin or a region of the skin or mucous membrane due to a right to left shunt permitting unoxygenated blood to reach the left side of the circulation.

tardive c., SYN cyanose *tardive.*

toxic c., c. due to methemoglobin formation resulting from the action of certain drugs, *e.g.,* nitrites.

cy·a·not·ic (sī-ă-not'ik). Relating to or marked by cyanosis. SYN cyanochroic, cyanochrous, cyanosed.

cy·a·nu·ria (sī-ă-nū'rē-ă). The presence of blue urine. [cyano- + G. *ouron,* urine]

cy·a·nu·ric ac·id (sī-ă-nūr'ik). 2,4,6-Trihydroxy-1,3,5-triazine; a cyclic product formed by heating urea; used industrially and as an herbicide.

Cy·a·tho·sto·ma (sī-ă-thos'tō-mă). A genus of gapeworms of poultry in the nematode family Syngamidae, so called because of the gaping habit of fowl infected by these worms in their upper respiratory tract. [G. *kyathos,* cup, cup-shaped, + *stoma,* mouth]

C. bronchia'lis, a species found in wild geese and domestic ducks, geese, and swans; occurs in the larynx, trachea, and bronchi and causes distress and symptoms similar to those produced by the chicken gapeworm, *Syngamus trachea;* its life cycle is thought to be similar to that of *Syngamus trachea.*

Cy·a·tho·sto·mum (sī-ă-thos'tō-mŭm). A genus of strongyle nematodes (family Cyasthostomidae, formerly part of the family Strongylidae); it includes many of the small strongyles of horses formerly placed in the genus *Trichonema,* which have been variously divided into a number of genera and subgenera. [see *Cyathostoma*]

cy·ber·net·ics (sī-ber-net'iks). 1. The comparative study of electronic calculators and the human nervous system, with intent to explain the functioning of the brain. 2. The science of control and communication in both living and nonliving systems; characteristically, control is governed by feedback, that is, by communication within the system concerning the difference between the actual and the desired result, action then being modified so as to minimize this difference. SEE ALSO feedback. [G. *kybernētica,* things pertaining to control or piloting]

cy·brid (sī'brid). A cell with cytoplasm from two different cells as a result of cell hybridization. [cell + hybrid]

△cycl-. SEE cyclo-.

cy·cla·mate (sī'klă-māt). A salt or ester of cyclamic acid; the calcium and sodium are noncaloric artificial sweetening agents.

cy·clam·ic ac·id (sī-klam'ik). A sweetening agent, usually used as sodium or calcium cyclamate. SYN cyclohexanesulfamic acid, cyclohexylsulfamic acid.

cy·cla·mide (sī'klă-mīd). SYN glycyclamide.

cy·clan·de·late (sī-klan'de-lāt). 3,3,5-Trimethylcyclohexyl mandelate; an antispasmodic similar in action to papaverine; used for obliterative vascular diseases and vasospastic conditions.

cy·clar·ba·mate (sī-klar'bă-māt). 1,1-cyclopentanedimethanol dicarbanilate; a tranquilizer with antispasmodic properties. SYN cyclopentaphene.

cy·clar·thro·di·al (sī-klar-thrō'dē-ăl). Relating to a cyclarthrosis.

cy·clar·thro·sis (sī-klar-thrō'sis). A joint capable of rotation. [cyclo- + G. *arthrōsis,* articulation]

cy·clase (sī'klās). Descriptive name applied to an enzyme that forms a cyclic compound; *e.g.,* adenylate cyclase.

CYCLE

cy·cle (sī'kl). 1. A recurrent series of events. 2. A recurring period of time. 3. One successive compression and rarefaction of a wave, as of a sound wave. [G. *kyklos,* circle]

anovulatory c., a sexual c. in which no ovum is discharged.

brain wave c., the complete upward and downward excursion of a single wave, complex, or impulse as seen on an electroencephalogram.

carbon dioxide c., carbon c., the circulation of carbon as CO_2 from the expired air of animals and decaying organic matter to plant life where it is synthesized (through photosynthesis) to carbohydrate material, from which, as a result of catabolic processes in all life, it is again ultimately released to the atmosphere as CO_2.

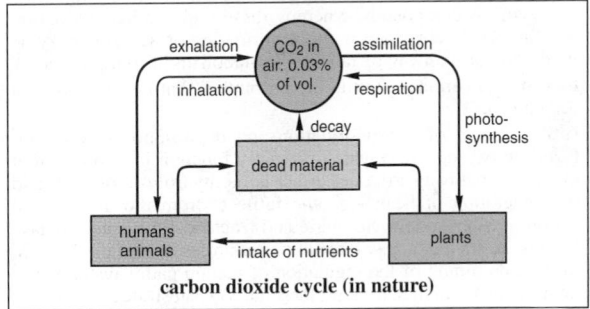

carbon dioxide cycle (in nature)

cardiac c., the complete round of cardiac systole and diastole with the intervals between, or commencing with, any event in the heart's action to the moment when that same event is repeated.

cell c., the periodic biochemical and structural events occurring during proliferation of cells such as in tissue culture; the c. is divided into periods called: G_0, Gap$_1$ (G_1), synthesis (S_1), Gap$_2$ (G_2), and mitosis (M). The period runs from one division to the next. SYN mitotic c.

chewing c., a complete course of movement of the mandible during a single masticatory stroke.

citric acid c., SYN tricarboxylic acid c.

Cori c., the phases in the metabolism of carbohydrate: 1) glycogenolysis in the liver; 2) passage of glucose into the circulation; 3) deposition of glucose in the muscles as glycogen; 4) glycogen-

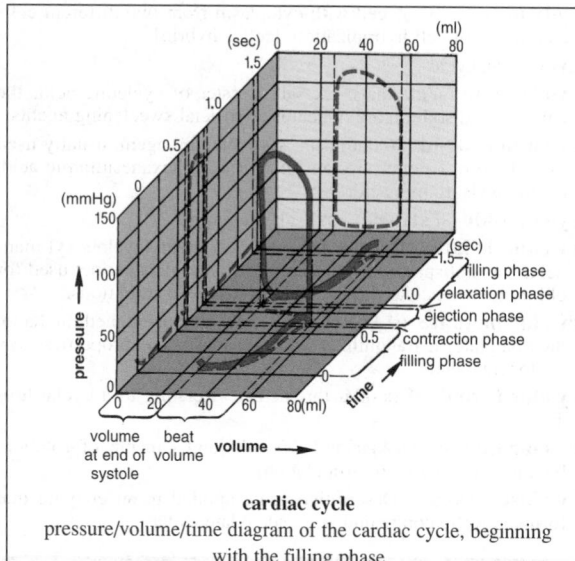

cardiac cycle

pressure/volume/time diagram of the cardiac cycle, beginning
with the filling phase

acid to form citric acid in the tricarboxylic acid c.). SYN Krebs-Kornberg c.

gonadotrophic c. (gŏ'nad-ō-trŏf'ik), one complete round of ovarian development in the insect vector from the time when the blood meal is taken to the time when the fully developed eggs are laid.

hair c., the cyclical phases of growth (anagen), regression (catagen), and quiescence (telogen) in the life of a hair.

Krebs c., SYN tricarboxylic acid c.

Krebs-Henseleit c., Krebs ornithine c., Krebs urea c., SYN urea c.

Krebs-Kornberg c., SYN glyoxylic acid c.

life c., the entire life history of a living organism.

masticating c.'s, the patterns of mandibular movements formed during the chewing of food.

menstrual c., the period in which an ovum matures, is ovulated, and enters the uterine lumen via the fallopian tubes; ovarian hormonal secretions effect endometrial changes such that, if fertilization occurs, nidation will be possible; in the absence of fertilization, ovarian secretions wane, the endometrium sloughs, and menstruation begins; this c. lasts an average of 28 days, with day 1 of the c. designated as that day on which menstrual flow begins.

olysis during muscular activity and conversion to lactate, which is converted to glycogen in the liver.

dicarboxylic acid c., (1) that portion of the tricarboxylic acid c. involving the dicarboxylic acids (succinic, fumaric, malic, and oxaloacetic acids); (2) a cyclic scheme in which certain steps of the tricarboxylic acid c. are used with the glyoxylate c.; important in the utilization of glyoxylic acid in microorganisms.

endogenous c., the portion of a parasitic life cycle occurring within the host.

estrous c., the series of physiologic uterine, ovarian, and other changes that occur in higher animals, consisting of proestrus, estrus, postestrus, and anestrus or diestrus.

exoerythrocytic c., that nonpathogenic portion of the vertebrate phase of the life cycle of malarial organisms that takes place in liver cells, outside of the blood cells.

exogenous c., the portion of a parasitic life cycle occurring outside the host.

fatty acid oxidation c., a series of reactions involving acyl-coenzyme A compounds, whereby these undergo beta oxidation and thioclastic cleavage, with the formation of acetyl-coenzyme A; the major pathway of fatty acid catabolism in living tissue.

forced c., a cardiac c. (atrial or ventricular) that is cut short by a forced beat.

futile c., a c. of phosphorylation and dephosphorylation catalyzed by two enzymes which normally function in two different metabolic pathways; the net effect is the hydrolysis of ATP and the generation of heat; *e.g.,* the futile c. from the unregulated action of 6-phosphofructokinase and fructose-1,6-bisphosphatase in muscle; such c.'s may have important roles in heat production, in the fine tuning of the regulation of certain pathways and may be a factor in malignant hyperthermia. SYN substrate c.

genesial c., the reproductive period of a woman's life.

γ-glutamyl c., a proposed pathway for the glutathione-dependent transport of certain amino acids (most notably L-cystine, L-methionine, and L-glutamine) and dipeptides into certain cells; this c. requires the formation of γ-glutamyl amino acids and γ-glutamyl dipeptides as well as a protein for the translocation of these di- and triisopeptides into the cells.

glycine-succinate c., a series of metabolic steps in which glycine is condensed with succinyl-CoA and is then oxidized to CO_2 and H_2O with regeneration of the succinyl-CoA; important in the synthesis of δ-aminolevulinic acid and in the metabolism of red blood cells. SYN Shemin c.

glyoxylic acid c., a catabolic c. in plants and microorganisms like that of the tricarboxylic acid c. in animals; its key reaction is the condensation of acetyl-CoA with glyoxylic acid to malic acid (analogous to the condensation of acetyl-CoA and oxaloacetic

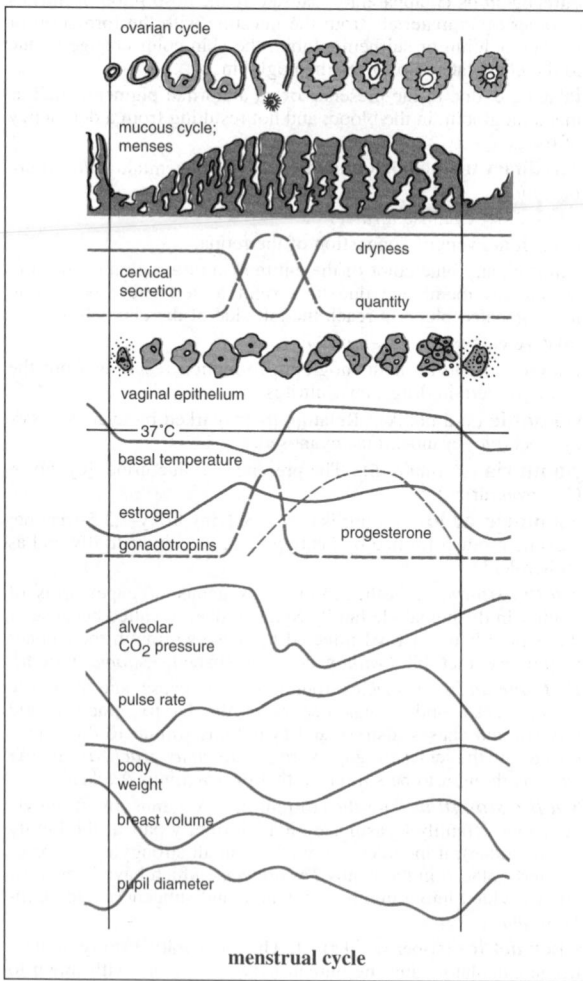

menstrual cycle

mitotic c., SYN cell c.

nitrogen c., the series of events in which the nitrogen of the atmosphere is fixed, thus made available for plant and animal life, and is then returned to the atmosphere: nitrifying bacteria convert N_2 and O_2 to NO_2^- and NO_3^-, the latter being absorbed by plants and converted to protein; if plants decay, the nitrogen is in part given up to the atmosphere and the remainder is converted by microorganisms to ammonia, nitrites, and nitrates; if the plants are eaten, the animals' excreta or bacterial decay return the nitrogen to the soil and air.

ornithine c., SYN urea c.

ovarian c., the normal sex c. which includes development of an ovarian (graafian) follicle, rupture of the follicle with discharge of the ovum, and formation and regression of a corpus luteum.

pentose phosphate c., SYN pentose phosphate *pathway.*

reproductive c., the c. which begins with conception and extends through gestation and parturition.

restored c., an atrial or ventricular cardiac c. that follows the returning c. and resumes the normal rhythm.

returning c., an atrial or ventricular cardiac c. that begins with an extrasystole or a forced beat.

Ross c., the life c. of the malaria parasite.

Shemin c., SYN glycine-succinate c.

substrate c., SYN futile c.

succinic acid c., a series of oxidation reduction reactions in which succinic acid and other 4-carbon atoms acids (fumaric, malic, oxaloacetic) take part in the oxidation of pyruvic acid as part of the tricarboxylic acid c. SEE ALSO dicarboxylic acid c.

tricarboxylic acid c., together with oxidative phosphorylation, the main source of energy in the mammalian body and the end toward which carbohydrate, fat, and protein metabolism are directed; a series of reactions, beginning and ending with oxaloacetic acid, during the course of which a two-carbon fragment is completely oxidized to carbon dioxide and water with the production of 12 high-energy phosphate bonds. So called because the first four substances involved (citric acid, *cis*-aconitic acid, isocitric acid, and oxalosuccinic acid) are all tricarboxylic acids; from oxalosuccinate, the others are, in order, α-ketoglutarate, succinate, fumarate, L-malate, and oxaloacetate, which condenses with acetyl-CoA (from fatty acid degradation) to form citrate (citric acid) again. SYN citric acid c., Krebs c.

urea c., the sequence of chemical reactions, occurring primarily in the liver, that results in the production of urea; the key reaction is the hydrolysis of L-arginine by arginase to L-ornithine and urea; L-ornithine is then converted to L-citrulline by a carbamoylation and then to L-arginine again by an amination reaction involving L-aspartic acid. SYN Krebs-Henseleit c., Krebs ornithine c., Krebs urea c., ornithine c.

visual c., the transformation of carotenoids involved in the bleaching and regeneration of the visual pigment.

---

cy·clec·to·my (sī-klek′tō-mē, sik-lek′tō-mē). Excision of a portion of the ciliary body. SYN ciliectomy. [cyclo- + G. *ektomē*, excision]

cy·clen·ceph·a·ly, cy·clen·ce·pha·lia (sī-klen-sef′ă-lē, -se-fā′lē-ă). Condition in a malformed fetus characterized by poor development and a varying degree of fusion of the two cerebral hemispheres. SYN cyclocephaly, cyclocephalia. [cyclo- + G. *enkephalos,* brain]

cy·cles per sec·ond (cps). The number of successive compressions and rarefactions per second of a sound wave. The preferred designation for this unit of frequency is hertz.

cy·clic (sī′klik, sik′lik). **1.** Pertaining to, or characteristic of, a cycle; occurring periodically, denoting the course of the symptoms in certain diseases or disorders. **2.** In chemistry, continuous, without end, as in a ring; denoting a c. compound.

cy·clic AMP. SYN adenosine 3′,5′-cyclic monophosphate.

3′,5′-cy·clic AMP syn·the·tase. SYN *adenylate* cyclase.

cy·clic GMP. SYN cyclic *guanosine* 3′,5′-monophosphate.

cy·cli·tis (sī-klī′tis). Inflammation of the ciliary body. [G. *kyklos,* circle (ciliary body), + *-itis,* inflammation]

Fuchs' heterochromic c., SYN Fuchs' *syndrome.*

heterochromic c., a chronic inflammatory c. in which the iris of the affected eye becomes atrophic.

plastic c., inflammation of the ciliary body, and usually of the entire uveal tract, with a fibrinous exudation into the anterior and vitreous chambers.

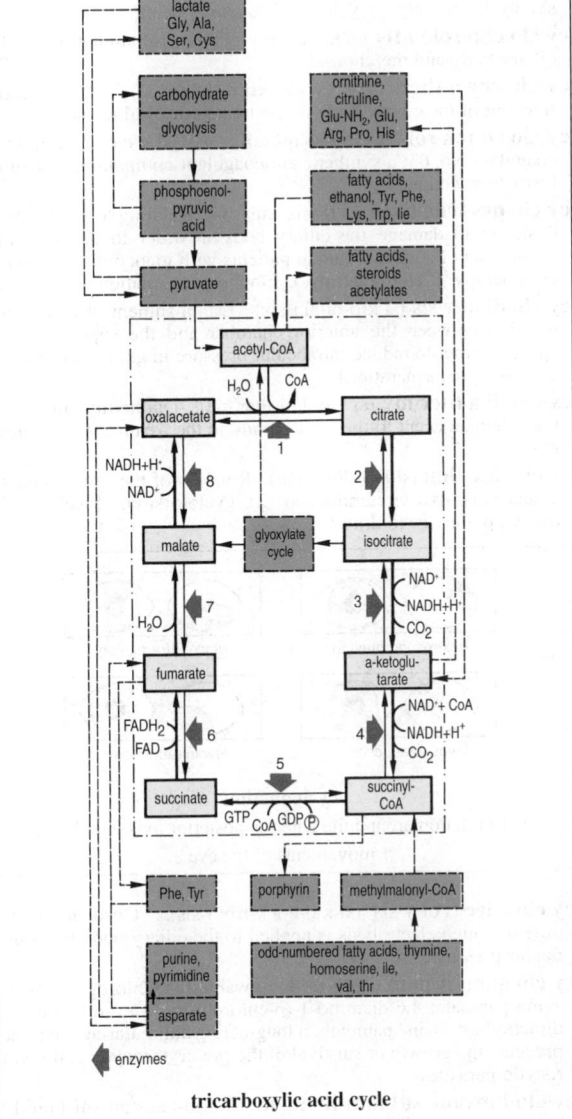

tricarboxylic acid cycle

1 = citrate synthetase	5 = succinate-CoA ligase
2 = aconitase	6 = succinate dehydrogenase
3 = isocitrate-dehydrogenase	7 = fumarase
4 = α-ketoglurate-dehydrogenase	8 = malate-dehydrogenase

purulent c., suppurative inflammation of the ciliary body.

cy·cli·zine hy·dro·chlo·ride (sī′kli-zēn). 1-Diphenylmethyl-4-methylpiperazine hydrochloride; an antihistamine agent useful in the prevention and relief of motion sickness and symptoms caused by vestibular disorders.

cy·cli·zine lac·tate. An agent with the same use and action as the hydrochloride.

cyclo-, cycl-. 1. Combining forms relating to a circle or cycle; or denoting an association with the ciliary body. **2.** In chemistry, a combining form indicating a continuous molecule, without end, or the formation of such a structure between two parts of a molecule. [G. *kyklos,* circle]

cy·clo·ben·za·prine hy·dro·chlo·ride (sī-klō-ben′ză-prēn). 1-Propanamine, 3-(5*H*-dibenzo[*a,d*]cyclohepten-5-ylidene)-*N,N*-diemthyl-, hydrochloride; a centrally acting skeletal muscle relaxant used to relieve acute muscular spasms.

cy·clo·ceph·a·ly, cy·clo·ce·pha·lia (sī-klō-sef′ă-lē, -sĕ-fā′lē-ă). SYN cyclencephaly. [cyclo- + G. *kephalē,* head]

cy·clo·cho·roid·i·tis (sī′klō-kō-roy-dī′tis). Inflammation of the ciliary body and the choroid.

cy·clo·cry·o·ther·a·py (sī′klō-krī′ō-thār′ă-pē). Transscleral freezing of the ciliary body in the treatment of glaucoma.

cy·clo·cu·ma·rol (sī-klō-kyū′mă-rol). 4-Hydroxycoumarin anticoagulant No. 63; a synthetic anticoagulant compound, related to bishydroxycoumarin.

cy·clo·des·truc·tive (sī′klō-dis-truk′tiv). Relating to a procedure designed to damage the ciliary body in order to diminish the production of aqueous fluid in patients with glaucoma. SEE cyclocryotherapy, cyclodiathermy, cyclophotocoagulation.

cy·clo·di·al·y·sis (sī′klō-dī-al′i-sis). Establishment of a communication between the anterior chamber and the suprachoroidal space in order to reduce intraocular pressure in glaucoma. [cyclo- + G. *dialysis,* separation]

cy·clo·di·a·ther·my (sī′klō-dī-ă-ther′mē). Diathermy applied to the sclera adjacent to the ciliary body in the treatment of glaucoma.

cy·clo·duc·tion (sī-klō-dŭk′shŭn). Rotation of the eye around its visual axis. SYN circumduction (2), cyclotorsion. [cyclo- + L. *duco,* pp. *ductus,* to draw]

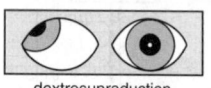
dextrosupraduction   dextroinfraduction
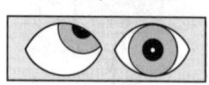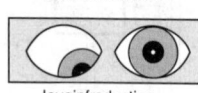
levosupraduction   levoinfraduction

cycloduction
with rotation around the anterior-posterior axis; combined movements of the eye

cy·clo·e·lec·trol·y·sis (sī′klō-ē-lek-trōl′i-sis). Obsolete procedure in which electrolysis is applied to the ciliary body to reduce ocular pressure.

cy·clo·guan·il pam·o·ate (sī-klō-gwahn′il). Chloroguanide triazine pamoate; 4,6-diamino-1-(*p*-chlorophenyl)-1,2-dihydro-2,2-dimethyl-*s*-triazine pamoate; a long-acting antimalarial agent that prevents the growth or survival of the pre-erythrocytic and erythrocytic parasites.

cy·clo·hex·ane·sul·fam·ic ac·id (sī-klō-heks′an-sŭl-fam′ik). SYN cyclamic acid.

cy·clo·hex·a·tri·ene (sī′klō-heks-ă-trī′ēn). Obsolete term for benzene.

cy·clo·hex·i·mide (sī-klō-heks′i-mīd). 3-[2-(3,5-Dimethyl-2-oxocyclohexyl)-2-hydroxyethyl]glutarimide; an antibiotic obtained from certain strains of *Streptomyces griseus;* used in biochemical research to inhibit *in vitro* protein synthesis; also a fungicide and rat repellent.

cy·clo·hex·i·tol (sī-klō-heks′i-tol). SYN inositol.

cy·clo·hex·yl·sul·fam·ic ac·id (sī-klō-hek′sil-sŭl-fam′ik). SYN cyclamic acid.

cy·cloid (sī′kloyd). Suggesting cyclothymia; a term applied to a person who tends to have periods of marked swings of mood, but within normal limits. [cyclo- + G. *eidos,* resembling]

cy·clol (sī′klol). A cyclic dipeptide postulated as occurring in proteins; it does occur in some of the ergot alkaloids.

cy·clo·na·mine (sī-klō-nā′mēn). SYN ethamsylate.

cy·clo·ox·y·gen·ase (sī′klō-oks′ē-jen-ās). SYN *prostaglandin* endoperoxide synthase.

cy·clo·pea (sī-klō′pē-ă). SYN cyclopia.

cy·clo·pe·an (sī-klō′pē-an). SYN cyclopian.

cy·clo·pent·a·mine hy·dro·chlo·ride (sī-klō-pent′ă-mēn). *N*,α-dimethylcyclopentaneethylamine hydrochloride; 1-cyclopentyl-2-methylaminopropane hydrochloride; a sympathomimetic amine, similar in action to ephedrine.

cy·clo·pen·tane (sī-klō-pen′tān). A closed ring hydrocarbon containing five carbon atoms, isomeric with pentene.

cy·clo·pen·ta[*a*]phen·an·threne. Phenanthrene, to the *a* side of which a three-carbon fragment is fused; as the perhydro (saturated) derivative, it is the basic structure of the steroids.

cy·clo·pen·ta·phene (sī-klō-pen′tă-fēn). SYN cyclarbamate.

cy·clo·pen·thi·a·zide (sī′klō-pen-thī′ă-zīd). $C_{13}H_{18}ClN_3O_4S_2$; a benzothiadiazide diuretic.

cy·clo·pen·to·late hy·dro·chlo·ride (sī-klō-pen′tō-lāt). 2-(Dimethylamino)ethyl-1-hydroxy-α-phenylcyclopentaneacetate hydrochloride; an anticholinergic, spasmolytic drug, used in refraction determinations; causes cycloplegia and mydriasis; an atropine-like agent with brief duration of action.

cy·clo·pep·tide (sī-klō-pep′tīd). A polypeptide lacking terminal —NH₂ and —COOH groups by virtue of their combination to form another peptide link, forming a ring.

cy·clo·phen·a·zine hy·dro·chlo·ride (sī-klō-fen′ă-zēn). 10-[3-(4-Cyclopropyl-1-piperazinyl)propyl]-2-(trifluoromethyl)-phenothiazine dihydrochloride; a tranquilizing drug.

cy·clo·pho·ras·es (sī-klō-fōr′ās-ez). The group of enzymes in mitochondria that catalyze the complete oxidation of pyruvic acid to carbon dioxide and water; essentially, those enzymes and coenzymes involved in the tricarboxylic acid cycle.

cy·clo·pho·ria (sī-klō-fō′rē-ă). Abnormal tendency for each eye to rotate around its anteroposterior axis, the rotation being prevented by visual fusional impulses. [cyclo- + G. *phora,* movement]

cy·clo·phos·pha·mide (sī-klō-fos′fă-mīd). *N,N*-Bis-(2-chloroethyl)-*N′*-(3-hydroxypropyl)phosphordiamidic acid cyclic ester monohydrate; an alkylating agent with antitumor activity and uses similar to those of its parent compound, nitrogen mustard (mechlorethamine hydrochloride); also a suppressor of B-cell activity and antibody formation, used to treat autoimmune diseases.

cy·clo·pho·to·co·ag·u·la·tion (sī′klō-fō′tō-kō-ag-yū-lā′shŭn). Photocoagulation of the ciliary processes to reduce the secretion of aqueous humor in glaucoma. [cyclo- + photocoagulation]

cy·clo·phre·nia (sī-klō-frē′nē-ă). Obsolete term for manic-depressive *psychosis.* [cyclo- + G. *phrēn,* the mind]

Cy·clo·phyl·li·dae (sī-klō-fil′i-dē). An order of tapeworms that includes most of the common parasites of humans and domestic animals. [cyclo- + G. *phyllon,* leaf]

cy·clo·pia (sī-klō′pē-ă). A congenital defect in which the two orbits merge to form a single cavity containing one eye, its origin evidenced by fusion of the right and left optic primordia, and in which the nose is absent; usually combined with cyclencephaly. SYN cyclopea, synophthalmia, synophthalmus. [G. *Kyklōps,* fr. *kyklos,* circle, + *ōps,* eye]

cy·clo·pi·an (sī-klō′pē-an). Denoting or relating to cyclopia. SYN cyclopean.

cy·clo·ple·gia (sī-klō-plē′jē-ă). Loss of power in the ciliary muscle of the eye; may be by denervation or by pharmacologic action. [cyclo- + G. *plēgē,* stroke]

cy·clo·ple·gic (sī-klō-plē′jik). **1.** Relating to cycloplegia. **2.** A drug that paralyzes the ciliary muscle and thus the power of accommodation.

cy·clo·pro·pane (sī-klō-prō′pān). (CH₂)₃; an explosive gas of characteristic odor; in the past, widely used for producing general anesthesia. SYN trimethylene.

cy·clops (sī′klops). An individual with cyclopia. SYN monoculus (1), monophthalmus, monops. [see cyclopia]

cy·clo·ser·ine (sī-klō-ser′ēn). D-4-amino-3-isoxazolidinone; cyclic anhydride of serine amide; an antibiotic produced by strains of *Streptomyces orchidaceus* or *S. garyphalus* with a wide spectrum of antibacterial activity. SYN orientomycin.

cy·clo·sis (sī-klō′sis). The movement of the protoplasm and contained plastids within the protozoan cell. [G., fr. *kykloō,* to move around]

Cy·clo·spo·ra (sī-klō-spōr′ah). A *Cryptosporidium*-like genus of coccidian parasites reported from millipedes, reptiles, insectivores, and a rodent species. C. is characterized by acid-fast oocysts with two sporocysts, each with two sporozoites. C. species is an undescribed but distinct species of C. that is implicated as the cause of a widespread, prolonged but self-limited human diarrhea in patients in North, Central, and South America; Caribbean countries; Southeast Asia; and eastern Europe previously reported as caused by cyanobacterium-like bodies. SYN cyanobacterium-like bodies.

cy·clo·spor·in A (sī-klō-spōr'in). SYN cyclosporine.

cy·clo·spor·ine (sī-klō-spōr'ēn). $C_{62}H_{111}N_{11}O_{12}$; a cyclic oligopeptide immunosupressant produced by the fungus *Tolypocladium inflatum Gams;* used to inhibit organ transplant rejection. SYN cyclosporin A.

cy·clo·thi·a·zide (sī-klō-thī'ă-zīd). 6-Chloro-3,4-dihydro-3-(2-norbornen-5-yl)-2*H*-1,2,4-benzothiadiazine-7-sulfonamide 1,1-dioxide; a diuretic and antihypertensive.

cy·clo·thy·mia (sī-klō-thī'mē-ă). A mental disorder characterized by marked swings of mood from depression to hypomania but not to the degree that occurs in bipolar disorder. [cyclo- + G. *thymos,* rage]

cy·clo·thy·mi·ac, cy·clo·thy·mic (sī-klō-thī'mē-ăk, -thī'mik). Relating to cyclothymia.

cy·clot·o·my (sī-klot'ō-mē). Operation of cutting the ciliary muscle. [cyclo- + G. *tomē,* incision]

cy·clo·tor·sion (sī'klō-tōr'shun). SYN cycloduction.

cy·clo·tron (sī'klō-tron). An accelerator that produces high-speed ions (*e.g.,* protons and deuterons) under the influence of an alternating magnetic field, for bombardment and disruption of atomic nuclei. Used to produce clinically useful positron-emitting radionuclides. [cyclo- + G. *-tron,* instrumental suffix]

cy·clo·tro·pia (sī-klō-trō'pē-;a). A disparity of ocular position in which one eye is rotated around its visual axis, with respect to the other eye. [cyclo- + G. *trope,* a turn, turning]

cy·clo·zo·o·no·sis (sī'klō-zō-ō-nō'sis). A zoonosis that requires more than one vertebrate host (but no invertebrate) for completion of the life cycle; *e.g.,* various taenioid cestodes such as *Taenia saginata* and *T. solium* in which humans are an obligatory host; hydatid disease, a c. in which man is not an obligatory host. [cyclo- + G. *zōon,* animal, + *nosos,* disease]

cy·cri·mine hy·dro·chlo·ride (sī'kri-mēn). 1-Phenyl-1-cyclopentyl-3-piperidino-1-propanol hydrochloride; an anticholinergic drug used in the treatment of parkinsonism.

Cyd Symbol for cytidine.

cy·e·sis (sī-ē'sis). Obsolete term for pregnancy. [G. *kyēsis*]

cy·hep·ta·mide (sī-hep'tă-mīd). 10,11-Dihydro-5*H*-dibenzo-[*a,d*]cycloheptene-5-carboxamide; an anticonvulsant.

cyl. Abbreviation for cylinder, or cylindrical *lens.*

cyl·in·der (**cyl., C**) (sil'in-der). **1.** A cylindrical *lens.* **2.** A cylindrical or rodlike renal cast. **3.** A cylindrical metal container for gases stored under high pressure. [G. *kylindros,* a roll]

axis c., obsolete term for axon.

Bence Jones c.'s, slightly irregular, relatively smooth, rod-shaped or cylindroid bodies of fairly tenacious, viscid proteinaceous material in the fluid of the seminal vesicles.

crossed c.'s, a lens used in refraction to determine the strength and axis of a cylindrical lens to correct astigmatism; a combination of concave and convex cylinders of like power whose axes are at right angles to each other.

Külz's c., SYN coma *cast.*

cyl·in·drax·is (sil-in-drak'sis). Historical precursor of the term axon, based on an interpretation of the myelinated nerve fiber as a cylinder of which the axon formed the axis.

cy·lin·dri·cal (si-lin'dri-kăl). Shaped like a cylinder; referring to a cylinder.

cyl·in·dro·ad·e·no·ma (sil'in-drō-ad-ĕ-nō'mă). SYN cylindroma.

cyl·in·droid (sil'in-droyd). SYN false *cast.* [G. *kylindrōdēs,* fr. *kylindros,* roll, cylinder, + *eidos,* appearance]

cyl·in·dro·ma (sil-in-drō'mă). A histologic type of epithelial neoplasm, frequently malignant, characterized by islands of neoplastic cells embedded in a hyalinized stroma which may represent a thickened basement membrane; may form from ducts of

glands, especially in salivary glands, skin, and bronchi; in the salivary glands, also termed adenoid cystic carcinoma. SYN cylindroadenoma. [G. *kylindros,* cylinder, *-oma,* tumor]

cyl·in·dro·sar·co·ma (sil'in-drō-sar-kō'mă). Obsolete term for a sarcoma that manifests several foci of hyaline degenerative changes, such as those observed in cylindromas.

cyl·in·dru·ria (sil-in-drū'rē-ă). The presence of renal cylinders or casts in the urine.

cyl·lo·so·ma (sil-ō-sō'mă). One-sided congenital defect of the lower abdominal wall (eventration) with defective development of the corresponding lower limb. [G. *kyllos,* deformed, esp. club-footed or bandylegged, + *sōma,* body]

cy·ma·rin (sī'mă-rin). K-Strophanthin-α, a glycoside of cymarose present in the seeds of *Strophanthus kombé;* the aglycone is strophanthin; a cardiotonic.

cym·ba con·chae (sim'bă kong'kē) [NA]. The upper, smaller part of the external ear lying above the crus helicis. [G. *kymbē,* the hollow of a vessel, a cup, bowl, a boat]

cym·bo·ce·phal·ic, cym·bo·ceph·a·lous (sim-bō-se-fal'ik, -sef'ă-lŭs). Relating to cymbocephaly.

cym·bo·ceph·a·ly (sim-bō-sef'ă-lē). SYN scaphocephaly. [G. *kymbē,* the hollow of a vessel, a boat-shaped structure, + *kephalē,* head]

cy·nan·thro·py (sī-nan'thrō-pē). A delusion in which one barks and growls, imagining himself to be a dog. [G. *kyōn,* dog, + *anthrōpos,* man]

cyn·ic (sin'ik). Doglike, denoting a spasm of the muscles of the face as in risus caninus. [G. *kynikos,* doglike]

cy·no·ceph·a·ly (sī-nō-sef'ă-lē). Craniostenosis in which the skull slopes back from the orbits, producing a resemblance to the head of a dog. [G. *kyōn,* dog, + *kephalē,* head]

cyn·o·dont (sī'nō-dont). **1.** A canine tooth. **2.** A tooth having one cusp or point. [G. *kyōn,* dog, + *odous* (*odont-*), tooth]

cy·no·pho·bia (sī-nō-fō'bē-ă). Morbid fear of dogs. [G. *kyōn,* dog, + *phobos,* fear]

Cyon, Elie de, Russian physiologist, 1843–1912. SEE C.'s *nerve.*

cy·pri·do·pho·bia (sī'pri-dō-fō'bē-ă). Morbid fear of venereal disease or of sexual intercourse. [G. *Kypris,* Aphrodite, + *phobos,* fear]

Cy·prin·i·dae (sī-prin'i-dē). A family of bony freshwater fishes including the goldfishes, carp, chubs, and minnows. [G. *kyprinos,* a carp]

cy·pro·hep·ta·dine hy·dro·chlo·ride (sī-prō-hep'tă-dēn). 1-Methyl-4-(5-dibenzo-[a,e]-cycloheptatrienylidine)-piperidine; a potent antagonist of histamine and serotonin, with antihistaminic and antipruritic actions.

cy·pro·ter·one ac·e·tate (sī-prō'ter-ōn). 6-Chloro-1β,2β-dihydro-17-hydroxy-3'*H*-cyclopropa[1,2]pregna-1,4,6-triene-3,20-dione acetate; a synthetic steroid capable of inhibiting the biological effects exerted by endogenous or exogenous androgenic hormones; an antiandrogen.

Cys Symbol for cysteine (half-cystine) or its mono- or diradical.

CYST

cyst (sist). **1.** A bladder. **2.** An abnormal sac containing gas, fluid, or a semisolid material, with a membranous lining. SEE ALSO pseudocyst. [G. *kystis,* bladder]

adventitious c., SYN pseudocyst (1).

allantoic c., SYN urachal c.

alveolar hydatid c., a hydatid c. of a multiloculate type, usually in the liver, caused by *Echinococcus multilocularis,* adults of which are in foxes; larvae (alveolar hydatid) are found chiefly in microtine rodents, but also among humans such as trappers and others handling pelts of infected foxes and other carnivores; growth is by exogenous budding and is not limited by an outer laminated membrane as in the hydatid c. from *E. granulosus;*

necrosis, cavitation, contiguous spread, and death usually ensue. SYN multilocular hydatid c., multiloculate hydatid c.

aneurysmal bone c., a solitary benign osteolytic lesion expanding a long bone or within a vertebra, consisting of blood-filled spaces, and separated by fibrous tissue containing multinucleated giant cells; such c.'s cause swelling, pain, and tenderness. SYN benign bone aneurysm.

angioblastic c., mesenchymal tissue capable of forming blood in the embryo.

apical periodontal c., an inflammatory odontogenic c. derived histogenetically from Malassez' epithelial rests surrounding the root apex of a nonvital tooth. SYN periapical c., radicular c., root end c.

apoplectic c., a pseudocyst formed of extravasated blood as in a stroke.

arachnoid c., a fluid-filled c. lined with arachnoid membrane, frequently situated near the lateral aspect of the fissure of Sylvius; usually congenital in origin. SYN leptomeningeal c.

Baker's c., a collection of synovial fluid which has escaped from the knee joint or a bursa and formed a new synovial-lined sac in the popliteal space; seen in degenerative or other joint diseases.

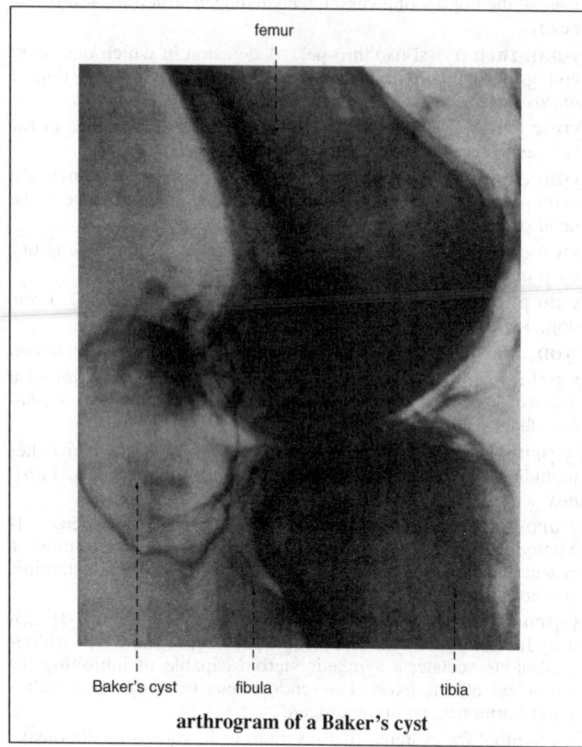

femur

Baker's cyst   fibula   tibia

arthrogram of a Baker's cyst

Bartholin's c., a c. arising from the major vestibular gland or its ducts.

bile c., SYN gallbladder.

blood c., SYN hemorrhagic c.

blue dome c., (1) one of a number of small dark blue nodules or c.'s in the vaginal fornix due to retained menstrual blood in endometriosis affecting this region; **(2)** a benign retention c. of the mammary gland in fibrocystic disease, containing a pale slightly yellow fluid which gives a blue color to the c. when seen through the surrounding fibrous tissue.

bone c., SEE solitary bone c.

botryoid odontogenic c., a type of lateral periodontal c. that shows a multilocular growth pattern.

Boyer's c., a subhyoid c.

branchial c., a cervical c. arising from developmental persistence of ectodermal branchial grooves or endodermal pharyngeal pouches. SYN branchial cleft c., cervical c. (1).

branchial cleft c., SYN branchial c.

bronchogenic c., a c. lined by ciliated columnar epithelium believed to represent bronchial differentiation; smooth muscle and mucous glands may be present.

bursal c., a retention c. in a bursa.

calcifying and keratinizing odontogenic c., SYN calcifying odontogenic c.

calcifying odontogenic c., a mixed radiolucent-radiopaque lesion of the jaws with features of both a c. and a solid neoplasm; characterized microscopically by an epithelial lining showing a palisaded layer of columnar basal cells, presence of ghost cell keratinization, dentinoid, and calcification. SYN calcifying and keratinizing odontogenic c., Gorlin c.

cerebellar c., a c. usually occurring in the lateral cerebellar white matter; often a part of cerebellar astrocytoma.

cervical c., (1) SYN branchial c. **(2)** SYN thyroglossal duct c.

chocolate c., c. of the ovary with intracavitary hemorrhage and formation of a hematoma containing old brown blood; often seen with endometriosis of the ovary but occasionally with other types of c.'s.

choledochal c., c. originating from common bile duct; usually becomes apparent early in life as a right upper abdominal mass in association with jaundice.

chyle c., a circumscribed dilation of a lymphatic channel of the mesentery, containing chyle.

colloid c., a c. with gelatinous contents.

compound c., SYN multilocular c.

corpora lutea c.'s, persistent corpora lutea with c. formation.

Cowper's c., a retention c. of a bulbourethral gland.

daughter c., a secondary c., usually multiple, derived from a mother c.

dental lamina c., a small keratin-filled c., usually multiple, on the alveolar ridge of newborn infants; derived from remnants of the dental lamina.

dentigerous c., an odontogenic c. derived from the reduced enamel epithelium surrounding the crown of an impacted or embedded tooth. SYN follicular c. (2).

dermoid c., a tumor consisting of displaced ectodermal structures along lines of embryonic fusion, the wall being formed of epithelium-lined connective tissue, including skin appendages and containing keratin, sebum, and hair. SYN dermoid tumor, dermoid (2), inclusion dermoid, sequestration c.

dermoid c. of ovary, a common benign cystic teratoma of the ovary, lined for the most part by skin, and containing hair and sebum, but also usually containing a variety of other well differentiated structures within a small inwardly projecting mass of solid tissue.

distention c., SYN retention c.

duplication c., a congenital cystic malformation attached to or originating from any part of the alimentary canal, from the base of the tongue to the anus, which reproduces the structure of the adjacent alimentary tract.

echinococcus c., SYN hydatid c.

endometrial c., a c. resulting from endometrial implantation outside the uterus, as in endometriosis.

endothelial c., a serous c. whose sac is lined with endothelium.

enterogenous c.'s, mediastinal cysts derived from cells sequestered from the primitive foregut; may be classified histologically as bronchogenic, esophageal, or gastric.

ependymal c., a circumscribed distention of some portion of the central canal of the spinal cord or of the cerebral ventricles. SYN neural c.

epidermal c., a c. formed of a mass of epidermal cells which, as a result of trauma, has been pushed beneath the epidermis; the c. is lined with stratified squamous epithelium and contains concentric layers of keratin. SYN implantation c., inclusion c. (1).

epidermoid c., a spherical, unilocular c. of the dermis, comprised of encysted keratin and sebum; the c. is lined by a keratinizing epithelium resembling the epidermis derived from the follicular infundibulum.

epithelial c., a c. lined with epithelium.

eruption c., a form of dentigerous c. in the soft tissues in conjunction with an erupting tooth; seen on the alveolar ridge of children.

extravasation c., obsolete term for hemorrhagic c.

exudation c., a c. resulting from distention of a closed cavity, such as a bursa, by an excessive secretion of its normal fluid contents.

false c., SYN pseudocyst (1).

fissural c., a c. derived from epithelial remnants entrapped along the fusion line of embryonal processes. SYN inclusion c. (2).

follicular c., (1) a cystic graafian follicle; (2) SYN dentigerous c.

Gartner's c., a c. of the principal duct in the vestigial structures of the paroöphoron in the cervix or anterolateral vaginal wall, corresponding to the sexual portion of mesonephros in the male.

gas c., a c. with gaseous instead of the ordinary liquid or pultaceous contents.

gingival c., a c. derived from remnants of the dental lamina situated in the attached gingiva, occasionally producing superficial erosion of the cortical plate of bone; most are located in the cuspid-premolar region.

globulomaxillary c. (glō′bū-lō-maks′il-lar-ē), a c. of odontogenic origin found between the roots of the maxillary lateral incisor and canine teeth.

glomerular c.'s, c.'s formed by dilatation of Bowman's capsules, found in rare cases of congenital polycystic kidneys.

Gorlin c., SYN calcifying odontogenic c.

granddaughter c., a tertiary c. sometimes developed within a daughter c., as in the hydatid cyst of *Echinococcus.*

hemorrhagic c., a c. containing blood or resulting from the encapsulation of a hematoma. SYN blood c., hematocele (1), hematocyst, sanguineous c.

hepatic c.'s, congenital c.'s thought to originate from an obstruction of biliary ductules; they may be solitary and range in size from small to enormous; polycystic disease may also occur.

heterotrophic oral gastrointestinal c., a c. of the oral cavity lined by gastric or intestinal mucosa from misplaced embryonic rests.

hydatid c., a c. formed in the liver, or, less frequently, elsewhere, by the larval stage of *Echinococcus,* chiefly in ruminants; two morphological forms caused by *Echinococcus granulosus* are found in humans: the unilocular hydatid c. and the osseous hydatid c.; a third form in humans is the alveolar hydatid c., caused by *Echinococcus multilocularis.* SYN echinococcus c., hydatid (1).

implantation c., SYN epidermal c.

incisive canal c., a c. in or near the incisive canal, arising from proliferation of epithelial remnants of the nasopalatine duct; the most common maxillary development c. SYN median anterior maxillary c., nasopalatine duct c.

inclusion c., (1) SYN epidermal c. (2) SYN fissural c.

involution c., a mammary c. occurring at the menopause, due to fibrocystic disease.

iodine c.'s, obsolete term used to indicate the c.'s of *Iodamoeba butschlii,* characterized by a large iodine-positive glycogen vacuole.

junctional c., a c. of the testis arising from the structures connecting the rete testis with the epididymis.

keratinous c., an epithelial c. containing keratin.

Klestadt's c., SYN nasoalveolar c.

lacteal c., a retention c. in the mammary gland resulting from closure of a lactiferous duct. SYN milk c.

lateral periodontal c., an intraosseous c., usually encountered in the cuspid-premolar region of the mandible, derived from the remnants of the dental lamina and representing the intraosseous counterpart of the gingival c.

leptomeningeal c., SYN arachnoid c.

lymphoepithelial c., a cervical c. arising from salivary gland epithelium entrapped in lymph nodes during embryogenesis. Also seen within the oral cavity.

median anterior maxillary c., SYN incisive canal c.

median palatal c., a developmental c. located in the midline of the hard palate.

median raphe c. of the penis, a c. of the raphe penis resulting from incomplete closure of the urethral groove, becoming clinically evident in childhood or later.

meibomian c., SYN chalazion.

milk c., SYN lacteal c.

morgagnian c., SYN vesicular *appendices* of uterine tube, under *appendix.*

mother c., a hydatid c. from the inner, or germinal, layer, from which secondary c.'s containing scoleces (daughter c.'s) are developed; sometimes tertiary c.'s (granddaughter c.'s) are developed within the daughter c.'s; occurs most frequently in the liver, but may be found in other organs and tissues; symptoms are those of a tumor of the part affected. SYN parent c.

mucous c., a retention c. resulting from obstruction in the duct of a mucous gland. SYN mucocele.

multilocular c., a c. containing several compartments formed by membranous septa. SYN compound c.

multilocular hydatid c., multiloculate hydatid c., SYN alveolar hydatid c.

myxoid c., SYN ganglion (2).

nabothian c., a retention c. that develops when a mucous gland of the cervix uteri is obstructed; of no pathologic significance. SYN nabothian follicle.

nasoalveolar c., a soft tissue c. located near the attachment of the ala over the maxilla; probably derived from the lower anterior part of the nasolacrimal duct. SYN Klestadt's c., nasolabial c.

nasolabial c., SYN nasoalveolar c.

nasopalatine duct c., SYN incisive canal c.

nasopalatine c., a c. due to a circumscribed encapsulated area of necrosis with subsequent liquefaction of the dead tissue.

necrotic c., a c. due to a circumscribed encapsulated area of necrosis with subsequent liquefaction of the dead tissue.

neural c., SYN ependymal c.

neurenteric c.'s, paravertebral c.'s commonly connected to the meninges or a portion of the gastrointestinal tract that develop due to incomplete separation of endoderm from the notochord during early fetal life; often symptomatic.

odontogenic c., a c. derived from odontogenic epithelium. [odont- + G. *genos,* birth, origin, + suffix *-ic,* pertaining to]

oil c., a c. resulting from loss of the epithelial lining of a sebaceous, dermoid, or lacteal c., or from the subcutaneous injection of oil or fat material.

omphalomesenteric c., cystic lesion found within the umbilical cord, presumed to develop from remnants of the omphalomesenteric duct early in gestation. May be found on antenatal ultrasound. SYN omphalomesenteric duct c.

omphalomesenteric duct c., SYN omphalomesenteric c.

oophoritic c., SYN ovarian c.

osseous hydatid c., a morphological form of hydatid c. caused by *Echinococcus granulosus,* and found in the long bones or the pelvic arch of humans if the embryo is filtered out in bony tissue; in this site no limiting membrane forms and the c. grows in an uncontrolled fashion, producing cancellous structures and inducing fracture, followed by spread to new sites.

ovarian c., a cystic tumor of the ovary, either non-neoplastic (follicle, lutein, germinal inclusion, or endometrial) or neoplastic; usually restricted to benign c.'s, *i.e.,* mucinous serous cystadenoma, or dermoid c.'s. SYN oophoritic c.

paraphysial c.'s, c.'s arising from vestigial remnants of the paraphysis; they are the possible origin of some third ventricular colloid c.'s.

parasitic c., a c. formed by the larva of a metazoan parasite, such as a hydatid or trichinal c.

parent c., SYN mother c.

paroophoritic c., a c. arising from the paroöpheron.

parvilocular c., a tumor composed of multiple small c.'s.

pearl c., a mass of epithelial cells introduced into the interior of the eye by a perforating injury.

periapical c., SYN apical periodontal c.

phaeomycotic c., a subcutaneous cystic granuloma caused by pigmented fungi, usually solitary and located on the extremities.

pilar c., a common c. of the skin and subcutis which contains sebum and keratin, and is lined by pale-staining stratified epithelial cells derived from follicular trichilemma. SYN trichilemmal c.

piliferous c., a dermoid c. containing hair.

pilonidal c., SEE pilonidal *sinus.*

pineal c., a c. of the pineal gland; rarely of clinical importance.

posttraumatic leptomeningeal c., a persistent cystic accumulation of cerebrospinal fluid with progressive loss of bone and dura, occurring at the site of a previous fracture.

primordial c., a c. which develops in place of a tooth through cystic degeneration of the enamel organ prior to formation of calcified odontogenic tissue.

proliferating tricholemmal c., SYN pilar *tumor* of scalp.

proliferation c., proliferative c., proliferous c., a mother c. containing daughter c.'s; a c. with tumorous formation at one portion of the sac.

protozoan c., infectious form of many protozoan parasites such as *Entamoeba histolytica, Giardia lamblia, Balantidium coli,* etc., usually passed in the feces and provided with a highly condensed cytoplasm and resistant cell wall.

pseudomucinous c., a c. containing a gelatinous fluid, formerly thought to differ significantly from mucin, occurring especially in the ovary.

radicular c., SYN apical periodontal c.

Rathke's cleft c., an intrasellar or suprasellar c. lined by cuboidal epithelium derived from remnants of Rathke's pouch.

residual c., the persistence of an apical periodontal c. that remains after tooth extraction.

retention c., a c. resulting from some obstruction to the excretory duct of a gland. SYN distention c., secretory c.

rete c. of ovary, a c. derived from the germinal cords in the hilum of the ovary.

root end c., SYN apical periodontal c.

sanguineous c., SYN hemorrhagic c.

sebaceous c., a common c. of the skin and subcutis containing sebum and keratin, and lined by epithelium derived from the pilosebaceous follicle. SEE epidermoid c., pilar c.

secretory c., SYN retention c.

seminal vesical c., a c., usually congenital, of the seminal vesicle.

sequestration c., SYN dermoid c.

serous c., a c. containing clear serous fluid, such as a hygroma.

simple bone c., SYN solitary bone c.

solitary bone c., a unilocular c. containing serous fluid and lined with a thin layer of connective tissue, occurring usually in the shaft of a long bone in a child. SYN idiopathic bone cavity, osteocystoma, simple bone c., traumatic bone c., unicameral bone c.

Stafne bone c., SYN lingual salivary gland *depression.*

static bone c., SYN lingual salivary gland *depression.*

sterile c., a hydatid c. without brood capsules or viable scoleces.

sublingual c., SYN ranula (2).

suprasellar c., SYN craniopharyngioma.

surgical ciliated c., a c. that arises from maxillary sinus epithelium implanted along a line of surgical entry.

synovial c., SYN ganglion (2).

Tarlov's c., a perineural c. found in the proximal radicles of the lower spinal cord; it is usually productive of symptoms.

tarry c., a c. or collection of old blood having a tarry or black, sticky appearance; usually due to endometriosis.

tarsal c., SYN chalazion.

teratomatous c., a c. containing structures derived from all three of the primary germ layers of the embryo.

thyroglossal duct c., thyrolingual c., a c. in the midline of the neck resulting from nonclosure of a segment of the ductus thyroglossus. SYN cervical c. (2).

Tornwaldt's c., SYN pharyngeal *bursa.*

traumatic bone c., SYN solitary bone c.

trichilemmal c., SYN pilar c.

tubular c., SYN tubulocyst.

umbilical c., SYN vitellointestinal c.

unicameral c., SYN unilocular c.

unicameral bone c., SYN solitary bone c.

unilocular c., a c. having a single sac. SYN unicameral c.

unilocular hydatid c., the commonest form of hydatid c. in man, caused by *Echinococcus granulosus* and found in the liver, lungs, or any other site where the hexacanth embryo may settle if it passes the hepatic or pulmonary capillary filters; characterized by large balloon-like forms lined internally with a germinative membrane, enclosed externally in a laminated membrane within a host-parasite capsule, and filled with fluid (hydatid fluid) and infectious scoleces of the young tapeworms (hydatid sand).

urachal c., a c. of the urachus which may communicate with the umbilicus or bladder, or give rise to a mid-line swelling. SYN allantoic c.

urinary c., a c. containing extravasated urine.

utricular c., dilatation of the utricular lumen; usually unilocular.

vitellointestinal c., a small red sessile or pedunculated tumor at the umbilicus or in an infant; it is due to the persistence of a segment of the vitellointestinal duct. SYN umbilical c.

wolffian c., a c. lying in the broad ligaments of the uterus and arising from any mesonephric structures.

---

cyst-. SEE cysto-.

cys·ta·canth (sis′tă-kanth). The fully developed larva of Acanthocephala, infective to the final host and with an inverted fully formed proboscis characteristic of the adult worm. [cyst- + G. *akantha,* thorn or spine]

cyst·ad·e·no·car·ci·no·ma (sist-ad′en-ō-kar-si-nō′mă). A malignant neoplasm derived from glandular epithelium, in which cystic accumulations of retained secretions are formed; the neoplastic cells manifest varying degrees of anaplasia and invasiveness, and local extension and metastases occur; c.'s develop frequently in the ovaries, where pseudomucinous and serous types are recognized.

cyst·ad·e·no·ma (sist′ad-ĕ-nō′mă). A histologically benign neoplasm derived from glandular epithelium, in which cystic accumulations of retained secretions are formed; in some instances, considerable portions of the neoplasm, or even the entire mass, may be cystic. SYN cystoadenoma.

papillary c. lymphomato′sum, SYN adenolymphoma.

cyst·al·gia (sist-al′jē-ă). Pain in a bladder, especially the urinary bladder. [cyst- + G. *algos,* pain]

cys·ta·mine (sis′tă-mēn). $(H_2NCH_2CH_2)_2S_2$; Decarboxycystine; forms when cystine is distilled. The disulfide of cysteamine.

cys·ta·thi·o·nase (sis-tă-thī′ō-nās). SYN cystathionine γ-lyase.

β-cys·ta·thi·o·nase. SYN cystathionine β-lyase.

γ-cys·ta·thi·o·nase. SYN cystathionine γ-lyase.

cys·ta·thi·o·nine (sis-tă-thī′ō-nēn). ⁻OOC-CH (NH₃⁺) CH₂- S-CH₂ CH ₂-CH(NH₃)⁺ COO⁻; the L-isomer is an intermediate in the conversion of L-methionine to L-cysteine; cleaved by cystathionases.

cys·ta·thi·o·nine β-ly·ase. An enzyme catalyzing the hydrolysis of L-cystathionine to pyruvate, L-homocysteine, and NH_3. SEE ALSO cystathionine γ-lyase. SYN β-cystathionase, cystine lyase.

cys·ta·thi·o·nine γ-ly·ase. A liver enzyme, requiring pyridoxal phosphate as coenzyme, that catalyzes the hydrolysis of L-cystathionine to L-cysteine and 2-ketobutyrate, releasing NH_3; also catalyzes formation of 2-ketobutyrate from L-homoserine, of pyruvate (and NH_3 and H_2S) from L-cysteine, and of thiocysteine, pyruvate, and NH_3 from cystine. A deficiency of this enzyme results in cystathioninuria. A step in methionine catabolism and in cysteine biosynthesis. SEE ALSO cystathionine β-lyase. SYN cystathionase, cysteine desulfhydrase, cystine desulfhydrase, γ-cystathionase, homoserine deaminase, homoserine dehydratase.

cys·ta·thi·o·nine β-syn·thase. An enzyme catalyzing the reversible hydrolysis of L-cystathionine to L-serine and L-homocysteine. A step in cysteine biosynthesis and in methionine catabolism. A deficiency of this enzyme leads to vascular thrombosis, dislocation of ocular lens, and abnormal development. SEE ALSO cystathionine γ-synthase. SYN β-thionase, cysteine synthase, serine sulfhydrase.

cys·ta·thi·o·nine γ-syn·thase. SYN *O*-succinylhomoserine (thiol)-lyase.

cys·ta·thi·o·nin·u·ria (sis′tă-thī′ō-nin-ū′rē-ă) [MIM*219500]. A disorder characterized by inability to metabolize cystathionine, normally due to deficiency of cystathionase, with high concentration of the amino acid in blood, tissue, and urine; mental retardation is an associated condition; autosomal recessive inheritance.

cys·te·a·mine (sis-tā′a-mēn). Sulfhydryl compound used experimentally to produce ulcers in rats and as a radioprotective agent; antidote to acetaminophen.

cys·tec·ta·sia, cys·tec·ta·sy (sis-tek-tā′zē-ă, sis-tek′tă-sē). Dilation of the bladder. [cyst- + G. *ektasis*, a stretching]

cys·tec·to·my (sis-tek′tō-mē). **1.** Excision of the the urinary bladder. **2.** Excision of the gallbladder (cholecystectomy). **3.** Removal of a cyst. [cyst- + G. *ektomē*, excision]

    Bartholin's c., removal of a cyst of a major vestibular gland. SYN vulvovaginal c.

    partial c., removal of a part or segment of the bladder.

    radical c., removal of the entire bladder, surrounding fatty tissues, and regional lymph nodes.

    salvage c., removal of the bladder.

    total c., removal of the entire bladder.

    vulvovaginal c., SYN Bartholin's c.

cys·te·ic ac·id (sis-tā′ik). $HOOC-CH(NH_2)CH_2-SO_3H$; an oxidation product of cysteine, and a precursor of taurine and isethionic acid. SYN 3-sulfoalanine.

cys·te·ine (C, Cys) (sis′ta-ēn). $HS-CH_2CH(NH_3)^+COO^-$; 2-amino-3-mercaptopropionic acid; the L-isomer is found in most proteins; especially abundant in keratin.

    c. desulfhydrase, SYN cystathionine γ-lyase.

    c. synthase, SYN cystathionine β-synthase.

cys·te·ine sul·fin·ic ac·id (sis′tē-ēn-sul-fin′ik). $^-O_2S-CH_2CH(NH_3)^+COO^-$; a natural oxidation product of cysteine; an intermediate in the formation of taurine (via cysteic acid).

cys·tein·yl (sis′tēn-il). Aminoacyl radical of cysteine.

△**cysti-.** SEE cysto-.

cys·tic (sis′tik). **1.** Relating to the urinary bladder or gallbladder. **2.** Relating to a cyst. **3.** Containing cysts. SYN cystous.

cys·ti·cer·coid (sis-ti-ser′koyd). A larval tapeworm resembling a cysticercus but having a smaller bladder, containing little or no fluid, in which scolex of the future adult tapeworm is found; the larval form is typically found in insect intermediate hosts. [cysti- + G. *kerkos*, tail, + *eidos*, resemblance]

cys·ti·cer·co·sis (sis′ti-ser-kō′sis). **1.** Disease caused by encystment of cysticercus larvae (*e.g., Taenia solium* or *T. saginata*) in subcutaneous, muscle, or central nervous system tissues; c. is typically developed in swine and cattle, producing measly pork and beef. In humans, it results from the hatching of the eggs of *Taenia solium* in the intestines or by accidental ingestion of eggs from human feces; encystment in the brain may cause serious nervous damage, and encystment in the eye (usually the rear chamber) may cause ophthalmic damage. **2.** Larval infections in animals with other taeniid tapeworm larvae. SYN cysticercus disease.

Cys·ti·cer·cus (sis-ti-ser′kŭs). Originally described as a genus of bladderworms, now known to be the encysted larvae of various taenioid tapeworms; the generic name is, however, retained as a convenience in referring to the larval encysted forms. SEE cysticercus. SYN bladderworm. [G. *kystis*, bladder, + *kerkos*, tail]

    C. bo'vis, the cysticercus larva of *Taenia saginata* in cattle; the cause of measly beef.

    C. cellulo'sae, the cysticercus larva of *Taenia solium* in pigs; also the cause of human cysticercosis.

    C. fasciola'ris, the strobilocercus larva of *Taenia taeniaeformis*, found in the liver of mice, rats, and other rodents; adult worms infect cats and canids.

    C. pisifor'mis, the larva of *Taenia pisiformis;* it occurs in the liver and abdominal cavity of rabbits and hares; adult worms are found in dogs and other canids.

    C. tenuicol'lis, the cystic form of *Taenia hydatigena;* it is found in the liver and peritoneal cavity of sheep, cattle, pigs, and wild ruminants; adults are found in various predators.

cys·ti·cer·cus, pl. **cys·ti·cer·ci** (sis-ti-ser′kŭs, -ser′sē). The larval form of certain *Taenia* species, typically found in muscles of

mammalian intermediate hosts that serve as a prey of various predators; it consists of a fluid-filled bladder in which the invaginated cestode scolex develops. SEE ALSO *Taenia saginata*, *Taenia solium*. [G. *kystis*, bladder, + *kerkos*, tail]

cys·ti·des (sis′ti-dēz). Plural of cystis.

cys·ti·fel·le·ot·o·my (sis′ti-fel-ē-ot′-ō-mē). Obsolete term for cholecystotomy. [cysti- + L. *felleus*, pertaining to bile, + G. *tomē*, incision]

cys·ti·form (sis′ti-fōrm). SYN cystoid (1).

cys·tig·er·ous (sis-tij′er-ŭs). SYN cystopherous.

cys·tine (sis′tīn). $HOOC-CH(NH_2)-CH_2-S-S-CH_2-CH(NH_2)COOH$; 3,3′-dithiobis(2-aminopropionic acid); the disulfide product of two cysteines in which two –SH groups become one –S–S– group; if two cysteinyl residues in polypeptide chains form a disulfide linkage, then the two polymers are cross-linked; sometimes occurs as a deposit in the urine, or forming a vesical calculus. Cf. *meso*-cystine. SYN dicysteine.

    c. desulfhydrase, SYN cystathionine γ-lyase.

    half c., refers to one-half of a cystine molecule or of a cystinyl residue in a protein or peptide.

    c. lyase, SYN cystathionine β-lyase.

meso-**cys·tine.** An isomer of cystine in which the configuration about one of the α-carbons is D, about the other, L, so that the molecule as a whole possesses a plane of symmetry and is optically inactive. Note that *meso*-cystine is not DL-cystine. DL-cystine is a racemic mixture of DD-cystine and LL-cystine.

cys·ti·ne·mia (sis-ti-nē′mē-ă). The presence of cystine in the blood. [cystine + G. *haima*, blood]

cys·ti·no·sis (sis-ti-nō′sis). The most common of a group of diseases with characteristic renal tubular dysfunction disorders, termed collectively Fanconi's *syndrome* (2). There are various forms. An autosomal recessive hereditary disease of early childhood [MIM*219800] characterized by widespread deposits of cystine crystals throughout the body, including bone marrow and other tissues, with slight increase in the level of plasma cystine and cystinuria; this apparent abnormality in cystine metabolism is associated with a marked generalized aminoaciduria, glycosuria, polyuria, chronic acidosis, hypophosphatemia with vitamin D-resistant rickets, and often with hypokalemia; the latter abnormalities are probably due to deficient tubular reabsorption and are accompanied by a characteristic abnormality of the proximal convoluted tubule, shown by microdissection to be narrowed at the glomerular junction (swan-neck deformity). There is a milder form with onset in adolescence [MIM* 219900] and one with adult onset without kidney damage [MIM*219750]. Due to a defect in the transport of cystine across lysosomal membranes. SYN cystine disease, cystine storage disease, De Toni-Fanconi syndrome, Lignac-Fanconi syndrome. [cystine + G. *-osis*, condition]

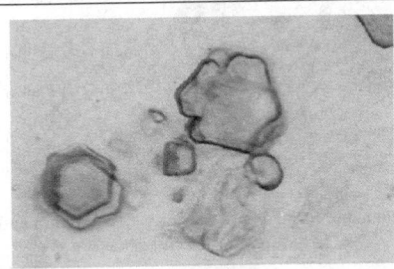

cystinosis
microscopic view of cystine crystals in the urine

cys·ti·nu·ria (sis-ti-nū′rē-ă) [MIM*220100]. Excessive urinary excretion of cystine, along with lysine, arginine, and ornithine, arising from defective transport systems for these acids in the kidney and intestine; renal function is sometimes compromised by cystine crystalluria and nephrolithiasis; occurs in certain heritable diseases, such as Fanconi's syndrome (cystinosis) and hepatoIenticular degeneration. There are several forms, all with autosomal recessive inheritance. [cystine + G. *ouron*, urine]

cys·tin·yl (sis′tin-il). Aminoacyl radical of cystine.

cys·tiph·or·ous (sis-tif′er-ŭs). SYN cystopherous.

cys·tis, pl. **cys·ti·des** (sis′tis, sis′ti-dēz). SEE cyst, pouch, sac. [G. *kystis*]

  c. fel′lea, SYN gallbladder.

  c. urina′ria, SYN urinary *bladder.*

cys·ti·stax·is (sis-ti-stak′sis). Obsolete term for oozing of blood from the mucous membrane of the bladder. [cysti- + G. *staxis*, trickling]

cys·ti·tis (sis-tī′tis). Inflammation of the urinary bladder. [cyst- + G. *-itis*, inflammation]

  bacterial c., bladder inflammation caused by bacteria.

  c. col′li, inflammation of the neck of the bladder.

  c. cys′tica, c. glandularis with the formation of cysts.

  emphysematous c., inflammation of the bladder wall caused by gas-forming bacteria, usually secondary to diabetes mellitus.

  eosinophilic c., bladder inflammation with many eosinophils in urinary sediment as well as bladder wall.

  follicular c., chronic c. characterized by small mucosal nodules due to lymphocytic infiltration.

  c. glandula′ris, chronic c. with glandlike metaplasia of transitional epithelium.

  hemorrhagic c., bladder inflammation with macroscopic hematuria. Generally the result of a chemical or other traumatic insult to the bladder (chemotherapy, radiation therapy).

  incrusted c., bladder inflammation with deposition of inorganic minerals on luminal wall. There generally is evidence of chronic inflammation.

  interstitial c., a chronic inflammatory condition of unknown etiology involving the mucosa and muscularis of the bladder, resulting in reduced bladder capacity, pain relieved by voiding, and severe bladder irritative symptoms. SEE ALSO Hunner's *ulcer.*

  viral c., bladder inflammation due to a viral infection.

⌂**cysto-, cysti-, cyst-.** Combining forms relating to: **1.** The bladder. **2.** The cystic duct. **3.** A cyst. Cf. vesico-. [G. *kystis*, bladder, pouch]

cys·to·ad·e·no·ma (sis′tō-ad-ĕ-nō′mă). SYN cystadenoma.

cys·to·car·ci·no·ma (sis′tō-kar-si-nō′mă). A carcinoma in which cystic degeneration has occurred; sometimes used incorrectly as a term for cystadenocarcinoma. SYN cystoepithelioma.

cys·to·cele (sis′tō-sēl). Hernia of the bladder usually into the vagina and introitus. SYN colpocystocele, vesicocele. [cysto- + G. *kēlē*, hernia]

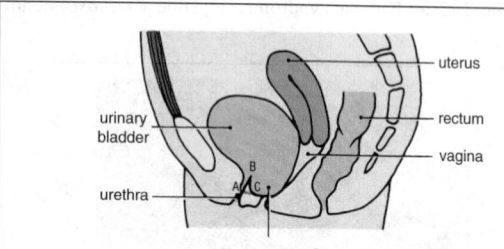

cystocele
ABC, acute angle formed by posterior wall of urethra and anterior wall of urinary bladder

cys·to·chro·mos·co·py (sis′tō-krō-mos′kŏ-pē). Examination of the interior of the bladder after administration of a colored dye to aid in the identification or study of the function of the ureteral orifices. SYN chromocystoscopy. [cysto- + G. *chrōma*, color + *skopeō*, to view]

cys·to·co·los·to·my (sis-tō-kō-los′tō-mē). SYN cholecystocolostomy. [cysto- + G. *kolon*, colon, + *stoma*, mouth]

cys·to·du·o·de·nos·to·my (sis-tō-dū′ō-dē-nos′tō-mē). Drainage of a cyst, usually pancreatic pseudocyst, into duodenum. SYN

duodenocystostomy (2). [cysto- + duodenum, + G. *stoma*, mouth]

  pancreatic c., surgical or endoscopic drainage of pancreatic pseudocyst into duodenum. SYN duodenocystostomy (3).

cys·to·en·ter·o·cele (sis-tō-en′ter-ō-sēl). Hernial protrusion of portions of the bladder and of the intestine, usually into the vagina and introitus. [cysto- + G. *enteron*, intestine, + *kēlē*, hernia]

cys·to·en·ter·os·to·my (sis′tō-en-ter-os′tō-mē). Internal drainage of pancreatic pseudocysts into some portion of the intestinal tract. [cysto- + G. *enteron*, intestine, + *stoma*, mouth]

cys·to·e·pip·lo·cele (sis-tō-e-pip′lō-sēl). Hernial protrusion of portions of the bladder and of the omentum. [cysto- + G. *epiploon*, omentum, + *kēlē*, tumor]

cys·to·ep·i·the·li·o·ma (sis′tō-ep-i-thē-lē-ō′mă). SYN cystocarcinoma.

cys·to·fi·bro·ma (sis′tō-fī-brō′mă). A fibroma in which cysts or cystlike foci have formed.

cys·to·gas·tros·to·my (sis′tō-gas-tros′tō-mē). Drainage of a cyst, usually pancreatic pseudocyst, into the stomach. [cysto- + G. *gastēr*, stomach, + *stoma*, mouth]

cys·to·gram (sis′tō-gram). Radiographic demonstration of the bladder filled with contrast medium.

  voiding c., SYN cystourethrogram.

cys·tog·ra·phy (sis-tog′ră-fē). Radiography of the bladder following injection of a radiopaque substance. [cysto- + G. *graphō*, to write]

  antegrade c., antegrade urography in which the contrast medium is injected into the urinary bladder.

cys·toid (sis′toyd). **1.** Bladder-like, resembling a cyst. SYN cystiform, cystomorphous. **2.** A tumor resembling a cyst, with fluid, granular, or pulpy contents, but without a capsule. [cysto- + G. *eidos*, appearance]

cys·to·je·ju·nos·to·my (sis′tō-je-jū-nos′tō-mē). Drainage of a cyst, usually pancreatic pseudocyst, into the jejunum. [cysto- + jejunum, + G. *stoma*, mouth]

cys·to·lith (sis′tō-lith). SYN vesical *calculus.* [cysto- + G. *lithos*, stone]

cy·sto·lith·a·lo·paxy. Removal of bladder calculi by intravesical crushing and then irrigating to remove fragments. [cysto- + G. *lithos*, stone, + *lapaxis*, and emptying out]

cys·to·li·thi·a·sis (sis′tō-li-thī′ă-sis). The presence of a vesical calculus. SYN vesicolithiasis. [cysto- + G. *lithos*, stone, + *-iasis*, condition]

cys·to·lith·ic (sis-tō-lith′ik). Relating to a vesical calculus.

cys·to·li·thot·o·my (sis′tō-li-thot′ō-mē). Removal of a stone from the bladder through an incision in its wall. SYN vesical lithotomy. [cysto- + G. *lithos*, stone, + *tomē*, incision]

cys·to·ma (sis-tō′mă). A cystic tumor; a new growth containing cysts. [cyst- + G. *-oma*, tumor]

cys·tom·e·ter (sis-tom′ĕ-ter). A device for studying bladder function by measuring capacity, sensation, intravesical pressure, and residual urine. [cysto- + G. *metron*, measure]

cys·to·met·ro·gram (CMG) (sis-tō-met′rō-gram). A graphic recording of urinary bladder pressure at various volumes. [cysto- + G. *metron*, measure, + *gramma*, a writing]

cys·to·me·trog·ra·phy (sis′tō-mĕ-trog′ră-fē). SYN cystometry.

cys·tom·e·try (sis-tom′ĕ-trē). A method for measurement of the pressure/volume relationship of the bladder. SYN cystometrography. [see cystometer]

cys·to·mor·phous (sis-tō-mōr′fŭs). SYN cystoid (1). [cysto- + G. *morphē*, form]

cys·to·my·o·ma (sis′tō-mī-ō′mă). A myoma in which cysts or cystlike foci have developed.

cys·to·myx·o·ad·e·no·ma (sis-tō-mik′sō-ad-ĕ-nō′mă). An adenoma in which there are cysts or cystlike foci in association with myxomatous change in the stroma.

cys·to·myx·o·ma (sis′tō-mik-sō′mă). A myxoma in which cysts or cystlike foci have formed.

cys·to·pan·en·dos·co·py (sis′tō-pan-en-dos′kŏ-pē). Inspection of the interior of the bladder and urethra by means of specially designed endoscopes introduced in retrograde fashion through the urethra and into the bladder. [cysto- + panendoscope]

cys·to·pa·ral·y·sis (sis-tō-pă-ral′i-sis). SYN cystoplegia.

cys·to·pexy (sis′tō-pek-sē). Surgical attachment of the gallbladder or of the urinary bladder to the abdominal wall or to other supporting structures. SYN ventrocystorrhaphy. [cysto- + G. *pēxis*, fixation]

cys·toph·er·ous (sis-tof′er-ŭs). Containing cysts. SYN cystigerous, cystiphorous. [cysto- + G. *phoreō*, to carry]

cys·to·pho·tog·ra·phy (sis′tō-fō-tog′ră-fē). Photographing the interior of the bladder.

cys·to·plas·ty (sis′tō-plas-tē). Any reconstructive operation on the urinary bladder. Cf. ileocystoplasty, colocystoplasty. [cysto- + G. *plastos*, formed]

cys·to·ple·gia (sis-tō-plē′jē-ă). Paralysis of the bladder. SYN cystoparalysis. [cysto- + G. *plēgē*, a stroke]

cysto·pros·ta·tec·to·my (sis′tō-pros-tă-tek′tō-mē). Surgical removal of bladder, prostate, and seminal vesicles simultaneously.

cys·to·py·e·li·tis (sis′tō-pī-el-ī′tis). Inflammation of both the bladder and the pelvis of the kidney. [cysto- + G. *pyelos*, trough (pelvis), + *-itis*, inflammation]

cys·to·py·e·lo·ne·phri·tis (sis-tō-pī′el-ō-nef-rī′tis). Inflammation of the bladder, the pelvis of the kidney, and the kidney parenchyma. [cysto- + G. *pyelos*, trough (pelvis), + *nephros*, kidney, + *-itis*, inflammation]

cys·to·ra·di·o·gram (sis′tō-rā′dē-ō-gram). Radiographic demonstration of the bladder and ureters.

cys·to·ra·di·og·ra·phy (sis′tō-rā-dē-og′ră-fē). Radiography of the urinary bladder.

cys·tor·rha·phy (sis-tōr′ă-fē). Suture of a wound or defect in the urinary bladder. [cysto- + G. *rhaphē*, a sewing]

cys·tor·rhea (sis′tō-rē-ă). A mucous discharge from the bladder. [cysto- + G. *rhoia*, a flow]

cys·to·sar·co·ma (sis′tō-sar-kō′mă). A sarcoma in which the formation of cysts or cystlike foci has occurred.

   c. phyllo′des, a circumscribed or infiltrating fibroadenomatous tumor of the breast or other organs that may be partly cystic; the stroma is cellular and resembles a fibrosarcoma; the tumor can be either benign or malignant.

cys·to·scope (sis′tō-skōp). A lighted tubular endoscope for examining the interior of the bladder. [cysto- + G. *skopeō*, to examine]

cys·tos·co·py (sis-tos′kŏ-pē). The inspection of the interior of the bladder by means of a cystoscope.

cys·to·spasm (sis′tō-spazm). Bladder spasm, unintentional, painful contraction of the bladder, often without micturition.

cys·tos·to·my (sis-tos′tō-mē). Creation of an opening into the urinary bladder. SYN vesicostomy. [cysto- + G. *stoma*, mouth]

cys·to·tome (sis′tō-tōm). **1.** An instrument for incising the urinary bladder or gallbladder. **2.** A surgical instrument used for incising the capsule of a lens. SYN capsulotome.

cys·tot·o·my (sis-tot′ō-mē). Incision into urinary bladder or gallbladder. SYN vesicotomy. [cysto- + G. *tomē*, incision]

   suprapubic c., opening into the bladder through an incision or puncture above the symphysis pubis.

cys·to·u·re·ter·i·tis (sis′tō-yū-rē-ter-ī′tis). Inflammation of the bladder and of one or both ureters.

cys·to·u·re·ter·o·gram (sis′tō-yū-rē′ter-ō-gram). Radiographic demonstration of the bladder and ureters.

cys·to·u·re·ter·og·ra·phy (sis′tō-ū-rē′ter-og′ră-fē). Radiography of the bladder and ureters.

cys·to·u·re·thri·tis (sis′tō-yū-rē-thrī′tis). Inflammation of the bladder and of the urethra.

cys·to·u·re·thro·cele (sis′tō-yū-rē′thrō-sēl). Hernia of the urinary bladder and urethra. [cysto- + urethra + G. *kēlē*, hernia]

cys·to·u·re·thro·gram (sis-tō-yū-reth′rō-gram). An x-ray image made during voiding and with the bladder and urethra filled with contrast medium to demonstrate the urethra. SYN voiding cystogram.

cys·to·u·re·throg·ra·phy (sis′tō-yū′rē-throg′ră-fē). Radiogra-

phy of the bladder and urethra during voiding, following filling of the bladder with a radiopaque contrast medium either by intravenous injection or retrograde catheterization.

cys·to·u·re·thro·scope (sis-tō-yū-rē′thrō-skōp). An instrument combining the uses of a cystoscope and a urethroscope, whereby both the bladder and urethra can be visually inspected.

cyst·ous (sis′tŭs). SYN cystic.

Cys·to·vir·i·dae (sis′tō-vir′i-dē). Provisional name for a family of monotypic bacterial viruses, the type species of which is phage Φ6. Virions are 73 nm in diameter, isometric, have lipid envelopes, and adsorb to the sides of pili of *Pseudomonas* species. Capsids are of cubic symmetry, and the genomes are of double-stranded RNA in three pieces (MW 13×10^6). [G. *kystis*, bladder]

cys·tyl·a·mi·no·pep·ti·dase (sis′til-am-i-nō-pep′ti-dās). Oxytocinase; an enzyme that degrades cystine-containing peptides, such as oxytocin.

Cyt Symbol for cytosine.

△**cyt-.** SEE cyto-.

cy·ta·pher·e·sis (sī′tă-fě-rē′sis). A procedure in which various cells can be separated from the withdrawn blood and retained, with the plasma and other formed elements retransfused into the donor. [cyt- + G. *aphairesis*, a withdrawal]

cy·tar·a·bine (sī′tar-ă-bēn). SYN arabinosylcytosine.

cy·tase (sī′tās). An obsolete term, coined by Metchnikoff, for alexin or complement, which he held to be a digestive secretion of the leukocyte.

Cy·taux·zo·on (sī-tawk′zō-on). SYN *Theileria*. [cyt- + G. *zōon*, animal]

   C. fe′lis, SYN *Theileria felis*.

cy·taux·zo·on·o·sis (sī-tawks′zō-ō-nō′sis). Former name for theileriosis.

△**-cyte.** Suffix meaning cell. [G. *kyton*, a hollow (cell)]

cyt·i·dine (C, Cyd) (sī′ti-dēn). A major component of ribonucleic acids. SYN 1-β-D-ribofuranosylcytosine, cytosine ribonucleoside.

   c. diphosphate choline, SYN cytidine diphosphocholine.

   c. phosphate, SEE cytidylic acid.

cyt·i·dine 5′-di·phos·phate (CDP). An ester, at the 5′ position, between cytidine and diphosphoric acid.

cyt·i·dine di·phos·pho·cho·line (CDP-cho·line) (sī′ti-dēn-dī′fos-fō-kō′lēn). An intermediate in the formation of phosphatidylcholine (lecithin); formed by the action of cytidine 5′-triphosphate on phosphocholine, linking the choline phosphate group to the α-phosphate of the cytidine 5′-triphosphate to give a pyrophosphate. SYN activated choline, cytidine diphosphate choline.

cyt·i·dine di·phos·pho·glyc·er·ide (CDP-glyc·er·ide) (sī′ti-dēn dī′fos-fō-gli′cer-īd). An intermediate in the formation of phospholipids (*e.g.*, cardiolipin formed by the action on CTP and 1,2-diacylglycerols by a cytidyl transferase, releasing CDP-glyceride and pyrophosphate.

cyt·i·dine di·phos·pho·sug·ar (CDP-sug·ar). An activated form of a sugar.

cyt·i·dine 5′-tri·phos·phate (CTP). An ester, at the 5′ position, between cytidine and triphosphoric acid.

cyt·i·dyl·ic ac·id (sī-ti-dil′ik). Cytidine monophosphate (five are possible, depending on the site of attachment of the phosphate to the ribosyl OH's); a constituent of ribonucleic acids.

cy·ti·sine (sit′i-sin). A toxic selective nicotinic cholinergic alkaloid from the seed of *Laburnum anagyroides* and other Leguminosae. Used in pharmacological studies of nicotinic cholinergic receptors in the brain. SYN baptitoxine.

△**cyto-, cyt-.** A cell. [G. *kytos*, a hollow (cell)]

cy·to·an·a·lyz·er (sī-tō-an′ă-lī-zer). An electronic optical machine that screens smears containing cells suspected of malignancy. [cyto- + analyzer]

cy·to·ar·chi·tec·ton·ics (sī′tō-ar-ki-tek-ton′iks). SYN cytoarchitecture. [cyto- + G. *architektonikē*, architectural]

cy·to·ar·chi·tec·tur·al (sī-tō-ar-ki-tek′chŭr-ăl). Pertaining to cytoarchitecture.

cy·to·ar·chi·tec·ture (sī′tō-ar′ki-tek-chŭr). The arrangement of cells in a tissue; the term commonly refers to the arrangement of nerve-cell bodies in the brain, especially the cerebral cortex. SYN architectonics, cytoarchitectonics.

cy·to·bi·ol·o·gy (sī'tō-bī-ol'ō-jē). SYN cytology.

cy·to·bi·o·tax·is (sī'tō-bī-ō-tak'sis). SYN cytoclesis. [cyto- + G. *bios*, life, + *taxis*, arrangement]

cy·to·cen·trum (sī-tō-sen'trŭm). A zone of cytoplasm containing one or two centrioles but devoid of other organelles; usually located near the nucleus of a cell. SYN cell center, central body, centrosome, cinocentrum, kinocentrum, microcentrum. [cyto- + G. *kentron*, center]

cy·to·chal·a·sins (sī-tō-kal'ă-zinz). A group of substances derived from molds that disaggregate the microfilaments of the cell and interfere with the division of cytoplasm, inhibit cell movement, and cause extrusion of the nucleus; used for investigations in cell biology. [cyto- + G. *chalasis*, a relaxing]

cy·to·chem·is·try (sī'tō-kem-is-trē). The study of intracellular distribution of chemicals, reaction sites, enzymes, etc., often by means of staining reactions, radioactive isotope uptake, selective metal distribution in electron microscopy, or other methods. SYN histochemistry.

cy·to·chrome (sī'tō-krōm). A class of hemoprotein whose principal biological function is electron and/or hydrogen transport by virtue of a reversible valency change of the heme iron. C.'s are classified in four groups (*a*, *b*, *c*, and *d*) according to spectrochemical characteristics; many variants exist, particularly among bacteria and in green plants and algae, one being a variant of the *c* type cytochrome called cytochrome *f*. The mitochondrial system of c.'s provides electron transport through cytochrome *c* oxidase to molecular oxygen as the terminal electron acceptor (respiration). [cyto- + G. *chrōma*, color]

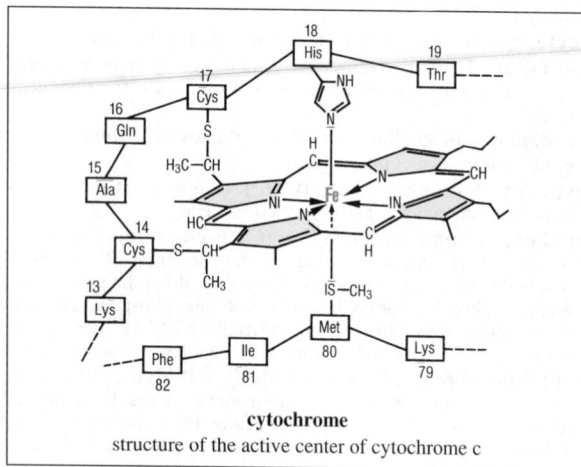

cytochrome
structure of the active center of cytochrome c

cy·to·chrome aa₃. SYN cytochrome *c* oxidase.

cy·to·chrome b. A cytochrome of the respiratory chain. A deficiency of this cytochrome leads to chronic granulomatous disease.

cy·to·chrome b₅. A cytochrome in the endoplasmic reticulum; a deficiency of this cytochrome results in a form of hereditary methemoglobinemia.

cy·to·chrome b₅ re·duc·tase. An enzyme catalyzing the reduction of 2ferricytochrome b_5 to 2ferrocytochrome b_5 at the expense of NADH; has a role in fatty acid desaturation; a deficiency can lead to hereditary methemoglobinemia (type I, only observed in erythrocyte cytosol; type II, deficiency in all tissues; type III, deficiency in all hematopoetic cells).

cy·to·chrome c. The mobile cytochrome that transports electrons from Complex III to Complex IV of the respiratory chain.

cy·to·chrome cd. SYN cytochrome oxidase (*Pseudomonas*).

cy·to·chrome c₃ hy·dro·gen·ase. A hydrogenase enzyme catalyzing reduction of 2ferricytochrome c_3 by H_2 to 2ferrocytochrome c_3 and $2H^+$.

cy·to·chrome c ox·i·dase. A cytochrome of the *a* type, containing copper, that catalyzes the oxidation of 4ferrocytochrome *c* by molecular oxygen to 4ferricytochrome *c* and $2H_2O$. A part of Complex IV of the respiratory chain. A deficiency of one or more of the polypeptides of this complex results in neuronal loss in brain leading to psychomotor retardation and neurodegenerative disease. SYN cytochrome aa_3, indophenol oxidase, indophenolase.

cy·to·chrome c re·duc·tase. SYN *NADH*-dehydrogenase.

cy·to·chrome c₂ re·duc·tase. SYN NADPH-cytochrome c_2 reductase.

cy·to·chrome ox·i·dase (Pseu·do·mo·nas). An enzyme with action identical to that of cytochrome *c* oxidase, but acting on ferrocytochrome c_2. SYN cytochrome *cd*.

cy·to·chrome P-450SCC. Cholesterol monooxygenase (side chain cleaving). [*450 nm*, the absorption maximum that the CO compound of the reduced pigment exhibits]

cy·to·chrome per·ox·i·dase. A hemoprotein enzyme catalyzing the reaction between H_2O_2 and 2 ferrocytochrome *c* to yield 2ferricytochrome *c* and $2H_2O$.

cy·to·chrome re·duc·tase. SYN NADPH-ferrihemoprotein reductase.

cy·to·chy·le·ma (sī'tō-kī-lē'mă). The more fluid portion of the cytoplasm. [cyto- + G. *chylos*, juice]

cy·toc·i·dal (sī-tō-sī'dăl). Causing the death of cells. [cyto- + L. *caedo*, to kill]

cy·to·cide (sī'tō-sīd). An agent that is destructive to cells. [cyto- + L. *caedo*, to kill]

cy·toc·la·sis (sī-tok'lă-sis). Fragmentation of cells. [cyto- + G. *klasis*, a breaking]

cy·to·clas·tic (sī-tō-klas'tik). Relating to cytoclasis.

cy·to·cle·sis (sī-tō-klē'sis). The influence of one cell on another. SYN biotaxis (2), cytobiotaxis. [cyto- + G. *klēsis*, a call]

cy·to·cu·pre·in (sī-tō-kū'prē-in). Former terms for copper-containing proteins found in human erythrocytes and other tissues. SEE *superoxide* dismutase, ceruloplasmin. SYN cerebrocuprein, erythrocuprein, hemocuprein, hepatocuprein.

cy·to·cyst (sī'tō-sist). Rarely used term for the bladder-like remains of the red blood cell or tissue cell that encloses a mature schizont. [cyto- + G. *kystis*, bladder]

cy·to·di·ag·no·sis (sī'tō-dī-ag-nō'sis). Diagnosis of the type and, when feasible, the cause of a pathologic process by means of microscopic study of cells in an exudate or other form of body fluid.

cy·to·di·er·e·sis (sī'tō-dī-er'ĕ-sis). SYN cytokinesis. [cyto- + G. *diairesis*, division]

cy·to·gene (sī'tō-jēn). SYN plasmagene.

cy·to·gen·e·sis (sī-tō-jen'ĕ-sis). The origin and development of cells. [cyto- + G. *genesis*, origin]

cy·to·ge·net·i·cist (sī'tō-jĕ-net'i-sist). A specialist in cytogenetics.

cy·to·ge·net·ics (sī'tō-jĕ-net'iks). The branch of genetics concerned with the structure and function of the cell, especially the chromosomes.

The field arose as a fusion of 19th century cytology and 20th century genetics (which properly began in 1903 with articulation of the chromosome theory of inheritance). Subsequently, the field concerned itself with detailing the behavior of chromosomes and their functional subunits—the genes—during reproduction, and with relating that behavior statistically to characteristics of the resulting cells or animals. Modern molecular cytogenetics involves the microscopic study of chromosomes that have been arranged as karyotypes. Individuals can be classified according to characteristic banding patterns that appear when the karyotypes are exposed to certain dyes. In addition, DNA probes may be applied to locate specific gene sequences. Cytogenetic techniques are used to test for inborn errors of metabolism, for disorders such as Down syndrome, and to determine sex in cases where anatomy is inconclusive.

cy·to·gen·ic (sī-tō-jen′ik). Relating to cytogenesis.

cy·tog·e·nous (sī-toj′ĕ-nŭs). Cell-forming.

cy·to·glu·co·pe·nia (sī′tō-glū-kō-pē′nē-ă). An intracellular deficiency of glucose. [cyto- + glucose + G. *penia,* poverty]

cy·to·hy·a·lo·plasm (sī-tō-hī′ă-lō-plazm). Obsolete term for hyaloplasm.

cy·toid (sī′toyd). Resembling a cell. [cyto- + G. *eidos,* resemblance]

cy·to·ker·a·tins (sī-to-ker-a-tinz). A class of intermediate filament proteins; several are associated with the epithelium that lines internal body cavities while others are specific for hard tissue such as nails and hair.

cy·to·kine (sī′tō-kīn). Hormone-like low molecular weight proteins, secreted by many different cell types, which regulate the intensity and duration of immune responses and are involved in cell-to-cell communication. SEE interferon, interleukin, lymphokines. See entries under various growth factors. [cyto- + G. *kinēsis,* movement]

c. network, a group of c.'s which together modulate and regulate key cellular functions.

Cytokines are released by stromal cells of the spleen and thymus; by epithelial, endothelial, and mast cells; and by fibroblasts and lymphocytes. They are involved in mediating immunity and regulating lymph activity, and themselves act as hemopoietic growth factors, so in this sense can be said to serve both antiviral and antitumor functions. They also promote allergic reactions. Because T-cell function is boosted by cytokines, these proteins are used to evaluate immune activity.

cy·to·ki·ne·sis (sī′tō-ki-nē′sis). Changes occurring in the protoplasm of the cell outside the nucleus during cell division. SYN cytodieresis. [cyto- + G. *kinēsis,* movement]

cy·to·lem·ma (sī-tō-lem′mă). SYN cell *membrane.* [cyto- + G. *lemma,* husk]

cy·to·lip·in (sī-tō-lip′in). A glycosphingolipid, specifically a ceramide oligosaccharide; **c. H,** a lactosylceramide, may display immunological properties under certain conditions; **c. K** is probably identical with globoside. Cf. *ceramide* lactosidase.

cy·to·log·ic (sī-tō-loj′ik). Relating to cytology.

cy·tol·o·gist (sī-tol′ō-jist). One who specializes in cytology.

cy·tol·o·gy (sī-tol′ō-jē). The study of the anatomy, physiology, pathology, and chemistry of the cell. SYN cellular biology, cytobiology. [cyto- + G. *logos,* study]

exfoliative c., the examination, for diagnostic purposes, of cells denuded from a neoplasm (or other type of lesion) and recovered from the sediment of the exudate, secretions, or washings from the tissue (*e.g.,* sputum, vaginal secretion, gastric washings, urine). SYN cytopathology (2).

cy·to·lymph (sī′tō-limf). Obsolete term for hyaloplasm.

cy·tol·y·sin (sī-tol′i-sin). A substance *i.e.,* an antibody that effects partial or complete destruction of an animal cell; may require complement. SEE ALSO perforin.

cy·tol·y·sis (sī-tol′i-sis). The dissolution of a cell. [cyto- + G. *lysis,* loosening]

cy·to·ly·so·some (sī-tō-lī′sō-sōm). A variety of secondary lysosome that contains the remnants of mitochondria, ribosomes, or other organelles. SYN autophagic vacuole.

cy·to·lyt·ic (sī-tō-lit′ik). Pertaining to cytolysis; possessing a solvent or destructive action on cells.

cy·to·ma (sī-tō′mă). An obsolete and undesirable general term to indicate any neoplasm composed almost entirely of neoplastic cells, with virtually no stroma or formation of histologic structures. [cyto- + G. *-ōma,* tumor]

cy·to·ma·trix (sī-tō-mā′triks). SYN cytoplasmic *matrix.*

cy·to·me·ga·lic (sī-tō-meg′ă-lik). Denoting or characterized by markedly enlarged cells. [cyto- + G. *megas,* big]

cy·to·meg·a·lo·vi·rus (CMV) (sī-tō-meg′ă-lō-vī′rŭs). A group of viruses in the family Herpesviridae infecting man and other animals, many of the viruses having special affinity for salivary glands, and causing enlargement of cells of various organs and development of characteristic inclusions in the cytoplasm or nucleus. Infection of embryo in utero may result in malformation and fetal death. They are all species-specific and include salivary gland virus, inclusion body rhinitis virus of pigs, and others. SYN visceral disease virus. [cyto- + G. *megas,* big]

diagnosis of cytomegalovirus (CMV)	
histology	liver, kidney, lung (salivary glands) and other organs
cytology	urine; inclusion bodies in epithelial cells, especially in children up to three mos.; saliva
immuno-fluorescence	specific intranuclear and intracytoplasmic inclusions in tissue sections
virus culture	tissue cultures from urine, throat cultures, lymphocytes, cervical secretion, biopsy and necropsy materials (sperm, breast milk)
hybridization treatment	separation of cellular from viral DNA
serological antibody evidence	complement binding reaction (CBR), passive hemoagglutination, immunofluorescence, neutralization test in tissue cultures, determination of IgM antibodies if active infection is suspected

cy·to·mem·brane (sī-tō-mem′brān). SYN cell *membrane.*

cy·to·mere (sī′tō-mēr). The structure separating the portions of the contents of a large schizont in the course of schizogony, as in some of the sporozoans undergoing exoerythrocytic asexual division. C.'s are caused by complex invaginations of the surface of the schizont, which isolates them; ultimately, c.'s complete the budding process in the formation of large numbers of merozoites. [cyto- + G. *meros,* part]

cy·to·met·a·pla·sia (sī′tō-met-ă-plā′zē-ă). Change of form or function of a cell, other than that related to neoplasia. [cyto- + G. *metaplasis,* transformation]

cy·tom·e·ter (sī-tom′ĕ-ter). A standardized, usually ruled glass slide or small glass chamber of known volume, used in counting and measuring cells, especially blood cells. [cyto- + G. *metron,* measure]

cy·tom·e·try (sī-tom′ĕ-trē). The counting of cells, especially blood cells, using a cytometer or hemocytometer.

flow c., a method of measuring fluorescence from stained cells that are in suspension and flowing through a narrow orifice, usually in combination with one or two lasers to activate the dyes; used to measure cell size, number, viability, and nucleic acid content with the aid of acridine orange, Kasten's fluorescent Feulgen stain, ethidium bromide, trypan blue, and other selected staining reagents. SYN flow cytophotometry.

cy·to·mi·cro·some (sī-tō-mī′krō-sōm). SEE microsome. [cyto- + G. *mikros,* small, + *sōma,* body]

cy·to·mor·phol·o·gy (sī′tō-mōr-fol′ō-jē). The study of the structure of cells.

cy·to·mor·pho·sis (sī-tō-mōr-fō′sis). Changes that the cell undergoes during the various stages of its existence. SEE ALSO prosoplasia. [cyto- + G. *morphōsis,* a shaping]

cy·ton (sī′ton). Obsolete term for perikaryon.

cy·to·path·ic (sī-tō-path′ik). Pertaining to or exhibiting cytopathy.

cy·to·path·o·gen·ic (sī′tō-path-ō-jen′ik). Pertaining to an agent or substance that causes a diseased condition in cells, in contrast to histologic changes; used especially with reference to effects observed in cells in tissue cultures.

cy·to·path·o·log·ic, cy·to·path·o·log·i·cal (sī′tō-pa-thō-loj′ik,

cy

-loj′i-kăl). **1.** Denoting cellular changes in disease. **2.** Relating to cytopathology.

cy·to·pa·thol·o·gist (sī′tō-pa-thol′ō-jist). A physician, usually skilled in anatomical pathology, who is specially trained and experienced in cytopathology.

cy·to·pa·thol·o·gy (sī′tō-pa-thol′ō-jē). **1.** The study of disease changes within individual cells or cell types. **2.** SYN exfoliative *cytology.*

cy·top·a·thy (sī-top′ă-thē). Any disorder of a cell or anomaly of any of its constituents. [cyto- + G. *pathos,* disease]

cy·to·pemp·sis (sī-tō-pemp′sis). SYN transcytosis. [cyto- + G. *pempis,* sending through]

cy·to·pe·nia (sī-tō-pē′nē-ă). A reduction, *i.e.,* hypocytosis, or a lack of cellular elements in the circulating blood. [cyto- + G. *penia,* poverty]

cy·toph·a·gous (sī-tof′ă-gŭs). Devouring, or destructive to, cells.

cy·toph·a·gy (sī-tof′ă-jē). Devouring of other cells by phagocytes. [cyto- + G. *phagō,* to devour]

cy·to·phan·ere (sī′tō-fă-nēr). A radial spine seen in certain cysts of *Sarcocystis,* as in rabbit and sheep tissue cysts. [cyto- + G. *phaneros,* visible, evident, open]

cy·to·phar·ynx (sī′tō-far′inks). An organelle in certain flagellates and ciliates that serves as a gullet through which food material passes from the cytostome to the cell interior; food passed is collected in food vacuoles, into which digestive enzymes are secreted.

cy·to·phil·ic (sī-tō-fil′ik). SYN cytotropic. [cyto- + G. *philos,* fond]

cy·to·pho·tom·e·try (sī′tō-fō-tom′ĕ-trē). A method of measuring the absorption of monochromatic light by stained microscopic structures (*e.g.,* chromosomes, nuclei, whole cells) with the aid of a photoelectric cell; also used to measure emitted light from such objects by fluorescence in combination with selected fluorochrome dyes. [cyto- + G. *phōs,* light + *metron,* measure]

flow c., SYN flow *cytometry.*

cy·to·phy·lac·tic (sī′tō-fī-lak′tik). Relating to cytophylaxis.

cy·to·phy·lax·is (sī′tō-fī-lak′sis). Protection of cells against lytic agents. [cyto- + G. *phylaxis,* a guarding]

cy·to·phy·let·ic (sī′tō-fī-let′ik). Relating to the genealogy of a cell. [cyto- + G. *phylē,* a tribe]

cy·to·pi·pette (sī′tō-pi-pet′). A slightly curved, blunt end pipette usually made of glass and fitted with a rubber bulb to provide gentle negative pressure for the collection of vaginal secretions for cytological examination.

cy·to·plasm (sī′tō-plazm). The substance of a cell, exclusive of the nucleus, which contains various organelles and inclusions within a colloidal protoplasm. SEE ALSO protoplasm, hyaloplasm, cytosol. [cyto- + G. *plasma,* thing formed]

ground-glass c., uniform finely granular eosinophilic c. seen in hepatocytes in carriers of hepatitis B virus, and also in epidermal cells in keratoacanthoma.

cy·to·plas·mic (sī-tō-plaz′mik). Relating to the cytoplasm.

cy·to·plas·mon (sī-tō-plaz′mon). The total extranuclear genetic information of a eukaryotic cell excluding that of mitochondria and plastids.

cy·to·plast (sī′tō-plast). The living intact cytoplasm that remains following cell enucleation. [cyto- + G. *plastos,* formed]

cy·to·poi·e·sis (sī-tō-poy-ē′sis). Formation of cells. [cyto- + G. *poiēsis,* a making]

cy·to·prep·a·ra·tion (sī′tō-prep-a-rā′shŭn). Laboratory preparation of a cellular specimen for cytologic examination.

cy·to·py·ge (sī-tō-pī′jē). The anal orifice (cell "anus") found in certain structurally complex protozoa, such as the rumen-dwelling ciliates of herbivores, through which waste matter is ejected. [cyto- + G. *pygē,* buttocks]

cy·to·ryc·tes, cy·tor·rhyc·tes (sī-tō-rik′tēz). Old term for inclusion *bodies,* under *body.* [cyto- + G. *oryktēs,* a digger]

cy·to·sides (sī′tō-sīdz). Ceramide disaccharides. SEE glycosphingolipid.

cy·to·sine (Cyt) (sī′tō-sēn). 4-Amino-2(1*H*)-pyrimidinone; a pyrimidine found in nucleic acids.

c. arabinoside (CA, AraC), (1) a synthetic nucleoside used as an antimetabolite in the treatment of neoplasms. **(2)** incorrect term for arabinosylcytosine.

c. ribonucleoside, SYN cytidine.

cy·to·sis (sī-tō′sis). **1.** A condition in which there is more than the usual number of cells, as the c. of spinal fluid in acute leptomeningitis. **2.** Frequently used with a prefixed combining form as a means of describing certain features pertaining to cells; *e.g.,* isocytosis, equality in size; polycytosis, abnormal increase in number. [cyto- + G. *-osis,* condition]

cy·to·skel·e·ton (sī-tō-skel′ĕ-ton). The tonofilaments, keratin, desmin, neurofilaments, or other intermediate filaments serving to act as supportive cytoplasmic elements to stiffen cells or to organize intracellular organelles.

cy·to·smear (sī′tō-smēr). SYN cytologic *smear.*

cy·to·sol (sī′tō-sol). Cytoplasm exclusive of the mitochondria, endoplasmic reticulum, and other membranous components. [cyto- + "sol," abbrev. of soluble]

cy·to·sol·ic (sī-tō-sol′ik). Relating to or contained in the cytosol.

cy·to·some (sī-tō-sōm). **1.** The cell body exclusive of the nucleus. **2.** One of the osmiophilic bodies that are 1 μm or less in diameter, have concentric lamellae, and occur in the great alveolar cells of the lung. SYN multilamellar body. [cyto- + G. *sōma,* body]

cy·tos·ta·sis (sī-tos′tă-sis). The slowing of movement and accumulation of blood cells, especially polymorphonuclear leukocytes, in the capillaries, as in a region of inflammation; obstruction of a capillary as the result of accumulated leukocytes. [cyto- + G. *stasis,* standing]

cy·to·stat·ic (sī-tō-stat′ik). Characterized by cytostasis.

cy·to·stome (sī′tō-stōm). The cell "mouth" of certain complex protozoa, usually with a short gullet or cytopharynx leading food into the organism, where it is collected into food vacuoles, then circulated inside the body, eventually to be excreted through the cytopyge. [cyto- + G. *stoma,* mouth]

cy·to·tac·tic (sī-tō-tak′tik). Relating to cytotaxis.

cy·to·tax·is, cy·to·tax·ia (sī-tō-tak′sis, -tak′sē-ă). The attraction (**positive c.**) or repulsion (**negative c.**) of cells for one another. [cyto- + G. *taxis,* arrangement]

cy·toth·e·sis (sī-toth′ĕ-sis). The repair of injury in a cell; the restoration of cells. [cyto- + G. *thesis,* a placing]

cy·to·tox·ic (sī-tō-tok′sik). Detrimental or destructive to cells; pertaining to the effect of noncytophilic antibody on specific antigen, frequently, but not always, mediating the action of complement.

cy·to·tox·ic·i·ty (sī′tō-tok-sis′i-tē). The quality or state of being cytotoxic.

antibody-dependent cell-mediated c. (ADCC), a form of lymphocyte-mediated cytotoxicity that functions only if antibodies are bound to the target cell.

lymphocyte-mediated c., the toxic or lytic activity of T-lymphocytes, which may or may not be mediated by antibodies. Cytotoxic T lymphocytes may cause lysis of cells by production of cytolytic proteins such as perforin. B cells may cause lysis of cells by antibody-complement binding to a target cell. Natural killer cells are cytotoxic without prior sensitization. Toxicity by lymphocytes may also be mediated by antibodies; there are three kinds of cytotoxic T-lymphocytes: those that are antigen-specific as a result of previous allergization (immunization), killer cells, and natural killer cells. SEE ALSO antibody-dependent cell-mediated c.

cy·to·tox·in (sī′tō-tok′sin). A specific substance, which may or may not be antibody, that inhibits or prevents the functions of cells, causes destruction of cells, or both. [cyto- + G. *toxikon,* poison]

cy·to·tro·pho·blast (sī-tō-trof′ō-blast). The inner layer of the trophoblast. SYN Langhans' layer.

cy·to·tro·pic (sī-tō-trop′ik). Having an affinity for cells. SYN cytophilic.

cy·tot·ro·pism (sī-tot′rō-pizm). **1.** Affinity for cells. **2.** Affinity

cytotoxicity (cellular immune reaction with specific effect)				
type of immune reaction	effector cell	specificity		mechanism
cytotoxicity of sensitized lymphocytes	T-lymphocyte	MHL restriction*	membrane-receptor	lysis through cell contact
Ab-dependent cytotoxicity (ADCC)	monocytes/ macrophages	no restriction	Ab	lysis through cell contact
	K-lymphocytes			phagocytosis (?)
* specificity is determined by antigen *and* the membranous structures of the targeted cell, which are coded by MHC (major histocompatibility complex)				

for specific cells, especially the ability of viruses to localize in and damage specific cells. [cyto- + G. *tropos,* a turning]

cy·to·zo·ic (sī-tō-zō′ik). Living in a cell; denoting certain parasitic protozoa.

cy·to·zo·on (sī-tō-zō′on). A protozoan cell or organism. [cyto- + G. *zōon,* animal]

cy·to·zyme (sī′tō-zīm). An obsolete term for thromboplastin. [cyto- + G. *zymē,* leaven]

cy·tu·ria (sī-tū′rē-ă). The passage of cells in unusual numbers in the urine. [G. *kytos,* cell, + *ouron,* urine]

Czapek, Friedrich J.F., Czechoslovakian botanist, 1868–1921. SEE C.'s solution *agar;* C.-Dox *medium.*

CZE Abbreviation for capillary zone *electrophoresis.*

Czerny, Vincenz, German surgeon, 1842–1916. SEE C.'s *suture;* C.-Lembert *suture.*

Cz

D

Δ, δ. **1.** Fourth letter of the Greek alphabet, delta. **2.** In chemistry, denotes a double bond, usually with a superscript to indicate position in a chain (Δ^5); application of heat in a reaction (A $\xrightarrow{\Delta}$ B); absence of heat treatment ($\cancel{\Delta}$); distance between two atoms in a molecule; or position of a substituent located on the fourth atom from the carboxyl or other primary functional group (δ); change (Δ); thickness (δ); chemical shift in NMR (δ).

δ-ami·no·bu·tyr·ic ac·id. An enzyme catalyzing the reversible transfer of an amino group from δ-aminobutyric acid to 2-oxoglutarate, thus forming a L-glutamic acid and succinate semialdehyde. An important step in the catabolism of δ-aminobutyric acid.

D 1. Symbol for the vitamin D potency of cod liver oil, multiples of which (5D, 100D, etc.) are used to designate the vitamin D potency of irradiated ergosterol (viosterol) or other substances; for deuterium; for dihydrouridine in nucleic acids; for diffusing capacity; for aspartic acid; dihydrouridine; diffusion *coefficient* (in italics). **2.** In optics, abbreviation for diopter; for dexter (right). **3.** In electrodiagnosis, abbreviation for duration, the current flowing and the circuit being closed. **4.** In dental formulas, abbreviation for deciduous (2). **5.** As a subscript, refers to dead *space*. SEE physiologic dead *space*. **6.** D line in Na emission spectra.

2,4-D Abbreviation for (2,4-dichlorophenoxy) acetic acid.

d Symbol for deci-; abbreviation for *dexter* [L], right; diameter; day.

◬D-. Prefix indicating that a chemical compound is sterically related to D-glyceraldehyde, the basis of stereochemical nomenclature. Cf. Λ.

◬d-. Prefix indicating a chemical compound to be dextrorotatory; should be avoided when (+) or (−) could be used. Cf. L-.

◬-d. Suffix indicating the presence of deuterium in a compound in concentrations above normal, thus labelling the compound; subscripts (d_2, d_3, etc.) indicate the number of such atoms so fortified.

DA Abbreviation for developmental *age* (2).

Da. Symbol for dalton.

dA, dAdo Abbreviation for deoxyadenosine.

da Symbol for deca-.

Daae, Anders, Norwegian physician, 1838–1910. SEE D.'s *disease.*

DAB Abbreviation for 3′3-diaminobenzidine HCl; in the immunoperoxidase technique, used to produce a colored complex at the site of peroxidase activity; carcinogenic.

da·car·ba·zine (DTIC) (dă-kar′bă-zēn). 5-(3,3-Dimethyl-1-triazenyl)-1*H*-imidazole-4-carboxamide; an antineoplastic agent used in the treatment of malignant melanoma and Hodgkin's disease.

DaCosta, Jacob M., U.S. surgeon, 1833–1900. SEE DaC.'s's *syndrome.*

◬dacry-. SEE dacryo-.

dac·ry·ad·e·ni·tis (dak′rē-ad-ĕ-nī′tis). SYN dacryoadenitis.

◬dacryo-, dacry-. Tears; lacrimal sac or duct. [G. *dakryon*, tear]

dac·ry·o·ad·e·ni·tis (dak-rē-ō-ad-ĕ-nī′tis). Inflammation of the lacrimal gland. SYN dacryadenitis. [dacryo- + G. *adēn*, gland, + *-itis*, inflammation]

dac·ry·o·blen·nor·rhea (dak-rē-ō-blen-ō-rē′ă). A chronic discharge of mucus from a lacrimal sac. [dacryo- + G. *blenna*, mucus, + *rhoia*, flow]

dac·ry·o·cele (dak′rē-ō-sēl). SYN dacryocystocele.

dac·ry·o·cyst (dak′rē-ō-sist). SYN lacrimal *sac*. [dacryo- + G. *kystis*, sac]

dac·ry·o·cys·tal·gia (dak′rē-ō-sis-tal′jē-ă). Pain in the lacrimal sac. [dacryocyst + G. *algos*, pain]

dac·ry·o·cys·tec·to·my (dak′rē-ō-sis-tek′tō-mē). Surgical removal of the lacrimal sac. [dacryocyst + G. *ektomē*, excision]

dac·ry·o·cys·ti·tis (dak′rē-ō-sis-tī′tis). Inflammation of the lacrimal sac. [dacryocyst + G. *-itis*, inflammation]

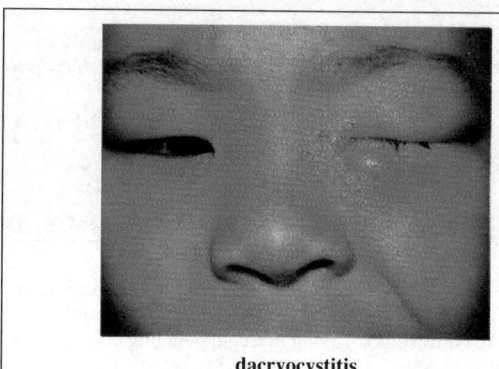

dacryocystitis

dac·ry·o·cys·to·cele (dak′rē-ō-sis′tō-sēl). Enlargement of the lacrimal sac with fluid. SYN dacryocele. [dacryocyst + G. *kēlē*, hernia]

dac·ry·o·cys·to·gram (dak′rē-ō-sis′tō-gram). A radiograph of the lacrimal apparatus obtained (after injection of radiopaque substances) for the purpose of determining the presence of and localizing a site of obstruction; this procedure has been largely replaced by the CT and MRI. [dacryocyst + G. *gramma*, a writing]

dac·ry·o·cys·to·rhi·nos·to·my (dak′rē-ō-sis′tō-rī-nos′tō-mē). An operation providing an anastomosis between the lacrimal sac and the nasal mucosa through an opening in the lacrimal bone. [dacryocyst + G. *rhis (rhin-)*, nose, + *stoma*, mouth]

dac·ry·o·cys·tot·o·my (dak′rē-ō-sis-tot′ō-mē). Incision of the lacrimal sac. [dacryocyst + G. *tomē*, incision]

dac·ry·o·hem·or·rhea (dak′rē-ō-hem-ō-rē′ă). Bloody tears. [dacryo- + G. *haima*, blood, + *rhoia*, flow]

dac·ry·o·lith (dak′rē-ō-lith). A concretion in the lacrimal apparatus. SYN lacrimal calculus, ophthalmolith, tear stone. [dacryo- + G. *lithos*, stone]

Desmarres' d.'s, SYN Nocardia d.'s.

Nocardia d.'s, white pseudoconcretions, composed of masses of *Nocardia* species found in the lacrimal canaliculi. SYN Desmarres' d.'s.

dac·ry·o·li·thi·a·sis (dak′rē-ō-li-thī′ă-sis). The formation and presence of dacryoliths.

dac·ry·on (dak′rē-on). The point of junction of the frontomaxillary and lacrimomaxillary sutures on the medial wall of the orbit. See figure under craniometric *points*, under *point*. [G. a tear]

dac·ry·ops (dak′rē-ops). **1.** Excess of tears in the eye. **2.** A cyst of a duct of the lacrimal gland. [dacryo- + G. *ōps*, eye]

dac·ry·o·py·or·rhea (dak′rē-ō-pī-ō-rē′ă). The discharge of tears containing leukocytes. [dacryo- + G. *pyon*, pus, + *rhoia*, flow]

dac·ry·or·rhea (dak′rē-ō-rē′ă). An excessive secretion of tears. [dacryo- + G. *rhoia*, flow]

dac·ry·o·ste·no·sis (dak′rē-ō-ste-nō′sis). Stricture of a lacrimal or nasal duct. [dacryo- + G. *stenōsis*, narrowing]

dac·ti·no·my·cin (dak′ti-nō-mī′sin). Produced by several species of *Streptomyces* (*e.g.*, *S. parvulus*); an antineoplastic antibiotic used especially for Ewing's sarcoma, rhabdomyosarcoma, and Wilms' tumor in children and for trophoblastic disease in women. SEE ALSO actinomycin. SYN actinomycin D.

dac·tyl (dak′til). SYN digit. [G. *daktylos*]

◬dactyl-. SEE dactylo-.

dac·ty·lag·ra (dak-ti-lag′ră). Obsolete term meaning gout for the fingers. [dactyl- + G. *agra*, seizure]

dac·ty·lal·gia (dak-ti-lal'jē-ă). Pain in the fingers. SYN dactylodynia. [dactyl- + G. *algos,* pain]

Dac·ty·la·ria (dak-ti-lā'rē-ă). A genus of dematiaceous soil-dwelling fungi. *D. gallopava* is a causative agent of phaeohyphomycosis in chickens and turkeys. [G. *daktylos,* finger]

dac·tyl·e·de·ma (dak'til-e-dē'mă). Edema of the finger. [dactyl- + G. *oidema,* swelling]

dac·ty·li·tis (dak-ti-lī'tis). Inflammation of one or more fingers.
  blistering distal d., infection of the volar fat pad of the distal phalanx of the finger by group A β-hemolytic streptococci.
  sickle cell d., SYN hand-and-foot *syndrome.*

⊘**dactylo-, dactyl-.** The fingers, and (less often) toes. See entries under digit. [G. *daktylos,* finger]

dac·ty·lo·camp·sis (dak'ti-lō-kamp'sis). Permanent flexion of the fingers. [dactylo- + G. *kampsis,* bending]

dac·ty·lo·camp·so·dyn·ia (dak'ti-lō-kamp'sō-din'ē-ă). Painful contraction of one or more fingers. [dactylo- + G. *kampsis,* a bending, + *odynē,* pain]

dac·ty·lo·dyn·ia (dak'tĭ-lō-din'ē-ă). SYN dactylalgia.

dac·ty·lo·gry·po·sis (dak'ti-lō-gri-pō'sis). Contraction of the fingers. [dactylo- + G. *grypōsis,* a crooking]

dac·ty·lol·o·gy (dak'ti-lol'ō-jē). The use of the finger alphabet in talking. SYN cheirology, chirology, chirology. [dactylo- + G. *logos,* word]

dac·tyl·o·meg·a·ly (dak'til-ō-meg'ă-lē). SYN megadactyly. [dactylo- + G. *megas,* large]

dac·ty·los·co·py (dak-ti-los'kŏ-pē). An examination of the markings in prints made from the fingertips; employed as a method of personal identification. SEE Galton's system of classification of *fingerprints,* under *fingerprint.* [dactylo- + G. *skopeō,* to examine]

dac·ty·lo·spasm (dak'ti-lō-spazm). Spasmodic contraction of the fingers or toes.

dac·ty·lus, pl. **dac·ty·li** (dak'ti-lŭs, -lī). SYN digit. [G. *daktylos*]

dac·u·ro·ni·um (dak-yū-rō'nē-ŭm). A nondepolarizing steroid neuromuscular blocking agent with more rapid onset and shorter duration of action than pancuronium.

Da Fano, Corrado D., Italian-American anatomist, 1879–1927. SEE Da F.'s *stain.*

DAG Abbreviation for diacylglycerol.

dag·ga (dag'ă). Leaves of *Leonotis leonurus,* a plant found in South Africa, where it is smoked like tobacco with mild sedative effect; a term mistakenly applied to Indian hemp, *Cannabis sativa.* [aborigines' term]

Dagnini, Giuseppe, Italian physician, 1866–1928. SEE Aschner-D. *reflex.*

DAH Abbreviation for disordered action of heart.

dah·lia (dal'yah). A violet dye, methyl-triethyl-amino-triphenyl-carbinol chloride. Also called Hoffman's violet.

dah·lin. SYN inulin. [fr. *dahlia,* after A. *Dahl,* Swedish botanist, 1751–1789]

dahll·ite (dah'līt). CaCO₃·2Ca₃(PO₄)₂; a naturally occurring calcium phosphate, similar in structure to the mineral portions of bones and teeth. SYN podolite.

dai·sy (dā'zē). Colloquial term descriptive of the segmented forms (merozoites) of the mature schizont of *Plasmodium malariae.*

Dakin, Henry, U.S. chemist, 1880–1952. SEE D.'s *fluid, solution;* D.-Carrel *treatment.*

Dale, Sir Henry Hallett, English physiologist and Nobel laureate, 1875–1968. SEE D. *reaction;* D.-Feldberg *law;* Schultz-D. *reaction.*

Dalen, Johan A., Swedish ophthalmologist, 1866–1940. SEE D.-Fuchs *nodules,* under *nodule.*

Dalgarno, Lynn, contemporary Australian molecular biologist.

Dalrymple, John, English oculist, 1804–1852. SEE D.'s *sign.*

Dalton, John, English chemist, mathematician, and natural philosopher, 1766–1844. SEE D.'s *law;* D.-Henry *law;* daltonian; daltonism.

dal·ton (Da) (dawl'tŏn). Term unofficially used to indicate a unit of mass equal to ¹/₁₂ the mass of a carbon-12 atom, 1.0000 in the atomic mass scale; numerically, but not dimensionally, equal to molecular or particle weight (atomic mass units). [J. *Dalton*]

dal·to·ni·an (dawl-tō'nē-ăn). **1.** Attributed to or described by John Dalton. **2.** Pertaining to daltonism.

dal·ton·ism (dawl'tŏn-izm). A color vision deficiency, especially deuteranomaly or deuteranopia. [J. *Dalton*]

DAM Abbreviation for diacetylmonoxime.

Dam, C.P. Henrik, Danish biochemist and Nobel laureate, 1895–1976. SEE D. *unit.*

dam. **1.** Any barrier to the flow of fluid. **2.** In surgery and dentistry, a sheet of thin rubber arranged so as to shut off the part operated upon from the access of fluid. [A.S. *fordemman,* to stop up]
  post d., SYN posterior palatal *seal.*
  rubber d., (1) in surgery, thin strips of rubber used as a surgical drain or barrier; (2) a thin sheet of rubber with holes that is placed over teeth to isolate them from the oral cavity.

Dam·a·lin·ia (dam-ă-lin'ē-ă). A genus of biting lice containing a number of species found on domestic and wild animals; they are all highly host-specific, one species being confined to each species of mammal. SEE ALSO *Bovicola, Trichodectes.*

dam·mar. A resin resembling copal, obtained from various species of *Shorea* (family Dipterocarpaceae) in the East Indies; used, dissolved in chloroform, for mounting microscopic specimens. [Hind. *dāmar,* resin]

dam meth·yl·ase. an enzyme responsible for the methylation of adenine residues in specific sequences. SYN deoxyadenosine methylase.

dAMP Abbreviation for deoxyadenylic acid.

damp. **1.** Humid; moist. **2.** Atmospheric moisture. **3.** Foul air in a mine; air charged with carbon oxides (black or choke d.) or with various explosive hydrocarbon vapors (firedamp).

damp·ing. Bringing a mechanism to rest with minimal oscillation; *e.g.,* in echocardiography, electrical or mechanical loading to reduce duration of echo, transmitter pulse, and transmitter complex. [M.E. *damp,* poisonous vapor]

Damus-Kaye-Stancel pro·ce·dure. See under procedure.

Dana, Charles L., U.S. neurologist, 1852–1935. SEE D.'s *operation;* Putnam-D. *syndrome.*

da·na·zol (dā'nă-zol). 17α-Pregna-2,4-dien-20-yno[2,3-*d*]-isoxazol-17-ol; an anterior pituitary suppressant.

Dance, Jean B.H., French physician, 1797–1832. SEE D.'s *sign.*

dance (dans). Involuntary movements related to brain damage.
  hilar d., vigorous pulmonary arterial pulsations due to increased blood flow, often seen fluoroscopically in patients with congenital left-to-right shunts, especially atrial septal defects.
  Saint Anthony's d., Saint John's d., Saint Vitus d., obsolete eponyms for Sydenham's *chorea.*

dan·der. **1.** A fine scaling of the skin and scalp. SEE ALSO dandruff. **2.** A normal effluvium of animal hair or coat capable of causing allergic responses in atopic persons.

dan·druff (dan'drŭf). The presence, in varying amounts, of white or gray scales in the hair of the scalp, due to excessive or normal branny exfoliation of the epidermis. SEE ALSO seborrheic *dermatitis.* SYN branny tetter (1), pityriasis capitis, pityriasis sicca, scurf, seborrhea sicca (2).

Dandy, Walter E., U.S. surgeon, 1886–1946. SEE D. *operation;* D.-Walker *syndrome.*

Dane, D.S., 20th century British virologist. SEE D. *particles,* under *particle.*

Dane's stain. See under stain.

Danforth, William Clark, U.S. obstetrician-gynecologist, 1878–1949. SEE D.'s *sign.*

Danielssen, Daniel C., Norwegian physician, 1815–1894. SEE D.'s *disease;* D.-Boeck *disease.*

Danlos, Henri A., French dermatologist, 1844–1912. SEE Ehlers-D. *syndrome.*

DANS Abbreviation for 1-dimethylaminonaphthalene-5-sulfonic acid; a green fluorescing compound used in immunohistochemistry to detect antigens.

DA

dan·syl (Dns, DNS) (dan'sil). The 5-dimethylami-nonaphthalene-1-sulfonyl radical; a blocking agent for NH$_2$ groups, used in peptide synthesis.

dan·thron. 1,8-dihydroxyanthraquinone; an anthraquinone laxative. SYN chrysazine.

dan·tro·lene so·di·um (dan'trō-lēn). 1-{[5-(p-Nitrophenyl)-furfurylidene]amino}hydantoin sodium hydrate; a synthetic skeletal muscle relaxant which acts directly on muscle by uncoupling electrical from mechanical events; also, the specific agent for prevention and treatment of malignant hyperthermia.

Danysz, Jean, Polish pathologist in France, 1860–1928. SEE D. *phenomenon.*

DAPI Abbreviation for 4'6-diamidino-2-phenylindole·2HCl, a fluorescent probe for DNA. SEE DAPI *stain.*

dap·sone (dap'sōn). 4,4'Sulfonylbisbenzeneamine; 4,4'-sulfobisaniline; it is used in the treatment of leprosy and certain cutaneous diseases such as dermatitis herpetiformis, and is active against the tubercle bacillus; it is also used in the treatment of bovine coccidiosis and streptococcal mastitis.

d'Arcet, Jean, French chemist, 1725–1801. SEE d'A.'s *metal.*

Darier, Jean F., French dermatologist, 1856–1938. SEE D.'s *disease, sign.*

Darkschewitsch (Darkshevich), Liverij O., Russian neurologist, 1858–1925. SEE *nucleus* of D.

Darling, Samuel Taylor, U.S. physician in Panama, 1872–1925. SEE D.'s *disease.*

Darrow red. A basic oxazin dye, C$_{18}$H$_{14}$N$_3$O$_2$Cl, used as a substitute for cresyl violet acetate in the staining of Nissl substance. [Mary A. *Darrow,* U.S. stain technologist, 1894–1973]

d'Arsonval, Jacques Arsène, French biophysicist, 1851–1940. SEE d'A. *current, galvanometer.*

dar·to·ic, dar·toid (dar-tō'ik, dar'toyd). Resembling tunica dartos in its slow involuntary contractions. [G. *dartos,* flayed]

dar·tos (dar'tōs). SEE dartos *fascia.* [G. skinned or flayed, fr. *derō,* to skin]

  d. mulieb'ris, a very thin layer of smooth muscle in the integument of the labia majora; less well-developed than the tunica dartos of the scrotum.

Darwin, Charles R., English biologist and evolutionist, 1809–1882. SEE darwinian *ear;* Darwinian *evolution;* darwinian *reflex;* darwinian *theory;* darwinian *tubercle.*

dar·win·i·an (dar-win'e-an). Relating to or ascribed to Darwin.

Das·y·proc·ta (das'e-prok'tă). A genus of rodents of the guinea pig family, a reservoir host of *Trypanosoma cruzi.* SYN *agouti.* [G. *dasyprōktos,* having hairy buttocks]

da·ta. Multiple facts (usually but not necessarily empirical) used as a basis for inference, testing, models, etc. The word is plural and takes a plural verb.

da·ta pro·cess·ing. Conversion of crude information into usable or storable form; statistical analysis of data by a computer program.

da·tum (dā'tŭm). An individual piece of information used in a scholarly field. [L., *given,* fr. *do, pp. datum,* to give]

Da·tu·ra (da-tū'ră). A genus of solanaceous plants. Several species (*D. arborea, D. fastuosa, D. ferox,* and *D. sanguinea*) are used in Brazil, India, and Peru to produce unconsciousness. The seeds contain hyoscine (scopolamine), an alkaloid with an anticholinergic action similar to that of atropine. [Hind.]

  D. me'tel, *D. fastuosa* L. var. *alba;* a species that contains scopolamine as its chief alkaloid and traces of hyoscyamine and atropine.

  D. stramo'nium, a species that is the main source of stramonium. SYN Jamestown weed, jimson weed, stink weed, thorn apple.

da·tu·rine (da-tū'rin, -rēn). SYN hyoscyamine.

Daubenton (D'Aubenton), Louis J.M., French physician, 1716–1799. SEE D.'s *angle, line, plane.*

Dau·er·schlaf (dow'er-shlahf). Rarely used term for prolonged sleep induced by drugs as a treatment for certain mental disorders. [Ger.]

daugh·ter (daw'ter). In nuclear medicine, an isotope that is the disintegration product of a radionuclide. SEE daughter *isotope,* radionuclide *generator.* [O.E. *dohtor*]

dau·no·my·cin (daw-nō-mī'sin). SYN daunorubicin.

dau·no·ru·bi·cin (daw-nō-rū'bi-sin). An antibiotic of the rhodomycin group, obtained from *Streptomyces peucetius;* used in the treatment of acute leukemia; also used in cytogenetics to produce Q-type chromosome bands. SYN daunomycin.

Davidoff, M. von, German histologist, †1904. SEE D.'s *cells,* under *cell.*

Davidson, Edward C., U.S. surgeon, 1894–1933. SEE D. *syringe.*

Daviel, Jacques, French oculist, 1696–1762. SEE D.'s *operation, spoon.*

Davies, J.N.P., U.S. pathologist, *1915. SEE D.'s *disease.*

Davis, David M., U.S. urologist, *1886.

Davis, John Staige, U.S. surgeon, 1872–1946. SEE D. *grafts,* under *graft;* D.-Crowe mouth *gag.*

Davis in·ter·lock·ing sound. See under sound.

Dawbarn, Robert Hugh Mackay, U.S. surgeon, 1860–1915. SEE D.'s *sign.*

Dawson, James R., U.S. pathologist, *1908. SEE D.'s *encephalitis.*

Day, Richard H., U.S. physician, 1813–1892. SEE D.'s *test.*

Day, Richard L., U.S. pediatrician, *1905. SEE Riley-D. *syndrome.*

daz·z·ling. The consequence of illumination too intense for adaptation by the eye; in contrast to glare, d. is alleviated by appropriate tinted glasses.

dB, db Abbreviation for decibel.

DBP Abbreviation for vitamin D-binding *protein.*

DC Abbreviation for direct *current.*

D & C Abbreviation for dilation and curettage.

D.C. Abbreviation for Doctor of Chiropractic.

DCI Symbol for dichloroisoproterenol.

dCMP Abbreviation for deoxycytidylic acid.

DDA Abbreviation for dideoxyadenosine.

DDI Abbreviation for dideoxyinosine.

D.D.S. Abbreviation for Doctor of Dental Surgery.

DDT Abbreviation for dichlorodiphenyltrichloroethane.

D & E Abbreviation for dilation and evacuation.

de-. 1. Away from, cessation, without; sometimes has an intensive force. 2. For names with this prefix not found here, see under the principal part of the name. [L. *de,* from, away]

de·a·cid·i·fi·ca·tion (dē-a-sid'i-fi-kā'shŭn). The removal or neutralization of acid.

de·ac·ti·va·tion (dē-ak-ti-vā'shŭn). The process of rendering or of becoming inactive.

de·ac·yl·ase (dē-as'il-ās). 1. A member of the subclass of hydrolases (EC class 3), especially of that subclass of esterases, lipases, lactonases, and hydrolases (EC subclass 3.1). 2. Any enzyme catalyzing the hydrolytic cleavage of an acyl group (R-CO-) in an ester linkage; also includes enzymes cleaving amide linkages (EC subclass 3.5) and similar acyl compounds.

dead (ded). 1. Without life. SEE ALSO death. 2. Numb.

DEAE-cel·lu·lose. SYN *O*-diethylaminoethyl *cellulose.*

deaf (def). Unable to hear; hearing indistinctly; hard of hearing. [A.S. *déaf*]

de·af·fer·en·ta·tion (dē-af'er-en-tā'shŭn). A loss of the sensory input from a portion of the body, usually caused by interruption of the peripheral sensory fibers. [L. *de,* from, + afferent]

deaf-mute (def'myūt). An individual with deafmutism.

deaf·mut·ism (def-myū'tizm). Inability to speak, due to congenital or early acquired profound deafness.

  endemic d., d. in individuals living in regions where goiter is prevalent, due to severe thyroid deficiency.

deaf·ness (def'nes). General term for loss of the ability to hear, without designation of the degree or cause of the loss.

  acoustic trauma d., sensorineural hearing loss due to overexposure to high intensity noise levels. SYN boilermaker's d., industrial d., occupational d.

Alexander's d. [MIM*203500], high frequency d. due to membranous cochlear dysplasia.

boilermaker's d., SYN acoustic trauma d.

central d., d. due to disorder of the auditory system of the brainstem or cerebral cortex.

conductive d., hearing impairment caused by interference with sound or transmission through the external canal, middle ear, or ossicles.

cortical d., d. resulting from bilateral lesions of the primary receptive area of the temporal lobe.

functional d., SYN psychogenic d.

high frequency d., selective loss of hearing acuity for high frequencies, usually associated with neurosensory damage; common in acoustic trauma.

hysterical d., SYN psychogenic d.

industrial d., SYN acoustic trauma d.

low tone d., inability to hear low notes or frequencies.

Mondini d., the hearing loss resulting from the structural aberration of Mondini dysplasia.

nerve d., neural d., former terms for sensorineural d.

noise–induced d., a type of sensorineural d. caused by prolonged exposure to loud sounds, *e.g.,* jet engines.

occupational d., SYN acoustic trauma d.

organic d., d. due to a pathologic process or an organic etiology, as opposed to psychogenic d.

perceptive d., former term for sensorineural d.

postlingual d., hearing impairment occurring after speech and language skills have been developed.

prelingual d., hearing impairment occurring before development of speech and language skills.

psychogenic d., hearing loss without evidence of organic cause or malingering; often follows severe psychic shock. SYN functional d., hysterical d.

retrocochlear d., former term for sensorineural d.; suggesting a lesion proximal to the cochlea.

Scheibe's d., d. (may be unilateral) due to cochleosaccular dysplasia; usually autosomal recessive inheritance.

sensorineural d., hearing impairment due to disorders of the cochlear division of the 9th cranial nerve (auditory nerve), the cochlea, or the retrocochlear nerve tracts, as opposed to conductive d.

word d., SYN auditory *aphasia.*

de·al·ba·tion (dē-al-bā'shŭn). The act of whitening, bleaching, or blanching. [L. *de-albo,* pp. *-atus,* to whiten]

de·al·co·hol·i·za·tion (dē-al'kō-hol-i-zā'shŭn). The removal of alcohol from a fluid; in histologic technique, the removal of alcohol from a specimen that has been previously immersed in this fluid.

de·al·ler·gize (dē-al'er-jīz). SYN desensitize (1).

de·am·i·das·es (dē-am'i-dā-sez). SYN amidohydrolases.

de·am·i·da·tion, de·am·i·di·za·tion (dē-am-i-dā'shŭn, dē-am'i-di-zā'shŭn). The hydrolytic removal of an amide group.

de·am·i·dize (dē-am'i-dīz). To perform deamidation. SYN desamidize.

de·am·i·nas·es (dē-am'i-nā-sez) [EC group 3.5.4]. Enzymes catalyzing simple hydrolysis of C—NH_2 bonds of purines, pyrimidines, and pterins, usually named in terms of the substrate, *e.g.,* guanine d., adenosine d., AMP d., pterin d. and thus producing ammonia; not generally used for deamination of noncyclic amides. D. are distinguished from ammonia-lyases (EC group 4.3.1) in that the latter produce an unsaturation at the point of NH_3 removal. SYN deaminating enzymes.

de·am·i·na·tion, de·am·i·ni·za·tion (dē-am-i-nā'shŭn, dē-am'i-ni-zā'shŭn). Removal, usually by hydrolysis, of the NH_2 group from an amino compound.

oxidative d., d. by enzymes that uses flavin or pyridine nucleotides (such as FAD or NAD^+).

de·am·in·ize (dē-am'i-nīz). To perform deamination.

Dean, Henry Trendley, U.S. dentist and epidemiologist, 1893–1962. SEE D.'s fluorosis *index.*

de·a·nol ac·et·a·mi·do·ben·zo·ate (dē'ă-nol as-ĕ-tam'i-dō-ben'

deafness

type of inner-ear defect	principal characteristics	morphologic changes
Michel type (1863)	complete aplasia	aplasia of pars petrosa of temporal bone or osseous labyrinth
Mondini type (1791)	severe hypoplasia of osseous and membranous labyrinth	absence of spiral lamina in proximal part of cochlea; widening of endolymphatic sac and duct; defect of Corti's organ
Sceibe type (1892)	aplasia of membranous labyrinth (cochlea and sacculus)	sacculus is widened or collapsed; cochlear duct is widened; Corti's organ is aplastic or hypoplastic, with defective supporting or hair cells

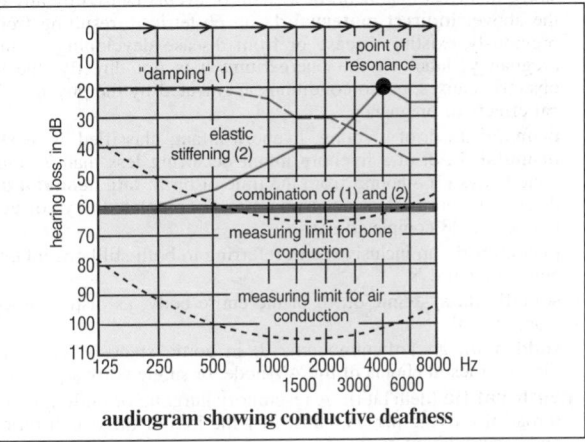

audiogram showing conductive deafness

zō-āt). The *p*-acetamidobenzoic acid salt of 2-dimethylaminoethanol; a central nervous system stimulant.

de·ar·te·ri·al·i·za·tion (dē-ar-tēr'ē-ăl-i-zā'shŭn). Changing the character of arterial blood to that of venous blood; *i.e.,* deoxygenation of blood.

death (deth). The cessation of life. In lower multicellular organisms, d. is a gradual process at the cellular level, because tissues vary in their ability to withstand deprivation of oxygen; in higher organisms, a cessation of integrated tissue and organ functions; in humans, manifested by the loss of heartbeat, by the absence of spontaneous breathing, and by cerebral d. SYN mors. [A.S. *dēath*]

black d., term applied to the worldwide epidemic of the 14th century, of which some 60 million persons are said to have died; the descriptions indicate that it was pneumonic plague.

brain d., SYN cerebral d.

cerebral d., a clinical syndrome characterized by the permanent loss of cerebral and brain stem function, manifested by absence of responsiveness to external stimuli, absence of cephalic reflexes, and apnea. An isoelectric electroencephalogram for at least 30 minutes in the absence of hypothermia and poisoning by central nervous system depressants supports the diagnosis. SYN brain d.

d. certificate, official, legal document and vital record, signed by a licensed physician or other designated authority, that includes cause of d., decedent's name, sex, place of residence, date of d.; other information, *e.g.,* birth date, birth place, occupation may be included; the immediate cause of d. is recorded on the first line of the certificate, followed by the condition(s) giving rise to this, with the underlying cause on the last line; the underlying cause is coded and tabulated in official publications of mortality.

cot d., SYN sudden infant death *syndrome*.

crib d., SYN sudden infant death *syndrome*.

crude d. rate, SYN death *rate*.

fetal d., d. prior to the complete expulsion or extraction from the mother of a product of conception, irrespective of the duration of pregnancy. Fetal death is considered *early* if it takes place in the first 20 weeks of gestation; *middle* (intermediate) if it takes place from 21 to 28 weeks of gestation, and *late* if it takes place after 28 weeks.

genetic d., d. of the bearer of a gene at any age before generating living offspring. May be compatible with good health and long life. SEE ALSO genetic *lethal*.

infant d., d. of a liveborn infant within the first year.

local d., d. of a part of the body or of a tissue by necrosis.

maternal d., d. of a woman while pregnant or within 42 days after the termination of gestation, irrespective of the duration and site of pregnancy and the cause of d.; two periods are recognized in the 42-day interval: period 1 includes day 1 to day 7; period 2 includes day 8 to day 42. Maternal d.'s are further classified as: **direct maternal d.,** d. resulting from obstetric complications of the gestation, labor, or puerperium, and from interventions, omissions, incorrect treatment, or a chain of events caused by any of the above; **indirect maternal d.,** an obstetric d. resulting from previously existing disease or from disease developing during pregnancy, labor, or the puerperium; it is not directly due to obstetric causes, but to conditions aggravated by the physiological effects of pregnancy.

neonatal d., d. of a young, liveborn infant; classified as: **early neonatal d.,** d. of a liveborn infant occurring less than 7 completed days (168 hours) from the time of birth; **late neonatal d.,** d. of a liveborn infant occurring after 7 completed days of age but before 28 completed days.

perinatal d., an inclusive term referring to both stillborn infants and neonatal d.'s.

somatic d., systemic d., d. of the entire body, as distinguished from local d.

sudden d., an arrhythmogenic d. in aortic stenosis, coronary disease, mesothelioma of the AV node, or single coronary artery.

death-rat·tle (deth′rat′l). A respiratory gurgling or rattling in the throat of a dying person, caused by the loss of the cough reflex and accumulation of mucus.

Deaver, John B., U.S. surgeon, 1855–1931. SEE D.'s *incision*.

DeBakey, Michael Ellis, U.S. heart surgeon, *1908. SEE DeBakey's *classification*, DeBakey *forceps*.

de·band·ing (dē-band′ing). The removal of fixed orthodontic appliances.

de·bil·i·tant (dē-bil′i-tant). **1.** Weakening; causing debility. **2.** Obsolete term for a quieting agent or one that subdues excitement. [L. *debilito*, to weaken, fr. *de*, neg., + *habilis*, able]

de·bil·i·tat·ing (dĕ-bil′i-tāt-ing). Denoting or characteristic of a morbid process that causes weakness.

de·bil·i·ty (dĕ-bil′i-tē). Weakness. [L. *debilitas*, fr. *debilis*, weak, fr. *de*- priv. + *habilis*, able]

de·bouch (dĕ-būsh′). To open or empty into another part. [Fr. *bouche*, mouth]

dé·bouche·ment (dā-būsh-mon′). Opening or emptying into another part. [Fr.]

Debré, Robert, French pediatrician and bacteriologist, *1882. SEE D. *phenomenon*; D.-Sémélaigne *syndrome*; Kocher-D.-Sémélaigne *syndrome*.

dé·bride·ment (dā-brēd-mon′). Excision of devitalized tissue and foreign matter from a wound. [Fr. unbridle]

de·bris·o·quine sul·fate (dĕ-bris′ō-kwin). 3-4-Dihydro-2(1*H*)-isoquinolinecarboxamidine sulfate; an antihypertensive agent resembling guanethidine; used in drug metabolism studies.

debt (det). A deficit; a liability. [L. *debitum*, debt]

alactic oxygen d., that part of the oxygen d. that is not lactacid oxygen d.; during recovery, stores of ATP and creatine phosphate must be replenished by oxidative metabolism, and a small amount of oxygen is also needed to restore the normal oxyhemoglobin levels throughout the circulating blood.

lactacid oxygen d., that part of an oxygen d. represented by the production of lactic acid by anaerobic glycolysis during exercise and, therefore, by the need to eliminate it by oxidative metabolism during recovery.

oxygen d., the extra oxygen, taken in by the body during recovery from exercise, beyond the resting needs of the body; sometimes used as if synonymous with oxygen deficit.

△**deca- (da).** Prefix used in the SI and metric systems to signify 10. Also spelled deka-. [G. *deka*, ten]

dec·a·gram (dek′ă-gram). Ten grams.

de·cal·ci·fi·ca·tion (dē′kal-si-fi-kā′shŭn). **1.** Removal of lime salts, chiefly tricalcium phosphate, from bones and teeth, either *in vitro* or as a result of a pathologic process. **2.** Precipitation of calcium from blood as by oxalate or fluoride, or the conversion of blood calcium to an un-ionized form as by citrate, thus preventing or delaying coagulation. [L. *de*-, away, + *calx* (*calc*-), lime, + *facio*, to make]

de·cal·ci·fy (dē-kal′si-fī). To remove lime or calcium salts, especially from bones or teeth.

de·cal·ci·fy·ing (dē-kal′si-fī-ing). Denoting an agent, measure, or process that causes decalcification.

dec·a·li·ter (dek′ă-lē-ter). Ten liters.

de·cal·vant (dē-kal′vant). Removing the hair; making bald. [L. *decalvare*, to make bald]

dec·a·me·ter (dek′ă-mē-ter). Ten meters.

dec·a·me·tho·ni·um bro·mide (dek-ă-me-thō′nē-ŭm). Decamethylene-1,10-bis-trimethylammonium dibromide; a synthetic nondepolarizing neuromuscular blocking agent used to produce muscular relaxation during general anesthesia.

dec·a·mine (dek′ă-mēn). SYN dequalinium acetate.

n-**dec·ane** (dek′ān). A paraffin hydrocarbon, CH_3-$(CH_2)_8$-CH_3.

n-**dec·a·no·ic ac·id** (dek-ă-nō′ik). SYN *n*-capric acid.

dec·a·no·in (dek-ă-nō′in). SYN caprin.

dec·a·nor·mal (dek-ă-nōr′măl). Rarely used term denoting the concentration of a solution 10 times that of normal.

de·cant (dē-kant′). To pour off gently the upper clear portion of a fluid, leaving the sediment in the vessel. [Mediev. L. *decantho*, fr. *de*- + *canthus*, the beak of a jug, fr. G. *kanthos*, corner of the eye]

de·can·ta·tion (dē-kan-tā′shŭn). Pouring off the clear upper portion of a fluid, leaving a sediment or precipitate.

de·ca·pac·i·ta·tion (dē′kă-pas-i-tā′shŭn). Prevention of spermatozoa from undergoing capacitation and thus from becoming able to fertilize ova. SEE ALSO decapacitation *factor*.

dec·a·pep·tide (dek′ă-pep′tīd). An oligopeptide containing 10 amino acids.

de·cap·i·tate (dē-kap′i-tāt). **1.** To cut off the head; specifically, to remove the head of a fetus to facilitate delivery in cases of irremediable dystocia; to cut off the head of an animal in preparation for certain physiologic experiments; obsolete term. **2.** Relating to an experimental animal with the head removed. [L. *de*-, away, + *caput*, head]

de·cap·i·ta·tion (dē-kap-i-tā′shŭn). Removal of a head. SEE decapitate.

de·cap·su·la·tion (dē-kap-sū-lā′shŭn). Incision and removal of a capsule or enveloping membrane.

d. of kidney, removing or stripping off the capsule of the kidney.

de·car·bo·ni·za·tion (dē-kar′bon-i-zā′shŭn). Rarely used term denoting the process of arterialization of the blood by oxygenation and the removal of carbon dioxide in the lungs.

de·car·box·yl·ase (dē-kar-boks′ē-lās). Any enzyme (EC subclass 4.1.1) that removes a molecule of carbon dioxide from a carboxylic group (*e.g.*, from an α-amino acid, converting it into an amine).

de·car·box·yl·a·tion (dē′kar-boks-ē-lā′shŭn). A reaction involving the removal of a molecule of carbon dioxide from a carboxylic acid.

oxidative d., d. requiring the participation of coenzymes such as NAD^+, $NADP^+$, FAD, or FMN.

de·cay (dē-kā′). **1.** Destruction of an organic substance by slow combustion or gradual oxidation. **2.** SYN putrefaction. **3.** To deteriorate; to undergo slow combustion or putrefaction. **4.** In dentistry, caries. **5.** In psychology, loss of information registered by the senses and processed into short-term memory. SEE ALSO memory. **6.** Loss of radioactivity with time; spontaneous emission of radiation or charged particles or both from an unstable nucleus. [L. *de,* down, + *cado,* to fall]

free induction d. (FID), in magnetic resonance imaging, the d. curve that is detected by the radiofrequency coil after the application of an excitation pulse, without additional pulses (free).

de·cel·er·a·tion (dē-sel-er-ā′shŭn). **1.** The act of decelerating. **2.** The rate of decrease in velocity per unit of time.

early d., slowing of the fetal heart rate early in the uterine contraction phase, denoting compression of the fetal head.

late d., any transient fetal bradycardia, the nadir of which occurs after the peak of the uterine contraction.

variable d., transient fetal bradycardia usually denoting compression of the umbilical cord which may occur at any time in relation to a uterine contraction.

de·cen·tra·tion (dē-sen-trā′shŭn). Removal from the center.

de·cer·e·brate (dē-ser′ĕ-brāt). **1.** To cause decerebration. **2.** Denoting an animal so prepared, or a patient whose brain has suffered an injury which renders him in his neurologic behavior comparable to a decerebrate animal.

de·cer·e·bra·tion (dē-ser′ĕ-brā′shŭn). Removal of the brain above the lower border of the corpora quadrigemina, or a complete section of the brain at this level or somewhat below.

bloodless d., destroying the function of the cerebrum by tying the basilar artery at about the middle of the pons and the common carotid arteries in the neck.

de·cer·e·brize (dē-ser′ĕ-brīz). To remove the brain.

de·chlo·ri·da·tion (dē′klōr-i-dā′shŭn). Reduction of sodium chloride in the tissues and fluids of the body by reducing its intake or increasing its excretion. SYN dechlorination, dechloruration.

de·chlo·ri·na·tion (dē′klōr-i-nā′shŭn). SYN dechloridation.

de·chlo·ru·ra·tion (dē′klōr-ū-rā′shŭn). SYN dechloridation.

de·cho·les·ter·ol·i·za·tion (dē′kō-les′ter-ol-i-zā′shŭn). Therapeutic reduction of the cholesterol concentration of the blood.

♻**deci- (d).** Prefix used in the SI and metric systems to signify one-tenth (10⁻). [L. *decimus,* tenth]

dec·i·bel (dB, db) (des′i-bel). One-tenth of a bel; unit for expressing the relative loudness of sound on a logarithmic scale. [L. *decimus,* tenth, + bel]

de·cid·ua (dē-sid′yū-ă). SYN deciduous *membrane.* [L. *deciduus,* falling off (qualifying *membrana,* membrane, understood)]

d. basa′lis [NA], the area of endometrium between the implanted chorionic vesicle and the myometrium, which develops into the maternal part of the placenta. SYN d. serotina.

d. capsula′ris [NA], the layer of endometrium overlying the implanted chorionic vesicle; it becomes progressively attenuated as the chorionic vesicle enlarges and, by the fourth month, is squeezed against the d. parietalis and thereafter undergoes rapid regression. SYN d. reflexa, membrana adventitia (2).

ectopic d., decidual cells which may be found in the cervix, appendix, or areas other than the endometrium.

d. menstrua′lis, the succulent mucous membrane of the non-pregnant uterus at the menstrual period.

d. parieta′lis [NA], the altered mucous membrane lining the main cavity of the pregnant uterus other than at the site of attachment of the chorionic vesicle. SYN d. vera.

d. polypo′sa, d. parietalis showing polypoid projections of the endometrial surface.

d. reflex′a, SYN d. capsularis.

d. seroti′na, SYN d. basalis.

d. spongio′sa, the portion of the d. basalis attached to the myometrium.

d. ve′ra, SYN d. parietalis.

de·cid·u·al (dē-sid′yū-ăl). Relating to the decidua.

de·cid·u·ate (dē-sid′yū-āt). Relating to those mammals (*e.g.,* man, dog, rodent) that shed maternal uterine tissue when expelling the placenta at birth, in contrast to indeciduate mammals (horse, pig). [see deciduation]

de·cid·u·a·tion (dē-sid-yū-ā′shŭn). Shedding of endometrial tissue during menstruation. [L. *deciduus,* falling off]

de·cid·u·i·tis (dē-sid-yū-ī′tis). Inflammation of the decidua.

de·cid·u·o·ma (dē-sid-yū-ō′mă). An intrauterine mass of decidual tissue, probably the result of hyperplasia of decidual cells retained in the uterus. SYN placentoma.

Loeb's d., mass of decidual tissue produced in the uterus, in the absence of a fertilized ovum, by means of mechanical or hormonal stimulation.

de·cid·u·ous (dē-sid′yū-ŭs). **1.** Not permanent; denoting that which eventually falls off. **2 (D)** (in dental formulas). In dentistry, often used to designate the first or primary dentition. SEE deciduous *tooth.* [L. *deciduus,* falling off]

dec·i·gram (des′i-gram). One-tenth of a gram.

dec·i·li·ter (des′i-lē-ter). One-tenth of a liter.

dec·i·me·ter (des′i-mē-ter). One-tenth of a meter.

dec·i·mor·gan (des′i-mōr-găn). SEE morgan.

dec·i·nor·mal (des-i-nōr′măl). One-tenth of normal, denoting the concentration of a solution.

de·ci·sion tree. Alternative choices available at each stage of deciding how to manage a clinical problem, displayed graphically; at each branch or decision node, the probabilities of each outcome that can be predicted are shown; the relative worth of each outcome is described in terms of its utility or quality of life, *e.g.,* as measured by probability of life expectancy or freedom from disability.

de Clerambault, G., French psychiatrist, 1872–1934. SEE de C. *syndrome.*

dec·li·na·tion (dek-li-nā′shŭn). A bending, sloping, or other deviation from a normal vertical position. [L. *declinatio,* a bending aside]

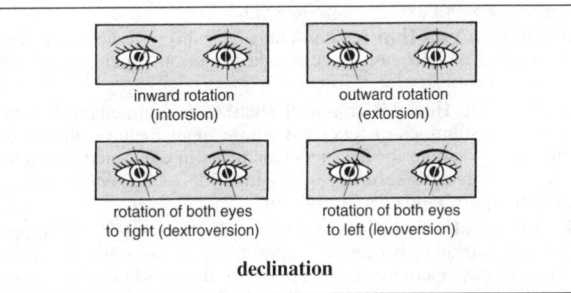

inward rotation (intorsion) — outward rotation (extorsion)

rotation of both eyes to right (dextroversion) — rotation of both eyes to left (levoversion)

declination

dec·lin·a·tor (dek′lin-ā-ter, -tōr). A retractor that holds certain structures out of the way during an operation.

de·clive (dē-klīv′) [NA]. The posterior sloping portion of the monticulus of the vermis of the cerebellum; vermal lobule caudal to the primary fissure. SYN declivis, lobulus clivi. [L. *declivis,* sloping downward, fr. *clivus,* a slope]

de·cli·vis (dē-klī′vis). SYN declive.

de·coc·tion (dē-kok′shŭn). **1.** The process of boiling. **2.** The pharmacopeial name for preparations made by boiling crude vegetable drugs, and then straining, in the proportion of 50 g of the drug to 1000 ml of water. SYN apozem, apozema. [L. *decoctio,* fr. *de-coquo,* pp. *-coctus,* to boil down]

dé·colle·ment (dā-kŭl-mon′). Rarely used term for surgical separation of tissues or organs which are adherent, either normally or pathologically. [Fr. ungluing]

de·com·pen·sa·tion (de′kom-pen-sā′shŭn). **1.** A failure of compensation in heart disease. **2.** The appearance or exacerbation of a mental disorder due to failure of defense mechanisms.

corneal d., corneal edema resulting from failure of the corneal endothelium to maintain deturgescence.

de·com·pose (dē′kom-pōz). **1.** To resolve a compound into its component parts; to disintegrate. **2.** To decay; to putrefy. [L. *de,* from, down, + *com-pono,* pp. *-positus,* to put together]

de·com·po·si·tion (dē′kom-pō-zish′ŭn). SYN putrefaction.

de·com·pres·sion (dē′kom-presh-ŭn). Removal of pressure. [L. *de-,* from, down, + *com-primo,* pp. *-pressus,* to press together]

cardiac d., incision into the pericardium or aspiration of fluid from pericardium to relieve pressure due to blood or other fluid in the pericardial sac. SYN pericardial d.

cerebral d., removal of a piece of the cranium, usually in the subtemporal region, with incision of the dura, to relieve intracranial pressure.

explosive d., SYN rapid d.

internal d., removal of intracranial tissue, usually tumor or brain tissue. to relieve pressure.

nerve d., release of pressure on a nerve trunk by the surgical excision of constricting bands or widening of a bony canal.

optic nerve sheath d., a venting of the optic nerve sheath into the retrobulbar space, by slitting or by fenestrating the sheath. SEE optic nerve sheath *fenestration*.

orbital d., removal of a portion of the bony orbit, usually superior (Naffziger operation), lateral (Krönlein operation), or inferior (Ogura operation).

pericardial d., SYN cardiac d.

rapid d., sudden severe expansion of gases due to a reduction in ambient pressure. SYN explosive d.

spinal d., the removal of pressure upon the spinal cord as created by a tumor, cyst, hematoma, nucleus pulposus, abscess, or bone.

suboccipital d., d. of the posterior fossa by occipital craniectomy and opening of the dura.

subtemporal d., d. of the brain by temporal craniectomy and opening of the dura over the inferolateral surface of the temporal lobe.

trigeminal d., d. of the trigeminal nerve root.

de·con·ges·tant (dē-kon-jes′tant). **1.** SYN decongestive. **2.** An agent that possesses this action.

de·con·ges·tive (dē-kon-jes′tiv). Having the property of reducing congestion. SYN decongestant (1).

de·con·tam·i·na·tion (dē′kon-tam-i-nā′shŭn). Removal or neutralization of poisonous gas or other injurious agents from the environment.

de·con·vo·lu·tion (dē-con-vō-lū′shŭn). A mathematical technique for solutions of functions whose input includes their output; used to solve for the image elements in computed tomography or magnetic resonance imaging. [de- + L. *convulutio,* a rolling up, fr. *convolvo,* to roll up]

de·cor·ti·ca·tion (dē-kōr-ti-kā′shŭn). **1.** Removal of the cortex, or external layer, beneath the capsule from any organ or structure. **2.** An operation for removal of the residual clot and/or newly organized scar tissue that form after a hemothorax or neglected empyema. [L. *decortico,* pp. *-atus,* to deprive of bark, fr. *de,* from, + *cortex,* rind, bark]

cerebral d., destruction of the cerebral cortex, usually due to anoxia.

reversible d., a temporary loss of function of the cerebral cortex.

dec·re·ment (dek′rĕ-ment). **1.** Decrease. **2.** Decrease in conduction velocity at a particular point; a result of altered properties at that point. SEE ALSO decremental *conduction.* [L. *decrementum,* fr. *decresco,* to decrease]

de·crep·i·ta·tion (dē-krep-i-tā′shŭn). Crackling; the snapping of certain salts when heated. [L. *de,* from, + *crepo,* pp. *crepitus,* to crackle]

de·cru·des·cence (dē-krū-des′ens). Abatement of the symptoms of disease. [L. *de,* from, + *crudesco,* to become worse, fr. *crudus,* crude]

de·cu·ba·tion (dē-kū-bā′shŭn). Rarely used term for the final period of an infectious disease from the disappearance of the specific symptoms to complete restoration of health and the end of the infectious period. [L. *de,* from, + *cubo,* to lie down]

de·cu·bi·tal (dē-kyū′bi-tăl). Relating to a decubitus ulcer.

de·cu·bi·tus (dē-kyū′bi-tŭs). **1.** The position of the patient in bed; *e.g.,* dorsal d., lateral d. SEE decubitus *film.* **2.** Sometimes used in referring to a decubitus ulcer. [L. *decumbo,* to lie down]

Andral's d., position assumed by the patient who lies on the sound side in cases of beginning pleurisy.

ventral d., pressure sores (decubitus ulceration) occurring in ventral locations, such as the abdominal wall or the anterior surface of an extremity.

de·cur·rent (dē-kŭr′ent). Extending downward. [L. *de-curro,* pp. *-cursus,* to run down]

de·cus·sate (dē′kŭ-sāt, dē-kŭs′āt). **1.** To cross. **2.** Crossed like the arms of an X. [L. *decusso,* pp. *-atus,* to make in the form of an X, fr. *decussis,* a large, bronze Roman (2nd c. BC), 10-unit coin marked with an X to indicate its denomination]

de·cus·sa·tio, pl. **de·cus·sa·ti·o·nes** (dē-kŭ-sā′shē-ō, -ō′nēz) [NA]. **1.** In general, any crossing over or intersection of parts. **2.** The intercrossing of two homonymous fiber bundles as each crosses over to the opposite side of the brain in the course of its ascent or descent through the brainstem or spinal cord. SYN decussation. [L. (see decussate)]

d. bra′chii conjuncti′vi, SYN *decussation* of superior cerebellar peduncles.

d. fontina′lis, SEE decussationes tegmenti.

d. lemnisco′rum [NA], SYN *decussation* of medial lemniscus.

d. moto′ria [NA], ✫official alternate term for pyramidal *decussation.*

d. nervo′rum trochlear′ium [NA], SYN *decussation* of trochlear nerves.

d. pedunculo′rum cerebella′rium superio′rum [NA], SYN *decussation* of superior cerebellar peduncles.

d. pyram′idum [NA], SYN pyramidal *decussation.*

d. senso′ria [NA], ✫official alternate term for *decussation* of medial lemniscus.

decussatio′nes tegmen′ti [NA], SYN tegmental *decussations,* under *decussation.*

de·cus·sa·tion (dē-kŭ-sā′shŭn). SYN decussatio. [L. *decussatio*]

d. of brachia conjunctiva, SYN d. of superior cerebellar peduncles.

dorsal tegmental d., SEE tegmental d.'s (1).

d. of the fillet, SYN d. of medial lemniscus.

Forel's d., SEE tegmental d.'s (2).

fountain d., SEE tegmental d.'s (1).

Held's d., the crossing of some of the fibers arising from the cochlear nuclei to form the lateral lemniscus.

d. of medial lemniscus, the intercrossing of the fibers of the left and right medial lemniscus ascending from the gracile and cuneate nuclei, immediately rostral to the level of the decussation of the pyramidal tracts in the medulla oblongata. SYN decussatio lemniscorum [NA], decussatio sensoria✫ [NA], d. of the fillet, sensory d. of medulla oblongata.

Meynert's d., SEE tegmental d.'s (1).

motor d., SYN pyramidal d.

optic d., SYN optic *chiasm.*

pyramidal d., the intercrossing of the bundles of the pyramidal tracts at the lower border region of the medulla oblongata. SYN decussatio pyramidum [NA], decussatio motoria✫ [NA], motor d.

rubrospinal d., SEE tegmental d.'s (2).

sensory d. of medulla oblongata, SYN d. of medial lemniscus.

d. of superior cerebellar peduncles, the decussation of the left and right superior cerebellar peduncles in the tegmentum of the caudal mesencephalon. SYN decussatio pedunculorum cerebellarium superiorum [NA], decussatio brachii conjunctivi, d. of brachia conjunctiva, Wernekinck's d.

tectospinal d., SEE tegmental d.'s (1).

tegmental d.'s, (1) the dorsal tegmental decussation (fountain or Meynert's decussation, d. fontinalis) of the left and right tectospinal and tectobulbar tracts; **(2)** the ventral tegmental d. (rubrospinal or Forel's d.) of the left and right rubrospinal and rubrobulbar tracts; both are located in the mesencephalon. SYN decussationes tegmenti [NA].

d. of trochlear nerves, the crossing of the two trochlear nerves at their exit through the velum medullare anterius. SYN decussatio nervorum trochlearium [NA].

ventral tegmental d., SEE tegmental d.'s (2).

Wernekinck's d., SYN d. of superior cerebellar peduncles.

de·cus·sa·ti·o·nes (dē-kŭs-ā-shē-ō′nēz). Plural of decussatio.

de·den·ti·tion (dē-den-tish′ŭn). Obsolete term denoting loss of teeth.

de·dif·fer·en·ti·a·tion (dē-dif′er-en-shē-ā′shŭn). **1.** The return of parts to a more homogeneous state. **2.** SYN anaplasia.

de·do·la·tion (dē-dō-lā′shŭn). A slicing wound made by a sharp instrument grazing the surface. [L. *de-dolo,* pp. *-atus,* to hew away]

de·duc·tion (dē-duk′shun). The logical derivation of a conclusion from certain premises. The conclusion will be true if the premises are true and the deductive argument is valid. Cf. induction (9).

de·ef·fer·en·ta·tion (dē-ef-er-en-tā′shŭn). A loss of the motor nerve fibers to an area of the body. [L. *de,* from, + efferent]

deep (dēp). SYN profundus.

de·ep·i·car·di·al·i·za·tion (dē-ep-i-kar′dē-al-i-zā′shŭn). Surgical destruction of the epicardium, usually by the application of phenol, designed to promote collateral circulation to the myocardium.

Deetjen, Hermann, German physician, 1867–1915. SEE D.'s *bodies,* under body.

def, DEF Abbreviation for decayed, extracted, and filled tooth. SEE def caries *index.*

de·fat·i·ga·tion (dē-fat-i-gā′shŭn). Weariness, exhaustion, or extreme fatigue. [L. *de-fatigo,* pp. *-atus,* to tire out]

def·e·cate (def′ĕ-kāt). To perform defecation.

def·e·ca·tion (def-ĕ-kā′shŭn). The discharge of feces from the rectum. SYN motion (2), movement (3). [L. *defaeco,* pp. *-atus,* to remove the dregs, purify]

de·fec·og·ra·phy (de-fĕ-kog′ră-fē). Radiographic examination of the act of defecation of a radiopaque stool. [defecation + G. *graphō,* to write]

de·fect (dē′fekt). An imperfection, malformation, dysfunction, or absence; an attribute of quality, in contrast with deficiency, which is an attribute of quantity. [L. *deficio,* pp. *-fectus,* to fail, to lack]

aortic septal d., aorticopulmonary septal d., a small congenital opening between the aorta and pulmonary artery about 1 cm above the semilunar valves, *e.g.,* aorticopulmonary window. SYN aorticopulmonary window.

atrial septal d., a congenital d. in the septum between the atria of the heart, due to failure of the foramen primum or secundum to close normally; may involve atrioventricular canal cushions; occasionally there is strong evidence of autosomal dominant inheritance [MIM*108800]. In varying degree, it is also a common feature of the autosomal recessive Ellis-van Creveld *syndrome* [MIM*225500] and the autosomal dominant Holt-Oram *syndrome* [MIM*142900].

atrial ventricular canal d., a d. caused by deficient or absent septal tissue immediately above and below the normal level of the atrioventricular valves, including the region normally occupied by the A-V septum in hearts with two ventricles. The A-V valves are abnormal to a varying degree.

birth d., d. present at birth; sometimes referred to as congenital d.

congenital ectodermal d., incomplete development of the epidermis and skin appendages; the skin is smooth and hairless, the facies abnormal, and the teeth and nails may be affected; sweating may be deficient. SYN congenital ectodermal dysplasia.

coupling d., SEE familial *goiter.*

Eisenmenger's d., SYN Eisenmenger's *complex.*

endocardial cushion d., SYN persistent atrioventricular *canal.*

fibrous cortical d., a common 1 to 3 cm d. in the cortex of a bone, most commonly the lower femoral shaft of a child, filled with fibrous tissue. Nonosteogenic or nonossifying *fibroma* by convention refers to lesions greater than 3 cm in diameter. SEE ALSO nonossifying *fibroma.* SYN nonosteogenic fibroma.

filling d., displacement of contrast medium by a space-occupying lesion in a radiographic study of a contrast-filled hollow

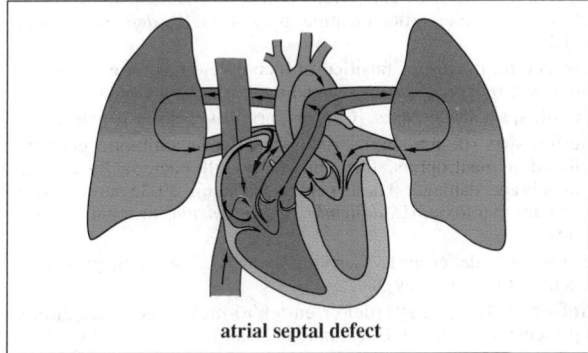

atrial septal defect

viscus, such as a polyp on a barium enema; also applied to defects in the otherwise uniform distribution of radionuclide in an organ, such as a metastasis in the liver on a ^{99m}Tc-sulfur colloid scan.

Gerbode d., a defect in the interventricular portion of the membranous septum, associated with a communication between the right ventricle and the right atrium through an abnormality in the tricuspid valve.

iodide transport d., SEE familial *goiter.*

iodotyrosine deiodinase d., SEE familial *goiter.*

luteal phase d., a condition characterized by inadequate secretion of progesterone during the luteal phase of the menstrual cycle, with resultant sterility; subnormal luteal function commonly attributed to abnormal pituitary gonadotropin secretion. SYN luteal phase deficiency.

metaphysial fibrous cortical d., a small (less than 2 to 3 cm in diameter) fibrous cortical d.

organification d., SEE familial *goiter.*

osteoporotic marrow d. (ŏs′tē-ō-pō-ro′tik), focal osteoporotic bone marrow d. of the jaw; a focal radiolucent d. composed of normal marrow.

postinfarction ventricular septal d., a d. developed in the ventricular septum resulting from rupture of an acute myocardial infarction.

salt-losing d., renal tubular abnormality causing loss of sodium in the urine.

ventricular septal d., a congenital d. in the septum (membranous or muscular) between the cardiac ventricles, usually resulting from failure of the spiral septum to close the interventricular foramen.

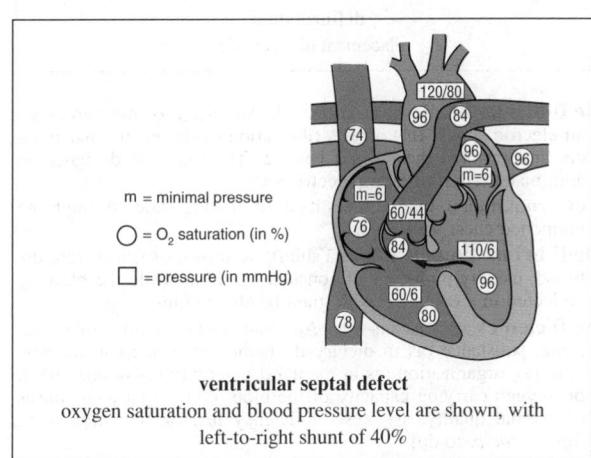

m = minimal pressure

◯ = O₂ saturation (in %)

▢ = pressure (in mmHg)

ventricular septal defect
oxygen saturation and blood pressure level are shown, with left-to-right shunt of 40%

de·fec·tive (dē-fek′tiv). Denoting or exhibiting a defect; imperfect; a failure of quality.

de·fem·i·na·tion (dē-fem-i-nā′shŭn). A weakening or loss of feminine characteristics. [L. *de-,* away, + *femina,* woman]

de·fense (dē-fens′). The psychological mechanisms used to control anxiety, *e.g.*, rationalization, projection. [L. *defendo,* to ward off]

  screen d., the use of falsified or incomplete memories or affects to cover repressed but associated memories and affects.

  ur-d.'s, SEE ur-defenses. [Ger. *ur-,* primitive, earliest, + defenses]

de·fen·sins (dē-fen-sinz). A class of basic antibiotic peptides, found in neutrophils, that apparently kill bacteria by causing membrane damage. These peptides contain 29-35 amino acids and are cytotoxic. [L. *de-fendo,* pp. *de-fensum,* to repel, avert, + -in]

def·er·ent (def′er-ent). Carrying away. [L. *deferens,* pres. p. of *defero,* to carry away]

def·er·en·tec·to·my (def′er-en-tek′tō-mē). SYN vasectomy. [(ductus) deferens, + G. *ektomē,* excision]

def·er·en·tial (def-er-en′shăl). Relating to the ductus deferens.

def·er·en·ti·tis (def′er-en-tī′tis). Inflammation of the ductus deferens. SYN vasitis.

de·fer·ox·a·mine mes·y·late (de-fer-ok′să-mēn). methanesulfonate of 30-amino-3,14,25-trihydroxy-3,9,14,20,25-penta-aza-triacontane-2,10,13,21,24-pentaone; chelate used in the treatment of iron poisoning. SYN desferrioxamine mesylate.

de·fer·ves·cence (def-er-ves′ens). Falling at an elevated temperature; abatement of fever. [L. *de-fervesco,* to cease boiling, fr. *de-* neg. + *fervesco,* to begin to boil]

de·fi·bril·la·tion (dē-fib-ri-lā′shŭn). The arrest of fibrillation of the cardiac muscle (atrial or ventricular) with restoration of the normal rhythm.

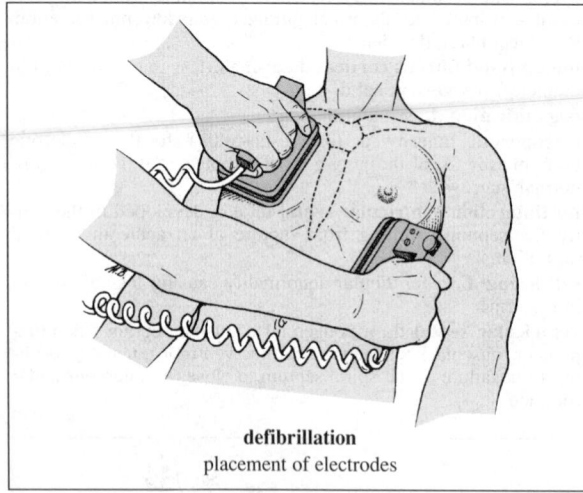

defibrillation
placement of electrodes

de·fi·bril·la·tor (dē-fib′ri-lā-ter). **1.** Any agent or measure, *e.g.,* an electric shock, that arrests fibrillation of the ventricular muscle and restores the normal beat. **2.** The machine designed to administer a defibrillating electric shock.

  external d., a d. that delivers its defibrillating shock through the unopened·chest wall.

de·fi·bri·na·tion (dē-fī-bri-nā′shŭn). Removal of fibrin from the blood, usually by means of constant agitation while the blood is collected in a container with glass beads or chips.

de·fi·cien·cy (dē-fish′en-sē). An insufficient quantity of something, substance (as in dietary d., hemoglobin d. as in marrow aplasia), organization (as in mental d.), activity (as in enzyme d. or oxygen-carrying capacity of the blood), etc., that available is of normal quality. SEE ALSO deficiency *disease.* [L. *deficio,* to fail, fr. *facio,* to do]

  adult lactase d., onset of lactase d., with resulting milk intolerance and malabsorption, in adulthood. Inherited forms may not be manifested until adulthood; any process that damages the intestinal lining cells can cause lactase d. in adults.

  antitrypsin d., d. of α₁-antitrypsin, a glycoprotein of the postalbumin region of human serum. Many forms are known which

may be moderate (40 to 60% of normal activity) or severe (less than 10% of normal), all autosomal dominant; the severe form is often associated with familial emphysema or hepatic cirrhosis.

  arch length d., the difference between the available circumference of the dental arch and that required to accommodate the succedaneous teeth in proper alignment.

  debrancher d., SYN brancher glycogen storage *disease.*

  familial high density lipoprotein d., SYN analphalipoproteinemia.

  galactokinase d. [MIM*230200], an inborn error of metabolism due to congenital d. of galactokinase, resulting in increased blood galactose concentration (galactosemia), cataracts, hepatomegaly, and mental deficiency; autosomal recessive inheritance. Galactose epimerase d. [MIM 230350] and galactose-1-phosphate uridyl transferase d. [MIM 230400] produce much the same clinical picture.

  glucose-6-phosphate dehydrogenase d., a d. of glucose-6-phosphate dehydrogenase, an enzyme important for maintaining cellular concentrations of reduced nucleotides. An X-linked disorder with various polymorphic forms, it can cause a variety of anemias including favism, primaquine sensitivity and other drug sensitivity anemias, anemia of the newborn, and chronic nonspherocytic hemolytic anemia.

  glucosephosphate isomerase d. [MIM*172400], an enzyme d. characterized by chronic nonspherocytic hemolytic anemia; autosomal recessive inheritance. SYN phosphohexose isomerase d.

  β-*d*-glucuronidase d., a rare d. of β-*d*-glucuronidase; an autosomal recessive disorder with several allelic forms, characterized by abnormal mucopolysaccharide metabolism leading to progressive mental deterioration, splenic and hepatic enlargement, and dysostosis multiplex. SYN mucopolysaccharidase.

  glutathione synthetase d., an inborn error of metabolism associated with massive urinary excretion of 5-oxyproline, elevated levels of 5-oxyproline in the blood and cerebrospinal fluid, severe metabolic acidosis, tendency toward hemolysis, and defective central nervous systems function. Glutathione synthetase d. has been reported as a generalized condition or with a d. restricted to erythrocytes.

  hypoxanthine guanine phosphoribosyltransferase d., a sex-linked inherited metabolic disorder; complete d. results in Lesch-Nyhan syndrome; incomplete d. is associated with acute gouty arthritis and renal stones.

  immune d., SYN immunodeficiency.

  immunity d., SYN immunodeficiency.

  immunological d., SYN immunodeficiency.

  LCAT d., a rare condition characterized by corneal opacities, hemolytic anemia, proteinuria, renal insufficiency, and premature atherosclerosis, and very low levels of lecithin cholesterol acyltransferase (LCAT) activity; results in accumulation of unesterified cholesterol in plasma and tissues.

  d. adhesion deficiency (LAD), an inherited disorder (autosomal recessive) in which there is a defective CD18 adherence complex that disturbs d. chemotaxis. It is characterized by recurrent bacterial infections and impaired wound healing.

  luteal phase d., SYN luteal phase *defect.*

  mental d., SYN mental *retardation.*

  muscle phosphorylase d., type V glycogen storage disease, affecting muscle, caused by d. of muscle phosphorylase.

  phosphohexose isomerase d., SYN glucosephosphate isomerase d.

  placental sulfatase d., an enzyme defect in the placenta which results in failure of conversion of 16α-hydroxydehydroepiandrosterone to estriol; women with this condition rarely enter into spontaneous labor.

  α-1-proteinase d., absence of a serum proteinase inhibitor that may cause nodular non-suppurative panniculitis.

  proximal femoral focal d. (PFFD), a congenital defect in which variable portions of the upper end of the femur are reduced or absent.

  pseudocholinesterase d. [MIM*177400], an autosomal dominant disorder manifested by exaggerated responses to drugs ordinarily hydrolyzed by serum pseudocholinesterase (*e.g.,* succinylcholine); believed to entail production of a variant enzyme that is less active than the normal enzyme in hydrolyzing appropriate substrates, but also abnormally resistant to the effects of anticholinesterases.

pyruvate kinase d. [MIM*166200], a disorder in which there is a d. of pyruvate kinase in red blood cells; characterized by hemolytic anemia varying in degree from one patient to another; autosomal recessive inheritance.

riboflavin d., SEE ariboflavinosis.

secondary antibody d., SYN secondary *immunodeficiency.*

taste d. [MIM*171200], reduced or absent ability to detect a bitter taste in a group of compounds of which phenylthiocarbamide is the prototype, due to the homozygous state of a common allele. SEE ALSO phenylthiourea.

def·i·cit (def′i-sit). The result of temporarily using up something faster than it is being replenished. [L. *deficio,* to fail]

base d., a decrease in the total concentration of blood buffer base, indicative of metabolic acidosis or compensated respiratory alkalosis.

oxygen d., the difference between oxygen uptake of the body during early stages of exercise and during a similar duration in a steady state of exercise; sometimes considered as the formation of the oxygen debt.

pulse d., (1) the absence of palpable pulse waves in a peripheral artery for one or more heart beats, as is often seen in atrial fibrillation; **(2)** the number of such missing pulse waves (usually expressed as heart rate minus pulse rate per minute).

def·i·ni·tion (def′i-nish′ŭn). In optics, the power of a lens to give a distinct image. SEE ALSO resolving *power.* [L. *de-finio,* pp. *-finitus,* to bound, fr. *finis,* limit]

de·flec·tion (dē-flek′shŭn). **1.** A moving to one side. **2.** In the electrocardiogram, a deviation of the curve from the isoelectric base line; any wave or complex of the electrocardiogram. [L. *de-flecto,* pp. *-flexus,* to bend aside]

intrinsic d., with the electrode in direct contact with the muscle fiber, a rapid downward d. from the peak of maximum positivity, signifying that the activation front has reached the subjacent muscle.

intrinsicoid d., the abrupt downstroke from maximum positivity when the electrode is placed not directly on the muscle but at a distance, as in the unipolar chest leads in clinical electrocardiography.

de·flex·ion (dē′fleks-shŭn). Term used to describe the position of the fetal head in relation to the maternal pelvis in which the head is descending in a nonflexed or extended attitude. [de- + L. *flexio,* a bending, fr. *flecto,* pp. *flexum,* to bend]

def·lo·res·cence (dē-flō-res′ens). Disappearance of the eruption in scarlet fever or other exanthemas. [L. *de-floresco,* to fade, wither, fr. *flos (flor-),* flower]

de·flu·o·ri·da·tion (dē-flŭr′i-dā′shŭn). Removal of excess fluorides from a community water supply.

de·flu·vi·um (dē-flŭ′vē-ŭm). SYN defluxion. [L., fr. *de-fluo,* pp. *-fluxus,* to flow down]

d. capillo′rum, a falling (or loss) of hair.

d. ung′uium, a falling (or loss) of nails.

de·flux·ion (dē-flŭk′shŭn). **1.** A falling down or out, as of the hair. SEE ALSO effluvium (1). **2.** A flowing down or discharge of fluid. SYN defluvium. [L. *defluxio, de-fluo,* pp. *-fluxus,* to flow down]

de·for·ma·bi·li·ty (dē-form′ă-bil′i-tē). The ability of cells, such as erythrocytes, to change shape as they pass through narrow spaces, such as the microvasculature.

de·for·ma·tion (dē-fōr-mā′shŭn). **1.** Deviation of form from the normal; specifically, an alteration in shape and/or structure of a previously normally formed part. It occurs after organogenesis and often involves the musculoskeletal system (*e.g.,* clubfoot). **2.** SYN deformity. **3.** In rheology, the change in the physical shape of a mass by applied stress. [L. *de-formo,* pp. *-atus,* to deform, fr. *forma,* form]

de·form·ing (dē-fōrm′ing). Causing a deviation from the normal form.

de·for·mi·ty (dē-fōr′mi-tē). A permanent structural deviation

from the normal shape or size, resulting in disfigurement; may be congenital or acquired. SYN deformation (2).

Åkerlund d., indentation (incisura) with niche of duodenal cap as demonstrated radiographically.

Arnold-Chiari d. [MIM*207950], SYN Arnold-Chiari *malformation.*

bell clapper d., a testis and epididymis free of the usual posterior attachment of the tunica vaginalis such that the tunic inserts high on the spermatic cord leaving the gonad more likely to undergo torsion.

boutonnière d., flexion of the proximal interphalangeal joint with hyperextension of the distal interphalangeal joint of the finger, caused by splitting of the extensor hood and protrusion of the head of the proximal phalanx through the resulting "buttonhole."

contracture d., d. of a limb without discernable primary changes of bone.

Erlenmeyer flask d., a d. at the distal end of the femur caused by a failure of the shaft of the bone to develop to its normal tubular shape, with the result that the bone is wide for a much longer distance up the shaft than normal. [resemblance to an E. flask]

gunstock d., a form of cubitus varus resulting from condylar fracture at the elbow in which the axis of the extended forearm is not continuous with that of the arm but is displaced toward midline.

Haglund's d., SYN Haglund's *disease.*

J-sella d., pear-shaped or J-shaped d. of sella turcica caused by increased pressure on growing sphenoid bone; noted in the mucopolysaccharide storage diseases.

keyhole d., mucosal ectropion at the posterior edge of the anus following sphincterotomy at that location.

lobster-claw d., SEE ectrodactyly.

Madelung's d., a distal radioulnar subluxation due to a relative deficiency of axial growth of the medial side of the distal radius, which, as a consequence, is abnormally inclined proximally and ulnarwards. SYN carpus curvus.

mermaid d., SYN sirenomelia.

parachute d., SYN parachute mitral *valve.*

reduction d., congenital absence or attenuation of one or more body parts; usually of the limbs or limb components.

seal-fin d., deflection outward of the fingers in rheumatoid arthritis.

silver-fork d., the d. resembling the curve of the back of a fork seen in Colles' fractures.

Sprengel's d., congenital elevation of the scapula. SYN scapula elevata.

swan-neck d., narrowing of the first part of the renal proximal convoluted tubule adjoining the glomerulus, seen in cystinosis and occasionally in other renal diseases.

torsional d., in orthopedics, a d. caused by rotation of a portion of an extremity with relationship to the long axis of the entire extremity.

whistling d., d. caused by insufficient tissue in the lower border of a repaired cleft lip, giving the appearance of whistling.

Whitehead d., circumferential mucosal ectropion at the anus following Whitehead's operation.

de·fur·fur·a·tion (dē-fer-fer-ā′shŭn). The shedding of the epidermis in the form of fine scales. SYN branny desquamation. [L. *de,* away from, + *furfur,* bran]

de·gan·gli·on·ate (dē-gang′glē-on-āt). To deprive of ganglia.

de·gen·er·a·cy (dē-jen′er-ă-sē). **1.** A condition marked by deterioration of mental, physical, or moral processes. **2.** The fact that several different triplet codons encode the same amino acid. [L. *de,* from, + *genus, (gener-),* race]

de·gen·er·ate. 1 (dē-jen′er-āt). To pass to a lower level of mental, physical, or moral state; to fall below the normal or acceptable type or state. **2** (dē-jen′ĕ-răt). Below the normal or acceptable; that which has passed to a lower level.

de·gen·er·a·tio (dē-jen-er-ā′shē-ō). SYN degeneration. [L. *degenero,* pp. *-atus,* fr. *de,* from, + *genus,* race]

de

DEGENERATION

de·gen·er·a·tion (dē-jen-er-ā'shŭn). **1.** Degeneration; passing from a higher to a lower level or type. **2.** A worsening of mental, physical, or moral qualities. **3.** A retrogressive pathologic change in cells or tissues, in consequence of which their functions often are impaired or destroyed; sometimes reversible, in the early stages necrosis results. SYN retrograde metamorphosis. SYN degeneratio. [L. *degeneratio*]

adipose d., SYN fatty d.

adiposogenital d., SYN *dystrophia* adiposogenitalis.

age-related macular d., a common macular d. beginning with drusen of the macula and pigment disruption and sometimes leading to severe loss of central vision.

albuminoid d., albuminous d., obsolete terms for cloudy *swelling*.

amyloid d., infiltration of amyloid between cells and fibers of tissues and organs. SYN waxy d. (1).

angiolithic d., calcareous d. of the walls of the blood vessels.

ascending d., (1) retrograde d. of an injured nerve fiber; *i.e.,* toward the nerve cell of the fiber; **(2)** d. cephalad to a spinal cord lesion.

atheromatous d., focal accumulation of lipid material (atheroma) in the intima and subintimal portion of arteries, eventually resulting in fibrous thickening or calcification.

axon d., SYN axonal d.

axonal d., a type of peripheral nerve fiber response to insult, wherein axon death and subsequent breakdown occurs, with secondary breakdown of the myelin sheath associated; caused by focal injury to peripheral nerve fibers; often referred to as wallerian d. SYN axon d.

ballooning d., a phenomenon observed especially in cells that are infected with certain viruses, resulting in conspicuous swelling of the cell and cytoplasmic vacuolation.

basophilic d., blue staining of connective tissues when hematoxylin-eosin stain is used; found in such conditions as solar elastosis.

calcareous d., in a precise sense, not a degenerative process *per se*, but the deposition of insoluble calcium salts in tissue that has degenerated and become necrotic, as in dystrophic calcification.

carneous d., SYN red d.

caseous d., SYN caseous *necrosis*.

colliquative d., obsolete term for liquefaction d.

colloid d., a d. similar to mucoid d., in which the material is inspissated.

cone d., SYN cone *dystrophy*.

Crooke's hyaline d., SYN Crooke's hyaline *change*.

descending d., (1) orthograde (wallerian) d. of an injured nerve fiber; *i.e.,* distal to the lesion; **(2)** d. caudal to the level of a spinal cord lesion.

disciform d., foveal or parafoveal subretinal neovascularization with retinal separation and hemorrhage leading finally to a circular mass of fibrous tissue with marked loss of visual acuity. SYN disciform macular d.

disciform macular d., SYN disciform d.

ectatic marginal d. of cornea, SYN marginal corneal d.

elastoid d., (1) SYN elastosis (2). **(2)** hyaline d. of the elastic tissue of the arterial wall, seen during involution of the uterus.

elastotic d., SYN elastosis (2).

familial pseudoinflammatory macular d. [MIM*136900], macular d. that occurs during the fifth decade of life, with sudden development of a central scotoma in one eye followed rapidly by a similar lesion in the opposite eye; autosomal dominant inheritance. SYN Sorsby's macular d.

fascicular d., muscular d. due to loss of motor neurons in the spinal cord or brainstem.

fatty d., abnormal formation of microscopically visible droplets of fat in the cytoplasm of cells, as a result of injury. SYN adipose d., steatosis (2).

fibrinoid d., fibrinous d., a process resulting in poorly defined, deeply acidophilic, homogeneous refractile deposits with some staining reactions that resemble fibrin, occurring in connective tissue, blood vessel walls, and other sites.

fibrous d., not a d. *per se*, but rather a reparative process; cells and foci of tissue previously affected with degenerative processes, and necrosis, are replaced by cellular fibrous tissue.

granular d., SYN cloudy *swelling*.

granulovacuolar d., d. of hippocampal brain cells in elderly persons, characterized by basophilic granules surrounded by a clear zone in hippocampal neurons; occurs more frequently in Alzheimer's disease.

gray d., d. of the white substance of the spinal cord, the fibers of which lose their myelin sheaths and become darker in color.

hepatolenticular d., (1) a familial disorder characterized by copper deposition in the liver, causing chronic hepatitis and eventually cirrhosis; d. of the lenticular (pallidal and putaminal) nuclei, and marked hyperplasia of astrocytes in the cerebral cortex, cerebellum, basal ganglia, and brainstem nuclei; plasma levels of ceruloplasmins and copper are decreased, urinary excretion of copper is increased, and the amounts of copper in the liver, brain, and kidneys is high; clinical features include deposition of golden brown pigment in the cornea (Kayser-Fleischer rings), dysphasia and dysarthria, rigidity, and a coarse resting tremor, which increases when the limbs are outstretched ("wing-beating" tremor); autosomal recessive inheritance; **(2)** SYN Wilson's *disease* (1).

hyaline d., a group of several degenerative processes that affect various cells and tissues, resulting in the formation of rounded masses ("droplets") or relatively broad bands of substances that are homogeneous, translucent, refractile, and moderately to deeply acidophilic; may occur in the collagen of old fibrous tissue, smooth muscle of arterioles or the uterus, and as droplets in parenchymal cells.

hyaloideoretinal d. [MIM*163200], progressive liquefaction and destruction of the vitreous humor with grayish-white preretinal membranes, myopia, cataract, retinal detachment, and hyper- and hypopigmentation; autosomal dominant inheritance. SYN Wagner's disease, Wagner's syndrome.

hydropic d., SYN cloudy *swelling*.

infantile neuronal d., degenerative disorder of infants with widespread neuronal loss in thalamus, cerebellum, pons, and spinal cord, resembling infantile muscular atrophy.

Kuhnt-Junius d., an obsolete eponym for disciform d. SYN Kuhnt-Junius disease.

lenticular progressive d., SYN Wilson's *disease* (1).

liquefaction d., (1) necrosis with softening, as in ischemic brain tissue; **(2)** dissolution of the basal epidermal layer by necrosis of scattered cells with edema, observed in lichen planus, lupus erythematosus, and other dermatologic conditions.

macular d., any ocular d. affecting predominantly the posterior fundus, but most commonly age-related macular d.

marginal corneal d., bilateral opacification and vascularization of the periphery of the cornea, progressing to formation of a gutter and ectasia. SYN ectatic marginal d. of cornea.

Mönckeberg's d., SYN Mönckeberg's *arteriosclerosis*.

mucinoid d., a term including both mucoid and colloid d., the essential cellular changes in both being similar, the only difference being that, in colloid d., the substance is firmer and more inspissated than in mucoid d., in which it is thin and jelly-like.

mucoid d., a conversion of any of the connective tissues into a gelatinous or mucoid substance. SYN myxoid d., myxomatous d., myxomatosis (2).

mucoid medial d., SYN cystic medial *necrosis*.

myelinic d., formation of myelin figures in the cytoplasm of cells, possibly by degradation or hydration of lipoprotein of self-digested organelles.

myopic d., association of crescent of the optic disk, atrophy of the choroid and macular pigment, subretinal neovascularization, hemorrhage, and pigment proliferation in pathologic myopia.

myxoid d., myxomatous d., SYN mucoid d.

neurofibrillary d., formation of coarse, argentophilic, intracytoplasmic fibers, often in complex tangles within intracranial nerve cells that are undergoing aging. SEE ALSO Alzheimer's *disease.*

Nissl d., d. of the cell body occurring after transection of the axon; characterized by dispersion of the granular endoplasmic reticulum, swelling of the soma, and an eccentric position of the nucleus of the cell.

olivopontocerebellar d., SYN olivopontocerebellar *atrophy.*

orthograde d., SYN wallerian d.

parenchymatous d., SYN cloudy *swelling.*

primary neuronal d., SYN Alzheimer's *disease.*

primary pigmentary d. of retina, SYN tapetoretinal d.

primary progressive cerebellar d., a familial ataxic condition related to cerebellar d.

pseudotubular d., a form of d. observed in adrenal glands, especially those of patients with febrile infectious disease; the shrunken, lipid-depleted cells of the zona fasciculata (and sometimes the zona glomerulosa) are arranged in a circular pattern about spaces that may be empty or partly filled with fibrin, necrotic cells, or amorphous material.

red d., necrosis, with staining by hemoglobin, which may occur in uterine myomas, especially during pregnancy; marked by softening and a red color resembling partly cooked meat. SYN carneous d.

reticular d., severe epidermal edema resulting in multilocular bullae.

retrograde d., retrograde cell d. with chromatolysis of Nissl bodies and peripheral displacement of the nucleus of the cell of origin of a nerve fiber injured or sectioned.

Salzmann's nodular corneal d., large and prominent nodules of a solid, opaque material that stands out from the surface of the cornea; occurs occasionally in persons previously affected by phlyctenular keratitis.

secondary d., SYN wallerian d.

senile d., the process of involution occurring in old age.

Sorsby's macular d., SYN familial pseudoinflammatory macular d.

spongy d. of infancy [MIM*271900], SYN Canavan's *disease.*

subacute combined d. of the spinal cord, a subacute or chronic disorder of the spinal cord, such as that occurring in certain patients with vitamin B_{12} deficiency, characterized by a slight to moderate degree of gliosis in association with spongiform degeneration of the posterior and lateral columns. SYN combined sclerosis, combined system disease, funicular myelitis (2), Putnam-Dana syndrome, vitamin B_{12} neuropathy.

tapetoretinal d. [MIM*272600], a hereditary disorder of the retina mainly affecting photoreceptors and retinal pigment epithelium; a miscellaneous category including Friedreich's *ataxia,* Refsum's *disease,* and abetalipoproteinemia. SYN primary pigmentary d. of retina.

Terrien's marginal d., a form of marginal corneal d.

transsynaptic d., an atrophy of nerve cells following damage to the axons that make synaptic connection with them; noted especially in the lateral geniculate body. SYN transneuronal atrophy, transsynaptic chromatolysis.

Türck's d., d. of a nerve fiber and its sheath distal to the point of injury or section of the axon; usually applied to d. within the central nervous system.

vacuolar d., formation of nonlipid vacuoles in cytoplasm, most frequently due to accumulation of water by cloudy swelling.

vitelliform d. [MIM*153700], d. in Best's disease, with the macular region of each eye occupied by a bright orange-yellow circular deposit resembling an egg yolk, followed by scarring; autosomal dominant inheritance. SYN vitelliruptive d.

vitelliruptive d., SYN vitelliform d.

wallerian d., the degenerative changes the distal segment of a peripheral nerve fiber (axon and myelin) undergoes when its continuity with its cell body is interrupted by a focal lesion. SYN orthograde d., secondary d.

waxy d., (1) SYN amyloid d. (2) SYN Zenker's d.

xerotic d., scarring of the conjunctiva associated with keratinized epithelium.

Zenker's d., a form of severe hyaline d. or necrosis in skeletal muscle, occurring in severe infections. SYN waxy d. (2), Zenker's necrosis.

de·gen·er·a·tive (dē-jen′er-ă-tiv). Relating to degeneration.

de·glov·ing (dē-glov′ing). **1.** Intraoral surgical exposure of the anterior mandible used in various orthognathic surgical operations such as genioplasty or mandibular alveolar surgery. **2.** SEE degloving *injury.*

deglut. Abbreviation for L. *deglutiatur,* swallow.

de·glu·ti·tion (dē-glū-tish′ŭn). The act of swallowing. [L. *de-glutio,* to swallow]

de·glu·ti·tive (dē-glū′ti-tiv). Relating to deglutition.

Degos, R., French dermatologist, *1904. SEE D.'s *acanthoma, disease, syndrome;* Kohlmeier-D. *syndrome.*

deg·ra·da·tion (deg-ră-dā′shŭn). The change of a chemical compound into a less complex compound. [L. *degradatus,* degrade]

de·gran·u·la·tion (dē-gran-yū-lā′shŭn). Disappearance of cytoplasmic granules (lysosomes) from a cell.

de·gree (dĕ-grē′). **1.** One of the divisions on the scale of a measuring instrument such as a thermometer, barometer, etc. See Comparative Temperature Scales appendix. SEE scale. **2.** The 360th part of the circumference of a circle. **3.** A position or rank within a graded series. **4.** A measure of damage to tissue. [Fr. *degré;* L. *gradus,* a step]

d.'s of freedom, in statistics, the number of independent comparisons that can be made between the members of a sample (*e.g.,* subjects, test items and scores, trials, conditions); in a contingency table it is on e less than the number of row categories multiplied by one less than the number of column categories.

de·gus·ta·tion (dē-gŭs-tā′shŭn). **1.** The act of tasting. **2.** The sense of taste. [L. *degustatio,* fr. *de-gusto,* pp. *-atus,* to taste]

de·hal·o·gen·ase (dē-hal′ō-jen-ās). Any enzyme (EC subclass 3.8) removing halogen atoms from organic halides.

Dehio, Karl K., Russian physician, 1851–1927. SEE D.'s *test.*

de·his·cence (dē-his′ens). A bursting open, splitting, or gaping along natural or sutured lines. [L. *dehisco,* to split apart or open]

iris d., a defect of the eye characterized by multiple holes in the iris.

root d., a loss of the buccal or lingual bone overlaying the root portion of a tooth, leaving that area covered by soft tissue only.

wound d., disruption of apposed surfaces of a wound.

de·hu·man·i·za·tion (dē-hyū′măn-i-zā′shŭn). Loss of human characteristics; brutalization by either mental or physical means; stripping one of self-esteem. [*de-* + *humanus,* human, fr. *homo,* man]

de·hy·drase (dē-hī′drās). Former name for dehydratase.

de·hy·dra·tase (dē-hī′drā-tās). A subclass (EC 4.2.1) of lyases (hydro-lyases) that remove H and OH as H_2O from a substrate, leaving a double bond, or add a group to a double bond by the elimination of water from two substances to form a third; synthase is sometimes used when the synthetic aspect of the reaction is emphasized. Some trivial names of enzymes in this subclass bear the generic term hydratase, emphasizing the reverse reaction.

de·hy·drate (dē-hī′drāt). **1.** To extract water from. **2.** To lose water. [L. *de,* from + G. *hydōr* (*hydr-*), water]

de·hy·dra·tion (dē-hī-drā′shŭn). **1.** Deprivation of water. SYN anhydration. **2.** Reduction of water content. **3.** SYN exsiccation (2). **4.** SYN desiccation.

absolute d., actual water deficit as measured by a difference from the normal or from a given water content.

relative d., water deficit relative to content of solutes contributing effective osmotic pressure; a state of increased effective osmotic pressure of body fluids.

voluntary d., that physiologic lag or deficit that results when sensations of thirst are not strong enough to bring about complete replacement of water loss, as in rapid sweating.

△**dehydro-.** Prefix used in the names of those chemical compounds that differ from other and more familiar compounds in the absence of two hydrogen atoms; *e.g.*, dehydroascorbic acid, which resembles ascorbic acid in all structural features except for its lack of two hydrogen atoms that are present in the ascorbic acid molecule. In systematic nomenclature, didehydro- is preferred as being more exact.

de·hy·dro·a·ce·tic ac·id (dē-hī′drō-ă-sē′tik). 3-Acetyl-6-methyl-2*H*-pyran-2,4-(3*H*)-dione; an antimicrobial agent used as a preservative in cosmetics.

L-**de·hy·dro·a·scor·bic ac·id** (dē-hī′drō-as-kōr′bik). The reversibly oxidized form of ascorbic acid; it is antiscorbutic, but is converted in the body to 2,3-diketo-L-gulonic acid, which has no vitamin C activity.

de·hy·dro·bil·i·ru·bin (dē-hī′drō-bil-ĕ-rū′bin). SYN biliverdin.

de·hy·dro·cho·late (dē-hī-drō-kō′lāt). A salt or ester of dehydrocholic acid.

7-de·hy·dro·cho·les·ter·ol (dē-hī′drō-kō-les′ter-ol). cholesta-5,7-dien-3β-ol; a zoosterol in skin and other animal tissues that upon activation by ultraviolet light becomes antirachitic and is then referred to as cholecalciferol (vitamin D_3). SYN provitamin D_3.

24-de·hy·dro·cho·les·ter·ol. SYN desmosterol.

de·hy·dro·cho·lic ac·id (dē-hī-drō-kol′ik). 3,7,12-Trioxo-5β-cholan-24-oic acid; has a stimulating effect upon the secretion of bile by the liver (choleretic), and improves the absorption of essential food materials in states associated with deficient bile formation.

11-de·hy·dro·cor·ti·co·ster·one (dē-hī′drō-kōr-ti-kos′ter-ōn). 21-Hydroxypregn-4-ene-3,11,20-trione; principally a metabolite of corticosterone, found in the adrenal cortex.

de·hy·dro·em·e·tine (dē-hī-drō-em′ĕ-tēn). A synthetic derivative of emetine; used in the treatment of intestinal amebiasis.

    d. resinate, a derivative of emetine.

de·hy·dro-3-ep·i·an·dros·ter·one (dē-hī′drō-ep-i-an-dros′ter-ōn). 3β-hydroxyandrost-5-ene-17-one; a weakly androgenic steroid secreted largely by the adrenal cortex, but also by the testes; one of the principal components of urinary 17-ketosteroids; a precursor of testosterone. SYN androstenolone, dehydroisoandrosterone.

de·hy·dro·gen·ase (dē-hī′drō-jen-ās). Class name for those enzymes that oxidize substrates by catalyzing removal of hydrogen from metabolites (hydrogen donors) and transferring it to other substances (hydrogen acceptors), which are thus reduced; most of the oxidative enzymes (oxidoreductases, EC class 1) perform their oxidations in this manner.

    aerobic d., an enzyme (usually a metalloflavoenzyme) catalyzing the transfer of hydrogen from some metabolite to oxygen, forming hydrogen peroxide in the process; usually a metalloflavoenzyme; *e.g.*, xanthine oxidase and others in several sub-subclasses (*e.g.*, EC 1.1.3, 1.2.3, 1.7.3, 1.8.3, 1.10.3).

    α-**keto acid d.,** SEE α-keto acid dehydrogenase.

    anaerobic d., an enzyme (usually a pyridinoenzyme) catalyzing the transfer of hydrogen from some metabolite to some acceptor molecule (*e.g.*, NAD$^+$, cytochrome) other than oxygen; *e.g.*, lactate d.'s, isocitrate d.'s, and others in EC class 1, excluding those listed under aerobic d.

    Robison ester d., SYN glucose-6-phosphate dehydrogenase.

de·hy·dro·gen·ate (dē-hī′drō-jen-āt). To subject to dehydrogenation.

de·hy·dro·gen·a·tion (dē-hī′drō-jen-ā′shŭn). Removal of a pair of hydrogen atoms from a compound by the action of enzymes (dehydrogenases) or other catalysts.

de·hy·dro·i·so·an·dros·ter·one (dē-hī′drō-ī-sō-an-dros′ter-ōn). SYN dehydro-3-epiandrosterone.

de·hy·dro·pep·ti·dase II (dē-hī-drō-pep′ti-dās). SYN aminoacylase.

de·hy·dro·ret·i·nal·de·hyde (dē-hī′drō-ret-i-nal′dĕ-hīd). 3-Dehydroretinaldehyde; dehydroretinol with –CHO instead of –CH$_2$OH at the terminal carbon of the side chain. SYN retinene-2, vitamin A$_2$ aldehyde.

de·hy·dro·ret·i·no·ic ac·id (dē-hī′drō-ret-i-nō′ik). 3-Dehydro-

retinoic acid; dehydroretinol with –COOH in place of –CH$_2$OH at the terminal carbon of the side chain.

de·hy·dro·ret·i·nol (dē-hī-drō-ret′i-nol). 3-Dehydroretinol; retinol with an additional double bond in the 3-4 position of the cyclohexane ring. SYN vitamin A$_2$.

de·hy·dro·sug·ars (dē-hī′drō-shug-erz). SYN anhydrosugars.

de·hy·dro·tes·tos·ter·one (dē-hī′drō-tes-tos′ter-ōn). SYN boldenone.

de·hyp·no·tize (dē-hip′nō-tīz). To bring out of the hypnotic state.

de·im·i·nas·es (dē-im′i-nās-ez). SYN iminohydrolases.

de·in·sti·tu·tion·al·i·za·tion (dē′in-sti-tū′shŭn-ăl-i-zā-shŭn). The discharge of institutionalized patients from a mental hospital into treatment programs in half-way houses and other community-based programs.

de·i·on·i·za·tion (dē-ī′-on-ī-zā′shŭn). The production of a mineral-free state by the removal of ions.

Deiters, Otto F.K., German anatomist, 1834–1863. SEE D.'s *cells*, under *cell*, terminal *frames*, under *frame*, *nucleus*.

dé·jà vou·lu (dā-zhă′ vū-lū′). A term for a type of disturbance of memory in which the individual believes that his or her present desires are exactly the same as the desires the individual had some time before.

dé·jà vu (dā-zhah-vū′). Feeling of having been in a place before. SEE déjà vu *phenomenon*. SEE phenomenon. [Fr. already seen]

de·jec·ta (dē-jek′tă). SYN dejection (3). [L. neut, pl. of *de-jectus*, fr. *de-jicio*, to cast down]

de·jec·tion (dē-jek′shŭn). **1.** SYN depression (4). **2.** The discharge of excrementitious matter. **3.** The matter so discharged. SYN dejecta. [L. *dejectio*, fr. *de- jicio*, pp. *-jectus*, to cast down]

Dejerine, Joseph J., Paris neurologist, 1849–1917. SEE D.'s *disease*, hand *phenomenon*, *reflex*, *sign*; D.-Lichtheim *phenomenon*; D.-Roussy *syndrome*; D.-Sottas *disease*; D.-Klumpke *syndrome*; Landouzy-D. *dystrophy*.

Dejerine-Klumpke, Augusta, French neurologist (born in the U.S.), 1859–1927. SEE Klumpke *palsy*; Klumpke's *paralysis*; Dejerine-Klumpke *palsy*; Dejerine-Klumpke *syndrome*.

△**deka-.** SEE deca-.

Delafield, Francis, U.S. physician and pathologist, 1841–1915. SEE D.'s *hematoxylin*.

de·lam·i·na·tion (dē-lam-i-nā′shŭn). Division into separate layers. [L. *de*, from, + *lamina*, a thin plate]

Delaney clause. A clause of the Food Additive Amendment of the U.S. Federal law specifying that no substance that has been found to induce cancer in any animal may be incorporated into food. [James F. *Delaney*, U.S. Congressman]

de Lange, Cornelia, Dutch pediatrician, 1871–1950. SEE de L. *syndrome*.

Delbet, Pierre, French surgeon, 1861–1925. SEE D.'s *sign*.

Del Castillo, E.B., 20th century Argentinian physician. SEE Del C. *syndrome*; Argonz-Del C. *syndrome*; Ahumada-Del C. *syndrome*.

de·lead (dē-led′). To cause the mobilization and excretion of lead deposited in the bones and other tissues, as by the administration of a chelating agent.

DeLee, Joseph B., U.S. obstetrician and gynecologist, 1869–1942. SEE DeL.'s *maneuver*.

del·e·te·ri·ous (del-ĕ-tēr′ē-ŭs). Injurious; noxious; harmful. [G. *dēlētērios*, fr. *dēleomai*, to injure]

de·le·tion (dĕ-lē′shŭn). In genetics, any spontaneous elimination of part of the normal genetic complement, whether cytogenetically visible (chromosomal d.) or inferred from phenotypic evidence (point d.). [L. *deletio*, destruction]

    chromosomal d., a microscopically evident loss of part of a chromosome. SEE ALSO monosomy.

    gene d., d. of a segment of a chromosome too small to be detected cytogenetically, inferred from the phenotype at one particular locus.

    interstitial d., d. that does not involve the terminal parts of a chromosome.

nucleotide d., d. of a single nucleotide, which in a transcribed gene will lead to a frame-shift mutation. SYN point d. (2).

point d., (1) d. involving a submicroscopic loss of genetic material too small to be resolved by linkage analysis; **(2)** SYN nucleotide d.

terminal d., d. involving the terminal part of a chromosome and leading to a adhesive terminus.

del·i·cate (del'i-kăt). Of feeble resisting power. [L. *delicatus,* soft, luxurious, fr. *de,* from, + *lacio,* to entice]

de·lim·i·ta·tion (dē-lim-i-tā'shŭn). Marking off; putting bounds or limits; preventing the spread of a morbid process in the body or of a disease in the community. [L. *de-limito,* pp. *-atus,* to bound, fr. *limes,* boundary]

del·i·quesce (del-i-kwes'). To undergo deliquescence.

del·i·ques·cence (del-i-kwes'ens). Becoming damp or liquid by absorption of water from the atmosphere; a property of certain salts, such as $CaCl_2$. [L. *de-liquesco,* to melt or become liquid]

del·i·ques·cent (del-i-kwes'ent). Denoting a solid capable of deliquescence.

de·li·ria (dē-lir'ē-ă). Plural of delirium.

de·lir·i·ant (de-lir'ē-ant). **1.** Causing delirium. **2.** A toxic agent that produces delirium.

de·lir·i·ous (de-lir'ē-ŭs). In a state of delirium.

de·lir·i·um, pl. **de·li·ria** (dē-lir'ē-ŭm, dē-lir'ē-ă). An altered state of consciousness, consisting of confusion, distractibility, disorientation, disordered thinking and memory, defective perception (illusions and hallucinations), prominent hyperactivity, agitation and autonomic nervous system overactivity; caused by a number of toxic structural and metabolic disorders. [L. fr. *deliro,* to be crazy, fr. *de-* + *lira,* a furrow (*i.e.,* go out of the furrow)]

acute d., d. of recent, rapid onset.

alcohol withdrawal d., the d. experienced by an alcohol-habituated individual caused by the abrupt cessation of alcohol intake.

anxious d., d. in which the predominating symptom is an incoherent apprehension or anxiety.

collapse d., d. caused by extreme physical depression induced by a shock, profuse hemorrhage, exhausting labor, etc.

d. cor'dis, obsolete term for atrial *fibrillation.*

low d., d. in which there is little excitement, either mental or motor, the ideas being confused and incoherent, but following each other slowly.

d. mus'sitans, muttering d., d. common in low fevers in which the subject is unconscious, but constantly mutters incoherently.

posttraumatic d., d. caused by a structural traumatic brain injury.

senile d., d. associated with senile dementia.

toxic d., d. caused by the action of a poison.

d. tre'mens (DT), a severe, sometimes fatal, form of d. due to alcoholic withdrawal following a period of sustained intoxication. [L. pres. p. of *tremo,* to tremble]

del·i·tes·cence (del-i-tes'ens). Rarely used term for: **1.** Sudden subsidence of symptoms; disappearance of a tumor or a cutaneous lesion. **2.** Period of incubation of an infectious disease. [L. *delitesco,* to lie hidden away]

de·liv·er (dē-liv'er). **1.** To assist a woman in childbirth. **2.** To extract from an enclosed place, as the fetus from the womb, an object or foreign body, *e.g.,* a tumor from its capsule or surroundings, or the lens of the eye in cases of cataract. [fr. O. Fr. fr. L. *de-* + *liber,* free]

de·liv·ery (dē-liv'er-ē). Passage of the fetus and the placenta from the genital canal into the external world.

assisted cephalic d., extraction of a fetus that presents by the head.

breech d., extraction or expulsion of a fetus that presents by the buttocks or feet.

forceps d., assisted birth of the child by an instrument designed to grasp the fetal head.

high forceps d., d. by forceps applied to the fetal head before engagement has taken place.

low forceps d., d. by forceps applied to the fetal head after it is

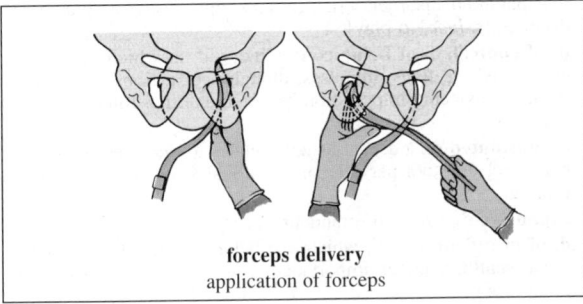

forceps delivery
application of forceps

clearly visible, the skull has reached the perineal floor, and plus 2 (+2) station. This classification of forceps delivery may be with or without rotation of the fetal head.

midforceps d., d. by forceps applied to the fetal head before the criteria of low forceps d. have been met, but after engagement has taken place.

outlet forceps d., d. by forceps applied to the fetal head when it has reached the perineal floor and is visible between contractions.

perimortem d., SYN postmortem d.

postmortem d., extraction of the fetus after the death of its mother. SYN perimortem d.

premature d., birth of a fetus before its proper time. SEE ALSO premature *birth.*

spontaneous cephalic d., unassisted expulsion of a fetus that presents by the head.

del·le (del'eh). The central lighter-colored portion of the erythrocyte, as observed in a stained film of blood. [D. *delle,* low ground, pit]

del·len. Shallow, saucer-like, clearly defined excavations at the margin of the cornea, about 1.5 by 2 mm, due to localized dehydration; also called Fuchs' dellen. [D. pl. of *delle,* low ground, pit]

del·o·mor·phous (del-ō-mōr'fŭs). Of definite form and shape; a term applied in the past to the parietal cells of the gastric glands. [G. *dēlos,* manifest, + *morphē,* form]

de·louse (dē-lows'). To remove lice from; to free from infestation with lice; used especially of prophylaxis of louse-borne diseases.

del·phi·nine (del'fin-ēn). A toxic alkaloid, an aconine derivative, from *Delphinium staphisagria;* it resembles aconitine in its action and chemical structure.

Del·phin·i·um aja·cis (del-fin'ē-ŭm ă-jā'sis). A species of plant (family Ranunculaceae) containing the alkaloids ajacine and ajaconine; the dried ripe seeds have been used externally as a parasiticide in pediculosis; rarely used now because of its toxicity. SYN larkspur. [G. *delphinion,* larkspur]

del·ta (del'tă). **1.** Fourth letter of the Greek alphabet, Δ (capital), δ (lower case). **2.** In anatomy, a triangular surface.

d. for'nicis, SYN *commissura* fornicis.

Galton's d., (1) a more or less well-marked triangle, in a fingerprint, on either side where the straight ridges near the joint of the distal phalanx are succeeded by arches, loops, or whorls; SEE ALSO Galton's system of classification of *fingerprints,* under *fingerprint.* **(2)** SYN triradius.

d. mesoscap'ulae, the flat triangular surface at the vertebral extremity of the spine of the scapula over which glides the tendon for the lower fibers of the trapezius muscle.

del·ta check. a comparison of consecutive values for a given test in a patient's laboratory file used to detect abrupt changes, usually generated as a part of computer-based quality control programs. SYN Δ check.

del·toid (del'toyd). **1.** Resembling the Greek letter delta (Δ); triangular. **2.** SYN deltoid *muscle.* [G. *deltoeidēs,* shaped like the letter *delta*]

de·lu·sion (dē-lū'zhŭn). A false belief or wrong judgment held with conviction despite incontrovertible evidence to the contrary.

de

SYN paranoid disorder. [L. *de-ludo,* pp. *-lusus,* to play false, deceive, fr. *ludo,* to play]

d. of control, d. of being controlled, a d. in which one experiences one's feelings, impulses, thoughts, or actions as not one's own, but as being imposed on by some external force. SYN d. of passivity.

encapsulated d., a d. that usually relates to one specific topic or belief but does not pervade an individual's life or level of functioning.

expansive d., SYN d. of grandeur.

d. of grandeur, a d. in which one believes oneself possessed of great wealth, intellect, importance, power, etc. SYN expansive d., grandiose d.

grandiose d., SYN d. of grandeur.

d. of negation, a d. in which one imagines that the world and all that relates to it have ceased to exist. SYN nihilistic d.

nihilistic d., SYN d. of negation.

organic d.'s, false beliefs experienced in the delirium associated with dementia in conjunction with traumatic injury to the brain, or an organic change in the brain such as in Alzheimer's syndrome, or in cocaine or other drug intoxication.

d. of passivity, SYN d. of control.

d. of persecution, persecutory d., a false notion that one is being persecuted; characteristic symptom of paranoid schizophrenia.

d. of reference, a delusional idea that external events, etc., refer to the self.

somatic d., a d. having reference to a nonexistent lesion or alteration of some organ or part of the body; sometimes indistinguishable from hypochondriasis.

systematized d., a d. that is logically constructed from a false premise and embraces a specific sector of the patient's life.

unsystematized d., one of a group of apparently discrete, disconnected d.'s.

de·lu·sion·al (dē-lū'zhŭn-ăl). Relating to a delusion.

de·mand (dē-mand'). A quantity of a substance, commodity, or service wanted or required.

biochemical oxygen d. (BOD), the rate at which dissolved oxygen is consumed by an organism (often, a microorganism) or a culture of cells.

de·mar·ca·tion (dē-mar-kā'shŭn). A setting of limits; a boundary. [Fr. fr. L. *de,* from, + Mediev. L. *marco,* to mark]

Demarquay, Jean N., French surgeon, 1811–1875. SEE D.'s *symptom.*

de·mas·cu·lin·iz·ing (dē-mas'kyū-lin-īz'ing). Depriving of male characteristics or inhibiting development of such characteristics.

De·mat·i·a·ce·ae (dē-mat-ē-ā'sē-ē). A family of soil-inhabiting, brown or black melanin-producing fungi found in decaying vegetables, rotting wood, and forest carpets, and including several of the dark-colored genera that cause chromoblastomycosis in man, such as *Phialophora, Fonsecaea,* and *Cladosporium.*

de·mat·i·a·ceous (dē-mat-ē-ā'shŭs). Denoting dark conidia and/or hyphae, usually brown or black; used frequently to denote dark-colored fungi.

deme (dēm). A local, small, highly inbred group or kinship. Cf. isolate. [G. *dēmos,* people]

dem·e·car·i·um bro·mide (dem-ĕ-kar'ē-ŭm). A potent cholinesterase inhibitor used in the treatment of glaucoma and accommodative esotropia; it is stable in aqueous solution.

dem·e·clo·cy·cline (dem'ē-klō-sī'klēn). Demethylchlortetracycline; 7-chloro-6-demethyltetracycline; a broad-spectrum antibiotic that is more slowly excreted and more stable in acid and alkali than are other forms of the tetracyclines; available as the hydrochloride.

dem·e·col·cine (dem-ĕ-kol'sēn). *N*-Desacetyl-*N*-methylcolchicine; an alkaloid from *Colchicum autumnale* (family Liliaceae) similar chemically to colchicine except that the acetyl group is replaced by a methyl group; used for gout and leukemia, is said to be less toxic than colchicine, and has an action upon mitosis similar to that of colchicine.

de·ment·ed (dē-ment'ed). Suffering from dementia.

de·men·tia (dē-men'shē-ă). The loss, usually progressive, of cognitive and intellectual functions, without impairment of perception or consciousness; caused by a variety of disorders, most commonly structural brain disease. Characterized by disorientation, impaired memory, judgment, and intellect, and a shallow labile affect. SYN amentia (2). [L. fr. *de-* priv. + *mens,* mind]

AIDS d., SYN AIDS dementia *complex.*

Alzheimer's d., SYN Alzheimer's *disease.*

catatonic d., d. with catatonic symptoms.

dialysis d., SYN dialysis encephalopathy *syndrome.*

epileptic d., d. occurring in an individual afflicted with epilepsy, and thought to be a result of prolonged seizures, the epileptogenic brain lesion, or antiepileptic drugs.

hebephrenic d., d. with hebephrenic symptoms.

multi-infarct d., SYN vascular d.

paralytic d., d. and paralysis resulting from a chronic syphilitic meningoencephalitis. SYN d. paralytica.

d. paralytica, SYN paralytic d.

d. paranoi'des, d. with paranoid features.

posttraumatic d., d. caused by traumatic brain injury.

d. prae'cox, any one of the group of psychotic disorders known as the schizophrenias; formerly used to describe schizophrenia as a single entity. [L. precocious]

presenile d., d. preseni'lis, (1) d. of Alzheimer's disease developing before age 65; **(2)** SYN Alzheimer's *disease.*

primary d., d. occurring independently as a mental disorder.

primary senile d., SYN Alzheimer's *disease.*

secondary d., chronic d. following and due to a psychosis or some other underlying disease process.

senile d., d. of Alzheimer's disease developing after age 65.

toxic d., d. caused by an exogenous agent.

transmissible d., SYN Creutzfeldt-Jakob *disease.*

vascular d., a step-like deterioration in intellectual functions with focal neurological signs, as the result of multiple infarctions of the cerebral hemispheres. SYN multi-infarct d.

de·meth·yl·ase (dē-meth'i-lās). SYN methyltransferase.

de·meth·yl·a·tion. The enzymatic removal of methyl groups.

△**demi-.** Half, lesser. SEE ALSO hemi-, semi-. [Fr. fr. L. *dimidius,* half]

dem·i·gaunt·let (dem-ē-gawnt'let). A glovelike bandage for the fingers and hand. [demi- + *gauntlet,* armored glove, fr. M.E., fr. O. Fr., fr. Germanic]

dem·i·lune (dem'ē-lūn). **1.** A small body with a form similar to that of a half-moon or a crescent. **2.** Term frequently used for the gametocyte of *Plasmodium falciparum.* [Fr. half-moon]

Giannuzzi's d.'s, SYN serous d.'s.

Heidenhain's d.'s, SYN serous d.'s.

serous d.'s, the serous cells at the distal end of a mucous, tubuloalveolar secretory unit of certain salivary glands. SYN Giannuzzi's crescents, Giannuzzi's d.'s, Heidenhain's crescents, Heidenhain's d.'s.

de·min·er·al·i·za·tion (dē-min'er-ăl-ī-zā'shŭn). A loss or decrease of the mineral constituents of the body or individual tissues, especially of bone.

dem·i·pen·ni·form (dem'ē-pen'i-fōrm). SYN unipennate.

Dem·o·dex (dem'ō-deks). A genus of very minute (0.1 to 0.4 mm) follicular mites (family Demodicidae) that inhabit the skin and are usually found in the sebaceous glands and hair follicles of mammals, including humans. [G. *dēmos,* tallow, + *dēx,* a woodworm]

D. bo'vis, a species that causes large swellings in the skin, filled with fluid or a cheezy material containing mites, which damages the hide of cattle.

D. ca'nis, species causing red or demodectic mange in dogs, characterized by alopecia and commonly associated with staphylococcal pyoderma.

D. ca'ti, a species causing mange in cats.

D. folliculo'rum, a very common, universally distributed, and usually nonpathogenic species of mite that inhabits the hair follicles and sebaceous glands of humans, commonly around the nose and scalp margins. SYN *Acarus folliculorum, Simonea folliculorum.*

de·mog·ra·phy (dĕ-mog′ră-fē). The study of populations, especially with reference to size, density, fertility, mortality, growth rate, age distribution, migration, and vital statistics. [G. *demos,* people, + *graphō,* to write]

dynamic d., a study of the functioning of a community, including statistical records.

Demoivre, Abraham, English mathematician, 1667–1754. SEE D.'s *formula.*

de·mo·ni·ac (dē-mō′nē-ak). Frenzied, fiendish, as if possessed by evil spirits. [G. *daimōn,* a spirit]

dem·on·stra·tor (dem′on-strā-ter, -tōr). An assistant to a professor of anatomy, surgery, etc., who prepares for the lecture by dissections, collection of patients, etc., or who instructs small classes supplementary to the regular lectures; a d. corresponds in a general way to the Dozent of a German university. [L. *de-monstro,* pp. *-atus,* to point out]

De Morgan, Campbell, English physician, 1811–1876. SEE De M.'s *spots,* under *spot.*

de·mor·phin·i·za·tion (dē-mōr′fin-i-zā′shŭn). **1.** Removal of morphine from an opiate. **2.** Gradual withdrawal of morphine as a method of overcoming morphine dependence.

de Morsier, G., 20th century Swiss neurologist. SEE de M.'s *syndrome.*

de·mu·co·sa·tion (dē-myū-kō-sā′shŭn). Rarely used term for excision or stripping of the mucosa of any part.

de·mul·cent (de-mŭl′sent). **1.** Soothing; relieving irritation. **2.** An agent, such as a mucilage or oil, that soothes and relieves irritation, especially of the mucous surfaces. [L. *de-mulceo,* pp. *-mulctus,* to stroke lightly, to soften]

de Musset, Alfred. SEE Musset.

de·my·e·li·na·tion, de·my·e·lin·i·za·tion (dē-mī′ĕ-li-nā′shŭn, dē-mī′ĕ-lin-i-za′shŭn). Loss of myelin with preservation of the axons or fiber tracts. Central demyelination occurs within the central nervous system (*e.g.,* the demyelination seen with multiple sclerosis); peripheral demyelination affects the peripheral nervous system (*e.g.,* the demyelination seen with Guillain-Barré syndrome).

de·nar·co·tize (dē-nar′kō-tīz). To remove narcotic properties from an opiate; to deprive of narcotic properties.

de·na·to·ni·um ben·zo·ate (dē-nă-tō′nē-ŭm). Benzyldiethyl[(2,6-xylylcarbamoyl)methyl]ammonium benzoate; an alcohol denaturant.

de·na·tur·a·tion (dē-na-tyū-rā′shŭn). The process of becoming denatured.

de·na·tured (dē-nā′tyūrd). **1.** Made unnatural or changed from the normal in any of its characteristics; often applied to proteins or nucleic acids heated or otherwise treated to the point where tertiary structural characteristics are altered. **2.** Adulterated, as by addition of methanol to ethanol.

den·drax·on (den-drak′son). Obsolete term for telodendron. [G. *dendron,* tree, + *axōn,* axis]

den·dri·form (den′dri-fōrm). Tree-shaped, or branching. SYN arborescent, dendritic (1), dendroid. [G. *dendron,* tree, + L. *forma,* form]

den·drite (den′drīt). **1.** One of the two types of branching protoplasmic processes of the nerve cell (the other being the axon). SYN dendritic process, dendron, neurodendrite, neurodendron. **2.** A crystalline treelike structure formed during the freezing of an alloy. [G. *dendritēs,* relating to a tree]

apical d., SYN apical *process.*

den·drit·ic (den-drit′ik). **1.** SYN dendriform. **2.** Relating to the dendrites of nerve cells.

den·dro·gram (den′drō-gram). A treelike figure used to represent graphically a hierarchy. [*dendron,* tree, + *gramma,* a drawing]

den·droid (den′droyd). SYN dendriform. [G. *dendron,* tree, + *eidos,* appearance]

den·dron. SYN dendrite (1). [G. a tree]

de·ner·vate (dē-ner′vāt). To cause denervation.

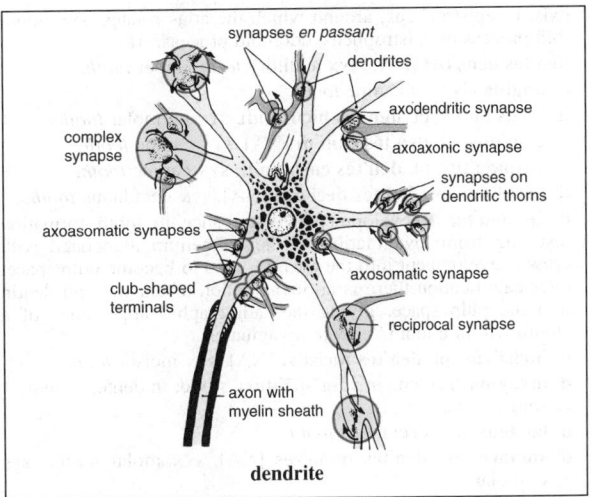

synapses *en passant*
dendrites
axodendritic synapse
complex synapse
axoaxonic synapse
synapses on dendritic thorns
axoasomatic synapses
axosomatic synapse
club-shaped terminals
reciprocal synapse
axon with myelin sheath

dendrite

de

de·ner·va·tion (dē-ner-vā′shŭn). Loss of nerve supply.

den·gue (den′gā). A disease of tropical and subtropical regions that occurs epidemically, is caused by dengue virus, a member of the family Flaviviridae. There are 4 antigenic types, and they are transmitted by a mosquito of the genus *Aedes* (usually *A. aegypti,* but frequently *A. albopictus*). Four grades of severity are recognized: grade I, fever and constitutional symptoms; grade II, grade I plus spontaneous bleeding (of skin, gums, or gastrointestinal tract); grade III, grade II plus agitation and circulatory failure; grade IV, profound shock. SYN Aden fever, bouquet fever, breakbone fever, dandy fever, date fever, dengue fever, dengue hemorrhagic fever, exanthesis arthrosia, polka fever, scarlatina rheumatica, solar fever (1). [Sp. corruption of "dandy" fever]

hemorrhagic d., a more severe epidemic form of d. characterized by hemorrhagic skin lesions, which has erupted in a number of epidemic outbreaks in the Pacific basin.

de·ni·al (dē-nī′ăl). An unconscious defense mechanism used to allay anxiety by denying the existence of important conflicts or troublesome impulses. SYN negation. [M.E., fr, O. Fr., fr. L. *denegare,* to say no]

den·i·da·tion (den-i-dā′shŭn). Exfoliation of the superficial portion of the mucous membrane of the uterus; stripping off of the menstrual decidua. [L. *de,* from, + *nidus,* nest]

de·ni·tra·tion (dē-nī-trā′shŭn). SYN denitrification.

de·ni·tri·fi·ca·tion (dē-nī′tri-fi-kā′shŭn). **1.** Removal of nitrogen from any material or chemical compound; especially from the soil, as by certain (denitrifying) bacteria that render the nitrogen unavailable for plant growth. **2.** Withdrawal of nitrogen from soil by plant growth. SYN denitration.

de·ni·tri·fy (dē-nī′tri-fī). To remove nitrogen from any material or chemical compound.

de·ni·tro·gen·a·tion (dē-nī′trō-jĕ-nā′shŭn). Elimination of nitrogen from lungs and body tissues by breathing gases devoid of nitrogen.

Denman, Thomas, English obstetrician, 1733–1815. SEE D.'s spontaneous *evolution.*

Dennie, Charles Clayton, U.S. dermatologist, 1883–1971. SEE D.'s infraorbital *fold, line.*

de·nom·in·a·tor (dē-nōm′i-nā-tor). The lower portion of a fraction used to calculate a rate or ratio; the population at risk in the calculation of a rate or ratio.

Denonvilliers, Charles P., French surgeon, 1808–1872. SEE D.'s *aponeurosis, ligament.*

de novo (di-nō′vō). Anew; often applied to particular biochemical pathways in which metabolites are newly biosynthesized (*e.g., de novo* purine biosynthesis). [L.]

dens, pl. **den·tes** (denz, den′tēz) [NA]. **1.** SYN Tooth. **2.** A strong toothlike process projecting upward from the body of the axis, or epistropheus, around which the atlas rotates. SYN odontoid process of epistropheus, odontoid process. [L.]

den·tes acus′tici [NA], SYN auditory *teeth*, under *tooth*.

d. angula′ris, SYN canine *tooth*.

d. bicus′pidus, pl. **den′tes bicus′pidi**, SYN premolar *tooth*.

d. cani′nus, pl. **den′tes cani′ni** [NA], SYN canine *tooth*.

d. cuspida′tus, pl. **den′tes cuspida′ti**, SYN canine *tooth*.

d. decid′uus, pl. **den′tes deci′dui** [NA], SYN deciduous *tooth*.

d. in den′te, a developmental disturbance in tooth formation resulting from invagination of the epithelium associated with crown development into the area destined to become pulp space; after calcification there is an invagination of enamel and dentin into the pulp space, giving the radiographic appearance of a "tooth within a tooth." SYN d. invaginatus.

d. incisi′vus, pl. **den′tes incisi′vi** [NA], SYN incisor *tooth*.

d. invaginatus (denz in′vă-gē-nā′-tus), SYN d. in dente. [Mediev. L. folded inward, fr. L. *vagina*, sheath]

d. lac′teus, SYN deciduous *tooth*.

d. molaris, pl. **den′tes mola′res** [NA], SYN molar *tooth*. SEE ALSO molar.

d. per′manens, pl. **den′tes permanen′tes** [NA], SYN permanent *tooth*.

d. premola′ris, pl. **den′tes premola′res** [NA], SYN premolar *tooth*.

d. sapien′tiae, SYN third *molar*. [L. *sapientia*, wisdom]

d. seroti′nus [NA], SYN third *molar*.

d. succeda′neus, SYN permanent *tooth*.

den·sim·e·ter (den-sim′ĕ-ter). SYN densitometer (1). [L. *densitas*, density, + G. *metron*, measure]

den·si·tom·e·ter (den-si-tom′ĕ-ter). **1.** An instrument for measuring the density of a fluid. SYN densimeter. **2.** An instrument for measuring, by virtue of relative turbidity, the growth of bacteria in broth; useful in microbiologic assay of nutrients and antibiotics, phage studies, etc. **3.** An instrument for measuring the density of components (*e.g.*, protein fractions) separated by electrophoresis or chromatography, utilizing light absorption or reflection. **4.** An electronic instrument for measuring the blackening of radiographic film by x-ray exposure; used for film sensitometry, bone densitometry, measurement of line spread function (microdensitometer). [L. *densitas*, density, + G. *metron*, measure]

den·si·tom·e·try (den-si-tom′ĕ-trē). A procedure utilizing a densitometer.

den·si·ty (den′si-tē). **1.** The compactness of a substance; the ratio of mass to unit volume, usually expressed as g/cm^3 (kg/m^3 in the SI system). **2.** The quantity of electricity on a given surface or in a given time per unit of volume. **3.** In radiological physics, the opacity to light of an exposed radiographic or photographic film; the darker the film, the greater the measured d. **4.** In clinical radiology, a less-exposed area on a film, corresponding to a region of greater x-ray attenuation (radiopacity) in the subject; the more light transmitted by the film, the greater the d. of the subject; this is not actually the opposite of the prior definition, since one concerns film d. and the other subject d. [L. *densitas*, fr. *densus*, thick]

buoyant d., the d. that allows a substance to float in some standard fluid.

count d., SYN photon d.

flux d., **(1)** SYN flux (4). **(2)** either particle flux d., the particle fluence rate, or energy flux d., the energy fluence rate of intensity. Cf. fluence.

incidence d., the person-time incidence rate.

optical d. (OD), SYN absorbance.

photon d., the number of counted events recorded in scintigraphy per square centimeter or per square inch of imaged area. SYN count d.

spin d., the number of nuclear dipoles per unit volume.

vapor d., the mass per unit volume of a vapor; since the vapor d. changes with temperature and pressure, it is commonly expressed as a specific gravity, *i.e.*, the weight of the vapor divided by the weight of an equal volume of a reference gas (*e.g.*, oxygen or hydrogen) at the same temperature and pressure.

◊dent-, denti-, dento-. Teeth; dental. SEE ALSO odonto-. [L. *dens*, tooth]

den·tal (den′tăl). Relating to the teeth. [L. *dens*, tooth]

den·tal en·gine. The motive power of a dental handpiece that causes it to rotate.

den·tal·gia (den-tal′jē-ă). SYN toothache. [L. *dens*, tooth, + G. *algos*, pain]

den·tate (den′tāt). Notched; toothed; cogged. [L. *dentatus*, toothed]

den·ta·tec·to·my (den-tă-tek′tō-mē). Surgical destruction of the dentate nucleus of the cerebellum. [dentate (nucleus) + G. *ectomē*, excision]

den·ta·tum (den-tā′tŭm, den-tah′tŭm). SYN dentate *nucleus* of cerebellum. [L. neut. of *dentatus*, toothed]

den·tes (den′tēz). Plural of dens. [L.]

◊denti-. SEE dent-.

den·tia (den-tē′a). The process of tooth development or eruption. Also serves to denote a relationship to the teeth. [dent- + suffix *-ia*, condition, process]

d. praecox (den-tē′a prē-coks), Premature tooth eruption. [L. premature]

d. tarda (den-tēa′ tar′dă), Delayed tooth eruption. [L. delayed]

den·ti·cle (den′ti-kl). **1.** SYN endolith. **2.** A toothlike projection from a hard surface. [L. *denticulus*, a small tooth]

den·tic·u·late, den·tic·u·lat·ed (den-tik′yū-lāt, -lāt-ed). **1.** Finely dentated, notched, or serrated. **2.** Having small teeth.

den·ti·form (den′ti-fōrm). Tooth-shaped; pegged. SEE ALSO odontoid (1). [denti- + L. *forma*, form]

den·ti·frice (den′ti-fris). Any preparation used in the cleansing of the teeth, *e.g.*, a tooth powder, toothpaste, or tooth wash. [L. *dentifricium*, fr. *dens*, tooth, + *frico*, pp. *frictus*, to rub]

den·tig·er·ous (den-tij′er-ŭs). Arising from or associated with teeth, as a d. cyst. [denti- + L. *gero*, to bear]

den·ti·la·bi·al (den′ti-lā′bē-ăl). Relating to the teeth and lips. [denti- + L. *labium*, lip]

den·ti·lin·gual (den-ti-ling′gwăl). Relating to the teeth and tongue. [denti- + L. *lingua*, tongue]

den·tin (den′tin). The ivory forming the mass of the tooth. About 20% is organic matrix, mostly collagen, with some elastin and a small amount of mucopolysaccharide; the inorganic fraction (70%) is mainly hydroxyapatite, with some carbonate, magnesium, and fluoride. The d. is traversed by a large number of fine tubules running from the pulp cavity outward; within the tubules are processes from the odontoblasts. SYN dentinum [NA], dentine, ebur dentis, substantia eburnea. [L. *dens*, tooth]

hereditary opalescent d., (1) SYN *dentinogenesis* imperfecta. **(2)** SYN opalescent d.

hypersensitive d., exposed d. at the cervical portion of a tooth, painful to touch, sweetness, or temperature changes.

interglobular d., imperfectly calcified matrix of d. situated between the calcified globules near the dentinal periphery.

irregular d., irritation d., SYN tertiary d.

opalescent d., d. usually associated with dentinogenesis imperfecta. It gives an unusual opalescent or translucent appearance to the teeth. SYN hereditary opalescent d. (2).

peritubular d., an electron-dense layer of d. observed adjacent to the odontoblastic process.

primary d., d. which forms until the root is completed.

reparative d., SYN tertiary d.

sclerotic d., d. characterized by calcification of the dentinal tubules as a result of injury or normal aging. SYN transparent d.

secondary d., d. formed by normal pulp function after root end formation is complete.

tertiary d., morphologically irregular d. formed in response to an irritant. SYN irregular d., irritation d., reparative d.

transparent d., SYN sclerotic d.

vascular d., SYN vasodentin.

den·ti·nal (den′ti-năl). Relating to dentin.

den·ti·nal·gia (den-ti-nal′jē-ă). Dentinal sensitivity or pain. [dentin + G. *algos*, pain]

den·tine (den'tēn). SYN dentin.

den·tin·o·ce·ment·al (den'ti-nō-se-men'tăl). Relating to the dentin and cementum of teeth. SYN cementodentinal.

den·tin·o·e·nam·el (den'ti-nō-ē-nam'ĕl). Relating to the dentin and enamel of teeth. SYN amelodentinal.

den·tin·o·gen·e·sis (den'ti-nō-jen'ĕ-sis). The process of dentin formation in the development of teeth. [dentin + G. *genesis*, production]

d. imperfec'ta [MIM*125490 & MIM*125500], an autosomal dominant disorder of the teeth characterized clinically by translucent gray to yellow-brown teeth involving both primary and permanent dentition; the enamel fractures easily, leaving exposed dentin which undergoes rapid attrition; radiographically, the pulp chambers and canals appear obliterated and the roots are short and blunted; sometimes occurs in association with osteogenesis imperfecta; autosomal dominant inheritance. SYN hereditary opalescent dentin (1).

den·ti·noid (den'ti-noyd). **1.** Resembling dentin. **2.** SYN dentinoma. [dentin + G. *eidos*, resembling]

den·ti·no·ma (den'ti-nō'mă). A rare benign odontogenic tumor consisting microscopically of dysplastic dentin and strands of epithelium within a fibrous stroma. SYN dentinoid (2). [dentin + G. *-oma*, tumor]

den·ti·num (den'ti-nŭm) [NA]. SYN dentin. [L. *dens*, tooth]

den·tip·a·rous (den-tip'ă-rŭs). Tooth-bearing. [denti- + L. *pario*, to bear]

den·tist. A legally qualified practitioner of dentistry.

den·tis·try (den'tis-trē). The healing science and art concerned with the embryology, anatomy, physiology, and pathology of the oral-facial complex, and with the prevention, diagnosis, and treatment of deformities, pathoses, and traumatic injuries thereof. SYN odontology, odontonosology.

community d., public health d., with an academic base, emphasizing the professional obligation to foster the delivery of prevention, education, and care to populations.

esthetic d., a field of d. concerned especially with the appearance of a dental restoration as achieved through its form and color.

forensic d., (1) the relation and application of dental facts to legal problems, as in using the teeth for identifying the dead; **(2)** the law in its bearing on the practice of dentistry. SYN dental jurisprudence, forensic odontology, legal d.

legal d., SYN forensic d.

operative d., usually, the individual restoration of teeth by means of metallic or nonmetallic materials. SYN restorative d.

pediatric d., SYN pedodontics.

preventive d., a philosophy and method of dental practice which seeks to prevent the initiation, progression, and recurrence of dental caries.

prosthetic d., SYN prosthodontics.

public health d., that specialty of d. concerned with the prevention and control of dental diseases and promotion of oral health through organized community efforts.

restorative d., SYN operative d.

den·ti·tion (den-tish'ŭn). The natural teeth, as considered collectively, in the dental arch; may be deciduous, permanent, or mixed. [L. *dentitio*, to teethe]

artificial d., SYN denture (1).

deciduous d., SYN deciduous *tooth.*

delayed d., delayed eruption of the teeth.

first d., SYN deciduous *tooth.*

mandibular d., SYN inferior dental *arch.*

maxillary d., SYN superior dental *arch.*

natural d., SEE dentition.

primary d., SYN deciduous *tooth.*

retarded d., d. in which growth phenomena such as calcification, elongation, and eruption occur later than in the average range of normal variation as a result of some systemic metabolic dysfunction (*e.g.*, hypothyroidism).

secondary d., SYN permanent *tooth.*

succedaneous d., SYN permanent *tooth.*

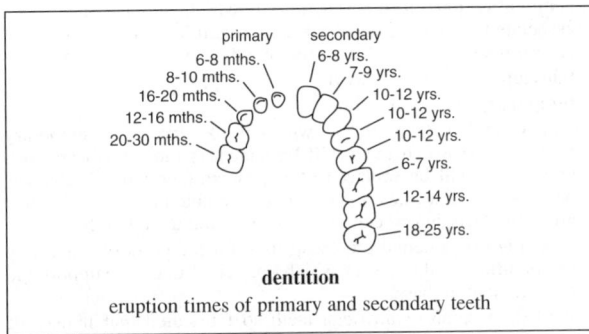

dentition
eruption times of primary and secondary teeth

△**dento-.** SEE dent-.

den·to·al·ve·o·lar (den'to-al-vē'ō-lăr). Usually, denoting that portion of the alveolar bone immediately about the teeth; used also to denote the functional unity of teeth and alveolar bone.

den·tode (den'tōd). An exact reproduction of a tooth on a gnathographically mounted cast.

den·toid (den'toyd). SYN odontoid (1). SEE ALSO dentiform. [dent- + G. *eidos*, resemblance]

den·to·le·gal (den-tō-lē'găl). Relating to both dentistry and the law. SEE forensic *dentistry.*

den·to·li·va (den-tō-lī'vă). Rarely used term for oliva. [L. *dens*, tooth, + *oliva*, olive]

den·tu·lous (den'tyū-lŭs). Having natural teeth present in the mouth.

den·ture (den'tyūr). **1.** An artificial substitute for missing natural teeth and adjacent tissues. SYN artificial dentition. **2.** Sometimes used to denote the dentition of animals.

bar joint d., SYN overlay d.

complete d., a dental prosthesis which is a substitute for the lost natural dentition and associated structures of the maxillae or mandible. SYN full d.

design d., a planned visualization of the form and extent of a dental prosthesis, made after a study of all factors involved.

fixed partial d., a restoration of one or more missing teeth which cannot be readily removed by the patient or dentist; it is permanently attached to natural teeth or roots which furnish the primary support to the appliance. SYN bridge (3).

full d., SYN complete d.

immediate d., a complete or partial d. constructed for insertion immediately following the removal of natural teeth. SYN immediate insertion d.

immediate insertion d., SYN immediate d.

implant d., a d. that receives its stability and retention from a substructure which is partially or wholly implanted under the soft tissues of the d. basal seat. SEE ALSO implant denture *substructure*, implant denture *superstructure*, subperiosteal *implant*.

interim d., a dental prosthesis to be used for a short interval of time for reasons of esthetics, mastication, occlusal support, or convenience, or to condition the patient to accept an artificial substitute for missing natural teeth until more definite prosthetic dental treatment can be provided. SYN provisional d., temporary d.

overlay d., a complete d. that is supported by both soft tissue and natural teeth that have been altered so as to permit the d. to fit over them. The altered teeth may have been fitted with short or long copings, locking devices, or connecting bars. SYN bar joint d., hybrid prosthesis, overdenture, telescopic d.

partial d., a dental prosthesis which restores one or more, but less than all, of the natural teeth and/or associated parts and which is supported by the teeth and/or the mucosa; it may be removable or fixed. SYN bridgework.

partial d., distal extension, a removable partial d. that is retained by natural teeth at one end of the d. base segments only, and in which a portion of the functional load is carried by the residual ridge.

provisional d., SYN interim d.

removable partial d., a partial d. which supplies teeth and associated structures on a partially edentulous jaw, and which can be readily removed from the mouth. SYN removable bridge.

telescopic d., SYN overlay d.

temporary d., SYN interim d.

transitional d., a partial d. which is to serve as a temporary prosthesis to which teeth will be added as more teeth are lost, and which will be replaced after postextraction tissue changes have occurred; a transitional d. may become an interim d. when all of the teeth have been removed from the dental arch.

treatment d., a dental prosthesis used for the purpose of treating or conditioning the tissues which are called upon to support and retain a denture base.

trial d., a setup of artificial teeth so fabricated that it may be placed in the patient's mouth to verify esthetics, for the making of records, or for any other operation deemed necessary before final completion of the d. SYN wax model d.

wax model d., SYN trial d.

den·ture ser·vice. Those procedures performed in the diagnosis, construction, and maintenance of artificial substitutes for missing natural teeth.

den·tur·ist (den'tyūr-ist). A dental technician who fabricates and fits dentures without supervision of a dentist.

Denucé, Jean L.P., French surgeon, 1824–1889. SEE D.'s *ligament.*

de·nu·cle·at·ed (dē-nū'klē-ā-ted). Deprived of a nucleus.

de·nu·da·tion (den-yū-dā'shŭn). Depriving of a covering or protecting layer; the act of laying bare, as in the removal of the epithelium from an underlying surface. [L. *de-nudo,* to lay bare, fr. *de,* from, + *nudus,* naked]

de·nude (dē'nūd). To perform denudation.

Denys, Joseph, Belgian bacteriologist, 1857–1932. SEE D.-Leclef *phenomenon.*

de·ob·stru·ent (dē-ob'strū-ent). **1.** Obsolete term for relieving or removing obstruction. **2.** Obsolete term for an agent that removes an obstruction to flow. [L. *de-* priv. + *obstruo,* pp. *-structus,* to build against, obstruct]

de·o·dor·ant (dē-ō'der-ant). **1.** Eliminating or masking a smell, especially an unpleasant one. **2.** An agent having such an action; especially a cosmetic combined with an antiperspirant. SYN deodorizer. [L. *de-* priv. + *odoro,* pp. *-atus,* to give an odor to, fr. *odor,* a smell]

de·o·dor·ize (dē-ō'der-īz). To use a deodorant.

de·o·dor·iz·er (dē-ō'der-īz-er). SYN deodorant (2).

de·on·tol·o·gy (dē-on-tol'ō-jē). A study of the field of professional ethics and duties. [G. *deon* (*deont-*), that which is binding, pr. part. ntr. of *dei,* (impers.) it behooves, fr. *deō,* to bind, + *logos,* study]

de·op·pi·la·tive (dē-op'pi-lā-tiv). Obsolete term for deobstruent. [L. *de-* priv. + *op-pilo,* pp. *-atus,* to stop up, fr. *ob-* against, + *pilo,* to ram down]

de·or·sum·duc·tion (dē-ōr'sŭm-dŭk'shŭn). Rotation of one eye downward. SYN infraduction. [L. *deorsum,* downward, + *duco,* to lead]

de·os·si·fi·ca·tion (dē-os'i-fi-kā'shŭn). Removal of the mineral constituents of bone. [L. *de,* from, + *os,* bone, + *facio,* to make]

de·ox·i·da·tion (dē'oks-i-dā'shŭn). Depriving a chemical compound of its oxygen.

de·ox·i·dize (dē-oks'i-dīz). To remove oxygen from its chemical combination.

△**deoxy-.** Prefix to chemical names of substances to indicate replacement of an —OH by an H. The older desoxy- has been retained in some instances.

de·ox·y·a·den·o·sine (dA, dAdo) (dē-oks'ē-ă-den'ō-sēn). 2'-Deoxyribosyladenine, one of the four major nucleosides of DNA (the others being deoxycytidine, deoxyguanosine, and thymidine). The 5′ derivative is also an important component of one form of vitamin B$_{12}$. D. accumulates in individuals with severe combined immunodeficiency disease.

de·ox·y·a·den·o·sine meth·yl·ase. SYN dam *methylase.*

5′-de·ox·y·ad·e·no·syl·co·bal·a·min (dē-oks'ē-ă-den-ō-sil-kō-

bal'ă-min). An active coenzyme form of vitamin B$_{12}$; required in the conversion of methylmalonyl-CoA to succinyl-CoA. A deficiency of 5′-d. will result in methylmalonic acidemia.

de·ox·y·ad·e·nyl·ic ac·id (dAMP) (dē-oks'ē-ad-en-il'ik). Deoxyadenosine monophosphate, a hydrolysis product of DNA, differing from adenylic acid in containing deoxyribose in place of ribose. SYN adenine deoxyribonucleotide.

de·ox·y·bar·bi·tu·rate (dē-oks-ē-bar-bit'yūr-āt). A barbiturate compound lacking the oxygen atom at the #2 position in the ring; example of a deoxybarbiturate is the antiepileptic drug, primidone. SEE ALSO barbiturate.

de·ox·y·cho·late (DOC) (dē-oks-ē-kō'lāt). A salt or ester of deoxycholic acid.

de·ox·y·cho·lic ac·id (dē-oks-ē-kō'lik). 7-Deoxycholic acid; 3α,12α-dihydroxy-5β-cholanic acid; a bile acid and choleretic; used in biochemical preparations as a detergent.

de·ox·y·co·for·my·cin (dē-oks-ē-cō-fōr-mī'sin). A purine analog which acts as an antimetabolite; potent inhibitor of adenosine deaminase. Used as an antineoplastic agent. SEE ALSO pentostatin.

2-de·ox·y·co·for·my·cin. SYN pentostatin.

de·ox·y·cor·ti·cos·ter·one (DOC) (dē-oks'ē-kōr-ti-kos'ter-ōn). 11-Deoxycorticosterone; 21-hydroxypregn-4-ene-3,20-dione; an adrenocortical steroid, principally a biosynthetic precursor of corticosterone and possibly aldosterone, that rarely appears in adrenocortical secretions; a potent mineralocorticoid with no appreciable glucocorticoid activity. SYN 21-hydroxyprogesterone, cortexone, deoxycortone, desoxycortone.

d. acetate, desoxycorticosterone acetate; acetate salt used for intramuscular injection for replacement therapy of the adrenocortical steroid.

d. pivalate, desoxycorticosterone pivalate; pivalate salt of the steroid.

de·ox·y·cor·tone (dē-oks-ē-kōr'tōn). SYN deoxycorticosterone.

de·ox·y·cyt·i·dine (dē-oks-ē-sī'ti-dēn). 2′-Deoxyribosylcytosine, one of the four major nucleosides of DNA (the others being deoxyadenosine, deoxyguanosine, and thymidine).

de·ox·y·cyt·i·dyl·ic ac·id (dCMP) (dē-oks'ē-sī-ti-dil'ik). Deoxycytidine monophosphate, a hydrolysis product of DNA.

de·ox·y·ep·i·neph·rine (dē-oks'ē-ep-i-nef'rēn). 4-[2-(Methylamino)ethyl]pyrocatechol; a sympathomimetic amine used as a vasoconstrictor.

de·ox·y·gua·no·sine (dē-oks-ē-gwan'ō-sēn). 2′-Deoxyribosylguanine, one of the four major nucleosides of DNA (the others being deoxyadenosine, deoxycytidine, and thymidine). Found to accumulate in individuals with purine nucleoside phosphorylase deficiency.

de·ox·y·gua·nyl·ic ac·id (dGMP) (dē-oks-ē-gwan-il'ik). Deoxyguanosine monophosphate, a hydrolysis product of DNA. SYN guanine deoxyribonucleotide.

de·ox·y·hex·ose (dē-oks-ē-heks'ōs). A 6-carbon deoxy-sugar in which one OH is replaced by H.

de·ox·y·nu·cle·o·side (dē-oks'ē-nū'klē-ō-sīd). SEE deoxyribonucleoside.

de·ox·y·nu·cle·o·tide (dē-oks'ē-nū'klē-ō-tīd). SEE deoxyribonucleoside.

de·ox·y·pen·tose (dē-oks-ē-pen'tōs). A 5-carbon deoxy-sugar in which one OH is replaced by H.

de·ox·y·ri·bo·al·dol·ase (dē-oks'ē-rī-bō-al'dō-lās). SYN deoxyribosephosphate aldolase.

de·ox·y·ri·bo·di·py·rim·i·dine pho·to·ly·ase (dē-oks'ē-rī'bō-dī-pī-rim'i-dēn). An enzyme in yeast which is activated by light, whereupon it can reverse a previous photochemical reaction by cleaving the cyclobutane ring of the thymine dimer. SYN dipyrimidine photolyase, photoreactivating enzyme.

de·ox·y·ri·bo·nu·cle·ase (DNAse, DNAase, DNase) (de-oks'ē-rī-bō-nū'klē-ās). Any enzyme (phosphodiesterase) hydrolyzing phosphodiester bonds in DNA. SEE ALSO endonuclease, nuclease.

acid d., SYN d. II.

d. I, DNase I, an endonuclease that cleaves primarily double-stranded DNA to a mixture of oligodeoxyribonucleotides, each ending in a 5′-phosphate; streptodornase is a similar enzyme.

Under appropriate conditions, it can produce single-strand nicks in DNA; used in nick translation and in the mapping of hypersensitive sites. SYN pancreatic d., thymonuclease.

d. II, DNase II, an endonuclease that cleaves both strands of native DNA (as well as single-stranded DNA) to produce a mixture of oligodeoxynucleotides, each ending in a 3′-phosphate. SYN acid d.

pancreatic d., SYN d. I.

d. S₁, SYN endonuclease S₁ *Aspergillus.*

spleen d., former name for micrococcal *endonuclease.*

de·ox·y·ri·bo·nu·cle·ic ac·id (DNA) (dē-oks′ē-rī′bō-nū-klē′ik). The type of nucleic acid containing deoxyribose as the sugar component and found principally in the nuclei (chromatin, chromosomes) and mitochondria of animal and vegetable cells, usually loosely bound to protein (hence the term deoxyribonucleoprotein); considered to be the autoreproducing component of chromosomes and of many viruses, and the repository of hereditary characteristics. Its linear macromolecular chain consists of deoxyribose molecules esterified with phosphate groups between the 3′ and 5′ hydroxyl groups; linked to this structure are the purines adenine (A) and guanine (G) and the pyrimidines cytosine (C) and thymine (T). DNA may be open-ended or circular, single- or double-stranded, and many forms are known, the most comonly described of which is double-stranded, wherein the pyrimidines and purines cross-link through hydrogen bonding in the schema A-T and C-G, bringing two antiparallel strands into a double helix. Chromosomes are composed of double-stranded DNA; mitochondrial DNA is circular.

A-DNA, a form of DNA in which the helix is right-handed and the overall appearance is short and broad.

antisense DNA, the strand of DNA complementary to the one bearing the genetic message and from which it may be reconstructed. A DNA sequence complementary to a portion of mRNA.

B-DNA, a form of DNA in which the helix is right-handed and the overall appearance is long and thin.

blunt-ended DNA, double-stranded DNA in which at least one of the ends has no unpaired bases.

competitor DNA, DNA from a test organism that is denatured and then used in *in vitro* hybridization experiments in which it competes with DNA (homologous) from a reference organism; used to determine the relationship of the test organism to the reference organism.

complementary DNA (cDNA), (1) single-stranded DNA that is complementary to messenger RNA; **(2)** DNA that has been synthesized from mRNA by the action of reverse transcriptase.

extrachromosomal DNA, DNA that occurs naturally outside of the nucleus (*e.g.,* mitochondrial DNA).

genomic DNA, DNA that contains both introns and exons.

junk DNA, that portion of DNA which is not transcribed and expressed, comprising about 90% of the 3 billion base pairs of the human genome; its function is not known.

DNA ligase, an enzyme that leads to the formation of a phosphodiester bond at a break of one strand in duplex DNA; a part of the DNA repair system.

linker DNA, the DNA found between nucleosomes on chromatin; since it is not complexed to proteins as strongly as other forms of DNA, it is accessible to exonuclease hydrolysis.

DNA nucleotidylexotransferase, an enzyme that can catalyze the addition of a nucleotide, presented as a nucleoside triphosphate, on a DNA or similar polydeoxynucleotide; has been used in DNA recombination studies to add nucleotides to form homopolymer tails. SYN terminal addition enzyme, terminal deoxynucleotidyltransferase.

palindromic DNA, a segment of DNA in which the sequence is symmetrical about its midpoint.

DNA polymerase, SEE nucleotidyltransferases.

recombinant DNA, SEE recombinant DNA.

repetitive DNA, a segment of DNA that consists of a linear array of multiple copies of the same sequence of nucleotides.

satellite DNA, DNA in the satellite regions of acrocentric chromosomes.

sticky-ended DNA, double-stranded DNA in which one of the

strands protrudes from the other strand (*i.e.,* has a number of unpaired bases) at one end or more.

Z-DNA, a form of DNA in which the helix is left-handed, and the overall appearance is elongated and slim.

zero time-binding DNA, DNA that has become the duplex form at the start of a reassociation process.

de·ox·y·ri·bo·nu·cle·o·pro·tein (DNP, Dnp) (dē-oks′ē-rī-bō-nū′klē-ō-prō′tēn). The complex of DNA and protein in which DNA is usually found upon cell disruption and isolation.

de·ox·y·ri·bo·nu·cle·o·side (dē-oks′ē-rī-bō-nū′klē-ō-sīd). A nucleoside component of DNA containing 2-deoxy-D-ribose; the condensation product of deoxy-D-ribose with purines or pyrimidines.

de·ox·y·ri·bo·nu·cle·o·tide (dē-oks′ē-rī-bō-nū′klē-ō-tīd). A nucleotide component of DNA containing 2-deoxy-D-ribose; the phosphoric ester of deoxyribonucleoside; formed in nucleotide biosynthesis.

de·ox·y·ri·bose (dē-oks-ē-rī′bōs). A deoxypentose, 2-deoxy-D-ribose being the most common example, occurring in DNA and responsible for its name.

d. phosphate, SEE deoxyribonucleotide.

de·ox·y·ri·bose·phos·phate al·dol·ase (dē-oks′ē-rī-bōs-fos′fāt). An enzyme catalyzing cleavage of 2-deoxy-D-ribose 5-phosphate to D-glyceraldehyde 3-phosphate and acetaldehyde. SYN deoxyriboaldolase.

de·ox·y·ri·bo·side (dē-oks-ē-rī′bō-sīd). Deoxyribose combined via its 1-O atom with a radical derived from an alcohol; not to be confused with deoxyribosyl compounds such as deoxyribonucleosides. Cf. deoxyribosyl.

de·ox·y·ri·bo·syl (dē-oks-ē-rī′bō-sil). The radical formed from deoxyribose by removal of the OH from the C1 carbon; *e.g.,* deoxyadenosine. Cf. deoxyriboside.

de·ox·y·ri·bo·syl·trans·fer·ases (dē-oks′ē-rī′bō-sil-trans′fer-ās-es). Enzymes that catalyze the transfer of 2-deoxy-D-ribose from deoxyribosides to free bases.

de·ox·y·ri·bo·tide (dē-oks-ē-rī′bō-tīd). Misnomer for deoxyribonucleotide or deoxynucleotide derived, by analogy with nucleoside-nucleotide, from incorrect usage of deoxyriboside.

de·ox·y·thy·mi·dine (dT) (dē-oks′ē-thi′mi-dēn). SYN thymidine.

de·ox·y·thy·mi·dyl·ic ac·id (dTMP) (dē-oks′ē-thī-mi-dil′ik). A component of DNA; originally and properly called thymidylic acid, but use of deoxy- is less ambiguous, as ribothymidylic acid is now known to exist. SYN thymine deoxyribonucleotide.

de·ox·y·ur·i·dine (dē-oks′ē-yūr′i-dēn). A derivative of uridine in which one or more of the hydroxyl groups on the ribose moiety has been replaced by a hydrogen; *e.g.,* 2′-deoxyuridine is a rare naturally occurring deoxynucleoside.

de·ox·y·vi·rus (dē-ok′sē-vī′rŭs). SYN DNA *virus.*

de·o·zon·ize (dē-ō′zō-nīz). To deprive of ozone.

de·pen·dence (dē-pen′dens). The quality or condition of relying upon, being influenced by, or being subservient to a person or object reflecting a particular need. [L. *dependeo,* to hang from]

anchorage d., the need of normal cells to have an appropriate surface to attach to in order for them to grow in culture.

substance d., a pattern of behavioral, physiologic, and cognitive symptoms that develop due to substance use or abuse; usually indicated by tolerance to the effects of the substance and withdrawal symptoms that develop when use of the substance is terminated.

de·pen·den·cy (dē-pen′dens-ē). The state of being dependent.

pyridoxine d. with seizure, an inherited disorder (autosomal recessive) apparently associated with deficient brain type I glutamate decarboxylase; seizures can be controlled with vitamin B₆.

De·pen·do·vi·rus (dē-pen′dō-vī-rŭs). A genus of small defective single-stranded DNA viruses in the family Parvoviridae that depend on adenoviruses for replication. SYN adeno-associated virus, adenosatellite virus. [L. *dependeo,* to be dependent upon, + virus]

de·per·son·al·i·za·tion (dē-per′sŏn-ăl-i-zā′shŭn). A state in which a person loses the feeling of his own identity in relation to others in his family or peer group, or loses the feeling of his own reality. SYN depersonalization syndrome.

de Pezzer, O., 19th century French physician. SEE de P. *catheter.*

de·phas·ing. In the magnetic resonance, following alignment by a radiofrequency pulse, the gradual loss of orientation of the magnetic atomic nuclei due to random molecular energy transfer or relaxation.

de·phos·pho·ryl·a·tion (dē-fos′fōr-i-lā′shŭn). Removal of a phosphoric group, usually hydrolytically and by enzyme action, from a compound.

de·pig·men·ta·tion (dē-pig-men-tā′shŭn). Loss of pigment which may be partial or complete. SEE ALSO achromia (1).

dep·i·late (dep′i-lāt). To remove hair by any means. Cf. epilate. [L. *de-pilo,* pp. *-atus,* to deprive of hair, fr. *de-* neg. + *pilo,* to grow hair]

dep·i·la·tion (dep-i-lā′shŭn). SYN epilation.

de·pil·a·to·ry (dē-pil′ă-tō-rē). **1.** SYN epilatory (1). **2.** An agent that causes the falling out of hair. SYN epilatory (2).

chemical d., a topically applied d. substance.

de·ple·tion (dē-plē′shŭn). **1.** The removal of accumulated fluids or solids. **2.** A reduced state of strength from too many free discharges. **3.** Excessive loss of a constituent, usually essential, of the body, *e.g.,* salt, water, etc.

chloride d., SYN salt d.

salt d., excessive loss of sodium chloride from the body in urine, sweat, etc.; a cause of secondary dehydration. SYN chloride d.

water d., reduction in the total volume of body water; dehydration.

de·po·lar·i·za·tion (dē-pō′lăr-i-zā′shŭn). The destruction, neutralization, or change in direction of polarity.

dendritic d., the loss of a negative charge in the dendrites of a nerve cell.

de·po·lar·ize (dē-pō′lăr-īz). To deprive of polarity.

de·pol·y·mer·ase (dē-pol′i-mer-ās). Name used originally, before hydrolytic action was understood, for an enzyme catalyzing the hydrolysis of a macromolecule to simpler components. SEE nuclease.

de·pop·u·la·tion (dē-pop-yū-lā′shŭn). Humane destruction of all animals on a premises during a disease eradication program; in the U.S., used primarily in national programs established to eradicate newly introduced diseases (*e.g.,* foot-and-mouth disease) that pose serious economic threats to the livestock industries.

de·pos·it (dē-poz′it). **1.** A sediment or precipitate. **2.** A pathological accumulation of inorganic material in a tissue. [L. *de-pono,* pp. *-positus,* to lay down]

brickdust d., a sediment of urates in the urine. SYN sedimentum lateritium.

dep·ra·va·tion (dep′ră-vā′shŭn). SYN depravity. [L. *depravatio,* fr. *depravo,* pp. *-atus,* to corrupt]

de·praved (dē-prāvd′). Deteriorated or degenerate; corrupt. [L. *depravo,* to corrupt]

de·prav·i·ty (dē-prav′i-tē). A depraved act or the condition of being depraved. SYN depravation.

de·pre·nyl (dē′pren-il). An inhibitor of monoamine oxidase selective for the type B isozyme. The drug is used as an antiparkinsonian agent. It does not give rise to the hypertensive crisis that can occur when nonselective monoamine oxidase inhibitors are taken in the presence of dietary sources of tyramine. SYN selegiline.

de·pres·sant (dē-pres′ănt). **1.** Diminishing functional tone or activity. **2.** An agent that reduces nervous or functional activity, such as a sedative or anesthetic. [L. *de-primo,* pp. *-pressus,* to press down]

de·pressed (dē-prest′). **1.** Flattened from above downward. **2.** Below the normal level or the level of the surrounding parts. **3.** Below the normal functional level. **4.** Dejected; lowered in spirits.

de·pres·sion (dē-presh′ŭn). **1.** Reduction of the level of functioning. **2.** A hollow or sunken area. **3.** Displacement of a part

downward or inward. **4.** A temporary mental state or chronic mental disorder characterized by feelings of sadness, loneliness, despair, low self-esteem, and self-reproach; accompanying signs include psychomotor retardation or less frequently agitation, withdrawal from social contact, and vegetative states such as loss of appetite and insomnia. SYN dejection (1). SYN depressive reaction, depressive syndrome. [L. *depressio,* fr. *deprimo,* to press down]

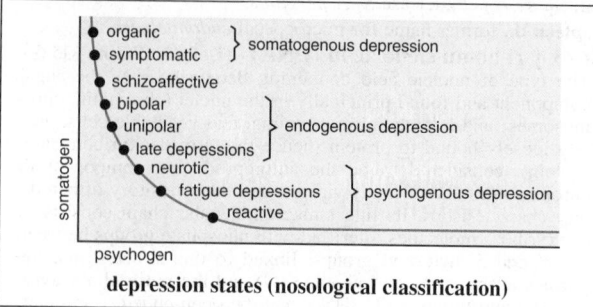

depression states (nosological classification)

agitated d., d. with excitement and restlessness.

anaclitic d., impairment of an infant's physical, social, and intellectual development following separation from its mother or from a mothering surrogate; characterized by listlessness, withdrawal, and anorexia. SEE ALSO hospitalism.

endogenous d., endogenomorphic d., a descriptive syndrome for a cluster of symptoms and features occurring in the absence of external precipitants and believed to have a biologic origin; *e.g.,* anhedonia, psychomotor agitation or retardation, diurnal mood variation with increased severity in the morning, early morning awakening and insomnia in the middle of the night, weight loss, self-reproach or guilt, and lack of reactivity to one's environment. SYN nonreactive d.

Annually, approximately 20 million people in the U.S. suffer from depression. Major strides in treatment of endogenous depression and other mood disorders have been made since the 1970s, in large measure because of psychopharmacological advances. The tricyclics and monoamine oxidase inhibitors, effective in reversing only a fraction of clinical depressions, have been joined by the serotonin and dopamine re-uptake inhibitors, classes of drugs that act to increase the amounts of those neurotransmitters available in the synapses. The selective serotonin reuptake inhibitors (SSRIs), including fluoxetine (Prozac), sertraline (Zoloft), and paroxetine (Paxil), are widely prescribed, and some 6 million people in the U.S. have taken Prozac since its introduction in 1987. SSRIs also have scored successes against panic attacks, bulimia, and obsessive-compulsive disorder, and may alleviate shyness, chronic feelings of emptiness, and fear of rejection. Depression can be masked by substance abuse (depressives may attempt to self-medicate with alcohol or drugs), and among the elderly is often confused with senile dementia. Timely diagnosis may be critical, because those suffering a major depressive episode run a higher risk than average of attempting suicide (the overall rate of suicides in the U.S. is 20 per 100,000, mainly in the 15–35 age group). Of the traditional talk therapies, the one that has demonstrated greatest success in reversing depression is cognitive therapy, developed by Aaron Beck. Refined methods of electroconvulsive shock therapy (ECT) have been used with increasing frequency since the 1980s, generally for cases that do not respond to other treatment. To minimize memory loss, a barbiturate is administered before the procedure, and muscle relaxants lessen convulsions. With severely depressed patients, ECT has a cure rate of 80%.

exogenous d., similar signs and symptoms as endogenous d. but the precipitating factors are social or environmental and outside the individual.

involutional d., depression or psychosis first occurring in the involutional years (40 to 55 for women, 50 to 65 for men).

lingual salivary gland d., an indentation on the lingual surface of the mandible within which a portion of the submandibular gland lies; it appears radiographically as a sharply circumscribed ovoid radiolucency between the mandibular canal and the inferior or border of the posterior mandible. SYN Stafne bone cyst, static bone cyst.

major d., a mental d. characterized by depressed or irritable mood, pervasive loss of interest in usually pleasurable activities, sleep and appetite disturbance, fatigue, suicidal thoughts, hopelessness, worthlessness, and guilt. SEE endogenous d., exogenous d., bipolar *disorder.*

nonreactive d., SYN endogenous d.

d. of optic disk, SYN *excavation* of optic disc.

pacchionian d.'s, SYN granular *pits*, under *pit.*

postdrive d., slowing of the heart, often with a rate-dependent blockade of A-V and/or V-A conduction following rapid atrial stimulation.

pterygoid d., SYN pterygoid *fovea.*

reactive d., a psychological state occasioned directly by an intensely sad external situation (frequently loss of a loved person), relieved by the removal of the external situation (*e.g.,* reunion with a loved person).

spreading d., a decrease of activity evoked by local stimulation of the cerebral cortex and spreading slowly over the whole cortex.

de·pres·sive (dē-pres'iv). **1.** Pushing down. **2.** Pertaining to or causing depression.

de·pres·sor (dē-pres'ŏr). **1.** A muscle that flattens or lowers a part. **2.** Anything that depresses or retards functional activity. **3.** An instrument or device used to push certain structures out of the way during an operation or examination. **4.** An agent producing decreased blood pressure. SYN hypotensor. [L. *de-primo*, pp. *-pressus*, to press down]

tongue d., an instrument with a broad flat extremity used for pressing down the tongue to facilitate examination of the oral cavity and pharynx.

dep·ri·va·tion (dep'ri-vā'shŭn). Absence, loss, or withholding of something needed.

emotional d., lack of adequate and appropriate interpersonal or environmental experiences, or both, usually in the early developmental years.

sensory d., diminution or absence of usual external stimuli or perceptual experiences, commonly resulting in psychological distress and aberrant functioning if continued too long.

dep·si·pep·tide (dep'sē-pep'tīd). An oligo- or polypeptide containing one or more ester bonds as well as peptide bonds. SEE ALSO peptolide. [G. *deseō*, to knead, blend, + peptide]

depth. Distance from the surface downward.

anesthetic d., the degree of central nervous system depression produced by a general anesthetic agent; a function of potency of the anesthetic and the concentration in which it is administered.

focal d., d. of focus, the greatest distance through which an object point can be moved while maintaining a clear image. SYN penetration (3).

dep·tro·pine cit·rate (dep'trō-pēn). 3α-[(10,11-dihydro-5*H*-dibenzo[*a,d*]cyclohepten-5-yl)oxy]1α*H*,5α*H*-tropane citrate; an antihistaminic agent with anticholinergic properties. SYN dibenzheptropine citrate.

de·pu·li·za·tion (dē-pyū'li-zā'shŭn). Destruction of fleas which convey the plague bacillus from animals to humans. [L. *de,* from, + *pulex* (*pulic-*), flea]

dep·u·rant (dep'yū-rant). **1.** An agent or means used to effect purification. **2.** An agent that promotes the excretion and removal of waste material. [L. *de-* intens. + *puro,* pp. *-atus,* to make pure]

dep·u·ra·tion (dep-yū-rā'shŭn). Purification; removal of waste products or foul excretions.

dep·u·ra·tive (dep'yū-ră-tiv). Tending to depurate; depurant.

de·qua·lin·i·um ac·e·tate (dē-kwah-lin'ē-ŭm). 1,1'-

decamethylenebis[4-aminoquinaldinium acetate]; an antimicrobial agent. SYN decamine.

de·qua·lin·i·um chlo·ride. Dequalinium acetate, with chloride replacing acetate, used as an antimicrobial agent primarily in lozenges for the treatment of mouth and throat infections.

de Quervain, Fritz, Swiss surgeon, 1868–1940. SEE de Q.'s *disease, fracture, thyroiditis.*

der·a·del·phus (dār-ă-del'fŭs). Conjoined twins with a single head and neck and separate bodies below the thoracic level. SEE conjoined *twins*, under *twin.* [G. *derē*, neck, + *adelphos*, brother]

de·rail·ment (dē-rāl'ment). A symptom of a thought disorder in which one constantly gets "off the track" in his thoughts and speech; similar to loosening of association.

der·an·en·ceph·a·ly, der·an·en·ce·pha·lia (dār-an'en-sef'ă-lē, -se-fā'lē-ă). **1.** Congenital malformation in which the head is absent, although there is a rudimentary neck. **2.** Defect of the brain and upper part of the spinal cord. [G. *derē,* neck, + *an-,* priv., + *kephalē,* head]

de·range·ment (dē-rānj'ment). **1.** A disturbance of the regular order or arrangement. **2.** Rarely used term for a mental disturbance or disorder. [Fr.]

Hey's internal d., dislocation of the semilunar cartilages of the knee joint.

Dercum, Francis X., U.S. neurologist, 1856–1931. SEE D.'s *disease.*

de·re·al·i·za·tion (dē-rē'ă-li-zā'shŭn). An alteration in one's perception of the environment such that things that are ordinarily familiar seem strange, unreal, or two-dimensional.

de·re·ism (dē'rē-izm). Mental activity in fantasy in contrast to reality. [L. *de,* away, + *res,* thing]

de·re·is·tic (dē-rē-is'tik). Living in imagination or fantasy with thoughts that are incongruent with logic or experience.

der·en·ce·pha·lia (dār-en-se-fā'lē-ă). SYN derencephaly.

der·en·ceph·a·lo·cele (dār-en-sef'ă-lō-sēl). In derencephaly, protrusion of the rudimentary brain through a defect in the upper cervical spinal canal. [G. *derē,* neck, + *enkephalos,* brain, + *kēlē,* hernia]

der·en·ceph·a·ly (dār-en-sef'ă-lē). Cervical rachischisis and anencephaly, a malformation involving an open cranial vault with a rudimentary brain usually crowded back toward bifid cervical vertebrae. SYN derencephalia. [G. *derē,* neck, + *enkephalos,* brain]

de·re·pres·sion (dē-rē-presh'ŭn). A homeostatic mechanism for regulating enzyme production in an inducible enzyme system: an inducer, usually a substrate of a specific enzyme pathway, by combining with an active repressor (produced by a regulator gene) deactivates it; the release of the previously repressed operator is followed by enzyme production.

der·i·va·tion (dār-i-vā'shŭn). **1.** The drawing of blood or the body fluids to one part to relieve congestion in another. SYN revulsion (2). **2.** The source or process of an evolution. [L. *derivatio,* fr. *derivo,* pp. *-atus,* to draw off, fr. *rivus,* a stream]

de·riv·a·tive (dĕ-riv'ă-tiv). **1.** Relating to or producing derivation. **2.** Something produced by modification of something preexisting. **3.** Specifically, a chemical compound that may be produced from another compound of similar structure in one or

de *(tab marker)*

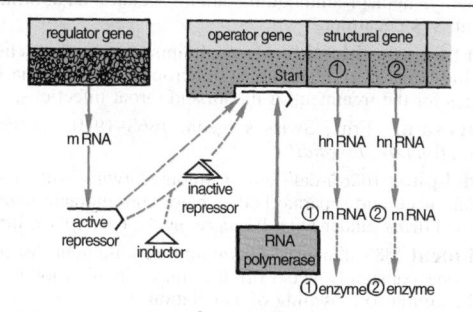

derepression

diagram of an operon showing the derepression effect of a hormone ("inductor"); inactivation of repressor enables the polymerase to "read" the structural genes; protein synthesis cascade can then be resumed (hn RNA, heterogenous RNA, a precursor of messenger (m) RNA)

more steps, as in replacement of H by an alkyl, acyl, or amino group.

derm-, derma-. The skin; corresponds to the L. *cut-*. See entries under cut. [G. *derma*]

der·ma·brad·er (derm'ă-brād-er). A motor-driven device used in dermabrasion.

der·ma·bra·sion (der-mă-brā'zhŭn). Operative procedure used to remove acne scars or pits performed with sandpaper, rotating wire brushes, or other abrasive materials. SYN mechanical abrasion, planing.

Der·ma·cen·tor (der-mă-sen'ter). An ornate, characteristically marked genus of hard ticks (family Ixodidae) that possess eyes and 11 festoons; it consists of some 20 species whose members commonly attack dogs, humans, and other mammals. [derm- + G. *kentōr*, a goader]

D. albopic'tus, the winter tick, a species found principally on horses, cattle, elk, moose, and deer in Canada and the northern and western United States; it is a one-host tick, but humans are sometimes attacked when skinning or dressing deer.

D. anderso'ni, the Rocky Mountain spotted-fever, or wood tick; a species that is the vector of spotted fever in the Rocky Mountain regions, and also transmits tularemia and causes tick paralysis; there are characteristic black and white markings on the large scutum of the male.

D. ni'tens, the tropical horse tick, a species found primarily on horses, mules, and asses (usually on the ears), chiefly in southern Florida, southern Texas, Mexico, Central America, and the West Indies.

D. occidenta'lis, the Pacific Coast tick, a species found on all domestic herbivores, deer, dogs, humans, and other animals in California and western Oregon.

D. reticula'tus, a common species attacking sheep, oxen, goats, and deer, and sometimes troublesome to humans; it is found in Europe, Asia, and America.

D. variabi'lis, the American dog tick, a species that is a common pest of dogs along the eastern seaboard of the U.S., a vector of tularemia, and a principal vector of *Rickettsia rickettsii* which causes Rocky Mountain spotted fever in the central and eastern U.S.; may also cause tick paralysis.

der·mad (der'mad). In the direction of the outer integument. [derm- + L. *ad*, to]

der·mag·ra·phy (der-mag'ră-fē). SYN dermatographism.

der·ma·he·mia (der-mă-hē'mē-ă). Hyperemia of the skin. [derma- + G. *haima*, blood]

der·mal (der'măl). Relating to the skin. SYN dermatic, dermatoid (2), dermic.

der·ma·lax·ia (der-mă-lak'sē-ă). SYN cutis laxa. [derm- + G. *malaxis*, softening]

der·ma·met·rop·a·thism (der'mă-me-trop'ă-thizm). A system that measures the intensity and nature of certain cutaneous disorders by observing the markings made by drawing a blunt instru-

ment across the skin. [derm- + G. *metron*, measure, + *pathos*, disease]

Der·ma·nys·sus gal·li·nae (der-mă-nis'ŭs ga-lē'-nē). The red hen-mite, a parasite of chickens, pigeons, and other birds; it sometimes attacks humans and causes an itching eruption, especially in sensitized individuals. SYN *Acarus gallinae*. [derm- + G. *nyssō*, to prick; L. *gallina*, hen]

dermat-. The skin. SEE ALSO derm-, dermato-, dermo-. [G. *derma*]

der·ma·tal·gia (der-mă-tăl'jē-ă). Localized pain, usually confined to the skin. SYN dermatodynia. [dermat- + G. *algos*, pain]

der·mat·ic (der-mat'ik). SYN dermal.

der·ma·ti·tis, pl. **der·ma·tit·i·des** (der-mă-tī'tis, -tit'i-dēz). Inflammation of the skin. [derm- + G. *-itis*, inflammation]

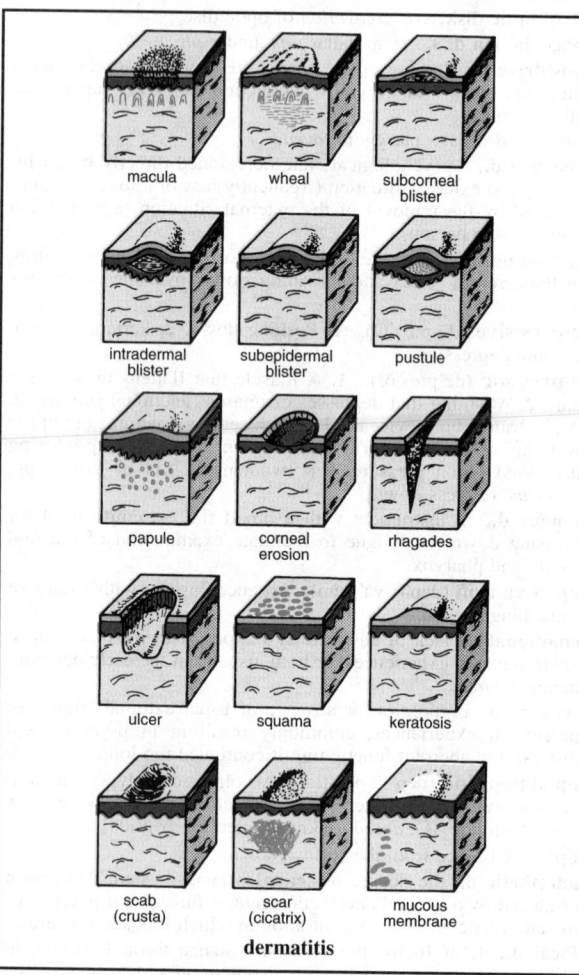

dermatitis

actinic d., SYN photodermatitis.

d. aestiva'lis, eczema recurring during the summer.

allergic contact d., a delayed type IV allergic reaction of the skin with varying degrees of erythema, edema, and vesiculation resulting from cutaneous contact with a specific allergen. SYN contact allergy.

d. ambustio'nis, inflammation of the skin resulting from the action of heat. SYN d. calorica, uritis.

ancylostoma d., SYN cutaneous *ancylostomiasis*.

d. artefac'ta, self-induced skin lesions resulting from habitual rubbing, scratching or hair-pulling, malingering, or mental disturbance. SYN d. autophytica, factitial d., feigned eruption.

atopic d., d. characterized by the distinctive phenomena of atopy, including infantile and flexural eczema. SYN atopic eczema.

d. atroph′icans, a diffuse idiopathic atrophy of the skin involving the appendages.

d. autophy′tica, SYN d. artefacta.

berloque d., berlock d., a type of photosensitization resulting in deep brown pigmentation on exposure to sunlight after application of bergamot oil and other essential oils in perfume.

blastomycetic d., d. blastomycot′ica, a cutaneous form of blastomycosis.

bubble gum d., allergic contact d. developing about the lips in children who chew bubble gum; caused by plastics in the gum substance.

d. calor′ica, SYN d. ambustionis.

caterpillar d., allergic contact d. caused by the larva of the browntail moth, puss caterpillar, gypsy moths and other caterpillars. SYN caterpillar rash.

chemical d., allergic contact d. or primary irritation d. due to application of chemicals; usually characterized by erythema, edema, and vesiculation of the exposed or contacted site.

d. combustio′nis, inflammation of the skin following a burn.

d. congelatio′nis, SYN frostbite.

contact d., d. resulting from cutaneous contact with a specific allergen (allergic contact d.) or irritant (irritant contact d.). SYN contact hypersensitivity (1).

contact-type d., d. resembling contact d. or eczema, but caused by an ingested or injected allergen, usually a drug, and with a widespread or generalized distribution.

contagious pustular d., SYN orf.

cosmetic d., a cutaneous eruption that results from the application of a cosmetic; due to allergic sensitization or primary irritation.

dhobie mark d., an allergic contact d. due to hypersensitivity to ingredients in laundry marking ink. SYN dhobie mark, washerman's mark.

diaper d., colloquially referred to as diaper, ammonia, or napkin rash; d. of thighs and buttocks resulting from exposure to urine and feces in infants' diapers. Formerly attributed to ammonia formation; moisture, bacterial growth, and alkalinity may all induce lesions. SYN ammonia rash, diaper rash, Jacquet's erythema, napkin rash.

d. exfoliati′va, SYN exfoliative d.

d. exfoliati′va infan′tum, d. exfoliati′va neonato′rum, a generalized pyoderma accompanied by exfoliative d., with constitutional symptoms, affecting young infants, which may result from atopic d., Leiner's disease or staphylococcal scalded skin syndrome. SYN impetigo neonatorum (1).

exfoliative d., generalized exfoliation with scaling of the skin and usually with erythema (erythroderma); may be a drug reaction or associated with various benign dermatoses, lupus erythematosus, lymphomas, or of undetermined cause. SYN d. exfoliativa, pityriasis rubra, Wilson's disease (2).

exudative discoid and lichenoid d., SYN Sulzberger-Garbe *disease.*

factitial d., SYN d. artefacta.

d. gangreno′sa infan′tum, a bullous or pustular eruption, of uncertain origin, followed by necrotic ulcers or extensive gangrene in children under 2 years of age; if untreated, death may result from hematogenous infection, such as liver abscess. SYN disseminated cutaneous gangrene, ecthyma gangrenosum, pemphigus gangrenosus (1), rupia escharotica.

d. herpetifor′mis, a chronic disease of the skin marked by a symmetric itching eruption of vesicles and papules that occur in groups; relapses are common; associated with gluten-sensitive enteropathy and IgA immune complexes beneath the epidermis of lesioned and normal-appearing skin. SYN d. multiformis, Duhring's disease, herpes circinatus bullosus, hydroa herpetiforme.

d. hiema′lis, a recurrent eczema appearing with the advent of cold weather. SYN frost itch, lumberman's itch, pruritus hiemalis, winter itch.

infectious eczematoid d., an inflammatory reaction of skin adjacent to the site of a pyogenic infection; *e.g.,* purulent otitis, the area around a colostomy, or intranasal infection; thought to be due to a local sensitization to the resident organisms.

dermatitis – division into types	
endogenous	contact (or exogenous) dermatitis

atopic
seborrheic
coin-shaped
chronic hand and foot
  dermatitis
exfoliative
congestion-influenced
circumscribed
  neurodermatitis
pruritus of anus / vulva
drug eruption
	direct irritation
	  not photosensitive
	  phototoxic
	allergic
	  not photosensitive
	  photoallergic

de

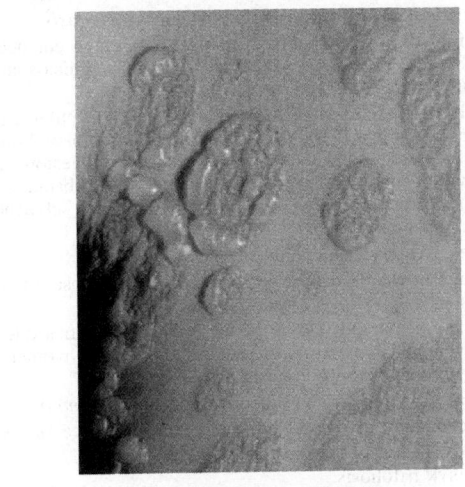

dermatitis herpetiformis

irritant contact d., skin reactions ranging from erythema and scaling to necrotic burns resulting from nonimmunologic damage by chemicals in contact with the skin immediately or repeatedly.

livedoid d., a reddish blue mottled condition of the skin due to affection of the cutaneous vascular apparatus.

mango d., a perioral d. resulting from a sensitization reaction to the resinous coating on the peel of the mango fruit.

meadow d., meadow grass d., a photoallergic reaction to contact with a plant containing furocoumarin in which the bizarre configuration of the eruption is that of the streaky pattern of the plant contact; often occurs after sunbathing. SYN phytophlyctodermatitis.

d. medicamento′sa, SYN drug *eruption.*

d. multifor′mis, SYN d. herpetiformis.

nickel d., allergic d. due to contact with, or in some cases ingestion of, nickel or other metals containing nickel (*e.g.,* stainless steel) as a diluent.

d. nodo′sa, a papular eruption on the legs, related to craw-craw.

d. nodula′ris necrot′ica, a recurrent eruption of vesicles, papules, and papulonecrotic lesions on the buttocks and extensor surfaces of the extremities, accompanied by fever, sore throat, diarrhea, and eosinophilia; probably a variant of vasculitis, it can be of varying and increasing severity and duration, and can occasionally involve the heart, kidneys, and gastrointestinal tract. SYN Werther's disease.

nummular d., SYN nummular *eczema.*

d. papilla′ris capillit′ii, SYN acne *keloid.*

papular d. of pregnancy, intensely pruritic papular eruption of torso and extremities occurring throughout pregnancy, with no systemic toxicity; may be similar to pruritic urticarial papules and plaques of pregnancy.

d. pediculoi′des ventrico′sus, SYN straw *itch*.

plant d., SEE d. venenata.

primary irritant d., a frequently cumulative reaction of irritation on exposure of the skin to substances which are toxic to epidermal or connective tissue cells; lesions are usually erythematous and papular, but can be purulent or necrotic, depending on the nature of the toxic material applied.

proliferative d., SYN dermatophilosis.

rat mite d., an eruption of wheals, papules, or vesicles caused by the rat mite.

d. re′pens, SYN *pustulosis* palmaris et plantaris. [L. creeping]

rhus d., contact d. caused by cutaneous exposure to urushiol from species of *Toxicodendron* (*Rhus*), such as poison ivy, oak, or sumac.

sandal strap d., allergic contact on the dorsal surfaces of the feet, caused by synthetic rubber sandal straps or additives to natural rubber.

Schamberg's d., SYN progressive pigmentary *dermatosis*.

schistosomal d., a sensitization response to repeated cutaneous invasion by cercariae of bird, mammal, or human schistosomes. SYN swimmer's itch (2), water itch (2).

seborrheic d., d. seborrhe′ica, a common scaly macular eruption that occurs primarily on the face, scalp (dandruff), and other areas of increased sebaceous gland secretion; the lesions are covered with a slightly adherent oily scale. SYN dyssebacia, dyssebacea, seborrhea corporis, seborrheic dermatosis, seborrheic eczema, Unna's disease.

d. sim′plex, SYN *erythema* simplex.

solar d., a d. in photosensitive persons caused by exposure to the sun's rays.

stasis d., erythema and scaling of the lower extremities due to impaired venous circulation, seen commonly in older women or secondary to deep vein thrombosis.

subcorneal pustular d., SYN subcorneal pustular *dermatosis*.

traumatic d., any d. caused by an irritant substance or by a physical agent.

trefoil d., SYN trifoliosis.

d. veg′etans, a benign fungating granulomatous mass caused by chronic pyogenic infection. SYN pyoderma vegetans.

d. venena′ta, obsolete term for a cutaneous eruption due to contact with a sensitizing agent such as urushiol in poison ivy, resins, chemicals, cosmetics, etc.; the eruption is edematous, erythematous, and vesicular.

d. verruco′sa, obsolete term for chromoblastomycosis.

△**dermato-.** SEE derm-. [G. *derma,* skin]

der·mat·o·al·lo·plas·ty (der′ma-tō-al′ō-plas-tē). Obsolete term for allografting of skin. [dermato- + G. *allos,* other, + *plastos,* formed]

der·mat·o·ar·thri·tis (der′mă-tō-ar-thrī′tis). Associated skin disease and arthritis.

lipoid d., a multicentric *reticulohistiocytosis*.

der·mat·o·au·to·plas·ty (der′ma-tō-aw′tō-plas-tē). Obsolete term for autografting of skin taken from another part of the patient's own body. [dermato- + G. *autos,* self, + *plastos,* formed]

Der·ma·to·bia (der-mă-tō′bē-ă). A genus of flies (family Oestridae) found in tropical America. [dermato- + G. *bios,* way of living]

D. cyaniven′tris, SYN *D. hominis.*

D. hom′inis, a large, blue, brown-winged species whose larvae develop in open boil-like lesions in the skin of humans, many domestic animals, and some fowl. It is a very serious and damaging cattle parasite and frequently attacks small children in Central and South America. Its eggs are laid on the legs or abdomen of another insect, such as the mosquito; the eggs later hatch, when stimulated by warmth or other factors, to release the botfly larvae on the skin of the mosquito's bloodmeal host, and the larvae quickly invade the skin to initiate myiasis. SYN *D. cyaniventris,* human botfly, skin botflies, warble botfly.

der·ma·to·bi·a·sis (der′mă-tō-bī′ă-sis). Infection of man and animals with larvae of the fly *Dermatobia hominis.* SYN human botfly myiasis.

der·mat·o·cel·lu·li·tis (der′mă-tō-sel-yū-lī′tis). Inflammation of the skin and subcutaneous connective tissue.

der·mat·o·cha·la·sis (der′mă-tō-kă-lā′sis). SYN *cutis* laxa. [dermato- + G. *chalaō,* to loosen]

der·mat·o·co·ni·o·sis (der′mă-tō-kō-nī-o′sis). An occupational dermatitis caused by local irritation from dust. [dermato- + G. *konis,* dust, + *-osis,* condition]

der·mat·o·cyst (der′mă-tō-sist). A cyst of the skin.

der·mat·o·dyn·ia (der′mă-tō-din′ē-ă). SYN dermatalgia. [dermato- + G. *odynē,* pain]

der·mat·o·fi·bro·ma (der′mă-tō-fī-brō′mă). A slowly growing benign skin nodule consisting of poorly demarcated cellular fibrous tissue enclosing collapsed capillaries, with scattered hemosiderin-pigmented and lipid macrophages. The following terms are considered by some to be synonymous with, and by others to be varieties of, d.: sclerosing hemangioma, fibrous histiocytoma, nodular subepidermal fibrosis.

der·mat·o·fi·bro·sar·co·ma pro·tu·ber·ans (der′mă-tō-fī′brō-sar-kō′mă prō-tū′ber-anz). A relatively slowly growing dermal neoplasm consisting of one or several firm nodules that are usually covered by dark red-blue skin, which tends to be fixed to the palpable masses; histologically, the neoplasm resembles a cellular dermatofibroma with a pronounced storiform pattern; metastases are unusual, but the incidence of recurrence is fairly high.

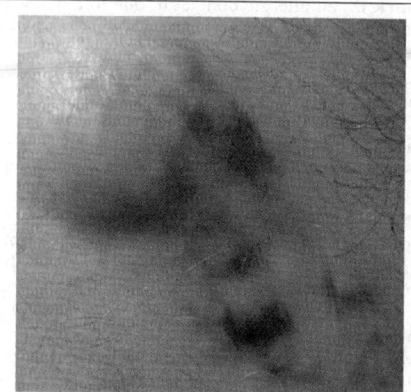

dermatofibrosarcoma protuberans
regrowth on scar of prior excision

pigmented d. p., an uncommon variant of d. p. containing heavily pigmented dendritic melanocytes scattered between spindle cells of the tumor. SYN Bednar tumor, storiform neurofibroma.

der·ma·to·fi·bro·sis len·tic·u·lar·is dis·sem·i·na·ta (der′mă-tō-fī-brō′sis len-tik-yū-lā′ris di-sem-i-nă′tă) [MIM*166700]. Small papules or discs of increased dermal elastic tissue appearing in early life; when osteopoikilosis is also present, the condition is called osteodermatopoikilosis or Buschke-Ollendorf syndrome; autosomal dominant inheritance.

der·mat·o·glyph·ics (der′mă-tō-glif′iks). **1.** The configurations of the characteristic ridge patterns of the volar surfaces of the skin; in the hand of man, the distal segment of each digit has three types of configurations: whorl, loop, and arch. SEE ALSO fingerprint. **2.** The science or study of these configurations or patterns. [dermato- + *glyphē,* carved work]

der·mat·o·graph (der-mat′ō-graf). The linear wheal made in the skin in dermatographism.

der·ma·tog·ra·phism (der-mă-tog′ră-fizm). A form of urticaria in which whealing occurs in the site and in the configuration of application of stroking (pressure, friction) of the skin. SYN autographism, dermagraphy, dermatography, dermographia, dermography, dermography, factitious urticaria, skin writing, urticaria factitia. [dermato- + G. *graphō,* to write]

der·ma·tog·ra·phy (der-mă-tog′ră-fē). SYN dermatographism.

der·mat·o·het·er·o·plas·ty (der′ma-tō-het′er-ō-plas-tē). Rarely used term for dermatoxenoplasty. [dermato- + G. *heteros,* another, + *plastos,* formed]

der·mat·o·ho·mo·plas·ty (der′mă-tō-hō′mō-plas-tē). Obsolete term for dermatoalloplasty. [dermato- + G. *homos,* same, + *plastos,* formed]

der·ma·toid (der′mă-toyd). **1.** Resembling skin. SYN dermoid (1). **2.** SYN dermal.

der·ma·tol·o·gist (der-mă-tol′ō-jist). A physician who specializes in the diagnosis and treatment of cutaneous diseases and related systemic diseases.

der·ma·tol·o·gy (der-mă-tol′ō-jē). The branch of medicine concerned with the study of the skin, diseases of the skin, and the relationship of cutaneous lesions to systemic disease. [dermato- + G. *logos,* study]

der·ma·tol·y·sis (der-mă-tol′i-sis). Loosening of the skin or atrophy of the skin by disease; erroneously used as a synonym for cutis laxa. SYN dermolysis. [dermato- + G. *lysis,* a loosening]

der·ma·to·ma (der-mă-tō′mă). A circumscribed thickening or hypertrophy of the skin. [dermato- + G. *-oma,* tumor]

der·ma·tome (der′mă-tōm). **1.** An instrument for cutting thin slices of skin for grafting, or excising small lesions. **2.** The dorsolateral part of an embryonic somite. SYN cutis plate. **3.** The area of skin supplied by cutaneous branches from a single spinal nerve; neighboring d.'s may overlap. SYN dermatomal distribution, dermatomic area. [dermato- + G. *tomē,* a cutting]

electric d., SEE electrodermatome.

der·mat·o·meg·a·ly (der′mă-tō-meg′a-lē). Congenital or acquired defect in which the skin hangs in folds; may be part of a syndrome or may occur in isolation as cutis laxa, dermatochalasis, or dermatolysis. [dermato- + G. *megas,* large]

der·mat·o·mere (der′mă-tō-mēr). A metameric area of the embryonic integument. [dermato- + G. *meros,* part]

der·mat·o·my·co·sis (der′mă-tō-mī-kō′sis). Fungus infection of the skin caused by dermatophytes, yeasts, and other fungi. Cf. dermatophytosis.

d. ped′is, SYN tinea pedis.

der·mat·o·my·o·ma (der′mă-tō-mī-ō′mă). SYN *leiomyoma* cutis. [dermato- + G. *mys,* muscle, + *-oma,* tumor]

der·mat·o·my·o·si·tis (der′mă-tō-mī-ō-sī′tis). A progressive condition characterized by symmetric proximal muscular weakness with elevated muscle enzyme levels and a skin rash, typically a purplish-red or heliotrope erythema on the face, and edema of the eyelids and periorbital tissue; affected muscle tissue shows degeneration of fibers with a chronic inflammatory reaction; occurs in children and adults, and in the latter may be associated with visceral cancer. [dermato- + G. *mys,* muscle, + *-itis,* inflammation]

der·mat·o·neu·ro·sis (der′mă-tō-nū-ro′sis). Any cutaneous eruption due to emotional stimuli. SYN dermoneurosis.

der·mat·o·no·sol·o·gy (der′mă-tō-nō-sol′ō-jē). The science of the nomenclature and classification of diseases of the skin. SYN dermonosology. [dermato- + G. *nosos,* disease, + *logos,* treatise]

der·mat·o·path·ia (der′mă-tō-path′ē-ă). SYN dermatopathy.

d. pigmento′sa reticula′ris, SYN *livedo* reticularis.

der·mat·o·pa·thol·o·gy (der′mă-tō-pa-thol′ō-jē). Histopathology of the skin and subcutis, and study of the causes of skin disease.

der·ma·top·a·thy (der′mă-top′ă-thē). Any disease of the skin. SYN dermatopathia, dermopathy. [dermato- + G. *pathos,* suffering]

Der·ma·toph·a·goi·des pter·o·nys·si·nus (der-mă-tof-ă-goy′dēz ter-ō-ni-sī′nŭs). A common species of cosmopolitan mites found in house dust and a common contributory cause of atopic asthma. [dermato- + G. *phagō,* to eat; ptero- + G. *nyssō,* to prick, stab]

der·ma·to·phi·lo·sis (der′mă-tō-fi-lō′sis). An infectious exuda-tive dermatitis of cattle, sheep, goats, horses, and other animals (occasionally man) caused by *Dermatophilus congolensis;* severe (sometimes fatal) d. is seen in cattle in the Caribbean, invariable in association with *Amblyomma variegatum* infestations. SYN proliferative dermatitis, streptothrichosis, streptotrichiasis, strep-totrichosis.

Der·ma·toph·i·lus con·go·len·sis (der-mă-tof′i-lŭs kon-gō-len′ sis). A species of motile, nonacid fast, aerobic to facultatively anaerobic, Gram-positive bacteria that is the etiologic agent of dermatophilosis; also causes proliferative dermatitis. [dermato- + G. *philos,* fond]

der·mat·o·pho·bia (der′mă-tō-fō′bē-ă). Morbid fear of acquiring a skin disease. [dermatosis + G. *phobos,* fear]

der·mat·o·phone (der′mă-tō-fōn). An instrument used for listening to blood flow in the skin.

der·mat·o·phy·lax·is (der′mă-tō-fī-lak′sis). Protection of the skin against potentially harmful agents; *e.g.,* infection, excessive sunlight, noxious agents. [dermato- + G. *phylaxis,* protection]

der·mat·o·phyte (der′mă-tō-fīt). A fungus that causes superficial infections of the skin, hair, and/or nails, *i.e.,* keratinized tissues. Species of *Epidermophyton, Microsporum,* and *Trichophyton* are regarded as dermatophytes, but causative agents of tinea versicolor, tinea nigra, and cutaneous candidiasis are not so classified. [dermato- + G. *phyton,* plant]

der·mat·o·phy·tid (der′mă-tof′i-tid). An allergic manifestation of dermatophytosis at a site distant from that of the primary fungous infection. The lesions, usually small vesicles on the hands and/or arms, are devoid of the fungus and may become extensive, covering wide areas of the body and causing extreme discomfort to the patient. SEE ALSO -id (1), id *reaction.*

der·mat·o·phy·to·sis (der′mă-tō-fī-tō′sis). An infection of the hair, skin, or nails caused by any one of the dermatophytes. The lesions may occur at any site on the body and, on the skin, are characterized by erythema, small papular vesicles, fissures, and scaling. Common sites of infection are the feet (tinea pedis), nails (onychomycosis), and scalp (tinea capitis). Cf. dermatomycosis.

der·mat·o·plas·tic (der′ma-tō-plas′tik). Obsolete term relating to dermatoplasty.

der·mat·o·plas·ty (der′ma-tō-plas-tē). Plastic surgery of the skin, as by skin grafting. SYN dermoplasty. [dermato- + G. *plastos,* formed]

der·mat·o·pol·y·neu·ri·tis (der′mă-tō-pol′ē-nū-rī′tis). SYN acrodynia (2).

der·ma·tor·rha·gia (der′mă-tō-rā′jē-ă). Hemorrhage from or into the skin. [dermato- + G. *rhēgnymi,* to break forth]

d. parasit′ica, a disease of the horse marked by numerous localized hemorrhages into and through the skin from small nodules, due to the presence of the parasitic filarial nematode, *Parafilaria multipapillosa.*

der·ma·tor·rhea (der′mă-tō-rē′ă). An excessive secretion of the sebaceous or sweat glands of the skin. [dermato- + G. *rhoia,* flow]

der·ma·tor·rhex·is (der′mă-tō-rek′sis). Rupture of the skin; *e.g.,* as is seen in striae cutis distensae or in Ehlers-Danlos syndrome. [dermato- + G. *rhēxis,* rupture]

der·mat·o·scle·ro·sis (der′mă-tō-skler-ō′sis). SYN scleroderma. [dermato- + G. *sklēroō,* to harden]

der·ma·tos·co·py (der′mă-tos′kŏ-pē). Inspection of the skin, usually with the aid of a lens. [dermato- + G. *skopeō,* to view]

der·ma·to·sis, pl. **der·ma·to·ses** (der′mă-tō′sis, -sēz). Nonspecific term used to denote any cutaneous abnormality or eruption. [dermato- + G. *-osis,* condition]

acarine d., an eruption caused by one of the acarine parasites.

acute febrile neutrophilic d., a rare d., predominant in women, of rapid onset and characterized by plaque-like lesions, usually multiple, on the face, neck, and upper extremities, accompanied by conjunctivitis, mucosal lesions, fever, malaise, arthralgia, and peripheral blood neutrophilia in many cases; biopsy reveals polymorphonuclear infiltrate of the dermis; rapid remission occurs with systemic steroid therapy. SYN Sweet's disease.

ashy d., SYN *erythema* dyschromicum perstans.

Bowen's precancerous d., SYN Bowen's *disease*.

chick nutritional d., d. in chicks, with eruptions about the eyes, mouth, and feet; responds to pantothenic acid.

chronic bullous d. of childhood, a rare self-limiting bullous disease, chiefly of the trunk, perioral, and pelvic areas, with onset in the first decade, successively less severe recurrences, and total remission at adolescence; linear epidermal basement membrane zone deposit of IgA is found in involved and in normal skin. SYN linear IgA bullous disease in children.

dermolytic bullous d., SYN *epidermolysis* bullosa dystrophica.

digitate d., SEE *parapsoriasis* en plaque. SYN small plaque parapsoriasis.

filarial d., a disease of sheep on high mountain ranges during the summer caused by larvae of the filarial worm, *Elaeophora schneideri*, which localize chiefly on the head, causing intense itching and loss of wool. SYN sorehead.

lichenoid d., any chronic skin eruption, characterized clinically by induration and thickening of the skin with accentuation of skin markings, and microscopically by a band-like lymphocytic infiltration of the papillary dermis.

d. medicamento'sa, SYN drug *eruption*.

d. papulo'sa ni'gra, dark brown papular lesions, observed in blacks, on the face and upper trunk; histologically and clinically, they resemble seborrheic keratoses.

pigmented purpuric lichenoid d., an eruption comprised of lichenoid papules variously pigmented from the hemosiderin of the associated purpura; found on the legs, usually in men over 40 years of age. SYN Gougerot and Blum disease.

progressive pigmentary d., chronic purpura, especially of the legs in men, spreading to form brownish patches; associated microscopically with perivascular lymphatic infiltration, diapedesis, and hemosiderosis. SYN Schamberg's dermatitis.

radiation d., skin changes at the site of ionizing radiation, particularly erythema in the acute stage, temporary or permanent epilation, and chronic changes in the epidermis and dermis resembling actinic keratosis.

seborrheic d., SYN seborrheic *dermatitis*.

subcorneal pustular d., a pruritic chronic annular eruption of sterile vesicles and pustules beneath the stratum corneum; bears a considerable clinical resemblance to dermatitis herpetiformis. SYN Sneddon-Wilkinson disease, subcorneal pustular dermatitis.

transient acantholytic d., a pruritic papular eruption, with histologic suprabasal acantholysis, of the chest, with scattered lesions of the back and lateral aspects of the extremities, lasting from a few weeks to several months; seen predominantly in males over 40. SYN Grover's disease.

ulcerative d., an infectious disease of sheep characterized by crusted ulcers on the skin of the face, feet, and external genitalia; thought to be caused by the orf virus. SYN lip and leg ulceration.

der·mat·o·ther·a·py (der'mă-tō-thār'ă-pē). Treatment of skin diseases.

der·mat·o·thla·si·a (der'mă-tō-thlā'zē-ă). An uncontrollable impulse to pinch and bruise the skin. [dermato- + G. *thlasis*, a bruising]

der·mat·o·tro·pic (der'mă-tō-trop'ik). Having an affinity for the skin. SYN dermotropic. [dermato- + G. *trope*, a turning]

der·ma·to·xen·o·plas·ty (der'mă-tō-zē'nō-plas-tē). Obsolete term for xenografting of skin. [dermato- + G. *xenos*, stranger, + *plastos*, formed]

der·mat·o·zo·i·a·sis (der'mă-tō-zō-ī'ă-sis). Obsolete term for dermatozoonosis. [dermato- + G. *zōon*, animal, + *-iasis*, condition]

der·mat·o·zo·on (der'mă-tō-zō'on). An animal parasite of the skin. [dermato- + G. *zōon*, animal]

der·mat·o·zo·o·no·sis (der'mă-tō-zō-ō-nō'sis, -zō-on'ō-sis). Infestation of the skin by an animal parasite. [dermato- + G. *zōon*, animal, + *nosos*, disease]

der·ma·tro·phia, der·mat·ro·phy (der-mă-trō'fē-ă, der-mat' rō-fē). Atrophy or thinning of the skin.

der·men·chy·sis (der-men'ki-sis). Rarely used term for subcutaneous administration of remedies. [derm- + G. *enchysis*, a pouring in]

der·mic (der'mik). SYN dermal.

der·mis [NA]. A layer of skin composed of a superficial thin layer that interdigitates with the epidermis, the stratum papillare, and the stratum reticulare; it contains blood and lymphatic vessels, nerves and nerve endings, glands, and, except for glabrous skin, hair follicles. SYN corium [NA], cutis vera. [G. *derma*, skin]

dermo-. SEE derm-. [G. *derma*, skin]

der·mo·blast (der'mō-blast). One of the mesodermal cells from which the corium is developed. [dermo- + G. *blastos*, germ]

der·mo·cy·ma (der'mō-sī'mă). Unequal conjoined twins in which the smaller parasite is buried in the integument of the autosite. [dermo- + G. *kyma*, fetus]

der·mo·graph·ia, der·mog·ra·phism, der·mog·ra·phy (der-mō-graf'ē-ă, -mog'ră-fizm, -mog'ră-fē). SYN dermatographism.

der·moid (der'moyd). 1. SYN dermatoid (1). 2. SYN dermoid *cyst*. [dermo- + G. *eidos*, resemblance]

inclusion d., SYN dermoid *cyst*.

sequestration d., obsolete term for epidermal *cyst*.

der·moi·dec·to·my (der-moy-dek'tō-mē). Rarely used term for operative removal of a dermoid cyst. [dermoid + G. *ektomē*, excision]

der·mol·y·sis (der-mol'i-sis). SYN dermatolysis.

der·mo·ne·crot·ic (der'mō-nĕ-krot'ik). Pertaining to any application or illness which may cause necrosis of the skin.

der·mo·neu·ro·sis (der'mō-nū-rō'sis). SYN dermatoneurosis.

der·mo·no·sol·o·gy (der'mō-nō-sol'ō-jē). SYN dermatonosology.

der·mop·a·thy (der-mop'ă-thē). SYN dermatopathy.

diabetic d., small macules and papules of the extensor surfaces of the extremities, most commonly the shins of diabetics, which become atrophic, hyperpigmented, and occasionally undergo ulceration with scarring; may be a manifestation of microangiopathy.

der·mo·phle·bi·tis (der'mō-flĕ-bī'tis). Inflammation of the superficial veins and the surrounding skin. [dermo- + G. *phleps*, vein, + *-itis*, inflammation]

der·mo·plas·ty (der'mō-plas-tē). SYN dermatoplasty.

der·mo·skel·e·ton (der-mō-skel'ĕ-tŏn). SYN exoskeleton (1).

der·mo·ste·no·sis (der'mō-stĕ-nō'sis). Pathologic contraction of the skin. [dermo- + G. *stenōsis*, a narrowing]

der·mos·to·sis (der'mos-tō'sis). SYN *osteoma* cutis. [derm- + G. *osteon*, bone, + *-osis*, condition]

der·mo·syph·i·lop·a·thy (der'mō-sif-i-lop'ă-thē). Cutaneous lesions of syphilis; any syphilid.

der·mo·tox·in (der-mō-tok'sin). A substance elaborated by a living agent, especially an exotoxin formed by bacteria, and characterized by its ability to cause pathologic changes in skin, *e.g.,* erythema, degenerative changes, necrosis.

der·mo·tro·pic (der-mō-trop'ik). SYN dermatotropic.

der·mo·vas·cu·lar (der-mō-vas'kyū-lăr). Pertaining to the blood vessels of the skin. [dermo- + L. *vasculus*, small vessel]

der·o·did·y·mus (dăr'ō-did'i-mŭs). SYN *dicephalus* diauchenos. [G. *derē*, neck, + *didymos*, twin]

de·ro·ta·tion (dē-rō-tā'shŭn). 1. A turning back. 2. In orthopedics, the correction of a rotation deformity by turning or rotating the deformed structure toward a normal position. [L. *de*, away, + *rotatio*, turning]

DES Abbreviation for diethylstilbestrol.

des-. In chemistry, a prefix indicating absence of some component of the principal part of the name; largely replaced by de- (*e.g.,* deoxyribonucleic acid, dehydro-) but retained where "de" could be taken for D or *d*, as part of "desmo" (*e.g.,* desmosterol), and in such terms as desoxycortone.

des·am·i·dize (dē-sam'i-dīz). SYN deamidize.

De Sanctis, Carlo, Italian psychiatrist, *1888. SEE De S.-Cacchione *syndrome*.

de·sat·u·rate (dē-sat'yū-rāt). To produce desaturation.

de·sat·u·ra·tion (dē'sat-yū-rā'shŭn). The act, or the result of the act, of making something less completely saturated; more specifically, the percentage of total binding sites remaining unfilled, *e.g.,* when hemoglobin is 70% saturated with oxygen and nothing else, its d. is 30%. Cf. saturation (5).

Desault, Pierre J., French surgeon, 1744–1795. SEE D.'s *bandage.*

Descartes (Cartesius), René, French philosopher, mathematician, physiologist, 1596–1650. The founder of modern philosophy and proponent of the mechanistic *school* or iatromathematical *school.* SEE D.'s *law.*

Descemet, Jean, French physician, 1732–1810. SEE D.'s *membrane.*

des·ce·me·ti·tis (des′ĕ-mĕ-tī′tis). Inflammation of Descemet's membrane.

des·ce·met·o·cele (des-ĕ-met′ō-sēl). A bulging forward of Descemet's membrane caused by the destruction of the substance of the cornea by infection.

de·scen·dens (dē-sen′denz). SYN descending. [L.]

  d. cervica′lis, SYN inferior *root* of ansa cervicalis.

  d. hypoglos′si, SYN superior *root* of ansa cervicalis.

de·scend·ing (dē-send′ing). Running downward or toward the periphery. SYN descendens. [L. *de-scendo,* pp. *-scensus,* to come down, fr. *scando,* to climb]

de·scen·sus (dē-sen′sŭs). A falling away from a higher position. SEE ALSO ptosis, procidentia. SYN descent (1). [L.]

  d. tes′tis [NA], descent of the testis from the abdomen into the scrotum during the seventh and eighth months of intrauterine life.

  d. u′teri, SYN *prolapse* of the uterus.

  d. ventric′uli, SYN gastroptosis.

de·scent (dē-sent′). **1.** SYN descensus. **2.** In obstetrics, the passage of the presenting part of the fetus into and through the birth canal. [L. descensus]

Deschamps, Joseph F.L., French surgeon, 1740–1824. SEE D. *needle.*

de·sen·si·tiz·a·tion (dē-sen′si-ti-zā′shŭn). **1.** The reduction or abolition of allergic sensitivity or reactions to the specific antigen (allergen). SYN ananaphylaxis, antianaphylaxis. **2.** The act of removing an emotional complex. SYN hyposensitization.

  heterologous d., stimulation by one agonist which leads to a broad pattern of unresponsiveness to further stimulation by a variety of other agonists.

  homologous d., loss of sensitivity only to the class of agonist used to desensitize the tissue.

  systematic d., a type of behavior therapy for eliminating phobias or anxieties: the patient and therapist construct a list of imagined scenes eliciting the phobia, ranked from least to most anxiety-producing; the patient then is trained in deep muscle relaxation, and is repeatedly asked to imagine himself in the presence of the least anxiety-producing scene on the list until he feels fully relaxed while doing so; the procedure is repeated for each scene on the list until the patient develops the capacity to feel relaxed with any of the anxiety-producing scenes; real life scenes are then substituted for the imagined scenes. SYN reciprocal inhibition (2).

de·sen·si·tize (dē-sen′si-tīz). **1.** To reduce or remove any form of sensitivity. SYN deallergize. **2.** To effect desensitization (1). **3.** In dentistry, to eliminate or subdue the painful response of exposed, vital dentin to irritative agents or thermal changes.

de·ser·pi·dine (dē-ser′pi-dēn). 11-Desmethoxyreserpine; ester alkaloid isolated from *Rauwolfia canescens* (family Apocynaceae) with the same actions and uses as reserpine.

des·e·tope (dē′se-tōp). That part of the Class II major histocompatibility molecule that interacts with the antigen. The term desetope is derived from determinant selection. [*de*terminant *sel*ection + -tope]

des·fer·ri·ox·a·mine mes·y·late (des′făr-ē-ok′să-mēn). SYN deferoxamine mesylate.

des·flu·rane (des′flŭr′ān). 1-Fluoro-2,2,2-trifluoro-ethyl difluoromethyl ether; an inhalation anesthesia with physical characteristics that provide rapid induction of and recovery from anesthesia.

des·hy·dre·mia (des′hī-drē′mē-ă). Hemoconcentration due to the loss of water from blood plasma. [L. *de-,* away from, + G. *hydor,* water, + *haima,* blood + -ia]

des·ic·cant (des′i-kant). **1.** Drying; causing or promoting dryness. SYN desiccative. **2.** An agent that absorbs moisture; a drying agent. SYN desiccator (1). SYN exsiccant. [L. *de-sicco,* pp. *-siccatus,* to dry up]

des·ic·cate (des′i-kāt). To dry thoroughly; to render free from moisture. SYN exsiccate.

des·ic·ca·tion (des-i-kā′shŭn). The process of being desiccated. SYN dehydration (4), exsiccation (1).

des·ic·ca·tive (des-i-kā′tiv). SYN desiccant (1).

des·ic·ca·tor (des′i-kā-ter, tōr). **1.** SYN desiccant (2). **2.** An apparatus, such as a glass chamber containing calcium chloride, sulfuric acid, or other drying agent, in which a material is placed for drying.

  vacuum d., a d. that can be evacuated.

de·si·pra·mine hy·dro·chlo·ride (des-ip′ră-mēn). Desmethylimipramine hydrochloride; norimipramine hydrochloride; a dibenzazepine derivative; an antidepressant similar to imipramine hydrochloride.

des·lan·o·side (des-lan′ō-sīd). Desacetyllanatoside C; a rapidly acting steroid glycoside obtained from lanatoside C (*Digitalis lanata*) by alkaline hydrolysis; a cardiotonic.

△**desm-.** SEE desmo-.

Desmarres, Louis A., French ophthalmologist, 1810–1882. SEE D.'s *dacryoliths,* under *dacryolith.*

des·mec·ta·sis, des·mec·ta·sia (dez-mek′tă-sis, -mek-tā′zē-ă). Ectasia of a ligament. [desm- + G. *ektasis,* a stretching]

des·mins (dez′minz). Certain proteins found in intermediate filaments that copolymerizes with vimentin to form constituents of connective tissue, cell walls, filaments, etc.

des·mi·tis (dez-mī′tis). Inflammation of a ligament. [desm- + G. *-itis,* inflammation]

△**desmo-, desm-.** Fibrous connection; ligament. [G. *desmos,* a band]

des·mo·cra·ni·um (dez-mō-krā′nē-ŭm). The mesenchymal primordium of the cranium.

Des·mo·dus (dez′mō-dŭs). A blood-feeding genus of Chiroptera, known generally as vampire bats, found in Trinidad, Mexico, and Central and South America; *D. artibaeus, D. rotundus,* and *D. rufus,* three species present in Trinidad and South America, are reservoir hosts of rabies virus. [desmo- + G. *odous,* tooth]

des·mo·dyn·ia (dez-mō-din′ē-ă). Pain in a ligament. [desmo- + G. *odynē,* pain]

des·mog·e·nous (dez-moj′ĕ-nŭs). Of connective tissue or ligamentous origin or causation; *e.g.,* denoting a deformity due to contraction of ligaments, fascia, or a scar. [desmo- + G. *-gen,* producing]

des·mog·ra·phy (dez-mog′ră-fē). A description of, or treatise on, the ligaments. [desmo- + G. *graphō,* to describe]

des·moid (dez′moyd). **1.** Fibrous or ligamentous. **2.** A nodule or relatively large mass of unusually firm scarlike connective tissue resulting from active proliferation of fibroblasts, occurring most frequently in the abdominal muscles of women who have borne children; the fibroblasts infiltrate surrounding muscle and fascia. SYN abdominal fibromatosis, desmoid tumor. [desmo- + G. *eidos,* appearance, form]

  extra-abdominal d., a deep-seated firm tumor, most frequently occurring on the shoulders, chest, or back of young men or women, consisting of collagenous fibrous tissue that infiltrates surrounding muscle; frequently recurs but does not metastasize.

des·mo·las·es (dez′mō-lā′sez). Old and nonspecific term for enzymes catalyzing reactions other than those involving hydrolysis; *e.g.,* those involving oxidation and reduction, isomerization, the breaking of carbon-carbon bonds.

des·mol·o·gy (dez-mol′ō-jē). The branch of anatomy concerned with the ligaments. [desmo- + G. *logos,* study]

des·mon (dez′mon). An old term for complement-fixing antibody. [G. *desmos,* band, bond]

des·mop·a·thy (dez-mop′ă-thē). Any disease of the ligaments. [desmo- + G. *pathos,* suffering]

des·mo·pla·sia (dez-mō-plā′zē-ă).   Hyperplasia of fibroblasts and disproportionate formation of fibrous connective tissue, especially in the stroma of a carcinoma. [desmo- + G. *plasis,* a molding]

des·mo·plas·tic (des-mō-plas′tik).   1. Causing or forming adhesions. 2. Causing fibrosis in the vascular stroma of a neoplasm.

des·mo·pres·sin (des-mō-pres′in).   An analog of vasopressin (antidiuretic hormone, ADH) possessing powerful antidiuretic activity.

 d. acetate, 1-(3-Mercaptopropionic acid)-8-D-arginine-vasopressin monoacetate trihydrate; a synthetic analog of vasopressin and an antidiuretic hormone.

des·mo·pres·sin ac·e·tate.   See under desmopressin.

des·mo·sine (dez′mō-sēn).   A cross-linking amino acid formed from lysyl residues found in elastin. [G. *desmos,* bond, fr. *deō,* to bind, + -ine]

des·mo·some (dez′mō-sōm).   A site of adhesion between two epithelial cells, consisting of a dense attachment plaque separated from a similar structure in the other cell by a thin layer of extracellular material. SYN bridge corpuscle, macula adherens. [desmo- + G. *sōma,* body]

des·mos·te·rol (dez-mos′ter-ol).   5α-cholesta-5,24-diene-3β-ol; postulated intermediate in cholesterol biosynthesis from lanosterol via zymosterol; accumulates after prolonged administration of substances interfering with cholesterol biosynthesis. SYN 24-dehydrocholesterol.

des·o·nide (des′ō-nīd).   Pregna-1,4-diene-3,20-dione, 11,21-dihydroxy-16,17-[(1-methylethylidene)bis(oxy)]-, (11β,16α)-; an anti-inflammatory corticosteroid used in topical preparations.

des·ox·i·met·a·sone (des-ok-si-met′ă-sōn).   Pregna-1,4-diene-3,20-dione, 9-fluoro-11,21-dihydroxy-16-methyl-, (11β,16α)-; an anti-inflammatory corticosteroid used in topical preparations.

⚠**desoxy-.**   SEE deoxy-.

des·ox·y·cor·ti·cos·ter·one (dēs-oks-ē-kōr′tĭ-ōs-ter-ōn).   A steroid derived from the adrenal cortex with strong mineralocorticoid activity.

des·ox·y·cor·tone (des-oks-ē-kōr′tōn).   SYN deoxycorticosterone.

de·spe·ci·a·tion (dē-spē′shē-ā′shŭn).   1. Alteration of, or loss of species characteristics. 2. Removal of species-specific antigenic properties from a foreign protein.

D'Éspine,   Jean H.A., French physician, 1846–1930. SEE D.'s *sign.*

des·pu·ma·tion (des-pyū-mā′shŭn).   1. The rising of impurities to the surface of a liquid. 2. The skimming off of impurities on the surface of a liquid. [L. *de-spumo,* pp. *-atus,* to skim, fr. *spumo,* to foam, fr. *spuma,* foam]

des·qua·mate (des′kwă-māt).   To shred, peel, or scale off, as the casting off of the epidermis in scales or shreds, or the shedding of the outer layer of any surface. [L. *desquamo,* pp. *-atus,* to scale off, fr. *squama,* a scale]

des·qua·ma·tion (des-kwă-mā′shŭn).   The shedding of the cuticle in scales or of the outer layer of any surface.

 branny d., SYN defurfuration.

des·qua·ma·tive (des-kwam′ă-tiv).   Relating to or marked by desquamation.

des·thi·o·bi·o·tin (des′thī-ō-bī′ō-tin).   A compound derived from biotin by the removal of the sulfur atom; a precursor of biotin in bacteria and molds; it can substitute for biotin in some microorganisms, but is without effect on or is inhibitory to the growth of others.

de·stru·do (dē-strū′dō).   Energy associated with the death or destructive instinct. [coinage on the analogy of *libido* fr. L. *destruo,* to destroy]

de·sulf·hy·dras·es (dē′sulf-hī′dră-sez).   Enzymes or groups of enzymes catalyzing the removal of a molecule of H_2S or substituted H_2S from a compound, as in the conversion of cysteine to pyruvic acid by cysteine desulfhydrase (cystathionine γ-lyase). SYN desulfurases.

de·sul·fi·nase (dē-sŭl′fin-ās).   Term sometimes applied to the enzyme (aspartate-4-decarboxylase) removing sulfite: 1) from cysteinesulfinate, an intermediate in cysteine degradation, yield-

ing alanine; 2) from sulfinylpyruvate, previously postulated to be formed by deamination of cysteinesulfinate, yielding pyruvate; degradation of sulfinylpyruvate is now considered to be spontaneous, not requiring an enzyme.

De·sul·fo·to·ma·cu·lum.   A genus of rod-shaped (straight or curved), anaerobic, chemoorganotrophic motile bacteria that stain Gram-negative but have Gram-positive cell walls. Found in soil, the rumen and elsewhere. The type species is *D. nigrificans.*

 D. nigri′ficans, a species found in canned corn showing "sulfur stinker spoilage." It is not pathogenic.

de·sul·fu·ras·es (dē-sŭl′fyūr-ās-ez).   SYN desulfhydrases.

de·syn·chro·nous (de-sin′kron-ŭs).   Lack of synchrony, as in brain waves. [de- + G. *syn,* with, + *chronos,* time]

DET   Abbreviation for diethyltryptamine.

det.   Abbreviation for L. *detur,* give. [let it be given]

de·tach·ment (dē-tach′ment).   1. A voluntary or involuntary feeling or emotion that accompanies a sense of separation from normal associations or environment. 2. Separation of a structure from its support.

 exudative retinal d., d. of the retina without retinal breaks, arising from inflammatory disease of choroid, retinal tumors, and retinal angiomatosis.

 retinal d., d. of retina, loss of apposition between the sensory retina and the retinal pigment epithelium. SYN detached retina, separation of retina.

 rhegmatogenous retinal d., retinal separation associated with a break, a hole, or a tear in the sensory retina.

 vitreous d., separation of the peripheral vitreous humor from the retina.

de·tec·tion (dē-tek′shun).   The act of discovery. 2. In chromatography, visualization of the separated material.

de·tec·tor (dē-tek′ter, -tōr).   The component of a laboratory instrument which detects the chemical or physical signal indicating the presence or quantity of the substance of interest.

 solid-state d., a d. that uses a crystalline scintillating material rather than an ionization chamber to detect or measure radiation.

de·ter·gent (dē-ter′jent).   1. Cleansing. 2. A cleansing or purging agent, usually salts of long-chain aliphatic bases or acids (*e.g.,* quaternary ammonium or sulfonic acid compounds) which, through a surface action that depends on their possessing both hydrophilic and hydrophobic properties, exert cleansing (oil-dissolving) and antibacterial effects; acridine derivatives (*e.g.,* acriflavine, proflavine) as well as other dyes (*e.g.,* brilliant green, crystal violet) have d. properties for the same reasons. SYN detersive. [L. *de-tergeo,* pp. *-tersus,* to wipe off]

 anionic d.'s, d.'s, such as soaps (alkali metal salts of long-chain fatty acids), that carry a negative electric charge on a lipid-like molecule and exert a limited antibacterial effect.

 cationic d.'s, d.'s, such as the amine salts or quaternary ammonium or pyridinium compounds of long-chain fatty acids, that have positively charged groups attached to the larger hydrophobic portions.

 zwitterionic d., SYN zwittergents.

de·te·ri·o·ra·tion (dē-tēr′i-ō-rā′shŭn).   The process or condition of becoming worse. [L. *deterior,* worse]

 alcoholic d., dementia occurring in persons chronically addicted to alcohol. SEE chronic *alcoholism.*

 senile d., a slowly progressing decline in physical and mental health, apparently due to natural causes attendant upon the processes of aging. SEE Alzheimer's *disease.*

de·ter·mi·nant (dē-ter′mi-nănt).   The factor that contributes to the generation of a trait. [L. *determans,* determining, limiting]

 allotypic d.'s, antigenic d.'s of allotypes.

 antigenic d., the particular chemical group of a molecule that determines immunological specificity. SYN determinant group.

 disease d.'s, any variables that directly or indirectly influence the frequency of occurrence and/or the distribution of any given disease; they include specific disease agents, host characteristics, and environmental factors.

 genetic d., any antigenic d. or identifying characteristic, particularly those of allotypes. SYN genetic marker.

 idiotypic antigenic d., SYN idiotype.

isoallotypic d.'s, genetic d.'s that are both isotypic and allotypic in that they appear in all members of at least one subclass of immunoglobulin but only in some members of another subclass of the same species.

mathematical d., a formal algebraic operation on the terms of a square matrix of quantities, fundamental in solving multiple simultaneous equations and widely used in regression analysis, notably in epidemiology and quantitative genetics. If d. is zero, the equations have no unambiguous solution.

de·ter·mi·na·tion (dē-ter-mi-nā'shŭn). 1. A change, for the better or for the worse, in the course of a disease. 2. A general move toward a given point. 3. The measurement or estimation of any quantity or quality in scientific or laboratory investigation. 4. Discernment of a state or category (*e.g.,* in diagnosis). 5. A process, both necessary and sufficient, whereby an effect is caused. [L. *de-termino,* pp. *-atus,* to limit, determine, fr. *terminus,* a boundary]

cell d., the process by which embryonic cells, previously undifferentiated, take on a specific developmental character. SEE morphogenesis, induction, evocator.

> Although the mechanism is not fully understood, homeotic proteins coded for by certain gene sequences (the homeobox) appear to trigger the process. Genes for homeotic proteins show remarkable similarity among species.

sex d., d. of the sex of a fetus *in utero* by identification of fetal chromosomes.

de·ter·mi·nism (dē-ter'mi-nizm). The proposition that all behavior is caused exclusively by genetic and environmental influences with no random components, and independent of free will. [L. *determino,* to limit, fr. *terminus,* boundary + -ism]

psychic d., in psychoanalysis, the concept that all psychological and behavioral phenomena result from antecedent, unconsciously operating causes.

de·ter·sive (dē-ter'siv). SYN detergent.

De Toni, Giovanni, Italian pediatrician, *1895. SEE De T.-Fanconi *syndrome.*

de·tox·i·cate (dē-tok'si-kāt). To diminish or remove the poisonous quality of any substance; to lessen the virulence of any pathogenic organism. SYN detoxify. [L. *de,* from, + *toxicum,* poison]

de·tox·i·ca·tion (dē-tok-si-kā'shŭn). 1. Recovery from the toxic effects of a drug. 2. Removal of the toxic properties from a poison. 3. Metabolic conversion of pharmacologically active principles to pharmacologically less active principles. SYN detoxification.

ammonia d., the d. of ammonia and ammonium ion by the formation of ammonium salts, specific nitrogen-excretion products, or L-glutamine.

de·tox·i·fi·ca·tion (dē-tok'si-fi-kā'shŭn). SYN detoxication.

de·tox·i·fy (dē-tok'si-fī). SYN detoxicate.

de·tri·tion (dē-trish'ŭn). A wearing away by use or friction. [L. *de-tero,* pp. *-tritus,* to rub off]

de·tri·tus (dē-trī'tŭs). Any broken-down material, carious or gangrenous matter, gravel, etc. [L. (see detrition)]

de·tru·sor (dē-trū'ser, -sōr). A muscle that has the action of expelling a substance. [L. *detrudo,* to drive away]

de·tu·mes·cence (dē-tū-mes'ens). Subsidence of a swelling. [L. *de,* from, + *tumesco,* to swell up, fr. *tumeo,* to swell]

de·tur·ges·cence (dē-tūr-ges'ens). The mechanism by which the stroma of the cornea remains relatively dehydrated. [L. *de,* from, + *turgesco,* to begin to swell]

⌂**deut-.** SEE deutero-.

deu·ten·ceph·a·lon (dū'ten-sef'ă-lon). Rarely used term for diencephalon. [G. *deuteros,* second, + *enkephalos,* brain]

deu·ter·a·nom·a·ly (dū'ter-ă-nom'ă-lē). A form of anomalous trichromatism due to a defect of the green-sensitive retinal cones. [G. *deuteros,* second, + *anōmalia,* anomaly]

deu·ter·an·ope (dū'ter-ă-nōp). A person affected with deuteranopia.

deu·ter·an·o·pia (dū'ter-ă-nō'pē-ă). A congenital abnormality of the retina in which there are two rather than three retinal cone pigments (dichromatism) and complete insensitivity to middle wavelengths (green). [G. *deuteros,* second, + anopia]

⌂**deuterio-.** Prefix indicating "containing deuterium."

deu·te·ri·um (D) (dū-tēr'ē-ŭm). SYN hydrogen-2. [G. *deuteros,* second]

d. oxide, SYN heavy *water.*

⌂**deutero-, deut-, deuto-.** Combining forms meaning two, or second (in a series); secondary. [G. *deuteros,* second]

deu·ter·o·my·ce·tes (du'ter-ō-mī-se'tēz). Members of the class Deuteromycetes or the phylum Deuteromycota.

Deu·ter·o·my·cota (dū'ter-ō-mī-kō-tă). A phylum in which the sexual (teleomorph or perfect) part of the life cycle has not been discovered; only the asexual (anamorph or imperfect) part of the life cycle has been found. SEE ALSO Fungi Imperfecti.

deu·ter·on (dū'ter-on). The nucleus of hydrogen-2, composed of one neutron and one proton; it thus has the one positive charge characteristic of a hydrogen nucleus. SYN deuton, diplon.

deu·ter·o·path·ic (dū'ter-ō-path'ik). Relating to a deuteropathy.

deu·ter·op·a·thy (dū-ter-op'ă-thē). A secondary disease or symptom. [deutero- + G. *pathos,* suffering]

deu·ter·o·plasm (dū'ter-ō-plazm). SYN deutoplasm. [deutero- + G. *plasma,* thing formed]

deu·ter·o·por·phy·rin (dū'ter-ō-pōr'fi-rin). A porphyrin derivative resembling the protoporphyrins except that the two vinyl side chains are replaced by hydrogen.

deu·ter·o·some (dū'ter-ō-sōm). Dense spherical fibrous granules that occur in the centrosphere and act in the development of centrioles or basal bodies. SYN procentriole organizer.

deu·ter·o·to·cia (dū'ter-ō-tō'sē-ă). A form of parthenogenesis in which the female has offspring of both sexes. SYN deuterotoky. [deutero- + G. *tokos,* childbirth]

deu·ter·ot·o·ky (dū-ter-ot'ō-kē). SYN deuterotocia.

⌂**deuto-.** SEE deutero-.

deu·to·gen·ic (dū-tō-jen'ik). Of secondary origin following an inductive influence. [deuto- + G. *-gen,* production]

deu·tom·er·ite (dū-tom'er-īt). The posterior nucleated portion of an attached cephalont in a gregarine protozoan, separated by an ectoplasmic septum from the anterior portion, or protomerite. [deuto- + L. *meros,* part]

deu·ton (dū'ton). SYN deuteron.

deu·to·plasm (dū'tō-plazm). The yolk of a meroblastic egg; the nonliving material in the cytoplasm, especially that stored in the ovum as food for the developing embryo, the commonest types being lipoid droplets and yolk granules. SYN deuteroplasm. [deuto- + G. *plasma,* thing formed]

deu·to·plas·mic (dū-tō-plaz'mik). Relating to the deutoplasm.

deu·to·plas·mi·gen·on (dū'tō-plaz-mi-jen'on). That which produces or gives rise to deutoplasm. [deutoplasm + G. *genos,* birth]

deu·to·plas·mol·y·sis (dū'tō-plaz-mol'i-sis). The disintegration of deutoplasm. [deutoplasm + G. *lysis,* dissolution]

Deutschländer, Carl E. W., German surgeon, 1872–1942. SEE D.'s *disease.*

DEV. Abbreviation for duck embryo origin *vaccine.*

de·vas·cu·lar·i·za·tion (dē-vas'kyū-lăr-i-zā'shŭn). Occlusion of all or most of the blood vessels to any part or organ. [L. *de,* away, + *vasculus,* small vessel, + G. *izo,* to cause]

de·vel·op (dē-vel'ŏp). To process an exposed photographic or radiographic film in order to turn the latent image into a permanent one. [O. Fr. *desveloper,* to unwrap, fr. *voloper,* to wrap]

de·vel·op·er (dē-vel'ŏp-er). 1. An individual or procedure that develops. 2. SYN eluent. 3. The chemicals used to develop film by reducing the light-activated silver halide molecules to atomic silver.

de·vel·op·ment (dē-vel'ŏp-ment). 1. The act or process of natural progression in physical and psychological maturation from a previous, lower, or embryonic stage to a later, more complex, or adult stage. **2.** The process of chromatography.

cognitive d., the evolving d. of the infant's and child's intellectual functions.

life-span d., development and mastery (or loss) of differing biologic, intellectual, behavioral, and social skills in different epochs of the life-span from the prenatal through the gerontological periods of growth.

psychosexual d., maturation and development of the psychic and behavioral phases of sexuality from birth to adult life through the oral, anal, phallic, latency, and genital phases.

Deventer, Hendrik van, Dutch obstetrician, 1651–1724. SEE D.'s *pelvis.*

de·vi·ance (dē'vē-ans). SYN deviation (3).

de·vi·ant (dē'vē-ant). **1.** Denoting or indicative of deviation. **2.** An individual exhibiting deviation, especially sexual.

de·vi·a·tion (dē-vē-ā'shŭn). **1.** A turning away or aside from the normal point or course. **2.** An abnormality. **3.** In psychiatry and the behavioral sciences, a departure from an accepted norm, role, or rule. SYN deviance. **4.** A statistical measure representing the difference between an individual value in a set of values and the mean value in that set. [L. *devio,* to turn from the straight path, fr. *de,* from, + *via,* way]

axis d., deflection of the electrical axis of the heart to the right or left of the normal. SEE ALSO left axis d., right axis d., axis. SYN axis shift.

conjugate d. of the eyes, (1) rotation of the eyes equally and simultaneously in the same direction, as occurs normally; (2) a condition in which both eyes are turned to the same side as a result of either paralysis or muscular spasm.

immune d., modification of an immune response to an antigen after prior exposure to that antigen. SYN split tolerance.

d. to the left, SYN *shift* to the left (1).

left axis d., a mean electrical axis of the heart pointing to −30° or more negative. SEE hexaxial reference *system.*

primary d., the ocular deviation seen in paralysis of an ocular muscle when the nonparalyzed eye is used for fixation.

d. to the right, SYN *shift* to the right (1).

right axis d., a mean electrical axis of the heart pointing to the right of +90°. SEE hexaxial reference *system.*

secondary d., ocular deviation seen in paralysis of an ocular muscle when the paralyzed eye is used for fixation.

sexual d., a sexual practice that is biologically atypical, considered morally wrong, or legally prohibited. SEE bestiality, pedophilia. SYN sexual perversion.

skew d., a hypertropia in which the eyes move in opposite directions equally; an acquired hypertropia, often fairly comitant, not fitting the characteristic pattern of trochlear nerve damage or of ocular muscle abnormality; often due to a brainstem or cerebellar lesion.

standard d. (SD, σ), (1) statistical index of the degree of d. from central tendency, namely, of the variability within a distribution; the square root of the average of the squared d.'s from the mean. (2) a measure of dispersion or variation used to describe a characteristic of a frequency distribution.

Devic, Eugène, French physician, 1869–1930. SEE D.'s *disease.*

de·vice (dē-vīs'). An appliance, usually mechanical, designed to perform a specific function, such as prosthesis or orthesis. [M.E., fr. O. Fr. *devis,* fr. L. *divisum,* divided]

central-bearing d., in dentistry, a d. which provides a central point of bearing, or support, between upper and lower record bases; it consists of a contacting point which is attached to one base and a plate attached to the other which provides the surface on which the bearing point rests or moves.

central-bearing tracing d., in dentistry, a central-bearing d. used for making a tracing and/or for support between upper and lower bases.

contraceptive d., a d. used to prevent pregnancy; *e.g.,* occlusive diaphragm, condom, intrauterine d.

intra-aortic d., an externally and intermittently inflatable balloon placed into the descending aorta and which, on activation during diastole, augments blood pressure and organ perfusion by its pulsatile thrust; then, on deflation, decreases the cardiac work with each systole—the so-called counterpulsation principle—by reducing cardiac afterload.

intrauterine d.'s (IUD), pieces of plastic or metal of various shapes (*e.g.,* coil, loop, bow) inserted into the uterus to exert a contraceptive effect. SYN intrauterine contraceptive devices.

left-ventricular assist d., mechanical pump inserted at some point in the circulation to parallel the activity of the left ventricle and thereby reduce its load.

ventricular assist d., a d. that supports or replaces the function of a ventricle (LVAD or RVAD indicates which ventricle). The patient's heart remains in place when this device or system is used. The device is used in patients with potentially salvageable myocardium, where centrifugal or pneumatic devices can be placed in either heterotopic or orthotopic positions (the latter is termed a total artificial heart). The function of either the left, right, or both ventricles can thus be supported for days to weeks. Either recovery of heart function or need for transplantation then becomes apparent.

Devine, Sir Hugh B., Australian surgeon, 1878–1959. SEE D. *exclusion.*

de·vi·om·e·ter (dē-vē-om'ě-ter). A form of strabismometer.

de·vi·tal·i·za·tion (dē-vi'tăl-i-zā'shŭn). **1.** Deprivation of vitality or of vital properties. **2.** In dentistry, the process by which tooth pulp is destroyed; *e.g.,* by chemical means, by infection, or by extirpation.

de·vi·tal·ize (dē-vī'tăl-īz). To deprive of vitality or of vital properties.

de·vi·tal·ized (dē-vī'tăl-īzd). Devoid of life; dead.

dev·o·lu·tion (dev-ō-lū'shŭn). A continuing process of degeneration or breaking down, in contrast to evolution. SEE ALSO involution, catabolism. [L. *de-volvo,* pp. *-volutus,* to roll down]

Dewar, Sir James, English chemist, 1842–1923. SEE D. *flask.*

de Wecker, Louis H., French physician, 1832–1906. SEE de W.'s *scissors.*

dew·lap (doo'lap). The loose fold of skin hanging below the neck of cattle and similar animals.

dex·a·meth·a·sone (dek-să-meth'ă-sōn). 9α-Fluoro-16α-methylprednisolone; a potent synthetic analogue of cortisol, with similar biological action; used as an anti-inflammatory agent and as a test material for adrenal cortical function.

dex·am·phet·a·mine (deks-am-fet'ă-mēn). SYN dextroamphetamine sulfate.

d. sodium phosphate, the water-soluble ester of d., with the same actions and uses.

dex·brom·phen·ir·a·mine ma·le·ate (deks'brom-fen-ir'ă-mēn). *d*-2-[*p*-Bromo-α-(2-dimethylaminoethyl)benzyl]pyridine maleate; the dextrorotatory isomer of brompheniramine; an antihistamine.

dex·chlor·phen·ir·a·mine ma·le·ate (deks'klōr-fen-ir'ă-mēn). *d*-2-[*p*-Chloro-α-(2-dimethylaminoethyl)benzyl]pyridine maleate; the dextrorotatory isomer of chlorpheniramine; an antihistamine.

dex·i·o·car·dia (deks-ē-ō-kar'dē-ă). SYN dextrocardia.

dex·pan·the·nol (deks-pan'thě-nol). D-(+)-2,4-dihydroxy-*N*-(3-hydroxypropyl)-3,3-dimethylbutyramide; pantothenic acid with −CH$_2$OH replacing the terminal −COOH; a cholinergic agent and a dietary source of pantothenic acid. SYN panthenol, pantothenyl alcohol.

dex·ter (D) (deks'ter) [NA]. Located on or relating to the right side. [L. fr. *dextra,* neut. *dextrum*]

dextr-. SEE dextro-.

dex·trad (deks'trad). Toward the right side. [L. *dexter,* right, + *ad,* to]

dex·tral (deks'trăl). SYN right-handed.

dex·tral·i·ty (deks-tral'i-tē). Right-handedness; preference for the right hand in performing manual tasks.

dex·tran (deks'tran). **1.** Any of several water-soluble high molecular weight glucose polymers (average MW 75,000; ranging between 10,000 and 40,000,000) produced by the action of *Leuconostoc mesenteroides* and certain other microorganisms on sucrose; used in isotonic sodium chloride solution for the treatment of shock, and in distilled water for the relief of the edema of nephrosis; lower molecular weight d. (*e.g.,* MW 40,000) improves blood flow in areas of stasis by reducing cellular aggregation. **2.** Poly α(1,6-glucose); α-1,6-Glucan with branch points (1.2; 1.3; 1.4) and spacing of these characteristic of the species; used as plasma substitutes or expanders. SEE dextransucrase.

d. 40, d. (average MW 40,000) used as a plasma volume expander and blood flow adjuvant.

d. 70, d. (average MW 70,000) used as a plasma volume expander.

d. 75, d. (average MW 75,000) used as a plasma volume expander.

d. 110, d. (average MW 110,000) available as 5% solution in water or saline solution; used as a plasma volume expander.

acid d., the product of acid and heat treatment of d.

animal d., SYN glycogen.

blue d., high molecular weight d. containing a blue chlorotriazine dye, Cibacron Blue; used to measure the void volumes in gel filtration columns.

d. sulfate, the sodium salt of sulfuric acid esters of the polysaccharide d.; it contains not less than 10 units per mg and not less than 14% of sulfate; an anticoagulant.

dex·tran·ase (deks'tran-ās). An enzyme hydrolyzing 1,6-α-D-glucosidic linkages in dextran; used in the prevention of caries.

dex·tran·su·crase (deks-tran-su'krās). A glucosyltransferase that builds poly(1,6-α-D-glucosyl), *i.e.,* polyglucoses, dextrans, or α-glucans, from sucrose, releasing D-fructose residues.

dex·trase (deks'trās). Nonspecific term for the complex of enzymes that converts dextrose (D-glucose) into lactic acid.

dex·tri·fer·ron (deks-tri-fer'on). A colloidal solution of ferric hydroxide in complex with partially hydrolyzed dextrin, used in the treatment of iron-deficiency anemia; it is suitable for intravenous administration and contains 20 mg of iron per ml.

dex·trin (deks'trin). A mixture of oligo(α-1,4-D-glucose) molecules formed during the enzymic or acid hydrolysis of starch, amylopectin, or glycogen; on further hydrolysis they are converted into D-glucose. D.'s are of much lower molecular weight than dextrans, hence are not suitable as plasma expanders; d. (usually white d.) is used in pharmaceutical preparations. SYN starch gum.

acid dextrin, the product of acid and heat treatment of d.

limit d., the polysaccharide fragments remaining at the end (limit) of exhaustive hydrolysis of amylopectin or glycogen by α-1,4-glucan maltohydrolase, which cannot hydrolyze the α-1,6 bonds at branch points; accumulates in individuals with type III glycogen storage disease. SYN dextrin limit.

Schardinger d.'s, cyclic rings of glucose monomer (usually 6 to 8) linked α-1,4; the result of action of *Bacillus macerans* on starch.

dex·tri·nase (deks'tri-nās). Any of the enzymes catalyzing the hydrolysis of dextrins; *e.g.,* amylo-1,6-glucosidase, dextrin dextranase.

limit d., (1) SYN α-dextrin endo-1,6-α-glucosidase. **(2)** SYN oligo-α1,6-glucosidase.

dex·trin dex·tran·ase. A glucosyltransferase transferring 1,4-α-D-glucosyl residues, thus catalyzing the synthesis of dextrans (with 1,6 links between monosaccharide units) from dextrins (with 1,4 links) by glucose transfer. SYN dextrin → dextran transglucosidase, dextrin 6-glucosyltransferase.

dex·trin → dex·tran trans·glu·co·si·dase. SYN dextrin dextranase.

α-dex·trin en·do-1,6-α-glu·co·si·dase. An enzyme with action similar to that of isoamylase; it cleaves 1,6-α-glucosidic linkages in pullalan, amylopectin, and glycogen, and in α- and β-amylase limit-dextrins of amylopectin and glycogen. Cf. isoamylase. SYN limit dextrinase (1), pullulanase, R enzyme.

dex·trin 6-α-D-glu·co·si·dase. SYN amylo-1,6-glucosidase.

dex·trin 6-glu·co·syl·trans·fer·ase. SYN dextrin dextranase.

dex·trin gly·co·syl·trans·fer·ase. SYN 4-α-D-glucanotransferase.

dex·trin lim·it. SYN limit *dextrin.*

dex·trin·o·gen·ic (deks'trin-ō-jen'ik). Capable of producing dextrin.

dex·tri·no·sis (deks-trin-ō'sis). SYN glycogenosis.

debranching deficiency limit d., limit d., SYN type 3 *glycogenosis.*

dex·trin trans·gly·co·syl·ase. SYN 4-α-D-glucanotransferase.

dex·tri·nu·ria (deks-tri-nū'rē-ă). The passage of dextrin in the urine.

⌂**dextro-, dextr-. 1.** Prefixes meaning right, toward, or on the right side. **2.** Chemical prefixes meaning dextrorotatory. [L. *dexter,* on the right-hand side]

dex·tro·am·phet·a·mine phos·phate (deks'trō-am-fet'ă-mēn). monobasic *d*-α-methylphenethylamine phosphate; same actions and uses as dextroamphetamine sulfate. SYN *d*-amphetamine phosphate.

dex·tro·am·phet·a·mine sul·fate. (+)-α-methylphenethylamine sulfate; similar in action to racemic amphetamine sulfate, but is more stimulating to the central nervous system; sympathomimetic and appetite depressant. SYN *d*-amphetamine sulfate, dexamphetamine.

dex·tro·car·dia (deks'trō-kar'dē-ă). Displacement of the heart to the right, either as dextroposition, with simple displacement to the right, or as cardiac heterotaxia, with complete transposition of the right and left chambers, resulting in a heart that is the mirror image of a normal heart. SYN dexiocardia. [dextro- + G. *kardia,* heart]

corrected d., displacement and rotation of the heart into the right side of the chest but without mirror transposition of the cardiac chambers. SYN dextroversion of the heart, false d., type 3 d.

false d., SYN corrected d.

isolated d., d. with mirror transposition of the cardiac chambers but without displacement of the abdominal viscera. SYN type 2 d.

mirror image d., perfect right to left congenital reversal of the heart sometimes with other congenital abnormalities, sometimes normal except for position.

secondary d., dextroposition of the heart by some disease of the lungs, pleura, or diaphragm. SYN type 4 d.

type 1 d., SYN d. with situs inversus.

type 2 d., SYN isolated d.

type 3 d., SYN corrected d.

type 4 d., SYN secondary d.

d. with si'tus inver'sus, displacement of the heart to the right side of the chest with mirror transposition of the cardiac chambers together with transposition of the abdominal viscera. SYN type 1 d.

dex·tro·car·di·o·gram (deks'trō-kar'dē-ō-gram). That part of the electrocardiogram that is derived from the right ventricle.

dex·tro·ce·re·bral (deks'trō-ser'ĕ-brăl). Having a dominant right cerebral hemisphere.

dex·tro·cli·na·tion (deks'trō-kli-nā'shŭn). Obsolete term for dextrotorsion. SYN dextrotorsion (2).

dex·troc·u·lar (deks-trok'yū-lăr). Rarely used term for indicating right ocular dominance; denoting one who prefers the right eye in monocular work, such as microscopy. SYN right-eyed. [dextro- + L. *oculus,* eye]

dex·tro·cy·clo·duc·tion (deks'trō-sī-klō-dŭk'shŭn). Rotation of the upper pole of the cornea to the right. SEE excycloduction. [dextro- + cyclo- + L. *duco,* pp. *ductus,* to lead]

dex·tro·duc·tion (deks'trō-dŭk'shŭn). Seldom-used term for rotation of one eye to the right. [dextro- + L. *duco,* pp. *ductus,* to lead]

dex·tro·gas·tria (deks'trō-gas'trē-ă). Condition in which the stomach is displaced to the right; may represent either simple displacement or situs inversus. Usually associated with dextrocardia. [dextro- + G. *gastēr,* stomach]

dex·tro·glu·cose (deks'trō-glū'kōs). SEE D-glucose.

dex·tro·gram (deks'trō-gram). Electrocardiographic record in an experimental animal representing spread of impulse through the right ventricle alone.

dex·tro·gy·ra·tion (deks'trō-jī-rā'shŭn). A twisting to the right. [dextro- + L. *gyro,* pp. *-atus,* to turn in a circle, fr. *gyrus,* circle]

de

dex·tro·man·u·al (deks-trō-man′yū-ăl). SYN right-handed. [dextro- + L. *manus,* hand]

dex·tro·meth·or·phan hy·dro·bro·mide (deks′trō-meth-ōr′ fan hī-drō-brō′mīd). Hydrobromide of *d*-racemethorphan; *d*-3-methoxy-*N*-methylmorphinan hydrobromide; a synthetic morphine derivative used as an antitussive agent. It has weak central depressant action, and appears to have little addiction liability.

dex·tro·mor·a·mide tar·trate (deks-trō-mōr′ă-mīd). A narcotic analgesic related chemically and pharmacologically to methadone.

dex·trop·e·dal (deks-trop′ĕ-dăl). Denoting one who uses the right leg in preference to the left. SYN right-footed. [dextro- + L. *pes* (*ped*-), foot]

dex·tro·po·si·tion (deks′trō-pō-zi′shŭn). Abnormal right-sided location or origin of a normally left-sided structure, *e.g.,* origin of the aorta from the right ventricle.
   d. of the heart, SEE dextrocardia.

dex·tro·pro·pox·y·phene hy·dro·chlo·ride (deks′trō-prō-pok′ sē-fēn). SYN propoxyphene hydrochloride.

dex·tro·pro·pox·y·phene nap·syl·ate. SYN propoxyphene napsylate.

dex·tro·ro·ta·tion (deks′trō-rō-tā′shŭn). A turning or twisting to the right; especially, the clockwise twist given the plane of plane-polarized light by solutions of certain optically active substances. Cf. levorotation.

dex·tro·ro·ta·to·ry (deks-trō-rō′tă-tōr-ē). Denoting dextrorotation, or certain crystals or solutions capable of so doing; as a chemical prefix, usually abbreviated *d*-. Cf. levorotatory.

dex·trose (deks′trōs). SEE D-glucose.

dex·tro·si·nis·tral (deks′trō-si-nis′trăl). In a direction from right to left. [dextro- + L. *sinister,* left]

dex·tro·su·ria (deks-trō-sū′rē-ă). Obsolete term for glycosuria.

dex·tro·thy·rox·ine so·di·um (deks-trō-thī-roks′ēn). D-Thyroxine sodium salt; an antihypercholesterolemic agent.

dex·tro·tor·sion (deks-trō-tōr′shŭn). **1.** A twisting to the right. **2.** In ophthalmology, a seldom-used term for a conjugate rotation of the upper pole of both corneas to the right. SYN dextroclination. [dextro- + L. *torsio,* a twisting]

dex·tro·tro·p·ic (dek-trō-trop′ik). Turning to the right. [dextro- + G. *tropos,* a turn]

dex·tro·ver·sion (deks′trō-ver′zhŭn). **1.** Version toward the right. **2.** In ophthalmology, a conjugate rotation of both eyes to the right. [dextro- + L. *verto,* pp. *versus,* to turn]
   d. of the heart, SYN corrected *dextrocardia.*

d.f.. Abbreviation for *degrees* of freedom, under *degree.*

df, DF Abbreviation for decayed and filled teeth. SYN df caries *index.*

DFP Abbreviation for diisopropyl fluorophosphate.

dGlc Abbreviation for 2-deoxyglucose.

1,4-α-D-glu·can branch·ing en·zyme. amylo-(1,4→1,6)-transglucosylase or transglucosidase; an enzyme in muscle and in plants (Q enzyme) that cleaves α-1,4 linkages in glycogen or starch, transferring the fragments into α-1,6 linkages, creating branches in the polysaccharide molecules; in plants, it converts amylose to amylopectin; this enzyme is deficient in individuals with glycogen storage disease type IV. SYN α-glucan branching glycosyltransferase, amylo-1,4:1,6-glucantransferase, amylo-(1,4→1,6)-transglucosidase, amylo-(1,4→1,6)-transglucosylase, branching enzyme.

dGMP Abbreviation for deoxyguanylic acid.

DHAP Abbreviation for *dihydroxyacetone* phosphate.

Dharmendra an·ti·gen. See under antigen.

d'Herelle, Felix H., Canadian physician and bacteriologist, 1873–1949. SEE d'H. *phenomenon;* Twort-d'H. *phenomenon.*

DHF Abbreviation for dihydrofolic acid.

DHFR Abbreviation for dihydrofolate reductase.

D. Hy. Abbreviation for Doctor of Hygiene.

DI Abbreviation for dental *index.*

△**di-.** **1.** Two, twice. **2.** In chemistry, often used in place of bis-

when not likely to be confusing; *e.g.,* dichloro- compounds. Cf. bi-, bis-. [G. *dis,* two]

△**dia-.** Through, throughout, completely. [G. *dia,* through]

di·a·be·tes (dī-ă-bē′tēz). Either d. insipidus or d. mellitus, diseases having in common the symptom polyuria; when used without qualification, refers to d. mellitus. [G. *diabētēs,* a compass, a siphon, diabetes]

---

diabetes mellitus: etiologic classification

I. Primary (essential, familiar diabetes) type I = insulin-dependent d.m. (IDDM) and type II = non insulin-dependent d.m. (NIDDM)

II. Secondary (nonessential) diabetes

  A. pancreatic diabetes:
    – after total or partial pancreatectomy
    – with extensive destruction of pancreas
    – through tumor or wound
    – pancreatitis; hemochromatosis

  B. extrapancreatic/endocrine diabetes
    – with hypersomatotropism (acromegaly)
    – with hyperadrenalism (Cushing syndrome; Conn syndrome, pheochromocytoma)
    – with hyperthyroidism
    – with glucagonoma

  C. drug-induced diabetes
    – after exogenous hormone intake (STH; ACTH Corticoid hormone [steroid diabetes]; thyroid hormone)
    – after benzothiadiazides

III. Rare, exceptional forms of diabetes
    e.g., lipoatrophic diabetes (Lawrence); myatonic diabetes (Prader-Labhart-Willi); disturbance of insulin receptors; d.m. with certain genetic syndromes

---

adult-onset d., non-insulin-dependent d. mellitus.

alimentary d., SYN alimentary *glycosuria.*

alloxan d., experimental d. mellitus produced in animals by the administration of alloxan, which damages the insulin-producing islet cells of the pancreas.

brittle d., d. mellitus in which there are marked fluctuations in blood glucose concentrations that are difficult to control.

bronze d., d. mellitus associated with hemochromatosis, with iron deposits in the skin, liver, pancreas, and other viscera, often with severe liver damage and glycosuria. SEE ALSO hemochromatosis. SYN bronzed d., bronzed disease.

bronzed d., SYN bronze d.

calcinuric d., SYN hypercalciuria.

chemical d., SYN latent d.

galactose d., SYN galactosemia.

gestational d., carbohydrate intolerance during pregnancy usually resolving after delivery.

growth-onset d., SYN insulin-dependent d. mellitus.

d. in′nocens, SYN renal *glycosuria.*

d. insip′idus, chronic excretion of very large amounts of pale urine of low specific gravity, causing dehydration and extreme thirst; ordinarily results from inadequate output of pituitary antidiuretic hormone; the urine abnormalities may be mimicked as a result of excessive fluid intake, as in psychogenic polydipsia. Several types exist: central, neurohypophyseal, and nephrogenic. Autosomal dominant [MIM*125700, *125800, *192340], X-linked [MIM*304800 and *304900], and even autosomal recessive forms [MIM*222000] have been described. SEE ALSO nephrogenic d. insipidus.

insulin-dependent d. mellitus (IDDM), severe d. mellitus, often brittle, usually of abrupt onset during the first two decades of life but can develop at any age; characterized by polydipsia, polyuria, increased appetite, weight loss, low plasma insulin levels, and episodic ketoacidosis; immune-medicated destruction of pancreatic B cells; insulin therapy and dietary regulation are necessary. SYN growth-onset d., juvenile-onset d., type I d.

insulinopenic d., any form of d. mellitus resulting from inadequate secretion of insulin.

d. intermit′tens, d. mellitus in which there are periods of relatively normal carbohydrate metabolism followed by relapses to the previous diabetic state.

juvenile d., d. mellitus appearing in a child or adolescent; often fatal, usually of abrupt onset during first or second decaces of life; characterized by polyuria, polydipsia, weight loss; usually severe, insulin-dependent and prone to periods of ketoacidosis; can be familial, follow a viral infection such as mumps; thought to be due to viral-induced or immune destruction of pancreatic islets. SYN type I d. mellitus.

juvenile-onset d., SYN insulin-dependent d. mellitus.

ketosis-prone d., type I or juvenile d. mellitus, in which inadequate treatment leads to development of ketoacidosis.

ketosis-resistant d., type II or adult onset d. mellitus, in which episodes of ketoacidosis rarely occur.

latent d., a mild form of d. mellitus in which the patient displays no overt symptoms, but displays certain abnormal responses to diagnostic procedures, such as an elevated fasting blood glucose concentration or reduced glucose tolerance. SYN chemical d.

lipoatrophic d., SYN lipoatrophy.

lipogenous d., d. and obesity combined.

maturity-onset d., non-insulin-dependent d. mellitus.

maturity onset d. of youth, a relatively mild, non-insulin requiring form of d. mellitus beginning at a younger age than usual.

d. mel′litus (DM), a metabolic disease in which carbohydrate utilization is reduced and that of lipid and protein enhanced; it is caused by an absolute or relative deficiency of insulin and is characterized, in more severe cases, by chronic hyperglycemia, glycosuria, water and electrolyte loss, ketoacidosis, and coma; long-term complications include development of neuropathy, retinopathy, nephropathy, generalized degenerative changes in large and small blood vessels, and increased susceptibility to infection. SEE ALSO insulin-dependent d. mellitus, non-insulin-dependent d. mellitus. [L. sweetened with honey]

> Of the 14 million Americans with diabetes, roughly 90% have Type II (non–insulin-dependent) and roughly 10% have Type I (insulin-dependent) disease. Previously, it was thought diabetics were bound to suffer from chronic complications. However, in 1993, the results of a 10-year multicenter study found that by rigorously managing blood sugar levels, diabetics could substantially minimize long-term complications, including retinopathy, neuropathy, and nephropathy. The American Diabetes Association now recognizes that there can be no universal guidelines; rather, it recommends that dietary regimens and weight goals be tailored for each diabetic. This requires both greater commitment on the part of diabetics themselves, and greater involvement of medical professionals, particularly dieticians.

metahypophysial d., (1) d. mellitus caused by large quantities of endogenous or exogenous pituitary growth hormone; (2) term used to designate the irreversible phase of d. mellitus in acromegaly.

Mosler's d., inosituria with excretion of large quantities of water.

nephrogenic d. insipidus [MIM*304800], d. insipidus due to inability of the kidney tubules to respond to antidiuretic hormone; X-linked inheritance, with full expression in males and partial defect in heterozygous females. SYN vasopressin-resistant d.

non-insulin-dependent d. mellitus (NIDDM), an often mild form of d. mellitus of gradual onset, usually in obese individuals

stages of diabetes mellitus

stage	glucose tolerance test
prediabetes	normal
latent diabetes pregnancy diabetes }	pathological by now (or sooner)
manifest diabetes (hyperglycemia > 120 mg/dl, glycosuria)	not required

over age 35; absolute plasma insulin levels are normal to high, but relatively low in relation to plasma glucose levels; ketoacidosis is rare, but hyperosmolar coma can occur; responds well to dietary regulation and/or oral hypoglycemic agents, but diabetic complications and degenerative changes can develop.

pancreatic d., (1) d. mellitus demonstrably dependent upon a pancreatic lesion; (2) d. following removal of the pancreas in an animal.

phlorizin d. (flō-rid′zin), SYN phlorizin *glycosuria.*

phosphate d., excessive secretion of phosphate in the urine due to a defect in tubular reabsorption; usually part of a more generalized abnormality, such as Fanconi syndrome.

piqûre d., SYN puncture d. [Fr.]

pregnancy d., SEE subclinical d.

puncture d., experimental d. produced in animals by puncture of the floor of the fourth ventricle of the brain. SYN piqûre d.

renal d., SYN renal *glycosuria.*

starvation d., after prolonged fasting, glycosuria following the ingestion of carbohydrate or glucose because of reduced output of insulin and/or reduced rate of glucose metabolism with a reduced ability to form glycogen.

steroid d., d. mellitus produced by pharmacological doses of steroid hormones, particularly glucocorticoids or estrogens; characterized by one or more of the typical manifestations of d. mellitus.

steroidogenic d., abnormal glucose tolerance, often frank d. mellitus, induced by the metabolic effects of adrenocortical steroid hormones such as cortisone or therapeutic analogues such as prednisone. The effect may be temporary, resolving when the steroid therapy is discontinued, or d. mellitus may persist.

subclinical d., a form of d. mellitus that is clinically evident only under certain circumstances, such as pregnancy or extreme stress; persons so afflicted may, in time, manifest more severe forms of the disease.

thiazide d., impaired carbohydrate metabolism associated with the use of thiazide diuretic drugs; severe manifestations are seen in persons having d. mellitus, but impairment is mild or absent in nondiabetic individuals.

type I d., SYN insulin-dependent d. mellitus.

type II d., non-insulin-dependent d. mellitus.

type I d. mellitus, SYN juvenile d.

vasopressin-resistant d., SYN nephrogenic d. insipidus.

di·a·bet·ic (dī-ă-bet′ik). **1.** Relating to or suffering from diabetes. **2.** One who suffers from diabetes.

di·a·be·to·gen·ic (dī′ă-bet-ō-jen′ik, -bē-tō-jen′ik). Causing diabetes.

di·a·be·tog·en·ous (dī′ă-bĕ-toj′en-ŭs). Caused by diabetes.

di·a·be·tol·o·gy (dī′ă-be-tol′ō-jē). The field of medicine concerned with diabetes.

di·a·cele (dī′ă-sēl). SYN third *ventricle.* [G. *dia-,* through, + *koilia,* a hollow]

di·a·ce·tal (dī-as′ĕ-tal). SEE diacetyl.

di·a·ce·tate (dī-as′ĕ-tāt). **1.** SYN acetoacetate. **2.** A compound containing two acetate residues.

di·ac·e·te·mia (dī-as-ĕ-tē′mē-ă). A form of acidosis resulting from the presence of acetoacetic (diacetic) acid in the blood.

di·a·ce·tic ac·id (dī-ă-sē′tik, -set′ik). SYN acetoacetic acid.

di·ac·e·ton·u·ria (dī-as′ĕ-tō-nū′rē-ă). SYN diaceturia.

di

di·ac·e·tu·ria (dī-as-ĕ-tū′rē-ă). The urinary excretion of acetoacetic (diacetic) acid. SYN diacetonuria.

di·ace·tyl, di·ac·e·tal (dī-as′ĕ-til, dī-as′ĕ-tal). 2,3-Butanedione; a yellow liquid, $(CH_3CO)_2$, having the pungent odor of quinone and carrying the aromas of coffee, vinegar, butter, and other foods; a byproduct of carbohydrate degradation.

di·a·ce·tyl·cho·line (dī-as′ĕ-til-kō′lēn). SYN succinylcholine.

di·a·ce·tyl·mon·ox·ime (DAM) (dī-as′ĕ-til-mon-ok′sīm). A 2-oxo-oxime that can reactivate phosphorylated acetylcholinesterase *in vitro* and *in vivo*; it penetrates the blood-brain barrier.

di·a·ce·tyl·mor·phine (dī-as′ĕ-til-mōr′fēn). SYN heroin.

di·a·ce·tyl·tan·nic ac·id (dī-as′ĕ-til-tan′ik). SYN acetyltannic acid.

di·a·chron·ic (dī-ă-kron′ik). Systematically observed over time in the same subjects throughout as opposed to synchronic or cross-sectional; the inferences are equivalent only where there is strict stability of all elements. [dia- + G. *chronos,* time]

di·ac·id (dī-as′id). Denoting a substance containing two ionizable hydrogen atoms per molecule; more generally, a base capable of combining with two hydrogen ions per molecule.

di·ac·la·sis, di·a·cla·sia (dī-ak′lă-sis, dī-ă-klā′zē-ă). SYN osteoclasis. [G. *diaklasis,* a breaking up, fr. *dia,* through, + *klasis,* a breaking]

di·ac·ri·nous (dī-ak′ri-nŭs). Excreting by simple passage through a gland cell. [G. *dia-krinō,* to separate one from another]

di·ac·ri·sis (dī-ak′ri-sis). SYN diagnosis. [G. *dia-,* through, + *krisis,* a judgment]

di·a·crit·ic, di·a·crit·i·cal (dī-ă-krit′ik, -krit′i-kăl). Distinguishing; diagnostic; allowing of distinction. [G. *diakritikos,* able to distinguish]

di·ac·tin·ic (dī′ak-tin′ik). Having the property of transmitting light capable of bringing about chemical reactions. [G. *dia,* through, + *aktis,* ray]

di·ac·yl·glyc·er·ol (DAG) (dī′as-il-glis′er-ol). Glycerol with two esterified acyl moieties, either 1,3-d. or 1,2-d.; if the two acyl groups are nonidentical, there are four possible stereoisomers; 1,2-d. is an intermediate in the synthesis of triacylglycerols and of lecithin; also serves as a second messenger in stimulating the activity of protein kinase C.
  d. acyltransferase, an enzyme, in fat biosynthesis, that catalyzes the transfer of an acyl moiety from acyl-CoA to 1,2-d. thus forming free coenzyme A and triacylglycerol.
  d. lipase, SYN lipoprotein lipase.

di·ad (dī′ad). **1.** The transverse tubule and a cisterna in cardiac muscle fibers. **2.** SYN dyad (1).

di·a·der·mic (dī-ă-der′mik). SYN percutaneous. [G. *dia,* through, + *derma,* skin]

di·ad·o·cho·ci·ne·sia (dī-ad′ō-kō-si-nē′zē-ă). SYN diadochokinesia.

di·ad·o·cho·ki·ne·sia, di·ad·o·cho·ki·ne·sis (dī-ad′ō-kō-ki-nē′zē-ă, -ki-nē′sis). The normal power of alternately bringing a limb into opposite positions, as of flexion and extention or of pronation and supination. SYN diadochocinesia. [G. *diadochos,* working in turn, + *kinēsis,* movement]

di·ad·o·cho·ki·net·ic (dī-ad′ō-kō-ki-net′ik). Relating to diadochokinesia.

di·ag·nose (dī-ag-nōs′). To make a diagnosis.

di·ag·no·sis (dī-ag-nō′sis). The determination of the nature of a disease. SYN diacrisis. [G. *diagnōsis,* a deciding]
  antenatal d., SYN prenatal d.
  clinical d., a d. made from a study of the signs and symptoms of a disease.
  differential d., the determination of which of two or more diseases with similar symptoms is the one from which the patient is suffering, by a systematic comparison and contrasting of the clinical findings. SYN differentiation (2).
  d. by exclusion, a d. made by excluding those diseases to which only some of the patient's symptoms might belong, leaving one disease as the most likely d., although no definitive tests or findings establish that d.
  laboratory d., a d. made by a chemical, microscopic, microbiologic, immunologic, or pathologic study of secretions, discharges, blood, or tissue.
  neonatal d., systematic evaluation of the newborn for evidence of disease or malformations, and the conclusion reached.
  pathologic d., a d., sometimes postmortem, made from an anatomic and/or histologic study of the lesions present.
  physical d., a d. made by means of physical examination of the patient, or the process of a physical examination.
  prenatal d., d. utilizing procedures available for the recognition of diseases and malformations *in utero,* and the conclusion reached. SYN antenatal d.

di·ag·no·sis-re·lat·ed group (DRG). A classification of patients by diagnosis or surgical procedure (sometimes including age) into major diagnostic categories (each containing specific diseases, disorders, or procedures) for the purpose of determining payment of hospitalization charges, based on the premise that treatment of similar medical diagnoses generate similar costs.

di·ag·nos·tic (dī-ag-nos′tik). **1.** Relating to or aiding in diagnosis. **2.** Establishing or confirming a diagnosis.

di·ag·nos·ti·cian (dī′ag-nos-tish′ăn). One who is skilled in making diagnoses; formerly, a name for specialists in internal medicine.

Diagnostic and Statistical Manual. An American Psychiatric Association publication which classifies mental illnesses.

  Currently in its fourth edition (DSM-IV) and first published in 1980, the manual provides health practitioners with a comprehensive system for diagnosing mental illnesses based on specific ideational and behavioral symptoms. The DSM approach supplants older, less rigorous methods of diagnosis, and as such represents a major step forward for the field of psychiatry. It consists of five axes covering clinical syndromes, developmental and personality disorders, physical disorders, severity of psychosocial stressors, and global assessment of functioning. It is used primarily in the U.S.; elsewhere, the World Health Organization's International Classification of Diseases is preferred.

di·a·gram. a simple, graphic depiction of an idea or object.
  Dieuaide d., SYN triaxial reference *system.*
  Venn d., pictorial representation of the extent to which two or more quantities or concepts are mutually inclusive and exclusive.

di·a·ki·ne·sis (dī′ă-ki-nē′sis). Final stage of prophase in meiosis I, in which the chiasmata present during the diplotene stage disappear, the chromosomes continue to shorten, and the nucleolus and nuclear membrane disappear. [G. *dia,* through, + *kinēsis,* movement]

dial (dī′ăl, dīl). A clock face or instrument resembling a clock face. [L. *dies,* day]
  astigmatic d., a diagram of radiating lines, used to test for astigmatism.

Di·a·lis·ter (dī-ăl-is′ter). An obsolete genus of bacteria, the type species of which, *D. pneumosintes,* is now placed in the genus *Bacteroides.*

di·al·lyl (dī-al′il). A compound containing two allyl groups.

di·al·y·sance (dī-al′i-sans). The number of milliliters of blood completely cleared of any substance by an artificial kidney or by peritoneal dialysis in a unit of time; conventional clearance formulas are expressed as mm/min. [fr. dialysis]

di·al·y·sate (dī-al′i-sāt). That part of a mixture that passes through a dialyzing membrane. SYN diffusate.

di·al·y·sis (dī-al′i-sis). A form of filtration to separate crystalloid from colloid substances (or smaller molecules from larger ones) in a solution by interposing a semipermeable membrane between the solution and water; the crystalloid (smaller) substances pass through the membrane into the water on the other side, the colloids do not. SYN diffusion (2). [G. a separation, fr. *dia- lyo,* to separate]
  continuous ambulatory peritoneal d. (CAPD), method of peritoneal d. performed in ambulatory patients with influx and efflux of dialysate during normal activities.

equilibrium d., in immunology, a method for determination of association constants for hapten-antibody reactions in a system in which the hapten (dialyzable) and antibody (nondialyzable) solutions are separated by semipermeable membranes. Since at equilibrium the quantity of free hapten will be the same in the two compartments, quantitative determinations can be made of hapten-bound antibody, free antibody, and free hapten.

extracorporeal d., hemodialysis performed through an apparatus outside the body.

peritoneal d., removal from the body of soluble substances and water by transfer across the peritoneum, utilizing a d. solution which is intermittently introduced into and removed from the peritoneal cavity; transfer of diffusable solutes and water between the blood and the peritoneal cavity depends on the concentration gradient between the two fluid compartments.

d. ret′inae, congenital or traumatic separation of the peripheral sensory retina from the retinal pigment epithelium at the ora serrata, often causing a retinal detachment. SYN retinodialysis.

di·a·lyze (dī′ă-līz). To perform dialysis; to separate a substance from a solution by means of dialysis.

di·a·lyz·er (dī′ă-lī-zer). The apparatus for performing dialysis; a membrane used in dialysis.

di·a·mag·net·ic (dī′ă-mag-net′ik). Having the property of diamagnetism.

di·a·mag·net·ism (dī-ă-mag′nĕ-tizm). The property of zero magnetic movement, given by molecules in which all electrons are paired; an unpaired electron yields a magnetic movement, hence the molecule containing such exhibits paramagnetism.

di·a·me·lia (dī-ă-mē′lē-ă). Absence of two limbs.

di·am·e·ter (dī-am′ĕ-ter). **1.** A straight line connecting two opposite points on the surface of a more or less spherical or cylindrical body, or at the boundary of an opening or foramen, passing through the center of such body or opening. **2.** The distance measured along such a line. [G. *diametros,* fr. *dia,* through, + *metron,* measure]

anteroposterior d. of the pelvic inlet, SYN *conjugate* of pelvic inlet.

Baudelocque's d., SYN external *conjugate.*

biparietal d., the d. of the fetal head between the two parietal eminences.

buccolingual d., the d. of the crown of a tooth measured from the buccal to the lingual surfaces.

conjugate d. of pelvic inlet, SYN *conjugate* of pelvic inlet.

conjugate d. of pelvic outlet, SYN *conjugate* of pelvic outlet.

diagonal conjugate d., SYN diagonal *conjugate.*

external conjugate d., SYN external *conjugate.*

d. media′na, SYN *conjugate* of pelvic inlet.

d. obli′qua [NA], SYN oblique d.

oblique d., a measurement across the pelvic inlet from the sacroiliac joint of one side to the opposite iliopectineal eminence. SYN d. obliqua [NA].

obstetric conjugate d., SYN obstetric *conjugate.*

occipitofrontal d., the d. of the fetal head from the external occipital protuberance to the most prominent point of the frontal bone in the midline.

occipitomental d., the d. of the fetal head from the external occipital protuberance to the midpoint of the chin.

posterior sagittal d., distance from the sacrococcygeal junction to the middle of an imaginary line running between the left and right ischial tuberosities.

suboccipitobregmatic d., the d. of the fetal head from the lowest posterior point of the occipital bone to the center of the anterior fontanelle.

total end-diastolic d. (TEDD), cross sectional d. of the left ventricle including the septum and posterior wall thicknesses in diastole.

total end-systolic d. (TESD), cross sectional d. of the left ventricle including the septum and posterior wall thicknesses in systole.

trachelobregmatic d., the d. of the fetal head from the middle of the anterior fontanelle to the neck.

d. transver′sa [NA], SYN transverse d.

transverse d., the transverse d. of the pelvic inlet, measured between the terminal lines. SYN d. transversa [NA].

zygomatic d., the extreme breadth of the skull at the zygomatic arches.

di·am·ide (dī′am-id, -īd). A compound containing two amide groups.

di·am·i·dines (dī-am′i-dēnz). A group of compounds containing two amidine groups; *e.g.,* stilbamidine, propamidine.

di·a·mine (dī′ă-mēn, -min). An organic compound containing two amine groups per molecule; *e.g.,* ethylenediamine, $NH_2CH_2CH_2NH_2$.

d. oxidase, SYN *amine* oxidase (copper-containing), *amine* oxidase (flavin-containing).

di·a·mi·no ox·y·hy·drase (dī-am′i-nō oks-ē-hī′drās). SYN *amine* oxidase (copper-containing).

di·am·ni·ot·ic (dī-am-nē-ot′ik). Exhibiting two amniotic sacs.

Diamond, Louis K., U.S. physician, *1902. SEE D.-Blackfan *anemia, syndrome;* Gardner-D. *syndrome.*

di·am·tha·zole di·hy·dro·chlo·ride (dī-am′thă-zōl). 6-(2-diethylaminoethoxy)-2-dimethylaminobenzothiazole dihydrochloride; an antifungal agent for topical use. SYN dimazole dihydrochloride.

di·an·dry, di·an·dria (dī′an-drē, dī-an′drē-ă). The phenomenon in which a single ovum is fertilized by a diploid sperm and hence produces a triploid fetus. Cf. digyny. [di- + G. *andros,* male]

di·a·no·et·ic (dī′ă-nō-et′ik). Of or pertaining to reason or other intellectual functions. [G. *dia,* through, + *noeō,* to think]

di·a·pause (dī′ă-pawz). A period of biological quiescence or dormancy with decreased metabolism; an interval in which development is arrested or greatly slowed. [dia- + G. *pausis,* pause]

embryonic d., a d. in the course of embryogenesis; postulated to occur in instances of double parturition and possibly of delayed implantation.

di·a·pe·de·sis (dī′ă-pĕ-dē′sis). The passage of blood, or any of its formed elements, through the intact walls of blood vessels. SYN migration (2). [G. *dia,* through, + *pēdēsis,* a leaping]

di·a·phan·og·ra·phy (dī-ă-fă-nog′ră-fē). Examination of a body part by transillumination, especially for the detection of breast cancer. [G. *diaphanēs,* transparent, + *graphō,* to write]

di·aph·a·nos·cope (dī-af′ă-nō-skōp). An instrument for illuminating the interior of a cavity to determine the translucency of its walls. SYN polyscope. [G. *diaphanēs,* transparent, + *skopeō,* to examine]

di·aph·a·nos·co·py (dī-af-ă-nos′kŏ-pē). Examination of a cavity with a diaphanoscope.

di·a·phe·met·ric (dī′ă-fē-met′rik). Relating to the determination of the degree of tactile sensibility. [G. *dia,* through, + *haphē,* touch, + *metron,* measure]

di·a·phen hy·dro·chlo·ride (dī′ă-fen). 2-Diethylaminoethyl α-chlorodiphenylacetate hydrochloride; an antihistaminic agent with anticholinergic properties.

di·aph·o·rase (dī-af′ōr-ās). Originally, a series of flavoproteins with reductase activity in mitochondria; now dihydrolipoamide dehydrogenase.

di·a·pho·re·sis (dī′ă-fō-rē′sis). SYN perspiration (1). [G. *diaphorēsis,* fr. *dia,* through, + *phoreō,* to carry]

di·a·pho·ret·ic (dī-ă-fō-ret′ik). **1.** Relating to, or causing, perspiration. **2.** An agent that increases perspiration.

di·a·phragm (dī′ă-fram). **1.** The musculomembranous partition between the abdominal and thoracic cavities. SYN diaphragma (2) [NA], interseptum, midriff, phren (1). **2.** A thin disk pierced with an opening, used in a microscope, camera, or other optical instrument in order to shut out the marginal rays of light, thus giving a more direct illumination. **3.** A flexible ring covered with a dome-shaped sheet of elastic material used in the vagina to prevent pregnancy. **4.** In radiography, a grid (2). [G. *diaphragma*]

aperture d., a metal device that limits the area of the beam emerging from an x-ray tube.

Bucky d., in radiography, a d. with a moving grid that avoids grid shadows. SYN Potter-Bucky d.

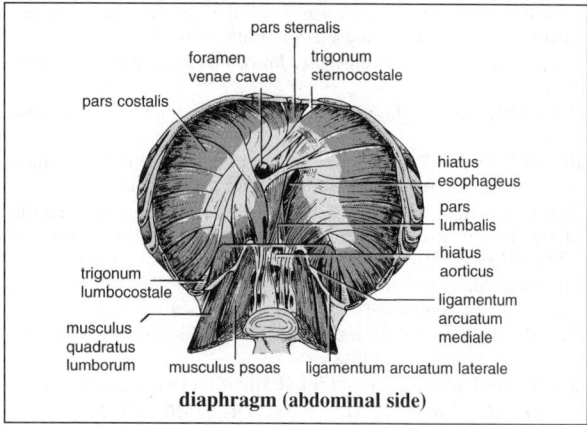

diaphragm (abdominal side)

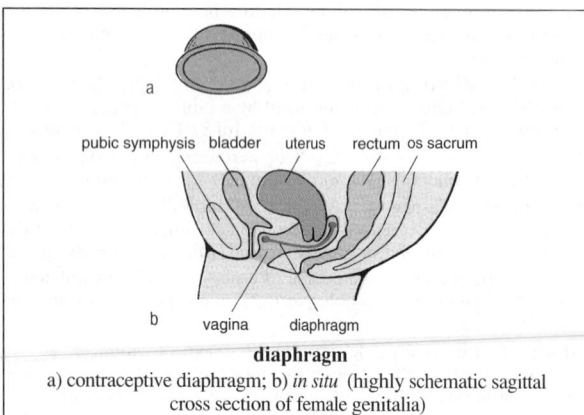

diaphragm

a) contraceptive diaphragm; b) *in situ* (highly schematic sagittal cross section of female genitalia)

pelvic d., d. of pelvis, the paired levator ani and coccygeus muscles together with the fascia above and below them. SYN diaphragma pelvis [NA].

Potter-Bucky d., SYN Bucky d.

d. of sella, a fold of dura mater extending transversely across the sella turcica and roofing over the hypophyseal fossa; it is perforated in its center for the passage of the infundibulum. SYN diaphragma sellae [NA], d. sellae, tentorium of hypophysis.

d. sellae, SYN d. of sella.

urogenital d., a triangular sheet of muscle between the ischiopubic rami; composed of the sphincter urethrae, and the deep transverse perineal muscles. SYN diaphragma urogenitale [NA].

di·a·phrag·ma, pl. **di·a·phrag·ma·ta** (dī-ă-frag'mă, -frag'mă-tă) [NA]. **1.** A thin partition separating adjacent regions. **2.** SYN diaphragm (1). [G. *diaphragma,* a partition wall, midriff]

d. pel'vis [NA], SYN pelvic *diaphragm.*

d. sel'lae [NA], SYN *diaphragm* of sella.

d. urogenita'le [NA], SYN urogenital *diaphragm.*

di·a·phrag·mal·gia (dī'ă-frag-mal'jē-ă). Rarely used term for a pain in the diaphragm. SYN diaphragmodynia. [diaphragm + G. *algos,* pain]

di·a·phrag·mat·ic (dī'ă-frag-mat'ik). Relating to a diaphragm. SYN phrenic (1).

di·a·phrag·mat·o·cele (dī'ă-frag-mat'ō-sēl). Rarely used term for diaphragmatic *hernia.* [diaphragm + G. *kēlē,* hernia]

di·a·phrag·mo·dyn·ia (dī'ă-frag-mō-din'ē-ă). SYN diaphragmalgia. [diaphragm + G. *odynē,* pain]

di·aph·y·se·al (dī-ă-fiz'ē-ăl). SYN diaphysial.

di·a·phy·sec·to·my (dī'ă-fī-sek'tō-mē). Partial or complete removal of the shaft of a long bone. [diaphysis + G. *ektomē,* excision]

di·a·phys·i·al (dī-ă-fiz'ē-ăl). Relating to a diaphysis. SYN diaphyseal.

di·aph·y·sis, pl. **di·aph·y·ses** (dī-af'i-sis, -sēz) [NA]. SYN shaft. [G. a growing between]

di·aph·y·si·tis (dī-af-i-sī'tis). Inflammation of the shaft of a long bone.

di·a·pi·re·sis (dī'ă-pī-rē'sis). Passage of colloidal or other small particles of suspended matter through the unruptured walls of the blood vessels. SEE ALSO diapedesis. [G. *diapeirō,* to drive through, fr. *peirō,* to pierce]

di·a·pla·cen·tal (dī'ă-pla-sen'tăl). Passing through or "across" the placenta.

di·ap·la·sis (dī-ap'lă-sis). Obsolete term for setting of a fracture or reduction of a dislocation. [G. a putting in shape]

di·a·plas·tic (dī-ă-plas'tik). Pertaining to diaplasis.

di·a·plex·us (dī-ă-plek'sŭs). Rarely used term for choroid *plexus* of third ventricle. [G. *dia,* through, + L. *plexus,* a plaiting]

di·ap·no·ic, di·ap·not·ic (dī-ap-nō'ik, -not'ik). **1.** Relating to, or causing perspiration, especially insensible perspiration. **2.** A mild sudorific.

di·a·poph·y·sis (dī'ă-pof'i-sis). A transverse process of a thoracic vertebra or the portion of a cervical or lumber vertebra homologous thereto. Cf. pleurapophysis. [G. *dia,* through, + *apophysis,* an offshoot]

Di·ap·to·mus (dī-ap'tō-mŭs). A genus of copepod crustacea, the principal intermediate host for *Diphyllobothrium latum* in North America.

di·ar·rhea (dī-ă-rē'ă). An abnormally frequent discharge of semisolid or fluid fecal matter from the bowel. [G. *diarrhoia,* fr. *dia,* through, + *rhoia,* a flow, a flux]

d. al'ba, SYN pullorum *disease.*

bovine virus d., a specific infectious disease of cattle, caused by a togavirus; characterized by ulceration of the mouth, pharynx, esophagus, and sometimes the stomachs and intestines; may or may not be accompanied by severe d. SYN mucosal disease.

cachectic d., d. occurring in patients with severe wasting. Usually due to underlying gastrointestinal disease.

choleraic d., SYN summer d.

chronic bacillary d., prolonged diarrhea occurring in association with bacterial infection, usually occurring in patients with gastrointestinal stasis, allowing bacterial proliferation in the intestine with secondary malabsorption. Occurs in blind-loop syndrome after intestinal surgery, following vagotomy, and occasionally in scleroderma or diabetes.

Cochin China d., obsolete term for tropical *sprue.*

colliquative d., d. associated with excessive discharge of fluid.

dientamoeba d., d. thought to be due to infection with the flagellate, *Dientamoeba fragilis.*

dysenteric d., d. in bacillary or amebic dysentery.

fatty d., d. seen in malabsorption syndromes including chronic pancreatic disease, characterized by foul smelling stools with increased fat content that usually float in water. SYN pimelorrhea.

flagellate d., d. due to infection with flagellate *Giardia lamblia.*

gastrogenous d., a d. that may occur in achylia gastrica, or that is caused by excess secretion of gastric and other intestinal juices.

lienteric d., d. in which undigested food appears in the stools.

morning d., a form in which there are several loose stools in the early morning and during the forenoon, the bowels being quiet during the remainder of the day and night.

mucous d., d. with the presence of considerable mucus in the stools.

nocturnal d., d. that occurs chiefly at night, usually in association with diabetic autonomic neuropathy.

pancreatic d., SYN d. pancreatica.

d. pancreatica (pan-krē-a'ti-kă), d. characterized by severe, watery, secretory d. and hyperkalemia; most patients have hypercalcemia, many have hyperglycemia; results from excessive secretion of VIP (vasoactive intestinal peptide) by an islet cell tumor of the pancreas. Sometimes called WDHA *syndrome.* SEE Verner-Morrison *syndrome*, WDHA *syndrome*. SYN pancreatic cholera, pancreatic d.

pancreatogenous d., d. in which the stools are bulky, pale, foul, greasy, and oily, as a result of malabsorption of fat due to deficient secretion of pancreatic enzymes in chronic pancreatitis.

porcine epidemic d., a disease of pigs caused by the porcine epidemic d. virus and characterized by acute d., with high mortality in piglets.

serous d., d. characterized by watery stools.

summer d., d. of infants in hot weather, usually an acute gastroenteritis due to the presence of *Shigella* or *Salmonella*. SYN choleraic d.

traveler's d., d. of sudden onset, often accompanied by abdominal cramps, vomiting, and fever, occurring sporadically in travelers usually during the first week of a trip; most commonly caused by unfamiliar strains of enterotoxigenic *Escherichia coli*.

tropical d., SYN tropical *sprue*.

white d., SYN pullorum *disease*.

di·ar·rhe·al, di·ar·rhe·ic (dī-ă-rē′ăl, -rē′ik). Relating to diarrhea.

di·ar·thric (dī-ar′thrik). Relating to two joints. SYN biarticular, diarticular. [G. *di-*, two, + *arthron*, joint]

di·ar·thro·sis, pl. **di·ar·thro·ses** (dī-ar-thrō′sis, -sēz). SYN synovial *joint*. [G. articulation]

di·ar·tic·u·lar (dī-ar-tik′yū-lăr). SYN diarthric.

di·as·chi·sis (dī-as′ki-sis). A sudden inhibition of function produced by an acute focal disturbance in a portion of the brain at a distance from the original seat of injury, but anatomically connected with it through fiber tracts. [G. a splitting]

di·a·scope (dī′ă-skōp). A flat glass plate through which one can examine superficial skin lesions by means of pressure. [G. *dia*, through, + *skopeō*, to view]

di·as·co·py (dī-as′kŏ-pē). Examination of superficial skin lesions with a diascope. [G. *dia*, through, + *skopeō*, to see]

di·a·stal·sis (dī-ă-stal′sis). The type of peristalsis in which a region of inhibition precedes the wave of contraction, as seen in the intestinal tract. [G. an arrangement]

di·a·stal·tic (dī-ă-stal′tik). Pertaining to diastalsis.

di·a·stase (dī′as-tās). A mixture, obtained from malt and containing amylolytic enzymes (principally α- and β-amylases), that converts starch into dextrin and maltose; used to make soluble starches, to aid in digestion of starches in certain types of dyspepsia, and to digest glycogen in histologic sections. [Fr., fr. G. *diastasis*, separation, fr. *dia*, apart + *histēmi*, to make to stand]

di·as·ta·sis (dī-as′tă-sis). **1.** Any simple separation of normally joined parts. SYN divarication. **2.** The mid-portion of diastole when the blood enters the ventricle slowly or ceases to enter prior to atrial systole. Diastasis duration is in inverse proportion to heart rate and is absent at very high heart rates. [G. a separation]

d. rec′ti, separation of rectus abdominis muscles away from the midline, sometimes seen during or following pregnancy.

di·as·tas·u·ria (dī-as-tās-yū′rē-ă). SYN amylasuria.

di·a·stat·ic (dī-ă-stat′ik). Relating to a diastasis.

di·a·ste·ma, pl. **di·a·ste·ma·ta** (dī′ă-stē′mă, -stē′mă-tă). **1.** Fissure or abnormal opening in any part, especially if congenital. **2** [NA]. Space between two adjacent teeth in the same dental arch. **3.** Cleft or space between the maxillary lateral incisor and canine teeth, into which the lower canine is received when the jaws are closed; abnormal in man but normal in dogs and many other animals. [G. *diastēma*, an interval]

di·a·ste·ma·to·cra·nia (dī-ă-stē′mă-tō-krā′nē-ă). Congenital sagittal fissure of the skull. [G. *diastēma*, an interval, + *kranion*, skull]

di·a·ste·ma·to·my·e·lia (dī-ă-stē′mă-tō-mī-e′lē-ă). Complete or incomplete sagittal division of the spinal cord by an osseous or fibrocartilaginous septum. [G. *diastēma*, interval, + *myelon*, marrow]

di·as·ter (dī′as-ter). SYN amphiaster. [G. *di-*, two, + *astēr*, star]

di·a·ste·re·o·i·so·mers (dī′ă-stār-ē-ō-ī′sō-merz). Optically active isomers that are not enantiomorphs (mirror images); *e.g.*, D-glucose and D-galactose.

di·as·to·le (dī-as′tō-lē). Normal postsystolic dilation of the heart cavities, during which they fill with blood; d. of the atria precedes that of the ventricles; d. of either chamber alternates rhythmically with systole or contraction of that chamber. [G. *diastolē*, dilation]

atrial d., period of relaxation and repolarization of the atrial muscle.

electrical d., period from end of T wave to beginning of next Q wave.

gastric d., a phase of relaxation of stomach peristalsis seen fluoroscopically or with the gastroscope.

late d., SYN presystole.

ventricular d., period of relaxation and repolarization of the ventricular muscle.

di·a·stol·ic (dī-ă-stol′ik). Relating to diastole.

di·as·tro·phism (dī-as′trof-izm). Distortion that occurs in objects as a result of bending. [G. *diastrophē*, fr. *diastrephein*, distortion]

di·a·tax·ia (dī′ă-tak′sē-ă). Ataxia affecting both sides of the body.

cerebral d., the ataxic type of cerebral birth palsy.

di·a·te·la (dī-ă-tē′lă). Rarely used term for choroid *tela* of third ventricle. [G. *dia*, through, between, + L. *tela*, web]

di·a·ther·mal (dī-ă-ther′mal). SYN diathermic. [G. *dia*, through, + *thermē*, heat]

di·a·ther·man·cy (dī-ă-ther′man-sē). The condition of being diathermic.

di·a·ther·ma·nous (dī-ă-ther′man-ŭs). Permeable by heat rays. SYN transcalent. [G. *dia-thermaino*, to heat through, fr. *thermos*, hot]

di·a·ther·mic (dī-ă-ther′mik). Relating to, characterized by, or affected by diathermy. SYN diathermal.

di·a·ther·mo·co·ag·u·la·tion (dī-ă-ther′mō-kō-ag-yū-lā′shŭn). SYN surgical *diathermy*.

di·a·ther·my (dī′ă-ther-mē). Local elevation of temperature within the tissues, produced by high frequency current, ultrasonic waves, or microwave radiation. SYN transthermia. [G. *dia*, through, + *thermē*, heat]

medical d., d. of mild degree causing no destruction of tissue. SYN thermopenetration.

short wave d., therapeutic elevation of temperature in the tissues by means of an oscillating electric current of extremely high frequency (10 to 100 million Hz) and short wavelength of 3 to 30 meters.

surgical d., electrocoagulation with a high frequency electrocautery, resulting in local tissue destruction; usually used to seal blood vessels and arrest bleeding. SYN diathermocoagulation.

ultrashortwave d., shortwave d. in which the wavelength is under 10 meters.

di·ath·e·sis (dī-ath′ĕ-sis). The constitutional or inborn state disposing to a disease, group of diseases, or metabolic or structural anomaly. [G. arrangement, condition]

contractural d., a tendency to have contractures in hysteria.

cystic d., a condition in which multiple cysts form in the liver, kidneys, and other organs.

gouty d., a state of susceptibility to attacks of gout or development of tophi, usually associated with hyperuricemia or hyperexcretion of urate in urine.

hemorrhagic d., any tendency to spontaneous bleeding or bleeding from trivial trauma caused by a defect in clotting or a flaw in the structure of blood vessels.

spasmophilic d., a condition in which there is an abnormal excitability of the motor nerves, shown by a tendency to tetany, laryngeal spasm, or general convulsions.

di·a·thet·ic (dī-ă-thet′ik). Relating to a diathesis.

di·a·tom (dī′ă-tom). An individual of microscopic unicellular algae, the shells of which compose a sedimentary infusorial earth. [G. *diatomos*, cut in two]

di·a·to·ma·ceous (dī'ă-tō-mā'shŭs). Pertaining to diatoms or their fossil remains.

di·a·tom·ic (dī-ă-tom'ik). **1.** Denoting a compound with a molecule made up of two atoms. **2.** Denoting any ion or atomic grouping composed of two atoms only.

di·a·tor·ic (dī'ă-tōr'ik). **1.** The vertical cylindric aperture formed in the base of artificial porcelain teeth and extending into the body of the tooth, serving as a mechanical means of attaching the tooth to the denture base. **2.** Denoting teeth that contain a d. [G. *diatoros,* pierced]

di·a·tri·zo·ate. Sodium 3,5-diacetamido-2,4,6-triiodobenzoate SEE *sodium* diatrizoate.

di·az·e·pam (dī-az'ĕ-pam). 7-Chloro-1,3-dihydro-1-methyl-5-phenyl-2*H*-1,4-benzodiazepin-2-one; a skeletal muscle relaxant, sedative, and antianxiety agent; also used as an anticonvulsant, particularly in the treatment of status epilepticus by the parenteral route.

di·a·zines (dī'ă-zēnz). A group of synthetic tuberculostatic drugs, such as pyrazine carboxamide and pyridazine-3-carboxamide.

di·az·in·on (dī-az'in-on). A sulfur-containing organophosphate compound used as an insecticide and cholinesterase inhibitor.

⚠**diazo-.** Prefix denoting a compound containing the ≡C–N=N–X grouping, where X is not carbon (except for CN), or the grouping N_2 attached by one atom to carbon (*e.g.,* diazomethane, CH_2N_2). Cf. azo-. [G. *di-,* two, + Fr. *azote,* nitrogen]

di·az·o·tize (dī-az'ō-tīz). To introduce the diazo group into a chemical compound, usually through the treatment of an amine with nitrous acid.

di·az·ox·ide (dī-ă-zok'sīd). 7-Chloro-3-methyl-2*H*-1,2,4-benzothiadiazine 1,1-dioxide; an antihypertensive agent.

di·ba·sic (dī-bā'sik). Having two replaceable hydrogen atoms, denoting an acid with two ionizable hydrogen atoms. SYN bibasic.

di·ben·a·mine (dī-ben'ă-mēn). A nonspecific and irreversible antagonist at alpha adrenergic receptors. Prevents vasoconstriction produced by epinephrine and norepinephrine and similar agents causing vasoconstriction by an action on alpha adrenergic receptors. Similar to dibenzyline.

di·benz·e·pin hy·dro·chlo·ride (dī-benz'ĕ-pin). 10-[2-(Dimethylamino)ethyl]-5,10-dihydro-5-methyl-11*H*-dibenzo-[*b,e*][1,4]diazepin-11-one hydrochloride; an antidepressant.

di·benz·hep·tro·pine cit·rate (dī-benz-hep'trō-pēn). SYN deptropine citrate.

di·ben·zo·pyr·i·dine (dī-ben'zō-pir'i-dēn). SYN acridine.

di·ben·zo·thi·a·zine (dī-ben'zō-thī'ă-zēn). SYN phenothiazine.

di·benz·thi·one (dī-benz-thī'ōn). 3,5-dibenzyltetrahydro-2*H*-1,3,5-thiadiazine-2-thione; an antifungal antiseptic. SYN sulbentine.

Di·both·ri·o·ceph·a·lus (dī-both'rē-ō-sef'ă-lŭs). Former name for *Diphyllobothrium.* [G. *di-,* two, + *bothrion,* dim. of *bothros,* a pit, + *kephalē,* head]

D. la'tus, SYN *Diphyllobothrium latum.*

di·bro·mo·pro·pam·i·dine is·e·thi·o·nate (dī-brō'mō-prō-pam'i-dēn). 2-Hydroxyethanesulfonic acid, a compound with 4,4'-(trimethylenedioxy)bis(3-bromobenzamidine); an antiseptic.

di·brom·sa·lan (dī-brom'să-lan). 4',5-Dibromosalicylanilide; a disinfectant.

di·bu·caine. A potent local anesthetic with a long duration of action used by injection or topically on skin or mucous membranes.

di·bu·caine hy·dro·chlo·ride (dī-byū'kān). 2-*n*-Butoxy-*N*-[2-(diethylamino)ethyl]cinchoninamide monohydrochloride; a potent local anesthetic (surface and spinal anesthesia).

di·bu·caine num·ber (DN). A test for differentiation of one of several forms of atypical pseudocholinesterases that are unable to inactivate succinylcholine at normal rates; based upon percent inhibition of the enzymes by dibucaine, normal enzyme has a DN of 75 and above, heterozygous atypical enzyme has a DN of 40-70, and homozygous atypical enzyme has a DN of less than 20. SEE ALSO fluoride number.

di·bu·to·line sul·fate (dī-byū'tō-lēn). Dibutyl urethane of

dimethylethyl-β-hydroxyethylammonium sulfate; an anticholinergic agent used as a mydriatic, a cycloplegic, and a gastrointestinal antispasmodic.

di·bu·tyl phthal·ate (dī-byū'til thal'āt). *n*-Butyl phthalate; di-*n*-butyl ester of benzene-*o*-dicarboxylic acid; an insect repellent.

DIC Abbreviation for disseminated intravascular *coagulation.*

di·cac·o·dyl (dī-kak'ō-dil). SYN cacodyl.

di·ce·lous (dī-sē'lŭs). Having two cavities or excavations on opposite surfaces. [G. *di-,* two, + *koilos,* hollow]

di·cen·tric (dī-sen'trik). Having two centromeres, an abnormal state.

di·ceph·a·lous (dī-sef'ă-lŭs). Having two heads.

di·ceph·a·lus (dī-sef'ă-lŭs). Symmetrical conjoined twins with two separate heads. SEE conjoined *twins,* under *twin.* SYN bicephalus, diplocephalus. [G. *di-,* two, + *kephalē,* head]

d. di'auchenos, a d. with separate necks. SYN derodidymus.

d. di'pus dibra'chius, a d. in which the merging of the bodies has obliterated the appendages on the side of the union, leaving only two arms and two legs for the double body.

d. di'pus tetrabra'chius, a d. with two legs and four separate arms.

d. di'pus tribra'chius, a d. with two legs and three arms.

d. dip'ygus, SYN anakatadidymus. SEE conjoined *twins,* under *twin.*

d. mon'auchenos, a d. in which fusion has involved the cervical region so that the two heads are on a single neck.

di·chei·lia, di·chi·lia (dī-kī'lē-ă). A lip appearing to be double because of the presence of an abnormal fold of mucosa. [G. *di-,* two, + *cheilos,* lip]

di·chei·ria, di·chi·ria (dī-kī'rē-ă). Complete or incomplete duplication of the hand. SEE ALSO polydactyly. SYN diplocheiria, diplochiria. [G. *di-,* two, + *cheir,* hand]

Di·chel·o·bac·ter no·do·sus. SYN *Bacteroides nodosus.*

di·chlo·ra·mine-T (dī-klōr'ă-mēn). $CH_3C_6H_4SO_2NCl_2$; *p*-Toluenesulfonic acid dichloramide; used as an antiseptic in surgical dressings.

di·chlo·ride (dī-klōr'īd). A compound with a molecule containing two atoms of chlorine to one of another element. SYN bichloride.

di·chlo·ri·sone (dī-klōr'i-sōn). 9α,11β-Dichloro-17α,21-dihydroxy-1,4-pregnadiene-3,20-dione; 9,11-dichloropredisolone; a topical antipruritic agent.

di·chlor·i·so·pro·ter·e·nol (dī-klōr'is-ō-prō-tār'ĕ-nol). SYN dichloroisoproterenol.

di·chlo·ro·ben·zene (dī-klōr'ō-ben'zēn). ClC_6H_4Cl; an insecticide used chiefly as a moth repellent.

di·chlo·ro·di·flu·o·ro·meth·ane (dī-klōr'ō-dī-flū-rō-meth'ān). CF_2Cl_2; an easily liquefiable gas used as a refrigerant and aerosol propellant.

***p,p'*-di·chlo·ro·di·phen·yl meth·yl car·bi·nol (DMC)** (dī-chlōr'ō-dī-fen'il). A synthetic compound found effective as a miticide.

di·chlo·ro·di·phen·yl·tri·chlo·ro·eth·ane (DDT) (dī-chlōr'ō-dī-fen'il-trī-klōr-ō-eth'ān). 1,1,1-Trichloro-2,2-*bis*(p-chlorophenyl)ethane; an insecticide that came into prominence during and after World War II. For a time it proved very effective, but insect populations rapidly developed tolerance for it, hence much of its original effectiveness has been lost; general usage is now widely discouraged because of the toxicity that results from the environmental persistence of this agent. SYN chlorophenothane, dicophane.

di(2-chlo·ro·eth·yl)sul·fide. SYN mustard *gas.*

di·chlo·ro·for·mox·ime. SYN *phosgene* oxime.

di·chlo·ro·hy·drin (dī-klōr-ō-hī'drin). A colorless, odorless fluid prepared by heating anhydrous glycerin with sulfur monochloride; a solvent of resins. SYN dichloroisopropyl alcohol.

2,6-di·chlo·ro·in·do·phe·nol (dī-klōr'ō-in-dō-fē'nol). A reagent for the chemical assay of ascorbic acid which depends upon the reducing properties of the latter. It is red in acid solution; in the presence of the vitamin C it undergoes reduction and becomes colorless, the vitamin being oxidized to dehydroascorbic acid. Often misnamed dichlorophenol-indophenol.

di·chlo·ro·i·so·pro·pyl al·co·hol (dī-klōr'ō-is-ō-prō'pil). SYN dichlorohydrin.

di·chlo·ro·i·so·pro·ter·e·nol (DCI) (dī-klōr'ō-is-ō-prō-tār'ĕ-nol). *dl*-1-[3,4-dichlorophenyl]-2-isopropylaminoethanol; the congener of the adrenergic beta receptor stimulant, isoproterenol; it blocks the responses, involving beta receptors, to epinephrine and other sympathomimetic drugs. SYN dichlorisoproterenol.

di·chlo·ro·phen (dī-klōr'ō-fen). 2,2'-Dihydroxy-5,5' methylenebix(4-chlorophenol); used topically as a fungicide and bactericide, and internally in the treatment of infections by tapeworms of man and domestic animals.

di·chlo·ro·phen·ar·sine hy·dro·chlo·ride (dī-klōr'ō-fen-ar' sēn). (3-Amino-4-Hydroxyphenyl)dichloroarisine hydrochloride, formerly used as an arsenical antisyphilitic.

2,6-di·chlo·ro·phe·nol-in·do·phe·nol (dī'klōr-ō-fē'nol-in-dō-fē'nol). Misnomer for 2,6-dichloroindophenol.

(2,4-di·chlo·ro·phen·oxy) ace·tic ac·id (2,4-D). A herbicide, more toxic to broad-leaved dicotyledonous plants (weeds) than to monocotyledonous ones (grains and grass), used with (2,4,5-trichlorophenoxy)acetic acid as a constituent of Agent Orange.

di·chlo·ro·vos (dī-klōr'ō-vos). SYN dichlorvos.

di·chlor·phen·a·mide (dī-klōr-fen'ă-mīd). 4,5-Dichloro-*m*-benzenedisulfonamide; a carbonic anhydrase inhibitor with actions similar to those of acetazolamide.

di·chlor·vos (dī-klōr'vos). phosphoric acid 2,2-dichlorovinyl dimethyl phosphate; an anthelmintic in veterinary and human medicine. SYN dichlorovos.

di·cho·ri·al, di·cho·ri·on·ic (dī-kō'rē-ăl, dī-kō-rē-on'ik). Showing evidence of two chorions. [G. *di-*, two, + chorion]

di·chot·ic (dī-kot'ik). SYN dichotomous.

di·chot·o·mous (dī-kot'ō-mŭs). Denoting or characterized by dichotomy. SYN dichotic.

di·chot·o·my (dī-kot'ō-mē). Division into two parts. [G. *dichotomia*, a cutting in two, fr. *dicha*, in two, + *tomē*, a cutting]

di·chro·ic (dī-krō'ik). Relating to dichroism.

di·chro·ism (dī'krō-izm). The property of seeming to be differently colored when viewed from emitted light and from transmitted light. [G. *di-*, two, + *chrōa*, color]

circular d. (CD), the change from circular polarization to elliptical polarization of monochromatic, circularly polarized light in the immediate vicinity of the absorption band of the substance through which the light passes. SEE ALSO Cotton *effect*.

di·chro·mat (dī'krō-mat). An individual with dichromatism.

di·chro·mate (dī-krō'māt). A compound containing the radical $Cr_2O_7^=$. SYN bichromate.

di·chro·mat·ic (dī-krō-mat'ik). 1. Having or exhibiting two colors. 2. Relating to dichromatism (2).

di·chro·ma·tism (dī-krō'mă-tizm). 1. The state of being dichromatic (1). 2. The abnormality of color vision in which only two of the three retinal cone pigments are present, as in protanopia, deuteranopia, and tritanopia. SYN dichromatopsia. [G. *di-*, two, + *chrōma*, color]

di·chro·ma·top·sia (dī-krō-mă-top'sē-ă). SYN dichromatism (2). [G. *di-*, two, + *chrōma*, color, + *opsis*, vision]

di·chro·mic (dī-krō'mik). Having, or relating to, two colors.

di·chro·mo·phil, di·chro·mo·phile (dī-krō'mō-fil, dī-krō'mō-fīl). Taking a double stain; denoting a tissue or cell taking both acid and basic dyes in different parts. [G. *di-*, two, + *chrōma*, color, + *philos*, fond]

Dick, George Frederick, U.S. internist, 1881–1967. SEE D. *method*, *test*, test *toxin*.

Dick, Gladys R.H., U.S. internist, 1881–1963. SEE D. *method*, *test*, test *toxin*.

Dickens, Frank, British biochemist, *1899. SEE D. *shunt;* Warburg-Lipmann-D.-Horecker *shunt*.

di·clo·fen·ac (dī-clō'fén-ák). One of several nonsteroidal antiinflammatory drugs used in the treatment of rheumatic disorders

such as rheumatoid arthritis; also used in osteoarthritis and other conditions. Acts by preventing prostaglandin synthesis.

di·clox·a·cil·lin so·di·um (dī-klok-să-sil'in). Sodium salt of 3-(2,6-dichlorophenyl)-5-methyl-4-isoazolylpenicillin; a semisynthetic penicillin resistant to penicillinase.

di·co·phane (dī'kō-fān). SYN dichlorodiphenyltrichloroethane.

di·co·ria (dī-kō'rē-ă). SYN diplocoria. [G. *di-*, two, + *korē*, pupil]

di·cot·yl·ed·on. Plant (shrub, herb, or tree) whose seeds consist of two cotyledons, *i.e.*, the primary or rudimentary leaf of the embryo of seed plants.

di·cro·coe·li·o·sis (dī'krō-sē-li-ō'sis). Infection of animals and rarely man with trematodes of the genus *Dicrocoelium*.

Di·cro·coe·li·um (dīk-rō-sē'lē-ŭm). A genus of digenetic trematodes inhabiting the bile ducts and gallbladder of herbivores. The species *D. dentriticum* (lancet fluke) is rarely found in humans, but is an important parasite of sheep in some localities. [G. *dikroos*, forked, + *koilia*, belly]

di·crot·ic (dī-krot'ik). Relating to dicrotism. [G. *dikrotos*, double-beating]

di·cro·tism (dī'krō-tizm). That form of the pulse in which a double beat can be appreciated at any arterial pulse for each beat of the heart; due to accentuation of the dicrotic wave. [G. *di-*, two, + *krotos*, a beat]

dicta- (dik'ta). Prefix used to signify two hundred. [G.]

Dic·ty·o·cau·lus (dik'tē-ō-kaw'lŭs). A genus of thin elongate metastrongylid nematode lungworms (subfamily Dictyocaulinae) that inhabit the air passages of herbivorous animals; the life cycle is direct, infection occurring from ingestion of infective larvae. [G. *diktyon*, net, + *kaulos*, stalk]

D. arnfiel'di, species that occurs in the bronchi of horses, mules, and donkeys; generally produces few or no symptoms, except with heavy infection.

D. fila'ria, the large or thread lungworm, a species that is the common lungworm of sheep, goats, camels, and many wild ruminants; it causes much damage, especially in younger heavily infected animals, which cough and suffer from dyspnea; emaciation and anemia often occur.

D. vivip'arus, species that is the common lungworm of cattle, deer, and other ruminants, usually found in the trachea, bronchi, and bronchioles; the chronic cough caused by this parasite is sometimes called hoose or husk, especially in Great Britain.

dic·ty·o·ma (dik-tē-ō'mă). A benign tumor of the ciliary epithelium with a net-like structure resembling embryonic retina. [G. *dikyton*, net (retina), + *-oma*, tumor]

dic·ty·o·some (dik'tē-ō-sōm). SYN Golgi *apparatus*. [G. *diktyon*, net, + *-some*]

dic·ty·o·tene (dik'tē-ō-tēn). The state of meiosis at which the oocyte is arrested during the several years between late fetal life and menarche. [G. *diktyon*, net, + *tainia*, band]

di·cu·ma·rol (dī-kū'mă-rol). 3,3'-methylene-bis(4-hydroxycoumarin); an anticoagulant that inhibits the formation of prothrombin in the liver. SYN bishydroxycoumarin.

di·cy·clo·mine hy·dro·chlo·ride (dī-sī'klō-mēn). 2-Diethylaminoethyl bicyclohexyl-1-carboxylate hydrochloride; an anticholinergic agent.

di·cys·te·ine (dī-sis'tēn). SYN cystine.

di·dac·tic (dī-dak'tik). Instructive; denoting medical teaching by lectures or textbooks, as distinguished from clinical demonstrations with patients or laboratory exercises. [G. *didaktikos*, fr. *didaskō*, to teach]

di·dac·ty·lism (dī-dak'ti-lizm). Congenital condition of having two fingers on a hand or two toes on a foot. [G. *di-*, two, + *daktylos*, finger or toe]

di·del·phic (dī-del'fik). Having or relating to a double uterus. [G. *di-*, two, + *delphys*, womb]

Di·del·phis (dī-del'fis). A genus of marsupials, commonly called opossums, that serve as reservoir hosts of *Trypanosoma cruzi*. *D. marsupialis* is the common North American variety; *D. paraguayensis* is a South American form. [G. *di-*, two, + *delphys*, womb]

di

di·de·ox·y·aden·o·sine (DDA) (dī′dē-oks′ē-ă-den′ō-sēn). An antiviral agent that has been tried in AIDS, similar to DDC.

di·de·ox·y·cy·ti·dine (dī′-dē-ok′-sē-sī′-ti-dñ). Pyrimidine nucleoside analog with antiviral activity; has been tried in AIDS.

di·de·ox·y·in·o·sine (DDI) (dī′-dē-oks-ē-ī′-nō-sēn). Antiviral agent; has been used in treatment of AIDS.

⬭**didym-, didymo-.** The didymus, testis. [G. *didymos,* twin]

did·y·mus (did′ē-mŭs). SYN testis. [G. *didymos,* a twin, pl. *didymoi,* testes]

⬭**-didymus.** A conjoined twin, with the first element of the complete word designating fused parts. SEE ALSO -dymus, -pagus. [G. *didymos,* twin]

die (dī). In dentistry, the positive reproduction of the form of a prepared tooth in any suitable hard substance, usually in metal or specially prepared artificial stone. SEE ALSO counterdie.

dieb. alt. Abbreviation for L. *diebus alternis,* every other day.

di·e·cious (dī-ē′shŭs). Denoting animals or plants that are sexually distinct, the individuals being of one or the other sex. [G. *di-,* two, + *oikia,* house]

Dieffenbach, Johann F., German surgeon, 1792–1847. SEE D.'s *method.*

Diego blood group, Di blood group. See Blood Groups appendix.

di·el (dī′el). Term frequently used synonymously with diurnal (2) or circadian. [irreg., fr. L. *dies,* day]

di·el·drin (dī-el′drin). A chlorinated hydrocarbon used as an insecticide; may cause toxic effects in persons and animals exposed to its action through skin contact, inhalation, or food contamination.

di·e·lec·trog·ra·phy (dī-ē-lek-trog′ră-fē). SYN impedance *plethysmography.*

di·e·lec·trol·y·sis (dī′ē-lek-trol′i-sis). SYN electrophoresis.

Diels, Otto, German chemist and Nobel laureate, 1876–1954. SEE D. *hydrocarbon.*

di·en·ceph·a·lo·hy·po·phy·si·al (dī-en-sef′ă-lō-hī-pō-fiz′ē-ăl). Relating to the diencephalon and hypophysis.

di·en·ceph·a·lon, pl. **di·en·ceph·a·la** (dī-en-sef′ă-lon, -sef′ă-lă) [NA]. That part of the prosencephalon composed of the epithalamus, dorsal thalamus, subthalamus, and hypothalamus. [G. *dia,* through, + *enkephalos,* brain]

die·ner (dē′ner). A laboratory worker who assists in cleaning. [Ger. *Diener,* servant]

di·en·es·trol (dī-en-es′trol). 3,4-bis(*p*-hydroxyphenyl)-2,4-hexadiene; an estrogenic agent. SYN estrodienol.

Di·ent·a·moe·ba frag·i·lis (dī-ent-ă-mē′bă fraj′i-lis). A species of small ameba-like flagellates, formerly considered a true ameba, now recognized as an amebo-flagellate related to *Trichomonas,* parasitic in the large intestine of humans and certain monkeys; usually nonpathogenic, but believed to be capable of sometimes causing low-grade inflammation with mucous diarrhea and gastrointestinal disturbance in humans. SEE ALSO *Histomonas meleagridis.*

di·er·e·sis (dī-er′ē-sis). SYN *solution* of continuity. [G. *diairesis,* a division]

di·e·ret·ic (dī-er-et′ik). 1. Relating to dieresis. 2. Dividing; ulcerating; corroding.

di·es·ter·ase (dī-es′ter-ās). SEE phosphodiesterases.

di·es·trous (dī-es′trŭs). Pertaining to diestrus.

di·es·trus (dī-es′trŭs). A period of sexual quiescence intervening between two periods of estrus. [G. *dia,* between, + *oistros,* desire]

di·et (dī′et). 1. Food and drink in general. 2. A prescribed course of eating and drinking in which the amount and kind of food, as well as the times at which it is to be taken, are regulated for therapeutic purposes. 3. Reduction of caloric intake so as to lose weight. 4. To follow any prescribed or specific d. [G. *diaita,* a way of life; a diet]

acid-ash d., SYN alkaline-ash d.

alkaline-ash d., a d. consisting mainly of fruits, vegetables, and milk (with minimal amounts of meat, fish, eggs, cheese, and cereals), which, when catabolized, leave an alkaline residue to be excreted in the urine. SYN acid-ash d., basic d.

balanced d., a d. containing the essential nutrients with a reasonable ration of all the major food groups.

basal d., (1) a d. having a caloric value equal to the basal heat production and sufficient quanties of essential nutrients to meet basic needs; **(2)** in experiments in nutrition, a d. from which a given constituent (*e.g.,* a vitamin, mineral, or amino acid), the nutritional value of which is to be determined, is omitted for a period and the effects observed; the subject is observed for a second period during which the ingredient being studied is added to the d.

basic d., SYN alkaline-ash d.

bland d., a regular d. omitting foods that mechanically or chemically irritate the gastrointestinal tract.

challenge d., a d. in which one or more specific substances are included for the purpose of determining whether an abnormal reaction occurs.

clear liquid d., a d., often used postoperatively, consisting usually of water, tea, coffee, gelatin preparations, and clear soups or broth.

diabetic d., a dietary adjustment for patients with *diabetes* mellitus intended to decrease the need for insulin or oral diabetic agents and control weight by adjusting caloric and carbohydrate intake.

elimination d., a d. designed to detect what ingredient of the food causes allergic manifestations in the patient; food items to which the patient may be sensitive are withdrawn separately and successively from the d. until that which causes the symptoms is discovered.

full liquid d., a d. consisting only of liquids but including cream soups, ice cream, and milk.

Giordano-Giovannetti d., a d. designed for patients with renal failure; it provides small amounts of protein, primarily as essential amino acids, along with alpha-keto derivatives of amino acids; breakdown of protein in skeletal muscle is retarded and, because transaminase reactions are reversible, a small proportion of the ammonia released by urea breakdown is used for synthesis of nonessential amino acids. SYN Giovannetti d.

Giovannetti d., SYN Giordano-Giovannetti d.

gluten-free d., elimination of all wheat, rye, barley, and oat gluten from the d.; treatment for gluten-sensitive enteropathy (celiac disease). SEE celiac *disease.*

gout d., a d. containing a minimal quantity of purine bases (meats); liver, kidney, and sweetbread especially are excluded and replaced by dairy products, fruits, and cereals; alcoholic beverages also are excluded. SYN purine-free d.

high-calorie d., a d. containing upward of 4,000 calories per day.

high-fat d., a d. containing large amounts of fat.

high-fiber d., a d. high in the nondigestible part of plants, which is fiber. Fiber is found in fruits, vegetables, whole grains, and legumes. Insoluble fiber increases stool bulk, decreases transit time of food in the bowel, and decreases constipation and the risk of colon cancer. Soluble fiber delays absorption of glucose, which helps to control blood sugar in diabetes mellitus, and delays absorption of lipids, which helps to control hyperlipidemia. Recommended in treatment of diverticular disease of the colon.

Kempner d., SYN rice d.

ketogenic d., a high-fat, low-carbohydrate, and normal protein d. causing ketosis.

low-calorie d., a d. of 1,200 calories or less per day.

low-fat d., a d. containing minimal amounts of fat.

Diets containing low amounts of fat and cholesterol are designed to reduce the risk of heart disease and, in some cases, cancer. Dozens of such diets have been promulgated, both by medical and lay advisors. Their popularity can be attributed in part to clinical studies that have, since the 1980s, revealed, on the one hand, the hazards of eating high-fat, high-cholesterol foods and, on the other, the benefits of ingesting less saturated fat and LDL (low density lipoprotein) cholesterol. Although coronary deaths have been reduced by roughly 30% since 1970, the aim of health officials is to further reduce heart attack rates. The average cholesterol level among adult Americans has fallen from 213 to 205 mg/dl since 1978. However, the National Cholesterol Education Program recommends that individuals maintain a total cholesterol level of no more than 200 mg/dl, with LDL at less than 130 mg/dl and HDL (high density lipoprotein) around 60 mg/dl. About one-half of American adults exceed those recommendations. Low-fat, low-cholesterol diets are rich in whole grains, fresh fruits and vegetables, and legumes, and limit or exclude consumption of processed oils, dairy products, nuts and seeds, and meats. See atherosclerosis, free radicals.

low purine d., a d. low in precursors of purines (such as tissues rich in cells with abundant nuclei, as in liver, glandular meats, etc.) to minimize formation of uric acid. Useful in treatment of patients with gout or urate-containing renal calculi.

low residue d., a d. that leaves minimal unabsorbed components in the intestine, to minimize functional stress on the colon.

low salt d., a d. with restricted amounts of sodium chloride, necessary in the treatment of some cases of hypertension, heart failure, and other syndromes characterized by fluid retention and/or edema formation.

macrobiotic d., a d. claimed to promote longevity, often by promoting an emphasis on natural foods and restrictions on non-cereal foods, as well as liquids.

Meulengracht's d., a feeding program for patients with peptic ulcer disease, containing a relatively full diet free of acidic or highly seasoned food.

Minot-Murphy d., the use of large amounts of raw liver in the treatment of pernicious *anemia*. First successes in the treatment of this disease occurred with this diet and led to development of liver extract for treatment.

Ornish prevention d.'s, relaxed versions of the Ornish reversal d., which is designed to prevent coronary artery disease. These d.'s reduce dietary fat in proportion to blood cholesterol level.

Ornish reversal d., a d. designed by Dean Ornish, who has evidence that it will reverse coronary artery disease. It consists of 10% of calories from fat (mostly polyunsaturated or monounsaturated, with 5 mg cholesterol per day), 70 to 75% from carbohydrate, and 15 to 20% from protein.

purine-free d., SYN gout d.

purine-restricted d., SEE gout d.

rachitic d., a d. that will induce rickets in susceptible experimental animals.

reducing d., a d. in which caloric expenditure is greater than caloric intake.

rice d., a d. of rice, fruit, and sugar, plus vitamin and iron supplements, devised by Kempner to treat hypertension. In 2,000 calories, the d. contains 5 gm or less of fat, about 20 gm of protein, and not more than 150 mg of sodium. SYN Kempner d.

Schmidt d., SYN Schmidt-Strassburger d.

Schmidt-Strassburger d., an obsolete d. designed to facilitate examination of the stools in patients with diarrhea, consisting of milk, zwieback, oatmeal gruel, eggs, butter, small amounts of beef and potato. SYN Schmidt d.

sippy d., a d. formerly used in the initial stages of treatment of peptic ulcer, beginning with milk and cream every hour or two to keep gastric acid neutralized, gradually increasing to include cereal, eggs and crackers after three days, pureed vegetables later.

smooth d., a d. containing little roughage; used primarily in diseases of the colon.

soft d., a normal d. limited to soft foods for those who have difficulty chewing or swallowing; there are no restrictions on seasoning or method of food preparation.

subsistence d., a meager d. providing barely enough for sustenance.

Wilder's d., obsolete d., low in potassium, for treating Addison's *disease*.

di·e·tary (dī′ĕ-tār-ē). Relating to the diet.

Dieterle's stain. See under stain.

di·e·tet·ic (dī′ĕ-tet′ik). **1.** Relating to the diet. **2.** Descriptive of food that, naturally or through processing, has a low caloric content.

di·e·tet·ics (dī-ĕ-tet′iks). The practical application of diet in the prophylaxis and treatment of disease.

di·eth·a·di·one (dī-eth-ă-dī′ōn). 5,5-Diethyldihydro-2*H*-1,3-oxazine-2,4(3*H*)-dione; an analeptic.

di·eth·a·nol·a·mine (dī-eth-ă-nol′ă-mēn). bis(hydroxyethyl)-amine; 2,2′-iminodiethanol; used as an emulsifier and as a dispersing agent in cosmetics and pharmaceuticals. SYN diethylolamine.

di·eth·a·zine (dī-eth′ă-zēn). 10-(2-Diethylaminoethyl)-phenothiazine; an anticholinergic agent.

di·eth·yl (dī-eth′il). A compound containing two ethyl radicals.

5,5-di·eth·yl·bar·bi·tu·ric ac·id (dī-eth′il-bar-bi-tyū′rik). SYN barbital.

di·eth·yl·car·bam·a·zine cit·rate (dī-eth′il-kar-bam′ă-zēn). *N,N*-Diethyl-4-methyl-1-piperazinecarboxamide citrate; an effective microfilaricide, although relatively ineffective against the adult filariae.

di·eth·yl·ene·di·a·mine (dī-eth′il-ēn-dī′ă-mēn). SYN piperazine.

1,4-di·eth·yl·ene di·ox·ide (dī-eth′il-ēn). SYN dioxane.

di·eth·yl·ene gly·col (dī-eth′il-ēn). An organic solvent chemically related to ethylene glycol. Upon metabolic conversion it becomes oxalic acid, which is toxic to the kidney. A sweet, viscous liquid that was used to make the infamous elixir of sulfanilamide that proved fatal to over 100 children in 1937, leading to the establishment of the FDA to monitor drug safety.

di·eth·yl·ene·tri·a·mine pen·ta·a·ce·tic ac·id (DTPA) (dī-eth′il-ēn-trī′ă-mēn pen-tă-a-sē′tik). An important chelating agent used in therapy (*e.g.,* in therapy for lead poisoning), and in metal-containing diagnostic agents for magnetic resonance imaging and nuclear scanning.

di·eth·yl ether. $CH_3CH_2OCH_2CH_3$; a flammable, volatile organic solvent used in extraction procedures; formerly widely used as an inhalation anesthetic; shortcomings include: irritating vapor, slow onset and prolonged recovery phase, explosion hazard. SYN ethyl ether, ethyl oxide, sulfuric ether.

di·eth·y·lol·a·mine (dī-eth-i-lol′ă-mēn). SYN diethanolamine.

di·eth·yl·pro·pi·on hy·dro·chlo·ride (dī-eth-il-prō′pē-on). 1-Phenyl-2-diethylaminopropanone-1 hydrochloride; a sympathomimetic drug resembling amphetamine in its actions and used as an appetite suppressant. Increases blood pressure, heart rate.

di·eth·yl·stil·bes·trol (DES) (dī-eth′il-stil-bes′trol). A synthetic nonsteroidal estrogenic compound. Sometimes used as a postcoital antipregnancy agent to prevent implantation of the fertilized ovum. The first demonstrated transplacental carcinogen responsible for a delayed clear cell vaginal carcinoma in female offspring of mothers who took the drug during pregnancy when the drug was erroneously thought to prevent threatened abortion. SYN stilbestrol.

di·eth·yl·tol·u·am·ide (dī-eth′il-tō-lū′ă-mīd). *m*-Delphene; *N,N*-diethyl-*m*-toluamide; an insect repellent.

di·eth·yl·tryp·ta·mine (DET) (dī-eth-il-trip′tă-mēn). *N,N*-Di-

di

ethyltryptamine; a hallucinogenic agent similar to dimethyltryptamine.

di·e·ti·tian (dī-ĕ-tish'ŭn). An expert in dietetics.

Dietl, Józef, Polish physician, 1804–1878. SEE D.'s *crisis.*

Dieuaide di·a·gram. See under diagram.

Dieulafoy, Georges, French physician, 1839–1911. SEE D.'s *erosion, theory.*

di·far·ne·syl group (di-far'nĕ-sil). A 30-carbon open chain hexaisoprenoid hydrocarbon radical; occurs as a side chain in vitamin K_2.

di·fen·ox·in (dī-fen-ok'sin). 1-(3-cyano-3,3-diphenylpropyl)-4-phenylisonipecotic acid; an antidiarrheal agent with actions similar to those of diphenoxylate. SYN difenoxylic acid.

di·fen·ox·y·lic ac·id (dī-fen-ok'si-lik). SYN difenoxin.

dif·fer·ence (dif'er-ens). The magnitude or degree by which one quality or quantity differs from another of the same kind.

alveolar-arterial oxygen d., the d. or gradient between the partial pressure of oxygen in the alveolar spaces and the arterial blood: $P_{(A-a)}O_2$. Normally in young adults this value is less than 20 mm Hg. SEE ALSO alveolar gas *equation.*

arteriovenous carbon dioxide d., the d. in carbon dioxide content (in ml per 100 ml blood) between arterial and venous blood.

arteriovenous oxygen d., the d. in the oxygen content (in ml per 100 ml blood) between arterial and venous blood.

arteriovenous differences		
	vol. %	
	O_2	CO_2
arterial blood	20	48
venous blood		
when calm	14	53
in vigorous exertion	7	60
arteriovenous differences		
when calm	+ 6	− 5
in vigorous exertion	+13	−12

A-V d., abbreviation for arteriovenous difference of concentration of a substance.

cation-anion d., SYN anion *gap.*

individual d.'s, in clinical psychology, deviations of individuals from the group average or from each other.

light d., (1) the d. in light sensitivity of the two eyes; **(2)** SYN brightness difference *threshold.*

standard error of d., a statistical index of the probability that a d. between two sample means is greater than zero.

dif·fer·en·tial (dif-er-en'shăl). Relating to, or characterized by, a difference; distinguishing. [L. *dif-fero,* to carry apart, differ, fr. *dis,* apart]

threshold d., SYN differential *threshold.*

dif·fer·en·ti·at·ed (dif-er-en'shē-ā-ted). Having a different character or function from the surrounding structures or from the original type; said of tissues, cells, or portions of the cytoplasm.

dif·fer·en·ti·a·tion (dif'er-en-shē-ā'shŭn). **1.** The acquisition or possession of one or more characteristics or functions different from that of the original type. SYN specialization (2). **2.** SYN differential *diagnosis.* **3.** Partial removal of a stain from a histologic section to accentuate the staining differences of tissue components.

correlative d., d. due to the interaction of different parts of an organism.

echocardiographic d., the processing of a signal so that the output depends upon the rate of change of the input; *e.g.,* it will display changes in amplitude but will reduce the duration of the waveform.

invisible d., SYN chemodifferentiation.

dif·flu·ence (dif'lū-ens). The process of becoming fluid. [L. *diffluo,* to flow in different directions, dissolve]

dif·frac·tion (di-frak'shŭn). Deflection of the rays of light from a straight line in passing by the edge of an opaque body or in passing an obstacle of about the size of the wavelength of the light. [L. *dif- fringo,* pp. *-fractus,* to break in pieces]

dif·frac·tion grat·ing. A variety of filter composed of lined grooves in a thin layer of aluminum-copper alloy on a glass surface. SEE monochromator.

dif·fu·sate (dif-fyū'zāt). SYN dialysate. [L. *dif-fundo,* pp. *-fusus,* to pour in different directions]

dif·fuse (di-fyūs). **1** (di-fyūz'). To disseminate; to spread about. **2** (di-fyūs'). Disseminated; spread about; not restricted. [L. *dif-fundo,* pp. *-fusus,* to pour in different directions]

dif·fus·i·ble (di-fyūz'i-bl). Capable of diffusing.

dif·fu·sion (di-fyū'zhŭn). **1.** The random movement of molecules or ions or small particles in solution or suspension under the influence of brownian (thermal) motion toward a uniform distribution throughout the available volume; the rate is relatively rapid among liquids and gases, but takes place very slowly among solids. **2.** SYN dialysis.

facilitated d., SEE facilitated *transport.*

gel d., d. in a gel, as in the case of gel d. precipitin tests in which the immune reactants diffuse in agar. SEE ALSO immunodiffusion.

passive d., SEE facilitated *transport.*

di·flor·a·sone di·ac·e·tate (dī-flōr'ă-sōn). Pregna-1,4-diene-3,20-dione, 17,21-bis(acetyloxy)-6,9-difluoro-11-hydroxy-16-methyl-, (6α,11β,16β)-; an anti-inflammatory corticosteroid used in topical preparations.

di·flu·cor·to·lone (dī-flū-kōr'ti-lōn). 6α,9-Difluoro-11β,21-dihydroxy-16α-methylpregna-1,4-diene-3,20-dione; a synthetic glucocorticoid steroid analog.

di·flu·ni·sal (dī-flū'ni-saul). [1-1'-Biphenyl]-3-carboxylic acid, 2',4'-difluoro-4-hydroxy-; a salicyclic acid derivative with anti-inflammatory, analgesic, and antipyretic actions.

di·ga·met·ic (dī-gă-met'ik). SYN heterogametic.

di·gas·tric (dī-gas'trik). **1.** Having two bellies; denoting especially a muscle with two fleshy parts separated by an intervening tendinous part. SYN biventral. SEE digastric *muscle.* **2.** Relating to the d. muscle; denoting a fossa or groove with which it is in relation and a nerve supplying its posterior belly. SYN digastricus (1). [G. *di-,* two, + *gastēr,* belly]

di·gas·tri·cus (dī-gas'tri-kŭs). **1.** SYN digastric. **2.** Denoting the *musculus* digastricus. [L.]

Di·ge·nea (dī-jē'nē-ă). Subclass of parasitic flatworms (class Trematoda) characterized by a complex life cycle involving developmental multiplying stages in a mollusk intermediate host, an adult stage in a vertebrate, and often involving an additional transport host or an additional intermediate host; includes all of the common flukes of humans and other mammals. [G. *di-,* two, + *genesis,* generation]

di·gen·e·sis (dī-jen'ĕ-sis). Reproduction in distinctive patterns in alternate generations, as seen in the nonsexual (invertebrate) and the sexual (vertebrate) cycles of digenetic trematode parasites. [G. *di-,* two, + G. *genesis,* generation]

di·ge·net·ic (dī-jĕ-net'ik). **1.** Pertaining to or characterized by digenesis. SYN heteroxenous. **2.** Pertaining to the digenetic fluke.

DiGeorge, Angelo M., U.S. pediatrician, *1921. SEE DiG. *syndrome.*

di·gest. 1 (di-jest', dī-). To soften by moisture and heat. **2** (di-jest', dī-). To hydrolyze or break up into simpler chemical compounds by means of hydrolyzing enzymes or chemical action, as in the action of the secretions of the alimentary tract upon food. **3** (dī'jest). The materials resulting from digestion or hydrolysis. [L. *digero,* pp. *-gestus,* to force apart, divide, dissolve]

di·ges·tant (di-jes'tănt, dī-). **1.** Aiding digestion. **2.** An agent that favors or assists the process of digestion. SYN digestive (2).

di·ges·tion (di-jes'chŭn, dī-). **1.** The process of making a digest. **2.** The mechanical, chemical, and enzymatic process whereby ingested food is converted into material suitable for assimilation for synthesis of tissues or liberation of energy. [L. *digestio.* See digest]

buccal d., that part of d. carried on in the mouth; *e.g.,* the action of salivary amylases.

duodenal d., that part of d. carried on in the duodenum.

gastric d., that part of d., chiefly of the proteins, carried on in the stomach by the enzymes of the gastric juice. SYN peptic d.

intercellular d., d. in a cavity by means of secretions from the surrounding cells, such as occurs in the metazoa.

intestinal d., that part of d. carried on in the intestine; it affects all the foodstuffs: starches, fats, and proteins.

intracellular d., d. within the boundaries of a cell, such as occurs in the protozoa and in phagocytes.

pancreatic d., d. in the intestine by the enzymes of the pancreatic juice.

peptic d., SYN gastric d.

primary d., d. in the alimentary tract.

salivary d., the conversion of starch into sugar by the action of salivary amylase.

secondary d., the change in the chyle effected by the action of the cells of the body, whereby the final products of d. are assimilated in the process of metabolism.

di·ges·tive (di-jes′tiv, dī-). **1.** Relating to digestion. **2.** SYN digestant (2).

dig·in (dij′in). SYN gitogenin.

dig·it (dij′it). A finger or toe. SYN digitus [NA], dactyl, dactylus. [L. *digitus*]

   binary d., (1) The smallest unit of digital information expressed in the binary system of notation (either 0 or 1). (2) The signal in computing.

   clubbed d.'s, SEE clubbing.

dig·i·tal (dij′i-tăl). Relating to or resembling a digit or digits or an impression made by them; based on numerical methodology.

dig·i·tal·in (dij-i-tal′in). $C_{36}H_{56}O_{14}$; a standardized mixture of digitalis glycosides used as a cardiotonic.

   crystalline d., SYN digitoxin.

Dig·i·tal·is (dij-i-tal′is, -ta′lis). A genus of perennial flowering plants of the family Schrophulariaceae. *D. lanata,* a European species, and *D. purpurea,* purple foxglove, are the main sources of cardioactive steroid glycosides used in the treatment of certain heart diseases, especially congestive heart failure; also used to treat tachyarrhythmias of atrial origin. SYN foxglove. [L. *digitalis,* relating to the fingers; in allusion to the finger-like flowers]

dig·i·tal·ism (dij′i-tal-izm). The symptoms caused by digitalis poisoning or overdosage.

dig·i·tal·i·za·tion (dij′i-tal-i-zā′shŭn). Administration of digitalis by any one of a number of schedules until sufficient amounts are present in the body to produce the desired therapeutic effects.

dig·i·tate (dij′i-tāt). Marked by a number of finger-like processes or impressions. [L. *digitatus,* having fingers, fr. *digitus,* finger]

dig·i·ta·tion (dij-i-tā′shŭn). A process resembling a finger. [Mod. L. *digitatio*]

dig·i·ta·ti·o·nes hip·po·cam·pi (dij-i-tā-shē-ō′nēz hip-ō-kam′pē). SYN *foot* of hippocampus. [Mod. L. pl. of *digitatio*]

di·gi·ti (dij′i-tī). Plural of digitus. [L.]

dig·i·ti·grade (dij′i-ti-grād). Animals whose weight is borne on the digits only, such as the dog and cat. Cf. plantigrade. [L. *digitus,* finger, + *gradior,* to walk]

dig·i·tin (dij′i-tin). SYN digitonin.

dig·i·to·nin (dij-i-tō′nin). **1.** A steroid glycoside obtained from *Digitalis purpurea* that has no cardiac action; used as a reagent in the determination of plasma cholesterol and steroids having a 3-hydroxyl group in beta configuration. **2.** A mixture of four different steroids found in the seeds of *Digitalis purpurea;* a strong hemolytic poison. SYN digitin.

dig·i·tox·ic·i·ty (dij′i-tok-sis′i-tē). Colloquialism for digitalis toxicity.

dig·i·tox·i·gen·in (dij′i-toks′ĭ-jen-in). The aglycon derived from digitoxin; can be prepared by refluxing digitoxin in a mixture of water, alcohol, and hydrochloric acid.

dig·i·tox·in (dij-i-tok′sin). A cardioactive glycoside obtained from the leaves of *Digitalis purpurea;* it is more completely absorbed from the gastrointestinal tract than is digitalis. SYN crystalline digitalin.

dig·i·tox·ose (dij′ĭ-toks′ōs). The sugar moiety obtained by mild acid hydrolysis of the glycosides digitoxin, gitoxin, and digoxin. The hydrolysis yields 3 moles of d. for each mole of the respective aglycon.

D-dig·i·tox·ose (dij′i-toks′ōs). The carbohydrate moiety found in digitalis glycosides.

dig·i·tus, pl. **di·gi·ti** (dij′i-tŭs, -tī) [NA]. SYN digit. [L.]

   d. annula′ris [NA], SYN ring *finger.*

   d. auricula′ris, SYN little *finger.*

   dig′iti hippocrat′ici, obsolete term for clubbed digits or fingers. SEE clubbing.

   d. ma′nus [NA], SYN finger.

   d. me′dius [NA], SYN middle *finger.*

   d. min′imus [NA], SYN little *finger.*

   dig′itus ped′is [NA], SYN toe.

   d. pri′mus [NA], SYN thumb.

   d. quin′tus [NA], SYN little *finger.*

   d. secun′dus [NA], SYN index *finger.*

   d. ter′tius [NA], SYN middle *finger.*

   d. val′gus, permanent deviation of one or more fingers to the radial side.

   d. va′rus, permanent deviation of one or more fingers to the ulnar side.

di·glos·sia (dī-glos′ē-ă). A developmental condition that results in a longitudinal split in the tongue. SEE bifid *tongue.* [G. *di-,* two, + *glōssa,* tongue]

di·glyc·er·ide li·pase (dī-glis′er-īd). SYN lipoprotein lipase.

di·gly·co·coll hy·dro·i·o·dide·io·dine (dī-glī′kō-kol hī-drō-ī′ō-dīd-ī′ō-dīn). Two moles of diglycocoll hydroiodide combined with two atomic weights of iodine; an antibacterial agent used in tablet form to disinfect drinking water.

di·gna·thus (dī-nath′ŭs). A malformed fetus with a double mandible. SYN augnathus. [G. *di-,* two, + *gnathos,* jaw]

di·gox·i·gen·in (dī-joks′ĭ-jen-in). The aglycon of digoxin which is joined by 3 moles of digitoxose to form the glycoside, digoxin.

di·gox·in (dī-jok′sin). A cardioactive steroid glycoside obtained from *Digitalis lanata.*

Di Guglielmo, Giovanni, Italian physician, 1886–1961. SEE Di G.'s's *disease, syndrome.*

di·gy·ny, di·gyn·ia (dī′ji-nē, dī-jin′ē-ă). Fertilization of a diploid ovum by a sperm, which results in a triploid zygote. Cf. diandry. [di- + G. *gynē,* woman]

di·het·er·o·zy·gote (dī-het′er-ō-zī′gōt). An individual heterozygous at two loci of interest, especially in genetic linkage analysis.

di·hy·brid (dī-hī′brid). The offspring of parents differing in two characters. [G. *di-,* two, + L. *hybrida,* offspring of a tame sow and a wild boar]

di·hy·dral·a·zine (dī-hī-drăl′ă-zēn). 1,4-Dihydrazinophthalazine; an antihypertensive agent.

di·hy·drate (dī-hī′drāt). A compound with two molecules of water of crystallization.

di·hy·dra·zone (dī-hī′dră-zōn). SYN osazone.

△**dihydro-.** Prefix indicating the addition of two hydrogen atoms. [G. *di,* two + *hydr,* water]

di·hy·dro·a·scor·bic ac·id (di-hī′drō-as-kōr′bik). SYN L-gulonolactone.

di·hy·dro·bi·op·ter·in (di-hī′drō-bī-op′ter-in). Precursor to tetrahydrobiopter, a required cofactor for a number of enzymes, including the biosynthesis of L-tyrosine; the inability to synthesize d. can result in a form of malignant hyperphenylalaninemia.

   d. reductase, SYN dihydropteridine reductase.

di·hy·dro·co·deine tar·trate (dī-hī-drō-kō′dēn). 6-Hydroxy-3-methoxy-*N*-methyl-4,5-epoxymorphinan bitartrate; an analgesic derivative of codeine, about one-sixth as potent as morphine; a narcotic antitussive.

di·hy·dro·co·de·i·none (dī-hī-drō-kō′dēn-ōn). SYN hydrocodone.

di

4,5α-di·hy·dro·cor·ti·sol (dī-hī-drō-kōr′ti-sol). SYN hydrallostane.

di·hy·dro·cor·ti·sone (dī-hī-drō-kōr′ti-sōn). 17α,21-Dihydroxy-5β-pregnane-3,11,20-trione; a metabolite of cortisone, reduced at the 4,5 double bond.

di·hy·dro·er·go·cor·nine (dī-hī′drō-er-gō-kōr′nīn). An ergot alkaloid derivative prepared by the hydrogenation of ergocornine and less toxic than the latter. SEE dihydroergotoxine mesylate.

di·hy·dro·er·go·cris·tine (dī-hī′drō-er-gō-kris′tēn). An ergot alkaloid derivative prepared by the hydrogenation of ergocristine and less toxic than the latter. SEE dihydroergotoxine mesylate.

di·hy·dro·er·go·cryp·tine (dī-hī′drō-er-gō-krip′tēn). An ergot alkaloid derivative prepared by the hydrogenation of ergocryptine and less toxic than the latter. SEE dihydroergotoxine mesylate.

di·hy·dro·er·got·a·mine (dī-hī′drō-er-got′ă-mēn). An ergot alkaloid derivative prepared by the hydrogenation of ergotamine; used in the treatment of migraine; less toxic and less oxytocic than ergotamine.

di·hy·dro·er·go·tox·ine mes·y·late (dī-hī′drō-er-gō-tok′sēn). A mixture of dihydroergocornine methanesulfate, dihydroergocristine methanesulfate, and dihydroergocryptine methane sulfate; used as an α-adrenergic blocking agent for relief of cardiovascular insufficiency.

di·hy·dro·fo·late re·duc·tase (DHFR) (dī-hī-drō-fō′lāt). An enzyme reversibly oxidizing tetrahydrofolate to 7,8-dihydrofolate with NADP⁺. A crucial enzyme in one-carbon metabolism; used as a marker of drug resistance to methotrexate. SYN 5,6,7,8-tetrahydrofolate dehydrogenase.

7,8-di·hy·dro·fo·lic ac·id (dī-hī-drō-fō′lik). Intermediate between folic acid and 5,6,7,8-tetrahydrofolic acid, oxidation of the latter requiring NADP⁺ and dehydrofolate reductase.

di·hy·dro·lip·o·am·ide ace·tyl·trans·fer·ase (dī-hī′drō-lip-ō-am′id ă-sē-til-trans′fer-āz). An enzyme transferring acetyl from S⁶-acetyldihydrolipoamide to coenzyme A. A part of many enzyme complexes (e.g., pyruvate dehydrogenase complex). SYN lipoate acetyltransferase, thioltransacetylase A.

di·hy·dro·lip·o·am·ide de·hy·dro·gen·ase (dī-hī′drō-lip-ō-am′id dī-hī-dro′jen-āz). An enzyme oxidizing dihydrolipoamide at the expense of NAD⁺; completes the oxidative decarboxylation of pyruvate; a part of several enzyme complexes (e.g., α-ketoglutarate dehydrogenase complex). Decreased activity leads to neuronal loss in brain resulting in psychomotor retardation. SYN coenzyme factor, lipoamide dehydrogenase, lipoamide reductase (NADH), lipoyl dehydrogenase.

di·hy·dro·li·po·ic ac·id (dī-hī′drō-lip-ō′ik). Reduced lipoic acid, formed by cleavage of the —S—S— bond as a result of the acceptance of two hydrogens. Cf. lipoic acid.

di·hy·dro·mor·phi·none hy·dro·chlo·ride (dī-hī-drō-mōr′fi-nōn). SYN hydromorphone hydrochloride.

di·hy·dro-or·o·tase (dī-hī′drō-ōr-ō′tās). An enzyme catalyzing ring closure of N-carbamoyl-L-aspartate to form L-5,6-dihydroorotate and water; an enzyme in pyrimidine biosynthesis. SYN carbamoylaspartate dehydrase.

di·hy·dro-or·o·tate (dī-hī′drō-ōr-ō′tāt). L-5,6-dihydroorotate; an intermediate in the biosynthesis of pyrimidines.

di·hy·dro·pter·i·dine re·duc·tase. An enzyme that catalyzes the reversible formation of tetrahydrobiopterin from dihydrobiopterine using NADPH; a deficiency of this enzyme can result in malignant hyperphenylalaninemia. SYN dihydrobiopterin reductase.

di·hy·dro·pte·ro·ic ac·id (dī-hī′drō-te-rō′ik). An intermediate in the formation of folic acid; a compound of 6-hydroxymethylpterin and p-aminobenzoic acid, the combining of which is inhibited by sulfonamides.

di·hy·dro·py·rim·i·dine de·hy·dro·gen·ase (dī-hī-drō′pī-rim′ĭ-dēn dē-hī-dro′jen-ās). An enzyme in pyrimidine biosynthesis that reacts 5,6-dihydrouracil with NADP⁺ to form uracil and NADPH; it also acts on dihydrothymine; a deficiency of this enzyme can result in hyperuracil thyminuria. SYN dihydrouracil dehydrogenase.

di·hy·dro·strep·to·my·cin (dī-hī′drō-strep-tō-mī′sin). An aminoglycoside antibiotic similar in action to streptomycin but with a higher risk of ototoxicity.

di·hy·dro·ta·chys·ter·ol (dī-hī′drō-tă-kis′ter-ōl). SEE tachysterol.

di·hy·dro·tes·tos·ter·one (dī-hī′drō-tes-tos′ter-ōn). SYN stanolone.

di·hy·dro·ur·a·cil (dī-hī-drō-yūr′ă-sil). 5,6-Dihydrouracil; a reduction product of uracil and one of the intermediates of uracil catabolism.

di·hy·dro·ur·a·cil de·hy·dro·gen·ase. SYN dihydropyrimidine dehydrogenase.

di·hy·dro·ur·i·dine (hU, hu, D) (dī-hī-drō-yūr′i-dēn). Uridine in which the 5,6- double bond has been saturated by addition of two hydrogen atoms; a rare constituent of transfer ribonucleic acids.

⌂**dihydroxy-.** Prefix denoting addition of two hydroxyl groups; as a suffix, becomes -diol.

di·hy·drox·y·ac·e·tone (dī′hī-drok-sē-as′e-tōn). HOCH₂–CO–CH₂OH; 1,3-dihydroxy-2-propanone; the simplest ketose. SYN glycerone, glycerulose.

d. phosphate (DHAP), HOCH₂-CO-CH₂-O-PO₃ ²⁻; one of the intermediates in the glycolytic pathway and in fat biosynthesis.

d. phosphate acyltransferase, an enzyme that catalyzes an important step in plasmalogen biosynthesis; an acyl group from acyl-CoA is transferred to d. phosphate producing free coenzyme A and 1-acyldihydroxyacetone phosphate.

2,8-di·hy·drox·y·ad·en·ine (di-hī-drok′sē-ad′ĕ-nēn). An insoluble minor product of adenine catabolism that is elevated in individuals with an absence of adenine phosphoribosyltransferase.

di·hy·drox·y·a·lu·mi·num ami·no·ac·e·tate (dī-hī-drok′sē-ă-lū′mi-nŭm am′i-nō-as′ĕ-tāt). Dihydroxy(glycinato)aluminum; (glycinato-N,O) dihydroxyaluminum; basic aluminum glycinate, a basic aluminum salt of aminoacetic acid containing small amounts of aluminum hydroxide and aminoacetic acid; used as an antacid in hyperchlorhydria and peptic ulcer.

di·hy·drox·y·a·lu·mi·num so·di·um car·bon·ate. Aluminum sodium carbonate hydroxide; a gastric antacid.

1α,25-di·hy·drox·y·cho·le·cal·cif·er·ol (dī-hī-drok′sē-ko′lē-kal-si′fer-ol). An active form of vitamin D formed in the proximal convoluted tubules of the kidney. A deficiency of the receptor for 1α,25-dihydroxycholecalciferol results in all of the features of a vitamin D₃ deficiency.

1,25-di·hy·drox·y·er·go·cal·cif·er·ol (dī-hī-drok′sē-er′gō-kal-sif′er-ol). A biologically active metabolite of vitamin D₂. SYN ercalcitriol.

3,4-di·hy·drox·y·phen·yl·al·a·nine (dī-hī-droks′e-fen-il-al′ă-nēn). SYN dopa.

di·i·o·dide (dī-ī′ō-dīd). A compound containing two atoms of iodine per molecule.

⌂**diiodo-.** Prefix indicating two atoms of iodine. [G. di, + ioeidēs, violet flower color]

di·i·o·do·hy·drox·y·quin (dī-ī-ō′dō-hī-drok′si-kwin). C₉H₅I₂NO; 5,7-diiodo-8-quinolinol; diiodohydroxyquinoline; an antiprotozoal agent, used in the treatment of intestinal amebiasis. SYN diodoquin.

di·i·o·do·ty·ro·sine (DIT) (di′ī-ō-dō-tī′rō-sēn). An intermediate in the biosynthesis of thyroid hormone.

di·i·so·pro·mine (dī-ī-sō-prō′mēn). N,N-diisopropyl-3,3-diphenylpropylamine; a cholagogue. SYN disopromine.

di·i·so·pro·pyl flu·o·ro·phos·phate (DFP) (dī-ī-sō-prō′pil flŭr-ō-fos′fāt). SYN isofluorphate.

di·i·so·pro·pyl im·in·o·di·ace·tic ac·id (DISIDA) (dī-ē-sō-prō′pil im′i- nō-dī-ă-sē-tik). A radiopharmaceutical labeled with ⁹⁹ᵐTc, used for cholescintigraphy. SYN disofenin.

2,6-diisopropyl phenol. SYN propofol.

2,3-di·ke·to-L-gul·on·ate. A product of catabolism of vitamin C; formed from L-dehydroascorbate; it has no vitamin C activity.

di·ke·to·hy·drin·dyl·i·dene-di·ke·to·hy·drin·da·mine (dī-kē′tō-hī-drin-dil′i-dēn dī-kē′tō-hī-drind′ă-mēn). The colored product formed in the reaction of an α-amino acid and ninhydrin (triketohydrindene hydrate); a reaction used in the quantitative assay of α-amino acids.

di·ke·tone (dī-kē′tōn). A molecule containing two carbonyl groups; *e.g.,* acetylacetone ($CH_3COCH_2COCH_3$).

di·ke·to·pi·per·a·zines (dī-kē′tō-pī-per′ă-zēnz). A class of organic compounds with a closed ring structure formed from two α-amino acids by the joining of the α-amino group of each to the carboxyl group of the other, with the loss of two molecules of water.

dil. Abbreviation for L. *dilue,* dilute, or L. *dilutus,* diluted.

di·lac·er·a·tion (dī-las-er-ā′shŭn). Displacement of some portion of a developing tooth which is then further developed in its new relation, resulting in a tooth with sharply angulated root(s). [L. *di-lacero,* pp. *laceratus,* to tear in pieces, fr. *lacer,* mangled]

di·la·tan·cy (dī-lā′tan-sē). An increasing viscosity with increasing rate of shear accompanied by volumetric expansion. [L. *dilato,* to dilate]

dil·a·ta·tion (dil-ă-tā′shŭn). SYN dilation.

    digital d., use of the finger or finger-tip to enlarge an orifice or opening, such as enlarging the orifice of a sclerosed mitral valve surgically.

dil·a·ta·tor (dil′ă-tā-tĕr, -tōr). SYN dilator.

di·late (dī′lāt). To perform or undergo dilation.

di·la·tion (dī-lā′shŭn). **1.** Physiologic or artificial enlargement of a hollow structure or opening. **2.** The act of stretching or enlarging an opening or the lumen of a hollow structure. SYN dilatation. [L. *dilato,* pp. *dilatatus,* to spread out, dilate]

    post-stenotic d., d. of an artery, most commonly the pulmonary artery or the aorta, distal to an area of narrowing.

    urethral d., increasing the caliber of the urethra by passage of a dilator.

di·la·tion and cu·ret·tage (D & C). Dilation of the cervix and curettement of the endometrium.

di·la·tion and evac·u·a·tion (D & E). Dilation of the cervix and removal of the products of conception.

di·la·tor (dī′lā-tĕr). **1.** An instrument designed for enlarging a hollow structure or opening. **2.** A muscle that pulls open an orifice. **3.** A substance that causes dilation or enlargement of an opening or the lumen of a hollow structure. SYN dilatator.

    Chevalier-Jackson d., an esophageal dilator that passes through a rigid endoscope.

    Goodell's d., obsolete term for a uterine d. used for dilating the cervix.

    Hanks d.'s, uterine d.'s of solid metal construction.

    Hegar's d.'s, a series of cylindrical bougies of graduated sizes used to dilate the cervical canal.

    hydrostatic d., an instrument for dilating esophageal strictures; fluid pressure is delivered into a flexible area of the instrument placed in the stricture to establish a uniform dilating pressure.

    d. ir′idis, SYN dilator pupillae *muscle.*

    Kollmann's d., a metallic expandable instrument used to dilate urethral strictures.

    Plummer's d., an instrument for dilating the lower end of the esophagus in cardiospasm; it consists of a rubber tube with a perforated metal tip, and a dilatable elongated balloon near its lower end; in difficult cases the tube is threaded along a guiding thread swallowed by the patient.

    Pratt d.'s, cylindrical metal rods of graduated sizes used to dilate the cervical canal.

    d. of pupil, SYN dilator pupillae *muscle.*

    d. tu′bae, SYN tensor veli palati *muscle.*

    Walther's d., a gently curved instrument that tapers to an increased diameter, used to dilate the female urethra.

dil·do, dil·doe (dil′dō). An artificial penis; an object having the approximate shape and size of an erect penis, and commonly made of wood, plastic, or rubber; utilized for sexual pleasure.

dill oil. A volatile oil distilled from the fruit of *Anethum graveolens* (family Umbelliferae); a carminative.

di·lox·a·nide fu·ro·ate (dī-lok′să-nīd fyū′rō-āt). 2,2-Dichloro-4′-hydroxy-*N*-methylacetanilide furoate; an amebicide used in the treatment of dysentery.

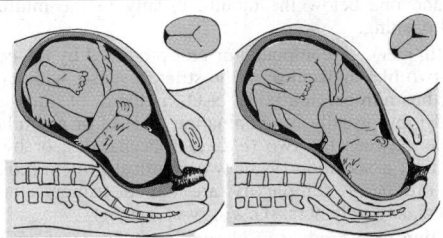

dilation (with forward occipital presentation)
a) the head enters the pelvic strait; b) it moves deeper and rotates

dil·ti·a·zem hy·dro·chlo·ride (dil-tī′ă-zem). 1,5-Benzothiazepin-4(5*H*)one,3-(acetyloxy)-5-[2-(dimethylamino)-ethyl]-2,3-dihydro-2-(4-methoxyphenyl)-monohydrochloride, (+)-*cis*-; a calcium channel blocking agent used as a coronary vasodilator and antihypertensive.

dil·u·ent. 1. Ingredient in a medicinal preparation which lacks pharmacological activity but is pharmaceutically necessary or desirable. In tablet or capsule dosage forms this may be lactose or starch; it is particularly useful in increasing the bulk of potent drug substances whose mass is too small for dosage form manufacture or administration. May be a liquid for the dissolution of drug(s) to be injected, ingested, or inhaled. **2.** Diluting; denoting that which dilutes.

di·lute (dī-lūt′). **1.** To reduce a solution or mixture in concentration, strength, quality, or purity. **2.** Diluted; denoting a solution or mixture so effected. [L. *di-luo,* to wash away, dilute]

di·lu·tion (dī-lū′shŭn). **1.** The act of being diluted. **2.** A diluted solution or mixture. **3.** In microbiologic techniques, a method for counting the number of viable cells in a suspension; a sample is diluted to the point where an aliquot, when plated, yields a countable number of separate colonies.

dim. Abbreviation for L. *dimidus,* one-half.

di·ma·zole di·hy·dro·chlo·ride (dī′mă-zōl). SYN diamthazole dihydrochloride.

di·ma·zon (dī-mā′zon). 4-*o*-Tolylazo-*o*-diacetotoluide; an azo compound occurring in red crystals; used with petrolatum as an ointment to stimulate epithelial cell proliferation and thus promote the healing of superficial wounds.

di·me·lia (dī-mē′lē-ă). Congenital duplication of the whole or a part of a limb. [G. *di-,* two, + *melos,* limb]

di·men·hy·dri·nate (dī-men-hī′dri-nāt). The 8-chlorotheophylline salt of the antihistamine, diphenhydramine; used for the prevention of motion sickness, as an antihistamine and mild sedative. SYN dramamine(R).

di·men·sion (di-men′shŭn). Scope, size, magnitude; denoting, in the plural, linear measurements of length, width, and height.

    buccolingual d., the diameter or d. of a premolar or molar tooth from buccal to lingual surface.

    occlusal vertical d., the vertical d. of the face when the teeth or occlusion rims are in contact in centric occlusion; *decrease* in occlusal vertical d. may result from modification of tooth form by attrition or grinding, drifting of teeth, or, in edentulous patients, by resorption of residual ridges; *increase* may result from modifications of tooth form, tooth position, height of occlusion rims, rebasing or relining, or occlusal splints.

    rest vertical d., the vertical d. of the face with the jaws in rest relation; *decrease* in rest vertical d. may or may not accompany a decrease in occlusal vertical d.; it may occur without a decrease in occlusal vertical d. in patients with a preponderant activity of the jaw-closing musculature, as in patients with muscular hypertenseness or in chronic gum chewers; *increase* in rest vertical d. may or may not accompany an increase in occlusal vertical d.; it sometimes occurs after the removal of remaining occlusal contacts, perhaps as a result of the removal of noxious reflex stimuli.

    vertical d., a vertical measurement of the face between any two arbitrarily selected points which are conveniently located, one above and one below the mouth, usually in the midline. SYN vertical opening.

di·mer (dī′mer). A compound or unit produced by the combination of two like molecules; in the strictest sense, without loss of atoms (thus nitrogen tetroxide, N_2O_4, is the d. of nitrogen dioxide, NO_2), but usually by elimination of H_2O or a similar small molecule between the two (*e.g.,* a disaccharide), or by simple noncovalent association (as of two identical protein molecules); higher orders of complexity are called trimers, tetramers, oligomers, and polymers. [G. *di-,* two, + -mer]

pyrimidine d., a product of ultraviolet radiation of pyrimidines in nucleic acids; most frequently thymidine d.'s.

thymine d., a product of ultraviolet irradiation of thymine (free in ice or bound in nucleic acids) in which two thymine residues become linked by formation of a cyclobutane ring involving both C-5's and both C-6's at the expense of the two double bonds; several stereoisomeric forms are possible.

di·mer·cap·rol (dī-mer-kap′rol). $HSCH_2CH(SH)CH_2OH$; 2,3-dimercaptopropanol; a chelating agent, developed as an antidote for lewisite and other arsenical poisons. It acts by competing for the metal with the essential —SH groups in the pyruvate oxidase system of the cells and forms, with arsenic, a stable, relatively nontoxic cyclic compound, the metal having a greater affinity for it than for the —SH groups of the cell proteins; also used as an antidote for antimony, bismuth, chromium, mercury, gold, and nickel. SYN antilewisite, British anti-Lewisite.

di·mer·cur·i·on (dī-mer′kyūr-ī′on). The mercuric ion, Hg^{2+}.

di·mer·ic (dī′mer-ik). Having the characteristics of a dimer.

dim·er·ous (dim′er-ŭs). Consisting of two parts. [G. *di-,* two, + *meros,* part]

di·met·a·crine tar·trate (dī-met′ă-krēn). 10-[3-(Dimethylamino)propyl]-9,9-dimethylacridan tartrate; an antidepressant.

di·meth·a·di·one (dī-meth-ă-dī′ōn). The active metabolite formed by the N-demethylation of trimethadione, an oxazolidinedione type antiepileptic agent. Can be used for *in vivo* measurement of intracellular pH.

di·meth·i·cone (dī-meth′i-kōn). A silicone oil consisting of dimethylsiloxane polymers, usually incorporated into a petrolatum base or a nongreasy preparation and used for the protection of normal skin against various, chiefly industrial, skin irritants; may also be used to prevent diaper dermatitis.

di·meth·in·dene ma·le·ate (dī-meth′in-dēn). 2-[1-[2-(2-Dimethylaminoethyl)inden-3-yl]ethyl]pyridine maleate; an antihistamine also used as an antipruritic.

di·me·this·ter·one (dī-me-this′ter-ōn). 6α-Methyl-17-(1-propynyl)testosterone; 6α,21-dimethylethisterone; a modified testosterone or ethisterone; an orally effective synthetic progestin used alone or in combination with ethynyl estradiol as a contraceptive agent.

di·meth·o·thi·a·zine mes·y·late (dī-meth-ō-thī′ă-zēn). SYN fonazine mesylate.

di·me·thox·a·nate hy·dro·chlo·ride (dī′me-thok′să-nāt). 2-Dimethylaminoethoxyethyl phenothiazine-10-carboxylate hydrochloride; a non-narcotic antitussive agent, less effective than codeine.

di·me·thox·y·am·phet·a·mine (DMA). A hallucinogen with properties resembling *lysergic acid* diethylamide (LSD).

2,5-di·me·thox·y·4·meth·yl·am·phet·a·mine (DOM). An hallucinogenic agent chemically related to amphetamine and mescaline, a drug of abuse.

di·meth·yl·al·lyl·py·ro·phos·phate (di-meth′il-ăl′lil-pī′rō -fos′fāt). An intermediate in steroid and terpene biosynthesis.

di·meth·yl·a·mi·no·az·o·ben·zene (dī-meth′il-ă-mē-nō-az-ō-ben′zēn) [C.I. 11160]. SYN butter yellow.

di·meth·yl·ar·sin·ic ac·id (dī-meth′il-ar-sin′ik). SYN cacodylic acid.

di·meth·yl·ben·zene (dī-meth-il-ben′zēn). SYN xylol.

5,6-di·meth·yl·benz·im·id·a·zole (dī-meth′il-benz-ē-mid-a-zōl). A structural moiety found in one of the cobalamins.

di·meth·yl·car·bi·nol (dī-meth-il-kar′bi-nol). SYN isopropyl alcohol.

di·meth·yl·1·car·bo·me·thox·y·1·pro·pen·2·yl phosphos·phate. An organic phosphorus compound used as a systemic poison for the extermination of such pests as mites, aphids, and houseflies.

β, β-di·meth·yl·cys·teine (dī-meth-il-sis′tē-ēn). SYN penicillamine.

di·meth·yl im·in·o·di·ace·tic ac·id (HIDA) (dī-meth′il im′i-nō-dī-ă-sē-tik). A radiopharmaceutical labeled with ^{99m}Tc, an early agent used for cholescintigraphy.

di·meth·yl ke·tone (dī-meth′il kē′tōn). SYN acetone.

di·meth·yl·mer·cu·ry (dī-meth-il-mer′kyū-rē). A contaminant of seafood products synthesized in sediments from mercury and mercury-containing chemicals dumped in waters supporting marine life. The methylmercury is concentrated in aquatic life forms and can thus be deposited in fishes intended for human consumption. Probable cause of Minimata disease, a teratogenic condition characterized by multiple birth defects. An inorganic reagent. SEE ALSO Minamata *disease.* SYN methylmercury.

di·meth·yl·phe·nol (dī-meth-il-fē′nol). SYN xylenol.

di·meth·yl·phen·yl·pi·per·a·zin·i·um (DMPP) (dī-meth′il-fen′il-pi-pār-ă-zin′ē-ŭm). A highly selective stimulant of autonomic ganglionic cells; used experimentally.

di·meth·yl phthal·ate (dī-meth′il thal′āt). An insect repellent.

di·meth·yl·pi·per·a·zine tar·trate (dī-meth′il-pi-pār′ă-zēn). A diuretic, also used as a uric acid solvent.

di·meth·yl sul·fate. An industrial chemical (sulfuric acid dimethyl ester $(CH_3)_2SO_4$), used in synthesis as an alkylating agent; it causes nystagmus, convulsions, and death from pulmonary complications.

di·meth·yl sulf·ox·ide (DMSO) (dī-meth′il). Me_2SO; Methyl sulfoxide; a penetrating solvent, enhancing absorption of therapeutic agents from the skin; an industrial solvent that has been proposed as an effective analgesic and anti-inflammatory agent in arthritis and bursitis.

N,N-di·meth·yl·tryp·ta·mine (DMT) (dī-meth′il-trip′tă-mēn). A psychotomimetic agent present in several South American snuffs (*e.g.,* cohoba snuff) and in the leaves of *Prestonia amazonica* (family Apocynaceae). Effects are similar to those of LSD, but with more rapid onset, greater likelihood of a panic reaction, and a shorter duration (1 to 2 hours, "businessman's trip"); it produces pronounced autonomic effects, including a marked increase in blood pressure.

di·meth·yl *d*-tu·bo·cu·ra·rine. SYN metocurine iodide.

di·meth·yl tu·bo·cu·ra·rine chlo·ride. Dimethyl ether of *d*-tubocurarine chloride; a skeletal muscle relaxant. SEE tubocurarine chloride.

di·meth·yl tu·bo·cu·ra·rine io·dide. SYN metocurine iodide.

di·me·tria (dī-mē′trē-ă). Obsolete term for *uterus* didelphys. [G. *di-,* two, + *mētra,* womb]

Dimmer, Friedrich, Austrian ophthalmologist, 1855–1926. SEE D.'s *keratitis.*

di·mor·phic (dī-mōr′fik). 1. In fungi, a term referring to growth and reproduction in two forms: mold and yeast. SYN dimorphous (2). 2. SYN dimorphous (1).

di·mor·phism (dī-mōr′fizm). Existence in two shapes or forms; denoting a difference of crystaline form exhibited by the same substance, or a difference in form or outward appearance between individuals of the same species. [G. *di-,* two, + *morphē,* shape]

sexual d., the somatic differences within species between male and female individuals that arise as a consequence of sexual maturation; inclusive of, but not restricted to, the secondary sexual characters.

di·mor·phol·a·mine (dī-mōr-fol′ă-mēn). *N,N'*-1,2-Ethanediylbis [*N*-butyl-4-morpholinecarboxamide]; an analeptic.

di·mor·phous (dī-mōr′fŭs). 1. Having the property of dimorphism. SYN dimorphic (2). 2. SYN dimorphic (1).

dim·ple (dim′pl). 1. A natural indentation, usually circular and of small area, in the chin, cheek, or sacral region. 2. A depression of similar appearance to a d., resulting from trauma or the contraction of scar tissue. 3. To cause d.'s.

coccygeal d., SYN coccygeal *foveola.*

dimp·ling. 1. Causing dimples. 2. A condition marked by the formation of dimples, natural or artificial.

di·ner·ic (dī-ner′ik). Denoting the interface between two mutually immiscible liquids (*e.g.,* oil and water) in the same container. [di- + G. *nerōn,* water]

di·ni·tro·cel·lu·lose (dī-nī-trō-sel′yū-lōs). SYN pyroxylin.

4,6-di·ni·tro-o-cre·sol. 2-Methyl-4,6-dinitrophenol; an insecticide used against mites in the form of a spray or dust; also used as a weed killer.

di·ni·tro·gen mon·ox·ide (dī-nī′trō-jen). SYN nitrous oxide.

2,4-di·ni·tro·phe·nol (DNP, Dnp, Dnp) (dī-nī-trō-fē′nol). N_2pH-OH; a toxic dye, chemically related to trinitrophenol (picric acid), used in biochemical studies of oxidative processes where it uncouples oxidative phosphorylation; it is also a metabolic stimulant.

di·no·flag·el·late (dī′nō-flaj′ĕ-lāt). A plantlike flagellate of the subclass Phytomastigophorea, some species of which (*e.g., Gonyaulax cantanella*) produce a potent neurotoxin that may cause severe food intoxication following ingestion of parasitized shellfish. [G. *dinos,* whirling, + L. *flagellum,* a whip]

di·no·prost (dī′nō-prost). 7-[3α,5α-dihydroxy-2β-[(3S)-hydroxy-*trans*-1-octenyl]cyclopentyl]-*cis*-5-heptenoic acid; an oxytocic agent. SYN prostaglandin $F_{2\alpha}$.

d. tromethamine, an oxytocic agent. SYN prostaglandin $F_{2\alpha}$ tromethamine.

di·no·pros·tone (dī-nō-pros′tōn). Prosta-5,13-dien-1-oic acid, 11,15-dihydroxy-9-oxo, (5Z,11α,13E,15S)-; an oxytocic agent used as an abortifacient. SYN prostaglandin E_2.

di·nor·mo·cy·to·sis (dī-nōr′mō-sī-tō′sis). Obsolete term for isonormocytosis.

di·nu·cle·o·tide (dī-nū′klē-ō-tīd). A compound containing two nucleotides; *e.g.,* NAD^+, ApGp.

Di·oc·to·phy·ma (dī-ok-tō-fī′mă). A genus of very large nematode worms infecting the kidney. [L. fr. G. *dionkoō,* to distend, + *phyma,* growth]

D. rena′le, a large blood red nematode found in the pelvis of the kidney and the peritoneal cavity of the dog; fairly common in wild carnivores like the mink, but rarely found in man; the life cycle is via leeches ectoparasitic on crayfish, which are then eaten by various fishes and finally by man or any of a number of other mammalian fish-eating hosts.

di·oc·to·phy·mi·a·sis (dī-ok′tō-fi-mī′ă-sis). Infection of animals and rarely humans with the giant kidney worm, *Dioctophyma renale.*

di·oc·tyl cal·ci·um sul·fo·suc·ci·nate (dī-ok′til kal′sē-ŭm sŭl-fō-sŭk′si-nāt). SYN docusate calcium.

di·oc·tyl so·di·um sul·fo·suc·ci·nate. SYN docusate sodium.

Di·o·don (dī′ō-don). A genus of porcupine fishes related to balloon fish, globefish, and puffers. Although the common puffer is widely eaten as "sea squab" in the United States, many puffers, especially in the Pacific, are poisonous because of the presence of a neurotoxin, tetrodotoxin, in the liver and ovary. [G. *di-,* two, + *odous* (*odont-*), tooth]

di·o·done (dī′ō-dōn). SYN iodopyracet.

di·o·do·quin (dī-ō′dō-kwin). SYN diiodohydroxyquin.

Diogenes, Of Sinope, Greek philosopher, 412–323 B.C. SEE D. *cup; poculum* diogenis.

△**-diol** (dī′ol). 1. Suffix form of the prefix dihydroxy. 2. A member of a class of compounds containing two hydroxyl groups.

gym-diol, a compound in which both hydroxyl groups are attached to the same carbon atom; an intermediate in many reactions.

di·ol·a·mine (dī-ōl′ă-mēn). USAN-approved contraction for diethanolamine.

di·op·ter (D) (dī-op′ter). The unit of refracting power of lenses, denoting the reciprocal of the focal length expressed in meters. [G. *dioptra,* a leveling instrument]

prism d. (p.d.), the unit of measurement of the deviation of light in passing through a prism, being a deflection of 1 cm at a distance of 1 m.

di·op·trics (dī-op′triks). The branch of optics concerned with the refraction of light.

di·or·tho·sis (dī′ōr-thō′sis). Obsolete term for setting of a fracture or reduction of a dislocation. [G. a making straight, fr. *di-orthoō,* to make straight, fr. *orthos,* straight]

di·os·cin (dī-ōs-in). A steroid saponin found in yams (Dioscorea) and trilliums.

di·ose (dī′ōs). SYN glycolaldehyde.

di·os·gen·in (dī′os-jen′in). (25R)-Spirost-5-en-3β-ol; the aglycon of dioscing a sapogenin derived from the saponins dioscin and trillin found in the roots of plants such as the yam; its steroid portion serves as a source from which pregnenolone and progesterone can be prepared.

di·ov·u·lar (dī′ov-yū-lar). Relating to two ova. SYN biovular. [di- + Mod. L. *ovulum,* dim. of L. *ovum,* egg]

di·ov·u·la·to·ry (dī-ō′vyū-lă-tō′rē). Releasing two ova in one ovarian cycle.

di·ox·ane (dī-oks′ān). 1,4-dioxane; a colorless liquid used as a solvent for cellulose esters and in histology as a drying agent. SYN 1,4-diethylene dioxide.

di·ox·ide (dī-oks′īd). A molecule containing two atoms of oxygen; *e.g.,* carbon dioxide, CO_2.

di·ox·in (dī-oks′in). 1. A ring consisting of two oxygen atoms, four CH groups, and two double bonds; the positions of the oxygen atoms are specified by prefixes, as in 1,4-dioxin. 2. Abbreviation for dibenzo[b,e][1,4]dioxin which may be visualized as an anhydride of two molecules of 1,2 benzenediol (pyrocatechol), thus forming two oxygen bridges between two benzene moieties, or as a 1,4-dioxin with a benzene ring fused to catch each of the two CH=CH groups. 3. 2,3,7,8-Tetrachlorodibenzo[b,e][1,4]dioxin; a contaminant in the herbicide, 2,4,5-T; it is potentially toxic, teratogenic, and carcinogenic.

di·ox·y·ben·zone (dī-ok-sē-ben′zōn). 2,2′-Dihydroxy-4-methoxybenzophenone; an ultraviolet screen for topical application to the skin.

di·ox·y·gen·ase (dī-oks′ē-jen-ās). An oxidoreductase that incorporates two atoms of oxygen (from one molecule of O_2) into the (reduced) substrate.

D.I.P. Abbreviation for desquamative interstitial *pneumonia.*

dip. 1. A downward inclination or slope. 2. A preparation for coating a surface by submersion, as for the destruction of skin parasites. [M.E. *dippen*]

Cournand's d., in constrictive pericarditis, rapid early diastolic fall and reascent of the ventricular pressure curve to an elevated plateau.

type I d., early deceleration of the fetal heart rate at the height of uterine contraction, as displayed on a fetal monitor graph.

type II d., late deceleration of the fetal heart rate, 30 seconds or more after the height of uterine contraction, as displayed on a fetal monitor graph.

di·pep·ti·dase (dī-pep′ti-dās) [EC 3.4.13.11.]. A hydrolase catalyzing the hydrolysis of a dipeptide to its constituent amino acids.

methionyl d., a hydrolase catalyzing the hydrolysis of an L-methionyl-amino acid to L-methionine and an amino acid.

di·pep·tide (dī-pep′tīd). A combination of two amino acids by means of a peptide (–CO–NH–) link.

di·pep·ti·dyl car·box·y·pep·ti·dase (dī-pep′ti-dil). SYN peptidyl dipeptidase A.

di·pep·ti·dyl pep·ti·dase. A hydrolase occurring in two forms: **dipeptidyl peptidase I,** dipeptidyl transferase, cleaving dipeptides from the amino end of polypeptides; **dipeptidyl peptidase II,** with properties similar to those of I, has a different specificity.

di·pep·ti·dyl trans·fer·ase. Cleaving dipeptides from the amino end of polypeptides. SEE dipeptidyl peptidase.

Di·pet·a·lo·ne·ma (dī-pet′ă-lō-nē′mă). A genus of nematode filariae with species in man and many other mammals; as with other filarial worms, it produces microfilariae in blood or tissue fluids, with adults found in deep connective tissue, membranes, or visceral surfaces. [G. *di-*, two, + *petalon*, leaf, + *nēma*, thread]

D. recondi′tum, a filarial species found in dogs, transmitted by fleas and lice, in contrast to the canine heartworm, *Dirofilaria immitis*, which is transmitted by mosquitoes.

D. streptocer′ca, former name for *Mansonella streptocerca*.

di·phal·lus (dī-fal′ŭs). A rare congenital anomaly in which the penis is partly or completely duplicated; may be symmetrical, or placed one above the other; often there are associated urogenital or other anomalies; occurs when two genital tubercles develop. May also be associated with exstrophy of the urinary bladder. SYN bifid penis. [G. *di-*, two, + *phallos*, penis]

di·pha·sic (dī-fā′zik). Occurring in or characterized by two phases or stages.

di·phe·ma·nil meth·yl·sul·fate (dī-fē′mă-nil). 4-Diphenylmethylene-1,1-dimethyl piperidinium methyl sulfate; an anticholinergic agent.

di·phem·e·thox·i·dine (dī-fem-ě-thok′si-dēn). 2-(Diphenylmethyl)-1-piperidineethanol; an anorexigenic drug.

di·phen·a·di·one (dī-fen-ă-dī′ōn). 2-Diphenylacetyl-1,3-indandione; an orally effective anticoagulant with actions and uses similar to those of bishydroxycoumarin.

di·phen·an (dī′fen-ān, dī-fen′an). *p*-Benzylphenylcarbamate; used as a vermicide in oxyuriasis.

di·phen·hy·dra·mine hy·dro·chlo·ride (dī-fen-hī′dră-mēn). 2-(Diphenylmethoxy)-*N*,*N*-dimethylethylamine hydrochloride; an antihistaminic with anticholinergic and sedative properties.

di·phen·i·dol (dī-fen′i-dol). α,α-Diphenyl-1-piperidinebutanol; an antiemetic.

o-di·phe·no·lase (dī-fen′ō-lās). SYN *catechol* oxidase.

di·phe·nol ox·i·dase (dī-fen′ol). SYN *catechol* oxidase.

di·phe·nox·y·late hy·dro·chlo·ride (dī-fen-ok′si-lāt). 1-(3-Cyano-3,3-diphenylpropyl)-4-phenylpiperidine-4-carboxylic acid ethyl ester hydrochloride; an antidiarrheal agent, chemically related to meperidine, that inhibits rhythmic contraction of smooth muscle; it has modest addiction liability.

di·phen·yl (dī-fen′il). Phenylbenzene; colorless liquid; used as heat transfer agent, frequently as polychlorinated biphenyls (PCBs); as fungistat for oranges (applied to inside of shipping container or wrappers); and in organic syntheses. Produces convulsions and central nervous system depression. SYN biphenyl, phenylbenzene.

△**diphenyl-.** Prefix denoting two independent phenyl groups attached to a third atom or radical, as in diphenylamine.

di·phen·yl·chlor·ar·sine (dī-fen′il-klōr-ar′sēn). $(C_6H_5)_2A_5Cl$; a sternutator, inhalation of which causes violent sneezing, cough, salivation, headache, and retrosternal pain; a common vomiting agent used in mob and riot control.

di·phen·yl·cy·an·o·ar·sine (dī-fen′il-sī-an-ō-ar-sēn). A common vomiting agent used for mob and riot control.

di·phen·yl·en·i·mine (dī′fen-il-ēn′i-mēn). SYN carbazole.

di·phen·yl·hy·dan·to·in (dī′fen-il-hī-dan′tō-in). SEE phenytoin.

5,5-di·phen·yl·hy·dan·to·in (dī-fen′il-hī-dan′tō-in). SYN phenytoin.

2,5-di·phen·yl·ox·a·zole (PPO) (dī′fen-il-oks′ă-zōl). A scintillator used in radioactivity measurements by scintillation counting.

di·phen·yl·pyr·a·line hy·dro·chlo·ride (dī-fen-il-pir′ă-lēn). 4-Diphenylmethoxy-1-methylpiperidine hydrochloride; an antihistaminic similar in action and use to diphenhydramine.

di·phos·gene (dī-fos′jēn). $ClCOOCCl_3$; Trichloromethyl chloroformate; a poison gas used in World War I; it is also slightly lacrimatoric.

di·phos·phate. SYN pyrophosphate.

1,3-di·phos·pho·glyc·er·ate (1,3-P$_2$Gri) (dī-fos′fō-glis′er-āt). An intermediate in glycolysis which enzymatically reacts with ADP to generate ATP and 3-phosphoglycerate.

2,3-di·phos·pho·glyc·er·ate (2,3-P$_2$Gri). An intermediate in the Rapoport-Luebering shunt, formed between 1,3-P$_2$Gri and 3-phosphoglycerate; an important regulator of the affinity of hemoglobin for oxygen; an intermediate of phosphoglycerate mutase.

2,3-diphosphoglycerate mutase, an enzyme of the Rapaport-Leubering shunt; catalyzes the reversible interconversion of 1,3-diphosphoglycerate to 2,3-diphosphoglycerate; it also has a phosphatase activity, converting 2,3-diphosphoglycerate to P$_i$ and 3-phosphoglycerate; a deficiency of 2,3-diphosphoglycerate mutase can result in mild erythrocytosis.

di·phos·pho·pyr·i·dine nu·cle·o·tide (DPN) (dī′fos-fō-pir′i-dēn). SYN nicotinamide adenine dinucleotide.

di·phos·pho·thi·a·min (dī′fos-fō-thī′ă-min). SYN *thiamin* pyrophosphate.

diph·the·ria (dif-thēr′ē-ă). A specific infectious disease due to *Corynebacterium diphtheriae* and its highly potent toxin; marked by severe inflammation that can form a membranous coating, with formation of a thick fibrinous exudate of the mucous membrane of the pharynx, the nose, and sometimes the tracheobronchial tree; the toxin produces degeneration in peripheral nerves, heart muscle, and other tissues. Had a high fatality rate, especially in children; now rare due to an effective vaccine. SYN diphtheritis. [G. *diphthera*, leather]

avian d., an infection by the fowlpox virus in which tracheal involvement is especially severe. SEE ALSO fowlpox. SYN fowl d.

calf d., a necrotic oropharyngolaryngitis of calves associated with *Fusobacterium necrophorum* infection that may spread to the lungs.

cutaneous d., an ulcer resulting from infection of the skin by *Corynebacterium diphtheriae;* systemic manifestations are the same as those of pharyngeal d.

false d., SYN diphtheroid (1).

faucial d., severe pharyngitis affecting the fauces, the usual site affected by infection with *Corynebacterium diphtheriae*.

fowl d., SYN avian d.

laryngeal d., d. affecting the larynx, usually with asphyxiation due to obstruction of the airway by the membrane that forms, with fatal outcome. SYN laryngotracheal d.

laryngotracheal d., SYN laryngeal d.

diph·the·ri·al, diph·the·rit·ic (dif-thēr′ē-ăl, dif-thě-rit′ik). Relating to diphtheria, or the membranous exudate characteristic of this disease. SYN diphtheric.

diph·ther·ic. SYN diphtherial.

diph·the·ri·tis (dif-thě-rī′tis). SYN diphtheria.

diph·the·roid (dif′thě-royd). **1.** One of a group of local infections suggesting diphtheria, but caused by microorganisms other than *Corynebacterium diphtheriae*. SYN Epstein's disease, false diphtheria, pseudodiphtheria. **2.** Any microorganism resembling *Corynebacterium diphtheriae*. [diphtheria + G. *eidos*, resemblance]

diph·the·ro·tox·in (dif′thēr-ō-tok′sin). The toxin of diphtheria.

di·phyl·lo·both·ri·a·sis (dī-fil′ō-both-rī′ă-sis). Infection with the cestode *Diphyllobothrium latum;* human infection is caused by ingestion of raw or inadequately cooked fish infected with the plerocercoid larva. Leukocytosis and eosinophilia may occur; if the worm is high enough in the alimentary canal, it may preempt the supply of vitamin B_{12} or alter its absorption, leading to hyperchromic macrocytic anemia resembling pernicious anemia, although the condition is rare, even in hyperendemic areas. SYN bothriocephaliasis.

Di·phyl·lo·both·ri·um (dī-fil-lō-both′rē-ŭm). A large genus of tapeworms (order Pseudophyllidea) characterized by a spatulate scolex with dorsal and ventral sucking grooves or bothria. Several species are found in humans, although only one, *D. latum*, is of widespread importance. [G. *di-*, two, + *phyllon*, leaf, + *bothrion*, little ditch]

D. corda′tum, a species found in dogs, sea mammals, and occasionally man, in Greenland.

D. la′tum, the broad or broad fish tapeworm, a species that causes diphyllobothriasis, found in man and fish-eating mammals in many parts of northern Europe, Japan and elsewhere in Asia, and in Scandinavian populations of the American north central states; it often has 3 or 4 thousand segments, broader than long; the head has typical bothria characteristic of the genus. SYN *Dibothriocephalus latus*.

D. linguloi′des, SYN *Spirometra mansoni*.

D. man′soni, SYN *Spirometra mansoni.*

D. mansonoi′des, SYN *Spirometra mansonoides.*

di·phy·o·dont (dif′ē-ō-dont). Possessing two sets of teeth, as occurs in humans and most other mammals. [G. *di-,* two, + *phyō,* to produce, + *odous* (*odont-*), tooth]

di·pi·pro·ver·ine (dī-pī-prō′ver-ēn). α-Phenyl-1-piperidineacetic acid 2-piperidinoethyl ester; an intestinal antispasmodic.

di·piv·e·frin hy·dro·chlo·ride (dī-piv′ĕ-frin). Propanoic acid, 2,2-dimethyl-, 4-[1-hydroxy-2-methylamino)ethyl]-1,2-phenylene ester, hydrochloride, (±)-; an adrenergic epinephrine prodrug used in drop form in initial therapy for control of intraocular pressure in chronic open-angle glaucoma.

dip·la·cu·sis (dip-lă-kū′sis). Abnormal perception of sound, either in time or in pitch, so that one sound is heard as two. [G. *diplous,* double, + *akousis,* a hearing]

d. binaura′lis, a condition in which the same sound is heard differently by the two ears.

d. dysharmon′ica, a condition in which the same sound is heard with a different pitch in each ear.

d. echo′ica, a condition in which sound heard in the affected ear is repeated.

d. monaura′lis, a condition in which one sound is perceived as two in the same ear.

di·ple·gia (dī-plē′jē-ă). Paralysis of corresponding parts on both sides of the body. SYN double hemiplegia. [G. *di-,* two, + *plēgē,* a stroke]

congenital facial d., SYN Möbius′ *syndrome.*

facial d., paralysis of both sides of the face.

infantile d., SYN spastic d.

masticatory d., paralysis of all the muscles of mastication.

spastic d., a type of cerebral palsy in which there is bilateral spasticity, with the lower extremities more severely affected. Cf. flaccid *paralysis.* SYN Erb-Charcot disease (1), infantile d., Little′s disease, spastic spinal paralysis, tabes spasmodica.

◬**diplo-.** Double, twofold. SEE haplo-. [G. *diploos,* double]

dip·lo·al·bu·mi·nu·ria (dip′lō-al-byū-mi-nū′rē-ă). The coexistence of nephritic, or pathologic, and nonnephritic, or physiologic, albuminuria.

dip·lo·ba·cil·lus (dip′lō-bă-sil′ŭs). Two rod-shaped bacterial cells linked end to end. [diplo- + bacillus]

Morax-Axenfeld d., SYN *Moraxella lacunata.*

dip·lo·bac·te·ria (dip′lō-bak-tēr′ē-ă). Bacterial cells linked together in pairs.

dip·lo·blas·tic (dip-lō-blas′tik). Formed of two germ layers. [diplo- + G. *blastos,* germ]

dip·lo·car·dia (dip-lō-kar′dē-ă). An anomaly in which the two lateral halves of the heart are separated to varying degrees by a central fissure. [diplo- + G. *kardia,* heart]

dip·lo·ceph·a·lus (dip-lō-sef′ă-lŭs). SYN dicephalus.

dip·lo·chei·ria, dip·lo·chi·ria (dip′lō-kī′rē-ă). SYN dicheiria. [diplo- + G. *cheir,* hand]

dip·lo·coc·ce·mia (dip-lō-kok-sē′mē-ă). The presence of diplococci in the blood; used especially in referring to *Neisseria meningitidis* (meningococci) in circulating blood.

dip·lo·coc·ci (dip′lō-kok′sī). Plural of diplococcus.

dip·lo·coc·cin (dip-lō-kok′sin). HAn antibiotic crystalline substance isolated from cultures of lactic acid-producing cocci present in milk active against lactobacilli and certain Gram-positive cocci, but inactive against Gram-negative bacteria.

Dip·lo·coc·cus (dip′lō-kok′ŭs). Species of this genus of bacteria are now assigned to other genera. *Diplococcus pneumoniae,* the type species of *D.,* is a member of the genus *Streptococcus.* SEE *Neisseria, Peptococcus, Streptococcus.* [diplo- + G. *kokkos,* berry]

dip·lo·coc·cus, pl. **dip·lo·coc·ci** (dip′lō-kok′ŭs, -kok′sī). **1.** Spherical or ovoid bacterial cells joined together in pairs. **2.** Common name of any organism belonging to the bacterial genus *Diplococcus.* [diplo- + G. *kokkos,* berry]

dip·lo·co·ri·a (dip-lō-kō′rē-ă). The occurrence of two pupils in the eye. SYN dicoria. [diplo- + G. *korē,* pupil]

dip·loë (dip′lō-ē) [NA]. The central layer of spongy bone between the two layers of compact bone, outer and inner plates, or tables, of the flat cranial bones. [G. *diploē,* fem. of *diplous,* double]

dip·lo·gen·e·sis (dip-lō-jen′ĕ-sis). Production of a double fetus or of one with some parts doubled. [diplo- + G. *genesis,* production]

Dip·lo·go·nop·o·rus (dip′lō-gō-nop′ŏ-rŭs). A genus of tapeworms found in Japan (*D. grandis*) and probably also in Rumania (*D. brauni*) [diplo- + G. *gonos,* seed, + *poros,* pore]

di·plo·ic (dip-lō′ik). Relating to the diploë.

dip·loid (dip′loyd). Denoting the state of a cell containing two haploid sets derived from the father and from the mother respectively; the normal chromosome complement of somatic cells (in man, 46 chromosomes). [diplo- + G. *eidos* resemblance]

dip·lo·kar·y·on (dip′lō-kar′ē-on). A cell nucleus containing four haploid sets; *i.e.,* a tetraploid nucleus. SEE ALSO polyploidy. [diplo- + G. *karyon,* nut (nucleus)]

dip·lo·mel·i·tu·ria (dip′lō-mel-i-tū′rē-ă). The occurrence of diabetic and nondiabetic glycosuria in the same individual. [diplo- + G. *meli,* honey, + *ouron,* urine]

dip·lo·my·e·lia (dip-lō-mī-ē′lē-ă). Complete or incomplete doubling of the spinal cord; may be accompanied by a bony septum of the vertebral canal. [diplo- + G. *myelon,* marrow]

dip·lon (dip′lon). SYN deuteron.

dip·lo·ne·ma (dip-lō-nē′mă). The doubled form of the chromosome strand visible at the diplotene stage of meiosis. [diplo- + G. *nēma,* thread]

dip·lo·neu·ral (dip-lō-nū′răl). Supplied by two nerves from different sources, said of certain muscles. [diplo- + G. *neuron,* nerve]

dip·lop·a·gus (dip-lop′ă-gŭs). General term for conjoined twins, each with fairly complete bodies, although one or more internal organs may be in common. SEE conjoined *twins,* under twin. [diplo- + G. *pagos,* something fixed]

di·plo·pia (di-plō′pē-ă). The condition in which a single object is perceived as two objects. SYN double vision. [diplo- + G. *ōps,* eye]

crossed d., d. in which the image seen by the right eye is to the left of the image seen by the left eye. SYN heteronymous d.

heteronymous d., SYN crossed d.

homonymous d., SYN homonymous *images,* under *image.*

monocular d., a double image or an extra ghost image produced in one eye, almost always by an aberration of the ocular media; for example, a corneal or lenticular irregularity, an uncorrected astigmatism or an irregularity of the vitreous or the retina. If a similar process occurs in both eyes (bilateral monocular diplopia), that is, the doubling is still present with either eye covered, the patient may still only see two images; seeing multiple images (polyopia) is rare.

simple d., SYN homonymous *images,* under *image.*

uncrossed d., SYN homonymous *images,* under *image.*

dip·lo·po·dia (dip-lō-pō′dē-ă). Duplication of digits of the foot. [diplo- + G. *pous,* foot]

dip·lo·some (dip′lō-sōm). Paired allosomes; the pair of centrioles of mammalian cells. SYN paired allosome. [diplo- + G. *sōma,* body]

dip·lo·so·mia (dip-lō-sō′mē-ă). Condition in which twins who seem functionally independent are joined at one or more points. SEE conjoined *twins,* under twin. [diplo- + G. *sōma,* body]

dip·lo·tene (dip′lō-tēn). The late stage of prophase in meiosis in which the paired homologous chromosomes begin to repel each other and move apart, but are usually held together by chiasmata. The chiasmata are associated with breakage of two chromatids at corresponding points followed by refusion of the broken ends with exchange of segments between the chromatids; this is considered to be the cytologic basis for the crossing-over of genes. [diplo- + G. *tainia,* band]

dip·lo·ter·a·tol·o·gy (dip′lō-tār-ă-tol′ō-jē). The division of teratology concerned with conjoined twins.

di·po·dia (dī-pō′dē-ă). **1.** A developmental anomaly involving complete or incomplete duplication of a foot. **2.** In conjoined twins and sirenomelia, a degree of fusion leaving two feet evident. [G. *di-*, two, + *pous* (*pod-*), foot]

di·pole (dī'pōl). A pair of separated electrical charges, one or more positive and one or more negative; or a pair of separated partial charges. SYN doublet (2).

di·po·tas·si·um phos·phate (dī-pō-tas'ē-ŭm). SYN *potassium* phosphate.

di·pre·nor·phine (dī-pren'ōr-fēn). A narcotic antagonist resembling naloxone but more potent.

di·pro·pyl·tryp·ta·mine (dī-prō-pil-trip'tă-mēn). *N,N*-Dipropyltryptamine; a hallucinogenic agent similar to dimethyltryptamine.

di·pro·so·pus (dī-pros'ō-pŭs, dī-prō-sō'pus). Conjoined twins with almost complete fusion of the bodies and with normal limbs. Part or all of the face may be duplicated. SEE conjoined *twins*, under *twin*. [G. *di-*, two + *prosōpon*, face]

dip·se·sis (dip-sē'sis). An abnormal or excessive thirst, or a craving for unusual forms of drink. SYN dipsosis, morbid thirst. [G. *dipseō*, to thirst]

dip·so·gen (dip'sō-jen). A thirst-provoking agent. [G. *dipsa*, thirst, + *-gen*, producing]

dip·so·ma·nia (dip-sō-mā'nē-ă). A recurring compulsion to drink alcoholic beverages to excess. SEE alcoholism. [G. *dipsa*, thirst, + *mania*, madness]

dip·so·sis (dip-sō'sis). SYN dipsesis. [G. *dipsa*, thirst, + *-osis*, condition]

dip·so·ther·a·py (dip'sō-thār'ă-pē). Treatment of certain diseases by abstention, as far as possible, from liquids.

Dip·tera (dip'ter-ă). An important order of insects (the two-wing flies and gnats), including many significant disease vectors such as the mosquito, tsetse fly, sandfly, and biting midge. [G. *di-*, two, + *pteron*, wing]

dip·ter·an (dip'ter-an). Denoting insects of the order Diptera.

dip·ter·ous (dip'ter-ŭs). Relating to or characteristic of the order Diptera.

Di·pus sa·git·ta (dī'pŭs saj'i-tă). A small rodent of southern Russia that serves as a vector, through fleas, of *Yersinia pestis* (plague bacillus). [G. *dipous*, jerboa, two-footed; L. *sagitta*, arrow]

di·py·gus (dī-pī'gŭs, dip'ē-gŭs). Conjoined twins with the head and thorax completely merged, and the pelvis and lower extremities duplicated; when the duplications of the lower parts are symmetrical, usually called duplicitas posterior. SEE conjoined *twins*, under *twin*. [G. *di-*, two, + *pyge*, buttocks]

dip·y·li·di·a·sis (dip'i-li-dī'ă-sis). Infection of carnivores and man with the cestode *Dipylidium caninum*.

Dip·y·lid·i·um ca·ni·num (dip-ĭ-lid'ē-ŭm kā-nī'nŭm). The commonest species of dog tapeworm, the double-pored tapeworm, the larvae of which are harbored by dog fleas or lice; the worm occasionally infects humans, especially children licked by dogs that have recently nipped infected fleas. [G. *dipylos*, with two entrances; L. ntr. of *caninus*, pertaining to *canis*, dog]

di·py·rid·am·ole (dī-pī-rid'ă-mōl). 2,2',2'',2''-[4,8-Dipiperidinopyrimidino [5,4-d]pyrimidino-2,6-diyldinitrilo]tetraethanol; a coronary vasodilator that also has a weak action to reduce platelet aggregation; commonly used in place of exercise for radionuclide studies of the myocardium.

di·py·rim·i·dine pho·to·ly·ase (dī-pi-rim'i-dēn). SYN deoxyribodipyrimidine photolyase.

di·py·rine (dī-pī'rēn). SYN aminopyrine.

di·py·rone (dī-pī'rōn). $C_{13}H_{16}N_3NaO_4S \cdot H_2O$; an analgesic, antiinflammatory, and antipyretic agent rarely used because of a high incidence of agranulocytosis. SYN methampyrone.

di·rec·tor (di-rek'ter, -tōr, dī-). 1. A smoothly grooved instrument used with a knife to limit the incision of tissues. SYN staff (2). 2. The head of a service or specialty division. [L. *dirigo*, pp. *-rectus*, to arrange, set in order]

dir·i·ga·tion (dir'i-gā'shŭn). Development of voluntary control over functions that are ordinarily involuntary. [irreg., fr. L. *dirigo*, to direct, control]

dir·i·go·mo·tor (dir'i-gō-mō'ter). Directing muscular movement.

Di·ro·fil·a·ria (dī-rō-fi-lā'rē-ă). A genus of filaria (family Onchocercidae, superfamily Filarioidea); *D.* species are usually found in mammals other than man, but rare examples of human infection are known, as by *D. immitis*. [L. *dirus*, dread, + *filum*, thread]

D. conjuncti'vae, name assigned to filarial worms removed from tumors and abscesses in various sites in human cases, especially palpebral conjunctivae and other eye tissues, but also subcutaneous tissues from other sites; probably caused by a number of species of animal origin.

D. im'mitis, a species of filarial worms of dogs and other canids in tropical and subtropical areas, found chiefly in the right ventricle and pulmonary arteries of dogs; sometimes a serious pathogen of racing and show dogs, especially in the southern U.S. where mosquito vectors are common; *D. immitis* and its canine host have been used to test chemotherapeutic agents, and an extract of *D. immitis* may be used as a nonspecific intradermal antigen in the diagnosis of human filariasis and in complement-fixation tests. SEE ALSO *Dipetalonema reconditum*. SYN heartworm.

di·ro·fil·a·ri·a·sis (dir'ō-fil-ă-rī'ă-sis). Infection of animals and rarely man with nematodes of the genus *Dirofilaria*.

dir. prop. Abbreviation for L. *directione propria*, with proper direction.

dirt-eat·ing. SYN geophagia.

△**dis-.** In two, apart; un-, not; very. Cf. dys-. [L. separation]

dis·a·bil·i·ty (dis-ă-bil'i-tē). 1. According to the "International Classification of Impairments, Disabilities and Handicaps" (World Health Organization), any restriction or lack of ability to perform an activity in a manner or within the range considered normal for a human being. The term disability reflects the consequences of impairment in terms of functional performance and activity by the individual; disabilities thus represent disturbances at the level of the person; 2. An impairment or defect of one or more organs or members.

developmental d., loss of function brought on by prenatal and postnatal events in which the predominant disturbance is in the acquisition of cognitive, language, motor, or social skills; *e.g.,* mental retardation, autistic disorder, learning disorder, and attention-deficit hyperactivity disorder.

learning d., a disorder in one or more of the basic cognitive and psychological processes involved in understanding or using written or spoken language; may be manifested in age-related impairment in the ability to read, write, spell, speak, or perform mathematical calculations.

di·sac·cha·rid·as·es (dī-sak'ă-rid-ăs-ez). A group of enzymes that catalyze the hydrolysis of disaccharides, producing two monosaccharides.

di·sac·cha·ride (dī-sak'ă-rīd). A condensation product of two monosaccharides by elimination of water (usually between an alcoholic OH and a hemiacetal OH); *e.g.,* sucrose, lactose, maltose. SYN bioside.

dis·ag·gre·ga·tion (dis'ag-grĕ-gā'shŭn). 1. A breaking up into component parts. 2. An inability to coordinate various sensations and failure to comprehend their mutual relations. [L. *dis-*, separating, + *ag- grego* (*adg-*), pp. *-gregatus*, to add to something]

dis·ar·tic·u·la·tion (dis-ar-tik-yū-lā'shŭn). Amputation of a limb through a joint, without cutting of bone. SYN exarticulation. [L. *dis-*, apart, + *articulus*, joint]

dis·as·sim·i·la·tion (dis'ă-sim-i-lā'shŭn). Destructive or retrograde metabolism. SYN dissimilation (1).

dis·as·so·ci·a·tion (dis'ă-sō-sē-ā'shŭn). SYN dissociation (1).

disc (disk). 1. A round, flat plate; any approximately flat circular structure. 2. SYN lamella (2).

articular d., a plate or ring of fibrocartilage attached to the joint capsule and separating the articular surfaces of the bones for a varying distance, sometimes completely; it serves to adapt two articular surfaces that are not entirely congruent. SYN discus articularis [NA], articular disk, fibrocartilago interarticularis, fibroplate, interarticular fibrocartilage, intra-articular cartilage (1).

articular d. of acromioclavicular joint, the articular disk of fibrocartilage usually found between the acromial end of the clavicle and the medial border of the acromion. SYN discus articularis acromioclavicularis [NA], acromioclavicular disk, Weitbrecht's cartilage.

articular d. of distal radioulnar joint, the disk that holds together the distal ends of the radius and ulna; it is attached by its apex to a depression between the styloid process and distal surface of the head of the ulna, and by its base to the ridge separating the ulnar notch from the carpal surface of the radius. SYN discus articularis radioulnaris [NA], radioulnar disk, radioulnar articular disk, triangular cartilage, triangular disk of wrist, triquetrous cartilage (1).

articular d. of sternoclavicular joint, the fibrocartilaginous disk that subdivides the sternoclavicular joint into two cavities. SYN discus articularis sternoclavicularis [NA], sternoclavicular disk, sternoclavicular articular disk.

interpubic d., the disk of fibrocartilage that unites the pubic bones at the pubic symphysis. SYN discus interpubicus [NA], interpubic disk, lamina fibrocartilaginea interpubica.

intervertebral d., a disk interposed between the bodies of adjacent vertebrae. It is composed of an outer fibrous part (annulus fibrosus) that surrounds a central gelatinous mass (nucleus pulposus). SYN discus intervertebralis [NA], fibrocartilago intervertebralis, intervertebral cartilage, intervertebral disk.

sacrococcygeal d., a thin plate of fibrocartilage interposed between the sacrum and coccyx.

⚠**disc-.** SEE disco-.

disc·ec·to·my (dis-ek'tō-mē). Excision, in part or whole, of an intervertebral disk. SYN discotomy. [disco- + G. *ektomē,* excision]

dis·charge (dis'charj). **1.** That which is emitted or evacuated, as an excretion or a secretion. **2.** The activation or firing of a neuron.

after-d., SEE afterdischarge.

Dische, Zacharias, 20th century Austrian-U.S. biochemist, *1895. SEE D. *reaction, reagent;* D.-Schwarz *reagent.*

dis·chro·na·tion (dis-krō-nā'shŭn). A disturbance in the consciousness of time. [L. *dis-,* apart, + G. *chronos,* time]

dis·ci (dis'kī). Plural of discus.

dis·ci·form (dis'i-fōrm). Disk-shaped.

dis·cis·sion (di-sish'ŭn). **1.** Incision or cutting through a part. **2.** In ophthalmology, opening of the capsule and breaking up of the cortex of the lens with a needle knife or laser. [L. *di- scindo,* pp. *-scissus,* to tear asunder]

dis·ci·tis (dis-kī'tis). Nonbacterial inflammation of an intervertebral disk or disk space. SYN diskitis.

⚠**disco-, disc-.** A disk; disk-shaped. [G. *diskos*]

dis·co·blas·tic (dis-kō-blas'tik). Denoting a discoblastula.

dis·co·blas·tu·la (dis'kō-blas'tyū-lă). A blastula of the type produced by the meroblastic discoidal cleavage of a large-yolked ovum.

dis·co·gas·tru·la (dis'kō-gas'trū-lă). A gastrula of the type formed after the discoidal cleavage of a large-yolked ovum.

dis·co·gen·ic (dis'kō-gen'ik). Denoting a disorder originating in or from an intervertebral disk. [disco- + G. *genesis,* origin]

dis·coid (dis'koyd). **1.** Resembling a disk. **2.** In dentistry, an excavating or carving instrument having a circular blade with a cutting edge around the periphery. [disco- + G. *eidos,* appearance]

dis·con·ju·gate (dis-cŏn'jū-gāt). Not paired in action or joined together; the opposite of conjugate. SEE disconjugate *movement* of eyes. [L. *dis-,* apart, + *jugatus,* yoked]

dis·cop·a·thy (dis-kop'ă-thē). Disease of a disk, particularly of an invertebral disk. [disco- + G. *pathos,* disease]

traumatic cervical d., an injury characterized by fissuration, laceration and/or fragmentation of a cervical disk or surrounding ligaments, with or without displacement of fragments against spinal cord, nerve roots, or ligaments.

dis·co·pla·cen·ta (dis-kō-pla-sen'tă). A placenta of discoid shape.

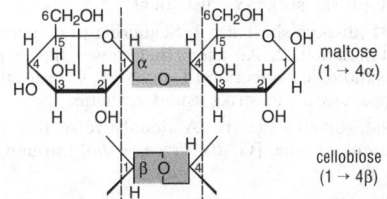

disaccharide	components	linkage
gentiobiose	glucose – glucose	(1 → 6β)
isomaltose	glucose – glucose	(1 → 6α)
kojibiose	glucose – glucose	(1 → 2α)
lactose (milk sugar)	galactose – glucose	(1 → 4β)
maltose (malt sugar)	glucose – glucose	(1 → 4α)
melibiose	galactose – glucose	(1 → 6α)
nigerose	glucose – glucose	(1 → 3α)
primverose	xylose – glucose	(1 → 6β)
rutinose	rhamnose – glucose	(1 → 6β)
saccharose (cane sugar, sugar, sucrose)	glucose – fructose	(1 → 2β)
trehalose (mycose)	glucose – glucose	(1 → 1α)
cellobiose	glucose – glucose	(1 → 4β)

disaccharide

dis·cor·dance (dis-kōr'dans). Dissociation of two characteristics in the members of a sample from a population; used as a measure of dependence. Cf. concordance.

dis·cot·o·my (dis-kot'ō-mē). SYN discectomy. [disco- + G. *tomē,* incision]

dis·crete (dis-krēt'). Separate; distinct; not joined to or incorporated with another; denoting especially certain lesions of the skin. [L. *dis- cerno,* pp. *-cretus,* to separate]

dis·crim·i·na·tion (dis'krim-i-nā'shŭn). In conditioning, responding differentially, as when an organism makes one response to a reinforced stimulus and a different response to an unreinforced stimulus. [L. *discrimino,* pp. *-atus,* to separate]

dis·cus, pl. **dis·ci** (dis'kŭs, -kī) [NA]. SYN lamella (2). [L. fr. G. *diskos,* a quoit, disk]

d. articula'ris [NA], SYN articular *disc.*

d. articula'ris acromioclavicula'ris [NA], SYN articular *disc* of acromioclavicular joint.

d. articula'ris radioulna'ris [NA], SYN articular *disc* of distal radioulnar joint.

d. articula'ris sternoclavicula'ris [NA], SYN articular *disc* of sternoclavicular joint.

d. articula'ris temporomandibula'ris [NA], SYN articular *disc* of temporomandibular joint.

d. interpu'bicus [NA], SYN interpubic *disc.*

d. intervertebra'lis [NA], SYN intervertebral *disc.*

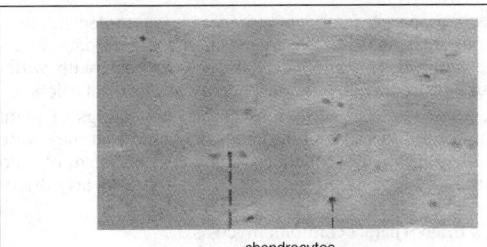

chondrocytes
discus intervertebralis
fibrous cartilage with single or double chondrocytes

d. lentifor'mis, rarely used term for subthalamic *nucleus.*

d. ner'vi op'tici [NA], SYN optic *disk.*

d. prolig'erus, SYN *cumulus* oöphorus.

di

dis·cus·sive (di-skŭ′siv). SYN discutient.

dis·cu·ti·ent (di-skyū′shē-ent). **1.** Scattering or dispersing a pathologic accumulation. **2.** An agent that causes the dispersal of a tumor or pathologic collection of any sort. SYN discussive. [L. *dis-cutio,* pp. *-cussus,* to strike asunder, shatter]

dis·di·a·clast (dis-dī′ă-klast). A doubly refractive element in striated muscular tissue. [G. *dis,* twice, + *dia,* through, + *klastos,* broken]

DISEASE

dis·ease (di-zēz′). **1.** An interruption, cessation, or disorder of body functions, systems, or organs. SYN illness, morbus, sickness. **2.** A morbid entity characterized usually by at least two of these criteria: recognized etiologic agent(s), identifiable group of signs and symptoms, or consistent anatomical alterations. SEE ALSO syndrome. **3.** Literally, dis-ease, the opposite of ease, when something is wrong with a bodily function. [Eng. *dis-* priv. + ease]

aaa d., endemic anemia of ancient Egypt, ascribed in the Papyrus Ebers to intestinal infestation with ancylostoma; now called ancylostomiasis.

ABO hemolytic d. of the newborn, erythroblastosis fetalis due to maternal-fetal incompatibility with respect to an antigen of the ABO blood group; the fetus possesses A or B antigen which is lacking in the mother, and the mother produces immune antibody which causes hemolysis of fetal erythrocytes.

accumulation d., a disease characterized by abnormal accumulation of a metabolic product in certain cells and tissues; examples include the mucopolysaccharidoses, lipoidoses.

Acosta's d., SYN altitude *sickness* (1).

Adams-Stokes d., SYN Adams-Stokes *syndrome.*

adaptation d.'s, d.'s falling theoretically into Selye's concept of the general-adaptation syndrome.

Addison-Biermer d., SYN pernicious *anemia.*

Addison's d., SYN chronic adrenocortical *insufficiency.*

Akabane d., a d. of cattle, sheep and goats, caused by the Akabane virus and characterized by fetal or neonatal arthrogryposis and hydranencephaly, abortions, and fetal death; the causative virus is transmitted by mosquitoes in Japan and by the midge *Culicoides brevitarsis* in Australia.

akamushi d. (ak-kă-mū′shē), SYN tsutsugamushi d.

Akureyri d., SYN epidemic *neuromyasthenia.*

Albers-Schönberg d., SYN osteopetrosis.

Albert's d., achillobursitis involving inflammation of the bursa between the Achilles tendon and the os calcis. SYN Swediauer's d.

Albright's d., SYN McCune-Albright *syndrome.*

Aleutian mink d., a chronic immune-complex d. of mink caused by a parvovirus.

Alexander's d., a rare, fatal central nervous system degenerative disease of infants, characterized by psychomotor retardation, seizures, and paralysis; megaloencephaly is associated with widespread leukodystrophic changes, especially in the frontal lobes.

alkali d., a term applied to various animal poisonings of plant and mineral origin in arid regions under the belief that they were caused by the ingestion of alkaline waters; *e.g.,* botulism of wild ducks, caused by feeding on decayed vegetation in nearly dried-up lakes.

Almeida's d., SYN paracoccidioidomycosis.

Alpers d., SYN *poliodystrophia* cerebri progressiva infantilis.

altitude d., SYN altitude *sickness.*

Alzheimer's d., progressive mental deterioration manifested by loss of memory, ability to calculate, and visual-spatial orientation; confusion; disorientation. Begins in late middle life and results in death in 5–10 years. Pathologically, the brain is atrophic, especially in the frontal occipital and temporal regions; histo-
logically, there is distortion of the intracellular neurofibrils (neurofibrillary tangles) and senile plaques composed of granular or filamentous argentophilic masses with an amyloid core, found predominantly in the cerebral cortex, amygdala, and hippocampus; the cerebral cortex has few and shrunken neurons which may contain cytoplasmic vacuoles and argentophilic granules displacing the nucleus to the periphery; the most common degenerative brain disorder. SYN Alzheimer's dementia, presenile dementia (2), dementia presenilis, primary neuronal degeneration, primary senile dementia.

Alzheimer's accounts for some 60–70% of senile dementias, which in the U.S. afflict 5–10% of those over age 65, and 20% of those over age 80. In recent years, clinicians have instituted a protocol for monitoring the progress of the disease, known as FAST (*f*unctional *a*ssessment *stag*es). Basic understanding of the brain changes brought about by Alzheimer's has been greatly aided by MRI and PET scanning; however, the cause of the disease is not yet clear. Arguments have been advanced for genetic, environmental, viral, neurochemical, and immunological causes. With the aging of the post-WW2 generation, the ranks of Alzheimer's patients are expected to swell, making the need for adequate diagnostic techniques and therapies more pressing. Treatments being explored include drugs to correct neurochemical imbalances. Some researchers are investigating repairing or augmenting damaged nerves through application of nerve growth factor or neural tissue transplants, but this approach remains highly experimental.

anarthritic rheumatoid d., rheumatoid d. without arthritis.

Anders' d., SYN *adiposis* dolorosa.

Andersen's d., SYN type 4 *glycogenosis.*

antibody deficiency d., SYN antibody deficiency *syndrome.*

aortoiliac occlusive d., obstruction of the abdominal aorta and its main branches by atherosclerosis.

Aran-Duchenne d., SYN amyotrophic lateral *sclerosis.*

Aujeszky's d., SYN pseudorabies.

Australian X d., SYN Murray Valley *encephalitis.*

autoimmune d., any disorder in which loss of function or destruction of normal tissue arises from humoral or cellular immune responses of the individual to his own tissue constituents; may be systemic, as systemic lupus erythematosus, or organ specific, as thyroiditis.

aviator's d., syndrome resembling decompression sickness occurring in occupants of airplanes that reach very high altitudes without adequate pressurization of the cabin. SEE ALSO decompression *sickness.*

Ayerza's d., SYN Ayerza's *syndrome.*

Azorean d., SYN Machado-Joseph.

Baelz' d., SYN *cheilitis* glandularis.

Baló's d., SYN *encephalitis* periaxialis concentrica.

Baltic myoclonus d., one of the familial light sensitive myoclonic epilepsies. Unlike Lafora body polymyoclonus, where inclusion bodies are seen in the brain cells, the prognosis is often favorable. Probably an autosomal recessive disorder.

Bamberger-Marie d., SYN hypertrophic pulmonary *osteoarthropathy.*

Bamberger's d., (1) SYN saltatory *spasm.* (2) SYN polyserositis.

Bang's d., SYN bovine *brucellosis.*

Bannister's d., SYN angioedema.

Banti's d., SYN Banti's *syndrome.*

Barclay-Baron d., SYN vallecular *dysphagia.*

Barlow's d., SYN infantile *scurvy.*

Barraquer's d., SYN progressive *lipodystrophy.*

Basedow's d., SYN Graves' d.

Batten d., cerebral *sphingolipidosis,* late juvenile type.

Batten-Mayou d., cerebral *sphingolipidosis,* late infantile and juvenile types.

Bayle's d., SYN paresis (2).

Bazin's d., SYN *erythema* induratum.

Bechterew's d., SYN *spondylitis* deformans.

di

Becker's d., an obscure South African cardiomyopathy leading to rapidly fatal congestive heart failure and idiopathic mural endomyocardial d.

Begbie's d., localized chorea.

Béguez César d., SYN Chédiak-Steinbrinck-Higashi *syndrome.*

Behçet's d., SYN Behçet's *syndrome.*

Behr's d., SYN Behr's *syndrome.*

Berger's d., SYN focal *glomerulonephritis.*

Bernard-Soulier d. (ber-nar′-sool-ya), an autosomal recessive disorder of absent or decreased platelet membrane glycoproteins Ib, IX, and V (the receptor for factor VIII R. This deficiency can lead to a failure to bind von Willebrand factor, causing moderate bleeding.

Bernhardt's d., SYN *meralgia* paraesthetica.

Besnier-Boeck-Schaumann d., SYN sarcoidosis.

Best's d. [MIM*153700], autosomal dominant retinal degeneration beginning during the first years of life. SEE ALSO vitelliform *degeneration.*

Bielschowsky's d., early childhood type of lipofuscinosis.

Biermer's d., SYN pernicious *anemia.*

big liver d., SEE avian *lymphomatosis.*

Binswanger's d., one of the causes of multiinfarct dementia, in which there are many infarcts and lacunes in the white matter, with relative sparing of the cortex and basal ganglia. SYN Binswanger's encephalopathy, encephalitis subcorticalis chronica, subcortical arteriosclerotic encephalopathy.

bird-breeder's d., SYN bird-breeder's *lung.*

black d., SYN infectious necrotic *hepatitis* of sheep.

black-tongue d., a d. of dogs similar to human pellagra and due to niacin deficiency.

blinding d., SYN onchocerciasis.

Bloch-Sulzberger d., SYN *incontinentia* pigmenti.

Blocq's d., SYN astasia-abasia.

Blount-Barber d., SYN Blount's d.

Blount's d., tibia vara; nonrachitic bowlegs in children. SYN Blount-Barber d.

blue d., SYN Rocky Mountain spotted *fever.*

bluecomb d. of chickens, an acute or subacute d. of young laying chickens characterized by lowered egg production, diarrhea, frequently cyanosis of the head, and pathologic changes involving chiefly the liver and kidney; etiology is not definitely established. SYN avian monocytosis.

bluecomb d. of turkeys, an acute or chronic d. of young turkeys caused by bluecomb virus, with diarrhea, loss of weight, and often cyanosis of the head. SYN mud fever (2), transmissible enteritis.

Boeck's d., SYN sarcoidosis.

border d., a congenital disorder of lambs caused by a pestivirus and characterized by low birth weight and viability, tremor, and an excessively hairy coat. SYN hairy shaker d.

Borna d., an infectious encephalomyelitis of horses, cattle, and sheep caused by Borna disease virus and occurring in Germany and several other European countries; affected animals show depression, then excitement and spasms, and finally paralysis. SYN enzootic encephalomyelitis. [*Borna,* Saxony where a severe epidemic occurred]

Bornholm d., SYN epidemic *pleurodynia.* [*Bornholm,* Danish island in the Baltic where the d. was first described]

Bosin's d., SYN subacute sclerosing *panencephalitis.*

Bouchard's d., myopathic dilation of the stomach.

Bouillaud's d., obsolete eponym for acute rheumatic fever with carditis.

Bourneville-Pringle d., facial lesions with tuberous sclerosis, first reported as adenoma sebaceum, but now recognized as angiofibromas.

Bourneville's d., SYN tuberous *sclerosis.*

Bowen's d., a form of intraepidermal carcinoma characterized by the development of pinkish or brownish papules covered with a thickened horny layer; microscopically, there is dyskeratosis with large round epidermal cells with large nuclei and pale-staining cytoplasm which are scattered through all levels of the epidermis. SYN Bowen's precancerous dermatosis.

Brailsford-Morquio d., SYN Morquio's *syndrome.*

brancher glycogen storage d., type of glycogen storage d., due to deficiency of amylo-1,4-1,6-transglucosidase (brancher enzyme). SYN brancher deficiency glycogenosis, debrancher deficiency.

Breda's d., SYN espundia.

Bright's d., nonsuppurative nephritis with albuminuria and edema, associated in fatal cases with large white kidneys; or with hematuria and red kidneys; or with contracted granular kidneys, corresponding to the stages of glomerulonephritis now termed subacute or membranous, acute, and chronic, respectively.

Brill's d., SYN Brill-Zinsser d.

Brill-Symmers d., obsolete term for nodular *lymphoma.*

Brill-Zinsser d., an endogenous reinfection associated with the "carrier state" in persons who previously had epidemic typhus fever; it is a rather mild d. and may be mistaken for endemic (murine) typhus; first described by Brill in New York City but not recognized as a recrudescent form of epidemic typhus until after the work of Zinsser. SYN Brill's d., recrudescent typhus fever, recrudescent typhus.

Briquet's d., hysterical neurosis, conversion type.

brisket d., a d. of cattle, characterized by edematous swelling of the brisket and the tissues of the neck; the body cavities also contain large quantities of clear straw-colored transudate; this d. results from right heart failure as a consequence of increased pulmonary resistance, which is in some way associated with movement of animals to high altitudes. SYN mountain sickness (2).

Brissaud's d., SYN tic.

broad beta d., type III familial hyperlipoproteinemia.

Brocq's d., a variety of parapsoriasis.

Brodie's d., (1) SYN Brodie's *knee.* (2) hysterical spinal neuralgia, simulating Pott's disease, following a trauma.

bronzed d., SYN bronze *diabetes.* SEE hemochromatosis.

Brooke's d., (1) trichoepithelioma; (2) SYN *keratosis* follicularis contagiosa.

Bruck's d., a d. marked by osteogenesis imperfecta, ankylosis of the joints, and muscular atrophy.

Brushfield-Wyatt d., a familial disorder characterized by unilateral nevus, contralateral hemiplegia, hemianopia, cerebral angioma, and mental retardation; possibly a variant of Sturge-Weber syndrome. SYN nevoid amentia.

Buerger's d., SYN *thromboangiitis* obliterans.

bulging eye d., SYN gedoelstiosis.

Bürger-Grütz d., obsolete term for idiopathic *hyperlipemia.*

Bury's d., SYN *erythema* elevatum diutinum.

Buschke's d., (1) SYN *scleredema* adultorum. (2) obsolete eponym for cryptococcosis.

Busquet's d., an osteoperiostitis of the metatarsal bones, leading to exostoses on the dorsum of the foot.

Buss d., SYN bovine sporadic *encephalomyelitis.*

Busse-Buschke d., SYN cryptococcosis.

Byler d. [MIM*211600], familial intrahepatic cholestasis, with early onset of loose, foul-smelling stools, jaundice, hepatosplenomegaly, and dwarfism, due to an error in conjugated bile salt metabolism; autosomal recessive inheritance. [*Byler,* an Amish kindred]

Caffey's d., SYN infantile cortical *hyperostosis.*

caisson d. (kā′son), SYN decompression *sickness.* [Fr. *caisson* (fr. *caisse,* a chest) a water-tight box or cylinder containing air under high pressure used in sinking structural pilings underwater]

calcium pyrophosphate deposition d. (CPPD), a crystal deposition arthritis that may simulate gout.

Calvé-Perthes d., SYN Legg-Calvé-Perthes d.

Canavan's d., autosomal recessive degenerative d. of infancy; mostly in Jewish infants; onset typically within first 3–4 months of birth, consisting of blindness, psychomotor regression, enlarged head, optic atrophy, hypotonia, spasticity, increased N-acetylaspartic acid urinary excretion. MRI shows enlarged brain, decreased attenuation of cerebral and cerebellar white matter, and normal ventricles. Pathologically, there is increased brain volume and weight, and spongy degeneration in the subcortical white matter. SEE ALSO leukodystrophy. SYN Canavan's sclerosis, Canavan-van Bogaert-Bertrand d., spongy degeneration of infancy.

Canavan-van Bogaert-Bertrand d., SYN Canavan's d.

canine parvovirus d., an acute d. of dogs with a variable mortality rate caused by the canine parvovirus; seen in three distinct clinical forms; a generalized neonatal d., a severe nonsuppurative myocarditis, and a frequently fatal enteritis.

Caroli's d. [MIM*263200], congenital cystic dilation of the intrahepatic bile ducts, sometimes associated with intrahepatic stones and biliary obstruction; a part of the phenotype of infantile polycystic kidney.

Carrington's d., SYN chronic eosinophilic *pneumonia.*

Carrión's d., SYN Oroya *fever.*

Castleman's d., SYN benign giant lymph node *hyperplasia.*

cat-bite d., rat-bite fever, presumably spread from rats to cats and thus to humans. SYN cat-bite fever.

cat-scratch d., a chronic benign adenopathy, especially in children and young adults, commonly associated with a recent cat scratch or bite and caused by bacteria including *Rochalimaea henselae* and *Alipia felis;* the lymphadenopathy usually resolves spontaneously within a period of several months, but complications involving central nervous system, liver, spleen, lung, and skin have been seen. SYN benign inoculation lymphoreticulosis, benign inoculation reticulosis, cat-scratch fever, regional granulomatous lymphadenitis.

celiac d., a disease occurring in children and adults characterized by sensitivity to gluten, with chronic inflammation and atrophy of the mucosa of the upper small intestine; manifestations include diarrhea, malabsorption, steatorrhea, and nutritional and vitamin deficiencies. SYN celiac sprue, celiac syndrome, gluten enteropathy.

central core d. [MIM*117000], a congenital myopathy characterized by hypotonia, delay of motor development in infancy, and nonprogressive or slowly progressive muscle weakness; on biopsy the central core of muscle fibers stains abnormally, myofibrils are abnormally compact, and there is virtual absence of mitochondria and sarcoplasmic reticulum; histochemically, the cores are devoid of oxidative enzyme, phosphorylase, and ATPase activity; autosomal dominant inheritance, often subclinical.

central Recklinghausen's disease type II, type 1 neurofibromatosis. SEE neurofibromatosis.

cerebrovascular d., general term for a brain dysfunction caused by an abnormality of the cerebral blood supply.

Chagas' d., SYN South American *trypanosomiasis.*

Chagas-Cruz d., SYN South American *trypanosomiasis.*

α chain d., a vague or indefinite term; could be used for α-heavy-chain d. (a lymphoplasma cell proliferative d. usually seen in Mediterranean men, characterized by intestinal involvement with steatorrhea, often progressive with fatal outcome) or α *thalassemia* (a genetic abnormality in the alpha globin chain of hemoglobin).

Charcot-Marie-Tooth d., SYN peroneal muscular *atrophy.*

Charcot's d., SYN amyotrophic lateral *sclerosis.*

Charlouis' d., SYN yaws.

Cheadle's d., SYN infantile *scurvy.*

Chédiak-Higashi d., SYN Chédiak-Steinbrinck-Higashi *syndrome.*

Chiari's d., SYN Chiari's *syndrome.*

Chicago d., obsolete term for North American *blastomycosis.*

cholesterol ester storage d. [MIM*278000], a lipidosis caused by a deficiency of lysosomal acid lipase activity resulting in widespread accumulation of cholesterol esters and triglycerides in viscera with xanthomatosis, adrenal calcification, hepatosplenomegaly, foam cells in bone marrow and other tissues, and vacuolated lymphocytes in peripheral blood; autosomal recessive inheritance.

Christensen-Krabbe d., SYN *poliodystrophia* cerebri progressiva infantilis.

Christian's d., (1) SYN Hand-Schüller-Christian d. **(2)** SYN relapsing febrile nodular nonsuppurative *panniculitis.*

Christmas d., SYN *hemophilia* B.

chronic active liver d., SYN chronic *hepatitis.*

chronic granulomatous d., a congenital defect in the killing of phagocytosed bacteria by polymorphonuclear leukocytes, which cannot increase their oxygen metabolism either because of defective cytochrome [MIM*233710 and MIM*233690] or other specific factor deficiencies [MIM*233700 and MIM*306400]. As a result there is an increased susceptibility to severe infection; inheritance is usually autosomal recessive or X-linked. SYN congenital dysphagocytosis, granulomatous d.

chronic hypertensive d., the chronic accumulative effects of long-standing high blood pressure on such vital organs as the heart, kidney, and brain.

chronic obstructive pulmonary d. (COPD), general term used for those diseases with permanent or temporary narrowing of small bronchi, in which forced expiratory flow is slowed, especially when no etiologic or other more specific term can be applied.

chronic respiratory d. (CRD), a common and serious d. of the respiratory tract of chickens caused by the bacterium *Mycoplasma gallinarum;* secondary infection with *Escherichia coli* is common.

chylomicron retention d., an inherited disorder in which apolipoprotein B-48 is retained in intestine and absent in plasma; results in fat malabsorption.

circling d., listeriosis in sheep.

Civatte's d., SYN *poikiloderma* of Civatte.

clover d., SYN trifoliosis.

Coats' d., SYN exudative *retinitis.*

Cockayne's d., SYN Cockayne's *syndrome.*

cold hemagglutinin d., a condition associated with the presence of hemagglutinating autoantibody active *in vivo* but *in vitro* particularly or solely active in the cold; when the concentration of IgM antibody is high there may be increased serum viscosity, but clinical manifestations (due to hemagglutination) usually appear following exposure to cold; hemolysis usually is mild but may be severe, resulting in autoimmune hemolytic anemia, cold antibody type.

collagen d.'s, collagen-vascular d.'s, a group of generalized d.'s affecting connective tissue and frequently characterized by fibrinoid necrosis or vasculitis; in some collagen d.'s, auto-immunization, particularly antinuclear antibodies, has been shown and circulating immune complexes are found. The term is not entirely acceptable because there is no evidence that collagen is primarily involved; "collagen" was once synonymous with "connective tissue" rather than describing a specific fibrinous protein in that tissue. SEE ALSO connective-tissue d.'s.

combined system d., SYN subacute combined *degeneration* of the spinal cord.

communicable d., any d. that is transmissible by infection or contagion directly or through the agency of a vector.

Concato's d., SYN polyserositis.

connective-tissue d.'s, a group of generalized d.'s affecting connective tissue, especially those not inherited as mendelian characteristics; rheumatic fever and rheumatoid arthritis were first proposed as such d.'s, and other so-called collagen d.'s have been added.

Conradi's d. [MIM*215100 & MIM*302950], congenital shortening of the humerus and femur, with stippled epiphyses, high-arched palate, cataracts, erythroderma in the newborn, and scaling followed by follicular atrophoderma; there is also an autosomal dominant inheritance pattern [MIM*118650 and MIM*118651]. SYN chondrodystrophia congenita punctata.

contagious d., an infectious d. transmissible by direct or indirect contact; now used synonymously with communicable d.

Cori's d., SYN type 3 *glycogenosis.*

cornmeal d., SEE *Besnoitia tarandi.*

corridor d., a highly pathogenic disease of cape buffaloes (*Syncerus caffer*) and cattle in eastern and southern Africa caused by the protozoan *Theileria parva lawrencei* and transmitted primarily by the tick *Rhipicephalus appendiculatus;* lesions and symptoms are similar to those of East Coast fever.

Corrigan's d., SYN aortic *regurgitation.*

Cotunnius d., SYN sciatica.

Cowden's d. [MIM*158350], hypertrichosis and gingival fibromatosis from infancy, accompanied by postpubertal fibroadenomatous breast enlargement; papules of the face are characteristic of multiple trichilemmomas. SYN multiple hamartoma syndrome.

crazy chick d., SYN nutritional *encephalomalacia* of chicks.

Creutzfeldt-Jakob d. (CJD), a type of subacute spongiform encephalopathy caused by a transmissible agent termed a prion. Affects adults, especially older adults, and is characterized by progressive dementia, myoclonic jerks, ataxia, and dysarthria; rapidly progressive and invariably fatal, usually within one year of onset. Often accompanied by a distinctive EEG pattern: burst suppression, consisting of intermittent sharp and slow wave complexes on a flat background. Pathologically, nerve cell degeneration and loss with associated astroglial proliferation are confined primarily to the cerebral and cerebellar cortices. SYN Jakob-Creutzfeldt d., transmissible dementia.

Crigler-Najjar d., SYN Crigler-Najjar *syndrome.*

Crocq's d., SYN acrocyanosis.

Crohn's d., SYN regional *enteritis.*

Crouzon's d., SYN craniofacial *dysostosis.*

Cruveilhier-Baumgarten d., SYN Cruveilhier-Baumgarten *syndrome.*

Cruveilhier's d., SYN amyotrophic lateral *sclerosis.*

Csillag's d., chronic atrophic and lichenoid dermatitis.

Curschmann's d., SYN frosted *liver.*

Cushing's d., adrenal hyperplasia (Cushing's syndrome) caused by an ACTH-secreting basophil adenoma of the pituitary. SYN Cushing's pituitary basophilism.

cystic d. of the breast, fibrocystic condition of the breasts.

cystic d. of renal medulla [MIM*256100], presence of small cysts in the renal medulla associated with anemia, sodium depletion, and chronic renal failure. It is of two types: 1) fatal autosomal recessive or juvenile type (also called familial juvenile nephrophthisis), beginning at about age 10 with an average duration of 6 to 8 years; 2) autosomal dominant or adult type, beginning at about age 30 but with a more fulminant course. SYN microcystic d. of renal medulla.

cysticercus d., SYN cysticercosis.

cystine d., SYN cystinosis.

cystine storage d., SYN cystinosis.

cytomegalic inclusion d., the presence of inclusion bodies within the cytoplasm and nuclei of enlarged cells of various organs of newborn infants dying with jaundice, hepatomegaly, splenomegaly, purpura, thrombocytopenia, and fever; the condition also occurs, at all ages, as a complication of other d.'s in which immune mechanisms are severely depressed, and has been found incidentally in salivary gland epithelium, apparently as a localized or mild infection (salivary gland virus d.). SYN cytomegalovirus d., inclusion body d.

cytomegalovirus d., SYN cytomegalic inclusion d.

Daae's d., SYN epidemic *pleurodynia.*

Danielssen-Boeck d., SYN anesthetic *leprosy.*

Danielssen's d., SYN anesthetic *leprosy.*

Darier's d., SYN *keratosis* follicularis.

Darling's d., SYN histoplasmosis.

Davies' d., SYN endomyocardial *fibrosis.*

decompression d., SYN decompression *sickness.*

deer-fly d., SYN tularemia.

deficiency d., any d. resulting from undernutrition or an inadequacy of calories, proteins, essential amino acids, fatty acids, vitamins, or trace minerals.

degenerative joint d., SYN osteoarthritis.

Degos' d., SYN malignant atrophic *papulosis.*

Dejerine's d., SYN Dejerine-Sottas d.

Dejerine-Sottas d., a familial type of demyelinating sensorimotor polyneuropathy that begins in early childhood and is slowly progressive; clinically characterized by foot pain and paresthe-

sias, followed by symmetrical weakness and wasting of the distal limbs; one of the causes of stork legs; patients are wheelchair bound at an early age; peripheral nerves are palpably enlarged and non-tender; pathologically, onion bulb formation is seen in the nerves: whorls of overlapping, intertwined Schwann cell processes that encircle bare axons; usually autosomal recessive inheritance. SYN Dejerine's d., progressive hypertrophic polyneuropathy.

demyelinating d., generic term for a group of d.'s, of unknown cause, in which there is extensive loss of the myelin in the central nervous system, as in multiple sclerosis and Schilder's disease.

dense-deposit d., SEE membranoproliferative *glomerulonephritis.*

de Quervain's d., fibrosis of the sheath of a tendon of the thumb. SYN radial styloid tendovaginitis.

Dercum's d., SYN *adiposis* dolorosa.

Derzsy's d., SYN goose viral *hepatitis.*

Deutschländer's d., (1) tumor of one of the metatarsal bones; (2) SYN march *fracture.*

Devic's d., SYN *neuromyelitis* optica.

diamond skin d., a form of swine erysipelas, caused by the bacterium *Erysipelothrix rhusiopathiae,* in which rhomboidal erythematous areas appear on the skin.

Di Guglielmo's d., the acute form of erythremic myelosis.

disappearing bone d., extensive decalcification of a single bone; of unknown cause, sometimes associated with angioma. SYN Gorham's d.

diverticular d., symptomatic congenital or acquired diverticula of any portion of the gastrointestinal tract. Such diverticula occur in about 15% of the population but rarely cause symptoms.

dog d., SYN phlebotomus *fever.*

dominantly inherited Lévi's d., SYN snub-nose *dwarfism.*

Donohue's d., SYN leprechaunism.

drug-induced d., a toxic reaction to or morbid condition resulting from the administration of a drug.

Dubois' d., SYN Dubois' *abscesses,* under *abscess.*

Duchenne-Aran d., SYN amyotrophic lateral *sclerosis.*

Duchenne's d., (1) SYN Duchenne *dystrophy.* (2) SYN progressive bulbar *paralysis.*

Duhring's d., SYN *dermatitis* herpetiformis.

Dukes' d., an exanthem-producing infectious d. of childhood; unknown etiology.

Duncan's d. [MIM*308240], an X-linked recessive immunodeficiency and lymphoproliferative disease occurring in boys.

Duplay's d., SYN subacromial *bursitis.*

Dupuytren's d. of the foot, SYN plantar *fibromatosis.*

Duroziez' d., congenital stenosis of the mitral valve.

Dutton's d., African tick-borne relapsing fever caused by *Borrelia duttonii* and spread by the soft tick, *Ornithodoros moubata.* SYN Dutton's relapsing fever.

dynamic d., SYN functional *disorder.*

Eales' d., peripheral retinal periphlebitis causing recurrent retinal or intravitreous hemorrhages in young adults.

Ebstein's d., SYN Ebstein's *anomaly.*

echinococcus d., SYN echinococcosis. SYN echinococciasis.

edema d., an acute, highly fatal d. of young pigs caused by toxins of the bacterium *Escherichia coli* and characterized by edema of various parts of the body but particularly the walls of the gastrointestinal tract.

Eisenmenger's d., SYN Eisenmenger's *complex.*

elephant man's d., (1) SYN Proteus *syndrome.* (2) SYN neurofibromatosis (2).

elevator d., respiratory distress arising in persons who work in grain elevators resulting from inhalation of dusts or insects.

emotional d., SEE mental *illness.*

endemic d., continued prevalence of a d. in a specific population or area. SEE ALSO endemic, enzootic.

Engelmann's d., SYN diaphysial *dysplasia.*

English d., obsolete term for rickets.

English sweating d., a d. of unknown nature that appeared in

di

England and spread over Europe in 1485, 1508 and 1528–30 and was characterized by heavy sweats, prostration, and a high fatality rate. SYN sudor anglicus.

eosinophilic endomyocardial d., a restrictive cardiomyopathy associated with hyperproduction of eosinophiles and their cardiac infiltration, clinically characterized by diastolic and later systolic ventricular failure.

epidemic d., marked increase in prevalence of a d. in a specific population or area, usually with an environmental cause, such as an infectious or toxic agent.

epizootic hemorrhagic d. of deer, a hemorrhagic disease of certain deer of the central and eastern United States, caused by an orbivirus, a member of the Reoviridae, and characterized by multiple hemorrhages, shock, and trauma; infection is thought to be arthropod-borne. SYN hemorrhagic d. of deer.

Epstein's d., SYN diphtheroid (1).

Erb d., SYN progressive bulbar *paralysis*.

Erb-Charcot d., (**1**) SYN spastic *diplegia*. (**2**) SYN spastic *paraplegia*.

Erdheim d., SYN cystic medial *necrosis*.

ergot alkaloid-associated heart d., heart d. caused by endomyocardial fibrosis which extends into valve structures, producing stenosis and/or regurgitation, associated with ergot alkaloid use.

Eulenburg's d., SYN congenital *paramyotonia*.

exanthematous d., SEE exanthema.

extramammary Paget d., an intraepidermal form of mucinous adenocarcinoma, most commonly in the anogenital region. SYN Paget's d. (3).

extrapyramidal d., a general term for a number of disorders caused by abnormalities of the basal ganglia or certain brain stem or thalamic nuclei; characterized by motor deficits, loss of postural reflexes, bradykinesia, tremor, rigidity, and various involuntary movements. SYN extrapyramidal motor system d.

extrapyramidal motor system d., SYN extrapyramidal d.

Fabry's d. [MIM*301500], an X-linked recessive disorder due to deficiency of α-galactosidase and characterized by abnormal accumulations of neutral glycolipids (*e.g.,* globotriaosylceramide) in endothelial cells in blood vessel walls, with angiokeratomas on the thighs, buttocks, and genitalia, hypohidrosis, paresthesia in extremities, cornea verticillata, and spokelike posterior subcapsular cataracts; death results from renal, cardiac, or cerebrovascular complications. SYN diffuse angiokeratoma, glycolipid lipidosis.

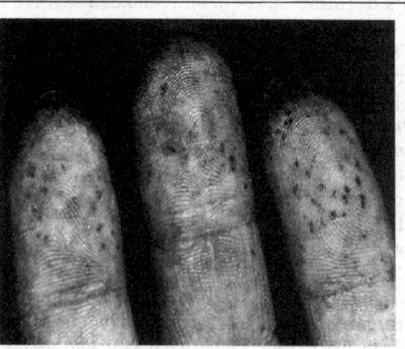

Fabry's disease
appearance of the skin in Fabry's disease

Fahr's d., progressive calcific deposition in the walls of blood vessels of the basal ganglia, in young to middle-aged persons; occasionally associated with mental retardation and extrapyramidal symptoms.

Farber's d., SYN disseminated *lipogranulomatosis*.

Favre-Durand-Nicholas d., SYN *lymphogranuloma* venereum.

Favre-Racouchet's d., comedones developing on sun-damaged skin due to obstruction of pilosebaceous follicles by solar elastosis.

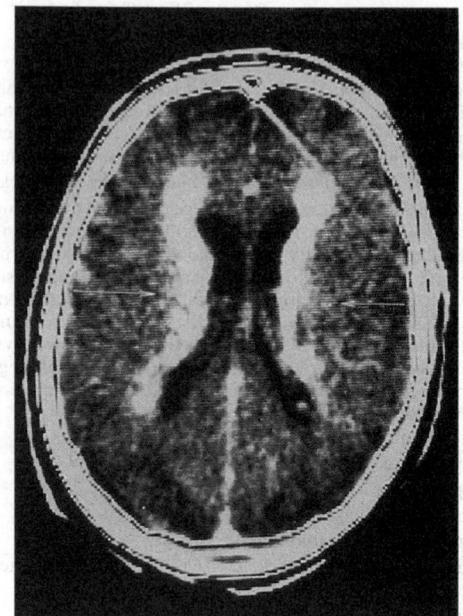

Fahr's disease
arteriosclerotic calcification of the basal ganglia, on both sides
(computed tomogram)

Feer's d., SYN acrodynia (2).

femoropopliteal occlusive d., obstruction of the femoral and popliteal arteries by atherosclerosis.

Fenwick's d., idiopathic gastric atrophy. SEE atrophic *gastritis*.

fibrocystic d. of the breast, a benign d. common in women of the third, fourth, and fifth decades characterized by formation, in one or both breasts, of small cysts containing fluid which may appear as blue dome cysts; associated with stromal fibrosis and with variable degrees of intraductal epithelial hyperplasia and sclerosing adenosis. SYN cystic hyperplasia of the breast.

fibrocystic d. of the pancreas, SYN cystic *fibrosis*.

fifth d., SYN *erythema* infectiosum. [after scarlatina, morbilli, rubella, and fourth d.]

Filatov Dukes' d., an exanthem-producing infectious disease of childhood of unknown etiology. SYN Filatov's d., fourth d., parascarlatina, scarlatinella.

Filatov's d., SYN Filatov Dukes' d.

fish eye d., an inherited disorder resulting in low HDL cholesterol and corneal opacities; also, low LCAT activity.

Flatau-Schilder d., SYN Schilder's d.

flax-dresser's d., chronic obstructive pulmonary d. caused by inhalation of particles of unprocessed flax; a form of byssinosis. SEE ALSO byssinosis.

Flegel's d., SYN *hyperkeratosis* lenticularis perstans.

flint d., SYN chalicosis.

flip-over d., a d. of young, fast-growing broiler chickens which causes them to die suddenly with a short, terminal, wing-beating convulsion, whereby they often flip over and die on their backs.

focal metastatic d., presence of a single area of metastasis of a malignant tumor or infection distant from the primary lesion.

Folling's d., SYN phenylketonuria.

foot-and-mouth d. (FMD), a highly infectious disease of wide distribution and great economic importance, occurring in cattle, swine, sheep, goats and all wild and domestic cloven-footed animals caused by a picornavirus (genus *Rhinovirus*) and characterized by vesicular eruptions in the mouth, tongue, hoofs, and udder; humans are rarely affected. SYN aftosa.

Forbes' d., SYN type 3 *glycogenosis*.

Fordyce's d., SYN Fordyce's *spots*, under *spot*.

Forestier's d., SYN diffuse idiopathic skeletal *hyperostosis*.

Fothergill's d., (1) SYN trigeminal *neuralgia*. **(2)** SYN anginose *scarlatina*.

Fournier's d., infective gangrene involving the scrotum. SYN Fournier's gangrene, syphiloma of Fournier.

fourth d., SYN Filatov Dukes' d. SYN scarlatinoid (2).

Fox-Fordyce d., a rare chronic pruritic eruption of dry papules and distended ruptured apocrine glands, with follicular hyperkeratosis of the nipples, axillae, and pubic and sternal regions. SYN apocrine miliaria.

Franklin's d., SYN γ-heavy-chain d.

Freiberg's d., epiphysial ischemic (aseptic) necrosis of second metatarsal head.

Friend d., mouse leukemia caused by the Friend leukemia virus, a member of the family Retroviridae.

functional d., SYN functional *disorder*.

functional cardiovascular d., a euphemism for cardiovascular symptoms deemed to be psychogenic. More generally, sometimes used for abnormal cardiac function.

fusospirochetal d., infection of the mouth and/or pharynx associated with fusiform bacilli and spirochetes, commonly part of the normal flora of the mouth. SEE ALSO necrotizing ulcerative *gingivitis*.

Gairdner's d., attacks of cardiac distress accompanied by apprehension. SYN angina pectoris sine dolore, angor pectoris (1).

Gamna's d., a form of chronic splenomegaly characterized by conspicuous thickening of the capsule and the presence of multiple, small, rustlike, brown foci (Gamna-Gandy bodies), which contain iron; this condition may be observed in fibrocongestive splenomegaly, sickle cell d., and some examples of hemochromatosis.

Gandy-Nanta d., siderotic splenomegaly, probably the same as Gamna's d.

garapata d., tick fever occurring in Spain.

Garré's d., SYN sclerosing *osteitis*.

gasping d., SYN infectious avian *bronchitis*.

Gaucher's d., a lysosomal storage d. resulting from glycocerebroside accumulation due to a genetic deficiency of glucocerebrosidase; may occur in adults but occurs most severely in infants; marked by hepatosplenomegaly, regression of neurological maturation, and characteristic histiocytes (Gaucher cells) in the viscera; autosomal recessive inheritance. There are three main types: the noncerebral juvenile [MIM*230800], the cerebral juvenile [MIM* 230900], and the adult cerebral [MIM*231000]. SYN cerebroside lipidosis, familial splenic anemia, Gaucher disorder.

Gerhardt-Mitchell d., SYN erythromelalgia.

Gerhardt's d., SYN erythromelalgia.

Gerlier's d., SYN vestibular *neuronitis*.

Gierke's d., SYN type 1 *glycogenosis*.

Gilbert's d., SYN familial nonhemolytic *jaundice*.

Gilchrist's d., SYN blastomycosis.

Gilles de la Tourette's d., SYN Tourette *syndrome*.

Glanzmann's d., SYN Glanzmann's *thrombasthenia*.

Glasser's d., a fibrinous polyserositis, polyarthritis, and meningitis of pigs caused by the bacterium *Haemophilus parasuis*.

glycogen-storage d., SYN glycogenosis.

Goldflam d., SYN *myasthenia* gravis.

Gorham's d., SYN disappearing bone d.

Gougerot and Blum d., SYN pigmented purpuric lichenoid *dermatosis*.

Gougerot-Sjögren d., SYN Sjögren's *syndrome*. [Sjögren, Henrik S.C.]

Gowers d., (1) SYN saltatory *spasm*. **(2)** a distal type of progressive muscular dystrophy.

graft versus host d., an incompatibility reaction (which may be fatal) in a subject (host) of low immunological competence (deficient lymphoid tissue) who has been the recipient of immunologically competent lymphoid tissue from a donor who lacks at least one antigen possessed by the recipient host; the reaction, or disease, is the result of action of the transplanted cells against those host tissues that possess the antigen not possessed by the donor. Seen most commonly following bone marrow transplantation, acute d. is seen after 5-40 days and chronic d. weeks to months after transplantation, affecting, principally, the gastrointestinal tract, liver, and skin. SYN GVH d.

granulomatous d., SYN chronic granulomatous d.

Graves' d., (1) toxic goiter characterized by diffuse hyperplasia of the thyroid gland, a form of hyperthyroidism; exophthalmos is a common, but not invariable, concomitant; **(2)** thyroid dysfunction and all or any of its clinical associations; **(3)** an organ-specific autoimmune disease of the thyroid gland. SEE thyrotoxicosis, Hashimoto's *thyroiditis*, goiter, myxedema. SYN Basedow's d., ophthalmic hyperthyroidism, Parry's d.

greasy pig d., a generalized exudative epidermitis of young pigs, characterized by high mortality and caused by staphylococcal bacteria.

Greenhow's d., SYN parasitic *melanoderma*.

Griesinger's d., bilious typhoid of Griesinger, a severe form of louse-borne relapsing fever caused by *Borrelia recurrentis* and causing high fever, epistaxis, dyspnea, intense jaundice, purpura, and splenomegaly.

Grover's d., SYN transient acantholytic *dermatosis*.

Gumboro d., SYN infectious bursal d.

GVH d., SYN graft versus host d.

Haff d., hemoglobinuria, muscular weakness, and pains in the limbs, occurring in persons living in the vicinity of the Haff inlet, caused by arsenic poisoning from waste in a celluloid factory. [*Haff*, an arm of the Baltic Sea in East Prussia]

Haglund's d., an abnormal prominence of the posterior superior lateral aspect of the os calcis, caused by a gait disorder. SYN Haglund's deformity.

Hailey-Hailey d., SYN benign familial chronic *pemphigus*.

hairy shaker d., SYN border d.

Hallervorden-Spatz d., SYN Hallervorden-Spatz *syndrome*.

Hallopeau's d., (1) SYN *pustulosis* palmaris et plantaris. **(2)** SYN *pemphigus* vegetans (2).

Hamman's d., SYN Hamman's *syndrome*.

Hammond's d., SYN athetosis.

hand-foot-and-mouth d., an exanthematous eruption of small, pearl-gray vesicles of the fingers, toes, palms, and soles, accompanied by often painful vesicles and ulceration of the buccal mucous membrane and the tongue and by slight fever; the d. lasts 4 to 7 days, and is usually caused by Coxsackie virus type A-16, but other types have been identified.

Hand-Schüller-Christian d., the chronic disseminated form of Langerhans cell histiocytosis. The classic triad of signs consists of diabetes insipidus, exophthalmus, and bony lesions composed of histiocytes. SYN Christian's d. (1), Christian's syndrome, normal cholesteremic xanthomatosis, Schüller's d., Schüller's syndrome.

Hansen's d., SYN leprosy (2).

Harada's d., SYN Harada's *syndrome*.

hard pad d., a form of canine distemper characterized by hyperkeratosis of the foot pads and nose. SEE canine *distemper*.

hardware d., SYN traumatic *gastritis*.

Hartnup d. [MIM*234500], a congenital metabolic disorder consisting of aminoaciduria due to a defect in renal tubular absorption of neutral α-amino acids and urinary excretion of tryptophan derivatives, because defective intestinal absorption leads to bacterial degradation of unabsorbed tryptophan in the gut; characterized by a pellagra-like, light-sensitive skin rash with temporary cerebellar ataxia; autosomal recessive inheritance. SYN Hartnup disorder, Hartnup syndrome.

Hashimoto's d., SYN Hashimoto's *thyroiditis*.

heavy chain d., a term used for a group of d.'s, the paraproteinemias, characterized by production of homogenous immunoglobulins or fragments, and associated with malignant disorders of the plasmacytic and lymphoid cell series. Three types have been recognized: γ-heavy-chain d., α-heavy-chain d., and μ-heavy-chain d.; each is diagnosed by the finding of the appropriate heavy-chain fragment in the serum, urine, or both.

di

α-heavy-chain d., the most common form of heavy-chain d., characterized by a finding in the serum of a protein reactive with antisera to α-chains but not light chains; clinical features include diarrhea, steatorrhea, and severe malabsorption.

γ-heavy-chain d., heavy-chain d. characterized by a finding in the serum and urine of a broad protein peak that is reactive with antisera to γ-chains and unreactive with antisera to light chains; common features include anemia, lymphocytosis, eosinophilia, thrombocytopenia, hyperuricemia, lymphadenopathy, and hepatosplenomegaly. SYN Franklin's d.

μ-heavy-chain d., the rarest form of heavy-chain d., primarily seen in patients with long-standing chronic lymphatic leukemia; diagnosis is made on immunoelectrophoresis by finding a component reactive with antisera to μ-chains but not to light chains.

Hebra's d., (1) SYN *erythema* multiforme. (2) SYN familial nonhemolytic *jaundice.*

Heck's d., SYN focal epithelial *hyperplasia.*

Heerfordt's d., SYN uveoparotid *fever.*

hemoglobin C d., the homozygous state of hemoglobin C.

hemoglobin H d., SEE *hemoglobin* H.

hemolytic d. of newborn, SYN *erythroblastosis* fetalis.

hemorrhagic d. of deer, SYN epizootic hemorrhagic d. of deer.

hemorrhagic d. of the newborn, a syndrome characterized by spontaneous internal or external bleeding accompanied by hypoprothrombinemia, slightly decreased platelets, and markedly elevated bleeding and clotting times, usually occurring between the third and sixth days of life and effectively treated with vitamin K.

hepatolenticular d., SYN Wilson's d. (1).

herring-worm d., SYN anisakiasis.

Hers' d., SYN type 6 *glycogenosis.*

hidebound d., scleroderma (usually applied to extensive involvement).

Hirschsprung's d., SYN congenital *megacolon.*

Hjärre's d., a granulomatous d. of the intestines and liver of chickens, due to coliform organisms. SYN coli granuloma.

Hodgkin's d., a d. marked by chronic enlargement of the lymph nodes, often local at the onset and later generalized, together with enlargement of the spleen and often of the liver, no pronounced leukocytosis, and commonly anemia and continuous or remittent (Pel-Ebstein) fever; considered to be a malignant neoplasm of lymphoid cells of uncertain origin (Reed-Sternberg cells), associated with inflammatory infiltration of lymphocytes and eosinophilic leukocytes and fibrosis; can be classified into lymphocytic predominant, nodular sclerosing, mixed cellularity, and lymphocytic depletion type; a similar disease occurs in domestic cats. SYN Hodgkin's lymphoma, lymphadenoma (2).

stages of Hodgkin's disease

stage	1971 Ann Arbor classification
I	affects one anatomical lymph node region (I) or has a localized extralymphatic focus (IE)
II	affects two or more anatomical regions on same side of diaphragm (II) or solitary extralymphatic focus and/or one or more lymph node regions on same side of diaphragm (IIE); spleen can also be affected if on lower side of diaphragm
III	affects anatomical regions on both sides of diaphragm (III); spleen (IIIS) or localized extralymphatic foci (IIIE) or both (IIISE) are involved
IV	generalized or disseminated attack on one or several extralymphatic organs or tissues, with or without concurrent lymph node involvement

Hodgson's d., dilation of the arch of the aorta associated with insufficiency of the aortic valve.

holoendemic d. (hol'ō-en-dem'ik), a d. for which a high prevalent level of infection begins early in life and affects most or all of the child population, leading to a state of equilibrium, such that the adult population shows evidence of the disease much less frequently than do the children.

hoof-and-mouth d., obsolete term for foot-and-mouth d.

hookworm d., SEE ancylostomiasis, necatoriasis.

Huntington's d. [MIM*143100], SYN Huntington's *chorea.*

Hurler's d., SYN Hurler's *syndrome.*

Hutchinson-Gilford d., SYN progeria.

hyaline membrane d. of the newborn, a d. seen especially in premature neonates with respiratory distress; characterized postmortem by atelectasis and alveolar ducts lined by an eosinophilic membrane; also associated with reduced amounts of lung surfactant. SYN hyaline membrane syndrome, respiratory distress syndrome of the newborn.

hydatid d., infection of humans, sheep, and most other herbivorous and omnivorous mammals with larvae of the tapeworm *Echinococcus.*

Hyde's d., SYN *prurigo* nodularis.

hyperendemic d. (hī'per-en-dem'ik), a d. that is constantly present at a high incidence and/or prevalence rate and affects all age groups equally.

Iceland d., SYN epidemic *neuromyasthenia.*

I-cell d., SYN *mucolipidosis* II.

idiopathic d., a d. of unknown cause or mechanism.

immune complex d., an immunologic category of d.'s evoked by the deposition of antigen-antibody or antigen-antibody-complement complexes on cell surfaces, with subsequent involvement of breakdown products of complement, platelets, and polymorphonuclear leukocytes, and development of vasculitis; nephritis is common. Arthus phenomenon and serum sickness are classic examples, but many other disorders, including most of the connective tissue d.'s, may belong in this immunologic category; immune complex d.'s can also occur during a variety of d.'s of known etiology, such as subacute bacterial endocarditis. SEE ALSO autoimmune d. SYN immune complex disorder, type III hypersensitivity reaction.

immunoproliferative small intestinal d., diffuse lymphoplasmacytic infiltration of the proximal small bowel mucosa and mesenteric lymph nodes resulting in diarrhea, weight loss, abdominal pain, and clubbing of fingers and toes; seen in poor people in developing countries. SYN Mediterranean lymphoma.

inborn lysosomal d., inherited disorder of one or more degradative enzymes normally located in lysosomes leading to accumulation (storage) of abnormal quantities of a substance, such as a glycosaminoglycan as in Hurler's *syndrome* or a lipopolysaccharide as in Gaucher's d.

inclusion body d., SYN cytomegalic inclusion d.

inclusion cell d., SYN *mucolipidosis* II.

industrial d., a morbid condition resulting from exposure to an agent discharged by a commercial enterprise into the environment. Cf. occupational d.

infantile celiac d., gluten-sensitive enteropathy appearing in infancy, often before the age of 9 months and characterized by acute onset, diarrhea, abdominal pain, and "failure to thrive."

infectious d., infective d., a d. resulting from the presence and activity of a microbial agent.

infectious bursal d., a highly contagious acute d. of chickens caused by the infectious bursal disease virus and characterized by whitish diarrhea, dehydration, prostration, and destruction of the bursa of Fabricius, compromising the bird's immune system. SYN Gumboro d.

intercurrent d., a new d. occurring during the course of another d., not related to the primary disease process.

interstitial d., a d. occurring chiefly in the connective-tissue framework of an organ, the parenchyma suffering secondarily.

iron-storage d., the storage of excess iron in the parenchyma of many organs, as in idiopathic hemochromatosis or transfusion hemosiderosis.

island d., SYN tsutsugamushi d.

Itai-Itai d., a form of cadmium poisoning described in Japanese people, characterized by renal tubular dysfunction, osteomalacia, pseudofractures, and anemia, caused by ingestion of contaminated shellfish or other sources containing cadmium.

Jaffe-Lichtenstein d., obsolete term for fibrous *dysplasia* of bone.

Jakob-Creutzfeldt d., SYN Creutzfeldt-Jakob d.

Jansky-Bielschowsky d., cerebral *sphingolipidosis*, early juvenile type.

Jembrana d., a febrile d. of cattle thought to be caused by a rickettsia of the genus *Ehrlichia*. [*Jembrana*, county in Bali, Indonesia, where disease was first recognized]

Jensen's d., SYN *retinochoroiditis* juxtapapillaris.

Johne's d., a d. occurring in cattle and sheep, usually manifested by thickening of the wall of the intestine, particularly of the ileum; caused by infection with *Mycobacterium paratuberculosis*. SYN chronic dysentery of cattle, paratuberculosis.

jumping d., jumper d., one of the pathological startle syndromes found in isolated parts of the world, characterized by greatly exaggerated responses, such as jumping, flinging the arms and yelling, to minimal stimuli. SYN jumping Frenchmen of Maine d., jumper d. of Maine.

jumping Frenchmen of Maine d., jumper d. of Maine, SYN jumping d.

Jüngling's d., SYN *osteitis* tuberculosa multiplex cystica.

Kashin-Bek d., a form of generalized osteoarthrosis limited to areas of Asia, including the Urov river; believed to result from ingestion of wheat infected with the fungus *Fusarium sporotrichiella*.

Katayama d., acute early egg-laying phase of schistosomiasis, a toxemic syndrome in heavy primary infections, rarely seen in chronic cases. It is considered a form of immune complex d. or serum sickness-like condition. Described for *schistosomiasis* japonica, but observed with other forms as well. SYN Katayama fever. [town in Japan where the d. is common]

Kawasaki's d., SYN mucocutaneous lymph node *syndrome*.

Kennedy's d., an X-linked recessive disorder characterized by progressive spinal and bulbar muscular atrophy; associated features include distal degeneration of sensory axons, and signs of endocrine dysfunction, including diabetes mellitus, gynecomastia, and testicular atrophy.

Kienböck's d., osteolysis of the lunate bone following trauma to the wrist. SYN lunatomalacia.

Kimmelstiel-Wilson d., SYN Kimmelstiel-Wilson *syndrome*.

Kimura's d., SYN angiolymphoid *hyperplasia* with eosinophilia.

kinky-hair d., kinky hair d. [MIM*309400], congenital defect of copper metabolism manifested in short, sparse, poorly pigmented kinky hair; associated with failure to thrive, physical and mental retardation, and progressive severe deterioration of the brain; apparently a defect of copper transport; X-linked recessive inheritance. SYN kinky-hair disorder, Menkes' syndrome, trichopoliodystrophy.

Köhler's d., epiphysial aseptic necrosis of the tarsal navicular bone or of the patella.

Krabbe's d., SYN globoid cell *leukodystrophy*.

Kufs d., cerebral *sphingolipidosis*, adult type.

Kugelberg-Welander d., SYN juvenile spinal muscular *atrophy*.

Kuhnt-Junius d., SYN Kuhnt-Junius *degeneration*.

Kussmaul's d., SYN *polyarteritis* nodosa.

Kyasanur Forest d., a d. occurring among forest workers in the Kyasanur Forest and in Mysore, India, caused by a group B arbovirus (*Flavivirus*) transmitted chiefly by *Haemaphysalis spinigera*, although other ticks have been implicated as well; symptoms include fever, headache, back and limb pains, diarrhea, and intestinal bleeding; central nervous system symptoms do not occur.

Kyrle's d., SYN *hyperkeratosis* follicularis et parafollicularis.

Lafora body d. [MIM*254780], a form of progressive myoclonus epilepsy beginning from age 6 to 19; characterized by generalized tonic-clonic seizures, resting and action myoclonus, ataxia, dementia, and classic EEG findings, including polyspike and wave discharges; basophilic cytoplasmic inclusion bodies present in portions of the brain, the liver, and skin, as well as the duct

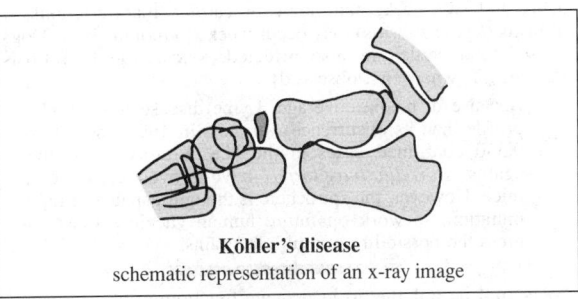

Köhler's disease
schematic representation of an x-ray image

cells of the sweat glands. Death usually occurs within 10 years of onset; autosomal recessive inheritance. SYN Lafora's d.

Lafora's d., SYN Lafora body d.

Lane's d., SYN *erythema* palmare hereditarium.

Larrey-Weil d., SYN Weil's d.

Lasègue's d., obsolete eponym for delusions of persecution.

laughing d., (1) a disabling state of hypnosis or narcosis induced by witch doctors and characterized by involuntary laughing; (2) the compulsive mirthless laughter of schizophrenics.

L-chain d., SYN Bence Jones *myeloma*.

Legg-Calvé-Perthes d., Legg's d., Legg-Perthes d., epiphysial aseptic necrosis of the upper end of the femur. SYN Calvé-Perthes d., coxa plana, osteochondritis deformans juvenilis, Perthes d., pseudocoxalgia, quiet hip d.

Legionnaire's d., an acute infectious d., caused by *Legionella pneumophila*, with prodromal influenza-like symptoms and a rapidly rising high fever, followed by severe pneumonia and production of usually nonpurulent sputum, mental confusion, hepatic fatty changes, and renal tubular degeneration. It has a high case-fatality rate. Acquired from water systems rather than person to person. SYN legionellosis. [American *Legion* convention, 1976, at which many delegates were so affected]

Leigh's d., subacute encephalomyelopathy affecting infants, causing dementia, spasticity, and optic atrophy; autosomal recessive inheritance. SYN necrotizing encephalomyelopathy, necrotizing encephalopathy.

Leiner's d., SYN *erythroderma* desquamativum.

Lenègre's d., SYN Lenègre's *syndrome*.

Leri-Weill d., SYN dyschondrosteosis.

Letterer-Siwe d., the acute disseminated form of Langerhans cell histiocytosis. SYN nonlipid histiocytosis.

Lev's d., SYN Lev's *syndrome*.

Lindau's d., SYN von Hippel-Lindau *syndrome*.

linear IgA bullous d. in children, SYN chronic bullous *dermatosis* of childhood.

Little's d., SYN spastic *diplegia*.

Lobo's d., SYN lobomycosis.

locoweed d., SYN loco.

Löffler's d., SYN Löffler's *endocarditis*.

Lorain's d., SYN idiopathic *infantilism*.

Lou Gehrig's d., SYN amyotrophic lateral *sclerosis*.

Luft's d. [MIM*238800], a metabolic d. due to relative uncoupling of phosphorylation in skeletal muscle causing myopathy and general hypermetabolism; a mitochondial myopathy.

lumpy skin d., an infectious d. of cattle in Africa, manifested by an acute febrile illness followed by the appearance of lumps and plaques under the skin and on some of the mucous membranes; caused by the lumpy skin disease virus.

lung fluke d., infection with the lung fluke, *Clonorchis sinensis*.

Lutz-Splendore-Almeida d., SYN paracoccidioidomycosis.

Lyell's d., SYN staphylococcal scalded skin *syndrome*.

Lyme d., an inflammatory disorder typically occurring during the summer months and caused by *Borrelia burgdorferi*, a nonpyogenic, penicillin-sensitive spirochete transmitted by *Ixodes dammini* in the eastern U.S. and *I. pacificus* in the western U.S.; the characteristic skin lesion, erythema chronicum migrans, usually is preceded or accompanied by fever, malaise, fatigue, head-

di

ache, and stiff neck; neurologic or cardiac manifestations, or arthritis (Lyme arthritis) may occur weeks to months later. Dogs, horses, and cattle are also affected. SYN Lyme borreliosis. [Lyme, CT, where first observed]

> Because of media coverage, Lyme disease has a higher profile than its occurrence warrants. In 1993, there were 9,350 confirmed cases in the U.S. Prototype vaccines against *Borrelia burgdorferi* have proved effective in mice. However, the spirochete is thought capable of rapid mutation, so work on future human vaccines must address the possibility of multiple strains.

lysosomal d., a d. due to inadequate functioning of a lysosomal enzyme; most such d.'s are associated with a storage d.

Machado-Joseph [MIM*109150], a rare form of hereditary ataxia, characterized by onset in early adult life of progressive, spinocerebellar and extrapyramidal disease with external ophthalmoplegia, rigidity dystonia symptoms, and, often, peripheral amyotrophy; found predominantly in people of Azorean ancestry; autosomal dominant inheritance. SYN Azorean d., Portuguese-Azorean d. [Surnames of two families studied in major descriptions of the disease.]

mad cow d., SYN bovine spongiform *encephalopathy*.

Madelung's d., SYN multiple symmetric *lipomatosis*.

Majocchi's d., SYN *purpura* annularis telangiectodes.

Manson's d., SYN *schistosomiasis* mansoni.

maple bark d., hypersensitivity pneumonitis caused by spores of *Cryptostroma corticale* growing under the bark of stacked maple logs.

maple syrup urine d. [MIM*248600], a disorder caused by deficient oxidative decarboxylation of α-keto acid metabolites of leucine, isoleucine, and valine which are present in blood and urine in high concentrations, the urine having an odor similar to that of maple syrup; neonatal death is common; survivors usually exhibit gross brain damage; autosomal recessive inheritance. SYN branched chain ketoaciduria, branched chain ketonuria, ketoacidemia.

marble bone d., SYN osteopetrosis.

Marburg d., infection with an unusual rhabdovirus composed of RNA and lipid, tentatively assigned to the family of Filoviridae. Virus is "pantropic" and affects most organ systems. The disease is characterized by a prominent rash and hemorrhages in many organs and is often fatal. First seen among laboratory workers in Marburg, Germany, exposed to African green monkeys. Some person-to-person spread has been observed. Attempts to isolate virus should be done only in high-security laboratories. SYN Marburg virus d.

Marburg virus d., SYN Marburg d.

Marchiafava-Bignami d., a disorder recognized primarily by its pathological features, consisting of demyelination of the corpus callosum and cortical laminar necrosis involving the frontal and temporal lobes. Occurs predominantly in chronic alcoholics, particularly wine drinkers.

Marek's d., SEE avian *lymphomatosis*.

Marfan's d., SYN Marfan's *syndrome*.

margarine d., erythema multiforme caused by an emulsifying agent used in the manufacture of margarine.

Marie's d., a hypertrophic osteopathy of dogs in which osseous changes of the limbs are associated with intrathoracic lesions such as pulmonary neoplasms; also occurs in horses, cattle, and sheep.

Marie-Strümpell d., SYN ankylosing *spondylitis*.

Marion's d., a congenital obstruction of the posterior urethra.

Martin's d., a periosteoarthritis of the foot from excessive walking.

McArdle's d., SYN type 5 *glycogenosis*.

McArdle-Schmid-Pearson d., SYN type 5 *glycogenosis*.

mechanobullous d. (mek'an-ō-bul-ous), SYN *epidermolysis* bullosa. [G. *mechanē*, machine, + bullous]

Meige's d. [MIM*153200], autosomal dominant lymphedema with onset at about the age of puberty.

Ménétrier's d., gastric mucosal hyperplasia, either mucoid or glandular; the latter type may be associated with the Zollinger-Ellison syndrome. SYN giant hypertrophy of gastric mucosa, hypertrophic gastritis, Ménétrier's syndrome.

Ménière's d., an affection characterized clinically by vertigo, nausea, vomiting, tinnitus, and progressive deafness due to swelling of the endolymphatic duct. SYN auditory vertigo, endolymphatic hydrops, labyrinthine vertigo, Ménière's syndrome.

mental d., SEE mental *illness*.

Merzbacher-Pelizaeus d., SYN Pelizaeus-Merzbacher d.

metabolic d., generic term for disease caused by an abnormal metabolic process. It can be a congenital due to inherited enzyme abnormality or acquired due to disease of an endocrine organ or failure of function of a metabolic important organ such as the liver.

Meyenburg's d., SYN relapsing *polychondritis*.

Meyer-Betz d., SYN myoglobinuria.

mianeh d., SYN Persian relapsing *fever*.

Mibelli's d., SYN porokeratosis.

microcystic d. of renal medulla, SYN cystic d. of renal medulla.

micrometastatic d., the condition of a patient who has had all clinically evident cancer removed, but who may be expected to have a recurrence from metastases that are too small to be apparent.

Mikulicz' d., benign swelling of the lacrimal, and usually also of the salivary glands in consequence of an infiltration of and replacement of the normal gland structure by lymphoid tissue. SEE ALSO Mikulicz' *syndrome*, Sjögren's *syndrome*.

Milian's d., SYN ninth-day *erythema*.

Milroy's d. [MIM*153100], the congenital type of autosomal dominant lymphedema.

Milton's d., SYN angioedema.

Minamata d., a neurologic disorder caused by methyl mercury intoxication; first described in the inhabitants of Minamata Bay, Japan, resulting from their eating fish contaminated with mercury industrial waste. Characterized by peripheral sensory loss, tremors, dysarthria, ataxia, and both hearing and visual loss.

miner's d., (1) SYN ancylostomiasis, miner's *nystagmus*.

minimal-change d., SYN lipoid *nephrosis*.

Mitchell's d., SYN erythromelalgia.

mixed connective-tissue d., d. with overlapping features of various systemic connective-tissue d.'s and with serum antibodies to nuclear ribonucleoprotein.

molecular d., a d. in which the manifestations are due to alterations in molecular structure and function.

Mondor's d., thrombophlebitis of the thoracoepigastric vein of the breast and chest wall.

Monge's d., SYN chronic mountain *sickness*.

Morgagni's d., SYN Adams-Stokes *syndrome*.

Morquio's d., SYN Morquio's *syndrome*.

Morquio-Ullrich d., SYN Morquio's *syndrome*.

Morvan's d., SYN syringomyelia.

Moschcowitz' d., SYN thrombotic thrombocytopenic *purpura*.

motor neuron d. (MND), a general term including progressive spinal muscular atrophy (infantile, juvenile, and adult), amyotrophic lateral sclerosis, progressive bulbar paralysis, and primary lateral sclerosis; frequently a familial d. SYN motor system d.

motor system d., SYN motor neuron d.

mountain d., a term that can mean acute altitude sickness; also used for chronic disease characterized by low oxygen saturation of hemoglobin, due to low partial pressure of oxygen in inspired air plus alveolar hypoventilation that develops in some individuals, especially older people. Polycythemia leads to florid skin color but cyanosis appears on mild exertion, along with dyspnea, fatigue, headache, and mental torpor. A person so afflicted returns to normal shortly after return to normal altitude.

moyamoya d., a cerebrovascular disorder occurring predominantly in the Japanese, in which the vessels of the base of the brain become occluded and revascularized with a fine network of vessels; it occurs commonly in young children and is manifested by convulsions, hemiplegia, mental retardation, and subarachnoid hemorrhage; the diagnosis is made by the angiographic picture. [Jap. addlebrained]

Mucha-Habermann d., SYN *pityriasis* lichenoides et varioliformis acuta.

mucosal d., SYN bovine virus *diarrhea.*

multicore d., nonprogressive congenital myopathy characterized by weakness of proximal muscles, multifocal degeneration of the muscle fibers, and eccentric areas of decreased or absent oxidative enzyme activity in muscles.

Nairobi sheep d., a d. of sheep in East Africa caused by Nairobi sheep d. virus, a member of the family Bunyaviridae, transmitted by *Rhipicephalus appendiculatus,* and characterized by hemorrhagic gastroenteritis with high fever.

navicular d., a common cause of lameness in horses, especially light racing animals; it is essentially a chronic osteitis of the navicular bone associated with bursitis and inflammation of the plantar aponeurosis; occurs most frequently in the forefeet and is believed to be due to damage from frequent and severe strain. SYN navicularthritis.

Neftel's d., paresthesia of the head and trunk, and extreme discomfort in any but the recumbent position.

Neumann's d., SYN *pemphigus* vegetans (1).

neutral lipid storage d., SYN Dorfman-Chanarin *syndrome.*

Newcastle d., an acute febrile, and contagious d. of fowls resembling fowl plague, caused by a *Paramyxovirus* (Newcastle d. virus) and characterized by high infectivity and respiratory and nervous symptoms; it is readily transmissible to man, in whom it causes a severe but transient conjunctivitis. SYN Ranikhet d. [*Newcastle* upon Tyne, England, where first reported]

new duck d., SYN infectious *serositis.*

Nicolas-Favre d., SYN venereal *lymphogranuloma.*

Niemann d., SYN Niemann-Pick d.

Niemann-Pick d. [MIM*257200], lipid histiocytosis with accumulation of sphingomyelin in histiocytes in the liver, spleen, lymph nodes, and bone marrow; cerebral involvement may occur at a late stage, with red macular spots less common than in Tay-Sachs d.; occurs most commonly in Jewish infants and leads to early death; a more benign form may occur rarely in adults; autosomal recessive inheritance. Type I Niemann-Pick d. is due to a deficiency of sphingomyelinase; the cause of Type II Niemann-Pick d. (or, secondary Niemann-Pick d.) is unknown. SYN Niemann d., sphingomyelin lipidosis.

nil d., SYN lipoid *nephrosis.*

nodular d., oesophagostomiasis in herbivores and primates, characterized by nodules in the wall of the large intestine, cecum, and occasionally, the ileum; the nodules are filled with caseous material and result from host response to encystment of the larvae of *Oesophagostomum* species.

Norrie's d. [MIM*310600], congenital bilateral masses of tissue arising from the retina or vitreous and resembling glioma (pseudoglioma), usually with atrophy of iris and development of cataract; associated mental retardation and deafness; X-linked recessive inheritance.

notifiable d., a d. that, by statutory requirements, must be reported to the public health or veterinary authorities when the diagnosis is made because of its importance to human or animal health. SYN reportable d.

oasthouse urine d. [MIM*250900], an inherited metabolic defect in the absorption of methionine which is converted by intestinal bacteria to α-hydroxybutyric acid; characterized by diarrhea, tachypnea, and marked urinary excretion of α-hydroxybutyric acid (causing an odor like that of an oasthouse). [*oast,* kiln for drying hops, malt, or tobacco]

occupational d., a morbid condition resulting from exposure to an agent during the usual performance of one's occupation. Cf. industrial d.

Ofuji's d., SYN eosinophilic pustular *folliculitis.*

Oguchi's d. [MIM*258100], a rare, congenital, nonprogressive night blindness with yellow or gray coloration of fundus; after 2 or 3 hours in total darkness, normal color of fundus returns; autosomal recessive inheritance.

Ollier's d., SYN enchondromatosis.

Ondiri d., SYN bovine petechial *fever.*

Oppenheim's d., SYN *amyotonia* congenita (1).

organic d., a d. in which there are anatomical or pathophysio-

logical changes in some bodily tissue or organ, in contrast to a functional disorder; particularly one of psychogenic origin.

Ormond's d., SYN retroperitoneal *fibrosis.*

orphan d., a d. for which no treatment has been developed because of its rarity (affecting no more than 200,000 persons in the U.S.). SEE ALSO orphan *products,* under *product.*

Osgood-Schlatter d., epiphysial aseptic necrosis of the tibial tubercle. SYN apophysitis tibialis adolescentium, Schlatter's d., Schlatter-Osgood d.

Osler's d., (1) SYN *polycythemia* vera.

Osler-Vaquez d., SYN *polycythemia* vera.

Otto's d., a d. characterized by an inward bulging of the acetabulum into the pelvic cavity, resulting from arthritis of the hip joints, usually due to rheumatoid arthritis. SYN arthrokatadysis, Otto pelvis, protrusio acetabuli.

Owren's d. [MIM*227400], a congenital deficiency of factor V, resulting in prolongation of prothrombin time and coagulation time.

Paas' d., a familial skeletal deformation marked by coxa valga, double patella, shortening of the middle and terminal phalanges of fingers and toes, deformities of the elbows, scoliosis, and spondylitis deformans of the lumbar vertebrae; all of these manifestations may be unilateral or bilateral.

Pacheco's d., a highly contagious, acute d. of psittacine birds caused by a herpesvirus and characterized by bright yellow urates with scant feces, icterus, and terminal anorexia.

Paget's d., (1) a generalized skeletal disease, frequently familial, of older persons in which bone resorption and formation are both increased, leading to thickening and softening of bones (*e.g.,* the skull), and bending of weight-bearing bones; SYN osteitis deformans. **(2)** a d. of elderly women, characterized by an infiltrated, somewhat eczematous lesion surrounding and involving the nipple and areola, and associated with subjacent intraductal cancer of the breast and infiltration of the lower epidermis by malignant cells; **(3)** SYN extramammary Paget d.

Panner's d., epiphysial aseptic necrosis of the capitellum of the humerus.

paper mill worker's d., extrinsic allergic alveolitis caused by moldy wood pulp containing spores of *Alternaria* fungi.

parasitic d., a d. due to the presence and vital activity of a parasite, or as a reaction to a parasite.

Parkinson's d., SYN parkinsonism (1).

parrot d., SYN psittacosis.

Parrot's d., (1) pseudoparalysis in infants, due to syphilitic osteochondritis; **(2)** SYN marasmus.

Parry's d., SYN Graves' d.

Pauzat's d., osteoplastic periostitis or fatigue fractures of the metatarsal bones, caused by excessive marching.

Pavy's d., cyclic or recurrent physiologic albuminuria.

Paxton's d., SYN *trichomycosis* axillaris.

pearl-worker's d., inflammatory hypertrophy of the bones affecting grinders of mother-of-pearl.

Pel-Ebstein d., SYN Pel-Ebstein *fever.*

Pelizaeus-Merzbacher d. [MIM*260600], a sudanophilic leukodystrophy with a tigroid appearance of the myelin resulting from patchy demyelination. Type 1-classic, nystagmus and tremor appearing in the first few months of life, followed by slow motor development sometimes with choreoathetosis, spasticity, optic

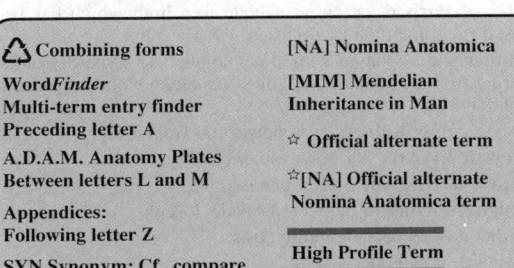

♻ Combining forms	[NA] Nomina Anatomica
Word*Finder* Multi-term entry finder Preceding letter A	**[MIM] Mendelian Inheritance in Man**
A.D.A.M. Anatomy Plates Between letters L and M	☆ **Official alternate term**
Appendices: Following letter Z	☆[NA] Official alternate Nomina Anatomica term
SYN Synonym; Cf., compare	**High Profile Term**

di

atrophy and seizures, with death in early adulthood, X-linked recessive inheritance; type 2-contralateral form with death in months to years after birth, X-linked recessive inheritance; type 3-transitional, with death in the first decade; type 4-adult form associated with involuntary movements, ataxia and hyperreflexia, but without nystagmus; type 5-variant forms. Cockayne is sometimes included as a sixth form. SYN Merzbacher-Pelizaeus d.

Pellegrini's d., a calcific density in the medial collateral ligament and/or bony growth at the internal condyle of the femur. SYN Pellegrini-Stieda d.

Pellegrini-Stieda d., SYN Pellegrini's d.

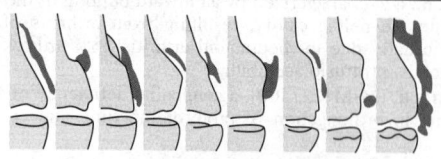

Pellegrini-Stieda disease
calcification shadows as seen by x-ray

pelvic inflammatory d. (PID), acute or chronic inflammation in the pelvic cavity, particularly, suppurative lesions of the upper female genital tract; *e.g.,* salpingitis and its complications.

PID is most commonly caused by sexually transmitted diseases, including chlamydia and gonorrhea, that have ascended into the uterus, fallopian tubes, or ovaries as a result of intercourse or childbirth, or of surgical procedures, including insertion of IUDs or abortion. It may be either symptomatic (acute phase, 5–10 days and subsequently symptom free) or asymptomatic. The rate of PID varies with age group, with the highest rate reported in women 20–29 years old. Because of scarring damage, PID accounts for a share of tubal infertility (estimated at 1.7% in the U.S., based on 1988 figures). It also may raise the risk of ectopic pregnancy (about a 1 in 16 chance for women who have had PID, versus 1 in 147 for all women).

periodic d., any condition or d. in which episodes tend to recur at regular intervals; many such cases are manifestations of familial Mediterranean fever; the cause of the periodicity is usually unknown.

perna d., halogen or chloric acne occurring in workers in perchlornaphthalin. [*per*chlor*na*phthalin]

Perthes d., SYN Legg-Calvé-Perthes d.

Pette-Döring d., SYN nodular *panencephalitis.*

Peyronie's d., a d. of unknown cause in which there are plaques or strands of dense fibrous tissue surrounding the corpus cavernosum of the penis, causing deformity and painful erection; sometimes associated with Dupuytren's contracture. SYN penile fibromatosis, van Buren's d.

Pick's d., progressive circumscribed cerebral atrophy; a rare type of cerebrodegenerative disorder manifested primarily as dementia, in which there is striking atrophy of portions of the frontal and temporal lobes. SYN Pick's syndrome. [F. Pick]

pink d., SYN acrodynia (2).

plaster of Paris d., atrophy of bone in a limb which has been encased for some time in a plaster of Paris splint.

Plummer's d., eponym sometimes applied to hyperthyroidism resulting from a nodular toxic goiter, usually not accompanied by exophthalmos.

polycystic d. of kidneys, SYN polycystic *kidney.*

polycystic liver d., SYN polycystic *liver.*

Pompe's d., SYN type 2 *glycogenosis.*

Portuguese-Azorean d., SYN Machado-Joseph.

Posadas d., SYN coccidioidomycosis.

Potter's d., SYN Potter's *facies.*

Pott's d., SYN tuberculous *spondylitis.*

poultry handler's d., extrinsic allergic alveolitis similar to bird-

breeder's lung, caused by inhalation of particulate emanations from domesticated fowl such as chickens and turkeys.

pregnancy d. of sheep, a highly fatal metabolic d. of well-nourished ewes in the late stages of pregnancy, especially in ewes carrying twin lambs; it is caused by carbohydrate depletion of the blood and tissues, and is characterized by hypoglycemia, ketonuria, fatty infiltration of the liver, rapid emaciation, coma, and a high death rate. SYN lambing paralysis, lambing sickness.

primary d., a d. that arises spontaneously and is not associated with or caused by a previous disease, injury, or event, but which may lead to a secondary d.

Pringle's d., SYN *adenoma* sebaceum.

pseudo-Hurler d., SYN infantile, generalized G_{M1} *gangliosidosis.*

pullorum d., an infectious d. of chicks and other young birds caused by the bacterium *Salmonella pullorum,* which is carried in the ovaries of adult hens and appears in the eggs; in incubator-hatched birds, the d. usually involves the lungs and air sacs, but often spreads in flocks of young birds as an alimentary tract infection manifested by severe diarrhea followed by septicemia and death. SYN diarrhea alba, white diarrhea.

pulpy kidney d., an enterotoxemia of sheep caused by the bacterium *Clostridium perfringens* type D and characterized by sudden death preceded in some cases by excitement, incoordination, and convulsions; also occurs in goats and rarely in cattle.

pulseless d., SYN Takayasu's *arteritis.*

Purtscher's d., SYN Purtscher's *retinopathy.*

pyramidal d., SYN buttress *foot.*

quiet hip d., SYN Legg-Calvé-Perthes d.

Quincke's d., SYN angioedema.

rabbit hemorrhagic d., a highly infectious d. of rabbits, caused by a calicivirus and characterized by hemorrhagic lesions, particularly affecting the lungs and liver; since it was first identified in China in 1984, it has been reported from Korea, it has spread through Europe, and it has reached North Africa and Mexico.

ragpicker's d., SYN pulmonary *anthrax.*

ragsorter's d., rag-sorter's d., SYN pulmonary *anthrax.*

rag-sorter's d.,

railroad d., SYN transport *tetany.*

Ranikhet d., SYN Newcastle d. [Ranikhet, town in northern India]

rat-bite d., SYN rat-bite *fever.*

Raussly d., a rare autosomal dominant neurological disorder with many of the clinical features of hereditary hypertrophic sensorimotor polyneuropathy combined with an essential tremor. SYN hereditary areflexic dystasia.

Rayer's d., SYN biliary *xanthomatosis.*

Raynaud's d., SYN Raynaud's *syndrome.*

Recklinghausen's d. of bone, SYN *osteitis* fibrosa cystica.

Recklinghausen's d. type I, SYN neurofibromatosis (2).

Refsum's d. [MIM*266500] a rare degenerative disorder transmitted as an autosomal recessive trait and caused by the absence of phytanic acid α-hydroxylase; clinically characterized by retinitis pigmentosa, demyelinating polyneuropathy, deafness, nystagmus, and cerebellar signs; infantile Refsum's d. [MIM*266510] is an impaired peroxisomal function with accumulation of phytanic acid, pipecolic acid, etc; autosomal recessive inheritance. SYN heredopathia atactica polyneuritiformis, Refsum's syndrome.

Reiter's d., SYN Reiter's *syndrome.*

reportable d., SYN notifiable d.

rhesus d., sensitization of the mother during pregnancy to Rh factor in fetal blood, leading to erythroblastosis fetalis.

rheumatic d., SEE rheumatism.

rheumatic heart d., d. of the heart resulting from rheumatic fever, chiefly manifested by abnormalities of the valves.

rheumatoid d., rheumatoid *arthritis,* referring particularly to nonarticular lesions such as subcutaneous nodules.

Ribas-Torres d., a mild form of smallpox. SEE ALSO *variola* minor.

rice d., beriberi, the original outbreaks of which were caused by feeding people rice from which the husks had been removed (polished rice), decreasing the vitamin B1 content of the rice.

Riedel's d., SYN Riedel's *thyroiditis.*

Riga-Fede d., ulceration of the lingual frenum in teething infants, related to abrasion of the tissue against the new central incisors.

Robinson's d., ohbsolete term for hidrocystoma(s) occurring in the skin of the face, especially in the region of the eyes.

Roger's d., a congenital cardiac anomaly consisting of a small, isolated, asymptomatic defect of the interventricular septum. SYN maladie de Roger.

Rokitansky's d., (1) SYN acute yellow *atrophy* of the liver. **(2)** SYN Chiari's *syndrome.*

Romberg's d., SYN facial *hemiatrophy.*

Rosai-Dorman d., SYN sinus *histiocytosis* with massive lymphadenopathy.

Rosenbach's d., (1) SYN Heberden's *nodes,* under *node.* **(2)** SYN erysipeloid.

Roth-Bernhardt d., SYN *meralgia* paraesthetica.

Roth's d., SYN *meralgia* paraesthetica.

Rougnon-Heberden d., SYN *angina* pectoris.

round heart d., a spontaneous cardiomyopathy of unknown etiology that affects young turkeys; characterized by sudden death due to cardiac arrest.

Roussy-Lévy d. [MIM*180800], a type of cerebellar ataxia regularly associated with wasting of the calves and intrinsic muscles of the hands and with absent tendon reflexes; pes cavus and claw toes develop; autosomal dominant inheritance. SYN Roussy-Lévy syndrome.

Rubarth's d., SYN infectious canine *hepatitis.*

runt d., a graft versus host reaction in mice first observed following intravenous injection of allogeneic spleen cells into newborn animals. SYN wasting d.

Rust's d., tuberculosis of the two upper cervical vertebrae and their articulations. SYN malum vertebrale suboccipitale, spondylarthrocace (2), spondylocace (2).

salivary gland d., disorder of salivary glands; *i.e.,* Sjögren's *syndrome.*

salivary gland virus d., SEE cytomegalic inclusion d.

Salla d. (sal'ya), an autosomal recessive disorder in which there is a defect in the transport of free sialic acid across lysosomal membranes.

salmon d., SYN salmon *poisoning.*

Sandhoff's d. [MIM*268800], an infantile form of G_{M2} gangliosidosis characterized by a defect in the production of hexosaminidases A and B; it resembles Tay-Sachs disease, but occurs predominantly (if not entirely) in non-Jewish children; accumulation of glucoside and ganglioside G_{m2}.

sandworm d., an inflammatory eruption on the inner side of the sole, observed in certain parts of Australia, marked by a patch of erythema spreading in spirals, and disappearing spontaneously; probably a form of creeping eruption similar to larva migrans.

San Joaquin Valley d., SYN primary *coccidioidomycosis.*

Schenck's d., SYN sporotrichosis.

Scheuermann's d., epiphysial aseptic necrosis of vertebral bodies. SYN adolescent round back, juvenile kyphosis, osteochondritis deformans juvenilis dorsi.

Schilder's d., term used to describe at least two separate disorders described by Schilder: 1) Diffuse sclerosis or encephalitis periaxialis diffusa; a nonfamilial disorder affecting primarily children and young adults and characterized by progressive dementia, visual disturbances, deafness, pseudobulbar palsy, and hemiplegia or quadriplegia. Most patients die within a few years of onset; pathologically, there is a large, asymmetrical area of myelin destruction, sometimes involving an entire cerebral hemisphere, and typically with extension across the corpus callosum. 2) The leukodystrophies. SYN encephalitis periaxialis diffusa, Flatau-Schilder d.

Schindler d. (shind'ler), an autosomal recessive disorder with deficient activity of α-*N*-acetylgalactosaminidase resulting in accumulation of glycoproteins and other substrates which are deposited in terminal axons, primarily in gray matter.

Schlatter's d., Schlatter-Osgood d., SYN Osgood-Schlatter d.

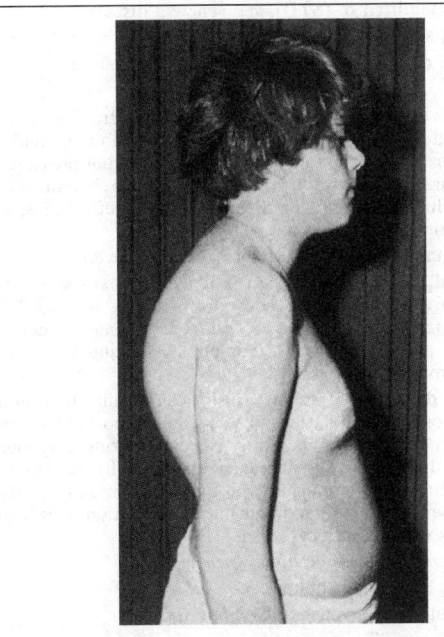

Scheuermann's disease
kyphosis of 13-yr.-old girl

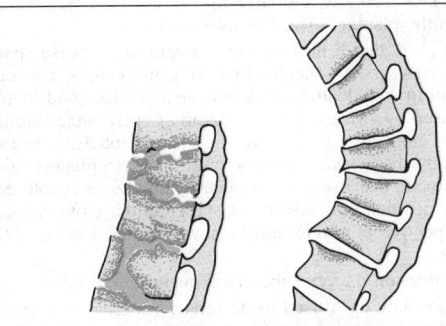

Scheuermann's disease
schematic representation of x-ray view of spinal column in Scheuermann's disease

Scholz' d., former eponym for the juvenile form of metachromatic leukodystrophy.

Schönlein's d., SYN Henoch-Schönlein *purpura.*

Schottmueller's d., SYN paratyphoid *fever.*

Schüller's d., SYN Hand-Schüller-Christian d.

sclerocystic d. of the ovary, SYN polycystic ovary *syndrome.*

sea-blue histiocyte d. [MIM*269600], splenomegaly and mild thrombocytopenia, with histiocytes in the bone marrow which contain cytoplasmic granules that stain bright blue; sometimes familial; perhaps a lipidosis; autosomal recessive inheritance.

secondary d., (1) a d. that follows and results from an earlier disease, injury, or event; **(2)** a wasting disorder that follows successful transplantation of bone marrow into a lethally irradiated host; frequently severe and usually associated with fever, anorexia, diarrhea, dermatitis, and desquamation. SEE ALSO graft versus host d.

self-limited d., a d. process that resolves spontaneously with or without specific treatment.

Senear-Usher d., SYN *pemphigus* erythematosus.

senile hip d., SYN *malum* coxae senile.

serum d., SYN serum *sickness.*

sexually transmitted d. (STD), SEE venereal disease.

Shaver's d., SYN bauxite *pneumoconiosis*.

shimamushi d. (shē-mă-mū'shē), SYN tsutsugamushi d.

sickle cell d., SYN sickle cell *anemia*.

sickle cell C d. [MIM*141900], a d. resulting from abnormal sickle-shaped erythrocytes (containing hemoglobin C and S) which appear in response to a lowering of the partial pressure of oxygen; characterized by anemia, crises due to hemolysis or vascular occlusion, chronic leg ulcers and bone deformities, and infarcts of bone or of the spleen.

sickle cell-thalassemia d., SYN microdrepanocytic *anemia*.

silo-filler's d., a pulmonary lesion produced by oxides of nitrogen due to fresh silage; in its acute form it may lead to death from pulmonary edema or may go on to a subacute or chronic proliferative pulmonary disease sometimes leading to chronic pulmonary invalidism.

Simmonds' d., anterior pituitary insufficiency due to trauma, vascular lesions, or tumors; usually developing postpartum as a result of pituitary necrosis caused by ischemia during a hypotensive episode during delivery; characterized clinically by asthenia, loss of weight and body hair, arterial hypotension, and manifestations of thyroid, adrenal, and gonadal hypofunction. SYN hypophysial cachexia, pituitary cachexia.

Simons' d., SYN progressive *lipodystrophy*.

sixth d., SYN *exanthema* subitum.

sixth venereal d., SYN venereal *lymphogranuloma*.

Sjögren's d., SYN Sjögren's *syndrome*.

skinbound d., scleroderma (usually applied to extensive involvement).

slipped tendon d., a manganese-deficiency perosis in the young chick, which allows the tendons on the caudal aspect of the tarsus to displace medially and laterally, so that the chick squats and walks on the plantar surface of the limbs.

slow virus d., a d. that follows a slow, progressive course spanning months to years, frequently involving the central nervous system, and ultimately leading to death, such as visna and maedi of sheep, caused by viruses of the subfamily Lentivirinae (family Retroviridae), and subacute sclerosing panencephalitis, seemingly caused by the measles virus; spongiform encephalopathies including kuru of man, scrapie of sheep, and transmissible encephalopathy of mink may also be classified under slow virus d. but their respective etiologic agents have not been adequately characterized.

Sneddon-Wilkinson d., SYN subcorneal pustular *dermatosis*.

social d.'s, obsolete term used to designate venereal d.'s, especially gonorrhea and syphilis.

specific d., a d. produced by the action of a special pathogenic microorganism.

Spielmeyer-Sjögren d., cerebral *sphingolipidosis*, late juvenile type.

Spielmeyer-Stock d., retinal atrophy in amaurotic familial idiocy.

Spielmeyer-Vogt d., cerebral *sphingolipidosis*, late juvenile type. SYN Vogt-Spielmeyer d.

Stargardt's d. [MIM*248200], fundus flavimaculatus initiated with atrophic macular lesions.

Steele-Richardson-Olszewski d., SYN progressive supranuclear *palsy*.

Steinert's d., SYN myotonic *dystrophy*.

Sticker's d., SYN *erythema* infectiosum.

stiff lamb d., a muscular dystrophy occurring in young lambs fed on ewe's milk or on feed that is deficient in vitamin E or selenium, or both. SEE ALSO white muscle d.

Still's d., a form of juvenile chronic arthritis (formerly juvenile rheumatoid arthritis) characterized by high fever and signs of systemic illness that can exist for months before the onset of arthritis.

Stokes-Adams d., SYN Adams-Stokes *syndrome*.

stone-mason's d., SYN silicosis.

storage d., a generic term that includes any accumulation of a specific substance within tissues, generally because of congenital deficiency of an enzyme necessary for further metabolism of the substance; *e.g.*, glycogen-storage d.'s.

Strümpell-Marie d., SYN ankylosing *spondylitis*.

Strümpell's d., (**1**) SYN *spondylitis* deformans. (**2**) SYN acute epidemic *leukoencephalitis*.

Strümpell-Westphal d., SYN Wilson's d. (1).

Sturge-Weber d., SYN Sturge-Weber *syndrome*.

Stuttgart d., the uremic form of canine leptospirosis. SYN canine typhus.

Sulzberger-Garbe d., d. resembling an exudative form of nummular eczema described in Jewish males with oval lesions on the penis, trunk, and face. SYN exudative discoid and lichenoid dermatitis, Sulzberger-Garbe syndrome.

Sutton's d., (**1**) SYN halo *nevus*. [R. L. Sutton] (**2**) SYN *aphthae* major, under *aphtha*. [R. L. Sutton, Jr.]

Swediauer's d., SYN Albert's d.

sweet clover d., a hemorrhagic d., due to dicumarol which causes marked reduction in prothrombin, occurring in cattle fed on sweet clover fodder, spoiled during curing.

Sweet's d., SYN acute febrile neutrophilic *dermatosis*.

Swift's d., SYN acrodynia (2).

swineherd's d., a leptospirosis caused by a leptospira occurring in those who attend swine or who are occupied in the slaughtering or processing of pork, and characterized by aches and pains throughout the body, fever, headache, dizziness, and nausea.

swine vesicular d., a contagious disease of swine caused by a porcine enterovirus of the family Picornaviridae, closely related to the human enterovirus Coxsackie B-5, and characterized by vesicular lesions and erosions of the epithelium of the mouth, nares, snout, and feet; human infections have been reported in laboratory workers.

swollen belly d., a fatal d. of infants infected with *Strongyloides fuelleborni* subsp. *kellyi*; appears in localized areas of New Guinea. SYN swollen belly syndrome.

Sydenham's d., SYN Sydenham's *chorea*.

Sylvest's d., SYN epidemic *pleurodynia*.

systemic autoimmune d.'s, a group of connective tissue d.'s characterized by the presence of autoantibodies responsible for immunopathologically mediated tissue lesions; systemic lupus erythematosus is the prototype.

systemic febrile d.'s, generic term for diseases characterized by fever.

Takahara's d., SYN acatalasia.

Takayasu's d., SYN Takayasu's *arteritis*.

Tangier d., SYN analphalipoproteinemia. [an island in the Chesapeake Bay, home of the family of first cases described]

Taussig-Bing d., SYN Taussig-Bing *syndrome*.

Taylor's d., diffuse idiopathic cutaneous atrophy.

Tay-Sachs d., a lysosomal storage disease, resulting from hexosaminidase A deficiency. The monosialoganglioside is stored in central and peripheral neuronal cells. Infants present with hyperacusis and irritability, hypotonia, and failure to develop motor skills. Blindness with macular cherry red spots and seizures are evident in the first year. Death occurs within a few years. Autosomal-recessive transmission; found primarily in Jewish populations. SYN infantile G_{M2} gangliosidosis.

Teschen d., porcine polioencephalomyelitis; a d. of swine caused by porcine enterovirus 1 and resembling human poliomyelitis; it is characterized by stiffness, convulsions, paralysis, and prostration, and is widespread in Europe, with most serious losses occurring in Poland and the Czech Republic and Slóvakia. SYN infectious porcine encephalomyelitis, porcine polioencephalomyelitis. [*Teschen*, Silisia]

Theiler's d., (**1**) SYN mouse *encephalomyelitis*. (**2**) SYN equine serum *hepatitis*.

Thiemann's d., SYN Thiemann's *syndrome*.

third d., SYN rubella.

Thomsen's d., SYN *myotonia* congenita.

Thygeson's d., SYN superficial punctate *keratitis*.

thyrocardiac d., heart d. resulting from hyperthyroidism.

thyrotoxic heart d., cardiac symptoms, signs, and physiologic impairment due to overactivity of the thyroid gland usually due to excessive sympathetic stimulation.

Tommaselli's d., hemoglobinuria and pyrexia due to quinine intoxication.

Tornwaldt's d., inflammation or obstruction of the pharyngeal bursa or an adenoid cleft with the formation of a cyst containing pus.

torsion d. of childhood, SYN *dystonia* musculorum deformans.

Tourette's d., SYN Tourette *syndrome*.

Trevor's d., SYN tarsoepiphyseal *aclasis*.

tropical d.'s, infectious and parasitic d.'s endemic in tropical and subtropical zones, including Chagas' disease, leishmaniasis, leprosy, malaria, onchocerciasis, schistosomiasis, sleeping sickness, yellow fever, and others; often water- or insect-borne. SEE ALSO emerging *viruses*, under *virus*.

tsutsugamushi d. (sū'sū-gă-mū'shē), an acute infectious disease, caused by *Rickettsia tsutsugamushi* and transmitted by *Trombicula akamushi* and *T. deliensis*, that occurs in harvesters of hemp in some parts of Japan; characterized by fever, painful swelling of the lymphatic glands, a small blackish scab on the genitals, neck, or axilla, and an eruption of large dark red papules. SYN akamushi d., flood fever, inundation fever, island d., island fever, Japanese river fever, kedani fever, mite typhus, scrub typhus, shimamushi d., tropical typhus, tsutsugamushi fever.

tunnel d., SYN ancylostomiasis.

Tyzzer's d., an acute d. of many animal species (especially laboratory animals such as mice and rabbits) caused by the bacterium *Bacillus piliformis* and characterized by depression, diarrhea, and sudden death.

Underwood's d., SYN *sclerema* neonatorum.

Unna's d., SYN seborrheic *dermatitis*.

Unverricht's d. [MIM*254800], a progressive myoclonic epilepsy; one of the degenerative gray matter disorders characterized by myoclonus and generalized seizures, with progressive neurological and intellectual decline; age of onset between 8 and 13 years of age; autosomal recessive inheritance.

Urbach-Wiethe d., SYN lipoid *proteinosis*.

vagabond's d., SYN parasitic *melanoderma*.

vagrant's d., SYN parasitic *melanoderma*.

van Buren's d., SYN Peyronie's d.

Vaquez' d., SYN *polycythemia* vera.

veldt d., SYN heartwater.

venereal d., any contagious d. acquired during sexual contact; *e.g.,* syphilis, gonorrhea, chancroid.

veno-occlusive d. of the liver, obliterating endophlebitis of small hepatic vein radicles, described in Jamaican children, associated with ingestion of toxic plant substances in bush tea; causes ascites, which may progress to cirrhosis.

Vidal's d., obsolete term for *lichen* simplex chronicus.

Vincent's d., SYN necrotizing ulcerative *gingivitis*.

Virchow's d., SYN megacephaly.

virus X d., a term applied to a number of virus d.'s of obscure etiology, *e.g.,* Australian X d. (Murray Valley encephalitis).

Vogt-Spielmeyer d., SYN Spielmeyer-Vogt d.

Voltolini's d., d. of the labyrinth, leading to deafmutism, in young children.

von Economo's d., A unique encephalitis, presumably viral in origin, which followed the influenza pandemic of 1914–1918. Symptoms included ophthalmoplegia and marked somnolence, and in many survivors, the delayed development of Parkinson's disease; the basis for postencephalitic Parkinsonism. SYN encephalitis lethargica, polioencephalitis infectiva.

von Gierke's d., SYN type 1 *glycogenosis*.

von Meyenburg's d., SYN relapsing *polychondritis*.

von Recklinghausen d., SYN neurofibromatosis.

von Willebrand's d. [MIM*193400], a hemorrhagic diathesis characterized by tendency to bleed primarily from mucous membranes, prolonged bleeding time, normal platelet count, normal clot retraction, partial and variable deficiency of factor VIIIR, and possibly a morphologic defect of platelets; autosomal dominant inheritance with reduced penetrance and variable expressivity. Type III von Willebrand's d. is a more severe disorder with

markedly reduced factor VIIIR levels. There is a recessive version of this disease [MIM*277480] which has the remarkable property that it represents a mutation at the same locus as the undominant form.

Voorhoeve's d., SYN *osteopathia* striata.

Wagner's d., SYN hyaloideoretinal *degeneration*.

Wardrop's d., SYN *onychia* maligna.

wasting d., SYN runt d.

Weber-Christian d., SYN relapsing febrile nodular nonsuppurative *panniculitis*.

Wegner's d., SYN syphilitic *osteochondritis*.

Weil's d., A form of leptospirosis generally caused by *Leptospira interrogans* serogroup *icterohaemorrhagiae*, believed to be acquired by contact with the urine of infected rats; characterized clinically by fever, jaundice, muscular pains, conjunctival congestion, and albuminuria; agglutinins regularly appear in the serum. SYN infectious icterus, infectious jaundice (1), Larrey-Weil d.

Weir Mitchell's d., SYN erythromelalgia.

Werdnig-Hoffmann d., SYN infantile spinal muscular *atrophy*.

Werlhof's d., obsolete term for idiopathic thrombocytopenic *purpura*.

Wernicke's d., SYN Wernicke's *syndrome*.

Werther's d., SYN *dermatitis* nodularis necrotica.

Wesselsbron d., SYN Wesselsbron *fever*.

Westphal's d., SYN Wilson's d. (1).

Whipple's d., a rare d. characterized by steatorrhea, frequently generalized lymphadenopathy, arthritis, fever, and cough; many "foamy" macrophages are found in the jejunal lamina propria; lymph nodes contain periodic acid-Schiff positive particles that appear bacilliform by electron microscopy.

white muscle d., a nutritional myopathy of young animals, manifested by stiffness and soreness; cardiac muscle damage is frequent, and affected muscles exhibit whitish, chalklike streaks, which are degenerated fibers; it is due to a deficiency of vitamin E or selenium, or both, and is seen most frequently in calves and lambs but has also been reported in other species.

white spot d., SYN *morphea* guttata.

Whitmore's d., SYN melioidosis.

Wilkie's d., SYN superior mesenteric artery *syndrome*.

Wilson's d., (1) disorder characterized by cirrhosis, d. in the basal ganglia of the brain, and deposition of green pigment in the periphery of the cornea; the plasma levels of ceruloplasmin and copper are decreased, urinary excretion of copper is increased, and the amounts of copper in the liver, brain, kidneys, and lenticular nucleus are unusually high, while cytochrome oxidase is reduced; autosomal recessive inheritance; SYN hepatolenticular degeneration (2), hepatolenticular d., lenticular progressive degeneration, pseudosclerosis (2), Strümpell-Westphal d., Westphal's d., Westphal's pseudosclerosis, Westphal-Strümpell pseudosclerosis, Wilson's syndrome. SEE ALSO Kayser-Fleischer *ring*. [S. A. K. Wilson] **(2)** SYN exfoliative *dermatitis*. [Sir W.J.E. Wilson]

Winiwarter-Buerger d., SYN *thromboangiitis* obliterans.

Winkler's d., SYN chondrodermatitis nodularis chronica helicis.

Wohlfart-Kugelberg-Welander d., SYN juvenile spinal muscular *atrophy*.

Wolman's d., SEE cholesterol ester storage d. Cf. cholesterol ester storage d.

woolsorter's d., wool-sorter's d., SYN pulmonary *anthrax*.

Woringer-Kolopp d., a benign localized form of lymphoma with solitary or closely grouped cutaneous tumors consisting of predominantly epidermal infiltration of mononuclear cells resembling those found in mycosis fungoides. SYN pagetoid reticulosis.

X d., one of several viral d.'s of obscure etiology.

X d. of cattle, SYN bovine *hyperkeratosis*.

yellow d., SYN xanthochromia.

Ziehen-Oppenheim d., SYN *dystonia* musculorum deformans.

---

dis·en·gage·ment (dis-en-gāj'ment). **1.** The act of setting free or extricating; in childbirth, the emergence of the head from the vulva. **2.** Ascent of the presenting part from the pelvis after the inlet has been negotiated. [Fr.]

dis·e·qui·lib·ri·um (dis-ē′kwi-lib′rē-ŭm). A disturbance or absence of equilibrium.

genetic d., a state in the genetic composition of a population which under selection may be expected to change toward an equilibrium or absorbing state.

linkage d., a state involving two loci in which the probability of a joint gamete is not equal to the product of the probabilities of the constituent genes. The difference between these quantities is the increase of the d.; there are many causes of the d.

dis·ger·mi·no·ma (dis-jer-mi-nō′mă). SYN dysgerminoma.

DISH Abbreviation for diffuse idiopathic skeletal *hyperostosis*.

dish. A shallow container, usually concave.

Petri d., a small, shallow, circular d. made of thin glass or clear plastic with a loosely fitting, overlapping cover used especially in microbiology for the cultivation of microorganisms on solid media; it is frequently referred to as a plate.

Stender d., a flat shallow vessel used in staining sections.

dis·har·mo·ny (dis-har′mŏ-nē). The state of being deranged or lacking in orderliness.

occlusal d., (1) contacts of opposing occlusal surfaces of teeth which are not in harmony with other tooth contacts and with the anatomic and physiologic control of the mandible; **(2)** occlusions which do not coincide with their respective jaw relations. SEE ALSO deflective occlusal *contact*.

DISIDA Abbreviation for diisopropyl iminodiacetic acid or disofenin.

dis·im·pac·tion (dis′im-pak′shŭn). Separation of impaction in a fractured bone. **2.** Removal of feces, usually manually, in fecal impaction.

dis·in·fect (dis-in-fekt′). To destroy pathogenic microorganisms in or on any substance or to inhibit their growth and vital activity.

dis·in·fec·tant (dis-in-fek′tănt). **1.** Capable of destroying pathogenic microorganisms or inhibiting their growth activity. **2.** An agent that possesses this property.

complete d., a d. that kills both vegetative forms and spores.

incomplete d., a d. that kills only the vegetative forms, leaving the spores uninjured.

dis·in·fec·tion (dis-in-fek′shŭn). Destruction of pathogenic microorganisms or their toxins or vectors by direct exposure to chemical or physical agents.

concurrent d., application of disinfective measures as soon as possible after discharge of infectious material from the body of an infected person, or after soiling of articles with such infectious discharges.

terminal d., application of disinfective measures after the patient has been removed, *e.g.,* by death, or has ceased to be a source of infection.

dis·in·fes·ta·tion. Physical or chemical process to destroy or remove small undesirable animal forms, particularly arthropods or rodents, present upon the person, clothing, or environment of an individual or domestic animals.

dis·in·hi·bi·tion (dis′in-hi-bish′ŭn). Inhibition of an inhibition; removal of an inhibitory effect by a stimulus, as when a conditioned reflex has undergone extinction but is restored by some extraneous stimulus.

dis·in·sec·tion, dis·in·sec·ti·za·tion (dis-in-sek′shŭn, dis′in-sek-ti-zā′shŭn). Freeing an area from insects. [L. *dis-,* apart, + insect]

dis·in·te·gra·tion (dis-in-tĕ-grā′shŭn). **1.** Loss or separation of the component parts of a substance, as in catabolism or decay. **2.** Disorganization of psychic and behavioral processes. [dis- + L. *integer,* whole, intact]

dis·in·vag·i·na·tion (dis′in-vaj-i-nā′shŭn). Relieving an invagination.

dis·junc·tion (dis-jŭnk′shŭn). The normal separation of pairs of chromosomes at the anaphase stage of meiosis I or II. [dis- + L. *junctio,* a joining, fr. *jungo,* pp. *junctum,* to join]

disk. 1. SYN lamella (2). **2.** In dentistry, a circular piece of thin paper or other material, coated with an abrasive substance, used for cutting and polishing teeth and fillings. [L. *discus;* G. *diskos,* a quoit, disk]

A d.'s, SYN A *bands,* under band.

acromioclavicular d., SYN articular *disc* of acromioclavicular joint.

anisotropic d.'s, SYN A *bands,* under band.

articular d., SYN articular *disc*.

articular d. of temporomandibular joint, the fibrocartilaginous plate that separates the joint into upper and lower cavities. SYN discus articularis temporomandibularis [NA], mandibular d., temporomandibular articular d.

blastodermic d., the aggregation of blastomeres of a telolecithal ovum after cleavage has occurred.

blood d., SYN platelet.

Bowman's d.'s, d.'s resulting from transverse segmentation of striated muscular fiber treated with weak acids, certain alkaline solutions, or freezing.

Burlew d., an abrasive-impregnated rubber wheel used in dentistry for polishing. SYN Burlew wheel.

choked d., SYN papilledema.

ciliary d., SYN orbiculus ciliaris.

cone d.'s, membranous d.'s of flattened sacs about 14 nm thick that occur in the outer segment of cones of the retina.

cuttlefish d., a circle of paper or thin plastic coated with ground cuttlefish bone; used, when attached to a mandrel and rotated by a dental handpiece, for fine smoothing and finishing of dental materials and tooth.

diamond d., a steel d. with the cutting surface(s) covered with fine diamond chips, for use in a dental handpiece.

embryonic d., SYN germinal d.

emery d.'s, d.'s of paper or other materials coated with emery powder used to abrade or smooth the surface of teeth or fillings.

germinal d., germ d., the point in a telolecithal ovum where the embryo begins to be formed. SYN embryonic d., germinal area, area germinativa.

H d., SYN H *band*.

hair d., a richly innervated area of skin around a hair follicle, consisting of a thickened layer of epithelial cells in which ramify unmyelinated terminals of a single axon.

Hensen's d., SYN H *band*.

herniated d., protrusion of a degenerated or fragmented intervertebral d. into the intervertebral foramen with potential compression of a nerve root or into the spinal canal with potential compression of the cauda equina in the lumbar region or the spinal cord at higher levels. SYN protruded d., ruptured d.

I d., SYN I *band*.

intercalated d., a specialized intercellular attachment of cardiac muscle comprising gap junctions, fascia adherens, and occasionally desmosomes.

intermediate d., SYN Z *line*.

interpubic d., SYN interpubic *disc*.

intervertebral d., SYN intervertebral *disc*.

isotropic d., SYN I *band*.

mandibular d., SYN articular d. of temporomandibular joint.

Merkel's tactile d., SYN tactile *meniscus*.

Newton's d., a d. on which are seven colored sectors, each occupying proportionally the same space as the corresponding primary color in the spectrum; when the disk is rapidly rotated it appears white.

optic d., an oval area of the ocular fundus devoid of light receptors where the axons of the retinal ganglion cell converge to form the optic nerve head; SYN discus nervi optici [NA], blind spot (3), Mariotte's blind spot, optic nerve head, optic papilla, papilla nervi optici, porus opticus.

Placido da Costa's d., SYN keratoscope.

proligerous d., SYN *cumulus* oöphorus.

protruded d., SYN herniated d.

Q d.'s, SYN A *bands,* under *band*.

radioulnar d., radioulnar articular d., SYN articular *disc* of distal radioulnar joint.

Ranvier's d.'s, tactile nerve endings, of cupped disklike form, in the skin.

rod d.'s, membranous d.'s of flattened sacs about 14 nm thick that occur in the outer segment of rods of the retina.

ruptured d., SYN herniated d.

sandpaper d.'s, d.'s of paper coated with various grits of silica; used to abrade or smooth the surface of teeth or dental materials.

stenopeic d., stenopaic d., a metallic or other opaque d. with a narrow slit through which one looks; used as a test for astigmatism.

sternoclavicular d., sternoclavicular articular d., SYN articular *disc* of sternoclavicular joint.

stroboscopic d., a revolving d. that gives successive views of a moving object.

tactile d., SYN tactile *meniscus.*

temporomandibular articular d., SYN articular d. of temporomandibular joint.

transverse d., one of the dark transverse bands seen on examining a striated muscular fiber under the microscope.

triangular d. of wrist, SYN articular *disc* of distal radioulnar joint.

Z d., SYN Z *line.*

dis·ki·tis (dis-kī'tis). SYN discitis.

⊘**disko-.** SEE disco-.

dis·ko·gram (dis'kō-gram). The graphic record, usually radiographic, of diskography.

dis·kog·ra·phy (dis-kog'ră-fē). Radiographic demonstration of intervertebral disk by injection of contrast media into the nucleus pulposus. [disco- + G. *graphō,* to write]

dis·lo·cate (dis'lō-kāt). To luxate; to put out of joint.

dis·lo·ca·tio (dis-lō-kā'shē-ō). SYN dislocation. [L.]

d. erec'ta, a subglenoid dislocation of the shoulder in which, when the arm is held vertically with the hand on top of the head, the head of the humerus is inferiorly placed.

dis·lo·ca·tion (dis-lō-kā'shŭn). Displacement of an organ or any part; specifically a disturbance or disarrangement of the normal relation of the bones entering into the formation of a joint. SYN dislocatio, luxation (1). [L. *dislocatio,* fr. *dis-,* apart, + *locatio,* a placing]

d. of articular processes, complete d. of one or both articular processes, usually with overriding of the inferior articular process of the vertebra above into a position anterior to the superior articular process of the vertebra below. SYN locked facets.

closed d., a d. not complicated by an external wound. SYN simple d.

compound d., SYN open d.

fracture d., dislocation associated with or accompanied by a fracture.

Kienböck's d., d. of semilunar bone.

Nélaton's d., wedging of the astragalus between the widely separated tibia and fibula, usually complicated with fracture.

open d., a d. complicated by a wound opening from the surface down to the affected joint. SYN compound d.

perilunar d., d. of carpal bones around the lunate, which remains in relation to the radius; distinguish from d. of lunate, Kienböck's d.

simple d., SYN closed d.

dis·mem·ber (dis-mem'ber). To amputate an arm or leg.

dis·mu·tase (dis'myū-tās). Generic name for enzymes catalyzing the reaction of two identical molecules to produce two molecules in differing states of oxidation (*e.g.,* superoxide dismutase) or of phosphorylation (*e.g.,* glucose 1-phosphate phosphodismutase).

dis·mu·ta·tion (dis'myū-tā'shŭn). A reaction involving a single substance but producing two products; *e.g.,* two molecules of acetaldehyde may react, producing an oxidation product (acetic acid) and a reduction product (ethyl alcohol).

diso·bli·ter·a·tion (dis'ob-lit-er-ā'shŭn). Opening of a pathologically closed channel.

di·so·fen·in (dī'sō-fen-in). SYN diisopropyl iminodiacetic acid.

di·so·mic (dī-sō'mik). Relating to disomy.

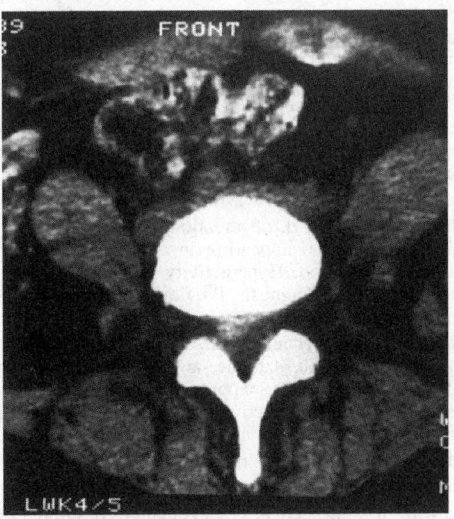

herniated disk
at the fourth and fifth lumbar vertebrae, right mediolateral
(computed tomography)

di·so·my (dī'sō-mē). The state of an individual or cell having two members of a pair of homologous chromosomes; the normal state in humans, in contrast to monosomy and trisomy. **2.** An abnormal chromosome represented twice in a single cell. [G. *dis,* two, + *sōma,* body]

di·so·pro·mine (di-sō-prō'mēn). SYN diisopromine.

di·so·pyr·a·mide (dī-sō-pir'ă-mīd). α-[2-(Diisopropylamino)-ethyl]-α-phenyl-2-pyridineacetamide; an antiarrhythmic drug.

dis·or·der (dis-ōr'der). A disturbance of function, structure, or both, resulting from a genetic or embryologic failure in development or from exogenous factors such as poison, trauma, or disease.

adjustment d.'s, (1) a class of mental and behavioral d.'s in which the development of symptoms is related to the presence of some environmental stressor or life event and is expected to remit when the stress ceases; (2) a d. whose essential feature is a maladaptive reaction to an identifiable psychological stress, or stressors, that occurs within weeks of the onset of the stressors and persists for up to six months; the maladaptive nature of the reaction is indicated by impairment in occupational (including school) functioning, or in usual social activities or relationships with others, or with symptoms that are in excess of a normal or expectable reaction to the stressor.

affective d.'s, a class of mental d.'s characterized by a disturbance in mood.

affective personality d., a disturbance of feelings or mood expressed as a milder form of depression and related emotional features that color the whole psychic life and for which psychosocial stressors are believed to play the major role.

antisocial personality d., a personality d. characterized by a history of continuous and chronic antisocial behavior with disregard for and violation of the rights of others, beginning before the age of 15; early childhood signs include chronic lying, stealing, fighting, and truancy; in adolescence there may be unusually early or aggressive sexual behavior, excessive drinking, and use of illicit drugs, such behavior continuing in adulthood.

anxiety d.'s, a category of interrelated mental illnesses involving anxiety reactions in response to stress. The types include: 1) generalized anxiety, by far the most prevalent condition, which strikes slightly more females than males, mostly in the 20–35 age group; 2) panic d., in which a person suffers repeated panic attacks. Some 2–5 percent of Americans are subject to this ailment, about twice as many women as men; 3) obsessive-compulsive d., afflicting 2–3 percent of the U.S. population. About two-thirds of these patients go on to experience a major depressive episode; 4) posttraumatic stress disorder, most frequent among combat veterans or survivors of major physical trauma; and 5) the phobias (*e.g.*, fear of snakes, crowds, confinement, heights, etc.), which on a minor scale affect about one in eight people in the U.S. Drugs that have proven effective against anxiety d.'s are beta blockers, which act on adrenaline receptors; anxiolytics; antidepressants; and serotonergic drugs. Regular exercise has also proved beneficial.

asthenic personality d., SYN asthenic *personality.*

attention deficit d., a d. of attention and impulse control with specific DSM criteria, appearing in childhood and sometimes persisting to adulthood. Hyperactivity may be a feature, but is not necessary for the diagnosis. Previously erroneously identified as minimal brain dysfunction.

attention deficit hyperactivity d., a disorder of childhood and adolescence manifested at home, in school, and in social situations by developmentally inappropriate degrees of inattention, impulsiveness, and hyperactivity; also called hyperactivity or hyperactive child syndrome. SYN hyperactive child syndrome.

autistic d., SYN autism, infantile *autism.*

autonomic d., disorganization of autonomic processes.

avoidant d. of adolescence, SYN avoidant d. of childhood.

avoidant d. of childhood, a mental d. occurring in childhood or adolescence characterized by an excessive shrinking away from contact with people who are unfamiliar. SYN avoidant d. of adolescence.

avoidant personality d., SEE avoidant *personality.*

behavior d., general term used to denote mental illness or psychological dysfunction, specifically those mental, emotional, or behavioral subclasses for which organic correlates do not exist. SEE antisocial personality d.

bipolar d., an affective d. characterized by the occurrence of alternating periods of euphoria (mania) and depression. SYN manic-depressive psychosis.

body dysmorphic d., a psychosomatic (somatoform) d. characterized by preoccupation with some imagined defect in appearance in a normal-appearing person. SYN dysmorphophobia.

borderline personality d., a mental d. in which the symptoms are not continually psychotic yet are not strictly neurotic: may include impulsivity and unpredictability, unstable interpersonal relationships, inappropriate or uncontrolled anger, identity disturbances, rapid shifts of mood, suicidal acts, self-mutilations, job and marital instability, chronic feelings of emptiness or boredom, and intolerance of being alone.

character d., a term referring to a group of behavioral d.'s, now replaced by a more general term, personality d., of which character d.'s are now a subclass.

conduct d., a mental d. of childhood or adolescence characterized by a persistent pattern of of violating societal norms and the rights of others; children with the d. may exhibit physical aggression, cruelty to animals, vandalism and robbery, along with truancy, cheating, and lying. SEE borderline personality d.

conversion d., a mental d. in which an unconscious emotional conflict is expressed as an alteration or loss of physical functioning, usually controlled by the voluntary nervous system.

cumulative trauma d.'s (CTD), chronic d.'s involving muscle inflammation and nerve damage, often resulting from work-related physical activities.

CTDs now account for half of all occupational illnesses in the U.S. The ailments, including repetitive motion disorders and carpal tunnel syndrome, result when the body is subjected to direct pressure, vibration, or repetitive movements for prolonged periods of time, as in the use of computer keyboards for data entry or order processing. Carpal tunnel syndrome, a swelling of the tendons in the wrist sheathing the median nerve, now accounts for 40% of all worker compensation claims and was called "the occupational disease of the 1980s." It results in temporary or permanent numbness, pain in the fingers, and loss or impairment of the ability to grasp. Generally CTDs are treated with heat or cold, corticosteroid injections, immo-

bilization, or physical therapy, but surgery is also performed—over 100,000 operations each year for carpal tunnel syndrome alone. Prevention appears to be the best approach. Workers at risk of CTDs are advised to suspend the responsible activity for 15 minutes every 2 hours. Physicans can play a role by becoming involved in ergonomic assessments of the workplace.

cyclothymic d., an affective d. characterized by mood swings including periods of hypomania and depression; a form of depressive disorder.

cyclothymic personality d., SYN cyclothymic *personality.*

delusional d., a severe mental d. characterized by the presence of delusions. The delusions may be related to paranoid, grandiose, somatic, or erotic themes.

dependent personality d., SYN asthenic *personality.*

depersonalization d., SYN schizophrenia.

dissociative d.'s, a group of mental d.'s characterized by a disturbance in functions of identity, memory, and consciousness; includes multiple personality d., psychogenic fugue, psychogenic amnesia, and depersonalization d.

dysthymic d., a chronic disturbance of mood characterized by mild depression or loss of interest in usual activities. SEE depression.

eating d.'s, a class of mental d.'s including anorexia nervosa, bulimia nervosa, pica, and rumination d. of infancy.

emotional d., SEE mental *illness,* behavior d.

erotomanic type of paranoid d., the false belief that one is loved by another such as a movie star or a casual acquaintance.

factitious d., a mental d. in which the individual intentionally produces symptoms of illness or feigns illness for psychological reasons rather than for environmental goals.

familial bipolar mood d., bipolar mood d. commonly inherited as an autosomal dominant [MIM*125480] trait and also occasionally as an X-linked one [MIM*309200].

functional d., a physical d. with no known or detectable organic basis to explain the symptoms. SEE behavior d., neurosis. SYN dynamic disease, functional disease, functional illness.

Gaucher d., SYN Gaucher's *disease.*

gender identity d.'s, a class of mental d.'s characterized by an incongruity between an assigned culturally determined set of attitudes, behavior patterns, and physical characteristics associated with masculinity or femininity and gender identity. SEE ALSO transsexualism.

generalized anxiety d., chronic, repeated episodes of anxiety reactions; a psychological d. in which anxiety or morbid fear and dread accompanied by autonomic changes are prominent features. SEE anxiety.

grandiose type of paranoid d., a delusion in which the person believes that he or she possesses some great but unrecognized talent or insight, or has made an important discovery, with subsequent efforts toward official or public recognition.

Hartnup d., SYN Hartnup *disease.*

histrionic personality d., a d. characterized by a persuasive pattern of excessive and shallow emotionality, attention-seeking, demanding of approval and reassurance, beginning in early childhood and present in a variety of contexts; also called hysterical personality disorder.

identity d., a mental d. of childhood or adolescence in which one suffers severe distress regarding one's ability to reconcile aspects of the self into a coherent acceptable sense of self.

immune complex d., SYN immune complex *disease.*

immunoproliferative d.'s, d.'s in which there is a continuing proliferation of cells of the immunocyte complex associated with autoallergic disturbances and γ-globulin abnormalities such as in chronic lymphocytic leukemia, "macroglobulinemias," and multiple myeloma.

impulse control d., a class of mental d.'s characterized by an individual's failure to resist an impulse to perform some act harmful to himself or to others; includes pathological gambling, pedophilia, kleptomania, pyromania, trichotillomania, intermittent and isolated explosive d.'s.

induced psychotic d., a severe mental disorder brought about by a toxic agent such as a drug or hallucinogen. SEE psychosis.

intermittent explosive d., an uncommon disorder that begins in early childhood, characterized by repeated acts of violent, aggressive behavior in otherwise normal persons that is markedly out of proportion to the event that provokes it. SYN dyscontrol, episodic dyscontrol syndrome.

isolated explosive d., a d. of impulse control characterized by a single episode of failure to resist a violent, externally directed act which had serious impact on others.

jealous type of paranoid d., the false belief that one's spouse or lover is unfaithful and leading to repeated confrontation, or the taking of extraordinary steps to intervene in the imagined infidelity.

kinky-hair d., SYN kinky-hair *disease.*

late luteal phase dysphoric d., SYN premenstrual *syndrome.*

LDL receptor d., abnormality in clearance of LDL from the plasma due to abnormality in LDL receptor activity; causes hypercholesterolemia.

major mood d., SEE bipolar d., affective *psychosis,* endogenous *depression,* dysthymia.

manic-depressive d., obsolete term for one of the mood disorders; *i.e.,* bipolar disorder, depression; affective psychosis, affective disorder, bipolar disorder, and endogenous depression.

mental d., a psychological syndrome or behavioral pattern that is associated with either subjective distress or objective impairment. SEE ALSO mental *illness,* behavior d.

---

mood d.'s, a group of mental disorders involving a disturbance of mood, accompanied by either a full or partial manic or depressive syndrome that is not due to any other physical or mental disorder. Mood refers to a prolonged emotion that colors the whole psychic life; it generally involves either depression or elation; *e.g.,* manic episode, major depressive episode, bipolar disorders, and depressive disorder (see separate entries for each).

> Established in 1987 for the revised edition of the Diagnostic and Statistical Manual III, this category includes types of depression (formerly unipolar depression) and manic depression (formerly bipolar depression), as well as conditions with cyclic patterns, such as seasonal affective disorder (SAD). Many of the mood disorders, which have proven unresponsive to traditional psychological talk therapies, are highly responsive to treatment with drugs.

---

multiple personality d., a sudden, gradual, transient, or chronic psychological disorder whose essential feature is a disturbance or alteration in the normally integrated functions of identity, memory, or consciousness. SEE ALSO multiple *personality.*

narcissistic personality d., a psychological d. with a pervasive pattern of grandiosity (in fantasy or behavior), hypersensitivity to the evaluation of others, and lack of empathy that begins by early adulthood and is manifested in a variety of contexts.

neuropsychologic d., a disturbance of mental function due to brain trauma, associated with one of more of the following: neurocognitive, psychotic, neurotic, behavioral, or psychophysiologic manifestations, or mental impairment. SEE ALSO mental *illness.*

obsessive-compulsive d., a type of anxiety d. whose essential feature is recurrent obsessions, persistent, intrusive ideas, thoughts, impulses or images, or compulsions (repetitive, purposeful, and intentional behaviors performed in response to an obsession) sufficiently severe to cause marked distress, be time-consuming, or to significantly interfere with the individual's normal routine, occupational functioning, or usual social activities or relationships with others. SEE ALSO obsessive-compulsive personality d. SYN obsessive-compulsive neurosis.

obsessive-compulsive personality d., a psychological d. with a pervasive pattern of inflexible perfectionism which begins by early adulthood as indicated by many of the following symptoms: (1) an unattainable perfectionism with overly strict standards which often make it impossible to complete a task; (2) preoccupation with details, rules, lists, order, organization, or

scheduling to the extent that the major point of the activity is lost; (3) unreasonable insistence that others submit to exactly his or her way of doing things; (4) an unnecessary, excessive devotion to work and productivity to the exclusion of leisure activities and friendships; (5) rumination to the point of indecisiveness; (6) overconscientiousness about matters of morality, ethics, or values; (7) restricted expression of affection; (8) lack of generosity in giving time, money, or gifts when no personal gain is likely to result; and (9) an inability to discard worn-out or worthless objects even when they have no sentimental value. SYN obsessional neurosis.

oppositional d., a mental d. of childhood or adolescence marked by a pattern of disobedient, negativistic, and provocative opposition to authority figures.

organic mental d., a psychological, cognitive, or behavioral abnormality associated with transient or permanent dysfunction of the brain, usually characterized by the presence of an organic mental *syndrome.*

overanxious d., a mental d. of childhood or adolescence marked by excessive worrying and fearful behavior not related specifically to separation or due to recent stress.

panic d., recurrent panic attacks that occur unpredictably. SEE generalized anxiety d.

paranoid d., SYN delusion.

paranoid personality d., a personality d. that is less debilitating than is the paranoid or delusional paranoid d.; the essential feature is a pervasive and unwarranted tendency, beginning in early adulthood and present in a variety of contexts, to misinterpret the actions of others as deliberately exploitive, harmful, demeaning, or threatening.

persecutory type of paranoid d., one of the most common of the types of paranoid disorders, it involves a single theme or series of connected themes, such as being conspired against, cheated, spied on, followed, poisoned or drugged, maligned, harassed, or obstructed in the pursuit of long-term goals; small slights may be exaggerated and become the focus of a delusional system. SEE paranoia. Cf. paranoid personality d.

personality d., general term for a group of behavioral d.'s characterized by usually lifelong, ingrained, maladaptive patterns of deviant behavior, life style, and social adjustment that are different in quality from psychotic and neurotic symptoms; former designations for individuals with these personality d.'s were psychopath and sociopath. SEE ALSO antisocial personality d.

pervasive developmental d., a class of mental disorders of infancy, childhood, or adolescence characterized by distortions in the development of the multiple basic psychological functions involved in the development of social skills and language.

plasma iodoprotein d., SEE familial *goiter.*

posttraumatic stress d., development of characteristic symptoms following a psychologically traumatic event that is generally outside the range of usual human experience; symptoms include numbed responsiveness to environmental stimuli, a variety of autonomic and cognitive dysfunctions, and dysphoria.

psychogenic pain d., a d. in which the principal complaint is pain that is out of proportion to objective findings and that is related to psychological factors.

psychosomatic d., psychophysiologic d., a d. characterized by physical symptoms of psychic origin, usually involving a single organ system innervated by the autonomic nervous system; physiological and organic changes stem from a sustained disturbance.

reactive attachment d., a mental d. of infancy or early childhood characterized by disturbed social relatedness; thought to be caused by grossly pathologic care.

REM behavior d., a d. characterized by lack of the atonia of voluntary muscles that normally occurs in REM sleep.

rumination d., a mental d. occurring in infancy characterized by repeated regurgitation of food; usually accompanied by weight loss or failure to gain weight.

schizophreniform d. (skiz′ō-fren′ĭ-fōrm), a d. whose essential features are identical with those of schizophrenia, with the exception that the duration including prodromal, active, and residual phases is less than six months.

seasonal affective d. (SAD), a depressive mood disorder that

di

occurs at approximately the same time year after year and spontaneously remits at the same time each year. The most common type is winter depression and it is characterized by morning hypersomnia, low energy, increased appetite, weight gain, and carbohydrate craving, all of which remit in the spring.

separation anxiety d., a mental d. occurring in childhood characterized by excessive anxiety when the child is separated from someone to whom the child is attached, usually a parent.

shared psychotic d., SYN *folie* à deux.

sleep terror d., SEE night-terrors.

somatization d., a mental d. characterized by presentation of a complicated medical history and of physical symptoms referring to a variety of organ systems, but without a detectable or known organic basis. SEE conversion, hysteria.

somatoform d., a group of d.'s in which physical symptoms suggesting physical d.'s for which there are no demonstrable organic findings or known physiologic mechanisms, and for which there is positive evidence, or a strong presumption that the symptoms are linked to psychological factors; *e.g.,* hysteria, conversion disorder, hypochondriasis, and pain disorder.

substance abuse d.'s, a class of mental d.'s in which behavioral and biological changes are associated with regular use of alcohol, drugs, and related substances that affect the central nervous system and personal and social functioning.

substance-induced organic mental d.'s, mental d.'s caused by use of drugs, *e.g.,* cocaine.

thought process d., an intellectual function symptom of schizophrenia, manifested by irrelevance and incoherence of verbal productions ranging from simple blocking and mild circumstantiality to total loosening of associations.

visceral d., nomenclature used in reference to psychosomatic d.

dis·or·ga·ni·za·tion (dis-ōr′gan-i-zā′shŭn). Destruction of an organ or tissue with consequent loss of function.

dis·o·ri·en·ta·tion (dis′ōr-ē-en-tā′shŭn). Loss of the sense of familiarity with one's surroundings (time, place, and person); loss of one's bearings.

dis·par·ate (dis′pa-răt). Unequal; not alike. [L. *dis-paro,* pp. -*atus,* to separate, fr. *paro,* to prepare]

dis·par·i·ty (dis-par′i-tē). The condition of being disparate. [L. *dispar,* dissimilar]

fixation d., the amount of heterophoria possible with fusion present.

retinal d., the slight difference in retinal images that arises because of the lateral separation of the two eyes that stimulates stereoscopic vision.

dis·pen·sa·ry (dis-pen′ser-ē). **1.** A physician's office, especially the office of one who dispenses medicines. **2.** The office of a hospital pharmacist, where medicines are given out on physicians' orders. **3.** An outpatient department of a hospital. [L. *dis-penso,* pp. -*atus,* to distribute by weight, fr. *penso,* to weigh]

Dis·pen·sa·to·ry (dis-pen′să-tō-rē). A work originally intended as a commentary on the Pharmacopeia, but now more of a supplement to that work, which contains an account of the sources, mode of preparation, physiologic action, and therapeutic uses of most of the agents, official and nonofficial; used in the treatment of disease. [L. *dispensator,* a manager, steward; see dispensary]

dis·pense (dis-pens′). To give out medicine and other necessities to the sick; to fill a medical prescription.

di·sper·my, di·sperm·ia (dī′sper-mē, dī-sperm′ē-ă). Entrance of two spermatozoa into one ovum.

dis·per·sal (dis-per′săl). SYN dispersion (1).

flash d., the property of rapid disintegration of a tablet when placed on the tongue.

dis·perse (dis-pers′). To dissipate, to cause disappearance of, to scatter, to dilute.

dis·per·sion (dis-per′zhŭn). **1.** The act of dispersing or of being dispersed. SYN dispersal. **2.** Incorporation of the particles of one substance into the mass of another, including solutions, suspensions, and colloidal dispersions (solutions). **3.** Specifically, what is usually called a colloidal *solution.* [L. *dispersio*]

coarse d., SYN suspension (4).

colloidal d., SYN colloidal *solution.*

molecular d., d. in which the dispersed phase consists of individual molecules; if the molecules are of less than colloidal size, the result is a true solution.

optical rotatory d. (ORD), the change in optical rotation with the wavelength of the incident monochromatic polarized light; the displacement of the former from zero within the absorption band is known as the Cotton *effect.*

temporal d., asynchronous repolarization of myocardial fibers that predisposes to abnormal current flow and ectopic rhythms (especially with bradyarrhythmias).

dis·per·si·ty (dis-per′si-tē). The extent to which the dimensions of particles have been reduced in colloid formation.

dis·per·soid (dis-per′soyd). A colloidal solution in which the dispersed phase can be concentrated by centrifugation. SYN dispersion colloid, molecular dispersed solution.

di·spi·reme (dī-spī′rēm). The double chromatin skein in the telophase of mitosis. [G. *di-,* twice, + *speirēma,* coil, convolution]

dis·place·a·bil·i·ty (dis-plās-ă-bil′i-tē). The capability of, or susceptibility to, displacement.

tissue d., the property of tissue that permits it to be moved from an initial or relaxed position or form. SYN compression of tissue.

dis·place·ment (dis-plās′ment). **1.** Removal from the normal location or position. **2.** The adding to a fluid (particularly a gas) in an open vessel one of greater density whereby the first is expelled. **3.** In chemistry, a change in which one element, radical, or molecule is replaced by another, or in which one element exchanges electric charges with another by reduction or oxidation. **4.** In psychiatry, the transfer of impulses from one expression to another, as from fighting to talking.

affect d., a shift of feeling from the object originally arousing it to some associated object.

mesial d., SYN mesioversion.

tissue d., the change in the form or position of tissues as a result of pressure.

Disse, Josef, German anatomist, 1852–1912. SEE D.'s *space.*

dis·sect (di-sekt′, dī-). **1.** To cut apart or separate the tissues of the body for study. **2.** In an operation, to separate the different structures along natural lines by dividing the connective tissue framework. [L. *dis-seco,* pp. -*sectus,* to cut asunder]

dis·sec·tion (di-sek′shŭn, dī-). The act of dissecting. SYN anatomy (3), necrotomy (1).

aortic d., a pathologic process, characterized by splitting of the media layer of the aorta, which leads to formation of a dissecting aneurysm. Classified according to location as follows: type I involves the ascending aorta, transverse arch, and distal aorta; type II is confined to the ascending aorta; type III extends distally in the descending aorta.

dis·sem·i·nat·ed (di-sem′i-nā-ted). Widely scattered throughout an organ, tissue, or the body. [L. *dis-semino,* pp. -*atus,* to scatter seed, fr. *semen* (-*min-*), seed]

dis·sep·i·ment (di-sep′i-ment). A separating tissue, partition, or septum. [L. *dis- sepio,* pp. -*septus,* to divide by a fence]

dis·sim·i·la·tion (di-sim-i-lā′shŭn). **1.** SYN disassimilation. **2.** SYN catabolism.

dis·sim·u·la·tion (di-sim-yū-lā′shŭn). Concealment of the truth about a situation, especially about a state of health or during a mental status examination, as by a malingerer or someone with a factitious disorder. [L. *dissimulatio,* fr. *dissimulo,* to feign, fr. *dis,* apart, + *similis,* same]

dis·so·ci·a·tion (di-sō-sē-ā′shŭn, -shē-ā′shŭn). **1.** Separation, or a dissolution of relations. SYN disassociation. **2.** The change of a complex chemical compound into a simpler one by any lytic reaction or by ionization. **3.** An unconscious process by which a group of mental processes is separated from the rest of the thinking processes, resulting in an independent functioning of these processes and a loss of the usual relationships; for example, a separation of affect from cognition. SEE multiple *personality.* [L. *dis-socio,* pp. -*atus,* to disjoin, separate, fr. *socius,* partner, ally]

albuminocytologic d., increased protein in the cerebrospinal fluid without increase in cell count, characteristic of the Guillain-Barré syndrome; it is also associated with spinal block and with intracranial neoplasia, and is seen in the last phases of poliomyelitis.

atrial d., mutually independent beating of the two atria or of parts of the atria.

atrioventricular d. (AVD), A-V d., (1) any situation in which atria and ventricles are activated and contract independently, as in complete A-V block; **(2)** more specifically, the d. between atria and ventricles that results from slowing of the atrial pacemaker or acceleration of the ventricular pacemaker at nearly equal (rarely equal) rates, each depolarizing its own chamber, thus interfering with depolarization by the other (interference-dissociation).

complete atrioventricular d., complete A-V d., (1) A-V d. not interrupted by ventricular captures; **(2)** SYN complete A-V *block*.

electromechanical d., persistence of electrical activity in the heart without associated mechanical contraction; often a sign of cardiac rupture.

incomplete atrioventricular d., incomplete A-V d., A-V d. interrupted by ventricular captures.

interference d., the simultaneous operation of two separate cardiac pacemaking foci that are unassociated because of interference (a normal physiologic phenomenon) due to rendering their respective territories refractory to each other. Usually atrioventricular d. is indicated, the rates being quite close to each other with the atrial rate slightly faster than that of the pacemaker in control of the ventricles. Capture is in either direction, usually the ventricle by the atrium, in incomplete d. h SYN d. by interference.

d. by interference, SYN interference d.

isorhythmic d., A-V d. characterized by equal or closely similar atrial and ventricular rates.

light-near d., SYN *pupillary* light-near dissociation.

longitudinal d., d. between parallel chambers of the heart, as between one atrium and the other or between one ventricle and the other, in contrast to d. between atria and ventricles.

sleep d., SYN sleep *paralysis*.

syringomyelic d., loss of pain and temperature sensation with relative retention of tactile sensation, related to a cavity in the central portion of the cord interrupting the decussation of nerve fibers.

tabetic d., loss of proprioceptive sensation with retained pain and temperature sensation due to involvement of the posterior columns of the spinal cord.

dis·solve (di-zolv). To change or cause to change from a solid to a dispersed form by immersion in a fluid of suitable properties. [L. *dis-solvo,* pp. *-solutus,* to loose asunder, to dissolve]

dis·so·nance (di′sō-nans). In social psychology and attitude theory, an aversive state which arises when an individual is minimally aware of inconsistency or conflict within himself. SEE cognitive dissonance *theory.* [L. *dissonus,* discordant, confused]

cognitive d., a motivational state studied by social and clinical psychologists which exists when a person's attitudes, perceptions, and related d. state are inconsistent with each other, *e.g.,* hating blacks but admiring Martin Luther King.

dis·sym·me·try (di-sim′ĕ-trē). SYN asymmetry. [dis- + symmetry]

dis·tad (dis′tad). Toward the periphery; in a distal direction.

dis·tal (dis′tăl). **1.** Situated away from the center of the body, or from the point of origin; specifically applied to the extremity or distant part of a limb or organ. **2.** In dentistry, away from the median sagittal plane of the face, following the curvature of the dental arch. SYN distalis [NA]. [L. *distalis*]

dis·ta·lis (dis-tā′lis) [NA]. SYN distal.

dis·tance (dis′tans). The measure of space between two objects. [L. *distantia,* fr. *di-sto,* to stand apart, be distant]

focal d., the d. from the center of a lens to its focus.

infinite d., the limit of distant vision, the rays entering the eyes from an object at that point being practically parallel. SYN infinity.

interarch d., (1) the vertical d. between the maxillary and mandibular arches under conditions of vertical dimensions which must be specified; **(2)** the vertical d. between maxillary and mandibular ridges. SYN interalveolar space, interridge d.

interocclusal d., (1) the vertical d. between the opposing occlusal surfaces, assuming rest relation unless otherwise designated; SYN interocclusal rest space (1). **(2)** SYN freeway *space*.

interridge d., SYN interarch d.

large interarch d., a large d. between the maxillary and mandibular arches; may also imply an excessive vertical dimension. SYN open bite (1).

pupillary d., the d. between the center of each pupil; the major reference points in measuring for fitting of spectacle frames and lenses.

reduced interarch d., an occluding vertical dimension which results in an excessive interocclusal d. when the mandible is in rest position, and in a reduced interridge d. when the teeth are in contact.

small interarch d., a small d. between the maxillary and mandibular arches. SYN close bite.

sociometric d., some measurable degree of mutual or social perception, acceptance, and understanding; hypothetically, greater sociometric d. is associated with more inaccuracy in evaluating a relationship (*e.g.,* it is easier to understand and deal with a native than a foreigner).

dis·tem·per (dis-tem′per). **1.** SYN canine d. **2.** SYN panleukopenia. [L. *dis-* priv. + *tempero,* to qualify, temper, fr. *tempus,* time]

canine d., a highly contagious systemic disease of dogs caused by the canine d. virus and characterized by a diphasic fever, leukopenia, gastrointestinal and respiratory catarrh and, frequently, pneumonic and neurological complications; the disease also occurs in foxes, wolves, ferrets, mink, skunks, and raccoons. SYN distemper (1).

feline d., SYN panleukopenia.

dis·ten·si·bil·i·ty (dis-ten-si-bil′i-tē). The capability of being distended or stretched. [L. *dis- tendo,* to stretch apart]

dis·ten·tion, dis·ten·sion (dis-ten′shŭn). The act or state of being distended or stretched. SEE ALSO dilation. [L. *dis-tendo,* to stretch apart]

dis·ti·chi·a·sis (dis′tĭ-kī′ă-sis). A congenital, abnormal, accessory row of eyelashes. [G. *di-* double, + *stichos,* row]

dis·till (dis-til′). To extract a substance by distillation.

dis·til·late (dis′ti-lāt). The product of distillation.

dis·til·la·tion (dis-ti-lā′shŭn). Volatilization of a liquid by heat and subsequent condensation of the vapor; a means of separating the volatile from the nonvolatile, or the more volatile from the less volatile, part of a liquid mixture. [L. *de-(di-)stillo,* pp. *-atus,* to drop down]

destructive d., SYN dry d.

dry d., submission of an organic substance to heat in a closed vessel so that oxygen is absent and combustion prevented, with the objective of effecting its decomposition with release of volatile constituents and the formation of new substances. SYN destructive d.

fractional d., d. of a compound liquid at varying degrees of heat whereby the components of different boiling points are collected separately.

molecular d., d. in high vacuum, intended to make possible use of low temperatures to minimize damage to thermally labile molecules that would be decomposed by boiling at higher temperatures.

dis·to·buc·cal (dis-tō-bŭk′kăl). Relating to the distal and buccal surfaces of a tooth; denoting the angle formed by their junction.

dis·to·buc·co·oc·clu·sal (dis′tō-bŭk′ŏ-ō-klū′săl). Relating to the distal, buccal, and occlusal surfaces of a bicuspid or molar tooth; denoting especially the angle formed by the junction of these surfaces.

dis·to·buc·co·pul·pal (dis′tō-bŭk′ŏ-pŭl′păl). Relating to the point (trihedral) angle formed by the junction of a distal, buccal, and pulpal wall of a cavity.

dis·to·cer·vi·cal (dis-tō-ser′vi-kăl). Relating to the line angle formed by the junction of the distal and cervical (gingival) walls of a class V cavity.

di

dis·to·clu·sal (dis-tō-klū'săl). **1.** Relating to or characterized by distoclusion. **2.** Denoting a compound cavity or restoration involving the distal and occlusal surfaces of a tooth. **3.** Denoting the line angle formed by the distal and occlusal walls of a class V cavity. SYN disto-occlusal.

dis·to·clu·sion (dis-tō-klū'zhŭn). A malocclusion in which the mandibular arch articulates with the maxillary arch in a position distal to normal; in Angle's classification, a Class II malocclusion. SYN distal occlusion (2).

dis·to·gin·gi·val (dis-tō-jin'ji-văl). Relating to the junction of the distal surface with the gingival line of a tooth.

dis·to·in·ci·sal (dis'tō-in-sī'zăl). Relating to the line (dihedral) angle formed by the junction of the distal and incisal walls of a class V cavity in an anterior tooth.

dis·to·la·bi·al (dis-tō-lā'bē-ăl). Relating to the distal and labial surfaces of a tooth; denoting the angle formed by their junction.

dis·to·la·bi·o·pul·pal (dis'tō-lā'bē-ō-pŭl'păl). Relating to the point (trihedral) angle formed by the junction of distal, labial and pulpal walls of the incisal part of a class IV (mesioincisal) cavity.

dis·to·lin·gual (dis-tō-ling'gwăl). Relating to the distal and lingual surfaces of a tooth; denoting the angle formed by their junction.

dis·to·lin·guo·oc·clu·sal (dis'tō-ling'gwō-ŏ-klū'zăl). Relating to the distal, lingual, and occlusal surfaces of a bicuspid or molar tooth; denoting especially the angle formed by the junction of these surfaces.

Dis·to·ma (dis'tō-mă). Obsolete term for various digenetic flukes, now referred to other genera; *e.g., Fasciola, Fasciolopsis, Paragonimus, Opisthorchis, Clonorchis, Dicrocoelium, Heterophyes,* and *Schistosoma.* SYN *Distomum.* [G. *di-,* two, + *stoma,* mouth]

dis·to·mi·a·sis, dis·to·ma·to·sis (dis'tō-mī'ă-sis, -mă-tō'sis). Presence in any of the organs or tissues of digenetic flukes formerly classified as Distoma or Distomum; in general, infection by any parasitic trematode or fluke.

hemic d., SYN schistosomiasis.

pulmonary d., SYN paragonimiasis.

dis·to·mo·lar (dis-tō-mō'lăr). A supernumerary tooth located in the region posterior to the third molar tooth.

Dis·to·mum (dis'tō-mŭm). SYN *Distoma.*

dis·to·oc·clu·sal (dis'tō-ŏ-klū'săl). SYN distoclusal.

dis·to·oc·clu·sion (dis'tō-ŏ-klū'zhŭn). SYN distal *occlusion* (1).

dis·to·place·ment (dis'tō-plās-ment). SYN distoversion.

dis·to·pul·pal (dis-tō-pŭl'păl). Relating to the line (dihedral) angle formed by the junction of the distal and pulpal walls of a cavity.

dis·tor·tion (dis-tōr'shŭn). **1.** In psychiatry, a defense mechanism that helps to repress or disguise unacceptable thoughts. **2.** In dental impressions, the permanent deformation of the impression material after the registration of an imprint. **3.** A twisting out of normal shape or form. [L. *distortio,* fr. *dis-torqueo,* to wrench apart]

parataxic d., an attitude toward another person based on a distorted evaluation, usually because of too close an identification of that person with emotionally significant figures in the patient's past life.

dis·to·ver·sion (dis'tō-ver-zhŭn). Malposition of a tooth distal to normal, in a posterior direction following the curvature of the dental arch. SYN distoplacement.

dis·tract·i·bil·i·ty (dis-trak-tī-bil'i-tē). A disorder of attention in which the mind is easily diverted by inconsequential occurrences; seen in mania and attention deficit disorder.

dis·trac·tion (dis-trak'shŭn). **1.** Difficulty or impossibility of concentration or fixation of the mind. **2.** Extension of a limb to separate bony fragments or joint surfaces. [L. *dis-traho,* pp. *-tractus,* to pull in different directions]

dis·tress (dis-tres'). Mental or physical suffering or anguish. [L. *distringo,* to draw asunder]

fetal d., any threatening or adverse condition of the fetus, caused by stress; some of the criteria for recognition of fetal d. are cardiac arrhythmia, bradycardia, and tachycardia.

dis·tri·bu·tion (dis-tri-byū'shŭn). **1.** The passage of the branches of arteries or nerves to the tissues and organs. **2.** The area in which the branches of an artery or a nerve terminate, or the area supplied by such an artery or nerve. **3.** The relative numbers of individuals in each of various categories or populations such as in different age, sex, or occupational samples. SEE frequency d. [L. *dis-tribuo,* pp. *-tributus,* to distribute, fr. *tribus,* a tribe]

Bernoulli d., the probability d. associated with two mutually exclusive and exhaustive outcomes, *e.g.,* death or survival.

binomial d., (1) a probability d. associated with two mutually exclusive outcomes, *e.g.,* presence or absence of a clinical sign. **(2)** the possible array of the number of successes in the outcomes from a fixed number, *n,* of independent Bernoulli trials; the probabilities associated with each constitute a binomial process of order *n.*

chi-square d. (kī), a variable is said to have a chi-square d. with *K* degrees of freedom if it is distributed like the sum of the squares of *K* independent random variables, each of which has a normal (gaussian) d. with mean zero and variance one. The chi square d. is the basis for many variations of the chi-square(d) test, perhaps the most widely used test for statistical significance in biology and medicine.

countercurrent d., a method of separation of two or more substances by repeated distribution between two immiscible liquid phases that move past each other in opposite directions; a form of liquid-liquid chromatography.

dermatomal d., SYN dermatome (3).

epidemiological d., SEE histogram.

exponential d., the time until failure of a process at constant hazard.

f d., the d. of the ratio of two independent quantities each of which is distributed like a variance in normally distributed samples. So named in honor of the English statistician and geneticist R.A. Fisher.

frequency d., a statistical description of raw data in terms of the number or frequency of items characterized by each of a series or range of values of a continuous variable.

gaussian d., SYN normal d.

lognormal d., if a variable y is such that x = log y, it is said to have a lognormal d.; this is a skew d.

multinomial d., probability distribution associated with the classification of each of a sample of individuals into one of several mutually exclusive and exhaustive categories.

normal d., a specific bell-shaped frequency d. commonly assumed by statisticians to represent the infinite population of measurements from which a sample has been drawn; characterized by two parameters, the mean (x) and the standard deviation (σ), in the equation: SYN gaussian curve, gaussian d.

Poisson d., (1) a discontinuous d. important in statistical work and defined by the equation $p(x) = e^{-\mu}\mu^x / x!$, where *e* is the base of natural logarithms, *x* is the sequence of integers, μ is the mean, and *x!* represents the factorial of *x.* **(2)** a d. function used to describe the occurrence of rare events, or the sampling d. of isolated counts in a continuum of time or space.

skew d., an asymmetrical frequency d.; in biology and medicine it is usually a lognormal d.

***t* d.,** the d. of the quotient of independent random variables, the numerator of which is a standardized normal variate and the denominator the positive square root of the quotient of a chi-square distributed variate and its number of degrees of freedom.

dis·tri·chi·a·sis (dis-tri-kī'ă-sis). Growth of two hairs in a single follicle. [G. *dis,* double, + *thrix* (trich-), hair]

dis·trix (dis'triks). Splitting of the hairs at their ends. [G. *dis,* twice, + *thrix,* hair]

dis·tur·bance (dis-ter'bans). Deviation from, interruption of, or interference with a normal state.

emotional d., mental d., SEE mental *illness,* behavior *disorder.*

di·sulf·am·ide (dī-sul'fă-mīd). 5-Chlorotoluene-2,4-disulfonamide; a diuretic.

di·sul·fate (dī-sŭl'fāt). A molecule containing two sulfates.

di·sul·fide (dī-sŭl'fīd). **1.** A molecule containing two atoms of sulfur to one of the reference element, *e.g.*, CS_2, carbon disulfide. **2.** A compound containing the –S–S– group, *e.g.*, cystine.

asymmetric d., SYN mixed d.

mixed d., d. which is not symmetric on both sides of the –s–s– linkage; *e.g.*, the d. formed between coenzyme A and glutathione or between cysteine and coenzyme A or glutathione. SYN asymmetric d.

symmetric d., d. that is symmetric on both sides of the –s–s– linkage; *i.e.*, d. formed from identical thiol-containing compounds; *e.g.*, cystine, glutathione disulfide.

di·sul·fi·ram (dī-sŭl′fi-ram). bis(diethylthiocarbamyl)disulfide; an antioxidant that interferes with the normal metabolic degradation of alcohol in the body, resulting in increased acetaldehyde concentrations in blood and tissues. Used in the treatment of chronic alcoholism; when a small quantity of alcohol is consumed an unpleasant reaction results. Also used as a chelator in copper and nickel poisoning. SYN tetraethylthiuram disulfide.

DIT Abbreviation for diiodotyrosine.

di·ter·penes (dī-ter′pēnz). Hydrocarbons or their derivatives containing 4 isoprene units, hence containing 20 carbon atoms and 4 branched methyl groups; *e.g.*, vitamin A, retinene, aconitine.

di·thi·az·a·nine io·dide (dī-thī-az′ă-nēn). 3-Ethyl-2-[5-(3-ethyl-2(3*H*)-benzothiazolylidene)-1,3-pentadienyl]benzothiazolium iodide; a broad spectrum anthelmintic, effective against *Strongyloides*.

di·thi·o·thre·i·tol (dī-thē′ō-thrē-tol). A donor of thiol groups used in biochemical and pharmacological studies. SYN Cleland's reagent.

di·thra·nol (dith′ră-nol). SYN anthralin.

Dittrich, Franz, German pathologist, 1815–1859. SEE D.'s *plugs*, under *plug, stenosis*.

di·u·re·sis (dī-yū-rē′sis). Excretion of urine; commonly denotes production of unusually large volumes of urine. [G. *dia*, throughout, completely, + *ourēsis*, urination]

alcohol d., d. following the ingestion of alcoholic beverages; due, in part, to inhibition of the output of antidiuretic hormone by the neurohypophysis.

osmotic d., d. due to a high concentration of osmotically active substances in the renal tubules (*e.g.*, urea, sodium sulfate), which limit the reabsorption of water.

water d., d. following the drinking of water; due to reduced secretion of the antidiuretic hormone of the neurohypophysis in response to the lowered osmotic pressure of the blood.

di·u·ret·ic (dī-yū-ret′ik). **1.** Promoting the excretion of urine. **2.** An agent that increases the amount of urine excreted.

cardiac d., a d. which acts by increasing function of the heart, and thereby improves renal perfusion.

direct d., a d. whose primary effect is on renal tubular function.

indirect d., a d. that acts by increasing cardiac function or by increasing the state of hydration.

loop d., a class of d. agents (*e.g.*, furosemide, ethacrynic acid) that act by inhibiting reabsorption of sodium and chloride, not only in the proximal and distal tubules but also in Henle's loop.

mercurial d.'s, d. drugs containing organic mercury (*e.g.*, Mercuhydrin) which promote substantial salt and water loss through the kidney. Among the first potent d. agents used in congestive heart failure, but now obsolescent.

osmotic d.'s, drugs, such as mannitol, which by their osmotic effects retain water during urine formation and thus dilute electrolytes in the urine, making resorption less efficient; they promote the elimination of water and electrolytes in the urine.

potassium sparing d.'s, d. agents that, unlike most d.'s, retain potassium; examples are triamterene and amiloride. Often used together with d.'s that promote the loss of both sodium and potassium. Used in hypertension and in congestive heart failure.

di·ur·nal (dī-er′năl). **1.** Pertaining to the daylight hours; opposite of nocturnal. **2.** Repeating once each 24 hours, *e.g.*, a d. variation or a d. rhythm. Cf. circadian. [L. *diurnus*, of the day]

di·ur·nule (dī-er′nūl). A pill, tablet, or capsule containing the maximum daily dose of a drug. [L. *diurnus*, daily, fr. *dies*, day]

di·va·lence, di·va·len·cy (dī-vā′lens, dī-vā′len-sē). SYN bivalence.

di·va·lent (dī-vā′lent, div′ă-). SYN bivalent (1).

di·val·pro·ex so·di·um (dī-val′prō-eks). Pentanoic acid, 2-propyl-, sodium salt (2:1); an anticonvulsant used in absence seizures and related seizure disorders.

di·var·i·ca·tion (dī′var-i-kā′shŭn). SYN diastasis (1). [L. *divaricare*, to spread asunder]

di·ver·gence (dī-ver′jens). **1.** A moving or spreading apart or in different directions. **2.** The spreading of branches of the neuron to form synapses with several other neurons. [L. *di-*, apart, + *vergo*, to incline]

di·ver·gent (dī-ver′jent). Moving in different directions; radiating.

di·ver·tic·u·la (dī-ver-tik′yū-lă). Plural of diverticulum.

di·ver·tic·u·lar (dī-ver-tik′yū-lăr). Relating to a diverticulum.

di·ver·tic·u·lec·to·my (dī′ver-tik-yū-lek′tō-mē). Excision of a diverticulum.

di·ver·tic·u·li·tis (dī′ver-tik-yū-lī′tis). Inflammation of a diverticulum, especially of the small pockets in the wall of the colon which fill with stagnant fecal material and become inflamed; rarely, they may cause obstruction, perforation, or bleeding.

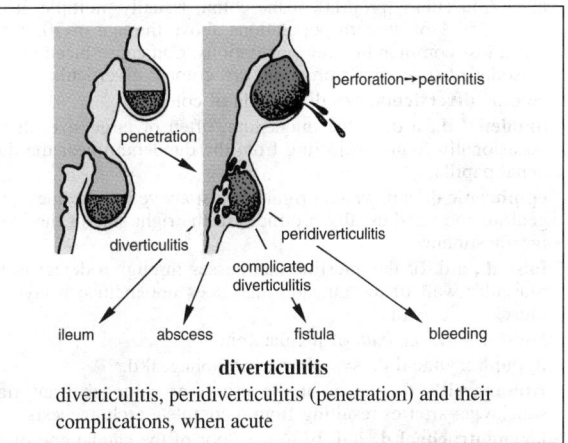

diverticulitis
diverticulitis, peridiverticulitis (penetration) and their complications, when acute

di·ver·tic·u·lo·ma (dī′ver-tik-yū-lō′mă). Development of a granulomatous mass in the wall of the colon. [diverticulum + G. *-oma*, tumor]

di·ver·tic·u·lo·pexy (dī-ver-tik′yū-lō-pek-sē). A plastic operation to obliterate a diverticulum. [diverticulum + G. *pēxis*, fixation]

di·ver·tic·u·lo·sis (dī′ver-tik-yū-lō′sis). Presence of a number of diverticula of the intestine, common in middle age; the lesions are acquired pulsion diverticula.

di·ver·tic·u·lum, pl. **di·ver·tic·u·la** (dī-ver-tik′yū-lŭm, yū-lă) [NA]. A pouch or sac opening from a tubular or saccular organ, such as the gut or bladder. [L. *deverticulum* (or *di-*), a by-road, fr. *de-verto*, to turn aside]

allantoenteric d., SYN allantoic d.

allantoic d., an endoderm-lined outpouching of the hindgut (in humans, the yolk sac of a very young embryo) representing the primordium of the allantois; in most amniotes, it grows into the extraembryonic celom; in humans, the distal part of the allantoic lumen is rudimentary, not extending beyond the body stalk. SYN allantoenteric d.

diverticula of ampulla of ductus deferens, the irregular sacculations of the ampullary part of the ductus deferens near its termination in the ejaculatory duct. SYN diverticula ampullae ductus deferentis [NA].

diverticula ampul′lae duc′tus deferen′tis [NA], SYN diverticula of ampulla of ductus deferens.

cervical d., a d. in the neck derived from retention of part of one of the pharyngeal pouches (endodermal) or branchial grooves (ectodermal) of the embryo.

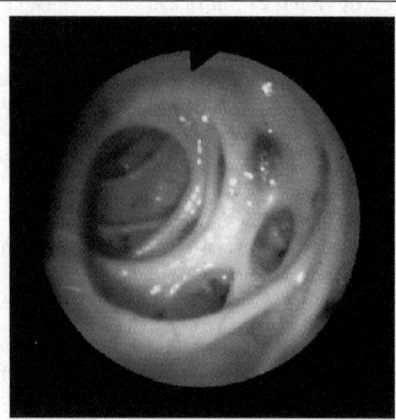

diverticulosis (large intestine, endoscopic finding)

diverticula of colon, diverticula, which are herniations of mucosa and submucosa through or between fibers of the major muscle layer (muscularis propria) of the colon. Usually multiple, it occurs in 50% of western populations above the age of 70, but is much less common in other populations. Can cause bleeding and episodes of severe inflammation. SYN colonic diverticula.

colonic diverticula, SYN diverticula of colon.

duodenal d., a d. of the duodenum, often of large size, that is occasionally found projecting from the duodenum near the duodenal papilla.

epiphrenic d., a d. which originates just above the cardioesophageal junction and usually protrudes to the right side of the lower meadiastinum.

false d., a d. of the intestine that passes through a defect in the muscular wall of the gut and thus does not include a layer of muscle in its wall.

Heister's d., SEE *bulb* of jugular vein.

hypopharyngeal d., SYN pharyngoesophageal d.

Kommerell's d., the d. at the origin of some aberrant right subclavian arteries resulting from incomplete arch agenesis.

laryngotracheal d., a d. from the floor of the caudal end of the pharynx which gives rise to the epithelium and glands of the larynx, trachea, bronchi, and lungs. Once this d. separates from the foregut, it is referred to as a tube.

Meckel's d., the remains of the yolk stalk of the embryo, which, when persisting abnormally as a blind sac or pouch in the adult, is located on the ileum a short distance above the cecum; it may be attached to the umbilicus and, if the lining includes gastric mucosa, peptic ulceration and bleeding may result.

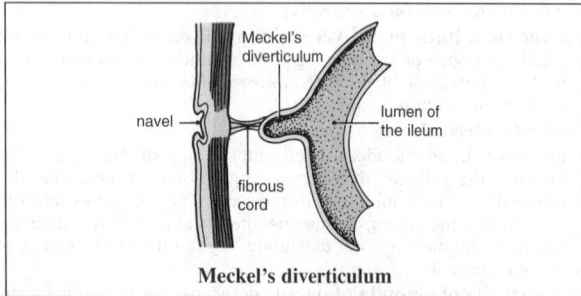

Meckel's diverticulum

metanephric d., an outgrowth from the caudal portion of the mesonephric duct on either side, which grows cephalodorsally to make contact with the masses of metanephrogenous tissue (nephric blastemas) that give rise to the epithelial lining of the ureter and of the pelvis and the collecting ducts of the kidney.

Nuck's d., SYN *processus* vaginalis of peritoneum.

pancreatic diverticula, the ventral and dorsal endodermal buds

from the embryonic foregut that constitute the primordia of the parenchyma of the pancreas.

Pertik's d., an abnormally deep recessus pharyngeus.

pharyngoesophageal d., most common d. of the esophagus; arises between the inferior pharyngeal constrictor and the cricopharyngeus muscle. SYN hypopharyngeal d., Zenker's d.

pituitary d., a tubular outgrowth of ectoderm from the stomodeum of the embryo; it grows dorsad toward the infundibular process of the diencephalon, around which it forms a cup-like mass, giving rise to the pars distalis and pars juxtaneuralis of the hypophysis. SYN craniopharyngeal canal, hypophyseal pouch, Rathke's d., Rathke's pocket, Rathke's pouch.

pulsion d., a d. formed by pressure from within, frequently causing herniation of mucosa through the muscularis.

Rathke's d., SYN pituitary d.

thyroid d., thyroglossal d., the endodermal bud from the floor of the embryonic pharynx; the primordium of the parenchyma of the thyroid gland.

tracheobronchial d., the endodermal lung primordium which will give rise to the epithelial lining of the respiratory tract. SYN lung bud.

traction d., a d. formed by the pulling force of contracting bands of adhesion, occurring mainly in the distal esophagus, from tuberculous hilar or mediastinal lymphadenitis.

true d., a term denoting a d. that includes all the layers of the wall from which it protrudes.

urethral d., a sac-like outpouching of the urethral wall, either from a congenital defect or, more commonly, as a result of chronic penetrating inflammation.

ventricular d., a congenital outpouching of the right or left ventricle.

vesical d., a d. of the bladder wall; may be either true or false type.

Zenker's d., SYN pharyngoesophageal d.

di·vic·ine (dī'vis-ēn). A base with alkaloidal properties present in *Lathyrus sativus* which is responsible, in part at least, for the latter's poisonous action. SEE lathyrism.

di·vi·nyl ether (dī-vī'nil). O(CH=CH$_2$)$_2$; a volatile liquid, the vapor of which produces rapid induction of general anesthesia; prolonged administration is associated with adverse side effects on the liver and central nervous system; an obsolete agent. SYN vinyl ether.

di·vi·sion (di-vizh'ŭn). A separating into two or more parts.

anterior primary d., SYN ventral primary *ramus* of spinal nerve.

cleavage d., the rapid mitotic d. of the zygote with decrease in size of individual cells or blastomeres and the formation of a morula. SEE ALSO cleavage (1).

conjugate d., simultaneous d. of haploid nuclei, as in Basidiomycota.

direct nuclear d., SYN amitosis.

equatorial d., nuclear d. in which each chromosome divides equally.

indirect nuclear d., SYN mitosis.

meiotic d., SYN meiosis.

mitotic d., SYN mitosis.

multiplicative d., reproduction by simultaneous d. of a mother cell into a number of daughter cells. If the process occurs without fertilization of the mother cell, or encystment, the daughter cells are called merozoites; if they develop within a cyst, and usually after fertilization, they are called sporozoites.

posterior primary d., SYN dorsal primary *ramus* of spinal nerve.

reduction d., SEE *reduction* of chromosomes.

Remak's nuclear d., SYN amitosis.

div. in p. aeg. Abbreviation for L. *divide in partes aequales,* divide into equal parts.

di·vulse (di-vŭls'). To tear away or apart. [L. *di-vello,* pp. *di-vulsus,* to pull apart]

di·vul·sion (di-vŭl'shŭn). **1.** Removal of a part by tearing. **2.** Forcible dilation of the walls of a cavity or canal.

di·vul·sor (di-vŭl'sĕr, -sōr). An instrument for forcible dilation of the urethra or other canal or cavity.

di·xyr·a·zine (dī-zir′ă-zēn). 2-{2-[4-(2-Methyl-3(10*H*-Phenothiazin-10-yl)propyl)-1-piperazinyl]ethoxy}ethanol; a phenothiazine compound used as an antipsychotic.

di·zy·got·ic, di·zy·gous (dī′zī-got′ik, dī-zī′gŭs). Relating to twins derived from two separate zygotes, *i.e.,* bearing the same genetic relationship as full sibs but sharing a common intrauterine environment. [G. *di-*, two, + *zygotos,* yoked together]

diz·zi·ness (diz′i-nes). Imprecise term commonly used by patients in an attempt to describe various symptoms such as faintness, giddiness, light-headedness, or unsteadiness. SEE ALSO vertigo. [A. S. *dyzig,* foolish]

djen·kol·ic ac·id (jeng-kol′ik). CH$_2$[S–CH$_2$CH (NH$_3$)$^+$COO$^+$]$_2$; *S,S′*-Methylenebiscysteine; a sulfur-containing amino acid, resembling cystine but with a methylene bridge between the two sulfur atoms; very insoluble. [*djenkol,* bean, bean in which first isolated]

ᴅᴌ-. Prefix (in small capital letters) denoting a substance consisting of equal quantities of the two enantiomorphs, ᴅ and ʟ; replaces the older *dl-* (in lower case italics) as a more exact definition of structure.

DM Abbreviation for adamsite; *diabetes* mellitus; diastolic *murmur;* dopamine.

DMA Abbreviation for dimethoxyamphetamine.

DMC Abbreviation for *p,p,′*-dichlorodiphenyl methyl carbinol.

D.M.D. Abbreviation for Doctor of Dental Medicine.

dmf, DMF Abbreviation for decayed, missing, and filled teeth. SEE ALSO dmfs caries *index.*

dmfs, DMFS Abbreviation for decayed, missing, and filled surfaces. SEE ALSO dmfs caries *index.*

DMPP Abbreviation for dimethylphenylpiperazinium.

DMSO Abbreviation for dimethyl sulfoxide.

DMT Abbreviation for *N,N*-dimethyltryptamine.

DN Abbreviation for dibucaine number.

DNA Abbreviation for deoxyribonucleic acid. For terms bearing this abbreviation, see subentries under deoxyribonucleic acid.

DNA diagnostics. Identifying fetuses or infants afflicted with hereditary diseases or conditions, and carriers of recessive disorders by means of DNA analysis. SEE DNA markers, familial *screening,* prenatal *screening.* SYN genetic testing.

DNA fin·ger·print·ing. See under fingerprint.

dnaG. SYN primase.

DNA markers. Segments of chromosomal DNA known to be linked with heritable traits or diseases. Although the markers themselves to not produce the conditions, they exist in concert with the genes responsible and are passed on with them. Certain markers, restriction fragment length polymorphisms, consist of segments of DNA that can be identified on autoradiographs (produced after digestion of the DNA by restriction enzymes and segregation of the resulting fragments through gel electrophoresis).

DNA profiling. SYN DNA fingerprinting.

DNAse, DNAase, DNase Abbreviations for deoxyribonuclease.

DNA typing. SYN DNA fingerprinting.

DNP, Dnp 1. Abbreviation for 2,4-dinitrophenol. **2.** Abbreviation for deoxyribonucleoprotein.

DNR Abbreviation for "do not resuscitate."

Dns, DNS Abbreviations for dansyl.

D.O. Abbreviation for Doctor of Osteopathy.

DOA Abbreviation for dead on arrival.

do·bu·ta·mine (dō-byū′tă-mēn). (±)-4-[2-[[(3-(*p*-Hydroxyphenyl)-1-methylpropyl]amino]ethyl]pyrocatechol hydrochloride; a synthetic derivative of dopamine characterized by prominent inotropic but weak chronotropic and arrhythmogenic properties; a cardiotonic agent.

DOC Abbreviation for deoxycorticosterone; deoxycholate.

d'Ocagne, Philbert M., French mathematician, 1862–1938. SEE d'O. *nomogram.*

dock (dok). **1.** The amputation of a part of the tail of horses, sheep, or dogs. **2.** The base of the tail left after docking.

n-doc·o·sa·no·ic ac·id (dō′kō-san-ō′ik). SYN behenic acid.

doc·tor (dok′ter). **1.** A title conferred by a university on one who has followed a prescribed course of study, or given as a title of distinction; as d. of medicine, laws, philosophy, etc. **2.** A physician, especially one upon whom has been conferred the degree of M.D. by a university or medical school. [L. a teacher, fr. *doceo,* pp. *doctus,* to teach]

doc·trine (dok′trin). A particular system of principles taught or advocated. [L. *doceo,* to teach]

Arrhenius d., the theory of electrolytic dissociation (1887) that became the basis of our modern understanding of electrolytes: in an electrically conductive solution (*e.g.,* acid, base, or salt), free ions are present before electrolysis, and the proportion of molecules dissociated into ions can be calculated from measurements of electrical conductivity as well as of osmotic pressure. SYN Arrhenius law.

humoral d., the ancient Greek theory of the four body humors (blood, yellow and black bile, and phlegm) that determined health and disease. The humors were associated with the four elements (air, fire, earth, and water), which in turn corresponded to a pair of the qualities (hot, cold, dry, and moist). A proper and evenly balanced mixture of the humors was characteristic of health of body and mind; an imperfect balance resulted in disease. Temperament of body or mind also was supposed to be determined, *e.g.,* sanguine (blood), choleric (yellow bile), melancholic (black bile), or phlegmatic (phlegm). SYN fluidism, humoralism, humorism.

Monro-Kellie d., SYN Monro's d.

Monro's d., a d. that states that the cranial cavity is a closed rigid box and that therefore a change in the quantity of intracranial blood can occur only through the displacement of or replacement by cerebrospinal fluid. SYN Monro-Kellie d.

doc·u·sate cal·ci·um (dok′yū-sāt). calcium salt of bis(2-ethylhexyl)sulfosuccinate; a surface-active agent used in the treatment of constipation as a nonlaxative fecal softener. SYN dioctyl calcium sulfosuccinate.

doc·u·sate so·di·um. bis-2-ethylhexyl sodium sulfosuccinate; a surface-active agent used as a dispersing agent in topically applied preparations. After oral administration it lowers the surface tension of the gastrointestinal tract and is used in the treatment of constipation. SYN dioctyl sodium sulfosuccinate.

do·de·cane (dō′dĕ-kān). *n*-C$_{12}$H$_{26}$; a straight, unbranched, saturated hydrocarbon containing 12 carbon atoms; the 12th member of the alkane series that begins with methane.

n-do·dec·a·no·ic ac·id (dō-dek′ă-nō-ik). SYN lauric acid.

do·dec·an·o·yl-CoA syn·the·tase (dō-dek′ăn-ō-il-kō-ā-sin ′thetās). SYN long-chain fatty acid-CoA ligase.

do·de·car·bo·ni·um chlo·ride (dō-dē-kar-bō′nē-ŭm). Benzyl-(dodecylcarbamoylmethyl)dimethyl ammonium chloride; an antiseptic.

do·de·cyl (dō′dĕ-sil). The radical of dodecane.

d. gallate, dodecyl 3,4,5-trihydroxybenzoate; an antioxidant.

d. sulfate, SEE *sodium* dodecyl sulfate.

Döderlein, Albert, S.G., German obstetrician, 1860–1941. SEE D.'s *bacillus.*

Doerfler, Leo, U.S. audiologist, *1919. SEE D.-Stewart *test.*

Dogiel, Alexander S., Russian histologist, 1852–1922. SEE D.'s *corpuscle.*

Dogiel, Jan von, Russian anatomist and physiologist, 1830–1905. SEE D.'s *cells,* under cell.

dog·ma. A theory or belief that is formally stated, defined, and thought to be true.

central d., the proposition that while genetic information is transferred from parent to offspring via DNA duplication, within the cell genetic information is transferred from DNA to mRNA (transcription) and then to protein (translation); proposed by Francis Crick.

dog·mat·ic (dog-mat′ik). SEE dogmatic *school.* [G. *dogmatikos,* concerning opinions; d. *iatroi,* physicians who go by general principles; fr. *dogma,* an opinion]

do

dog·ma·tist (dog′mă-tist). A follower of the dogmatic *school*.

Döhle, Karl G.P., German histologist and pathologist, 1855–1928. SEE D. *bodies*, under *body*, *inclusions*, under *inclusion*.

Doisy, Edward A., U.S. biochemist and Nobel laureate, 1893–1986. SEE Allen-D. *test*, *unit*.

dol (dōl). A unit measure of pain. [L. *dolor*, pain]

⌂**dolicho-.** Long. [G. *dolichos*]

dol·i·cho·ce·phal·ic, dol·i·cho·ceph·a·lous (dol-i-kō-sĕ-fal′ik, -sef′ă-lŭs). Having a disproportionately long head; denoting a skull with a cephalic index below 75. SYN dolichocranial. [dolicho- + G. *kephalē*, head]

dol·i·cho·ceph·a·ly, dol·i·cho·ceph·a·lism (dol-i-kō-sef′ă-lē, sef′ă-lizm). The condition of being dolichocephalic.

dol·i·cho·co·lon (dol-i-kō-kō′lŏn). A colon of abnormal length. [dolicho- + G. *kōlon*, colon]

dol·i·cho·cra·ni·al (dol-i-kō-krā′nē-ăl). SYN dolichocephalic.

dol·i·cho·fa·cial (dol-i-kō-fā′shăl). SYN dolichoprosopic.

dol·i·chol (dol′i-kol). Polyisoprenes in which the terminal member is saturated and oxidized to an alcohol, usually phosphorylated and often glycosylated; found in endoplasmic reticulum, but not in mitochondrial or plasma membranes; urinary levels are elevated in disorders exhibiting abnormal skin, rectal, or brain profiles in electron microscopy of biopsies.

d. phosphate, an intermediate in the glycosylation of proteins and lipids; contains 11 to 24 isoprene units; a product of the isoprenylation pathway; participates in the formation of glycosylphosphatidylinositol anchors of proteins in biomembranes.

dol·i·cho·pel·lic, dol·i·cho·pel·vic (dol-i-kō-pel′ik, -pel′vik). Having a disproportionately long pelvis; denoting a pelvis with a pelvic index above 95. [dolicho- + G. *pellis*, bowl (pelvis)]

dol·i·cho·pro·sop·ic, dol·i·cho·pro·so·pous (dol-i-kō-pros-ō′pik, -kō-pros′ō-pŭs). Having a disproportionately long face. SYN dolichofacial. [dolicho- + G. *prosōpikos*, facial]

dol·i·cho·sten·o·me·lia (dol′i-kō-sten′ō-mē′lē-ă). Narrow body habitus which, like arachondactyly, is a common feature of several kinds of hereditary disorders of connective tissue. [dolicho- + G. *stenos*, narrow, + *melos*, limb]

dol·i·cho·u·ran·ic, dol·i·chu·ran·ic (dol′i-kō-yū-ran′ik, dol-ik-yū-). Having a long palate, with a palatal index below 110. [dolicho- + G. *ouranos*, vault of the palate]

do·lor (dō′lōr). Pain, as one of the four signs of inflammation (d., calor, rubor, tumor) enunciated by Celsus. [L.]

d. cap′itis, headache, especially due to changes in the scalp or bones rather than in the intracranial structures.

do·lo·rif·ic (dō-lōr-if′ik). Pain-producing.

do·lo·rim·e·try (dō-lō-rim′ĕ-trē). The measurement of pain. [L. *dolor*, pain, + G. *metron*, measure]

do·lor·ol·o·gy (dō-lōr-ol′ŏ-jē). The study and treatment of pain. [L. *dolor*, pain, + G. *logos*, study]

DOM Abbreviation for 2,5-dimethoxy-4-methylamphetamine.

do·main (dō-mān′). An independently folded, globular structure composed of one section of a polypeptide chain. A d. may interact with another d.; it may be associated with a particular function. D.'s can vary in size.

dinucleotide d., SYN dinucleotide *fold*.

do·mains (dō-mānz′). **1.** Homologous units of approximately 110 to 120 amino acids each which comprise the light and heavy chains of the immunoglobulin molecule and which serve specific functions. The light chain has two d.'s, one in the variable region and one in the constant region of the chain; the heavy chain has four to five d.'s, depending upon the class of immunoglobulin, one in the variable region and the remaining ones in the constant region. **2.** A region of a protein having some distinctive physical feature or role. [Fr. *domaine*, fr. L. *dominium*, property, dominion]

Dombrock blood group. See Blood Groups appendix.

do·mes·tic vi·o·lence. intentionally inflicted injury perpetrated by and on family member(s); varieties include spouse abuse, child abuse, and sexual abuse, including incest. Various kinds of abuse, such as sexual abuse, also happen outside of the family

unit. The American Medical Association, like similar organizations in other countries, has issued advisory notices to physicians on the detection and treatment of domestic d. v.

dom·i·cil·i·at·ed (dō-mi-sil′ē-āt-ed). A state of close association of an organism within human abodes or activities, such that partial domestication results, leading to the organism's dependence on continued association with the human environment; this frequently results in the d. organism becoming a noxious pest, a vector, or an intermediate host of human disease. [L. *domicilium*, a dwelling]

dom·i·nance (dom′i-nans). The state of being dominant.

cerebral d., the fact that one hemisphere is dominant over the other and will exercise greater influence over certain functions; the left cerebral hemisphere is usually dominant in the control of speech, language and analytical processing, and mathematics, while the right hemisphere (usually nondominant) processes spatial concepts and language as related to certain types of visual images; handedness (right-handed people have left cerebral d.) is considered a general example of cerebral d.

false d., SYN quasidominance.

genetic d., denoting a pattern of inheritance of an autosomal mendelian trait due to a gene that always manifests itself phenotypically; generally, the phenotype in the homozygote is more severe than in the heterozygote, but details depend on what criterion of phenotyping is used.

d. of traits, an expression of the apparent physiologic relationship existing between two or more genes that may occupy the same chromosomal locus (alleles). At a specific locus there are three possible combinations of two allelic genes, *A* and *a*: two homozygous (*AA* and *aa*) and one heterozygous (*Aa*). If a heterozygous individual presents only the hereditary characteristic determined by gene *A*, but not *a*, *A* is said to be dominant and *a* recessive; in this case, *AA* and *Aa*, although genotypically distinct, should be phenotypically indistinguishable. If *AA*, *Aa*, and *aa* are distinguishable, each from the others, *A* and *a* are codominant.

dom·i·nant (dom′i-nant). **1.** Ruling or controlling. **2.** In genetics, denoting an allele possessed by one of the parents of a hybrid which is expressed in the latter to the exclusion of a contrasting allele (the recessive) from the other parent. [L. *dominans*, pres. p. of *dominor*, to rule, fr. *dominus*, lord, master, fr. *domus*, house]

do·mi·o·dol (do-mē′ō-dol). An organic form of iodine complexed with glycerol; used as a mucolytic/expectorant.

do·mi·phen bro·mide (dō′mi-fen). Dodecyldimethyl(2-phenoxyethyl)ammonium bromide; an antiseptic.

dom·per·i·done (dom-per′ĭ-dōn). A dopamine antagonist (like chlorpromazine) with antiemetic properties.

Donath, Julius, German physician, 1870–1950. SEE D.-Landsteiner *phenomenon*, cold *autoantibody*; Landsteiner-D. *test*.

Donders, Franz C., Dutch ophthalmologist, 1818–1889. SEE D.'s *glaucoma*, *law*, *pressure*, *rings*, under *ring*; *space* of D.

Don Juan (don wahn). In psychiatry, a term used to denote males with compulsive sexual or romantic overactivity, usually with a succession of female partners. [legendary Spanish nobleman]

Don Juan·ism (don wăn′izm). SEE Don Juan.

Donnan, Frederick G., English physical chemist, 1870–1956. SEE D. *equilibrium*; Gibbs-D. *equilibrium*.

Donné, Alfred, French physician, 1801–1878. SEE D.'s *corpuscle*.

Donohue, William L., Canadian pathologist, *1906. SEE D.'s *disease*.

do·nor (dō′ner). **1.** An individual from whom blood, tissue, or an organ is taken for transplantation. **2.** A compound that will transfer an atom or a radical to an acceptor; *e.g.*, methionine is a methyl d.; glutathione is a glutamyl d. **3.** An atom that readily yields electrons to an acceptor; *e.g.*, nitrogen, which will donate both electrons to a shared pool in forming a coordinate bond. [L. *dono*, pp. *donatus*, to donate, to give]

hydrogen d., a metabolite from which hydrogen is removed (by a dehydrogenase system) and transferred by a hydrogen carrier to another metabolite, which is thus reduced.

universal d., in blood grouping, a person belonging to group O; *i.e.,* one whose erythrocytes do not contain either agglutinogen A or B and are, therefore, not agglutinated by plasma containing either of the ordinary isoagglutinins, alpha or beta.

Donovan, Charles, Irish surgeon, 1863–1951. SEE D.'s *bodies,* under *body;* Leishman-D. *body.*

don·o·va·no·sis (don′ō-vă-nō′sis). SYN *granuloma* inguinale.

Doose, H., 20th century German pediatrician and epileptologist. SEE D. *syndrome.*

do·pa, DO·PA, Do·pa (dō′pă). An intermediate in the catabolism of L-phenylalanine and L-tyrosine, and in the biosynthesis of norepinephrine, epinephrine, and melanin; the L form, levodopa, is biologically active. SYN 3,4-dihydroxyphenylalanine.

alpha methyl d., SYN methyldopa.

d. decarboxylase, SYN aromatic D-amino-acid decarboxylase.

decarboxylated d., SYN dopamine.

d. oxidase, provisional name given the enzyme(s) catalyzing the formation of melanins from d.; it now appears that the copper-containing monophenol monooxygenases and/or catechol oxidases are responsible for the oxidation of L-tyrosine to d. and d. quinone.

d. quinone, an oxidation product of d. and an intermediate in the formation of melanin from tyrosine.

L-dopa. SYN levodopa.

do·pa·mine (DM) (dō′pă-mēn). 3,4-dihydroxyphenylethylamine; an intermediate in tyrosine metabolism and precursor of norepinephrine and epinephrine; it accounts for 90% of the catecholamines; its presence in the central nervous system and localization in the basal ganglia (caudate and lentiform nuclei) suggest that d. may have other functions. SYN 3-hydroxytyramine, decarboxylated dopa.

d. hydrochloride, a biogenic amine and neural transmitter substance, used as a vasopressor agent for treatment of shock.

do·pa·mine β-hy·drox·y·lase. SYN dopamine β-monooxygenase.

do·pa·mine β-mon·o·ox·y·gen·ase. A copper-containing enzyme catalyzing oxidation of ascorbate and 3,4-dihydroxyphenylethylamine simultaneously by O_2 to yield norepinephrine, dehydroascorbate, and water; a crucial step in catecholamine metabolism. SYN dopamine β-hydroxylase.

do·pa·min·er·gic (dō′pă-min-er′jik). Relating to nerve cells or fibers that employ dopamine as their neurotransmitter. [dopamine + G. *ergon,* work]

dope (dōp). 1. Any drug, either stimulating or depressing, administered for its temporary effect, or taken habitually or addictively. 2. To administer or take such a drug. [Dutch, *doop,* sauce]

dop·ing (dōp′ing). The administration of foreign substances to an individual; often used in reference to athletes who try to stimulate physical and psychological strength.

Doppler, Christian J., Austrian mathematician and physicist in U.S., 1803–1853. SEE D. *echocardiography, effect, phenomenon, shift, ultrasonography.*

dop·pler. A diagnostic instrument that emits an ultrasonic beam into the body; the ultrasound reflected from moving structures changes its frequency (Doppler effect). Of diagnostic value in peripheral vascular and cardiac disease.

do·ra·pho·bia (dō-ră-fō′bē-ă). Morbid fear of touching the skin or fur of animals. [G. *dora,* hide, skin, + *phobos,* fear]

Dorello, P., Italian anatomist, *1872. SEE D.'s *canal.*

Dorendorf, H., German physician, *1866. SEE D.'s *sign.*

Dorfman, Maurice L., 20th century Israeli dermatologist. SEE D.-Chanarin *syndrome.*

Döring, G., German neurologist. SEE Pette-D. *disease.*

dor·nase (dōr′nās). Obsolete contraction of deoxyribonuclease. SEE ALSO streptodornase.

pancreatic d., a stabilized deoxyribonuclease preparation from beef pancreas; used by inhalation in the form of aerosols to reduce thick mucopurulent secretions in certain bronchopulmonary infections.

Dorno, Carl, Swiss climatologist, 1865–1942. SEE D. *rays,* under *ray.*

do·ro·ma·ni·a (dō-rō-mā′nē-ă). An abnormal desire to give presents. [G. *dōron,* gift, + *mania,* insanity]

dor·sa (dōr′să). Plural of dorsum.

dor·sab·dom·i·nal (dōr-sab-dom′i-nal). Relating to the back and the abdomen.

dor·sad (dor′sad). Toward or in the direction of the back. [L. *dorsum,* back, + *ad,* to]

dor·sal (dōr′săl). 1. Pertaining to the back or any dorsum. SYN tergal. 2. SYN posterior (2). 3. In veterinary anatomy, pertaining to the back or upper surface of an animal. Often used to indicate the position of one structure relative to another; *i.e.,* nearer the back surface of the body. 4. Old term meaning thoracic, in a limited sense; *e.g.,* d. vertebrae. [Mediev. L. *dorsalis,* fr. *dorsum,* back]

dor·sal·gia (dōr-sal′jē-ă). Pain in the upper back. SYN dorsodynia. [L. *dorsum,* back, + G. *algos,* pain]

dor·sa·lis (dōr-sā′lis) [NA]. SYN posterior (2). [L.]

Dorset, Marion, U.S. bacteriologist, 1872–1935. SEE D.'s culture egg *medium.*

dor·si·duct (dōr′si-dŭkt). To draw backward or toward the back. [L. *dorsum,* back, + *duco,* pp. *ductus,* to draw]

dor·si·flex·ion (dōr-si-flek′shŭn). Turning upward of the foot or toes or of the hand or fingers.

dor·si·scap·u·lar (dōr′si-skap′yū-lăr). Relating to the dorsal surface of the scapula.

dor·si·spi·nal (dōr′si-spī′năl). Relating to the vertebral column, especially to its dorsal aspect.

dor·so·ceph·a·lad (dōr′sō-sef′ă-lad). Toward the occiput, or back of the head. [L. *dorsum,* back, + G. *kephalē,* head, + L. *ad,* to]

dor·so·dyn·ia (dōr-sō-din′ē-ă). SYN dorsalgia. [L. *dorsum,* back, + G. *odynē,* pain]

dor·so·lat·er·al (dōr-sō-lat′er-ăl). Relating to the back and the side.

dor·so·lum·bar (dōr-sō-lŭm′bar). Referring to the back in the region of the lower thoracic and upper lumbar vertebrae.

dor·so·ven·trad (dōr-sō-ven′trad). In a direction from the dorsal to the ventral aspect.

dor·sum, gen. **dor·si,** pl. **dor·sa** (dōr′sŭm, -sī, -să) [NA]. 1. The back of the body. 2. The upper or posterior surface, or the back, of any part. SYN tergum. [L. back]

d. ephip′pii, SYN d. sellae.

d. of foot, the back, or upper surface, of the foot. SYN d. pedis [NA].

d. lin′guae [NA], SYN d. of tongue.

d. ma′nus [NA], SYN *dorsum* of hand.

d. na′si [NA], SYN d. of nose.

d. of nose, the external ridge of the nose, looking forward and upward. SYN d. nasi [NA].

d. pe′dis [NA], SYN d. of foot.

d. of penis, the aspect of the penis opposite to that of the urethra. SYN d. penis [NA].

d. pe′nis [NA], SYN d. of penis.

d. scap′ulae, the posterior surface of the scapula.

d. sel′lae [NA], a square portion of bone on the body of the sphenoid posterior to the sella turcica or hypophysial fossa. SYN d. ephippii.

d. of tongue, the back of the tongue; the upper surface of the tongue divided by the sulcus terminalis into an anterior two-thirds, the pars presulcalis (presulcal part), and a posterior one-third, the pars postsulcalis (postsulcal part). SYN d. linguae [NA].

dos·age (dō′sij). 1. The giving of medicine or other therapeutic agent in prescribed amounts. 2. The determination of the proper dose of a remedy. Cf. dose.

dose (dōs). The quantity of a drug or other remedy to be taken or applied all at one time or in fractional amounts within a given period. Cf. dosage (2). [G. *dosis* see dosis]

absorbed d., the amount of energy absorbed per unit mass of irradiated material at the target site; in radiation therapy, the former unit for absorbed d. is the rad; the current (S.I.) unit is the gray.

air d., SYN exposure d.

bone marrow d., the cumulative d. to the blood-forming organ from therapeutic or nuclear fallout irradiation; the presumed leukemogenic d.

booster d., a d. given at some time after an initial d. to enhance the effect, said usually of antigens for the production of antibodies.

cumulative d., the total d. resulting from repeated exposures to radiation of the same part of the body or of the whole body.

curative d. (CD, CD^{50}), (1) the quantity of any substance required to effect the cure of a disease or that will correct the manifestations of a deficiency of a particular factor in the diet; **(2)** effective d. used with therapeutically applied compounds. SYN therapeutic d.

daily d., the total amount of a remedy that is to be taken within 24 hours.

depth d., the d. of radiation at a distance beneath the surface, including secondary radiation or scatter, in proportion to the d. at the surface.

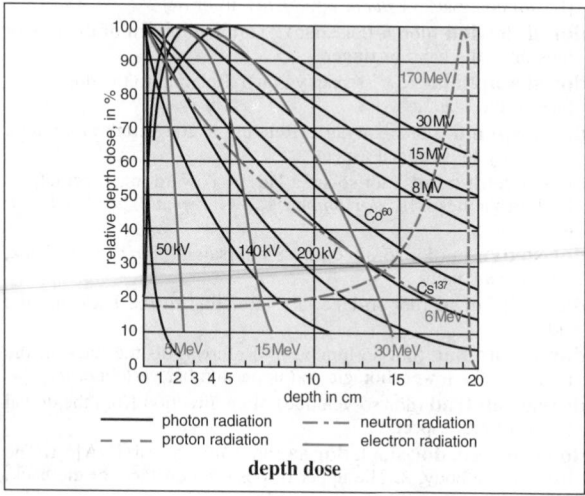

depth dose

divided d., a definite fraction of a full d.; given repeatedly at short intervals so that the full d. is taken within a specified period, usually one day. SYN fractional d.

effective d. (ED), (1) the d. that produces the desired effect; when followed by a subscript (generally "ED$_{50}$"), it denotes the d. having such an effect on a certain percentage (*e.g.,* 50%) of the test animals; ED$_{50}$ is the median effective dose; **(2)** in radiation protection, the sum of the equivalent d.'s in all tissues and organs of the body weighted for tissue effects of radiation. The unit of effective d. is the sievert (Sv);

epilation d., the minimum amount of radiation sufficient to produce hair loss, usually in 10 to 14 days.

equianalgesic d., the qualitative ratio between actual milligram potency of comparable analgesics required to achieve the equivalent therapeutic effect.

equivalent d., in radiation protection, the absorbed d. averaged over a tissue or organ and weighted for the quality of the radiation of interest. The unit of equivalent d. is the sievert.

erythema d., the minimum amount of x-rays or other form of radiation sufficient to produce erythema; historically, this d. was indicated by the Sabouraud meter as the B tint, the Holzknecht as 5(5H), the Hampson as 4, and the Kienbock as 10.

exit d., the exposure dose of radiation leaving a body opposite the portal of entry.

exposure d., the radiation d., expressed in roentgens, delivered at a point in free air. SYN air d.

fractional d., SYN divided d.

gonad d., the exposure d. to the male or female gonad, usually from incidental secondary radiation in diagnostic or therapeutic irradiation, or from whole-body irradiation. SYN gonadal d.

gonadal d., SYN gonad d.

initial d., a comparatively large d. given at the beginning of treatment to get the patient under the influence of the drug. SYN loading d.

integral d., the total energy absorbed by the body, the product of the mass of tissue irradiated and the absorbed d.; unit, the gram rad.

L d.'s, a group of terms that indicate the relative activity or potency of diphtheria toxin; the L d.'s are distinctly different from the minimal lethal d. and minimal reacting d., inasmuch as the latter two represent the direct effects of toxin, whereas the L d.'s pertain to the combining power of toxin with specific antitoxin. ["L" for *limes*]

L$^+$ d., L$_+$ d., alternatives for L†, the limes tod d. of diphtheria toxin, *i.e.,* the smallest amount of toxin that, when mixed with one unit of antitoxin and injected subcutaneously into a 250-g guinea pig, results in death of the animal within 96 hours (based on the average in a series); on theoretical grounds, one might expect that the difference between the L$_+$ and L$_0$ d.'s would be identical to 1 MLD, but this is not so in actual practice; with various toxic filtrates, the difference may range from several to more than 100 MLD's, indicating that the toxin-antitoxin combination is *not* a firm chemical union that occurs in constant proportions.

lethal d. (LD), the d. of a chemical or biologic preparation (*e.g.,* a bacterial exotoxin or a suspension of bacteria) that is likely to cause death; it varies in relation to the type of animal and the route of administration; when followed by a subscript (generally "LD$_{50}$" or median lethal d.), it denotes the d. likely to cause death in a certain percentage (*e.g.,* 50%) of the test animals; median lethal d. is LD$_{50}$, absolute lethal d. is LD$_{100}$, and minimal lethal d. is LD$_{05}$.

Lf d., L$_f$ d., the limes flocculation d. of diphtheria toxin, *i.e.,* the smallest amount of toxin that, when mixed with one unit of antitoxin, yields the most rapid flocculation in the Ramon test (*in vitro*); in general, the L$_f$ d. is slightly less than the L$_r$ d.

Lo d., L$_0$ d., the limes nul d. of diphtheria toxin, *i.e.,* the largest amount of toxin that, when mixed with one unit of antitoxin and injected subcutaneously into a 250-g guinea pig, yields no recognizable reaction in the average of a series; actually, the L$_0$d. is usually recorded as the one that causes a barely perceptible local edema at the site of inoculation.

loading d., SYN initial d.

Lr d., L$_r$ d., the limes reacting d. of diphtheria toxin, *i.e.,* the smallest amount of toxin that, when mixed with one unit of antitoxin and injected intracutaneously in the shaved skin of a susceptible guinea pig, yields a minimal, positive reaction and inflammation localized to the region of the injection; the L$_r$d. closely approximates the L$_0$d., as would be expected, inasmuch as a slight excess of unneutralized toxin results in a reaction.

maintenance d., SEE maintenance drug *therapy*.

maximal d., the largest amount of a drug or physical procedure that an adult can take with safety.

maximal permissible d., SEE maximum permissible d.

maximum permissible d. (MPD), defined by the International Commission on Radiological Protection as the greatest d. of radiation which, in the light of present knowledge, is not expected to cause detectable bodily injury to a person at any time during his lifetime. This d. has been reduced with each Commission report. The MPD is given in terms of acute or chronic exposure of the whole body or of organs, systems, or regions of the body, and differs for persons who are occupationally exposed versus the public at large.

median effective dose (ED$_{50}$), SEE effective d.

minimal d., the smallest amount of a drug or physical procedure that will produce a desired physiologic effect in an adult.

minimal infecting d. (M.I.D.), the smallest quantity of infectious material regularly producing infection; usually expressed as I.D.$_{50}$, the quantity causing infection in 50% of a suitable series of animals or cells (cell cultures).

minimal lethal d. (MLD, mld), (1) the minimal d. of a toxic substance or infectious agent that is lethal, as assayed in various experimental animals (*e.g.,* the least amount of diphtheria toxin that, on an average, kills a 250-g guinea pig within 96 hours after subcutaneous inoculation); when followed by a subscript (generally "MLD_{50}"), denotes the minimal dose that is lethal to a certain percentage (*e.g.,* 50%) of animals so assayed; **(2)** LD_{05}. SEE lethal d.

minimal reacting d. (MRD, mrd), the minimal d. of a toxic substance causing a reaction, as manifested in the skin of a series of susceptible test animals; the assay is based on the development of a characteristic, minimal but definite, "standard," focal inflammation (congestion and edema, induration, degenerative changes, and desquamation of epidermal cells).

optimum d., the d. of a drug or radiation that will produce the desired effect with minimum likelihood of undesirable symptoms.

preventive d., the smallest amount of any substance that will prevent occurrence of symptoms of a disease or the consequences of a lack of a particular factor in the diet.

sensitizing d., in experimental anaphylaxis, the antigenic inoculum that renders an animal susceptible (sensitive) to anaphylactic shock following a subsequent inoculum (shocking d.) of the same antigen (anaphylactogen).

shocking d., in experimental anaphylaxis, the inoculum of antigen that causes anaphylactic shock in an animal sensitized by a previous inoculum (sensitizing d.) of the same antigen.

skin d., the quantity of radiation delivered to the skin surface.

therapeutic d., SYN curative d.

tissue culture infectious d. ($TCID_{50}$, TCD_{50}), the quantity of a cytopathogenic agent, such as a virus, that will produce a cytopathic effect in 50% of the cultures inoculated.

tolerance d., the largest d. of a remedy that can be accepted without the production of injurious symptoms.

dos·im·e·ter (dō-sim′ĕ-ter). A device for measuring radiation, especially x-rays. [G. *dosis,* dose, + *metron,* measure]

do·sim·e·try (dō-sim′ĕ-trē). Measurement of radiation exposure, especially x-rays or gamma rays; calculation of radiation dose from internally administered radionuclides.

thermoluminescence d., the calculation of a radiation dose by measuring the light output after heating a special absorbent material (*e.g.,* lithium fluoride) placed in the radiation beam; the light output is proportional to the amount of radiation exposure.

x-ray d., SYN roentgenometry.

dot. A small spot.

Gunn's d.'s, minute, highly glistening, white or yellowish specks usually seen in the posterior part of the fundus; nonpathologic.

Horner-Trantas d.'s, evanescent white cellular infiltrates occurring in the bulbar form of vernal keratoconjunctivitis.

Maurer's d.'s, finely granular precipitates or irregular cytoplasmic particles that usually occur diffusely in red blood cells infected with the trophozoites of *Plasmodium falciparum,* occasionally those of *P. malariae;* rarely observed in *P. falciparum* blood smears because its trophozoites seldom are seen in peripheral blood. SYN Maurer's clefts.

Schüffner's d.'s, fine, round, uniform red or red-yellow d.'s (as colored with Romanovsky stains) characteristically observed in erythrocytes infected with *Plasmodium vivax* and *P. ovale,* but not ordinarily found in *P. malariae* and *P. falciparum* infections. SYN Schüffner's granules.

Trantas' d.'s, pale, grayish red, uneven nodules of gelatinous aspect at the limbal conjunctiva in vernal conjunctivitis.

Ziemann's d.'s, fine d.'s seen in erythrocytes in malariae malaria. SYN Ziemann's stippling.

dot·age (dō′tij). The deterioration of previously intact mental powers, common in old age. SYN dotardness.

dot·ard·ness (dō′tard-nes). SYN dotage.

dou·blet (dŭb′let). **1.** A combination of two lenses designed to correct the chromatic and spherical aberration. **2.** SYN dipole.

Wollaston's d., a combination of two planoconvex lenses in the eyepiece of a microscope designed to correct the chromatic aberration.

douche (dūsh). **1.** A current of water, gas, or vapor directed against a surface or projected into a cavity. **2.** An instrument for giving a d. **3.** To apply a d. [Fr. fr. *doucher,* to pour]

Douglas, Beverly, U.S. surgeon, *1891. SEE D. graft.

Douglas, Claude G., English physiologist, 1882–1963. SEE D. *bag.*

Douglas, James, Scottish anatomist in London, 1675–1742. SEE D. *abscess;* D.'s *cul-de-sac, fold, line, pouch; cavum* douglasi.

Douglas, John C., Irish obstetrician, 1777–1850. SEE D.'s spontaneous *evolution;* D. *mechanism.*

dou·rine (dū′ren). A venereally transmitted trypanosomiasis of horses caused by *Trypanosoma equiperdum* and characterized by inflammation of the genitals, glandular swelling, and paralysis of the hind quarters. SYN equine syphilis. [Fr.]

dove·tail (dŭv′tāl). A widened portion of a cavity preparation usually established to increase the retention and resistance form.

dow·el (dow′l). **1.** A cast gold or preformed metal pin placed into a root canal for the purpose of providing retention for a crown. **2.** A preformed metal pin placed in a copper-plated die to provide a die stem.

Down, John Langdon H., English physician, 1828–1896. SEE D.'s *syndrome.*

Downey, H., U.S. hematologist, 1877–1959. SEE D. *cell.*

down·reg·u·la·tion. Development of a refractory or tolerant state consequent upon repeated administration of a pharmacologically or physiologically active substance; often accompanied by an initial decrease in affinity of receptors for the agent and a subsequent diminution in the number of receptors.

Downs, William B., U.S. orthodontist, 1899–1966. SEE D.'s *analysis.*

Dox, Arthur W., U.S. chemist, *1882. SEE Czapek-D. *medium.*

dox·a·cu·ri·um chlo·ride (doks′a-kū′rē-um). A nondepolarizing neuromuscular blocking drug similar to pancuronium but without cardiovascular side effects.

dox·a·pram hy·dro·chlo·ride (doks′ă-pram). 1-Ethyl-4-(2-morpholinoethyl)-3,3-diphenyl-2-pyrrolidone monohydrochloride (or hydrochloride hydrate); a central nervous system stimulant, advocated but infrequently used as a respiratory stimulant in anesthesia.

dox·a·zo·cin. An antihypertensive agent that selectively blocks the α_1 (postjunctional) subtype of α-adrenergic receptors; resembles prazocin in pharmacologic actions. Prevents the blood pressure elevating effects of norepinephrine, phenylephrine, and other agonists at vascular α_1-receptors.

dox·e·pin hy·dro·chlo·ride (dok′sĕ-pin). *N,N*-Dimethyldibenz-[*b,e*]oxepin-$\Delta^{11(6H)},\gamma$-propylamine hydrochloride; an antidepressant agent.

dox·o·phyl·line (dok′ō-fil′in). A theophylline-like drug used as a bronchodilator in asthma and chronic obstructive pulmonary disease.

dox·o·ru·bi·cin (dok′sō-rū′bi-sin). An antineoplastic antibiotic isolated from *Streptomyces peucetius;* also used in cytogenetics to produce Q-band chromosome bands. SYN adriamycin.

dox·y·cy·cline (dok-sē-sī′klēn). α-6-Deoxy-5-hydroxytetracycline; an antibiotic.

dox·yl·a·mine suc·ci·nate (dok-sil′ă-mēn). 2-[α-(2-dimethylaminoethoxy)-α-methylbenzyl]pyridine succinate; an antihistaminic. SYN mereprine.

Doyère, Louis, French physiologist, 1811–1863. SEE D.'s *eminence.*

Doyle, J.B., U.S. gynecologist, *1907. SEE D.'s *operation.*

Doyne, Robert Walter, English ophthalmologist, 1857–1916. SEE D.'s honeycomb *choroidopathy.*

D.P. Abbreviation for Doctor of Podiatry.

D.P.H. Abbreviation for Department of Public Health; Doctor of Public Health.

D.P.M. Abbreviation for Doctor of Podiatric Medicine.

DPN Abbreviation for diphosphopyridine nucleotide.

DPN⁺ Abbreviation for oxidized diphosphopyridine nucleotide.

DPNase SYN *NAD⁺* nucleosidase.

DPNH Abbreviation for reduced diphosphopyridine nucleotide.

DPNH → al·de·hyde trans·hy·dro·gen·ase. SYN alcohol dehydrogenase (NADP⁺).

DPT. Abbreviation for diphtheria-pertussis-tetanus (vaccine). SEE diphtheria toxoid, tetanus toxoid, and pertussis *vaccine.*

DR Abbreviation for *reaction* of degeneration.

dr Abbreviation for dram.

drachm (dram). SYN dram. [G. *drachmē,* an ancient Greek weight, equivalent to about 60 gr]

drac·on·ti·a·sis (drak-on-tī′ă-sis). Former term for dracunculiasis. [G. *drakōn (drakont-),* dragon]

dra·cun·cu·li·a·sis, dra·cun·cu·lo·sis (dra-kŭng-kyū-lī′ă-sis, -kyū-lō′sis). Infection with *Dracunculus medinensis.*

Dra·cun·cu·lus (dra-kŭng′kyū-lŭs). A genus of nematodes (superfamily Dracunculoidea) that have some resemblances to true filarial worms; however, adults are larger (females being as long as 1 m), and the intermediate host is a freshwater crustacean rather than an insect. [L. dim. of *draco,* serpent]

D. lova, old incorrect term for *Loa loa.*

D. medinen′sis, a species of skin-infecting, yard-long nematodes, formerly incorrectly classed as *Filaria;* adult worms live anywhere in the body of humans and various semi-aquatic mammals; the females migrate along fascial planes to subcutaneous tissues, where troublesome chronic ulcers are formed in the skin; when the host enters water, larvae are discharged from the ulcers, from which the head of the female worm protrudes; these larvae, if ingested by *Cyclops* species, develop in the intermediate host to the infective stage; humans and various animals contract the infection from accidental ingestion of infected *Cyclops* in drinking water. Popularly known as guinea, Medina, serpent, or dragon worm, and frequently thought to be the "fiery serpent" that plagued the Israelites. [L. of Medina]

D. oc′uli, old incorrect term for *Loa loa.*

D. persa′rum, old term for *D. medinensis.* [L. of the Persians]

draft. 1. A current of air in a confined space. 2. A quantity of liquid medicine ordered as a single dose. SYN draught.

drag. 1. The lower or cast side of a denture flask. 2. Any tendency for one moving thing to pull something else along with it.

solvent d., the influence exerted by a flow of solvent through a membrane on the simultaneous movement of a solute through the membrane.

dra·gée (dra-zhā′). A sugar-coated pill or capsule. [Fr.]

Dragendorff, Georg J.N., German physician and pharmaceutical chemist, 1836–1898. SEE D.'s *test.*

Drager, Glenn A., U.S. neurologist, *1917. SEE Shy-D. *syndrome.*

Dräger, Heinrich, German manufacturer of industrial and diving respiratory apparatus, *1898. SEE D. *respirometer.*

drain (drān). 1. To draw off fluid from a cavity as it forms. 2. A device, usually in the shape of a tube or wick, for removing fluid as it collects in a cavity, especially a wound cavity. [A. S. *drehnian,* to draw off]

cigarette d., a wick of gauze wrapped in rubber tissue, providing capillary drainage.

Mikulicz′ d., a d. made of several strings of gauze held together by a single layer of gauze.

Penrose d., a soft tube-shaped rubber drain.

stab d., a d. passed into a cavity through a puncture made at a dependent part away from the wound of operation, designed to prevent infection of the wound.

sump d., a d. consisting of an outer tube with a smaller tube within it which is attached to a suction pump; the outer tube has multiple perforations that allow fluid and air to pass into its interior and be carried away through the suction tube.

drain·age (drān′ij). Continuous withdrawal of fluids from a wound or other cavity.

capillary d., d. by means of a wick of gauze or other material.

closed d., d. of a body cavity via a water- or air-tight system.

dependent d., d. from the lowest part and into a receptacle at a level lower than the structure being drained. SYN downward d.

downward d., SYN dependent d.

infusion-aspiration d., a type of d. in which antibiotics are continuously infused into a cavity at the same time fluid is being drained (aspirated) from the cavity. SYN drip-suck irrigation.

open d., d. allowing air to enter.

postural d., d. used in bronchiectasis and lung abscess. The patient's body is positioned so that the trachea is inclined downward and below the affected chest area.

suction d., closed drainage of a cavity, with a suction apparatus attached to the drainage tube.

through d., d. obtained by the passage of a perforated tube, open at both extremities, through a cavity; in addition, the cavity can be washed out by a solution passed through the tube.

tidal d., d. of the urinary bladder by means of an intermittent filling and emptying apparatus.

Wangensteen d., continuous d. by suction through an indwelling gastric or duodenal tube.

dram (dr). A unit of weight: $\frac{1}{8}$ oz.; 60 gr, apothecaries' weight; $\frac{1}{16}$ oz., avoirdupois weight. SYN drachm. [see drachm]

dra·ma·mine(R). SYN dimenhydrinate.

drape (drāp). 1. To cover parts of the body other than those to be examined or operated upon. 2. The cloth or materials used for such cover. [M.E., fr. L.L. *drappus,* cloth]

Draper, John W., English chemist, 1811–1882. SEE D.'s *law.*

drap·e·to·ma·nia (drap′ĕ-tō-mā′nē-ă). An uncontrollable desire to run away from home. [G. *drapetēs,* runaway, + *mania,* insanity]

draught (draft). SYN draft.

draw-sheet (draw′shēt). A narrow sheet placed crosswise on the bed under the patient, with a rubber sheet of the same width beneath it; used to assist in moving the patient or in changing soiled bed coverings.

dream (drēm). Mental activity during sleep in which events, thought, emotions, and images are experienced as real.

anxiety d., a d. (or nightmare) in which morbid fear and anxiety form an important part.

wet d., a true physiologic orgasm during sleep including, in males, a nocturnal seminal emission (oneirogmus), usually accompanying a d. with sexual content.

dream-work. In psychoanalysis, the process by which the change from latent to manifest content of a dream is effected.

Drechs·lera (dresh′ler-ă). A saprobic genus of fungi, frequently recovered in the clinical laboratory, characterized by conidia attached to a zigzagged conidiophore. Species in the genus may cause phaeohyphomycosis in humans, cats, and horses.

Dreifuss, F. E. SEE Emery-D. muscular *dystrophy.*

drench. 1. The pouring of a liquid medicinal agent from a bottle into the mouth of an animal while holding its head high, thus forcing it to swallow. 2. The liquid medicinal agent intended for giving to an animal by drenching. [M.E. *drenchen,* to drown, fr. O.E. *drencan,* to give a drink]

drep·a·nid·i·um (drep-ă-nid′ē-ŭm). A young sickle-shaped or crescentic form of a gregarine. [G. *drepanē,* a sickle]

drep·a·no·cyte (drep′ă-nō-sīt). SYN sickle *cell.* [G. *drepanē,* sickle, + *kytos,* a hollow (cell)]

drep·a·no·cyt·ic (drep′ă-nō-sit′ik). Relating to or resembling a sickle cell.

dress·er (dres′ĕr). In Great Britain, a surgical assistant whose primary duty is bandaging and dressing wounds.

dress·ing (dres′ing). The material applied, or the application itself of material, to a wound for protection, absorbance, drainage, etc.

adhesive absorbent d., a sterile individual d. consisting of a plain absorbent compress affixed to a film of fabric coated with a pressure-sensitive adhesive.

antiseptic d., a sterile d. of gauze impregnated with an antiseptic.

bolus d., SYN tie-over d.

dry d., dry gauze or other material applied to a wound.

fixed d., a d. stiffened with a substance that produces immobilization when it dries.

Lister's d., the first type of antiseptic d., one of gauze impregnated with carbolic acid.

occlusive d., a d. that hermetically seals a wound.

pressure d., a d. by which pressure is exerted on the area covered to prevent the collection of fluids in the underlying tissues; most commonly used after skin grafting and in the treatment of burns.

tie-over d., a d. placed over a skin graft or other sutured wound and tied on by the sutures which have been left of sufficient length for that purpose. SYN bolus d.

water d., an application of gauze or other material that is kept wet with sterilized water or saline solution.

Dressler, William, U.S. physician, 1890–1969. SEE D. *beat;* D.'s *syndrome.*

Dreyer, Georges, English pathologist, 1873–1934. SEE D.'s *formula.*

DRG Abbreviation for diagnosis-related group.

drib·ble (drĭ′bl). **1.** To drool, slaver, drivel. **2.** To fall in drops, as the urine from a distended bladder.

drift. A gradual movement, as from an original position. **2.** A gradual change in the value of a random variable over time as a result of various factors, some random and some systematic effects of trend, manipulation, etc.

antigenic d., the process of "evolutionary" changes in molecular structure of DNA/RNA in microorganisms during their passage from one host to another; it may be due to recombination, deletion, or insertion of genes, point mutations or combinations of these events; it leads to alteration (usually slow and progressive) in the antigenic composition, and therefore in the immunologic responses of individuals and populations to exposure to the microorganism concerned.

genetic d., a change in the frequencies of genetic traits over generations.

pure random d., that which has random components only with an average value of zero and no systematic effects. Brownian movement in a still container shows pure random d. but in the Mississippi shows a steady downstream tendency.

drift·ing. Random movement of a tooth to a position of greater stability.

drifts. Slow ocular movements of greater amplitude than flicks, occurring during ocular fixation. SYN drift movements.

Drigalski, Wilhelm von, German bacteriologist, 1871–1950. SEE D.-Conradi *agar;* Conradi-D. *agar.*

drill. **1.** To make a hole in bone or other hard substance. **2.** An instrument for making or enlarging a hole in bone or in a tooth. [Middle Dutch *drillen,* to bore]

bur d., SEE bur.

dental d., a rotary power-driven instrument into which cutting points may be inserted. SEE ALSO handpiece.

Drinker, Philip, U.S. industrial hygienist, 1894–1972. SEE D. *respirator.*

drip. **1.** To flow a drop at a time. **2.** A flowing in drops.

alkaline milk d., a variable mixture of sodium bicarbonate in whole milk dripped into the stomach through a small oral or nasal tube to produce constant achlorhydria; used in the treatment of certain ulcers.

intravenous d., the slow but continuous introduction of solutions intravenously, a drop at a time.

Murphy d., SYN proctoclysis.

postnasal d., term sometimes used to describe sensation of excessive mucoid or mucopurulent discharge from the posterior nares.

drive. **1.** A basic compelling urge. **2.** In psychology, classified as either innate (*e.g.,* hunger) or learned (*e.g.,* hoarding) and appetitive (*e.g.,* hunger, thirst, sex) or aversive (*e.g.,* fear, pain, grief). SEE ALSO motive, motivation.

acquired d.'s, SYN secondary d.'s.

exploratory d., the d. typical of toddlers and some animals to investigate the unfamiliar or unknown.

learned d., SYN motive (1).

meiotic d., differential fitness in males and females.

physiological d.'s, those d.'s such as hunger and thirst which stem from the biological needs of an organism. SYN primary d.'s.

primary d.'s, SYN physiological d.'s.

secondary d.'s, those d.'s not directly related to biological needs; a secondary d. can be learned as an offshoot of a primary d., in which case it is often referred to as a motive. SYN acquired d.'s.

driv·ing (drīv′ing). The induction of a frequency in the electroencephalogram by sensory stimulation at this frequency.

photic d., a normal EEG phenomenon whereby the frequency of the activity recorded over the parieto-occipital regions is time-locked to the flash frequency during photic stimulation.

drom·ic (drŏ′mik). SYN orthodromic. [G. *dromos,* a running, race-course]

drom·o·graph (drŏm′ō-graf). An instrument for recording the rapidity of the blood circulation. [G. *dromos,* a running, + *graphō,* to record]

drom·o·ma·nia (drŏm-ō-mā′nē-ă). An uncontrollable impulse to wander or travel. [G. *dromos,* a running, + *mania,* insanity]

dro·mo·stan·o·lone pro·pi·o·nate (drō-mos′tan-ō-lōn, drō-mō-stan′ō-lōn). 17β-Hydroxy-2α-methyl-5α-androstan-3-one propionate; an antineoplastic agent.

dro·mo·tro·pic (drō-mō-trop′ik). Influencing the velocity of conduction of excitation, as in nerve or cardiac muscle fibers. [G. *dromos,* a running, + *tropē,* a turn]

negatively d., acting to diminish conduction velocity.

positively d., acting to increase conduction velocity.

dro·nab·i·nol (drō-nab′i-nol). 6*H*-Dibenzo[*b,d*]pyran-l-ol, 6a,7,8,10a-tetrahydro-6,6,9-trimethyl-3-pentyl-, (6a*R-trans*)-; the principal psychoactive substance present in *Cannabis sativa,* used therapeutically as an antinauseant to control the nausea and vomiting associated with cancer chemotherapy. SEE ALSO tetrahydrocannabinol.

drop. **1.** To fall, or to be dispensed or poured in globules. **2.** A liquid globule. **3.** A volume of liquid regarded as a unit of dosage, equivalent in the case of water to about 1 minim. SEE ALSO drops. **4.** A solid confection in globular form, usually directed to be allowed to dissolve in the mouth. [A.S. *droppan*]

enamel d., SYN enameloma.

hanging d., a d. of liquid on the undersurface of the object glass for examination under the microscope.

dro·per·i·dol (drō-per′i-dol). A butyrophenone drug used in neuroleptanalgesia and preanesthetic medication; the pharmacology is similar to that of haloperidol; a dopamine receptor blocker.

drop·let (drop′let). A diminutive drop, such as a particle of moisture discharged from the mouth during coughing, sneezing, or speaking; these may transmit infections to others by their airborne passage. [drop + *-let,* dim. suffix]

drop·per. SYN instillator.

drops. A popular term for a medicine taken in doses measured by d.'s, usually a tincture, or applied by dropping, as an eyewash.

eye d., SEE eyewash, ophthalmic *solutions,* under *solution.*

knock-out d., a popular name for chloral alcoholate given with criminal intent to produce unconsciousness rapidly; it is formed by adding chloral hydrate to beer or some stronger alcoholic liquor.

nose d., a liquid preparation intended for intranasal administration with a medicine dropper. Most frequently used for decongestion of the nasal passages but can be used for any other appropriate indication.

stomach d., a stomachic tonic, usually tincture of gentian, alone or with other stomachics.

drop·si·cal (drop'si-kăl). SYN hydropic.

drop·sy (drop'sē). Old term for edema. [G. *hydrōps*]

abdominal d., SYN ascites.

cardiac d., edema due to heart failure.

epidemic d., a disease causing occasional epidemics in India and Mauritius; marked by edema, anemia, eruptive angiomatosis, and mild fever; may be associated with nutritional deficiency.

famine d., edema occurring with the hypoproteinemia of low protein intake occurring as starvation of a large population group.

nutritional d., edema due to hypoproteinemia secondary to malnutrition.

d. of pericardium, SYN pericardial *effusion.*

drown·ing. Death within 24 hours of immersion in liquid, either due to anoxia or cardiac arrest caused by sudden extreme lowering of temperature (immersion syndrome). SEE ALSO near d.

dry d., d. in an individual whose laryngeal reflexes are brisk, resulting in spasm that prevents inhalation of water; may be associated with the highest recovery rate.

near d., initial survival following immersion in liquid; the victim may die more than 24 hours later, *e.g.,* from ARDS.

secondary d., pulmonary edema and resulting asphyxia, resulting from hypoxia and increased permeability of pulmonary capillaries occurring in a patient who has been immersed in and aspirated some water.

drows·i·ness (drow'zē-nes). A state of impaired awareness associated with a desire or inclination to sleep. SYN hypnesthesia.

Dr.P.H. Abbreviation of Doctor of Public Health.

drug (drŭg). **1.** Therapeutic agent; any substance, other than food, used in the prevention, diagnosis, alleviation, treatment, or cure of disease. For types or classifications of d.'s, see the specific name. SEE ALSO agent. **2.** To administer or take a d., usually implying an overly large quantity or a narcotic. **3.** General term for any substance, stimulating or depressing, that can be habituating or addictive, especially a narcotic. [M.E. *drogge*]

addictive d., any d. that creates a certain degree of euphoria and has a strong potential for addiction.

crude d., an unrefined preparation, usually of plant origin, that occurs either in the entire, nearly entire, broken, cut, or powdered state.

d. holidays, intervals when a chronically medicated patient temporarily stops taking the medication; used to allow some recuperation of normal functions and/or to maintain sensitivity to the drug(s).

nonsteroidal anti-inflammatory d.'s (NSAID), a large number of d.'s exerting anti-inflammatory (and also usually analgesic and antipyretic) actions; examples include aspirin, acetaminophen, diclofenac, ibuprofen, and naproxen. A contrast is made with steroidal compounds (such as hydrocortisone or prednisone) exerting anti-inflammatory activity.

orphan d.'s, SYN orphan *products,* under *product.*

psychedelic d., SYN hallucinogen.

psychodysleptic d., SYN hallucinogen.

psycholytic d., SYN hallucinogen.

psychotomimetic d., SYN hallucinogen.

psychotropic d., any d. that affects the mind.

recreational d., SYN street d.

scheduled d., a d. assigned to any of the five schedules in the Controlled Substances Act (1970). SEE ALSO controlled *substance.*

street d., a controlled substance taken for non-medical purposes. Street d.'s comprise various amphetamines, anesthetics, barbiturates, opiates, and psychoactive drugs, and many are derived from natural sources (*e.g.,* the plants *Papaver somniferum, Can-*

nibis sativa, Amanita pantherina, Lophophora williamsii). Slang names include acid (lysergic acid diethylamide), angel dust (phencyclidine), coke (cocaine), downers (barbiturates), grass (marijuana), hash (concentrated tetrahydrocannibinol), magic mushrooms (psilocybin), mescaline (peyote), speed (amphetamines). During the 1980s, a new class of "designer drugs" arose, mostly analogs of psychoactive substances intended to escape regulation under the Controlled Substances Act. Also, crack cocaine, a potent, smokable form of cocaine, emerged as a major public health problem. In the U.S. illicit use of drugs such as cocaine, marijuana, and heroin historically has occurred in cycles. SYN recreational d.

drug-fast. Pertaining to microorganisms that resist or become tolerant to an antibacterial agent.

drug·gist (drŭg'ist). Old common term for pharmacist.

drug in·ter·ac·tions. The pharmacological result, either desirable or undesirable, of drugs interacting with themselves or other drugs, with endogenous physiologic chemical agents (*e.g.,* MAOI with epinephrine), with components of the diet, and with chemicals used in diagnostic tests or the results of such tests.

drum, drum·head (drŭm, drŭm'hed). SYN tympanic *membrane.*

Drummond, Sir David, English physician, 1852–1932. SEE *artery* of D.; D.'s *sign.*

drunk·en·ness (drŭnk'en-nes). Intoxication, usually alcoholic. SEE ALSO acute *alcoholism.*

sleep d., a half-waking condition in which the faculty of orientation is in abeyance, and under the influence of nightmare-like ideas the person may become actively excited and violent. SYN somnolentia (2).

dru·sen (drū'sen). Small bright structures seen in the retina and in the optic disc. [Ger. pl. of *druse,* stony nodule, geode]

giant d., obsolete term for a glial hamartoma of the optic nerve head or the peripapillary retina, seen in tuberous sclerosis.

intrapapillary d., SYN d. of the optic nerve head.

d. of the macula, excrescences of Bruch's membrane that produce a window in the retinal pigment epithelium and are a feature of age-related macular retinal degeneration. SYN macular d.

macular d., SYN d. of the macula.

optic nerve d., basophilic, calcareous, laminated acellular bodies within the optic nerve anterior to the scleral lamina cribrosa.

d. of the optic nerve head, basophilic, laminated, calcareous acellular masses that resemble crystals within the nerve head, anterior to the lamina cribrosa, that may simulate papilledema and/or cause visual field defects. SYN intrapapillary d.

dry ice (drī īs). SYN *carbon* dioxide snow.

ds Abbreviation for double-stranded.

DSA Abbreviation for digital subtraction *angiography.*

DT Abbreviation for *delirium* tremens; duration *tetany.*

dT Abbreviation for deoxythymidine.

DT-di·aph·o·rase. SYN NADPH dehydrogenase (quinone).

dTDP Abbreviation for thymidine 5'-diphosphate.

dTDP-sug·ars. Sugars or sugar derivatives bonded to dTDP.

DTH Abbreviation for delayed-type hypersensitivity.

dThd Abbreviation for thymidine.

DTIC Abbreviation for dacarbazine.

dTMP Abbreviation for deoxythymidylic acid; thymidine 5'-monophosphate.

DTP Abbreviation for distal *tingling* on percussion; diphtheria toxoid, tetanus toxoid, and pertussis *vaccine.*

DTPA Abbreviation for diethylenetriamine pentaacetic acid.

DTR Abbreviation for deep tendon reflex.

dTTP Abbreviation for thymidine 5'-triphosphate.

du·al·ism (dū'ăl-izm). **1.** In chemistry, a theory advanced by J.J. Berzelius (Swedish chemist, 1779–1848) that every compound, no matter how many elements enter into it, is composed of two parts, one electrically negative, the other positive; still applicable, with modification, to polar compounds, but inapplicable to nonpolar compounds. **2.** In hematology, the concept that blood cells have two origins, *i.e.,* lymphogenous or myelogenous. **3.**

The theory that the mind and body are two distinct systems, independent and different in nature. [L. *dualis,* relating to two, fr. *duo,* two]

Duane, Alexander, U.S. ophthalmologist, 1858–1926. SEE D.'s *syndrome.*

Dubin, I. Nathan, U.S. pathologist, 1913–1980. SEE D.-Johnson *syndrome.*

DuBois, Eugene F., U.S. physiologist, 1882–1959. SEE DuB.'s *formula;* Aub-DuB. *table.*

Dubois, Paul, French obstetrician, 1795–1871. SEE D.'s *abscesses,* under *abscess, disease.*

du·boi·sine (dū-boy′sēn). An alkaloid obtained from the leaves of *Duboisia myoporoides* (family Solanaceae). SEE hyoscyamine.

Du Bois-Reymond, Emil H., German physiologist, 1818–1896. SEE Du Bois-Reymond's *law.*

Duboscq, Jules, French optician, 1817–1886. SEE D.'s *colorimeter.*

Dubowitz, Victor, South African-English pediatrician, *1931. SEE D. *score.*

Dubreuil-Chambardel, Louis, French dentist, 1879–1927. SEE Dubreuil-Chambardel *syndrome.*

Dubreuilh, M.W., 20th century French dermatologist. SEE precancerous *melanosis* of D.

Duchenne, Guillaume B.A., French neurologist, 1806–1875. SEE D.'s *disease, sign, syndrome;* D.-Aran *disease;* Aran-D. *disease;* D.-Erb *paralysis;* D. *dystrophy.*

Duckworth, Sir Dyce, English physician, 1840–1928. SEE D.'s *phenomenon.*

Ducrey, Augusto, Italian dermatologist, 1860–1940. SEE D.'s *bacillus;* D. *test.*

DUCT

duct (dŭkt). A tubular structure giving exit to the secretion of a gland, or conducting any fluid. SEE ALSO canal. SYN ductus [NA]. [L. *duco,* pp. *ductus,* to lead]

aberrant d.'s, SYN aberrant *ductules,* under *ductule.*

aberrant bile d.'s, small d.'s occasionally present in the ligaments of the liver or originating from the surface of the liver.

accessory pancreatic d., the excretory duct of the head of the pancreas, one branch of which joins the pancreatic duct, the other opening independently into the duodenum at the lesser duodenal papilla. SYN ductus pancreaticus accessorius [NA], Bernard's canal, Bernard's d., ductus dorsopancreaticus, Santorini's canal, Santorini's d.

alveolar d., (1) the part of the respiratory passages distal to the respiratory bronchiole; from it arise alveolar sacs and alveoli; **(2)** the smallest of the intralobular d.'s in the mammary gland, into which the secretory alveoli open. SYN ductulus alveolaris [NA].

amniotic d., the transitory opening between the seroamniotic folds in birds just before they fuse to form the seroamniotic raphe.

anal d.'s, short d.'s lined with simple columnar to stratified columnar epithelium that extend from the valvulae anales to the sinus anales.

arterial d., SYN *ductus* arteriosus.

Bartholin's d., SYN major sublingual d.

Bellini's d.'s, SYN papillary d.'s.

Bernard's d., SYN accessory pancreatic d.

bile d., any of the d.'s conveying bile between the liver and the intestine, including hepatic, cystic, and common bile d. SYN biliary d.

biliary d., SYN bile d.

Blasius' d., SYN parotid d.

Botallo's d., SYN *ductus* arteriosus.

bucconeural d., SYN craniopharyngeal d.

d. of bulbourethral gland, the long slender duct on each side

passing down through the inferior fascia of the urogenital diaphragm to enter the bulb of the penis and course forward 2 or 3 cm before terminating in the urethra. SYN ductus glandulae bulbourethralis [NA].

canalicular d.'s, (1) SYN lactiferous d.'s. **(2)** SYN biliary *ductules,* under *ductule.*

carotid d., SYN *ductus* caroticus.

cervical d., SEE cervical *diverticulum.*

choledoch d., SYN common bile d.

cochlear d., a spirally arranged membranous tube suspended within the cochlea, occupying the lower portion of the scala vestibuli; it begins by a blind extremity, the vestibular cecum, in the cochlear recess of the vestibule, terminating in another blind extremity, the cecum cupulare or lagena, at the cupola of the cochlea; it contains endolymph and communicates with the sacculus by the ductus reuniens; the spiral organ (of Corti), the neuroepithelial receptor organ for hearing, occupies the floor of the duct. SYN ductus cochlearis [NA], Löwenberg's canal, Löwenberg's scala, membranous cochlea, scala media.

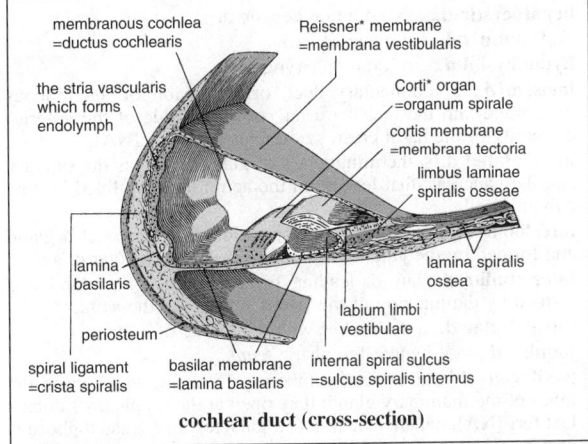

cochlear duct (cross-section)

common bile d., a duct formed by the union of the hepatic and cystic ducts; it discharges at the duodenal papilla. SYN ductus choledochus [NA], choledoch d., choledoch, choledochus.

common hepatic d., the part of the biliary duct system that is formed by the confluence of right and left hepatic ducts. At the porta hepatis it is joined by the cystic duct to become the common bile duct. SYN ductus hepaticus communis [NA], hepatocystic d.

craniopharyngeal d., the slender tubular part of the hypophysial diverticulum; the stalk of Rathke's pocket. SYN bucconeural d., hypophysial d.

Cuvier's d.'s, obsolete term for the common cardinal veins.

cystic d., cystic gall d., the d. leading from the gallbladder; it joins the hepatic duct to form the common bile duct. SYN ductus cysticus [NA].

deferent d., SYN *ductus* deferens.

efferent d., SYN efferent *ductules* of testis, under *ductule.*

ejaculatory d., the duct formed by the union of the deferent duct and the excretory duct of the seminal vesicle, which opens into the prostatic urethra. SYN ductus ejaculatorius [NA], spermiduct (2).

endolymphatic d., a small membranous canal, connecting with both saccule and utricle of the membranous labyrinth, passing through the aqueduct of vestibule, and terminating in a dilated blind extremity, the endolymphatic sac, on the posterior surface of the petrous portion of the temporal bone beneath the dura mater. SYN ductus endolymphaticus [NA].

d. of epididymis, a convoluted tube into which the efferent ductules open and which itself terminates in the ductus deferens. SYN ductus epididymidis [NA].

excretory d., a d. carrying the secretion from a gland or a fluid from any reservoir. SYN ductus excretorius.

excretory d.'s of lacrimal gland, the multiple (6 to 10) excretory ducts of the lacrimal gland that open into the superior fornix of the conjunctival sac. SYN ductuli excretorii glandulae lacrimalis [NA], excretory ductules of lacrimal gland.

excretory d. of seminal vesicle, the passage leading from a seminal vesicle to the ejaculatory duct. SYN ductus excretorius vesiculae seminalis [NA].

frontonasal d., the passage that leads downward from the frontal sinus to open into the ethmoidal infundibulum.

galactophorous d.'s, SYN lactiferous d.'s.

gall d., Obsolete term for bile d.

Gartner's d., SYN longitudinal d. of epoöphoron.

genital d., SYN genital *tract*.

guttural d., SYN auditory *tube*.

hemithoracic d., an accessory thoracic duct, usually emptying into the thoracic duct but sometimes discharging independently into the right subclavian vein. SYN ductus hemithoracicus.

Hensen's d., SYN uniting d.

hepatic d., SEE common hepatic d., right hepatic d., left hepatic d.

hepatocystic d., SYN common hepatic d.

Hoffmann's d., SYN pancreatic d.

hypophysial d., SYN craniopharyngeal d.

incisive d., a rudimentary duct, or protrusion of the mucous membrane into the incisive canal, on either side of the anterior extremity of the nasal crest. SYN ductus incisivus [NA].

intercalated d.'s, the minute d.'s of glands, such as the salivary and the pancreas, that lead from the acini; they are lined by low cuboidal cells.

interlobar d., a d. draining the secretion of the lobe of a gland and formed by the junction of a number of interlobular d.'s.

interlobular d., any d. leading from a lobule of a gland and formed by the junction of the fine d.'s draining the acini.

intralobular d., a d. that lies within a lobule of a gland.

jugular d., SYN jugular lymphatic *trunk*.

lactiferous d.'s, the ducts, numbering 15 or 20, which drain the lobes of the mammary gland; they open at the nipple. SYN ductus lactiferi [NA], canalicular d.'s (1), galactophore, galactophorous canals, galactophorous d.'s, mamillary d.'s, mammary d.'s, milk d.'s, tubuli galactophori, tubuli lactiferi.

left d. of caudate lobe, a tributary to the left hepatic duct draining bile from the left half of the caudate lobe. SYN ductus lobi caudati sinister [NA].

left hepatic d., the duct that drains bile from the left half of the liver, including the quadrate lobe and the left part of the caudate lobe. SYN ductus hepaticus sinister [NA].

longitudinal d. of epoöphoron, a rudimentary vestige of the mesonephric duct in the female into which the tubules of the epoöphoron open; it is located in the broad ligament of the uterus, parallel with the lateral part of the uterine tube, and in the lateral walls of the cervix and vagina. SYN ductus epoöphori longitudinalis [NA], ductus deferens vestigialis, Gartner's canal, Gartner's d.

Luschka's d.'s, glandlike tubular structures in the wall of the gallbladder, especially in the part covered with peritoneum.

lymphatic d., one of the two large lymph channels, right lymphatic d. or thoracic d.

major sublingual d., the duct that drains the anterior portion of the sublingual gland; it opens at the sublingual papilla. SYN ductus sublingualis major [NA], Bartholin's d.

mamillary d.'s, SYN lactiferous d.'s.

mammary d.'s, SYN lactiferous d.'s.

mesonephric d., a duct in the embryo draining the mesonephric tubules; in the male it becomes the ductus deferens; in the female it becomes vestigial. SEE ALSO longitudinal d. of epoöphoron. SYN ductus mesonephricus [NA], wolffian d.

metanephric d., the slender tubular portion of the metanephric diverticulum; the primordium of the epithelial lining of the ureter. SEE epoöphoron, longitudinal d. of epoöphoron.

milk d.'s, SYN lactiferous d.'s.

minor sublingual d.'s, from 8 to 20 small ducts of the sublingual salivary gland that open into the mouth on the surface of the

sublingual fold; a few join the submandibular ducts. SYN ductus sublinguales minores [NA], Rivinus' d.'s, Walther's canals, Walther's d.'s.

Müller's d., müllerian d., SYN paramesonephric d.

nasal d., SYN nasolacrimal d.

nasolacrimal d., the passage leading downward from the lacrimal sac on each side to the anterior portion of the inferior meatus of the nose, through which tears are conducted into the nasal cavity. SYN ductus nasolacrimalis [NA], nasal d.

nephric d., SYN pronephric d.

omphalomesenteric d., obsolete term for yolk *stalk*.

pancreatic d., the excretory duct of the pancreas that extends through the gland from tail to head where it empties into the duodenum at the greater duodenal papilla. SYN ductus pancreaticus [NA], Hoffmann's d., Wirsung's canal, Wirsung's d.

papillary d.'s, the largest straight excretory d.'s in the kidney medulla and papillae whose openings form the area cribrosa; they are a continuation of the collecting tubules. SYN Bellini's d.'s.

paramesonephric d., either of the two paired embryonic tubes extending along the mesonephros roughly parallel to the mesonephric duct and emptying into the cloaca; in the female, the upper parts of the ducts form the uterine tubes, while the lower fuse to form the uterus and part of the vagina; in the male, vestiges of the ducts form the vagina masculina and the appendix testis. SYN ductus paramesonephricus [NA], Müller's d., müllerian d.

paraurethral d.'s, inconstant ducts along the side of the female urethra that convey the mucoid secretion of Skene's glands to the vestibule. SYN ductus paraurethrales [NA], d.'s of Skene's glands, Schüller's d.'s.

parotid d., the duct of the parotid gland opening from the cheek into the vestibule of the mouth opposite the neck of the superior second molar tooth. SYN ductus parotideus [NA], Blasius' d., Stensen's d., Steno's d.

Pecquet's d., SYN thoracic d.

perilymphatic d., a fine canal connecting the perilymphatic space of the cochlea with the subarachnoid space. SYN ductus perilymphaticus [NA], aqueductus cochleae, cochlear aqueduct.

pharyngobranchial d.'s, SEE *ductus* pharyngobranchialis III, *ductus* pharyngobranchialis IV.

pronephric d., the d. of the pronephros; serves as the mesonephric duct. SYN nephric d.

prostatic d.'s, SYN prostatic *ductules*, under *ductule*.

right d. of caudate lobe, the bile duct from the right half of the caudate lobe, a tributary to the right hepatic duct. SYN ductus lobi caudati dexter [NA].

right hepatic d., the duct that transmits bile to the common hepatic duct from the right half of the liver and the right part of the caudate lobe. SYN ductus hepaticus dexter [NA].

right lymphatic d., one of the two terminal lymph vessels, a short trunk, about 2 cm in length, formed by the union of the right jugular lymphatic vessel and vessels from the lymph nodes of the right superior limb, thoracic wall, and both lungs; it lies on the right side of the root of the neck and empties into the right brachiocephalic vein. SYN ductus lymphaticus dexter [NA], ductus thoracicus dexter [NA].

Rivinus' d.'s, SYN minor sublingual d.'s.

salivary d., SYN striated d.

Santorini's d., SYN accessory pancreatic d.

Schüller's d.'s, SYN paraurethral d.'s.

secretory d., SYN striated d.

semicircular d.'s, three small membranous tubes in the bony semicircular canals that lie within the bony labyrinth and form loops of about two-thirds of a circle. The three (anterior semicircular d., lateral semicircular d., and posterior semicircular d.) lie in planes at right angles to each other and open into the vestibule by five openings of which one is common to the anterior and lateral ducts. Each duct has an ampulla at one end within which filaments of the vestibular nerve terminate. SYN ductus semicirculares [NA].

seminal d., any one of the d.'s conveying semen from the epididymis to the urethra, ductus deferens, or ejaculatory d. SYN gonaduct (1).

d.'s of Skene's glands, SYN paraurethral d.'s.

spermatic d., SYN *ductus* deferens.

Stensen's d., Steno's d., SYN parotid d.

striated d., a type of intralobular d. found in some salivary glands that modifies the secretory product; it derives its name from extensive infolding of the basal membrane. SYN salivary d., secretory d.

subclavian d., SYN subclavian lymphatic *trunk.*

submandibular d., the duct of the submandibular salivary gland; it opens at the sublingual papilla near the frenulum of the tongue. SYN ductus submandibularis [NA], ductus submaxillaris, submaxillary d., Wharton's d.

submaxillary d., SYN submandibular d.

sudoriferous d., SYN d. of sweat glands.

sweat d., SYN d. of sweat glands.

d. of sweat glands, the superficial portion of the sweat gland that passes through the corium and epidermis, opening on the surface by the porus sudoriferus or sweat pore. SYN ductus sudoriferus, sudoriferous d., sweat d.

testicular d., SYN *ductus* deferens.

thoracic d., the largest lymph vessel in the body, beginning at the cisterna chyli at about the level of the second lumbar vertebra; the abdominal part extends superiorly to pass through the aortic opening of the diaphragm, where it becomes the thoracic part and crosses the posterior mediastinum to form the arch of thoracic duct and discharge into the left venous angle (origin of the brachiocephalic vein). SYN ductus thoracicus [NA], Pecquet's d., van Horne's canal.

thyroglossal d., a transitory endodermal tube in the embryo, carrying thyroid-forming tissue at its caudal end; normally, the duct disappears after the thyroid has moved to its definitive location in the neck; its point of origin is regularly marked on the root of the adult tongue by the foramen cecum; occasionally, its incomplete regression results in the formation of cysts along its embryonic course. SEE ALSO pyramidal *lobe* of thyroid gland. SYN ductus thyroglossus, thyrolingual d.

thyrolingual d., SYN thyroglossal d.

umbilical d., SYN yolk *stalk.*

uniting d., a short membranous tube passing from the lower end of the saccule to the cochlear duct of the membranous labyrinth. SYN ductus reuniens [NA], canaliculus reuniens, canalis reuniens, Hensen's canal, Hensen's d., uniting canal.

utriculosaccular d., a duct that connects the inner aspect of the utricle with the endolymphatic duct a short distance from its origin from the saccule. SYN ductus utriculosaccularis [NA], Böttcher's canal.

vitelline d., vitellointestinal d., SYN yolk *stalk.*

Walther's d.'s, SYN minor sublingual d.'s.

Wharton's d., SYN submandibular d.

Wirsung's d., SYN pancreatic d.

wolffian d., SYN mesonephric d.

---

duc·tal (dŭk′tăl). Relating to a duct.

duc·tile (dŭk′tĭl). Denoting the property of a material that allows it to be bent, drawn out (as a wire), or otherwise deformed without breaking. [L. *ductilis,* capable of being led or drawn]

duc·tion (dŭk′shŭn). **1.** The act of leading, bringing, conducting. **2.** In ophthalmology, ocular rotations with reference to one eye; usually additionally designating direction of movement of the eye; *e.g.,* rotation toward the nose, adduction; toward the temple, abduction; upward, supra- or sursumduction; downward, deorsumduction; of the upper pole of one cornea, cycloduction; of the upper pole of one cornea outward, excycloduction; of the upper pole of one cornea inward, incycloduction. [L. *duco,* to lead]

F d., transfer of chromosomal fragments from one bacterium to another by means of F′ carriers. SYN sexduction.

forced d., a maneuver to determine whether a mechanical obstruction is present in the eye; with forceps grasping an eye

muscle, an attempt is made to passively move the eyeball in the direction of restricted rotation. SYN passive d.

passive d., SYN forced d.

duct·less (dŭkt′les). Having no duct; denoting certain glands having only an internal secretion.

duc·tu·lar (dŭk′tū-lăr). Relating to a ductule.

duc·tule (dŭk′tūl). A minute duct. SYN ductulus [NA].

aberrant d.'s, the superior or inferior diverticula of the epididymis. SYN ductuli aberrantes [NA], aberrant ducts, ductus aberrantes, vasa aberrantes.

biliary d.'s, the excretory ducts of the liver that connect the interlobular ductules to the right (or left) hepatic duct. SYN ductuli biliferi [NA], canalicular ducts (2), ductus biliferi, tubuli biliferi.

efferent d.'s of testis, one of 12 to 14 small seminal ducts leading from the testis to the head of the epididymis. SYN ductulus efferens testis [NA], vas efferens (3) [NA], efferent duct.

excretory d.'s of lacrimal gland, SYN excretory *ducts* of lacrimal gland, under *duct.*

inferior aberrant d., a narrow, coiled tubule frequently connected to the first part of the ductus deferens or to the lower part of the ductus epididymitis. SYN ductulus aberrans inferior, Haller's vas aberrans.

interlobular d.'s, bile ductules occupying portal canals between hepatic lobules that open into the ductuli biliferi. SYN ductuli interlobulares [NA].

prostatic d.'s, about 20 minute canals that receive the prostatic secretion from the glandular tubules and discharge it through openings on either side of the urethral crest in the posterior wall of the urethra. SYN ductuli prostatici [NA], ductus prostatici, prostatic ducts.

superior aberrant d., a diverticulum from the head of the epididymis. SYN ductulus aberrans superior.

transverse d.'s of epoöphoron, a series of 10 to 15 short tubules that open into the longitudinal duct of the epoöphoron and represent vestiges of the mesonephric duct. SYN ductuli transversi epoöphori [NA], tubuli epoöphori.

duc·tu·lus, pl. **duc·tu·li** (dŭk′tū-lŭs, -tū-lī) [NA]. SYN ductule. [Mod. L. dim. of L. *ductus,* duct]

ductuli aber′rantes [NA], SYN aberrant *ductules,* under *ductule.*

d. aberrans infe′rior, SYN inferior aberrant *ductule.*

d. aberrans supe′rior, SYN superior aberrant *ductule.*

d. alveola′ris, pl. **duc′tuli alveola′res** [NA], SYN alveolar *duct.*

duc′tuli bilif′eri [NA], SYN biliary *ductules,* under *ductule.*

d. ef′ferens tes′tis, pl. **duc′tuli efferen′tes tes′tis** [NA], SYN efferent *ductules* of testis, under *ductule.*

duc′tuli excreto′rii glan′dulae lacrima′lis [NA], SYN excretory *ducts* of lacrimal gland, under *duct.*

duc′tuli interlobula′res [NA], SYN interlobular *ductules,* under *ductule.*

duc′tuli paroöph′ori, tubular remnants of the embryonic mesonephros forming the paroöphoron. SYN tubuli paroöphori.

duc′tuli prostat′ici [NA], SYN prostatic *ductules,* under *ductule.*

duc′tuli transver′si epoöph′ori [NA], SYN transverse *ductules* of epoöphoron, under *ductule.* SEE ALSO epoöphoron.

DUCTUS

---

duc·tus, gen. and pl. **duc·tus** (dŭk′tŭs) [NA]. SYN duct. [L. a leading, fr. *duco,* pp. *ductus,* to lead]

d. aber′rantes, SYN aberrant *ductules,* under *ductule.*

d. arterio′sus [NA], a fetal vessel connecting the left pulmonary artery with the descending aorta; in the first two months after birth, it normally changes into a fibrous cord, the ligamentum arteriosum; occasional postnatal failure to close causes a surgically correctable cardiovascular handicap. SYN arterial canal, arterial duct, Botallo's duct.

d. bilif′eri, SYN biliary *ductules,* under *ductule.*

du

d. carot'icus, a portion of the embryonic dorsal aorta between points of juncture with the third and fourth arch arteries; it disappears early in development. SYN carotid duct.

d. choled'ochus [NA], SYN common bile *duct.*

d. cochlea'ris [NA], SYN cochlear *duct.*

d. cys'ticus [NA], SYN cystic *duct.*

d. def'erens [NA], the secretory duct of the testicle, running from the epididymis, of which it is the continuation, to the prostatic urethra where it terminates as the ejaculatory duct. SYN deferent canal, deferent duct, spermatic duct, spermiduct (1), testicular duct, vas deferens.

d. def'erens vestigia'lis, SYN longitudinal *duct* of epoöphoron.

d. dorsopancreat'icus, SYN accessory pancreatic *duct.*

d. ejaculato'rius [NA], SYN ejaculatory *duct.*

d. endolymphat'icus [NA], SYN endolymphatic *duct.*

d. epididym'idis [NA], SYN *duct* of epididymis.

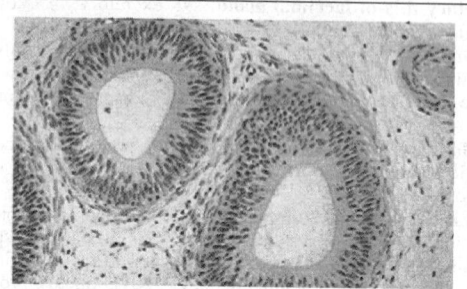

duct of epididymis
histology: two-tiered, highly prismatic
epithelium with stereocilia

d. epoöph'ori longitudina'lis [NA], SYN longitudinal *duct* of epoöphoron. SEE ALSO epoöphoron.

d. excreto'rius, SYN excretory *duct.*

d. excreto'rius vesic'ulae semina'lis [NA], SYN excretory *duct* of seminal vesicle.

d. glan'dulae bulbourethra'lis [NA], SYN *duct* of bulbourethral gland.

d. hemithorac'icus, SYN hemithoracic *duct.*

d. hepat'icus commu'nis [NA], SYN common hepatic *duct.*

d. hepat'icus dex'ter [NA], SYN right hepatic *duct.*

d. hepat'icus sinis'ter [NA], SYN left hepatic *duct.*

d. incisi'vus [NA], SYN incisive *duct.*

d. lactif'eri [NA], SYN lactiferous *ducts,* under *duct.*

d. lingua'lis, a pit on the upper surface of the tongue at the apex of the sulcus terminalis; it marks the point of origin of the d. thyroglossus of the embryo; known more commonly as the foramen cecum.

d. lo'bi cauda'ti dex'ter [NA], SYN right *duct* of caudate lobe.

d. lo'bi cauda'ti sinis'ter [NA], SYN left *duct* of caudate lobe.

d. lymphat'icus dex'ter [NA], SYN right lymphatic *duct.*

d. mesoneph'ricus [NA], SYN mesonephric *duct.* SEE ALSO longitudinal *duct* of epoöphoron.

d. nasolacrima'lis [NA], SYN nasolacrimal *duct.*

d. pancreat'icus [NA], SYN pancreatic *duct.*

d. pancreat'icus accesso'rius [NA], SYN accessory pancreatic *duct.*

d. paramesoneph'ricus [NA], SYN paramesonephric *duct.*

d. paraurethra'les [NA], SYN paraurethral *ducts,* under *duct.*

d. parotid'eus [NA], SYN parotid *duct.*

patent d. arterio'sus, SEE d. arteriosus.

d. perilymphat'icus [NA], SYN perilymphatic *duct.*

d. pharyngobranchia'lis III, a narrow communication between the third branchial pouch and the pharynx in the embryo.

d. pharyngobranchia'lis IV, a narrow communication between the fourth branchial pouch and the pharynx in the embryo.

d. prostat'ici, SYN prostatic *ductules,* under *ductule.*

d. reun'iens [NA], SYN uniting *duct.*

d. semicircula'res [NA], SYN semicircular *ducts,* under *duct.*

d. sublingua'les mino'res [NA], SYN minor sublingual *ducts,* under *duct.*

d. sublingua'lis ma'jor [NA], SYN major sublingual *duct.*

d. submandibula'ris [NA], SYN submandibular *duct.*

d. submaxilla'ris, SYN submandibular *duct.*

d. sudorif'erus, SYN *duct* of sweat glands.

d. thorac'icus [NA], SYN thoracic *duct.*

d. thorac'icus dex'ter [NA], SYN right lymphatic *duct.*

d. thyroglos'sus, SYN thyroglossal *duct.*

d. utric'ulosaccula'ris [NA], SYN utriculosaccular *duct.*

d. veno'sus [NA], in the fetus, continuation of the left umbilical vein through the liver to the vena cava inferior; after birth, its lumen becomes obliterated, forming the ligamentum venosum.

d. veno'sus aran'tii, rarely used term for d. venosus.

Duddell, Benedict, 18th century British oculist. SEE D.'s *membrane.*

Duffy blood group. See Blood Groups appendix.

Dugas, Louis A., U.S. physician, 1806–1884. SEE D.'s *test.*

Duhring, Louis A., U.S. dermatologist, 1845–1913. SEE D.'s *disease.*

Dührssen, Alfred, German obstetrician-gynecologist, 1862–1933. SEE D.'s *incisions,* under *incision.*

Duke, William Waddell Duke, U.S. pathologist, 1883–1945. SEE D. bleeding time *test.*

Dukes, Clement, English physician, 1845–1925. SEE D.'s *disease;* Filatov D. *disease.*

Dukes, Cuthbert E., British pathologist, 1890–1977. SEE D.'s *classification.*

dul·cin (dŭl'sin). *p*-Phenetol carbamide; 4-ethoxyphenylurea; has been used as a substitute for sugar, being 200 times as sweet as cane sugar. Because of hydrolysis to aminophenol, it may produce an injurious effect when used over long periods of time.

dul·cite, dul·ci·tol, dul·cose (dŭl'sīt, -si'tol, -kōs). Galactitol.

dull (dŭl). Not sharp or acute, in any sense; qualifying a surgical instrument, the action of the mind, pain, a sound (especially the percussion note), etc. [M.E. *dul*]

dull·ness, dul·ness (dŭl'nes). The character of the sound obtained by percussing over a solid part incapable of resonating; usually applied to an area containing less air than those which can resonate.

shifting d., a sign of free peritoneal fluid wherein the d. of percussion shifts, generally from one to the other, as the patient is turned from side to side.

Dulong, Pierre L., French chemist, 1785–1838. SEE D.-Petit *law.*

du·mas (dū'mas). SYN foot *yaws.*

dum·my (dŭm'ē). SYN pontic.

Dumontpallier, Alphonse, French physician, 1827–1899. SEE D.'s *pessary.*

dump·ing (dŭmp'ing). SEE dumping *syndrome.*

Duncan, James M., Scottish gynecologist, 1826–1890. SEE Duncan's *folds,* under *fold,* Duncan's *mechanism,* Duncan's *ventricle.*

Duncan. Surname of boys afflicted with what is now known as Duncan's *disease.*

Dunn, R.L. SEE Lison-D. *stain.*

du·o·crin·in (dū-ō-krin'in). A postulated gastrointestinal hormone that is liberated by the contact of gastric contents with the intestine and that stimulates the secretory activity of the duodenal glands (Brunner's glands). [duodenum + G. *krinō,* to secrete, + -in]

du·o·de·nal (dū'ō-dē'năl, dū-od'ĕ-năl). Relating to the duodenum.

du·o·de·nec·to·my (dū-ō-dĕ-nek'tō-mē). Excision of the duodenum. [duodenum + G. *ektomē,* excision]

du·o·de·ni·tis (dū-od-ĕ-nī'tis). Inflammation of the duodenum.

⌂**duodeno-.** Combining form relating to the duodenum. [L. *duodenum, scil., digitorum* breadth of 12 fingers]

du·o·de·no·cho·lan·gi·tis (dū-ō-dē′nō-kō-lan-jī′tis). Inflammation of the duodenum and common bile duct. [duodeno- + G. *cholē,* bile, + *angeion,* vessel, + *-itis,* inflammation]

du·o·de·no·cho·le·cys·tos·to·my (dū-ō-dē′nō-kō-lē-sis-tos′tō-mē). SYN cholecystoduodenostomy. [duodeno- + G. *cholē,* bile, + *kystis,* bladder, + *stoma,* mouth]

du·o·de·no·cho·led·o·chot·o·my (dū-ō-dē′nō-kō-led-ō-kot′ō-mē). Incision into the common bile duct and the adjacent portion of the duodenum. [duodeno- + G. *cholèdochus,* bile duct, + *tomē,* incision]

du·o·de·no·cys·tos·to·my (dū-ō-dē′nō-sis-tos′tō-mē). **1.** SYN cholecystoduodenostomy. **2.** SYN cystoduodenostomy. **3.** SYN pancreatic *cystoduodenostomy.*

du·o·de·no·en·ter·os·to·my (dū-ō-dē′nō-en-ter-os′tō-mē). Establishment of communication between the duodenum and another part of the intestinal tract. [duodeno- + G. *enteron,* intestine, + *stoma,* mouth]

du·o·de·no·je·ju·nos·to·my (dū-ō-dē′nō-jĕ-jū-nos′tō-mē). Operative formation of an artificial communication between the duodenum and the jejunum. [duodeno- + jejunum, + G. *stoma,* mouth]

du·o·de·nol·y·sis (dū-ō-dĕ-nol′i-sis). Incision of adhesions to the duodenum. [duodeno- + G. *lysis,* a freeing]

du·o·de·nor·rha·phy (dū-ō-dĕ-nōr′ă-fē). Suture of a tear or incision in the duodenum. [duodeno- + G. *rhaphē,* a seam]

du·o·de·nos·co·py (dū-ō-dĕ-nos′kŏ-pē). Inspection of the interior of the duodenum through an endoscope. [duodeno- + G. *skopeō,* to examine]

du·o·de·nos·to·my (dū-ō-dĕ-nos′tō-mē). Establishment of a fistula into the duodenum. [duodeno- + G. *stoma,* mouth]

du·o·de·not·o·my (dū-ō-dĕ-not′ō-mē). Incision of the duodenum. [duodeno- + G. *tomē,* incision]

du·o·de·num, gen. **du·o·de·ni,** pl. **du·o·de·na** (dū-ō-dē′nŭm, dū-od′ĕ-nŭm; -od′ĕ-nă, -dē′nă) [NA]. The first division of the small intestine, about 25 cm or 12 fingerbreadths (hence the name) in length, extending from the pylorus to the junction with the jejunum at the level of the first or second lumbar vertebra on the left side. It is divided into the superior part, the first part of which is the duodenal cap, the descending part, into which the bile and pancreatic ducts open, the horizontal (inferior) part and the ascending part, terminating at the duodenojejunal junction. [Mediev. L. fr. L. *duodeni,* twelve]

du·o·vi·rus (dū′ō-vī′rŭs). SYN rotavirus.

Duplay, Emanuel Simon, French surgeon, 1836–1924. SEE D.'s *disease.*

du·plex (dū′pleks). Providing two functions. SEE duplex *ultrasonography.*

du·pli·ca·tion (dū-pli-kā′shŭn). **1.** A doubling. SEE ALSO reduplication. **2.** Inclusion of two copies of the same genetic material in a genome; an important step in diversification of genomes, as in the evolution of the (non-allelic) hemoglobin chains from a common ancestor. SYN gene d. [L. *duplicatio,* a doubling, fr. *duplico,* to double]

  d. of chromosomes, a chromosome aberration resulting from unequal crossing over or exchange of segments between two homologous chromosomes; one chromosome of the pair loses a small segment, while the other gains this segment; the chromosome gaining the segment has undergone d. while its homologue has undergone deletion. SEE *hemoglobin* Lepore.

  gene d., SYN duplication (2).

du·plic·i·tas (dū-plis′i-tahs). Doubling of a part. [L. a doubling, fr. *duplex* (*duplic-*), two-fold]

  d. ante′rior, conjoined twins in which fusion has united the pelvis and lower extremities, leaving the thoraces and heads separate. SEE conjoined *twins,* under *twin.* SEE ALSO cephalodidymus, ileadelphus, iliadelphus. SYN catadidymus.

  d. poste′rior, conjoined twins in which the heads and upper parts of the bodies have become fused, leaving the buttocks and legs separate. SEE conjoined *twins,* under *twin.* SEE ALSO dipygus. SYN anadidymus, ileadelphus, iliadelphus.

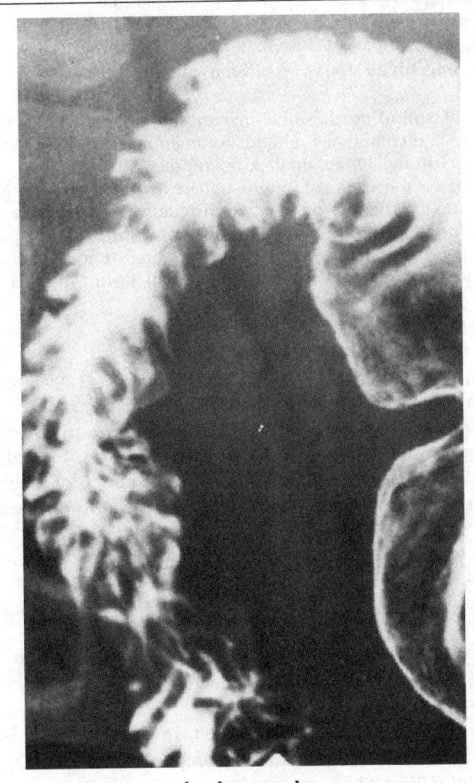

duodenography

Dupré, 17th Century Paris surgeon and anatomist. SEE D.'s *muscle.*

Dupuy-Dutemps, Louis, French ophthalmologist, 1871–1946. SEE Dupuy-Dutemps *operation.*

Dupuytren, Baron Guillaume, French surgeon and surgical pathologist, 1777–1835. SEE D.'s *amputation, canal, contracture, disease* of the foot, *fascia, fracture, hydrocele, sign, suture, tourniquet.*

du·ra (dū′ră). SYN dura mater. [L. fem. of *durus,* hard]

  d. mater cranialis [NA], SYN *dura mater* of brain.

dur·a·en·ceph·a·lo·syn·an·gi·o·sis (door′a-en-sef′a-lō-sin-anj-ē- ō′sis). Surgical transposition of the superficial temporal artery with attached galea to the underlying dura with hope for cerebral revascularization; most commonly used in moyamoya syndrome. SYN encephaloduroarteriosynangios.

du·ral (dū′răl). Relating to the dura mater. SYN duramatral.

du·ral·u·min (dūr-al′ū-min). An alloy of aluminum slightly heavier than this metal but nearly as strong as steel and noncorrodible; used in the manufacture of surgical and orthopedic appliances, *e.g.,* splints; not for internal use in the body as screws, plates.

du·ra mat·er (dū′ră mā′ter). Pachymeninx (as distinguished from leptomeninx, the combined pia mater and arachnoid); a tough, fibrous membrane forming the outer covering of the central nervous system. SYN dura. [L. hard mother]

  d. m. of brain, the intracranial d. m., consisting of two layers: the outer *periosteal layer* which normally always adheres to the periosteum of the bones of the cranial vault; and the inner *meningeal layer* which in most places is fused with the outer. The two layers separate to accommodate meningeal vessels and large venous (dural) sinuses. The meningeal layer is also involved in the formation of the various dural folds, such as the falx cerebri and tentorium cerebelli and is comparable to and continuous with the dural mater of the spinal cord. The cranial epidural space is then a potential space between the bone and the combined periosteum/periosteal layer of the d. m. realized only pathologically and is neither continuous with or comparable to the vertebral epidural space. SYN dura mater cranialis [NA], d. m. encephali☆ [NA], cerebral part of dura mater, cranial epidural space.

d. m. enceph′ali [NA], ☆official alternate term for d. m. of brain.

d. m. of spinal cord, single-layered strong membrane, comparable to and continuous with (at foramen magnum) the meningeal layer of the intracranial d. m. of the brain. It does not (in contrast to the d. m. of brain) adhere to the enveloping bony structures (vertebrae) or their periosteum, being separated from the latter by a considerable space, the vertebral epidural space—a true space containing the internal vertebral venous plexus embedded in a matrix of epidural fat. SYN d. m. spinalis [NA], endorrhachis, theca vertebralis.

d. m. spina′lis [NA], SYN d. m. of spinal cord.

du·ra·ma·tral (dū-ră-mā′trăl). SYN dural.

Duran-Reynals, Francisco, U.S. bacteriologist, 1899–1958. SEE Duran-Reynals permeability *factor.*

du·ra·plas·ty (dū′ră-plas-tē). A plastic or reconstructive operation on the dura mater. [dura (mater) + G. *plastos,* formed]

du·ra·tion (D) (dū-rā′shŭn). A continuous period of time.

half amplitude pulse d., the time, in milliseconds, required for a wave form to reach half of its full magnitude.

pulse d., the interval between onset of the leading edge and the end of the trailing edge of a pulse wave.

Dürck, Hermann, German pathologist, 1869–1941. SEE D.'s *nodes,* under *node.*

dur. dolor. Abbreviation for L. *duarte dolare,* while pain lasts.

Duret, Henri, French neurosurgeon, 1849–1921. SEE D.'s *lesion, hemorrhage.*

Durham, Arthur E., English surgeon, 1834–1895. SEE D.'s *tube.*

Duroziez, Paul L., French physician, 1826–1897. SEE D.'s *disease, murmur, sign.*

dUTP. Abbreviation for deoxyuridine 5-triphosphate.

Dutton, Joseph Everett, English physician, 1877–1905. SEE D.'s *disease,* relapsing *fever.*

Duverney, Joseph G., French anatomist, 1648–1730. SEE D.'s *fissures,* under *fissure, foramen, gland, muscle.*

D.V.M. Abbreviation for Doctor of Veterinary Medicine.

dwarf (dwōrf). An abnormally undersized person with disproportion among the bodily parts. SEE dwarfism. [A.S. *dweorh*]

hypophysial d., dwarfism as result of failure of growth hormone production because of hypothalamic or pituitary abnormality. SYN pituitary d.

hypothyroid d., dwarfism associated with lack of thyroid function.

pituitary d., SYN hypophysial d.

dwarf·ish·ness (dwōrf′ish-nes). SYN dwarfism.

dwarf·ism (dwōrf′izm). The condition of being abnormally undersized. SYN dwarfishness.

achondroplastic d., SEE achondroplasia.

acromelic d., SYN acromesomelia.

aortic d., underdevelopment of physical stature associated with severe aortic stenosis.

asexual d., d. in which adult sexual development is deficient.

ateliotic d., SYN panhypopituitarism.

camptomelic d., d. with shortening of the lower limbs due to anterior bending of the femur and tibia.

chondrodystrophic d., SEE chondrodystrophy.

diastrophic d. [MIM*222600], an autosomal recessive form of d. characterized in its complete form by scoliosis, hitchhiker thumb, absent interphalangeal joints, cleft palate, chondritis followed by calcification of the ears, shortening of the Achilles tendon, clubbed foot, and characteristic radiologic findings; a milder variant may be allelic.

disproportionate d., d. in which the limbs and trunk are not of proportional length for age or stage of development.

Fröhlich's d., d. with Fröhlich's syndrome.

hypothyroid d., SYN infantile *hypothyroidism.*

infantile d., SYN infantilism (1).

Laron type d., d. associated with an absent or very low levels of somatomedin C (insulin-like growth factor I) or abnormalities in receptor activity.

lethal d., d. leading to intrauterine or neonatal death.

Lorain-Lévi d., SYN pituitary d.

mesomelic d., d. with shortness of the forearms and lower legs.

metatropic d. [MIM*250600], congenital disproportionate dwarfism in which the trunk is long relative to the limbs at birth but undergoes reversal of this proportion with subsequent development.

micromelic d., d. with abnormally short or small limbs.

panhypopituitary d., type I is an autosomal recessive disorder with deficient human growth hormone, ACTH, FSH, etc., having delayed sexual development, hypothyroidism, and adrenal insufficiency; type II is similar but is an X-linked disorder.

phocomelic d., d. in which the diaphyses of the long bones are abnormally short or the intermediate parts of the limbs are absent.

physiologic d., d. characterized by normal development that is at a strikingly lesser rate than that for members of the same family, race, or other races. SYN primordial d., true d.

pituitary d., a rare form of d. caused by the absence of a functional anterior pituitary gland; may be present at birth or develop during early childhood. SYN Lorain-Lévi d., Lorain-Lévi infantilism, Lorain-Lévi syndrome, pituitary infantilism.

polydystrophic d., SYN Maroteaux-Lamy *syndrome.*

primordial d., SYN physiologic d.

Robinow d., d. associated with fetal face, acral dysostosis, and genital anomalies; there is also an autosomal recessive form [MIM*268310].

Seckel d., SYN Seckel *syndrome.*

senile d., d. characterized by craniofacial anomalies with progeroid appearance.

sexual d., d. with normal sexual development.

Silver-Russell d., SYN Silver-Russell *syndrome.*

snub-nose d. [MIM*127100], d. characterized by low birth weight, snub nose, and stocky build; autosomal dominant inheritance. There is a similar autosomal recessive phenotype [MIM*223600]. SYN dominantly inherited Lévi's disease.

thanatophoric d., a lethal d. characterized by micromelia, bowed long bones, enlarged head, flattened vertebral bodies, and muscular hypotonia; lack of pulmonary ventilation causes respiratory difficulties with cyanosis leading to death within the first few hours or days after birth.

true d., SYN physiologic d.

Dy Symbol for dysprosium.

dy·ad (dī′ad). **1.** A pair. SYN diad (2). **2.** In chemistry, a bivalent element. **3.** A pair of persons in an interactional situation, *e.g.,* patient and therapist, husband and wife. **4.** The double chromosome resulting from the splitting of a tetrad during meiosis. [G. *dyas,* the number two, duality]

dy·clo·nine hy·dro·chlo·ride (dī′klō-nēn). 4′-Butoxy-3-piperidino-propiophenone hydrochloride; a topical local anesthetic.

dy·dro·ges·ter·one (dī-drō-jes′ter-ōn). 9β,10α-pregna-4,6-diene-3,20-dione; a synthetic steroid, derived from retroprogesterone, with progestational effects.

dye (dī). A stain or coloring matter; a compound consisting of chromophore and auxochrome groups attached to one or more benzene rings, its color being due to the chromophore and its dyeing affinities to the auxochrome. D.'s are used for intravital coloration of living cells, staining tissues and microorganisms, as antiseptics and germicides, and some as stimulants of epithelial growth. For individual d.'s, see the specific names. Commonly but improperly used for radiographic contrast medium. [A.S. *deah, deag*]

acidic d.'s, d.'s which ionize in solution to produce negatively charged ions or anions; they consist of sodium salts of phenols and carboxylic acid dyes; their solutions tend to be neutral or slightly alkaline; examples are eosin and aniline blue.

acridine d.'s, derivatives of the compound acridine which is closely related to xanthene; important as fluorochromes in histology, cytochemistry, and chemotherapy; examples include acriflavine, acridine orange, and quinacrine mustard.

azin d.'s, d. derivatives of phenazine, $C_6H_4 \cdot N_2 \cdot C_6H_4$ that include important histologic stains, such as neutral red, azocarmine G., and safranin O.

azo d.'s, d.'s in which the azo group is the chromophore and joins benzene or naphthalene rings; they include a large number of biologic stains, such as Congo red and oil red O; also used clinically to promote epithelial growth in the treatment of ulcers, burns, and other wounds; many have anticoagulant action.

azocarmine d.'s, d.'s giving a dark purplish red color as histologic stains.

basic d.'s, d.'s which ionize in solution to give positively charged ions or cations; the auxochrome group is an amine which can form a salt with an acid like HCl; solutions are usually slightly acidic; examples include basic fuchsin and toluidine blue O.

chlorotriazine d.'s, d.'s containing one or more chlorotriazine moieties that react with polysaccharides.

diphenylmethane d.'s, d.'s in which the central carbon connecting two phenyl groups lacks an amino or imino group; the chromophore is the quinoid ring; an alternative formulation is as a ketonimide; the most common example is auramine O.

ketonimine d.'s, d.'s in which the chromophore is $=C=NH$ connected to two benzene rings; alkylamino groups are added para to the methane carbon on both rings. The most important member for biological purposes is auramine O; an alternative formulation is as a diphenylmethane dye.

natural d.'s, d.'s obtained from animals or plants; examples include carmine, obtained from cochineal in the dried female insect *Dactylopius cacti* of Central America, and hematoxylin, extracted from the bark of the logwood tree *Haematoxylon campechianum* in the Caribbean area.

nitro d.'s, d.'s in which the chromophore is -NO_2, which is so acidic that all dyes in this group are of the acid type; important examples in cytoplasmic staining are picric acid and naphthol yellow S.

oxazin d.'s, similar to azin d.'s except that one of the connecting N atoms is replaced by O; most important representatives are brilliant cresyl blue, orcein, litmus, and cresyl violet.

rosanilin d.'s, several triaminotriphenylmethane d.'s or mixtures of them often sold under the name of basic fuchsin; rosanilin d.'s differ from other triphenylmethane d.'s in that the amino groups are unsubstituted, and they may have methyl groups introduced directly onto the benzene rings; the four possible such dyes are pararosanilin, rosanilin, new fuchsin, and magenta II.

salt d., SYN neutral *stain*.

synthetic d.'s, organic d. compounds originally derived from coal-tar derivatives; presently produced by synthesis from benzene and its derivatives; examples include eosin, methylene blue, and fluorescein.

thiazin d.'s, similar to azin d.'s except that one of the connecting N atoms is replaced by S; includes many important biological stains, especially in hematology, *e.g.,* azure A, azure B, and methylene blue.

triphenylmethane d.'s, a group of d.'s that includes pararosanilin, as well as many others used in histology and cytology; employed as nuclear, cytoplasmic, and connective tissue stains; important in histochemistry as in the preparation of Schiff's reagent.

xanthene d.'s, derivatives of the compound xanthene; include the pyronins, rhodamines, and fluoresceins.

Dyggve, Holger, Danish pediatrician, 1913–1984. SEE D.-Melchior-Clausen *syndrome*.

△-dymus. **1.** Suffix to be combined with number roots; *e.g.,* didymus, tridymus, tetradymus. **2.** Occasionally used shortened form for -didymus. [G. *-dymos,* fold]

dy·nam·ics (dī-nam′iks). **1.** The science of motion in response to forces. **2.** In psychiatry, the determination of how emotional and mental disorders develop. **3.** In the behavioral sciences, any of the numerous intrapersonal and interpersonal influences or phenomena associated with personality development and interpersonal processes. [G. *dynamis,* force]

group d., a term used to represent the study of underlying features of group behavior, *e.g.,* motives, attitudes; it is concerned with group change rather than with static characteristics.

△dynamo-. Combining form, force, energy. [G. *dynamis,* power]

dy·na·mo·gen·e·sis (dī′nă-mō-jen′ĕ-sis). The production of force, especially of muscular or nervous energy. SYN dynamogeny. [dynamo- + G. *genesis,* production]

dy·na·mo·gen·ic (dī′nă-mō-jen′ik). Producing power or force, especially nervous or muscular power or activity.

dy·na·mog·e·ny (dī-nă-moj′ĕ-nē). SYN dynamogenesis.

dy·nam·o·graph (dī-nam′ō-graf). An instrument for recording the degree of muscular power. [dynamo- + G. *graphō,* to write]

dy·na·mom·e·ter (dī-nă-mom′ĕ-ter). An instrument for measuring the degree of muscular power. SYN ergometer. [dynamo- + G. *metron,* measure]

dy·nam·o·scope (dī-nam′ō-skōp). A modified stethoscope for auscultation of the muscles. [dynamo- + G. *skopeō,* to examine]

dy·na·mos·co·py (dī-nă-mos′kŏ-pē). Auscultation of a contracting muscle.

dy·na·therm (dī′nă-therm). An apparatus for inducing diathermy. [G. *dynamis,* force, + *thermē,* heat]

dyne (dīn). The unit of force in the CGS system, replaced in the SI system by the newton (1 newton = 10^5 dynes), that gives a body of 1 g mass an acceleration of 1 cm/sec²; expressed as F (dynes) = m (grams) $\times a$ (cm/sec²). [G. *dynamis,* force]

dyn·ein (dīn′ēn). A protein associated with motile structures, exhibiting adenosine triphosphatase activity; it forms "arms" on the outer tubules of cilia and flagella. SEE ALSO tubulin, dynein *arm.* [dyne + protein]

dy·nor·phin (dī′nōr-fin). An endogenous opioid ligand which acts as an agonist at opiate receptors. Extremely potent, widely distributed neuropeptide that has 17 amino acid residues and contains leu⁵-enkephalin as its NH_2-terminal sequence.

dy·phyl·line (dī-fil′in). 7-(2,3-Dihydroxypropyl)theophylline; exhibits characteristic peripheral vasodilator and bronchodilator actions of other theophylline compounds.

△dys-. Bad, difficult, un-, mis; opposite of eu-. Cf. dis-. [G.]

dys·a·cou·sia, dys·a·cu·sia (dis-ă-kū′sē-ă). SYN dysacusis.

dys·a·cu·sis (dis-ă-kū′sis). **1.** Any impairment of hearing involving difficulty in processing details of sound as opposed to any loss of sensitivity to sound. **2.** Pain or discomfort in the ear from exposure to sound. SYN dysacousia, dysacusia. [dys- + G. *akousis,* hearing]

dys·ad·ap·ta·tion (dis′ad-ap-tā′shŭn). Inability of the retina and iris to accommodate well to varying intensities of light.

dys·an·ti·graph·ia (dis′an-tē-graf′ē-ă). A form of agraphia in which the subject is unable to copy written or printed matter. [dys- + G. *antigraphō,* to write back]

dys·a·phia (dis-ā′fē-ă, dis-af′ē-ă). Impairment of the sense of touch. [dys- + G. *haphē,* touch]

dys·a·phic (dis-ā′fik). Relating to impaired tactile sensibility.

dys·ar·te·ri·ot·o·ny (dis-ar-tēr-ē-ot′ō-nē). Abnormal blood pressure, either too high or too low. [dys- + G. *artēria,* artery, + *tonos,* tension]

dys·ar·thria (dis-ar′thrē-ă). A disturbance of speech and language due to emotional stress, to brain injury, or to paralysis, incoordination, or spasticity of the muscles used for speaking. SYN dysarthrosis (1). [dys- + G. *arthroō,* to articulate]

ataxic d., d. caused by cerebellar lesions.

hyperkinetic d., d. caused by chorea and myoclonus.

hypokinetic d., d. caused by the rigid types of extrapyramidal *disease.*

d. litera′lis, seldom used term for stammering.

lower motor neuron d., d. caused by dysfunction of the motor nuclei and the lower pons or medulla, or other neural connections, central and peripheral to the muscles of articulation.

rigid d., SYN spastic d.

spastic d., d. caused by lesions along the corticobulbar tracts. SYN rigid d.

d. syllaba′ris spasmod′ica, seldom used term for stuttering.

dys·ar·thric (dis-ar′thrik). Relating to dysarthria.

dys·ar·thro·sis (dis-ar-thrō′sis). **1.** SYN dysarthria. **2.** Malformation of a joint. **3.** A false joint. [dys- + G. *arthrōsis*, joint]

dys·au·to·no·mia (dis′aw-tō-nō′mē-ă). Abnormal functioning of the autonomic nervous system. [dys- + G. *autonomia*, self-government]

canine d., a newly recognized disease of dogs characterized by dysfunction of the autonomic nervous system. SYN Key-Gaskell syndrome.

familial d. [MIM*223900], a congenital syndrome with specific disturbances of the nervous system and aberrations in autonomic nervous system function such as indifference to pain, diminished lacrimation, poor vasomotor homeostasis, motor incoordination, labile cardiovascular reactions, hyporeflexia, frequent attacks of bronchial pneumonia, hypersalivation with aspiration and difficulty in swallowing, hyperemesis, emotional instability, and an intolerance for anesthetics; autosomal recessive inheritance. SYN Riley-Day syndrome.

dys·ba·rism (dis′bar-izm). General term for the symptom complex resulting from exposure to decreased or changing barometric pressure, including all physiologic effects resulting from such changes with the exception of hypoxia, and including the effects of rapid decompression. [dys- + G. *baros*, weight]

dys·ba·sia (dis-bā′zē-ă). **1.** Difficulty in walking. **2.** The difficult or distorted walking that occurs in persons with certain mental disorders. [dys- + G. *basis*, a step]

d. angiosclerot′ica, d. angiospas′tica, obsolete terms meaning intermittent difficulty in walking due to peripheral vascular causes.

d. lordot′ica progressi′va, an affection characterized by lordoscoliosis of the lower portion of the vertebral column, occurring when the patient stands or walks and usually disappearing when the patient lies down. SYN torsion neurosis.

dys·be·ta·lip·o·pro·tei·ne·mia (dis-bā′tă-lip-ō-prō′tēn-ē′mē-a). SYN type III familial *hyperlipoproteinemia*.

dys·bo·lism (dis′bō-lizm). Abnormal, but not necessarily morbid, metabolism, as in alkaptonuria. [dys- + G. *bolē* (*metabolē*), + *-ismos*, metabolism]

dys·bu·lia (dis-bū′lē-ă). Weakness and uncertainty of volition. [dys- + G. *boulē*, will]

dys·bu·lic (dis-bū′lik). Relating to, or characterized by, dysbulia.

dys·cal·cu·lia (dis-kal-kyū′lē-ă). Difficulty in performing simple mathematical problems; commonly seen in parietal lobe lesions. [dys- + L. *calculo*, to compute, fr. *calculus*, pebble, counter]

dys·ce·pha·lia (dis-sĕ-fā′lē-ă). Malformation of the head and face. SYN dyscephaly. [dys- + G. *kephalē*, head]

d. mandib′ulo-oculofacia′lis [MIM*234100], a syndrome of bony anomalies of the calvaria, face, and jaw, with brachygnathia, narrow curved nose, and multiple ocular defects including microphthalmia, microcornea, and cataract, often with alopecia overlying skull sutures, or alopecia areata and hypoplasia, or absence of eyebrows. The pattern of inheritance is undecided. SYN congenital sutural alopecia, Hallermann-Streiff syndrome, Hallermann-Streiff-François syndrome, mandibulo-oculofacial syndrome, oculomandibulodyscephaly, oculomandibulofacial syndrome, progeria with cataract, progeria with microphthalmia.

dys·ceph·a·ly (dis-sef′ă-lē). SYN dyscephalia.

dys·chei·ral, dys·chi·ral (dis-kī′răl). Relating to dyscheiria.

dys·chei·ria, dys·chi·ria (dis-kī′rē-ă). A disorder of sensibility in which, although there is no apparent loss of sensation, the patient is unable to tell which side of the body has been touched (acheiria), or refers it to the wrong side (allocheiria), or to both sides (syncheiria). [dys- + G. *cheir*, hand]

dys·che·zia (dis-kē′zē-ă). Difficulty in defecation. [dys- + G. *chezō*, to defecate]

dys·chon·dro·gen·e·sis (dis-kon-drō-jen′ĕ-sis). Abnormal development of cartilage. [dys- + G. *chondros*, cartilage, + *genesis*, production]

dys·chon·dro·pla·sia (dis-kon-drō-pla′zē-ă). SYN enchondromatosis. [dys- + G. *chondros*, cartilage, + *plasis*, a forming]

d. with hemangiomas, SYN Maffucci's *syndrome*.

dys·chon·dros·te·o·sis (dis′kon-dros-tē-ō′sis) [MIM*127300].

A bone dysplasia characterized by bowing of the radius, dorsal dislocation of the distal ulna and proximal carpal bones, and mesomelic dwarfism; autosomal dominant inheritance. SYN Leri's pleonosteosis, Leri-Weill disease, Leri-Weill syndrome. [dys- + G. *chondros*, cartilage, + *osteon*, bone, + *-osis*, condition]

dys·chroia, dys·chroa (dis-kroy′ă, -krō′ă). A bad complexion; discoloration of the skin. [dys- + G. *chroia, chroa*, color]

dys·chro·ma·top·sia (dis′krō-mă-top′sē-ă). A condition in which the ability to perceive colors is not fully normal. Cf. anomalous *trichromatism*, dichromatism, monochromatism, chromatopsia. [dys- + G. *chrōma*, color, + *opsis*, vision]

dys·chro·ma·to·sis (dis-krō-mă-tō′sis). An asymptomatic anomaly of pigmentation occurring among the Japanese; may be localized or diffuse. [dys- + G. *chrōma*, color, + *-osis*, condition]

dys·chro·mia (dis-krō′mē-ă). Any abnormality in the color of the skin.

dys·ci·ne·sia (dis′si-nē′zē-ă). SYN dyskinesia.

dys·coi·me·sis (dis-koy-mē′sis). A form of insomnia marked by difficulty or delay in falling asleep. [dys- + G. *koimēsis*, a sleeping, fr. *koimaō*, to put to sleep]

dys·con·trol (dis-kon-trōl′). SYN intermittent explosive *disorder*.

dys·co·ria (dis-kō′rē-ă). Abnormality in the shape of the pupil. [dys- + G. *korē*, pupil of eye]

dys·cra·sia (dis-krā′zē-ă). **1.** A morbid general state resulting from the presence of abnormal material in the blood, usually applied to diseases affecting blood cells or platelets. **2.** Old term indicating disease. [G. bad temperament, fr. dys- + *krasis*, a mixing]

blood d., a diseased state of the blood; usually refers to abnormal cellular elements of a permanent character.

dys·cra·sic, dys·crat·ic (dis-krā′sik, krat′ik). Pertaining to or affected with dyscrasia.

dys·di·ad·o·cho·ki·ne·sia, dys·di·ad·o·cho·ci·ne·sia (dis-dī-ad′ō-kō-ki-nē′zē-ă). Impairment of the ability to perform rapidly alternating movements. [dys- + G. *diadochos*, working in turn, + *kinēsis*, movement]

dys·di·a·do·cho·ki·ne·sis (dis′dī-ad-ō-kō-ki-nē′sis). SYN adiadochokinesis.

dys·em·bry·o·ma (dis-em-brē-ō′mă). A teratoid tumor with its tissues showing more irregular arrangement than the typical embryoma.

dys·em·bry·o·pla·sia (dis-em′brē-ō-plā′zē-ă). Prenatal malformation. [dys- + G. *embryon*, fetus, + *plasis*, a molding]

dys·e·mia (dis-ē′mē-ă). Any abnormal condition or disease of the blood. [dys- + G. *haima*, blood]

dys·en·ce·pha·lia splanch·no·cys·ti·ca (dis′en-se-fā′lē-ă splangk-nō-sis′ti-kă) [MIM*249000]. A malformation syndrome, lethal in the perinatal period, and characterized by intrauterine growth retardation, sloping forehead, occipital exencephalocele, ocular anomalies, cleft palate, polydactyly, polycystic kidney, and other malformations; autosomal recessive inheritance. SYN Meckel syndrome, Meckel-Gruber syndrome.

dys·en·ter·ic (dis-en-tār′ik). Relating to or suffering from dysentery.

dys·en·ter·y (dis-en-tār-ē). A disease marked by frequent watery stools, often with blood and mucus, and characterized clinically by pain, tenesmus, fever, and dehydration. [G. *dysenteria*, fr. *dys-*, bad, + *entera*, bowels]

amebic d., diarrhea resulting from ulcerative inflammation of the colon, caused chiefly by infection with *Entamoeba histolytica*; may be mild or severe and also may be associated with amebic infection of other organs.

bacillary d., infection with *Shigella dysenteriae, S. flexneri*, or other organisms. SYN Japanese d.

balantidial d., a type of colitis resembling in many respects amebic d.; caused by the parasitic ciliate, *Balantidium coli*.

bilharzial d., d. due to infection with *Schistosoma mansoni, S. haematobium*, or *S. japonicum*.

chronic d. of cattle, SYN Johne's *disease*.

fulminating d., SYN malignant d.

helminthic d., d. caused by infection with parasitic worms.

Japanese d., SYN bacillary d.

lamb d., enterotoxemia of lambs caused by type B toxins of *Clostridium perfringens.*

malignant d., d. in which the symptoms are intensely acute, leading to prostration, collapse, and often death. SYN fulminating d.

Sonne d., d. due to infection by *Shigella sonnei;* sometimes milder than other types of bacterial d. caused by *Shigella.*

spirillar d., a form of d. or diarrhea, described as occurring in the south of France, believed to be caused by a spirillum present in great numbers in the intestinal epithelia.

swine d., an acute hemorrhagic colitis of swine, often accompanied by gastritis; the small intestines usually are not involved; its primary cause is *Treponema hyodysenteriae,* and it has a high mortality rate, especially among feeder pigs.

viral d., profuse watery diarrhea due to, or thought to be due to, infection by a virus.

winter d. of cattle, a specific, highly contagious and severe disease of unknown origin; the disease is seen in the cold months of the year, outbreaks generally abate after a few days; the death rate is low, but the loss in flesh and milk is often high.

dys·er·e·thism (dis-er'ĕ-thizm). A condition of slow response to stimuli. [dys- + G. *erethismos,* irritation]

dys·er·gia (dis-er'jē-ă). Lack of harmonious action between the muscles concerned in executing any definite voluntary movement. [dys- + G. *ergon,* work]

dys·es·the·sia (dis-es-thē'zē-ă). **1.** Impairment of sensation short of anesthesia. **2.** A condition in which a disagreeable sensation is produced by ordinary stimuli; caused by lesions of the sensory pathways, peripheral or central. **3.** Abnormal sensations experienced in the absence of stimulation. [G. *dysaisthesia,* fr. *dys-,* hard, difficult, + *aisthēsis,* sensation]

dys·fi·brin·o·ge·ne·mia (dis'fī-brin'ō-jĕ-nē'mē-ă) [MIM* 134820]. An autosomal dominant disorder of qualitatively abnormal fibrinogens of various types; each type is named for the city in which the abnormal fibrinogen was discovered. Examples include: 1) Amsterdam, Bethesda II, Cleveland, Los Angeles, Saint Louis, Zurich I and II: major defect, aggregation of fibrin monomers; thrombin time prolonged; inhibitory effect on normal clotting; asymptomatic; 2) Bethesda I and Detroit: major defect, fibrinopeptide release; thrombin time prolonged; inhibitory effect on normal clotting; abnormal bleeding; 3) Baltimore: major defect, fibrinopeptide release; thrombin time prolonged; no inhibitory effect on normal clotting; bleeding and thrombosis; 4) Leuven: major defect, questionable aggregation of fibrin monomers; thrombin time prolonged; slight inhibitory effect on normal clotting; abnormal bleeding; 5) Metz: major defect unreported; thrombin time infinite; effect on normal clotting unreported; abnormal bleeding; 6) Nancy: major defect, aggregation of fibrin monomers; thrombin time prolonged; slight inhibitory effect on normal clotting; asymptomatic; 7) Oklahoma: major defect unreported; thrombin time normal; no effect on normal clotting; abnormal bleeding; 8) Oslo: major defect unreported; thrombin time shortened; effect on normal clotting unreported; abnormal thrombosis; 9) Parma: major defect unreported; thrombin time infinite; no inhibitory effect on normal clotting; abnormal bleeding; 10) Paris I: major defect unreported; thrombin time infinite; inhibitory effect on normal clotting; asymptomatic; 11) Paris II: major defect unreported; thrombin time prolonged; inhibitory effect on normal clotting; asymptomatic; 12) Troyes: major defect unreported; thrombin time prolonged; effect on normal clotting unreported; asymptomatic; 13) Vancouver: major defect unreported; thrombin time prolonged; no effect on normal clotting; abnormal bleeding; 14) Wiesbaden: major defect, aggregation of fibrin monomers; thrombin time prolonged; inhibitory effect on normal clotting; bleeding and thrombosis.

dys·func·tion (dis-fŭnk'shŭn). Difficult or abnormal function.

constitutional hepatic d., SYN familial nonhemolytic *jaundice.*

dental d., abnormal functioning of dental structures.

Le Fort III craniofacial d., SYN craniofacial dysjunction *fracture.*

minimal brain d., SEE attention deficit *disorder.*

papillary muscle d., impaired function of a papillary muscle,

usually due to ischemia or infarction, with resulting incompetence of the mitral valve. SYN papillary muscle syndrome.

phagocyte d. (fā'gō-sīt), disorder in which the ability of the phagocyte to engulf and ingest particles may be impaired.

placental d., SYN dysmature (3).

psychosexual d., sexual d., a disturbance of sexual functioning, *e.g.,* impotence, premature ejaculation, anorgasmia, presumed to be of psychological rather than physical etiology.

sphincter of Oddi d., structural or functional abnormality of the sphincter of Oddi that interferes with bile drainage. SYN biliary dyskinesia.

temporomandibular joint d. (TMD, TMJ), chronic or impaired function of the temporomandibular articulation. SEE temporomandibular *arthrosis,* myofacial pain-dysfunction *syndrome.*

dys·gam·ma·glob·u·lin·e·mia (dis-gam'ă-glob'yū-li-nē'mē-ă) [MIM*308230]. An immunoglobulin abnormality, especially a disturbance of the percentage distribution of γ-globulins.

dys·gen·e·sis (dis-jen'ĕ-sis). Defective development. [dys- + G. *genesis,* generation]

gonadal d., defective gonadal development, varying types and degrees of which have been identified, including gonadal aplasia or agenesis, rudimentary gonads, congenitally defective gonads, and true hermaphroditism; the character of the external genitalia, genital ducts, and secondary sexual development are only sometimes uniquely related to a given type of gonadal d. **XO gonadal d.** consists of monosomy X with a gonadal streak rather than a true ovary, notably seen in Turner's syndrome; **XX gonadal d.** is an autosomal recessive disorder with a female karyotype, streaked gonads, and primary amenorrhea, but with no body features of Turner's syndrome; **XY gonadal d.** is an X-linked disorder associated with a male karyotype and a female habitus, streaked gonads, and absence of secondary sexual characteristics.

iridocorneal mesodermal d., mesodermal d. of cornea and iris, producing pupillary anomalies, posterior embryotoxon, and secondary glaucoma. SYN Rieger's anomaly.

seminiferous tubule d., a disorder in which the seminiferous tubules exhibit an abnormal cytoarchitecture and extensive hyalinization; the testes are small, and few spermatozoa are formed; the body habitus may be eunuchoid, and gynecomastia may be present; urinary gonadotropin output is usually high, and the incidence of mental deficiency and illness increased; sex chromatin may be male or female, and androgen secretion ranges from subnormal to normal. It is a constant feature of (and is often used synonymously with) Klinefelter's *syndrome.* SYN germinal aplasia.

testicular d. [MIM*305700], a congenital derangement of seminiferous tubular structure and function, resulting in male infertility; the defect in spermatogenesis may be incomplete, as in maturational arrest or premature sloughing, or spermatogenesis may be completely absent, as in the Sertoli-cell-only syndrome.

dys·gen·ic (dis-jen'ik). Applying to factors that have a detrimental effect upon hereditary qualities, physical or mental.

dys·ger·mi·no·ma (dis-jer-mi-nō'mă). A rare malignant neoplasm of the ovary (counterpart of seminoma of the testis), composed of undifferentiated gonadal germinal cells and occurring more frequently in patients less than 20 years of age. The neoplasms are gray-yellow and firm, contain foci of necrosis and hemorrhage, and tend to be encapsulated; characteristically, they spread by way of lymphatic vessels, but widespread metastases also occur. SYN disgerminoma. [dys- + L. *germen,* a bud or sprout, + *-ōma,* tumor]

dys·geu·sia (dis-gū'sē-ă). Impairment or perversion of the gustatory sense. [dys- + G. *geusis,* taste]

dys·gna·thia (dis-nath'ē-ă). Any abnormality that extends beyond the teeth and includes the maxilla or mandible, or both. [dys- + G. *gnathos,* jaw]

dys·gnath·ic (dis-nath'ik). Pertaining to or characterized by abnormality of the maxilla and mandible.

dys·gno·sia (dis-nō'sē-ă). Any cognitive disorder, *i.e.,* any mental illness. [G. *dysgnōsia,* difficulty of knowing]

dys·gon·ic (dis-gon'ik). A term used to indicate that the growth of a bacterial culture is slow and relatively poor; used especially in reference to the growth of cultures of the bovine tubercle

dy

bacillus (*Mycobacterium bovis*) SEE ALSO eugonic. [dys- + G. *gonikos,* relating to the seed or offspring]

dys·graph·ia (dis-graf′ē-ă). **1.** Difficulty in writing. **2.** SYN writer's *cramp.* [dys- + G. *graphē,* writing]

dys·hem·a·to·poi·e·sis (dis-hē′mă-tō-poy-ē′sis). Defective formation of the blood. SYN dyshemopoiesis. [dys- + G. *haima* (*haimat-*), blood, + *poiēsis,* making]

dys·hem·a·to·poi·et·ic (dis-hē′mă-tō-poy-et′ik). Pertaining to or characterized by dyshematopoiesis. SYN dyshemopoietic.

dys·he·mo·poi·e·sis (dis-hē′mō-poy-ē′sis). SYN dyshematopoiesis.

dys·he·mo·poi·et·ic (dis-hē′mō-poy-et′ik). SYN dyshematopoietic.

dys·hid·ria (dis-hid′rē-ă). SYN dyshidrosis.

dys·hi·dro·sis (dis-i-drō′sis). A vesicular or vesicopustular eruption of multiple causes that occurs primarily on the volar surfaces of the hands and feet; the lesions spread peripherally but have a tendency to central clearing. SYN cheiropompholyx, chiropompholyx, chiropompholyx, dyshidria, dysidria, dysidrosis, pompholyx. [dys- + G. *hidrōs,* sweat]

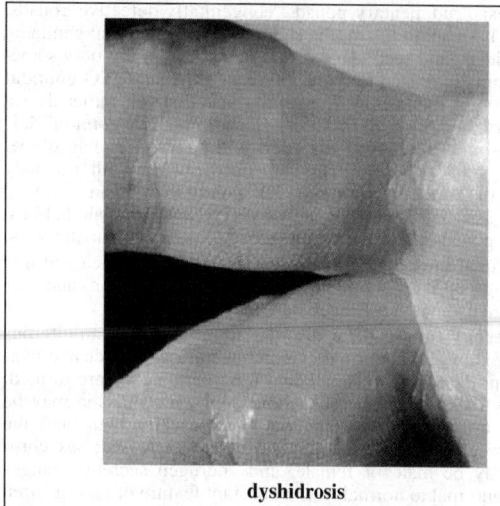

dyshidrosis

dys·id·ria (dis-id′rē-ă). SYN dyshidrosis.
dys·i·dro·sis (dis-i-drō′sis). SYN dyshidrosis.
dys·kar·y·o·sis (dis-kar-ē-ō′sis). Abnormal maturation seen in exfoliated cells that have normal cytoplasm but hyperchromatic nuclei, or irregular chromatin distribution; may be followed by the development of a malignant neoplasm. [dys- + G. *karyon,* nucleus, + *-ōsis,* condition]

dys·kar·y·ot·ic (dis-kar-ē-ot′ik). Pertaining to or characterized by dyskaryosis.

dys·ker·a·to·ma (dis-ker-ă-tō′mă). A skin tumor exhibiting dyskeratosis. [dys- + G. *keras,* horn, + *-oma,* tumor]
warty d., a benign solitary tumor of the skin, usually of the scalp, face, or neck, with a central keratotic plug; it appears to arise from a hair follicle, and microscopically resembles a lesion of keratosis follicularis but is larger, with more extensive epithelial downgrowth. SYN isolated dyskeratosis follicularis.

dys·ker·a·to·sis (dis′ker-ă-tō′sis). **1.** Premature keratinization of epithelial cells that have not reached the keratinizing surface layer; dyskeratotic cells generally become rounded and they may break away from adjacent cells and fall off. **2.** Epidermalization of the conjunctival and corneal epithelium. **3.** A disorder of keratinization. [dys- + G. *keras,* horn, + *-osis,* condition]
benign d., d. that may occur in congenital and bullous diseases of the skin.
d. congen′ita [MIM*305000], nail dystrophy, oral leukoplakia, and reticular pigmentation of the skin, with anemia progressing to pancytopenia; X-linked recessive inheritance.
hereditary benign intraepithelial d., SYN intraepithelial d.

intraepithelial d. [MIM*127600], **(1)** an autosomal dominant condition consisting of white spongy lesions of the buccal mucosa, floor of the mouth, ventral lateral tongue, gingiva and palate. Transient gelatinous plaques form over the cornea, which may produce temporary blindness; **(2)** hereditary benign intraepithelial d. SYN hereditary benign intraepithelial d.
isolated d. follicula′ris, SYN warty *dyskeratoma.*
malignant d., d. that may occur in precancerous or malignant lesions.

dys·ker·a·tot·ic (dis′ker-a-tot′ik). Relating to or characterized by dyskeratosis.

dys·ki·ne·sia (dis-ki-nē′zē-ă). Difficulty in performing voluntary movements. Term usually used in relation to various extrapyramidal disorders. SYN dyscinesia. [dys- + G. *kinēsis,* movement]
d. al′gera, a hysterical condition in which active movement causes pain.
biliary d., SYN sphincter of Oddi *dysfunction.*
extrapyramidal d.'s, abnormal involuntary movements attributed to pathological states of one or more parts of the striate body and characterized by insuppressible, stereotyped, automatic movements that cease only during sleep; *e.g.,* Parkinson's disease; chorea; athetosis; hemiballism.
d. intermit′tens, intermittent disability of the limbs due to impairment of circulation.
lingual-facial-buccal d., SYN tardive d.
tardive d., involuntary movements of the facial muscles and tongue, often persistent, that develop as a late complication of some neuroleptic therapy (especially phenothiazine). SYN lingual-facial-buccal d.
tracheobronchial d., degeneration of elastic and connective tissue of bronchi and trachea.

dys·ki·net·ic (dis-ki-net′ik). Denoting or characteristic of dyskinesia.

dys·lex·ia (dis-lek′sē-ă). Impaired reading ability with a competence level below that expected on the basis of the individual's level of intelligence, and in the presence of normal vision and letter recognition and normal recognition of the meaning of pictures and objects. SYN incomplete alexia. [dys- + G. *lexis,* word, phrase]

dys·lex·ic (dis-lek′sik). Relating to, or characterized by, dyslexia.

dys·lo·gia (dis-lō′jē-ă). Impairment of speech and reasoning as the result of a mental disorder. [dys- + G. *logos,* speaking, reason]

dys·ma·se·sis (dis-mă-sē′sis). Difficulty in mastication. [dys- + G. *masēsis,* chewing]

dys·ma·ture (dis′mă-tyūr). **1.** Denoting faulty development or ripening; often connoting structural and/or functional abnormalities. **2.** In obstetrics, denoting an infant whose birth weight is inappropriately low for its gestational age. **3.** Immature development of the placenta so that normal function does not occur. SYN placental dysfunction.

dys·ma·tu·ri·ty (dis′mă-chūr-i-tē). Syndrome of an infant born with relative absence of subcutaneous fat, wrinkling of the skin, prominent finger and toe nails, and meconium staining of the infant's skin and of the placental membranes; often associated with postmaturity or placental insufficiency.

dys·me·lia (dis-mē′lē-ă). Congenital abnormality characterized by missing or foreshortened limbs, sometimes with associated spine abnormalities; caused by metabolic disturbance at the time of primordial limb development. SEE amelia, phocomelia. [dys- + G. *melos,* limb]

dys·men·or·rhea (dis-men-ōr-ē′ă). Difficult and painful menstruation. SYN menorrhalgia. [dys- + G. *mēn,* month, + *rhoia,* a flow]
essential d., SYN primary d.
functional d., SYN primary d.
intrinsic d., SYN primary d.
mechanical d., d. due to obstruction of discharge of menstrual blood, as in cervical stenosis. SYN obstructive d.
membranous d., d. accompanied by an exfoliation of the menstrual decidua.
obstructive d., SYN mechanical d.

ovarian d., a form of secondary d. due to disease of an ovary.

primary d., d. due to a functional disturbance and not due to inflammation, new growths, or anatomic factors. SYN essential d., functional d., intrinsic d.

secondary d., d. due to inflammation, infection, tumor, or anatomical factors.

spasmodic d., d. accompanied by painful contractions of the uterus.

tubal d., a form of secondary d. due to stenosis or other abnormal condition of the fallopian tubes.

ureteric d., a form of secondary d. characterized by pain due to spasm of the ureter occurring at the time of the menses.

uterine d., a form of secondary d. resulting from disease of the uterus.

vaginal d., a form of secondary d. due to obstruction or other abnormal condition in the vagina.

dys·met·ria (dis-me′trē-ă, -met′rē-ă). An aspect of ataxia, in which the ability to control the distance, power, and speed of an act is impaired. Usually used to describe abnormalities of movement caused by cerebellar disorders. SEE ALSO hypermetria, hypometria. [dys- + G. *metron,* measure]

ocular d., abnormality of ocular movements in which the eyes overshoot on attempting to fixate an object.

dys·mim·ia (dis-mim′ē-ă). Obsolete term for an impairment of expression by gestures or of imitation. [dys- + G. *mimeomai,* to mimic]

dys·mne·sia (dis-nē′zē-ă). Obsolete term for a naturally poor or an impaired memory. [dys- + G. *mnēmē, mnēsi-,* memory]

dys·mor·phia (dis-mōr′fē-ă). SYN dysmorphism.

dys·mor·phism (dis-mōr′fizm). Abnormality of shape. SYN dysmorphia. [G. *dysmorphia,* badness of form]

dys·mor·pho·gen·e·sis (dis′mōr-fō-jen′ĕ-sis). The process of abnormal tissue formation. [dys- + G. *morphē,* form, + *genesis,* production]

dys·mor·phol·o·gy (dis-mōr-fol′ō-jē). General term for the study of, or the subject of, abnormal development of tissue form. A branch of clinical genetics. [dys- + G. *morphē,* form, + *logos,* study]

dys·mor·pho·pho·bia (dis′mōr-fō-fō′bē-ă). SYN body dysmorphic *disorder.* [dys- + G. *morphē,* form, + *phobos,* fear]

dys·my·e·li·na·tion (dis-mī-ĕ-li-nā′shŭn). Improper laying down or breakdown of a myelin sheath of a nerve fiber, caused by abnormal myelin metabolism.

dys·my·o·to·nia (dis-mī-ō-tō′nē-ă). Abnormal muscular tonicity (either hyper- or hypo-). SEE dystonia. [dys- + G. *mys,* muscle, + *tonos,* tension, tone]

dys·nys·tax·is (dis-nis-tak′sis). A condition of half sleep. SYN light sleep. [dys- + G. *nystaxis,* drowsiness]

dys·o·don·ti·a·sis (dis′ō-don-tī′ă-sis). Difficulty or irregularity in the eruption of the teeth. [dys- + G. *odous,* tooth, + *-iasis,* condition]

dys·on·to·gen·e·sis (dis′on-tō-jen′ĕ-sis). Defective embryonic development. [dys- + G. *ōn,* being, + *genesis,* origin]

dys·on·to·ge·net·ic (dis′on-tō-jĕ-net′ik). Characterized by dysontogenesis.

dys·o·rex·ia (dis-ō-rek′sē-ă). Diminished or perverted appetite. [dys- + G. *orexis,* appetite]

dys·os·mia (dis-oz′mē-ă). Altered sense of smell. [dys- + G. *osmē,* smell]

dys·os·te·o·gen·e·sis (dis′os-tē-ō-jen′ĕ-sis). Defective bone formation. SYN dysostosis. [dys- + G. *osteon,* bone, + *genesis,* production]

dys·os·to·sis (dis-os-tō′sis). SYN dysosteogenesis. [dys- + G. *osteon,* bone, + *-osis,* condition]

acrofacial d., mandibulofacial d. associated with malformations of the extremities such as defective radius and thumbs, and radioulnar synostosis. SEE ALSO Treacher Collins' *syndrome.* SYN acrofacial syndrome.

cleidocranial d., clidocranial d. [MIM*119600 & MIM*216330], a development defect characterized by absence or rudimentary development of the clavicles, abnormal shape of the skull with depression of the sagittal suture, frontal bosses, many wormian bones, and aplasia or hypoplasia of teeth; autosomal dominant inheritance, and perhaps an autosomal recessive form. SYN cleidocranial dysplasia, clidocranial dysplasia, craniocleido-dysostosis.

craniofacial d. [MIM*123500], craniostosis with widening of the skull and high forehead, ocular hypertelorism, exophthalmos, beaked nose, and hypoplasia of the maxilla; usually autosomal dominant inheritance. There may also be an autosomal recessive form [MIM*218500]. SYN Crouzon's disease, Crouzon's syndrome.

mandibuloacral d. [MIM*248370], an autosomal recessive disorder characterized by dental crowding, acro-osteolysis, stiff joints, and atrophy of the skin of the hands and feet; clavicles are hypoplastic, cranial sutures are wide, and multiple wormian bones are present.

mandibulofacial d., a variable syndrome of malformations primarily of derivatives of the first branchial arch; characterized by palpebral fissures sloping outward and downward with notches or colobomas in the outer third of the lower lids, bony defects or hypoplasia of malar bones and zygoma, hypoplasia of the mandible, macrostomia with high or cleft palate and malposition and malocclusion of teeth, low-set malformed external ears, atypical hair growth, and occasional pits or clefts between mouth and ear. SEE ALSO Treacher Collins' *syndrome.* SYN mandibulofacial dysotosis syndrome, mandibulofacial dysplasia.

metaphysial d., a rare developmental abnormality of the skeleton in which metaphyses of tubular bones are expanded by deposits of cartilage.

d. mul′tiplex, SYN Hurler's *syndrome.*

orodigitofacial d., an inherited syndrome, lethal in males, with varying combinations of defects of the oral cavity, face, and hands, including lobulated or bifid tongue, cleft or pseudocleft palate, tongue tumors, missing or malpositioned teeth, hypoplastic nasal alar cartilage, depressed nasal bridge, brachydactyly, clinodactyly, incomplete syndactyly, and, frequently, mental retardation; autosomal recessive [MIM 252100] and [MIM 258850] or X-linked [MIM 311200] inheritance. SYN OFD syndrome, orofaciodigital syndrome, Papillon-Léage and Psaume syndrome.

otomandibular d., hypoplasia of the mandible, often with malformation of the temporomandibular joint, associated with malformations of the ear but not eye malformations or malar defects. SYN otomandibular syndrome.

peripheral d. [MIM*170700], d. of the metacarpals and metatarsals, accompanied by variable facial features; possibly autosomal dominant inheritance.

dys·pal·lia (dis-pal′ē-ă). Developmental distortion of the brain mantle. [dys- + L. *pallium,* cloak]

dys·pa·reu·nia (dis-pa-rū′nē-ă). Occurrence of pain during sexual intercourse. [dys- + G. *pareunos,* lying beside, fr. *para,* beside, + *eunē,* a bed]

dys·pep·sia (dis-pep′sē-ă). Impaired gastric function or "upset stomach" due to some disorder of the stomach; characterized by epigastric pain, sometimes burning, nausea, and gaseous eructation. SYN gastric indigestion. [dys- + G. *pepsis,* digestion]

acid d., d. associated with excess gastric acidity.

adhesion d., pain, d., and other symptoms alleged to result from perigastric adhesions.

atonic d., d. with impaired tone in the muscular walls of the stomach. SYN functional d. (1).

fermentative d., d. accompanied by fermentation of the contents of the stomach, usually occurring in gastric dilation.

flatulent d., d. with frequent eructations of swallowed air, sometimes without underlying organic disease.

functional d., (1) SYN atonic d. **(2)** SYN nervous d.

nervous d., d. associated with nervousness, tension, or anxiety. SYN functional d. (2).

reflex d., functional d. excited by reflex irritation from disease elsewhere than in the stomach or intestines.

dys·pep·tic (dis-pep′tik). Relating to or suffering from dyspepsia.

dy

dys·pha·gia, dys·pha·gy (dis-fā′jē-ă, dis′fă-jē). Difficulty in swallowing. SYN aglutition. [dys- + G. *phagō*, to eat]

d. luso′ria, d. said to be due to compression by the right subclavian artery arising abnormally from the thoracic aorta and passing behind the esophagus. [coinage from L. *lusus naturae,* a sport of nature]

d. nervo′sa, nervous d., SYN esophagism.

sideropenic d., SYN Plummer-Vinson *syndrome.*

vallecular d., d. caused by food becoming lodged above the epiglottis. SYN Barclay-Baron disease.

dys·pha·go·cy·to·sis (dis-fag′ō-sī-tō′sis). Disordered phagocytosis, especially failure of cells to ingest and digest bacteria.

congenital d., SYN chronic granulomatous *disease.*

dys·pha·sia (dis-fā′zē-ă). Impairment in the production of speech and failure to arrange words in an understandable way; caused by an acquired lesion of the brain. SYN dysphrasia. [dys- + G. *phasis,* speaking]

dys·phe·mia (dis-fē′mē-ă). Disordered phonation, articulation, or hearing due to emotional or mental deficits. [dys- + G. *phēmē,* speech]

dys·pho·nia (dis-fō′nē-ă). Altered voice production. [dys- + G. *phōnē,* voice]

d. pli′cae ventricula′ris, phonation with the ventricular bands rather than with the vocal cords.

spastic d., SYN d. spastica.

d. spas′tica, a spasmodic contraction of the intrinsic muscles of the larynx excited by attempted phonation, producing either adductor or abductor subtypes caused by central nervous system disease. A localized form of movement disorder. SYN phonic spasm, spastic d.

dys·pho·ria (dis-fōr′ē-ă). A mood of general dissatisfaction, restlessness, depression, and anxiety; a feeling of unpleasantness or discomfort. [dys- + G. *phora,* a bearing]

dys·phra·sia (dis-frā′zē-ă). SYN dysphasia. [dys- + G. *phrasis,* speaking]

dys·phy·lax·ia (dis-fī-lak′sē-ă). A form of insomnia marked by awakening too early. [dys- + G. *phylaxis,* watching]

dys·pig·men·ta·tion (dis′pig-men-tā′shŭn). Any abnormality in the formation or distribution of pigment, especially in the skin; usually applied to an abnormal reduction in pigmentation (depigmentation).

dys·pin·e·al·ism (dis-pin′ē-ăl-izm). Obsolete term for the syndrome supposed to result from the deficiency of pineal gland secretion.

dys·pi·tu·i·tar·ism (dis-pi-tū′i-ter-izm). The complex of phenomena due to excessive or deficient secretion by the pituitary gland.

dys·pla·sia (dis-plā′zē-ă). Abnormal tissue development. SEE ALSO heteroplasia. [dys- + G. *plasis,* a molding]

anhidrotic ectodermal d. [MIM*305100], congenitally defective or absent sweat glands, smooth, finely wrinkled skin, sunken nose, malformed and missing teeth, sparse fragile hair, and associated with deformed nails, absent breast tissue, mental retardation, syndactyly; associated X-linked recessive inheritance. SYN Christ-Siemens-Touraine syndrome, hypohidrotic ectodermal d.

anterofacial d., anteroposterior facial d., anteroposterior d., abnormal growth of the face or cranium in an anteroposterior direction as seen and measured with a cephalogram.

asphyxiating thoracic d. [MIM*208500], hereditary hypoplasia of the thorax, associated with pelvic skeletal abnormality. SYN asphyxiating thoracic chondrodystrophy, Jeune's syndrome, thoracic-pelvic-phalangeal dystrophy.

bronchopulmonary d., chronic pulmonary insufficiency arising from long-term artificial pulmonary ventilation; seen more frequently in premature infants than in mature infants.

cerebral d., abnormal development of the telencephalon.

cervical d., d. of the uterine cervix, epithelial atypia involving part or all of the thickness of cervical squamous epithelium, occurring most often in young women; appears to regress frequently, but may progress over a long period to carcinoma; severe d. may be microscopically indistinguishable from carcinoma in situ.

chondroectodermal d. [MIM*225500], triad of chondrodysplasia, ectodermal d., and polydactyly, with congenital heart defects in over half of patients; autosomal recessive inheritance. SYN Ellis-van Creveld syndrome.

cleidocranial d., clidocranial d., SYN cleidocranial *dysostosis.*

congenital ectodermal d., SYN congenital ectodermal *defect.*

cortical d., a malformative disorganization of the cytoarchitecture of the cortex relative to neurons.

craniocarpotarsal d., SYN craniocarpotarsal *dystrophy.*

craniodiaphysial d. [MIM*218300], small stature and thickening of the cranial bones with sclerosis and diaphysial widening of tubular bones; autosomal recessive inheritance.

craniometaphysial d., syndrome of metaphysial d. associated with severe sclerosis and overgrowth of bones of the skull (leontiasis ossea) and with hypertelorism.

dentin d., a hereditary disorder of the teeth, involving both primary and permanent dentition, in which the clinical morphology and color of the teeth are normal, but the teeth radiographically exhibit short roots [MIM125400], obliteration of the pulp chambers and canals, and mobility and premature exfoliation; autosomal dominant inheritance. In another type of d. the teeth are opalescent [MIM 125420].

diaphysial d., progressive, symmetrical fusiform enlargement of the shafts of long bones characterized by the formation of excessive new periosteal and endosteal bone and irregular conversion of this cortical bone into cancellous bone; anemia does not occur as a rule, as in osteopetrosis. SYN Engelmann's disease.

ectodermal d., a congenital defect of the ectodermal tissues, including the skin and its appendages. SEE anhidrotic ectodermal d., hidrotic ectodermal d.

enamel d., SYN *amelogenesis* imperfecta.

d. epiphysia′lis hemime′lia, SYN tarsomegaly.

d. epiphysia′lis mul′tiplex, SYN multiple epiphysial d.

d. epiphysia′lis punc′ta′ta, a developmental error of the epiphyses characterized by severe deformities, epiphyses ossified from several discrete centers and with a stippled appearance, and thickened shafts of the long bones; congenital cataract and mental retardation are often present. There is an autosomal dominant form [MIM *118650] and an autosomal recessive form [MIM*215100]. SYN chondrodysplasia punctata, chondrodystrophia calcificans congenita, hypoplastic fetal chondrodystrophy, stippled epiphysis.

epithelial d., a disorder of differentiation of epithelial cells which may regress, remain stable, or progress to invasive carcinoma.

faciodigitogenital d., a syndrome of ocular hypertelorism, anteverted nostrils, broad upper lip, saddle-bag scrotum, and laxity of ligaments resulting in genu recurvatum, flat feet, and hyperextensible fingers; X-linked [MIM*305400] and autosomal dominant [MIM*100050] forms. SYN Aarskog-Scott syndrome.

familial white folded d., SYN white sponge *nevus.*

fibromuscular d., idiopathic nonatherosclerotic disease leading to stenosis of arteries, usually the renal arteries, and hypertension; two varieties are fibromuscular hyperplasia and perimuscular fibrosis.

fibrous d. of bone, a disturbance of medullary bone maintenance in which bone undergoing physiologic lysis is replaced by abnormal proliferation of fibrous tissue, resulting in asymmetric distortion and expansion of bone; may be confined to a single bone (monostotic fibrous d.) or involve multiple bones (polyostotic fibrous d.).

fibrous d. of jaws, SYN cherubism.

florid osseous d., cemental d., SYN sclerotic cemental *mass.*

hidrotic ectodermal d. [MIM*129500], congenital dystrophy of the nails and hair with thickened nails and sparse or absent scalp hair; often associated with keratoderma of the palms and soles; teeth and sweat gland function are normal; autosomal dominant inheritance.

hip d., a developmental disease of dogs in which joint instability due to disconformity of the head of the femur and the acetabulum allows excessive movement of the femoral head.

hypohidrotic ectodermal d., SYN anhidrotic ectodermal d.

lymphopenic thymic d., obsolete term for thymic *alymphoplasia.*

mammary d., obsolete term for fibrocystic *condition* of the breast.

mandibulofacial d., SYN mandibulofacial *dysostosis.*

metaphysial d., an abnormality that occurs when new bone at the metaphyses of long bones fails to undergo remodeling to the normal tubular structure; the ends of long bones appear to be expanded and porotic, with thin cortex; there may be an associated overgrowth of cranial bones (craniometaphysial d.).

Mondini d., congenital anomaly of osseus and membranous labyrinth characterized by aplastic cochlea, and deformity of the vestibule and semicircular canals with partial or complete loss of auditory and vestibular function; may be associated with spontaneous cerebrospinal fluid otorrhoea resulting in meningitis. SEE ALSO Mondini *deafness.*

monostotic fibrous d., fibrous d. of a single bone. SYN localized osteitis fibrosa, osteitis fibrosa circumscripta.

mucoepithelial d. [MIM*158310], an epithelial cell dishesive disease characterized by red, periorificial mucosal lesions of oral, nasal, vaginal, urethral, anal, bladder, and conjunctival mucosa, with cataracts, follicular keratosis, non-scarring alopecia, frequent pulmonary infections, pneumothorax, and sometimes cor pulmonale; autosomal dominant inheritance.

multiple epiphysial d., a dominantly inherited abnormality of epiphyses [MIM*132400] characterized by difficulty in walking, pain and stiffness of joints, stubby fingers, and often dwarfism of short-limb type; on x-ray examination, the epiphyses are mottled and irregular; ossification centers are late in appearance and may be multiple, but the vertebrae are normal. There is also an autosomal recessive form [MIM *226900]. SYN d. epiphysialis multiplex.

neuronal intestinal d., SYN neuronal *hyperplasia.*

oculoauriculovertebral d., OAV d. [MIM*257700], a syndrome characterized by epibulbar dermoids, preauricular appendages, micrognathia, and vertebral and other anomalies. SYN Goldenhar's syndrome, OAV syndrome.

oculodentodigital d. [MIM*164200], microphthalmia, coloboma, or anomalies of the iris associated with malformed and malpositioned teeth and with anomalies of the fingers including syndactyly, campylodactyly, or absent phalanges; autosomal dominant inheritance.

oculovertebral d., microphthalmia, colobomas, or anophthalmia with small orbit, twisted face due to unilateral d. of maxilla, macrostomia with malformed teeth and malocclusion, vertebral malformations, and branched and hypoplastic ribs. SYN oculovertebral syndrome, Weyers-Thier syndrome.

odontogenic d., SYN odontodysplasia.

ophthalmomandibulomelic d. [MIM*164900], an autosomal dominant disorder with corneal clouding and multiple abnormalities of the mandible and limbs.

periapical cemental d., a benign, painless, non-neoplastic condition of the jaws which occurs almost exclusively in middle-aged black females; lesions are usually multiple, most frequently involve vital mandibular anterior teeth, surround the root apices, and are initially radiolucent (becoming more opaque as they mature). SYN periapical osteofibrosis.

polyostotic fibrous d., the occurrence of lesions of fibrous d. in multiple bones, commonly on one side of the body; may occur with areas of pigmentation and endocrine dysfunction (McCune-Albright syndrome). SYN multifocal osteitis fibrosa, osteitis fibrosa disseminata.

pseudoachondroplastic spondyloepiphysial d., a group of severe dwarfisms with short limbs, a relatively long trunk, joint laxity especially in hands and knees. Autosomal dominant [MIM*177150 and MIM* 177170] and recessive [MIM*264150 and *264160] forms exist.

retinal d., an overgrowth of glial tissue compensating for aplasia of sensory elements.

septo-optic d., congenital optic nerve hypoplasia associated with midline cerebral anomalies. SYN de Morsier's syndrome.

spondyloepiphysial d., a group of conditions characterized by growth insufficiency of the vertebral column, with flattening of vertebrae, and often involving the epiphyses at the hip and shoulder; results in dwarfism of the short trunk type, often also with short extremities, sometimes with other malformations; types with dominant [MIM *183850], recessive [[MIM*208230 and MIM 271600], and X-linked recessive [MIM *313400 and MIM*313420] inheritance have been described in different families.

ventriculoradial d., a congenital syndrome consisting of a ventricular septal defect with associated absence of thumb or radius.

dys·plas·tic (dis-plas'tik). Pertaining to or marked by dysplasia.

dysp·nea (disp-nē'ă). Shortness of breath, a subjective difficulty or distress in breathing, usually associated with disease of the heart or lungs; occurs normally during intense physical exertion or at high altitude. [G. *dyspnoia,* fr. *dys-,* bad, + *pnoē,* breathing]
cardiac d., shortness of breath of cardiac origin.
exertional d., excessive shortness of breath after exercise.
expiratory d., difficulty with the expiratory phase of breathing, often due to obstruction in the larynx or large bronchi, such as by a foreign body.
functional d., shortness of breath without apparent underlying disease.
nocturnal d., d. occurring at night, several hours after assuming recumbent position. Occurs in heart failure and results from reabsorption of water from dependent areas after removal of effect of gravity, causing hypervolemia, aggravating left-ventricular failure.
paroxysmal nocturnal d., acute d. appearing suddenly at night, usually waking the patient after an hour or two of sleep; caused by pulmonary congestion with or without edema that results from left-sided heart failure following immobilization of fluid from dependent areas after lying down.
Traube's d., obsolete eponym for inspiratory d. with maximal expansion of the chest and a slow respiratory rhythm.

dysp·ne·ic (disp-nē'ik). Out of breath; relating to or suffering from dyspnea.

dys·prax·ia (dis-prak'sē-ă). Impaired or painful functioning in any organ. [dys- + G. *praxis,* a doing]

dys·pro·si·um (Dy) (dis-prō'sē-ŭm). A metallic element of the lanthanide (rare earth) series, atomic no. 66, atomic wt. 162.50. [G. *dysprosits,* hard to get at]

dys·pro·tein·e·mia (dis-prō'tēn-ē'mē-ă, -prō'tē-in-). An abnormality in plasma proteins, usually in immunoglobulins.

dys·pro·tein·e·mic (dis-prō-tēn-ē'mik). Relating to dysproteinemia.

dys·ra·phism, dys·raph·ia (dis'ră-fizm, dis-raf'ē-ă). Defective fusion, especially of the neural folds, resulting in status dysraphicus. [dys- + G. *rhaphē,* suture]

dys·rhyth·mia (dis-rith'mē-ă). Defective rhythm. See also entries under rhythm. Cf. arrhythmia. [dys- + G. *rhythmos,* rhythm]
cardiac d., any abnormality in the rate, regularity, or sequence of cardiac activation.
electroencephalographic d., a diffusely irregular brain wave tracing.
esophageal d., abnormal motility of the muscular layers of the esophageal wall, such as occurs in esophageal spasm.
paroxysmal cerebral d., a diffusely abnormal electroencephalogram often seen with epilepsy.

dys·se·ba·cia, dys·se·ba·cea (dis-sĕ-bā'shē-ă, dis'sē-bă'shē-ă). SYN seborrheic *dermatitis.* [dys- + L. *sebum,* grease]

dys·som·nia (dis-som'nē-ă). Disturbance of normal sleep or rhythm pattern.

dys·spon·dy·lism (dis-spon'di-lizm). An abnormality of development of the spine or vertebral column. [dys- + G. *spondylos,* vertebra]

dys·sta·sia (dis-stā'sē-ă). Difficulty in standing. SYN dystasia. [dys- + G. *stasis,* standing]

dys·stat·ic (dis-tat'ik). Marked by difficulty in standing.

dys·syl·la·bia (dis-il-lā'bē-ă). SYN syllable-stumbling. [dys- + G. *syllabē,* syllable]

dys·syn·er·gia (dis-in-er'jē-ă). An aspect of ataxia, in which an act is not performed smoothly or accurately because of lack of harmonious association of its various components; usually used to describe abnormalities of movement caused by cerebellar disorders. [dys- + G. *syn*, with, + *ergon*, work]

d. cerebellaris myoclonica, a familial disorder beginning in late childhood, characterized by progressive cerebellar ataxia, action myoclonus and preserved intellect. Probably due to multiple causes, mitochondrial abnormalities being one. SYN dentatorubral cerebellar atrophy with polymyoclonus.

detrusor sphincter d., a disturbance of the normal relationship between bladder (detrusor) contraction and sphincter relaxation during voluntary or involuntary voiding efforts.

dys·tas·ia. SYN dysstasia.

hereditary areflexic dystasia, SYN Raussly *disease.*

dys·tel·e·pha·lan·gy (dis-tel′ē-fă-lan′jē). Bowing of the distal phalanx of the little finger. [dys- + G. *telos*, end, + phalanx]

dys·thy·mia (dis-thī′mē-ă). A chronic mood disorder manifested as depression for most of the day, more days than not, accompanied by some of the following symptoms: poor appetite or overeating, insomnia or hypersomnia, low energy or fatigue, low self-esteem, poor concentration, difficulty making decisions, and feelings of hopelessness. SEE mood *disorders*, under *disorder*, endogenous *depression*, exogenous *depression*. [dys- + G. *thymos*, mind, emotion]

dys·thy·mic (dis-thī′mik). Relating to dysthymia.

dys·to·cia (dis-tō′sē-ă). Difficult childbirth. [G. *dystokia*, fr. *dys-*, difficult, + *tokos*, childbirth]

fetal d., d. due to an abnormality of the fetus.

maternal d., d. caused by an abnormality or physical problem in the mother.

placental d., retention or difficult delivery of the placenta.

dys·to·nia (dis-tō′nē-ă). A state of abnormal (either hypo- or hyper-) tonicity in any of the tissues. SYN torsion spasm. [dys- + G. *tonos*, tension]

d. lenticula′ris, d. resulting from a lesion of the lenticulate nucleus.

d. musculo′rum defor′mans, a genetic, environmental, or idiopathic disorder, usually beginning in childhood or adolescence, marked by muscular contractions that distort the spine, limbs, hips, and sometimes the cranial-innervated muscles. The abnormal movements are increased by excitement and, at least initially, abolished by sleep. The musculature is hypertonic when in action, hypotonic when at rest. Hereditary forms usually begin with involuntary posturing of the foot or hand (autosomal recessive form [MIM*224500]) or of the neck or trunk (autosomal dominant form [MIM*128100]); both forms may progress to produce contortions of the entire body. SYN progressive torsion spasm, torsion disease of childhood, torsion d., Ziehen-Oppenheim disease.

torsion d., SYN d. musculorum deformans.

dys·ton·ic (dis-ton′ik). Pertaining to dystonia.

dys·to·pia (dis-tō′pē-ă). Faulty or abnormal position of a part or organ. SYN allotopia, malposition. [dys- + G. *topos*, place]

dys·top·ic (dis-top′ik). Pertaining to, or characterized by, dystopia. SEE ALSO ectopic.

dys·tro·phia (dis-trō′fē-ă). SYN dystrophy. [L. fr. G. *dys-*, bad, + *trophē*, nourishment]

d. adipo′sogenita′lis, a disorder characterized primarily by obesity and hypogonadotrophic hypogonadism in adolescent boys; dwarfism is rare, and when present is thought to reflect hypothyroidism. Visual loss, behavioral abnormalities, and diabetes insipidus may occur. Fröhlich's syndrome often is used synonymously for this disorder, although the original case involved a pituitary tumor; most cases are thought to result from hypothalamic dysfunction in areas regulating appetite and gonadal development. The most common causes are pituitary and hypothalamic neoplasms. SYN adiposis orchica, adiposogenital degeneration, adiposogenital dystrophy, adiposogenital syndrome, hypophysial syndrome, hypothalamic obesity with hypogonadism.

d. brevicol′lis, a condition marked by symptoms of d. adiposogenitalis together with a deforming shortness of the neck, but without synostosis of the cervical vertebrae seen in Klippel-Feil syndrome.

d. myoton′ica, SYN myotonic *dystrophy.*

d. un′guium, dystrophy of the nails.

d. un′gulae, SYN seedy *toe.*

dys·tro·phic (dis-trof′ik). Relating to dystrophy.

dys·tro·phin (dis-trō′fin). A protein found in the sarcolemma of normal muscle; it is missing in individuals with pseudohypertrophic muscular dystrophy and in other forms of muscular dystrophy; its role may be in the linkage of the cytoskeleton of the muscle cell to extracellular protein.

dys·tro·phy (dis′trō-fē). Progressive changes that may result from defective nutrition of a tissue or organ. SYN dystrophia. [dys- + G. *trophē*, nourishment]

adiposogenital d., SYN *dystrophia* adiposogenitalis.

adult pseudohypertrophic muscular d. [MIM*310200.0002], muscular d. of late onset, often in the second or third decade, with relatively mild course; X-linked recessive inheritance; perhaps allelic with Duchenne's d., but milder and not a genetic lethal. Cf. Duchenne d. SYN Becker type tardive muscular d.

Barnes' d., a rare type of muscular d., in which muscles are often hypertrophic and stronger than normal, but later become weak and atrophic.

Becker type muscular d., a muscular dystrophy that has many of the clinical features of Duchenne muscular dystrophy *e.g.,* symmetrical involvement of first the pelvicrural muscles and then the pectoral girdle and proximal upper extremity muscles; pseudohypertrophy, especially of the calf muscles but with a much later age of onset (35–45 years), and more benign course. X-linked inheritance.

Becker type tardive muscular d., SYN adult pseudohypertrophic muscular d.

childhood muscular d., SYN Duchenne d.

cone d., a retinal abnormality in which color perception is severely deficient and typical changes occur in electroretinogram. SEE achromatopsia. SYN cone degeneration.

corneal d. [MIM*217600], central corneal opacification, usually bilateral, symmetrical, and often autosomal recessive, involving predominantly epithelial, stromal, or endothelial layers, often in a typical pattern.

craniocarpotarsal d. [MIM*193700], congenital association of skeletal defects (ulnar deviation of hands with camptodactyly, talipes equinovarus, and frontal bone defects) and characteristic facies (protrusion of lips as in whistling, sunken eyes with hypertelorism, and small nose); autosomal dominant inheritance. SYN craniocarpotarsal dysplasia, Freeman-Sheldon syndrome, whistling face syndrome.

Duchenne d., the most common childhood muscular d., with onset usually before age 6. Characterized by symmetrical weakness and wasting of first the pelvic and crural muscles and then the pectoral and proximal upper extremity muscles; pseudohypertrophy of some muscles, especially the calf; heart involvement; sometimes mild mental retardation; progressive course and early death, usually in adolescence. X-linked inheritance (affects males and transmitted by females). SYN childhood muscular d., Duchenne's disease (1), pseudohypertrophic muscular d.

Emery-Dreifuss muscular d., a generally benign type of muscular d., with onset in childhood or early adulthood. Weakness begins with the pectoral girdle and proximal upper extremity muscles and spreads to the pelvic girdle and distal lower extremity muscles. Contractures of the elbow, flexors, neck flexors, and calf muscles often occur; muscle pseudohypertrophy and mental retardation do not occur. A cardiomyopathy is common. An X-linked inherited disorder, nonallelic to Duchenne's muscular d.

endothelial d. of cornea, spontaneous loss of corneal endothelium leading to edema of the corneal stroma and epithelium.

epithelial d., corneal d. affecting primarily the epithelium and its basement membrane. SEE ALSO juvenile epithelial corneal d.

facioscapulohumeral muscular d. [MIM*158900], a relatively benign type of muscular d. commencing in childhood and slowly progressive; characterized by wasting and weakness, sometimes asymmetrical, mainly of the muscles of the face, shoulder girdle, and arms; autosomal dominant inheritance. SYN facioscapulohumeral atrophy, Landouzy-Dejerine d.

Favre's d., SYN vitreo-tapetoretinal d.

fingerprint d., a condition wherein fine parallel lines in a fingerprint configuration area are seen in the basal epithelial layer and basement membrane of the corneal epithelium. SEE ALSO map-dot-fingerprint d.

fleck d. of cornea [MIM*121850], a bilateral occurrence of subtle spots in the corneal stroma; the spots vary in size and shape, and have sharp margins and clear centers; photophobia may occur; autosomal dominant inheritance.

Fuchs' epithelial d., epithelial edema secondary to endothelial d. of the cornea.

Groenouw's corneal d., (1) a granular type of corneal d., with autosomal dominant inheritance [MIM*121900]; (2) a macular type of corneal d., with autosomal recessive inheritance [MIM*217800].

gutter d. of cornea, a marginal furrow usually inferiorly about 1 mm from the limbus; and sometimes bilateral. SYN keratoleptynsis (1).

hypertrophic d., SYN squamous cell *hyperplasia*.

infantile neuroaxonal d., a rare, familial disorder of early childhood manifested as progressive psychomotor deterioration, increased reflexes, Babinski sign, hypotonia and progressive blindness. Pathologically, eosinophilic spheroids of swollen axoplasm are found in various central nervous system nuclei.

juvenile epithelial corneal d. [MIM*122100], epithelial d. characterized by progressive cysts and opacities of the corneal epithelium, with onset in infancy; autosomal dominant inheritance with incomplete penetrance. SYN Meesman d.

Landouzy-Dejerine d., SYN facioscapulohumeral muscular d.

lattice corneal d. [MIM*122200], a corneal d. due to localized accumulation of amyloid in a reticular pattern; manifest at puberty and progressing slowly until eventually useful vision is lost; autosomal dominant inheritance.

Leyden-Möbius muscular d., SYN limb-girdle muscular d.

limb-girdle muscular d. [MIM*253600], one of the less well-defined types of muscular d., probably heterogenous in nature. Onset usually in childhood or early adulthood and both sexes affected. Characterized by weakness and wasting, usually symmetrical, of the pelvic girdle muscles, the shoulder girdle muscles, or both, but not the facial muscles. Muscle pseudohypertrophy, heart involvement, and mental retardation are absent. Variable inheritance. SYN Leyden-Möbius muscular d., pelvofemoral muscular d., scapulohumeral muscular d.

macular d., a group of disorders involving predominately the posterior portion of the ocular fundus, due to degeneration in the sensory layer of the retina, retinal pigment epithelium, Bruch's membrane, choroid, or a combination of these tissues. SEE Stargardt's *disease*, Best's *disease*.

map-dot-fingerprint d., fingerprint d. accompanied by map-like patterns and microcystic epithelial inclusions.

Meesman d., SYN juvenile epithelial corneal d.

microcystic epithelial d., bilateral, symmetrical intraepithelial cysts in the central area of the cornea of healthy women, without hereditary predisposition.

mucopolysaccharide keratin d., a histologic finding seen in the surface epithelium of oral inflammatory fibrous hyperplasia, consisting of homogeneous eosinophilic pools of material in the superficial spinous layer.

muscular d., a general term for a number of hereditary, progressive degenerative disorders affecting skeletal muscles, and often other organ systems as well. SYN myodystrophy, myodystrophia.

myotonic d. [MIM*160900], the most common adult muscular dystrophy, characterized by progressive muscle weakness and wasting of some of the cranial innervated muscles, as well as the distal limb muscles; myotonia; cataracts; hypogonadism; cardiac abnormalities; and frontal balding. Onset usually in the third decade; autosomal dominant inheritance. SYN dystrophia myotonica, myotonia atrophica, myotonia dystrophica, Steinert's disease.

neuroaxonal d., a rare disorder that begins in the second year of life and is relentlessly progressive; clinically characterized initially by walking difficulties, weakness, and areflexia, later followed by corticospinal and pseudobulbar findings, blindness, loss of pain appreciation, and mental deterioration; pathologically, eosinophilic spheroids of swollen axoplasm are found in various central nuclei; autosomal recessive inheritance.

oculopharyngeal d., a dominantly inherited form of chronic progressive external *ophthalmoplegia* usually presenting in middle life or old age with chronic ptosis and/or difficulty swallowing. Many sufferers have French-Canadian ancestry.

pelvofemoral muscular d., SYN limb-girdle muscular d.

progressive muscular d., a form of progressive muscular atrophy in which the disease begins in the muscle and not in the spinal centers. SYN Erb atrophy, idiopathic muscular atrophy.

progressive tapetochoroidal d., SYN choroideremia.

pseudohypertrophic muscular d., SYN Duchenne d.

reflex sympathetic d. (RSD), diffuse persistent pain usually in an extremity often associated with vasomotor disturbances, trophic changes, and limitation or immobility of joints; frequently follows some local injury. SEE ALSO causalgia. SYN shoulder-hand syndrome, sympathetic reflex d.

reticular d. of cornea, bilateral, progressive, superficial degeneration of the corneal epithelium and adjacent Bowman's membrane.

ring-like corneal d. [MIM*121900], thread-like opacities of the anterior corneal stroma, with acute, painful onset followed by decreased vision; autosomal dominant inheritance.

scapulohumeral muscular d., SYN limb-girdle muscular d.

sympathetic reflex d., SYN reflex sympathetic d.

thoracic-pelvic-phalangeal d., SYN asphyxiating thoracic *dysplasia*.

twenty-nail d., longitudinal ridging of all of the nails; seen in alopecia areata and lichen planus.

vitreo-tapetoretinal d. [MIM*268100], autosomal recessive bilateral peripheral and central retinoschisis with pigmentary degeneration of the retina, chorioretinal atrophy, vitreous degeneration, and night blindness. SYN Favre's d.

vulvar d., a spectrum of vulvar eruptions consisting of white atrophic papules, including lichen sclerosus et atrophicus, squamous cell hyperplasia (hypertrophic dystrophy), or a combination of these (mixed dystrophy). SEE ALSO *lichen* sclerosus et atrophicus.

dys·tro·py (dis′trō-pē). Abnormal or eccentric behavior. [dys- + G. *tropos*, a turning]

dys·u·ria (dis-yū′rē-ă). Difficulty or pain in urination. SYN dysury. [dys- + G. *ouron*, urine]

dys·u·ric (dis-yū′rik). Relating to or suffering from dysuria.

dys·u·ry (dis′yū-rē). SYN dysuria.

dys·ver·sion (dis-ver′zhŭn). A turning in any direction, less than inversion; particularly d. of the optic nerve head (situs inversus of the optic disk). [dys- + L. *verto*, to turn]

E

ε **1.** Fifth letter of the Greek alphabet, epsilon. **2.** Symbol for molar absorption *coefficient* or extinction *coefficient*. For terms beginning with this prefix, see the specific term. **3.** In chemistry, denotes a position of a substituent located on the fifth atom from the carboxyl or other primary functional group. For terms beginning with this prefix, see the specific term.

E 1. Symbol for exa-; extraction *ratio*; glutamic acid; energy; electromotive *force*; glutamyl; internal *energy*. **2.** As a subscript, refers to expired *gas*; obsolete symbol for einsteinium.

E_0^+, E^0, E_h Symbols for oxidation-reduction potential.

E_1 Symbol for estrone.

E_2 Symbol for estradiol.

E Abbreviation for entgegen.

e Symbol for elementary charge; base of natural logarithms (2,71828...).

EAE Abbreviation for experimental allergic *encephalitis*.

Eagle, Harry, U.S. physician and cell biologist, 1905–1992. SEE E.'s basal *medium*, minimum essential *medium*.

Eagle, W., 20th century U.S. otolaryngologist. SEE E. *syndrome*.

Eales, Henry, English ophthalmologist, 1852–1913. SEE E.'s *disease*.

ear (ēr). The organ of hearing: composed of the **external e.**, which includes the auricle and the external acoustic, or auditory, meatus; the **middle e.**, or the tympanic cavity with its ossicles; and the **internal e.** or **inner e.**, or labyrinth, which includes the semicircular canals, vestibule, and cochlea. SEE ALSO auricle. SYN auris [NA]. [A.S. *eáre*]

aviator's e., SYN aerotitis media.

Aztec e., an auricle with the lobule absent.

bat e., SYN lop-ear.

Blainville e.'s, asymmetry in size or shape of the auricles.

boxer's e., SYN cauliflower e.

Cagot e. (kǎ-gō′), an auricle having no lobulus. [a people in the Pyrenees among whom physical stigmata are common]

cauliflower e., thickening and induration of the e. with distortion of contours following extravasation of blood within its tissues. SYN boxer's e.

darwinian e., an auricle in which the upper border is not rolled over to form the helix, but projects upward as a flat, sharp edge.

dog e., redundant corner of skin, usually the result of mismatch in a wound closure, leaving an excessive hump or triangular bit of tissue.

glue e., middle e. inflammation with thick mucoid effusion caused by long-standing eustachian tube obstruction.

lop e., SEE lop-ear.

Morel's e., a large, misshapen, outstanding auricle, with obliterated grooves and thinned edges.

Mozart e., a deformity of the pinna where the two crura of the antihelix and the crus of the helix are fixed, giving a bulging appearance of the superior part of the pinna. [Wolfgang Amadeus Mozart, 1756–1791, composer, said to have had this deformity]

scroll e., a deformity of the external e. in which the pinna is rolled forward.

Stahl's e., a deformed external e., in which the fossa ovalis and upper portion of the scaphoid fossa are covered by the helix; regarded as a stigma of degenerate constitution.

swimmer's e., SYN otitis externa.

Wildermuth's e., an e. in which the helix is turned backward and the antihelix is prominent.

ear·ache (ēr′āk). Pain in the ear. SYN otalgia, otodynia.

ear·drum (ēr′drŭm). SYN tympanic *membrane*.

Earle, Wilton R., U.S. pathologist, 1902–1962. SEE E. L *fibrosarcoma*.

Earle's so·lu·tion. See under solution.

earth (erth). **1.** Soil; the soft substance of the land, as opposed to

rock and sand. **2.** An easily pulverized mineral. **3.** An insoluble oxide of aluminum or of certain other elements characterized by a high melting point. [A.S. *eorthe*]

alkaline e.'s, SEE alkaline earth *elements*, under *element*.

diatomaceous e., a powder made of desiccated diatom material; used as a filtering agent, adsorbent, and abrasive in many chemical operations.

fuller's e., **(1)** an amorphous variety of kaolin of varying composition, containing an aluminum magnesium silicate. The name is derived from an ancient process of cleansing or "fulling" wool to remove the oil and dirt particles with a water slurry of e. or clay. **(2)** a refined clay sometimes used as a dusting powder or applied moistened with water as a form of poultice. Currently refers to any clay that can be used for the purpose of decolorizing in oil refining. Used as decolorizer for oils and other liquids, filtering medium, filler for rubber, and in agricultural formulations. [fr. *fulling*, an old process of cleaning wool, with earth or clay]

rare e.'s, SEE lanthanides.

earth-eat·ing. SYN geophagia.

ear·wax (ēr′waks). SYN cerumen.

eat (ēt). **1.** To take solid food. **2.** To chew and swallow any substance as one would food. **3.** To corrode. [A.S. *etan*]

Eaton, Lee M., U.S. neurologist, 1905–1958. SEE E.-Lambert *syndrome*.

Eaton, Monroe D., U.S. microbiologist, *1904. SEE E. *agent*, agent *pneumonia*.

E.B., EB Abbreviation for elementary *bodies* (1), under *body*.

Ebbinghaus, Hermann, German, 1850–1909. SEE E. *test*.

Eberth, Karl J., German physician, 1835–1926. SEE E.'s *bacillus*, *lines*, under *line*, *perithelium*.

Ebner, Victor von. SEE von Ebner.

e·bo·na·tion (ē-bō-nā′shŭn). Removal of loose fragments of bone from a wound. [L.]

ébran·le·ment (ā-brahn-la-mon′). Twisting a polyp on its stalk to cause atrophy. [Fr.]

Ebstein, Wilhelm, German physician, 1836–1912. SEE E.'s *anomaly*, *disease*, *sign*; Armanni-E. *change*, *kidney*; Pel-E. *disease*, *fever*.

eb·ul·lism (eb′yū-lizm). Formation of water vapor bubbles in the tissues brought on by an extreme reduction in barometric pressure; occurs if the body is exposed to pressures which are found above an altitude of 63,000 feet. [L. *ebullire*, to boil out]

e·bur (ē′bŭr). A tissue resembling ivory in outward appearance or structure. [L. ivory]

e. den·tis, SYN dentin.

eb·ur·na·tion (ē-bŭr-nā′shŭn). A change in exposed subchondral bone in degenerative joint disease in which it is converted into a dense substance with a smooth surface like ivory. SYN bone sclerosis. [L. *eburneus*, of ivory]

e. of dentin, a condition observed in arrested dental caries wherein decalcified dentin is burnished and takes on a polished, often brown-stained appearance.

ebur·ne·ous (ē-bŭr′nē-ŭs). Resembling ivory, especially in color.

ebur·ni·tis (ē-bŭr-nī′tis). Increased density and hardness of dentin, which may occur after the dentin is exposed. [L. *eburneus*, of ivory, + G. -itis, inflammation]

EBV Abbreviation for Epstein-Barr *virus*.

EC Abbreviation for Enzyme Commission of the International Union of Biochemistry, used in conjunction with a unique number to define a specific enzyme in the Enzyme Commission's list [*Enzyme Nomenclature*], (1984); *e.g.*, EC 1.1.1.1 defines an alcohol dehydrogenase; EC 2.6.1.1 defines aspartate aminotransferase, popularly known as glutamic-oxalacetic transaminase (GOT).

ec-. Out of, away from. [G.]

E-cad·her·in (Ē-cǎd-hěr′in). SYN uvomorulin.

538

écar·teur (ā-kar-ter'). A type of retractor. [Fr. *écarter*, to separate]

ecau·date (ē-kaw'dāt). Tailless. [L. *e*- priv. + *cauda*, tail]

ec·bo·line (ek'bŏ-lēn). SYN ergotoxine.

ec·cen·tric (ek-sen'trik). **1.** Abnormal or peculiar in ideas or behavior. SYN erratic (1). **2.** Proceeding from a center. Cf. centrifugal (2). **3.** SYN peripheral. [G. *ek*, out, + *kentron*, center]

ec·cen·tro·chon·dro·pla·sia (ek-sen'trō-kon-drō-plā'zē-ă). Abnormal epiphysial development from eccentric centers of ossification. [G. *ek*, out + *kentron*, center, + *chondros*, cartilage, + *plasis*, a molding]

ec·cen·tro·pi·e·sis (ek-sen'trō-pī-ē'sis). Pressure exerted from within outward. [G. *ek*, out, + *kentron*, center, + *piesis*, pressure]

ec·chon·dro·ma (ek-kon-drō'mă). **1.** A cartilaginous neoplasm arising as an overgrowth from normally situated cartilage, as a mass protruding from the articular surface of a bone, in contrast to enchondroma. **2.** An enchondroma which has burst through the shaft of a bone and become pedunculated. SYN ecchondrosis. [G. *ek*, from, + *chondros*, cartilage, + *-oma*, tumor]

ec·chon·dro·sis (ek-kon-drō'sis). SYN ecchondroma.

ec·chon·dro·tome (ek-kon'drō-tōm). SYN chondrotome. [G. *ek*, out, + *chondros*, cartilage, + *tomē*, incision]

ec·chor·do·sis phy·sa·li·for·'mis. A notochordal rest of the cranial clivus which may form a small tumor.

ec·chy·mo·ma (ek-i-mō'mă). A slight hematoma following a bruise. [G. *ek*, out, + *chymos*, juice, + *-oma*, tumor]

ec·chy·mosed (ek'i-mōsd). Characterized by or affected with ecchymosis.

ec·chy·mo·sis (ek-i-mō'sis). A purplish patch caused by extravasation of blood into the skin, differing from petechiae only in size (larger than 3 mm diameter). [G. *ekchymōsis*, ecchymosis, fr. *ek*, out, + *chymos*, juice]

bilateral medial orbital e.'s, SYN raccoon *eyes*, under *eye*.

Tardieu's e.'s, subpleural and subpericardial petechiae or ecchymoses (or both), as observed in the tissues of persons who have been strangled, or otherwise asphyxiated. SYN Tardieu's petechiae, Tardieu's spots.

ec·chy·mot·ic (ek-i-mot'ik). Relating to an ecchymosis.

Eccleston. SEE Paget-Eccleston *stain*.

ec·crine (ek'rin). **1.** SYN exocrine (1). **2.** Denoting the flow of sweat. [G. *ek-krino*, to secrete]

ec·cri·nol·o·gy (ek-ri-nol'ō-jē). The branch of physiology and of anatomy concerned with the secretions and the secreting (exocrine) glands. [G. *ek-drino*, to secrete, + *logos*, study]

ec·cri·sis (ek'ri-sis). **1.** The removal of waste products. **2.** Any waste product; excrement. [G. separation]

ec·crit·ic (ek-krit'ik). **1.** Promoting the expulsion of waste matters. **2.** An agent that promotes excretion.

ec·cy·e·sis (ek-sī-ē'sis). SYN ectopic *pregnancy*. [G. *ek*, out, + *kyēsis*, pregnancy]

ec·dem·ic (ek-dem'ik). Denoting a disease brought into a region from without. [G. *ekdēmos*, foreign, from home, fr. *dēmos*, people]

ec·dys·i·asm (ek-diz'ē-azm). A morbid tendency to undress to produce sexual desire in others. [fr. G. *ekdyō*, to remove one's clothes]

ec·dy·sis (ek'di-sis). Desquamation, sloughing, or molting as a necessary phenomenon to permit growth in arthropods and skin renewal in amphibians and reptiles. [G. *ekdysis*, shedding]

ECF Abbreviation for extracellular *fluid*.

ECF-A Abbreviation for eosinophil chemotactic factor of anaphylaxis.

ECFV Abbreviation for extracellular fluid *volume*.

ECG Abbreviation for electrocardiogram.

ec·go·nine (ek'gō-nēn, -nin). 3β-Hydroxy-1αH,5α H-tropane-2β-carboxylic acid; the important part of the cocaine molecule; a topical anesthetic; basis of many coca alkaloids.

ecgonine e., SYN benzoylecgonine.

ech·e·o·sis (ek-ē-ō'sis). Rarely used term for a mental distur-

bance caused by continuous disturbing noises. [G. *ēchein*, to suffer from noises in ears]

Echid·noph·a·ga gal·li·na·cea (ek-id-nof'ă-gă gal-i-nā'sē-ă). The sticktight flea, a serious pest of poultry in subtropical America; also frequently attacks domestic mammals and humans.

Ɔechin-. SEE echino-.

echi·nate (ek'i-nāt). SYN echinulate.

Ɔechino-, echin-. Prickly, spiny. [G. *echinos*, hedgehog, sea urchin]

Echi·no·chas·mus (ĕ-kī-nō-kaz'mŭs). A genus of digenetic flukes (family Echinostomatidae), particularly common in wading and fish-eating birds; the species *E. perfoliatus* var. *japonicus* is reported as a rare intestinal parasite of humans in Japan. [echino- + G. *chasma*, open mouth]

echi·no·coc·ci·a·sis (ĕ-kī'nō-kok-sē'ā-sis). SYN echinococcus *disease.*

echi·no·coc·co·sis (ĕ-kī'nō-kok-kō'sis). Infection with *Echinococcus;* larval infection is called hydatid *disease.* SYN echinococcus disease.

Echi·no·coc·cus (ĕ-kī'nō-kok'ŭs). A genus of very small taeniid tapeworms, two to five segments in adult worms; adults are found in various carnivores but not in humans; larvae, in the form of hydatid cysts, are found in the liver and other organs of ruminants, pigs, horses, rodents, and, under certain epidemiological circumstances, humans (*e.g.,* sheep herders living closely with their infected dogs). [echino- + G. *kokkos*, a berry]

E. granulo'sus, hydatid tapeworm, a species in which adults infect canids and the larval form (osseous and unilocular hydatid cysts) infects sheep and other ruminants, pigs, and horses; may also occur in humans, giving rise to a large cyst in the liver or other organs and tissues.

E. multilocula'ris, a north temperate and Arctic species that occurs, in the adult form, in foxes; the larva (alveolar hydatid cyst) is found in the liver of microtine rodents and in humans; it produces a proliferative, often slow-growing cyst in the liver that, in humans, is usually fatal.

E. voge'li, a species reported from humid tropical forests of Panama and northern South America causing a polycystic form of human hydatid disease intermediate between cystic and alveolar hydatid disease; the typical cycle involves domestic dogs and wild canids as host of the adult tapeworm, and rodents such as the paca (*Cuniculus paca*) as the intermediate host for the cystic form.

echi·no·cyte (ek'i-nō-sīt). A crenated red blood cell. [echino- + G. *kytos*, cell]

echi·no·derm (e-kī'nō-derm). A member of the phylum Echinodermata.

Echi·no·der·ma·ta (e-kī-nō-der'mă-tă). A phylum of Metazoa which includes starfish, sea urchins, sea lilies, and other classes. All but the sea cucumbers (Holothuroidea) are basically radially symmetrical and most possess a calcareous endoskeleton with external spines. They inhabit the sea bottom, some near shore, others in deep water. [echino- + G. *derma*, skin]

Echi·no·rhyn·chus (e-kī-nō-ring'kŭs). A genus of acanthocephalid (thorny-headed) worms which originally included species now contained in *Macracanthorhynchus, Gigantorhynchus,* and other genera. [echino- + G. *rhynchos,* snout]

ech·i·no·sis (ek-i-nō'sis). A condition in which the red blood cells have lost their smooth outlines, resembling an echinus or sea urchin. [echino- + G. *-osis*, condition]

Echi·no·sto·ma (ĕ-kī-nō-stō'mă, ek-i-nos'tō-mă). A genus of digenetic flukes (family Echinostomatidae) with characteristic oral spines; widely distributed and parasitic in a broad range of bird and mammal hosts; several species have been reported in man from Southeast Asia. [echino- + G. *stoma,* mouth]

E. iloca'num, a species reported from man in the Philippines.

E. malay'anum, a species typically found in the pig, but reported occasionally from man in Malaysia; infection results from ingestion of snails with infective cysts (metacercariae).

echi·no·sto·mi·a·sis (ĕ-kī'nō-stō-mī'ă-sis). Infection of birds and mammals, including humans, with trematodes of the genus *Echinostoma.*

ec

echin·u·late (e-kin'yū-lāt). Prickly or spinous. Covered with small spines. SYN echinate. [Mod. L. *echinulus,* dim. of L. *echinus,* hedgehog]

Ech·is (ek'is, ē'kis). The saw-scaled or carpet viper, a genus of small (under 1 m), irritable, and alert snakes with a highly toxic venom; they are responsible for numerous snakebite cases with many fatalities. [G. *echis,* a viper]

ech·o (ek'ō). **1.** A reverberating sound sometimes heard during auscultation of the chest. **2.** In ultrasonography, the acoustic signal received from scattering or reflecting structures or the corresponding pattern of light on a CRT or ultrasonogram. **3.** In magnetic resonance imaging, the signal detected following an inverting pulse. [G.]

atrial e., electrical reactivation of the atrium by a retrograde impulse returning from the A-V node while the antegrade impulse continues to the ventricle; characterized electrocardiographically, by a pair of P waves enclosing a QRS complex, the second P wave being inverted, indicating that it is the reverse (the retrograde pathway) of the pathway of the first P wave (the antegrade pathway).

nodus sinuatrialis e., NS e., a postectopic sinus beat occurring earlier than would be expected from the preceding sinus node discharge interval; *i.e.,* the interval following a premature beat of supraventricular origin is less than the ordinary cycle length between sinus beats, whereas ordinarily the interval would be expected to exceed cycle length.

e. planar, a method of magnetic resonance imaging that allows rapid image acquisition during free induction decay, using technically difficult rapidly oscillating radiofrequency gradients.

spin e., a commonly used technique to recover T^2 relaxation signals in magnetic resonance imaging, by using a 180° inverting pulse in the pulse sequence to compensate for loss of transverse magnetization caused by magnetic field inhomogeneities.

ech·o·a·cou·sia (ek'ō-ă-kū'zē-ă). A subjective disturbance of hearing in which a sound appears to be repeated. [echo + G. *akouō,* to hear]

ech·o·a·or·tog·ra·phy (ek'ō-ā-ōr-tog'ră-fē). Application of ultrasound techniques to the diagnosis and study of the aorta. [echo + aortography]

ech·o·car·di·o·gram (ek-ō-kar'dē-ō-gram). The ultrasonic record obtained by echocardiography. SEE ultrasonography.

ech·o·car·di·og·ra·phy (ek'ō-kar-dē-og'ră-fē). The use of ultrasound in the investigation of the heart and great vessels and diagnosis of cardiovascular lesions. SYN ultrasonic cardiography, ultrasound cardiography. [echo + cardiography]

B-mode e., SYN two-dimensional e.

contrast e., the injection of contrast media of high echo reflectants (*e.g.,* bubbles) to outline a chamber or delineate a shunt within the heart.

cross-sectional e., SYN two-dimensional e.

Doppler e., use of Doppler ultrasonography techniques to augment two-dimensional e. by allowing velocities to be registered within the echocardiographic image. SEE duplex *ultrasonography,* Doppler *ultrasonography.* SYN duplex e.

duplex e., SYN Doppler e.

stress e., echocardiographic monitoring of a circulatory challenge, usually exercise.

transesophageal e., recording of the echocardiogram from a transducer swallowed by the patient to predetermined distances in the esophagus and stomach.

transthoracic e., the standard e. recorded from echocardiographic "windows" on the precordium.

two-dimensional e., e. in which an image is reconstructed from the echoes stimulated and detected by a linear array or moving transducers. SYN B-mode e., cross-sectional e.

ech·o·en·ceph·a·log·ra·phy (ek'ō-en-sef-ă-log'ră-fē). The use of reflected ultrasound in the diagnosis of intracranial processes. [echo + encephalography]

echo-free (ek'ō-frē). SYN anechoic.

ech·o·gen·ic (ek-ō-jen'ik). a structure or medium (*e.g.,* tissue) that is capable of producing echoes. Contrast with the terms hypoechoic, hyperechoic, and anechoic, which refer to the

plaucity, abundance, and absence of echoes displayed on the image.

ech·o·gram (ek'ō-gram). A record obtained using high frequency acoustic reflection techniques in any one of the various display modes, especially an echocardiogram. SEE ALSO ultrasonogram. [echo + G. *gramma,* a diagram]

echog·ra·pher (e-kog'ră-fer). SYN ultrasonographer.

ech·o·graph·ia (ek-ō-graf'ē-ă). A form of agraphia in which one cannot write spontaneously, but can write from dictation or copy. [echo + G. *graphō,* to write]

echog·ra·phy (e-kog'ră-fē). SYN ultrasonography. [echo + G. *graphō,* to write]

ech·o·ki·ne·sis, ech·o·ki·ne·sia (ek'ō-ki-nē'sis, -nē'zē-ă). SYN echopraxia. [echo + G. *kinēsis,* movement]

ech·o·la·lia (ek-ō-lā'lē-ă). Involuntary parrot-like repetition of a word or sentence just spoken by another person. Usually seen with schizophrenia. SYN echo reaction, echo speech, echophrasia. [echo + G. *lalia,* a form of speech]

ech·o·lo·ca·tion (ek'ō-lō-kā'shŭn). Term applied to the method by which bats direct their flight and avoid solid objects. The creatures emit high-pitched cries which, though inaudible to human ears, are heard by the bats themselves as reflected sounds (echoes) from objects in their path.

e·cho·ma·tism (e-kō'mă-tizm). SYN echopraxia. [echo + G. *matizō,* to strive to do]

ech·o·mim·ia (ek-ō-mim'ē-ă). SYN echopathy. [echo + G. *mimēsis,* imitation]

ech·o·mo·tism (ek'ō-mō'tizm). SYN echopraxia. [echo + L. *motio,* motion]

e·chop·a·thy (ĕ-kop'ă-thē). A form of psychopathology, usually associated with schizophrenia, in which the words (echolalia) or actions (echopraxia) of another are imitated and repeated. SYN echomimia. [echo + G. *pathos,* suffering]

e·choph·o·ny, ech·o·pho·nia (ĕ-kof'ō-nē, ek-ō-fō'nē-ă). A duplication of the voice sound occasionally heard during auscultation of the chest. [echo + G. *phōnē,* voice]

ech·o·phot·o·ny (ek-ō-fot'ō-nē). The mental association of sound tones with particular colors. [echo + G. *phōs* (*phōt*-), light, + *tonos,* tone]

ech·o·phra·sia (ek-ō-frā'zē-ă). SYN echolalia. [echo + *phrasis,* speech]

ech·o·prax·ia (ek'ō-prak'sē-ă). Involuntary imitation of movements made by another. SEE echopathy. SYN echokinesis, echokinesia, echomatism, echomotism. [echo + G. *praxis,* action]

ech·o·scope (ek'ō-skōp). Instrument for displaying echoes by means of ultrasonic pulses on an oscilloscope to demonstrate structures lying at depths within the body. [echo + G. *skopeō,* to view]

ech·o·thi·o·phate io·dide (ek-ō-thī'ō-fāt). Diethoxyphosphorylthiocholine iodide; a potent organophosphorus compound and cholinesterase inhibitor, used in the treatment of glaucoma.

Ec·ho·vi·rus 28 (ek'ō-vī'rŭs). Reclassified as Rhinovirus type 1.

ech·o·vi·rus (ek'ō-vī'rŭs). SYN ECHO *virus.*

Eck, Nikolai V., Russian physiologist, 1849–1917. SEE E. *fistula;* reverse E. *fistula.*

Ecker, Alexander, German anatomist, 1816–1887. SEE E.'s *fissure.*

Ecker, Enrique E., U.S. bacteriologist, 1887–1966. SEE Rees-E. *fluid.*

ec·la·bi·um (ek-lā'bē-ŭm). Eversion of a lip. [G. *ek,* out, + L. *labium,* lip]

ec·lamp·sia (ek-lamp'sē-ă). Occurrence of one or more convulsions, not attributable to other cerebral conditions such as epilepsy or cerebral hemorrhage, in a patient with preeclampsia. [G. *eklampsis,* a shining forth]

puerperal e., convulsions and coma associated with hypertension, edema, or proteinuria occurring in a woman following delivery. SYN puerperal convulsions.

superimposed e., SYN superimposed *preeclampsia.*

ec·lamp·tic (ek-lamp'tik). Relating to eclampsia.

ec·lamp·to·gen·ic, ec·lamp·tog·e·nous (ek-lamp-tō-jen'ik, -tog'ĕ-nŭs). Causing eclampsia.

ec·lec·tic (ek-lek'tik). Picking out from different sources what appears to be the best or most desirable. [G. *eklektikos,* selecting, fr. *ek,* out, + *lego,* to select]

ec·lec·ti·cism (ek-lek'ti-sizm). **1.** A now defunct system of medicine that advocated use of indigenous plants to effect specific cures of certain signs and symptoms. **2.** A system of medicine practiced by ancient Greek and Roman physicians who were not affiliated with a medical sect but who adopted the practice and teachings which they considered best from other systems.

ec·mne·sia (ek-nē'zē-ă). Obsolete term for a loss of memory for recent events. [G. *ek,* out, + *mnēsios,* relating to memory]

△**eco-.** The environment. [G. *oikos,* house, household, habitation]

eco·en·do·cri·nol·o·gy (ē'kō-en'dō-kri-nol'ō-jē). The study of the interactions of endocrine systems with the environment.

ECoG Abbreviation for electrocorticography.

e·coid (e'koyd). The framework of a red blood cell. [eco- + G. *eidos,* resemblance]

ec·o·log·i·cal fal·la·cy. the bias that may occur because an association observed between variables at an aggregate level does not necessarily represent an association that exists at an individual level; an error of inference due to failure to distinguish between different levels of organization.

e·col·o·gy (ē-kol'ō-jē). The branch of biology concerned with the total complex of interrelationships among living organisms, encompassing the relations of organisms to each other, to the environment, and to the entire energy balance within a given ecosystem. SYN bioecology, bionomics (2). [eco- + G. *logos,* study]

   human e., the relations of persons to their total (biologic and social) environment.

eco·ma·ni·a (ē-kō-mā'nē-ă). Obsolete term for a syndrome of domineering behavior at home and humility toward persons in authority. [eco- + G. *mania,* frenzy]

econ·a·zole (e-kōn'ă-zōl). 1-2-[(4-chlorophenyl)methoxy]-2-(2,4-dichlorophenyl)ethyl]-1*H*-imidazole; a broad spectrum antifungal agent used in the treatment of tinea pedis and related fungal infections.

Economo. SEE von Economo.

econ·o·my (ē-kon'ō-mē). system; the body regarded as an aggregate of functioning organs. [G. *oikonomia,* management of the house, fr. *oikos,* house, + *nomos,* usage, law]

eco·pho·bia (ē-kō-fō'bē-ă). Obsolete term for a morbid fear of one's home surroundings. SEE ALSO nostophobia. [eco- + G. *phobos,* fear]

ec·o·spe·cies (ē-kō-spē'shēz). Two or more populations of a species isolated by ecological barriers, theoretically able to exchange genes and interbreed, but partially separated from one another by differences in habitat or behavior.

ec·o·sys·tem (ē'kō-sis-tem). **1.** The fundamental unit in ecology, comprising the living organisms and the nonliving elements that interact in a defined region. **2.** A biocenosis (biotic community) and its biotope. SYN ecological system.

   parasite-host e., SYN parasitocenose.

ec·o·tax·is (ē-kō-tak'sis). Migration of lymphocytes "homing" from the thymus and bone marrow into tissues possessing an appropriate microenvironment. [eco- + G. *taxis,* order, arrangement]

écou·teur (ā-kū-ter'). One who obtains erotic gratification through listening to sexual accounts. [Fr. a listener-in]

écou·vil·lon (ā-kū-vē-yōhn'). A brush with firm bristles for freshening sores or abrading the interior of a cavity. [Fr., cleaning brush]

ec·pho·ria (ek-fōr'ē-ă). The recall of memory. [G. *ek,* out, + *phora,* a carrying]

ec·pho·rize (ek'fōr-īz). To revive a memory. [see ecphoria]

ec·phy·ma (ek-fī'mă). A warty growth or protuberance. [G. a pimply eruption]

écra·seur (ā-krah-zer'). Obsolete term for a snare, especially one of enough strength to cut through the base or pedicle of a tumor. [Fr. *écraser,* to crush]

ECS Abbreviation for electrocerebral silence.

ec·sta·sy (ek'stă-sē). Mental exaltation, with some degree of sensory anesthesia and a rapturous expression. [G. *ekstasis,* astonishment]

ec·stat·ic (ek-stat'ik). Relating to or marked by ecstasy.

ec·stro·phe (ek'strō-fē). SYN exstrophy.

ECT Abbreviation for electroconvulsive *therapy,* electroshock *therapy.*

△**ect-.** SEE ecto-.

ec·ta·co·lia (ek-tă-kō'lē-ă). Obsolete term for colectasia. [G. *ektasis,* a stretching, + *kolon,* colon]

ec·tad (ek'tad). Outward. [G. *ektos,* outside, + L. *ad,* to]

ec·tal (ek'tăl). Outer; external. [G. *ektos,* outside]

ec·ta·sia, ec·ta·sis (ek-tā'zē-ă, ek'tă-sis). Dilation of a tubular structure. [G. *ektasis,* a stretching]

   annuloaortic e., supravalvular dilation of the aorta involving both its wall and the valve ring, which, however, remains of smaller diameter than the more distal ectatic wall; many cases are related to Marfan's syndrome. SYN aortoannular e.

   aortoannular e., SYN annuloaortic e.

   e. cor'dis, dilation of the heart.

   corneal e., SYN keratoectasia.

   diffuse arterial e., spontaneous enlargement with dilation of the vessels in a circumscribed area.

   familial aortic e. (ek'tā-zē-ă), SYN familial aortic ectasia *syndrome.*

   hypostatic e., dilation of a blood vessel, usually a vein, in a dependent portion of the body, as in varicose veins of the leg.

   mammary duct e., dilation of mammary ducts by lipid and cellular debris in older women; rupture of ducts may result in granulomatous inflammation and infiltration by plasma cells. SEE ALSO plasma cell *mastitis.*

   papillary e., obsolete term for senile *hemangioma.*

   scleral e., SYN sclerectasia.

   senile e., obsolete term for senile *hemangioma.*

   e. ventric'uli paradox'a, SYN hourglass *stomach.*

△**-ectasia, -ectasis.** Dilation, expansion. [G. *ektasis,* a stretching]

ec·tat·ic (ek-tat'ik). Relating to, or marked by, ectasis.

ec·ten·tal (ek-ten'tăl). Relating to both ectoderm and endoderm; denoting the line where these two layers join. SYN ectoental. [G. *ektos,* outside, + *entos,* within]

ect·eth·moid (ekt-eth'moyd). SYN ethmoidal *labyrinth.* [G. *ektos,* outside, + ethmoid]

ec·thy·ma (ek-thī'mă). A pyogenic infection of the skin initiated by β-hemolytic streptococci and characterized by adherent crusts beneath which ulceration occurs; the ulcers may be single or multiple, and heal with scar formation. [G. a pustule]

   contagious e., SYN orf.

   e. gangreno'sum, SYN *dermatitis* gangrenosa infantum.

ec·thy·mat·i·form, ec·thy·mi·form (ek-thī-mat'i-fōrm, ek-thī'mi-fōrm). Resembling ecthyma.

ec·ti·ris (ek-tī'ris). The outer layer of the iris. [G. *ektos,* outside, + iris]

△**ecto-, ect-.** Outer, on the outside. SEE ALSO exo-. [G. *ektos,* outside]

△ Combining forms	[NA] Nomina Anatomica
Word*Finder* **Multi-term entry finder** **Preceding letter A**	**[MIM] Mendelian Inheritance in Man**
A.D.A.M. Anatomy Plates	☆ **Official alternate term**
Between letters L and M	☆**[NA] Official alternate Nomina Anatomica term**
Appendices: Following letter Z	
SYN Synonym; Cf., compare	**High Profile Term**

ec

ec·to·an·ti·gen (ek-tō-an'ti-jen). Any toxin or other excitor of antibody formation, separate or separable from its source. SYN exoantigen.

ec·to·blast (ek'tō-blast). **1.** SYN ectoderm. **2.** As used by some experimental embryologists, the original outer cell layer from which the primary germ layers are formed; in this sense, synonymous with protoderm. **3.** A cell wall. [ecto- + G. *blastos*, germ]

ec·to·car·dia (ek-tō-kar'dē-ă). Congenital displacement of the heart. SYN exocardia. [ecto- + G. *kardia*, heart]

ec·to·cer·vi·cal (ek'tō-ser'vi-kăl). Pertaining to the pars vaginalis of the cervix uteri lined with stratified squamous epithelium.

ec·to·cho·roi·dea (ek'tō-kō-roy'dē-ă). SYN suprachoroid *lamina*.

ec·to·cor·nea (ek-tō-kōr'nē-ă). The outer layer of the cornea.

ec·to·crine (ek'tō-krin). **1.** Relating to substances, either synthesized or arising by decomposition of organisms, that affect plant life. **2.** A compound with ectocrine properties. **3.** An ectohormone. Cf. endocrine, exocrine. [ecto- + G. *krinō*, to separate]

   ecological e., a chemical substance that undergoes biosynthesis in one species and that exerts an effect on the function of another species through mechanisms of the external environment; *e.g.,* the biosynthesis of vitamins by ruminants and their subsequent ingestion by other animals. SEE ALSO ectohormone.

ec·to·cyst (ek'tō-sist). The outer layer of a hydatid cyst. [ecto- + G. *kystis*, bladder]

ec·to·derm (ek'tō-derm). The outer layer of cells in the embryo, after establishment of the three primary germ layers (ectoderm, mesoderm, endoderm). SYN ectoblast (1). [ecto- + G. *derma*, skin]

   amniotic e., inner layer of the amnion continuous with body ectoderm.

   blastodermic e., external layer of the blastula.

   chorionic e., SYN trophoblast.

   epithelial e., that part of the e. separating from the neuroectoderm at about the fourth week of embryonic life; the epidermis and its specialized derivatives develop from it. SYN superficial e.

   extraembryonic e., derivative of epiblast outside the embryo's body.

   superficial e., SYN epithelial e.

ec·to·der·mal (ek-tō-der'măl). Relating to the ectoderm. SYN ectodermic.

ec·to·der·ma·to·sis (ek'tō-der-mă-tō'sis). SYN ectodermosis.

ec·to·der·mic (ek-tō-der'mik). SYN ectodermal.

ec·to·der·mo·sis (ek'tō-der-mō'sis). A disorder of any organ or tissue developed from the ectoderm. SYN ectodermatosis.

   e. ero'siva plu'riorifica'lis, SYN Stevens-Johnson *syndrome*.

ec·to·en·tad (ek-tō-en'tad). From without inward.

ec·to·en·tal (ek-tō-en'tăl). SYN ectental.

ec·to·en·zyme (ek-tō-en'zīm). An enzyme that is excreted externally and that acts outside the organism.

ec·to·eth·moid (ek-tō-eth'moyd). SYN ethmoidal *labyrinth*.

ec·tog·e·nous (ek-toj'e-nŭs). SYN exogenous. [ecto- + G. *-gen*, producing]

ec·to·glob·u·lar (ek-tō-glob'yū-lăr). Not within a globular body; specifically not within a red blood cell.

ec·to·hor·mone (ek'tō-hōr-mōn). A parahormonal chemical mediator of ecological significance which is secreted, largely by an organism (usually an invertebrate) into its immediate environment (air or water); it can alter the behavior or functional activity of a second organism, often of the same species as that secreting the e. SEE ALSO ecological *ectocrine*.

ec·to·mere (ek'tō-mēr). One of the blastomeres involved in formation of ectoderm. [ecto- + G. *meros*, part]

ec·to·me·rog·o·ny (ek'tō-mě-rog'ō-nē). The production of merozoites in the asexual reproduction of sporozoan parasites at the surface of schizonts and of blastophores, or by infolding into the schizont, as contrasted with endomerogony; e. has been observed in various species of *Eimeria*. [ecto- + G. *meros*, part, + *gonē*, generation]

ec·to·mes·en·chyme (ek-tō-mes'en-kīm). SYN mesectoderm (2). [ecto- + G. *mesos*, middle, + *enkyma*, infusion]

ec·to·morph (ek'tō-mōrf). A constitutional body type or build (biotype or somatotype) in which tissues originating from the ectoderm predominate; from a morphological standpoint, the limbs predominate over the trunk. SYN longitype. [ecto- + G. *morphē*, form]

ec·to·mor·phic (ek-tō-mōrf'ik). Relating to, or having the characteristics of, an ectomorph.

△**-ectomy.** Removal of an anatomical structure. SEE ALSO -tomy. [G. *ektomē*, a cutting out]

ec·top·a·gus (ek-top'ă-gŭs). Conjoined twins in which the bodies are joined laterally. SEE conjoined *twins*, under *twin*. [ecto- + G. *pagos*, something fixed]

ec·to·par·a·site (ek-tō-par'ă-sīt). A parasite that lives on the surface of the host body.

ec·to·par·a·sit·i·cide (ek-tō-par-ă-sit'i-sīd). An agent that is applied directly to the host to kill ectoparasites. [ectoparasite + L. *caedo*, to kill]

ec·to·par·a·sit·ism (ek-tō-par'ă-sī-tizm). SYN infestation.

ec·to·per·i·to·ni·tis (ek'tō-pār-i-tō-nī'tis). Inflammation beginning in the deeper layer of the peritoneum which is next to the viscera or the abdominal wall.

ec·to·phyte (ek'tō-fīt). A plant parasite of the skin. [ecto- + G. *phyton*, plant]

ec·to·pia (ek-tō'pē-ă). Congenital displacement or malposition of any organ or part of the body. SYN ectopy, heterotopia (1). [G. *ektopos*, out of place, fr. *ektos*, outside, + *topos*, place]

   e. cloa'cae, SYN *exstrophy* of the cloaca.

   e. cor'dis, congenital condition in which the heart is exposed on the chest wall because of maldevelopment of the sternum and pericardium.

   crossed renal e., ectopic kidney located on opposite (contralateral) side of midline from its ureteral insertion into bladder. In most instances, the two renal moieties are fused (crossed fused ectopia).

   crossed testicular e., testis that has crossed the midline to join its contralateral mate in the contralateral inguinal canal or hemiscrotum.

   e. len'tis, displacement of the lens of the eye. SYN dislocation of lens.

   e. mac'ulae, a condition in which one macula is displaced so that the two foveas are not at corresponding retinal points. SYN heterotopia maculae.

   e. pupil'lae congen'ita, displacement of the pupil present at birth.

   e. re'nis, displacement of the kidney.

   e. tes'tis, SYN testis e.

   testis e., testis that is malpositioned other than along the normal path of descent. SYN e. testis, parorchidium.

   e. vesi'cae, SYN *exstrophy* of the bladder.

ec·top·ic (ek-top'ik). **1.** Out of place; said of an organ not in its proper position, or of a pregnancy occurring elsewhere than in the cavity of the uterus. SYN aberrant (3), heterotopic (1), imperforate anus (2). **2.** In cardiography, denoting a heartbeat that has its origin in some abnormal focus; developing from a focus other than the sinoatrial node. [see ectopia]

ec·to·pla·cen·tal (ek'tō-pla-sen'tăl). **1.** Outside, beyond, or surrounding the placenta; in primates, referring especially to the parts of the trophoblast not directly involved in the formation of the placenta. **2.** In rodents, referring to the actively growing part of the trophoblast involved in the formation of the placenta.

ec·to·plasm (ek'tō-plazm). The peripheral, more viscous cytoplasm of a cell; it contains microfilaments but is lacking in other organelles. SYN exoplasm. [ecto- + G. *plasma*, something formed]

ec·to·plas·mat·ic, ek·to·plas·mic, ek·to·plas·tic (ek-tō-plas-mat'ik, -plas'mik, -plas'tik). Relating to the ectoplasm.

ec·to·py (ek'tō-pē). SYN ectopia.

ec·to·ret·i·na (ek'tō-ret'i-nă). SYN pigmented *layer* of retina.

ec·to·sarc (ek'tō-sark). The outer membrane, or ectoplasm, of a protozoon. [ecto- + G. *sarx*, flesh]

ec·tos·co·py (ek-tos'kŏ-pē). An obsolete method of diagnosis of disease of any of the internal organs by a study of movements of the abdominal wall or thorax caused by phonation. [ecto- + G. *skopeō*, to examine]

ec·tos·te·al (ek-tos'tē-ăl). Relating to the external surface of a bone. [ecto- + G. *osteon*, bone]

ec·tos·to·sis (ek-tos-tō'sis). Ossification in cartilage beneath the perichondrium, or formation of bone beneath the periosteum. [ecto- + G. *osteon*, bone, + *-osis*, condition]

ec·to·thrix (ek'tō-thriks). A sheath of spores (conidia) on the outside of a hair. [ecto- + G. *thrix*, hair]

ec·to·tox·in (ek-tō-tok'sin). SYN exotoxin.

ec·to·zo·on (ek-tō-zō'on). An animal parasite living on the surface of the body. [ecto- + G. *zōon*, animal]

ectro-. Congenital absence of a part. [G. *ektrōsis*, miscarriage]

ec·tro·chei·ry, ec·tro·chi·ry (ek-trō-kī'rē). Total or partial absence of a hand. [ectro- + G. *cheir*, hand]

ec·tro·dac·ty·ly, ec·tro·dac·tyl·ia, ec·tro·dac·tyl·ism (ek-trō-dak'ti-lē, -dak-til'i-ă, -dak'ti-lizm). Congenital absence of all or part of one or more fingers or toes. Known also as split-hand/foot deformity, lobster claw. There are several varieties and the pattern of inheritance, which though lasting through multiple generations, is usually somewhat irregular; may be autosomal dominant [MIM*183600-802], autosomal recessive [MIM*225290-300], or X-linked [MIM*313350]. [ectro- + G. *daktylos*, finger]

ec·tro·gen·ic (ek-trō-jen'ik). Relating to ectrogeny.

ec·trog·e·ny (ek-troj'ĕ-nē). Congenital absence or defect of any bodily part. [ectro- + G. *-gen*, producing]

ec·tro·me·lia (ek-trō-mē'lē-ă). **1.** Congenital hypoplasia or aplasia of one or more limbs. **2.** A disease of mice caused by the ectromelia virus; characterized by gangrenous loss of feet and necrotic areas in the internal organs; in laboratory mouse colonies, it usually results in high mortality rates. SYN mousepox. [ectro- + G. *melos*, limb]

ec·tro·mel·ic (ek-trō-mel'ik). Pertaining to, or characterized by, ectromelia.

ec·tro·pi·on, ec·tro·pi·um (ek-trō'pē-on, -pē-ŭm). A rolling outward of the margin of a part, *e.g.,* of an eyelid. [G. *ek*, out, + *tropē*, a turning]

atonic e., e. of the lower eyelid following paralysis of the orbicularis oculi muscle. SYN flaccid e., paralytic e.

cicatricial e., e. of the eyelids after burns, lacerations, or skin infection.

flaccid e., SYN atonic e.

paralytic e., SYN atonic e.

spastic e., e. of the lower eyelid as a result of ocular irritation.

e. u'veae, eversion of the pigmented posterior epithelium of the iris at the pupillary margin.

ec·trop·o·dy (ek-trop'ō-dē). Total or partial absence of a foot. [ectro- + G. *pous*, foot]

ec·tro·syn·dac·ty·ly (ek'trō-sin-dak'ti-lē). Congenital deformity marked by the absence of one or more digits and the fusion of others. [ectro- + G. *syn*, together, + *daktylos*, finger]

ec·trot·ic (ek-trot'ik). Obsolete term for abortive (1). [G. *ektrō-tikos*, relating to abortion, fr. *ektrōsis*, miscarriage]

ec·tyl·u·rea (ek'til-yū-rē'ă). 2-Ethyl-*cis*-crotonylurea; a mild obsolete sedative used in the treatment of nervous tension and anxiety.

ec·type (ek'tīp). Extreme somatotype, such as ectomorph (longitype) or endomorph (brachytype). [G. *ek*, out, + *typos*, stamp, model]

ec·u·re·sis (ek-yū-rē'sis). A condition in which urinary excretion and intake of water act to produce an absolute dehydration of the body. SEE ALSO emuresis. [G. *ek*, out, + *ourēsis*, urination]

ec·ze·ma (ek'zĕ-mă, eg'zĕ-mă, eg-zē'mă). Generic term for inflammatory conditions of the skin, particularly with vesiculation in the acute stage, typically erythematous, edematous, papular, and crusting; followed often by lichenification and scaling and occasionally by duskiness of the erythema and, infrequently, hyperpigmentation; often accompanied by sensations of itching and burning; the vesicles form by intraepidermal spongiosis.

Sometimes referred to colloquially as tetter, dry tetter, scaly tetter. [G. fr. *ekzeō*, to boil over]

allergic e., macular, papular, or vesicular eruption due to an allergic reaction.

atopic e., SYN atopic *dermatitis*.

baker's e., allergic e. due to contact with flour, yeast, or other ingredients handled by bakers.

chronic e., SYN lichenoid e.

e. craquelé, SYN winter e.

e. diabetico'rum, e. occurring in diabetes.

e. ep'ilans, e. with hair loss.

e. erythemato'sum, a dry form of e. marked by extensive areas of redness with scaly desquamation.

facial e., a photosensitivity disease of sheep in New Zealand associated with ingestion of plants during periods when autumn rains produce lush growth following seasons of dryness and close grazing; the predisposing cause is hepatic disease, which results from toxins of the fungus *Pithomyces chartarum*, which grows on the plants.

flexural e., e. of skin at the flexures of elbow, knees, wrists, etc., associated with atopy persisting through childhood.

hand e., e. that predominantly and persistently affects the hands; of multiple causation, including allergic, industrial, irritant, dyshidrotic, bacterial, and atopic mechanisms.

e. herpet'icum, a febrile condition caused by cutaneous dissemination of herpesvirus type 1, occurring most commonly in children, consisting of a widespread eruption of vesicles rapidly becoming umbilicated pustules; clinically indistinguishable from a generalized vaccinia. The two may be distinguished by electron microscopy or demonstration of inclusion bodies in smears, which are intranuclear in e. herpeticum and intracytoplasmic in e. vaccinatum. SYN pustulosis vacciniformis acuta.

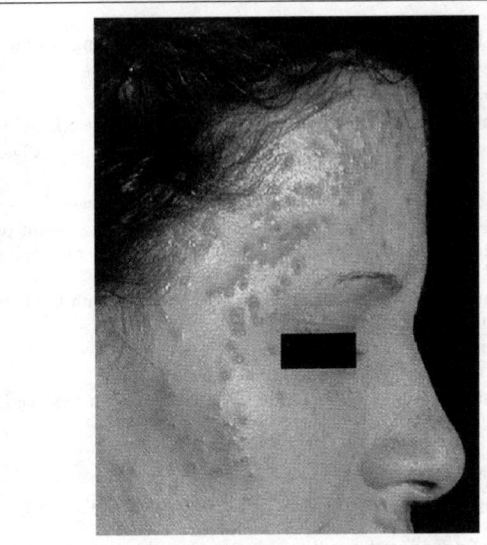

eczema herpeticum

e. hypertroph'icum, SYN lichenoid e.

infantile e., e. in infants; the clinical appearance varies according to the dominant causative mechanism, *e.g.,* contact-type hypersensitivity, candidiasis, atopy, seborrhea, or a combination including intertrigo and diaper dermatitis.

e. intertri'go, SEE intertrigo.

lichenoid e., thickening of skin with accentuated skin lines in e. SYN chronic e., e. hypertrophicum.

e. margina'tum, SYN *tinea* cruris.

nummular e., discrete, coin-shaped patches of e. SYN e. nummulare, nummular dermatitis.

e. nummula're, SYN nummular e.

e. papulo′sum, a dermatitis marked by an eruption of discrete or aggregated reddish excoriated papules.

e. parasit′icum, eczematous eruption precipitated by parasite infestation.

e. pustulo′sum, a later stage of vesicular e., in which the vesicles have become secondarily infected; the lesions become covered with purulent crusts. SYN impetigo eczematodes.

e. ru′brum, a stage of vesicular e., presenting red, excoriated, weeping areas.

seborrheic e., SYN seborrheic *dermatitis.*

e. squamo′sum, a form of dry, scaly e.

stasis e., eczematous eruption on legs due to or aggravated by vascular stasis.

tropical e., e. occurring in plaques on extensors of the extremities; of common occurrence and unknown etiology.

e. tylot′icum, hyperkeratotic hand and foot eczema.

e. vaccina′tum, SYN Kaposi's varicelliform *eruption.*

varicose e., e. occurring over areas in which the skin has been compromised by varicosities.

e. verruco′sum, e. with hyperkeratosis; chronic lichenified e.

e. vesiculo′sum, dermatitis marked by an eruption of vesicles upon erythematous patches that rupture and exude serum.

weeping e., a moist, eczematous dermatitis.

winter e., e. resulting from accelerated evaporation of moisture (including insensitive sweat) from the cutaneous surface; occurs as dry cracked plaques, usually on the extremities, but not infrequently also on the trunk in any season under circumstances (occupational, environmental) of excessively rapid drying out of the skin. SYN e. craquelé.

ec·zem·a·ti·za·tion (ek-zem′ă-ti-zā′shŭn). **1.** Formation of an eruption resembling eczema. **2.** Occurrence of eczema secondary to a preexisting dermatosis.

ec·ze·ma·toid (ek-zem′ă-toyd). Resembling eczema in appearance.

ec·ze·ma·tous (ek-zem′ă-tŭs). Marked by or resembling eczema.

ED Abbreviation for effective *dose*; ethyldichloroarsine.

ED₅₀ Abbreviation for median effective dose.

edath·a·mil (ĕ-dath′ă-mil). SYN ethylenediaminetetraacetic acid.

EDC Abbreviation for estimated date of confinement. SEE Nägele's *rule.*

edea (e-dē′ă). The external genitals. [G. *aidoia,* genitals]

ede·ma (e-dē′mă). An accumulation of an excessive amount of watery fluid in cells, tissues, or serous cavities. [G. *oidēma,* a swelling]

ambulant e., e. forming during periods of walking with the legs dependent.

angioneurotic e., SYN angioedema.

Berlin's e., retinal e. after blunt trauma to the globe.

blue e., the swelling and cyanosis of an extremity in hysterical paralysis.

brain e., SYN cerebral e.

brawny e., SYN nonpitting e.

brown e., e. of the lungs associated with chronic passive congestion.

bullous e., a reddened, swollen appearance of the ureteral orifice in the bladder wall, frequently observed with distal ureteral calculi or in tuberculosis of the ureter.

bullous e. vesi′cae, a prominent area of focal e. involving the bladder mucosa, consisting of elevated masses of edematous tissue or clusters of clear fluid-filled vesicles; often associated with chronic inflammation or irritation secondary to tubes, foreign bodies, or perivesical inflammation.

cachectic e., e. occurring in diseases characterized by wasting and hypoproteinemia; due to low plasma oncotic pressure. SYN marantic e.

cardiac e., e. resulting from congestive heart failure.

cerebral e., brain swelling due to increased volume of the extravascular compartment from the uptake of water in the neuropile and white matter. SEE ALSO brain *swelling.* SYN brain e.

cystoid macular e., e. of the posterior pole of the eye secondary

to abnormal permeability of capillaries of the central sensory retina.

dependent e., a clinically detectable increase in extracellular fluid volume localized in a dependent area, as of a limb, characterized by swelling or pitting.

gestational e., occurrence of a generalized and excessive accumulation of fluid in the tissues of greater than 1+ pitting after 12 hours' bed rest, or of a weight gain of 5 pounds or more in 1 week due to the influence of pregnancy.

e. glot′tidis, e. of the larynx.

heat e., e. caused by excessively high external temperature.

hereditary angioneurotic e. (HANE) [MIM*106100], a relatively rare hereditary form of angioneurotic e. characterized by onset, usually in adolescence, of erythema followed by asymptomatic e. associated with either a deficiency of C1 esterase inhibitor or a functionally inactive form of the inhibitor; there is uncontrolled activation of early complement components and production of a kinin-like factor which induces the angioedema; autosomal dominant inheritance. Death may occur due to upper respiratory tract e. and asphyxia. There are many families in which there is an autosomal dominant pattern of inheritance [MIM*106100]; males outnumber females by about 2 to 1.

hydremic e., obsolete term for e. occurring in states marked by pronounced hydremia.

infantile acute hemorrhagic e. of the skin, a generally benign form of cutaneous vasculitis, characterized by ecchymotic purpura, often in a cockade pattern, and inflammatory e. in infants.

inflammatory e., a swelling due to effusion of fluid in the soft parts surrounding a focus of inflammation.

lymphatic e., e. due to stasis in the lymph channels. SYN leukophlegmasia.

malignant e., an acute toxemia of cattle, horses, sheep, goats, and pigs caused by the bacterium *Clostridium septicum* and characterized by edematous swellings around the entry wound, anorexia, high fever, and death.

marantic e., SYN cachectic e.

menstrual e., retention of water and increase in weight, which occurs during or preceding menstruation.

e. neonato′rum, a diffuse, firm, and commonly fatal e. occurring in the newborn, usually beginning in the legs and spreading upward.

nephrotic e., e. resulting from renal dysfunction.

noninflammatory e., e. due to mechanical or other causes, not marked by inflammation or congestion.

nonpitting e., swelling of subcutaneous tissues which cannot be indented by compression easily. Usually due to metabolic abnormality, such as increased glycosaminoglycan content, like that which occurs in Graves' *disease* (pretibial myxedema) or in early phase of scleroderma. SYN brawny e.

nutritional e., a form of swelling caused by insufficient protein intake resulting in hypoproteinemia and low plasma oncotic pressure.

periodic e., SYN angioedema.

pitting e., e. that retains for a time the indentation produced by pressure.

premenstrual e., SEE menstrual e.

pulmonary e., e. of lungs usually resulting from mitral stenosis or left ventricular failure.

Quincke's e., SYN angioedema.

salt e., e. from excessive intake or retention of sodium chloride.

solid e., infiltration of the subcutaneous tissues by mucoid material, as in myxedema.

Yangtze e., SYN gnathostomiasis.

edem·a·ti·za·tion (e-dem′ă-ti-zā′shŭn). Making edematous.

edem·a·tous (e-dem′ă-tŭs). Marked by edema.

eden·tate (ē-den′tāt). SYN edentulous. [L. *edentatus*]

eden·tu·lous (ē-den′tyū-lŭs). Toothless, having lost the natural teeth. SYN edentate. [L. *edentulus,* toothless]

edes·tin (ĕ-des′tin). A hexameric globulin derived from the castor oil bean, hemp seed, and other seeds.

ed·e·tate (ed′ĕ-tāt). USAN-approved contraction for ethylenediaminetetraacetate, the anion of ethylenediaminetetraacetic acid; various e.'s are used as chelating agents to carry cations in (*e.g.,* ferric sodium e. as an iron ion carrier) or out (*e.g.,* sodium e. for calcium or heavy metal ion removal).

ed·e·tate cal·ci·um di·so·di·um. Contracted name for a salt of ethylenediaminetetraacetate, an agent used as a chelator of lead and some other heavy metals. Available in several forms: disodium, sodium, and trisodium.

edet·ic ac·id (ĕ-det'ik). SYN ethylenediaminetetraacetic acid.

edge (ej). A line at which a surface terminates. SEE ALSO border, margin, border.

  cutting e., (1) the beveled, knifelike, sharpened working angle of a dental hand instrument; **(2)** SYN incisal e.

  denture e., SYN denture *border.*

  incisal e., the part of an anterior tooth farthest from the apex of the root. SYN margo incisalis [NA], cutting e. (2), incisal margin, incisal surface, shearing e.

  leading e., the initial part of a wave form at maximum slope.

  shearing e., SYN incisal e.

Edinger, Ludwig, German anatomist, 1855–1918. SEE E.-Westphal *nucleus.*

edis·y·late (e-dis'i-lāt). USAN-approved contraction for 1,2-ethanedisulfonate, $^-O_3S(CH_2)_2SO_3^-$.

Edlefsen, Gustav J.F., German physician, 1842–1910. SEE E.'s *reagent.*

Edman, Pehr, Australian scientist, 1916–1977. SEE E. *method;* E.'s *reagent.*

EDRF Abbreviation for endothelium-derived relaxing *factor.*

Edridge-Green, Frederick W., English ophthalmologist, 1863–1953. SEE Edridge-Green *lamp.*

ed·ro·pho·ni·um chlo·ride (ed-rō-fō'nē-ŭm). Dimethylethyl (3-hydroxyphenyl)ammonium chloride; a competitive antagonist of skeletal muscle relaxants (curare derivatives and gallamine triethiodide) and an anticholinesterase, used as an antidote for curariform drugs, as a diagnostic agent in myasthenia gravis, and in myasthenic crisis.

EDTA Abbreviation for ethylenediaminetetraacetic acid.

educt (ē'dŭkt). An extract.

edul·co·rant (e-dŭl'kō-rant). Sweetening.

edul·co·rate (e-dŭl'kō-rāt). To sweeten or render less acrid. [L. *e-* intensive, + *dulcoro,* to sweeten, fr. *dulcor,* sweetness, fr. *dulcis,* sweet]

Edwards, James Hilton, English physician and medical geneticist, *1928. SEE E.'s *syndrome.*

Edwards, M.L., U.S. physician, *1906. SEE Carpentier-Edwards *valve;* Starr-Edwards *valve.*

Ed·ward·si·el·la (ed'ward-sē-el'lă). A genus of Gram-negative, facultatively anaerobic bacteria (family Enterobacteriaceae) containing motile, peritrichous, nonencapsulated rods. The type species is *E. tarda,* which is occasionally isolated from the stools of healthy humans and those with diarrhea, from the blood of humans and other animals, and from human urine. *E. tarda* is an etiologic agent of gastroenteritis in humans. The two other species in this genus are *E. hoshinae* and *E. ictaluri.*

EEE Abbreviation for eastern equine *encephalomyelitis.*

EEG Abbreviation for electroencephalogram; electroencephalography.

EENT Abbreviation for eye, ear, nose, and throat. See also ENT.

ef·fect (e-fekt'). The result or consequence of an action. [L. *ef-ficio,* pp. *effectus,* to accomplish, fr. *facio,* to do]

  abscopal e., a reaction produced following irradiation but occurring outside the zone of actual radiation absorption.

  additive e., an e. wherein two or more substances or actions used in combination produce a total e. the same as the arithmetic sum of the individual e.'s.

  after-e., SEE aftereffect.

  Anrep e., a small transient positive inotropic e. of abrupt increases of systolic aortic and left ventricular pressures related to recovery from transient subendocardial ischemia (*e.g.,* cold pressor test).

  Arias-Stella e., SYN Arias-Stella *phenomenon.*

  autokinetic e., in psychology, the apparent drifting about of a small, fixed, spot of light which is being observed in a dark room.

  Bernoulli e., the decrease in fluid pressure that occurs in converting potential to kinetic energy when motion of the fluid is accelerated, in accordance with Bernoulli's law; applied in water aspirators, atomizers, and humidifiers in which a gas is accelerated across the end of a narrow, fluid-filled orifice.

  Bohr e., the influence exerted by carbon dioxide on the oxygen dissociation curve of blood, *i.e.,* the curve is shifted to the right, which means a reduction in the affinity of hemoglobin for oxygen. Cf. Haldane e.

  Bowditch e., homeometric autoregulation of cardiac function induced by changing heart rate.

  Circe e., an e. observed in enzyme catalysis in which accelerated diffusion of the substrate occurs through attractive forces of the enzyme's active site.

  clasp-knife e., SYN clasp-knife *spasticity.*

  Compton e., in electromagnetic radiations of medium energy, a decrease in energy of the bombarding photon with the dislodgement of an orbital electron, usually from an outer shell. SYN Compton scattering.

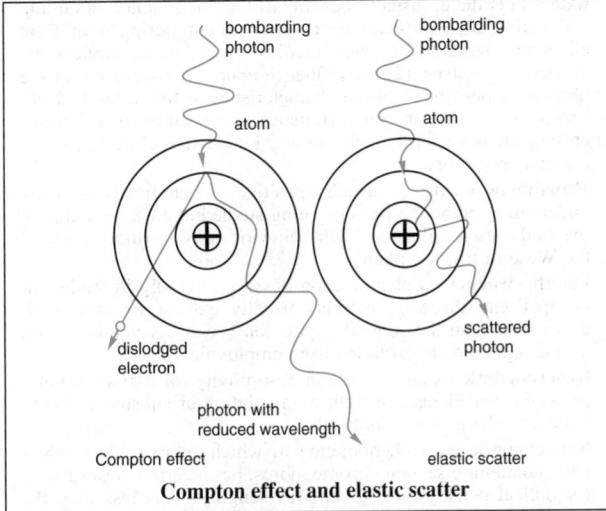

        Compton effect and elastic scatter

  Cotton e., the positive and negative displacement from zero of the rotation of plane polarized monochromatic light and the change of monochromatic circularly polarized light into elliptically polarized light in the immediate vicinity of the absorption band of the substance through which the light passes. SEE ALSO optical rotatory *dispersion,* circular *dichroism.*

  Crabtree e., inhibition of cellular respiration of isolated systems by high concentrations of glucose; a "reciprocal" of Pasteur's e.; due, in part, to the inhibition of hexokinase by elevated glucose 6-phosphate. Cf. Pasteur's e.

  cumulative e., the condition in which repeated administration of a drug may produce e.'s that are more pronounced than those produced by the first dose. SYN cumulative action.

  Cushing e., SYN Cushing *phenomenon.*

  cytopathic e., degenerative changes in cells (especially in tissue culture) associated with the multiplication of certain viruses; when, in tissue culture, spread of virus is restricted by an overlay of agar (or other suitable substance) the cytopathic e. may lead to formation of plaque.

  Doppler e., a change in frequency observed when the sound and observer are in relative motion away from or toward each other. SEE ALSO Doppler *shift.* SYN Doppler phenomenon.

  electrophonic e., the sensation of hearing produced when an alternating current of suitable frequency and magnitude is passed from an external source through a person.

  experimenter e.'s, the influence of the experimenter's behavior, personality traits, or expectancies on the results of that person's own research. SEE double blind *study.*

Fahraeus-Lindqvist e., the decrease in apparent viscosity that occurs when a suspension, such as blood, is made to flow through a tube of smaller diameter; observed in tubes less than about 0.3 mm in diameter. SYN sigma e.

Fenn e., the increased liberation of heat in a stimulated muscle when it is allowed to do mechanical work; the amount of heat liberated is increased in proportion to the distance the muscle is allowed to shorten and in proportion to the tension it must develop (*e.g.*, the weight it lifts) during shortening; thus increased chemical energy is consumed both to liberate increased heat and to do increased mechanical work.

founder e., an unusually high frequency of a gene in a particular population derived from a small set of unrepresentative ancestors.

gene dosage e., in codominant alleles, the more or less linear relationship between the phenotypic value and the number of genes of one type substituted by another type.

generation e., variation in health status arising from the different causal factors of disease to which each successive generation born is exposed as it passes through life.

Haldane e., the promotion of carbon dioxide dissociation by oxygenation of hemoglobin.

halo e., (1) the e. (usually beneficial) that the manner, attention, and caring of a provider have on a patient during a medical encounter, regardless of what medical procedure or services the encounter involves; **(2)** the influence upon an observation of the observer's perception of the characteristics of the individual observed (other than the characteristics under study) or the influence of the observer's recollection or knowledge of findings on a previous occasion.

Hawthorne e., the e. (usually positive or beneficial) of being under study, upon the persons being studied; their knowledge of the study often influences their behavior. [city in Illinois; site of the Western Electric plant]

healthy worker e., phenomenon observed initially in studies of occupational diseases; workers usually exhibit lower overall death rates than the general population because severely ill and disabled people are excluded from employment.

hyperchromic e., an increase in absorptivity (or extinction) at a particular wavelength of light by a solution or substance due to structural changes in a molecule.

hypochromic e., a phenomenon in which an individual molecule, containing several chromophores, has a certain absorptivity (or optical density) at a given wavelength that is less than the sum of the optical densities of the individual chromophores (at that same wavelength).

Mach e., the appearance of a light or dark line on a radiograph where there is a concave or convex interface in the subject, a physiological optical form of edge enhancement. SEE ALSO Mach's *band*.

e. modifier, a factor that modifies the e. of a putative causal factor under study; *e.g.,* age is an e. modifier for many conditions.

nuclear Overhauser e. (NOE), an e. seen in nuclear magnetic resonance in which there is a through-space nearest neighbor interaction.

Orbeli e., the fatigue of a muscle stimulated by its nerve (*i.e.*, indirectly) is reduced by concurrent stimulation of sympathetic fibers to the muscle; thought to be caused by norepinephrine diffusing from adrenergic fibers which innervate blood vessels in the muscle.

oxygen e., enhancement of radiosensitivity of cells in a high concentration of oxygen.

Pasteur's e., the inhibition of fermentation by oxygen, first observed by Pasteur; either not observed, or only slightly observed, in malignant tumors. Cf. Crabtree e.

photechic e., the ability of an agent, other than light, to make a developable latent image in a photographic film emulsion. SYN Russell e.

photoelectric e., the loss of electrons from the surface of a metal upon exposure to light; a mode of interaction of radiation with matter in which all of the energy of the incident photon is absorbed, with ejection of a photoelectron and characteristic ra-

diation from filling the vacancy from another shell; since the energy absorption per gram of tissue is proportional to the cube of the atomic number, this mode is important in diagnostic radiography.

piezoelectric e., the property of certain crystalline or ceramic materials to emit electricity when deformed and to deform when an electric current is passed across them, a mechanism of interconverting electrical and acoustic energy; an ultrasound transducer sends and receives acoustic energy using this e.

position e., a change in the phenotypic expression of one or more genes due to a change in its physical location with respect to other genes; may result from change in chromosome structure or from crossing-over.

Purkinje e., SYN Purkinje's *phenomenon*.

Raman e., a change in frequency undergone by monochromatic light scattered in passage through a transparent substance whose characteristics determine the amount of change, yielding a spectrum in which the incident wavelength band is flanked by small satellite bands of greater and lesser wavelengths.

Rivero-Carvallo e., inspiratory increase in the systolic murmur of tricuspid insufficiency; the characteristic distinguishing tricuspid insufficiency from mitral insufficiency.

Russell e., SYN photechic e.

second gas e., when a constant concentration of an anesthetic like halothane is inspired, the increase in alveolar concentration is accelerated by concomitant administration of nitrous oxide, because alveolar uptake of the latter creates a potential subatmospheric intrapulmonary pressure that leads to increased tracheal inflow.

sigma e., SYN Fahraeus-Lindqvist e.

Somogyi e., in diabetes, a rebound phenomenon of reactive hyperglycemia in response to a preceding period of relative hypoglycemia that has increased secretion of hyperglycemic agents (epinephrine, norepinephrine, glucagon, cortisol, and growth hormone); described in diabetic patients given too much insulin who developed unrecognized nocturnal hypoglycemia that made them hyperglycemic (suggesting insufficient insulin) when tested the next morning.

Staub-Traugott e., in normal persons, a drop in blood glucose which follows a second oral dose of glucose given 30 minutes or so after the first.

Stiles-Crawford e., light that enters through the center of the pupil produces a greater visual effect than light that enters obliquely.

synergistic e., SYN synergism.

Tyndall e., SYN Tyndall *phenomenon*.

Venturi e., term applied to the operation of a Venturi tube and similar systems.

Wedensky e., a relatively long enhancing e. following application of a maximal shock or stimulus to a neuromuscular preparation during which a subthreshold stimulation, otherwise too small to evoke a response, will produce a response; a relatively prolonged lowered threshold of excitability following a maximal shock.

Wolff-Chaikoff e., SYN Wolff-Chaikoff *block*.

Zeeman e., the splitting of spectral lines into three or more symmetrically placed lines when the light source is subjected to a magnetic field.

ef·fec·tive·ness. 1. A measure of the accuracy or success of a diagnostic or therapeutic technique when carried out in an average clinical environment; Cf. efficacy. **2.** The extent to which a treatment achieves its intended purpose.

relative biological effectiveness, A factor used to compare the biological effectiveness of absorbed radiation doses due to different types and energies of ionizing radiation. It is determined by the ratio of an absorbed dose of the particular radiation in question to the absorbed dose of a reference radiation required to produce an identical biological effect in a specific organism, organ, or tissue.

ef·fec·tor (ē-fek'tŏr, -tōr). **1.** C. Sherrington's term for a peripheral tissue that receives nerve impulses and reacts by contraction (muscle), secretion (gland), or a discharge of electricity (electric organ of certain bony fishes). **2.** A small metabolic molecule that by combining with a repressor gene depresses the activity of an operon. **3.** A small molecule that binds to a protein and, in so doing, alters the activity of that protein. **4.** A substance, technique, procedure, or individual that causes an effect. [L. *producer*]

ef·fem·i·na·tion (e-fem-i-nā′shŭn). Acquisition of feminine characteristics, either physiologically as part of female maturation, or pathologically by individuals of either sex. [L. *ef-femino*, pp. *-atus*, to make feminine, fr. *ex*, out, + *femina*, woman]

ef·fer·ent (ef′er-ent). Conducting (fluid or a nerve impulse) outward from a given organ or part thereof; *e.g.*, the efferent connections of a group of nerve cells, efferent blood vessels, or the excretory duct of an organ. [L. *efferens*, fr. *effero*, to bring out]

   gamma e., the thin axon of a gamma motor neuron innervating the intrafusal muscle fibers of a muscle spindle.

ef·fer·vesce (ef-er-ves′). To boil up or form bubbles rising to the surface of a fluid in large numbers, as in the evolution of CO_2 from aqueous solution when the pressure is reduced. [L. *ef-fervesco*, to boil up, from *ferveo*, to boil]

ef·fer·ves·cent (ef-er-ves′ent). **1.** Boiling; bubbling; effervescing. **2.** Causing to effervesce, as an e. powder. **3.** Tending to effervesce when freed from pressure, as an e. solution.

ef·fi·ca·cy. The extent to which a specific intervention, procedure, regimen, or service produces a beneficial result under ideal conditions. [L. *efficacia*, fr, *ef-ficio*, to perform, accomplish]

ef·fi·cien·cy (ĕ-fish′en-sē). **1.** The production of the desired effects or results with minimum waste of time, effort, or skill. **2.** A measure of effectiveness; specifically, the useful work output divided by the energy input.

   quantum e., SYN quantum *yield*.

   visual e., a rating used in computing compensation for industrial ocular injuries, incorporating measurements of central acuity, visual field, and ocular motility.

ef·fleu·rage (e-fler-ahz′). A stroking movement in massage. [Fr. *effleurer*, to touch lightly]

ef·flo·resce (e-flōr-es′). To become powdery by losing the water of crystallization on exposure to a dry atmosphere. [L. *ef-floresco* (*exf-*), to blossom, fr. *flos* (*flor-*), flower]

ef·flo·res·cent (e-flōr-es′ent). Denoting a crystalline body that gradually changes to a powder by losing its water of crystallization on exposure to a dry atmosphere.

ef·flu·vi·um, pl. **ef·flu·via** (e-flū′vē-ŭm, -ē-ă). **1.** Shedding of hair. SEE ALSO defluxion (1), *defluvium* capillorum. **2.** Obsolete term for an exhalation, especially one of bad odor or injurious influence. [L. a flowing out, fr. *ef-fluo*, to flow out]

   anagen e. (ă′nā-jen ef-flū′vē- ŭm), sudden diffuse hair shedding with cancer chemotherapy or radiation, usually reversible when treatment ends.

   telogen e., increased transient shedding of normal club hairs by premature development of telogen in anagen follicles, resulting from various kinds of stress, *e.g.*, childbirth, shock, drug intake or cessation of an oral contraceptive, fever, and dieting with marked weight loss.

ef·fort (ef′ert). Deliberate exertion of physical or mental power.

   distributed e., in psychology, learning that involves small units of work and interpolated rest periods, as contrasted with massed learning, in which the individual works continually until the skill is mastered.

ef·fuse (e-fūs′). Thin and widely spread; denoting the surface character of a bacterial culture. [L. *ef-fundo*, pp. *-fusus;* to pour out]

ef·fu·sion (e-fū′zhŭn). **1.** The escape of fluid from the blood vessels or lymphatics into the tissues or a cavity. **2.** The fluid effused. [L. *effusio*, a pouring out]

   joint e., increased fluid in synovial cavity of a joint.

   pericardial e., increased amounts of fluid within the pericardial sac, usually due to inflammation. SYN dropsy of pericardium.

   pleural e., increased amounts of fluid within the pleural cavity, usually due to inflammation.

   subpulmonic e., a collection of fluid in the pleural space princi-

pally hidden between the diaphragm and the caudal surface of the lung.

eflor·ni·thine hy·dro·chlo·ride (ē-flōr′ni-thēn). 2-(Difluoromethyl)-DL-ornithine monohydrochloride, monohydrate; an antineoplastic and antiprotozoal orphan drug used in the treatment of *Pneumocystis carinii* pneumonia in AIDS and of *Trypanosoma brucei gambiense* sleeping sickness.

EGD Abbreviation for esophagogastroduodenoscopy.

eger·sis (ē-ger′sis). Extremely alert wakefulness. [G. a waking]

eges·ta (ē-jes′tă). Unabsorbed food residues that are discharged from the digestive tract. [L. *e-gero*, pp. *-gestus*, to carry out, discharge]

EGF Abbreviation for epidermal growth *factor*.

egg (eg). The female sexual cell or gamete; after fertilization and fusion of the pronuclei it is a zygote and no longer an egg, although some authors refer to a 2-celled or 4-celled "egg." In reptiles and birds, the egg is provided with a protective shell, membranes, albumin, and yolk for the nourishment of the embryo. SEE ALSO oocyte, ovum. [A.S. *aeg*]

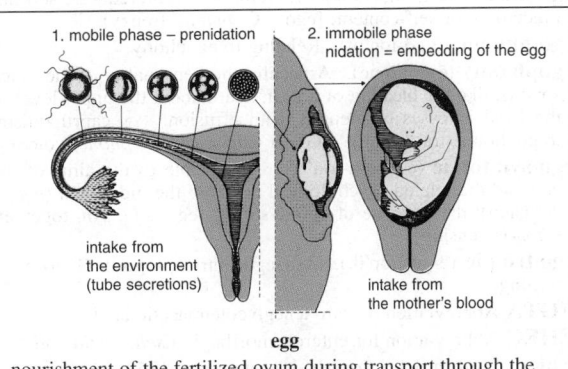

egg

nourishment of the fertilized ovum during transport through the fallopian tube, and after implantation in the endometrium

   centrolecithal e., an e. in which the yolk is concentrated near the center of the e. cell, as is the case in many of the insects.

   homolecithal e., an e. in which the total amount of yolk is small and fairly uniformly distributed throughout the cytoplasm. SYN isolecithal e.

   isolecithal e., SYN homolecithal e.

   microlecithal e., an e. containing a small amount of deutoplasm.

   telolecithal e., an e. containing a relatively large quantity of deutoplasm concentrated at the abapical pole; *e.g.*, e.'s of reptiles and birds.

egg clus·ter. One of the clumps of cells resulting from the breaking up of the gonadal cords in the ovarian cortex; these clumps later develop into primary ovarian follicles.

Egger, Fritz, Swiss internist, 1863–1938. SEE E.'s *line*.

Eggleston, Cary, U.S. physician, 1884–1966. SEE E. *method*.

egg·shell. The calcareous envelope of a bird's egg. SYN testa (1).

eglan·du·lous (ē-glan′dū-lŭs). Without glands. [L. *e*, without, + gland or glandula]

Eglis' glands. See under gland.

e·go (ē′gō). In psychoanalysis, one of the three components of the psychic apparatus in the freudian structural framework, the other two being the id and superego. Although the e. has some conscious components, many of its functions are learned and automatic. It occupies a position between the primal instincts (pleasure principle) and the demands of the outer world (reality principle), and therefore mediates between the person and external reality by performing the important functions of perceiving the needs of the self, both physical and psychological, and the qualities and attitudes of the environment. It evaluates, coordinates, and integrates these perceptions so that internal demands can be adjusted to external requirements, and is also responsible for certain defensive functions to protect the person against the demands of the id and superego. [L. I]

ego·al·ien (ē′gō-ā′lē-en). syn ego-dystonic.

ego·bron·choph·o·ny (ē′gō-brong-kof′ō-nē). Egophony with bronchophony. [G. *aix* (*aig*-), goat, + *bronchos,* bronchus, + *phōnē,* voice]

ego·cen·tric (ē-gō-sen′trik). Marked by extreme concentration of attention upon oneself, *i.e.,* self-centered. Cf. allocentric. syn egotropic. [ego + G. *kentron,* center]

ego·cen·tric·i·ty (ē′gō-sen-tris′i-tē). The condition of being egocentric.

ego·dys·ton·ic (ē′gō-dis-ton′ik). Repugnant to or at variance with the aims of the ego and related psychological needs of the individual (*e.g.,* an obsessive thought or compulsive behavior); the opposite of ego-syntonic. syn ego-alien. [ego + G. *dys,* bad, + *tonos,* tension]

ego-ideal. In psychoanalysis, a more or less conscious ideal of personal excellence toward which an individual strives, and that is derived from a composite image of the personal characteristics of a parent, public figure, or one or more other individuals the person admires.

ego·ma·nia (ē-gō-mā′nē-ă). Extreme self-centeredness, self-appreciation, or self-content. [ego + G. *mania,* frenzy]

ego·phon·ic (ē-gō-fon′ik). Relating to egophony.

egoph·o·ny (ē-gof′ō-nē). A peculiar broken quality of the voice sounds, like the bleating of a goat, heard about the upper level of the fluid in cases of pleurisy with effusion. syn capriloquism, tragophonia, tragophony. [G. *aix* (*aig*-), goat, + *phōnē,* voice]

ego-syn·ton·ic (ē′gō-sin-ton′ik). Acceptable to the aims of the ego and the related psychological needs of the individual (*e.g.,* a delusion); the opposite of ego-dystonic. [ego + G. *syn,* together, + *tonos,* tension]

ego·tro·pic (ē-gō-trop′ik). syn egocentric. [ego + G. *tropē,* a turning]

EGTA Abbreviation for ethyleneglycotetraacetic acid.

EHEC Abbreviation for enterohemorrhagic *Escherichia coli.*

Ehlers, Edward L., Danish dermatologist, 1863–1937. see E.-Danlos *syndrome.*

Ehrenritter, Johann, Austrian anatomist, †1790. see E.'s *ganglion.*

Ehret, Heinrich, German physician, *1870. see E.'s *phenomenon.*

Ehrlich, Paul, German bacteriologist, immunologist, and Nobel laureate, 1854–1915. see *Ehrlichia;* E.'s *anemia,* inner *body, phenomenon, postulate,* diazo *reagent, theory,* side-chain *theory;* E.-Türk *line.* See entries under stain; reaction.

Ehr·lich·ia (er-lik′ē-ă). A genus of small, often pleomorphic, coccoid to ellipsoidal, nonmotile, Gram-negative bacteria (order Rickettsiales) that occur either singly or in compact inclusions in circulating mammalian leukocytes; species are the etiologic agents of ehrlichiosis and are transmitted by ticks. The type species is *E. canis.* [P. *Ehrlich*]

E. ca′nis, the species causing the tick borne disease canine ehrlichiosis in dogs (transmitted by the tick *Rhipicephalus sanguineus*); it is the type species of the genus *E.* Occasionally causes tick borne infection in humans.

E. chaffee′nsis, a recently described species associated with human ehrlichiosis and carried by the tick vector, *Amblyomma americanum,* the Lone Star tick.

E. on′diri, the species causing bovine petechial fever.

E. pla′tys, the species causing canine infectious cyclic thrombocytopenia in dogs.

E. ristic′ii, the species causing equine monocytic ehrlichiosis.

E. sennet′su, the species causing Sennetsu fever in humans. syn *Rickettsia sennetsu.*

Ehr·lic·hi·eae. Members of the Rickettsiaceae family; obligate intracellular parasites of peripheral blood leukocytes.

ehr·lich·i·o·sis (er-lik-ē-ō′sis). Infection with parasitic leukocytic rickettsiae of the genus *Ehrlichia;* in man, especially by *E. sennetsu* which produces manifestations similar to those of Rocky Mountain spotted fever.

canine e., a fatal disease of dogs in Asia, Africa, and the U.S. caused by *Ehrlichia canis,* transmitted by the tick *Rhipicephalus*

sanguineus, and characterized by hemorrhage, pancytopenia, and emaciation. syn tropical canine pancytopenia.

equine monocytic e., a febrile disease of horses in North America caused by *Ehrlichia risticii* and characterized by anorexia, leukopenia, and occasional diarrhea. syn Potomac horse fever.

human e., a form of e. that presents clinically as a undifferentiated acute febrile illness characterized by fever, chills, diarrhea, and headache, following tick bite(s), probably by the Lone Star Tick, *Amblyomma americanum.* Caused by *Ehrlichia chaffeensis.* First described in 1987. (Thought to be predominantly a monocytic form of ehrlichiosis.)

human granulocytic e., a form of e. in a patient with a history of tick bite. Characterized by leukopenia, thrombocytopenia, and mild liver damage. (Thought to be predominantly a granulocytic form of e.) The species of *Ehrlichia* that is the agent of this disease is unknown at present.

Eichhorst, Hermann L., Swiss physician, 1849–1921. see E.'s *corpuscles,* under *corpuscle, neuritis.*

Eicken, Karl von, German laryngologist, 1873–1960. see E.'s *method.*

n-**ei·co·sa·no·ic ac·id** (ī′kō-să-nō′ik). syn arachidic acid.

ei·co·sa·noids (ī′kō-să-noydz). The physiologically active substances derived from arachidonic acid, *i.e.,* the prostaglandins, leukotrienes, and thromboxanes; synthesized via a cascade pathway. [G. *eicosa-,* twenty, + *eidos,* form]

9-ei·co·se·no·ic ac·id (ī′kō-sĕ-nō′ik). syn gadoleic acid.

ei·det·ic (ī-det′ik). **1.** Relating to the power of visualization of and memory for objects previously seen which reaches its height in children aged 8 to 10. **2.** A person possessing this power to a high degree. [G. *eidon,* saw (aorist of verb)]

EIEC Abbreviation for enteroinvasive *Escherichia coli.*

Ei·ken·el·la cor·ro·dens (ī-kĕ-nel′ă kōr-rō′denz). A species of nonmotile, rod-shaped, Gram-negative, facultatively anaerobic bacteria that is part of the normal flora of the adult human oral cavity but may be an opportunistic pathogen, especially in immunocompromised hosts. [M. *Eiken,* 1958]

ei·ko·nom·e·ter (ī-kō-nom′ĕ-ter). **1.** An instrument for determining the magnifying power of a microscope, or the size of a microscopic object. **2.** An instrument for determining the degree of aniseikonia. [G. *eikon,* image, + *metron,* measure]

ei·loid (ī′loyd). Resembling a coil or roll. [G. *eilō,* to roll up, + *eidos,* appearance]

Eimer, Gustav Heinrich Theodor, German zoologist, 1843–1898. see *Eimeria.*

Ei·me·ria (ī-mē′rē-ă). The largest, most economically important, and most widespread genus of the coccidial protozoa (family Eimeriidae, class Sporozoea). The mature oocyst contains four sporocysts, each of which contains two sporozoites. *E.* may be highly pathogenic, especially in young hosts. Many species are known that infect wild vertebrates; domesticated mammals and birds commonly are infected with one or more species. Domestic animals and fowl suffer from *E.* infections (coccidiosis) most acutely under conditions of overcrowding with fecal contamination. [G.H.T. *Eimer*]

E. of cattle, *E. zuernii,* the species most often associated with clinical cases of coccidiosis in calves and young adults; found in the cecum and lower bowel, and sometimes in the small intestine. *E. bovis,* a species that occurs principally in the small intestine causes clinically recognizable disease; many less common species have been described. syn coccidia of cattle.

E. of chickens, *E. tenella,* a species producing cecal coccidiosis of young chicks; *E. necatrix,* producing severe disease in the small intestine and ceca; *E. acervulina, E. hagani,* and *E. praecox,* which localize in the duodenum; *E. mitis* localizes in the small intestine, *E. brunetti* in the lower small intestine and rectum, and *E. maxima* in the lower small intestine. syn coccidia of chickens.

E. of geese, *E. truncata,* a species occurring in the kidney tubules where it causes much damage and considerable mortality in young birds; *E. anseris, E. nocens,* and *E. parvula,* occurring in the small intestine where *E. anseris* can produce hemorrhagic enteritis. syn coccidia of geese.

E. of pheasants, *E. phasiani* and *E. dispersa,* species which infect the small intestine; coccidiosis of pheasants in captivity under overcrowded conditions may be very destructive. SYN coccidia of pheasants.

E. of rabbits, *E. stiedae,* the most common species in rabbits, affecting the bile ducts; *E. perforans,* affecting the small intestine and cecum; *E. media, magna,* and *E. irresidua* which infect the small intestine. SYN coccidia of rabbits.

E. sardi′nae, species that occurs in sardines and herring, and has been found in the feces of humans who have eaten these fish; it was once erroneously believed to be a coccidium of humans.

E. of sheep and goats, *E. ovina (arloingi),* the most common and destructive species in sheep, principal losses being in young lambs; *E. minakolyakimovae,* a highly pathogenic parasite of sheep; *E. parva* and *E. pallida* are frequently found but believed to be of low virulence; *E. faurei, E. intricata, E. granulosa, E. ahsata, E. hawkins, E. gilruthi, E. gonzalezi, E. christenseni, E. punctata, E. crandallis,* and *E. honessi,* are found in sheep or goats, and are probably of low pathogenicity. All of these species invade the epithelium of the small intestine. SYN coccidia of sheep and goats.

E. of swine, *E. debliecki,* the most common and most pathogenic species, involving the small intestine, cecum, and colon; *E. scabra,* involving the small intestine; *E. perminuta, E. spinosa, E. scrofae, E. suis, E. cerdonis, E. porci,* and *E. neodebliecki* believed to have little pathogenicity. SEE *Isospora.* SYN coccidia of swine.

E. of turkeys, *E. meleagridis,* a species which localizes in the cecum, *E. dispersa* and *E. innocua* in the small intestine, *E. adenoeides* in the lower ileum, cecum, and rectum, and *E. gallopavonis* in the ileum and rectum. SYN coccidia of turkeys.

Ei·me·ri·i·dae (ī-mēr-ī′i-dē). A family of sporozoan coccidia; important genera are *Eimeria* and *Isospora,* infections by *Eimeria* being by far the most common and most serious in domesticated animals. [see *Eimeria*]

Einarson's gal·lo·cy·a·nin-chrome al·um stain. See under stain.

ein·stein (īn′stīn). A unit of energy equal to 1 mol quantum, hence to 6.0221367×10^{23} quanta. The value of e., in kJ, is dependent upon the wavelength. [A. *Einstein,* German-born theoretical physicist and Nobel laureate in U.S., 1879–1955]

ein·stein·i·um (Es) (īn-stīn′ē-ŭm). An artificially prepared transuranium element, atomic no. 99, atomic wt. 252.0; it has many isotopes, all of which are radioactive (^{252}Es has the longest known half-life, 1.29 years).

Einthoven, Willem, Dutch physiologist and Nobel laureate, 1860–1927. SEE E.'s *equation, law,* string *galvanometer, triangle.*

Eisenlohr, Carl, German physician, 1847–1896. SEE E.'s *syndrome.*

Eisenmenger, Victor, German physician, 1864–1932. SEE E.'s *complex, defect, disease, syndrome, tetralogy.*

ei·sod·ic (ī-sod′ik). Rarely used term for afferent. [G. *eis,* into, + *hodos,* a way]

ejac·u·late (ē-jak′yū-lāt). 1. To expel suddenly, as of semen. 2. Semen expelled in ejaculation. [see ejaculation]

ejac·u·la·tio (ē-jak-yū-lā′shē-ō). SYN ejaculation.
  e. defic′iens, absence of ejaculation.
  e. prae′cox, SYN premature *ejaculation.*
  e. retarda′ta, unusually delayed ejaculation.

ejac·u·la·tion (ē-jak-yū-lā′shŭn). Emission of seminal fluid. SYN ejaculatio. [L. *e-iaculo,* pp. *-atus,* to shoot out]
  premature e., during sexual intercourse, too rapid achievement of climax and e. in the male relative to his own or his partner's wishes. SYN ejaculatio praecox.

ejac·u·la·to·ry (ē-jak′yū-lă-tōr-ē). Relating to an ejaculation.

ejec·ta (ē-jek′tă). SYN ejection (2). [L. ntr. pl. of *ejectus,* pp. of *ejicio,* to throw out]

ejec·tion (ē-jek′shŭn). 1. The act of driving or throwing out by physical force from within. 2. That which is ejected. SYN ejecta. [L. *ejectio,* from *ejicio,* to cast out]

ejec·tor (ē-jek′tŏr, -tōr). A device used for forcibly expelling (ejecting) a substance.

saliva e., a hollow, perforated suction tube used in the evacuation of saliva or liquid debris from the oral cavity. SYN dental pump, saliva pump.

EJP Abbreviation for excitatory junction *potential.*

Ejrup, Erick, 20th century Swedish internist. SEE E. *maneuver.*

△**eka-.** Prefix used to denote an undiscovered or just discovered element in the periodic system before a proper and official name is assigned by authorities; *e.g.,* eka-osmium, now plutonium. [Sanskrit *eka,* one]

Ekbom, K. A., Swedish neurologist, *1907. SEE E. *syndrome.*

EKG Abbreviation for electrocardiogram.

eki·ri (ē-kī′rī). An acute, toxic form of dysentery of infants seen in Japan and due to *Shigella sonnei.* [Jap.]

EKY Abbreviation for electrokymogram.

elab·o·ra·tion (ē-lab′ōr-ā′shŭn). The process of working out in detail by labor and study. [L. *e-laborō,* pp. *-atus,* to labor, endeavor, fr. *labor,* toil, to work out]
  secondary e., the mental process occurring partly during dreaming and partly during the recalling or telling of a dream by means of which the latent (relatively disorganized and psychologically painful) content of the dream is brought into increasingly more coherent and logical order, resulting in the manifest content of the dream; an aspect of dream work.

Elae·oph·o·ra schnei·deri (ē-lē-of′ŏ-ră schnī′der-ī). The bloodworm of sheep; a species of nematodes causing filarial dermatosis. [Mod. L. *elaea,* fr. G. *elaia,* olive, + *agnos,* sheep, + *phoros,* to bear]

el·a·id·ic ac·id (el-ā-id′ik). $CH_3(CH_2)_7CH=CH(CH_2)_7COOH$; *trans*-9-octadecenoic acid; an unsaturated monobasic *trans*-isomer of oleic acid; found in ruminant fats. Cf. oleic acid.

elai·o·path·ia (el′ā-ō-path′ē-ă). SYN eleopathy. [G. *elaion,* oil, + *pathos,* suffering]

E-LAM Abbreviation for endothelial-leukocyte adhesion *molecule.*

el·a·pid (el′ă-pid). Any member of the snake family Elapidae.

Elap·i·dae (ē-lap′i-dē). A family of highly venomous snakes characterized by a pair of comparatively short, permanently erect deeply grooved fangs at the front of the mouth. There are over 150 species, including the cobra, krait, mamba, and coral snakes. [G. *elops,* a serpent]

elas·mo·branch (ē-las′mō-brank). Cartilaginous fish of the class Chondrichthyes that have platelike gills, with each gill slit opening independently on the body surface. [G. *elasmos,* a metal plate, + *branchia,* gills]

elas·tance (ē-las′tans). A measure of the tendency of a structure to return to its original form after removal of a deforming force. In medicine and physiology, usually a measure of the tendency of a hollow viscus (*e.g.,* lung, urinary bladder, gallbladder) to recoil toward its original dimensions upon removal of a distending or compressing force, the recoil pressure resulting from a unit distention or compression of the viscus; the reciprocal of compliance. The relationship between elasticity and e. is of the same nature as that between the specific inductive capacity of an insulator material and the capacitance of a particular condenser made from that material.

elas·tase (ĕ-las′tās). A serine proteinase hydrolyzing elastin; other e.-like enzymes have been identified (*e.g.,* pancreatic e. [pancreatopeptidase E] and leukocyte e. [lysosomal or neutrophil e.]) with different sequences and kinetic parameters; all have fairly broad specificities.

elas·tic (ĕ-las′tik). 1. Having the property of returning to the original shape after being compressed, bent, or otherwise distorted. 2. A rubber or plastic band used in orthodontics as either a primary or adjunctive source of force to move teeth. The term is generally modified by an adjective to describe the direction of the force or the location of the terminal connecting points. [G. *elastreō,* epic form of *elaunō,* drive, push]
  intermaxillary e., material used to provide e. traction between the upper and lower teeth.
  vertical e., e. material used in a direction perpendicular to the occlusal plane, connecting one arch wire to the other, and usually used to improve intercuspation.

el

elas·ti·ca (ĕ-las′ti-kă). **1.** The elastic layer in the wall of an artery. **2.** SYN elastic *tissue.*

elas·ti·cin (ĕ-las′ti-sin). SYN elastin.

elas·tic·i·ty (ĕ-las-tis′i-tē). The quality or condition of being elastic.

physical e. of muscle, the quality of muscle that enables it to yield to passive physical stretch.

physiologic e. of muscle, the biologic quality, unique for muscle, of being able to change and resume size under neuromuscular control.

total e. of muscle, the combined effect of physical and physiologic e. of muscle.

elas·tin (ĕ-las′tin). A yellow elastic fibrous mucoprotein that is the major connective tissue protein of elastic structures (*e.g.,* large blood vessels); tendons, ligaments, etc.); e.'s precursor is tropoelastin. SYN elasticin.

elas·to·fi·bro·ma (ĕ-las′tō-fī-brō′mă). A nonencapsulated slow-growing mass of poorly cellular, collagenous, fibrous tissue and elastic tissue; occurs usually in subscapular adipose tissue of old persons. [G. *elastos,* beaten, + L. *fibra, -oma* tumor]

elas·toi·din (ĕ-las′toy-din). A complex collagen.

elas·tol·y·sis. Dissolution of elastic fibers. [elasto- + G. *lysis,* loosening, fr. *luō,* to loosen]

generalized e., SYN *cutis* laxa.

elas·to·ma (ĕ-las-tō′mă). A tumor-like deposit of elastic tissue.

juvenile e., a connective tissue nevus characterized by an increase in the number and size of the elastic fibers. SEE ALSO osteodermatopoikilosis.

Miescher's e., circinate groups of hyperkeratotic papules that become dislodged, leaving a small bloody depression; associated with pseudoxanthoma elasticum.

elas·tom·e·ter (ĕ-las-tom′ĕ-ter). A device for measuring the elasticity of any body or of the animal tissues.

elas·to·mu·cin (ĕ-las-tō-myū′kin). The mucoprotein of connective tissue; *e.g.,* elastin.

elas·tor·rhex·is (ĕ-las-tō-rek′sis). Fragmentation of elastic tissue in which the normal wavy strands appear shredded and clumped, and take a basophilic stain. [G. *rhēxis,* rupture]

elas·to·sis (ĕ-las-tō′sis). **1.** Degenerative change in elastic tissue. **2.** Degeneration of collagen fibers, with altered staining properties resembling elastic tissue, or formation by fibroblast-activated ultraviolet or mast cell mediators of abnormal fibers. SYN elastoid degeneration (1), elastotic degeneration.

e. colloida′lis conglomera′ta, SYN colloid milium.

e. dystroph′ica, SYN *angioid* streaks.

e. per′forans serpigino′sa, circinate groups of asymptomatic keratotic papules; the epidermis is thickened around a central plug of dermal elastic tissue which is extruded through the epidermis.

solar e., e. seen histologically in the sun-exposed skin of the elderly or in those who have chronic actinic damage.

ela·tion (ē-lā′shŭn). The feeling or expression of excitement or gaiety; if prolonged and inappropriate, a characteristic of mania. [L. *elatio,* fr. *ef-fero,* pp. *e-latus,* to lift up]

Elaut, Leon J.S., 20th century Belgian pathologist. SEE E.'s *triangle.*

el·bow (el′bō). **1.** The joint between the arm and the forearm. SYN cubitus (1) [NA], ancon. **2.** An angular body resembling a flexed e. [A.S. *elnboga*]

capped e., SYN shoe *boil.*

Little Leaguer's e., an epicondylitis of the medial epicondyle at the origin of the flexor muscles of the forearm; related to throwing and usually seen in children or adolescents.

miner's e., inflammation with fluid distention of the olecranon bursa.

nursemaid's e., longitudinal subluxation of the radial head from the annular ligament. SYN Malgaigne's luxation.

tennis e., chronic inflammation at the origin of the extensor muscles of the forearm from the lateral epicondyle of the humerus, as a result of unusual strain (not necessarily from playing tennis). SYN epicondylalgia externa, lateral humeral epicondylitis.

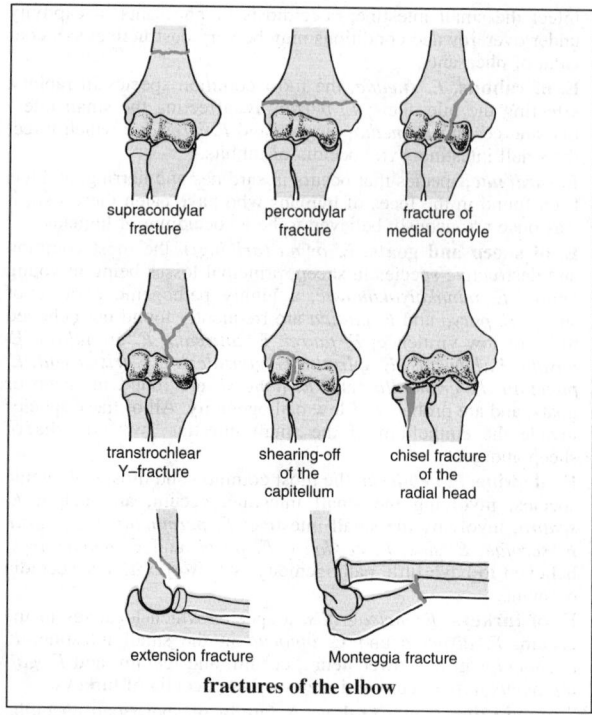

supracondylar fracture   percondylar fracture   fracture of medial condyle

transtrochlear Y–fracture   shearing-off of the capitellum   chisel fracture of the radial head

extension fracture   Monteggia fracture

fractures of the elbow

el·bowed (el′bōd). Angular; kneed.

el·der, el.′der flow·ers. SYN sambucus.

electro-. Electric, electricity. [G. *ēlektron,* amber (on which static electricity can be generated by friction)]

elec·tro·an·al·ge·sia (ē-lek′trō-an-ăl-jē′zē-ă). Analgesia induced by the passage of an electric current.

elec·tro·a·nal·y·sis (ē-lek′trō-ă-nal′i-sis). Quantitative analysis of metals by electrolysis.

elec·tro·an·es·the·sia (ē-lek′trō-an-es-thē′zē-ă). Anesthesia produced by an electric current.

elec·tro·ax·on·og·ra·phy (ē-lek′trō-ak-son-og′ră-fē). SYN axonography.

elec·tro·ba·so·graph (ē-lek-trō-bā′sō-graf). An apparatus for recording gait. [electro- + G. *basis,* walking, + *graphō,* to write]

elec·tro·ba·sog·ra·phy (ē-lek-trō-bā-sog′ră-fē). The graphic process by which an electrobasograph is made; used for gait analysis.

elec·tro·bi·os·co·py (ē-lek′trō-bī-os′kŏ-pē). Rare term for use of electricity as a means of determining whether life is present or not. [electro- + G. *bios,* life, + *skopeō,* to examine]

elec·tro·car·di·o·gram (ECG, EKG) (ē-lek-trō-kar′dē-ō-gram). Graphic record of the heart's integrated action currents obtained with the electrocardiograph. [electro- + G. *kardia,* heart, + *gramma,* a drawing]

scalar e. (skāl′ar), electrocardiographic lead output that can be displayed on one plane of the body in contradistinction to vector electrocardiogram in which the display is on two or more planes.

unipolar e., an e. taken with the exploring electrode placed on the chest overlying the heart or upon a single limb, the indifferent ("zero") potential electrode being the central terminal.

elec·tro·car·di·o·graph (ē-lek-trō-kar′dē-ō-graf). An instrument for recording the potential of the electrical currents that traverse the heart and initiate its contraction.

elec·tro·car·di·og·ra·phy (ē-lek-trō-kar-dē-og′ră-fē). **1.** A method of recording electrical currents traversing the heart muscle just prior to each heart beat. **2.** The study and interpretation of electrocardiograms.

fetal e., recording the electrocardiogram of the fetus *in utero.*

precordial e., recording of electrocardiographic signals from the anterior left chest; conventionally six electrode positions are used but any number may be applied.

elec·tro·car·di·o·pho·no·gram (ē-lek′trō-kar-dē-ō-fōn′ō-gram). The record obtained by electrocardiophonography.

elec·tro·car·di·o·pho·nog·ra·phy (ē-lek′trō-kar-dē-ō-fō-nog′ră-fē). Method of electrically recording the heart sounds. [electro- + G. *kardia*, heart, + *phōnē*, sound, + *graphō*, to write]

elec·tro·cau·ter·i·za·tion (ē-lek′trō-caw′ter-i-zā′shŭn). Cauterization by passage of high frequency current through tissue or by metal that has been electrically heated.

elec·tro·cau·tery (ē-lek′trō-caw′ter-ē). **1.** An instrument for directing a high frequency current through a local area of tissue. **2.** A metal cauterizing instrument heated by an electric current. SYN electric cautery.

elec·tro·ce·re·bral in·ac·tiv·i·ty. SYN electrocerebral silence.

elec·tro·ce·re·bral si·lence (ECS) (ē-lek′trō-ser-ē′brăl sī′lens). Flat or isoelectric encephalogram; an electroencephalogram with absence of cerebral activity over 2 μv from symmetrically placed electrode pairs 10 or more centimeters apart, and with interelectrode resistance between 100 and 10,000 ohms; if such a record is present for 30 minutes in a clinically brain dead adult and if drug intoxication, hypothermia, and recent hypotension have been excluded, the diagnosis of cerebral death is supported. SYN electrocerebral inactivity, flat electroencephalogram, isoelectric electroencephalogram.

elec·tro·chem·i·cal (ē-lek′trō-kem′i-kăl). Denoting chemical reactions involving electricity, and the mechanisms involved.

elec·tro·cho·le·cys·tec·to·my (ē-lek′trō-kō-lē-sis-tek′tō-mē). Rarely used term for removal of the gallbladder by electrosurgery.

elec·tro·cho·le·cys·to·cau·sis (ē-lek′trō-kō-lē-sis′tō-kaw-sis). Rarely used term for cauterization of gallbladder mucosa by electrosurgery.

elec·tro·co·ag·u·la·tion (ē-lek′trō-kō-ag-yū-lā′shŭn). Coagulation produced by an electrocautery.

elec·tro·co·chle·o·gram (ē-lek′trō-kok′lē-ō-gram). The record obtained by electrocochleography.

elec·tro·co·chle·og·ra·phy (ē-lek′trō-kok-lē-og′ră-fē). A measurement of the electrical potentials generated in the inner ear as a result of sound stimulation. [electro- + L. *cochlea*, snail shell, + G. *graphō*, to write]

elec·tro·con·trac·til·i·ty (ē-lek′trō-kon-trak-til′i-tē). The power of contraction of muscular tissue in response to an electrical stimulus.

elec·tro·con·vul·sive (ē-lek′trō-kon-vŭl′siv). Denoting a convulsive response to an electrical stimulus. SEE electroshock *therapy*.

elec·tro·cor·ti·co·gram (ē-lek-trō-kōr′ti-kō-gram). A record of electrical activity derived directly from the cerebral cortex.

elec·tro·cor·ti·cog·ra·phy (ECoG) (ē-lek′trō-kōr-ti-kog′ră-fē). The technique of recording the electrical activity of the cerebral cortex by means of electrodes placed directly on it.

elec·tro·cute (ē-lek′trō-kyūt). To cause death by the passage of an electric current through the body. [electro- + execute]

elec·tro·cu·tion (ē-lek-trō-kyū′shŭn). Death caused by electricity. SEE electrocute. SYN electrothanasia.

elec·tro·cys·tog·ra·phy (ē-lek′trō-sis-tog′ră-fē). Recording of electric currents or changes in electric potential from the urinary bladder.

elec·trode (ē-lek′trōd). **1.** One of the two extremities of an electric circuit; one of the two poles of an electric battery or of the end of the conductors connected thereto. **2.** An electrical terminal specialized for a particular electrochemical reaction. [electro- + G. *hodos,* way]

active e., a small e. whose exciting effect is used to stimulate or record potentials from a localized area. SYN exciting e., localizing e., therapeutic e.

calomel e., an e. in which the wire is connected through a pool of mercury to a paste of mercurous chloride (Hg_2Cl_2, calomel) in a potassium chloride solution covered by more potassium chloride solution; commonly used as a reference e.

carbon dioxide e., a glass e. in a film of bicarbonate solution

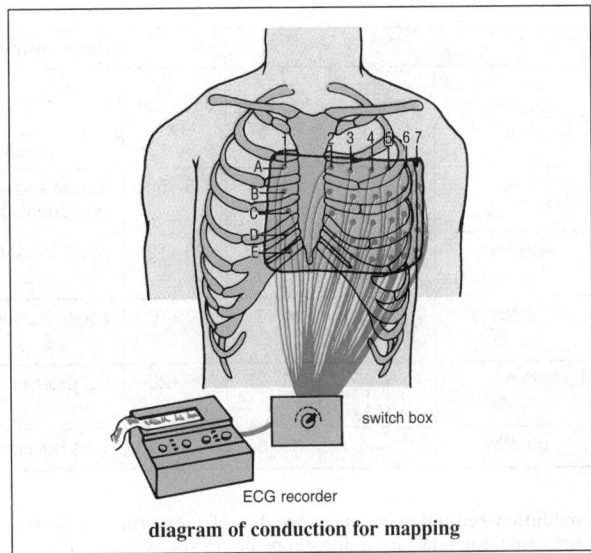

diagram of conduction for mapping

covered by a thin plastic membrane permeable to carbon dioxide but impermeable to water and electrolytes; the carbon dioxide pressure of a gas or liquid sample quickly equilibrates through the membrane and is measured in terms of the resulting pH of the bicarbonate solution, as sensed by the glass e.; commonly used to analyze arterial blood samples. SYN Severinghaus e.

central terminal e., in electrocardiography, an e. in which connections from the three limbs (right arm, left arm, and left leg) are joined and led to the electrocardiograph to form the indifferent e., theoretically at zero potential for the system.

Clark e., an oxygen e. consisting of the tip of a platinum wire exposed to a thin film of electrolyte covered by a plastic membrane permeable to oxygen but not to water or the electrolyte. When a certain voltage is applied, oxygen is destroyed at the platinum surface; the flow of current is then proportional to the rate at which oxygen can diffuse to the platinum surface from the gas or liquid sample outside the membrane, and is thus a measure of the oxygen pressure in the sample; commonly used to measure oxygen pressure in arterial blood samples.

dispersing e., SYN indifferent e.

exciting e., SYN active e.

exploring e., an e. placed on or near an excitable tissue; in unipolar electrocardiography, the e. is placed on the chest in the region of the heart and paired with an indifferent electrode.

glass e., a thin-walled glass bulb containing a standard buffer solution, quinhydrone, and a platinum wire; when immersed in an unknown solution, a potential difference develops that varies with the pH of the unknown solution; this difference can be made to give the pH; used in pH meters.

hydrogen e., the ultimate standard of reference in all pH determinations, limited and technically difficult to use, consisting of a piece of spongy platinum black partly immersed in a solution in a small glass tube; the tube above the solution is filled with hydrogen gas that is bubbled through the solution and absorbed by the platinum; the electrode thus measures the potential between H_2 and H^+, the "standard" potential of which (1 atmosphere, 1 molar) is taken as zero; hence, the hydrogen e. potential measures $[H^+]$ or pH.

indifferent e., in unipolar electrocardiography, a remote e. placed either upon a single limb or connected with the central terminal and paired with an exploring e.; the indifferent e. is supposed to contribute little or nothing to the resulting record. SYN dispersing e., silent e.

ion-selective e.'s, glass, liquid ion-exchange, or solid state e.'s used to measure electrolyte and calcium ion activity in biological fluids.

localizing e., SYN active e.

negative e., SYN cathode.

electroencephalogram						
type of wave	shape	frequency per sec.	amplitude in µV	physiological variations of potential		
				in waking EEG		in sleeping EEG
				adult	child	all ages
beta		14–30	5–50	frontal and precentral prominent, in clusters	seldom prominent	beta-activity ("spindles") sign of light sleep
alpha		8–13	20–120	predominant activity	predominant activity, age 5 and above	not a sign of sleep
theta		4–7	20–100	constant, not prominent	predominant activity, from 18 mos. to 5 yrs.	normal sign of sleep
delta		0.5–3	5–250	not prominent	predominant activity until 18 mos.	concomitant sign of deep sleep
gamma	—	31–60	–10	laws governing predominance and localization not fully known		

oxidation-reduction e., an e. capable of measuring oxidation-reduction potential. SEE quinhydrone e. SYN redox e.

oxygen e., an e., usually consisting of a platinum wire or dropping mercury, used to measure the oxygen concentration in a solution by polarography.

positive e., SYN anode.

quinhydrone e., one of several oxidation-reduction e.'s in which the ratio of the two forms (quinone-quinhydrone), determined by the hydrogen ion concentration, sets up a potential that can be measured and converted to a pH value (fails above pH 8).

redox e., SYN oxidation-reduction e.

reference e., an e. expected to have a constant potential, such as a calomel e., and used with another e. to complete an electrical circuit through a solution; *e.g.,* when a reference e. is used with a glass e. for pH measurement, changes in voltage between the two e.'s can be attributed to the effects of pH on the glass e. alone.

Severinghaus e., SYN carbon dioxide e.

silent e., SYN indifferent e.

therapeutic e., SYN active e.

elec·tro·der·mal (ē-lek′trō-der′măl). Pertaining to electric properties of the skin, usually referring to altered resistance. [electro- + G. *derma,* skin]

e·lec·tro·der·ma·tome (ē-lek′trō-der′mă-tōm). Any dermatome powered by electricity.

elec·tro·des·ic·ca·tion (ē-lek′trō-des-i-kā′shŭn). Destruction of lesions or sealing off of blood vessels (usually of the skin, but also of available surfaces of mucous membrane) by monopolar high frequency electric current. [electro- + L. *desicco,* to dry up]

elec·tro·di·ag·no·sis (ē-lek′trō-dī-ag-nō′sis). 1. The use of electronic devices for diagnostic purposes. 2. By convention, the studies performed in the EMG laboratory, *i.e.,* nerve conduction studies and needle electrode examination (EMG proper). SYN electroneurography. 3. Determination of the nature of a disease through observation of changes in electrical activity.

elec·tro·di·al·y·sis (ē-lek′trō-dī-al′i-sis). In an electric field, the removal of ions from larger molecules and particles. Cf. electro-osmosis.

elec·tro·en·ceph·a·lo·gram (EEG) (ē-lek′trō-en-sef′ă-lō-gram). The record obtained by means of the electroencephalograph.

flat e., SYN electrocerebral silence.

isoelectric e., SYN electrocerebral silence.

elec·tro·en·ceph·a·lo·graph (ē-lek′trō-en-sef′ă-lō-graf). A system for recording the electric potentials of the brain derived from electrodes attached to the scalp. [electro- + G. *encephalon,* brain, + *graphō,* to write]

elec·tro·en·ceph·a·log·ra·phy (EEG) (ēlek′trō-en-sef′ă-log′ră-fē). Registration of the electrical potentials recorded by an electroencephalograph.

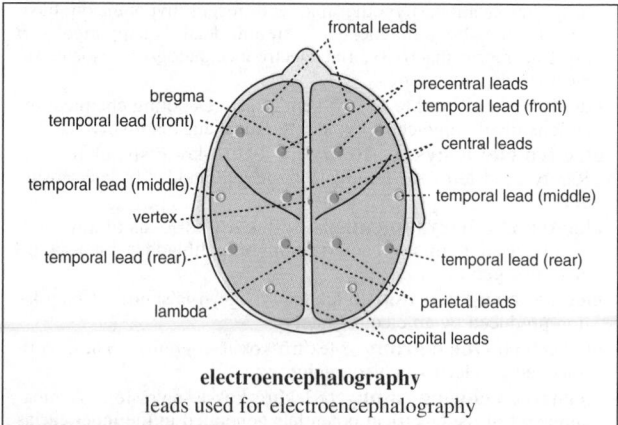

electroencephalography
leads used for electroencephalography

elec·tro·en·dos·mo·sis (ē-lek′trō-en-dos-mō′sis). Endosmosis produced by means of an electric field.

elec·tro·focus·ing (ē-lek′trō-fō-kus-ing). The process of separating macromolecules or small molecules via electrophoresis in a pH gradient.

elec·tro·gas·tro·gram (ē-lek′trō-gas′trō-gram). The record obtained with the electrogastrograph.

elec·tro·gas·tro·graph (ē-lek′trō-gas′trō-graf). An instrument used in electrogastrography. [electro- + G. *gastēr,* stomach, + *graphō,* to write]

elec·tro·gas·trog·ra·phy (ē-lek′trō-gas-trog′ră-fē). The recording of the electrical phenomena associated with gastric secretion and motility.

elec·tro·gram (ē-lek′trō-gram). 1. Any record on paper or film made by an electrical event. 2. In electrophysiology, a recording taken directly from the surface by unipolar or bipolar leads.

His bundle e. (HBE), an e. recorded from the His bundle, either in the experimental animal or in man during cardiac catheterization.

elec·tro·he·mo·sta·sis (ē-lek′trō-hē-mos′tă-sis, -hē-mō-stā′sis). Arrest of hemorrhage by means of an electrocautery. [electro- + G. *haima,* blood, + *stasis,* halt]

elec·tro·hys·ter·o·graph (ē-lek′trō-his′ter-ō-graf). Instrument that records uterine electrical activity. [electro- + G. *hystera,* womb, + *graphō,* to write]

elec·tro·im·mu·no·dif·fu·sion (ē-lek′trō-im′yū-nō-di-fyū′zhŭn). An immunochemical method that combines electrophoretic separation with immunodiffusion by incorporating antibody into the support medium.

elec·tro·ky·mo·gram (EKY) (ē-lek-trō-kī′mō-gram). An obsolete technique for making a graphic record of the heart's movements produced by the electrokymograph.

elec·tro·ky·mo·graph (ē-lek-trō-kī′mō-graf). An obsolete apparatus for recording, from changes in the x-ray silhouette, the movements of the heart and great vessels; consists of a fluoroscope, x-ray tube, and a photomultiplier tube together with an electrocardiograph.

elec·trol·y·sis (ē-lek-trol′i-sis). **1.** Decomposition of a salt or other chemical compound by means of an electric current. **2.** Destruction of certain hair follicles by means of galvanic electricity. [electro- + G. *lysis,* dissolution]

elec·tro·lyte (ē-lek′trō-līt). Any compound that, in solution, conducts electricity and is decomposed (electrolyzed) by it; an ionizable substance in solution. [electro- + G. *lytos,* soluble]

amphoteric e., an e. that can either give up or take on a hydrogen ion and can thus behave as either an acid or a base. SYN ampholyte.

elec·tro·lyt·ic (ē-lek-trō-lit′ik). Referring to or caused by electrolysis.

elec·tro·lyze (ē-lek′trō-līz). To decompose chemically by means of an electric current.

elec·tro·lyz·er (ē-lek′trō-līz-er). An obsolete apparatus for the treatment of strictures, fibromas, etc., by electrolysis.

elec·tro·mag·net (ē-lek-trō-mag′net). A bar of soft iron rendered magnetic by an electric current encircling it.

elec·tro·mas·sage (ē-lek′trō-mas-sazh′). Massage combined with the application of electricity.

elec·tro·mic·tu·ra·tion (ē-lek′trō-mik-tū-rā′shŭn). Electrical stimulation of the conus medullaris to empty the urinary bladder of paraplegics. [electro- + L. *micturio,* to desire to make water]

e·lec·tro·morph (ē-lek′trō-mōrf). A mutant form of a protein, phenotypically distinguished by its electrophoretic mobility. [electro- + G. *morphē,* form, shape]

elec·tro·my·o·gram (EMG) (ē-lek-trō-mī′ō-gram). A graphic representation of the electric currents associated with muscular action.

elec·tro·my·o·graph (ē-lek-trō-mī′ō-graf). An instrument for recording electrical currents generated in an active muscle.

elec·tro·my·og·ra·phy (ē-lek′trō-mī-og′ră-fē). **1.** The recording of electrical activity generated in muscle for diagnostic purposes; both surface and needle recording electrodes can be used, although characteristically the latter is employed, so that the procedure is also called needle electrode examination. **2.** Umbrella term for the entire electrodiagnostic study performed in the EMG laboratory, including not only the needle electrode examination, but also the nerve conduction studies. [electro- + G. *mys,* muscle, + *graphō,* to write]

elec·tron (ē-lek′tron). One of the negatively charged subatomic particles that are distributed about the positive nucleus and with it constitute the atom; in mass they are estimated to be 1/1836.15 of a proton; when emitted from inside the nucleus of a radioactive substance, e.'s are called beta particles. [electro- + -on]

Auger e., an e. ejected from a lower energy orbital after a photoelectric interaction of an x-ray photon with a K-shell e. by the characteristic radiation photon; the Auger e. recoils with energy equal to the characteristic radiation less the difference in shell binding energies. SEE photoelectric *effect.*

conversion e., an internal conversion e.

emission e., a beta particle resulting from radioactive decay.

internal conversion e., an e., similar to an Auger e., released from one of the e. orbits of the atom upon activation by a gamma-ray from that atom's nucleus; the e. has kinetic energy equal to the net energy transition of the disintegration.

positive e., SYN positron.

transition e., an e. that moves from one energy level to another to fill a vacancy in a shell, with the emission of characteristic radiation.

valence e., one of the e.'s that take part in chemical reactions of an atom.

elec·tro·nar·co·sis (ē-lek′trō-nar-kō′sis). Production of insensibility to pain by the use of electrical current.

elec·tro·neg·a·tive (ē-lek′trō-neg′ă-tiv). Relating to or charged

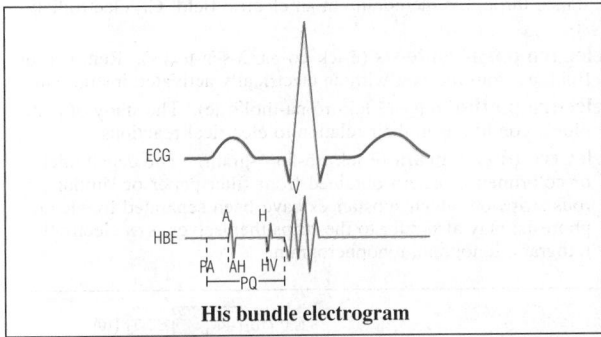

His bundle electrogram

with negative electricity; referring to an element whose uncharged atoms have a tendency to ionize by adding electrons, thus becoming anions (*e.g.,* oxygen, fluorine, chlorine).

elec·tro·neu·rog·ra·phy (ē-lek′trō-nū-rog′ră-fē). SYN electrodiagnosis (2).

elec·tro·neu·rol·y·sis (ē-lek′trō-nū-rol′i-sis). Destruction of nerve tissue by electricity.

elec·tro·neu·ro·my·og·ra·phy (ē-lek′trō-nūr′ō-mī-og′ră-fē). A method of measuring changes in a peripheral nerve by combining electromyography of a muscle with electrical stimulation of the nerve trunk carrying fibers to and from the muscle.

elec·tron·ic (ē-lek-tron′ik). **1.** Pertaining to electrons. **2.** Denoting devices or systems utilizing the flow of electrons in a vacuum, gas, or semiconductor.

elec·tron-volt (eV, ev). The energy imparted to an electron by a potential of 1 volt; equal to 1.60218×10^{-12} erg in the CGS system, or 1.60218×10^{-19} joule in the SI system.

elec·tro·nys·tag·mog·ra·phy (ENG) (ē-lek′trō-nis′tag-mog′ră-fē). A method of nystagmography based on electro-oculography; skin electrodes are placed at outer canthi to register horizontal nystagmus or above and below each eye for vertical nystagmus. [electro- + nystagmus + G. *graphō,* to write]

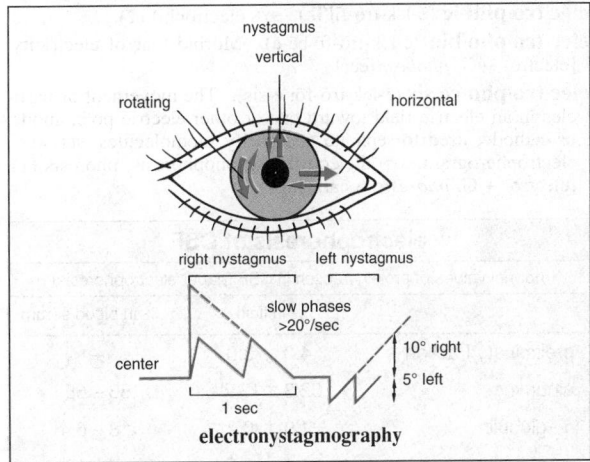

electronystagmography

elec·tro·oc·u·lo·gram (ē-lek′trō-ok′yū-lō-gram). A record of electric currents in electro-oculography.

elec·tro·oc·u·log·ra·phy (EOG) (ē-lek′trō-ok′yū-log′ră-fē). Oculography in which electrodes placed on the skin adjacent to the eyes measure changes in standing potential between the front and back of the eyeball as the eyes move; a sensitive electrical test for detection of retinal pigment epithelium dysfunction.

elec·tro·ol·fac·to·gram (EOG) (ē-lek′trō-ol-fak′tō-gram). An electronegative wave of potential occurring on the surface of the olfactory epithelium in response to stimulation by an odor. SYN osmogram, Ottoson potential.

elec·tro·os·mo·sis (ē-lek′trō-os-mō′sis). The diffusion of a sub-

el

stance through a membrane in an electric field. Cf. electrodialysis.

elec·tro·para·cen·te·sis (ē-lek′tro-par′ă-sen-tē′sis). Removal of fluid, as from the eye, with an electrically activated instrument.

elec·tro·pa·thol·o·gy (ē-lek-trō-pa-thol′ō-jē). The study of pathologic conditions in their relation to electrical reactions.

elec·tro·pher·o·gram (ē-lek-trō-fer′ō-gram). The densitometric or colorimetric pattern obtained from filter paper or similar porous strips on which substances have been separated by electrophoresis; may also refer to the strips themselves. SYN electrophoretogram, ionogram, ionopherogram.

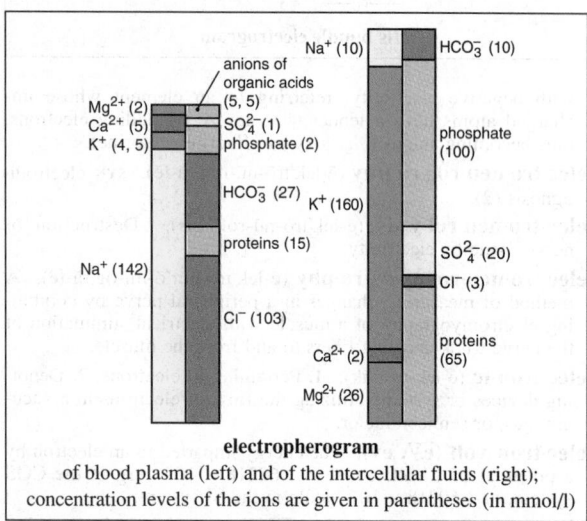

electropherogram

of blood plasma (left) and of the intercellular fluids (right); concentration levels of the ions are given in parentheses (in mmol/l)

·**elec·tro·phil, elec·tro·phile** (ē-lek′trō-fil, -fīl). **1.** The electron-attracting atom or agent in an organic reaction. Cf. nucleophil. **2.** Relating to an electrophil. SYN electrophilic. [electro- + G. *philos,* fond]

elec·tro·phil·ic (ē-lek-trō-fil′ik). SYN electrophil (2).

elec·tro·pho·bia (ē-lek-trō-fō′bē-ă). Morbid fear of electricity. [electro- + G. *phobos,* fear]

elec·tro·pho·re·sis (ē-lek-trō-fōr′ē-sis). The movement of particles in an electric field toward one or other electric pole, anode, or cathode; used to separate and purify biomolecules. SEE ALSO electropherogram. SYN dielectrolysis, ionophoresis, phoresis (1). [electro- + G. *phorēsis,* a carrying]

electrophoresis of CSF

normal values of protein fraction in CSF (paper electrophoresis)		
	% in fluid	% in blood serum
preliminary fraction	4.3 ± 3.0	–
albumins	62.3 ±13.2	53 – 65
$α_1$-globulin	4.9 ± 0.2	2.8 – 6.4
$α_2$-globulin	5.4 ± 2.5	7 – 10
β-globulin	8.6 ± 2.4	9 – 13
τ-globulin	5.9 ± 2.9	–
γ-globulin	9.5 ± 3.7	1 – 18

capillary zone e. (CZE), a method for separating molecules extremely rapidly based on their electrophoretic mobility.

carrier e., e. done on a carrier (such as paper, polyacrylamide gel, etc.).

disc e., a modification of gel e. in which a discontinuity (pH, gel pore size) is introduced near the origin to produce a lamina (disc)

of the materials being separated; the separating bands retain their disc-like shape as they move through the gel.

free e., e. of substances placed in a solution in a U-shaped tube.

gel e., e. through a gel, usually a cylindrical tube or on a slab gel.

isoenzyme e., electrophoretic separation of serum enzymes; separation of lactate dehydrogenase and creatine phosphokinase is commonly used for diagnosis of acute myocardial infarction.

lipoprotein e., electrophoretic separation of plasma lipoproteins.

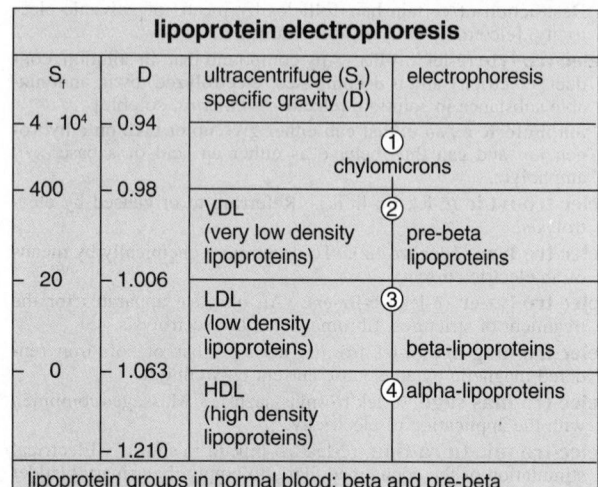

lipoprotein electrophoresis

S_f	D	ultracentrifuge (S_f) specific gravity (D)	electrophoresis
– 4 - 10^4	– 0.94		
		① chylomicrons	
– 400	– 0.98		
		VDL (very low density lipoproteins)	② pre-beta lipoproteins
– 20	– 1.006		
		LDL (low density lipoproteins)	③ beta-lipoproteins
– 0	– 1.063		
		HDL (high density lipoproteins)	④ alpha-lipoproteins
	– 1.210		

lipoprotein groups in normal blood; beta and pre-beta lipoproteins are reversed in electrophoretic separation (S_f = Svedberg unit = flotation unit)

polyacrylamide gel e. (PAGE), a gel formed by cross-linking of acrylamide that is used for the separation of proteins or nucleic acids. These substances are separated on the basis of both size and charge.

pulsed-field gel e., SYN pulse-field gel e.

pulse-field gel e., gel e. in which, after electrophoretic migration has begun, the current is briefly stopped and reapplied in a different orientation; allows for the purification of long DNA molecules. SYN pulsed-field gel e.

thin-layer e. (TLE), electrophoretic migrations (separations) through a thin layer of inert material, such as cellulose, supported on a glass or plastic plate.

elec·tro·pho·ret·ic (ē-lek′trō-phōr-et′ik). Relating to electrophoresis, as an e. separation. SYN ionophoretic.

elec·tro·pho·ret·o·gram (ē-lek′trō-fōr-et′ō-gram). SYN electropherogram.

elec·tro·pho·to·ther·a·py (ē-lek′trō-fō′tō-ther′ă-pē). Phototherapy in which the source of the rays is the electric light.

elec·tro·phren·ic (ē-lek′trō-fren′ik). Denoting electrical stimulation of the phrenic nerve usually at its motor point in the neck. SEE ALSO electrophrenic *respiration.*

elec·tro·phys·i·ol·o·gy (ē-lek′trō-fiz-ē-ol′ō-jē). The branch of science concerned with electrical phenomena that are associated with physiologic processes. Electrical phenomena are prominent in neurons and effectors.

elec·tro·pneu·mo·graph (ē-lek-trō-nū′mō-graf). An obsolete electric apparatus used for recording breathing. SEE pneumograph.

elec·tro·por·a·tion (ē-lek′trō-pōr-ā-shŭn). A technique in which a brief electric shock is applied to cells; momentary holes open briefly in the plasma membrane, allowing the entry of macromolecules (*e.g.,* a way of introducing new DNA into a cell).

elec·tro·pos·i·tive (ē-lek-trō-pos′i-tiv). Relating to or charged with positive electricity; referring to an element whose atoms tend to lose electrons; *e.g.,* sodium, potassium, calcium.

elec·tro·punc·ture (ē-lek-trō-pŭnk′chŭr). Passage of an electrical current through needle electrodes piercing the tissues.

elec·tro·ra·di·ol·o·gy (ē-lek′trō-rā-dē-ol′ō-jē). Archaic term for the use of electricity and x-ray in treatment.

elec·tro·ra·di·om·e·ter (ē-lek′trō-rā-dē-om′ĕ-ter). A modified electroscope designed for the differentiation of radiant energy. [electro- + L. *radius,* ray, + G. *metron,* measure]

elec·tro·ret·i·no·gram (ERG) (ē-lek′trō-ret′i-nō-gram). A record of the retinal action currents produced in the retina by an adequate light stimulus. [electro- + retina + G. *gramma,* something written]

elec·tro·ret·i·nog·ra·phy (ē-lek′trō-ret′i-nog′ră-fē). The recording and study of the retinal action currents.

elec·tro·scis·sion (ē-lek′trō-si-shŭn). Division of tissues by means of an electrocautery knife. [electro- + L. *scissio,* a splitting, fr. *scindo,* to split]

elec·tro·scope (ē-lek′trō-skōp). An instrument for the detection of electrical charges or ionization of gas by β or x-rays; consists of two strips of gold leaf suspended from an insulated conductor and enclosed in an airtight container viewed with a low-power microscope. [electro- + G. *skopeō,* to examine]

elec·tro·shock (ē-lek′trō-shok). SEE electroshock *therapy.*

elec·tro·sol (ē-lek′trō-sol). SYN colloidal *metal.*

elec·tro·spec·trog·ra·phy (ē-lek′trō-spek-trog′ră-fē). The recording, study, and interpretation of electroencephalographic wave patterns.

elec·tro·spi·no·gram (ē-lek-trō-spī′nō-gram). The record obtained by electrospinography.

elec·tro·spi·nog·ra·phy (ē-lek′trō-spī-nog′ră-fē). The recording of spontaneous electrical activity of the spinal cord.

elec·tro·ste·nol·y·sis (ē-lek′trō-stĕ-nol′i-sis). The precipitation of metals in membrane pores in the course of electrolysis.

elec·tro·steth·o·graph (ē-lek′trō-steth′ō-graf). Electrical instrument that amplifies or records the respiratory and cardiac sounds of the chest. [electro- + G. *stēthos,* chest, + *graphō,* to record]

elec·tro·stric·tion (ē-lek-trō-strik′shŭn). The contraction in volume in a protein solution during proteolysis due to the formation of new charged groups.

elec·tro·sur·gery (ē-lek-trō-ser′jer-ē). Division of tissues by high frequency current applied locally with a metal instrument or needle. SEE ALSO electrocautery. SYN electrotomy.

elec·tro·tax·is (ē-lek-trō-tak′sis). Reaction of plant or animal protoplasm to either an anode or a cathode. SEE ALSO tropism. SYN electrotropism, galvanotaxis, galvanotropism. [electro- + G. *taxis,* orderly arrangement]

    negative e., e. by which an organism is attracted toward an anode or repelled from a cathode.

    positive e., e. by which an organism is attracted toward a cathode or repelled from an anode.

elec·tro·tha·na·sia (ē-lek′trō-thă-nā′zē-ă). SYN electrocution. [electro- + G. *thanatos,* death]

elec·tro·ther·a·peu·tics, elec·tro·ther·a·py (ē-lek′trō-thār-ă-pyū′tiks, -thār′ă-pē). Use of electricity in the treatment of disease.

elec·tro·therm (ē-lek′trō-therm). A flexible sheet of resistance coils used for applying heat to the surface of the body. [electro- + G. *thermē,* heat]

elec·tro·tome (ē-lek′trō-tōm). An electric scalpel.

elec·trot·o·my (ē-lek-trot′ō-mē). SYN electrosurgery. [electro- + G. *tomē,* incision]

elec·tro·ton·ic (ē-lek-trō-ton′ik). Relating to electrotonus.

elec·trot·o·nus (ē-lek-trot′ō-nŭs). Changes in excitability and conductivity in a nerve or muscle cell caused by the passage of a constant electric current. SEE ALSO catelectrotonus, anelectrotonus. SYN galvanotonus (1). [electro- + G. *tonos,* tension]

elec·trot·ro·pism (ē-lek-trot′rō-pizm, ē-lek-trō-trō′pizm). SYN electrotaxis. [electro- + G. *tropē,* a turning]

elec·tu·ar·y (ē-lek′chū-ā-rē). SYN confection. [G. *eleikton,* a medicine that melts in the mouth, fr. *ekleichō,* to lick up]

el·e·doi·sin (el-ĕ-doy′sin). An undecapeptide toxin that is formed in the venom gland of cephalopods of the genus *Eledone* and causes vasodilation and contraction of extravascular smooth muscle.

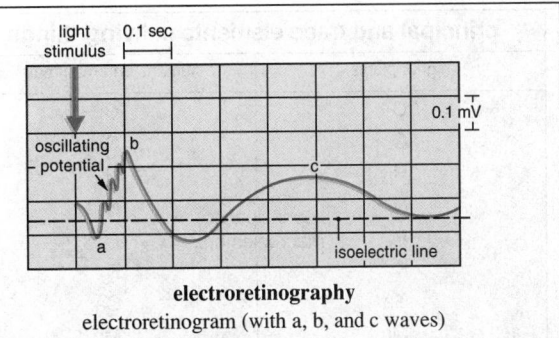

electroretinography
electroretinogram (with a, b, and c waves)

ele·i·din (ē-lē′ī-din). A refractile and weakly staining keratin present in the cells of the stratum lucidum of the palmar and plantar epidermis.

el·e·ment (el′ĕ-ment). **1.** A substance composed of atoms of only one kind, *i.e.,* of identical atomic (proton) number, that therefore cannot be decomposed into two or more e.'s, and that can lose its chemical properties only by union with some other e. or by a nuclear reaction changing the proton number. **2.** An indivisible structure or entity. **3.** A functional entity, frequently exogenous, within a bacterium, such as an extrachromosomal e. [L. *elementum,* a rudiment, beginning]

    actinide e.'s, SYN actinides.

    alkaline earth e.'s, those e.'s in the family Be, Mg, Ca, Sr, Ba, and Ra, the hydroxides of which are highly ionized and hence alkaline in water solution.

    amphoteric e., an e. one or more of whose oxides unite with water to form hydroxides that may act as acids or as bases (*e.g.,* aluminum).

    anatomical e., any anatomical unit, such as a cell. SYN morphologic e.

    copia e.'s, a mobile genetic e. with retrovirus-like sequence organization.

    electronegative e., an e. whose atoms have a tendency to accept electrons and form negative ions (*e.g.,* oxygen, sulfur, chlorine, etc.).

    electropositive e., an e. whose atoms have a tendency to lose electrons and form positive ions (*e.g.,* sodium).

    extrachromosomal e., extrachromosomal genetic e., SYN plasmid.

    fold-back e.'s, a type of transposable e. that possesses long inverted repeats, such that when denatured, loops are formed.

    labile e.'s, tissue cells, as of epithelium, connective tissue, etc., that continue to multiply by mitosis during the life of the individual.

    long interspersed e.'s (LINES), long repetitive sequences in DNA with terminal repeats seen in human and mouse DNA.

    morphologic e., SYN anatomical e.

    neutral e., an e. of the zero group of the periodic system comprising the rare gases, He, Ne, Ar, Kr, Xe, Rn. SYN noble e. (2).

    noble e., (1) SYN noble *metal.* **(2)** SYN neutral e.

    P e.'s, a class of transposable e.'s in Drosophila responsible for hybrid dysgenesis; utilized as tools for introducing genes into new locations in the genome.

    picture e., SEE pixel.

    rare earth e.'s, SYN lanthanides.

    short interspersed e.'s (SINES), repetitive sequences of DNA of about 300 base pairs in length that occur about every 3000–5000 bp in the genome.

    trace e.'s, e.'s present in minute amounts in the body, many of which are essential in metabolism or for the manufacture of essential compounds; *e.g.,* Zn, Se, V, Ni, Mg, Mn, etc.. SYN microelements, microminerals.

    transposable e., a DNA sequence that can move from one location in the genome to another; the transposition event can involve both recombination and replication, producing two copies of the moving piece of DNA; the insertion of these DNA fragments can

el

principal and trace elements in living things	
higher plants	humans and mammals
*C	C
*O	O
*H	H
N	N
P	P
K	K
Ca	Ca
Mg	Mg
S	S
	Na
Fe	Fe
B	F
Cl	Cl
Cu	Cu
Mn	Co
Mo	I
Zn	Mn
	Mo
	Zn

principal or macroelements

trace or microelements

*elements present in every organic substance

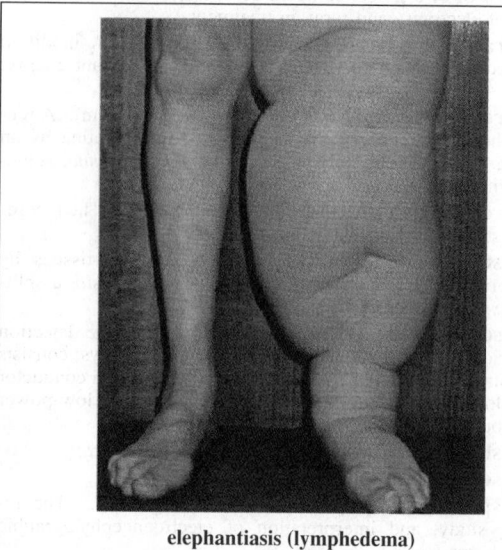

elephantiasis (lymphedema)

lymphatic obstruction. SYN chyloderma, lymph scrotum, parasitic chylocele.

e. telangiecto′des, hypertrophy of the skin and subcutaneous tissues accompanied by and dependent upon dilation of the blood vessels.

e. vul′vae, SYN chronic hypertrophic *vulvitis.*

eleu·ther·o·ma·nia (ē-lū′ther-ō-mā′nē-ă). Rarely used term for an excessive passion for freedom. [G. *eleutheros,* free, + *mania,* madness]

el·e·va·tion (el-ĕ-vā′shŭn). A raised place. SEE ALSO eminence, eminentia.

tactile e.'s, small areas in the skin of the palms and soles especially rich in sensory nerve endings. SYN toruli tactiles [NA].

el·e·va·tor (el′ĕ-vā-tĕr). **1.** An instrument for prying up a sunken part, as the depressed fragment of bone in fracture of the skull, or for elevating tissues. **2.** A surgical instrument used to luxate and remove teeth and roots that cannot be engaged by the beaks of a forceps, or to loosen teeth and roots prior to forceps application. SYN dental lever. [L. fr. *e-levo,* pp. *-atus,* to lift up]

periosteal e., an instrument used for separating the periosteum from the bone. SYN rugine (1).

screw e., a dental instrument with a threaded extremity used for extracting the root of a broken tooth.

elim·i·nant (ē-lim′i-nant). **1.** An evacuant that promotes excretion or the removal of waste. **2.** An agent that increases excretion.

elim·i·na·tion (ē-lim-i-nā′shŭn). Expulsion; removal of waste material from the body; the getting rid of anything. [L. *elimino,* pp. *-atus,* to turn out of doors, fr. *limen,* threshold]

carbon dioxide e. ($\dot{V}_{CO_2}$) ($\dot{V}_{CO_2}$), the rate at which carbon dioxide enters the alveolar gas from the blood, equal in the steady state to the metabolic production of carbon dioxide by tissue metabolism throughout the body; units: ml/min STPD or mmol/min.

elin·gua·tion (ē-ling-gwā′shŭn). SYN glossectomy. [L. *e,* out, + *lingua,* tongue]

el·i·nin (el′i-nin). A lipoprotein fraction of red blood cells that contains the Rh and A and B factors.

ELISA Abbreviation for enzyme-linked immunosorbent *assay.*

elix·ir (ē-lik′ser). A clear, sweetened, hydroalcoholic liquid intended for oral use; e.'s contain flavoring substances and are used either as vehicles or for the therapeutic effect of the active medicinal agents. [Mediev. L., fr. Ar. *al- iksir,* the philosopher's stone]

phenobarbital e., a palatable, colored hydroalcoholic (12–15%

disrupt the integrity of the target gene, possibly causing activation of dormant genes, deletions, inversions, and a variety of chromosomal aberrations.

volume e., SEE voxel.

eleo-. Oil. SEE ALSO oleo-. [G. *elaion,* olive oil]

el·e·o·ma (el-ē-ō′mă). SYN lipogranuloma. [G. *elaion,* oil, + *-oma,* tumor]

el·e·om·e·ter (el-ē-om′ĕ-ter). SYN oleometer. [G. *elaion,* oil, + *metron,* measure]

el·e·op·a·thy (el-ē-op′ă-thē). A rare condition in which there is boggy swelling of the joints, said to be due to a fatty deposit following contusion; or possibly a condition resulting from the injection of paraffin oil as a form of malingering. SYN elaiopathia.

el·e·o·stear·ic ac·id (el-ē-ō-stē′ă-rik, -stēr′ik). An 18-carbon fatty acid with three double bonds (at carbons 9, 11, and 13); isomeric with linolenic acid; found in plant fats.

el·e·o·ther·a·py (el-ē-ō-thār′ă-pē). SYN oleotherapy. [G. *elaion,* oil]

el·e·phan·ti·ac, el·e·phan·ti·as·ic (el-ĕ-fan′tē-ak, fan-tē-as′ik). Relating to elephantiasis.

el·e·phan·ti·a·sis (el-ĕ-fan-tī′ă-sis). Hypertrophy and fibrosis of the skin and subcutaneous tissue, especially of the lower extremities and genitalia, due to long-standing obstructed lymphatic vessels, most commonly after years of infection by the filarial worms *Wuchereria bancrofti* or *Brugia malayi.* SYN Barbados leg, elephant leg, mal de Cayenne, mal de San Lazaro, Malabar leprosy, phlegmasia malabarica. [G. fr. *elephas,* elephant]

congenital e., congenital enlargement of one or more of the limbs or other parts, due to dilation of the lymphatics.

gingival e., a fibrous hyperplasia of the gingiva.

e. neuromato′sa, enlargement of a limb due to diffuse neurofibromatosis of the skin and subcutaneous tissue.

nevoid e., thickening of skin, usually unilateral, involving a small area or the entire extremity, due to congenital enlargement of lymph vessels and lymph vessel obstruction.

e. scro′ti, brawny swelling of the scrotum as a result of chronic

alcohol) mixture containing 20 mg of phenobarbital per 5 ml (teaspoonful); useful in administering the drug to persons who have difficulty swallowing tablets; used as an anticonvulsant and sedative.

Ellik, Milo, U.S. urologist, *1905. SEE E. *evacuator.*

Elliot, John W., U.S. surgeon, 1852–1925. SEE E.'s *position.*

Elliot, Robert H., British ophthalmologist, 1864–1936. SEE E.'s *operation.*

Elliott, Thomas R., British physician, 1877–1961. SEE E.'s *law.*

el·lip·sis (ē-lip′sis). Omission of words or ideas, leaving the whole to be completed by the reader or listener. [G. *ek-,* out, + *leipsis,* leaving]

el·lip·soid (ē-lip′soyd). 1. A spherical or spindle-shaped condensation of phagocytic macrophages in a reticular stroma investing the wall of the splenic arterial capillaries shortly before they release their blood in the cords of red pulp. 2. The outer end of the inner segment of the retinal rods and cones. 3. Having the shape of an ellipse or oval. SYN sheath of Schweigger-Seidel. [G. *ellips,* oval, + *eidos,* form]

el·lip·to·cyte (ē-lip′tō-sīt). An elliptical red blood corpuscle found normally in the lower vertebrates with the exception of Cyclostomata; in mammals it occurs normally only among the camels (family Camelidae), hence cameloid cell. SYN cameloid cell, ovalocyte. [G. *elleipsis,* a leaving out, an ellipse, + *kytos,* cell]

el·lip·to·cy·to·sis (ē-lip′tō-sī-tō′sis). A hereditary abnormality of hemopoiesis in which 50 to 90% of the red blood cells consist of rod forms and elliptocytes, often with an associated hemolytic anemia. There are several autosomal dominant forms [MIM*130500, *130600, and *179650] and one autosomal recessive [MIM*177650] form known. SEE ALSO elliptocytic *anemia.* SYN ovalocytosis.

Ellis, Richard W.B., English physician, 1902–1966. SEE E.-van Creveld *syndrome.*

Ellison, Edwin H., U.S. physician, 1918–1970. SEE Zollinger-E. *syndrome, tumor.*

Ellis type 2 ne·phri·tis. SYN Ellis type 2 *glomerulonephritis.*

Ellis types 1 and 2 glo·mer·u·lo·ne·phri·tis or ne·phri·tis. SEE Ellis type 1 *glomerulonephritis,* Ellis type 2 *glomerulonephritis,* Ellis type 1 *nephritis,* Ellis type 2 *nephritis.*

Ellsworth, Read McLane, U.S. physician, 1899–1970. SEE E.-Howard *test.*

Eloesser, Leo, U.S. thoracic surgeon, 1881–1976. SEE E. *procedure.*

elon·ga·tion (ē-lon-gā′shŭn). 1. The increase in the gauge length measured after fracture in tension within the gauge length, expressed in percentage of original gauge length. 2. The lengthening of a macromolecule; *e.g.,* in the synthesis of long-chain fatty acids or in the synthesis of a protein.

Elschnig, Anton, German ophthalmologist, 1863–1939. SEE E. *pearls,* under *pearl;* E.'s *spots,* under *spot.*

el·u·ant (el′yū-ant). The material that has been eluted.

el·u·ate (el′yū-āt). The solution emerging from a column or paper in chromatography. [see elution]

el·u·ent (el′yū-ent). The mobile phase in chromatography. SYN developer (2), elutant. [see elution]

elu·tant (ē-lū′tant). SYN eluent.

elute (ē-lūt′). To perform or accomplish an elution. SYN elutriate.

elu·tion (ē-lū′shŭn). 1. The separation, by washing, of one solid from another. 2. The removal, by means of a suitable solvent, of one material from another that is insoluble in that solvent, as in column chromatography. 3. The removal of antibodies absorbed onto the erythrocyte surface. SYN elutriation. [L. *e-luo,* pp. lutus, to wash out]

    gradient e., e. in column chromatography in which a changing pH or ionic strength is used to separate substances.

elu·tri·ate (ē-lū′trē-āt). SYN elute.

elu·tri·a·tion (ē-lū-trē-ā′shŭn). SYN elution. [L. *elutrio,* pp. *-atus,* to wash out, decant, fr. *e-luo,* to wash out]

△**elytro-.** Obsolete combining form meaning the vagina. SEE ALSO colpo-, vagino-. [G. *elytron,* sheath (vagina)]

△**em-.** SEE en-.

ema·ci·a·tion (ē-mā-sē-ā′shŭn). Becoming abnormally thin from extreme loss of flesh. SYN wasting (1). [L. *e-macio,* pp. *-atus,* to make thin]

emac·u·la·tion (ē-mak-yū-lā′shŭn). Removal of spots or other blemishes from the skin. [L. *emaculo,* pp. *-atus,* to clear from spots, fr. *e-,* out, + *macula,* spot]

em·a·na·tion (em-ă-nā′shŭn). 1. Any substance that flows out or is emitted from a source or origin. 2. The radiation from a radioactive element. [L. *e- mano,* pp. *-atus,* to flow out]

    actinium e., radon-219. SEE emanon.

    radium e., radon-222. SEE emanon.

    thorium e., radon-220. SEE emanon.

em·a·na·tor·i·um (em′ă-nā-tōr′ē-ŭm). An institution where, formerly, radiation treatment now considered dangerous (using radioactive waters and the inhalation of radium emanations) was administered.

eman·ci·pa·tion (ē-man-si-pā′shŭn). In embryology, delimitation of a specific area in an organ-forming field, giving definite shape and limits to the organ primordium.

em·a·non (em′ă-non). Archaic term once used to denote all radon isotopes collectively, when the term radon was restricted to the isotope radon-222, the naturally occurring intermediate of the uranium-238 radioactive series; so called because original names for radon-219, radon-220, and radon-222 were, respectively, "actinium emanation," "thorium emanation," and "radium emanation." [L. *emano,* to flow out + *-on*]

em·a·no·ther·a·py (em′ă-nō-thār′ă-pē). An obsolete treatment of various diseases by means of radium emanation (radon), or other emanation.

emar·gi·nate (ē-mar′ji-nāt). Nicked; with broken margin. SYN notched. [L. *emargino,* to deprive of its edge, fr. *e-* priv. + *margo* (*margin-*), edge]

emar·gi·na·tion (ē-mar′ji-nā′shŭn). SYN notch.

emas·cu·la·tion (ē-mas-kyū-lā′shŭn). Castration of the male by removal of the testis and/or penis. SYN eviration (1). [L. *emasculo,* pp. *-atus,* to castrate, fr. *e-* priv. + *masculus,* masculine]

EMB. Abbreviation for eosin-methylene blue. SEE eosin-methylene blue *agar.*

Em·ba·dom·o·nas (em-bă-dom′ō-nas, em′bă-dō-mō′nas). Old name for *Retortamonas.* [G. *embadon,* surface, + *monas,* unit, monad]

em·balm (em-bahlm′). To treat a dead body with balsams or other chemicals to preserve it from decay. [L. *in,* in, + *balsamum,* balsam]

Embden, Gustav G., German biochemist, 1874–1933. SEE E. *ester;* Robison-E. *ester;* E.-Meyerhof *pathway;* E.-Meyerhof-Parnas *pathway.*

em·bed (em-bed′). To surround a pathological or histological specimen with a firm and sometimes hard medium such as paraffin, wax, celloidin, or a resin, in order to make possible the cutting of thin sections for microscopic examination. SYN imbed.

em·be·lin (em′bĕ-lin). 2,5-Dihydroxy-3-undecyl-*p*-benzoquinone; the active principle from the dried fruit of *Embelia ribes* and *E. robusta* (family Myrsinaceae); has been used as a teniacide.

em·boite·ment (awm-bwaht-mawn′). SYN preformation *theory.* [Fr., encasement]

em·bo·la·lia (em-bō-lā′lē-ă). SYN embololalia.

em·bo·le (em′bō-lē). 1. Reduction of a limb dislocation. SYN embolia. 2. Formation of the gastrula by invagination. SYN emboly. [G. *embolē,* insertion]

em·bo·lec·to·my (em-bō-lek′tō-mē). Removal of an embolus. [G. *embolos,* a plug (embolus), + *ektomē,* excision]

em·bo·le·mia (em-bō-lē′mē-ă). The presence of emboli in the circulating blood. [G. *embolos,* a plug (embolus), + *haima,* blood]

em·bo·li (em′bō-lī). Plural of embolus.

em·bo·lia (em-bō′lē-ă). SYN embole (1).

em·bol·ic (em-bol′ik). Relating to an embolus or to embolism.

em·bol·i·form (em-bol'i-fōrm). Shaped like an embolus. [G. *embolos,* plug (embolus), + L. *forma,* form]

em·bo·lism (em'bō-lizm). Obstruction or occlusion of a vessel by an embolus. [G. *embolisma,* a piece or patch; lit. something thrust in]

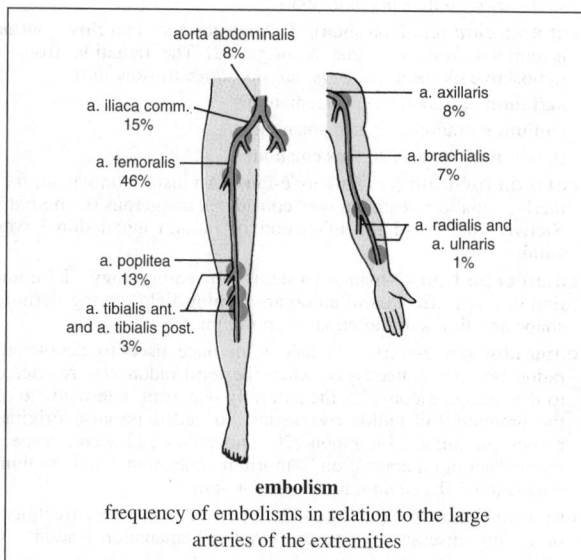

embolism
frequency of embolisms in relation to the large arteries of the extremities

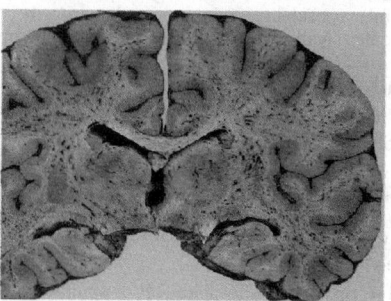

fat embolism
in the brain, following multiple fractures

air e., e. of air that can occur during cardiopulmonary bypass or with lung injury; either the pulmonary arteries or the systemic arteries can be filled with air. SYN gas e.

amniotic fluid e., obstruction and constriction of pulmonary blood vessels by amniotic fluid entering the maternal circulation, causing obstetric shock. SEE ALSO amniotic fluid *syndrome.*

atheroma e., SYN cholesterol e.

bland e., e. by simple nonseptic material.

bone marrow e., obstruction of a vessel by bone marrow, usually following fracture of a bone.

cellular e., e. due to a mass of cells transported from disintegrating tissue.

cholesterol e., e. of lipid debris from an ulcerated atheromatous deposit, generally from a large artery to small arterial branches; it is usually small and rarely causes infarction. SYN atheroma e.

cotton-fiber e., e. by cotton fibers from sterile gauze used in intravenous medication or transfusion; may form as foreign body granulomas in small pulmonary arteries.

crossed e., (1) obstruction of a systemic artery by an embolus originating in the venous system which passes through a septal defect, patent foramen ovale, or other shunt to the arterial system; **(2)** obstruction by a minute embolism that passes through the pulmonary capillaries from the venous to the arterial system. SYN paradoxical e.

direct e., e. occurring in the direction of the blood current.

fat e., the occurrence of fat globules in the circulation following fractures of a long bone, in burns, in parturition, and in association with fatty degeneration of the liver; the emboli most commonly block pulmonary or cerebral vessels when symptoms referable to either or both of these regions appear. SYN oil e.

gas e., SYN air e.

hematogenous e., e. occurring in a blood vessel.

infective e., SYN pyemic e.

lymph e., lymphogenous e., e. occurring in a lymphatic vessel.

miliary e., e. occurring simultaneously in a number of capillaries. SYN multiple e. (1).

multiple e., (1) SYN miliary e. **(2)** e. caused by the arrest of a number of small emboli.

obturating e., complete closing of the lumen of a vessel by an embolism.

oil e., SYN fat e.

pantaloon e., SYN saddle e.

paradoxical e., SYN crossed e.

pulmonary e., e. of pulmonary arteries, most frequently by detached fragments of thrombus from a leg or pelvic vein, commonly when thrombosis has followed an operation or confinement to bed.

pyemic e., plugging of an artery by an embolus detached from a suppurating thrombus. SYN infective e.

retinal e., e. of an artery of the retina.

retrograde e., e. of a vein by an embolus carried in a direction opposite to that of the normal blood current, after being diverted into a smaller vein. SYN venous e.

riding e., SYN straddling e.

saddle e., a straddling e. at any vascular bifurcation, *e.g.,* of the aorta which occludes both common iliac arteries. SYN pantaloon e.

straddling e., e. occurring at the bifurcation of an artery and blocking more or less completely both branches. SYN riding e.

tumor e., e. by neoplastic tissue transported from a tumor site and which may grow as a metastasis.

venous e., SYN retrograde e.

em·bo·li·za·tion (em'bol-i-zā'shŭn). Therapeutic introduction of various substances into the circulation to occlude vessels, either to arrest or prevent hemorrhaging or to devitalize a structure or organ by occluding its blood supply.

em·bo·lo·la·lia (em'bō-lō-lā'lē-ă). Interjection of meaningless words into a sentence when speaking. SYN embolalia, embolophasia, embolophrasia. [G. *embolos,* something thrown in, fr. *emballo,* to throw in, + *lalia,* speaking]

em·bo·lo·my·cot·ic (em'bō-lō-mī-kot'ik). Relating to or caused by an infective embolus. [G. *embolos,* a plug (embolus), + *mykēs,* fungus]

em·bo·lo·pha·sia (em'bō-lō-fā'zē-ă). SYN embolalia. [G. *embolos,* something thrown in, + *phasis,* a saying]

em·bo·lo·phra·sia (em'bō-lō-frā'zē-ă). SYN embolalia. [G. *embolos,* something thrown in, + *phrasis,* phrase]

em·bo·lo·ther·a·py (em-bō-lō-thăr'ă-pē). Occlusion of arteries by insertion of blood clots, Gelfoam, coils, balloons, etc., with an angiographic catheter; used for control of inoperable hemorrhage or preoperative management of highly vascular neoplasms. [G. *embolos,* plug, + *therapeia,* medical treatment]

em·bo·lus, pl. **em·bo·li** (em'bō-lŭs, -lī). **1.** A plug, composed of a detached thrombus or vegetation, mass of bacteria, or other foreign body, occluding a vessel. **2.** SYN emboliform *nucleus.* [G. *embolos,* a plug, wedge or stopper]

catheter e., coiled worm-shaped platelet and fibrin aggregates produced during vascular catheterization, originating on the catheter or its guide wire; embolization of the catheter itself.

em·bo·ly (em'bō-lē). SYN embole (2).

em·bouche·ment (ahm-būsh-mon'). The opening of one blood vessel into another. [Fr.]

em·bra·sure (em-brā'shūr). In dentistry, an opening that widens outwardly or inwardly; specifically, that space adjacent to the interproximal contact area that spreads toward the facial, gingival, lingual, occlusal, or incisal aspect. [Fr. an opening in a wall for cannon]

buccal e., a space existing on the facial aspect of the interproximal contact area between adjacent posterior teeth.

gingival e., a space existing cervical to the interproximal contact area between adjacent teeth.

incisal e., a space existing on the incisal aspect of the interproximal contact area between adjacent anterior teeth.

labial e., a space existing on the facial aspect of the interproximal contact area between adjacent anterior teeth.

lingual e., a space existing on the lingual aspect of the interproximal contact area between adjacent teeth.

occlusal e., a space existing on the occlusal aspect of the interproximal contact areas between adjacent posterior teeth.

em·bro·ca·tion (em-brō-kā′shŭn). Rarely used term for liniment or for the application of a liniment. [G. *embrochē*, a fomentation]

△**embry-.** SEE embryo-.

em·bry·at·rics (em-brē-at′riks). Rarely used term for fetology. [embryo- + G. *iatros*, physician]

em·bryo (em′brē-ō). **1.** An organism in the early stages of development. **2.** In humans, the developing organism from conception until approximately the end of the second month; developmental stages from this time to birth are commonly designated as fetal. **3.** A primordial plant within a seed. [G. *embryon*, fr. *en*, in, + *bryō*, to be full, swell]

heterogametic e., a male e. with XY karyotype.

hexacanth e., the e. of tapeworms of the subclass Cestoda, such as *Taenia saginata*, characterized by three pairs of hooks used for penetration through the gut of an intermediate host. SYN oncosphere e.

homogametic e., a female e. with XX karyotype.

oncosphere e., SYN hexacanth e.

presomite e., an e. prior to the appearance of the first pair of somites, about 20 to 21 days after fertilization in humans.

previllous e., the e. of a placental mammal prior to the formation of chorionic villi.

△**embryo-, embry-.** The embryo. [G. *embryon,* a young one]

em·bry·o·blast (em′brē-ō-blast). The cells at the embryonic pole of the blastocyst concerned with formation of the body of the embryo *per se.* SYN inner cell mass. [embryo- + G. *blastos,* germ]

em·bry·o·car·dia (em′brē-ō-kar′dē-ă). A condition in which the cadence of the heart sounds resembles that of the fetus, the first and second sounds becoming alike and evenly spaced; a sign of serious myocardial disease. SYN pendulum rhythm, tic-tac rhythm, tic-tac sounds. [embryo- + G. *kardia,* heart]

jugular e., SYN atrial *flutter.*

em·bry·o·gen·e·sis (em′brē-ō-jen′ĕ-sis). That phase of prenatal development involved in establishment of the characteristic configuration of the embryonic body; in humans, e. is usually regarded as extending from the end of the second week, when the embryonic disk is formed, to the end of the eighth week, after which the conceptus is usually spoken of as a fetus. [embryo- + G. *genesis,* origin]

em·bry·o·gen·ic, em·bry·o·ge·net·ic (em-brē-ō-jen′ik, -jĕ-net′ik). Producing an embryo; relating to the formation of an embryo.

em·bry·og·e·ny (em-brē-oj′ĕ-nē). The origin and growth of the embryo.

em·bry·oid (em′brē-oyd). SYN embryonoid.

em·bry·ol·o·gist (em-brē-ol′ō-jist). One who specializes in embryology.

em·bry·ol·o·gy (em-brē-ol′ōjē). Science of the origin and development of the organism from fertilization of the ovum to the end of the eighth week. Sometimes used to include all stages of the life cycle. [embryo- + G. *logos,* study]

em·bry·o·ma (em-brē-ō′mă). SYN embryonal *tumor.*

e. of the kidney, SYN Wilms′ *tumor.*

em·bry·o·mor·phous (em′brē-ō-mōr′fŭs). **1.** Relating to the formation and structure of the embryo. **2.** Applied to structures or

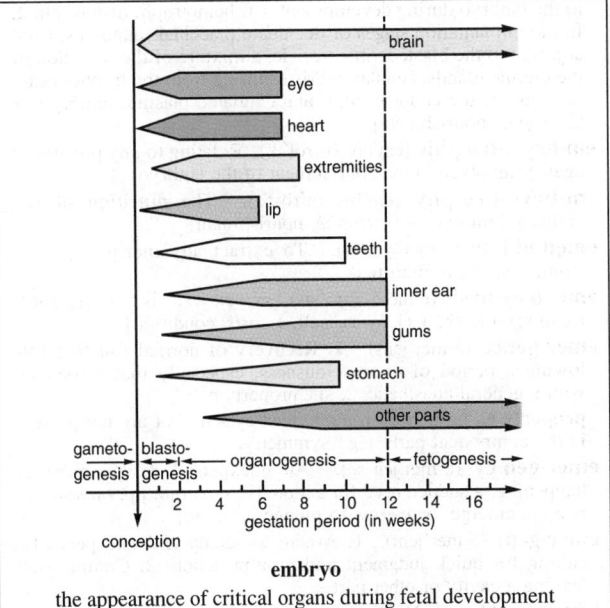

embryo
the appearance of critical organs during fetal development

tissues in the body similar to those in the embryo, or embryonal rests. [embryo- + G. *morphē,* shape]

em·bry·o·nal (em′brē-ō-năl). Relating to an embryo. SYN embryonate (1).

em·bry·o·nate (em′brē-ō-nāt). **1.** SYN embryonal. **2.** Containing an embryo. **3.** Impregnated.

em·bry·on·ic (em-brē-on′ik). Of, pertaining to, or in the condition of an embryo.

em·bry·on·i·form (em-brē-on′i-fōrm). SYN embryonoid.

em·bry·on·i·za·tion (em′brē-on-i-zā′shŭn). Reversion of a cell or tissue to an embryonic form.

em·bry·o·noid (em′brē-ō-noyd). Resembling an embryo or a fetus. SYN embryoid, embryoniform. [embryo- + G. *eidos,* appearance]

em·bry·o·ny (em′brē-ō-nē). The forming of an embryo.

em·bry·op·a·thy (em-brē-op′ă-thē). A morbid condition in the embryo or fetus. SYN fetopathy. [embryo- + G. *pathos,* disease]

em·bry·o·phore (em′brē-ō-fōr). A membrane or wall around the hexacanth embryo of tapeworms, forming the inner portion of the eggshell. In the genus *Taenia,* the e. is exceptionally thick, with radial striations that form a highly protective structure; in the genus *Diphyllobothrium,* the e. is ciliated and enhances the aquatic life cycle of this and other pseudophyllid cestodes. SEE ALSO coracidium. [embryo- + G. *phoros,* bearing]

em·bry·o·plas·tic (em-brē-ō-plas′tik). **1.** Producing an embryo. **2.** Relating to the formation of an embryo. [embryo- + G. *plassō,* to form]

em·bry·o·scope (em′brē-ō-skōp). An instrument for examining the embryos in hens′ eggs at different stages of development. [embryo- + G. *skopeō,* to examine]

em·bry·ot·o·my (em-brē-ot′ō-mē). Any mutilating operation on the fetus to make possible its removal when delivery is impossible by natural means. [embryo- + G. *tomē,* cutting]

em·bry·o·tox·ic·i·ty (em′brē-ō-tok-sis′i-tē). Injury to the embryo, which may result in death or in abnormal development of a part, owing to substances that enter the placental circulation.

em·bry·o·tox·on (em′brē-ō-tok′son). Congenital opacity of the periphery of the cornea, a feature of osteogenesis imperfecta. [embryo- + G. *toxon,* bow]

anterior e., SYN *arcus* cornealis.

posterior e., a developmental abnormality marked by a prominent white ring of Schwalbe and iris strands that partially obscure the chamber angle.

em·bry·o·troph (em′brē-ō-trōf). **1.** Nutritive material supplied to the embryo during development. Cf. hemotroph, histotroph. **2.** In the implantation stages of deciduate placental mammals, fluid adjacent to the blastodermic vesicle; a mixture of the secretion of the uterine glands, cellular debris resulting from the trophoblastic invasion of the endometrium, and exudated plasma. [embryo- + G. *trophē,* nourishment]

em·bry·o·tro·phic (em′brē-ō-trof′ik). Relating to any process or agency involved in the nourishment of the embryo.

em·bry·ot·ro·phy (em′brē-ot′rō-fē). The nutrition of the embryo. [embryo- + G. *trophē,* nourishment]

emed·ul·late (ē-med′yū-lāt). To extract any marrow. [L. *e-,* from, + *medulla,* marrow]

emei·o·cy·to·sis (ē′mē-ō-sī-tō′sis). SYN exocytosis (2). [L. *emitto,* to send forth, + G. *kytos,* cell, + *-osis,* condition]

emer·gence (ē-mer′jens). **1.** Recovery of normal function following a period of unconsciousness, especially that associated with a general anesthetic. **2.** SEE property e.

property e., properties in a complex system that are not present in the component parts, *e.g.,* symmetry.

emer·gen·cy (ē-mer′jen-sē). An unexpected development or happening; a sudden need for action. [L. *e-mergo,* pp. *-mersus,* to rise up, emerge, fr. *mergo,* to plunge into, dip]

emer·gent (ē-mer′jent). **1.** Arising suddenly and unexpectedly, calling for quick judgment and prompt action. **2.** Coming out; leaving a cavity or other part.

Emery, Alan E. H., Contemporary British physician. SEE E.-Dreifuss muscular *dystrophy.*

em·ery (em′er-ē). An abrasive containing aluminum oxide and iron. [O.Fr. *emeri,* fr. L.L. *smericulum,* fr. G. *smiris*]

em·e·sis (em′ĕ-sis). **1.** SYN vomiting. **2.** Combining form, used in the suffix position, for vomiting. [G. fr. *emeō,* to vomit]

emet·ic (ĕ-met′ik). **1.** Relating to or causing vomiting. **2.** An agent that causes vomiting. [G. *emetikos,* producing vomiting, fr. *emeō,* to vomit]

em·e·tine (em′ĕ-tēn). $C_{29}H_{40}N_2O_4$; Cephaeline methyl ether; the principal alkaloid of ipecac, used as an emetic; its salts are used in amebiasis; available as the hydrochloride.

em·e·to·ca·thar·tic (em′ĕ-tō-kă-thar′tik). **1.** Both emetic and cathartic. **2.** An agent that causes vomiting and purging of the lower intestines.

eme·to·gen·ic. Having the capacity to induce emesis (vomiting), a common property of anticancer agents, narcotics, and amorphine.

e·me·to·ge·nic·i·ty. The property of being emetogenic.

EMF Abbreviation for electromotive *force.*

EMG Abbreviation for electromyogram.

△-emia. Blood. [G. *haima*]

emic·tion (ē-mik′shŭn). Rarely used term for urination.

em·i·gra·tion (em-i-grā′shŭn). The passage of white blood cells through the endothelium and wall of small blood vessels. [L. *e-migro,* pp. *-atus,* to emigrate]

em·i·nence (em′i-nens). A circumscribed area raised above the general level of the surrounding surface, particularly on a bone surface. SYN eminentia [NA]. [L. *eminentia*]

abducens e., SYN facial *colliculus.*

arcuate e., a prominence on the anterior surface of the petrous portion of the temporal bone indicating the position of the superior or semicircular canal. SYN eminentia arcuata [NA].

articular e. of temporal bone, SYN articular *tubercle* of temporal bone.

canine e., an elevation on the maxilla corresponding to the socket of the canine tooth. SYN canine prominence.

collateral e., a longitudinal elevation of the floor of the collateral trigone of the lateral ventricle of the brain, between the hippocampus and the calcar avis, caused by the proximity of the floor of the collateral fissure. SYN eminentia collateralis [NA].

e. of concha, the prominence on the cranial surface of the auricle corresponding to the concha. SYN eminentia conchae [NA], apophysis conchae.

cruciate e., SYN cruciform e.

cruciform e., bony cross-like elevation on the internal aspect of

the squamous portion of the occipital bone formed by the intersection of the groove for the transverse sinuses and the internal occipital crest, with the internal occipital protuberance at the center of the "cross." SYN eminentia cruciformis [NA], cruciate e.

deltoid e., SYN deltoid *tuberosity.*

Doyère's e., the slightly elevated area of the striated muscle fiber's surface that corresponds to the site of the motor *endplate.*

facial e., SYN facial *colliculus.*

forebrain e., SYN frontonasal *prominence.*

frontal e., the most prominent portion of the frontal bone on either side. SYN tuber frontale [NA], eminentia frontalis★ [NA], frontal tuber.

genital e., in very young embryos, the vaguely outlined median elevation immediately cephalic to the proctodeum; its central part develops into the genital tubercle.

hypobranchial e., a median elevation in the floor of the embryonic pharynx caudal to the tuberculum impar; it merges laterally with the ventral part of the second and third branchial arches, and in later development is incorporated in the root of the tongue. SYN copula linguae, His' copula.

hypoglossal e., SYN hypoglossal *trigone.*

hypothenar e., the fleshy mass at the medial side of the palm. SYN eminentia hypothena′ris★, antithenar, hypothenar prominence, hypothenar (1).

ileocecal e., SYN ileocecal *valve.*

iliopectineal e., SYN iliopubic e.

iliopubic e., a rounded elevation on the superior surface of the hip bone at the junction of the ilium and the superior ramus of the pubis. SYN eminentia iliopubica [NA], iliopectineal e.

intercondylar e., intercondyloid e., an elevation on the proximal extremity of the tibia between the two articular surfaces. SYN eminentia intercondylaris [NA], eminentia intercondyloidea, spinous process of tibia.

maxillary e., SYN maxillary *tuberosity.*

medial e., longitudinal elevation of the rhomboid fossa, extending along either side of the midline throughout the length of the rhombencephalon; made up of named elevations such as the facial colliculus and the hypoglossal and vagal trigones. SYN eminentia medialis [NA], eminentia teres, funiculus teres, round e.

median e., the slightly prominent lower segment of the infundibulum of the hypothalamus, immediately proximal to the hypophysial stalk; the region is characterized by the capillary tufts of the infundibular arteries, from which the hypothalamohypophysial portal system of veins arises. SYN eminentia mediana.

olivary e., SYN oliva.

orbital e. of zygomatic bone, SYN orbital *tubercle* of zygomatic bone.

parietal e., a prominent portion of the parietal bone, a little above the center of its external surface, usually corresponding to the point of maximum width of the head. SYN tuber parietale [NA], eminentia parietalis, parietal tuber.

pyramidal e., SYN *eminentia* pyramidalis.

radial e. of wrist, a rather large flat e. on the radial side of the palmar aspect of the wrist, due to the tuberosity of scaphoid and the ridge on the trapezium. SYN eminentia carpi radialis.

restiform e., a prominence of the dorsolateral surface of the medulla oblongata corresponding to the larger lateral part of the inferior cerebellar peduncle. SYN eminentia restiformis.

round e., SYN medial e.

e. of scapha, the prominence on the cranial surface of the auricle corresponding to the scapha. SYN eminentia scaphae [NA].

thenar e., the fleshy mass on the lateral side of the palm; the radial palm; the ball of the thumb. SYN eminentia thena′ris★, thenar prominence, thenar (1).

thyroid e., SYN laryngeal *prominence.*

e. of triangular fossa of auricle, the prominence on the cranial surface of the auricle corresponding to the triangular fossa. SYN eminentia fossae triangularis auricularis [NA], agger perpendicularis, eminentia triangularis.

ulnar e. of wrist, an e. smaller than the radial, on the ulnar side of the palmar aspect of the wrist, due to presence of the pisiform bone. SYN eminentia carpi ulnaris.

EMINENTIA

em·i·nen·tia, pl. **em·i·nen·ti·ae** (em-i-nen′shē-ă, -shē-ē) [NA]. SYN eminence. [L. prominence, fr. *e-mineo,* to stand out, project]
e. abducen′tis, SYN facial *colliculus.*
e. arcua′ta [NA], SYN arcuate *eminence.*
e. articula′ris os′sis tempora′lis, SYN articular *tubercle* of temporal bone.
e. car′pi radia′lis, SYN radial *eminence* of wrist.
e. car′pi ulna′ris, SYN ulnar *eminence* of wrist.
e. collatera′lis [NA], SYN collateral *eminence.*
e. con′chae [NA], SYN *eminence* of concha.
e. crucifor′mis [NA], SYN cruciform *eminence.*
e. facia′lis, SYN facial *colliculus.*
e. fos′sae triangula′ris auricula′ris [NA], SYN *eminence* of triangular fossa of auricle.
e. fronta′lis [NA], ☆official alternate term for frontal *eminence,* frontal *eminence.*
e. hypoglos′si, SYN hypoglossal *trigone.*
e. hypothena′ris, ☆official alternate term for hypothenar *eminence.*
e. iliopu′bica [NA], SYN iliopubic *eminence.*
e. intercondyla′ris [NA], SYN intercondylar *eminence.*
e. intercondyloid′ea, SYN intercondylar *eminence.*
e. maxil′lae [NA], ☆official alternate term for maxillary *tuberosity,* maxillary *tuberosity.*
e. media′lis [NA], SYN medial *eminence.*
e. media′na, SYN median *eminence.*
e. orbita′lis ossis zygoma′tici [NA], SYN orbital *tubercle* of zygomatic bone.
e. parieta′lis, SYN parietal *eminence.*
e. pyramida′lis [NA], a conical projection posterior to the vestibular window in the middle ear; it is hollow and contains the stapedius muscle. SYN pyramid of tympanum, pyramidal eminence, pyramis tympani.
e. restifor′mis, SYN restiform *eminence.*
e. sca′phae [NA], SYN *eminence* of scapha.
e. sym′physis, SYN mental *tubercle.*
e. te′res, SYN medial *eminence.*
e. thena′ris, ☆official alternate term for thenar *eminence.*
va′gi e., SYN vagal *trigone.*

---

em·i·o·cy·to·sis (ē′mē-ō-sī-tō′sis). SYN exocytosis (2). [L. *emitto,* to send forth, + G. *kytos,* cell, + *-osis,* condition]
em·is·sar·i·um (em-i-sā′rē-ŭm). SYN emissary *vein.* [L. an outlet, fr. *e-mitto,* pp. *-missus,* to send out]
e. condyloid′eum, SYN condylar emissary *vein.*
e. mastoid′eum, SYN mastoid emissary *vein.*
e. occipita′le, SYN occipital emissary *vein.*
e. parieta′le, SYN parietal emissary *vein.*
em·is·sary (em′i-sār-ē). **1.** Relating to, or providing, an outlet or drain. **2.** SYN emissary *vein.* [see emissarium]
emis·sion (ē-mish′ŭn). A discharge; referring usually to a seminal discharge occurring during sleep (**nocturnal e.**). [L. *emissio,* fr. *e- mitto,* to send out]
characteristic e., SYN characteristic *radiation.*
emis·siv·i·ty (ē-mi-siv′i-tē). The giving off of heat rays; a perfect "black body" has an e. of 1, a highly polished metallic surface may have an e. as low as 0.02.
EMIT Abbreviation for enzyme-multiplied *immunoassay* technique.

em·men·a·gog·ic (ĕ-men′ă-goj′ik). Relating to or acting as an emmenagogue.
em·men·a·gogue (ĕ-men′ă-gog). An agent that induces or increases menstrual flow. SYN hemagogue (2). [G. *emmēnos,* monthly, fr. *en,* in, + *mēn,* month, + *agōgos,* leading]
em·men·ia (ĕ-men′ē-ă, ĕ-mē′nē-ă). SYN menses. [G. *emmēnos,* monthly]
em·men·ic (ĕ-men′ik). SYN menstrual.
em·men·i·op·a·thy (ĕ-men′ē-op′ă-thē). Any disorder of menstruation. [G. *emmēnos,* monthly, + *pathos,* suffering]
em·me·nol·o·gy (em-ĕ-nol′ō-jē). Obsolete term for the branch of medicine concerned with the physiology and pathology of menstruation. [G. *emmēnos,* monthly, + *logos,* study]
Emmet, Thomas A., U.S. gynecologist, 1828–1919. SEE E.'s *needle, operation.*
em·me·tro·pia (em-ĕ-trō′pē-ă). The state of refraction of the eye in which parallel rays, when the eye is at rest, are focused exactly on the retina. [G. *emmetros,* according to measure, + *ōps,* eye]
em·me·tro·pic (em-ĕ-trop′ik). Pertaining to or characterized by emmetropia.
em·me·trop·i·za·tion (em′ĕ-trōp-i-zā′shŭn). The process by which the refraction of the anterior ocular segment and the axial length of the eye tend to balance each other to produce emmetropia.
Em·mon·si·el·la cap·su·la·ta (e-mon-sī-el′ă kap-sū-lā′tă). SYN Ajellomyces capsulatum.
em·o·din (em′ō-din). 1,3,8-trihydroxy-6-methylanthraquinone; a crystalline substance (cathartic) found in rhubarb, senna, cascara sagrada, and other purgative drugs. SYN archin, frangulic acid.
emol·lient (ē-mol′ē-ent). **1.** Soothing to the skin or mucous membrane. **2.** An agent that softens the skin or soothes irritation in the skin or mucous membrane. SYN malactic. [L. *emolliens,* pres. p. of *e- mollio, emollire,* to soften]
emo·tion (ē-mō′shŭn). A strong feeling, aroused mental state, or intense state of drive or unrest directed toward a definite object and evidenced in both behavior and in psychologic changes, with accompanying autonomic nervous system manifestations. [L. *e-moveo,* pp. *-motus,* to move out, agitate]
emo·tion·al (ē-mō′shŭn-ăl). Relating to or marked by an emotion.
emo·ti·o·vas·cu·lar (ē-mō′shē-ō-vas′kyū-ler). Relating to the vascular changes, such as pallor and blushing, caused by emotions of various kinds.
e.m.p. Abbreviation for L. *ex modo praescripto,* in the manner prescribed.
em·pasm, em·pas·ma (em′pazm, em-paz′mă). A dusting powder. [G. *empasma,* fr. *em-passo,* to sprinkle on]
em·path·ic (em-path′ik). Relating to or marked by empathy.
em·pa·thize (em′pă-thīz). To feel empathy in relation to another person; to put oneself in another's place.
em·pa·thy (em′pă-thē). **1.** The ability to intellectually and emotionally sense the emotions, feelings, and reactions that another person is experiencing and to effectively communicate that understanding to the individual. Cf. sympathy (3). **2.** The anthropomorphization or humanizing of objects and the feeling of oneself as being in and part of them. [G. *en (em),* in, + *pathos,* feeling]

△ Combining forms	[NA] Nomina Anatomica
Word*Finder*	[MIM] Mendelian
Multi-term entry finder	**Inheritance in Man**
Preceding letter A	
A.D.A.M. Anatomy Plates	☆ **Official alternate term**
Between letters L and M	
Appendices:	☆[NA] **Official alternate**
Following letter Z	**Nomina Anatomica term**
SYN **Synonym; Cf., compare**	**High Profile Term**

generative e., the inner experience of sharing in and comprehending the momentary psychologic state of another person.

em·per·i·po·le·sis (em-pār'i-pō-lē'sis). Active penetration of one cell by another, which remains intact; observed in tissue cultures in which polymorphonuclear leukocytes have entered macrophages and subsequently left. [G. *en* (*em*), inside, + *peri,* around, + *poleomai,* to wander about]

em·phly·sis (em'fli-sis). Obsolete term for a vesicular eruption, such as pemphigus. [G. *en,* in, + *phlysis,* an eruption, fr. *phlyō,* to boil over]

em·phrac·tic (em-frak'tik). Relating to emphraxis.

em·phrax·is (em-frak'sis). **1.** A clogging or obstruction of the mouth of the sweat gland. **2.** An impaction. [G. a stoppage]

em·phy·se·ma (em-fi-sē'mă). **1.** Presence of air in the interstices of the connective tissue of a part. **2.** A condition of the lung characterized by increase beyond the normal in the size of air spaces distal to the terminal bronchiole (those parts containing alveoli), with destructive changes in their walls and reduction in their number. Clinical manifestation is undue breathlessness on exertion, due to the combined effect (in varying degrees) of reduction of alveolar surface for gas exchange, ventilation-perfusion imbalance, and collapse of smaller airways with trapping of alveolar gas occurring predominantly in expiration; this causes the chest to be held in the position of inspiration ("barrel chest"), with prolonged expiration and increased residual volume; symptoms of chronic bronchitis often, but not necessarily, coexist. Two structural varieties are described: panlobular e. and centrilobular e. SYN pulmonary e. [G. inflation of stomach, etc. fr. *en,* in, + *physēma,* a blowing, fr. *physa,* bellows]

---

morphological classification of pulmonary emphysema

1. panlobular/panacinar emphysema: affecting the entire lung from periphery inward

2. centrilobular/centriacinar emphysema: beginning near terminal bronchioli in center of lobule

3. irregular emphysema: extensive loss of lobular structures (so-called "empty lobules"); both pan- and centrilobular emphysema can develop into this final condition

---

alveolar duct e., e. in which the primary involvement is in the alveolar ducts and respiratory bronchioles, as opposed to panacinar e.

---

pathological classification of pulmonary emphysema

1. physiologic atrophy of old age (senile emphysema)

2. volumen pulmonum auctum (expanded lung volume; acute emphysema)

3. chronic destructive emphysema
   a) primary (broncho-) obstructive emphysema
   b) emphysematous sclerosis of lungs

4. special forms of pulmonary emphysema
   a) congenital, so-called lobar emphysema
   b) scar emphysema
   c) emphysema bullosum
   d) marginal emphysema

---

bullous e., e. in which the enlarged airspaces are one to several cm in diameter, often visible on chest radiographs. Thin-walled air sacs under tension compress pulmonary tissue, either single or multiple. Sometimes amenable to surgical resection with improvement in pulmonary function.

centri-acinar e., SYN centrilobular e.

centrilobular e., e. affecting the lobules around their central bronchioles, causally related to bronchiolitis, and seen in coalminer's pneumoconiosis. SYN centri-acinar e.

compensating e., compensatory e., increase in the air capacity of a portion of the lung when another portion is consolidated, shrunken, or unable to perform its respiratory function; the alveoli are distended, but there is no destruction of alveolar walls, and hence, no true e., as this term is now defined.

congenital lobar e., common cause of neonatal respiratory distress which usually involves the left upper lobe.

cutaneous e., SYN subcutaneous e.

diffuse e., SYN panlobular e.

diffuse obstructive e., the major component of chronic obstructive lung disease.

ectatic e., obstructive airway disease with areas of dilatation of alveoli acini. Seen primarily in association with inherited deficiency of alpha-1 protease inhibitor. SEE panlobular e.

familial e., e. inherited in association with severe α-1 antitrypsin deficiency. It may occur as an isolated feature [MIM*130700, 130710] or with *cutis* laxa and hemolytic *anemia* [MIM*225360].

gangrenous e., SYN gas *gangrene.*

generalized e., SYN panlobular e.

increased markings e., a term applied to mixed obstructive lung disease in which radiographic findings of emphysema coexist with nonvascular shadows, probably related to bronchial inflammation.

interlobular e., interstitial e. in the connective tissue septa between the pulmonary lobules.

interstitial e., (**1**) presence of air in the pulmonary tissues consequent upon rupture of the air cells; (**2**) presence of air or gas in the connective tissue.

intestinal e., SYN *pneumatosis* cystoides intestinalis.

irregular e., e. that shows no consistent relationship to any portion of the acinus; always associated with fibrosis.

mediastinal e., deflection of air, usually from a ruptured emphysematous bleb in the lung, into the mediastinal tissue.

panacinar e., SYN panlobular e.

panlobular e., e. affecting all parts of the lobules, in part, or usually the whole, of the lungs, and usually associated with α$_1$-antiprotease deficiency e. SYN diffuse e., generalized e., panacinar e.

paraseptal e., e. involving the periphery of the pulmonary lobules.

pulmonary e., SYN emphysema (2).

senile e., e. consequent upon the physiologic atrophy of old age.

subcutaneous e., the presence of air or gas in the subcutaneous tissues. SYN aerodermectasia, cutaneous e., pneumoderma, pneumohypoderma.

subgaleal e., collection of air or gas between the inner layer of the scalp and the cranium.

surgical e., subcutaneous e. from air trapped in the tissues by an operation or injury.

unilateral lobar e., a state in which the roentgenographic density of one lung (or one lobe) is markedly less than the density of the other(s) because of the presence of air trapped during expiration. SYN Macleod's syndrome, Swyer-James syndrome (1).

em·phy·sem·a·tous (em-fi-sem'ă-tŭs). Relating to or affected with emphysema.

em·pir·ic (em-pir'ik). **1.** SYN empirical. **2.** A member of a school of Graeco-Roman physicians, late B.C. to early A.D., who placed their confidence in and based their practice purely on experience, avoiding all speculation, theory, or abstract reasoning; they were little concerned with causes or with correlating symptoms in order to gain a true understanding of a disease, even holding basic knowledge, physiology, pathology, and anatomy in low esteem and of no value in practice. **3.** Modern: testing a hypothesis by careful observation, hence rationally based on experience. [see empirical]

em·pir·i·cal (em-pir'i-kăl). **1.** Founded on practical experience, rather than on reasoning alone, but not proved scientifically, in contrast to rational (1). **2.** Relating to an empiric (2). **3.** Based on careful observational testing of a hypothesis; rational. SYN empiric (1). [G. *empeirikos; fr. empeiria,* experience, fr. *en,* in, + *peira,* a trial]

em·pir·i·cism (em-pir'ĭ-sizm). A looking to experience as a guide to practice or to the therapeutic use of any remedy.

em·pros·thot·o·nos (em'pros-thot'ŏ-nŭs). A tetanic contraction of the flexor muscles, curving the back with concavity forward. SYN tetanus anticus. [G. *emprosthen,* forward, + *tonos,* tension]

em·py·ec·to·my (em-pī-ek'tō-mē). Resection of the empyema and its capsule.

em·py·e·ma (em-pī-ē'mă, -pi-ē'mă). Pus in a body cavity; when used without qualification, refers specifically to pyothorax. [G. *empyēma,* suppuration, fr. *en,* in, + *pyon,* pus]

e. artic'uli, obsolete term for suppurative *arthritis.*

e. benig'num, SYN latent e.

e. of gallbladder, severe acute cholecystitis with purulent inflammation of the gallbladder.

latent e., the presence of pus in a cavity, especially one of the accessory sinuses, unattended by subjective symptoms. SYN e. benignum.

loculated e., pyothorax in which pleural adhesions form one or more pockets containing pus.

mastoid e., SYN mastoiditis.

e. necessita'tis, a form of pyothorax in which the pus burrows to the outside, producing a subcutaneous abscess which finally ruptures; it may result in spontaneous recovery without requiring an operation.

e. of the pericardium, SYN pyopericardium.

pneumococcal e., infection of the pleural cavity by *Streptococcus pneumoniae,* the pneumococcus, with pus formation.

pulsating e., a large, tense collection of pus in the pleural cavity through which the cardiac pulsations are transmitted to the chest wall.

streptococcal e., purulent exudation into the pleural cavity caused by infection with *Streptococcus hemolyticus.*

em·py·e·mic (em-pī-ē'mik). Relating to empyema.

em·py·e·sis (em-pī-ē'sis). A pustular eruption. [G. suppuration]

em·py·o·cele (em'pī-ō-sēl). A suppurating hydrocele; a collection of pus in the scrotum. [G. *en,* in, + *pyon,* pus, + *kēlē,* tumor]

em·py·reu·ma (em-pī-rū'mă). Characteristic odor given off by organic substances when charred or subjected to destructive distillation in closed vessels. [G. a banked fire]

emu Abbreviation for electromagnetic *unit.*

emul·gent (ē-mŭl'jent). Denoting a straining, extracting, or purifying process. [L. *e- mulgeo,* pp. *-mulsus,* to milk out, drain out]

emul·si·fi·er (ē-mŭl'si-fī-er). An agent, such as gum arabic or the yolk of an egg, used to make an emulsion of a fixed oil. Soaps, detergents, steroids, and proteins can act as emulsifiers; they stabilize 2-phase systems af oil and aqueous phases.

emul·si·fy (ē-mŭl'si-fī). To make in the form of an emulsion.

emul·sin (ē-mŭl'sin). **1.** A preparation, derived from almonds, that contains β-glucosidase. **2.** Sometimes used as a synonym for β-glucosidase.

emul·sion (ē-mŭl'shŭn). A system containing two immiscible liquids in which one is dispersed, in the form of very small globules (internal phase), throughout the other (external phase) (*e.g.,* oil in water (milk) or water in oil (mayonnaise)). [Mod. L. fr. *e-mulgeo,* pp. *-mulsus,* to milk or drain out]

emul·sive (ē-mŭl'siv). **1.** Denoting a substance that can be made into an emulsion. **2.** Denoting a substance, such as a mucilage, by which a fat or resin can be emulsified. **3.** Making soft or pliant. **4.** Yielding a fixed oil on pressure.

emul·soid (ē-mŭl'soyd). A colloidal dispersion in which the dispersed particles are more or less liquid and exert a certain attraction on and absorb a certain quantity of the fluid in which they are suspended. SYN emulsion colloid, hydrophil colloid, hydrophilic colloid, lyophilic colloid.

em·u·re·sis (em-yū-rē'sis). A condition in which urinary excretion and intake of water act to produce an absolute hydration of the body. SEE ALSO ecuresis. [G. *en (em),* in, + *ourēsis,* urination]

emyl·ca·mate (ĕ-mil'kă-māt, em-il-kam'āt). 1-Ethyl-1-methyl-

propyl carbamate; a mild sedative, used to control tension and anxiety and to relieve pain and muscular spasm.

△**en-.** In; appears as em- before b, p, or m. [G.]

en·al·a·pril·at (ē-nal'ă-pril-āt). The active metabolite of enalapril, an ACE inhibitor used to treat hypertension and congestive heart failure.

enal·a·pril ma·le·ate (e-nal'ă-pril). L-Proline, 1-[*N*-[1-(ethoxycarbonyl)-3-phenylpropyl]-L-alanyl]-,(*S*)-, (*Z*)-2-butenedioate (1:1); a prodrug for enalaprilat, an angiotensin converting enzyme inhibitor used as an anti-hypertensive agent.

enam·el (ē-nam'ĕl). The hard glistening substance covering the exposed portion of the tooth. In its mature form, it is composed of an inorganic portion made up of 90% hydroxyapatite and 6-8% calcium carbonate, calcium fluoride, and magnesium carbonate, the remainder comprising an organic matrix of protein and glycoprotein; structurally, it is made up of oriented rods each of which consists of a stack of rodlets encased in an organic prism sheath. SYN enamelum [NA], substantia adamantina, substantia vitrea. [M.E., fr. Fr. *enamailer,* to apply enamel, fr. *en,* on, + *amail,* enamel, fr. Germanic]

dwarfed e., SYN nanoid e.

mottled e., alterations in e. structure due to excessive fluoride ingestion during tooth formation; varies in appearance from small white opacities to yellow and black spotting.

nanoid e., a condition of abnormal thinness of the e. SYN dwarfed e.

whorled e., e. in which the rods assume a spiral or twisting course.

enam·el·o·blast (en-am'el-ō-blast). SYN ameloblast.

enam·el·o·gen·e·sis (ē-nam'ĕl-ō-jen'ĕ-sis). SYN amelogenesis.

e. imperfec'ta, SYN *amelogenesis* imperfecta.

enam·el·o·ma (ē-nam-ĕl-ō'mă). A developmental anomaly in which there is a small nodule of enamel below the cementoenamel junction, usually at the bifurcation of molar teeth. SYN enamel drop, enamel nodule, enamel pearl.

enam·e·lum (ē-nam'ĕ-lŭm) [NA]. SYN enamel.

enan·thal (ē-nan'thăl). SYN heptanal.

enan·thate (e-nan'thāt). USAN-approved contraction for heptanoate, $CH_3(CH_2)_5COO^-$.

en·an·them, en·an·the·ma (en-an'them, en-an-thē'mă). A mucous membrane eruption, especially one occurring in connection with one of the exanthemas. [G. *en,* in, + *anthēma,* bloom, eruption, fr. *antheō,* to bloom]

en·an·them·a·tous (en-an-them'ă-tŭs). Relating to an enanthem.

en·an·the·sis (en-an-thē'sis). The skin eruption of a general disease, such as scarlatina or typhoid fever. [G. *en,* in, + *anthēsis,* full bloom]

△**enantio-.** Combining form meaning opposite, opposed, or opposing. [G. *enantios,* opposite]

en·an·ti·o·mer (ē-nan'tē-ō-mer). One of a pair of molecules that are nonsuperimposable mirror images of each other; neither molecule has an internal plane of symmetry. SYN antimer, optical antipode. [enantio- + G. *meros,* part]

en·an·ti·o·mer·ic (ē-nan'tē-ō-mer'ik). Pertaining to enantiomerism.

en·an·ti·om·er·ism (ē-nan-tē-om'er-izm). In chemistry, isomerism in which the molecules in their configuration are related to one another like an object and its mirror image (enantiomers), and consequently are not superimposable; e. entails optical activity, both enantiomers rotating the plane of polarized light equally, but in opposite directions.

en·an·ti·o·morph (ē-nan'tē-ō-mōrf). An enantiomer in crystal form.

en·an·ti·o·mor·phic (ē-nan'tē-ō-mōr'fik). **1.** Relating to two objects, each of which is the mirror image of the other. **2.** In chemistry, relating to isomers, the optical activities of which are equal in magnitude but opposite in sign. SYN enantiomorphous. [enantio- + G. *morphē,* form]

en·an·ti·o·mor·phism (ē-nan'tē-ō-mōr'fizm). The relation of two objects similar in form but not superimposable, as the two hands or an object and its mirror image. [enantio- + G. *morphē*, form]

en·an·ti·o·mor·phous (ē-nan'tē-ō-mōr'fŭs). SYN enantiomorphic.

en·ar·thro·di·al (en-ar-thrō'dē-al). Relating to an enarthrosis.

en·ar·thro·sis (en-ar-thrō'sis). SYN ball-and-socket *joint*. [G. *en-arthrōsis*, a jointing where the ball is deep set in the socket]

en bloc (ăhn blok). In a lump; as a whole; used to refer to autopsy techniques in which visceral organs are removed in large blocks allowing the prosector to retain a continuity in organ architecture during the subsequent dissection. [Fr., in a lump]

en·cai·nide hy·dro·chlo·ride (en-kā'nīd). Benzamide, 4-methoxy-*N*-[2-[2-(1-methyl-2-piperidinyl)ethyl]phenyl]-, monohydrochloride, (±)-; an anti-arrhythmic.

en·cap·su·lat·ed (en-kap'sū-lā-ted). Enclosed in a capsule or sheath. SYN encapsuled.

en·cap·su·la·tion (en-kap-sū-lā'shŭn). Enclosure in a capsule or sheath. [L. *in* + capsula, dim. of *capsa*, box]

en·cap·suled (en-kap'sŭld). SYN encapsulated.

en·car·di·tis (en-kar-dī'tis). SYN endocarditis.

en·ca·tar·rha·phy (en-kă-tar'ră-fē). Obsolete term for the artificial implantation of an organ or tissue in a part where it does not naturally occur. [G. *enkatarrhaptō*, to sew in]

en·ce·li·tis, en·ce·li·i·tis (en-sē-lī'tis, -lē-ī'tis). Inflammation of any of the abdominal viscera. [G. *en*, in, + *koilia*, belly, + *-itis*, inflammation]

△**encephal-**. SEE encephalo-.

en·ceph·a·lal·gia (en-sef-ă-lal'jē-ă). SYN headache. [encephalo- + G. *algos*, pain]

en·ceph·a·la·tro·phic (en-sef-ă-lă-trof'ik). Relating to encephalatrophy.

en·ceph·a·lat·ro·phy (en-sef-ă-lat'rō-fē). Atrophy of the brain. [encephalo- + G. *a-* priv. + *trophē*, nourishment]

en·ceph·a·lauxe (en-sef-ă-lawk'sē). Hypertrophy of the brain. [encephalo- + G. *auxē*, increase]

en·céph·ale iso·lé (ahn-sef-al' ē-sō-lā'). An animal with its caudal medulla transected and its respiration maintained artificially; it remains alert, has sleep-wake cycles, normal pupillary reactions, and a normal electroencephalogram. Cf. cerveau isolé. [Fr. isolated brain]

en·ceph·a·le·mia (en-sef-ă-lē'mē-ă). SYN brain congestion. [encephalo- + G. *haima*, blood]

en·ce·phal·ic (en'se-fal'ik). Relating to the brain, or to the structures within the cranium.

en·ceph·a·lit·ic (en-sef-ă-lit'ik). Relating to encephalitis.

en·ceph·a·li·tis, pl. **en·ceph·a·lit·i·des** (en-sef-ă-lī'tis, en-sef-ă-lit'i-dēz). Inflammation of the brain. SYN cephalitis. [G. *enkephalos*, brain, + *-itis*, inflammation]

acute hemorrhagic e., e. of apoplectoid character due to blood extravasation. SYN e. hemorrhagica.

acute inclusion body e., SYN herpes simplex e.

acute necrotizing e., an acute form of e., characterized by destruction of brain parenchyme.

Australian X e., SYN Murray Valley e.

bacterial e., e. of bacterial etiology. SYN e. pyogenica, purulent e., suppurative e.

bunyavirus e., e. of abrupt onset, with severe frontal headache and low-grade to moderate fever, caused by members of the genus *Bunyavirus* (Bunyaviridae family); infections also occur in rodents, lagomorphs, and domestic animals. SYN California e.

California e., SYN bunyavirus e.

Coxsackie e., a viral e., seen mainly in infants and involving principally the gray matter of the medulla and cord, caused by *Enterovirus* Coxsackie B.

Dawson's e., SYN subacute sclerosing *panencephalitis*.

epidemic e., a viral e. occurring epidemically, such as in Japanese B e., St. Louis e., and lethargic e.

equine e., SYN equine *encephalomyelitis*.

experimental allergic e. (EAE), SYN experimental allergic *encephalomyelitis*.

Far East Russian e., tick-borne e. (Eastern subtype).

fox e., e. in foxes, caused by the infectious canine hepatitis virus, a member of the family Adenoviridae family, and characterized by paralysis and death.

e. hemorrhag'ica, SYN acute hemorrhagic e.

herpes e., SYN herpes simplex e.

herpes simplex e., the most common acute encephalitis, caused by HSV-1; affects persons of any age; preferentially involves the inferomedial portions of the temporal lobe and the orbital portions of the frontal lobes; pathologically, severe hemorrhagic necrosis is present along with, in the acute stages, intranuclear eosinophilic inclusion bodies in the neurons and glial cells. SYN acute inclusion body e., herpes e.

hyperergic e., e. as a result of an immunologic allergic reaction of the nervous system to antigenic stimuli.

Ilhéus e., an e. caused by the Ilhéus virus (genus *Flavivirus*) and endemic to eastern Brazil and other parts of South and Central America; transmitted by mosquitoes.

inclusion body e., SYN subacute sclerosing *panencephalitis*.

Japanese B e., an epidemic e. or encephalomyelitis of Japan, Siberian Russia, and other parts of Asia; due to the Japanese B e. virus (genus *Flavivirus*) and transmitted by mosquitoes; can occur as a symptomless, subclinical infection but may cause an acute meningoencephalomyelitis. SYN e. japonica, Russian autumn e.

e. japon'ica, SYN Japanese B e.

lead e., SYN lead *encephalopathy*.

e. lethar'gica, SYN von Economo's *disease*.

Mengo e., an e. occurring in Africa, due to the Mengo strain of encephalomyocarditis virus, a member of the Picornaviridae.

Murray Valley e., a severe e. with a high mortality rate occurring in the Murray Valley of Australia; the disease is most severe in children and is characterized by headache, fever, malaise, drowsiness or convulsions, and rigidity of the neck; extensive brain damage may result; it is caused by the Murray Valley encephalitis virus (genus *Flavivirus*). SYN Australian X disease, Australian X e.

necrotizing e., any e. in which extensive brain necrosis occurs, *e.g.*, acute necrotizing hemorrhagic encephalomyelitis.

e. neonato'rum, e. of the newborn, described by R. Virchow as marked by the presence of fat-laden cells in the brain.

opossum e., e. of opossum caused by *Chlamydia psittaci*.

e. periaxia'lis concen'trica, e. that is clinically similar to adrenoleukodystrophy, but pathologically characterized by concentric globes or circles of demyelination of cerebral white matter separated by normal tissue. SYN Baló's disease.

encephalitis periaxialis diffusa, SYN Schilder's *disease*.

postvaccinal e., SYN postvaccinal *encephalomyelitis*.

Powassan e., an acute disease of children varying clinically from undifferentiated febrile illness to e.; caused by the Powassan virus, a member of the Flaviviridae family, and transmitted by ixodid ticks; most frequently seen in Canada.

purulent e., SYN bacterial e.

e. pyogen'ica, SYN bacterial e.

Russian autumn e., SYN Japanese B e.

Russian spring-summer e. (Eastern subtype), a tick-borne e. virus belonging to the family Flaviviridae.

Russian spring-summer e. (Western subtype), SYN tick-borne e. (Central European subtype).

Russian tick-borne e., SYN tick-borne e. (Eastern subtype).

secondary e., collective term for post-infectious, post-exanthem, and post-vaccinal encephalitides.

subacute inclusion body e., SYN subacute sclerosing *panencephalitis*.

e. subcortical'is chron'ica, SYN Binswanger's *disease*.

suppurative e., SYN bacterial e.

tick-borne e. (Central European subtype), tick-borne meningoencephalitis caused by a flavivirus closely related to the virus causing the Far Eastern type; it is transmitted by *Ixodes ricinus*, also by infected raw milk, especially that of goats. SYN biundulant meningoencephalitis, Central European tick-borne fever, diphasic milk fever, Russian spring-summer e. (Western subtype).

tick-borne e. (Eastern subtype), a severe form of e. caused by a flavivirus, a virus belonging to the Flaviviridae family, and transmitted by ticks (*Ixodes pertulcatus* and *I. ricinus*). SYN Russian tick-borne e.

Van Bogaert e., SYN subacute sclerosing *panencephalitis.*

varicella e., e. occurring as a complication of chickenpox.

vernal e., tick-borne e. (Eastern subtype).

woodcutter's e., tick-borne e. (Eastern subtype).

en·ceph·a·li·to·gen (en-sef'ă-lī'tō-jen). An agent which evokes encephalitis, particularly with reference to the antigen which produces experimental allergic encephalomyelitis. [encephalitis + G. *-gen,* producing]

en·ceph·a·li·to·gen·ic (en-sef'ă-li-tō-jen'ik). Producing encephalitis; typically by hypersensitivity mechanisms. SEE encephalitogen.

En·ceph·a·li·to·zo·on (en-sef'ă-li-tō-zō'on). A genus of protozoan parasites, formerly considered part of the family Toxoplasmatidae, class Sporozoea, but now recognized as a member of the protozoan phylum Microspora, family Nosematidae. *E. cuniculi* is considered the primary microsporan parasite of mammals, commonly found in the brain and kidney tubules of rodents and carnivores and causing nosematosis in rabbits. [encephalitis + G. *zōon,* animal]

E. cuniculi, a common cryptic infection of most mammals and some birds, transmitted in urine-contaminated food and by transplacental transmission. Disseminated human infection has been reported among immunosuppressed individuals. Latent infection seen by serodiagnosis suggests widespread nonsymptomatic infection in tropical regions.

E. hellum, a species of E. described from human ophthalmic infections causing punctate keratopathy and corneal ulceration in AIDS patients.

en·ceph·a·li·za·tion (en-sef'ă-li-zā'shŭn). SYN corticalization.

encephalo-, encephal-. The brain. Cf. cerebro-. [G. *enkephalos,* brain]

en·ceph·a·lo·cele (en-sef'ă-lō-sēl). A congenital gap in the skull with herniation of brain substance. SYN craniocele, cranium bifidum, bifid cranium. [encephalo- + G. *kēlē,* hernia]

en·ceph·a·lo·cys·to·cele. SYN hydrencephalocele.

en·ceph·a·lo·dur·o·ar·te·ri·o·syn·an·gi·o·s (en-sef'a-lō-door-ō-ar-tēr'ē-ō-sin-anj-ē-ō'sis). SYN duraencephalosynangiosis.

en·ceph·a·lo·dyn·ia (en-sef'ă-lō-din'ē-ă). SYN headache. [encephalo- + G. *odynē,* pain]

en·ceph·a·lo·dys·pla·sia (en-sef'ă-lō-dis-plā'zē-ă). Any congenital abnormality of the brain. [encephalo- + G. *dys,* bad, + *plastos,* formed]

en·ceph·a·lo·gram (en-sef'ă-lō-gram). The record obtained by encephalography. [encephalo- + G. *gramma,* a drawing]

en·ceph·a·log·ra·phy (en-sef-ă-log'ră-fē). Radiographic representation of the brain. SEE pneumoencephalography. [encephalo- + G. *graphō,* to write]

gamma e., imaging of the encephalon by the administration of small amounts of gamma-emitting radionuclides; commonly called a brain scan; superseded by computed tomography and magnetic resonance imaging.

en·ceph·a·loid (en-sef'ă-loyd). Resembling brain substance; denoting a carcinoma of soft, brainlike consistency, with reference to gross features. [encephalo- + G. *eidos,* resemblance]

en·ceph·a·lo·lith (en-sef'ă-lō-lith). A concretion in the brain or one of its ventricles. SYN cerebral calculus. [encephalo- + G. *lithos,* stone]

en·ceph·a·lol·o·gy (en-sef-ă-lol'ō-jē). The branch of medicine dealing with the brain in all its relations. [encephalo- + G. *logos,* study]

en·ceph·a·lo·ma (en-sef-ă-lō'mă). Herniation of brain substance. SYN cerebroma.

en·ceph·a·lo·ma·la·cia (en-sef'ă-lō-mă-lā'shē-ă). Abnormal softness of the cerebral parenchyma often due to ischemia or infarction. SYN cerebromalacia. [encephalo- + G. *malakia,* softness]

nutritional e. of chicks, a disease of young chicks caused by vitamin E deficiency. SYN crazy chick disease.

en·ceph·a·lo·men·in·gi·tis (en-sef'ă-lō-men-in-jī'tis). SYN meningoencephalitis. [encephalo- + G. *mēninx,* membrane, + *-itis,* inflammation]

en·ceph·a·lo·me·nin·go·cele (en-sef'ă-lō-me-nin'gō-sēl). SYN meningoencephalocele. [encephalo- + G. *mēninx,* membrane, + *kēlē,* hernia]

en·ceph·a·lo·men·in·gop·a·thy (en-sef'ă-lō-men-in-gop'ă-thē). SYN meningoencephalopathy.

en·ceph·a·lo·mere (en-sef'ă-lō-mēr). A neuromere. [encephalo- + G. *meros,* a part]

en·ceph·a·lom·e·ter (en-sef-ă-lom'ĕ-ter). An apparatus for indicating on the skull the location of the cortical centers. [encephalo- + G. *metron,* measure]

en·ceph·a·lo·my·e·li·tis (en-sef-ă-lō-mī'ĕ-lī'tis). Inflammation of the brain and spinal cord. [encephalo- + G. *myelon,* marrow, + *-itis,* inflammation]

acute disseminated e., an acute demyelinating disorder of the central nervous system, in which focal demyelination is present throughout the brain and spinal cord. This process is common to postinfectious, postexanthem, and postvaccinal encephalomyelitis.

acute necrotizing hemorrhagic e., a fulminating demyelinating disorder of the central nervous system that affects mainly children and young adults. Almost always preceded by a respiratory infection, characterized by the abrupt onset of fever, headache, confusion, and nuchal rigidity, soon followed by focal seizures, hemiplegia, or quadriplegia, brainstem findings, and coma; the CSF shows evidence of an inflammatory process; due to the massive destruction of the white matter of one or both hemispheres, often accompanied by similar destruction of the white matter of the brainstem and cerebellar peduncles; of unknown etiology. SYN acute hemorrhagic leukoencephalitis, acute necrotizing hemorrhagic leukoencephalitis.

e. associated with carcinoma, SYN paraneoplastic *encephalomyelopathy.*

avian infectious e., a disease of very young chicks caused by a picornavirus and characterized by tremor, ataxia, somnolence, and finally death. SYN epidemic tremor.

benign myalgic e., SYN epidemic *neuromyasthenia.*

bovine sporadic e., an acute, septic e., pleuritis, and peritonitis of cattle caused by *Chlamydia psittaci;* it occurs in the north central United States. SYN Buss disease.

caprine arthritis-e. (CAE), a worldwide disease of goats caused by the caprine e. virus; two syndromes are recognized, encephalomyelitis in kids and more commonly arthritis in adults.

eastern equine e. (EEE), a form of mosquito-borne equine e. seen in the eastern U.S. and caused by the eastern equine e. virus, a species of *Alphavirus,* which belongs to the family Togaviridae; initial fever and viremia are followed by signs of central nervous system involvement (excitement, then somnolence, paralysis, and death); the incidence of clinical infection in man is low but case fatality may be high.

enzootic e., SYN Borna *disease.*

epidemic myalgic e., SYN epidemic *neuromyasthenia.*

equine e., an acute, often fatal, virus disease of horses and mules transmitted by mosquitoes and characterized by central nervous system disturbances; in the U.S., this disease is typically caused by one of two arthropod-borne viruses, and their resulting diseases are designated western equine or eastern equine e.; these viruses belong to the family Togaviridae and can also cause neurologic disease in humans. SYN equine encephalitis.

experimental allergic e., a demyelinating allergic e. produced by the injection of brain tissue, usually with an adjuvant. SYN experimental allergic encephalitis.

granulomatous e., an e. in which granulomas occur.

herpes B e., a frequently lethal disease of humans caused by infection with a normally latent monkey herpesvirus.

infectious porcine e., SYN Teschen *disease.*

mouse e., e. due to the mouse encephalomyelitis virus (a species of *Enterovirus*) which is not pathogenic in monkeys or in man,

en

but attacks mouse colonies and causes a flaccid paralysis, usually of the hind limbs. SYN mouse poliomyelitis, Theiler's disease (1).

postvaccinal e., a severe type of encephalomyelitis that can follow the rabies vaccination. SYN postvaccinal encephalitis.

sporadic bovine e., a disease of cattle caused by the bacterium *Chlamydia psittaci* and characterized by fever, depression, excessive salivation, diarrhea, anorexia, and incoordination.

Venezuelan equine e. (VEE), a form of mosquito-borne equine e. found in parts of South America, Panama, and Trinidad, caused by the Venezuelan equine e. virus (a species of *Alphavirus* in the family Togaviridae), and characterized by less central nervous system involvement than occurs in either eastern or western equine e.; fever, diarrhea, and depression are common; in man, there is fever and severe headache after an incubation period of 2 to 5 days, and in a few cases there has been central nervous system involvement.

viral e., virus e., an e. due to a neurotropic virus.

western equine e. (WEE), an equine e. found in the western U.S. and parts of South America, transmitted by mosquitoes and caused by the western equine e. virus (a species of *Alphavirus* in the family Togaviridae); the infection is similar to but milder than eastern equine e. in man and is, as a rule, inapparent, but some cases with central nervous system involvement have been fatal.

zoster e., inflammation of the brain and spinal cord caused by varicella-zoster virus, a member of the family Herpesviridae.

en·ceph·a·lo·my·e·lo·cele (en-sef′ă-lō-mī′ĕ-lō-sēl). Congenital defect usually in the occipital region (foramen magnum) and cervical vertebrae, with herniation of the meninges, medulla, and spinal cord. [G. *enkephalos,* brain, + *myelon,* marrow, + *kēlē,* hernia]

en·ceph·a·lo·my·e·lo·neu·rop·a·thy (en-sef′ă-lō-mī′ĕ-lō-nū-rop′ă-thē). A disease involving the brain, spinal cord, and peripheral nerves.

en·ceph·a·lo·my·e·lop·a·thy (en-sef′ă-lō-mī-ĕ-lop′ă-thē). Any disease of both brain and spinal cord. [G. *enkephalos,* brain, + *myelon,* marrow, + *pathos,* suffering]

carcinomatous e., SYN paraneoplastic e.

epidemic myalgic e., a disease superficially resembling poliomyelitis, characterized by diffuse involvement of the nervous system associated with myalgia.

necrotizing e. [MIM*256000], SYN Leigh's *disease.*

paracarcinomatous e., SYN paraneoplastic e.

paraneoplastic e., an encephalomyelopathy as a remote effect of carcinoma, most often oat cell carcinoma of the lung; characterized by extensive nerve cell loss, which may be diffuse, but often predominates in particular portions of the central nervous system, particularly the limbic lobes, medulla, cerebellum, and gray matter of the spinal cord. SYN carcinomatous e., encephalomyelitis associated with carcinoma, paracarcinomatous e.

subacute necrotizing e. (SNE), a rare fatal disorder, primarily of children, being both acute and chronic in onset, manifested primarily as brainstem dysfunction, with ataxia, cranial nerve palsies, pseudobulbar palsy, hemi- or quadriplegia, mental deterioration, and involuntary movements; deficiencies of pyruvate dehydrogenase or cytochrome C oxydase have been found in some patients; pathologically, there is widespread symmetric necrosis involving much of the brainstem; these changes are similar to those seen with Wernicke encephalopathy.

en·ceph·a·lo·my·e·lo·ra·dic·u·li·tis (en-sef′ă-lō-mī′ĕ-lō-ră-dik′yū-lī-tis). SYN encephalomyeloradiculopathy.

en·ceph·a·lo·my·e·lo·ra·dic·u·lop·a·thy (en-sef′ă-lō-mī′ĕ-lō-ră-dik′yū-lop-ă-thē). A disease process involving the brain, spinal cord, and spinal roots. SYN encephalomyeloradiculitis.

en·ceph·a·lo·my·o·car·di·tis (en-sef′ă-lō-mī′ō-kar-dī′tis). Associated encephalitis and myocarditis; often caused by a viral infection such as in polio myelitis.

en·ceph·a·lon, pl. **en·ceph·a·la** (en-sef′ă-lon, lă) [NA]. That portion of the cerebrospinal axis contained within the cranium, comprised of the prosencephalon, mesencephalon, and rhombencephalon. [G. *enkephalos,* brain, fr. *en,* in, + *kephalē,* head]

en·ceph·a·lo·nar·co·sis (en-sef′ă-lō-nar-kō′sis). Stupor brought on by a brain disease.

en·ceph·a·lo·path·ia (en-sef′ă-lō-path′ē-ă). SYN encephalopathy.

e. addiso′nia, reversible disturbance in mentation, occurring in the course of Addison's disease, probably related to electrolyte imbalance.

en·ceph·a·lop·a·thy (en-sef′ă-lop′ă-thē). Any disorder of the brain. SYN cephalopathy, cerebropathia, cerebropathy, encephalopathia, encephalosis. [encephalo- + G. *pathos,* suffering]

bilirubin e., SYN kernicterus.

Binswanger's e., SYN Binswanger's *disease.*

bovine spongiform e. (BSE), a new disease of cattle, first reported in 1986 in Great Britain, characterized clinically by apprehensive behavior, hyperesthesia, and ataxia and histopathologically by spongiform changes in the gray-matter neuropil of the brain stem; it is thought to be caused by an agent, possibly a prion, similar to that observed as the cause of scrapie. SYN mad cow disease.

demyelinating e., extensive idiopathic loss of myelin sheaths in the brain, as occurs in leukodystrophy.

hepatic e., SYN portal-systemic e.

HIV encephalopathy, SYN AIDS dementia *complex.*

hypernatremic e., subarachnoid and subdural effusions in infants with hypernatremic dehydration.

hypertensive e., a metabolic e. caused by diffuse cerebral edema; follows an abrupt elevation of blood pressure in a long-term hypertensive patient.

hypoxic-hypercarbic e., SYN hypoventilation *coma.*

lead e., a metabolic e., caused by the ingestion of lead compounds and seen particularly in early childhood; it is characterized pathologically by extensive cerebral edema, status spongiosus, neurocytolysis, and some reactive inflammation; clinical manifestations include convulsions, delirium, and hallucinations. SEE ALSO lead *poisoning.* SYN lead encephalitis, saturnine e.

metabolic e., e. characterized by memory loss, vertigo, and generalized weakness, due to metabolic brain disease including hypoxia, ischemia, hypoglycemia, or secondary to other organ failure such as liver or kidney.

necrotizing e., SYN Leigh's *disease.*

palindromic e., a relatively mild form which tends to recur.

pancreatic e., a metabolic e. associated with extensive pancreatic necrosis.

portal-systemic e., an e. associated with cirrhosis of the liver, attributed to the passage of toxic nitrogenous substances from the portal to the systemic circulation; cerebral manifestations may include coma. SYN hepatic e.

progressive subcortical e., SYN progressive multifocal *leukoencephalopathy.*

pulmonary e., SYN hypoventilation *coma.*

recurrent e. [MIM*130950], a progressive form of e. occurring in young members of the same family; characterized by headache, vertigo, truncal ataxia, drowsiness and stupor, speech impairments, choreic-athetoid movements, and sometimes convulsions.

saturnine e., SYN lead e.

severe postanoxic e., SYN delayed *coma* after hypoxia.

spongiform e., an e. characterized by vacuolation within nerve and glial cells.

subacute spongiform e., a form of spongiform e. that is associated with a "slow virus", which to date has not been adequately described, is transmissible, and has a rapidly progressive, fatal course; e.g., Creutzfeldt-Jakob disease, kuru, Gerstmann-Sträussler syndrome, scrapie. SEE prion.

subcortical arteriosclerotic e., SYN Binswanger's *disease.*

thyrotoxic e., a metabolic e. arising in severe cases of thyrotoxicosis.

transmissible mink e., a transmissible disease in mink caused by an agent similar to that observed as a cause of scrapie in sheep.

traumatic e., an e. resulting from structural brain injury.

traumatic progressive e., chronic progressive brain damage resulting from multiple brain injuries, *e.g.,* dementia pugilistica.

Wernicke-Korsakoff e., SEE Wernicke's *syndrome,* Korsakoff's *syndrome.*

Wernicke's e., SYN Wernicke's *syndrome.*

en·ceph·a·lop·sy (en-sef′ă-lop-sē). The association of special colors with words or other sensory data. [encephalo- + G. *opsis,* sight]

en·ceph·a·lo·py·o·sis (en-sef′ă-lō-pī-ō′sis). Archaic term for purulent inflammation of the brain. [encephalo- + G. *pyōsis,* suppuration]

en·ceph·a·lor·rha·chid·i·an (en-sef′ă-lō-ră-kid′ē-an). SYN cerebrospinal. [encephalo- + G. *rhachis,* spine]

en·ceph·a·lor·rha·gia (en-sef′ă-lō-rā′jē-ă). Archaic term for cerebral *hemorrhage.* [encephalo- + G. *rhēgnymi,* to burst forth]

en·ceph·a·los·chi·sis (en-sef-ă-los′ki-sis). Developmental failure of closure of the rostral part of the neural tube. [encephalo- + G. *schisis,* fissure]

en·ceph·a·lo·scle·ro·sis (en-sef′ă-lō-sklēr-o′sis). A sclerosis, or hardening, of the brain. SEE ALSO cerebrosclerosis. [encephalo- + G. *sklērōsis,* hardening]

en·ceph·a·lo·scope (en-sef′ă-lō-skōp). Any instrument used to view the interior of a brain abscess or other cerebral cavity through an opening in the skull. [encephalo- + G. *skopeō,* to view]

en·ceph·a·los·co·py (en-sef-ă-los′kŏ-pē). Examination of the brain or the cavity of a cerebral abscess by direct inspection.

en·ceph·a·lo·sis. SYN encephalopathy.

equine e., a disease of horses, caused by the equine e. virus and characterized by peracute death preceded by alternating periods of hyperexcitement and depression; only reported from South Africa.

en·ceph·a·lo·spi·nal (en-sef′ă-lō-spī′năl). SYN cerebrospinal.

en·ceph·a·lo·thlip·sis (en-sef′ă-lō-thlip′sis). Compression of the brain. [encephalo- + G. *thlipsis,* pressure]

en·ceph·a·lo·tome (en-sef′ă-lō-tōm). An instrument for use in performing encephalotomy.

en·ceph·a·lot·o·my (en-sef-ă-lot′ō-mē). Dissection or incision of the brain. [encephalo- + G. *tomē,* incision]

en·chon·dral (en-kon′drăl). SYN intracartilaginous.

en·chon·dro·ma (en-kon-drō′mă). A benign cartilaginous growth starting within the medullary cavity of a bone originally formed from cartilage; e.'s may distend the cortex, especially of small bones, and may be solitary or multiple (endochondromatosis). [Mod. L. fr. G. *en,* in, + *chondros,* cartilage, + *-oma,* tumor]

en·chon·dro·ma·to·sis (en-kon′drō-ma-tō′sis) [MIM*166000]. A rarely familial, and probably hamartomatous proliferation of cartilage in the metaphyses of several bones, most commonly of the hands and feet, causing distorted growth in length or pathological fractures; chondrosarcoma frequently develops. When combined with hemangiomas in the cutaneous or visceral regions, called Maffucci's *syndrome.* The pattern of inheritance is like that of an irregular autosomal dominant. SYN asymmetrical chondrodystrophy, dyschondroplasia, hereditary deforming chondrodystrophy (2), Ollier's disease.

en·chon·drom·a·tous (en-kon-drō′mă-tŭs). Relating to or having the elements of enchondroma.

en·chon·dro·sar·co·ma (en-kon′drō-sar-kō′mă). Obsolete term for a malignant neoplasm of cartilage cells derived from an enchondroma, as may occur in enchondromatosis.

en·clave (en-klāv, ahn-klahv′). An enclosure; a detached mass of tissue enclosed in tissue of another kind; seen especially in the case of isolated masses of gland tissue detached from the main gland. [Fr. fr. L. *clavis,* key]

en·cod·ing (en-kōd′ing). The first stage in the memory process, followed by storage and retrieval, involving processes associated with receiving or briefly registering stimuli through one or more of the senses and modifying that information; a decay process or loss of this information (a type of forgetting) occurs rapidly unless the next two stages, storage and retrieval, are activated.

en·cop·re·sis (en-kō-prē′sis). The repeated, generally involuntary passage of feces into inappropriate places (*e.g.,* clothing);

considered a mental disorder if it occurs in a child more than 4 years old. [G. *enkopros,* full of manure]

en·cra·ni·al (en-krā′nē-ăl). SYN endocranial.

en·cra·ni·us (en-krā′nē-ŭs). In conjoined twins, a form of fetal inclusion in which the smaller parasite lies partly or wholly within the cranial cavity of the larger autosite. [G. *en,* in, + *kranion,* skull]

encu Acronym for *e*quivalent *n*ormal *c*hild *u*nit, an amount of information from any source (linkage analysis, parental, and collateral phenotypes, biochemistry of the carrier state, etc.) that will have the same impact on the probability as one usual progeny does that a consultand is a carrier for an autosomal dominant trait; *e.g.,* each normal child contributes one encu. Cf. ensu.

en·cyst·ed (en-sis′ted). Encapsulated by a membranous bag. [G. *kystis,* bladder]

en·cyst·ment (en-sist′ment). The condition of being or becoming encysted.

end. An extremity, or the most remote point of an extremity.
acromial e. of clavicle, SYN acromial *extremity* of clavicle.
distal e., the posterior extremity of a dental appliance. SYN heel (2).
sternal e. of clavicle, SYN sternal *extremity* of clavicle.

△ **end-.** SEE endo-.

end·a·del·phos (end′ā-del′fos). Unequal conjoined twins in which the parasitic member is included in the body of the host. [end- + G. *adelphos,* brother]

End·a·moe·ba (end′ă-mē′bă). A genus of amebae parasitic in invertebrates; originally described from cockroaches. [endo- + G. *amoibē,* change]

end·an·gi·i·tis, end·an·ge·i·tis (end-an-jē-ī′tis). Inflammation of the intima of a blood vessel. SYN endoangiitis, endovasculitis. [endo- + G. *angeion,* vessel, + *-itis,* inflammation]

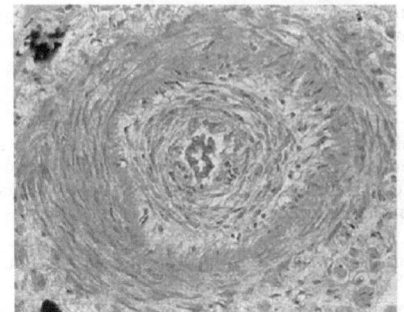
endangiitis
note narrowing of lumen of vessel by fibrous thickening

e. oblit′erans, inflammation of the intima of a vessel with resulting occlusion of its lumen.

end·a·or·ti·tis (end′ā-ōr-tī′tis). Inflammation of the intima of the aorta. SYN endo-aortitis.

end·ar·ter·ec·to·my (end-ar-ter-ek′tō-mē). Excision of diseased endothelial and media or most of the media of an artery, and also of occluding atheromatous deposits, so as to leave a smooth lining, mostly consisting of adventitia. [endo- + artery + G. *ektomē,* excision]
carotid e., excision of occluding material, including intima and most of the media, from the carotid a.
coronary e., excision of occluding material, including intima and most of the media, from the coronary artery.

end·ar·te·ri·tis (end′ar-ter-ī′tis). Inflammation of the intima of an artery. SYN endoarteritis.
bacterial e., implantation and growth of bacteria with formation of vegetations on the arterial wall, such as may occur in a patent ductus arteriosus or arteriovenous fistula.
e. defor′mans, e. with atheromatous patches and calcareous deposits.

e. oblit′erans, obliterating e., an extreme degree of e. proliferans closing the lumen of the artery. SYN arteritis obliterans, obliterating arteritis.

e. prolif′erans, proliferating e., chronic e. accompanied by a marked increase of fibrous tissue in the intima.

end·au·ral (end-aw′răl). Within the ear. [endo- + L. *auris*, ear]

end·brain. SYN telencephalon.

end·brush (end′brŭsh). SYN telodendron.

end·bulb. SEE end *bulb.*

end-di·a·stol·ic (end′dī-ă-stol′ik). **1.** Occurring at the end of diastole, immediately before the next systole, as in end-diastolic pressure. **2.** Interrupting the final moments of diastole, barely premature, as in end-diastolic extrasystole.

en·de·mia (en-dē′mē-ă). Rarely used term for an endemic disease.

en·dem·ic (en-dem′ik). **1.** Present in a community or among a group of people; said of a disease prevailing continually in a region. Cf. epidemic, sporadic. **2.** SYN enzootic. [G. *endēmos,* native, fr. *en,* in, + *dēmos,* the people]

en·dem·o·ep·i·dem·ic (en-dem′ō-ep-i-dem′ik). Denoting a temporary large increase in the number of cases of an endemic disease.

end·er·gon·ic (en-der-gon′ik). Referring to a chemical reaction that takes place with absorption of energy from its surroundings (*i.e.,* a positive change in Gibbs free energy). Cf. exergonic. [endo- + G. *ergon,* work]

en·der·mic, en·der·mat·ic (en-der′mik, en-der-mat′ik). In or through the skin; denoting a method of treatment, as by inunction; the remedy produces its constitutional effect when absorbed through the skin surface to which it is applied. [G. *en,* in, + *derma* (*dermat-*), skin]

en·der·mism (en-der′mizm). Treatment with endermic medication.

en·der·mo·sis (en-der-mō′sis). Any eruptive disease of the mucous membrane.

end-feet. SYN axon *terminals,* under *terminal.*

end-gut. SYN hindgut.

end·ing. 1. A termination or conclusion. **2.** A nerve e.

annulospiral e., one of two types of sensory nerve e. associated with a neuromuscular spindle (the other being the flower-spray e.); after entering the muscle spindle, the fiber divides into two flat ribbon-like branches that wind themselves in rings or spirals about the intrafusal muscle fibers. SYN annulospiral organ.

calyciform e., caliciform e., a synaptic e. in relation to certain neuroepithelial hair cells of the inner ear.

epilemmal e., a nerve e. in close relation to the outer surface of the sarcolemma.

flower-spray e., one of the two types of sensory nerve e. associated with the neuromuscular spindle (the other being the annulospiral e.); in this type, the fiber branches spread out upon the surface of the intrafusal fibers like a spray of flowers. SYN flower-spray organ of Ruffini.

free nerve e.'s, a form of peripheral ending of sensory nerve fibers in which the terminal filaments end freely in the tissue. SYN terminationes nervorum liberae [NA].

grape e.'s, an autodescriptive term applied to synaptic terminals at the ends of short, stalklike axon branches.

hederiform e., a type of free sensory ending in the skin.

nerve e., any one of the specialized terminations of peripheral sensory or motor nerve fibers. SEE motor *endplate,* corpuscle, bulb.

sole-plate e., SYN motor *endplate.*

synaptic e.'s, SYN axon *terminals,* under *terminal.*

Endo, Shigeru, Japanese bacteriologist, 1869–1937. SEE E. *agar;* E.'s fuchsin *agar, medium.*

endo-, end-. Prefixes indicating within, inner, absorbing, or containing. SEE ALSO ento-. [G. *endon,* within]

en·do·ab·dom·i·nal (en′dō-ab-dom′i-năl). Within the abdomen.

en·do·am·y·lase (en′dō-am′il-ās). A glucanohydrolase acting on internal glycosidic bonds (*e.g.,* α-amylase).

en·do·an·eu·rys·mo·plas·ty (en′dō-an-yū-riz′mō-plas-tē). SYN aneurysmoplasty.

en·do·an·eu·rys·mor·rha·phy (en′dō-an-yū-riz-mōr′ă-fē). SYN aneurysmoplasty. [endo- + G. *aneurysma,* aneurysm, + *rhaphē,* suture]

en·do·an·gi·i·tis (en′dō-an-jē-ī′tis). SYN endangiitis.

en·do·a·or·ti·tis (en′dō-ā-ōr-tī′tis). SYN endaortitis.

en·do·ap·pen·di·ci·tis (en′dō-ă-pen-di-sī′tis). Simple catarrhal inflammation, limited more or less strictly to the mucosal surface of the vermiform appendix.

en·do·ar·te·ri·tis (en′dō-ar-ter-ī′tis). SYN endarteritis.

en·do·aus·cul·ta·tion (en′dō-aws-kŭl-tā′shŭn). Auscultation of the thoracic organs, especially the heart, by means of a stethoscopic tube passed into the esophagus or into the heart.

en·do·bag. SYN endosac.

en·do·ba·si·on (en′dō-bā′sē-on). A cephalometric and craniometric point located in the midline at the most posterior point of the anterior border of the foramen magnum on the contour of the foramen; it is slightly posterior and internal to basion.

en·do·bi·ot·ic (en-dō-bī-ot′ik). Living as a parasite within the host.

en·do·blast (en′dō-blast). Entoderm. [endo- + G. *blastos,* germ]

en·do·bron·chi·al (en-dō-brong′kē-ăl). SYN intrabronchial.

en·do·car·di·ac, en·do·car·di·al (en-dō-kar′dē-ak, -dē-ăl). **1.** SYN intracardiac. **2.** Relating to the endocardium.

en·do·car·di·og·ra·phy (en′dō-kar-dē-og′ră-fē). Electrocardiography with the exploring electrode within the chambers of the heart. SEE ALSO intracardiac *catheter.*

en·do·car·dit·ic (en′dō-kar-dit′ik). Relating to endocarditis.

en·do·car·di·tis (en′dō-kar-dī′tis). Inflammation of the endocardium. SYN encarditis.

abacterial thrombotic e., SYN nonbacterial thrombotic e.

acute bacterial e., a type of bacterial endocarditis caused by pyogenic organisms such as hemolytic streptococci or staphylococci.

atypical verrucous e., SYN Libman-Sacks e.

bacteria-free stage of bacterial e., e. described prior to the antibiotic era and presumably due to spontaneous healing of the bacterial vegetations.

bacterial e., e. caused by the direct invasion of bacteria and leading to deformity and destruction of the valve leaflets. Two types are acute bacterial endocarditis and subacute bacterial endocarditis.

cachectic e., SYN nonbacterial thrombotic e.

e. chorda′lis, e. affecting particularly the chordae tendineae.

constrictive e., thickening of the endocardium due to inflammation of any origin that restricts the diastolic relaxation of one or both ventricles producing diastolic ventricular failure.

infectious e., infective e., e. due to infection by microorganisms.

isolated parietal e., fibrous thickening of the endocardium of the left ventricle without valvular involvement.

Libman-Sacks e., verrucous e. sometimes associated with disseminated lupus erythematosus. SYN atypical verrucous e., Libman-Sacks syndrome, nonbacterial verrucous e.

Löffler's e., Löffler's fibroplastic e., fibroplastic parietal e. with eosinophilia, an e. of obscure cause characterized by progressive congestive heart failure, multiple systemic emboli, and eosinophilia. SYN Löffler's disease, Löffler's syndrome (2).

Loffler's parietal fibroplastic e., sclerosis of the endocardium in the presence of a high eosinophile count.

malignant e., acute bacterial e., usually secondary to suppuration elsewhere and running a fulminating course. SYN septic e.

marantic e., nonbacterial thrombotic e. associated with cancer and other debilitating diseases.

mural e., inflammation of the endocardium involving the walls of the chambers of the heart.

mycotic e., e. due to infection by fungi.

nonbacterial thrombotic e., verrucous endocardial lesions occurring in the terminal stages of many chronic infectious and wasting diseases. SYN abacterial thrombotic e., cachectic e., terminal e., thromboendocarditis.

nonbacterial verrucous e., SYN Libman-Sacks e.

polypous e., bacterial e. with the formation of pedunculated masses of fibrin, or thrombi, attached to the ulcerated valves.

rheumatic e., endocardial involvment as part of rheumatic heart disease, recognized clinically by valvular involvement; in the acute stage, there may be tiny fibrin vegetations along the lines of closure of the valve leaflets, with subsequent fibrous thickening and shortening of the leaflets.

septic e., SYN malignant e.

subacute bacterial e. (SBE), subacute bacterial endocarditis is usually due to *Streptococcus viridans* or *S. fecalis.*

terminal e., SYN nonbacterial thrombotic e.

valvular e., inflammation confined to the endocardium of the valves.

vegetative e., verrucous e., e. associated with the presence of fibrinous clots (vegetations) forming on the ulcerated surfaces of the valves.

en·do·car·di·um, pl. **en·do·car·dia** (en-dō-kar′dē-ŭm, -ē-ă) [NA]. The innermost tunic of the heart, which includes endothelium and subendothelial connective tissue; in the atrial wall, smooth muscle and numerous elastic fibers also occur. [endo- + G. *kardia,* heart]

en·do·ce·li·ac (en-dō-sē′lē-ak). Within one of the body cavities. [endo- + G. *koilia,* cavity, ventricle]

en·do·cer·vi·cal (en′dō-ser′vi-kăl). **1.** Within any cervix, specifically within the cervix uteri. SYN intracervical. **2.** Relating to the endocervix.

en·do·cer·vi·ci·tis (en′dō-ser-vi-sī′tis). Inflammation of the mucous membrane of the cervix uteri. SYN endotrachelitis.

en·do·cer·vix (en-dō-ser′viks). The mucous membrane of the cervical canal.

en·do·chon·dral (en-dō-kon′drăl). SYN intracartilaginous. [endo- + G. *chondros,* cartilage]

en·do·co·li·tis (en′dō-kō-lī′tis). Simple catarrhal inflammation of the colon.

en·do·col·pi·tis (en′dō-kol-pī′tis). Inflammation of the vaginal mucous membrane. [endo- + G. *colpos,* vagina, + *-itis,* inflammation]

en·do·cra·ni·al (en-dō-krā′nē-ăl). **1.** Within the cranium. **2.** Relating to the endocranium. SYN encranial, entocranial.

en·do·cra·ni·um (en′dō-krā′nē-ŭm). The lining membrane of the cranium, or dura mater of the brain. SYN entocranium.

en·do·crine (en′dō-krin). **1.** Secreting internally, most commonly into the systemic circulation; of or pertaining to such secretion. Cf. paracrine. **2.** The internal or hormonal secretion of a ductless gland. **3.** Denoting a gland that furnishes an internal secretion. [endo- + G. *krinō,* to separate]

en·do·cri·nol·o·gist (en′dō-kri-nol′ō-jist). One who specializes in endocrinology.

en·do·cri·nol·o·gy (en′dō-kri-nol′ō-jē). The science and medical specialty concerned with the internal or hormonal secretions and their physiologic and pathologic relations. [endocrine + G. *logos,* study]

en·do·cri·no·ma (en′dō-kri-nō′mă). A tumor with endocrine tissue that retains the function of the parent organ, usually to an excessive degree.

en·do·crin·o·path·ic (en′dō-kri-nō-path′ik). Relating to or suffering from an endocrinopathy.

en·do·cri·nop·a·thy (en′dō-kri-nop′ă-thē). A disorder in the function of an endocrine gland and the consequences thereof. [endocrine + G. *pathos,* disease]

en·do·cri·no·ther·a·py (en′dō-kri-nō-thār′ă-pē). Treatment of disease by the administration of extracts of endocrine glands. [endocrine + G. *therapeia,* medical treatment]

en·do·cy·clic (en-dō-sī′klik, -sik′lik). Within a cycle or ring; *e.g.,* the 6 C atoms of the benzene ring in toluene. Cf. exocyclic.

en·do·cyst (en′dō-sist). The inner layer of a hydatid cyst.

en·do·cys·ti·tis (en′dō-sis-tī′tis). Inflammation of the mucous membrane of the bladder. [endo- + G. *kystis,* bladder, + *-itis,* inflammation]

en·do·cy·to·sis (en′dō-sī-tō′sis). Internalization of substances from the extracellular environment through the formation of vesicles formed from the plasma membrane. There are two forms: (a) fluid phase (pinocytosis), and (b) receptor mediated. SEE ALSO phagocytosis. Cf. exocytosis (2). [endo- + G. *kytos,* cell, + *-osis,* condition]

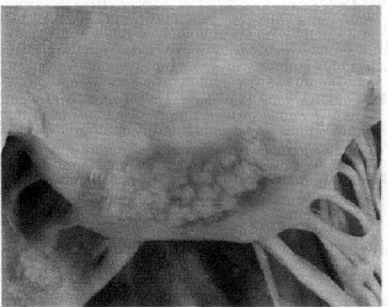
vegetative endocarditis (shown here on the mitral valve)

en·do·derm (en′dō-derm). The innermost of the three primary germ layers of the embryo (ectoderm, mesoderm, endoderm); from it is derived the epithelial lining of the primitive gut tract and the epithelial component of the glands and other structures (*e.g.,* lower respiratory system) that developed as outgrowths from the gut tube. SYN entoderm, hypoblast. [endo- + G. *derma,* skin]

En·do·der·mo·phy·ton (en′dō-der-mof′i-ton). Former name for *Trichophyton,* especially for the species causing tinea imbricata, *T. concentricum.* [endo- + G. *derma,* skin, + *phyton,* plant]

en·do·di·a·scope (en′dō-dī′ă-skōp). An x-ray tube that may be placed within a cavity of the body; an archaic device.

en·do·di·as·co·py (en′dō-dī-as′kŏ-pē). X-ray visualization by means of an endodiascope; an archaic procedure. [endo- + G. *dia,* through, + *skopeō,* to view]

en·do·don·tia (en-dō-don′shē-ă). SYN endodontics.

en·do·don·tics (en-dō-don′tiks). A field of dentistry concerned with the biology and pathology of the dental pulp and periapical tissues, and with the prevention, diagnosis, and treatment of pathoses and traumatic injuries in these tissues. SYN endodontia, endodontology. [endo- + G. *odous,* tooth]

en·do·don·tist (en-dō-don′tist). One who specializes in the practice of endodontics. SYN endodontologist.

en·do·don·tol·o·gist (en′dō-don-tol′ō-jist). SYN endodontist.

en·do·don·tol·o·gy (en′do-don-tol′ō-jē). SYN endodontics.

en·do·dy·o·cyte (en′dō-dī′ō-sīt). **1.** A trophozoite formed by endodyogeny. **2.** SYN merozoite. [endo- + G. *dys,* two, + *kytos,* cell]

en·do·dy·og·e·ny (en′dō-dī-oj′ĕ-nē). A process of asexual development seen among certain coccidia, such as *Toxoplasma* and *Frenkelia,* in which no separate nuclear division occurs, as in schizogony; the two daughters develop internally within the parent, without nuclear conjugation. [endo- + G. *dys,* two, + *genesis,* creation]

en·do·en·ter·i·tis (en′dō-en-ter-ī′tis). Inflammation of the intestinal mucous membrane. [endo- + G. *enteron,* intestine, *-itis,* inflammation]

en·do·en·zyme (en-dō-en′zīm). SYN intracellular *enzyme.*

en·do·e·soph·a·gi·tis (en′dō-ē-sof-ă-jī′tis). Inflammation of the internal lining of the esophagus.

en·do·far·a·dism (en-dō-far′ă-dizm). Application of an alternating electric current to the interior of any cavity of the body. SEE fulguration.

en·do·gal·va·nism (en-dō-gal′van-izm). Application of a direct electric current to the interior of any cavity of the body. SEE fulguration.

en·dog·a·my (en-dog′ă-mē). Reproduction by conjugation between sister cells, the descendants of one original cell. [endo- + G. *gamos,* marriage]

en

en·do·gas·tric (en-dō-gas'trik). Within the stomach.

en·do·gas·tri·tis (en'dō-gas-trī'tis). Inflammation of the mucous membrane of the stomach. [endo- + G. *gastēr*, stomach, + *-itis*, inflammation]

en·do·gen·ic (en-dō-jen'ik). SYN endogenous.

en·do·ge·note (en-dō-jē'nōt). In microbial genetics, the recipient cell's genome. [endo- + genote]

en·dog·e·nous (en-doj'ĕ-nŭs). Originating or produced within the organism or one of its parts. SYN endogenic. [endo- + G. *-gen*, production]

en·do·glob·u·lar, en·do·glo·bar (en-dō-glob'yū-lăr, -glō'bar). Within a globular body; specifically, within a red blood cell.

en·do·gnath·i·on (en-dog-nath'ē-on, en-dō-nā'thē-on). The medial of the two segments constituting the incisive bone. SEE mesognathion. [endo- + G. *gnathos*, jaw]

en·do·her·ni·ot·o·my (en'dō-her-nē-ot'ō-mē). An obsolete procedure for closure, by sutures, of the interior lining of a hernial sac.

en·do·in·tox·i·ca·tion (en'dō-in-tok-si-kā'shŭn). Poisoning by an endogenous toxin.

en·do·la·ryn·ge·al (en'dō-lă-rin'jē-ăl). Within the larynx.

En·do·li·max (en-dō-lī'maks). A genus of small nonpathogenic amebae parasitic in the large intestine of man and other animals. [endo- + G. *leimax*, a meadow or garden]

en·do·lith (en'dō-lith). A calcified body found in the pulp chamber of a tooth; may be composed of irregular dentin (true denticle) or due to ectopic calcification of pulp tissue (false denticle). SYN denticle (1), pulp calcification, pulp calculus, pulp nodule, pulp stone. [endo- + G. *lithos*, stone]

en·do·lymph (en'dō-limf). The fluid contained within the membranous labyrinth of the inner ear; endolymph resembles intracellular fluid in composition (potassium is the main positively-charged ion). SYN endolympha [NA], Scarpa's fluid, Scarpa's liquor.

en·do·lym·pha (en'dō-lim'fă) [NA]. SYN endolymph. [endo- + L. *lympha*, a clear fluid]

en·do·lym·phic (en-dō-lim'fik). Relating to the endolymph.

en·do·me·rog·o·ny (en'dō-me-rog'ō-nē). Production of merozoites in the asexual reproduction of sporozoan protozoa by a process originating in the interior of the schizont (as contrasted with ectomerogony); observed in species of *Eimeria*. [endo- + G. *meros*, part, + *gonē*, generation]

en·do·me·tria (en-dō-mē'trē-ă). Plural of endometrium.

en·do·me·tri·al (en-dō-mē'trē-ăl). Relating to or composed of endometrium.

en·do·me·tri·oid (en-dō-mē'trē-oyd). Microscopically resembling endometrial tissue.

en·do·me·tri·o·ma (en'dō-mē-trē-ō'mă). Circumscribed mass of ectopic endometrial tissue in endometriosis. [endometrium + *-oma*, tumor]

en·do·me·tri·o·sis (en'dō-mē-trē-ō'sis). Ectopic occurrence of endometrial tissue, frequently forming cysts containing altered blood. [endometrium + *-osis*, condition]

en·do·me·tri·tis (en'dō-mē-trī'tis). Inflammation of the endometrium. [endometrium + *-itis*, inflammation]

decidual e., inflammation of the decidual mucous membrane of the gravid uterus.

e. dis'secans, e. with ulceration and exfoliation of the mucous membrane.

en·do·me·tri·um, pl. **en·do·me·tria** (en'dō-mē'trē-ŭm, -trē-ă) [NA]. The mucous membrane comprising the inner layer of the uterine wall; it consists of a simple columnar epithelium and a lamina propria that contains simple tubular uterine glands. The structure, thickness, and state of the endometrium undergo marked change with the menstrual cycle. SYN tunica mucosa uteri [NA]. [endo- + G. *mētra*, uterus]

Swiss cheese e., glandular hyperplasia of the e. with cyst formation, so-called because of the appearance of the cysts in histologic sections.

en·do·me·tro·pic (en'dō-mē-trop'ik). Denoting an external stim-

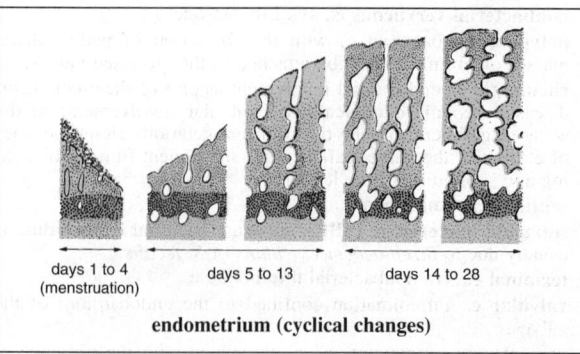

days 1 to 4 (menstruation) days 5 to 13 days 14 to 28

endometrium (cyclical changes)

ulus capable of producing a response of the uterus, specifically the endometrium. [endo- + G. *mētra*, uterus, + *tropē*, a turning]

en·do·mi·to·sis (en'dō-mī-tō'sis). SYN endopolyploidy.

en·do·morph (en'dō-mōrf). A constitutional body type or build (biotype or somatotype) in which tissues that originated in the endoderm prevail; from a morphological standpoint, the trunk predominates over the limbs. SYN brachytype. [endo- + G. *morphē*, form]

en·do·mor·phic (en'dō-mōr'fik). Relating to, or having the characteristics of, an endomorph.

en·do·mo·tor·sonde (en'dō-mō'tŏr-sond'). Radiotelemetering capsule for studying the interior of the gastrointestinal tract. [endo- + L. *motor*, mover, + Fr. *sonde*, sounding line]

En·do·my·ces ge·ot·ri·chum (en-dō-mī'sez jē-ot'ri-kŭm). A species of yeastlike fungus that is the perfect state of *Geotrichum candidum* and the cause of geotrichosis.

En·do·my·ce·ta·les (en'dō-mī-sē-tā'lēz). An order of Ascomycota that includes the yeasts. SYN Saccharomycetales.

en·do·my·o·car·di·al (en'dō-mī-ō-kar'dē-ăl). Relating to the endocardium and the myocardium.

en·do·my·o·car·di·tis (en-dō-mī'ō-kar-dī'tis). Inflammation of both endocardium and myocardium.

en·do·my·o·me·tri·tis (en'dō-mī-ō-mē-trī'tis). Sepsis involving the tissues of the uterus. [endo- + G. *mys*, muscle, + *mētra*, uterus, + *-itis*, inflammation]

en·do·mys·i·um (en'dō-miz'ē-ŭm, -mis'ē-ŭm). The fine connective tissue sheath surrounding a muscle fiber. [endo- + G. *mys*, muscle]

en·do·neu·ri·tis (en'dō-nū-rī'tis). Obsolete term for inflammation of the endoneurium.

en·do·neu·ri·um (en-dō-nū'rē-ŭm). The innermost connective tissue supportive structure present in peripheral nerve trunks, found within the fascicles. With the perineurium and epineurium, composes the peripheral nerve stroma. SYN Henle's sheath, sheath of Key and Retzius. [endo- + G. *neuron*, nerve]

en·do·nu·cle·ase (en-dō-nū'klē-ās). A nuclease (phosphodiesterase) that cleaves polynucleotides (nucleic acids) at interior bonds, thus producing poly- or oligonucleotide fragments of varying size. Cf. exonuclease.

microccocal e., an enzyme that cleaves nucleic acids to oligonucleotides terminating in 3'-phosphates. SYN micrococcal nuclease, spleen e., spleen phosphodiesterases.

nucleate e., SYN endonuclease *Serratia marcescens*.

restriction e., one of many e.'s isolated from bacteria that hydrolyze (cut) double-stranded DNA chains at specific sequences, thus inactivating a foreign (viral or other) DNA and restricting its activity; these e.'s have become standard laboratory devices for making specific cuts in DNA as a first step in deducing sequences and are sometimes referred to as a "chemical knife;" usually named by a three- or four-letter abbreviation of the name of the organism from which isolated (*e.g.,* EcoB from *Escherichia coli*, strain B). SYN restriction enzyme.

single-stranded nucleate e., endonuclease S₁ *Aspergillus*.

spleen e., SYN micrococcal e.

en·do·nu·cle·ase S₁ *As·per·gil·lus*. An enzyme cleaving RNA or DNA to 5′-ended mono- or oligonucleotides; prefers single stranded polynucleic acids. SYN deoxyribonuclease S₁.

en·do·nu·cle·ase *Ser·ra·tia mar·ces·cens.* A nuclease (a nucleate oligonucleotidohydrolase) that forms oligonucleotides ending in 5′-phosphates from RNA and DNA; hydrolyzes both double-stranded and single-stranded polynucleic acids. SYN nucleate endonuclease.

en·do·nu·cle·o·lus (en′dō-nū-klē′ō-lŭs). A minute unstainable spot near the center of a nucleolus.

en·do·par·a·site (en-dō-par′ă-sīt). A parasite living within the body of its host.

en·do·par·a·sit·ism (en-dō-par′ă-sī-tizm). SYN infection.

en·do·pep·ti·dase (en-dō-pep′ti-dās). An enzyme catalyzing the hydrolysis of a peptide chain at points well within the chain, not near termini; *e.g.,* pepsin, trypsin. Cf. exopeptidase. SYN proteinase.

en·do·per·i·ar·te·ri·tis (en′dō-pār′i-ar-ter-ī′tis). SYN panarteritis. [endo- + G. *peri,* around, + arteritis]

en·do·per·i·car·di·ac (en′dō-pār-ē-kar′dē-ak). SYN intrapericardiac.

en·do·per·i·car·di·tis (en′dō-pār′i-kar-dī′tis). Simultaneous inflammation of the endocardium and pericardium. [endo- + G. *peri,* around, + *kardia,* heart, + *-itis,* inflammation]

en·do·per·i·my·o·car·di·tis (en′dō-pār′i-mī′ō-kar-dī′tis). Simultaneous inflammation of the heart muscle and of the endocardium and pericardium. [endo- + G. *peri,* around, + *mys,* muscle, + *kardia,* heart, + *-itis,* inflammation]

en·do·per·i·neu·ri·tis (en′dō-pār′i-nū-rī′tis). Obsolete term for inflammation of both endoneurium and perineurium.

en·do·per·i·to·ni·tis (en′dō-pār′i-tō-nī′tis). Superficial inflammation of the peritoneum.

en·do·per·ox·ide (en′dō-per-ok′sīd). A peroxide (–O–O–) group that bridges two atoms that are both parts of a larger molecule.

en·do·phle·bi·tis (en′dō-fle-bī′tis). Inflammation of the intima of a vein. [endo- + G. *phleps (phleb-),* vein, + *-itis,* inflammation]

en·doph·thal·mi·tis (en-dof-thal-mī′tis). Inflammation of the tissues within the eyeball. [endo- + G. *ophthalmos,* eye, + *-itis,* inflammation]

granulomatous e., a diffuse, chronic inflammation of intraocular tissues.

e. ophthal′mia nodo′sa, e. due to intraocular caterpillar hairs. SEE *ophthalmia* nodosa.

e. phacoanaphylac′tica, inflammation of the uveal tract as a result of sensitization by the lens cortex; simulates sympathetic ophthalmia.

en·doph·thal·mo·do·nes·is (en′dof-thal-mō-dō-nē′sis). Tremulousness of any intraocular structure, especially of an implanted lens (pseudophakodonesis). [endo- + ophthalmo- + G. *doneō,* to shake]

en·do·phyte (en′dō-fīt). A plant parasite living within another organism. [endo- + G. *phyton,* plant]

en·do·phyt·ic (en-dō-fit′ik). **1.** Pertaining to an endophyte. **2.** Referring to an infiltrative, invasive tumor.

en·do·plasm (en′dō-plazm). The inner or medullary part of the cytoplasm, as opposed to the ectoplasm, containing the cell organelles. SYN entoplasm.

en·do·plas·mic (en′dō-plas′mik). Referring to the endoplasm.

en·do·plast (en′dō-plast). Former name for endosome. [endo- + G. *plastos,* formed]

en·do·plas·tic (en-dō-plas′tik). Relating to the endoplasm.

en·do·po·lyg·e·ny (en′dō-pō-lij′ĕ-nē). Asexual reproduction in which more than two offspring are formed within the parent organism and in which two or possibly more nuclear divisions occur before merozoite formation begins; a form of internal budding observed in *Toxoplasma gondii.* Cf. endodyogeny. [endo- + G. *polys,* many, + *genesis,* creation]

en·do·pol·y·ploid (en-dō-pol′ē-ployd). Relating to endopolyploidy.

en·do·pol·y·ploi·dy (en-dō-pol′ē-ploy-dē). The process or state of duplication of the chromosomes without accompanying spin-

---

examples of restriction endonucleases, with cleaving sites

length of known sequence	formation of fragments, the ends of which are:	name[1]	known palindrome (with cleaving sites[2])	number of cleaving sites in λ-DNA
hexanucleotide	cohesive	Bam HI	G/GATCC	5
	smooth	Hpa I	GTT/AAC	11
tetranucleotide	cohesive	Hha I	GCG/C	> 50
	smooth	Alu I	AG/CT	> 50

[1] abbreviation for source bacteria
[2] only 5′–3′ strand given

---

dle formation or cytokinesis, resulting in a polyploid nucleus. SYN endomitosis. [endo- + polyploidy]

en·do·re·du·pli·ca·tion (en′dō-rē-dū′pli-kā′shŭn). A form of polyploidy or polysomy by redoubling of chromosomes, giving rise to four-stranded chromosomes at prophase and metaphase.

end or·gan. See under organ.

en·dor·phin·er·gic (en′dōr-fin-er′jik). Relating to nerve cells or fibers that employ an endorphin as their neurotransmitter. [endorphin + G. *ergon,* work]

en·dor·phins (en′dōr-finz). Opioid peptides originally isolated from the brain but now found in many parts of the body; in the nervous system, e.'s bind to the same receptors that bind exogenous opiates. A variety of e.'s (*e.g.,* alpha and beta) that vary not only in their physical and chemical properties but also in physiologic action have been isolated. SEE ALSO enkephalins. [fr. *endogenous morphine*]

en·dor·rha·chis (en-dō-rā′kis). SYN *dura mater* of spinal cord. [endo- + G. *rhachis,* the spine]

en·do·sac (en′dō-sak). A sac or bag used in laparoscopic surgery in which tissue is placed to facilitate removal or morcellation. SYN endobag.

en·do·sal·pin·gi·o·sis (en′dō-sal-pin-jē-ō′sis). Aberrant mucous membrane in the ovary or elsewhere consisting of ciliated tubal mucosa without stroma of endometrial type.

en·do·sal·pin·gi·tis (en′dō-sal-pin-jī′tis). Inflammation of the lining membrane of the eustachian or the fallopian tube. [endo- + G. *salpinx (salping-),* tube, + *-itis,* inflammation]

en·do·sal·pinx (en′dō-sal′pinks). The mucosa of the fallopian tube. [endo + G. *salpinx,* tube]

en·do·sarc (en′dō-sark). The endoplasm of a protozoan. SYN entosarc. [endo- + G. *sarx (sark-),* flesh]

en·do·scope (en′dō-skōp). An instrument for the examination of the interior of a canal or hollow viscus. [endo- + G. *skopeō,* to examine]

en·dos·co·pist (en-dos′kŏ-pist). A specialist trained in the use of an endoscope.

en·dos·co·py (en-dos′kŏ-pē). Examination of the interior of a canal or hollow viscus by means of a special instrument, such as an endoscope. [see endoscope]

peroral e., visual examination of interior sections of the body by introduction of an instrument (an endoscope) through the mouth; examples include esophagoscopy, gastroscopy, bronchoscopy.

en·do·skel·e·ton (en-dō-skel′ĕ-tŏn). The internal bony framework of the body; the skeleton in its usual context as distinguished from exoskeleton.

en·dos·mo·sis (en-dos-mō′sis). Obsolete term for osmosis in a direction toward the interior of a cell or a cavity; the inward direction is not self-evident in all systems.

en·do·some (en′dō-sōm). A more or less central body in the vesicular nucleus of certain Feulgen-negative (DNA-) protozoa (*e.g.,* trypanosomes, parasitic amebae, and phytoflagellates), with the chromatin (DNA₊) lying between the nuclear membrane and the e. Cf. nucleolus. [endo- + G. *sōma,* body]

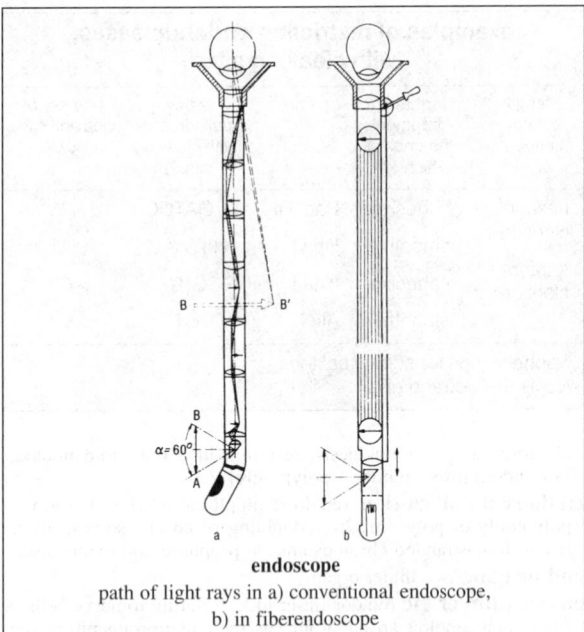

endoscope
path of light rays in a) conventional endoscope,
b) in fiberendoscope

en·do·son·og·ra·phy (en'dō-sō-nog'ră-fē). Ultrasonography performed using an ultrasound transducer mounted on a fiberoptic endoscope.

en·do·so·nos·co·py (en-dō-son'ŏ-skŏ-pē). A sonographic study carried out by transducers inserted into the body as miniature probes in the esophagus, urethra, bladder, vagina, or rectum.

en·do·sperm (en'dō-sperm). A storage tissue found in many seeds that nourishes the embryo of a plant.

en·do·spore (en'dō-spōr). 1. A resistant body formed within the vegetative cells of some bacteria, particularly those belonging to the genera *Bacillus* and *Clostridium.* 2. A fungus spore borne within a cell or within the tubular end of a sporophore as in the spherale of *Coccidioides immitis.* [endo- + G. *sporos,* seed]

en·dos·te·al (en-dos'tē-ăl). Relating to the endosteum.

en·dos·te·i·tis, en·dos·ti·tis (en'dos-tē-ī'tis, en'dos-tī'tis). Inflammation of the endosteum or of the medullary cavity of a bone. SYN central osteitis (2), perimyelitis. [endo- + G. *osteon,* bone, + *-itis,* inflammation]

en·dos·te·o·ma (en-dos'tē-ō'mă). A benign neoplasm of bone tissue in the medullary cavity of a bone. SYN endostoma. [endo- + G. *osteon,* bone, + *-ōma,* tumor]

en·do·steth·o·scope (en-dō-steth'ŏ-skōp). A stethoscopic tube used in endoauscultation. [endo- + G. *stēthos,* chest, + *skopeō,* to examine]

en·dos·te·um (en-dos'tē-ŭm) [NA]. A layer of cells lining the inner surface of bone in the central medullary cavity. SYN medullary membrane, perimyelis. [endo- + G. *osteon,* bone]

en·dos·to·ma (en-dō-stō'mă). SYN endosteoma.

en·do·ten·din·e·um (en'dō-ten-din'ē-ŭm). The fine connective tissue surrounding secondary fascicles of a tendon. [endo- + L. *tendon,* tendon, + *-eus,* adj.; the whole, in its neuter form, used substantively]

en·do·the·li·a (en-dō-thē'lē-ă). Plural of endothelium.

en·do·the·li·al (en-dō-thē'lē-ăl). Relating to the endothelium.

en·do·the·lin. A 21-amino acid peptide originally derived from endothelial cells. It is an extremely potent vasoconstrictor. Three different gene products have been identified, endothelin 1, endothelin 2, and endothelin 3; they are found in brain, kidney, and endothelium (endothelin 1), intestine (endothelin 2), and intestine and adrenal gland (endothelin 3).

en·do·the·li·o·cyte (en-dō-thē'lē-ō-sīt). SYN endothelial *cell.*

en·do·the·li·oid (en-dō-thē'lē-oyd). Resembling endothelium.

en·do·the·li·o·ma (en'dō-thē-lē-ō'mă). Generic term for a group of neoplasms, particularly benign tumors, derived from the endothelial tissue of blood vessels or lymphatic channels; e.'s may be benign or malignant. [endothelium + *-oma,* tumor]

en·do·the·li·o·sis (en'dō-thē-lē-ō'sis). Proliferation of endothelium.

en·do·the·li·um, pl. **en·do·the·li·a** (en-dō-thē'lē-ŭm, -lē-ă). A layer of flat cells lining especially blood and lymphatic vessels and the heart. [endo- + G. *thēlē,* nipple]

e. of anterior chamber, a single layer of large, squamous cells that covers the posterior surface of the cornea. SYN e. camerae anterioris [NA].

e. cam'erae anterio'ris [NA], SYN e. of anterior chamber.

en·do·ther·mic (en-dō-ther'mik). Denoting a chemical reaction during which heat (enthalpy) is absorbed. Cf. exothermic (1). [endo- + G. *thermē,* heat]

en·do·thrix (en'dō-thriks). Fungal spores (conidia) invading the interior of a hair shaft; there is no conspicuous external sheath of spores, as there is with ectothrix. [endo- + G. *thrix,* hair]

en·do·tox·e·mia (en'dō-tok-sē'mē-ă). Presence in the blood of endotoxins, which, if derived from Gram-negative rod-shaped bacteria, may cause a generalized Shwartzman phenomenon with shock.

en·do·tox·ic (en-dō-tok'sik). Denoting an endotoxin.

en·do·tox·i·co·sis (en'dō-tok-si-kō'sis). Poisoning by an endotoxin.

en·do·tox·in (en-dō-tok'sin). 1. A bacterial toxin not freely liberated into the surrounding medium, in contrast to exotoxin. 2. The complex phospholipid-polysaccharide macromolecules which form an integral part of the cell wall of a variety of relatively avirulent as well as virulent strains of Gram-negative bacteria. The toxins are relatively heat-stable, are less potent than most exotoxins, are less specific, and do not form toxoids; on injection, they may cause a state of shock accompanied by severe diarrhea, and, in smaller doses, fever and leukopenia followed by leukocytosis; they have the capacity of eliciting the Shwartzman and the Sanarelli-Shwartzman phenomena. SYN intracellular toxin.

en·do·tra·che·al (en'dō-trā'kē-ăl). Within the trachea.

en·do·tra·che·li·tis (en'dō-trak-el-ī'tis). SYN endocervicitis.

en·do·u·rol·o·gy (en-dō-yūr-ol'ŏ-jē). Genitourinary operative procedures (diagnostic and therapeutic) performed through instruments. These may be cystoscopic, pelviscopic, celioscopic, or laparoscopic.

en·do·vac·ci·na·tion (en'dō-vak-si-nā'shŭn). Oral administration of vaccines.

en·do·vas·cu·li·tis (en'dō-vas'kyū-lī'tis). SYN endangiitis.

hemorrhagic e., endothelial and medial hyperplasia of placental blood vessels with thrombosis, fragmentation, and diapedesis of red blood cells resulting in stillbirth or fetal developmental disorders.

en·do·ve·nous (en-dō-vē'nŭs). SYN intravenous.

end-piece. The terminal part of the tail of a spermatozoon consisting of the axoneme and the flagellar membrane.

end·plate, end-plate (end'plāt). The ending of a motor nerve fiber in relation to a skeletal muscle fiber.

motor e., the large and complex end-formation by which the axon of a motor neuron establishes synaptic contact with a striated muscle fiber (cell); several terminal branches of a motor axon end in irregular, club-shaped synaptic end-formations that are bedded in a single trough-like depression of the muscle fiber's surface; the postsynaptic membrane, the sarcolemma that forms the bottom of the trough, is greatly increased in surface area by deep infoldings protruding into the underlying cytoplasm of the muscle fiber; the subsynaptic interval between the plasma membrane of the axon terminals and the sarcolemma is filled with an amorphous substance; the trough is closed off toward the surface by the Schwann sheath, which peels away from the axons as the latter enter the trough and thus forms a lid over the trough; the slight bulge of this closure plate corresponds to Doyère's eminence. SYN sole-plate ending.

end-tid·al (end-tī'dăl). At the end of a normal expiration.

en·dy·ma (en'di-mă). SYN ependyma. [G. a garment]

E.N.E. Abbreviation for ethylnorepinephrine.

-ene. Suffix applied to a chemical name indicating the presence of a carbon-carbon double bond; *e.g.,* propene (unsaturated propane, CH_3—CH=CH_2). [G. *enos,* origin]

ene·di·ol (ēn-dī'ōl). The atomic arrangement —C(OH)=C(OH)— produced by proton migration from the CH of a —CHOH group that is attached to a —CO— group to the oxygen of the —CO— group (usually induced by alkali), giving rise to doubly bonded carbon atoms (the -ene group), each bearing a –CHOH group (a diol); a special case of enolization.

en·e·ma (en'ĕ-mă). A rectal injection for clearing out the bowel, or administering drugs or food. [G.]

air contrast e., a double contrast e. in which air is introduced after coating of the colon with a dense barium suspension for radiographic study. SYN air contrast barium e.

air contrast barium e., SYN air contrast e.

analeptic e., an e. of a pint of lukewarm water with one-half teaspoonful of table salt.

barium e., a type of contrast enema; administration of barium, a radiopaque medium, for radiographic and fluoroscopic study of the lower intestinal tract.

blind e., the introduction into the rectum of a rubber tube to facilitate the expulsion of flatus.

contrast e., e. using barium or another contrast medium.

double contrast e., after evacuation of a barium e. and injection of air into the rectum, radiographs show fine details of mucosa of the rectum and colon.

flatus e., an e. of magnesium sulfate in glycerin and warm water.

high e., an e. instilled high up into the colon. SYN enteroclysis (1).

Hypaque e., e. with water-soluble radiographic contrast material, whether diatrizoate or other.

nutrient e., a rectal injection of predigested food.

oil retention e., a rectal injection of mineral oil, introduced at low pressure and retained for several hours before expelling, to soften feces.

small bowel e., radiographic examination of the small intestine, by retrograde filling from the contrast-filled large bowel.

soapsuds e., an e. of shredded or powdered soap in warm water.

turpentine e., an e. of turpentine and olive oil in soapsuds.

en·e·ma·tor (en-ĕ-mā'ter, -tōr). An appliance used to give an enema.

en·e·mi·a·sis (en-ĕ-mī'ă-sis). The use of enemas.

en·er·get·ics (en-er-jet'iks). The study of the energy changes involved in physical and chemical reaction, changes, and systems.

en·er·gom·e·ter (en-er-gom'ĕ-ter). An apparatus for measuring blood pressure. [G. *energeia,* energy, + *metron,* measure]

en·er·gy (en'er-jē). The exertion of power; the capacity to do work, taking the forms of kinetic e., potential e., chemical e., electrical e., etc. SYN dynamic force. [G. *energeia,* fr. *en,* in, + *ergon,* work]

e. of activation, e. that must be added to that already possessed by a molecule or molecules in order to initiate a reaction; usually expressed in the Arrhenius equation relating a rate constant to absolute temperature.

binding e., e. that would be released if a particular atomic nucleus were formed through the combination of individual protons and neutrons. SYN fusion e.

chemical e., e. liberated or absorbed by a chemical reaction, *e.g.,* oxidation of carbon, or absorbed in the formation of a chemical compound.

free e. (F), a thermodynamic function symbolized as *F,* or *G* (Gibbs free e.), =$H - TS$, where *H* is the enthalpy of a system, *T* the absolute temperature, and *S* the entropy; chemical reactions proceed spontaneously in the direction that involves a net decrease in the free e. of the system (*i.e.,* $\Delta G < 0$).

fusion e., SYN binding e.

Gibbs e. of activation, the Gibbs e. that must be added to that

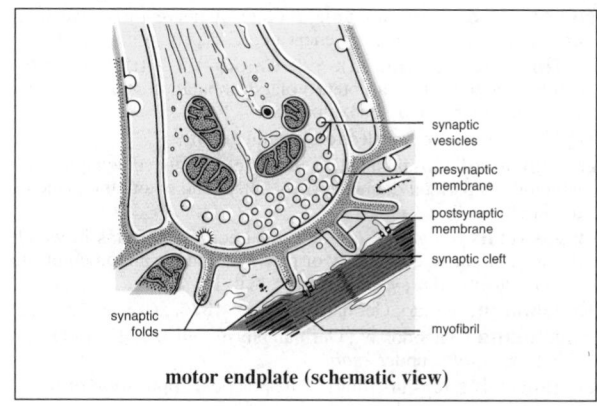
motor endplate (schematic view)

synaptic vesicles
presynaptic membrane
postsynaptic membrane
synaptic cleft
myofibril
synaptic folds

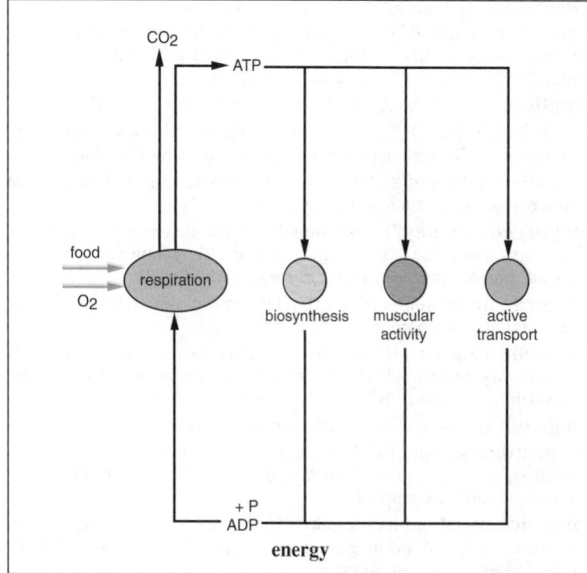
energy

CO_2
ATP
food
O_2
respiration
biosynthesis
muscular activity
active transport
+ P
ADP

already possessed by a molecule or molecules in order to initiate a reaction.

Gibbs free e. (G), SEE free e.

Helmholtz e. (A), e. equivalent to the internal energy minus the entropy contribution (TS).

internal e. (U), e. of a system measured by the heat absorbed from the system's surroundings and the amount of work done on the system by its surroundings.

kinetic e., the e. of motion.

latent e., SYN potential e.

nuclear e., e. given off in the course of nuclear reaction or stored in the formation of an atomic nucleus.

nutritional e., SYN trophodynamics.

e. of position, SYN potential e.

potential e., the e., existing in a body by virtue of its position or state of existence, which is not being exerted at the time. SYN e. of position, latent e.

psychic e., in psychoanalysis, a hypothetical mental force, analogous to the physical concept of e., which enables and vitalizes an individual's psychological activity. SEE ALSO libido. SYN psychic force.

radiant e., e. contained in light rays or any other form of radiation.

solar e., e. derived from sunlight.

total e., the sum of kinetic and potential e.'s.

en

en·er·va·tion (en-er-vā′shŭn). Failure of nerve force; weakening. [L. *enervo,* pp. *-atus,* to enervate, fr. *e-* priv. + *nervus,* nerve]

en·flu·rane (en-flūr′ān). 2-Chloro-1,1,2-trifluoroethyl difluoromethyl ether; a potent volatile inhalation anesthetic that is nonflammable and nonexplosive.

ENG Abbreviation for electronystagmography.

en·gage·ment (en-gāj′ment). In obstetrics, the mechanism by which the biparietal diameter of the fetal head enters the plane of the inlet.

en·gas·tri·us (en-gas′trē-ŭs). Unequal conjoined twins in which the smaller parasite is wholly or partly within the abdomen of the larger autosite. [G. *en,* in, + *gastēr,* belly]

Engelmann, Guido, German surgeon, *1876. SEE E.'s *disease.*

Engelmann, Theodor W., German physiologist, 1843–1909. SEE E.'s basal *knobs,* under *knob.*

en·gi·neer·ing (en-jin-ēr′ing). The practical application of physical, mechanical, and mathematical principles.

  biomedical e., application of e. principles to obtain solutions to biomedical problems.

  dental e., application of e. principles to dentistry.

  genetic e., internal manipulation of basic genetic material of an organism to modify biologic heredity or to produce peptides of high purity, such as hormones or antigens.

Englisch, Josef, Austrian physician, 1835–1915. SEE E.'s *sinus.*

en·globe (en-glōb′). To take in by a spheroidal body; said of the ingestion of bacteria and other foreign bodies by the phagocytes.

en·globe·ment (en-glōb′ment). The process of inclusion by a spheroidal body, such as by a phagocyte.

en·gorged (en-gōrjd′). Absolutely filled; distended with fluid. SEE ALSO congested, hyperemic. [O. Fr. fr. Mediev. L. *gorgia,* throat, narrow passage, fr. L. *gurges,* a whirlpool]

en·gorge·ment (en-gōrj′ment). Distention with fluid or other material. SEE ALSO congestion, hyperemia.

en·gram (en′gram). In the mnemic hypothesis, a physical habit or memory trace made on the protoplasm of an organism by the repetition of stimuli. [G. *en,* in, + *gramma,* mark]

en·graph·ia (en-graf′ē-ă). The formation of engrams.

en grappe (ahn-grap′). Denoting the grapelike cluster arrangement of microconidia of certain dermatophytes. [Fr. *en,* in, + *grappe,* bunch of grapes]

en·hance·ment (en-hans′ment). 1. The act of augmenting. 2. In immunology, the prolongation of a process or event by suppressing an opposing process.

  acoustic e., a manifestation of increased acoustic signal amplitude returning from regions beyond an object which causes little or no attenuation of the sound beam. Cf. acoustic *shadow.*

  contrast e., the intravenous administration of water-soluble iodinated contrast material, which increases the CT number of the vascular pool, as well as some lesions (particularly in the brain), due to abnormal leakage into the interstitium; the property of showing increased radiopacity from concentration of contrast medium.

  edge e., using analogue or digital image processing to increase the contrast of each interface; equivalent to using a high-pass filter.

  immunological e., SYN immunoenhancement.

  ring e., in computed tomography, when a bright circle appears on an image made after injection of contrast medium, characteristic of localization of the contrast in the wall of an abscess.

en·hanc·ers. Genetic elements important in the function of a specific promoter. [M.E. *enhauncen,* raise, increase, fr. O. Fr. *enhaucier,* fr. L.L. *inalto,* fr. *altus,* high, + *-er,* agent suffix]

en·he·ma·to·spore, en·he·mo·spore (en-hem′ă-tō-spōr, en-hem′ō-spōr). Obsolete terms for merozoite. [G. *en,* in, + *haima,* blood, + *sporos,* seed]

en·keph·a·lin·er·gic (en-kef′ă-lin-er′jik). Relating to nerve cells or fibers that employ an enkephalin as their neurotransmitter. [enkephalin + G. *ergon,* work]

en·keph·a·lins (en-kef′ă-linz). Pentapeptide endorphins, found in many parts of the brain, that bind to specific receptor sites, some of which may be pain-related opiate receptors; hypoth-

esized as endogenous neurotransmitters and nonaddicting analgesics. Metenkephalin is Tyr-Gly-Gly-Phe-Met; leuenkephalin has Leu in place of Met; proenkephalin has Pro in place of Met.

en·large·ment (en-larj′ment). 1. An increase in size; an anatomical swelling, enlargement, or prominence. 2. An intumescence or swelling. SYN intumescentia [NA], intumescence (1).

  cervical e., a spindle-shaped swelling of the spinal cord extending from the third cervical to the second thoracic vertebra, with maximum thickness opposite the fifth or sixth cervical vertebra, consequential to the innervation of the upper limb. SYN intumescentia cervicalis [NA], cervical e. of spinal cord.

  cervical e. of spinal cord, SYN cervical e.

  gingival e., an overgrowth (localized or diffuse) of gingival tissue, nonspecific in nature. SEE ALSO gingival *hyperplasia.*

  lumbar e., a spindle-shaped swelling of the spinal cord beginning at the level of the tenth thoracic vertebra and tapering into the medullary cone, with maximum thickness opposite the last thoracic vertebra, consequential to the innervation of the lower limb. SYN intumescentia lumbalis [NA], lumbar e. of spinal cord.

  lumbar e. of spinal cord, SYN lumbar e.

  tympanic e., a swelling, not ganglionic, on the tympanic branch of the glossopharyngeus nerve; it is regarded as possibly similar to the carotid glomus. SYN intumescentia tympanica, tympanic intumescence.

△ **-enoic.** Suffix indicating an unsaturated acid. [-ene + -ic]

enol (ē′nol). A compound possessing a hydroxyl group (alcohol) attached to a doubly bonded (ethylenic) carbon atom (–CH=CH(OH)–); properly italicized when attached as a prefix or infix to an otherwise complete name; *e.g., enol* pyruvate; phospho*enol*pyruvate; usually in equilibrium with its keto tautomer. [-ene + -ol]

eno·lase (ē′nol-ās). An enzyme catalyzing the reversible dehydration of 2-phospho-D-glycerate to phospho*enol*pyruvate and water; a step in both glycolysis and gluconeogenesis; several isozymes exist; inhibited by F⁻. SYN phosphopyruvate hydratase.

eno·li·za·tion (ē′nol-i-zā′shŭn). Conversion of a keto to an enol form; *e.g.,* CH_3-CO-COOH → CH_2=C(OH)COOH.

enol **py·ru·vate** (ē-nol-pī′rū-vāt). CH_2=C(OH)–COO⁻ᵘⁿ, the form of pyruvate encountered in the biologically important phospho*enol*pyruvate (*enol* pyruvate phosphate), not in the free form.

en·oph·thal·mia (en-of-thal′mē-ă). SYN enophthalmos.

en·oph·thal·mos (en′of-thal′mos). Recession of the eyeball within the orbit. SYN enophthalmia. [G. *en,* in, + *ophthalmos,* eye]

en·or·gan·ic (en-ōr-gan′ik). Rarely used term denoting that which occurs as an innate characteristic of an organism.

en·o·si·ma·nia (en′ō-si-mā′nē-ă). Rarely used term for the obsessive belief of having committed an unpardonable offense. [G. *enosis,* a quaking, + *mania,* insanity]

en·os·to·sis (en-os-tō′sis). A mass of proliferating bone tissue within a bone. [G. *en,* in, + *osteon,* bone, + *-osis,* condition]

en·o·yl (ēn′ō-il). The acyl radical of an unsaturated aliphatic acid. [-ene + -oyl]

en·o·yl-ACP re·duc·tase. An enzyme catalyzing hydrogenation of acyl-ACP complexes to 2,3-dehydroacyl-ACP's, with NAD⁺ as hydrogen acceptor; important in fatty acid metabolism. SYN crotonyl-ACP reductase.

en·o·yl-ACP re·duc·tase (NADPH). An enzyme carrying out the same reaction as enoyl-ACP reductase, but with NADP⁺ as hydrogen acceptor. SYN acyl-ACP dehydrogenase, acyl-ACP reductase.

en·o·yl-CoA hy·dra·tase. Δ²-enoyl-CoA hydratase; an enzyme catalyzing a reversible reaction between an L-3-hydroxyacyl-CoA and a 2,3- (or 3,4) *trans*-enoyl-CoA in fatty acid degradation. SYN crotonase, enoyl hydrase.

eno·yl-CoA re·duc·tase. SYN *acyl-CoA* dehydrogenase (NADPH⁺).

2-en·o·yl-CoA re·duc·tase. Acyl-CoA dehydrogenase (NADP⁺).

en·o·yl hy·drase. SYN enoyl-CoA hydratase.

en·pro·fyl·line (eb-prō-fī-lin). A derivative of theophylline which shares with the latter agent bronchodilator properties. A xanthine derivative containing a propyl but lacking the methyl groups usually found in theophylline, caffeine and theobromine preparations. Used in asthma and chronic obstructive pulmonary disease.

E.N.S. Abbreviation for ethylnorepinephrine.

en·si·form (en′si-fōrm). SYN xiphoid. [L. *ensis,* sword, + *forma,* appearance]

en·sis·ter·num (en′sis-ter′nŭm). SYN xiphoid *process.* [L. *ensis,* sword, + sternum]

en·stro·phe (en′strō-fē). Obsolete term for entropion. [G. *en,* in, + *strophē,* a turning]

ensu Acronym for equivalent *n*ormal *s*on *u*nit, that amount of information (from any source linkage carrier phenotype, etc.) that will have the same impact on the conditional probability that a female consultand is a carrier for an X-linked trait as one normal son does; each normal son contributes one ensu. Cf. encu.

ENT Abbreviation for ears, nose, and throat. SEE otorhinolaryngology.

△**ent-.** SEE ento-.

en·tac·tin (ent-ak′tin). A glycoprotein that binds to laminin in the basal lamina of the renal glomerulus and is a major cell attachment factor. SYN nidogen.

en·tad. Toward the interior. [G. *entos,* within, + L. *ad,* to]

en·tal (en′tăl). Relating to the interior; inside. [G. *entos,* within]

ent·am·e·bi·a·sis (ent-ă-mē-bi′ă-sis). Infection with *Entamoeba histolytica.* SEE amebiasis, amebic *dysentery.*

Ent·a·moe·ba (ent-ă-mē′bă). A genus of ameba parasitic in the cecum and large bowel of man and other primates and in many domestic and wild mammals and birds; with the exception of *E. histolytica,* members of the genus appear to be relatively harmless inhabitants of the host. [G. *entos,* within + *amoibē,* change]

E. bucca′lis, former name for *E. gingivalis.*

E. co′li, nonpathogenic species that occurs in the large intestine of man, other primates, dogs, and possibly pigs; often confused with *E. histolytica,* but distinguished by nuclear details and by the number of nuclei and the form of chromatoidals in the cyst.

E. gingiva′lis, a species found in the oral cavity of man, other primates, dogs, and cats; in man, it is frequently associated with poor oral hygiene and its resultant diseases.

E. hartman′ni, species found in the large intestine of man, other primates, and dogs; now considered to be a distinct strain or species that is nonpathogenic and smaller than *E. histolytica* but otherwise indistinguishable from it; formerly called the "small race" of *E. histolytica.*

E. histoly′tica, a species that is the only distinct pathogen of the genus, the so-called "large race" of *E. histolytica,* causing tropical or amebic dysentery in man and also in dogs (man is the reservoir for canine infections). In man, the organism, though usually nonpathogenic, may penetrate the epithelial tissues of the colon, causing ulceration (amebic dysentery); in a small proportion of these cases, the organism may reach the liver by the portal bloodstream and produce abscesses (hepatic amebiasis); in a fraction of these cases it may then spread to other organs, such as the lungs, brain, kidney, or skin and frequently be fatal.

E. moshkov′skii, a species of ameba very similar to *E. histolytica,* probably not infective to man, but a cause of diagnostic difficulties since it has been recovered from human sewage and may be responsible for false-positive results in tests of sewage plant effluents.

En·te·mo·pox·vi·rus (en′tē-mō-poks-vī′rŭs). The genus of viruses (family Poxviridae) that comprises the poxviruses of insects; they seem not to multiply in vertebrates. [G. *entomon,* insect]

△**enter-.** SEE entero-.

en·ter·al (en′ter-ăl). Within, or by way of, the intestine or gastrointestinal tract, especially as distinguished from parenteral. [G. *enteron,* intestine]

en·ter·al·gia (en-ter-al′jē-ă). Enterdynia; severe abdominal pain accompanying spasm of the bowel. SYN enterdynia, enterodynia. [entero- + G. *algos,* pain]

en·ter·a·mine (en-ter-am′ēn). SYN serotonin.

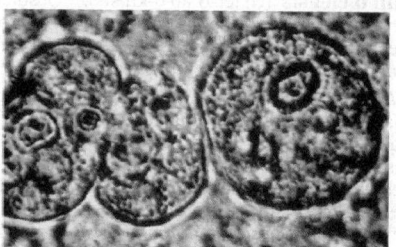

Entamoeba histolytica **(large form, in stool)**

en·ter·dy·nia (en-ter-din′ē-ă). SYN enteralgia.

en·ter·ec·ta·sis (en-ter-ek′tă-sis). Dilation of the bowel. [entero- + G. *ektasis,* a stretching]

en·ter·ec·to·my (en-ter-ek′tō-mē). Resection of a segment of the intestine. [entero- + G. *ektomē,* excision]

en·ter·el·co·sis (en-ter-el-kō′sis). Ulceration of the bowel. [entero- + G. *helkos,* ulcer]

en·ter·ic (en-ter′ik). Relating to the intestine. [G. *enterikos,* from *entera,* bowels]

en·ter·i·tis (en-ter-ī′tis). Inflammation of the intestine, especially of the small intestine. [entero- + G. *-itis,* inflammation]

e. anaphylac′tica, a hemorrhagic and necrotizing inflammation developing in the ileum (and also the colon) of sensitized dogs when they are fed a second dose of the sensitizing material. SYN chronic anaphylaxis.

chronic cicatrizing e., SYN regional e.

diphtheritic e., e. with the formation of a membrane or a false membrane. SEE ALSO pseudomembranous *enterocolitis.*

duck viral e., SYN duck *plague.*

feline infectious e., SYN panleukopenia.

granulomatous e., SYN regional e.

hemorrhagic e., a disease of turkeys caused by an adenovirus and characterized by splenomegaly and intestinal hemorrhage.

e. of mink, a highly contagious enteric disease of mink similar to panleukopenia and caused by mink enteritis virus.

mucomembranous e., an affection of the intestinal mucous membrane characterized by constipation or diarrhea (sometimes alternating), colic, and the passage of pseudomembranous shreds or incomplete casts of the intestine. SYN mucoenteritis (2).

e. necrot′icans, e. with necrosis of the bowel wall caused by *Clostridium welchii.*

phlegmonous e., severe acute inflammation of the intestine, with edematous bowel wall infiltrated with pus.

e. polypo′sa, e. associated with polyp formation.

pseudomembranous e., SYN pseudomembranous *enterocolitis.*

regional e., a subacute chronic e., of unknown cause, involving the terminal ileum and less frequently other parts of the gastrointestinal tract; characterized by patchy deep ulcers that may cause fistulas, and narrowing and thickening of the bowel by fibrosis and lymphocytic infiltration, with noncaseating tuberculoid granulomas that also may be found in regional lymph nodes; symptoms include fever, diarrhea, cramping abdominal pain, and weight loss. SYN chronic cicatrizing e., Crohn's disease, distal ileitis, regional ileitis, terminal ileitis, granulomatous e.

transmissible e., SYN bluecomb *disease* of turkeys.

tuberculous e., enteric tuberculosis that may occur in the absence of obvious pulmonary t.; may be caused by bovine tuberculosis contracted through drinking of unpasteurized milk or swallowing of tubercle bacilli expectorated from cavitary lesions in the lung.

ulcerative e., an e. of quail and chickens caused by the bacterium *Clostridium colinum.*

△**entero-, enter-.** The intestines. [G. *enteron,* intestine]

en·ter·o·a·nas·to·mo·sis (en′ter-ō-an-as-tō-mō′sis). SYN enteroenterostomy.

en·ter·o·an·the·lone (en′ter-ō-an′thĕ-lōn). SYN enterogastrone.

en

en·ter·o·ap·o·clei·sis (en'ter-ō-ap'ō-klī'sis). Obsolete term for exclusion of a segment of the intestine by forming an anastomosis between the parts above and below. [entero- + G. *apokleisis*, exclusion, fr. *apo*, from, + *kleiō*, to close]

En·ter·o·bac·ter (en'ter-ō-bak'ter). A genus of aerobic, facultatively anaerobic, nonsporeforming, motile bacteria (family Enterobacteriaceae) containing Gram-negative rods. The cells are peritrichous, and some strains have encapsulated cells. Glucose is fermented with the production of acid and gas. The Voges-Proskauer test is usually positive. Gelatin is slowly liquefied by the most commonly occurring forms (*E. cloacae*). These organisms occur in the feces of man and other animals and in sewage, soil, water, and dairy products; recognized as an agent of common nosocomial infections of the urinary tract, lungs, or blood. Somewhat resistant to antibiotics. The type species is *E. cloacae*.

E. aerog'enes, a species found in water, soil, sewage, dairy products, and the feces of man and other animals. Organisms previously identified as motile strains of *Aerobacter aerogenes* are now placed in this species. SYN *Klebsiella mobilis*.

E. cloa'cae, a species found in the feces of man and other animals and in sewage, soil, and water; it is occasionally found in urine and pus and in other pathologic materials from animals; it is the type species of the genus *E.*

en·ter·o·bac·te·ria (en'ter-ō-bak-tēr'ē-ă). Plural of enterobacterium.

En·ter·o·bac·te·ri·a·ce·ae (en'ter-ō-bak-tēr-ē-ā'sē-ē). A family of aerobic, facultatively anaerobic, nonsporeforming bacteria (order Eubacteriales) containing Gram-negative rods. Some species are nonmotile, and nonmotile variants of motile species occur; the motile cells are peritrichous. These organisms grow well on artificial media. They reduce nitrates to nitrites and utilize glucose fermentatively with the production of acid or acid and gas. Indophenol oxidase is not produced by these organisms. They do not liquefy alginate, and pectate is liquefied only by members of one genus, *Pectobacterium*. This family includes many animal parasites and some plant parasites causing blights, galls, and soft rots. Some of these organisms occur as saprophytes which decompose carbohydrate-containing plant materials. The type genus is *Escherichia*.

en·ter·o·bac·te·ri·um, pl. **en·ter·o·bac·te·ria** (en'ter-ō-bak-tēr'ē-ŭm, -ă). A member of the family Enterobacteriaceae.

en·ter·o·bi·a·sis (en'ter-ō-bī'ă-sis). Infection with *Enterobius vermicularis*, the human pinworm.

En·te·ro·bi·us (en-ter-ō'bī-ŭs). A genus of nematode worms, formerly included with the genus *Oxyuris*, which includes the pinworms (*E. vermicularis*) of man and primates. [entero- + G. *bios*, life]

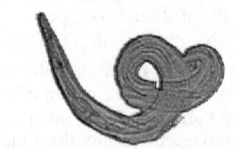

Enterobius vermicularis (pinworm, adult male)

en·ter·o·bro·sis, en·ter·o·bro·sia (en'ter-ō-brō'sis, -brō'zhē-ă). Obsolete term for perforation of the intestine. [entero- + G. *brōsis*, corrosion]

en·ter·o·cele (en'ter-o-sēl). **1.** A hernial protrusion through a defect in the rectovaginal or vesicovaginal pouch. [entero- + G. *kēlē*, hernia] **2.** SYN abdominal *cavity*. [entero- + G. *koilia*, a hollow] **3.** An intestinal hernia. [see 1]

partial e., SYN parietal *hernia*.

en·ter·o·cen·te·sis (en'ter-ō-sen-tē'sis). Puncture of the intestine with a hollow needle (trocar and cannula) to withdraw substances. [entero- + G. *kentēsis*, puncture]

en·ter·o·cho·le·cys·tos·to·my (en'ter-ō-kō-lē-sis-tos'tō-mē). SYN cholecystenterostomy. [entero- + G. *cholē*, bile, + *kystis*, bladder, + *stoma*, mouth]

en·ter·o·cho·le·cys·tot·o·my (en'ter-ō-kō-lē-sis-tot'ō-mē). SYN

cholecystenterotomy. [entero- + G. *cholē*, bile, + *kystis*, bladder, + *tomē*, a cutting]

en·ter·o·clei·sis (en-ter-ō-klī'sis). Occlusion of the lumen of the alimentary canal. [entero- + G. *kleisis*, a closing]

omental e., use of omentum to aid closure of an opening in intestine.

en·ter·oc·ly·sis (en-ter-ok'li-sis). **1.** SYN high *enema*. **2.** In radiography of the small intestine, filling by introduction of contrast medium through a catheter advanced into the duodenum or jejunum from above. [entero- + G. *klysis*, a washing out]

radiological e., method of imaging the duodenum and small intestine by intubation of the duodenum and installation of dilute barium; also known as small bowel enema.

en·ter·o·coc·cem·ia (en'ter-ō-kok-sēm'ē-ah). A blood-borne disease, occasionally leading to septicemia, caused by members of the group D streptococci, *Enterococcus faecalis* or *Enterococcus faecium*.

En·ter·o·coc·cus. Genus of facultatively anaerobic, generally nonmotile, non-spore forming, Gram-positive bacteria belonging to the family Streptococcaceae, formerly classified as part of the genus *Streptococcus*. Found in the intestinal tract of humans and animals, enterococci cause intraabdominal, wound and urinary tract infections. Type species is *E. faecalis*. *E. faecium* is also clinically significant.

en·ter·o·coc·cus, pl. **en·ter·o·coc·ci** (en'ter-ō-kok'ŭs, -kok'sī). A streptococcus that inhabits the intestinal tract. [entero- + G. *kokkos*, a berry]

en·ter·o·co·li·tis (en'ter-ō-kō-lī'tis). Inflammation of the mucous membrane of a greater or lesser extent of both small and large intestines. SYN coloenteritis. [entero- + G. *kolon*, colon, + *-itis*, inflammation]

antibiotic e., e. caused by oral administration of broad spectrum antibiotics, resulting from overgrowth of antibiotic-resistant staphylococci or yeasts and fungi, when the normal fecal Gram-negative organisms are suppressed, resulting in diarrhea or pseudomembranous disease.

necrotizing e., extensive ulceration and necrosis of the ileum and colon in premature infants in the neonatal period; possibly due to perinatal intestinal ischemia and bacterial invasion.

pseudomembranous e., e. with the formation and passage of pseudomembranous material in the stools; occurs most commonly as a sequel to antibiotic therapy; caused by a necrolytic exotoxin made by *Clostridium difficile*. SYN pseudomembranous colitis, pseudomembranous enteritis.

regional e., the changes of regional enteritis involving both the colon and the small intestine.

en·ter·o·co·los·to·my (en'ter-ō-kō-los'tō-mē). Establishment of an artificial opening between the small intestine and the colon. [entero- + G. *kōlon*, colon, + *stoma*, mouth]

en·ter·o·cyst (en'ter-ō-sist). A cyst of the wall of the intestine. SYN enterocystoma. [entero- + G. *kystis*, bladder]

en·ter·o·cys·to·cele (en'ter-ō-sis'tō-sēl). A hernia of both intestine and bladder wall. [entero- + G. *kystis*, bladder, + *kēlē*, hernia]

en·ter·o·cys·to·ma (en'ter-ō-sis-tō'mă). SYN enterocyst.

En·ter·o·cy·to·zo·on (en'ter-ō-sī'tō-zō'on). A genus in the protozoan phylum Microspora, all of which are obligate intracellular spore-forming parasites.

E. bieneusi, agent of microsporidian infection, primarily infecting the small intestine, especially in immunocompromised individuals. It is the microsporidian most frequently reported in AIDS patients, where it has been implicated in chronic diarrhea and weight loss; suggested treatment has been with octreotide with albendazole. SEE ALSO microsporidia.

en·ter·o·dyn·ia (en'ter-ō-din'ē-ă). SYN enteralgia. [entero- + G. *odynē*, pain]

en·ter·o·en·ter·os·to·my (en'ter-ō-en-ter-os'tō-mē). Establishment of a new communication between two segments of intestine. SYN enteroanastomosis, intestinal anastomosis.

en·ter·o·gas·tri·tis (en'ter-ō-gas-trī'tis). SYN gastroenteritis. [entero- + G. *gastēr*, belly, + *-itis*, inflammation]

en·ter·o·gas·trone (en'ter-ō-gas'trōn). A hormone, obtained from intestinal mucosa, that inhibits gastric secretion and motility; secretion of e. is stimulated by exposure of duodenal mucosa to dietary lipids. SYN anthelone E, enteroanthelone.

en·ter·og·e·nous (en-ter-oj′ĕ-nŭs). Of intestinal origin. [entero- + G. *-gen,* producing]

en·ter·o·graph (en′ter-ō-graf). An instrument designed for use in enterography.

en·ter·og·ra·phy (en-ter-og′ră-fē). The making of a graphic record delineating the intestinal muscular activity. [entero- + G. *graphō,* to write]

en·ter·o·hep·a·ti·tis (en′ter-ō-hep-ă-tī′tis). Inflammation of both the intestine and the liver. [entero- + G. *hēpar (hēpat-),* liver, + *-itis,* inflammation]

infectious e., SYN histomoniasis.

en·ter·o·hep·a·to·cele (en′ter-ō-hep′ă-tō-sēl). Congenital umbilical hernia containing intestine and liver. SEE omphalocele. [entero- + G. *hēpar (hēpat-),* liver, + *kēlē,* hernia]

en·ter·oi·dea (en-ter-oy′dē-ă). Fevers due to infection caused by any of the intestinal bacteria, including the enteric fevers (typhoid and paratyphoid A and B) and the parenteric fevers. [entero- + G. *eidos,* resemblance]

en·ter·o·ki·nase (en′tĕr-ō-kī′nās). SYN enteropeptidase.

en·ter·o·ki·ne·sis (en′ter-ō-ki-nē′sis). Muscular contraction of the alimentary canal. SEE ALSO peristalsis. [entero- + G. *kinēsis,* movement]

en·ter·o·ki·net·ic (en′ter-ō-ki-net′ik). Relating to, or producing, enterokinesis.

en·ter·o·lith (en′ter-ō-lith). An intestinal calculus formed of layers of soaps and earthy phosphates surrounding a nucleus of some hard body such as a swallowed fruit stone or other indigestible substance. [entero- + G. *lithos,* stone]

en·ter·o·li·thi·a·sis (en′ter-ō-li-thī′ă-sis). Presence of calculi in the intestine.

en·ter·ol·o·gy (en-ter-ol′ō-jē). The branch of medical science concerned especially with the intestinal tract. [entero- + G. *logos,* study]

en·ter·ol·y·sis (en-ter-ol′i-sis). Division of intestinal adhesions. [entero- + G. *lysis,* dissolution]

en·ter·o·meg·a·ly, en·ter·o·me·ga·lia (mak-rō-mēr, -ō-me-gā′lē-ă). SYN megaloenteron. [entero- + G. *megas,* great]

en·ter·o·me·nia (en-ter-ō-mē′nē-ă). Vicarious menstruation due to presence of tissue sensitive to effects of estrogen/progesterone in the intestine. [entero- + G. *emmēnos,* monthly]

en·ter·o·mer·o·cele (en′ter-ō-mēr′ō-sēl). Rarely used term for femoral *hernia.* [entero- + G. *mēros,* thigh, + *kēlē,* hernia]

en·ter·om·e·ter (en-ter-om′ĕ-ter). An instrument used in measuring the diameter of the intestine. [entero- + G. *metron,* measure]

En·te·ro·mo·nas (en′ter-ō-mō′nas, en-ter-om′ŏ-nas). A genus of flagellate protozoa, one species of which, *E. hominis,* is found as a rare nonpathogenic resident in the human large intestine. [entero- + G. *monas,* monad]

en·ter·o·my·co·sis (en′ter-ō-mī-kō′sis). An intestinal disease of fungal origin. [entero- + G. *mykēs,* fungus, + *-osis,* condition]

en·ter·o·pa·re·sis (en′ter-ō-pă-rē′sis, -par′i-sis). Rarely used term for a state of diminished or absent peristalsis with flaccidity of the muscles of the intestinal walls. [entero- + G. *paresis,* slackening, relaxation]

en·ter·o·path·o·gen (en′ter-ō-path′ō-jen). An organism capable of producing disease in the intestinal tract.

en·ter·o·path·o·gen·ic (en′ter-ō-path-ō-jen′ik). Capable of producing disease in the intestinal tract.

en·ter·op·a·thy (en-ter-op′ă-thē). An intestinal disease. [entero- + G. *pathos,* suffering]

gluten e., SYN celiac *disease.*

protein-losing e., increased fecal loss of serum protein, especially albumin, causing hypoproteinemia.

en·ter·o·pep·ti·dase (en′ter-ō-pep′ti-dās). An intestinal proteolytic glycoenzyme from the duodenal mucosa that converts trypsinogen into trypsin (removes a hexapeptide from trypsinogen). SYN enterokinase.

en·ter·o·pex·y (en′ter-ō-pek-sē). Fixation of a segment of the intestine to the abdominal wall. [entero- + G. *pēxis,* fixation]

en·ter·o·plas·ty (en′ter-ō-plas-tē). Obsolete term for plastic surgery of the intestine. [entero- + G. *plastos,* formed]

en·ter·o·ple·gia (en′ter-ō-plē′jē-ă). Rarely used term for adynamic *ileus.* [entero- + G. *plēgē,* stroke]

en·ter·o·plex (en-ter-ō-pleks). Obsolete term for an instrument for use in effecting union of the divided ends of the intestine.

en·ter·o·plexy (en′ter-ō-plek-sē). Obsolete term for joining the divided ends of the intestine. [entero- + G. *plexis,* weaving]

en·ter·o·proc·tia (en′ter-ō-prok′shē-ă). Rarely used term for the presence of an artifical anus, as by a colostomy. [entero- + G. *prōktos,* anus]

en·ter·op·to·sis, en·ter·op·to·sia (en′ter-ō-tō′sis, -tō′sē-ă). Abnormal descent of the intestines in the abdominal cavity, usually associated with falling of the other viscera. [entero- + G. *ptōsis,* a falling]

en·ter·op·tot·ic (en′ter-ō-tot′ik). Relating to or suffering from enteroptosis.

en·ter·o·re·nal (en′ter-ō-rē′năl). Relating to both the intestines and the kidneys.

en·ter·or·rha·gia (en-ter-ō-rā′jē-ă). Bleeding within the intestinal tract. [entero- + G. *rhēgnymi,* to burst forth]

en·ter·or·rha·phy (en-ter-ōr′ă-fē). Suture of the intestine. [entero- + G. *rhaphē,* suture]

en·ter·or·rhex·is (en′ter-ō-rek′sis). Rarely used term for rupture of the gut or bowel. [entero- + G. *rhēxis,* rupture]

en·ter·o·scope (en′ter-ō-skōp). A speculum for inspecting the inside of the intestine in operative cases. [entero- + G. *skopeō,* to view]

en·ter·o·sep·sis (en′ter-ō-sep′sis). Sepsis occurring in or derived from the alimentary canal. [entero- + G. *sēpsis,* putrefaction]

en·ter·o·spasm (en′ter-ō-spazm). Increased, irregular, and painful peristalsis. [entero- + G. *spasmos,* spasm]

en·ter·o·sta·sis (en-ter-os′tă-sis). Intestinal stasis; a retardation or arrest of the passage of the intestinal contents. SYN intestinal stasis. [entero- + G. *stasis,* a standing]

en·ter·o·stax·is (en′ter-ō-stak′sis). Obsolete term for oozing of blood from the mucous membrane of the intestine. [entero- + G. *staxis,* a dripping]

en·ter·o·ste·no·sis (en′ter-ō-sten-ō′sis). Narrowing of the lumen of the intestine. [entero- + G. *stenōsis,* narrowing]

en·ter·os·to·my (en-ter-os′tō-mē). An artificial anus or fistula into the intestine through the abdominal wall. [entero- + G. *stoma,* mouth]

double e., e. in which both proximal and distal openings of divided intestine are sutured to the abdomen wall.

en·ter·o·tome (en′ter-ō-tōm). An instrument for incising the intestine, especially in the creation of an artificial anus. [entero- + G. *tomē,* a cutting]

en·ter·ot·o·my (en-ter-ot′ō-mē). Incision into the intestine.

en·ter·o·tox·e·mia (en′ter-ō-tok-sē′mē-ă). Acute, highly fatal diseases, chiefly of cattle and sheep, caused by toxins produced in the intestine by various types of *Clostridium perfringens.* SYN milk colic. [entero- + toxemia]

en·ter·o·tox·i·ca·tion (en′ter-ō-tok-si-kā′shŭn). SYN autointoxication.

en·ter·o·tox·i·gen·ic (en′ter-ō-tok-si-jen′ik). Denoting an organism containing or producing a toxin specific for cells of the intestinal mucosa.

en·ter·o·tox·in (en′ter-ō-tok′sin). A cytotoxin specific for the cells of the intestinal mucosa. SYN intestinotoxin.

cytotonic e., an e. which morphologically changes, but does not kill, the target cell.

***Escherichia coli* e.,** e. produced by certain strains (serotypes) of *Escherichia coli,* seemingly associated with a transferable plasmid.

staphylococcal e., a soluble exotoxin produced by some strains of *Staphylococcus aureus,* and a cause of food poisoning.

en·ter·o·tox·ism (en′ter-ō-tok′sizm). SYN autointoxication.

en·ter·o·tro·pic (en'ter-ō-trop'ik). Attracted by or affecting the intestine. [entero- + G. *tropikos*, turning]

En·te·ro·vi·rus (en'ter-ō-vī'rŭs). A large and diverse group of viruses (family Picornaviridae) that includes poliovirus types 1 to 3, Coxsackievirus A and B, echoviruses, and the enteroviruses identified since 1969 and assigned type numbers. They are transient inhabitants of the alimentary canal and are stable at low pH.
   porcine E., a picornavirus causing Teschen disease in swine.

en·ter·o·zo·ic (en'ter-ō-zō'ik). Relating to an enterozoon.

en·ter·o·zo·on (en'ter-ō-zō'on). An animal parasite in the intestine. [entero- + G. *zōon*, animal]

ent·ge·gen (*E*) (ent'ge-gen). Term used when the two higher ranking groups, attached to different carbon atoms in a carbon-carbon double bond, are on opposite sides of the double bond (hence, analogous to trans-). [Ger. opposite]

en·thal·py (*H*) (en'thal-pē). Heat content, symbolized as *H;* a thermodynamic function, defined as $E + PV$, where E is the internal energy of a system, P the pressure, and V the volume; the heat of a reaction, measured at constant pressure, is ΔH. SYN heat (3). [G. *enthalpein*, to warm in]

en·the·sis (en'thĕ-sis). Obsolete term for the insertion of synthetic or other inorganic material to replace lost tissue. [G. an insertion, fr. *en*, in, + *thesis*, a placing]

en·the·si·tis (en-thĕ-sī'tis). Traumatic disease occurring at the insertion of muscles where recurring concentration of muscle stress provokes inflammation with a strong tendency toward fibrosis and calcification. [G. *enthetos*, implanted, + *-itis*, inflammation]

en·the·so·path·ic (en-thē-sō-path'ik). Denoting or characteristic of enthesopathy.

en·the·sop·a·thy (en-thē-sop'ă-thē). A disease process occurring at the site of insertion of muscle tendons and ligaments into bones or joint capsules. [G. *en*, in, + *thesis*, a placing, + *pathos*, suffering]

en·thet·ic (en-thet'ik). Obsolete term denoting both enthesis and exogenous.

en·thla·sis (en'thlă-sis). Depressed fracture of the skull. [G. a dent, fr. *en*, in, + *thlaō*, to crush]

en thyrse (ahn tirs'). Microconidia of certain dermatophytes arranged singly along both sides of a hypha. [Fr., fr. G. *en-*, in, + *thyrsos*, a stalk, wand]

en·tire (en-tīr'). Having a smoothly continuous edge or border without indentations or projections; denoting a margin, as of a bacterial colony.

en·ti·ty (en'ti-tē). An independent thing; that which contains in itself all the conditions essential to individuality; that which forms of itself a complete whole; medically, denoting a separate and distinct disease or condition. [L. *ens* (*ent-*), being, pres. p. of *esse*, to be]

⌂**ento-, ent-.** Inner, or within. SEE ALSO endo-. [G. *entos*, within]

en·to·blast (en'tō-blast). **1.** Pertaining to entoderm. **2.** Cell nucleolus. [ento- + G. *blastos*, germ]

en·to·cele (en'tō-sēl). An internal hernia. [ento- + G. *kēlē*, hernia]

en·to·cho·roi·dea (en'tō-kō-roy'dē-ă). SYN choriocapillary *layer.* [ento- + G. *chorioeidēs*, choroid]

en·to·cone (en-tō-kōn). The mesiolingual cusp of a maxillary molar tooth. [ento- + G. *kōnos*, cone]

en·to·co·nid (en-tō-kō'nid). The inner posterior cusp of a mandibular molar tooth. [ento- + G. *kōnos*, cone]

en·to·cor·nea (en-tō-kōr'nē-ă). SYN posterior limiting *layer* of cornea.

en·to·cra·ni·al (en'tō-krā'nē-ăl). SYN endocranial.

en·to·cra·ni·um (en'tō-krā'nē-ŭm). SYN endocranium.

en·to·derm (en'tō-derm). SYN endoderm. [ento- + G. *derma*, skin]

en·to·ec·tad (en-tō-ek'tad). From within outward. [G. *entos*, within, + *ektos*, without, + L. *ad*, to]

En·to·lo·ma si·nu·a·tum (en-tō-lō'mă sī-nyū-ā'tum). A species of mushroom capable of producing mycetismus gastrointestinalis.

en·to·mi·on (en-tō'mē-on). The tip of the mastoid angle of the parietal bone. [G. *entomē*, notch]

en·to·mol·o·gy (en-tō-mol'ō-jē). The science concerned with the study of insects. [G. *entomon*, insect, + *logos*, study]

en·to·mo·pho·bia (en'tō-mō-fō'bē-ă). Morbid fear of insects. [G. *entomon*, insect, + *phobos*, fear]

en·to·moph·tho·ra·my·co·sis (en-tō-mof'thō-ră-mī-kō'sis). A disease caused by fungi of the genera *Basidiobolus* or *Conidiobolus;* tissues are invaded by broad nonseptate hyphae that become surrounded by eosinophilic material. A form of zygomycosis. SEE zygomycosis. SYN rhinomucormycosis, rhinophycomycosis, subcutaneous phycomycosis. [Entomophthorales (order name) + G. *mykēs*, fungus + *-osis*, condition]
   e. basidiobo'lae, a subcutaneous phycomycosis due to the fungus *Basidiobolus ranarum*, characterized by the development of flat, firm subcutaneous fibrotic granulomas which do not ulcerate; occasionally, lesions may extend to muscles and lymph nodes and other deep tissues; the disease is found in Indonesia and in Uganda and other tropical African countries, but has not been seen in tropical America. A form of zygomycosis.
   e. conidiobo'lae, a zygomycosis caused by *Conidiobolus coronatus*, characterized by large nasal polyps and granulomas of the nasal cavity; it has been reported from Texas, the West Indies, Zaire, Nigeria, and other African states, Colombia, and Brazil. A form of zygomycosis.

en·top·ic (ent-op'tik). Placed within; occurring or situated in the normal place; opposed to ectopic. [G. *en*, within, + *topos*, place]

en·to·plasm (en'tō-plasm). SYN endoplasm.

ent·op·tic (en-top'tik). Within the eyeball. Often used to describe visual phenomena generated by mechanical or electrical stimulations of the retina. [ento- + G. *optikos*, relating to vision]

en·to·ret·i·na (en-tō-ret'i-nă). The layers of the retina from the outer plexiform to the nerve fiber layer inclusive. SYN Henle's nervous layer.

en·to·sarc (en'tō-sark). SYN endosarc.

En·to·zoa (en-tō-zō'ă). A nontaxonomic name for the branch of the kingdom Animalia, whose members possess a digestive cavity or tract; includes all vertebrates and higher invertebrate forms. [ento- + G. *zōon*, animal]

en·to·zo·al (en-tō-zō'ăl). Relating to entozoa.

en·to·zo·on, pl. **en·to·zoa** (en-tō-zō'on, -ă). An animal parasite whose habitat is any of the internal organs or tissues. [ento- + G. *zōon*, animal]

en·trails (en'trālz). The viscera of an animal.

en·tro·pi·on, en·tro·pi·um (en-trō'pē-on, -pē-ŭm). **1.** Inversion or turning inward of a part. **2.** The infolding of the margin of an eyelid. [G. *en*, in, + *tropē*, a turning]
   atonic e., e. that follows loss of tone of the orbicularis oculi muscle or elasticity of the skin.
   cicatricial e., e. that follows scarring of the palpebral conjunctiva.
   spastic e., e. that arises from excessive contracture of the orbicularis oculi muscle.

en·tro·pi·on·ize (en-trō'pē-on-īz). To invert a part.

en·tro·py (en'trō-pē). That fraction of heat (energy) content not available for the performance of work, usually because (in a chemical reaction) it has been used to increase the random motion of the atoms or molecules in the system; thus, e. is a measure of randomness or disorder. E. occurs in the Gibbs free energy (*G*) equation: $\Delta G = \Delta H - T\Delta S$ (ΔH, change in enthalpy or heat content; *T*, absolute temperature; ΔS, change in entropy). SEE ALSO second *law* of thermodynamics. [G. *entropia*, a turning towards]

en·ty·py (en'ti-pē). A type of gastrulation seen in some early mammalian embryos in which the endoderm covers the embryonic and amniotic ectoderm; part of the preplacental trophoblast may also be covered. [G. *entypē*, pattern]

enu·cle·ate (ē-nū'klē-āt). To remove entirely; to shell like a nut, as in the removal of an eye from its capsule or a tumor from its enveloping capsule.

enu·cle·a·tion (ē-nū-klē-ā'shŭn). **1.** Removal of an entire structure (such as an eyeball or tumor), without rupture, as one shells the kernel of a nut. **2.** Removal or destruction of the nucleus of a cell. [L. *enucleo,* to remove the kernel, fr. *e,* out, + *nucleus,* nut, kernel]

en·u·re·sis (en-yū-rē´sis). Urinary incontinence; may be intentional or involuntary but not due to a physical disorder. [G. *en-oureō,* to urinate in]

diurnal e., urinary accidents during wakefulness.

nocturnal e., urinary incontinence during sleep. SYN bedwetting.

en·ve·lope (en´vĕ-lōp). In anatomy, a structure that encloses or covers.

corneocyte e., an electron-dense, 10-15 nm thick layer of highly cross-linked protein on the cytoplasmic surface of the cell membrane of epidermal corneocytes; it is highly resistant to proteolytic agents. SYN subplasmalemmal dense zone.

nuclear e., the double membrane at the boundary of the nucleoplasm; it has regularly spaced pores covered by a disklike nuclear pore complex and a space or cisterna about 150 Å wide between the two layers; the outer membrane is continuous at intervals with the endoplasmic reticulum. SYN caryotheca, karyotheca, nuclear membrane.

viral e., the outer structure that encloses the nucleocapsids of some viruses; may contain host material.

en·ven·om·a·tion (en-ven-ō-mā´shŭn). The act of injecting a poisonous material (venom) by sting, spine, bite, or other venom apparatus.

en·vi·ron·ment (en-vī´ron-ment). The milieu; the aggregate of all of the external conditions and influences affecting the life and development of an organism. It can be divided into physical, biological, social, cultural, etc., any or all of which can influence the health status of the population. [Fr. *environ,* around]

en·vy (en´vē). One's feeling of discontent or jealousy resulting from comparison with another person.

penis e., the psychoanalytic concept in which a female envies male characteristics or capabilities, especially the possession of a penis.

en·zo·ot·ic (en-zō-ot´ik). Denoting a temporal pattern of disease occurrence in an animal population in which the disease occurs with predictable regularity with only relatively minor fluctuations in its frequency over time. SEE epizootic, sporadic. Cf. epizootic, sporadic. SYN endemic (2). [G. *en,* in, + *zōon,* animal]

en·zy·got·ic (en-zī-got´ik). Derived from a single fertilized ovum; denoting twins so derived. [G. *eis (en),* one, + zygote]

en·zy·mat·ic (en-zī-mat´ik). Relating to an enzyme. SYN enzymic.

en·zyme (en´zīm). A protein that acts as a catalyst to induce chemical changes in other substances, itself remaining apparently unchanged by the process. E.'s, with the exception of those discovered long ago (*e.g.,* pepsin, emulsin), are generally named by adding -ase to the name of the substrate on which the e. acts (*e.g.,* glucosidase), the substance activated (*e.g.,* hydrogenase), and/or the type of reaction (*e.g.,* oxidoreductase, transferase, hydrolase, lyase, isomerase, ligase or synthetase—these being the six main groups in the Enzyme Nomenclature Recommendations of the International Union of Biochemistry). For individual enzymes not listed below, see the specific name. SYN organic catalyst (1). [G. + L. *en,,* in, + *zymē,* leaven]

acetyl-activating e., SYN *acetyl-CoA* ligase.

acyl-activating e., (1) SYN long-chain fatty acid-CoA ligase. **(2)** SYN butyrate-CoA ligase.

adaptive e., SYN induced e.

allosteric e., an e. that exhibits the property of allosterism.

amino acid activating e., SYN *aminoacyl-tRNA* synthetases.

angiotensin-converting e. (ACE), a hydrolase responsible for the conversion of angiotensin I to the vasoactive angiotensin II by removal of a dipeptide (histidylleucine) from angiotensin I. Drugs that inhibit ACE are used to treat hypertension and congestive heart failure.

antitumor e., an e. that stimulates the degradation of a particular metabolite that cannot be synthesized by tumor cells, inhibits the synthesis of a metabolite needed by tumor cells, or inhibits tumor-specific DNA utilization; *e.g.,* asparaginase.

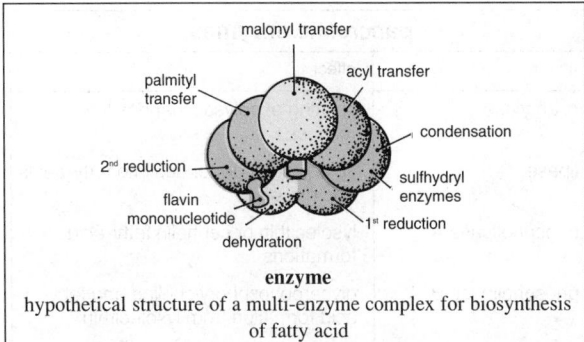

enzyme
hypothetical structure of a multi-enzyme complex for biosynthesis of fatty acid

examples of secretion enzymes	
inactive	active
plasma	
prothrombin	thrombin
plasminogen	plasmin
prekallikrein	kallikrein
lipoprotein lipase	lipoprotein lipase + apolipoprotein CII (as cofactor)
digestive tract	
trypsinogen	α-amylase
chymotrypsinogen	pancrelipase
	trypsin
	chymotrypsin

autolytic e., an e. capable of causing lysis of the cell forming it.

branching e., SYN 1,4-α-D-glucan branching enzyme.

β-carotene cleavage e., SYN β-carotene 15,15′-dioxygenase.

citrate cleavage e., SYN ATP *citrate (pro-3S)*-lyase.

cold sensitive e., an e. that loses its stability as the temperature is lowered.

condensing e., SYN *citrate* synthase.

constitutive e., an e. that is constantly produced by the cell regardless of the growth conditions. Cf. induced e.

cooperative e., an e. that exhibits the property of cooperativity.

D e., SYN 4-α-D-glucanotransferase.

deamidizing e.'s, SYN amidohydrolases.

deaminating e.'s, SYN deaminases.

debranching e.'s, e.'s that bring about destruction of branches in glycogen; formerly considered to be one enzyme, now known to be a mixture of transferases (4-α-D-glucanotransferase) and hydrolases (amylo-1,6-glucosidase). SYN debranching factors.

digestive e.'s, (1) e.'s that are utilized in the digestive system; **(2)** e.'s that are hydrolases of macromolecules (*e.g.,* amylases, proteinases).

disproportionating e., SYN 4-α-D-glucanotransferase.

extracellular e., an e. performing its functions outside a cell; *e.g.,* the various digestive e.'s. SYN exoenzyme, lyoenzyme.

heat-stable e., SYN thermostable e.

hydrolyzing e.'s, SYN hydrolases.

immobilized e., an e. that has been bound, usually covalently, to an insoluble organic or inorganic matrix or has been encapsulated.

induced e., inducible e., an e. that can be detected in a growing culture of a microorganism, after the addition of a particular substance (inducer) to the culture medium, but was not detect-

pancreatic enzymes	
name	effect
α-amylase	splitting of polysaccharides into maltose
lipase	splitting of triglycerides into fatty-acids and glycerin
phospholipase A	lysolecithin or cephalin fatty-acid formations
phospholipase B	glycerophosphorylcholine and fatty-acid formation from lysolecithin
trypsin	splitting (especially) of denatured proteins; secreted as trypsinogen
chymotrypsins	similar to trypsin
carboxypeptidases	release of terminal amino acids
ribonuclease	divides 3′-phosphates
desoxyribonuclease	specific phosphodiesterase end products: oligodesoxynucleotide
elastase collagenase	digestion of elastic or collagenous fibers
kallikrein	release of kinins
sterolesterhydrolase	divides sterol fatty-acid esters

able prior to the addition and can act on the inducer. A prototype is the β-galactosidase of *Escherichia coli*, synthesized upon the addition of various galactosides, whether or not these are good substrates. Cf. constitutive e. SYN adaptive e.

intracellular e., an e. that performs its functions within the cell that produces it; most e.'s are intracellular e.'s. SYN endoenzyme.

Kornberg e., DNA polymerase I from *Escherichia coli*.

malate-condensing e., SYN *malate* synthase.

malic e., SYN *malate* dehydrogenase.

marker e., an e. that is used to identify a specific cell type, cell organelle, or cell component.

membrane e., an e. present or embedded in a biomembrane.

methionine-activating e., SYN *methionine* adenosyltransferase.

new yellow e., the D-amino-acid oxidase found in yeast, a flavoenzyme, which contains FAD as coenzyme instead of FMN as does NADPH dehydrogenase; so-called to distinguish it from Warburg's old yellow e. Cf. *amino acid* oxidases.

old yellow e., SYN NADPH dehydrogenase.

P e., SYN phosphorylase.

pantoate-activating e., SYN *pantothenate* synthetase.

phosphorylase-rupturing e. (PR e.), SYN *phosphorylase* phosphatase.

photoreactivating e. (PR e.), SYN deoxyribodipyrimidine photolyase.

PR e., abbreviation for phosphorylase-rupturing e.; photoreactivating e.

Q e., 1,4-α-glucan branching e. in plants.

R e., SYN α-dextrin endo-1,6-α-glucosidase.

reducing e., SYN reductase.

repair e., an e. that can catalyze the repair of damaged DNA; *e.g.,* DNA ligase.

repressible e., an e. that is produced continuously unless production is repressed by excess of an inhibitor (corepressor). SEE ALSO inactive *repressor*.

respiratory e., one of those e.'s in tissues that is a part of an oxidation-reduction system accomplishing the conversion of substrates to CO_2 and H_2O and the transfer of the electrons removed to O_2.

restriction e., SYN restriction *endonuclease*.

RNA e., SYN ribozyme.

Schardinger e., SYN *xanthine* oxidase.

splitting e.'s, e.'s that, like aldolases, catalyze the conversion of a molecule into two smaller molecules without the addition or subtraction of any atoms.

T e., 1,4-α-D-glucan 6-α-D-glucosyltransferase.

terminal addition e., SYN DNA nucleotidylexotransferase.

thermostable e., an e. that is not readily subject to destruction or alteration by heat. SYN heat-stable e.

thiol e., an e. whose activity depends on a free thiol group.

transferring e.'s, SYN transferases.

Warburg's old yellow e., SYN NADPH dehydrogenase. SEE ALSO new yellow e., yellow e.

Warburg's respiratory e., SYN Atmungsferment.

yellow e., SYN flavoenzyme. SEE ALSO Warburg's old yellow e., new yellow e.

En·zyme Com·mis·sion. SEE EC.

en·zy·mic (en-zī'mik). SYN enzymatic.

en·zy·mol·o·gist (en-zī-mol'ō-jist). A specialist in enzymology.

en·zy·mol·o·gy (en-zī-mol'ō-jē). The branch of chemistry concerned with the properties and actions of enzymes. [enzyme + G. *logos,* study]

en·zy·mol·y·sis (en-zī-mol'i-sis). **1.** The splitting or cleavage of a substance into smaller parts by means of enzymatic action. **2.** Lysis by the action of an enzyme. [enzyme + G. *lysis,* dissolution]

en·zy·mop·a·thy (en-zī-mop'ă-thē). Any disturbance of enzyme function, including genetic deficiency or defect in specific enzymes. [enzyme + G. *pathos,* disease]

EOG Abbreviation for electro-oculography; electro-olfactogram.

eo·sin (ē'ō-sin). A derivative of fluorescein used as a fluorescent acid dye for cytoplasmic stains and counterstains in histology and in Romanovsky-type blood stains. [G. *ēōs,* dawn]

alcohol-soluble e., SYN ethyl e.

e. B, the disodium salt of 4′,5′-dibromo-2′,7′-dinitrofluorescein. SYN acid red 91, e. I bluish. [C.I. 45400]

ethyl e., SEE ethyl e. SYN alcohol-soluble e.

e. I bluish, SYN e. B.

e. y, e. Ys, the disodium salt of 2′,4′,5′,7′-tetrabromofluorescein. SYN acid red 87, e. yellowish. [C.I. 45380]

e. yellowish, SYN e. y.

eo·sin·o·cyte (ē-ō-sin'ō-sīt). SYN eosinophilic *leukocyte*.

eo·sin·o·pe·ni·a (ē'ō-sin-ō-pē'nē-ă). The presence of eosinophils in an abnormally small number in the peripheral bloodstream. SYN hypoeosinophilia. [eosino(phil) + G. *penia,* poverty]

eo·sin·o·phil, eo·sin·o·phile (ē-ō-sin'ō-fil, -fīl). SYN eosinophilic *leukocyte*. [eosin + G. *philos,* fond]

eo·sin·o·phil·ia (ē'ō-sin-ō-fil'ē-ă). SYN eosinophilic *leukocytosis*.

simple pulmonary e., pulmonary infiltrates seen as transient migratory shadows on the chest x-ray, accompanied by blood e.; often symptomless, but there may be cough, fever, and breathlessness; most cases are due to worm infestation, especially by *Ascaris lumbricoides;* a few cases follow administration of drugs. SYN Löffler's syndrome (1).

tropical e., e. associated with cough and asthma, caused by occult filarial infection without evidence of microfilaremia, occurring most frequently in India and Southeast Asia.

eo·sin·o·phil·ic (ē-ō-sin-ō-fil'ik). Staining readily with eosin dyes; denoting such cell or tissue elements.

eo·sin·o·phil·u·ria (ē-ō-sin'ō-fil-yū'rē-ă). Presence of eosinophils in the urine.

eo·sin·o·tac·tic (ē'ō-sin-ō-tak'tik). Exerting a force of attraction or repulsion on eosinophile cells. [eosino(phile) + G. *taktikos,* in orderly arrangement]

eo·sin·o·tax·is (ē'ō-sin-ō-tak'sis). Movement of eosinophils with reference to a stimulus which attracts or repels them.

eo·so·pho·bia (ē-ō-sō-fō'bē-ă). Morbid dread of the dawn. [G. *ēōs,* dawn, + *phobos,* fear]

EP Abbreviation for endogenous *pyrogen.*

epac·tal (ē-pak'tăl). SYN supernumerary. [G. *epaktos,* imported, fr. *epagō,* to bring on or in]

ep·am·ni·ot·ic (ep′am-nē-ot′ik). Upon or above the amnion. [G. *epi,* upon, + amnion]

ep·ar·sal·gia (ep-ar-sal′jē-ă). Pain and soreness from overuse or unaccustomed use of a part, as a joint or muscle. SYN epersalgia. [G. *epairo,* to lift up, + *algos,* pain]

ep·ar·te·ri·al (ep′ar-tēr-ē-ăl). Upon or superior to an artery. [G. *epi,* upon, + *artēia,* artery]

ep·ax·i·al (ep-ak′sē-ăl). Above or behind any axis, such as the spinal axis or the axis of a limb. [G. *epi,* upon, + L. *axis,* axis]

EPEC. Abbreviation for enteropathogenic *Escherichia coli.*

ep·en·dy·ma (ep-en′di-mă) [NA]. The cellular membrane lining the central canal of the spinal cord and the brain ventricles. SYN endyma. [G. *ependyma,* an upper garment]

ep·en·dy·mal (ep-en′di-măl). Relating to the ependyma.

ep·en·dy·mi·tis (ep-en-di-mī′tis). Inflammation of the ependyma.

ep·en·dy·mo·blast (ep-en′di-mō-blast). An embryonic ependymal cell. [ependyma + G. *blastos,* germ]

ep·en·dy·mo·blas·to·ma (ep-en′di-mō-blas-tō′mă). A glial neoplasm of the central nervous system, occurring typically in childhood; the prototype tumor cells resemble ependymoblasts. [ependymoblast + G. *-ōma,* tumor]

ep·en·dy·mo·cyte (ep-en′di-mō-sīt). An ependymal cell. [ependyma + G. *kytos,* cell]

ep·en·dy·mo·ma (ep-en-di-mō′mă). A glioma derived from relatively undifferentiated ependymal cells, comprising approximately 1 to 3% of all intracranial neoplasms; e.'s occur in all age groups and may originate from the lining of any of the ventricles or, more commonly, from the central canal of the spinal cord; histologically, the neoplastic cells tend to be arranged radially about blood vessels, to which they are attached by means of fibrillary processes.

myxopapillary e., a slow-growing e. of the filum terminale, occurring most often in young adults, consisting of cuboidal cells in papillary arrangement around a mucinous vascular core.

ep·er·sal·gia (ep-er-sal′jē-ă). SYN eparsalgia.

Ep·e·ryth·ro·zo·on (ep′ĕ-rith′rō-zō′on). A genus of minute rickettsiae (family Bartonellaceae, order Rickettsiales) of animals occurring upon the surface of erythrocytes and in the plasma; they appear as rings, coccoids, and short rods when clustered on the surface of the red cells in stained films. Some species cause anemia and icterus. [G. *epi,* upon + *erythros,* red, + *zōon,* animal]

E. coccoi′des, a species present in mice, but usually requiring splenectomy to reveal infections; rats and hamsters may be artificially infected; bloodsucking arthropods, especially lice, have been implicated as biological vectors, and mechanical transmission by bloodsucking flies has been demonstrated; the pathogenic effect is slight except when combined with other disease-producing agents.

E. o′vis, a species found in sheep, rarely causing disease.

E. su′is, a species that produces icterus and anemia in young pigs and icteroanemia of swine.

E. wenyo′ni, a species found in cattle, rarely causing disease.

ep·e·ryth·ro·zo·on·o·sis (ep′ĕ-rith′rō-zō-ō-nō′sis). Infection with any species of *Eperythrozoon.*

eph·apse (ef′aps). A place where two or more nerve cell processes (axons, dendrites) touch without forming a typical synaptic contact; some form of neural transmission may occur at such nonsynaptic contact sites. [G. *ephapsis,* contact]

eph·ap·tic (e-fap′tik). Relating to an ephapse.

ephe·bic (ĕ-fē′bik). Rarely used term relating to the period of puberty or to a youth. [G. *ephēbikos,* relating to youth, fr. *hēbē,* youth]

eph·e·bol·o·gy (ef-ĕ-bol′ō-jē). Rarely used term for the study of the morphologic and other changes incidental to puberty. [G. *ephēbos,* puberty, + *logos,* study]

ephed·ra (ē-fed′răh). *Ephedra equisetina* (family Gnetaceae). Ma Huang; the plant source for the alkaloid ephedrine. Indigenous to China and India, it is 0.75 to over 1% ephedrine; also contains some pseudoephedrine.

ephed·rine (ĕ-fed′rin, ef′ĕ-drin). 2-Methylamino-1-phenyl-1-propanol; an alkaloid from the leaves of *Ephedra equisetina,* E. sinica, and other species (family Gnetaceae), or produced synthetically; an adrenergic (sympathomimetic) agent with actions similar to those of epinephrine; used as a bronchodilator, mydriatic, pressor agent, and topical vasoconstrictor. Generally used salts are e. hydrochloride and e. sulfate.

ephe·lis, pl. **ephe·li·des** (ef-ē′lis, ef-ē′li-dēz). SYN freckle. [G.]

⚠**epi-.** Upon, following, or subsequent to. [G.]

ep·i·an·dros·ter·one (ep′i-an-dros′ter-ōn). 3β-hydroxy-5α-androstan-17-one; inactive isomer (3β instead of 3α) of androsterone; found in urine and in testicular and ovarian tissue. SYN isoandrosterone.

ep·i·bati·dine (ep′ĭ-băt′tĭ-dīn). A toxic alkaloid extracted from the venom of a South American frog, *Epipedobates tricolor.* The venom has been used as an arrow poison by native hunters; exerts analgesia by a mechanism other than activation of opiate receptors or cyclooxygenase inhibition.

ep·i·blast (ep′i-blast). Gives rise to ectoderm and mesoderm. The mesoderm then displaces the hypoblast cells and forms the entodermal cell layer on its inner surface. [epi- + G. *blastos,* germ]

ep·i·blas·tic (ep-i-blas′tik). Relating to epiblast.

ep·i·bleph·a·ron (ep′i-blef′ă-ron). A congenital horizontal skin fold near the margin of the eyelid, caused by abnormal insertion of muscle fibers. In the upper lid, it simulates blepharochalasis; in the lower lid, it causes a turning inward of the lashes. [epi- + G. *blepharon,* eyelid]

epib·o·ly, epib·o·le (ē-pib′ō-lē). 1. A process involved in gastrulation of telolecithal eggs in which, as a result of differential growth, some of the cells of the protoderm move over the surface toward the lips of the blastopore. 2. Growth of epithelium in an organ culture to surround the underlying mesenchymal tissue. [G. *epibolē,* a throwing or laying on]

ep·i·bul·bar (ep-i-bŭl′bar). Upon a bulb of any kind; specifically, upon the eyeball.

ep·i·can·thus (ep-i-kan′thŭs). SYN epicanthal *fold.* [epi- + G. *kanthos,* canthus]

e. inver′sus, a crescentic upward fold of skin from the lower eyelid at the inner canthus; frequent in congenital blepharoptosis.

e. palpebra′lis, e. arising from the upper lid above the tarsal portion and extending to the lower portion of the orbit.

e. supracilia′ris, e. arising from the region of the eyebrows and extending toward the tear sac.

e. tarsa′lis, e. arising from the tarsal fold and disappearing in the skin close to the inner canthus.

ep·i·car·dia (ep-i-kar′dē-ă). The portion of the esophagus from where it passes through the diaphragm to the stomach. [epi- + G. *kardia,* heart]

ep·i·car·di·al (ep-i-kar′dē-ăl). 1. Relating to the epicardia. 2. Relating to the epicardium.

ep·i·car·di·um (ep-i-kar′dē-ŭm) [NA]. SYN visceral *layer* of serous pericardium. [epi- + G. *kardia,* heart]

ep·i·chord·al (ep-i-kōr′dăl). On the dorsal side of the notochord; applicable particularly to that part of the brain developing dorsal to the cephalic part of the notochord. [epi- + G. *chordē,* a chord]

ep·i·cil·lin (ep-ĭ-sil′in). Semisynthetic beta-lactam antibiotic related to penicillin; an antibacterial.

ep·i·co·mus (ep-i-kō′mŭs, ē-pik′ō-mŭs). Unequal conjoined twins in which the smaller parasite is joined to the larger autosite at the top of the head. SEE conjoined *twins*, under *twin*. [epi- + G. *komē*, hair of the head]

ep·i·con·dy·lal·gia (ep′i-kon-di-lal′jē-ă). Pain in an epicondyle of the humerus or in the tendons or muscles originating therefrom. [epicondyle + G. *algos*, pain]

  e. exter′na, SYN tennis *elbow.*

ep·i·con·dyle (ep-i-kon′dīl). A projection from a long bone near the articular extremity above or upon the condyle. SYN epicondylus [NA]. [epi- + G. *kondylos*, a knuckle]

  lateral e. of femur, the e. located proximal to the lateral condyle. SYN epicondylus lateralis ossis femoris [NA], lateral femoral tuberosity.

  lateral e. of humerus, the e. situated at the lateral side of the distal end of the bone. SYN epicondylus lateralis humeri [NA].

  medial e. of femur, the e. located proximal to the medial condyle. SYN epicondylus medialis ossis femoris [NA], medial femoral tuberosity.

  medial e. of humerus, the e. situated proximal and medial to the condyle. SYN epicondylus medialis humeri [NA], epitrochlea.

ep·i·con·dy·li (ep-i-kon′di-lī). Plural of epicondylus.

ep·i·con·dyl·i·an (ep-i-kon-dil′ē-an). SYN epicondylic.

ep·i·con·dyl·ic (ep-i-kon-dil′ik). Relating to an epicondyle or to the part above a condyle. SYN epicondylian.

ep·i·con·dy·li·tis (ep′i-kon-di-lī′tis). Infection or inflammation of an epicondyle.

  lateral humeral e., SYN tennis *elbow.*

ep·i·con·dy·lus, pl. **ep·i·con·dy·li** (ep-i-kon′di-lŭs, -lī) [NA]. SYN epicondyle. [L.]

  e. latera′lis hu′meri [NA], SYN lateral *epicondyle* of humerus.

  e. latera′lis os′sis fem′oris [NA], SYN lateral *epicondyle* of femur.

  e. media′lis hu′meri [NA], SYN medial *epicondyle* of humerus.

  e. media′lis os′sis fem′oris [NA], SYN medial *epicondyle* of femur.

ep·i·cor·a·coid (ep-i-kōr′ă-koyd). Upon or above the coracoid process.

ep·i·cra·ni·al. Relating to the epicranium.

ep·i·cra·ni·um (ep-i-krā′nē-ŭm). The muscle, aponeurosis, and skin covering the cranium. [epi- + G. *kranion*, skull]

ep·i·cri·sis (ep-i-krī′sis). A secondary crisis; a crisis terminating a recrudescence of morbid symptoms following a primary crisis.

ep·i·crit·ic (ep-i-krit′ik). That aspect of somatic sensation which permits the discrimination and the topographical localization of the finer degrees of touch and temperature stimuli. Cf. protopathic. [G. *epikritikos*, adjudicatory, fr. *epi*, on, + *krinō*, to separate, judge]

ep·i·cys·ti·tis (ep′i-sis-tī′tis). Inflammation of the cellular tissue around the bladder. [epi- + G. *kystis*, bladder, + *-itis*, inflammation]

ep·i·cyte (ep′i-sīt). A cell membrane, especially of protozoa; the external layer of cytoplasm in gregarines. [epi- + G. *kytos*, cell]

ep·i·dem·ic (ep-i-dem′ik). The occurrence in a community or region of cases of an illness, specific health-related behavior, or other health-related events clearly in excess of normal expectancy; the word also is used to describe outbreaks of disease in animals or plants. Cf. endemic, sporadic. [epi- + G. *dēmos*, the people]

  behavioral e., an e. originating in behavioral patterns (in contrast to invading microorganisms); examples include medieval dancing mania, episodes of crowd panic.

  outbreak e., localized epidemic.

  point e., an e. where a pronounced clustering of cases of disease occurs within a very short period of time (within a few days or even hours) due to exposure of persons or animals to a common source of infection such as food or water.

ep·i·dem·ic·i·ty (ep′i-dem-is′i-tē). The state of prevailing disease in epidemic form.

ep·i·de·mi·og·ra·phy (ep′i-dem-ē-og′ră-fē). A descriptive trea-

tise of epidemic diseases or of any particular epidemic. [G. *epidēmios*, epidemic, + *graphē*, a writing]

ep·i·de·mi·ol·o·gist (ep-i-dē-mē-ol′ō-jist). An investigator who studies the occurrence of disease or other health-related conditions, states, or events in specified populations; one who practices epidemiology; the control of disease is usually also considered to be a task of the epidemiologist.

ep·i·de·mi·ol·o·gy (ep-i-dē-mē-ol′ō-jē). The study of the distribution and determinants of health-related states or events in specified populations, and the application of this study to control of health problems. [G. *epidēmios*, epidemic, + *logos*, study]

The study of the distribution and determinants of health-related states in human and other animal populations. Epidemiological studies involve surveillance, observation, hypothesis-testing, and experiment. Distribution is established by analyzing the time, place, and class of person affected by a disease. Determinants may include physical, biological, social, cultural, and behavioral factors. Epidemiological methods are most commonly applied to the study of disease; however, they also may be used to examine causes of death (e.g., homicides of various sorts) or behaviors (e.g., tobacco or alcohol use, practice of safe sex, use of health services). Epidemiology plays a key role in formulation and implementation of public health policy.

  clinical e., the field concerned with applying epidemiological principles in a clinical setting.

Whereas classical epidemiology studies populations in an attempt to assess causes and distribution of disease and to formulate statistical measures of risk, clinical epidemiology focuses on medically defined populations (patients).

ep·i·derm, ep·i·der·ma (ep′i-derm, ep-i-der′mă). SYN epidermis.

ep·i·der·mal, ep·i·der·mat·ic (ep-i-der′măl, -der-mat′ik). Relating to the epidermis. SYN epidermic.

ep·i·der·mal·i·za·tion (ep-i-der′mal-i-zā′shŭn). SYN squamous *metaplasia.*

ep·i·der·mat·o·plas·ty (ep-i-der′ma-tō-plas-tē). Rarely used term for skin grafting by means of strips or small patches of epidermis with the underlying outer layer of the corium. [epidermis + G. *plastos*, formed]

ep·i·der·mic (ep-i-der′mik). SYN epidermal.

ep·i·der·mi·do·sis (ep′i-der-mi-dō′sis). SYN epidermosis.

ep·i·der·mis, pl. **ep·i·derm·i·des** (ep-i-derm′is, -derm′i-dēz) [NA]. **1.** The superficial epithelial portion of the skin (cutis). The e. of the palms and soles has the following strata: stratum corneum (horny layer), stratum lucidum (clear layer), stratum granulosum (granular layer), stratum spinosum (prickle cell layer), and stratum basale (basal cell layer); in other parts of the body, the stratum lucidum may be absent. **2.** In botany, the outermost layer of cells in leaves and the young parts of plants. SYN cuticle (3), cuticula (2), epiderm, epiderma. [G. *epidermis*, the outer skin, fr. *epi*, on, + *derma*, skin]

ep·i·der·mi·tis (ep-i-der-mī′tis). Inflammation of the epidermis or superficial layers of the skin.

ep·i·der·mi·za·tion (ep′i-der-mi-zā′shŭn). **1.** Rarely used term for skin grafting. **2.** Rarely used term for the covering of an area with epidermis.

ep·i·der·mo·dys·pla·sia (ep-i-der′mō-dis-plā′zē-ă). Faulty growth or development of the epidermis. [epidermis + G. *dys-*, bad, + *plasis*, a molding]

  e. verrucifor′mis [MIM*226400], numerous flat warts on the hands and feet, in patients with inherited defects in cell-mediated immunity and increased susceptibility to human papilloma virus infections; skin carcinoma sometimes develops. The genetic component in the etiology is suspect, but is, if anything, autosomal recessive.

ep·i·der·moid (ep-i-der′moyd). **1.** Resembling epidermis. **2.** A cholesteatoma or other cystic tumor arising from aberrant epidermal cells. [epidermis + G. *eidos,* appearance]

ep·i·der·mol·y·sis (ep'i-der-mol'i-sis). A condition in which the epidermis is loosely attached to the corium, readily exfoliating or forming blisters. [epidermis + G. *lysis,* loosening]

e. bullo'sa [MIM*131800], a group of inherited chronic noninflammatory skin diseases in which large bullae and erosions result from slight mechanical trauma; a dominant form localized on the hands and feet is also called Weber-Cockayne syndrome. SYN mechanobullous disease.

e. bullosa, dermal type, SYN e. bullosa dystrophica.

e. bullo'sa dystroph'ica [MIM*131705], a form of e. bullosa in which scarring develops after separation of the entire epidermis with blistering; it is inherited as a dominant (appearing in infancy or childhood) or recessive (present at birth or appearing in early infancy) trait, the latter including lethal and nonlethal types. SYN dermolytic bullous dermatosis, e. bullosa, dermal type.

e. bullosa, epidermal type (bu'lō-să), SYN e. bullosa simplex.

e. bullosa, junctional type, SYN e. bullosa lethalis.

e. bullo'sa letha'lis, e. bullosa in which the bullae are persistent, nonhealing, and often present in the oral mucosa and trachea, but not on the palms and soles, leading to death. SYN e. bullosa, junctional type, Herlitz syndrome.

e. bullo'sa sim'plex [MIM*131900], e. bullosa in which lesions heal rapidly without scarring and there is separation through the cytoplasm of basal epidermal cells; occurs most frequently on the feet in adults after unaccustomed trauma such as long marches; autosomal dominant inheritance. SYN e. bullosa, epidermal type.

Ep·i·der·mo·phy·ton (ep'i-der-mof'i-ton, -der'mō-fī'ton). A genus of fungi, separated by Sabouraud from *Trichophyton* on the basis that it never invades the hair follicles, whose macroconidia are clavate and smooth-walled. The only species, *E. floccosum,* is an anthropophilic species that is a common cause of tinea pedis and tinea cruris. [epidermis + G. *phyton,* plant]

ep·i·der·mo·sis (ep-i-der-mō'sis). A skin disease affecting only the epidermis. SYN epidermidosis.

ep·i·der·mot·ro·pism (ep-i-der-mot'rō-pizm). Movement towards the epidermis, as in the migration of T lymphocytes into the epidermis in mycosis fungoides. [epidermis + G. *tropē,* a turning]

ep·i·di·al·y·sis (ep'i-dī-al'i-sis). Obsolete term for dehiscence of the pigmentary layer of the iris. [epi- + G. *dialysis,* a separation]

ep·i·di·a·scope (ep-i-dī'ă-skōp). A projector by which images are reflected by a mirror through a lens, or lenses, onto a screen, using reflected light for opaque objects and transmitted light for translucent or transparent ones. SYN overhead projector. [epi- + G. *dia,* through, + *skopeō,* to view]

ep·i·did·y·mal (ep-i-did'i-măl). Relating to the epididymis.

ep·i·did·y·mec·to·my (ep'i-did-i-mek'tō-mē). Operative removal of the epididymis. [epididymis + G. *ektomē,* excision]

ep·i·did·y·mis, gen. **ep·i·did·y·mi·dis,** pl. **ep·i·did·y·mi·des** (ep-i-did'i-mis, -di-dim'i-dis, -di-dim'i-dēz) [NA]. An elongated structure connected to the posterior surface of the testis, consisting of the head of the epididymis, body of epididymis, and tail of epididymis, which turns sharply upon itself to become the ductus deferens; the main component is the very convoluted duct of the epididymis which in the tail and the beginning of the ductus deferens is a reservoir for spermatozoa. The e. transports, stores, and matures spermatozoa between testis and ductus deferens (vas deferens). SYN parorchis. [Mod. L. fr. G. *epididymis,* fr. *epi,* on, + *didymos,* twin, in pl. testes]

caput e., SYN *head* of epididymis.

cauda e., SYN *tail* of epididymis.

corpus e., body of e.

ep·i·did·y·mi·tis (ep-i-did-i-mī'tis). Inflammation of the epididymis.

ep·i·did·y·mo-or·chi·tis (ep-i-did'i-mō-ōr-kī'tis). Simultaneous inflammation of both epididymis and testis. [epididymis + G. *orchis,* testis]

ep·i·did·y·mo·plas·ty (ep-i-did'i-mō-plas-tē). Surgical repair of the epididymis. [epididymis + G. *plastos,* formed]

ep·i·did·y·mot·o·my (ep'i-did-i-mot'ō-mē). Incision into the epididymis, as in preparation for epididymovasostomy or for drainage of purulent material. [epididymis + G. *tomē,* a cutting]

ep·i·did·y·mo·vas·ec·to·my (ep-i-did'i-mō-va-sek'tō-mē). Surgical removal of the epididymis and vas deferens, usually proximal to its entry into the inguinal canal. [epididymis + vasectomy]

ep·i·did·y·mo·va·sos·to·my (ep-i-did'i-mō-va-sos'tō-mē). Surgical anastomosis of the vas deferens to the epididymis. [epididymis + vasostomy]

ep·i·du·ral (ep-i-dū'răl). Upon (or outside) the dura mater. SYN peridural.

ep·i·du·rog·ra·phy (ep-i-dū-rog'ră-fē). Radiographic visualization of the epidural space following the regional instillation of a radiopaque contrast medium.

ep·i·es·tri·ol (ep-i-es'trē-ol). SEE estriol.

ep·i·fas·cial (ep-i-fash'ē-ăl). Upon the surface of a fascia, denoting a method of injecting drugs in which the solution is put on the fascia lata instead of injected into the substance of the muscle.

ep·i·gas·tral·gia (ep'i-gas-tral'jē-ă). Pain in the epigastric region. [epigastrium + G. *algos,* pain]

ep·i·gas·tric (ep-i-gas'trik). Relating to the epigastrium.

ep·i·gas·tri·um (ep-i-gas'trē-ŭm) [NA]. SYN epigastric *region,* epigastric *region.* [G. *epigastrion*]

ep·i·gas·tri·us (ep-i-gas'trē-ŭs). Unequal conjoined twins in which the smaller parasite is attached to the larger autosite in the epigastric region. SEE conjoined *twins,* under *twin.*

ep·i·gas·tro·cele (ep-i-gas'trō-sēl). Obsolete term for a hernia in the epigastric region. [epigastrium + G. *kēlē,* hernia]

ep·i·gen·e·sis (ep-i-jen'ě-sis). **1.** Development of offspring from a zygote. Cf. preformation *theory.* **2.** Regulation of the expression of gene activity without alteration of genetic structure. [epi- + G. *genesis,* creation]

ep·i·ge·net·ic (ep'i-jě-net'ik). Relating to epigenesis.

ep·i·glot·tic, ep·i·glot·tid·e·an (ep-i-glot'ik, ep-i-glo-tid'ē-an). Relating to the epiglottis.

ep·i·glot·ti·dec·to·my (ep'i-glot-i-dek'tō-mē). Excision of the epiglottis. [epiglottis + G. *ektomē,* excision]

ep·i·glot·ti·di·tis (ep'i-glot-i-dī'tis). SYN epiglottitis.

ep·i·glot·tis (ep-i-glot'is) [NA]. A leaf-shaped plate of elastic cartilage, covered with mucous membrane, at the root of the tongue, which serves as a diverter valve over the superior aperture of the larynx during the act of swallowing; it stands erect when liquids are being swallowed, but is passively bent over the aperture by solid foods being swallowed. [G. *epiglōttis,* fr. *epi,* on, + *glōttis,* the mouth of the windpipe]

ep·i·glot·ti·tis (ep-i-glot-ī'tis). Inflammation of the epiglottis, which may cause respiratory obstruction, especially in children; frequently due to infection by *Haemophilus influenzae* type b. SYN epiglottiditis.

epig·na·thus (e-pig'nă-thŭs). Unequal conjoined twins in which the smaller, incomplete parasite is attached to the larger autosite at the lower jaw. SEE conjoined *twins,* under *twin.* [epi- + G. *gnathos,* jaw]

ep·i·hy·al (ep-i-hī'ăl). Above the hyoid arch.

ep·i·hy·oid (ep-i-hī'oyd). Upon the hyoid bone; denoting certain accessory thyroid glands lying above the geniohyoid muscle.

ep·i·ker·a·to·phak·ia (ep'i-ker'ă-tō-phak'ē-ă). Modification of refractive error by application of a donor cornea to the anterior surface of the patient's cornea from which epithelium has been removed. SYN epikeratophakic keratoplasty. [epi- + G. *keras,* horn, + *phakos,* lens]

ep·i·ker·a·to·pros·the·sis (ep'i-ker'ă-tō-pros'thē-sis). A contact lens attached to the corneal stroma to replace the epithelium. [epi- + G. *keras,* horn, + *prosthesis,* an addition]

ep·i·la·mel·lar (ep'i-lă-mel'ăr). Upon or above a basement membrane. [epi- + L. *lamella,* dim. of *lamina,* a thin metal plate]

ep·i·late (ep'i-lāt). To extract a hair; to remove the hair from a part by forcible extraction, electrolysis, or loosening at the root by chemical means. Cf. depilate. [L. *e,* out, + *pilus,* a hair]

ep

ep·i·la·tion (ep-i-lā'shŭn). The act or result of removing hair. SYN depilation.

epil·a·to·ry (e-pil'ă-tō-rē). **1.** Having the property of removing hair; relating to epilation. SYN depilatory (1), psilotic (2). SEE ALSO decalvant. **2.** SYN depilatory (2).

ep·i·lem·ma (ep-i-lem'ă). The connective tissue sheath of nerve fibers near their termination. [epi- *lemma*, husk]

ep·i·lep·i·do·ma (ep'i-lep-i-dō'mă). A tumor resulting from hyperplasia of tissue derived from the true epiblast. [epi- + G. *lepis*, rind, + *-ōma*, tumor]

ep·i·lep·sia (ep-i-lep'sē-ă). SYN epilepsy. [G.]
e. partia'lis contin'ua, (1) a form of epilepsy marked by repetitive clonic muscular contractions with or without major convulsions; **(2)** simple partial motor status epilepticus of the rolandic cortex, often with myoclonic features; **(3)** a seizure type seen commonly with Rasmussen Syndrome. SYN Kojewnikoff's epilepsy.

ep·i·lep·sy (ep'i-lep'sē). A chronic disorder characterized by paroxysmal brain dysfunction due to excessive neuronal discharge, and usually associated with some alteration of consciousness. The clinical manifestations of the attack may vary from complex abnormalities of behavior including generalized or focal convulsions to momentary spells of impaired consciousness. These clinical states have been subjected to a variety of classifications, none universally accepted to date and, accordingly, the terminologies used to describe the different types of attacks remain purely descriptive and nonstandardized; they are variously based on 1) the clinical manifestations of the seizure (motor, sensory, reflex, psychic or vegetative), 2) the pathological substrate (hereditary, inflammatory, degenerative, neoplastic, traumatic, or cryptogenic), 3) the location of the epileptogenic lesion (rolandic, temporal, diencephalic regions), and 4) the time of life at which the attacks occur (nocturnal, diurnal, menstrual, etc.). SYN convulsive state, epilepsia, falling sickness, fit (3), status convulsivus. [G. *epilēpsia*, seizure]
anosognosic e., epilepsy characterized by attacks of which the person is unaware. SYN anosognosic seizures.
automatic e., SYN psychomotor e.
autonomic e., episodes of autonomic dysfunction presumably due to diencephalic irritation. SYN diencephalic e., vasomotor e., vasovagal e.
benign childhood e. with centrotemporal spikes, a specific epilepsy syndrome beginning in childhood and remitting in adolescence, characterized by nocturnal simple partial motor seizures or generalized tonic-clonic seizures. EEG shows centrotemporal spikes that are activated by sleep and an otherwise normal EEG background.
centrencephalic e., an imprecise term referring to e. characterized electroencephalographically by bilateral synchronous discharges, and clinically by absence or generalized tonic-clonic seizures.
childhood absence e., a generalized e. syndrome characterized by the onset of absence seizures in childhood, typically at age six or seven years. There is a strong genetic predisposition and girls are affected more often than boys. EEG reveals generalized 3 Hz spike-wave activity on a normal background. Prognosis for remission is good if the patient does not also have generalized tonic-clonic seizures. SEE ALSO absence. SYN petit mal e., pyknolepsy.
childhood e. with occipital paroxysms, a benign e. syndrome characterized by frequent occipital spikes often activated by eye closure. It has a seizure semiology that includes visual manifestations; not always remitting later in life.
complex precipitated e., a form of reflex e. initiated by specialized sensory stimuli, *e.g.,* certain visual patterns.
cortical e., SYN focal e.
cryptogenic e., SYN generalized tonic-clonic *seizure.*
diencephalic e., SYN autonomic e.
early posttraumatic e., seizures beginning within one week after severe head injury.
eating e., epileptic, often generalized, seizures provoked by eating; a type of reflex e.
focal e., e. of various etiologies characterized by focal seizures

or secondarily generalized tonic-clonic seizures. Ictal symptoms are often related to the brain region where the seizure begins focally. SYN cortical e., local e., partial e.
frontal lobe e., a localization-related e. with seizures originating in the frontal lobe. A variety of clinical syndromes exist depending on the exact localization of seizures and clinical semiology of the seizure type. Frontal lobe epilepsies have been divided into several specific syndromes including the syndrome of supplementary motor seizures, cingulate seizures, anterior frontal polar region seizures, orbital frontal seizures, dorsolateral seizures, opercular seizures, and seizures of the motor cortex.
generalized e., a major category of e. syndromes characterized by one or more types of generalized seizures.
generalized tonic-clonic e., SYN generalized tonic-clonic *seizure.*
grand mal e., older term for e. characterized by generalized tonic-clonic *seizure.*
idiopathic e., (1) an e. without evident cause; term often used to describe the genetic e.'s; **(2)** SYN generalized tonic-clonic *seizure.*
intractable e., e. not adequately controlled by medication. SYN pharmacoresistent e.
jacksonian e., SYN Jacksonian *seizure.*
juvenile absence e., a generalized e. syndrome with onset around puberty, characterized by absence seizures and generalized tonic-clonic seizures. EEG often shows a greater than 3 Hz generalized spike wave pattern.
juvenile myoclonic e., an e. syndrome typically beginning in early adolescence, and characterized by early morning myoclonic jerks that may progress into a generalized tonic-clonic seizure. A genetic disorder: some families have had gene linkage to chromosome-6. The EEG is characterized by generalized polyspike and wave discharges at 4–6 Hz.
Kojewnikoff's e., SYN *epilepsia* partialis continua.
laryngeal e., a form of reflex e. precipitated by coughing.
local e., SYN focal e.
localization related e., SYN myoclonus e.
major e., SYN generalized tonic-clonic *seizure.*
masked e., a form of e. characterized by a paroxysmal disturbance, such as headache or vomiting, associated with an epileptic electroencephalographic pattern.
matutinal e., a form of e. which occurs on awakening.
myoclonic astatic e., a petit mal variant characterized by atonic (drop attacks) and tonic or tonic-clonic attacks in neurologically disabled (hemiplegic, ataxic, etc.) children with mental retardation; characterized in EEG by 2/sec spike and wave discharges; usually progresses in spite of medication.
myoclonus e. [MIM*159800], a clinically diverse group of epilepsy syndromes, some benign, some progressive. Many are hereditary with mendelian and nonmendelian mitochondrial inheritance. All are characterized by the occurrence of myoclonus, which may be limited or predominate in the condition. Specific syndromes include cherry red spot myoclonus syndrome, ceroid lipofuscinosis, myoclonic e. with ragged red fibers, and Baltic myoclonus. SYN localization related e.
nocturnal e., an e. syndrome characterized by nocturnal seizures only.
occipital lobe e., a localization-related e. where seizures originate from the occipital lobe. Symptoms commonly include visual abnormalities during seizures.
parietal lobe e., a localization-related e. where seizures originate within the parietal lobe. Seizure semiology may involve abnormalities of sensation.
partial e., SYN focal e.
pattern sensitive e., a form of reflex e. precipitated by viewing certain patterns.
petit mal e., SYN childhood absence e.
pharmacoresistent e., SYN intractable e.
photogenic e., a form of reflex e. precipitated by light.
posttraumatic e., a convulsive state following and causally related to head injury; with brain damage either manifested clinically or ascertained by special examinations such as computed tomography. To assume causal relationship, the individual must have had no previous epilepsy, no cerebral disease, and no other

brain trauma. The attacks should have started, depending on the severity of the wounding, within 3 months to 2 years of the alleged trauma and be of a type compatible with the site of injury and the EEG abnormalities.

primary generalized e., e. without evidence of focal or multifocal central nervous system disease. Seizures are generalized from onset, both by EEG and clinical criteria. Often a pure genetic form of e. SEE ALSO generalized tonic-clonic *seizure.*

procursive e., a psychomotor attack initiated by whirling or running.

psychomotor e., attacks with elaborate and multiple sensory, motor, and/or psychic components, the common feature being a clouding or loss of consciousness and amnesia for the event; clinical manifestations may take the form of automatisms; emotional outbursts of temper, anger or show of fear; motor or psychic disturbances; or may be related to any sphere of human activity. Electroencephalographically, the attack is characterized by spike discharges in the temporal lobe, especially in sleep. SEE ALSO procursive e., visceral e., uncinate e. SYN automatic e., psychomotor seizure.

reflex e., seizures which are induced by peripheral stimulation; *e.g.,* audiogenic, laryngeal, photogenic, or other stimulation. SYN sensory precipitated e.

rolandic e., a benign, autosomal, dominant form of e. occurring in children, characterized clinically by arrest of speech, by muscular contractions of the side of the face and arm and epileptic discharges electroencephalographically. [Luigi *Rolando*]

secondary generalized e., a group of e. syndromes of diverse etiologies with diffuse or multifocal cerebral involvement. Patients typically have a variety of generalized seizure types, including tonic, atonic, myoclonic, atypical absence, and generalized tonic-clonic seizures. Partial seizures may also occur. One classic syndrome is the Lennox-Gastaut syndrome. SYN symptomatic e.

sensory e., focal e. initiated by a somatosensory phenomenon.

sensory precipitated e., SYN reflex e.

sleep e., incorrect term for narcolepsy.

somnambulic e., postictal automatism in which the patient walks or runs about exhibiting natural behavior of which he or she has no subsequent remembrance.

startle e., a form of reflex e. precipitated by sudden noises.

supplementary motor area e., a localization-related epilepsy syndrome in which seizures originate from the supplementary motor area of the mesial frontal lobe. Typical seizure semiology includes sudden bilateral tonic movements, vocalization, and preservation of consciousness. Attacks are often nocturnal.

symptomatic e., SYN secondary generalized e.

temporal lobe e., a localization-related e. with seizures originating from the temporal lobe, most commonly the mesial temporal lobe. The most common pathology is hippocampal sclerosis. SYN uncinate fit.

tonic e., an attack in which the body is rigid.

tornado e., a type of focal e. or partial seizure with an aura of severe vertigo and a feeling of being drawn up into space.

uncinate e., a form of psychomotor e. or complex partial seizure initiated by a dreamy state and hallucinations of smell and taste, usually the result of a medial temporal lesion. SYN uncinate attack.

vasomotor e., SYN autonomic e.

vasovagal e., SYN autonomic e.

visceral e., e., usually psychomotor, in which the attacks are initiated by visceral symptoms or sensations; most cases have their focus in the temporal lobe.

e. with grand mal seizures on awakening, generalized e. syndrome characterized by onset in the second decade of life, typically with generalized tonic-clonic seizures, of which most occur shortly after awakening (regardless of the time of day) and are exacerbated by sleep deprivation. There is a genetic predisposition and EEG shows one of several generalized patterns of interictal discharges; photosensitivity is common.

e. with myoclonic absences, a form of generalized e. characterized by absence seizures, severe bilateral rhythmic clonic jerks often associated with tonic contraction, and an EEG 3 Hz spike

and wave pattern. Age of onset is usually around seven years and males are more often affected.

ep·i·lep·tic (ep-i-lep'tik). Relating to, characterized by, or suffering from epilepsy.

ep·i·lep·ti·form (ep-i-lep'ti-fōrm). SYN epileptoid.

ep·i·lep·to·gen·ic, ep·i·lep·tog·e·nous (ep-i-lep-tō-jen'ik, ep-i-lep-toj'ĕ-nŭs). Causing epilepsy.

ep·i·lep·toid (ep-i-lep'toyd). Resembling epilepsy; denoting certain convulsions, especially of functional nature. SYN epileptiform. [G. *epilēpsia,* seizure, epilepsy, + *eidos,* resemblance]

ep·i·loia (ep-i-loy'ă). SYN tuberous *sclerosis.* [term coined by Sherloc (1911)]

ep·i·man·dib·u·lar (ep-i-man-dib'yū-lăr). Upon the lower jaw. [epi- + L. *mandibulum,* mandible]

ep·i·mas·ti·cal (ep-i-mast'i-kăl). Increasing steadily until an acme is reached, then declining; said of a fever. [G. *epakmastikos,* coming to a height]

ep·i·mas·ti·gote (ep-i-mas'ti-gōt). Term replacing "crithidial stage," to avoid confusion with the insect-parasitizing flagellates of the genus *Crithidia.* In the e. stage the flagellum arises from the kinetoplast alongside the nucleus and emerges from the anterior end of the organism; an undulating membrane is present. [epi- + G. *mastix,* whip]

ep·i·men·or·rha·gia (ep-i-men-ō-rā'jē-ă). Prolonged and profuse menstruation occurring at any time, but most frequently at the beginning and end of menstrual life.

ep·i·men·or·rhea (ep-i-men-ō-rē'ă). Too frequent menstruation, occurring at any time, but particularly at the beginning and end of menstrual life.

ep·i·mer (ep'i-mer). One of two molecules (having more than one chiral center) differing only in the spatial arrangement about a single chiral atom; *e.g.,* α-D-glucose and α-D-galactose (with respect to carbon-4). SEE sugars. Cf. anomer. [epi- + G. *meros,* part]

ep·i·mer·ase (ep'i-mer-ās) [EC 5.1]. A class of enzymes catalyzing epimeric changes.

ep·i·mere (ep'i-mēr). The dorsal part of the myotome. SEE myotome (3). [epi- + G. *meros,* part]

ep·im·er·ite (ep-i-mēr'īt). The hooklike anchoring structure at the anterior end of a cephaline gregarine sporozoan; it is left embedded in tissues when the rest of the cephalont is freed in the lumen of the intestine of the invertebrate host. [epi- + G. *meros,* part]

ep·i·mi·cro·scope (ep-i-mī'krō-skōp). A microscope with a condenser built around the objective; used for the investigation of opaque, or only slightly translucent, minute specimens. SYN opaque microscope.

ep·i·mor·pho·sis (ep'i-mōr-fō'sis). Regeneration of a part of an organism by growth at the cut surface. [epi- + G. *morphē,* shape]

ep·i·mys·i·ot·o·my (ep'i-mis-ē-ot'ō-mē). Incision of the sheath of a muscle. [epimysium + G. *tomē,* a cutting]

ep·i·mys·i·um (ep-i-mis'ē-ŭm). The fibrous connective tissue envelope surrounding a skeletal muscle. SYN perimysium externum. [epi- + G. *mys,* muscle]

ep·i·neph·rine (ep'i-nef'rin). 4-[1-hydroxy-2-(methylamino)-ethyl]-1,2-benzenediol; a catecholamine that is the chief neurohormone of the adrenal medulla of most species. The L-isomer is the most potent stimulant (sympathomimetic) of adrenergic α- and β-receptors, resulting in increased heart rate and force of contraction, vasoconstriction or vasodilation, relaxation of bronchiolar and intestinal smooth muscle, glycogenolysis, lipolysis, and other metabolic effects; used in the treatment of bronchial asthma, acute allergic disorders, open-angle glaucoma, and heart block, and as a topical and local vasoconstrictor. Generally used salts are e. hydrochloride and e. bitartrate, the latter most frequently used in topical preparations. SYN adrenaline. [epi- + G. *nephros,* kidney, + -ine]

ep·i·neph·ros (ep-i-nef'ros). SYN suprarenal *gland.* [epi- + G. *nephros,* kidney]

ep·i·neu·ral (ep-i-nū'răl). On a neural arch of a vertebra.

ep·i·neu·ri·al (ep-i-nū'rē-ăl). Relating to the epineurium.

ep·i·neu·ri·um (ep-i-nū′rē-ŭm). The outermost supporting structure of peripheral nerve trunks, consisting of a condensation of areolar connective tissue; subdivided into those layers that surround the whole nerve trunk (epifascicular e.), and those layers which extend between the nerve fascicles (interfascicular e.). With the endoneurium and perineurium, the e. composes the peripheral nerve stroma. [epi- + G. *neuron,* nerve]

epifascicular e., the portion of the e. which surrounds the whole nerve trunk, in contrast to interfascicular e., which passes down between the nerve fascicles.

ep·i·no·sic (ep-i-nō′sik). Relating to epinosis.

ep·i·no·sis (ep-i-nō′sis). An imaginary feeling of illness following a real illness. [epi- + G. *nosos,* disease]

ep·i·o·nych·i·um (ep-i-ō-nik′ē-ŭm). SYN eponychium.

ep·i·ot·ic (ep′i-ot′ik, -ō′tik). One of the components of the otic capsule of some vertebrates; in the mammal the petrosal or petrous temporal bone incorporates the various otic elements seen in lower vertebrates. [epi- + G. *ous,* ear]

ep·i·pas·tic (ep-i-pas′tik). **1.** Usable as a dusting powder. **2.** A dusting powder. [G. *epi-passō,* to sprinkle over]

ep·i·per·i·car·di·al (ep′i-per-i-kar′dē-ăl). Upon or about the pericardium.

ep·i·phar·ynx (ep′i-far′ingks). SYN nasopharynx. [G. *epi,* on, over, + pharynx]

ep·i·phe·nom·e·non (ep′i-fĕ-nom′ĕ-non). A symptom appearing during the course of a disease, not of usual occurrence, and not necessarily associated with the disease.

epiph·o·ra (ē-pif′ō-ră). An overflow of tears upon the cheek, due to imperfect drainage by the tear-conducting passages. SYN tearing, watery eye (1). [G. a sudden flow, fr. *epi,* on, + *pherō,* to bear]

atonic e., e. arising from weakness of the orbicularis oculi muscle.

ep·i·phren·ic, ep·i·phre·nal (ep′i-fren′ik, -frē′năl). Upon or above the diaphragm. [epi- + G. *phrēn,* diaphragm]

ep·i·phys·i·al, epiph·y·se·al (ep-i-fiz′ē-ăl). Relating to an epiphysis.

epiph·y·si·od·e·sis (ep′i-fiz-ē-od′e-sis). **1.** Premature union of the epiphysis with the diaphysis, resulting in cessation of growth. **2.** An operative procedure that partially or totally destroys an epiphysis and may incorporate a bone graft to produce fusion of the epiphysis or premature cessation of its growth; generally undertaken to equalize leg length. [epiphysis + G. *desis,* binding]

epiph·y·si·ol·y·sis (ep-i-fiz-ē-ol′i-sis). **1.** Loosening or separation, either partial or complete, of an epiphysis from the shaft of a bone. **2.** Arrest of growth by ablation of the growth plate cartilage. [epiphysis + G. *lysis,* loosening]

ep·i·phys·i·op·a·thy (ep-i-fiz-ē-op′ă-thē). Any disorder of an epiphysis of the long bones. [epiphysis + G. *pathos,* suffering]

epiph·y·sis, pl. **epiph·y·ses** (e-pif′i-sis, -sēz) [NA]. A part of a long bone developed from a center of ossification distinct from that of the shaft and separated at first from the latter by a layer of cartilage. [G. an excrescence, fr. *epi,* upon, + *physis,* growth]

atavistic e., a bone that is independent phylogenetically but is now fused with another bone, *e.g.,* the coracoid process of the scapula.

e. cer′ebri, SYN pineal *body.*

pressure e., a secondary center of ossification in the articular end of a long bone.

stippled e., SYN *dysplasia* epiphysialis punctata.

traction e., a secondary center of ossification at the site of attachment of a tendon.

epiph·y·si·tis (e-pif-i-sī′tis). Inflammation of an epiphysis.

ep·i·pi·al (ep′i-pī′ăl). On the pia mater.

epiplo-. Omentum. SEE ALSO omento-. [G. *epiploon*]

epip·lo·cele (e-pip′lō-sēl). Rarely used term for hernia of the omentum. [epiplo- + G. *kēlē,* hernia]

ep·i·plo·ic (ep′i-plō′ik). SYN omental.

epip·lo·on (e-pip′lō-on). SYN greater *omentum.* [G.]

epip·lo·pexy (e-pip′lō-pek-sē). Obsolete synonym of omentopexy. [epiplo- + G. *pēxis,* fixation]

ep·i·pter·ic (ep′i-ter′ik). In the neighborhood of the pterion.

ep·i·py·gus (ep-i-pī′gŭs). Unequal conjoined twins in which the smaller, incomplete parasite is attached to the buttock of the larger autosite. SEE pygomelus, conjoined *twins,* under *twin.* [epi- + G. *pygē,* buttocks]

D-ep·i·rham·nose (ep-i-ram′nōz). 6-deoxy-D-glucose; occurs in plants and bacteria in combination with diacylglycerol and is often sulfated (at C-6) in glycolipids. SYN quinovose.

ep·i·scle·ra (ep′i-sklēr′ă). The connective tissue between the sclera and the conjunctiva. [epi- + sclera]

ep·i·scle·ral (ep-i-sklēr′ăl). **1.** Upon the sclera. **2.** Relating to the episclera.

ep·i·scle·ri·tis (ep-i-skle-rī′tis). Inflammation of the episcleral connective tissue. SEE ALSO scleritis.

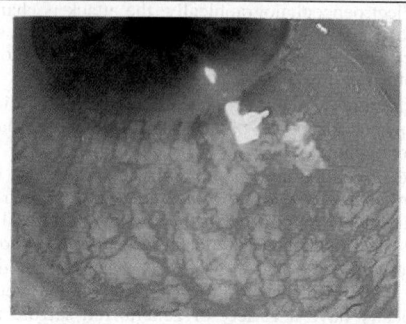

episcleritis (with rheumatoid arthritis)

e. multinodula′ris, e. with numerous nodules near the corneoscleral limbus.

nodular e., e. with localized inflammation foci in episcleral tissues.

e. periodi′ca fu′gax, diffuse transient e., with a tendency to recur at regular intervals. SYN subconjunctivitis.

episio-. The vulva. SEE ALSO vulvo-. [G. *episeion,* pubic region]

ep·i·si·o·per·i·ne·or·rha·phy (e-piz′ē-ō-per′i-nē-ōr′ă-fē, e-pis′). Repair of an incised or a ruptured perineum and lacerated vulva or repair of a surgical incision of the vulva and perineum. [episio- + G. *perinaion,* perineum, + *rhaphē,* a stitching]

ep·i·si·o·plas·ty (e-piz′ē-ō-plas-tē, e-pis′). Plastic surgery of the vulva. [episio- + G. *plastos,* formed]

ep·i·si·or·rha·phy (e-piz-i-ōr′ră-fē, e-pis-). Repair of a lacerated vulva or an episiotomy. [episio- + G. *rhaphē,* a stitching]

ep·i·si·o·ste·no·sis (e-piz′i-ō-stĕ-nō′sis, e-pis′). Narrowing of the vulvar orifice. [episio- + G. *stenōsis,* narrowing]

ep·i·si·ot·o·my (e-piz-ē-ot′ō-mē, e-pis-). Surgical incision of the vulva to prevent laceration at the time of delivery or to facilitate vaginal surgery. [episio- + G. *tomē,* incision]

ep·i·so·de (ep′i-sōd). An important event or series of events taking place in the course of continuous events *e.g.,* an episode of depression.

acute schizophrenic e., SYN acute *schizophrenia.*

manic e., manifestation of a major mood disorder in which there is a distinct period during which the predominant mood of the individual is either elevated, expansive, or irritable, and there are associated symptoms of the excited or manic phase of the bipolar disorder. SEE affective *disorders,* under *disorder,* endogenous *depression.*

ep·i·some (ep′i-sōm). An extrachromosomal element (plasmid) that may either integrate into the bacterial chromosome of the host or replicate and function stably when physically separated from the chromosome. [epi- + G. *sōma,* body (chromosome)]

resistance-transferring e.'s, SYN resistance *plasmids,* under *plasmid.*

ep·i·spa·di·as (ep-i-spā′dē-ăs). A malformation in which the urethra opens on the dorsum of the penis; frequently associated with estrophy of the bladder. [epi- + G. *spadōn* a rent]

balanitic e., excessively proximal position of meatus on dorsum of glans penis.

coronal e., excessively proximal position of meatus in coronal sulcus.

penile e., proximal position of urethral meatus on the dorsum of the penile shaft.

penopubic e., position of the urethral meatus at junction of base of penis and lower abdominal wall.

ep·i·spas·tic (ep-i-spas′tik). SYN vesicant.

ep·i·spi·nal (ep-i-spī′năl). Upon the vertebral column or spinal cord, or upon any structure resembling a spine.

ep·i·sple·ni·tis (ep-i-splē-nī′tis). Inflammation of the capsule of the spleen.

epis·ta·sis (e-pis′tă-sis). **1.** The formation of a pellicle or scum on the surface of a liquid, especially as on standing urine. **2.** Phenotypic interaction of non-allelic genes. **3.** A form of gene interaction whereby one gene masks or interferes with the phenotypic expression of one or more genes at other loci; the gene whose phenotype is expressed is said to be "epistatic," while the phenotype altered or suppressed is then said to be "hypostatic". SYN epistasy. [G. scum; epi- + G. *stasis,* a standing]

epis·ta·sy (e-pis′tă-sē). SYN epistasis.

ep·i·stat·ic (ep-is-tat′ik). Relating to epistasis.

ep·i·stax·is (ep′i-stak′sis). Profuse bleeding from the nose. SYN nasal hemorrhage, nosebleed. [G. fr. *epistazō,* to bleed at the nose, fr. *epi,* on, + *stazō,* to fall in drops]

renal e., hematuria occurring without a detectable lesion.

epis·te·mol·o·gy (ĕ-pis′tō-mol′ō-gē). The study of knowledge and rules of evidence involved. Traditionally a branch of philosophy, it is now coming to be used also as a discipline incorporated in, and in some respects peculiar to, individual fields of scholarship (medicine, science, history, etc.).

epis·te·mo·phil·ia (ĕ-pis′tē-mō-fil′ē-ă). Love, especially excessive, of knowledge. [G. *epistēmē,* knowledge, + *philos,* fond]

ep·i·ster·nal (ep-i-ster′năl). **1.** Over or on the sternum. **2.** Relating to the episternum.

ep·i·ster·num (ep-i-ster′nŭm). SYN *manubrium* of sternum. [epi- + L. *sternum,* chest]

ep·i·stro·phe·us (ep-i-strō′fē-ŭs). SYN axis (5). [G. the pivot]

ep·i·tar·sus (ep-i-tar′sŭs). A fold of conjunctiva arising on the tarsal surface of the lid and losing itself in the skin close to the medial angle of the eye. [epi- + G. *tarsos,* flat mat, edge of eyelid]

ep·i·taxy (ep-i-tak′sē). The growth of one crystal in one or more specific orientations on the substrate of another kind of crystal, with a close geometric fit between the networks in contact; seen in the alternating layers of different composition in stones from the kidney and gallbladder, indicating an abrupt change of composition during formation. [epi- + G. *taxis,* arrangement]

ep·i·ten·din·e·um (ep′i-ten-din′ē-ŭm). The white fibrous sheath surrounding a tendon. SYN epitenon. [L.]

epit·e·non (ĕ-pit′ĕ-non, ep-i-ten′on). SYN epitendineum.

17-ep·i·tes·tos·ter·one (ep′i-tes-tos′ter-ōn). 17α-Hydroxyandrost-4-en-3-one; 17α-epimer of testosterone; a biologically inactive steroid found in testes and ovaries; may be a metabolite of 4-androstene-3,17-dione and a precursor of 17α-estradiol.

ep·i·thal·a·mus (ep′i-thal′ă-mŭs) [NA]. A small dorsomedial area of the thalamus corresponding to the habenula and its associated structures, the medullary stria, pineal body, and habenular commissure. [epi- + thalamus]

ep·i·tha·lax·i·a (ep′i-thă-lak′sē-ă). Shedding of any surface epithelium, but especially of that lining the intestine. [epithelium + G. *allaxis,* exchange]

ep·i·the·lia (ep-i-thē′lē-ă). Plural of epithelium.

ep·i·the·li·al (ep-i-thē′lē-ăl). Relating to or consisting of epithelium.

ep·i·the·li·al·i·za·tion (ep-i-thē′lē-ăl-i-zā′shŭn). Formation of epithelium over a denuded surface. SYN epithelization.

ep·i·the·li·o·cyte (ep-i-thē′lē-ō-sīt). An *in vitro* tissue culture epithelial cell. [epithelium + G. *kytos,* cell]

ep·i·the·li·o·fi·bril (ep-i-thē′lē-ō-fī′bril). SYN tonofibril.

ep·i·the·li·o·glan·du·lar (ep-i-thē′lē-ō-glan′dyū-lăr). Relating to glandular epithelium.

ep·i·the·li·oid (ep-i-thē′lē-oyd). Resembling or having some of the characteristics of epithelium. [epithelium + G. *eidos,* resemblance]

ep·i·the·li·o·lyt·ic (ep-i-thē′lē-ō-lit′ik). Destructive to epithelium.

ep·i·the·li·o·ma (ep′i-thē-lē-ō′mă). **1.** An epithelial neoplasm or hamartoma of the skin, especially of skin appendage origin. **2.** A carcinoma of the skin derived from squamous, basal, or adnexal cells. [epithelium + G. *-ōma,* tumor]

e. adenoi′des cys′ticum, SYN trichoepithelioma.

basal cell e., SYN basal cell *carcinoma.*

Borst-Jadassohn type intraepidermal e., precancerous lesions clinically suggestive of actinic or seborrheic keratosis, with nests of immature or abnormal keratinocytes within the epidermis.

chorionic e., obsolete term for choriocarcinoma.

e. contagio′sum, SYN fowlpox.

e. cunicula′tum, verrucous carcinoma occurring uncommonly on the sole of the foot, forming a slowly growing warty mass that may invade deeply but which rarely metastasizes.

Malherbe's calcifying e., SYN pilomatrixoma.

malignant ciliary e., malignant hyperplasia of ciliary epithelium with frequent involvement of the pigmented layer. SYN adult medulloepithelioma.

multiple self-healing squamous e. [MIM*132800], multiple skin tumors, most frequently on the head, each resembling a well-differentiated squamous carcinoma or keratoacanthoma; individual tumors resolve spontaneously after several months, leaving deep-pitted scars with irregular crenellated borders, and are usually replaced by additional new tumors; autosomal dominant inheritance.

sebaceous e., a benign tumor of the sebaceous gland epithelium in which small basaloid or germinative cells predominate.

ep·i·the·li·om·a·tous (ep-i-thē-lē-ō′mă-tŭs). Pertaining to epithelioma.

ep·i·the·li·op·a·thy (ep′i-thē-lē-op′ă-thē). Disease involving epithelium. [epithelium + G. *pathos,* suffering]

pigment e., an acute disease manifested by rapid loss of vision, and multifocal, cream-colored placoid lesions of the retinal pigment epithelium; resolves with restoration of vision.

ep·i·the·li·o·sis (ep-i-thē-lē-ō′sis). Proliferation of epithelial cells, as seen in ducts of the breast in fibrocystic disease.

ep·i·the·li·o·tro·pic (ep-ē-thē′lē-ō-trō′pik). Having an affinity for epithelium.

ep·i·the·lite (ep-i-thē′līt). Obsolete term for a skin lesion resulting from excessive irradiation. [epithelium + -ite]

ep·i·the·li·um, pl. **ep·i·the·lia** (ep-i-thē′lē-ŭm, -ă) [NA]. The purely cellular avascular layer covering all the free surfaces, cutaneous, mucous, and serous, including the glands and other structures derived therefrom. [G. *epi,* upon, + *thēlē,* nipple, a term applied originally to the thin skin covering the nipples and the papillary layer of the border of the lips]

anterior e. of cornea, the stratified squamous e. covering the outer surface of the cornea; it is smooth, consists usually of five layers of cells, and contains numerous free nerve endings. SYN e. anterius corneae [NA].

e. ante′rius cor′neae [NA], SYN anterior e. of cornea.

Barrett's e., columnar esophageal e. seen in Barrett's *syndrome.*

ciliated e., any e. having motile cilia on the free surface.

columnar e., e. formed of a single layer of prismatic cells taller than they are wide. SYN cylindrical e.

crevicular e., the stratified squamous e. lining the inner aspect of the soft tissue wall of the gingival sulcus. SYN sulcular e.

cuboidal e., simple e. with cells appearing as cubes in a vertical section but as polyhedra in surface view.

cylindrical e., SYN columnar e.

e. duc′tus semicircula′ris [NA], SYN e. of semicircular duct.

enamel e., the several layers of the enamel organ remaining on the enamel surface after formation of enamel is completed. SYN reduced enamel e.

ep

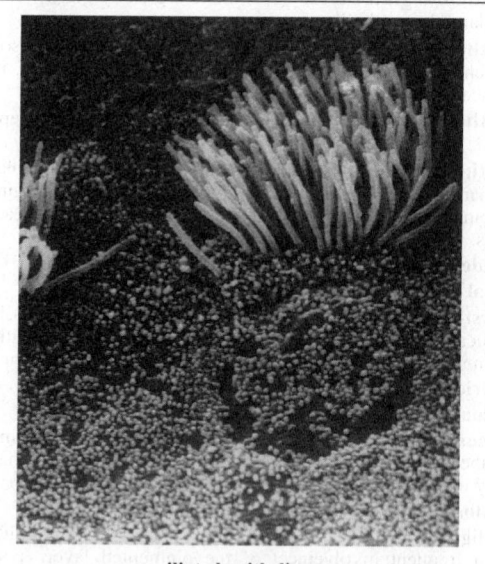

ciliated epithelium
cilia of epithelium (scanning electron microscopy)

external dental e., external enamel e., the cuboidal cells of the outer layer of the odontogenic organ of a developing tooth.

germinal e., a cuboidal layer of peritoneal e. covering the gonads, once thought to be the source of germ cells.

gingival e., a stratified squamous e. that undergoes some degree of keratinization and covers the free and attached gingiva.

glandular e., e. composed of secretory cells.

inner dental e., inner enamel e., the columnar epithelial layer of enamel matrix, secreting ameloblasts, of the odontogenic organ of a developing tooth.

junctional e., a collar of epthelial cells attached to the tooth surface and subepithelial connective tissue found at the base of the gingival crevice. SYN epithelial attachment.

laminated e., SYN stratified e.

e. of lens, the layer of cuboidal cells lying on the anterior surface of the crystalline lens inside the lens capsule. At the equator the cells elongate and give rise to the lens fibers. SYN e. lentis [NA].

e. lentis [NA], SYN e. of lens.

mesenchymal e., the flat e. derived from mesenchymal cells found lining certain connective tissue spaces such as the anterior chamber of eye, perilymph spaces in the ear, and subdural and subarachnoid spaces.

muscle e., SYN myoepithelium.

olfactory e., an e. of the pseudostratified type that contains olfactory, receptor, nerve cells whose axons extend to the olfactory bulb of the brain.

pavement e., SYN simple squamous e.

pigment e., e. composed of cells containing granules of pigment or melanin, as in the retinal or iris pigment layer.

pigment e. of optic retina, SYN *pars* pigmentosa. SEE retina.

pseudostratified e., an e. that gives a superficial appearance of being stratified because the cell nuclei are at different levels, but in which all cells reach the basement membrane, hence it is classed as a simple e.

reduced enamel e., SYN enamel e.

respiratory e., the pseudostratified ciliated e. that lines the conducting portion of the airway, including part of the nasal cavity and larynx, the trachea, and bronchi.

e. of semicircular duct, the simple squamous e. of the semicircular ducts. SYN e. ductus semicircularis [NA].

seminiferous e., the e. lining the convoluted tubules of the testis where spermatogenesis and spermiogenesis occur.

simple e., an e. having one layer of cells.

simple squamous e., e. composed of a single layer of flattened scalelike cells, such as mesothelium, endothelium, and that in the pulmonary alveoli. SYN pavement e.

stratified e., a type of e. composed of a series of layers, the cells of each varying in size and shape. It is named more specifically according to the type of cells at the surface, *e.g.,* stratified squamous e., stratified columnar e., stratified ciliated columnar e. SYN laminated e.

stratified ciliated columnar e., an e. consisting of several layers of cells with the deeper cells being polyhedral in form and the surface ones columnar with motile cilia, such as that which lines the fetal esophagus.

stratified squamous e., an e. consisting of several layers of keratin containing cells in which the surface cells are flattened and scale-like and the deeper cells are polyhedral in form. Keratin filaments become progressively more abundant toward the surface, which on the dry surfaces of the body may consist of a layer of dead corneocytes.

sulcular e., SYN crevicular e.

surface e., (1) a layer of celomic epithelial cells covering the gonadal ridges as they are formed on the medial border of the mesonephroi near the root of the mesentery; (2) the mesothelial covering of the definitive ovary.

transitional e., a highly distensible pseudostratified e. with large polyploid superficial cells that are cuboidal in the relaxed state but broad and squamous in the distended state; occurs in the kidney, ureter, and bladder.

ep·i·the·li·za·tion (ep-i-thē-li-zā'shŭn). SYN epithelialization.

ep·i·them (ep'i-them). An external application, such as a poultice, but not a plaster or ointment. [G. *epithēma,* a cover]

epith·e·sis (ĕ-pith'ĕ-sis). **1.** Orthopedic correction of a deformed extremity. **2.** A splint or other apparatus applied to an extremity. [epi- + G. *tithēmi,* to place]

ep·i·thet (ep'i-thet). Characterizing term or name. [G. *epithetos,* added, fr. epi- + *tithēmi,* to place]

specific e., in bacteriology, the second part of the name of a species; it is not, by itself, a name; the name of a bacterial species consists of two parts, the generic name and the specific e.

ep·i·thi·a·zide (ep-i-thī'ă-zīd). 6-Chloro-3,4-dihydro-3-{[(2,2,2-trifluoroethyl)-thio]methyl}-2*H*-1,2,4-benzothiadiazine-7-sulfonamide 1,1-dioxide; a diuretic.

ep·i·tope (ep'i-tōp). The simplest form of an antigenic determinant, on a complex antigenic molecule, which can combine with antibody or T cell receptor. [epi- + -tope]

ep·i·tox·oid (ep-i-tok'soyd). A toxoid that has less affinity for specific antitoxin than that manifested by the toxin.

ep·i·trich·i·al (ep-i-trik'ē-ăl). Relating to the epitrichium.

ep·i·trich·i·um (ep-i-trik'ē-ŭm). SYN periderm. SEE dome *cell.* [epi- + G. *trichion,* dim. of *thrix,* (trich-), hair]

ep·i·troch·lea (ep-i-trok'lē-ă). SYN medial *epicondyle* of humerus. [epi- + L. *trochlea,* a pulley, block, contr. fr. G. *trochilia*]

ep·i·troch·le·ar (ep-i-trok'lē-ăr). Relating to the epitrochlea.

ep·i·tu·ber·cu·lo·sis (ep'i-tū-ber-kyū-lō'sis). The occurrence of glandular swelling or pulmonary infiltration in an area near a focus of pulmonary tuberculosis or of enlarged bronchial glands.

ep·i·tym·pan·ic (ep-i-tim-pan'ik). Above, or in the upper part of, the tympanic cavity or membrane.

ep·i·tym·pa·num (ep'i-tim'pă-nŭm). SYN epitympanic *recess.*

ep·i·typh·li·tis (ep'ĭ-tif-lī'tis). Inflammation of tissues around or near the cecum. SEE appendicitis. [epi- + G. *typhlon,* cecum, + -itis, inflammation]

ep·i·zo·ic (ep-i-zō'ik). Living as a parasite on the skin surface.

ep·i·zo·ol·o·gy (ep'i-zō-ol'ō-jē). SYN epizootiology. [epi- + G. *zōon,* animal, + *logos,* study]

ep·i·zo·on, pl. **ep·i·zoa** (ep-i-zō'on, -zō'ă). An animal parasite living on the body surface. [epi- + G. *zōon,* animal]

ep·i·zo·ot·ic (ep'i-zō-ot'ik). **1.** Denoting a temporal pattern of disease occurrence in an animal population in which the disease occurs with a frequency clearly in excess of the expected frequency in that population during a given time interval. **2.** An outbreak (epidemic) of disease in an animal population; often with the implication that it may also affect human populations. [epi- + G. *zōon*, animal]

ep·i·zo·ot·i·ol·o·gy (ep'i-zō-ot'ē-ol'ō-jē). Epidemiology of disease in animal populations. SYN epizoology. [epi- + G. *zōon*, animal, + *logos*, study]

éplu·chage (ā-plū-shazh'). Rarely used term for the removal of all contaminated tissue in infected wounds. [F. picking, cleaning]

EPN. O-ethyl O-p-nitrophenyl phenylphosphonothiolate; a sulfur-containing organophosphate-anticholinsterase used as an insecticide and acaricide.

epo·e·tin al·fa (ē-pō'ĕ-tin). Recombinant human erythropoietin, a powerful stimulator of red blood cell synthesis. Often used in patients with anemia and in those undergoing renal transplants and AZT treatment.

ep·o·nych·ia (ep-ō-nik'ē-ă). Infection involving the proximal nail fold.

ep·o·nych·i·um (ep-ō-nik'ē-ŭm). **1.** The thin, condensed, eleidin-rich layer of epidermis which procedes and initially covers the nail plate in the embryo. It normally degenerates by the eighth month except at the nail base where it remains as the cuticle of the nail. **2** [NA]. The corneal layer of epidermis overlapping and in direct contact with the nail root proximally or the sides of the nail plate laterally, forming the undersurface of the nail wall or nail folds of nail. SYN hidden nail skin, perionychium. **3.** The thin skin adherent to the nail at its proximal portion. SYN epionychium. [G. *epi*, upon, + *onyx* (*onych-*), nail]

ep·o·nym (ep'ō-nim). The name of a disease, structure, operation, or procedure, usually derived from the name of the person who discovered or described it first. [G. *epōnymos*, named after]

ep·o·nym·ic (ep-ō-nim'ik). **1.** Relating to an eponym. **2.** An eponym.

ep·o·oph·o·rec·to·my (ep-ō-of'ō-rek'tō-mē). Removal of the epoophoron. [G. *epi*, upon, + *ōophoros*, bearing eggs, + *ektomē*, excision]

ep·o·öph·o·ron (ep'ō-of'ŏ-ron) [NA]. A collection of rudimentary tubules in the mesosalpinx between the ovary and the uterine tube; composed of two portions, the longitudinal duct of epoöphoron and the transverse ductules of epoöphoron, they are the vestiges of tubules of the middle portion of the mesonephros and the homologue of the aberrant ductules and proximal duct of epididymis in the male. SEE *ductus* epoöphori longitudinalis. SYN corpus pampiniforme, organ of Rosenmüller, pampiniform body. [epi- + G. *ōophoros*, egg-bearing]

epo·prost·en·ol, epo·prost·en·ol so·di·um (e-pō-prost'en-ol). SYN prostacyclin.

epor·nit·ic (ep'or-nit'ik). Referring to an outbreak of disease in a bird population. [epi- + G. *ornithos*, bird + -ic]

ep·ox·y (ē-pok'sē). Chemical term describing an oxygen atom bound to two linked carbon atoms

$$-CH-CH-$$
$$\diagdown O \diagup$$

generally, any cyclic ether, but commonly applied to a 3-membered ring; specifically, a three-membered ring is an oxirane, a four-membered ring is an oxetane, a five-membered ring is an oxolane, and a six membered ring is an oxane; oxiranes are commonly produced from peracids acting on alkenes. E.'s are important chemical intermediates, and the basis of e. resins (polymers) formed from e. monomers.

2,3-epox·y·squa·lene (ĕ-pok'sē-skwā'lēn). An oxirane derivative of squalene; a precursor to all of the steroids.

Epple, Associate of Leonard S. Fosdick. SEE Fosdick-Hansen-E. *test*.

EPR Abbreviation for electron paramagnetic *resonance*.

EPS Abbreviation for exophthalmos-producing *substance*.

ep·si·lon (ep'si-lon). Fifth letter of the Greek alphabet, ε.

EPSP Abbreviation for excitatory postsynaptic *potential*.

Epstein, Alois, German pediatrician, 1849–1918. SEE E.'s *disease, pearls*, under *pearl, sign, symptom*.

Epstein, Michael Anthony, English virologist, *1921. SEE E.-Barr *virus*.

epu·lis (ep-yū'lis). A nonspecific exophytic gingival mass. [G. *epoulis*, a gumboil]

congenital e. of newborn, a congenital benign nodular tumor of the alveolar ridge, of unknown histogenesis; histologically, it is composed of large cells with a granular cytoplasm similar to that of a granular cell tumor (myoblastoma).

e. fissura'tum, SYN inflammatory fibrous *hyperplasia*.

giant cell e., SYN giant cell *granuloma*.

e. gravida'rum, a gingival pyogenic granuloma that develops during pregnancy.

pigmented e., SYN melanotic neuroectodermal *tumor* of infancy.

ep·u·loid (ep'yū-loyd). A gingival mass that resembles an epulis.

Eq, eq Abbreviation for equivalent.

equa·tion (ē-kwā'zhŭn). A statement expressing the equality of two things, usually with the use of mathematical or chemical symbols. [L. *aequare*, to make equal]

alveolar gas e., the e. defining the steady state relation of the alveolar oxygen pressure to the barometric pressure, inspired gas composition, alveolar carbon dioxide pressure, and respiratory exchange ratio; the e. is used in various forms depending upon which simplifying assumptions are acceptable for different applications.

Arrhenius e., an e. relating chemical reaction rate (k) to the absolute temperature (T) by the e.: $d(\ln k)/dT) = \Delta E_a/RT^2$ where E_a is the activation energy and R is the universal gas constant.

Bohr's e., an e. to calculate the respiratory dead space from the fact that gas expired from the lungs is a mixture of gas from the dead space and gas from the alveoli, *i.e.*, the dead space volume divided by the tidal volume equals the difference between alveolar and mixed expired gas composition, divided by the difference between alveolar and inspired gas composition; gas composition can be expressed in any consistent units of concentration or partial pressure of oxygen or carbon dioxide.

chemical e., an e. on one side of which are the reactants and on the other side the products of a chemical reaction; the two halves may be separated by an equal sign or by arrows.

constant field e., SYN Goldman e.

Einthoven's e., SYN Einthoven's *law*.

Gay-Lussac's e., the overall chemical e. for alcoholic fermentation; $C_6H_{12}O_6 = 2CO_2 + 2CH_3CH_2OH$.

Gibbs-Helmholtz e., an e. expressing the relationship in a galvanic cell between the chemical energy transformed and the maximal electromotive force obtainable.

Goldman e., an e. derived to predict membrane potentials in terms of the membrane's permeability to ions and their concentrations on either side. SYN constant field e., Goldman-Hodgkin-Katz e., GHK e.

Goldman-Hodgkin-Katz e., GHK e., SYN Goldman e.

Henderson-Hasselbalch e., a formula relating the pH value of a solution to the pK_a value of the acid in the solution and the ratio of the acid and the conjugate base concentrations: $pH = pK_a + \log([A^-]/[HA])$ where $[A^-]$ is the concentration of the conjugate base and $[HA]$ is the concentration of the protonated acid. For the bicarbonate buffer system in blood, $pH = pK' + \log([HCO_3^-]/[CO_2]$. The value of pK' for blood plasma is 6.10 and includes the first dissociation constant of H_2CO_3, the relation between $[H_2CO_3]$ and $[CO_2]$ and other corrections. The partial pressure of CO_2 multiplied by its solubility in plasma at 38°C (0.0301 mM/mm Hg) is commonly substituted for $[CO_2]$; *e.g.*, when the plasma bicarbonate concentration is 24 mEq/liter and the P_{CO_2} is 40 mm Hg, the pH value is $6.10 + \log(24/0.0301 \times 40) = 7.40$.

Hill's e., the e.,$y(1-y) = [S]^n/K_d$, where y is the fractional degree of saturation, $[S]$ is the binding ligand concentration, n is the Hill coefficient, and K_d is the dissociation constant for the ligand. The Hill coefficient is a measure of the cooperativity of the protein; the larger the value, the higher the cooperativity. This coefficient cannot be higher than the number of binding sites. For the oxygen binding curve of hemoglobin, an association constant, K_a, is used and the e. becomes $y/(1-y) = K_a[S]^n$. For human blood, n equals 2.5. Cf. Hill *plot*.

Hüfner's e., an e. expressing the relationship between myoglobin dissociation and oxygen partial pressure: $([MBO_2]/[Mb]) = (K \times pO_2)$.

equation 590 **equivalence**

Lineweaver-Burk e., a rearrangement of the Michaelis-Menten e., $1/v = 1/V_{max} + (K_m/V_{max})(1/[S])$. Cf. double-reciprocal *plot*.

Michaelis-Menten e., an initial-rate e. for a single-substrate noncooperative enzyme-catalyzed reaction relating the intial velocity to the initial substrate concentration; $v = V_{max}$ [S]/$(K_m + [S])$, where v is the initial velocity of the reaction, V_{max} is the maximum velocity, [S] is the initial substrate concentration, and K_m is the Michaelis constant. Similar equations can be derived for conditions in which the product is present and for multisubstrate enzymes. SYN Victor-Michaelis-Menten e.

Nernst's e., the e. relating the equilibrium potential of electrodes to ion concentrations; the e. relating the electrical potential and concentration gradient of an ion across a permeable membrane at equilibrium: $E = [RT / nF]$ [ln (C_1/C_2)], where E = potential, R = absolute gas constant, T = absolute temperature, n = valence, F = the Faraday, ln = the natural logarithm, and C_1 and C_2 are the ion concentrations on the two sides; in nonideal solutions, concentration should be replaced by activity. SEE ALSO Nernst's *theory*, activity (2).

personal e., a slight error in judgment, perceptual response, or action peculiar to the individual and so constant that it is usually possible to allow for it in accepting the person's statements or conclusions, thus arriving at approximate exactness; observed in persons whose work involves readings of events in time, such as navigators and air traffic controllers.

rate e., a mathematical expression for a chemical, radiochemical, or enzyme-catalyzed reaction.

Rayleigh e., a ratio of red to green required by each observer to match spectral yellow. SYN Rayleigh test.

Svedberg e., SEE sedimentation *constant*.

van't Hoff's e., (1) e. for osmotic pressure of dilute solutions. SEE van't Hoff's *law*. **(2)** for any reaction, d(ln K_{eq}/d(1/T) equals $-\Delta H/R$ where K_{eq} is the equilibrium constant, T the absolute temperature, R is the universal gas constant, and ΔH is the change in enthalpy; thus, plotting ln K_{eq} *vs.* 1/T allows the determination of ΔH.

Victor-Michaelis-Menten e., SYN Michaelis-Menten e.

equa·tor (ē-kwā′ter) [NA]. A line encircling a globular body, equidistant at all points from the two poles; the periphery of a plane cutting a sphere at the midpoint of, and at right angles to, its axis. [Mediev. L. *aequator,* fr. L. *aequo,* to make equal]

e. bul′bi oc′uli [NA], SYN e. of eyeball.

e. of eyeball, an imaginary line encircling the globe of the eye equidistant from the anterior and posterior poles. SYN e. bulbi oculi [NA].

e. of lens, the periphery of the lens lying between the two layers of the ciliary zonule. SYN e. lentis [NA].

e. len′tis [NA], SYN e. of lens.

equa·to·ri·al (ē-kwă-tō′rē-ăl). Situated, like the earth's equator, equidistant from each end.

equi·ax·i·al (ē′kwi-ak′sē-ăl). Having axes of equal length.

equi·ca·lor·ic (ē′kwi-kă-lōr′ik). Equal in heat value. SEE ALSO isodynamic. [L. *aequus,* equal, + *calor,* heat]

eq·ui·len·in (ek-wi-len′in). 3-Hydroxyestra-1,3,5(10),6,8-pentaen-17-one; an estrogenic steroid isolated from pregnant mare's urine. [L. *equa,* mare]

equil·i·bra·tion (ē′kwi-li-brā′shŭn, e-kwil-ĭ-). **1.** The act of maintaining an equilibrium or balance. **2.** The act of exposing a liquid, *e.g.,* blood or plasma, to a gas at a certain partial pressure until the partial pressures of the gas within and without the liquid are equal. **3.** In dentistry, modification of occlusal forms of the teeth by grinding, with the intent of equalizing occlusal stress, producing simultaneous occlusal contacts, or harmonizing cuspal relations. **4.** In chromatography, the saturation of the stationary phase with the vapor of the elution solvent to be used.

equi·lib·ri·um (ē-kwi-lib′rē-ŭm). **1.** The condition of being evenly balanced; a state of repose between two or more antagonistic forces that exactly counteract each other. **2.** In chemistry, a state of apparent repose created by two reactions proceeding in opposite directions at equal speed; in chemical equations, sometimes indicated by two opposing arrows (↔) instead of the equal sign. SYN dynamic e. SEE ALSO equilibrium *constant*. [L. *ae-*

quilibrium, a horizontal position, fr. *aequus,* equal, + *libra,* a balance]

acid-base e., SYN acid-base *balance.*

Donnan e., when a semipermeable membrane or its equivalent (*e.g.,* a solid ion-exchanger) separates a nondiffusible substance, such as protein, from diffusible substances, the diffusible anions and cations are distributed on the two sides of the membrane so that 1) the products of their concentrations are equal, and 2) the sum of the diffusible and nondiffusible anions on either side of the membrane is equal to the sum of the concentrations of diffusible and nondiffusible cations; the unequal distribution of diffusible ions thus produced creates a potential difference across the membrane (membrane potential). SYN Gibbs-Donnan e.

dynamic e., SYN equilibrium (2).

genetic e., the condition of a dynamic genetic system in which the several rates of change between all possible pairs of parts are such that the composition is invariant.

Gibbs-Donnan e., SYN Donnan e.

Hardy-Weinberg e., that state in which the genetic structure of the population conforms to the prediction of the Hardy-Weinberg law; it is not a stable e., although for a large mating population it may be approximated. SYN random mating e.

homeostatic e., SEE homeostasis.

nitrogenous e., a condition in which the amount of nitrogen excreted from the body equals that taken in with the food; nutritive e. so far as protein is concerned.

nutritive e., condition in which there is a perfect balance between intake and excretion of nutritive material, so that there is no increase or loss in weight. SYN physiologic e.

physiologic e., SYN nutritive e.

radioactive e., a situation (not a true e.) in which a particular atom is being produced by the radioactive breakdown of a precursor while it is itself breaking down, the two breakdowns matching so that after a period of time the ratio of radioactivity of product and precursor is constant with time.

random mating e., SYN Hardy-Weinberg e.

secular e., a type of radioactive e. in which the half-life of the precursor (parent) radioisotope is so much longer than that of the product (daughter) that the radioactivity of the daughter becomes equal to that of the parent with time.

stable e., e. in which, after every small perturbation, the original state will tend to be restored.

transient e., a type of radioactive e. in which the half-life of the parent radioisotope is longer than that of the daughter so that the ratio of activities of parent and daughter become constant as they decrease with time.

unstable e., e. in which the response to a small perturbation will tend to make the perturbation greater (*e.g.,* a logged feedback process of zero order).

eq·ui·lin (ek′wi-lin). 3-Hydroxyestra-1,3,5(10),7-tetraen-17-one; an estrogenic steroid occurring in the urine of pregnant mares. [L. *equa,* mare]

equi·mo·lar (ē-kwi-mō′ler). Containing an equal number of moles or having the same molarity, as in two or more substances.

equi·mo·lec·u·lar (ē′kwi-mō-lek′yū-ler). Containing an equal number of molecules, as in two or more solutions.

e·quine (ē′kwīn). Relating to, derived from, or resembling the horse, mule, ass, or other members of the genus *Equus.* [L. *equinus,* fr. *equus,* horse]

equine leu·ko·en·ceph·a·lo·ma·la·cia. a mycotoxic disease of horses, mules, and donkeys associated with eating moldy corn containing the fungus *Fusarium moniliforme;* the causative toxin is fumonisin B_1, which produces apathy, pharyngeal paralysis, blindness, staggering, and recumbency.

equi·no·val·gus (ē-kwī-nō-val′gŭs, ek′wi-nō-). SYN *talipes* equinovalgus.

equi·no·var·us (ē-kwī-nō-vā′rŭs, ek′wi-nō-). SYN *talipes* equinovarus.

equi·se·to·sis (ē′kwi-se-tō′sis). A toxicosis in horses caused by eating horsetail (*Equisetum arvense,* a weed).

equi·tox·ic (ē-kwi-tok′sik). Of equivalent toxicity.

equiv·a·lence, equiv·a·len·cy (ē-kwiv′ă-lens, -len-sē). The property of an element or radical of combining with or displacing, in definite and fixed proportion, another element or radical in a compound. [L. *aequus,* equal, + *valentia,* strength (valence)]

equiv·a·lent (Eq, eq) (ē-kwiv′ă-lent). **1.** Equal in any respect. **2.** That which is equal in size, weight, force, or any other quality to something else. [see equivalence]

combustion e., the heat value of a gram of carbohydrate or fat oxidized outside the body.

gold e., a unit of power of the protective colloids; the number of milligrams of protective colloid just sufficient to prevent the precipitation of 10 ml of a 0.0053 to 0.0058% gold solution by the action of 1 ml of a 10% sodium chloride solution. SYN gold number.

gram e., **(1)** the weight in grams of an element that combines with or replaces 1 gram of hydrogen; **(2)** the atomic or molecular weight in grams of an atom or group of atoms involved in a chemical reaction divided by the number of electrons donated, taken up, or shared by the atom or group of atoms in the course of that reaction; **(3)** the weight of a substance contained in 1 liter of 1 normal solution; a variant of (1). SYN combining weight, equivalent weight.

Joule's e. (J), the dynamic e. of heat; the amount of work converted to heat that will raise the temperature of 1 pound of water 1°F is 778 foot-pounds; in metric units, 1 calorie, which raises 1 gram of water 1°C, equals 4.184×10^7 dyne-centimeters, which equals 4.184 joules.

lethal e., **(1)** a combination of selective effects that on average have the same impact on the composition of the gene pool as one death; *e.g.,* two carriers at 50% risk of dying would be the lethal e. of one carrier at 100% risk; **(2)** in the population genetics of recessive traits lethal e. is expressed as twice the sum of the expected number of deaths ascribable to the genetic load.

metabolic e. (MET), the oxygen cost of energy expenditure measured at supine rest (1 MET = 3.5 ml O_2 per kg of body weight per minute); multiples of MET are used to estimate the oxygen cost of activity, *e.g.,* 3 to 5 METs for light work; more than 9 METs for heavy work.

nitrogen e., the nitrogen content of protein; used in calculating the protein breakdown in the body from the nitrogen excreted in the urine, 1 g of nitrogen considered as having originated in 6.25 g of protein catabolized.

starch e., the amount of oxygen consumed in the combustion of a given weight of fat as compared with that consumed in the combustion of an equal weight of starch; the figure is about 2.38, that for starch being taken as 1.

toxic e., the amount of toxin or other poison per kilogram of body weight necessary to kill an animal.

ER Abbreviation for endoplasmic *reticulum.*

Er Symbol for erbium.

ERA Abbreviation for evoked response *audiometry.*

erad·i·ca·tion. Referring to disease, the termination of all transmission of infection by extermination of the infectious agent through surveillance and containment; global eradication has been achieved for smallpox, regional eradication for malaria and perhaps in some places for measles.

Eranko, Eino, Finnish anatomist, *1924. SEE E.'s fluorescence *stain.*

era·sion (ē-rā′zhŭn). Obsolete term for the scraping away of tissue, especially of bone. [L. *e-rado,* pp. *e-rasum,* to scrape away]

Erb, Wilhelm H., German neurologist, 1840–1921. SEE E. *atrophy, disease, palsy, paralysis,* spinal *paralysis, sign;* E.-Charcot *disease;* Duchenne-E. *paralysis;* E.-Westphal *sign;* Westphal-E. *sign.*

ERBF Abbreviation for effective renal blood *flow.*

er·bi·um (Er) (er′bē-ŭm). A rare earth (lanthanide) element, atomic no. 68, atomic wt. 167.26. [from Ytterby, a village in Sweden]

er·cal·cid·i·ol (er-kal-sid′ē-ol). SYN 25-hydroxyergocalciferol.

er·cal·ci·ol (er-kal′sē-ol). SYN ergocalciferol.

er·cal·cit·ri·ol (er-kal-sit′rē-ol). SYN 1,25-dihydroxyergocalciferol.

ERCP Abbreviation for endoscopic retrograde *cholangiopancreatography.*

Erdheim, Jakob, Austrian physician, 1874–1937. SEE E. *disease, tumor.*

Erdmann, Hugo, German chemist, 1862–1910. SEE E.'s *reagent.*

erec·tile (ē-rek′tīl). Capable of erection.

erec·tion (ē-rek′shŭn). The condition of erectile tissue when filled with blood, which then becomes hard and unyielding; denoting especially this state of the penis. [L. *erectio,* fr. *erigo,* pp. *erectus,* to set up]

erec·tor (ērek′tŏr, -tōr). **1.** One who or that which raises or makes erect. **2.** Denoting specifically certain muscles having such action. SYN arrector. [Mod. L.]

er·e·mo·phil·ia (er′ē-mō-fil′ē-ă). Morbid desire to be alone. [G. *erēmia,* solitude, + *philos,* fond]

er·e·mo·pho·bia (er′ē-mō-fō′bē-ă). Morbid fear of deserted places or of solitude. [G. *erēmia,* solitude, + *phobos,* fear]

er·e·thism (er′ĕ-thizm). An abnormal state of excitement or irritation, either general or local. [G. *erethismos,* irritation]

er·e·this·mic, er·e·this·tic, er·e·thit·ic (er-ĕ-thiz′mik, -this′tik, -thit′ik). Excited; marked by or causing erethism; irritable.

er·eu·tho·pho·bi·a (er′ū-thō-fō′bē-ă). Morbid fear of blushing. [G. *ereuthos,* blushing, + *phobos,* fear]

ERG Abbreviation for electroretinogram.

erg. The unit of work in the CGS system; the amount of work done by 1 dyne acting through 1 cm, 1 g cm^2 s^{-2}; in the SI system, 1 erg equals 10^{-7} joule. [G. *ergon,* work]

er·ga·sia (er-gā′zē-ă). **1.** Any form of activity, especially mental. **2.** The total of functions and reactions of an individual. [G. work]

er·ga·si·o·ma·nia (er-gas′ē-ō-mā′nē-ă). Morbid or obsessive need to work. [G. *ergasia,* work, + *mania,* insanity]

er·ga·si·o·pho·bia (er-gas′ē-ō-fō′bē-ă). Aversion to work of any kind. [G. *ergasia,* work, + *phobos,* fear]

er·gas·the·ni·a (er-gas-thē′nē-ă). Rarely used term for debility or any morbid symptoms due to overexertion. [G. *ergasia,* work, + *astheneia,* weakness, disease]

er·gas·to·plasm (er-gas′tō-plazm). SYN granular endoplasmic *reticulum.* [G. *ergastēr,* a workman, + *plasma,* something formed]

erg·ine (erg′ēn). SYN *lysergic acid* amide.

ergo-. Work. [G. *ergon*]

er·go·ba·sine (er-gō-bā′sēn). SYN ergonovine.

er·go·cal·cif·er·ol (er′gō-kal-sif′er-ol). (5Z,7E,22E)-(3S)-9,10-secoergosta-5,7,10(19),22-tetraen-3-ol; activated ergosterol, the vitamin D of plant origin; it arises from ultraviolet irradiation of ergosterol, which is cleaved at the 9,10 bond and develops a double bond between C-10 and C-19; used in prophylaxis and treatment of vitamin D deficiency. SYN calciferol, ercalciol, viosterol, vitamin D_2.

er·go·cor·nine (er-gō-kōr′nēn). $C_{31}H_{39}N_5O_5$; an alkaloid isolated from ergot.

er·go·cris·tine (er′gō-kris′tēn). $C_{35}H_{39}N_5O_5$; an alkaloid isolated from ergot.

er·go·cryp·tine (er-gō-krip′tēn). $C_{32}H_{41}N_5O_5$; an alkaloid isolated from ergot.

er·go·dy·nam·o·graph (er′gō-dī-nam′ō-graf). An instrument for recording both the degree of muscular force and the amount of the work accomplished by muscular contraction. [ergo- + G. *dynamis,* force, + *graphō,* to write]

er·go·es·the·si·o·graph (er′gō-es-thē′zē-ō-graf). An apparatus for recording graphically muscular aptness as shown in the ability to counterbalance variable resistances. [ergo- + G. *aisthēsis,* sensation, + *graphō,* to record]

er·go·gen·ic (er-gō-jen′ik). Tending to increase work.

er·go·graph (er′gō-graf). An instrument for recording the amount of work done by muscular contractions, or the amplitude of contraction. [ergo- + G. *graphō,* to write]

Mosso's e., an instrument consisting of pulleys, weights, and a

er

recording lever, which is used to obtain a graphic record of flexion of a finger, hand, or arm.

er·go·graph·ic (er-gō-graf'ik). Relating to the ergograph and the record made by it.

er·go·lines (er'gō-linz). A class of drugs with prominent agonistic or antagonistic actions on dopamine receptors. Agents belonging to this group include bromocriptine, pergolide, and lisuride.

er·gom·e·ter (er-gom'ĕ-ter). SYN dynamometer. [ergo- + G. *metron,* measure]

er·go·met·rine (er-gō-met'rēn). SYN ergonovine.

e. maleate, SYN *ergonovine* maleate.

er·go·nom·ics (er-gō-nom'iks). A branch of ecology concerned with human factors in the design and operations of machines and the physical environment. [ergo- + G. *nomos,* law]

er·go·no·vine (er-gō-nō'vēn, -vin). An alkaloid from ergot; on hydrolysis it yields D-lysergic acid and L-2-aminopropanol. SYN ergobasine, ergometrine, ergostetrine.

e. maleate, a powerful oxytocic agent; this action is more prominent, and other actions of ergot (vasoconstriction, central nervous system stimulation, adrenergic blockade, etc.) are less prominent than for other ergot alkaloids; effective orally and parenterally. SYN ergometrine maleate.

er·go·sine (er'gō-sēn, -sin). An alkaloid from ergot with actions similar to those of ergotamine.

er·go·stat (er'gō-stat). A form of machine for exercising the muscles. [ergo- + G. *statos,* standing, placed]

er·gos·ter·in (er-gos'ter-in). SYN ergosterol.

er·gos·ter·ol (er-gos'ter-ol). 7,22-didehydrocholesterol; ergosta-5,7,22-trien-3β-ol; the most important of the provitamins D_2; ultraviolet irradiation converts e. to lumisterol, tachysterol, and ergocalciferol; main sterol in yeast. SYN ergosterin.

er·go·stet·rine (er-gō-stet'rēn, -rin). SYN ergonovine.

er·got (er'got). The resistant, overwintering stage of the parasitic ascomycetous fungus *Claviceps purpurea,* a pathogen of rye grass that transforms the seed of rye into a compact spurlike mass of fungal pseudotissue (the sclerotium) containing five or more optically isomeric pairs of alkaloids. The levorotary isomers induce uterine contractions, control bleeding, and alleviate certain localized vascular disorders (migraine headaches). E. exemplifies fungal products with profound toxic effects at appropriate levels. SYN rye smut. [O. Fr. *argot,* cock's spur]

corn e., SYN *Ustilago maydis.*

er·got·a·mine (er-got'ă-mēn). $C_{33}H_{35}N_5O_5$; an alkaloid from ergot, used for the relief of migraine; it is a potent stimulant of smooth muscle, particularly of the blood vessels and the uterus, and produces adrenergic blockade (chiefly of the alpha receptors); hydrogenated e., dihydroergotamine, is less toxic and has fewer side effects. Also available as e. tartrate.

er·got·am·i·nine (er-got-am'i-nēn). An isomer of ergotamine but practically inert.

er·go·ther·a·py (er-gō-thār'ă-pē). Treatment of disease by muscular exercise. [G. *ergon,* work, + *therapeia,* therapy]

er·go·thi·o·ne·ine (er'gō-thī-ō-nē'in). thiohistidylbetaine; 2'-thiolhistidine betaine; the betaine of a sulfur-containing derivative of histidine, present in blood and other mammalian tissue and in ergot. SYN thiolhistidylbetaine, thioneine.

er·got·ism (er'got-izm). Poisoning by a toxic substance contained in the sclerotia of the fungus, *Claviceps purpura,* growing on rye grass; characterized by necrosis of the extremities (gangrene) due to contraction of the peripheral vascular bed. SEE ALSO ergot *poisoning.* SYN Saint Anthony's fire (1).

er·go·tox·ine (er'gō-tok'sēn, -sin). A mixture of alkaloids obtained from ergot, consisting of 1:1:1 ergocristine, ergocornine and ergocryptine, more toxic than other natural and semisynthetic ergot alkaloids; a potent stimulant of smooth muscle, particularly of the blood vessels and uterus, and produces adrenergic blockade (chiefly of the alpha receptors). SYN ecboline.

er·go·tro·pic (er'gō-trop'ik). The term introduced by W.R. Hess to denote those mechanisms and the functional status of the nervous system that favor the organism's capacity to expend energy, as distinguished from the trophotropic mechanisms pro-

moting rest and reconstitution of energy stores. In general, the balance between ergotropic and trophotropic nervous mechanisms corresponds in large part to that between the sympathetic and parasympathetic subdivisions of the autonomic nervous system. [ergo- + G. *tropos,* a turning]

Erichsen, Sir John, English surgeon, 1818–1896. SEE E.'s *sign.*

er·i·o·dic·ty·on (ār'ē-ō-dik'tē-on). The dried leaves of *Eriodictyon californicum* (family Hydrophyllaceae); the fluidextract and the syrup have been used as an expectorant and to mask the taste of bitter substances. SYN mountain balm, yerba santa.

eris·o·phake (e-ris'ō-fāk). A surgical instrument designed to hold the lens by suction in cataract extraction; now seldom used. [G. *erysis,* a drawing, + *phakos,* lentil]

Erlenmeyer, Emil, German chemist, 1825–1909. SEE E. *flask,* flask *deformity.*

Ernst, Paul, German pathologist, 1859–1937. SEE Babès-E. *bodies,* under *body.*

erode (ē-rōd'). **1.** To cause, or to be affected by, erosion. **2.** To remove by ulceration. [L. *erodo,* to gnaw away]

erog·e·nous (ĕ-roj'ĕ-nŭs). Capable of producing sexual excitement when stimulated. [G. *eros,* love, + *genos,* birth]

eros (ē'ros, ār'os). In psychoanalysis, the life principle representing all instinctual tendencies toward procreation and life. See also entries under instinct. Cf. thanatos. [G. love]

erose (ē-rōs'). Denoting an edge or margin which is irregularly notched or indented, as if gnawed away; used especially in reference to bacterial colonies. [L. *erodo,* pp. *erosus,* to gnaw away]

ero·sion (ē-rō'zhŭn). **1.** A wearing away or a state of being worn away, as by friction or pressure. Cf. corrosion. **2.** A shallow ulcer; in the stomach and intestine, an ulcer limited to the mucosa, with no penetration of the muscularis mucosa. **3.** The wearing away of a tooth by chemical action or abrasive; when the cause is unknown, it is referred to as idiopathic e. SYN odontolysis. [L. *erosio,* fr. *erodo,* to gnaw away]

Dieulafoy's e., acute ulcerative gastroenteritis complicating pneumonia, possibly caused by overproduction of adrenal steroid hormones.

recurrent corneal e., repeated vesiculation followed by exfoliation of the corneal epithelium.

ero·sive (ē-rō'siv). **1.** Having the property of eroding or wearing away. **2.** An eroding agent.

erot·ic (ĕ-rot'ik). Lustful; relating to sexual passion; having the quality to produce sexual arousal. [G. *erōtikos,* relating to love, fr. *erōs,* love]

er·o·tism, erot·i·cism (er'ō-tizm, ĕ-rot'i-sizm). A condition of sexual excitement.

anal e., pleasurable experience centered around defecation and related activities associated with the anal zone, especially during the anal phase in one- to three-year-old children.

er·o·ti·za·tion (er'ō-ti-zā'shŭn). The act of sexual arousal or the state of being sexually excited. SYN libidinization.

ero·to·gen·e·sis (er'ō-tō-jen'ĕ-sis). The origin or genesis of sexual impulses. [G. *erōs,* love, + *genesis,* origin]

ero·to·gen·ic (er'ō-tō-jen'ik). Capable of causing sexual excitement or arousal. [G. *erōs,* love, + *-gen,* production]

ero·to·ma·nia (er'ō-tō-mā'nē-ă). **1.** Excessive or morbid inclination to erotic thoughts and behavior. **2.** The delusional belief that one is involved in a relationship with another, generally of higher socioeconomic status. [G. *erōs,* love, + *mania,* frenzy]

ero·to·path·ic (er'ō-tō-path'ik). Relating to erotopathy.

er·o·top·a·thy (er-ō-top'ă-thē). Any abnormality of the sexual impulse. [G. *erōs,* love, + *pathos,* suffering]

ero·to·pho·bia (er'ō-tō-fō'bē-ă). Morbid aversion to the thought of sexual love and to its physical expression. [G. *erōs,* love, + *phobos,* fear]

ERP Abbreviation for early receptor *potential.*

ERPF Abbreviation for effective renal plasma *flow.*

er·rat·ic (ĕ-rat'ik). **1.** SYN eccentric (1). **2.** Denoting symptoms that vary in intensity, frequency, or location. [L. *erro,* pp. *erratus,* to wander]

er·ror (er'ōr). **1.** A defect in structure or function. **2.** In biostatistics: 1) a mistaken decision, as in hypothesis testing or classification by a discriminant function; 2) the difference between the true value and the observed value of a variate, ascribed to randomness or misreading by an observer. **3.** A false or mistaken belief; in biomedical and other sciences, there are many varieties of e., for example due to bias, inaccurate measurements, or faulty instruments.

alpha e., SYN type I e.

beta e., SYN type II e.

experimental e., the total e. of measurement ascribed to the conduct of an empirical observation. It is commonly expressed as the standard deviation of replicated experiments. There may be many components, including those in the sampling procedure, the measurements, injudicious choice of a model, observer bias, etc.

e. of the first kind, in a Neyman-Pearson test of a statistical hypothesis the probability of rejecting the null hypothesis when it is true. SYN type I e.

inborn e.'s of metabolism, a group of disorders, each of which involves a disorder of a single unique enzyme, genetic in origin and operating from birth; effects are ascribable to accumulation of the substrate on which the enzyme normally acts (*e.g.,* phenylketonuria), to deficiency of the product of the enzyme (*e.g.,* albinism), or to forcing metabolism through an auxiliary pathway (*e.g.,* oxaluria).

interobserver e., the differences in interpretation by two or more individuals making observations of the same phenomenon.

intraobserver e., the differences in interpretation by an individual making observations of the same phenomenon at different times.

residual e., the estimated discrepancy between the actual measured datum and the value for that value computed after a model has been fitted to the set of the data by an estimator.

e. of the second kind, in a Neyman-Pearson test of a statistical hypothesis, the probability of accepting the null hypothesis when it is false; the complement of the power of the test. SYN type II e.

technical e., that component of experimental e. that is due to the conduct of the experiment and in principle estimated by replicate determinations on aliquots from the same specimen.

type I e., SYN e. of the first kind. SYN alpha e.

type II e., SYN e. of the second kind. SYN beta e.

er·ta·cal·ci·ol (er-tă-kal′sē-ol). SEE tachysterol.

er·u·bes·cence (er-ū-bes′ens). A reddening of the skin. [L. *erubescere,* to redden]

er·u·bes·cent (er-ū-bes′ent). Denoting reddening of the skin.

eru·cic ac·id (ĕ-rū′sik). 13-Docosenoic acid; a 22-carbon unsaturated fatty acid present in the seeds of nasturtium (Indian cress) and of several *Cruciferae* species (rape, mustard, and wallflower); thought to be toxic to cardiac muscle.

eruc·ta·tion (ē-rŭk-tā′shŭn). The voiding of gas or of a small quantity of acid fluid from the stomach through the mouth. SYN belching, ructus. [L. *eructo,* pp. -*atus,* to belch]

erup·tion (ē-rŭp′shŭn). **1.** A breaking out, especially the appearance of lesions on the skin. **2.** A rapidly developing dermatosis of the skin or mucous membranes, especially when appearing as a local manifestation of one of the exanthemata; an e. is characterized, according to the nature of the lesion, as macular, papular, vesicular, pustular, bullous, nodular, erythematous, etc. **3.** The passage of a tooth through the alveolar process and perforation of the gums. [L. *e-rumpo,* pp. -*ruptus,* to break out]

accelerated e., a dental e. pattern which is chronologically advanced in comparison with the average pattern of dental e.; e. of the first tooth occurs at an earlier age than the average, and the intervals of time between subsequent dental e.'s are shorter than the average.

butterfly e., SYN butterfly (2).

clinical e., development of the crown of a tooth that can be observed clinically.

continuous e., the e. of a tooth into the mouth and its continuous movement in a vertical direction.

creeping e., SYN cutaneous *larva migrans.*

delayed e., a dental e. pattern which is chronologically late in comparison with the average pattern of dental e.; e. of the first tooth occurs at a later age than the average, and the intervals of time between subsequent dental e.'s are longer than the average.

drug e., any e. caused by the ingestion, injection, or inhalation of a drug, most often the result of allergic sensitization; reactions to drugs applied to the cutaneous surface are not generally designated as drug e., but as contact-type dermatitis. SYN dermatitis medicamentosa, dermatosis medicamentosa, drug rash, medicinal e.

feigned e., SYN *dermatitis* artefacta.

fixed drug e., a type of drug e. that recurs at a fixed site (or sites) following the administration of a particular drug; the lesions usually consist of intensely erythematous and purplish, sharply demarcated macules, and occasionally of herpetic vesicles; the affected areas undergo gradual involution, but flare and enlarge on readministration of the offending drug and may become hyperpigmented.

iodine e., an acneform or follicular e. or granulomatous lesion caused by a reaction to systemic iodine or iodide administration.

Kaposi's varicelliform e., a now rare complication of vaccinia superimposed on atopic dermatitis, with generalized vesicles and vesicopapules and high fever. SYN eczema vaccinatum.

medicinal e., SYN drug e.

passive e., the apparent continued e. of the teeth, actually the result of regression of the gingivae and crestal bone.

polymorphous light e., a common pruritic papular e. appearing in a few hours and lasting up to several days on skin exposed to shortwave ultraviolet light; subepidermal edema and deep perivascular lymphocytic infiltration is seen microscopically.

e. sequestrum (sē′kwes-trum), spicule of bone overlying the central occlusal fossa of an erupting permanent molar.

serum e., urticaria seen in serum sickness.

surgical e., the uncovering of an unerupted tooth to permit its further e. into the oral cavity by surgically removing overlying soft tissue, bone, and sometimes teeth.

erup·tive (ē-rŭp′tiv). Characterized by eruption.

ERV Abbreviation for expiratory reserve *volume.*

er·y·sip·e·las (er-i-sip′ĕ-las). A specific, acute, cutaneous inflammatory disease caused by β-hemolytic streptococci and characterized by hot, red, edematous, brawny, and sharply defined eruptions; usually accompanied by severe constitutional symptoms. SYN rose (1). [G., fr. *erythros,* red + *pella,* skin]

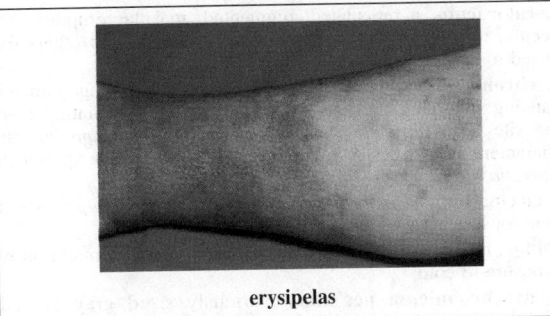

erysipelas

ambulant e., SYN e. migrans.

e. inter′num, an erysipelatous eruption in the vagina, uterus, and peritoneum, occurring in the puerperium.

e. mi′grans, a widely spreading form involving the entire face or body surface. SYN ambulant e., wandering e.

e. per′stans facie′i, chronic, dusky red eruption of erysipelas on the face.

phlegmonous e., a form marked by invasion of the subcutaneous tissues, with the formation of deep-seated abscesses.

e. pustulo′sum, development of pustules over the area of e.

surgical e., e. caused by infection of the wound following a surgical procedure.

swine e., a destructive disease of swine, occurring in both acute and chronic forms, caused by *Erysipelothrix rhusiopathiae.*

e. verruco′sum, development of verrucous or warty lesions on the area of e.

wandering e., SYN e. migrans.

er·y·si·pel·a·tous (er′i-si-pel′ă-tŭs). Relating to erysipelas.

er·y·sip·e·loid (er-i-sip′ĕ-loyd). A specific, usually self-limiting, cellulitis of the hand caused by *Erysipelothrix rhusiopathiae*; appears as a dusky erythema with diamondlike configuration of the skin at the site of a wound sustained in handling fish or meat and may become generalized, with plaques of erythema and bullae, and occasionally, severe toxemia. SYN blubber finger, crab hand, pseudoerysipelas, Rosenbach's disease (2), seal fingers, speck finger, whale fingers. [G. *erysipelas + eidos,* resemblance]

Er·y·sip·e·lo·thrix (ār-i-sip′ĕ-lō-thriks, -si-pel′ō-thriks). A genus of bacteria (family Corynebacteriaceae) containing nonmotile, Gram-positive, rod-shaped organisms which have a tendency to form long filaments; older cells tend to become Gram-negative. They produce acid but no gas from glucose. They are facultatively anaerobic and catalase-negative. Members of this genus are parasitic on mammals, birds, and fish. The type species is *E. rhusiopathiae.* [erysipelas + G. *thrix,* hair]

E. **insidio′sa,** SYN *E. rhusiopathiae.*

E. **rhusiopath′iae,** a species which causes swine erysipelas, human erysipeloid, non-suppurative polyarthritis in lambs, and septicemia in mice, and commonly infects fish handlers; it is the type species of the genus *E.* SYN *E. insidiosa.*

er·y·sip·e·lo·tox·in (ār-i-sip′ĕ-lō-tok′sin). A toxin produced by types of *Streptococcus pyogenes* (group A hemolytic streptococci), the bacterial cause of erysipelas.

er·y·the·ma (er-i-thē′mă). Redness of the skin due to capillary dilatation. [G. *erythēma,* flush]

e. ab ig′ne, SYN e. caloricum.

acrodynic e., SYN acrodynia (2).

e. annula′re, rounded or ringed lesions.

e. annula′re centrif′ugum, a chronic recurring erythematous eruption consisting of small and large annular lesions, with a scant marginal scale, usually of unknown cause. SYN e. figuratum perstans.

e. annula′re rheumat′icum, a variant of e. multiforme associated with rheumatic fever.

e. arthrit′icum epidem′icum, SYN Haverhill *fever.*

e. bullo′sum, e. multiforme with formation of large vesicles or bullae.

e. calor′icum, a reticulated, pigmented, macular eruption that occurs, mostly on the shins, of bakers, stokers, and others exposed to radiant heat. SYN e. ab igne, toasted shins.

e. chron′icum mi′grans, a raised erythematous ring with advancing indurated borders and central clearing, radiating from the site of a tick bite such as that by *Ixodes dammini;* the characteristic skin lesion of Lyme disease, due to the spirochete *Borrelia burgdorferi.*

e. circina′tum, e. multiforme in which the lesions are grouped in more or less circular fashion.

cold e., rash characterized by redness and itching, brought on by exposure to cold.

e. dyschro′micum per′stans, variously sized gray or red, slightly elevated macular lesions that tend to coalesce on the trunk, extremities, and face, commonly in dark-skinned Latin Americans; of unknown cause. SYN e. ashy dermatosis.

e. eleva′tum diu′tinum, a chronic symmetrical eruption of flattened nodules, of a pinkish or purplish color, occurring in plaques on the buttocks and extensors of wrists, elbows, and knees, becoming fibrotic and finally scarring; early lesions show necrotizing vasculitis with fibrinoid or lipid deposits in vessel walls. SYN Bury's disease.

e. exfoliati′va, SYN *keratolysis* exfoliativa.

e. figura′tum per′stans, SYN e. annulare centrifugum.

e. fu′gax, obsolete term for a diffuse and fleeting e. from emotional stimuli.

e. gyra′tum, e. circinatum in which the various ringed lesions overlap each other.

hemorrhagic exudative e., SYN Henoch-Schönlein *purpura.*

e. indura′tum, recurrent hard subcutaneous nodules that frequently break down and form necrotic ulcers, usually on the calves and less frequently on the thighs or arms of middle-aged women; they are associated with erythrocyanotic changes in cold weather; although microscopically granulomatous and necrotizing, the lesions are sterile; probably a form of nodular vasculitis. SYN Bazin's disease, nodular tuberculid.

e. infectio′sum, a mild infectious exanthema of childhood characterized by an erythematous maculopapular eruption, resulting in a lace-like facial rash or "slapped cheek" appearance. Fever and arthritis may also accompany infection; caused by Parvovirus B 19. SYN fifth disease, Sticker's disease.

e. intertri′go, SEE intertrigo.

e. i′ris, concentric rings of e. varying in intensity, characteristic of e. multiforme. SYN herpes iris (1).

Jacquet's e., SYN diaper *dermatitis.*

e. kerato′des, keratodermia with an erythematous border.

macular e., SYN roseola.

e. margina′tum, a variant of e. multiforme seen in rheumatic fever; occasionally has a configuration to suggest the designation e. migrans (geographic tongue).

e. mi′grans, e. mi′grans ling′uae, SYN geographic *tongue.*

Milian's e., SYN ninth-day e.

e. multifor′me, an acute eruption of macules, papules, or subdermal vesicles presenting a multiform appearance, the characteristic lesion being the target or iris lesion over the dorsal aspect of the hands and forearms; its origin may be allergic, seasonal, or from drug sensitivity, and the eruption, although usually self-limited (*e.g.,* multiforme minor), may be recurrent or may run a severe course, sometimes with fatal termination (*e.g.,* multiforme major or Stevens-Johnson syndrome). SYN e. polymorphe, Hebra's disease (1), herpes iris (2).

e. multifor′me bullo′sum, SYN Stevens-Johnson *syndrome.*

e. multifor′me exudati′vum, SYN Stevens-Johnson *syndrome.*

e. multifor′me ma′jor, SYN Stevens-Johnson *syndrome.*

necrolytic migratory e., an erythematous, scaling, and sometimes bullous and erosive dermatitis occurring irregularly in plaques chiefly on the lower trunk, buttocks, perineum, and thighs; associated with weight loss, anemia, stomatitis, and elevation of plasma glucagon in islet cell tumor (glucagonoma) of the pancreas. SEE ALSO glucagonoma *syndrome.*

e. neonato′rum, SYN e. toxicum neonatorum.

ninth-day e., obsolete term for a nontoxic eruption that simulates measles or a toxic erythema, occurring usually on the ninth day of a course of medication; first described as a reaction to arsenical treatment of syphilis. SYN Milian's disease, Milian's e.

e. nodo′sum, a panniculitis marked by the sudden formation of painful nodes on the extensor surfaces of the lower extremities, with lesions that are self-limiting but tend to recur; associated with arthralgia and fever; may be the result of drug sensitivity or associated with sarcoidosis and various infections. Deep biopsies show a septal panniculitis with infiltration by lymphocytes and scattered multinucleated giant cells. SYN nodal fever.

e. nodo′sum lepro′sum, an acute type of lepromatous reaction with generalized systemic involvement and tender deep cutaneous and subcutaneous nodules of the face, thighs, and arms; usually seen in undiagnosed, untreated, or neglected cases of leprosy.

e. nodo′sum mi′grans, SYN subacute migratory *panniculitis.*

e. palma′re heredita′rium [MIM*133000], a condition characterized by asymptomatic symmetrical palmar e.; autosomal dominant inheritance. SYN Lane's disease.

e. papula′tum, the papular form of e. multiforme.

e. paratrim′ma, e. due to stasis over pressure points.

e. per′nio, SYN chilblain.

e. per′stans, probably a chronic form of e. multiforme in which the relapses recur so persistently that the eruption is almost permanent.

e. polymor′phe, SYN e. multiforme.

scarlatiniform e., e. scarlatinoi′des, an erythematous macular eruption accompanied by slight constitutional symptoms and followed by desquamation.

e. sim′plex, blushing or redness of the skin caused by a toxic reaction or a neurovascular phenomenon. SYN dermatitis simplex.

e. sola′re, SYN sunburn.

symptomatic e., a general term applied to various e.'s associated with systemic disease, fevers, allergic states, etc.

e. tox′icum, flushing of the skin due to allergic reaction to some toxic substance.

e. tox′icum neonato′rum, a common transient idiopathic eruption of erythema, small papules, and occasionally pustules filled with eosinophilic leukocytes overlying hair follicles of the newborn. SYN e. neonatorum.

e. tubercula′tum, e. multiforme in which the papules are of large size.

er·y·them·a·tous (er-i-them′ă-tŭs, -thē′mă-tŭs). Relating to or marked by erythema.

er·y·the·ma·to·ve·sic·u·lar (er-i-thē′mă-tō-ve-sik′yū-lăr). Denoting a condition characterized by erythema and vesiculation, as in allergic contact dermatitis.

er·y·ther·mal·gia (er′i-ther-mal′jē-ă). SYN erythromelalgia.

♺**erythr-.** SEE erythro-.

er·y·thral·gia (ār-i-thral′jē-ă). Painful redness of the skin. SEE ALSO erythromelalgia. [erythro- + G. *algos*, pain]

ery·thras·ma (er-i-thraz′mă). An eruption of well-circumscribed reddish brown patches, in the axillae and groins especially, due to the presence of *Corynebacterium minutissimum* in the stratum corneum. [G. *erythrainō*, to redden]

eryth·re·de·ma (ĕ-rith-rē-dē′mă). SYN acrodynia (2). [erythro- + G. *oidēma*, swelling]

er·y·thre·mia (er-i-thrē′mē-ă). SYN *polycythemia* vera. [erythro- + G. *haima*, blood]

altitude e., SYN chronic mountain *sickness*.

er·y·thrism (er′i-thrizm, ĕ-rith′rizm). Redness of the hair with a ruddy, freckled complexion. [G. *erythros*, red]

er·y·thris·tic (er-i-thris′tik). Relating to or marked by erythrism; having a ruddy complexion and reddish hair. SYN rufous.

er·y·thrite (ĕ-rith′rīt). SYN erythritol.

eryth·ri·tol (ĕ-rith′ri-tol). tetrahydroxybutane (1,2,3,4-butanetetrol); the 4-carbon sugar alcohol obtained by the reduction of erythrose, notable for its sweetness (twice that of sucrose); found in lichens, algae, and fungi; a coronary vasodilator. SYN erythrite, erythrol.

eryth·ri·tyl tet·ra·ni·trate (ĕ-rith′ri-til tet-ră-nī′trāt). A vasodilator used in angina pectoris and hypertension. SYN erythrol tetranitrate, tetranitrol.

♺**erythro-, erythr-.** **1.** Combining form denoting red or red blood cell; corresponds to L. *rub-.* **2.** Indicates the structure of erythrose in a larger sugar; used as such, it is italicized (*e.g.,* 2-deoxy-D-*erythro*-pentose). [G. *erythros*, red]

eryth·ro·blast (ĕ-rith′rō-blast). Originally, a term denoting all forms of human red blood cells containing a nucleus, both pathologic (*i.e.,* megaloblastic) and normal (*e.g.,* normoblastic). The pathologic or megaloblastic series is observed in pernicious anemia in relapse. The term megaloblast is also used to indicate the first generation of cells in the red blood cell series that can be distinguished from precursor endothelial cells; hence with this usage, megaloblast denotes both a normal and an abnormal cell. In the *normoblastic series* of maturation four stages of development can be recognized: 1) pronormoblast, 2) basophilic normoblast, 3) polychromatic normoblast, and 4) orthochromatic normoblast. In the *megaloblastic series* of maturation, stages similar to those found in the normoblastic series are seen: 1) promegaloblast, 2) basophilic megaloblast, 3) polychromatic megaloblast, and 4) orthochromatic megaloblast. In the *normal series* of maturation, after loss of the nucleus, young erythrocytes are called *reticulocytes;* these cells may be recognized with supravital stains such as brilliant cresyl blue; ultimately the reticulocytes become erythrocytes, or mature red blood cells. SYN erythrocytoblast, Loevit's cell. [erythro- + G. *blastos*, germ]

eryth·ro·blas·te·mia (ĕ-rith′rō-blas-tē′mē-ă). The presence of nucleated red cells in the peripheral blood. [erythroblast + G. *haima*, blood]

eryth·ro·blas·to·pe·nia (ĕ-rith′rō-blas-tō-pē′nē-ă). A primary deficiency of erythroblasts in bone marrow, seen in aplastic anemia. [erythroblast + G. *penia,* poverty]

eryth·ro·blas·to·sis (ĕ-rith′rō-blas-tō′sis). The presence of erythroblasts in considerable number in the blood. [erythroblast + *-osis,* condition]

avian e., an expression of disease of the avian leukosis-sarcoma complex; characterized by severe anemia and large numbers of erythroblasts in the blood; chickens are most susceptible but fatal natural infections have been reported in guinea fowl. SYN fowl e.

fetal e., SYN e. fetalis.

e. feta′lis, a grave hemolytic anemia that, in most instances, results from development in the mother of anti-Rh antibody in response to the Rh factor in the (Rh-positive) fetal blood; it is characterized by many erythroblasts in the circulation, and often generalized edema (hydrops fetalis) and enlargement of the liver and spleen; the disease is sometimes caused by antibodies for antigens other than Rh. SEE ALSO hemolytic *anemia* of newborn (2). SYN anemia neonatorum, congenital anemia, fetal e., hemolytic anemia of newborn (1), hemolytic disease of newborn, neonatal anemia.

fowl e., SYN avian e.

eryth·ro·blas·tot·ic (ĕ-rith′rō-blas-tot′ik). Pertaining to erythroblastosis, especially erythroblastosis fetalis.

eryth·ro·ca·tal·y·sis (ĕ-rith′rō-kă-tal′i-sis). Phagocytosis of the red blood cells. [erythro- + G. *katalysis,* dissolution]

eryth·ro·chro·mia (ĕ-rith′rō-krō′mē-ă). A red coloration or staining. [erythro- + G. *chrōma,* color]

eryth·ro·cla·sis (er-i-throk′lă-sis). Fragmentation of the red blood cells. [erythro- + G. *klasis,* a breaking]

eryth·ro·clas·tic (ĕ-rith′rō-klas′tik). Pertaining to erythroclasis; destructive to red blood cells.

eryth·ro·cu·pre·in (ĕ-rith′rō-kū′prē-in). SYN cytocuprein.

eryth·ro·cy·a·no·sis (ĕ-rith′rō-sī-ă-nō′sis). A condition seen in girls and young women in which exposure of the limbs to cold causes them to become swollen and dusky red; it results from direct exposure to cold, but not freezing, temperatures. [erythro- + G. *kyanos,* blue, + *-osis,* condition]

eryth·ro·cyte (ĕ-rith′rō-sīt). A mature red blood cell. SYN red blood cell, red corpuscle. [erythro- + G. *kytos,* cell]

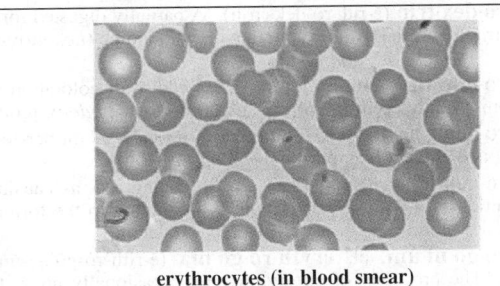

erythrocytes (in blood smear)

eryth·ro·cy·the·mia (ĕ-rith′rō-sī-thē′mē-ă). SYN polycythemia. [erythro- + G. *kytos,* cell, + *haima,* blood]

eryth·ro·cyt·ic (ĕ-rith-rō-sit′ik). Pertaining to an erythrocyte.

eryth·ro·cy·to·blast (ĕ-rith-rō-sī′tō-blast). SYN erythroblast. [erythro- + G. *kytos,* cell, + *blastos,* germ]

eryth·ro·cy·tol·y·sin (ĕ-rith′rō-sī-tol′i-sin). SYN hemolysin (1).

eryth·ro·cy·tol·y·sis (ĕ-rith′rō-sī-tol′i-sis). SYN hemolysis. [erythrocyte + G. *lysis,* loosening]

eryth·ro·cy·tom·e·ter (ĕ-rith′rō-sī-tom′ĕ-ter). An instrument for counting the red blood cells; Hayden used this term to denote an instrument to measure the diameter of red blood cells. [erythrocyte + G. *metron,* measure]

eryth·ro·cy·to·pe·nia (ĕ-rith′rō-sī-tō-pē′nē-ă). SYN erythropenia.

eryth·ro·cy·to·poi·e·sis (ĕ-rith′rō-sī′tō-poy-ē′sis). SYN erythropoiesis.

eryth·ro·cy·tor·rhex·is (ĕ-rith′rō-sī-tō-rek′sis). A partial erythrocytolysis in which particles of protoplasm escape from the red blood cells, which then become crenated and deformed. SYN erythrorrhexis. [erythrocyte + G. *rhēxis,* rupture]

eryth·ro·cy·tos·chi·sis (ĕ-rith′rō-sī-tos′ki-sis). A breaking up of the red blood cells into small particles that morphologically resemble platelets. [erythrocyte + G. *schisis,* a splitting]

eryth·ro·cy·to·sis (ĕ-rith′rō-sī-tō′sis). Polycythemia, especially that which occurs in response to some known stimulus.

eryth·ro·cy·tu·ria (ĕ-rith′rō-sī-tū′rē-ă). Red blood cells in urine.

eryth·ro·de·gen·er·a·tive (ĕ-rith′rō-de-jen′er-ă-tiv). Pertaining to or characterized by degeneration of the red blood cells.

eryth·ro·der·ma (ĕ-rith-rō-der′mă). A nonspecific designation for intense and usually widespread reddening of the skin from dilatation of blood vessels, often preceding, or associated with exfoliation. SYN erythrodermatitis. [erythro- + G. *derma,* skin]

   bullous congenital ichthyosiform e. (ik-thē-os′ē-form), diffusely red, eroded skin at birth, with subsequent scaling, tending to improve in later life, characterized by generalized epidermolytic hyperkeratosis and autosomal dominant inheritance. SEE ALSO epidermolytic *hyperkeratosis.* SYN generalized epidermolytic hyperkeratosis, ichthyismus hystrix, ichthyosis hystrix.

   congenital ichthyosiform e., a genodermatosis characterized by diffuse chronic erythema and scale formation which may be separated into bullous and nonbullous forms. SYN ichthyosiform e., ichthyosis spinosa, keratoma malignum.

   e. desquamati′vum, severe, extensive seborrheic dermatitis with exfoliative dermatitis, generalized lymphoadenopathy, and diarrhea in the newborn; frequently occurs in undernourished, cachectic children. SYN Leiner's disease.

   e. exfoliati′va, SYN *keratolysis* exfoliativa.

   ichthyosiform e., SYN congenital ichthyosiform e.

   nonbullous congenital ichthyosiform e., e. or a collodion membrane at birth, usually without improvement during childhood, characterized by proliferation of epidermal keratinocytes with lipid accumulation; autosomal recessive inheritance.

   e. psoriat′icum, extensive exfoliative dermatitis simulating psoriasis.

   Sézary e., SYN Sézary *syndrome.*

eryth·ro·der·ma·ti·tis (ĕ-rith′rō-der-mă-tī′tis). SYN erythroderma.

eryth·ro·dex·trin (ĕ-rith′rō-deks′trin). A partially digested form of dextrin identified by its color reaction with iodine (*i.e.,* turning red).

eryth·ro·don·tia (ĕ-rith′rō-don′shē-ă). Reddish discoloration of the teeth, as may occur in porphyria. [erythro- + G. *odous,* tooth]

eryth·ro·gen·e·sis im·per·fec·ta (ĕ-rith-rō-jen′ĕ-sis im-per-fek′tă). SYN congenital hypoplastic *anemia.*

eryth·ro·gen·ic (ĕ-rith-rō-jen′ik). **1.** Producing red, as causing an eruption or a red color sensation. **2.** Pertaining to the formation of red blood cells. [erythro- + *-gen,* producing]

eryth·ro·go·ni·um, pl. **eryth·ro·go·nia** (ĕ-rith-rō-gō′nē-ŭm, -nē-ă). The precursor of an erythrocyte; occasionally refers to the erythropoietic tissue as a whole. [erythro- + G. *gonē,* generation]

er·y·throid (er′i-throyd, ĕ-rith′royd). Reddish in color.

er·y·throid·in (er′i-thrōy′din). A nicotinic cholinergic antagonist which unlike most members of this group of agents, is a tertiary amine and hence enters the central nervous system.

eryth·ro·ker·a·to·der·mi·a (ĕ-rith′rō-kār-ă-tō-der′mēă) [MIM* 133190]. The association of erythoderma and hyperkeratosis, which may be symptomatic at sites of chronic injury or inherited; ataxia appears later in life; symmetrical progressive e. is inherited as an autosomal dominant gene and does not involve the palms and soles. [erythro- + G. *keras,* horn, + *derma,* skin, + *-ia,* condition]

   e. variabi′lis [MIM*133200], a dermatosis characterized by hyperkeratotic plaques of bizarre, geographic configuration, associated with erythrodermic areas that may vary remarkably in size, shape, and position from day to day; onset is usually in the first year of life; autosomal dominant inheritance. SYN keratosis rubra figurata.

eryth·ro·ki·net·ics (ĕ-rith′rō-ki-net′iks). A consideration of the kinetics of erythrocytes from their generation to destruction; erythrokinetic studies are sometimes made in cases of anemia to evaluate the balance between erythrocyte production and destruction. [erythro- + G. *kinēsis,* movement]

er·y·throl (er′i-throl). SYN erythritol.

   e. tetranitrate, SYN erythrityl tetranitrate.

eryth·ro·leu·ke·mia (ĕ-rith′rō-lū-kē′mē-ă). Simultaneous neoplastic proliferation of erythroblastic and leukoblastic tissues.

eryth·ro·leu·ko·sis (ĕ-rith′rō-lū-kō′sis). A condition resembling leukemia in which the erythropoietic tissue is affected in addition to the leukopoietic tissue.

er·y·throl·y·sin (er-i-throl′i-sin). SYN hemolysin (1).

er·y·throl·y·sis (er-i-throl′i-sis). SYN hemolysis.

eryth·ro·mel·al·gia (ĕ-rith′rō-mel-al′jē-ă). **1.** Paroxysmal throbbing and burning pain in the skin often precipitated by exertion or heat, affecting the hands and feet, accompanied by a dusky mottled redness of the parts with increased skin temperature; may be associated with myeloproliferative disorders. **2.** A rare disorder of middle age, characterized by paroxysmal attacks of severe burning pain, reddening, hyperalgesia and sweating, involving one or more extremities, usually both feet; the attacks can be triggered by warmth, and are usually relieved by cold and limb elevation. SYN erythermalgia, Gerhardt's disease, Gerhardt-Mitchell disease, Mitchell's disease, red neuralgia, rodonalgia, Weir Mitchell's disease. [erythro- + G. *melos,* limb, + *algos,* pain]

eryth·ro·me·lia (ĕ-rith-rō-mē′lē-ă). Diffuse idiopathic erythema and atrophy of the skin of the lower limbs. [erythro- + G. *melos,* limb]

eryth·ro·my·cin (ĕ-rith-rō-mī′sin). A macrolide antibiotic agent obtained from cultures of a strain of *Streptomyces erythraeus* found in soil; it is active against *Corynebacterium diphtheriae* and several other species of *Corynebacterium,* Group A hemolytic streptococci, *Streptococcus pneumoniae,* and *Bordetella pertussis;* Gram-positive bacteria are in general more susceptible to its action than are Gram-negative bacteria, although *neisseriae* and *brucellae* are susceptible to its action. Available as the estolate, ethylcarbonate, ethylsuccinate, gluceptate, lactobionate, stearate, and salts; active against *Legionella.* Often used as a substitute antibiotic in penicillin-allergic individuals.

   e. estolate, a salt of the macrolide antibiotic, erythromycin.

   e. glucoheptonate, A salt of the macrolide antibiotic, erythromycin.

   e. propionate, A salt of the macrolide antibiotic, erythromycin.

   e. stearate, A salt of the macrolide antibiotic, erythromycin.

er·y·thron (er′i-thron). The total mass of circulating red blood cells, and that part of the hematopoietic tissue from which they are derived.

eryth·ro·ne·o·cy·to·sis (ĕ-rith′rō-nē-ō-sī-tō′sis). The presence in the peripheral circulation of regenerative forms of red blood cells. [erythrocyte + G. *neos,* new, + *kytos,* cell, + *-osis,* condition]

eryth·ro·pe·nia (ĕ-rith-rō-pē′nē-ă). Deficiency in the number of red blood cells. SYN erythrocytopenia. [erythrocyte + G. *penia,* poverty]

eryth·ro·pha·gia (ĕ-rith-rō-fā′jē-ă). Phagocytic destruction of red blood cells. [erythrocyte + G. *phagō,* to eat, + *-ia*]

eryth·ro·phag·o·cy·to·sis (ĕ-rith′rō-fag′ō-sī-tō′sis). Phagocytosis of erythrocytes.

eryth·ro·phil (ĕ-rith′rō-fil). **1.** Staining readily with red dyes. SYN erythrophilic. **2.** A cell or tissue element that stains red. [erythro- + G. *philos,* fond]

eryth·ro·phil·ic (ĕ-rith-rō-fil′ik). SYN erythrophil (1).

eryth·ro·phore (ĕ-rith′rō-fōr). A chromatophore containing granules of a red or brown pigment. SYN allophore. [erythro- + G. *phoros,* bearing]

eryth·ro·pla·kia (ĕ-rith-rō-plā′kē-ă). A red velvety plaque-like lesion of mucous membrane which often represents malignant change. [erythro- + G. *plax,* plate]

eryth·ro·pla·sia (ĕ-rith-rō-plā′zē-ă). Erythema and dysplasia of the epithelium. [erythro- + G. *plassō,* to form]

   e. of Queyrat, carcinoma *in situ* of the glans penis.

Zoon's e., SYN plasma cell *balanitis.*

eryth·ro·poi·e·sis (ĕ-rith′rō-poy-ē′sis). The formation of red blood cells. SYN erythrocytopoiesis. [erythrocyte + G. *poiēsis,* a making]

eryth·ro·poi·et·ic (ĕ-rith′rō-poy-et′ik). Pertaining to or characterized by erythropoiesis.

eryth·ro·poi·e·tin (ĕ-rith-rō-poy′ĕ-tin). A sialic acid-containing protein that enhances erythropoiesis by stimulating formation of proerythroblasts and release of reticulocytes from bone marrow; it is secreted by the kidney, and possibly by other tissues, and can be detected in human plasma and urine. SYN erythropoietic hormone (2), hematopoietin, hemopoietin.

eryth·ro·pros·o·pal·gia (ĕ-rith′rō-pros-ō-pal′jē-ă). A disorder similar to erythromelalgia, but with the pain and redness occurring in the face. [erythro- + G. *prosōpon,* face, + *algos,* pain]

eryth·rop·sia (ĕ-rith-rop′sē-ă). An abnormality of vision in which all objects appear to be tinged with red. SYN red vision. [erythro- + G. *ōps,* eye]

eryth·ro·pyk·no·sis (ĕ-rith′rō-pik-nō′sis). Alteration of red blood cells to develop the so-called "brassy bodies," under the influence of the malarial parasite. [erythro- + G. *pyknos,* dense]

er·y·thror·rhex·is (er′i-thrō-rek′sis, ĕ-rith-rō-rek′sis). SYN erythrocytorrhexis. [erythrocyte + G. *rhēxis,* rupture]

er·y·throse (ĕ-rith′rōs). An aldotetrose epimeric with threose. The D-isomer plays a role in intermediary metabolism.

e. 4-phosphate, a phosphorylated derivative of e. that serves as an important intermediate in the pentose phosphate pathway.

eryth·ro·sin B (ĕ-rith′rō-sin) [C.I. 45430]. Tetraiodofluorescein, a fluorescent red acid dye, used as a counterstain in histology and as a fluorescent indicator.

er·y·throx·y·line (er-i-throk′si-lēn). Name given to cocaine by its discoverer, Gaedeke, in 1855.

eryth·ru·lose (ĕ-rith′rū-lōs). The 2-keto analog of erythrose; the only ketotetrose.

er·y·thru·ria (er-i-thrū′rē-ă). The passage of red urine. [erythro- + G. *ouron,* urine]

Es Symbol for einsteinium.

Esbach, Georges H., French physician, 1843–1890. SEE E.'s *reagent.*

es·cape (es-kāp′). Term used to describe the situation when a higher pacemaker defaults or A-V conduction fails and a lower pacemaker assumes the function of pacemaking for one or more beats.

junctional e., e. with the A-V node as pacemaker.

ventricular e., e. with an ectopic ventricular focus as pacemaker.

es·char (es′kar). A thick, coagulated crust or slough which develops following a thermal burn or chemical or physical cauterization of the skin. [G. *eschara,* a fireplace, a scab caused by burning]

es·char·ec·to·my (es′kar-rek-tō-mē). Excision of all or part of an eschar, usually following a burn.

es·cha·rot·ic (es-kă-rot′ik). Caustic or corrosive. [G. escharōtikos]

es·cha·rot·o·my (es-kă-rot′ō-mē). Surgical incision in an eschar to lessen constriction, as might be done following a burn. [eschar + G. *tomē,* incision]

Escherich, Theodor, German physician, 1857–1911. SEE *Escherichia coli; E.'s sign.*

Esch·e·rich·ia (esh-ĕ-rik′ē-ă). A genus of aerobic, facultatively anaerobic bacteria containing short, motile or nonmotile, Gram-negative rods. Motile cells are peritrichous. Glucose and lactose are fermented with the production of acid and gas. These organisms are found in feces; some are pathogenic to man, causing enteritis, peritonitis, cystitis, etc. It is the type genus of the family Enterobacteriaceae. The type species is *E. coli.* [T. *Escherich,* German pediatrician and bacteriologist, 1857–1911]

E. co′li, a species that occurs normally in the intestines of man and other vertebrates, is widely distributed in nature, and is a frequent cause of infections of the urogenital tract and of diarrhea in infants; enteropathogenic strains (serovars) of *E. coli* cause diarrhea due to enterotoxin, the production of which seems

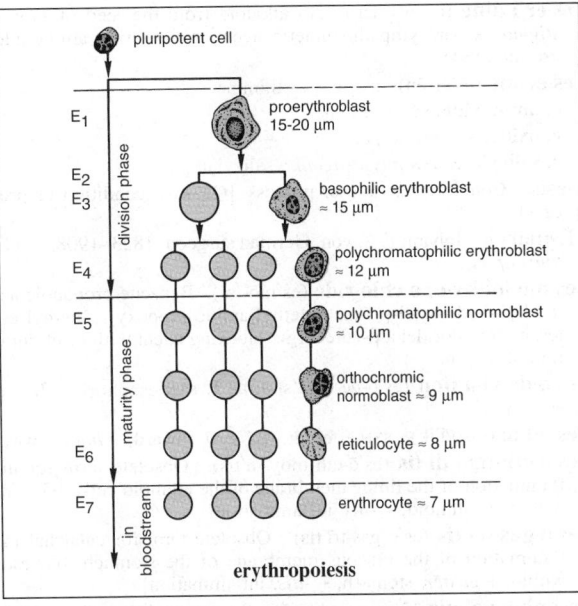

erythropoiesis

to be associated with a transferable episome; the type species of the genus. SYN colibacillus, colon bacillus.

enterohemorrhagic *E. coli* **(EHEC),** enterohemorrhagic strains of *E. coli,* usually of the serotype 0157:H7; produces a toxin resembling that produced by *Shigella;* associated with damage to the epithelium, ischemia of the bowel, and necrosis of the colon. Apparently responsible for a hemorrhagic form of colitis without fever, which can be very severe, spread primarily by contaminated beef. May also cause microangiopathic hemolytic anemia, renal failure, and the hemolytic uremic syndrome.

enteroinvasive *E. coli* **(EIEC),** enteroinvasive strain of *E. coli* penetrates gut mucosa and multiplies in colon epithelial cells, resulting in shigellosis-like changes of the mucosa. This strain produces a severe diarrheal illness that can resemble shigellosis except for the absence of vomiting and shorter duration of illness.

enteropathogenic *E. coli* **(EPEC),** enteropathogenic strain of *E. coli;* organisms adhere to small bowel mucosa and produce characteristic changes in the microvilli. This strain produces symptomatic, sometimes serious, gastrointestinal illnesses, especially severe in neonates and young children; typically it produces toxins, one of which is heat-labile, resembling that produced by *Vibrio cholerae,* the other heat-stable.

enterotoxigenic *E. coli* **(ETEC),** enterotoxigenic strain of *E. coli;* attaches to the duodenum or proximal small intestine mucosa, where it forms heat-stable and heat-labile toxins that activate adenylate cyclase, causing wasting diarrhea. Responsible for 40–70% of traveler's diarrhea; chiefly water-borne via human feces. Most important cause of diarrhea among infants living in tropical areas.

E. freun′dii, former name for *Citrobacter freundii.*

es·cor·cin, es·cor·cin·ol (es-kōr′sin, -sin-ol). A brown powder derived from esculetin, a substance derived from esculin; used for the detection of defects in the cornea and conjunctiva, which it marks by a red coloration.

es·cu·la·pi·an (es-kyū-lā′pē-ăn). SYN aesculapian.

es·cu·lent (es′kyū-lent). Edible; fit for eating. [L. *esculentus,* edible]

es·cu·lin (es′kyū-lin). bicolorin; enallachrome; esculoside; polychrome; 6,7-dihydroxycoumarin 6-glucoside; a glucoside from horse-chestnut bark; used as a sunburn protective. SYN aesculin. [L. *aesculus,* the Italian oak]

es·cutch·eon (es-kūch′ŭn). The region of the skin in quadrupeds (usually cattle) between the hind legs above the udder and below the anus; the hair in this region generally grows upward. [through O. Fr., fr. L. *scutum,* shield]

es·er·i·dine (es-er'i-dēn). An alkaloid from the seed of *Physostigma;* a parasympathomimetic agent. SYN eserine aminoxide, eserine oxide.

es·er·ine (es'er-ēn). SYN physostigmine.

e. aminoxide, SYN eseridine.

e. oxide, SYN eseridine.

e. salicylate, SYN *physostigmine* salicylate.

△**-esis.** Condition, action, or process. [G. *-esis,* condition or process]

Esmarch, Johann F.A. von, German surgeon, 1823–1908. SEE E. *tourniquet.*

es·mo·lol hy·dro·chlo·ride (es'mō-lol). Benzene propanoic acid, 4-[2-hydroxy-3-[(1-methylethyl)amino]propoxy]-, methyl ester, hydrochloride; a β-adrenergic blocking agent with brief duration of action.

es·o·de·vi·a·tion (es'ō-dē-vē-ā'shŭn). 1. SYN esophoria. 2. SYN esotropia.

es·od·ic (e-sod'ik). SYN afferent. [G. *esō,* inward, + *hodos,* way]

es·o·eth·moi·di·tis (es'ō-eth-moy-dī'tis). Obsolete term for inflammation of the lining membrane of the ethmoid cells. [G. *esō,* within, + ethmoid, + *-itis,* inflammation]

es·o·gas·tri·tis (es'ō-gas-trī'tis). Obsolete term for catarrhal inflammation of the mucous membrane of the stomach. [G. *esō,* within, + *gastēr,* stomach, + *-itis,* inflammation]

esoph·a·gal·gia (e-sof-ă-gal'jē-ă). Rarely used term for pain in the esophagus. SYN esophagodynia. [esophagus + G. *algos,* pain]

esoph·a·ge·al (ē-sof'ă-jē'ăl, ē'-sŏ-faj'ē-ăl). Relating to the esophagus.

esoph·a·gec·ta·sis, esoph·a·gec·ta·sia (ē-sof-ă-jek'tă-sis, -jek-tā'zē-ă). Dilation of the esophagus. [esophagus + G. *ektasis,* a stretching]

e·soph·a·gec·to·my (ē-sof-ă-jek'tō-mē). Excision of any part of the esophagus. [esophagus + G. *ektomē,* excision]

transhiatal e., resection of the esophagus by blunt dissection from a cervical incision from above and transhiatal approach through an abdominal incision.

transthoracic e., resection of the esophagus through a thoracotomy incision.

esoph·a·gi (ē-sof'ă-jī, -gī). Plural of esophagus.

esoph·a·gism (ē-sof'ă-jizm). Esophageal spasm causing dysphagia. SYN dysphagia nervosa, nervous dysphagia.

esoph·a·gi·tis (ē-sof-ă-jī'tis). Inflammation of the esophagus.

reflux e., peptic e., inflammation of the lower esophagus from regurgitation of acid gastric contents, usually due to malfunction of the lower esophageal sphincter; symptoms include substernal pain, heartburn, and regurgitation of acid juice.

esoph·a·go·car·di·o·plas·ty (ē-sof-ă-gō-kar'dē-ō-plas-tē). Plastic surgery of the esophagus and cardiac end of the stomach.

esoph·a·go·cele (ē-sof'ă-gō-sēl). Protrusion of the mucous membrane of the esophagus through a tear in the muscular coat. [esophagus + G. *kēlē,* hernia]

esoph·a·go·dyn·ia (ē-sof'ă-gō-din'ē-ă). SYN esophagalgia. [esophagus + G. *odynē,* pain]

esoph·a·go·en·ter·os·to·my (ē-sof'ă-gō-en-ter-os'tō-mē). Surgical formation of a direct communication between the esophagus and intestine. [esophagus + G. *enteron,* intestine, + *stoma,* mouth]

esoph·a·go·gas·trec·to·my (ē-sof'ă-gō-gas-trek'tō-mē). Removal of a portion of the lower esophagus and proximal stomach for treatment of neoplasms or strictures of those organs, especially those lesions located at or near the cardioesophageal junction.

esoph·a·go·gas·tro·a·nas·to·mo·sis (ē-sof'ă-gō-gas'trō-ă-nas-tō-mō'sis). SYN esophagogastrostomy.

esoph·a·go·gas·tro·du·o·de·nos·co·py (EGD) (ē-sof'ă-gō-gas'trō- dū'ō-den-os-kō-pē). Endoscopic examination of the esophagus, stomach and duodenum usually performed using a fiberoptic instrument.

esoph·a·go·gas·tro·my·ot·o·my (ē-sof'ă-gō-gas'trō-mī-ot'ō-mē). SYN esophagomyotomy.

esoph·a·go·gas·tro·plas·ty (ē-sof'ă-gō-gas'trō-plas-tē). SYN cardioplasty.

esoph·a·go·gas·tros·to·my (ē-sof'ă-gō-gas-tros'tō-mē). Anastomosis of esophagus to stomach, usually following esophagogastrectomy. SYN esophagogastroanastomosis, gastroesophagostomy. [esophagus + G. *gastēr,* stomach, + *stoma,* mouth]

esoph·a·go·gram (e-sof'ă-gō-gram). A roentgenogram of the esophagus.

esoph·a·gog·ra·phy (ē-sof-ă-gog'ră-fē). Radiography of the esophagus using swallowed or injected radiopaque contrast media; the technique of obtaining an esophagogram. [esophagus + G. *graphō,* to write]

esoph·a·gol·o·gy (ē-sof'ă-gol'ō-gē). Study of the structure, physiology, and diseases of the esophagus. [esophagus + G. *logos,* study]

esoph·a·go·ma·la·cia (ē-sof'ă-gō-mă-lā'shē-ă). Softening of the walls of the esophagus. [esophagus + G. *malakia,* softness]

esoph·a·go·my·co·sis (ē-sof'ă-gō-mī-kō'sis). A fungous infection of the esophagus. [esophagus + G. *mykēs,* fungus, + *-osis,* condition]

esoph·a·go·my·ot·o·my (ē-sof'ă-gō-mī-ot'ō-mē). Treatment of esophageal achalasia by longitudinal division of the lowest part of the esophageal muscle down to the submucosal layer; some muscle fibers of the cardia may also be divided. SYN cardiomyotomy, esophagogastromyotomy, Heller myotomy. [esophagus + G. *mys,* muscle, + *tomē,* incision]

esoph·a·go·plas·ty (ē-sof'ă-gō-plas-tē). Plastic surgery of the wall of the esophagus. [esophagus + G. *plastos,* formed]

esoph·a·go·pli·ca·tion (ē-sof'ă-gō-pli-kā'shŭn). Reduction in size of a dilated esophagus or of a pouch in it by making longitudinal folds or tucks in its wall. [esophagus + L. *plico,* to fold]

esoph·a·go·pto·sis, esoph·a·go·pto·sia (ē-sof'ă-gō-tō'sis, -tō'sē-ă). Relaxation and downward displacement of the walls of the esophagus. [esophagus + G. *ptōsis,* a falling]

esoph·a·go·scope (ē-sof'ă-gō-skōp). An endoscope for inspecting the interior of the esophagus. [esophagus + G. *skopeō,* to examine]

esoph·a·gos·co·py (ē-sof-ă-gos'kŏ-pē). Inspection of the interior of the esophagus by means of an endoscope. [esophagus + G. *skopeō,* to examine]

esoph·a·go·spasm (ē-sof'ă-gō-spazm). Spasm of the walls of the esophagus.

esoph·a·go·ste·no·sis (ē-sof'ă-gō-stĕ-nō'sis). Stricture or a general narrowing of the esophagus. [esophagus + G. *stenōsis,* a narrowing]

esoph·a·go·sto·mi·a·sis (ē-sof'ă-gō-stō-mī'ă-sis). SYN oesophagostomiasis. [esophagus + G. *stoma,* mouth, + *-iasis,* condition]

esoph·a·gos·to·my (ē-sof-ă-gos'tō-mē). Surgical formation of an opening directly into the esophagus from without. [esophagus + G. *stoma,* mouth]

esoph·a·got·o·my (ē-sof-ă-got'ō-mē). An incision through the wall of the esophagus. [esophagus + G. *tomē,* an incision]

esoph·a·gram (ē-sof'ă-gram). A radiographic record of contrast esophagography or barium swallow.

esoph·a·gus, pl. **esoph·a·gi** (ē-sof'ă-gŭs, -gī; -jī) [NA]. The portion of the digestive canal between the pharynx and stomach. It is about 25 cm long and consists of three parts: the cervical part, from the cricoid cartilage to the thoracic inlet; thoracic part, from thoracic inlet to the diaphragm; and abdominal part, below the diaphragm to the cardiac opening of the stomach. [G. *oisophagos,* gullet]

Barrett's e., SYN Barrett's *syndrome.*

es·o·pho·ria (es-ō-fō'rē-ă). A tendency for the eyes to turn inward, prevented by binocular vision. SYN esodeviation (1). [G. *esō,* inward, + *phora,* a carrying]

es·o·phor·ic (es-ō-fōr'ik). Relating to or marked by esophoria.

es·o·sphe·noid·i·tis (es'ō-sfē'noyd-ī'tis). Obsolete term for osteomyelitis of the sphenoid bone. [G. *esō,* within, + sphenoid, + *-itis,* inflammation]

es·o·tro·pia (es-ō-trō'pē-ă). The form of strabismus in which the visual axes converge; may be paralytic or concomitant, monocular or alternating, accommodative or nonaccommodative. SYN convergent squint, convergent strabismus, esodeviation (2), internal squint. [G. *esō,* inward, + *tropē,* turn]

A-e., convergent strabismus greater in upward than in downward gaze.

basic e., SYN nonaccommodative e.

consecutive e., e. that follows surgical correction of exotropia.

cyclic e., periodic convergent strabismus often occurring every 48 hours. SYN alternate day strabismus.

mixed e., that type of e. in which both accommodative and nonaccommodative factors are present.

nonaccommodative e., that type of e. not influenced by correction of refractive error. SYN basic e.

nonrefractive accommodative e., that type of e. in which an abnormality of the accommodative-convergence mechanism is not eliminated by correction of refractive error.

refractive accommodative e., that type of e. eliminated by correction of hypermetropic refractive error.

V-e., convergent strabismus greater in downward than in upward gaze.

X-e., decreasing convergence from the primary position in both upward and downward gaze.

es·o·tro·pic (es-ō-trop′ik). Relating to or marked by esotropia.

ESP Abbreviation for extrasensory *perception.*

es·pun·dia (es-pūn′dē-ă). A type of American leishmaniasis caused by *Leishmania braziliensis* that affects the mucous membranes, particularly in the nasal and oral region, resulting in grossly destructive changes; particularly common in Brazil where a significant proportion of persons infected with *L. braziliensis* develop this condition; may develop metastatically from sores originally found elsewhere on the body. SYN Breda's disease, bubas braziliana. [Sp., fr. L. *spongia,* sponge]

es·qui·nan·cea (es-kwi-nan′sē-ă). Sense of suffocation caused by an inflammatory swelling in the throat, as in suppurative tonsillitis or pharyngitis. [Fr. *esquinancie,* quinsy]

ESR Abbreviation for erythrocyte sedimentation *rate*; electron spin *resonance.*

es·sence (es′ens). **1.** The true characteristic or substance of a body. **2.** An element. **3.** A fluidextract. **4.** An alcoholic solution, or spirit, of the volatile oil of a plant. **5.** Any volatile substance responsible for odor or taste of the organism (usually a plant) producing it; by extension, synthetic perfumes or flavors. [L. *essentia,* fr. *esse,* to be]

essence of rose, SYN *oil* of rose.

es·sen·tial (ĕ-sen′shăl). **1.** Necessary, indispensable, (*e.g.,* e. amino acids, e. fatty acids). **2.** Characteristic of. **3.** Determining. **4.** Of unknown etiology. **5.** Relating to an essence (*e.g.,* e. oil). **6.** SYN intrinsic.

Esser, Johannes F.S., Dutch surgeon, 1877–1946. SEE E. *graft, operation.*

Essick, C., 20th century U.S. anatomist. SEE E.'s cell *bands,* under *band.*

Essig splint. See under splint.

es·taz·o·lam (ĕs-taz′-ō-lam). A benzodiazepine compound with sedative/hypnotic properties.

es·ter (es′ter). An organic compound containing the grouping, –X(O)–O–R (X = carbon, sulfur, phosphorus, etc.; R = radical of an alcohol), formed by the elimination of H_2O between the –OH of an acid group and the –OH of an alcohol group; usually written as in ethyl acetate (from acetic acid and ethyl alcohol), $CH_3CO—OC_2H_5$ or $CH_3COOC_2H_5$.

carboxylic acid e., specifically, an e. derived from a carboxylic acid and an alcohol; R–CO–R′.

Cori e., SYN D-glucose 1-phosphate.

Embden e., hexose phosphate; a mixture of D-glucose 6-phosphate and D-fructose 6-phosphate; significant in the understanding of sugar metabolism.

Harden-Young e., D-fructose 1,6-bisphosphate; important intermediate in sugar metabolism.

Neuberg e., SYN fructose 6-phosphate.

Robison e., SYN D-glucose 6-phosphate.

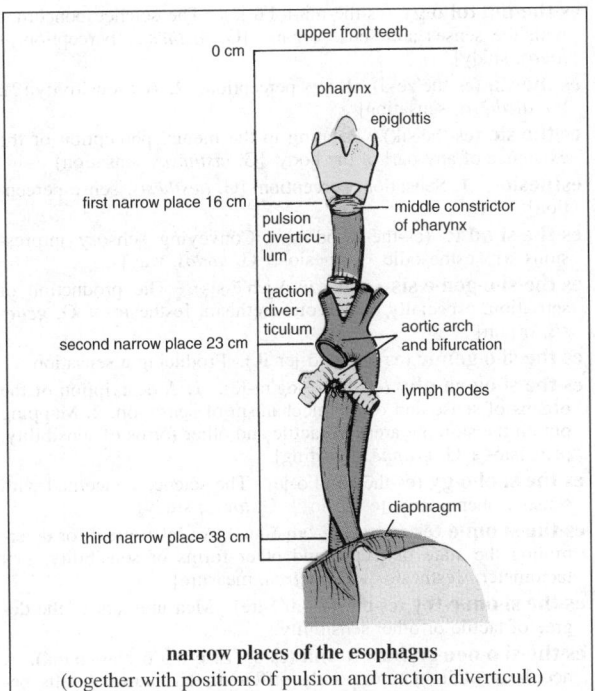

narrow places of the esophagus
(together with positions of pulsion and traction diverticula)

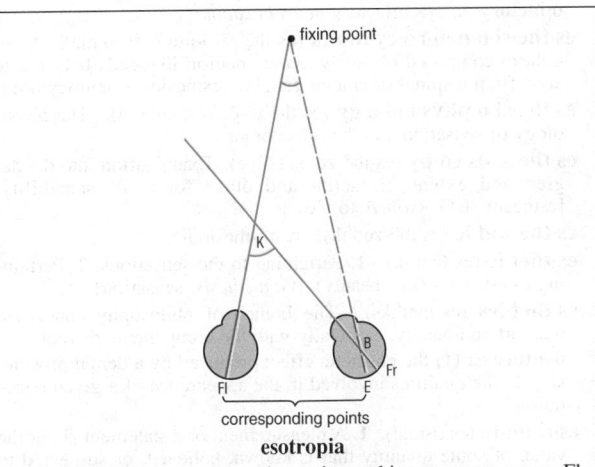

esotropia
anomalous retinal correspondence in strabismus convergens; Fl, foveola of the fixing eye; Fr, foveola of the deviating eye; E, extrafoveolar point of deviating eye corresponding to Fl; angle FlKFr, objective angle of deviation; angle FlAE, subjective angle of deviation; angle EBFr, angle of anomaly (difference between objective and subjective angle of deviation)

Robison-Embden e., SYN D-glucose 6-phosphate.

sugar e., e. of a sugar with an organic or inorganic acid; *e.g.,* D-glucose 6-phosphate.

thiol e., an e. formed from a carboxylic acid and a thiol (*i.e.,* RCO-SR′) *e.g.,* acetyl-coenzyme A.

es·ter·ase (es′ter-ās). A generic term for enzymes (EC class 3.1, hydrolases) that catalyze the hydrolysis of esters.

C1 e., the activated first component of complement (C1).

es·ter·i·fi·ca·tion (es′ter′i-fi-kā′shŭn). The process of forming an ester, as in the reaction of ethanol and acetic acid to form ethyl acetate.

Estes, William L., Jr., U.S. surgeon, 1885–1940. SEE E. *operation.*

es·the·ma·tol·o·gy (es-thē-mă-tol′ō-jē). The science concerned with the senses and sense organs. [G. *aisthēma*, perception, + *logos*, study]

es·the·sia (es-thē′zē-ă). **1.** SYN perception. **2.** SYN sensitivity (2). [G. *aisthēsis*, sensation]

es·the·sic (es-thē′sik). Relating to the mental perception of the existence of any part of the body. [G. *aisthēsis*, sensation]

♻**esthesio-.** **1.** Sensation, perception. [G. *aesthēsis*, sense perception]

es·the·si·od·ic (es-thē-zē-od′ik). Conveying sensory impressions. SYN esthesodic. [esthesio- + G. *hodos*, way]

es·the·si·o·gen·e·sis (es-thē′zē-ō-jen′ĕ-sis). The production of sensation, especially of nervous erethism. [esthesio- + G. *genesis*, origin]

es·the·si·o·gen·ic (es-thē-zē-ō-jen′ik). Producing a sensation.

es·the·si·og·ra·phy (es-thē-zē-og′ră-fē). **1.** A description of the organs of sense and of the mechanism of sensation. **2.** Mapping out on the skin the areas of tactile and other forms of sensibility. [esthesio- + G. *graphē*, a writing]

es·the·si·ol·o·gy (es-thē-zē-ol′ō-jē). The science concerned with sensory phenomena. [esthesio- + G. *logos*, study]

es·the·si·om·e·ter (es-thē-zē-om′ĕ-ter). An instrument for determining the state of tactile and other forms of sensibility. SYN tactometer. [esthesio- + G. *metron*, measure]

es·the·si·om·e·try (es-thē-zē-om′ĕ-trē). Measurement of the degree of tactile or other sensibility.

es·the·si·o·neu·ro·blas·to·ma (es-thē′zē-ō-nūr′ō-blas-tō′mă). A neoplasm of immature, poorly differentiated neuronal cells believed to arise from neuroepithelial elements. [esthesio- + neuroblastoma]

olfactory e., SYN olfactory *neuroblastoma.*

es·the·si·o·neu·ro·cy·to·ma (es-thē′zē-ō-nur′ō-sī-tō′mă). A neoplasm composed of nearly mature neuron-like cells believed to arise from a spinal or cranial ganglia. [esthesio- + neurocytoma]

es·the·si·o·phys·i·ol·o·gy (es-thē′zē-ō-fiz-ē-ol′ō-jē). The physiology of sensation and the sense organs.

es·the·si·os·co·py (es-thē-zē-os′kŏ-pē). Examination into the degree and extent of tactile and other forms of sensibility. [esthesio- + G. *skopeō*, to view]

es·the·sod·ic (es′thē-zod′ik). SYN esthesiodic.

es·thet·ic (es-thet′ik). **1.** Pertaining to the sensations. **2.** Pertaining to esthetics (*i.e.,* beauty). [G. *aisthēsis*, sensation]

es·thet·ics (es-thet′iks). The branch of philosophy concerned with art and beauty, especially with the components thereof.

denture e., **(1)** the cosmetic effect produced by a dental prosthesis; **(2)** the qualities involved in the appearance of a given restoration.

es·ti·mate (es′tĭ-māt). **1.** A measurement or a statement about the value of some quantity that is known, believed, or suspected to incorporate some degree of error. **2.** The result of applying any estimator to a random sample of data. It is not a random variable but a realization of one, a fixed quantity, and it has no variance although commonly it also furnishes an estimate of what the variance of the estimator is. (Not to be confused with an estimator, which is a prescription for obtaining an estimate.) [L. *aestimo*, pp. *aestimatum*, to appraise]

es·ti·ma·tion (es-tĭ-mā-shun). Any non-trivial statistical procedure that assigns to an unknown quantity (parameter) a plausible value on the basis of appropriate and pertinent data collected in a proper random sample.

es·ti·ma·tor (es′tĭ-mā-tor). A prescription for obtaining an estimate from a random sample of data. An e. is a procedure, not a result, and therefore is a random variable and has a variance. For instance an e. of the mean weight in adult men may consist of the prescription "Add up the weights of 100 men and divide by 100." The actual outcome (the estimate) will vary from sample to sample, but one answer will not be a random variable.

least squares e., the prescription "Assign to the unknown parameter the value that minimizes the mean of the squares of the residual errors".

maximum likelihood e., the prescription "Assign to the un-

known parameter that value that maximizes the likelihood for the sample". For many problems this procedure is an optimal one.

es·ti·val (es′ti-văl). Relating to or occurring in the summer. SYN aestival. [L. *aestivus,* summer (adj.)]

es·ti·va·tion (es-ti-vā′shŭn). Living through the summer in a quiescent, torpid state. Cf. hibernation.

es·ti·vo·au·tum·nal (es′ti-vō-aw-tŭm′năl). Relating to or occurring in summer and autumn. [L. *aestivus,* summer (adj.), + *autumnalis,* autumnal]

Estlander, Jakob A., Finnish surgeon, 1831–1881. SEE E. *flap, operation.*

es·tra·di·ol (E₂) (es-tră-dī′ol). β-estradiol; 17β-estradiol; 1,3,5(10)-estratriene-3,17β-diol; the most potent naturally occurring estrogen in mammals, formed by the ovary, placenta, testis, and possibly the adrenal cortex; therapeutic indications for e. are those typical of an estrogen. α-Estradiol, (17α-estradiol), exhibits considerably less biologic activity. E. is used in the treatment of menstrual disorders, menopause problems, etc. SYN estrogenic hormone, oestradiol.

e. benzoate, fatty acid esters of 17β-estradiol usually dissolved in oil for injection purposes; such esters exhibit a longer duration of action than does the unesterified steroid.

e. cypionate, has the same actions and uses as e. but a prolonged duration of action; administered in oil by intramuscular injection.

e. dipropionate, an esterified natural estrogen for parenteral use.

ethinyl e., SYN ethynyl e.

ethynyl e., 17α-ethynyl-1,3,5-estratriene-3,17-diol; a semisynthetic derivative of 17β-estradiol; active by mouth, with a long half-life, it is among the most potent of known estrogenic compounds; used in oral contraceptive preparations. SYN ethinyl e.

e. undecylate, an esterified natural estrogen for parenteral use.

e. valerate, estra-1,3,5(10)-triene-3,17β-diol 17-valerate; same actions and uses as e., but with a prolonged duration of action; administered in sesame oil by intramuscular injection.

es·tra·gon oil (es′tră-gon). SYN tarragon oil.

es·tra·mus·tine phos·phate so·di·um (es-tră-mŭs′tēn). Estra-1,3,5(10)-triene-3,17-diol(17β)-, 3-[bis(2-chloroethyl)carbamate] 17-(dihydrogen phosphate), disodium salt; an antineoplastic agent that combines the actions of estrogen and nitrogen mustard in the treatment of carcinoma of the prostate.

es·trane (es′trān). Hypothetical parent hydrocarbon of the (steroid) estrogenic compounds whose names begin with "estr-" (estradiol, estrone, estriol); conceived to establish a systematic nomenclature.

es·tra·tri·ene (es-tră-trī′ēn). 1,3,5(10)-Estratriene; the hypothetical triply-unsaturated estrane that is the nucleus of most naturally occurring estrogenic steroids in animals.

es·trin (es′trin). SYN estrogen.

es·tri·ol (es′trē-ol). estra-1,3,5(10)-triene-3,16α,17β-triol; an estrogenic metabolite of estradiol, usually the predominant estrogenic metabolite found in urine (especially during pregnancy); epimers at C-16, C-17, or both are known as 16-epiestriol, etc. SYN folliculin hydrate, oestriol, trihydroxyestrin.

es·tro·die·nol (es-trō-dē′nol). SYN dienestrol.

es·tro·gen (es′trō-jen). Generic term for any substance, natural or synthetic, that exerts biological effects characteristic of estrogenic hormones such as estradiol. E.'s are formed by the ovary, placenta, testes, and possibly the adrenal cortex, as well as by certain plants; stimulate secondary sexual characteristics, and exert systemic effects, such as growth and maturation of long bones; and are used therapeutically in any disorder attributable to e. deficiency or amenable to e. therapy, such as menstrual disorders and menopausal problems. They control the course of the menstrual cycle. Used in certain treatments of coronary disorders in women. SYN estrin, oestrogen. [G. *oistrus*, estrus, + *-gen*, producing]

catechol e., any 2-hydroxylated derivative of an e.; they, with their methylated derivatives, can account for up to one-half of all excreted e. metabolites.

conjugated e., an amorphous preparation of naturally occurring, water-soluble, conjugated forms of mixed e.'s obtained from the urine of pregnant mares; the principal e. present is sodium es-

e. oxide, a fumigant, used for sterilizing surgical instruments. SYN oxirane.

e. tetrachloride, SYN tetrachlorethylene.

eth·yl·ene·di·a·mine (eth'i-lēn-dī'ă-mēn). $H_2N(CH_2)_2NH_2$; a volatile colorless liquid of ammoniacal odor and caustic taste; the dihydrochloride is used as a urinary acidifier. SYN ethanediamine.

eth·yl·ene·di·a·mine·tet·ra·a·ce·tic ac·id (EDTA) (eth'il-ēn-dī'ă-mēn-tet-ră-ă-sē'tik). $(HOOC–CH_2)_2N(CH_2)_2N(CH_2–COOH)_2$; a chelating agent used to remove multivalent cations from solution as chelates, and used in biochemical research to remove Mg^{2+}, Fe^{2+}, etc., from reactions affected by such ions. As the sodium salt, used as a water softener, to stabilize drugs rapidly decomposed in the presence of traces of metal ions, and as an anticoagulant; as the sodium calcium salt, used to remove radium, lead, strontium, plutonium, and cadmium from the skeleton, forming stable un-ionized soluble compounds that are excreted by the kidneys. Cf. EGTA. SYN edathamil, edetic acid.

eth·yl·ene di·bro·mide. Compound used in antiknock gasolines. Severe skin irritant; may cause blistering. Inhalation causes delayed pulmonary lesions. Prolonged exposure may also result in liver and kidney injury. May be a human carcinogen.

eth·yl·ene gly·col. SEE glycol (2).

eth·yl·es·tre·nol (eth-il-es'tre-nol). 17α-Ethyl-4-estren-17β-ol; a semisynthetic orally effective anabolic steroid.

eth·yl ether. SYN diethyl ether.

eth·yl green. SYN brilliant green.

eth·yl·i·dene (eth-il-i'-dēn). The radical $CH_3CH=$. SYN ethidene.

eth·yl·i·dyne (eth-il-i'-dīn). The radical $CH_3C\equiv$.

eth·yl·mor·phine hy·dro·chlo·ride (eth-il-mōr'fēn). The ethyl ether of morphine; an antispasmodic, antitussive, and analgesic, used locally as an irritant lymphagogue in chronic catarrhal middle ear disease, atrophic rhinitis, and painful ocular diseases (iritis, corneal ulcer, etc.).

eth·yl·nor·ep·i·neph·rine (E.N.E., E.N.S.) (eth'il-nōr-ep-i-nef'rin). α-(1-Aminopropyl)-3,4-dihydroxybenzyl alcohol; a sympathomimetic, used in asthma; it does not raise the blood pressure.

eth·yl·pa·pav·er·ine hy·dro·chlo·ride (eth'il-pa-pav'er-ēn). SYN ethaverine hydrochloride.

eth·yl·par·a·ben (eth-il-par'ă-ben). Ethyl *p*-hydroxybenzoate; an antifungal preservative.

eth·yl·phen·ac·e·mide (eth-il-fen-as'ĕ-mīd). (2-Phenylbutyryl)-urea; an anticonvulsant.

eth·yl·phen·yl·eph·rine hy·dro·chlo·ride (eth'il-fen-il-ef'rēn). SYN etilefrine hydrochloride.

eth·yl·stib·a·mine (eth-il-stib'ă-mēn). A synthetic organic compound of antimony. SYN Fourneau 693.

ethy·no·di·ol (ĕ-thī-nō-dī'ōl). 17α-Ethynyl-4-estrene-3β, 17β-diol; a semisynthetic orally effective steroid with biological effects that largely resemble those of progesterone; in addition, it is weakly estrogenic and androgenic; administered in combination with an estrogen as an oral contraceptive.

e. diacetate, 3,17-diacetate of ethynodiol; an antifertility agent, usually used in combination with mestranol.

ethy·nyl (e-thī'nil). The monovalent radical $HC\equiv C–$. SYN acetenyl, ethinyl.

eti·do·caine (e-tī'dō-kān). $(\pm)$-2-(Ethylpropylamino)-2',6'-butyroxylidide; a local anesthetic.

eti·dro·nate di·so·di·um (e-ti-drō'nāt). Phosphoric acid, (1-hydroxyethylidene)-bis-, disodium salt; a drug that affects bone resorption, used in the treatment of Paget's disease, heterotopic ossification, and hypercalcemia of malignancy.

eti·dron·ic ac·id (e-ti-dron'ik). (1-Hydroxyethylidene)bis-(phosphonic acid); used as a calcium regulator, usually as the salt etidronate disodium.

et·il·ef·rine hy·dro·chlo·ride (et-il-ef'rin). A sympathomimetic amine vasopressor agent. SYN ethylphenylephrine hydrochloride.

⌂**etio-.** **1.** Prefix used with (for example) cholane to indicate replacement of the C-17 side chain by H; thus, etiocholane is the

5β isomer of androstane. **2.** Combining form meaning cause. [G. *aitia,* cause]

eti·o·cho·lan·o·lone (ē'tē-ō-kō-lan'ō-lōn). 3α-Hydroxy-5β-androstan-17-one; a metabolite of adrenocortical and testicular hormones, and an important urinary 17-ketosteroid; produces fever when given to human beings.

eti·o·gen·ic (ē'tē-ō-jen'ik). Of a causal nature. [G. *aitia,* cause, + *genesis,* production]

eti·o·lat·ed (ē'tē-ō-lāt-ed). Subjected to, or characterized by, etiolation.

eti·o·la·tion (ē-tē-ō-lā'shŭn). **1.** Paleness or pallor resulting from absence of light, as in persons confined because of illness or imprisonment, or in plants bleached by being deprived of light. **2.** The process of blanching, bleaching, or making pale by withholding light. [Fr. *étioler,* to blanch]

eti·o·log·ic (ē'tē-ō-loj'ik). Relating to etiology.

eti·ol·o·gy (ē-tē-ol'ō-jē). **1.** The science and study of the causes of disease and their mode of operation. Cf. pathogenesis. **2.** The science of causes, causality; in common usage, cause. [G. *aitia,* cause, + *logos,* treatise, discourse]

eti·o·path·ic (ē'tē-ō-path'ik). Relating to specific lesions concerned with the cause of a disease. [G. *aitia,* cause, + *pathos,* disease]

eti·o·pa·thol·o·gy (ē'tē-ō-pa-thol'ō-jē). Consideration of the cause of an abnormal state or finding. [G. *aitia,* cause, + pathology]

eti·o·por·phy·rin (ē'tē-ō-pōr'fi-rin). A porphyrin derivative characterized by the presence on each of the four pyrrole rings of one methyl group and one ethyl group; four isomeric forms are thus possible.

eti·o·tro·pic (ē'tē-ō-trop'ik). Directed against the cause; denoting a remedy that attenuates or destroys the causal factor of a disease. [G. *aitia,* cause, + *tropē,* a turning]

eto·fam·ide (ē-tō'fă-mīd). An intraluminal amebicide similar to teclozan and diloxanide.

etom·i·date (ē-tom'i-dāt). R-(+)-1-(α-Methylbenzyl)imidazole-5-carboxylate; a potent intravenous depressant.

eto·po·side (e-tō-pō'sīd). 4'-Demethylpipodophyllotoxin 9-[4,6-O-(R)-ethylidene-β-D-glucopyranoside]; a semisynthetic derivative of podophyllotoxin; a mitotic inhibitor used in the treatment of refractory testicular tumors and small cell lung cancer.

etor·phine (et-ōr'fēn). Tetrahydro-7α-(1-hydroxy-1-methylbutyl)-6,14-*endo*-ethenooripavine; a narcotic analgesic.

et·o·zo·lin (et-ō-zō'lin). 3-Methyl-4-oxo-5-piperidino-$\Delta^{2,\alpha}$-thiazolidineacetic acid ethyl ester; a diuretic.

ETP Abbreviation for electron transport *particles,* under *particle.*

etret·i·nate (e-tret'i-nāt). 2,4,6,8-Nonatetraenoic acid; a retinoid used in the treatment of severe recalcitrant psoriasis.

et·y·mem·a·zine (et-i-mem'ă-zēn). 10-(3-dimethylamino-2-methylpropyl)-2-ethylphenothiazine; an antihistaminic. SYN ethotrimeprazine.

Eu Symbol for europium.

⌂**eu-.** Good, well; opposite of dys-, caco-. [G.]

eu·al·leles (yū'ă-lēlz). Genes having different nucleotide substitutions at the same position. Cf. heteroalleles.

Eu·bac·te·ri·a·les (yū'bak-tē-rē-ā'lēz). An obsolete name for an order of bacteria which contained simple, undifferentiated, rigid cells which were either spheres or straight rods. It contained motile (peritrichous) and nonmotile, Gram-negative and Gram-positive, and sporeforming and nonsporeforming species. The order contained 13 families: Achromobacteriaceae, Azotobacteriaceae, Bacillaceae, Bacteroidaceae, Brevibacteriaceae, Brucellaceae, Corynebacteriaceae, Enterobacteriaceae, Lactobacillaceae, Micrococcaceae, Neisseriaceae, Propionibacteriaceae, and Rhizobacteriaceae.

Eu·bac·te·ri·um (yū'bak-tēr'ē-ŭm). A genus of anaerobic, nonsporeforming, nonmotile bacteria containing straight or curved Gram-positive rods which usually occur singly, in pairs, or in short chains. Usually these organisms attack carbohydrates. They may be pathogenic. Rarely associated with intraabdominal sepsis in humans. The type species is *E. limosum.*

Eu

E. aerofa′ciens, a species infrequently found in human intestines; pathogenic for mice.

E. bifor′me, a species that occurs infrequently in human intestines; pathogenic for rabbits but not for mice.

E. combe′si, a species from forest soil found in an area then called French West Africa; it is not pathogenic for guinea pigs or mice. Formerly called *Cillobacterium combesi.*

E. contor′tum, a species found in cases of putrid, gangrenous appendicitis and in the intestines.

E. crispa′tum, former name for *Lactobacillus crispatus.*

E. discifor′mans, a species found in cases of fetid suppurations in empyema, pulmonary gangrene, liver abscess, and dermatosis; occurs commonly in the respiratory system, the liver, and the skin; pathogenic for man, rabbits, guinea pigs, and mice.

E. ethyl′icum, a species found in a case of gastritis; occurs infrequently in the human stomach.

E. filamento′sum, former name for *Clostridium ramosum.*

E. len′tum, a species occurring commonly in the feces of normal persons.

E. limo′sum, a species that occurs in human feces and presumably in the feces of other warm-blooded animals. The type species of the genus.

E. minu′tum, a species that occurs infrequently in the intestines of breast-fed infants; it was originally found in a case of infant diarrhea; it is pathogenic for mice.

E. monilifor′me, a species found rarely in the human respiratory system; it is pathogenic for guinea pigs, causing death in eight days. Formerly called *Cillobacterium moniliforme.*

E. multifor′me, a species isolated from the feces of a dog and from soil from equatorial Africa; it is not pathogenic for guinea pigs. Formerly called *Cillobacterium multiforme.*

E. nio′sii, a species that occurs in the respiratory tract; pathogenic for rabbits and guinea pigs.

E. par′vum, a species found in the large intestine of a horse and in a case of acute appendicitis; it occurs infrequently in the intestines of foals and of humans, and is not pathogenic for laboratory animals.

E. plau′ti, SYN *Fusobacterium plauti.*

E. poeciloi′des, a species infrequently found in human intestines; originally found in a case of intestinal occlusion; it is pathogenic for guinea pigs and rabbits.

E. pseudotortuo′sum, a species found in a case of purulent, acute appendicitis; occurs uncommonly in the intestines.

E. quar′tum, a species found in cases of infantile diarrhea; occurs in the intestines of children, but is rather uncommon.

E. quin′tum, a species found in cases of infantile diarrhea; pathogenic for guinea pigs.

E. recta′le, a species found in association with a rectal ulcer; occurs in the rectum.

E. ten′ue, a species isolated from dog feces; its pathogenicity is unknown; formerly called *Cillobacterium tenue.*

E. tortuo′sum, a species found infrequently in the intestines of humans.

eu·bi·ot·ics (yū-bī-ot′iks). The science of hygienic living. [eu- + G. *biotikos,* relating to life]

eu·bo·lism (yū′bō-lizm). Obsolete word for normal body metabolism.

eu·caine (yū′kān). β-Eucaine; 2,2,6-trimethyl-4-piperidinol benzoate; a local anesthetic.

eu·ca·lyp·tol (yū-kă-lip′tol). SYN cineole.

eu·ca·lyp·tus (yū-kă-lip′tŭs). The dried leaves of *Eucalyptus globulus* (family Myrtaceae), the blue gum or Australian fever tree.

e. oil, the volatile oil distilled with steam from the fresh leaf of *Eucalyptus globulus* or some other species of *Eucalyptus;* contains not less than 70% of eucalyptol; used as an antiseptic and expectorant.

eu·cap·nia (yū-kap′nē-ă). A state in which the arterial carbon dioxide pressure is optimal. SEE ALSO normocapnia. [eu- + G. *kapnos,* vapor]

eu·car·y·ote (yū-kar′ē-ōt). SYN eukaryote. [eu- + G. *karyon,* kernel, nut]

eu·car·y·ot·ic (yū-kar-ē-ot′ik). SYN eukaryotic.

eu·ca·sin (yū-kā′sin). Ammonium caseinate prepared by passing ammonia gas over finely powdered dry casein; added as a concentrated food to bouillon, chocolate, etc.

eu·cat·ro·pine hy·dro·chlo·ride (yū-kat′rō-pēn). 1,2,2,6-Tetramethyl-4-piperidinol mandelate hydrochloride; a mydriatic; it produces no anesthesia, pain, or increased intraocular pressure.

Eu·ces·to·da (yū-ses-tō′dă). SYN Cestoda.

eu·chlor·hy·dria (yū-klōr-hi′drē-ă). A condition in which free hydrochloric acid exists in normal amount in the gastric juice. [eu- + cholohydric (acid) + -ia]

eu·cho·lia (yū-kō′lē-ă). A normal state of the bile as regards quantity and quality. [eu- + G. *cholē,* bile]

eu·chro·mat·ic (yū-krō-mat′ik). **1.** SYN orthochromatic. **2.** Characteristic of euchromatin.

eu·chro·ma·tin (yū-krō′mă-tin). The parts of chromosomes that, during interphase, are uncoiled dispersed threads and not stained by ordinary dyes; metabolically active, in contrast to the inert heterochromatin.

eu·chro·mo·some (yū-krō′mō-sōm). SYN autosome.

eu·cor·ti·cal·ism (yū-kōr′ti-kăl-izm). Normal functioning of the adrenal cortex.

eu·cra·sia (yū-krā′zhē-ă). **1.** Obsolete term for homeostasis. **2.** Obsolete term for a condition of reduced susceptibility to the adverse effects of certain drugs, articles of diet, etc. [G. *eukrasia,* good temperament, fr. *eu,* well, + *krasis,* a mixing]

eu·cu·pine (yū′kū-pēn). SYN euprocin hydrochloride.

eu·de·mo·nia (yū-dĕ-mō′nē-ă). A feeling of well-being or happiness. [eu- + G. *daimon,* destiny]

eu·di·a·pho·re·sis (yū-dī′ă-fō-rē′sis). Normal free sweating. [eu- + G. *diaphorēsis,* perspiration]

eu·dip·sia (yū-dip′sē-ă). Ordinary mild thirst. [eu- + G. *dipsa,* thirst]

Eu·flag·el·la·ta (yū-flaj′ĕ-lā′tă). Former term for the protozoan flagellates now included in the subphylum Mastigophora.

eu·gen·ic (yū-jen′ik). Relating to eugenics.

eu·gen·ic ac·id. SYN eugenol.

eu·gen·ics (yū-jen′iks). Practices and policies, as of mate selection or of sterilization, that tend to better the innate qualities of progeny and human stock. **2.** Practices and genetic counseling directed to anticipating genetic disability and disease. SYN orthogenics. [G. *eugeneia,* nobility of birth, fr. *eu,* well, + *genesis,* production]

eu·gen·ism (yū′jen-izm). "The aggregate of the most favorable conditions for healthy and happy existence" (Galton).

eu·ge·nol (yū′je-nol). 4-allyl-2-methoxyphenol; obtained from oil of cloves; used in dentistry with zinc oxide as an analgesic and as a base for impression materials; also used in perfumery as a substitute for oil of cloves. SYN eugenic acid.

Eu·gle·na (yū-glē′nă). A widespread genus of photosynthesizing free-living fresh water flagellates (family Euglinidae). [eu- + G. *glēnē,* eyeball]

E. grac′ilis, an abundant species sometimes used in assaying vitamin B_{12} concentrations of serum and urine in various types of anemia.

E. vir′idis, a species that inhabits stagnant pools, often in great numbers.

Eu·gle·ni·dae (yū-glē′ni-dē). A family of green (phytomonad) flagellates (subphylum Mastigophora, class Phytomastigophorea).

eu·glob·u·lin (yū-glob′yū-lin). That fraction of the serum globulin less soluble in $(NH_4)_2SO_4$ solution than the pseudoglobulin fraction.

eu·gly·ce·mia (yū-glī-sē′mē-ă). A normal blood glucose concentration. SYN normoglycemia. [eu- + G. *glykys,* sweet, + *haima,* blood]

eu·gly·ce·mic (yū-glī-sē′mik). Denoting, characteristic of, or promoting euglycemia. SYN normoglycemic.

eu·gna·thia (yū-nā'thē-ă, -nath'ē-ă). An abnormality that is limited to the teeth and their immediate alveolar supports. SYN eugnathic anomaly. [eu- + G. *gnathos,* jaw]

eu·gno·sia (yū-nō'sē-ă). Normal ability to synthesize sensory stimuli. [eu- + G. *gnōsis,* perception]

eu·gon·ic (yū-gon'ik). A term used to indicate that the growth of a bacterial culture is rapid and relatively luxuriant; used especially in reference to the growth of cultures of the human tubercle bacillus (*Mycobacterium tuberculosis*). SEE ALSO dysgonic. [G. *eugonos,* productive, fr. *eu,* well, + *gonos,* seed, offspring]

Eu·gre·ga·rin·i·da (yū'greg-ă-rin'i-dă). An order of gregarines (subclass Gregarinia), reproducing only by sporogony, in which schizogony is absent; they are parasites of annelids and arthropods. [eu- + L. *gregarius,* gregarious]

eu·hy·dra·tion (yū-hī-drā'shŭn). Normal state of body water content; absence of absolute or relative hydration or dehydration.

Eu·kar·y·o·tae, Eu·car·y·o·tae (yū-kar-ē-ō'tē). A superkingdom of organisms characterized by eukaryotic cells; acellular members (kingdom Protoctista) are characterized by a single eukaryotic unit; more complex (multicellular) members have been assigned to the kingdoms Fungi, Plantae, and Animalia.

eu·kar·y·ote (yū-kar'ē-ōt). **1.** A cell containing a membrane-bound nucleus with chromosomes of DNA, RNA, and proteins, mostly large (10-100 μm), with cell division involving a form of mitosis in which mitotic spindles (or some microtubule arrangement) are involved; mitochondria are present, and, in photosynthetic species, plastids are found; undulipodia (cilia or flagella) are of the complex 9+2 organization of tubulin and various proteins. Possession of a e. type of cell characterizes the four kingdoms above the Monera or prokaryote level of complexity: Protoctista, Fungi, Plantae, and Animalia, combined into the superkingdom Eukaryotae. **2.** Common name for members of the Eukaryotae. SYN eucaryote. [eu- + G. *karyon,* kernel, nut]

eu·kar·y·ot·ic (yū'kar-ē-ot'ik). Pertaining to or characteristic of a eukaryote. SYN eucaryotic.

eu·ker·a·tin (yū-kār'ă-tin). Hard keratin present in hair, wool, horn, nails, etc.

eu·ki·ne·sia (yū-ki-nē'zē-ă). Normal movement. [eu- + G. *kinesis,* movement]

Eulenburg, Albert, German neurologist, 1840–1917. SEE E.'s disease.

eu·mel·a·nin (yū-mel'ă-nin). The most abundant type of human melanin, found in brown and black skin and hair; cross-linked polymers of 5,6-dihydroxyindoles, usually linked to proteins; levels are decreased in certain types of albinism. [eu- + G. *melos* (*melan-*), black]

eu·mel·a·no·some (yū-mel'ă-nō-sōm). SYN melanosome.

eu·me·tria (yū-mē'trē-ă). Graduation of the strength of nerve impulses to match the need. [G. moderation, goodness of meter]

eu·mor·phism (yū-mōr'fizm). Preservation of the natural form of a cell. [eu- + G. *morphē,* shape]

eu·my·cetes (yū-mī-sē'tēz). The true fungi. [eu- + G. *mykēs,* fungus]

Eu·my·ce·to·zo·ea (yū'mī-sē-tō-zō'ē-ă). Microscopic animal forms, frequently known as slime animals, that consist of an irregular semifluid mass of multinucleated ameboid protoplasm; although grouped as a class of the superclass Rhizopoda (subphylum Sarcodina), some of the mycetozoan forms closely resemble certain species of pseudomycetes and are sometimes classified as members of the Myxomycetes, the slime molds. SEE ALSO Proteomyxidia. [eu- + G. *mykēs* (*mykēt-*), fungus, + *zōon,* animal]

eu·noia (yū-noy'ă). Rarely used term denoting a normal mental state. [G. goodwill, fr. *eu,* well, + *nous,* mind]

eu·nuch (yū'nŭk). A male individual whose testes have been removed or have never developed. [G. *eunouchos,* chamberlain, fr. *eunē,* bed, + *echein,* to have]

eu·nuch·ism (yū'nŭk-izm). **1.** The state of being a eunuch; absence of the testes or failure of the gonads to develop or function with consequent lack of reproductive and sexual function and of development of secondary sex characteristics. **2.** SYN eunuchoidism.

eu·nuch·oid (yū'nŭ-koyd). Resembling, or having the general characteristics of, a eunuch; usually indicating the physical habitus of a male in whom hypogonadism occurred before puberty. [G. *eunouchos,* eunuch, + *eidos,* resembling]

eu·nuch·oid·ism (yū'nŭ-koyd-izm). A state in which testes are present but fail to function normally; may be of gonadal or pituitary origin. SYN eunuchism (2), male hypogonadism.

  hypergonadotropic e., e. of gonadal origin, commonly accompanied by enhanced levels of pituitary gonadotropins in the blood and urine, as in Klinefelter's *syndrome.*

  hypogonadotropic e., SYN hypogonadotropic *hypogonadism.*

eu·os·mia (yū-oz'mē-ă). **1.** A pleasant odor. **2.** Normal olfaction. [eu- + G. *osmē,* smell]

eu·pan·cre·a·tism (yū-pan'krē-ă-tizm). The state of normal pancreatic digestive function.

eu·pa·ral (yū'pa-răl). A medium for mounting histologic specimens, composed of sandarac, eucalyptol, paraldehyde, camphor, and phenyl salicylate.

Eu·pa·ryph·i·um (yū-pa-rif'ē-ŭm). A genus of nonpathogenic flukes (family Echinostomatidae), several species of which have been reported from the intestines of humans. [eu- + G. *paryphē,* a border]

eu·pav·er·in (yū-pav'ē-rin). 1-Benzyl-3-ethyl-6,7-dimethoxyisoquinoline; a smooth muscle relaxant.

eu·pep·sia (yū-pep'sē-ă). Good digestion. [G., fr. *eu,* well, + *pepsis,* digestion]

eu·pep·tic (yū-pep'tik). Digesting well; having a good digestion.

eu·pep·tide (yū-pep'tīd). A peptide containing normal peptide bonds (between α-carboxyl groups and α-amino groups). Cf. isopeptide, peptide. [G. *eu-,* normal, usual + peptide]

eu·phen·ics (yū-fē'niks). Modification of the internal or external environment of an individual so as to prevent or modify the phenotypic expression of a genetic defect, without changing the genotype or the inheritance. [eu- + G. *phainō,* to show forth]

Eu·phor·bia pi·lu·lif·e·ra (yū-fōr'bē-ă pil-ŭ-lif'ē-ră). A species of plant (family Euphorbiaceae); the dried herb used in asthma, coryza and other respiratory affections, in angina pectoris, and as an antispasmodic. SYN asthma-weed (2).

eu·pho·ret·ic (yū-fō-ret'ik). SYN euphoriant.

eu·pho·ria (yū-fōr'ē-ă). A feeling of well-being, commonly exaggerated and not necessarily well founded. [eu- + G. *pherō,* to bear]

eu·pho·ri·ant (yū-fōr'ē-ant). **1.** Having the capability to produce a sense of well-being. **2.** An agent with such a capability. SYN euphoretic.

eu·pla·sia (yū-plā'zē-ă). The state of cells or tissue that is normal or typical for that particular type. [eu- + G. *plassō,* form]

eu·plas·tic (yū-plas'tik). **1.** Relating to euplasia. **2.** Healing readily and well. [G. *euplastos,* easily molded; *eu,* well, + *plastos,* formed]

eu·ploid (yū'ployd). Relating to euploidy.

eu·ploidy (yū'ploy-dē). The state of a cell containing whole haploid sets. [eu- + G. *-ploos,* -fold]

eup·nea (yūp-nē'ă). Easy, free respiration; the type observed in a normal individual under resting conditions. [G. *eupnoia,* fr. *eu,* well, + *pnoia,* breath]

eu·prax·ia (yū-prak'sē-ă). Normal ability to perform coordinated movements. [eu- + G. *praxis,* a doing]

eu·pro·cin hy·dro·chlo·ride (yū'prō-sin). Hydrocupreine isopentyl ether; a derivative of quinine. SYN eucupine.

Eu·proc·tis (yū-prok'tis). A genus of moths. The hairs of the cocoon and caterpillar of the species E. chrysorrhoea, the brown-tail moth, cause caterpillar dermatitis. [eu- + G. *prōktos,* rump]

eu·rhyth·mia (yū-rith'mē-ă). Harmonious body relationships of the separate organs. [eu- + G. *rhythmos,* rhythm]

eu·ro·pi·um (Eu) (yū-rō'pē-ŭm). An element of the rare earth (lanthanide) group, atomic no. 63, atomic wt. 151.965. [L. *Europa,* Europe]

eury-. Broad, wide; opposite of steno-. [G. *eurys,* wide]

eu·ry·ce·phal·ic, eu·ry·ceph·a·lous (yū'rē-se-fal'ik, -sef'ă-lŭs).

eu

Having an abnormally broad head; sometimes used in reference to a brachycephalic head. [eury- + G. *kephalē,* head]

eu·ryg·nath·ic (yū-rig-nath'ik). Having a wide jaw. SYN eurygnathous.

eu·ryg·na·thism (yū-rig'nă-thizm). The condition of having a wide jaw. [eury- + G. *gnathos,* jaw]

eu·ryg·na·thous (yū-rig'nă-thŭs). SYN eurygnathic.

eu·ry·on (yū'rē-on). The extremity, on either side, of the greatest transverse diameter of the head; a point used in craniometry. [G. *eurys,* broad]

eu·ry·op·ic. Wide-eyed. SEE blepharodiastasis. [eury- + G. *ops,* eye]

eu·ry·so·mat·ic (yū'rē-sō-mat'ik). Having a thick-set body. [eury- + G. *soma,* body]

eu·scope (yū'skōp). An instrument for showing on a screen an enlarged image from a microscope. [eu- + G. *skopeō,* to view]

Eu·sim·u·li·um (yū-si-myū'lē-ŭm). SYN *Simulium.* [eu- + L. *simulo,* to simulate]

eu·sta·chi·an (yū-stā'shŭn, yū-stā'kē-ăn). Described by or attributed to Eustachio.

Eustachio, Bartolommeo E., Italian anatomist, 1524–1574. SEE eustachian *catheter,* eustachian *cushion,* eustachian *tonsil, tuba* eustachiana, *tuba* eustachii, eustachian *tube,* eustachian *tuber,* eustachian *valve.*

eu·sta·chi·tis (yū-stā-kī'tis). Inflammation of the mucous membrane of the eustachian tube.

eus·the·nia (yū-sthē'nē-ă). Normal strength. [eu- + G. *sthenos,* strength]

Eu·stron·gy·lus (yū-stron'ji-lŭs). Former name for *Dioctophyma.* [eu- + G. *strongylos,* rounded]

eu·sys·to·le (yū-sis'tō-lē). A condition in which the cardiac systole is normal in force and time. [eu- + systole]

eu·sys·tol·ic (yū-sis-tol'ik). Relating to eusystole.

eu·tec·tic (yū-tek'tik). **1.** Easily melted; denoting specifically mixtures of certain chemical compounds that have a lower melting point than any of their individual ingredients; *e.g.,* a solid, such as menthol, that when triturated with another solid of the same class, such as camphor, unites with it to form a liquid, the mixture having a lower melting point than either of its components. **2.** The alloy that freezes at a constant temperature; the lowest of the series. [eu- + G. *tēxis,* a melting away]

eu·tha·na·sia (yū-thă-nā'zē-ă). **1.** A quiet, painless death. **2.** The intentional putting to death of a person with an incurable or painful disease intended as an act of mercy. [eu- + G. *thanatos,* death]

eu·then·ics (yū-then'iks). The science concerned with establishing optimum living conditions for plants, animals, or humans, especially through proper provisioning and environment. [G. *eutheneō,* to thrive]

eu·ther·a·peu·tic (yū'thār-ă-pyū'tik). Having excellent curative properties.

Eu·the·ria (yū-thē'rē-ă). A subclass of mammals, excluding monotremes and marsupials, having a placenta through which the young are nourished. [eu- + G. *thērion,* animal]

eu·ther·mic (yū-ther'mik). At an optimal temperature. [eu- + G. *thermos,* warm]

eu·thy·mia (yū-thī'mē-ă). **1.** Joyfulness; mental peace and tranquility. **2.** Moderation of mood, not manic or depressed. [eu- + G. *thymos,* mind]

eu·thy·mic (yū-thī'mik). Relating to or characterized by, euthymia.

eu·thy·roid·ism (yū-thī'roy-dizm). A condition in which the thyroid gland is functioning normally, its secretion being of proper amount and constitution.

eu·thy·scope (yū'thi-skōp). A modified ophthalmoscope, now seldom used, with which the site of excentric fixation may be dazzled by a bright light while the true fovea is simultaneously shielded by an opaque disk; used in pleoptics. [G. *euthys,* straight, + *skopeō,* to view]

eu·thys·co·py (yū-this'kŏ-pē). Examination with the euthyscope.

eu·ton·ic (yū-ton'ik). SYN normotonic (1). [eu- + G. *tonus,* tone]

eu·tri·cho·sis (yū-tri-kō'sis). A normal growth of healthy hair. [eu- + G. *thrix,* hair]

eu·tro·phia (yū-trō'fē-ă). A state of normal nourishment and growth. SYN eutrophy. [G. fr. *eu,* well, + *trophē,* nourishment]

eu·tro·phic (yū-trof'ik). Relating to, characterized by, or promoting eutrophia.

eu·tro·phy (yū'trō-fē). SYN eutrophia.

eu·vo·lia (yū-vō'lē-ă). Normal water content or volume of a given compartment; *e.g.,* extracellular e.

eV, ev Abbreviation for electron-volt.

evac·u·ant (ē-vak'yū-ant). **1.** Promoting an excretion, especially of the bowels. **2.** An agent that increases excretion, especially a cathartic.

evac·u·ate (ē-vak'yū-āt). To accomplish evacuation. [L. *e-vacuo,* pp. -*vacuatus,* to empty out]

evac·u·a·tion (ē-vak-yū-ā'shŭn). **1.** Removal of material, especially wastes from the bowels by defecation. **2.** SYN stool (2). **3.** Removal of air from a closed vessel; production of a vacuum.

evac·u·a·tor (ē-vak'yū-ā-tŏr). A mechanical evacuant; an instrument for the removal of fluid or small particles from a body cavity, or of impacted feces from the rectum.

Ellik e., a special instrument with glass receptacle, latex or plastic bulb, and flexible tubing, used to evacuate tissue fragments, blood clots, or calculi from the urinary bladder.

evag·i·na·tion (ē-vaj-i-nā'shŭn). Protrusion of some part or organ from its normal position. [L. *e,* out, + *vagina,* sheath]

eval·u·a·tion. Systematic, objective assessment of the relevance, effectiveness, and impact of activities in the light of specified objectives.

ev·a·nes·cent (ev-ă-nes'ent). Of short duration. [L. *e,* out, + *vanesco,* to vanish]

Evans, H.M., U.S. anatomist and physiologist, 1882–1971. SEE Evans blue.

Evans, Robert S., U.S. physician, *1912. SEE E.'s *syndrome.*

Evans blue [C.I. 23860]. $C_{34}H_{24}N_6Na_4O_{14}S_4$; tetrasodium salt of 4,4′-bis[7-(1-amino-8-hydroxy-2,4-disulfo)naphthylazo]-3,3′-bitolyl; a diazo dye used for the determination of the blood volume on the basis of the dilution of a standard solution of the dye in the plasma after its intravenous injection; it binds to proteins and is also used as a vital stain for following diffusion through blood vessel walls. SYN azovan blue.

Evans for·ceps. See under forceps.

e·vap·o·rate (ē-vap'ŏr-āt). To cause or undergo evaporation. SYN volatilize.

evap·o·ra·tion (ē-vap-ŏ-ra'shŭn). **1.** A change from liquid to vapor form. **2.** Loss of volume of a liquid by conversion into vapor. SYN volatilization. [L. *e,* out, + *vaporare,* to emit vapor]

eva·sion (ē-vā'zhŭn). The act of escaping, avoiding, or feigning. **macular e.,** SYN *horror* fusionis.

even·tra·tion (ē'ven-trā'shŭn). **1.** Protrusion of omentum and/or intestine through an opening in the abdominal wall. SYN evisceration (3). **2.** Removal of the contents of the abdominal cavity. [L. *e,* out, + *venter,* belly]

e. of the diaphragm, extreme elevation of a half or part of the diaphragm, which is usually atrophic and abnormally thin.

ever·sion (ē-ver'zhŭn). A turning outward, as of the eyelid or foot. [L. *e-everto,* pp. -*versus,* to overturn]

evert (ē-vert'). To turn outward. [L. *e-verto,* to overturn]

evide·ment (e-vēd-mon'). Obsolete term for the scraping out of morbid tissue from a natural or pathologic cavity. [Fr. *évider,* to scoop out]

evil (ē'vil). Disease, especially of animals.

joint e., SYN joint ill.

king's e., historic term for cervical tuberculous lymphadenitis (scrofula) which was formerly thought to be curable by the touch of a king.

poll e., suppurative inflammation of the cranial nuchal (atlantal) bursa that lies between the atlas and the cranial end of the ligamentum nuchae in the horse.

quarter e., SYN blackleg.

ev·i·ra·tion (ev-i-rā'shŭn, ē-vī-rā'shŭn). **1.** SYN emasculation. **2.** Loss or absence of the masculine, with acquisition of feminine characteristics; a type of effemination. **3.** Delusional belief of a man that he has become a woman. [L. *e,* out, + *vir,* man]

evis·cer·a·tion (ē-vis-er-ā'shŭn). **1.** SYN exenteration. **2.** Removal of the contents of the eyeball, leaving the sclera and sometimes the cornea. **3.** SYN eventration (1). [L. *eviscero,* to disembowel]

evis·cer·o·neu·rot·o·my (ē-vis'er-ō-nū-rot'ō-mē). Evisceration of the eye with division of the optic nerve. [L. *eviscero,* to disembowel, + G. *neuron,* nerve, + *tomē,* a cutting]

evo·ca·tion (ev-ō-kā'shŭn, ē-vō-kā'shŭn). Induction of a particular tissue produced by the action of an evocator during embryogenesis. [L. *evoco,* pp. *evocatus,* to call forth, evoke]

evo·ca·tor (ev'ō-kā-ter, -tōr). A factor in the control of morphogenesis in the early embryo.

ev·o·lu·tion (ev-ō-lū'shŭn). A continuing process of change from one state, condition or form to another. **2.** A progressive distancing between the genotype and the phenotype in a line of descent. [L. *e-volvo,* pp. *-volutus,* to roll out]

biologic e., the doctrine that all forms of animal or plant life have been derived by gradual changes from simpler forms and ultimately unicellular organisms. SYN organic e.

chemical e., the theory of the process by which life arose from inorganic matter.

coincidental e., SYN concerted e.

concerted e., the ability of two related genes to evolve together as though constituting a single locus. SYN coincidental e.

convergent e., the evolutionary development of similar structures in two or more species, often widely separated phylogenetically, in response to similarities of environment; for example, the wing-like structures in insects, birds, and flying mammals.

Darwinian e., the proposition that the phylogeny of all species is wholly ascribable to the combined effects of random variation (mutation) in genotypes of the members of a stock as a result of the operation of undirected accidents with consequences to their phenotypes and the operation of preferential (but by no means certain) survival of those resulting phenotypes most suited to survive in the contemporary environment. The proposed system survives largely because of genetic factors that avidly conserve the ontogeny of the stock.

Denman's spontaneous e., a mechanism of spontaneous molding of the fetus and impaction of the shoulder with prolapse of the arm noted in some cases of transverse lie; vaginal delivery is achieved with the breech appearing at the vulva immediately after the prolapsed shoulder.

divergent e., the process by which a species or gene product gives rise to two or more different products.

Douglas' spontaneous e., a mechanism whereby molding of the fetus and impaction of the shoulder and prolapsed arm occurs in transverse lie, allowing vaginal delivery with the lateral aspect of the thorax following the prolapsed shoulder.

emergent e., appearance of a property in a complex system *e.g.,* organism that could have been predicted only with difficulty, or perhaps not at all, from a knowledge and understanding of the individual genotype changes taken separately.

organic e., SYN biologic e.

saltatory e., the theory that e. of a new species from an older one may occur as a large jump, such as a major repatterning of chromosomes, rather than by gradual accumulation of small steps or mutations. Cf. emergent e.

spontaneous e., the unaided delivery of the fetus from a transverse lie.

evul·sion (ē-vŭl'shŭn). A forcible pulling out or extraction. Cf. avulsion. [L. *evulsio,* fr. *e-vello,* pp. *-vulsus,* to pluck out]

Ewart, William, English physician, 1848–1929. SEE E.'s *procedure, sign.*

ewe (yew). A female sheep of breeding age.

Ewing, James, U.S. pathologist, 1866–1943. SEE E.'s *sarcoma, tumor.*

Ewing, James H., pathologist, 1798–1827. SEE E.'s *sign.*

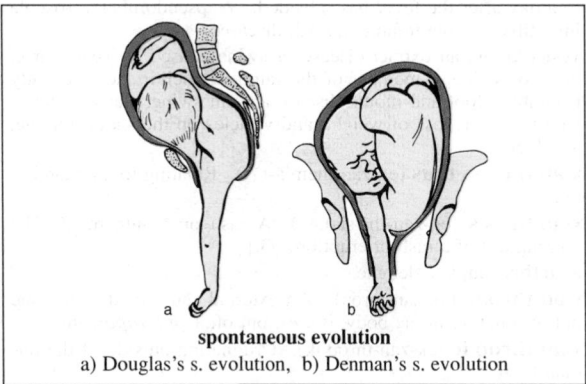

spontaneous evolution
a) Douglas's s. evolution, b) Denman's s. evolution

Ewin·gel·la (ū'ing-el'ah). Newly named genus of Enterobacteriaceae.

ex-. Out of, from, away from. [L. and G. out of]

exa- (E). Prefix used in the SI and metric systems to signify one quintillion (10^{18}).

ex·ac·er·ba·tion (eg-zas-er-bā'shŭn, -ek-sas-). An increase in the severity of a disease or any of its signs or symptoms. [L. *exacerbo,* pp. *-atus,* to exasperate, increase, fr. *acerbus,* sour]

ex·al·ta·tion (eks'al-tā'-shŭn). An utterance, discourse, or address conveying a marked level of joy, glee, and happiness.

ex·am·i·na·tion (eg-zam-i-nā'shŭn). Any investigation or inspection made for the purpose of diagnosis; usually qualified by the method used.

cytologic e., microscopic examination of cells, especially for diagnosis of disease.

EMG e., (1) needle electrode examination portion of the electrodiagnostic examination (limited sense); **(2)** synonym for entire electrodiagnostic examination, including not only the needle electrode examination (electromyogram proper), but the nerve conduction studies as well (expanded sense).

Papanicolaou e., SEE Pap *test.*

physical e., e. by means such as visual inspection, palpation, percussion, and auscultation to collect information for diagnosis.

postmortem e., SYN autopsy.

ex·am·in·er (eg-zam'in-er). One who performs an examination. [L. *examino,* to weigh, examine]

medical e., (1) a physician who examines a person and reports upon his physical condition to the company or individual at whose request the examination was made; **(2)** in states or municipalities where the office of coroner has been abolished, a physician appointed to investigate all cases of sudden, violent, or suspicious death.

ex·an·them (eg-zan'them). SYN exanthema.

ex·an·the·ma (eg-zan-thē'mă). A skin eruption occurring as a symptom of an acute viral or coccal disease, as in scarlet fever or measles. SYN anthema, exanthem. [G. efflorescence, an eruption, fr. *anthos,* flower]

Boston e., a viral disease resembling e. subitum, with the e., if it develops, appearing after the fever has subsided; it is caused by strain 16 of ECHO virus. [after the city in which an epidemic occurred]

epidemic e., SYN epidemic *polyarthritis.*

equine coital e., a disease of horses caused by equine herpesvirus 3 and characterized by pustular and ulcerative lesions on the vaginal and vestibular mucosa and on the skin of the penis, prepuce, and the perineal region.

keratoid e., a symptom occurring in the secondary stage of yaws: patches of fine, light colored, furfuraceous desquamation, scattered irregularly over limbs and trunk.

e. subi'tum, a disease due to herpes virus-6 of infants and young children, marked by sudden onset with fever lasting several days (sometimes with convulsions) and followed by a fine macular (sometimes maculopapular) rash that appears within a few hours

ex

to a day after the fever has subsided. SYN pseudorubella, roseola infantilis, roseola infantum, sixth disease.

vesicular e., an extinct disease of swine caused by vesicular e. virus of swine, a member of the family Caliciviridae; it closely resembled foot-and-mouth disease and, in swine, was characterized by fever, loss of weight, and vesicles on the snout, tongue, and feet.

ex·an·them·a·tous (eg-zan-them′ă-tŭs). Relating to an exanthema.

ex·an·the·sis (eg-zan-thē′sis). 1. A rash or exanthem. 2. The coming out of a rash or eruption. [G.]

e. arthro′sia, SYN dengue.

ex·an·thrope (ek′zan-thrōp). An external cause of disease, one not originating in the body. [G. *ex,* out of, + *anthrōpos,* man]

ex·an·throp·ic (ek-zan-throp′ik). Originating outside of the human body.

ex·ar·te·ri·tis (eks-ar-ter-ī′tis). SYN periarteritis.

ex·ar·tic·u·la·tion (eks-ar-tik-yū-lā′shŭn). SYN disarticulation. [L. *ex,* out, + *articulus,* joint]

ex·cal·a·tion (eks-kă-lā′shŭn). Absence, suppression, or failure of development of one of a series of structures, as of a digit or vertebra. [G. *ex,* from, + *chalaō,* to abate, release]

ex·ca·va·tio (eks-kă-vā′shē-ō) [NA]. SYN excavation (1). [L. fr. *ex-cavo,* pp. *-cavatus,* to hollow out, fr. *ex,* out, + *cavus,* hollow]

e. dis′ci [NA], SYN *excavation* of optic disc.

e. papil′lae, SYN *excavation* of optic disc.

e. rectouteri′na [NA], SYN rectouterine *pouch.*

e. rectovesica′lis [NA], SYN rectovesical *pouch.*

e. vesicouteri′na [NA], SYN uterovesical *pouch.*

ex·ca·va·tion (eks-kă-vā′shŭn). 1. A natural cavity, pouch, or recess. SYN excavatio [NA]. 2. A cavity formed artificially or as the result of a pathologic process.

atrophic e., an exaggeration of the normal or physiologic cupping of the optic disk caused by atrophy of the optic nerve.

glaucomatous e., SYN glaucomatous *cup.*

e. of optic disc, the normally occurring depression or pit in the center of the optic disc. SYN excavatio disci [NA], depression of optic disk, excavatio papillae, physiologic cup, physiologic e.

physiologic e., SYN e. of optic disc.

ex·ca·va·tor (eks′că-vā-tŏr, -tŏr). 1. An instrument like a large sharp spoon or scoop, used in scraping out pathologic tissue. 2. In dentistry, an instrument, generally a small spoon or curette, for cleaning out and shaping a carious cavity preparatory to filling.

hatchet e., SEE hatchet.

hoe e., a single-beveled dental e., with the blade at an angle to the axis of the handle and the cutting edge perpendicular to the plane of the angle.

ex·ce·men·to·sis (ek′sē-men-tō′sis). A nodular outgrowth of cementum on the root surface of a tooth.

ex·cen·tric (ek-sen′trik). Alternative spelling for eccentric (2, 3).

ex·cess (ek′ses). That which is more than the usual or specified amount.

antibody e., in a precipitation test, the presence of antibody in an amount greater than that required to combine with all of the antigen present.

antigen e., (1) in a precipitation test, the presence of uncombined antigen above that required to combine with all of the antibody; precipitation may be inhibited because the presence of excess antigen gives rise to soluble antigen-antibody complexes; **(2)** *in vivo* the resultant antigen-antibody interaction in such an antigen e. may give rise to immune complexes, which have a potential to induce cellular damage; such injury underlies the pathologic changes seen in certain immune complex diseases.

base e., a measure of metabolic alkalosis, usually predicted from the Siggaard-Andersen nomogram; the amount of strong acid that would have to be added per unit volume of whole blood to titrate it to pH 7.4 while at 37°C and at a carbon dioxide pressure of 40 mm Hg.

convergence e., that condition in which an esophoria or esotropia is greater for near vision than for far vision.

negative base e., a measure of metabolic acidosis, usually predicted from the Siggaard-Andersen nomogram; the amount of strong alkali that would have to be added per unit volume of whole blood to titrate it to pH 7.4 while at 37°C and at a carbon dioxide pressure of 40 mm Hg.

ex·change (eks-chānj′). To substitute one thing for another, or the act of such substitution.

sister chromatid e., the e. during mitosis of homologous genetic material between sister chromatids; increased as a result of inordinate chromosomal fragility due to genetic or environmental factors. SEE recombination.

ex·cip·i·ent (ek-sip′ē-ent). A more or less inert substance added in a prescription as a diluent or vehicle or to give form or consistency when the remedy is given in pill form; *e.g.,* simple syrup, aromatic powder, honey, and various elixirs. [L. *excipiens;* pres. p. of ex- *cipio,* to take out]

ex·cise (ek-sīz′). To cut out. SEE ALSO resect.

ex·ci·sion (ek-sizh′ŭn). 1. The act of cutting out; the surgical removal of part or all of a structure or organ. SYN resection (2). SEE ALSO resection. 2. In molecular biology, a recombination event in which a genetic element is removed. SYN exeresis. [L. *excido,* to cut out]

loop e., a diagnostic and therapeutic gynecological surgical technique for removing dysplastic cells from the cervix. SYN loop resection.

In this office procedure conducted with the aid of colposcopy, a small wire loop is used to excise visible patches of cervical intraepithelial neoplasia. Like cauterization, cryosurgery, and CO_2 laser procedures, loop excision can be done with local anaesthetic, and is an uncomplicated, relatively inexpensive way of removing dysplastic cells; in addition, it provides material for biopsy. It is not advised for cases of severe dysplasia or carcinoma in situ, which are better addressed by cervical conization, an inpatient procedure.

ex·cit·a·bil·i·ty (ek-sī′tă-bil′i-tē). Having the capability of being excitable.

supranormal e., at the end of phase three of the cardiac action potential, the successful stimulation threshold falls below (*i.e.,* less negative than) the level necessary to produce excitation during the rest of the phase of diastole, so that an ordinary subthreshold stimulus becomes effective. Cf. supranormal *conduction.*

ex·cit·a·ble (ek-sī′tă-bl). 1. Capable of quick response to a stimulus; having potentiality for emotional arousal. Cf. irritable. 2. In neurophysiology, referring to a tissue, cell, or membrane capable of undergoing excitation in response to an adequate stimulus.

ex·cit·ant (ek-sī′tănt). SYN stimulant. [L. *excito,* pp. *-atus,* pres. p. *-ans,* to arouse]

ex·ci·ta·tion (ek-sī-tā′shŭn). 1. The act of increasing the rapidity or intensity of the physical or mental processes. 2. In neurophysiology, the complete all-or-none response of a nerve or muscle to an adequate stimulus, ordinarily including propagation of e. along the membranes of the cell or cells involved. SEE ALSO stimulation.

anomalous atrioventricular e., ectopic atrial beat conducted to the ventricle.

ventricular pre-e., SEE Wolff-Parkinson-White *syndrome.*

ex·cit·a·to·ry (ek-sī′tă-tō-rē). Tending to produce excitation.

ex·cite·ment (ek-sīt′ment). An emotional state sometimes characterized by its potential for impulsive or poorly controlled activity.

catatonic e., an excited catatonic state seen in one of the schizophrenic disorders. SEE catatonia.

manic e., an excited mental state seen in a bipolar (manic-depressive) disorder characterized by hyperactivity, talkativeness, flight of ideas, pressured speech, grandiosity, and, occasionally, grandiose delusions. SEE mania, manic-depressive. SYN acute mania.

ex·ci·to·glan·du·lar (ek-sī′tō-glan′dyū-lăr). Increasing the secretory activity of a gland.

ex·ci·to·met·a·bol·ic (ek-sī′tō-met-ă-bol′ik). Increasing the activity of the metabolic processes.

ex·ci·to·mo·tor (ek-sī′tō-mō′ter). Causing or increasing the rapidity of motion. SYN centrokinetic (2).

ex·ci·to·mus·cu·lar (ek-sī′tō-mŭs′kyū-lăr). Causing muscular activity.

ex·ci·tor (ek-sī′ter, -tōr). SYN stimulant (2).

ex·ci·to·se·cre·to·ry (ek-sī′tō-sē-krē′tō-rē). Stimulating to secretion.

ex·ci·to·tox·ic (ek-sī′-tō-tok-sik). Possessing the property of exciting and then poisoning cells or tissues; examples include nerve injury produced by glutamate. [excite + G. *toxikon*, poison]

ex·citotox·ins (ek-sī′tō-toks′ins). Toxins that bind to certain receptors (*e.g.*, certain glutamate receptors) and may cause neuronal cell death; e.'s may be involved in brain damage associated with strokes.

ex·ci·to·vas·cu·lar (ek-sī′tō-vas′kyū-lăr). Increasing the activity of the circulation.

ex·clave (eks-klāv′). An outlying, detached portion of a gland or other part, such as the thyroid or pancreas; an accessory gland. [L. *ex*, out, + *-clave* (in enclave)]

ex·clu·sion (eks-klū′zhŭn). A shutting out; disconnection from the main portion. [L. *ex- cludo*, pp. *-clusus*, to shut out]

allelic e., in each cell of an individual heterozygous at an autosomal locus, the non-preferential suppression of the phenotypic manifestation of one or other of the alleles; the phenotype of the body is thus mosaic. Cf. lyonization.

Devine e., e. of the lower part of the stomach, followed by gastrojejunostomy, for treatment of duodenal ulcer.

e. of pupil, SYN seclusion of *pupil*.

ex·con·ju·gant (eks-kon′jū-gant). A member of a conjugating pair of protozoan ciliates after separation and prior to the subsequent mitotic division of each of the e.'s. SEE ALSO conjugant, conjugation (3). [ex- + L. *conjugo*, to join]

ex·co·ri·ate (eks-kō′rē-āt). To scratch or otherwise denude the skin by physical means.

ex·co·ri·a·tion (eks-kō′rē-ā′shŭn). A scratch mark; a linear break in the skin surface, usually covered with blood or serous crusts. [L. *excorio*, to skin, strip, fr. *corium*, skin, hide]

neurotic e., repeated self-induced e., with or without underlying skin lesions, associated with compulsive or neurotic behavioral problems.

ex·cre·ment (eks′krĕ-ment). Waste matter or any excretion cast out of the body; *e.g.*, feces. [L. *ex- cerno*, pp. *-cretus*, to separate]

ex·cre·men·ti·tious (eks′krĕ-men-tish′ŭs). Relating to any excrement.

ex·cres·cence (eks-kres′ens). Any outgrowth from a surface. [L. *ex- cresco*, pp. *-cretus*, to grow forth]

Lambl's e.'s, small pointed projections from the edges of the aortic cusps of unknown significance.

ex·cre·ta (eks-krē′tă). SYN excretion (2). [L. neut. pl. of *excretus*, pp. of *ex-cerno*, to separate]

ex·crete (eks-krēt′). To separate from the blood and cast out; to perform excretion.

ex·cre·tion (eks-krē′shŭn). **1.** The process whereby the undigested residue of food and the waste products of metabolism are eliminated, material is removed to regulate the composition of body fluids and tissues, or substances are expelled to perform functions on an exterior surface. **2.** The product of a tissue or organ that is material to be passed out of the body. SYN excreta. Cf. secretion. [see excrement]

ex·cre·to·ry (eks-krē′tō-rē). Relating to excretion.

ex·cur·sion (eks-ker′zhŭn). Any movement from one point to another, usually with the implied idea of returning again to the original position.

lateral e., movement of the mandible to the right or left side.

protrusive e., movement of the mandible to a position forward of the centric position.

retrusive e., the slight backward and return movement of the mandible between the position of closure and a slightly posterior position.

ex·cy·clo·duc·tion (ek-sī-klō-dŭk′shŭn). A cycloduction in which the upper pole of the cornea is rotated outward (laterally). [ex- + cyclo- + L. *duco*, pp. *ductus*, to lead]

ex·cy·clo·pho·ria (ek-sī-klō-fō′rē-ă). A cyclophoria in which the upper poles of each cornea tend to rotate laterally. [ex- + cyclo- + G. *phora*, a carrying]

ex·cy·clo·tor·sion (eks′sī-klō-tōr′shun). SYN extorsion (2). [ex- + cyclo- + L. *torqueo*, pp. *torsus*, to twist]

ex·cy·clo·tro·pia (eks′sī-klō-trō′pē-a). A cyclotropia in which the upper poles of the corneas are rotated outward (laterally) relative to each other. [ex- + cyclo- + G. *tropē*, a turning]

ex·cy·clo·ver·gence (ek-sī-klō-ver′jens). Rotation of the upper pole of each cornea outwards. [ex- + cyclo- + L. *vergo*, to bend, incline]

ex·cys·ta·tion (ek-sis-tā′shŭn). Removal from a cyst; denoting the action of certain encysted organisms in escaping from their envelope.

ex·duc·tion (eks-duk′shun). SYN lateroduction. [ex- + L. *duco*, pp. *ductus*, to lead]

ex·e·mia (ek-sē′mē-ă). A condition, as in shock, in which a considerable portion of the blood is removed from the main circulation but remains within blood vessels in certain areas where it is stagnant. [G. *ex*, out of, + *haima*, blood]

ex·en·ce·pha·lia (eks′en-se-fā′lē-ă). SYN exencephaly.

ex·en·ce·phal·ic (eks′en-se-fal′ik). Relating to exencephaly. SYN exencephalous.

ex·en·ceph·a·lo·cele (eks′en-sef′ă-lō-sēl). Herniation of the brain. [*ex*, out, + G. *enkephalos*, brain, + *kēlē*, tumor]

ex·en·ceph·a·lous (eks-en-sef′ă-lŭs). SYN exencephalic.

ex·en·ceph·a·ly (eks-en-sef′ă-lē). Condition in which the skull is defective with the brain exposed or extruding. SYN exencephalia. [G. *ex*, out, + *enkephalos*, brain]

ex·en·ter·a·tion (eks-en-ter-ā′shŭn). Removal of internal organs and tissues, usually radical removal of the contents of a body cavity. SYN evisceration (1). [G. *ex*, out, + *enteron*, bowel]

anterior pelvic e., removal of the urinary bladder, lower parts of the ureter, vagina, uterus, adnexa, and adjacent lymph nodes; a urinary diversion is necessary.

orbital e., removal of the entire contents of the orbit.

pelvic e., removal of all of the organs and adjacent structures of the pelvis; usually performed to surgically ablate cancer involving urinary bladder, uterine cervix, or rectum.

posterior pelvic e., removal of the vagina, uterus, adnexa, rectum, anus, and adjacent lymph nodes; a colostomy is necessary.

total pelvic e., removal of the urinary bladder, lower parts of the ureter, vagina, uterus, adnexa, rectum, anus, and adjacent lymph nodes; a colostomy and urinary diversion are necessary. SYN Brunschwig's operation.

ex·en·ter·i·tis (eks-en-ter-ī′tis). Inflammation of the peritoneal covering of the intestine. [G. *exō*, on the outside, + enteritis]

ex·er·cise (ek′ser-sīz). **1.** *Active:* bodily exertion for the sake of restoring the organs and functions to a healthy state or keeping them healthy. **2.** *Passive:* motion of limbs without effort by the patient.

isometric e., e. consisting of muscular contractions without movement of the involved parts of the body.

isotonic e., SYN isotonic *contraction*.

Kegel's e.'s, alternate contraction and relaxation of perineal muscles for treatment of urinary stress incontinence.

ex·er·e·sis (ek-ser′ĕ-sis). SYN excision. [G. *exairesis*, a taking out, fr. *haireō*, to take, grasp]

ex·er·gon·ic (ek-ser-gon′ik). Referring to a chemical reaction that takes place with release of Gibbs free energy to its surroundings. Cf. endergonic. [exo- + G. *ergon*, work]

ex·flag·el·la·tion (eks-flaj-ĕ-lā′shŭn). The extrusion of rapidly waving flagellum-like microgametes from microgametocytes; in the case of human malaria parasites, this occurs in the blood meal taken by the proper anopheline vector within a few minutes

ex

after ingestion of the infected blood by the mosquito. SYN polymitus.

ex·fo·li·a·tion (eks-fō-lē-ā'shŭn). **1.** Detachment and shedding of superficial cells of an epithelium or from any tissue surface. **2.** Scaling or desquamation of the horny layer of epidermis, which varies in amount from minute quantities to shedding the entire integument. **3.** Loss of deciduous teeth following physiological loss of root structure. [Mod. L. fr. L. *ex,* out, + *folium,* leaf]

e. of lens, sheetlike separation of the capsule of the lens; it may occur if the eyes are exposed to intense heat.

ex·fo·li·a·tive (eks-fō'lē-ā-tiv). Marked by exfoliation, desquamation, or profuse scaling. [Mod. L. *exfoliativus*]

ex·ha·la·tion (eks-hă-lā'shŭn). **1.** Breathing out. SYN expiration (1). **2.** The giving forth of gas or vapor. **3.** Any exhaled or emitted gas or vapor. [L. *ex-halo,* pp. *-halatus,* to breathe out]

ex·hale (eks'hāl). **1.** To breathe out. SYN expire (1). **2.** To emit a gas or vapor or odor.

ex·haus·tion (ek-zos'chŭn). **1.** Extreme fatigue; inability to respond to stimuli. **2.** Removal of contents; using up of a supply of anything. **3.** Extraction of the active constituents of a drug by treating with water, alcohol, or other solvent. [L. *ex-haurio,* pp. *-haustus,* to draw out, empty]

combat e., SEE battle *fatigue,* posttraumatic stress *disorder,* war *neurosis.*

heat e., a form of reaction to heat, marked by prostration, weakness, and collapse, resulting from severe dehydration.

ex·hi·bi·tion·ism (ek-si-bish'ŭn-izm). A morbid compulsion to expose a part of the body, especially the genitals, with the intent of provoking sexual interest in the viewer.

ex·hi·bi·tion·ist (ek-si-bish'ŭn-ist). One who engages in exhibitionism.

ex·hil·a·rant (eg-zil'ar-ant). Mentally stimulating. [L. *ex-hilaro,* pp. *-atus,* pres. p. *-ans,* to gladden]

ex·is·ten·tial (eg-zi-sten'shăl). Pertaining to a branch of philosophy, existentialism, concerned with the search for the meaning of one's own existence, that has been extended into existential *psychotherapy.* [L. *existentia,* existence]

ex·i·tus (eks'i-tŭs). An exit or outlet; death. [L. fr. *ex-eo,* pp. *-itus,* to go out]

Exner, Siegmund, Austrian physiologist, 1846–1926. SEE Call-E. *bodies,* under *body;* E.'s *plexus.*

⌂**exo-.** Exterior, external, or outward. SEE ALSO ecto-. [G. *exō,* outside]

ex·o·am·y·lase (ek-sō-am'il-ās). A glucanohydrolase acting on a glycosidic bond near an end of the polysaccharide; *e.g.,* β-amylase.

ex·o·an·ti·gen (ek-sō-an'ti-jen). SYN ectoantigen.

ex·o·car·dia (ek-sō-kar'dē-ă). SYN ectocardia.

ex·o·crine (ek'sō-krin). **1.** Denoting glandular secretion delivered to an apical or luminal surface. SYN eccrine (1). **2.** Denoting a gland that secretes outwardly through excretory ducts. [exo- + G. *krinō,* to separate]

ex·o·cy·clic (ek-sō-sī'klik, -sik'lik). Relating to atoms or groups attached to a cyclic structure but not themselves cyclic; *e.g.,* the —CH₃ group of toluene. Cf. endocyclic.

ex·o·cy·to·sis (ek'sō-sī-to'sis). **1.** The appearance of migrating inflammatory cells in the epidermis. **2.** The process whereby secretory granules or droplets are released from a cell; the membrane around the granule fuses with the cell membrane, which ruptures, and the secretion is discharged. SYN emeiocytosis, emiocytosis. Cf. endocytosis. [exo- + G. *kytos,* cell, + *-osis,* condition]

ex·o·de·vi·a·tion (ek'sō-dē-vē-ā'shŭn). **1.** SYN exophoria. **2.** SYN exotropia.

ex·o·don·tia (ek-sō-don'shē-ă). The branch of dental practice concerned with the extraction of teeth. [exo- + G. *odous,* tooth]

ex·o·don·tist (ek-sō-don'tist). One who specializes in the extraction of teeth.

ex·o·en·zyme (ek-sō-en'zīm). SYN extracellular *enzyme.*

ex·og·a·my (ek-sog'ă-mē). Sexual reproduction by means of

conjugation of two gametes of different ancestry, as in certain protozoan species. [exo- + G. *gamos,* marriage]

ex·o·gas·tru·la (eks-ō-gas'trū-lă). An abnormal embryo in which the primitive gut has been everted.

ex·o·ge·net·ic (ek'sō-je-net'ik). SYN exogenous.

ex·o·ge·note (ek-sō-jē'nōt). In microbial genetics, the fragment of genetic material that has been transferred from a donor to the recipient and, being homologous for a region of the recipient's original genome (endogenote), produces in the homologous region a condition analogous to diploidy. [exo + genote]

ex·og·e·nous (eks-oj'ě-nŭs). Originating or produced outside of the organism. SYN ectogenous, exogenetic. [exo- + G. *-gen,* production]

exo-1,4-α-D-glu·co·si·dase. A hydrolase removing terminal α-1,4-linked D-glucose residues from nonreducing ends of chains, with release of β-D-glucose. SYN acid maltase, amyloglucosidase, γ-amylase, glucoamylase.

ex·o·lev·er (ek'sō-lē'ver). A modified elevator for the extraction of tooth roots. [exo- + L. *levare,* to raise]

ex·om·pha·los (eks-om'fă-lŭs). **1.** Protrusion of the umbilicus. SYN exumbilication (1). **2.** SYN umbilical *hernia.* **3.** SYN omphalocele. [G. *ex,* out, + *omphalos,* umbilicus]

ex·on (ek'son). A portion of a DNA that codes for a section of the mature messenger RNA from that DNA, and is therefore expressed ("translated") into protein) at the ribosome. [ex- + on]

ex·on shuf·fle. The variation in the patterns by which RNA may produce diverse sets of exons from a single gene.

ex·o·nu·cle·ase (ek-sō-nū'klē-ās). A nuclease that releases one nucleotide at a time, serially, beginning at one end of a polynucleotide (nucleic acid); several have been prepared from *Escherichia coli,* designated e. I, e. II, etc.; e. III, which removes nucleotides from 3′ ends of DNA, is used in DNA sequencing. Cf. endonuclease.

ex·o·pep·ti·dase (ek-sō-pep'ti-dās). An enzyme that catalyzes the hydrolysis of the terminal amino acid of a peptide chain; *e.g.,* carboxypeptidase. Cf. endopeptidase.

Ex·o·phi·a·la (ek-sō-fī'ă-lă). A genus of pathogenic fungi having dematiaceous conidiophores with one- or two-celled annelloconidia. They cause mycetoma or phaeohyphomycosis; in cases of mycetoma, black granules develop in subcutaneous abscesses; in cases of phaeohyphomycosis, sclerotic bodies are found in tissues. [*exo* + G. *phiale,* a broad flat vessel]

E. jeansel'mei, a species found in cases of mycetoma or phaeohyphomycosis.

E. wernec'kii, a species that causes tinea nigra. SYN *Cladosporium werneckii.*

ex·o·pho·ria (ek'so-fō'rē-ă). Tendency of the eyes to deviate outward when fusion is suspended. SYN exodeviation (1). [exo- + G. *phora,* a carrying]

ex·o·phor·ic (ek-sō-fōr'ik). Relating to exophoria.

ex·oph·thal·mic (ek-sof-thal'mik). Relating to exophthalmos; marked by prominence of the eyeball.

ex·oph·thal·mom·e·ter (ek-sof-thal-mom'ě-ter). An instrument to measure the distance between the anterior pole of the eye and a fixed reference point, often the zygomatic bone. SYN orthometer, proptometer, statometer. [exophthalmos + G. *metron,* measure]

ex·oph·thal·mos, ex·oph·thal·mus (ek-sof-thal'mos). Protrusion of one or both eyeballs; can be congenital and familial, or due to pathology, such as a retro-orbital tumor (usually unilateral) or thyroid disease (usually bilateral). SYN proptosis. [G. *ex,* out, + *ophthalmos,* eye]

endocrine e., e. associated with thyroid gland disorders. SEE Graves' *ophthalmopathy,* Graves' *orbitopathy.*

malignant e., relentless, progressive protrusion of the eyeballs.

ex·o·phyte (ek'sō-fīt). An exterior or external plant parasite. [exo- + G. *phyton,* plant]

ex·o·phyt·ic (ek-sō-fit'ik). **1.** Pertaining to an exophyte. **2.** Denoting a neoplasm or lesion that grows outward from an epithelial surface.

ex·o·plasm (ek'sō-plazm). SYN ectoplasm.

ex·o·se·ro·sis (ek'sō-se-rō'sis). Serous exudation from the skin surface, as in eczema or abrasions.

ex·o·skel·e·ton (ek-sō-skel'ĕ-tŏn). **1.** All hard parts, such as hair, teeth, nails, feathers, dermal plates, scales, etc., developed from the ectoderm or somatic mesoderm in vertebrates. SYN dermoskeleton. **2.** Outer chitinous envelope of an insect, or the chitinous or calcareous covering of certain Crustacea and other invertebrates.

ex·o·spore (ek'sō-spōr). An exogenous spore, not encased in a sporangium. [exo- + G. *sporos,* seed]

ex·o·spo·ri·um (ek-sō-spō'rē-um). The outer envelope of a spore.

ex·os·tec·to·my (ek-sos-tek'tō-mē). Removal of an exostosis. SYN exostosectomy. [exostosis + G. *ektomē,* excision]

ex·os·to·sec·to·my (ek-sos-tō-sek'tō-mē). SYN exostectomy.

ex·os·to·sis, pl. **ex·os·to·ses** (eks-os-tō'sis, -sēz). A cartilage-capped bony projection arising from any bone that develops from cartilage. SEE ALSO osteochondroma. SYN hyperostosis (2), poroma (2). [exo- + G. *osteon,* bone, + *-osis,* condition]

e. bursa'ta, an e. arising from the joint surface of a bone and covered with cartilage and a synovial sac.

e. cartilagin'ea, an ossified chondroma arising from the epiphysis or joint surface of a bone.

hereditary multiple exostoses [MIM*133700], a disturbance of enchondral bone growth in which multiple, generally benign osteochondromas of long bones appear during childhood, commonly with shortening of the radius and fibula; the ill-effects are usually mechanical but malignant change is rare; autosomal dominant inheritance. SYN diaphysial aclasis, hereditary deforming chondrodystrophy (1), multiple e., osteochondromatosis.

ivory e., a small, rounded, eburnated tumor arising from a bone, usually one of the cranial bones.

multiple e., SYN hereditary multiple exostoses.

solitary osteocartilaginous e., SYN osteochondroma.

subungual e., painful osseous outgrowths that elevate the nail of the great toe or fingers in young people.

ex·o·ter·ic (ek-sō-tār'ik). Of external origin; arising outside the organism. [G. *exōterikos,* outer]

ex·o·ther·mic (ek-sō-ther'mik). **1.** Denoting a chemical reaction during which heat (*i.e.,* enthalpy) is emitted. Cf. endothermic. **2.** Relating to the external warmth of the body. [exo- + G. *thermē,* heat]

ex·o·tox·ic (ek-sō-tok'sik). **1.** Relating to an exotoxin. **2.** Relating to the introduction of an exogenous poison or toxin.

ex·o·tox·in (ek-sō-tok'sin). A specific, soluble, antigenic, usually heat labile, injurious substance elaborated by certain Gram-positive or Gram-negative bacteria; it is formed within the cell, but is released into the environment where it is rapidly active in extremely small amounts; most e.'s are protein in nature (MW 70,000 to 900,000) and can have the toxic portion of the molecule destroyed by heat, prolonged storage, or chemicals; the nontoxic but antigenic form is a toxoid. SYN ectotoxin, extracellular toxin.

ex·o·tro·pia (ek-sō-trō'pē-ă). That type of strabismus in which the visual axes diverge; may be paralytic or concomitant, monocular or alternating, constant or intermittent. SYN divergent squint, divergent strabismus, exodeviation (2), external squint, wall-eye (1). [exo- + G. *tropē,* turn]

A-e., divergent strabismus greater in downward than in upward gaze.

basic e., e. in which the strabismus is the same for near and far vision.

divergence excess e., e. in which the strabismus is notably greater for far vision than for near vision.

divergence insufficiency e., e. in which the strabismus is notably greater for near vision than for far vision.

V-e., divergent strabismus greater in upward than in downward gaze.

X-e., increasing divergence from primary position in both upward and downward gaze.

ex·pan·sion (eks-pan'shŭn). **1.** An increase in size as of chest or

lungs. **2.** The spreading out of any structure, as a tendon. **3.** An expanse; a wide area. [L. *ex-pando,* pp. -*pansus,* to spread out]

clonal e. (klō'nal), production of daughter cells all arising originally from a single cell.

extensor e., SYN extensor digital e.

extensor digital e., a triangular tendinous aponeurosis including the tendon of the extensor digitorum centrally, interosseus tendons on each side, and a lumbrical tendon laterally. It covers the dorsal aspect of the metacarpophalangeal joint and the proximal phalanx. SYN dorsal hood, extensor aponeurosis, extensor e.

hygroscopic e., (1) e. due to the absorption of moisture; **(2)** in dental casting, the addition of water to the surface of the casting investment during setting to increase the size of the mold.

perceptual e., development of an ability to recognize and interpret sensory stimuli through associations with past similar stimuli; perceptual e. by relaxation of defenses is a goal of psychotherapy.

setting e., the dimensional increase that occurs concurrently with the hardening of various materials, such as plaster of Paris.

wax e., in dentistry, a method of expanding wax patterns to compensate for the shrinkage of gold during the casting process.

ex·pan·sive·ness (ek-span'siv-nes). A state of optimism, loquacity, and reactivity.

ex·pec·ta·tion. In probability theory and statistics the true mean or average (of a sample distribution).

ex·pec·ta·tion of life. The average number of years of life an individual of a given age is expected to live if current mortality rates continue to apply; a statistical abstraction based on existing age-specific death rates.

e. o. l. at age x, The average number of additional years a person aged x would live if current mortality trends continue to apply, based on the age-specific death rates for a given year.

e. o. l. at birth, Average number of years of life a newborn baby can be expected to live if current mortality trends continue.

ex·pect·ed. In probability theory and statistics, interchangeable with mean or average; it need not be a probable or even possible value. For instance, the expected number of children in completed families may be 2.53, but that is not a possible size of any actual family.

ex·pec·to·rant (ek-spek'tō-rănt). **1.** Promoting secretion from the mucous membrane of the air passages or facilitating its expulsion. **2.** An agent that increases bronchial secretion and facilitates its expulsion. [L. *ex,* out, + *pectus,* chest]

ex·pec·to·rate (ek-spek'tō-rāt). To spit; to eject saliva, mucus, or other fluid from the mouth.

ex·pec·to·ra·tion (ek-spek-tō-rā'shŭn). **1.** Mucus and other fluids formed in the air passages and upper food passages (the mouth), and expelled by coughing. SEE ALSO sputum (1). **2.** The act of spitting; the expelling from the mouth of saliva, mucus, and other material from the air or upper food passages. SYN spitting.

prune-juice e., SYN prune-juice *sputum.*

ex·pe·ri·ence (ek-spēr'ē-ens). The feeling of emotions and sensations, as opposed to thinking; involvement in what is happening rather than abstract reflection on an event or interpersonal encounter. [L. *experientia,* fr. *experior,* to try]

corrective emotional e., reexposure under favorable circumstances to an emotional situation with which one could not cope in the past.

ex·per·i·ment (eks-per'i-ment). **1.** A study in which the investigator intentionally alters one or more factors under controlled conditions in order to study the effects of doing so. **2.** In nuclear magnetic resonance, the term applied to a pulse sequence. [L. *experimentum,* fr. *experior,* to test, try]

Carr-Purcell e., in magnetic resonance, the multiple spin echo technique.

control e., an e. used to check another, to verify the result, or to demonstrate what would have occurred had the factor under study been omitted. SEE ALSO control, control *animal.*

delayed reaction e., a method of measuring memory: a stimulus is presented and removed before the organism is permitted to respond to it; the interval during which the stimulus is absent,

ex

providing the organism responds correctly, is an indication of the length of memory.

double blind e., an e. conducted with neither experimenter nor subjects knowing which e. is the control; prevents bias in recording results. SEE ALSO double-masked e.

double-masked e., a double-blind study conducted so neither the subject nor the observer know the identity of the control or variable.

factorial e.'s, an experimental design in which two or more series of treatments are tried in all combinations.

hertzian e.'s, e.'s demonstrating that electromagnetic induction is propagated in waves, analogous to waves of light but not affecting the retina.

Mariotte's e., an e. in which one looks fixedly with one eye (the other being closed), at a black dot on a card, on which is also marked a black cross; as the card is moved to or from the eye, at a certain distance the cross becomes invisible but appears again as the card is moved further; this proves the absence of photoreceptors where the optic nerve enters the eye.

Nussbaum's e., exclusion of the glomeruli of the kidney from the circulation by ligation of the renal artery in animals, such as the frog, that have a renal portal system to maintain circulation to the tubules.

pulse-chase e., an e. in which an enzyme, a metabolic pathway, a culture of cells, etc., interacts with a brief addition (pulse) of a labeled compound followed by its removal and replacement (chase) by an excess of unlabeled compound.

Scheiner's e., a demonstration of accommodation; through two minute holes in a card, separated from each other by less than the diameter of the pupil, one looks at a pin; at a short distance from the eye the pin appears double; as it is moved from the eye a point is found where it appears single, and beyond which it remains single for the emmetropic eye, but for the myopic eye it soon again becomes double.

Stensen's e., compression of the abdominal aorta of an animal promptly causes paralysis of the posterior portions of the body since the blood supply to the lumbar cord is almost entirely shut off.

Weber's e., if the peripheral end of the divided vagus nerve is stimulated the heart is arrested in diastole.

ex·pi·ra·tion (eks-pi-rā'shŭn). **1.** SYN exhalation (1). **2.** a death. [L. *expiro* or *ex-spiro*, pp. *-atus*, to breathe out]

ex·pi·ra·to·ry (ek-spī'ră-tō-rē). Relating to expiration.

ex·pire (ek-spīr'). **1.** SYN exhale (1). **2.** To die.

ex·plant (eks'plant). Living tissue transferred from an organism to an artificial medium for culture.

ex·plan·ta·tion (eks-plan-tā'shŭn). The act of transferring an explant.

ex·plo·ra·tion (eks-plōr-ā'shŭn). An active examination, usually involving endoscopy or a surgical procedure, to ascertain conditions present as an aid in diagnosis. [L. *ex-ploro*, pp. *-ploratus*, to explore]

ex·plor·a·to·ry (eks-plōr'ă-tōr-ē). Relating to, or with a view to, exploration.

ex·plor·er (ek'splōr'er). A sharp pointed probe used to investigate natural or restored tooth surfaces in order to detect caries or other defects.

ex·plo·sion (eks-plō'zhŭn). A sudden and violent increase in volume accompanied by noise and release of energy, as from a chemical change, nuclear reaction, or escape of gases or vapors under pressure. [L. *explosio*, fr. *explodo*, to drive away by clapping]

ex·pose (eks-pōz'). To perform or undergo exposure. [O. Fr. *exposer*, fr. L. *ex-pono*, pp. *ex-positum*, to set out, expose]

ex·po·sure (eks-pō'zhŭr). **1.** A displaying, revealing, exhibiting, or making accessible. **2.** In dentistry, loss of hard tooth structure covering the dental pulp due to caries, dental instrumentation, or trauma. **3.** Proximity and/or contact with a source of a disease agent in such a manner that effective transmission of the agent or harmful effects of the agent may occur. **4.** The amount of a factor to which a group or individual was exposed, in contrast to the dose, the amount that enters or interacts with the organism.

ex·press (eks-pres'). To press or squeeze out. [L. *ex-premo*, pp. *-pressus*, to press out]

ex·pres·sion (eks-presh'ŭn). **1.** Squeezing out; expelling by pressure. **2.** Mobility of the features giving a particular emotional significance to the face. SYN facies (3). **3.** Any act by an individual. **4.** Something that manifests something else.

differential gene e., gene e. that responds to signals or triggers; a means of gene regulation; *e.g.,* effects of certain hormones on protein biosynthesis.

gene e., (1) the detectable effect of a gene. (2) appearance of an inherited trait; for many reasons genetic (*e.g.,* recessiveness, hypostasis, parastasis) and environmental (the absence of pertinent challenges), a gene may not be expressed at all. In those circumstances, it will have no impact on Darwinian evolution.

integrated rate e., an equation of a chemical or enzyme-catalyzed reaction for the entire progress curve.

e. library, a collection of plasmid or phage containing a representative sample of cDNA or genomic fragments that are constructed in such a way that they will be transcribed and translated by the host organism (usually bacteria).

ex·pres·siv·i·ty (eks-pres-siv'i-tē). In clinical genetics, the form in which a gene is manifested.

ex·pul·sive (eks-pŭl'siv). Tending to expel. [L. *ex-pello*, pp. *-pulsus*, to drive out]

ex·qui·site (eks-kwiz'it). Extremely intense, keen, sharp; said of pain or tenderness in a part. [L. *exquiro*, pp. *exquisitus*, to search out]

ex·san·gui·nate (ek-sang'gwi-nāt). **1.** To remove or withdraw the circulating blood; to make bloodless. **2.** SYN exsanguine. [L. *ex,* out, + *sanguis* (*-guin*), blood]

ex·san·gui·na·tion (ek-sang'gwi-nā'shŭn). Removal of blood; making exsanguine.

ex·san·guine (ek-sang'gwin). Deprived of blood. SYN exsanguinate (2).

ex·sect (ek-sekt'). Rarely used term for excise. [L. *ex- seco,* pp. *-sectus,* to cut out]

ex·sec·tion (ek-sek'shŭn). Rarely used term for excision.

ex·sic·cant (ek-sik'ant). SYN desiccant.

ex·sic·cate (ek'si-kāt). SYN desiccate.

ex·sic·ca·tion (ek-si-kā'shŭn). **1.** SYN desiccation. **2.** The removal of water of crystallization. SYN dehydration (3). [L. *ex sicco,* pp. *siccatus,* to dry up]

ex·so·ma·tize (ek-sō'mă-tīz). To remove from the body. [G. *ex,* out of, + *sōma,* body]

ex·sorp·tion (ek-sōrp'shŭn). Movement of substances from the blood into the lumen of the gut. [G. *ex,* out, + *sorbēre,* to suck]

ex·stro·phy (ek'strō-fē). Congenital eversion of a hollow organ. SYN ecstrophe. [G. *ex,* out, + *strophē,* a turning]

e. of the bladder, a congenital gap in the anterior wall of the bladder and the abdominal wall in front of it, the posterior wall of the bladder being exposed. SYN ectopia vesicae.

e. of the cloaca, a developmental anomaly in which an area of intestinal mucosa is interposed between two separate areas of the urinary bladder. SYN ectopia cloacae.

cloacal e., congenital anomaly with two exstrophied bladder units separated by an exstrophied segment of intestine, which is usually cecum, receiving ileum superiorly and continuing distally to blend microcolon. A number of variants of anatomic disarray can occur.

ex·tend (eks-tend'). To straighten a limb, to diminish or extinguish the angle formed by flexion; to place the distal segment of a limb in such a position that its axis is continuous with that of the proximal segment. [L. *ex- tendo,* pp. *-tensus,* to stretch out]

ex·ten·sion (eks-ten'shŭn). **1.** The act of bringing the distal portion of a joint in continuity (though only parallel) with the long axis of the proximal portion. **2.** A pulling or dragging force exerted on a limb in a distal direction. **3.** Obsolete term for traction. [L. *extensio,* to stretch out]

Buck's e., apparatus for applying longitudinal skin traction on the leg through contact between the skin and adhesive tape; friction between the tape and skin permits application of force, which is applied through a cord over a pulley, suspending a weight; elevation of the foot of the bed allows the body to act as a counterweight. SYN Buck's traction.

nail e., an obsolete method of e., by a weight on a nail or pin in the distal fragment of a fracture.

primer e., a technique for determining the 5'-untranslated region of a specific mRNA molecule. Uses an oligonucleotide complementary to the known RNA sequence as a primer for cDNA synthesis via reverse transcriptase.

ridge e., an intraoral surgical operation for deepening the labial, buccal, and/or lingual sulci; it is performed to increase the intraoral height of the alveolar ridge in order to assist denture retention.

skeletal e., SYN skeletal *traction.*

ex·ten·sor (eks-ten'ser, -sōr) [NA]. A muscle the contraction of which causes movement at a joint with the consequence that the limb or body assumes a more straight line, or so that the distance between the parts proximal and distal to the joint is increased or extended; the antagonist of a flexor. SEE muscle. [L. one who stretches, fr. *ex-tendo,* to stretch out]

ex·te·ri·or (eks-tē'rē-ōr). Outside; external. [L.]

ex·te·ri·or·ize (eks-tēr'ē-ōr-īz). 1. To direct a patient's interests, thoughts, or feelings into a channel leading outside the self, to some definite aim or object. 2. To expose an organ temporarily for observation, or permanently for purposes of physiologic experiment, *e.g.,* fixation of a segment of bowel with blood supply intact to the outer aspect of the abdominal wall.

ex·tern (eks'tern). An advanced student or recent graduate who assists in the medical or surgical care of hospital patients; formerly, one who lived outside of the institution. [F. *externe,* outside, a day scholar]

ex·ter·nal (eks-ter'năl). On the outside or farther from the center; often incorrectly used to mean lateral. SYN externus. [L. *externus*]

ex·ter·nus (eks-ter'nŭs). SYN external.

ex·ter·o·cep·tive (eks'ter-ō-sep'tiv). Relating to the exteroceptors; denoting the surface of the body containing the end organs adapted to receive impressions or stimuli from without. [L. *exterus,* outside, + *capio,* to take]

ex·ter·o·cep·tor (eks'ter-ō-sep'ter, -tōr). One of the peripheral end organs of the afferent nerves in the skin or mucous membrane, which respond to stimulation by external agents. [L. *exterus,* external, + *receptor,* receiver]

ex·ter·o·fec·tive (eks'ter-ō-fek'tiv). Pertaining to the response of the nervous system to external stimuli. [L. *extero,* from outside, + *affectus,* affected]

ex·tinc·tion (eks-tingk'shŭn). 1. In behavior modification or classical or operant conditioning, a progressive decrease in the frequency of a response that is not positively reinforced; the withdrawal of reinforcers known to maintain an undesirable behavior. SEE conditioning. 2. SYN absorbance. [L. *extinguo,* to quench]

specific e., SYN specific absorption *coefficient.*

visual e., SYN pseudo-*hemianopia.*

ex·tin·guish (eks-ting'gwish). 1. To abolish; to quench, as a flame; to cause loss of identity; to destroy. 2. In psychology, to progressively abolish a previously conditioned response. SEE conditioning. [L. *extinguo,* to quench]

ex·tir·pa·tion (eks-tir-pā'shŭn). Partial or complete removal of an organ or diseased tissue. [L. *extirpo,* to root out, fr. *stirps,* a stalk, root]

Exton, William G., U.S. physician, 1876–1943. SEE E. *reagent.*

ex·tor·sion (eks-tōr'shŭn). 1. Outward rotation of a limb or of an organ. 2. Conjugate rotation of the upper poles of each cornea outward. SYN excyclotorsion. [L. *extorsio,* fr. *ex- torqueo,* to twist out]

ex·tor·tor (eks-tōr'ter, -tōr). An outward rotator.

△**ex·tra-.** Without, outside of. [L.]

ex·tra-ar·tic·u·lar (eks-tră-ar-tik'yū-lăr). Outside of a joint.

ex·tra-ax·i·al (eks-tră-aks'ē-ăl). Off the axis; applied to intracerebral lesions that do not arise from the brain itself.

ex·tra·buc·cal (eks-tră-bŭk'ăl). Outside or not part of the cheek.

ex·tra·bul·bar (eks-tra-bul'bar). Outside of or unrelated to any bulb, such as the bulb of the urethra, or the medulla oblongata.

ex·tra·cal·i·ce·al (eks'tră-kă-lis'ē-ăl). Outside of a calix.

ex·tra·cap·su·lar (eks'tră-kap'sū-lăr). Outside of the capsule of a joint.

ex·tra·car·pal (eks-tră-kar'păl). 1. Outside of, having no relation to, the carpus. 2. On the outer side of the carpus.

ex·tra·cel·lu·lar (eks-tră-sel'yū-lăr). Outside the cells.

ex·tra·chro·mo·som·al (eks'tră-krō-mō-sōm'ăl). Outside of, or separated from, a chromosome.

ex·tra·cor·po·re·al (eks'tră-kōr-pō'rē-ăl). Outside of, or unrelated to, the body or any anatomical "corpus."

ex·tra·cor·pus·cu·lar (eks'tră-kōr-pŭs'kyū-lăr). Outside the corpuscles, especially the blood corpuscles.

ex·tra·cra·ni·al (eks-tră-krā'nē-ăl). Outside of the cranial cavity.

ex·tract (eks'trakt). 1 (ek'strakt). A concentrated preparation of a drug obtained by removing the active constituents of the drug with suitable solvents, evaporating all or nearly all of the solvent, and adjusting the residual mass or powder to the prescribed standard. 2 (ek-strakt'). To remove part of a mixture with a solvent. 3. To perform extraction. [L. *ex-traho,* pp. *-tractus,* to draw out]

alcoholic e., a solid e. obtained by extracting the alcohol-soluble principles of a drug, followed by the evaporation of the alcohol.

allergenic e., e. (usually containing protein) from various sources, *e.g.,* food, bacteria, pollen, and the like, suspected of specific action in stimulating manifestations of allergy; may be used for skin testing or desensitization. SYN allergic e.

allergic e., SYN allergenic e.

belladonna e., a powdered e. from the leaves and/or roots of *Atropa belladonna;* used to formulate various pharmaceutical dosage forms. Contains the alkaloids of belladonna (atropine and scopolamine) and has been used in the treatment of ulcers, diarrhea, and parkinsonism.

Büchner e., a cell-free e. of yeast, such as was prepared by Eduard and Hans Büchner and observed to catalyze alcoholic fermentation; this observation essentially eliminated "vitalism" as being responsible for biological chemical reactions and initiated the beginnings of modern biochemistry (enzymology).

equivalent e., a fluidextract of the same strength, weight for weight, as the original drug. SYN valoid.

fluid e., SEE fluidextract.

hydroalcoholic e., a solid e. obtained by extracting the soluble principles of the drug with alcohol and water, followed by evaporation of the solution.

liquid e., SYN fluidextract.

pollen e., liquid obtained by extracting the protein from the pollen of plants used for diagnostic testing or treatment.

ex·tract·ant (ek-strak'tant). An agent used to isolate or extract a substance from a mixture or combination of substances, from the tissues, or from a crude drug.

ex·trac·tion (ek-strak'shŭn). 1. Luxation and removal of a tooth from its alveolus. 2. Partitioning of material (solute) into a solvent. 3. The active portion of a drug; the making of an extract. 4. Surgical removal by pulling out. 5. Removal of the fetus from the uterus or vagina at or near the end of pregnancy, either manually or with instruments. 6. Removal by suction of the product of conception before a menstrual period has been missed. [L. *ex-traho,* pp. *-tractus,* to draw out]

Baker's pyridine e., hot pyridine treatment of tissues fixed in dilute Bouin's fixative, used to extract phospholipids from tissues as a control in the histochemical staining of this material.

breech e., obstetrical e. of the baby by the buttocks.

partial breech e., assisted breech delivery by the obstetrician with spontaneous delivery of the fetus to the level of the umbilicus.

podalic e., obstetrical e. of the baby by the feet.

serial e., the selective e. of certain deciduous or permanent teeth, or both, during the early years of dental development, usually with the eventual e. of the first, or occasionally the second,

ex

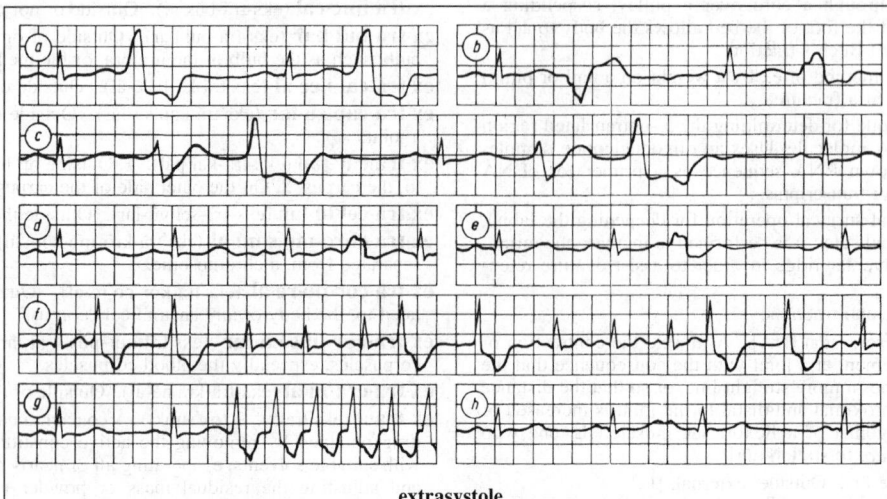

extrasystole

ventricular extrasystole: a) monomorphic (bigeminy); b) polymorphic (bigeminy); c) polymorphic (trigeminy); d) interpolated; e) compensatory; f) return; g) paroxysmal tachycardia; h) atrial extrasystole

premolars, to encourage autonomous adjustment of moderate to severe crowding of anterior teeth; it may or may not require subsequent orthodontic treatment.

spontaneous breech e., delivery of a fetus in the breech presentation without e. by the obstetrician.

total breech e., delivery of a fetus in breech presentation with complete e. of the entire fetal body from the uterus.

ex·trac·tives (ek-strak′tivs). Substances present in vegetable or animal tissue that can be separated by successive treatment with solvents and recovered by evaporation of the solution.

ex·trac·tor (ek-strak′ter, tōr). Instrument for use in drawing or pulling out any natural part, as a tooth, or a foreign body.

vacuum e., device for producing traction upon the head of a fetus by means of a soft cup held by a vacuum.

ex·tra·cys·tic (eks-strǎ-sis′tik). Outside of, or unrelated to, the gallbladder or urinary bladder or any cystic tumor.

ex·tra·du·ral (eks-strǎ-dū′răl). 1. On the outer side of the dura mater. 2. Unconnected with the dura mater.

ex·tra·em·bry·on·ic (eks′trǎ-em-brē-on′ik). Outside the embryonic body; e.g., those membranes involved with the embryo's protection and nutrition which are discarded at birth without being incorporated in its body.

ex·tra·ep·i·phy·si·al (eks′trǎ-ep-i-fiz′ē-ǎl). Not relating to, or connected with, an epiphysis.

ex·tra·gen·i·tal (eks′trǎ-jen′i-tǎl). Outside of, away from, or unrelated to, the genital organs.

ex·tra·he·pat·ic (eks-strǎ-he-pat′ik). Outside of, or unrelated to, the liver.

ex·tra·jec·tion (eks-strǎ-jek′shŭn). Attributing or projecting one's own psychic process to another person. [L. *ex*, out of, + *jacio*, to cast]

ex·tra·lig·a·men·tous (eks-strǎ-lig-ǎ-men′tŭs). Outside of, or unconnected with, a ligament.

ex·tra·mal·le·o·lus (eks-strǎ-mal-ē′ō-lŭs). SYN lateral *malleolus.*

ex·tra·med·ul·lary (eks-strǎ-med′yū-lār-ē). Outside of, or unrelated to, any medulla, especially the medulla oblongata.

ex·tra·mi·to·chon·dri·al (eks-strǎ-mī-tō-kon′drē-al). Outside of the mitochondria.

ex·tra·mu·ral (eks-strǎ-myū′răl). Outside, not in the substance of, the wall of a part. [extra- + L. *murus,* wall]

ex·tra·ne·ous (eks-trā′nē-ŭs). Outside of the organism and not belonging to it. [L. *extraneus*]

ex·tra·nu·cle·ar (eks-strǎ-nū′klē-er). Located outside, or not involving, a cell nucleus.

ex·tra·oc·u·lar (eks-strǎ-ok′yū-lǎr). Adjacent to but outside the eyeball.

ex·tra·o·ral (eks-strǎ-ō′răl). Outside of the oral cavity; external to the oral cavity. In its usual use it includes anything external to the lips and cheeks also.

ex·tra·ov·u·lar (eks′trǎ-ov′yū-lǎr, -ōv′yū-lǎr). Outside the egg; existence after hatching from the egg, as in reptiles and birds.

ex·tra·pap·il·lary (eks-strǎ-pap′i-lā-rē). Unconnected with any papillary structure.

ex·tra·pa·ren·chy·mal (eks′trǎ-pǎ-reng′kī-mǎl). Unrelated to the parenchyma of an organ.

ex·tra·per·i·ne·al (eks-strǎ-per-i-ne′al). Not connected with the perineum.

ex·tra·per·i·os·te·al (eks-strǎ-per-ē-os′tē-ǎl). Not connected with, or unrelated to, the periosteum.

ex·tra·per·i·to·ne·al (eks-strǎ-per-i-tō-nē′ǎl). Outside of the peritoneal cavity.

ex·tra·phys·i·o·log·ic (eks′trǎ-fiz-ē-ō-loj′ik). Outside of the domain of physiology; more than physiologic, therefore pathologic.

ex·tra·pla·cen·tal (eks-strǎ-pla-sen′tǎl). Unrelated to the placenta.

ex·tra·pros·tat·ic (eks-strǎ-pros-tat′ik). Outside of, or independent of, the prostate.

ex·tra·psy·chic (eks-strǎ-fiz′ik). Denoting the psychological dynamics that occur in the mind in association with the individual's exchanges with other persons or events. Cf. intrapsychic.

ex·tra·pul·mo·nary (eks-strǎ-pŭl′mō-nār-ē). Outside of, or having no relation to, the lungs.

ex·tra·py·ram·i·dal (eks-strǎ-pi-ram′i-dǎl). Other than the pyramidal tract. SEE extrapyramidal motor *system.*

ex·tra·sen·so·ry (eks-strǎ-sen′sōr-ē). Outside or beyond the ordinary senses; not limited to the senses, as in extrasensory *perception.*

ex·tra·se·rous (eks-strǎ-sē′rŭs). Outside a serous cavity.

ex·tra·so·mat·ic (eks-strǎ-sō-mat′ik). Outside of, or unrelated to, the body.

ex·tra·sys·to·le (eks′trǎ-sis′tō-lē). A nonspecific word for an ectopic beat from any source in the heart. SYN premature beat, premature systole.

atrial e., a premature contraction of the heart arising from an ectopic atrial focus.

atrioventricular e. (AVE), A-V e., an e. arising from the "junctional" tissues, either the A-V node or A-V bundle. SYN junctional e.

atrioventricular nodal e., A-V nodal e., a premature beat arising from the A-V junction and leading to a simultaneous or almost simultaneous contraction of atria and ventricles.

auricular e., SYN atrial e.

infranodal e., SYN ventricular e.

interpolated e., a ventricular e. which, instead of being followed by a compensatory pause, is sandwiched between two consecutive sinus cycles.

junctional e., SYN atrioventricular e.

lower nodal e., obsolete term for a nodal e. supposed to arise from the lower part of the A-V node, recognized in the electrocardiogram by the retrograde P wave that follows the QRS complex.

midnodal e., obsolete term for a nodal e. supposed to arise from the midportion of the A-V node and recognized in the electrocardiogram by absence of the P wave that is lost within the normal QRS complex.

return e., a form of reciprocal rhythm in which the impulse having arisen in the ventricle ascends toward the atria, but before reaching the atria is reflected back to the ventricles to produce a second ventricular contraction.

supraventricular e., an e. arising from a center above the ventricle, *i.e.,* arising from the atrium or A-V junction.

upper nodal e., obsolete term for a nodal e. supposed to arise from the upper part of the A-V node; recognized in the electrocardiogram by a retrograde P wave preceding the QRS complex by an abnormally short P-R interval.

ventricular e., a premature contraction of the ventricle. SYN infranodal e.

ex·tra·tar·sal (eks-tră-tar′săl). **1.** Outside, having no relation to, the tarsus. **2.** On the outer side of the tarsus.

ex·tra·tra·che·al (eks-tră-trā′kē-ăl). Outside of the trachea.

ex·tra·tub·al (eks-tră-tū′băl). Outside of any tube; specifically, not in the auditory (eustachian) or uterine (fallopian) tubes.

ex·tra·u·ter·ine (eks-tră-yū′ter-in). Outside of the uterus.

ex·tra·vag·i·nal (eks-tră-vaj′i-năl). Outside of the vagina.

ex·trav·a·sate (eks-trav′ă-sāt). **1.** To exude from or pass out of a vessel into the tissues, said of blood, lymph, or urine. **2.** The substance thus exuded. SYN extravasation (2), suffusion (4). [L. *extra,* out of, + *vas,* vessel]

ex·trav·a·sa·tion (eks-trav′ă-sā′shŭn). **1.** The act of extravasating. **2.** SYN extravasate (2). [extra- + L. *vas,* vessel]

ex·tra·vas·cu·lar (eks-tră-vas′kyŭ-lăr). Outside of the blood vessels or lymphatics or of any special blood vessel.

ex·tra·ven·tric·u·lar (eks-tră-ven-trik′yū-lăr). Outside of any ventricle, especially of one of the ventricles of the heart.

ex·tra·ver·sion (eks-tră-ver′zhŭn, -shŭn). SYN extroversion.

ex·tra·vert (eks′-tră-vert). SYN extrovert.

ex·tra·vi·su·al (ek-stră-vizh′ū-ăl). Outside the field of vision, or beyond the visible spectrum.

ex·trem·i·tal (eks-trem′i-tăl). Relating to an extremity. SEE ALSO distal.

ex·trem·i·tas (eks-trem′i-tas) [NA]. SYN extremity. SEE limb. [L. fr. *extremus,* last, outermost]

e. acromia′lis clavic′ulae [NA], SYN acromial *extremity* of clavicle.

e. ante′rior [NA], SYN anterior *extremity.*

e. infe′rior [NA], SYN inferior *pole.*

e. infe′rior ren′is [NA], SYN inferior *pole* of kidney.

e. infe′rior tes′tis [NA], SYN inferior *pole* of testis.

e. poste′rior [NA], SYN posterior *extremity.*

e. sterna′lis clavic′ulae [NA], SYN sternal *extremity* of clavicle.

e. supe′rior [NA], SYN superior *pole.*

e. supe′rior ren′is [NA], SYN superior *pole* of kidney.

e. supe′rior tes′tis [NA], SYN superior *pole* of testis.

e. tuba′ria ovar′ii [NA], SYN tubal *extremity* of ovary.

e. uteri′na ovar′ii [NA], SYN uterine *extremity* of ovary.

ex·trem·i·ty (eks-trem′i-tē). One of the ends of an elongated or pointed structure. Incorrectly used to mean limb. SYN extremitas [NA].

Lown classification of extrasystoles	
ventricular arrhythmia (type)	class
no VES	0
< 30 VES/hr.	I
> 30 VES/hr.	II
multiform VES bigeminus	III a III b
couplet (2 VES in a row) salve	IV a IV b
R-on-T phenomenon, VES	V
(VES = ventricular extrasystole)	

acromial e. of clavicle, the flattened lateral end of the clavicle that articulates with the acromion and is anchored to the coracoid process by the conoid and trapezoid ligaments. SYN extremitas acromialis claviculae [NA], acromial end of clavicle.

anterior e., specifically, the anterior end of the spleen (extremitas anterior splenis [NA]). SYN extremitas anterior [NA].

anterior e. of caudate nucleus, SYN *head* of the caudate nucleus.

inferior e., (1) SYN inferior *pole.* **(2)** incorrectly, but commonly used for lower *limb.*

lower e., SYN lower *limb.*

posterior e., specifically, the posterior end of the spleen (extremitas posterior splenis [NA]). SYN extremitas posterior [NA].

sternal e. of clavicle, the enlarged medial end of the clavicle that articulates with the manubrium sterni. SYN extremitas sternalis claviculae [NA], sternal end of clavicle.

superior e., (1) SYN superior *pole.* **(2)** incorrectly, but commonly used term for upper *limb.*

tubal e. of ovary, the rounded lateral end of the ovary, usually directed toward the infundibulum of the uterine tube. SYN extremitas tubaria ovarii [NA], lateral pole.

upper e., SYN upper *limb.*

upper e. of fibula, SYN *head* of fibula.

uterine e. of ovary, the rounded medial end of the ovary, usually directed toward the uterus. SYN extremitas uterina ovarii [NA], medial pole of ovary.

ex·trin·sic (eks-trin′sik). Originating outside of the part where found or upon which it acts; denoting especially a muscle, such as extrinsic muscles of hand. [L. *extrinsecus,* from without]

ex·tro·gas·tru·la·tion (eks′trō-gas-trū-lā′shŭn). Evagination of the primitive gut material during gastrulation instead of the normal invagination, as the result of some natural or experimental manipulation of the developing embryo or its environment.

ex·tro·spec·tion (eks-trō-spek′shŭn). Constant examination of the skin because of fear of parasites or dirt. [ex- + L. *spectō,* pp. *-atus,* to look at, inspect]

ex·tro·ver·sion (eks′trō-ver′zhŭn, -shŭn). **1.** A turning outward. **2.** A trait involving social intercourse, as practiced by an extrovert. Cf. introversion. SYN extraversion. [incorrectly formed fr. L. *extra,* outside, + *verto,* pp. *versus,* to turn]

ex·tro·vert (eks′trō-vert). A gregarious person whose chief interests lie outside the self, and who is socially self-confident and involved in the affairs of others. Cf. introvert. SYN extravert.

ex·trude (eks-trūd′). To thrust, force, or press out.

ex·tru·sion (eks-trū′zhŭn). **1.** A thrusting or forcing out of a normal position. **2.** The overeruption or migration of a tooth beyond its normal occlusal position.

e. of a tooth, elongation of a tooth; movement of a tooth in an occlusal or incisal direction.

ex·tu·bate (eks′tū-bāt). To accomplish extubation.

ex·tu·ba·tion (eks′tū-bā′shŭn). Removal of a tube from an organ, structure, or orifice; specifically, removal of the tube after intubation. [L. *ex,* out, + *tuba,* tube]

ex·u·ber·ant (ek-zū′ber-ănt). Denoting excessive proliferation or growth, as of a tissue or granulation. [L. *exubero,* to abound, be abundant]

ex·u·date (eks′ū-dāt). Any fluid that has exuded out of a tissue or its capillaries, more specifically because of injury or inflammation (*e.g.,* peritoneal pus in peritonitis, or the e. that forms a scab over a skin abrasion) in which case it is characteristically high in protein and white blood cells. Cf. transudate. SYN exudation (2). [L. *ex,* out, + *sudo,* to sweat]

ex·u·da·tion (eks-ū-dā′shŭn). **1.** The act or process of exuding. **2.** SYN exudate.

ex·ud·a·tive (eks-ū′dă-tiv). Relating to the process of exudation or to an exudate.

ex·ude (ek-zūd′). In general, to ooze or pass gradually out of a body structure or tissue; more specifically, restricted to a fluid or semisolid that so passes and may become encrusted or infected, because of injury or inflammation. [L. *ex,* out, + *sudo,* to sweat]

ex·ul·cer·ans (eks-ŭl′ser-anz). Ulcerating.

ex·um·bil·i·ca·tion (eks′ŭm-bil-i-kā′shŭn). **1.** SYN exomphalos (1). **2.** SYN umbilical *hernia.* **3.** SYN omphalocele. [L. *ex,* out, + *umbilicus,* navel]

ex·u·vi·ae (ex-ū′vē-ē). Obsolete term for any cast-off parts, as desquamated epidermis. [L. clothing, etc., stripped from the body, fr. *exuo,* pp. *exutus,* to strip off]

eye (ī). **1.** The organ of vision that consists of the eyeball and the optic nerve; SYN oculus [NA]. **2.** The area of the eye, including lids and other accessory organs of the eye; the contents of the orbit (common). [A.S. *eāge*]

amaurotic cat's e., a yellow reflex from the pupil in cases of retinoblastoma or pseudoglioma.

accommodation of eye age-related decrease in accommodative power (in diopters) for persons with normal vision	
8 years – 13.8 dptr	40 years – 5.8 dptr
16 years – 12.0 dptr	48 years – 2.5 dptr
24 years – 10.2 dptr	56 years – 1.25 dptr
32 years – 8.2 dptr	64 years – 1.1 dptr

aphakic e., the e. from which the lens is absent.

artificial e., a curved disk of opaque glass or plastic, containing an imitation iris and pupil in the center, inserted beneath the eyelids and supported by the orbital contents after evisceration or enucleation; it may be ready-made (stock) or custom-made.

black e., ecchymosis of the lids and their surroundings.

blear e., blepharitis accompanied by a viscid discharge that tends to cause the lid edges to cling together. SYN lippitude, lippitudo.

bleary e., sore, runny, watery e. with an associated lackluster appearance and, by extension, dimness of vision.

bovine cancer e., a malignant squamous cell carcinoma of cattle, especially the Hereford breed, that originates in the conjunctival mucous membranes or the surrounding skin; it occurs principally in range cattle having unpigmented skin around the eye and living in regions of intense sunlight.

compound e., the eye of arthropods, most highly developed in insects and crustaceans; the e. consists of a group of functionally related visual elements (ommatidia) whose corneal surfaces collectively form a segment of a sphere.

crossed e.'s, SYN strabismus.

cyclopian e., cyclopean e., SEE cyclopia.

dark-adapted e., an e. that has been in darkness or semidarkness and has undergone regeneration of rhodopsin (visual purple), which renders it more sensitive to reduced illumination. SYN scotopic e.

dominant e., the e. that is customarily used for monocular tasks. SYN master e.

epiphysial e., SYN pineal e.

exciting e., the injured e. in sympathetic ophthalmia.

fixing e., the e., in cases of strabismus, that is directed toward the object of regard.

hare's e., SYN lagophthalmia.

light-adapted e., an e. that has been exposed to light, with bleaching of rhodopsin (visual purple) and insensitivity to low illumination. SYN photopic e.

Listing's reduced e., a representation that simplifies calculations of retinal imagery: radius of anterior refracting surface, 5.1 mm; total length, 20 mm; distance of nodal point to retina, 15 mm.

master e., SYN dominant e.

parietal e., SYN pineal e.

phakic e., an e. containing the natural lens.

photopic e., SYN light-adapted e.

pineal e., a non-image-forming, photoreceptive e. in or near the median line in certain crustacea and lower vertebrates; homologue of pineal gland in higher forms. SYN epiphysial e., parietal e.

pink e., SEE pinkeye.

raccoon e.'s, descriptive term for the appearance produced by subconjunctival hemorrhages. SYN bilateral medial orbital ecchymoses.

reduced e., a simplified design of the ocular optical system, represented as having a single refracting surface and a uniform index of refraction; a model based on this concept is used in retinoscopy and ophthalmoscopy.

schematic e., the representation of the optical system of an ideal normal eye in which are listed the curvatures and indices of refraction of the refracting elements and their intervening distances.

scotopic e., SYN dark-adapted e.

spectacle e.'s, a condition in rats caused by pantothenic acid deficiency, and possibly lack of inositol as well, in which a hairless ring of inflamed skin surrounds the e.'s.

squinting e., the e., in cases of strabismus, that is not directed toward the object of regard.

sympathizing e., the uninjured e. in sympathetic ophthalmia that becomes involved later in the disease process.

watery e., (1) SYN epiphora. **(2)** excessive lacrimation.

web e., SYN pterygium (1).

eye·ball (ī′bawl). The eye proper without the appendages. SYN bulbus oculi [NA], bulb of eye, globe of eye.

eye bank. A place where corneas of eyes removed after death are preserved for subsequent keratoplasty.

eye·brow. The crescentic line of hairs at the superior edge of the orbit. SYN supercilium (1) [NA].

eye·glass·es. SYN spectacles.

eye·grounds (ī′growndz). The fundus of the eye as seen with the ophthalmoscope.

eye·lash. One of the stiff hairs projecting from the margin of the eyelid. SYN cilium (1).

ectopic e., the condition in which the e.'s grow from the eyelid at a site other than the lid margin. SYN canities poliosis.

piebald e., an isolated bundle of white e.'s among normally pigmented e.'s. SYN canities circumscripta, ciliary poliosis, poliosis.

eye·lid. One of the two movable folds covering the front of the eyeball when closed; formed of a fibrous core (tarsal plate) and the palpebral portions of the orbicularis oculi muscle covered with skin on the superficial, anterior surface and lined with conjunctiva on the deep, posterior surface; rapid contraction of the contained muscle fibers produces blinking; they each have fixed (orbital) and free margins, the latter separated centrally by the palpebral fissure, united at the lateral and medial palpebral commissures, and bearing eyelashes, the openings of tarsal and ciliary glands and (medially) the lacrimal puncta. SYN palpebra [NA], blepharon, lid.

lower e., the inferior, smaller and less mobile of the two e.'s; a check ligament from the inferior rectus muscle extends into it,

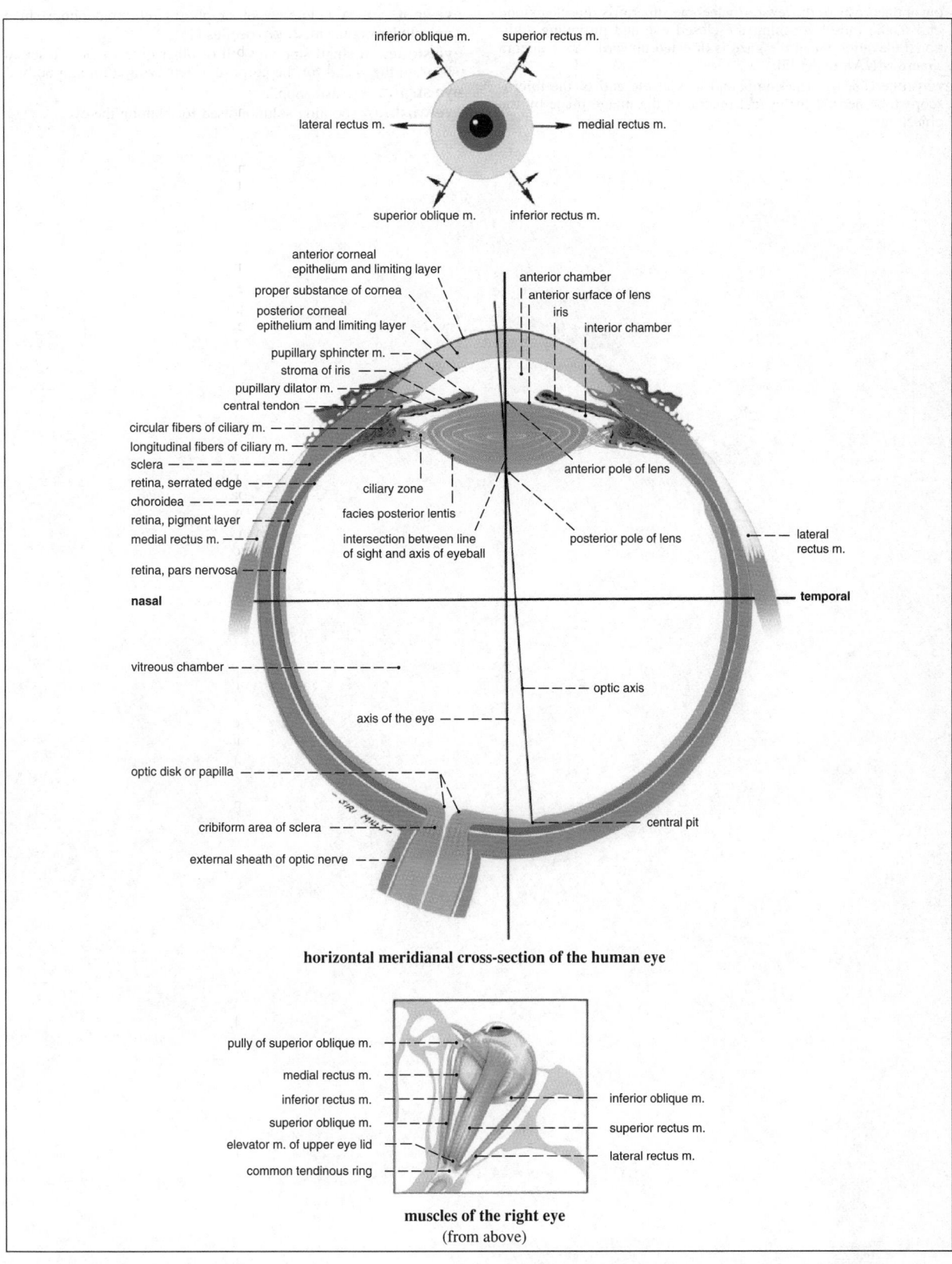

inferior oblique m.   superior rectus m.

lateral rectus m.   medial rectus m.

superior oblique m.   inferior rectus m.

anterior corneal epithelium and limiting layer
proper substance of cornea
posterior corneal epithelium and limiting layer
pupillary sphincter m.
stroma of iris
pupillary dilator m.
central tendon
circular fibers of ciliary m.
longitudinal fibers of ciliary m.
sclera
retina, serrated edge
choroidea
retina, pigment layer
medial rectus m.
retina, pars nervosa

anterior chamber
anterior surface of lens
iris
interior chamber

anterior pole of lens

ciliary zone
facies posterior lentis
intersection between line of sight and axis of eyeball

posterior pole of lens

nasal

temporal

lateral rectus m.

vitreous chamber

optic axis

axis of the eye

optic disk or papilla

cribiform area of sclera

external sheath of optic nerve

central pit

horizontal meridianal cross-section of the human eye

pully of superior oblique m.
medial rectus m.
inferior rectus m.
superior oblique m.
elevator m. of upper eye lid
common tendinous ring

inferior oblique m.
superior rectus m.
lateral rectus m.

muscles of the right eye
(from above)

pulling the lid inferiorly when the gaze is directed downward. SYN palpebra inferior [NA], lower lid.
third e., SYN *plica* semilunaris conjunctivae (2).

upper e., the superior, larger and more mobile of the two e.'s which covers most of the anterior surface of the eyeball, including the cornea, when closed; a portion of the lacrimal gland and the aponeurosis of the levator palpebrae superioris muscle extend into it, the muscle opening the closed eye and providing additional elevation when the gaze is directed upward. SYN palpebra superior [NA], upper lid.

eye·piece (ī′pēs). The compound lens at the end of the microscope tube nearest the eye; it magnifies the image made by the objective.

eye·spot. **1.** A colored spot or plastid (chromatophore) in a unicellular organism. **2.** SYN ocellus (1).

eye·stone. A small smooth shell or other object that is inserted beneath the eyelid for the purpose of removing a foreign body.

eye·strain. SYN asthenopia.

eye·wash. A soothing solution used for bathing the eye.

F 1. Symbol for fractional concentration, followed by subscripts indicating location and chemical species; free *energy*; Fahrenheit; farad; faraday; Faraday's *constant*; visual *field*; fluorine; force; filial *generation*, followed by subscript numerals indicating indicating specified matings; phenylalanine; variance *ratio*. **2.** Abbreviation for focus (1).

f Symbol for femto-; respiratory *frequency*; fugacity; formyl.

F.A.A.N. Abbreviation for Fellow of the American Academy of Nursing.

Fab. SEE Fab *fragment*.

fa·bel·la (fa-bel′lă). A sesamoid bone in the tendon of the lateral head of the gastrocnemius muscle. [Mod. L. dim. of *faba,* bean]

Faber, Knud H., Danish physician, 1862–1956. SEE F.'s *anemia, syndrome.*

fa·bism (fā′bizm). SYN favism. [L. *faba,* bean]

fab·ri·ca·tion (fab-ri-kā′shŭn). Telling false tales as true; *e.g.,* the malingering of symptoms or illness or feigning an incorrect response or calculation during a psychological or mental status examination. SYN fabulation.

Fabricius (Fabrizzi), Girolamo (Hieronymus ab Aquapendente), Italian anatomist and embryologist, 1537–1619. SEE *bursa* fabricii; F.'s *ship.*

Fabry, Johannes, German dermatologist, 1860–1930. SEE F.'s *disease.*

fab·u·la·tion (fab-yū-lā′shŭn). SYN fabrication. [L. *fabulatio,* fr. *fabulor,* pp. *-atus,* to speak]

F.A.C.C.P. Abbreviation for Fellow of the American College of Chest Physicians.

F.A.C.D. Abbreviation for Fellow of the American College of Dentists.

face (fās). **1.** The front portion of the head; the visage including eyes, nose, mouth, forehead, cheeks, and chin; excludes ears. SYN facies (1). **2.** SYN surface.

bird f., SYN brachygnathia.

cow f., SYN *facies* bovina.

dish f., SYN *facies* scaphoidea.

frog f., the appearance caused by broadening of the nose which occurs in certain cases of nasal polyps.

hippocratic f., SYN hippocratic *facies.*

masklike f., SYN Parkinson's *facies.*

moon f., the round, usually red face, with large jowls, seen in Cushing's disease or in exogenous hyperadrenocorticalism.

moon shaped f., moon *facies.*

face-bow. A caliper-like device used to record the relationship of the jaws to the temporomandibular joints; the record may then be used to orient a cast or model of the maxilla to the opening and closing axis of the articulator. SYN hinge-bow.

adjustable axis f., a f. whose caliper ends can be adjusted to permit location of the axis of rotation of the mandible. SYN kinematic f.

kinematic f., SYN adjustable axis f.

face-lift. SEE rhytidectomy.

fac·et, fa·cette (fas′et, fă-set′). **1.** A small smooth area on a bone or other firm structure. **2.** A worn spot on a tooth, produced by chewing or grinding. [Fr. *facette*]

articular f., a relatively small articular surface of a bone, especially a vertebra.

f. of atlas for dens, a circular facet on the posterior (inner) surface of the anterior arch of the atlas which articulates with the dens of the axis. SYN fovea dentis atlantis [NA], pit of atlas for dens.

clavicular f., SYN clavicular *notch* of sternum.

corneal f., a corneal depression following loss of stroma.

costal f.'s, articular surface on a vertebra for articulation with a rib.

inferior articular f. of atlas, one of two concave surfaces on the lateral masses of the atlas that articulate with corresponding surfaces on the axis. SYN facies articularis inferior atlantis [NA], fovea articularis inferior atlantis, inferior articular pit of atlas.

inferior costal f., demifacet on the lower edge of the body of a vertebra articulating with the head of a rib. SYN fovea costalis inferior [NA], inferior costal pit.

Lenoir's f., the medial articular surface of the patella.

locked f.'s, SYN *dislocation* of articular processes.

superior articular f. of atlas, one of two concave articular surfaces on the superior aspect of the lateral masses of the atlas that articulate with the occipital condyles. SYN facies articularis superior atlantis [NA], fovea articularis superior atlantis, superior articular pit of atlas.

superior costal f., a demifacet on the upper edge of the body of a vertebra articulating with the head of a rib; a single rib articulates with the inferior costal f. and superior costal f. of the adjacent vertebrae. SYN fovea costalis superior [NA], superior costal pit.

transverse costal f., a facet on the transverse process of a vertebra for articulation with the tubercle of a rib. SYN fovea costalis processus transversi [NA], costal pit of transverse process.

fac·e·tec·to·my (fas-ĕ-tek′tō-mē). Excision of a facet. [facet + G. *ektomē,* excision]

fa·cial (fā′shăl). Relating to the face. SYN facialis [NA].

fa·ci·a·lis (fā-shē-ā′lis) [NA]. SYN facial, facial. [L.]

◬-facient. Causing; one who or that which brings about. [L. *facio,* to make]

FACIES

fa·ci·es, pl. **fa·ci·es** (fā′shē-ēz, fash′ē-ēz). **1** [NA]. SYN face (1). **2** [NA]. SYN surface. **3.** SYN expression (2). [L.]

acromial articular f. of clavicle, SYN acromial articular *surface* of clavicle.

adenoid f., the open-mouthed and often dull appearance in children with adenoid hypertrophy, associated with a pinched nose.

f. antebrachia′lis ante′rior [NA], SYN anterior *region* of forearm.

f. antebrachia′lis poste′rior [NA], ⋆official alternate term for posterior *region* of forearm.

f. ante′rior [NA], SYN anterior *surface.*

f. ante′rior antebra′chii, SYN anterior *region* of forearm.

f. ante′rior bra′chii, SYN anterior *region* of arm.

f. ante′rior cor′neae [NA], SYN anterior *surface* of cornea.

f. ante′rior cor′poris maxil′lae [NA], SYN anterior *surface* of maxilla.

f. ante′rior cru′ris, SYN anterior *region* of leg.

f. ante′rior glan′dulae suprarena′lis [NA], SYN anterior *surface* of suprarenal gland.

f. ante′rior ir′idis [NA], SYN anterior *surface* of iris.

f. ante′rior latera′lis cor′poris hu′meri [NA], SYN anterolateral *surface* of shaft of humerus.

f. ante′rior len′tis [NA], SYN anterior *surface* of lens.

f. ante′rior media′lis cor′poris hu′meri [NA], SYN anteromedial *surface* of shaft of humerus.

f. ante′rior mem′bri inferio′ris, SYN anterior *surface* of lower limb.

f. ante′rior palpebra′rum [NA], SYN anterior surface of eyelids.

f. ante′rior pancrea′tis [NA], SYN anterior *surface* of pancreas.

f. ante′rior par′tis petro′sae os′sis tempora′lis [NA], SYN anterior *surface* of petrous part of temporal bone.

f. ante′rior patel′lae [NA], SYN anterior *surface* of patella.

f. ante′rior pros′tatae [NA], SYN anterior *surface* of prostate.

f. ante′rior ra′dii [NA], SYN anterior *surface* of radius.

f. ante′rior re′nis [NA], SYN anterior *surface* of kidney.

f. ante′rior ul′nae [NA], SYN anterior *surface* of ulna.

f. anterolatera′lis cor′poris hu′meri [NA], ⭐official alternate term for anterolateral *surface* of shaft of humerus.

f. anteromedia′lis cor′poris hu′meri [NA], ⭐official alternate term for anteromedial *surface* of shaft of humerus.

f. antoni′na, a facial expression due to alteration in the eyelids and anterior segment of the eye; found in leprosy.

aortic f., the pale sallow complexion of one suffering from incompetence of the aortic valve.

f. approxima′lis de′ntis [NA], SYN contact *surface* of tooth.

f. articular′is [NA], SYN articular *surface*.

f. articula′ris acromia′lis clavic′ulae [NA], SYN acromial articular *surface* of clavicle.

f. articula′ris acro′mii [NA], SYN articular *surface* of acromion.

f. articula′ris ante′rior den′tis [NA], SYN anterior articular *surface* of dens.

f. articula′ris arytenoi′dea cricoi′deae [NA], SYN arytenoidal articular *surface* of cricoid.

f. articula′ris calca′nea ta′li [NA], SYN calcaneal articular *surface* of talus.

f. articula′ris cap′itis cos′tae [NA], SYN articular *surface* of head of rib.

f. articula′ris cap′itis fib′ulae [NA], SYN articular *surface* of head of fibula.

f. articula′ris car′pi ra′dii [NA], SYN carpal articular *surface* of radius.

f. articula′ris cartila′ginis arytenoi′deae [NA], SYN articular *surface* of arytenoid cartilage.

f. articula′ris cuboi′dea calca′nei [NA], SYN cuboidal articular *surface* of calcaneus.

f. articula′ris fibula′ris tib′iae [NA], SYN fibular articular *surface* of tibia.

f. articula′ris infe′rior atlan′tis [NA], SYN inferior articular *facet* of atlas.

f. articula′ris infe′rior tib′iae [NA], SYN inferior articular *surface* of tibia.

f. articula′ris malle′oli fib′ulae [NA], SYN malleolar articular *surface* of fibula.

f. articula′ris malle′oli tib′iae [NA], SYN malleolar articular *surface* of tibia.

f. articula′ris navicula′ris ta′li [NA], SYN navicular articular *surface* of talus.

f. articula′ris os′sis tempora′lis [NA], SYN articular *surface* of temporal bone.

f. articula′ris patel′lae [NA], SYN articular *surface* of patella.

f. articula′ris poste′rior den′tis [NA], SYN posterior articular *surface* of dens.

f. articula′ris sterna′lis clavic′ulae [NA], SYN sternal articular *surface* of clavicle.

f. articula′ris supe′rior atlan′tis [NA], SYN superior articular *facet* of atlas.

f. articula′ris supe′rior tib′iae [NA], SYN superior articular *surface* of tibia.

f. articula′ris talaris ante′rior calcanei [NA], SYN anterior talar articular *surface* of calcaneus.

f. articula′ris tala′ris calca′nei [NA], SYN talar articular *surface* of calcaneus.

f. articula′ris talaris media calcanei [NA], SYN middle talar articular *surface* of calcaneus.

f. articularis talaris posterior calca′nei, SYN posterior talar articular *surface* of calcaneus.

f. articula′ris thyroi′dea cricoi′deae [NA], SYN thyroidal articular *surface* of cricoid.

f. articula′ris tuber′culi cos′tae [NA], SYN articular *surface* of tubercle of rib.

f. auricula′ris os′sis il′ii [NA], SYN auricular *surface* of ilium.

f. auricula′ris os′sis sac′ri [NA], SYN auricular *surface* of sacrum.

f. bovi′na, the cowlike face of ocular hypertelorism; typical of craniofacial dysostosis. SYN cow face.

f. brachia′lis ante′rior [NA], SYN anterior *region* of arm.

f. brachia′lis poste′rior [NA], SYN posterior *region* of arm.

f. bucca′lis, SYN vestibular *surface* of tooth.

f. cerebra′lis, SYN cerebral *surface*.

cherubic f., the characteristic child-like f. seen in cherubism; also seen in glycogenosis, particularly type 2.

f. co′lica sple′nis [NA], SYN colic *surface* of spleen.

f. contac′tus den′tis, SYN contact *surface* of tooth.

Corvisart's f., the characteristic f. seen in cardiac insufficiency or aortic regurgitation; a swollen, purplish, cyanotic face with shiny eyes and puffy eyelids.

f. costa′lis [NA], SYN costal *surface*.

f. costa′lis pulmo′nis [NA], SYN costal *surface* of lung.

f. costa′lis scap′ulae [NA], SYN costal *surface* of scapula.

f. crura′lis ante′rior [NA], SYN anterior *region* of leg.

f. crura′lis poste′rior [NA], SYN posterior *surface* of leg.

f. cubita′lis ante′rior [NA], SYN anterior *region* of elbow.

f. cubita′lis poste′rior [NA], SYN posterior *region* of elbow.

f. diaphragmat′ica [NA], SYN diaphragmatic *surface*.

f. digita′lis dorsa′lis [NA], SYN dorsal *surface* of digit.

f. digita′lis palma′ris [NA], ⭐official alternate term for palmar *surface* of fingers.

f. digita′lis planta′ris [NA], SYN plantar *surface* of toe.

f. digita′lis ventra′lis [NA], SYN palmar *surface* of fingers.

f. dista′lis den′tis [NA], SYN distal *surface* of tooth.

f. doloro′sa, facial expression of an unhappy person or one sick or in pain.

f. dorsa′lis [NA], SYN dorsal *surface*.

f. dorsa′lis os′sis sac′ri [NA], SYN dorsal *surface* of sacrum.

f. dorsa′lis scap′ulae [NA], SYN dorsal *surface* of scapula.

elfin f., f. characterized by a short, upturned nose, wide mouth, widely spaced eyes, and full cheeks; it may be associated with hypercalcemia, supravalvar aortic stenosis, and mental retardation.

f. exter′na [NA], SYN external *surface*.

f. exter′na os′sis fronta′lis [NA], SYN external *surface* of frontal bone.

f. exter′na os′sis parieta′lis [NA], SYN external *surface* of parietal bone.

f. facia′lis den′tis [NA], ⭐official alternate term for vestibular *surface* of tooth.

f. rena′lis lie′nis, SYN renal *surface* of spleen.

f. femora′lis ante′rior [NA], ⭐official alternate term for anterior *region* of thigh.

f. femora′lis poste′rior [NA], ⭐official alternate term for posterior *region* of thigh.

f. gas′trica sple′nis [NA], SYN gastric *surface* of spleen.

f. glu′tea os′sis il′ii [NA], SYN gluteal *surface* of ilium.

hippocratic f., f. hippocra′tica, a pinched expression of the face, with sunken eyes, concavity of cheeks and temples, relaxed lips, and leaden complexion; observed in one close to death after severe and prolonged illness. SYN hippocratic face.

hound-dog f., the facial appearance in cutis laxa, with loose facial skin hanging in folds.

Hutchinson's f., the peculiar facial expression produced by the drooping eyelids and motionless eyes in external ophthalmoplegia.

f. infe′rior cer′ebri [NA], SYN *base* of brain.

f. infe′rior hemisphe′rii cerebel′li [NA], SYN inferior *surface* of cerebellar hemisphere.

f. infe′rior lin′guae [NA], SYN inferior *surface* of tongue.

f. infe′rior pancre′tis [NA], SYN inferior *surface* of pancreas.

f. infe′rior par′tis petro′sae os′sis tempora′lis [NA], SYN inferior *surface* of petrous part of temporal bone.

f. inferolatera′lis pros′tatae [NA], SYN inferolateral *surface* of prostate.

f. infratempora′lis maxil′lae [NA], SYN infratemporal *surface* of maxilla.

f. interloba′res pulmo′nis [NA], SYN interlobar *surfaces* of lung, under *surface*.

f. inter′na [NA], SYN internal *surface*.

f. inter′na os′sis fronta′lis [NA], SYN internal *surface* of frontal bone.

f. inter′na os′sis parieta′lis [NA], SYN internal *surface* of parietal bone.

f. intestina′lis u′teri [NA], SYN intestinal *surface* of uterus.

f. labia′lis, SYN vestibular *surface* of tooth.

f. latera′lis [NA], SYN lateral *surface*.

f. latera′lis bra′chii, SYN lateral *surface* of arm.

f. latera′lis cru′ris, SYN lateral *surface* of leg.

f. latera′lis dig′iti ma′nus, SYN lateral *surface* of finger.

f. latera′lis dig′iti pe′dis, SYN lateral *surface* of toe.

f. latera′lis fib′ulae [NA], SYN lateral *surface* of fibula.

f. latera′lis mem′bri inferior′is, SYN lateral *surface* of lower limb.

f. latera′lis os′sis zygomat′ici [NA], SYN lateral *surface* of zygomatic bone.

f. latera′lis ova′rii [NA], SYN lateral *surface* of ovary.

f. latera′lis tes′tis [NA], SYN lateral *surface* of testis.

f. latera′lis tib′iae [NA], SYN lateral *surface* of tibia.

leonine f., SYN leontiasis.

f. lingua′lis den′tis [NA], SYN lingual *surface* of tooth.

f. luna′ta acetab′uli [NA], SYN lunate *surface* of acetabulum.

f. malleola′ris latera′lis ta′li [NA], SYN lateral malleolar *surface* of talus.

f. malleola′ris media′lis ta′li [NA], SYN medial malleolar *surface* of talus.

f. masticato′ria, SYN denture occlusal *surface*.

f. maxilla′ris a′lae majo′ris, SYN maxillary *surface* of greater wing of sphenoid bone.

f. maxilla′ris os′sis palati′ni [NA], SYN maxillary *surface* of palatine bone. **(2)** the part of the anterior surface of the greater wing of the sphenoid bone that is perforated by the foramen rotundum and forms the posterior boundary of the pterygopalatine fossa.

f. media′lis [NA], SYN medial *surface*.

f. media′lis cartilag′inis arytenoi′deae [NA], SYN medial surface of arytenoid cartilage.

f. media′lis cer′ebri [NA], SYN medial *surface* of cerebral hemisphere.

f. media′lis dig′iti pe′dis, SYN medial *surface* of toes.

f. media′lis fib′ulae [NA], SYN medial surface of fibula.

f. media′lis ova′rii [NA], SYN medial *surface* of ovary.

f. media′lis pulmo′nis, SYN medial *surface* of lung.

f. media′lis tes′tis [NA], SYN medial surface of testis.

f. media′lis tib′iae [NA], SYN medial surface of tibia.

f. media′lis ul′nae [NA], SYN medial surface of ulna.

f. mediastinalis pulmonis, SYN mediastinal *surface* of lung.

f. mesia′lis den′tis [NA], SYN mesial *surface* of tooth.

mitral f., the pink, slightly cyanosed cheeks of patients with mitral valve disease.

moon f., roundness of the face due to increased fat deposition laterally seen in patients with hyperadrenocorticalism, either of endogenous (*e.g.*, Cushing's disease) or exogenous origin, such as the use of cortisone-like drugs as therapy.

myasthenic f., the facial expression in myasthenia gravis, caused by drooping of the eyelids and corners of the mouth, and weakness of the muscles of the face.

myopathic f., facial appearance of some patients with myopathies and with myasthenia gravis, consisting of bilateral ptosis and inability to elevate the corners of the mouth, due to muscle weakness.

f. nasa′lis maxil′lae [NA], SYN nasal *surface* of maxilla.

f. nasa′lis os′sis palati′ni [NA], SYN nasal *surface* of palatine bone.

f. occlusa′lis den′tis [NA], SYN denture occlusal *surface*.

f. orbita′lis [NA], SYN orbital *surface*.

f. palati′na la′minae horizonta′lis os′sis pala′tini [NA], SYN palatine *surface* of horizontal plate of palatine bone.

Parkinson's f., the expressionless or masklike f. characteristic of parkinsonism (1). SYN masklike face.

f. patella′ris fem′oris [NA], SYN patellar *surface* of femur.

f. pelvi′na os′sis sa′cri [NA], SYN pelvic *surface* of sacrum.

f. poplit′ea fem′oris [NA], SYN popliteal *surface* of femur.

f. poste′rior [NA], SYN posterior *surface*.

f. poste′rior cartilag′inis arytenoi′deae [NA], the posterior surface of the arytenoid cartilage.

f. poste′rior cor′neae [NA], SYN posterior *surface* of cornea.

f. poste′rior corporis hu′meri [NA], SYN posterior *surface* of shaft of humerus.

f. poste′rior cru′ris, SYN posterior *surface* of leg.

f. poste′rior fib′ulae [NA], SYN posterior *surface* of fibula.

f. poste′rior glan′dulae suprarena′lis [NA], SYN posterior *surface* of suprarenal gland.

f. poste′rior ir′idis [NA], SYN posterior *surface* of iris.

f. poste′rior len′tis [NA], SYN posterior *surface* of lens.

f. poste′rior mem′bri inferio′ris, SYN posterior *surface* of lower limb.

f. poste′rior palpebra′rum [NA], SYN posterior *surface* of eyelids.

f. poste′rior pancrea′tis [NA], SYN posterior *surface* of pancreas.

f. poste′rior par′tis petro′sae os′sis tempora′lis [NA], SYN posterior *surface* of petrous part of temporal bone.

f. poste′rior pros′tatae [NA], SYN posterior *surface* of prostate.

f. poste′rior ra′dii [NA], SYN posterior *surface* of radius.

f. poste′rior re′nis [NA], SYN posterior *surface* of kidney.

f. poste′rior tib′iae [NA], SYN posterior *surface* of tibia.

f. poste′rior ul′nae [NA], SYN posterior *surface* of ulna.

Potter's f., characteristic f. seen in bilateral renal agenesis and other severe renal malformations, exhibiting ocular hypertelorism, low-set ears, receding chin, and flattening of the nose. SEE ALSO Potter's *syndrome*. SYN Potter's disease.

f. pulmona′lis cor′dis [NA], SYN pulmonary *surface* of heart.

f. rena′lis glan′dulae suprarena′lis [NA], the surface of the suprarenal gland in contact with the kidney. SYN renal surface of the suprarenal gland.

f. rena′lis sple′nis, SYN renal *surface* of spleen.

f. sacropelvi′na os′sis il′ii [NA], SYN sacropelvic *surface* of ilium.

f. scaphoi′dea, a facial malformation characterized by protuberant forehead, depressed nose and maxilla, and prominent chin. SYN dish face.

f. sternocosta′lis cor′dis [NA], SYN sternocostal *surface* of heart.

f. supe′rior hemisphe′rii cerebel′li [NA], SYN superior *surface* of cerebellar hemisphere.

f. supe′rior ta′li [NA], SYN superior *surface* of talus.

f. superolatera′lis cer′ebri [NA], SYN superolateral *surface* of cerebrum.

f. symphy′sialis [NA], SYN symphysial surface of pubis.

f. tempora′lis [NA], SYN temporal *surface*.

f. urethra′lis pe′nis [NA], SYN urethral *surface* of penis.

f. vesica′lis u′teri [NA], SYN vesical *surface* of uterus.

f. vestibula′ris den′tis [NA], SYN vestibular *surface* of tooth.
f. viscera′lis hep′atis [NA], SYN visceral *surface* of liver.
f. viscera′lis sple′nis [NA], SYN visceral *surface* of the spleen.
SEE ALSO colic *surface* of spleen, gastric *surface* of spleen, renal *surface* of spleen.

---

fa·cil·i·ta·tion (fă-sil′i-tā′shŭn). Enhancement or reinforcement of a reflex or other nervous activity by the arrival at the reflex center of other excitatory impulses. [L. *facilitas,* fr. *facilis,* easy]
Wedensky f., the arrival of an impulse at a blocked zone, enhancing the excitability of the nerve beyond the block and indicating that the neuromuscular preparation distal to the block has been changed even though the enhancing stimulus is not conducted through the blocked zone.
fac·ing (fās′ing). A tooth-colored material (usually plastic or porcelain) used to hide the buccal or labial surface of a metal crown to give the outward appearance of a natural tooth.
⌂**facio-.** The face. SEE ALSO prosopo-. [L. *facies*]
fa·ci·o·lin·gual (fā′shē-ō-ling′gwăl). Relating to the face and the tongue, often denoting a paralysis affecting these parts.
fa·ci·o·plas·ty (fā′shē-ō-plas-tē). Plastic surgery involving the face. [facio- + G. *plastos,* formed]
fa·ci·o·ple·gia (fā′shē-ō-plē′jē-ă). SYN facial *palsy.* [facio- + G. *plēgē,* a stroke]
F.A.C.N.M. Abbreviation for Fellow of the American College of Nuclear Medicine.
F.A.C.N.P. Abbreviation for Fellow of the American College of Nuclear Physicians.
F.A.C.O.G. Abbreviation for Fellow of the American College of Obstetricians and Gynecologists.
F.A.C.P. Abbreviation for Fellow of the American College of Physicians, or of Prosthodontists.
F.A.C.R. Abbreviation for Fellow of the American College of Radiology.
FACS Abbreviation for fluorescence-activated cell sorter.
F.A.C.S. Abbreviation for Fellow of the American College of Surgeons.
F.A.C.S.M. Abbreviation for Fellow of the American College of Sports Medicine.
F-ac·tin. See under actin.
fac·ti·tious (fak-tish′ŭs). Artificial; self-induced; not naturally occurring. [L. *factitius,* made by art, fr. *facio,* to make]

FACTOR

---

fac·tor (fak′ter). **1.** One of the contributing causes in any action. **2.** One of the components that by multiplication makes up a number or expression. **3.** SYN gene. **4.** A vitamin or other essential element. **5.** An event, characteristic, or other definable entity that brings about a change in a health condition. **6.** A categorical independent variable, used to identify, by means of numerical codes, membership in a qualitatively identifiable group; for example, "overcrowding is a factor in disease transmission." [L. maker, causer, fr. *facio,* to make]
f. 3, (1) operational name given to an incompletely characterized selenium-containing natural product which, in minute amounts, prevents liver damage in rats due to deficiency of vitamin E; **(2)** f. III in the vitamin B_{12} series, 5-hydroxybenzimidazole, analogue of the usual B_{12} nucleotide components.
f. A, SEE properdin f. A.
ABO f.'s, see Blood Groups appendix.
accelerator f., SYN f. V.
acetate replacement f., SYN lipoic acid.
adrenal weight f., a postulated substance of adenohypophysial origin responsible for maintenance of the weight of the adrenal cortex.

adrenocorticotropic releasing f., hormone produced by hypothalamus that causes pituitary to secrete adrenocorticotropic hormone.
angiogenesis f., a substance of 2000 to 20,000 MW which is secreted by macrophages and stimulates neovascularization in healing wounds or in the stroma of tumors.
animal protein f. (APF), SYN *vitamin* B_{12}.
antialopecia f., SYN inositol.
antianemic f., SYN *vitamin* B_{12}.
antiberiberi f., SYN thiamin.
anti-black-tongue f., SYN nicotinic acid.
anticomplementary f., a f. that interferes with the action or function of complement.
antidermatitis f., SYN pantothenic acid.
antihemophilic f. A (AHF), SYN f. VIII.
antihemophilic f. B, SYN f. IX.
antihemorrhagic f., SYN *vitamin* K.
antineuritic f., SYN thiamin.
antinuclear f. (ANF), a f., usually antibodies, present in serum with strong affinity for nuclei and detected by fluorescent antibody technique; present in lupus erythematosus, rheumatic arthritis, and certain other autoimmune conditions; may also be present at lower levels in normal individuals.
antipellagra f., SYN nicotinic acid.
antipernicious anemia f. (APA), (1) SYN *vitamin* B_{12}. **(2)** specifically, cyanocobalamin.
antisterility f., SYN *vitamin* E (2).
atrial natriuretic f. (ANF), an early name given to a natriuretic f. derived from cardiac atria. The term is no longer correct because the f. is now known to be a peptide.
f. B, SEE properdin f. B.
B_T f., SYN carnitine.
bacteriocin f.'s, SYN bacteriocinogenic *plasmids,* under *plasmid.*
B-cell differentiating f., SYN interleukin-4.
B cell differentiation/growth f.'s, various substances, usually obtained from the supernatant of T cell cultures, such as interleukin 4, 5, and 6. These substances are necessary for B cell growth, maturation, and differentiation into plasma cells or B memory cells.
B-cell stimulatory f. 2, SYN interleukin-6.
bifidus f., an unidentified substance associated with *Lactobacillus bifidus* subsp. *pennsylvanicus,* present in mammalian milk.
biotic f.'s, environmental f.'s or influences resulting from the activities of living organisms, as contrasted to those resulting from climatic, geological, or other f.'s.
Bittner's milk f., SYN mammary tumor *virus* of mice.
branching f., 1,4-α-glucan-branching enzyme.
C f.'s, SYN coupling f.'s.
CAMP f., SEE CAMP *test.*
capillary permeability f., SYN *vitamin* P.
Castle's intrinsic f., SYN intrinsic f.
Christmas f., SYN f. IX.
citrovorum f. (CF), SYN folinic acid.
clearing f.'s, lipoprotein lipases that appear in plasma during lipemia and catalyze hydrolysis of triglycerides only when the latter are bound to protein and when an acceptor (*e.g.,* serum albumin) is present, thus "clearing" the plasma.
clotting f., any of the various plasma components involved in the clotting process. SYN coagulation f.
coagulation f., SYN clotting f.
cobra venom f., a component of cobra venom that renders C3 proactivator (properdin factor B) susceptible to factor D of the properdin system, leading to activation of C3 and other components of complement and lysis of unsensitized erythrocytes.
coenzyme f., SYN dihydrolipoamide dehydrogenase.
colony-stimulating f.'s (CSF), a group of glycoprotein growth f.'s regulating differentiation in mycloid cell lines. These substances act in either paracrine or autocrine fashion on marrow cells, appear to act synergistically in complex and poorly understood ways; each appears to have the ability to exert actions on

several lines of progenitor cells, and to influence end cell function.

complement chemotactic f., the activated complex of the fifth, sixth, and seventh components of complement (C567) which induces chemotaxis in the case of polymorphonuclear leukocytes.

complement f. I, a heterodimeric glycoprotein; a deficiency results in uncontrolled activation of C3.

corticotropin releasing f. (CRF), (1) SYN corticoliberin. **(2)** SYN corticotropin releasing *hormone.*

coupling f.'s, proteins that restore phosphorylating ability to mitochondria that have lost it, *i.e.,* have become "uncoupled" so that oxidation and electron transport no longer produces ATP. Usually termed coupling factor F_1, F_2, etc. SYN C f.'s.

f. D, SEE properdin f. D.

debranching f.'s, SYN debranching *enzymes,* under *enzyme.*

decapacitation f., a f., postulated to be present in epididymal fluid and seminal plasma, that prevents the capacitation of spermatozoa.

diabetogenic f., rarely used term for a f. in crude extracts of the anterior lobe of the hypophysis that produces degenerative changes in the islet cells of the pancreas and causes permanent diabetes.

diffusing f., SYN hyaluronidase (1).

direct lytic f. of cobra venom, SYN cobrotoxin.

Duran-Reynals permeability f., Duran-Reynals spreading f., SYN hyaluronidase (1).

f. E, SEE properdin f. E.

elongation f., proteins that catalyze the elongation of peptide chains during protein biosynthesis. SYN transfer f. (3).

endothelial relaxing f. (en'dō-thē'li-al), a molecule functioning as a neurotransmitter and produced by activated macrophages. It is capable of killing tumor cells, parasites, and intracellular bacteria.

endothelium-derived relaxing f. (EDRF), diffusible substances produced by endothelial cells that cause vascular smooth muscle relaxation; nitric oxide (NO) is one such substance.

eosinophil chemotactic f. of anaphylaxis, a peptide (MW 500 to 600) that is chemotactic for eosinophilic leukocytes and is released from disrupted mast cells.

epidermal growth f. (EGF), a heat-stable antigenic protein isolated from the submaxillary glands of male mice; when injected into newborn animals it accelerates eyelid opening and tooth eruption, stimulates epidermal growth and keratinization, and, in larger doses, inhibits body growth and hair development and produces fatty livers.

erythrocyte maturation f., SYN *vitamin* B_{12}.

essential food f.'s, those substances required in the diet: certain amino acids and unsaturated fatty acids, vitamins, essential minerals, etc.

extrinsic f., dietary vitamin B_{12}.

F f., SYN F *plasmid.*

fermentation *Lactobacillus casei* f., SYN pteropterin.

fertility f., SYN F *plasmid.*

fibrin-stabilizing f., SYN f. XIII.

filtrate f., former term for pantothenic acid.

Fitzgerald f., SYN high molecular weight *kininogen.*

Flaujeac f., SYN high molecular weight *kininogen.*

Fletcher f., SYN prekallikrein.

follicle-stimulating hormone-releasing f. (FRF, FSH-RF), SYN folliberin.

G f., (1) the single common variance or f. that is common to (*i.e.,* empirically intercorrelates with) different intelligence tests (general). **(2)** a substance required for the growth of a specific organism.

galactagogue f., a f. in extracts of the posterior lobe of the hypophysis that, by stimulating the smooth muscle of the lobuloalveolar system of the mammary gland, causes a flow of milk from the nipple.

galactopoietic f., SYN prolactin.

glass f., SYN f. XII.

glucose tolerance f., a water-soluble complex containing chromium needed for normal glucose tolerance.

glycotropic f., a principle in extracts of the anterior lobe of the hypophysis that raises the blood sugar and antagonizes the action of insulin; purified pituitary growth hormone produces an identical effect. SYN insulin-antagonizing f.

f. Gm, a f. that determines certain of the allotypes of human immunoglobulins; found only on the γ chains of IgG (γ-globulin).

gonadotropin-releasing f., SYN gonadoliberin (1).

granulocyte colony-stimulating f. (G-CSF) (gran'yū-lō-sīt), glycoproteins that are synthesized by a variety of cells and are involved in growth and differentiation of hematopoietic stem cells. In addition, these f.'s stimulate the end-cell functional activity of stem cells. SEE ALSO colony-stimulating f.'s.

granulocyte-macrophage colony-stimulating f. (GM-CSF) (gran'ū-lō-sīt), a glycoprotein secreted by macrophages or bone stromal cells that functions as a growth factor for myeloid progenitor cells such as granulocytes, macrophages, and eosinophils. SEE ALSO colony-stimulating f.'s.

---

growth f.'s, proteins involved in cell differentiation and growth.

> Growth factors are essential to the normal cell cycle, and are thus vital elements in the life of animals from conception to death. Among other things, they mediate fetal development, play a role in maintenance and repair of tissues, stimulate production of blood cells, and, gone awry, participate in cancerous processes.

---

growth hormone-releasing f. (GHRF, GH-RF), SYN somatoliberin.

f. H, (1) former designation for biotin; **(2)** vitamin B_{12} analogue or precursor; **(3)** a glycoprotein that regulates the activity of complement factor C3b; a deficiency results in the lack of inhibition of the alternative hemolytic pathway leading to continuous activation and consumption of factor C3 (hemolytic uremic syndrome).

Hageman f., SYN f. XII.

HG f., SYN glucagon.

human antihemophilic f., a lyophilized concentrate of f. VIII, obtained from fresh normal human plasma; used as a hemostatic agent in hemophilia. SYN antihemophilic globulin (2), human antihemophilic fraction.

hyperglycemic-glycogenolytic f. (HGF), SYN glucagon.

f. I, in the clotting of blood a f. that is converted to fibrin through the action of thrombin. SEE ALSO fibrinogen.

f. II, a glycoprotein converted in the clotting of blood to thrombin by factor Xa, platelets, calcium ions, and factor V. SEE ALSO prothrombin.

f. IIa, SYN thrombin.

f. III, in the clotting of blood, tissue f. or thromboplastin; it initiates the extrinsic pathway by reacting with f. VII and calcium to form f. VIIa. SEE thromboplastin.

inhibition f., SYN migration-inhibitory f.

initiation f. (IF), one of several soluble proteins involved in the initiation of protein or RNA synthesis.

insulin-antagonizing f., SYN glycotropic f.

insulin-like growth f.'s (IGF), peptides whose formation is stimulated by growth hormone. These peptides bring about peripheral tissue effects of that hormone and have high (about 70%) homology to human insulin. SYN somatomedins.

intrinsic f. (IF), a relatively small mucoprotein (MW about 50,000) secreted by the neck cell of the gastric glands and required for adequate absorption of vitamin B_{12}; deficiency results in pernicious anemia. SYN Castle's intrinsic f.

f. Inv, a f. that determines certain of the allotypes of human immunoglobulins; found on the κ chains of IgG, IgA, IgM, and Bence Jones protein.

ischemia-modifying f.'s, various factors that play a role in determining the extent of necrosis with cerebral stroke; these include blood viscosity and osmolality, the blood pressure, and the anatomy of the neck and intracranial arteries.

fa

f. IV, in the clotting of blood, calcium ions.

f. IX, in the clotting of blood, also known as: Christmas f. (Biggs and Macfarlane), plasma thromboplastin component (Aggeler), antihemophilic globulin B (Cramer), plasma thromboplastin f. B (Aggeler), plasma f. X (Shulman), antihemophilic f. B, and platelet cofactor II. F. IX is required for the formation of intrinsic blood thromboplastin and affects the amount formed (rather than the rate). Its active form, f. IXa (EC 3.4.21.22) is a serine proteinase converting f. X to f. Xa by cleaving an arginine-isoleucine bond. Deficiency of f. IX causes hemophilia B. SYN antihemophilic f. B, antihemophilic globulin B, Christmas f., plasma f. X, plasma thromboplastin component, plasma thromboplastin f. B, platelet cofactor II.

labile f., SYN f. V.

Lactobacillus bulgaricus **f. (LBF),** SYN pantetheine.

Lactobacillus casei **f.,** SYN folic acid (2).

lactogenic f., SYN prolactin.

Laki-Lorand f., SYN f. XIII.

LE f.'s, antinuclear immunoglobulins in plasma of persons with disseminated lupus erythematosus, associated with positive LE tests.

lethal f., SEE genetic *lethal.*

leukocytosis-promoting f., a substance obtained by Menkin from inflammatory exudates; it stimulates leukocytosis.

leukopenic f., a principle obtained by Menkin from inflammatory exudates; it causes leukopenia when injected into normal animals.

lipotropic f., SYN choline.

liver filtrate f., former term for pantothenic acid.

liver *Lactobacillus casei* **f.,** SYN folic acid (2).

L-L f., SYN f. XIII.

luteinizing hormone/follicle-stimulating hormone-releasing f. (LH/FSH-RF), SYN gonadoliberin (2).

luteinizing hormone-releasing f. (LH-RF, LRF), former name for luteinizing *hormone*-releasing *hormone.*

lymph node permeability f. (LNPF), a substance, released by lymphocytes when stimulated or damaged, that increases capillary permeability and the accumulation of mononuclear cells.

macrophage-activating f. (MAF) (mak′rō-fāj), group of lymphokines that induces macrophage activation. Two major macrophage activating f.'s are interferon gamma and interleukin-4.

macrophage colony-stimulating f. (M-CSF), a glycoprotein growth f. that causes the committed cell line to proliferate and mature into macrophages. SEE ALSO colony-stimulating f.'s.

maize f., SYN zeatin.

mammotropic f., SYN prolactin.

maturation f., SYN *vitamin* B_{12}.

melanotropin-releasing f., SYN melanoliberin.

mesodermal f., a protein that can induce the formation of kidney and muscle primordia in embryos.

migration-inhibitory f. (MIF), a soluble, nondialyzable substance that is produced by sensitized lymphocytes (*i.e.,* lymphocytes from a sensitized animal) when exposed to the specific antigen, and that causes adherence and inhibition of migration of macrophages. SYN inhibition f.

milk f., SYN mammary tumor *virus* of mice.

monocyte derived neutrophil chemotactic f. (MDNCF), SYN interleukin-8.

mouse antialopecia f., SYN inositol.

müllerian inhibiting f., SYN müllerian inhibiting *substance.*

müllerian regression f., müllerian duct inhibitory f., a nonsteroidal substance of fetal testicular origin that acts unilaterally to inhibit development of the paramesonephric (müllerian) ducts and acts with testosterone to promote development of the vas deferens and related structures.

multi-colony-stimulating f. (multi-CSF), SYN interleukin-3.

myocardial depressant f. (MDF), a toxic f. in shock that impairs cardiac contractility; probably a peptide released with underperfusion of the splanchnic area at the release of proteolytic enzymes from the pancreas.

natural killer cell stimulating f. (NKSF), SYN interleukin-12.

nephritic f., a serum protein (possibly an IgG autoantibody), found in some patients with membranoproliferative glomerulonephritis and hypocomplementemia, which, together with the cofactors of the alternate pathway of complement activation, cleaves the third component of complement (C3).

nerve growth f. (NGF), a protein (MW about 26,000) that controls the development of sympathetic postganglionic neurons and possibly also sensory (dorsal root) ganglion cells in mammals; similar, but not identical, factors have been isolated from the venoms of several species of snakes; it has been isolated from the submaxillary glands of male mice, and when injected into newborn animals, sympathetic ganglia become hyperplastic and hypertrophic; stimulates synthesis of nucleic acids and protein.

neural f., a protein that can induce the formation of notochord tissue in embryos.

neutrophil activating f. (NAF), SYN interleukin-8.

neutrophil chemotactant f. (nū′trō-fil kē′mō-tak-tant), SYN interleukin-8. SEE interleukin-8.

osteoclast activating f., a lymphokine that stimulates bone resorption and inhibits bone-collagen synthesis.

ψ f., SYN psi f.

f. P, a chemical (postulated by T. Lewis), formed in ischemic skeletal or cardiac muscle, held to be responsible for the pain of intermittent claudication and angina pectoris.

P f., see P blood group, Blood Groups appendix.

pellagra-preventing f. (p-p f.), SYN nicotinic acid.

plasma labile f., SYN f. V.

plasma thromboplastin f. (PTF), SYN f. VIII.

plasma thromboplastin f. B, SYN f. IX.

plasma f. X, SYN f. IX.

plasmin prothrombins conversion f. (PPCF), SYN f. V.

platelet f. 3, a blood coagulation factor derived from platelets; chemically, a phospholipid lipoprotein that acts with certain plasma thromboplastin f.'s to convert prothrombin to thrombin.

platelet-activating f. (PAF), SYN platelet-aggregating f.

platelet-aggregating f. (PAF), phospholipid mediator of platelet aggregation, inflammation, and anaphylaxis. Produced in response to specific stimuli by a variety of cell types, including neutrophils, basophils, platelets, and endothelial cells. Several molecular species of PAF have been identified which vary in the length of the *O*-alkyl side chain. It is an important mediator of bronchoconstriction. SYN platelet-activating f.

platelet-derived growth f. (PDGF), a f. in platelets that is mitogenic for cells at the site of a wound, *e.g.,* causing endothelial proliferation; cationic glycoprotein mitogen for fibroblasts, smooth muscle cells, and glial cells. Principal f. in serum required for the growth and proliferation of mesenchymal derived cells in tissue culture.

platelet tissue f., SYN thromboplastin.

p-p f., abbreviation for pellagra-preventing f.

predisposing f.'s, attitudinal, personality, and related f.'s that motivate and guide an individual to take certain health actions.

prolactin-inhibiting f. (PIF), SYN prolactostatin.

prolactin-releasing f. (PRF), SYN prolactoliberin.

properdin f. A, a component of the properdin system; a hydrazine-sensitive β_1-globulin (mw about 180,000), now known to be C3 (third component of complement).

properdin f. B, a normal serum protein (mw 95,000) and a component of the properdin system. SYN β_2-glycoprotein II, C3 proactivator, cobra venom cofactor, glycine-rich β-glycoprotein.

properdin f. D, a normal serum α-globulin (mw about 25,000) required in the properdin system. SYN C3 proactivator convertase, glycine-rich β-glycoproteinase.

properdin f. E, a serum protein (mw 160,000) required for activation of C3 (third component of complement) by cobra venom factor. SEE ALSO properdin *system.*

protein f., the f. (6.25) by which the nitrogen content of a protein is multiplied to give the amount of protein.

psi f., a protein responsible for the specific initiation of the RNA polymerase-catalyzed reaction at the promoter sites of genes. SYN ψ f.

pyruvate oxidation f., SYN lipoic acid.

quality f. (QF), (1) a f. by which absorbed radiation doses are multiplied; **(2)** to obtain, for radiation protection purposes, a quantity that expresses the approximate biological effectiveness of the absorbed dose.

ρ f., SYN rho f.

R f.'s, SYN resistance *plasmids*, under *plasmid*.

radiation weighting f., in radiation protection, a f. weighting the absorbed dose of radiation of a specific type and energy for its effect on tissue. SEE equivalent *dose*.

recognition f.'s, f.'s which effect "recognition" of target antigens by polymorphonuclear leukocytes; apparently the Fc portion of antibody molecules and the activated third component of complement (C3), for both of which phagocytes have receptor sites.

relaxation f., substance presumably involved in the return of muscle fibrils to the resting state after nervous stimulation ceases, postulated to act by withdrawing Ca^{2+} from myosin-ATPase sites.

releasing f. (RF), (1) substances, usually of hypothalamic origin, capable of accelerating the rate of secretion of a given hormone by the anterior pituitary gland; **(2)** f.'s required in the termination phase of either RNA biosynthesis or protein biosynthesis. SYN termination f. SYN liberins, releasing hormone, statins.

resistance f.'s, SYN resistance *plasmids*, under *plasmid*.

resistance-inducing f. (RIF), an agent from normal chick embryos that interferes with multiplication of the avian leukosis-sarcoma virus, and is seemingly an avirulent leukosis virus antigenically related to the avian leukosis-sarcoma virus.

resistance-transfer f., the transfer gene of the resistance plasmid.

Rh f., the antigen of the Rh blood group system. See Blood Groups Appendix. SYN Rhesus f.

Rhesus f., see Blood Groups Appendix. SYN Rh f.

rheumatoid f.'s (RF), antibodies in the serum of individuals with rheumatoid arthritis that react with antigenic determinants or immunoglobulins that enhance agglutination of suspended particles coated with pooled human γ-globulin. Rheumatoid f.'s also occur in other autoimmune and certain infectious diseases.

rho f., a termination f. that releases RNA from the DNA template. SYN ρ f.

risk f., a single characteristic statistically associated with, although not necessarily causally related to, an increased risk of morbidity or mortality *e.g.,* smoking as a risk f. for heart disease.

σ f., SYN sigma f.

S f., the individual variables, or empirically most minute subclusters of intercorrelations or common variance, found in different intelligence tests (specific).

secretor f., the capacity to secrete antigens of the ABO blood group in saliva and other body fluids, controlled by a pair of allelic genes designated *Se* and *se* (or *S* and *s*), with the *Se* phenotype dominant to *se;* the saliva of genotypes *SeSe* and *Sese* contains the blood group substances A, B, or H found in their erythrocytes; the saliva of nonsecretors (genotype *sese*) contains no blood group substance; tests for ABH secretion are useful in genetic linkage and population studies; the secretor phenomenon is also closely associated with the Lewis blood group.

sex f., SYN F *plasmid*.

sigma f., a f. that inhibits the nonspecific DNA binding of RNA polymerase, as well as helping to identify the starting point of transcription. SYN σ f.

slow-reacting f. of anaphylaxis (SRF-A), SYN slow-reacting *substance* of anaphylaxis.

SLR f., *Streptococcus lactis* R f., SYN rhizopterin.

somatotropin release-inhibiting f. (SRIF, SIF), SYN somatostatin.

somatotropin-releasing f. (SRF), SYN somatoliberin.

spreading f., SYN hyaluronidase (1).

stable f., SYN f. VII.

stringent f., the gene product (an enzyme) that is crucial to the cellular response of decreased ribosome production as a result of amino acid starvation. SEE ALSO stringent *response*.

Stuart f., Stuart-Prower f., SYN f. X.

sulfation f., SYN somatomedin.

sun protection f. (SPF), the ratio of the minimal ultraviolet dose required to produce erythema with and without a sunscreen; highly effective sunscreens have an SPF of 15 or more.

T-cell growth f., SYN interleukin-2.

T-cell growth f.-1, SYN interleukin-2.

T-cell growth f.-2, SYN interleukin-4.

termination f., SYN releasing f. (2).

testis-determining f. (TDF), the product of a gene on the short arm of the Y chromosome that is responsible for production of testes.

thymic lymphopoietic f., a glycoprotein (MW about 12,000) that has been extracted from thymus; this thymus-produced hormone(s) confers immunological competence on thymus-dependent cells and induces lymphopoiesis.

thyroid-stimulating hormone-releasing f. (TSH-RF), SYN thyroliberin.

thyrotoxic complement-fixation f., a form of thyrotoxin; an antigen found most readily in thyroid tissue from thyrotoxic individuals; known to be chemically and immunologically distinct from thyroglobulin, and fixes complement when combined with antibody related to the γ-globulin fraction of serum. With the exception of extremely small concentrations, the antigen is rarely found in normal glands or in diseased glands that are not associated with thyrotoxicosis; it is probably an intracellular substance (possibly a constituent of the "microsomal fraction"), and does not contain iodine in significant quantity. Not related to the complement-fixation reaction occurring with serum in Hashimoto's disease, in which the antigen is thyroglobulin.

thyrotropin-releasing f. (TRF), former name for thyrotropin-releasing *hormone*.

tissue f., SYN thromboplastin.

tissue weighting f., in radiation protection, a f. weighting the equivalent dose in a particular tissue or organ in terms of its relative contribution to the total deleterious effects resulting from uniform irradiation of the whole body. SEE effective *dose*.

transfer f., (1) the transfer gene of a conjugative plasmid, especially of the resistance plasmid; **(2)** a dialyzable extract that is obtained from the leukocytes of a person with a delayed-type sensitivity and that, following injection into the skin of a nonsensitive person, transfers the specific sensitivity to the recipient; **(3)** SYN elongation f.

transforming f., the DNA responsible for bacterial transformation.

transforming growth f.'s (TGF), two polypeptide growth f.'s; TGF-α stimulates growth of many epidermal and epithelial cells and is obtained from conditioned media of transformed or tumor cells; TGF-β is obtained from kidney and platelets and may even have inhibitory effects on certain cells.

transforming growth f. α (TGF), a cytokine made by tumor and transformed cells that is associated with growth and differentiation. It is also made in normal tissues during embryogenesis and in certain adult tissues.

transforming growth f. β (TGF), a cytokine that has multifunctional properties including interfering with other cytokines. It is produced by platelets and bone cells but can be made by many other cell types.

transmethylation f., SYN choline.

tumor angiogenic f. (TAF), a substance released by solid tumors which induces formation of new blood vessels to supply the tumor.

tumor necrosis f. (TNF), SYN cachectin.

tumor necrosis f.-beta, A cytolytic factor that is produced by CD4 and CD8 T cells after their exposure to an antigen.

uncoupling f.'s, SYN uncouplers.

uterine relaxing f. (URF), SYN relaxin.

f. V, in the clotting of blood, also known as: proaccelerin (Owren), labile or plasma labile f. (Quick), plasma accelerator globulin (Ware and Seegars), thrombogene (Nolf), prothrombokinase (Milstone), plasmin prothrombins conversion f. (Stefanini), component A of prothrombin (Quick), prothrombin accelerator (Fantl and Nance), cofactor of thromboplastin (Honorato), and accelerator f. F. V does not have enzymatic action itself but participates in the common pathway of coagulation by binding f. Xa to platelet surfaces. Deficiency of this f. leads to a rare hemorrhagic tendency known as parahemophilia or hypoproaccelerinemia, with autosomal recessive inheritance; heterozygous individuals are recognized by reduced levels of f. V but have no bleeding tendency. SYN accelerator f., labile f., plasma accelerator globulin, plasma labile f., plasmin prothrombins conversion f., proaccelerin, prothrombin accelerator, prothrombokinase, thrombogene.

f. V$_{1a}$, SYN cobyric acid.

f. V$_a$, in the clotting of blood, accelerin.

f. VII, in the clotting of blood, also known as: proconvertin (Owren), convertin, serum prothrombin conversion accelerator (de Vries, Alexander), stable f. (Stefanini), cofactor V (Owren), prothrombinogen (Quick), cothromboplastin (Mann and Hurn), serum accelerator (Jacox). F. VII forms a complex with tissue thromboplastin and calcium to activate f. X. F. VII is known to be involved in: 1) the congenital deficiency of f. VII, with purpura and bleeding from mucous membranes, autosomal recessive inheritance; 2) the acquired deficiency of f. VII in association with a deficiency of vitamin K, the neonatal period, and the administration of prothrombinopenic drugs; 3) the acquired excess of f. VII in some patients with thromboembolism. It accelerates the conversion of prothrombin to thrombin, in the presence of tissue thromboplastin, calcium, and f. V. SYN proconvertin, prothrombinogen, serum accelerator, serum prothrombin conversion accelerator, stable f.

f. VIII, in the clotting of blood, also known as: antihemophilic f. A (Brinkhous), antihemophilic globulin (1) (Patek and Taylor), antihemophilic globulin A (Cramer), plasma thromboplastin f. (Ratnoff), plasma thromboplastin f. A (Aggeler), thromboplastic plasma component (Shinowara), thromboplastinogen (Quick), prothrombokinase (Feissly), platelet cofactor (Johnson), plasmokinin (Laki), thrombokatilysin (Leggenhager), and proserum prothrombin conversion accelerator. F. VIII participates in the clotting of the blood by forming a complex with f. IXa, platelets, and calcium and enzymatically catalyzing the activation of f. X. Deficiency of f. VIII is associated with classic hemophilia A. **F. VIII:C** is the coagulant component of f. VIII which, in normal persons, circulates in the plasma complexed with **f. VIIIR** (von Willebrand f.), the plasma f. VIII related protein, a large glycoprotein component that is synthesized by endothelial cells and megakaryocytes, and circulates in the plasma where it binds to arteries that have lost their endothelial cell linings, creating a surface to which platelets adhere. Disorders involving f. VIIIR form a heterogenous group of abnormalities called von Willebrand's disease. A deficiency of f. can lead to impaired blood coagulation. SYN antihemophilic f. A, antihemophilic globulin A, antihemophilic globulin (1), plasma thromboplastin f., plasmokinin, platelet cofactor I, proserum prothrombin conversion accelerator, prothrombokinase, thrombokatilysin, thromboplastinogen.

von Willebrand f., SEE f. VIII.

W f., SYN biotin.

Williams f., SYN high molecular weight *kininogen*.

f. X, in the clotting of blood, also known as: Stuart f., Stuart-Prower f., prothrombase, and prothrombinase. Its active form, f. Xa (EC 3.4.21.6), is formed from f. X by limited proteolysis and assists in the conversion of prothrombin to thrombin. A deficiency of f. X will lead to impaired blood coagulation. SYN prothrombinase, Stuart f., Stuart-Prower f.

f. X for *Haemophilus*, SYN hemin.

f. XI, in the clotting of blood, also known as plasma thromboplastin antecedent, a component of the contact system which is absorbed from plasma and serum by glass and similar surfaces. Its active form, f. XIa (EC 3.4.21.27), is a serine proteinase converting f. IX to f. IXa. Deficiency of f. XI results in a hemorrhagic tendency and is caused by an autosomal recessive gene. SYN plasma thromboplastin antecedent.

f. XII, in the clotting of blood, also known as glass f. and Hageman f. When activated by glass or otherwise to its active form, f. XIIa (EC 3.4.21.38), a serine proteinase, it activates f.'s VII and XI and converts f. XI to its active form, f. XIa. Deficien-

cy of f. XII results in great prolongation of the clotting time of venous blood, but only rarely in a hemorrhagic tendency; deficiency is caused by an autosomal recessive gene. SYN glass f., Hageman f.

f. XIII, in the clotting of blood, also known as: fibrin-stabilizing f., Laki-Lorand f., and L-L f. It is catalyzed by thrombin into its active form, f. XIIIa, which cross-links subunits of the fibrin clot to form insoluble fibrin. SYN fibrin-stabilizing f., L-L f., Laki-Lorand f.

fac·to·ri·al (fak-tōr′ē-ăl). **1.** Pertaining to a statistical factor or factors. **2.** Of an integer, that integer multiplied by each smaller integer in succession down to one; *e.g.,* 5! equals $5 \times 4 \times 3 \times 2 \times 1 = 120$.

fac·ul·ta·tive (fak-ŭl-tā′tiv). Able to live under more than one specific set of environmental conditions; possessing an alternative pathway.

fac·ul·ty (fak′ŭl-tē). A natural or specialized power of a living organism.

FAD Abbreviation for *flavin* adenine dinucleotide.

Faget, Jean C., French physician, 1818–1884. SEE F.'s *sign*.

fag·o·py·rism (fag-ō-pī′rizm, fă-gop′i-rizm). Photosensitization, mainly in cattle and sheep, caused by ingestion of buckwheat (*Fagopyrum esculentum*) and characterized by irritation of the skin, edema, and a serous exudate.

Fahr, Theodore, German physician, 1877–1945. SEE F.'s *disease*.

Fahraeus, Robert (Robin) Sanno, Swedish pathologist, 1888–1968. SEE F.-Lindqvist *effect*.

Fahrenheit (F), Gabriel D., German-Dutch physicist, 1686–1736. SEE Fahrenheit *scale*.

fail·ure (fāl′yūr). The state of insufficiency or nonperformance.

acute respiratory f. (ARF), loss of pulmonary function either acute or chronic that results in hypoxemia or hypercarbia.

backward heart f., a concept (formerly considered mutually exclusive of forward heart f.) that maintains that the phenomena of congestive heart f. result from passive engorgement of the veins caused by a "backward" rise in pressure proximal to the failing cardiac chambers. Cf. forward heart f.

cardiac f., SYN heart f. (1).

congestive heart f., SYN heart f. (1).

coronary f., acute coronary insufficiency.

electrical f., f. in which the cardiac inadequacy is secondary to disturbance of the electrical impulse.

forward heart f., a concept (formerly considered mutually exclusive of backward heart f.) that maintains that the phenomena of congestive heart f. result from the inadequate cardiac output, and especially from the consequent inadequacy of renal blood flow with resulting retention of sodium and water. Cf. backward heart f.

heart f., (1) inadequacy of the heart so that as a pump it fails to maintain the circulation of blood, with the result that congestion and edema develop in the tissues; SYN cardiac f., cardiac insufficiency, congestive heart f., myocardial insufficiency. SEE ALSO forward heart f., backward heart f., right ventricular f., left ventricular f. **(2)** resulting clinical syndromes including shortness of breath, pitting edema, enlarged tender liver, engorged neck veins, and pulmonary rales in various combinations.

high output f., heart f. in which, despite relative myocardial insufficiency and consequent congestive heart f., the cardiac output is maintained at normal or supernormal levels, as is sometimes seen in emphysema, thyrotoxicosis, etc.

left-sided heart f., inability of the left heart to maintain its circulatory load with corresponding rise in pressure in the pulmonary circulation usually with pulmonary congestion and ultimately pulmonary edema.

left ventricular f., congestive heart f. manifested by signs of pulmonary congestion and edema, *i.e.,* dyspnea, rales, pulmonary edema, etc.

low output f., heart f. in which the cardiac output is subnormal, as is usually seen in f. due to coronary, hypertensive, or valvular heart disease.

pacemaker f., f. of an artificial pacemaker to generate or deliver effective stimuli to the myocardium.

power f., SYN pump f.

pump f., a term used to emphasize mechanical default of the heart as a pump; in acute myocardial infarction, pump f. signifies congestive heart failure, pulmonary edema, or cardiogenic shock. Cf. electrical f. SYN power f.

renal f., loss of renal function, either acute or chronic, that results in increased severe urea and creatinine.

right ventricular f., congestive heart f. manifested by distention of the neck veins, enlargement of the liver, and dependent edema due to pump f. of the right ventricle.

secondary f., (1) f. of the function of an organ as a result of antecedent pathology elsewhere; (2) decreasing responsiveness to a drug after an initial satisfactory response, usually occurring several months after initiation of treatment.

f. to thrive, a condition in which an infant's weight gain and growth is far below usual levels for age.

faint (fānt). **1.** Extremely weak; threatened with syncope. **2.** An episode of syncope. SEE ALSO syncope. [M.E., fr. O. Fr. *feindre*, to feign]

fal·cate (fal′kāt). SYN falciform.

fal·ces (fal′sēz). Plural of falx.

fal·cial (fal′shăl). Relating to the falx cerebelli or falx cerebri. SYN falcine.

fal·ci·form (fal′si-fōrm). Having a crescentic or sickle shape. SYN falcate. [L. *falx*, sickle, + *forma*, form]

fal·cine (fal′sēn). SYN falcial.

fal·cu·la (fal′kyū-lă). SYN *falx* cerebelli. [L. dim. of *falx*]

fal·cu·lar (fal′kyū-lăr). **1.** Resembling a sickle or falx. **2.** Relating to the falx cerebelli or cerebri.

fal·lo·pi·an (fa-lō′pē-an). Described by or attributed to Fallopius.

Fallopius (Fallopio), Gabriele, Italian anatomist, 1523–1562. SEE fallopian *aqueduct;* fallopian *arch;* fallopian *canal;* fallopian *hiatus;* fallopian *ligament;* fallopian *neuritis;* fallopian *pregnancy;* fallopian *tube; aqueductus* fallopii; *tuba* fallopiana; *tuba* fallopii; fallopian *tube.*

Fallot, Étienne-Louis A., French physician, 1850–1911. SEE *pentalogy* of F.; F.'s *tetrad, triad; trilogy* of F.

false neg·a·tive (fawls neg′ă-tiv). **1.** A test result which erroneously excludes an individual from a specific diagnostic or reference group, due particularly to insufficiently exact methods of testing. **2.** An individual whose test results exclude him from a particular diagnostic group though he may truly belong to such a group. **3.** Term used to denote a false-negative *result.*

false pos·i·tive (fawls pos′i-tiv). **1.** A test result which erroneously assigns an individual to a specific diagnostic or reference group, due particularly to insufficiently exact methods of testing. **2.** An individual whose test results include him in a particular diagnostic group though he may not truly belong to such a group. **3.** Term used to denote a false-positive *result.*

fal·si·fi·ca·tion (fawl′si-fi-kā′shŭn). The deliberate act of misrepresentation so as to deceive. SEE Munchausen *syndrome.* [L. *falsus*, false, + *facio*, to make]

retrospective f., unconscious distortion of past experience to conform to present psychological needs.

falx, pl. **fal·ces** (falks, fal′sēz) [NA]. A sickle-shaped structure. [L. sickle]

f. aponeurot′ica, SYN conjoint *tendon.*

f. cerebel′li [NA], a short process of dura mater projecting forward from the internal occipital crest below the tentorium; it occupies the posterior cerebellar notch and the vallecula, and bifurcates below into two diverging limbs passing to either side of the foramen magnum. SYN falcula.

f. cer′ebri [NA], the scythe-shaped fold of dura mater in the longitudinal fissure between the two cerebral hemispheres; it is attached anteriorly to the crista galli of the ethmoid bone and caudally to the upper surface of the tentorium.

f. inguina′lis [NA], SYN conjoint *tendon.*

f. sep′ti [NA], ☆official alternate term for *valve* of foramen ovale.

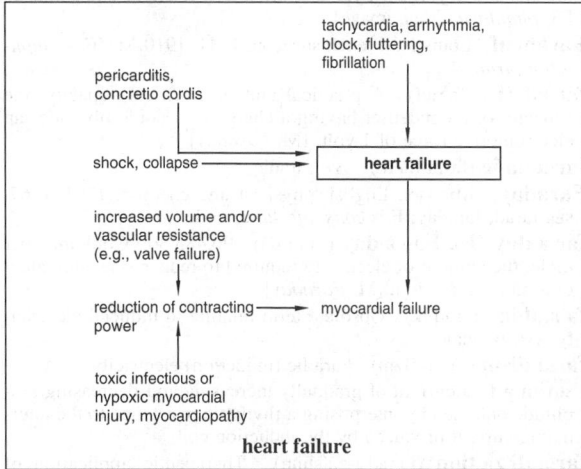

heart failure

fa·mil·i·al (fa-mil′ē-ăl). Affecting more members of the same family than can be accounted for by chance, usually within a single sibship; commonly but incorrectly used to mean genetic. [L. *familia*, family]

fa·mil·i·al neu·ro·vis·cer·o·lip·i·do·sis. SYN infantile, generalized G_{M1} *gangliosidosis.*

fam·i·ly (fam′ĭ-lē). **1.** A group of two or more persons united by blood, adoptive or marital ties, or the common law equivalent. **2.** In biologic classification a taxonomic grouping at the level intermediate between the order and the tribe or genus. [L. *familia*]

alu f., a set of dispersed sequences in the human genome having Alu cleavage sites at each end.

alu-equivalent f., a set of sequences in a mammalian genome that is related to the human Alu f.

cancer f., a group of blood relatives of whom several have had cancer; the mode of aggregation may be genetic and homogeneous, as in familial polyposis of the colon; diverse as in neurofibromatosis; or due to common exposure to a carcinogenic or oncogenic agent, such as a virus.

extended f., a group of persons comprising members of several generations united by blood, adoptive, marital or equivalent ties.

nuclear f., in genetics, two parents and their progeny in common.

fa·mo·ti·dine (fă-mō′ti-dēn). Propanimidamide, *N*′-(aminosulfonyl)-3-[[[2-[(diaminomethylene)amino]-4-thiazdyl]-methyl]thio]-; a histamine H_2 antagonist used in the treatment of duodenal ulcers to reduce hydrochloric acid secretion.

fam·o·tine hy·dro·chlo·ride (fam′ō-tēn). 1-[(*p*-Chlorophenoxy)methyl]-3,4-dihydroisoquinoline hydrochloride; an antiviral agent.

Fañanás, J., Spanish physician. SEE F. *cell.*

Fanconi, Guido, Swiss pediatrician, 1892–1979. SEE F.'s *anemia, pancytopenia, syndrome;* De Toni-F. *syndrome;* Lignac-F. *syndrome.*

fang. 1. A long tooth or tusk, usually a canine. **2.** The hollow tooth of a snake through which the venom is ejected. [A.S. *fōhan*, to seize]

fan·go (fang′gō). Mud from the Battaglio thermal springs in Italy, applied externally in the treatment of rheumatism and other diseases of the joints and muscles. [It. mud]

Fan·nia (fan′ē-ă). A genus of flies of the family Muscidae. Species include *F. canicularis* (the lesser housefly), commonly observed in kitchens or near food, which resembles *Musca domestica* (the common housefly) but is somewhat smaller and has three brown stripes on the thorax, and *F. scalaris* (the latrine fly) which commonly lays eggs in liquid feces of humans and animals and is distinguished from *F. canicularis* by two brown stripes on its thorax.

fan·ta·sy (fan′tă-sē). Imagery that is more or less coherent, as in dreams and daydreams, yet unrestricted by reality. SYN phantasia. [G. *phantasia,* idea, image]

Farabeuf, Louis H., French surgeon, 1841–1910. SEE F.'s *amputation, triangle.*

far·ad (F) (fa'rad). A practical unit of electrical capacity; the capacity of a condenser having a charge of 1 coulomb under an electromotive force of 1 volt. [M. *Faraday*]

far·a·da·ic (fa-ră-dā'ik). SYN faradic.

Faraday, Michael, English physicist and chemist, 1791–1867. SEE farad; faraday; F.'s *constant, laws,* under *law.*

far·a·day (F), Fa·ra·day (fa'ră-dā). 96,485.309 Coulombs per mole, the amount of electricity required to reduce one equivalent of a monovalent ion. [M. *Faraday*]

fa·rad·ic (fa-rad'ik). Obsolete term relating to induced electricity. SYN faradaic.

far·a·dism (fa'ră-dizm). Faradic (induction) electricity.

   surging f., a current of gradually increasing and decreasing amplitude obtained by interposing a rhythmic resistance to the alternating current produced by the induction coil.

far·a·di·za·tion (fa'rad-i-zā'shŭn). Therapeutic application of the faradic (induced) electrical current.

fa·ra·do·con·trac·til·i·ty (fa'ră-dō-kon'trak-til'i-tē). Contractility of muscles under the stimulus of a faradic (induced) electric current.

fa·ra·do·mus·cu·lar (fa'ră-dō-mŭs'kyū-lăr). Denoting the effect of applying a faradic (induced) electric current directly to a muscle.

far·a·do·pal·pa·tion (fa'ră-dō-pal-pā'shŭn). Esthesiometry by means of a sharp-pointed electrode through which a feeble alternating current passes to an indifferent electrode.

far·a·do·ther·a·py (fa'ră-dō-thār'ă-pē). Treatment of disease or paralysis by means of faradic (induced) electric current.

Farber, Sidney, U.S. pediatric pathologist, 1903–1973. SEE F.'s *disease, syndrome.*

far·cy (far'sē). **1.** A lymphatic disease of cattle caused by *Nocardia farcinica.* **2.** The skin form of glanders. [L. *farcio,* to stuff]

far·del (far-del'). The total measurable penalty that is incurred as a result of the occurrence of a genetic disease in one individual; one of two major quantitative considerations in the prognostic aspects of genetic counseling, the other being risk of occurrence. The f. roughly measures the duration and the severity of the penalty, *i.e.,* the integral of the total time-intensity function; *e.g.,* color blindness has a low intensity of penalty throughout life, anencephaly causes intense distress for a brief time, Alzheimer's disease is intermediate in both respects but the f. is greater. [M.E., fr. O. Fr., fr. Ar. *fardah,* bundle]

far·fa·ra (far'far-ă). The dried leaves of *Tussilago farfara* (family Compositae); a demulcent. [L. *farfarus,* coltsfoot]

fa·ri·na (fă-rē'nă). Flour or meal, as prepared from cereal grains such as *Avena sativa* (oats) or *Triticum sativum* (wheat); used as a starchy food. [L.]

   f. avenae (fă-rē'nă ă-vē-nă), oatmeal flour.

   f. tritici (fă-rē'nă trit'ĭ-sē), wheat flour.

far·i·na·ceous (far-i-nā'shŭs). **1.** Relating to farina or flour. **2.** Starchy.

α-far·ne·sene (far'nĕ-sēn). 3,7,11-Trimethyl-1,3,6,10-dodecatetraene; a straight open-chain hydrocarbon built up of three isoprene units; one of the four isomeric forms occurs in the natural coating of apples.

β-far·ne·sene. 7,11-Dimethyl-3-methylene-1,6,10-dodecatriene; one of the two isomers (*trans*) that occurs in the alarm pheromone of some aphids and also in various essential oils.

far·ne·sene al·co·hol. SYN farnesol.

far·ne·sol (far'nĕ-sol). A difarnesyl group that occurs in the side chain of vitamin K$_2$ and constitutes squalene; found in oil of citronella; a sesquiterpene alcohol. SYN farnesene alcohol.

far·nes·yl py·ro·phos·phate (far'nĕ-sil pī'rō-fos'fāt). The pyrophosphoryl derivative of farnesol; a key intermediate in the synthesis of steroids, dolichol, ubiquinone, prenylated proteins, and heme a.

far·no·qui·none (far'nō-kwin'ōn). SYN menaquinone-6.

Farnsworth, Dean, U.S. naval officer, 1902–1959. SEE F.-Munsell color *test.*

Farr, William, English medical statistician, 1807–1883. SEE F.'s *law.*

Farrant's mount·ing flu·id. See under fluid.

Farre, Arthur, English obstetrician and gynecologist, 1811–1887. SEE F.'s *line.*

far·sight·ed·ness (far'sīt'ed-nes). SYN hyperopia.

FASCIA

fas·cia, fas·ci·as, pl. **fas·ci·ae, fas·ci·as** (fash'ē-ă, -ē-ē) [NA]. A sheet of fibrous tissue that envelops the body beneath the skin; it also encloses muscles and groups of muscles, and separates their several layers or groups. [L. a band or fillet]

   Abernethy's f., a layer of subperitoneal areolar tissue in front of the external iliac artery. SEE iliac f.

   f. adhe'rens, a broad intercellular junction in the intercalated disk of cardiac muscle that anchors actin filaments.

   anal f., SYN inferior f. of pelvic diaphragm.

   antebrachial f., it is continuous with the brachial f.; in the region of the wrist it forms two thickened bands, the extensor and flexor retinacula. SYN f. antebrachii [NA], deep f. of forearm, f. of forearm.

   f. antebra'chii [NA], SYN antebrachial f.

   f. axilla'ris [NA], SYN axillary f.

   axillary f., the f. that forms the floor of the axilla. It is continuous with the pectoral and clavipectoral f. anteriorly, with the brachial f. laterally, and with the f. of the latissimus dorsi and serratus anterior muscles posteriorly and medially. SYN f. axillaris [NA].

   bicipital f., SYN bicipital *aponeurosis.*

   brachial f., the deep f. of the arm; it is continuous proximally with the pectoral f. and the f. covering the deltoid; distally it is continuous with the antebrachial f. SYN f. brachii [NA], deep f. of arm.

   f. bra'chii [NA], SYN brachial f.

   broad f., SYN deep f. of thigh.

   f. buc'copharyn'gea [NA], SYN buccopharyngeal f.

   buccopharyngeal f., the f. that covers the muscular layer of the pharynx and is continued forward onto the buccinator muscle. SYN f. buccopharyngea [NA].

   Buck's f., SYN deep f. of penis.

   f. bul'bi, SYN fascial *sheath* of eyeball.

   Camper's f., the more superficial, fatty part of the superficial fascia of the lower anterior abdominal wall. SYN fatty layer of superficial fascia.

   f. cervica'lis [NA], SYN deep cervical f.

   f. cervicalis profunda, SYN deep cervical f.

   f. cine'rea, SYN fasciolar *gyrus.*

   clavipectoral f., a f. that extends between the coracoid process, the clavicle, and the thoracic wall. It includes the muscular f. which envelops the subclavius and pectoralis minor muscles and the strong membrane (costocoracoid membrane) formed in the interval between them, and the suspensory ligament of the axilla. The clavipectoral fascia (and the muscles it envelopes) constitute the deep anterior wall of the axilla. SYN f. clavipectoralis [NA].

   f. clavipectora'lis [NA], SYN clavipectoral f.

   f. clitor'idis [NA], SYN f. of clitoris.

   f. of clitoris, fibrous tissue comparable to the f. of the penis. SYN f. clitoridis [NA].

   Colles' f., SYN superficial f. of perineum.

   Cooper's f., SYN cremasteric f.

   cremasteric f., h; one of the coverings of the spermatic cord, formed of delicate connective tissue and of muscular fibers derived from the internal oblique muscle (cremaster muscle). SEE

ALSO *aponeurosis* of internal abdominal oblique muscle. SYN f. cremasterica [NA], Cooper's f., Scarpa's sheath.

f. cremaster′ica [NA], SYN cremasteric f.

cribriform f., the part of the superficial f. of the thigh that covers the saphenous opening. SYN f. cribrosa [NA], Hesselbach's f.

f. cribro′sa [NA], SYN cribriform f.

crural f., f. of the leg; it is continuous with the f. lata and is attached proximally to the patella, ligamentum patellae, the tubercle and condyles of the tibia, and the head of the fibula; distally it is thickened to form the flexor and extensor retinacula. SYN f. cruris [NA], deep f. of leg, f. of leg.

f. cru′ris [NA], SYN crural f.

Cruveilhier's f., SYN superficial f. of perineum.

dartos f., a layer of smooth muscular tissue in the integument of the scrotum. SEE ALSO *dartos* muliebris. SYN tunica dartos [NA], dartos muscle, membrana carnosa, tunica carnea.

deep f., a thin fibrous membrane, devoid of fat, that invests the muscles, separating the several groups and the individual muscles, forms sheaths for the nerves and vessels, becomes specialized around the joints to form or strengthen ligaments, envelops various organs and glands, and binds all the structures together into a firm compact mass. SYN f. profunda [NA].

deep f. of arm, SYN brachial f.

deep cervical f., f. of the neck; it is divided into an external or investing layer (superficial lamina) that surrounds the neck and encloses the trapezius and sternocleidomastoid muscles, a middle or pretracheal layer in relation to the infrahyoid muscles, and a deep or prevertebral layer applied to the vertebrae and axial muscles. SYN f. cervicalis [NA], deep f. of neck, f. cervicalis profunda.

deep f. of forearm, SYN antebrachial f.

deep f. of leg, SYN crural f.

deep f. of neck, SYN deep cervical f.

deep f. of penis, a deep layer which surrounds the three erectile bodies of the penis. SYN Buck's f., f. penis profunda.

deep f. of thigh, the strong deep f. of the thigh, enveloping the muscles of the thigh and thickened laterally as the iliotibial track. SYN f. lata [NA], broad f.

f. denta′ta hippocam′pi, SYN dentate *gyrus.*

dentate f., SYN dentate *gyrus.*

f. diaphrag′matis pel′vis infe′rior [NA], SYN inferior f. of pelvic diaphragm.

f. diaphrag′matis pel′vis supe′rior [NA], SYN superior f. of pelvic diaphragm.

f. diaphrag′matis urogenita′lis infe′rior [NA], ☆official alternate term for inferior f. of urogenital diaphragm.

f. diaphrag′matis urogenita′lis supe′rior, SYN superior f. of urogenital diaphragm.

dorsal f. of foot, the f. that encloses the extensor tendons of the toes and blends with the inferior extensor retinaculum. SYN f. dorsalis pedis [NA].

dorsal f. of hand, the deep f. of the back of the hand continuous proximally with the extensor retinaculum. SYN f. dorsalis manus [NA].

f. dorsa′lis ma′nus [NA], SYN dorsal f. of hand.

f. dorsa′lis pe′dis [NA], SYN dorsal f. of foot.

Dupuytren's f., SYN palmar *aponeurosis.*

endopelvic f., SYN visceral pelvic f.

endothoracic f., the extrapleural f. that lines the wall of the thorax; it extends over the cupula of the pleura as the suprapleural membrane and also forms a thin layer between the diaphragm and pleura (phrenicopleura f.) SYN f. endothoracica [NA].

f. endothora′cica [NA], SYN endothoracic f.

external spermatic f., the outer fascial covering of the spermatic cord; it is continuous at the superficial inguinal ring with the f. covering the external oblique muscle. SEE ALSO *aponeurosis* of external abdominal oblique muscle. SYN f. spermatica externa [NA].

f. of extraocular muscles, SYN fascial *sheaths* of extraocular muscles, under *sheath.*

extraperitoneal f., the thin layer of f. and adipose tissue between the peritoneum and f. transversalis. SYN f. subperitonealis [NA], subperitoneal f.

f. of forearm, SYN antebrachial f.

Gerota's f., SYN renal f.

Godman's f., an extension of the pretracheal f. into the thorax and on to the pericardium.

Hesselbach's f., SYN cribriform f.

iliac f., the f. covering the iliacus and psoas muscles, continuous with transversalis fascia anterolaterally and with femoral sheath inferiorly. SYN f. iliaca [NA].

f. ili′aca [NA], SYN iliac f.

iliopectineal f., a f. formed by the union of the fasciae covering the iliacus and pectinus muscles which cover the floor of the iliopectineal fossa. SEE iliopectineal *arch.*

inferior f. of pelvic diaphragm, the f. that covers the inferior aspect of the levator ani and coccygeus muscles. SYN f. diaphragmatis pelvis inferior [NA], anal f.

inferior f. of urogenital diaphragm, the layer of fascia extending between the ischiopubic rami inferior to the sphincter urethrae and the deep transverse perineal muscles. SYN membrana perinei [NA], f. diaphragmatis urogenitalis inferior☆ [NA], Camper's ligament, ligamentum triangulare, perineal membrane, triangular ligament.

infraspinatus f., f. in′fraspina′ta, the f. attached to the borders of the infraspinous fossa and covering the infraspinatus muscle; it is continuous with the f. covering the deltoid.

infundibuliform f., SYN internal spermatic f.

intercolumnar fasciae, SYN intercrural *fibers,* under *fiber.*

internal spermatic f., the inner covering of the spermatic cord, continuous above the deep inguinal ring with f. transversalis. SYN f. spermatica interna [NA], infundibuliform f., tunica vaginalis communis.

interosseous f., the f. covering the interosseous muscles of the hand or foot; it consists of a dorsal layer and a palmar or plantar layer.

investing f., SYN investing *layer* of deep cervical fascia.

lacrimal f., that part of the periorbita that bridges across the fossa or lacrimal sac.

f. la′ta [NA], SYN deep f. of thigh.

f. of leg, SYN crural f.

lumbodorsal f., SYN thoracolumbar f.

masseteric f., the f. that covers the lateral surface of the masseter muscle. SYN f. masseterica [NA].

f. massete′rica [NA], SYN masseteric f.

middle cervical f., SYN pretracheal f.

muscular f. of extraocular muscle, SYN fascial *sheaths* of extraocular muscles, under *sheath.*

f. muscula′ris musculo′rum bul′bi [NA], SYN fascial *sheaths* of extraocular muscles, under *sheath.*

f. nu′chae [NA], SYN nuchal f.

nuchal f., the f. that encloses the posterior muscles of the neck. SYN f. nuchae [NA].

obturator f., the portion of the pelvic f. that covers the obturator internus muscle. SYN f. obturatoria [NA].

f. obturato′ria [NA], SYN obturator f.

orbital fasciae, the fascial layers in the orbit consisting of periorbita, septum orbitale, f. muscularis musculorum bulbi, and vagina bulbi. SYN fasciae orbitales [NA].

fas′ciae orbita′les [NA], SYN orbital fasciae.

palmar f., SYN palmar *aponeurosis.*

parietal pelvic f., including the obturator f., covers the muscles that pass from the interior of the pelvis to the thigh. SYN f. pelvis parietalis.

parotid f., the part of the investing cervical f. that ensheaths the parotid gland and is fixed above to the zygomatic arch. SYN f. parotidea [NA], fibrous capsule of parotid gland, parotid sheath.

f. parotid′ea [NA], SYN parotid f.

parotideomasseteric f., a dense membrane covering both the lateral and medial surfaces of the parotid gland, continuous anteriorly with the f. covering the masseter muscle. SEE parotid f., masseteric f. SYN f. parotideomasseterica.

f. parotideomasseter'ica, SYN parotideomasseteric f.

pectoral f., the f. that covers the pectoralis major muscle; it is attached to the sternum and to the clavicle; laterally and below it is continuous with the f. of the shoulder, axilla, and thorax. SYN f. pectoralis [NA].

f. pectora'lis [NA], SYN pectoral f.

pelvic f., it includes parietal and visceral components: fascia pelvis parietalis and fascia pelvis visceralis. SYN f. pelvis [NA].

f. pel'vis [NA], SYN pelvic f.

f. pel'vis parieta'lis, SYN parietal pelvic f.

f. pel'vis viscera'lis, SYN visceral pelvic f.

f. pe'nis [NA], SYN f. of penis.

f. of penis, it is divided into two layers: deep f. of penis and of f. superficial penis. SYN f. penis [NA].

f. pe'nis profun'da, SYN deep f. of penis.

f. pe'nis superficia'lis, SYN superficial f. of penis.

f. perine'i superficia'lis [NA], SYN superficial f. of perineum.

perirenal f., SYN renal f.

pharyngobasilar f., the fibrous coat of the pharyngeal wall situated between the mucous and muscular coats; it is attached above to the basilar part of the occipital bone, and the petrous part of the temporal bone. This layer and the mucosa which lines it forms the wall of the non-muscular pharynx (pharyngeal vault) above the superior pharyngesl constrictor muscle. SYN f. pharyngobasilaris [NA], aponeurosis pharyngea, tela submucosa pharyngis.

f. pharyngobasila'ris [NA], SYN pharyngobasilar f.

phrenicopleural f., the thin layer of endothoracic f. intervening between the diaphragmatic pleura and the diaphragm. SYN f. phrenicopleuralis [NA].

f. phrenicopleura'lis [NA], SYN phrenicopleural f.

plantar f., SYN plantar *aponeurosis*.

popliteal f., the f. that covers the popliteal fossa, continuous with fascia lata superiorly and crural fascia inferiorly.

Porter's f., SYN pretracheal f.

pretracheal f., the layer of fascia investing the infrahyoid muscles and contributing to the formation of the carotid sheath. SYN lamina pretrachealis [NA], middle cervical f., Porter's f., pretracheal layer.

prevertebral f., the part of the cervical fascia which covers the bodies of the cervical vertebrae and the muscles attaching to them and to the anterior parts of their transverse processes. SYN lamina prevertebralis [NA], prevertebral layer.

f. profun'da [NA], SYN deep f.

f. pros'tatae [NA], SYN f. of prostate.

f. of prostate, the condensation of pelvic visceral f. that encloses the prostate gland. SYN f. prostatae [NA].

rectovesical f., SYN rectovesical *septum*.

renal f., the condensation of the fibroareolar tissue and fat surrounding the kidney to form a sheath for the organ. SYN f. renalis [NA], Gerota's capsule, Gerota's f., perirenal f.

f. rena'lis [NA], SYN renal f.

Scarpa's f., the deeper, membranous or lamellar part of the subcutaneous tissue of the lower abdominal wall; it is continuous with the superficial perineal (Colles') f. SYN membranous layer of superficial fascia (2).

semilunar f., SYN bicipital *aponeurosis*.

Sibson's f., SYN suprapleural *membrane*.

f. spermat'ica exter'na [NA], SYN external spermatic f.

f. spermat'ica inter'na [NA], SYN internal spermatic f.

subperitoneal f., SYN extraperitoneal f.

f. subperitonea'lis [NA], SYN extraperitoneal f.

subsartorial f., dense fascial triangle extending from the inferior medial border of the adductor magnus muscle to the vastus medialis muscle. Along with the sartorius muscle, this dense f. forms the roof of the lower 1/2 of the adductor canal and, as the femoral vessels pass deep to it, is often mistaken for the adductor hiatus. SYN vastoadductor f.

superficial f., a loose fibrous envelope beneath the skin, containing fat in its meshes (panniculus adiposus) or fasciculi of muscular tissue (panniculus carnosus); it contains the cutaneous vessels

and nerves and is in relation by its undersurface with the deep fascia. SYN f. superficialis [NA], tela subcutanea [NA], hypoderm, hypodermis, stratum subcutaneum, subcutis.

f. superficia'lis [NA], SYN superficial f.

superficial f. of penis, a superficial layer continuous with f. perinei superficialis. SYN f. penis superficialis.

superficial f. of perineum, the membranous layer of the subcutaneous tissue in the urogenital region attaching posteriorly to the border of the urogenital diaphragm, at the sides to the ischiopubic rami, and continuing anteriorly onto the abdominal wall. SYN f. perinei superficialis [NA], Colles' f., Cruveilhier's f., membranous layer of superficial fascia (1).

superior f. of pelvic diaphragm, the f. on the superior aspect of the levator ani and coccygeus muscles. SYN f. diaphragmatis pelvis superior [NA].

superior f. of urogenital diaphragm, a layer of f. that has been described on the superior surface of the sphincter urethrae and the deep transverse perineal muscles. Its presence is doubted by some anatomists. SYN f. diaphragmatis urogenitalis superior.

temporal f., the f. covering the temporal muscle; it is composed of two layers, lamina superficialis and lamina profunda; both attach above to the superior temporal line but diverge inferiorly to attach to the lateral and medial surfaces of the zygomatic arch. SYN f. temporalis [NA], temporal aponeurosis.

f. tempora'lis [NA], SYN temporal f.

thoracolumbar f., the f. which covers the deep muscles of the back; it is attached to the angles of the ribs and to the spines of the thoracic, lumbar, and sacral vertebrae, to the transverse processes of the lumbar vertebrae, to the lower border of the twelth rib and to the iliac crest, as well as to the lumbocostal, iliolumbar, intertransverse, and supraspinous ligaments. SYN f. thoracolumbalis [NA], lumbodorsal f., thoracolumbar aponeurosis.

f. thoracolumba'lis [NA], SYN thoracolumbar f.

Toldt's f., continuation of Treitz's f. behind the body of the pancreas.

f. transversa'lis [NA], SYN transversalis f.

transversalis f., the lining f. of the abdominal cavity, between the inner surface of the abdominal musculature and the peritoneum. SYN f. transversalis [NA].

Treitz's f., f. behind the head of the pancreas.

triangular f., SYN reflected inguinal *ligament*.

f. triangula'ris abdom'inis, SYN reflected inguinal *ligament*.

Tyrrell's f., SYN rectovesical *septum*.

umbilical prevesical f., the thin fascial layer interposed between the transversalis f. and the umbilicovesical f. It extends between the medial umbilical ligaments from the umbilicus downward in front of the bladder, forming the posterior boundary of the retropubic space.

umbilicovesical f., a thin fascial layer that extends between the medial umbilical ligaments and is continuous with f. enclosing the bladder.

vastoadductor f., SYN subsartorial f.

visceral pelvic f., covers the pelvic organs and surrounds vessels and nerves in the subperitoneal space. SYN endopelvic f., f. pelvis visceralis.

Zuckerkandl's f., the posterior layer of the renal f.

---

fas·cial (fash'ē-ăl). Relating to any fascia.

fas·ci·as. SEE fascia.

fas·ci·cle (fas'i-kl). A band or bundle of fibers, usually of muscle or nerve fibers; a nerve fiber tract. SYN fasciculus [NA].

muscle f., a bundle of muscle fibers surrounded by perimysium.

nerve f., a bundle of nerve fibers surrounded by perineurium.

fas·cic·u·lar (fa-sik'yū-lăr). Relating to a fasciculus; arranged in the form of a bundle or collection of rods. SYN fasciculate, fasciculated.

fas·cic·u·late, fas·cic·u·lat·ed (fa-sik'yū-lāt, -lā-ted). SYN fascicular.

fas·cic·u·la·tion (fa-sik-yū-lā'shŭn). **1.** An arrangement in the form of fasciculi. **2.** Involuntary contractions, or twitchings, of groups (fasciculi) of muscle fibers, a coarser form of muscular contraction than fibrillation.

fas·cic·u·li (fa-sik′yū-lī). Plural of fasciculus.

FASCICULUS

fas·cic·u·lus, gen. and pl. **fas·cic·u·li** (fă-sik′yū-lŭs, fă-sik′yū-lī) [NA]. SYN fascicle. [L. dim. of *fascis*, bundle]

f. ante′rior pro′prius, the ground bundle of the anterior column of the spinal cord. SEE fasciculi proprii. SYN anterior ground bundle.

anterior pyramidal f., SYN anterior pyramidal *tract*.

arcuate f., (1) SYN superior longitudinal f. **(2)** SYN uncinate f.

f. at′rioventricula′ris [NA], SYN atrioventricular *bundle*.

Burdach's f., SYN cuneate f.

calcarine f., a group of short association fibers beneath the calcarine fissure of the occipital lobe of the cerebrum.

central tegmental f., SYN central tegmental *tract*.

f. cir′cumoliva′ris pyram′idis, an anomalous bundle of nerve fibers on the anterior surface of the medulla oblongata that emerges from the pyramid and curves forward and dorsally over the lower pole of the olive; it is variously interpreted as an aberrant bundle of pontocerebellar fibers or corticopontine fibers.

f. corticospina′lis ante′rior, SYN anterior pyramidal *tract*.

f. corticospina′lis latera′lis, SYN lateral pyramidal *tract*.

cuneate f., the larger lateral subdivision of the posterior funiculus. SYN f. cuneatus [NA], Burdach's column, Burdach's f., Burdach's tract, cuneate funiculus, wedge-shaped f.

f. cunea′tus [NA], SYN cuneate f.

dorsal longitudinal f., a bundle of thin, poorly myelinated nerve fibers reciprocally connecting the periventricular zone of the hypothalamus with ventral parts of the central gray substance of the midbrain. SYN f. longitudinalis dorsalis [NA], Schütz' bundle, tract of Schütz.

dorsolateral f., a longitudinal bundle of thin, unmyelinated and poorly myelinated fibers capping the apex of the posterior horn of the spinal gray matter, composed of posterior root fibers and short association fibers that interconnect neighboring segments of the posterior horn. SYN f. dorsolateralis [NA], tractus dorsolateralis [NA], dorsolateral tract, f. marginalis, Lissauer's bundle, Lissauer's column, Lissauer's f., Lissauer's marginal zone, Lissauer's tract, marginal f., Spitzka's marginal tract, Spitzka's marginal zone, Waldeyer's tract, Waldeyer's zonal layer.

f. dorsolatera′lis [NA], SYN dorsolateral f.

Flechsig's fasciculi, f. anterior proprius and f. lateralis proprius. SEE fasciculi proprii.

Foville's f., SYN terminal *stria*.

fronto-occipital f., SYN occipitofrontal f.

gracile f., the smaller medial subdivision of the posterior funiculus. SYN f. gracilis [NA].

f. grac′ilis [NA], SYN gracile f. SYN funiculus gracilis, Goll's column, posterior pyramid of the medulla, slender f., tract of Goll.

hooked f., SYN uncinate f.

inferior longitudinal f., a well marked bundle of long association fibers running the whole length of the occipital and temporal lobes of the cerebrum, in part parallel with the inferior horn of the lateral ventricle. SYN f. longitudinalis inferior [NA].

interfascicular f., SYN semilunar f.

f. interfascicula′ris [NA], ✩official alternate term for semilunar f.

intersegmental fasciculi, SYN fasciculi proprii.

f. latera′lis plex′us brachia′lis [NA], SYN lateral *cord* of brachial plexus.

f. latera′lis pro′prius, SEE fasciculi proprii.

lateral pyramidal f., SYN lateral pyramidal *tract*.

lenticular f., the pallidal efferent fibers that cross the internal capsule and are insinuated between the subthalamic nucleus and

zona incerta; they join in the formation of the thalamic fasciculus. SEE ALSO lenticular *loop*. SYN f. lenticularis.

f. lenticula′ris, SYN lenticular f.

Lissauer's f., SYN dorsolateral f.

fasciculi longitudina′les ligamen′ti crucifor′mis atlan′tis [NA], SYN longitudinal *bands* of cruciform ligament, under *band*.

fascic′uli longitudina′les pon′tis, SYN longitudinal pontine fasciculi.

f. longitudina′lis dorsa′lis [NA], SYN dorsal longitudinal f.

f. longitudina′lis infe′rior [NA], SYN inferior longitudinal f.

f. longitudina′lis media′lis [NA], SYN medial longitudinal f.

f. longitudina′lis supe′rior [NA], SYN superior longitudinal f.

longitudinal pontine fasciculi, the massive bundles of corticofugal fibers passing longitudinally through the ventral part of pons; they are composed of corticopontine, corticobulbar, and corticospinal fibers. SYN fasciculi longitudinales pontis, longitudinal pontine bundles.

macular f., the collection of fibers in the optic nerve directly connected with the macula lutea. SYN f. macularis.

f. macula′ris, SYN macular f.

mamillotegmental f., a small bundle of fibers that passes dorsalward from the mamillary body for a short distance with the mamillothalamic tract, then turns down the brainstem to reach the dorsal and ventral tegmental nuclei of the mesencephalon. SYN f. mamillotegmentalis [NA].

f. mamillotegmenta′lis [NA], SYN mamillotegmental f.

mamillothalamic f., a compact, thick bundle of nerve fibers that passes dorsalward from the mamillary body on either side to terminate in the anterior nucleus of the thalamus. SYN f. mamillothalamicus [NA], f. thalamomamillaris, mamillothalamic tract, Vicq d'Azyr's bundle.

f. mamillothalam′icus [NA], SYN mamillothalamic f.

marginal f., SYN dorsolateral f.

f. margina′lis, SYN dorsolateral f.

f. media′lis plex′us brachia′lis [NA], SYN medial *cord* of brachial plexus.

medial longitudinal f., a longitudinal bundle of fibers extending from the upper border of the mesencephalon into the cervical segments of the spinal cord, located close to the midline and ventral to the central gray matter; it is composed largely of fibers from the vestibular nuclei ascending to the motor neurons innervating the external eye muscles (abducens, trochlear, and oculomotor nuclei), and descending to spinal cord segments innervating the musculature of the neck. SYN f. longitudinalis medialis [NA], Collier's tract, medial longitudinal bundle, posterior longitudinal bundle.

Meynert's f., SYN retroflex f.

oblique pontine f., a bundle of fibers in the ventral surface of the pons running from the anterior mesial portion outward and backward. SYN f. obliquus pontis, oblique bundle of pons.

f. obli′quus pon′tis, SYN oblique pontine f.

occipitofrontal f., a bundle of association fibers extending from the frontal to the occipital lobes of the cerebrum. SYN f. occipitofrontalis, fronto-occipital f.

f. occip′itofronta′lis, SYN occipitofrontal f.

oval f., SEE semilunar f.

f. pedun′culomamilla′ris, SYN *peduncle* of mamillary body.

pedunculomamillary f., SYN *peduncle* of mamillary body.

perpendicular f., a bundle of association fibers running vertically and interconnecting regions of the temporal, occipital, and parietal lobes.

f. poste′rior plex′us brachia′lis [NA], SYN posterior *cord* of brachial plexus.

proper fasciculi, SYN fasciculi proprii.

fascic′uli pro′prii [NA], Flechsig's fasciculi or ground bundles (f. anterior proprius and f. lateralis proprius or lateral ground bundle); intersegmental fasciculi; ascending and descending association fiber systems of the spinal cord which lie deep in the anterior, lateral, and posterior funiculi adjacent to the gray matter. SYN ground bundles, intersegmental fasciculi, proper fasciculi.

f. pyramida′lis ante′rior, SYN anterior pyramidal *tract*.

fa

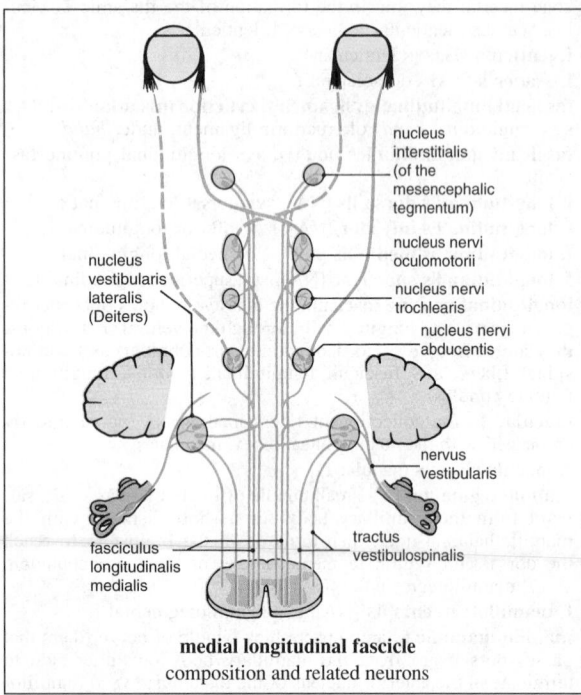

nucleus interstitialis (of the mesencephalic tegmentum)

nucleus nervi oculomotorii

nucleus nervi trochlearis

nucleus nervi abducentis

nucleus vestibularis lateralis (Deiters)

nervus vestibularis

fasciculus longitudinalis medialis

tractus vestibulospinalis

medial longitudinal fascicle
composition and related neurons

f. pyramida′lis latera′lis, SYN lateral pyramidal *tract*.

retroflex f., a compact bundle of fibers arising in the habenula and passing ventralward to the interpeduncular nucleus at the base of the midbrain; part of its fibers bypass this nucleus and terminate in the raphe nuclei of the caudal mesencephalic tegmentum. SYN f. retroflexus [NA], habenulointerpeduncular tract, Meynert's f., Meynert's retroflex bundle.

f. retroflex′us [NA], SYN retroflex f.

f. rotun′dus, SYN solitary *tract*.

round f., SYN solitary *tract*.

rubroreticular fasciculi, bundles of fibers that connect the red nucleus to the pontine and midbrain reticular nuclei. SYN fasciculi rubroreticulares [NA].

fasciculi rubroreticula′res [NA], SYN rubroreticular fasciculi.

semilunar f., a compact bundle composed of descending branches of posterior root fibers located near the border between the fasciculi gracilis and cuneatus of the cervical and thoracic spinal cord; it corresponds to the septomarginal f., Hoche's tract, or oval area of Flechsig in the lumbar, and to the triangle of Philippe-Gombault in the sacral spinal segments; like these, it can be demonstrated only in cases of demyelination resulting from dorsal root lesions. SYN f. semilunaris [NA], f. interfascicularis✶ [NA], comma bundle of Schultze, comma tract of Schultze, interfascicular f.

f. semiluna′ris [NA], SYN semilunar f.

septomarginal f., septomarginal f. or tract. SEE semilunar f. SYN f. septomarginalis [NA].

f. septomargina′lis [NA], SYN septomarginal f.

slender f., SYN f. gracilis.

f. solita′rius, SYN solitary *tract*.

solitary f., SYN solitary *tract*.

subcallosal f., a bundle of thin nerve fibers running longitudinally beneath the corpus callosum in the angle between the latter and the caudate nucleus; it forms an anterior continuation of the tapetum of the temporal lobe and appears to consist largely of fibers projecting from the cerebral cortex to the caudate nucleus. SYN f. subcallosus [NA].

f. subcallo′sus [NA], SYN subcallosal f.

subthalamic f., nerve fibers crossing the internal capsule between the subthalamic nucleus and the globus pallidus; this f. contains pallidosubthalamic and subthalamopallidal fibers.

superior longitudinal f., long association fiber bundle lateral to the centrum ovale of the cerebral hemisphere, connecting the frontal, occipital, and temporal lobes; the fibers pass from the frontal lobe through the operculum to the posterior end of the lateral sulcus where many fibers radiate into the occipital lobe and others turn downward and forward around the putamen and pass to anterior portions of the temporal lobe. SYN f. longitudinalis superior [NA], arcuate f. (1).

thalamic f., nerve fibers forming a composite bundle containing cerebellothalamic (crossed) and pallidothalamic (uncrossed) fibers that is insinuated between the thalamus and zona incerta. SEE ALSO *fields* of Forel, under *field*. SYN f. thalamicus.

f. thalam′icus, SYN thalamic f.

f. thal′amomamilla′ris, SYN mamillothalamic f.

transverse fasciculi, SYN fasciculi transversi.

fascic′uli transver′si [NA], the transversely directed fibers in the distal portions of the palmar and plantar aponeuroses. SYN transverse fasciculi.

unciform f., uncinate f., a band of long association fibers reciprocally connecting the frontal and temporal lobes of the cerebrum, running caudally through the white matter of the frontal lobe, sharply curving ventrally under the stem of the sylvian fissure, and then fanning out to the cortex of the anterior half of the superior and middle temporal gyri.

uncinate f. of Russell, SYN uncinate *bundle* of Russell.

f. uncina′tus [NA], SYN uncinate f.

wedge-shaped f., SYN cuneate f.

fas·ci·ec·to·my (fash-ē-ek′tō-mē). Excision of strips of fascia. [fascia + G. *ektomē*, excision]

fas·ci·i·tis (fas-ē-ī′tis, fash-). **1.** Inflammation in fascia. **2.** Reactive proliferation of fibroblasts in fascia. SYN fascitis.

eosinophilic f., induration and edema of the connective tissues of the extremities, usually appearing following exertion; associated with elevated sedimentation rate, elevated IgG, and eosinophilia. SYN Shulman's syndrome.

group A streptococcal necrotizing f., a complication of infection with GAS (group A streptococci) in which the bacteria attacks and destroys muscle tissue. According to the CDC, 5–10% of people with severe GAS infection develop necrotizing f. Though the infection can be treated with antibiotics, the fatality rate is close to 30%. This complication often develops as a wound infection after surgery or injury.

necrotizing f., a rare soft-tissue infection primarily involving the superficial fascia and resulting in extensive undermining of surrounding tissues; progress is often fulminant and may involve all soft-tissue components, including the skin; usually occurs postoperatively, after minor trauma, or after inadequate care of abscesses or cutaneous ulcers. SEE ALSO group A streptococcal necrotizing f.

nodular f., a rapidly-growing tumor-like proliferation of fibroblasts, not thought to be neoplastic, with mild inflammatory exudation occurring in fascia; the fibrosis may infiltrate surrounding tissue but does not progress indefinitely or metastasize. SYN pseudosarcomatous f.

parosteal f., a rare form of nodular f. arising from the periosteum, and which may be associated with reactive cortical bone formation.

proliferative f., a benign rapidly-growing subcutaneous nodule characterized by proliferation of fibroblasts and basophilic giant cells slightly resembling ganglion cells.

pseudosarcomatous f., SYN nodular f.

△**fascio-.** A fascia. [L. *fascia*, a band or fillet]

fas·ci·od·e·sis (fas-ē-od′ĕ-sis, fas-). Surgical attachment of a fascia to another fascia or a tendon. [fascio- + G. *desis*, a binding together]

Fas·ci·o·la (fa-sē′ō-lă, fa-sī′ō-lă). A genus of large, leaf-shaped, digenetic liver flukes (family Fasciolidae, class Trematoda) of mammals. [L. dim. of *fascia*, a band]

F. gigan′tica, a species, resembling *F. hepatica* but of larger size, found in herbivores, especially in Africa, where it also infects humans.

F. hepat'ica, the common liver fluke inhabiting the bile ducts of sheep and cattle; the intermediate hosts are aquatic snails, *Lymnaea* or related genera; after the cercariae escape, they become encysted on water plants by which they gain access to the intestinal canal; rarely, this fluke is reported from humans, in whom it may cause considerable biliary damage.

fas·ci·o·la, pl. **fas·ci·o·lae** (fa-sē′ō-lă, fa-sī′ō-lă; -ō-lē). A small band or group of fibers. [L. dim. of *fascia,* band, fillet]

  f. cine′rea, SYN fasciolar *gyrus.*

fas·ci·o·lar (fa-sē′ō-lăr, fa-sī′). Relating to the gyrus fasciolaris.

fas·ci·o·li·a·sis (fas′ē-ō-lī′ă-sis, fa-sī′ō-lī′ă-sis). Infection with a species of *Fasciola.*

fas·ci·o·lid (fa-sē′ō-lid, fa-sī′). A member of the family Fasciolidae.

Fas·ci·o·loi·des mag·na (fas′ē-ō-loy′dēz mag′nă, fa-sī′o-). A species of fasciolid flukes found in the lungs and liver of deer and sometimes cattle in North America; it is not known to infect humans.

fas·ci·o·lop·si·a·sis (fas′ē-ō-lop-sī′ă-sis, fa-sī′o-). Parasitization by any of the flukes of the genus *Fasciolopsis.*

Fas·ci·o·lop·sis (fas′ē-ō-lop′sis, fa-sī′ō-). A genus of very large intestinal fasciolid flukes. [*Fasciola* + G. *opsis,* form, appearance]

  F. bus′ki, the large intestinal fluke, a species found in the intestine of humans in eastern and southern Asia; transmitted via ingestion of water chestnuts or other vegetation contaminated with infective metacercariae.

  F. rathoui′si, a species reported from China in a few cases in the intestine or liver; possibly the same as *F. buski.*

fas·ci·o·plas·ty (fash′ē-ō-plas-tē). Plastic surgery of a fascia. [fascia + G. *plastos,* formed]

fas·ci·or·rha·phy (fash-ē-ōr′ă-fē). Suture of a fascia or aponeurosis. SYN aponeurorrhaphy. [fascio- + G. *rhaphē,* suture]

fas·ci·ot·o·my (fash-ē-ot′ō-mē). Incision through a fascia; used in the treatment of certain vascular disorders and injuries when marked swelling is anticipated which could compromise blood flow; f. may be combined with embolectomy in the treatment of acute arterial embolism. [fascio- + G. *tomē,* incision]

fas·ci·tis (fa-sī′tis). SYN fasciitis.

fast. **1.** Durable; resistant to change; applied to stained microorganisms which cannot be decolorized. SEE ALSO acid-fast. **2.** Not eating. [A.S. *foest,* firm, fixed]

fast green FCF [C.I. 42053]. An acid arylmethane dye widely used in histology and cytology and less subject to fading than light green FCF which it has replaced in many procedures; used as a quantitative cytochemical stain for histones at alkaline pH after acid extraction of DNA, and also in electrophoresis as a protein stain.

fas·tid·i·ous (fas-tid′ē-ŭs). In bacteriology, having complex nutritional requirements.

fas·tid·i·um ci·bi (fas-tid′ē-ŭm kib′ī). Rarely used term for fickle or finicky appetite, caused by distaste for food. [L.]

fas·ti·ga·tum (fas-ti-gā′tŭm). SYN fastigial *nucleus.* [L. *fastigatus,* pointed]

fas·tig·i·um (fas-tij′ē-ŭm). **1.** Apex of the roof of the fourth ventricle of the brain, an angle formed by the anterior and posterior medullary vela extending into the substance of the vermis. **2.** The acme or period of full development of a disease. [L. top, as of a gable; a pointed extremity]

fast·ness (fast′nes). The state of tolerance exhibited by bacteria to a drug or other agent. SEE fast.

fat. **1.** SYN adipose *tissue.* **2.** Common term for obese. **3.** A greasy, soft-solid material, found in animal tissues and many plants, composed of a mixture of glycerol esters; together with oils they comprise the homolipids. **4.** SYN triacylglycerol. [A.S. *faet*]

  brown f., thermogenic tissue that is composed of cells containing numerous small fat droplets; lobular masses are found in the interscapular and mediastinal regions and other locations; although found most frequently in certain hibernating animals, it is also found in pigs, rodents, and the newborn of humans. SYN brown adipose tissue, hibernating gland, interscapular gland, in-

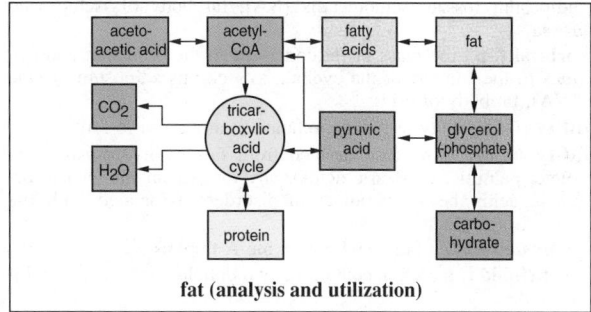

fat (analysis and utilization)

terscapular hibernoma, multilocular adipose tissue, multilocular f.

  multilocular f., SYN brown f.

  neutral f., a triester of fatty acids and glycerol (*i.e.,* triacylglycerol).

  saturated f., SEE saturated *fatty acid.*

  split f., free fatty acids, as reduced by the action of lipases, neutral f.'s, or phospholipids.

  unilocular f., adipose tissue in which the fat is present in a single droplet within the fat cells. SYN white f. (2).

  unsaturated f., SEE unsaturated *fatty acid.*

  white f., (1) SYN adipose *tissue.* (2) SYN unilocular f.

  wool f., SYN lanolin.

fa·tal (fā′tăl). Pertaining to or causing death; denoting especially inevitability or inescapability of death. [L. *fatalis,* of or belonging to fate]

fa·tal·i·ty (fā-tal′i-tē). **1.** A condition, disease, or disaster ending in death. **2.** An individual instance of death.

fate. The ultimate outcome.

  prospective f., the normal development by any part of the egg or embryo without interference.

fat·i·ga·bil·i·ty (fat′i-gă-bil′i-tē). A condition in which fatigue is easily induced.

fa·ti·ga·ble (fat′i-gă-bl). Tiring on very slight exertion. [L. *fatigabilis,* easily tired, fr. *fatigo,* to tire]

fa·tigue (fă-tēg′). **1.** That state, following a period of mental or bodily activity, characterized by a lessened capacity for work and reduced efficiency of accomplishment, usually accompanied by a feeling of weariness, sleepiness, or irritability; may also supervene when, from any cause, energy expenditure outstrips restorative processes and may be confined to a single organ. **2.** Sensation of boredom and lassitude due to absence of stimulation, monotony, or lack of interest in one's surroundings. [Fr., fr. L. *fatigo,* to tire]

  auditory f., temporary shift of threshold sensitivity following exposure to sound.

  battle f., a term used to denote psychiatric illness consequent to the stresses of battle. SEE ALSO war *neurosis,* neurocirculatory *asthenia.* SYN shell shock.

  functional vocal f., SYN phonasthenia.

fat-pad. An accumulation of somewhat encapsulated adipose tissue. SYN corpus adiposum [NA].

  Bichat's f.-p., SYN buccal f.-p.

  buccal f.-p., an encapsuled mass of fat in the cheek on the outer side of the buccinator muscle, especially marked in the infant; supposed to strengthen and support the cheek during the act of sucking. SYN corpus adiposum buccae [NA], Bichat's f.-p., Bichat's protuberance, fat body of cheek, sucking cushion, sucking pad, suctorial pad.

  Imlach's f.-p., fat surrounding the round ligament of the uterus in the inguinal canal.

  infrapatellar f.-p., the fatty mass that occupies the area between the patellar ligament and the infrapatellar synovial fold of the knee joint. SYN corpus adiposum infrapatellare [NA], infrapatellar fat body.

  ischiorectal f.-p., the fat within the ischiorectal fossa. SYN corpus

fa

adiposum fossae ischiorectalis [NA], fat body of ischiorectal fossa.

orbital f.-p., the mass of fat contained in the orbit that contributes to the support of the eyeball. SYN corpus adiposum orbitae [NA], fat body of orbit.

fat·ty (fat′ē). Oily or greasy; relating in any sense to fat.

fat·ty ac·id. Any acid derived from fats by hydrolysis (*e.g.,* oleic, palmitic, or stearic acids); any long-chain monobasic organic acid; they accumulate in disorders associated with the peroxisomes.

activated f. a., a fatty acyl-coenzyme A thiol ester.

diethenoid f. a., a f. a. containing two double bonds, *e.g.,* linoleic acid.

essential f. a., a f. a. that is nutritionally essential; *e.g.,* linoleic acid, linolenic acid.

ω3 f. a.'s, a class of f. a.'s that have a double bond three carbons from the methyl moiety; reportedly, they play a role in lowering cholesterol and LDL levels. SYN omega-3 f. a.'s.

omega-3 f. a.'s, SYN ω3 f. a.'s.

saturated f. a., a f. a., the carbon chain of which contains no ethylenic or other unsaturated linkages between carbon atoms (*e.g.,* stearic acid and palmitic acid); called saturated because it is incapable of absorbing any more hydrogen.

f. a. synthase complex, the multienzyme complex that catalyzes the formation of palmitate from acetylcoenzyme A, malonylcoenzyme A, and NADPH.

f. a. thiokinase, (1) long chain: long-chain fatty acid–CoA ligase; **(2)** medium chain: butyrate-CoA ligase.

unesterified free f. a. (UFA, FFA), free f. a.'s which occur in plasma as a result of lipolysis in adipose tissue or when plasma triacylglycerols are taken into tissues.

unsaturated f. a., a f. a., the carbon chain of which possesses one or more double or triple bonds (*e.g.,* oleic acid, with one double bond in the molecule, and linoleic acid, with two); called unsaturated because it is capable of absorbing additional hydrogen.

fau·ces, gen. **fau·ci·um** (faw′sēz, faw′sē-ŭm) [NA]. The space between the cavity of the mouth and the pharynx, bounded by the soft palate and the base of the tongue. SEE ALSO *isthmus* of fauces. SYN oropharyngeal passage. [L. the throat]

fau·cial (faw′shăl). Relating to the fauces.

fau·na (faw′nă). The animal forms of a continent, district, locality, or habitat. [Mod. L. application of *Fauna,* sister of *Faunus,* a rural deity]

fa·ve·o·late (fă-vē′ō-lāt). Pitted.

fa·ve·o·lus, pl. **fa·ve·o·li** (fă-vē′ō-lŭs, -ō-lī). A small pit or depression. [Mod. L. dim. of *favus,* honeycomb]

fa·vic chan·de·liers (fā′vik shan-dĕ-lērz′). Specialized fungal hyphae that are curved, branched, and antler-like in appearance, formed by the pathogens *Trichophyton schoenleinii* and *T. concentricum.*

fa·vid (fā′vid). An allergic reaction in the skin observed in patients who have favus.

fa·vism (fā′vizm). An acute condition seen chiefly in Italy, following the ingestion of certain species of beans, *e.g., Vicia faba,* or inhalation of the pollen of its flower; characterized by fever, headache, abdominal pain, severe anemia, prostration, and coma; it occurs in certain individuals with genetic erythrocytic deficiency of glucose 6-phosphate dehydrogenase. Chance exposure to the *Vicia fava,* by its impact on the phenotype of glucose-6-phosphate dehydrogenase, impinges on the expression or the gene, an example of incomplete penetrance. SYN fabism. [Ital. *favismo,* from *fava,* bean]

Favre, Maurice, French physician, 1876–1954. SEE Gamna-F. *bodies,* under *body;* Nicolas-F. *disease.*

Favre's dys·tro·phy. See under dystrophy.

fa·vus (fā′vŭs, fah′vŭs). A severe type of chronic ringworm of the scalp and nails caused by three dissimilar dermatophytes, *Trichophyton schoenleinii, T. violaceum,* and *Microsporum gypseum;* it occurs more frequently in the Mediterranean countries, southeastern Europe, southern Asia, northern Africa, and the Orient. Differences in severity are related to hygiene. SYN crusted

ringworm, honeycomb ringworm, porrigo favosa, porrigo lupinosa, porrigo scutulata, tinea favosa. [L. honeycomb]

Fc. SEE Fc *fragment.*

F.C.A.P. Abbreviation for Fellow of the College of American Pathologists.

F.C.C.P. Abbreviation for Fellow of the College of Chest Physicians.

Fd Abbreviation for ferredoxin.

FDA Abbreviation for Food and Drug Administration of the United States Department of Health and Human Services.

FDNB Abbreviation for fluoro-2,4-dinitrobenzene.

FDP Abbreviation for fibrin/fibrinogen degradation *products,* under *product.*

Fe Symbol for iron. [L. *ferrum,* iron]

^{52}**Fe.** Symbol for iron-52.

^{55}**Fe.** Symbol for iron-55.

^{59}**Fe.** Symbol for iron-59.

fear (fēr). Apprehension; dread; alarm; by having an identifiable stimulus, f. is differentiated from anxiety which has no easily identifiable stimulus. [A.S. *faer*]

fea·tures (fē′chŭrz). The various parts of the face, forehead, eyes, nose, mouth, chin, cheeks, and ears, that give to it its individuality and character. [through O. Fr., fr. L. *factura,* a making, fr. *facio,* to do]

feb·ri·cant (feb′ri-kant). SYN febrifacient.

fe·bric·u·la (fĕ-brik′yu-lă). A simple continued fever; a mild fever of short duration, of indefinite origin, and without any distinctive pathology. [L. dim. of *febris,* fever]

feb·ri·fa·cient (feb-ri-fā′shĕnt). **1.** Causing or favoring the development of fever. SYN febriferous, febrific. **2.** Anything that produces fever. SEE ALSO pyrogenic. SYN febricant. [L. *febris,* fever, + *facio,* to make]

fe·brif·er·ous (fĕ-brif′er-ŭs). SYN febrifacient (1). [L. *febris,* fever, + *fero,* to bear, + *-ous*]

fe·brif·ic (fĕ-brif′ik). SYN febrifacient (1).

fe·brif·u·gal (fĕ-brif′yū-găl). SYN antipyretic (1).

feb·ri·fuge (feb′ri-fyūj). SYN antipyretic (2). [L. *febris,* fever, + *fugo,* to put to flight]

feb·rile (feb′ril, fē′brīl). Denoting or relating to fever. SYN feverish (1), pyretic, pyrexic.

fe·bris (fē′bris). SYN fever. [L.]

f. melitensis (fē′bris mel-ĭ-ten′sis), infection with *Brucella melitensis;* SEE ALSO *Brucella melitensis.*

f. undulans (fē′bris ŭn-dū-lanz′), SYN brucellosis.

fe·cal (fē′kăl). Relating to feces.

fe·ca·lith (fē′kă-lith). SYN coprolith. [L. *faeces,* feces, + G. *lithos,* stone]

fe·cal·oid (fē′kă-loyd). Resembling feces. [L. *faeces,* feces, + G. *eidos,* resemblance]

fe·ca·lo·ma (fē′kă-lō-mă). SYN coproma.

fe·ca·lu·ria (fē-kă-lū′rē-ă). The commingling of feces with urine passed from the urethra in persons with a fistula connecting the intestinal tract and bladder, often noticed most dramatically by the passage of flatus through the urethra. [L. *faeces,* feces, + G. *ouron,* urine]

fe·ces (fē′sēz). The matter discharged from the bowel during defecation, consisting of the undigested residue of the food, epithelium, the intestinal mucus, bacteria, and waste material from the food. SYN stercus. [L., pl. of *faex* (faec-), dregs]

Fechner, Gustav T., German physicist, 1801–1887. SEE Weber-F. *law;* F.-Weber *law.*

fec·u·lent (fek′yū-lent). Foul. [L. *faeculentus,* full of excrement, fr. *faeces,* dregs, feces]

fe·cund (fē′kŭnd, fek′ŭnd). SYN fertile (1). [L. *fecundus,* fruitful]

fec·un·date (fē′kŭn-dāt). To impregnate; to make fertile. [L. *fecundo,* pp. *-atus,* to make fruitful, fertilize]

fec·un·da·tion (fē-kŭn-dā′shŭn). The act of rendering fertile. SEE ALSO fertilization, impregnation.

fe·cun·di·ty (fē-kŭn′di-tē). The ability to produce live offspring.

Fede, Francesco, Italian physician, 1832–1913. SEE Riga-F. *disease.*

feed·back (fēd′bak). **1.** In a given system, the return, as input, of some of the output, as a regulatory mechanism; *e.g.,* regulation of a furnace by a thermostat. **2.** An explanation for the learning of motor skills: sensory stimuli set up by muscle contractions modulate the activity of the motor system. **3.** The feeling evoked by another person's reaction to oneself. SEE biofeedback.

negative f., that which occurs if the sign or sense of the returned signal results in reduced amplification.

positive f., that which occurs when the sign or sense of the returned signal results in increased amplification or leads to instability.

feed·ing (fēd′ing). Giving food or nourishment.

fictitious f., SYN sham f.

forced f., forcible f., (1) giving liquid food through a nasal tube passed into the stomach; **(2)** forcing a person to eat more food than desired. SYN forced alimentation.

gastric f., giving of nutriment directly into the stomach by means of a tube inserted via the nasopharynx and esophagus or directly through the abdominal wall.

nasal f., the giving of nourishment through a flexible tube passed through the nasal passages into the stomach.

sham f., a procedure used in the study of the psychic phase of gastric secretion: in experiments on dogs, the food, after being eaten, does not enter the stomach but issues from an esophageal fistula made in the neck; the chewing and swallowing of food causes an abundant secretion of gastric juice. SYN fictitious f.

feel·ing (fēl′ing). **1.** Any kind of conscious experience of sensation. **2.** The mental perception of a sensory stimulus. **3.** A quality of any mental state or mood, whereby it is recognized as pleasurable or the reverse.

Feer, Emil, Swiss pediatrician, 1864–1955. SEE F.'s *disease.*

FEF Abbreviation for forced expiratory *flow.*

Fehling, Hermann von, German chemist, 1812–1885. SEE F.'s *reagent, solution.*

Feil, André, French physician, *1884. SEE Klippel-F. *syndrome.*

Feiss, Henry O., 20th century American orthopedic surgeon. SEE F. *line.*

fel·bam·ate (fel′bă-māt). An anticonvulsant/antiepileptic agent chemically related to meprobamate; useful in complex partial seizures.

Feldberg, Wilhelm, British physiologist, *1900. SEE Dale-F. *law.*

Feldman, Harry Alfred, U.S. epidemiologist, *1914. SEE Sabin-F. dye *test.*

Fe·li·dae (fē′li-dē). A family of Carnivora embracing domestic and wild cats such as lions and tigers. [L. *felis,* cat]

fe·line (fē′līn). Pertaining or relating to cats. [L. *felis,* cat]

Felix, Arthur, Polish bacteriologist, 1887–1956. SEE Weil-F. *reaction, test.*

fel·la·tio (fĕ-lā′shē-ō). Oral stimulation of the penis; a type of oral-genital sexual activity; contrasted with cunnilingus, which is the oral stimulation of the vulva or clitoris. SYN fellation, fellatorism, irrumation. [L.]

fel·la·tion (fĕ-lā′shŭn). SYN fellatio.

fel·la·tor·ism (fel′ă-tōr-izm). SYN fellatio.

fel·la·trix (fel-ă-triks′). A female who takes the oral part in fellatio.

fel·o·dip·ine (fē-lō′dī-pēn). A calcium blocking agent of the dihydropyridine class resembling nifedipine.

fel·on (fel′ŏn). A purulent infection or abscess involving the bulbous distal end of a finger. SYN whitlow. [M.E. *feloun,* malignant]

Fel·son. Benjamin, U.S. radiologist, 1913–1988. SEE silhouette *sign* of Felson.

felt·work. **1.** A fibrous network. **2.** A close plexus of nerve fibrils. SEE neuropile.

Felty, Augustus R., U.S. physician, 1895–1963. SEE F.'s *syndrome.*

FeLV Abbreviation for feline leukemia *virus.*

fel·y·pres·sin (fel-i-pres′in). [Phe^2,Lys^8]vasopressin; lysine vasopressin with L-phenylalanine at position 2. SYN octapressin.

fe·male (fē′māl). In zoology, denoting the sex that bears the young or the ovum.

genetic f., (1) an individual with a normal female karyotype, including two X chromosomes; **(2)** an individual whose cell nuclei contain Barr sex chromatin bodies, which are normally absent in males.

XO f., the genetic f. in Turner's syndrome, where the criterion is the macroscopic appearance of the external genitals.

XXX f., SEE triple X *syndrome.*

fem·i·ni·za·tion (fem′i-ni-zā′shŭn). Development of what are superficially external female characteristics by a male.

testicular f., SEE testicular feminization *syndrome.*

fem·o·ral (fem′ŏ-răl). Relating to the femur or thigh.

fem·o·ro·cele (fem′ŏ-rō-sēl). SYN femoral *hernia.* [L. *femur,* thigh, + G. *kēlē,* hernia]

fem·o·ro·tib·i·al (fem′ŏ-rō-tib′ē-ăl). Relating to the femur and the tibia.

femto- (f). SI and metric systems to signify one-quadrillionth (10^{-15}). [Danish and Norwegian *femten,* fifteen]

fe·mur, gen. **fe·mo·ris,** pl. **fem·o·ra** (fē′mŭr, fem′ŏ-ris, -ă) [NA]. **1.** The thigh. **2.** The long bone of the thigh, articulating with the hip bone proximally and the tibia and patella distally. SYN os femoris [NA], thigh bone. [L. thigh]

fen·bu·fen (fen-bū′fen). A nonsteroidal anti-inflammatory agent resembling ibuprofen.

fen·ca·mine (fen′kă-mēn). 8-({2-[Methyl(α-methylphenethyl)-amino]ethyl}amino)caffeine; a central nervous system stimulant.

fen·clo·fen·ac (fen-klō′fen-ak). A nonsteroidal anti-inflammatory drug used in the treatment of joint disorders; similar to diclofenac.

fen·clo·nine (fen′klō-nēn). DL-3-(*p*-Chlorophenyl)alanine; a serotonin inhibitor.

Fendt, H., 19th century Austrian dermatologist. SEE Spiegler-F. *pseudolymphoma, sarcoid.*

fe·nes·tra, pl. **fe·nes·trae** (fe-nes′tră, -trē). **1** [NA]. An anatomical aperture, often closed by a membrane. **2.** An opening left in a plaster of Paris or other form of fixed dressing in order to permit access to a wound or inspection of the part. **3.** The opening in one of the blades of an obstetrical forceps. **4.** A lateral opening in the sheath of an endoscopic instrument that allows lateral viewing or operative maneuvering through the sheath. **5.** Openings in the wall of a tube, catheter, or trocar designed to promote better flow of air or fluids. SYN window. [L. window]

f. of the cochlea, SYN f. cochleae.

f. coch′leae [NA], an opening on the medial wall of the middle ear leading into the cochlea, closed in life by the secondary tympanic membrane. SYN cochlear window, f. of the cochlea, f. rotunda, round window.

f. nov-ova′lis, artificial opening through the otic capsule of the lateral semicircular canal, connecting the membranous labyrinth with the mastoid cavity produced during fenestration surgery.

f. ova′lis, SYN f. vestibuli.

f. rotun′da, SYN f. cochleae.

f. of the vestibule, SYN f. vestibuli.

f. vestib′uli [NA], an oval opening on the medial wall of the tympanic cavity leading into the vestibule, closed in life by the foot of the stapes. SYN f. of the vestibule, f. ovalis, oval window, vestibular window.

fen·es·trat·ed (fen′es-trā′ted). Having fenestrae or window-like openings.

fen·es·tra·tion (fen-es-trā′shŭn). **1.** The presence of openings or fenestrae in a part. **2.** Making openings in a dressing to allow inspection of the parts. **3.** In dentistry, a surgical perforation of the mucoperiosteum and alveolar process to expose the root tip of a tooth to permit drainage of tissue exudate.

optic nerve sheath f., the cutting of a window in the dura of the optic nerve sheath to relieve papilledema and prevent further loss of optic nerve fibers.

tracheal f., a surgical procedure to create an epithelialized mucocutaneous opening from the neck into the trachea.

fen·eth·yl·line hy·dro·chlo·ride (fen-eth′ĭ-lēn). 7-{2-[(α-Methylphenethyl)amino]ethyl}theophylline hydrochloride; an analeptic.

fen·flur·a·mine hy·dro·chlo·ride (fen-flū′ră-mēn). *N*-Ethyl-α-methyl-*m*-(trifluoromethyl)phenethylamine hydrochloride; an anorexigenic agent.

Fenn, Wallace Osgood, U.S. physiologist, 1893–1971. SEE F. *effect.*

fen·nel (fen′l). Fennel seed, the dried ripe fruit of cultivated varieties of *Foeniculum vulgare* (family Umbelliferae), an herb native to southern Europe and Asia, a diaphoretic and carminative; a volatile oil distilled from the fruit is used as a flavoring. [through O. Fr., fr. L. *faeniculum,* fennel, dim. of *faenum,* hay]

fen·o·pro·fen cal·ci·um (fen-ō-prō′fen). Calcium (±)-*m*-phenoxyhydratropate dihydrate; an anti-inflammatory analgesic used for treatment of mild to moderate pain and for osteoarthritis.

fen·o·ter·ol (fen′ō-ter′ŏl). A β₂ agonist inhalation bronchodilator.

fen·pip·ra·mide (fen-pip′ră-mīd). α,α-Diphenyl-1-piperidinebutyramide; an antispasmodic.

fen·ta·nyl cit·rate (fen′tă-nil). *N*-(1-Phenethyl-4-piperidyl)-propionanilide citrate; a short-acting narcotic analgesic used as a supplementary analgesic in general anesthesia.

fen·ti·clor (fen′ti-klōr). 2,2′-Thiobis[4-chlorophenol]; a topical anti-infective agent.

fen·u·greek (fen′yū-grēk). *Trigonella faenumgraecum* (family Leguminosae); an annual plant indigenous to western Asia and cultivated in Africa and parts of Europe; the mucilaginous seeds are used as food and in the preparation of culinary spices (curry). [L. *faenum graecum,* fenugreek, fr. *faenum,* hay, + *Graecus,* Greek]

Fenwick, Edwin Hurry, British urologist, 1856–1944. SEE F.-Hunner *ulcer.*

Fenwick, Samuel, British physician, 1821–1902. SEE F.'s *disease.*

fer·al (fer′il). Denoting an animal that is wild and untamed.

Féréol, Louis H.F., Paris physician, 1825–1891.

Fergusson, Sir William, Scottish surgeon, 1808–1877. SEE F.'s *incision.*

fer·ment (fer-ment′). To cause or to undergo fermentation. [L. *fermentum,* leaven]

fer·ment·a·ble (fer-ment′ă-bl). Capable of undergoing fermentation.

fer·men·ta·tion (fer-men-tā′shŭn). **1.** A chemical change induced in a complex organic compound by the action of an enzyme, whereby the substance is split into simpler compounds. **2.** In bacteriology, the anaerobic dissimilation of substrates with the production of energy and reduced compounds; the mechanism of f. does not involve a respiratory chain or cytochrome, hence oxygen is not the final electron acceptor as it is in oxidation. [L. *fermento,* pp. *-atus,* to ferment, from L. *fermentum,* yeast]

acetic f., acetous f., f., as of wine or beer, whereby the alcohol is oxidized to acetic acid (vinegar).

alcoholic f., the anaerobic formation of ethanol and CO_2 from D-glucose. Cf. Gay-Lussac's *equation.*

amylic f., f. of potato or corn mash, or other starchy material, by which fusel oil is produced.

lactic acid f., the production of lactic acid in milk, or other carbohydrate-containing media, caused by the presence of any one of a number of lactic acid bacteria.

fer·ment·a·tive (fer-ment′ă-tiv). Causing or having the ability to cause fermentation.

fer·ment·er (fer-ment′er). A large container used in cultures of microorganisms.

fer·mi·um (Fm) (fer′mē-ŭm). Radioactive element, artificially prepared in 1955, atomic no. 100, atomic wt. 257.095; [257]Fm has the longest known half-life (100.5 days). [E. *Fermi,* It.-U.S. physicist and Nobel laureate, 1901–1954]

Fernandez re·ac·tion. See under reaction.

Fernbach, Auguste, French microbiologist, 1860–1939. SEE F. *flask.*

fern·ing. A term used to describe the pattern of arborization produced by cervical mucus, secreted at midcycle, upon crystallization, which resembles somewhat a fern or a palm leaf.

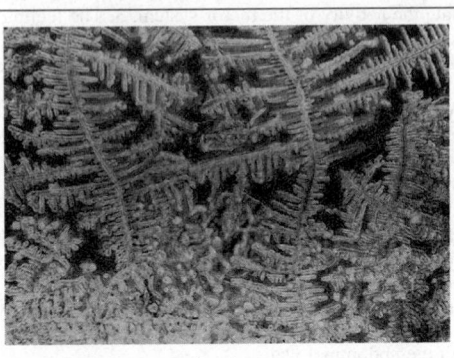

ferning

fer·ra·tin (fer′ă-tin). Sodium iron albuminate; a hematinic.

fer·re·dox·ins (fer-ĕ-dok′sinz). Proteins containing iron and (labile) sulfur in equal amounts, displaying electron-carrier activity but no classical enzyme function; differentiated from rubredoxins but, generally, not from high potential iron-sulfur proteins. F.'s are found in green plants, algae, and anaerobic bacteria, and are involved in several oxidation-reduction reactions in living organisms (*e.g.,* nitrogen fixation).

Ferrein, Antoine, French anatomist, 1693–1769. SEE F.'s canal, cords, under *cord, foramen, ligament, pyramid, tube, vasa* aberrantia, under *vas; processus* ferreini.

♻**ferri-.** Prefix designating the presence of a ferric ion in a compound. [L. *ferrum,* iron]

fer·ric (fer′ik). Relating to iron, especially denoting a salt containing iron in its higher (triad) valence, Fe^{3+}.

fer·ric am·mo·ni·um cit·rate. Soluble ferric citrate; a compound used in hypochromic anemia; it is relatively free of astringent and irritant action.

fer·ric am·mo·ni·um cit·rate, green. A compound used in hypochromic anemia.

fer·ric am·mo·ni·um sul·fate. An astringent and styptic. SYN ammonium ferric sulfate, ferric alum, iron alum.

fer·ric chlo·ride. An astringent and styptic.

fer·ric fruc·tose. A potassium-iron-fructose; a hematinic drug.

fer·ric glyc·er·o·phos·phate. A tonic and a source of iron.

fer·ric hy·drox·ide. Hydrated iron oxide; a compound previously used, freshly prepared, as an antidote to arsenic poisoning.

fer·ric ox·ide. A compound used as a coloring material.

fer·ric phos·phate. A compound used as a feed and as a food supplement.

soluble f. p., f. p. with sodium citrate; a hematinic.

fer·ric sul·fate. Iron persulfate, tersulfate, or sesquisulfate; an astringent and styptic.

fer·ri·cy·a·nide (fe-rī-sī′ă-nīd, fer-ē-). The anion $Fe(CN)_6^{3-}$.

fer·ri·cy·to·chrome (fe-rī-sī′tō-krōm, fer-ē-). A cytochrome containing oxidized (ferric) iron.

fer·ri·heme (fe′rī-hēm, fer′ē-). SYN hematin.

f. chloride, SYN hemin.

fer·ri·he·mo·glo·bin (fer′ĭ-hē-mō-glō′bin, fer′ē-). SYN methemoglobin.

fer·ri·por·phy·rin (fe-rī-pōr′fi-rin, fer-ē-). The compound formed between a ferric ion and a porphyrin; *e.g.,* ferriprotoporphyrin (hemin).

f. chloride, SYN hemin.

fer·ri·pro·to·por·phy·rin (fer′i-prō-tō-pōr′fi-rin, fer′ē-). SYN hemin.

fer·ri·tin (fer′ĭ-tin, fer′ă-). An iron protein complex, containing up to 23% iron, formed by the union of ferric iron with apoferritin; it is found in the intestinal mucosa, spleen, bone marrow, reticulocytes, and liver, and regulates iron storage and transport from the intestinal lumen to plasma.

ferro-. Prefix designating the presence of metallic iron or of the divalent ion Fe^{2+}. [L. *ferrum,* iron]

fer·ro·che·la·tase (fār-ō-kē′lă-tās). A lyase that catalyzes the reversible acid hydrolysis of heme, forming protoporphyrin IX and free ferrous iron; inhibited by lead; a deficiency of f. results in erythropoietic protoporphyria.

fer·ro·cho·li·nate (fār-ō-kō′li-nāt). Iron choline citrate chelate, used for oral administration in the treatment and prevention of iron deficiency anemias.

fer·ro·cy·a·nide (fār-ō-sī′ă-nīd). A compound containing the anion $Fe(CN)_6^{4-}$.

fer·ro·cy·to·chrome (fār-ō-sī′tō-krōm). A cytochrome containing reduced (ferrous) iron.

fer·ro·heme (fār′ō-hēm). SYN heme.

fer·ro·ki·net·ics (fār-ō-ki-net′iks). The study of iron metabolism using radioactive iron. [L. *ferrum,* iron, + G. *kinēsis,* movement]

fer·ro·por·phy·rin (fār-ō-pōr′fi-rin). The compound formed between a ferrous ion and a porphyrin; *e.g.,* ferroprotoporphyrin (heme).

fer·ro·pro·teins (fār-ō-prō′tēnz). Proteins containing iron in a prosthetic group; *e.g.,* heme, cytochrome.

fer·ro·pro·to·por·phy·rin (fār′ō-prō-tō-pōr′fi-rin). SYN heme.

fer·ro·so·fer·ric (fār-ō-sō-fār′ik). Denoting a combination of a ferrous compound with a ferric compound, as in Fe_3O_4.

fer·ro·ther·a·py (fār′ō-thār′ă-pē). Therapeutic use of iron. [L. *ferrum,* iron]

fer·rous (fār′ŭs). Relating to iron, especially denoting a salt containing iron in its lowest valence state, Fe^{2+}. [L. *ferreus,* made of iron]

fer·rous cit·rate. A compound that occurs in several forms, two of which are monoferrous acid citrate monohydrate and triferrous dicitrate decahydrate; a hematinic.

fer·rous fu·ma·rate. Iron fumarate, a hematinic.

fer·rous glu·co·nate. Iron gluconate; a hematinic.

fer·rous lac·tate. Iron lactate; a hematinic.

fer·rous suc·ci·nate. Iron succinate; a hematinic.

fer·rous sul·fate. SYN iron *sulfate.*

dried f. s., exsiccated iron sulfate; a hematinic.

fer·ru·gi·na·tion (fe-rū′ji-nā′shŭn). Deposition of mineral deposits including iron in the walls of small blood vessels and at the site of a dead neuron. [L. *ferrugo,* iron-rust]

fer·ru·gi·nous (fe-rū′ji-nŭs). 1. Iron-bearing; associated with or containing iron. 2. Of the color of iron rust. [L. *ferrugineus,* iron rust, rust-colored]

fer·rule (fer′ŭl). A metal band or ring used around the crown or root of a tooth. [corrupted through O. Fr. and Medieval L., fr. L. *viriola,* a small bracelet]

Ferry, Erwin S., U.S. physicist, 1868–1956. SEE F.-Porter *law.*

fer·tile (fer′til). 1. Fruitful; capable of conceiving and bearing young. SYN fecund. 2. Impregnated; fertilized. [L. *fertilis,* fr. *fero,* to bear]

fer·til·i·ty (fer-til′i-tē). The actual production of live offspring, *i.e.,* does not include stillbirths.

fer·til·i·za·tion (fer′til-i-zā′shŭn). The process beginning with penetration of the secondary oocyte by the spermatozoon and completed by fusion of the male and female pronuclei.

in vitro **f. (IVF),** a process whereby (usually multiple) ova are placed in a medium to which sperm are added for fertilization, the zygote thus produced then being introduced into the uterus and allowed to develop to term.

in vivo **f.,** f. of a ripe egg within the distal fallopian tube of a fertile donor female (rather than in an artificial medium), for subsequent nonsurgical transfer to an infertile recipient.

fer·til·i·zin (fer-til′i-zin). An acid polysaccharide-amino acid complex associated with the female gamete membrane of several organisms; provides receptor groups that agglutinate sperm and bind them to ova.

Fer·u·la (fār′ū-lă). A genus of plants of the family Umbelliferae. *F. assa-foetida, F. rubricaulis* and *F. foetida* furnish asafetida; *F. galbaniflua* and *F. rubricaulis,* galbanium; and *F. sumbul,* sumbul. [L. giant plant]

fer·ves·cence (fer-ves′ens). An increase of fever. [L. *fervesco,* to begin to boil, fr. *ferveo,* to boil]

fes·ter. 1. To form pus or putrefy. 2. To make inflamed. [L. *fistula*]

fes·ti·nant (fes′ti-nant). Rapid; hastening; accelerating. [L. *festino,* to hasten]

fes·ti·na·tion (fes-ti-nā′shŭn). SYN festinating *gait.* [L. *festino,* to hasten]

fes·toon (fes-tūn′). 1. A carving in the base material of a denture that simulates the contours of the natural tissue that is being replaced by the denture. 2. A distinguishing characteristic of certain hard tick species, consisting of small rectangular areas separated by grooves along the posterior margin of the dorsum of both males and females. [thr. Fr. fr. L. *festum,* festival, hence festive decorations]

gingival f., an arcuate enlargement of the marginal gingiva.

fes·toon·ing (fes-tūn′ing). Undulating, like the pattern of dermal papillae beneath a subepidermal blister.

FET Abbreviation for forced expiratory *time.*

fe·tal (fē′tăl). 1. Relating to a fetus; 2. In utero development after the eighth week.

fe·tal·ism (fē′tăl-izm). Presence of certain fetal structures or characteristics in the body after birth.

fe·tal re·tic·u·la·ris (fē′tăl re-tik-yū-lā′ris). 1. SYN fetal adrenal *cortex.* 2. SYN androgenic *zone* (2). 3. SYN X *zone* (2).

fe·ta·tion (fē-tā′shŭn). SYN pregnancy.

fe·ti·cide (fē′ti-sīd). Destruction of the embryo or fetus in the uterus. [L. *fetus* + *caedo,* to kill]

fet·id (fet′id, fē′tid). Foul-smelling. [L. *foetidus*]

fet·ish (fet′ish, fē′tish). An inanimate object or nonsexual body part that is regarded as endowed with magic or erotic qualities. [Fr. *fétiche,* fr. L. *factitius,* made by art, artificial]

fet·ish·ism (fet′ish-izm, fē′tish-). The act of worshipping or using for sexual arousal and gratification that which is regarded as a fetish.

fet·lock (fet′lok). The metacarpophalangeal and metatarsophalangeal joints of ungulates; also the cushion-like caudal projection above the hoof of the horse and similar animals, and the tuft of hair in this region.

fe·to·glob·u·lins (fē-tō-glob′yū-linz). One of a number of proteins found in fetal blood of unknown function. α-F. occurs in small amounts in normal adults and in larger amounts in the fetus and pregnant mother, especially in the second trimester; elevated levels are also detected in adult patients with liver disease and neoplasms.

fe·tog·ra·phy (fē-tog′ră-fē). Radiography of the fetus *in utero,* using contrast medium; an obsolete technique. Cf. amniography. [L. *fetus* + G. *graphō,* to write]

fe·tol·o·gy (fē-tol′ō-jē). SYN fetal *medicine.* [L. *fetus* + G. *logos,* study]

fe·tom·e·try (fē-tom′ĕ-trē). Estimation of the size of the fetus, especially of its head, prior to delivery. [L. *fetus* + G. *metron,* measure]

fe·top·a·thy (fē-top′ă-thē). SYN embryopathy. [L. *fetus* + G. *pathos,* suffering, disease]

diabetic f., f. resulting from maternal diabetes, which may cause macrosomia and fetal death.

fe·to·pla·cen·tal (fē′tō-pla-sen′tăl). Relating to the fetus and its placenta.

fe·to·pro·teins (fē-tō-prō′tēnz). Fetal proteins found in small amounts in adults in the following forms: α-**f.** (AFP) increases in maternal blood during pregnancy and, when detected by amniocentesis, is an important indicator of open neural tube defects and is also used as a tumor marker in adults with hepatocellular carcinoma; β-**f.,** although a fetal liver protein, has been detected in adult patients with liver disease; γ-**f.** occurs in various neoplasms. SEE ALSO fetoglobulins.

α **f.,** a protein normally produced during the 12th to 15th week of gestation, decreasing thereafter, but appearing in the blood in certain tumors, such as embryonal carcinomas of the testis and ovary, hepatoma, and less often in patients with carcinomas of the pancreas, stomach, colon, or lung. When present, a useful marker in following the course of a tumor.

fe·tor (fē′tōr). A very offensive odor. [L. an offensive smell, fr. *feteo,* to stink]

f. hepat′icus, a peculiar odor to the breath in persons with severe liver disease; caused by volatile aromatic substances that accumulate in the blood and urine due to defective hepatic metabolism. SYN liver breath.

f. o′ris, SYN halitosis.

fe·to·scope (fē′tō-skōp). **1.** A fiberoptic endoscope used in fetology. **2.** A stethoscope designed for listening to fetal heart sounds.

fe·tos·co·py (fē-tos′kŏ-pē). Use of a fiberoptic endoscope to view the fetus and the fetal surface of the placenta transabdominally, and also for collection of fetal blood from the umbilical vein for antenatal diagnosis of fetal disorders.

fe·tus, pl. **fe·tus·es** (fē′tŭs, fē′tŭs-ez). **1.** The unborn young of a viviparous animal after it has taken form in the uterus. **2** [NA]. In humans, the product of conception from the end of the eighth week to the moment of birth. [L. offspring]

development of the fetus

week of pregnancy	length (in cm.)	weight (in g.)	particular changes noted
12th	7.5–10		stump-formed extremities, sexual differences outwardly visible; anal opening, eye brows present
16th	16		body fully shaped; eyelids "sewn" shut; skin crab-red; down on forehead and chin; beginning of skeletal articulation, dental structures, blood formation in the liver
20th	25		vernix caseosa on forehead and chin; meconium; cecum descends in process of intestinal rotation; digestive enzyme is present, blood formation in the spine
24th	30–32		down (lanugo) on whole body; finished epidermis on palms of hands and soles of feet
28th	35–40	1000	attainment of ability to live outside the womb; fat cushioning still incomplete; grimacing face, hair on head is .5 cm in length; scrotum descends, eyes "unsewn"; whining voice
32nd	46	1800	increase of vernix caseosa, red skin
36th	51	2500	greater cushion of fat; fingernails reach finger ends; a strong voice if born
40th	49–53	3200	completely developed

f. in fe′tu, condition in which a small, imperfectly formed fetus is contained within a fetus.

harlequin f., a severe autosomal recessive form of collodian baby in a newborn, usually premature, infant; *i.e.,* a form of ichthyosiform erythroderma characterized by encasement of the body in grayish brown, often fissured plaques resembling plates of armor, and by grotesque deformity of the face, hands, and feet; usually fatal within a few days, although treatment with 13-cis-retinoic acid has been successful in some cases. SYN ichthyosis fetalis (1).

impacted f., a f. which, because of its large size or narrowing of the pelvic canal, has become wedged and incapable of spontaneous advance or recession.

f. papyra′ceus, one of twin f.'s that has died and been pressed flat against the uterine wall by the growth of the living f.

f. sanguinolentis (san-gwi′nō-len′tis), dead f. that has become macerated.

Feulgen, Robert, German nucleic acid biochemist and cytochemist, 1884–1955. First to detect DNA in cells by a specific cytochemical test.

FEV Abbreviation for forced expiratory *volume,* with subscript indicating time interval in seconds.

FEVER

fe·ver (fē′ver). A complex physiologic response to disease mediated by pyrogenic cytokines and characterized by a rise in core temperature, generation of acute phase reactants and activation of immunologic systems. SYN febris, pyrexia. [A.S. *fefer*]

absorption f., an elevation of temperature often occurring, without other untoward symptoms, shortly after childbirth, assumed to be due to absorption of uterine discharges through abrasions of the vaginal wall.

acclimating f., elevated temperature with malaise that occurs upon working in a very hot environment.

Aden f., SYN dengue.

aestivoautumnal f., SYN falciparum *malaria.*

African hemorrhagic f., hemorrhagic f. associated with the morphologically similar but antigenically distinct Marburg and Ebola viruses. SEE ALSO viral hemorrhagic f.

African swine f. (ASF), a highly fatal disease of swine caused by African swine f. virus, which has not been classified to date. It has its reservoir in wild wart hogs and bush pigs; it is characterized by high f., cough, diarrhea, and high mortality; clinically, it closely resembles hog cholera (swine f.), but the viruses of these diseases do not cross-immunize.

African tick f., SYN Crimean-Congo hemorrhagic f.

algid pernicious f., a pernicious malarial attack in which the patient presents symptoms of collapse and shock.

ardent f., a term sometimes applied to hyperpyrexia occurring in intermittent malarial f. SYN heat apoplexy (2).

Argentinean hemorrhagic f., a form of hemorrhagic f. observed in South America, seemingly transmitted by contact from rodents to man and caused by the Junin virus, a member of the family Arenaviridae.

artificial f., SYN pyretotherapy.

aseptic f., f. accompanied by malaise due to absorption of dead but not infected tissue following an injury.

Assam f., SYN visceral *leishmaniasis.*

Australian Q f., a variety of Q f. occurring in Australia; an acute infectious rickettsial infection caused by *Coxiella burnetii* and transmitted by ticks, enzootic in animals in Australia, especially bandicoots.

autumn f., (**1**) a f. resembling dengue occurring at the end of the summer in India; SYN seven-day f. (1). (**2**) SYN hasamiyami.

biliary f. of dogs, a form of babesiosis (piroplasmosis) of the dog characterized by fever and icterus and caused by *Babesia canis.*

biliary f. of horses, SYN equine *babesiosis.*

bilious remittent f., (**1**) old term for relapsing f.; (**2**) malarial

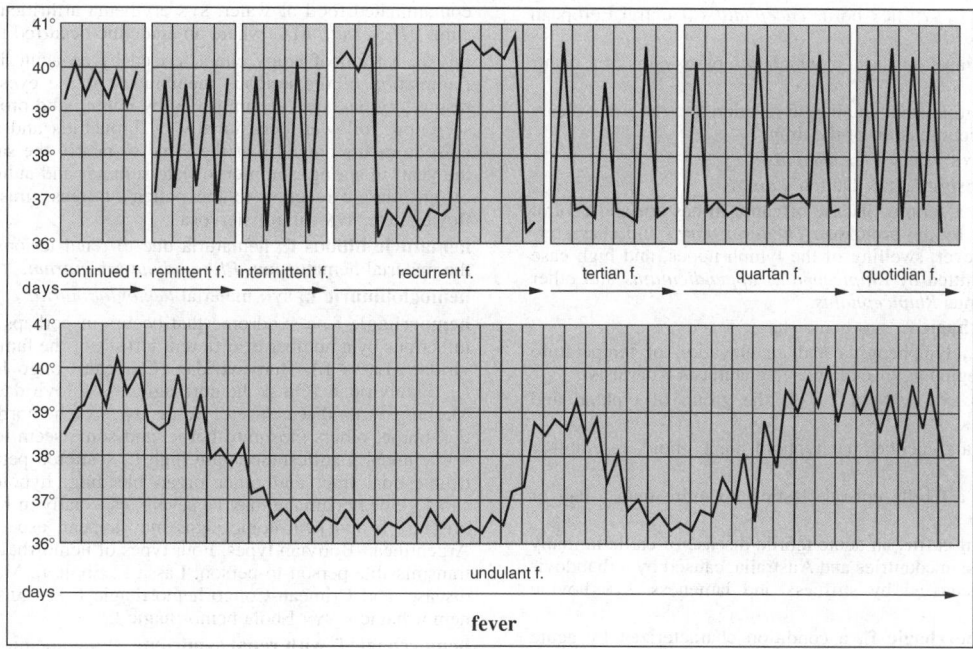

"bilious" vomiting associated with marked increase of serum bilirubin.

black f., SYN Rocky Mountain spotted f.

blackwater f., hemoglobinuria resulting from severe hemolysis occurring in falciparum malaria. SYN malarial *hemoglobinuria.*

blue f., SYN Rocky Mountain spotted f.

Bolivian hemorrhagic f., a disease similar to Argentinian hemorrhagic f. but caused by the Machupo virus, a member of the family Arenaviridae.

bouquet f., SYN dengue.

boutonneuse f., tick-borne infection with *Rickettsia conorii* seen in Africa, Europe, the Middle East, India, and known by different names in different areas *e.g.,* Marseille fever, Crimean fever, Indian tick typhus, and Kenya fever. SYN Crimean f., eruptive f., fièvre boutonneuse, Indian tick typhus, Kenya f., Marseilles f., tick typhus.

bovine ephemeral f., SYN ephemeral f. of cattle.

bovine petechial f., a disease of cattle in Kenya caused by the rickettsia *Ehrlichia ondiri* and characterized by hemorrhage and edema. SYN Ondiri disease.

brass founder's f., an occupational disease, characterized by malaria-like symptoms, due to inhalation of particles and fumes of metallic oxides. Fumes are formed by evaporation at very high temperature and condensation in air into fine particles. SYN brass founder's ague, foundryman's f., metal fume f., zinc fume f.

Brazilian hemorrhagic f., SYN Brazilian spotted f.

Brazilian purpuric f., SYN Brazilian spotted f.

Brazilian spotted f., fulminating sepsis, usually beginning with conjunctivitis, characterized by purpuric skin lesions, a high fatality rate; thought to be due to *Hemophilus aegyptius.* SYN Brazilian hemorrhagic f., Brazilian purpuric f.

breakbone f., SYN dengue.

bullous f., SYN *pemphigus* acutus.

Bunyamwera f., a febrile illness of humans in Africa caused by the Bunyamwera virus and transmitted by culicine mosquitoes.

Burdwan f., SYN visceral *leishmaniasis.*

Bwamba f., a febrile illness of humans in Africa caused by a virus of the family Bunyaviridae and transmitted by mosquitoes.

cachectic f., SYN visceral *leishmaniasis.*

camp f., (1) SYN typhus. **(2)** any epidemic febrile illness affecting troops in an encampment.

canefield f., SYN field f.

canicola f., a disease of man caused by the *canicola* serovar of *Leptospira interrogans* and transmitted by infective urine, usually from dogs but rarely from cattle and swine.

Carter's f., an Asiatic relapsing f. caused by *Borrelia carteri.*

catarrhal f., old term for the group of respiratory tract diseases including the common cold, influenza, and lobular and lobar pneumonia.

cat-bite f., SYN cat-bite *disease.*

cat-scratch f., SYN cat-scratch *disease.*

catheter f., SYN urinary f.

Central European tick-borne f., SYN tick-borne *encephalitis* (Central European subtype).

cerebrospinal f., SYN meningococcal *meningitis.*

Charcot's intermittent f., f., chills, right upper quadrant pain, and jaundice associated with intermittently obstructing common duct stones.

childbed f., SYN puerperal f.

Colorado tick f., an infection caused by Colorado tick f. virus and transmitted to humans by *Dermacentor andersoni;* the symptoms are mild, there is no rash, the temperature is not excessive, and the disease is rarely, if ever, fatal. SYN tick f. (5).

Congolian red f., SYN murine *typhus.*

continued f., obsolete term for a febrile illness without the intermittency of malaria. Many cases were typhoid f., but included many types of febrile illnesses.

cotton-mill f., SYN byssinosis.

Crimean f., SYN boutonneuse f.

Crimean-Congo hemorrhagic f., a form of hemorrhagic f. distinct from Omsk hemorrhagic f., occurring in central Russia, transmitted by species of the tick *Hyalomma,* and caused by Crimean-Congo hemorrhagic f. virus, a member of the Bunyaviridae family; horses are the chief reservoir of human infection; characterized by abrupt onset, high f., headache, myalgia, widespread petechia hemorrhagic lesions, gastrointestinal bleeding, high fatality rate. SYN African tick f.

dandy f., SYN dengue.

date f., SYN dengue.

deer-fly f., SYN tularemia.

dehydration f., SYN thirst f.

dengue f., SYN dengue.

dengue hemorrhagic f., SYN dengue.

desert f., SYN primary *coccidioidomycosis.*

digestive f., a slight rise of body temperature occurring during the period of digestion.

diphasic milk f., SYN tick-borne *encephalitis* (Central European subtype).

double quotidian f., malaria in which two paroxysms of f. occur daily.

drug f., f. resulting from an allergic reaction to a drug that clears rapidly on discontinuation of the drug.

Dumdum f., SYN visceral *leishmaniasis.*

Dutton's relapsing f., SYN Dutton's *disease.*

East Coast f., a serious disease of cattle in eastern and central Africa, caused by the protozoan *Theileria parva* and characterized by high fever, swelling of the lymph nodes, and high case fatality; transmitted by *Rhipicephalus appendiculatus* and other ticks of the genus *Rhipicephalus.*

Ebola hemorrhagic f., SYN hemorrhagic f.

elephantoid f., lymphangitis and an elevation of temperature marking the beginning of endemic elephantiasis (filariasis).

enteric f., (1) SYN typhoid f. **(2)** the group of typhoid and paratyphoid f.'s.

entericoid f., a f., neither paratyphoid nor typhoid, resembling the latter.

ephemeral f., a febrile episode lasting no more than a day or two.

ephemeral f. of cattle, an acute febrile disease of cattle in many African and Asian countries and Australia, caused by a rhabdovirus and characterized by stiffness and lameness. SYN bovine ephemeral f.

epidemic hemorrhagic f., a condition characterized by acute onset of headache, chills and high f., sweating, thirst, photophobia, coryza, cough, myalgia, arthralgia, and abdominal pain with nausea and vomiting; this phase lasts from three to six days and is followed by capillary and renal interstitial hemorrhages, edema, oliguria, azotemia, and shock; most varieties are caused by arboviruses (togaviruses, arenaviruses, flaviviruses, and bunyaviruses), and are rodent-borne. SYN hemorrhagic f. with renal syndrome, Songo f.

epimastical f., a f. increasing steadily until its acme is reached, then declining by crisis or lysis.

equine biliary f., SYN equine *babesiosis.*

eruptive f., SYN boutonneuse f.

essential f., f. without known infectious disease.

exanthematous f., fever associated with an exanthem.

exsiccation f., SYN thirst f.

falciparum f., SYN falciparum *malaria.*

familial Mediterranean f., SYN familial paroxysmal *polyserositis.*

famine f., SYN relapsing f.

Far East hemorrhagic f., tick-borne infection with *Rickettsia sibirica,* seen primarily in Siberia and Mongolia.

fatigue f., an elevation of the body temperature, lasting sometimes several days, following excessive and long continued muscular exertion.

field f., a leptospirosis caused by *leptospira.* SYN canefield f.

five-day f., SYN trench f.

flood f., SYN tsutsugamushi *disease.*

food f., a disorder seen primarily in childhood, consisting of a sudden rise of temperature accompanied by marked digestive disturbances, which lasts from a few days to several weeks; believed to be a form of food poisoning.

Fort Bragg f., SYN pretibial f.

foundryman's f., SYN brass founder's f.

Gambian f., an irregular relapsing f., lasting one to four days with intermissions of two to five days, marked by enlargement of the spleen, rapid pulse, and breathing; due to the presence in the blood of *Trypanosoma brucei gambiense,* the pathogenic microorganism of Gambian or West African sleeping sickness.

glandular f., SYN infectious *mononucleosis.*

Haverhill f., an infection by *Streptobacillus moniliformis* marked by initial chills and high f. (gradually subsiding), by arthritis usually in the larger joints and spine, and by a rash occurring chiefly over the joints and on the extensor surfaces of the extremities; "Haverhill f." is used to indicate *Streptobacillus moniliformis* infections not associated with rat bite resulting from

contaminated food or water. SYN erythema arthriticum epidemicum. [*Haverhill, MA,* where an epidemic occurred in 1926]

hay f., a form of atopy characterized by an acute irritative inflammation of the mucous membranes of the eyes and upper respiratory passages accompanied by itching and profuse watery secretion, followed occasionally by bronchitis and asthma; the episode recurs annually at the same or nearly the same time of the year, in spring, summer, or late summer and autumn, caused by an allergic reaction to the pollen of trees, grasses, weeds, flowers, etc. SYN rhinitis nervosa.

hematuric bilious f., hematuria due to renal lesions caused by the malarial hematozoon, *Plasmodium falciparum.*

hemoglobinuric f., SYN malarial *hemoglobinuria.*

hemorrhagic f., a syndrome that occurs in perhaps 20–40% of infections by a number of different viruses of the families Arenaviridae (Lassa f.), Bunyaviridae (Crimean-Congo hemorrhagic f.), Flaviviridae (Omsk hemorrhagic f.), Filoviridae (Ebola f., Marburg virus disease), etc. Some types of hemorrhagic f. are tick-borne, others mosquito-borne, and some seem to be zoonoses; clinical manifestations are high f., scattered petechiae, gastrointestinal tract and other organ bleeding, hypotension, and shock; kidney damage may be severe, especially in Korean hemorrhagic f. and neurologic signs may appear, especially in the Argentinean-Bolivian types. Four types of hemorrhagic fever are transmissible person-to-person: Lassa f., Ebola f., Marburg virus disease, and Crimean-Congo hemorrhagic f. SEE ALSO epidemic hemorrhagic f. SYN Ebola hemorrhagic f.

hemorrhagic f. with renal syndrome, SYN epidemic hemorrhagic f.

hepatic intermittent f., ague-like paroxysms of f. occurring in cases of one or more stones in the common bile duct.

herpetic f., a disease of short duration, apparently infectious, marked by chills, nausea, elevation of temperature, sore throat, and a herpetic eruption on the face and other areas; primary infection is with herpes simplex virus.

hospital f., SYN epidemic *typhus.*

icterohemorrhagic f., infection with the variety of *Leptospira interrogans* serotype known as icterohemorrhagiae, characterized by fever, jaundice, hemorrhagic lesions, azotemia, and central nervous system manifestations. SYN leptospirosis icterohemorrhagica.

Ilhéus f., a febrile illness caused by the Ilhéus virus, an arborvirus (genus *Flavivirus*), and transmitted by a mosquito. SEE ALSO Ilhéus *encephalitis.*

inanition f., SYN thirst f.

induced f., SYN pyretotherapy.

intermittent malarial f., SEE intermittent *malaria.*

inundation f., SYN tsutsugamushi *disease.*

island f., SYN tsutsugamushi *disease.*

jail f., SYN typhus.

Japanese river f., SYN tsutsugamushi *disease.*

jungle f., SYN malaria.

jungle yellow f., a form occurring in South America, transmitted by *Aedes leucocelaenus* and various treetop mosquitoes of the *Haemagogus* complex; transmitted normally to primates, occasionally by chance to man to set off a human outbreak of classical yellow fever transmitted by *Aedes aegypti.*

Katayama f., SYN Katayama *disease.*

kedani f., SYN tsutsugamushi *disease.*

Kenya f., SYN boutonneuse f.

Kew Gardens f., SYN rickettsialpox. [*Kew Gardens,* area in Queens, NYC, where first reported]

Kinkiang f., SYN *schistosomiasis* japonica.

Korean hemorrhagic f., a form of epidemic hemorrhagic f. caused by the Hantaan virus. SYN Manchurian hemorrhagic f.

Lassa f., a severe form of epidemic hemorrhagic f. which is highly fatal. It was first recognized in Lassa, Nigeria, is caused by the Lassa virus, a member of the Arenaviridae family, and is characterized by high f., sore throat, severe muscle aches, skin rash with hemorrhages, headache, abdominal pain, vomiting, and diarrhea; the multimammate rat *Mastomys natalensis* serves as reservoir, but person-to-person transmission also is common. SYN Lassa hemorrhagic f.

Lassa hemorrhagic f., SYN Lassa f.

laurel f., an affection of the same nature as hay f., occurring at the time of flowering of laurel.

malarial f., SEE malaria.

malignant catarrhal f., a highly fatal, sporadic disease of cattle caused by alcelaphine herpesvirus 1 (a member of the Herpesviridae family) and characterized by inflammation, ulceration, and exudation of the oral and upper respiratory mucous membranes, and sometimes eye lesions and nervous system disturbances. SYN malignant catarrh of cattle.

malignant tertian f., SYN falciparum *malaria.*

Malta f., SYN brucellosis.

Manchurian f., a f. closely resembling typhus that prevails from September to December in South Manchuria; the probable pathogen is *Rickettsia manchuriae.*

Manchurian hemorrhagic f., SYN Korean hemorrhagic f.

Marseilles f., SYN boutonneuse f.

marsh f., SYN malaria.

Mediterranean f., (1) SYN brucellosis. **(2)** SYN familial paroxysmal *polyserositis.*

Mediterranean exanthematous f., an affection occurring sporadically in the Mediterranean littoral marked by a severe chill with abrupt rise of temperature, pains in the joints, tonsillitis, diarrhea, vomiting, and, on the third to fifth day, a rash of elevated nonconfluent macules beginning on the thighs and spreading to the entire body; lasts from ten days to two weeks and then disappears by rapid lysis without desquamation; probably caused by *Rickettsia conorii,* like Boutonneuse fever.

meningotyphoid f., typhoid f. marked by symptoms of irritation or inflammation of the cerebral or spinal meninges.

metal fume f., SYN brass founder's f.

Mexican spotted f., SYN Rocky Mountain spotted f.

mianeh f., SYN Persian relapsing f.

miliary f., (1) an infectious disease characterized by profuse sweating and the production of sudamina, occurring formerly in severe epidemics; **(2)** SYN miliaria.

milk f., (1) a slight elevation of temperature following childbirth, said to be due to the establishment of the secretion of milk, but probably the same as absorption f.; **(2)** an afebrile metabolic disease, occurring shortly after parturition in dairy cattle, characterized by hypocalcemia and manifested by loss of consciousness and general paralysis. SYN parturient paralysis, parturient paresis.

mill f., SYN byssinosis.

miniature scarlet f., a reaction consisting of f., nausea, vomiting, and a transient scarlatiniform rash that appears in a susceptible person when injected with the toxin of *Streptococcus pyogenes.* [L. *minio,* pp. *atus,* to color with *minium,* red-lead]

monoleptic f., a continued f. having but one paroxysm. Cf. polyleptic f.

Mossman f., a f., noted especially among sugar cane cutters in the Mossman District of North Queensland, caused by a leptospira.

mud f., (1) a leptospirosis caused by the *grippotyphosa* serovar of *Leptospira interrogans;* **(2)** SYN bluecomb *disease* of turkeys.

mumu f., Samoan term for elephantoid f.

nanukayami f., a form of leptospirosis known in Japan and caused by a leptospira normally found in the field mouse or vole. SYN nanukayami.

nine mile f., SYN Q f.

nodal f., SYN *erythema* nodosum.

North Queensland tick f., a mild form of tick-borne typhus with eschar, adenopathy, rash, and fever, caused by *Rickettsia australis* and thought to be transmitted by the tick, *Ixodes holocyclus.*

Omsk hemorrhagic f., a form of epidemic hemorrhagic fever found in central Russia, caused by the Omsk hemorrhagic f. virus, a member of the family Flaviviridae, and transmitted by *Dermacentor* ticks; associated with gastrointestinal symptoms and hemorrhages but little or no central nervous system involvement.

o'nyong-nyong f., a dengue-like disease caused by the o'nyong-nyong virus, a member of the family Togaviridae, and transmitted by a mosquito, characterized by joint pains and notable lymphadenopathy followed by a maculopapular eruption of the face which extends to the trunk and extremities but fades in several days without desquamation.

Oroya f., a generalized, acute, febrile, endemic, and systemic form of bartonellosis; marked by high fever, rheumatic pains, progressive, severe anemia, and albuminuria. SYN Carrión's disease.

Pahvant Valley f., SYN tularemia.

paludal f., SYN malaria.

pappataci f., SYN phlebotomus f.

papular f., an affection characterized by mild f., rheumatoid pains, and a maculopapular eruption.

paratyphoid f., an acute infectious disease with symptoms and lesions resembling those of typhoid f., though milder in character; associated with the presence of the paratyphoid organism of which at least three varieties (types A, B, and C) have been described. SYN paratyphoid, Schottmueller's disease.

parenteric f., one of a group of f.'s clinically resembling typhoid and paratyphoid A and B, but caused by bacteria differing specifically from those of either of these diseases.

parrot f., SYN psittacosis.

Pel-Ebstein f., the remittent fever common in Hodgkin's disease. SYN Pel-Ebstein disease.

periodic f., an obsolete term introduced to describe the intermittent febrile episodes seen in disease later recognized and named familial Mediterranean f.

Persian relapsing f., a tick-borne relapsing f., occurring in the Middle East, caused by *Borrelia persica* and transmitted by *Ornithodoros tholozani* and possibly by *Ornithodoros lahorensis.* SYN mianeh disease, mianeh f.

petechial f., SYN *purpura* hemorrhagica (2).

pharyngoconjunctival f., a disease characterized by fever, pharyngitis, and conjunctivitis, and caused by adenoviruses, often type 3 but occasionally other types.

Philippine hemorrhagic f., severe arbovirus infection with hemorrhagic manifestations, considerable mortality, probably due to mosquito borne dengue *virus;* seen in tropical and subtropical urban areas of southeast Asia, South Pacific, Australia, Central and South America, and the Caribbean islands.

phlebotomus f., an infectious but not contagious disease occurring in the Balkan Peninsula and other parts of southern Europe, caused by an arbovirus (family Bunyaviridae) apparently introduced by the bite of the sandfly, *Phlebotomus papatasii;* symptoms resemble those of dengue but are less severe and of shorter duration. SYN dog disease, pappataci f., Pym's f., sandfly f., three-day f.

pinta f., a term used in Mexico for Rocky Mountain spotted f.

polka f., SYN dengue.

polyleptic f., a f. occurring in two or more paroxysms; *e.g.,* smallpox, relapsing f., intermittent f. Cf. monoleptic f.

polymer fume f., an occupational disease marked by f., pain in the chest, and cough caused by the inhalation of fumes given off by a plastic, polytetrafluorethylene, when heated.

Potomac horse f., SYN equine monocytic *ehrlichiosis.*

pretibial f., a mild disease first observed among military personnel at Fort Bragg, North Carolina, characterized by f., moderate

fe

prostration, splenomegaly, and a rash on the anterior aspects of the legs; due to the *autumnalis* serovar of *Leptospira interrogans*. SYN Fort Bragg f.

protein f., f. produced by the injection of foreign protein, such as milk.

puerperal f., postpartum sepsis with a rise in f. after the first 24 hours following delivery, but before the eleventh postpartum day. SYN childbed f., puerperal sepsis.

Pym's f., SYN phlebotomus f.

pyogenic f., SYN pyemia.

Q f., a disease caused by the rickettsia *Coxiella burnetii*, which is propagated in sheep and cattle, where it produces no symptoms; human infections occur as a result of contact not only with such animals but also with other infected humans, air and dust, wild reservoir hosts, and other sources. SYN nine mile f. [*Q*, for "query," so named because etiologic agent was unknown]

quartan f., SYN malariae *malaria*.

quintan f., SYN trench f.

quotidian f., SYN quotidian *malaria*.

rabbit f., SYN tularemia.

rat-bite f., a single designation for two bacterial diseases associated with rat bites, one caused by *Streptobacillus moniliformis* (*e.g.,* Haverhill f.), the other by *Spirillum minus* (*e.g.,* sodoku); both diseases are characterized by relapsing f., chills, headache, arthralgia, lymphadenopathy, and a maculopapular rash on the extremities. SYN rat-bite disease, sodoku, sokosho.

recrudescent typhus f., SYN Brill-Zinsser *disease*.

recurrent f., SYN relapsing f.

red f., red f. of the Congo, SYN murine *typhus*.

redwater f., (1) SYN bovine *babesiosis*. (2) a highly fatal disease of cattle and occasionally of sheep caused by infection with *Clostridium haemolyticum*.

relapsing f., an acute infectious disease caused by any one of a number of strains of *Borrelia*, marked by a number of febrile attacks lasting about six days and separated from each other by apyretic intervals of about the same length; the microorganism is found in the blood during the febrile periods but not during the intervals, the disappearance being associated with specific antibodies and previously evoked antibodies. There are two epidemiologic varieties: 1) the louse-borne variety, occurring chiefly in Europe, northern Africa, and India, and caused by strains of *B. recurrentis;* 2) the tick-borne variety, occurring in Africa, Asia, and North and South America, caused by various species of *Borrelia*, each of which is transmitted by a different species of the soft tick, *Ornithodoros*. SYN bilious typhoid of Griesinger, famine f., recurrent f., spirillum f., typhinia.

remittent f., a f. pattern in which temperature varies during each 24 hour period, but never reaches normal. Most f.'s are remittent and the pattern is not characteristic of any disease, although in the 19th century it was considered a diagnostic term.

remittent malarial f., SEE remittent *malaria*.

rheumatic f., f. following infection of the throat with group A streptococci, occurring primarily in children and young adults, and inducing an immunopathy variably associated with acute migratory polyarthritis, Sydenham's chorea, subcutaneous nodules over bony prominences (myocarditis with formation of Aschoff bodies) which may cause acute cardiac failure, and endocarditis (frequently followed by scarring of valves, causing stenosis or incompetence); relapses are common if repeated streptococcal infections occur.

rice-field f., a febrile illness affecting workers in rice fields, reported in Po valley in Italy and in Sumatra, caused by infection with a species of *Leptospira*.

Rift Valley f., a fatal endemic disease of sheep, caused by Rift Valley f. virus, a member of the family Bunyaviridae, which is also pathogenic for man and cattle, producing in man f. of an undifferentiated type. [*Rift Valley* in Kenya]

Rocky Mountain spotted f., an acute infectious disease of high mortality, characterized by frontal and occipital headache, intense lumbar pain, malaise, a moderately high continuous f., and a rash on wrists, palms, ankles, and soles from the second to the fifth day, later spreading to all parts of the body; it occurs in the spring of the year primarily in the southeast U.S. and the Rocky

Mountain region, although it is also endemic elsewhere in the U.S., in parts of Canada, in Mexico, and in South America; the pathogenic organism is *Rickettsia rickettsii*, transmitted by two or more tick species of the genus *Dermacentor;* in the U.S. it is spread by *D. andersoni* in the western states and *D. variabilis* (a dog tick) in the eastern states. SYN black f., black measles (2), blue disease, blue f., Mexican spotted f., São Paulo f., tick f. (4), Tobia f.

Roman f., malignant tertian, falciparum, or aestivoautumnal f., formerly prevalent in the Roman Campagna and in the city of Rome; caused by *Plasmodium falciparum*.

Ross River f., SYN epidemic *polyarthritis*.

sakushu f., SYN hasamiyami.

Salinem f., infection with *Leptospira pyrogenes*, reported in Salinem. SYN Salinem infection.

salt f., elevated temperature in an infant, following a rectal injection of a salt solution. SEE ALSO thirst f.

sandfly f., SYN phlebotomus f.

San Joaquin f., SYN primary *coccidioidomycosis*.

San Joaquin Valley f., SYN primary *coccidioidomycosis*.

São Paulo f., SYN Rocky Mountain spotted f.

scarlet f., SYN scarlatina.

Sennetsu f., a disease of man in western Japan caused by the rickettsia *Ehrlichia sennetsu* and characterized by fever, malaise, anorexia, backache, and lymphadenopathy.

septic f., SYN septicemia.

seven-day f., (1) SYN autumn f. (1). **(2)** SYN hasamiyami.

shin bone f., SYN trench f.

ship f., SYN typhus.

shipping f., (1) in horses, synonymous with pinkeye or influenza; **(2)** in cattle, a common syndrome seen especially during or after shipping in cold weather or other stressful circumstances, manifested by acute inflammation of the upper respiratory tract usually terminating in pneumonia; associated with parainfluenza virus type 3, although some of the infections are associated with *Pasteurella*.

shoddy f., febrile disease occurring in workers in shoddy factories, with cough, dyspnea and headache, caused by inhalation of dust.

simian hemorrhagic f., a highly fatal disease of macaque monkeys caused by the simian hemorrhagic f. virus and characterized by fever, facial edema, anorexia, adipsia, skin petechiae, diarrhea, hemorrhages, and death.

Sindbis f., a febrile illness of humans in Africa, Australia, and other countries, characterized by arthralgia, rash, and malaise; caused by the Sindbis virus, a member of the family Togaviridae, and transmitted by culicine mosquitoes.

slime f., leptospiral infection with jaundice, presumably infection by *Leptospira icterohemorrhagica*.

slow f., a continued f. of long duration.

smelter's f., metal fume f., occurring in workers in zinc smelters. SYN smelter's chills, smelter's shakes.

snail f., SYN schistosomiasis.

solar f., (1) SYN dengue. **(2)** SYN sunstroke.

Songo f., SYN epidemic hemorrhagic f.

South African tick-bite f., a typhus-like f. of South Africa caused by *Rickettsia rickettsii* and usually characterized by primary eschar and regional adenitis, rigors, and maculopapular rash on the fifth day, often with severe central nervous system symptoms.

spirillum f., SYN relapsing f.

spotted f., tick typhus caused by *Rickettsia rickettsii* in North and South America and Siberia.

steroid f., f. presumably caused by elevated plasma concentrations of certain pyrogenic steroids; can be produced by administration of etiocholanolone.

swamp f., (1) SYN equine infectious *anemia*. **(2)** SYN malaria.

swine f., SYN hog *cholera*.

symptomatic f., SYN traumatic f.

syphilitic f., the elevation of temperature often present in the early roseolous stage of secondary syphilis.

tertian f., SYN vivax *malaria*.

Texas f., SYN bovine *babesiosis*.

therapeutic f., SYN pyrotherapy.

thermic f., SYN heatstroke.

thirst f., an elevation of temperature in infants after reduction of fluid intake, diarrhea, or vomiting; probably caused by reduced available body water, with reduced heat loss by evaporation; an analogous condition in adults is seen when exertion is continued in the face of dehydration. SYN dehydration f., exsiccation f., inanition f.

three-day f., SYN phlebotomus f.

tick f., (1) any infectious disease of man or the lower animals caused by a protozoan blood parasite, a bacterium, a rickettsia, or a virus, and transmitted by a tick; **(2)** the tick-borne variety of relapsing f.; **(3)** SYN bovine *babesiosis*. **(4)** SYN Rocky Mountain spotted f. **(5)** SYN Colorado tick f.

tick-borne f., a rickettsial disease of ruminants transmitted by the tick *Ixodes ricinus* in Europe and *Rhipicephalus haemaphysaloides supina* in India and characterized by pyrexia, depression, and anorexia.

Tobia f., SYN Rocky Mountain spotted f.

traumatic f., elevation of temperature following an injury. SYN symptomatic f., wound f.

trench f., an uncommon rickettsial f. caused by *Rochalimaea quintans* and transmitted by the louse *Pediculus humanus*, first appearing as an epidemic during the trench warfare of World War I; characterized by the sudden onset of chills and f., myalgia (especially of the back and legs), headache, and general malaise that typically lasts five days but may recur. SYN five-day f., quintan f., shin bone f.

trypanosome f., the febrile stage of sleeping sickness.

tsutsugamushi f., SYN tsutsugamushi *disease*.

typhoid f., an acute infectious disease caused by *Salmonella typhi* and characterized by a continued f. rising in a steplike curve the first week, severe physical and mental depression, an eruption of rose-colored spots on the chest and abdomen, tympanites, often diarrhea, and sometimes intestinal hemorrhage or perforation of the bowel; average duration is four weeks, although aborted forms and relapses are not uncommon; the lesions are located chiefly in the lymph follicles of the intestines (Peyer's patches), the mesenteric glands, and the spleen; antibody titer of the Widal test rises during the infection, and early positive blood and urine cultures become negative. SYN abdominal typhoid, enteric f. (1), typhoid (2).

undifferentiated type f.'s, a term applied to illnesses resulting from infection by any one of the arboviruses pathogenic for man, in which the only constant manifestation is f.; rash, lymphadenopathy, or arthralgia (alone or in combination) may occur in some individuals but not in others; some arboviruses may induce infections in which undifferentiated type f. is the only manifestation, whereas other arboviruses may induce in some persons only undifferentiated f., and in other persons similar f. followed by secondary manifestations, *e.g.,* a hemorrhagic f. or encephalitis.

undulant f., SYN brucellosis. [referring to the wavy appearance of the long temperature curve]

undulating f., SYN brucellosis.

urethral f., SYN urinary f.

urinary f., an elevation of temperature, usually slight and transitory, following catheterization of the urethra, or the passage of blood clots, gravel, or a calculus. SYN catheter f., urethral f.

urticarial f., SYN *schistosomiasis* japonica.

uveoparotid f., chronic enlargement of the parotid glands and inflammation of the uveal tract accompanied by a long-continued f. of low degree; now recognized as a form of sarcoidosis. SYN Heerfordt's disease.

Uzbekistan hemorrhagic f., a viral f. in central Asia probably transmitted by *Hyalomma anatolicum*.

valley f., SYN primary *coccidioidomycosis*.

viral hemorrhagic f., an epidemic disease, and associated with fever, malaise, muscular pain, respiratory tract symptoms, vomiting, and diarrhea; epistaxis, hemoptysis, hematemesis, and subconjunctival hemorrhages occur in severe cases, and body rash and tremors occur in some instances; a disease caused by a number of different viruses in the families Arenoviridae, Bunyviridae, Flaviviridae, Filoviridae, etc. SEE ALSO hemorrhagic f.

vivax f., SYN vivax *malaria*.

Wesselsbron f., a mosquito-borne disease of sheep and man caused by the Wesselsbron disease virus, a member of the family Flaviviridae, and characterized by abortion and lamb mortality in sheep and by fever, headache, muscular pains, and mild rash in humans. SYN Wesselsbron disease. [*Wesselsbron,* town in South Africa where causative agent first isolated]

West African f., SYN malarial *hemoglobinuria*.

West Nile f., a febrile illness caused by West Nile virus, a member of the family Flaviviridae, and characterized by headache, fever, maculopapular rash, myalgia, lymphadenopathy, and leukopenia; spread by *Culex* mosquitoes from a reservoir in birds.

wound f., SYN traumatic f.

Yangtze Valley f., SYN *schistosomiasis* japonica.

yellow f., a tropical mosquito-borne viral hepatitis, due to yellow f. virus, a member of the family Flaviviridae, with an urban form transmitted by *Aedes aegypti*, and a rural, jungle, or sylvatic form from tree-dwelling mammals by various mosquitoes of the *Haemagogus* species complex; characterized clinically by fever, slow pulse, albuminuria, jaundice, congestion of the face, and hemorrhages, especially hematemesis; immunity to reinfection accompanies recovery.

Zika f., an acute disease, probably transmitted by mosquitoes, clinically resembling dengue; caused by Zika virus, a member of the family Flaviviridae.

zinc fume f., SYN brass founder's f.

---

fe·ver·ish (fē′ver-ish). **1.** SYN febrile. **2.** Having a fever.

Fevold, Harry Leonard, U.S. biochemist, *1902. SEE test.

Fevold test. See under test.

FF Abbreviation for filtration *fraction*.

FFA Abbreviation for unesterified free *fatty acid*.

FFP. Abbreviation for fresh frozen *plasma*.

F.F.R. Abbreviation for Fellow of the Faculty of Radiologists.

FGAR Abbreviation for *N*-formylglycinamide ribotide.

FH₄ Abbreviation for tetrahydrofolic acid. SEE 5,6,7,8-tetrahydrofolate dehydrogenase, tetrahydrofolate methyltransferase.

FIA Abbreviation for feline infectious *anemia*.

FIBER

fi·ber (fī′ber). A slender thread or filament. **1.** Extracellular filamentous structures such as collagenic or elastic connective tissue f.'s. **2.** The nerve cell axon with its glial envelope. **3.** Elongated, hence threadlike, cells such as muscle cells and the epithelial cells composing the major part of the eye lens. SYN fibra [NA], fibre. [L. *fibra*]

A f.'s, myelinated nerve f.'s in somatic nerves, measuring 1 to 22 μm in diameter, conducting nerve impulses at a rate of 6 to 120 m/sec.

accelerator f.'s, postganglionic sympathetic nerve f.'s originating in the superior, middle, and inferior cervical ganglia of the sympathetic trunk, conveying nervous impulses to the heart that increase the rapidity and force of the cardiac pulsations. SYN augmentor f.'s.

adrenergic f.'s, nerve f.'s that transmit nervous impulses to other nerve cells (or smooth muscle or gland cells) by the medium of the adrenaline-like transmitter substance norepinephrine (noradrenaline).

afferent f.'s, those that convey impulses to a ganglion or to a nerve center in the brain or spinal cord.

fiber groups				
diameter of fiber	histology	fiber group	conduction speed	function
3–20 μm thick	thick fibers with relatively thick myelin sheaths	A α	80–120 m/sec	motor impulses, afferent impulses from muscle spindles and tendon organs
		β	60 m/sec	tactile impulses of the skin
		γ	40 m/sec	efferent impulses to the contractile portions of intrafusal muscle fibers
		δ	20 m/sec	mechanoreceptor impulses; cold, warm and pain sensations of the skin (fast)
1–3 μm thick	thin fibers or thin myelin sheaths	B	10 m/sec	preganglionic vegetative fibers
1 μm thick	fibers without sheaths	C	1 m/sec	postganglionic vegetative fibers and afferent fibers of the sympathetic trunk, impulses of mechanoreceptors, cold and warm receptors (slow)

alpha f.'s, large somatic motor or proprioceptive nerve f.'s conducting impulses at rates near 100 m/sec.

anastomosing f.'s, anastomotic f.'s, individual f.'s passing from one nerve trunk or muscle bundle to another.

arcuate f.'s, nervous or tendinous f.'s passing in the form of an arch from one part to another. SEE arcuate f.'s of cerebrum, external arcuate f.'s, internal arcuate f.'s.

arcuate f.'s of cerebrum, short association fibers that connect adjacent gyri in the cerebral cortex. SYN fibrae arcuatae cerebri [NA].

argyrophilic f.'s, reticular connective tissue f.'s that react with silver salts and appear black microscopically.

association f.'s, nerve f.'s interconnecting subdivisions of the cerebral cortex of the same hemisphere or different segments of the spinal cord on the same side. SYN endogenous f.'s, intrinsic f.'s.

astral f.'s, f.'s (fibrils) radiating from the centrosphere toward the periphery of the cell as seen with a light microscope; revealed as microtubules under the electron microscope. Cf. kinetochore f.'s, polar f.'s.

augmentor f.'s, SYN accelerator f.'s.

B f.'s, myelinated f.'s autonomic nerves, with a diameter of 2 μm or less, conducting at a rate of 3 to 15 m/sec.

Bergmann's f.'s, filamentous glia f.'s traversing the cerebellar cortex perpendicular to the surface.

beta f.'s, nerve f.'s having conduction velocities of about 40 m/sec.

C f.'s, unmyelinated f.'s, 0.4 to 1.2 μm in diameter, conducting nerve impulses at a velocity of 0.7 to 2.3 m/sec.

cerebellohypothalamic f.'s, nerve f.'s originating from cells of the cerebellar nuclei and projecting, via the superior cerebellar peduncle, to the contralateral hypothalamus, mainly its dorsal, lateral, and posterior areas and dorsomedial nucleus.

cerebellospinal f.'s, SEE fastigiospinal f.'s.

cholinergic f.'s, nerve f.'s that transmit impulses to other nerve cells, muscle fibers, or gland cells by the medium of the transmitter substance acetylcholine.

chromatic f., SYN chromonema.

circular f.'s, the circular f.'s of the ciliary muscle. SYN fibrae circulares [NA], Müller's f.'s (1), Müller's muscle (2), Rouget's muscle.

climbing f.'s, nerve f.'s in the cerebellar cortex that synapse upon smooth branchlets of Purkinje cell dendrites.

collagen f., collagenous f., an individual f. that varies in diameter from less than 1 μm to about 12 μm and is composed of fibrils; the f.'s, which are usually arranged in bundles, undergo some branching and are of indefinite length; chemically the f. is a glycoprotein, collagen, which yields gelatin upon boiling; they make up the principal element of irregular connective tissue, tendons, aponeuroses, and most ligaments, and occur in the matrix of cartilage and osseous tissue. SYN white f. (2).

commissural f.'s, nerve f.'s crossing the midline and connecting two corresponding parts or regions of the nervous system.

cone f., a part of the cone cell of the retina; the **inner cone f.** is a slender axon-like part of the cone extending from the cell body to the pedicle located in the outer plexiform layer of the retina; in the outer fovea, where the cones are much elongated, they narrow to an **outer cone f.,** located between the inner segment and the cell body.

corticobulbar f.'s, nerve f.'s projecting from the motor and somatic sensory cortex to the rhombencephalon; included in this corticofugal f. system are corticoreticular f.'s terminating in the reticular formation of the rhombencephalon, and corticonuclear f.'s to the motor nuclei innervating the musculature of the face, tongue, and jaws, and to some f.'s of the rhombencephalic sensory relay nuclei. SEE ALSO corticobulbar *tract*.

corticonuclear f.'s, descriptive term connoting f.'s from a cortical structure (cerebral or cerebellar) passing to subcortical cell groups; f.'s comprising the tractus corticobulbaris; cerebellar corticonuclear f.'s (Purkinje cell axons to the cerebellar nuclei). SYN fibrae corticonucleares [NA].

corticopontine f.'s, the f.'s that compose the corticopontine *tract*. SYN fibrae corticopontinae.

corticoreticular f.'s, corticofugal f.'s distributed to the reticular formation of the mesencephalon and rhombencephalon. SEE ALSO corticobulbar f.'s. SYN fibrae corticoreticulares [NA].

corticorubral f.'s, nerve f.'s projecting from the cerebral cortex (primarily precentral and premotor regions) to the red nucleus of the midbrain.

corticospinal f.'s, SYN pyramidal f.'s.

corticothalamic f.'s, a general term designating nerve f.'s originating from any area of the cerebral cortex and terminating in the nuclei of the thalamus.

dentatorubral f.'s, nerve f.'s arising in the dentate nucleus of the cerebellum and projecting, via the superior cerebellar peduncle and its decussation, to the contralateral red nucleus of the midbrain. SYN fibrae dentatorubrales.

dentatothalamic f.'s, nerve f.'s projecting from the dentate nucleus of the cerebellum to the contralateral thalamus via the superior cerebellar peduncle (and its decussation); enter the thalamus as one component of the thalamic fasciculus.

dentinal f.'s, dental f.'s, (1) the processes of the pulpal cells, the odontoblasts, which extend in radial fashion through the dentin to the dentoenamel junction and are contained within the dentinal tubules; SYN Tomes' f.'s. **(2)** the intertubular fine collagenous f.'s that with the dentinal ground substance infiltrated with calcium salts constitutes the dentinal matrix.

depressor f.'s, sensory nerve f.'s having pressure-sensitive nerve endings in the wall of certain arteries capable of activating blood pressure-lowering brainstem mechanisms when stimulated by an increase in intra-arterial pressure.

dietary f., the plant polysaccharides and lignin that are resistant to hydrolysis by the digestive enzymes in humans.

efferent f.'s, those f.'s conveying impulses to effector tissues (muscle: smooth, cardiac or striated; or glands) in the periphery; those f.'s exiting a specific cell group (*i.e.,* efferent fibers of the basilar pons), used in reference to a cell group.

elastic f.'s, f.'s that are 0.2 to 2 μm in diameter but may be larger in some ligaments; they branch and anastomose to form networks and fuse to form fenestrated membranes; the f.'s and membranes consist of microfibrils about 10 nm wide and an amorphous substance containing elastin. SYN yellow f.'s.

enamel f.'s, SYN *prismata* adamantina, under *prisma*.

endogenous f.'s, SYN association f.'s.

exogenous f.'s, nerve f.'s by which a given region of the central nervous system is connected with other regions; the term applies to both afferent and efferent fiber connections.

external arcuate f.'s, they include: 1) dorsal external arcuate f.'s that arise from cells in the accessory or lateral cuneate nucleus and pass to the cerebellum; 2) ventral external arcuate f.'s that arise from the arcuate nuclei at the base of the medulla oblongata and pass around the lateral surface of the medulla; both enter the cerebellum as components of the restiform portion of the inferior cerebellar peduncle. SYN fibrae arcuatae externae [NA].

fastigiobulbar f.'s, nerve f.'s projecting from the fastigial nuclei of the cerebellum to the brain stem; crossed and uncrossed f.'s that terminate mainly in the vestibular and reticular nuclei, and in the medial accessory olivary nucleus.

fastigiospinal f.'s, crossed descending f.'s originating in the fastigial nucleus of the cerebellum and ending in the spinal cord gray matter at cervical, and possibly lower, levels.

gamma f.'s, nerve f.'s that have a conduction rate of about 20 m/sec. SEE ALSO gamma *efferent.*

Gerdy's f.'s, SYN superficial transverse metacarpal *ligament.*

Gratiolet's f.'s, SYN optic *radiation.*

gray f.'s, SYN unmyelinated f.'s.

hypothalamocerebellar f.'s, nerve f.'s originating from cells in the hypothalamus and projecting to the cerebellar cortex and nuclei.

inhibitory f.'s, nerve f.'s that inhibit the activity of the nerve cells with which they have synaptic connections, or of the effector tissue (smooth muscle, heart muscle, glands) in which they terminate.

intercolumnar f.'s, SYN intercrural f.'s.

intercrural f.'s, horizontal arched fibers that pass from the inguinal ligament across the medial and lateral crura of the superficial inguinal ring. SYN fibrae intercrurales [NA], intercolumnar fasciae, intercolumnar f.'s.

internal arcuate f.'s, f.'s that arise in the cuneate and gracile nuclei, pass in a curving course across the midline of the medulla oblongata, and form the contralateral medial lemniscus; also designates other f.'s such as those of the olivocerebellar tract that arch through the substance of the medulla and form sensory decussation. SYN fibrae arcuatae internae [NA].

intrafusal f.'s, muscle f.'s present within a neuromuscular spindle.

intrinsic f.'s, SYN association f.'s.

James f.'s, atrio-His bundle connections thought to be the basis for the short P-R interval syndrome; these f.'s should be distinguished from the internodal tracts of the atrium, sometimes referred to as "James tracts." SYN James tracts.

kinetochore f.'s, f.'s of the mitotic spindle attached to the centromere and extending toward the poles. Cf. astral f.'s, polar f.'s.

Korff's f.'s, argyrophilic f.'s that pass between odontoblasts at the periphery of the dental pulp and fan out into the dentin.

Kühne's f., artificial muscle f. made by filling the intestine of an insect with a growth of myxomycetes; used to demonstrate the contractility of protoplasm.

f.'s of lens, the elongated cells of ectodermal origin forming the

substance of the crystalline lens of the eye. SYN fibrae lentis [NA].

Mahaim f.'s, paraspecific f.'s originating from the A-V node, the His bundle, or the bundle branches and inserting into the ventricular myocardium; they are potential pathways for reentrant dysrhythmias. SYN nodoventricular f.'s.

medullated nerve f., SYN myelinated nerve f.

meridional f.'s, the longitudinal fibers of the ciliary muscle. SYN fibrae meridionales [NA].

mossy f.'s, highly branched nerve f.'s in the cerebellar cortex that terminate in rosette formations and synapse upon granule cell dendrites.

motor f.'s, nerve f.'s that transmit impulses that activate effector cells, *e.g.,* in muscle or gland tissue.

Müller's f.'s, (1) SYN circular f.'s. **(2)** sustentacular neuroglial cells of the retina, running through the thickness of the retina from the internal limiting membrane to the bases of the rods and cones where they form a row of junctional complexes. SYN Müller's radial cells, sustentacular f.'s of retina.

myelinated nerve f., an axon enveloped by a myelin sheath formed by oligodendroglia cells (in brain and spinal cord) or Schwann cells (in peripheral nerves). SYN medullated nerve f.

Nélaton's f.'s, SYN Nélaton's *sphincter.*

nerve f., the axon of a nerve cell, ensheathed by oligodendroglia cells in brain and spinal cord, and by Schwann cells in peripheral nerves.

nodoventricular f.'s, SYN Mahaim f.'s.

nonmedullated f.'s, SYN unmyelinated f.'s.

nuclear bag f., the largest type of intrafusal muscle f.'s in a neuromuscular spindle, containing a central aggregation of nuclei (nuclear bag).

nuclear chain f., the shortest and most numerous type of intrafusal muscle f.'s in a neuromuscular spindle, containing a single row of centrally positioned nuclei.

nucleocortical f.'s, general term for projections from a nucleus to an overlying cortical structure; specifically used to designate axons of cerebellar nuclear cells that project to the cerebellar cortex (cerebellar nucleocortical f.'s) where they end as mossy f.'s.

oblique f.'s of stomach, the smooth muscle fibers of the innermost layer of the muscular coat of the stomach; the fibers occur chiefly at the cardiac end of the stomach and spread over the anterior and posterior surfaces. SYN fibrae obliquae gastrici [NA].

olivocochlear f.'s, SYN olivocochlear *bundle.*

osteocollagenous f.'s, fine collagenous f.'s in the matrix of osseous tissue.

osteogenetic f.'s, the f.'s in the osteogenetic layer of the periosteum.

pectinate f.'s, SYN pectinate *muscles,* under *muscle.*

perforating f.'s, bundles of collagenous f.'s that pass into the outer circumferential lamellae of bone or the cementum of teeth. SYN Sharpey's f.'s.

periodontal ligament f.'s, the collagen f.'s, running from the cementum to the alveolar bone, that suspend a tooth in its socket; they include apical, oblique, horizontal, and alveolar crest f.'s, indicating that the orientation of the f.'s varies at different levels.

periventricular f.'s, a heterogeneous system of thin nerve f.'s in the periventricular gray matter of the hypothalamus; the dorsal longitudinal fasciculus is a caudal continuation of the system. SYN fibrae periventriculares [NA].

pilomotor f.'s, nerve f.'s that innervate the erector muscles of hair follicles responsible for piloerection.

polar f.'s, those f.'s of the mitotic spindle extending from the two poles of the spindle toward the equator. Cf. astral f.'s, kinetochore f.'s.

postganglionic f.'s, a f. whose cell body is located in an autonomic (motor) ganglion and whose peripheral process will terminate on smooth muscle, cardiac muscle, or glandular epithelium; associated with sympathetic or parasympathetic parts of the autonomic nervous system.

precollagenous f.'s, immature, argyrophilic f.'s.

preganglionic f.'s, a f. whose cell body is located in an autonomic nucleus in the spinal cord or brain stem and whose axon terminates in an autonomic (motor) ganglion; found in nerves conveying sympathetic or parasympathetic f.'s.

pressor f.'s, sensory nerve f.'s whose stimulation causes vasoconstriction and rise of blood pressure.

projection f.'s, nerve f.'s connecting the cerebral cortex with other centers in the brain or spinal cord; fibers arising from cells in the central nervous system that pass to distant loci.

Prussak's f.'s, elastic and connective tissue f.'s bounding the pars flaccida membranae tympani.

Purkinje's f.'s, interlacing f.'s formed of modified cardiac muscle cells with central granulated protoplasm containing one or two nuclei and a transversely striated peripheral portion; they are the terminal ramifications of the conducting system of the heart found beneath the endocardium of the ventricles. SEE ALSO conducting *system* of heart.

pyramidal f.'s, the f.'s that compose the pyramidal tract (corticospinalis). SYN fibrae corticospinales [NA], corticospinal f.'s, fibrae pyramidales.

raphespinal f.'s, nerve f.'s originating from cells of the nuclei raphe magnus, pallidus, and obscurus of the pons and medulla and terminating in the spinal cord gray matter; f.'s involved in the descending inhibition of nociceptive input in the dorsal (posterior) horn; they contain serotonin.

red f.'s, red striated muscle f.'s that are rich in sarcoplasm, myoglobin, and mitochondria; they are smaller in diameter and contract more slowly than white f.'s.

Reissner's f., a rodlike, highly refractive f. running caudally from the subcommissural organ throughout the length of the central canal of the brainstem and spinal cord.

Remak's f.'s, SYN unmyelinated f.'s.

reticular f.'s, the collagen (type III) f.'s forming the distinctive loose connective tissue stroma of embryonic tissues, mesenchyme, red pulp of the spleen, cortex and medulla of lymph nodes, and the hematopoietic compartments of bone marrow and comprising a substantial portion of the collagen f.'s of the skin, blood vessels, synovial membrane, uterine tissue, and granulation tissue; characterized by its organization as a reticular meshwork of fine filaments and an affinity for silver and for periodic acid-Schiff stains.

Retzius' f.'s, stiff f.'s in Deiters' cells.

rod f., a part of the rod cell of the retina that extends to either side of the cell body; the inner rod f. terminates in the spherule, a synaptic ending located in the outer plexiform layer.

Rosenthal f., an oval or elongated eosinophilic mass believed to represent a modified process of an astrocyte; seen in large numbers in certain slowly growing astrocytomas and areas of chronic reactive gliosis.

Sappey's f.'s, nonstriated muscular f.'s in the check ligaments of the eyeball.

Sharpey's f.'s, SYN perforating f.'s.

skeletal muscle f.'s, multinucleated contractile cells varying from less than 10 to 100 μm in diameter and from less than 1 mm to several centimeters in length; the f. consists of sarcoplasm and cross-striated myofibrils, which in turn consist of myofilaments; human skeletal muscles are a mixture of red, white, and intermediate type f.'s.

spindle f., SEE mitotic *spindle*.

spinoreticular f.'s, nerve f.'s originating from the spinal cord and terminating in the reticular formation of the brainstem. SYN spinoreticular tract.

stress f.'s, long bundles of microfilaments made up of actin; believed to be involved in the attachment of cultured cells to a substratum and also in the determination of the shape of cells such as fibroblasts; may be involved in cellular mobility.

striatonigral f.'s, SYN strionigral f.'s.

strionigral f.'s, nerve f.'s originating from cells of the caudate and putamen and terminating mainly in the pars reticulata of the substantia nigra; they utilize GABA and substance P. SYN striatonigral f.'s.

sudomotor f.'s, postganglionic and cholinergic sympathetic nerve f.'s that innervate the sweat glands.

sustentacular f.'s of retina, SYN Müller's f.'s (2).

T f., a f. that branches at right angles to the right and left; term used to describe the branching patterns of granular cell axons in the molecular layer of the cerebellum.

tautomeric f.'s, nerve f.'s of the spinal cord that do not extend beyond the limits of the spinal cord segment in which they originate.

thalamocortical f.'s, a general term identifying nerve f.'s arising from nuclei of the thalamus and projecting to, and terminating in, the cerebral cortex.

Tomes' f.'s, SYN dentinal f.'s (1).

transseptal f.'s, nonelastic f.'s running from tooth to tooth over the crest of the alveolus.

transverse pontine f.'s, f.'s arising from the pontine nuclei, decussate and pass into the cerebellum as the middle cerebellar peduncles. SYN fibrae pontis transversae [NA].

unmyelinated f.'s, a f. having no myelin covering (CNS); a naked axon; in the PNS represented by all axons lying in troughs in a single Schwann cell (Schwann cell unit); a slow conducting f. SYN gray f.'s, nonmedullated f.'s, Remak's f.'s.

vasomotor f.'s, postganglionic visceral efferent f.'s innervating the smooth muscles of vessel walls.

Weitbrecht's f.'s, SYN *retinaculum* of articular capsule of hip.

white f., (1) white mammalian muscle f.'s; larger in diameter than red f.'s they have less myoglobin, sarcoplasm, and mitochondria, and contract more quickly; (2) SYN collagen f.

yellow f.'s, SYN elastic f.'s.

zonular f.'s, delicate fibers that pass from the equator of the lens to the ciliary body, collectively known as the ciliary zonule. SYN fibrae zonulares [NA].

---

fi·ber·op·tic (fī-ber-op′tik). Pertaining to fiberoptics.

fi·ber·op·tics (fī-ber-op′tiks). An optical system in which the image is conveyed by a compact bundle of small diameter, flexible, glass or plastic fibers.

fi·ber·scope (fī′ber-skōp). An optical instrument that transmits light and carries images back to the observer through a flexible bundle of small (about 10 micron) glass or plastic fibers. It is used to inspect of interior portions of the body. SEE ALSO fiberoptics.

△**fibr-.** SEE fibro-.

fi·bra, pl. **fi·brae** (fī′bră, fī′brē) [NA]. SYN fiber, fiber. [L.]

   fi′brae arcua′tae cer′ebri [NA], SYN arcuate *fibers* of cerebrum, under *fiber.*

   fi′brae arcua′tae exter′nae [NA], SYN external arcuate *fibers,* under *fiber.*

   fi′brae arcua′tae inter′nae [NA], SYN internal arcuate *fibers,* under *fiber.*

   fi′brae circula′res [NA], SYN circular *fibers,* under *fiber.*

   fi′brae corticonuclea′res [NA], SYN corticonuclear *fibers,* under *fiber.*

   fi′brae corticopon′tinae, SYN corticopontine *fibers,* under *fiber.*

   fi′brae corticoreticula′res [NA], SYN corticoreticular *fibers,* under *fiber.*

   fi′brae corticospina′les [NA], SYN pyramidal *fibers,* under *fiber.*

   fi′brae dentatorubra′les [na], SYN dentatorubral *fibers,* under *fiber.* SEE dentatorubral *fibers,* under *fiber.*

   fi′brae intercrura′les [NA], SYN intercrural *fibers,* under *fiber.*

   fi′brae len′tis [NA], SYN *fibers* of lens, under *fiber.*

   fi′brae meridiona′les [NA], SYN meridional *fibers,* under *fiber.*

   fi′brae obli′quae gastri′ci [NA], SYN oblique *fibers* of stomach, under *fiber.*

   fi′brae periventricula′res [NA], SYN periventricular *fibers,* under *fiber.*

   fi′brae pon′tis transver′sae [NA], SYN transverse pontine *fibers,* under *fiber.*

   fi′brae pyramida′les, SYN pyramidal *fibers,* under *fiber.*

   fi′brae zonula′res [NA], SYN zonular *fibers,* under *fiber.*

fi·bre (fī′ber). SYN fiber.

fi·bre·mia (fī-brē′mē-ă). Presence of formed fibrin in the blood, causing thrombosis or embolism. SYN inosemia (2). [fibrin + G. *haima,* blood]

fi·bril (fi′bril). A minute fiber or component of a fiber. SYN fibrilla. [Mod. L. *fibrilla*]

collagen f.'s, SYN unit f.'s.

muscular f., SYN myofibril.

subpellicular f., SYN subpellicular *microtubule.*

unit f.'s, the f.'s that comprise a collagen fiber, ranging from 20 to 200 nm and averaging about 100 nm in diameter (substantially larger in tendons), with cross-striations averaging 64 nm. SYN collagen f.'s.

fi·bril·la, pl. **fi·bril·lae** (fī-bril′ă, -ē). SYN fibril. [Mod. L. dim. of L. *fibra,* a fiber]

fi·bril·lar, fi·bril·lary (fi′bri-lăr, -lar-ē). **1.** Relating to a fibril. **2.** Denoting the fine rapid contractions or twitchings of fibers or of small groups of fibers in skeletal or cardiac muscle. SYN filar (1).

fi·bril·late (fi′bri-lāt). **1.** To make or to become fibrillar. **2.** SYN fibrillated. **3.** To be in a state of fibrillation (3).

fi·bril·lat·ed (fi′bri-lā-ted). Composed of fibrils. SYN fibrillate (2).

fi·bril·la·tion (fī-bri-lā′shŭn, fib-rĭ-). **1.** The condition of being fibrillated. **2.** The formation of fibrils. **3.** Exceedingly rapid contractions or twitching of muscular fibrils, but not of the muscle as a whole. **4.** Vermicular twitching, usually slow, of individual muscular fibers; commonly occurs in atria or ventricles of the heart as well as in recently denervated skeletal muscle fibers.

atrial f., auricular f., f. in which the normal rhythmical contractions of the cardiac atria are replaced by rapid irregular twitchings of the muscular wall; the ventricles respond irregularly to the dysrhythmic bombardment from the atria. SYN ataxia cordis.

ventricular f., coarse or fine, rapid, fibrillary movements of the ventricular muscle that replace the normal contraction.

fi·bril·lin (fi′bril-in). A protein in connective tissue with a wide distribution in the body; molecular weight about 350,000. There is good evidence that at least some forms of the Marfan syndrome are due to mutations of f. [MIM*134794]. [Mod. L. *fibrilla,* fibril, + -in]

fi·bril·lo·flut·ter (fib′ril-ō-flut′er). SYN impure *flutter.*

fi·bril·lo·gen·e·sis (fi′bril-ō-jen′ě-sis). The development of fine fibrils (as seen with the electron microscope) normally present in collagenous fibers of connective tissue.

fi·brin (fi′brin). An elastic filamentous protein derived from fibrinogen by the action of thrombin, which releases fibrinopeptides A and B from fibrinogen in coagulation of the blood; a component of thrombi, vegetations, and acute inflammatory exudates such as in diphtheria and lobar pneumonia. [L. *fibra,* fiber]

fi·brin·ase (fi′brin-ās). **1.** Former term for *factor* XIII. **2.** SYN plasmin.

⚕fibrino-. Fibrin. [L. *fibra,* fiber]

fi·bri·no·cel·lu·lar (fi′bri-nō-sel′yū-lăr). Composed of fibrin and cells, as in certain types of exudates resulting from acute inflammation.

fi·brin·o·gen (fī-brin′ō-jen). A globulin of the blood plasma that is converted into fibrin by the action of thrombin in the presence of ionized calcium to produce coagulation of the blood; the only coagulable protein in the blood plasma of vertebrates; it is absent in afibrinogenemia and is defective in dysfibrinogenemia.

human f., f. prepared from normal human plasma; a coagulant (clotting factor), used as an adjunct in the management of acute, congenital, or acquired chronic hypofibrinogenemia.

fi·brin·og·e·nase (fī-brin′ō-je-nās). SYN thrombin.

fi·brin·o·ge·ne·mia (fī-brin′ō-jě-nē′mē-ă). SYN hyperfibrinogenemia.

fi·bri·no·gen·e·sis (fi′bri-nō-jen′ě-sis). Formation or production of fibrin.

fi·bri·no·gen·ic, fi·bri·nog·e·nous (fi′brin-ō-jen′ik, fi′brin-noj′ě-nŭs). **1.** Pertaining to fibrinogen. **2.** Producing fibrin.

fi·brin·o·gen·ol·y·sis (fī-brin′ō-jen-ol′i-sis). The inactivation or dissolution of fibrinogen in the blood. [fibrinogen + G. *lysis,* dissolution]

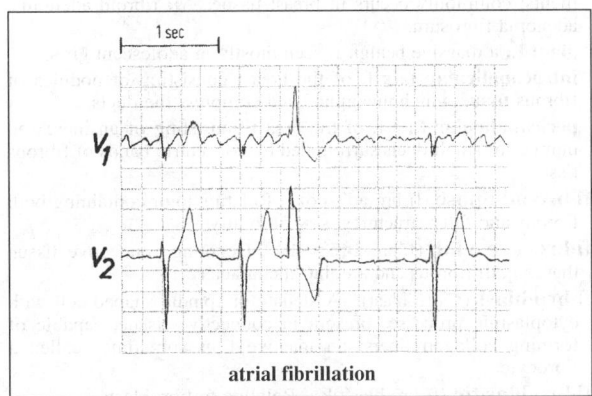

atrial fibrillation

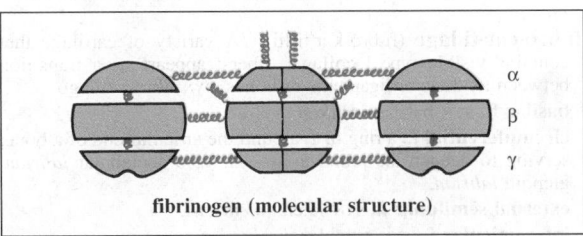

fibrinogen (molecular structure)

fi·brin·o·gen·o·pe·nia (fī-brin′ō-jen-ō-pē′nē-ă). A concentration of fibrinogen in the blood that is less than the normal. [fibrinogen + G. *penia,* poverty]

fi·brin·oid (fi′bri-noyd). **1.** Resembling fibrin. **2.** A deeply or brilliantly acidophilic, homogeneous, refractile, proteinaceous material that: 1) is frequently formed in the walls of blood vessels and in connective tissue of patients with such diseases as disseminated lupus erythematosus, polyarteritis nodosa, scleroderma, dermatomyositis, and rheumatic fever; 2) is sometimes observed in healing wounds, chronic peptic ulcers, the placenta, necrotic arterioles of malignant hypertension, and other unrelated conditions. [fibrin + G. *eidos,* resemblance]

fi·bri·no·ki·nase (fi′brin-ō-ki′nās). Name proposed for the enzyme that converts plasminogen to plasmin; subsequently called urokinase, but now called plasminogen *activator.* SYN fibrinolysokinase.

fi·bri·nol·y·sin (fī-brin-ō-lī′sin). SYN plasmin.

streptococcal f., SYN streptokinase.

fi·bri·nol·y·sis (fī-bri-nol′i-sis). Hydrolysis of fibrin. [fibrino- + G. *lysis,* dissolution]

fi·bri·no·ly·so·ki·nase (fi′brin-ō-lī-sō-ki′nās). SYN fibrinokinase.

fi·bri·no·lyt·ic (fī-brin-ō-lit′ik). Denoting, characterized by, or causing fibrinolysis.

fi·brin·o·pep·tide (fi′brin-ō-pep′tīd). One of two pairs of peptides (A and B) released from the amino-terminal ends of 2α- and 2β-chains of fibrinogen by the action of thrombin to form fibrin; they have a vasoconstrictive effect.

fi·bri·no·pu·ru·lent (fi′bri-nō-pyū′rū-lent). Pertaining to pus or suppurative exudate that contains a relatively large amount of fibrin.

fi·bri·nos·co·py (fī-bri-nos′kŏ-pē). The chemical and physical examination of the fibrin of exudates, blood clots, etc. [fibrino- + G. *skopeō,* to view]

fi·brin·ous (fi′brin-ŭs). Pertaining to or composed of fibrin.

fi·bri·nu·ria (fī-bri-nū′rē-ă). The passage of urine that contains fibrin. [fibrin + G. *ouron,* urine]

⚕fibro-, fibr-. Fiber. [L. *fibra*]

fi·bro·ad·e·no·ma (fi′brō-ad-ě-nō′mă). A benign neoplasm derived from glandular epithelium, in which there is a conspicuous stroma of proliferating fibroblasts and connective tissue elements; commonly occurs in breast tissue. SYN fibroid adenoma, adenoma fibrosum.

giant f., a massive benign f. seen mostly in adolescent girls.

intracanalicular f., a f. of the breast consisting of nodules of fibrous tissue which invaginate and compress the ducts.

pericanalicular f., a f. of the breast consisting of an increased number of small ducts surrounded by concentric bands of fibrous tissue.

fi·bro·ad·i·pose (fī-brō-ad´i-pōz). Relating to or containing both fibrous and fatty structures. SYN fibrofatty.

fi·bro·a·re·o·lar (fī´brō-ă-rē´ō-lăr). Denoting connective tissue that is both fibrous and areolar in character.

fi·bro·blast (fī´brō-blast). A stellate or spindle-shaped cell with cytoplasmic processes present in connective tissue, capable of forming collagen fibers; an inactive f. is sometimes called a fibrocyte.

fi·bro·blas·tic (fī-brō-blas´tik). Relating to fibroblasts.

fi·bro·car·ci·no·ma (fī´brō-kar-si-nō´mă). SYN scirrhous *carcinoma*.

fi·bro·car·ti·lage (fī-brō-kar´ti-lij). A variety of cartilage that contains visible type I collagen fibers; appears as a transition between tendons or ligaments or bones. SYN fibrocartilago.

basilar f., SYN basilar *cartilage.*

circumferential f., a ring of f. around the articular end of a bone, serving to deepen the joint cavity. SEE ALSO acetabular *labrum,* glenoid *labrum.*

external semilunar f., SYN lateral *meniscus.*

interarticular f., SYN articular *disc.*

internal semilunar f. of knee joint, SYN medial *meniscus.*

semilunar f., SEE lateral *meniscus,* medial *meniscus.*

stratiform f., a layer of f. in the bottom of a groove in a bone through which a tendon runs.

fi·bro·car·ti·lag·i·nous (fī´brō-kar-ti-laj´i-nŭs). Relating to or composed of fibrocartilage.

fi·bro·car·ti·la·go (fī´brō-kar-ti-lā´gō). SYN fibrocartilage.

f. basa´lis, SYN basilar *cartilage.*

f. interarticula´ris, SYN articular *disc.*

f. intervertebra´lis, SYN intervertebral *disc.*

fi·bro·cel·lu·lar (fī-brō-sel´yū-lăr). Both fibrous and cellular.

fi·bro·chon·dri·tis (fī´brō-kon-drī´tis). Inflammation of a fibrocartilage.

fi·bro·chon·dro·ma (fī´brō-kon-drō´mă). A benign neoplasm of cartilaginous tissue, in which there is a relatively unusual amount of fibrous stroma.

fi·bro·con·ges·tive (fī´brō-kon-jes´tiv). Term sometimes used to indicate the general condition of an organ or tissue in which acute or chronic, persistent congestion has resulted in degeneration and necrosis of cells and replacement with connective tissue elements, as in chronic congestive splenomegaly.

fi·bro·cyst (fī´brō-sist). Any cystic lesion circumscribed by or situated within a conspicuous amount of fibrous connective tissue.

fi·bro·cys·tic (fī-brō-sis´tik). Pertaining to or characterized by the presence of fibrocysts.

fi·bro·cys·to·ma (fī´brō-sis-tō´mă). A benign neoplasm, usually derived from glandular epithelium, characterized by cysts within a conspicuous fibrous stroma.

fi·bro·cyte (fī´brō-sīt). Designation sometimes applied to an inactive fibroblast. [fibro- + G. *kytos,* cell]

fi·bro·dys·pla·sia (fī´brō-dis-plā´zē-ă). Abnormal development of fibrous connective tissue.

f. ossif´icans progres´siva [MIM*135100], a generalized disorder of connective tissue in which bone replaces tendons, fasciae, and ligaments; a lethal genetic disorder inferred from indirect evidence to have autosomal dominant inheritance. SEE ALSO fibrous *dysplasia* of bone.

fi·bro·e·las·tic (fī´brō-ē-las´tik). Composed of collagen and elastic fibers.

fi·bro·e·las·to·sis (fī´brō-ē-las-tō´sis). Excessive proliferation of collagenous and elastic fibrous tissue.

endocardial f., **endomyocardial f.,** (1) a congenital condition characterized by thickening of the left ventricular wall endocardium (chiefly due to fibrous and elastic tissue), thickening and malformation of the cardiac valves, subendocardial changes in the myocardium, and hypertrophy of the heart; chief symptoms are cyanosis, dyspnea, anorexia, and irritability; SYN endocardial sclerosis (1). (2) SYN endomyocardial *fibrosis.*

fi·bro·en·chon·dro·ma (fī´brō-en-kon-drō´mă). An enchondroma in which the neoplastic cartilage cells are situated within an abundant fibrous stroma.

fi·bro·ep·i·the·li·o·ma (fī´brō-ep-i-thē-lē-ō´mă). A skin tumor composed of fibrous tissue intersected by thin anastomosing bands of basal cells of the epidermis; may give rise to basal cell carcinoma of the nodular type. SYN Pinkus tumor.

fi·bro·fat·ty (fī-brō-fat´ē). SYN fibroadipose.

fi·bro·fol·lic·u·lo·ma (fī´brō-fŏ-lik-yū-lō´mă). Neoplastic proliferation of the fibrous sheath of the hair follicle, with solid extensions of the epithelium of the follicular infundibulum; multiple f.'s may be familial.

fi·bro·gen·e·sis (fī-brō-jen´ĕ-sis). The production or development of fibers.

fi·bro·gli·o·sis (fī´brō-glī-ō´sis). A cellular reaction within the brain, usually in response to a penetrating injury, in which both astrocytes and fibroblasts participate and which culminates in a fibrous and glial scar. [fibro- + G. *glia,* glue, + *-osis,* condition]

fi·broid (fī´broyd). **1.** Resembling or composed of fibers or fibrous tissue. **2.** Old term for certain types of leiomyoma, especially those occurring in the uterus. **3.** SYN fibroleiomyoma. [fibro- + G. *eidos,* resemblance]

fi·broid·ec·to·my (fī-broy-dek´tō-mē). Removal of a fibroid tumor. SYN fibromectomy. [fibroid + G. *ektomē,* excision]

fi·bro·in (fī´brō-in). A white insoluble protein forming the primary constituent (70%) of cobweb and silk.

fi·bro·ker·a·to·ma (fī´brō-ker-ă-tō´mă). A keratotic cutaneous polyp containing abundant connective tissue.

fi·bro·lei·o·my·o·ma (fī´brō-lī´ō-mī-ō´mă). A leiomyoma containing non-neoplastic collagenous fibrous tissue, which may make the tumor hard; f. usually arises in the myometrium, and the proportion of fibrous tissue increases with age. SYN fibroid (3), leiomyofibroma.

fi·bro·li·po·ma (fī´brō-li-pō´mă). A lipoma with an abundant stroma of fibrous tissue. SYN lipoma fibrosum.

fi·bro·ma (fī-brō´mă). A benign neoplasm derived from fibrous connective tissue. [fibro- + G. *-oma,* tumor]

ameloblastic f., a benign mixed odontogenic tumor characterized by neoplastic proliferation of both epithelial and mesenchymal components of the tooth bud without the production of dental hard tissue; presents clinically as a slow-growing painless radiolucency occurring most commonly in the mandible of children and adolescents.

aponeurotic f., a calcifying recurrent non-metastasizing but infiltrating f. seen most frequently on the palms of young people as a small firm nodule not attached to the overlying skin.

central cementifying f., a microscopic variant of a central ossifying f.

central ossifying f., a painless, slow-growing, expansile, sharply circumscribed benign fibro-osseus tumor of the jaws that is derived from cells of the periodontal ligament; presents initially as a radiolucency that becomes progressively more opaque as it matures. SEE ALSO central cementifying f.

chondromyxoid f., an uncommon benign bone tumor, occurring most frequently in the tibia of adolescents and young adults, composed of lobulated myxoid tissue with scanty chondroid foci. SYN chondrofibroma, chondromyxoma.

concentric f., a benign neoplasm, actually a leiomyoma, that occupies the entire circumference of the wall of the uterus.

desmoplastic f., a benign fibrous tumor of bone affecting children and young adults; cortical destruction may result.

giant cell f., a tumor of the oral mucosa composed of fibrous connective tissue with large stellate and multinucleate fibroblasts; shares a similar histology with the retrocuspid papilla, fibrous papule of the nose, pearly penile papule, and the ungual fibroma.

irritation f., a slow-growing nodule on the oral mucosa, composed of fibrous tissue covered by epithelium, resulting from mechanical irritation by dentures, fillings, cheek biting, etc.

f. mol′le, SYN skin *tag.*

f. mol′le gravida′rum, skin tags or polyps that develop on women during pregnancy and often disappear at term.

f. myxomato′des, SYN myxofibroma.

nonossifying f., a loculated osteolytic focus of cellular fibrous tissue, slightly expanding a bone, usually near the end of a long bone in older children; similar to fibrous cortical *defect*, although larger.

nonosteogenic f., SYN fibrous cortical *defect.*

odontogenic f., a rare odontogenic tumor found in soft tissue or as a central bony lesion. The tumor is composed of fibrous connective tissue, odontogenic epithelium, and sometimes calcification.

peripheral ossifying f., a reactive focal gingival overgrowth derived histogenetically from cells of the periodontal ligament and usually developing in response to local irritants (plaque and calculus) on associated teeth; consists microscopically of a hyperplastic cellular fibrous stroma supporting deposits of bone, cementum, or dystrophic calcification.

periungual f., multiple smooth firm nodules formed at the nail folds, often over 10 mm in length, which appear at or after puberty in some patients with tuberous sclerosis. SYN Koenen's tumor.

rabbit f., SYN Shope f.

recurring digital f.'s of childhood, multiple fibrous flesh-colored nodules on the extensor aspect of the terminal phalanges of adjacent digits of infants and young children which often recur after attempted excision, do not metastasize, and may spontaneously regress in two to three years; composed of spindle cells containing cytoplasmic inclusions believed to be derived from myofibrils. SYN infantile digital fibromatosis.

senile f., SYN skin *tag.*

Shope f., a connective tissue tumor of cottontail rabbits caused by a poxvirus of the genus *Leporipoxvirus* and found by Shope to be transmissible with cellular suspensions or Berkefeld filtrates; it is related to myxomatosis and is used in Europe as a source of vaccine to protect against the myxoma virus. SYN rabbit f.

telangiectatic f., a benign neoplasm of fibrous tissue in which there are numerous, small and large, frequently dilated, vascular channels. SYN angiofibroma.

fi·bro·ma·toid (fī-brō′mă-toyd). A focus, nodule, or mass (of proliferating fibroblasts) that resembles a fibroma but is not regarded as neoplastic.

fi·bro·ma·to·sis (fī′brō-mă-tō′sis). **1.** A condition characterized by the occurrence of multiple fibromas, with a relatively large distribution. **2.** Abnormal hyperplasia of fibrous tissue.

abdominal f., SYN desmoid (2).

aggressive infantile f., a childhood counterpart of abdominal or extra-abdominal desmoid tumors, characterized by firm subcutaneous nodules that grow rapidly in any part of the body that invade locally and recur but do not metastasize.

f. col′li, a fibrous mass in the midportion of the sternocleidomastoid muscle; the mass may be a hematoma resulting from a birth injury and may cause torticollis.

congenital generalized f. [MIM*228550], multiple subcutaneous and visceral fibrous tumors present at birth; a rare disorder often fatal in the first week of life, although sometimes undergoing spontaneous remission; probable autosomal recessive inheritance.

gingival f., f. that may be associated with trichodiscomas. Several genetic forms are known, all autosomal dominant [MIM*135300, *135400, *135500, *135550].

infantile digital f., SYN recurring digital *fibromas* of childhood, under *fibroma.*

juvenile hyalin f. [MIM*228600], a rare recessively inherited deforming disorder of head, neck, and generalized cutaneous nodules or tumors in children with normal mentality; the lesions

consist of fibroblasts separated by an eosinophilic hyalin stroma composed mostly of glycosaminoglycans. SYN systemic hyalinosis.

juvenile palmo-plantar f., f. that occurs in children from birth to adolescence as a single poorly demarcated nodule of the thenar or hypothenar eminence or overlying the calcaneus of the mid-sole.

palmar f., nodular fibroplastic proliferation in the palmar fascia of one or both hands, preceding or associated with Dupuytren's contracture.

penile f., SYN Peyronie's *disease.*

plantar f., nodular fibroblastic proliferation in plantar fascia of one or both feet; rarely associated with contracture. SYN Dupuytren's disease of the foot.

fi·bro·ma·tous (fī-brō′mă-tŭs). Pertaining to, or of the nature of, a fibroma.

fi·bro·mec·to·my (fī-brō-mek′tō-mē). SYN fibroidectomy.

fi·brom·e·ter (fī′brō-mē′ter). An instrument that measures clot formation (as in tests for blood clotting *in vitro*) by mechanical detection of the clot by a moving probe.

fi·bro·mus·cu·lar (fī′brō-mŭs′kyū-lăr). Both fibrous and muscular; relating to both fibrous and muscular tissues.

fi·bro·my·ec·to·my (fī′brō-mī-ek′tō-mē). Excision of a fibromyoma.

fi·bro·my·o·ma (fī′brō-mī-ō′mă). A leiomyoma that contains a relatively abundant amount of fibrous tissue.

fi·bro·my·o·si·tis (fī′brō-mī-ō-sī′tis). Chronic inflammation of a muscle with an overgrowth, or hyperplasia, of the connective tissue. [fibro- + G. *mys,* muscle, + *-itis,* inflammation]

fi·bro·myx·o·ma (fī′brō-mik-sō′mă). A myxoma that contains a relatively abundant amount of mature fibroblasts and connective tissue. [fibro- + G. *myxa,* mucus, + *-ōma,* tumor]

fi·bro·nec·tins (fī-brō-nek′tins). High molecular weight multifunctional glycoproteins found on cell surface membranes and in blood plasma and other body fluids. f. are thought to function as adhesive ligand-like molecules. This class of proteins is under investigation for possible roles in other processes, including transformation to malignancy; a deficiency of fibronectin is associated with Ehlers-Danlos syndrome type X. Autosomal dominant anomalies of fibronectin are numerous [MIM* 135600-135631]. SYN zetaprotein. [L. *fibra,* fiber, + *nexus,* interconnection]

plasma f., a circulating α_2-glycoprotein that functions as an opsonin, mediating reticuloendothelial and macrophage clearance of fibrin microaggregates, collagen debris, and bacterial particulates, protecting microvascular perfusion and lymphatic drainage.

fi·bro·neu·ro·ma (fī′brō-nū-rō′mă). SYN neurofibroma.

fi·bro·os·te·o·ma (fī′brō-os-tē-ō′mă). An osteoma in which the neoplastic bone-forming cells are situated within a relatively abundant stroma of fibrous tissue.

fi·bro·pap·il·lo·ma (fī′brō-pap-i-lō′mă). A papilloma characterized by a conspicuous amount of fibrous connective tissue at the base and forming the cores upon which the neoplastic epithelial cells are massed.

fi·bro·pla·sia (fī-brō-plā′zē-ă). Production of fibrous tissue, usually implying an abnormal increase of non-neoplastic fibrous tissue. [fibro- + G. *plasis,* a molding]

retrolental f., SYN *retinopathy* of prematurity.

fi·bro·plas·tic (fī-brō-plas′tik). Producing fibrous tissue. [fibro- + G. *plastos,* formed]

fi·bro·plate (fī′brō-plāt). SYN articular *disc.*

fi·bro·pol·y·pus (fī-brō-pol′i-pŭs). A polyp composed chiefly of fibrous tissue.

fi·bro·re·tic·u·late (fī′brō-re-tik′yū-lāt). Relating to or consisting of a network of fibrous tissue.

fi·bro·sar·co·ma (fī′brō-sar-kō′mă). A malignant neoplasm derived from deep fibrous tissue, characterized by bundles of immature proliferating fibroblasts arranged in a distinctive herringbone pattern with variable collagen formation, which tends to invade locally and metastasize by the bloodstream.

ameloblastic f., a rapidly growing, painful, destructive, radiolucent odontogenic tumor that usually arises through malignant change in the mesenchymal component of a pre-existing ameloblastic fibroma. SYN ameloblastic sarcoma.

Earle L f., a transplantable f. derived from subcutaneous tissue of a mouse of C3H strain, grown in tissue culture to which 20-methylcholanthrene had been added.

infantile f., a rapidly growing but infrequently metastasizing f. which usually appears on the extremities in the first year of life.

fi·brose (fī-brōs'). To form fibrous tissue.

fi·bro·se·rous (fī-brō-sē'rŭs). Composed of fibrous tissue with a serous surface; denoting any serous membrane.

fi·bro·sis (fī-brō'sis). Formation of fibrous tissue as a reparative or reactive process, as opposed to formation of fibrous tissue as a normal constituent of an organ or tissue.

African endomyocardial f., f. of the inner layers of the myocardium, often including the endocardium, causing diastolic restriction of the heart; indigenous to East Africa.

congenital f. of the extraocular muscles [MIM*135700], an autosomal dominant disorder associated with blepharoptosis and absence of eye movements.

cystic f., cystic f. of the pancreas [MIM*219700], a congenital metabolic disorder, inherited as an autosomal trait, in which secretions of exocrine glands are abnormal; excessively viscid mucus causes obstruction of passageways (including pancreatic and bile ducts, intestines, and bronchi), and the sodium and chloride content of sweat are increased throughout the patient's life; symptoms usually appear in childhood and include meconium ileus, poor growth despite good appetite, malabsorption and foul bulky stools, chronic bronchitis with cough, recurrent pneumonia, bronchiectasis, emphysema, clubbing of the fingers, and salt depletion in hot weather. Detailed genetic mapping and molecular biology have been accomplished by the methods of reverse genetics. SYN Clarke-Hadfield syndrome, fibrocystic disease of the pancreas, mucoviscidosis, viscidosis.

endocardial f., scarring or collaginosis of the endocardium. SYN endocardial sclerosis (2).

endomyocardial f., thickening of the ventricular endocardium by f., involving the subendocardial myocardium, and sometimes the atrioventricular valves, with mural thrombosis, leading to progressive right and left ventricular failure with mitral and tricuspid insufficiency; occurs in adults and is endemic in parts of Africa. SYN Davies' disease, endocardial fibroelastosis (2), endomyocardial fibroelastosis.

idiopathic interstitial f., SYN usual interstitial *pneumonia* of Liebow.

idiopathic pulmonary f. (IPF), subacute form also called Hamman-Rich syndrome; an acute to chronic inflammatory process of the lungs, the healing stage of diffuse alveolar damage or acute interstitial pneumonia, either completely idiopathic or associated with collagen-vascular diseases. SYN chronic fibrosing alveolitis, interstitial pulmonary f.

interstitial pulmonary f., SYN idiopathic pulmonary f.

leptomeningeal f., a fibrous reaction within the subarachnoid space; sometimes a sequel to infectious or chemical meningitis. SEE ALSO adhesive *arachnoiditis.*

mediastinal f., f. that may obstruct the superior vena cava, pulmonary arteries, veins, or bronchi; most common cause is histoplasmosis; less commonly tuberculosis or unknown. SYN fibrosing mediastinitis, idiopathic fibrous mediastinitis.

nodular subepidermal f., SEE dermatofibroma.

oral submucous f., a precancerous condition of the oral mucosa and upper aerodigestive tract characteristically in a native of India.

pericentral f., f. occurring around the central veins in the hepatic lobules.

perimuscular f., f. in the outer media of arteries, usually the renal arteries of young women, where it causes segmental stenosis and hypertension; a variety of fibromuscular dysplasia. SYN subadventitial f.

pipestem f., a characteristic pipe-shaped f. formed around hepatic portal veins in some cases of long-continued heavy infection with *Schistosoma mansoni;* thought to be induced by the pres-

ence of large numbers of schistosome eggs in the hepatic tissues. SYN Symmers' clay pipestem f., Symmers' f.

replacement f., the formation of fibrous tissue that occupies sites where various other cells and tissues have become atrophied, or degenerated and necrotic.

retroperitoneal f., f. of retroperitoneal structures commonly involving and often obstructing the ureters; the cause is usually unknown. SYN idiopathic fibrous retroperitonitis, Ormond's disease, periureteritis plastica.

subadventitial f., SYN perimuscular f.

Symmers' clay pipestem f., Symmers' f., SYN pipestem f.

fi·bro·si·tis (fī-brō-sī'tis). 1. Inflammation of fibrous tissue. 2. Term used to denote aching, soreness, or stiffness, with multiple tender foci (trigger points); unknown etiology; thought by some to be due to a sleep disturbance preventing normal muscle relaxation. SYN muscular rheumatism. [fibro- + G. -*itis,* inflammation]

cervical f., SYN posttraumatic neck *syndrome.*

fi·bro·tho·rax (fī-brō-thō'raks). Fibrosis of the pleural space.

fi·brot·ic (fī-brot'ik). Pertaining to or characterized by fibrosis.

fi·brous (fī'brŭs). Composed of or containing fibroblasts, and also the fibrils and fibers of connective tissue formed by such cells.

fi·bro·xan·tho·ma (fī'brō-zan-thō'mă). A fibrohistiocytic neoplasm.

atypical f., a solitary, often ulcerated, small cutaneous benign tumor composed of foamy histiocytes, spindle cells, and bizarre giant cells; usually found on the exposed skin of older people; microscopically, atypical f. closely resembles malignant fibrous histiocytoma, but originates in the dermis.

fib·u·la (fib'yū-lă) [NA]. The lateral and smaller of the two bones of the leg; it is not-weight bearing and articulates with the tibia above and the tibia and talus below. SYN calf bone, calfbone (1), perone, peroneal bone, splint bone (2). [L. *fibula* (contr. fr. *figibula),* that which fastens, a clasp, buckle, fr. *figo,* to fix, fasten]

fib·u·lar (fib'yū-lăr). Relating to the fibula. SYN fibularis [NA]. [L. *fibularis*]

fib·u·la·ris (fib-yū-lā'ris) [NA]. SYN fibular, fibular. [Mod. L.]

fib·u·lo·cal·ca·ne·al (fib'yū-lō-kal-kā'nē-ăl). Relating to the fibula and the calcaneus.

fi·cin (fī'sin). A proteolytic enzyme isolated from figs (*Ficus carica, globata,* and *doliaria*); used in industry as a protein digestant; f. has a wide specificity for protein substrates; an anthelmintic.

Fick, Adolf, German physician, 1829–1901. SEE F. *principle, method.*

fi·co·sis (fī-kō'sis). SYN sycosis. [L. *ficus,* fig]

FID Abbreviation for free induction *decay.*

Fiedler, Carl L.A., German physician, 1835–1921. SEE F.'s *myocarditis.*

field (fēld). A definite area of plane surface, considered in relation to some specific object. [A.S. *feld*]

auditory f., the space included within the limits of hearing of a definite sound, as of a tuning fork.

Broca's f., SYN Broca's *center.*

Cohnheim's f., SYN Cohnheim's *area.*

f. of consciousness, SEE field of *consciousness.*

f. of fixation, in ophthalmology, the angular distance around which the line of fixation can be turned.

f.'s of Forel, three circumscript, myelin-rich regions of the subthalamus known as H fields (from Haubenfelder); 1) field H_1, corresponding to the thalamic fasciculus, a horizontal fiber stratum at the junction of the subthalamus and the overlying thalamus, is composed of pallidothalamic and cerebellothalamic fibers (brachium conjunctivum) and is separated by the zona incerta from the more ventrally placed field H_2; 2) field H_2, formed by the lenticular fasciculus and arching over the dorsal border of the subthalamic nucleus, is composed largely of pallidothalamic fibers; 3) field H_3 or prerubral field, is a large field of intermingling gray and white matter immediately rostral to the red nucleus, uniting fields H$_1$ and H$_2$ around the medial margin of the zona incerta; its gray matter forms the prerubral nucleus. SEE ALSO lenticular *loop*. SYN campi foreli, tegmental f.'s of Forel.

free f., a f. (three-dimensional space) in a homogeneous, isotropic medium free from boundaries; in practice, a f. in which boundary effects are negligible.

H f.'s, SEE f.'s of Forel.

individuation f., the f. within which an organizer can bring about the rearrangement of primordial tissues in such a manner that a complete embryo is formed.

magnetic f., the sphere of influence of a magnet.

microscopic f., the area within which objects are visible with microscope oculars and objectives of various magnifying powers.

nerve f., the regional distribution of nerve terminals.

prerubral f., SEE f.'s of Forel.

tegmental f.'s of Forel, SYN f.'s of Forel.

visual f. (F), the area simultaneously visible to one eye without movement; often measured by means of a bowl perimeter located 330 mm from the eye.

Wernicke's f., SYN Wernicke's *center*.

Fielding, George H., British anatomist, 1801–1871. SEE F.'s *membrane*.

Field's rap·id stain. See under stain.

field-vole. A species of field mouse (*Microtus montebelloi*), normal host of *Leptospira hebdomadis*, the cause of a type of leptospirosis resembling infectious mononucleosis.

Fiessinger, Noël Armand, French physician, 1881–1946. SEE F.-Leroy-Reiter *syndrome*.

fièv·re. (fē-evr′) French term for fever.

f. boutonneuse (fē-evr′ bū-ton-nŭz′), SYN boutonneuse *fever*.

fig. Ficus, the partially dried fruit of *Ficus carica* (family Moraceae); used as a nutrient, mild laxative, and demulcent. [L. *ficus;* A.S. *fic*]

FIGLU Abbreviation for formiminoglutamic acid.

Figueira, Fernandes, Brazilian pediatrician, †1928. SEE F.'s *syndrome*.

fig·u·ra·tus (fig-yū-rā′tŭs). Figured; a term descriptive of certain skin lesions. [L. *figuro,* pp. *-atus,* to form, fashion]

fig·ure (fig′ūr). **1.** A form or shape. **2.** A person representing the essential aspects of a particular role (*e.g.,* relating to one's male boss as a father figure or to one's female teacher as a mother figure). **3.** A form, shape, outline, or representation of an object or person. [L. *figura,* fr *fingo,* to shape, fashion]

authority f., a real or projected person in a position of power; one's parents, police, and boss are authority figures to some people; during the transference phase of psychoanalysis, the psychoanalyst becomes an authority f.

flame f., a small area of dermal or subcutaneous necrosis with intense eosinophil staining of collagen bundles; seen in the lesions of Well's syndrome.

fortification f.'s, SYN fortification *spectrum*.

mitotic f., the microscopic appearance of a cell undergoing mitosis; a cell of which the chromosomes are visible by the light microscope.

myelin f., a rolled-up or scroll-like arrangement of a lipid bilayer within a cell, superficially resembling the myelin sheath of nerves; observed with the electron microscope in the cytoplasm or as inclusion in mitochondria and autophagic vacuoles where they may represent artifacts of lipid fixation. SYN myelin body.

Purkinje's f.'s, shadows of the retinal vessels, seen as dark lines on a reddish field when a light enters the eye through the sclera and not the pupil.

fig·ure and ground. That aspect of perception wherein the perceived is separated into at least two parts, each with different attributes but influencing one another. Figure is the most distinct; ground the least formed; *e.g.,* a bird or tree (figure) seen against the sky (ground).

fi·la (fī′lă). Plural of filum. [L.]

fi·la·ceous (fī-lā′shŭs). SYN filamentous. [L. *filum,* a thread]

fil·ag·grin (fil-ag′grin). A major protein of the keratohyalin

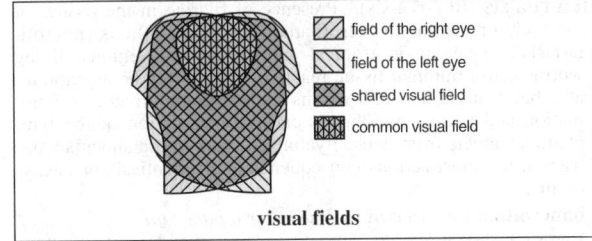

visual fields

granule, composed mostly of L-histadyl, lysyl, and arginyl residues (stratum corneum basic proteins). [*fil*ament + *aggreg*ating]

fil·a·men (fil′ă-men). A high-molecular-weight, actin-binding protein that is part of the intracellular filamentous structure of fibroblastic cells; its distribution in cells is derived from its interaction with polymerized actin.

fil·a·ment (fil′ă-ment). **1.** SYN filamentum. **2.** In bacteriology, a fine threadlike form, unsegmented or segmented without constrictions. [L. *filamentum,* fr. *filum,* a thread]

actin f., one of the contractile elements in muscular fibers and other cells; in skeletal muscle, the actin f.'s are about 5 nm wide and 100 μm long, and attach to the transverse Z f.'s.

axial f., the central f. of a flagellum or cilium; with the electron microscope it is seen as a complex of nine peripheral diplomicrotubules and a central pair of microtubules. SYN axoneme (2).

cytokeratin f.'s, SYN keratin f.'s.

intermediate f.'s, a class of tough protein f.'s (including keratin f.'s, neurofilaments, desmin, and vimentin) that measure 8-10 nm in thickness and comprise part of the cytoskeleton of the cytoplasm of most eukaryotic cells; so named because they are intermediate in thickness between actin f.'s and microtubules.

keratin f.'s, a class of intermediate f.'s that form a network within epithelial cells and anchor to desmosomes, thus imparting tensile strength to the tissue. SYN cytokeratin f.'s.

myosin f., one of the contractile elements in skeletal, cardiac, and smooth muscle fibers; in skeletal muscle, the f. is about 10 nm thick and 1.5 μm long.

parabasal f., term formerly used for rhizoplast.

root f.'s, SYN radicular *fila*, under *filum*.

spermatic f., a spermatozoon, especially the tail of a spermatozoon.

Z f., the thin zig-zag structure at the Z line of striated muscle fibers to which the actin f.'s attach.

fil·a·men·tous (fil-ă-men′tŭs). **1.** Threadlike in structure. SYN filiform (1). **2.** Composed of filaments or threadlike structures. SYN filaceous, filar (2).

fil·a·men·tum, pl. **fil·a·men·ta** (fil-ă-men′tŭm, -tă). A fibril, fine fiber, or threadlike structure. SYN filament (1). [L.]

fi·lar (fī′lăr). **1.** SYN fibrillar. **2.** SYN filamentous. [L. *filum,* a thread]

Fi·lar·ia (fī-lar′ē-ă). Former genus of nematodes now classified in several genera and species of the family Onchocercidae; *e.g., Wuchereria bancrofti* (*F. bancrofti, F. diurna,* or *F. nocturna*), *Brugia malayi* (*F. malaya*), *Onchocerca volvulus* (*F. volvulus*), *Mansonella perstans* (*F. perstans* or *F. sanguinis hominis*), *M. streptocerca, M. ozzardi* (*F. demarquayi* or *F. ozzardi*), *Loa loa* (*F. extraocularis, F. lentis, F. loa,* or *F. oculi humani*), and *Dracunculus medinensis* (*F. medinensis*) SEE ALSO filaria.

fi·lar·ia, pl. **fi·lar·i·ae** (fī-lar′ē-ă, -ē-ē). Common name for nematodes of the family Onchocercidae, which live as adults in the blood, tissue fluids, tissues, or body cavities of many vertebrates. The females lay partially embryonated eggs, the embryos uncoil and circulate in blood or tissue fluids as microfilariae; if ingested by an appropriate bloodsucking arthropod, larval stages develop; later, infective larvae may be deposited on another vertebrate host's skin when the arthropod seeks another blood meal. [L. *filum,* a thread]

fi·lar·i·al (fī-lā′rē-ăl). Pertaining to a filaria (or filariae), including the microfilaria stage.

fil·a·ri·a·sis (fil-ă-rī′ă-sis). Presence of filariae in the tissues of the body or in blood (microfilaremia) or tissue fluids (microfilariasis), occurring in tropical and subtropical regions; living worms cause minimal tissue reaction, which may be asymptomatic, but death of the adult worms leads to granulomatous inflammation and permanent fibrosis causing obstruction of the lymphatic channels from dense hyalinized scars in the subcutaneous tissues; the most serious consequence is elephantiasis or pachyderma.

bancroftian f., f. caused by *Wuchereria bancrofti*.

Brug's f., infection with filarial organism *Brugia malayi*, which causes adenitis, fever, lymphangitis, and sometimes elephantiasis; occurs primarily in southeast Asia, India, Indonesia, China, Japan, Korea, and the Philippines.

periodic f., a form of f. in which microfilariae appear in the peripheral blood at regular 24-hr intervals; usually refers to the nocturnal periodicity of bancroftian filariasis.

fi·lar·i·ci·dal (fi-lar-i-sī′dăl). Fatal to filariae.

fi·lar·i·cide (fi-lar′i-sīd). An agent that kills filariae. [filaria + L. *caedo,* to kill]

fi·lar·i·form (fi-lar′i-fōrm). **1.** Resembling filariae or other types of small nematode worms. SEE ALSO filariform *larva.* **2.** Thin or hairlike.

Fil·a·ri·i·cae (fi-lar′ē-i-sē). SYN Filarioidea.

Fi·lar·i·oi·dea (fi-lar′ē-oy′dē-ă). A superfamily of filarial nematodes parasitic in many animal species, including man; includes the families Filariidae, Diplotraenidae, Onchocercidae, and Stephanofilariidae. SEE *Filaria.* SEE ALSO *Dipetalonema, Dirofilaria, Loa loa, Mansonella, Onchocerca, Wuchereria, Brugia.* SYN Filariicae.

Fi·lar·oi·des (fil′ă-roy′dēz). A genus of nematode parasites occurring in the lungs, bronchi, and trachea of dogs. *F. osleri* is a small, widely distributed species that causes a chronic disease of dogs, manifested by small (usually less than 1 cm in diameter), gray-white or pink nodules; the most marked symptom is a harsh cough.

Filatov, Nil, Russian pediatrician, 1847–1902. SEE F.'s *disease, spots,* under *spot.*

Filatov, Vladimir P., Russian ophthalmologist, 1875–1956. SEE F. *flap;* F.'s *operation;* F.-Gillies *flap,* tubed *pedicle.*

file (fīl). A tool for smoothing, grinding, or cutting.

Hedström f., a coarse root canal f. similar to a rasp.

periodontal f., an instrument with a series of ridges or points arranged in rows on its surface, used for scaling or removing dental calculus from the teeth.

root canal f., a pointed, flexible, steel intracanal instrument used in rasping canal walls.

fil·i·al (fil′ē-ăl). Denoting the relationship of offspring to parents. SEE filial *generation.* [L. *filialis,* fr. *filius,* son, *filia,* daughter]

fi·li·form (fil′i-fōrm). **1.** SYN filamentous (1). **2.** In bacteriology, denoting an even growth along the line of inoculation, either stroke or stab. [L. *filum,* thread]

fi·li·form ad·na·tum. SYN congenital *ankyloblepharon.*

fil·i·o·pa·ren·tal (fil′ē-ō-pă-ren′tăl). Pertaining to a child-parent relationship. [L. *filius,* son, + *parens,* parent, fr. *pario,* to give birth]

fil·let (fil′et). **1.** SYN lemniscus. **2.** A skein, loop of cord, or tape used for making traction on a part of the fetus. [Fr. *filet,* a band]

lateral f., SYN lateral *lemniscus.*

medial f., SYN medial *lemniscus.*

fill·ing (fil′ing). Lay term for a dental restoration.

film. **1.** A light-sensitive or x-ray-sensitive substance used in taking photographs or radiographs. **2.** A thin layer or coating. **3.** A radiograph (colloq.).

absorbable gelatin f., a sterile, nonantigenic, absorbable, water-insoluble, thin sheet of gelatin prepared by drying a gelatin-formaldehyde solution on plates; used in the closure and repair of defects in membranes such as the dura mater or the pleura; it undergoes absorption over a period of 1 to 6 months.

bitewing f., a special packaging of radiographic f. that allows appendage of the f. package to be held between the occlusal surfaces of the teeth.

decubitus f., a radiograph exposed with the subject in the decubitus position; named for the side that is dependent. SYN right or left lateral decubitus f.

horizontal beam f., a radiograph made with the central axis of the x-ray beam parallel to the floor, able to show an air-fluid level.

latitude f., SYN wide-latitude f.

panoramic x-ray f., in dentistry, a radiograph taken to give a panoramic view of the entire upper and lower dental arch as well as the temporomandibular joints.

plain f., a radiograph made without use of a contrast medium.

precorneal f., a protective f., 7 to 9 nm thick, consisting of external oily, intermediate watery, and deep mucoprotein layers. SYN tear f.

right or left lateral decubitus f., SYN decubitus f.

scout f., a radiograph exposed before contrast medium is given, such as the preliminary film for an angiogram, urogram, or barium contrast gastrointestinal examination. SYN scout radiograph.

f. speed, the relative sensitivity of f. emulsion to light or radiation exposure; speed is inversely related to detail resolution.

spot f., a radiograph made during the course of an examination under fluoroscopic control, with a device attached to the fluoroscope.

tear f., SYN precorneal f.

wide-latitude f., f. that does not show large contrast differences with differences in exposure; the slope of the H and D curve is low. SYN latitude f.

film chang·er. A device that moves film for radiographic studies that require rapid serial x-ray exposures, such as angiography. SYN rapid f. c., serial f. c.

rapid f. c., SYN film changer.

serial f. c., SYN film changer.

Fil·mer, David L., U.S. biochemist, *1932. SEE Adair-Koshland-Némethy-Filmer *model;* Koshland-Némethy-Filmer *model.*

fil·o·po·dia (fil-ō-pō′dē-ă). Plural of filopodium.

fil·o·po·di·um, pl. **fil·o·po·dia** (fī-lō-pō′dē-ŭm, -ă). A slender filamentous pseudopodium of certain free-living amebae. [L. *filum,* thread, + G. *pous,* foot]

fi·lo·pres·sure (fī-lō-presh′ŭr). Temporary pressure on a blood vessel by a ligature, which is removed when the flow of blood has ceased. [L. *filum,* thread]

fi·lo·var·i·co·sis (fī′lō-var-ē-kō′sis). A series of swellings along the course of the axon of a nerve fiber. [L. *filum,* thread, + *varix,* dilation of vein]

Fil·o·vi·ri·dae (fī′lō-vī′rā-dā). A family of filamentous, single-stranded, negative sense RNA viruses with an enveloped nucleocapsid. Formerly classified with the Rhabdoviridae. SEE Ebola *virus.* [L. *filum,* thread, + virus]

Fil·o·vi·rus (fī′lō-vī-rŭs). A genus in the family Filoviridae that includes Marburg and Ebola viruses.

fil·ter (fil′ter). **1.** A porous substance through which a liquid or gas is passed in order to separate it from contained particulate matter or impurities. SYN filtrum. **2.** To use or to subject to the action of a f. **3.** In diagnostic or therapeutic radiology, a plate made of one or more metals such as aluminum and copper that, placed in the x- or gamma-ray beam, permits passage of a greater proportion of higher energy radiation and attenuation of lower and less desirable energy radiation, raising the average energy or hardening the beam. **4.** A device used in spectrophotometric analysis to isolate a segment of the spectrum. **5.** A mathematical algorithm applied to image data for the purpose of enhancing image quality, usually by suppression of high spatial frequency noise. [Mediev. L. *filtro,* pp. *-atus,* to strain through felt, fr. *filtrum,* felt]

bandpass f., a device that allows a limited range of frequencies to pass.

Berkefeld f., a bacterial f. used in 1891, made of earth known as Kieselguhr taken from the name of the mine in Hanover, Germany, from which the earth was found. Ground water at this mine

f. media′na ante′rior medul′lae oblonga′tae [NA], SYN anterior median *fissure* of medulla oblongata.

f. media′na ante′rior medul′lae spina′lis [NA], SYN anterior median *fissure* of spinal cord.

f. obli′qua pulmon′is [NA], SYN oblique *fissure* of lung.

f. orbita′lis infe′rior [NA], SYN inferior orbital *fissure.*

f. orbita′lis supe′rior [NA], SYN superior orbital *fissure.*

f. parietooccipita′lis, SYN parieto-occipital *sulcus.*

f. petro-occipita′lis [NA], SYN petro-occipital *fissure.*

f. petrosquamo′sa [NA], SYN petrosquamous *fissure.*

f. petrotympan′ica [NA], SYN petrotympanic *fissure.*

f. posterolatera′lis [NA], SYN posterolateral *fissure.*

f. pri′ma cerebel′li [NA], SYN primary *fissure* of cerebellum.

f. pterygoid′ea, SYN pterygoid *fissure.*

f. pterygomaxilla′ris [NA], SYN pterygomaxillary *fissure.*

f. pterygopalati′na, SYN pterygomaxillary *fissure.*

f. puden′di, SYN pudendal *cleft.*

f. secun′da cerebel′li [NA], SYN secondary *fissure* of cerebellum.

f. sphenopetro′sa [NA], SYN sphenopetrosal *fissure.*

f. transver′sa cerebel′li, SYN transverse *fissure* of cerebellum.

f. transver′sa cer′ebri [NA], SYN transverse *fissure* of cerebrum.

f. tympanomastoid′ea [NA], SYN tympanomastoid *fissure.*

f. tympanosquamo′sa [NA], SYN squamotympanic *fissure.*

---

fis·sur·al (fish′ŭ-răl). Relating to a fissure.

fis·su·ra·tion (fish′ŭ-rā′shŭn). State of being fissured.

FISSURE

---

fis·sure (fish′ŭr). **1.** A deep furrow, cleft, or slit. (For most of the brain fissures, see entries under sulcus). **2.** In dentistry, a developmental break or fault in the tooth enamel. SYN fissura (1) [NA]. [L. *fissura*]

abdominal f., congenital failure of the ventral body wall to close. SEE ALSO celosomia, gastroschisis.

Ammon's f., a pearl-shaped opening in the sclera during early embryogenesis.

anal f., a crack or slit in the mucous membrane of the anus, very painful and difficult to heal.

anterior median f. of medulla oblongata, the longitudinal groove in the midline of the anterior aspect of the medulla oblongata; it is the medullary equivalent of the anterior median f. of the spinal cord and ends at the foramen cecum posterius; its caudal part is obliterated by the decussation of the pyramids. SYN fissura mediana anterior medullae oblongatae [NA], anteromedian groove (1).

anterior median f. of spinal cord, a deep median f. on the anterior surface of the spinal cord. SYN fissura mediana anterior medullae spinalis [NA], anteromedian groove (2), sulcus ventralis.

antitragohelicine f., a fissure in the auricular cartilage between the cauda helicis and the antitragus. SYN fissura antitragohelicina [NA].

ape f., SYN lunate cerebral *sulcus.*

auricular f., SYN tympanomastoid f.

azygos f., the four-layered pleural fold that separates the lobus azygos from the rest of the right upper lobe of the lung, seen as an oblique line pointing downward toward the mediastinal shadow in the upper right lung field on a chest radiograph.

Bichat's f., the nearly circular f. corresponding to the medial margin of the cerebral (pallial) mantle, marking the hilus of the cerebral hemisphere, consisting of the callosomarginal f. and choroidal f. along the hippocampus, both of which are continuous with the stem of the f. of Sylvius at the anterior extremity of the temporal lobe.

branchial f., a persistent branchial cleft.

Broca's f., the f. surrounding Broca's convolution.

calcarine f., SYN calcarine *sulcus.*

callosomarginal f., SYN cingulate *sulcus.*

caudal transverse f., SYN *porta* hepatis.

cerebellar f.'s, the deep furrows which divide the lobules of the cerebellum. SEE ALSO postcentral f., primary f. of cerebellum, secondary f. of cerebellum. SYN fissurae cerebelli [NA].

cerebral f.'s, the variously named fissures of the cerebral hemispheres. SEE ALSO *sulci* cerebri, under *sulcus.*

choroid f., (1) SYN optic f. **(2)** SYN optic f.

choroidal f., (1) SYN optic f. **(2)** the narrow cleft along the medial wall of the lateral ventricle along the margins of which the choroid plexus is attached; it lies between the upper surface of the thalamus and lateral edge of the fornix in the central part of the ventricle and between the terminal stria and fimbria hippocampi in the inferior horn; SYN fissura choroidea (1).

Clevenger's f., SYN inferior temporal *sulcus.*

collateral f., SYN collateral *sulcus.*

decidual f., a cleft in the decidua basalis or placenta.

dentate f., SYN hippocampal *sulcus.*

Duverney's f.'s, SYN *notches* in cartilage of external acoustic meatus, under *notch.*

Ecker's f., SYN petro-occipital f.

enamel f., a deep cleft between adjoining cusps affording retention to caries-producing agents.

glaserian f., SYN petrotympanic f.

great horizontal f., SYN horizontal f. of cerebellum.

great longitudinal f., SYN longitudinal f. of cerebrum.

Henle's f.'s, minute spaces filled with connective tissue between the muscular fasciculi of the heart.

hippocampal f., SYN hippocampal *sulcus.*

horizontal f. of cerebellum, horizontal f. that divides the ansiform lobule into its major parts, crus I (superior semilunar lobule) and crus II (inferior semilunar lobule). SYN fissura horizontalis cerebelli [NA], great horizontal f.

horizontal f. of right lung, SYN transverse f. of the lung.

inferior accessory f., the f. that commonly separates the medial basal segment of the right lower lobe of the lung from the other basal segments, seen as an oblique line near the right heart border on chest radiographs.

inferior orbital f., a cleft between the greater wing of the sphenoid and the orbital plate of the maxilla, through which pass the maxillary division and the orbital branch of the trigeminal nerve, fibers from the pterygopalatine (Meckel's) ganglion, and the infraorbital vessels. SYN fissura orbitalis inferior [NA], sphenomaxillary f.

lateral cerebral f., SYN lateral cerebral *sulcus.*

left sagittal f., a sagittal groove on the undersurface of the liver formed by the fissura ligamenti teretis anteriorly and the fissura ligamenti venosi posteriorly.

f. for ligamentum teres, SYN f. of round ligament of liver.

f. of ligamentum venosum, a deep cleft extending from the porta hepatis and the inferior vena cava between the left lobe and the caudate lobe; it lodges the ligamentum venosum and is thus a vestige of the fossa of the ductus venosus. SYN fissura ligamenti venosi [NA], f. of venous ligament.

linguogingival f., a f. sometimes occurring on the lingual surface of one of the upper incisors and extending into the cementum.

f.'s of liver, SEE left sagittal f., right sagittal f., *porta* hepatis, f. of round ligament of liver, f. of ligamentum venosum.

longitudinal f. of cerebrum, the deep cleft separating the two hemispheres of the cerebrum. SYN fissura longitudinalis cerebri [NA], great longitudinal f.

lunate f., SYN lunate cerebral *sulcus.*

f.'s of lung, SEE transverse f. of the lung, oblique f. of lung.

major f., SYN oblique f. of lung.

minor f., SYN transverse f. of the lung.

oblique f., SYN oblique f. of lung.

oblique f. of lung, the deep fissure in each lung that runs obliquely downward and forward. It divides the upper and lower lobes of the left lung and separates the upper and middle lobes

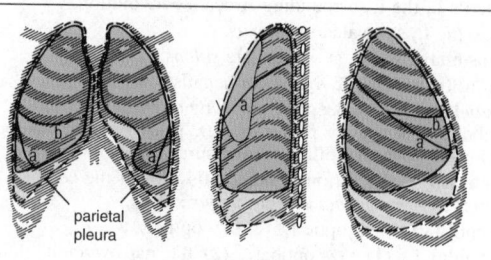

fissures of the lung
interlobular fissures of the lungs (projected onto ribcage):
a) oblique f.; b) horizontal f.

from the lower lobe of the right lung. SYN fissura obliqua pulmonis [NA], major f., oblique f.

optic f., in the embryo, the temporary gap in the ventral margin of the developing optic cup. SYN choroid f. (1), choroid f. (2), choroidal f. (1).

oral f., SYN *rima* oris.

palpebral f., SYN *rima* palpebrarum.

Pansch's f., a cerebral f. (sulcus) running from the lower extremity of the central f. (sulcus) nearly to the end of the occipital lobe.

paracentral f., a curved f. (sulcus) on the medial surface of the cerebral hemisphere, bounding the paracentral gyrus and separating it from the precuneus and the cingulate gyrus.

parieto-occipital f., SYN parieto-occipital *sulcus*.

petro-occipital f., a fissure between the petrous part of the temporal bone and the basilar part of the occipital bone that extends anteromedially from the jugular foramen; includes the jugular foramen (at its posterior end). SYN fissura petro-occipitalis [NA], Ecker's f.

petrosquamous f., a shallow fissure indicating externally the line of fusion of the petrous and squamous portions of the temporal bone. SYN fissura petrosquamosa [NA].

petrotympanic f., a fissure between the tympanic and petrous portions of the temporal bone; it transmits the chorda tympani nerve through a small patent portion, the anterior canaliculus of the chorda tympani. SYN fissura petrotympanica [NA], glaserian f.

portal f., SYN *porta* hepatis.

postcentral f., a f. on the superior surface of the cerebellum separating the culmen from the central lobule.

posterior median f. of the medulla oblongata, SYN posterior median *sulcus* of medulla oblongata.

posterior median f. of spinal cord, SYN posterior median *sulcus* of spinal cord.

posterolateral f., the earliest f. to appear in the development of the cerebellum; it separates the flocculus and nodulus from the uvula and tonsil. SYN fissura posterolateralis [NA], prenodular f.

posthippocampal f., SYN calcarine *sulcus*.

postlingual f., a transverse f. on the superior vermis of the cerebellum separating the lingula from the central lobule.

postlunate f., a transverse f. on the superior vermis of the cerebellum separating the posterior lunate lobule in front from the ansiform lobule behind.

postpyramidal f., a f. that separates the pyramid of the cerebellum from the tuber.

postrhinal f., a f. separating the hippocampal from the collateral gyrus.

prenodular f., SYN posterolateral f.

primary f. of cerebellum, the deepest f. of the cerebellum; demarcates the division of anterior and posterior lobes of the cerebellum; second to appear embryologically. SYN fissura prima cerebelli [NA].

pterygoid f., the cleft between the medial and lateral laminae of the pterygoid process of the sphenoid bone into which the py-

ramidal process of the palatine bone is fitted. SYN incisura pterygoidea [NA], fissura pterygoidea, pterygoid notch.

pterygomaxillary f., the narrow gap between the lateral pterygoid plate and the infratemporal surface of the maxilla through which the infratemporal fossa communicates with the pterygopalatine fossa; gives passage to the third part of the maxillary artery and the posterior superior alveolar arteries, veins and nerves. SYN fissura pterygomaxillaris [NA], fissura pterygopalatina.

rhinal f., SYN rhinal *sulcus*.

right sagittal f., a sagittal groove on the undersurface of the liver formed by the fossa vesicae felleae anteriorly and the sulcus venae cavae posteriorly.

f. of Rolando, SYN central *sulcus*.

f. of round ligament of liver, a cleft on the inferior surface of the liver, running from the inferior border to the left extremity of the porta hepatis; it lodges the round ligament of the liver. SYN fissura ligamenti teretis [NA], f. for ligamentum teres, fossa venae umbilicalis, umbilical f., umbilical fossa.

Santorini's f.'s, SYN *notches* in cartilage of external acoustic meatus, under *notch*.

secondary f. of cerebellum, a f. that separates the uvula of the inferior vermis of the cerebellum from the pyramid. SYN fissura secunda cerebelli [NA].

simian f., SYN lunate cerebral *sulcus*.

sphenoidal f., SYN superior orbital f.

sphenomaxillary f., SYN inferior orbital f.

sphenopetrosal f., a narrow fissure between the undersurface of the greater wing of the sphenoid and the petrous portion of the temporal bone. SYN fissura sphenopetrosa [NA].

squamotympanic f., the f. separating the tympanic part of the temporal bone from the squamous part; it is continuous medially with the petrotympanic f. and the petrosquamous f. SYN fissura tympanosquamosa [NA], tympanosquamous f.

superior orbital f., a cleft between the greater and the lesser wings of the sphenoid establishing a channel of communication between the middle cranial fossa and the orbit, through which pass the oculomotor and trochlear nerves, the ophthalmic division of the trigeminal nerve, the abducens nerve, and the ophthalmic veins. SYN fissura orbitalis superior [NA], foramen lacerum anterius, sphenoidal f.

superior temporal f., SYN superior temporal *sulcus*.

sylvian f., f. of Sylvius, SYN lateral cerebral *sulcus*.

transverse f. of cerebellum, the cleft caused by the protrusion of the anterior lobe of the cerebellum over the superior and middle cerebellar peduncles. SYN fissura transversa cerebelli.

transverse f. of cerebrum, the triangular space between the corpus callosum and fornix above and the dorsal surface of the thalamus below, which is bounded laterally by the choroid f. of the lateral ventricle, lined by pia mater, and opens caudally into the cistern of the great cerebral vein of the subarachnoid space. SYN fissura transversa cerebri [NA].

transverse f. of the lung, the deep fissure that separates the upper and middle lobes of the right lung. SYN fissura horizontalis pulmonis dextri [NA], horizontal f. of right lung, minor f.

tympanomastoid f., a fissure separating the tympanic portion from the mastoid portion of the temporal bone; it transmits the auricular branch of the vagus nerve. SYN fissura tympanomastoidea [NA], auricular f., tympanomastoid suture.

tympanosquamous f., SYN squamotympanic f.

umbilical f., SYN f. of round ligament of liver.

f. of venous ligament, SYN f. of ligamentum venosum.

vestibular f. of cochlea, a fine f. in the lower part of the first turn of the cochlea, formed by a spiral lamina which projects from the outer wall of the cochlea but does not quite reach the osseous spiral lamina, thus leaving a narrow gap.

zygal f., a figure formed by two nearly parallel cerebral f.'s connected by a short f. at right angles, forming an H.

FISTULA

fis·tu·la, pl. **fis·tu·lae**, **fis·tu·las** (fis′tyū-lă, -tyū-lē, -tyū-lăs). An abnormal passage from one epithelialized surface to another epithelialized surface. [L. a pipe, a tube]

abdominal f., a tract leading from one of the abdominal viscera to the external surface.

amphibolic f., amphibolous f., a complete anal f. opening both externally and internally.

anal f., a f. opening at or near the anus; usually, but not always, opening into the rectum above the internal sphincter.

arteriovenous f., an abnormal communication between an artery and a vein, usually resulting in the formation of an arteriovenous aneurysm.

f. au′ris congen′ita, a congenital f. resulting from a defect in the formation of the auricle of the ear.

biliary f., a f. leading to some portion of the biliary tract.

f. bimuco′sa, a complete f., both ends of which open on the mucous surface.

blind f., a f. that ends in a cul-de-sac, being open at one extremity only. SYN incomplete f.

B-P f., SYN bronchopleural f.

branchial f., a congenital f. in the neck resulting from incomplete closure of a branchial cleft.

Brescia-Cimino f., a direct, surgically created, arteriovenous f.; used to facilitate chronic hemodialysis.

bronchobiliary f., communication between a bronchus and the bile duct, *e.g.*, after a ruptured hepatic abscess.

bronchocavitary f., a communication between the bronchus and a lung abscess cavity.

bronchoesophageal f., communication between a bronchus and the esophagus; may occur in association with either infection or tumors involving a bronchus or the esophagus.

bronchopleural f., communication between a bronchus and the pleural cavity; usually caused by necrotizing pneumonia or empyema; also may follow pulmonary surgery or irradiation. SYN B-P f.

carotid-cavernous f., a fistulous communication, of spontaneous or traumatic origin, between the cavernous sinus and the traversing internal carotid artery; a pulsating unilateral exophthalmos and a detectable cranial bruit are common manifestations.

cholecystoduodenal f., communication between gallbladder and duodenum secondary to severe cholecystitis with perforation and abscess formation; stones erode through adjacent duodenal wall, and large stones may cause gallstone ileus.

coccygeal f., a fistulous opening of a dermoid cyst in the coccygeal region.

f. col′li congen′ita, a congenital f. of the neck leading to the pharynx, larynx, or trachea.

colocutaneous f., a f. between the colon and the skin.

coloileal f., a f. between the colon and the ileum.

colonic f., (1) internal, a f. between the colon and a hollow viscus; **(2)** external, a f. between the colon and the skin.

colovaginal f., a f. between colon and vagina.

colovesical f., a f. between colon and urinary bladder. SYN vesicocolic f.

complete f., a f. that is open at both ends.

congenital pulmonary arteriovenous f., abnormal congenital communication between pulmonary arteries and veins usually found in the lung parenchyma.

dental f., SYN gingival f.

duodenal f., an opening through the duodenal wall and into the peritoneal cavity, into another organ, or through the abdominal wall.

Eck f., transposition of the portal circulation to the systemic by making an anastomosis between the vena cava and portal vein and then ligating the latter close to the liver.

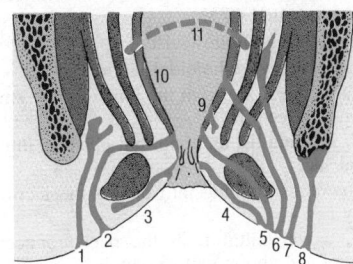

anal fistula (types)

1. incomplete ischiorectal f. 2. complete ischiorectal f. 3. incomplete subcutaneous f. 4. complete subcutaneous f. 5. complete transsphincteral f. 6. complete pelvirectal f. 7. incomplete pelvirectal f. 8. pelvic bone f. 9. incomplete submucosal f. 10. complete submucosal f. (f. bimucosa) 11. commissural f.

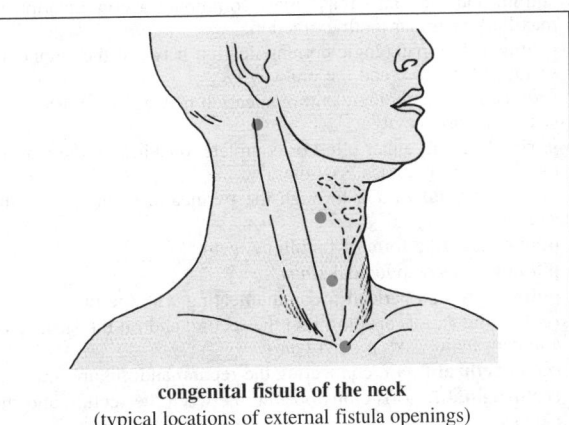

congenital fistula of the neck
(typical locations of external fistula openings)

enterocutaneous f., a f. between the intestine and skin of the abdomen.

enterovaginal f., a fistulous passage connecting the intestine and the vagina.

enterovesical f., a f. connecting the intestine and the bladder.

ethmoidal-lacrimal f., a fistulous communication between the lacrimal sac and the ethmoidal sinus. SYN internal lacrimal f.

external f., a f. between a hollow viscus and the skin.

fecal f., SYN intestinal f.

gastric f., a fistulous tract from the stomach to the abdominal wall.

gastrocolic f., a fistulous communication between the stomach and the colon.

gastrocutaneous f., a f. between the stomach and the skin.

gastroduodenal f., an abnormal opening between the stomach and the duodenum.

gastrointestinal f., a fistulous tract connecting the stomach with the intestine.

genitourinary f., a fistulous opening into the urogenital tract. SYN urogenital f.

gingival f., a sinus tract originating in a peripheral abscess and opening into the oral cavity on the gingiva. SYN dental f.

hepatic f., a f. leading to the liver.

hepatopleural f., a f. between the liver and the pleural space.

horseshoe f., an anal f. partially encircling the anus and opening at both extremities on the cutaneous surface.

H-type f., a rare form of congenital tracheoesophageal f. in which there is no esophageal atresia, manifest as aspiration pneumonias. SYN H-type tracheoesophageal f.

fi

H-type tracheoesophageal f., SYN H-type f.

incomplete f., SYN blind f.

internal f., a f. between hollow viscera.

internal lacrimal f., SYN ethmoidal-lacrimal f.

intestinal f., a tract leading from the lumen of the small intestine to the exterior. SYN fecal f.

lacrimal f., f. lacrima′lis, an abnormal opening into a tear duct or the lacrimal sac.

lacteal f., a fistulous opening into one of the lactiferous ducts. SYN mammary f.

lymphatic f., a congenital f. in the neck connecting with a lymphatic vessel and giving exit to lymph.

mammary f., SYN lacteal f.

Mann-Bollman f., a f. used in experimental investigations; a loop of ileum is isolated, the distal (aboral) end is anastomosed laterally to the duodenum or the small intestine, and the open proximal (oral) end is sutured to the abdominal wall; peristaltic waves travel from oral to aboral end, with leakage to the exterior thus reduced to a minimum.

metroperitoneal f., SYN uteroperitoneal f.

oroantral f., a pathologic communication between the maxillary antrum and the oral cavity, most commonly a complication of maxillary or molar tooth extraction.

orofacial f., a pathologic communication between the cutaneous surface of the face and the oral cavity.

oronasal f., a pathologic communication between the nasal cavity and the oral cavity.

parietal f., a f., either blind or complete, opening on the wall of the thorax or abdomen. SYN thoracic f.

perineovaginal f., a f. through the perineum, opening into the vagina.

pharyngeal f., a form of f. colli congenita.

pilonidal f., SYN pilonidal *sinus.*

pulmonary f., a parietal f. communicating with the lung.

rectolabial f., a f. opening into the rectum and on the surface of a labium majus. SYN rectovulvar f.

rectourethral f., a f. connecting the rectum and the urethra.

rectovaginal f., a fistulous opening between the rectum and the vagina.

rectovesical f., a fistulous communication between the rectum and the bladder.

rectovestibular f., a f. between rectum and vestibule of the vagina.

rectovulvar f., SYN rectolabial f.

reverse Eck f., side-to-side anastomosis of the portal vein with the inferior vena cava and ligation of the latter above the anastomosis but below the hepatic veins; the blood from the lower part of the body is thus directed through the hepatic circulation.

salivary f., a pathologic communication between a salivary duct or gland and the cutaneous surface or the oral mucus.

sigmoidovesical f., a f. between sigmoid colon and urinary bladder.

spermatic f., a f. communicating with the testis or any of the seminal passages.

T-E f., SYN tracheoesophageal f.

Thiry's f., an artificial f. for collecting the intestinal secretions of a dog or other animal for experimental purposes; a loop of intestine is isolated, its vascular and nervous connections are preserved, and the continuity of the intestinal tract is restored by anastomosis; one end of the isolated segment is closed, the other attached to the skin of the abdomen.

Thiry-Vella f., experimental isolation of a segment of intestine in a dog or other animal; the mesenteric attachment is preserved, the divided intestine at each end of the segment is joined by anastomosis, and the ends of the segment are stitched to openings in the abdominal wall. SYN Vella's f.

thoracic f., SYN parietal f.

tracheal f., a form of f. colli congenita.

tracheobiliary fistula, a rare congenital anastomosis between an accessory bronchus and aberrant biliary duct system.

tracheoesophageal f., congenital abnormality involving a communication between the trachea and esophagus; often associated with esophageal atresia, but may also be acquired; in the adult, etiology is similar to that of bronchoesophageal f. SYN T-E f.

umbilical f., a f. of intestine or urachus at the umbilicus.

urachal f., a f. connecting the urachus with a hollow organ.

ureterocutaneous f., a f. between the ureter and the skin.

ureterovaginal f., a f. between the lower ureter and vagina.

urethrovaginal f., a f. between the urethra and the vagina.

urinary f., a f. resulting in abnormal drainage of urine to the skin or into another organ.

urogenital f., SYN genitourinary f.

uteroperitoneal f., a fistulous tract through the uterine wall opening into the peritoneal cavity. SYN metroperitoneal f.

Vella's f., SYN Thiry-Vella f.

vesical f., a f. from the urinary bladder.

vesicocolic f., SYN colovesical f.

vesicocutaneous f., a f. between the bladder and the skin.

vesicointestinal f., a f. between the urinary bladder and the small intestine.

vesicouterine f., a f. between the bladder and the uterus.

vesicovaginal f., f. between the bladder and the vagina.

vesicovaginorectal f., an abnormal opening between the vagina and the bladder and rectum.

vitelline f., a f. between the umbilicus and the terminal ileum along the course of a persistent vitelline cord. SEE Meckel's *diverticulum.*

fis·tu·la·tion, fis·tu·li·za·tion (fis-tyū-lā′shŭn, -tyū-li-zā′shŭn). Formation of a fistula in a part; becoming fistulous.

fis·tu·la·tome (fis′tyū-lă-tōm). A long, thin-bladed, probe-pointed knife for slitting open a fistula. SYN fistula knife, syringotome. [fistula + G. *tomē,* a cutting]

fis·tu·lec·to·my (fis-tyū-lek′tō-mē). Excision of a fistula. SYN syringectomy. [fistula + G. *ektomē,* excision]

fis·tu·lo·en·ter·os·to·my (fis′tyū-lō-en-ter-os′tō-mē). An operation connecting a fistula with the intestine. [fistula + G. *enteron,* intestine, + *stoma,* mouth]

fis·tu·lot·o·my (fis-tyū-lot′ō-mē). Incision or surgical enlargement of a fistula. SYN syringotomy. [fistula + G. *tomē,* incision]

fis·tu·lous (fis′tyū-lŭs). Relating to or containing a fistula.

fit. 1. An attack of an acute disease or the sudden appearance of some symptom, such as coughing. 2. A convulsion. 3. SYN epilepsy. 4. In dentistry, the adaptation of any dental restoration, *e.g.,* of an inlay to the cavity preparation in a tooth, or of a denture to its basal seat. [A.S. *fitt*]

induced f., a conformational change in a macromolecule (*e.g.,* protein) as a result of multiple weak interactions with a ligand or substrate.

uncinate f., SYN temporal lobe *epilepsy.*

FITC Abbreviation for fluorescein isothiocyanate.

fit·ness (fit′nes). 1. Well-being. 2. Suitability. 3. In population genetics, a measure of the relative survival and reproductive success of a given individual or phenotype, or of a population subgroup. 4. A set of attributes, primarily respiratory and cardiovascular, relating to ability to perform tasks requiring expenditure of energy.

clinical f., absence of frank disease or of subclinical precursors.

evolutionary f., the probability that the line of descent from an individual with a specific trait will not eventually die out.

genetic f., in a phenotype, the mean number of surviving offspring that it generates in its lifetime, usually expressed as a fraction or percentage of the average genetic f. of the population.

physical f., a state of well-being in which performance is optimal.

Fitz-Hugh, T., Jr., U.S. physician, 1894–1963. SEE Fitz-Hugh and Curtis *syndrome.*

FIV Abbreviation for feline immunodeficiency *virus.*

fix·a·tion (fik-sā′shŭn). 1. The condition of being firmly attached or set. 2. In histology, the rapid killing of tissue elements and their preservation and hardening to retain as nearly as possible the same relations they had in the living body. SYN fixing. **3.** In chemistry, the conversion of a gas into solid or liquid form by chemical reactions, with or without the help of living tissue. **4.** In psychoanalysis, the quality of being firmly attached to a particular person or object or period in one's development. **5.** In physiological optics, the coordinated positioning and accommodation of both eyes that results in bringing or maintaining a sharp image of a stationary or moving object on the fovea of each eye. [L. *figo*, pp. *fixus*, to fix, fasten]

ammonia f., SYN ammonia *assimilation*.

bifoveal f., SYN binocular f.

binocular f., a condition in which both eyes are simultaneously directed to the same target. SYN bifoveal f.

circumalveolar f., stabilization of a fracture segment or surgical splint by wire passed through and around the dental alveolar process.

circummandibular f., stabilization of a fracture segment or surgical splint by wire passed around the mandible.

circumzygomatic f., stabilization of a fracture segment or surgical splint by wire passed around the zygomatic arch.

complement f., f. of complement in a serum by an antigen-antibody combination whereby it is rendered unavailable to complete a reaction in a second antigen-antibody combination for which complement is necessary; the second system usually serves as an indicator (red blood cells plus specific hemolysin); if complement is fixed with the first antigen-antibody union, hemolysis does not occur, but, if complement is not so removed, it causes hemolysis in the second system. SEE ALSO Bordet-Gengou *phenomenon*, Wassermann *test*. SYN CF test.

craniofacial f., stabilization of facial fractures to the cranial base by direct wiring or by external skeletal pin fixation.

crossed f., in convergent strabismus, the use of the right inturned eye to look at objects to the left and the left inturned eye to look at objects to the right, in order to avoid ocular rotation.

eccentric f., a monocular condition in which the line of sight connects the object and an extrafoveal retinal area.

elastic band f., the stabilization of fractured segments of the jaws by means of intermaxillary elastics applied to splints or appliances.

external f., f. of fractured bones by splints, plastic dressings, or transfixion pins.

external pin f., in oral surgery, stabilization of fractures of the mandible, maxilla, or zygoma by pins or screws drilled into the bony part through the overlying skin and connected by a metal bar.

external pin f., biphase, pin f. by replacing the rigid metal bar connector with an acrylic bar adapted at the time of reduction of the fracture.

freudian f., SEE fixation (4).

genetic f., the increase of the frequency of a gene by genetic drift until no other allele is preserved in a specific finite population.

intermaxillary f., f. of fractures of the mandible or maxilla by applying elastic bands or stainless steel wire between the maxillary and mandibular arch bars or other types of splint. SYN mandibulomaxillary f., maxillomandibular f.

internal f., stabilization of fractured bony parts by direct f. to one another with surgical wires, screws, pins, rods, plates, or methylmethacrylate. SYN intraosseous f.

intraosseous f., SYN internal f.

mandibulomaxillary f., SYN intermaxillary f.

maxillomandibular f., SYN intermaxillary f.

nasomandibular f., mandibular immobilization, especially for edentulous jaws, with maxillomandibular splints, attached by connecting a circum-mandibular wire with an intraoral interosseous wire passed through a hole drilled into the anterior nasal spine of the maxillae.

nitrogen f., process in which atmospheric nitrogen is converted to ammonia.

fix·a·tive (fik′să-tiv). **1.** Serving to fix, bind, or make firm or stable. **2.** A substance used for the preservation of gross and histologic specimens of tissue, or individual cells, usually by denaturing and precipitating or cross-linking the protein constituents. SEE ALSO fluid, solution.

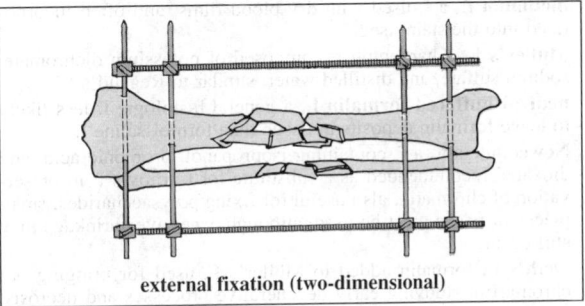

external fixation (two-dimensional)

acetone f., acetone used at low temperatures to fix enzymes, particularly phosphatases; it removes fat and glycogen.

Altmann's f., a bichromate-osmic acid f.

Bouin's f., a solution of glacial acetic acid, formalin, and picric acid, useful for soft and delicate tissues (as those of embryos) and small pieces of tissues; it preserves glycogen and nuclei and permits brilliant staining, but penetrates slowly, distorts kidney tissue and mitochondria, and does not permit Feulgen stain for DNA.

Carnoy's f., ethanol, chloroform, and acetic acid (6:3:1) or ethanol and acetic acid (3:1), an extremely rapid f. used for glycogen preservation and as a nuclear f.

Champy's f., a mixture of potassium bichromate, chromic acid, and osmic acid, considered an excellent cytologic f. with advantages and disadvantages similar to those of Flemming's f.; it differs from Flemming's f. in substituting bichromate for acetic acid.

Flemming's f., a mixture of chromic acid, osmic acid, and acetic acid that makes an excellent cytoplasmic and chromosomal f., especially when acetic acid is omitted; disadvantages are that it penetrates poorly, requires lengthy washing, and deteriorates rapidly.

formaldehyde f., a widely used fixing agent for pathologic histology; the commercial solution is 37-40% formaldehyde and is known as 100% formalin or formol; a common impurity is formic acid, which must be neutralized or the f. made in buffer solution; tissues fixed may have a pigment artifact precipitated.

formol-calcium f., a f. for preservation of lipids.

formol-Müller f., Müller's f. containing 2% commercial formalin.

formol-saline f., a general f. for histologic and histochemical preparations.

formol-Zenker f., Zenker's f. in which glacial acetic acid has been replaced by formalin.

glutaraldehyde f., a f. used in phosphate or cacodylate buffer for electron microscopy, and as a chromatin and enzyme f.; may be used preceding osmic acid as a second f. to add membrane preservation for electron microscopy.

Golgi's osmiobichromate f., an osmic-bichromate mixture used to demonstrate nerve cells and their processes.

Helly's f., a combination of potassium dichromate, mercuric chloride, formaldehyde, and distilled water, used as a microanatomic f. for cytoplasmic granules and nuclear staining; has the same disadvantages as Zenker's f.

Hermann's f., a hardening f. of glacial acetic acid, osmic acid, and platinum chloride.

Kaiserling's f., a method of preserving histologic and pathologic specimens without altering the color, by immersing them in an aqueous solution of potassium nitrate, potassium acetate, and formalin.

Luft's potassium permanganate f., a f. useful in electron microscopy for cytologic preservation of lipoprotein complexes in membranes and myelin, because of its oxidative properties.

Marchi's f., a mixture of Müller's f. with osmium tetroxide, with potassium chlorate substituted for the potassium dichromate of Müller's f. for better results; used to demonstrate degenerating myelin. SEE ALSO Marchi's *stain*.

fi

methanol f., a f. used with dry blood films, and often incorporated into the stain used.

Müller's f., a hardening f. composed of potassium dichromate, sodium sulfate, and distilled water, similar to Regaud's f.

neutral buffered formalin f., a general histologic f. less likely to leave formalin deposits in tissue than formol-saline f.

Newcomer's f., a f. containing isopropanol, propionic acid, and dioxane, recommended as a substitute for Carnoy's f. in preservation of chromatin; also useful for fixing polysaccharides; small pieces of tissue must be used, although excessive shrinkage may still occur.

Orth's f., formalin added to Müller's f., used for bringing out chromaffin, studying early degenerative processes and necrosis, and for demonstrating rickettsiae and bacteria.

osmic acid f., a f. used alone in buffer or as a postfixative after a glutaraldehyde f. in electron microscopy; an excellent membrane f. but a poor preservative of chromatin.

Park-Williams f., a f. for spirochetes, comprised of a 2% solution of osmic acid to the fumes of which the bacteria are exposed for a few seconds.

picroformol f., a f. containing formalin and picric acid.

Regaud's f., a f. containing formaldehyde and sodium dichromate, used to preserve mitochondria but not fat; requires afterchroming and extensive washing.

Schaudinn's f., a solution of mercuric chloride, sodium chloride, alcohol, and glacial acetic acid, used on wet smears for cytologic fixation.

Thoma's f., nitric acid in 95% alcohol, used for decalcifying bone in the preparation of histologic specimens.

Zenker's f., a rapid f. consisting of mercuric chloride, potassium dichromate, sodium sulfate, glacial acetic acid, and water, useful for trichrome stains; must be washed to remove potassium dichromate and treated with iodine solution to remove mercuric chloride; tissues tend to become brittle if left in the f. for more than 24 hours.

fix·a·tor (fik-sā′ter). A device providing rigid immobilization through external skeletal fixation by means of rods (f.'s) attached to pins which are placed in or through the bone.

fix·ing (fik′sing). SYN fixation (2).

flac·cid (flak′sid, flas′id). Relaxed, flabby, or without tone. [L. *flaccidus*]

flac·cid·i·ty (flă-sid′i-tē). The condition or state of being flaccid.

Flack, Martin, British physiologist, 1882–1931. SEE F.'s *node;* Keith and F. *node.*

fla·gel·la (flă-jel′ă). Plural of flagellum.

fla·gel·lar (fla-jel′ăr). Relating to a flagellum or to the extremity of a protozoan.

Flag·el·la·ta (flaj′ĕ-lā′tă). Former name for Mastigophora.

flag·el·late (flaj′ĕ-lāt). **1.** Possessing one or more flagella. **2.** Common name for a member of the class Mastigophora.

collared f., SYN choanomastigote.

flag·el·lat·ed (flaj′ĕ-lā-ted). Possessing one or more flagella.

flag·el·la·tion (flaj′ĕ-lā′shŭn). **1.** Whipping either one's self or another as a means of arousing or heightening sexual feeling. **2.** The pattern of formation of flagella. [L. *flagellatus,* fr. *flagello,* to whip or scourge]

fla·gel·lin (flaj′ĕ-lin). A protein (MW about 20,000) containing the amino acid, ε-*N*-methyllysine; the main protein component of the flagella of bacteria.

flag·el·lo·sis (flaj′ĕ-lō′sis). Infection with flagellated protozoa in the intestinal or genital tract, *e.g.,* trichomoniasis.

fla·gel·lum, pl. **fla·gel·la** (flă-jel′ŭm, -ă). A whiplike locomotory organelle of constant structural arrangement consisting of nine double peripheral microtubules and two single central microtubules; it arises from a deeply staining basal granule, often connected to the nucleus by a fiber, the rhizoplast. Though characteristic of the protozoan class Mastigophora, comparable structures are commonly found in many other groups, *e.g.,* in spermatozoa. [L. dim. of *flagrum,* a whip]

flam·ma·ble (flam′ă-bl). The property of burning readily and quickly. SYN inflammable. [L. *flamma,* flame]

flange (flanj). That part of the denture base which extends from the cervical ends of the teeth to the border of the denture.

buccal f., the portion of the f. of a denture that occupies the buccal vestibule of the mouth.

denture f., (1) the essentially vertical extension from the body of the denture into one of the vestibules of the oral cavity; also, on the lower denture, the essentially vertical extension along the lingual side of the alveololingual sulcus; (2) the buccal and labial vertical extension of the upper or lower denture base, and the lingual vertical extension of the lower one; the buccal and labial denture f.'s have two surfaces: the buccal or labial surface and the basal seat surface; the lower lingual f. also has two surfaces: the basal seat surface and the lingual surface.

labial f., the portion of the f. of a denture which occupies the labial vestibule of the mouth.

lingual f., the portion of the f. of a mandibular denture that occupies the space adjacent to the tongue.

flank. SYN latus.

flap. 1. Mass or tongue of tissue for transplantation, vascularized by a pedicle or stem; specifically, a pedicle f. **2.** An uncontrolled movement, as of the hands. SEE asterixis. [M.E. *flappe*]

Abbe f., a full-thickness f. of the middle portion of the lower lip that is transferred into the upper lip, or vice versa.

advancement f., SYN sliding f.

arterial f., SYN axial pattern f.

axial pattern f., a f. that includes a direct specific artery within its longitudinal axis. SYN arterial f.

bilobed f., a f. consisting of two lobes at approximately right angles, based on a common pedicle.

bipedicle f., a f. with two pedicles, one at each end. SYN double pedicle f.

bone f., portion of cranium removed but left attached to overlying soft tissue structures.

buried f., a f. denuded of both surface epithelium and superficial dermis and transferred into the subcutaneous tissues.

caterpillar f., a tubed f. transferred end-over-end (in stages) from the donor area to a distant recipient area. SYN waltzed f.

cellulocutaneous f., a f. of skin and subcutaneous tissue.

composite f., compound f., a f. of 2 or more elements incorporating underlying muscle, bone, or cartilage.

cross f., a skin f. transferred from one part of the body to a corresponding part, as from one arm to the other.

delayed f., a f. raised in its donor area in two or more stages to increase its chances of survival after transfer.

deltopectoral f., an axial pattern skin f. of the deltoid and pectoral regions, based on the internal mammary vessels.

direct f., a f. raised completely and transferred at the same stage. SYN immediate f.

distant f., a f. in which the donor site is distant from the recipient area.

double pedicle f., SYN bipedicle f.

envelope f., a mucoperiosteal f. retracted from a horizontal incision along the free gingival margin.

Estlander f., a full-thickness f. of the lip, transferred from the side of one lip to the same side of the other lip.

Filatov f., SYN tubed f.

Filatov-Gillies f., SYN tubed f.

flag f., a flag-shaped f. on a proximal pedicle, transferred from one surface to another of the same finger or from one finger to an adjacent finger.

flat f., a f. in which during transfer the pedicle is left flat or open, *i.e.,* untubed.

free f., island f. in which the donor vessels are severed proximally, the f. is transported as a free object to the recipient area, and the f. is revascularized by anastomosing its supplying vessels to vessels there.

free bone f., portion of cranium removed and detached from overlying soft tissue structures.

French f., SYN sliding f.

full-thickness f., a f. of the full thickness of mucosa and submucosa or of skin and subcutaneous tissues.

gingival f., a portion of the gingiva whose coronal margin is surgically detached from the tooth and the alveolar process.

hinged f., a turnover f. transferred by lifting it over on its pedicle as though the pedicle was a hinge.

immediate f., SYN direct f.

Indian f., f. from a contiguous area, such as cheek or forehead, used to rebuild the nose.

interpolated f., f. that is rotated into an adjoining area.

island f., a f. in which the pedicle consists solely of the supplying artery and vein(s), sometimes including a nerve.

Italian f., f. from a distant area; usually used in reference to a f. from the upper arm to rebuild a nose.

jump f., a distant f. transferred in stages via an intermediate carrier; *e.g.,* an abdominal f. is attached to the wrist, then at a later stage the wrist is brought to the face.

lined f., a f. covered with epithelium on both sides; *e.g.,* a folded skin f.

lingual f., SYN tongue f.

liver f., SEE asterixis.

local f., a f. transferred to an adjacent area.

mucoperichondrial f., a f. composed of mucosa and perichondrium, as from the nasal septum.

mucoperiosteal f., a f. composed of mucosa and periosteum, as from the hard palate or gingiva.

musculocutaneous f., SYN myocutaneous f.

myocutaneous f., a pedicle skin f., often an island f., with an attached subjacent muscle and its investments and blood supply. SYN musculocutaneous f., myodermal f.

myodermal f., SYN myocutaneous f.

neurovascular f., a f. containing a sensory nerve, one purpose of which is to restore sensation to the recipient area.

open f., SYN flat f.

parabiotic f., a skin f. bridging from one animal to another.

partial-thickness f., SYN split-thickness f.

pedicle f., (1) a skin f. sustained by a blood-carrying stem from the donor site during transfer; (2) in periodontal surgery, a f. used to increase the width of attached gingiva, or to cover a root surface, by moving the attached gingiva, which remains joined at one side, to an adjacent position and suturing the free end.

pericoronal f., a f. of gingiva covering an unerupted tooth, especially the lower third molar.

permanent pedicle f., a pedicle f. in which the pedicle is not severed at the time of transfer, so that it continues to supply blood from the donor site to the recipient area.

pharyngeal f., a f. from the posterior wall of the pharynx to the soft palate, as a speech aid in cleft palate.

random pattern f., a f. in which the pedicle blood supply is derived randomly from the network of vessels in the area, rather than from a single longitudinal artery as in an axial pattern f.

rope f., SYN tubed f.

rotation f., a pedicle f. that is rotated from the donor site to an adjacent recipient area, usually as a direct f.

sickle f., a sickle-shaped f. from the anterior scalp and one side of the forehead, based on the opposite temporal artery.

skin f., a f. comprised of skin and its subjacent subcutaneous tissue.

sliding f., a rectangular f. raised in an elastic area, with its free end adjacent to a defect; the defect is covered by stretching the f. longitudinally until the end comes over it. SYN advancement f., French f.

split-thickness f., a f. of a portion of the skin, *i.e.,* the epidermis and part of the dermis, or of part of the mucosa and submucosa, but not including the periosteum. SYN partial-thickness f.

subcutaneous f., a pedicle f. in which the pedicle is denuded of epithelium and buried in the subcutaneous tissue of the recipient area.

tongue f., a f. derived from the tongue; used to close a defect in an adjacent part, such as the lip or palate. SYN lingual f.

tubed f., a f. in which the sides of the pedicle are sutured together to create a tube, with the entire surface covered by skin.

SYN Filatov f., Filatov-Gillies f., Filatov-Gillies tubed pedicle, rope f., tubed pedicle f.

tubed pedicle f., SYN tubed f.

turnover f., a hinged f. that is turned over 180°, usually to receive a second (covering) f.

von Langenbeck's bipedicle mucoperiosteal f., an operation to close a cleft of the palate using lateral incisions designed to move medially where they are sutured together.

V-Y f., a f. in which the incision is made in a V shape and sutured in a Y shape to gain additional tissue. SYN V-Y plasty, V-Y plasty.

waltzed f., SYN caterpillar f.

Zimany's bilobed f., a surgical f. that is transposed into a defect with a smaller f. transposed to fill the secondary defect caused by the rotation of the larger f.

flare (flār). **1.** A gradual tapering or spreading outward. **2.** A diffuse redness of the skin extending beyond the local reaction to the application of an irritant; it is due to dilation of the arterioles and capillaries; depends upon an axon reflex set up by the liberation of a histamine-like substance in skin when injured. SEE ALSO triple *response.*

aqueous f., Tyndall phenomenon observed in the fluid of the anterior chamber of the eye.

fla·rim·e·ter (flă-rim′ĕ-ter). Obsolete device for use in evaluating cardiopulmonary fitness; pulse rate and blood pressure were measured during attempts to expire the vital capacity through calibrated orifices while maintaining a mouth pressure of 20 mm Hg. [L. *flare,* to blow, + G. *metron,* measure]

flash. 1. A sudden and brief burst of light or heat. **2.** Excess material extruded between the sections of a flask in the process of molding denture bases or other dental restorations.

hot f., colloquialism for one of the vasomotor symptoms of the climacteric that may involve the whole body as a f. of heat; also used interchangeably with hot *flush.*

flash·back. An involuntary recurrence of some aspect of a hallucinatory experience or perceptual distortion occurring some time after taking the hallucinogen that produced the original effect and without subsequent ingestion of the substance.

flask. A small receptacle, usually of glass, used for holding liquids, powder, or gases. [M.E. keg, fr. Fr. *flasque,* fr. Germanic]

casting f., SYN refractory f.

crown f., SYN denture f.

denture f., a sectional metal boxlike case in which a sectional mold is made of plaster of Paris or artificial stone for the purpose of compressing and curing dentures or other resinous restorations. SYN crown f.

Dewar f., a glass vessel, often silvered, with two walls, the space between which is evacuated; used for maintaining materials at constant temperature or, more usually, at low temperature. SYN vacuum f.

Erlenmeyer f., a f. with a broad base, conical body, and narrow neck; so shaped that its liquid content can be shaken laterally without spilling.

Fernbach f., a f. used in microbial fermentations where a large surface area of the liquid substrate is required.

Florence f., a globular long-necked bottle of thin glass used for holding water or other liquid in laboratory work.

♻ Combining forms	[NA] Nomina Anatomica
Word*Finder* **Multi-term entry finder** Preceding letter A	[MIM] Mendelian Inheritance in Man
A.D.A.M. Anatomy Plates Between letters L and M	☆ Official alternate term
Appendices: Following letter Z	☆[NA] Official alternate Nomina Anatomica term
SYN Synonym; Cf., compare	**High Profile Term**

injection f., a denture f. designed so as to permit the forced flow of denture base material from a reservoir into the mold after the flask is closed and during curing.

refractory f., a metal tube in which a refractory mold is made for casting metal dental restorations or appliances. SYN casting f., casting ring.

vacuum f., SYN Dewar f.

volumetric f., a f. calibrated to contain or to deliver a definite amount of liquid.

flask·ing. The process of investing the cast and a wax denture in a flask preparatory to molding the denture-base material into the form of the denture.

Flatau, Edward, Polish neurologist, 1869–1932. SEE F.-Schilder *disease;* F.'s *law.*

flat·foot (flat'fut). SYN *pes* planus.

flat·u·lence (flat'yū-lens). Presence of an excessive amount of gas in the stomach and intestines. [Mod. L. *flatulentus,* fr. L. *flatus,* a blowing, fr. *flo,* pp. *flatus,* to blow]

flat·u·lent (flat'yū-lent). Relating to or suffering from flatulence.

fla·tus (flā'tŭs). Gas or air in the gastrointestinal tract which may be expelled through the anus. [L. a blowing]

f. vagina'lis, expulsion of gas from the vagina.

flat·worm (flat'werm). A member of the phylum Platyhelminthes, including the parasitic tapeworms and flukes.

fla·ve·do (fla-vē'dō). Yellowness or sallowness of the skin. [L. *flavus,* yellow]

fla·vi·an·ic ac·id (flā-vē-an'ik) [C.I. 10316]. A naphthol derivative dye, 8-hydroxy-5,7-dinitro-2-naphthalenesulfonic acid, useful in the precipitation (and subsequent determination) of arginine and other basic substances.

fla·vin, fla·vine (flā'vin, -vēn, flav'in, -ēn). **1.** SYN riboflavin. **2.** A yellow acridine dye, preparations of which are used as antiseptics. [L. *flavus,* yellow]

f. adenine dinucleotide (FAD), a condensation product of riboflavin and adenosine 5'-diphosphate; the coenzyme of various aerobic dehydrogenases, *e.g.,* D-amino-acid oxidase and aldehyde dehydrogenase; strictly speaking, FAD is not a dinucleotide since it contains a sugar alcohol.

electron transfer f., flavoproteins that participate in the electron transport pathway.

f. mononucleotide (FMN), riboflavin 5'-phosphate; the coenzyme of a number of oxidation-reduction enzymes; *e.g.,* NADH dehydrogenase and L-amino acid oxidase. Strictly speaking, FMN is not a nucleotide since it contains a sugar alcohol instead of a sugar. SYN riboflavin 5'-phosphate.

Fla·vi·vi·ri·dae (flā'vī-vī'rā-dā). A family of enveloped single-stranded positive sense RNA viruses formerly classified as the "group B" arboviruses, including yellow fever and dengue viruses.

Fla·vi·vi·rus (flā'vi-vī'rŭs). A genus in the family Flaviviridae that includes yellow fever, dengue, and St. Louis encephalitis viruses. [L. *flavus,* yellow, + virus]

Fla·vo·bac·te·ri·um (flā-vō-bak-tēr'ē-ŭm). A genus of aerobic to facultatively anaerobic, nonsporeforming, motile and nonmotile bacteria (family Achromobacteraceae) containing Gram-negative rods; motile cells are peritrichous. These organisms characteristically produce yellow, orange, red, or yellow-brown pigments. They are found in soil and fresh and salt water. Some species are pathogenic. The type species is *F. aquatile.* [L. *flavus,* yellow]

F. aqua'tile, a species found in water containing a high percentage of calcium carbonate; it is the type species of *F.*

F. bre've, a species found in sewage; pathogenic for laboratory animals.

F. piscici'da, former name for *Pseudomonas piscicida.*

fla·vo·en·zyme (flā-vō-en'zīm). Any enzyme that possesses a flavin nucleotide as coenzyme; *e.g.,* xanthine oxidase, succinate dehydrogenase. SYN yellow enzyme.

fla·vo·ki·nase (flā-vō-kī'nās). SYN *riboflavin* kinase.

fla·vone (flā'vōn). **1.** 2-Phenyl-4*H*-1-benzopyran-4-one; or 2-

phenylchromone; a plant pigment that is the basis of the flavonoids. **2.** One of a class of compounds based on f. (1).

fla·vo·noids (flā'vō-noydz). Substances of plant origin containing flavone in various combinations (anthoxanthins, apigenins, flavones, quercitins, etc.) and with varying biological activities.

fla·vo·nol (flā'vō-nol). **1.** Reduced flavone. **2.** flavone (1) hydroxylated at position 3; a member of a class of vascular pigments.

fla·vo·pro·tein (flā'vō-prō'tēn). A compound protein possessing a flavin as prosthetic group. Cf. flavoenzyme.

fla·vor (flā'ver). **1.** The quality affecting the taste or odor of any substance. **2.** A therapeutically inert substance added to a prescription to give an agreeable taste to the mixture. [M.E., fr. O. Fr., fr. L.L. *flator,* aroma, fr. *flo,* to blow]

fla·vox·ate hy·dro·chlo·ride (flā-vok'sāt). 2-Piperidinoethyl 3-methyl-4-oxo-2-phenyl-4*H*-1-benzopyran-8-carboxylate hydrochloride; a smooth muscle relaxant for the urinary tract.

fla·vus (flā'vŭs). Latin for yellow. [L.]

flax·seed (flaks'sēd). SYN linseed.

f. oil, SYN *linseed* oil.

flea (flē). An insect of the order Siphonaptera, marked by lateral compression, sucking mouthparts, extraordinary jumping powers, and ectoparasitic adult life in the hair and feathers of warm-blooded animals. Important f.'s include *Ctenocephalides felis* (cat f.), or *C. canis* (dog f.), *Pulex irritans* (human f.), *Tunga penetrans* (chigger, chigoe, or sand f.), *Echidnophaga gallinacea* (sticktight f.), *Xenopsylla* (rat f.), and *Ceratophyllus.* SEE ALSO Copepoda.

fle·cai·nide ac·e·tate (flĕ-kā'nīd). *N*-(2-Piperidylmethyl)-2,5-bis(2,2,2-trifluoroethoxy)benzamide monoacetate; a member of the membrane-stabilizing group of antiarrhythmics, with local anesthetic activity, used in the treatment of refractory ventricular arrhythmias.

Flechsig, Paul E., German neurologist, 1847–1929. SEE F.'s *areas,* under *area,* ground *bundles,* under *bundle,* *fasciculi,* under *fasciculus, tract;* oval *area* of F.; semilunar *nucleus* of F.

flec·tion (flek'shŭn). SYN flexion.

Flegel, H., 20th century German dermatologist. SEE F.'s *disease.*

Fleisch, Alfred, Swiss physician and physiologist, *1892. SEE F. *pneumotachograph.*

Fleischer, Bruno, German ophthalmologist, 1874–1965. SEE F.'s *ring, vortex;* Kayser-F. *ring;* Fleischer-Strumpell *ring.*

Fleischmann, Friedrich Ludwig, 19th century German anatomist. SEE sublingual *bursa.*

Fleischner, Felix, Austrian-American radiologist, 1893–1969. SEE F. *lines,* under *line.*

Fleitmann, Theodore, 19th century German chemist. SEE F.'s *test.*

Flemming, Walther, German anatomist, 1843–1905. SEE intermediate *body* of F.; germinal *center* of F.; F.'s *fixative,* triple *stain.*

Flesch, Rudolf, Austrian educator, *1911. SEE F. *formula.*

flesh. **1.** The meat of animals used for food. **2.** SYN muscular *tissue.* [A.S. *flaesc*]

goose f., SYN *cutis* anserina.

proud f., exuberant granulations in the granulation tissue on the surface of a wound.

flesh·flies (flesh'flīz). Members of the order Diptera, whose larvae (maggots) develop in putrefying or living tissues. Maggots of the latter group produce myiasis; these include screw-worms (both primary and secondary invaders); wool maggots of sheep; botflies or skin maggots of man and domestic animals (including warble or heel flies); head or nasal botflies of sheep and goats, horses, camels, and deer; and horse botflies (or gadflies) whose larvae develop in the stomach, duodenum, or rectum of horses.

flex (fleks). To bend; to move a joint in such a direction as to approximate the two parts which it connects. [L. *flecto,* pp. *flexus,* to bend]

flex·i·bil·i·tas ce·rea (flek-si-bil'i-tas sē'rē-ă). The rigidity of catalepsy which may be overcome by slight external force, but which returns at once, holding the limb firmly in the new position. [L. waxy flexibility]

flex·im·e·ter (flek-sim′ĕ-ter). SYN goniometer (3).

flex·ion (flek′shŭn). **1.** The act of flexing or bending, *e.g.*, bending of a joint so as to approximate the parts it connects; bending of the spine so that the concavity of the curve looks forward. **2.** The condition of being flexed or bent. SYN flection. [L. *flecto*, pp. *flexus*, to bend]

palmar f., turning the hand or fingers toward the palmar surface.

plantar f., turning the foot or toes toward the plantar surface.

Flexner, Simon, U.S. pathologist, 1863–1946. SEE F.'s *bacillus*.

flex·or (flek′ser, -sōr). A muscle the action of which is to flex a joint.

flex·u·ra, pl. **flex·u·′rae** (flek-shyūr′ă, -shyūr′ē) [NA]. SYN flexure. [L. a bending]

  f. co′li dex′tra [NA], SYN right colic *flexure.*

  f. co′li sinis′tra [NA], SYN left colic *flexure.*

  f. duode′ni infe′rior [NA], SYN inferior *flexure* of duodenum.

  f. duode′ni supe′rior [NA], SYN superior *flexure* of duodenum.

  f. duode′nojejuna′lis [NA], SYN duodenojejunal *flexure.*

  f. perinea′lis rec′ti [NA], SYN perineal *flexure* of rectum.

  f. sacra′lis rec′ti [NA], SYN sacral *flexure* of rectum.

  f. sigmoid′ea, SYN sigmoid *colon.*

flex·ur·al (flek′sher-ăl). Relating to a flexure.

flex·ure (flek′sher). A bend, as in an organ or structure. SYN flexura [NA]. [L. *flexura*]

  anorectal f., SYN perineal f. of rectum.

  basicranial f., SYN pontine f.

  caudal f., the bend in the lumbosacral region of the embryo. SYN sacral f.

  cephalic f., the sharp, ventrally concave bend in the developing midbrain of the embryo. SYN cerebral f., cranial f., mesencephalic f.

  cerebral f., SYN cephalic f.

  cervical f., the ventrally concave bend at the juncture of the brainstem and spinal cord in the embryo.

  cranial f., SYN cephalic f.

  dorsal f., a f. in the mid-dorsal region in the embryo.

  duodenojejunal f., an abrupt bend in the small intestine at the junction of the duodenum and jejunum. SYN flexura duodenojejunalis [NA], duodenojejunal angle.

  hepatic f., SYN right colic f.

  inferior f. of duodenum, the bend at the junction of the descending and horizontal parts of the duodenum. Occasionally a bend, the left inferior duodenal flexure, occurs at the junction of the horizontal and ascending parts. SYN flexura duodeni inferior [NA].

  left colic f., the bend at the junction of the transverse and descending colon. SYN flexura coli sinistra [NA], splenic f.

  lumbar f., the normal ventral curve of the vertebral column in the lumbar region.

  mesencephalic f., SYN cephalic f.

  perineal f. of rectum, the anteroposterior curve with convexity anteriorward of the last portion of the rectum. SYN flexura perinealis recti [NA], anorectal angle (2), anorectal f.

  pontine f., the dorsally concave curvature of the rhombencephalon in the embryo; appearance indicates division of rhombencephalon into myelencephalon and metencephalon. SYN basicranial f., transverse rhombencephalic f.

  right colic f., the bend of the colon at the juncture of its ascending and transverse portions. SYN flexura coli dextra [NA], hepatic f.

  sacral f., SYN caudal f.

  sacral f. of rectum, the anteroposterior curve with concavity anteriorward of the first portion of the rectum. SYN flexura sacralis recti [NA].

  sigmoid f., SYN sigmoid *colon.*

  splenic f., SYN left colic f.

  superior f. of duodenum, the flexure at the junction of the

superior and descending parts of the duodenum. SYN flexura duodeni superior [NA].

  telencephalic f., a f. appearing in the embryonic forebrain region.

  transverse rhombencephalic f., SYN pontine f.

flick·er. The visual sensation caused by stimulation of the retina by a series of intermittent light flashes occurring at a certain rate. SEE ALSO flicker *fusion*, critical flicker fusion *frequency*.

flicks. Rapid, involuntary fixation movements of the eye of 5 to 10 minutes of arc. SYN flick movements.

Flieringa, Henri J., Dutch ophthalmologist, *1891. SEE F.'s *ring*.

flight in·to dis·ease. Gain through falling ill or assuming the sick role. SEE primary *gain*, secondary *gain*.

flight in·to health. In dynamic psychotherapy, the early but often only temporary disappearance of the symptoms that ostensibly brought the patient into therapy; a defense against the anxiety engendered by the prospect of further psychoanalytic exploration of the patient's conflicts.

Flint, Austin, U.S. physician, 1812–1886. SEE Austin F. *murmur;* F.'s *murmur;* Austin F. *phenomenon.*

Flint, Austin, Jr., U.S. physiologist, 1836–1915. SEE F.'s *arcade.*

flint dis·ease. See under disease.

flint glass. See under glass.

flip. A burn occurring on one side only of the entrance site in a gunshot wound of the soft parts.

float·er (flōt′er). An object in the field of vision that originates in the vitreous body. SEE ALSO muscae volitantes.

float·ing (flōt′ing). **1.** Free or unattached. **2.** Unduly movable; out of the normal position; denoting an occasional abnormal condition of certain organs, such as the kidneys, liver, spleen, etc.

floc (flok). A colloquial term for the product of a flocculation, *i.e.*, the separation of the disperse phase of a colloidal suspension into discrete, usually visible particles, as in certain serologic precipitin tests.

floc·cil·la·tion (flok-si-lā′shŭn). An aimless plucking at the bedclothes, as if one were picking off threads or tufts of cotton. SYN carphologia, carphology, crocidismus. [Mod. L. *flocculus*]

floc·cose (flok′ōs). In bacteriology, applied to a growth of short, curving filaments or chains closely but irregularly disposed. [L. *floccus*, a flock of wool]

floc·cu·la·ble (flok′yū-lă-bl). Capable of undergoing flocculation.

floc·cu·lar (flok′yū-lăr). Relating to a flocculus of any sort; specifically to the flocculus of the cerebellum.

floc·cu·late (flok′yū-lāt). To become flocculent.

floc·cu·la·tion (flok-yū-lā′shŭn). Precipitation from solution in the form of fleecy masses; the process of becoming flocculent. SYN flocculence.

floc·cule (flok′yūl). SYN flocculus.

floc·cu·lence (flok′yū-lens). SYN flocculation.

floc·cu·lent (flok′yū-lent). **1.** Resembling tufts of cotton or wool; denoting a fluid, such as the urine, containing numerous shreds or fluffy particles of gray-white or white mucus or other material. **2.** In bacteriology, denoting a fluid culture in which there are numerous colonies either floating in the fluid medium or loosely deposited at the bottom.

floc·cu·lo·nod·u·lar (flok′yū-lō-nod′yū-lăr). SEE flocculonodular *lobe.*

floc·cu·lus, pl. **floc·cu·li** (flok′yū-lŭs, -lī). **1.** A tuft or shred of cotton or wool or anything resembling it. **2** [NA]. A small lobe of the cerebellum at the posterior border of the middle cerebellar peduncle anterior to the biventer lobule; it is associated with the nodulus of the vermis; together, these two structures compose the vestibular part of the cerebellum. SYN floccule. [Mod. L. dim. of L. *floccus*, a tuft of wool]

  accessory f., an occasional small lobule of the cerebellum adjacent to the flocculus.

Flocks, Milton, U.S. ophthalmologist, *1914. SEE Harrington-F. *test.*

Fl

Flood, Valentine, Irish anatomist and surgeon, 1800–1847. SEE F.'s *ligament*.

flood (flŭd). **1.** To bleed profusely from the uterus, as after childbirth or in cases of menorrhagia. **2.** Colloquialism for a profuse menstrual discharge. [A.S. *flōd*]

flood·ing (flŭd'ing). **1.** Bleeding profusely from the uterus, especially after childbirth or in severe cases of menorrhagia. **2.** Profuse uterine hemorrhage. **3.** A type of behavior therapy; a therapeutic strategy at the beginning of therapy, in which the patients imagine the most anxiety-producing scene and fully immerse (flood) themselves in it. Cf. systematic *desensitization*.

floor (flōr). The lower inner surface of an open space or hollow organ.

f. of orbit, the floor of the orbit; the shortest of the four walls of the orbit, sloping upward from the orbital margin; it is comprised of the maxilla and orbital process of the palatine bone. SYN paries inferior orbitae [NA], inferior wall of orbit.

f. of tympanic cavity, the floor of the tympanic cavity; a thin plate of bone separating the tympanic cavity from the jugular fossa. SYN paries jugularis cavi tympani [NA], fundus tympani, inferior wall of tympanic cavity, jugular wall of middle ear.

flo·ra (flō'ră). **1.** Plant life, usually of a certain locality or district. **2.** The population of microorganisms inhabiting the internal and external surfaces of healthy conventional animals. SYN microbial associates. [L. *Flora*, goddess of flowers, fr. *flos* (*flor-*), a flower]

flor·an·ty·rone (flor-an'ti-rōn). γ-Oxy-γ-(8-fluoranthene)butyric acid; an agent which increases the volume of bile without increasing the quantity of bile solids or stimulating evacuation of the gallbladder.

Florence, Albert, French physician, 1851–1927. SEE F.'s *crystals*, under *crystal*.

Florence flask. See under flask.

Florey, Sir Howard W., Australian-British pathologist and Nobel laureate, 1898–1968. SEE F. *unit*.

flor·id (flor'id). **1.** Of a bright red color; denoting certain cutaneous lesions. **2.** Fully developed. [L. *floridus*, flowery]

Florschütz, Georg, German physician, *1859. SEE F.'s *formula*.

floss. 1. SYN dental f. **2.** To use dental f. in oral hygiene.

dental f., an untwisted thread made from fine, short, silk or synthetic fibers, frequently waxed; used for cleansing interproximal spaces and between contact areas of the teeth. SYN floss silk, floss (1).

flo·ta·tion (flō-tā'shŭn). A process for separating solids by their tendency to float upon or sink into a liquid.

Flourens, Marie J.P., French physiologist, 1794–1867. SEE F.'s *theory*.

flow (flō) **1.** To bleed from the uterus less profusely than in flooding. **2.** The menstrual discharge. **3.** Movement of a liquid or gas; specifically, the volume of liquid or gas passing a given point per unit of time. In respiratory physiology, the symbol for gas flow is V̇ and for blood flow is Q̇, followed by subscripts denoting location and chemical species. **4.** In rheology, a permanent deformation of a body which proceeds with time. [A.S. *flōwan*]

Bingham f., the f. characteristics exhibited by a Bingham plastic.

Doppler color f., a computer-generated color image produced by Doppler ultrasonography in which different directions of f. are represented by different hues. SEE Doppler *ultrasonography*.

> This technique is typically used to examine blood flow when evaluating heart disease. Where obstructions (for instance, arterial plaques) exist, blood flow will alter according to the principles of fluid mechanics. Eddies and reversals are readily apparent on the color image.

effective renal blood f. (ERBF), the amount of blood flowing to the parts of the kidney that are involved with production of constituents of urine.

effective renal plasma f. (ERPF), the amount of plasma flowing to the parts of the kidney that have a function in the production of constituents of urine; the clearance of substances such as

iodopyracet and *p*-aminohippuric acid, assuming that the extraction ratio in the peritubular capillaries is 100%.

forced expiratory f. (FEF), expiratory f. during measurement of forced vital capacity; subscripts specify the exact parameter measured, *e.g.,* peak instantaneous f., the instantaneous f. at some specified point on the curve of volume expired versus time, or on the flow-volume curve, the mean f. between two expired volumes.

gene f., changes over time in the genetic composition of a population as a result of migration rather than of mutation and selection.

laminar f., the relative motion of elements of a fluid along smooth parallel paths, which occurs at lower values of Reynolds number.

newtonian f., the type of f. characteristic of a newtonian fluid.

peak expiratory f., the maximum f. at the outset of forced expiration, which is reduced in proportion to the severity of airway obstruction, as in asthma.

shear f., a f. of a material in which parallel planes in the material are displaced in a direction parallel to each other.

Flower, Sir William H., English surgeon and anatomist, 1831–1899. SEE F.'s *bone*, dental *index*.

flow·er bas·ket of Bochdalek. Part of the choroid plexus of the fourth ventricle protruding through Luschka's foramen and resting on the dorsal surface of the glossopharyngeal nerve.

flow·ers (flow'erz). A mineral substance in a powdery state after sublimation.

f. of antimony, SYN *antimony* trioxide.

f. of benzoin, SYN benzoic acid.

f. of sulfur, SYN sublimed *sulfur*.

f. of zinc, SYN *zinc* oxide.

flow·me·ter (flō'mē-ter). A device for measuring velocity or volume of flow of liquids or gases.

electromagnetic f., a f. in which a magnetic field is applied to a blood vessel to measure flow in terms of the voltage developed by the blood as a conductor moving through the magnetic field.

flox·a·cil·lin (flok'să-sil'in). A penicillin antibiotic resistant to β-lactamase (penicillinase).

flox·ur·i·dine (flok-sū'ri-dēn). 5-Fluoro-2'-deoxyuridine (5-FUDR); the deoxynucleoside of fluorouracil; an antineoplastic agent. Fluorouracil is metabolized to f. and this, in turn, to 5-fluoro-2'-deoxyuridine 5'-monophosphate. The latter agent inhibits thymidylic synthetase; uridine phosphatase is also inhibited.

flu (flū). SYN influenza.

flu·an·i·sone (flū-an'i-sōn). 4'-fluoro-4-[4-(*o*-methoxyphenyl)-1-piperazinyl]butyrophenone; an antianxiety agent. SYN haloanisone.

flu·cry·late (flū'kri-lāt). 2,2,2-Trifluoro-1-methylethyl-2-cyanoacrylate; a surgical tissue adhesive.

fluc·tu·ate (flŭk'tyū-āt). **1.** To move in waves. **2.** To vary, to change from time to time, as in referring to any quantity or quality, *e.g.,* height of blood pressure, concentration of substance in urine or blood, secretory activity, etc. [L. *fluctuo*, pp. *-atus*, to flow in waves]

fluc·tu·a·tion (flŭk-tyū-ā'shŭn). **1.** The act of fluctuating. **2.** A wavelike motion felt on palpating a cavity with nonrigid walls, especially one containing fluid.

flu·cy·to·sine (flū-sī'tō-sēn). 5-Fluorocytosine; an antifungal drug.

flu·dro·cor·ti·sone ac·e·tate (flū-drō-kōr'ti-sōn). 9α-fluoro-17-hydroxycorticosterone 9α-fluoro-11β,17α,21-trihydroxypregn-4-en e-3,20-dione 21-acetate; a potent mineralocorticoid. SYN 9α-fluorocortisol, 9α-fluorohydrocortisone acetate.

flu·ence (flū'ens). A measure of the quantity of x-radiation in a beam in diagnostic radiology, either particle f., the number of photons entering a sphere of unit cross-sectional area, or energy f., the sum of the energies of the photons passing through a unit area. Cf. flux. [L. *fluentia*, a flowing, fr. *fluo*, to flow]

flu·fen·am·ic ac·id (flū-fen-am'ik). *N*-(α,α,α-Trifluoro- *m*-tolyl)anthranilic acid; an anti-inflammatory agent.

flu·id (flū'id). **1.** Consisting of particles or distinct entities that can readily change their relative positions; *i.e.,* tending to move or capable of flowing. **2.** A nonsolid substance, such as a liquid or gas, that tends to flow or conform to the shape of the container. [L. *fluidus,* fr. *fluo,* to flow]

allantoic f., the f. within the allantoic cavity.

amniotic f., a liquid within the amnion that surrounds the fetus and protects it from mechanical injury. SYN liquor amnii.

Brodie f., an aqueous salt solution used in manometers designed for testing gas evolution or uptake, as in cell respiration.

Callison's f., a diluting f. for counting red blood cells, consisting of 1 ml of Loeffler's alkaline methylene blue, 1 ml of formalin, 10 ml of glycerol, 1 g of neutral ammonium oxalate, and 2.5 g of sodium chloride added to 90 ml of distilled water, mixed well, and permitted to stand until the solids are dissolved and the reagent is clear; the preparation is filtered prior to use.

cerebrospinal f. (CSF), a fluid largely secreted by the choroid plexuses of the ventricles of the brain, filling the ventricles and the subarachnoid cavities of the brain and spinal cord. SYN liquor cerebrospinalis [NA].

crevicular f., SYN gingival f.

Dakin's f., SYN Dakin's *solution.*

dentinal f., the lymph or f. of dentin which appears on the surface of freshly cut dentin, especially in young teeth; it is a transudate of extracellular f., mainly cytoplasm of odontoblastic processes, from the dental pulp via the dentinal tubules. SYN dental lymph.

extracellular f. (ECF), (1) the interstitial f. and the plasma, constituting about 20% of the weight of the body; **(2)** sometimes used to mean all f. outside of cells, usually excluding transcellular f.

extravascular f., all f. outside the blood vessels, *i.e.,* intracellular, interstitial, and transcellular f.'s; it constitutes about 48 to 58% of the body weight.

Farrant's mounting f., an aqueous solution containing gum arabic, arsenic trioxide, glycerol, and water, used in mounting histologic sections directly from water; some modifications involve addition of potassium acetate to bring the pH up to neutrality and substitution of other preservatives like cresol or thymol for arsenic trioxide.

gingival f., f. containing plasma proteins, which is present in increasing amounts in association with gingival inflammation. SYN crevicular f., sulcular f.

infranatant f., clear f. that, after the settling out of an insoluble liquid or solid by the action of normal gravity or of centrifugal force, takes up the lower portion of the contents of a vessel.

interstitial f., the f. in spaces between the tissue cells, constituting about 16% of the weight of the body; closely similar in composition to lymph. SYN tissue f.

intracellular f. (ICF), the f. within the tissue cells, constituting about 30 to 40% of the body weight.

intraocular f., SYN aqueous *humor.*

newtonian f., a f. in which flow and rate of shear are always proportional to the applied stress; such f. precisely obeys Poiseuille's law. Cf. non-newtonian f.

non-newtonian f., a f. in which flow and rate of shear are not always proportional to the applied stress and which does not obey Poiseuille's law. As in anomalous *viscosity;* Fahraeus-Lindqvist *effect;* Bingham *plastic.* Cf. newtonian f.

pleural f., the thin film of f. between the visceral and parietal pleurae.

prostatic f., succus prostaticus; a whitish secretion that is one of the constituents of the semen.

pseudoplastic f., a f. which exhibits shear thinning.

Rees-Ecker f., an aqueous solution of sodium citrate, sucrose, and brilliant cresyl blue used in platelet counts.

Scarpa's f., SYN endolymph.

seminal f., SYN semen (1).

sulcular f., SYN gingival f.

supernatant f., clear f. that, after the settling out of an insoluble liquid or solid by the action of normal gravity or of centrifugal force, takes up the upper portion of the contents of a vessel.

synovial f., a clear thixotropic fluid, the main function of which

human cerebrospinal fluid (average measurements, mg/dl)	
volume	120–200 ml
specific gravity	1.006–1.008
reaction	pH ca. 7.5
reduction of freezing point	0.55° (0.52°–0.58°)
pressure (lumbar, subject reclining)	70–220 mm H$_2$O
protein	15–25
glucose	40–60 (up to 80)
phosphatidic acid	ca. 1.0
cholesterol	0.3–0.6
chloride	730–740
phosphate	3–5

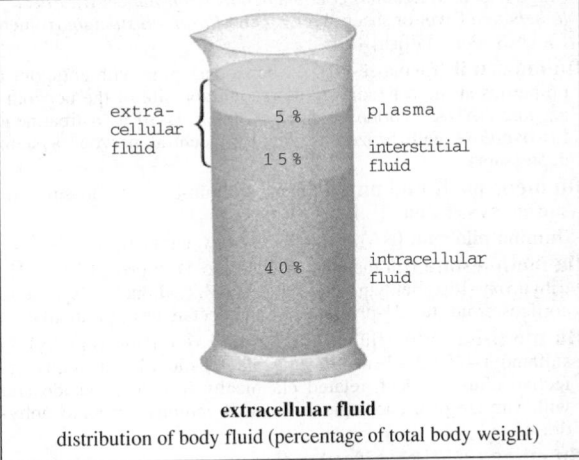

extracellular fluid
distribution of body fluid (percentage of total body weight)

is to serve as a lubricant in a joint, tendon sheath, or bursa; consists mainly of mucin with some albumin, fat, epithelium, and leukocytes; synovial f. also helps to nourish the avascular articular cartilage. SYN synovia [NA], joint oil.

thixotropic f., a liquid that tends to turn into a gel when left standing, but which turns back into a liquid if agitated, as by vibrations or subjection to adequate shear.

tissue f., SYN interstitial f.

transcellular f.'s, the f.'s that are not inside cells, but are separated from plasma and interstitial f. by cellular barriers; *e.g.,* cerebrospinal f., synovial f., pleural f.

ventricular f., the portion of the cerebrospinal f. that is contained in the ventricles of the brain.

flu·id·ex·tract (flū-id-eks'trakt). Pharmacopeial liquid preparation of vegetable drugs, made by percolation, containing alcohol as a solvent or as a preservative, or both, and so made that each milliliter contains the therapeutic constituents of 1 g of the standard drug that it represents. SYN liquid extract.

flu·id·glyc·er·ates (flū-id-glis'er-āts). Pharmaceutical preparations, formerly official in the NF, containing approximately 50% by volume of glycerin but no alcohol, and of the same drug strength as fluidextracts.

flu·id·ism (flū'i-dizm). SYN humoral *doctrine.*

flu·id·i·ty (flū-id'i-tē). The reciprocal of viscosity; unit: rhe = poise^{-1}.

flu·id·ounce (flū'id-owns'). A measure of capacity: 8 fluidrams. The imperial f. is a measure containing 1 avoirdupois ounce, 437.5 grains, of distilled water at 15.6°C, and equals 28.4 ml; the

U.S. f. is $^1/_{128}$ gallon, contains 454.6 grains of distilled water at 25°C, and equals 29.57 ml.

flu·i·drachm, flu·i·dram (flŭ'i-dram'). A measure of capacity: ⅛ of a fluidounce; a teaspoonful. The imperial f. contains 54.8 grains of distilled water, and equals 3.55 ml; the U.S. f. contains 57.1 grains of distilled water and equals 3.70 ml.

fluke (flūk). Common name for members of the class Trematoda (phylum Platyhelminthes). All f.'s of mammals (subclass Digenea) are internal parasites in the adult stage and are characterized by complex digenetic life cycles involving a snail initial host, in which larval multiplication occurs, and the release of swimming larvae (cercariae) which directly penetrate the skin of the final host (as in schistosomes), encyst on vegetation (as in *Fasciola*), or encyst in or on another intermediate host (as in *Clonorchis* and other fish-borne f.'s). F.'s of lower vertebrates (order Monogenea), especially fish, are frequently monogenetic ectoparasites or gill parasites. Blood f.'s live in the mesenteric-portal bloodstream and associated vesical and pelvic venous plexuses; they include *Schistosoma haematobium* (the vesical blood f.), *S. mansoni* (Manson's intestinal blood f.), and *S. japonicum* (the Oriental blood f.). Other important f.'s are *Paragonimus westermani* (bronchial or lung f.), *Opisthorchis felineus* (cat liver f.), *Clonorchis sinensis* (Chinese liver or Oriental f.), *Heterophyes heterophyes* (Egyptian or small intestinal f.), *Fasciolopsis buski* (large intestinal f.), *Dicrocoelium dendriticum* (lancet f.), *Fasciola hepatica* (liver or sheep liver f.), and *Paramphistomum* (rumen f.). [A.S. *flōc*, flatfish]

flu·maz·en·il (flŭ'mā-zē-nil). A benzodiazepine with antagonist properties at the benzodiazepine recognition site of the benzodiazepine-GABA-chloride channel complex. Used as a treatment for overdose with benzodiazepine-type central nervous system depressants.

flu·men, pl. **flu·mi·na** (flŭ'men, flŭ'min-ă). A flowing, or stream. SYN stream. [L.]

flumina pilo'rum [NA], SYN hair *streams*, under *stream*.

flu·meth·a·sone (flŭ-meth'ă-sōn). 6α,9α-Difluoro-11β,17α,21-trihydroxy-16α-methylpregna-1,4-diene-3,20-dione; a synthetic corticosteroid; the 21-pivalate salt and acetate are also available.

flu·me·thi·a·zide (flŭ'me-thī'ă-zīd). 6-Trifluoromethyl-7-sulfamoyl-4*H*-1,2,4-benzothi adiazine 1,1-dioxide; an orally effective diuretic agent, related chemically to chlorothiazide and with similar pharmacologic actions; it inhibits carbonic anhydrase.

flu·mi·na (flŭ'mi-nă). Plural of flumen.

flu·nar·i·zine (flŭ-nar'ĭ-zēn). A calcium-blocking agent with anticonvulsant properties.

flu·nis·o·lide (flŭ-nis'ō-lid). Pregna-1,4-diene-3,20-dione, 6-fluoro-11,21-dihydroxy-16,17[(1-methylethylidene)bis(oxy)]-, hemihydrate, (6α,11β,16α)-; an anti-inflammatory corticosteroid used intranasally or by inhalation in the treatment of allergies and asthma.

flu·ni·traz·e·pam (flŭ'nī-trāz'ĕ-pam). A benzodiazepine compound with sedative/hypnotic properties.

△**fluo-**. 1. Combining form denoting flow. 2. Prefix often used to denote fluorine (used in the generic names of drugs). SEE ALSO fluor-. [L. *fluo*, pp. *fluxus*, to flow]

flu·o·cin·o·lone ac·e·to·nide (flŭ-ō-sin'ō-lōn as'ĕ-tō-nīd). 6α,9α-Difluoro-11β,16α,17α,21-tetrahydroxy-1,4-pregnadiene-3,20-dione cyclic 16,17-acetal with acetone; 6α,9α-difluoro-16α-hydroxyprednisolone 16,17-acetonide; a fluorinated corticosteroid for topical use in the treatment of selected dermatoses.

flu·o·cin·o·nide (flŭ-ō-sin'ō-nīd). Pregna-1,4-diene-3,20-dione, 21-(acetyloxy)-6,9-difluoro-11-hydroxy-16,17-[(methylethylidene)-bis(oxy)]-, (6α,11β,16β)-; an anti-inflammatory corticosteroid used in topical preparations.

flu·o·cor·to·lone (flŭ-ŏ-kōr'tō-lōn). 6α-Fluoro-11β,21-dihydroxy-16α-methylpreg na-1,4-diene-3,20-dione; a glucocorticoid.

f. caproate, ester of f. used topically in the treatment of skin diseases. SYN f. hexanoate.

f. hexanoate, SYN f. caproate.

f. pivalate, an ester of f.

△**fluor-, fluoro-**. Fluorine.

flu·or·ap·a·tite (flūr-ap'ă-tīt). $3Ca_3(PO_4)_2 \cdot CaF_2$; a naturally occurring fluorophosphate of calcium.

9*H*-flu·o·rene (flūr'ēn). Diphenylenemethane; parent compound of 2-acetylaminofluorene; occurs in coal tar.

flu·o·res·ca·mine (flūr-es'ka-mēn). $C_{17}H_{10}O_4$; A nonfluorescent reagent that reacts with primary amines to form fluorescent compounds.

flu·o·resce (fluō-res'). 1. To produce or exhibit fluorescence. 2. 4-phenyl[furan[2*H*(3*H*)-1'-phthalane]-3,3'-dione; a reagent that reacts with amino acids to procude a fluorescing compound.

flu·o·res·ce·in (flūr-es'ē-in) [C.I. 45350]. 9-(*o*-carboxyphenyl)-6-hydroxy-3*H*-xanthen-3-one; an orange-red crystalline powder that yields a bright green fluorescence in solution, and is reduced to fluorescin; a nontoxic, water-soluble indicator used diagnostically to trace water flow. SYN resorcinol phthalic anhydride, resorcinolphthalein.

f. sodium, a dye used for diagnosis of certain ocular diseases, differentiation or delineation of organ parts in surgery, and determination of circulation time. SYN resorcinolphthalein sodium, uranin.

flu·o·res·ce·in iso·thi·o·cy·a·nate (FITC) (ī'sō-thī-ō-sī'ă-nāt). A fluorochrome dye frequently coupled to antibodies which are used to locate and identify specific antigens.

flu·o·res·cence (flūr-es'ens). Emission of a longer wavelength radiation by a substance as a consequence of absorption of energy from a shorter wavelength radiation, continuing only as long as the stimulus is present; distinguished from phosphorescence in that, in the latter, emission persists for a perceptible period of time after the stimulus has been removed. SEE photoelectric *effect*. [*fluor*spar + *-escence*, inchoative suffix]

flu·o·res·cence-ac·ti·vat·ed cell sort·er (FACS) (flūr-es'ens). A machine that can separate and analyze cells, such as lymphocytes, which are labeled with fluorochrome-conjugated antibody, by their fluorescence and light scattering patterns.

flu·o·res·cent (flūr-es'ent). Possessing the quality of fluorescence.

flu·o·res·cin (flūr'-es-in). Reduced fluorescein, with similar uses as fluorescein.

flu·o·ri·da·tion (flūr'i-dā'shŭn). Addition of fluorides to a community water supply, usually 1 ppm, to reduce incidence of dental decay.

flu·o·ride (flūr'īd). A compound of fluorine with a metal, a nonmetal, or an organic radical; the anion of fluorine; inhibits enolase; found in bone and tooth apatite; f. has a cariostatic effect; high levels are toxic.

flu·o·ride num·ber. The percent inhibition of pseudocholinesterase produced by fluorides; used to differentiate normal from atypical pseudocholinesterases. SEE ALSO dibucaine number.

flu·o·ri·di·za·tion (flūr'i-di-zā'shŭn). Therapeutic use of fluorides to reduce the incidence of dental decay; sometimes used to refer to the topical application of fluoride agents to the teeth.

flu·o·rine (F) (flūr'ēn). A gaseous chemical element, atomic no. 9, atomic weight 18.9984032; ^{18}F (half-life of 1.83 hours) is used as a diagnostic aid in various tissue scans. [L. *fluere*, flow]

△**fluoro-**. SEE fluor-.

flu·o·ro·chrome (flūr'ō-krōm). Any fluorescent dye used to label or stain.

flu·or·o·chrom·ing (flūr'ō-krōm-ing). 1. Tagging or "labeling" of antibody with a fluorescent dye so that it may be observed with a microscope (using ultraviolet light), as a means of studying the origin, distribution, and sites of reaction (with antigen) in tissues. 2. Microscopic detection of cellular and tissue chemical components (DNA, RNA, proteins, polysaccharides) with the aid of fluorochromes bound to these components.

9α-flu·o·ro·cor·ti·sol (flūr-ō-kōr'ti-sol). SYN fludrocortisone acetate.

flu·o·ro·cyte (flūr'ō-sīt). Term used occasionally for a reticulocyte that exhibits fluorescence.

flu·o·ro-2,4-di·ni·tro·ben·zene (FDNB) (flūr'ō-dī-nī-trō-ben'zēn). A reagent used to combine with the free NH_2 group of the

NH₂-terminal amino acid residue in a peptide, thus marking this residue; the combined forms are known as DNP-proteins, Dnp-aminoacyl, etc., the fluorine having been replaced to leave a dinitrophenyl residue (DNP, Dnp, or N₂Ph-) attached to the NH₂ group. SYN Sanger's reagent.

flu·o·rog·ra·phy (flūr-og′ră-fē). SYN photofluorography.

9α-flu·o·ro·hy·dro·cor·ti·sone ac·e·tate (flūr′ō-hī-drō-kōr′ti-sōn). SYN fludrocortisone acetate.

flu·o·rom·e·ter (flūr-om′ĕ-ter). A device employing an ultraviolet source, monochromators for selection of wavelength, and a detector of visible light; used in fluorometry.

flu·o·ro·meth·o·lone (flūr-ō-meth′ŏ-lōn). 9α-Fluoro-11β,17α-dihydroxy-6α-methyl-1,4-pregnadiene-3,20-dione; a glucocorticoid for topical use.

flu·o·rom·e·try (flūr-om′ĕ-trē). An analytic method for determining fluorescent compounds, using a beam at ultraviolet light that excites the compounds and causes them to emit visible light. [fluoro- + G. *metron*, measure]

flu·o·ro·pho·tom·e·try (flūr′ō-fō-tom′ĕ-trē). Photomultiplier tube measurement of fluorescence emitted from the interior of the eye after intravenous administration of fluorescein; used to measure the rate of formation of aqueous humor or integrity of the retinal vasculature.

flu·o·ro·quin·o·lones. A class of antibiotics with a broad spectrum of antimicrobial activity; well-absorbed orally, with good tissue penetration and relatively long duration of effect. Members of this class are derived from nalidixic acid and include norfloxacin, ciprofloxacin and ofloxacin. These agents bind to DNA and impair its replication.

flu·o·ro·roent·gen·og·ra·phy (flūr′ō-rent-gen-og′ră-fē). SYN photofluorography.

flu·o·ro·scope (flūr′ō-skōp). An apparatus for rendering visible the patterns of x-rays which have passed through a body under examination, by interposing a glass plate coated with fluorescent materials, such as calcium tungstate; to examine a patient by fluoroscopy. SYN roentgenoscope. [fluorescence + G. *skopeō*, to examine]

flu·o·ro·scop·ic (flūr-ō-skop′ik). Relating to or effected by means of fluoroscopy.

flu·o·ros·co·py (flūr-os′kŏ-pē). Examination of the tissues and deep structures of the body by x-ray, using the fluoroscope. SYN roentgenoscopy.

video f., f. using an image intensifier and television camera for image detection and a video monitor for display.

flu·o·ro·sis (flūr-ō′sis). 1. A condition caused by an excessive intake of fluorides (2 or more p.p.m. in drinking water), characterized mainly by mottling, staining, or hypoplasia of the enamel of the teeth, although the skeletal bones are also affected. 2. Chronic poisoning of livestock with fluorides which blacken and soften developing teeth and reduce bones to a chalky brittleness; most often caused by ingestion of forage contaminants near large aluminum plants.

chronic endemic f., f. caused by excessive fluorine in the natural water supply, as seen in parts of India; osteosclerosis with ankylosis of the spine may develop.

flu·o·ro·u·ra·cil (flūr-ō-yū′ră-sil). 5-Fluorouracil; a pyrimidine analogue; an antineoplastic effective in the treatment of some carcinomas; the cells of certain neoplasms incorporate uracil into ribonucleic acid more readily than do normal tissue cells. SEE ALSO floxuridine.

flu·o·sol-DA (flu′ō-sol). Experimental perfluorochemical solution under investigation as an artificial blood substitute.

flu·ox·e·tine hy·dro·chlo·ride (flū-oks′ĕ-tēn). Benzenepropanamine, *N*-methyl-γ-[4-(trifluoromethyl)-phenoxy]-; an oral antidepressant chemically unrelated to other antidepressants; prevents serotonin reuptake.

flu·ox·y·mes·ter·one (flū-ok-sē-mes′ter-ōn). 9α-Fluoro-11β,17β-dihydroxy-17α-methyl-4-androstene-3-one; an orally effective synthetic halogenated steroid, related in chemical structure and pharmacologic action to methyltestosterone, but more potent.

flu·pen·tix·ol (flū-pen-tik′sol). 4-{3-[2-(Trifluoromethyl)-thioxanthen-9-ylidene]propyl}-1-piperazineethanol; a neuroleptic.

flu·per·o·lone ac·e·tate (flū-per′ŏ-lōn). 9α-Fluoro-11β,17α,21-trihydroxy-21-methyl pregna-1,4-diene-3,20-dione 21-acetate; a synthetic corticosteroid.

flu·phen·a·zine (flū-fen′ă-zēn). 4-[3-[2-(Trifluoromethyl)-phenothiazin-10-yl]propyl]-1-piperazine ethanol; a phenothiazine-piperazine compound; a tranquilizer used as an antipsychotic and neuroleptic agent.

f. enanthate, a long-acting antipsychotic, used parenterally.

f. hydrochloride, an antipsychotic, used in the management of acute and chronic schizophrenia, involutional, senile, and toxic psychoses, and the manic phase of manic-depressive psychosis.

flu·pred·nis·o·lone (flū-pred-nis′ŏ-lōn). 6α-Fluoro-11β,17α,21-trihydroxy-1,4-pregnadiene-3,20-dione; a glucocorticoid with anti-inflammatory activity and toxicity similar to those of cortisol.

flur·an·dren·o·lide (flūr-an-dren′ŏ-līd). Pregn-4-ene-3,20-dione, 6-fluoro-11,21-dihydroxy-16,17-[(1-methylethylidene)bis-(oxy)]-, (6α,11β,16α)-; an anti-inflammatory glucocorticoid used in topical preparations.

flur·az·e·pam hy·dro·chlo·ride (flūr-az′ĕ-pam). 7-Chloro-1-[2-(diethylamino)ethyl]-5-(*o*-fluorophenyl)-1,3-dihydro-2*H*-1,4-benzodiazepin-2-one dihydrochloride; an oral hypnotic and sedative of the benzodiazepine series.

flur·bi·pro·fen (flūr-bi′prō-fen). [1,1′-Biphenyl]-4-acetic acid, 2-fluoro-α-methyl-, (±)-; a nonsteroidal anti-inflammatory agent with analgesic, anti-inflammatory, and antipyretic actions.

flur·o·ges·tone ac·e·tate (flūr-ō-jes′tōn). 9-Fluoro-11β,17-dihydroxypregn-4-ene-3,20-dione 17-acetate; a progestational agent.

flur·oth·yl (flūr′ō-thil). Bis(2,2,2-trifluoroethyl) ether; an inhalant convulsant; produces grand mal convulsions.

flur·ox·ene (flūr-ok′sēn). 2,2,2-Trifluoroethyl vinyl ether; a volatile, halogenated inhalation anesthetic. SYN 2,2,2-trifluoroethyl vinyl.

flush (flŭsh). **1.** To wash out with a full stream of fluid. **2.** A transient erythema due to heat, exertion, stress, or disease. **3.** Flat, or even with another surface, as a f. stoma.

carcinoid f., periodic hyperemia (flushing) of the skin of the face and other parts of the body seen in patients with a carcinoid tumor; the mediator has not been identified but it is not serotonin; flush can be precipitated by alcohol, food, stress, or palpation of the liver.

hectic f., redness of the face associated with a rise of temperature in various fevers.

histamine f., vasodilatation and erythema occurring as a result of release of histamine; thought to be a factor in genesis of f. of carcinoid syndrome.

hot f., colloquialism for a vasomotor symptom of the climacteric characterized by sudden vasodilation with a sensation of heat, usually involving the face and neck, and upper part of the chest. Cf. hot *flash.*

malar f., localized hectic f. and warmth of the malar eminences, often occurring in tuberculosis and sometimes seen in rheumatic fever.

flu·tam·ide (flū′tă-mīd). A nonsteroidal synthetic antiandrogen used in the treatment of prostatic cancer; antineoplastic (hormonal).

flut·ter (flŭt′er). Agitation; tremulousness. [A.S. *floterian,* to float about]

atrial f., auricular f., rapid regular atrial contractions occurring usually at rates between 250 and 350 per minute and often producing "saw-tooth" waves in the electrocardiogram, particularly leads II, III, and aVF. SYN jugular embryocardia.

diaphragmatic f., rapid rhythmical contractions (average, 150 per minute) of the diaphragm, simulating atrial f. clinically and sometimes electrocardiographically.

impure f., mixture of atrial flutter (FF) waves and fibrillation (ff) waves in the electrocardiogram. SYN fibrilloflutter, flutter-fibrillation.

ocular f., a spontaneous, brief, intermittent, horizontal oscillation

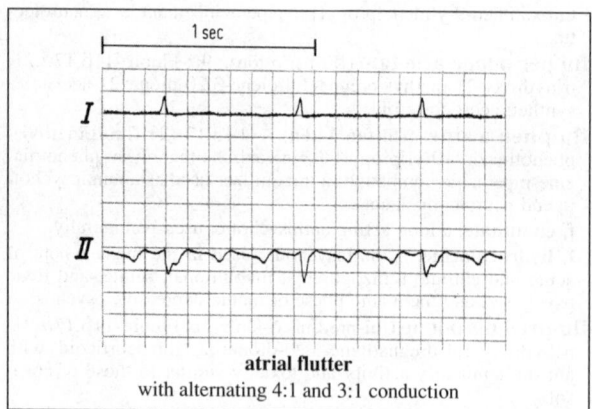

atrial flutter
with alternating 4:1 and 3:1 conduction

of the eyes occurring during fixation; it often coexists with ocular dysmetria in cerebellar syndromes.

pure f., consistent registration of atrial f. waves unmixed with other signals.

ventricular f., a form of rapid ventricular tachycardia in which the electrocardiographic complexes assume a regular undulating pattern without distinct QRS and T waves.

flut·ter-fi·bril·la·tion. SYN impure *flutter.*

flux (flŭks). **1.** The discharge of a fluid material in large amount from a cavity or surface of the body. SEE ALSO diarrhea. **2.** Material discharged from the bowels. **3.** A material used to remove oxides from the surface of molten metal and to protect it when casting; serves a similar purpose in soldering operations. Also, an ingredient in dental porcelain that by its lower melting temperature helps to bond the silica particles. **4** (*J*). The moles of a substance crossing through a unit area of a boundary layer or membrane per unit of time. SYN flux density (1). **5.** Bidirectional movement of a substance at a membrane or surface. **6.** In diagnostic radiology, photon fluence per unit time. [L. *fluxus,* a flow]

luminous f., the quantity of light emitted from a point source in a given time; its unit is the lumen.

net f., the difference between the two unidirectional f.'s.

unidirectional f., the f. of a substance from one surface of a boundary layer or membrane to the other, disregarding any counterbalancing f. in the other direction, as measured by tracer technique.

fly (flī). A two-winged insect in the order Diptera. Typical flies of the housefly type and similar forms are in the family Muscidae. Important f.'s include *Simulium* (black f.), *Calliphora* (bluebottle f.), *Piophila casei* (cheese f.), *Chrysops* (deer f.), *Siphona irritans* (horn f.), *Fannia scolaris* (latrine f.), *Oestrus ovis* and *Gasterophilus hemorrhoidalis* (nose f.), *Cochliomyia hominivorax* (primary screw-worm f.) and *C. macellaria* (secondary screw-worm f.), *Stomoxys calcitrans* (stable f.), *Glossina* (tsetse f.), and members of the insect order Trichoptera. For some types of flies not listed as subentries here (usually written as one word), see the full name (*e.g.,* blowfly, botfly, gadfly, horsefly, housefly). [A.S. *fleóge*]

heel f., SEE botfly.

horn f., a major pest of cattle in the Northern Hemisphere that transmits the filarial parasite *Stephanofilaria stilesi.* SYN *Haematobia irritans.*

louse f.'s, pupiparous, dorsoventrally flattened dipterous ectoparasites of the family Hippoboscidae. SEE ALSO *Hippobosca, Melophagus.*

mangrove f., species of *Chrysops* in Africa, vectors of *Loa loa; e.g., Chrysops silacea.*

Russian f., Spanish f., SYN cantharis.

warble f., SEE botfly.

Flynn, P., U.S. physician. SEE F.-Aird *syndrome;* F. *phenomenon.*

Fm Symbol for fermium.

FMD Abbreviation for foot-and-mouth *disease.*

fMet Abbreviation for formylmethionine.

fMet-tRNA Abbreviation for formylmethionyl tRNA.

FMN Abbreviation for *flavin* mononucleotide.

FNA Abbreviation for fine needle aspiration biopsy.

foam (fōm). **1.** Masses of small bubbles on the surface of a liquid. **2.** To produce such bubbles. **3.** Masses of air cells in a solid or semisolid, as in f. rubber.

human fibrin f., a dry artificial sponge of human fibrin prepared by clotting with thrombin a f. of a solution of human fibrinogen; the clotted f. is dried from the frozen state and heated; used as a topical anticoagulant.

fo·cal (fō′kăl). **1.** Denoting a focus. **2.** Relating to a localized area.

fo·cal spot size. the measured size of a focal spot, a function of its actual size and the angulation of the anode surface. SEE focal *spot.*

fo·ci (fō′sī). Plural of focus.

fo·cim·e·ter (fō-sim′ĕ-ter). SYN lensometer.

fo·cus, pl. **fo·ci** (fō′kŭs, fō′sī). **1** (**F**). The point at which the light rays meet after passing through a convex lens. **2.** The center, or the starting point, of a disease process. [L. a hearth]

conjugate foci, two points so related to a lens or concave mirror that an image at one point is focused at the other, and vice versa.

Ghon's f., SYN Ghon's *tubercle.*

natural f. of infection, an ecosystem in which an infectious agent normally persists in nature; *e.g.,* yellow fever virus in a jungle monkey-*Haemagogus* mosquito ecosystem.

principal f., the real or virtual meeting point of rays passing into a lens parallel to its axis.

real f., the point of meeting of convergent rays.

virtual f., the point from which divergent rays seem to proceed, or that at which they would meet if prolonged backward.

fo·drin (fō′drin). A spectrin-like protein that cross-links adjacent actin filaments in vertebrate cells.

Fogarty, Thomas J., U.S. thoracic surgeon, *1934. SEE F. *catheter, clamp.*

fog·ging (fog′ing). A method of refraction in which accommodation is relaxed by overcorrection with a convex spherical lens.

fo·go sel·va·gem (fō′gō sel′vă-jem). A form of pemphigus foliaceus, occurring in southern Brazil, in which the lesions are bullous, appear localized to the face and upper trunk, become widespread, variegated, erythrodermic, and exfoliative, and are immunologically indistinguishable from pemphigus foliaceus or vulgaris. SYN Brazilian pemphigus, wildfire. [Pg. wild fire]

foil (foyl). An extremely thin pliable sheet of metal.

Foix, Charles, French neurologist, 1882-1927. SEE F.-Alajouanine *myelitis, syndrome;* F.-Cavany-Marie *syndrome.*

fo·la·cin (fō′lă-sin). An obsolete and now unapproved term for folic acid or any derivative thereof that has the biological (vitamin) activity of folic acid.

fo·late (fō′lāt). A salt or ester of folic acid.

FOLD

fold (fōld). **1.** A ridge or margin apparently formed by the doubling back of a lamina. SEE ALSO plica. **2.** In the embryo, a transient elevation or reduplication of tissue in the form of a lamina.

adipose f.'s of the pleura, SYN *plicae* adiposae, under *plica.*

alar f.'s, winglike lateral fringes or expansions of the f. synovialis infrapatellaris. SYN ligamenta alaria [NA], plicae alares [NA], alar ligaments (2), odontoid ligament.

amniotic f., a f. of amniotic membrane enclosing the yolk stalk and extending from the point of insertion of the umbilical cord to the yolk sac; in reptiles and birds it is the reflected edge of the amnion where it folds over to cover the embryo during early development. SYN Schultze's f.

ampullary f.'s of uterine tube, one of the f.'s of mucous membrane at the fimbriated extremity of the uterine tube. SYN plicae ampullares tubae uterinae.

anterior axillary f., bounds axilla anteriorly; formed by skin and fascia overlying inferior border of pectoralis major muscle.

aryepiglottic f., arytenoepiglottidean f., a prominent fold of mucous membrane stretching between the lateral margin of the epiglottis and the arytenoid cartilage on either side; it encloses the aryepiglottic muscle. SYN plica aryepiglottica [NA].

axillary f., one of the folds of skin and muscular tissue bounding the axilla anteriorly and posteriorly. SYN plica axillaris.

caval f., a f. near the base on the right side of the dorsal mesentery, in which a primordial segment of the inferior vena cava develops between the right subcardinal vein and vessels within the liver.

cecal f.'s, the two peritoneal folds that border the retrocecal fossa. SYN plicae cecales [NA].

f. of chorda tympani, the fold of mucosa that surrounds the chorda tympani nerve in its course through the tympanic cavity. SYN plica chordae tympani [NA].

ciliary f.'s, a number of low ridges in the furrows between the ciliary processes; together with the processes they constitute the corona ciliaris. SYN plicae ciliares [NA].

circular f.'s, SYN *plicae* circulares, under *plica.*

Dennie's infraorbital f., SYN Dennie's *line.*

dinucleotide f., a structural domain in certain proteins that binds NAD$^+$ or NADP$^+$. SYN dinucleotide domain.

Douglas' f., SYN sacrouterine f.

Duncan's f.'s, the f.'s on the peritoneal surface of the uterus immediately after delivery.

duodenojejunal f., SYN superior duodenal f.

duodenomesocolic f., SYN inferior duodenal f.

epicanthal f., a fold of skin extending from the root of the nose to the medial termination of the eyebrow, overlapping the medial angle of the eye; its presence is normal in fetal life and in Orientals. SYN plica palpebronasalis [NA], epicanthus, mongolian f., palpebronasal f.

epigastric f., SYN lateral umbilical f.

epiglottic f.'s, one of the three f.'s of mucous membrane passing between the tongue and the epiglottis, lateral glossoepiglottic f. on either side, and median glossoepiglottic f. centrally. SYN plicae epiglottica.

falciform retinal f., a congenital f. from the disk to the ciliary region in the inferior temporal quadrant of the retina.

fimbriated f., SYN *plica* fimbriata.

gastric f.'s, SYN *rugae* of stomach, under *ruga.*

gastropancreatic f.'s, the folds of peritoneum in the omental bursa that encase the hepatic and left gastric arteries as these vessels pass toward their destinations. SYN plicae gastropancreaticae [NA].

genital f., SYN urogenital *ridge.*

giant gastric f.'s, enlarged gastric submucosal ridges covered by hyperplastic mucosa, as seen in Zollinger-Ellison syndrome, Ménétrier's disease, and hypertrophic hypersecretory gastropathy.

glossopalatine f., SYN palatoglossal *arch.*

gluteal f., a prominent f. that marks the upper limit of the thigh from the lower limit of the buttock; it coincides with the lower border of the gluteus maximus muscle; the furrow between the buttock and thigh. SYN sulcus gluteus [NA], gluteal furrow.

Guérin's f., SYN *valve* of navicular fossa.

Hasner's f., SYN lacrimal f.

head f., a ventral folding of the cephalic extremity in the embryonic disk, so that the brain lies rostrad to the mouth and pericardium.

Houston's f.'s, SYN transverse rectal f.'s.

ileocecal f., a fold of peritoneum bounding the ileocecal or ileoappendicular fossa. SYN plica ileocecalis [NA], Treves' f.

incudal f., a variable fold of mucosa that passes from the roof of the tympanic cavity to the body and short limb of the incus. SYN plica incudis [NA].

inferior duodenal f., a fold of peritoneum bounding the inferior

duodenal recess. SYN plica duodenalis inferior [NA], plica duodenomesocolica⁎ [NA], duodenomesocolic f.

infrapatellar synovial f., a fold of synovial membrane extending from below the level of the articular surface of the patella to the anterior part of the intercondylar fossa. SYN plica synovialis infrapatellaris [NA], plica synovialis patellaris.

inguinal f., SYN *plica* inguinalis.

inguinal aponeurotic f., SYN conjoint *tendon.*

interdigital f.'s, SYN *web* of fingers/toes.

interureteric f., a fold of mucous membrane extending from the orifice of the ureter of one side to that of the other side. SYN plica interureterica [NA], bar of bladder, Mercier's bar, plica ureterica, torus uretericus, ureteric f.

f.'s of iris, numerous very fine, almost microscopic, radial folds on the posterior surface of the iris that extend around the pupillary margin. SYN plicae iridis [NA].

Kerckring's f.'s, SYN *plicae* circulares, under *plica.*

labioscrotal f.'s, lateral f.'s at either side of the embryonic cloacal membrane that develop into either the scrotum or the labia majora.

lacrimal f., a fold of mucous membrane guarding the lower opening of the nasolacrimal duct. SYN plica lacrimalis [NA], Bianchi's valve, Hasner's f., Hasner's valve, Huschke's valve, Rosenmüller's valve.

f. of laryngeal nerve, SYN f. of superior laryngeal nerve.

lateral f.'s, ventral foldings of the lateral margins of the embryonic disk, the development of which establishes the definitive embryonic body form.

lateral glossoepiglottic f., the fold of mucous membrane that extends from the margin of the epiglottis to the pharyngeal wall and base of the tongue on each side, forming the lateral boundary of the epiglottic valleculae. SYN plica glossoepiglottica lateralis [NA], pharyngoepiglottic f.

lateral nasal f., SYN lateral nasal *prominence.*

lateral umbilical f., the ridge on the peritoneal surface of the anterior abdominal wall formed by the inferior epigastric vessels. SYN plica umbilicalis lateralis [NA], epigastric f., plica epigastrica.

f. of left vena cava, a pericardial fold lying between the left oblique vein of the atrium and the left superior pulmonary vein containing the obliterated remains of the left superior vena cava. SYN plica venae cavae sinistrae [NA], Marshall's vestigial f., vestigial f.

longitudinal f. of duodenum, a fold of mucosa on the medial wall of the descending part of the duodenum above the major duodenal papilla, probably caused by the relation to the common bile duct. SYN plica longitudinalis duodeni [NA].

malar f., an ill-defined groove in the skin that extends downward and medially from the lateral canthus.

mallear f., one of two ligamentous bands, anterior and posterior, making folds on the tympanic side of the tympanic membrane extending from each extremity of the tympanic notch to the malleolar prominence; they mark the boundary between the tense and the flaccid portions of the tympanic membrane. SYN plica mallearis [NA], plica membranae tympani, Tröltsch's f.

mammary f., SYN mammary *ridge.*

Marshall's vestigial f., SYN f. of left vena cava.

medial nasal f., SYN medial nasal *prominence.*

medial umbilical f., a fold of peritoneum on the lower part of the anterior abdominal wall that covers the obliterated umbilical artery on either side of the urachus. SYN plica umbilicalis medialis [NA], plica hypogastrica.

median glossoepiglottic f., a fold of mucous membrane in the midline that extends from the back of the tongue to the epiglottis, forming the medial boundary of the epiglottic valleculae. SYN plica glossoepiglottica mediana [NA], frenulum epiglottidis, middle glossoepiglottic f.

median umbilical f., a fold of peritoneum on the anterior wall of the abdomen covering the urachus, or remains of the allantoic stalk. SYN plica umbilicalis mediana [NA], middle umbilical f., plica umbilicalis media, plica urachi, urachal f.

medullary f.'s, SYN neural f.'s.

fo

mesonephric f., SYN mesonephric *ridge.*

middle glossoepiglottic f., SYN median glossoepiglottic f.

middle transverse rectal f., SEE transverse rectal f.'s.

middle umbilical f., SYN median umbilical f.

mongolian f., SYN epicanthal f.

Morgan's f., a crease or f. beneath the margin of the lower lid of both eyes, present from birth (or shortly thereafter) in patients with atopic dermatitis.

mucobuccal f., the line of flexure of the mucous membrane as it passes from the mandible or maxillae to the cheek.

mucosal f.'s of gallbladder, the interlacing folds of the mucosa that produce a honeycomb appearance in the interior of the gallbladder. SYN plicae tunicae mucosae vesicae felleae [NA].

nail f., the fold of skin overlapping the lateral and proximal margins of the nail. SYN vallum unguis [NA], wall of nail.

nasojugal f., a shallow groove in the skin that extends downward and laterally from the medial canthus.

Nélaton's f., SEE transverse rectal f.'s.

neural f.'s, the elevated margins of the neural groove. SYN medullary f.'s.

opercular f., tissue forming a bridge or an adhesion between the tonsil and the anterior pillar of the fauces.

palmate f.'s, the two longitudinal ridges, anterior and posterior, in the mucous membrane lining the cervix uteri, from which numerous secondary folds, or rugae, branch off. SYN plicae palmatae [NA], arbor vitae uteri, lyra uterina.

palpebronasal f., SYN epicanthal f.

paraduodenal f., a sickle-shaped fold of peritoneum sometimes found arching between the left side of the duodenojejunal flexure and the medial border of the left kidney; its right free edge contains the ascending branch of the left colic artery and inferior mesenteric vein; forms anterior boundary of the paraduodenal recess. SEE ALSO paraduodenal *recess.* SYN plica paraduodenalis [NA], Treitz' arch.

pharyngoepiglottic f., SYN lateral glossoepiglottic f.

pleuropericardial f., a tissue f. jutting into the right or left embryonic pericardioperitoneal canal; it separates the developing pericardium from the pleural cavity and is formed by the growth of the common cardinal veins to the midline of the body. SYN pericardiopleural membrane, pleuropericardial membrane.

pleuroperitoneal f., a tissue f. jutting into the caudal portion of the embryonic pericardioperitoneal canal; it develops into the dorsal portion of the definitive diaphragm and is formed by the lungs growing caudally and the liver expanding cranially. SYN pleuroperitoneal membrane.

posterior axillary f., bounds axilla posteriorly; formed by skin and fascia overlying latissimus dorsi and teres major muscles and tendons of insertion.

presplenic f., a fan-shaped f. of peritoneum that passes from the gastrosplenic ligament near the lower end of the spleen to the phrenicocolic ligament with which it blends. It contains branches of the splenic or the left gastroepiploic artery.

rectal f.'s, SYN transverse rectal f.'s.

rectouterine f., SYN sacrouterine f.

rectovesical f., SYN sacrovesical f.

retinal f., a congenital or secondary f., consequent to membrane contraction, producing star-shaped, meridional, or circular f.'s on the retina.

retrotarsal f., SYN conjunctival *fornix.*

Rindfleisch's f.'s, semilunar f.'s of the serous surface of the pericardium, embracing the beginning of the aorta.

sacrogenital f.'s, peritoneal f.'s that extend backward from the sides of the bladder of the male or uterus of the female on either side of the rectum to the sacrum, forming the lateral boundaries of the rectovesical pouch. SEE sacrouterine f., sacrovesical f.

sacrouterine f., a fold of peritoneum, containing the rectouterine muscle, passing from the sacrum to the base of the broad ligament on either side, forming the lateral boundary of the rectouterine (Douglas') pouch. SYN plica rectouterina [NA], Douglas' f., Jarjavay's ligament, Petit's ligament, rectouterine f., uterosacral ligament.

sacrovaginal f., the lower part of the sacrouterine f. SYN plica rectovaginalis.

sacrovesical f., the f. of peritoneum in the male that bounds the rectovesical pouch laterally. SYN rectovesical f.

salpingopalatine f., a ridge of mucous membrane passing from the anterior border of the opening of the auditory (eustachian) tube to the palate. SYN plica salpingopalatina [NA], plica tubopalatina.

salpingopharyngeal f., a ridge of mucous membrane extending from the lower end of the tubal elevation along the wall of the pharynx overlying the salpingopharyngeus muscle. SYN plica salpingopharyngea [NA].

Schultze's f., SYN amniotic f.

semilunar f., the curved fold connecting the palatoglossal arch and palatopharyngeal arch above the supratonsillar fossa; it always contains lymphoid tissue. SYN plica semilunaris [NA].

semilunar f. of colon, SYN *plica* semilunaris of colon.

semilunar conjunctival f., SYN *plica* semilunaris conjunctivae.

spiral f. of cystic duct, a series of crescentic folds of mucous membrane in the upper part of the cystic duct, arranged in a somewhat spiral manner. SYN plica spiralis ductus cystici [NA], Amussat's valve, Heister's valve, spiral valve of cystic duct, valvula spiralis.

stapedial f., a reflection of the delicate mucous membrane from the posterior wall of the tympanic cavity that covers the stapes. SYN plica stapedis [NA].

sublingual f., an elevation in the floor of the mouth beneath the tongue, on either side, marking the site of the sublingual gland. SYN plica sublingualis [NA].

superior duodenal f., a fold of peritoneum bounding the superior or duodenal recess. SYN plica duodenalis superior [NA], plica duodenojejunalis☆ [NA], duodenojejunal f.

f. of superior laryngeal nerve, the slight fold of mucosa in the piriform recess of the pharynx that encloses the superior laryngeal nerve. SYN plica nervi laryngei [NA], f. of laryngeal nerve.

synovial f., a projection from the synovial membrane of a joint extending toward or between the two articular surfaces. SYN plica synovialis [NA].

tail f., the ventral folding of the caudal extremity of the embryonic disk.

tarsal f., the f. marking the attachment of the levator palpebrae superioris muscle into the skin of the upper eyelid.

transverse palatine f., a masticatory vestige on the hard palate; one of several irregular, sometimes branching, crests of soft tissue that radiate from the region of the incisive papillae at their most anterior parts and extend a slight distance backward, crossing the hard palate and reaching laterally for variable distances. SYN plica palatina transversa [NA], ruga palatina, transverse palatine ridge.

transverse rectal f.'s, the three or four crescentic f.'s placed horizontally in the rectal mucous membrane; the superior rectal f. is situated near the beginning of the rectum on the left side; the middle rectal f. (Nélaton's f.) is most prominent and consistent and projects from the right side about 8 cm above the anus (approximately the level of the floor of the rectouterine or rectovesical pouch); the inferior rectal f. is on the left side about 5 cm above the anus. SYN plicae transversales recti [NA], Houston's f.'s, Houston's valves, Kohlrausch's valves, plicae recti, rectal f.'s, rectal valves.

transverse vesical f., a duplication of peritoneum passing over the empty bladder, but obliterated when the viscus is full. SYN plica vesicalis transversa [NA].

Treves' f., SYN ileocecal f.

triangular f., a f. of mucous membrane anterior to the palatine tonsil arising from the palatoglossal arch. SYN plica triangularis [NA].

Tröltsch's f., SYN mallear f.

tubal f.'s of uterine tubes, many longitudinal folds in the mucous membrane of the uterine (fallopian) tube. SYN plicae tubariae tubae uterinae [NA].

urachal f., SYN median umbilical f.

ureteric f., SYN interureteric f.

urorectal f., SYN urorectal *septum*, urorectal *membrane*.

uterovesical f., SYN uterovesical *ligament*.

vascular f. of the cecum, a peritoneal fold that arches over a branch of the ileocolic artery and bounds in front a narrow recess, the superior ileocecal (or ileocolic) recess. SYN plica cecalis vascularis [NA].

Vater's f., a f. of mucous membrane in the duodenum just above the greater duodenal papilla.

ventricular f., SYN vestibular f.

vestibular f., one of the pair of folds of mucous membrane stretching across the laryngeal cavity from the angle of the thyroid cartilage to the arytenoid cartilage; they enclose a space called the rima vestibuli or false glottis. SYN plica vestibularis [NA], false vocal cord, plica ventricularis, ventricular band of larynx, ventricular f.

vestigial f., SYN f. of left vena cava.

vocal f., one of Ferrein's cords; the sharp edge of a fold of mucous membrane overlying the vocal ligament and stretching along either wall of the larynx from the angle between the laminae of the thyroid cartilage to the vocal process of the arytenoid cartilage; the vocal folds are the agents concerned in voice production. SYN plica vocalis [NA], chorda vocalis, labium vocale, true vocal cord, vocal cord, vocal shelf.

Foley, Frederic E.B., U.S. urologist, 1891–1966. SEE F. *catheter*, *operation*, Y-plasty *pyeloplasty*.

fo·lia (fō'lē-ă). Plural of folium.

fo·li·a·ceous (fō-lē-ā'shŭs). SYN foliate.

fo·li·ar (fō'lē-ăr). SYN foliate.

fo·li·ate (fō'lē-āt). Pertaining to or resembling a leaf or leaflet. SYN foliaceous, foliar, foliose.

fo·lic ac·id (fō'lik). **1.** Collective term for pteroylglutamic acids and their oligoglutamic acid conjugates. **2.** *N*-[*p*-[[(2-Amino-4-hydroxypteridin-6- yl)methyl]amino]benzoyl]-L(+)-glutamic acid; specifically, pteroylmonoglutamic acid; the growth factor for *Lactobacillus casei*, and a member of the vitamin B complex necessary for the normal production of red blood cells. It is a hemopoietic vitamin present, with or without L(+)-glutamic acid moieties, in peptide linkages in liver, green vegetables, and yeast; used to treat folate deficiency and megaloblastic anemia. SYN *Lactobacillus casei* factor, liver *Lactobacillus casei* factor, pteroylmonoglutamic acid.

fo·lie (fō-lē'). Old term for madness or insanity. [Fr. folly]

f. à deux (ă-du), identical or similar mental disorders, such as a paranoid fixation, usually affecting two members of the same family living together. SYN shared psychotic disorder. [Fr. two]

f. du doute (du-dūt), an excessive doubting about all the affairs of life and a morbid scrupulousness concerning minutiae. [Fr. from doubt]

f. du pourquoi (pūr-kwah'), a psychopathologic tendency to ask questions. [Fr. why]

f. gémellaire (zha-mel-ār'), a psychosis appearing simultaneously, or nearly so, in twins, who are not necessarily living together or intimately associated at the time. [Fr. relating to twins]

Folin, Otto K.O., U.S. biochemist, 1867–1934. SEE F.'s *reaction*, *test;* F.-Looney *test*.

fo·li·nate (fō'li-nāt). A salt or ester of folinic acid.

fo·lin·ic ac·id (fō-lin'ik). N^5Formyl-5,6,7,8- tetrahydrofolic acid; the active form of folic acid which acts as a formyl group carrier in transformylation reactions; the calcium salt, leucovorin calcium, has therapeutic use. SYN citrovorum factor, leucovorin.

fo·li·ose (fō'lē-ōs). SYN foliate.

fo·li·um, pl. **fo·lia** (fō'lē-ŭm, -lē-ă) [NA]. A broad, thin, leaflike structure. [L. a leaf]

cerebellar folia, the narrow, leaf-like gyri of the cerebellar cortex. SEE ALSO vermis f. SYN folia cerebelli [NA].

fo'lia cerebel'li [NA], SYN cerebellar folia.

fo'lia lin'guae, SYN foliate *papillae*, under *papilla*.

f. ver'mis [NA], SYN vermis f.

vermis f., a small posterior subdivision of the superior vermis of the cerebellum. SYN f. vermis [NA].

Folli, Folius. Cecilio (Caesilius), Venitian anatomist, 1615–1660. SEE Folli's *process*, follian *process*.

fol·lib·er·in (fol-lib'er-in). A decapeptide of hypothalamic origin capable of accelerating pituitary secretion of follitropin. SYN follicle-stimulating hormone-releasing factor, follicle-stimulating hormone-releasing hormone. [follicle-stimulating hormone + L. *libero*, to free, + -in]

fol·li·cle (fol'i-kl). **1.** A more or less spherical mass of cells usually containing a cavity. **2.** A crypt or minute cul-de-sac or lacuna, such as the depression in the skin from which the hair emerges. SYN folliculus [NA]. [L. *folliculus,* a small sac, dim. of *follis,* a pair of bellows]

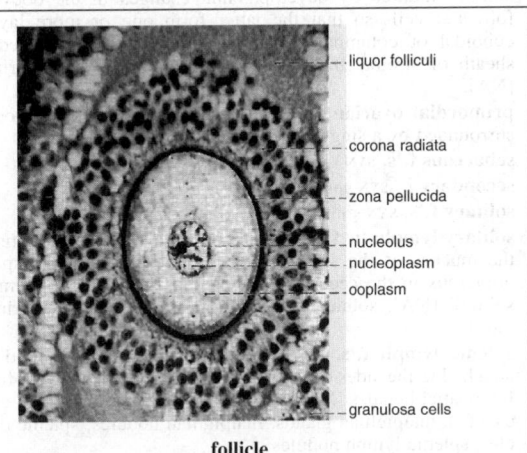

liquor folliculi

corona radiata

zona pellucida

nucleolus

nucleoplasm

ooplasm

granulosa cells

follicle
egg cell and corona radiata, from an ovarian follicle (tertiary)

aggregated lymphatic f.'s, SYN Peyer's *patches*, under *patch*.

aggregated lymphatic f.'s of vermiform appendix, masses of lymphoid tissue in the submucous coat of the vermiform appendix. SYN folliculi lymphatici aggregati appendicis vermiformis [NA].

anovular ovarian f., a f. that does not contain an ovum.

atretic ovarian f., a f. that degenerates before coming to maturity; great numbers of such atretic f.'s occur in the ovary before puberty; in the sexually mature woman, several are formed each month. SYN corpus atreticum.

dental f., the dental sac with its enclosed odontogenic organ and developing tooth.

gastric f.'s, SYN gastric *glands*, under *gland*.

gastric lymphatic f.'s, lymphoid tissue within the lamina propria which, especially in early life, collect in small masses similar to intestinal solitary lymphatic f.'s. SYN folliculi lymphatici gastrici.

graafian f., SYN vesicular ovarian f.

growing ovarian f., a f. having several layers of proliferating follicular cells surrounding the ovum, but separated from it by an extracellular glycoprotein layer (zona pellucida).

hair f., a tube-like invagination of the epidermis from which the hair shaft develops and into which the sebaceous glands open; the follicle is lined by a cellular inner and outer root sheath of epidermal origin and is invested with a fibrous sheath derived from the dermis. SYN folliculus pili [NA].

intestinal f.'s, SYN intestinal *glands*, under *gland*.

laryngeal lymphatic f.'s, small f.'s located on the posterior aspect of the epiglottis and in the ventricle of the larynx. SYN folliculi lymphatici laryngei [NA].

Lieberkühn's f.'s, SYN intestinal *glands*, under *gland*.

lingual f.'s, SYN *folliculi* linguales, under *folliculus*.

lymph f., lymphatic f., one of the spherical masses of lymphoid cells, frequently having a more lightly staining center. SEE solitary lymphatic f.'s, Peyer's *patches*, under *patch*. SYN folliculus lymphaticus, lymph nodule, nodulus lymphaticus.

lymphatic f.'s of larynx, SYN *folliculi* lymphatici laryngei, under *folliculus*.

fo

lymphatic f.'s of rectum, SYN *folliculi* lymphatici recti, under *folliculus.*

mature ovarian f., a f. ready for ovulation; in the human ovary its antrum attains a diameter of 6 to 8 mm and presents a surface bulge; a first maturation (meiotic) division of the ovum usually occurs just prior to the rupture of the f.

Montgomery's f.'s, SYN areolar *glands,* under *gland.*

nabothian f., SYN nabothian *cyst.*

ovarian follicle, one of the spheroidal cell aggregations in the ovary containing an ovum.

polyovular ovarian f., a f. containing more than one ovum.

primary ovarian f., an ovarian f. before the appearance of an antrum; marked by developmental changes in the oocyte and follicular cells so that the latter form one or more layers of cuboidal or columnar cells; the f. becomes surrounded by a sheath of stroma, the theca. SYN folliculus ovaricus primarius [NA].

primordial ovarian f., a f. in which the primordial oocyte is surrounded by a single layer of flattened follicular cells.

sebaceous f.'s, SYN sebaceous *glands,* under *gland.*

secondary f., SYN vesicular ovarian f.

solitary f.'s, SYN solitary lymphatic f.'s.

solitary lymphatic f.'s, minute collections of lymphoid tissue in the mucosa of the small and large intestines, being especially numerous in the cecum and appendix. SYN folliculi lymphatici solitarii [NA], solitary f.'s, solitary glands, solitary nodules of intestine.

splenic lymph f.'s, small nodular masses of lymphoid tissue attached to the sides of the smaller arterial branches. SYN folliculi lymphatici lienales [NA], malpighian bodies, malpighian corpuscles (2), malpighian glands, malpighian nodules, splenic corpuscles, splenic lymph nodules.

f.'s of thyroid gland, SYN *folliculi* glandulae thyroideae, under *folliculus.*

vesicular ovarian f., a f. in which the oocyte attains its full size and is surrounded by an extracellular glycoprotein layer (zona pellucida) that separates it from a peripheral layer of follicular cells permeated by one or more fluid-filled antra; the theca of the f. develops into internal and external layers. SYN folliculus ovaricus vesiculosus [NA], graafian f., secondary f.

fol·lic·u·lar (fŏ-lik′yū-lăr). Relating to a follicle or follicles.

fol·lic·u·li (fŏ-lik′yū-lī). Plural of folliculus.

fol·lic·u·lin (fŏ-lik′ū-lin). SYN estrone.

folliculin hydrate. SYN estriol.

fol·lic·u·li·tis (fŏ-lik-yū-lī′tis). An inflammatory reaction in hair follicles; the lesions may be papules or pustules.

f. absce′dens et suffo′diens, a chronic progressive follicular-pustular eruption in the scalp.

f. bar′bae, SYN *tinea* barbae.

f. decal′vans, a papular or pustular inflammation of the hair follicles of the scalp seen mostly in men, resulting in scarring and loss of hair in the affected area. SYN acne decalvans, alopecia follicularis.

eosinophilic pustular f., a dermatosis characterized by sterile pruritic papules and pustules that coalesce to form plaques with papulovesicular borders; spontaneous exacerbations and remissions may be accompanied by peripheral leukocytosis, eosinophilia, or both, and may result in eventual destruction of hair follicles and formation of eosinophilic abscesses. The disease has been reported in AIDS, and a possibly separate form of eosinophilic pustular f. occurs in infants. SYN Ofuji's disease.

f. keloida′lis, SYN acne *keloid.*

f. na′res per′forans, inflammation of a hair follicle in the nose; the infection extends to, and perforates, the cutaneous surface.

perforating f., erythematous papules with a central keratin plug which are scattered on the arms, thighs, and buttocks; seen especially in diabetics on hemodialysis. SEE ALSO *hyperkeratosis* follicularis et parafollicularis.

f. ulerythemato′sa reticula′ta, erythematous "ice-pick" or pitted scars on the cheeks; a scarring type of folliculitis, associated with keratosis pilaris and commonly inherited as an autosomal dominant trait. SYN atrophoderma vermiculatum.

fol·lic·u·lo·ma (fŏ-lik-yū-lō′mă). **1.** SYN granulosa cell *tumor.* **2.** Cystic enlargement of a graafian follicle.

fol·lic·u·lo·sis (fŏ-lik-yū-lō′sis). Presence of lymph follicles in abnormally great numbers.

fol·lic·u·lus, pl. **fol·lic·u·li** (fŏ-lik′yū-lŭs, -yū-lī) [NA]. SYN follicle. [L. a small sac, dim. of *follis,* bellows]

follic′uli glan′dulae thyroi′deae, the small spherical vesicular components of the thyroid gland lined with epithelium and containing colloid in varying amounts; the colloid serves for storage of the thyroid hormone precursor, thyroglobulin. SYN follicles of thyroid gland.

follic′uli lingua′les, collections of lymphoid tissue in the mucosa of the pharyngeal part of the tongue posterior to the terminal sulcus collectively forming the lingual tonsil. SYN lenticular papillae, lingual follicles.

follic′uli lymphat′ici aggrega′ti [NA], SYN Peyer's *patches,* under *patch.*

follic′uli lymphat′ici aggrega′ti appen′dicis vermifor′mis [NA], SYN aggregated lymphatic *follicles* of vermiform appendix, under *follicle.*

folliculi lymphat′ici gas′trici, SYN gastric lymphatic *follicles,* under *follicle.*

follic′uli lymphat′ici laryn′gei [NA], SYN laryngeal lymphatic *follicles,* under *follicle.* SYN laryngeal tonsils, lymphatic follicles of larynx.

follic′uli lymphat′ici liena′les [NA], SYN splenic lymph *follicles,* under *follicle.*

follic′uli lymphat′ici rec′ti, scattered collections of lymphoid tissue in the wall of the rectum. SYN lymphatic follicles of rectum.

follic′uli lymphat′ici solita′rii [NA], SYN solitary lymphatic *follicles,* under *follicle.*

f. lymphat′icus, SYN lymph *follicle.*

f. ovar′icus prima′rius [NA], SYN primary ovarian *follicle.*

f. ovar′icus vesiculo′sus [NA], SYN vesicular ovarian *follicle.*

f. pi′li [NA], SYN hair *follicle.*

Folling, Ivar A., Norwegian physician, 1888–1973. SEE F.'s *disease.*

fol·li·tro·pin (fol-i-trō′pin). An acidic glycoprotein hormone of the anterior pituitary that stimulates the graafian follicles of the ovary and assists subsequently in follicular maturation and the secretion of estradiol; in the male, it stimulates the epithelium of the seminiferous tubules and is partially responsible for inducing spermatogenesis. SYN follicle-stimulating hormone, follicle-stimulating principle, gametokinetic hormone. [follicle + G. *trope,* a turning, + -in]

Foltz, Jean C.E., French anatomist and ophthalmologist, 1822–1876. SEE F.'s *valvule.*

fo·men·ta·tion (fō-men-tā′shŭn). **1.** A warm application. SEE ALSO poultice, stupe. **2.** Application of warmth and moisture in the treatment of disease. [L. *fomento,* pp. *-atus,* to foment, fr. *fomentum,* a poultice, fr. *foveo,* to keep warm]

fo·mes, pl. **fom·i·tes** (fō′mēz, fōm′i-tēz). Objects, such as clothing, towels, and utensils that possibly harbor a disease agent and are capable of transmitting it; usually used in the plural. SYN fomite. [L. tinder, fr. *foveo,* to keep warm]

fo·mite (fō′mīt). SYN fomes.

fom·i·tes (fō′mi-tēz). Plural of fomes.

fo·na·zine mes·y·late (fō′nă-zēn). 10-[2-(Dimethylamino)propyl]-*N,N*-dimethylphenot hiazine-2-sulfonamide monomethanesulfonate; a serotonin inhibitor. SYN dimethothiazine mesylate.

Fonio, Anton, Swiss physician, *1889. SEE F.'s *solution.*

Fonsecaea (fon-sē-sē′ă). A genus of fungi of which at least two species, *F. pedrosoi* and *F. compacta,* cause chromoblastomycosis.

Fontan, Francois, French thoracic surgeon, *1929. SEE F. *procedure, operation.*

Fontana, Arturo, Italian dermatologist, 1873–1950. SEE F.'s *stain;* F.-Masson silver *stain;* Masson-F. ammoniacal silver *stain.*

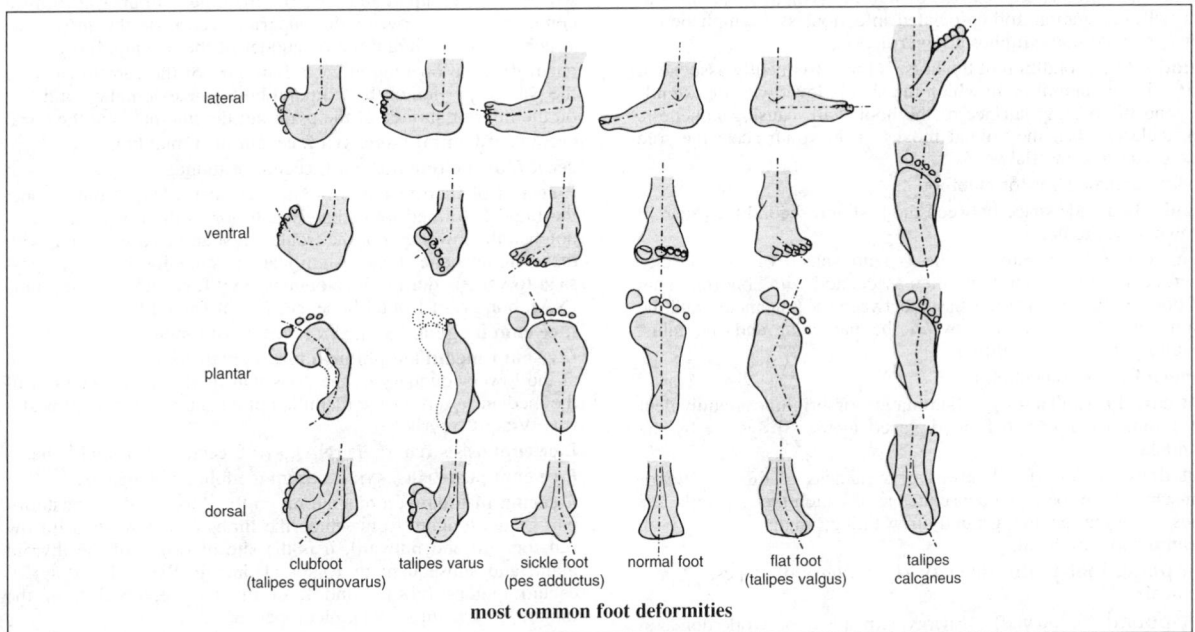

| | clubfoot (talipes equinovarus) | talipes varus | sickle foot (pes adductus) | normal foot | flat foot (talipes valgus) | talipes calcaneus |

most common foot deformities

Fontana, Felice, Italian physiologist, 1730–1805. SEE F.'s *canal, spaces,* under *space.*

fon·ta·nel, fon·ta·nelle (fon'tă-nel'). One of several membranous intervals at the angles of the cranial bones in the infant. SEE cranial f.'s. SYN fonticulus [NA]. [Fr. dim. of *fontaine,* fountain, spring]

anterior f., a diamond-shaped membranous interval at the junction of the coronal, sagittal, and metopic sutures where the frontal angles of the parietal bones meet the two ununited halves of the frontal bone. SYN fonticulus anterior [NA], bregmatic f., frontal f.

anterolateral f., SYN sphenoidal f.

bregmatic f., SYN anterior f.

Casser's f., SYN mastoid f.

cranial f.'s, the membranous intervals between the angles of the cranial bones in the infant; they include the midline anterior f. and posterior f., and the paired sphenoidal f. and mastoid f. SYN fonticuli cranii [NA].

frontal f., SYN anterior f.

Gerdy's f., SYN sagittal f.

mastoid f., the membranous interval on either side between the mastoid angle of the parietal bone, the petrous portion of the temporal bone, and the occipital bone. SYN fonticulus mastoideus [NA], fonticulus posterolateralis☆ [NA], Casser's f., posterolateral f.

occipital f., SYN posterior f.

posterior f., a triangular interval at the union of the lambdoid and sagittal sutures where the occipital angles of the parietal bones meet the occipital. SYN fonticulus posterior [NA], occipital f.

posterolateral f., SYN mastoid f.

sagittal f., an occasional f.-like defect in the sagittal suture in the newborn. SYN Gerdy's f.

sphenoidal f., an irregularly shaped interval on either side where the frontal, sphenoidal angle of the parietal, squamous portion of the temporal and greater wing of the sphenoid meet. SYN fonticulus sphenoidalis [NA], fonticulus anterolateralis☆ [NA], anterolateral f.

fon·tic·u·lus, pl. **fon·tic·u·li** (fon-tik'yū-lŭs, -lī) [NA]. SYN fontanel. SEE cranial *fontanels,* under *fontanel.* [L. dim. of *fons* (*font-*), fountain, spring]

f. ante'rior [NA], SYN anterior *fontanel.*

f. anterolatera'lis [NA], ☆official alternate term for sphenoidal *fontanel.*

fontic'uli cra'nii [NA], SYN cranial *fontanels,* under *fontanel.*

f. mastoi'deus [NA], SYN mastoid *fontanel.*

f. poste'rior [NA], SYN posterior *fontanel.*

f. posterolatera'lis [NA], ☆official alternate term for mastoid *fontanel.*

f. sphenoida'lis [NA], SYN sphenoidal *fontanel.*

food (fūd). That which is eaten to supply necessary nutritive elements. [A.S. *fōda*]

Foot, N.C., 20th century U.S. pathologist. SEE F.'s reticulin impregnation *stain.*

foot (fut). **1.** The lower, pedal, podalic, extremity of the leg. SYN pes (1). **2.** A unit of length, containing 12 inches, equal to 30.48 cm. [A.S. *fōt*]

athlete's f., SYN *tinea* pedis.

buttress f., a condition of the horse's f. in which there is exostosis of the extensor process of the third phalanx, with swelling and chronic inflammation at the coronary band on the anterior surface of the f. SYN pyramidal disease.

claw f., SEE clawfoot.

club f., SEE *talipes* equinovarus.

contracted f., (1) SYN *talipes* cavus. **(2)** a condition of the horse in which a part of the foot, often a heel, is contracted and shrunken as a result of loss of moisture in the hoof. SYN contracted heel.

drop f., SEE foot-drop.

fescue f., poisoning by a toxic principle in tall fescue grass; mainly a disease of cattle, but sheep are sometimes affected; lameness in the hind feet is first noticed, followed by necrosis of the extremities. SYN fescue poisoning.

fungous f., SYN mycetoma (1).

f. of hippocampus, the anterior thickened extremity of the hippocampus. SYN pes hippocampi [NA], digitationes hippocampi.

Hong Kong f., SYN *tinea* pedis.

immersion f., a condition resulting from prolonged exposure to damp and cold; the extremity is initially cold and anesthetic, but on rewarming becomes hyperemic, paresthetic, and hyperhidrotic; recovery is often slow. SYN trench f.

Madura f., SYN mycetoma (1).

Morand's f., a f. having eight toes.

mossy f., a profuse velvety papillomatous growth that develops large warty projections; caused by chronic lymphedema and stasis with maceration and associated infection. SYN lymphedematous keratoderma, lymphostatic verrucosis.

pumiced f., a condition of the horse's hoof, frequently associated with chronic laminitis, in which the sole is level with or extends beyond the bearing surface of the hoof wall, causing lameness, particularly when the animal moves on hard surfaces; the sole becomes thick and flaky.

reel f., archaic term for clubfoot.

sandal f., a wide space between the first and second toes seen in Down's syndrome.

spastic flat f., eversion of the f. with spasm of the muscles (peroneal) on the outer side; often associated with abnormal bars of bone cartilage or fibrous tissue between the calcaneum and the navicular (scaphoid) or between the navicular and the talus, resulting in a tarsal coalition.

trench f., SYN immersion f.

foot·can·dle (fut′kan-dl). Illumination or brightness equivalent to 1 lumen per square foot; replaced in the SI system by the candela.

foot-drop (fut′drop). Paralysis or weakness of the dorsiflexor muscles of the foot, as a consequence of which the foot falls, the toes dragging on the ground in walking; many causes, both central and peripheral.

foot·plate, foot-plate (fut′plāt). **1.** SYN *base* of stapes. **2.** SYN pedicel.

foot-pound (fut′pownd). Energy expended, or work done, in raising a mass of 1 pound a height of 1 foot vertically against gravitational force.

foot-pound·al (fut′pownd-ăl). Energy exerted, or work done, when a force of 1 poundal displaces a body 1 foot in the direction of the force; equal to about 0.01 calorie.

foot·print·ing (fŭt′print-ing). A method for determining the area of DNA covered by protein binding; accomplished by nuclease digestion of the protein-DNA complex followed by analysis of the region of DNA protected by the interaction with protein.

for·age (fōr-ahzh′). The operation of cutting a channel by surgical diathermy through an enlarged prostate. [Fr. boring]

FORAMEN

fo·ra·men, pl. **fo·ram·i·na** (fō-rā′men, fō-ram′i-nă) [NA]. An aperture or perforation through a bone or a membranous structure. SYN trema (1). [L. an aperture, fr. *foro*, to pierce]

alveolar foramina, openings of the posterior dental canals on the infratemporal surface of the maxilla. SYN foramina alveolaria [NA].

foram′ina alveola′ria [NA], SYN alveolar foramina.

anterior condyloid f., SYN hypoglossal *canal.*

anterior palatine f., SYN greater palatine f.

aortic f., SYN aortic *hiatus.*

apical dental f., SYN apical f. of tooth.

apical f. of tooth, the opening at the apex of the root of a tooth that gives passage to the nerve and blood vessels. SYN f. apicis dentis [NA], apical dental f., root f.

f. ap′icis den′tis [NA], SYN apical f. of tooth.

arachnoid f., SYN medial *aperture* of the fourth ventricle.

f. of Arnold, SYN petrosal f.

Bichat's f., SYN *cistern* of great cerebral vein.

blind f. of frontal bone, SYN f. cecum of frontal bone.

blind f. of the tongue, SYN f. cecum of tongue.

Bochdalek's f., SYN pleuroperitoneal *hiatus.*

Botallo's f., the orifice of communication between the two atria of the fetal heart. SEE ALSO f. ovale.

f. bur′sae omenta′lis major′is, a f. produced by two folds of peritoneum, that covering the common/proper hepatic artery on the right and that covering the left gastric artery on the left,

which encroach upon and constrict the omental bursa; it forms a communication between the superior recess of the lesser sac which lies above it and the remainder of the omental bursa.

carotid f., the opening at each extremity of the carotid canal in the petrous portion of the temporal bone; the external carotid f. is on the inferior surface of the pyramid; the internal is at the apex.

cecal f. of frontal bone, SYN f. cecum of frontal bone.

cecal f. of the tongue, SYN f. cecum of tongue.

f. cecum of frontal bone, blind or cecal f. of the frontal bone; the blind f. formed immediately anterior to the crista galli by a notch at the lower end of the frontal crest and its articulation with the ethmoid bone. It is insignificant postnatally, but gives passage to vessels during development. SYN f. cecum ossis frontalis [NA], blind f. of frontal bone, cecal f. of frontal bone.

f. ce′cum lin′guae [NA], SYN f. cecum of tongue.

f. ce′cum medul′lae oblonga′tae, a small triangular depression at the lower boundary of the pons that marks the upper limit of the median fissure of the medulla oblongata. SYN f. cecum posterius, Vicq d'Azyr's f.

f. ce′cum os′sis fronta′lis [NA], SYN f. cecum of frontal bone.

f. ce′cum poste′rius, SYN f. cecum medullae oblongatae.

f. cecum of tongue, a median pit on the dorsum of the posterior part of the tongue, from which the limbs of a V-shaped furrow run forward and outward; it is the site of origin of the thyroid gland and subsequent thyroglossal duct in the embryo. SYN f. cecum linguae [NA], blind f. of the tongue, cecal f. of the tongue, Morgagni's f. (1), pleuroperitoneal f.

conjugate f., a f. formed by the notches of two bones in apposition.

f. costotransversa′rium [NA], SYN costotransverse f.

costotransverse f., an opening between the neck of a rib and the transverse process of a vertebra, occupied by the costotransverse ligament. SYN f. costotransversarium [NA].

f. diaphrag′matis sel′lae, a hole in the center of the diaphragm of the sella turcica giving passage to the infundibulum of the hypothalamus.

Duverney's f., SYN epiploic f.

emissary sphenoidal f., SYN f. venosum.

epiploic f., the passage, below and behind the portal hepatis, connecting the two sacs of the peritoneum; it is bounded anteriorly by the hepatoduodenal ligament and posteriorly by a peritoneal fold over the inferior vena cava. SYN f. omentale [NA], f. epiploicum☆, aditus ad saccum peritonei minorem, Duverney's f., Winslow's f.

f. epiplo′icum, ☆official alternate term for epiploic f.

ethmoidal f., either of two foramina formed by grooves on either edge of the ethmoidal notch of the frontal bone, and completed by similar grooves on the ethmoid bone: anterior ethmoidal f., located in an anterior position; posterior ethmoidal f. located in a posterior position. SYN f. ethmoidale [NA].

f. ethmoida′le [NA], SYN ethmoidal f.

external acoustic f., SYN *opening* of external acoustic meatus.

external auditory f., SYN *opening* of external acoustic meatus.

Ferrein's f., SYN *hiatus* of facial canal.

frontal f., an occasional small opening in the supraorbital margin of the frontal bone medial to the supraorbital foramen. SYN f. frontale [NA].

f. fronta′le [NA], SYN frontal f. SEE ALSO frontal *notch.*

great f., SYN f. magnum.

greater palatine f., an opening in the posterolateral corner of the hard palate opposite the last molar tooth, marking the lower end of the pterygopalatine canal. SYN f. palatinum majus [NA], anterior palatine f.

Huschke's f., an opening in the floor of the bony part of the external acoustic meatus near the tympanic membrane, normally closed in the adult.

Hyrtl's f., SYN *porus* crotaphytico-buccinatorius.

incisive f., one of several (usually four) openings of the incisive canals into the incisive fossa. SYN f. incisivum [NA], incisor f., Stensen's f.

f. incisi′vum [NA], SYN incisive f.

incisor f., SYN incisive f.

inferior dental f., SYN mandibular f.

infraorbital f., the external opening of the infraorbital canal, on the anterior surface of the body of the maxilla. SYN f. infraorbitale [NA].

f. infraorbita′le [NA], SYN infraorbital f.

interatrial f. pri′mum, (1) in the embryonic heart, the temporary opening between right and left atria situated between the lower margin of the septum primum and the atrioventricular canal cushions; **(2)** in an adult heart, the abnormal persistence of the so-named communication which is normal in young embryos. SYN f. subseptale, ostium primum, primary interatrial f.

interatrial f. secun′dum, a secondary opening appearing in the upper part of the septum primum in the sixth week of embryonic life, just prior to the closure of the interatrial f. primum. SYN ostium secundum, secondary interatrial f.

internal acoustic f., SYN *opening* of internal acoustic meatus.

internal auditory f., SYN *opening* of internal acoustic meatus.

interventricular f., the short, often slitlike passage that, on both the left and right side, connects the third brain ventricle (of the diencephalon) with the lateral ventricles (of the cerebral hemispheres); the passage is bounded anteriomedially by the column of fornix and posterolaterally by the anterior pole of the thalamus. SYN f. interventriculare [NA], Monro's f., porta (2).

f. interventricula′re [NA], SYN interventricular f.

intervertebral f., one of a number of openings into the vertebral canal bounded by the pedicles of adjacent vertebrae above and below, the vertebral body (mostly of the superior vertebra) and intervertebral disc anteriorly, and the articular processes forming the zygopophyseal joint posteriorly. SYN f. intervertebrale [NA].

f. intervertebra′le [NA], SYN intervertebral f.

f. ischiad′icum [NA], SYN sciatic f.

jugular f., a passage between the petrous portion of the temporal bone and the jugular process of the occipital, sometimes divided into two by the intrajugular processes; it contains the internal jugular vein, inferior petrosal sinus, the glossopharyngeal, vagus, and accessory nerves, and meningeal branches of the ascending pharyngeal and occipital arteries. SYN f. jugulare [NA], f. lacerum posterius.

f. jugula′re [NA], SYN jugular f.

f. of Key-Retzius, SYN lateral *aperture* of the fourth ventricle.

lacerated f., SYN f. lacerum.

f. lac′erum [NA], an irregular aperture, filled with cartilage (basilar cartilage) in the living, located between the apex of the petrous part of the temporal bone, the body of the sphenoid, and the basilar part of the occipital bones. Several structures pass along the margins of the f. in a nearly horizontal direction but no structures pass through vertically. SYN f. lacerum medium, lacerated f., sphenotic f.

f. lac′erum ante′rius, SYN superior orbital *fissure*.

f. lac′erum me′dium, SYN f. lacerum.

f. lac′erum poste′rius, SYN jugular f.

Lannelongue's foramina, SYN foramina of the venae minimae.

f. latera′lis ventric′uli quar′ti, SYN lateral *aperture* of the fourth ventricle.

lesser palatine foramina, openings on the hard palate of palatine canals passing vertically through the tuberosity of the palatine bone and transmitting the smaller palatine nerves and vessels. SYN foramina palatina minora [NA], posterior palatine foramina.

f. of Luschka, SYN lateral *aperture* of the fourth ventricle.

Magendie's f., SYN medial *aperture* of the fourth ventricle.

f. mag′num [NA], the large opening in the basal part of the occipital bone through which the spinal cord becomes continuous with the medulla oblongata. SYN great f.

malar f., SYN zygomaticofacial f.

f. mandib′ulae [NA], SYN mandibular f.

mandibular f., the opening into the mandibular canal on the medial surface of the ramus of the mandible giving passage to the inferior alveolar nerve, artery, and vein. SYN f. mandibulae [NA], inferior dental f.

mastoid f., an opening at the posterior portion of the mastoid process, transmitting the mastoid branch of the occipital artery to the dura and an emissary vein to the sigmoid sinus. SYN f. mastoideum [NA].

f. mastoi′deum [NA], SYN mastoid f.

mental f., the anterior opening of the mandibular canal on the body of the mandible lateral to and above the mental tubercle giving passage to the mental artery and nerve. SYN f. mentale [NA], mental canal.

f. menta′le [NA], SYN mental f.

Monro's f., SYN interventricular f.

Morgagni's f., (1) SYN f. cecum of tongue. **(2)** congenital defect in the fusion of sternal and costal elements of the diaphragmatic anlage that is the site of a parasternal hernia. SYN parasternal hernia.

nasal f., vascular f. opening on the outer surface of each nasal bone.

foram′ina nervo′sa [NA], the perforations along the tympanic lip of the spiral lamina giving passage to the cochlear nerves. SYN habenulae perforata, zona perforata.

f. nutric′ium [NA], SYN nutrient f.

nutrient f., the external opening of the nutrient canal in a bone. SYN f. nutricium [NA].

obturator f., a large, oval or irregularly triangular aperture in the hip bone, the margins of which are formed by the pubis and the ischium; it is closed in the natural state by the obturator membrane, except for a small opening for the passage of the obturator vessels and nerve. SYN f. obturatum [NA].

f. obtura′tum [NA], SYN obturator f.

olfactory f., one of the openings in the cribriform plate of the ethmoid bone, transmitting the olfactory nerves.

f. omentale [NA], SYN epiploic f.

optic f., SYN optic *canal*.

f. op′ticum, SYN optic *canal*.

f. ova′le, oval f., (1) [NA] in the fetal heart, the oval opening in the septum secundum; the persistent part of the septum primum acts as a valve for this interatrial communication during fetal life and normally postnatally becomes fused to the septum secundum to close it; **(2)** [NA] a large oval opening in the base of the greater wing of the sphenoid bone, transmitting the mandibular nerve and a small meningeal artery; **(3)** valvular incompetence of the f. ovale of the heart; a condition contrasting with probe patency of the f. ovale in that the valvula foraminis ovalis has abnormal perforations in it, or is of insufficient size to afford adequate valvular action at the f. ovale prenatally, or effect a complete closure postnatally.

foram′ina palati′na mino′ra [NA], SYN lesser palatine foramina.

f. palati′num ma′jus [NA], SYN greater palatine f.

foram′ina papilla′ria re′nis [NA], SYN papillary foramina of kidney.

papillary foramina of kidney, numerous minute openings, the apertures of the papillary ducts converging on the apical pole of each renal papilla. SYN foramina papillaria renis [NA].

parietal f., an inconstant f. in the parietal bone occasionally found bilaterally near the sagittal margin posteriorly; when present it transmits an emissary vein to the superior sagittal sinus. SYN f. parietale [NA].

f. parieta′le [NA], SYN parietal f.

petrosal f., an occasional opening in the greater wing of the sphenoid bone, between the f. spinosum and f. ovale, which transmits the lesser petrosal nerve. SYN f. petrosum [NA], canaliculus innominatus, f. of Arnold.

f. petro′sum [NA], SYN petrosal f.

pleuroperitoneal f., SYN f. cecum of tongue.

posterior condyloid f., SYN condylar *canal*.

posterior palatine foramina, SYN lesser palatine foramina.

postglenoid f., a small f. that is sometimes present in the temporal bone immediately in front of the external acoustic meatus.

primary interatrial f., SYN interatrial f. primum.

f. proces′sus transver′si [NA], SYN transverse f.

f. quadra′tum, SYN vena caval f.

Retzius' f., SYN lateral *aperture* of the fourth ventricle.

root f., SYN apical f. of tooth.

fo

f. rotun′dum [NA], an opening in the base of the greater wing of the sphenoid bone, transmitting the maxillary nerve. SYN round f.

round f., SYN f. rotundum.

sacral f., one of the openings between the fused sacral vertebrae transmitting the sacral nerves. The anterior sacral foramina transmit ventral primary rami of the sacral nerves. The posterior sacral foramina give passage to dorsal primary rami of the sacral nerves. SYN f. sacrale [NA].

f. sacra′le [NA], SYN sacral f.

Scarpa's foramina, two openings in the line of the intermaxillary suture; the anterior f. transmits the left nasopalatine nerve, the posterior the right.

sciatic f., either of two foramina formed by the sacrospinous and sacrotuberous ligaments crossing the sciatic notches of the hip bone: greater sciatic f. and lesser sciatic f. SYN f. ischiadicum [NA].

secondary interatrial f., SYN interatrial f. secundum.

f. singula′re [NA], SYN solitary f.

foramina of the smallest veins of heart, SYN foramina of the venae minimae.

solitary f., a f. in the internal acoustic meatus, posterior to the cochlear area, that transmits the nerves to the ampulla of the posterior semicircular duct. SYN f. singulare [NA].

sphenopalatine f., the f. formed from the sphenopalatine notch of the palatine bone in articulation with the sphenoid bone; it transmits the sphenopalatine artery and accompanying nerves. SYN f. sphenopalatinum [NA].

f. sphenopalati′num [NA], SYN sphenopalatine f.

sphenotic f., SYN f. lacerum.

f. spino′sum [NA], an opening in the base of the greater wing of the sphenoid bone, anterior to the spine of the sphenoid, transmitting the middle meningeal artery.

Stensen's f., SYN f. incisive f.

stylomastoid f., the distal or external opening of the facial canal on the inferior surface of the petrous portion of the temporal bone, between the styloid and mastoid processes; it transmits the facial nerve and stylomastoid artery. SYN f. stylomastoideum [NA].

f. stylomastoid′eum [NA], SYN stylomastoid f.

f. subsepta′le, SYN interatrial f. primum.

supraorbital f., a f. in the supraorbital margin of the frontal bone at the junction of the medial and intermediate thirds. SYN f. supraorbitale [NA].

f. supraorbita′le [NA], SYN supraorbital f. SEE ALSO supraorbital notch.

thebesian foramina, SYN foramina of the venae minimae.

thyroid f., an opening occasionally existing in one or both of the plates of the thyroid cartilage. SYN f. thyroideum [NA].

f. thyroid′eum [NA], SYN thyroid f.

f. transversa′rium [NA], SYN transverse f.

transverse f., f. processus transversus. SYN f. processus transversi [NA], f. transversarium [NA], f. vertebroarterialis [NA], f. of transverse process, vertebroarterial f.

f. of transverse process, SYN transverse f.

f. of vena cava, SYN vena caval f.

vena caval f., an opening in the right lobe of the central tendon of the diaphragm which transmits the inferior vena cava and branches of the right phrenic nerve. SYN f. venae cavae [NA], f. of vena cava, f. quadratum.

f. ve′nae ca′vae [NA], SYN vena caval f.

foramina of the venae minimae, a number of fossae in the wall of the right atrium, containing the openings of minute intramural veins. SYN foramina venarum minimarum cordis [NA], foramina of the smallest veins of heart, Lannelongue's foramina, thebesian foramina, Vieussens' foramina.

foram′ina vena′rum minima′rum cordis [NA], SYN foramina of the venae minimae.

f. veno′sum [NA], a minute inconstant f. in the greater wing of the sphenoid bone, anterior and medial to the f. ovale, transmitting a small emissary vein from the cavernous sinus. SYN emissary sphenoidal f., venous f., Vesalius' f.

venous f., SYN f. venosum.

vertebral f., the f. formed by the union of the vertebral arch with the body; in the articulated vertebral column, the vertebral f. collectively form the vertebral column. SYN f. vertebrale [NA].

f. vertebra′le [NA], SYN vertebral f.

vertebroarterial f., SYN transverse f.

f. vertebroarteria′lis [NA], SYN transverse f.

Vesalius' f., SYN f. venosum.

Vicq d'Azyr's f., SYN f. cecum medullae oblongatae.

Vieussens' foramina, SYN foramina of the venae minimae.

Weitbrecht's f., an opening in the articular capsule of the shoulder joint, communicating with the subtendinous bursa of the subscapularis muscle.

Winslow's f., SYN epiploic f.

zygomaticofacial f., the opening on the lateral surface of the zygomatic bone below the orbital margin that transmits the zygomaticofacial nerve. SYN f. zygomaticofaciale [NA], malar f.

f. zygomaticofacia′le [NA], SYN zygomaticofacial f.

zygomatico-orbital f., the common opening on the orbital surface of the zygomatic bone of the canals transmitting the zygomaticofacial and zygomaticotemporal nerves; sometimes each of these canals has a separate opening on the orbital surface. SYN f. zygomatico-orbitale [NA].

f. zygomat′ico-orbita′le [NA], SYN zygomatico-orbital f.

zygomaticotemporal f., the opening, on the temporal surface of the zygomatic bone, of the canal that gives passage to the zygomaticotemporal nerve. SYN f. zygomaticotemporale [NA].

f. zygomat′icotempora′le [NA], SYN zygomaticotemporal f.

---

fo·ram·i·na (fō-ram′i-nă). Plural of foramen.

Fo·ram·i·nif·e·ra (fō-ram-i-nif′er-ă, for′ă-mi-nif′er-ă). A subclass of Rhizopoda possessing anastomosing pseudopodia; these form a network around the cell which usually develops into a complex calcareous shell; an important component of the ocean bottom and of rockbeds overlying oil deposits. [L. *foramen,* aperture, + *fero,* to carry]

fo·ram·i·nif·er·ous (fō-ram-i-nif′er-ŭs, fōr′ă-mi-nif′er-ŭs). **1.** Possessing openings or foramina. **2.** Relating to the Foraminifera.

for·am·i·not·o·my (fōr′am-i-not′ō-mē). An operation upon an aperture, usually to open it, *e.g.,* surgical enlargement of the intervertebral foramen. [L. *foramen,* aperture, + G. *tomē,* a cutting]

fo·ra·min·u·lum, pl. **fo·ra·min·u·la** (fōr′ă-min′yū-lŭm, yū-lă). A very minute foramen. [Mod. L. dim. of *foramen*]

Forbes, A.P., 20th century U.S. physician. SEE F.-Albright *syndrome.*

Forbes, Gilbert B., U.S. pediatrician, *1915. SEE F.'s *disease.*

Forbes, Thomas R. SEE Hooker-F. *test.*

force (F) (fōrs). That which tends to produce motion in a body. [L. *fortis,* strong]

animal f., muscular power.

chewing f., SYN masticatory f.

dynamic f., SYN energy.

electromotive f. (EMF), the f. (measured in volts) that causes the flow of electricity from one point to another.

G f., inertial f. produced by accelerations or gravity, expressed in gravitational units; one G is equal to the pull of gravity at the earth's surface at sea level and 45° North latitude (32.1725 ft/sec^2; 980.621 cm/sec^2). SEE ALSO γ.

London f.'s, SYN van der Waals' f.'s.

f. of mastication, the motive f. created by the dynamic action of the muscles during the physiologic act of mastication. SYN biting strength, masticatory f.

masticatory f., SYN f. of mastication. SYN chewing f.

nerve f., nervous f., obsolete terms denoting the property of nerve tissue to conduct stimuli.

occlusal f., the result of muscular f. applied on opposing teeth.

psychic f., SYN psychic *energy.*

reciprocal f.'s, in dentistry, f.'s whereby the resistance of one or more teeth is utilized to move one or more opposing teeth.

reserve f., the energy residing in the organism or any of its parts above that required for its normal functioning.

van der Waals' f.'s, first postulated by van der Waals in 1873 to explain deviations from ideal gas behavior seen in real gases; the attractive f.'s between atoms or molecules other than electrostatic (ionic), covalent (sharing of electrons), or hydrogen bonding (sharing a proton); generally ascribed to dipolar and dispersion effects, π-electrons, etc.; these relatively nondescript f.'s contribute to the mutual attraction of organic molecules. SYN London f.'s.

vital f., SEE vitalism.

force plat·form. A device used to measure the strength, symmetry, and latency of compensatory postural movements when visual, vestibular, and somatosensory stimuli are varied.

for·ceps (fōr'seps). **1.** An instrument for seizing a structure, and making compression or traction. Cf. clamp. **2** [NA]. Bands of white fibers in the brain, major f. and minor f. [L. a pair of tongs]

Adson f., a small thumb f. with two teeth on one tip and one tooth on the other.

alligator f., a long f. with a small hinged jaw on the end.

Allis f., a straight grasping f. with serrated jaws, used to forcibly grasp or retract tissues or structures.

f. anterior, SYN minor f.

Arruga's f., f. for the intracapsular extraction of a cataract.

arterial f., a locking f. with sloping blades for grasping the end of a blood vessel until a ligature is applied.

axis-traction f., obstetrical f. provided with a second handle so attached that traction can be made in the line in which the head must move in the axis of the pelvis.

Barton's f., an obstetrical f. with one fixed curved blade and a hinged anterior blade for application to a high transverse head.

bayonet f., f. with offset blades, such as those for use through an otoscope.

bone f., a strong f. used for seizing or removing fragments of bone.

Brown-Adson f., an Adson f. with about 16 delicate teeth on each tip.

bulldog f., a f. for occluding a blood vessel.

bullet f., a f. with thin curved blades with serrated grasping surfaces, for extracting a bullet from tissues.

capsule f., f. used for removing the capsule of the lens in extracapsular extraction of a cataract.

Chamberlen f., the original obstetrical f., without a curvature.

clamp f., a f. with pronged jaws designed to engage the jaws of a rubber dam clamp so that they may be separated to pass over the widest buccolingual contour of a tooth. SYN rubber dam clamp f.

clip f., a small f. with spring catch to hold a bleeding vessel.

cup biopsy f., a slender flexible f. with movable cup-shaped jaws, used to obtain biopsy specimens by introduction through a specially designed endoscope.

cutting f., SYN labitome.

DeBakey f., nontraumatic f. used to pick up blood vessels.

dental f., f. used to luxate teeth and remove them from the alveolus. SYN extracting f.

dressing f., a f. for general use in dressing wounds, removing fragments of necrosed tissue, small foreign bodies, etc.

Evans f., a thumb f. with points designed to resemble a needle holder, used to grasp curved needles during various suture procedures.

extracting f., SYN dental f.

Graefe f., a small thumb f. with one horizontal row of six or eight delicate teeth across each tip.

hemostatic f., a f. with a catch for locking the blades, used for seizing the end of a blood vessel to control hemorrhage.

jeweller's f., a small thumb f. with very fine pointed blades, used to grasp tissues in microsurgical procedures.

Kjelland's f., an obstetrical f. having a sliding lock, and little pelvic curve.

Lahey f., thyroid f. used to deliver the uterus in vaginohysterectomy.

Laplace's f., a f. for approximating intestines during surgical anastomosis.

Levret's f., a modification of the Chamberlen f., curved to correspond to the curve of the parturient passage.

lion-jaw bone-holding f., a sturdy f. with strong sharp teeth in the jaws, used for holding bone fragments.

Löwenberg's f., f. with short curved blades ending in rounded grasping extremities devised for the removal of adenoid growths in the nasopharynx.

f. ma'jor [NA], SYN major f.

major f., occipital radiation of the corpus callosum; that part of the fiber radiation of the corpus callosum which bends sharply backward into the occipital lobe of the cerebrum. SYN f. major [NA], f. posterior, occipital part of corpus callosum, pars occipitalis corporis callosi.

f. mi'nor [NA], SYN minor f.

minor f., frontal radiation of the corpus callosum; that part of the fiber radiation of the corpus callosum which bends forward toward the frontal pole of the cerebrum. SYN f. minor [NA], f. anterior, frontal part of corpus callosum, pars frontalis corporis callosi.

mosquito f., SYN mosquito *clamp*.

mouse-tooth f., a f. with one or two fine points at the tip of each blade, fitting into hollows between the points on the opposite blade.

needle f., SYN needle-holder.

nonfenestrated f., obstetrical f. without openings in the blades, thus facilitating rotation of the head.

obstetrical f., f. used for grasping and applying traction to or for rotation of the fetal head; the blades are introduced separately into the genital canal, permitting the fetal head to be grasped firmly but with minimal compression, and then are articulated after being placed in correct position.

O'Hara f., two slender clamp f.'s held together by a serrefine, once used in intestinal anastomosis; now obsolete.

Piper's f., obstetrical f. used to facilitate delivery of the head in breech presentation.

f. poste'rior, SYN major f.

Randall stone f., a f. with variably curved slender blades and serrated jaws, used to extract calculi from the renal pelvis or calices.

rubber dam clamp f., SYN clamp f.

Simpson's f., an obstetrical f.

speculum f., a tubular f. for use through a speculum.

Tarnier's f., a type of axis-traction f.

tenaculum f., a f. with jaws armed each with a sharp, straight hook like a tenaculum.

thumb f., a spring f. used by compression with thumb and forefinger.

tubular f., a long slender f. intended for use through a cannula or other tubular instrument.

Tucker-McLean f., a type of axis-traction f.

vulsella f., vulsellum f., a f. with hooks at the tip of each blade. SYN volsella, vulsella, vulsellum.

Willett's f., obsolete term for a traction f. used to treat placenta previa by pulling the fetal head down against the placenta.

Forchheimer, Frederick, U.S. physician, 1853–1913. SEE F.'s *sign*.

for·ci·pate (fōr'si-pāt). Shaped like a forceps.

for·ci·pres·sure (fōr'si-presh-ŭr). A method of arresting hemorrhage by compressing a blood vessel with forceps.

Fordyce, John A., U.S. dermatologist, 1858–1925. SEE F.'s *angiokeratoma, disease, granules,* under *granule, spots,* under *spot;* Fox-F. *disease.*

fore·arm (fōr'arm). The segment of the upper limb between the elbow and the wrist. SYN antebrachium [NA].

fore·brain (fōr'brān). SYN prosencephalon.

fore·con·scious (fōr'kon-shŭs). Denoting memories, not at present in the consciousness, which can be evoked from time to time, or an unconscious mental process which becomes conscious only on the fulfillment of certain conditions. Cf. preconscious.

fore·fin·ger (fōr'fing'ger). SYN index *finger*.

fore·foot (fōr'fut). A front foot of a quadruped.

fore·gut (fōr'gŭt). The cephalic portion of the primitive digestive tube in the embryo. From its endoderm arises the epithelial lining of the pharynx, trachea, lungs, esophagus, and stomach, the first part and cranial half of the second part of the duodenum, and the parenchyma of the liver, gallbladder, and pancreas. SYN headgut.

fore·head (fōr'ed, fōr'hed). The part of the face between the eyebrows and the hairy scalp. SYN frons [NA], brow (2).

olympian f., the abnormally prominent, high, and broad f. in hereditary syphilis.

fore·kid·ney (fōr'kid-nē). SYN pronephros.

Forel, Auguste H., Swiss neurologist, 1848–1931. SEE F.'s *decussation; fields* of F., under *field; tegmental fields* of F. under *field*.

fore·lock (fō'lok). The lock of hair that grows just above the forehead.

white forelock, a triangular or diamond-shaped depigmented macule with white hairs, usually located in the anterior midline of the scalp, seen in piebaldism.

fore·milk (fōr'milk). SYN colostrum.

fo·ren·sic (fō-ren'sik). Pertaining or applicable to personal injury, murder, and other legal proceedings. [L. *forensis,* of a forum]

fore·play (fōr'plā). Stimulative sexual activity preceding sexual intercourse.

fore·pleas·ure (fōr'plezh'er, plā'zher). Sexual pleasure resulting from the foreplay that precedes the genital-orgastic pleasure in sexual intercourse.

fore·skin (fōr'skin). SYN prepuce.

Forestier, Jacques, French rheumatologist, *1890. SEE F.'s *disease*.

fore·stom·ach (fōr'stŭm'ŭk). SYN antrum cardiacum.

fore·wa·ters (fōr'wah-terz). Colloquialism for the bulging fluid-filled amniotic membrane presenting in front of the fetal head.

for·get·ting. Being unable to retrieve or recall information that was once registered, learned, and stored in short- or long-term memory.

fork (fōrk). **1.** A pronged instrument used for holding or lifting. **2.** An instrument resembling a f. in that it has tines or prongs.

bite f., SYN face-bow f.

face-bow f., that part of the face-bow assemblage used to attach the maxillary trial base to the face-bow proper. SYN bite f.

tuning f., a steel or magnesium-alloy instrument roughly resembling a two-pronged f., the vibrations of the prongs of which, when struck, give a musical note of restricted band width; used to test the hearing and vibratory sensation.

form (fōrm). Shape; mold. [L. *forma*]

accolé f.'s (ak-ōlā'), SYN appliqué f.'s.

appliqué f.'s (ap-li-kā'), a term applied to the manner in which the ring stage of *Plasmodium falciparum* parasitizes the marginal portion of erythrocytes. SYN accolé f.'s.

arch f., the shape and contour of the dental arch, or of an orthodontic wire formed to the shape of that arch.

boat f., the less stable of two conformations assumed by 6-membered cyclic sugars (pyranoses) or cyclohexane derivatives, as opposed to chair f. SEE ALSO Haworth conformational formulas of cyclic *sugars*.

cavity preparation f., the configuration or shape of a cavity preparation.

chair f., the more stable of two conformations assumed by 6-membered cyclic sugars (*e.g.,* the pyranoses) or cyclohexane derivatives, as opposed to boat f. SEE ALSO Haworth conformational formulas of cyclic *sugars*.

convenience f., the changes needed outside the basic outline f. to enable proper instrumentation for the cavity preparation and insertion of a dental restoration.

extension f., the extension of the cavity preparation outline f. to include areas of incipient carious lesions; this extension provides

a dental restoration with margins that are self-cleansing or easily cleaned.

face f., (1) the outline f. of the face; **(2)** the outline f. of the face from an anterior view.

half-chair f., SEE Haworth conformational formulas of cyclic *sugars*.

involution f., an irregular or atypical bacterial cell produced as a result of exposure to unfavorable conditions.

L f., SEE L-phase *variants,* under *variant*.

occlusal f., the f. of the occlusal surface of a tooth or a row of teeth. SYN occlusal pattern.

outline f., the shape of the area of the tooth surface included within the cavosurface margins of the cavity preparation of a dental restoration.

posterior tooth f., the distinguishing contours of the occlusal surface of the various posterior teeth.

replicative f. (RF), (1) an intermediate stage in the replication of either DNA or RNA viral genomes that is usually double stranded; **(2)** the altered, double-stranded f. to which single-stranded coliphage DNA is converted after infection of a susceptible bacterium, formation of the complementary ("minus") strand being mediated by enzymes that were present in the bacterium before entrance of the viral ("plus") strand.

resistance f., the shape given to a cavity preparation that enables the dental restoration to withstand masticatory forces.

retention f., the shape of a cavity preparation that prevents displacement of the dental restoration by lateral or tipping forces as well as masticatory forces.

sickle f., SYN malarial *crescent*.

skew f., SEE Haworth conformational formulas of cyclic *sugars*.

tooth f., the characteristics of the curves, lines, angles, and contours of various teeth which permit their identification and differentiation.

twist f., SEE Haworth conformational formulas of cyclic *sugars*.

wave f., the f. of a pulse; *e.g.,* an arterial pressure or displacement wave; or of the pacemaker pulse as demonstrated on the oscilloscope under a specified load. SYN waveshape.

wax f., SYN wax *pattern*.

△**-form.** In the form, shape of; equivalent to -oid. SEE morpho-. [L. -*formis*]

Formad, Henry, U.S. physician, 1847–1892. SEE F.'s *kidney*.

form·al·de·hyde (fōr-mal'dĕ-hīd). A pungent gas, HCHO; used as an antiseptic, disinfectant, and histologic fixative. SYN formic aldehyde, methyl aldehyde. [form(ic) + aldehyde]

active f., (1) a hydroxymethyl derivative of tetrahydrofolate or thiamin pyrophosphate; **(2)** N^5,N^{10}-methylenetetrahydrofo late.

for·ma·lin (fōr'mă-lin). A 37% aqueous solution of formaldehyde. SYN formol.

for·ma·lin·ize (fōr-mă-li-nīz). To add formalin solution to inactivate vaccines without destroying their immunizing power.

for·mam·i·dase (fōr-mam'i-dās). An enzyme catalyzing the hydrolysis of N-formyl-L-kynurenine to L-kynurenine and formate, a reaction of significance in L-tryptophan catabolism. SYN formylase, kynurenine formamidase.

5-for·mam·i·do·im·id·a·zole-4-car·box·im·ide ri·bo·tide. An intermediate in purine biosynthesis.

for·mate (fōr'māt). A salt or ester of formic acid; *i.e.,* the monovalent radical HCOO– or the anion HCOO⁻.

active f., N^{10}-formyltetrahydrofolate or an equivalent oxidation product of tetrahydrofolate.

for·ma·tio, pl. **for·ma·ti·o·nes** (fōr-mā'shē-ō, -ō'nēz) [NA]. **1.** SYN formation. **2.** A structure of definite shape or cellular arrangement. [L. fr. *formo,* pp. -*atus,* to form]

f. hippocampa'lis, hippocampal formation. SEE hippocampus.

f. reticula'ris [NA], SYN reticular *formation*.

for·ma·tion (fōr-mā'shŭn). **1.** A formation; a structure of definite shape or cellular arrangement. **2.** That which is formed. **3.** The act of giving form and shape. SYN formatio (1) [NA].

concept f., in psychology, the learning to conceive and respond in terms of abstract ideas based upon an action or object.

personality f., the life history associated with the development of individual patterns and of one's individuality.

reaction f., in psychoanalysis, a postulated defense mechanism in which attitudes and behaviors that are adopted are the opposites of that which the individual would ordinarily be expected to express and actually feel at an unconscious level.

reticular f. (RF), a massive but vaguely delimited neural apparatus composed of closely intermingled gray and white matter and extending throughout the central core of the brainstem into the diencephalon; the term refers to the large neuronal population of the brainstem that does not compose motoneuronal cell groups or cell groups forming part of specific sensory conduction systems; its neurons generally have long dendrites and heterogeneous afferent connections, the reason why the f. is often called "nonspecific"; the reticular f. has complex, largely polysynaptic ascending and descending connections that play a role in the central control of autonomic (respiration, blood pressure, thermoregulation, etc.) and endocrine functions, as well as in bodily posture, skeletomuscular reflex activity, and general behavioral states such as alertness and sleep. SYN formatio reticularis [NA], reticular substance (2), substantia reticularis (2).

rouleaux f., the arrangement of red blood cells in fluid blood (or in diluted suspensions) with their biconcave surfaces in apposition, thereby forming groups that resemble stacks of coins. SYN false agglutination (2), pseudoagglutination (2). [Fr. pl. of *rouleau,* a roll]

symptom f., SYN symptom *substitution.*

for·ma·ti·o·nes (fōr-mā′shē-ō′nēz). Plural of formatio.

for·ma·zan (fōr′mă-zan). A water-insoluble colored compound of the general structure, RNH—N=CR′—N=NR″, formed by reduction of a tetrazolium salt in the histochemical demonstration of oxidative enzymes; the R's are usually phenyl groups; examples include neotetrazolium, blue tetrazolium, and nitro blue tetrazolium.

form·board (fōrm′bōrd). A board containing cut-outs in various shapes, into which blocks of corresponding shape are to be fitted; a neuropsychological test of which the Tactual Performance Test of the Halstead-Reitan Battery is an example. SEE Halstead-Reitan *battery.*

forme fruste, pl. **formes frustes** (fōrm′ frŭst′). A partial, arrested, or inapparent form of disease. [Fr. unfinished form]

for·mic (fōr′mik). **1.** Pertaining to f. acid. **2.** Relating to ants. [L. *formica,* ant]

for·mic ac·id. HCOOH; the smallest carboxylic acid; a strong caustic, used as an astringent and counterirritant.

for·mic al·de·hyde. SYN formaldehyde.

for·mi·ca·tion (fōr-mi-kā′shŭn). A form of paresthesia or tactile hallucination; a sensation as if small insects are creeping under the skin. [L. *formica,* ant]

for·mim·i·no·glu·tam·ic ac·id (FIGLU) (fōr-mim′i-nō-glū-tam′ik). HN=CH–NH–CH(COOH)CH₂CH₂ COOH; an intermediate metabolite in L-histidine catabolism in the conversion of L-histidine to L-glutamic acid, with the formimino group being transferred to tetrahydrofolic acid; it may appear in the urine of patients with folic acid or vitamin B_{12} deficiency, or liver disease.

***N*-for·mim·i·no·tet·ra·hy·dro·fo·late** (for-mim′i-nō-tet′ră-hī-drō-fō′lāt). A derivative of one-carbon tetrahydrofolate formed via L-histidine catabolism.

for·mo·cre·sol (fōr-mō-krē′sol). An aqueous solution containing cresol, formaldehyde, and glycerine, used in vital primary teeth needing coronal pulpotomy.

for·mol (fōr′mol). SYN formalin.

for·mo·sul·fa·thi·a·zole (fōr′mō-sŭl-fă-thī′ă-zol). N^1-(2-Thiazolyl)sulfanilamide condensation product with formaldehyde; an antimicrobial agent for treatment of intestinal infections.

FORMULA

for·mu·la, pl. **for·mu·las, for·mu·lae** (fōr′myū-lă, -lăz, -lē). **1.** A recipe or prescription containing directions for the compounding of a medicinal preparation. **2.** In chemistry, a symbol or collection of symbols expressing the number of atoms of the element or elements forming one molecule of a substance, together with, on occasion, information concerning the arrangement of the atoms within the molecule, their electronic structure, their charge, the nature of the bonds within the molecule, etc. **3.** An expression by symbols and numbers of the normal order or arrangement of parts or structures. [L. dim. of *forma,* form]

Arneth f., the normal, approximate ratio of polymorphonuclear neutrophils, based on the number of lobes in the nuclei, as follows: 1 lobe, 5%; 2 lobes, 35%; 3 lobes, 41%; 4 lobes, 17%; 5 lobes, 2%.

Bazett's f., a f. for correcting the observed Q-T interval in the electrocardiogram for cardiac rate: corrected Q-T = Q-T sec/√R − R sec.

Bernhardt's f., a f. used to calculate the ideal weight, in kilograms, for an adult; it is the height in centimeters times the chest circumference in centimeters divided by 240.

Black's f., a translation of Pignet's f. into British measurements: $F = (W + C) − H$; F is the empirical factor, W is the weight in pounds, C the chest girth in inches at full inspiration, and H the height in inches; a man is classed as very strong when F is over 120, strong between 110 and 120, good 100 to 110, fair 90 to 100, weak 80 to 90, very weak under 80.

Broca's f., a fully developed man (30 years old) should weigh as many kilograms as he is centimeters in height over and above 1 meter.

chemical f., a statement of the structure of a molecule expressed in chemical symbols.

Christison's f., SYN Häser's f.

constitutional f., SYN structural f.

Demoivre's f., an obsolete f. for calculating life expectancy.

dental f., a statement in tabular form of the number of each kind of teeth in the jaw; the dental f. for man is, for the deciduous teeth:

$$i. \frac{2-2}{2-2}, c. \frac{1-1}{1-1}, m. \frac{2-2}{2-2} = 20$$

for the permanent teeth:

$$i. \frac{2-2}{2-2}, c. \frac{1-1}{1-1}, bic. \frac{2-2}{2-2}, m. \frac{3-3}{3-3} = 32.$$

Dreyer's f., an obsolete f. indicating relationship between vital capacity and body surface area.

DuBois' f., a f. for predicting a man's surface area from weight and height: $A = 71.84W^{0.425} H^{0.725}$, where A = surface area in cm², W = weight in kg, and H = height in cm.

electrical f., a graphic representation by means of symbols of the reaction of a muscle to an electrical stimulus.

empirical f., in chemistry, a f. indicating the kind and number of atoms in the molecules of a substance, or its composition, but not the relation of the atoms to each other or the intimate structure of the molecule. SYN molecular f.

Fischer's projection formulas, SEE Fischer projection formulas of *sugars.*

Flesch f., a method of determining the difficulty of a written passage by a formulation that provides an estimate of how many people in the U.S. would be able to read and understand the passage; used in determining patient comprehension of hospital consent forms.

Florschütz' f., the correct relation of height to the abdominal circumference: $L: (2B − L)$, L representing the individual's height, and B the circumference of the abdomen; the normal value so determined would be 5, and any below that would indicate obesity.

Gorlin f., a f. for calculating the area of the orifice of a cardiac valve, based on flow across the valve and the mean pressures in the chambers on either side of the valve.

graphic f., SYN structural f.

Hamilton-Stewart f., SYN Hamilton-Stewart *method.*

Häser's f., a f. to determine the number of grams of urinary solids per liter, obtained by multiplying 2.33 by the last two figures of the specific gravity of the urine. SYN Christison's f., Trapp's f., Trapp-Häser f.

Haworth perspective and conformational formulas, SEE Haworth perspective formulas of cyclic *sugars.*

Jellinek f., a method of estimating the prevalence of alcoholism in a nation's population, based on the assumption that a predictable proportion of persons addicted to alcohol die of cirrhosis of the liver.

Ledermann f., a f. to calculate alcohol dependancy levels. Ledermann showed empirically that the distribution of alcohol consumption in a population is log normal; the formula used this observation to estimate the prevalence of various degrees of alcohol dependency. Some questions have been raised about the validity of Ledermann's observations.

Long's f., a f. for estimating from the specific gravity of a specimen of urine the approximate amount of solids in grams per liter; the last two figures of the value for specific gravity are multiplied by 2.6. SYN Long's coefficient.

Mall's f., a f. for determining the age (in days) of a human embryo; calculated as the square root of its length (measured from vertex to breech) in millimeters multiplied by 100.

Meeh f., SYN Meeh-Dubois f.

Meeh-Dubois f., a f. for predicting surface area, assuming that it is proportional to the 2/3 power of the body weight. SYN Meeh f.

molecular f., SYN empirical f.

official f., a f. contained in the Pharmacopeia or the National Formulary.

Pignet's f., SEE Black's f.

Poisson-Pearson f., a f. to determine the statistical error in calculating the endemic index of malaria: let N = total number of children under 15 years in a locality; n = total number examined for the spleen-rate; x = number found with enlarged spleen; $(x/n)100$ = spleen-rate; $e\%$ = percentage of error; the percentage error will be, by this f.:

$$e\% = \frac{200}{n}\sqrt{\frac{2x(n-x)}{n}}\sqrt{1-\frac{n-1}{N-1}}.$$

Ranke's f., A = grams of albumin per liter of a serous fluid: then, A = (sp. gr. - 1000) × 0.52 - 5.406.

rational f., in chemistry, a f. that indicates the constitution as well as the composition of a substance.

Reuss' f., a means of estimating the approximate amount of albumin in a transudate or exudate; 3/8 (sp. gr. - 1.000) - 2.8 results in a value that is a practicable indication of the percentage of albumin in the fluid.

Runeberg's f., a f. for estimating the percentage of albumin in a serous fluid, similar to Reuss' f. except that, instead of 2.8, 2.73 is subtracted in the instance of a transudate, and 2.88 in that of an inflammatory exudate.

spatial f., SYN stereochemical f.

stereochemical f., a chemical f. in which the arrangement of the atoms or atomic groupings in space are indicated. SYN spatial f.

structural f., a f. in which the connections of the atoms and groups of atoms, as well as their kind and number, are indicated. SYN constitutional f., graphic f.

Toronto f. for pulmonary artery banding, a technique that provides a general guide for the size of the band relative to the patient's weight.

Trapp-Häser f., SYN Häser's f.

Trapp's f., SYN Häser's f.

Van Slyke's f., SYN standard urea *clearance.*

vertebral f., a f. indicating the number of vertebrae in each segment of the spinal column; for man it is C. 7, T. 12, L. 5, S. 5, Co. 4 = 33, the letters standing for cervical, thoracic, lumbar, sacral, and coccygeal.

for·mu·lary (fōr'myū-lā-rē). A collection of formulas for the compounding of medicinal preparations. SEE National Formulary, Pharmacopeia.

hospital f., a continually revised compilation of approved pharmaceuticals, plus important ancillary information, that reflects the current clinical judgment of the institution's medical staff.

for·myl (f) (fōr'mil). The radical, HCO–.

active f., the f. group taking part in transformylation reactions with a folic acid derivative in the role of carrier.

formyl-methionyl-f., SYN initiation tRNA.

for·my·lase (fōr'mi-lās). SYN formamidase.

N-**for·myl·gly·cin·a·mide ri·bo·tide (FGAR).** An intermediate in purine biosynthesis.

N-**for·myl·ky·nur·e·nine** (en-fōr'mil-ki-nūr'ĕ-nēn). The product of the oxidative cleavage of the indole ring in L-tryptophan; the intermediate first formed in L-tryptophan catabolism.

for·myl·me·thi·o·nine (fMet) (fōr'mil-me-thī'ō-nēn). Methionine acylated on the NH_2 group by a formyl (–CHO) group. This is the starting amino acid residue for virtually all bacterial polypeptides. SEE ALSO initiating *codon.* SYN *N*-formylmethionine.

N-**for·myl·meth·i·o·nine.** SYN formylmethionine.

for·myl·me·thi·o·nyl-tRNA. Initiation tRNA in certain organisms.

N^{10}-**for·myl·tet·ra·hy·dro·fo·late.** A formyl derivative of tetrahydrofolate that serves as a one-carbon source in metabolism.

Forney, William R., U.S. pediatrician, *1931.

for·ni·cate (fōr'ni-kāt). **1.** Vaulted or arched; resembling a fornix. [L. *fornicatus,* arched, fr. *fornix,* vault, arch] **2.** To have sexual intercourse. [see fornication]

for·ni·ca·tion (fōr-ni-kā'shŭn). Sexual intercourse, especially between unmarried partners. [L. *fornicatio,* an arched or vaulted basement (brothel)]

for·ni·ces (fōr'ni-sēz). Plural of fornix.

for·nix, gen. **for·ni·cis,** pl. **for·ni·ces** (fōr'niks, -ni-sis, -ni-sēz). **1** [NA]. In general, an arch-shaped structure; often the arch-shaped roof (or roof portion) of an anatomical space. **2** [NA]. The compact, white fiber bundle by which the hippocampus of each cerebral hemisphere projects to the contralateral hippocampus and to the septum, anterior nucleus of the thalamus, and mamillary body. Arising from pyramidal cells of Ammon's horn, the fibers of the f. form the alveus hippocampi and the fimbria hippocampi, and in their further course compose, sequentially, the crus fornicis, body of fornix, commissura fornicis, and column of fornix; the f. fibers to the septum issue from the upper part of the column of fornix, passing in part anterior to the anterior commissure as the precommissural f., while all others follow the compact postcommissural f. bundle to the anterior thalamic nucleus and mamillary body. SYN trigonum cerebrale. SYN cerebral trigone. [L. arch, vault]

f. conjuncti'vae [NA], SYN conjunctival f.

conjunctival f., the space formed by the junction of the bulbar and palpebral portions of the conjunctiva, that of the upper lid being the f. conjunctivae superior and that of the lower lid the f. conjunctivae inferior. SYN f. conjunctivae [NA], conjunctival cul-de-sac, retrotarsal fold.

f. of the lacrimal sac, fornix of the lacrimal sac; the upper, blind end of the lacrimal sac that extends above the openings of the lacrimal canaliculi. SYN f. sacci lacrimalis [NA].

pharyngeal f., the non-muscular upper end of the nasopharynx where the pharyngeal mucosa is firmly applied to the body of the sphenoid bone and to pharyngobasilar fascia. SYN f. pharyngis [NA].

f. pharyn'gis [NA], SYN pharyngeal f.

f. sac'ci lacrima'lis [NA], SYN f. of the lacrimal sac.

transverse f., SYN *commissura* fornicis.

f. u'teri, SYN vaginal f.

f. vagi'nae [NA], SYN vaginal f.

vaginal f., the recess at the vault of the vagina; it is divided into an anterior part, posterior part, and lateral part with respect to its relation to the cervix of the uterus. The posterior part is clinically significant as the site for culdocentesis and culdoscopy. The proximity of the ureter (below) and the uterine artery (above) adjacent to the lateral fornix is important clinically. SYN f. vaginae [NA], f. uteri.

Forssman, Hans, Swedish physician, *1912. SEE Börjeson-F.-Lehmann *syndrome.*

Forssman, John, Swedish bacteriologist and pathologist, 1868–1947. SEE F. *antibody, antigen, reaction,* antigen-antibody *reaction.*

Förster, Richard, German ophthalmologist, 1825–1902. SEE F.'s *uveitis.*

fos·car·net (fos-kar′net). Trisodium phosphonoformate; a pyrophosphate analogue antiviral drug.

Fosdick, Leonard S., U.S. chemist, *1903. SEE F.-Hansen-Epple *test.*

Foshay, Lee, U.S. bacteriologist, 1896–1961. SEE F. *test.*

FOSSA

fos·sa, gen. and pl. **fos·sae** (fos′ă, fos′ē) [NA]. A depression usually more or less longitudinal in shape below the level of the surface of a part. [L. a trench or ditch]

acetabular f., a depressed area in the floor of the acetabulum superior to the acetabular notch. SYN f. acetabuli [NA].

f. acetab′uli [NA], SYN acetabular f.

adipose fossae, subcutaneous spaces containing accumulations of fat in the breast.

amygdaloid f., SYN tonsillar f.

anconal f., SYN olecranon f.

anterior cranial f., the portion of the internal base of the skull, anterior to the sphenoidal ridges and limbus, in which the frontal lobes of the brain rest. SYN f. cranii anterior [NA], anterior cranial base.

f. anthel′icis [NA], SYN f. of anthelix.

f. of anthelix, the depression on the medial surface of the auricle that corresponds to the anthelix. SYN f. anthelicis [NA], periconchal sulcus.

articular f. of temporal bone, SYN mandibular f.

f. axilla′ris [NA], SYN axilla.

axillary f., SYN axilla.

Bichat's f., SYN pterygopalatine f.

Biesiadecki's f., SYN iliacosubfascial f.

Broesike's f., SYN parajejunal f.

f. cani′na [NA], SYN canine f.

canine f., a depression on the anterior surface of the maxilla below the infraorbital foramen and on the lateral side of the canine eminence. SYN f. canina [NA].

f. carot′ica, SYN carotid *triangle.*

cerebellar f., the large concave impressions on the inner surface of the occipital bone on either side of the foramen magnum and internal occipital crest, housing the cerebellar hemispheres; a part of the posterior cranial f.

Claudius' f., SYN ovarian f.

condylar f., a depression behind the condyle of the occipital bone in which the posterior margin of the superior facet of the atlas lies in extension. SYN f. condylaris [NA].

f. condyla′ris [NA], SYN condylar f.

coronoid f. of humerus, a hollow on the anterior surface of the distal end of the humerus, just above the trochlea, in which the coronoid process of the ulna rests when the elbow is flexed. SYN f. coronoidea humeri [NA].

f. coronoi′dea humeri [NA], SYN coronoid f. of humerus.

f. cra′nii ante′rior [NA], SYN anterior cranial f.

f. cra′nii me′dia [NA], SYN middle cranial f.

f. cra′nii poste′rior [NA], SYN posterior cranial f.

crural f., SYN femoral f.

Cruveilhier's f., SYN scaphoid f. (1).

cubital f., the f. in front of the elbow, bounded laterally and medially by the humeral origins of the extensors and flexors of the forearm, respectively, and superiorly by an imaginary line connecting the humeral condyles. SYN f. cubitalis [NA], antecubital space, chelidon, triangle of elbow.

f. cubita′lis [NA], SYN cubital f.

digastric f., a hollow on the posterior surface of the base of the mandible, on either side of the median plane, giving attachment to the anterior belly of the digastric muscle. SYN f. digastrica [NA].

f. digas′trica [NA], SYN digastric f.

digital f., (1) SYN trochanteric f. (2) SYN f. of lateral malleolus.

f. duc′tus veno′si, SYN f. of ductus venosi.

f. of ductus venosus, a wide groove located posteriorly on the undersurface of the fetal liver between the caudate and left lobes; it lodges the ductus venosus and becomes the fissure of the ligamentum venosum in the adult. SYN f. ductus venosi.

duodenal fossae, SEE inferior duodenal *recess,* superior duodenal *recess.*

duodenojejunal f., SYN superior duodenal *recess.*

epigastric f., the slight depression in the midline just inferior to the xiphoid process of the sternum. SYN f. epigastrica, pit of stomach, scrobiculus cordis.

f. epigas′trica, SYN epigastric f.

femoral f., a depression on the peritoneal surface of the abdominal wall, inferior to the inguinal ligament, corresponding to the situation of the femoral ring. SYN crural f., fovea femoralis.

floccular f., SYN subarcuate f.

gallbladder f., SYN f. for gallbladder.

f. for gallbladder, a depression on the visceral surface of the liver anteriorly, between the quadrate and the right lobes, lodging the gallbladder. SYN f. vesicae biliaris [felleae] [NA], gallbladder f.

Gerdy's hyoid f., SYN carotid *triangle.*

f. glan′dulae lacrima′lis [NA], SYN lacrimal f.

glenoid f., (1) the hollow in the head of the scapula that receives the head of the humerus to make the shoulder joint; (2) SYN mandibular f.

greater supraclavicular f., SYN supraclavicular *triangle.*

Gruber-Landzert f., SYN inferior duodenal *recess.*

f. of helix, SYN scapha (1).

hyaloid f., a depression on the anterior surface of the vitreous body in which lies the lens. SYN f. hyaloidea [NA], lenticular f., patellar f. of vitreous.

f. hyaloi′dea [NA], SYN hyaloid f.

hypophysial f., f. of the sphenoid bone housing the pituitary gland. SEE ALSO *sella* turcica. SYN f. hypophysialis [NA], pituitary f.

f. hypophysia′lis [NA], SYN hypophysial f.

iliac f., the smooth inner surface of the ilium above the arcuate line, giving attachment to the iliacus muscle. SYN f. iliaca [NA].

f. ili′aca [NA], SYN iliac f.

iliacosubfascial f., a peritoneal recess between the psoas muscle and the crest of the ilium. SYN Biesiadecki's f., f. iliacosubfascialis.

f. iliacosubfascia′lis, SYN iliacosubfascial f.

iliopectineal f., a hollow between the iliopsoas and pectineus muscles in the center of the femoral triangle, lodging the femoral vessels and nerve.

f. incisi′va [NA], SYN incisive f.

⟳ **Combining forms**	**[NA] Nomina Anatomica**
Word*Finder* Multi-term entry finder Preceding letter A	**[MIM] Mendelian Inheritance in Man**
A.D.A.M. Anatomy Plates Between letters L and M	☆ **Official alternate term**
Appendices: Following letter Z	☆[NA] **Official alternate Nomina Anatomica term**
SYN Synonym; Cf., compare	**High Profile Term**

fo

incisive f., the depression in the midline of the bony palate behind the central incisors into which the incisive canals open. SYN f. incisiva [NA].

incudal f., SYN f. incudis.

f. incu'dis [NA], a small depression in the lower and posterior part of the epitympanic recess that lodges the short limb of the incus. SYN f. for incus, incudal f.

f. for incus, SYN f. incudis.

inferior duodenal f., SYN inferior duodenal *recess.*

infraclavicular f., a triangular depression bounded by the clavicle and the adjacent borders of the deltoid and pectoralis major muscles. SYN f. infraclavicularis [NA], deltoideopectoral triangle, deltoideopectoral trigone, infraclavicular triangle, Mohrenheim's f., Mohrenheim's space, regio infraclavicularis, trigonum deltoideopectorale.

f. infraclavicula'ris [NA], SYN infraclavicular f.

infraduodenal f., SYN retroduodenal *recess.*

f. infraspina'ta [NA], SYN infraspinous f.

infraspinous f., the hollow on the dorsal aspect of the scapula inferior to the spine, giving attachment chiefly to the infraspinatus muscle. SYN f. infraspinata [NA].

infratemporal f., the cavity on the side of the skull bounded laterally by the zygomatic arch and ramus of the mandible, medially by the lateral pterygoid plate, anteriorly by the zygomatic process of the maxilla, posteriorly by the articular tubercle of the temporal bone and the posterior border of the lateral pterygoid plate, and above by the squama of the temporal bone and the infratemporal crest on the greater wing of the sphenoid bone. SYN f. infratemporalis [NA], zygomatic f.

f. infratempora'lis [NA], SYN infratemporal f.

inguinal f., SEE lateral inguinal f., medial inguinal f.

f. inguina'lis latera'lis [NA], SYN lateral inguinal f.

f. inguina'lis media'lis [NA], SYN medial inguinal f.

f. innomina'ta, SYN innominate f.

innominate f., a shallow depression between the false vocal cord and the aryepiglottic fold on either side. SYN f. innominata.

intercondylar f., the deep f. between the femoral condyles in which the cruciate ligaments are attached. SYN f. intercondylaris [NA], intercondyloid f. (2), intercondylic f., intercondyloid notch, popliteal notch.

f. intercondyla'ris [NA], SYN intercondylar f.

intercondyloid f., intercondylic f., (1) SEE *area* intercondylaris anterior tibiae, *area* intercondylaris posterior tibiae. **(2)** SYN intercondylar f.

f. intermesocol'ica transver'sa, a f. occupying the position of the superior duodenal recess but extending transversely from right to left for a few cms.

interpeduncular f., deep depression on the inferior surface of the mesencephalon, between the crura cerebri, the floor of which is formed by the posterior perforated substance. SEE interpeduncular *cistern.* SYN f. interpeduncularis [NA].

f. interpeduncula'ris [NA], SYN interpeduncular f.

intrabulbar f., the dilated commencement of the spongy part of the male urethra lying within the bulb of the penis.

ischioanal f., SYN ischiorectal f.

ischiorectal f., a wedge-shaped space with its base toward the perineum and lying between the tuberosity of the ischium and the obturator internus muscle laterally and the external anal sphincter and the levator ani muscle medially. SYN f. ischiorectalis [NA], ischioanal f., Velpeau's f.

f. ischiorecta'lis [NA], SYN ischiorectal f.

Jobert de Lamballe's f., the hollow just above the knee formed by the adductor magnus and the sartorius and gracilis.

Jonnesco's f., SYN superior duodenal *recess.*

jugular f., an oval depression near the posterior border of the petrous portion of the temporal bone, medial to the styloid process, in which lies the beginning of the internal jugular vein (jugular bulb); SYN f. jugularis.

f. jugula'ris, SYN jugular f.

lacrimal f., a hollow in the orbital plate of the frontal bone, formed by the overhanging margin and zygomatic process, lodging the lacrimal gland. SYN f. glandulae lacrimalis [NA], f. of lacrimal gland.

f. of lacrimal gland, SYN lacrimal f.

f. of lacrimal sac, a f. formed by the lacrimal bone and the frontal process of the maxilla, lodging the lacrimal sac. SYN f. sacci lacrimalis [NA].

Landzert's f., a f. formed by two peritoneal folds, enclosing the left colic artery and the inferior mesenteric vein, respectively, at the side of the duodenum; it is smaller than the paraduodenal recess which is sometimes found in the same region.

lateral f. of brain, SYN lateral cerebral f.

lateral cerebral f., the deep depression of the basal surface of the forebrain that corresponds in position to the anterior perforated substance. Bounded medially by the optic tract and rostrally by the orbital surface of the frontal lobe, it extends laterally around the overhanging pole of the temporal lobe into the Sylvian fissure (sulcus lateralis). SYN f. lateralis cerebri [NA], f. of Sylvius, lateral f. of brain, vallecula sylvii.

lateral inguinal f., a depression on the peritoneal surface of the anterior abdominal wall lateral to the ridge formed by the inferior epigastric artery; it corresponds to the position of the deep inguinal ring, and is the site of an indirect inguinal hernia. SYN f. inguinalis lateralis [NA].

f. latera'lis cer'ebri [NA], SYN lateral cerebral f.

f. of lateral malleolus, a large rough depression on the medial aspect of the lower end of the fibula just behind the articular facet for the talus giving attachment to the posterior talofibular and the transverse tibiofibular ligaments. SYN f. malleoli lateralis [NA], digital f. (2), f. malleoli fibulae.

lenticular f., SYN hyaloid f.

lesser supraclavicular f., a triangular space between the two heads of origin of the sternocleidomastoid muscle. SYN f. supraclavicularis minor [NA].

little f. of the cochlear window, SYN *fossula* fenestrae cochleae.

little f. of the vestibular window, little f. of the vestibular round window, SYN *fossula* fenestrae vestibuli.

Malgaigne's f., SYN carotid *triangle.*

f. malle'oli fib'ulae, SYN f. of lateral malleolus.

f. malle'oli latera'lis [NA], SYN f. of lateral malleolus.

mandibular f., a deep hollow in the squamous portion of the temporal bone at the root of the zygoma, in which rests the condyle of the mandible. SYN cavitas glenoidalis [NA], f. mandibularis [NA], articular f. of temporal bone, glenoid cavity, glenoid f. (2), glenoid surface.

f. mandibula'ris [NA], SYN mandibular f.

mastoid f., f. mastoi'dea, SYN suprameatal *pit.*

medial inguinal f., a depression on the peritoneal surface of the anterior abdominal wall between the ridges formed by the inferior epigastric artery and the medial umbilical ligament; it corresponds to the position of the superficial inguinal ring and is the site of a direct inguinal hernia. SYN f. inguinalis medialis [NA], fovea inguinalis interna.

Merkel's f., a groove in the posterolateral wall of the vestibule of the larynx between the corniculate and cuneiform cartilages.

mesentericoparietal f., SYN parajejunal f.

middle cranial f., a butterfly-shaped portion of the internal base of the skull posterior to the sphenoidal ridges and limbus and anterior to the crests of the petrous part of the temporal bones and dorsum sellae; it lodges the temporal lobes of the brain in the lateral portions, and the hypophysis centrally. SYN f. cranii media [NA].

Mohrenheim's f., SYN infraclavicular f.

Morgagni's f., SYN navicular f. of urethra.

mylohyoid f., SYN mylohyoid *groove.*

f. navicula'ris auric'ulae, SYN triangular f.

f. navicula'ris au'ris, outmoded term for scapha (1).

f. navicula'ris Cruveil'hier, SYN scaphoid f. (1).

f. navicula'ris ure'thrae [NA], SYN navicular f. of urethra.

f. navicula'ris vestib'ulae vagi'nae, SYN f. of vestibule of vagina.

navicular f. of urethra, the terminal dilated portion of the urethra in the glans penis. SYN f. navicularis urethrae [NA], f. terminalis urethrae, Morgagni's f., Morgagni's fovea.

f. olecra′ni [NA], SYN olecranon f.

olecranon f., a hollow on the dorsum of the distal end of the humerus, just above the trochlea, in which the olecranon process of the ulna rests when the elbow is extended. SYN f. olecrani [NA], anconal f.

oval f., SEE f. ovalis.

f. ova′lis, (1) [NA], an oval depression on the lower part of the septum of the right atrium; it is a vestige of the foramen ovale, and its floor corresponds to the septum primum of the fetal heart; **(2)** SYN saphenous *opening.*

ovarian f., a depression in the parietal peritoneum of the pelvis; it is bounded in front by the obliterated umbilical artery, and behind by the ureter and the uterine vessels; it lodges the ovary. SYN f. ovarica [NA], Claudius' f.

f. ova′rica [NA], SYN ovarian f.

paraduodenal f., SYN paraduodenal *recess.*

parajejunal f., a peritoneal f. that has been seen in a few cases in which the jejunum has no mesentery but is attached to the posterior parietal peritoneum; the f. begins at the point where the mesentery ends, and is seen on raising up the knuckle of free intestine. SYN Broesike's f., f. parajejunalis, mesentericoparietal f., mesentericoparietal recess.

f. parajejuna′lis, SYN parajejunal f.

pararectal f., a peritoneal depression on either side of the rectum formed by peritoneal (sacrogenital) folds passing from the posterolateral pelvic wall to the central pelvic viscera. The f. is a lateral extension of the male rectovesical pouch or the female rectouterine pouch. SYN pararectal pouch.

paravesical f., a peritoneal depression formed by the reflection of the peritoneum from the lateral pelvic wall onto the roof of the bladder; in the female, it is the lateral portion of the uterovesical pouch, separated from the pararectal pouch by the broad ligament. SYN f. paravesicalis [NA], paracystic pouch, paravesical pouch.

f. paravesica′lis [NA], SYN paravesical f.

patellar f. of vitreous, SYN hyaloid f.

peritoneal fossae, depressions or pouches formed between various peritoneal folds; they may be the sites of internal hernias.

petrosal f., SYN petrosal *fossula.*

piriform f., a recess in the anterolateral wall of the nasopharynx on each side of the vestibule of the larynx separated from it by the aryepiglottic folds. SYN recessus piriformis [NA], piriform recess, piriform sinus.

pituitary f., SYN hypophysial f.

f. poplit′ea [NA], SYN popliteal f.

popliteal f., the diamond-shaped space posterior to the knee joint bounded superficially by the diverging biceps femoris and semimembranosus muscles above and inferiorly by the two heads of the gastrocnemius muscle; deeply, the f. is bound superiorly by the diverging supracondylar lines of the femur and the soleal line of the tibia inferiorly. Contents: tibial nerve, popliteal artery, vein, fat. SYN f. poplitea [NA], poples [NA], ham (1), popliteal region, popliteal space, popliteus (2).

posterior cranial f., the internal base of the skull posterior to the crest of the petrous part of the temporal bones and the dorsum sellae and anterior to the grooves for the transverse sinuses, where the cerebellum, pons, and medulla oblongata rest. SYN f. cranii posterior [NA].

f. provesica′lis, SYN Hartmann's *pouch.*

pterygoid f., the f. formed by the divergence posteriorly of the plates of the pterygoid process of the sphenoid bone; it lodges the origin of medial pterygoid and the tensor palati muscles. SYN f. pterygoidea [NA].

f. pterygoi′dea [NA], SYN pterygoid f.

pterygomaxillary f., SYN pterygopalatine f.

f. pterygopalati′na [NA], SYN pterygopalatine f.

pterygopalatine f., sphenomaxillary f., a small pyramidal space, housing the pterygopalatine ganglion, between the pterygoid process, the maxilla, and the palatine bone. SYN f. pterygopalatina [NA], Bichat's f., pterygomaxillary f., sphenomaxillary f.

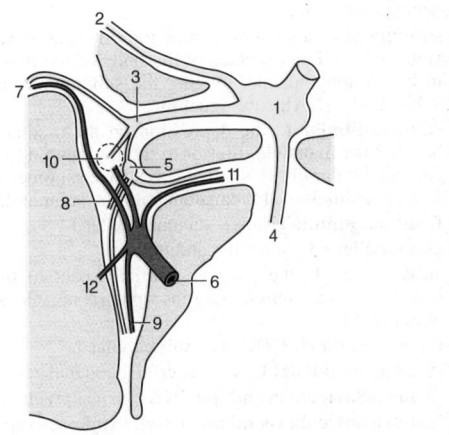

pterygopalatine fossa

in lateral projection: 1. ganglion trigeminale 2. nervus ophthalmicus 3. nervus maxillaris 4. nervus mandibularis 5. ganglion pterygopalatinum 6. arteria maxillaris 7. nervus and arteria infraorbitalis 8. ramus alveolaris posterior 9. nervus palatinus and arteria palatina 10. ramus nasalis posterior and a. sphenopalatina in the foramen sphenopalatinum 11. nervus petrosus superficialis major with the nervus petrosus profundus and the arteria canalis pterygoidei 12. arteria alveolaris superior posterior

radial f. of humerus, a shallow depression on the anterior aspect of the distal humerus, superior to the capitulum of the humerus and lateral to the coronoid fossa, in which the margin of the head of the radius rests when the elbow is in extreme flexion. SYN f. radialis humeri [NA].

f. radia′lis hu′meri [NA], SYN radial f. of humerus.

retroduodenal f., SYN retroduodenal *recess.*

retromandibular f., the depression inferior to the auricle and posterior to the ramus and angle of the mandible. SYN f. retromandibularis.

f. retromandibula′ris, SYN retromandibular f.

retromolar f., a triangular depression in the mandible posterior to the third molar tooth.

rhomboid f., the floor of the fourth ventricle of the brain, formed by the ventricular surface of the rhombencephalon. SYN f. rhomboidea [NA].

f. rhomboi′dea [NA], SYN rhomboid f.

Rosenmüller's f., SYN pharyngeal *recess.*

f. sac′ci lacrima′lis [NA], SYN f. of lacrimal sac.

scaphoid f., a boat-shaped hollow. **(1)** a longitudinal hollow on the posterior surface of the superior portion (root) of the medial pterygoid plate; it gives origin to the tensor veli palati muscle; SYN f. scaphoidea ossis sphenoidalis [NA], Cruveilhier's f., f. navicularis Cruveilhier, scaphoid f. of sphenoid bone. **(2)** SYN scapha (1).

f. scaphoid′ea ossis sphenoidalis [NA], SYN scaphoid f. (1).

scaphoid f. of sphenoid bone, SYN scaphoid f. (1).

f. scar′pae ma′jor, SYN femoral *triangle.*

sigmoid f., SYN *groove* for sigmoid sinus.

sphenomaxillary f., SYN pterygopalatine f.

f. subarcua′ta [NA], SYN subarcuate f.

subarcuate f., an irregular depression on the posterior surface of the petrous portion of the temporal bone just below its crest and above and lateral to the internal acoustic meatus. In the fetus, the flocculus of the cerebellum rests here; in the adult, a small vein enters the bone here. SYN f. subarcuata [NA], floccular f., hiatus subarcuatus.

subcecal f., an inconstant depression in the peritoneum extending posterior to the cecum. SYN Treitz's f.

fo

subinguinal f., the depression on the anterior surface of the thigh beneath the groin.

sublingual f., a shallow depression on either side of the mental spine, on the inner surface of the body of the mandible, superior to the mylohyoid line, lodging the sublingual gland. SYN fovea sublingualis [NA], sublingual pit.

submandibular f., the depression on the medial surface of the body of the mandible inferior to the mylohyoid line in which the submandibular gland is lodged. SYN fovea submandibularis [NA], f. submandibularis, fovea submaxillaris, submaxillary f.

f. submandibula′ris, SYN submandibular f.

submaxillary f., SYN submandibular f.

subscapular f., the concave ventral aspect of the body of the scapula giving origin to the subscapularis muscle. SYN f. subscapularis [NA].

f. subscapula′ris [NA], SYN subscapular f.

superior duodenal f., SYN superior duodenal *recess*.

f. supraclavicula′ris ma′jor [NA], SYN supraclavicular *triangle*.

f. supraclavicula′ris mi′nor [NA], SYN lesser supraclavicular f.

supramastoid f., SYN suprameatal *pit*.

f. supraspina′ta [NA], SYN supraspinous f.

supraspinous f., the hollow on the dorsal aspect of the scapula above the spine, lodging the supraspinatus muscle. SYN f. supraspinata [NA].

supratonsillar f., the interval between the palatoglossal and palatopharyngeal arches above the tonsil, most obvious after the tonsil has regressed in the adult. SYN f. supratonsillaris [NA], supratonsillar recess, Tourtual's sinus.

f. supratonsilla′ris [NA], SYN supratonsillar f.

supravesical f., the depression on the peritoneal surface of the anterior abdominal wall above the bladder and between the median and medial umbilical folds. Its level, relative to the pubis, changes with filling of the bladder. SYN f. supravesicalis [NA], fovea supravesicalis.

f. supravesica′lis [NA], SYN supravesical f.

f. of Sylvius, SYN lateral cerebral f.

temporal f., the space on the side of the cranium bounded by the temporal lines and terminating below at the level of the zygomatic arch. SYN f. temporalis [NA].

f. tempora′lis [NA], SYN temporal f.

f. termina′lis ure′thrae, SYN navicular f. of urethra.

tonsillar f., the depression between the palatoglossal and palatopharyngeal arches occupied by the palatine tonsil. SYN f. tonsillaris [NA], amygdaloid f., sinus tonsillaris.

f. tonsilla′ris [NA], SYN tonsillar f.

Treitz's f., SYN subcecal f.

triangular f., the depression at the upper part of the auricle between the two crura of the anthelix. SYN f. triangularis [NA], f. navicularis auriculae.

f. triangula′ris [NA], SYN triangular f.

trochanteric f., a depression at the root of the neck of the femur beneath the curved tip of the great trochanter; it gives attachment to the tendon of the obturator externus. SYN f. trochanterica [NA], digital f. (1).

f. trochanter′ica [NA], SYN trochanteric f.

trochlear f., SYN trochlear *fovea*.

f. trochlea′ris, SYN trochlear *fovea*.

umbilical f., SYN *fissure* of round ligament of liver.

Velpeau's f., SYN ischiorectal f.

f. ve′nae ca′vae, SYN *groove* for inferior venae cava.

f. ve′nae umbilica′lis, SYN *fissure* of round ligament of liver.

f. veno′sa, SYN paraduodenal *recess*.

vermian f., a small depression near the lower part of the internal occipital crest which lodges part of the inferior vermis of the cerebellum.

f. vesi′cae bilia′ris [fel′leae] [NA], SYN f. for gallbladder.

vestibular f., SYN f. of vestibule of vagina.

f. of vestibule of vagina, the portion of the vestibule of the vagina between the frenulum of the labia minora and the posterior labial commissure of the vulva. SYN f. vestibuli vaginae [NA], f. navicularis vestibulae vaginae, vestibular f.

f. vestib′uli vagi′nae [NA], SYN f. of vestibule of vagina.

Waldeyer's fossae, SEE inferior duodenal *recess*, superior duodenal *recess*.

zygomatic f., SYN infratemporal f.

fos·sette (fo-set′). **1.** SYN fossula. **2.** A seldom-used term for corneal ulcer of small diameter. [Fr. dim. of *fosse*, a ditch]

fos·su·la, pl. **fos·su·lae** (fos′yū-lă, -lē). **1** [NA]. A small fossa. **2.** A minor fissure or slight depression on the surface of the cerebrum. SYN fossette (1). [L. dim. of *fossa*, ditch]

f. fenes′trae coch′leae [NA], a depression on the medial wall of the middle ear which has the fenestra cochleae (round window) in its lower portion. SYN f. rotunda, little fossa of the cochlear window.

f. fenes′trae vestib′uli [NA], a depression on the medial wall of the middle ear which has the fenestra vestibulae (oval window) in its lower portion. SYN Huguier's sinus, little fossa of the vestibular window, little fossa of the vestibular round window.

f. petro′sa [NA], SYN petrosal f.

petrosal f., a small and often only faintly marked depression on the inferior surface of the petrous portion of the temporal bone, between the jugular fossa and the opening of the carotid canal; here opens the canaliculus tympanicus transmitting the tympanic nerve. SYN f. petrosa [NA], petrosal fossa, receptaculum ganglii petrosi.

f. rotun′da, SYN f. fenestrae cochleae.

tonsillar fossulae, the small pits at the openings of the tonsillar crypts onto the medial surface of the tonsil. SYN fossulae tonsillares [NA].

fos′sulae tonsilla′res [NA], SYN tonsillar fossulae.

fos·su·late (fos′yū-lāt). Grooved; containing a fossula or small fossa; hollowed out.

Foster frame. See under frame.

Foster Kennedy. SEE Kennedy.

Fothergill, John, English physician, 1712–1780. SEE F.'s *disease, neuralgia, sign.*

Fothergill, William E., English gynecologist, 1865–1926. SEE F.'s *operation.*

Fouchet, A., French physician, *1894. SEE F.'s *reagent, stain.*

fou·lage (fū-lahzh′). Kneading and pressure of the muscles, constituting a form of massage. [Fr. impression]

foun·da·tion (fown-dā′shŭn). A base; a supporting structure.

denture f., that portion of the oral structures which is available to support a denture. SEE ALSO denture foundation *area*, denture foundation *surface*, mean foundation *plane*.

found·er (fown′der). **1.** A person who contributes to the initial genetic structure of a population and is liable to contribute to a large proportion of the genes in the descendants from it. **2.** SYN laminitis (2).

four·chette (fūr-shet′). SYN *frenulum* of the labia minora. [Fr. dim. of *fourché*, fr. L. *furca*, fork]

Fou·ri·er, J. B. J., French mathematician and administrator, 1768–1830. SEE Fourier *analysis*, Fourier transform.

Fou·ri·er trans·form. SYN Fourier *analysis*.

Fourneau, Ernest F.A., French chemist and pharmacologist, 1872–1949. SEE F. 693, 710, 933.

Fourneau 693. SYN ethylstibamine. [Ernest F.A. *Fourneau*]

Fourneau 710. A synthetic quinoline; an antimalarial agent. [Ernest F.A. *Fourneau*]

Fourneau 933. SYN piperoxan hydrochloride. [Ernest F.A. *Fourneau*]

Fournier, Jean A., French syphilographer, 1832–1914. SEE F.'s *disease, gangrene; syphiloma* of F.

fo·vea, pl. **fo·ve·ae** (fō′vē-ă, fō′vē-ē) [NA]. A relatively small cup-shaped depression or pit. [L. a pit]

f. ante′rior, SYN superior f.

anterior f., SYN superior f.

f. articula′ris cap′itis ra′dii [NA], SYN f. of the radial head.

f. articula′ris infe′rior atlan′tis, SYN inferior articular *facet* of atlas.

f. articula′ris supe′rior atlan′tis, SYN superior articular *facet* of atlas.

f. cap′itis os′sis fem′oris [NA], SYN f. of the femoral head.

f. cardi′aca, anterior intestinal portal; the opening of the foregut into the midgut. SEE ALSO epigastric *fossa.* SYN anterior intestinal portal.

f. centra′lis ret′inae [NA], SYN central retinal f.

central retinal f., a depression in the center of the macula retinae containing only cones and lacking blood vessels. SYN f. centralis retinae [NA], central pit.

f. coc′cygis, it marks the site where the embryonic spinal cord attaches to the skin. SYN postnatal pit of the newborn.

f. costa′lis infe′rior [NA], SYN inferior costal *facet.*

f. costa′lis proces′sus transver′si [NA], SYN transverse costal *facet.*

f. costa′lis supe′rior [NA], SYN superior costal *facet.*

f. den′tis atlan′tis [NA], SYN *facet* of atlas for dens.

f. ellip′tica, SYN elliptical *recess.*

f. ethmoida′lis, the roof of the ethmoid air cells.

f. of the femoral head, a depression on the extremity of the head of the femur giving attachment to the ligamentum teres femoris. SYN f. capitis ossis femoris [NA], pit of head of femur.

f. femora′lis, SYN femoral *fossa.*

f. hemiellip′tica, SYN elliptical *recess.*

f. hemisphe′rica, SYN spherical *recess.*

f. infe′rior [NA], SYN inferior f.

inferior f., a small depression in the limiting sulcus of the rhomboidal fossa below the medullary striae of either side, generally lateral to the hypoglossal and vagal trigones. SYN f. inferior [NA].

f. inguina′lis inter′na, SYN medial inguinal *fossa.*

Morgagni's f., SYN navicular *fossa* of urethra.

f. oblon′ga cartilag′inis arytenoid′eae [NA], SYN oblong f. of arytenoid cartilage.

oblong f. of arytenoid cartilage, a broad shallow depression on the anterolateral surface of the arytenoid cartilage, for attachment of the thyroarytenoid muscle. SYN f. oblonga cartilaginis arytenoideae [NA], oblong pit of arytenoid cartilage.

pterygoid f., a depression on the antero-medial side of the neck of the condylar process of the mandible, giving attachment to the lateral pterygoid muscle. SYN f. pterygoidea [NA], pterygoid depression, pterygoid pit.

f. pterygoid′ea [NA], SYN pterygoid f.

f. of the radial head, the depression on the top (superior surface) of the head of the radius for articulation with the capitulum of the humerus. SYN f. articularis capitis radii [NA], articular pit of head of radius.

f. sphe′rica, SYN spherical *recess.*

f. sublingua′lis [NA], SYN sublingual *fossa.*

f. submandibula′ris [NA], SYN submandibular *fossa.*

f. submaxilla′ris, SYN submandibular *fossa.*

f. supe′rior [NA], SYN superior f.

superior f., a slight depression in the limiting sulcus on either side of the rhomboidal fossa, above the medullary striae and lateral to the facial colliculus. SYN f. superior [NA], anterior f., f. anterior.

f. supravesica′lis, SYN supravesical *fossa.*

triangular f. of arytenoid cartilage, a deep depression in the upper portion of the anterolateral surface of the arytenoid cartilage, lodging glands. SYN f. triangularis cartilaginis arytenoideae [NA], triangular pit of arytenoid cartilage.

f. triangula′ris cartilag′inis arytenoid′eae [NA], SYN triangular f. of arytenoid cartilage.

trochlear f., a shallow depression in the roof of the orbit close to the medial margin to which is attached the pulley for the superior oblique tendon. SYN f. trochlearis [NA], fossa trochlearis, trochlear fossa, trochlear pit.

f. trochlea′ris [NA], SYN trochlear f.

fo·ve·ate, fo·ve·at·ed (fō′-vē-āt, -ā-ted). Pitted; having foveas or depressions on the surface.

fo·ve·a·tion (fō-vē-ā′shŭn). Pitted scar formation, as in smallpox, chickenpox, or vaccinia. [L. *fovea,* a pit]

fo·ve·o·la, pl. **fo·ve·o·lae** (fō-vē′ō-lă, -lē) [NA]. A minute fovea or pit. [Mod. L. dim. of L. *fovea,* pit]

f. coccy′gea [NA], SYN coccygeal f.

coccygeal f., a depression in the skin over the coccyx caused by the caudal retinaculum. SYN f. coccygea [NA], coccygeal dimple.

f. gas′trica [NA], SYN gastric *pit.*

foveolae granula′res [NA], SYN granular *pits,* under *pit.*

f. ocula′ris, SYN f. retinae.

f. papilla′ris, the minute depression sometimes seen at the apex of a papilla of the kidney where a papillary duct opens into a calix.

f. retinae [NA], the central portion of the central retinal fovea that contains cones only. SYN f. ocularis.

f. supramea′tica [NA], SYN suprameatal *pit.*

fo·ve·o·lar (fō-vē′ō-lăr). Pertaining to a foveola.

fo·ve·o·late (fō′vē-ō-lāt, fō-vē′ō-lāt). Having minute pits (foveolae) or small depressions on the surface.

Foville, Achille L., French neurologist, 1799–1878. SEE F.'s *fasciculus, syndrome.*

Fowler, George R., U.S. surgeon, 1848–1906. SEE F.'s *position.*

fowl·pox (fowl′poks). A disease of fowl, worldwide in distribution, caused by fowlpox virus, a member of the family Poxviridae, and characterized by proliferative nodular dermal lesions followed by scabbing, chiefly on the head but sometimes involving the feet and vent; there may also be eye lesions or involvement of the trachea (so-called fowl diphtheria); transmission is by contact, or mechanically by mosquitoes. SYN epithelioma contagiosum.

Fox, George H., U.S. dermatologist, 1846–1937. SEE F.-Fordyce *disease.*

Fox, Lewis, U.S. periodontist, *1903. SEE Goldman-F. *knives,* under *knife.*

fox·glove (foks′glŭv). SYN *Digitalis.*

FPLC Abbreviation for fast protein liquid chromatography.

FPS, fps Abbreviation for foot-pound-second. SEE foot-pound-second *system,* foot-pound-second *unit.*

Fr 1. Symbol for francium. **2.** Abbreviation for French *scale.*

Fraccaro, M., Italian physician. SEE Schmid-F. *syndrome.*

F.R.A.C.P. Abbreviation for Fellow of the Royal Australasian College of Physicians.

frac·tion (frak′shŭn). **1.** The quotient of two quantities. **2.** An aliquot portion or any portion.

amorphous f. of adrenal cortex, noncrystalline residue of an acetone extract of the adrenal cortex after crystalline steroids, *e.g.,* corticosterone, deoxycorticosterone, etc., have been isolated.

blood plasma f.'s, portions of the blood plasma as separated by electrophoresis or other technique.

f. collector, a device used to collect the eluate from a column in column chromatography.

dried human plasma protein f., freeze-dried human plasma protein f.

ejection f., systolic ejection f., the f. of the blood contained in the ventricle at the end of diastole that is expelled during its contraction, *i.e.,* the stroke volume divided by end-diastolic volume, normally 0.67 or greater; with the onset of congestive heart failure, the ejection f. decreases, sometimes to 0.10 or even less in severe cases.

filtration f. (FF), the f. of the plasma entering the kidney that filters into the lumen of the renal tubules, determined by dividing the glomerular filtration rate by the renal plasma flow; normally, it is around 0.17.

human antihemophilic f., SYN human antihemophilic *factor.*

human plasma protein f., a sterile solution of selected proteins derived from the blood plasma of adult human donors, containing 4.5 to 5.5 g of protein per 100 ml, of which 83 to 90% is albumin and the remainder is α- and β-globulins; used as a blood volume supporter.

mole f., the ratio of the moles of one component of a system to the total moles of all the components present.

recombination f., the proportion of progeny of a mating pair of specific genotype and coupling phase that are recombinant; there must be no differential selection among the possible types of progeny, and the recombination f. should be the same regardless of the alleles involved or their coupling phase.

regurgitant f., the amount of blood regurgitated into a cardiac chamber divided by the stroke output; normally, no blood regurgitates; in patients with severe valvular lesions such as mitral or aortic insufficiency, regurgitation can approach 80%; this f. affords a quantitative measure of the severity of the valvular lesion.

frac·tion·a·tion (frak-shŭn-ā′shŭn). **1.** To separate components of a mixture. **2.** The administration of a course of therapeutic radiation of a neoplasm in a planned series of fractions of the total dose, most often once a day for several weeks, in order to minimize radiation damage of contiguous normal tissues.

FRACTURE

frac·ture (frak′chūr). **1.** To break. **2.** A break, especially the breaking of a bone or cartilage. [L. *fractura*, a break]

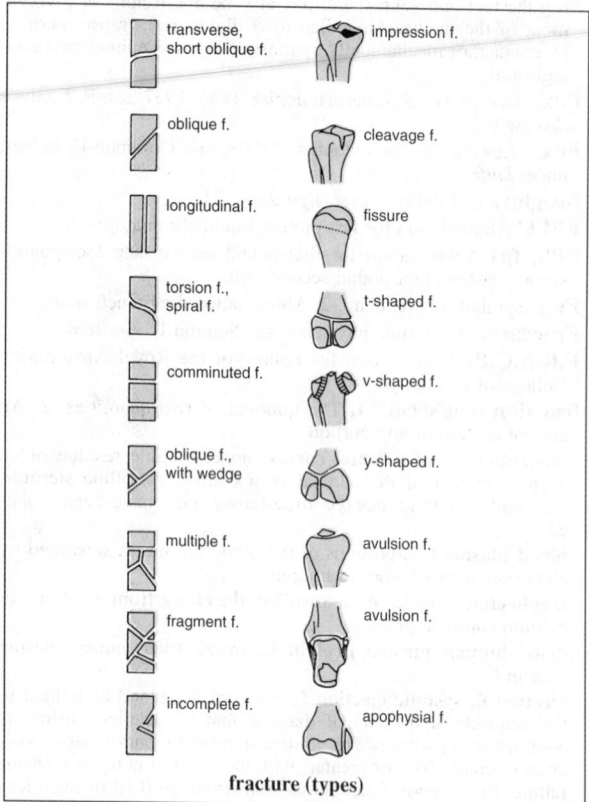

transverse, short oblique f.

oblique f.

longitudinal f.

torsion f., spiral f.

comminuted f.

oblique f., with wedge

multiple f.

fragment f.

incomplete f.

impression f.

cleavage f.

fissure

t-shaped f.

v-shaped f.

y-shaped f.

avulsion f.

avulsion f.

apophysial f.

fracture (types)

apophysial f., separation of apophysis from bone.

articular f., a f. involving the joint surface of a bone.

avulsion f., a f. that occurs when a joint capsule, ligament, or muscle insertion of origin is pulled from the bone as a result of a sprain dislocation or strong contracture of the muscle against resistance; as the soft tissue is pulled away from the bone, a fragment or fragments of the bone may come away with it.

Barton's f., f. of the distal radius with dislocation of the radio-carpal joint.

basal skull f., a f. involving the base of the cranium.

bending f., an injury in which a long bone or bones, usually the radius and ulna, are bent due to multiple microfractures, none of which can be seen by x-ray imaging.

Bennett's f., f. dislocation of the first metacarpal bone at the carpal-metacarpal joint.

birth f., f. occurring during the trauma of delivery or, occasionally, before delivery in infants with osteogenesis imperfecta.

blow-out f., a f. of the floor of the orbit, without a fracture of the rim, produced by a blow on the globe with the force being transmitted via the globe to the orbital floor.

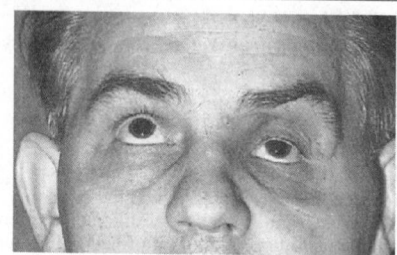

blow-out fracture
on left, with enophthalmos and recession of globe

boxer's f., f. of the neck of a metacarpal bone—typically of the fifth metacarpals.

capillary f., SYN hairline f.

Chance f., a transverse f., usually in the thoracic or lumbar spine, through the body of the vertebra extending posteriorly through the pedicles and the spinous process.

clay shoveler's f., an avulsion f. of the base of spinous processes of C-7, C-6, or T-1 (in order of prevalence).

closed f., a f. in which skin is intact at site of f. SYN simple f.

closed skull f., f. with intact overlying scalp and/or mucous membranes. SYN simple skull f.

Colles' f., a f. of the lower end of the radius with displacement of the distal fragment dorsally; sometimes called a reversed Colles' f., or Smith's f. when volar displacement of the distal fragment occurs in the same location.

comminuted f., a f. in which the bone is broken into pieces.

comminuted skull f., a f. of the skull with fragmentation of bone.

complicated f., a f. with significant soft tissue injury.

compound f., SYN open f.

compound skull f., SYN open skull f.

f. by contrecoup, skull f. at a point distant from the site of impact.

cough f., a f. of a rib or cartilage, usually the fifth or seventh, from vigorous coughing.

craniofacial dysjunction f., a complex f. in which the facial bones are separated from the cranial bones. SYN Le Fort III craniofacial dysjunction, Le Fort III f., transverse facial f.

dentate f., a f. in which the opposing surfaces are rough, with toothed or serrate projections fitting into corresponding indentations.

depressed f., SYN depressed skull f.

depressed skull f., a f. with inward displacement of a part of the calvarium; may or may not be associated with disruption of the underlying dura or cerebral cortex. SYN depressed f.

de Quervain's f., f. of navicular bone with dislocation of lunar bone.

derby hat f., regular cranial concavity in infants; may or may not be associated with f. SYN dishpan f.

diastatic skull f., (1) separation of cranial bones at a suture; (2) f. with marked separation of bone fragments.

direct f., a f., especially of the skull, occurring at the point of injury.

dishpan f., SYN derby hat f.

dislocation f., a f. of a bone near an articulation with its concomitant dislocation from that joint.

double f., SYN segmental f.

Dupuytren's f., f. of lower part of fibula, with dislocation of ankle.

dyscrasic f., obsolete term for a f. occurring in general malnutrition.

epiphysial f., epiphyseal f., separation of the epiphysis of a long bone, caused by trauma. SEE Salter-Harris *classification* of epiphysial plate injuries.

expressed skull f., a f. with outward displacement of a part of the cranium.

extracapsular f., a f. at the articular extremity of a bone, but outside of the line of attachment of the capsular ligament of the joint.

fatigue f., f. that occurs in bone subject to repeated or unusual subliminal, endogenous stress, most often transverse in configuration.

fetal f., SYN intrauterine f.

fissured f., SYN linear f.

folding f., SYN torus f.

freeze f., a procedure for preparing cells or other biological samples for electron microscopy in which the sample is frozen quickly and then broken with a sharp blow.

Galeazzi's f., f. of the shaft of the radius with dislocation of the distal radioulnar joint.

Gosselin's f., v-shaped f. of distal end of tibia.

greenstick f., the bending of a bone with incomplete f. involving the convex side of the curve only.

growing f., linear skull f. in a young child which increases in size, usually as the result of an associated dural tear and arachnoid cyst formation within the f. line.

Guérin's f., a f. of the facial bones in which there is a horizontal f. at the base of the maxillae above the apices of the teeth. SYN horizontal f., Le Fort I f.

gutter f., a long, narrow, depressed f. of the skull.

hairline f., a f. without separation of the fragments, the line of break being hairlike, as seen sometimes in the skull. SYN capillary f.

hangman's f., a f. of the cervical spine through the pedicles of C_2; may be associated with an anterior dislocation of the C_2 vertebral body with respect to C_3.

horizontal f., SYN Guérin's f.

impacted f., a f. in which one of the fragments is driven into the cancellous tissue of the other fragment.

incomplete f., a f. in which the line of f. does not include the entire bone.

indirect f., a f., especially of the skull, that occurs at a point not at the site of impact.

intra-articular f., f. occurring within a joint capsule.

intracapsular f., a f. at the articular extremity of a bone within the line of insertion of the capsular ligament of the joint.

intraperiosteal f., a f. in which the periosteum is not ruptured.

intrauterine f., a f. of one or more bones of a fetus occurring before birth. SYN fetal f.

Le Fort I f., SYN Guérin's f.

Le Fort II f., SYN pyramidal f.

Le Fort III f., SYN craniofacial dysjunction f.

linear f., a f. running parallel with the long axis of the bone. SYN fissured f.

linear skull f., a skull f. resembling a line.

longitudinal f., a f. involving the bone in the line of its axis.

march f., a fatigue f. of one of the metatarsals. SYN Deutschländer's disease (2).

Monteggia's f., f. of the ulna with dislocation of the head of the radius.

multiple f., (1) f. at two or more places in a bone; SEE segmental f. **(2)** f. of several bones occurring simultaneously.

neurogenic f., a f. in bone weakened by disease of the nerve supply.

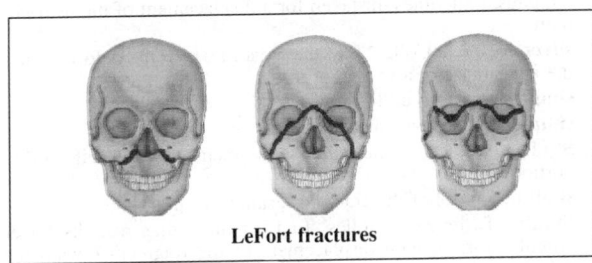

LeFort fractures

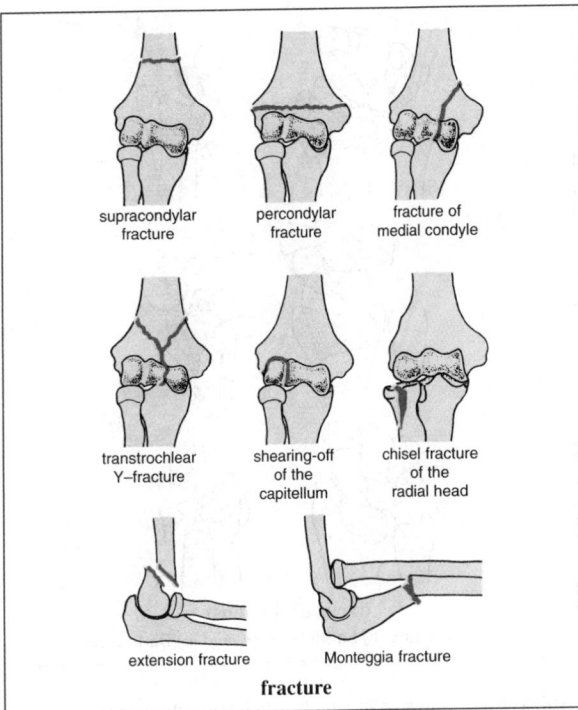

supracondylar fracture

percondylar fracture

fracture of medial condyle

transtrochlear Y–fracture

shearing-off of the capitellum

chisel fracture of the radial head

extension fracture

Monteggia fracture

fracture

oblique f., a f. the line of which runs obliquely to the axis of the bone.

occult f., a condition in which there are clinical signs of f. but no x-ray evidence; after 3 or 4 weeks x-ray imaging shows new bone formation.

open f., f. in which the skin is perforated and there is an open wound down to the f. SYN compound f.

open skull f., a f. with laceration of overlying scalp and/or mucous membrane. SYN compound skull f.

parry f., rarely used synonym for Monteggia's f.

pathologic f., a f. occurring at a site weakened by preexisting disease, especially neoplasm or necrosis, of the bone.

pertrochanteric f., a f. through the great trochanter of the femur; a form of extracapsular hip f.

pilon f., a f. of the distal metaphysis of the tibia extending into the ankle joint.

ping-pong f., SEE derby hat f.

pond f., a circular depressed skull f.

Pott's f., f. of the lower part of the fibula and of the malleolus of the tibia, with outward displacement of the foot.

pyramidal f., a f. of the midfacial skeleton with the principal f. lines meeting at an apex at or near the superior aspect of the nasal bones. SYN Le Fort II f.

segmental f., a f. in two parts of the same bone. SYN double f.

sentinel spinous process f., f. of the spinous process with undetected deeper f.'s of the vertebral arch.

Shepherd's f., a f. of the external tubercle (posterior process) of

fr

the talus, sometimes mistaken for a displacement of the os trigonum.

silver-fork f., a Colles' f. of the wrist in which the deformity has the appearance of a fork in profile.

simple f., SYN closed f.

simple skull f., SYN closed skull f.

Skillern's f., f. of distal radius with greenstick f. of neighboring portion of ulna.

skull f., a break of the cranium resulting from trauma.

Smith's f., reversed Colles' f.; f. of the radius near its lower articular surface with displacement of the fragment toward the palmar (volar) aspect.

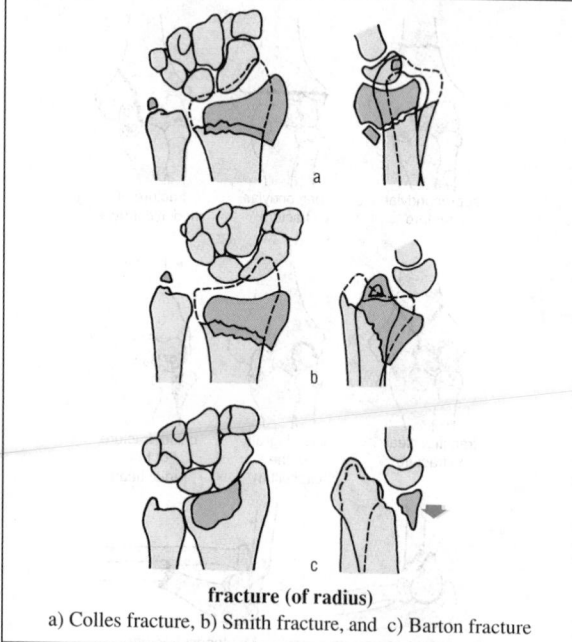

fracture (of radius)
a) Colles fracture, b) Smith fracture, and c) Barton fracture

spiral f., a f. the line of which is helical in the bone.

splintered f., a comminuted f. in which the fragments are long and sharp-pointed.

spontaneous f., a f. occurring without any external injury.

sprain f., an avulsion f. in which a small portion of adjacent bone has been pulled or pushed off.

stable f., a f. that does not tend to displace once it has been reduced and immobilized.

stellate f., a f. in which the lines of break radiate from a central point.

stellate skull f., a skull f. with multiple linear fractures radiating from the site of impact.

strain f., the tearing off, by a sudden force, of a piece of bone attached to a tendon, ligament, or capsule; the force may be exogenous or endogenous.

stress f., a f. resulting from force on a bony structure during use as opposed to one resulting from exogenous trauma.

subcapital f., an intracapsular f. of the neck of the femur, at the point where the neck of the femur joins the head.

subperiosteal f., a f. occurring beneath the periosteum, and without displacement.

supracondylar f., a f. of the distal end of the humerus or femur.

torsion f., a f. resulting from twisting of the limb.

torus f., a deformity in children consisting of a local bulging caused by the longitudinal compression of the soft bone; it occurs commonly in the radius or ulna or both. SYN folding f.

transcervical f., a f. through the neck of the femur.

transcondylar f., a f. through condyles of the humerus or femur.

transverse f., a f. the line of which forms a right angle with the axis of the bone.

transverse facial f., SYN craniofacial dysjunction f.

trimalleolar f., a f. through both malleoli and the posterior process of the tibia.

tripod f., a facial f. involving the three supports of the malar prominence, the arch of the zygomatic bone, the zygomatic process of the frontal bone, and the zygomatic process of the maxillary bone.

unstable f., a f. with an intrinsic tendency to slip out of place after reduction.

ununited f., a f. in which union fails to occur, the ends of the bone becoming rounded and eburnated, and a false joint occurs.

Wagstaffe's f., f., with displacement, of the medial malleolus.

Fraenkel, Albert, German physician, 1848–1916. SEE F.'s *pneumococcus;* F.-Weichselbaum *pneumococcus.*

fra·gil·i·tas (fră-jil'i-tas). SYN fragility. [L.]

f. crin′ium, brittleness of the hair; a condition in which the hair of the head or face tends to split or break off.

f. san′guinis, SYN osmotic *fragility.*

fra·gil·i·ty (fră-jil'i-tē). Brittleness; liability to break, burst, or disintegrate. SYN fragilitas. [L. *fragilitas*]

f. of the blood, SYN osmotic f.

capillary f., the susceptibility of capillaries to breakage and extravasation of red cells under conditions of increased stress.

osmotic f., the susceptibility of erythrocytes to hemolyze when exposed to increasingly hypotonic saline solutions. SYN fragilitas sanguinis, f. of the blood.

fra·gil·o·cyte (fra-jil'ō-sīt). A red blood cell that is unusually fragile when subjected to a hypotonic salt solution. [L. *fragilis*, brittle, + G. *kytos*, hollow (cell)]

fra·gil·o·cy·to·sis (fra-jil'ō-sī-tō'sis). A condition of the blood in which the red blood cells are abnormally fragile.

frag·ment (frag'ment). A small part broken from a larger entity.

acentric f., SYN acentric *chromosome.*

Brimacombe f., a ribonucleoprotein f. obtained by mild ribonuclease treatment of ribosomes.

butterfly f., a broad triangular f. that is commonly present in comminuted fractures of the diaphysis.

Fab f., the antigen-binding f. of an immunoglobulin molecule, consisting of both a light chain and part of a heavy chain. SYN Fab piece.

Fc f., the crystallizable f. of an immunoglobulin molecule composed of part of the heavy chains and responsible for binding to antibody receptors on cells and the Clq component of complement. SYN Fc piece.

Klenow f., carboxyl terminal fragment of DNA polymerase I, contains polymerase as well as $3' \rightarrow 5'$ exonuclease activity to edit out mismatches.

Okazaki f., a relatively short (100–1000 bp) fragment of DNA that is later joined by DNA ligase to allow for $3' \rightarrow 5'$ overall chain growth during replication.

one-carbon f., the formyl group or the methyl group that takes part in transformylation or transmethylation reactions; by means of these reactions, a group containing a single carbon atom is added to a compound being biosynthesized, adding a methyl group (as in thymidine formation), adding a hydroxymethyl group (as in serine biosynthesis), or closing a ring (as in purine formation).

two-carbon f., the acetyl group (CH_3CO-) that takes part in transacetylation reactions with coenzyme A as carrier; commonly referred to as acetate or acetic acid, from which it is derived.

frag·men·ta·tion (frag-men-tā'shŭn). The breaking of an entity into smaller parts. SYN spallation (1).

f. of the myocardium, a transverse rupture of the muscular fibers of the heart, especially those of the papillary muscles.

fraise (frāz). A burr in the shape of a hemispherical button with cutting edges, used to enlarge a trephine opening in the skull or to cut osteoplastic flaps; the smooth convexity of the button prevents injury to the dura. [Fr. strawberry]

Fraley, Elwin E., U.S. urologist, *1934. SEE F. *syndrome.*

fram·be·sia tro·pi·ca (fram-ē′zē-ă trop′ĭ-kă). SYN yaws. [Fr. *framboise,* raspberry]

fram·be·si·form (fram-bē′zi-fōrm). Resembling the lesion of frambesia.

fram·be·si·o·ma (fram-bē-zē-ō′mă). SYN mother *yaw.* [frambesia + *-oma,* tumor]

frame (frām). A structure made of parts fitted together.

  Balkan f., an overhead f., supported on uprights attached to the bedposts or to a separate stand, from which a splinted limb is slung in the treatment of fracture or joint disease. SYN Balkan beam, Balkan splint.

  Bradford f., an oblong rectangular f. made of pipe, over which are stretched transversely two strips of canvas; permits trunk and lower extremities of a bed-ridden patient to move as a unit.

  Deiters' terminal f.'s, platelike structures in the organ of Corti uniting the outer phalangeal cells with Hensen's cells.

  Foster f., a reversible bed similar to a Stryker f.

  occluding f., SYN articulator.

  Stryker f., a f. that holds the patient and permits turning in various planes without individual motion of parts.

  trial f., a type of spectacle f. with variable adjustments, for holding trial lenses during refraction.

  Whitman's f., a f. similar to the Bradford f., but with curved sides.

frame·shift (frām′shift). As used in genetics: a mutation that causes a sequence such that the reading frame groups of three bases in mRNA become out of register; the insertion or deletion of one or two bases, for example, would lead to an altered grouping of three bases causing incorrect amino acid residues to be incorporated into growing polypeptide chains.

frame·work (frām′wŏrk). **1.** SEE stroma. **2.** In dentistry, the skeletal prosthesis (usually metal) around which and to which are attached the remaining portions of the prosthesis to produce the finished appliance (partial denture).

Franceschetti, Adolphe, Swiss ophthalmologist, 1896–1968. SEE F.'s *syndrome;* F.-Jadassohn *syndrome.*

Francisella (fran′si-sel′lă). A genus of nonmotile, nonsporeforming, aerobic bacteria that contain small, Gram-negative cocci and rods. Capsules are rarely produced and the cells may show bipolar staining. These organisms are highly pleomorphic; they do not grow on plain agar or in liquid media without special enrichment; they are pathogenic and cause tularemia in humans. The type species is *F. tularensis.*

  F. novici′da, a species pathogenic for white mice, guinea pigs, and hamsters but not known to infect human beings. It produces lesions in experimental animals similar to those found in tularemia.

  F. tularen′sis, a species that causes tularemia in man, transmitted to man from wild animals by bloodsucking insects or by contact with infected animals such as ticks; main sources of infection are rabbits and ticks; it can penetrate unbroken skin to cause infection; it is the type species of the genus *F.* SYN *Pasteurella tularensis.*

fran·ci·um (Fr) (fran′sē-ŭm). Radioactive element of the alkali metal series; atomic no. 87; half-life of most stable known isotope, [223]Fr, is 21.8 minutes. [*France,* native country of Mlle. M. Perey, the discoverer]

Francke, Karl E., German physician, 1859–1920. SEE F.'s *needle.*

fran·gu·la (frang′gū-lă). The bark of *Rhamnus frangula* (family Rhamnaceae); a laxative or cathartic.

fran·gu·lic ac·id (frang′yū-lik). SYN emodin. [see frangula]

fran·gu·lin (frang′yū-lin). $C_{21}H_{20}O_9$; emodine-*l*-rhamnoside; a glycoside from frangula; has been used as a purgative. SYN rhamnoxanthin.

Frank, Otto, German physiologist, 1865–1944. SEE F.-Starling *curve.*

frank. Unmistakable; manifest; clinically evident.

Frankenhäuser, Ferdinand, German gynecologist, 1832–1894. SEE F.'s *ganglion.*

Frankfort. SEE Frankfort horizontal *plane,* Frankfort-mandibular incisor *angle.* [*Frankfurt*-am-Main, Germany]

frank·in·cense (frangk′in-sens). SYN olibanum. [Mediev. L. *francum incensum,* pure incense]

Franklin, Benjamin, U.S. physicist and statesman, 1706–1790. SEE franklinic; F. *spectacles.*

Franklin, Edward C., U.S. physician, *1928. SEE F.'s *disease.*

frank·lin·ic (frank′lin-ik). Denoting static or frictional electricity. [B. *Franklin*]

Fräntzel (fränt′zel), Oscar Maximilian Victor, German physician, 1838–1894.

Fräntzel's mur·mur. See under murmur.

Fraser, Alexander, Canadian pathologist, 1869–1939. SEE F.-Lendrum *stain* for fibrin.

Fraser, G. R., 20th century British geneticist. SEE F.'s *syndrome.*

Fraumeni, Joseph F., Jr., 20th century epidemiologist. SEE Li-F. cancer *syndrome.*

Fraunhofer, Joseph von, German optician, 1787–1826. SEE F.'s *lines,* under *line.*

Frazier, Charles H., U.S. surgeon, 1870–1936. SEE F.'s *needle;* F.-Spiller *operation.*

FRC Abbreviation for functional residual *capacity.*

F.R.C.P. Abbreviation for Fellow of the Royal College of Physicians (of England).

F.R.C.P.(C) Abbreviation for Fellow of the Royal College of Physicians (Canada).

F.R.C.P.(E), F.R.C.P.(Edin) Abbreviation for Fellow of the Royal College of Physicians (Edinburgh).

F.R.C.P.(I) Abbreviation for Fellow of the Royal College of Physicians (Ireland).

F.R.C.S. Abbreviation for Fellow of the Royal College of Surgeons (of England).

F.R.C.S.(C) Abbreviation for Fellow of the Royal College of Surgeons (Canada).

F.R.C.S.(E), F.R.C.S.(Edin) Abbreviation for Fellow of the Royal College of Surgeons (Edinburgh).

F.R.C.S.(I) Abbreviation for Fellow of the Royal College of Surgeons (Ireland).

freck·le (frek′l). Yellowish or brownish macules developing on the exposed parts of the skin, especially in persons of light complexion; the lesions increase in number on exposure to the sun; the epidermis is microscopically normal except for increased melanin. SEE ALSO lentigo. SYN ephelis. [O. E. *freken*]

  Hutchinson's f., SYN *lentigo* maligna.

  iris f.'s, small, pigmented clusters of uveal melanocytes on the surface of the iris.

  melanotic f., SYN *lentigo* maligna.

Fredet, Pierre, French surgeon, 1870–1946. SEE F.-Ramstedt *operation.*

Freeman, E.A. SEE F.-Sheldon *syndrome.*

free·mar·tin (frē′mar-tin). A masculinized, sterile female twin calf, developing from twin fetuses of opposite sexes in which the chorionic blood vessels become fused at an early stage of embryonic development, with the result that the hormones of the male twin are conveyed in the circulation to the female twin and influence its sexual development. F.'s are a type of hermaphrodite with underdeveloped uterus, enlarged penis-like clitoris, and, sometimes, structures resembling the ductus deferens and seminal vesicles. [(?) Sc. *fear* or *fearr,* sterile and dry cow, + *martin,* fr. Martinmas when cattle, especially if sterile and unproductive of milk, were slaughtered]

freeze-dry·ing (frēz′drī-ing). SYN lyophilization.

freez·ing (frē′zing). Congealing, stiffening, or hardening by exposure to cold. SYN congelation (1).

  gastric f., formerly used treatment for peptic ulcer designed to reduce or eliminate the production of acid gastric juice by freezing the secretory cells with a supercooled fluid introduced into a balloon positioned in the stomach.

Frei, Wilhelm S., German dermatologist, 1885–1943. SEE F. *test;* F.-Hoffmann *reaction.*

Freiberg, Albert Henry, U.S. surgeon, 1869–1940. SEE F.'s *disease.*

Frejka, B., 20th century Czech orthopedist. SEE F. pillow *splint.*

fré·mis·se·ment cat·taire (frā-mēs′mon kat′air). SYN purr.

frem·i·tus (frem′i-tŭs). A vibration imparted to the hand resting on the chest or other part of the body. SEE ALSO thrill. [L. a dull roaring sound, fr. *fremo,* pp. *-itus,* to roar, resound]

bronchial f., adventitious pulmonary sounds or voice sounds perceptible to the hand resting on the chest, as well as by the ear.

hydatid f., SYN hydatid *thrill.*

pericardial f., vibration in the chest wall produced by the friction of opposing roughened surfaces of the pericardium. SEE ALSO pericardial *rub.*

pleural f., vibration in the chest wall produced by a friction rub resulting from the rubbing together of the roughened inflamed opposing surfaces of the pleura.

rhonchal f., f. produced by vibrations from the passage of air in the bronchial tubes partially obstructed by mucous secretion.

subjective f., vibration felt within the chest by the patient himself, when humming with the mouth closed; or f. felt when there is a rough, pericardial or pleural friction rub, particularly when pain is minimal.

tactile f., vibration felt with the hand on the chest during vocal f.

tussive f., a form of f. similar to the vocal, produced by a cough.

vocal f., the vibration in the chest wall, felt on palpation, produced by the spoken voice.

fre·na (frē′nă). Plural of frenum.

fre·nal (frē′năl). Relating to any frenum.

French. SEE French *scale.*

fre·nec·to·my (frē-nek′tō-mē). Removal of any frenum. [frenum + G. *ektomē,* excision]

Frenkel, Heinrich S., Swiss neurologist, 1860–1931. SEE F.'s *symptom.*

Frenkel, Henri, French ophthalmologist, 1864–1934. SEE F.'s anterior ocular traumatic *syndrome.*

fre·no·plas·ty (frē′nō-plas-tē). Correction of an abnormally attached frenum by surgically repositioning it. [frenum + G. *plastos,* formed]

fre·not·o·my (frē-not′ō-mē). Division of any frenum or frenulum, especially that of the tongue. [frenum + G. *tomē,* a cutting]

fren·u·lum, pl. **fren·u·la** (fren′yū-lŭm, -lă) [NA]. A small frenum or bridle. SYN habenula (1). [Mod. L. dim. of L. *frenum,* bridle]

cerebellar f., SYN f. of superior medullary velum.

f. cerebell′i, SYN f. of superior medullary velum.

f. clitor′idis [NA], SYN f. of clitoris.

f. of clitoris, the line of union of the inner-laminae portions of the labia minora on the undersurface of the glans clitoridis. SYN f. clitoridis [NA], f. preputii clitoridis.

f. epiglot′tidis, SYN median glossoepiglottic *fold.*

f. of Giacomini, SYN uncus *band* of Giacomini.

f. of ileocecal valve, a fold, more evident in cadavers, running from the junction of the two commissures of the ileocecal valve on either side along the inner wall of the cecocolic junction. SYN f. valvae ileocecalis [NA], f. of Morgagni, Morgagni's frenum, Morgagni's retinaculum.

f. of the labia minora, the fold connecting the two labia minora posteriorly. SYN f. labiorum pudendi [NA], fourchette, f. labiorum minorum, f. of pudendal lips, f. pudendi.

f. la′bii inferio′ris, f. la′bii superio′ris [NA], SYN f. of lower lip, f. of upper lip.

f. labio′rum mino′rum, SYN f. of the labia minora.

f. labio′rum puden′di [NA], SYN f. of the labia minora.

f. lin′guae [NA], SYN lingual f.

lingual f., a fold of mucous membrane extending from the floor of the mouth to the midline of the undersurface of the tongue. SYN f. linguae [NA], f. of tongue, vinculum linguae.

f. of lower lip, f. of upper lip, SYN f. labii inferioris et superioris; f. of the lower lip; f. of the upper lip; the folds of mucous membrane extending from the gingiva to the midline of the lower and

upper lips, respectively. SYN f. labii inferioris, f. labii superioris [NA].

f. of M'Dowel, tendinous fasciculi passing from the tendon of the pectoralis major muscle across the bicipital groove.

f. of Morgagni, SYN f. of ileocecal valve.

f. of prepuce, a fold of mucous membrane passing from the undersurface of the glans penis to the deep surface of the prepuce. SYN f. preputii [NA], vinculum preputii.

f. prepu′tii [NA], SYN f. of prepuce.

f. prepu′tii clitor′idis, SYN f. of clitoris.

f. of pudendal lips, SYN f. of the labia minora.

f. puden′di, SYN f. of the labia minora.

f. of superior medullary velum, a band passing from the longitudinal groove between the quadrigeminal bodies on to the superior medullary velum. SYN f. veli medullaris superioris [NA], cerebellar f., f. cerebelli.

synovial frenula, SYN *vincula* of tendons, under *vinculum.*

f. of tongue, SYN lingual f.

f. val′vae ileoceca′lis [NA], SYN f. of ileocecal valve.

f. ve′li medulla′ris superio′ris [NA], SYN f. of superior medullary velum.

fre·num, pl. **fre·na, fre·nums** (frē′nŭm, -nă, -nŭmz). **1.** A narrow reflection or fold of mucous membrane passing from a more fixed to a movable part, serving to check undue movement of the part. **2.** An anatomical structure resembling such a fold. SYN bridle (1). [L. a bridle, curb]

Morgagni's f., SYN *frenulum* of ileocecal valve.

synovial frena, SYN *vincula* of tendons, under *vinculum.*

fren·zy (fren′zē). Extreme mental or emotional excitement. [thr. Old Fr. and L. fr. G. *phrenēsis,* inflammation of the brain, fr. *phrēn,* mind]

fre·quen·cy (v) (frē′kwen-sē). The number of regular recurrences in a given time, *e.g.,* heartbeats, sound vibrations. [L. *frequens,* repeated, often, constant]

critical flicker fusion f., the minimal number of flashes of light per second at which an intermittent light stimulus no longer stimulates a continuous visual sensation.

f. domain, the expression of a function by its amplitude and phase at each component f., usually as determined by Fourier analysis.

dominant f., the f. occurring most often in an electroencephalogram.

f. encoding, in magnetic resonance imaging, a method of varying the magnetic field strength with location to encode the location of each voxel uniquely in one direction.

fundamental f., (1) the principal component of a sound wave, which has the greatest wavelength; **(2)** tone produced by the vibration of the vocal folds before the air reaches any cavities.

gene f., (1) the probability that a gene picked at random from a defined population is of a particular type; **(2)** epidemiologically, the proportion of genes in a population that are of the particular type; **(3)** statistically, the estimate of either of the foregoing two quantities.

Larmor f., in magnetic resonance, the precessional f., n_0, of magnetic nuclei in a plane perpendicular to the direction of the external magnetic field; $v_0 = \gamma B_0/2\ \pi$, where B_0 is the magnetic field strength and γ is the magnetogyric ratio.

f. of micturition, micturition at short intervals; it may result from increased urine formation, decreased bladder capacity, or lower urinary tract irritation.

mutational f., the proportions of mutations in a population.

nearest neighbor f., the f. by which certain types of entities or structures are immediately adjacent to a given structure.

resonant f., the f. at which individual magnetic nuclei absorb or emit radiofrequency energy in magnetic resonance studies. SYN resonance (6).

respiratory f. (f), the number of breaths per minute.

Frerichs, Friedrich T. von, German pathologist and clinician, 1819–1885. SEE F.'s *theory.*

fresh·en·ing (fresh′ĕn-ing). Preparation of an open, partially healed wound for secondary closure by removal of fibrin, granulations, and early scar tissue.

Fresnel, Augustin Jean, French physicist, 1788–1827. SEE F. *lens, prism.*

fress·re·flex (fres're-fleks). Sucking and chewing movements elicited by stimulation of the face and lips. [Ger fr. *fressen,* to feed, said of animals]

fret·ting (fret'ing). Abrasive polishing and wear of two metallic surfaces at their interface due to repetitive motion. [M.E., fr. O.E. *fretan,* to devour]

fre·tum, pl. **fre·ta** (frē'tŭm, -tă). A strait; a constriction. [L.]

Freud, Sigmund, Austrian neurologist and psychiatrist, 1856–1939, founder of psychoanalysis. SEE freudian; freudian *fixation;* freudian *psychoanalysis; freudian* slip; F.'s *theory.*

freud·i·an (froyd'ē-ăn). Relating to or described by Freud.

f. slip, A mistake in speech or deed which presumably suggests some underlying motive, often sexual or aggressive in nature.

Freund, Jules, U.S. bacteriologist, 1891–1960. SEE F.'s complete *adjuvant,* incomplete *adjuvant.*

Freund, Wilhelm A., German gynecologist, 1833–1918. SEE F.'s *anomaly, operation.*

Frey, Lucie, Polish physician, 1852–1932. SEE F.'s *syndrome.*

Frey, Max von, German physician, 1852–1932. SEE F.'s *hairs,* under *hair.*

FRF Abbreviation for follicle-stimulating hormone-releasing *factor.*

FRH. Abbreviation for follitropin-releasing hormone.

fri·a·ble (frī'ă-bl). 1. Easily reduced to powder. 2. In bacteriology, denoting a dry and brittle culture falling into powder when touched or shaken. [L. *friabilis,* fr. *frio,* to crumble]

fric·a·tive (frik'ă-tiv). Speech sound made by forcing the air stream through a narrow orifice.

fric·tion (frik'shŭn). 1. The act of rubbing the surface of an object against that of another; especially rubbing the limbs of the body to aid the circulation. 2. The force required for relative motion of two bodies that are in contact. [L. *frictio,* fr. *frico,* to rub]

dynamic f., the force that must be overcome to maintain steady motion of one body relative to another because they remain in contact. Cf. starting f.

starting f., the force that must be overcome to initiate the motion of one body relative to another because they have been resting in contact. Cf. dynamic f. SYN static f.

static f., SYN starting f.

Fridenberg, Percy H., U.S. ophthalmologist, 1868–1960. SEE F.'s stigmometric card *test.*

Fridenberg's stig·o·met·ric card test. See under test.

Friderichsen, Carl, Danish physician, *1886. SEE Waterhouse-F. *syndrome;* Friderichsen-Waterhouse *syndrome.*

Friedländer, Carl, German pathologist, 1847–1887. SEE F.'s *bacillus, pneumonia, stain* for capsules.

Friedman, Emanuel A., U.S. obstetrician, *1926. SEE F. *curve.*

Friedreich, Nikolaus, German neurologist, 1825–1882. SEE F.'s *ataxia, phenomenon, sign.*

Friend, Charlotte, U.S. microbiologist, *1921. SEE F. *disease, virus,* leukemia *virus.*

frig·id (frij'id). 1. SYN cold. 2. Temperamentally, especially sexually, cold or irresponsive. [L. *frigidus,* cold]

fri·gid·i·ty (fri-jid'i-tē). 1. Impotence in the female. 2. The state of being frigid (2); female sexual inadequacy ranging from the freudian concept of inability to achieve orgasm to any degree of sexual response considered unsatisfactory by either the female or her partner.

frig·o·rif·ic (frig-ō-rif'ik). Producing cold. [L. *frigus,* cold, + *facio,* to make]

frig·o·rism (frig'ō-rizm). SYN cryopathy. [L. *frigus,* cold]

fringe (frinj). SYN fimbria (1).

costal f., an irregularly disposed collection of visible veins seen in the skin of people usually of or past middle age; it has no specific connection with any deep structure, such as the diaphragm, and no necessary connection with underlying visceral disease. SYN zona corona.

Richard's f.'s, SYN *fimbriae* of uterine tube, under *fimbria.*

synovial f., SYN synovial *villi,* under *villus.*

frit (frit). 1. The material from which the glaze for artificial teeth is made. 2. A powdered pigment material used in coloring the porcelain of artificial teeth. [Fr. *frit,* fried]

Fritsch, Heinrich, German gynecologist, 1844–1915. SEE Bozeman-F. *catheter.*

Froehde, A., 19th century German chemist. SEE F.'s *reagent.*

frog (frŏg). 1. An amphibian in the order Anura, which includes the toads; the commonest frog genera are *Rana* (grass frogs) and *Hyla* (tree frogs). 2. A specialized portion of the hoof of the horse; a wedge-shaped, horny mass lying between the bars and the sole on the ground surface of the foot. [A.S. *frogge*]

Fröhlich, Alfred, Austrian neurologist and pharmacologist, 1871–1953. SEE F.'s *dwarfism, syndrome.*

Frohn, Damianus, German physician, *1843. SEE F.'s *reagent.*

Froin, Georges, French physician, 1874–1932. SEE F.'s *syndrome.*

frôle·ment (frol-mon'). 1. Light friction or massage with the palm of the hand. 2. A rustling sound heard in auscultation. [Fr.]

Froment, Jules, Lyon physician, 1878–1946. SEE F.'s *sign.*

Frommel, Richard, German gynecologist, 1854–1912. SEE Chiari-F. *syndrome.*

frons, gen. **fron·tis** (fronz, fron'tis) [NA]. SYN forehead. [L.]

front (frŭnt). The position of the leading edge of the solvent in chromatography.

front·ad (frŭn'tad). Toward the front.

fron·tal (frŭn'tăl). 1. In front; relating to the anterior part of a body. 2. Referring to the frontal (coronal) plane or to the frontal bone or forehead. SYN frontalis [NA].

fron·ta·lis (frŭn-tā'lis) [NA]. SYN frontal. [L.]

fron·to·ma·lar (frŭn'tō-mā'lăr). SYN frontozygomatic.

fron·to·max·il·lary (frŭn'tō-mak'si-lā-rē). Relating to the frontal and the maxillary bones.

fron·to·na·sal (frŭn'tō-nā'săl). Relating to the frontal and the nasal bones.

fron·to·oc·cip·i·tal (frŭn'tō-ok-sip'i-tăl). Relating to the frontal and the occipital bones, or to the forehead and the occiput.

fron·to·pa·ri·e·tal (frŭn'tō-pa-rī'ĕ-tăl). Relating to the frontal and the parietal bones.

fron·to·tem·po·ral (frŭn-tō-tem'pŏ-răl). Relating to the frontal and the temporal bones.

fron·to·tem·po·ra·le (frŭn'tō-tem-pō-rā'lē). A craniometric point located at the most anterior point of the temporal line on the frontal bone.

fron·to·zy·go·mat·ic (frŭn'tō-zī'gō-mat'ik). Relating to the frontal and zygomatic bones. SYN frontomalar.

Froriep, August von, German anatomist, 1849–1917. SEE F.'s *ganglion, induration.*

Frost, Albert D., U.S. ophthalmologist, 1889–1945. SEE F. *suture.*

Frost, William A., English ophthalmologist, 1853–1935.

frost. A deposit resembling that of frozen vapor or dew.

urea f., uremic f., powdery deposits on the skin, especially the face, of urea and uric acid salts due to excretion of nitrogenous compounds in the sweat; seen in severe uremia. SYN uridrosis crystallina.

frost·bite (frost'bīt). Local tissue destruction resulting from exposure to extreme cold; in mild cases, it results in superficial, reversible freezing followed by erythema and slight pain; in severe cases, it can be painless or paresthetic and result in blistering, persistent edema, and gangrene. F. is currently treated by rapid rewarming. SYN dermatitis congelationis.

frot·tage (frō-tahzh'). 1. The rubbing movement in massage. 2. Production of sexual excitement by rubbing against someone. [F. a rubbing]

frot·teur (frō-tuhr'). One who gets sexual excitement through frottage.

FRS Abbreviation for first rank *symptoms,* under *symptom.*

F.R.S. Abbreviation for Fellow of the Royal Society.

F.R.S.C. Abbreviation for Fellow of the Royal Society (Canada).

Fru Symbol for fructose.

fruc·tans (frŭk′tanz). High-molecular weight polysaccharides of fructose; *e.g.*, inulin.

⌂fructo-. Chemical prefix denoting the fructose configuration. [L. *fructus,* fruit]

fruc·to·fu·ra·nose (frŭk-tō-fūr′ă-nōs, fruk-). Fructose in furanose form.

β-fruc·to·fu·ran·o·sid·ase (frŭk′tō-fūr-ă-nō-sīd′ās, fruk-). β-*h*-Fructosidase; an enzyme hydrolyzing β-D-fructofuranosides and releasing free D-fructose; if the substrate is sucrose, the product is D-glucose plus D-fructose (invert sugar); invert sugar is more easily digestible than sucrose. SYN invertase, invertin, saccharase.

fruc·to·ki·nase (frŭk-tō-kī′nās, fruk-). A liver enzyme that catalyzes the reaction of ATP and D-fructose to form fructose 6-phosphate and ADP; deficient in individuals with essential fructosuria (hepatic f. deficiency).

fruc·tol·y·sis (fruk-to′lĭ-sis). The conversion of fructose to lactate; analogous to glycolysis.

fruc·to·san (frŭk′tō-san, fruk-). A polysaccharide of fructose (*e.g.*, inulin) containing small amounts of other sugars; present in certain tubers. SYN levan, levulan, levulin, levulosan, polyfructose.

fruc·tose (Fru) (frŭk′tōs, fruk-). D-*arabino*-2-Hexulose; the D-isomer (also referred to as fruit sugar, levoglucose, levulose, and D-*arabino*-2-hexulose, is a 2-ketohexose that in D form is physiologically the most important of the ketohexoses and one of the two products of sucrose hydrolysis, and is metabolized or converted to glycogen in the absence of insulin. [L. *fructus,* fruit, + -ose]

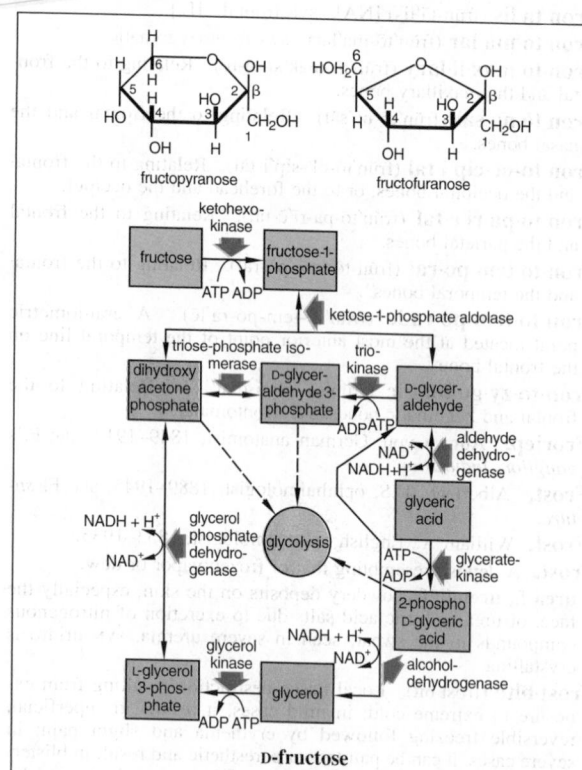

D-fructose

fruc·tose-bis·phos·pha·tase. A hydrolase that catalyzes conversion of fructose 1,6-bisphosphate to D-fructose 6-phosphate and phosphate in gluconeogenesis; AMP is an allosteric inhibitor; f.-b. deficiency results in problems with impaired gluconeogenesis; there is a similar enzyme that acts on fructose 2,6-bisphosphate.

fruc·tose 1,6-bis·phos·phate. A key intermediate in glycolysis and gluconeogenesis. SYN hexosebisphosphatase, hexosediphosphatase.

fruc·tose 2,6-bis·phos·phate. An analog of fructose 1,6-bisphosphate that plays a key role in the regulation of glycolysis and gluconeogenesis; activates phosphofructokinase and inhibits fructose 1,6-bisphosphatase.

fruc·tose-bis·phos·phate al·dol·ase. Fructose-1,6-bisphosphate triphosphate-lyase; an enzyme reversibly cleaving fructose 1,6-bisphosphate to dihydroxyacetone phosphate and glyceraldehyde 3-phosphate; also acts on certain ketose 1-phosphates; deficient in individuals with hereditary fructose intolerance (aldolase B); a deficiency of aldolase A leads to erythrocyte aldolase deficiency with nonspherocytic hemolytic anemia. Cf. hereditary fructose *intolerance.* SYN 1-phosphofructaldolase, fructosediphosphate aldolase.

fruc·tose-di·phos·phate al·dol·ase. SYN fructose-bisphosphate aldolase.

fruc·to·se·mia (frŭk-tō-sē′mē-ă, fruk-). Presence of fructose in the circulating blood. SEE ALSO hereditary fructose *intolerance.* SYN levulosemia.

fruc·tose 1-phos·phate. A fructose derivative that accumulates in individuals with hereditary fructose intolerance.

fruc·tose 6-phos·phate. An intermediate in glycolysis and in transketolation of erythrose 4-phosphate. SYN Neuberg ester.

fruc·to·side (frŭk′tō-sīd, fruk′). Fructose in -C-O- linkage where the -C-O- group is the original 2 group of the fructose.

fruc·to·su·ria (frŭk-tō-sū′rē-ă, fruk-). Excretion of fructose in the urine. SYN levulosuria. [fructose + G. *ouron,* urine]

essential f. [MIM*229800], a benign, asymptomatic inborn error of metabolism due to deficiency of fructokinase, the first enzyme in the specific fructose pathway; fructose appears in the blood and urine, but is simply excreted unchanged; autosomal recessive inheritance. A fructokinase deficiency. SEE ALSO hereditary fructose *intolerance.*

⌂fructosyl-. Chemical prefix indicating fructose in -C-R- (not -C-O-R-) linkage through its carbon-2 (R usually C).

fru·se·mide (frū′sĕ-mīd). SYN furosemide.

frus·tra·tion (frŭs′trā′shŭn). A psychologic or psychiatric term indicating the thwarting of or inability to gratify a desire or to satisfy an urge or need. [L. *frustro,* pp. *-atus,* to deceive, disappoint, fr. *frustra* (adv.), in vain]

FSH Abbreviation for follicle-stimulating *hormone.*

FSH-RF Abbreviation for follicle-stimulating hormone-releasing *factor.*

FSH-RH Abbreviation for follicle-stimulating hormone-releasing *hormone.*

ft. Abbreviation for L. *fiat,* let it be done (made); abbreviation for foot or feet.

FTA-ABS. Abbreviation for fluorescent treponemal antibody absorption. SEE fluorescent treponemal antibody-absorption *test.*

FTI Abbreviation for free thyroxine *index.*

Fuc Abbreviation for fucose.

Fuchs, Ernst, Austrian ophthalmologist, 1851–1930. SEE F.'s *adenoma; angle* of F.; F.'s heterochromic *cyclitis, coloboma,* epithelial *dystrophy,* black *spot, spur, stomas,* under *stoma, syndrome, uveitis;* Dalen-F. *nodules,* under *nodule.*

fuch·sin (fuk′sin). A nonspecific term referring to any of several red rosanilin dyes used as stains in histology and bacteriology. [Leonhard *Fuchs,* German botanist, 1501–1506]

acid f. [C.I. 42685], a mixture of the sodium salts bi- and trisulfonic acids of rosanilin and pararosanilin; used as an indicator dye and for staining of cytoplasm and collagen. SYN rubin S, rubine.

aldehyde f., a stain developed by Gomori, utilizing basic f. paraldehyde and hydrochloric acid; it produces violet staining of elastic fibers, mast cell granules, gastric chief cells, beta cells of the pancreatic islets, and certain hypophyseal beta granules; other pituitary granules and cells stain in other colors. SEE ALSO Gomori's aldehyde fuchsin *stain.*

aniline f., a mixture of aniline and basic f. in 30% ethanol with a trace of phenol, as in Goodpasture's stain.

basic f. [C.I. 42500], a triphenylmethane dye whose dominant component is pararosanilin; an important stain in histology, histochemistry, and bacteriology. SYN diamond f.

carbol f., SEE carbol-fuchsin paint, Ziehl's stain.

diamond f., SYN basic f.

fuch·sin·o·phil (fuk'si-nō-fil). **1.** Staining readily with fuchsin dyes. SYN fuchsinophilic. **2.** A cell or histologic element that stains readily with fuchsin. [fuchsin + G. *philos,* fond]

fuch·sin·o·phil·ia (fuk'si-nō-fil'ē-ă). The property of staining readily with fuchsin.

fuch·sin·o·phil·ic (fuk'si-nō-fil'ik). SYN fuchsinophil (1).

fu·cose (Fuc) (fyū'kōs). 6-Deoxygalactose; a methylpentose, the L-configuration of which occurs in the mucopolysaccharides of the blood group substances, in human milk (as a polysaccharide), and elsewhere in nature. The D-configuration has been found in certain antibiotics. SYN rhodeose.

α-fu·co·si·dase (fyū-kōs'i-dās). An enzyme that catalyzes the hydrolysis of an an α-L-fucoside, producing an alcohol and L-fucose; a deficiency of the lysosomal enzyme will result in fucosidosis.

fu·co·si·do·sis (fyū'kō-sī-dō'sis) [MIM*230000]. A metabolic storage disease characterized by accumulation of fucose-containing glycolipids and deficiency of the enzyme α-fucosidase; progressive neurologic deterioration begins after the first year of life, accompanied by spasticity, tremor, and mild skeletal changes; autosomal recessive inheritance.

FUDR Abbreviation for fluorodeoxyuridine. SEE floxuridine.

fu·gac·i·ty (f) (fū-gas'i-tē). The tendency of the molecules in a fluid, as a result of all forces acting on them, to leave a given site in the body; the escaping tendency of a fluid, as in diffusion, evaporation, etc. [L. *fuga,* flight]

△**-fugal.** Movement away from the part indicated by the main portion of the word. [L. *fugio,* to flee]

△**-fuge.** Flight, denoting the place from which flight takes place or that which is put to flight. [L. *fuga* a running away]

fu·gi·tive (fyū'ji-tiv). **1.** Temporary; transient. **2.** Fleeting; denoting certain inconstant symptoms. [L. *fugitivus,* fleeing, fr. *fugio,* pp. *fugitus,* to flee]

fugue (fūg). A condition in which an individual suddenly abandons a present activity or lifestyle and starts a new and different one for a period of time, often in a different city; afterward, the individual alleges amnesia for events occurring during the f. period, although earlier events are remembered and habits and skills are usually unaffected. [Fr. fr. L. *fuga,* flight]

fu·gu·tox·in (fū'gū-tok-sin). The potent poison derived from the ovaries and skin of the Pacific pufferfish. SEE ALSO tetradotoxin.

ful·crum, pl. **ful·cra, ful·crums** (ful'krŭm, -kră, -krŭmz). A support or the point thereon on which a lever turns. [L. a bedpost, fr. *fulcio,* to prop up]

ful·gu·rant (ful'gŭ-rănt). Sharp and piercing. Cf. fulminant. SYN fulgurating (1). [L. *fulgur,* flashing lightning]

ful·gu·rat·ing (ful'gŭ-rā-ting). **1.** SYN fulgurant. **2.** Relating to fulguration.

ful·gu·ra·tion (ful-gŭ-rā'shŭn). Destruction of tissue by means of a high-frequency electric current: **direct f.** utilizes an insulated electrode with a metal point, which is connected to the uniterminal of the high-frequency apparatus, from which a spark of electricity is allowed to impinge on the area to be treated; **indirect f.** involves directly connecting the patient by a metal handle to the uniterminal and utilizing an active electrode to complete an arc from the patient. [L. *fulgur,* lightning stroke]

ful·mi·nant (ful'mi-nănt). Occurring suddenly, with lightning-like rapidity, and with great intensity or severity; applied to certain pains, *e.g.,* those of tabes dorsalis. Cf. fulgurant. [L. *fulmino,* pp. *-atus,* to hurl lightning, fr. *fulmen,* lightning]

ful·mi·nat·ing (ful'mi-nā'ting). Running a speedy course, with rapid worsening.

fu·ma·rase (fyū'mă-rās). SYN fumarate hydratase.

fu·ma·rate hy·dra·tase (fyū'mă-rāt). An enzyme catalyzing the reversible interconversion of fumaric acid and water to malic acid, a reaction of importance in the tricarboxylic acid cycle. A deficiency will lead to mental retardation. SYN fumarase.

fu·ma·rate re·duc·tase (NADH) [EC 1.3.1.6]. SYN *succinate* dehydrogenase.

fu·mar·ic ac·id (fyū-mar'ik). *trans*-Butanedioic acid; an unsaturated dicarboxylic acid occurring as an intermediate in the tricarboxylic acid cycle. SYN allomaleic acid.

fu·mar·ic ac·i·de·mia. Elevated levels of fumarate in blood plasma; due to a decrease in activity of fumarate hydratase.

fu·mar·ic am·i·nase. SYN *aspartate* ammonia-lyase.

fu·mar·ic hy·dro·gen·ase. SYN *succinate* dehydrogenase.

fum·ar·yl·ac·e·to·ac·e·tate (fyū-mă'ril-as-ē'tō-ăs-ē-tāt). $HOOCCH=CHCOCH_2COCH_2COOH$; an intermediate in phenylalanine and tyrosine catabolism; elevated in tyrosinemia IA.

f. hydrolase, an enzyme that catalyzes the hydrolysis of f. to fumarate and acetoacetate; a deficiency indicates tyrosinemia IA.

fu·mi·gant (fyū'mi-gănt). A substance utilized in fumigation.

fu·mi·gate (fyū'mi-gāt). To expose to the action of smoke or of fumes of any kind as a means of disinfection or eradication. [L. *fumigo* pp. *-atus,* to fumigate, fr. *fumus,* smoke, + *ago,* to drive]

fu·mi·ga·tion (fyū-mi-gā'shŭn). The act of fumigating; the use of a fumigant.

fum·ing (fyūm'ing). Giving forth a visible vapor, a property of concentrated nitric, sulfuric, and hydrochloric acids, and certain other substances. [L. *fumus,* smoke]

func·tio lae·sa (fŭngk'shē-ō lē'să). Loss of function; a fifth sign of inflammation added by Galen to those enunciated by Celsus (rubor, tumor, calor, and dolor). [L.]

func·tion (fŭngk'shŭn). **1.** The special action or physiologic property of an organ or other part of the body. **2.** To perform its special work or office, said of an organ or other part of the body. **3.** The general properties of any substance, depending on its chemical character and relation to other substances, according to which it may be grouped among acids, bases, alcohols, esters, etc. **4.** A particular reactive grouping in a molecule; *e.g.,* a functional group, such as the —OH group of an alcohol. **5.** A quality, trait, or fact that is so related to another as to be dependent upon and to vary with this other. [L. *functio,* fr. *fungor,* pp. *functus,* to perform]

allomeric f., the combined f. of the several segments of the spinal cord and medulla, communicating with each other by means of the white matter.

arousal f., the ability of a sensory event to arouse the cortex to vigilance or readiness.

atrial transport f., the role of the atria in filling and stretching the ventricles by their presystolic contraction, without which the force of ventricular contraction and hence the cardiac output may significantly decrease.

discriminant f., a particular combination of continuous variable test results designed to achieve separation of groups; *e.g.,* a single number representing a combination of weighted laboratory test results designed to discriminate between clinical classes.

isomeric f., the individual f. of an isolated segment of the spinal cord.

line spread f. (LSF), a measure of the ability of a system to form sharp images; in radiology, determined by measuring the spatial density distribution on film of the x-ray image of a narrow slit in a dense metal, such as uranium; from this can be calculated the modulation transfer f.

modulation transfer f. (MTF), in depicting radionuclide distribution or radiographic systems, the efficiency, at a given spatial frequency, of transferring the modulation of the object to that of the image; it is a more complete expression of spatial resolution and is used to evaluate imaging systems and their components; also known as the frequency response function or contrast transmission f.; usually given as a plot of percent amplitude response versus frequency in cycles per mm.

func·tion·al (fŭnk'shŭn-ăl). **1.** Relating to a function. **2.** Not organic in origin; denoting a disorder with no known or detectable organic basis to explain the symptoms. SEE neurosis.

func·tion·al·ism (fŭnk'shŭn-ăl-izm). A branch of psychology

fu

concerned with the function of mental processes in man and animals, especially the role of the mind, intellect, emotions, and behavior in an individual's adaptation to the environment. Cf. structuralism.

func·tion cor·rec·tor. A removable orthodontic appliance utilizing oral and facial muscle forces to move teeth and possibly change the relationship of the dental arches.

fun·da·ment (fŭn'dă-ment). **1.** A foundation. **2.** The anus. [L. *fundamentum*, foundation, fr. *fundus*, bottom]

fun·dec·to·my (fŭn-dek'tō-mē). SYN fundusectomy. [fundus + G. *ektomē*, excision]

fun·dic (fŭn'dik). Relating to a fundus.

fun·di·form (fŭn'di-fōrm). Looped; sling-shaped. [L. *funda*, a sling, + *forma*, shape]

fun·do·pli·ca·tion (fŭn'dō-pli-kā'shŭn). Suture of the fundus of the stomach around the esophagus to prevent reflux in repair of hiatal hernia. SYN Nissen's operation. [fundus + L. *plico*, to fold]

Fun·du·lus (fŭn'dŭ-lŭs). A genus of marine and freshwater fish, of many species, native to the U.S.; commonly called killifish, mumichog, or mudfish. They are widely used as bait fish, experimental fish, or in mosquito-control programs. [Mod. L. fr. L. *fundus*, bottom]

fun·dus, pl. **fun·di** (fŭn'dŭs, dī) [NA]. The bottom or lowest part of a sac or hollow organ; that part farthest removed from the opening or exit; occasionally a broad cul-de-sac. [L. bottom]

f. albipuncta'tus [MIM*136880], a nonprogressive disorder of the retinal pigment epithelium characterized by numerous discrete, white dots; night blindness is a feature; the genetics involved are unclear.

f. diabet'icus, SYN diabetic *retinopathy.*

f. flavimacula'tus [MIM*230100], a genetic disorder of the pigment epithelium of the retina manifested by yellowish white flecks; some loss of central vision is involved; probably autosomal recesssive.

f. of gallbladder, the wide closed end of the gallbladder situated at the inferior border of the liver. SYN f. vesicae biliaris (felleae) [NA].

f. gastricus [NA], SYN f. of stomach.

f. of internal acoustic meatus, the thin cribriform plate of bone separating the cochlea and vestibule from the internal acoustic meatus; a transverse crest divides it into two regions; in the superior region are located the area nervi facialis and the area vestibularis superior; in the inferior region are located the area cochleae, area vestibularis inferior, and foramen singulare. SYN f. meatus acustici interni [NA], f. of internal auditory meatus.

f. of internal auditory meatus, SYN f. of internal acoustic meatus.

leopard f., SYN tessellated f.

f. mea'tus acus'tici inter'ni [NA], SYN f. of internal acoustic meatus.

mosaic f., SYN tessellated f.

f. oc'uli, the portion of the interior of the eyeball around the posterior pole, visible through the ophthalmoscope. SEE eyegrounds.

pepper and salt f., ophthalmoscopic appearance of the f. caused by choriocapillaris atrophy and pigment proliferation.

f. polycythe'micus, the engorged, dilated veins, with cyanotic retina, occurring in erythremia.

f. of stomach, the portion of the stomach that lies above the cardiac notch. SYN f. gastricus [NA], f. ventriculi✩, greater cul-de-sac.

tessellated f., a normal f. to which a deeply pigmented choroid gives the appearance of dark polygonal areas between the choroidal vessels, especially in the periphery. SYN f. tigré, leopard f., leopard retina, mosaic f., tigroid f., tigroid retina.

f. tigré, SYN tessellated f.

tigroid f., SYN tessellated f.

f. tym'pani, SYN *floor* of tympanic cavity.

f. of urinary bladder, the f. is formed by the posterior wall which is somewhat convex. SYN f. vesicae urinariae [NA], basfond, base of bladder.

f. u'teri [NA], SYN f. of uterus.

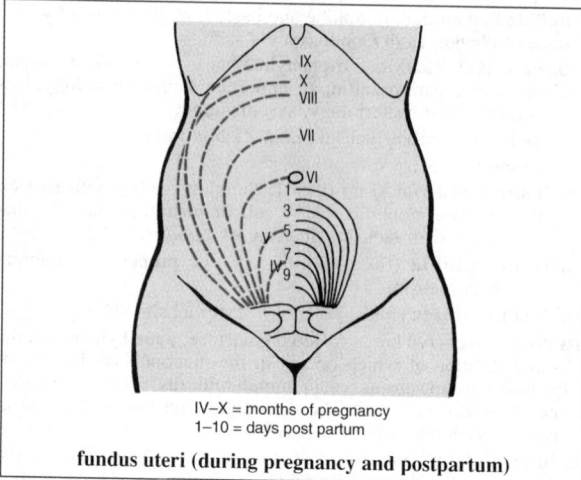

IV–X = months of pregnancy
1–10 = days post partum

fundus uteri (during pregnancy and postpartum)

f. of uterus, the upper rounded extremity of the uterus above the openings of the uterine (fallopian) tubes. SYN f. uteri [NA].

f. ventric'uli, ✩official alternate term for f. of stomach.

f. vesi'cae biliaris (fel'leae) [NA], SYN f. of gallbladder.

f. vesi'cae urina'riae [NA], SYN f. of urinary bladder.

fun·du·scope (fŭn'dŭs-skōp). SYN ophthalmoscope. [L. *fundus*, bottom, + G. *skopeō*, to view]

fun·dus·co·py (fŭn-dŭs'kŏ-pē). SYN ophthalmoscopy.

fun·du·sec·to·my (fŭn-dŭ-sek'tō-mē). Excision of the fundus of an organ. SYN fundectomy. [L. *fundus*, + G. *ektomē*, excision]

fun·gal (fŭng'găl). SYN fungous.

fun·gate (fŭng'gāt). To grow exuberantly like a fungus or spongy growth.

fun·ge·mia (fŭn-jē'mē-ă). Fungal infection disseminated by way of the bloodstream.

Fun·gi (fŭn'jī). A division of eukaryotic organisms that grow in irregular masses, without roots, stems, or leaves, and are devoid of chlorophyll or other pigments capable of photosynthesis. Each organism (thallus) is unicellular to filamentous, and possesses branched somatic structures (hyphae) surrounded by cell walls containing cellulose or chitin or both, and containing true nuclei. They reproduce sexually or asexually (spore formation), and may obtain nutrition from other living organisms as parasites or from dead organic matter as saprobes (saprophytes). [L. *fungus*, a mushroom]

fun·gi (fŭn'jī). Plural of fungus.

fun·gi·ci·dal (fŭn-ji-sī'dăl). Having a killing action on fungi. [fungus + L. *caedo*, to kill]

fun·gi·cide (fŭn'ji-sīd). Any substance that has a destructive killing action upon fungi. SYN mycocide.

fun·gi·ci·din (fŭn-ji-sī'din). SYN nystatin.

fun·gi·form (fŭn'ji-fōrm). Shaped like a fungus or mushroom; applied to any structure with a broad, often branched, free portion and a narrower base. SYN fungilliform.

Fun·gi Im·per·fec·ti (fŭn'jī im-per-fek'tī). A phylum of fungi in which sexual reproduction is not known or in which one of the mating types has not yet been discovered. Formerly, most fungi causing disease in humans were considered asexual and were placed in this class, but studies have revealed that they are not imperfect and that in their sexual forms they can be classified as ascomycetes or basidiomycetes.

fun·gil·li·form (fŭn-jil'i-fōrm). SYN fungiform. [Mod L. *fungillus*, dim. of L. *fungus*]

fun·gi·stat (fŭn'ji-stat). An agent having fungistatic action.

fun·gi·stat·ic (fŭn-ji-stat'ik). Having an inhibiting action upon the growth of fungi. SYN mycostatic. [fungus + G. *statos*, standing]

fun·gi·tox·ic (fŭn-ji-tok'sik). Poisonous or in any way deleterious to the growth of fungi.

fun·gi·tox·ic·i·ty (fŭn′ji-tok-sis′i-tē). The property of being fungitoxic.

fun·goid (fŭng′goyd). Resembling a fungus; denoting an exuberant morbid growth on the surface of the body.

fun·gos·i·ty (fŭng-gos′i-tē). A fungoid growth.

fun·gous (fŭng′gŭs). Relating to a fungus. SYN fungal.

fun·gus, pl. **fun·gi** (fŭng′gŭs, fŭn′jī). A general term used to encompass the diverse morphological forms of yeasts and molds. Originally classified as primitive plants without chlorophyll, the fungi are placed in the kingdom Fungi and some in the kingdom Protista, along with the algae (all but the blue-green algae), the protozoa, and the slime molds. Fungi share with bacteria the important ability to break down complex organic substances of almost every type (cellulose) and are essential to the recycling of carbon and other elements in the cycle of life. Fungi are important as foods and to the fermentation process in the development of substances of industrial and medical importance, including alcohol, the antibiotics, other drugs, and antitoxins. Relatively few fungi are pathogenic for humans, whereas most plant diseases are caused by fungi. [L. *fungus*, a mushroom]

f. cer′ebri, an ulcerated cerebral hernia with granulation tissue protruding from scalp wound.

dematiaceous fungi (de-măt′ē-ā-cē-ous), dark f. that form melanin. [Mod. L. *Dematium* (genus name), fr. g. *demation*, fine strand, fr. *dema*, band, fr. *deō*, to bind + suffix *-aceous*, characterized by]

fission fungi, SYN Schizomycetes.

imperfect f., a f. in which the means of sexual reproduction is not yet recognized; these fungi generally reproduce by means of conidia.

perfect f., a f. possessing both sexual and asexual means of reproduction, and in which both mating forms are recognized.

ray f., a bacterium which is a member of the order Actinomycetales.

thrush f., SYN *Candida albicans*.

umbilical f., a mass of granulation tissue on the stump of the umbilical cord in the newborn.

yeast f., obsolete term for *Saccharomyces*.

fu·nic (few′nik). Relating to the funis, or umbilical cord. SYN funicular (2).

fu·ni·cle (fyū′ni-kl). SYN cord.

fu·nic·u·lar (fyū-nik′yū-lăr). 1. Relating to a funiculus. 2. SYN funic.

fu·nic·u·li·tis (fyū-nik′yū-lī′tis). Inflammation of a funiculus, especially of the spermatic cord. 3. Inflammation of the umbilical cord usually associated with chorioamnionitis. [funiculus + G. *-itis*, inflammation]

endemic f., SYN filarial f.

filarial f., cellulitis of the spermatic cord due to filariasis; occurs endemically in Sri Lanka and Egypt, and probably elsewhere in the East. SYN endemic f.

fu·nic·u·lo·pexy (fyū-nik′yū-lō-pek-sē). Suturing of the spermatic cord to the surrounding tissue in the correction of an undescended testicle. [funiculus + G. *pēxis*, a fixing]

fu·nic·u·lus, pl. **fu·nic·u·li** (fyū-nik′yū-lŭs, -lī) [NA]. SYN cord. [L. dim. of *funis*, cord]

f. am′nii, amniotic cord found in several domestic animals.

anterior f., anterior white column of spinal cord, a column or bundle of white matter on either side of the anterior median fissure, between that and the anterolateral sulcus. SYN f. anterior [NA].

f. ante′rior [NA], SYN anterior f.

cuneate f., SYN cuneate *fasciculus*.

dorsal f., SYN posterior f.

f. dorsa′lis, SYN posterior f.

f. gra′cilis, SYN *fasciculus* gracilis.

lateral f., the lateral white column of the spinal cord between the lines of exit and entrance of the anterior and posterior nerve roots. SYN f. lateralis [NA], anterolateral column of spinal cord, lateral f. of spinal cord.

f. latera′lis [NA], SYN lateral f.

lateral f. of spinal cord, SYN lateral f.

funic′uli medu′llae spina′lis [NA], any of the columns of the spinal cord.

posterior f., posterior white column of the spinal cord, the large wedge-shaped fiber bundle lying between the posterior gray column and the posterior median septum, and composed largely of dorsal root fibers. SYN f. posterior [NA], dorsal f., f. dorsalis.

f. poste′rior [NA], SYN posterior f.

f. sep′arans, an oblique ridge in the floor of the fourth ventricle of the brain, separating the area postrema from the vagal trigone.

f. solita′rius, SYN solitary *tract*.

f. spermat′icus [NA], SYN spermatic *cord*.

f. te′res, SYN medial *eminence*.

f. umbilica′lis [NA], SYN umbilical *cord*.

fu·ni·form (fyū′ni-fōrm). Ropelike. [L. *funis*, cord, + *forma*, shape]

fu·ni·punc·ture (fyū-nē-pŭnk-chŭr). SYN cordocentesis. [L. *funis*, cord, + puncture]

fu·nis (fyū′nis). 1. SYN umbilical *cord*. 2. A cordlike structure. [L. a rope, cord]

fun·nel (fŭn′ĕl). 1. A hollow conical vessel with a tube of variable length proceeding from its apex, used in pouring fluids from one container to another, in filtering, etc. 2. In anatomy, an infundibulum.

Büchner f., a porcelain f. that contains a perforated porcelain plate upon which filter paper can be laid.

Martegiani's f., the funnel-shaped dilation on the optic disk that indicates the beginning of the hyaloid canal. SYN Martegiani's area.

pial f., the pia-lined channel in which each blood vessel entering the brain lies suspended; essentially, the pial f.'s are perivascular extensions of the subarachnoid space.

FUO Abbreviation for fever of unknown origin.

fur (fer). 1. The coat of soft, fine hair of some mammals. 2. A layer of epithelium, mucus, and debris on the dorsum of the tongue. Its relation to underlying disease or disturbance of the alimentary canal is not proved. [M.E. *furre*, fr. O.Fr., fr. Germanic]

fura-2 (fū′ra). A fluorescent indicator which binds calcium; it is excited at longer wavelengths when free of calcium than when calcium is bound; the ratio of fluorescence intensity at two excitation wavelengths provides a measure of free calcium ion concentration; may be injected into cells to monitor moment-to-moment changes in intracellular free calcium ion concentration. SEE ALSO aequorin.

fu·ral·ta·done (fyū-ral′tă-dōn). Furmethonol; nitrofurmethone; a complex morpholino-furfuryl-oxazolidone; an antibacterial agent.

fu·ran (fyūr′an). A cyclic compound found, usually in saturated form, in those sugars with an oxygen bridge between carbon atoms 1 and 4, or 2 and 5, or 3 and 7, for which reason they are known as furanoses.

fu·ra·nose (fyūr′ă-nōs). A saccharide unit or molecule containing the furan grouping; specific examples are preceded by prefixes indicating the configuration, *e.g.*, fructofuranose, ribofuranose. [furan + -ose(1)]

fu·ra·zol·i·done (fyū-ră-zol′i-dōn). 3-(5-Nitro-2-furfurylideneamino)-2-oxazolidione; has antibacterial and antiprotozoal activity against enteric organisms; used in the treatment of bacterial enteritis and diarrhea.

fur·cal (fer′kăl). Forked.

fur·ca·tion (fŭr-kā′shŭn). 1. A forking, or a forklike part or branch. 2. In dental histology, the region of a multirooted tooth at which the roots divide. [L. *furca*, fork]

fur·cu·la (fer′kyū-lă). 1. The fused clavicles, which form the V-shaped bone (wishbone) of the bird's skeleton. 2. In the embryo, an inverted U-shaped elevation that appears on the ventral wall of the pharynx, being formed by the two linear ridges and the caudal part of the hypobranchial eminence; the depression enclosed by the U is the laryngotracheal groove. [L. a forked prop, dim. of *furca*, a fork]

fu

fur·fur, pl. **fur·fu·res** (fer′fer, fer′fyū-rēz). An epidermal scale; *e.g.,* dandruff. [L. bran]

fur·fu·ra·ceous (fer-fyū-rā′shŭs). Branny, or composed of small scales; denoting a form of desquamation. SYN pityroid. [L. *furfuraceus,* fr. *furfur,* bran]

fur·fu·ral (fer′fyūr-ăl). C_4H_3O-CHO; C_4H_3O-CHO; a colorless, aromatic, irritating fluid obtained in the distillation of bran with dilute sulfuric acid; used in the manufacture of medicinal agents.

fur·fu·rol (fer′fyūr-ol). Misnomer for furfural and furfuryl alcohol.

fur·fu·ryl (fer′fyū-ril). The monovalent radical derived from f. alcohol by loss of the OH group.

   f. alcohol, 2-furanmethanol; 2-hydroxymethylfuran; a solvent and wetting agent.

fur·nace (fŭr′năs). A stovelike apparatus containing a chamber for heating, melting, or fusing.

   dental f., (1) a f. used to eliminate the wax pattern from the investment mold prior to casting in metal; **(2)** a f. used to fuse and glaze dental porcelains.

   muffle f., (1) an electric f. heated by direct transfer of heat from a resistant muffle; **(2)** a dental f. heated by a muffle.

fu·ror ep·i·lep·ti·cus (fyū′rōr ep-i-lep′ti-kŭs). Attacks of anger to which epileptic individuals are occasionally subject, occurring without apparent provocation and without disturbance of consciousness.

fu·ro·se·mide (fyū-rō′sĕ-mid, -mīd). 4-Chloro-*N*-furfuryl-5-sulfamoylanthranilic acid; a diuretic used in edematous states and hypertension. SYN frusemide.

fur·row (fer′rō). A groove or sulcus. [A.S. *furh*]

   digital f., SYN digital *crease.*

   genital f., a groove on the genital tubercle in the embryo, appearing toward the end of the second month.

   gluteal f., SYN gluteal *fold.*

   mentolabial f., SYN mentolabial *sulcus.*

   primitive f., SYN primitive *groove.*

   skin f.'s, the numerous grooves of variable depth on the surface of the epidermis. SYN sulci cutis [NA], skin grooves.

fu·run·cle (fyū′rŭng-kl). A localized pyogenic infection, most frequently by *Staphylococcus aureus,* originating deep in a hair follicle. SYN boil, furunculus. [L. *furunculus,* a petty thief]

fu·run·cu·lar (fyū-rŭng′kyū-lăr). Relating to a furuncle. SYN furunculous.

fu·run·cu·loid (fyū-rŭng′kyū-loyd). Resembling a furuncle. [furunculus + G. *eidos,* resemblance]

fu·run·cu·lo·sis (fyū-rŭng-kyū-lō′sis). A condition marked by the presence of furuncles, often chronic and recurrent.

   f. orienta′lis, the lesion occurring in cutaneous leishmaniasis.

fu·run·cu·lous (fyū-rŭng′kyū-lŭs). SYN furuncular.

fu·run·cu·lus, pl. **fu·run·cu·li** (fyū-rŭng′kyū-lŭs, -lī). SYN furuncle. [L. a petty thief, a boil, dim. of *fur,* a thief]

Fu·sar·i·um (fyū-zā′rē-ŭm). A genus of rapidly growing fungi producing characteristic sickle-shaped, multiseptate macroconidia which can be mistaken for those produced by some dermatophytes. Usually saprobic, a few species such as *F. oxysporum* and *F. solani,* *F. moniliforme,* and other species can produce corneal ulcers; some species are common colonizers of burned skin and some species may cause disseminated hyalohyphomycosis. [L. *fusus,* spindle]

   F. graminearum, a species producing the toxin zearalenone, which causes estrogenism in pigs.

   F. moniliforme, a species producing the toxin fumonisin B_1, which causes equine leukoencephalomalacia in horses and other Equidae.

fu·seau (fĕ-zō). A fusiform or spindle-shaped, multiseptate macroconidium. [Fr. *spindle* fr. L. *fusus*]

fu·si·date so·di·um (fyū′si-dāt). The sodium salt of fusidic acid; has antibacterial properties. SYN sodium fusidate.

fu·sid·ic ac·id (fyū-sid′ik). 3α,11α,16β-Trihydroxy-4α,8, 14-trimethyl-18-nor-5α,8α,9β,13α, 14β-cholesta-17(20),24-dien-21-oic 16-acetate; a fermentation product of *Fusidium coccine-*

um, a parasitic fungus on the plant *Veronica;* inhibits protein synthesis. SEE fusidate sodium.

fu·si·form (fyū′zi-fōrm, fyū′si-). Spindle-shaped; tapering at both ends. [L. *fusus,* a spindle, + *forma,* form]

Fu·si·for·mis (fyū-si-fōr′mis). An obsolete generic name sometimes used for the anaerobic fusiform bacteria found in the human mouth; these organisms are closely related to the anaerobic organisms found in the human intestine and have been placed in the genus *Fusobacterium.* [see fusiform]

fu·si·mo·tor (fyū′zē-mō′ter). Pertaining to the efferent innervation of intrafusal muscle fibers by gamma motor neurons. SEE ALSO neuromuscular *spindle.* [L. *fusus,* spindle, + *moveo,* to move]

fu·sion (fyū′zhŭn). **1.** Liquefaction, as by melting by heat. **2.** Union, as by joining together. **3.** The blending of slightly different images from each eye into a single perception. **4.** The joining of two or more adjacent teeth during their development by a dentinal union. SEE ALSO concrescence. **5.** Joining of two genes, often neighboring genes. [L. *fusio,* a pouring, fr. *fundo,* pp. *fusus,* to pour]

   cell f., the merging of the contents of two cells by artificial means without the destruction of either, resulting in a heterokaryon that, for at least a few generations, will reproduce its kind; an important method in assignment of loci to chromosomes.

   centric f., SYN robertsonian *translocation.*

   flicker f., SEE critical flicker fusion *frequency.*

   nuclear f., the formation of more complex atomic nuclei from less complex nuclei with release of energy, as in the formation of helium nuclei from hydrogen nuclei (hydrogen f.).

   spinal f., spine f., an operative procedure to accomplish bony ankylosis between two or more vertebrae. SYN spondylosyndesis, vertebral f.

   splenogonadal f., the formation of a mass consisting of splenic and testicular or ovarian tissue.

   vertebral f., SYN spinal f.

Fu·so·bac·te·ri·um (fyū′zō-bak-tēr′ē-ŭm). A genus of bacteria (family Bacteroidaceae) containing Gram-negative, nonsporeforming, obligately anaerobic rods which produce butyric acid as a major metabolic product. Nonmotile and motile organisms occur; motile cells are peritrichous. These organisms are found in cavities of humans and other animals; some species are pathogenic. The type species is *F. nucleatum.* [L. *fusus,* a spindle, + bacterium]

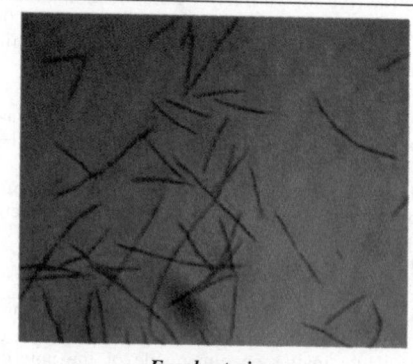

Fusobacterium

   F. morti′ferum, *Sphaerophorus mortiferus*; a species found in various infections in humans.

   F. necro′phorum, *Sphaerophorus necrophorus*; a bacterial species causing or associated with several necrotic conditions in animals, such as calf diphtheria, labial necrosis of rabbits, necrotic rhinitis of pigs, foot rot of cattle, sheep, and goats, and occasionally necrotic lesions in humans. SYN necrosis bacillus, Schmorl's bacillus.

   F. nuclea′tum, a species (probably Plaut's or Vincent's bacillus) found in the mouth and in infections of the upper respiratory tract, pleural cavity, and occasionally the lower intestinal tract; it is the type species of the genus *F.*

F. plau'ti, a species found in the buccal cavity; also found in cultures of *Entamoeba histolytica.* SYN *Eubacterium plauti.*

fu·so·cel·lu·lar (fyū′zō-sel′yū-lăr). Spindle-celled.

fu·so·spi·ro·chet·al (fyū-zō-spī-rō-kē′tăl). Referring to the associated fusiform and spirochetal organisms such as those found in the lesions of Vincent's angina.

fus·tic (fŭs′tik). A complex of natural dyes derived from certain West Indian, Central, and South American trees, *Rhus cotinus* and *Chlorophora tinctoria;* used as mordant dyes for textiles. An important dye in the complex is morin, which is associated with the dye maclurin.

fus·ti·ga·tion (fŭs′ti-gā′shŭn). A form of massage consisting in beating the surface with light rods. [L. *fustigo,* pp. *-atus,* to beat with a cudgel]

Futcher, Palmer Howard, U.S.-Canadian physician, *1910. SEE F.'s *line.*

Futcher's line. See under line.

FVC Abbreviation for forced vital *capacity.*

Fy blood group. See Duffy blood group, Blood Groups Appendix.

Fy

γ **1.** Third letter in the Greek alphabet, gamma. **2.** In chemistry, denotes the third in a series, the fourth carbon in an aliphatic acid, or position 2 removed from the α position in the benzene ring. **3.** Symbol for 10^{-4} gauss; surface *tension*; activity *coefficient*. **4.** Symbol for photon. For terms having this prefix, see the specific term.

G Abbreviation or symbol for Newtonian *constant* of gravitation, gravitational *units*, under *unit*; gap (3); gauss; giga-; D-glucose, as in UDPG; guanosine, as in GDP; glycine; guanine.

G Symbol for Gibbs free *energy*; G_{act} or $G^{\ddagger}$, Gibbs *energy* of activation.

g Abbreviation for gram.

g. Unit of acceleration based on the acceleration produced by the earth's gravitational attraction, where 1 *g* = 980.621 cm/sec^2 (about 32.1725 ft/sec^2) at sea level and 45° latitude. At 30° latitude, *g* equals 979.329 cm/sec^2.

G1. Symbol for *gap* 1.

G2. Symbol for *gap* 2.

Ga Symbol for gallium.

^{67}**Ga.** Symbol for gallium-67.

^{68}**Ga.** Symbol for gallium-68.

GABA Abbreviation for γ-aminobutyric acid.

G ac·id. 2-Naphthol-6,8-disulfonic acid.

G-ac·tin. See under actin.

GAD Abbreviation for *glutamate* decarboxylase.

Gaddum, John H., English biochemist, *1900. SEE G. and Schild *test*.

gad·fly (gad′flī). SEE *Tabanus*.

gad·o·di·am·ide (gad-ō-dī′ă-mid). GdDTPA-BMA, diethylenetriaminepentaacetatobis(methylamide)gadolinium (III); a nonionic structural analog of gadolinium DPTA; used as a paramagnetic contrast medium in magnetic resonance imaging.

gad·o·le·ic ac·id (gad-ō-lē′ik). An unsaturated fatty acid from cod liver oil and other sources. SYN 9-eicosenoic acid.

gad·o·lin·i·um (Gd) (gad-ō-lin′ē-ŭm). An element of the lanthanide group, atomic no. 64, atomic wt. 157.25. The pramagnetic properties of this element are used in contrast media for magnetic resonance imaging. [mineral, gadolinite, from Johan *Gadolin,* Finnish chemist, 1760–1852]

gad·o·pen·te·tate (gad-ō-pen′tĕ-tāt). (NMG)2[GdDTPA], dimeglumine diethylenetriaminepentaacetatogadolinate (III); the methylglucamine salt of dianionic gadolinium DPTA, an acyclic chelate; used as a paramagnetic contrast medium in magnetic resonance imaging.

gad·o·ter·i·dol (gad-ō-ter′i-dol). GdHP-DO3A; a gadolinium (III) chelate of 10-(2-hydroxypropyl)-1,4,7,10-tetraaza-cyclododecane-1,4,7-triacetic acid; a nonionic macrocyclic analog of gadolinium DOTA; used as a paramagnetic contrast medium in magnetic resonance imaging.

Gaenslen, Frederick J., U.S. surgeon, 1877–1937. SEE G.'s *sign*.

Gaffky, Georg T.A., German hygienist, 1850–1918. SEE G. *scale, table*.

gag. 1. To retch; to cause to retch or heave. **2.** To prevent from talking. **3.** An instrument adjusted between the teeth to keep the mouth from closing during operations in the mouth or throat.

Davis-Crowe mouth g., instrument used for opening the mouth, depressing the tongue, maintaining the airway, and transmitting volatile anesthetics during tonsillectomy or oropharyngeal surgery.

gage (gāj). SYN gauge.

gain (gān). **1.** Profit; advantage. **2.** The ratio of output to input of an amplifying system, generally expressed in decibels in ultrasound. [M.E. *gayne*, booty, fr. O.Fr., fr. Germanic]

primary g., interpersonal, social, or financial advantages from the conversion of emotional stress directly into demonstrably organic illnesses (*e.g.,* hysterical blindness or paralysis). Cf. secondary g.

secondary g., interpersonal or social advantages (*e.g.,* assistance, attention, sympathy) gained indirectly from organic illness. Cf. primary g.

time-compensated g., SYN time-gain *compensation*.

time compensation g. (TCG), SYN time-gain *compensation*.

time-varied g. (TVG), SYN time-gain *compensation*.

Gairdner, Sir William T., Scottish physician, 1824–1907. SEE G.'s *disease*.

Gaisböck, Felix, German physician, 1868–1955. SEE G.'s *syndrome*.

gait (gāt). Manner of walking.

antalgic g., a characteristic g. resulting from pain on weightbearing in which the stance phase of g. is shortened on the affected side.

ataxic g., SYN cerebellar g.

calcaneal g., a g. disturbance, characterized by walking on heel, due to paralysis of the calf muscles, seen following poliomyelitis and in some other neurologic diseases.

cerebellar g., wide-based gait with lateral veering, unsteadiness, and irregularity of steps; often with a tendency to fall to one or other side, forward or backward. SYN ataxic g.

Charcot's g., the g. of hereditary ataxia.

circumduction g., SYN hemiplegic g.

equine g., SYN high steppage g.

festinating g., g. in which the trunk is flexed, legs are flexed at the knees and hips, but stiff, while the steps are short and progressively more rapid; characteristically seen with parkinsonism (1) and other neurologic diseases. SYN festination.

gluteus maximus g., compensatory backward propulsion of trunk to maintain center of gravity over the supporting lower extremity.

gluteus medius g., compensatory list of body (or throw of trunk) to weak gluteal side, to put center of gravity over the supporting lower extremity.

helicopod g., a g., seen in some conversion reactions or hysterical disorders, in which the feet describe half circles. SYN helicopodia.

hemiplegic g., g. in which the leg is stiff, without flexion at knee and ankle, and with each step is rotated away from the body, then towards it, forming a semicircle. SYN circumduction g., spastic g.

high steppage g., a g. in which the foot is raised high to avoid catching a drooping foot and brought down suddenly in a flapping manner; often seen in peroneal nerve palsy and tabes. SYN equine g.

hysterical g., a variety of bizarre g.'s seen with hysteria-conversion reaction; usually the foot is dragged or pushed ahead, instead of lifted, while walking; frequently the foot is held dorsiflexed and inverted.

scissor g., one leg swings across the other instead of straight forward, producing a criss-cross motion of the legs in walking, with the foot imprints reversed; bilateral hemiplegic g.

spastic g., SYN hemiplegic g.

steppage g., a g. in which the advancing foot is lifted higher than usual so that it can clear the ground, because it cannot be dorsiflexed. Seen with peroneal neuropathies and other disorders causing foot dorsiflexion weakness. SEE high steppage g. SYN steppage.

toppling g., a g. in which the steps are uncertain and hesitant, and the patient totters and sometimes falls; probably due to a balance disorder; may be seen in elderly patients after a stroke.

waddling g., rolling g. in which the weight-bearing hip is not stabilized; it bulges outward with each step, while the opposite side of the pelvis drops, resulting in alternating lateral trunk movements; due to gluteus medius muscle weakness, and seen with muscular dystrophies, among other disorders. SYN waddle.

Gal Symbol for galactose.

⌂**galact-.** SEE galacto-.

ga·lac·ta·cra·sia (gă-lak′tă-krā′zē-ă). Abnormal composition of mother's milk. [galact- + G. *akrasia,* bad mixture, fr. *a-* priv. + *krasis,* a mixing]

ga·lac·ta·gogue (gă-lak′tă-gog). An agent that promotes the secretion and flow of milk. [galact- + G. *agōgos,* leading]

ga·lac·tans (gă-lak′tanz). Polymers of galactose occurring naturally, along with galacturonans and arabans, in pectins; *e.g.,* agar. SYN galactosans.

ga·lac·tic (gă-lak′tik). Pertaining to milk; promoting the flow of milk.

ga·lac·ti·dro·sis (gă-lak-ti-drō′sis). Sweating of a milky fluid. [galact- + G. *hidrōs,* sweat, + *-osis,* condition]

ga·lac·ti·tol (gă-lak′ti-tol). A sugar alcohol derived from galactose; g. accumulates in transferase deficiency galactosemia.

⌂**galacto-, galact-.** Milk. Cf. lact-. [G. *gala*]

ga·lac·to·blast (gă-lak′tō-blast). SYN colostrum *corpuscle.* [galacto- + *blastos,* germ]

ga·lac·to·bol·ic (gă-lak-tō-bol′ik). Obsolete term for causing the release or ejection of milk from the breast. [galacto- + G. *bolē* throwing]

ga·lac·to·cele (gă-lak′tō-sēl). Retention cyst caused by occlusion of a lactiferous duct. SYN lactocele. [galacto- + G. *kēlē,* tumor]

ga·lac·to·gen (gă-lak′tō-jen). A polysaccharide containing galactose in various forms. [galacto- + G. *-gen,* producing]

ga·lac·to·ki·nase (gă-lak-tō-kī′nās). An enzyme (phosphotransferase) that, in the presence of ATP, catalyzes the phosphorylation of D-galactose to D-galactose 1-phosphate, the first step in the metabolism of D-galactose; g. is deficient in one form of galactosemia.

ga·lac·tom·e·ter (gal′ak-tom′ě-ter). A form of hydrometer for determining the specific gravity of milk as an indication of its fat content. SYN lactometer. [galacto- + G. *metron,* measure]

ga·lac·to·pha·gia (gal-ak-tō-fāj′ē-a). A behavioral anomaly in which animals suck other than their own natural or foster mother.

gal·ac·toph·a·gous (gal′ak-tof′ă-gŭs). Subsisting on milk. [galacto- + G. *phagō,* to eat]

ga·lac·to·phore (gă-lak′tō-fōr). SYN lactiferous *ducts,* under *duct.* [galacto- + G. *phoros,* bearing]

ga·lac·to·pho·ri·tis (gă-lak′tō-fō-rī′tis). Inflammation of the milk ducts. [galacto- + G. *phoros,* carrying, + -itis, inflammation]

gal·ac·toph·o·rous (gal-ak-tof′ŏ-rŭs). Conveying milk.

ga·lac·to·poi·e·sis (gă-lak′tō-poy-ē′sis). Milk production. [galacto- + G. *poiēsis,* forming]

ga·lac·to·poi·et·ic (gă-lak′tō-poy-et′ik). Pertaining to galactopoiesis.

ga·lac·to·pyr·a·nose (gă-lak-tō-pir′ă-nōs). Galactose in pyranose form.

ga·lac·tor·rhea (gă-lak-tō-rē′ă). **1.** Any white discharge from the nipple that is persistent and looks like milk. **2.** Continued discharge of milk from the breasts between intervals of nursing or after the child has been weaned. SYN incontinence of milk, lactorrhea. [galacto- + G. *rhoia,* a flow]

ga·lac·tos·a·mine (gă-lak-tō-sam′ēn). The 2-amino-2-deoxy derivative of galactose, in which the NH_2 replaces the 2-OH group; the D-isomer occurs in various mucopolysaccharides, notably of chondroitin sulfuric acid and of B blood group substance; usually found as the *N*-acetyl derivative.

ga·lac·tos·am·i·no·gly·can (gă-lak′tōs-am-i-nō-glī′kan). SEE mucopolysaccharide.

ga·lac·to·sans (gă-lak′tō-sanz). SYN galactans.

ga·lac·to·scope (gă-lak′tō-skōp). An instrument for judging of the richness and purity of milk by the translucency of a thin layer. SYN lactoscope. [galacto- + G. *skopeō,* to examine]

ga·lac·tose (Gal) (gă-lak′tōs). An aldohexose found (in D form) as a constituent of lactose, cerebrosides, gangliosides, mucoproteins, etc., in galactoside or galactosyl combination; an epimer of D-glucose. SYN cerebrose.

ga·lac·to·se·mia (gă-lak-tō-sē′mē-ă) [MIM*230400]. An inborn error of galactose metabolism due to congenital deficiency of the enzyme galactosyl-1-phosphate uridyltransferase, resulting in tissue accumulation of galactose 1-phosphate; manifested by nutritional failure, hepatosplenomegaly with cirrhosis, cataracts, mental retardation, galactosuria, aminoaciduria, and albuminuria which regress or disappear if galactose is removed from the diet; autosomal recessive inheritance. SYN galactose diabetes. [galactose + G. *haima,* blood]

epimerase deficiency g., an inborn error in metabolism in which there is a deficiency of uridine diphosphate galactose 4-epimerase; galactose 1-phosphate accumulates.

galactokinase deficiency g., an autosomal recessive disorder resulting in an accumulation of galactose and galactitol.

transferase deficiency g., an autosomal recessive disorder in which there is a deficiency of galactose- 1-phosphate uridylyltransferase (see main entry for g.).

ga·lac·tose-1-phos·phate. A phosphorylated derivative of galactose that is key in galactose metabolism; accumulates in certain types of galactosemia.

g.-1-p. uridyltransferase, an enzyme catalyzing the reaction of UTP and α-D-g.-1-p. to form UDPgalactose and pyrophosphate, the second and most important step in the metabolism of D-galactose; a deficiency of this enzyme results in an accumulation of galactose, g.-1-p., and galactitol.

ga·lac·tose-6-sul·fa·tase. An enzyme that eliminates sulfur from the galactose-6-sulfate residues of certain mucopolysaccharides, producing 3,6-anhydrogalactose residues; it is absent in Morquio's syndrome type A. SYN galactose-6-sulfurase.

ga·lac·tose-6-sul·fu·rase. SYN galactose-6-sulfatase.

α-D-ga·lac·to·sid·ase (gă-lak-tō-sīd′ās). An enzyme catalyzing the hydrolysis of α-D-galactosides to release free D-galactose. A deficiency of type A α-D-galactosidase is associated with Fabry's disease. SYN melibiase.

β ga·lac·to·sid·ase (ga-lak′tō-si′dās). an enzyme that hydrolyzes the beta galactoside linkage in lactose-producing glucose and galactose; also hydrolyzes the chromogenic substrate IPTG (isopropylthiogalactoside) and thus is used as an indicator of fused genes and gene expression.

β-D-ga·lac·to·sid·ase. A sugar-splitting enzyme that catalyzes the hydrolysis of lactose into D-glucose and D-galactose, and that of other β-D-galactosides; it also catalyzes galactotransferase reactions; a deficiency of β-D -galactosidase leads to problems in the intestinal digestion of lactose; used in the production of milk products for adults who do not have the intestinal enzyme; a defect of one isozyme of β-D-galactosidase is associated with Morquio's syndrome type B. Cf. lactase *persistence,* lactase *restriction.* SYN lactase.

ga·lac·to·side (gă-lak′tō-sīd). A compound in which the H of the OH group on carbon-1 of galactose is replaced by an organic radical.

ga·lac·to·sis (gal-ak-tō′sis). Formation of milk by the lacteal glands. [galacto- + G. *-osis,* condition]

ga·lac·tos·u·ria (gă-lak-tō-sū′rē-ă). The excretion of galactose in the urine. [galactose + G. *ouron,* urine]

ga·lac·to·syl (gă-lak′tō-sil). A compound in which the –OH attached to carbon-1 of galactose is replaced by an organic radical.

β-ga·lac·to·syl·cer·am·i·dase. An enzyme that participates in the catabolism of certain ceramides; a deficiency of β-galactosylceramidase is associated with Krabbe's disease.

ga·lac·to·syl·cer·a·mide (gă-lak′tō-sil-ser′ă-mīd). A sphingolipid that accumulates in individuals with Krabbe's disease.

ga·lac·to·ther·a·py (gă-lak′tō-thār′ă-pē). Treatment of disease by means of an exclusive or nearly exclusive milk diet. SYN lactotherapy.

ga·lac·tur·o·nan (gă-lak′tūr-ō-nan). A polysaccharide that yields galacturonic acid on hydrolysis; a constituent of some pectins.

D-ga·lac·tu·ron·ic ac·id (gă-lak-tūr-on′ik). The D-isomer is an oxidation product of D-galactose, in which the $6-CH_2OH$ group has become a –COOH group; occurs in many natural products (*e.g.,* pectins). SYN pectic acid.

ga·lan·gal, ga·lan·ga (ga-lan′găl, -gă). The rhizome of *Alpinia* *offcinarum* (family Zingiberaceae); an aromatic stimulant and carminative. SYN Chinese ginger. [Mediev. L. *galanga,* mild ginger, fr. Chinese]

Galant, Nikolay Fedorovich, Russian hygienist, *1893. SEE G.'s *reflex.*

ga·lan·tha·mine (gă-lan'thă-mēn). An alkaloid derived from Caucasian snowdrops (a white flower of early spring) *Galanthus woronowii* (family Amaryllidaceae); from *Narcissus* spp. An alkaloid with anticholinesterase properties; enjoys use in Eastern Europe.

Galassi's pu·pil·lary phe·nom·e·non. See under phenomenon.

ga·lea (gā'lē-ă). **1** [NA]. A structure shaped like a helmet. **2.** SYN epicranial *aponeurosis.* **3.** A form of bandage covering the head. **4.** SYN caul (1). [L. a helmet]

g. aponeurot'ica [NA], SYN epicranial *aponeurosis.*

Galeati, Domenico, Italian physician, 1686–1775. SEE G.'s *glands,* under *gland.*

ga·le·at·o·my (gā-lē-at'ō-mē). Incision of the galea aponeurotica. [galea + G. *tomē,* incision]

Galeazzi, Riccardo, Italian surgeon, 1886–1952. SEE G.'s *fracture.*

Galen (Galenius, Galenos), Claudius, Greek physician and medical scientist in Rome, *c.* 130–201 A.D. SEE G.'s *anastomosis, nerve; veins* of G., under *vein; great vein* of G.

ga·le·na (gā-lē'nă). SYN *lead* sulfide. [L.]

ga·len·ic (gā-len'ik). Relating to Galen or to his theories.

ga·len·i·cals (gā-len'i-kălz). **1.** Herbs and other vegetable drugs, as distinguished from the mineral or chemical remedies. **2.** Crude drugs and the tinctures, decoctions, and other preparations made from them, as distinguished from the alkaloids and other active principles. **3.** Remedies prepared according to an official formula. [Claudius *Galen*]

Gall, Franz J., German-Austrian anatomist, 1758–1828. SEE G.'s *craniology.*

gall (gawl). **1.** SYN bile. **2.** An excoriation or erosion. **3.** SYN nutgall. [A.S. *gealla*]

gal·la (gal'ă). SYN nutgall. [L.]

gal·la·mine tri·eth·i·o·dide (gal'ă-mēn trī-eth-ī'ō-dīd). [v-Phenenyltris(oxyethylene)]tris[triethylammonium iodide]; a triple quaternary ammonium compound with action comparable to that of curarine.

Gallavardin, Louis, French physician, 1875–1957. SEE G.'s *phenomenon.*

gall·blad·der (gawl'blad-er). A pear-shaped receptacle on the inferior surface of the liver, in a hollow between the right lobe and the quadrate lobe; it serves as a storage reservoir for bile. SYN vesica biliaris [NA], vesica fellea✶ [NA], bile cyst, cholecyst, cholecystis, cystis fellea, gall bladder, vesicula fellis.

Courvoisier's g., an enlarged, often palpable g. in a patient with carcinoma of the head of the pancreas. It is associated with jaundice due to obstruction of the common bile duct. SEE Courvoisier's *law.*

porcelain g., intramural calcification of the g. commonly associated with g. cancer.

sandpaper g., a roughened condition of the mucous membrane of the g., associated usually with the presence of gallstones.

strawberry g., a g. of which the mucosa is dotted with yellowish cholesterol deposits contrasting with the red hyperemic background.

Gallego's dif·fer·en·ti·at·ing so·lu·tion. See under solution.

gal·le·in (gal'ē-in). 3′,4′,5′,6′-Tetrahydroxyfluoran; structurally related to fluorescein and used as an aniline dye indicator, turning rose red above pH 6.6, yellowish brown below pH 4. SYN pyrogallolphthalein.

gal·lic ac·id (gal'ik). 3,4,5-Trihydroxybenzoic acid; usually made from tannic acid or nutgalls; used locally as an astringent, for the same purpose as tannic acid.

Gallie, William E., Canadian surgeon, 1882–1959. SEE G.'s *transplant.*

Gal·li·for·mes (gal-i-fōr'mēz). An order of birds embracing the pheasant, turkey, and chicken. [L. *gallus,* a cock, + *forma,* form]

gal·li·na·ceous (gal-i-nā'shŭs). Pertaining to the order Galliformes. [L. *gallinaceus,* fr. *gallina,* a hen]

gal·li·um (Ga) (gal'ē-ŭm). A rare metal, atomic no. 31, atomic wt. 69.723. [L. *Gallia,* France]

gal·li·um-67 (⁶⁷Ga). A cyclotron-produced radionuclide with a half-life of 3.260 days and major gamma ray emissions of 93, 185, and 300 kiloelectron volts; used in the citrate form as a tumor- and inflammation-localizing radiotracer.

gal·li·um-68 (⁶⁸Ga). A positron emitter with a radioactive half-life of 1.130 hours.

gal·lo·cy·a·nin, gal·lo·cy·a·nine (gal-ō-sī'ă-nin, ă-nēn) [C.I. 51030]. A blue phenoxazin dye, $C_{15}H_{13}N_2O_5Cl$, used as a stain for nucleic acids after boiling with chrome alum, and is applicable for quantitative cytophotometric determination of these moieties.

gal·lon (gal'ŭn). A measure of U.S. liquid capacity containing 4 quarts, 231 cubic inches, or 8.3293 pounds of distilled water at 20° C; it is the equivalent of 3.785412 liters. The British imperial g. contains 277.4194 cubic inches. [O.Fr. *galon*]

gal·lop (gal'op). A triple cadence to the heart sounds; due to an abnormal third or fourth heart sound being heard in addition to the first and second sounds, and usually indicative of serious disease. SYN bruit de galop, cantering rhythm, gallop rhythm, Traube's bruit.

atrial g., SYN presystolic g.

presystolic g., g. rhythm in which the g. sound follows atrial systole in late diastole and is an audible fourth heart sound due to forceful ventricular filling. SYN atrial g.

protodiastolic g., g. rhythm in which the g. sound occurs in early diastole and is an abnormal third heart sound.

S₇ g., SYN summation g.

summation g., g. rhythm in which the g. sound is due to superimposition of third and fourth heart sounds; sometimes heard in normal subjects with tachycardia, but usually indicative of myocardial disease. SYN S₇ g., S₇.

systolic g., obsolete term for a triple cadence to the heart sounds in which the extra sound occurs during systole, usually in the form of a systolic "click."

gall·stone (gal'stōn). A concretion in the gallbladder or a bile duct, composed chiefly of a mixture of cholesterol, calcium bilirubinate, and calcium carbonate, occasionally as a pure stone composed of just one of these substances. SYN biliary calculus, cholelith.

opacifying g.'s, g.'s becoming roentgenographically opaque after prolonged exposure to cholecystographic contrast mediums.

silent g.'s, g.'s that cause no symptoms and are discovered by radiographic or ultrasound examination, at the time of operation, or autopsy.

Gal·lus (gal'ŭs). A genus of gallinaceous birds including *G. domestica,* the domestic chicken. [L. *gallus,* a cock]

GALT Abbreviation for gut-associated lymphoid *tissue.*

Galton, Sir Francis, English scientist, 1822–1911. SEE G.'s *delta,* system of classification of *fingerprints,* under *fingerprint, law, whistle.*

gal·to·ni·an (gahl-tō'nē-ăn). Attributed to or described by Sir Francis Galton.

Gal·vani, Luigi, Italian physician and anatomist, 1737-1798. SEE galvanism.

gal·van·ic (gal-van'ik). Pertaining to galvanism. SYN voltaic.

gal·va·nism (gal'vă-nizm). **1.** Direct current electricity produced by chemical action, as by a battery. **2.** Oral manifestations of direct current electricity occurring when dental restorations with dissimilar electric potentials (such as silver and gold) are placed in the mouth; characterized by pain or development of small areas of leukoplakia. SYN voltaism.

gal·va·ni·za·tion (gal'va-ni-zā'shŭn). Application of direct current (galvanic) electricity, as in galvanizing (electroplating).

△**galvano-.** Prefix denoting electrical, primarily direct current. [see galvanism]

gal·va·no·cau·tery (gal′vă-nō-kaw′ter-ē). A form of electrocautery using a wire heated by a galvanic current.

gal·va·no·con·trac·til·i·ty (gal′vă-nō-kon-trak-til′i-tē). The capability of a muscle of contracting under the stimulus of a galvanic (direct) current.

gal·va·no·far·a·di·za·tion (gal′vă-nō-far′ă-di-zā′shŭn). Simultaneous application of a galvanic and a faradic current.

gal·va·nom·e·ter (gal′vă-nom′ĕ-ter). An instrument for measuring the strength of an electric current.

d'Arsonval g., a sensitive g. consisting of a moving coil suspended in a permanent magnetic field between delicate metallic wires or ribbons that serve as both torsion springs and conductors; a mirror on the coil deflects a beam of light along the scale.

Einthoven's string g., the original instrument on which Einthoven developed the first electrocardiogram.

gal·va·no·mus·cu·lar (gal′vă-nō-mŭs′kyū-lăr). Denoting the effect of the application of a galvanic (direct) current to a muscle.

gal·va·no·pal·pa·tion (gal′vă-nō-pal-pā′shŭn). Esthesiometry by means of a sharp-pointed electrode through which a feeble direct current passes to the cathode applied to an indifferent part.

gal·va·no·scope (gal′vă-nō-skōp). An instrument for detecting the presence of a galvanic current. [galvano- + G. *skopeō,* to view]

gal·va·no·sur·gery (gal′vă-nō-ser′jer-ē). An operation in which direct electric current is utilized.

gal·va·no·tax·is (gal′vă-nō-tak′sis). SYN electrotaxis.

gal·va·no·ther·a·py (gal′van-ō-thār′ă-pē). Treatment of disease by application of direct (galvanic) current.

gal·va·not·o·nus (gal-vă-not′ō-nŭs). **1.** SYN electrotonus. **2.** Tonic muscular contraction in response to a galvanic stimulus. [galvano- + G. *tonos,* tension]

gal·va·not·ro·pism (gal-vă-not′rō-pizm). SYN electrotaxis. [galvano- + G. *tropē,* a turning]

gam·a·bu·fa·gin (gam-ă-bū′fă-jin). SYN gamabufotalin.

gam·a·bu·fo·gen·in (gam-ă-bū′fō-jen-in). SYN gamabufotalin.

gam·a·bu·fo·tal·in (gam-ă-bū′fō-tal-in). A trihydroxybufadienolide, present in the venoms of toads (family Bufonidae), which chemically and pharmacologically resembles digitalis. SYN gamabufagin, gamabufogenin.

gam·bir (gam′bēr). An extract from the leaves of *Uncaria* (*Ourouparia*) gambier (family Rubiaceae); an astringent. Commercial g. is known as terra japonica.

game (gām). A contest, physical or mental, conducted according to set rules, played for amusement or for a stake. [M.E. fr. O.E. *gamen*]

language g., in philosophy, all the operations and behaviors contained in and expressed by symbols, language rules, and the social customs concerning language use.

model g., the use of g.'s, especially of g.'s of strategy, for the explanation of human behavior (both normal and abnormal).

ga·me·tan·gi·um (gam′ĕ-tan′jē-ŭm). A structure in which gametes are produced.

gam·ete (gam′ēt). **1.** One of two haploid cells undergoing karyogamy. **2.** Any germ cell, whether ovum or spermatozoon. [G. *gametēs,* husband; *gametē,* wife]

joint g., the haploid set of (nonallelic) genes inherited in a single germinal cell.

△gameto-. A gamete. [G. *gametēs,* husband, *gametē,* wife, fr. *gameō,* to marry]

ga·me·to·cide (gă-mē′tō-sīd). An agent destructive of gametes, specifically the malarial gametocytes. [gameto- + L. *caedo,* to kill]

ga·me·to·cyst (ga-mē′tō-sist). A cyst formed around a pair of united gregarine gamonts in which gametes are produced. [gameto- + G. *kystis,* bladder]

ga·me·to·cyte (gă-mē′tō-sīt). A cell capable of dividing to produce gametes, *e.g.,* a spermatocyte or oocyte. SYN gamont. [gameto- + G. *kytos,* cell]

ga·me·to·gen·e·sis (gam′ĕ-tō-jen′ĕ-sis). The process of formation and development of gametes. [gameto- + G. *genesis,* production]

ga·me·to·go·nia (gam′ĕ-tō-gō′nē-ă). SYN gametogony.

gam·e·tog·o·ny (gam-ĕ-tog′ō-nē). A stage in the sexual cycle of sporozoans in which gametes are formed, often by schizogony. SYN gametogonia, gamogony. [gameto- + G. *gonē,* a begetting]

gam·e·toid (gam′ĕ-toyd). Pertaining to certain biologic features that resemble those characteristic of gametes or reproductive cells.

ga·me·to·ki·net·ic (gam′ĕ-tō-ki-net′ik). Promoting or causing karyogamy or true conjugation. [gameto- + G. *kinēsis,* movement]

gam·e·to·pha·gia (gam′ĕ-tō-fā′jē-ă). The disappearance of the male or female element in zygosis. SYN gamophagia. [gameto- + G. *phagō,* to eat]

Gamgee, Joseph Sampson, British surgeon, 1828–1886. SEE Gamgee *tissue.*

gam·ic (gam′ik). Relating to or derived from sexual union; usually used as a suffix. [G. *gamikos,* pert. to marriage]

gam·ma (gam′ă). **1.** Third letter of the Greek alphabet, γ. **2.** A unit of magnetic field intensity equal to 10^{-9} tesla. [G.]

gam·ma·cism (gam′ă-sizm). Mispronunciation of, or trouble articulating, the "g" sound. [G. *gamma,* equivalent of the letter g]

gam·ma·gram (gam′ă-gram). Archaic term for scintiscan.

gam·mop·a·thy (gă-mop′ă-thē). A primary disturbance in immunoglobulin synthesis.

biclonal g., a g. in which the serum contains two distinct monoclonal immunoglobulins.

monoclonal g., any one of a group of disorders due to proliferation of a single clone of lymphoid or plasma cells (visible on electrophoresis as a single peak) and characterized by the presence of monoclonal immunoglobulin in serum or urine.

polyclonal g., a g. in which there is a heterogeneous increase in immunoglobulins involving more than one cell line; may be caused by any of a variety of inflammatory, infectious, or neoplastic disorders.

Gamna, Carlos, Italian physician, 1896–1950. SEE G.'s *disease;* G.-Favre *bodies,* under *body;* Gandy-G. *bodies,* under *body;* G.-Gandy *bodies,* under *body,* nodules, under *nodule.*

gam·o·gen·e·sis (gam-ō-jen′ĕ-sis). SYN sexual *reproduction.* [G. *gamos,* marriage, + *genesis,* production]

gam·og·o·ny (gam-og′ō-nē). SYN gametogony.

gam·ont. SYN gametocyte. [G. *gamos,* marriage, + *ōn* (*ont-*), being]

gam·o·pha·gia (gam-ō-fā′jē-ă). SYN gametophagia.

gam·o·pho·bia (gam-ō-fō′bē-ă). Morbid fear of marriage. [G. *gamos,* marriage, + *phobos,* fear]

gan·ci·clo·vir (gan-sī′klō-vir). 9-[[Hydroxy-1-(hydroxymethyl)-ethoxy]methyl]guanine; an antiviral agent used in the treatment of opportunistic cytomegalovirus infections.

Gandy, Charles, French physician, *1872. SEE Gamna-G. *bodies,* under *body,* nodules, under *nodule;* G.-Gamna *bodies,* under *body;* G.-Nanta *disease.*

gan·ga (gang′gă). An extract of the flowers of *Cannabis sativa* (Indian hemp or hashish) which grows in India, Persia, and Arabia. SEE ALSO cannabis.

gan·glia (gang′glē-ă). Plural of ganglion.

gan·gli·al (gang′glē-ăl). SYN ganglionic.

△ Combining forms	[NA] Nomina Anatomica
Word*Finder* Multi-term entry finder Preceding letter A	[MIM] Mendelian Inheritance in Man
A.D.A.M. Anatomy Plates Between letters L and M	☆ Official alternate term
Appendices: Following letter Z	☆[NA] Official alternate Nomina Anatomica term
SYN Synonym; Cf., compare	High Profile Term

ga

gan·gli·ate, gan·gli·at·ed (gang'glē-āt, gang'glē-ā-ted). Having ganglia. SYN ganglionated.

gan·gli·ec·to·my (gang-glē-ek'tō-mē). SYN ganglionectomy.

gan·gli·form (gang'glē-fōrm). Having the form or appearance of a ganglion. SYN ganglioform.

gan·gli·i·tis (gang-glē-ī'tis). SYN ganglionitis.

gan·gli·o·blast (gang'glē-ō-blast). An embryonic cell from which develop ganglion cells. [ganglion + G. *blastos,* germ]

gan·gli·o·cyte (gang'glē-ō-sīt). SYN ganglion *cell.*

gan·gli·o·cy·to·ma (gang'glē-ō-sī-tō'mă). A rare lesion that contains neuronal (ganglion) cells in a sparse glial stoma. SYN central ganglioneuroma. [ganglion + G. *kytos,* cell, + -*oma,* tumor]

gan·gli·o·form (gang'glē-ō-fōrm). SYN gangliform.

gan·gli·o·gli·o·ma (gang'glē-ō-glē-ō'mă). A rare tumor comprised of a glioma component and an atypical neuronal (ganglion) cell component; in younger patients often associated with seizures.

gan·gli·ol·y·sis (gang-glē-ol'i-sis). The dissolution or breaking up of a ganglion.

  percutaneous radiofrequency g., g. produced by radiofrequency currents applied to a ganglion by a needle passed through the skin.

gan·gli·o·ma (gang-glē-ō'mă). SYN ganglioneuroma.

GANGLION

---

gan·gli·on, pl. **gan·glia, gan·gli·ons** (gang'glē-on, -glē-ă, -glē-onz). **1** [NA]. Originally, any group of nerve cell bodies in the central or peripheral nervous system; currently, an aggregation of nerve cell bodies located in the peripheral nervous system. SYN nerve g., neural g., neuroganglion. **2.** A cyst containing mucopolysaccharide-rich fluid within fibrous tissue or, occasionally, muscle bone or a semilunar cartilage; usually attached to a tendon sheath in the hand, wrist, or foot, or connected with the underlying joint. SYN myxoid cyst, peritendinitis serosa, synovial cyst. [G. a swelling or knot]

aberrant g., a collection of nerve cells sometimes found on a posterior spinal nerve root between the spinal g. and the spinal cord.

acousticofacial g., a primordial ganglionic cell mass in young embryos which later separates into the acoustic or spiral g. of the vestibulocochlear (eighth cranial) nerve and the geniculate g. of the facial (seventh cranial) nerve.

Acrel's g., (**1**) pseudoganglion on the posterior interosseous nerve on the dorsal aspect of the wrist joint; (**2**) a cyst on a tendon of an extensor muscle at the level of the wrist.

Andersch's g., SYN inferior g. of glossopharyngeal nerve.

aorticorenal ganglia, a semidetached portion of the celiac ganglia, at the origin of each renal artery; contains the sympathetic neurons innervating the vasculature of the kidney. SYN ganglia aorticorenalia [NA].

gang'lia aorticorena'lia [NA], SYN aorticorenal ganglia.

Arnold's g., SYN otic g.

auditory g., SYN spiral g. of cochlea.

Auerbach's ganglia, collections of parasympathetic nerve cells in the myenteric plexus. SEE myenteric *plexus.*

auricular g., SYN otic g.

autonomic ganglia, visceral ganglia. SEE autonomic nervous *system.*

ganglia of autonomic plexuses, autonomic ganglia lying in plexuses of autonomic fibers, *e.g.,* the celiac and inferior mesenteric ganglia of the sympathetic, and the small parasympathetic ganglia of the myenteric plexus. SYN ganglia plexuum autonomicorum [NA].

basal ganglia, originally, all of the large masses of gray matter at the base of the cerebral hemisphere; currently, the striate body (caudate and lentiform nuclei) and cell groups associated with

the striate body, such as the subthalamic nucleus and substantia nigra.

Bezold's g., an aggregation of nerve cells in the interatrial septum.

Bochdalek's g., a g. of the plexus of the dental nerve lying in the maxilla just above the root of the canine tooth.

Bock's g., SYN carotid g.

Böttcher's g., g. on the cochlear nerve in the internal acoustic meatus.

cardiac ganglia, parasympathetic ganglia of the cardiac plexus lying between the arch of the aorta and the bifurcation of the pulmonary artery. SYN ganglia cardiaca [NA], Wrisberg's ganglia.

gang'lia cardi'aca [NA], SYN cardiac ganglia.

carotid g., a small ganglionic swelling on filaments from the internal carotid plexus, lying on the undersurface of the carotid artery in the cavernous sinus. SYN Bock's g., Laumonier's g.

celiac ganglia, the largest and highest group of prevertebral sympathetic ganglia, located on the superior part of the abdominal aorta, on either side of the origin of the celiac artery; contains sympathetic neurons whose unmyelinated postganglionic axons innervate the stomach, liver, gallbladder, spleen, kidney, small intestine, and ascending and transverse colon. h SYN ganglia celiaca [NA], semilunar g. (2), solar ganglia, Vieussens' ganglia, Willis' centrum nervosum.

gang'lia celi'aca [NA], SYN celiac ganglia.

g. cervica'le infe'rius, SYN inferior cervical g.

g. cervica'le me'dium [NA], SYN middle cervical g.

g. cervica'le supe'rius [NA], SYN superior cervical g.

cervicothoracic g., a sympathetic trunk g. lying behind the subclavian artery near the origin of the vertebral artery, it is formed by the fusion of the inferior cervical ganglion, at the level of the seventh cervical vertebra, with the first thoracic g. SYN g. stellatum* [NA], stellate g.

g. cer'vicothora'cicum [NA], a sympathetic trunk g. lying behind the subclavian artery near the origin of the vertebral artery, at the level of the seventh cervical vertebra, close to the first thoracic g. with which it is usually fused.

g. cilia're [NA], SYN ciliary g.

ciliary g., a small parasympathetic g. lying in the orbit between the optic nerve and the lateral rectus muscle; it receives preganglionic innervation from the Edinger-Westphal nucleus by way of the oculomotor nerve, and in turn gives rise to postganglionic fibers that innervate the ciliary muscle and the sphincter of the iris (sphincter pupillae muscle). SYN g. ciliare [NA], lenticular g., Schacher's g.

coccygeal g., SYN g. impar.

cochlear g., SYN spiral g. of cochlea.

Corti's g., SYN spiral g. of cochlea.

craniospinal ganglia, a term collectively designating the sensory ganglia on the dorsal (posterior) roots of spinal nerves and on those cranial nerves that contain general sensory and taste fibers; also called encephalospinal ganglia. SYN craniospinalia ganglia.

craniospinal'ia gan'glia, SYN craniospinal ganglia.

diffuse g., a cystic swelling due to inflammatory effusion into one or several adjacent tendon sheaths.

dorsal root g., SYN spinal g.

Ehrenritter's g., SYN superior g. of glossopharyngeal nerve.

extracranial ganglia, SYN inferior g. of glossopharyngeal nerve.

g. extracrania'le, SYN inferior g. of glossopharyngeal nerve.

g. of facial nerve, SYN geniculate g.

Frankenhäuser's g., SYN uterovaginal *plexus.*

Froriep's g., a temporary collection of nerve cells on the dorsal aspect of the hypoglossal nerve in the embryo; it represents a rudimentary sensory g.

gasserian g., SYN trigeminal g.

geniculate g., a g. of the nervus intermedius fibers conveyed by the facial nerve, located within the facial canal at the genu of the canal and containing the sensory neurons innervating the taste buds on the anterior two-thirds of the tongue and a small area on the external ear. SYN g. geniculi [NA], g. of facial nerve, g. of intermediate nerve, g. of nervus intermedius, intumescentia gan-glioformis.

g. genic′uli [NA], SYN geniculate g.

Gudden's g., SYN interpeduncular *nucleus.*

g. haben′ulae, SYN habenular *nucleus.*

hypogastric ganglia, SYN pelvic ganglia.

g. im′par [NA], the most inferior, unpaired g. of the sympathetic trunk; inconstant. SYN coccygeal g., Walther's g.

inferior cervical g., inferior-most of the three ganglia of the cervical portion of the sympathetic trunk, occurring at the C7 vertebral level. Most commonly, it is fused to the first thoracic sympathetic ganglion to form a stellate ganglion. SYN g. cervicale inferius.

inferior g. of glossopharyngeal nerve, the lower of two sensory g.'s on the glossopharyngeal nerve as it traverses the jugular foramen. SYN g. inferius nervi glossopharyngei [NA], Andersch's g., extracranial ganglia, g. extracraniale, petrosal g., petrous g.

inferior mesenteric g., the lowest of the sympathetic preverte-bral ganglia, located at the origin of the inferior mesenteric artery from the aorta and containing the sympathetic neurons innervat-ing the descending and sigmoid colon. SYN g. mesentericum inferius [NA].

inferior g. of vagus nerve, a large sensory g. of the vagus, anterior to the internal jugular vein. SYN g. inferius nervi vagi [NA], g. of trunk of vagus, nodose g.

g. infe′rius ner′vi glossopharyn′gei [NA], SYN inferior g. of glossopharyngeal nerve.

g. infe′rius ner′vi va′gi [NA], SYN inferior g. of vagus nerve.

intercrural g., SYN interpeduncular *nucleus.*

gang′lia interme′dia [NA], SYN intermediate ganglia.

intermediate ganglia, small sympathetic ganglia most com-monly found on the communicating branches in the cervical and lumbar region. SYN ganglia intermedia [NA].

g. of intermediate nerve, SYN geniculate g.

interpeduncular g., SYN interpeduncular *nucleus.*

intervertebral g., SYN spinal g.

intracranial g., SYN superior g. of glossopharyngeal nerve.

g. isth′mi, SYN interpeduncular *nucleus.*

jugular g., (1) SYN superior g. of glossopharyngeal nerve. **(2)** SYN superior g. of vagus nerve.

Laumonier's g., SYN carotid g.

Lee's g., SYN uterovaginal *plexus.*

lenticular g., SYN ciliary g.

Lobstein's g., SYN splanchnic g.

Ludwig's g., a small collection of parasympathetic nerve cells in the interatrial septum.

gang′lia lumba′lia [NA], SYN lumbar ganglia.

lumbar ganglia, four or more ganglia on the medial border of the psoas major muscle on either side; they form, with the sacral and coccygeal ganglia and their interganglionic rami, the abdom-inopelvic sympathetic trunk. SYN ganglia lumbalia [NA].

Meckel's g., SYN pterygopalatine g.

g. mesenter′icum infe′rius [NA], SYN inferior mesenteric g.

g. mesenter′icum supe′rius [NA], SYN superior mesenteric g.

middle cervical g., a sympathetic g., of small size and some-times absent; located at the level of the cricoid cartilage. SYN g. cervicale medium [NA].

nasal g., SYN pterygopalatine g.

nerve g., neural g., SYN ganglion (1).

g. of nervus intermedius, SYN geniculate g.

nodose g., SYN inferior g. of vagus nerve.

otic g., an autonomic g. situated below the foramen ovale medial to the mandibular nerve; its postganglionic, parasympathetic fi-bers are distributed to the parotid gland. SYN g. oticum [NA], Arnold's g., auricular g., otoganglion.

g. o′ticum [NA], SYN otic g.

parasympathetic ganglia, those ganglia of the autonomic ner-vous system composed of cholinergic neurons receiving afferent fibers from preganglionic visceral motor neurons in either the brainstem or the middle sacral spinal segments (S2 to S4); on the basis of their location with respect to the organs they innervate,

most parasympathetic ganglia, at least outside the head, can be categorized as juxtamural or intramural ganglia. SEE ALSO auto-nomic nervous *system.*

paravertebral ganglia, SYN ganglia of sympathetic trunk.

pelvic ganglia, the parasympathetic ganglia scattered through the pelvic plexus on either side. SYN ganglia pelvina [NA], hypogas-tric ganglia.

gang′lia pelvi′na [NA], SYN pelvic ganglia.

periosteal g., a flattened subperiosteal cavity containing clear, yellow, viscous, synovial-like fluid.

petrosal g., petrous g., SYN inferior g. of glossopharyngeal nerve.

phrenic ganglia, several small autonomic ganglia contained in the plexuses accompanying the inferior phrenic arteries. SYN gan-glia phrenica [NA].

gang′lia phren′ica [NA], SYN phrenic ganglia.

gang′lia plex′uum autonomico′rum [NA], SYN ganglia of auto-nomic plexuses.

prevertebral ganglia, the sympathetic ganglia (celiac, aorticore-nal, superior and inferior mesenteric) lying in front of the verte-bral column, as distinguished from the ganglia of the sympathetic trunk (paravertebral ganglia); these ganglia occur mostly around the origin of the major branches of the abdominal aorta; all are in the abdomino-pelvic cavity, concerned with innervation of abdomino-pelvic viscera.

pterygopalatine g., a small parasympathetic g. in the upper part of the pterygopalatine fossa whose postsynaptic fibers supply the lacrimal, nasal, palatine and pharyngeal glands. SYN g. pterygo-palatinum [NA], Meckel's g., nasal g., sphenopalatine g.

g. pterygopalati′num [NA], SYN pterygopalatine g.

Remak's ganglia, (1) groups of nerve cells in the wall of the venous sinus where it joins the right atrium of the heart; **(2)** autonomic ganglia in nerves of the stomach.

renal ganglia, small scattered sympathetic ganglia along the renal plexus. SYN ganglia renalia [NA].

gang′lia rena′lia [NA], SYN renal ganglia.

Ribes' g., a small sympathetic g. situated on the anterior commu-nicating artery of the brain.

sacral ganglia, three or four ganglia on either side constituting, with the g. impar and the interganglionic rami, the pelvic portion of the sympathetic trunk. SYN ganglia sacralia [NA].

gang′lia sacra′lia [NA], SYN sacral ganglia.

Scarpa's g., SYN vestibular g.

Schacher's g., SYN ciliary g.

semilunar g., (1) SYN trigeminal g. **(2)** SYN celiac ganglia.

sensory g., a cluster of primary sensory neurons forming a usu-ally visible swelling in the course of a peripheral nerve or its dorsal root; such nerve cells establish the sole afferent neural connection between the sensory periphery (skin, mucous mem-branes of the oral and nasal cavities, muscle tissue, tendons, joint capsules, special sense organs, blood vessel walls, tissues of the internal organs) and the central nervous system; they are the cells of origin of all sensory fibers of the peripheral nervous system.

Soemmerring's g., SYN *substantia* nigra.

solar ganglia, SYN celiac ganglia.

sphenopalatine g., SYN pterygopalatine g.

spinal g., the g. of the posterior root of each spinal segmental nerve; contains the cell bodies of the pseudounipolar primary sensory neurons whose peripheral axonal branches become part of the mixed segmental nerve, while the central axonal branches enter the spinal cord as a component of the sensory posterior root. SYN g. spinale [NA], dorsal root g., intervertebral g.

g. spina′le [NA], SYN spinal g.

spiral g. of cochlea, an elongated g. of bipolar sensory nerve cell bodies on the cochlear part of the vestibulocochlear nerve in the spiral canal of the modiolus; each g. cell gives rise to a periphe-ral process that passes between the layers of the bony spiral lamina to the organ of Corti, and a central axon that enters the hindbrain as a component of the inferior (cochlear) root of the eighth nerve. SYN g. spirale cochleae [NA], auditory g., cochlear g., Corti's g., spiral cochlear g.

spiral cochlear g., SYN spiral g. of cochlea.

ga

g. spira'le coch'leae [NA], SYN spiral g. of cochlea.

splanchnic g., ha small sympathetic g. often present in the course of the greater splanchnic nerve. SYN g. splanchnicum [NA], Lobstein's g.

g. splanch'nicum [NA], SYN splanchnic g.

stellate g., SYN cervicothoracic g.

g. stella'tum [NA], ⋆official alternate term for cervicothoracic g.

sublingual g., a tiny g. occasionally found anterior to the submandibular g., of which it is a displaced portion; innervates the sublingual gland. SYN g. sublinguale.

g. sublingua'le, SYN sublingual g.

submandibular g., a small parasympathetic g. suspended from the lingual nerve; its postganglionic branches go to the submandibular and sublingual glands; its preganglionic fibers come from the superior salvatory nucleus by way of the chorda tympani. SYN g. submandibulare [NA], submaxillary g.

g. submandibula're [NA], SYN submandibular g.

submaxillary g., SYN submandibular g.

superior cervical g., the uppermost and largest of the ganglia of the sympathetic trunk, lying near the base of the skull between the internal carotid artery and the internal jugular vein. SYN g. cervicale superius [NA].

superior g. of glossopharyngeal nerve, the upper and smaller of two ganglia on the glossopharyngeal nerve as it traverses the jugular foramen. SYN g. superius nervi glossopharyngei [NA], Ehrenritter's g., intracranial g., jugular g. (1).

superior mesenteric g., a paired sympathetic g. located at the origin of the superior mesenteric artery from the aorta. SYN g. mesentericum superius [NA].

superior g. of vagus nerve, a small sensory g. on the vagus as it traverses the jugular foramen. SYN g. superius nervi vagi [NA], jugular g. (2).

g. supe'rius ner'vi glossopharyn'gei [NA], SYN superior g. of glossopharyngeal nerve.

g. supe'rius ner'vi va'gi [NA], SYN superior g. of vagus nerve.

sympathetic ganglia, those ganglia of the autonomic nervous system that receive efferent fibers originating from preganglionic visceral motor neurons in the intermediolateral cell column of thoracic and upper lumbar spinal segments (T1–L2). On the basis of their location, the sympathetic ganglia can be classified as paravertebral ganglia (ganglia trunci sympathici) and prevertebral ganglia (ganglia celiaca). SEE ALSO autonomic nervous *system.*

ganglia of sympathetic trunk, the clusters of postganglionic neurons located at intervals along the sympathetic trunks, including the superior cervical, middle cervical, and cervicothoracic (stellate) g., the thoracic, lumbar, and sacral ganglia, and the g. impar. SYN ganglia trunci sympathici [NA], paravertebral ganglia.

terminal g., (1) one of the cells located along the terminal nerves; **(2)** one of the scattered postganglionic autonomic neurons located in or close to the wall of the organ innervated; they are usually parasympathetic. SYN g. terminale [NA].

g. termina'le [NA], SYN terminal g.

thoracic ganglia, ganglia, 11 or 12 on either side, at the level of the head of each rib, constituting with the interganglionic rami the thoracic portion of the sympathetic trunk. SYN ganglia thoracica [NA].

gang'lia thorac'ica [NA], SYN thoracic ganglia.

trigeminal g., the large flattened sensory g. of the trigeminal nerve lying close to the cavernous sinus along the medial part of the middle cranial fossa in the trigeminal cavity of the dura mater. SYN g. trigeminale [NA], gasserian g., semilunar g. (1).

g. trigemina'le [NA], SYN trigeminal g.

Troisier's g., historic term for a lymph node immediately above the clavicle, especially on the left side, that is palpably enlarged as the result of a metastasis from a malignant neoplasm; the presence of such a node indicates that the probable site of primary involvement is in an abdominal organ. SEE ALSO signal *node.* SYN Troisier's node.

gang'lia trun'ci sympath'ici [NA], SYN ganglia of sympathetic trunk.

g. of trunk of vagus, SYN inferior g. of vagus nerve.

tympanic g., a small g. on the tympanic nerve during its passage through the petrous portion of the temporal bone. SYN g. tympanicum [NA].

g. tympan'icum [NA], SYN tympanic g.

Valentin's g., a g. on the superior alveolar nerve.

vertebral g., a small g. located along the sympathetic trunk or one of the nerve cords connecting the middle cervical g. and the cervicothoracic g.; it usually lies near the vertebral artery. SYN g. vertebrale [NA].

g. vertebra'le [NA], SYN vertebral g.

vestibular g., a collection of bipolar nerve cell bodies forming a swelling on the vestibular part of the eighth nerve in the internal acoustic meatus; consists of a superior part and an inferior part connected by a narrow isthmus. SYN g. vestibulare [NA], Scarpa's g.

g. vestibula're [NA], SYN vestibular g.

Vieussens' ganglia, SYN celiac ganglia.

Walther's g., SYN g. impar.

Wrisberg's ganglia, SYN cardiac ganglia.

---

gan·gli·on·at·ed (gang'glē-ō-nā'ted). SYN gangliate.

gan·gli·on·ec·to·my (gang'glē-ō-nek'tō-mē). Excision of a ganglion. SYN gangliectomy. [ganglion + G. *ektomē,* excision]

gan·glio·neu·ro·ma (gang'glē-ō-nū-rō'mă). A benign neoplasm composed of mature ganglionic neurons, in varying numbers, scattered singly or in clumps within a relatively abundant and dense stroma of neurofibrils and collagenous fibers; usually found in the posterior mediastinum and retroperitoneum, sometimes in relation to the adrenal glands. SYN ganglioma. [ganglion + G. *neuron,* nerve, + *-oma,* tumor]

central g., SYN gangliocytoma.

dumbbell g., a g. in which the gross configuration resembles a dumbbell, *e.g.,* two spheroidal masses connected by a narrow portion, usually the result of the neoplasm being somewhat molded by a resistant structure such as two ribs.

gan·glio·neu·ro·ma·to·sis (gang'glē-ō-nūr'ō-mă-tō'sis). The condition of having many widespread ganglioneuromas.

gan·gli·on·ic (gang-glē-on'ik). Relating to a ganglion. SYN ganglial.

gan·gli·on·i·tis (gang'glē-ō-nī'tis). **1.** Inflammation of a lymphatic ganglion. **2.** Inflammation of a nerve ganglion. SYN ganglitis.

gan·gli·o·nos·to·my (gang'glē-ō-nos'tō-mē). Making an opening into a ganglion (2). [ganglion + G. *stoma,* mouth]

gan·gli·o·ple·gic (gang'glē-ō-plē'jik). A pharmacologic compound that paralyzes an autonomic ganglion, usually for a relatively short period of time. [ganglion + G. *plēgē,* stroke, shock]

gan·gli·os·i·a·li·do·sis (gang'glē-ō-sī-al-ē-dō'sis). SYN gangliosidosis.

gan·gli·o·side (gang'glē-ō-sīd). A glycosphingolipid chemically similar to cerebrosides but containing one or more sialic (*N*-acetylneuraminic or *N*-glycolylneuraminic) acid residues; found principally in nerve tissue, spleen, and thymus; G_{M1} accumulates in generalized gangliosidosis; G_{M2} accumulates in Tay-Sachs disease. SYN sialoglycosphingolipid.

gan·gli·o·si·do·sis (gang'glē-ō-si-dō'sis). Any disease characterized, in part, by the abnormal accumulation within the nervous system of specific gangliosides, *e.g.,* G_{M2} gangliosidosis, Tay-Sachs disease, caused by hexosaminidase A enzyme deficiency with accumulation of G_{M2} ganglioside. SYN gangliosialidosis, ganglioside lipidosis.

G_{M1} **g.,** three forms exist: infantile, generalized; juvenile; and adult; g. characterized by accumulation of a specific monosialoganglioside, G_{M1}; due to deficiency of G_{M1}-β-galactosidase. SYN generalized g.

G_{M2} **g.,** one of the hereditary metabolic disorders; several forms exist, including Tay-Sachs *disease,* Sandhoff's *disease,* AV variant and adult onset; characterized by accumulation of a specific metabolite, G_{M2} ganglioside, due to deficiency of hexosaminidase A or B, or G_{M2} activator factor.

generalized g., SYN G_{M1} g.

infantile G_{M2} g., SYN Tay-Sachs *disease.*

infantile, generalized G_{M1} g., one of the hereditary metabolic diseases of infancy; resembles Tay-Sachs *disease*, except other organ systems (bone, liver, kidney) are affected. SYN familial neuroviscerolipidosis, pseudo-Hurler disease, Type 1 G_{M1} g.

Type 1 G_{M1} g., SYN infantile, generalized G_{M1} g.

gan·go·sa (gang-gō′să). A destructive ulceration beginning on the soft palate and extending thence to the hard palate, nasopharynx, and nose, resulting in mutilating cicatrices. The disease, so far as is known, occurs only in certain portions of the tropics, especially the islands of the Pacific, and is generally regarded as a sequel to yaws. [Sp. *gangoso,* snuffling; fem. to agree with *enfermedad* disease]

gan·grene (gang′grēn). **1.** Necrosis due to obstruction, loss, or diminution of blood supply; it may be localized to a small area or involve an entire extremity or organ (such as the bowel), and may be wet or dry. SYN mortification. **2.** Extensive necrosis from any cause, *e.g.,* gas gangrene. [G. *gangraina,* an eating sore, fr. *graō,* to gnaw]

arteriosclerotic g., dry g. resulting from sclerotic changes in the arteries, with subsequent occlusion, as in the aged.

cold g., SYN dry g.

cutaneous g., g. of the skin characterized by sloughing; may occur in shingles or in any acute infection that interferes with superficial circulation.

decubital g., SYN decubitus *ulcer.*

diabetic g., g. resulting from arteriosclerosis associated with diabetes.

disseminated cutaneous g., SYN *dermatitis* gangrenosa infantum.

dry g., a form of g. in which the involved part is dry and shriveled. SYN cold g., mummification necrosis, mummification (1).

embolic g., g. resulting from obstruction of an artery by an embolus.

emphysematous g., SYN gas g.

Fournier's g., SYN Fournier's *disease.*

gas g., g. occurring in a wound infected with various anaerobic sporeforming bacteria, especially *Clostridium perfringens* and *C. novyi,* which cause crepitation of the surrounding tissues, due to gas liberated by bacterial fermentation, and constitutional septic symptoms. SYN clostridial myonecrosis, emphysematous g., emphysematous phlegmon, gangrenous emphysema, gas phlegmon, progressive emphysematous necrosis.

hemorrhagic g., (1) SYN hemorrhagic *infarct.* **(2)** g. occurring rarely in advanced meningococcal septicemia.

hospital g., SYN decubitus *ulcer.*

hot g., g. following inflammation of the part.

Meleney's g., SYN Meleney's *ulcer.*

moist g., SYN wet g.

nosocomial g., SYN decubitus *ulcer.*

Pott's g., SYN senile g.

presenile spontaneous g., g. occurring in middle life as a result of thromboangiitis obliterans.

pressure g., SYN decubitus *ulcer.*

progressive bacterial synergistic g., SYN Meleney's *ulcer.*

senile g., dry g. occurring in the aged in consequence of occlusion of an artery, particularly affecting the extremities. SYN Pott's g.

spontaneous g. of newborn, g. due to vascular occlusion of unknown cause, usually in marasmic or dehydrated infants.

static g., moist g. due to obstruction in the return circulation. SYN venous g.

symmetrical g., g. affecting the extremities of both sides of the body; it is seen particularly in severe arteriosclerosis, myocardial infarction, and ball-valve thrombus.

thrombotic g., g. due to occlusion of an artery by a thrombus.

trophic g., SYN trophic *ulcer.*

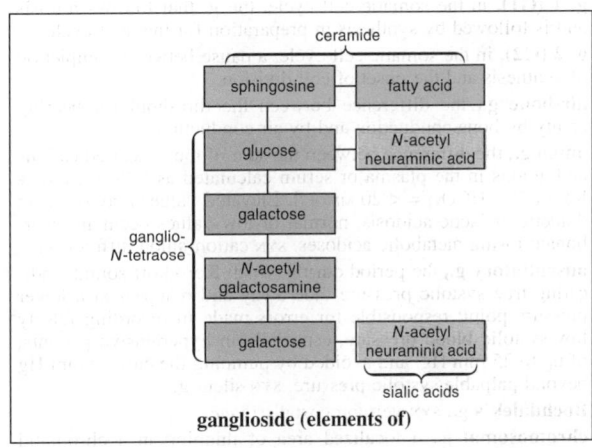

ganglioside (elements of)

gangliosidosis		
disease	storage substance	missing enzyme
G_{M1}–gangliosidosis type I: generalized form type II: juvenile form	ganglioside G_{M1}	β galactosidase (isoenzyme A, B and C differ)
G_{M2}–gangliosidosis type 1: Tay-Sachs disease	ganglioside G_{M2}	hexosaminidase A
type 2: Sandhoff-Jatzkewitz variant		hexosaminidase A and B
type 3: juvenile form		hexosaminidase A (partial)
G_{M3}–gangliosidosis	ganglioside G_{M3}	(N-acetyl-galactosaminyl transferase)

venous g., SYN static g.

wet g., ischemic necrosis of an extremity with bacterial infection, producing cellulitis adjacent to the necrotic areas. SYN moist g.

white g., death of a part accompanied by the formation of grayish white sloughs. SYN leukonecrosis.

gan·gre·nous (gang′grĕ-nŭs). Relating to or affected with gangrene. SYN mortified.

gan·o·blast (gan′o-blast). SYN ameloblast.

Ganong, William F., U.S. physiologist, *1924. SEE Lown-G.-Levine *syndrome.*

Ganser, Siegbert J.M., German psychiatrist, 1853–1931. SEE G.'s *commissures,* under *commissure, syndrome; nucleus* basalis of G.

Gant, Samuel, U.S. surgeon, 1870–1944. SEE G.'s *clamp.*

gan·try (gan′trē). A frame housing the x-ray tube, collimators, and detectors in a CT machine, with a large opening into which the patient is inserted; a mechanical support for mounting a device to be moved in a circular path. [M.E., fr. O.Fr., fr. L. *cantherius,* wooden frame, fr. G. *kanthēlia,* pack saddle, fr. *kanthos,* pack ass]

Gantzer, Carol F.L., 17th century German anatomist. SEE G.'s accessory *bundle, muscle.*

Ganz, William, U.S. cardiologist, *1919. SEE Swan-G. *catheter.*

gap. 1. A hiatus or opening in a structure. **2.** An interval or discontinuity in any series or sequence. **3 (G).** A period in the cell cycle.

ga

g. 1 (G1), in the somatic cell cycle, the g. that follows mitosis and is followed by synthesis in preparation for the next cycle.

g. 2 (G2), in the somatic cell cycle, a pause between completion of synthesis and the onset of cell division.

air-bone g., the difference between the threshold for hearing acuity by bone conduction and by air conduction.

anion g., the difference between the sum of the measured cations and anions in the plasma or serum calculated as follows: (Na + K) − (Cl + HCO$_3$) = < 20 mmol/l. Elevated values may occur in diabetic or lactic acidosis; normal or low values occur in bicarbonate-losing metabolic acidoses. SYN cation-anion difference.

auscultatory g., the period during which Korotkoff sounds indicating true systolic pressure fade away and reappear at a lower pressure point; responsible for errors made in recording falsely low systolic blood pressure, especially in hypertensive patients, of up to 25 mm Hg, and avoided by pumping the cuff 30 mm Hg beyond palpable systolic pressure. SYN silent g.

Bochdalek's g., SYN vertebrocostal *trigone.*

chromosomal g., a localized area of thinning in a chromatid which may simulate a complete break.

DNA g., a localized loss of one of the two strands in the double helix of DNA.

excitable g., SYN gap *phenomenon.*

interocclusal g., SYN freeway *space.*

silent g., SYN auscultatory g.

gapes (gāps). A disease of young chickens, turkeys, and other birds caused by the gapeworm, *Syngamus trachea*, which localizes in the trachea and causes gasping and choking; infection is either direct, by ingestion of infective eggs, or indirect, by ingestion of transport hosts such as land snails, slugs, or earthworms.

gape·worm (gāp'wŏrm). SEE *Syngamus.*

Garbe, William, Canadian dermatologist, *1908. SEE Sulzberger-G. *disease, syndrome.*

Gardner, Eldon J., U.S. geneticist, *1909. SEE G.'s *syndrome.*

Gardner, F.H. SEE G.-Diamond *syndrome.*

Gard·ner·el·la (gărd'ner-el'ă). A genus of facultatively anaerobic, oxidase- and catalase-negative, nonsporeforming, nonencapsulated, nonmotile, pleomorphic bacteria with Gram-variable rods.

G. vaginalis, a species that is the etiologic agent of bacterial vaginosis in humans.

gar·gle (gar'gl). **1.** To rinse the fauces with fluid in the mouth through which expired breath is forced to produce a bubbling effect while the head is held far back. **2.** A medicated fluid used for gargling; a throat wash. [O. Fr. fr. L. *gurgulio,* gullet, windpipe]

Gariel, Maurice, French physician, 1812–1878. SEE G.'s *pessary.*

Garland, Hugh, British neurologist. SEE Marinesco-Garland *syndrome.*

Garland, M., U.S. physician, 1848–1926. SEE G.'s *triangle.*

gar·lic (gar'lik). SYN allium.

g. oil, a volatile oil from the bulb or entire plant of *Allium sativum* (family Liliaceae); contains diallyl disulfide and allyl propyl disulfide; has been used as an anthelmintic and rubefacient.

Garré, Carl, Swiss surgeon, 1857–1928. SEE G.'s *disease;* Garré's *osteomyelitis.*

Gärtner, August, German physician, 1848–1934. SEE G.'s *bacillus, method,* vein *phenomenon, tonometer.*

Gartner, Herman T., Danish anatomist and surgeon, 1785–1827. SEE G.'s *canal, cyst, duct.*

GAS Abbreviation for group A *streptococci,* under *streptococcus.*

gas. 1. A thin fluid, like air, capable of indefinite expansion but convertible by compression and cold into a liquid and, eventually, a solid. **2.** In clinical practice, a liquid entirely in its vapor phase at one atmosphere of pressure because ambient temperature is above its boiling point. [coined by J.B. van Helmont, Flemish chemist, 1577–1644]

alveolar g. (symbol subscript A), the g. in the pulmonary alveoli, where O_2-CO_2 exchange with pulmonary capillary blood occurs. SYN alveolar air.

anesthetic g., SEE inhalation *anesthetic.*

blood g.'s, a clinical expression for the determination of the partial pressures of oxygen and carbon dioxide in blood.

carbonic acid g., SYN *carbon* dioxide.

expired g., (1) any g. that has been expired from the lungs; **(2)** often used synonymously with mixed expired g.

hemolytic g., a poisonous g., such as arsine, inhalation of which causes hemolysis with hemoglobinuria, jaundice, gastroenteritis, and nephritis.

ideal alveolar g., the uniform composition of g. that would exist in all alveoli for a given total respiratory exchange if all alveoli had identical ventilation-perfusion ratios and achieved perfect equilibrium with the blood leaving the pulmonary capillaries.

inert g.'s, SYN noble g.'s.

inspired g. (I) (symbol subscript I), **(1)** any g. that is being inhaled; **(2)** specifically, that g. after it has been humidified at body temperature.

laughing g., a historical term for nitrous oxide. [so called because its inhalation sometimes excites a hilarious delirium preceding insensibility]

marsh g., SYN methane.

mixed expired g., one or more complete breaths of expired g. coming thoroughly mixed from the dead space and the alveoli.

mustard g. (HD), S(CH$_2$CH$_2$Cl)$_2$; bis- or di(2-chloroethyl)-sulfide; a poisonous vesicating gas introduced in World War I; it is the progenitor of the so-called nitrogen mustards; used in chemical warfare; a known carcinogen. SYN di(2-chloroethyl)sulfide, mustard (2), sulfur mustard.

noble g.'s, elements in the zero group in the periodic series: helium, neon, argon, krypton, xenon, and radon. SYN inert g.'s.

sewer g., g., probably mostly methane, resulting from decomposition of organic matter in sewers; potentially explosive and toxic.

sneezing g., SYN sternutator.

suffocating g., a g., such as chlorine or phosgene, that causes intense irritation of the bronchial tubes and lungs, resulting in pulmonary edema.

tear g., a g., such as acetone, benzene bromide, and xylol, that causes irritation of the conjunctiva and profuse lacrimation. SEE ALSO lacrimator.

vesicating g., a g., such as mustard g., which upon contact with the skin causes vesication and sloughing; inhalation may result in bronchopneumonia.

vomiting g., a g., such as chloropicrin, that can cause vomiting and gastrointestinal disorders such as colic and diarrhea.

water g., an illuminating and fuel g. produced by passing steam over red-hot coal; consists chiefly of hydrogen, hydrocarbons, and carbon monoxide.

gas·e·ous (gas'ē-ŭs). Of the nature of gas.

Gaskell, Walter H., English physiologist, 1847–1914. SEE G.'s *bridge, clamp.*

gas·om·e·ter (gas-om'ĕ-ter). A calibrated instrument or vessel for measuring the volumes of gases. SEE ALSO spirometer.

gas·o·met·ric (gas-ō-met'rik). Relating to gasometry.

gas·om·e·try (gas-om'ĕ-trē). Measurement of gases; determination of the relative proportion of gases in a mixture.

Gass, J. Donald M., U.S. ophthalmologist, *1928. SEE Irvine-G. *syndrome.*

Gasser (Gas·ser·i·o), Johann L., Austrian anatomist, 1723–1765. SEE gasserian *ganglion.*

gas·ser·i·an (ga-ser'ē-an). Relating to or described by Johann L. Gasser.

gas·sing (gas'ing). Poisoning by irrespirable or otherwise noxious gases.

Gastaut, Henri, French biologist, *1915. SEE Lennox-G. *syndrome.*

gas·ter (gas'ter) [NA]. SYN stomach. [G. *gastēr,* belly]

Gas·ter·o·phil·i·dae (gas'ter-ō-fil'i-dē). A family of botflies (or warble flies) that produce enteric myiasis in members of the horse family (genus *Gasterophilus*), in rhinoceroses (genus *Gyrostigma*), and in elephants (genera *Cobboldia*, *Platycobboldia*, and *Rodhainomyia*) SYN Gastrophilidae. [G. *gastēr*, belly, stomach, + *philos*, fond]

Gas·ter·oph·i·lus (gas-ter-of′i-lŭs). A genus of botflies (horse botflies or warble flies) that cause enteric myiasis in domestic and wild horses and other equids. The bee-like adult attaches eggs to the hairs of the legs or body of the horse; infective eggs hatch when contacted by the lips of the horse, and the larvae attach to, penetrate, and are swallowed or burrow through the tissues to the stomach, where they adhere. After some months, the larvae pass out with the feces, pupate, and emerge as adults. Moderate infection produces little or no symptomatology; heavy infection can cause severe digestive disorders. Important species include *G. hemorrhoidalis* (the redtailed botflies, a nose fly); *G. intestinalis* (the common horse botfly or nit fly), whose larvae are found in the esophageal portion of the stomach; *G. nasalis* or *G. veterinus* (chin fly or throat botfly), found in the throat or under the jaws of the horse, the larvae migrating to the pyloric portion of the stomach or the anterior duodenum; and *G. pecuorum* (the dark-winged horsefly), the most common and pathogenic species in Europe (absent in the U.S.). SYN *Gastrophilus*. [G. *gastēr*, belly, stomach, + *philos*, fond]

⌂**gastr-.** SEE gastro-.

gas·trad·e·ni·tis (gas′trad-ĕ-nī′tis). Inflammation of the glands of the stomach. SYN gastroadenitis. [gastr- + G. *adēn*, gland, + *-itis*, inflammation]

gas·tral·gia (gas-tral′jē-ă). SYN stomach *ache*. [gastr- + G. *algos*, pain]

gas·trec·ta·sis, gas·trec·ta·sia (gas-trek′tă-sis, gas-trek-tā′zē-ă). Dilation of the stomach. [gastr- + G. *ektasis*, extension]

gas·trec·to·my (gas-trek′tō-mē). Excision of a part or all of the stomach. [gastr- + G. *ektomē*, excision]

Hofmeister g., Hofmeister's operation in which a portion of the stomach is removed and a retrocolic gastrojejunostomy is constructed in an end-to-side fashion to only the greater curvature portion of the transected stomach.

Pólya g., operation in which a portion of the stomach is removed and a retrocolic gastrojejunostomy is constructed in an end-to-side fashion to the entire cut end of the stomach. SYN Pólya's operation.

gas·tric (gas′trik). Relating to the stomach. SYN gastricus [NA].

gas·tric car·dia (gas′trik kar′dē-ă). SYN cardiac *part* of stomach.

gas·tric·sin (gas-trik′sin). Former term for a human peptidase now termed pepsin C.

gas·tri·cus (gas′tri-kŭs) [NA]. SYN gastric. [L.]

gas·trin·o·ma (gas-tri-nō′mă). A gastrin-secreting tumor associated with the Zollinger-Ellison syndrome.

gas·trins (gas′trinz). Hormones secreted in the pyloric-antral mucosa of the mammalian stomach that stimulate secretion of HCl by the parietal cells of the gastric glands; there are two types (one sulfated [type II], the other not [type I]), both heptadecapeptides, the terminal tetrapeptide (Trp-Met-Asp-Phe-NH₂) (often termed tetragastrin) being as active as the whole molecule; a competitive inhibitor of g. is cholecystokinin. [G. *gastēr*, stomach, + -in]

gas·tri·tis (gas-trī′tis). Inflammation, especially mucosal, of the stomach. [gastr- + G. *-itis*, inflammation]

alkaline reflux g., SYN bile g.

atrophic g., chronic g. with atrophy of the mucous membrane and destruction of the peptic glands, sometimes associated with pernicious anemia or gastric carcinoma; also applied to gastric atrophy without inflammatory changes.

bile g., an inflammation of the gastric mucosa believed to be caused by irritating factors in bile. SYN alkaline reflux g.

catarrhal g., g. with excessive secretion of mucus.

g. cys′tica polypo′sa, large sessile mucosal polyps arising in the stomach proximal to an old gastroenterostomy.

eosinophilic g., SYN eosinophilic *gastroenteritis*.

exfoliative g., g. with excessive shedding of mucosal epithelial cells.

g. fibroplas′tica, obsolete term for g. with fibrosis and sclerosis.

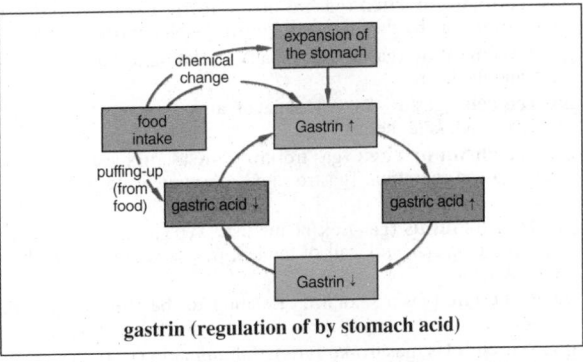

gastrin (regulation of by stomach acid)

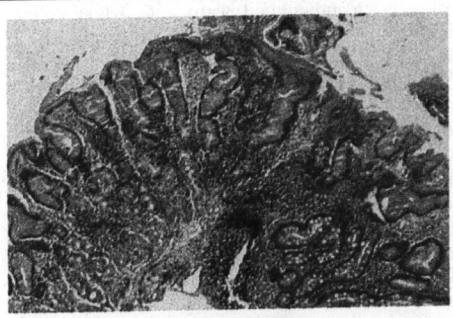

atrophic gastritis
chronic gastritis, with advanced atrophy of the mucous membrane, and with intestinal metaplasia

hypertrophic g., SYN Ménétrier's *disease*.

interstitial g., inflammation of the stomach involving the submucosa and muscle coats.

phlegmonous g., obsolete term for severe inflammation, chiefly of the submucous coat, with purulent infiltration of the wall of the stomach.

polypous g., a form of chronic g., in which there is irregular atrophy of the mucous membrane with cystic glands giving rise to a knobby or polypous appearance of the surface.

pseudomembranous g., g. characterized by the formation of a false membrane.

sclerotic g., a fibrous thickening of the walls of the stomach with diminution in the capacity of the organ.

traumatic g., a condition of cattle, caused by the penetration of the stomach wall, usually the reticulum, by any kind of sharp object (usually metallic) which has been swallowed. SYN hardware disease, traumatic reticuloperitonitis.

⌂**gastro-, gastr-.** The stomach, abdomen. [G. *gastēr*, the belly]

gas·tro·a·ceph·a·lus (gas′trō-ă-sef′ă-lŭs). Unequal conjoined twins in which an acephalous parasite is attached to the abdomen of the autosite. SEE conjoined *twins*, under twin. [gastro- + G. *a*-priv. + *kephalē*, head]

gas·tro·ad·e·ni·tis (gas′trō-ad-ĕ-nī′tis). SYN gastradenitis.

gas·tro·al·bum·or·rhea (gas′trō-al-byū-mō-rē′ă). Loss of albumin into the stomach. [gastro- + albumin, + G. *rhoia*, flow]

gas·tro·a·mor·phus (gas′trō-ă-mōr′fŭs). An included amorphous parasitic twin within the abdomen of the autosite. [gastro- + G. *amorphos*, unshapely]

gas·tro·a·nas·to·mo·sis (gas′trō-an-as-tō-mō′sis). Anastomosis of the cardiac and antral segments of the stomach, for relief from marked hour-glass contraction of the stomach. SYN gastrogastrostomy.

gas·tro·a·to·nia (gas′trō-ă-tō′nē-ă). Obsolete term for loss of tone in the stomach musculature. [gastro- + G. *atonia*, languor]

ga

gas·tro·blen·nor·rhea (gas′trō-blen-ō-rē′ă). Excessive proliferation of mucus by the stomach. [gastro- + blennorrhea]

gas·tro·car·di·ac (gas′trō-kar′dē-ak). Relating to both the stomach and the heart.

gas·tro·cele (gas′trō-sēl). Hernia of a portion of the stomach. [gastro- + G. *kēlē*, hernia]

gas·tro·chron·or·rhea (gas′trō-kron-ō-rē′ă). Excessive continuous gastric secretion. [gastro- + G. *chronos*, time (chronic), + *rhoia*, a flow]

gas·troc·ne·mi·us (gas-trok-nē′mē-ŭs). SYN gastrocnemius *muscle*. [G. *gastroknēmia*, calf of the leg, fr. *gaster* (*gastr*-), belly, + *knēmē*, leg]

gas·tro·co·lic (gas′trō-kol′ik). Relating to the stomach and the colon.

gas·tro·co·li·tis (gas′trō-kō-lī′tis). Inflammation of both stomach and colon.

gas·tro·co·lop·to·sis (gas′trō-kō-lō-tō′sis). Displacement downward of stomach and colon. [gastro- + G. *kōlon*, colon, + *ptōsis*, a falling]

gas·tro·co·los·to·my (gas′trō-kō-los′tō-mē). Establishment of a communication between stomach and colon. [gastro- + G. *kōlon*, colon, + *stoma*, mouth]

gas·tro·cys·to·plas·ty (gas′trō-sis′tō-plas-tē). Augmentation of the bladder by a patch or piece of vascularized gastric tissue.

gas·tro·di·al·y·sis (gas′trō-dī-al′i-sis). Dialysis across the mucous membrane of the stomach.

Gas·tro·dis·coi·des hom·i·nis (gas′trō-dis-koy′dēz hom′i-nis). A species of trematode sometimes found in the intestinal canal of man in India, Southeast Asia, and China; its normal host is the pig. SYN *Gastrodiscus hominis*. [gastro- + G. *diskos*, disk; L. *homo*, gen. *hominis*, man]

Gas·tro·dis·cus hom·i·nis (gas-trō-dis′kŭs). SYN *Gastrodiscoides hominis.*

gas·tro·du·o·de·nal (gas′trō-dū′ō-dē′năl, -du-od′ĕ-nal). Relating to the stomach and duodenum.

gas·tro·du·o·de·ni·tis (gas′trō-dū-ō-dē-nī′tis). Inflammation of both stomach and duodenum.

gas·tro·du·o·de·nos·co·py (gas′trō-dū-ō-dĕ-nos′kŏ-pē). Visualization of the interior of the stomach and duodenum by a gastroscope. [gastro- + duodenum, + G. *skopeō*, to view]

gas·tro·du·o·de·nos·to·my (gas′trō-dū-ō-dĕ-nos′tō-mē). Establishment of a communication between the stomach and the duodenum. [gastro- + duodenum + G. *stoma*, mouth]

gas·tro·dyn·ia (gas-trō-din′ē-ă). SYN stomach *ache*. [gastro- + G. *odynē*, pain]

gas·tro·en·ter·ic (gas′trō-en-ter′ik). SYN gastrointestinal.

gas·tro·en·ter·i·tis (gas′trō-en-ter-ī′tis). Inflammation of the mucous membrane of both stomach and intestine. SYN enterogastritis. [gastro- + G. *enteron*, intestine, + *-itis*, inflammation]

acute infectious nonbacterial g., SYN epidemic nonbacterial g.

endemic nonbacterial infantile g., an endemic viral g. of young children (6 months to 12 years) that is especially widespread during winter, caused by strains of rotavirus; the incubation period is 2 to 4 days, with symptoms lasting 3 to 5 days, including abdominal pain, diarrhea, fever, and vomiting. SYN infantile g.

eosinophilic g., gastroenteritis with abdominal pain, malabsorption, often obstructive symptoms, associated with peripheral eosinophilia and areas of eosinophilic infiltration of the stomach, small intestine and/or colon with eosinophiles. May be an allergic etiology and responds to elimination diet in some patients; corticosteroid therapy is also effective. SYN eosinophilic gastritis.

epidemic nonbacterial g., an epidemic, highly communicable but rather mild disease of sudden onset, caused by the epidemic gastroenteritis virus (especially Norwalk agent), with an incubation period of 16 to 48 hours and a duration of 1 to 2 days, which affects all age groups; infection is associated with some fever, abdominal cramps, nausea, vomiting, diarrhea, and headache, one or another of which may be predominant. SYN acute infectious nonbacterial g.

infantile g., SYN endemic nonbacterial infantile g.

porcine transmissible g., SYN transmissible g. of swine.

transmissible g. of swine (TGE), a rapidly spreading disease of swine, caused by a coronavirus (of the family Coronaviridae) and characterized by severe diarrhea and vomiting; case fatality rate in pigs younger than 10 days is high; in older pigs it is low. SYN porcine transmissible g.

viral g., SEE endemic nonbacterial infantile g., epidemic nonbacterial g.

gas·tro·en·ter·o·a·nas·to·mo·sis (gas′trō-en-ter-ō-an-as-tō-mō′sis). SYN gastroenterostomy.

gas·tro·en·ter·o·co·li·tis (gas′trō-en′ter-ō-kō-lī′tis). Inflammatory disease involving the stomach and intestines. [gastro- + G. *enteron*, intestine, + *kōlon*, colon, + *-itis*, inflammation]

gas·tro·en·ter·o·co·los·to·my (gas′trō-en-ter-ō-kō-los′tō-mē). Formation of direct communication between the stomach and the large and small intestines. [gastro- + G. *enteron*, intestine, + *kōlon*, colon + *stoma*, mouth]

gas·tro·en·ter·ol·o·gist (gas′trō-en-ter-ol′ō-jist). A specialist in gastroenterology.

gas·tro·en·ter·ol·o·gy (gas′trō-en-ter-ol′ō-jē). The medical specialty concerned with the function and disorders of the gastrointestinal tract, including stomach, intestines, and associated organs. [gastro- + G. *enteron*, intestine, + *logos*, study]

gas·tro·en·ter·op·a·thy (gas′trō-en-ter-op′ă-thē). Any disorder of the alimentary canal. [gastro- + G. *enteron*, intestine, + *pathos*, suffering]

gas·tro·en·ter·o·plas·ty (gas′trō-en-ter-ō-plas′tē). Operative repair of defects in the stomach and intestine. [gastro- + G. *enteron*, intestine, + *plassō*, to form]

gas·tro·en·ter·op·to·sis (gas′trō-en-ter-ō-tō′sis). Downward displacement of the stomach and a portion of the intestine. [gastro- + G. *enteron*, intestine, + *ptōsis*, a falling]

gas·tro·en·ter·os·to·my (gas′trō-en-ter-os′tō-mē). Establishment of a new opening between the stomach and the intestine, either anterior or posterior to the transverse colon. SYN gastroenteroanastomosis. [gastro- + G. *enteron*, intestine, + *stoma*, mouth]

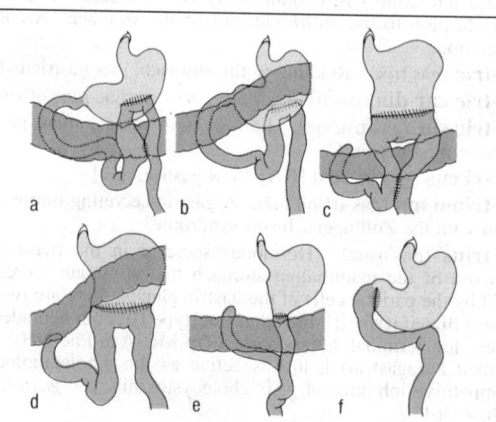

gastroenterostomy

a: frontal gastroenterostomy (anterior to the colon) with Braun's anastomosis; b: rear gastroenterostomy (posterior to the colon); c: Billroth II anastomosis (with Kroenlein's modification); d: Billroth II anastomosis (with Reichel-Polya modification: retrocolic gastrojejunostomy); e: Billroth II anastomosis (with Roux modification (Y)); f: Finney pyloroplasty (or gastroduodenostomy)

gas·tro·en·ter·ot·o·my (gas′trō-en-ter-ot′ō-mē). Section into both stomach and intestine. [gastro- + G. *enteron*, intestine, + *tomē*, incision]

gas·tro·ep·i·plo·ic (gas′trō-ep′i-plō′ik). Relating to the stomach and the greater omentum (epiploon).

gas·tro·e·soph·a·ge·al (gas′trō-ē-sof′ă-jē′ăl). Relating to both stomach and esophagus. [gastro- + G. *oisophagos,* gullet (esophagus)]

gas·tro·e·soph·a·gi·tis (gas'trō-ē-sof-ă-jī'tis). Inflammation of the stomach and esophagus.

gas·tro·e·soph·a·gos·to·my (gas'trō-ē-sof-ă-gos'tō-mē). SYN esophagogastrostomy. [gastro- + G. *oisophagos,* gullet (esophagus), + *stoma,* mouth]

gas·tro·gas·tros·to·my (gas'trō-gas-tros'tō-mē). SYN gastroanastomosis.

gas·tro·ga·vage (gas-trō-gă-vahzh'). SYN gavage (1).

gas·tro·gen·ic (gas-trō-jen'ik). Deriving from or caused by the stomach.

gas·tro·graph (gas'trō-graf). An instrument for recording graphically the movements of the stomach. SYN gastrokinesograph. [gastro- + G. *graphē,* a writing]

gas·tro·he·pat·ic (gas'trō-he-pat'ik). Relating to the stomach and the liver. [gastro- + G. *hēpar* (*hēpat-*), liver]

gas·tro·hy·dror·rhea (gas'trō-hī-drō-rē'ă). Excretion into the stomach of a large amount of watery fluid containing neither hydrochloric acid, chymosin nor pepsin ferments. [gastro- + G. *hydōr,* water, + *rhoia,* a flow]

gas·tro·il·e·i·tis (gas'trō-il-ē-ī'tis). Inflammation of the alimentary canal in which the stomach and ileum are primarily involved.

gas·tro·il·e·os·to·my (gas'trō-il-ē-os'tō-mē). A surgical joining of stomach to ileum; a technical error in which the ileum instead of jejunum is selected for the site of a gastrojejunostomy.

gas·tro·in·tes·ti·nal (GI) (gas'trō-in-tes'tin-ăl). Relating to the stomach and intestines. SYN gastroenteric.

gas·tro·je·ju·no·co·lic (gas'trō-jē-jū'nō-kol'ik). Referring to the stomach, jejunum, and colon.

gas·tro·je·ju·nos·to·my (gas'trō-jē-jū-nos'tō-mē). Establishment of a direct communication between the stomach and the jejunum. SYN gastronesteostomy. [gastro- + jejunum G. *stoma,* mouth]

gas·tro·ki·ne·so·graph (gas'trō-ki-nē'sō-graf). SYN gastrograph. [gastro- + G. *kinēsis,* motion, + *graphē,* a writing]

gas·tro·la·vage (gas-trō-lă-vahzh'). Lavage of the stomach.

gas·tro·li·e·nal (gas-trō-lī'ē-năl). SYN gastrosplenic. [gastro- + L. *lien,* spleen]

gas·tro·lith (gas'trō-lith). A concretion in the stomach. SYN gastric calculus. [gastro- + G. *lithos,* stone]

gas·tro·li·thi·a·sis (gas'trō-li-thī'ă-sis). Presence of one or more calculi in the stomach. [gastro- + G. *lithos,* stone + *-iasis,* condition]

gas·trol·o·gist (gas-trol'ō-jist). A specialist in gastrology.

gas·trol·o·gy (gas-trol'ō-jē). The branch of medicine concerned with the stomach and its diseases. [gastro- + G. *logos,* study]

gas·trol·y·sis (gas-trol'i-sis). Division of perigastric adhesions. [gastro- + G. *lysis,* loosening]

gas·tro·ma·la·cia (gas'trō-mă-lā'shē-ă). Softening of the walls of the stomach. [gastro- + G. *malakia,* softness]

gas·tro·meg·a·ly (gas'trō-meg'ă-lē). **1.** Enlargement of the stomach. **2.** Enlargement of the abdomen. [gastro- + G. *megas* (*megal-*), large]

gas·trom·e·lus (gas-trom'ĕ-lŭs). A condition in which an individual has a supernumerary limb attached to the abdomen. SEE conjoined *twins,* under *twin.* [gastro- + G. *melos,* a limb]

gas·tro·myx·or·rhea (gas'trō-mik-sō-rē'ă). Excessive secretion of mucus in the stomach. SYN myxorrhea gastrica. [gastro- + G. *myxa,* mucus, + *rhoia,* a flow]

gas·tro·ne·ste·os·to·my (gas'trō-nes-tē-os'tō-mē). SYN gastrojejunostomy. [gastro- + G. *nēstis,* jejunum, + *stoma,* mouth]

gas·trop·a·gus (gas-trop'ă-gŭs). Conjoined twins united at the abdomen. SEE conjoined *twins,* under *twin.* [gastro- + *-pagus*]

gas·tro·pa·ral·y·sis (gas'trō-pă-ral'i-sis). Paralysis of the muscular coat of the stomach.

gas·tro·par·a·si·tus (gas'trō-par-ă-sī'tŭs). Unequal conjoined twins in which the incomplete parasite is attached to, or within, the abdomen of the autosite. SEE conjoined *twins,* under *twin.*

gas·tro·pa·re·sis (gas-trō-pă-rē'sis, -par'ĕ-sis). A slight degree of gastroparalysis. [gastro- + G. *paresis,* a letting go, paralysis]

g. diabetico'rum, dilation of the stomach with gastric retention in diabetics, commonly seen in association with severe acidosis or coma.

gas·tro·path·ic (gas-trō-path'ik). Denoting gastropathy.

gas·trop·a·thy (gas-trop'ă-thē). Any disease of the stomach. [gastro- + G. *pathos,* disease]

hypertrophic hypersecretory g., nodular thickenings of gastric mucosa with acid hypersecretion and frequently peptic ulceration, not associated with a gastrin-secreting tumor.

gas·tro·pex·y (gas'trō-pek-sē). Attachment of the stomach to the abdominal wall or diaphragm. [gastro- + G. *pēxis,* fixation]

Gas·tro·phil·i·dae (gas-trō-fil'i-dē). SYN Gasterophilidae.

Gas·troph·i·lus (gas-trof'i-lŭs). SYN *Gasterophilus.*

gas·tro·phren·ic (gas'trō-fren'ik). Relating to the stomach and the diaphragm. [gastro- + G. *phrēn,* diaphragm]

gas·tro·plas·ty (gas'trō-plas-tē). Operative treatment of a defect in the stomach or lower esophagus which utilizes the stomach wall for the reconstruction. [gastro- + G. *plastos,* formed]

Collis g., a technique for lengthening a "short" esophagus; a full-thickness incision of the gastric cardia is made parallel to the lesser curvature, to allow transverse closure and so lengthen the esophagus by making tubular the upper part of the stomach.

vertical banded g., a g. for treatment of morbid obesity in which an upper gastric pouch is formed by a vertical staple line, with a cloth band applied to prevent dilation at the outlet into the main pouch.

gas·tro·pli·ca·tion (gas'trō-pli-kā'shŭn). An operation for reducing the size of the stomach by suturing a longitudinal fold with the peritoneal surfaces in apposition. SYN gastroptyxis, gastrorrhaphy (2), stomach reefing. [gastro- + L. *plico,* to fold]

gas·tro·pneu·mon·ic (gas'trō-nū-mon'ik). SYN pneumogastric. [gastro- + G. *pneumōn,* lung]

gas·tro·pod (gas'trō-pod). Common name for members of the class Gastropoda.

Gas·trop·o·da (gas-trop'ŏ-dă). A class of the phylum Mollusca that includes the snails, whelks, slugs, and limpets. [gastro- + G. *pous* (*pod-*), foot]

gas·trop·to·sis, gas·trop·to·sia (gas-trop-tō'sis, -tō'sē-ă). Downward displacement of the stomach. SYN bathygastry, descensus ventriculi, ventroptosis, ventroptosia. [gastro- + G. *ptosis,* a falling]

gas·tro·ptyx·is (gas-trō-tik'sis). SYN gastroplication. [gastro- + G. *ptyxis,* a fold]

gas·tro·pul·mo·nary (gas-trō-pŭl'mo-nar-ē). SYN pneumogastric.

gas·tro·py·lor·ec·to·my (gas'trō-pī-lōr-ek'tō-mē). SYN pylorectomy.

gas·tro·py·lor·ic (gas'trō-pī-lōr'ik). Relating to the stomach as a whole and to the pylorus.

gas·tror·rha·gia (gas-trō-rā'jē-ă). Hemorrhage from the stomach. SYN gastric hemorrhage. [gastro- + G. *rhēgnymi,* to burst forth]

gas·tror·rha·phy (gas-trōr'ă-fē). **1.** Suture of a perforation of the stomach. **2.** SYN gastroplication. [gastro- + G. *rhaphē,* a stitching]

gas·tror·rhea (gas-trō-rē'ă). Excessive secretion of gastric juice or of mucus (gastromyxorrhea) by the stomach. [gastro- + G. *rhoia,* a flow]

gas·tror·rhex·is (gas'trō-rek'sis). A tear or bursting of the stomach. [gastro- + G. *rhēxis,* a bursting]

gas·tros·chi·sis (gas-tros'ki-sis). A defect in the abdominal wall resulting from rupture of the amniotic membrane during physiological gut-loop herniation or, later, owing to delayed umbilical ring closure; usually accompanied by protrusion of viscera. [gastro- + G. *schisis,* a fissure]

gas·tro·scope (gas'trō-skōp). An endoscope for inspecting the inner surface of the stomach. [gastro- + G. *skopeō,* to examine]

fiberoptic g., instrument using fiberoptic system for inspection of the interior of the stomach.

ga

gas·tro·scop·ic (gas-trō-skop'ik). Relating to gastroscopy.

gas·tros·co·py (gas-tros'kŏ-pē). Inspection of the inner surface of the stomach through an endoscope.

gas·tro·spasm (gas'trō-spazm). Spasmodic contraction of the walls of the stomach.

gas·tro·splen·ic (gas-trō-splen'ik). Relating to the stomach and the spleen. SYN gastrolienal.

gas·tro·stax·is (gas'trō-stak'sis). Rarely used term for oozing of blood from the mucous membrane of the stomach. [gastro- + G. *staxis,* trickling]

gas·tro·ste·no·sis (gas-trō-ste-nō'sis). Diminution in size of the cavity of the stomach. [gastro- + G. *stenōsis,* narrowing]

gas·tros·to·ga·vage (gas-tros'tō-gă-vahzh'). SYN gavage (1).

gas·tros·to·la·vage (gas-tros'tō-lă-vahzh'). Lavage of the stomach through a gastric fistula.

gas·tros·to·my (gas-tros'tō-mē). Establishment of a new opening into the stomach. [gastro- + G. *stoma,* mouth]

 percutaneous endoscopic g., a g. performed without opening the abdominal cavity; usually involves puncture of abdominal wall and stomach after distention of the stomach by endoscopic methods.

gas·tro·tho·ra·cop·a·gus (gas'trō-thōr-ă-kop'ă-gŭs). Conjoined twins united at thorax and abdomen. SEE conjoined *twins,* under *twin.* [gastro- + G. *thōrax,* chest, + *pagos,* something fixed]

gas·tro·tome (gas'trō-tōm). A knife for incising the stomach.

gas·trot·o·my (gas-trot'ō-mē). Incision into the stomach. [gastro- + G. *tomē,* incision]

gas·tro·to·nom·e·ter (gas'trō-tō-nom'ĕ-ter). An apparatus used in gastrotonometry.

gas·tro·to·nom·e·try (gas'trō-tō-nom'ĕ-trē). The measurement of intragastric pressure. [gastro- + G. *tonos,* tension, + *metron,* measure]

gas·tro·tox·ic (gas-trō-tok'sik). Poisonous to the stomach.

gas·tro·tox·in (gas-trō-tok'sin). A cytotoxin specific for the cells of the mucous membrane of the stomach.

gas·tro·tro·pic (gas-trō-trop'ik). Affecting the stomach. [gastro- + G. *tropikos,* turning]

gas·trox·ia (gas-trok'sē-ă). Rarely used term for gastroxynsis. [gastro- + G. *oxys,* keen, acid]

gas·trox·yn·sis (gas-trok-sin'sis). Rarely used term for intermittent excessive secretion of the gastric juice. [gastro- + G. *oxynō,* to make sharp, acid]

gas·tru·la (gas'trū-lă). The embryo in the stage of development following the blastula; in lower forms with minimal yolk, it is a simple double-layered structure consisting of ectoderm and endoderm enclosing the archenteron, which opens to the outside by way of the blastopore; in forms with considerable yolk, the configuration of the g. is greatly modified owing to the persistence of the yolk throughout the gastrulation process; in the human embryo, the absence of yolk allows for a more rapid, direct "putting in place" of the germ layers, which are derived from the pluripotential embryonic disc. SYN invaginate planula. [Mod. L. dim. of G. *gastēr,* belly]

gas·tru·la·tion (gas-trū-lā'shŭn). Transformation of the blastula into the gastrula; the development and invagination of the embryonic germ layers.

Gatch, Willis D., U.S. surgeon, 1878–1961. SEE G. *bed.*

gate (gāt). **1.** To close an ion channel by electrical (*e.g.,* membrane potential) or chemical (*e.g.,* neurotransmitter) action. **2.** Action of a special nerve fiber to block the transmission of impulses through a synapse, *e.g.,* gating of pain impulses at synapses in the dorsal horns. **3.** A device which can be switched electronically to control the passage of a signal. **4.** To use a physiological signal, such as an ECG, to trigger an event such as an x-ray exposure or to partition continuously collected data. SEE gated radionuclide *angiocardiography.* SEE ALSO cardiac *gating.* [O.E. *geat*]

gate·keep·er (gāt'kēp-er). A health professional, typically a physician or nurse, who has the first encounter with a patient and who thus controls the patient's entry into the health care system.

gat·ing (gāt'ing). **1.** In a biological membrane, the opening and closing of a channel, believed to be associated with changes in integral membrane proteins. **2.** A process in which electrical signals are selected by a gate, which passes such signals only when the gate pulse is present to act as a control signal, or passes only the signals that have certain characteristics. SEE gate.

 cardiac gating, using an electronic signal from the cardiac cycle to trigger an event, such as in imaging separate phases of cardiac contraction.

Gaucher, Philippe C.E., French physician, 1854–1918. SEE G. *cells,* under *cell;* G.'s *disease;* pseudo-G. *cell.*

Gauer, Otto Hans, German physiologist, 1909–1979. SEE Henry-G. *response.*

gauge (gāj). A measuring device. SYN gage.

 bite g., SYN gnathodynamometer.

 Boley g., a caliper-type g. graduated in millimeters used to measure the thickness of various dental materials.

 catheter g., a metal plate with holes of graduated diameter used to determine the size of a catheter.

 strain g., a device, employing the Wheatstone bridge principle, used for accurate measurement of forces such as strain, stress, or pressure.

 undercut g., a device, used with a surveyor, to precisely locate areas for the placement of the retentive components of clasps when designing removable partial dentures.

gaul·the·ria oil (gawl-thēr'ē-ă). SYN *methyl* salicylate.

gaul·the·rin (gawl'thĕ-rin). A glycoside from the bark of several species of *Betula* (birch); it yields methyl salicylate, D-glucose, and D-xylose on hydrolysis.

gaunt·let (gawnt'let). A glove. SEE bandage.

Gauss, Johann K.F., German physicist, 1777–1855. SEE gauss, gaussian *curve,* gaussian *distribution.*

Gauss, Karl J., German gynecologist, 1875–1957. SEE G's *sign.*

gauss (G) (gows). A unit of magnetic field intensity, equal to 10^{-4} tesla. [J.K.F. *Gauss*]

Gaussel, A., French physician, 1871–1937. SEE Grasset-G. *phenomenon.*

gaus·si·an (gows'ē-ăn). Relating to or described by Johann K.F. Gauss. SEE gaussian *curve.*

gauze (gawz). A bleached cotton cloth of plain weave, used for dressings, bandages, and absorbent sponges; petrolatum g. is saturated with petrolatum. [Fr. *gaze,* fr. Ar. *gazz,* raw silk]

ga·vage (gă-vahzh'). **1.** Forced feeding by stomach tube. SYN gastrogavage, gastrostogavage. **2.** Therapeutic use of a high-potency diet administered by stomach tube. [Fr. *gaver,* to gorge fowls]

Gavard, Hyacinthe, French anatomist, 1753–1802. SEE G.'s *muscle.*

Gay, Alexander H., Russian anatomist, 1842–1907. SEE G.'s *glands,* under *gland.*

gay (gā). **1.** A homosexual, especially male. **2.** Denoting a homosexual individual or the male homosexual lifestyle. SEE lesbian.

Gay-Lussac, Joseph L., French naturalist, 1778–1850. SEE Gay-Lussac's *equation;* Gay-Lussac's *law.*

gaze (gāz). The act of looking steadily at an object.

 conjugate g., movement of both eyes with the visual axes parallel.

 dysconjugate g., failure of the eyes to turn together in the same direction.

G-band·ing. SEE G-banding *stain.*

GBG Abbreviation for gonadal steroid-binding *globulin.*

GBH Abbreviation for gamma benzene *hexachloride.*

GC Abbreviation for the guanine and cytosine base pair in polynucleic acids.

G-CSF Abbreviation for granulocyte colony-stimulating *factor.*

Gd Symbol for gadolinium.

GDP Abbreviation for guanosine 5'-diphosphate.

GDPman·nose phos·pho·ryl·ase. SYN mannose-1-phosphate guanylyltransferase (GDP).

Ge Symbol for germanium.

Ge·doel·stia (ge-del'stē-ă). A genus of nasal botflies (family

Oestridae) that includes the species *G. cristata* and *G. haessleri* which parasitize wildebeest, hartebeeste, and other African antelopes, and may also cause an ophthalmomyiasis in sheep and humans.

ge·doel·sti·o·sis (ge-del-sti-ō′sis). Infection of herbivores and rarely man with larvae of flies of the genus *Gedoelstia*, causing ophthalmomyiasis in humans. SYN bulging eye disease.

Geh·rig, Henry Louis, U.S. baseball player; 1903–1941, victim of Lou Gehrig's *disease*. SEE Lou Gehrig's *disease*.

Geigel, Richard, German physician, 1859–1930. SEE G.'s *reflex*.

Geiger, Hans, German physicist, 1882–1945. SEE G.-Müller *counter, tube.*

gel (jel). **1.** A jelly, or the solid or semisolid phase of a colloidal solution. SYN gelatum. **2.** To form a g. or jelly; to convert a sol into a g. [Mod. L. *gelatum*]

colloidal g., a colloid that has developed resistance to flow because of chemical or thermal change.

pharmacopeial g., a suspension, in a water medium, of an insoluble drug in hydrated form wherein the particle size approaches or attains colloidal dimensions.

ge·las·mus (jĕ-laz′mŭs). Rarely used term for spasmodic, hysterical laughter. [Gr. *gelasma*, a laugh, fr. *gelaō*, to laugh]

gel·ate (jel′āt). SYN gelatinize.

gel·a·tin (jel′ă-tin). A derived protein formed from the collagen of tissues by boiling in water; it swells up when put in cold water, but dissolves only in hot water; used as a hemostat, plasma substitute, and protein food adjunct in malnutrition. [L. *gelo*, pp. *gelatus*, to freeze, congeal]

glycerinated g., a preparation made of equal parts of g. and glycerin; a firm mass liquefying at gentle heat; it is used as a vehicle for suppositories and urethral bougies. SYN glycerin jelly, glycerogelatin, glycogelatin.

Irish moss g., g. extracted from Irish moss; used to make the mucilage of Irish moss that is used as a substitute for gum arabic in making emulsions.

vegetable g., a substance similar to g., obtained from gluten.

zinc g., SEE *zinc* gelatin.

gel·a·tin·ase (jel′ă-tin-ās). pepsin B; a proteolytic enzyme which hydrolyzes gelatin. SEE pepsin.

ge·la·ti·nif·er·ous (jel′ă-ti-nif′er-ŭs). Producing or containing gelatin. [gelatin + L. *fero*, to bear]

ge·lat·i·ni·za·tion (jĕ-lat′i-ni-zā′shŭn). Conversion into gelatin or a substance resembling it.

ge·lat·i·nize (jĕ-lat′i-nīz). **1.** To convert into gelatin. **2.** To become gelatinous. SYN gelate.

ge·lat·i·noid (jĕ-lat′i-noyd). SYN gelatinous (2).

ge·lat·i·nous (jĕ-lat′i-nŭs). **1.** Pertaining to or characteristic of gelatin. **2.** Jelly-like or resembling gelatin. SYN gelatinoid.

ge·la·tion (jĕ-lā′shŭn). In colloidal chemistry, the transformation of a sol into a gel.

ge·la·tum (jĕ-lā′tŭm). SYN gel (1). [Mod. L.]

Gélineau, Jean Baptiste Edouard, French physician, 1859–1906. SEE G.'s *syndrome*.

Gell, P.G., British immunologist. SEE G. and Coombs *reactions*, under *reaction*.

Gellé, Marie-Ernst, French otologist, 1834–1923. SEE G. *test*.

Gellerstedt, Nils, *1896. SEE Ceelen-G. *syndrome*.

ge·lo·sis (jĕ-lō′sis). An extremely firm mass in tissue (especially in a muscle), with a consistency resembling that of frozen tissue. [L. *gelo*, to freeze, congeal, + G. *-osis*, condition]

gel·o·trip·sy (jel′ō-trip-sē). Rubbing away an indurated swelling or tender point in neuralgia and myalgia. [gelosis + G. *tripsis*, a rubbing, fr. *tribō*, to rub]

gel·se·mine (jel′sĕ-mēn). A crystallizable alkaloid derived from gelsemium (yellow jasmine); a mydriatic and central nervous system stimulant. [Mod. L. *gelsemium*, fr. Pers. *yāsmin*, jasmine]

gel·so·lin (jel-sol′in). An actin-binding protein; a Ca^{2+}-triggered actin-filament-severing protein.

Gély, Jules A., French surgeon, 1806–1861. SEE G.'s *suture*.

△**gem-.** Prefix denoting twin substitutions on a single atom; *e.g.,*

the *gem*-dimethyl substitution on carbon-4 of lanosterol. [shortened form of L. *geminus*, twin]

Ge·mel·la (jĕ-mel′ă). A genus of motile, aerobic, facultatively anaerobic, coccoid bacteria (family Streptococcaceae) which occur singly or in pairs, with flattened adjacent sides. They are Gram-indeterminate but have a cell wall like that of Gram-positive bacteria, and are parasitic on mammals. The type species is *G. haemolysans*, which is found in bronchial secretions and in mucus from the respiratory tract. [L. dim. of *geminus*, twin]

gem·el·lip·a·ra (jem-ĕ-lip′ăr-ă). Obsolete term for a woman who has given birth to twins. [L. *gemellus*, twin, + *pario*, to bear]

ge·mel·lol·o·gy (jem-el-ol′ō-jē). The study of twins and the phenomenology of twinning. [L. *gemellus*, twin-born, + G. *logos*, study]

ge·mel·lus (jĕ-mel′ŭs). SYN inferior gemellus *muscle*, superior gemellus *muscle*. [L. dim. of *geminus*, twin]

gem·fi·bro·zil (jem-fī′brō-zil). 5-(2,5-Dimethylphenoxy)-2,2-dimethyl, pentanoic acid;; an antihyperlipidemic agent.

gem·i·nate (jem′i-nāt). Occurring in pairs. SYN geminous. [L. *gemino*, pp. *-atus*, to double, fr. *geminus*, twin]

gem·i·na·tion (jem-i-nā′shŭn). Embryologic partial division of a primordium. For example, g. of a single tooth germ results in two partially or completely separated crowns on a single root. [L. *geminatio*, a doubling]

gem·i·nous (jem′i-nŭs). SYN geminate.

ge·mis·to·cyte (jĕ-mis′tō-sīt). SYN gemistocytic *astrocyte*. [G. *gemistos*, loaded, fr. *gemizō*, to fill, + *-cyte*]

ge·mis·to·cy·to·ma (jĕ-mis′tō-sī-tō′mă). SYN gemistocytic *astrocytoma*.

gem·ma (jem′ă). Any budlike or bulblike body, especially a taste bud or end bulb. [L. bud]

gem·ma·tion (jem-ā′shŭn). A form of fission in which the parent cell does not divide, but puts out a small budlike process (daughter cell) with its proportionate amount of chromatin; the daughter cell then separates to begin independent existence. SYN bud fission, budding. [L. *gemma*, a bud]

gem·mule (jem′yūl). **1.** A small bud that projects from the parent cell, and finally becomes detached, forming a cell of a new generation. **2.** SYN dendritic *spines*, under *spine*. [L. *gemmula*, dim. of *gemma*, bud]

Hoboken's g.'s, SYN Hoboken's *nodules*, under *nodule*.

△**gen-.** Being born, producing, coming to be. [G. *genos*, birth]

△**-gen.** Suffix denoting "precursor of." SEE ALSO pro- (2).

ge·na (jē′nă). SYN cheek. [L.]

ge·nal (jē′năl). Relating to the gena, or cheek.

gen·der (jen′der). Category to which an individual is assigned by self or others, on the basis of sex. Cf. sex, gender *role*.

gene (jēn). A functional unit of heredity which occupies a specific place (locus) on a chromosome, is capable of reproducing itself exactly at each cell division, and directs the formation of an enzyme or other protein. The g. as a functional unit consists of a discrete segment of a giant DNA molecule containing the purine (adenine and guanine) and pyrimidine (cytosine and thymine) bases in the correct sequence to code the sequence of amino acids of a specific peptide. Protein synthesis is mediated by molecules of messenger-RNA formed on the chromosome with the g. acting as template. The RNA then passes into the cytoplasm and becomes oriented on the ribosomes where it in turn acts as template to organize a chain of amino acids to form a peptide. G.'s normally occur in pairs in all cells except gametes, as a consequence of the fact that all chromosomes are paired except the sex chromosomes (X and Y) of the male. SYN factor (3). [G. *genos*, birth]

allelic g., SEE allele, *dominance* of traits.

autosomal g., a g. located on any chromosome other than the sex chromosomes (X or Y).

C g., the g. coding for the constant regions of immunoglobulin chains.

codominant g., a set of two or more alleles, each expressed phenotypically in the presence of the other.

control g., SEE operator g., regulator g.

ge

dominant g., SEE *dominance* of traits.

extrachromosomal g., a g. located outside of the nucleus (*e.g.,* mitochondrial genes).

H g., SYN histocompatibility g.

histocompatibility g., in laboratory animals, a g. which can elicit an immune response and thereby cause rejection of a homograft when tissue is transplanted from one individual to another; in humans, histocompatibility g.'s control HLA antigens. SYN H g.

holandric g., SYN Y-linked g.

homeotic g.'s, a group of g.'s that regulate the development of the body parts by defining the boundaries of the several regions.

housekeeping g.'s, g.'s that are generally always expressed and thought to be involved in routine cellular metabolism.

immune response g.'s, g.'s in the HLA-D region of the histocompatibility complex of human chromosome 6 which control the immune response to specific antigens.

jumping g., a g. associated with transposable elements. SEE transposon.

lethal g., a g. that produces a genotype that leads to death of the organism before reproduction is possible or that precludes reproduction; for a recessive g. the homozygous or hemizygous state is lethal.

mimic g.'s, nonallelic (independent) g.'s with closely similar effects, *e.g.,* elliptocytosis.

mitochondrial g., a functioning g. located not in the nucleus of a cell but in the mitochondrial chromosome.

modifier g., a nonallelic g. that controls or changes the manifestation of a g. by interfering with its transcription.

mutant g., a g. that has been changed from an ancestral type, not necessarily in the current generation. SEE ALSO mutant, mutation.

operator g., a g. with the function of activating the production of messenger RNA by one or more adjacent structural loci; part of the feedback system for determining the rate of production of an enzyme.

pleiotropic g., a g. that has multiple, apparently unrelated, phenotypic manifestations. SYN polyphenic g.

polyphenic g., SYN pleiotropic g.

regulator g., a g. that produces a repressor substance that inhibits an operator g. when combined with it. It thus prevents production of a specific enzyme. When the enzyme is again in demand, a specific regulatory metabolite inhibits the repressor substance.

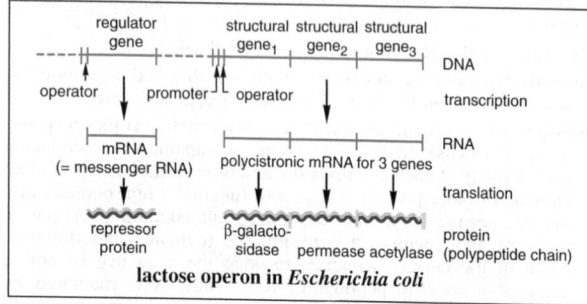

lactose operon in *Escherichia coli*

repressor g., a g. that prevents a nonallele from being transcribed.

SOS g.'s, a group of g.'s involved in DNA repair, often induced by damage severe enough to cause stoppage of DNA synthesis.

split g.'s, g.'s where the genomic sequences are interrupted by intervening sequences (introns) that are spliced out of the mRNA prior to translation.

structural g., a g. that codes for a specific protein or peptide.

transfer g.'s, g.'s carried by a conjugative plasmid, essential for fertility and establishment of the bacterial donor state.

transforming g., SYN oncogene.

V g., the g. coding for the major part of the variable region of an immunoglobulin chain.

X-linked g., a g. located on an X chromosome.

Y-linked g., a g. located on a Y chromosome. SYN holandric g.

Z g., the structural g. for β-galactosidase.

ge·ne·al·o·gy (jē-nē-awl′ō-jē). **1.** Heredity. **2.** The explicit assembly of the descent of a person or family; it may be of any length. [G. *genea,* descent, + *logos,* study]

gene li·brary. A haphazard assembly of cloned DNA fragments inside of a vector which may contain genetic information about a species.

gene map·ping. SEE genetic map.

gen·era (jen′er-ă). Plural of genus.

gen·er·al·ist (jen′er-ăl-ist). A general physician or family physician; a physician trained to take care of the majority of nonsurgical diseases, sometimes including obstetrics.

gen·er·al·i·za·tion (jen′er-ăl-i-zā′shŭn). **1.** Rendering or becoming general, diffuse, or widespread, as when a primarily local disease becomes systemic. **2.** The reasoning by which a basic conclusion is reached, which applies to different items, each having some common factor.

stimulus g., in Pavlovian conditioning, the eliciting of a conditioned response by stimuli never before experienced but which are similar to a particular conditioned stimulus. SEE conditioning, classical *conditioning*.

gen·er·al·ized (jen′er-ă-līzd). Involving the whole of an organ, as opposed to a focal or regional process.

gen·er·ate (jen′er-āt). **1.** To produce. **2.** To procreate. [L. *genero,* pp. *-atus,* to beget]

gen·er·a·tion (jen-er-ā′shŭn). **1.** SYN reproduction (2). **2.** A discrete stage in succession of descent; *e.g.,* father, son, and grandson are three g.'s. It may not be a unique designation, *e.g.,* the offspring of an uncle-niece marriage is in the third generation in the paternal line but the fourth in the maternal line. [L. *generatio,* fr. *genero,* pp. *-atus,* to beget]

asexual g., reproduction by fission, gemmation, or in any other way without union of the male and female cell, or conjugation. SEE ALSO parthenogenesis. SYN heterogenesis (2), nonsexual g.

filial g. (F), the offspring of a genetically specified mating: first filial g. (symbol F_1), the offspring of parents of contrasting genotypes; second filial g. (F_2), the offspring of two F_1 individuals; third filial g. (F_3), fourth filial g. (F_4), etc., the offspring in succeeding g.'s of continued inbreeding of F_1 descendents.

nonsexual g., SYN asexual g.

parental g. (P_1), the parents of a mating, commonly experimental, involving contrasting genotypes; the original mating of a genetic experiment; parents of the F_1 g.

sexual g., reproduction by conjugation, or the union of male and female cells, as opposed to asexual g.

skipped g., a phenomenon of pedigrees in which a gene is transmitted from one affected person to another through a phenotypically unaffected person, as by recessivity (especially for X-linked traits), epistasis, variable expressivity, or absence of an environmental challenge such as a toxin. Except at a crass phenotypic level (*e.g.,* clinical or commercial) this term becomes progressively less useful as the mechanisms are elucidated.

spontaneous g., the false concept according to which living matter can arise by the vitalization of nonliving matter. SEE ALSO biogenesis. SYN heterogenesis (3).

virgin g., SYN parthenogenesis.

gen·er·a·tion·al. Pertaining to generations, *i.e.,* the discrete staging in genealogical descent.

gen·er·a·tive (jen′er-ă-tiv). Pertaining to the process of generating.

gen·er·a·tor (jen′er-ā-ter). An apparatus for conversion of chemical, mechanical, atomic, or other forms of energy into electricity. [*generator,* a begetter, producer]

aerosol g., a device for producing airborne suspensions of small particles for inhalation therapy or experimental work; *e.g.,* a La Mer g., spinning disk, or vibrating reed, each of which produces a monodisperse aerosol.

asynchronous pulse g., a g. in which the rate of discharge is independent of the natural activity of the heart. SYN fixed rate pulse g.

atrial synchronous pulse g., a ventricular stimulating pulse whose rate of discharge is directly determined by the atrial rate. SYN atrial triggered pulse g.

atrial triggered pulse g., SYN atrial synchronous pulse g.

demand pulse g., SYN ventricular inhibited pulse g.

fixed rate pulse g., SYN asynchronous pulse g.

pulse g., a device that produces an electrical discharge with a regular or rhythmic wave form in which the electromotive force varies in a specific pattern in relation to time; *e.g.,* in an electronic pacemaker, it produces an electric discharge at regular intervals, and these intervals may be modified by a sensory circuit which can reset the time-base for subsequent discharge on the basis of other electrical activity, such as that produced by spontaneous cardiac beating.

radionuclide g., a column containing a large amount of a particular radionuclide (mother radionuclide) that decays down to a second radionuclide of shorter physical half-life; the daughter radionuclide is separated from the parent by the process of elution and affords a continuing supply of relatively short-lived radionuclides for laboratory use; the elution is loosely termed "milking" with the generator referred to as a "radioactive cow."

standby pulse g., SYN ventricular inhibited pulse g.

ventricular inhibited pulse g., a g. which suppresses its output in response to natural ventricular activity but which, in the absence of such activity, functions as an asynchronous pulse g. SYN demand pulse g., standby pulse g.

ventricular synchronous pulse g., a pulse which delivers its output synchronously with naturally occurring ventricular activity but which, in the absence of such activity, functions as an asynchronous pulse g. SYN ventricular triggered pulse g.

ventricular triggered pulse g., SYN ventricular synchronous pulse g.

x-ray g., the electronic device that controls production of x-rays in radiography; a key function is rectification of line voltage to produce a smooth direct current voltage to the x-ray tube.

ge·ner·ic (jĕ-năr′ik). **1.** Relating to or denoting a genus. **2.** General. **3.** Characteristic or distinctive. [L. *genus* (*gener-*), birth]

ge·ner·ic name. 1. In chemistry, a noun that indicates the class or type of a single compound; *e.g.,* salt, saccharide (sugar), hexose, alcohol, aldehyde, lactone, acid, amine, alkane, steroid, vitamin. "Class" is more appropriate and more often used than is "generic." **2.** In the pharmaceutical and commercial fields, a misnomer for nonproprietary name. **3.** In the biologic sciences, the first part of the scientific name (Latin binary combination or binomial) of an organism; written with an initial capital letter and in italics. In bacteriology, the species name consists of two parts (comprising one name): the g. n. and the specific epithet; in other biologic disciplines, the species name is regarded as being composed of two names: the g. n. and the specific name.

ge·ne·si·al (je-nē′sē-ăl). Relating to generation.

ge·ne·si·ol·o·gy (je-nē-sē-ol′ō-jē). The branch of science concerned with generation or reproduction. [G. *genesis,* generation, + *logos,* study]

gen·e·sis (jen′ĕ-sis). An origin or beginning process; also used as combining form in suffix position. [G.]

gene splic·ing. SYN splicing (1).

ge·net·ic (jĕ-net′ik). Pertaining to genetics; genetical.

ge·net·i·cist (jĕ-net′i-sist). A specialist in genetics.

ge·net·ic map. An abstract representation of the ordered array of genetic loci such that the interval between entries has algebraic signs and magnitude proportional to the expected number of crossings over between them and distances are algebraically additive; *e.g.,* on a g. m. the combined distance between locus A and locus C is the algebraic sum of the two distances between loci A and B, and B and C. SYN linkage map.

ge·net·ics (jĕ-net′iks). The branch of science concerned with the means and consequences of transmission and generation of the components of biological inheritance. [G. *genesis,* origin or production]

behavioral g., the study of heritable factors in behavioral patterns, as by pedigree analysis, biochemical abnormality, or karyotypic analysis.

biochemical g., the study of g. in terms of the chemical (biochemical) events involved, as in the manner in which DNA molecules replicate and control the synthesis of specific enzymes by the genetic code.

classical g., that body of method and analysis that perceives g. as the study of the transmission of genotype from parent to offspring; the study of multiple individuals is essential to it.

clinical g., g. applied to the diagnosis, prognosis, management, and prevention of genetic diseases. Cf. medical g.

epidemiological g., the study of g. as a phenomenon of defined populations by the criteria, methods, and objectives of epidemiology rather than of population g.

galtonian g., the study of traits by analysis of the first two moments of metrical data; the preferred method for analysis of traits following the multivariate gaussian distribution.

Galtonian-Fisher g., the g. of measurable traits determined by multiple loci which make contributions that are independent, additive, and approximately equal. SYN multilocal g.

human g., the study of the genetic aspects of humans as a species. Cf. medical g.

mathematical g., the study of genetic traits by formal analysis, *e.g.,* quantitative g., population dynamics, genetic epidemiology, modeling.

medical g., the study of the etiology, pathogenesis, and natural history of human diseases which are at least partially genetic in origin. Cf. clinical g., human g.

mendelian g., the study of the pattern of segregation of phenotypes under the control of genetic loci taken one at a time.

microbial g., the study of hereditary mechanisms of microbes.

modern g., that body of method and analysis that perceives g. as the study of the economy of nucleic acids and associated compounds.

molecular g., molecular biology applied to g.

multilocal g., SYN Galtonian-Fisher g.

population g., the study of genetic influences on the components of cause and effect in the somatic characteristics of populations.

quantitative g., the formal study of measurable genetic traits, traditionally but not necessarily confined to galtonian g.

reverse g., term referring to methods in molecular biology directed to tracing existent protein back to the gene that generated it in contrast with the classical path which was to argue from the gene to the protein. The usage of this term is not wholly standardized.

somatic cell g., the study of the structure, organization, and function of a genome by the techniques of cell hybridization.

statistical g., the study of the applications of principles of statistics to problems in genetics.

transplantation g., g. as applied to the transplanting of tissues from one animal to another.

ge·net·o·tro·phic (jĕ-net-ō-trof′ik). Relating to inherited individual distinctions in nutritional requirements. [G. *genesis,* origin, + *trophē,* nourishment]

Ge·ne·va Con·ven·tion. An international agreement formed at meetings in Geneva, Switzerland, in 1864 and 1906, relating (among medical subjects) to the safeguarding of the wounded in battle, of those having the care of them, and of the buildings in which they are being treated. The direct outcome of the first of these meetings was the establishment of the Red Cross Society.

Ge·ne·va lens mea·sure. A device for measuring the radii of the curvature of a spectacle lens. SYN lens clock. [*Geneva,* Switzerland]

Gengou, Octave, French bacteriologist, 1875–1957. SEE G. *phenomenon;* Bordet-G. potato blood *agar, bacillus, phenomenon;* Bordet and G. *reaction.*

ge·ni·al, ge·ni·an (jĕ-nī′ăl, -nī′an). SYN mental (2). [G. *geneion,* chin]

-genic. Producing, forming; produced, formed by. [G. *genos,* birth]

ge·nic·u·la (je-nik′yū-lă). Plural of geniculum.

ge·nic·u·lar (je-nik′yū-lăr). Commonly used to mean genual.

ge·nic·u·late (je-nik′yū-lāt). **1.** Bent like a knee. SYN geniculated. **2.** Referring to the geniculum of the facial nerve, denoting the ganglion there present. **3.** Denoting the lateral or medial geniculate body. [L. *geniculo,* pp. *-atus,* to bend the knee, fr. *genu,* knee]

ge·nic·u·lat·ed (je-nik′yū-lā-ted). SYN geniculate (1).

ge·nic·u·lum, pl. **ge·nic·u·la** (je-nik′yū-lŭm, -lă). **1** [NA]. A small genu or angular kneelike structure. **2.** A knotlike structure. [L. dim. of *genu,* knee]

g. cana′lis facia′lis [NA], SYN g. of facial canal.

g. of facial canal, the bend in the facial canal linking the medial and lateral crura of the horizontal port of the canal and corresponding to the location of the geniculate ganglion of the facial nerve. SYN g. canalis facialis [NA].

g. of facial nerve, (1) a rectangular bend of the facial nerve in the facial canal where it turns posterior in the medial wall of the middle ear (external g.); **(2)** complex loop of facial nerve fibers around the abducens nucleus (internal g.). SYN g. nervi facialis [NA].

g. ner′vi facia′lis [NA], SYN g. of facial nerve.

△**-genin.** Suffix used to denote the basic steroid unit of the toxic substance, usually a steroid glycoside (*e.g.,* the aglycon portion).

ge·ni·o·glos·sus (jĕ′nī-ō-glos′ŭs). SYN genioglossus *muscle.* [G. *geneion,* chin, + *glōssa,* tongue]

ge·ni·o·hy·oid (jĕ′nī′ō-hī′oyd). SYN geniohyoid *muscle.*

ge·ni·o·hy·oi·de·us (jĕ′nī′ō-hī-oyd′ē-ŭs). SYN geniohyoid *muscle.* [G. *geneion,* chin, + *hyoeidēs,* y-shaped, hyoid]

ge·ni·on (jĕ′nī′on). The tip of the mental spine, a point in craniometry. [G. *geneion,* chin]

ge·ni·o·plas·ty (jĕ′nī-ō-plas′tē). SYN mentoplasty. [G. *geneion,* chin, cheek, + *plastos,* formed]

gen·i·tal (jen′i-tăl). **1.** Relating to reproduction or generation. **2.** Relating to the primary female or male sex organs or genitals. **3.** Relating to or characterized by genitality. [L. *genitalis,* pertaining to reproduction, fr. *gigno,* to bring forth]

gen·i·ta·lia (jen′i-tā′lē-ă). SYN genital *organs,* under *organ.* [L. neut. pl. of *genitalis,* genital]

ambiguous external g., external g. not clearly of either sex; most commonly designates external g. that are incompletely masculinized.

external g., the vulva in the female, and the penis and scrotum in the male.

indifferent g., reproductive organs of the embryo prior to the definitive sex formation.

gen·i·tal·i·ty (jen-i-tal′i-tē). In psychoanalysis, a term referring to the genital components of sexuality (*i.e.,* the penis and vagina), as opposed, for example, to orality and anality.

gen·i·tals (jen′i-tălz). SYN genital *organs,* under *organ.* [see genitalia]

gen·i·to·cru·ral (jen′i-tō-krū′răl). SYN genitofemoral.

gen·i·to·fem·o·ral (jen′i-tō-fem′ŏ-răl). Relating to the genitalia and the thigh; denoting the g. nerve. SYN genitocrural.

gen·i·to·u·ri·nary (GU) (jen′i-tō-yū′ri-nar-ē). Relating to the organs of reproduction and urination. SYN urinogenital, urinosexual, urogenital.

ge·nius (jēn′yŭs, jēn′ē-ŭs). **1.** Markedly superior intellectual or artistic abilities or exceptional creative power. **2.** A person so endowed. **3.** In psychology, an individual who ranks in the top 1 percent of all individuals on a test of intelligence. [L.]

ge·nius ep·i·dem·i·cus (ep-i-dem′i-kŭs). The influence, atmospheric, telluric, or cosmic, or the combination of any two or three, anciently regarded as the cause of epidemic and endemic diseases. [Mod. L.]

Gennari, Francesco, Italian anatomist, 1750–1795. SEE G.'s *band, stria; line* of G.; *stripe* of G.

gen·o·blast (jen′ō-blast). The nucleus of the fertilized ovum.

gen·o·copy (jen′ō-kop-e). A genotype at one locus that produces a phenotype which at some levels of resolution is indistinguishable from that produced by another genotype; *e.g.,* two types of elliptocytosis that are g.'s of each other, but are distinguished by the fact that one is linked to the Rh blood group locus and the other is not.

ge·no·der·ma·tol·o·gy (jen′ō-der-mă-tol′ō-jē). Study of the he-

reditary aspects of cutaneous disorders. [G. *genos,* birth, descent, + *derma,* skin, + *logos,* theory]

ge·no·der·ma·to·sis (jen′ō-der-mă-tō′sis). A skin condition of genetic origin.

ge·nome (je′nōm, -nom). **1.** A complete set of chromosomes derived from one parent, the haploid number of a gamete. **2.** The total gene complement of a set of chromosomes found in higher life forms (the haploid set in a eukaryotic cell), or the functionally similar but simpler linear arrangements found in bacteria and viruses. SEE ALSO Human Genome Project. [gene + chromosome]

ge·nom·ic (jĕ-nom′ik). Relating to a genome.

ge·no·spe·cies (jē′nō-spē-sēz, jen′). A group of organisms in which interbreeding is possible, as evidenced by genetic transfer and recombination.

ge·note (jē′nōt). In microbial genetics, an element of recombination in which one of the pair is not a complete chromosome; commonly used as a suffix (*e.g.,* endogenote, exogenote, F genote). [gene + G. *-ōtēs,* toponymic suffix]

F g., F-g., SYN F *plasmid.*

ge·no·tox·ic (jē′nō-toks′ik). Denoting a substance that by damaging DNA may cause mutation or cancer. [gene + toxic]

gen·o·type (jen′ō-tīp). **1.** The genetic constitution of an individual. **2.** Gene combination at one specific locus or any specified combination of loci. For specific blood group genotypes, see Blood Groups appendix. [G. *genos,* birth, descent, + *typos,* type] **ZZ g.,** individuals who have a deficiency of α₁-antitrypsin and have emphasemia.

gen·o·typ·ic (jēn′ō-tip-ik). SYN genotypical.

gen·o·typ·i·cal (jen-ō-tip′i-kăl). Relating to the genotype. SYN genotypic.

gen·ta·mi·cin, gen·ta·my·cin (jen-tă-mī′sin). A broad spectrum antibiotic complex, obtained from *Micromonospora purpurea* and *M. echinospora,* that inhibits the growth of both Gram-positive and Gram-negative bacteria; the sulfate salt is used medicinally.

gen·tian, gen·tian root (jen′shŭn). The dried rhizome and roots of *Gentiana lutea* (family Gentianaceae), an herb of southern and central Europe; a simple bitter.

gen·tian·o·phil, gen·tian·o·phile (jen′shŭn-o-fil, -fīl). Staining readily with gentian violet. SYN gentianophilous. [gentian + G. *philos,* fond]

gen·tian·oph·i·lous (jen-shŭn-of′i-lŭs). SYN gentianophil.

gen·tian·o·pho·bic (jen′shŭn-ō-fō′bik). Not taking a gentian violet stain, or taking it poorly. [gentian + G. *phobos,* fear]

gen·tian root. SEE gentian.

gen·tian vi·o·let. An unstandardized dye mixture of violet rosanilins, now superseded by crystal violet or methyl violet 2B. SEE crystal violet.

gen·ti·o·bi·ase (jen′shi-o-bī′ās). SYN β-D-glucosidase.

gen·ti·o·bi·o·se (jen′tē-ō-bī′ōs). A disaccharide containing two D-glucopyranose molecules linked β-1,6; a structural moiety in many compounds (*e.g.,* amygdalin).

gen·tis·ic ac·id (jen-tis′ik). 2,5-Dihydroxybenzoic acid; 5-hydroxysalicylic acid; this compound is chemically related to salicylate and aspirin (acetylsalicylate) and shares with the latter agent analgesic and anti-inflammatory properties.

genu, gen. **ge·′nus,** pl. **gen·ua** (jē′nū, jē′nŭs, jen′ū-ă) [NA]. **1.** The place of articulation between the thigh and the leg. SYN knee (1). SEE ALSO knee *joint,* geniculum. **2.** Any structure of angular shape resembling a flexed knee. [L.]

g. cap′sulae inter′nae [NA], SYN g. of internal capsule.

g. cor′poris callo′si [NA], SYN g. of corpus callosum.

g. of corpus callosum, the anterior extremity of the corpus callosum that folds downward and backward on itself, terminating in the rostrum. SYN g. corporis callosi [NA].

g. of facial canal, a sharp bend in the facial canal where the geniculate ganglion is located.

g. of facial nerve, the curve which the fibers of the root of the facial nerve describe around the abducens nucleus in the pontine tegmentum; the internal g. of the facial nerve. SYN g. nervi facialis [NA].

g. of internal capsule, the obtuse angle, opening laterally in the horizontal plane, formed by the union of the two limbs (crus anterius and crus posterius) of the internal capsule. SYN g. capsulae internae [NA].

g. ner′vi facia′lis [NA], SYN g. of facial nerve.

g. recurva′tum, hyperextension of the knee, the lower extremity having a forward curvature. SYN back-knee.

g. val′gum, a deformity marked by lateral angulation of the leg in relation to the thigh. SYN knock-knee, tibia valga.

g. va′rum, a deformity marked by medial angulation of the leg in relation to the thigh; an outward bowing of the legs. SYN bandyleg, bowleg, bow-leg, tibia vara.

gen·u·al (jen′yū-ăl). Relating to the knee. [L. *genu,* knee]

ge·nus, pl. **gen·era** (jē′nŭs, jen′er-ă). In natural history classification, the taxonomic level of division between the family, or tribe, and the species; a group of species alike in the broad features of their organization but different in detail, and incapable of fertile mating. [L. birth, descent]

gen·y·an·trum (jen-ē-an′trŭm). SYN maxillary *sinus.* [G. *genys,* cheek, + *antron,* cave]

geo-. The earth, soil. [G. *gē,* earth]

ge·ode (jē′ōd). A cystlike space (or spaces) with or without an epithelial lining, observed radiologically in subarticular bone, usually in arthritic disorders. [Fr., fr. L. *geodes,* precious stone, fr. G. *gē,* earth, + *-ōdēs,* appearance]

ge·o·med·i·cine (jē-ō-med′i-sin). The science concerned with the influence of climatic and environmental conditions on health and disease. SYN nosochthonography, nosogeography.

ge·o·pa·thol·o·gy (jē′ō-pă-thol′ō-jē). The study of disease in relation to regions, climates, and other environmental influences.

ge·o·pha·gia, ge·oph·a·gism, ge·oph·a·gy (jē-ō-fā′jē-ă, jē-of′ă-jizm, -of′ă-jē). The practice of eating dirt or clay. SYN dirt-eating, earth-eating. [geo- + G. *phagō,* to eat]

ge·o·phil·ic. Terrestrial, soil inhabiting. [geo- + G. *philos,* love, attraction, + -ic]

Ge·oph·i·lus (jē-of′i-lŭs). A genus of centipedes, characterized by very large numbers of legs (47 to 67 pairs); includes *G. californius, G. rubens,* and *G. umbraticus,* in the U.S.

Georgi, Walter, German bacteriologist, 1889–1920. SEE Sachs-G. *test.*

ge·o·tax·is (jē-ō-tak′sis). A form of positive barotaxis in which there is a tendency to growth or movement toward or into the earth. SYN geotropism. [geo- + G. *taxis,* orderly arrangement]

ge·ot·ri·cho·sis (jē′ō-tri-kō′sis). An opportunistic systemic hyalohyphomycosis caused by *Geotrichum candidum;* ascribed symptoms are diverse and suggestive of secondary or mixed infections. [geo- + G. *thrix,* hair, + -*osis,* condition]

Ge·ot·ri·chum (jē-ot′ri-kŭm). A genus of yeastlike fungi which produce arthroconidia but rarely blastoconidia. One species, *G. candidum* (perfect state *Endomyces geotrichum*), may cause lesions in the pulmonary and alimentary tracts of humans; however these lesions may be secondary to an underlying condition unrelated to *G. candidum.* SEE ALSO geotrichosis.

ge·ot·ro·pism (jē-ot′rō-pizm). SYN geotaxis. [geo- + G. *trope,* a turning]

geph·y·ro·pho·bia (jĕ-fī-rō-fō′bē-ă). Fear of crossing a bridge. [G. *gephyra,* bridge, + *phobos,* fear]

gep·i·rone (je-pī′rōn). A nonbenzodiazepine anxiolytic which resembles buspirone both chemically and pharmacologically. Acts on serotonergic receptors rather than benzodiazepine receptors. Lacks dependence-producing properties and tolerance of benzodiazepine-type agents.

Geraghty, John T., U.S. physician, 1876–1924. SEE G.'s *test;* Rowntree and G. *test.*

ge·ran·i·ol (jĕ-ra′nē-ol). An olefinic terpene alcohol that is the principal constituent of oil of rose and oil of palmarosa; also found in many other volatile oils, such as citronella and lemon grass. An isomer of linalool; an oily liquid with sweet rose odor used in perfumery. Also used as an insect attractant.

ger·a·nyl·ger·a·nyl py·ro·phos·phate (jer′a-nil-jer-a-nil pī-rō-fos′fāt). A key intermediate in the biosynthesis of many terpenes.

ger·a·nyl py·ro·phos·phate (jer′a-nil-pī-rō-fos′fāt). a key intermediate in the biosynthesis of sterols, dolichols, ubiquinone, and prenylated proteins.

ger·a·tol·o·gy (jār-ă-tol′ō-jē). SYN gerontology.

Gerbich an·ti·gen. See under antigen.

ger·bil (jer′bil). A name applied to any of 13 genera of small rodents (subfamily Gerbillinae) from Africa and Asia; they resemble jerboas or kangaroo rats and can survive without drinking water. [Mod. L. *gerbillus,* fr. Arab.]

Ger·bode, Frank SEE Gerbode *defect.*

Gerdy, Pierre N., French surgeon, 1797–1856. SEE G.'s *fibers,* under *fiber, fontanel,* hyoid *fossa, ligament,* interatrial *loop,* tubercle.

Gerhardt, Carl J., German physician, 1833–1902. SEE G.'s *disease, reaction, sign, test* for acetoacetic acid; G.-Semon *law.*

Gerhardt, Charles F., French chemist, 1816–1856. SEE G.'s *test* for urobilin in the urine.

ger·i·at·ric (jār-ē-at′rik). Relating to old age or to geriatrics.

ger·i·at·rics (jār-ē-at′riks). The branch of medicine concerned with the medical problems and care of the aged. [G. *gēras,* old age, + *iatrikos,* healing]

dental g., treatment of dental problems peculiar to advanced age. SYN gerodontics, gerodontology.

Gerlach, Joseph, German anatomist, 1820–1896. SEE G.'s annular *tendon, tonsil; valve* of vermiform appendix; G.'s *valvula.*

Gerlier, Felix, Swiss physician, 1840–1914. SEE G.'s *disease.*

germ (jerm). **1.** A microbe; a microorganism. **2.** A primordium; the earliest trace of a structure within an embryo. [L. *germen,* sprout, bud, germ]

dental g., SYN tooth g.

enamel g., the enamel organ of a developing tooth; one of a series of knoblike projections from the dental lamina, later becoming bell-shaped and receiving in its hollow the dental papilla.

reserve tooth g., enamel organ and papilla of a permanent tooth.

tooth g., the enamel organ and dentin papilla, constituting the developing tooth. SYN dental g.

wheat g., the embryo of wheat; contains thiamine, riboflavin, and other vitamins.

ger·ma·ni·um (Ge) (jer-mān′ē-ŭm). A metallic element, atomic no. 32, atomic wt. 72.61. [L. *Germania,* Germany]

ger·mi·ci·dal (jer-mi-sī′dăl). SYN germicide (1).

ger·mi·cide (jer′mi-sīd). **1.** Destructive to germs or microbes. SYN germicidal. **2.** An agent with this action. [germ + L. *caedo,* to kill]

ger·mi·nal (jer′mi-năl). Relating to a germ or, in botany, to germination.

ger·mine (jer′mīn). An alkaloid that occurs in *Veratrum* and *Zygandenus* species. The drug, like veratrine and veratridine, induces repetitive discharges in nerve cells, seemingly due to derangements in sodium channel function. Often used as the acetate or diacetate derivative.

ger·mi·no·ma (jer-mi-nō′mă). A neoplasm of the germinal tissue of gonads, mediastinum, or pineal region such as seminoma. [L. *germen,* bud, + -*oma,* tumor]

gero-, geront-, geronto-. Old age. SEE ALSO presby-. [G. *gerōn,* old man]

ger·o·der·ma (jār-ō-der′mă). **1.** The atrophic skin of the aged. **2.** Any condition in which the skin is thinned and wrinkled, resembling the integument of old age. [gero- + G. *derma,* skin]

ger·o·don·tics, ger·o·don·tol·o·gy (jār-ō-don′tiks, -don-tol′ō-jē). SYN dental *geriatrics.* [gero- + G. *odous,* tooth]

ger·o·ma·ras·mus (jār′ō-mă-raz′mŭs). SYN senile *atrophy.* [gero- + G. *marasmos,* a wasting]

ger·on·tal (jār-on′tăl). Relating to old age.

ger·on·tine (jār′on-tēn). SYN spermine.

geronto-. SEE gero-.

ger·on·tol·o·gist (jār-on-tol′ō-jist). One who specializes in gerontology.

ger·on·tol·o·gy (jār-on-tol'ō-jē). The scientific study of the process and problems of aging. SYN geratology. [geronto- + G. *logos,* study]

ge·ron·to·phil·ia (jār'on-tō-fil'ē-ă). Morbid love for old persons. [geronto- + G. *philos,* fond]

ge·ron·to·pho·bia (jār'on-tō-fō'bē-ă). Morbid fear of old persons. [geronto- + G. *phobos,* fear]

ge·ron·to·ther·a·peu·tics (jār-on'tō-thār-ă-pyū'tiks). The science concerned with treatment of the aged.

ge·ron·to·ther·a·py (jār-on'tō-thār-ă-pē). Treatment of disease in the aged. SYN geriatric therapy.

ger·on·tox·on (jār'on-tok'son). SYN *arcus* cornealis. [geronto- + G. *toxon,* bow]

Gerota, Dimitru, Roumanian anatomist and surgeon, 1867–1939. SEE G.'s *capsule, fascia, method.*

Gersh, Isidore, U.S. histologist, *1907. SEE Altmann-G. *method.*

Gerstmann, Josef, Austrian neurologist, 1887–1969. SEE G. *syndrome;* G.-Sträussler *syndrome.*

ges·ta·gen (jes'tă-jen). Inclusive term used to denote any one of several gestagenic substances, which are usually steroid hormones. SYN gestin, progestin (3).

ges·ta·gen·ic (jes-tă-jen'ik). Inducing progestational effects in the uterus.

ge·stalt (ge-stahlt). A perceived entity so integrated as to constitute a functional unit with properties not derivable from its parts. SEE gestaltism. [Ger. shape]

ge·stalt·ism (ge-stahlt'izm). The theory in psychology that the objects of mind come as complete forms or configurations which cannot be split into parts; *e.g.,* a square is perceived as such rather than as four discrete lines. [see gestalt]

ges·ta·tion (jes-tā'shŭn). SYN pregnancy. [L. *gestatio,* from *gesto,* pp. *gestatus,* to bear]

ges·tin (jes'tin). SYN gestagen.

ges·to·sis, pl. **ges·to·ses** (jes-tō'sis, -sēz). Any disorder of pregnancy. [L. *gesto,* to carry, to bear, + G. *-osis,* condition]

ges·ture (jes'chŭr). **1.** Any movement expressive of an idea, opinion, or emotion. **2.** An act. [L. *gestus,* movement, gesture]

suicide g., an apparent attempt at suicide by someone wishing to attract attention, gain sympathy, or achieve some goal other than self-destruction.

Gey, George O., U.S. physician and researcher, *1899. SEE G.'s *solution.*

Gey's so·lu·tion. See under solution.

GFR Abbreviation for glomerular filtration *rate.*

GH Abbreviation for growth *hormone.*

ghee (gē). A clarified butter in India made from cow or buffalo milk that has been coagulated before churning; used as an emollient, a dressing for wounds, and a food. [Eng. spelling of Hind. *ghi*]

Gheel col·o·ny. See under colony.

Ghon, Anton, Czechoslovakian pathologist, 1866–1936. SEE G.'s *complex, focus,* primary *lesion, tubercle;* G.-Sachs *bacillus.*

ghost (gōst). A hemoglobin-depleted erythrocyte that has also lost most, if not all, of its internal proteins.

GHRF, GH-RF Abbreviation for growth hormone-releasing *factor.*

GHRH, GH-RH Abbreviation for growth *hormone*-releasing *hormone.*

GHz Abbreviation for gigahertz, equal to one billion (10^9) hertz; used in ultrasound.

GI Abbreviation for gastrointestinal; Gingival Index.

Giacomini, Carlo, Italian anatomist, 1841–1898. SEE band of G.; *frenulum* of G.; uncus *band* of G.

Giannuzzi, Italian anatomist, 1839–1876. SEE G.'s *crescents,* under *crescent, demilunes,* under *demilune.*

Gianotti, F., 20th century Italian dermatologist. SEE G.-Crosti *syndrome.*

gi·ant·ism (jī'an-tizm). SYN gigantism.

Gi·ar·dia (jē-ar'dē-ă). A genus of parasitic flagellates that parasi-

tize the small intestine of many mammals, including most domestic animals and humans; *e.g., G. bovis* in cattle, *G. canis* in dogs, and *G. cati* in cats. Many species have been described, but recent workers have suggested that these should be reduced to only two or three. [Alfred *Giard,* Fr. biologist, 1846–1908]

G. intestinalis, SYN *G. lamblia.*

G. lam'blia, a flattened, heart-shaped organism (10 to 20 μm in length) with 8 flagella; it attaches itself to the intestinal mucosa by means of a pair of sucking organs; it is usually asymptomatic except in heavy infections, when it may interfere with absorption of fats and produce flatulence, steatorrhea, and acute discomfort; it is the common species of *G.* in man, but is also found in pigs. SYN *G. intestinalis.*

gi·ar·di·a·sis (jē-ar-dī'ă-sis). Infection with the protozoan parasite *Giardia; Giardia lamblia* may cause diarrhea, dyspepsia, and occasionally malabsorption in humans. SYN lambliasis.

chinchilla g., an intestinal infection of chinchilla characterized by diarrhea, anorexia, lassitude, and frequently death, believed to be caused by the presence of large numbers of *Giardia.*

gib·ber·el·lic ac·id (jib'er-el-ik). An auxin, *i.e.,* a plant hormone which stimulates growth; most prominent of the plant-growth-promoting metabolites of *Gibberella fujikuroi.* Used as a plant growth regulator and promoter, especially the growth of seedlings. Used also as a food additive in the malting of barley.

gib·ber·el·lins. A class of plant growth hormones (auxins) of which over 60 are known; these were first isolated in 1938 from cultures of *Gibberella fujikuroi,* the fungus causing Bakanese disease in rice. Also found in higher plants; diterpenoid acids available commercially.

gib·bon (gib'on). A genus of anthropoid apes, *Hylobates,* of the superfamily Hominoidea. [Fr.]

gib·bous (gib'ŭs). Humped; humpbacked; denoting a sharp angle in the flexion of the spine. [L. *gibbosus*]

Gibbs, J. Willard, U.S. mathematician and physicist, 1839–1903. SEE G.-Donnan *equilibrium;* G.-Helmholtz *equation;* Helmholtz-G. *theory;* G.'s *theorem;* G. free *energy, energy* of activation.

gib·bus (gib'ŭs). Extreme kyphosis, hump, or hunch; a deformity of spine in which there is a sharply angulated segment, the apex of the angle being posterior. [L. a hump]

Gibney, Virgil P., U.S. orthopedist, 1847–1927. SEE G.'s fixation *bandage, boot.*

Gibson, George A., Scottish physician, 1854–1913. SEE G. *murmur.*

Gibson, Kasson C., U.S. dentist, 1849–1925. SEE G.'s *bandage.*

gid. SYN staggers (2).

Giemsa, Gustav, German bacteriologist, 1867–1948. SEE G. *stain,* chromosome banding *stain.*

Gierke, Edgar von, German pathologist, 1877–1945. SEE G.'s *disease;* von G. *disease.*

Gierke, Hans P.B., German anatomist, 1847–1886. SEE G.'s respiratory *bundle.*

Gifford, Harold, U.S. ophthalmologist, 1858–1929. SEE G.'s *reflex.*

△**giga-** (G). Prefix used in the SI and metric systems to signify one billion (10^9). [G. *gigas,* giant]

gi·gan·tism (jī'gan-tizm). A condition of abnormal size or overgrowth of the entire body or of any of its parts. SYN giantism. [G. *gigas,* giant]

acromegalic g., a form of pituitary g. in which the signs of acromegaly accompany abnormal height.

cerebral g., a syndrome characterized by increased birth weight and length (above 90th percentile), accelerated growth rate for the first 4 or 5 years without elevation of serum growth hormone levels, and then reversion to normal growth rate; characteristic facies include prognathism, hypertelorism, antimongoloid slant, and dolichocephalic skull; moderate mental retardation and impaired coordination are also associated. SEE Sotos' *syndrome.*

eunuchoid g., g. with deficient development of sexual organs; may be of pituitary or gonadal origin; g. accompanied by body proportions typical of hypogonadism during adolescence.

fetal g., excessive fetal or newborn size, *e.g.,* cerebral g. and infants of diabetic mothers.

pituitary g., a form of g. caused by hypersecretion of pituitary growth hormone; a rare disorder commonly the result of a pituitary adenoma.

primordial g., unusually large size from birth due to familial or genetic factors or intrauterine environment (*e.g.,* maternal prediabetic state) and not to hyperpituitarism.

△**giganto-.** Huge, gigantic. [G. *gigas,* one of the race of giants]

gi·gan·to·mas·tia (jī-gan'tō-mas'tē-ă). Massive hypertrophy of the breast. [giganto- + G. *mastos,* breast]

Gi·gan·to·rhyn·chus (ji-gan'to-ring'kŭs). A genus of very large acanthocephalan worms. SEE ALSO *Macracanthorhynchus, Moniliformis.* [giganto- + G. *rhynchos,* snout]

Gigli, Leonardo, Italian gynecologist, 1863–1908. SEE G.'s *operation, saw.*

GIH Abbreviation for growth hormone inhibiting *hormone.*

Gi·la mon·ster (hē'lă). A large poisonous lizard, *Heloderma suspectum* and *H. horridum,* of New Mexico, Arizona, and northern Mexico. [*Gila,* a river in Arizona]

Gilbert, Nicholas A., French physician, 1858–1927. SEE G.'s *disease, syndrome.*

Gilbert, Walter, U.S. microbiologist and Nobel laureate, *1932. SEE Maxim-G. *sequencing.*

gil·bert. The unit of magnetomotive force or magnetic potential. [W. *Gilbert,* English physicist, 1544–1603]

Gilchrist, Thomas C., U.S. physician, 1862–1927. SEE G.'s *disease, mycosis.*

Gilford, Hastings, English physician, 1861–1941. SEE Hutchinson-G. *disease, syndrome.*

Gilles de la Tourette, Georges, French physician, 1857–1904. SEE G. de la T.'s *disease, syndrome;* Tourette's *disease;* Tourette *syndrome.*

Gillette, Eugène P., French surgeon, 1836–1886. SEE G.'s suspensory *ligament.*

Gilliam, David Tod, U.S. gynecologist, 1844–1923. SEE G.'s *operation.*

Gillies, Sir Harold D., British plastic surgeon, 1882–1960. SEE G.'s *operation;* Filatov-G. *flap,* tubed *pedicle.*

Gillmore nee·dle. See under needle.

Gilmer, Thomas L., U.S. oral surgeon, 1849–1931. SEE G. *wiring.*

Gil-Vernet, Jose Maria Vila, Spanish urologist, *1922. SEE Gil-Vernet *operation.*

Gimbernat, Don Manuel L.A. de, Spanish anatomist and surgeon, 1734–1816. SEE G.'s *ligament.*

gin·ger (jin'jer). The dried rhizome of *Zingiber officinale* (family Zingiberaceae), known in commerce as Jamaica g., African g., and Cochin g. The outer cortical layers are often either partially or completely removed; used as a carminative and flavoring agent. SYN zingiber.

Chinese g., SYN galangal.

Indian g., SYN *Asarum* canadense.

g. oleoresin, a carminative, stimulant, and flavoring agent.

wild g., SYN *Asarum* canadense.

gin·gi·li oil (jin'ji-lē). SYN *sesame* oil.

gin·gi·va, gen. and pl. **gin·gi·vae** (jin'ji-vă, -vē) [NA]. The dense fibrous tissue, covered by mucous membrane, that envelops the alveolar processes of the upper and lower jaws and surrounds the necks of the teeth. SYN gum (2). [L.]

alveolar g., gingival tissue applied to the alveolar bone.

attached g., that part of the oral mucosa which is firmly bound to the tooth and alveolar process.

buccal g., that portion of the g. that covers the buccal surfaces of the teeth and alveolar process.

free g., that portion of the g. that surrounds the tooth and is not directly attached to the tooth surface; the outer wall of the gingival sulcus.

labial g., that portion of the g. that covers the labial surfaces of the teeth and the alveolar process.

lingual g., that portion of the g. that covers the lingual surfaces of the teeth and the alveolar process.

septal g., that portion of the g. that covers the interdental septum.

gin·gi·val (jin'ji-văl). Relating to the gums.

Gin·gi·val In·dex (GI). An index of periodontal disease based upon the severity and location of the lesion.

Gin·gi·val-Per·i·o·don·tal In·dex (GPI). An index of gingivitis, gingival irritation, and advanced periodontal disease.

gin·gi·vec·to·my (jin-ji-vek'tō-mē). Surgical resection of unsupported gingival tissue. SYN gum resection. [gingiva + G. *ektomē,* excision]

gin·gi·vi·tis (jin-ji-vī'tis). Inflammation of the gingiva as a response to bacterial plaque on adjacent teeth; characterized by erythema, edema, and fibrous enlargement of the gingiva without resorption of the underlying alveolar bone. [gingiva + G. *-itis,* inflammation]

acute necrotizing ulcerative g. (ANUG), SEE necrotizing ulcerative g.

atypical g., SYN plasma cell g.

chronic desquamative g., a clinical term for a gingival condition of unknown etiology, usually encountered in middle-aged and older women, characterized by erythema, mucosal atrophy, and desquamation, and usually accompanied by a burning sensation and pain; diagnosis is usually made by biopsy and direct immunofluorescence. SYN gingivosis.

diabetic g., g. in which the host response to bacterial plaque is presumably modified by the metabolic alterations encountered in the uncontrolled diabetic patient.

dilantin g., SYN diphenylhydantoin g.

diphenylhydantoin g., g. exacerbated by long-term therapy with diphenylhydantoin; the host response to bacterial plaque is characterized by marked hyperplasia of the fibrous connective tissue and, to a lesser degree, of the surface epithelium, resulting in gross enlargement of interdental papillae which may coalesce and obscure the clinical crowns of the teeth. SYN dilantin g.

fusospirochetal g., SYN necrotizing ulcerative g.

hormonal g., g. in which the host response to bacterial plaque is presumably exacerbated by hormonal alterations occurring during puberty, pregnancy, oral contraceptive use, or menopause.

hyperplastic g., g. of long-standing duration in which the gingiva becomes enlarged and firm due to proliferation of fibrous connective tissue.

leukemic hyperplastic g., enlarged gingiva due to infiltration of leukemic cells and infection from local factors in the face of diminshed host response.

marginal g., g. in which the clinical alterations are confined to the marginal gingiva and do not involve the attached gingiva.

necrotizing ulcerative g. (NUG), an acute or recurrent g. of young and middle-aged adults characterized clinically by gingival erythema and pain, fetid odor, and necrosis and sloughing of interdental papillae and marginal gingiva which gives rise to a gray pseudomembrane; fever, regional lymphadenopathy, and other systemic manifestations also may be present. A fusiform bacillus and *Treponema vincentii* can be isolated from the gingival tissues in large numbers and are felt to play a significant but poorly defined role in the pathogenesis. SYN fusospirochetal g., trench mouth, ulceromembranous g., Vincent's disease, Vincent's infection.

plasma cell g., intense hyperemic edema and inflammation of the gingiva resulting from a hypersensitivity reaction. A dense plasma cell infiltrate is seen in the lamina propria. SYN atypical g.

proliferative g., inflammatory changes in the gingiva characterized by proliferation of the gingival components.

suppurative g., g. in which a purulent exudate can be expressed from the gingival surface.

ulceromembranous g., SYN necrotizing ulcerative g.

△**gingivo-.** The gingivae, the gums of the mouth. [L. *gingiva*]

gin·gi·vo·ax·i·al (jin'ji-vō-ak'sē-ăl). Pertaining to the line angle formed by the gingival and axial walls of a cavity.

gin·gi·vo·glos·si·tis (jin'ji-vō-glos-sī'tis). Inflammation of both the tongue and gingival tissues. SEE ALSO stomatitis.

gin·gi·vo·la·bi·al (jin'ji-vō-lā'bē-ăl). Referring to the line angle formed by the junction of the gingival and labial walls of a (class III or IV) cavity.

gi

gin·gi·vo·lin·guo·ax·i·al (jin′ji-vō-ling′gwō-ak′sē-ăl). Referring to the point angle formed by the gingival, lingual, and axial walls of a cavity.

gin·gi·vo-os·se·ous (jin′ji-vō-os′ē-ŭs). Referring to the gingiva and its underlying bone.

gin·gi·vo·plas·ty (jin′ji-vō-plas-tē). A surgical procedure that reshapes and recontours the gingival tissue in order to attain esthetic, physiologic, and functional form.

gin·gi·vo·sis (jin-ji-vō′sis). SYN chronic desquamative *gingivitis*.

gin·gi·vo·sto·ma·ti·tis (jin′ji-vō-stō′mă-tī′tis). Inflammation of the gingiva and other oral mucous membranes. [gingivo- + G. *stoma*, mouth, + *-itis*, inflammation]

gin·gly·form (jing′gli-fōrm, ging-). SYN ginglymoid. [G. *ginglymos*, a hinge joint, + L. *forma*, form]

gin·glym·o·ar·thro·di·al (jing′gli-mō-ar-thrō′dē-ăl, ging-). Denoting a joint having the form of both ginglymus and arthrodia, or hinge joint and sliding joint.

gin·gly·moid (jing′gli-moyd, ging-). Relating to or resembling a hinge joint. SYN ginglyform. [G. *ginglymos*, a hinge joint, + *eidos*, resembling]

gin·gly·mus (jing′gli-mŭs, ging-) [NA]. SYN hinge *joint*. [G. *ginglymos*]

helicoid g., SYN pivot *joint*.

lateral g., SYN pivot *joint*.

gin·seng (jin′seng). The roots of several species of *Panax* (family Araliaceae), esteemed as of great medicinal virtue by the Chinese, but not often used in western medicine. [Ch.]

Giordano-Giovannetti di·et. See under diet.

GIP Abbreviation for gastric inhibitory *polypeptide*; gastric inhibitory *peptide*.

Girard, A., Swiss-born U.S. surgeon, 1841–1914. SEE G.'s *reagent*.

gir·dle (ger′dl). A belt; a zone. A structure that has the form of a belt or girdle. SYN cingulum (1) [NA]. [A.S. *gyrdel*]

Hitzig's g., SYN tabetic *cuirass*.

Neptune's g., a wet pack applied around the abdomen.

pectoral g., SYN shoulder g.

pelvic g., the bony ring formed by the hip bones and the sacrum, to which the lower limbs are attached. SYN cingulum membri inferioris [NA].

shoulder g., the bony ring, incomplete behind, that serves for the attachment and support of the upper limbs. It is formed by the manubrium sterni, the clavicles, and the scapulae. SYN cingulum membri superioris [NA], pectoral g., thoracic g.

thoracic g., SYN shoulder g.

Girdlestone, Gathorne Robert, British orthopedist, *1881. SEE G. *procedure*.

gi·tal·in (jit′ă-lin). An extract of *Digitalis purpurea* containing a mixture of glycosides and aglycons, with action and uses similar to those of digitalis.

gith·a·gism (gith′ă-jizm). A disease similar to lathyrism, believed to be due to poisoning by seeds of the corn cockle, *Lychnis githago*. [L. *gith*, a plant, Roman coriander, + *ago*, to drive]

gi·tog·e·nin (jit′ō-jen-in). (25*R*)-5α-Spirostan-2α,3β-diol; the genin of gitonin; a cardiotonic agent. SYN digin.

gi·to·nin (jit′ō-nin). A gitogenin tetraglycoside composed of two galactoses, one glucose, and one xylose; F-gitogenin has one galactose, two glucoses, and one xylose. Both are cardiotonic agents.

gi·tox·i·gen·in (ji-toks′ē-jen-in). The aglycon of gitoxin.

gi·tox·in (ji-tok′sin). $C_{41}H_{64}O_{14}$; a secondary cardiac glycoside from *Digitalis purpurea* and *D. lanata*. SYN anhydrogitalin, bigitalin, pseudodigitoxin.

git·ter·zel·le (git′er-zel-e). SYN compound granule *cell*. [Ger. fr. *Gitter*, lattice, + *Zelle*, cell]

Gla Abbreviation for 4-carboxyglutamic acid.

gla·bel·la (glă-bel′ă). **1** [NA]. A smooth prominence, most marked in the male, on the frontal bone above the root of the nose. **2.** The most forward projecting point of the forehead in the midline at the level of the supraorbital ridges. SYN mesophryon. SEE ALSO antinion. SYN intercilium. [L. *glabellus*, hairless, smooth, dim. of *glaber*]

gla·bel·lad (glă-bel′ad). Toward the glabella.

gla·brous, gla·brate (glā′brŭs, glā′brāt). Smooth or hairless; denoting areas of the body where hair does not normally grow, *i.e.*, palms or soles. [L. *glaber*, smooth]

glad·i·ate (glad′ē-āt). SYN xiphoid. [L. *gladius*, a sword]

glad·i·o·lus (glă-dī′ō-lŭs, glad′ē-ō′lŭs). SYN body of sternum. [L. dim. of *gladius*, a sword]

GLAND

---

gland. An organized aggregation of cells functioning as a secretory or excretory organ. SYN glandula (1). [L. *glans*, acorn]

accessory g., a small mass of glandular structure, detached from but lying near another and larger g., to which it is similar in structure and probably in function.

accessory lacrimal g.'s, small, compound, branched, tubular glands located in the middle part of the lid (Wolfring's glands, 1872, or Ciaccio's glands, 1874) and along the superior and inferior fornices of the conjunctival sac (Krause's g.'s, 1854). These accessory g.'s are just scattered scraps of lacrimal g. tissue; all of them produce the same kind of tears and debouch on to the conjunctival surface. Henle's and Baumgarten's "glands" are in fact not g.'s at all, but mere epithelial invaginations. SYN glandulae lacrimales accessoriae [NA].

accessory parotid g., an occasional islet of parotid tissue separate from the mass of the gland, lying anteriorly just above the commencement of the parotid duct. SYN glandula parotidea accessoria [NA], admaxillary g., glandula parotis accessoria, socia parotidis.

accessory suprarenal g.'s, isolated, often minute, masses of suprarenal tissue sometimes found near the main glands or in the broad ligament or the epididymis. SYN glandulae suprarenales accessoriae [NA].

accessory thyroid g., an isolated mass, or one of several such masses, of thyroid tissue, sometimes present in the side of the neck, or just above the hyoid bone (suprahyoid accessory thyroid gland), or even as low as the arch of the aorta. SYN glandula thyroidea accessoria [NA], accessory thyroid, prehyoid g., suprahyoid g., thyroidea accessoria, thyroidea ima, Wölfler's g.

acid g., one of the gastric g.'s secreting the hydrochloric acid of the gastric juice. SYN oxyntic g.

acinotubular g., SYN tubuloacinar g.

acinous g., a g. in which the secretory unit(s) has a grapelike shape and a very small lumen; *e.g.*, the exocrine part of the pancreas.

admaxillary g., SYN accessory parotid g.

adrenal g., SYN suprarenal g.

aggregate g.'s, SYN Peyer's *patches*, under *patch*.

agminate g.'s, agminated g.'s, SYN Peyer's *patches*, under *patch*.

Albarran's g.'s, minute submucosal glands or branching tubules in the subcervical region of the prostate g., emptying for the most part into the posterior portion of the urethra. SYN Albarran y Dominguez' tubules.

albuminous g., a g. that secretes a watery fluid.

alveolar g., a g. in which the secretory unit(s) has a saclike form and an obvious lumen; *e.g.*, the active mammary gland.

anal g., **(1)** one of a number of large sudoriferous g.'s in the mucous membrane of the anus; **(2)** an incorrect synonym for anal *sac*.

anterior lingual g., one of the small mixed glands deeply placed near the apex of the tongue on each side of the frenulum. SYN glandula lingualis anterior [NA], apical g., Bauhin's g., Blandin's g., Nuhn's g.

apical g., SYN anterior lingual g.

apocrine g., a g. whose secretory product includes an apical portion of the secretory cell such as the secretion of lipid droplets in lactation.

apocrine sweat g.'s, sudoriferous g.'s that develop in association with hair follicles and undergo enlargement and secretory development at puberty; they secrete a viscous and odorless sweat that supports the growth of bacteria leading to an acrid odor; secretion is by an eccrine, not apocrine, mechanism. SYN axillary sweat g.'s.

areolar g.'s, a number of small mammary glands forming small rounded projections from the surface of the areola of the breast; they enlarge with pregnancy and during lactation secrete a substance presumed to resist chapping. SYN glandulae areolares [NA], Montgomery's follicles, Montgomery's g.'s.

arteriococcygeal g., SYN coccygeal *body.*

arytenoid g.'s, a large number of mixed glands in the mucous membrane of the larynx; they are called, according to their situation, anterior, middle, and posterior. SYN glandulae laryngeae [NA], laryngeal g.'s.

Aselli's g., a single large lymph node ventral to the abdominal aorta that receives all the lymph from the intestines in many smaller mammals. SYN Aselli's pancreas.

g.'s of auditory tube, SYN mucous g.'s of auditory tube.

axillary g.'s, SYN axillary *lymph nodes,* under *lymph node.*

axillary sweat g.'s, SYN apocrine sweat g.'s.

Bartholin's g., SYN greater vestibular g.

basal g., SYN hypophysis.

Bauhin's g., SYN anterior lingual g.

Baumgarten's g.'s, SYN Henle's g.'s.

g.'s of biliary mucosa, small, mucous, tubuloalveolar glands in the mucosa of the larger bile ducts and especially in the neck of the gallbladder. SYN glandulae mucosae biliosae [NA], Luschka's cystic g.'s, Theile's g.'s.

Blandin's g., SYN anterior lingual g.

Boerhaave's g.'s, SYN sweat g.'s.

Bowman's g., SEE olfactory g.'s.

brachial g., one of the lymph nodes of the arm.

bronchial g.'s, (1) SYN bronchopulmonary *lymph nodes,* under *lymph node.* **(2)** mucous and seromucous glands whose secretory units lie outside the muscle of the bronchi.

Bruch's g.'s, lymph nodes in the palpebral conjunctiva. SYN trachoma g.'s.

Brunner's g.'s, SYN duodenal g.'s.

buccal g.'s, numerous racemose, mucous, or serous glands in the submucous tissue of the cheeks. SYN glandulae buccales [NA], genal g.'s.

bulbourethral g., one of two small compound racemose glands, that produce a mucoid secretion, lying side by side along the membranous urethra just above the bulb of the corpus spongiosum; they discharge through a small duct into the spongy portion of the urethra. SYN glandula bulbourethralis [NA], Cowper's g., Méry's g.

cardiac g., a coiled tubular g. located in the cardiac region of the stomach; secretes primarily mucus.

cardiac g.'s of esophagus, g.'s located in the lamina propria of the uppermost and lowermost levels of the esophagus; they resemble cardiac g.'s of the stomach in that they are branched tubules of mucous cells.

celiac g.'s, SYN celiac *lymph nodes,* under *lymph node.*

ceruminous g.'s, apocrine sudoriferous glands in the external acoustic meatus. SYN glandulae ceruminosae (1) [NA].

cervical g.'s, (1) SEE anterior cervical *lymph nodes,* under *lymph node,* lateral deep cervical *lymph nodes,* under *lymph node,* lateral superficial cervical *lymph nodes,* under *lymph node.* **(2)** branched mucus-secreting glands in the mucosa of the cervix. SYN glandulae cervicales uteri [NA], cervical g.'s of uterus.

cervical g.'s of uterus, SYN cervical g.'s (2).

Ciaccio's g.'s, SEE accessory lacrimal g.'s.

ciliary g.'s, a number of modified apocrine sudoriferous glands in the eyelids, with ducts that usually open into the follicles of the eyelashes. SYN glandulae ciliares [NA], Moll's g.'s.

circumanal g.'s, large apocrine sweat glands surrounding the anus. SYN glandulae circumanales [NA], Gay's g.'s.

coccygeal g., SYN coccygeal *body.*

coil g., a g. whose secretory part is convoluted. SYN convoluted g.

compound g., a g. whose larger excretory ducts branch repeatedly into smaller ducts, which ultimately drain secretory units.

conjunctival g.'s, clusters of mucous cells in the conjunctival epithelium, most numerous on the bulbar conjunctiva. SYN glandulae conjunctivales [NA], Terson's g.'s.

convoluted g., SYN coil g.

Cowper's g., SYN bulbourethral g.

crop g., cells in the crop of male and female pigeons and doves that secrete a caseous or milklike material with which the bird feeds its young; it is stimulated to secrete by prolactin, the lactogenic hormone of the anterior hypophysis, and is used as a test object for assaying the activity of this hormone.

cutaneous g.'s, any of the glands of the skin. SYN glandulae cutis [NA].

ductless g.'s, SYN endocrine g.'s.

duodenal g.'s, small, branched, coiled tubular glands that occur mostly in the submucosa of the first third of the duodenum; they secrete an alkaline mucoid substance that serves to neutralize gastric juice. SYN glandulae duodenales [NA], Brunner's g.'s, Wepfer's g.'s.

Duverney's g., SYN greater vestibular g.

Ebner's g.'s, serous g.'s of the tongue opening in the bottom of the trough surrounding the circumvallate papillae.

eccrine g., a coiled tubular sweat g. (other than apocrine g.'s) that occurs in the skin on almost all parts of the body.

ecdysial g.'s, insect structures that originate from the ectoderm of the ventrocaudal part of the head and serve as a source of ecdysone. SYN peritracheal g.'s, prothoracic g.'s, thoracic g.'s, ventral g.'s.

Eglis' g.'s, small, inconstant mucous g.'s of the ureter and renal pelvis.

endocrine g.'s, glands that have no ducts, their secretions being absorbed directly into the blood. SYN glandulae endocrinae [NA], glandulae sine ductibus [NA], ductless g.'s, g.'s of internal secretion.

esophageal g.'s, a variable number of small compound mucous glands in the submucosa of the esophagus. SYN glandulae esophageae [NA].

g.'s of eustachian tube, SYN mucous g.'s of auditory tube.

excretory g., a g. separating excrementitious or waste material from the blood.

exocrine g., a g. from which secretions reach a free surface of the body by ducts.

external salivary g., SYN parotid g.

g.'s of the female urethra, numerous mucous g.'s in the wall of the female urethra. SYN glandulae urethrales femininae, Guérin's g.'s, paraurethral g.'s, Skene's g.'s.

follicular g., a g. consisting of follicles.

fundus g.'s, SYN gastric g.'s.

Galeati's g.'s, SYN intestinal g.'s.

gastric g.'s, branched tubular glands lying in the mucosa of the fundus and body of the stomach; such glands contain parietal cells that secrete hydrochloric acid, zymogen cells that produce pepsin, and mucous cells. SYN glandulae gastricae [NA], glandulae propriae* [NA], fundus g.'s, gastric follicles, Wasmann's g.'s.

Gay's g.'s, SYN circumanal g.'s.

genal g.'s, SYN buccal g.'s.

genital g., (1) SYN testis. **(2)** SYN ovary.

Gley's g.'s, SEE parathyroid g.

glomiform g.'s, SYN glomus (2).

greater vestibular g., one of two mucoid-secreting tubuloalveolar glands on either side of the lower part of the vagina, the equivalent of the bulbourethral glands in the male; ensheathed with vestibular bulbs by ischiocavernosus muscles. Thus erection and muscle contraction cause secretion into vestibule of vagina. SYN glandula vestibularis major [NA], Bartholin's g., Duverney's g., Tiedemann's g., vulvovaginal g.

gl

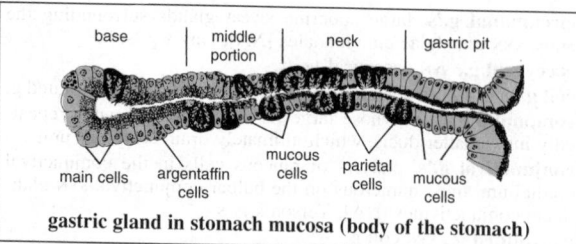

base | middle portion | neck | gastric pit

main cells | argentaffin cells | mucous cells | parietal cells | mucous cells

gastric gland in stomach mucosa (body of the stomach)

Guérin's g.'s, SYN g.'s of the female urethra.

Harder's g., harderian g., (1) the deep g. of the semilunar conjunctival fold or "third eyelid" found in animals such as the pig and deer; **(2)** misnomer for the superficial g. of the semilunar conjunctival fold in the dog; not present in humans.

Havers' g.'s, collections of adipose tissue in the hip, knee, and other joints, covered by synovial membrane, thought by Havers to be g.'s secreting the synovia. SYN synovial g.'s.

hemal g., SYN hemal *node*.

hematopoietic g., a blood-forming organ, such as the spleen.

hemolymph g., SYN hemal *node*.

Henle's g.'s, accessory lacrimal g.'s located near the fornices in the medial part of the palpebral conjunctiva; they open on the conjunctiva surface. SYN Baumgarten's g.'s.

hibernating g., SYN brown *fat*.

holocrine g., a g. whose secretion consists of disintegrated cells of the g. itself, *e.g.,* a sebaceous g., in contrast to a merocrine g.

inguinal g.'s, SEE deep inguinal *lymph nodes,* under *lymph node,* superficial inguinal *lymph nodes,* under *lymph node.*

internal salivary g., the sublingual and submandibular g.'s regarded as one.

g.'s of internal secretion, SYN endocrine g.'s.

interrenal g.'s, SYN interrenal *bodies,* under *body.*

interscapular g., SYN brown *fat.*

interstitial g., SEE interstitial *cells,* under *cell.*

intestinal g.'s, the tubular glands in the mucous membrane of the small and large intestines. SYN glandulae intestinales [NA], Galeati's g.'s, intestinal follicles, Lieberkühn's crypts, Lieberkühn's follicles, Lieberkühn's g.'s.

intraepithelial g.'s, accumulations of glandular cells that lie within an epithelium, as those of the urethra.

jugular g., SYN signal *node.*

Knoll's g.'s, g.'s in the ventricular folds of the larynx (false vocal cords).

Krause's g.'s, (1) SEE accessory lacrimal g.'s. **(2)** g.'s in the mucous membrane of the tympanic cavity. SEE accessory lacrimal g.'s.

labial g.'s, mucous glands in the submucous tissue of the lips. SYN glandulae labiales [NA].

lacrimal g., the gland that secretes tears; it consists of 6 to 12 separate compound tubuloalveolar serous glands, located in the upper lateral part of the orbit, and is partially divided into a smaller palpebral part and a larger orbital part by the aponeurosis of the levator palpebrae muscle. SYN glandula lacrimalis [NA].

lactiferous g., SYN mammary g.

laryngeal g.'s, SYN arytenoid g.'s.

lesser vestibular g.'s, a number of minute mucous glands opening on the surface of the vestibule between the orifices of the vagina and urethra. SYN glandulae vestibulares minores [NA].

Lieberkühn's g.'s, SYN intestinal g.'s.

Littré's g.'s, SYN g.'s of the male urethra.

Luschka's g., (1) SYN pharyngeal *tonsil.* **(2)** former name for *corpus* coccygeum.

Luschka's cystic g.'s, SYN g.'s of biliary mucosa.

lymph g., SYN lymph node.

major salivary g.'s, a category of salivary g.'s that includes the three largest g.'s of the oral cavity that also secrete most of the saliva: the parotid, submandibular, and sublingual g.'s.

g.'s of the male urethra, numerous mucous glands in the wall of

the penile urethra. SYN glandulae urethrales masculinae, Littré's g.'s.

malpighian g.'s, SYN splenic lymph *follicles,* under *follicle.*

mammary g., the compound alveolar apocrine secretory gland that forms the breast. It consists of 15 to 24 lobes, each consisting of many lobules, separated by adipose tissue and fibrous septa; the parenchyma of the resting gland consists of ducts; the alveoli develop only during pregnancy [NA], lactiferous g., milk g.

marrow-lymph g., a type of hemal node, resembling the bone marrow in structure and probable function.

master g., SYN hypophysis.

maxillary g., SYN submandibular g.

meibomian g.'s, SYN tarsal g.'s.

merocrine g., a g. that releases only an acellular secretory product, in contrast to a holocrine g.

Méry's g., SYN bulbourethral g.

mesenteric g.'s, SEE mesenteric *lymph nodes,* under *lymph node.*

metrial g., collections of granular epithelial cells in the uterine muscle beneath the placenta that develop during pregnancy in certain animals (*e.g.,* mouse, rat). The cells are thought to disintegrate and pass (as a holocrine secretion) into the afferent placental vessels to furnish nutriment for the embryo.

milk g., SYN mammary g.

minor salivary g.'s, the smaller, largely mucous-secreting, exocrine g.'s of the oral cavity, consisting of the labial, buccal, molar, lingual, and palatine g.'s.

mixed g., (1) a g. that contains both serous and mucous secretory units; **(2)** a g. that is both exocrine and endocrine, *e.g.,* the pancreas.

molar g.'s, four or five large buccal glands in the neighborhood of the last molar tooth. SYN glandulae molares [NA].

Moll's g.'s, SYN ciliary g.'s.

Montgomery's g.'s, SYN areolar g.'s.

g.'s of mouth, glands that empty into the oral cavity. SYN glandulae oris [NA].

mucilaginous g., one of the synovial villi, supposed by Havers to secrete the synovia.

muciparous g., SYN mucous g.

mucous g., a gland that secretes mucus. SYN glandula mucosa [NA], muciparous g.

mucous g.'s of auditory tube, glands located principally near the pharyngeal end of the auditory tube. SYN glandulae tubariae [NA], g.'s of auditory tube, g.'s of eustachian tube.

nasal g.'s, seromucous glands in the respiratory region of the nasal mucous membrane. SYN glandulae nasales [NA].

Nuhn's g., SYN anterior lingual g.

odoriferous g., (1) a g., such as Tyson's g., the secretion of which has a strong odor; **(2)** SEE sweat g.'s.

oil g.'s, (1) SYN sebaceous g.'s. **(2)** SYN uropygial g.

olfactory g.'s, branched tubuloalveolar serous secreting glands (of Bowman) in the mucous membrane of the olfactory region of the nasal cavity. SYN glandulae olfactoriae [NA].

oxyntic g., SYN acid g.

pacchionian g.'s, SYN arachnoid *granulations,* under *granulation.*

palatine g.'s, a number of racemose mucous glands in the posterior half of the submucous tissue covering the hard palate. SYN glandulae palatinae [NA].

palpebral g.'s, SYN tarsal g.'s.

parathyroid g., one of Gley's glands or Sandström's bodies; one of two small paired endocrine glands, superior and inferior, usually found embedded in the connective tissue capsule on the posterior surface of the thyroid gland; they secrete parathyroid hormone that regulates the metabolism of calcium and phosphorus. The parenchyma is composed of chief and oxyphilic cells arranged in anastomosing cords. Inadvertant removal of all parathyroid g.'s, as during thyroidectomy, produces tetany and death. SYN glandula parathyroidea [NA], epithelial body, parathyroid (2).

paraurethral g.'s, SYN g.'s of the female urethra.

parotid g., the largest of the salivary glands, one of two compound acinous glands situated inferior and anterior to the ear, on either side, extending from the angle of the jaw to the zygomatic arch and posteriorly to the sternocleidomastoid muscle; it is subdivided into a superficial part and a deep part by emerging branches of the facial nerve, and discharges through the parotid duct. SYN glandula parotidea [NA], external salivary g., glandula parotis.

pectoral g.'s, SEE axillary *lymph nodes,* under *lymph node.*

peptic g., a pepsin-secreting g. SEE gastric g.'s.

perianal odoriferous g.'s, SEE scent g.'s.

peritracheal g.'s, SYN ecdysial g.'s.

perspiratory g.'s, SYN sweat g.'s.

Peyer's g.'s, SYN Peyer's *patches,* under *patch.*

pharyngeal g.'s, racemose mucous glands beneath the mucous membrane of the pharynx. SYN glandula pharyngeae [NA].

Philip's g.'s, enlarged deep g.'s just above the clavicle, found in children with pulmonary tuberculosis and occasionally in others.

pileous g., a sebaceous g. emptying into the hair follicle.

pineal g., SYN pineal *body.*

pituitary g., SYN hypophysis.

Poirier's g., a lymph node on the uterine artery where it crosses the ureter.

preen g., SYN uropygial g.

prehyoid g., SYN accessory thyroid g.

preputial g.'s, sebaceous glands of the corona glandis and inner surface of the prepuce, which produce an odiferous substance called smegma. SYN glandulae preputiales [NA], Tyson's g.'s.

prostate g., SYN prostate.

prothoracic g.'s, SYN ecdysial g.'s.

pyloric g.'s, the coiled, tubular glands of the pylorus whose cells secrete mucus. SYN glandulae pyloricae [NA].

racemose g., a g. that has the appearance of a bunch of grapes if viewed as a three-dimensional reconstruction; *e.g.,* a compound acinous or alveolar g.

Rivinus' g., SYN sublingual g.

Rosenmüller's g., SYN *node* of Cloquet.

saccular g., a single alveolar g.

salivary g., any of the saliva-secreting exocrine glands of the oral cavity. SYN glandula salivaria [NA].

scent g.'s, cutaneous g.'s producing odoriferous secretions (pheromones or recognition odors); they may be located on different parts of the body, *e.g.,* under the chin (rabbit); between the digits (goat); on the medial surface of the metatarsus (deer), in the preorbital fold (antelope); in the occipital region (camel); on the flank (hamster); in the perianal region and on the dorsum of the tail base (carnivores).

sebaceous g.'s, numerous holocrine glands in the dermis that usually open into the hair follicles and secrete an oily semifluid sebum. SYN glandulae sebaceae [NA], oil g.'s (1), sebaceous follicles.

seminal g., SYN seminal *vesicle.*

sentinel g., a single enlarged lymph node in the omentum that may be an indication of an ulcer opposite to it in the greater or lesser curvature of the stomach.

seromucous g., (1) a gland in which some of the secretory cells are serous and some mucous; (2) a gland whose cells secrete a fluid intermediate between a watery and a viscous mucoid substance. SYN glandula seromucosa [NA].

serous g., a gland that secretes a watery substance that may or may not contain an enzyme. SYN glandula serosa [NA].

Serres' g.'s, epithelial cell rests found in the subepithelial connective tissue in the palate of the newborn, similar to those found in the gingivae.

sexual g., SEE testis, ovary.

Skene's g.'s, SYN g.'s of the female urethra.

solitary g.'s, SYN solitary lymphatic *follicles,* under *follicle.*

sublingual g., one of two salivary glands in the floor of the mouth beneath the tongue, discharging through the sublingual ducts; most of the secretory units in the human gland are mucus-secreting with serous demilunes. SYN glandula sublingualis [NA], Rivinus' g.

submandibular g., one of two salivary glands in the neck, located in the space bounded by the two bellies of the digastric muscle and the angle of the mandible; it discharges through the submandibular duct; the secretory units are predominantly serous although a few mucous alveoli, some with serous demilunes, occur. SYN glandula submandibularis [NA], maxillary g., submaxillary g.

submaxillary g., SYN submandibular g.

sudoriferous g.'s, SYN sweat g.'s.

suprahyoid g., SYN accessory thyroid g.

suprarenal g., a flattened, roughly triangular body resting upon the upper end of each kidney; it is one of the ductless glands furnishing internal secretions (epinephrine and norepinephrine from the medulla and steroid hormones from the cortex). SYN glandula suprarenalis [NA], adrenal body, adrenal capsule, adrenal g., atrabiliary capsule, epinephros, glandula atrabiliaris, paranephros, suprarenal body, suprarenal capsule.

Suzanne's g., a small mucous g. in the floor of the mouth.

sweat g.'s, the coil glands of the skin that secrete the sweat. SYN glandulae sudoriferae [NA], Boerhaave's g.'s, perspiratory g.'s, sudoriferous g.'s.

synovial g.'s, SYN Havers' g.'s.

target g., the effector that functions when stimulated by the internal secretion of another gland or by some other stimulus.

tarsal g.'s, sebaceous glands embedded in the tarsal plate of each eyelid, discharging at the edge of the lid near the posterior border. Their secretions create a lipid barrier along the margin of the eyelids which contains the normal secretions in the conjunctival sac by preventing the watery fluid from spilling over the barrier when the eye is open. SYN glandulae tarsales [NA], meibomian g.'s, palpebral g.'s.

Terson's g.'s, SYN conjunctival g.'s.

Theile's g.'s, SYN g.'s of biliary mucosa.

thoracic g.'s, SYN ecdysial g.'s.

thymus g., SYN thymus.

thyroid g., a ductless gland, consisting of irregularly spheroidal follicles, lying in front and to the sides of the upper part of the trachea, and of horseshoe shape, with two lateral lobes connected by a narrow central portion, the isthmus; occasionally an elongated offshoot, the pyramidal lobe, passes upward from the isthmus in front of the trachea. It is supplied by branches from the external carotid and subclavian arteries, and its nerves are derived from the middle cervical and cervicothoracic ganglia of the sympathetic system. It secretes thyroid hormone and calcitonin. SYN glandula thyroidea [NA], thyroid body, thyroidea.

Tiedemann's g., SYN greater vestibular g.

tracheal g.'s, numerous tubuloalveolar mixed glands located principally in the submucosa of the trachea; they open into the tracheal lumen through short ducts. SYN glandulae tracheales [NA].

trachoma g.'s, SYN Bruch's g.'s.

tubular g., a g. composed of one or more tubules ending in a blind extremity.

tubuloacinar g., a g. whose secretory elements are elongated acini. SYN acinotubular g.

tubuloalveolar g., a g. that has secretory units of short tubules.

tympanic g., one of the mucous g.'s in the mucosa of the tympanic cavity. SYN tympanic body.

⚠ **Combining forms**	**[NA] Nomina Anatomica**
Word*Finder*	**[MIM] Mendelian**
Multi-term entry finder	**Inheritance in Man**
Preceding letter A	
A.D.A.M. Anatomy Plates	☆ **Official alternate term**
Between letters L and M	
	☆**[NA] Official alternate**
Appendices:	**Nomina Anatomica term**
Following letter Z	
SYN Synonym; Cf., compare	**High Profile Term**

Tyson's g.'s, SYN preputial g.'s.

unicellular g., a single secretory cell such as a mucous goblet cell.

urethral g.'s, SEE g.'s of the female urethra, g.'s of the male urethra.

uropygial g., a compound alveolar g. of birds located on the dorsum of the tail or pygostyle; the secretion of this g. (fatty acids and wax) exits from a papilla on the dorsal surface at the base of the tail feathers; the bird applies the substance to its feathers by means of the bill when preening. The uropygial g. is lacking in some species but its waterproofing ability is essential to water birds. SYN glandula uropygius, oil g.'s (2), preen g.

uterine g.'s, numerous simple tubular glands in the uterine mucosa that secrete a glycogen-rich mucous fluid during the luted phase of the menstrual cycle. SYN glandulae uterinae [NA].

vaginal g., one of the mucous g.'s in the mucous membrane of the vagina.

vascular g., SYN hemal *node*.

ventral g.'s, SYN ecdysial g.'s.

vesical g., one of a number of mucous follicles, not true g.'s, in the mucous membrane near the neck of the bladder.

vestibular g.'s, SEE greater vestibular g., lesser vestibular g.'s.

vulvovaginal g., SYN greater vestibular g.

Waldeyer's g.'s, coil g.'s near the margins of the eyelids.

Wasmann's g.'s, SYN gastric g.'s.

Weber's g.'s, muciparous g.'s at the border of the tongue on either side posteriorly.

Wepfer's g.'s, SYN duodenal g.'s.

Wölfler's g., SYN accessory thyroid g.

Wolfring's g.'s, SEE accessory lacrimal g.'s.

Zeis' g.'s, sebaceous g.'s opening into the follicles of the eyelashes.

---

glan·ders (glan´derz). A chronic debilitating disease of horses and other equids, as well as some members of the cat family, caused by *Pseudomonas mallei* and transmissible to humans. It attacks the mucous membranes of the nostrils of the horse, producing an increased and vitiated secretion and discharge of mucus, and enlargement and induration of the glands of the lower jaw. [O. Fr. *glandres*, glands]

glan·des (glan´dēz). Plural of glans.

glan·di·lem·ma (glan-di-lem´ă). The capsule of a gland. [L. *glandula*, gland, + G. *lemma*, sheath]

GLANDULA

glan·du·la, pl. **glan·du·lae** (glan´dū-lă, -lē). **1** [NA]. SYN gland. **2.** SYN glandule. [L. gland, dim. of *glans*, acorn]

glan´dulae areola´res [NA], SYN areolar *glands*, under *gland*.

g. atrabilia´ris, SYN suprarenal *gland*.

g. basila´ris, SYN hypophysis.

glan´dulae bronchia´les [NA], SYN bronchopulmonary *lymph nodes*, under *lymph node*.

glan´dulae bucca´les [NA], SYN buccal *glands*, under *gland*.

g. bulbourethra´lis [NA], SYN bulbourethral *gland*.

glan´dulae cerumino´sae [NA], **(1)** SYN ceruminous *glands*, under *gland*. **(2)** tubuloalveolar glands of the external auditory meatus believed to be modified apocrine sweat glands; they secrete the waxy substance cerumen.

glan´dulae cervica´les uteri [NA], SYN cervical *glands* (2), under *gland*.

glan´dulae cilia´res [NA], SYN ciliary *glands*, under *gland*.

glan´dulae circumana´les [NA], SYN circumanal *glands*, under *gland*.

glan´dulae conjunctiva´les [NA], SYN conjunctival *glands*, under *gland*.

glan´dulae cu´tis [NA], SYN cutaneous *glands*, under *gland*.

glan´dulae duodena´les [NA], SYN duodenal *glands*, under *gland*.

glan´dulae endocri´nae [NA], SYN endocrine *glands*, under *gland*.

glan´dulae esopha´geae [NA], SYN esophageal *glands*, under *gland*.

glan´dulae gas´tricae [NA], SYN gastric *glands*, under *gland*.

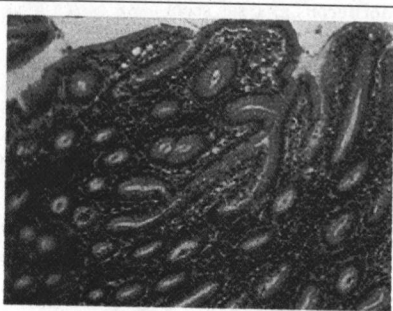

glandulae gastricae
branched, tubular glands in the tunica mucosa of the stomach

glan´dulae glomifor´mes [NA], **(1)** SYN glomus (2). **(2)** tubular glands of the skin, the blind extremity of which is coiled in the form of a ball or glomerulus; collective term for small eccrine and large apocrine sweat glands.

glan´dulae intestina´les [NA], SYN intestinal *glands*, under *gland*.

glan´dulae labia´les [NA], SYN labial *glands*, under *gland*.

glan´dulae lacrima´les accesso´riae [NA], SYN accessory lacrimal *glands*, under *gland*.

g. lacrima´lis [NA], SYN lacrimal *gland*.

glan´dulae laryn´geae [NA], SYN arytenoid *glands*, under *gland*.

g. lingua´lis ante´rior [NA], SYN anterior lingual *gland*.

g. mamma´ria [NA], SYN mammary *gland*. SEE ALSO breast.

glan´dulae mola´res [NA], SYN molar *glands*, under *gland*.

g. muco´sa, SYN mucous *gland*.

glan´dulae muco´sae bilio´sae [NA], SYN *glands* of biliary mucosa, under *gland*.

glan´dulae nasa´les [NA], SYN nasal *glands*, under *gland*.

glan´dulae olfacto´riae [NA], SYN olfactory *glands*, under *gland*.

glan´dulae o´ris [NA], SYN *glands* of mouth, under *gland*.

glan´dulae palati´nae [NA], SYN palatine *glands*, under *gland*.

g. parathyroi´dea [NA], SYN parathyroid *gland*.

g. parotid´ea [NA], SYN parotid *gland*.

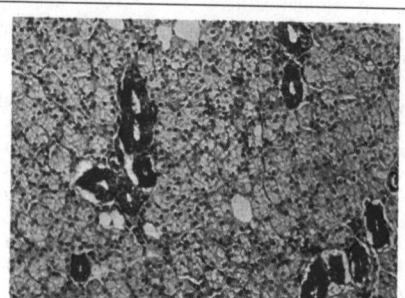

acinous glands (glandula parotidea)
note multiple branching of secretory units

g. parotid´ea accesso´ria [NA], SYN accessory parotid *gland*.

g. paro´tis, SYN parotid *gland*.

g. paro´tis accesso´ria, SYN accessory parotid *gland*.

glan′dulae pharyn′geae [NA], SYN pharyngeal *glands*, under *gland*.

g. pituita′ria [NA], SYN hypophysis.

glan′dulae preputia′les [NA], SYN preputial *glands*, under *gland*.

glan′dulae pro′priae [NA], *official alternate term for gastric *glands*, under *gland*.

g. prosta′tica, SYN prostate.

glan′dulae pylor′icae [NA], SYN pyloric *glands*, under *gland*.

g. saliva′ria [NA], SYN salivary *gland*. SEE major salivary *glands*, under *gland*, minor salivary *glands*, under *gland*.

glan′dulae seba′ceae [NA], SYN sebaceous *glands*, under *gland*.

g. semina′lis [NA], SYN seminal *vesicle*, seminal *vesicle*.

g. seromuco′sa [NA], SYN seromucous *gland*.

g. sero′sa [NA], SYN serous *gland*.

glan′dulae sine duc′tibus [NA], SYN endocrine *glands*, under *gland*.

g. sublingua′lis [NA], SYN sublingual *gland*.

g. submandibula′ris [NA], SYN submandibular *gland*.

glan′dulae sudorif′erae [NA], SYN sweat *glands*, under *gland*.

glan′dulae suprarena′les accesso′riae [NA], SYN accessory suprarenal *glands*, under *gland*.

g. suprarena′lis [NA], SYN suprarenal *gland*.

glan′dulae tarsa′les [NA], SYN tarsal *glands*, under *gland*.

g. thyroi′dea [NA], SYN thyroid *gland*.

g. thyroi′dea accesso′ria, pl. **glan′dulae thyroi′deae accesso′riae** [NA], SYN accessory thyroid *gland*.

glan′dulae trachea′les [NA], SYN tracheal *glands*, under *gland*.

glan′dulae tuba′riae [NA], SYN mucous *glands* of auditory tube, under *gland*.

glandulae urethra′les femini′nae, SYN *glands* of the female urethra, under *gland*.

glandulae urethra′les masculi′nae, SYN *glands* of the male urethra, under *gland*.

g. uropy′gius, SYN uropygial *gland*.

glan′dulae uteri′nae [NA], SYN uterine *glands*, under *gland*.

glan′dulae vestibula′res mino′res [NA], SYN lesser vestibular *glands*, under *gland*.

g. vestibula′ris ma′jor [NA], SYN greater vestibular *gland*.

---

glan·du·lar (glan′dū-lăr). Relating to a gland. SYN glandulous.

glan·dule (glan′dūl). A small gland. SYN glandula (2). [L. *glandula*]

glan·du·lous (glan′dū-lŭs). SYN glandular.

glans, pl. **glan·des** (glanz, glan′dēz) [NA]. A conical acorn-shaped structure. [L. acorn]

g. clitor′idis [NA], SYN g. of clitoris.

g. of clitoris, a small mass of highly-sensitized erectile tissue capping the body of the clitoris. SYN g. clitoridis [NA].

g. pe′nis [NA], the conical expansion of the corpus spongiosum which forms the head of the penis. SYN balanus.

Glanzmann, Eduard, Swiss clinician, 1887–1959. SEE G.'s *disease, thrombasthenia*.

gla·phen·ine (gla-fen′ēn). *N*-(7-Chloro-4-quinolyl)anthranilic acid 2,3-dihydroxypropyl ester; an anti-inflammatory agent with analgesic properties.

glare (glār). A sensation caused by brightness within the visual field that is sufficiently greater than the luminance to which the eyes are adapted; results in annoyance, discomfort, and decreased visual performance.

blinding g., g. resulting from excessive illumination. SYN veiling g.

dazzling g., g. produced by excessive illumination in the peripheral field.

peripheral g., g. occurring when the surrounding brightness is greater than the brightness of the object of attention.

specular g., g. arising from specularly reflected light.

veiling g., SYN blinding g.

gla·rom·e·ter (glā-rom′ĕ-ter). An instrument that measures sensitivity to central glare from the headlights of an approaching vehicle.

Glaser (Glaserius), Johann H., Swiss anatomist, 1629–1675. SEE glaserian *artery;* glaserian *fissure*.

gla·se·ri·an (gla-ser′ē-an). Relating to or described by Johann H. Glaser.

Glasgow, William C., U.S. physician, 1845–1907. SEE G.'s *sign*.

Glasgow co·ma scale. SEE coma *scale*.

Glasgow coma scale		
eye opening	spontaneous	4
	open when spoken to	3
	open at pain stimulus	2
	no reaction	1
verbal performance	coherent	5
	confused, disoriented	4
	disconnected words	3
	unintelligible sounds	2
	no verbal reaction	1
motor responsiveness	follows instructions	6
	intentional pain-avoidance	5
	large motor movement	4
	flexor synergism	3
	extensor synergism	2
	no reaction	1

glass. A transparent substance composed of silica and oxides of various bases. [A.S. *glaes*]

cover g., a thin g. disk or plate covering an object examined under the microscope. SYN coverslip.

Crookes′ g., a spectacle lens combined with metallic oxides to absorb ultraviolet or infrared rays.

crown g., a compound of lime, potash, alumina, and silica; commonly used in lenses; has a low dispersion (52.2) relative to index of refraction (1.523).

cupping g., a g. vessel, from which the air has been exhausted by heat or a special suction apparatus, formerly applied to the skin in order to draw blood to the surface. SEE ALSO cupping, cup. SYN cup (2).

flint g., g. that contains lead oxide instead of lime to increase index of refraction; used in reading segments of fused bifocal lenses.

object g., SYN objective (1).

quartz g., a transparent, colorless crystal, made by fusing pure quartz sand, which transmits ultraviolet light.

soluble g., a silicate of potassium or sodium, soluble in hot water but solid at ordinary temperatures; used for fixed dressings. SYN water g.

vita g., a specially prepared g. that is transparent to ultraviolet rays of the spectrum.

water g., SYN soluble g.

Wood′s g., a g. containing nickel oxide, used in Wood's lamp.

glass·es (glas′ez). **1.** SYN spectacles. **2.** Lenses for correcting refractive errors in the eyes.

Glauber, Johann R., German chemist, 1604–1668. SEE G.'s *salt*.

glau·cine (glaw′sēn). 5,6,6a,7-Tetrahydro-1,2,9,10-tetramethoxy-6-methyl-4H-dibenzo[*de,g*]quinoline; *d*-Form prevalent in nature. Found in *Glaucium flavum*, (*G. luteum scop.*), *Papaveraceae* and in *Dicentra* and *Corydalis* species, family *Fumariceae*. Antitussive agent. SYN 1,2,9,10-tetramethoxyaporphine, boldine dimethyl ether.

glau·co·ma (glaw-kō′mă). A disease of the eye characterized by increased intraocular pressure, excavation, and atrophy of the optic nerve; produces defects in the field of vision. [G.

glaukōma, opacity of the crystalline lens, fr. glaukos, bluish green]

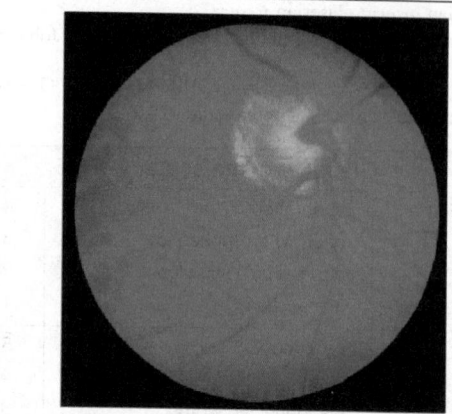

glaucoma (with atrophy of the optic nerve)

absolute g., the final stage of blindness in g.

acute g., SYN angle-closure g.

angle-closure g., primary g. in which contact of the iris with the peripheral cornea excludes aqueous humor from the trabecular drainage meshwork. SYN acute g., closed-angle g., narrow-angle g.

aphakic g., g. following cataract removal.

capsular g., g. occurring in association with widespread deposition of cellular organelles on the lens capsule, ocular blood vessels, iris, and ciliary body. SEE ALSO *pseudoexfoliation* of lens capsule.

chronic g., SYN open-angle g.

α-chymotrypsin-induced g., transient secondary g. following the use of α-chymotrypsin in cataract extraction.

closed-angle g., SYN angle-closure g.

combined g., g. with angle-closure and open-angle mechanisms in the same eye.

compensated g., SYN open-angle g.

congenital g., SYN buphthalmia.

corticosteroid-induced g., g. caused by a hereditary predisposition in which local instillation of eyedrops containing corticosteroid causes increased intraocular pressure.

Donders' g., obsolete eponym for open-angle g.

g. ful'minans, acute angle-closure g. rapidly followed by blindness.

ghost cell g., g. occurring after vitrectomy, arising from erythrocyte membranes blocking outflow channels of aqueous humor.

hemorrhagic g., secondary g. after formation of new blood vessels in the iris.

hypersecretion g., g. caused by excessive formation of the aqueous humor.

low tension g., optic nerve atrophy and excavation with typical field defects of g. but without abnormal increase in intraocular pressure.

malignant g., secondary g. caused by forward displacement of the iris and lens, obliterating the anterior chamber; usually follows a filtering operation for primary glaucoma.

narrow-angle g., SYN angle-closure g.

neovascular g., g. occurring in rubeosis iridis.

open-angle g., primary g. in which the aqueous humor has free access to the trabecular meshwork. SYN chronic g., compensated g., simple g., simplex.

phacogenic g., SYN phacomorphic g.

phacolytic g., g. secondary to hypermature cataract and occlusion of the trabecular drainage meshwork by lens material.

phacomorphic g., secondary g. caused by either excessive size or spherical shape of the lens. SYN phacogenic g.

pigmentary g., g. associated with erosion of pigment from the posterior iris, and with an accumulation of pigment particles in the trabecular meshwork.

pseudoexfoliative capsular g., secondary g. incident to a degenerative cyclitis producing deposits on anterior lens capsule.

pupillary block g., g. secondary to failure of the aqueous humor to pass through the pupil to the anterior chamber.

secondary g., g. occurring as a sequel of preexisting ocular disease or injury.

simple g., g. sim'plex, SYN open-angle g.

glau·co·ma·to·cy·clit·ic (glaw-kō′mă-tō-si-klit′ik). Denoting increased intraocular pressure associated with evidences of cyclitis. SEE ALSO glaucomatocyclitic *crisis*.

glau·co·ma·tous (glaw-kō′mă-tŭs). Relating to glaucoma.

glau·co·su·ria (glaw′kō-sū′rē-ă). Obsolete term for indicanuria. [G. *glaukos,* bluish green, + *ouron,* urine]

GLC Abbreviation for gas-liquid *chromatography*.

Glc, GlcA, GlcN, GlcNAc, GlcUA. Symbols for the radicals of D-glucose, gluconic and glucuronic acid, glucosamine, *N*-acetylglucosamine, and glucuronic acid, respectively.

Gleason, Donald F., U.S. pathologist, *1920. SEE G.'s tumor *grade, score.*

gleet (glēt). Obsolete term for a slight chronic discharge of thin mucus from the urethra, following gonorrhea. [M.E. *glet,* slime, fr. O.Fr. *glette,* fr. L. *glittus,* sticky]

Glenn. William W., *1914. SEE Glenn *shunt.*

Glenner, George B., U.S. pathologist and histologist, *1927. SEE G.-Lillie *stain* for pituitary.

gle·no·hu·mer·al (glē′nō-hyū′mer-ăl). Relating to the glenoid cavity and the humerus.

gle·noid (glē′noyd, glen′oyd). Resembling a socket; denoting the articular depression of the scapula entering into the formation of the shoulder joint. [G. *glēnoeidēs,* fr. *glēnē,* pupil of eye, socket of joint, honeycomb, + *eidos,* appearance]

Gley, Marcel E.E., French physiologist, 1857–1930. SEE G.'s *glands,* under *gland.*

glia (glī′ă). SYN neuroglia. [G. glue]

gli·a·cyte (glī′ă-sīt). A neuroglia cell. SEE neuroglia. [G. *glia,* glue, + *kytos,* cell]

gli·a·din (glī′ă-din). A class of protein, separable from wheat and rye glutens, that contains up to 40% L-glutamine; a member of the prolamins, which are insoluble in water, absolute alcohol, and neutral solvents, but soluble in 50 to 90% alcohol.

gli·al (glī′ăl). Pertaining to glia or neuroglia.

gli·cla·zide (glī′klă-zīd). A sulfonylurea oral antidiabetic agent used for the treatment of type II diabetes mellitus. The drug releases endogenous insulin from beta cells of the islands of Langerhans located in the pancreas; resembles glipizide and tolbutamide.

glide (glīd). A smooth, or effortless, continuous movement.

mandibular g., the side-to-side, protrusive, and intermediate movement of the mandible occurring when the teeth or other occluding surfaces are in contact.

△**glio-.** Glue, gluelike (relating specifically to the neuroglia). [G. *glia,* glue]

gli·o·blast (glī′ō-blast). An early neural cell developing, like the neuroblast, from the early ependymal cell of the neural tube; gives rise to neuroglial and ependymal cells, astrocytes, and oligodendrocytes. SEE ALSO spongioblast. [glio- + G. *blastos,* germ]

gli·o·blas·to·ma multiforme (glī′ō-blas-tō′mă). A glioma consisting chiefly of undifferentiated anaplastic cells of glial origin that show marked nuclear pleomorphism, necrosis, and vascular endothelial proliferation; frequently, tumor cells are arranged radially about an irregular focus of necrosis; these neoplasms grow rapidly, invade extensively, and occur most frequently in the cerebrum of adults. SYN grade IV astrocytoma. [G. *glia,* glue, + *blastos,* germ, + *-oma,* tumor]

gli·o·blas·to·sis ce·re·bri. SYN *gliomatosis* cerebri.

gli·o·ma (glī-ō′mă). Any neoplasm derived from one of the various types of cells that form the interstitial tissue of the brain, spinal cord, pineal gland, posterior pituitary gland, and retina. [G. *glia,* glue, + *-oma,* tumor]

brainstem g., a g., generally an astrocytoma, arising in the medulla, pons, or midbrain.

gigantocellular g., a histologic form of glioblastoma with large, often multinucleated, bizarre, tumor cells. SYN giant cell monstrocellular sarcoma of Zülch.

mixed g., a glioma comprised of two or more malignant elements, most frequently astrocytoma and oligodendroglioma.

nasal g., term for a lesion that is probably not a true neoplasm, but an unusual anomaly consisting of glial tissue with reactive astrocytes, ganglionic neurons, and ependymal cells in small nodules at the base of the nose.

g. of optic chiasm, a slow-growing tumor, usually an astrocytoma, of the optic chiasm in children.

optic nerve g., a g., generally an astrocytoma, involving the optic nerve or chiasm.

g. of the spinal cord, a glial tumor of the spinal cord, commonly an ependymoma; neoplasms of the spinal cord are relatively rare, but g.'s constitute approximately one-fourth of the total.

telangiectatic g., g. telangiecto′des, a g. in which the stroma has numerous, conspicuous, frequently dilated small blood vessels and capillaries, as well as large, endothelium-rimmed lakes of blood.

gli·o·ma·to·sis (glī-ō-mă-tō′sis). Neoplastic growth of neuroglial cells in the brain or spinal cord; the term is used especially with reference to a relatively large neoplasm or to multiple foci. SYN neurogliomatosis.

g. cerebri (glī′ō-blas-tō′sis ser′ĕ-brī), a diffuse intracranial neoplasm of astrocytic origin. SYN astrocytosis cerebri, glioblastosis cerebri.

gli·o·ma·tous (glī-ō′mă-tŭs). Pertaining to or characterized by a glioma.

gli·o·myx·o·ma (glī′ō-mik-sō′mă). A myxoma that contains a considerable amount of proliferating glial cells and fibers.

gli·o·neu·ro·ma (glī′ō-nū-rō′mă). A ganglioneuroma derived from neurons, with numerous glial cells and fibers in the matrix.

gli·o·sar·co·ma (glī′ō-sar-kō′mă). A glioblastoma multiforme with an associated malignant mesenchymal component. Sometimes used as a term for a malignant neoplasm derived from connective tissue (*e.g.,* that associated with blood vessels in the brain) in which there are proliferating glial cells.

gli·o·sis (glī-ō′sis). Overgrowth of the astrocytes in an area of damage in the brain or spinal cord.

isomorphous g., a gliosis in which there is a regular and ordered arrangement of glial fibers.

piloid g., an area of chronic, reactive astrocytosis composed of thin, hairlike cells in vaguely parallel array.

g. u′teri, fetal neural tissue persisting or recurring locally as a benign condition in the endometrium or cervix; possibly derived from a homograft of fetal glial stroma.

glip·i·zide (glip′i-zīd). 1-Cyclohexyl-3-[[*p*-[2-(5-methylpyrazinecarboxamido)ethyl]phenyl]sulfonyl]urea; an oral sulfonylurea used in the treatment of type II diabetes.

Glisson, Francis, English physician, anatomist, physiologist and pathologist, 1597–1677. SEE G.'s *capsule, cirrhosis, sphincter.*

glis·so·ni·tis (glis-ŏ-nī′tis). Inflammation of Glisson's capsule, or the connective tissue surrounding the portal vein and the hepatic artery and bile ducts.

Gln Symbol for glutamine or its acyl radical, glutaminyl.

glob·al (glō′băl). The complete, generalized, overall, or total aspect.

globe (glōb). SYN globus.

g. of eye, SYN eyeball.

pale g., SYN *globus* pallidus.

glo·bi (glō′bī). **1.** Plural of globus. **2.** Brown bodies sometimes found in the granulomatous lesions of leprosy, in addition to the macrophages that contain the acid-fast bacilli; thought to be degenerate forms of such cells, in which the organisms are no longer viable and have become granular or amorphous.

glo·bin (glō′bin). The protein of hemoglobin; α-g. and β-g. represent the two types of chains found in adult hemoglobin. SYN hematohiston.

Glo·bo·ceph·a·lus (glō-bō-sef′ă-lŭs). A genus of hookworm (subfamily Uncinariinae, family Ancylostomatidae) consisting of about five species, found chiefly in the small intestine of pigs. The species *G. urosubalatus,* of worldwide distribution, is a common hookworm of wild and domestic pigs.

glo·bo·side (glō′bō-sīd). A glycosphingolipid; specifically, a ceramide tetrasaccharide (tetraglycosylceramide), isolated from kidney and erythrocytes, of the structure: *N*-acetylgalactosaminyl-(β1→3)galactosyl(α1→4)galactosyl(β1→4)glucosylceramide; accumulates in individuals with Sandhoff's disease.

glo·bo·tri·a·o·syl·cer·a·mide (glō′bō-trī-ă-ō-sil-ser-a-mīd). A sphingolipid containing three sugar moieties that accumulates in individuals with Fabry's disease. SYN trihexosylceramide.

glob·ule (glob′yūl). **1.** A small spherical body of any kind. **2.** A fat droplet in milk. SYN globulus. [L. *globulus,* dim. of *globus,* a ball]

dentin g., calcospherites formed by calcification or mineralization of the dentin occurring in globular areas.

Morgagni's g.'s, vesicles beneath the capsule and between lens fibers in early cataract. SYN Morgagni's spheres.

polar g., SYN polar *body.*

glob·u·lif·er·ous (glob-yū-lif′er-ŭs). Containing globules or corpuscles, especially red blood cells. [L. *globulus,* globule, + *fero,* to bear]

glob·u·lin (glob′yū-lin). Name for a family of proteins precipitated from plasma (or serum) by half-saturation with ammonium sulfate (*i.e.,* addition of an equal volume of saturated ammonium sulfate). G.'s may be further fractionated by solubility, electrophoresis, ultracentrifugation, and other separation methods into many subgroups, the main groups being α-, β-, and γ-g.; these differ with respect to associated lipids or carbohydrates and in their content of many physiologically important factors. Among the latter are immunoglobulins (antibodies) in the β and γ fractions, lipoproteins in the α and β fractions, gluco- or mucoproteins (orosomucoid, haptoglobin), and metal-binding and metal-transporting proteins (transferrin, siderophilin, ceruloplasmin). Other substances found in g. fractions are: macroglobulin, plasminogen, prothrombin, euglobulin, antihemophilic g., fibrinogen, cryoglobulin. [L. *globulus,* globule]

accelerator g. (AcG, ac-g) [MIM*227300], g. in serum that promotes the conversion of prothrombin to thrombin in the presence of thromboplastin and ionized calcium. SEE *factor* V$_a$, *factor* V, serum accelerator g.

antihemophilic g. (AHG), (1) SYN *factor* VIII. **(2)** SYN human antihemophilic *factor.*

antihemophilic g. A, SYN *factor* VIII.

antihemophilic g. B, SYN *factor* IX.

antihuman g., serum from a rabbit or other animal previously immunized with purified human g. to prepare antibodies directed against IgG and complement; used in the direct and indirect Coombs' tests. SYN Coombs' serum.

antilymphocyte g. (ALG), SYN antilymphocyte *serum.*

β$_{1C}$ g., the third component (C3) of complement. SEE *component* of complement.

β$_{1E}$ g., the fourth component (C4) of complement. SEE *component* of complement.

β$_{1F}$ g., the fifth component (C5) of complement. SEE *component* of complement.

chickenpox immune g. (human), g. fraction of serum from persons recently recovered from herpes zoster infection; used to prevent infection of high-risk children. SYN chickenpox immunoglobulin.

corticosteroid-binding g. (CBG), SYN transcortin.

gonadal steroid-binding g. (GBG), a protein that transports 65% of the testosterone in plasma. SYN sex steroid-binding g.

human gamma g., a preparation of the proteins of liquid human plasma, containing the antibodies of normal adults; it is obtained

gl

from pooled liquid human plasma from a number of donors and may be prepared by precipitation with organic solvents under controlled conditions of pH, ionic strength, and temperature. SYN human normal immunoglobulin.

immune serum g., a sterile solution of g.'s that contains many antibodies normally present in adult human blood; a passive immunizing agent frequently used for prophylaxis against hepatitis A.

measles immune g. (human), a sterile solution of g.'s derived from the blood plasma of normal adult human donors; it is prepared from immune serum g. that complies with the measles antibody reference standard; a passive immunizing agent. SYN measles immunoglobulin.

pertussis immune g., a sterile solution of g.'s derived from the plasma of adult human donors who have been immunized with pertussis vaccine; used both prophylactically and therapeutically. SYN pertussis immunoglobulin.

plasma accelerator g., SYN *factor* V.

poliomyelitis immune g. (human), a sterile solution of g.'s that contains those antibodies normally present in adult human blood; it is a passive immunologic agent that attenuates or prevents poliomyelitis, measles, and infectious hepatitis, and confers temporary but significant protection against paralytic polio. SYN poliomyelitis immunoglobulin.

rabies immune g. (human), g. fraction of pooled plasma of high anti-rabies virus titer from immunized persons. SYN rabies immunoglobulin.

$RH_o(D)$ immune g., a g. fraction of antibody, derived from human donors, specific for the most common antigen, $Rh_o(D)$, of the Rh group; used to prevent Rh-sensitization of an Rh-negative woman after delivery of an Rh-positive fetus. SYN anti-D immunoglobulin, $Rh_o(D)$ immunoglobulin.

serum accelerator g., a substance in serum that accelerates the conversion of prothrombin to thrombin in the presence of thromboplastin and calcium; produced by the action of traces of thrombin upon plasma accelerator g.

sex hormone-binding g. (SHBG), a plasma β-g., produced by the liver, that binds testosterone and, with a weaker affinity, estrogen; serum levels of SHBG in women are twice the levels seen in men; serum concentrations are increased in certain types of liver disease and in hyperthyroidism; are decreased with advancing age, by androgens, and in hypothyroidism. SYN testosterone-estrogen-binding g.

sex steroid-binding g., SYN gonadal steroid-binding g.

specific immune g. (human), g. fraction of pooled serums (or plasma) selected for high titer of antibodies specific for a particular antigen, or from persons specifically immunized.

testosterone-estrogen-binding g., SYN sex hormone-binding g.

tetanus immune g., a sterile solution of g.'s derived from the blood plasma of adult human donors who have been immunized with tetanus toxoid; a passive immunizing agent. SYN tetanus immunoglobulin.

thyroxine-binding g. (TBG), an α-globulin of blood with a strong binding affinity for thyroxine; triiodothyronine is bound to it much less firmly; a deficiency or excess of this protein may occur as a rare benign X-linked disorder. SYN thyroxine-binding protein (1).

zoster immune g., a g. fraction of pooled plasma from individuals who have recovered from herpes zoster; used prophylactically and therapeutically for varicella.

glob·u·li·nu·ria (glob′yū-li-nū′rē-ă). The excretion of globulin in the urine, usually, if not always, in association with serum albumin.

glob·u·lus (glob′yū-lŭs). SYN globule. [L.]

glo·bus, pl. **glo·bi** (glō′bŭs, -bī). **1** [NA]. A round body; ball. **2.** SEE globi. SYN globe. [L.]

g. hyster′icus, difficulty in swallowing; a sensation as of a ball in the throat or as if the throat were compressed; a symptom of conversion *disorder.*

g. ma′jor, SYN *head* of epididymis.

g. mi′nor, SYN *tail* of epididymis.

g. pal′lidus [NA], the inner and lighter gray portion of the lentiform nucleus. SEE ALSO paleostriatum. SYN pale globe, pallidum.

glo·mal (glō′măl). Relating to or involving a glomus.

glo·man·gi·o·ma (glō-man-jē-ō′mă). A variant of glomus *tumor,* characterized by multiple tumors resembling cavernous hemangioma.

glo·man·gi·o·sis (glō-man-jē-ō′sis). The occurrence of multiple complexes of small vascular channels, each resembling a glomus.

pulmonary g., g. occurring within small pulmonary arteries in severe pulmonary hypertension and congenital heart disease.

glome (glōm). SYN glomus.

glo·mec·to·my (glō-mek′tō-mē). Excision of a glomus tumor. [L. *glomus* + G. *ektomē,* cutting out]

glom·era (glom′er-ă). Plural of glomus.

glom·era aor·ti·ca. SYN para-aortic *bodies,* under *body.*

glo·mer·u·lar (glō-mār′yū-lăr). Relating to or affecting a glomerulus or the glomeruli. SYN glomerulose.

glom·er·ule (glom′er-yūl). SYN glomerulus.

glo·mer·u·li·tis (glō-mār′yū-lī′tis). Inflammation of a glomerulus, specifically of the renal glomeruli, as in glomerulonephritis.

glo·mer·u·lo·ne·phri·tis (glō-mār′yū-lō-nef-rī′tis). Renal disease characterized by bilateral inflammatory changes in glomeruli which are not the result of infection of the kidneys. SYN glomerular nephritis. [glomerulus + G. *nephros,* kidney, + *-itis,* inflammation]

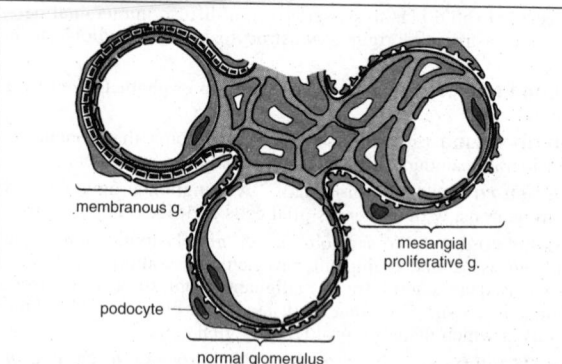

membranous g.

mesangial proliferative g.

podocyte

normal glomerulus

glomerulonephritis (schematic view of two typical forms)
left: membranous g., with spikes of basement membrane material, deposits of immunoglobulins, and loss of foot processes; right: mesangial proliferative g., with increase in mesangial cells and matrix, and narrowing of the capillary lumina

acute g., g. that frequently occurs as a late complication of pharyngitis, especially due to type 12 β-hemolytic streptococci, characterized by abrupt onset of hematuria, edema of the face, oliguria, and variable azotemia and hypertension; the renal glomeruli usually show cellular proliferation or infiltration by polymorphonuclear leukocytes. SYN acute hemorrhagic g., acute nephritis, acute post-streptococcal g.

acute crescentic g., SYN rapidly progressive g.

acute hemorrhagic g., SYN acute g.

acute post-streptococcal g., SYN acute g.

anti-basement membrane g., g. resulting from anti-basement membrane antibodies, characterized by smooth linear deposits of IgG and C3 along glomerular capillary walls; includes rapidly progressive g. and g. in Goodpasture's syndrome.

Berger's focal g., SYN focal g.

chronic g., g. that presents with persisting proteinuria, chronic renal failure, and hypertension, of insidious onset or as a late sequel of acute g.; the kidneys are symmetrically contracted and granular, with scarring and loss of glomeruli and the presence of tubular atrophy and interstitial fibrosis. SYN chronic nephritis.

diffuse g., g. affecting most of the renal glomeruli; it may lead to azotemia.

Ellis type 1 g., obsolete designation for g. presenting as acute g., followed by complete recovery in most cases, or the development of rapidly progressive g., or incomplete remission with persistent proteinuria and subsequent development of chronic g. SYN Ellis type 1 nephritis.

Ellis type 2 g., obsolete designation for g. which is usually not related to preceding bacterial infection; characterized by an insidious onset of the nephrotic syndrome, failure of complete remission, and eventual development of chronic renal failure. The kidneys usually show membranous g. SYN Ellis type 2 nephritis.

exudative g., g. with infiltration of glomeruli by polymorphonuclear leukocytes, occurring in acute g.

focal g., g. affecting a small proportion of renal glomeruli which commonly presents with hematuria and may be associated with acute upper respiratory infection in young males, not usually due to streptococci; associated with IgA deposits in the glomerular mesangium and may also be associated with systemic disease, as in Henoch-Schönlein purpura. SYN Berger's disease, Berger's focal g., focal nephritis, IgA nephropathy.

focal embolic g., g. associated with subacute bacterial endocarditis, frequently producing microscopic hematuria without azotemia.

hypocomplementemic g., SYN membranoproliferative g.

immune complex g., immune complexes are deposited in the renal glomerulus where they bind complement and initiate an inflammatory process attracting neutrophils and macrophages resulting in an alteration of the basement layer of the kidney. The disease state can lead to ultimate destruction of the glomerulus and renal failure.

lobular g., SYN membranoproliferative g.

local g., SYN segmental g.

membranoproliferative g., chronic g. characterized by mesangial cell proliferation, increased lobular separation of glomeruli, thickening of glomerular capillary walls and increased mesangial matrix, and low serum levels of complement; occurs mainly in older children, with a variably slow progressive course, episodes of hematuria or edema, and hypertension. It is classified into three types: type 1, the commonest, in which there are subendothelial electron-dense deposits; type 2, dense-deposit disease, in which the lamina densa is greatly thickened by extremely electron-dense material; type 3, in which there are both subendothelial and subepithelial deposits. SYN hypocomplementemic g., lobular g., mesangiocapillary g.

membranous g., g. characterized by diffuse thickening of glomerular capillary basement membranes, due in part to subepithelial deposits of immunoglobulins separated by spikes of basement membrane material, and clinically by an insidious onset of the nephrotic syndrome and failure of disappearance of proteinuria; the disease is most commonly idiopathic but may be secondary to malignant tumors, drugs, infections, or systemic lupus erythematosus.

mesangial proliferative g., g. characterized clinically by the nephrotic syndrome and histologically by diffuse glomerular increases in endocapillary and mesangial cells and in mesangial matrix; in some cases, there are mesangial deposits of IgM and complement. SYN diffuse mesangial proliferation, IgM nephropathy.

mesangiocapillary g., SYN membranoproliferative g.

proliferative g., g. with hypercellularity of glomeruli due to proliferation of endothelial or mesangial cells, occurring in acute g. and membranoproliferative g.

rapidly progressive g., g. usually presenting insidiously, without preceding streptococcal infection, with increasing renal failure leading to death within a few months; at autopsy the kidneys are normal in size, numerous glomerular capsular epithelial crescents are present, and antiglomerular basement membrane antibodies are frequently found. SYN acute crescentic g.

segmental g., g. affecting only part of a glomerulus or glomeruli. SYN local g.

subacute g., undesirable term for g. with proteinuria, hematuria

and azotemia persisting for many weeks; renal changes are variable, including those of rapidly progressive and membranoproliferative g. SYN subacute nephritis.

glo·mer·u·lop·a·thy (glō-mār-yū-lop′ă-thē). Glomerular disease of any type. [glomerulus + G. *pathos,* suffering]

focal sclerosing g., focal, segmental glomerulosclerosis reported in adults and children with normal serum complement, progressing to chronic glomerulonephritis.

glo·mer·u·lo·scle·ro·sis (glo-mār′yū-lō-sklĕ-rō′sis). Hyaline deposits or scarring within the renal glomeruli, a degenerative process occurring in association with renal arteriosclerosis or diabetes. SYN glomerular sclerosis. [glomerulus + G. *sklērōsis,* hardness]

diabetic g., rounded hyaline or laminated nodules in the periphery of the glomeruli with capillary basement membrane thickening and increased mesangial matrix occurring in long-standing diabetes, proteinuria, and ultimately renal failure. SYN intercapillary g.

focal segmental g., segmental collapse of glomerular capillaries with thickened basement membranes and increased mesangial matrix; seen in some glomeruli of patients with nephrotic syndrome or mesangial proliferative glomerulonephritis.

intercapillary g., SYN diabetic g.

glo·mer·u·lose (glō-mār′yū-lōs). SYN glomerular.

glo·mer·u·lus, pl. **glo·mer·u·li** (glō-mār′yū-lŭs, -yū-lī) [NA]. **1.** A plexus of capillaries. **2.** A tuft formed of capillary loops at the beginning of each nephric tubule in the kidney; this tuft with its capsule (Bowman's capsule) constitutes the corpusculum renis (malpighian body). SYN malpighian g., malpighian tuft. **3.** The twisted secretory portion of a sweat gland. **4.** A cluster of dendritic ramifications and axon terminals forming a complex synaptic relationship and surrounded by a glial sheath. SYN glomerule. [Mod. L. dim. of L. *glomus,* a ball of yarn]

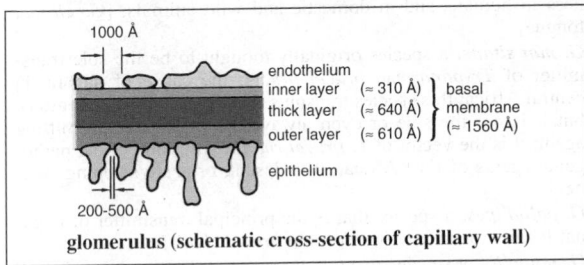

glomerulus (schematic cross-section of capillary wall)

juxtamedullary g., a g. close to the medullary border.

malpighian g., SYN glomerulus (2).

g. of mesonephros, one of the tufts of capillary vessels within the mesonephros derived from a lateral branch of the primary aorta; each g. is connected to a tubule.

olfactory g., one of the small spherical territories in the olfactory bulb in which dendrites of mitral and tufted cells synapse with axons of olfactory receptor cells.

g. of pronephros, one of the tufts of capillary vessels in the pronephros derived from a lateral branch of the aorta.

glo·mus, pl. **glom·era** (glō′mŭs, glom′er-ă). **1** [NA]. A small globular body. **2.** A highly organized arteriolovenular anastomosis forming a tiny nodular focus in the nailbed, pads of the fingers and toes, ears, hands, and feet and many other organs of the body. The afferent arteriole enters the connective tissue capsule of the g., becomes devoid of an internal elastic membrane, and develops a relatively thick epithelioid muscular wall and small lumen; the anastomosis may be branched and convoluted, richly innervated with sympathetic and myelinated nerves, and connected with a short, thin-walled vein that drains into a periglomic vein and then into one of the veins of the skin. The g. functions as a shunt- or bypass-regulating mechanism in the flow of blood, temperature, and conservation of heat in the part as well as in the indirect control of the blood pressure and other functions of the circulatory system. SYN glandulae glomiformes (1) [NA], glomiform glands, glomus body. SYN glome. [L. *glomus,* a ball]

g. carot'icum [NA], SYN carotid *body*.

choroid g., a marked enlargement of the choroid plexus of the lateral ventricle at the junction of the central part with the inferior horn. SYN g. choroideum [NA], choroid skein.

g. choroide'um [NA], SYN choroid g.

g. coccy'geum, SYN coccygeal *body*.

intravagal g., a minute collection of chemoreceptor cells on the auricular branch of the vagus nerve. A tumor of this g. may cause deafness and tinnitus. SYN g. intravagale.

g. intravaga'le, SYN intravagal g.

jugular g., a microscopic collection of chemoreceptor tissue in the adventitia of the jugular bulb; a tumor of this g. may cause paralysis of the vocal cords, attacks of dizziness, blackouts, and nystagmus. SYN g. jugulare.

g. jugula're, SYN jugular g.

g. pulmona'le, SYN pulmonary g.

pulmonary g., a structure similar to the carotid body, found in relation to the pulmonary artery. SYN g. pulmonale.

glo·no·in (glō'nō-in). SYN nitroglycerin.

⌂gloss-. SEE glosso-.

glos·sa (glos'ă). SYN tongue (1). [G.]

glos·sag·ra (glos-ag'ră). Glossalgia of gouty origin. [gloss- + G. *agra*, a seizure]

glos·sal (glos'ăl). SYN lingual (1).

glos·sal·gia (glos-al'jē-ă). SYN glossodynia. [gloss- + G. *algos*, pain]

glos·sec·to·my (glo-sek'tō-mē). Resection or amputation of the tongue. SYN elinguation, glossosteresis, lingulectomy (1). [gloss- + G. *ektomē*, excision]

Glos·si·na (glo-sī'nă). A genus of bloodsucking Diptera (tsetse flies) confined to Africa; they serve as vectors of the pathogenic trypanosomes that cause various forms of African sleeping sickness in humans and in domestic and wild animals. [G. *glōssa*, tongue]

G. mor'sitans, a species originally thought to be the sole transmitter of *Trypanosoma brucei brucei*, the cause of nagana in central Africa; this species transmits this disease in some regions, but it is not the sole or even always the principal transmitting agent; it is the vector of *T. brucei rhodesiense*, one of the pathogenic agents of East African, Rhodesian, or acute sleeping sickness.

G. pallid'ipes, a species that is the principal transmitter of nagana; it also transmits *Trypanosoma brucei rhodesiense*.

G. palpa'lis, a species of *G.* that transmits *Trypanosoma brucei gambiense*, one of the pathogenic parasites of West African, Gambian, or chronic sleeping sickness.

glos·si·tis (glo-sī'tis). Inflammation of the tongue. [gloss- + G. *-itis*, inflammation]

g. area'ta exfoliati'va, SYN geographic *tongue*.

atrophic g., an erythematous, edematous, and painful tongue which appears smooth due to loss of the filiform and sometimes the fungiform papillae secondary to certain nutritional deficiencies, especially B-vitamin deficencies, as seen in pellagra, thiamin deficiency, and disorders such as pernicious anemia (Hunter's or Moeller's g.). SYN bald tongue.

benign migratory g., SYN geographic *tongue*.

g. desic'cans, a painful affection of the tongue, of unknown origin, in which the surface becomes raw and fissured.

Hunter's g., SEE atrophic g.

median rhomboid g., an asymptomatic, ovoid or rhomboid, macular or mamellated, erythematous lesion with papillary atrophy on the dorsum of the tongue just anterior to the circumvallate papillae; thought to represent a persistent tuberculum impar.

Moeller's g., SEE atrophic g.

⌂glosso-, gloss-. Language; corresponds to L. *linguo-*. Cf. linguo-. [G. *glōssa*, tongue]

glos·so·cele (glos'ō-sēl). Protrusion of the tongue from the mouth, owing to its excessive size. SEE ALSO macroglossia. [glosso- + G. *kēlē*, tumor, hernia]

glos·so·cin·es·thet·ic (glos'ō-sin-es-thet'ik). SYN glossokinesthetic.

glos·so·don·to·tro·pism (glos-ō-don'tō-trō-pizm). A manifestation of tension or anxiety in which the tongue is attracted to the teeth or to dental faults. [glosso- + G. *odous (odont-)*, tooth, + *tropē*, a turning]

glos·so·dy·na·mom·e·ter (glos'ō-dī-nă-mom'ĕ-ter). An apparatus for estimating the contractile force of the tongue muscles. [glosso- + G. *dynamis*, power, + *metron*, measure]

glos·so·dyn·ia (glos'ō-din'ē-ă). A condition characterized by burning or painful tongue. SYN glossalgia, glossopyrosis. [glosso- + G. *odynē*, pain]

glos·so·dyn·i·o·tro·pism (glos-ō-din'ē-ō-trō-pizm). Apparent satisfaction from subjecting the tongue to a pain-inducing dental fault; considered by some to be a masochistic behavior or manifestation. [glosso- + G. *odynē*, pain, + *tropē*, a turning]

glos·so·ep·i·glot·tic, glos·so·ep·i·glot·tid·e·an (glos'ō-ep-i-glot'ik, glos'ō-ep-i-glo-tid'ē-an). Relating to the tongue and the epiglottis.

glos·so·graph (glos'ō-graf). An instrument for recording the movements of the tongue in speaking. [glosso- + G. *graphō*, to write]

glos·so·hy·al (glos-ō-hī'ăl). SYN hyoglossal.

glos·so·kin·es·thet·ic (glos'ō-kin-es-thet'ik). Denoting the subjective sensation of the movements of the tongue. SYN glossocinesthetic. [glosso- + G. *kinēsis*, movement, + *aisthētikos*, perceptive]

glos·so·la·lia (glos-ō-lā'lē-ă). Rarely used term for unintelligible jargon or babbling. [glosso- + G. *lalia*, talk, chat]

glos·sol·o·gy (glos-ol'ō-jē). The branch of medical science concerned with the tongue and its diseases. SYN glottology. [glosso- + G. *logos*, study]

glos·sol·y·sis (glos-ol'i-sis). Paralysis of the tongue. SYN glossoplegia. [glosso- + G. *lysis*, a loosening]

glos·son·cus (glos-ong'kŭs). Any swelling involving the tongue, including neoplasms. [glosso- + G. *onkos*, mass, tumor]

glos·so·pal·a·ti·nus (glos'ō-pal-ă-tī'nŭs). SYN palatoglossus *muscle*. [glosso- + Mod. L. *palatinus*, fr. L. *palatum*, palate]

glos·sop·a·thy (glos-op'ă-thē). A disease of the tongue. [glosso- + G. *pathos*, suffering]

glos·so·pha·ryn·ge·al (glos'ō-fă-rin'jē-ăl). Relating to the tongue and the pharynx.

glos·so·pha·ryn·ge·us (glos'ō-fă-rin'jē-ŭs). SEE superior constrictor *muscle* of pharynx.

glos·so·plas·ty (glos'ō-plas-tē). Plastic surgery of the tongue. [glosso- + G. *plastos*, formed]

glos·so·ple·gia (glos-ō-plē'jē-ă). SYN glossolysis. [glosso- + G. *plēgē*, stroke]

glos·sop·to·sis, glos·sop·to·sia (glos-op-tō'sis, -op-tō'sē-ă). Downward displacement of the tongue. [glosso- + G. *ptōsis*, a falling]

glos·so·py·ro·sis (glos-ō-pī-rō'sis). SYN glossodynia. [glosso- + G. *pyrōsis*, a burning]

glos·sor·rha·phy (glo-sōr'ă-fē). Suture of a wound of the tongue. [glosso- + G. *rhaphē*, suture]

glos·so·spasm (glos'ō-spazm). Spasmodic contraction of the tongue.

glos·so·ste·re·sis (glos-ō-ste-rē'sis). SYN glossectomy.

glos·sot·o·my (glo-sot'ō-mē). Any cutting operation on the tongue, usually to obtain access to further reaches of the pharynx. [glosso- + G. *tomē*, incision]

glos·so·trich·ia (glos-ō-trik'ē-ă). SYN hairy *tongue*. [glosso- + G. *thrix*, hair]

glot·tal (glot'ăl). Relating to the glottis.

glot·tic (glot'ik). Relating to (1) the tongue or (2) the glottis.

glot·ti·do·spasm (glot'i-dō-spazm). SYN laryngospasm.

glot·tis, pl. **glot·ti·des** (glot'is, glot'i-dēz) [NA]. The vocal apparatus of the larynx, consisting of the vocal folds of mucous membrane investing the vocal ligament and vocal muscle on each side, the free edges of which are the vocal cords, and of a median fissure, the rima glottidis. [G. *glōttis*, aperture of the larynx]

false g., SYN *rima* vestibuli.

g. respirato'ria, SYN intercartilaginous *part* of rima glottidis.

g. spu'ria, SYN *rima* vestibuli.

true g., SYN *rima* glottidis.

g. ve'ra, SYN *rima* glottidis.

g. voca'lis, SYN intermembranous *part* of rima glottidis.

glot·ti·tis (glo-tī'tis). Inflammation of the glottic portion of the larynx.

glot·tol·o·gy (glo-tol'ŏ-jē). SYN glossology. [G. *glōssa, glōtta,* tongue, + *logos,* study]

Glo·ver. J.A., 20th century British physician.

Glp Abbreviation for 5-oxoproline.

Glu Symbol for glutamic acid or its acyl radical, glutamyl.

glu·ca·gon (glū'kă-gon). A hormone consisting of a straight-chain polypeptide of 29 amino acid residues (bovine g.), extracted from pancreatic alpha cells. Parenteral administration of 0.5 to 1 mg results in prompt mobilization of hepatic glycogen, thus elevating blood glucose concentration. It activates hepatic phosphorylase, thereby increasing glycogenolysis, decreases gastric motility and gastric and pancreatic secretions, and increases urinary excretion of nitrogen and potassium; it has no effect on muscle phosphorylase. As the hydrochloride, it is used in the treatment of glycogen storage disease (von Gierke's) and hypoglycemia, particularly hypoglycemic coma due to exogenously administered insulin. SYN HG factor, hyperglycemic-glycogenolytic factor, pancreatic hyperglycemic hormone. [glucose + G. *agō,* to lead]

gut g., a substance of intestinal origin that is secreted into the blood following ingestion of glucose and is a potent stimulus to the secretion of insulin; its chemical structure and the biologic effects that it produces are different from those of g., and it cross-reacts with antibodies to g.

glu·ca·gon·o·ma (glu'kă-gon-ō'mă). A glucagon-secreting tumor, usually derived from pancreatic islet cells.

glu·cal (glū'kăl). SYN glycal.

glu·can (glū'kan). A polyglucose; *e.g.,* callose, cellulose, starch amylose, glycogen amylose.

α-glu·can branch·ing gly·co·syl·trans·fer·ase. SYN 1,4-α-D-glucan branching enzyme.

1,4-α-D-glu·can 6-α-D-glu·co·syl·trans·fer·ase. A glucosyltransferase that transfers an α-glucosyl residue in a 1,4-α-glucan to the primary hydroxyl group of glucose in a 1,4-α-glucan. SEE ALSO 1,4-α-D-glucan branching enzyme. SYN oligoglucan-branching glycosyltransferase.

4-α-D-glu·can·o·trans·fer·ase. Dextrin transglycosylase or glycosyltransferase; a 4-glycosyltransferase converting maltodextrins into amylose and glucose by transferring parts of 1,4-glucan chains to new 4-positions on glucose or other 1,4-glucans. SYN amylomaltase, D enzyme, dextrin glycosyltransferase, dextrin transglycosylase, disproportionating enzyme.

α-glu·can phos·pho·ryl·ase. SYN phosphorylase.

glu·cas·es (glū'cās-ez). Obsolete term for enzymes cleaving starch to glucose.

glu·ce·mia (glū-sē'mē-ă). Obsolete term for glycemia.

glu·cep·tate (glū-sep'tat). USAN-approved contraction for glucoheptonate.

glu·ci·phore (glū'si-fōr). Term coined for chemical groups believed to be responsible for sweet taste. [G. *glykys,* sweet, + *phoros,* bearing]

⌂**gluco-.** Combining form denoting relationship to glucose. SEE ALSO glyco-. [G. *gleukos,* sweet new wine, sweetness]

glu·co·am·y·lase (glū-kō-am'i-lās). SYN exo-1,4-α-D-glucosidase.

glu·co·a·scor·bic ac·id (glū'kŏ-as-kōr'bik). 3-Keto-D-glucoheptonofuranolactone; a compound resembling ascorbic acid but with an additional –CHOH– between C-5 and C-6 of ascorbic acid; shows toxic effects on addition to diet which apparently are not caused by ascorbic acid antagonism.

β-glu·co·cer·e·bro·sid·ase (glū'kō-ser'ĕ-brō-sīd-ās). An enzyme that hydrolyzes β-glucosides in cerebrosides; a deficiency of this enzyme results in Gaucher disease.

glu·co·cer·e·bro·side (glū-kō-ser'ĕ-brō-sīd). SYN glucosylceramide.

glu·co·cor·ti·coid (glū-kō-kōr'ti-koyd). **1.** Any steroid-like compound capable of significantly influencing intermediary metabolism such as promotion of hepatic glycogen deposition, and of exerting a clinically useful anti-inflammatory effect. Cortisol is the most potent of the naturally occurring g.'s; most semisynthetic g.'s are cortisol derivatives. **2.** Denoting this type of biological activity. SYN glycocorticoid.

glu·co·cor·ti·co·tro·phic (glū'kō-kōr'ti-kō-trōf'ik). Denoting a principle of the anterior hypophysis that stimulates the production of glucocorticoid hormones of the adrenal cortex; no hormone exerting only this effect has been identified, but ACTH does stimulate adrenal corticoid production.

glu·co·cy·a·mine (glū-kō-sī'ă-mēn). SYN glycocyamine.

glu·co·fu·ra·nose (glū-kō-fūr'ă-nōs). Glucose in furanose form.

glu·co·gen·e·sis (glū-kō-jen'ĕ-sis). Formation of glucose. [gluco- + G. *genesis,* production]

glu·co·gen·ic (glū-kō-jen'ik). Giving rise to or producing glucose. SYN glucoplastic.

glu·co·he·mia (glū-kō-hē'mē-ă). Obsolete term for glycemia.

glu·co·in·vert·ase (glū-kō-in'ver-tās). SYN α-D-glucosidase.

glu·co·ki·nase (glū-kō-kī'nās). Phosphotransferase that catalyzes the conversion of D-glucose and ATP D-glucose 6-phosphate and ADP; the liver enzyme has a higher K_m value for D-glucose than does hexokinase.

glu·co·ki·net·ic (glū'kō-ki-net'ik). Tending to mobilize glucose; usually evidenced by a reduction of the glycogen stores in the tissues to produce an increase in the concentration of glucose circulating in the blood.

glu·co·lip·ids (glū-kō-lip'idz). Glycosphingolipids that contain D-glucose.

glu·col·y·sis (glū-kol'i-sis). SYN glycolysis.

glu·co·ne·o·gen·e·sis (glū'kō-nē-ō-jen'ĕ-sis). The formation of glucose from noncarbohydrates, such as protein or fat. Cf. glyconeogenesis.

glu·con·ic ac·id (glū-kon'ik). The hexonic (aldonic) acid derived from glucose by oxidation of the –CHO group to –COOH.

glu·con·o·lac·to·nase (glū'kon-o-lak'tō-nās). An enzyme catalyzing the hydrolysis of D-glucono-δ-lactone to D-gluconic acid. SYN lactonase.

glu·co·pe·nia (glū-kō-pē'nē-ă). SYN hypoglycemia. [gluco- + G. *penia,* poverty]

glu·co·plas·tic. SYN glucogenic.

glu·co·pro·tein (glū-kō-prō'tēn). A glycoprotein in which the sugar is glucose.

glu·co·pyr·a·nose (glū-kō-pir'ă-nōs). Glucose in its pyranose form.

glu·co·sa·mine (glū'kō-să-mēn). 2-Amino-2-deoxyglucose; an amino sugar found in chitin, cell membranes, and mucopolysaccharides generally; used as a pharmaceutic aid.

glu·cos·a·mi·no·gly·cans (glū-kō-smen-ō-glī'kans). Glycosaminoglycans (or mucopolysaccharides) in which all of the constituent sugar amines are glucosamines.

glu·co·sans (glū'kō-sanz). Polysaccharides yielding glucose upon hydrolysis; *e.g.,* cellulose, glycogen, starch, dextrins.

D-glu·cose (G, Glc) (glū'kōs). D-Glucose; a dextrorotatory monosaccharide (hexose) found in the free state in fruits and other parts of plants, and combined in glucosides, disaccharides (often with fructose in sugars), oligosaccharides, and polysaccharides; it is the product of complete hydrolysis of cellulose, starch, and glycogen. Free g. also occurs in the blood (normal human concentration, 70 to 110 mg per 100 ml); in diabetes mellitus, it appears in the urine. The epimers of D-g. are D-allose, D-mannose, D-galactose, and L-idose. Dextrose should not be confused with the L-isomer which is sinistrose. SYN cellohexose.

activated g., a nucleoside diphosphoglucose such as UDP glucose.

g. dehydrogenase, converts β-D-glucose to D-glucono-δ-lactone, transferring hydrogen to NAD^+ or $NADP^+$. Cf. g. oxidase.

liquid g., a pharmaceutic aid consisting of dextrose, dextrins,

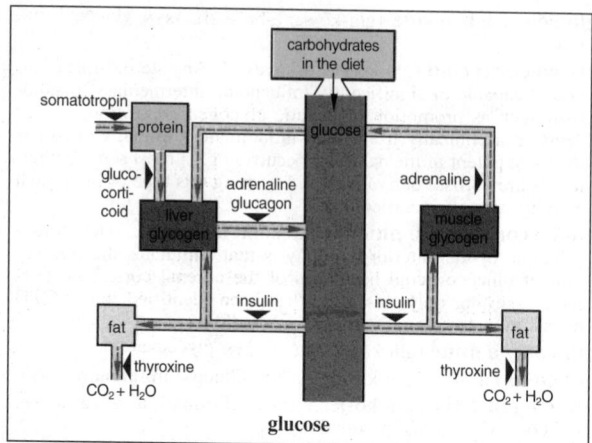

glucose

maltose, and water, obtained by the incomplete hydrolysis of starch.

g. oxidase, an antibacterial flavoprotein enzyme, obtained from *Penicillum notatum* and other fungi, which is antibacterial only in the presence of glucose and oxygen, its effect being due to the oxidation of D-glucose to D-glucono-δ-lactone, with the coconversion of O_2 to H_2O_2; used in the preservation of food and in assays for glucose levels. SYN corylophyline, g. oxyhydrase, microcide.

g. oxyhydrase, SYN g. oxidase.

g. phosphomutase, SYN phosphoglucomutase.

D-glu·cose 1,6-bis·phos·phate. A bisphosphorylated derivative of D-glucose that is a required intermediate in the interconversion of D-glucose 1-phosphate and D-glucose 6-phosphate.

glu·cose-6-phos·pha·tase. A liver enzyme catalyzing the hydrolysis of D-glucose 6-phosphate to D-glucose and inorganic phosphate; this enzyme is deficient in glycogen storage disease Ia.

glu·cose 6-phos·phate. An ester of glucose with phosphoric acid; made in the course of glucose metabolism by mammalian and other cells; a normal constituent of resting muscle, probably always existing in equilibrium with fructose 6-phosphate.

D-glu·cose 1-phos·phate. An important intermediate in glycogenesis and glycogenolysis. SYN Cori ester.

D-glu·cose 6-phos·phate. A key intermediate in glycolysis, glycogenolysis, pentose phosphate shunt, etc.; elevated levels inhibit brain hexokinase and glycolysis. SYN Robison ester, Robison-Embden ester.

glu·cose-6-phos·phate de·hy·dro·gen·ase. An NADP+ enzyme catalyzing the dehydrogenation (oxidation) of D-glucose 6-phosphate to 6-phospho-D-glucono-δ-lactone, this reaction initiating the Dickens shunt. A deficiency of this enzyme can lead to severe hemolytic anemia and favism. A deficiency of the leukocyte enzyme prevents neutrophils expressing respiratory burst. SYN Robison ester dehydrogenase, Zwischenferment.

glu·cose-phos·phate isom·er·ase. An enzyme that catalyzes the reversible interconversion of D-fructose 6-phosphate and D-glucose 6-phosphate; a part of glycolysis and gluconeogenesis; g.-p. i. deficiency is an inherited disorder resulting in liver glycogenesis and hemolytic anemia. SYN hexosephosphate isomerase, phosphohexomutase, phosphohexose isomerase.

glu·cose-1-phos·phate ki·nase. SYN phosphoglucokinase.

glu·cose-1-phos·phate phos·pho·dis·mu·tase. A phosphotransferase catalyzing the reversible transfer of a phosphate residue from one D-glucose 1-phosphate to another, yielding D-glucose 1,6-bisphosphate and D-glucose. This enzyme provides a crucial intermediate needed for glucose-phosphate isomerase.

glu·cose-6-phos·phate trans·lo·case. A transport protein in the membrane of the endoplasmic reticulum; a deficiency of this protein is associated with glycogen storage disease type Ib.

glu·cose-1-phos·phate uri·dyl·yl·trans·fer·ase. An enzyme that activates D-glucose by reacting D-glucose 1-phosphate with

UTP, producing pyrophosphate and UDP glucose; a crucial step in glycogen biosynthesis.

α-D-glu·co·si·dase (glū′kō-si-dās). A glucohydrolase removing terminal nonreducing 1,4-linked α-glucose residues by hydrolysis, yielding α-glucose; a deficiency of the lysosomal enzyme is associated with glycogen storage disease type II. There are at least five isozymes of maltase. SYN glucoinvertase.

β-D-glu·co·si·dase. A glucohydrolase similar to α-D-glucosidase, but attacking β-glucosides and releasing β-D-glucose. SYN amygdalase, cellobiase, gentiobiase.

glu·co·si·das·es (glū′kō-sid-ās-ez). Enzymes that hydrolyze glucosides.

glu·co·side (glū′kō-sīd). A compound of glucose with an alcohol or other R–OH compound involving loss of the H atom of the 1-OH (hemiacetal) group of the glucose, yielding a –C–O–R link from the C-1 of the glucose; a glycoside of glucose.

glu·co·sone (glū′kō-sōn). A 2-dehydrogenation (2-keto) product of glucose; a possible intermediate in the formation of glucosamine from glucose. [glucose + -one]

glu·co·sul·fone so·di·um (glū-kō-sŭl′fōn). p,p′-Sulfonyldianiline N,N′-diglucoside disodium; a chemotherapeutic agent used in the treatment of leprosy; parenteral administration is better tolerated than oral administration.

glu·cos·u·ria (glū-kō-sū′rē-ă). The urinary excretion of glucose, usually in enhanced quantities. SYN glycosuria (1), glycuresis (1). [glucose + G. ouron, urine]

glu·co·syl (glū′kō-sil). The radical of glucose that has lost its hemiacetal (C-1) OH.

glu·co·syl·cer·a·mide (glū′kō-sil-ser′ă-mīd). A neutral glycolipid containing equimolar amounts of fatty acid, glucose, and sphingosine (or a derivative thereof); accumulates in individuals with Gaucher disease. SYN glucocerebroside.

glu·co·syl·trans·fer·ase (glū′kō-sil-trans′fer-ās). Any enzyme transferring glucosyl groups from one compound to another; g.'s are in EC subclass 2.4 (glycosyltransferases). SYN transglucosylase.

glu·cu·ro·nate (glū-kūr′ō-nāt). A salt or ester of glucuronic acid.

glu·cu·rone (glū′kū-rōn). SYN D-glucuronolactone.

glu·cu·ron·ic ac·id (glū-kū-ron′ik). The uronic acid of glucose in which C-6 is oxidized to a carboxyl group; the D-isomer detoxicates or inactivates various substances (e.g., benzoic acid, phenol, camphor, and the female sex hormones) undergoing conjugation with such substances in the liver, the glucuronides so formed being excreted in the urine.

β-D-glu·cu·ron·i·dase (glū-kū-ron′i-dās). An enzyme catalyzing the hydrolysis of various β-D-glucuronides, liberating free D-glucuronic acid and an alcohol; a deficiency of this enzyme is associated with Sly syndrome. SYN glusulase, glycuronidase.

glu·cu·ro·nide (glū-kū′ron-īd). A glycoside of glucuronic acid; many foreign chemicals, as well as catabolic products of normal body constituents (e.g., steroid hormones), are commonly excreted in the urine as D-g.'s, the conjugation taking place in the liver.

D-glu·cu·ron·o·lac·tone (glū′kū-rō′nō-lak′tōn). Lactone of D-glucofuranuronic acid; used as a means of orally administering glucuronic acid in the management of collagen and joint diseases. SYN glucurone.

glu·cu·ron·ose (glū-kū′ron-ōs). Obsolete term for glucuronic acid.

glu·cu·ron·o·syl·trans·fer·ase (glū-kū-ron′ō-sil-trans′fer-ās). Any of a family of enzymes that transfer D-glucuronate to the acceptor named, forming glucuronosides; e.g., UDPglucuronate-bilirubin glucuronosyltransferase.

glue-sniff·ing (glū′snif-ing). Inhalation of fumes from plastic cements; the solvents, which include toluene, xylene, and benzene, induce central nervous system stimulation followed by depression. SEE ALSO solvent *inhalation*.

Gluge, Gottlieb, German histologist, 1812–1898. SEE G.'s *corpuscles*, under *corpuscle*.

glu·sul·ase (glū′sŭl-ās). SYN β-D-glucuronidase.

glu·ta·con·ic ac·id (glū′ta-kon-ik). $HOOCCH_2CH=CHCOOH$; dicarboxylic acid that accumulates in individuals with glutaric acidemia type I.

glu·ta·mate (glū'tă-māt). A salt or ester of glutamic acid.

g. acetyltransferase, an enzyme catalyzing transfer of an acetyl group from N^2-acetylornithine to L-g. forming L-ornithine and N-acetyl-L-glutamate, an activator of the urea cycle. SYN ornithine acetyltransferase.

g. decarboxylase (GAD), a carboxy-lyase converting L-g. to 4-aminobutyrate and CO_2 as well as L-aspartate to 3-aminopropanoate and CO_2; a defect in the binding of this protein's coenzyme is believed to be the cause of pyridoxine dependency with seizures. SYN aspartate 1-decarboxylase.

g. dehydrogenases, enzymes that catalyze the reaction of L-g., H_2O, and NAD^+ (or $NADP^+$ in some cases) producing α-ketoglutarate (2-oxoglutarate), ammonia, and NADH; in mammals, this is the prime contributor to oxidative deamination. SYN glutamic acid dehydrogenases.

g. formiminotransferase, an enzyme that catalyzes the transfer of the formimino moiety of N-formimino-L-glutamate to tetrahydrofolate; a deficiency of this enzyme will lead to elevated formiminoglutamate levels.

g. γ-semialdehyde, $^-OOCCH(NH_3)^+CH_2CH_2CHO$; an intermediate in L-proline and L-ornithine metabolism; becomes elevated in type II hyperprolinemia.

g. synthase, an enzyme that converts L-glutamine, α-ketoglutarate, and NADH (in some cases, NADPH) to two L-g.'s and NAD^+ (or, $NADP^+$); apparently, a nonmammalian enzyme.

γ-glu·ta·mate (glu·ta·mate γ-) car·box·y·pep·ti·dase. SYN γ-glutamyl hydrolase.

glu·tam·ic ac·id (E, Glu) (glū-tam'ik). An amino acid, $HOOC–CH_2–CH_2–CH(NH_2)–COOH$ the L-isomer; occurs in proteins; the sodium salt is monosodium glutamate. Cf. glutamate.

g. a. dehydrogenases, SYN *glutamate* dehydrogenases.

g. a. hydrochloride, a gastric acidifier alleged to aid in digestion; also used for gastric HCl replacement therapy.

glu·tam·ic-as·par·tic trans·am·i·nase. SYN *aspartate* aminotransferase.

glu·tam·ic-ox·a·lo·ace·tic trans·am·i·nase (GOT). SYN *aspartate* aminotransferase.

glu·tam·ic-py·ru·vic trans·am·i·nase (GPT). SYN alanine aminotransferase.

glu·ta·min·ase (glū-tam'in-ās). An enzyme in kidney and other tissues that catalyzes the hydrolysis of L-glutamine to ammonia and L-glutamic acid; an important enzyme for urinary ammonia formation.

glu·ta·min·ate (glū-tam'in-āt). The anion form of glutamine.

glu·ta·mine (Gln, Q) (glū'tă-mēn, -tă-min, glū-tam'in). The δ-amide of glutamic acid, derived by oxidation from proline in the liver or by the combination of glutamic acid with ammonia; the L-isomer is present in proteins and in blood and other tissues, and is an important source of urinary ammonia, being broken down in the kidney by the action of the enzyme glutaminase; nonenzymatically, it is converted to 5-oxoproline.

g. aminotransferase, an enzyme that reversibly converts L-glutamine, α-ketoglutaramate, and L-glutamate; α-ketoglutaramate is elevated in certain cases of hepatocoma. SYN g. transaminase.

g. synthetase, an enzyme that catalyzes the reaction of L-glutamic acid, ammonia, and ATP to g., ADP, and orthophosphate; one of the few known mammalian enzymes that uses ammonium ion as a substrate under physiological conditions.

g. transaminase, SYN g. aminotransferase.

glu·tam·i·nyl (Gln, Q) (glū-tam'i-nil). The acyl radical of glutamine.

glu·tam·o·yl (glū-tam'ō-il). The radical of glutamic acid from which both α- and δ-hydroxyl groups have been removed.

glu·tam·yl (E, Glu) (glū-tam'il, glū'tă-mil). The radical of glutamic acid from which either the α- or the δ-hydroxyl group has been removed.

γ-glu·tam·yl car·box·yl·ase. An enzyme that catalyzes the formation of γ-carboxyglutamyl residues in many proteins, several appearing in the blood clotting cascade.

γ-glu·ta·myl·cys·teine (glū'tă-mil-sis'te-in). A necessary precursor in the biosynthesis of glutathione; contains an isopeptide rather than a eupeptide bond.

γ-g. synthetase, an enzyme that catalyzes the first step in glutathione biosynthesis, reacting L-glutamate, L-cysteine, and ATP to form γ-g., ADP, and orthophosphate; inhibited by thiols such as glutathione.

γ-L-glu·ta·myl·-L-cysteinylglycine. SYN glutathione.

γ-glu·tam·yl hy·dro·lase. N-Pteroyl-L-glutamate hydrolase; an enzyme cleaving L-glutamyl residues from pteridine oligoglutamates; used in certain antitumor treatments. SYN carboxypeptidase G, conjugase, γ-glutamate (glutamate γ-) carboxypeptidase.

γ-glu·tam·yl·trans·fer·ase (glū-tam'il-trans'fer-ās). An enzyme that catalyzes the transfer of a γ-glutamyl group from a γ-glutamyl peptide (usually glutathione) to another peptide, certain amino acids, or water; a deficiency of this enzyme will result in glutathionuria. SYN γ-glutamyl transpeptidase.

γ-glu·tam·yl trans·pep·ti·dase. SYN γ-glutamyltransferase.

glu·ta·ral (glū'tă-ral). SYN glutaraldehyde.

glu·tar·al·de·hyde (glū-tă-ral'dĕ-hīd). $C_5H_8O_2$; a dialdehyde used as a fixative for electron microscopy, especially for nuclear morphology and for localization of enzyme activity; also used as a germicidal agent for disinfection and sterilization of instruments or equipment that cannot be heat sterilized. SYN glutaral.

glu·tar·ic ac·id (glū-tar'ik). $HOOC(CH_2)_3COOH$; pentanedioic acid; an intermediate in tryptophan catabolism; accumulates in glutaric acidemia.

glu·ta·ryl-CoA (glū'tă-ril). The mono thiol ester of coenzyme A and glutaric acid; an intermediate in L-lysine and L-tryptophan catabolism.

g.-CoA dehydrogenase, an enzyme that catalyzes the reaction of g.-CoA with an acceptor to form crotonoyl-CoA, CO_2, and the reduced acceptor; a deficiency of this enzyme will lead to either glutaric acidemia type I or hyperoxaluria type II.

g.-CoA synthetase, an enzyme similar to acyl-CoA synthetase, but which splits ATP, GTP, or ITP to the nucleoside diphosphate and orthophosphate in acting on glutarate, thus forming g.-CoA.

glu·ta·thi·one (GSH) (glū-tă-thī'ōn). **1.** γ-L-Glutamyl-L-cysteinylglycine; a tripeptide of glycine, L-cysteine, and L-glutamate, with L-glutamate having an isopeptide bond with the amino moiety of L-cysteine. G. has a wide variety of roles in a cell; it is the most prevalent non-protein thiol. G. disulfide (GSSG) consists of two g.'s linked via a disulfide bridge; the term oxidized g. for GSSG should be avoided since it includes the sulfones and sulfoxides. The term reduced g. is not necessary since g. is the thiol form. A deficiency of g. can cause hemolysis with oxidative stress. SEE ALSO oxidized g., reduced g., g. reductase. **2.** The principal low molecular weight thiol compound of living plant cells; used in the course of intermediary metabolism as a donor of thiol (SH) groups; essential for detoxification of acetaminophen. SYN γ-L-glutamyl-L-cysteinylglycine.

oxidized g., g. acting in cells as a hydrogen acceptor; reduced by g. reductase.

g. peroxidase, an enzyme that catalyzes the reaction of two g.'s with H_2O_2 forming GSSG and two water molecules; a crucial enzyme in hydrogen peroxide detoxification.

reduced g., glutathione acting as a hydrogen donor.

g. reductase, an enzyme that catalyzes the reaction of GSSG with NADH (or NADPH) forming two g.'s and NAD^+ (or $NADP^+$); involved in many redox reactions; a deficiency can cause hemolysis with oxidative stress.

g. synthetase, an enzyme that catalyzes the formation of g., ADP, and orthophosphate from γ-glutamylcysteine, ATP, and glycine; a deficiency will lead to metabolic acidosis and progressive brain dysfunction.

g. S-transferase, a class of enzymes that catalyze the reaction of g. with an acceptor molecule (*e.g.,* an arene oxide) to form an S-substituted g.; a key step in detoxification of many substances; start of the mercapturic acid pathway. SYN ligandin.

glu·ta·thi·o·nu·ria (glū-tă-thī'ō-nur-ē-ă). Elevated glutathione and/or glutathione disulfide levels in the urine.

glu·te·al (glū'tē-ăl). Relating to the buttocks. [G. *gloutos,* buttock]

glu·te·lins (glū'tĕ-linz). A class of simple proteins occurring in the seeds of grain; soluble in dilute acids and bases, but not in neutral solutions (*e.g.,* glutenin from wheat and orycenin in rice).

glu·ten (glū'těn). The insoluble protein (prolamines) constituent of wheat and other grains; a mixture of gliadin, glutenin, and other proteins; the presence of g. allows flour to rise. SYN wheat gum. [L. *gluten,* glue]

g. casein, a protein resembling casein, present in g.

glu·te·nin (glū'tĕ-nin). A glutelin in wheat.

glu·te·o·fem·o·ral (glū'tē-ō-fem'ō-răl). Relating to the buttock and the thigh.

glu·te·o·in·gui·nal (glū'tē-ō-ing'gwi-năl). Relating to the buttock and the groin.

glu·teth·i·mide (glū-teth'i-mīd). 2-Ethyl-2-phenylglutarimide; a central nervous system depressant used as a hypnotic in simple insomnia and formerly as a daytime sedative.

glu·te·us (glū-tē'ŭs). SEE gluteus maximus *muscle,* gluteus medius *muscle,* gluteus minimus *muscle.*

glu·ti·noid (glū'ti-noyd). SYN albuminoid (3).

glu·ti·nous (glū'tin-ŭs). Sticky.

glu·ti·tis (glū-tī'tis). Inflammation of the muscles of the buttock. [G. *gloutos,* buttock, + *-itis,* inflammation]

Glx Symbol for glutamyl (Glu), glutaminyl (Gln), and/or any substance that would yield glutamate upon acid hydrolysis of a peptide (*e.g.,* 5-oxoproline, 4-carboxyglutamate) to denote uncertainty between them.

Gly Symbol for glycine or its acyl radical, glycyl.

gly·bu·ride (glī'byū-rīd). Glybenzycyclamide 1-[[*p*-[2-(5-chloro-*o*-anisamido)ethyl]phenyl]sulfonyl]-3-cyclohexylurea; an oral hypoglycemic drug used in the treatment of type II diabetes.

gly·cal (glī'kăl). An unsaturated sugar derivative in which the adjacent hydroxyl groups are removed, one of which is that upon the carbon-1 of the aldose (or carbon-2 of the ketose), yielding a CH=CH between these two positions. SYN glucal.

gly·can (glī'kan). SYN polysaccharide. SEE ALSO heteroglycan, homoglycan.

gly·can·o·hy·dro·las·es (glī'kan-ō-hī'drō-lā-sez) [EC group 3.2.1]. Hydrolases acting on glycans; *e.g.,* chitinase, hyaluronoglucosidase.

gly·cate (glī'kāt). The product of the nonenzymic reaction between a sugar and the free amino group(s) of proteins in which it is not known if the sugar is attached by a glycosyl or a glycoside linkage, or has formed a Schiff base.

gly·ca·tion (glī-kā'shŭn). The nonenzymic reaction that forms a glycate.

gly·ce·mia (glī-sē'mē-ă). The presence of glucose in the blood. [G. *glykys,* sweet, + *haima,* blood]

glyc·er·al·de·hyde (glis-er-al'dĕ-hīd). HOCH₂-CHOH-CHO; a triose and the simplest optically active aldose; the dextrorotatory isomer is taken as the structural reference point for all D compounds, the levorotatory isomer for all L compounds. SYN glyceric aldehyde.

glyc·er·al·de·hyde 3-phos·phate. HCO–CHOH–CH₂–OPO₃²⁻; an intermediate in the glycolytic breakdown of D-glucose; one of the products of the splitting of fructose 1,6-bisphosphate under the catalytic influence of fructose-bisphosphate aldolase.

gly·cer·ic ac·id (gli-ser'ik, glis'er-ik). HOCH₂-CHOH-COOH; the fatty acid analog of glycerol; occurs particularly in the form of phosphorylated derivatives, as an intermediate in glycolysis.

D-glyceric aciduria (gli-ser'i, as-id-ū-ē-ă). **1.** Elevated levels of D-glyceric acid in the urine. **2.** An inborn error in metabolism resulting in D-glyceric aciduria (1).

L-gly·cer·ic ac·i·du·ria. Excretion of L-glyceric acid in the urine; a primary metabolic error due to deficiency of D-glyceric dehydrogenase resulting in excretion of L-glyceric and oxalic acids, leading to the clinical syndrome of oxalosis with frequent formation of oxalate renal calculi.

gly·cer·ic al·de·hyde. SYN glyceraldehyde.

glyc·er·i·das·es (glis'er-ĭ-dās-ez). General term for enzymes catalyzing the hydrolysis of glycerol esters (glycerides); *e.g.,* triacylglycerol lipase.

glyc·er·ide (glis'er-id, -īd). An ester of glycerol. The term is usually used in combination with phospho- (phosphoglyceride). The use of mono-, di-, and triglyceride is being replaced by the more precise terms mono-, di-, and triacylglycerol, respectively.

mixed g.'s, g.'s which, on hydrolysis, yield more than one variety of fatty acid.

glyc·er·in (glis'er-in). SYN glycerol.

g. jelly, SYN glycerinated *gelatin.*

glyc·er·ite (glis'er-īt). **1.** SYN glycerol. **2.** A pharmaceutical preparation made by triturating the active medicinal substance with glycerol.

starch g., a preparation containing 100 g of starch, 2 g of benzoic acid, 200 ml of purified water, and 700 g of glycerin in each 1000 g; a topical emollient.

tannic acid g., g. of tannin, containing tannic acid, sodium citrate, exsiccated sodium sulfite, and glycerin; an astringent.

glyc·er·o·gel·a·tin (glis'er-ō-jel'ă-tin). SYN glycerinated *gelatin.*

glyc·er·o·ke·tone (glis'er-ō-kē'tŏn). Obsolete term for dihydroxyacetone.

glyc·er·o·ki·nase (glis'er-ō-kī'nās). SYN *glycerol* kinase.

glyc·er·ol (glis'er-ol). HOCH₂CH(OH)CH₂OH; a sweet oily fluid obtained by the saponification of fats and fixed oils; used as a solvent, as a skin emollient, by injection or in the form of suppository for constipation, orally to reduce ocular tension, and as a vehicle and sweetening agent. SYN 1,2,3-propanetriol, glycerin, glycerite (1), glyceryl alcohol.

iodinated g., a form of organically bound iodine which liberates iodine systemically. Has been used as a medicinal source of iodine and as an expectorant in place of inorganic iodides such as potassium iodide. SYN iodopropylidene glycerol, organidin.

g. kinase, an enzyme that catalyzes a reaction between ATP and glycerol to yield *sn*-glycerol 3-phosphate and ADP; in adipose tissue, the first step in the synthesis of triacylglycerols; deficiency results in the disruption of adrenal, muscle, and/or liver and brain function. SYN glycerokinase.

g. phosphate, the anion of a phosphoric ester of g.; the 3-derivative is the central component of phosphatidates (R-glycerol 3-phosphate). SYN glycerophosphate.

glyc·er·ol-3-phos·phate ac·yl·trans·fer·ase. An enzyme that participates in phospholipid biosynthesis, catalyzing the transfer of an acyl group from a fatty acyl-CoA to *sn*-glycerol-3-phosphate producing coenzyme A and lysophosphatidic acid.

glyc·er·ol-3-phos·phate de·hy·dro·gen·ase (NAD⁺). α-Glycerol phosphate dehydrogenase; 3-phosphoglycerol dehydrogenase; an oxidoreductase that catalyzes the interconversion of dihydroxyacetone phosphate and *sn*-glycerol 3-phosphate, with the participation of NAD⁺; its action provides the glycerol moiety from carbohydrate during lipogenesis.

glycerone. SYN dihydroxyacetone.

glyc·er·o·phos·phate (glis'er-ō-fos'făt). SYN *glycerol* phosphate.

glyc·er·o·phos·pho·cho·line (glis'er-ō-fos-fō-kō'lēn). HOCH₂–CHOH–CH₂–OP(O₂H)–OCH₂CH₂–[N(CH₃)₃]⁺; a component of phosphatidylcholines (lecithins), in which the two OH's of g. are esterified with fatty acids. SYN glycerophosphorylcholine.

glyc·er·o·phos·phor·ic ac·id (glis'er-ō-fos-fōr'ik). A phosphoric ester of glycerol. SEE ALSO *glycerol* phosphate.

glyc·er·o·phos·pho·ryl·cho·line (glis'er-ō-fos'fōr-il-kō'lēn). SYN glycerophosphocholine.

glyc·er·ul·ose (glis'er'ul-ōse). SYN dihydroxyacetone.

glyc·er·yl (glis'er-il). The trivalent radical, C₃H₅‴, of glycerol; often used in error for glycero- or glyceryl.

g. alcohol, SYN glycerol.

g. borate, SYN boroglycerin.

g. guaiacolate, SYN guaifenesin.

g. monostearate, the ester of glycerol and one molecule of stearic acid; used in the manufacture of cosmetic creams and dermatologic preparations.

g. triacetate, SYN triacetin.

g. tributyrate, SYN tributyrin.

g. tricaprate, SYN caprin.

g. trinitrate, SYN nitroglycerin.

glyc·er·yl io·dide. An organic form of iodine which slowly liberates iodine in the body after oral administration. Used primarily as an expectorant/mucolytic. SYN 3-iodo-1,2-propanediol, γ-iodopropyleneglycol.

gly·cin·am·ide ri·bo·nu·cle·o·tide (glī-sin'a-mīd). SEE glycineamide ribonucleotide.

gly·cin·ate (glī'sin-āt). **1.** A salt of glycine. **2.** Glycine anion.

gly·cine (G, Gly) (glī'sēn). $^+NH_3$–CH_2–COO^-; the simplest amino acid; a major component of gelatin and silk fibroin; used as a nutrient and dietary supplement, and in solution for irrigation; used in the treatment of sweaty feet syndrome. SYN aminoacetic acid, aminoethanoic acid, gelatin sugar.

g. acyltransferase, an enzyme catalyzing the reversible transfer of an acyl group from acyl-CoA to g., producing free coenzyme A and N-acylglycine; a step in a detoxification pathway.

g. amidinotransferase, an enzyme catalyzing the transfer of an amidine group from L-arginine to glycine, forming guanidinoacetate and L-ornithine; an important reaction in creatine synthesis; it can also act on canavanine. SYN g. transamidinase.

g. betaine, SYN betaine.

g. cleavage complex, a complex of several proteins that catalyze the reversible reaction of g. with tetrahydrofolate to produce CO_2, NH_3, and N^5,N^{10}-methylenetetrahydrofolate; a deficiency of this enzyme (or one of its subunits) will result in nonketotic hyperglycinemia. SYN g. synthase.

g. dehydrogenases, enzymes that catalyze the conversion of glycine to glyoxylate and ammonia, using either NAD^+ or ferricytochrome c.

g. synthase, SYN g. cleavage complex.

g. transamidinase, SYN g. amidinotransferase.

gly·cine·a·mide ri·bo·nu·cle·o·tide, gly·cin·am·ide ri·bo·nu·cle·o·tide (glī'sin-ă-mīd, glī-sin'a-mīd). An intermediate in purine biosynthesis, in which the amide N of glycineamide is linked to the C-1 of a ribosyl moiety.

gly·cine-rich β-gly·co·pro·tein. SYN properdin *factor* B.

gly·cine-rich β-gly·co·pro·tein·ase. SYN properdin *factor* D.

gly·cin·in (glī-sen'in). The chief protein of soybeans.

gly·ci·ni·um (glī-sen-ē-um). Glycine cation.

gly·ci·nu·ria (glī-si-nū'rē-ă). The excretion of glycine in the urine. [glycine + G. *ouron,* urine]

familial g. [MIM*138500], a metabolic disorder believed to be due to defective renal glycine reabsorption; it may or may not be accompanied by oxalate urolithiasis; may be the heterozygous state of iminoglycinuria; autosomal dominant inheritance.

△**glyco-.** Combining form denoting relationship to sugars (*e.g.,* glycogen), or to glycine (*e.g.,* glycocholate). SEE ALSO gluco-. [G. *glykys,* sweet]

gly·co·bi·ar·sol (glī-kō-bī'ar-sol). Oxo(hydrogen N-glycoloylarsanilato)bismuth; a pentavalent arsenical containing bismuth; used in the treatment of milder forms of intestinal amebiasis or as subsequent therapy.

gly·co·ca·lyx (glī-kō-kā'liks). A PAS-positive filamentous coating on the apical surface of certain epithelial cells, composed of carbohydrate moieties of proteins that protrude from the free surface of the plasma membrane. [glyco- + G. *kalyx,* husk, shell]

gly·co·cho·late (glī-kō-kō'lāt). A salt or ester of glycocholic acid.

g. sodium, a normal constituent of bile of man and herbivores; g. sodium from herbivores is purified and used as a choleretic and cholagogue.

gly·co·cho·lic ac·id (glī-kō-kō'lik). N-Cholylglycine; one of the major bile acid conjugates, formed by condensation of the —COOH group of cholic acid and the amino group of glycine; water-soluble and a powerful detergent.

gly·co·cor·ti·coid (glī'kō-kōr'ti-koyd). SYN glucocorticoid.

gly·co·cy·a·mine (glī-kō-sī'ă-mēn). HN=C(NH_2)NH-CH_2COOH; 2-guanidinoacetic acid; formed by the transfer of the amidine group from L-arginine to glycine. SYN glucocyamine.

gly·co·gel·a·tin (glī-kō-jel'ă-tin). SYN glycerinated *gelatin.*

gly·co·gen (glī'kō-jen). A glucosan of high molecular weight, resembling amylopectin in structure (with α(1,4 linkages) but even more highly branched (α(1,6 linkages), found in most of the tissues of the body, especially those of the liver and muscle; as the principal carbohydrate reserve, it is readily converted into glucose. SYN animal dextran, animal starch, hepatin, liver starch.

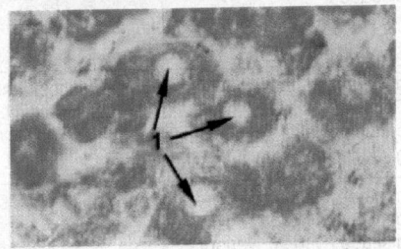

glycogen (in liver cells)
the glycogen appears red, the cell nuclei (1) colorless

g. phosphorylase, SYN phosphorylase.

g. synthase, g. starch synthase, a glucosyltransferase catalyzing the incorporation of D-glucose from UDP-D-glucose into 1,4-α-D-glucosyl chains. A deficiency of the liver enzyme may lead to a type of hypoglycemia.

gly·co·ge·nase (glī'kō-jĕ-nās). SYN α-amylase, β-amylase.

gly·co·gen·e·sis (glī-kō-jen'ĕ-sis). Formation of glycogen from D-glucose by means of glycogen synthase and dextrin dextranase; the first enzyme catalyzes formation of a polyglucose with α-1,4 links from UDPglucose, the second cleaves fragments from one chain and transfers them to an α-1,6 linkage in another. [glyco- + G. *genesis,* production]

gly·co·ge·net·ic (glī'kō-jĕ-net'ik). Glycogenic (2); relating to glycogenesis. SYN D-glycogenous.

gly·co·gen·ic (glī-ko-gen'ik). Giving rise to or producing glycogen.

gly·co·gen·ol·y·sis (glī'kō-jĕ-nol'i-sis). The hydrolysis of glycogen to glucose.

gly·co·ge·no·sis (glī'kō-jĕ-nō'sis). Any of the glycogen deposition diseases characterized by accumulation of glycogen of normal or abnormal chemical structure in tissue; there may be enlargement of the liver, heart, or striated muscle, including the tongue, with progressive muscular weakness. Seven types (Cori classification) are recognized, depending on the enzyme deficiency involved, all of autosomal recessive inheritance, but with a different gene for each enzyme deficiency. [MIM designations: I *232200, *232220, *232240; II *232300; III *232400; IV *232500; V *232600; VI *232700; VII *232800]. SYN dextrinosis, glycogen-storage disease.

brancher deficiency g., SYN brancher glycogen storage *disease.*

generalized g., SYN type 2 g.

glucose-6-phosphatase hepatorenal g., SYN type 1 g.

hepatophosphorylase deficiency g., SYN type 6 g.

myophosphorylase deficiency g., SYN type 5 g.

type 1 g., g. due to glucose 6-phosphatase deficiency, resulting in accumulation of excessive amounts of glycogen of normal chemical structure, particularly in liver and kidney. SYN Gierke's disease, glucose-6-phosphatase hepatorenal g., von Gierke's disease.

type 2 g., g. due to lysosomal α-1,4-glucosidase deficiency, resulting in accumulation of excessive amounts of glycogen of normal chemical structure in heart, muscle, liver, and nervous system. SYN generalized g., Pompe's disease.

type 3 g., g. due to amylo-1,6-glucosidase deficiency, resulting in accumulation of abnormal glycogen with short outer chains in liver and muscle. SYN Cori's disease, debranching deficiency limit dextrinosis, limit dextrinosis, Forbes' disease.

type 4 g., familial cirrhosis of the liver with storage of abnormal glycogen; g. due to deficiency of 1,4-α-glucan branching enzyme, resulting in accumulation of abnormal glycogen with long

gl

types of glycogenosis

type	glycogenosis	deficient enzyme	biochemical diagnosis	clinical symptoms
1	hepatorenal g., Gierke's disease	glucose-6-phosphatase	normal glycogen, in liver and kidneys in excessive amounts	hypoglycemia, hyperlipemia, ketosis, hyperuricemia, hepatomegaly, dwarfism
2	generalized, malign g.; Pompe's disease; cardiomegalia glycogenica	α-1.4-glucosidase	normal glycogen, excessive in all organs	muscle hypotonia, heart insufficiency, neurological symptoms, infant death
3	hepatomuscular, benign g.; Cori's disease, Forbes' disease (with subvariants 3b through f)	amylo-1.6-glucosidase	abnormal glycogen, with short outer chains, in liver and (more rarely) in muscles	hepatomegaly, hypoglycemia; mild course of disease
4	liver, cirrhotic, reticuloendothelial g.; Andersen's disease; amylopectinosis	α-1.4-glucan: α-1.4-glucan-6-glycosyltransferase	abnormal glycogen, with long outer chains, in liver, spleen, and lymphnodes	cirrhosis of the liver; hepatosplenomegaly
5	muscular g., McArdle's disease	α-glucanphosphorylase of the muscle	normal glycogen, in muscle in excessive amounts	generalized myasthemia and myalgia, myoglobinuria
6	hepatic g., Hers glycogenosis	α-glucanphosphorylase of the liver	normal glycogen, in liver in excessive amounts	hepatomegaly, relatively benign
7	muscular g.; Tarui's disease	phosphofructokinase of the muscle	normal glycogen, in the skeletal muscle	muscle cramping, myoglobinuria
8	hepatic g.; X-chromosome inheritance	phosphorylase-b kinase of the liver	normal glycogen, in the liver	clinically mild manifestation, hepatomegaly, hypoglycemia

inner and outer chains in liver, kidney, muscle, and other tissues. SYN Andersen's disease.

type 5 g., g. due to muscle glycogen phosphorylase deficiency, resulting in accumulation of glycogen of normal chemical structure in muscle. SYN McArdle's disease, McArdle's syndrome, McArdle-Schmid-Pearson disease, myophosphorylase deficiency g.

type 6 g., g. due to hepatic glycogen phosphorylase deficiency, resulting in accumulation of glycogen of normal chemical structure in liver and leukocytes. SYN hepatophosphorylase deficiency g., Hers' disease.

type 7 g., phosphofructokinase deficiency of muscle resulting in muscle cramps and myoglobinuria on extreme exertion. The clinical picture resembles type 5 g.

D-gly·cog·e·nous (glī-koj'ĕ-nŭs). SYN glycogenetic.

gly·co·geu·sia (glī-kō-gū'sē-ă). A subjective sweet taste. [glyco- + G. *geusis,* taste]

gly·co·gly·ci·nu·ria (glī'kō-glī-si-nū'rē-ă). A metabolic disorder characterized by glucosuria and hyperglycinuria; autosomal dominant inheritance.

gly·col (glī'kol). **1.** A compound containing adjacent alcohol groups. **2.** Ethylene g., $HOCH_2CH_2OH$, the simplest g.

gly·col·al·de·hyde (glī-kol-al'dĕ-hīd). $HOCH_2CHO$; the simplest (2-carbon) sugar; the aerobic deamination product of ethanolamine. SYN biose, diose.

active g., 2-(1,2-dihydroxyethyl)thiamin pyrophosphate; a derivative formed in carbohydrate metabolism.

gly·col·al·de·hyde·trans·fer·ase (glī-kol-al'dĕ-hīd-trans'fer-ās). SYN transketolase.

gly·co·late (glī-kō'lāt). A salt or ester of glycolic acid.

gly·col·leu·cine (glī'kō-lū-sin). SYN norleucine.

gly·col·ic ac·id (glī-kol'ik). $HOCH_2COOH$; an intermediate in the interconversion of glycine and ethanolamine. SYN hydroxyacetic acid.

gly·col·ic ac·i·du·ria. Excessive excretion of glycolic acid in the urine; a primary metabolic defect due to deficiency of 2-hydroxy-3-oxoadipate carboxylase, resulting in excretion of glycolic and oxalic acids, leading to the clinical syndrome of oxalosis.

gly·co·lip·id (glī-kō-lip'id). A lipid with one or more covalently attached sugars.

gly·co·lyl (glī'kō-lil). $HOCH_2CO-$; the acyl radical of glycolic acid, replacing acetyl in some sialic acids; the products are called *N*-glycolylneuraminic acids.

gly·col·yl·u·rea (glī'kō-lil-yū-rē'ă). SYN hydantoin.

gly·col·y·sis (glī-kol'i-sis). The energy-yielding conversion of D-glucose to lactic acid (instead of pyruvate oxidation products) in various tissues, notably muscle, when sufficient oxygen is not available (as in an emergency situation); since molecular oxygen is not consumed in the process, this is frequently referred to as "anaerobic g." Cf. Embden-Meyerhof-Parnas *pathway.* SYN glucolysis. [glyco- + G. *lysis,* a loosening]

gly·co·lyt·ic (glī-kō-lit'ik). Relating to glycolysis.

gly·co·ne·o·gen·e·sis (glī'kō-nē-ō-jen'ĕ-sis). The formation of glycogen from noncarbohydrates, such as protein or fat, by conversion of the latter to D-glucose. SEE ALSO glycogenesis. Cf. gluconeogenesis. [glyco- + G. *neos,* new, + *genesis,* production]

gly·con·ic ac·ids (glī-kon'ik). SYN aldonic acids.

gly·co·pe·nia (glī-kō-pē'nē-ă). A deficiency of any or all sugars in an organ or tissue. [glyco- + G. *penia,* poverty]

gly·co·pep·tide (glī-kō-pep'tīd). A compound containing sugar(s) linked to amino acids (or peptides), with the latter preponderant, as in bacterial cell walls. Cf. peptidoglycan.

Gly·co·pha·gus (glī-kof'ă-gŭs). A common genus of grain mites, frequently implicated in dermatitis among food handlers. SEE ALSO *Tyrophagus putrescentiae.* [glyco- + G. *phagō,* to eat]

gly·co·phil·ia (glī-kō-fil'ē-ă). A condition in which there is a distinct tendency to develop hyperglycemia, even after the ingestion of a relatively small quantity of glucose. [glyko- + G. *phileō,* to love]

gly·co·pho·rins (glī-kō-fōr'ins). A group of proteins found in erythrocyte membranes; certain glycophorins are associated with blood group antigens; glycophorin A is the major glycophorin; a deficiency of glycophorin C is observed in type 4 hereditary elliptocytosis.

gly·co·pro·tein (glī-kō-prō′tēn). **1.** One of a group of protein-carbohydrate compounds (conjugated proteins), among which the most important are the mucins, mucoid, and amyloid. **2.** Sometimes restricted to proteins containing small amounts of carbohydrate, in contrast to mucoids or mucoproteins, usually measured as hexosamine; such conjugated proteins are found in many places, notably γ-globulins, α_1-globulins, α_2-globulins, transferrin, etc., and are contained in mucus and mucins. SEE ALSO mucoprotein.

α_1-**acid g.,** SYN orosomucoid.

β_2-**gly·co·pro·tein II.** SYN properdin *factor* B.

gly·co·pty·a·lism (glī-kō-ptī′ă-lizm). SYN glycosialia. [glyco- + G. *ptyalon*, saliva]

gly·co·pyr·ro·late (glī-kō-pī′rō-lāt). 3-Hydroxy-1,1-dimethylpyrrolidinium bromide; a parasympatholytic compound used as premedication prior to general anesthesia, as an antagonist to the bradycardic effects of neostigmine during curare reversal, and as an adjunct in the treatment of peptic ulcer.

gly·cor·rha·chia (glī-kō-rā′kē-ă, -rak-ē-ă). Presence of sugar in the cerebrospinal fluid. [glyco- + G. *rhachis*, spine]

gly·cor·rhea (glī-kō-rē′ă). A discharge of sugar from the body, as in glucosuria, especially in unusually large quantities. [glyco- + G. *rhoia*, a flow]

gly·cos·am·i·no·gly·can (glī′kōs-am-i-nō-glī′kan). SEE mucopolysaccharide.

gly·co·se·cre·to·ry (glī′kō-sē-krē′tō-rē). Causing or involved in the secretion of glycogen.

gly·co·si·a·lia (glī′kō-sī-al′ē-ă, -ā′lē-ă). The presence of sugar in the saliva. SYN glycoptyalism. [glyco- + G. *sialon*, saliva]

gly·co·si·a·lor·rhea (glī′kō-sī′ă-lō-rē′ă). An excessive secretion of saliva that contains sugar. [glyco- + G. *sialon*, saliva, + *rhoia*, a flow]

gly·cos·i·dases (glī-kō-sīd-ās′ez). (glī-kō-sīd-ās′ez;) A class of hydrolytic enzymes that act on glycosides; α-glycosidases act on α-glycosidic linkages (*e.g.,* α-amylase) while β-glycosidases act on β-glycosidic linkages (*e.g.,* β-glucosidase).

gly·co·side (glī′kō-sīd). Condensation product of a sugar with any other radical involving the loss of the H of the hemiacetal or hemiketal OH of the sugar, leaving the O of this OH as the link; thus, the condensation through the O-1 with an alcohol, which loses its OH, yields an alcohol-glycoside (or a glycosido-alcohol); links involving loss of the entire sugar 1-OH, as in condensation with a purine or pyrimidine –NH– group, yield glycosyl (or N-glycosyl) compounds.

    cyanogenic g., a g. capable of generating CN⁻ upon metabolism (*e.g.,* amygdalin).

N-**gly·co·side.** Misnomer for glycosyl.

gly·co·sid·ic (glī-kō-sid′ik). Referring to or denoting a glycoside or glycoside linkage.

gly·co·sphin·go·lip·id (glī′kō-sfing-gō-lip′id). A ceramide linked to one or more sugars via the terminal OH group; included as g.'s are cerebrosides, gangliosides, and ceramide oligosaccharides (oligoglycosylceramides). The prefix glyc- may be replaced by gluc-, galact-, lact-, etc. SYN ceramide saccharide.

gly·co·stat·ic (glī-kō-stat′ik). Indicating the property of certain extracts of the anterior hypophysis that permits the body to maintain its glycogen stores in muscle, liver, and other tissues.

gly·cos·ur·ia (glī-kō-sū′rē-ă). **1.** SYN glucosuria. **2.** Urinary excretion of carbohydrates. SYN glycuresis (2). [glyco- + G. *ouron*, urine]

    alimentary g., g. developing after the ingestion of a moderate amount of sugar or starch, which normally is disposed of without appearing in the urine, because rate of intestinal absorption exceeds capacity of the liver and the other tissues to remove the glucose, thus allowing blood glucose levels to become high enough for renal excretion to occur. SYN alimentary diabetes, digestive g.

    benign g., g. not associated with diabetes mellitus but resulting from a low renal threshold for sugar.

    digestive g., SYN alimentary g.

    nondiabetic g., SYN nonhyperglycemic g.

    nonhyperglycemic g., presence of glucose in the urine without hyperglycemia due to abnormality in renal tubular reabsorption of filtered glucose. SYN nondiabetic g., orthoglycemic g.

    normoglycemic g., SYN renal g.

    orthoglycemic g. (ōr-thō-glī′cēm-ik), SYN nonhyperglycemic g.

    pathologic g., chronic excretion of relatively large amounts of sugar in the urine.

    phlorizin g., phloridzin g., the presence of sugar in the urine after the experimental administration of phlorizin, which results in a lower renal threshold for glucose reabsorption of glucose. SYN phlorizin diabetes.

    renal g., the recurring or persistent excretion of glucose in the urine, in association with blood glucose levels that are in the normal range; results from the failure of proximal renal tubules to reabsorb glucose at a normal rate from the glomerular filtrate (low renal threshold); defect in the glucose carrier in the nephron. SYN diabetes innocens, normoglycemic g., renal diabetes.

gly·co·syl (glī′kō-sil). The radical resulting from detachment of the OH of the hemiacetal or hemiketal of a saccharide. Cf. glycoside.

gly·co·sy·la·tion (glī′kō-si-lā′shŭn). Formation of linkages with glycosyl groups, as between D-glucose and the hemoglobin chain to form the fraction hemoglobin A_{Ic}, whose level rises in association with the raised blood D-glucose concentration in poorly controlled or uncontrolled diabetes mellitus. SEE ALSO glycosylated *hemoglobin*.

gly·co·syl·trans·fer·ase (glī′kō-sil-trans′fer-ās). Any enzyme (EC subclass 2.4) transferring glycosyl groups from one compound to another. SYN transglycosylase.

gly·co·tro·pic, gly·co·tro·phic (glī-kō-trop′ik, -trof′ik). Pertaining to a principle in extracts of the anterior lobe of the pituitary that antagonizes the action of insulin and causes hyperglycemia. SEE glycotropic *factor*. [glyco- + G. *trophē*, nourishment; *tropē*, a turning]

glyc·u·re·sis (glī-kū-rē′sis). **1.** SYN glucosuria. **2.** SYN glycosuria (2). [glyco- + G. *ourēsis*, urination]

gly·cu·ron·ate (glī-kūr′on-āt). A salt or ester of a glycuronic acid.

gly·cu·ron·ic ac·id (glī-kūr-on′ik). The uronic acid of a sugar in which the terminal carbon is oxidized to a carboxyl group.

gly·cu·ron·i·dase (glī-kūr-on′i-dās). SYN β-D-glucuronidase.

gly·cu·ro·nide (glī-kūr′on-īd). A glycoside of a uronic acid; *e.g.,* glucuronide.

gly·cu·ro·nu·ria (glī-kū-rō-nū′rē-ă). The presence of glucuronic acid in the urine.

gly·cy·cla·mide (glī-sī′klă-mīd). 1-Cyclohexyl-3-*p*-tolylsulfonylurea; an oral hypoglycemic agent. SYN cyclamide, tolcyclamide, tolhexamide.

gly·cyl (Gly) (glī′sil). The acyl radical of glycine.

    g. betaine, SYN betaine.

glyc·yr·rhi·za (glis-ĭ-rī′ză). The dried rhizome and root of *Glycyrrhiza glabra* (family Leguminoseae) and allied species; a demulcent, mild laxative, and expectorant; also used to disguise the taste of other remedies; its action appears to depend upon glycyrrhizic acid, a salt-retaining glycoside that mimics the action of aldosterone. SYN licorice, liquorice. [G. fr. *glykys*, sweet, + *rhiza*, root]

gly·ox·al (glī-oks′ăl). OHC–CHO; the simplest dialdehyde. SYN oxalaldehyde.

gly·ox·a·lase (glī-oks′ă-lās). An enzyme, lactoylglutathione lyase (g. I) or hydroxyacylglutathione hydrolase (g. II), in red cells and other tissues that converts glyoxal and substituted glyoxals bound to glutathione into the corresponding free hydroxy acids (g. II) or glyoxals (g. I).

gly·ox·y·late trans·a·cet·y·lase (glī-oks′i-lāt). SYN *malate* synthase.

gly·ox·yl·di·u·reide (glī-oks-il-dī′yū-rīd). SYN allantoin.

gly·ox·yl·ic ac·id (glī-oks-il′ik). OHC–COOH; produced by the action of glycine dehydrogenases upon glycine or sarcosine, or

gl

from allantoic acid by allantoicase or via alanine:glyoxylate aminotransferase. SYN oxoacetic acid.

gly·so·bu·zole (glī-sō-byū′zōl). SYN isobuzole.

gm Former abbreviation for gram.

GM-CSF Abbreviation for granulocyte-macrophage colony-stimulating *factor*.

Gmelin, Leopold, German physiologist and chemist, 1788–1853. SEE G.'s *test;* Rosenbach-G. *test.*

GMP Abbreviation for guanylic acid.

GMP re·duc·tase Abbreviation for *guanylic acid* reductase.

GMP syn·the·tase Abbreviation for *guanylic acid* synthetase.

GMS Abbreviation for Gomori's methenamine-silver *stain,* under *stain.*

gnash·ing (nash′ing). The grinding together of the teeth as a nonmasticatory function; sometimes associated with emotional tension. SEE ALSO bruxism.

gnat (nat). A midge; general term applied to several species of minute insects, including species of *Simulium* (buffalo g.) and *Hippelates* (eye g.). British authors sometimes include mosquitoes in this group, but this is not done in the U.S. [A.S. *gnaet*]

⚠ **gnath-.** SEE gnatho-.

gnath·ic (nath′ik). Relating to the jaw or alveolar process. [G. *gnathos,* jaw]

gnath·i·on (nath′ē-on) [NA]. The most inferior point of the mandible in the midline. In cephalometrics, it is the midpoint between the most anterior and inferior point on the bony chin, measured at the intersection of the mandibular baseline and the nasion-pogonion line. [G. *gnathos,* jaw]

⚠ **gnatho-, gnath-.** The jaw. [G. *gnathos*]

gnath·o·ceph·a·lus (nath-ō-sef′ă-lŭs). A fetal malformation with little of the head formed except the jaws. [*gnatho-* + G. *kephalē,* head]

gnath·o·dy·nam·ics (nath′ō-dī-nam′iks). The study of the relationship of the magnitude and direction of the forces developed by and upon the components of the masticatory system during function. [gnatho- + G. *dynamis,* power]

gnath·o·dy·na·mom·e·ter (nath′ō-dī-nă-mom′ĕ-ter). A device for measuring biting pressure. SYN bite gauge, occlusometer. [gnatho- + dynamometer]

gnath·og·ra·phy (nă-thog′ră-fē). The recording of the action of the masticatory apparatus in function.

gnath·o·log·ic·al (nath-ō-loj′i-kăl). Pertaining to gnathodynamics.

gnath·ol·o·gy (nă-thol′ō-jē). The science of the masticatory system, including physiology, functional disturbances, and treatment.

gnath·o·plas·ty (nath′ō-plas-tē). Plastic surgery of the jaw. [gnatho- + G. *plastos,* formed]

gnath·os·chi·sis (nă-thos′ki-sis). Cleft of the jaw. [gnatho- + G. *schisis,* a cleaving]

gnath·o·stat·ics (nath-ō-stat′iks). In orthodontic diagnosis, a technical procedure for orienting the dentition to certain cranial landmarks. [gnatho- + G. *statikos,* causing to stand]

Gna·thos·to·ma (nă-thos′tō-mă). A genus of spiruroid nematode worms (family Gnathostomatidae) characterized by several rows of cuticular spines about the head and by multiple-host aquatic life cycles; it includes pathogenic parasites of cats, cattle, and swine. [gnatho- + G. *stoma,* mouth]

G. siamen′se, invalid name for *G. spinigerum.*

G. spinig′erum, a parasite of cats, dogs, and wild carnivores, but it has occasionally been found in humans in the Far East; it is transmitted via copepods and fish; human infection is usually confined to the skin, but several cases have been reported of eye or brain infection with wandering larvae of this species.

gna·thos·to·mi·a·sis (nath-ō-stō-mī′ă-sis). A migrating edema, or creeping eruption, caused by cutaneous infection by larvae of *Gnathostoma spinigerum.* SYN Yangtze edema.

gnos·co·pine (nos′kō-pēn). α-Gnoscopine; an opium alkaloid, $C_{22}H_{23}NO_7$, obtained by racemization of noscapine; an antitussive. SYN *dl*-narcotine.

gno·sia (nō′sē-ă). The perceptive faculty enabling one to recognize the form and the nature of persons and things; the faculty of perceiving and recognizing. [G. *gnōsis,* knowledge]

gno·to·bi·ol·o·gy (nō′tō-bī-ol′ō-jē). The study of animals in the absence of contaminating microorganisms; *i.e.,* of "germ-free" animals. [G. *gnotos,* known, + *bios,* life, + *logos,* study]

gno·to·bi·o·ta (nō′tō-bī-ō′tă). Living colonies or species, assembled from pure isolates. [G. *gnotos,* known, + Mod. L. *biota,* fr. G. *bios,* life]

gno·to·bi·ote (nō-tō-bī′ōt). An individual organism from a group assembled from pure isolates (gnotobiota).

gno·to·bi·ot·ic (nō′tō-bī-ot′ik). Denoting germ-free or formerly germ-free organisms in which the composition of any associated microbial flora, if present, is fully defined. [see gnotobiota]

GnRH Abbreviation for gonadotropin-releasing *hormone.*

goal (gōl). In psychology, any object or objective that an organism seeks to attain or achieve. [M.E. *gol*]

goat·pox (gōt′poks). An acute infectious disease of goats caused by a strain of *Capripoxvirus* and characterized by generalized vesicular eruptions on the skin and frequently the respiratory mucous membranes; it occurs chiefly in southern and eastern Europe and North Africa.

Godélier, Charles P., French physician, 1813–1877. SEE G.'s *law.*

Godman, John D., U.S. anatomist, 1794–1830. SEE G.'s *fascia.*

Godwin, John T., U.S. pathologist, *1917. SEE G. *tumor.*

Goeckerman, William H., U.S. dermatologist, 1884–1954. SEE G. *treatment.*

Gofman, Moses, German physician, *1887. SEE G. *test.*

Goggia, Carlo P., 20th century Italian physician. SEE G.'s *sign.*

gog·gle (gog′gl). **1.** A screen cover for the eye. **2.** A type of spectacle with auxiliary shields for protecting the eyes. [M.E. *gogelen,* to squint]

plethysmographic g., a specially designed g. to serve as an ophthalmodynamometer while permitting subjective visual and objective ocular changes during transient increased intraocular pressure.

goi·ter (goy′ter). A chronic enlargement of the thyroid gland, not due to a neoplasm, occurring endemically in certain localities, especially mountainous regions, and sporadically elsewhere. SYN struma (1). [Fr. from L. *guttur,* throat]

aberrant g., enlargement of a supernumerary thyroid gland. SYN struma aberrata.

acute g., a g. that develops very rapidly.

adenomatous g., an enlargement of the thyroid gland due to the growth of one or more encapsulated adenomas or multiple nonencapsulated colloid nodules within its substance.

Basedow's g., colloid g. which becomes hyperfunctional after the ingestion of excess iodine, the Jod-Basedow *phenomenon.*

cabbage g., g. due to ingestion of cabbage or other goitrogenic foodstuff.

colloid g., a form of g. in which the contents of the follicles increase greatly, causing pressure atrophy of the epithelium so that the gelatinous matter predominates in the tumor. SYN struma colloides.

cystic g., an enlargement in the thyroid region due to the presence of one or more cysts within the gland.

diffuse g., g. in which the morbid process involves the whole gland, as opposed to nodular g. or thyroid adenoma.

diving g., a freely movable g. that is sometimes above and sometimes below the sternal notch. SYN wandering g.

endemic g., g., usually of simple type, prevalent in certain regions where dietary intake of iodine is suboptimal.

exophthalmic g., any of the various forms of hyperthyroidism in which the thyroid gland is enlarged and exophthalmos is present.

familial g., a group of heritable thyroid disorders in which g. is commonly apparent first during childhood; often associated with skeletal and/or mental retardation, and with other signs of hypothyroidism that may develop with age. Various types of familial g. have been identified: 1) iodide transport defect [MIM*274400], in which the gland is unable to concentrate iodide; 2) organification defect [MIM*274500 and *274600], in which the iodination of tyrosine is defective; 3) Pendred's *syndrome* [MIM*274600]; 4) coupling defect, in which cretinism results from defective coupling of iodotyrosines to form iodothyronines [MIM*274700]; 5) iodotyrosine deiodinase defect, in which deiodination of iodotyrosine is defective, considerable glandular loss of these hormonal precursors occurs, and cretinism may be present [MIM*274800]; 6) plasma iodoprotein disorder [MIM*274900], in which an abnormal iodinated serum protein that is insoluble in acidic butanol is present; 7) hereditary hyperthyroidism.

fibrous g., a firm hyperplasia of the thyroid and its capsule.

follicular g., SYN parenchymatous g.

lingual g., a tumor of thyroid tissue involving the embryonic rudiment at the base of the tongue.

lymphadenoid g., SYN Hashimoto's *thyroiditis.*

microfollicular g., g. in which the glandular tissue consists of unusually small colloid filled follicles and areas of undifferentiated tissue with indistinct follicle formation.

multinodular g., adenomatous g. with several colloid nodules.

nontoxic g., g. not accompanied by hyperthyroidism.

parenchymatous g., a form of g. in which there is a great increase in the follicles with proliferation of the epithelium. SYN follicular g.

simple g., thyroid enlargement unaccompanied by constitutional effects, *e.g.,* hypo- or hyperthyroidism, commonly caused by inadequate dietary intake of iodine.

substernal g., enlargement of the thyroid gland, chiefly of the lower part of the isthmus, palpable with difficulty or not at all.

suffocative g., a g. that by pressure causes extreme dyspnea.

thoracic g., enlargement of accessory thyroid tissue in the thorax with or without hyperthyroidism.

toxic g., a g. that forms an excessive secretion, causing signs and symptoms of hyperthyroidism.

wandering g., SYN diving g.

goi·tro·gen (goy′trō-jen). Any substance that induces goiter, *e.g.,* cabbage, rapeseed, etc.

goi·tro·gen·ic (goy-trō-jen′ik). Causing goiter.

goi·trous (goy′trŭs). Denoting or characteristic of a goiter.

gold (Au). A yellow metallic element, atomic no. 79, atomic wt. 196.96654; ^{198}Au (half-life of 2.694 days) is used in the treatment of certain tumors and in imaging. SYN aurum.

cohesive g., nearly pure g. so treated as to be free of adsorbed surface gases and impurities so that it will weld under pressure at room temperature; in dentistry, used as a restorative material placed directly into a prepared cavity and welded by pressure.

colloidal radioactive g., SYN radiogold colloid.

mat g., powdered g. formed by electrolytic precipitation, compressed into strips, and sintered.

noncohesive g., g. that will not weld because gases adsorb to the surface; some forms may be made cohesive by heat treatment; in dentistry, used as a direct filling material.

powdered g., g. formed by atomizing or by chemical precipitation, lightly precondensed, and wrapped with g. foil so as to form pellets.

g. sodium thiomalate, used in the treatment of rheumatoid arthritis. SYN sodium aurothiomalate.

g. sodium thiosulfate, used in the treatment of lupus erythematosus and some cases of rheumatoid arthritis. SYN sodium aurothiosulfate.

g. standard, term used to describe a method or procedure that is widely recognized as the best available. [jargon]

g. thioglucose, SYN aurothioglucose.

Goldblatt, Harry, U.S. pathologist, 1891–1977. SEE G.'s *clamp; G. hypertension, kidney, phenomenon, hypertension.*

Gol·den, Ross, U.S. radiologist, 1890–1975. SEE S *sign* of Golden.

Goldenhar, M., 20th century French physician. SEE G.'s *syndrome.*

gold·en seal (gold′n sēl). SYN hydrastis.

Goldflam, Samuel V., Polish neurologist, 1852–1932. SEE G. *disease.*

gold foil. Pure gold rolled into extremely thin sheets; used in the restoration of carious or fractured teeth. SEE ALSO cohesive *gold,* noncohesive *gold.*

Goldman, David E., U.S. physiologist, *1911. SEE G. *equation;* G.-Hodgkin-Katz *equation.*

Goldman, Henry M., U.S. periodontist, *1911. SEE G.-Fox *knives,* under *knife.*

Goldmann, Hans, Swiss ophthalmologist, *1899. SEE G. *perimeter;* G.'s applanation *tonometer.*

Goldscheider, J.K.A.E. Alfred, German neurologist, 1858–1935. SEE G.'s *test.*

Goldstein, Hyman I., U.S. physician, 1887–1954. SEE G.'s toe *sign.*

Goldthwait, Joel E., U.S. surgeon, 1866–1961. SEE G.'s *sign.*

Golgi, Camillo, Italian histologist and Nobel laureate, 1843–1926. SEE G. *apparatus, complex, corpuscle,* tendon *organ,* internal *reticulum, zone;* G.'s *cells,* under *cell,* osmiobichromate *fixative, stain;* G.-Mazzoni *corpuscle;* Holmgrén-G. *canals,* under *canal.*

gol·gi·o·ki·ne·sis (gol′jē-ō-ki-nē′sis). In mitosis, the process of division of the Golgi apparatus and its distribution to the two daughter cells.

Goll, Friedrich, Swiss anatomist, 1829–1903. SEE G.'s *column; nucleus* of G.; *tract* of G.

Goltz, Robert W., U.S. dermatologist, *1923. SEE G. *syndrome.*

Gombault, François A.A., French neurologist and pathologist, 1844–1904. SEE G.'s *triangle.*

go·me·nol (gō′mĕ-nol). An ethereal oil obtained from a plant, *Melaleuca viridiflora;* the chief constituent is cineole. It has germicidal action, is free from irritating properties, and has been used in chronic inflammations of the pulmonary mucous membrane and as a vermifuge. SYN oleogomenol. [*Gomen,* a locality in New Caledonia, + L. *oleum,* oil]

gom·i·to·li (gom-i′tō-lē). Intricately coiled and looped capillary vessels present largely in the upper infundibular stem of the stalk of the pituitary gland; they comprise a portion of the pituitary portal circulation. [It. *gomitolo,* coil]

gom·mel·in (gom′mē-lin). A form of dextrin.

Gomori, George, Hungarian histochemist in the U.S., 1904–1957. SEE Grocott-G. methenamine-silver *stain;* G.'s nonspecific alkaline phosphatase *stain,* one-step trichrome *stain,* silver impregnation *stain,* chrome alum hematoxylin-phloxine *stain.* See entries under stain.

Gompertz, Benjamin, English actuary, 1779–1865. SEE G.'s *hypothesis, law.*

gom·pho·sis (gom-fō′sis) [NA]. A form of fibrous joint in which a peglike process fits into a hole, as the root of a tooth into the socket in the alveolus. SYN articulatio dentoalveolaris⁂ [NA], dentoalveolar joint, gompholic joint, peg-and-socket articulation, peg-and-socket joint. [G. *gomphos,* bolt, nail, + *-osis,* condition]

go·nad (gō′nad). An organ that produces sex cells; a testis or an ovary. [Mod. L. fr. G. *gonē,* seed]

female g., SYN ovary.

indifferent g., the primordial organ in an embryo before its differentiation into testis or ovary. SEE indifferent *genitalia.*

male g., SYN testis.

streak g., SYN gonadal *streak.*

△**gonad-.** SEE gonado-.

go·nad·al (gō-nad′ăl). Relating to a gonad.

go·nad·ec·to·my (gō-nad-ek′tō-mē). Excision of ovary or testis. [gonado- + G. *ektomē,* excision]

△**gonado-, gonad-.** The gonads. [G. *gonē,* seed]

go·nad·o·crins (gō-nad′ō-krinz). Peptides that stimulate release of both follicle-stimulating hormone and luteinizing hormone from the pituitary; found in ovarian follicular fluid in rats. [gonad + G. *krinō,* to secrete]

go·nad·o·lib·er·in (gō′nad-ō-lib′er-in). **1.** A hypothalamic substance causing the release of gonadotropin. SYN gonadotropin-

go

releasing factor, gonadotropin-releasing hormone. **2.** A decapeptide from pig hypothalami that induces release of both lutropin and follitropin in constant proportions and thus acts as both luliberin and folliberin. SYN luteinizing hormone/follicle-stimulating hormone-releasing factor. [gonad + L. *libero,* to free, + -in]

gon·a·dop·athy (gon-ă-dop′ă-thē). Disease affecting the gonads. [gonado- + G. *pathos,* suffering]

go·nad·o·rel·in   **hy·dro·chlo·ride**   (gō-nad-ō-rel′in). $C_{55}H_{75}N_{17}O_{13} \cdot xHCl$; a gonadotropin-releasing hormone obtained from sheep, pigs, or other animals and used to evaluate the functional capacity of the gonadotrophs of the anterior pituitary. [*gonado*tropin-*rel*easing + -in]

go·nad·o·troph (gō-nad′ō-trōf, -gon′ă-dō-). An endocrine cell of the adenohypophysis that affects certain cells of the ovary or testis.

go·nad·o·tro·phic (gō′nad-o-trōf′ik, gon′ă-dō-). SYN gonadotropic. [gonado- + G. *trophē,* nourishment]

go·nad·o·tro·phin (gō′nad-ō-trō′fin, gon′ă-dō-). SYN gonadotropin. [for gonadotrophin, fr. gonad + G. *trophē,* nourishment]

go·nad·o·tro·pic (gō′nad-ō-trōp′ik, gon′ă-dō-). **1.** Descriptive of or relating to the actions of a gonadotropin. **2.** Promoting the growth and/or function of the gonads. SYN gonadotrophic. [gonado- + G. *tropē,* a turning]

go·nad·o·tro·pin (gō′nad-ō-trō′pin, gon′ă-dō-). A hormone capable of promoting gonadal growth and function; such effects, as exerted by a single hormone, usually are limited to discrete functions or histological components of a gonad, such as stimulation of follicular growth or of androgen formation; most g.'s exert their effects in both sexes, although the effect of a given g. will differ in males and females. SYN gonadotrophin, gonadotropic hormone.

composed of D-galactose and hexosamine, extracted from the urine of pregnant women and produced by the placental trophoblastic cells; its most important role appears to be stimulation, during the first trimester, of ovarian secretion of the estrogen and progesterone required for the integrity of conceptus; it appears to play no significant role in the last two trimesters of pregnancy, as the estrogen and progesterone are then formed by the placenta. SYN anterior pituitary-like hormone, choriogonadotropin, chorionic gonadotropic hormone, chorionic gonadotrophic hormone, placenta g., placentagonadotropin.

equine g., formed by the equine placenta. Its activity in animals is similar to that of the follicle-stimulating hormone; relatively ineffective in human beings. SYN pregnant mare's serum g.

human chorionic g. (HCG, hCG), SEE chorionic g.

human menopausal g. (HMG, hMG), a hormone of pituitary originally obtained from the urine of postmenopausal women now produced synthetically; used to induce ovulation. SEE ALSO menotropins.

placenta g. (plă-sen′tă-gō′nad-ō-trō-pin), SYN chorionic g.

pregnant mare's serum g. (PMSG), SYN equine g.

gon·a·duct (gon′ă-dŭkt). **1.** SYN seminal *duct.* **2.** SYN uterine *tube.* [gonado- + duct]

go·nal·gia (gō-nal′jē-ă). Pain in the knee. [G. *gony,* knee, + *algos,* pain]

gon·ane (gon′ān). The hypothetical parent hydrocarbon molecule of gonadal steroid hormones, such as estrane or androstane, which was conceived to achieve forms of systematic nomenclature.

gon·ar·thri·tis (gon-ar-thrī′tis). Inflammation of the knee joint. [G. *gony,* knee, + *arthron,* joint, + -*itis,* inflammation]

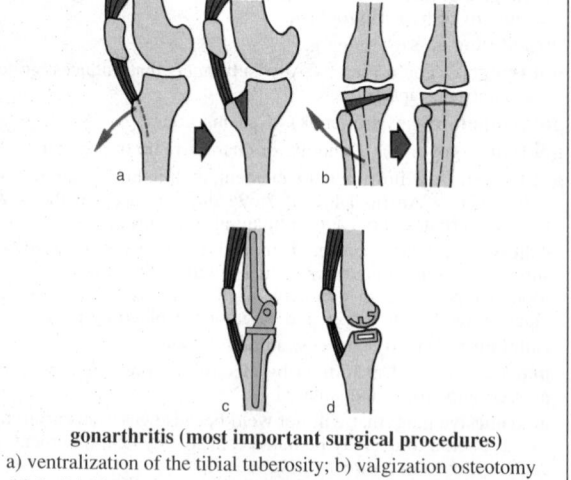

gonarthritis (most important surgical procedures)
a) ventralization of the tibial tuberosity; b) valgization osteotomy (high tibial head osteotomy) for bow-legged deformity; c) complete arthroplasty of the knee joint, with prosthesis; d) sliding prosthesis

gon·ar·throt·o·my (gon-ar-throt′ō-mē). Incision into the knee joint. [G. *gony,* knee, + *arthron,* joint, + *tomē,* incision]

gon·a·tag·ra (gon-ă-tag′ră). Obsolete term for gout in the knee. [G. *gony,* knee, + *agra,* seizure]

go·nat·o·cele (gō-nat′ō-sēl). Obsolete term for tumor of the knee. [G. *gony,* knee, + *kēlē,* tumor]

gon·e·cyst, gon·e·cys·tis (gon′ĕ-sist, gon-ĕ-sis′tis). SYN seminal *vesicle.* [G. *gonē,* seed, + *kystis,* bladder]

gon·e·cys·to·lith (gon-ĕ-sis′tō-lith). Obsolete term for a concretion or calculus in a seminal vesicle. [gonecyst + G. *kystis,* bladder, + *lithos,* stone]

Gon·gy·lo·ne·ma (gon′ji-lō-nē′mă). An important genus of spiruroid nematodes that parasitize the alimentary canal of birds and mammals; transmitted via various insects, especially beetles, carrying the encysted infective larvae. Several species are of veteri-

gonadotropins

anterior pituitary g., any g. of hypophysial origin; formerly used to designate a single hormone, because it was thought that the anterior hypophysis secreted only one g. SYN pituitary gonadotropic hormone.

chorionic g. (CG), a glycoprotein with a carbohydrate fraction

nary importance, and one is also known to parasitize humans. [Gr. *gongylos*, round, + *nēma*, thread]

G. ingluvic'ola, species parasitic in the mucosa of the crop, esophagus, and proventriculus of chickens, turkeys, and quail; transmitted by beetles, it tunnels into the crop wall but is relatively nonpathogenic.

G. neoplas'ticum, species parasitic in the stomach or esophagus epithelium of various rodents, rabbits, and sheep and transmitted by coprophagous beetles; it is often associated with benign proliferations, once thought to be neoplastic, in the stomach and esophagus of infected, malnourished rats.

G. pul'chrum, the gullet worm of cattle; a species that penetrates the submucosa of the esophagus or rumen of many domestic and wild ruminants, pigs, bears, and humans (human cases are chiefly caused by immature worms); it is transmitted by coprophagous beetles and is of worldwide distribution.

gon·gy·lo·ne·mi·a·sis (gon'ji-lō-nē-mī'ă-sis). Infection of animals and rarely humans with nematodes of the genus *Gongylonema.*

go·nia (gō'nē-ă). Plural of gonion.

gonio-. Angle. [G. *gōnia*]

go·ni·o·cra·ni·om·e·try (gō'nē-ō-krā-nē-om'ě-trē). Measurement of the angles of the cranium. [G. *gōnia*, angle, + *kranion*, skull, + *metron*, measure]

go·ni·o·dys·gen·e·sis (gō'nē-ō-dis-jen'ě-sis). Developmental aberration of the anterior ocular segment. [G. *gōnia*, angle, + dysgenesis]

go·ni·om·e·ter (gō-nē-om'ě-ter). **1.** An instrument for measuring angles. **2.** An appliance for the static test of labyrinthine disease, which consists of a plank, one end of which may be raised to any desired height; as one end of the plank is gradually raised, the point at which a patient loses balance is noted. **3.** A calibrated device designed to measure the arc or range of motion of a joint. SYN arthrometer, fleximeter, pronometer. [G. *gōnia*, angle, + *metron*, measure]

go·ni·on, pl. **go·nia** (gō'nē-on, gō'nē-ă) [NA]. The lowest posterior and most outward point of the angle of the mandible. In cephalometrics, it is measured by bisecting the angle formed by the tangents to the lower and the posterior borders of the mandible; when the angles of both sides of the mandible appear on the lateral radiograph, a point midway between the right and left side is used. [G. *gōnia*, an angle]

go·ni·o·punc·ture (gō'nē-ō-pŭnk-chūr). An operation for congenital glaucoma in which a puncture is made in the filtration angle of the anterior chamber.

go·ni·o·scope (gō'nē-ō-skōp). A lens designed to study the angle of the anterior chamber of the eye. [G. *gōnia*, angle, + *skopeō*, to examine]

go·ni·os·co·py (gō-nē-os'kŏ-pē). Examination of the angle of the anterior chamber of the eye with a gonioscope or with a contact prism lens.

go·ni·o·syn·ech·ia (gō'nē-ō-si-nek'ē-ă). Adhesion of the iris to the posterior surface of the cornea in the angle of the anterior chamber; associated with angle-closure glaucoma. SYN peripheral anterior synechia. [G. *gōnia*, angle, + *synechis*, holding together]

go·ni·ot·o·my (gō-nē-ot'ō-mē). Surgical opening of the trabecular meshwork in congenital glaucoma. [G. *gōnia*, angle, + *tomē*, incision]

go·ni·tis (gō-nī'tis). Obsolete term for inflammation of the knee. [G. *gony*, knee, + *-itis*, inflammation]

gon·o·cele (gon'ō-sēl). A cystic lesion of the epididymis or rete testis, resulting from obstruction and containing secretions from the testis. [G. *gonē*, seed, + *kēlē*, tumor]

gon·o·cho·rism, gon·o·cho·ris·mus (gon-ok'ō-rizm, -ō-riz'mŭs). Normal gonadal differentiation appropriate to the sex. [G. *gonē*, seed, sex, + *chōrizō*, to separate]

gon·o·cide (gon'ō-sīd). **1.** Destructive to the gonococcus. **2.** An agent that kills gonococci. SYN gonococcicide.

gon·o·coc·cal (gon'ō-kok'ăl). Relating to the gonococcus. SYN gonococcic.

gon·o·coc·ce·mia (gon'ō-kok-sē'mē-ă). The presence of gono-

cocci in the circulating blood. SYN gonohemia. [gonococcus + G. *haima*, blood]

gon·o·coc·ci (gon-ō-kok'sī). Plural of gonococcus.

gon·o·coc·cic (gon'ō-kok'sik). SYN gonococcal.

gon·o·coc·ci·cide (gon-ō-kok'si-sīd). SYN gonocide. [gonococcus + L. *caedo*, to kill]

gon·o·coc·cus, pl. **gon·o·coc·ci** (gon-ō-kok'ŭs, -sī). SYN *Neisseria gonorrhoeae.* [G. *gonē*, seed, + *kokkos*, berry]

gon·o·cyte (gon'ō-sīt). SYN primordial germ *cell.* [G. *gonē*, seed, + *kytos*, hollow (cell)]

gon·o·he·mia (gon-ō-hē'mē-ă). SYN gonococcemia.

gon·o·op·so·nin (gon-ō-op'sŏ-nin). A specific gonococcal opsonin.

gon·o·phage (gon'ō-fāj). A gonocidal bacteriophage.

gon·o·phore, gon·oph·o·rus (gon'ŏ-fōr, gō-nof'ŏ-rŭs). Any structure serving to store up or conduct the sexual cells; oviduct, spermatic duct, uterus, or seminal vesicle; an accessory generative organ. [G. *gonē*, seed, + *phoros*, bearing]

gon·or·rhea (gon-ō-rē'ă). A contagious catarrhal inflammation of the genital mucous membrane, transmitted chiefly by coitus and due to *Neisseria gonorrhoeae;* may involve the lower or upper genital tract, especially the urethra, endocervix, and uterine tubes, or spread to the peritoneum and rarely to the heart, joints, or other structures by way of the bloodstream. [G. *gonorrhoia,* fr. *gonē*, seed, + *rhoia*, a flow]

gon·or·rhe·al (gon-ō-rē'ăl). Relating to gonorrhea.

gon·o·some (gon'ō-sōm). SYN sex *chromosomes,* under *chromosome.* [G. *gonē*, seed + *sōma*, body]

gon·o·tox·e·mia (gon'ō-tok-sē'mē-ă). Toxic condition resulting from the hematogenous dissemination of gonococci and the effects of the absorbed endotoxin.

gon·o·tox·in (gon-ō-tok'sin). The endotoxin elaborated by the gonococcus, *Neisseria gonorrhoeae.*

gon·o·tyl (gon'ō-til). A sucker-like structure enclosing the genital pore of flukes of the family Heterophyidae. [G. *gonos,* offspring, + *tylē,* knob]

Go·ny·au·lax cat·a·nel·la (gon-ē-aw'laks kat-ă-nel'ă). A marine dinoflagellate protozoan that produces a powerful toxin that accumulates in the tissues of mussels and other filter-feeding shellfish and may cause fatal mussel poisoning in humans. [G. *gony,* knee, + *aulakos,* a furrow]

gon·y·camp·sis (gon-ē-kamp'sis). Ankylosis or any abnormal curvature of the knee. [G. *gony,* knee, + *kampsis,* a bending or curving]

Goodell, William, U.S. gynecologist, 1829–1894. SEE G.'s *dilator, sign.*

good·ness of fit. Degree of agreement between an empirically observed distribution and a mathematical or theoretical distribution.

Goodpasture, Ernest W., U.S. pathologist, 1886–1960. SEE G.'s *stain, syndrome.*

Goormaghtigh, Norbert, Belgian physician, 1890–1960. SEE G.'s *cells,* under *cell.*

goose·flesh (gūs'flesh). SYN *cutis* anserina.

Gopalan, C., 20th century Indian biochemist. SEE G.'s *syndrome.*

Gordius (gōr'dē-ŭs). An old name for the nematode genus *Dracunculus,* properly applied to members of the phylum Nematomorpha, commonly called the gordian or horsehair worms, hair worms, or hair snakes. [L., fr. G. *Gordios,* king of Gordium in Phrygia; an allusion to the knotlike twistings of these worms]

Gordon, Alfred, U.S. neurologist, 1874–1953. SEE G. *reflex;* G.'s *sign, symptom.*

Gordon and Sweet stain. See under stain.

gor·get (gōr'jet). A director or guide with wide groove for use in lithotomy.

probe g., a g. with a probe-pointed tip.

Gorham, Lemuel W., U.S. physician, 1885–1968. SEE G.'s *disease.*

Go

Goriaew's rule. See under rule.

Gorlin, Richard, U.S. physiologist and cardiologist, *1926. SEE G. formula.

Gorlin, Robert J., U.S. oral pathologist, *1923. SEE G.'s sign, syndrome; G.-Chaudhry-Moss syndrome.

Gorman's syn·drome. See under syndrome.

go·ron·dou (gō-ron′dū). SYN goundou.

Gosselin, Léon Athanese, French surgeon, 1815–1887. SEE G.'s fracture.

Gosset, William Sealy, British statistician and chemist who used the pseudonym Student, 1876–1937.

gos·sy·pol (gos′i-pol). $C_{30}H_{30}O_8$; a toxic principle isolated from the seed of the cotton plant (Gossypium) which reduces sperm count; used in China as an oral male contraceptive.

gos·sy·pose (gos′i-pōs). SYN raffinose.

GOT Abbreviation for glutamic-oxaloacetic transaminase.

Göthlin, Gustaf F., Swedish physiologist, 1874–1949. SEE G.'s test.

Gottron, H.A., German physician, 1890–1974. SEE Arndt-G. syndrome.

gouge (gowj). A strong curved chisel used in operation on bone.

Gougerot, Henri, French physician, 1881–1955. SEE G. and Blum disease; G.-Sjögren disease; G.-Carteaud syndrome.

Gould, Sir Alfred P., English surgeon, 1852–1922. SEE G.'s suture.

Gouley, John W.S., U.S. urologist, 1832–1920. SEE G.'s catheter.

goun·dou (gūn′dū). A disease, endemic in West Africa, characterized by exostoses from the nasal processes of the maxillary bones, producing a symmetrical swelling on each side of the nose; believed to be an osteitis connected with yaws. SYN anákhré, dog nose, gorondou, henpuye. [native name]

gout (gowt). A disorder of purine metabolism, occurring especially in men, characterized by a raised but variable blood uric acid level and severe recurrent acute arthritis of sudden onset resulting from deposition of crystals of sodium urate in connective tissues and articular cartilage; most cases are inherited, resulting from a variety of abnormalities of purine metabolism. The familial aggregation is for the most part galtonian with a threshold of expression determined by the solubility of uric acid. However, gout is a feature of the Lesch-Nyhan syndrome an X-linked disorder [MIM*308000]. [L. gutta, drop]

abarticular g., rarely used term for g. involving structures other than the joints.

articular g., the usual form of g. attacking one or more of the joints.

calcium g., SYN pseudogout.

idiopathic g., acute episodes of crystal-induced synovitis due to abnormality of purine metabolism; lower than normal urinary excretion of urate leading to hyperuricemia and acute episodes of joint inflammation. SYN primary g.

interval g., an asymptomatic phase between acute attacks of g.

latent g., hyperuricemia without symptoms of gout. Often used synonymously with interval g. SYN masked g.

lead g., SYN saturnine g.

masked g., SYN latent g.

primary g., SYN idiopathic g.

retrocedent g., obsolete term for the occurrence of severe gastric, cardiac, or cerebral symptoms during an attack of g., especially when the joint and other symptoms suddenly subside at the same time.

saturnine g., g. occurring in a person with lead poisoning. SYN lead g.

secondary g., g. resulting from increased serum uric acid levels as a result of an antecedent disease, such as a proliferative disease of the blood and bone marrow , lead poisoning, or prolonged chronic renal failure (on dialysis).

tophaceous g., g. in which deposits of uric acid and urates occur as gouty tophi.

gouty (gow′tē). Relating to or characteristic of gout.

Gowers, Sir William R., English neurologist, 1845–1915. SEE G.'s column, contraction; G. disease; G.'s syndrome, tract.

GPI Abbreviation for Gingival-Periodontal Index.

GPT Abbreviation for glutamic-pyruvic transaminase.

gr Abbreviation for grain (3).

Graaf, Reijnier de, Dutch physiologist and histologist, 1641–1673. SEE graafian follicle.

graafian. Relating to or described by R. de Graaf.

grac·i·lis (gras′i-lis). 1. Slender; denoting a thin or slender structure. 2. SYN gracilis muscle. [L.]

grad. Abbreviation for L. gradatim, by degrees, gradually.

grade (grād). 1. A rank, division, or level on the scale of a value system. 2. In cancer pathology, a classification of the degree of malignancy or differentiation of tumor tissue; e.g., well, moderately well, or poorly differentiated, and undifferentiated or anaplastic. 3. In exercise testing, the measurement of a vertical rise or fall as a percent of the horizontal distance traveled. [L. gradus, step]

Gleason's tumor g., a classification of adenocarcinoma of the prostate by evaluation of the pattern of glandular differentiation; the tumor g., know as Gleason's score, is the sum of the dominant and secondary patterns, each numbered on a scale of 1 to 5.

Heath-Edwards g.'s, a system that describes the pathology of hypertensive pulmonary vascular disease.

Gradenigo, Giuseppe, Italian physician, 1859–1926. SEE G.'s syndrome.

gra·di·ent (grā′dē-ent). Rate of change of temperature, pressure, or other variable as a function of distance, time, etc.

atrioventricular g., the diastolic pressure difference between the atrium and ventricle.

concentration g., SYN density g.

density g., a solution in which the concentration (density) of a solute increases in a continuous fashion from top to bottom, or end to end, of a container (e.g., the centrifuge tube in density-gradient centrifugation). SYN concentration g.

electrochemical g., a measure of the tendency of an ion to move passively from one point to another, taking into consideration the differences in its concentration and in the electrical potentials between the two points; commonly expressed as the additional voltage needed to achieve equilibrium.

g. encoding, SYN phase encoding.

field g., SYN magnetic field g.

magnetic field g., in magnetic resonance imaging, a magnetic field that varies with location, superimposed on the uniform field of the magnet, to alter the resonant frequency of nuclei and allow recovery of their spatial position. SYN field g.

mitral g., the diastolic pressure difference between the left atrium and left ventricle.

systolic g., the difference in pressure during systole between two communicating cardiovascular chambers, e.g., between the left ventricle and aorta in aortic stenosis.

ventricular g., the algebraic sum of (i.e., the net electrical difference between) the area enclosed within the QRS complex and that within the T wave in the electrocardiogram.

grad·u·ate (grad′yū-ăt). A vessel, usually of glass and suitably marked, used for measuring the volume of liquids. [Mediev. L. graduatus, fr. L. gradus, step]

grad·u·at·ed (grad′yū-āt′ed). 1. Marked by lines or in other ways to denote capacity, degrees, percentages, etc. 2. Divided or arranged in levels, grades, or successive steps.

Graefe, Albrecht von, German ophthalmologist, 1828–1870. SEE G. forceps; G.'s knife, operation, sign, spots, under spot; pseudo-G.'s phenomenon; G.'s sign; von G. sign.

Graefenberg, Ernst, German gynecologist in America, 1881–1957. SEE G. ring.

Graffi, Arnold, German pathologist, *1910. SEE G.'s virus.

graft. 1. Any free (unattached) tissue or organ for transplantation. 2. To transplant such structures. SEE ALSO flap, implant, transplant. [A.S. graef]

accordion g., a skin g. in which multiple slits have been made, so it can be stretched to cover a large area. SYN mesh g.

adipodermal g., SYN dermal-fat g.

allogeneic g., SYN allograft.

anastomosed g., a g. in which circulation is established by surgical anastomoses of blood vessels.

animal g., SYN zoograft.

augmentation g., a g. of material used to increase the size, shape, or volume of a structure.

autodermic g., a skin autograft.

autogeneic g., SYN autograft.

autologous g., SYN autograft.

autoplastic g., SYN autograft.

Blair-Brown g., a split-thickness g. of intermediate thickness.

bone g., bone transplanted from a donor site to a recipient site. SEE ALSO osteoplasty.

brephoplastic g., a g. from an embryo or newborn to an adult.

cable g., a multiple strand nerve g. arranged as a pathway for regeneration of axons.

chessboard g.'s, obsolete synonym for postage stamp g.'s.

chip g., a g. utilizing small pieces of cartilage or bone which is packed into a bone defect.

chorioallantoic g., transplanting of living material to the chorio-allantoic membrane of the embryonic chick.

composite g., a g. composed of several structures, such as skin and cartilage or a full-thickness segment of the ear.

corneal g., SYN keratoplasty.

cutis g., a g. of corium, from which epidermis and subcutaneous tissue have been separated.

Davis g.'s, small pieces (2 to 3 mm) of full-thickness skin.

delayed g., application of a skin g. after waiting several days for healthy granulations to form.

dermal g., a g. of dermis, made from skin by cutting away a thin split-thickness g.

dermal-fat g., a dermal g. with attached subcutaneous fat. SYN adipodermal g.

Douglas g., obsolete eponym for sieve g.

epidermic g., a g. supposed to contain only epidermis.

Esser g., SYN inlay g.

fascia g., a g. of fibrous tissue, usually the fascia lata.

fascicular g., a nerve g. in which each bundle of fibers is approximated and sutured separately.

fat g., a free g. of fat.

filler g., a g. used for the filling of defects, *e.g.,* filling a cyst with bone chips.

free g., a g. transplanted without its normal attachments, or a pedicle, from one site to another.

full-thickness g., a g. of the full thickness of mucosa and submucosa or of skin and subcutaneous tissue.

funicular g., a nerve g. in which each funiculus (composed of two or more fasciculi) is approximated and sutured separately.

H g., SYN H *shunt.*

heterologous g., SYN xenograft.

heteroplastic g., SYN xenograft.

heterospecific g., SYN xenograft.

heterotopic g., transplantation of a tissue or organ into a position it normally does not occupy.

homologous g., SYN allograft.

homoplastic g., SYN allograft.

hyperplastic g., a g. in active proliferation.

implantation g., placing of Davis g.'s deep into the interstices of granulation tissue.

infusion g., transplantation by injection of a suspension of cells.

inlay g., a skin g. wrapped (raw side out) around a bolus of dental compound and inserted into a prepared surgical pocket. SYN epithelial inlay, Esser g.

interspecific g., SYN xenograft.

isogeneic g., SYN syngraft.

isologous g., SYN syngraft.

isoplastic g., SYN syngraft.

Krause g., a full-thickness skin g. SYN Krause-Wolfe g.

Krause-Wolfe g., SYN Krause g.

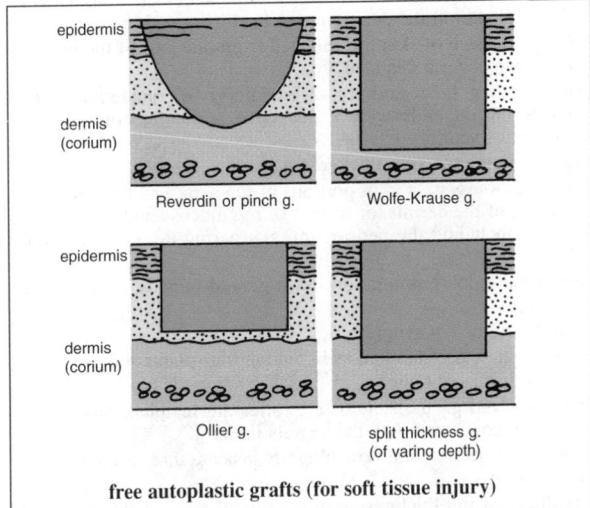

free autoplastic grafts (for soft tissue injury)

Reverdin or pinch g.

Wolfe-Krause g.

Ollier g.

split thickness g. (of varing depth)

epidermis

dermis (corium)

mesh g., SYN accordion g.

mucosal g., a g. of mucous membrane, usually the full-thickness of the lining of the cheek or lower lip.

nerve g., a nerve, or part of a nerve, used as a g.

Ollier g., a thin split-thickness g., usually in small pieces. SYN Ollier-Thiersch g., Thiersch g.

Ollier-Thiersch g., SYN Ollier g.

omental g., a segment of omentum, with its supplying blood vessels, transplanted as a free flap to a distant area and revascularized by arterial and venous anastomoses.

onlay g., a bone g. applied on the outside of the recipient bone(s).

orthotopic g., transplantation of a tissue or organ into its normal anatomical position.

osteoperiosteal g., a g. of bone with its attached periosteum.

partial-thickness g., SYN split-thickness g.

pedicle g., SEE pedicle *flap.*

periosteal g., a g. of periosteum, usually placed on bare bone.

Phemister g., an autogenous onlay bone graft used in treating delayed union of fractures.

pinch g., small bits of skin, of partial or full thickness, removed from a healthy area and seeded in a site to be covered. SYN Reverdin g.

porcine g., a split-thickness g. from a pig, applied to a raw area on a human as a temporary dressing.

postage stamp g.'s, small pieces cut from a sheet of split-thickness g.

primary skin g., a skin g. transferred immediately after the creation of a raw area.

punch g.'s, small full-thickness g.'s of the scalp, removed with a circular punch and transplanted to a bald area to grow hair.

Reverdin g., SYN pinch g.

sieve g., obsolete term for a full-thickness skin g. taken after

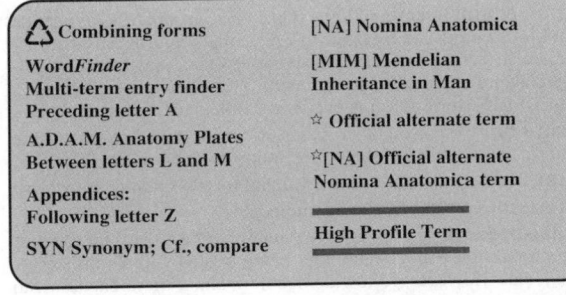

♻ **Combining forms**	**[NA] Nomina Anatomica**
Word*Finder*	**[MIM] Mendelian**
Multi-term entry finder	**Inheritance in Man**
Preceding letter A	
	☆ **Official alternate term**
A.D.A.M. Anatomy Plates	
Between letters L and M	☆**[NA] Official alternate**
	Nomina Anatomica term
Appendices:	
Following letter Z	
	High Profile Term
SYN Synonym; Cf., compare	

cutting multiple holes in it with a circular punch, thus leaving islands of skin in the donor area to heal it.

skin g., a piece of skin transplanted from one part of the body to another to cover a denuded area.

sleeve g., a g. for repairing a severed nerve by connecting central and peripheral ends with a sleevelike structure, commonly, a segment of vein.

split-skin g., SYN split-thickness g.

split-thickness g., a g. of portions of the skin, *i.e.,* the epidermis and part of the dermis, or of part of the mucosa and submucosa, but not including the periosteum. SYN partial-thickness g., split-skin g.

Stent g., an inlay skin g., or a skin g. held in place by a tie-over dressing.

syngeneic g., SYN syngraft.

tendon g., a g. of tendon, as in tendon transplantation.

Thiersch g., SYN Ollier g.

vascularized g., the state of a g. after the recipient vasculature has been connected with the vessels in the g.

white g., rejection of a skin allograft so acute that vascularization never occurs.

Wolfe g., a full-thickness skin g. without any subcutaneous fat. SYN Wolfe-Krause g.

Wolfe-Krause g., SYN Wolfe g.

xenogeneic g., SYN xenograft.

zooplastic g., SYN zoograft.

graft·ing. Transplanting a graft.

Graham, Evarts Ambrose, U.S. surgeon, 1883–1957. Reported with W. H. Cole the first successful cholecystography in 1924; In 1933, with J. J. Singer, reported first successful removal of a lung for cancer in one stage. SEE Graham-Cole *test*.

Graham, Thomas, English chemist, 1805–1869. SEE G.'s *law*.

Gra·ha·mel·la (grā-am-el′ă). A genus of aerobic, nonmotile microorganisms (order Rickettsiales) containing long or short, rod-shaped, Gram-negative cells which resemble those of *Bartonella* but which are less pleomorphic. These organisms occur within the erythrocytes of lower mammals, but they appear to be nonpathogenic and do not affect the health of the host. [G. S. Graham-Smith]

Graham Little, Sir Ernest Gordon, British physician, 1867–1950. SEE G. L. *syndrome*.

Graham Steell, SEE Steell.

grain (grān). 1. Cereal plants, such as corn, wheat, or rye, or a seed of one of them. 2. A minute, hard particle of any substance, as of sand. 3 **(gr).** A unit of weight, $\frac{1}{60}$ dram (apoth. or troy), $\frac{1}{437.5}$ avoirdupois ounce, $\frac{1}{480}$ troy ounce, $\frac{1}{5760}$ troy pound, $\frac{1}{7000}$ avoirdupois pound; the equivalent of 0.064799 g. [L. *granum*]

grains (grānz). Parakeratotic nuclei within the horny layer of the epidermis, found in keratosis follicularis.

Gram, Hans C.J., Danish bacteriologist, 1853–1938. SEE G.'s *iodine, stain;* Weigert-G. *stain*.

gram (g, gm). A unit of weight in the metric or centesimal system, the equivalent of 15.432358 grains or 0.03527 avoirdupois ounce.

△**-gram.** A recording, usually by an instrument. Cf. -graph. [G. *gramma,* character, mark]

gram-cen·ti·me·ter. The energy exerted, or work done, when a mass of 1 g is raised a height of 1 cm; equal to 9.807×10^{-5} joules or newton-meters.

gram·i·ci·din (gram-i-sī′din). One of a group of polypeptide antibiotics produced by *Bacillus brevis* that are primarily bacteriostatic in action against Gram-positive cocci and bacilli. Commercial preparations contain several g.'s known as g. A, B, C, and D; g. S (for Soviet) is cyclic, the others are linear.

gram-i·on. The weight in grams of an ion that is equal to the sum of the atomic weights of the atoms making up the ion.

gram-me·ter. A unit of energy equal to 100 gram-centimeters.

gram-mol·e·cule. See under molecule.

Gram-neg·a·tive. Refers to the inability of a bacterium to resist decolorization with alcohol after being treated with Gram's crystal violet. However, following decolorization, these bacteria can

be readily counterstained with safranin, imparting a pink or red color to the bacterium when viewed by light microscopy. This reaction is usually an indication that the outer structure of the bacterium consists of a cytoplasmic (inner) membrane surrounded by a relatively thin peptidoglycan layer, which in turn, is surrounded by an outer membrane. SEE Gram's *stain*.

Gram-pos·i·tive. Refers to the ability of a bacterium to resist decolorization with alcohol after being treated with Gram's crystal violet stain, imparting a violet color to the bacterium when viewed by light microscopy. This reaction is usually an indication that the outer structure of the bacterium consists of a cytoplasmic membrane surrounded by a thick, rigid bacterial cell wall comprised of peptidoglycan. SEE Gram's *stain*.

gra·na (grā′nă). Bodies within the chloroplasts of plant cells that contain layers composed of chlorophyll and phospholipids. [pl. of L. *granum,* grain]

gra·na·tum (gra-nā′tum). SYN pomegranate. [L. *granatus,* having many seeds]

gran·di·ose (gran′dē-ōs). Pertaining to feelings of great importance, expansiveness, or delusions of grandeur. [It. *grandioso,* fr. L. *grandis,* large]

Grandry, M., 19th century French anatomist. SEE G.'s *corpuscles,* under *corpuscle*.

Granger, Amedee, U.S. radiologist, 1879–1939. SEE G.'s *line*.

Granit, Ragnar A., Finnish-Swedish neurophysiologist and Nobel laureate, 1900–1991 SEE G.'s *loop*.

gran·u·lar (gran′yū-lăr). 1. Composed of or resembling granules or granulations. 2. Particles with strong affinity for nuclear stains, seen in many bacterial species.

gra·nu·la·tio, pl. **gran·u·la·ti·o·nes** (gran-yū-lā′shē-ō, -shē-o′ nēz). SYN granulation. [L.]

granulatio′nes arachnoidea′les [NA], SYN arachnoid *granulations,* under *granulation.* SEE ALSO arachnoid *villi,* under *villus*.

gran·u·la·tion (gran′yū-lā′shŭn). 1. Formation into grains or granules; the state of being granular. 2. A granular mass in or on the surface of any organ or membrane; or one of the individual granules forming the mass. 3. The formation of minute, rounded, fleshy connective tissue projections on the surface of a wound, ulcer, or inflamed tissue surface in the process of healing; one of the fleshy granules composing this surface. SEE ALSO granulation *tissue.* 4. In pharmacy, the formation of crystals by constant agitation of a supersaturated solution of a salt. SYN granulatio. [L. *granulatio*]

arachnoid g.'s, tufted prolongations of pia-arachnoid, composed of numerous arachnoid villi that penetrate dural venous sinuses and effect transfer of cerebrospinal fluid to the venous system. At advanced age these are more numerous and tend to calcify. SYN granulationes arachnoideales [NA], arachnoidal g.'s, pacchionian bodies, pacchionian corpuscles, pacchionian glands, pacchionian g.'s.

arachnoidal g.'s, SYN arachnoid g.'s.

pacchionian g.'s, SYN arachnoid g.'s.

gran·u·la·ti·o·nes (gran-yū-lā-shē-ō′nēz). Plural of granulatio.

gran·ule (gran′yūl). 1. A grain-like particle; a granulation; a minute discrete mass. 2. A very small pill, usually gelatin-coated or sugar-coated, containing a drug to be given in a small dose. 3. A colony of the bacterium or fungus causing a disease or simply colonizing the tissues of the patient. In compromised patients the differentiation is difficult. [L. *granulum,* dim. of *granum,* grain]

α g.'s, large, rodlike, or filamentous g.'s found in several types of cells, especially platelets where they are the most numerous type of g.; contain secretory proteins, including fibrinogen, fibronectin, fibrospondin, von Willebrand factor (collectively known as adhesive proteins) and other proteins (platelet factor 4, platelet-derived growth factor, coagulation factor V, etc.).

acidophil g., a g. that stains with an acid dye such as eosin. SYN oxyphil g.

acrosomal g., the single glycoprotein rich g. within an acrosomal vesicle, which results from the coalescence of proacrosomal g.'s.

alpha g., a g. of an alpha cell that was named as the first of several kinds or because it was acidophilic.

Altmann's g., (1) SYN fuchsinophil g. **(2)** SYN mitochondrion.

amphophil g., a g. that stains with both acid and basic dyes.

argentaffin g.'s, g.'s that reduce silver ions from an ammoniacal silver nitrate staining solution.

azurophil g., a g. that stains a reddish purple color with an azure dye; such g.'s are seen in dry smears of certain mature and developing blood cells, and are membrane-bound primary lysosomes containing enzymes. SYN kappa g.

basal g., SYN basal *body*.

basophil g., a g. that stains readily with a basic dye.

Bensley's specific g.'s, g.'s in the cells of the islands of Langerhans in the pancreas.

beta g., a g. of a beta cell.

Birbeck's g., SYN Langerhans' g.

Bollinger g.'s, (1) relatively small, but frequently microscopically visible, pale yellow or yellow-white g.'s observed in the granulomatous lesion, or the exudate, in botryomycosis; the g.'s consist of irregular aggregates or colonizations of Gram-positive cocci, usually staphylococci; **(2)** term sometimes incorrectly used synonymously with Bollinger bodies.

chromatic g., SYN chromophil g. (2).

chromophil g., (1) any readily stainable g.; **(2)** a g. of chromophil (Nissl) substance. SYN chromatic g.

chromophobe g.'s, g.'s that do not stain or stain poorly with the ordinary dyes; such g.'s are present in some cells in the anterior lobe of the pituitary.

cone g., nucleus of a retinal cell connecting with one of the cones.

Crooke's g.'s, lumpy masses of basophilic material in the basophil cells of the anterior lobe of the pituitary, associated with Cushing's disease, or following the administration of ACTH.

delta g., a g. of a delta cell.

elementary g., a particle of blood dust, or hemoconia.

eosinophil g., a g. that stains with eosin.

Fordyce's g.'s, SYN Fordyce's *spots*, under *spot*.

fuchsinophil g., a g. that has an affinity for fuchsin. SYN Altmann's g. (1).

glycogen g., glycogen occurring in cells as beta g.'s which average about 300 Å in diameter, or as alpha g.'s which are aggregates measuring 900 Å of smaller particles.

iodophil g., a g. that stains brown with iodine; found in many of the polymorphonuclear leukocytes in pneumonia, erysipelas, scarlet fever, and various other acute diseases.

juxtaglomerular g.'s, osmophilic secretory g.'s present in the juxtaglomerular cells, thought to contain renin.

kappa g., SYN azurophil g.

keratohyalin g.'s, irregularly shaped basophilic g.'s in the cells of the stratum granulosum of the epidermis.

lamellar g., SYN keratinosome.

Langerhans' g., a small tennis racket-shaped membrane-bound g. with characteristic cross-striated internal ultrastructure; first reported in Langerhans' cells of the epidermis. SYN Birbeck's g.

Langley's g.'s, g.'s in serous secreting cells.

membrane-coating g., SYN keratinosome.

metachromatic g.'s, (1) g.'s that stain a color different from that of the dye used; SEE ALSO metachromasia. **(2)** term sometimes used as a synonym for volutin.

mucinogen g.'s, g.'s that produce mucin, as in cells of the salivary glands and in the gastric and intestinal mucosae.

Neusser's g.'s, tiny basophilic g.'s sometimes observed in an indistinct zone about the nucleus of a leukocyte.

neutrophil g., a g. stainable with the neutral component of stains, *e.g.,* the Romanovsky-type blood stains.

Nissl g.'s, SYN Nissl *substance*.

oxyphil g., SYN acidophil g.

Palade g., SYN ribosome.

proacrosomal g.'s, small carbohydrate-rich g.'s appearing in vesicles of the Golgi apparatus of spermatids; they coalesce into a single acrosomal g. contained within an acrosomal vesicle.

prosecretion g.'s, g.'s in the cytoplasm of a cell indicative of a preliminary step in the formation of a secretory product.

rod g., the nucleus of a retinal cell connecting with one of the rods.

Schüffner's g.'s, SYN Schüffner's *dots*, under *dot*.

secretory g., a membrane-bound particle, usually protein, formed in the granular endoplasmic reticulum and the Golgi complex.

seminal g., one of the minute granular bodies present in the semen.

volutin g.'s, SYN volutin.

Zimmermann's g., SYN platelet.

zymogen g., secretory g. in pancreatic acinar cells.

△**granulo-.** Granular, granules. [L. *granulum,* a small grain.]

gran·u·lo·blast (gran′yū-lō-blast). Rarely used term for an immature hematopoietic cell capable of giving rise to granulocytes. [granulo- + G. *blastos,* germ]

gran·u·lo·blas·to·sis (gran′yū-lō-blas-tō′sis). A leukemic form of leukosis in the chicken characterized by an increase of immature, granular blood cells in the circulating blood and frequently infiltration of the parenchymatous organs.

gran·u·lo·cyte (gran′yū-lō-sīt). A mature granular leukocyte, including neutrophilic, acidophilic, and basophilic types of polymorphonuclear leukocytes, *i.e.,* respectively, neutrophils, eosinophils, and basophils. [granulo- + G. *kytos,* cell]

immature g., an immature neutrophil, except that it may be neutrophilic, acidophilic, or basophilic in character.

gran·u·lo·cy·to·pe·nia (gran′yū-lō-sī-tō-pē′nē-ă). Less than the normal number of granular leukocytes in the blood. SYN granulopenia, hypogranulocytosis. [granulocyte + G. *penia,* poverty]

gran·u·lo·cy·to·poi·e·sis (gran′yū-lō-sī′tō-poy-ē′sis). SYN granulopoiesis.

gran·u·lo·cy·to·poi·et·ic (gran′yū-lō-sī′tō-poy-et′ik). SYN granulopoietic. [granulocyte + G. *poieō,* to make]

gran·u·lo·cy·to·sis (gran′yū-lō-sī-tō′sis). A condition characterized by more than the normal number of granulocytes in the circulating blood or in the tissues.

gran·u·lo·ma (gran-yū-lō′mă). Indefinite term applied to nodular inflammatory lesions, usually small or granular, firm, persistent, and containing compactly grouped mononuclear phagocytes. SEE ALSO granulomatosis. [granulo- + G. *-oma,* tumor]

actinic g., an annular eruption on sun-exposed skin which microscopically shows phagocytosis of dermal elastic fibers by giant cells and histiocytes. SYN Miescher's g.

amebic g., SYN ameboma.

g. annula′re, a chronic or recurrent, usually self-limited papular eruption that tends to develop on the distal portions of the extremities and over prominences, although the condition may be generalized; waxy papules tend to form annular lesions characterized microscopically by foci of dermal necrosis with mucin deposits, bordered by histiocytes with palisaded nuclei. SYN lichen annularis.

apical g., SYN periapical g.

beryllium g., a sarcoid-like granulomatous reaction to exposure to inhaled beryllium, or skin cuts by fluorescent lamps.

bilharzial g., SYN schistosome g.

canine venereal g., a rapidly growing, soft, easily bleeding, infectious, connective tissue tumor occurring in the vagina of the female dog and on the penis and sheath of the male; ordinarily transmitted by coitus. SYN transmissible venereal tumor.

coccidioidal g., SYN secondary *coccidioidomycosis*.

coli g., SYN Hjärre's *disease*.

dental g., SYN periapical g.

g. endem′icum, the lesion occurring in cutaneous leishmaniasis.

eosinophilic g., a lesion observed more frequently in children and adolescents, occasionally in young adults, which occurs chiefly as a solitary focus in one bone, although multiple involvement is sometimes observed and similar foci may develop in the lung; characterized by numerous Langerhans cells and eosinophils, and occasional foci of necrosis; may be related to Hand-Schüller-Christian disease, possibly representing a benign clinical form.

g. facia′le, persistent well-demarcated nodules that usually ap-

gr

pear on the face and consist of a dense dermal infiltrate of eosinophils and neutrophils, separated from the epidermis and hair follicles, with fibrinoid vasculitis.

foreign body g., a g. caused by the presence of foreign particulate material in tissue, characterized by a histiocytic reaction with foreign body giant cells.

g. gangrenes'cens, SYN lethal midline g.

giant cell g., a non-neoplastic lesion characterized by a proliferation of granulation tissue containing numerous multinucleated giant cells; it occurs on the gingiva and alveolar mucosa (occasionally on other soft tissues) where it presents as a soft red-blue hemorrhagic nodular swelling; it also occurs within the mandible or maxilla as a unilocular or multilocular radiolucency; microscopically similar lesions occur in the tubular bones of the hands and feet, are considered neoplastic, and may have a malignant course. Identical bony lesions may be seen in hyperparathyroidism and cherubism. SEE ALSO giant cell *tumor* of bone. SYN giant cell epulis.

g. gravida'rum, a pyogenic g. developing on the gingiva during pregnancy; thought to be related to hormonally altered response of the oral mucous membranes to local irritants such as bacterial plaque on adjacent teeth. SYN pregnancy tumor.

infectious g., any granulomatous lesion known to be caused by a living agent; *e.g.,* bacteria, fungi, helminths.

g. inguina'le, a specific g., classified as a venereal disease and caused by *Calymmatobacterium granulomatis* observed in macrophages as Donovan bodies; the ulcerating granulomatous lesions occur in the inguinal regions and the genitalia; peripheral extension of the lesions produces extensive destruction. SYN donovanosis, g. pudendi, g. venereum, pudendal ulcer, ulcerating g. of pudenda.

g. inguina'le trop'icum, an elongated ulcer, with elevated papillary edges, sometimes occurring in the groin in persons in the tropics. SYN groin ulcer.

laryngeal g., a polypoid granulomatous projection of granulomatous tissue into the lumen of the larynx, commonly following a traumatic tracheal intubation.

lethal midline g., (1) destruction of the nasal septum, hard palate, lateral nasal walls, paranasal sinuses, skin of the face, orbit and nasopharynx by an inflammatory infiltrate with atypical lymphocytic and histiocytic cells; presumably a form of lymphoma in most cases. **(2)** obsolete term for polymorphic *reticulosis.* SYN g. gangrenescens, malignant g., midline malignant reticulosis granuloma.

lipoid g., g. characterized by aggregates or accumulations of fairly large mononuclear phagocytes that contain lipid.

lipophagic g., a lesion formed as a result of the inflammatory reaction provoked by foci of necrosis in subcutaneous fat, as in certain types of traumatic injury; the central focus of necrotic material is surrounded by an irregular zone of numerous macrophages, many of which become laden with tiny globules of lipid.

Majocchi g.'s, erythematous papules due to a deep follicular fungal infection with rupture of the hair follicles; most frequently seen on shaved legs of women. SYN tinea profunda.

malignant g., SYN lethal midline g.

Miescher's g., SYN actinic g.

g. multifor'me, a chronic granulomatous annular eruption of the skin on the upper body in older adults in central Africa; of unknown cause.

oily g., reaction to inclusion of a bulky, insoluble liquid (often an oily substance) which occurs several months, but sometimes years, after injection of the material.

paracoccidioidal g., SYN paracoccidioidomycosis.

parasitic g., cutaneous leishmaniasis manifested as warty papules affecting primarily the lower limbs.

periapical g., a proliferation of granulation tissue surrounding the apex of a nonvital tooth and arising in response to pulpal necrosis. SYN apical g., dental g., root end g.

g. puden'di, SYN g. inguinale.

pulse g., SYN giant cell hyaline *angiopathy.*

pyogenic g., g. pyogen'icum, an acquired small rounded mass of highly vascular granulation tissue, frequently with an ulcerated

surface, projecting from the skin or mucosa; histologically, the mass resembles a capillary hemangioma. SYN g. telangiectaticum.

reparative giant cell g., SEE giant cell g.

reticulohistiocytic g., obsolete term for reticulohistiocytoma.

root end g., SYN periapical g.

sarcoidal g., a non-necrotizing epithelioid cell g. similar to those seen in sarcoidosis.

schistosome g., a granulomatous lesion formed around schistosome eggs embedded in tissues in cases of schistosomiasis (bilharziasis); typically these granulomata are found in intestinal tissues (*Schistosoma japonicum* or *S. mansoni* infection), bladder tissue (*S. haematobium*), and hepatic tissue (all human schistosomes). SYN bilharzial g.

sea urchin g., granulomatous nodules, either foreign-body type or composed of epitheliod cells, from the retention of the spine of the sea urchin, occurring several months after the wounding of the skin.

silica g., eruption of granulomatous lesions due to traumatic inoculation of the skin with sand, or materials that contain silica; this condition may follow dermabrasion using sandpaper technique.

silicotic g., granulomatous nodule resulting from deposition of silica particles, usually occurring in lung.

swimming pool g., a chronic, verrucous lesion most commonly seen on the knees; due to infection by *Mycobacterium marinum.*

g. telangiecta'ticum, SYN pyogenic g.

g. trop'icum, SYN yaws.

ulcerating g. of pudenda, SYN g. inguinale.

g. vene'reum, SYN g. inguinale.

zirconium g., g. from zirconium salts, usually occurring in the axillae, from antiperspirants containing this material; may also be caused by intradermal injection of antigens containing the lactate salt.

gran·u·lo·ma·to·sis (gran'yū-lō-mă-tō'sis). Any condition characterized by multiple granulomas.

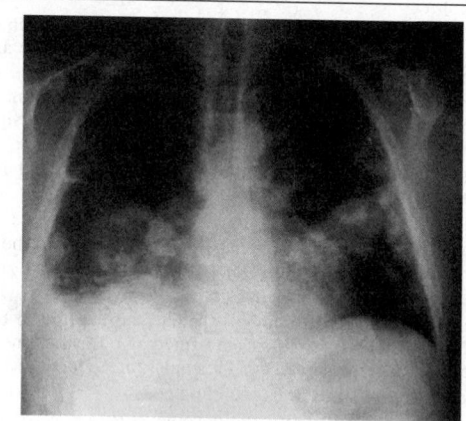

Wegener's granulomatosis (x-ray)
granulomas in both lungs

allergic g., SYN Churg-Strauss *syndrome.*

bronchocentric g., a severe form of allergic bronchopulmonary aspergillosis.

lipid g., lipoid g., SYN xanthomatosis.

lipophagic intestinal g., obsolete term for Whipple's *disease.*

lymphomatoid g., a disease related to Wegener's g., but more widespread and diffuse, most frequently affecting male adults; characterized initially by nodular lower lung lesions which are granulomatous proliferations of atypical lymphocytes, plasma cells, and histiocytes, notably perivascular with destruction of small arteries; eventually the skin, kidneys, and nervous system are often involved; pulmonary lymphomatoid g. may be followed by the development of malignant lymphoma. SEE ALSO polymorphic *reticulosis.*

g. siderot′ica, a form in which firm, brown foci that contain iron pigment (Gamna bodies) are present in an enlarged spleen.

Wegener's g., a disease, occurring mainly in the fourth and fifth decades, characterized by necrotizing granulomas and ulceration of the upper respiratory tract, with purulent rhinorrhea, nasal obstruction, and sometimes with otorrhea, hemoptysis, pulmonary infiltration and cavitation, and fever; exophthalmos, involvement of the larynx and pharynx, and glomerulonephritis may occur; the underlying condition is a vasculitis affecting small vessels, and is possibly due to an immune disorder. SEE ALSO lymphomatoid g.

gran·u·lom·a·tous (gran-yū-lom′ă-tŭs). Having the characteristics of a granuloma.

gran·u·lo·mere (gran′yū-lō-mēr). The central part of a blood platelet. SYN chromomere (2). [granulo- + G. *meros,* a part]

gran·u·lo·pe·nia (gran′yū-lō-pē′nē-ă). SYN granulocytopenia.

gran·u·lo·plasm (gran′yū-lō-plazm). The inner substance of an ameba, or other unicellular organism, within the ectoplasm and surrounding the nucleus.

gran·u·lo·plas·tic (gran′yū-lō-plas′tik). Forming granules.

gran·u·lo·poi·e·sis (gran′yū-lō-poy-ē′sis). Production of granulocytes. In adults, granulocytes are produced chiefly in the red bone marrow of flat bones. SYN granulocytopoiesis. [granulo- (cyte) + G. *poiēsis,* a making]

gran·u·lo·poi·et·ic (gran′yū-lō-poy-et′ik). Pertaining to granulopoiesis. SYN granulocytopoietic.

gran·u·lo·sa (gran-yū-lō′să). SYN *stratum* granulosum folliculi ovarici vesiculosi.

gran·u·lo·sis (gran-yū-lō′sis). A mass of minute granules of any character. SYN granulosity.

g. ru′bra na′si, erythema, papules, and occasional vesicles of the tip of the nose and extending upward and laterally to the cheeks, resulting from occlusion and chronic inflammation of sweat ducts.

gran·u·los·i·ty (gran-yū-los′i-tē). SYN granulosis.

gra·num (grā′nŭm). Singular of grana.

gran·zymes (gran′zīmz). Serine esterases that represent most of the granule content of T cytotoxic cells. It is not known if these enzymes are required for killing by the T cytotoxic cell. [granule + -zyme]

graph (graf). **1.** A line or tracing denoting varying values of commodities, temperatures, urinary output, etc.; more generally, any geometric or pictorial representation of measurements that might otherwise be expressed in tabular form. **2.** Visual display of the relationship between two variables, in which the values of one are plotted on the horizontal axis, the values of the other on the vertical axis; three-dimensional g.'s that show relationships between three variables can be depicted and comprehended visually in two dimensions. [G. *graphō,* to write]

△**-graph. 1.** Something written, as in monograph, radiograph. **2.** The instrument for making a recording, as in kymograph. Cf. -gram. [G. *graphō,* to write]

graph·an·es·the·sia (graf′an-es-thē′zē-ă). Tactual inability to recognize figures or letters written on the skin; may be due to spinal cord or brain disease. [G. *graphē,* writing + *anaisthēsia,* fr. *an-* priv. + *aisthēsis,* perception]

graph·es·the·sia (graf-es-thē′zē-ă). Tactual ability to recognize writing on the skin. [G. *graphē,* writing, + *aisthēsis,* perception]

graph·ite (graf′īt). A crystallizable soft black form of carbon. SYN black lead, plumbago.

△**grapho-.** A writing, description. [G. *graphō,* to write]

gra·phol·o·gy (grā-fol′ō-jē). The study of handwriting as an indication of temperament, character, or personality. [grapho- + G. *logos,* study]

graph·o·ma·nia (graf-ō-mā′ne-ă). Morbid and excessive impulse to write. [grapho- + G. *mania,* insanity]

graph·o·mo·tor (graf-ō-mō′ter). Relating to the movements used in writing. [grapho- + L. *motus,* fr. *movere,* to move]

graph·o·pa·thol·o·gy (graf′ō-path-ol′ō-jē). Interpretation of personality disorders from a study of handwriting. SEE graphology. [grapho- + pathology]

graph·o·pho·bia (graf-ō-fō′bē-ă). Morbid fear of writing. [grapho- + G. *phobos,* fear]

graph·or·rhea (graf-ō-rē′ă). Rarely used term for the writing of long lists of meaningless words, associated with a schizophrenic disorder. [grapho- + G. *rhoia,* flow]

graph·o·spasm (graf′ō-spazm). SYN writer's *cramp.*

△**-graphy.** A writing, a description. [G. *graphō,* to write]

grasp. The act of taking securely and holding firmly.

palm g., holding an object by wrapping the palm and the fingers around it.

pen g., a method, similar to that of holding a pen in writing, of grasping an instrument.

Grasset, Joseph, French physician, 1849–1918. SEE G.'s *law, phenomenon, sign;* G.-Gaussel *phenomenon;* Landouzy-G. *law.*

Gratiolet, Louis P., French anatomist, physiologist, and physician, 1815–1865. SEE G.'s *fibers,* under *fiber, radiation.*

grat·tage (grǎ-tazh′). Scraping or brushing an ulcer or surface with sluggish granulations to stimulate the healing process. [Fr. scraping]

Gräupner, Sigurd C., German physician, 1861–1916. SEE G.'s *method.*

grave (grāv). Denoting symptoms of a serious or dangerous character. [L. *gravis,* heavy, grave]

grav·el (grav′l). Small concretions, usually of uric acid, calcium oxalate, or phosphates, formed in the kidney and passed through the ureter, bladder, and urethra. SYN urocheras (1), uropsammus (1). [M.E., fr. O.Fr.]

Graves, Robert James, Irish physician remembered for his description of exophthalmic goiter in 1835, 1796–1853. SEE G.'s *disease, ophthalmopathy.*

grav·id. SYN pregnant.

grav·i·da (grav′i-dă). A pregnant woman. Gravida followed by a roman numeral or preceded by a Latin prefix (primi-, secundi-, etc.) designates the pregnant woman by number of pregnancies; *e.g.,* **gravida I,** primigravida; a woman in her first pregnancy; **gravida II,** secundigravida; a woman in her second pregnancy. Cf. para. [L. *gravidus* (adj.), fem. *gravida,* fr. *gravis,* heavy]

gra·vid·ic (grā-vid′ik). Relating to pregnancy or a pregnant woman.

grav·id·ism (grav′id-izm). SYN pregnancy.

gra·vid·i·tas (grav-vid′i-tas). SYN pregnancy. [L.]

g. examnia′lis, SYN extraamniotic *pregnancy.*

g. exochoria′lis, SYN extrachorial *pregnancy.*

gra·vid·i·ty (grā-vid′i-tē). The number of pregnancies (complete or incomplete) experienced by a woman. [L. *graviditas,* pregnancy]

gra·vim·e·ter (grā-vim′ĕ-ter). SYN hydrometer. [L. *gravis,* heavy, + G. *metron,* measure]

grav·i·met·ric (grav-i-met′rik). Relating to or determined by weight.

grav·i·re·cep·tors (grav′i-rē-sep′terz). Highly specialized receptor organs and nerve endings in the inner ear, joints, tendons, and muscles that give the brain information about body position, equilibrium, direction of gravitational forces, and the sensation of "down" or "up." [L. *gravis,* heavy, + receptor]

grav·i·ta·tion (grav-i-tā′shŭn). The force of attraction between any two bodies in the universe, varying directly as the product of their masses and inversely as the square of the distance between their centers; expressed as $F = Gm_1 m_2 l^{-2}$, where G (Newtonian constant of gravitation) $= 6.67259 \times 10^{-11}$ m^3 kg^{-1} s^{-2}. m_1 and m_2 are the masses (in kg) of the two bodies and l is the distance separating them in meters. [L. *gravitas,* weight]

grav·i·ty (grav′i-tē). The attraction toward the earth that makes any mass exert downward force or have weight. Strictly speaking, g. is the algebraic sum of the gravitational attraction of the earth and the opposing centrifugal effect of the mass's rotation around the earth; thus, g. equals gravitational attraction at the north and south poles but becomes progressively less as one approaches the equator. A satellite in a stable orbit has zero gravity because the centrifugal effect of orbital motion exactly balances the gravitational attraction of the earth. [L. *gravitas*]

gr

specific g. (sp. gr.), the weight of any body compared with that of another body of equal volume regarded as the unit; usually the weight of a liquid compared with that of distilled water.

zero g., SEE zero gravity.

Grawitz, Paul, German pathologist, 1850–1932. SEE G.'s *basophilia, tumor.*

gray (Gy) (grā). The SI unit of absorbed dose of ionizing radiation, equivalent to 1 J/kg of tissue; 1 Gy = 100 rad. SYN griseus. [Louis H. *Gray,* British radiologist, 1905–1965]

Greeff, C. Richard, German ophthalmologist, 1862–1938. SEE Prowazek-G. *bodies,* under *body.*

green (grēn). A color between blue and yellow in the spectrum. For individual green dyes, see specific names.

Scheele's g., SYN cupric arsenite.

Greenfield. L., American surgeon who designed the Greenfield filter. SEE Greenfield *filter.*

Greenhow, Edward H., British physician, 1814–1888. SEE G.'s *disease.*

gref·fo·tome (gref'ō-tōm). Obsolete term for an instrument for slicing off bits of epidermis to use in grafting. [Fr. *greff,* graft, + G. *tomē,* incision]

greg·a·loid (greg'ă-loyd). Denoting a loose colony of protozoa formed by the chance union of independent cells, especially among sarcodines with pseudopodial adherence. [L. *grex (greg-),* a flock]

Greg·a·ri·na (greg-ă-rī'nă). A genus of sporozoan protozoa (phylum Apicomplexa, subclass Gregarinia), parasitic in annelids and arthropods, and lacking schizogony and endodyogeny in the life cycle. [L. *gregarius,* gregarious, fr. *grex (greg-),* a flock]

greg·a·rine (greg'ă-rēn). A member of the subclass Gregarinia.

Greg·a·ri·nia (greg'ă-rin'i-ă). A sporozoan subclass consisting of a number of parasites of the body cavity and intestinal tract of invertebrates, especially annelids and arthropods; typical genera include *Gregarina* in insects and *Monocystis* in earthworms.

greg·a·ri·no·sis (greg'ă-ri-nō'sis). A disease due to the presence of gregarines.

Greig, David M., Scottish physician, 1864–1936. SEE G.'s *syndrome.*

gres·sion (gres'shŭn). Displacement of a tooth backward. [L. *grador,* pp. *gressus,* to walk, fr. *gradus,* a step]

Greville bath. See under bath.

grey mat·ter. SEE gray *matter.*

Grey Turner, SEE Turner.

GRH Abbreviation for gonadotropin-releasing *hormone.*

grid. **1.** A chart with horizontal and perpendicular lines for plotting curves. **2.** In x-ray imaging, a device formed of lead strips for preventing scattered radiation from reaching the x-ray film. [M.E. *gridel,* fr. L. *craticula,* lattice]

focused g., a g. (2) in which the divergent beam of x-rays from a particular distance range will be parallel to the lead strips.

Wetzel g., chart of growth, plotting height, weight, physical fitness and related aspects of young and adolescent children during growth.

Gridley, Mary F., U.S. medical technologist, 1908–1954. SEE G.'s *stain, stain* for fungi.

grief (grēf). A normal emotional response to an external loss; distinguished from a depressive disorder since it usually subsides after a reasonable time.

Griesinger, Wilhelm, German neurologist, 1817–1868. SEE G.'s *disease, symptom;* bilious *typhoid* of G.

grin·de·lia (grin-dē'lē-ă). The dried leaves and flowering tops of *G. camporum, G. humilius,* and *G. squarrosa* (family Compositae); used as an expectorant; a fluid extract has been used externally in the treatment of rhus poisoning. [David H. *Grindel,* German botanist, 1776–1836]

grind·ing (grīnd'ing). SYN abrasion (3).

selective g., the modification of the occlusal forms of teeth by g. according to a plan or by g. at selected places marked by articulating ribbon or paper.

grind·ing-in. A term used to denote the act of correcting occlusal disharmonies by grinding the natural or artificial teeth.

grip. **1.** SYN influenza. **2.** SEE grasp.

devil's g., SYN epidemic *pleurodynia.*

grippe (grip). SYN influenza. [Fr. *gripper,* to seize]

gris·e·o·ful·vin (gris'ē-ō-fŭl'vin). A fungistatic antibiotic produced by *Penicillium griseofulvin* and *Penicillium patulum;* used in the systemic treatment of superficial fungal infections caused by the dermatophytes *Microsporum, Trichophyton,* and *Epidermophyton;* inhibits microtubule assembly.

gris·e·us (gris'ē-ŭs). SYN gray. [L.]

Grisolle, Augustin, French physician, 1811–1869. SEE G.'s *sign.*

Gri·so·nel·la ra·tel·li·na (gri-sŏ-nel'ă ra-te-lī'nă). A South American weasel, a reservoir host of *Trypanosoma cruzi.*

gris·tle (gris'l). SYN cartilage. [A.S.]

Gritti, Rocco, Italian surgeon, 1828–1920. SEE G.'s *operation;* G.-Stokes *amputation.*

Grocco, Pietro, Italian physician, 1857–1916. SEE G.'s *sign, triangle;* Orsi-G. *method.*

Grocott-Gomori meth·en·a·mine-sil·ver stain. See under stain.

Groenouw, Arthur, German ophthalmologist, 1862–1945. SEE G.'s corneal *dystrophy.*

groin (groyn). **1.** SYN inguinal *region.* **2.** Sometimes used to indicate just the crease in the junction of the thigh with the trunk.

Grönblad, Ester E., Swedish ophthalmologist, *1898. SEE G.-Strandberg *syndrome.*

GROOVE

groove (grūv). A narrow elongated depression or furrow on any surface. SEE ALSO sulcus.

alveolobuccal g., the upper and lower half of the buccal vestibule on each side. SYN alveolobuccal sulcus, gingivobuccal g., gingivobuccal sulcus.

alveololabial g., (1) the upper and lower half of the labial vestibule; (2) in the embryo, the g. formed by the deepening of the labial sulcus; its inner wall becomes incorporated with the alveolar process of the mandible or the maxilla, and its outer wall with the lips and cheeks. SYN alveololabial sulcus, gingivolabial g., gingivolabial sulcus.

alveololingual g., (1) that part of the oral cavity proper, on each side of the frenulum linguae, between the tongue and the mandibular alveolar process or ridge; (2) in the embryo, the g. on each side between the lingual primordium and the alveolar elevations of the mandible. SYN alveololingual sulcus, gingivolingual g., gingivolingual sulcus.

anterior auricular g., SYN anterior *notch* of ear.

anterior intermediate g., SYN anterior intermediate *sulcus.*

anterior interventricular g., a groove on the anterosuperior surface of the heart, marking the location of the septum between the two ventricles. SYN sulcus interventricularis anterior [NA], crena cordis (1).

anterolateral g., SYN anterolateral *sulcus.*

anteromedian g., (1) SYN anterior median *fissure* of medulla oblongata. (2) SYN anterior median *fissure* of spinal cord.

g. for arch of aorta, a broad, deep sulcus arching superiorly over the hilus on the mediastinal surface of the left lung formed as a result of the aortic arch impressing or indenting the lung.

arterial g.'s, branching grooves on the interior surface of the cranial vault in which the meningeal arteries course, the most prominent of which are related to branches of the middle meningeal artery. SYN sulci arteriosi [NA].

atrioventricular g., SYN coronary g.

g. for auditory tube, a furrow on the inner surface of the posterior border of the greater wing of the sphenoid bone, for the cartilaginous auditory tube. SYN sulcus tubae auditivae [NA], pharyngotympanic g.

auriculoventricular g., SYN coronary g.

bicipital g., SYN intertubercular g.

branchial g., an external embryonic g. between contiguous branchial arches. SEE ALSO branchial *clefts*, under *cleft*.

carotid g., the groove on the body of the sphenoid bone in which the internal carotid artery lies in its course through the cavernous sinus. SYN sulcus caroticus [NA], carotid sulcus, cavernous g.

carpal g., the concavity on the anterior surface of the arch formed by the carpal bones. SYN sulcus carpi [NA], carpal canal (2).

cavernous g., SYN carotid g.

chiasmatic g., the groove on the upper surface of the sphenoid bone running transversely between the optic canals bounded anteriorly by the sphenoidal limbus and posteriorly by the tuberculum sellae; forms in relationship to the optic chiasm. SYN sulcus prechiasmatis [NA], chiasmatic sulcus, optic g., prechiasmatic sulcus.

coronary g., a groove on the outer surface of the heart marking the division between the atria and the ventricles. SYN sulcus coronarius [NA], atrioventricular g., atrioventricular sulcus, auriculoventricular g., coronary sulcus.

costal g., a groove in the lower inner border of the rib, lodging the intercostal vessels and nerve. SYN sulcus costae [NA], subcostal g.

costal g. for subclavian artery, a groove immediately posterior to the scalene tubercle on the upper surface of the first rib across which the subclavian artery passes. SYN sulcus costae arteriae subclaviae [NA].

g. of crus of the helix, a transverse fissure on the cranial surface of the auricle corresponding to the crus of the helix. SYN sulcus cruris helicis [NA].

dental g., a transitory depression in the gingival surface of the embryonic jaw along the line of ingrowth of the dental lamina.

g. for the descending aorta, a broad, deep, vertical sulcus immediately posterior to the hilus on the mediastinal surface of the left lung, formed as a result of the descending aorta impressing or indenting the lung.

developmental g.'s, fine lines found in the enamel of a tooth that mark the junction of the lobes of the crown in its development. SYN developmental lines.

digastric g., SYN mastoid g.

ethmoidal g., a groove on the inner surface of each nasal bone, lodging the external nasal branch of the anterior ethmoid nerve. SYN sulcus ethmoidalis [NA].

frontal g.'s, SEE inferior frontal *sulcus*, middle frontal *sulcus*, superior frontal *sulcus*.

gingivobuccal g., SYN alveolobuccal g.

gingivolabial g., SYN alveololabial g.

gingivolingual g., SYN alveololingual g.

greater palatine g., a groove on both the body of the maxilla and the perpendicular plate of the palatine bone; when the bones are articulated the grooves form the greater palatine canal. SYN sulcus palatinus major [NA], pterygopalatine g., sulcus for greater palatine nerve, sulcus pterygopalatinus.

g. of greater petrosal nerve, the groove on the anterior surface of the petrous part of the temporal bone that lodges the greater petrosal nerve. SYN sulcus nervi petrosi majoris [NA].

Harrison's g., a deformity of the ribs which results from the pull of the diaphragm on ribs weakened by rickets or other softening of the bone.

inferior petrosal g., SYN g. for inferior petrosal sinus.

g. for inferior petrosal sinus, a groove lodging the inferior petrosal sinus, formed by union of similarly named grooves in the petrous part of the temporal bone and the basilar part of the occipital bone. SYN sulcus sinus petrosi inferioris [NA], inferior petrosal g., inferior petrosal sulcus.

g. for inferior venae cava, a groove on the posterior surface of the liver between the caudate lobe and the right lobe which gives passage to the inferior vena cava. SYN sulcus venae cavae [NA], fossa venae cavae, sulcus for vena cava.

infraorbital g., a gradually deepening groove on the orbital surface of the maxilla, which leads to the infraorbital canal. SYN sulcus infraorbitalis [NA].

interosseous g., (1) SYN interosseous g. of calcaneus. **(2)** SYN interosseous g. of talus.

interosseous g. of calcaneus, the groove on the upper part of the calcaneus, which with a corresponding groove on the talus forms the sinus tarsi. SYN sulcus calcanei [NA], calcaneal sulcus, interosseous g. (1).

interosseous g. of talus, the groove on the inferior surface of the talus, which with a corresponding groove on the calcaneus forms the sinus tarsi. SYN sulcus tali [NA], interosseous g. (2), talar sulcus.

intertubercular g., a furrow running down the shaft of the humerus between the two tubercles, lodging the tendon of the long head of the biceps, and giving attachment in its floor to the latissimus dorsi muscle. SYN sulcus intertubercularis [NA], bicipital g., intertubercular sulcus.

interventricular g.'s, SEE anterior interventricular g., posterior interventricular g.

lacrimal g., (2) the groove in the nasal surface of the maxilla which, together with the lacrimal bone, forms the fossa for the lacrimal sac. SYN sulcus lacrimalis [NA].

laryngotracheal g., the depression in the floor of the caudal end of the pharynx, continued downward on the ventral wall of the foregut; from it are developed the lower part of the larynx and the trachea, bronchi, and lungs. SYN tracheobronchial g.

lateral bicipital g., at the cubital fossa, the groove separating the biceps brachii and brachialis muscles on the lateral side. SYN sulcus bicipitalis lateralis [NA].

g. of lesser petrosal nerve, the groove on the anterior surface of the petrous part of the temporal bone that accommodates the lesser petrosal nerve in its course to the otic ganglion. SYN sulcus nervi petrosi minoris [NA].

linguogingival g., a g. separating the embryonic mandibular portion of the tongue from the remainder of the mandibular process.

Lucas' g., SYN *stria* spinosa.

g. of lung for subclavian artery, a sulcus on the surface of the lung just below the apex, corresponding to the course of the subclavian artery. SYN sulcus subclavius.

major g., in a detailed analysis of DNA structure, there are two types of g.'s that can be seen; the major g. has the nitrogen and oxygen atoms of the base pairs pointing inward toward the helical axis, while in the minor g., the nitrogen and oxygen atoms point outwards; important because the major g. is more dependent on base composition and may be the site for protein recognition of specific DNA sequences or regions.

mastoid g., the groove medial to the mastoid process of the temporal bone from which the digastric muscle originates. SYN incisura mastoidea [NA], digastric g., digastric notch, mastoid notch.

medial bicipital g., at the cubital fossa, the groove separating the biceps brachii and brachialis muscles on the medial side. SYN sulcus bicipitalis medialis [NA].

median g. of tongue, median groove or median longitudinal raphe of tongue; raphe linguae; a slight longitudinal depression running forward on the dorsal surface of the tongue from the foramen cecum. SYN sulcus medianus linguae [NA], median longitudinal raphe of tongue, raphe linguae.

medullary g., SYN neural g.

middle meningeal artery g., a narrow g. on the inner table of the calvarium, seen on lateral radiographs as a thin dark line, which may be mistaken for a skull fracture. SEE *sulci* arteriosi, under *sulcus*.

g. for middle temporal artery, a vertical groove located above the external acoustic meatus on the external surface of the squamous part of the temporal bone. SYN sulcus arteriae temporalis mediae [NA], sulcus for middle temporal artery.

minor g., SEE major g.

musculospiral g., SYN g. for radial nerve.

mylohyoid g., a groove on the medial surface of the ramus of the mandible beginning at the lingula; it lodges the mylohyoid artery and nerve. SYN sulcus mylohyoideus [NA], mylohyoid fossa.

g. of nail matrix, SYN *sulcus* matricis unguis.

nasolabial g., a furrow between the wing of the nose and the lip. SYN sulcus nasolabialis.

nasopalatine g., a g. on the vomer lodging the nasopalatine nerve.

nasopharyngeal g., an indistinct line marking the boundary between the nasal cavities and the nasal part of the pharynx.

neural g., the gutter-like g. formed in the midline of the embryo's dorsal surface by the progressive elevation of the lateral margins of the neural plate; the ultimate dorsal fusion of the margins results in the formation of the neural tube. SYN medullary g.

obturator g., a deep groove on the inner surface of the superior ramus of the pubis. SYN sulcus obturatorius [NA].

occipital g., a narrow groove medial to the mastoid notch of the temporal bone that lodges the occipital artery. SYN sulcus arteriae occipitalis [NA], sulcus of occipital artery.

olfactory g., SYN olfactory *sulcus.*

optic g., SYN chiasmatic g.

palatine g., one of a number of grooves on the lower surface of the palatine process of the maxilla in which the palatine vessels and nerves lie. SYN sulcus palatinus [NA].

palatovaginal g., a furrow on the inferior aspect of the vaginal process of the sphenoid bone that is bridged below by the sphenoidal process of the palatine bone to form the palatovaginal canal. SYN sulcus palatovaginalis [NA].

paraglenoid g., SYN preauricular g.

pharyngeal g.'s, embryonic endodermal or ectodermal g.'s between successive pharyngeal arches.

pharyngotympanic g., SYN g. for auditory tube.

pontomedullary g., the transverse g. on the ventral aspect of the brainstem that demarcates the pons from the medulla oblongata; from its bottom the sixth, seventh, and eighth cranial nerves emerge.

popliteal g., a g. on the lateral condyle of the femur between the epicondyle and the articular margin. Its anterior end gives origin to the popliteus muscle; its posterior end lodges the tendon of the muscle when the knee is fully flexed. SYN sulcus popliteus.

posterior auricular g., the g. between the antitragus and cauda helicis overlying the antitragicohelicine fissure. SYN sulcus auriculae posterior [NA].

posterior intermediate g., SYN posterior intermediate *sulcus.*

posterior interventricular g., a g. on the diaphragmatic surface of the heart, marking the location of the septum between the two ventricles. SYN sulcus interventricularis posterior [NA], crena cordis (2).

posterolateral g., SYN posterolateral *sulcus.*

preauricular g., a g. on the pelvic surface of the ilium just lateral to the auricular surface; it is more pronounced in the female. SYN paraglenoid g., paraglenoid sulcus, preauricular sulcus, sulcus paraglenoidalis.

primary labial g., SYN labial *sulcus.*

primitive g., the median depression in the primitive streak flanked by the primitive ridges. SYN primitive furrow.

g. of pterygoid hamulus, a groove at the base of the hamular process which forms a pulley for the tendon of the tensor veli palatini muscle. SYN sulcus hamuli pterygoidei [NA], sulcus of pterygoid hamulus.

pterygopalatine g., SYN greater palatine g.

g. for radial nerve, the shallow groove that passes around the shaft of the humerus; it lodges the radial nerve and deep brachial artery. SYN sulcus nervi radialis [NA], musculospiral g., spiral g.

retention g., one of the g.'s forming opposing vertical constrictions in a tooth to aid in retention of a dental restoration.

rhombic g.'s, seven pairs of transverse furrows in the floor of the embryonic hindbrain.

sagittal g., SYN g. for superior sagittal sinus.

Sibson's g., a g. occasionally seen on the outer side of the thorax formed by the prominent lower border of the pectoralis major muscle.

sigmoid g., SYN g. for sigmoid sinus.

g. for sigmoid sinus, a broad groove in the posterior cranial fossa, first situated on the lateral portion of the occipital bone, then curving around the jugular process on to the mastoid portion of the temporal bone, and finally turning sharply on the posterior inferior angle of the parietal bone and becoming continuous with the transverse groove; it lodges the transverse sinus. SYN sulcus sinus sigmoidei [NA], sigmoid fossa, sigmoid g., sigmoid sulcus.

skin g.'s, SYN skin *furrows,* under *furrow.*

g. for spinal nerve, the laterally directed groove on the superior surface of the transverse processes of typical cervical vertebrae between the anterior and posterior tubercles along which the emerging spinal nerve passes. SYN sulcus nervi spinalis [NA].

spiral g., SYN g. for radial nerve.

subclavian g., a groove on the inferior surface of the body of the clavicle to which is attached the subclavius muscle. SYN sulcus musculi subclavii [NA], subclavian sulcus, sulcus subclavianus.

g. for subclavian vein, a groove just anterior to the scalene tubercle of the first rib marking the course of the subclavian vein across the rib. SYN sulcus venae subclaviae [NA].

subcostal g., SYN costal g.

g. for superior petrosal sinus, a groove on the crest of the petrous portion of the temporal bone in which rests the superior petrosal sinus. SYN sulcus sinus petrosi superioris [NA], superior petrosal sulcus.

g. for superior sagittal sinus, the groove in the midline of the inner table of the calvaria lodging the superior sagittal sinus. SYN sulcus sinus sagittalis superioris [NA], sagittal g., sagittal sulcus, superior longitudinal sulcus.

g. for superior vena cava, a g. on the surface of the right lung, above the hilum, in which runs the superior vena cava. SYN sulcus venae cavae cranialis.

supplemental g., a curvilinear depression normally found on each side of a triangular ridge (crista triangularis).

supra-acetabular g., a groove, posterosuperior to the acetabulum, that is the attachment for the reflected head of the rectus femoris muscle. SYN sulcus supra-acetabularis [NA], supra-acetabular sulcus.

g. for tendon of flexor hallucis longus, groove for tendon of the flexor hallucis longus; a vertical g. on the posterior process of the talus continuous with a similar groove on the underside of the sustentaculum tali of the calcaneus. SYN sulcus tendinis musculi flexoris hallucis longi [NA].

g. for tendon of peroneus longus muscle, (1) the g. below the peroneal trochlea of the calcaneus; **(2)** the g. distal to the tuberosity of the cuboid bone. SYN sulcus tendinis musculi peronei longi [NA], sulcus tendinis musculi fibularis longi ☆ [NA].

g. for tibialis posterior tendon, a broad groove on the posterior surface of the medial malleolus, through which the tendon of the tibialis posterior muscle runs. SYN sulcus malleolaris [NA], malleolar sulcus.

tracheobronchial g., SYN laryngotracheal g.

transverse anthelicine g., a deep groove on the cranial surface of the auricle separating the eminences of the triangular fossa and of the concha. SYN sulcus anthelicis transversus [NA].

transverse nasal g., SYN *stria* nasi transversa.

g. for transverse sinus, the groove on the inner surface of the occipital bone marking the course of the transverse sinus; the tentorium is attached to its margins. SYN sulcus sinus transversi [NA], sulcus for transverse sinus.

tympanic g., the g. on the inner aspect of the tympanic part of the temporal bone in which the tympanic membrane is fixed. SYN sulcus tympanicus [NA].

g. for ulnar nerve, a furrow on the posterior surface of the medial epicondyle of the humerus, lodging the ulnar nerve. SYN sulcus nervi ulnaris [NA].

urethral g., the g. on the ventral surface of the embryonic penis which ultimately is closed to form the penile portion of the urethra.

venous g.'s, grooves occasionally found on the internal surface of the parietal bone, in which veins lie. SYN sulci venosi [NA].

vertebral g., the depression bounded by the spinous processes and laminae of the vertebrae, in which lie the deep muscles of the back.

g. for vertebral artery, the g. on the superior aspect of the posterior arch of the atlas that transmits the vertebral artery medially toward the foramen magnum. SYN sulcus arteriae vertebralis [NA], sulcus for vertebral artery.

vomeral g., the groove on the anterior border of the vomer that receives the septal cartilage. SYN sulcus vomeralis [NA], sulcus vomeris [NA], vomeral sulcus.

vomerovaginal g., a g. on the inferior aspect of the vaginal process of the sphenoid bone that, together with ala of the vomer, forms the vomerovaginal canal. SYN sulcus vomerovaginalis [NA].

Gross, Ludwik, 20th century U.S. oncologist. SEE G.'s *virus,* leukemia *virus.*

gross (gros). Coarse or large; large enough to be visible to the naked eye. [L. *grossus,* thick]

group (grūp). **1.** A number of similar or related objects. **2.** In chemistry, a radical. For individual chemical groups, see the specific name.

blood g., SEE blood group.

characterizing g., a g. of atoms in a molecule that distinguishes the class of substances in which it occurs from all other classes; thus carbonyl (CO) is the characterizing g. of ketones; COOH, of organic acids, etc.

connective tissue g., a collective name for mucous tissue, dentin, bone, cartilage, and ordinary connective tissue, all derived from the mesenchyme.

control g., a g. of subjects participating in the same experiment as another g. of subjects, but which is not exposed to the variable under investigation. SEE ALSO experimental g.

cytophil g., the atom g. in the antibody (amboceptor) that binds it to the cell.

determinant g., SYN antigenic *determinant.*

diagnosis related g., a scheme for billing for medical and especially hospital services by combining diseases into g.'s according to the resources needed for care, arranged by diagnostic category. A dollar value is assigned to each g. as the basis of payment for all cases in that group, without regard to the actual cost of care or duration of hospitalization of any individual case, as a mechanism to motivate health-care providers to economize.

encounter g., a form of psychological sensitivity training that emphasizes the experiencing of individual relationships within the g. and minimizes intellectual and didactic input; the g. focuses on the present rather than concerning itself with the past or outside problems of its members. SEE ALSO sensitivity training g.

experimental g., a g. of subjects exposed to the variable of an experiment, as opposed to the control g.

functional g., SEE function (4).

HACEK g., a group of Gram-negative bacteria that includes *Haemophilus* spp., *Actinobacillus actinomycetemcomitans, Cardiobacterium hominis, Eikenella corrodens,* and *Kingella kingae.* Bacteria in this group have in common a culture requirement of an enhanced carbon dioxide atmosphere and ability to infect human heart valves.

linkage g., a set of two or more loci that have been shown by linkage analysis to be physically close in the genome but that have not yet been assigned to specific chromosomes. It is rapidly becoming an outmoded term.

matched g.'s, a method of experimental control in which subjects in one g. are matched on a one-to-one basis with subjects in other g.'s concerning all organism variables (*e.g.,* age, sex, height, weight) which the experimenter believes could influence the variable being investigated.

prosthetic g., a non-amino acid compound attached to a protein, often in a reversible fashion, that confers new properties upon the conjugated protein thus produced. SEE ALSO coenzyme.

sensitivity training g., a g. in which members seek to develop self-awareness and an understanding of g. processes rather than to obtain therapy for an emotional disturbance. SEE ALSO encounter g., personal growth *laboratory.*

symptom g., SEE syndrome, complex (1).

T g., abbreviation for training g.

therapeutic g., any g. of patients meeting together for mutual psychotherapeutic, personal development, and life change goals.

training g. (T g.), any g. emphasizing training in self-awareness and group dynamics. SEE sensitivity training g.

Grover, Ralph W., U.S. dermatologist, *1920. SEE G.'s *disease.*

growth (grōth). The increase in size of a living being or any of its parts occurring in the process of development.

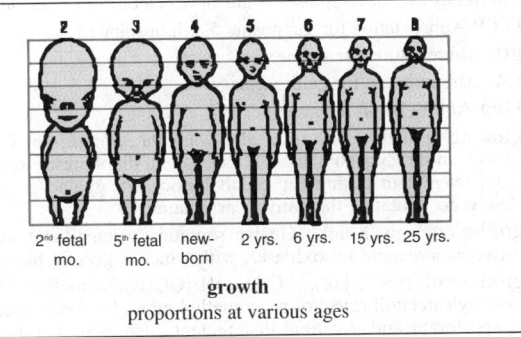

growth
proportions at various ages

accretionary g., g. by an increase of intercellular material.

appositional g., g. accomplished by the addition of new layers on those previously formed; *e.g.,* the addition of lamellae in the formation of bone; it is the characteristic method of g. when rigid materials are involved.

auxetic g., g. by increase in the size of component cells. SYN intussusceptive g.

bacterial g., g. of a bacterial culture either by increase in cell material or cell number.

differential g., different rates of g. in associated tissues or structures; used especially in embryology when the differences in g. rates result in changing the original proportions or relations.

exponential g., SEE logarithmic *phase.*

interstitial g., g. from a number of different centers within an area; in contrast with appositional g., it can occur only when the materials involved are nonrigid.

intussusceptive g., SYN auxetic g.

multiplicative g., g. by an increase in the number of cells.

new g., SYN neoplasm.

grub (grŭb). Wormlike larva or maggot of certain insects, particularly in the orders Coleoptera, Diptera, and Hymenoptera, and the genus *Hypoderma.*

Gruber, George B., German physician, 1884–1977. SEE Meckel-G. *syndrome;* Martin-G. *anastomosis.*

Gruber, Josef, Austrian otologist, 1827–1900. SEE G.'s *method.*

Gruber, Max von, German hygienist, 1853–1927. SEE G.'s *reaction;* G.-Widal *reaction.*

Gruber, Wenzel (Wenaslaus) L., Russian anatomist, 1814–1890. SEE G.'s *cul-de-sac;* G.-Landzert *fossa.*

gru·el (grū'ĕl). A semiliquid food of oatmeal or other cereal boiled in water; thin porridge. [thru O. Fr., fr. Mediev. L. *grutum,* meal]

gru·mous (grū'mŭs). Thick and lumpy, as clotting blood. [L. *grumus,* a little heap]

Grunert's spur. See under spur.

Grunstein-Hogness as·say. See under assay.

Grünwald. SEE May-Grünwald *stain.*

Grütz, O., German dermatologist, *1886. SEE Bürger-G. *syndrome.*

Grynfeltt, Joseph C., French surgeon, 1840–1913. SEE G.'s *triangle.*

gry·o·chrome (grī'ō-krōm). A term applied by Nissl to nerve cells in which the stainable portion is present in the form of minute granules without definite arrangement. [G. *gry,* something insignificant, + *chrōma,* color]

gr

gry·po·sis (gri-pō'sis). An abnormal curvature. [G. *grypos*, hooked, + *-osis*, condition]

g. un'guium, SYN onychogryposis.

GSH Abbreviation for glutathione.

GSR Abbreviation for galvanic skin *response*.

GSSG Abbreviation for glutathione disulfide.

G-stro·phan·thin. SEE ouabain.

gt. Abbreviation for gutta.

g-tol·er·ance. The tolerance of a person or a piece of equipment to forces that develop as a result of acceleration or deceleration.

GTP Abbreviation for guanosine 5'-triphosphate.

gtt. Abbreviation for guttae.

GU Abbreviation for genitourinary.

Gua Abbreviation for guanine.

guai·ac (gwī'ak). The resin of *Guaiacum officinale* or *G. sanctum* (family Zygophyllaceae); a nauseant, diaphoretic, stimulant, and reagent in testing for occult blood. SYN guaiac gum. [Sp. *guayaco,* imitating the native Carib name]

guai·a·cin (gwī'ă-sin). Guaiac saponin, a constituent of guiac used as a reagent for oxidases, with which it gives a blue color.

guai·a·col (gwī'ă-kol). $C_6H_4(OH)(OCH_3)$; *o*-methoxyphenol; methylcatechol; catechol-monomethyl ether; has been used as an expectorant and intestinal disinfectant; also available as g. carbonate.

g. glyceryl ether, SYN guaifenesin.

g. phosphate, phosphoric guaiacyl ether, a white crystalline powder, insoluble in water; used as an intestinal antiseptic and in fever.

guai·fen·e·sin (gwī-fen'ĕ-sin). 3-(*o*-Methoxyphenoxy)-1,2-propanediol; an expectorant that reduces the viscosity of sputum. SYN glyceryl guaiacolate, guaiacol glyceryl ether.

guan·a·benz ac·e·tate (gwahn-ă-benz). [(2,6-Dichlorobenzylidene)amino]guanidine monoacetate; a centrally acting antiadrenergic antihypertensive similar in action to clonidine.

gua·na·cline sul·fate (gwahn'ă-klēn). Cyclazenin sulfate; [2-(3,6-Dihydro-4-methyl-1(2*H*)-pyridinyl)ethyl]guanidine sulfate dihydrate; an antihypertensive.

gua·na·drel sul·fate (gwahn'ă-drel). (1,4-Dioxaspiro[4,5]dec-2-ylmethyl)guanidine sulfate; an antihypertensive drug similar in action to guanethidine.

gua·nase (gwahn'ās). SYN *guanine* deaminase.

guanazolo (gwahn-ă-zōl'ō). SYN 8-azaguanine.

gua·neth·i·dine sul·fate (gwahn-eth'i-dēn). [2-(Octahydro-1-azocinyl)ethyl]guanidine sulfate; a potent antihypertensive agent. It appears to interfere with the release of the chemical mediator (norepinephrine) at the sympathetic neuroeffector junction; it does not produce ganglionic or parasympathetic blockade with recommended doses. In ophthalmology, it is used topically for the treatment of glaucoma and to counteract eyelid retraction in Graves' disease.

guan·fa·cine (gwan'fă-sēn). An antihypertensive agent which is an α_2-adrenergic agonist acting in the central nervous system to reduce the output of the sympathetic nervous system; resembles clonidine in its pharmacologic profile.

gua·ni·dine (gwahn'i-dēn, -din). NH_2-$C(NH)$-NH_2; a strongly basic compound, usually found (in some plants and lower animals) as the hydrochloride; a constituent of creatine and arginine; administered as a cholinergic striated muscle stimulant.

guan·id·i·ni·um (gwahn'i-din-ē-um). Referring to a guanidine moiety in a molecule (*e.g.*, in arginine).

gua·ni·di·no·ac·e·tate (gwahn'i-din-ō-ăs-ē-tāt). H_2N–$C(NH)$ $NHCH_2COO^-$; an intermediate in creatine biosynthesis.

gua·ni·di·no·ac·e·tate meth·yl·trans·fer·ase. The enzyme catalyzing the transfer of a methyl group from *S*-adenosyl-L-methionine ("active methionine") to guanidinoacetate (glycocyamine), forming creatine and *S*-adenosyl-L-homocysteine.

gua·nine (Gua, G) (gwahn'ēn, -in). 2-Amino-6-oxypurine; one of the two major purines (the other being adenine) occurring in all nucleic acids.

g. aminase, SYN g. deaminase.

g. deaminase, a deaminase of the liver that catalyzes the hydrolysis of guanine into xanthine and ammonia; the first step in purine degradation. SYN guanase, g. aminase.

g. deoxyribonucleotide, SYN deoxyguanylic acid.

g. ribonucleotide, SYN guanylic acid.

gua·no·chlor sul·fate (gwahn'ō-klōr). {[2-(2,6-Dichlorophenoxy)ethyl]amino}guanidine sulfate; used as an α-adrenergic blocking agent for the treatment of essential hypertension.

gua·no·sine (G, Guo) (gwahn'ō-sēn, -sin). 9-β-D-Ribosylguanine (guanine combined through its N-9 with the C-1 of β-D-ribose); a major constituent of RNA and of guanine nucleotides. SYN 9-β-D-ribofuranosylguanine.

cyclic g. 3',5'-monophosphate (cGMP), an analog of cAMP; a second messenger for atrial natriuretic factor. SYN cyclic GMP.

gua·no·sine 5'-di·phos·phate (GDP). Guanosine esterified at its 5' position with diphosphoric acid; bound tightly in microtubules.

gua·no·sine 5'-monophos·phate. SYN guanylic acid.

gua·no·sine 5'-tri·phos·phate (GTP). An immediate precursor of guanine nucleotides in RNA; similar to ATP; has a crucial role in microtubule formation.

GTP cyclohydrolase, an enzyme that catalyzes the reaction of GTP and H_2O forming formate and a precursor of tetrahydrobiopterin; a deficiency of this enzyme will result in one form of malignant hyperphenylalaninemia.

guan·ox·an sul·fate (gwahn-ok'san). (1,4-Benzodioxan-2-ylmethyl)guanidine sulfate; an antihypertensive agent.

gua·nyl (gwahn'il). The radical of guanine.

g. cyclase, SYN guanylate cyclase.

guan·y·late cy·clase (gwahn'i-lāt). Analogous to adenylate (adenylyl) cyclase, but cyclizing guanosine 5'-triphosphate to guanosine 3':5'-cyclic monophosphate and also producing pyrophosphate; activated by nitric oxide. SYN guanyl cyclase, guanylyl cyclase.

gua·nyl·ic ac·id (GMP) (gwă-nil'ik). A major component of ribonucleic acids. SYN guanine ribonucleotide, guanosine 5'-monophosphate.

g. a. reductase (GMP reductase), an enzyme that catalyzes the reaction of GMP with NADPH producing IMP, NH_3, and $NADP^+$; a part of the purine salvage pathway.

g. a. synthetase (GMP synthetase), an enzyme catalyzing the reaction of L-glutamine, XMP, and ATP to produce GMP, L-glutamate, AMP, and pyrophosphate; a key step in purine biosynthesis.

gua·nyl·o·ri·bo·nu·cle·ase (gwahn'i-lō-rī-bō-nū'klē-ās). SYN RNase T₁. See entries under ribonuclease.

gua·nyl·yl (gwahn'i-lil). The radical of guanylic acid.

g. cyclase, SYN guanylate cyclase.

gua·ra·na (gwah-rah-nah'). A dried paste of the crushed seeds of *Paullinia cupana* (family Sapindaceae), a vine extensively cultivated in Brazil. It contains guaranine (caffeine), saponin, a volatile oil, and paullinitannic acid. Has been used for the relief of headache. [Native Brazilian word]

gua·ra·nine (gwahr'ă-nēn). SYN caffeine.

guard·ing (gard'ing). A spasm of muscles to minimize motion or agitation of sites affected by injury or disease.

abdominal g., a spasm of abdominal wall muscles, detected on palpation, to protect inflamed abdominal viscera from pressure; usually a result of inflammation of the peritoneal surface as in appendicitis, diverticulitis, or generalized peritonitis.

involuntary g., abdominal muscle spasm, caused by retroperitoneal inflammation, which cannot be willfully suppressed.

voluntary g., abdominal muscle spasm that can be willfully suppressed.

Guarnieri, Giuseppi, Italian physician, 1856–1918. SEE G.'s gelatin *agar;* G. *bodies,* under *body.*

gu·ber·nac·u·lum (gū'ber-nak'yū-lŭm). A fibrous cord connecting two structures. A mesenchymal column of tissue that connects the fetal testis to the developing scrotum; it appears to play a role in testicular descent. SYN g. testis [NA]. [L. a helm]

g. den′tis, a connective tissue band uniting the tooth sac with the gum.

Hunter's g., obsolete term for g. testis.

g. tes′tis [NA], SYN gubernaculum.

Gubler, Adolphe, French physician, 1821–1879. SEE G.'s *line, paralysis, syndrome, tumor;* Millard-G. *syndrome.*

Gudden, Bernhard A. von, German neurologist, 1824–1886. SEE G.'s *commissures,* under *commissure, ganglion,* tegmental *nuclei,* under *nucleus.*

Guéneau de Mussy, Noël F.O., French physician, 1813–1885. SEE G. de M.'s *point.*

Guérin, Alphonse F.M., French surgeon, 1816–1895. SEE G.'s *fold, fracture, glands,* under *gland, sinus, valve.*

Guérin, Camille, French bacteriologist, 1872–1961. SEE Bacille bilié de Calmette-Guérin; bacillus Calmette-Guérin *vaccine;* Calmette *test;* Calmette-Guérin *bacillus;* Calmette-Guérin *vaccine.*

guid·ance (gī′dăns). **1.** The act of guiding. **2.** A guide.

condylar g., the mechanical device on an articulator which is intended to produce g. in articulator movement, similar to those produced by the paths of the condyles in the temporomandibular joints. SEE ALSO condylar guidance *inclination.* SYN condylar guide.

incisal g., the influence on mandibular movements caused by the contacting surfaces of the mandibular and maxillary anterior teeth during eccentric excursions. SYN incisal path.

guide (gīd). **1.** To lead in a set course. **2.** Any device or instrument by which another is led into its proper course, *e.g.,* a grooved director, a catheter g. [M.E., fr. O.Fr. *guier,* to show the way, fr. Germanic]

anterior g., SYN incisal g.

catheter g., a flexible metallic wire or thin sound over which a catheter is passed to advance it into its proper position, as in a blood vessel or the urethra. SEE ALSO stylet.

condylar g., SYN condylar *guidance.*

incisal g., in dentistry, that part of an articulator on which the anterior g. pin rests to maintain the vertical dimension of occlusion and the incisal g. angle as established by the incisal guidance; may be adjustable, with a superior surface that may be changed to provide variations in the incisal g. angle, or customized, being individually formed in plastic to allow other than straight line incisal guidance in eccentric movements. SYN anterior g.

mold g., a g. used to specify the shape of artificial teeth, or of an artificial tooth.

guide·line (gīd′līn). A marking in the form of a line that serves as a guide or reference.

clasp g., SYN survey *line.*

Cummer's g., SYN survey *line.*

guide·wire (gīd′wīr). A long and flexible fine spring used to introduce and position an intravascular angiographic catheter (see Seldinger *technique*).

Guillain, Georges, French neurologist, 1876–1961. SEE G.-Barré *reflex, syndrome;* Landry-G.-Barré *syndrome.*

guil·lo·tine (gil′ŏ-tēn, gē′ŏ-tēn). An instrument in the shape of a metal ring through which runs a sliding knifeblade, used in cutting off an enlarged tonsil. [Fr. an instrument for execution by decapitation]

guin·ea green B (gin′ē) [C.I. 42085]. An acid diaminotriphenylmethane dye, used as an indicator for H-ion determinations (changing at pH 6.0 from magenta to green) and as a fiber cytoplasmic stain in certain Masson trichrome staining procedures.

guin·ea pig (gin′ē). SYN *Cavia* porcellus.

Guldberg, C., Norwegian chemist, 1862–1902. SEE G.-Waage *law.*

gul·let (gŭl′et). SYN throat (1). [L. *gula,* throat]

Gull·strand, Allvar, Swedish ophthalmologist and Nobel laureate, 1862–1930. SEE biomicroscope.

L-gu·lon·ic ac·id (gū-lon′ik). Reduction product of glucuronic acid (–CHO → –CH₂OH); oxidation product of L-gulose (–CHO

→ –COOH); a precursor (except in primates, guinea pigs, certain fishes, and the Indian fruit bat) of ascorbic acid via L-gulonolactone.

L-gu·lon·o·lac·tone (gū-lon′ō-lak-tōn). The immediate precursor of ascorbic acid in those animals capable of ascorbic acid biosynthesis. SYN dihydroascorbic acid, L-gulono-γ-lactone.

L-g. oxidase, the enzyme catalyzing the conversion of L-g. and O₂ to H₂O₂ and L-*xylo*-hexulonolactone, a precursor of ascorbic acid; absent in primates.

L-gul·o·no·-γ-lac·tone. SYN L-gulonolactone.

gu·lose (gū′lōs). One of the eight pairs (D and L) of aldoses; D-g. is an epimer of D-galactose.

gum (gŭm). **1.** The dried exuded sap from a number of trees and shrubs, forming an amorphous brittle mass; it usually forms a mucilaginous solution in water. [L. *gummi*] **2.** SYN gingiva. [A.S. *goma,* jaw]

g. arabic, SYN acacia. SEE ALSO arabin.

Bassora g., a g. from Iran and Turkey, resembling tragacanth, acacia, and the gummy exudate of cherry and plum trees; used in making storax.

g. benjamin, g. benzoin, SYN benzoin.

British g., a form of dextrin.

eucalyptus g., a dried gummy exudation from *Eucalyptus rostrata* and other species of *Eucalyptus* (family Myrtaceae); used as an astringent (in gargles and troches) and as an antidiarrheal agent. SYN red g.

ghatti g., SYN Indian g.

guaiac g., SYN guaiac.

guar g., the ground endosperms of *Cyamopsis tetragonolobus;* used in pharmaceutical jelly formulations.

Indian g., an exudation from *Anogeissus latifolia* (family Combrettaceae); the mucilage is used as a substitute for acacia mucilage. SYN ghatti g.

karaya g., SYN sterculia g.

locust g., SYN algaroba.

g. opium, SYN opium.

red g., SYN eucalyptus g.

senegal g., the g. of *Acacia senegal.* SEE acacia.

starch g., SYN dextrin.

sterculia g., the dried gummy exudation from *Sterculia urens, S. villosa, S. tragacantha,* or other species of *Sterculia,* or from *Cochlospermum gossypium* or other species of *Cochlospermum* (family Bixaceae); used as a hydrophilic laxative and in the manufacture of lotions and pastes. SYN karaya g.

wheat g., SYN gluten.

gum·boil (gŭm′boyl). SYN gingival *abscess.*

gum·ma, pl. **gum·ma·ta, gum·mas** (gŭm′ă, ă-tă, -ž). An infectious granuloma that is characteristic of tertiary syphilis, but does not always develop, and that may be solitary (as large as 8 to 10 cm in diameter) or multiple and diffusely scattered (1 mm or less in diameter). G.'s are characterized by an irregular central portion that is firm, sometimes partially hyalinized, and consisting of coagulative necrosis in which "ghosts" of structures may be recognized; a poorly defined middle zone of epithelioid cells, with occasional multinucleated giant cells; and a peripheral zone of fibroblasts and numerous capillaries, with infiltrated lymphocytes and plasma cells. As g.'s become older, an irregular scar or rounded fibrous nodule persists. SYN gummatous syphilid, nodular syphilid, syphiloma. [L. *gummi,* gum, fr. G. *kommi*]

gum·ma·tous (gŭm′ă-tŭs). Pertaining to or characterized by the features of a gumma. SYN syphilomatous.

gum·my (gŭm′ē). **1.** Resembling or of the consistency of gum. **2.** Pertaining to the gross consistency of or resembling a gumma.

Gumprecht, Ferdinand, German physician, *1864. SEE Klein-Gumprecht shadow *nuclei,* under *nucleus;* G.'s *shadows,* under *shadow.*

Gunn, Robert Marcus, British ophthalmologist, 1850–1909. SEE G. *phenomenon;* G.'s *dots,* under *dot, sign, syndrome;* Marcus G. *pupil.*

Gunning, Thomas B., U.S. dentist, 1813–1889. SEE G. *splint.*

Günning, Jan W., Dutch chemist, 1827–1901. SEE G.'s *reaction.*

Günz, Justus, German anatomist, 1714–1751. SEE G.'s *ligament.*

Günzberg, Alfred, German physician, *1861. SEE G.'s *reagent, test.*

Guo Symbol for guanosine.

gur·ney (gŭr'nē). A stretcher or cot with wheels used to transport hospital patients. [Scottish *gurn,* to grimace in pain; Sir Goldsworthy *Gurney,* British physician and inventor, 1793–1875]

Gussenbauer, Carl, German surgeon, 1842–1903. SEE G.'s *suture.*

gus·ta·tion (gŭs-tā'shŭn). **1.** The act of tasting. **2.** The sense of taste. [L. *gustatio,* fr. *gusto,* pp. *-atus,* to taste]

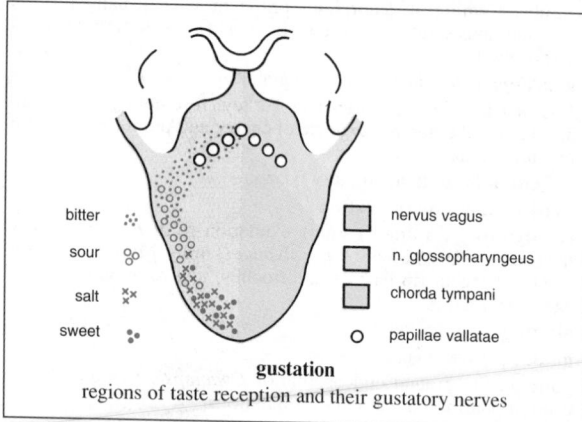

bitter

sour

salt

sweet

☐ nervus vagus

☐ n. glossopharyngeus

☐ chorda tympani

○ papillae vallatae

gustation
regions of taste reception and their gustatory nerves

gus·ta·to·ry (gŭs'tă-tōr-ē). Relating to gustation, or taste.

gust·duc·in (gŭst-dus-in). A protein messenger in taste buds that is activated in response to sweet tastes. [L. *gustus,* taste, + *duco,* to lead, induce, + -in]

gut (gŭt). **1.** SYN intestinum. **2.** Embryonic digestive tube. **3.** Abbreviated term for catgut. SEE ALSO suture. [A.S.]

blind g., SYN cecum (1).

postanal g., an extension of the hindgut caudal to the point at which the anal opening is formed. SYN postcloacal g., tailgut.

postcloacal g., SYN postanal g.

preoral g., SYN Seessel's *pocket.*

primitive g., a flat sheet of intraembryonic endoderm that will change into a tubular g. due to the folding of embryonic body— head, tail and lateral body folds. SYN archenteron, celenteron, endodermal canal, subgerminal cavity.

Guthrie, George J., English ophthalmologist, 1785–1856. SEE G.'s *muscle.*

Guthrie, R., U.S. pediatrician, *1916. SEE G. *test.*

Gutmann, Carl, German physician, *1872. SEE Michaelis-G. *body.*

gut·ta (gt.), pl. **gut·tae (gtt.)** (gŭt'ă, -ē). **1.** A drop. **2.** A rubber-like polyterpene found in gutta-percha. Cf. chicle, gutta-percha. [L.]

g. sere'na, former term for blindness of unknown etiology; the "serena" suggested that the anterior segment of the eye was clear and tranquil, that there was no visible cause for the blindness, no corneal scar, no inflammation, no cataract. Thus, g. serena became the code word for blindness due to some unfathomable posterior cause, some damage to retina, optic nerve, or brain. This was the name given to John Milton's blindness. With the opthalmoscope, in 1851, the diagnosis of g. serena suddenly became old-fashioned and inadequate.

gut·tae. Plural of gutta. [L.]

gut·ta-per·cha (gut'ă-per'chă). The coagulated, purified, dried, milky juice of trees of the genera *Palaguium* and *Payena* (family Sapotaceae); used as a filling material in dentistry, and in the manufacture of splints and electrical insulators; a solution is used as a substitute for collodion, as a protective, and to seal incised wounds. Cf. chicle, gutta. [Malay *gatah,* gum, + *percha,* the name of a tree]

guttat. Abbreviation for L. *guttatim,* drop by drop.

gut·tate (gŭt'tāt). Of the shape of, or resembling, a drop, characterizing certain cutaneous lesions.

gut·ter. Deep recess or grooves.

paracolic gutters, the grooves between the lateral aspect of the ascending or descending colon and the abdominal wall. SYN sulci paracolici [NA], paracolic recesses.

paravertebral gutter, the deep recess on either side of the vertebral column formed by the posterior sweep of the curvature of the ribs. SYN sulcus pulmonalis [NA], pulmonary sulcus.

gut·tur·al (gŭt'er-ăl). Relating to the throat.

gut·tur·o·tet·a·ny (gŭt'er-ō-tet'ă-nē). Laryngeal spasm causing a temporary stutter. [L. *guttur,* throat, + G. *tetanos,* convulsive tension]

Gutzeit, Max A.G., German chemist, 1847–1915. SEE G.'s *test.*

Guyon, Felix J.C., French surgeon, 1831–1920. SEE G.'s *amputation, isthmus, sign.*

GVH Abbreviation for graft versus host.

GVHR Abbreviation for graft versus host *reaction.*

Gy Abbreviation for gray.

gym·di·ol. SEE gym-*diol.*

Gym·na·moe·bi·da (jim-nă-mē'bi-dă). An order of naked amebae lacking a shell (testa), although there may be an enveloping layer of condensed ectoplasm; includes the genus *Amoeba.* [G. *gymnos,* naked, + *amoibē,* change (ameba)]

gym·nas·tics (jim-nas'tiks). Muscular exercise, performed indoors, as distinguished from athletics, and usually by means of special apparatus. [G. *gymnos,* naked]

Swedish g., SYN Swedish *movements,* under *movement.*

Gym·no·as·ca·ce·ae (jim'nō-as-kā'sē-ē). A family of fungi which includes the ascomycetous state of many of the dermatophytes and several of the systemic pathogens for humans (*Histoplasma capsulatum, Blastomyces dermatitidis,* etc.). Until the sexual forms were recognized, these pathogens were classified with Fungi Imperfecti.

gym·no·pho·bia (jim-nō-fō'bē-ă). Morbid dread of the sight of a naked person or of an uncovered part of the body. [G. *gymnos,* naked, + *phobos,* fear]

gym·no·the·ci·um (jim'nō-the'sē-um). An ascomycetous fruiting body composed of loosely interwoven hyphae. [G. *gymnos,* naked, + *thēkion,* case, dim. fr. *thēkē,* box]

GYN Abbreviation for gynecology.

gyn-, gyne-, gyneco-, gyno-. Female. [G. *gynē,* woman]

gy·nan·drism (ji-nan'drizm, gī'nan-drizm). A developmental abnormality characterized by hypertrophy of the clitoris and union of the labia majora, simulating in appearance the penis and scrotum. SEE hermaphroditism, female *pseudohermaphroditism.* [gyn- + G. *anēr* (*andr-*), man]

gy·nan·dro·blas·to·ma (ji-nan'drō-blas-tō'mă, gī-). **1.** SYN arrhenoblastoma. **2.** A rare variety of arrhenoblastoma of the ovary, containing granulosa or theca cell elements and producing simultaneous androgenic and estrogenic effects.

gy·nan·droid (gī-nan'droyd, jĭ-). An individual exhibiting gynandrism. [gyn- + G. *anēr* (*andr-*), man, + *eidos,* resemblance]

gy·nan·dro·mor·phism (gī-nan-drō-mōr'fizm, jĭ-). **1.** An abnormal combination of male and female characteristics. **2.** The presence of male and female sex chromosome complements in different tissues; sex chromosome mosaicism. [gyn- + G. *anēr* (*andr-*), a male human, + *morphē,* form]

gy·nan·dro·mor·phous (gī-nan-drō-mōr'fŭs, jĭ-). Having both male and female characteristics.

gy·na·tre·sia (gī-nă-trē'zē-ă, jĭ-). Occlusion of some part of the female genital tract, especially occlusion of the vagina by a thick membrane. [gyn- + G. *a-* priv. + *trēsis,* a hole]

gyne-. SEE gyn-.

gy·ne·cic (gī-nē'sik, jĭ-). Pertaining to or associated with women.

gy·ne·co·gen·ic (gī'nĕ-kō-jen'ik, jin'ĕ-). **1.** Giving birth predominantly to females. **2.** Obsolete term meaning productive of female characteristics.

gy·ne·cog·ra·phy (gī-nĕ-kog′ră-fē, jin′ĕ-). SYN hysterosalpingography. [gyne- + G. *graphō,* to write]

gy·ne·coid (gī′nĕ-koyd, jin′ĕ-). Resembling a woman in form and structure. [gyneco- + G. *eidos,* resemblance]

gy·ne·co·log·ic, gy·ne·co·log·i·cal (gī′nĕ-kō-loj′ik, jin′ĕ-; -loj′i-kăl). Relating to gynecology.

gy·ne·col·o·gist (gī-nĕ-kol′ō-jist, jǐ-nĕ-). A physician specializing in gynecology.

gy·ne·col·o·gy (GYN) (gī-nĕ-kol′ō-jē, jin′ĕ-). The medical specialty concerned with diseases of the female genital tract, as well as endocrinology and reproductive physiology of the female. [gyneco- + G. *logos,* study]

gy·ne·co·ma·nia (gī′nĕ-kō-mā′nē-ă, jin′ĕ-). Morbid or excessive desire for women. [gyneco- + G. *mania,* frenzy]

gy·ne·co·ma·stia, gy·ne·co·mas·ty (gī′nĕ-kō-mas′tē-ă, jin′ĕ-; -mas′tē). Excessive development of the male mammary glands, due mainly to ductal proliferation with periductal edema; frequently secondary to increased estrogen levels, but mild g. may occur in normal adolescence. [gyneco- + G. *mastos,* breast]

refeeding g., temporary breast enlargement seen in male patients who have been starving, when nutritional repletion is occurring. It probably represents an imbalance in endocrine function, as some systems increase function before others; seen most notably when concentration camp inmates and Allied prisoners of war were freed at the end of World War II.

gy·ne·pho·bia (gī-nĕ-fō′bē-ă, jin′ĕ-). Morbid fear of women or of the female sex. [gyne- + G. *phobos,* fear]

gy·ni·at·rics (gī-nē-at′riks, jin′ĕ-). Treatment of the diseases of women. SYN gyniatry. [gyn- + G. *iatrikos,* of medicine or surgery]

gy·ni·at·ry (gī-nē-at′rē, jin′ĕ-). SYN gyniatrics.

△**gyno-.** SEE gyn-.

gy·no·car·dia oil (gī-nō-kar′dē-ă). SYN chaulmoogra oil.

gy·no·gen·e·sis (gī-nō-jen′ĕ-sis, jin′ō-). Egg development activated by a spermatozoon, but to which the male gamete contributes no genetic material. [gyno- + G. *genesis,* production]

gy·nop·a·thy (gī-nop′ă-thē, jǐ-). Any disease peculiar to women. [gyno- + G. *pathos,* suffering]

gy·no·plas·ty, gy·no·plas·tics (gī′nō-plas-tē, jǐn′ō-, jin′ō-; gī′nō-plas-tiks). Reparative or plastic surgery of the female genital organs. [gyno- + G. *plassō,* to form]

gyp·sum (jip′sŭm). CaSO₄·2H₂O; the natural hydrated form of calcium sulfate; a component of the stones, plasters, and investments used in dentistry. [L. fr. G. *gypsos*]

gy·rase (gī′ras). The procaryotic topoisomerase II that utilizes ATP to generate negative supercoils of DNA. [L. *gyro,* to turn in a circle, fr. *gyrus,* G. *gyros,*]

gy·rate (jī′rāt). **1.** Of a convoluted or ring shape. **2.** To revolve. [L. *gyro,* pp. *gyratus,* to turn round in a circle, *gyrus*]

gy·ra·tion (jī-rā′shŭn). **1.** A circular motion or revolution. **2.** Arrangement of convolutions or gyri in the cerebral cortex.

gy·rec·to·my (jī-rek′tō-mē). Excision of a cerebral gyrus. [G. *gyros,* ring, + *ektomē,* excision]

gyr·en·ce·phal·ic (jī′ren-sĕ-fal′ik). Denoting brains, such as that of humans, in which the cerebral cortex has convolutions, in contrast to the lissencephalic (smooth) brains of small mammals such as the rodents. [G. *gyros,* ring (gyrus), + *enkaphalē,* brain]

gy·ri (jī′rī). Plural of gyrus. [L.]

gy·ro·chrome (jī′rō-krōm). Denoting a nerve cell in which the chromophil substance is arranged roughly in rings. [G. *gyros,* a ring, circle, + *chrōma,* a color]

Gy·ro·mi·tra es·cu·len·ta (gī-rō-mē′tră es-kyū-len′tă). A species of mushroom that may produce a monomethylhydrazine toxin which causes nausea, diarrhea, and other symptoms; in severe cases death may occur. SYN *Helvella esculenta.*

gy·ro·sa (jī-rō′să). SYN sham-movement *vertigo.* [L.]

gy·rose (jī′rōs). Marked by irregular curved lines like the surface of a cerebral hemisphere. [G. *gyros,* circle]

gy·ro·spasm (jī′rō-spazm). Spasmodic rotary movements of the head. [G. *gyros,* circle, + *spasmos,* spasm]

GYRUS

gy·rus, gen. and pl. **gy·′ri** (jī′rŭs, -rī) [NA]. One of the prominent rounded elevations that form the cerebral hemispheres, each consisting of an exposed superficial portion and a portion hidden from view in the wall and floor of the sulcus. [L. fr. G. *gyros,* circle]

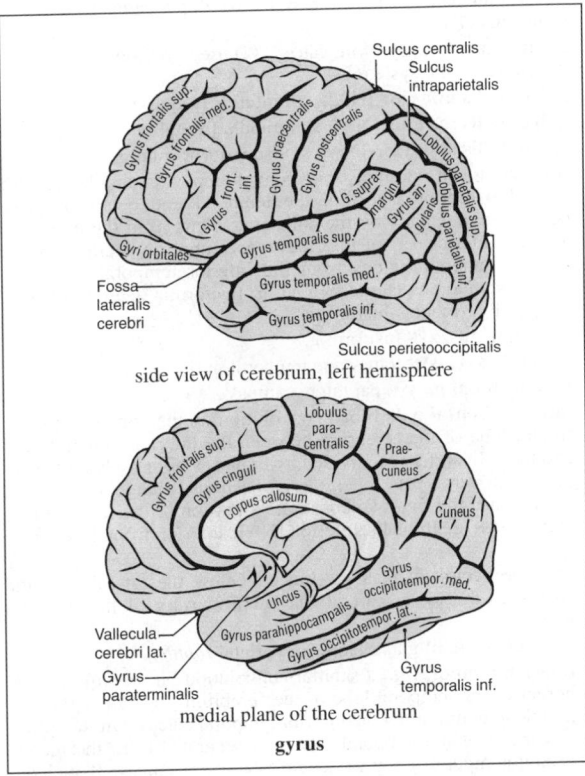

side view of cerebrum, left hemisphere

medial plane of the cerebrum

gyrus

angular g., a folded convolution in the inferior parietal lobule formed by the union of the posterior ends of the superior and middle temporal gyri. SYN g. angularis [NA], angular convolution.

g. angula′ris [NA], SYN angular g.

annectent g., SYN transitional g.

anterior central g., SYN precentral g.

anterior piriform g., SYN prepiriform g.

ascending frontal g., SYN precentral g.

ascending parietal g., SYN postcentral g.

gy′ri bre′ves in′sulae [NA], SYN short gyri of insula.

callosal g., SYN cingulate g.

central gyri, the precentral and postcentral gyri.

gy′ri cer′ebri, gyri of cerebrum [NA], the gyri or convolutions of the cerebral cortex.

cingulate g., a long, curved convolution of the medial surface of the cortical hemisphere, arched over the corpus callosum from which it is separated by the deep sulcus of corpus callosum; together with the parahippocampal g., with which it is continuous behind the corpus callosum, it forms the fornicate g. SYN g. cinguli [NA], callosal convolution, callosal g., cingulate convolution, falciform lobe, lobus falciformis.

g. cin′guli [NA], SYN cingulate g.

deep transitional g., the transverse g. of the embryo which in development becomes buried in the depth of the central sulcus of the cerebral hemisphere.

dentate g., one of the two interlocking gyri composing the hippocampus, the other one being the Ammon's horn. SYN g. dentatus [NA], dentate fascia, fascia dentata hippocampi.

g. denta'tus [NA], SYN dentate g.

fasciolar g., a small paired band that passes around the splenium of the corpus callosum from the lateral longitudinal stria to the dentate g. SYN g. fasciolaris [NA], fascia cinerea, fasciola cinerea.

g. fasciola'ris [NA], SYN fasciolar g.

fornicate g., the horseshoe-shaped cortical convolution bordering the hilus of the cerebral hemisphere; its upper limb is formed by the cingulate g., its lower by the parahippocampal g.; SYN g. fornicatus (1).

g. fornica'tus, (1) SYN fornicate g. **(2)** used previously to refer to the entire limbic system.

g. fronta'lis infe'rior [NA], SYN inferior frontal g.

g. fronta'lis me'dius [NA], SYN middle frontal g.

g. fronta'lis supe'rior [NA], SYN superior frontal g.

fusiform g., an extremely long convolution extending lengthwise over the inferior aspect of the temporal and occipital lobes, demarcated medially by the collateral sulcus from the lingual g. and the anterior part of the parahippocampal g., laterally by the inferior temporal sulcus from the inferior temporal g. SYN g. occipitotemporalis lateralis [NA], g. fusiformis, lateral occipitotemporal g., lobulus fusiformis.

g. fusifor'mis, SYN fusiform g.

Heschl's gyri, SYN transverse temporal gyri.

hippocampal g., SYN parahippocampal g.

inferior frontal g., a broad convolution on the convexity of the frontal lobe of the cerebrum between the inferior frontal sulcus and the sylvian fissure; divided by branches of the sylvian fissure into three parts: pars (opercularis) basilaris, triangular part, and orbital part; the first two constitute a portion of the frontal operculum. SYN g. frontalis inferior [NA], inferior frontal convolution.

inferior occipital g., a g. situated below the lateral occipital sulcus on the lower part of the lateral surface of the occipital lobe.

inferior parietal g., SYN inferior parietal *lobule.*

inferior temporal g., a sagittal convolution on the inferolateral border of the temporal lobe of the cerebrum, separated from the middle temporal g. by the inferior temporal sulcus. On the inferior surface of the temporal lobe it is separated from the medial occipitotemporal g. by the occipitotemporal sulcus. It includes the lateral occipitotemporal g. SYN g. temporalis inferior [NA], inferior temporal convolution, third temporal convolution.

gy'ri in'sulae [NA], SYN insular gyri.

insular gyri, the short gyri of insula and long g. of insula. SYN gyri insulae [NA].

interlocking gyri, several small gyri in the walls of the central sulcus of the hemisphere; the opposed gyri interlock with one another.

lateral occipitotemporal g., SYN fusiform g.

lingual g., a relatively short horizontal convolution on the inferomedial aspect of the occipital and temporal lobes, demarcated from the lateral occipitotemporal or fusiform g. by the deep collateral sulcus, from the cuneus by the calcarine sulcus; its anterior extreme abuts the isthmus of the parahippocampal g.; the medial or upper strip of the g. forming the lower bank of the calcarine sulcus corresponds to the inferior half of the striate area or primary visual cortex and represents the contralateral upper quadrant of the binocular field of vision. SYN g. lingualis [NA], g. occipitotemporalis medialis [NA], medial occipitotemporal g.

g. lingua'lis [NA], SYN lingual g.

long g. of insula, the most posterior and longest of the slender straight gyri that compose the insula. SYN g. longus insulae [NA].

g. lon'gus in'sulae [NA], SYN long g. of insula.

marginal g., SYN superior frontal g.

medial occipitotemporal g., SYN lingual g.

middle frontal g., a convolution on the convexity of each frontal lobe of the cerebrum running in an anteroposterior direction between the superior and inferior frontal sulci. SYN g. frontalis medius [NA], middle frontal convolution.

middle temporal g., a longitudinal g. on the lateral surface of the temporal lobe, between the superior and inferior temporal sulci. SYN g. temporalis medius [NA], middle temporal convolution, second temporal convolution.

occipital gyri, SEE inferior occipital g., superior occipital g.

g. occip'itotempora'lis latera'lis [NA], SYN fusiform g.

g. occip'itotempora'lis media'lis [NA], SYN lingual g.

orbital gyri, a number of small, irregular convolutions occupying the concave inferior surface of each frontal lobe of the cerebrum. SYN gyri orbitales [NA].

gy'ri orbita'les [NA], SYN orbital gyri.

parahippocampal g., a long convolution on the medial surface of the temporal lobe, forming the lower part of the fornicate g., extending from behind the splenium corporis callosi forward along the dentate g. of the hippocampus from which it is demarcated by the hippocampal fissure. The anterior extreme of the g. curves back upon itself, forming the uncus, the major location of the olfactory cortex. SEE ALSO entorhinal *area.* SYN g. parahippocampalis [NA], hippocampal convolution, hippocampal g.

g. par'ahippocampa'lis [NA], SYN parahippocampal g.

paraterminal g., SYN subcallosal g.

g. paratermina'lis [NA], SYN subcallosal g.

postcentral g., the anterior convolution of the parietal lobe, bounded in front by the central sulcus (fissure of Rolando) and posteriorly by the interparietal sulcus. SYN g. postcentralis [NA], ascending parietal convolution, ascending parietal g., posterior central convolution, posterior central g.

g. postcentra'lis [NA], SYN postcentral g.

posterior central g., SYN postcentral g.

precentral g., bounded posteriorly by the central sulcus and anteriorly by the precentral sulcus. SYN g. precentralis [NA], anterior central convolution, anterior central g., ascending frontal convolution, ascending frontal g.

g. precentra'lis [NA], SYN precentral g.

prepiriform g., a g. covering deeply placed amygdaloid nucleus; concerned with olfactory function. SYN anterior piriform g.

g. rec'tus [NA], SYN straight g.

Retzius' g., the intralimbic g. in the cortical portion of the rhinencephalon.

short gyri of insula, several short, radiating gyri converging toward the base of the insula, composing the anterior two-thirds of the insular cortex. SYN gyri breves insulae [NA].

splenial g., the band of cortex on the medial surface of the cerebral hemisphere which passes around the splenium of the corpus callosum, narrowing anteriorly and finally blending with the indusium griseum.

straight g., a g. running along the medial part of the orbital surface of the frontal lobe of the cerebral hemisphere. It is bounded laterally by the olfactory sulcus. SYN g. rectus [NA].

subcallosal g., a slender vertical whitish band immediately anterior to the lamina terminalis and anterior commissure; contrary to its name, it is not a cortical convolution but is the ventral continuation of the transparent septum. SYN area subcallosa [NA], g. paraterminalis [NA], g. subcallosus [NA], pedunculus corporis callosi [NA], corpus paraterminale, paraterminal body, paraterminal g., peduncle of corpus callosum, precommissural septal area, subcallosal area, Zuckerkandl's convolution.

g. subcallo'sus [NA], SYN subcallosal g.

superior frontal g., a broad convolution running in an anteroposterior direction on the medial edge of the convex surface and of each frontal lobe. SYN g. frontalis superior [NA], marginal g., superior frontal convolution.

superior occipital g., a g. lying above the lateral occipital sulcus on the lateral surface of the occipital lobe.

superior parietal g., SYN superior parietal *lobule.*

superior temporal g., a longitudinal g. on the lateral surface of the temporal lobe between the lateral (sylvian) fissure and the superior temporal sulcus. SYN g. temporalis superior [NA], first temporal convolution, superior temporal convolution.

supracallosal g., SYN *indusium* griseum.

supramarginal g., a folded convolution capping the posterior extremity of the lateral (sylvian) sulcus; together with the angular g., it forms the inferior half of the parietal lobe. SYN g. supramarginalis [NA], supramarginal convolution.

g. supramargina′lis [NA], SYN supramarginal g.

gy′ri tempora′les transver′si [NA], SYN transverse temporal gyri.

g. tempora′lis infe′rior [NA], SYN inferior temporal g.

g. tempora′lis me′dius [NA], SYN middle temporal g.

g. tempora′lis supe′rior [NA], SYN superior temporal g.

transitional g., a small convolution connecting two lobes or two main gyri in the depth of a sulcus. SYN annectent g., transitional convolution.

transverse temporal gyri, two or three convolutions running transversely on the upper surface of the temporal lobe bordering on the lateral (sylvian) fissure, separated from each other by the transverse temporal sulci. SYN gyri temporales transversi [NA], Heschl's gyri, transverse temporal convolutions.

uncinate g., SYN uncus (2).

gy

H

H Abbreviation or symbol for hyperopia or hyperopic; horizontal; Hauch; Holzknecht *unit*; henry, unit of electrical inductance; hydrogen; the Fraunhofer line at λ 3968 due to calcium; histidine; magnetic field strength; heroin.

H⁺ Symbol for hydrogen *ion*, the proton.

¹H, ²H, ³H Symbols for hydrogen-1, hydrogen-2, and hydrogen-3, respectively.

H Symbol for enthalpy, heat content, in the equation for free energy.

h Symbol for hecto-; height; hour.

hν. Symbol for photon.

h Symbol for Planck's *constant*; $h = h/2\pi$.

Ha. Symbol proposed for hahnium.

HAA Abbreviation for hepatitis-associated *antigen*.

Haab, Otto, Swiss ophthalmologist, 1850–1931.

Haase's rule. See under rule.

ha·be·na, pl. **ha·be·nae** (hă-bē'nă, -bē'nē). **1.** A frenum or restricting fibrous band. **2.** A restraining bandage. **3.** SYN habenula (2). [L. strap]

hab·e·nal, ha·be·nar (hab'ĕ-năl, hă-bē'năr). Relating to a habena.

ha·ben·u·la, pl. **ha·ben·u·lae** (ha-ben'yū-lă, -lē). **1.** SYN frenulum. **2** [NA]. In neuroanatomy, the term originally denoted the stalk of the pineal gland (pineal habenula; pedunculus of pineal body), but gradually came to refer to a neighboring group of nerve cells with which the pineal gland was believed to be associated, the habenular nucleus. Currently, the NA term refers exclusively to this circumscript cell mass in the dorsomedial thalamus, embedded in the posterior end of the medullary stria from which it receives most of its afferent fibers. By way of the retroflex fasciculus (habenulointerpeduncular tract) it projects to the interpeduncular nucleus and other paramedian cell groups of the midbrain tegmentum. Despite its proximity to the pineal stalk, no habenulopineal fiber connection is known to exist. It is a part of the epithalamus. SYN habena (3). [L.]

h. of cecum, extension of the mesocolic tenia, dorsal or ventral to the terminal ileum.

haben'ulae perfora'ta, SYN *foramina* nervosa, under *foramen*.

Haller's h., rarely used term for the cordlike remains of the vaginal process of the peritoneum. SYN Scarpa's h.

pineal h., the peduncle or stalk of the pineal gland. SEE habenula (2).

Scarpa's h., SYN Haller's h.

h. urethra'lis, one of two fine, whitish lines running from the meatus urethrae to the clitoris in girls and young women; the vestiges of the anterior part of the corpus spongiosum.

ha·ben·u·lar (hă-ben'yū-lăr). Relating to a habenula, especially the stalk of the pineal body.

Haber, Henry, 20th century British dermatologist. SEE H.'s *syndrome.*

Habermann, R., German dermatologist, 1884–1941. SEE Mucha-H. *disease, syndrome.*

hab·it. 1. An act, behavioral response, practice, or custom established in one's repertoire by frequent repetition of the same act. SEE ALSO addiction. **2.** A basic variable in the study of conditioning and learning used to designate a new response learned either by association or by being followed by a reward or reinforced event. SEE conditioning, learning. [L. *habeo*, pp. *habitus*, to have]

ha·bit·u·a·tion (ha-bit-chū-ā'shŭn). **1.** The process of forming a habit, referring generally to psychological dependence on the continued use of a drug to maintain a sense of well-being, which can result in drug addiction. **2.** The method by which the nervous system reduces or inhibits responsiveness during repeated stimulation.

hab·i·tus (hab'i-tŭs). The physical characteristics of a person. [L. habit]

fetal h., relationship of one fetal part to another. SYN fetal attitude.

gracile h., small stature, frail, underweight appearance.

hab·ro·ma·nia (hab-rō-mā'nē-ă). Rarely used term for a morbid impulse toward gaiety. [G. *habros*, graceful, + *mania*, insanity]

Hab·ro·ne·ma (ha-brō-nē'mă). A genus of spiruroid nematodes inhabiting the stomach of horses. The larvae develop in housefly and stable fly maggots living in manure, become infective when the fly larvae pupate, and are carried by adult flies to open wounds on horses, where they are left and cause cutaneous habronemiasis; reinfection of the horse's stomach by *H.* occurs by accidental ingestion of infected flies or from licking wounds in which infective larvae are found. [G. *habros*, graceful, delicate, + *nēma*, a thread]

H. ma'jus, one of two species (the other being *H. microstoma*) similar in appearance, hosts, distribution, and life cycle to *H. muscae;* the intermediate host is the stable fly, *Stomoxys calcitrans.*

H. megas'toma, a species that causes tumors in gastric mucosa containing large numbers of the small nematodes; the larvae cause cutaneous habronemiasis; the intermediate host is the common housefly, *Musca domestica.*

H. micros'toma, SEE H. majus.

H. mus'cae, a species that occurs in the stomach of the horse, mule, ass, or zebra; the intermediate host is the common housefly, *Musca domestica*, or related flies.

hab·ro·ne·mi·a·sis (hab'rō-nē-mī'ă-sis). Infection of horses with any nematodes of the genus *Habronema;* commonly denotes wound infections that contain the larvae of this worm.

cutaneous h., chronic granulomatous sores on the skin of horses caused by fly-borne larvae of *Draschia megastoma* (primarily), *Habronema muscae,* and *H. majus* which are deposited in skin wounds; the lesions are characterized by being pulpy and persistent but usually regress spontaneously in winter. SYN summer sores.

hack·ing (hak'ing). A chopping stroke made with the edge of the hand in massage.

Hadfield, Geoffrey, British physician, *1889. SEE Clarke-H. *syndrome.*

Ha·dru·rus (hă-drū'rŭs). A genus of scorpions found in the southwestern U.S., characterized by numerous setae on the stinger; the commonest species is *H. arizonensis,* the olive hairy scorpion. SEE ALSO Scorpionida. [G. *hadros*, thick, stout, + *ouro*, tail]

Haeckel, Ernst, German naturalist, 1834–1919. SEE H.'s gastrea *theory, law.*

△**haem-.** SEE hem-.

Hae·ma·dip·sa cey·lon·i·ca (hē-mă-dip'să să-lon'i-kă). A species of land leech found in Sri Lanka; it attaches itself to the skin of animals or humans. Its bite is painful, and numerous bites may cause anemia. [G. *haima*, blood, + *dipsa*, thirst]

Hae·ma·moe·ba (hē-mă-mē'bă). Old term for ameboid protozoa now classified in the suborder Haemosporina, blood parasites that include the genus *Plasmodium.* [G. *haima*, blood, + *amoibē*, change]

Hae·ma·phy·sa·lis (hē-mă-fī'să-lis). A genus of small, eyeless, inornate ticks. As larvae and nymphs, they are found chiefly on small mammals and birds; as adults, they are found on larger mammals and some birds. They are important as vectors of protozoa and viruses, (e.g., Kyasanur Forest disease virus). [G. *haima*, blood, + *physaleos*, full of wind]

H. chordei'lis, the bird tick, a common tick of turkeys and upland game birds in North America.

H. cinnabari'na, a tick that occurs chiefly in the dry district of British Columbia; this species can cause ascending paraplegia or tick paralysis in both humans and animals. [G. *kinnabarinos*, like cinnabar, vermilion]

H. cinnabari'na puncta'ta, a race of *H.* in Europe, north Africa, and Japan; larvae and nymphs feed on terrestrial reptiles, and adults on various domestic herbivores, rabbits, and hedgehogs; it transmits bovine babesiosis and anaplasmosis.

H. concin'na, common rodent tick species of the area formerly known as the U.S.S.R. that is a vector and reservoir of tick typhus.

H. leach'i, a species of Africa, Asia, and Australia that occurs on domestic and wild carnivores, on small rodents, and occasionally on cattle; it transmits canine babesiosis and boutonneuse fever.

H. lepo'ris-palus'tris, the rabbit tick, a tick species that occurs on all species of rabbits and on many wild birds in all parts of North America from Alaska to Mexico, and is important in the spread of Rocky Mountain spotted fever and tularemia among rabbits; it does not attack humans or most domestic animals and does not spread these diseases to them, but serves to maintain the infection in reservoir hosts. [L. fem. of *paluster,* marshy]

H. spinige'ra, a tropical forest species in India that is a vector of Kyasanur Forest disease; various rodents and insectivores serve as hosts of immature ticks of this species, which carry an arbovirus of the Russian spring-summer B group complex; monkeys act as reservoirs of human infection.

Hae·ma·to·bia. Genus of flies of the family Muscidae.

Haematobia irritans, SYN horn *fly.*

Hae·ma·to·pi·nus (hē'mă-tō-pī'nŭs). An important genus of sucking lice (family Haematopinidae) affecting swine and other domestic and wild animals; it is normally nonpathogenic. *H. asini* affects horses, mules, and asses; *H. eurysternus* and *H. quadripertusus,* cattle; and *H. suis,* swine. [G. *haima,* blood, + L. *pinus,* pine tree]

Hae·mo·bar·ton·el·la (hē'mō-bar-tō-nel'ă). A genus of parasitic bacteria (order Rickettsiales) found in and on the surface of erythrocytes, but which rarely produce disease in animals without splenectomy. They are identical to *Eperythrozoon* species, except that *H.* species are not found free in the plasma nor are ring forms seen on the surface of infected erythrocytes. Species are found in laboratory rats and in dogs, cats, and other domestic animals. The type species is *H. muris.* SYN *Hemobartonella.* [G. *haima,* blood, + dim. of A.S. *beretūn,* courtyard, grange, fr. *bere,* barley, + *tūn,* enclosure]

H. felis, the species causing feline infectious anemia.

H. mu'ris, a species found in rats, mice, and hamsters; ectoparasites such as the rat louse, the flea, and possibly the bedbug are vectors; it is the type species of *H.*

Hae·mo·coc·cid·i·um (hē'mō-kok-sid'ē-ŭm). Old name for *Plasmodium* species. [G. *haima,* blood, + *kokkos,* berry]

Hae·mo·dip·sus ven·tri·co·sus (hē-mō-dip'sŭs ven-tri-kō'sŭs). The rabbit louse, a transmitter of *Francisella tularensis.* [G. *haima,* blood, + *dipsos,* thirst; L. *venter* (*ventr*-), belly]

Hae·mo·greg·a·ri·na (hē'mō-greg-ă-rī'nă). A sporozoan coccidian genus (order Eucoccidiida, family Haemogregarinidae) that parasitizes the blood cells of cold-blooded animals and the digestive system of invertebrate primary hosts in an obligatory two-host cycle. [G. *haima,* blood, + L. *grex,* a flock]

Hae·mon·chus (hē-mong'kŭs). An economically important genus of nematode parasites (family Trichostrongylidae) occurring in the abomasum of ruminant animals and causing severe anemia, especially in younger or previously unexposed animals. Some significant species are *H. placei* (in cattle, sheep, and goats), *H. similis* (in cattle and sheep), and *H. contortus,* the stomach, barberpole, or twisted wire worm of cattle, sheep, goats, and other ruminants, of which a few cases have been reported from humans. [G. *haima,* blood, + *onchos,* spear]

Hae·moph·i·lus (hē-mof'i-lŭs). A genus of aerobic to facultatively anaerobic, nonmotile bacteria (family Brucellaceae) containing minute, Gram-negative, rod-shaped cells which sometimes form threads and are pleomorphic. These organisms are strictly parasitic, growing best, or only, on media containing blood. They may or may not be pathogenic. They occur in various lesions and secretions, as well as in normal respiratory tracts, of vertebrates. The type species is *H. influenzae.* [G. *haima,* blood, + *philos,* fond]

H. actinomycetemcomi'tans, SYN *Actinobacillus actinomycetemcomitans.*

H. aegyp'ticus, a species that causes acute or subacute infectious conjunctivitis in warm climates.

H. aphroph'ilus, a species found in the blood and, rarely, on the heart valve as a cause of endocarditis.

H. ducrey'i, a species which causes soft chancre (chancroid). SYN Ducrey's bacillus.

H. gallina'rum, former name for *H. paragallinarum.*

H. haemoglobinoph'ilus, a species which occurs in large numbers in preputial secretions of dogs.

H. haemolyt'icus, a species which is usually nonpathogenic but which, on rare occasions, causes subacute endocarditis.

H. influen'zae, a species found in the respiratory tract that causes acute respiratory infections; including pneumonia, acute conjunctivitis, bacterial meningitis, and purulent meningitis in children, rarely in adults; originally considered to be the cause of influenza, it is the type species of the genus *H.* SYN influenza bacillus, Koch-Weeks bacillus, Pfeiffer's bacillus, Weeks' bacillus.

H. paragallina'rum, a species that causes infectious coryza in chickens and other birds.

H. parahaemoly'ticus, a species found in the upper respiratory tract and associated frequently with pharyngitis; occasionally causes subacute endocarditis.

H. parainfluen'zae, a species which is usually nonpathogenic but which occasionally causes subacute endocarditis.

H. para'suis, a species causing Glasser's disease in pigs.

H. som'nus, a species causing thromboembolic meningoencephalitis in cattle.

H. su'is, a species, related to *H. influenzae,* found in swine and associated with influenza virus in the pneumonia of swine influenza.

Hae·mo·pro·te·us (hē'mō-prō'tē-ŭs). A genus of sporozoa (suborder Haemosporina) parasitic in birds and reptiles, combined with *Leucocytozoon, Hepatocystis,* and other genera in the family Haemoproteidae. Schizogony occurs in endothelial cells of blood vessels, especially in the lungs of the host, while halter-shaped gametocytes are found in the red blood cells. Infection is transmitted by pupiparous Diptera, such as louse flies (Hippoboscidae) and by bloodsucking midges (*Culicoides*) [G. *haima,* blood, + *Proteus,* a sea god who had the power of assuming different shapes]

Hae·mo·spo·ri·na (hē'mō-spō-rī'nă). A suborder of coccidia (class Sporozoea) that lack syzygy, with separate development of macrogamete and microgamont, the latter producing eight flagellated microgametes; heteroxenous with merogany in vertebrates and sporogony in bloodsucking insects; includes the genera *Haemoproteus, Leucocytozoon,* and *Plasmodium.* [G. *haima,* blood, + *sporos,* seed]

Hae·mo·stron·gy·lus va·so·rum (hē'mō-stron'ji-lŭs). SYN *Angiostrongylus vasorum.* [G. *haima,* blood, + *strongylos,* round]

Haenel, Hans G., German neurologist, 1874–1942. SEE H.'s *symptom.*

Haens·zel, William, U.S. epidemiologist/statistician, *1910. SEE Mantel-Haenszel *test.*

Haffkine, Waldemar M.W., Russian physician, 1860–1930. SEE H.'s *vaccine.*

Haf·nia (haf'nē-ah). Genus in the tribe *Klebsiella;* a rare cause of nosocomial infection. There is a single species, *Hafnia alvei.*

haf·ni·um (Hf) (haf'nē-ŭm). A rare chemical element, atomic no. 72, atomic wt. 178.49. [L. *Hafniae,* Copenhagen]

Hagedorn, Werner, German surgeon, 1831–1894. SEE H. *needle.*

Hageman. Surname of person in whom deficiency of Hageman *factor* (*q.v.,*) was first observed.

hag·i·o·ther·a·py (hag'ē-ō-thār'ă-pē). Treatment of the sick by contact with relics of the saints, visits to shrines, and other religious observances. [G. *hagios,* sacred]

Haglund, S.E. Patrick, Swedish orthopedist, 1870–1937. SEE H.'s *deformity, disease.*

Hahnemann, C.F.S., German physician and founder of homeopathy, 1755–1843. SEE hahnemannian.

hah·ne·man·ni·an (hah-ně-mahn′ē-an). Relating to homeopathy as taught by Hahnemann.

hahn·i·um (hahn′ē-ŭm). Name proposed for the artificially made element 105. [Otto *Hahn,* Ger. physical chemist and Nobel laureate, 1879–1968]

Hahn's ox·ine re·a·gent. See under reagent.

Haidinger, Wilhelm von, Austrian mineralogist, 1795–1871. SEE H.'s *brushes,* under *brush.*

Hailey, Hugh E., U.S. dermatologist, *1909. SEE H.-H. *disease.*

Hailey, W. Howard, U.S. dermatologist, 1898–1967. SEE H.-H. *disease.*

hair (hār). **1.** SYN pilus (1). **2.** One of the fine hairlike processes of the auditory cells of the labyrinth, and of other sensory cells, called auditory h.'s, sensory h.'s, etc. [A.S. *haer*]

auditory h.'s, cilia on the free surface of the auditory cells.

axillary h., h. of the armpit.

bamboo h., h. with regularly spaced nodules along the shaft caused by intermittent fractures with invagination of the distal h. into the proximal portion, with intervening lengths of normal h., giving the appearance of bamboo; seen in Netherton's syndrome; autosomal recessive trait. SYN trichorrhexis invaginata.

bayonet h., a spindle-shaped developmental defect occurring at the tapered end of the h.

beaded h., SYN monilethrix.

burrowing h.'s, SYN ingrown h.'s.

club h., a h. in resting state, prior to shedding, in which the bulb has become a club-shaped mass.

exclamation point h., the type of dystrophic anagen h. found at margins of patches of alopecia areata; the bulb is absent.

Frey's h.'s, short h.'s of varying degrees of stiffness, set at right angles into the end of a light wooden handle; used for assessing sensation.

ingrown h.'s, h.'s that grow at more acute angles than is normal, and in all directions; they incompletely clear the follicle, turn back in, and cause pseudofolliculitis. SYN burrowing h.'s.

kinky h., tightly curled or bent h. SEE kinky-hair *disease.*

lanugo h., SYN lanugo.

moniliform h., SYN monilethrix.

nettling h.'s, sharp-pointed barbed h.'s of certain caterpillars which cause a dermatitis when brought in contact with the skin.

ringed h., a rare condition in which the h. shows alternate pigmented and bright segments, the latter due to air cavities within the cortex. SYN leukotrichia annularis, pili annulati, thrix annulata, trichonosus versicolor.

scalp h., a hair of the head. SYN capillus [NA].

Schridde's cancer h.'s, thick lusterless h.'s scattered in the beard and the temporal region, said to occur in cancerous patients but found also in persons with other cachectic conditions.

stellate h., h. split in several strands at the free end.

tactile h., the vibrissae or whiskers of animals such as rats and cats which have especially well developed touch endings in the follicular wall.

taste h.'s, hairlike projections of gustatory cells of taste buds; electron micrographs show them to be clusters of microvilli.

terminal h., a mature pigmented, coarse h.

twisted h.'s, SYN *pili* torti, under *pilus.*

vellus h., colorless, soft, fine postnatal to adult h.

woolly h., tightly coiled h., oval in cross-section, with the texture of wool.

hair cast. A small, nodular accretion of epithelial cells and keratinous debris resulting from failure of the internal root sheath to disintegrate; it appears for 3 to 7 mm along the hair shaft.

hair·pin (hār′pin). The structure formed by a polynucleic acid by base-pairing between neighboring complementary sequences of a single strand of either DNA or RNA.

hair·worm (hār′werm). SEE *Trichostrongylus, Gordius.*

hairy (hār′ē). **1.** Of or resembling hair. **2.** Covered with hair. SEE ALSO hirsutism. SYN pilar, pilary, pileous, pilose.

ha·la·tion (hă-lā′shŭn). Blurring of the visual image by glare.

hal·az·e·pam (hal-az′e-pam). 7-Chloro-1,3-dihydro-5-phenyl-1-

(2,2,2-trifluoroethyl)-2*H*-1,4-benzodiazepin-2-one; a benzodiazepine used in the management of anxiety disorders and for short-term relief of symptoms of anxiety.

hal·a·zone (hal′ă-zōn). *N,N*-(*N,N*-Dichlorosulfamyl)benzoic acid; a chloramine used for the sterilization of drinking water.

Halbeisen, William A., U.S. physician, *1915. SEE Stryker-H. *syndrome.*

Halberstaedter, Ludwig, German physician, 1876–1949. SEE H.-Prowazek *bodies,* under *body.*

hal·cin·o·nide (hal-sin′ō-nīd). 21-Chloro-9-fluoro-11β-hydroxy-16α,17-[(1-methylethylidene)bis(oxy)]pregn-4-ene-3,20-dione; an anti-inflammatory corticosteroid used in topical preparations.

Haldane, John B.S., English biochemist and geneticist, 1892–1964. SEE H. *relationship.*

Haldane, John S., Scottish physiologist at Oxford, 1860–1936. SEE H.'s *apparatus;* H. *chamber, effect, transformation, tube;* H.-Priestley *sample.*

Hales, Stephen, English physiologist, 1677–1761. SEE H.'s *piesimeter.*

Hale's col·loi·dal iron stain. See under stain.

ha·leth·a·zole (hă-leth′ă-zōl). 5-Chloro-2-[*p*-(diethylaminoethoxy)phenyl]benzothiazole; an antiseptic with antifungal properties.

half-hap·ten (haf-hap′ten). A substance that elicits an antigen-antibody reaction, but no precipitation.

half-life (haf′līf). The period in which the radioactivity or number of atoms of a radioactive substance decreases by half; similarly applied to any substance whose quantity decreases exponentially with time. Cf. half-time.

biological h.-l., the time required for one-half of an amount of a substance to be lost through biological processes.

effective h.-l., the time required for the body burden of an administered quantity of radioactivity to decrease by half through a combination of radioactive decay and biological elimination.

physical h.-l., the time required for half the atoms of a radionuclide to undergo disintegration.

half-moon (haf′mūn). SYN lunula (1).

red h.-m., irregular red discoloration of the usually pale demilune at the base of the fingernail; may be seen in congestive failure, malignant disease, or liver disease, but not specific for any of these.

half-time (haf′tīm). The time, in a first-order chemical (or enzymic) reaction, for half of the substance (substrate) to be converted or to disappear. Cf. half-life.

half·way house (haf′wā hows). A facility for individuals who no longer require the complete facilities of a hospital or institution but are not yet prepared to return to independent living.

hal·i·but liv·er oil (hal′i-bŭt). The fixed oil obtained from the fresh or suitably preserved livers of halibut species of the genus *Hippoglossus* (family Pleuronectidae); a supplementary source of vitamins A and D.

hal·ide (hal′īd). A salt of a halogen.

hal·i·pha·gia (hal-i-fā′jē-ă). Ingestion of an excessive quantity of a salt or salts, especially of sodium chloride, calcium, magnesium, or potassium salts, or of sodium bicarbonate. [G. *hals,* salt, + *phagō,* to eat]

hal·i·ste·re·sis (hă-lis-ter-ē′sis). A deficiency of lime salts in the bones. SYN halosteresis. [G. *hals,* salt, + *sterēsis,* privation, fr. *stereō,* to deprive]

hal·i·ste·ret·ic (hă-lis-ter-et′ik). Relating to or marked by halisteresis.

hal·i·to·sis (hal-i-tō′sis). A foul odor from the mouth. SYN fetor oris, ozostomia, stomatodysodia. [L. *halitus,* breath, + G. *-osis,* condition]

hal·i·tus (hal′i-tŭs). Any exhalation, as of a breath or vapor. [L., fr. *halo,* to breathe]

hal·la·chrome (hal′ă-krōm). A quinone intermediate, derived from L-dopa, in the formation of melanin from L-tyrosine.

Hallé, Adrien J.M.N., French physician, 1859–1947. SEE H.'s *point.*

Haller, Albrecht von, Swiss physiologist, 1708–1777. SEE H.'s *ansa, annulus, arches,* under *arch, circle, cones,* under *cone, habenula, insula, line, plexus, rete,* vascular *tissue, tripod, tunica vasculosa, unguis, vas aberrans.*

Hallermann, Wilhelm, 20th century German ophthalmologist. SEE H.-Streiff *syndrome;* Hallermann-Streiff-François *syndrome.*

Hallervorden, Julius, German neurologist, 1882–1965. SEE H. *syndrome;* H.-Spatz *disease, syndrome.*

hal·lex, pl. **hal·li·ces** (hal′eks, hal′i-sēz). SYN hallux. [L.]

Hallgren, Bertil, 20th century Swedish geneticist. SEE H.'s *syndrome.*

Hallopeau, François H., French dermatologist, 1842–1919. SEE H.'s *disease.*

hal·lu·cal (hal′ū-kăl). Relating to the hallux.

hal·lu·ci·na·tion (ha-lū′si-nā′shŭn). The apparent, often strong subjective perception of an object or event when no such stimulus or situation is present; may be visual, auditory, olfactory, gustatory, or tactile. [L. *alucinor,* to wander in mind]

auditory h., a symptom frequently observed in a schizophrenic disorder consisting, in the absence of an external source, of hearing a voice or other auditory stimulus that other individuals do not perceive.

formed visual h., h. composed of scenes, often landscapes.

gustatory h., the sensation of taste in the absence of a gustatory stimulus; may be seen in temporal lobe epilepsy.

haptic h., the sensation of touch in the absence of stimuli; may be seen in alcoholic delirium tremens.

hypnagogic h., h. occurring in the period between wakefulness and sleep; one of the components of narcolepsy.

hypnopompic h., vivid hallucinations that occur when wakening from sleep; occurs with narcolepsy, but grouped with hypnagogic h.

lilliputian h., h. of reduced size of objects or persons.

mood-congruent h., h. in which the content is mood appropriate.

mood-incongruent h., h. that is not consistent with external stimuli; content is not consistent with either manic or depressed mood.

olfactory h., false perception in smell.

stump h., SYN phantom *limb.*

tactile h., false perception of movement or sensation, as from an amputated limb, or crawling sensation on the skin.

unformed visual h., h. composed of sparks, lights, or bursting spheres of light.

hal·lu·ci·no·gen (ha-lū′si-nō-jen). A mind-altering chemical, drug, or agent, specifically a chemical whose most prominent pharmacologic action is on the central nervous system (*e.g.,* mescaline); in normal subjects, it elicits optical or auditory hallucinations, depersonalization, perceptual disturbances, and disturbances of thought processes. SYN hallucinogenesis, psychedelic drug, psychodysleptic drug, psycholytic drug, psychotomimetic drug. [L. *alucinari,* to wander in mind, + G. *-gen,* producing]

hal·lu·ci·no·gen·e·sis (ha-lū′si-nō-jen′ĕ-sis). SYN hallucinogen.

hal·lu·ci·no·gen·ic (ha-lū′si-nō-jen′ik). SYN psychodelic.

hal·lu·ci·no·sis (ha-lū-si-nō′sis). A syndrome, usually of organic origin (*e.g.,* alcoholic h. characterized by more or less persistent hallucinations).

organic h., the state of experiencing a false sensory perception in the absence of external stimulus observed in individuals with one of the organic mental disorders (*e.g.,* the frightening sensations experienced in alcoholic hallucinosis or by a person who has ingested LSD or another of the mind-altering drugs). SEE hallucination.

hal·lus (hal′ŭs). SYN hallux.

hal·lux, pl. **hal·lu·ces** (hal′ŭks, hal′yū-sēz) [NA]. The great toe; the first digit of the foot. SYN great toe, hallex, hallus, pollex pedis. [a Mod. L. form for L. *hallex (hallic-),* great toe]

h. doloro′sus, a condition, usually associated with flatfoot, in which walking causes severe pain in the metatarsophalangeal joint of the great toe. SYN painful toe.

h. exten′sus, a deformity in which the great toe is held rigidly in the extended position.

h. flex′us, hammer toe involving the first toe.

h. mal′leus, hammer toe involving the first toe.

h. rig′idus, a condition in which there is stiffness in the first metatarsophalangeal joint; the joint may be the site of a osteoarthritis. SYN stiff toe.

h. val′gus, a deviation of the tip of the great toe, or main axis of the toe, toward the outer or lateral side of the foot.

h. va′rus, deviation of the main axis of the great toe to the inner side of the foot away from its neighbor.

ha·lo (hā′lō). **1.** A reddish yellow ring surrounding the optic disk, due to a widening of the scleral ring making the deeper structures visible. **2.** An annular flare of light surrounding a luminous body or a depigmented ring around a mole. SEE halo *nevus.* **3.** SYN areola (4). **4.** A circular metal band used in a h. cast or h. brace, attached to the skull with pins. [G. *halōs,* threshing floor on which oxen trod a circle; the halo round the sun or moon]

anemic h., pale, relatively avascular areas in the skin seen around vascular spiders, cherry angiomas, and sometimes in acute macular eruptions.

glaucomatous h., (1) a yellowish white ring surrounding the optic disk, indicating atrophy of the choroid in glaucoma; SYN glaucomatous ring. (2) a h. surrounding lights, caused by corneal edema in glaucoma. SYN rainbow symptom.

senile h., circumpapillary h. seen in choroidal atrophy of the aged.

hal·o·al·kyl·a·mines (hal-ō-al-kil′ă-mēnz). A class of drugs, including phenoxybenzamine and diabenamine, which binds alkylate α-adrenergic receptors so that they are irreversibly inactivated.

hal·o·an·i·sone (hal-ō-an′i-sōn). SYN fluanisone.

Hal·o·coc·cus. A genus of Gram variable, aerobic, chemoheterotrophic nonmotile bacteria. Found in seawater and saline soil. The type species is *Halococcus morrhuae.*

H. morrhu′ae, a species found in seawater brine, sea salt, and salt lakes; also found in association with red discoloration of salted fish.

hal·o·gen (hal′ō-jen). One of the chlorine group (fluorine, chlorine, bromine, iodine, astatine) of elements; h.'s form monobasic acids with hydrogen, and their hydroxides (fluorine forms none) are also monobasic acids. [G. *hals,* salt, + *-gen,* producing]

hal·o·gen·a·tion (hal′ō-jĕ-nā′shŭn). Incorporation of one or more halogen atoms into a molecule.

hal·o·gen·o·der·ma (hal-ō-gen′ō-der-mă). Dermatosis caused by ingestion or injection of halogens, most notably bromides and iodides. [halogen + G. *derma,* skin]

Hal·o·ge·ton (hal-ō-jē′ton). A genus of plants (family Chenopodiaceae) on range lands in the western U.S. and other arid regions of the world; it causes poisoning in cattle and sheep because of the presence of soluble oxalates.

ha·lom·e·ter (hal-om′ĕ-ter). An instrument used to measure the diffraction halo of a red blood cell; based on the premise that the halo of the large erythrocyte of pernicious anemia is smaller than that of the normal cell; the hazy colorless halo of normal size is characteristic of secondary anemia.

hal·o·per·i·dol (hal-ō-per′i-dol). A butyrophenone used as an antipsychotic; also used in Huntington's chorea and Gilles de la Tourette's disease; the drug blocks dopamine receptors.

hal·o·phil, hal·o·phile (hal′ō-fil, -fīl). A microorganism whose growth is enhanced by or dependent on a high salt concentration. [G. *hals,* salt, + *philos,* fond]

hal·o·phil·ic (hal-ō-fil′ik). Requiring a high concentration of salt for growth.

hal·o·pro·gin (hal-ō-prō′jin). 3-Iodo-2-propynyl 2,4,5-trichlorophenyl ether; an antifungal agent.

hal·o·ste·re·sis (hă-los-tĕ-rē′sis). SYN halisteresis.

hal·o·thane (hal′ō-thān). 2-Bromo-2-chloro-1,1,1-trifluoroethane; a widely used potent nonflammable and nonexplosive inhalation anesthetic, with rapid onset and reversal; side effects include respiratory and cardiovascular depression, and sensitization to epinephrine-induced arrhythmias.

Halstead, Ward C., U.S. psychologist, 1908–1968. SEE H.-Reitan *battery.*

Ha

Halsted, William Stewart, U.S. surgeon, 1852–1922. SEE H.'s *law, operation, suture.*

Hal·te·rid·i·um (hawl-tĕ-rid′ē-ŭm). Former name for *Haemoproteus.* [G. *haltēres,* weights held in the hand in leaping]

hal·zoun (hal′zŭn). Local name of a buccopharyngeal infection occurring in Lebanon, probably caused by pentastomid larvae of the dog tongue worm, *Linguatula serrata,* which wander into the throat of the human host after ingestion of infected raw sheep, or goat liver or lymph nodes. [Ar., snail]

Ham, Thomas Hale, U.S. physician, *1905. SEE H.'s *test.*

ham. **1.** SYN popliteal *fossa.* **2.** The buttock and back part of the thigh. [A.S.]

ham·a·me·lis (ham′ă-mē′lis). A shrub or small tree, *Hamamelis virginiana* (family Harmarmelidaceae), whose bark and dried leaves have been used externally as an application to contusions and other injuries, in headache, and for the cure of noninflammatory hemorrhoids; the water, popularly known as "extract of witch hazel," is made from the bark. SYN witch hazel. [Mod. L., fr. G. *hama- mēlis,* fr. *hama,* together with, + *mēlon,* apple]

ha·mar·tia (ha-mar′shē-ă). A localized developmental disturbance characterized by abnormal arrangement and/or combinations of the tissues normally present in the area. [G. *hamartion,* a bodily defect]

ham·ar·to·blas·to·ma (hă-mar′tō-blas-tō′mă). A malignant neoplasm of undifferentiated anaplastic cells thought to be derived from a hamartoma. [hamartoma + blastoma]

ham·ar·to·chon·dro·ma·to·sis (ham-ar′tō-kon′drō-mă-tō′sis). Neoplasm-like foci of cartilaginous tissue in sites where cartilage is a normal constituent, but in which the growth of cartilage cells is out of proportion to the other elements of the organ. [G. *hamartion,* bodily defect, + *chondros,* cartilage, + *-osis,* condition]

ham·ar·to·ma (ham-ar-tō′mă). A focal malformation that resembles a neoplasm, grossly and even microscopically, but results from faulty development in an organ; composed of an abnormal mixture of tissue elements, or an abnormal proportion of a single element, normally present in that site, which develop and grow at virtually the same rate as normal components, and are not likely to result in compression of adjacent tissue (in contrast to a neoplasm). [G. *hamartion,* a bodily defect, + *-oma,* tumor]

fibrous h. of infancy, a tumor appearing usually in the upper arm or shoulder in the first two years of life and consisting of cellular fibrous tissue infiltrating the subcutis.

pulmonary h., h. of the lung, producing a coin lesion composed primarily of cartilage and bronchial epithelium. SYN adenochondroma.

ham·ar·tom·a·tous (ham-ar-tō′mă-tŭs). Relating to hamartoma.

ham·ar·to·pho·bia (ham′ar-tō-fō′bē-ă). Morbid fear of error or sin. [G. *hamartia,* fault, + *phobos,* fear]

ha·ma·tum (ha-mā′tŭm). SYN hamate *bone.* [L. neut. of *hamatus,* hooked, fr. *hamus,* a hook]

ha·max·o·pho·bia (hă-maks′ō-fō′bē-ă). SYN amaxophobia.

Hamburger, Hartog J., Dutch physiologist, 1859–1924. SEE H.'s *law, phenomenon.*

Hamilton, Frank Hastings, U.S. surgeon, 1813–1886. SEE H.'s *pseudophlegmon.*

Hamman, Louis, U.S. physician, 1877–1946. SEE H.'s *disease, murmur, sign, syndrome;* H.-Rich *syndrome.*

Hammarsten, Olof, Swedish physiological chemist, 1841–1932. SEE H.'s *reagent.*

ham·mer (ham′er). SYN malleus.

Hammerschlag, Albert, Austrian physician, 1863–1935. SEE H.'s *method.*

Hammond, William A., U.S. neurologist, 1828–1900. SEE H.'s *disease.*

Hampton, Aubrey Otis, U.S. radiologist, 1900–1955. SEE H. *line, maneuver, technique;* H.'s *hump.*

ham·ster. Any of four genera (subfamily Cricetinae, family Muridae) of small rodents widely used in research and as pets: *Cricetus, Cricetulus, Mesocricetus,* and *Phodopus.* All hamsters are seed and plant feeders, store food, hibernate in winter, and breed throughout the year under laboratory conditions.

ham·string. **1.** One of the tendons bounding the popliteal space on either side; the **medial h.** comprises the tendons of the semimembranosus and semitendinosus, gracilis, and sartorius muscles; the **lateral h.** is the tendon of the biceps femoris muscle. H. muscles (a) have origin from the ischial tuberosity, (b) act across (at) both the hip and knee joints (producing extension and flexion, respectively), and (c) are innervated by the tibial portion of the sciatic nerve. The medial h. contributes to medial rotation of the leg at the flexed knee joint, while the lateral h. contributes to lateral rotation. **2.** In domestic animals, the combined tendons of the superficial digital flexor, triceps surae, biceps femoris, and semitendinosus muscles which are referred to as the common calcanean tendon (tendo calcaneus communis); it is attached to the tuber calcis of the hock.

ham·u·lar (ham′yū-lăr). Hook-shaped; unciform. [L. *hamulus, q.v.*]

ham·u·lus, gen. and pl. **ham·u·li** (ham′yū-lŭs, -lī) [NA]. Any hooklike structure. [L. dim. of *hamus,* hook]

h. coch′leae, SYN h. of spiral lamina.

lacrimal h., the hooklike lower end of the lacrimal crest, curving between the frontal process and orbital surface of the maxilla to form the upper aperture of the bony portion of the nasolacrimal canal. SYN h. lacrimalis [NA], hamular process of lacrimal bone.

h. lacrima′lis [NA], SYN lacrimal h.

h. lam′inae spira′lis [NA], SYN h. of spiral lamina.

h. os′sis hama′ti [NA], SYN *hook* of hamate bone.

pterygoid h., the inferior, hook-shaped extremity of the medial plate of the pterygoid process. SYN h. pterygoideus [NA], hamular process of sphenoid bone.

h. pterygoid′eus [NA], SYN pterygoid h.

h. of spiral lamina, the upper hooklike termination of the bony spiral lamina at the apex of the cochlea. SYN h. laminae spiralis [NA], h. cochleae, hook of spiral lamina.

Hancock, Henry, English surgeon, 1809–1880. SEE H.'s *amputation.*

Hand, Alfred, U.S. pediatrician, 1868–1949. SEE H.-Schüller-Christian *disease.*

hand. The portion of the upper limb distal to the radiocarpal joint, comprised of the wrist, palm, and fingers. SYN manus [NA], main. [A.S.]

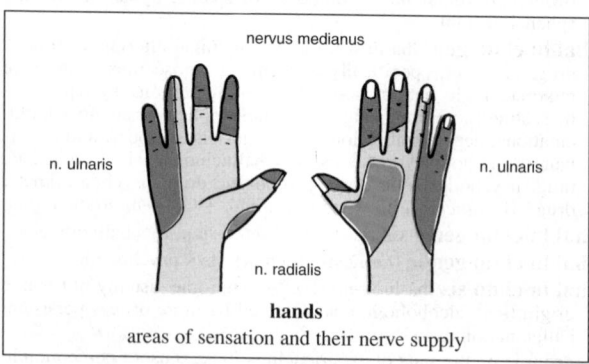

nervus medianus

n. ulnaris

n. ulnaris

n. radialis

hands
areas of sensation and their nerve supply

accoucheur's h., position of the h. in tetany or in muscular dystrophy; the fingers are flexed at the metacarpophalangeal joints and extended at the phalangeal joints, with the thumb flexed and adducted into the palm; in resemblance to the position of the physician's hand in making a vaginal examination. SYN main d'accoucheur, obstetrical h.

ape h., a deformity marked by extension of the thumb in the same plane as the palm and fingers. SYN monkey-paw.

claw h., SEE clawhand.

cleft h., a congenital deformity in which the division between the fingers, especially between the third and fourth, extends into the metacarpal region. SEE ALSO lobster-claw *deformity.* SYN main fourchée, split h.

club h., congenital or acquired angulation deformity of h. associated with partial or complete absence of radius or ulna; usually with intrinsic deformities of the h. in congenital variants. SEE *manus* valga, *manus* vara.

crab h., SYN erysipeloid.

drop h., SYN *wrist*-drop.

flat h., SYN *manus* plana.

ghoul h., a condition seen in African blacks, probably a manifestation of tertiary yaws, marked by depigmentation of the palms and contraction of the skin which give a clawlike and corpselike appearance to the h.'s.

h. of hand, the back of the hand. SYN dorsum manus [NA].

Marinesco's succulent h., edema of the h. with coldness and lividity of the skin, observed in syringomyelia. SYN main succulente.

monkey h., SYN monkey-paw.

obstetrical h., SYN accoucheur's h.

opera-glass h., a deformity of the h. seen in chronic absorptive arthritis, the fingers and wrists being shortened and the covering skin wrinkled into transverse folds; the phalanges appear to be retracted into one another like an opera glass or miniature telescope. SYN main en lorgnette.

simian h., deformity in which there is flattening of the thenar eminence, and the thumb lies adducted and extended; usually due to a median nerve lesion.

skeleton h., extension of fingers with atrophy of tissues; occurs in progressive muscular atrophy.

spade h., the coarse, thick, square h. of acromegaly or myxedema.

split h., SYN cleft h.

trench h., obsolete term for frostbite of the h.

trident h., a h. in which the fingers are of nearly equal length and deflected at the first interphalangeal joint, so as to give a forklike shape; seen in achondroplasia.

writing h., a contraction of the h. muscles in parkinsonism, bringing the fingers somewhat into the position of holding a pen.

hand·ed·ness (hand'ed-nes). Preference for the use of one hand, most commonly the right, associated with dominance of the opposite cerebral hemisphere; may also be the result of training or habit.

hand·i·cap (hand'i-kap). **1.** A physical, mental, or emotional condition that interferes with an individual's normal functioning. **2.** Reduction in a person's capacity to fulfill a social role as a consequence of an impairment, inadequate training for the role, or other circumstances. SEE ALSO disability. [fr. *hand in cap*, (game)]

hand·piece (hand'pēs). A powered dental instrument held in the hand, used to hold rotary cutting, grinding, or polishing implements while they are being revolved.

HANE Acronym for hereditary angioneurotic *edema*.

hang·nail (hang'nāl). A loose triangular tag of skin attached at the proximal portion in the medial or lateral nail fold.

Hanhart, Ernst, Swiss internist, 1891–1973. SEE H.'s *syndrome*.

Hanks, Horace Tracy, U.S. surgeon, 1837–1900. SEE H. *dilators*, under *dilator*.

Hanks' so·lu·tion. See under solution.

Hanlon, C. Rollins, U.S. cardiovascular and thoracic surgeon, *1915. SEE Blalock-H. *operation*.

Hannover, Adolph, Danish anatomist, 1814–1894. SEE H.'s *canal*.

Hanot, Victor C., French physician, 1844–1896. SEE H.'s *cirrhosis*.

Hansemann mac·ro·phage. See under macrophage.

Hansen, Gerhard A., Norwegian physician, 1841–1912. SEE H.'s *bacillus, disease*.

Han·ta·vi·rus (han'tā-vā-rŭs). A genus of Bunyaviridae responsible for pneumonia and hemorrhagic fevers. Four members of the genus are so far recognized: Hantaan, Puumala, Seoul, and Prospect Hill. The first three of these are known human pathogens; Hantaan virus causes Korean hemorrhagic fever. Various rodent species are the asumptomatic carriers of these viruses, which are shed in saliva, urine, and feces. Human infection is direct, or by the respiratory route from contaminated specimens; person-to-person spread has not been demonstrated. An outbreak of hantavirus infection, the Hantavirus Pulmonary Syndrome (HPS), causing severe and often fatal pulmonary symptoms was identified in the Four-Corners region of the USA in 1993.

hap·a·lo·nych·ia (hap'ă-lō-nik'ē-ă). Thinning of nails resulting in bending and breaking of the free edge, with longitudinal fissures. SYN egg shell nail. [hapalo- + G. *onyx* (onych-), nail]

haph·al·ge·sia (haf-al-jē'zē-ă). Pain or an extremely disagreeable sensation caused by the merest touch. SYN Pitres' sign (1). [G. *haphē*, touch, + *algēsis*, sense of pain]

haph·haz·ard. Lacking any coherent system, organization, or objective; not to be confused with random or chaotic.

haph·e·pho·bia (haf-ē-fō'bē-ă). A morbid dislike or fear of being touched. SYN aphephobia. [G. *haphē*, touch, + *phobos*, fear]

⌂**haplo-.** Simple, single. [G. *haplous*]

hap·lo·dont (hap'lō-dont). Having molar teeth with simple crowns, *i.e.,* simple conical teeth without ridges or tubercles. [haplo- + G. *odous*, tooth]

hap·loid (hap'loyd). Denoting the number of chromosomes in sperm or ova, which is half the number in somatic (diploid) cells; the h. number in normal human beings is 23. SYN monoploid. [G. *hapolls*, simple, + *eidos*, appearance]

hap·lol·o·gy (hap-lol'ō-jē). The omission of syllables because of excessive speed of utterance. [haplo- + G. *logos,* study]

hap·lo·pro·tein (hap-lō-prō'tēn). The functional complex between an apoprotein and the prosthetic group that together are responsible for biological activity.

hap·lo·scope (hap'lō-skōp). An instrument for presenting separate views to each eye so that they may be seen as one. [haplo- + G. *skopeō*, to view]

mirror h., a h. using mirrors to displace the field of view of the two eyes, as in Worth's amblyoscope and the synoptophore.

hap·lo·scop·ic (hap-lō-skop'ik). Relating to a haploscope.

Hap·lo·spo·rid·ia (hap'lō-spō-rid'ē-ă). An order of sporozoans, now placed in the protozoan phylum Ascetospora, class Stellatosporea, that reproduce asexually by schizogony and produce spores but no flagella, though pseudopodia may be present. [haplo- + G. *sporos,* seed]

hap·lo·type (hap'lō-tīp). **1.** The genetic constitution of an individual with respect to one member of a pair of allelic genes; individuals are of the same h. (but of different genotypes) if alike with respect to one allele of a pair but different with respect to the other allele of a pair. **2.** In immunogenetics, that portion of the phenotype determined by a set of closely linked genes inherited from one parent (*i.e.,* genes located on one of the pair of chromosomes). The human major histocompatability complex comprises 4 recognized loci (A, B, C, and D) for which there are more than 50 alleles. Similarly, the allotypic markers (antigens) of the immunoglobulin subclasses IgG1, IgG2, IgG3, and IgA2 occur in combinations and are inherited as units almost always unchanged in transmission; the alleles that control these various h.'s are not linked to those controlling the antigens of the κ type L chains. [haplo- + G. *typos*, impression, model]

hap·ten. A molecule that is incapable, alone, of causing the production of antibodies but can, however, combine with a larger

---

⌂ **Combining forms**	[NA] Nomina Anatomica
Word*Finder*	[MIM] Mendelian
Multi-term entry finder	Inheritance in Man
Preceding letter A	
A.D.A.M. Anatomy Plates	☆ **Official alternate term**
Between letters L and M	
	☆[NA] Official alternate
Appendices:	Nomina Anatomica term
Following letter Z	
	High Profile Term
SYN Synonym; Cf., compare	

ha

antigenic molecule called a carrier. SEE ALSO hapten *inhibition* of precipitation. SYN incomplete antigen, partial antigen. [G. *haptō,* to fasten, bind]

conjugated h., a h. that may cause the production of antibodies when it has been covalently linked to protein. SYN conjugated antigen.

Forssman h., a glycolipid from mammalian organs. Cf. Forssman *antibody,* Forssman *antigen.*

half h., SEE half-hapten.

hap·tics (hap'tiks). The science concerned with the tactile sense. [G. *haptō,* to grasp, touch]

hap·to·dys·pho·ria (hap'tō-dis-fō'rē-ă). An unpleasant sensation derived from touching certain objects. [G. *haptō,* to touch, + dysphoria]

hap·to·glo·bin (HP) (hap-tō-glō'bin) [MIM*140100 & MIM* 140210]. A group of α₂-globulins in human serum, so called because of their ability to combine with hemoglobin; variant types form a polymorphic system, with α- and β-polypeptide chains controlled by separate genetic loci. [G. *haptō,* to grasp, + hemoglobin]

hap·tom·e·ter (hap-tom'ĕ-ter). Instrument for measuring sensitivity to touch. [G. *haptō,* to touch, + *metron,* measure]

Har Abbreviation for homoarginine.

Harada, Einosuke, Japanese surgeon, 1892–1947. SEE H.'s *disease, syndrome.*

Harden, Sir Arthur, English biochemist and Nobel laureate, 1865–1940. SEE H.-Young *ester.*

Harder, Johann J., Swiss anatomist, 1656–1711. SEE H.'s *gland.*

har·di·ness. A health-enhancing behavior trait believed to increase one's resistance to illness, characterized by a high level of personal control, commitment, and action in responding to events of daily life. [M.E., fr. O.Fr. *hardi,* fr. Germanic]

Harding, Harold E., 20th century British pathologist. SEE H.-Passey *melanoma.*

hard·ness (hard'nes). **1.** The degree of firmness of a solid, as determined by its resistance to deformation, scratching, or abrasion. SEE ALSO hardness *scale,* number. **2.** The relative penetrating power of a beam of x-rays, used both within the diagnostic range of energy and in radiation therapy; expressed in terms of half-value layer.

indentation h., a number related to the size of the impression made by an indenter (or tool) of specific size and shape under a known load.

hard·ware. The electronic component of a computer.

Hardy, George H., English mathematician, 1877–1947. SEE H.-Weinberg *equilibrium, law.*

Hardy, LeGrand, U.S. ophthalmologist, 1895–1954. SEE H.-Rand-Ritter *test.*

hare·lip (hār'lip). SYN cleft *lip.*

har·ma·line (har'mă-līn). 4,9-dihydro-7-methoxy-1-methyl-3*H*-pyrido[3,4-*b*]indole; 3,4-dihydroharmine; an amine oxidase inhibitor and a central nervous system stimulant; obtained from the seeds of *Peganum harmala* (family Zygophyllaceae) and from *Banisteria caapi* (family Malpighiaceae); has been used in parkinsonism. SYN harmidine.

har·mi·dine (har'mi-dēn). SYN harmaline.

har·mine (har'mēn). 7-methoxy-1-methyl-9*H*-pyrido[3,4-*b*]-indole; obtained from *Peganum harmala* (family Zygophyllaceae) and *Banisteria caapi* (family Malpighiaceae); a central nervous system stimulant and potent monoamine oxidase inhibitor; psychic effects resemble those of LSD, but sedative and depressive qualities may predominate over hallucinatory manifestations. SYN banisterine, leucoharmine, telepathine. [G. *harmala,* harmal, fr. Ar. *harmalah,* + -ine]

har·mo·nia (har-mō'nē-ă). SYN plane *suture.* [L. and G. a joining]

har·mon·ic (har-mon'ik). A component of complex sound whose frequency is a multiple of the fundamental frequency of the sound. This fundamental frequency is called the first harmonic; the second harmonic has twice the frequency of the fundamental, and so forth.

har·mo·ny (har'mō-nē). Agreement; accord; in dentistry, denotes occlusal h.

functional occlusal h., such occlusal relationship of opposing teeth in all functional ranges and movements as will provide the greatest masticatory efficiency without causing undue strain or trauma upon the supporting tissues, teeth, and muscles.

occlusal h., occlusion without deflective or interceptive occlusal contacts in centric jaw relation as well as eccentric movements.

har·pax·o·pho·bia (har'paks-ō-fō'bē-ă). Morbid fear of robbers. [G. *harpax,* robber, + *phobos,* fear]

har·poon (har-pūn'). A small, sharp-pointed instrument with a barbed head used for extracting bits of tissue for microscopic examination.

Harrington, David O., U.S. ophthalmologist, *1904. SEE H.-Flocks *test.*

Harris, Henry A., English anatomist, 1886–1968. SEE H.'s *lines,* under *line.*

Harris, Henry F., U.S. physician, 1867–1926. SEE H.'s *hematoxylin.*

Harris, R.I., 20th century Canadian orthopedist. SEE Salter-H. *classification* of epiphysial plate injuries.

Harris. Seale, U.S. physician, 1870–1957, investigated food conditions and nutritional diseases. SEE Harris *syndrome.*

Harris, Wilfred, English physician, 1869–1960. SEE H.'s *migraine.*

Harrison, Edward, English physician, 1766–1838. SEE H.'s *groove.*

Harris and Ray test. See under *test.*

Hartel, Fritz, 20th century German surgeon. SEE H. *technique.*

Hartman, LeRoy L., U.S. dentist, 1893–1951. SEE H.'s *solution.*

Hartmann, Alexis F., U.S. pediatrician, 1898–1964. SEE H.'s *solution;* Shaffer-H. *method.*

Hartmann, Arthur, German laryngologist, 1849–1931. SEE H.'s *curette.*

Hartmann, Henri A.C.A., French surgeon, 1860–1952. SEE H.'s *operation, pouch.*

Hart·man·nel·la (hart-mă-nel'ă). A common free-living ameba found in soil, sewage, and water, known to invade invertebrates (snails, grasshoppers, oysters); suspected but not established as an agent of human primary amebic meningoencephalitis.

Hartnup. Surname of British family in which the disease was first described. SEE Hartnup *disease,* syndrome.

harts·horn (harts'hōrn). Crude ammonium carbonate; a mixture of ammonium bicarbonate and ammonium carbamate obtained from ammonium sulfate and calcium carbonate by sublimation; used as an expectorant and in smelling salts; so called because originally obtained from deer antlers.

har·vest bug. The larva of *Trombicula* species.

Harvey, William, 1578–1657. English anatomist, physiologist, and physician who first described the circulation of the blood in 1628. He understood that the interventricular septum is not porous so blood can not pass through it. He demonstrated the volume of blood which passes unidirectionally through a segment of a peripheral vein exceeds the volume of blood within the body, so blood must recirculate. He described the organization of the fetal circulation and the transition to the postnatal organization.

has·a·mi·ya·mi (has'ă-mē-yah'mē). A fever occurring in Japan in the autumn; resembles Weil's disease, but is milder and is caused by the *autumnalis* serovar of *Leptospira interrogans.* SYN akiyami, autumn fever (2), sakushu fever, seven-day fever (2).

Häser, Heinrich, German physician, 1811–1884. SEE H.'s *formula;* Trapp-H. *formula.*

Hashimoto, Japanese surgeon, 1881–1934. SEE H.'s *disease, struma, thyroiditis.*

hash·ish (hash'ish). A form of cannabis that consists largely of resin from the flowering tops and sprouts of cultivated female plants; contains the highest concentration of cannabinols among the preparations derived from cannabis. [Ar. hay]

Hasner, Joseph Ritter von, Czechoslovakian ophthalmologist, 1819–1892. SEE H.'s *fold, valve.*

Hassall, Arthur, British physician, 1817–1894. SEE H.'s *bodies*, under *body*, concentric *corpuscle*, under *corpuscle;* H.-Henle *bodies*, under *body;* Virchow-H. *bodies*, under *body*.

Hasselbalch, Karl, Danish biochemist and physician, 1874–1962. SEE Henderson-H. *equation*.

hatch·et. A dental instrument with an end cutting blade set at an angle to the axis of the handle and having one or two bevels; in the former case, made as right and left pairs called enamel h.'s; used for removing enamel and dentin on teeth.

Haubenfelder (how'ben-fel'der). SEE *fields* of Forel, under *field*. [Ger.]

Hauch (H) (howkh). A term used to designate the flagellar antigen of bacteria. SEE ALSO H *antigen*. [Ger. breath]

Haudek, Martin, Austrian roentgenologist, 1880–1931. SEE H.'s *niche*.

Hauser, G.A., 20th century German gynecologist. SEE Mayer-Rokitansky-Küster-H. *syndrome;* Rokitansky-Küster-H. *syndrome*.

haus·to·ri·um, pl. **haus·to·ria** (haw-stō'rē-ŭm, -stō'rē-ă). An organ for the absorption of nutriment. [Mod. L. fr. L. *haustus,* a drinking]

haus·tra (haw'stră). Plural of haustrum. [L.]

haus·tral (haw'străl). Relating to a haustrum.

haus·tra·tion (haw-stră'shŭn). **1.** The process of formation of a haustrum. **2.** An increase in prominence of the haustra.

h.'s of colon, SYN *haustra* of colon, under *haustrum*.

haus·trum, pl. **haus·tra** (haw'strŭm, haw'stră). One of a series of saccules or pouches, so called because of a fancied resemblance to the buckets on a water wheel. [L. a machine for drawing water, fr. *haurio,* pp. *haustus,* to draw up, drink up]

haus'tra co'li [NA], SYN haustra of colon. SYN cellulae coli.

haustra of colon, the sacculations of the colon, caused by the teniae, or longitudinal bands, which are slightly shorter than the gut so that the latter is thrown into tucks or pouches. SYN haustra coli [NA], haustrations of colon, sacculation of colon.

haus·tus (haws'tŭs). A potion or medicinal draft. [L. a drink, draft]

HAV Abbreviation for hepatitis A *virus*.

Ha·ver·hil·lia mul·ti·for·mis (ha-ver-hil'ē-ă mŭl-ti-fōr'mis). SEE *Streptobacillus moniliformis*.

Havers, Clopton, British anatomist, 1650–1702. SEE haversian *canals*, under *canal;* H.'s *glands*, under *gland;* haversian *lamella;* haversian *spaces*, under *space;* haversian *system*.

ha·ver·si·an (ha-ver'shan). Relating to Clopton Havers and the various osseous structures described by him.

Hawley, C.A., U.S. orthodontist. SEE H. *appliance*, *retainer*.

Haworth, Sir Walter Norman, British chemist and Nobel laureate, 1883–1950. SEE H. conformational formulas of cyclic *sugars*, perspective formulas of cyclic *sugars*.

Hayem, Georges, French physician, 1841–1933. SEE H.'s *hematoblast, solution;* H.-Widal *syndrome*.

Hayflick, Leonard, U.S. microbiologist, *1928. SEE H.'s *limit*.

Haygarth, John, English physician, 1740–1827. SEE H.'s *nodes*, under *node*, *nodosities*, under *nodosity*.

ha·zel·wort (hā'zel-wōrt). SYN *Asarum* europaeum.

Hb Abbreviation for hemoglobin.

Hb_Chesapeake_· Abbreviation for *hemoglobin* Chesapeake.

HB_cAb Abbreviation for antibody to the hepatitis B core *antigen*.

HB_eAb Abbreviation for antibody to the hepatitis B e *antigen*.

HB_sAb Abbreviation for antibody to the hepatitis B surface *antigen*.

HB_cAg Abbreviation for hepatitis B core *antigen*.

HB_sAg Abbreviation for hepatitis B surface *antigen*.

HbCO Abbreviation for carboxyhemoglobin.

HBE Abbreviation for His bundle *electrogram*.

HBe, HB_eAg Abbreviation for hepatitis B e *antigen*.

HbO_2 Abbreviation for oxyhemoglobin.

Hb S Abbreviation for sickle cell *hemoglobin*.

HBV Abbreviation for hepatitis B *virus*.

HCC Abbreviation for 25-hydroxycholecalciferol.

HCFA Abbreviation for Health Care Financing Administration.

HCG, hCG Abbreviation for human chorionic *gonadotropin*.

H chain. SYN heavy *chain*.

HCS Abbreviation for human chorionic somatomammotropic *hormone*; human chorionic *somatomammotropin*.

Hct Abbreviation for hematocrit.

HCV Abbreviation for hepatitis C *virus*.

Hcy Abbreviation for homocysteine.

HD Abbreviation for mustard *gas*.

h.d. Abbreviation for L. *hora decubitus*, at bedtime.

HDCV Abbreviation for human diploid cell *vaccine*; human diploid cell rabies *vaccine*.

HDL Abbreviation for high density lipoprotein. SEE lipoprotein.

HDV Abbreviation for hepatitis delta *virus*.

He Symbol for helium.

³He, ⁴He. Symbols for helium-3 and helium-4, respectively.

Head, Sir Henry, English neurologist, 1861–1940. SEE H.'s *areas*, under *area, lines,* under *line, zones,* under *zone*.

head (hed). SYN caput. [A.S. *heāfod*]

big h., an acute disease of young rams caused by the *Clostridium novyi, C. sordellii* or, rarely, *C. chauvoei* and characterized by a nongaseous, nonhemorrhagic, edematous swelling of the head and neck.

bulldog h., the broad h. with high vault occurring in achondroplasia.

h. of the caudate nucleus, the head or anterior extremity of the caudate nucleus projecting into the anterior horn of the lateral ventricle. SYN caput nuclei caudati [NA], anterior extremity of caudate nucleus.

clavicular h. of pectoralis major muscle, SYN clavicular *part* of pectoralis major muscle. SEE pectoralis major *muscle*.

deep h. of flexor pollicis brevis, the head of short flexor of the thumb that arises from the trapezoid and capitate bones and transverse carpal ligaments. It is innervated by the deep ulner nerve, and considered by many to be the first palmar interosseous muscle. SYN caput profundum musculi flexoris pollicis brevis [NA].

h. of epididymis, the upper and larger extremity of the epididymis. SYN caput epididymidis [NA], caput epididymis, globus major.

h. of femur, the hemispheric articular surface at the upper extremity of the thigh bone. SYN caput ossis femoris [NA], caput femoris, h. of thigh bone.

h. of fibula, the superior extremity of the fibula, which articulates by a facet with the undersurface of the lateral condyle of the tibia. SYN caput fibulae [NA], upper extremity of fibula.

hourglass h., in congenital syphilis, a skull with depressed coronal suture.

humeral h., the name applied to the heads of forearm muscles that attach to the humerus. Nomina Anatomica lists humeral heads (caput humerale ...) of the following: 1) flexor carpli ulnaris muscle (... musculi flexoris carpi ulnaris [NA]); 2) pronator teres muscle (... musculi pronatoris teretis [NA]). SYN caput humerale [NA].

humeroulnar h. of flexor digitorum superficialis muscle, the head of the superficial flexor of the digits that attaches to both the humerus and the ulna. SYN caput humeroulnare musculi flexoris digitorum superficialis [NA].

h. of humerus, the upper rounded extremity fitting into the glenoid cavity of the scapula. SYN caput humeri [NA].

lateral h., h. of origin farthest from the midline. Nomina Anatomica lists lateral h.'s (caput laterale ...) of the following: 1) triceps brachii muscle (... musculi tricipitis brachii [NA]); 2) gastrocnemius muscle (... musculi gastrocnemii [NA]). SYN caput laterale [NA].

little h. of humerus, SYN *capitulum* of humerus.

long h., the head that has the more proximal origin. Nomina Anatomica lists long h.'s (caput longum ...) of the following: 1) biceps brachii muscle (... musculi bicipitis brachii [NA]); 2) biceps femoris muscle (... musculi bicipitis femoris [NA]); 3) triceps brachii muscle (... musculi tricipitis brachii [NA]). SYN caput longum [NA].

h. of malleus, the rounded portion of the malleus articulating with the body of the incus. SYN caput mallei [NA].

h. of mandible, the expanded articular portion of the condylar process of the mandible. SYN caput mandibulae [NA].

medial h., the h. of origin closest to the midline. Nomina Anatomica lists medial h. of the following: 1) triceps brachii muscle (... musculi tricipitis brachii [NA]); 2) gastrocnemius muscle (... musculi gastrocnemii [NA]). SYN caput mediale [NA].

Medusa h., SYN *caput* medusae.

h. of metacarpal bone, the expanded distal end of a metacarpal that articulates with the proximal phalanx of the same digit. SYN caput ossis metacarpalis [NA].

h. of metatarsal bone, the expanded distal end of a metatarsal bone that articulates with the proximal phalanx of the same digit. SYN caput ossis metatarsalis [NA].

oblique h., h. of origin which is diagonally situated. Nomina Anatomica lists oblique h.'s (caput obliquum ...) of the following: 1) adductor hallucis muscle (... musculi adductoris hallucis [NA]); 2) adductor pollicis muscle (... musculi adductoris pollicis [NA]). SYN caput obliquum [NA].

optic nerve h., SYN optic *disk.*

h. of pancreas, that portion of the pancreas lying in the concavity of the duodenum. SYN caput pancreatis [NA].

h. of phalanx, the rounded articular surface at the distal end of the proximal and middle phalanx of each finger and toe. SYN caput phalangis [NA], trochlea phalangis* [NA].

radial h., the name applied to a head of origin of a muscle arising from the radius. Nomina Anatomica no longer lists any muscles as having radial heads, although formerly a radial head was listed for the flexor digitorum superficialis muscle SYN caput radiale [NA].

h. of radius, the disk-shaped upper extremity articulating with the capitulum of the humerus. SYN caput radii [NA].

h. of rib, the rounded medial extremity of a rib which, except for ribs 1, 10, 11, and 12, articulates by two facets with the bodies of two contiguous vertebrae. SYN caput costae [NA].

saddle h., SYN clinocephaly.

short h., for a muscle with two heads of origin (a "biceps" muscle), the head originating nearest the insertion. SEE short h. of biceps brachii muscle, short h. of biceps femoris muscle. SYN caput breve [NA].

short h. of biceps brachii muscle, h. of biceps brachii originating from coracoid process of scapula. SYN caput breve musculi bicipitis brachii [NA].

short h. of biceps femoris muscle, part of biceps femoris originating from linea aspera of distal half of femur. SYN caput breve musculi bicipitis femoris.

h. of stapes, the portion of the stapes that articulates with the lenticular process of the incus. SYN caput stapedis [NA].

sternocostal h. of pectoralis major muscle, SYN sternocostal *part* of pectoralis major muscle. SEE pectoralis major *muscle.*

superficial h. of flexor pollicis brevis muscle, the head of the short flexor of the thumb that arises from the transverse carpal ligament and the trapezium. It is innervated by the recurrent branch of the median nerve. SYN caput superficiale musculi flexoris pollicis brevis [NA].

h. of talus, the rounded anterior portion of the talus articulating with the navicular bone. SYN caput tali [NA].

h. of thigh bone, SYN h. of femur.

transverse h., h. of origin of a muscle which is transversely situated. Nomina Anatomica lists transverse h.'s (caput transversum ...) of the following: 1) adductor hallucis muscle (... musculi adductoris hallucis [NA]); 2) adductor pollicis muscle (... musculi adductoris pollicis [NA]). SYN caput transversum [NA].

h. of ulna, the small rounded distal extremity of the ulna articulating with the ulnar notch of the radius and the articular disk. SYN caput ulnae [NA].

ulnar h., the name applied to a h. of origin of a forearm muscle arising from the ulna. Nomina Antomica lists ulnar h.'s (caput ulnare ...) of the following: 1) flexor carpi ulnaris muscle (...

musculi flexoris carpi ulnaris [NA]); 2) pronator teres muscle (... musculi pronatoris teritis [NA]). SYN caput ulnare [NA].

head·ache (hed´āk). Pain in various parts of the head, not confined to the area of distribution of any nerve. SEE ALSO cephalodynia. SYN cephalalgia, cephalea, cerebralgia, encephalalgia, encephalodynia.

bilious h., SYN migraine.

blind h., SYN migraine.

cluster h., possibly due to a hypersensitivity to histamine; characterized by recurrent, severe, unilateral orbitotemporal h.'s associated with ipsilateral photophobia, lacrimation, and nasal congestion. SYN histaminic cephalalgia, histaminic h., Horton's cephalalgia, Horton's h.

fibrositic h., h. centered in the occipital region due to fibrositis of the occipital muscles; tender areas are present and, commonly, tender nodules are found in the scalp in the lower occipital region.

histaminic h., SYN cluster h.

Horton's h., SYN cluster h.

migraine h., SEE migraine.

nodular h., radiating pain in the head accompanied by nodular swellings in the splenius, frontalis, trapezius, and other muscles.

organic h., h. due to intracranial disease.

reflex h., SYN symptomatic h.

sick h., SYN migraine.

spinal h., h., usually frontal or occipital, following dural puncture; precipitated by sitting up, relieved by lying down; due to leakage of cerebrospinal fluid from subarachnoid space through the site of the puncture.

symptomatic h., a h. secondary to another organic condition. SYN reflex h.

tension h., h. associated with nervous tension, anxiety, etc., often related to chronic contraction of the scalp muscles. SEE ALSO posttraumatic neck *syndrome.*

vacuum h., h. due to closure of the frontal sinus.

vascular h., SYN migraine.

head·gear (hed´gēr). A removable extraoral appliance used as a source of traction to apply force to the teeth and jaws.

head·gut (hed´gŭt). SYN foregut.

head-nod·ding (hed´nod-ing). Head movements associated with congenital nystagmus, spasmus nutans, and miner's nystagmus. SYN head tremors.

head-tilt (hed´tilt). An abnormal position of the head adopted to prevent double vision resulting from underaction of the vertical ocular muscles.

heal (hēl). **1.** To restore to health, especially to cause an ulcer or wound to cicatrize or unite. **2.** To become well, to be cured; to cicatrize or close, said of an ulcer or wound. [A.S. *healan*]

heal·er (hē´ler). **1.** A physician; one who heals or cures. **2.** One who claims to cure by prayer, mysticism, new thought, or other form of suggestion.

heal·ing (hēl´ing). **1.** Restoring to health; promoting the closure of wounds and ulcers. **2.** The process of a return to health. **3.** Closing of a wound. SEE ALSO union.

faith h., a treatment utilized since antiquity based upon prayer and a profound belief in divine intervention in human affairs.

h. by first intention, h. by fibrous adhesion, without suppuration or granulation tissue formation. SYN primary adhesion, primary union.

h. by second intention, delayed closure of two granulating surfaces. SYN secondary adhesion, secondary union.

h. by third intention, the slow filling of a wound cavity or ulcer by granulations, with subsequent cicatrization.

---

health (helth). **1.** The state of the organism when it functions optimally without evidence of disease or abnormality. **2.** A state of dynamic balance in which an individual's or a group's capacity to cope with all the circumstances of living is at an optimum level. **3.** A state characterized by anatomical, physiological, and psychological integrity, ability to perform personally valued family, work, and community roles; ability to deal with physical, biological, psychological and social stress; a feeling of well-being; and freedom from the risk of disease and untimely death. [A.S. *haelth*]

From the Old English *hal,* meaning whole, the term has been variously defined among health specialists. In 1948, the World Health Organization described health as "a state of complete physical, mental, and social well-being and not merely the absence of disease." This definition was, in turn, criticized as unquantifiable. In 1984, WHO advanced a revised statement that any measure of health must take into account "the extent to which an individual or a group is able to realize aspirations and satisfy needs, and to change or cope with the environment." Health in this sense is seen as a "resource for everyday life." Health also involves an ability to perform within society, and to accommodate stresses, whether physical or mental. From an ecological viewpoint, the relative health of a group is evaluated according to whether that group might sustain its existence over time without major disruption to its own way of life or to the environment within which it functions.

behavioral h., an interdisciplinary field dedicated to promoting a philosophy of h. that stresses individual responsibility in the application of behavioral and biomedical science knowledge and techniques to the maintenance of h. and prevention of illness and dysfunction by a variety of self-initiated individual and shared activities.

h. education, process by which individuals and groups learn to behave in a manner conducive to promotion, maintenance, or restoration of health.

mental h., emotional, behavioral, and social maturity or normality; the absence of a mental or behavioral disorder; a state of psychological well-being in which the individual has achieved a satisfactory integration of his or her instinctual drives acceptable to both himself and his social milieu; an appropriate balance of love, work, and leisure pursuits.

public h., the art and science of community health, concerned with statistics, epidemiology, hygiene, and the prevention and eradication of epidemic diseases; an effort organized by society to promote, protect, and restore the people's health; public h. is a social institution, a service, and a practice.

Health Care Fi·nanc·ing Ad·min·is·tra·tion (HCFA). The federal agency that determines reimbursement for federal programs.

health cen·ter. An institution or group of institutions providing all types of medical care and preventive services to a population.

health main·te·nance or·ga·ni·za·tion (HMO). A comprehensive prepaid system of health care with emphasis on the prevention and early detection of disease, and continuity of care.

health risk h. r. a.. method of describing an individual's chance of falling ill or dying of a specified condition, based on actuarial calculations that allow for known exposure to risk; expressed as expected age at which death or disease will occur, and intended as a way of drawing an individual's attention to the probable consequences of risk behavior.

healthy (helth′ē). Well; in a state of normal functioning; free from disease.

Heaney, Noble Sproat, U.S. gynecological surgeon and obstetrician, 1880–1955. SEE H.'s *operation.*

hear (hēr). To perceive sounds; denoting the function of the ear. [A.S. *hēran*]

hear·ing (hēr′ing). The ability to perceive sound; the sensation of sound as opposed to vibration. SYN audition.

color h., a subjective perception of color produced by certain sounds. SYN chromatic audition, pseudochromesthesia (2).

normal h., SYN acusis.

hear·ing aid (hēr′ing ād). An electronic amplifying device designed to bring sound more effectively into the ear; it consists of a microphone, amplifier, and receiver.

hear·ing im·pair·ment, hear·ing loss. A reduction in the ability to perceive sound; may range from slight to complete deafness. SEE ALSO deafness, threshold *shift.*

heart (hart). A hollow muscular organ which receives the blood from the veins and propels it into the arteries. It is divided by a musculomembranous septum into two halves—right or venous and left or arterial—each of which consists of a receiving chamber (atrium) and an ejecting chamber (ventricle). SYN cor [NA], coeur. [A.S. *heorte*]

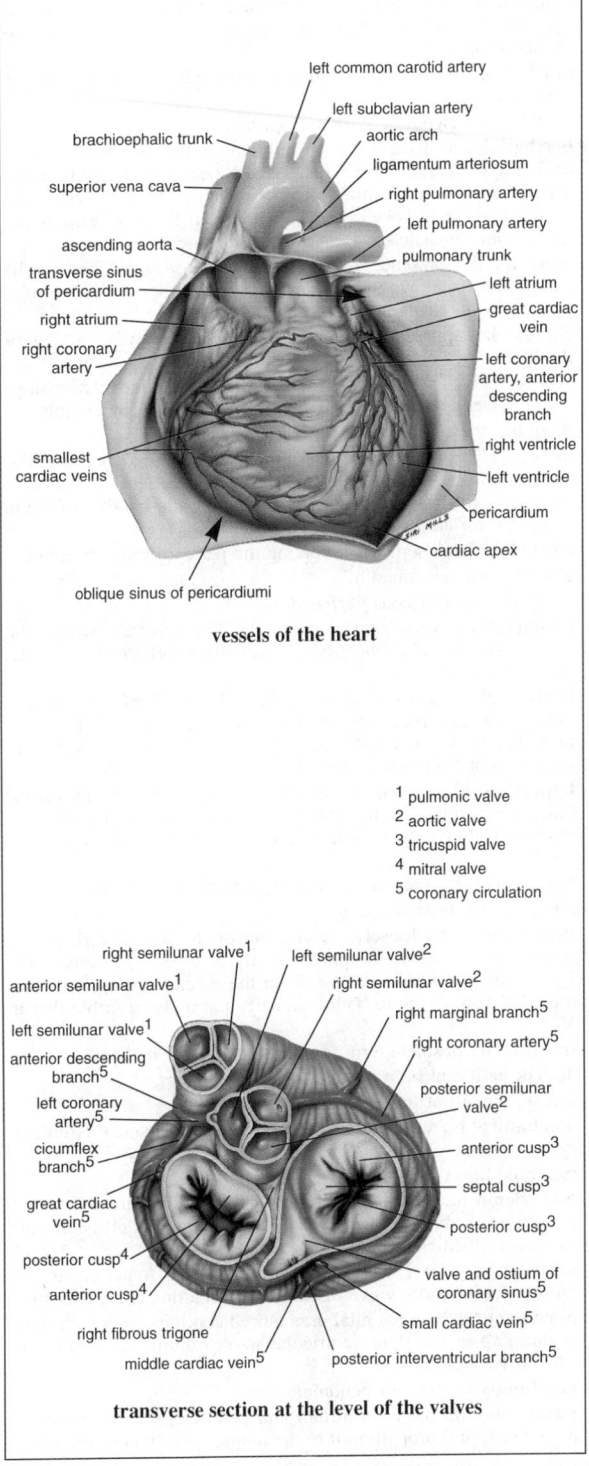

left common carotid artery
left subclavian artery
aortic arch
ligamentum arteriosum
brachioephalic trunk
right pulmonary artery
superior vena cava
left pulmonary artery
pulmonary trunk
ascending aorta
transverse sinus of pericardium
left atrium
right atrium
great cardiac vein
right coronary artery
left coronary artery, anterior descending branch
right ventricle
smallest cardiac veins
left ventricle
pericardium
cardiac apex
oblique sinus of pericardiumi

vessels of the heart

1 pulmonic valve
2 aortic valve
3 tricuspid valve
4 mitral valve
5 coronary circulation

right semilunar valve[1]
left semilunar valve[2]
anterior semilunar valve[1]
right semilunar valve[2]
right marginal branch[5]
left semilunar valve[1]
right coronary artery[5]
anterior descending branch[5]
posterior semilunar valve[2]
left coronary artery[5]
anterior cusp[3]
cicumflex branch[5]
septal cusp[3]
great cardiac vein[5]
posterior cusp[3]
posterior cusp[4]
valve and ostium of coronary sinus[5]
anterior cusp[4]
small cardiac vein[5]
right fibrous trigone
middle cardiac vein[5]
posterior interventricular branch[5]

transverse section at the level of the valves

armor h., extensive to complete calcification (rarely ossification) of the pericardium usually producing constrictive pericarditis.

armored h., calcareous deposits in the pericardium due to subacute or chronic pericarditis. SYN panzerherz.

artificial h., a mechanical pump used to replace the function of a damaged heart, either temporarily or as a permanent prosthesis.

athlete's h., a more or less loose designation for cardiac findings in healthy athletes that would be or could be abnormal in patients with disease, including atrioventricular blocks, left ventricular hypertrophy and, sometimes, benign arrhythmias and atrioventricular blocks.

athletic h., hypertrophy of the h. supposedly due to systematic athletic conditioning.

beer h., SYN alcoholic *cardiomyopathy.*

beriberi h., h. disease due to thiamine deficiency that may be epidemic or sporadic as characterized by cardiac metabolic damage and myocardial failure, often of the "high output" type, with edema (except in "dry" beri) and polyneuritis. The term is derived from Singhalese, "I am unable."

bony h., the presence of extensive calcareous patches in the pericardium and walls of the h., some of which chronically develop bony changes.

chaotic h., apparently totally uncoordinated cardiac action or rhythm.

crisscross h., an anomaly in which the ventricular relationships are not as expected for the given atrioventricular connection.

drop h., SYN cardioptosia.

fatty h., (**1**) fatty degeneration of the myocardium; (**2**) accumulation of adipose tissue on the external surface of the h. with occasional infiltration of fat between the muscle bundles of the h. wall. SYN cor adiposum.

frosted h., hyaloserositis involving the pericardium. SYN icing h.

globular h., SYN round h.

hairy h., SYN fibrinous *pericarditis.*

Holmes h., a variant of double inlet left ventricle where the ventricular-arterial connection is concordant and the right ventricle is rudimentary.

horizontal h., description of the h.'s electrical position; recognized in the electrocardiogram when the QRS in lead aVL resembles that in V_6 and QRS in aVF resembles that in V_1; also, loosely, when the electrical axis lies between $-30°$ and $+30°$.

hyperthyroid h., response of the h. to hyperthyroidism, essentially the result of sympathetic stimulation producing rapid h. rates and ultimately cardiac failure and atrial fibrillation if untreated.

hypoplastic h., a small h., as seen in Addison's disease.

icing h., SYN frosted h.

intermediate h., loosely, description of the h.'s electrical axis when this is directed at approximately between $+30°$ and $+60°$. For cardiac position, recognized in the electrocardiogram when the QRS complexes in both lead aVL and aVF resemble that in V_6.

irritable h., obsolete term for neurocirculatory *asthenia.*

Jarvik artificial h., a pneumatic artificial heart.

left h., the left atrium and left ventricle.

mechanical h., term loosely applied to any mechanical circulatory assist device.

movable h., SYN *cor* mobile.

myxedema h., the enlarged h. associated with untreated severe hypothyroidism, often accompanied by pericardial effusion; rare in modern medicine.

ox h., a very large h. usually due to chronic hypertension or, more often to aortic valve disease. SYN bucardia, cor bovinum.

parchment h., a congenital or acquired condition in which there is thinning of the right ventricular myocardium. SYN right ventricular hypoplasia.

pendulous h., SYN *cor* pendulum.

pulmonary h., the right atrium and ventricle, receiving the venous blood and propelling it to the lungs. SEE ALSO *cor* pulmonale.

right h., the right atrium and right ventricle.

round h., abnormally smooth arcuate contours of the heart due

either to disease of the ventricles or to a false cardiac appearance produced by excessive pericardial fluid. SYN globular h.

sabot h., SYN *coeur* en sabot.

semihorizontal h., loosely refers to the h.'s electrical axis when this is directed at approximately $0°$. As cardiac position, recognized in the electrocardiogram when the QRS complex in lead aVL resembles V_6 while that in aVF is small algebraically or absolutely.

semivertical h., loosely descriptive of the h.'s electrical axis when this is directed at approximately $+60°$. As cardiac position, recognized in the electrocardiogram when the QRS complex in lead aVF resembles V_6 while that in aVL is small algebraically or absolutely.

soldier's h., obsolete term for neurocirculatory *asthenia.*

stone h., SYN ischemic *contracture* of the left ventricle.

systemic h., the left atrium and ventricle, receiving the aerated blood from the lungs and propelling it throughout the body.

three-chambered h., congenital abnormality in which there may be a single atrium with two ventricles or a single ventricle with two atria. Rudimentary parts of the atrial and ventricular septa may be present but are incompetent to prevent a virtual single chamber in either case.

tiger h., a fatty degenerated h. in which the fat is disposed in the form of broken stripes in the subendocardial myocardium.

tobacco h., cardiac irritability marked by irregular action, palpitation, and sometimes pain, believed to occur as a result of the excessive use of tobacco.

univentricular h., an anomaly in which all blood flows through one ventricle or in which the arterioventricular valves are committed to empty into only one chamber in the ventricular mass.

venous h., the right side, including both the atrium and ventricle, of the h.

vertical h., loosely descriptive of the h.'s electrical axis when this is directed at approximately $+90°$. As a cardiac position, recognized in the electrocardiogram when the QRS complex in lead aVL resembles V_1 while that in aVF resembles V_6.

wooden-shoe h., SYN *coeur* en sabot.

heart·beat (hart'bēt). A single complete cycle of contraction and dilation of heart muscle.

heart·burn (hart'bern). SYN pyrosis.

heart·wa·ter (hart'wah-ter). An acute febrile disease of cattle, sheep, and goats in sub-Saharan Africa and certain areas in the Indian and Atlantic Oceans and in the Caribbean, caused by the rickettsial organism *Cowdria ruminantium* and transmitted by ticks of the genus *Amblyomma;* some species of African antelope and European and American deer also are susceptible. SYN cowdriosis, veldt disease.

heart·worm. SYN *Dirofilaria immitis.*

heat (hēt). **1.** A high temperature; the sensation produced by proximity to fire or an incandescent object, as opposed to cold. The basis of h. is the kinetic energy of atoms and molecules, which becomes zero at absolute zero. **2.** SYN estrus. **3.** SYN enthalpy. [A.S. *haete*]

atomic h., the amount of h. required to raise an atom from $0°$ to $1°C$; approximately the same for all elements (about 6 Cal/gram-atom).

h. of combustion, the quantity of h. liberated per gram-molecular weight when a substance undergoes complete oxidation.

h. of compression, h. produced when a gas is compressed.

conductive h., h. transmitted by direct contact, as by an electric pad or hot water bottle.

convective h., h. conveyed by a warm medium, such as air or water, in motion from its source.

conversive h., h. produced in a body by the absorption of waves that are not in themselves hot, such as the sun's rays or infrared radiation.

h. of crystallization, the quantity of h. liberated or absorbed per mol when a substance passes into the crystalline state.

h. of dissociation, the h. (expressed in calories or joules) expended in the dissociation of 1 mol of a substance into specified products.

h. of evaporation, the h. absorbed in the evaporation of water, sweat or other liquid; for water it amounts to 540 cal/g at 100°C. SYN h. of vaporization.

h. of formation, the h. (expressed in calories or joules) absorbed or liberated during the (hypothetical) reaction in which a mole of a compound is formed from the necessary elements, in elemental form.

initial h., the first burst of h. produced after the beginning of a muscle twitch, described by A. V. Hill.

innate h., in ancient Greek medicine, the h. of the heart sustained by the pneuma and distributed by the arteries throughout the body.

latent h., the amount of h. that a substance may absorb without an increase in temperature, as in conversion from solid to liquid state (ice to water at 0°C), or from liquid to gaseous state (water to steam at 100°C). Cf. sensible h.

molecular h., the product of the specific h. of a body multiplied by its molecular weight.

prickly h., SYN *miliaria* rubra.

radiant h., h. given off from any body in the form of waves, similar to light waves but of greater wavelength.

sensible h., the amount of h. that, when absorbed by a substance, causes a rise in temperature. Cf. latent h.

h. of solution, the quantity of h. absorbed or evolved when a solid is dissolved in a liquid.

specific h., the amount of h. required to raise any substance through 1°C of temperature, compared with that raising the same volume of water 1°C.

h. of vaporization, SYN h. of evaporation.

heat·la·bile (hēt′lā′bĭl). Destroyed or altered by heat.

heat·sta·ble (hēt′stā′bl). SYN thermostable.

heat·stroke (hēt′strōk). A severe and often fatal illness produced by exposure to excessively high temperatures, especially when accompanied by marked exertion; characterized by headache, vertigo, confusion, hot dry skin, and a slight rise in body temperature; in severe cases very high fever, vascular collapse, and coma develop. SYN heat apoplexy (1), heat hyperpyrexia, malignant hyperpyrexia, thermic fever.

heaves (hēvz). A chronic pulmonary emphysema of horses; symptoms include a wheezy cough and dyspnea, especially when exercised.

Heb·e·lo·ma (heb-ĕ-lō′mă). A genus of mushrooms that is a source of gastrointestinal toxins.

he·be·phre·nia (hē-bĕ-frē′nē-ă, heb′ē-). A syndrome characterized by shallow and inappropriate affect, giggling, and silly, regressive behavior and mannerisms; a subtype of schizophrenia now renamed disorganized *schizophrenia*. [G. *hēbē,* puberty, + *phrēn,* the mind]

he·be·phren·ic (hē-bĕ-frĕn′ik, heb-ē-). Relating to or characterized by hebephrenia.

Heberden, William, English physician, 1710–1801. SEE H.'s *angina, nodes,* under *node, nodosities,* under *nodosity;* Rougnon-H. *disease.*

he·bet·ic (hē-bet′ik). Pertaining to youth. [G. *hēbētikos,* youthful, fr. *hēbē,* youth]

heb·e·tude (heb′ĕ-tūd). SYN moria (1). [L. *hebetudo,* fr. *hebeo,* to be dull]

he·bi·at·rics (hē-bē-at′riks). SYN adolescent *medicine.* [G. *hēbē,* youth, + *iatrikos,* relating to medicine]

Hebra, Ferdinand von, Austrian dermatologist, 1816–1880. SEE H.'s *disease, prurigo.*

hec·a·ter·o·mer·ic (hek′ă-ter-ō-mer′ik). Denoting a spinal neuron whose axon divides and gives off processes to both sides of the cord; usually the same as a heteromeric neuron. SYN hecatomeral, hecatomeric. [G. *hekateros,* each of two, + *meros,* part]

hec·a·tom·er·al, hec·a·to·mer·ic (hek′ă-tom′er-ăl, hek′ă-tō-mer′ik). SYN hecateromeric.

Hecht, Victor, early 20th century Austrian pathologist. SEE H.'s *pneumonia.*

Heck, John W., U.S. dentist, *1923. SEE H.'s *disease.*

hec·tic (hek′tik). Denoting a daily afternoon rise of temperature, accompanied by a flush on the cheeks, occurring in active tuber-

culosis and other infections; use of the term is based on the appearance of the temperature chart. [G. *hektikos,* habitual, hectic, consumptive, fr. *hexis,* habit]

hecto- (h). Prefix used in the SI and metric systems to signify one hundred (10^2). [G. *hekaton,* one hundred]

hec·to·gram (hek′tō-gram). One hundred grams, the equivalent of 1543.7 grains.

hec·to·li·ter (hek′tō-lē-ter). One hundred liters, the equivalent of 105.7 quarts or 26.4 American (22 imperial) gallons.

hed·e·o·ma (he-dē-ō′mă). SEE pennyroyal.

hed·er·i·form (hed′er-i-fōrm). Ivy-shaped; a term used for certain sensory endings in the skin. [L. *hedera,* ivy, + *forma,* shape]

he·do·no·pho·bia (hē′dŏ-nō-fō′bē-ă). Morbid fear of pleasure. [G. *hēdonē,* delight, + *phobos,* fear]

hed·ro·cele (hed′rō-sēl). Prolapse of the intestine through the anus. [G. *hedra,* a seat, the fundament, + *kēlē,* hernia]

Hedström, Gustav, Swedish endodontist. SEE H. *file.*

heel (hēl). **1.** SYN calx (2). **2.** SYN distal *end.* [A.S. *hēla*]

black h., SYN calcaneal *petechiae.*

contracted h., SYN contracted *foot* (2).

cracked h., SYN *keratoderma* plantare sulcatum.

grease h., (1) initially, lesions of horsepox occurring in the skin of the flexor surface of the fetlock of the horse; **(2)** now frequently applied to any weeping, eczematous condition of that area. SYN scratches.

painful h., a condition in which bearing weight on the h. causes pain of varying severity. SYN calcaneodynia, calcodynia.

prominent h., a condition marked by a tender swelling on the os calcis due to a thickening of the periosteum or fibrous tissue covering the back of the os calcis.

Heerfordt, Christian Frederick, Danish ophthalmologist, *1871. SEE H.'s *disease.*

Hegar, Alfred, German gynecologist, 1830–1914. SEE H.'s *dilators,* under *dilator, sign.*

Hegglin, Robert M.P., Swiss physician, 20th century. SEE H.'s *anomaly, syndrome;* May-H. *anomaly.*

Hehner, Otto, British chemist, 1853–1924. SEE H. *number.*

Heidenhain, Rudolph P., German histologist and physiologist, 1834–1897. SEE H.'s *crescents,* under *crescent, demilunes,* under *demilune, law,* azan *stain,* iron hematoxylin *stain;* H. *pouch;* Biondi-H. *stain.*

height (h) (hīt). Vertical measurement.

anterior facial h. (AFH), in cephalometrics, the linear measurement from the nasion to the menton.

h. of contour, the line encircling a tooth or other structure at its greatest bulge or diameter with respect to a selected path of insertion.

cusp h., (1) the shortest distance between the tip of a cusp and its base plane; **(2)** the shortest distance between the deepest part of the central fossa of a posterior tooth and a line connecting the points of the cusps of the tooth.

facial h., the linear dimension in the midline from the hairline to the menton.

nasal h., the distance between the nasion and the lower border of the nasal aperture.

orbital h., the distance between the midpoints of the upper and lower margins of the orbit.

Heilbronner, Karl, Dutch physician, 1869–1914. SEE H.'s *thigh.*

Heim, Ernst L., German physician, 1747–1834. SEE H.-Kreysig *sign.*

Heimlich, Harry J., U.S. thoracic surgeon, *1920. SEE H. *maneuver.*

Heine, Leopold, German ophthalmologist, 1870–1940.

Heineke, Walter, German surgeon, 1834–1901. SEE H.-Mikulicz *pyloroplasty.*

Heinz, Robert, German pathologist, 1865–1924. SEE H. *bodies,* under *body,* body *test;* H.-Ehrlich *body;* H. body *anemia.*

Heister, Lorenz, German anatomist, 1683–1758. SEE H.'s *diverticulum, valve.*

HeLa (hē′la). Referring to cells of the first continuously cultured

He

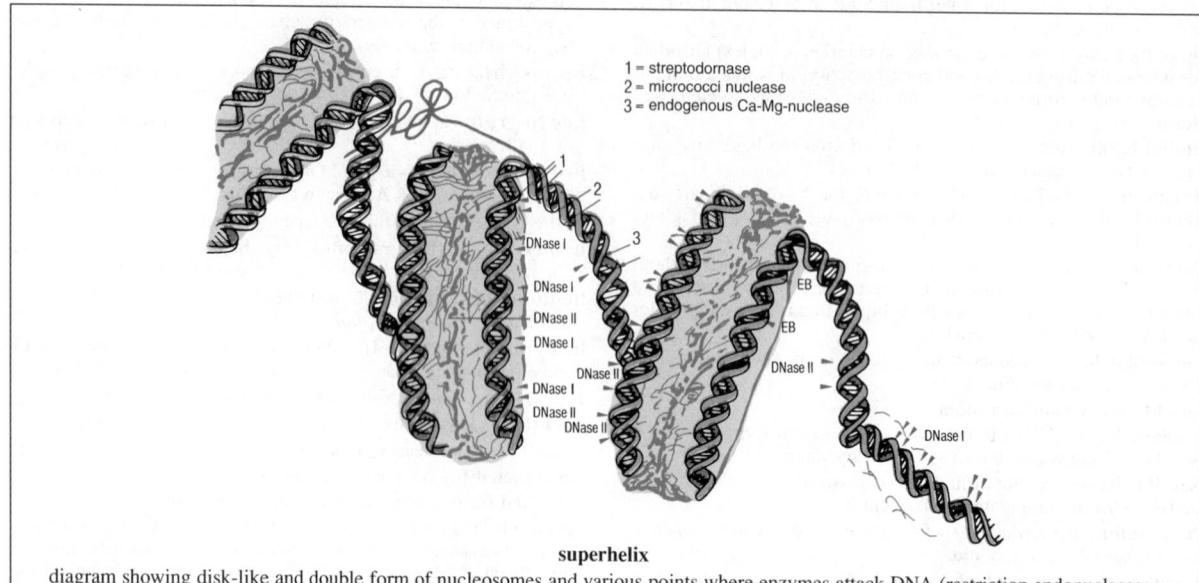

1 = streptodornase
2 = micrococci nuclease
3 = endogenous Ca-Mg-nuclease

superhelix
diagram showing disk-like and double form of nucleosomes and various points where enzymes attack DNA (restriction endonucleases, which cleave specific nucleotide sequences, are not indicated by arrows)

(human cervical) carcinoma strain. [*Henrietta Lacks* (d. 1951), whose cervical carcinoma was the source of the cell line]

Helbings' sign. See under sign.

hel·co·me·nia (hel-kō-mē'nē-ă). Occurrence of ulcers at the time of a menstruation. [G. *helkos*, ulcer, + *emmēnos*, monthly]

hel·co·plas·ty (hel'kō-plas-tē). Obsolete term for plastic surgery of ulcers. [G. *helkos*, ulcer, + *plastos*, formed]

Held, Hans, German anatomist, 1866–1942. SEE H.'s *bundle, decussation.*

he·li·an·thine (hē-li-an'thin). SYN methyl orange.

hel·i·cal (hel'i-kăl). **1.** Relating to a helix. SYN helicine (2). **2.** SYN helicoid. [G. *helix*, a coil]

hel·i·ces (hel'i-sēz). Plural of helix.

hel·i·cine (hel'i-sēn). **1.** Coiled. **2.** SYN helical (1). [G. *helix*, a coil]

Hel·i·co·bac·ter (hel'ĭ-kō-bak'ter). A genus of helical, curved, or straight microaerophilic bacteria with rounded ends and multiple sheathed flagella (unipolar or bipolar and lateral) with terminal bulbs. Form nonpigmented, translucent colonies, 1–2 mm in diameter. Catalase and oxidase positive. Found in gastric mucosa of primates, including human beings and ferrets. Some species are associated with gastric and peptic ulcers. The type species is *Helicobacter pylori.*

H. pylo'ri, a recently identified species that produces urease and is associated with several gastroduodenal diseases including gastritis and gastric, duodenal, and peptic ulcers. The type species of the genus *Helicobacter.* SYN *Campylobacter pylori.*

hel·i·coid (hel'i-koyd). Resembling a helix. SYN helical (2). [G. *helix*, a coil, + *eidos*, resemblance]

hel·i·co·po·dia (hel'i-kō-pō'dē-ă). SYN helicopod *gait.* [G. *helix*, a coil, + *pous*, foot]

hel·i·co·tre·ma (hel'i-kō-trē'mă) [NA]. A semilunar opening at the apex of the cochlea through which the scala vestibuli and the scala tympani of the cochlea communicate with one another. SYN Breschet's hiatus, Scarpa's hiatus. [G. *helix*, a spiral, + *trēma*, a hole]

Helie, Louis T., French gynecologist, 1804–1867. SEE H.'s *bundle.*

he·li·en·ceph·a·li·tis (hē-lē-en-sef-ă-lī'tis). Inflammation of the brain following sunstroke. [G. *helios*, sun, + *enkephalos*, brain, + *-itis*, inflammation]

helio-. The sun. [G. *hēlios*]

he·li·o·aer·o·ther·a·py (hē'lē-ō-ār-ō-thār'ă-pē). Treatment of disease by exposure to sunshine and fresh air.

he·li·op·a·thy (hē-lē-op'ă-thē). Injury from exposure to sunlight. [helio- + G. *pathos*, suffering]

he·li·o·pho·bia (hē'lē-ō-fō'bē-ă). Morbid fear of exposure to the sun's rays. [helio- + G. *phobos*, fear]

he·li·o·sis (hē-lē-ō'sis). SYN sunstroke. [helio- + G. *-osis*, condition]

he·li·o·tax·is (hē-lē-ō-tak'sis). A form of phototaxis, and perhaps of thermotaxis, in which there is a tendency to growth or movement toward (positive h.) or away from (negative h.) the sun or the sunlight. SYN heliotropism. [helio- + G. *taxis*, orderly arrangement]

he·li·ot·ro·pism (hē-lē-ot'rō-pizm). SYN heliotaxis. [helio- + G. *trope*, a turning]

He·li·o·zo·ea (hē'lē-ō-zō'ē-ă). A class of protozoans (subphylum Sarcodina) distinguished by stiff radiating axopodia on all sides, usually naked, though some have a skeleton of siliceous scales and spines, but without a central capsule. They are mostly fresh water dwellers, and colonial forms are common. [helio- + G. *zōon*, animal]

he·li·um (He) (hē'lē-ŭm). A gaseous element present in minute amounts in the atmosphere (0.000524% of dry volume); atomic no. 2, atomic wt. 4.002602; used as a diluent of medicinal gases; used as a diluent of oxygen principally in non-medical applications, and in its liquid form as the coolant for super-conducting magnets (as in magnetic resonance imaging). [G. *hēlios*, the sun]

he·li·um-3. The rare stable isotope of helium (1.37 parts per million of ordinary helium); produced by the beta decay of tritium.

he·li·um-4. The common helium isotope, making up 99.999% of natural helium; it is emitted in the form of alpha rays (which are helium nuclei), from a variety of radionuclides.

he·lix, pl. **hel·i·ces** (hē'liks, hel'i-sēz). **1** [NA]. The margin of the auricle; a folded rim of cartilage forming the upper part of the anterior, the superior, and the greater part of the posterior edges of the auricle. **2.** A line in the shape of a coil (or a spring, or the threads on a bolt), each point being equidistant from a straight line that is the axis of the cylinder in which each point of the h. lies; often, mistakenly, applied to a spiral (the threads on a screw). [L. fr. G. *helix*, a coil]

3_{10} **h.,** a type of right-handed h. found in small pieces in a number of proteins; has three amino acid residues per turn.

3.6_{13} **h.,** SYN α h.

α **h.,** the helical (commonly right-handed) form present in many proteins, deduced by Pauling and Corey from x-ray diffraction studies of proteins such as α-keratin; the h. is stabilized by hydrogen bonds between, *e.g.,* =C=O and HN= groups (symbolized by the center dot in =CO·HN=) of different eupeptide bonds. In a true α h., there are 3.6 amino acid residues per turn of the h. SYN 3.6_{13} h., Pauling-Corey h.

collagen h., an extended left-handed h. resulting from the high levels of glycine, L-proline, and L-hydroxyproline present in the collagens. There are 3.3 amino acids per turn of the helix. Three of those left-handed helices form a triple superhelix that is right-handed.

DNA h., SYN Watson-Crick h.

double h., SYN Watson-Crick h.

π **h.,** a rare right-handed h. found only in small portions of certain proteins. Stabilized by similar hydrogen bonds as in an α h.; there are 4.3 amino acid residues per turn of the h.

Pauling-Corey h., SYN α h.

triple h., the superhelix formed (right-handed) from three individual collagen helices (each being left-handed).

twin h., SYN Watson-Crick h.

Watson-Crick h., the helical structure assumed by two strands of deoxyribonucleic acid, held together throughout their length by hydrogen bonds between bases on opposite strands, referred to as Watson-Crick base pairing. SEE base *pair.* SYN DNA h., double h., twin h.

hel·le·bore (hel'ĕ-bōr). A plant of the genus *Helleborus,* especially *H. niger* (black h.). SEE ALSO *Veratrum* album, *Veratrum* viride. [G. *helleboros*]

false h., SYN adonis.

hel·leb·o·rin (hĕ-leb'o-rin, hel-ĕ-bō'rin). A toxic glycoside from *Veratrum viride* (green hellebore); a narcotic.

hel·le·bor·ism (hel'ĕ-bōr-izm). A condition resulting from poisoning by *Veratrum Helleborus.*

hel·leb·o·rus (he-leb'o-rŭs). Black hellebore, the dried rhizome and roots of *Helleborus niger* (family Ranunculaceae); used as a cardiac and arterial tonic, diuretic, and cathartic. [G. *helleboros*]

Heller, Arnold L.G., German pathologist, 1840–1913. SEE H.'s *plexus.*

Heller, Ernst, German surgeon, 1877–1964. SEE H. *operation.*

Hellin, Dyonizy, Polish pathologist, 1867–1935. SEE H.'s *law.*

Helly, Konrad, Swiss pathologist, *1875. SEE H.'s *fixative.*

Helmholtz, Hermann L.F. von, German physician, physicist, and physiologist, 1821–1894. SEE H.'s axis *ligament;* H. *energy, theory* of accommodation, *theory* of color vision, *theory* of hearing; H.-Gibbs *theory;* Gibbs-H. *equation;* Young-H. *theory* of color vision.

hel·minth. An intestinal vermiform parasite, primarily nematodes, cestodes, trematodes, and acanthocephalans. [G. *helmins,* worm]

hel·min·tha·gogue (hel-minth'ă-gog). SYN anthelmintic (1). [G. *helmins,* worm, + *agōgos,* leading]

hel·min·them·e·sis (hel-min-them'ĕ-sis). The vomiting or expulsion through the mouth of intestinal worms. [G. *helmins,* a worm, + *emesis,* vomiting]

hel·min·thi·a·sis (hel-min-thī'ă-sis). The condition of having intestinal vermiform parasites. SYN helminthism, invermination.

hel·min·thic (hel-min'thik). SYN anthelmintic (1).

hel·min·thism (hel'min-thizm). SYN helminthiasis.

hel·min·thoid (hel-min'thoyd). Wormlike. [G. *helminthōdēs,* wormlike, fr. *helmins,* worm, + *eidos,* resemblance]

hel·min·thol·o·gy (hel-min-thol'ō-jē). The branch of science concerned with worms; especially the branch of zoology and of medicine concerned with intestinal vermiform parasites. SYN scolecology. [G. *helmins,* worm, + *logos,* study]

hel·min·tho·ma (hel-min-thō'mă). A discrete nodule of granulomatous inflammation (including the healed stage) caused by a helminth or its products, so termed on the basis of certain gross resemblances to a neoplasm. [G. *helmins,* worm, + *-oma,* tumor]

hel·min·tho·pho·bia (hel'min-thō-fō'bē-ă). Morbid fear of worms. [G. *helmins,* worm, + *phobos,* fear]

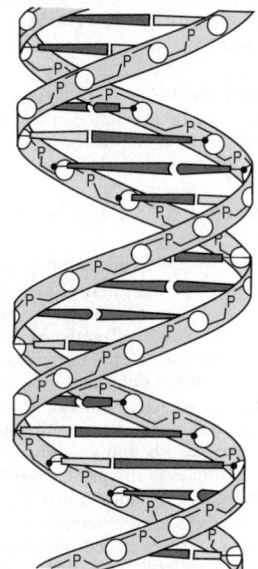

Watson-Crick helix (the "double helix" of DNA)
spiral ribbons indicate the deoxyribosephosphate (P) chains; the longer cross bars are purine bases (adenine, guanine), the shorter are pyrimidine (cytosine, thymine)

Hel·min·tho·spo·ri·um (hel-min-thō-spōr'ē-ŭm). A saprobic fungus, commonly misapplied to isolates of *Drechslera,* which is usually isolated in clinical laboratories; it has determinant parallel-walled conidiophores.

hel·min·tic (hel-min'tik). SYN anthelmintic (1).

He·lo·der·ma (hē-lō-der'mă). The only genus of poisonous lizards, such as the Gila monster, so named because of the tubercular scales which cover their bodies. They are native to Mexico and the southwestern U.S. [G. *hēlos,* nail, + *derma,* skin]

he·lo·ma (hē-lō'mă). SYN clavus (1). [G. *hēlos,* nail, + *-oma,* tumor]

h. dur'um, SYN hard *corn.*

h. mol'le, SYN soft *corn.*

he·lo·sis (hē-lō'sis). Rarely used term denoting the condition of having corns. [G. *hēlousthai,* to become callous]

he·lot·o·my (hē-lot'ō-mē). Surgical treatment of corns. [heloma + G. *tomē,* cutting]

Hel·vel·la es·cu·len·ta (hel-vel'ă es-kyū-len'tă). SYN *Gyromitra esculenta.*

Helweg, Hans K.S., Danish physician, 1847–1901. SEE H.'s *bundle.*

Helweg-Larssen, Helweg-Larssen, Hans F., 20th century Danish dermatologist. SEE Helweg-Larssen *syndrome.*

△**hem-, hema-.** Blood. SEE ALSO hemat-, hemato-, hemo-. [G. *haima*]

he·ma·chrome (hē'mă-krōm, hem'ă-). The coloring matter of the blood, hemoglobin or hematin. [hema- + G. *chrōma,* color]

he·ma·chro·sis (hē-mă-krō'sis, hem-ă). An intensified redness of the blood. [hema- + G. *chrōsis,* coloration]

he·ma·cy·tom·e·ter (hē'mă-sī-tom'ĕ-ter, hem'ă-). SYN hemocytometer.

he·ma·cy·to·zo·on (hē'mă-sī-tō-zō'on, hem'ă). SYN hemocytozoon.

he·ma·do·ste·no·sis (hē'mă-dō-ste-nō'sis, hem'ad-ŏ). Contraction of the arteries. [G. *haimas (haimad-),* a stream of blood, + *stenōsis,* a narrowing]

he·ma·drom·e·ter (hē-mă-drom'ĕ-ter, hem-ă). SYN hemodromometer.

he

he·ma·dro·mo·graph (hē-mă-drō′mō-graf, hem-ă-). SYN hemodromograph. [hema- + G. *dromos,* a course + *graphō,* to record]

he·ma·dro·mom·e·ter (hē′mă-drō-mom′ĕ-ter, hem-ă-). SYN hemodromometer.

he·mad·sorp·tion (hē′mad-sōrp-shŭn, hem′ad-). A phenomenon manifested by an agent or substance adhering to or being adsorbed on the surface of a red blood cell, as tuberculin (for example) can be adsorbed on red blood cells under certain conditions.

he·ma·dy·na·mom·e·ter (hē′mă-dī-nă-mom′ĕ-ter, hem′ă-). SYN hemodynamometer.

he·ma·fa·ci·ent (hē-mă-fā′shē-ent, hem-ă-). SYN hemopoietic.

he·mag·glu·ti·na·tion (hē-mă-glū′ti-nā′shŭn). The agglutination of red blood cells; may be immune as a result of specific antibody either for red blood cell antigens per se or other antigens which coat the red blood cells, or may be nonimmune as in h. caused by viruses or other microbes. SYN hemoagglutination.

passive h., a kind of passive agglutination in which erythrocytes, usually modified by mild treatment with tannic acid or other chemicals, are used to adsorb soluble antigen onto their surface, and which then agglutinate in the presence of antiserum specific for the adsorbed antigen. SYN indirect hemagglutination test.

reverse passive h., a diagnostic technique for virus infection using agglutination by viruses of red blood cells that previously have been coated with antibody specific to the virus.

viral h., the nonimmune agglutination of suspended red blood cells by certain of a wide range of otherwise unrelated viruses, usually by the virion itself but in some instances by products of viral growth, the species of erythrocyte agglutinated differing with the different viruses. SEE ALSO hemagglutination *inhibition.*

he·mag·glu·ti·nin (hē′mă-glū′ti-nin, hem-). A substance, antibody or other, that causes hemagglutination. SYN hemoagglutinin.

he·ma·gog·ic (hē-mă-goj′ik, hem-ă-). Promoting a flow of blood.

he·ma·gogue (hē′mă-gog, hem′ă-). **1.** An agent that promotes a flow of blood. **2.** SYN emmenagogue. [hem- + G. *agōgos,* leading]

he·mal (hē′măl). **1.** Relating to the blood or blood vessels. **2.** Referring to the ventral side of the vertebral bodies or their precursors, where the heart and great vessels are located, as opposed to neural (2). [G. *haima,* blood]

he·mal·um (hē-mal′ŭm, hem-). A solution of hematoxylin and alum used as a nuclear stain in histology, especially with eosin as a counterstain.

he·mam·e·bi·a·sis (hē′mă-mē-bī′ă-sis, hem′ă-). Any infection with ameboid forms of parasites in red blood cells, as in malaria.

he·ma·nal·y·sis (hē-mă-nal′ĭ-sis, hem-). Analysis of the blood; an examination of blood, especially with reference to chemical methods. [G. *haima,* blood, + analysis]

he·man·gi·ec·ta·sis, he·man·gi·ec·ta·sia (hē-man-jē-ek′tăsis, hem-an-; -ek-tā′zē-ă). Dilation of blood vessels. [G. *haima,* blood, + *angeion,* vessel, + *ektasis,* a stretching]

⚠hemangio-. The blood vessels. [G. *haima,* blood, + *angeion,* vessel]

he·man·gi·o·blast (he-man′jē-ō-blast). A primitive embryonic cell of mesodermal origin producing cells from which are derived vascular endothelium, reticuloendothelial elements, and blood-forming cells of all types. [hemangio- + G. *blastos,* germ]

he·man·gi·o·blas·to·ma (he-man′jē-ō-blas-tō′mă). A benign cerebellar neoplasm composed of capillary vessel-forming endothelial cells and stromal cells; a slowly growing tumor that affects, primarily, middle-aged individuals; increased incidence in von Hippel-Lindau disease. SYN angioblastoma, Lindau's tumor.

he·man·gi·o·en·do·the·li·o·blas·to·ma (he-man′jē-ō-en-dō-thē′-lē-ō-blas-tō′mă). Hemangioendothelioma in which the endothelial cells seem to be especially immature forms. [hemangio- + endothelium + G. *blastos,* germ, + *-oma,* tumor]

he·man·gi·o·en·do·the·li·o·ma (he-man′jē-ō-en-dō-thē-lē-ō′mă). A neoplasm derived from blood vessels, characterized by numerous prominent endothelial cells that occur singly, in aggregates, and as the lining of congeries of vascular tubes or channels; in the elderly, may be malignant (angiosarcoma or hemangiosarcoma), but in children are benign and probably represent a growing stage of capillary hemangioma. SYN hemendothelioma. [hemangio- + endothelium + G. *-oma,* tumor]

h. tubero′sum mul′tiplex, an eruption of pinkish papules, caused by hyperplasia of the endothelium of the superficial blood vessels.

he·man·gi·o·fi·bro·ma (he-man′jē-ō-fī-brō′mă). A hemangioma with an abundant fibrous tissue framework.

juvenile h., SYN juvenile *angiofibroma.*

he·man·gi·o·ma (he-man′jē-ō′mă). A congenital anomaly, in which proliferation of blood vessels leads to a mass that resembles a neoplasm; it can occur anywhere in the body but is most frequently noticed in the skin and subcutaneous tissues. SEE ALSO nevus. [hemangio- + G. *-oma,* tumor]

capillary h., an overgrowth of capillary blood vessels, seen most commonly in the skin, at or soon after birth, as a soft bright red to purple nodule or plaque that usually disappears by the fifth year. The most common type of h. SYN capillary angioma, capillary h. of infancy, nevus angiectodes, nevus sanguineus, nevus vascularis, nevus vasculosus, superficial angioma.

capillary h. of infancy, SYN capillary h.

cavernous h., a vascular malformation containing large blood-filled spaces, due apparently to dilation and thickening of the walls of the capillary loops; in the skin, extends more deeply than a capillary h. and is less likely to regress spontaneously.

h. pla′num exten′sum, a benign, flat, cutaneous hemangioma of considerable size.

racemose h., SYN cirsoid *aneurysm.*

sclerosing h., a benign lung or bronchial lesion, often subpleural, sometimes multiple, which forms hyalinized connective tissue. SYN fibrous histiocytoma.

senile h., a red papule due to weakening of the capillary wall, seen mostly in persons over 30 years of age. SYN cherry angioma, De Morgan's spots, ruby spots.

spider h., SYN spider *angioma.*

strawberry h., hyperproliferation of immature capillary vessels, usually on the head and neck, present at birth or within the first 2 to 3 months postnatally, which commonly regresses without scar formation.

verrucous h., a variant of the angiomatous nevus, appearing at birth or in early childhood, situated on the lower extremities with bluish-red nodules and warty surface; they enlarge and sometimes have satellite lesions.

he·man·gi·o·ma·to·sis (he-man′jē-ō-mă-tō′sis). A condition in which there are numerous hemangiomas.

he·man·gi·o·per·i·cy·to·ma (he-man′jē-ō-per′i-sī-tō′mă). An uncommon vascular, usually benign, neoplasm composed of round and spindle cells that are derived from the pericytes and surround endothelium-lined vessels; malignant h.'s are difficult to distinguish microscopically from the benign. [hemangio- + pericyte + G. *-oma,* tumor]

he·man·gi·o·sar·co·ma (he-man′jē-ō-sar-kō′mă). A rare malignant neoplasm characterized by rapidly proliferating, extensively infiltrating, anaplastic cells derived from blood vessels and lining irregular blood-filled or lumpy spaces.

he·ma·phe·ic (hē-mă-fē′ik, hem-ă-). Pertaining to or containing hemaphein.

he·ma·phe·in (hē-mă-fē′in, hem-ă-). A brown pathologic pigment derived from hemoglobin; said to be a combination of indican and urobilin. [G. *haima,* blood, + *phaios,* dusky]

he·ma·phe·ism (hē-mă-fē′izm, hem-ă-). The presence of hemaphein in the blood plasma and urine.

he·mar·thron, he·mar·thros (he-mar′thron, he-mar′thrōs). SYN hemarthrosis.

he·mar·thro·sis (hē′mar-thrō′sis, hem′ar-). Blood in a joint. SYN hemarthron, hemarthros. [G. *haima,* blood, + *arthron,* joint]

he·ma·stron·ti·um (hē-mă-stron′shē-ŭm, hem-ă-). A stain made by adding strontium chloride to a solution of hematein and aluminum chloride in citric acid and alcohol; used in histology.

⚠hemat-. Blood. SEE ALSO hem-, hemato-, hemo-. [G. *haima (haimat-)*]

he·ma·ta·chom·e·ter (hē′mă-tă-kom′ĕ-ter, hem′ă-). SYN hemotachometer.

he·mat·ap·os·te·ma (hē′mat-ă-pos-tē′mă, hem′at-). An abscess into which blood has effused. [hemat- + G. *apostēma,* abscess]

he·ma·te·in (hē-mă-tē′in, hem-ă). An oxidation product of hematoxylin.
    Baker's acid h., an acidic solution of oxidized hematoxylin used on frozen sections for staining phospholipids.

he·ma·tem·e·sis (hē-mă-tem′ĕ-sis, hem-ă-). Vomiting of blood. SYN vomitus cruentes. [hemat- + G. *emesis,* vomiting]

he·mat·en·ceph·a·lon (hē′mat-en-sef′ă-lon, hem′at-). SYN cerebral *hemorrhage.* [hemat- + G. *enkephalos,* brain]

he·ma·ther·a·py (hē′mă-thār′ă-pē, hem′ă-). SYN hemotherapy.

he·ma·therm (hē′mă-therm, hem′ă-). SYN homeotherm. [G. *haima,* blood, + *thermos,* warm]

he·ma·ther·mal (hē-mă-ther′măl, hem′ă-). SYN homeothermic. [G. *haima,* blood, + *thermos,* warm]

he·ma·ther·mous (hē-mă-ther′mŭs, hem-ă-). SYN homeothermic.

he·mat·hi·dro·sis (hē′mat-hī-drō′sis, hem′at-). SYN hematidrosis.

he·ma·tho·rax (hē-mă-thōr′aks, hem-ă-). SYN hemothorax.

he·mat·ic (hē-mat′ik). **1.** Relating to blood. SYN hemic. **2.** SYN hematinic (2).

he·ma·tid (hē′mă-tid, hem′ă-). **1.** A red blood cell. **2.** Obsolete term for a cutaneous eruption presumed to be caused by a substance in the circulating blood. [hemat- + *-id*]

he·ma·ti·dro·sis (hē′mat-i-drō′sis, hem′at-). Excretion of blood or blood pigment in the sweat; an extremely rare disorder. SYN hemathidrosis, hemidrosis (1), sudor sanguineus. [hemat- + G. *hidrōs,* sweat]

he·ma·tim·e·ter (hē-mă-tim′ĕ-ter, hem-ă-). SYN hemocytometer.

hem·a·tin (hē′mă-tin, hem′ă-). Heme in which the iron is Fe(III) (Fe³⁺); the prosthetic group of methemoglobin. SYN ferriheme, hematosin, hydroxyhemin, oxyheme, oxyhemochromogen, phenodin.
    h. chloride, SYN hemin.
    reduced h., SYN heme.

he·ma·ti·ne·mia (hē′mă-ti-nē′mē-ă, hem′ă-). The presence of heme in the circulating blood. [hematin + G. *haima,* blood]

hem·a·tin·ic (hē-mă-tin′ik, hem-a-). **1.** Improving the condition of the blood. **2.** An agent that improves the quality of blood by increasing the number of erythrocytes and/or the hemoglobin concentration. SYN hematic (2). SYN hematonic.

⟳**hemato-.** Combining form denoting blood. SEE ALSO hem-, hemat-, hemo-. [G. *haima (haimat-)*]

he·ma·to·bil·ia (hē′mă-tō-bil′ē-ă, hem′ă-). SYN hemobilia.

he·ma·to·bi·um (hē-mă-tō′bē-ŭm, hem-ă-). Any microorganism that is parasitic in the blood, especially an animal form or hemozoon. [hemato- + G. *bios,* life]

he·ma·to·blast (hē′mă-tō-blast, hem′ă-). A primitive, undifferentiated form of blood cell from which erythroblasts, lymphoblasts, myeloblasts, and other immature blood cells are derived; probably identical or closely similar to hemocytoblast and hemohistioblast; in normal bone marrow, present only in small numbers and difficult to identify in smears, inasmuch as h.'s are fragile and easily disintegrated; when marrow is hyperplastic, they may be observed in small groups. [hemato- + G. *blastos,* germ]
    Hayem's h., SYN platelet.

he·ma·to·cele (hē′mă-tō-sēl, hem′ă-). **1.** SYN hemorrhagic *cyst.* **2.** Effusion of blood into a canal or a cavity of the body. **3.** Swelling due to effusion of blood into the tunica vaginalis testis. [hemato- + G. *kēlē,* tumor]
    pelvic h., intraperitoneal effusion of blood into the pelvis.
    pudendal h., effusion of blood into the labium majus.

hem·a·to·ceph·a·ly (hē′mă-tō-sef′ă-lē, hem′ă-). Intracranial effusion of blood, commonly in a fetus. [hemato- + G. *kephalē,* head]

he·ma·to·che·zia (hē′mă-tō-kē′zē-ă, hem′ă-). Passage of bloody stools, in contradistinction to melena, or tarry stools. [hemato- + G. *chezō,* to go to stool]

he·ma·to·chlo·rin (hē′mă-tō-klō′rin, hem′ă). A green coloring matter derived from hemoglobin obtained from the placenta. [hemato- + G. *chlōros,* light green + -in]

he·ma·to·chy·lu·ria (hē′mă-tō-kī-lū′rē-ă, hem′a-). Presence of blood as well as chyle in the urine. [hemato- + G. *chylos,* juice, + *ouron,* urine]

he·ma·to·col·po·me·tra (hē′mă-tō-kol′pō-mē′tră, hem′ă-). Accumulation of blood in the uterus and vagina resulting from an imperforate hymen or other lower vaginal obstruction. [hemato- + G. *kolpos,* vagina, + *mētra,* womb]

he·ma·to·col·pos (hē′mă-tō-kol′pos, hem′ă-). An accumulation of menstrual blood in the vagina in consequence of imperforate hymen or other obstruction. SYN retained menstruation. [hemato- + G. *kolpos,* vagina]

he·mat·o·crit (Hct) (hē′mă-tō-krit, hem′ă-). **1.** Percentage of the volume of a blood sample occupied by cells. Cf. plasmacrit. **2.** Obsolete term for a centrifuge or device for separating the cells and other particulate elements of the blood from the plasma. [hemato- + G. *krinō,* to separate]

he·ma·toc·ry·al (hē-mă-tok′rē-ăl, hem-ă-). SYN poikilothermic. [hemato- + G. *kryos,* cold]

he·ma·to·cyst (hē′mă-tō-sist, hem′ă-). SYN hemorrhagic *cyst.*

he·ma·to·cys·tis (hē′mă-tō-sis′tis, hem′ă-). An effusion of blood into the bladder. [hemato- + G. *kystis,* bladder]

he·ma·to·cyte (hē′mă-tō-sīt, hem′ă-). SYN hemocyte.

he·ma·to·cy·to·blast (hē′mă-tō-sī′tō-blast, hem′ă-). SYN hemocytoblast.

he·ma·to·cy·tol·y·sis (hē′mă-tō-sī-tol′ĕ-sis, hem′ă-). SYN hemocytolysis.

he·ma·to·cy·tom·e·ter (hē′mă-tō-sī-tom′ĕ-ter, hem′ă-). SYN hemocytometer.

he·ma·to·cy·to·zo·on (hē′mă-tō-sī′tō-zō′on, hem′ă-). SYN hemocytozoon.

he·ma·to·dys·cra·sia (hē′mă-tō-dis-krā′zē-ă, hem′ă-). SYN hemodyscrasia.

he·ma·to·dys·tro·phy (hē′mă-tō-dis′trō-fē, hem′ă-). SYN hemodystrophy.

he·ma·to·gen·e·sis (hē′mă-tō-jen′ĕ-sis, hem′ă-). SYN hemopoiesis. [hemato- + G. *genesis,* production]

he·ma·to·gen·ic, he·ma·tog·e·nous (hē′mă-tō-jen′ik, hem′ă-; hem-ă-toj′en-ŭs). **1.** SYN hemopoietic. **2.** Pertaining to anything produced from, derived from, or transported by the blood.

he·ma·to·his·ti·o·blast (hē′mă-tō-his′tē-ō-blast, hem′ă-). SYN hemohistioblast.

he·ma·to·his·ton (hē′mă-tō-his′tŏn, hem′ă-). SYN globin.

he·ma·toid (hē′mă-toyd, hem′ă-). Resembling blood. [hemato- + G. *eidos,* resemblance]

he·ma·toi·din (hē-mă-toy′din). A pigment derived from hemoglobin which contains no iron but is closely related to or similar to bilirubin. H. is formed intracellularly, presumably within reticuloendothelial cells, but is often found extracellularly after 5 to 7 days in foci of previous hemorrhage. It occurs as refractile, yellow-brown and orange-red granules, but more characteristically as rhomboid plates arranged in a radial pattern, so-called h. burrs. SYN blood crystals, hematoidin crystals. [hemato- + G. *eidos,* resemblance, + -in]

he·ma·tol·o·gist (hē-mă-tol′ō-jist, hem-ă-). A physician trained and experienced in hematology, *i.e.,* skilled in performing diagnostic examinations of blood and bone marrow, or in treatment of such diseases, or both.

he·ma·tol·o·gy (hē-mă-tol′ō-jē, hem-ă-). The medical specialty that pertains to the anatomy, physiology, pathology, symptomatology, and therapeutics related to the blood and blood-forming tissues. SYN hemology. [hemato- + G. *logos,* study]

he·ma·to·lymph·an·gi·o·ma (hē′mă-tō-limf′an-jē-ō′-mă, hem′ă-). A congenital anomaly consisting of numerous, closely packed, variably sized lymphatic vessels and larger channels, in association with a moderate number of blood vessels of a similar type.

he

he·ma·tol·y·sis (hē-mă-tol′ĭ-sis, hem-ă-). SYN hemolysis.

he·ma·to·lyt·ic (hē′ma-tō-lit′ik, hem′ă). SYN hemolytic.

he·ma·to·ma (hē-mă-tō′mă, hem-ă-). A localized mass of extravasated blood that is relatively or completely confined within an organ or tissue, a space, or a potential space; the blood is usually clotted (or partly clotted), and, depending on how long it has been there, may manifest various degrees of organization and decolorization. [hemato- + G. -oma, tumor]

communicating h., SYN pseudoaneurysm.

corpus luteum h., SYN *corpus* hemorrhagicum.

epidural h., SYN extradural *hemorrhage.*

intracranial h., SEE intracranial *hemorrhage.*

intramural h., a h. in the wall of a structure, such as the bowel or bladder, usually resulting from trauma.

pulsatile h., SYN pseudoaneurysm.

subdural h., SYN subdural *hemorrhage.*

he·ma·to·ma·nom·e·ter (hē′mă-tō-mă-nom′ĕ-ter, hem′ă-). SYN hemomanometer.

he·ma·to·me·tra (hē′mă-tō-mē′tră, hem′ă-). A collection or retention of blood in the uterine cavity. SYN hemometra. [hemato- + G. *mētra,* uterus]

he·ma·tom·e·try (hē-mă-tom′ĕ-trē, hem-ă). Examination of the blood in order to determine any or all of the following: 1) the total number, types, and relative proportions of various blood cells; 2) the number or proportion of other formed elements; 3) the percentage of hemoglobin. In some instances, h. is used to include a determination of blood pressure. SYN hemometry. [hemato- + G. metron, measure]

he·mat·om·pha·lo·cele (hē′mat-om-fal′ō-sēl, hem′at-). Umbilical hernia into which an effusion of blood has taken place. [hemato- + G. *omphalos,* umbilicus, + *kēlē,* hernia]

he·ma·to·my·e·lia (hē′mă-tō-mī-ē′lē-ă, hem′ă-). Hemorrhage into the substance of the spinal cord; it is usually a posttraumatic lesion but may also be encountered in instances of spinal cord capillary telangiectases. SYN hematorrhachis interna, myelapoplexy, myelorrhagia. [hemato- + G. *myelos,* marrow]

he·ma·to·my·e·lo·pore (hē′mă-tō-mī′ĕ-lō-pōr, hem′ă-). Formation of porosities in the spinal cord as a result of hemorrhages. [hemato- + G. *myelos,* marrow, + *poros,* a pore]

he·ma·ton·ic (hē-mă-ton′ik, hem-ă-). SYN hematinic.

he·ma·to·pa·thol·o·gy (hē′mă-tō-path-ol′ō-jē, hem′ă-). The division of pathology concerned with diseases of the blood and of hemopoietic and lymphoid tissues. SYN hemopathology. [hemato- + G. *pathos,* suffering, + *logos,* study]

he·ma·top·a·thy (hē-mă-top′ă-thē, hem-ă-). SYN hemopathy.

he·ma·to·pe·nia (hē′mă-tō-pē′nē-ă, hem′ă-). Deficiency of blood, including hypocytosis or cytopenia. [hemato- + G. *penia,* poverty]

he·ma·to·pha·gia (hē′mă-tō-fā′jē-ă, hem′ă-). Living on the blood of another animal, as does the vampire bat or a leech. SYN hemophagia. [hemato- + G. *phagō,* to eat]

he·ma·toph·a·gous (hē′mă-tof′ă-gŭs, hem′ă-). Subsisting on blood. [hemato- + G. *phagō,* to eat]

he·ma·toph·a·gus (hē′mă-tof′ă-gŭs, hem′ă-). A blood eater, especially bloodsucking insects. [hemato- + G. *phagō,* to eat]

he·ma·to·plas·tic (hē′mă-tō-plas′tik, hem′ă). SYN hemopoietic. [hemato- + G. *plassō,* to form]

he·ma·to·poi·e·sis (hē′mă-tō-poy-ē′sis, hem′ă-). SYN hemopoiesis.

cyclic h., an autosomal recessive, inherited immunodeficiency of gray collie dogs characterized by overwhelming recurrent bacterial infections, bleeding, and coat color dilution. SYN gray collie syndrome.

he·ma·to·poi·et·ic (hē′mă-tō-poy-et′ik). SYN hemopoietic.

he·ma·to·poi·e·tin (hē′mă-tō-poy′ĕ-tin, hem′ă-). SYN erythropoietin.

he·ma·to·por·phyr·ia (hē′mă-tō-pōr-fir′ē-ă, hem′ă-). Obsolete term for any disorder of porphyrin metabolism, regardless of the cause. [hemato- + G. *porphyra,* purple]

he·ma·to·por·phy·rin (hē′mă-tō-pōr′fi-rin, hem′ă-). 3,8-Bis(α-hydroxyethyl)-2,7,12,18-tetramethylporphyrin-13,17-bispropion-

ic acid; a dark red, almost purple, porphyrin resulting from the decomposition of hemoglobin; chemical composition is that of heme with the iron removed and the two vinyl (–CH=CH₂) groups hydrated to hydroxyethyl (–CH(OH)–CH₃). SYN hemoporphyrin.

he·ma·to·por·phy·ri·ne·mia (hē′mă-tō-pōr′fi-ri-ne′mē-ă, hem′ă-). Older term used to designate the occurrence of hematoporphyrin in the circulating blood.

he·ma·to·por·phy·rin·u·ria (hē′mă-tō-pōr′fi-ri-nū′rē-ă, hem′ă-). Older term used to designate enhanced urinary excretion of porphyrins.

he·ma·top·sia (hē-mă-top′sē-ă, hem-ă-). SYN hemophthalmia. [hemato- + G. *opsis,* vision]

he·ma·tor·rha·chis (hē-mă-tōr′ă-kis, hem-ă-). A spinal hemorrhage. SYN hemorrhachis. [hemato- + G. *rhachis,* spine]

h. exter′na, hemorrhage into the spinal canal external to the cord, either within or outside the dura. SYN extradural h., subdural h.

extradural h., SYN h. externa.

h. inter′na, SYN hematomyelia.

subdural h., SYN h. externa.

he·ma·to·sal·pinx (hē′mă-tō-sal′pinks, hem′ă-). Collection of blood in a tube, often associated with a tubal pregnancy. SYN hemosalpinx. [hemato- + G. *salpinx,* a trumpet]

he·ma·to·sep·sis (hē′mă-tō-sep′sis, hem′ă). SYN septicemia.

he·ma·to·sin (hē-mă-tō′sin, hem-ă-). SYN hematin.

he·ma·to·sis (hē-mă-tō′sis, hem-ă-). **1.** SYN hemopoiesis. **2.** Oxygenation of the venous blood in the lungs.

he·ma·to·spec·tro·scope (hē′mă-tō-spek′trō-skōp, hem′ă-). A spectroscope especially adapted to examination of the blood.

he·ma·to·spec·tros·co·py (hē′mă-tō-spek-tros′kō-pē, hem′ă-). Examination of the blood by means of a spectroscope.

he·ma·to·sper·mat·o·cele (hē′mă-tō-sper′mă-tō-sēl, hem′ă-). A spermatocele that contains blood.

he·ma·to·sper·mia (hē′mă-tō-sper′mē-ă, hem′ă-). SYN hemospermia.

he·ma·to·stat·ic (hē′mă-tō-stat′ik, hem′ă-). **1.** Variant of hemostatic. **2.** Due to stagnation or arrest of blood in the vessels of the part.

he·ma·to·stax·is (hē′mă-tō-stak′sis, hem′ă-). Spontaneous bleeding due to a disease of the blood. [hemato- + G. *staxis,* a dripping]

he·ma·tos·te·on (hē-mă-tos′tē-on, hem-ă). Bleeding in the medullary cavity of a bone. [hemato- + G. *osteon,* bone]

he·ma·to·ther·mal (hē′mă-tō-ther′măl, hem′ă-). SYN homeothermic.

he·ma·to·tox·in (hē′mă-tō-toks′in, hem′ă-). SYN hemotoxin.

he·ma·to·trach·e·los (hē′mă-tō-tră-kē′lŭs, hem′ă-). Obsolete term for distention of the cervix uteri with accumulated blood. [hemato- + G. *trachēlos,* neck]

he·ma·to·tro·pic (hē′mă-tō-trop′ik, hem′ă-). SYN hemotropic.

he·ma·to·tym·pa·num (hē′mă-tō-tim′pan-ŭm, hem′ă-). SYN hemotympanum.

he·ma·tox·in (hē′mă-toks′in, hem-ă). SYN hemotoxin.

he·ma·tox·y·lin (hē′mă-toks′i-lin, hem-ă-) [C.I. 75290]. A crystalline compound, $C_{16}H_{14}O_6 \cdot 3H_2O$, containing the coloring matter of *Haematoxylon campechianum* (logwood), from which it is obtained by extraction with ether. It is used as a dye in histology, especially for cell nuclei and chromosomes, muscle cross-striations, and enterochromaffin cells; its staining properties depend upon its oxidation to hematein and mordanting with chrome and iron alums. It is also used as an indicator (red to yellow at pH 0.0 to 1.0, yellow to violet at pH 5.0 to 6.0).

Boehmer's h., an alum type of h. in which natural ripening occurs in about 8 to 10 days, and the solution is good for many months.

Delafield's h., an alum type of h. used in histology; natural ripening takes about 2 months and the solution is good for years.

Harris' h., an alum type of h. similar to Delafield's h., but which uses chemical ripening to produce oxidation of h. for immediate use.

iron h., unique ferric lakes of hematein that produce deep blue-black stains; useful for studies of cytologic detail, such as chromosomes, spindle fibers, Golgi apparatus, myofibrils, and mitochrondria; also useful to demonstrate *Entamoeba histolytica.* SEE ALSO Heidenhain's iron hematoxylin *stain,* Weigert's iron hematoxylin *stain.*

phosphotungstic acid h. (PTAH), a stain with broad application in cytology and histology; nuclei, mitochrondria, fibrin, neuroglial fibrils, and cross-striations of skeletal and cardiac muscle stain blue; cartilage ground substance, bone reticulum, and elastin appear in shades of yellow-orange and brownish red; also useful for demonstrating abnormal or diseased astrocytes, often in combination with periodic acid-Schiff stain and Luxol fast blue. SYN Mallory's phosphotungstic acid hematoxylin stain.

he·ma·to·zo·ic (hē′ma-tō-zō′ik, hem′ă). SYN hemozoic.

he·ma·to·zo·on (hē′ma-tō-zō′on, hem′ă-). SYN hemozoon.

he·ma·tu·ria (hē-mă-tū′-rē-ă, hem-ă-). Any condition in which the urine contains blood or red blood cells. [hemato- + G. *ouron,* urine]

Egyptian h., SYN *schistosomiasis* haematobium.

endemic h., SYN *schistosomiasis* haematobium.

enzootic h., a disease of cattle caused by long-term, low-level consumption of the bracken fern (*Pteridium aquilinum*) and characterized by hemorrhages or tumors in the bladder. SYN bracken poisoning.

false h., SYN pseudohematuria.

gross h., the presence of blood in the urine in sufficient quantity to be visible to the naked eye.

initial h., the presence of blood only in the first fraction of voided urine, usually indicating a urethral or prostatic source of bleeding.

microscopic h., presence of blood cells in uncatheterized urine, visible only under the microscope.

painful h., h. associated with dysuria, usually indicating the coexistence of infection, trauma, calculi, or foreign bodies within the lower urinary tract.

painless h., h. not associated with dysuria, often connoting a vascular or neoplastic etiology.

renal h., h. resulting from extravasation of blood into the glomerular spaces, or tubules, or pelves of the kidneys.

terminal h., the presence of blood only in the last fraction of voided urine, usually indicating a prostatic source of bleeding.

total h., uniform mixing of blood in the entire voided urine, commonly indicating an upper or mid-urinary tract source of bleeding.

urethral h., h. in which the site of bleeding is in the urethra.

vesical h., h. in which the site of bleeding is in the urinary bladder.

heme (hēm). **1.** The porphyrin chelate of iron in which the iron is Fe(II) (Fe^{2+}); the oxygen-carrying, color-furnishing, prosthetic group of hemoglobin. **2.** Iron complexed with nonporphyrins but related tetrapyrrole structures (*e.g.,* biliverdin heme). SYN ferroheme, ferroprotoporphyrin, reduced hematin. [G. *haima,* blood]

h. a, a derivative of h. found in cytochrome aa_3.

h. c, a derivative of h. found in cytochromes c, b_4, and f.

he·men·do·the·li·o·ma (hē-men′dō-thē-lē-ō′mă, hem′en-dō-). SYN hemangioendothelioma.

hem·er·a·lo·pia (hem′er-al-ō′pē-ă). Inability to see as distinctly in a bright light as in reduced illumination; seen in patients with impaired cone function. SYN day blindness, hemeranopia, night sight. [G. *hēmera,* day, + *alaos,* obscure, + *ōps,* eye]

hem·er·a·no·pia (hem′er-ă-nō′pē-ă). SYN hemeralopia. [G. *hemera,* day, + *an-,* priv., + *ōps,* eye]

he·me·ryth·rins (hē-mĕ-rith′rinz, hem-ĕ-). Iron-containing, oxygen-binding proteins in some worms, with molecular weights approximately that of hemoglobin but differing from hemoglobin in that the molecules do not contain porphyrin groups. Oxygenated h. is oxyhemerythrin. [G. *haima,* blood, + G. *erythros,* red, + -in]

△**hemi-.** One-half. Cf. semi-. [G.]

hem·i·a·car·di·us (hem′ē-ă-kar′dē-ŭs). One of twin fetuses, in which only a part of the circulation is effected by its own heart,

the rest by the heart of the other twin. [hemi- + G. *a-* priv. + *kardia,* heart]

hem·i·ac·e·tal (hem′ē-as′e-tăl). RCH(OH)OR′, a product of the addition of an alcohol to an aldehyde (an acetal is formed by the addition of an alcohol to a hemiacetal). In the aldose sugars, the h. formation is internal and labile, brought about by the 4-OH or 5-OH attack on the carbonyl O, yielding the furanose or pyranose structures; the h. forms of the sugars are involved in all polysaccharides, as glycosyls or glycosides. SEE ALSO hemiketal, acetal.

hem·i·ac·ro·so·mia (hem′ē-ak-rō-sō′mē-ă). A congenital form of hemihypertrophy of an extremity. [hemi- + G. *akron,* extremity, + *sōma,* body]

hem·i·a·geu·sia (hem′ē-ă-gū′sē-ă). Loss of taste from one side of the tongue. SYN hemiageustia, hemigeusia. [hemi- + G. *a-* priv. + *geusis,* taste]

hem·i·a·geus·tia (hem′ē-ă-gūs′tē-ă). SYN hemiageusia.

hem·i·al·gia (hem-ē-al′jē-ă). Pain affecting one entire half of the body. [hemi- + G. *algos,* pain]

hem·i·an·al·ge·sia (hem′ē-an′al-jē′zē-ă). Analgesia affecting one side of the body.

hem·i·an·en·ceph·a·ly (hem′ē-an-en-sef′ă-lē). Anencephaly on one side only, or involving one side much more extensively than the other.

hem·i·an·es·the·sia (hem′ē-an-es-thē′-zē-ă). Anesthesia on one side of the body. SYN unilateral anesthesia.

alternate h., h. affecting the head on one side and the body and extremities on the other side. SYN crossed h.

crossed h., SYN alternate h.

hem·i·a·no·pia (hem′ē-ă-nō′pē-ă). Loss of vision for one half of the visual field of one or both eyes. SYN hemianopsia.

absolute h., h. in which the affected field is totally insensitive to all visual stimuli. SYN complete h.

altitudinal h., a defect in the visual field in which the upper or lower half is lost; may be unilateral or bilateral.

binasal h., blindness in the nasal field of vision of both eyes.

bitemporal h., blindness in the temporal field of vision of both eyes.

complete h., SYN absolute h.

congruous h., h. in which the visual field defects in both eyes are completely symmetrical in extent and intensity.

crossed h., SYN heteronymous h.

heteronymous h., attitudinal h. involving the upper field of one eye and the lower field of the other; or a binasal or bitemporal h. SYN crossed h.

homonymous h., blindness in the corresponding (right or left) field of vision of each eye.

incomplete h., h. involving less than half the visual field of each eye.

incongruous h., an incomplete or asymmetric homonymous h.

pseudo-h., a condition in which individual stimuli are seen correctly, but when the nasal visual field of one eye and the temporal visual field of the fellow eye are stimulated simultaneously, one field is blind. SYN visual extinction.

quadrantic h., SYN quadrantanopia.

unilateral h., uniocular h., loss of sight in one-half of the visual field of one eye only.

hem·i·a·nop·ic (hem′ē-an-op′tik). Pertaining to hemianopia.

hem·i·a·nop·sia (hem′ē-an-op′sē-ă). SYN hemianopia. [hemi- + G. *an-* priv. + *opsis,* vision]

hem·i·an·os·mia (hem′ē-an-oz′mē-ă). Loss of the sense of smell on one side. [hemi- + G. *an-* priv. + *osmē,* smell]

hem·i·a·pla·sia (hem′ē-ă-plā′zē-ă). Absence of one lobe of a bilobed organ; used especially with reference to the thyroid gland. [hemi- + *aplasia*]

hem·i·a·prax·ia (hem′ē-ă-prak′sē-ă). Apraxia affecting one side of the body.

hem·i·ar·thro·plas·ty (hem-ē-ar′thrō-plas-tē). Arthroplasty in which one joint surface is replaced with artificial material, usually metal.

he

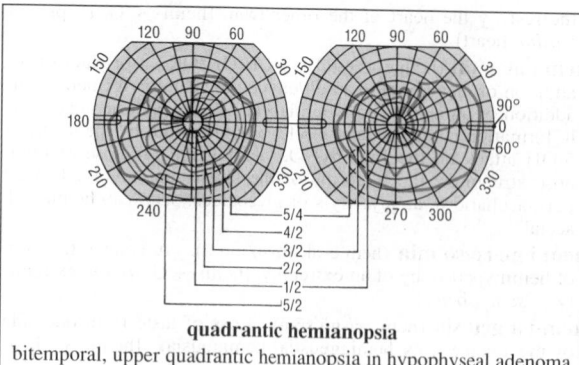

quadrantic hemianopsia

bitemporal, upper quadrantic hemianopsia in hypophyseal adenoma

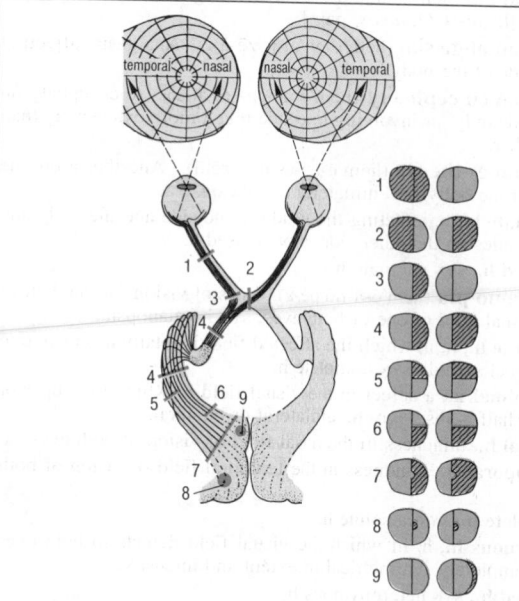

hemianopsia

loss of vision in various injuries to the nerve connection between the eye and the visual center of the cerebral cortex (red line equals interruption); the areas of loss are depicted on right with grey shading (1-9):
1. complete loss in left eye by interruption of left optic nerve; 2. bitemporal h., by interruption of the nerves that cross the optic chiasm; 3. nasal h. of the left eye, by interruption of the nerves that pass on the left side without crossing; 4. homonymous h. of the right side, by interruption of the optic tract; 5. quadrantic h. of the upper right side; 6. quadrantic h. of the lower right side; 7. complete homonymous h. of the right side (with the exception, at times, of the center, since the macula retinae is shown in the visual cortex as two-sided); 8. homonymous h. in the area of the macula retinae (lesion of the occipital pole); 9. segmental temporal h. of the right eye (only the outermost periphery of one field is affected)

hem·i·a·sy·ner·gia (hem′ē-ă-sin-er′jē-ă). Asynergia affecting one side of the body.

hem·i·a·tax·ia (hem′ē-ă-tak′sē-ă). Ataxia affecting one side of the body.

hem·i·ath·e·to·sis (hem′ē-ath′ĕ-tō′sis). Athetosis affecting one hand, or one hand and foot, only.

hem·i·at·ro·phy (hem-ē-at′rō-fē). Atrophy of one lateral half of a part or of an organ, as the face or tongue.

facial h., atrophy, usually progressive, affecting the tissues of one side of the face; saber-cut depression on forehead, heterochromia iridis, or bullous keratopathy may be present. SYN facial h. of Romberg, facial trophoneurosis, Romberg's disease, Romberg's syndrome, Romberg's trophoneurosis.

facial h. of Romberg, SYN facial h.

lingual h., atrophy of one lateral half of the tongue. SYN lingual trophoneurosis.

hem·i·bal·lism (hem-ē-bal′izm). SYN hemiballismus. [hemi- + G. *ballismos,* jumping about]

hem·i·bal·lis·mus (hem-ē-bal-iz′mŭs). Ballism involving one side of the body. SYN hemiballism. [hemi- + G. *ballismos,* jumping about]

hem·i·block (hem′ē-blok). Arrest of the impulse in one of the two main divisions of the left branch of the bundle of His; *i.e.,* in either the anterior (superior) division or the posterior (inferior) division.

he·mic (hē′mik). SYN hematic (1).

hem·i·car·dia (hem-ē-kar′dē-ă). **1.** Either lateral half, including atrium and ventricle, of the heart. **2.** A congenital malformation of the heart in which only two of the usual four chambers are formed. [hemi- + G. *kardia,* heart]

h. dex′tra, right side of the heart.

h. sinis′tra, left side of the heart.

hem·i·cel·lu·lose (hem-ē-sel′yū-lōs). Plant cell-wall polysaccharides closely associated with cellulose, such as xylans, mannans, and galactans. SYN cellulosan.

hem·i·cen·trum (hem′ē-sen′trŭm). One of the two lateral halves of the body of the vertebra. [hemi- + G. *kentron,* center]

hem·i·ceph·a·lal·gia (hem′ē-sef′ă-lal′jē-ă). The unilateral headache characteristic of typical migraine. SYN hemicrania (2). [hemi- + G. *kephalē,* head, + *algos,* pain]

hem·i·ce·pha·lia (hem-ē-se-fā′lē-ă). Congenital failure of the cerebrum to develop normally; usually the cerebellum and basal ganglia are represented at least in rudimentary form. SYN partial anencephaly. [hemi- + G. *kephalē,* head]

hem·i·cer·e·brum (hem′ē-ser′ē-brŭm). A cerebral hemisphere.

hem·i·cho·lin·i·um (hem-ē-kō-lin′ē-ŭm). A chemical which interferes with the synthesis of acetylcholine in cholinergic nerve terminals.

Hem·i·chor·da (hem-ē-kōr′dă). SYN Hemichordata.

Hem·i·chor·da·ta (hem′ē-kōr-dā′tă). A phylum comprised of soft-bodied, bilaterally symmetrical wormlike marine animals with gill-slits to the pharynx and a conical proboscis; a ciliated larval stage resembles that of echinoderms. SYN Hemichorda. [hemi- + Mod. L. *chordata,* having a notochord, fr. G. *chordē,* string]

hem·i·cho·rea (hem′ē-kōr-ē′ă). Chorea involving the muscles on one side only. SYN chorea dimidiata, hemilateral chorea.

hem·i·col·ec·to·my (hem′ē-kō-lek′tō-mē). Removal of the right or left side of the colon. [hemi- + G. *kolon,* colon, + *ektomē,* excision]

hem·i·cor·po·rec·to·my (hem′ē-kōr-pō-rek′tō-mē). Surgical removal of the lower half of the body, including the lower extremities, bony pelvis, genitalia, and various of the pelvic contents including the lower part of the rectum to the anus. [hemi- + L. *corpus,* body, + G. *ektomē,* excision]

hem·i·cra·nia (hem-ē-krā′nē-ă). **1.** SYN migraine. **2.** SYN hemicephalalgia. [hemi- + G. *kranion,* skull]

hem·i·cra·ni·ec·to·my (hem′ē-krā-nē-ek′tōmē). SYN hemicraniotomy. [hemi- + G. *kranion,* skull, + *ektomē,* excision]

hem·i·cra·ni·o·sis (hem′ē-krā-nē-ō′sis). Enlargement of one side of the cranium.

hem·i·cra·ni·ot·o·my (hem′ē-krā-nē-ot′ō-mē). Separation and reflection of the greater part or all of one half of the cranium, as a preliminary to an operation upon the brain. SYN hemicraniectomy. [hemi- + G. *kranion,* skull, + *tomē,* cut]

hem·i·des·mo·somes (hem-ē-des′mō-sōmz). Half desmosomes that occur on the basal surface of the stratum basalis of stratified squamous epithelium.

hem·i·di·a·pho·re·sis (hem′ē-dī-ă-fō-rē′sis). Diaphoresis, or sweating, on one side of the body. SYN hemidrosis (2), hemihidrosis.

hem·i·dro·sis (hem-ē-drō′sis). **1.** SYN hematidrosis. **2.** SYN hemidiaphoresis.

hem·i·dys·es·the·sia (hem′ē-dis-es-thē′-zē-ă). Dysesthesia affecting one side of the body.

hem·i·dys·tro·phy (hem-ē-dis′trō-fē). Underdevelopment of one lateral half of the body. [hemi- + G. *dys-*, ill, + *trophē*, nourishment, growth]

hem·i·ec·tro·me·lia (hem′ē-ek-trō-mē′lē-ă). Defective development of the limbs on one side of the body. [hemi- + ectromelia]

hem·i·fa·cial (hem-ē-fā′shăl). Pertaining to one side of the face.

hem·i·gas·trec·to·my (hem′ē-gas-trek-tō-mē). Excision of the distal one-half of the stomach.

hem·i·geu·sia (hem′ē-gū′sē-ă). SYN hemiageusia.

hem·i·glos·sal (hem′ē-glos′ăl). SYN hemilingual. [hemi- + G. *glōssa*, tongue]

hem·i·glos·sec·to·my (hem′ē-glos-ek′tō-mē). Surgical removal of one-half of the tongue. [hemi- + G. *glōssa*, tongue, + *ektomē*, excision]

hem·i·glos·si·tis (hem′ē-glos-ī′tis). A vesicular eruption on one side of the tongue and the corresponding inner surface of the cheek, probably herpetic. [hemi- + G. *glōssa*, tongue, + *-itis*, inflammation]

hem·i·gna·thia (hem-ē-nath′ē-ă). Defective development of one side of the mandible. [hemi- + G. *gnathos*, jaw]

hem·i·hep·a·tec·to·my (hem′ē-hep-ă-tek′tō-mē). Surgical removal of one-half or a lobe of the liver.

hem·i·hi·dro·sis (hem′ē-hī-drō′sis). SYN hemidiaphoresis.

hem·i·hy·dran·en·ceph·a·ly (hem-ē-hī′dran-en-sef′ă-lē). A unilateral form of hydranencephaly.

hem·i·hyp·al·ge·sia (hem′ē-hī-pal-je′zē-ă). Hypalgesia affecting one side of the body.

hem·i·hy·per·es·the·sia (hem′ē-hī′per-es-thē′zē-ă). Hyperesthesia, or increased tactile and painful sensibility, affecting one side of the body.

hem·i·hy·per·hi·dro·sis (hem′ē-hī-per-hī-drō′sis). Excessive sweating confined to one side of the body. [hemi- + G. *hyper*, over, + *hidrōsis*, sweating]

hem·i·hy·per·i·dro·sis (hem′ē-hī-per-i-drō′sis). Hemihyperhidrosis.

hem·i·hy·per·to·nia (hem′ē-hī-per-tō′nē-ă). Exaggerated muscular tonicity on one side of the body. SYN hemitonia. [hemi- + G. *hyper*, over, + *tonos*, tone]

hem·i·hy·per·tro·phy (hem′ē-hī-per′trō-fē). Muscular or osseous hypertrophy of one side of the face or body.

hem·i·hyp·es·the·sia (hem′ē-hī-pes-thē′zē-ă). Diminished sensibility in one side of the body. SYN hemihypoesthesia. [hemi- + G. *hypo*, under, + *aesthēsis*, sensation]

hem·i·hy·po·es·the·sia (hem′ē-hī-pō-es-thē′zē-ă). SYN hemihypesthesia. [hemi- + G. *hypo*, under, + *aisthēsis*, sensation]

hem·i·hy·po·to·nia (hem′ē-hī-pō-tō′nē-ă). Partial loss of muscular tonicity on one side of the body. [hemi- + G. *hypo*, under, + *tonos*, tone]

hem·i·kar·y·on (hem-i-kar′i-on). A cell nucleus containing a haploid set of chromosomes. [hemi- + G. *karyon*, nut (nucleus)]

hem·i·ke·tal (hem′ē-kē-tăl). RC(R′)(OH)OR″, a product of the addition of an alcohol to a ketone. In the ketose sugars, the h. formation is from an attack by an internal OH on the ketone carbonyl leading to intramolecular cyclization (furanose or pyranose); the h. forms of the sugars are involved in polysaccharide formation, as glycosyls or glycosides. SEE ALSO hemiacetal, ketal.

hem·i·lam·i·nec·to·my (hem′ē-lam-i-nek′tō-mē). Removal of a portion of a vertebral lamina, usually performed for exploration of, access to, or decompression of the intraspinal contents. [hemi- + L. *lamina*, layer, + G. *ektomē*, excision]

hem·i·lar·yn·gec·to·my (hem′ē-lar-in-jek′tō-mē). Excision of one lateral half of the larynx. [hemi- + G. *larnyx* (*laryng-*), larynx, + *ektomē*, excision]

hem·i·lat·er·al (hem-ē-lat′er-ăl). Relating to one lateral half.

hem·i·le·sion (hem-ē-lē′zhŭn). A unilateral lesion.

hem·i·lin·gual (hem-ē-ling′gwăl). Relating to one lateral half of the tongue. SYN hemiglossal. [hemi- + L. *lingua*, tongue]

hem·i·mac·ro·glos·sia (hem′ē-mak′rō-glos′ē-ă). Enlargement of half the tongue. [hemi- + G. *makros*, large, + *glōssa*, tongue]

hem·i·man·dib·u·lec·to·my (hem′ē-man-dib′yū-lek′tō-mē). Resection of one-half of the mandible.

hem·i·me·tab·o·lous (hem′ē-me-tab′ŏ-lŭs). Pertaining to a member of the series of insect orders, the Hemimetabola, in which simple or incomplete metamorphosis is found. [hemi- + G. *metabolē*, change]

he·min (hēm′in). Chloride of heme in which Fe^{2+} has become Fe^{3+}. H. crystals are called Teichmann's *crystals*, under *crystal*. SYN chlorohemin, factor X for *Haemophilus*, ferriheme chloride, ferriporphyrin chloride, ferriprotoporphyrin, hematin chloride.

hem·i·o·pal·gia (hem′ē-ō-pal′jē-ă). Pain in one eye, usually accompanied by hemicrania. [hemi- + G. *ōps*, eye, + *algos*, pain]

hem·ip·a·gus (hem-ip′ă-gŭs). Conjoined twins that are united laterally at the thorax; the zone of union may also involve the neck and jaws. SEE conjoined *twins*, under *twin*. [hemi- + G. *pagos*, something fixed]

hem·i·pan·cre·at·ec·to·my (hem′ē-pan′-krē-ă- tek′tō-mē). Surgical resection of half of the pancreas.

hem·i·pa·re·sis (hem-ē-pa-rē′sis, -par′ĕ-sis). Weakness affecting one side of the body.

hem·i·pel·vec·to·my (hem′ē-pel-vek′tō-mē). Amputation of an entire leg together with the os coxae. SYN hindquarter amputation, interilioabdominal amputation, interpelviabdominal amputation, Jaboulay's amputation. [hemi- + L. *pelvis*, basin (pelvis), + G. *ektomē*, excision]

hem·i·ple·gia (hem-ē-plē′jē-ă). Paralysis of one side of the body. [hemi- + G. *plēgē*, a stroke]

alternating h., h. on one side with contralateral cranial nerve palsies. SYN crossed h., crossed paralysis.

contralateral h., paralysis occurring on the side opposite to the causal central lesion.

crossed h., SYN alternating h.

double h., SYN diplegia.

facial h., paralysis of one side of the face, the muscles of the extremities being unaffected.

infantile h., SYN birth *palsy*.

spastic h., a h. with increased tone in the antigravity muscles of the affected side.

hem·i·ple·gic (hem-ē-plē′jik). Relating to hemiplegia.

He·mip·te·ra (hem-ip′ter-ă). An arthropod order of the class Insecta that includes many plant lice and other true bugs; those of the subfamily Triatominae are bloodsuckers and of medical importance. The best known species is *Cimex lectularius*, the common bedbug. [hemi- + G. *pteron*, wing]

hem·i·sec·tion (hem-ē-sek′shŭn). Surgical removal of a root of a multirooted tooth and its related coronal portion.

hem·i·sen·so·ry (hem′ē-sen′sōr-ē). Loss of sensation on one side of the body. Cf. hemianesthesia.

hem·i·sep·tum (hem-ē-sep′tŭm). A lateral half of any septum.

hem·i·spasm (hem′ē-spazm). A spasm affecting one or more muscles of one side of the face or body.

hem·i·sphere (hem′i-sfēr). Half of a spherical structure. SYN hemispherium cerebri [NA], cerebral h. (1). SYN hemispherium (1) [NA]. [hemi- + G. *sphaira*, ball, globe]

h. of bulb of penis, one of the lateral halves of the bulb of the penis that are separated by a median groove on the posterior part of the undersurface. SYN hemispherium bulbi urethrae.

cerebellar h., the large part of the cerebellum lateral to the vermis cerebelli. SYN hemispherium cerebelli [NA], hemispherium (2) [NA].

cerebral h., (1) SYN hemisphere. **(2)** the large mass of the telencephalon, on either side of the midline, consisting of the cerebral cortex and its associated fiber systems, together with the deeper-lying subcortical telencephalic nuclei (*i.e.*, basal ganglia [nuclei]).

dominant h., that cerebral hemisphere containing the representation of speech and controlling the arm and leg used preferentially in skilled movements; usually the left hemisphere.

hem·i·spher·ec·to·my (hem′ē-sfēr-ek′tō-mē). Excision of one cerebral hemisphere; undertaken for malignant tumors, intractable epilepsy usually associated with infantile hemiplegia due to birth injury, and other cerebral conditions.

hem·i·sphe·ri·um (hem′i-sfēr′ē-ŭm) [NA]. **1.** SYN hemisphere. **2.** SYN cerebellar *hemisphere*. [G. *hemisphairion*]

h. bul′bi ure′thrae, SYN *hemisphere* of bulb of penis.

h. cerebel′li [NA], SYN cerebellar *hemisphere*.

h. cer′ebri [NA], SYN hemisphere.

Hem·i·spo·ra (hem′ē-spō′ră). Generic name for certain species of *Fungi Imperfecti* in which chains of conidia develop from tubular structures that form as the result of a constriction at the end of each of a series of short hyphal branches; close septations divide the contents of the tube into relatively square, thick-walled, deeply staining segments that eventually separate and become rounded, thick-walled spores with rough surfaces. *H.* organisms occur fairly frequently as contaminants in cultures for other fungi; they are usually regarded as nonpathogenic forms, but there are a few reported instances in which they were apparently the causal agents of disease. [hemi- + G. *sporos*, seed]

hem·i·stru·mec·to·my (hem′ē-strū-mek′tō-mē). Rarely used term for excision of approximately one-half of a goiter. [hemi- + L. *struma*, + G. *ektomē*, excision]

hem·i·sub·stance (hem′ē-sŭb′stans). An amorphous substance found in cell walls.

hem·i·syn·drome (hem′ē-sin-drōm). **1.** A condition in which one-half of the body is atrophied or hypertrophied. **2.** Unilateral lesion of the spinal cord.

hem·i·sys·to·le (hem-ē-sis′tō-lē). Contraction of the left ventricle following every second atrial contraction only, so that there is but one pulse beat to every two heart beats. SYN systole alternans.

hem·i·ter·pene (hem-ē-ter′pēn). Isoprene or a derivative of a single isoprene.

hem·i·ther·mo·an·es·the·sia (hem′ē-ther′mō-an-es-thē′zē-ă). Loss of sensibility to heat and cold affecting one side of the body.

hem·i·tho·rax (hem-ē-thō′raks). One side of the thorax.

hem·i·to·nia (hem-ē-tō′nē-ă). SYN hemihypertonia.

hem·i·trem·or (hem′ē-trem′er, -trē′mer). Tremor affecting the muscles of one side of the body.

hem·i·trun·cus (hem′ē-trunk′us). A variant truncus arteriosus in which only one pulmonary artery originates from the truncal artery.

hem·i·ver·te·bra (hem-ē-ver′tĕ-bră). A congenital defect of the spine in which one side of a vertebra fails to develop completely.

hem·i·zy·gos·i·ty (hem′i-zī-gos′i-tē). The state of being hemizygous.

hem·i·zy·gote (hem-i-zī′gōt). An individual hemizygous with respect to one or more specified loci; *e.g.,* a normal male is a h. with respect to the gene for all X-linked or Y-linked genes in his genome. [hemi- + G. *zygōtos*, yoked]

hem·i·zy·got·ic (hem′i-zī-got′ik). SYN hemizygous.

hem·i·zy·gous (hem-i-zī′gŭs). Having unpaired genes in an otherwise diploid cell; males are normally h. for genes on both sex chromosomes. SYN hemizygotic.

hem·lock (hem′lok). SYN conium.

△**hemo-.** Combining form denoting blood. SEE ALSO hem-, hemat-, hemato-. [G. *haima*]

he·mo·ag·glu·ti·na·tion (hē′mō-ă-glū′ti-nā′shŭn). SYN hemagglutination.

he·mo·ag·glu·ti·nin (hē′mō-ă-glū′ti-nin). SYN hemagglutinin.

he·mo·an·ti·tox·in (hē′mō-an-ti-tok′sin). An antibody that neutralizes the effects of a hemotoxin, such as the hemolytic material in cobra venom.

He·mo·bar·to·nel·la. SYN *Haemobartonella.*

he·mo·bar·ton·el·lo·sis (hē′mō-bar-tō-nel-ō′sis). SYN feline infectious *anemia.*

he·mo·bil·ia (hē′mō-bil′ē-ă). Bleeding into the biliary passages,

usually as a result of hepatic trauma or a neoplasm in the liver or biliary tract. SYN hematobilia.

he·mo·blast (hēm′ō-blast). SYN hemocytoblast.

lymphoid h. of Pappenheim, SYN pronormoblast. SEE ALSO erythroblast.

he·mo·blas·to·sis (hē′mō-blas-tō′sis). A proliferative condition of the hematopoietic tissues in general.

he·mo·ca·thar·sis (hē′mō-kă-thar′sis). Cleansing the blood. [hemo- + G. *katharsis*, a cleansing]

he·mo·cath·e·re·sis (hē′mō-kath-e-rē′sis). Destruction of the blood cells, especially of erythrocytes (hemocytocatheresis). [hemo- + G. *kathairesis*, destruction]

he·mo·cath·e·re·tic (hē′mō-kath-ĕ-ret′ik). Pertaining to or characterized by hemocatheresis.

he·mo·cele (hē′mō-sēl). The system of blood-containing spaces pervading the body in arthropods. [hemo- + G. *koilōma*, cavity]

he·mo·cho·le·cyst (hē′mō-kō′lē-sist, -kol′ē-sist). **1.** Obsolete term for a cyst containing blood and bile. **2.** Obsolete term for nontraumatic hemorrhage or old blood accumulated in the gallbladder. [hemo- + G. *cholē*, bile, + *kystis*, bladder]

he·mo·cho·le·cys·ti·tis (hē′mō-kō′lē-sis-tī′tis). Hemorrhagic cholecystitis.

he·mo·chro·ma·to·sis (hē′mō-krō-mă-tō′sis). A disorder of iron metabolism characterized by excessive absorption of ingested iron, saturation of iron-binding protein, and deposition of hemosiderin in tissue, particularly in the liver, pancreas, and skin; cirrhosis of the liver, diabetes (bronze diabetes), bronze pigmentation of the skin, and, eventually heart failure may occur; also can result from administration of large amounts of iron orally, by injection, or in forms of blood transfusion therapy. [hemo- + G. *chrōma*, color, + *-osis*, condition]

exogenous h., hemosiderosis due to repeated blood transfusions; it can progress to pigmentary cirrhosis.

primary h. [MIM*235200], a specific inherited metabolic defect with increased absorption and accumulation of iron on a normal diet; autosomal dominant inheritance, less florid in females; juvenile h. may represent a homozygous state of the same gene.

secondary h., increased intake and accumulation of iron secondary to known cause, such as oral iron therapy or multiple transfusions.

he·mo·chrome (hē′mō-krōm). SYN hemochromogen.

he·mo·chro·mo·gen (hē-mō-krō′mō-jen). Term originally used for combinations of ferro- or ferriporphyrins with 2 mol of a nitrogenous base, *e.g.,* pyridine ferroporphyrin. SYN hemochrome. [hemo- + G. *chrōma*, color, + *-gen*, producing]

he·moc·la·sis, he·mo·cla·sia (hē-mok′lă-sis, hē′mō-klā′zē-ă). Rupture, dissolution (hemolysis), or other type of destruction of red blood cells. [hemo- + G. *klasis*, a breaking]

he·mo·clas·tic (hē′mō-klas′tik). Pertaining to hemoclasis.

he·mo·con·cen·tra·tion (hē′mō-kon-sen-trā′shŭn). Decrease in the volume of plasma in relation to the number of red blood cells; increase in the concentration of red blood cells in the circulating blood.

he·mo·co·nia (hē-mō-kō′nē-ă). Small refractive particles in the circulating blood, probably lipid material associated with fragmented stroma from red blood cells. SYN blood dust, blood motes, dust corpuscles. [hemo- + G. *konis*, dust]

he·mo·co·ni·o·sis (hē′mō-kō-nē-ō′sis). A condition in which there is an abnormal amount of hemoconia in the blood.

he·mo·cry·os·co·py (hē′mō-krī-os′kŏ-pē). Determination of the freezing point of blood. [hemo- + G. *kryos*, cold, + *skopeō*, to examine]

he·mo·cu·pre·in (hē-mō-kū′prē-in). SYN cytocuprein.

he·mo·cy·a·nin (hē-mō-sī′ă-nin). An oxygen-carrying pigment (molecular weights between 0.45 and 13×10^6) of lower sea animals (including molluscs and crustacea) and arthropods; copper is an essential component, but it contains no heme; used as an experimental antigen.

he·mo·cyte (hē′mō-sīt). Any cell or formed element of the blood. SYN hematocyte. [hemo- + G. *kytos*, a hollow (cell)]

he·mo·cy·to·blast (hē′mō-sī′tō-blast). A blood cell derived from embryonic mesenchyme, characterized by basophilic cytoplasm and a relatively large nucleus with a spongy, loose network of chromatin and several nucleoli; mitochondria are extremely fine and delicate. H.'s represent the primitive stem cells of the monophyletic theory of the origin of blood and have the potentiality of developing into erythroblasts, young forms of the granulocytic series, megakaryocytes, etc. SYN hematocytoblast, hemoblast. [hemo- + G. *kytos,* cell, + *blastos,* germ]

he·mo·cy·to·ca·ther·e·sis (hē′mō-sī′tō-kă-ther′ĕ-sis). Hemolysis, or other type of destruction of red blood cells. [hemo- + G. *kytos,* a hollow (cell), + *kathairesis,* destruction]

he·mo·cy·tol·y·sis (hē′mō-sī-tol′i-sis). The dissolution of blood cells, including hemolysis. SYN hematocytolysis. [hemo- + G. *kytos,* cell, + *lysis,* dissolution]

he·mo·cy·tom·e·ter (hē′mō-sī-tom′ĕ-ter). An apparatus for estimating the number of blood cells in a quantitatively measured volume of blood; it consists of a glass pipette with an ampulla for collecting and diluting the blood, and a counting chamber marked in squares. SYN hemacytometer, hematimeter, hematocytometer. [hemo- + G. *kytos,* cell, + *metron,* measure]

he·mo·cy·tom·e·try (hē′mō-sī-tom′ĕ-trē). The counting of red blood cells.

he·mo·cy·to·trip·sis (hē′mō-sī-tō-trip′sis). Fragmentation or disintegration of blood cells by means of mechanical trauma, *e.g.,* compression between hard surfaces. [hemo- + G. *kytos,* + *tripsis,* a grinding]

he·mo·cy·to·zo·on (hē′mō-sī-tō-zō′on). A protozoon parasite of the blood cells. SYN hemacytozoon, hematocytozoon. [hemo- + G. *kytos,* cell, + *zōon,* animal]

he·mo·di·ag·no·sis (hē′mō-dī-ag-nō′sis). Diagnosis by means of examination of the blood.

he·mo·di·al·y·sis (hē′mō-dī-al′i-sis). Dialysis of soluble substances and water from the blood by diffusion through a semipermeable membrane; separation of cellular elements and colloids from soluble substances is achieved by pore size in the membrane and rates of diffusion.

he·mo·di·a·lyz·er (hē-mō-dī′ă-lī-zer). A machine for hemodialysis in acute or chronic renal failure; toxic substances in the blood are removed by exposure to dialyzing fluid across a semipermeable membrane. SYN artificial kidney.

ultrafiltration h., a h. that uses fluid pressure differentials to bring about loss (usually) of protein-free fluid from the blood to the bath, as in certain edematous conditions.

he·mo·di·a·stase (hē-mō-dī′as-tās). Blood amylase.

he·mo·di·lu·tion (hē′mō-di-lū′shŭn). Increase in the volume of plasma in relation to red blood cells; reduced concentration of red blood cells in the circulation.

he·mo·drom·o·graph (hē-mō-drō′mō-graf). Rarely used term(s) for an instrument for recording the rapidity of the blood circulation. SYN hemadromograph. [hemo- + G. *dromos,* course, + *graphō,* to record]

he·mo·dro·mom·e·ter (hē′mō-drō-mom′ĕ-ter). Rarely used term(s) for an instrument for measuring the rapidity of the blood circulation. SYN hemadrometer, hemadromometer. [hemo- + G. *dromos,* course, + *metron,* measure]

he·mo·dy·nam·ic (hē′mō-dī-nam′ik). Relating to the physical aspects of the blood circulation.

he·mo·dy·nam·ics (hē′mō-dī-nam′iks). The study of the dynamics of the blood circulation. [hemo- + G. *dynamis,* power]

he·mo·dy·na·mom·e·ter (hē′mō-dī-nă-mom′ĕ-ter). An instrument for determining the blood pressure. SYN hemadynamometer. [hemo- + G. *dynamis,* force, + *metron,* measure]

he·mo·dys·cra·sia (hē′mō-dis-krā′zē-ă). Any abnormal condition or disorder of the blood and hemopoietic tissue, used especially with reference to those resulting in changes in the formed elements. SYN hematodyscrasia. [hemo- + G. *dyscrasia,* bad temperament]

he·mo·dys·tro·phy (hē-mō-dis′trō-fē). Any disease or abnormal condition of the blood and hemopoietic tissues, exclusive of simple transitory changes. SYN hematodystrophy.

he·mo·fil·tra·tion (hē′mō-fil-trā′shŭn). A process, similar to hemodialysis, by which blood is dialyzed using ultrafiltration and simultaneous reinfusion of physiologic saline solution.

he·mo·flag·el·lates (hē-mō-flaj′ĕ-lāts). Protozoan flagellates in the family Trypanosomatidae that are parasitic in the blood of many species of domestic and wild animals and birds, and of humans; they include the genera *Leishmania* and *Trypanosoma,* several species of which are important pathogens. [hemo- + L. *flagellum,* dim. of *flagrum,* a whip]

he·mo·fus·cin (hē-mō-fŭs′in). A brown pigment derived from hemoglobin that occurs in urine occasionally along with hemosiderin, usually indicative of increased red blood cell destruction; occurs also in the liver with hemosiderin in cases of hemochromatosis.

he·mo·gen·e·sis (hē-mō-jen′ĕ-sis). SYN hemopoiesis.

he·mo·gen·ic (hē-mō-jen′ik). SYN hemopoietic.

HEMOGLOBIN

he·mo·glo·bin (Hb) (hē-mō-glō′bin) [MIM*141800 to 142310]. The red respiratory protein of erythrocytes, consisting of approximately 3.8% heme and 96.2% globin, with a molecular weight of 64,450, which as oxyhemoglobin (HbO_2) transports oxygen from the lungs to the tissues where the oxygen is readily released and HbO_2 becomes Hb. When Hb is exposed to certain chemicals, its normal respiratory function is blocked; *e.g.,* the oxygen in HbO_2 is easily displaced by carbon monoxide, thereby resulting in the formation of fairly stable carboxyhemoglobin (HbCO), as in asphyxiation resulting from inhalation of exhaust fumes from gasoline engines. When the iron in Hb is oxidized from the ferrous to ferric state, as in poisoning with nitrates and certain other chemicals, a nonrespiratory compound, methemoglobin (MetHb), is formed.

In humans there are five kinds of normal Hb: two embryonic Hb's (Hb Gower-1, Hb Gower-2), fetal (Hb F), and two adult types (Hb A, Hb A_2). There are two α globin chains containing 141 amino acid residues, and two of another kind (β, γ, δ, ϵ, or ζ), each containing 146 amino acid residues in four of the Hb's. Hb Gower-1 has two ζ chains and two ϵ chains. The production of each kind of globin chain is controlled by a structural gene of similar Greek letter designation; normal individuals are homozygous for the normal allele at each loci. Substitution of any one amino acid for another in the polypeptide chain can occur at any codon in any of the five loci and have resulted in the production of many hundreds of abnormal Hb types, most of no known clinical significance. In addition, deletions of one or more amino acid residues are known, as well as gene rearrangements due to unequal crossing over between homologous chromosomes.

The Hb types below are the main abnormal types known to be of clinical significance. Newly discovered abnormal Hb types are first assigned a name, usually the location where discovered, and a molecular formula is added when determined. The formula consists of Greek letters to designate the basic chains, with subscript 2 if there are two identical chains; a superscript letter (^{A} if normal for adult Hb, etc.) is added, or the superscript may designate the site of amino acid substitution (numbering amino acid residues from the N terminus of the polypeptide) and specifying the change, using standard abbreviations for the amino acids. There is an exhaustive listing of variant h.'s in MIM where a composite numbering system is used.

h. A [MIM*141800], normal adult Hb (Hb A) with formula $\alpha_2^A\beta_2^A$ or $\alpha_2\beta_2$.

h. A_2 [MIM*141850], the normal Hb (Hb A_2) of the formula $\alpha_2^A\delta_2$ or $\alpha_2\delta_2$, which makes up approximately 2.5% of the total adult h. concentration. At least 18 mutant variants of the δ chain have been reported.

h. A_{Ic}, the major fraction of glycosylated h.

aberrant h., a mutant Hb that functions abnormally. Cf. variant h.

h. Anti-Lepore, a group of abnormal h.'s similar to h. Lepore. These h.'s have normal α chains, but the non-α chain consists of

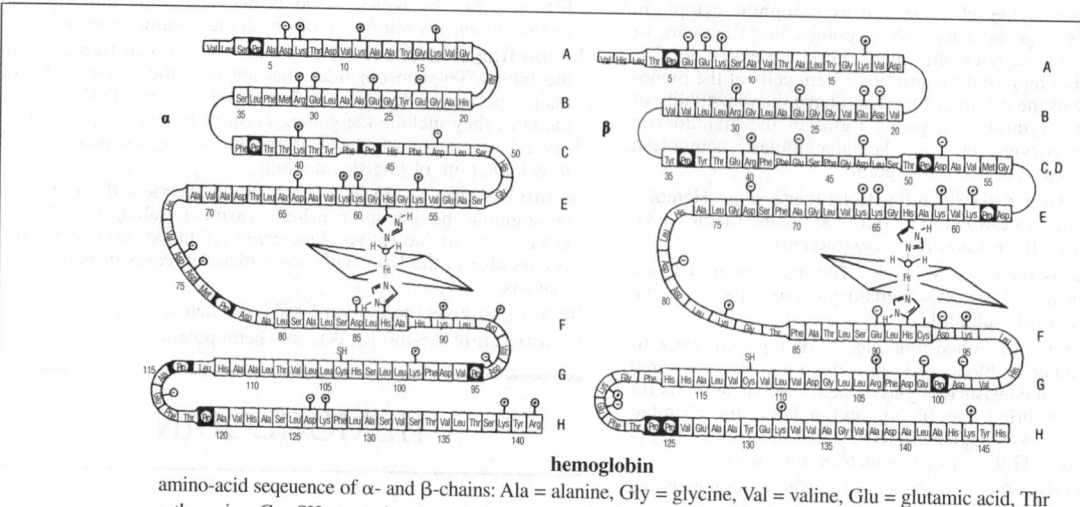

hemoglobin

amino-acid seqeuence of α- and β-chains: Ala = alanine, Gly = glycine, Val = valine, Glu = glutamic acid, Thr = threonine, Cys-SH = cysteine, His = histidine, Lys = lysine, Asp = aspartic acid, Leu = leucine, Pro = proline, Phe = phenylalanine, Met = methionine, Trp = tryptophan, Arg = arginine, Ser = serine, Tyr = tyrosine

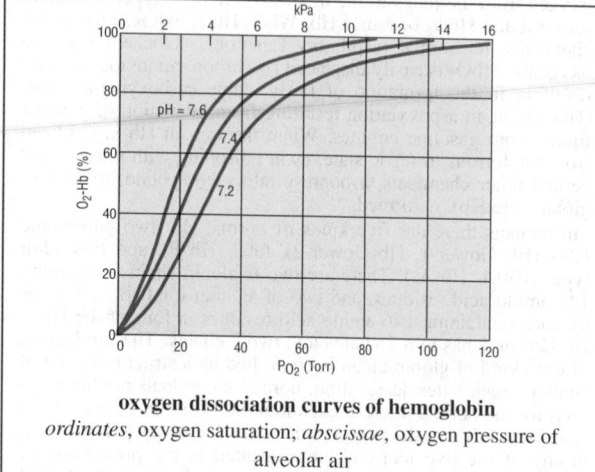

oxygen dissociation curves of hemoglobin

ordinates, oxygen saturation; *abscissae*, oxygen pressure of alveolar air

the N-terminal portion of the β chain joined to the C-terminal portion of the δ chain. This is the opposite crossing over pattern observed in h. Lepore. Examples of h. Anti-Lepore include Hb$_{Miyada}$, Hb P$_{Congo}$, Hb P$_{Nilotic}$, and Hb$_{Lincoln Park}$. There is also one variant that is both h. Lepore and h. Anti-Lepore (Hb$_{Parchman}$). Cf. h. Lepore.

h. Bart's [MIM*142309], a Hb homotetramer (all four polypeptides identical) of formula γ$_4$, found in the early embryo and in α-thalassemia 2; not effective in oxygen transport; does not display a Bohr effect.

bile pigment h., SYN choleglobin.

h. C [MIM*141900-0038], an abnormal Hb with substitution of lysyl residue for glutamyl at the 6th position of the β chain, of formula α$_2$2^{A}β$_2$$^{6Glu→Lys}$, this type reduces the normal plasticity of erythrocytes. Heterozygotes: Hb C trait, about 28 to 44% of total Hb is Hb C, no anemia; Homozygotes: nearly all Hb is Hb C, moderate normocytic hemolytic anemia; Individuals heterozygous for both Hb C and Hb S (Hb SC disease) and for Hb C and thalassemia are known, and have atypical hemolytic anemias; sickling is enhanced in Hb SC disease.

h. C$_{Georgetown}$, h. C$_{Harlem}$ [MIM*141900-0039], two abnormal Hb's, both with the substitution of a valyl residue for a glutamyl residue at the 6th position of the β chain as in Hb S, and in addition each has a second substitution; both have a second substitution of an asparaginyl residue for an aspartyl residue at

position 73 of the β chain; both types cause sickling of erythrocytes similar to Hb S.

carbon monoxide h., SYN carboxyhemoglobin.

h. Chesapeake (Hb$_{Chesapeake}$) [MIM*141800-0018], an abnormal Hb with a single α chain substitution, molecular formula α$_2$$^{92Arg-→Leu}$β$_2$^{A}; heterozygotes have polycythemia, apparently to compensate for the increased oxygen affinity of this Hb, resulting in decreased liberation of oxygen in the tissues.

h. Constant Spring, an abnormal hemoglobin having an extended polypeptide chain (31 additional amino acid residues) on the α chain (thus, the α chain is 172 amino acids long); approximately 20% of the individuals with Hb H disease also have this defect.

h. D$_{Punjab}$ [MIM*141900-0065], an abnormal Hb with a single β chain substitution, molecular formula α$_2$^{A}β$_2$$^{121Glu→Gln}$; heterozygotes are asymptomatic, homozygotes have mild hemolytic anemia; there is an increase in O$_2$ affinity; identical to h. D$_{Los Angeles}$, h. D$_{North Carolina}$, h. D$_{Portugal}$, h. D$_{Chicago}$, and h. Oak Ridge.

h. E [MIM*141900-0071], an abnormal Hb with a single β chain substitution, molecular formula α$_2$^{A}β$_2$$^{26Glu→Lys}$, common in Southeast Asia, especially Thailand; heterozygotes are asymptomatic with 35 to 45% Hb E; homozygotes have mild to moderate hemolytic anemia with 90 to 100% Hb E and the remainder Hb F.

embryonic h., SEE h. Gower-1, h. Gower-2.

h. F [MIM*142200], normal fetal Hb (Hb F) of molecular formula α$_2$^{A}γ$_2$^{F}, which is the major Hb component during intrauterine life, decreasing rapidly during infancy to reach a concentration of less than 0.5% in normal children and adults; the concentration of Hb F is increased in some hemoglobinopathies and in some cases of hypoplastic anemia, pernicious anemia, and leukemia; Hb F has a weaker affinity for 2,3-bisphosphoglycerate than does Hb A. More than 50 mutant variants of the γ chain have been reported. SYN fetal h.

h. F (hereditary persistence of) [MIM*142200-0026], a condition due to an allele that depresses synthesis of β and δ chains (as in thalassemia), but this is fully compensated by increased γ chain synthesis and there is no anemia; there are 3 types: 1) African type, no β or δ chain synthesis by the chromosome with the abnormal gene, heterozygotes have 20 to 30% Hb F and Hb A$_2$ slightly decreased, homozygotes form no Hb A or Hb A$_2$; 2) Greek type, reduced β and δ chain synthesis, heterozygotes have 10 to 20% Hb F and normal Hb A$_2$; 3) Swiss type, heterozygotes have only 1 to 3% Hb F and normal Hb A$_2$.

fetal h., SYN h. F.

glycosylated h., any one of four h. A fractions (A$_{Ia1}$, A$_{Ia2}$, A$_{Ib}$, or A$_{Ic}$) to which D-glucose and related monosaccharides bind; concentrations are increased in the erythrocytes of patients with diabetes mellitus and can be used as a retrospective index of glucose control over time in such patients.

h. Gower-1, a Hb of molecular formula $\zeta_2\epsilon_2$, found as a minor Hb in the early embryo; disappears by the third month of pregnancy in favor of h. Gower-2 and h. Portland and then by Hb F; the ζ chain has 141 amino acid residues. Synthesis of the ζ chain is deficient in cases of hydrops fetalis. Cf. h. Gower-2, h. Portland.

h. Gower-2, a normal Hb of molecular formula $\alpha_2{}^A\epsilon_2$, which is a major Hb component of the early embryo; production of ϵ chains normally ceases at about the third month of fetal development and is replaced by Hb F. Cf. h. Gower-1, h. Portland.

green h., SYN choleglobin.

h. H [MIM*142309], a homotetramer of Hb (all four polypeptides identical) of molecular formula β_4, found only when α chain synthesis is depressed and not effective in oxygen transport. Hb H disease (α-thalassemia intermedia) is a thalassemia-like syndrome in individuals heterozygous for both severe and mild genes for α-thalassemia; moderate anemia and red cell abnormalities with 25 to 35% Hb Bart's at birth, but with Hb Bart's later replaced by Hb H and with Hb A_2 decreased. Hb H shows no cooperativity with O_2 binding and does not exhibit a Bohr effect.

h. I [MIM*141800-0055], an abnormal Hb with a single α chain substitution, molecular formula $\alpha_2{}^{16Lys\rightarrow Glu}\beta_2{}^A$; a thalassemia-like syndrome has been found in individuals heterozygous for both Hb I and α-thalassemia genes, with formation of about 70% Hb I.

h. J$_{Capetown}$ [MIM*141800-0063], an abnormal Hb with a single α chain substitution, molecular formula $\alpha_2{}^{92Arg\rightarrow Gln}\beta_2{}^A$; heterozygotes have polycythemia because of increased oxygen affinity of this Hb.

h. Kansas [MIM*141900-0145], an abnormal Hb of molecular formula $\alpha_2{}^A\beta_2{}^{102Asn\rightarrow Thr}$; found in association with familial cyanosis due to decreased oxygen affinity of this Hb.

h. Lepore [MIM 142000-various], a group of abnormal Hb's with normal α chains, but the non-α chains consist of the N-terminal portion of the δ chain joined to the C-terminal portion of the β chain, apparently as the result of nonhomologous pairing and crossing over between the genes for β and δ chains. The major types are Hb Lepore$_{Boston}$ (identical to Hb Lepore$_{Washington}$), Hb Lepore$_{Hollandia}$, and Hb Lepore$_{Baltimore}$, which differ in the region of crossing over ($\delta 87$-$\beta 116$, $\delta 22$-$\beta 50$, and $\delta 50$-$\beta 86$, respectively). Heterozygotes form about 10% Hb Lepore, normal amounts of Hb A_2, and moderately increased amounts of Hb F and usually have mild anemia, microcytosis, and hypochromia; homozygotes form only Hb Lepore and Hb F and have severe anemia. Cf. h. Anti-Lepore.

h. M [MIM*142300 & various], a group of abnormal Hb's in which a single amino acid substitution favors the formation of methemoglobin in spite of normal quantities of methemoglobin reductase. Strictly speaking, Hb's M are h.'s with mutations at the proximal or distal histidyl residues. Other Hb's M tend to favor the Fe(III) state. Heterozygotes have congenital methemoglobinemia; the homozygous state of these genes is unknown and is presumably lethal. Specific types include: Hb M$_{Iwate}$, $\alpha^{87His\rightarrow Tyr}$ (α chain, position 87, histidine replaced by tyrosine); Hb M$_{Hyde\ Park}$, $\beta^{92His\rightarrow Tyr}$; Hb M$_{Boston}$, $\alpha^{58His\rightarrow Tyr}$; Hb M$_{Saskatoon}$, $\beta^{63His\rightarrow Tyr}$; Hb M$_{Milwaukee-1}$, $\beta^{67Val\rightarrow Glu}$.

mean corpuscular h. (MCH), the h. content of the average red cell, calculated from the h. therein and the red cell count, in erythrocyte indices.

muscle h., SYN myoglobin.

oxygenated h., SYN oxyhemoglobin.

h. Portland, a form of embryonic h. containing the ζ chains of h. Gower-1 and the γ chains of Hb F, thus having the formula $\zeta_2\gamma_2$; essentially disappears by the third month of pregnancy. Cf. h. Gower-1, h. Gower-2.

h. Rainier [MIM*141900-0232], an abnormal Hb of the molecular formula $\alpha_2{}^A\beta_2{}^{145Tyr\rightarrow Cys}$; heterozygotes have polycythemia because of increased oxygen affinity of this Hb.

reduced h., the form of Hb in red blood cells after the oxygen of oxyhemoglobin is released in the tissues.

h. S [MIM*141900], an abnormal Hb with substitution of valine for glutamic acid at the 6th position of the β chain; the formula is $\alpha_2{}^A\beta_2{}^S$, or, more specifically, $\alpha_2{}^A\beta_2{}^{6Glu\rightarrow Val}$. Heterozygous state: sickle cell trait, no anemia, Hb S 20 to 45% of total, the rest Hb A. Homozygous state: sickle cell anemia, Hb S 75 to 100% of total, the rest Hb F or Hb A_2. SYN sickle cell h.

sickle cell h. (Hb S), SYN h. S.

unstable h.'s, a group of rare Hb's with amino acid substitutions (or amino acid deletions in three types) that alter the three-dimensional shape of the globin in a manner that renders the molecule unstable; they have an increased but variable tendency to auto-oxidation and Heinz body formation and are associated with congenital nonspherocytic hemolytic anemia. The unstable β chain abnormalities include Hb's Genova, Gun Hill, Hammersmith, Köln, Philly, Sabine, Santa Ana, Sydney, Wien, and Zürich; unstable α chain abnormalities include Hb's Bibba, Sinai, and Torino.

variant h., a harmless mutant form of Hb.

h. Yakima [MIM*141900-0301], an abnormal Hb of the molecular formula $\alpha_2{}^A\beta_2{}^{99Asp\rightarrow His}$; heterozygotes have polycythemia because of increased oxygen affinity of this Hb.

---

he·mo·glo·bi·ne·mia (hē′mō-glo-bi-nē′mē-ă). The presence of free hemoglobin in the blood plasma, as when intravascular hemolysis occurs.

h. paralyt′ica, SYN *azoturia* of horses.

puerperal h., SYN postparturient *hemoglobinuria*.

he·mo·glo·bi·no·cho·lia (hē′mō-glō′bi-nō-kō′lē-ă). The presence of hemoglobin in the bile. [hemoglobin + G. *cholē*, bile]

he·mo·glo·bi·nol·y·sis (hē′mō-glō-bi-nol′i-sis). Destruction or chemical splitting of hemoglobin. SYN hemoglobinopepsia. [hemoglobin + G. *lysis*, dissolution]

he·mo·glo·bi·nop·a·thy (hē′mō-glō-bi-nop′ă-thē). A disorder or disease caused by or associated with the presence of hemoglobins in the blood, *e.g.*, sickle cell disease, thalassemia, hemoglobin C, D, E, H, or I disorders. Occasionally, combinations of abnormal hemoglobins are seen in hemoglobinopathies. [hemoglobin + G. *pathos*, disease]

he·mo·glo·bi·no·pep·sia (hē-mō-glō′bi-nō-pep′sē-ă). SYN hemoglobinolysis. [hemoglobin + G. *pepsis*, digestion]

he·mo·glo·bi·no·phil·ic (hē′mō-glō′bi-nō-fil′ik). Denoting certain microorganisms that cannot be cultured except in the presence of hemoglobin. [hemoglobin + G. *phileō*, to love]

he·mo·glo·bi·nu·ria (hē′mō-glō-bi-nū′rē-ă). The presence of hemoglobin in the urine, including certain closely related pigments that are formed from slight alteration of the hemoglobin molecule; when present in sufficient quantities, they result in the urine being colored varying shades from light red-yellow to fairly dark red. [hemoglobin + G. *ouron*, urine]

bacillary h., an acute toxemic disease of cattle caused by the bacterium *Clostridium haemolyticum* and characterized by severe depression, fever, abdominal pain, dyspnea, dysentery, hemoglobinuria, and rapid death; also occurs in sheep and, rarely, in dogs.

bovine h., SYN bovine *babesiosis*.

epidemic h., the presence of hemoglobin, or of pigments derived from it, in the urine of young infants, attended with cyanosis, jaundice, and other conditions; may be due to secondary methemoglobinemia; also called Winckel's disease.

intermittent h., recurrent episodic attacks of h. characteristic of paroxysmal nocturnal h. or paroxysmal cold h.

malarial h., a condition, now uncommon, resulting from *Plasmodium falciparum* infection (malignant tertian malaria with severe hemolysis); frequently seen in Caucasians after interrupted treatment with quinine. SYN blackwater fever, hemoglobinuric fever, West African fever.

march h., a form occurring after marathon races, protracted marching, or heavy physical exercise.

paroxysmal cold h., a rare disorder in which acute severe hemolysis follows exposure to cold.

paroxysmal nocturnal h., an infrequent disorder with insidious onset (usually in the third or fourth decade) and chronic course,

he

characterized by episodes of hemolytic anemia, hemoglobinuria (chiefly at night), pallor, icterus or bronzing of the skin, a moderate degree of splenomegaly, and sometimes hepatomegaly; red blood cells are usually macrocytic and vary considerably in size, but there is no evidence of spherocytosis, erythrophagocytosis, or abnormal leukocytes. The disorder is a result of an abnormality of the red cell membrane which makes the red cell unusually sensitive to lysis by complement. SYN Marchiafava-Micheli anemia, Marchiafava-Micheli syndrome.

postparturient h., a sudden, severe hemolytic disease that appears sporadically in well nourished dairy cows 2 to 4 weeks after calving, and usually occurs in stabled animals in the winter and early spring; the cause is not known, although the disease is often associated with hypophosphatemia. SYN puerperal hemoglobinemia, puerperal h.

puerperal h., SYN postparturient h.

toxic h., h. occurring after the ingestion of various poisons, in certain blood diseases, and in certain infections.

he·mo·glo·bi·nu·ric (hē′mō-glō-bi-nū′rik). Relating to or marked by hemoglobinuria.

he·mo·gram (hē′mō-gram). A complete detailed record of the findings in a thorough examination of the blood, especially with reference to the numbers, proportions, and morphologic features of the formed elements. [hemo- + G. *gramma,* a drawing]

he·mo·his·ti·o·blast (hē′mō-his′tē-ō-blast). A primitive mesenchymal cell believed to be capable of developing into all types of blood cells, including monocytes, and into histiocytes. SYN Ferrata′s cell, hematohistioblast. [hemo- + G. *histion,* web, + *blastos,* germ]

he·mo·la·mel·la (hē′mō-lă-mel′ă). SYN platelet.

he·mo·leu·ko·cyte (hē-mō-lū′kō-sīt). Obsolete term for leukocyte.

he·mo·li·pase (hē-mō-lip′ās). Blood lipase.

he·mo·lith (hē′mō-lith). A concretion in the wall of a blood vessel. [hemo- + G. *lithos,* stone]

he·mol·o·gy (hē-mol′ō-jē). SYN hematology.

he·mo·lymph (hē′mō-limf). **1.** The blood and lymph, in the sense of a "circulating tissue." **2.** The nutrient fluid of certain invertebrates. [hemo- + L. *lympha,* clear water]

he·mol·y·sate (hē-mol′i-sāt). Preparation resulting from the lysis of erythrocytes.

he·mo·ly·sin (hē-mol′i-sin). **1.** Any substance elaborated by a living agent and capable of causing lysis of red blood cells and liberation of their hemoglobin. SYN erythrocytolysin, erytholysin. **2.** A sensitizing (complement-fixing) antibody that combines with red blood cells of the antigenic type that stimulated formation of the h., affecting the cells in such a manner that complement fixes with the antibody-cell union and causes dissolution of the cells, with liberation of their hemoglobin.

α′ h., SEE α′ *hemolysis.*

β h., SEE β *hemolysis.*

bacterial h., any hemolytic agent elaborated by various species of bacteria, or by certain strains within a species.

cold h., SYN Donath-Landsteiner cold *autoantibody.*

heterophil h., a sensitizing antibody that can combine with red blood cells of various species (in addition to those used as the antigen in stimulating the formation of the h.), resulting in hemolysis when the proper amount of complement is present.

immune h., a sensitizing, complement-fixing, hemolytic antibody formed in an animal as the result of parenteral administration of red blood cells or whole blood from another species; immune h. may also be formed in human beings who are transfused with human blood that is antigenic in the recipient, *e.g.,* the formation of anti-Rh antibody in an Rh-negative person who is treated with Rh-positive red blood cells.

natural h., h. occurring in the plasma of an animal of one species, *e.g.,* a dog, which fixes complement with the red blood cells of some other species, *e.g.,* a rabbit, thereby causing hemolysis of the cells of the rabbit, although the dog was not previously exposed to antigenic stimulation with such cells.

specific h., a sensitizing, complement-fixing, hemolytic antibody

that reacts totally or completely with red blood cells of the antigenic type used to stimulate the formation of the h.

warm-cold h., h. which combines with red blood cells at temperatures below 20°C and are eluted at warmer temperatures, *e.g.,* 30 to 37°C. SEE Donath-Landsteiner cold *autoantibody,* hemagglutinating cold *autoantibody.*

he·mo·ly·sin·o·gen (hē′mō-lī-sin′ō-jen). The antigenic material in red blood cells that stimulates the formation of hemolysin.

he·mol·y·sis (hē-mol′i-sis). Alteration, dissolution, or destruction of red blood cells in such a manner that hemoglobin is liberated into the medium in which the cells are suspended, *e.g.,* by specific complement-fixing antibodies, toxins, various chemical agents, tonicity, alteration of temperature. SYN erythrocytolysis, erythrolysis, hematolysis. [hemo- + G. *lysis,* destruction]

α′ h., h. observed infrequently in blood agar cultures of occasional strains of streptococci; the zone of h. about the colony is not as clear, or wide, or distinctly outlined as it is in β h.; there are a few apparently intact erythrocytes throughout the zone, but they are more numerous in the immediate vicinity of the colony, and there is no discoloration as there is in α h.; the unique feature is that the zone becomes wider, *i.e.,* the process is stimulated, when the culture is incubated at refrigerator temperatures (not true for β h.); some strains of streptococci that are α′-hemolytic on horse blood agar cause typical α h. on rabbit blood agar.

β h., complete or "true" h. observed in blood agar cultures of various bacteria, especially hemolytic streptococci and staphylococci; virtually all of the erythrocytes are destroyed in a relatively wide, regularly circumscribed, circular zone about the colony, thereby resulting in a clear "halo" of transparent agar; the zone of h. is frequently much wider than the diameter of the colony; the degree of change varies with species of erythrocytes, *e.g.,* those of sheep and rabbits are usually more easily hemolyzed than those of man, and so on; the hemolysin acts extracellularly (in the absence of the bacterial cells) and may be quantitatively estimated by means of tube-dilution tests of a bacteria-free filtrate (containing the hemolytic substance) with a suspension of erythrocytes.

biologic h., h. caused by agents elaborated by various animal and plant forms.

conditioned h., SYN immune h.

γ h., a term sometimes used to indicate that there is no h. in relation to bacterial colonies in or on blood agar; thus, nonhemolytic organisms may be referred to as producing γ h.

immune h., h. caused by complement when erythrocytes have been sensitized by specific complement-fixing antibody. SYN conditioned h.

phenylhydrazine h. (fen′il-hī′-dră-zin), an *in vitro* test for G6PD deficiency; h. resulting from *in vitro* addition of phenylhydrazine to blood with red cells which are deficient in glucose-6-phosphate dehydrogenase (G6PD), with the appearance of Heinz-Ehrlich bodies.

venom h., that caused by hemolytic material in the venom of various species of snakes or other venomous animals.

viridans h., SEE α′ h.

he·mo·lyt·ic (hē-mō-lit′ik). Destructive to blood cells, resulting in dilation of hemoglobin. SYN hematolytic, hemotoxic (2), hematotoxic, hematoxic.

he·mo·ly·za·tion (hē′mol-i-zā′shŭn). The production or occurrence of hemolysis.

he·mo·lyze (hē′mō-līz). To produce hemolysis or liberation of the hemoglobin from red blood cells.

he·mo·ma·nom·e·ter (hē′mō-mă-nom′ĕ-ter). A manometer constructed and calibrated in such a manner that it is suitable for determining blood pressure. SYN hematomanometer.

he·mo·me·di·as·ti·num (hē′mō-mē-dē-ă-stī′nŭm). Blood in the mediastinum.

he·mo·me·tra (hē-mō-mē′tră). SYN hematometra.

he·mom·e·try (hē-mom′ĕ-trē). SYN hematometry.

he·mon·cho·sis (hē-mong-kō′sis). Infection of sheep or other ruminants with the nematode *Haemonchus contortus.*

he·mo·ne·phro·sis (hē′mō-ne-frō′sis). Obsolete term for blood in the pelvis of the kidney. [hemo- + G. *nephros,* kidney]

he·mo·pa·thol·o·gy (hē′mō-pa-thol′ō-jē). SYN hematopathology.

he·mop·a·thy (hē-mop′ă-thē). Any abnormal condition or disease of the blood or hemopoietic tissues. SYN hematopathy. [hemo- + G. *pathos,* suffering]

he·mo·per·fu·sion (hē′mō-per-fyū′zhŭn). Passage of blood through columns of adsorptive material, such as activated charcoal, to remove toxic substances from the blood. [hemo- + L. *perfusio,* to pass through]

he·mo·per·i·car·di·um (hē′mō-pār′-i-kar′dē-ŭm). Blood in the pericardial sac.

he·mo·per·i·to·ne·um (hē′mō-pār-i-tō-nē′ŭm). Blood in the peritoneal cavity.

he·mo·pex·in (hēm-ō-peks′in). A serum protein related to β-globulins, with molecular weight around 57,000, containing 22% carbohydrate; important in binding heme and porphyrins, preventing excretion, and perhaps regulating heme in drug metabolism. [hemo- + G. *pēxis,* fixation, + -in]

he·mo·pha·gia (hē-mō-fā′jē-ă). SYN hematophagia. [hemo- + G. *phagein,* to eat]

he·mo·phag·o·cy·to·sis (hē′mō-fag′ō-sī-tō′sis). The process of engulfment (and usually destruction) of blood cells by the various types of phagocytic cells; used especially with reference to the engulfment of erythrocytes and others of the erythroid series.

he·mo·phil, he·mo·phile (hē′mō-fil, -fīl). A microorganism growing preferably in media containing blood. [hemo- + G. *philos,* fond]

he·mo·phil·ia (hē-mō-fil′ē-ă). An inherited disorder of blood coagulation characterized by a permanent tendency to hemorrhages, spontaneous or traumatic, due to a defect in the blood coagulating mechanism. [hemo- + G. *philos,* fond]

  h. A [MIM*306900-various], h. due to deficiency of factor VIII; an X-linked recessive condition, occurring almost exclusively in human males and also affecting several breeds of dogs, characterized by prolonged clotting time, decreased formation of thromboplastin, and diminished conversion of prothrombin.

  h. B [MIM*306900-various], a clotting disorder resembling h. A, caused by hereditary deficiency of factor IX; also seen as an X-linked recessive condition in cairn terrier breed of dogs. SYN Christmas disease.

  h. C, h. due to deficiency of factor XI; clinically resembles h. A and B but is transmitted as an autosomal dominant inheritance.

  classical h., SEE h. A.

he·mo·phil·i·ac (hē-mō-fil′ē-ak). A person suffering from hemophilia.

he·mo·phil·ic (hē-mō-fil′ik). Relating to hemophilia.

he·mo·phil·o·sis (hē-mō-fil-ō′sis). Any disease caused by bacteria of the genus *Haemophilus.*

he·mo·pho·bia (hē-mō-fō′bē-ă). Morbid fear of blood or of bleeding. [hemo- + G. *phobos,* fear]

he·mo·pho·re·sis (hē′mō-fō-rē′sis). Blood convection or irrigation of tissues. [hemo- + G. *phoreō,* to bear]

he·moph·thal·mia, he·moph·thal·mus (hē-mof-thal′mē-ah, -mof-thal′mŭs). A blood-filled eye. SYN hematopsia. [hemo- + G. *ophthalmos,* eye]

he·moph·thi·sis (hē-mof′thi-sis, hē-mof-thī′sis). Anemia resulting from abnormal degeneration or destruction, or a deficiency in the formation of red blood cells. [hemo- + G. *phthisis,* a wasting away]

he·mo·plas·tic (hē-mō-plas′tik). SYN hemopoietic.

he·mo·plas·ty (hē′mō-plas-tē). Formation or elaboration of blood by the hemopoietic tissues. [hemo- + G. *plassō,* to form]

he·mo·pneu·mo·per·i·car·di·um (hē′mō-nū′mō-pār-i-kar′dē-ŭm). The occurrence of blood and air in the pericardium. SYN pneumohemopericardium. [hemo- + G. *pneuma,* air, + pericardium]

he·mo·pneu·mo·tho·rax (hē′mō-nū-mō-thō′raks). Accumulation of air and blood in the pleural cavity. SYN pneumohemothorax. [hemo- + G. *pneuma,* air, + thorax]

he·mo·poi·e·sis (hē′mō-poy-ē′sis). The process of formation and development of the various types of blood cells and other formed

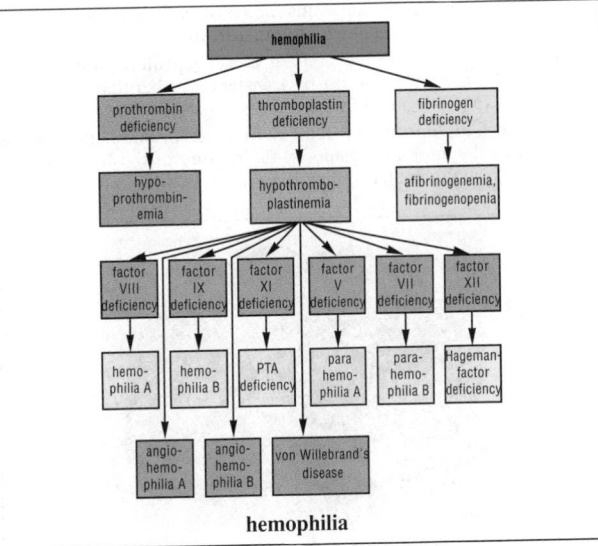

hemophilia

elements. SYN hematogenesis, hematopoiesis, hematosis (1), hemogenesis, sanguification. [hemo- + G. *poiēsis,* a making]

he·mo·poi·et·ic (hē′mō-poy-et′ik). Pertaining to or related to the formation of blood cells. SYN hemafacient, hematogenic (1), hematogenous, hematoplastic, hematopoietic, hemogenic, hemoplastic, sanguifacient.

he·mo·poi·e·tin (hē-mō-poy′ĕ-tin). SYN erythropoietin.

he·mo·por·phy·rin (hē-mō-pōr′fi-rin). SYN hematoporphyrin.

he·mo·pre·cip·i·tin (hē′mō-prē-sip′i-tin). An antibody that combines with and precipitates soluble antigenic material from erythrocytes.

he·mo·pro·tein (hē-mō-prō′tēn). Protein linked to a metal-porphyrin compound (*e.g.,* cytochromes, myoglobin, catalase).

he·mop·ty·sis (hē-mop′ti-sis). The spitting of blood derived from the lungs or bronchial tubes as a result of pulmonary or bronchial hemorrhage. [hemo- + G. *ptysis,* a spitting]

  cardiac h., h. secondary to heart disease or tachycardia.

  endemic h., SYN parasitic h.

  parasitic h., the clinical expression of paragonimiasis, marked by a cough and spitting of blood from the lungs. SYN endemic h.

he·mo·py·el·ec·ta·sis, he·mo·py·el·ec·ta·sia (hē′mō-pī′ĕ-lek′tă-sis, -lek-tā′zē-ă). Dilation of the pelvis of the kidney with blood and urine. [hemo- + pyelectasia]

he·mo·re·pel·lant (hē′mō-rē-pel′ant). **1.** A substance or surface that discourages the adherence of blood. **2.** Having such an action.

he·mo·rhe·ol·o·gy (he′mō-rē-ol′ō-jē). The science of the flow of blood in relation to the pressures, flow, volumes, and resistances in blood vessels, especially in terms of blood viscosity and red cell deformation in the microcirculation. [hemo- + G. *rheos,* stream, flow, + *logos,* study]

he·mor·rha·chis (hē-mōr′ă-kis). SYN hematorrhachis.

hem·or·rhage (hem′ŏ-rij). **1.** An escape of blood through rup-

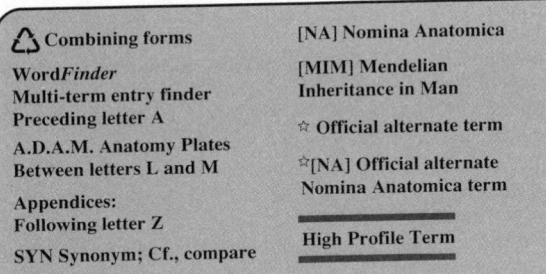

△ **Combining forms**

Word*Finder*
Multi-term entry finder
Preceding letter A

A.D.A.M. Anatomy Plates
Between letters L and M

Appendices:
Following letter Z

SYN Synonym; Cf., compare

[NA] **Nomina Anatomica**

[MIM] **Mendelian**
Inheritance in Man

☆ **Official alternate term**

☆[NA] **Official alternate**
Nomina Anatomica term

High Profile Term

he

tured or unruptured vessel walls. **2.** To bleed. [G. *haimorrhagia,* fr. *haima,* blood, + *rhēgnymi,* to burst forth]

brainstem h., h. into the pons or mesencephalon, often secondary to brainstem distortion by transentorial herniations due to rapidly expanding intracranial lesions.

cerebral h., h. into the substance of the cerebrum, usually in the region of the internal capsule by the rupture of the lenticulostriate artery. SYN hematencephalon, intracerebral h.

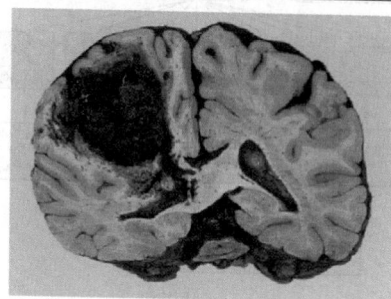

cerebral hemorrhage (left cerebrum)

concealed h., SYN internal h.

Duret's h., small brainstem h. resulting from brainstem distortion secondary to transentorial herniation.

extradural h., an accumulation of blood between the skull and the dura mater. SYN epidural hematoma.

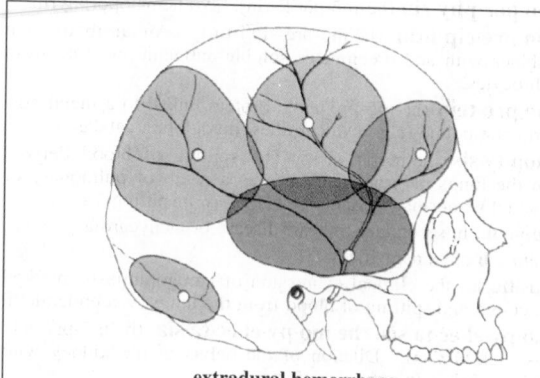

extradural hemorrhage
Krönlein diagram showing the position of drilling points for extradural hematomas in various places

gastric h., SYN gastrorrhagia.

intermediate h., h. that is recurrent.

internal h., bleeding into organs or cavities of the body. SYN concealed h.

intracerebral h., SYN cerebral h.

intracranial h., escape of blood within the cranium due to loss of integrity of vascular channels, frequently forming hematoma.

intrapartum h., h. occurring in the course of normal labor and delivery.

intraventricular h., extravasation of blood into the ventricular system of the brain.

nasal h., SYN epistaxis.

parenchymatous h., bleeding into the substance of an organ.

h. per rhex'is, h. due to the rupture of a blood vessel.

petechial h., capillary h. into the skin that forms petechiae. SYN punctate h.

pontine h., h. occurring in the substance of the pons, typically in hypertensive patients.

postpartum h., h. from the birth canal in excess of 500 ml after a vaginal delivery or 1000 ml after a cesarean delivery during the first 24 hours after birth.

primary h., h. immediately after an injury or operation, as distinguished from intermediate or secondary h.

punctate h., SYN petechial h.

renal h., gross hematuria, the source of which is in the kidney.

secondary h., h. at an interval after an injury or an operation.

serous h., obsolete term for a profuse transudation of plasma through the walls of the capillaries.

splinter h.'s, multiple tiny longitudinal subungual h.'s typically seen in but not diagnostic of bacterial endocarditis, trichinelliasis, etc.

subarachnoid h., extravasation of blood into the subarachnoid space, often due to aneurysm rupture and usually spreading throughout the cerebrospinal fluid pathways.

subdural h., extravasation of blood between the dural and arachnoidal membranes; acute and chronic forms occur; chronic hematomas may become encapsulated by neomembranes. SYN subdural hematoma.

subgaleal h., collection of blood beneath the galea aponeurotica.

syringomyelic h., h. into a syringomyelic cavity.

unavoidable h., obsolete term for h. occurring during labor in cases of placenta previa, as distinguished from accidental h.

hem·or·rhag·ic (hem-ŏ-raj'ik). Relating to or marked by hemorrhage.

hem·or·rhag·ins (hem-ŏ-raj'inz, -rā'jins). A group of toxins found in certain venoms and poisonous material from some plants, *e.g.,* rattlesnake venom and ricin; h. cause degeneration and lysis of endothelial cells in capillaries and small vessels, thereby resulting in numerous small hemorrhages in the tissues. [hemorrhage + -in]

hem·or·rhoid (hem'ŏ-royd). Denoting one of the tumors or varices constituting hemorrhoids.

external h., varicose dilatation of a vein of the external hemorrhoidal plexus, usually situated distal to the anal sphincter.

hem·or·rhoi·dal (hem-ŏ-roy'dăl). **1.** Relating to hemorrhoids. **2.** Formerly applied to certain arteries and veins supplying the region of the rectum and anus, currently replaced by "anal" or "rectal."

hem·or·rhoid·ec·to·my (hem'ŏ-roy-dek'tō-mē). Surgical removal of hemorrhoids; usually accomplished by excision of hemorrhoidal tissues by sharp dissection, or by application of elastic ligature at the base of the hemorrhoidal bundles to produce ischemic necrosis and ultimate ablation of the h. [hemorrhoids + G. *ektomē,* excision]

hem·or·rhoids (hem'ŏ-roydz). A varicose condition of the external hemorrhoidal veins causing painful swellings at the anus. SYN piles. [G. *haimorrhois,* pl. *haimorrhoides,* veins likely to bleed, fr. *haima,* blood, + *rhoia,* a flow]

cutaneous h., hyperplasia of the connective tissue in one or more of the normal radiating folds of the skin immediately surrounding the anus.

external h., dilated veins forming tumors at the outer side of the external sphincter.

internal h., dilated veins beneath the mucous membrane within the sphincter.

he·mo·sal·pinx (hē'mō-sal'pinks). SYN hematosalpinx.

he·mo·si·al·em·e·sis (hē'mō-sī-ăl-em'ĕ-sis). Vomiting of blood and saliva. [hemo- + G. *sialon,* saliva, + *emesis,* vomiting]

he·mo·sid·er·in (hē-mō-sid'er-in). A golden yellow or yellow-brown insoluble protein produced by phagocytic digestion of hematin; found in most tissues, especially in the liver, in the form of granules much larger than ferritin molecules (of which they are believed to be aggregates), but with a higher content, as much as 37%, of iron; stains blue with Perl's Prussian blue stain. [hemo- + G. *sidēros,* iron, + -in]

he·mo·sid·er·o·sis (hē'mō-sid-er-ō'sis). Accumulation of hemosiderin in tissue, particularly in liver and spleen. SEE hemochromatosis. [hemosiderin + -*osis,* condition]

idiopathic pulmonary h., repeated sudden attacks of dyspnea and hemoptysis leading to diffuse pulmonary h., seen most commonly in children; of unknown cause, but some cases may be associated with Goodpasture's syndrome. SYN Ceelen-Gellerstedt syndrome.

nutritional h., a disease seen in black South Africans that results from ingestion of iron in foodstuffs prepared in iron vessels; excessive absorption of iron affects the liver.

pulmonary h., h. usually associated with mitral stenosis and marked by an accumulation of macrophages loaded with hemosiderin within the alveoli.

he·mo·sper·mia (hē′mō-sper′mē-ă). The presence of blood in the seminal fluid. SYN hematospermia. [hemo- + G. *sperma,* seed]

h. spu′ria, h. occurring in the prostatic urethra.

h. ve′ra, h. in which the bleeding is from the seminal vesicles.

he·mo·spo·rid·i·um (hē′mō-spō-rid′ē-ŭm). A blood parasite of the order Haemosporidia. [hemo- + Mod. L. dim. of G. *sporos,* seed]

he·mo·spo·rines (hē′mō-spō-rēnz). Common term for members of the order Haemosporidia.

he·mo·sta·sia (hē-mō-stā′zē-ă). SYN hemostasis.

he·mo·sta·sis (hē′mō-stā-sis, hē-mos′tă-sis). **1.** The arrest of bleeding. **2.** The arrest of circulation in a part. **3.** Stagnation of blood. SYN hemostasia. [hemo- + G. *stasis,* a standing]

he·mo·stat (hē′mō-stat). **1.** Any agent that arrests, chemically or mechanically, the flow of blood from an open vessel. **2.** An instrument for arresting hemorrhage by compression of the bleeding vessel.

he·mo·stat·ic (hē-mō-stat′ik). **1.** Arresting the flow of blood within the vessels. **2.** SYN antihemorrhagic.

he·mo·styp·tic (hē-mo-stip′tik). SYN styptic (2). [hemo- + G. *styptikos,* astringent]

he·mo·suc·cus h. p.. bleeding into the pancreatic duct, usually as a result of trauma, tumor, inflammation, or pseudoaneurysm associated with pseudocyst.

he·mo·ta·cho·gram (hē-mō-ta′chō-gram). The record produced by hemotachometer. [hemo + tachos + G. *gramma,* something written]

he·mo·ta·chom·e·ter (hē′mō-tă-kom′ĕ-ter). An instrument for measuring the rapidity of the flow of blood in the arteries. SYN hematachometer. [hemo- + G. *tachos,* swiftness, + *metron,* measure]

he·mo·ther·a·py, he·mo·ther·a·peu·tics (hē′mō-thār′ă-pē, thār-ă-pyū′tiks). Treatment of disease by the use of blood or blood derivatives, as in transfusion. SYN hematherapy.

he·mo·tho·rax (hē-mō-thōr′aks). Blood in the pleural cavity. SYN hemathorax.

he·mo·thy·mia (hē-mō-thī′mē-ă). A passión for blood; a morbid impulse to commit murder. [hemo- + G. *thymos,* desire, anger]

he·mo·tox·ic, he·ma·to·tox·ic, he·ma·tox·ic (hē-mō-tok′sik; hē′mă-tō-toks′ik, hem′ă-; hē-mă-toks′ik, hem-ă-). **1.** Causing blood poisoning. **2.** SYN hemolytic.

he·mo·tox·in (hē-mō-tok′sin). Any substance that causes destruction of red blood cells, including various hemolysins; usually used with reference to substances of biologic origin, in contrast to chemicals. SYN hematotoxin, hematoxin.

cobra h., the constituent in cobra venom that hemolyzes the red blood cells of various species.

he·mo·troph, he·mot·ro·phe (hēm′ō-trof). The nutritive materials supplied to the embryos of placental mammals through the maternal bloodstream. Cf. embryotroph, histotroph. [hemo- + G. *trophē,* food]

he·mo·tro·pic (hē-mō-trop′ik). Pertaining to the mechanism by which a substance in or on blood cells, especially the erythrocytes, attracts phagocytic to the h. cells; the latter change direction and migrate toward the h. cells. SYN hematotropic. [hemo- + G. *tropos,* direction (or *trope,* a turning)]

he·mo·tym·pa·num (hē′mō-tim′pă-nŭm). The presence of blood in the middle ear. SYN hematotympanum.

he·mo·zo·ic (hē-mō-zō′ik). Parasitic in the blood of vertebrates; denoting certain protozoa. SYN hematozoic.

he·mo·zo·on (hē-mō-zō′on). A blood-dwelling parasitic animal

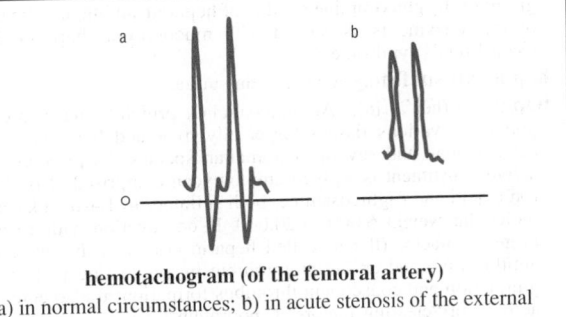

hemotachogram (of the femoral artery)
a) in normal circumstances; b) in acute stenosis of the external iliac artery

such as the trypanosomes or microfilariae of *Wuchereria* or *Brugia.* SYN hematozoon. [hemo- + G. *zöon,* animal]

HEMPAS Abbreviation for *h*ereditary *e*rythroblastic *m*ultinuclearity associated with *p*ositive *a*cidified *s*erum. SEE HEMPAS *cells,* under *cell.*

hen·bane (hen′bān). SYN hyoscyamus.

Henderson, Lawrence J., U.S. biochemist, 1879–1942. SEE H.-Hasselbalch *equation.*

Hen·der·so·nu·la to·ru·loi·dea (hen-der-sō-nyū′lă tōr-yū-loy′dē-ă). A species of black yeast capable of producing chronic infections of the nails as well as of the skin of the feet.

Henke, Wilhelm, German anatomist, 1834–1896. SEE H.'s *space.*

Henle, Friedrich G.J., German anatomist, pathologist, and histologist, 1809–1885. SEE *crypts* of H., under *crypt;* H.'s *ampulla, ansa, glands,* under *gland, fissures,* under *fissure, layer,* fiber *layer,* nervous *layer, loop, membrane,* fenestrated elastic *membrane, reaction, sheath, spine, tubules,* under *tubule, warts,* under *wart;* Hassall-H. *bodies,* under *body.*

hen·na (hen′ă). The leaves of the Egyptian privet, *Lawsonia inermis;* used as a cosmetic and hair dye. [Ar. *hennā*]

Hen·ne·bert. Camille, Belgian otologist, 1867–1958. SEE Hennebert's *sign.*

Henoch, Eduard H., German pediatrician, 1820–1910. SEE H.'s *chorea, purpura;* H.-Schönlein *purpura, syndrome;* Schönlein-H. *syndrome.*

hen·pu·ye (hen-pū′yē). SYN goundou. [native term on the Gold Coast (Ghana) meaning "dog-nose"]

Hen·ri, Victor, French 20th-century biochemist. SEE Michaelis-Menten *equation.*

Henry, James Paget, U. S. physiologist, *1914. SEE H.-Gauer *response.*

Henry, Joseph, U.S. physicist, 1797–1878. SEE Dalton-H. *law.*

Henry, William, British chemist, 1775–1837. SEE H.'s *law.*

hen·ry (H) (hen′rē). The unit of electrical inductance, when 1 volt is induced by a change in current of 1 ampere/sec. [Joseph *Henry*]

Henseleit, K., German internist, *1907. SEE Krebs-H. *cycle.*

Hensen, Victor, German anatomist and physiologist, 1835–1924. SEE H.'s *canal, cell, disk, duct, knot, line, node, stripe.*

Hensing, Friedrich W., German anatomist, 1719–1745. SEE H.'s *ligament.*

He·pad·na·vi·ri·dae (hē-pa′dnă-vī′rā-dā). A family of icosahedral DNA-containing viruses 42 mm in diameter whose genome is circular and mainly double-stranded, and is associated with hepatitis in a number of animal species. The principal genus *Hepadnavirus* is associated with hepatitis B. [*hep*atitis + DNA + virus]

he·par, gen. **hep·a·tis** (hē′par, hē′pah-tis) [NA]. SYN liver, liver. [L. borrowed fr. G. *hēpar,* gen. *hēpatos,* the liver]

h. loba′tum, a fissured liver, from the scars of healed syphilitic gummas.

hep·a·ran *N*-**sul·fa·tase** (hep′ă-ran). An enzyme that participates in the stepwise degradation of heparan sulfate; heparan *N*-sulfatase hydrolyzes the sulfate moiety attached to the amino group of the glucosamine residue of heparan sulfate; a deficiency of this enzyme is associated with mucopolysaccharidose IIIA (Sanfilippo's syndrome A).

hep·a·ran sul·fate. SYN heparitin sulfate.

hep·a·rin (hep'ă-rin). An anticoagulant principle that is a component of various tissues (especially liver and lung) and mast cells in man and several mammalian species; its principle and active constituent is a glycosaminoglycan comprised of D-glucuronic acid and D-glucosamine, both sulfated, in 1,4-α linkage, of molecular weight 6,000 to 20,000. In conjunction with a serum protein cofactor (the so-called heparin cofactor), h. acts as an antithrombin and an antiprothrombin by preventing platelet agglutination and consequent thrombus formation; it also enhances activity of "clearing factors" (lipoprotein lipases). SYN heparinic acid.

h. eliminase, SYN h. lyase.

h. lyase, an enzyme eliminating Δ-4,5-D-glucuronate residues from heparin and similar 1,4-linked polyglucuronates. SYN h. eliminase, heparinase.

h. sodium, a mixture of active principles (usually obtained from various tissues of domestic animals) having the properties of prolonging the clotting time of human blood; used in the treatment of angina pectoris, intermittent claudication, coronary thrombosis, and similar conditions.

hep·a·rin·ase (hep'ă-rin-ās). SYN *heparin* lyase.

hep·a·ri·ne·mia (hep'ă-ri-nē'mē-ă). The presence of demonstrable levels of heparin in the circulating blood.

hep·a·rin·ic ac·id (hep-ă-rin'ik). SYN heparin.

hep·a·rin·ize (hep'ă-rin-īz). To perform therapeutic administration of heparin.

hep·a·rit·in sul·fate (hep'ă-rit-in). A heteropolysaccharide that has the same repeating disaccharide as heparin but with fewer sulfates and more acetyl groups; accumulates in individuals with certain types of mucopolysaccharidosis. SYN heparan sulfate.

⌂**hepat-, hepatico-, hepato-.** The liver. [G. *hēpar* (*hēpat-*)]

hep·a·ta·tro·phia, hep·a·tat·ro·phy (hep'ă-tă-trō'fē-ă, hep-ă-tat'rō-fē). Atrophy of the liver.

hep·a·tec·to·my (hep-ă-tek'tō-mē). Removal of the liver, whole or in part. [hepat- + G. *ektomē*, excision]

he·pa·tic (he-pat'ik). Relating to the liver. [G. *hēpatikos*]

⌂**hepatico-.** SEE hepat-.

he·pat·i·co·do·chot·o·my (he-pat'i-kō-dō-kot'ō-mē). Combined hepaticotomy and choledochotomy.

he·pat·i·co·du·o·de·nos·to·my (he-pat'i-kō-dū'ō-de-nos'tō-mē). Establishment of a communication between the hepatic ducts and the duodenum. SYN hepatoduodenostomy. [hepatico- + duodenostomy]

he·pat·i·co·en·ter·os·to·my (he-pat'i-kō-en-ter-os'tō-mē). Establishment of a communication between the hepatic ducts and the intestine. SYN hepatocholangioenterostomy. [hepatico- + enterostomy]

he·pat·i·co·gas·tros·to·my (he-pat'i-kō-gas-tros'tō-mē). Establishment of a communication between the hepatic duct and the stomach. [hepatico- + gastrostomy]

he·pat·i·co·li·thot·o·my (he-pat'i-kō-li-thot'ō-mē). Removal of a stone from a hepatic duct. [hepatico- + G. *lithos*, stone, + *tomē*, a cutting]

he·pat·i·co·lith·o·trip·sy (he-pat'i-kō-lith'ō-trip-sē). The crushing or fragmentation of a biliary calculus in the hepatic duct. [hepatico- + G. *lithos*, stone, + *tripsis*, a rubbing]

he·pat·i·co·pul·mo·nary (he-pat'i-kō-pul'mŏ-nār-ē). SYN hepatopneumonic.

he·pat·i·cos·to·my (he-pat-i-kos'tō-mē). Establishment of an opening into the hepatic duct. [hepatico- + G. *stoma*, mouth]

he·pat·i·cot·o·my (he-pat-i-kot'ō-mē). Incision into the hepatic duct. [hepatico- + G. *tomē*, incision]

hep·a·tin (hep'ă-tin). SYN glycogen.

hep·a·tit·ic (hep-ă-tit'ik). Relating to hepatitis.

---

hep·a·ti·tis (hep-ă-tī'tis). Inflammation of the liver; usually from a viral infection, but sometimes from toxic agents. [hepat- + G. *-itis,* inflammation]

Previously endemic throughout much of the developing world, viral hepatitis now ranks as a major public health problem in industrialized nations. The three most common types of viral hepatitis—A, B, and C—afflict over 500,000 people in the U.S. each year, and millions worldwide. Hepatitis B alone ranks as the ninth leading killer in the world. Hepatitis A, an RNA enterovirus, spread by contact with fecal matter or blood, most often through ingestion of contaminated food. Rarely fatal, it cannot be treated except by bed rest for 1–4 weeks, during which time no alcohol should be consumed. It may recur after 3 months. Hepatitis B is shed through blood, semen, vaginal secretions, and saliva approximately 4–6 weeks after symptoms develop; the virus may take up to 6 months to incubate, and people may also become asymptomatic carriers. Hepatitis B may heal slowly, and is a leading cause of chronic liver disease and cirrhosis. Effective vaccines exist, but it is the fastest spreading form of the disease in the U.S., with some 300,000 cases reported annually. Rates were up 80% from 1981–1986 among IV drug users and up 38% during the same period among heterosexuals; among homosexuals, previously a high-risk group, rates held stable. Hepatitis C, infecting about 150,000 Americans annually, remains in the blood for years and accounts for a large percentage of cirrhosis, liver failure, and liver cancer cases. Its main mode of transmission is through blood transfusion, and possibly sexual intercourse. Types D and E are less frequently seen in the U.S.

---

h. A, SYN viral h. type A.

active chronic h., h. with chronic portal inflammation that extends into the parenchyma, with piecemeal necrosis and fibrosis which usually progresses to a coarsely nodular postnecrotic cirrhosis. SYN juvenile cirrhosis, posthepatitic cirrhosis, subacute h.

acute parenchymatous h., SYN acute yellow *atrophy* of the liver.

anicteric h., h. without jaundice.

anicteric virus h., a relatively mild h., without jaundice, due to a virus; the principal physical signs and symptoms are enlargement of the liver, lymph nodes, and often the spleen, together with headache, continuous fatigue, nausea, anorexia, sudden distaste for smoking, abdominal pains, and sometimes mild fever; labratory tests reveal evidence of hepatitis.

h. B, SYN viral h. type B.

hepatitis C, SYN viral h. type C.

cholangiolitic h., h. with inflammatory changes around small bile ducts, producing mainly obstructive jaundice; may be due to viral infection or bacterial infection ascending biliary tree because of obstruction.

cholestatic h., jaundice with bile stasis in inflamed intrahepatic bile ducts; usually due to toxic effects of a drug.

chronic h., any of several types of h. persisting for more than six months, often progressing to cirrhosis. SYN chronic active liver disease.

chronic interstitial h., obsolete term for cirrhosis of the liver.

chronic persistent h., SYN chronic persisting h.

chronic persisting h., a form of chronic h. that is usually benign, not progressing to cirrhosis, and usually asymptomatic without physical findings but with continuing abnormalities of tests of liver status. SYN chronic persistent h.

h. contagio'sa ca'nis, SYN infectious canine h.

h. D, SYN viral h. type D.

delta h., SYN viral h. type D.

drug-induced h., hepatocellular damage produced by a drug.

duck viral h., an acute, highly contagious disease of young ducklings caused by an enterovirus and characterized by lethargy, spasmodic paddling and rapid death.

h. E, SYN viral h. type E.

epidemic h., SYN viral h. type A.

equine serum h., an acute hepatic disease of the horse, often associated with prior administration of biological products; neurologic signs and jaundice are usually prominent signs; etiology is unknown. SYN Theiler's disease (2).

h. exter′na, SYN perihepatitis.

fulminant h., severe, rapidly progressive loss of hepatic function due to viral infection or other cause of inflammatory destruction of liver tissue.

giant cell h., SYN neonatal h.

goose viral h., an acute, highly fatal disease of goslings and Muscovy ducklings caused by the goose parvovirus and characterized by anorexia, feather loss, and tissue hemorrhages. SYN Derzsy's disease.

halothane h., hepatocellular damage said to result from the administration of halothane anesthesia.

infectious h. (IH), SYN viral h. type A.

infectious canine h., a disease of dogs, caused by canine adenovirus 1, and characterized by fever, depression, loss of appetite, vomiting, bloody diarrhea, petechial hemorrhages in the gums, pale mucous membranes, and jaundice. SYN h. contagiosa canis, Rubarth's disease.

infectious necrotic h. of sheep, a disease of sheep caused by the bacterium *Clostridium novyi*, which invades livers damaged by the fluke *Fasciola hepatica* and causes severe necrosis and death; this disease occurs in nearly all parts of the world, including the U.S. Sometimes called black disease because of the extensive hemorrhages seen on the inner surface of the pelt when it is removed. SYN black disease.

long incubation h., outdated name for h. B based on the longer incubation period (generally 30–180 days, usually 60–90) compared to h. A (15–45 days, mean 30).

lupoid h., jaundice with evidence of liver cell damage and positive antinuclear or LE cell tests, but without evidence of systemic lupus erythematosus; liver biopsies usually show active chronic h. with infiltration by plasma cells, or postnecrotic cirrhosis; serum is negative for h. B antigen. SYN plasma cell h.

mouse h., a form of h. in mice due to synergism between the mouse h. virus and *Eperythrozoon coccoides*. SYN murine h.

MS-1 h., SYN viral h. type A.

murine h., SYN mouse h.

NANB h., SYN non-A, non-B h.

NANBNC h., abbreviation for non-A, non-B, non-C h.

neonatal h., h. in the neonatal period presumed to be due to a variety of causes, chiefly viral; characterized by direct and indirect bilirubinemia, hepatocellular degeneration, and appearance of multinucleated giant cells; may be difficult to distinguish from biliary atresia, but is more likely to end with recovery, although cirrhosis may develop. SYN giant cell h.

non-A, non-B h., h. caused by two or more infectious agents not detectable by methods that reveal the presence of h. viruses A and B; one cause, now called type C h. has been identified; may follow blood transfusion and is often seen in chronic renal dialysis patients. SYN NANB h.

non-A, non-B, non-C h. (NANBNC h.), h. caused by viral organisms other than h. viruses A, B or C.

peliosis h., a rare condition in which the liver contains very numerous small blood-filled spaces, sometimes lined with endothelium; it may be found incidentally or rupture may cause intraperitoneal hemorrhage.

persistent chronic h., a benign chronic h. that may follow acute viral h. A or B, or complicate bowel diseases; after six months, liver biopsy changes are mild, unlike active chronic h.; rarely, if ever, progresses to cirrhosis, portal hypertension, or liver failure.

plasma cell h., SYN lupoid h.

serum h. (SH), SYN viral h. type B.

short incubation h., SYN viral h. type A.

subacute h., SYN active chronic h.

suppurative h., h. with abscess formation; often amebic in origin.

transfusion h., SYN viral h. type B.

viral h., (1) h. caused by any one of at least five immunologically unrelated viruses: h. A virus, h. B virus, h. C virus, h. D virus, h. E virus; **(2)** h. caused by a viral infection, including that by Epstein-Barr virus and cytomegalovirus. SYN virus h.

nomenclature of **hepatitis virus antigens** and the corresponding antibodies	
HA	hepatitis A
HAV	hepatitis A virus
HAA	hepatitis A antigen
anti-HAV	antibodies to HAV
anti-HAV-IgG	IgG antibodies to HAV
anti-HAV-IgM	IgM antibodies to HAV
HB	hepatitis B
HBV	hepatitis B virus
HBcAG	hepatitis B core antigen
HBeAG	hepatitis B e core antigen
HBsAG	hepatitis B s core antigen
anti-HBc	antibodies to HBcAG
anti-HBc-IgG	IgG antibodies to HBcAG
anti-HBc-IgM	IgM antibodies to HBcAG
anti-HBe	antibodies to HBeAG
anti-HBs	antibodies to HBsAG
HC	hepatitis C
HCV	hepatitis C virus
anti-HCV	antibodies to HCV
HD	hepatitis D
HDV	hepatitis D virus
anti-HDV	antibodies to HDV
delta-AG	delta antigen
anti-delta	antibodies to delta antigen
anti-delta-IgG	IgG antibodies to delta antigen
anti-delta-IgM	IgM antibodies to delta antigen
HE	hepatitis E
HEV	hepatitis E virus
anti-HEV-IgG	IgG antibodies to HEV
anti-HEV-IgM	IgM antibodies to HEV

viral hepatitis (incubation periods)	
hepatitis type	incubation period (days)
A	15–50
B	40–80
C	30–90
D	10–18
E	30–50

viral h. type A, a virus disease with a short incubation period (usually 15 to 50 days), caused by h. A virus, a member of the family Picornaviridae, often transmitted by fecal-oral route; may be inapparent, mild, severe, or occasionally fatal and occurs sporadically or in epidemics, commonly in school-age children and young adults; necrosis of periportal liver cells with lymphocytic and plasma cell infiltration is characteristic and jaundice is a common symptom. SYN epidemic h., h. A, infectious h., MS-1 h., short incubation h., virus A h.

viral h. type B, a virus disease with a long incubation period

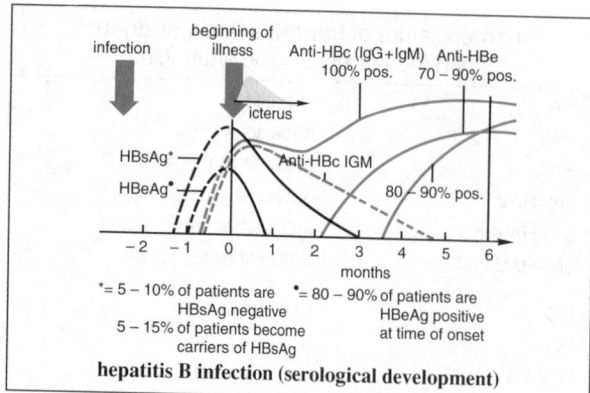

hepatitis B infection (serological development)

beginning of illness

infection

Anti-HBc (IgG+IgM) 100% pos. Anti-HBe 70 – 90% pos.

icterus

HBsAg*

HBeAg*

Anti-HBc IGM

80 – 90% pos.

−2 −1 0 1 2 3 4 5 6
months

*= 5 – 10% of patients are HBsAg negative
5 – 15% of patients become carriers of HBsAg

*= 80 – 90% of patients are HBeAg positive at time of onset

(usually 50 to 160 days), caused by hepatitis B virus, a DNA virus and member of the family Hepadnoviridae, usually transmitted by injection of infected blood or blood derivatives or by use of contaminated needles, lancets, or other instruments; clinically and pathologically similar to viral h. type A, but there is no cross-protective immunity; HB$_s$Ag is found in the serum and the hepatitis delta virus occurs in some patients. SYN h. B, serum h., transfusion h., virus B h.

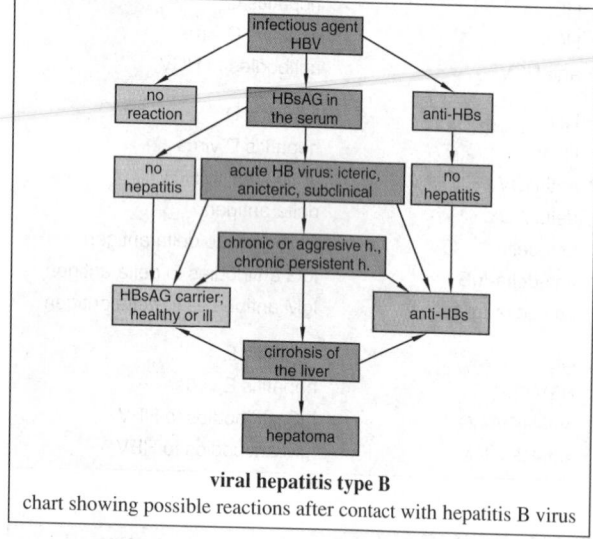

viral hepatitis type B

chart showing possible reactions after contact with hepatitis B virus

infectious agent HBV

no reaction

HBsAG in the serum

anti-HBs

no hepatitis

acute HB virus: icteric, anicteric, subclinical

no hepatitis

chronic or aggresive h., chronic persistent h.

HBsAG carrier; healthy or ill

anti-HBs

cirrohsis of the liver

hepatoma

viral h. type C, (NANB); principal cause of non-A, non-B posttransfusion h. caused by an RNA virus that may be related to Flaviviridae family. SYN hepatitis C, virus C h.

viral h. type D, acute or chronic h. caused by the h. delta virus, a defective RNA virus requiring HBV for replication. The acute type occurs in two forms: 1) coinfection, the simultaneous occurrence of h. B virus and h. delta virus infections, which usually is self-limiting; 2) superinfection, the appearance of h. delta virus infection in a h. B virus carrier, which often leads to chronic h. The chronic type appears to be more severe than other types of viral h. SYN delta h., h. D.

viral h. type E, h. caused by an RNA virus or possibly *Calicivirus*, and is the principal cause of enterically transmitted, waterborne, epidemic NANB hepatitis occurring primarily in Asia and Africa. SYN h. E.

virus h., SYN viral h.

virus A h., SYN viral h. type A.

virus B h., SYN viral h. type B.

virus C h., SYN viral h. type C.

virus h. of ducks, a disease of very young ducklings, caused by the duck h. virus (family Hepadnoviridae) and manifested as an acute illness of several days followed by death; the principal lesions are an enlarged necrotic liver filled with ecchymotic hemorrhages.

hep·a·ti·za·tion (hep′ă-ti-ză′shŭn). Conversion of a loose tissue into a firm mass like the substance of the liver macroscopically, denoting especially such a change in the lungs in the consolidation of pneumonia.

gray h., the second stage of h. in pneumonia, when the exudate is beginning to degenerate prior to breaking down; the color is a yellowish gray or mottled.

red h., the first stage of h. in which the exudate is blood-stained.

yellow h., the final stage of h. in which the exudate is becoming purulent.

△**hepato-.** SEE hepat-.

he·pa·to·blas·to·ma (hep′ă-tō-blas-tō′mă). A malignant neoplasm occurring in young children, primarily in the liver, composed of tissue resembling embryonal or fetal hepatic epithelium, or mixed epithelial and mesenchymal tissues.

he·pa·to·car·ci·no·ma (hep′ă-tō-kar-si-nō′mă). SYN malignant *hepatoma*.

he·pa·to·cele (hep′ă-tō-sēl, he-pat′ō-sēl). Protrusion of part of the liver through the abdominal wall or the diaphragm. [hepato- + G. *kēlē,* hernia]

he·pa·to·chol·an·gi·o·en·ter·os·to·my (hep′ă-tō-kō-lan′jē-ō-en-ter-os′tō-mē). SYN hepaticoenterostomy. [hepato- + G. *cholē,* bile, + *angeion,* vessel, + *enteron,* intestine, + *stoma,* mouth]

he·pa·to·chol·an·gi·o·je·ju·nos·to·my (hep′ă-tō-kō-lan′jē-ō-jē-jū-nos′tō-mē). Union of the hepatic duct to the jejunum. [hepato- + G. *cholē,* bile, + *angeion,* vessel, + jejunostomy]

he·pa·to·chol·an·gi·os·to·my (hep′ă-tō-kō-lan-jē-os′tō-mē). Creation of an opening into the common bile duct to establish drainage.

he·pa·to·chol·an·gi·tis (hep′ă-tō-kō-lan-jī′tis). Inflammation of the liver and biliary tree.

he·pa·to·cu·pre·in (hep′ă-tō-kū′prē-in). SYN cytocuprein.

he·pa·to·cys·tic (hep′ă-tō-sis′tik). Relating to the gallbladder, or to both liver and gallbladder. [hepato- + G. *kystis,* bladder]

He·pa·to·cys·tis (hep′ă-tō-sis′tis). A genus of blood-parasitizing hemosporines (family Plasmodiidae) with gametocytes in red cells and cystlike exoerythrocytic schizonts in the liver parenchyma; parasitic in Old World primates, bats, and squirrels, but not in domestic animals or in the western hemisphere. The species *H. kochi,* a common parasite of African baboons and other monkeys, is transmitted by the biting midge, *Culicoides.* [hepato- + G. *kystis,* bladder]

he·pa·to·cyte (hep′ă-tō-sīt). A parenchymal liver cell.

he·pa·to·du·o·de·nos·to·my (hep′ă-tō-dū-ō-de-nos′tō-mē). SYN hepaticoduodenostomy.

he·pa·to·dys·en·ter·y (hep′ă-tō-dis′en-ter-ē). Dysentery associated with liver disease.

he·pa·to·en·ter·ic (hep′ă-tō-en-tĕr′ik). Relating to the liver and the intestine. [hepato- + G. *enteron,* intestine]

hep·a·to·fu·gal (hep′ă-tō-fyū′găl). Away from the liver, usually referring to portal blood flow.

he·pa·to·gas·tric (hep′ă-tō-gas′trik). Relating to the liver and the stomach.

he·pa·to·gen·ic, he·pa·tog·e·nous (hep-ă-tō-jen′ik, -toj′en-ŭs). Of hepatic origin; formed in the liver.

he·pa·tog·ra·phy (hep-ă-tog′ră-fē). Radiography of the liver. [hepato- + G. *graphē,* a writing]

he·pa·to·he·mia (hep′ă-tō-hē′mē-ă). Rarely used term for congestion of the liver. [hepato- + G. *haima,* blood]

he·pa·toid (hep′ă-toyd). Resembling or like the liver. [hepato- + G. *eidos,* resemblance]

he·pa·to·jug·u·la·rom·e·ter (hep′ă-tō-jŭg′yū-lă-rom′ĕ-ter). An apparatus for the quantitative control and measurement of the pressure and force applied over the liver to test the hepatojugular reflux. [hepato- + L. *jugulum,* throat, + G. *metron,* measure]

he·pa·to·li·en·og·ra·phy (hep′ă-tō-lī-en-og′ră-fē). SYN hepatosplenography. [hepato- + L. *lien,* spleen, + G. *graphē,* a writing]

he·pa·to·li·en·o·meg·a·ly (hep'ă-tō-lī'ĕ-nō-meg'ă-lē). SYN hepatosplenomegaly.

he·pa·to·lith (hep'ă-tō-lith). A concretion in the liver. [hepato- + G. *lithos*, stone]

he·pa·to·li·thec·to·my (hep'ă-tō-li-thek'tō-mē). Removal of a calculus from the liver. [hepato- + G. *lithos*, stone, + *ektomē*, excision]

he·pa·to·li·thi·a·sis (hep'ă-tō-li-thī'ă-sis). Presence of calculi in the liver. [hepato- + G. *lithiasis*, presence of a calculus]

he·pa·tol·o·gist (hep-ă-tol'ō-jist). A specialist in hepatology.

he·pa·tol·o·gy (hep-ă-tol'ō-jē). The branch of medicine concerned with diseases of the liver. [hepato- + G. *logos*, study]

he·pa·tol·y·sin (hep-ă-tol'i-sin). A cytolysin that destroys parenchymal cells of the liver.

he·pa·to·ma (hep-ă-tō'mă). SEE malignant h. [hepato- + G. *-oma*, tumor]

malignant h., a carcinoma derived from parenchymal cells of the liver. SYN hepatocarcinoma, hepatocellular carcinoma, liver cell carcinoma.

he·pa·to·ma·la·cia (hep'ă-tō-mă-lā'shē-ă). Softening of the liver. [hepato- + G. *malakia*, softening]

he·pa·to·meg·a·ly, he·pa·to·me·ga·lia (hep'ă-tō-meg'ă-lē, -mĕ-gā'lē-ă). Enlargement of the liver. SYN megalohepatia. [hepato- + G. *megas*, large]

he·pa·to·mel·a·no·sis (hep'ă-tō-mel'ă-nō'sis). Heavy pigmentation of the liver. [hepato- + G. *melas*, black, + *-osis*, condition]

he·pa·tom·pha·lo·cele (hep'ă-tom-fal'ō-sēl, hep-ă-tom'fă-lō-sēl). Umbilical hernia with involvement of the liver. SYN hepatomphalos. [hepato- + omphalocele]

he·pa·tom·pha·los (hep-ă-tom'fă-lōs). SYN hepatomphalocele.

he·pa·to·ne·cro·sis (hep'ă-tō-ne-krō'sis). Death of liver cells.

he·pa·to·neph·ric (hep'ă-tō-nef'rik). SYN hepatorenal.

he·pa·to·neph·ro·meg·a·ly (hep'ă-tō-nef'rō-meg'ă-lē). Enlargement of both liver and kidney or kidneys. [hepato- + G. *nephros*, kidney, + *megas*, great]

he·pa·to·path·ic (hep'ă-tō-path'ik). Damaging the liver.

he·pa·top·a·thy (hep-ă-top'ă-thē). Disease of the liver. [hepato- + G. *pathos*, suffering]

he·pa·to·per·i·to·ni·tis (hep'ă-tō-pār'i-tō-nī'tis). SYN perihepatitis.

hep·a·to·pet·al (hep'ă-tō-pet'al). Toward the liver, usually referring to the normal direction of portal blood flow.

he·pa·to·pex·y (hep'ă-tō-pek-sē). Anchoring of the liver to the abdominal wall. [hepato- + G. *pēxis*, fixation]

he·pa·to·phy·ma (hep'ă-tō-fī'mă). Rounded or nodular tumor of the liver. [hepato- + G. *phyma*, tumor]

he·pa·to·pneu·mon·ic (hep'ă-tō-nū-mon'ik). Relating to the liver and the lungs. SYN hepaticopulmonary, hepatopulmonary. [hepato- + G. *pneumonikos*, pulmonary]

he·pa·to·por·tal (hep'ă-tō-pōr'tăl). Relating to the portal system of the liver.

he·pa·to·pto·sis (hep'ă-top-tō'sis, tō-tō'sis). A downward displacement of the liver. SYN wandering liver. [hepato- + G. *ptōsis*, a failing]

he·pa·to·pul·mo·nary (hep'ă-tō-pŭl'mō-nār'ē). SYN hepatopneumonic.

he·pa·to·re·nal (hep-ă-tō-rē'năl). Relating to the liver and the kidney. SYN hepatonephric. [hepato- + L. *renalis*, renal, fr. *renes*, kidneys]

he·pa·tor·rha·gia (hep'ă-tō-rā'jē-ă). Hemorrhage into or from the liver. [hepato- + G. *rhēgnymi*, to burst forth]

he·pa·tor·rha·phy (hep-ă-tōr'ă-fē). Suture of a wound of the liver. [hepato- + G. *rhaphē*, a suture]

he·pa·tor·rhex·is (hep'ă-tō-rek'sis). Rupture of the liver. [hepato- + G. *rhēxis*, rupture]

he·pa·tos·co·py (hep-ă-tos'kŏ-pē). Examination of the liver. [hepato- + G. *skopeō*, to examine]

he·pa·to·sple·ni·tis (hep'ă-tō-splē-nī'tis). Inflammation of the liver and spleen.

he·pa·to·sple·nog·ra·phy (hep'ă-tō-splē-nog'ră-fē). The use of a contrast medium to outline or depict the liver and spleen radiographically. SYN hepatolienography.

he·pa·to·splen·o·meg·a·ly (hep'ă-tō-splē-nō-meg'ă-lē). Enlargement of the liver and spleen. SYN hepatolienomegaly. [hepato- + G. *splēn*, spleen, + *megas*, large]

he·pa·to·sple·nop·a·thy (hep'ă-tō-splē-nop'ă-thē). Disease of the liver and spleen.

he·pa·tos·to·my (hep-ă-tos'tō-mē). Establishment of a fissure into the liver. [hepato- + G. *stoma*, mouth]

he·pa·to·ther·a·py (hep'ă-tō-thār'ă-pē). Rarely used term for: 1. Treatment of disease of the liver. 2. Therapeutic use of liver extract or of the raw substance of the liver.

he·pa·tot·o·my (hep-ă-tot'ō-mē). Incision into the liver. [hepato- + G. *tome*, incision]

he·pa·to·tox·e·mia (hep'ă-tō-tok-sē'mē-ă). Autointoxication assumed to be due to improper functioning of the liver. [hepato- + G. *toxikon*, poison, + *haima*, blood]

he·pa·to·tox·ic (hep'ă-tō-tok'sik). Relating to an agent that damages the liver, or pertaining to any such action.

he·pa·to·tox·ic·i·ty. The capacity of a drug, chemical, or other exposure to produce injury to the liver. Agents with recognized hepatotoxicity include carbon tetrachloride, alcohol, dantrolene sodium, valproic acid, isonicotinic acid hydrazide.

he·pa·to·tox·in (hep'ă-tō-tok'sin). A toxin that is destructive to parenchymal cells of the liver.

He·pa·to·zo·on (hep'ă-tō-zō'on). A genus of coccidian parasites (family Haemogregarinidae), in which schizogony occurs in the visceral organs, gametogony in the leukocytes or erythrocytes of vertebrate animals, and sporogony in certain ticks and other blood-sucking invertebrates. *H. canis* occurs in dogs, cats, jackals, and hyenas, but is most pathogenic in dogs, in which it may cause serious disease and death; other species have been described from rats, mice, rabbits, and squirrels. [hepato- + G. *zōon*, animal]

HEPES. 4-(2-Hydroxyethyl)-1-piperazineethanesulfonic acid; a compound lacking in pharmacological effects and widely used as a biological buffer in *in vitro* experiments.

hepta-. Prefix denoting seven. Cf. septi-, sept-. [G. *hepta*]

hep·ta·chlor (hep'tă-klōr). An insecticide for control of cotton boll weevil. It is a poison which may enter the body via skin contamination, inhalation or ingestion. Because of human toxicity concerns, this chemical has only limited application.

hep·tad (hep'tad). A septivalent chemical element or radical.

hep·tam·i·nol (hep-tam'i-nol). 6-Amino-2-methyl-2-heptanol; a sympathomimetic, vasoconstrictor, and cardiotonic.

hep·ta·nal (hep'tă-năl). $CH_3(CH_2)_5CHO$; heptaldehyde; obtained from the ricinoleic acid of castor oil by chemical means; used in the manufacture of ethyl oenanthate, a constituent of many artificial essences (flavors). SYN enanthal, oenanthal.

hep·ta·pep·tide (hep-tă-pep'tīd). A peptide containing seven amino acids.

hep·tose (hep'tōs). A sugar with seven carbon atoms in its molecule; *e.g.*, sedoheptulose.

hep·tu·lose (hep'tū-lōs). SYN ketoheptose.

D-*altro*-2-hep·tu·lose. SYN sedoheptulose.

D-*manno*-hep·tu·lose. A ketoheptose of the mannose configuration, occurring in the urine of individuals who have eaten a large quantity of avocados.

***n*-hep·tyl·pen·i·cil·lin** (hep'til-pen-ĭ-sil'in). Penicillin K.

Herbert, Herbert, English ophthalmic surgeon, 1865–1942.

her·biv·o·rous (her-biv'ŏ-rŭs). Feeding on plants. [L. *herba*, herb, + *voro*, to devour]

Herbst, Ernst F.G., German anatomist, 1803–1893. SEE H.'s *corpuscles*, under *corpuscle*.

herd. A group of people or animals in a given area. [O.E. *heord*]

he·red·i·tary (hĕ-red'i-ter-ē). Transmissible from parent to offspring by information encoded in the parental germ cell. [L. *hereditarius;* fr. *heres* (*hered*-), an heir]

he·red·i·ty (hĕ-red'i-tē). 1. The transmission of characters from parent to offspring by information encoded in the parental germ

he

cells. **2.** Genealogy. [L. *hereditas,* inheritance, fr. *heres* (*hered-*), heir]

⌂**heredo-.** Heredity. [L. *heres,* an heir]

her·e·do·path·ia atac·ti·ca pol·y·neu·ri·ti·for·mis (her′ĕ-dō-path′ē-ă ă-tak′ti-kă pol′ē-nū-rī-ti-fōr′mis). SYN Refsum's *disease.*

her·e·do·tax·ia. SYN hereditary spinal *ataxia.*

Herelle, Felix H. SEE d'Herelle.

He·rel·lea (hĕ-rel′ē-ă). A bacterial generic name which has been officially rejected because its type species, *H. vaginicola,* is a member of the genus *Acinetobacter.*

Hering, Heinrich Ewald, German physiologist, 1866–1948. SEE sinus *nerve* of H.; H.-Breuer *reflex;* Traube-H. *curves,* under *curve.*

Hering, Karl E.K., German physiologist, 1834–1918. SEE H.'s *test, theory* of color vision; *canal* of H.; Traube-H. *curves,* under *curve, waves,* under *wave;* Semon-Hering *theory.*

her·i·ta·bil·i·ty (her′i-tă-bil′i-tē). **1.** In psychometrics, a statistical term used to denote the extent of variance of an individual's total score or response which is attributable to a presumed genetic component, in contrast to an acquired component. **2.** In genetics, a statistical term used to denote the proportion of phenotypic variance due to variance in genotypes that is genetically determined, denoted by the traditional symbol h^2. [see heredity]

h. in the broad sense, the proportion of the total phenotypic variance that can be ascribed to genetic factors of any kind (additive, those due to dominance effects, epistasis and hypostasis, and interactions of all kinds).

h. in the narrow sense, the proportion of the total phenotypic variance that can be ascribed to additive genetic variance alone. It reflects the similarity between parent and offspring, and is related to the breeding value so important to commercial breeding.

her·i·tage (her′i-tij). The total of all the inherited characters. [O. Fr]

Herlitz, Gillis, Swedish pediatrician, *1902. SEE H. *syndrome.*

Herman. SEE Padykula-Herman *stain* for myosin ATPase.

Hermann, Friedrich, German anatomist, 1859–1920. SEE H.'s *fixative.*

Hermansky, F. Hermansky, 20th century Czech physician. SEE H.-Pudlak *syndrome;* H.-Pudlak *syndrome* type VI.

her·maph·ro·dism (her-maf′rō-dizm). SYN hermaphroditism.

her·maph·ro·dite (her-maf′rō-dīt). An individual with hermaphroditism. [G. *Hermaphroditos,* the son of *Hermēs,* Mercury, + *Aphroditē,* Venus]

her·maph·ro·dit·ism (her-maf′rō-dīt-izm). The presence in one individual of both ovarian and testicular tissue; *i.e.,* true h. SYN hermaphrodism.

adrenal h., altered appearance of the genitalia due to disorders of adrenocortical function, most often female virilization; not an example of true h.

bilateral h., true h. with an ovotestis on both sides.

dimidiate h., SYN lateral h.

false h., SYN pseudohermaphroditism.

female h., more correctly female pseudohermaphroditism, as the term is commonly used; however, it may designate true h., in which overt bodily characteristics are predominantly female.

lateral h., a form in which a testis is present on one side and an ovary on the other. SYN dimidiate h.

male h., more correctly designated as male pseudohermaphroditism, as the term is commonly used; however, it may designate an instance of true h. in which overt bodily characteristics are predominantly male.

transverse h., pseudohermaphroditism in which the external genitalia are characteristic of one sex and the gonads are characteristic of the other sex.

true h., h. in which both ovarian and testicular tissue are present. Somatic characteristics of both sexes are present; also called true intersex.

unilateral h., h. in which the doubling of sex characteristics occurs on one side only: ovotestis on one side and either ovary or testis on the other.

her·met·ic (her-met′ik). Airtight; denoting a vessel closed or sealed in such a way that air can neither enter it nor issue from it.

HERNIA

her·nia (her′nē-ă). Protrusion of a part or structure through the tissues normally containing it. SYN rupture (1). [L. rupture]

abdominal h., a h. protruding through or into any part of the abdominal wall. SYN laparocele.

Barth's h., a loop of intestine between a persistent vitelline duct and the abdominal wall.

Béclard's h., a h. through the opening for the saphenous vein.

bilocular femoral h., SYN Cooper's h.

h. en bissac, SYN properitoneal inguinal h.

Bochdalek's h., SYN congenital diaphragmatic h.

h. of the broad ligament of the uterus, a coil of intestine contained in a pouch projecting into the substance of the broad ligament.

cecal h., a h. containing cecum.

cerebral h., protrusion of brain substance through a defect in the skull.

Cloquet's h., a femoral h. perforating the aponeurosis of the pectineus and insinuating itself between this aponeurosis and the muscle, lying therefore behind the femoral vessels.

complete h., an indirect inguinal h. in which the contents extend into the tunica vaginalis.

concealed h., a h. not found on inspection or palpation.

congenital diaphragmatic h., absence of the pleuroperitoneal membrane (usually on the left) or an enlarged Morgagni's foramen which allows protrusion of abdominal viscera into the chest. SYN Bochdalek's h.

Cooper's h., a femoral h. with two sacs, the first being in the femoral canal, and the second passing through a defect in the superficial fascia and appearing immediately beneath the skin. SYN bilocular femoral h., Hey's h.

crural h., SYN femoral h.

diaphragmatic h., protrusion of abdominal contents into the chest through a weakness in the respiratory diaphragm; a common type is the hiatal h.

direct inguinal h., SEE inguinal h.

double loop h., SYN "w" h.

dry h., a h. with adherent sac and contents.

duodenojejunal h., a h. in the subperitoneal tissues. SYN retroperitoneal h., Treitz' h.

epigastric h., h. through the linea alba above the navel.

extrasaccular h., SYN sliding h.

fascial h., a bulging of muscle through a defect in its fascia.

fat h., h. in which the tissue protruding out of its normal location is composed only of fat.

fatty h., SYN pannicular h.

femoral h., h. through the femoral ring. SYN crural h., femorocele.

gastroesophageal h., a hiatal h. into the thorax.

gluteal h., SYN sciatic h.

Hesselbach's h., h. with diverticula through the cribriform fascia, presenting a lobular outline.

Hey's h., SYN Cooper's h.

hiatal h., hiatus h., h. of a part of the stomach through the esophageal hiatus of the diaphragm.

Holthouse's h., inguinal h. with extension of the loop of intestine along Poupart's ligament.

iliacosubfascial h., a h. the sac of which passes through the iliac fascia and lies in the iliac fossa in contact with the iliacus muscle.

incarcerated h., SYN irreducible h.

incisional h., h. occurring through a surgical incision or scar.

indirect inguinal h., SEE inguinal h.

infantile h., a h. in which an intestinal loop descends behind the tunica vaginalis, having, therefore, three peritoneal layers in front of it.

inguinal h., a h. at the inguinal region: direct inguinal h. involves the abdominal wall between the deep epigastric artery and the edge of the rectus muscle; indirect inguinal h. involves the internal inguinal ring and passes into the inguinal canal.

inguinocrural h., inguinofemoral h., a bilocular or double h., both inguinal and femoral.

inguinolabial h., an inguinal h. descending into the labium.

inguinoscrotal h., an inguinal h. descending into the scrotum.

inguinosuperficial h., an inguinal h. that has turned cephalad away from the scrotum and lies subcutaneously on the abdominal wall.

internal h., protrusion of an intraperitoneal viscus into a compartment within the abdominal cavity.

intersigmoid h., a h. into the intersigmoid fossa on the under surface of the root of the mesosigmoid near the inner border of the psoas magnus muscle.

interstitial h., a h. in which the protrusion is between any two of the layers of the abdominal wall.

intraepiploic h., a coil of intestine incarcerated in an omental sac.

intrailiac h., an interstitial h. projecting from the internal inguinal ring.

intrapelvic h., an interstitial h. projecting into the pelvis from the internal inguinal ring.

irreducible h., a h. that cannot be reduced without operation. SYN incarcerated h.

ischiatic h., a h. through the sacrosciatic foramen.

Krönlein's h., SYN properitoneal inguinal h.

labial h., h. through the canal of Nuck.

lateral ventral h., SYN spigelian h.

Laugier's h., a h. passing through an opening in the lacunar ligament.

levator h., SYN perineal h.

Littré's h., (1) SYN parietal h. **(2)** h. of Meckel's diverticulum.

lumbar h., a protrusion between the last rib and the iliac crest where the aponeurosis of the transversus muscle is covered only by the latissimus dorsi.

Malgaigne's h., infantile inguinal h. prior to the descent of the testis.

meningeal h., herniation of meninges through a spina bifida.

mesenteric h., h. through a hole in the mesentery.

obturator h., h. through the obturator foramen.

orbital h., displacement of orbital fat through a defect in the orbital septum or Tenon's capsule into the subcutaneous tissues of the eyelid or subconjunctivally.

pannicular h., the escape of subcutaneous fat through a gap in a fascia or an aponeurosis. SYN fatty h.

pantaloon h., an inguinal h. that involves both an indirect and a direct component.

paraduodenal h., a type of internal h., resulting from abnormal or incomplete midgut rotation, which involves one of several paraduodenal spaces.

paraesophageal h., a non-sliding hernia through or adjacent to the esophageal hiatus of the diaphragm; most commonly contains stomach and other abdominal viscera.

parahiatal h., a h. through the diaphragm that occurs at a point separate from the esophageal hiatus.

paraperitoneal h., a vesical h. in which only a part of the protruded organ is covered by the peritoneum of the sac.

parasaccular h., SYN sliding h.

parasternal h., SYN Morgagni's *foramen* (2).

parietal h., a h. in which only a portion of the wall of the intestine is engaged. SYN Littré's h. (1), partial enterocele, Richter's h.

perineal h., a h. protruding through the pelvic diaphragm. SYN levator h., pudendal h.

Petit's h., lumbar h., occurring in Petit's triangle.

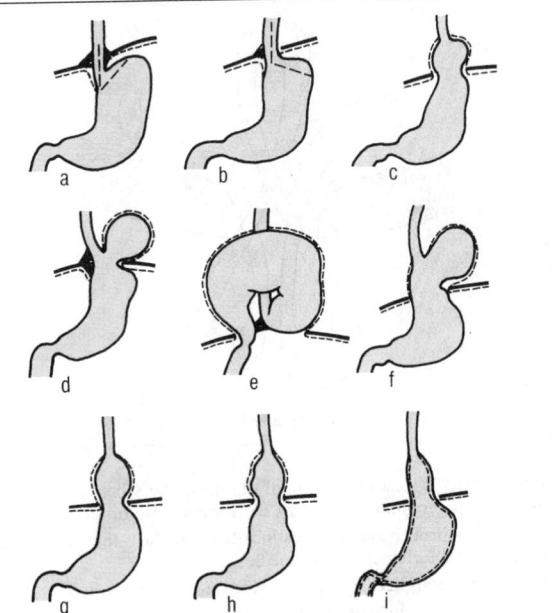

hiatal hernia (variants)

(dotted line = peritoneum) a) normal; b) cardiofundal displacement; c) sliding hiatal h.; d) paraesophageal h.; e) complete thoracic stomach ("upside-down stomach", the site of gastric volvulus; f) combined h.; g) congenital brachyesophagus in the form of a sliding hiatal h.; h) acquired from growth of hernial sac in persistent brachyesophagus; i) congenital endobrachyesophagus (sometimes with a sliding h.)

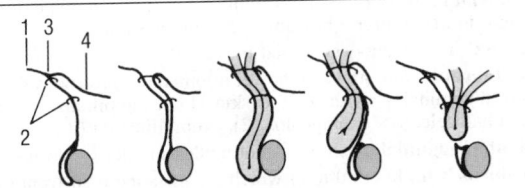

inguinal hernias (inguinal canal region)

(from left to right: normal; open vaginal process; inherited or acquired indirect h.; acquired direct h.) 1 = peritoneum; 2 = inguinal canal; 3 = lateral inguinal fossa; 4 = medial inguinal fossa

posterior vaginal h., downward displacement of Douglas' pouch.

properitoneal inguinal h., a complicated h. having a double sac, one part in the inguinal canal, the other projecting from the internal inguinal ring in the subperitoneal tissues. SYN h. en bissac, Krönlein's h.

pudendal h., SYN perineal h.

reducible h., a h. in which the contents of the sac can be returned to their normal location.

retrograde h., a double loop h. the central loop of which lies in the abdominal cavity.

retroperitoneal h., SYN duodenojejunal h.

retropubic h., a h. projecting downward, in the subperitoneal tissues, from the internal inguinal ring.

retrosternal h., a diaphragmatic h. protruding through Morgagni's foramen.

Richter's h., SYN parietal h.

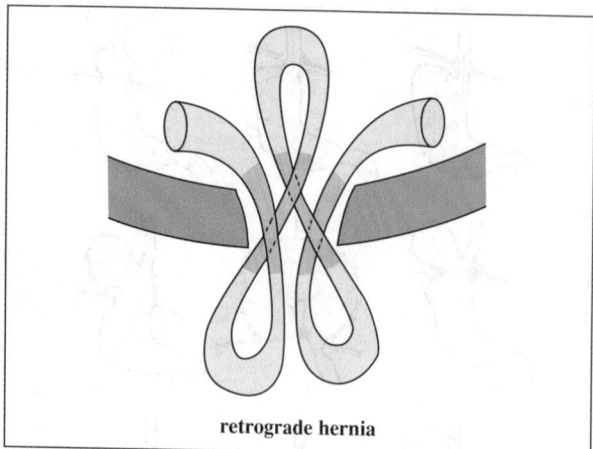

retrograde hernia

Rokitansky's h., a separation of the muscular fibers of the bowel allowing protrusion of a sac of the mucous membrane.

sciatic h., protrusion of intestine through the great sacrosciatic foramen. SYN gluteal h., ischiocele.

scrotal h., complete inguinal h., located in the scrotum.

sliding h., a h. in which an abdominal viscus forms part of the sac. SYN extrasaccular h., parasaccular h., slipped h.

sliding esophageal hiatal h., displacement of the cardioesophageal junction and the stomach through the esophageal hiatus.

sliding hiatal h., a h. of the esophagus through the diaphragm into the posterior mediastinum, with partial peritoneal sac anteriorly.

slipped h., SYN sliding h.

spigelian h., abdominal h. through the semilunar line. SYN lateral ventral h.

strangulated h., an irreducible h. in which the circulation is arrested; gangrene occurs unless relief is prompt.

synovial h., protrusion of a fold of the stratum synoviale through a rent in the stratum fibrosum of a joint capsule.

Treitz' h., SYN duodenojejunal h.

umbilical h., a h. in which bowel or omentum protrudes through the abdominal wall under the skin at the umbilicus. SEE ALSO omphalocele. SYN exomphalos (2), exumbilication (2).

h. uteri inguinale, SYN persistent müllerian duct *syndrome.*

Velpeau's h., femoral h. in which the intestine is in front of the blood vessels.

ventral h., an abdominal incisional h.

vesicle h., protrusion of a segment of the bladder through the abdominal wall or into the inguinal canal and into the scrotum.

vitreous h., prolapse of the vitreous humor into the anterior chamber; may follow removal or displacement of the lens from the lenticular space.

"w" h., the presence of two loops of intestine in a hernial sac. SYN double loop h.

her·nial (her′nē-ăl). Relating to hernia.

her·ni·at·ed (her′nē-ā-ted). Denoting any structure protruded through a hernial opening.

her·ni·a·tion (her-nē-ā′shŭn). Formation of a protrusion.

  caudal transtentorial h., displacement of medial temporal structures through the incisura, with or without rostrocaudal brainstem shift. SYN uncal h.

  cingulate h., displacement of the cingulate gyrus beneath the falx.

  foraminal h., displacement of cerebellar tonsils through the foramen magnum.

  rostral transtentorial h., displacement of anterior cerebellar structures through the incisura, with or without caudorostral brainstem shift.

  sphenoidal h., displacement of ventral frontal lobar tissue over the sphenoid ridge.

  subfalcial h., h. beneath the falx cerebri; usually of the cingulate gyrus.

  tonsillar h., h. of the cerebellar tonsils through the foramen magnum.

  transtentorial h., h. into the incisura, either from above (rostral h.) or below (caudal h.).

  uncal h., SYN caudal transtentorial h.

⚠**hernio-.** A hernia. [L. *hernia,* rupture]

her·ni·o·en·ter·ot·o·my (her′nē-ō-en-ter-ot′ō-mē). Incision of the intestine following the reduction of a hernia.

her·ni·og·ra·phy (her-nē-og′ră-fē). Radiographic examination of a hernia following injection of a contrast medium into the hernial sac. [hernia + G. *graphō,* to write]

her·ni·oid (her′nē-oyd). Resembling hernia. [hernio- + G. *eidos,* resemblance]

her·ni·o·lap·a·rot·o·my (her′nē-ō-lap-ă-rot′ō-mē). Laparotomy for correction of hernia.

her·ni·o·plas·ty (her′nē-ō-plas-tē). SYN herniorrhaphy. [hernio- + G. *plastos,* formed]

her·ni·o·punc·ture (her′nē-ō-pŭnk′chŭr). Insertion of a hollow needle into a hernia in order to reduce the size of the tumor by withdrawing gas or liquid.

her·ni·or·rha·phy (her′nē-ōr′ă-fē). Surgical repair of a hernia. SYN hernioplasty. [hernio- + G. *rhaphē,* a seam]

her·ni·o·tome (her′nē-ō-tōm). SYN hernia *knife.*

  Cooper's h., a slender bistoury with short cutting edge for dividing the constricting tissues at the neck of a hernial sac.

her·ni·ot·o·my (her-nē-ot′ō-mē). Surgical division of the constriction or strangulation of a hernia, often followed by herniorrhaphy. [hernio- + G. *tomē,* a cutting]

  Petit's h., h. without incision into the sac.

he·ro·ic (hē-rō′ik). Denoting an aggressive, daring procedure in a dangerously ill patient which in itself may endanger the patient but which also has a possibility of being successful, whereas lesser action would result in failure. [G. *hērōikos,* pertaining to a hero]

her·o·in (H) (her′ō-in). An alkaloid, $C_{17}H_{17}(OC_2H_3O)_2ON$, prepared from morphine by acetylation; formerly used for the relief of cough. Except for research, its use in the United States is prohibited by Federal law because of its potential for abuse. SYN diacetylmorphine.

He·roph·i·lus. Greek physician and anatomist of the Alexandrian school, circa 300 B.C. SEE torcular herophili.

her·pan·gi·na (her-pan′ji-nă, herp-an-jī′nă). A disease caused by types of coxsackievirus and marked by vesiculopapular lesions about 1 to 2 mm in diameter which are present around the fauces and soon break down to form grayish yellow ulcers; accompanied by sudden onset of fever, loss of appetite, dysphagia, pharyngitis, and sometimes abdominal pain, nausea, and vomiting. [G. *herpēs,* vesicular eruption, + L. *angina,* quinsy, fr. *ango,* to strangle]

her·pes (her′pēz). An inflammatory skin disease caused by herpesvirus; an eruption of groups of deep-seated vesicles on erythematous bases. SYN serpigo (2). [G. *herpēs,* a spreading skin eruption, shingles, fr. *herpō,* to creep]

  h. catarrha′lis, SYN h. simplex.

  h. circina′tus bullo′sus, SYN *dermatitis* herpetiformis.

  h. cor′neae, SYN herpetic *keratitis.*

  h. desqua′mans, SYN *tinea* imbricata.

  h. digita′lis, herpes simplex infection of the finger.

  h. facia′lis, SYN h. simplex.

  h. febri′lis, SYN h. simplex.

  h. generalisa′tus, generalized h. simplex virus infection.

  h. genita′lis, genital h., herpes simplex infection on the genitals, most commonly herpes simplex-1 virus.

  h. gestatio′nis, a polymorphous, bullous eruption, more common on the extremities than on the trunk, with the appearance of pemphigoid or dermatitis herpetiformis; beginning in the second or third trimester, flaring about the time of delivery and sub-

Human Herpesviruses

Official name	Common name	Subfamily	Genus
Human herpesvirus 1	Herpes simplex virus 1 (HSV-1)	*Alphaherpesvirinae*	*Simplexvirus*
Human herpesvirus 2	Herpes simplex virus 2 (HSV-2)		
Human herpesvirus 3	Varicella-zoster virus (VZV)		*Varicellovirus*
Human herpesvirus 4	Epstein-Barr virus (EBV)	*Gammaherpesvirinae*	*Lymphocryptovirus*
Human herpesvirus 5	Cytomegalovirus (CMV)	*Betaherpesvirinae*	*Cytomegalovirus*
Human herpesvirus 6	— (HHV-6)		*Roseolovirus*
Human herpesvirus 7	— (HHV-7)	—	—

sequently resolving; usually recurrent during subsequent pregnancy; etiology is unknown. SYN hydroa gestationis.

h. gladiato′rum, h. simplex infection associated with trauma to cutaneous tissue.

h. i′ris, (1) SYN *erythema* iris. **(2)** SYN *erythema* multiforme.

h. labia′lis, SYN h. simplex.

neonatal h., herpes simplex virus type 1 or 2 infection transmitted from the mother to the newborn infant, often during passage through an infected birth canal; severity varies from mild to fatal generalized infection, the latter especially with primary maternal genital h.

h. progenita′lis, genital h. infection caused by h. simplex virus.

h. sim′plex, a variety of infections caused by herpesvirus types 1 and 2; type 1 infections are marked most commonly by the eruption of one or more groups of vesicles on the vermilion border of the lips or at the external nares, type 2 by such lesions on the genitalia; both types often are recrudescent and reappear during other febrile illnesses or even physiologic states such as menstruation. SYN h. catarrhalis, h. facialis, h. febrilis, h. labialis, hydroa febrile.

traumatic h., h. simplex infection at the site of trauma or of a burn, sometimes accompanied by temperature elevation and malaise.

h. whitlow, herpes simplex inflammation at base of fingernail.

h. zos′ter, an infection caused by a herpesvirus (varicella-zoster virus), characterized by an eruption of groups of vesicles on one side of the body following the course of a nerve due to inflammation of ganglia and dorsal nerve roots resulting from activation of the virus which in many instances has remained latent for years; the condition is self-limited but may be accompanied by or followed by severe postherpetic pain. SYN shingles, zona ignea, zona serpiginosa, zona (2), zoster.

h. zos′ter ophthal′micus, a herpetic involvement of the ophthalmic branch of the trigeminal nerve, which may lead to corneal ulceration.

h. zos′ter o′ticus, a painful varicella virus infection presenting with a vesicular eruption on the pinna, with or without facial nerve paralysis. SYN geniculate zoster, Ramsay Hunt's syndrome (2).

h. zos′ter varicello′sus, h. zoster associated with disseminated varicelliform lesions.

Her·pes·vir·i·dae (her′pĕs-vir′i-dē). A heterogeneous family of morphologically similar viruses, all of which contain double-stranded DNA and which infect man and a wide variety of other vertebrates. Infections produce type A inclusion bodies; in many instances, infection may remain latent for many years, even in the presence of specific circulating antibodies. Virions are enveloped, ether-sensitive, and vary up to 200 nm in diameter; the nucleocapsids are 100 nm in diameter and of icosahedral symmetry, with 162 capsomeres. The family includes herpes simplex virus, varicella-zoster virus, cytomegalovirus, and EB virus (all of which infect humans), pseudorabies virus of swine, equine rhinopneumonitis virus, infectious bovine rhinotracheitis virus, canine herpesvirus, B virus of Old World monkeys, several vi-

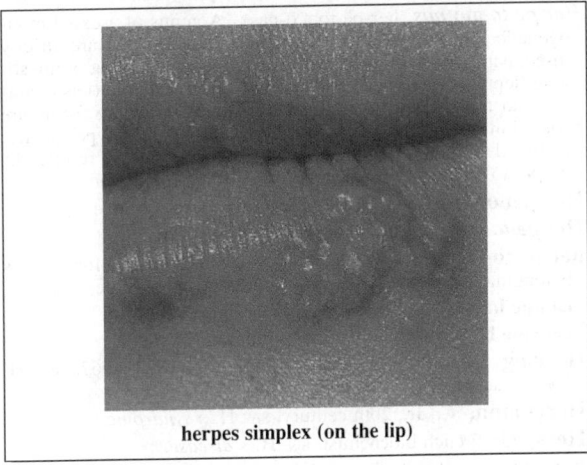

herpes simplex (on the lip)

ruses of New World monkeys, virus III of rabbits, infectious laryngotracheitis virus of fowl, Marek's disease virus of chickens, Lucké tumor virus of frogs, and many others.

her·pes·vi·rus (her′pēz-vī′rŭs). Any virus belonging to the family Herpesviridae.

alcelaphine h. 1, a virus causing malignant catarrhal fever in cattle and some wild ruminants (deer, buffalo, antelope).

anatid h. 1, a virus causing duck plague in ducks, geese, swans, and other waterfowl.

avian h. 1, a virus causing avian infectious *laryngotracheitis* in chickens.

avian h. 2, a virus causing Marek's disease in chickens.

bovine h. 1, a virus causing infectious bovine rhinotracheitis in cattle.

bovine h. 2, a virus causing bovine mammillitis in cattle.

canine h., a h. causing an upper respiratory tract infection which becomes generalized in puppies under 1 week of age, terminating invariably in death; infection is milder in older puppies and asymptomatic in adult dogs; the latter may become convalescent viral shedders.

caprine h., a h. that causes a severe generalized and fatal infection of newborn kids, characterized by fever, depression, inappetence, and mild to severe enteritis; the infection in adult goats is clinically mild, with abortion a frequent sequela.

equine h. 3, a virus causing equine coital exanthema in horses.

equine h. 4, a virus causing equine rhinopneumonitis in horses.

human h. 1, herpes simplex virus, type 1. SEE *herpes* simplex.

human h. 2, herpes simplex virus, type 2. SEE *herpes* simplex.

human h. 3, SYN varicella-zoster *virus*.

human h. 4, SYN Epstein-Barr *virus*.

human h. 5, SYN cytomegalovirus.

he

human h. 6, A recently discovered new human herpesvirus that was found in certain lymphoproliferative disorders, replicate in a number of different types of leukocytes, and is associated with the childhood disease roseola (exanthema subitum).

human h. 7, This virus has recently been discovered in association with human lymphocytes. However, a causal relationship to any known disease has not been determined.

porcine h. 1, a virus causing pseudorabies in swine and many other mammalian species including horses, cattle, sheep, goats, dogs, and cats.

porcine h. 2, a virus causing inclusion body rhinitis in pigs.

suid h., the causative agent of pseudorabies.

her·pet·ic (her-pet'ik). **1.** Relating to or characterized by herpes. **2.** Relating to or caused by a herpetovirus or herpesvirus.

her·pet·i·form (her-pet'i-fōrm). Resembling herpes.

her·pe·tol·o·gist (her-pet-ol'ō-jist). One who specializes in herpetology.

her·pe·tol·o·gy (her-pet-ol'ō-jē). The branch of zoology concerned with the study of reptiles and amphibians.

Her·pe·to·mo·nas (her-pĕ-tom'ō-nas). A genus of asexual monogenetic flagellates (family Trypanosomatidae) that are strictly insect parasites, with a variety of body forms including promastigote (leptomad), epimastigote (crithidial), amastigote (leishmanial), and trypomastigote (trypanosome-like); infective forms are passed in the host feces. *H. muscae domesticae,* the type species, is found in the common housefly. [G. *herpeton,* a reptile (fr. *herpō,* to creep), + *monas,* unit (one of the *Monadidae*)]

Her·pe·to·vir·i·dae. Obsolete term for Herpesviridae.

Her·pe·to·vi·rus. Obsolete term for herpesvirus.

her·pe·to·vi·rus (her'pĕ-tō-vī'rŭs). Obsolete name for a virus belonging to the family Herpesviridae. SEE ALSO herpesvirus.

canine h., obsolete term for canine *herpesvirus.*

caprine h., obsolete term for caprine *herpesvirus.*

Herring, Percy T., English physiologist, 1872–1967. SEE H. *bodies,* under *body.*

Herrmann, C., Jr., 20th century. SEE H.'s *syndrome.*

Hers, G., French biochemist. SEE H.'s *disease.*

her·sage (ār-sahzh'). Separating the individual fibers of a nerve trunk. [Fr. (from L. *hirpex,* a large rake), a harrowing]

Hertwig, Richard, German zoologist, 1850–1937. SEE Magendie-H. *sign, syndrome.*

Hertwig, Wilhelm A.O., German embryologist, 1849–1922. SEE H.'s *sheath.*

Hertz, Heinrich R., German physicist, 1857–1894. SEE hertz; hertzian *experiments,* under *experiment.*

hertz (Hz) (herts). A unit of frequency equivalent to 1 cycle per second; this term should not be used for radial (circular) frequency or for angular velocity, in which cases the term sec^{-1} should be used. [H.R. *Hertz*]

hertz·i·an (hert'zē-an). Attributed to or described by Heinrich R. Hertz.

Herxheimer, Karl, German dermatologist, 1861–1944. SEE H.'s *reaction;* Jarisch-H. *reaction.*

herz·stoss (hārz'stos). Cardiac systole characterized by a diffuse precordial heave with or without any definite point of maximal impulse. [Ger. heart thrust]

Heschl, Richard L., Austrian pathologist, 1824–1881. SEE H.'s *gyri,* under *gyrus.*

hes·i·tan·cy (hez'i-tăn-sē). An involuntary delay or inability in starting the urinary stream.

hes·per·i·din (hes-per'i-din). Hesperetin 7-rutinoside; hesperetin 7-rhamnoglucoside; a flavone diglycoside obtained from unripe citrus fruit, which reputedly possesses vitamin P activity. SYN cirantin.

Hess, Alfred F., U.S. physician, 1875–1933. SEE H.'s *test.*

Hess, Carl von, German ophthalmologist, 1863–1923. SEE H. *screen.*

Hess, Walter R., Swiss physiologist and Nobel laureate, 1881–1973. SEE trophotropic *zone* of H.

Hesselbach, Franz K., German anatomist and surgeon, 1759–1816. SEE H.'s *fascia, hernia, ligament, triangle.*

het·a·cil·lin (het-ă-sil'in). 6-(2,2-Dimethyl-5-oxo-4-phenyl-1-imidazolidinyl)penicillanic acid; a semisynthetic penicillin compound with antimicrobial properties. SYN phenazacillin.

het·a·starch (het'ă-starch). A carbohydrate starch derivative used as a cryoprotective agent for erythrocytes. Also used as an extender of blood plasma volume.

♻ **heter-.** SEE hetero-.

het·er·a·del·phus (het-er-ă-del'fŭs). Unequal conjoined twins in which the smaller incomplete parasite is attached to the larger, more nearly normal autosite. SEE conjoined *twins,* under *twin.* [heter- + G. *adelphos,* brother]

het·er·a·kid (het'er-ā'kid). Common name for members of the family Heterakidae.

Het·er·a·kis (het-er-ā'kis). A genus of important nematode parasites (family Heterakidae, order Ascaridida). *H. gallinarum* is the cecal worm of chickens, turkeys, and many gallinaceous birds, and is the vector of *Histomonas meleagridis,* a protozoan that causes histomoniasis. Other species include *H. brevispiculum, H. dispar, H. isolonche,* and *H. spumosa,* the latter an abundant cecal parasite of rats and other rodents.

het·er·a·li·us (het-er-ā'lē-ŭs). Unequal conjoined twins in which the parasite appears as little more than an excrescence on the autosite. SEE conjoined *twins,* under *twin.* [heter- + G. *halios,* useless]

het·er·ax·i·al (het-er-ak'sē-ăl). Having mutually perpendicular axes of unequal length.

het·er·e·cious (het-er-ē'shŭs). Having more than one host; said of a parasite passing different stages of its life cycle in different animals. SYN metoxenous. [heter- + G. *oikion,* home]

het·er·e·cism (het'er-ē-sizm). The occurrence, in a parasite, of two cycles of development passed in two different hosts. SYN metoxeny (1). [heter- + G. *oikion,* home]

het·er·es·the·sia (het-er-es-thē'zē-ă). A change occurring in the degree (either plus or minus) of the sensory response to a cutaneous stimulus as the latter crosses a certain line on the surface. [heter- + G. *aisthēsis,* sensation]

♻ **hetero-, heter-.** The other, different; opposite of homo- [G. *heteros,* other].

het·er·o·ag·glu·ti·nin (het'er-ō-ă-glū'ti-nin). A form of hemagglutinin, one that agglutinates the red blood cells of species other than that in which the h. occurs. SEE ALSO hemagglutinin.

het·er·o·al·leles (het'er-ō-ă-lēlz'). Genes that have undergone mutation at different nucleotide positions and therefore result from different mutational events. Cf. eualleles.

het·er·o·an·ti·body (het'er-ō-an'ti-bod-ē). Antibody that is heterologous with respect to antigen, in contradistinction to isoantibody.

het·er·o·an·ti·se·rum (het'er-ō-an'ti-sē-rŭm). Antiserum developed in one animal species against antigens or cells of another species.

het·er·o·at·om (het'er-ō-at'ŏm). An atom, other than carbon, located in the ring structure of an organic compound, as the N in pyridines or pyrimidines (heterocyclic compounds).

het·er·o·blas·tic (het-er-ō-blas'tik). Developing from more than a single type of tissue. [hetero- + G. *blastos,* germ]

het·er·o·cel·lu·lar (het'er-ō-sel'yū-lăr). Formed of cells of different kinds.

het·er·o·cen·tric (het'er-ō-sen'trik). **1.** Having different centers; said of rays that do not meet at a common focus. Cf. homocentric. **2.** SYN allocentric. [hetero- + G. *kentron,* center]

het·er·o·ceph·a·lus (het-er-ō-sef'ă-lŭs). Conjoined twins with heads of unequal size. SEE conjoined *twins,* under *twin.* [hetero- + G. *kephalē,* head]

het·er·o·chei·ral, het·er·o·chi·ral (het-er-ō-kī'răl). Relating to or referred to the other hand. [hetero- + G. *cheir,* hand]

het·er·o·chro·mat·ic (het'er-ō-krō-mat'ik). Characteristic of heterochromatin.

het·er·o·chro·ma·tin (het'er-ō-krō'mă-tin). The part of the chromonema that remains tightly coiled and condensed during interphase and thus stains readily. SYN heteropyknotic chromatin.

constitutive h., repetitive h. that lies in secondary constrictions in the nucleolar organizers.

facultative h., non-repetitive h. that comprises translatable sequences of DNA.

satellite-rich h., h. that codes for 18 S and 28 S components of ribosomal RNA and is located close to the centromeres of certain chromosomes.

het·er·o·chro·mia (het′er-ō-krō′mē-ă). A difference in coloration in two structures which are normally alike in color. [hetero- + G. *chrōma,* color]

atrophic h., h. iridis after trauma or inflammation, or in old age.

binocular h., an increase or decrease in pigmentation of one eye, with or without extraocular pigmentary defects.

h. i′ridis, h. of iris, a difference in coloration of the irides. SEE binocular h.

monocular h., SYN *iris* bicolor.

simple h., h. iridis appearing as a developmental defect, without any innervation defect.

sympathetic h., h. iridis occurring after lesions of the cervical sympathetic nerves.

het·er·o·chro·mo·some (het′er-ō-krō′mō-sōm). SYN allosome.

het·er·o·chro·mous (het′er-ō-krō′mŭs). Having an abnormal difference in coloration.

het·er·o·chron (het′er-ō-kron). Having varying chronaxies. [hetero- + G. *chronos,* time]

het·er·o·chro·nia (het-er-ō-krō′nē-ă). Origin or development of tissues or organs at an unusual time or out of the regular sequence. Cf. synchronia. [hetero- + G. *chronos,* time]

het·er·o·chron·ic (het-er-ō-kron′ik). SYN heterochronous.

het·er·och·ro·nous (het-er-ok′rō-nŭs). Relating to heterochronia. SYN heterochronic.

het·er·o·clad·ic (het′er-ō-klad′ik). Denoting an anastomosis between branches of different arterial trunks, as distinguished from homocladic. [hetero- + G. *klados,* a twig]

het·er·o·crine (het′er-ō-krin). Denoting the secretion of two or more kinds of material. [hetero- + G. *krinō,* to separate]

het·er·o·cri·sis (het-er-ō-krī′sis). Rarely used term for an irregular crisis, one occurring at an abnormal time or with unusual symptoms.

het·er·o·cy·to·tro·pic (het-er-ō-sī′tō-trop′ik). Having an affinity for cells of a different species. [hetero- + G. *kytos,* cell, + *tropē,* a turning toward]

het·er·o·der·mic (het′er-ō-der′mik). Obsolete term denoting skin grafting in which the grafts are taken from the skin of an animal of another species (dermatoheteroplasty). [hetero- + G. *derma,* skin]

het·er·o·dis·perse (het′er-ō-dis-pers′). Of varying size; describing aerosols whose particles are not uniform in size.

het·er·o·dont (het′er-ō-dont). Having teeth of varying shapes, such as those of humans and the majority of mammals, in contrast to homodont. [hetero- + G. *odous,* tooth]

Het·er·o·dox·us spi·ni·ger (het-er-ō-dok′sŭs spī′ni-ger). A biting louse of the dog, sometimes called the kangaroo louse.

het·er·od·ro·mous (het-er-ōd′rŏ-mŭs). Moving in the opposite direction. [hetero- + G. *dromos,* running]

het·er·o·du·plex (het′er-ō-dū′pleks). A DNA molecule, the two constitutive strands of which are derived from distinct sources and hence are likely to be somewhat mismatched. [hetero- + L. *duplex,* two-fold]

het·er·od·y·mus (het-er-od′i-mŭs). Unequal conjoined twins in which the incomplete parasite, consisting of head and neck and, to some extent, thorax, is attached to the anterior surface of the autosite. SEE conjoined *twins,* under *twin.* [hetero- + G. *didymos,* twin]

het·er·o·e·rot·ic (het′er-ō-ĕ-rot′ik). SYN alloerotic.

het·er·o·e·rot·i·cism. A condition of sexual excitement brought about by congress with a person of the opposite sex.

het·er·o·er·o·tism (het′er-ō-ār′ō-tizm). SYN alloerotism.

het·er·o·ga·met·ic (het′er-ō-gă-met′ik). Having sex gametes of

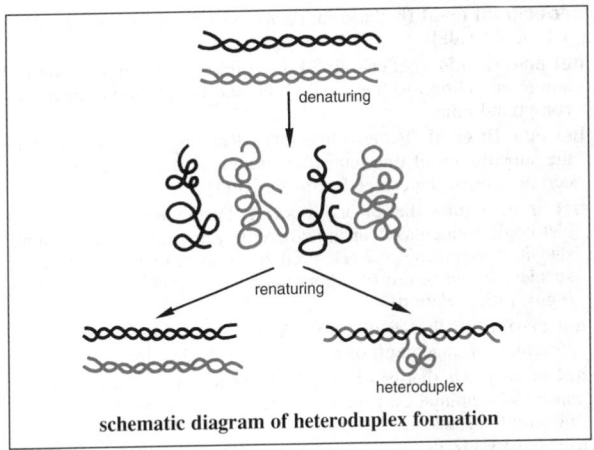

schematic diagram of heteroduplex formation

contrasting types; human males are h. SYN digametic. [hetero- + G. *gametikos,* connubial]

het·er·og·a·mous (het-er-og′ă-mŭs). Relating to heterogamy.

het·er·og·a·my (het-er-og′ă-mē). **1.** Conjugation of unlike gametes. **2.** Bearing different types of flowers. **3.** Reproduction by indirect methods of pollination. [hetero- + G. *gamos,* marriage]

het·er·o·ge·ne·i·ty (het′er-ō-jĕ-nē′i-tē). Heterogeneous state or quality.

genetic h., the character of a phenotype produced by diverse mechanisms which can be distinguished by special methods (such as linkage analysis) but are ordinarily indistinguishable. SEE genocopy.

het·er·o·ge·neous (het′er-ō-jē′nē-ŭs). Comprising elements with various and dissimilar properties.

het·er·o·gen·e·sis (het′er-ō-jen′ĕ-sis). **1.** Alternation of generations. **2.** SYN asexual *generation.* **3.** SYN spontaneous *generation.* [hetero- + G. *genesis,* production]

het·er·o·ge·net·ic (het′er-ō-jĕ-net′ik). Relating to heterogenesis.

het·er·o·gen·ic, het·er·o·ge·ne·ic (het′er-ō-jen′ik, -jĕ-nē′ik). Having different gene constitutions, especially in diverse species.

het·er·o·ge·note (het′er-ō-jē′nōt). In microbial genetics, an organism that contains exogenous genetic material that differs somewhat from the corresponding region of its own original genome, but in a very limited way resembles a heterozygote. [hetero- + genote]

het·er·og·e·nous (het-er-oj′ĕ-nŭs). Of foreign origin. Commonly confused with heterogeneous.

het·er·o·gly·can (het′er-ō-glī′kan). SYN heteropolysaccharide.

het·er·o·graft (het′er-ō-graft). SYN xenograft.

het·er·o·hyp·no·sis (het′er-ō-hip-nō′sis). Hypnosis induced by or in another, as opposed to autohypnosis.

het·er·o·kar·y·on (het′er-ō-kar′ē-on). A cell containing diverse nuclei inside a common cytoplasm, usually resulting from the artificial fusion of two cells from different species. [hetero- + G. *karyon,* kernel, nut]

het·er·o·kar·y·ot·ic (het′er-ō-kar-ē-ot′ik). Exhibiting the properties of a heterokaryon.

het·er·o·ker·a·to·plas·ty (het′er-ō-ker′ă-tō-plas-tē). Keratoplasty in which the cornea from one species of animal is grafted to the eye of another species.

het·er·o·ki·ne·sia (het′er-ō-ki-nē′zē-ă). Executing movements the reverse of those one is told to make. SYN heterokinesis (2). [hetero- + G. *kinēsis,* movement]

het·er·o·ki·ne·sis (het′er-ō-ki-nē′sis). **1.** Differential distribution of X and Y chromosomes during meiotic cell division. **2.** SYN heterokinesia. [hetero- + G. *kinēsis,* movement hetero- + G. *kinēsis,* movement]

het·er·o·la·lia (het′er-ō-lā′lē-ă). The habitual substitution of meaningless or inappropriate words for those intended; a form of aphasia. SYN heterophasia, heterophemia, heterophemy. [hetero- + G. *lalia,* speech]

het·er·o·lat·er·al (het′er-ō-lat′er-ăl). SYN contralateral. [hetero- + L. *latus*, side]

het·er·o·lip·ids (het′er-ō-lip′idz). Lipids containing N and P atoms in addition to the usual C, H, and O. Cf. homolipids. SYN compound lipids.

het·er·o·lit·er·al (het′er-ō-lit′er-ăl). Relating to stammering or the substitution of one letter for another in the pronunciation of certain words. [hetero- + L. *littera*, letter]

het·er·ol·o·gous (het-er-ol′ŏ-gŭs). **1.** Pertaining to cytologic or histologic elements occurring where they are not normally found. SEE ALSO xenogeneic. **2.** Derived from an animal of a different species, as the serum of a horse is h. for a rabbit. [hetero- + G. *logos*, ratio, relation]

het·er·ol·o·gy (het-er-ol′ŏ-jē). A departure from the normal in structure, arrangement, or mode or time of development.

het·er·o·ly·sin (het-er-ol′i-sin). A lysin that is formed in one species of animal and manifests lytic activity on the cells of a different species.

het·er·ol·y·sis (het-er-ol′i-sis). Dissolution or digestion of cells or protein components from one species by a lytic agent from a different species. [hetero- + G. *lysis*, a loosening]

het·er·o·lyt·ic (het′er-ō-lit′ik). Pertaining to heterolysis or to the effect of a heterolysin.

het·er·o·mas·ti·gote (het-er-ō-mas′ti-gōt). A flagellate having two flagella, one anterior and one posterior. [hetero- + G. *mastix*, a whip]

het·er·om·er·al (het′er-om′er-ăl). SYN heteromeric (2).

het·er·o·mer·ic (het′er-ō-mār′ik). **1.** Having a different chemical composition. **2.** Denoting spinal neurons that have processes passing over to the opposite side of the cord. SYN heteromeral, heteromerous. [hetero- + G. *meros*, part]

het·er·om·er·ous (het′er-om′er-ŭs). SYN heteromeric (2).

het·er·o·me·tab·o·lous (het′er-ō-me-tab′ŏ-lŭs). Pertaining to a member of the Heterometabola, a superorder sometimes used for a series of insect orders in which incomplete metamorphosis is found. [hetero- + G. *metabolē*, change]

het·er·o·met·a·pla·sia (het′er-ō-met-ă-plā′zē-ă). Tissue transformation resulting in production of a tissue foreign to the part where produced.

het·er·o·met·ric (het′er-ō-met′rik). Involving or depending upon a change in size. [hetero- + G. *metron*, measure]

het·er·o·me·tro·pia (het′er-ō-me-trō′pē-ă). A condition in which the refraction is different in the two eyes. [hetero- + G. *metron*, measure, + *ōps*, eye]

het·er·o·mor·phism (het′er-ō-mōrf′izm). In cytogenetics, a difference of shape or size in metaphase between the two homologous chromosomes. [hetero- + G. *morphē*, shape]

het·er·o·mor·pho·sis (het′er-ō-mōr-fō′sis). **1.** Development of one tissue from a tissue of another kind or type. **2.** Embryonic development of tissue or an organ inappropriate to its site. [hetero- + G. *morphōsis*, a molding]

het·er·o·mor·phous (het′er-ō-mōr′fŭs). Differing from the normal form.

het·er·on·o·mous (het-er-on′ō-mŭs). **1.** Different from the type; abnormal. **2.** Subject to the direction or control of another; not self-governing. Cf. autonomous. [hetero- + G. *nomos*, law]

het·er·on·o·my (het-er-on′ō-mē). The condition or state of being heteronomous. [hetero- + G. *nomos*, law]

het·er·o·nu·cle·ar (het′er-ō-nū′klē-er). Denoting a heterokaryon that has lost some of the nuclear material of which the cell line was originally constituted.

het·er·on·y·mous (het-er-on′i-mŭs). Having different names or expressed in different terms. [G. *heterōnymos*, having a different name, fr. *onyma*, or *onoma*, name]

het·er·o·os·te·o·plas·ty (het′er-ō-os′tē-ō-plas-tē). Bone transplantation from one species to another; formerly used to denote transplants from one person to another.

het·er·op·a·gus (het-er-op′ă-gŭs). Unequal conjoined twins in which the imperfectly developed parasite is attached to the ventral portion of the autosite. SEE conjoined *twins*, under *twin*. SEE ALSO epigastrius. [hetero- + G. *pagos*, fixed]

het·er·op·a·thy (het′er-op′ă-thē). **1.** Abnormal sensitivity to stimuli. **2.** SYN allopathy. [hetero- + G. *pathos*, suffering]

het·er·oph·a·gy (het-er-of′ă-jē). Digestion within a cell of an exogenous substance phagocytosed from the cell's environment. [hetero- + G. *phagein*, to eat]

het·er·o·pha·sia (het′er-ō-fā′zē-ă). SYN heterolalia. [hetero- + G. *phasis*, speech]

het·er·o·phe·mia, het·er·o·phe·my (het′er-ō-fē′mē-ă, het-er-of′ĕ-mē). SYN heterolalia. [hetero- + G. *phēmē*, a speech]

het·er·o·phil, het·er·o·phile (het′er-ō-fil, -fīl). **1.** The neutrophilic leukocyte in man; in some animals the granules vary in size and staining reaction. **2.** Pertaining to heterogenetic antigens occurring in different species or to antibodies directed against such antigens. [hetero- + G. *philos*, fond]

het·er·o·pho·nia (het′er-ō-fō′nē-ă). **1.** The change of voice at puberty. **2.** Any abnormality in the voice sounds. SYN heterophthongia. [hetero- + G. *phōnē*, voice]

het·er·o·pho·ria (het′er-ō-fō′rē-ă). A tendency for deviation of the eyes from parallelism, prevented by binocular vision. [hetero- + G. *phora*, movement]

het·er·oph·thal·mus (het′er-of-thal′mŭs). A seldom-used term for a difference in the appearance of the two eyes, usually due to heterochromia iridis. SYN allophthalmia. [hetero- + G. *ophthalmos*, eye]

het·er·oph·thon·gia (het-er-of-thon′jē-ă). SYN heterophonia. [G. *heterophthongos*, fr. *heteros*, different, + *phthongos*, sound, voice]

Het·er·o·phy·es (het-er-of′i-ēz). A genus of digenetic flukes (family Heterophyidae) parasitic in fish-eating birds and mammals, including man; cercariae from infected snails penetrate and encyst in fish, which are eaten by the final hosts. [hetero- + G. *phyē*, stature, form]

H. brevicae′ca, a species reported from man in the Philippines and implicated in heart lesions caused by the eggs of this minute fluke, carried from the intestinal mucosa to obstruct coronary capillaries.

H. heteroph′yes, the Egyptian intestinal or small intestinal fluke, a species infecting the small intestine and cecum in man and other fish-eating mammals in Egypt and the Far East.

H. katsura′dai, a species, somewhat smaller than *H. heterophyes*, found in Japan.

het·er·o·phy·i·a·sis (het′er-ō-fī-ī′ă-sis). Infection with a heterophyid trematode, particularly *Heterophyes heterophyes*. SYN heterophyidiasis.

het·er·o·phy·id (het′er-o-fī′id). Common name for a member of the family Heterophyidae.

Het·er·o·phy·i·dae (het′er-ō-fī′i-dē). A family of tiny fish-borne trematodes, including the genus *Heterophyes* and its common human parasite, *H. heterophyes*.

het·er·o·phy·id·i·a·sis (het′er-ō-fī-id-ī′ă-sis). SYN heterophyiasis.

het·er·o·pla·sia (het′er-ō-plā′zē-ă). **1.** Development of cytologic and histologic elements that are not normal for the organ or part in question, as the growth of bone in a site where there is normally fibrous connective tissue. **2.** Malposition of tissue or a part that is otherwise normal, as a ureter that develops at the lower pole of a kidney. SYN alloplasia. [hetero- + G. *plasis*, a forming]

het·er·o·plas·tic (het′er-ō-plas′tik). **1.** Pertaining to or manifesting heteroplasia. **2.** Relating to heteroplasty.

het·er·o·plas·tid (het′er-ō-plas′tid). The graft in heteroplasty.

het·er·o·plas·ty (het′er-ō-plas-tē). **1.** SYN heterotransplantation. **2.** Formerly, transplantation of any graft other than an autograft. [hetero- + G. *plastos*, formed]

het·er·o·ploid (het′er-ō-ployd). Relating to heteroploidy.

het·er·o·ploi·dy (het′er-ō-ploy′dē). The state of a cell possessing some number of complete haploid sets other than the normal. [hetero- + G. *ploides*, in form]

het·er·o·pol·y·sac·cha·ride (het′er-ō-pol-ē-sak′ă-rīd). A polysaccharide composed of two or more different types of monosaccharides. Cf. glycan, homoglycan. SYN heteroglycan.

het·er·o·pro·te·ose (het′er-ō-prō′tē-ōs). SEE primary *proteose*.

het·er·o·psy·cho·log·ic (het′er-ō-sī-kō-loj′ik). Relating to ideas developed from without or derived from another's consciousness.

het·er·o·pyk·no·sis (het′er-ō-pik-nō′sis). Any state of variable density or condensation, usually in different chromosomes or between different regions of the same chromosome; a region may be attentuated (**negative h**) or accentuated (**positive h**). [hetero- + G. *pyknos,* dense]

het·er·o·pyk·not·ic (het′er-ō-pik-not′ik). Relating to or characterized by heteropyknosis.

het·er·o·sac·cha·ride (het′er-ō-sak′ă-rīd). A glycoside in which a sugar group is attached to a nonsugar group; *e.g.,* amygdalin.

het·er·o·sced·as·tic·i·ty (het′er-o-skĕ-das-tis′ĭ- tē). Non-constancy of the variance of a measure over the levels of the factor under study. [hetero + G. *skedastikos,* pertaining to scattering, fr. *skedannumi,* to scatter]

het·er·o·sex·u·al (het′er-ō-sek′shū-ăl). **1.** A person whose sexual orientation is toward persons of the opposite sex. **2.** Relating to or characteristic of heterosexuality. **3.** One whose interests and behavior are characteristic of heterosexuality.

het·er·o·sex·u·al·i·ty (het′er-ō-sek-shū-al′i-tē). Erotic attraction, predisposition, or activity, including sexual congress between persons of the opposite sex.

het·er·o·side (het′er-ō-sīd). A compound containing two or more different carbohydrate residues that are covalently linked to a noncarbohydrate moiety.

het·er·o·sis (het-er-ō′sis). The beneficial effect on the phenotype of crossing (hybridization) upon growth, vigor, and physical or mental qualities in a strain of plants or in animal stock, as measured by the difference between the midparent mean phenotype and that of F₁. [hetero- + -*ōsis,* condition]

het·er·os·mia (het′er-os′mē-a). SYN allotriosmia.

het·er·o·some (het′er-ō-sōm). In genetics, the chromosome pair that is different in the two sexes. SEE sex *chromosomes,* under *chromosome.* [hetero- + G. *sōma,* body]

het·er·o·spe·cif·ic (het′er-ō-spe-sif′ik). Heterologous, as pertains to grafts.

het·er·o·sug·ges·tion (het′er-ō-sŭg-jes′chŭn). Hypnotic suggestion received from another person; opposed to autosuggestion.

het·er·o·tax·ia (het′er-ō-taks′ē-ă). Abnormal arrangement of organs or parts of the body in relation to each other. SYN heterotaxis, heterotaxy. [hetero- + G. *taxis,* arrangement]

  cardiac h., SEE dextrocardia.

het·er·o·tax·ic (het-er-ō-taks′ik). Abnormally placed or arranged.

het·er·o·tax·is, het·er·o·taxy (het-er-ō-taks′is, het′er-ō-taks-ē). SYN heterotaxia.

het·er·o·thal·lic (het′er-ō-thal′ik). In fungi, denoting a kind of sexual reproduction in which a sexual spore is produced only by fusion with a nucleus of another mating type. Cf. homothallic. [hetero- + G. *thallos,* a young shoot]

het·er·o·therm (het′er-ō-therm). A heterothermic animal.

het·er·o·ther·mic (het′er-ō-ther′mik). Having partial regulation of body temperature; between poikilothermic and homeothermic.

het·er·ot·ic (het-er-ot′ik). Relating to heterosis.

het·er·o·to·nia (het′er-ō-tō′nē-ă). Abnormality or variation in tension or tonus. [hetero- + G. *tonos,* tension]

het·er·o·to·pia (het-er-ō-tō′pē-ă). **1.** SYN ectopia. **2.** In neuropathology, displacement of gray matter, typically into the deep cerebral white matter. [hetero- + G. *topos,* place]

  h. mac′ulae, SYN *ectopia* maculae.

het·er·o·top·ic (het-er-ō-top′ik). **1.** SYN ectopic (1). **2.** Relating to heterotopia (2). [hetero- + *topos,* place, + suffix -*ic,* pertaining to]

het·er·ot·o·pous (het-er-ot′ō-pŭs). Heterotopic, especially in reference to teratomas composed of tissues that are out of place in the region where found.

het·er·o·trans·plan·ta·tion (het′er-ō-tranz-plan-tā′shŭn). Transfer of a heterograft (xenograft). SYN heteroplasty (1).

het·er·o·tri·cho·sis (het′er-ō-tri-kō′sis). A condition characterized by hair growth of variegated color. [hetero- + G. *trichōsis,* growth of hair]

het·er·o·troph (het′er-ō-trof, -trōf). A microorganism that obtains its carbon, as well as its energy, from organic compounds. SEE ALSO autotroph. [hetero- + G. *trophē,* nourishment]

het·er·o·tro·phic (het′er-ō-tro-fik). **1.** Relating to or exhibiting the properties of heterotrophy. **2.** Relating to a heterotroph.

het·er·ot·ro·phy (het′er-ō-trō-fē). The ability or requirement to synthesize all metabolites from organic compounds.

het·er·o·tro·pia, het·er·ot·ro·py (het′er-ō-trō′pē-ă, het-er-ot′ rō-pē). SYN strabismus. [hetero- + G. *tropē,* a turning]

het·er·o·typ·ic (het′er-ō-tip′ik). Of a different or unusual type or form.

het·er·o·xan·thine (het′er-ō-zan′thin). 7-Methylxanthine; one of the alloxuric bases in urine, representing end products of purine metabolism.

het·er·ox·e·nous (het-er-oks′ĕ-nŭs). SYN digenetic (1). [hetero- + G. *xenos,* stranger]

het·er·o·zo·ic (het-er-ō-zō′ik). Relating to another animal or another species of animal. [hetero- + G. *zōikos,* relating to an animal]

het·er·o·zy·gos·i·ty, het·er·o·zy·go·sis (het′er-ō-zī-gos′i-tē, -zī-gō′sis). The state of being heterozygous. [hetero- + G. *zygon,* a yoke]

het·er·o·zy·gote (het′er-ō-zī′gōt). A heterozygous individual. [hetero- + G. *zygotos,* yoked]

  compound h., in medical genetics, the presence of two different mutant alleles at the same loci. SYN genetic compound.

  manifesting h., an organism heterozygous for what is ordinarily a recessive condition which, as a result of special mechanisms (such as lyonization, allelic exclusion, or a deletion in the homologous chromosome), has phenotypic manifestations. SYN manifesting carrier.

het·er·o·zy·gous (het′er-ō-zī′gŭs). Having different allelic genes at one locus or (by extension) many loci; heterotic.

  doubly h., in the analysis of linkage between two loci, denoting that genotype in which a parent is h. at both loci, the state that on average contains the maximum information about the linkage.

Heubner, Johann O.L., German pediatrician, 1843–1926. SEE artery of H.; H.'s *arteritis.*

Heurenius, Johannes. SEE van Horne.

Heuser, Chester, U.S. embryologist, 1885–1965. SEE H.'s *membrane.*

HEV Abbreviation for hepatitis E *virus.*

hexa-, hex-. Prefix denoting six. [G. *hex*]

hex·a·canth (hek′să-kanth). The motile six-hooked first-stage larva of cyclophyllidean cestodes; it emerges from the egg and actively claws its way through the intermediate host's intestine prior to development into the next larval stage; *e.g.,* the h. of *Taenia saginata,* which penetrates the intestine of a cow that ingested the egg, then forms a cysticercus in the muscles of the intermediate host. SYN oncosphere. [hexa- + G. *akantha,* hook or thorn]

hex·a·chlo·ro·cy·clo·hex·ane (hek-să-klō′rō-sī-klō-hek′sān). SYN gamma benzene *hexachloride.*

hex·a·chlo·ro·phane (hek-să-klō′rō-fān). SYN hexachlorophene.

hex·a·chlo·ro·phene (hek-să-klo′rō-fēn). 2,2′-Methylene-bis(3,4,6-trichlorophenol); an antibacterial; used in soaps and detergents to inhibit bacterial growth; excessive use causes neurological lesions. SYN hexachlorophane.

hex·a·co·sa·no·ic ac·id (heks′ă-kō′sān-ō-ik). Systemic name for cerotinic acid.

hex·a·co·sa·nol (heks-ă-kō′să-nol). SEE ceryl.

hex·a·co·syl (heks-ă-kō′sil). SYN ceryl.

hex·ad (heks′ad). A sexivalent element or radical.

hex·a·dac·ty·ly, hex·a·dac·tyl·ism (hek′să-dak′ti-lē, -lizm). The presence of six fingers or six toes on one or both hands or feet. [hexa- + G. *daktylos,* finger]

hex·a·dec·a·no·ic ac·id (hek′să-dek-ă-nō′ik). SYN palmitic acid.

he

1-hex·a·dec·a·nol (hek-să-dek′ă-nol). SYN *cetyl* alcohol.

hex·a·di·phane (hek-să-dī′fān). SYN prozapine.

Hex·ad·no·vi·rus (hecks′-ad-nō-vī-rŭs). A genus in the family Hepadnaviridae, which is the cause of hepatitis B in man and certain animals.

hex·a·flu·o·ren·i·um bro·mide (hek′să-flū-rēn′ē-ŭm). Hexamethylenebis[fluoren-9-yldimethylammonium bromide]; a potentiator for succinylcholine in anesthesiology by producing a mild nondepolarizing neuromuscular blockade; also inhibits plasma cholinesterase.

hex·a·mer (hek′să-mer). **1.** SEE virion. **2.** A complex or compound containing six subunits or moieties (*e.g.,* a protein complex with six polypeptide chains or an oligopeptide with six amino acid residues). [hexa- + G. *meros,* part]

hex·a·mer·ic (heks′ă-mer-ik). Containing six subunits or moieties.

hex·a·met·a·zime (HMPAO). A lipophilic substance that readily crosses the blood-brain barrier; combined with ^{99m}Tc to produce a radiopharmaceutical for SPECT imaging or cerebral blood flow estimates. SYN hexamethylpropyleneamine oxime.

hex·a·meth·one bro·mide (hek-să-meth′ōn). SYN hexamethonium chloride.

hex·a·me·tho·ni·um chlo·ride (hek′să-me-thō′nē-ŭm). Hexamethylenebis(trimethylammonium chloride); a ganglionic blocking agent used in the treatment of hypertension, usually in combination with other hypotensive drugs; also used as the bromide and the tartrate. SYN hexamethone bromide, vegalysen.

hex·a·meth·yl·mel·a·mine (hek′să-meth′il-mel′ă-mēn). A drug which liberates formaldehyde in an acid urine; used as a urinary antiseptic.

hex·a·meth·yl·prop·yl·ene·a·mine ox·ime (heks′ă-meth′il-prō′pi-lēn- ă-mēn ok′sēm). SYN hexametazime.

hex·am·i·dine is·e·thi·o·nate (hek-sam′i-dēn). *p,p′-*(Hexamethylenedioxy)dibenzamidine bis(β-hydroxyethanesulfonate); a topical antiseptic.

hex·a·mine (hek′să-mēn). SYN methenamine.

Hex·am·i·ta (hek-sam′i-tă). A genus of protozoan flagellates (order Diplomonadida, class Zoomastigophorea), related to *Giardia;* they are parasitic in the small intestine of many gallinaceous birds and of certain mammals. *H. meleagridis* is a species that occurs in the turkey, peafowl, pheasant, quail, and Chukkar partridge; it is most pathogenic in turkeys, causing outbreaks of hexamitiasis. [hexa- + G. *mitos,* thread]

hex·am·i·ti·a·sis (hek-sam-i-tī′ă-sis). An infectious catarrhal enteritis of turkeys, quail, Chukkar partridges, and other gallinaceous birds caused by *Hexamita meleagridis* and manifested as diarrhea. Adult birds are symptomless carriers, but poults under 10 weeks often are severely affected.

hex·ane (hek′sān). A saturated hydrocarbon, C_6H_{14}, of the paraffin series (typically *n*-h., CH_3–$(CH_2)_4$–CH_3).

hex·a·no·ate (hek′să-nō-āt). SYN caproylate.

***n*-hex·a·no·ic ac·id** (hek-să-nō′ik). SYN *n*-caproic acid.

hex·a·no·yl (hek′să-nō-il). SYN caproyl.

hex·a·pep·tide (heks′a-pep′tīd). A peptide containing six amino acid residues.

hex·a·ploi·dy (heks′ă-ploy-dē). SEE polyploidy.

Hex·a·po·da (hek-sap′ō-dă). SYN Insecta. [hexa- + G. *pous,* foot]

hex·es·trol (hek-ses′trol). *p,p′-*(1,2-Diethylethylene)diphenol; dihydrodiethylstilbestrol; a synthetic *meso*-compound with estrogenic activity.

hex·et·i·dine (hek-set′i-dēn). 5-Amino-1,3-bis-(2-ethylhexyl)-hexahydro-5-methylpyrimidine; a local anti-infective agent used in the treatment of vaginitis and cervicitis due to fungal and protozoan organisms.

hex·i·tol (heks′i-tol). The polyol (sugar alcohol) obtained on the reduction of a hexose (*e.g.,* D-sorbitol).

hex·o·bar·bi·tal so·di·um (hek-sō-bar′bi-tal). Sodium 5-(1-cyclohexen-1-yl)-1,5-dimethylbarbiturate; a barbiturate sedative and hypnotic of short duration.

hex·o·ben·dine (hek-sō-ben′dēn). 3,4,5-Trimethoxybenzoic acid

ester with 3,3′-[ethylenebis(methylamino)]-di-1-propanol; a coronary and cerebral vasodilator.

hex·o·cyc·li·um meth·yl·sul·fate (hek-sō-sik′lē-ŭm meth′il-sŭl-fāt). N^4-(β-Cyclohexyl-β-hyd roxy-β-phenylethyl)-N^1-methylpiperazine dimethylsulfate; an anticholinergic agent.

hex·o·ki·nase (heks-ō-kī′nās). A phosphotransferase present in yeast, muscle, brain, and other tissues that catalyzes the phosphorylation of D-glucose and other hexoses to form D-glucose 6-phosphate (or other hexose 6-phosphate) (phosphate is transferred from ATP, which is converted to ADP); the first step in glycolysis; a deficiency of h. can result in hemolytic anemia and impaired glycolysis.

hex·on (heks′on). A hexagonal capsomere (hexamer unit) of adenovirus capsids. Antigenically, h.'s as a group differ from the penton base and also from its protruding fiber. [hex- + -on]

hex·on·ic ac·id (heks-on′ik). The aldonic acid obtained on the oxidation of the aldehyde group of an aldohexose to a carboxylic acid (*e.g.,* gluconic acid from glucose).

hex·os·a·mine (hek′sō-sam′ēn). The amine derivative (NH_2 replacing OH) of a hexose; *e.g.,* glucosamine.

hex·os·a·min·i·dase (hek′sō-sa-min′i-dās). General term for enzymes cleaving *N*-acetylhexose (*e.g.,* *N*-acetylglucosamine) residues from ganglioside-like oligosaccharides. At least four specific enzymes carrying out this type of reaction are known: α-*N*-acetyl-D-galactosaminidase, α-*N*-acetyl-D-glucosaminidase, β-*N*-acetyl-D-hexosaminidase, and β-*N*-acetyl-D-galactosaminidase, each being specific for the configuration and type of sugar included in the name.

h. A, a hydrolytic enzyme that acts on ganglioside G_{M2}, producing *N*-acetyl-D-galactosamine and ganglioside G_{M3}; a deficiency of this enzyme is associated with Tay-Sachs disease.

h. B, a hydrolytic enzyme that acts on ganglioside G_{M1}, producing ganglioside G_{M1} and galactose, as well as on globoside, producing *N*-acetylgalactosamine and trihexosylceramide; a deficiency of this enzyme is associated with Sandhoff's disease.

hex·o·sans (hek′sō-sanz). Polysaccharides with the general formula $(C_6H_{10}O_5)_x$ which, on hydrolysis, yield hexoses; included are glucosans (glucans), mannans, galactans, and fructosans (fructans). SYN polyhexoses.

hex·ose (hek′sōs). A monosaccharide containing six carbon atoms in the molecule ($C_6H_{12}O_6$); D-glucose is the principal h. in nature.

hex·ose·bis·phos·pha·tase, hex·ose·di·phos·pha·tase (hek′sōs-bis-fos′fă-tās, -dī-). SYN fructose 1,6-bisphosphate.

hex·ose phos·pha·tase. An enzyme catalyzing the hydrolysis of a hexose phosphate to a hexose (*e.g.,* glucose-6-phosphatase).

hex·ose·phos·phate isom·er·ase (hek-sōs-fos′fāt). SYN glucose-phosphate isomerase.

hex·ose-1-phos·phate uri·dyl·yl·trans·fer·ase. SYN UDPglucose–hexose-1-phosphate uridylyltransferase.

hex·u·lose (hek′syū-lōs). SYN ketohexose.

hex·u·ron·ic ac·id (hek-syūr-on′ik). The uronic acid of a hexose.

hex·yl (hek′sil). The radical of hexane, $CH_3(CH_2)_4CH_2^-$.

hex·yl·res·or·cin·ol (hek′sil-re-sōr′si-nol). 4-Hexyl-1,3-dihydroxybenzene; a broad spectrum anthelmintic.

Hey, William, English surgeon, 1736–1819. SEE H.'s *amputation,* internal *derangement, hernia,* ligament.

Heyer, W.T., U.S. scientist, *1902. SEE H.-Pudenz *valve.*

Heyns, O.S., 20th century South African obstetrician. SEE H.'s abdominal decompression *apparatus.*

Hf Symbol for hafnium.

Hg Symbol for mercury (hydrargyrum).

HGF Abbreviation for hyperglycemic-glycogenolytic *factor.*

HGH Abbreviation for human growth hormone. SEE somatotropin.

HGPRT Abbreviation for *hypoxanthine* guanine phosphoribosyltransferase.

HHV Abbreviation for human herpesvirus.

hi·a·tal (hī-ā′tăl). Relating to a hiatus.

hi·a·tus, pl. **hi·a·tus** (hī-ā′tŭs) [NA]. An aperture, opening, or foramen. [L. an aperture, fr. *hio,* pp. *hiatus,* to yawn]

adductor h., the aperture in the aponeurotic insertion of the adductor magnus that transmits the femoral artery and vein from the adductor canal to the popliteal space. SYN h. tendineus [NA], h. adductorius☆ [NA], femoral opening, tendinous opening.

h. adducto′rius [NA], ☆official alternate term for adductor h.

aortic h., the opening in the diaphragm bounded by the two crura, the vertebral column, and the median arcuate ligament, through which pass the aorta and thoracic duct. SYN h. aorticus [NA], aortic foramen, aortic opening.

h. aor′ticus [NA], SYN aortic h.

Breschet's h., SYN helicotrema.

h. of canal for greater petrosal nerve, SYN h. of facial canal.

h. cana′lis facia′lis, SYN h. of facial canal.

h. cana′lis ner′vi petro′si majo′ris [NA], SYN h. of facial canal.

h. cana′lis ner′vi petro′si mino′ris [NA], SYN h. of canal of lesser petrosal nerve.

h. of canal of lesser petrosal nerve, the small opening in the petrous bone lateral to the h. of facial canal that gives passage to the lesser petrosal nerve. SYN h. canalis nervi petrosi minoris [NA], Arnold's canal, canalis nervi petrosi superficialis minoris.

esophageal h., the opening in the right crus of the diaphragm, between the central tendon and the h. aorticus, through which pass the esophagus and the two vagus nerves. SYN h. esophageus [NA], esophageal opening.

h. esopha′geus [NA], SYN esophageal h.

h. ethmoida′lis, SYN semilunar h.

h. of facial canal, the opening on the anterior aspect of the petrous part of the temporal bone which leads to the facial canal and gives passage to the greater petrosal nerve. SYN h. canalis nervi petrosi majoris [NA], fallopian h., Ferrein's foramen, h. canalis facialis, h. of canal for greater petrosal nerve.

fallopian h., SYN h. of facial canal.

h. maxilla′ris [NA], SYN maxillary h.

maxillary h., the large opening into the maxillary sinus on the nasal surface of the maxilla. SYN h. maxillaris [NA].

pleuropericardial h., an opening connecting the pleural and pericardial cavities; usually the result of incomplete development of the pleuropericardial fold of the embryo.

pleuroperitoneal h., an opening through the diaphragm, connecting pleural and peritoneal cavities, usually the result of defective development of the pleuroperitoneal membrane in the embryo; if the defect is extensive there may be herniation of digestive organs into the pleural cavity. SEE ALSO diaphragmatic *hernia.* SYN Bochdalek's foramen.

sacral h., a normally-occurring gap at the lower end of the sacrum, exposing the vertebral canal, due to failure of the laminae of the last sacral segment to coalesce. It is closed by the sacrococcygeal ligament, and provides cannular access to the sacral epidural space for administration of anesthetics (caudal nerve blocks). SYN h. sacralis [NA].

h. sacra′lis [NA], SYN sacral h.

saphenous h., SYN saphenous *opening.*

h. saphe′nus [NA], SYN saphenous *opening.*

scalene h., triangular gap bounded by the scalenus anterior and scalenus medius muscles and the first rib to which the muscles attach; the h. provides passage for the subclavian artery and the roots of the brachial plexus. Compression of the structures passing through the h. by any means is manifest as "thoracic outlet syndrome." SYN interscalene triangle.

Scarpa's h., SYN helicotrema.

semilunar h., a deep, narrow groove in the lateral wall of the middle meatus of the nasal cavity, into which the maxillary sinus, the frontonasal duct, and the middle ethmoid cells open. SYN h. semilunaris [NA], h. ethmoidalis.

h. semiluna′ris [NA], SYN semilunar h.

h. subarcua′tus, SYN subarcuate *fossa.*

h. tendin′eus [NA], SYN adductor h.

h. tota′lis sacra′lis, developmental clefting in all sacral vertebrae; may also involve adjacent lumbar vertebrae.

hi·ber·na·tion (hī-ber-nā′shŭn). A torpid condition in which certain animals pass the cold months. True hibernators, such as woodchucks, ground squirrels, dormice, and some others, have body temperatures reduced to near the freezing point, with a very slow heartbeat, low metabolism, and infrequent respirations. Partial hibernators, such as bears, skunks, and raccoons, have reduced physiologic activity during the cold months, but they are not comatose. Cf. estivation. SYN winter sleep. [L. *hibernus,* relating to winter]

hi·ber·no·ma (hī′ber-nō′mă). A rare type of benign neoplasm in human beings, consisting of brown fat that resembles the fat in certain hibernating animals; individual tumor cells contain multiple lipid droplets. SEE ALSO brown *fat.* [L. *hibernus,* pertaining to winter, + G. *-ōma,* tumor]

interscapular h., SYN brown *fat.*

hic·cup, hic·cough (hik′ŭp). A diaphragmatic spasm causing a sudden inhalation which is interrupted by a spasmodic closure of the glottis, producing a noise.

epidemic h., a persistent h. occurring as a complication of influenza.

Hicks, John Braxton. SEE Braxton H.

HIDA Abbreviation for dimethyl iminodiacetic acid.

△**hidr-.** SEE hidro-.

hi·drad·e·ni·tis (hī-drad′ĕ-nī′tis). Inflammation of the sweat glands. SYN hidrosadenitis, hydradenitis, spiradenitis. [G. *hidrōs,* sweat, + *adēn,* gland, + *-itis,* inflammation]

h. axilla′ris of Verneuil, an axillary abscess.

h. suppurati′va, chronic suppurative folliculitis of apocrine sweat gland-bearing skin of the perianal, axillary, and genital areas or under the breasts, producing abscesses or sinuses with scarring.

hi·drad·e·no·ma (hī-drad-ĕ-nō′mă). A benign neoplasm derived from epithelial cells of sweat glands. SYN hydradenoma. [G. *hidrōs,* sweat, + *adēn,* gland, + *-oma,* tumor]

clear cell h., a tumor derived from eccrine sweat glands, composed of glycogen-rich clear cells. SYN eccrine acrospiroma, nodular h.

nodular h., SYN clear cell h.

papillary h., a solitary benign tumor occurring in women usually in the labia majora, cystic and papillary, and composed of epithelium resembling that of apocrine glands. SYN apocrine adenoma, h. papilliferum.

h. papillife′rum, SYN papillary h.

△**hidro-, hidr-.** Sweat, sweat glands. Cf. sudor-. [G. *hidrōs*]

hi·droa (hī-drō′ă). SYN hydroa.

hi·dro·cys·to·ma (hī′drō-sis-tō′mă). A cystic form of hidradenoma, usually apocrine. SYN hydrocystoma (2), syringocystoma. [hidro- + G. *kystis,* bladder, + *-ōma,* tumor]

hi·dro·mei·o·sis (hī′drō-mī-ō′sis). A decline in the rate of sweating during exposure to heat, especially that from warm baths. [hidro- + G. *meiōsis,* a lessening]

hi·dro·poi·e·sis (hī′drō-poy-ē′sis, hid′rō-). The formation of sweat. [hidro- + G. *poiēsis,* formation]

hi·dro·sad·e·ni·tis (hī′drō-sad-ĕ-nī′tis, hid′rō-). SYN hidradenitis.

hi·dros·che·sis (hī-dros′kē-sis, hid-ros′). Suppression of sweating. [hidro- + G. *schesis,* a checking]

hi·dro·sis (hi-drō′sis, hī-). The production and excretion of sweat. SYN idrosis. [G. *hidrōs,* sweat, + *-osis,* condition]

hi·drot·ic (hi-drot′ik, hī-). Relating to or causing hidrosis.

hi·er·ar·chy (hī′er-ar-kē, hī-rar′kē). **1.** Any system of persons or things ranked one above the other. **2.** In psychology and psychiatry, an organization of habits or concepts in which simpler components are combined to form increasingly complex integrations. [G. *hierarchia,* rule or power of the high priest]

dominance h., a social situation in which one organism dominates all below it, the next all below it, and so on down to the organism dominated by all; *e.g.,* the pecking order in apes, seals, barnyard hens, and other species.

Maslow's h., a ranking of needs which man presumably fills successively in the order of lowest to highest: physiological needs, love and belonging, self-esteem, and self-actualization.

response h., alternative reactions or modes of adjustment to a given situation arranged in the probable order of prior effectiveness; *e.g.,* a mother attempting to discipline an unruly child may first request, cajole, then plead, scold, and finally punish; her behaviors can be ordered along a response h. for further monitoring of effectiveness.

h. of terms, in radiology, the semantic concept of using different terms to describe anatomic or pathologic structures versus the resultant diagnostic images.

hi·er·o·ma·nia (hī'er-ō-mā'nē-ă). Obsolete term for pathologic religious fervor characterized by delusions with a religious content. [G. *hieros,* holy, + *mania,* insanity]

hi·er·o·pho·bia (hī'er-ō-fō'bē-ă). Morbid fear of religious or sacred objects. [G. *hieros,* holy, + *phobos,* fear]

hi·er·o·ther·a·py (hī'er-ō-thār'ă-pē). Treatment of disease by prayer and religious practices. [G. *hieros,* holy, + *therapeia,* therapy]

Higashi, Ototaka. Japanese physician. SEE Chédiak-H. *disease;* Chédiak-Steinbrinck-H. *anomaly, syndrome.*

Highmore, Nathaniel, British anatomist, 1613–1685. SEE *antrum* of H.; H.'s *body; corpus* highmori; *corpus* highmorianum.

Higoumenakia sign. See under sign.

hi·la (hī'lă). Plural of hilum.

hi·lar (hī'lăr). Pertaining to a hilum.

hi·li·tis (hī-lī'tis). Inflammation of the lining membrane of any hilus.

Hill, Archibald V., English biophysicist and Nobel laureate, 1886–1977. SEE H.'s *equation;* H. *plot.*

Hill, Harold A., 20th century U.S. radiologist. SEE H.-Sachs *lesion.*

Hill, Sir Leonard Erskine, English physiologist, 1866-1952. SEE H.'s *sign, phenomenon.*

Hill, Lucius, U.S. thoracic surgeon, *1921. SEE H. *operation.*

Hill, Robert, British plant physiologist, *1899. SEE H. *reaction.*

Hillis, David S., U.S. obstetrician-gynecologist, 1873–1942. SEE H.-Müller *maneuver.*

hil·lock (hil'lok). In anatomy, any small elevation or prominence.

axon h., the conical area of origin of the axon from the nerve cell body; it contains parallel arrays of microtubules and is devoid of Nissl substance. SYN implantation cone.

facial h., SYN facial *colliculus.*

seminal h., SYN seminal *colliculus.*

Hilton, John, English surgeon, 1804–1878. SEE H.'s *law,* white *line, method, sac.*

hi·lum, pl. **hi·la** (hī'lŭm, hī'lă) [NA]. **1.** The part of an organ where the nerves and vessels enter and leave. SYN porta (1). **2.** A depression or slit resembling the h. in the olivary nucleus of the brain. [L. a small bit or trifle]

h. of dentate nucleus, the mouth of the flasklike dentate nucleus of the cerebellum, directed inward, and giving exit to many of the fibers which compose the superior cerebellar peduncle or brachium conjunctivum. SYN h. nuclei dentati [NA].

h. of kidney, the depression on the medial border of the kidney through which pass the segmental renal vessels and renal nerves and where the apex of the renal pelvis occurs. SYN h. renalis [NA], porta renis.

h. li'enis, ☆official alternate term for h. of spleen.

h. of lung, a wedge-shaped depression on the mediastinal surface of each lung, where the bronchus, blood vessels, nerves, and lymphatics enter or leave the viscus. SYN h. pulmonis [NA], porta pulmonis.

h. of lymph node, the depressed area of the surface of a lymph node through which the efferent lymphatics emerge from the medulla and through which blood vessels enter and leave the node. SYN h. nodi lymphatici [NA].

h. no'di lympha'tici [NA], SYN h. of lymph node.

h. nu'clei denta'ti [NA], SYN h. of dentate nucleus.

h. nu'clei oliva'ris [NA], SYN h. of olivary nucleus.

h. of olivary nucleus, the medially oriented opening in the folded cell layer composing the inferior olivary nucleus through which the efferent fibers of the nucleus make their exit. SYN h. nuclei olivaris [NA].

h. ova'rii [NA], SYN h. of ovary.

h. of ovary, the depression along the mesovarian margin, at the insertion of the mesovarium, where vessels and nerves enter or leave the ovary. SYN h. ovarii [NA].

h. pulmo'nis [NA], SYN h. of lung.

h. rena'lis [NA], SYN h. of kidney.

h. of spleen, a fissure on the gastric surface of the spleen, giving passage to the splenic vessels and nerves. SYN h. splenicum [NA], h. lienis☆, porta lienis.

h. sple'nicum [NA], SYN h. of spleen.

hi·lus (hī'lŭs). Former incorrect NA designation for hilum. [an Eng. variant of L. *hilum*]

hi·man·to·sis (hī-man-tō'sis). An unusually long uvula. [G. *himas,* strap, + *-osis,* condition]

hind·brain (hīnd'brān). SYN rhombencephalon.

hind·gut (hīnd'gŭt). **1.** The caudal or terminal part of the embryonic gut. **2.** Descending and sigmoid colon, rectum and anal canal; some include entire large intestine. SYN endgut.

hind·wa·ter (hīnd'wah-ter). Colloquialism for amniotic fluid *in utero* behind the presenting part of the fetus.

hinge-bow (hinj'bō). SYN face-bow.

Hinman, Frank, Jr., U.S. urologist, *1915. SEE H. *syndrome.*

Hinton, William A., U.S. physician, 1883–1959. SEE H. *test;* Mueller-H. *agar.*

hip. 1. The lateral prominence of the pelvis from the waist to the thigh. **2.** Head, neck and greater trohantar of femur. It is this sense that is utilized in the common phrases "hip fracture" or "hip replacement." **3.** More strictly, the hip joint. [A.S. *hype*]

snapping h., a condition in which the fascia lata or gluteus maximus muscle under tension, moving over the greater trochanter of the proximal end of the femur, causes a click.

hip·ber·ries. SYN rose hips.

hip bone. See under bone.

Hippel, Eugen von. SEE von H.

Hip·pe·la·tes (hip-ĕ-lā'tēz). The eye gnats, a genus of flies in the family Chloropidae (fruit flies) that are attracted to the body secretions and fluids of animals and man, particularly those in the eyes. *H.* is suspected of transmitting certain types of conjunctivitis (such as pinkeye), bovine mastitis, and yaws (frambesia tropica). [G. *hippelatēs,* driver of horses]

Hip·po·bos·ca (hip-ō-bos'kă). A genus of pupiparous louse flies (family Hippoboscidae) related to the tsetse flies; they are ectoparasites on birds and mammals. SEE ALSO *Melophagus.* [G. *hippos,* horse, + *boskein,* to feed]

Hip·po·bos·ci·dae (hip-ō-bos'ki-dē, -bos'i-dē). A family of winged and wingless flies (order Diptera) that are parasitic on birds and mammals; it includes the genera *Hippobosca* and *Melophagus.*

hip·po·cam·pal (hip-ō-kam'păl). Relating to the hippocampus.

hip·po·cam·pus (hip-ō-kam'pŭs) [NA]. The complex, internally convoluted structure that forms the medial margin ("hem") of the cortical mantle of the cerebral hemisphere, bordering the choroid fissure of the lateral ventricle, and composed of two gyri (Ammon's horn and the dentate gyrus), together with their white matter, the alveus and fimbria hippocampi. In monkeys, apes, and humans the h. is confined to the temporal lobe by the massive development of the corpus callosum. Cytoarchitecturally a unique form of allocortex (archicortex), the h. forms part of the limbic system (formerly rhinencephalon). Its major afferent connections are with the entorhinal area of the parahippocampal gyrus, and transparent septum; by way of the fornix it projects to the septum, anterior nucleus of the thalamus, and mamillary body. SYN h. major, major h. [G. *hippocampos,* seahorse]

h. ma'jor, SYN hippocampus.

major h., SYN hippocampus.

h. mi'nor, SYN *calcar* avis.

minor h., SYN *calcar* avis.

Hippocrates of Cos. Greek physician, called the "Father of Medicine," circa 460–377 B.C. SEE hippocratic *facies,* hippocratic *fingers*, under *finger*, hippocratic *nails*, under *nail*, school, succussion.

hip·po·crat·ic (hip-ŏ-krat′ik). Relating to, described by, or attributed to Hippocrates.

Hip·po·crat·ic Oath. An oath demanded of physicians about to enter the practice of their profession, the composition of which, though usually attributed to Hippocrates of Cos, is probably an ancient oath of the Aesclepiads. It appears in a book of the hippocratic collection as follows:

"I swear by Apollo the physician, by Aesculapius, Hygeia, and Panacea, and I take to witness all the gods, all the goddesses, to keep according to my ability and my judgment the following Oath:

To consider dear to me as my parents him who taught me this art; to live in common with him and if necessary to share my goods with him; to look upon his children as my own brothers, to teach them this art if they so desire without fee or written promise; to impart to my sons and the sons of the master who taught me and the disciples who have enrolled themselves and have agreed to the rules of the profession, but to these alone, the precepts and the instruction. I will prescribe regimen for the good of my patients according to my ability and my judgment and never do harm to anyone. To please no one will I prescribe a deadly drug, nor give advice which may cause his death. Nor will I give a woman a pessary to procure abortion. But I will preserve the purity of my life and my art. I will not cut for stone, even for patients in whom the disease is manifest; I will leave this operation to be performed by practitioners (specialists in this art). In every house where I come I will enter only for the good of my patients, keeping myself far from all intentional ill-doing and all seduction, and especially from the pleasures of love with women or with men, be they free or slaves. All that may come to my knowledge in the exercise of my profession or outside of my profession or in daily commerce with men, which ought not to be spread abroad, I will keep secret and will never reveal. If I keep this oath faithfully, may I enjoy my life and practice my art, respected by all men and in all times; but if I swerve from it or violate it, may the reverse be my lot."

hip·poc·ra·tism (hi-pok′ră-tizm). A system of medicine, attributed to Hippocrates and his disciples, based on the imitation of nature's processes in the therapeutic management of disease.

hip·pu·rate (hip′yū-rāt). A salt or ester of hippuric acid.

hip·pu·ria (hi-pyū′rē-ă). The excretion of an abnormally large amount of hippuric acid in the urine.

hip·pu·ric ac·id (hi-pyūr′ik). *N*-Benzoylglycine; a detoxification and excretory product of benzoate found in the urine of man and many herbivorous animals; used therapeutically in the form of its salts (hippurates of calcium and ammonium). [G. *hippos*, horse, + *ouron*, urine]

hip·pu·ri·case (hi-pyūr′i-cās). SYN aminoacylase.

hip·pus (hip′ŭs). Intermittent pupillary dilation and constriction, independent of illumination, convergence, or psychic stimuli. [G. *hippos*, horse, from a fancied suggestion of galloping movements]

respiratory h., dilation of the pupils occurring during forced, voluntary inspiration, and contraction during expiration.

hir·ci (her′sī). Plural of hircus.

hir·cis·mus (her-siz′mŭs). Offensive odor of the axillae. [L. *hircus*, goat]

hir·cus, gen. and pl. **hir·ci** (her′kŭs, her′sī). **1.** The odor of the axillae. **2** [NA]. One of the hairs growing in the axillae. **3.** SYN tragus (1). [L. he-goat]

Hirschberg, Julius, German ophthalmologist, 1843–1925. SEE H.'s *method.*

Hirschfeld, Isador, U.S. dentist, 1881–1965. SEE H.'s *canals,* under *canal.*

Hirschowitz syn·drome. See under syndrome.

Hirsch-Peiffer stain. See under stain.

Hirschsprung, Harald, Danish physician, 1830–1916. SEE H.'s *disease.*

hir·sute (her-sūt′). Relating to or characterized by hirsutism. [L. *hirsutus*, shaggy]

hir·su·ti·es (her-su′tē-ēz). SYN hirsutism. [Mod. L. fr. L. *hirsutus*, shaggy]

hir·sut·ism (her′sū-tizm). Presence of excessive bodily and facial terminal hair, in a male pattern, especially in women; may be present in normal adults as an expression of an ethnic characteristic or may develop in children or adults as the result of androgen excess due to tumors or drugs, or nonandrogenetic drugs. SYN hirsuties, pilosis. [L. *hirsutus,* shaggy]

Apert's h., h. caused by a virilizing disorder of adrenocortical origin.

constitutional h., mild to moderate degree of h. present in an individual exhibiting otherwise normal endocrine and reproductive function.

idiopathic h., h. of uncertain origin in women, who may additionally exhibit menstrual abnormalities and infertility.

hir·tel·lous (hĭr′tĕ-lŭs). Having or resembling fine hairs; term describing the filamentous protein polysaccharide coating of microvilli. SEE glycocalyx. [L. *hirtus,* hairy, shaggy]

hir·u·di·cide (hi-rū′di-sīd). An agent that kills leeches. [L. *hirudo,* leech, + *caedo,* to kill]

hir·u·din (hir′yū-din). An antithrombin substance extracted from the salivary glands of the leech that has the property of preventing coagulation of the blood. [L. *hirudo,* leech]

Hir·u·din·ea (hir′ū-din′ē-ă). The leeches, a class of worms (phylum Annelida) with flat, segmented bodies, a sucker at the posterior end, and often a smaller sucker at the anterior end; they are predatory on invertebrate tissues, or feed on blood and tissue exudates of vertebrates. [L. *hirudo,* leech]

hir·u·di·ni·a·sis (hi-rū-di-nī′ă-sis). A condition resulting from leeches attaching themselves to the skin or being taken into the mouth or nose while drinking. [L. *hirudo,* leech, + G. *-iasis,* condition]

hir·u·din·i·za·tion (hi-rū′di-nī-zā′shŭn). **1.** The process of rendering the blood noncoagulable by the injection of hirudin. **2.** The application of leeches.

Hir·u·do (hi-rū′dō). A genus of leeches (class Hirudinea, family Gnathobdellidae). Species previously used in medicine are: *H. australis,* Australian leech; *H. decora,* American leech; *H. interrupta* or *H. troctina,* a leech of northern Africa; *H. medicinalis,* speckled, Swedish, or German leech, the species previously in most general use; *H. m. officinalis,* a variety of the preceding; *H. provincialis,* the green or Hungarian leech; *H. quinquestriata,* five-striped leech. [L. leech]

His, Wilhelm, Jr., German physician, 1863–1934. SEE H.'s *band, bundle;* H. bundle *electrogram;* H.'s *spindle;* Kent-H. *bundle;* H.-Tawara *system.*

His, Wilhelm, Sr., Swiss anatomist and embryologist in Germany, 1831–1904. SEE H.'s *copula, line, rule,* perivascular *space; isthmus* of H.

His- Symbol for histidyl.

-His Symbol for histidino.

His. Symbol for histidine.

Hiss, Philip, U.S. bacteriologist, 1868–1913. SEE H.'s *stain.*

his·ta·mi·nase (his-tam′i-nās). SYN *amine* oxidase (copper-containing).

his·ta·mine (his′tă-mēn). 2-(4-Imidazolyl)ethylamine; a depressor amine derived from histidine by histidine decarboxylase and present in ergot and in animal tissues. It is a powerful stimulant of gastric secretion, a constrictor of bronchial smooth muscle and a vasodilator (capillaries and arterioles) that causes a fall in blood pressure. H., or a substance indistinguishable in action from it, is liberated in the skin as a result of injury. When pricked into the skin in high dilution, it causes the triple response.

h. phosphate, used in the treatment of certain allergies, cephalalgia, and acute multiple sclerosis with varying results; also used to test gastric secretory function, in the diagnosis of pheochromocytoma and in the treatment of Ménière's disease; also available as h. acid phosphate.

his·ta·mine-fast. Indicating the absence of the normal response to histamine, especially in speaking of true gastric anacidity.

his·ta·mi·ne·mia (his′tă-mi-nē′mē-ă). The presence of histamine in the circulating blood. [histamine + G. *haima,* blood]

hi

histamine	
H₁ receptors	H₂ receptors
lung	
contraction of bronchial muscles (humans)	relaxation of bronchial muscles (sheep)
heart/circulatory system	
positive bathmotropic effect positive dromotropic effect vasoconstriction (vessels < 80 μm)	positive inotropic effect positive chronotropic effect
vasodilation (vessels > 80 μm)	
distribution of adrenaline	
endothelial contraction, and thereby increased permeability (edema of tissue)	
uterus	
contraction (guinea pig)	relaxation (rat)
intestine	
contraction	
stomach	
	increase of acid secretion

his·ta·mi·nu·ria (his'tă-mi-nū'rē-ă). The excretion of histamine in the urine. [histidine + G. *ouron,* urine]

his·tan·gic (his-tan'jik). SYN histoangic.

his·ti·dase (his'ti-dās). SYN *histidine* ammonia-lyase.

his·ti·din·al (his'ti-din-ăl). The aldehyde analogue of histidine (–CHO replacing –COOH).

his·ti·di·nase (his'ti-di-nās). SYN *histidine* ammonia-lyase.

his·ti·dine (His, H) (his'ti-dēn). α-Amino-β-(4-imidazolyl)-propionic acid; the L-isomer is a basic amino acid found in most proteins.

  h. ammonia-lyase, an enzyme catalyzing deamination of L-histidine to urocanate and ammonia; this enzyme is absent or deficient in individuals with histidinemia. SYN histidase, histidinase, h. deaminase.

  h. deaminase, SYN h. ammonia-lyase.

  h. decarboxylase, an enzyme catalyzing the decarboxylation of L-histidine to histamine and CO_2; thus, it plays a role in constriction of bronchial smooth muscle.

his·ti·di·ne·mia (his'ti-di-nē'mē-ă) [MIM*235800]. Elevation of blood histidine level and excretion of histidine and related imidazole metabolites in urine due to deficiency of histidine transport protein; speech defects and mild mental retardation are associated conditions in about half of the patients, growth retardation occurs in some; autosomal recessive inheritance. A deficiency of histidine ammonia lyase will also result in histidinemia. [histidine + G. *haima,* blood, + -ia]

his·ti·dino (-His) (his'ti-din-ō). The radical of histidine produced by removal of a hydrogen from a nitrogen atom; prefixed by N^α, N^τ, or N^π.

his·ti·di·nol (his'ti-di-nol). The alcohol analogue of histidine (–COOH becomes –CH₂OH).

his·ti·di·nu·ria (his'ti-di-nū'rē-ă). Excretion of considerable amounts of histidine in the urine; frequently observed in later months of pregnancy, and in histidinemia.

his·ti·dyl (His-) (his'ti-dil). The acyl radical of histidine.

△**histio-.** Tissue, especially connective tissue. [G. *histion,* web (tissue)]

his·ti·o·blast (his'tē-ō-blast). A tissue-forming cell. SYN histoblast. [histio- + G. *blastos,* germ]

his·ti·o·cyte (his'tē-ō-sīt). A macrophage present in connective tissue. SYN histocyte. [histio- + G. *kytos,* cell]

  cardiac h., a large mononuclear cell found in connective tissue of the heart wall in inflammatory conditions, especially in the Aschoff body. The ovoid nucleus contains a central chromatin mass appearing as a wavy bar in longitudinal section. SYN Anitschkow cell, Anitschkow myocyte, caterpillar cell.

  sea-blue h., a h. containing cytoplasmic granules that stain bright blue with hematologic stains such as Wright-Giemsa; found in bone marrow and in the spleen, associated with hepatosplenomegaly and thrombocytopenic purpura and in other blood diseases.

his·ti·o·cy·to·ma (his'tē-ō-sī-tō'mă). A tumor composed of histiocytes. [histio- + G. *kytos,* cell, + *-ōma,* tumor]

  fibrous h., SYN sclerosing *hemangioma.* SEE dermatofibroma.

  generalized eruptive h., a rare recurring generalized eruption in adults of flesh colored or erythematous papules remaining localized to the skin and consisting of dermal nodules of mononuclear histiocytes that do not stain for lipid. SYN nodular non-X histiocytosis.

  malignant fibrous h., a deeply situated tumor, especially on the extremities of adults, frequently recurring after surgery and metastasizing to the lungs; shows partial fibroblastic and histiocytic differentiation with a variable storiform pattern, myxoid areas, and giant cells.

his·ti·o·cy·to·sis (his'tē-ō-sī-tō'sis). A generalized multiplication of histiocytes. SYN histocytosis.

  lipid h., h. with cytoplasmic accumulation of lipid, either phospholipid (Niemann-Pick disease) or glucocerebroside (Gaucher's disease).

  malignant h., a rapidly fatal form of lymphoma, characterized by fever, jaundice, pancytopenia, and enlargement of the liver, spleen, and lymph nodes; the affected organs show focal necrosis and hemorrhage, with proliferation of histiocytes and phagocytosis of red blood cells.

  nodular non-X h., SYN generalized eruptive *histiocytoma.*

  nonlipid h., SYN Letterer-Siwe *disease.*

  regressing atypical h., a rare disease characterized clinically by multiple ulcerating cutaneous papules and nodules which show spontaneous regression; the skin is infiltrated by malignant-appearing histiocytes.

  sinus h. with massive lymphadenopathy, a chronic disease occurring in children and characterized by massive painless cervical lymphadenopathy due to distension of the lymphatic sinuses by macrophages containing ingested lymphocytes, and by capsular and pericapsular fibrosis. SYN Rosai-Dorman disease.

  h. X, proliferation of Langerhans' cells of undetermined clinical type, possibly Hand-Schüller-Christian d., Letterer-Siwe disease, and eosinophilic granuloma.

  h. Y, SYN verrucous *xanthoma.*

his·ti·o·gen·ic (his'tē-ō-jen'ik). SYN histogenous.

his·ti·oid (his'tē-oyd). SYN histoid.

his·ti·o·ma (his-tē-ō'mă). SYN histoma.

his·ti·on·ic (his-tē-on'ik). Relating to any tissue.

△**histo-.** Tissue. [G. *histos,* web (tissue)]

his·to·an·gic (his-tō-an'jik). Relating to the structure of blood vessels, especially in terms of their function. SYN histangic. [histo- + G. *angeion,* vessel]

his·to·blast (his'tō-blast). SYN histioblast.

his·to·chem·is·try (his'tō-kem'is-trē). SYN cytochemistry.

his·to·com·pat·i·bil·i·ty (his'tō-kom-pat-i-bil'i-tē). A state of immunologic similarity (or identity) that permits successful homograft transplantation.

his·to·com·pat·i·bil·i·ty test·ing. See under testing.

his·to·cyte (his'tō-sīt). SYN histiocyte.

his·to·cy·to·sis (his'tō-sī-tō'sis). SYN histiocytosis.

his·to·dif·fer·en·ti·a·tion (his'tō-dif-er-en-shē-ā'shŭn). The morphologic appearance of tissue characteristics during development.

his·to·flu·o·res·cence (his-tō-flŭr-es′ens). Fluorescence of the tissues under exposure to ultraviolet rays following the injection of a fluorescent substance or as a result of a natural fluorescing substance.

his·to·gen·e·sis (his-tō-jen′ĕ-sis). The origin of a tissue; the formation and development of the tissues of the body. SYN histogeny. [histo- + G. *genesis,* origin]

his·to·ge·net·ic (his-tō-jĕ-net′ik). Relating to histogenesis.

his·tog·e·nous (his-toj′ĕ-nŭs). Formed by the tissues; *e.g.,* the h. cells in an exudate arising from proliferation of the fixed tissue cells. SYN histogenic. [histo- + G. *-gen,* producing]

his·tog·e·ny (his-toj′ĕ-nē). SYN histogenesis.

his·to·gram (his′tō-gram). **1.** A graphic columnar or bar representation to compare the magnitudes of frequencies or numbers of items. **2.** Graphical representation of the frequency distribution of a variable, in which rectangles are drawn with their bases on a uniform linear scale representing intervals, and their heights are proportional to the values within each of the intervals. [histo- + G. *gramma,* a writing]

his·toid (his′toyd). **1.** Resembling in structure one of the tissues of the body. **2.** Sometimes used with reference to the histologic structure of a neoplasm derived from and consisting of a single, relatively simple type of neoplastic tissue that closely resembles the normal, as in certain fibromas and leiomyomas. SYN histioid. [histo- + G. *eidos,* resemblance]

his·to·in·com·pat·i·bil·i·ty (his′tō-in′kom-pat-i-bil′i-tē). A state of immunologic dissimilarity of tissues sufficient to cause rejection of a homograft when tissue is transplanted from one individual to another; implies a difference in histocompatibility genes in donor and recipient.

his·to·log·ic, his·to·log·i·cal (his-tō-loj′ik, i-kăl). Pertaining to histology.

his·tol·o·gist (his-tol′ō-jist). One who specializes in the science of histology. SYN microanatomist.

his·tol·o·gy (his-tol′ō-jē). The science concerned with the minute structure of cells, tissues, and organs in relation to their function. SEE microscopic *anatomy.* SYN microanatomy. [histo- + G. *logos,* study]

    pathologic h., SYN histopathology.

his·tol·y·sis (his-tol′i-sis). Disintegration of tissue. [histo- + G. *lysis,* dissolution]

his·to·ma (his-tō′mă). A benign neoplasm in which the cytologic and histologic elements are closely similar to those of normal tissue from which the neoplastic cells are derived. SYN histioma. [histo- + G. *-oma,* tumor]

his·to·met·a·plas·tic (his′tō-met-ă-plas′tik). Exciting tissue metaplasia.

His·to·mo·nas me·le·ag·ri·dis (hi-stom′ō-nas me-lē-ag′ri-dis). A protozoan flagellate (order Trichomonadida) parasitizing the intestine and liver of turkeys, chickens, and many other domestic and wild gallinaceous birds; it is nearly ubiquitous but rarely pathogenic in chickens; in the turkey, it causes histomoniasis. It is now considered to be in a family (Monocercomonadidae) that includes *Dientamoeba,* SYN *Amoeba meleagridis.*

his·tom·o·ni·a·sis (hi-stom′ō-nī′ă-sis). A disease chiefly affecting turkeys, caused by *Histomonas meleagridis* and characterized by ulcerative and necrotic lesions of the liver and cecum, acute onset, and a high mortality rate. It is transmitted inside the eggs of the nematode *Heterakis gallinae,* which is primarily responsible for maintaining and spreading the infection. SYN blackhead (2), infectious enterohepatitis.

his·to·mor·phom·e·try (his′tō-mōr-fom′ĕ-trē). The quantitative measurement and characterization of microscopical images using a computer; manual or automated digital image analysis typically involves measurements and comparisons of selected geometric areas, perimeters, length angle of orientation, form factors, center of gravity coordinates, as well as image enhancement. [histo- + G. *morphē,* shape, + *metron,* measure]

his·tone (his′tōn). One of a number of simple proteins (often found in the cell nucleus) that contains a high proportion of basic amino acids, are soluble in water, dilute acids, and alkalies, and

are not coagulable by heat; *e.g.,* the proteins associated with nucleic acids in the nuclei of plant and animal tissues.

his·to·nec·to·my (his-tō-nek′tō-mē). SYN periarterial *sympathectomy.* [histo- + G. *ektomē,* excision]

his·to·neu·rol·o·gy (his-tō-nū-rol′ō-jē). SYN neurohistology.

his·ton·o·my (his-ton′ō-mē). A law of the development and structure of the tissues of the body. [histo- + G. *nomos,* law]

his·to·nu·ria (his-tō-nū′rē-ă). The excretion of histone in the urine, as observed in certain instances of leukemia, febrile illnesses, and wasting diseases. [histone + G. *ouron,* urine]

his·to·path·o·gen·e·sis (his′tō-path-ō-jen′ĕ-sis). Abnormal embryonic development or growth of tissue. [histogenesis + pathogenesis]

his·to·pa·thol·o·gy (his′tō-pa-thol′ō-jē). The science or study dealing with the cytologic and histologic structure of abnormal or diseased tissue. SYN pathologic histology.

his·to·phys·i·ol·o·gy (his′tō-fiz-ē-ol′ŏ-jē). The microscopic study of tissues in relation to their functions.

His·to·plas·ma cap·su·la·tum (his-tō-plaz′mă kap-sū-lā′tŭm). A dimorphic fungus species of worldwide distribution that causes histoplasmosis in humans and other mammals; its ascomycetous state is *Ajellomyces capsulatum.* The organism's natural habitat is soil fertilized with bird and bat droppings, where it grows as a mold, fragments of which, following inhalation, produce the primary pulmonary infection; within the mammalian host tissues, inhaled mycelial fragments grow as uninuclear yeasts that reproduce by budding. This parasitic form may also be induced in the laboratory by culturing the mycelial phase at 37°C on a blood-enriched medium; growth reverts to the mycelial form when the temperature is below 37°C. *H. c.* var. *duboisii* causes a clinically distinct disease, African histoplasmosis, in which large yeast cells with thicker walls are found in tissues, in contrast to the small yeast cells of *H. c.* var. *farciminosum,* which causes epizootic lymphangitis. [histo- + G. *plasma,* something formed]

his·to·plas·min (his′tō-plas′min). An antigenic extract of *Histoplasma capsulatum,* used in immunological tests for the diagnosis of histoplasmosis; also used in skin test surveys of populations to determine the geographic distribution of the fungus and to predict those that are endemic for histoplasmosis.

his·to·plas·mo·ma (his′tō-plaz-mō′mă). An infectious granuloma caused by *Histoplasma capsulatum.*

his·to·plas·mo·sis (his′tō-plaz-mō′sis). A widely distributed infectious disease caused by *Histoplasma capsulatum* and occurring frequently in epidemics; usually acquired by inhalation of spores of the fungus in soil dust and manifested by a primary benign pneumonitis similar in clinical features to a mild form of primary tuberculosis; occasionally, the primary disease progresses to produce localized lesions in lung, such as pulmonary cavitation, or the typical disseminated disease of the reticuloendothelial system which is manifested by fever, emaciation, splenomegaly, and leukopenia. SYN Darling's disease.

    African h., a form of h. caused by *Histoplasma capsulatum* var. *duboisii,* observed only in tropical Africa; the organism grows chiefly in giant cells, causing lesions localized to skin, bone, or lacrimal glands, or is disseminated with multiple foci of osteomyelitis and visceral disorders; generalized forms produce le-

hi

⚠ **Combining forms**	**[NA] Nomina Anatomica**
Word*Finder*	**[MIM] Mendelian**
Multi-term entry finder	**Inheritance in Man**
Preceding letter A	
A.D.A.M. Anatomy Plates	☆ **Official alternate term**
Between letters L and M	
Appendices:	☆**[NA] Official alternate**
Following letter Z	**Nomina Anatomica term**
SYN Synonym; **Cf.,** compare	**High Profile Term**

sions in lymph nodes, spleen, liver, bone, and lungs, although lung involvement is uncommon.

presumed ocular h., subretinal neovascularization in the macular region associated with chorioretinal atrophy and pigment proliferation adjacent to the optic disk, and peripheral chorioretinal atrophy ("histo-spots").

his·to·ra·di·og·ra·phy (his'tō-rā-dē-og'ră-fē). Radiography of tissue, specifically microscopic sections; usually microradiography.

his·tor·rhex·is (his-tō-rek'sis). Breakdown of tissue by some agency other than infection. [histo- + G. *rhēxis*, rupture]

his·to·tome (his'tō-tōm). SYN microtome. [histo- + G. *tomē*, cut]

his·tot·o·my (his-tot'ō-mē). SYN microtomy.

his·to·tope (his'tō-tōp). That part of the Class II major histocompatibility molecule that interacts with the T cell receptor. [histo- + -tope]

his·to·tox·ic (his-tō-tok'sik). Relating to poisoning of the respiratory enzyme system of the tissues.

his·to·troph (his'tō-trof). The part of the nutrition of the embryo derived from cellular sources other than blood. Cf. embryotroph, hemotroph.

his·to·tro·phic (his-tō-trof'ik). Providing nourishment for or favoring the formation of tissue. [histo- + G. *trophē*, nourishment]

his·to·tro·pic (his-tō-trop'ik). Attracted toward the tissues; denoting certain parasites, stains, and chemical compounds. [histo- + G. *tropikos*, turning]

his·to·zo·ic (his-tō-zō'ik). Living in the tissues outside of a cell body; denoting certain parasitic protozoa. [histo- + G. *zōikos*, relating to an animal]

his·to·zyme (his'tō-zīm). SYN aminoacylase.

hitch·hik·er (hitch'hīk-er). A gene that has no selective advantage, or may even be harmful, but that nevertheless temporarily becomes widespread because it is closely linked and coupled with a highly advantageous gene that is strongly selected.

Hitzig, Eduard, German psychiatrist, 1838–1907. SEE H.'s *girdle*.

HIV Abbreviation for human immunodeficiency *virus*.

HIV-1. Abbreviation for human immunodeficiency virus-1. SEE human immunodeficiency *virus*.

HIV-2. Abbreviation for human immunodeficiency virus-2. SEE human immunodeficiency *virus*.

hives (hīvz). **1.** SYN urticaria. **2.** SYN wheal.

giant h., SYN angioedema.

Hjärre, A., German pathologist, 1897–1958. SEE H.'s *disease*.

HLA Abbreviation for human lymphocyte *antigens*, under *antigen*.

HLA typ·ing. Tests done in order to determine if a patient has antibodies against a potential donor's HLA antigens. The presence of antibodies means that a particular graft will be rapidly rejected.

HMG, hMG Abbreviation for human menopausal *gonadotropin*.

HMG-CoA Abbreviation for β-hydroxy-β-methylglutaryl-CoA.

HMO Abbreviation for hypothetical mean *organism*.

HMO Abbreviation for health maintenance organization.

> HMOs may be nonprofit or profit-making ventures, and along with PPOs and managed care plans have come to define the U.S. health care scene. HMOs generally offer a package of services; however, the choice of physician is frequently limited to those working within the HMO.

HMPAO Abbreviation for hexametazime or hexamethylpropyleneamine oxime.

HMS Abbreviation for hypothetical mean *strain*.

HN2 Symbol for nitrogen mustard. SEE nitrogen *mustards*, under *mustard*.

hnRNA Abbreviation for heterogeneous nuclear RNA.

Ho Symbol for holmium.

Hoagland's sign. See under sign.

hoarse (hōrs). Having a rough, harsh voice. [A.S. *hās*]

hoarse·ness (hōrs'nes). A harsh quality of the voice.

Hoboken, Nicholas van, Dutch anatomist and physician, 1632–1678. SEE H.'s *gemmules*, under *gemmule*, *nodules*, under *nodule*, *valves*, under *valve*.

HOCA Abbreviation for high osmolar contrast *agent*.

Hoche, Alfred E., German psychiatrist, 1865–1943. SEE H.'s *bundle*, *tract*.

hock (hok). The tarsus in the horse and other quadrupeds; the joint of the hind limb between the stifle and the fetlock; corresponds to the ankle in humans. [O.E. *hōh*, heel]

capped h., SYN calcaneal *bursitis*.

curby h., SYN curb.

HOCM Abbreviation for high osmolar contrast *medium*.

Hodge, Hugh L., U.S. gynecologist, 1796–1873. SEE H.'s *pessary*.

Hodgen, John T., U.S. surgeon, 1826–1882. SEE H. *splint*.

Hodgkin, Alan L., British physiologist and Nobel laureate, *1914. SEE Goldman-H.-Katz *equation*.

Hodgkin, Thomas, British physician, 1798–1866. SEE H.'s *disease*; H.-Key *murmur*; non-H.'s *lymphoma*.

Hodgson, Joseph, British physician, 1788–1869. SEE H.'s *disease*.

ho·do·neu·ro·mere (hō-dō-nū'rō-mēr). In embryology, obsolete term for a metameric segment of the neural tube with its pair of nerves and their branches. [G. *hodos*, path, + *neuron*, nerve, + *meros*, part]

ho·do·pho·bia (hō-dō-fō'bē-ă). Morbid fear of traveling. [G. *hodos*, path, + *phobos*, fear]

HOECHST 33258. A bisbenzimidazole dye employed in cytochemistry and fluorescence microscopy as a sensitive indicator of DNA in chromosomes, specifically constitutive heterochromatin.

Hoeppli, Reinhard J.C., German parasitologist, *1893. SEE Splendore-H. *phenomenon*.

hof (hōf). The hollow in the cytoplasm of a cell that lodges the nucleus. [Ger. court]

Hofbauer, J. Isfred I., U.S. gynecologist, 1878–1961. SEE H. *cell*.

Hoffa, Albert, German surgeon, 1859–1908. SEE H.'s *operation*.

Hoffman, August Wilhelm, German chemist, 1818–1892. SEE Frei-Hoffmann *reaction*, Hoffman's *violet*.

Hoffmann, Friedrich, German physician, 1660-1742. Professor of Anatomy and Surgery at Halle, noted for clinical observations of a variety of infectious diseases.

Hoffmann, Johann, German neurologist, 1857–1919. SEE H.'s muscular *atrophy, phenomenon, reflex, sign*; Werdnig-H. *disease*; Werdnig-Hoffmann muscular *atrophy*.

Hoffmann, Moritz, German anatomist, 1622–1698. SEE H.'s *duct*.

Hofmann (Hofmann-Wellenhof), Georg von, Austrian bacteriologist, 1843–1890. SEE H.'s *bacillus*.

Hofmeister, Franz, German biochemist, 1850–1922. SEE H. *series, gastrectomy*.

Hofmeister, Franz von, German surgeon, 1867–1926. SEE H.'s *operation*; H.-Pólya *anastomosis*.

Hog·ben, Lawrence, British mathematician, *1895. SEE H. *number*.

Hogness, D.S., U.S. molecular biologist, *1925. SEE Grunstein-H. *assay*; H. *box*.

hol·an·dric (hol-an'drik). Related to genes located on the Y chromosome. [G. *holos*, entire, + *aner*, human male]

hol·ar·thrit·ic (hol-ar-thrit'ik). Relating to holarthritis.

hol·ar·thri·tis (hol-ar-thrī'tis). Inflammation of all or a great number of the joints. [G. *holos*, entire, + *arthron*, joint, + *-itis*, inflammation]

Holden, Luther, English anatomist, 1815–1905. SEE H.'s *line*.

Holder. SEE Virchow-Holder *angle*.

hole in ret·i·na. A break in the continuity of the sensory retina, permitting separation between the retinal pigment epithelium and sensory retina.

ho·lism (hō'lizm). **1.** The principle that an organism, or one of its actions, is not equal to merely the sum of its parts but must be perceived or studied as a whole. **2.** The approach to the study of a psychological phenomenon through the analysis of a phenomenon as a complete entity in itself. Cf. atomism. [G. *holos,* entire]

ho·lis·tic (hō-lis'tik). Pertaining to the characteristics of holism or h. psychologies.

Holl, Mortiz, Austrian surgeon, 1852–1920. SEE H.'s *ligament.*

Hollander, Franklin, U.S. physiologist, 1899–1966. SEE H. *test.*

Hollenhorst, Robert W., U.S. ophthalmologist, *1913. SEE H. *plaques,* under *plaque.*

Hol·li·day, R. SEE H. *junction, structure.*

hol·low (hol'ō). A concavity or depression.

Sebileau's h., depression between the inferior aspect of the tongue and the sublingual glands.

Holmes, Sir Gordon M., English neurologist, 1876–1965. SEE H.-Adie *pupil, syndrome;* Stewart-H. *sign.*

Holmes, Oliver Wendell. American physician, identified the mode of spread and control of puerperal fever, thus saving innumerable young women's lives.

Holmes, Thomas, U.S. psychiatrist, *1918. SEE H.-Rahe *questionnaire.*

Holmes, W. SEE H.'s *stain.*

Holmgren, Alarik F., Swedish physiologist, 1831–1897. SEE H.'s wool *test.*

Holmgren, Emil A., Swedish histologist, 1866–1922. SEE Holmgrén-Golgi *canals,* under *canal.*

hol·mi·um (Ho) (hol'mē-ŭm). An element of the lanthanide group, atomic no. 67, atomic wt. 164.93032. [L. *Holmia,* for Stockholm]

◁**holo-.** Whole, entire, complete. [G. *holos*]

hol·o·a·car·di·us (hol'ō-ă-kar'dē-ŭs). A separate, grossly defective twin lacking a heart of its own, its blood supply being dependent on a shunt from the placental circulation of a more nearly normal twin; a placental parasitic twin or omphalosite. Cf. acardius. [holo- + G. *a-* priv. + *kardia,* heart]

h. aceph'alus, a h. also lacking a head.

h. amor'phus, a h. in which the body of the parasite is represented by only a shapeless mass. SEE ALSO anideus.

ho·lo-ACP syn·thase. An enzyme catalyzing transfer of the 4'-phosphopantetheinyl residue from CoA to a serine of apo-ACP (acyl carrier protein) to form holo-ACP, releasing adenosine 3',5'-bisphosphate; a required step if fatty acid biosynthesis is to function.

hol·o·a·cra·nia (hol'ō-ă-krā'nē-ă). A congenital skull defect in which bones of the vault are absent. [holo- + G. *a-* priv. + *kranion,* skull]

hol·o·an·en·ceph·a·ly (hol'ō-an-en-sef'ă-lē). Complete absence of cranium and brain. [holo- + G. *an-* priv. + *enkephalos,* brain]

hol·o·blas·tic (hol-ō-blas'tik). Denoting the involvement of the entire (isolecithal or moderately telolecithal) ovum in cleavage. [holo- + G. *blastos,* germ]

hol·o·car·box·y·lase syn·the·tase (hōl-ō-kar-boks'il-ās sen'thĕ-tās). One of several enzymes that biotinylate other proteins (*e.g.,* carboxylases); a deficiency of h. s. will result in organic acidemia.

hol·o·ce·phal·ic (hol'ō-sĕ-fal'ik). Denoting a fetus with a complete head but having deficiencies in other body parts. [holo- + G. *kephalē,* head]

hol·o·cord (hol'ō-kōrd). Relating to the entire spinal cord, extending from the cervico-medullary junction to the conus medullaris.

hol·o·crine (hol'ō-krin). SEE holocrine *gland.* [holo- + G. *krinō,* to separate]

hol·o·di·a·stol·ic (hol'ō-dī-ă-stol'ik). Relating to or occupying the entire diastolic period.

hol·o·en·dem·ic (hol'ō-en-dem'ik). Endemic in the entire population, as trachoma in the villages of Saudi Arabia.

hol·o·en·zyme (hol-ō-en'zīm). A complete enzyme, *i.e.,* apoenzyme plus coenzyme, cofactor, metal ion, and/or prosthetic group.

hol·o·gas·tros·chi·sis (hol'ō-gas-tros'ki-sis). A congenital malformation in which a cleft extends the entire length of the abdomen. [holo- + G. *gastēr,* belly, + *schisis,* cleaving]

hol·o·gram (hol'ō-gram). A three-dimensional image produced by wavefront reconstruction and recorded on a photographic plate. [holo- + G. *gramma,* something written]

hol·og·ra·phy (hō-log'ră-fē). The process of creating a hologram.

hol·o·gyn·ic (hol-ō-jin'ik). Related to characters manifest only in females. [holo- + G. *gynē,* woman]

hol·o·mas·ti·gote (hol-ō-mas'ti-gōt). Possessing flagella over the entire surface. [holo- + G. *mastix,* whip]

hol·o·me·tab·o·lous (hol'ō-me-tab'ō-lŭs). Pertaining to a member of the Holometabola, a series of insect orders in which complex or complete metamorphosis is found. [holo- + G. *metabolē,* change]

hol·o·mi·ant·ic (in·fec·tion) (hol'ōm-ī-an-tik). Infectious outbreak due to exposure of a group of persons to an agent that affects or is common to all members of the group. [holo + C. *miantos,* defiled, fr. *miainō.* to defile, + -ic]

hol·o·mor·pho·sis (hol'ō-mōr-fō'sis). Rarely used term for attainment or reestablishment of physical wholeness. [holo- + G. *morphosis,* shaping]

hol·o·phyt·ic (hol-ō-fit'ik). Having a plantlike mode of obtaining nourishment; denoting certain photosynthesizing protozoans, *e.g.,* Euglena. [holo- + G. *phyton,* plant]

hol·o·pros·en·ceph·a·ly (hol'ō-pros-en-sef'ă-lē). Failure of the forebrain or prosencephalon to divide into hemispheres or lobes; cycloplia occurs in the severest form. It is often accompanied by a deficit in midline facial development. [holo- + G. *prosō,* forward, + *enkephalos,* brain]

hol·o·pro·tein (hō-lō-prō-tēn). A complete protein; *i.e.,* apoprotein plus metal ion and/or prosthetic group.

hol·o·ra·chis·chi·sis (hol'ō-ră-kis'ki-sis). Spina bifida of the entire spinal column. SYN araphia, rachischisis totalis. [holo- + G. *rhachis,* spine, + *schisis,* fissure]

hol·o·side (hōl'ō-sīd). A compound containing one or more identical glycosidically linked carbohydrates.

hol·o·sys·tol·ic (hol'ō-sis-tol'ik). SYN pansystolic.

hol·o·tel·en·ceph·a·ly (hol'ō-tel-en-sef'ă-lē). Holoprosencephaly associated with arrhinencephaly. [holo- + telencephalon]

hol·o·thur·ins (hōl-ō-thu'rins). A class of highly toxic sulfated steroid glycosides secreted by sea cucumbers (*Holothurioidea*).

ho·lot·ri·chous (ho-lot'ri-kŭs). Possessing cilia over the entire surface. [holo- + G. *thrix,* hair]

hol·o·zo·ic (hol-ō-zō'ik). Animal-like in mode of obtaining nourishment, lacking photosynthetic capacity; denoting certain protozoans, in distinction to others that are holophytic. [holo- + G. *zōon,* animal]

Holt, Mary, 20th century English cardiologist. SEE H.-Oram *syndrome.*

Holter, Norman, U.S. biophysicist, 1914–1983. SEE H. *monitor.*

Holthouse, Carsten, British surgeon, 1810–1901. SEE H.'s *hernia.*

Holzknecht, Guido, Austrian radiologist, 1872–1931. SEE H. *unit.*

hom·a·lo·ceph·a·lous (hom'ă-lō-sef'ă-lŭs). Having a flattened head. [G. *homalos,* level, + *kephalē,* head]

Ho·ma·lo·my·ia (hom'ă-lō-mī'yă). A genus of flies the larvae of which sometimes infect human or animal intestines. [G. *homalos,* even, + *myia,* a fly]

hom·a·lu·ria (hom-a-lū're-ă). Rarely used term for normal urine flow. [G. *homalos,* level, + *ouron,* urine]

Homans, John, U.S. surgeon, 1877–1954. SEE H.'s *sign.*

ho·mat·ro·pine (hō-mat'rō-pēn). An anticholinergic, mydriatic, and cycloplegic agent; available as the hydrobromide and the methylbromide. SYN mandelytropine, tropine mandelate.

ho

hom·ax·i·al (hō-mak'sē-ăl). Having all the axes alike, as a sphere. [G. *homos,* the same, + axis]

Home, Sir Everard, English surgeon, 1756–1832. SEE H.'s *lobe.*

⌂**homeo-.** The same, alike. SEE ALSO homo- (1). [G. *homoios,* similar]

ho·me·o·met·ric (hō'mē-ō-met'rik). Without change in size. [homeo- + G. *metron,* measure]

ho·me·o·mor·phous (hō'mē-ō-mōr'fŭs). Of similar shape, but not necessarily of the same composition. [homeo- + G. *morphē,* shape]

ho·me·o·path (hō'mē-ō-path). SYN homeopathist.

ho·me·o·path·ic (hō'mē-ō-path'ik). **1.** Relating to homeopathy. SYN homeotherapeutic (1). **2.** Denoting an extremely small dose of a pharmacological agent, such as might be used in homeopathy; more generally, a dose believed to be too small to produce the effect usually expected from that agent. Cf. pharmacologic (2), physiologic (4), supraphysiologic. [homeo- + G. *pathos,* disease]

ho·me·op·a·thist (hō-mē-op'ă-thist). A medical practitioner of homeopathy. SYN homeopath.

ho·me·op·a·thy (hō-mē-op'ă-thē). A system of therapy developed by Samuel Hahnemann based on the "law of similia," from the aphorism, *similia similibus curantur* (likes are cured by likes), which holds that a medicinal substance that can evoke certain symptoms in healthy individuals may be effective in the treatment of illnesses having symptoms closely resembling those produced by the substance. [homeo- + G. *pathos,* suffering]

ho·me·o·pla·sia (hō'mē-ō-plā'zē-ă). The formation of new tissue of the same character as that already existing in the part. SYN homoioplasia. [homeo- + G. *plasis,* a molding]

ho·me·o·plas·tic (hō'mē-ō-plas'tik). Relating to or characterized by homeoplasia.

ho·me·or·rhe·sis (hō'mē-ō-rē'sis). The set of processes by which imbalances and other defects in ontogeny are corrected before development is completed. SYN ontogenic homeostasis, waddingtonian homeostasis. [homeo- + G. *rheos,* stream, current]

ho·me·o·sis (hō-mē-ō'sis). Formation of a body part having characteristics normally found in a related or homologous part at another location in the body. [homeo- + G. *-osis,* condition]

ho·me·o·sta·sis (hō'mē-ō-stā'sis, -os'tă-sis). **1.** The state of equilibrium (balance between opposing pressures) in the body with respect to various functions and to the chemical compositions of the fluids and tissues. **2.** The processes through which such bodily equilibrium is maintained. [homeo- + G. *stasis,* a standing]

Bernard-Cannon h., the set of mechanisms responsible for the cybernetic adjustment of physiological and biochemical states in postnatal life. SYN physiological h.

genetic h., SYN Lerner h.

Lerner h., the restorative mechanisms that tend to correct perturbations in the genetic composition of a population. SYN genetic h.

ontogenic h., SYN homeorrhesis.

physiological h., SYN Bernard-Cannon h.

waddingtonian h., SYN homeorrhesis.

ho·me·o·stat·ic (hō'mē-ō-stat'ik). Relating to homeostasis.

ho·me·o·ther·a·peu·tic (hō'mē-ō-thār-ă-pyū'tik). **1.** SYN homeopathic (1). **2.** Relating to homeotherapy.

ho·me·o·ther·a·py, ho·me·o·ther·a·peu·tics (hō'mē-ō-thār'ă-pē, -thār-ă-pyū'tiks). Treatment or prevention of a disease using the principles of homeopathy.

ho·me·o·therm (hō'mē-ō-therm). Any of the animals, including mammals and birds, that tend to maintain a constant body temperature. SYN hematherm, warm-blooded animal. [homeo- + G. *thermos,* warm]

ho·me·o·ther·mal (hō'mē-ō-ther'măl). SYN homeothermic.

ho·me·o·ther·mic (hō'mē-ō-ther'mik). Pertaining to, or having the essential characteristic of, homeotherms. Cf. poikilothermic, heterothermic. SYN hemathermal, hemathermous, hematothermal, homeothermal, homoiothermal, homothermal, warm-blooded.

ho·me·ot·ic (hō-mē-ot'ik). Pertaining to or characterized by homeosis.

ho·me·o·typ·i·cal (hō'mē-ō-tip'i-kăl). Of or resembling the usual type.

hom·er·gy (hom'er-jē). Obsolete term for normal metabolism and its results. [G. *homos,* same, + *ergon,* work]

hom·i·cid·al (hom-i-sī'dăl). Having a tendency toward homicide.

hom·i·cide (hom'i-sīd). The killing of one human being by another. [L. *homo,* man, + *caedo,* to kill]

ho·mid·i·um bro·mide (hō-mid'ē-ŭm). A trypanocide used in veterinary medicine. SYN ethidium.

Ho·min·i·dae (hō-min'i-dē). The Primate family which includes modern man (*Homo sapiens*) and several groups of fossil men.

Ho·mi·noi·dea (hom-i-noy'dē-ă). A superfamily of the Primates including the anthropoid apes and man. Divided into the families Pongidae (anthropoid apes) and Hominidae (humans). [L. *homo* (*homin-*), man, + G. *eidos,* form]

Ho·mo (hō'mō). The genus of Primates that includes humans. [L. man]

H. sa'piens, modern human beings. [L. wise man]

⌂**homo-.** **1.** Combining form meaning the same, alike; opposite of hetero-. SEE ALSO homeo-. **2.** In chemistry, prefix used to indicate insertion of one more carbon atom in a chain (*i.e.,* insertion of a methylene moiety). [G. *homos,* the same]

ho·mo·ar·gi·nine (Har) (hō-mō-ar'ji-nēn). A homolog of arginine having an additional methylene group.

ho·mo·bi·o·tin (hō-mō-bī'ō-tin). A compound resembling biotin except for the substitution of an oxygen atom for the sulfur and the presence of an additional CH_2 group in the side chain; an active biotin antagonist.

ho·mo·blas·tic (hō-mō-blas'tik). Developing from a single type of tissue. [homo- + G. *blastos,* germ]

ho·mo·car·no·sine (hō-mō-kar'nō-sēn). N^2-(4-Aminobutyryl)-L-histidine; a constituent of the brain formed from L-histidine and γ-aminobutyric acid.

ho·mo·car·no·sin·o·sis (hō-mō-kar'nō-sēn-ō-sis). An inborn error in metabolism in which homocarnosine levels are elevated, particularly in the cerebral spinal fluid.

ho·mo·cen·tric (hō'mō-sen'trik). Having the same center; denoting rays that meet at a common focus. Cf. heterocentric (1).

ho·mo·chlor·cy·cli·zine (hō'mō-klōr-sī'kli-zēn). 1-[(4-Chlorophenyl)phenylmethyl]hexahydro-4-methyl-1*H* -1,4-diazepine; an antihistaminic with antiserotonin properties.

ho·moch·ro·nous (hō-mōk'rō-nŭs). **1.** SYN synchronous. **2.** Occurring at the same age in each generation. [homo- + G. *chronos,* time]

ho·mo·cit·rul·li·nu·ria (hō-mō-sit'ru-lēn-ūr'ē-ă). An inherited disorder associated with elevated urinary levels of homocitrulline.

ho·mo·clad·ic (hō-mō-klad'ik). Denoting an anastomosis between branches of the same arterial trunk, as distinguished from heterocladic. [homo- + G. *klados,* a branch]

ho·mo·cys·te·ine (Hcy) (hō-mō-sis'tē-ēn). $HSCH_2CH_2CH$ $(NH_3)^+COO^-$; a homolog of cysteine, produced by the demethylation of methionine, and an intermediate in the biosynthesis of L-cysteine from L-methionine via L-cystathionine.

ho·mo·cys·tine (hō-mō-sis'tēn). The disulfide resulting from the mild oxidation of homocysteine; an analog of cystine.

ho·mo·cys·ti·ne·mia (hō-mō-sis-ti-nē'mē-ă). Presence of an excess of homocystine in the plasma, as in homocystinuria.

ho·mo·cys·ti·nu·ria (hō'mō-sis-ti-nū're-ă) [MIM*236200]. A disorder characterized by excretion of homocystine in urine, mental retardation, ectopia lentis, sparse blond hair, genu valgum, failure to thrive, thromboembolic episodes, and fatty changes of liver; associated with defective formation of cystathionine synthetase. There are also two other known varieties [MIM*236250 and *236270]. There are a number of inborn errors in metabolism that wil exhibit homocystinuria. It is also seen in certain types of methylmalonic acidemia.

ho·mo·cy·to·tro·pic (hō'mō-sī'tō-trop'ik). Having an affinity for cells of the same or a closely related species. [homo- + G. *kytos,* cell, + *trope,* a turning toward]

ho·mo·dont (hō′mō-dont). Having teeth all alike in form, as those of the lower vertebrates, in contrast to heterodont. [homo- + G. *odous,* tooth]

ho·mod·ro·mous (hō-mod′rō-mŭs). Moving in the same direction. [homo- + G. *dromos,* running]

◁**homoeo-.** SEE homeo-.

ho·mo·er·ot·ism, ho·mo·e·rot·i·cism (hō-mō-er′ō-tizm, -ĕ-rot′ i-sizm). SYN homosexuality. [homo- + G. *erōs,* love]

ho·mo·ga·met·ic (hō′mō-gă-met′ik). Producing only one type of gamete with respect to sex chromosomes; in humans and most animals, the female is h. SYN monogametic. [homo- + G. *gametikos,* connubial]

ho·mog·a·my (hō-mog′ă-mē). Similarity of husband and wife in a specific trait. [homo- + G. *gamos,* marriage]

ho·mog·e·nate (hŏ-moj′ĕ-nāt). Tissue ground into a creamy consistency in which the cell structure is disintegrated (so-called "cell-free"). Cf. brei.

ho·mo·ge·neous (hō-mō-jē′nē-ŭs). Of uniform structure or composition throughout. [homo- + G. *genos,* race]

ho·mo·gen·e·sis (hō-mō-jen′ĕ-sis). Production of offspring similar to the parents, in contrast to heterogenesis. SYN homogeny. [homo- + G. *genesis,* production]

ho·mog·e·ni·za·tion (hŏ-moj′ĕ-ni-zā′shŭn). The process by which a material is made homogeneous.

ho·mog·e·nize (hŏ-moj′ĕ-nīz). To make homogeneous.

ho·mog·e·nous (hō-moj′ĕ-nŭs). Having a structural similarity because of descent from a common ancestor. Commonly confused with homogeneous. [homo- + G. *genos,* family, kind]

ho·mo·gen·tis·ate 1,2-di·ox·y·gen·ase (hō-mō-jen′tis-āt). An iron-containing enzyme that catalyzes the oxidative cleavage of the benzene ring in homogentisic acid by O_2, forming 4-maleylacetoacetate; an absence or deficiency of this enzyme will result in alcaptonuria. SYN homogentisic acid oxidase.

ho·mo·gen·tis·ic ac·id (hō′mō-jen-tis′ik). Glycosuric acid; (2,5-dihydroxyphenyl)acetic acid; an intermediate in L-phenylalanine and L-tyrosine catabolism; if made alkaline, it oxidizes rapidly in air to a quinone that polymerizes to a melanin-like material; elevated levels are observed in individuals having alcaptonuria. SYN alcapton, alkapton.

h. a. oxidase, SYN homogentisate 1,2-dioxygenase.

ho·mog·e·ny (hō-moj′ĕ-ne). SYN homogenesis.

ho·mo·gly·can (hō-mō-glī′kan). A polysaccharide consisting of only one type of monosaccharide subunit (*e.g.,* glucan). Cf. heteroglycan, glycan.

ho·mo·graft (hō′mō-graft). SYN allograft *rejection.*

ho·moi·o·pla·sia (hō′moy-ō-plā′zē-ă). SYN homeoplasia.

ho·moi·o·ther·mal (hō-moy-ō-ther′măl). SYN homeothermic.

ho·mo·kar·y·on (hō-mō-kar′ē-on). Genetically identical multiple nuclei in a common cytoplasm, usually resulting from fusion of two cells from the same species. [homo- + G. *karyon,* kernel, nut]

ho·mo·kar·y·ot·ic (hō′mō-kar-ē-ot′ik). Exhibiting the properties of a homokaryon.

ho·mo·ker·a·to·plas·ty (hō′mō-ker′ă-tō-plas-tē). Corneal transplant between members of the same species.

ho·mo·lat·er·al (hō-mō-lat′er-ăl). SYN ipsilateral. [homo- + L. *latus,* side]

ho·mo·lip·ids (hō-mō-lip′idz). Lipids containing only C, H, and O. Cf. heterolipids. SYN simple lipids.

ho·mo·log, ho·mo·logue (hom′ō-log). A member of a homologous pair or series. [homo- + G. *logos,* word, ratio, relation]

ho·mol·o·gous (hŏ-mol′ō-gŭs). Corresponding or alike in certain critical attributes. **1.** In biology or zoology, denoting organs or parts corresponding in evolutionary origin and similar to some extent in structure, but not necessarily similar in function. **2.** In chemistry, denoting a single chemical series, differing by fixed increments. **3.** In genetics, denoting chromosomes or chromosome parts identical with respect to their construction and genetic content. **4.** In immunology, denoting serum or tissue derived

from members of a single species, or an antibody with respect to the antigen that produced it. [see homologue]

ho·mol·o·gy (hŏ-mol′ō-jē). The state of being homologous.

h. of chains, the degree of similarity between the base sequences of strands of two DNAs. SYN h. of strands.

DNA h., the degree (or percentage) of hybridization capable between the DNA of different microorganisms.

h. of strands, SYN h. of chains.

ho·mol·y·sin (hō-mol′i-sin). A sensitizing hemolytic antibody (hemolysin) formed as the result of stimulation by an antigen derived from an animal of the same species. [homo- + hemolysin]

ho·mol·y·sis (hō-mol′i-sis). Lysis of red blood cells by a homolysin and complement.

ho·mo·mor·phic (hō-mō-mōr′fik). Denoting two or more structures of similar size and shape. [homo- + G. *morphē,* shape, appearance]

ho·mon·o·mous (hō-mon′ō-mŭs). Denoting parts, having similar form and structure, arranged in a series, as the fingers or toes. [G. *homonemos,* under the same laws, fr. *homos,* same, + *nomos,* law]

ho·mon·o·my (hō-mon′ō-mē). The condition of being homonomous.

ho·mo·nu·cle·ar (hō-mō-nū′klē-er). Denoting a cell line that retains the original chromosome complement.

ho·mon·y·mous (hō-mon′i-mŭs). Having the same name or expressed in the same terms, *e.g.,* the corresponding halves (right or left, superior or inferior) of the retinas. [G. *homōnymous,* of the same name, fr. *onyma,* name]

ho·mo·phenes (hō′mō-fēnz). Words in which the visible organs of speech behave the same, *e.g.,* tug, tongue, tuck.

ho·mo·phil (hō′mō-fil). Denoting an antibody that reacts only with the specific antigen which induced its formation. [homo- + G. *philos,* fond]

ho·mo·plas·tic (hō-mō-plas′tik). Similar in form and structure, but not in origin. [homo- + G. *plastos,* formed]

ho·mo·plas·ty (hō′mō-plas′tē). Repair of a defect by a homograft.

ho·mo·pol·y·mer (hō-mō-pol′i-mer). A polymer composed of a series of identical radicals; *e.g.,* polylysine, poly(adenylic acid), polyglucose.

ho·mo·pro·line (hō-mō-prō′lēn). SYN pipecolic acid.

ho·mo·pro·to·cat·e·chu·ic ac·id (hō′mō-prō′tō-kat-ĕ-chū′ik). (3,4-Dihydroxyphenyl)acetic acid; an isomer of homogentisic acid found in urine; a degradation product of L-tyrosine, L-dopa, and hydroxytyramine.

hom·or·gan·ic (hom-ōr-gan′ik). Produced by the same organs, or by homologous organs.

ho·mo·sal·ate (hō-mō-sal′āt). 3,3,5-Trimethylcyclohexyl salicylate; an ultraviolet screening agent for topical application to the skin.

ho·mo·sced·as·tic·i·ty (hō′mō-skĕ-das-tis′ĭ-tē). Constancy of the variance of a measure over the levels of the factor under study.

ho·mo·ser·ine (hō-mō-ser′ēn). $HOCH_2CH_2CH(NH_2^+)COO^-$; 2-amino-4-hydroxybutyric acid; a hydroxyamino acid differing from serine in the possession of an additional CH_2 group; formed in the conversion of L-methionine to L-cysteine.

h. deaminase, SYN cystathionine γ-lyase.

h. dehydratase, SYN cystathionine γ-lyase.

h. lactone, the cyclic ester (*i.e.,* the δ-lactone) of h.; formed by the reaction of cyanogen bromide on methionyl residues in peptides and proteins.

ho·mo·sex·u·al (hō-mō-sek′shū-ăl). **1.** Relating to or characteristic of homosexuality. **2.** One whose interests and behavior are characteristic of homosexuality. SEE Gay, lesbian.

ho·mo·sex·u·al·i·ty (hō′mō-sek-shū-al′ĭ-tē). Erotic attraction, predisposition, or activity, including sexual congress, between individuals of the same sex, especially past puberty. SYN homoerotism, homoeroticism.

ego-dystonic h., a psychological or psychiatric disorder in which

ho

an individual experiences persistent distress associated with same-sex preference and a strong need to change the behavior or, at least, to alleviate the distress associated with the h.

female h., erotic predisposition, or activity, including sexual congress, between two women past the age of puberty.

latent h., an erotic inclination toward members of the same sex not consciously experienced or expressed in overt action, as opposed to overt h. Use of this term is disappearing because of both its potentially iatrogenic effect and the inability to validate the phenomenon by techniques outside of psychoanalytic theory. SYN unconscious h.

male h., erotic predisposition, or activity, including sexual congress, between two men, past the age of puberty.

overt h., homosexual inclinations consciously experienced and expressed in actual homosexual behavior.

unconscious h., SYN latent h.

D-ho·mo·ster·oid (hō-mō-stēr′oyd). A steroid in which the D ring is made up of six carbon atoms instead of the usual five.

ho·mo·ster·oid. A steroid that has had at least one of the rings in its structure expanded.

4-ho·mo·sul·fa·nil·a·mide (hō′mō-sŭl-fă-nil′ă-mīd). SYN mafenide.

ho·mo·thal·lic (hō-mō-thal′ik). In fungi, denoting a kind of sexual reproduction in which a nucleus of a thallus is capable of fusing with another nucleus from the same thallus or mating type. Cf. heterothallic. [homo- + G. *thallos*, a young shoot]

ho·mo·ther·mal (hō-mō-ther′măl). SYN homeothermic. [homo- + G. *thermē*, heat]

ho·mo·ton·ic (hō-mō-ton′ik). Of uniform tension or tonus.

ho·mo·top·ic (hō-mō-top′ik). Pertaining to or occurring at the same place or part of the body. [homo- + G. *topos*, place]

ho·mo·trans·plan·ta·tion (hō′mō-tranz-plan-tā′shŭn). SYN allotransplantation.

ho·mo·tro·pic (hō-mō-trō-pik). Referring to the binding of the same ligand to a macromolecule; *e.g.*, the binding of four O_2 to hemoglobin is homotropic cooperativity.

ho·mo·type (hō′mō-tīp). Any part or organ of the same structure or function as another, especially as one on the opposite side of the body. [homo- + G. *typos*, type]

ho·mo·typ·ic, ho·mo·typ·i·cal (hō-mō-tip′ik, i-kăl). Of the same type or form; corresponding to the other one of two paired organs or parts.

ho·mo·va·nil·lic ac·id (HVA) (hō′mō-vă-nil′ik). A phenol found in human urine; produced through the methylation of homoprotocatechuic acid on the *meta*-OH group.

ho·mo·zo·ic (hō-mō-zō′ik). Relating to the same animal or the same species of animal. [homo- + G. *zōikos*, relating to an animal]

ho·mo·zy·gos·i·ty, ho·mo·zy·go·sis (hō′mō-zī-gos′i-tē, -zī-gō′sis). The state of being homozygous. [homo- + G. *zygon*, yoke]

ho·mo·zy·gote (hō-mō-zī′gōt). A homozygous individual. [homo- + G. *zygōtos*, yoke]

ho·mo·zy·gous (hō-mō-zī′gŭs). Having identical genes at one or more loci.

ho·mo·zy·gous by de·scent. Possessing two genes at a given locus that are descended from a single source, as may occur in consanguineous mating.

ho·mun·cu·lus (hō-mŭngk′yū-lŭs). **1.** An exceedingly minute body which, according to the views of development held by medical scientists of the 16th and 17th centuries, was contained in a sex cell. From this preformed but infinitely small structure the human body was supposed to be developed. SEE ALSO preformation *theory*, animalcule. **2.** The figure of a human sometimes superimposed on pictures of the surface of the brain to represent the motor or sensory regions of the body represented there. [L. dim. of *homo*, man]

Hon·du·ras bark (hon-dū′răs). SYN *cascara* amara.

hon·ey (hŏn′ē). Clarified h., a saccharine substance deposited in the honeycomb by the honeybee, *Apis mellifera;* used as an excipient, as a flavor in gargles and cough remedies, and as a food. SYN mel (1). [A.S. *hunig*]

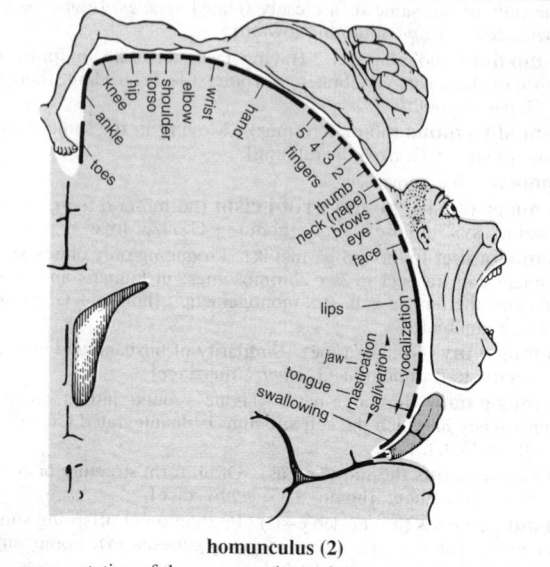

homunculus (2)
representation of the motor regions of the body in the anterior central gyrus

honk (hawnk). **1.** In medical terms, a sound that can be likened to the call of a goose. **2.** Sometimes specifically used to denote a sound of laryngeal origin which is often due to redundant vocal cords vibrating in a forced expiration, due to a congenital vascular ring surrounding the trachea or larynx. [echoic]

systolic h., a somewhat musical systolic murmur likened to the honking of a goose; sometimes of innocent but unexplained origin, at other times a sign of mitral insufficiency. SYN systolic whoop.

hood (hud). The anterior part of the integument of soft ticks (family Argasidae) that extends over the capitulum and forms the roof of the camerostome. [O.E. *hōd*, hat]

dorsal h., SYN extensor digital *expansion.*

hoof (huf). The horny covering of the ends of the digits or feet in many animals; it consists, like nails and horns, of thickened and modified epidermis or cuticle. [A.S. *hōf*]

hook (huk). **1.** An instrument curved or bent near its tip, used for fixation of a part or traction. **2.** A hooklike structure. [A.S. *hōk*]

calvarial h., an instrument used in prying off the top of the skull after it has been sawed around, at autopsies and dissections.

h. of hamate bone, a hooklike process on the distal and medial part of the palmar surface of the hamate bone. SYN hamulus ossis hamati [NA].

palate h., an instrument for pulling forward the soft palate in order to facilitate posterior rhinoscopy.

sliding h., a movable attachment used on an orthodontic wire for the application of elastic traction or headgear force.

h. of spiral lamina, SYN *hamulus* of spiral lamina.

squint h., a surgical instrument used to lift ocular muscles.

tracheotomy h., right-angled h. used in holding the trachea steady during tracheotomy.

Hooke, Robert, British experimental physicist, 1635–1703. SEE hookean *behavior;* H.'s *law.*

Hooker, Charles W. SEE H.-Forbes *test.*

hook·lets (huk′letz). **1.** Clawlike, retractile chitinous hooks that encircle or line the rostellum of the scolex of certain taenioid tapeworms for attachment to the intestinal mucosa, with the additional aid of suckers; the h.'s can be withdrawn and the rostellum inverted when the tapeworm moves. Various arrangements and forms of the h.'s characterize the families of taenioid cestodes. **2.** H.'s of degenerated scoleces of *Echinococcus* species in the fluids of the hydatid cyst. **3.** The h.'s of the oncosphere, by which it claws out of its membrane sheath after hatching and penetrates the host gut wall; these h.'s can later be found in the cercomer of the procercoid or cysticercoid.

hook·worm (huk'werm). Common name for bloodsucking nematodes of the family Ancyclostomatidae, chiefly members of the genera *Ancylostoma* (the Old World hookworm), *Necator,* and *Uncinaria,* and including the species *A. caninum* (dog h.) and *N. americanus* (New World h.).

hoose (hūs). SYN verminous *bronchitis.*

Hoover, Charles F., U.S. physician, 1865–1927. SEE H.'s *signs,* under *sign.*

Hopkins, Sir Frederick G., English biochemist and Nobel laureate, 1861–1947. SEE Benedict-H.-Cole *reagent.*

Hop·lop·syl·lus anom·a·lus (hop-lō-sil'ŭs ă-nom'ă-lŭs). A species of flea parasitic on ground squirrels of the western U.S., and a vector of plague. [G. *hoplo,* tool, weapon, + *psyll,* flea]

Hopmann, Carl M., German rhinologist, 1849–1925. SEE H.'s *papilloma, polyp.*

hops. SYN humulus.

ho·quet di·a·bo·lique (hō-kā', hok'et dē-ab-ō-leek'). long-lasting intractable hiccups that persist for months or years. [*hoque,* Fr., hiccough]

hor. decub. Abbreviation for L. *hora decubitus,* at bedtime.

hor·de·nine (hōr'den-ēn). A biogenic amine first isolated from barley; increases blood pressure. SYN anhaline. [L. *hordeum,* barley, + -in]

hor·de·o·lum (hōr-dē'ō-lŭm). A suppurative inflammation of a gland of the eyelid. [Mod. L., *hordeolus,* a sty in the eye, dim. of *hordeum,* barley]

h. exter'num, inflammation of the sebaceous gland of an eyelash. SYN sty, stye.

h. inter'num, an acute purulent infection of a meibomian (tarsal) gland. SYN acute chalazion, h. meibomianum, meibomian sty.

h. meibomia'num, SYN h. internum.

Hor·ec·ker, Bernard L., U.S. biochemist, *1914. SEE Warburg-Dickens-Horecker *shunt.*

hore·hound, hoar·hound (hōr-hound). *Marrubium vulgare* (family Labitae); bitter principle is marrubium, a volatile oil. A compound alleged to have expectorant properties and often found in cough drops and other patent medicines. [O.E. *hār,* hoary, + *hūne,* herb]

hor·i·zon·ta·lis (hōr-i-zon-tā'lis) [NA]. Horizontal, referring to the plane of the body, perpendicular to the vertical plane, at right angles both to the median and coronal planes, that separates the body into upper and lower parts. [L.]

hor·me·sis (hōr-mē'sis). The stimulating effect of subinhibitory concentrations of any toxic substance on any organism. [Gr. *hormēsis,* rapid motion]

hor·mi·on (hōr'mē-on). A craniometric point at the junction of the posterior border of the vomer with the sphenoid bone. [G. *hormos,* cord, chain, necklace]

hor·mo·gon·al (hōr-mō'gō-nal). Referring to a class of Cyanobacteria in which the cells grow in filaments.

hor·mo·nal (hōr-mōn'ăl). Pertaining to hormones.

HORMONE

hor·mone (hōr'mōn). A chemical substance, formed in one organ or part of the body and carried in the blood to another organ or part; depending on the specificity of their effects, h.'s can alter the functional activity, and sometimes the structure, of just one organ or of various numbers of them. A number of h.'s are formed by ductless glands, but secretin and pancreozymin, formed in the gastrointestinal tract, by definition are also h.'s. For h.'s not listed below, see specific names. [G. *hormōn,* pres. part. of *hormaō,* to rouse or set in motion]

adipokinetic h., SYN adipokinin.

adrenal androgen-stimulating h. (AASH), a putative pituitary

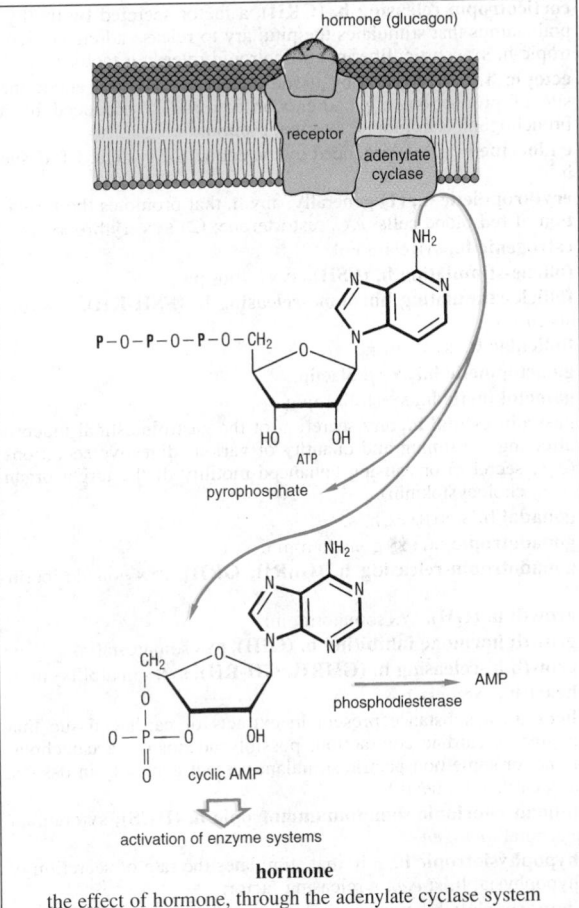

hormone
the effect of hormone, through the adenylate cyclase system

h. that may be responsible for increased secretion of adrenal androgens at the time of puberty.

adrenocortical h.'s, h.'s secreted by the human adrenal cortex; *e.g.,* cortisol, aldosterone, corticosterone.

adrenocorticotropic h. (ACTH), the h. of the anterior lobe of the hypophysis which governs the nutrition and growth of the adrenal cortex, stimulates it to functional activity, and also possesses extraadrenal adipokinetic activity; it is a polypeptide containing 39 amino acids, but exact structure varies from one species to another; sometimes prefixed by α to distinguish it from β-corticotropin. The first thirteen amino acids at the *N*-terminal region are identical to α-melanotropin. SYN adrenocorticotropin, adrenotropic h., adrenotropin, corticotropic h., corticotropin (1).

adrenomedullary h.'s, h.'s produced by the adrenal medulla, particularly the catecholamines, epinephrin, and norepinephrine.

adrenotropic h., SYN adrenocorticotropic h.

androgenic h., any h. that produces a masculinizing effect; of the naturally occurring androgenic h.'s, testosterone is the most potent.

anterior pituitary-like h., SYN chorionic *gonadotropin.*

antidiuretic h. (ADH), SYN vasopressin.

cardiac h., SYN herz h.

chorionic gonadotropic h., chorionic gonadotrophic h., SYN chorionic *gonadotropin.*

chorionic "growth h.-prolactin" (CGP), SYN human placental *lactogen.*

chromatophorotropic h., SEE melanotropin.

corpus luteum h., SYN progesterone.

cortical h.'s, steroid h.'s produced by the adrenal cortex.

corticotropic h., SYN adrenocorticotropic h.

corticotropin releasing h. (CRH), a factor secreted by the hypothalamus that stimulates the pituitary to release adrenocorticotropic h. SYN corticoliberin, corticotropin releasing factor (2).

ectopic h., a h. formed by tissue outside the normal endocrine site of production; *e.g.,* adrenocorticotropic h. produced by a bronchogenic carcinoma. SYN inappropriate h.

endocrine h.'s, h.'s produced by the endocrine system. Cf. tissue h.'s.

erythropoietic h., (1) generally, any h. that promotes the formation of red blood cells, *e.g.,* testosterone; **(2)** SYN erythropoietin.

estrogenic h., SYN estradiol.

follicle-stimulating h. (FSH), SYN follitropin.

follicle-stimulating hormone-releasing h. (FSH-RH), SYN folliberin.

follicular h., SYN estrone.

galactopoietic h., SYN prolactin.

gametokinetic h., SYN follitropin.

gastrointestinal h., any secretion of the gastrointestinal mucosa affecting the timing and quantity of various digestive secretions (*e.g.,* secretin) or causing enhanced motility of the target organ (*e.g.,* cholecystokinin).

gonadal h.'s, SYN sex h.'s.

gonadotropic h., SYN gonadotropin.

gonadotropin-releasing h. (GnRH, GRH), SYN gonadoliberin (1).

growth h. (GH), SYN somatotropin.

growth hormone inhibiting h. (GIH), SYN somatostatin.

growth h.-releasing h. (GHRH, GH-RH), SYN somatoliberin.

heart h., SYN herz h.

herz h., a substance present in extracts of cardiac tissue that augments cardiac contraction; possibly adenosine, a catecholamine, or some nonspecific stimulant present generally in tissues. SYN cardiac h., heart h.

human chorionic somatomammotropic h. (HCS), SYN human placental *lactogen.*

hypophysiotropic h., a h. that stimulates the rate of secretion of hypophysial h.'s; *e.g.,* a releasing factor.

inappropriate h., SYN ectopic h.

interstitial cell-stimulating h., SYN lutropin.

lactation h., SYN prolactin.

lactogenic h., SYN prolactin.

lipid-mobilizing h., SYN lipotropin.

lipotropic h. (LPH), lipotropic pituitary h., SYN lipotropin.

local h., a metabolic product secreted by one set of cells that affects the function of nearby cells; an autacoid; *e.g.,* prostaglandins and neurotransmitters.

luteinizing h. (LH), SYN lutropin.

luteinizing h.-releasing h. (LH-RH, LRH), SYN luliberin.

luteotropic h. (LTH), SYN luteotropin.

mammotropic h., SYN prolactin.

melanocyte-stimulating h. (MSH), SYN melanotropin.

melanotropin release-inhibiting h. (MIH), SYN melanostatin.

melanotropin-releasing h. (MRH), SYN melanoliberin.

neurotrophic h., inflammation of the cornea occurring after corneal anesthesia. SYN neuroparalytic keratitis.

ovarian hormone, SYN relaxin.

pancreatic hyperglycemic h., SYN glucagon.

parathyroid h. (PTH), a peptide h. formed by the parathyroid glands; it raises the serum calcium when administered parenterally by causing bone resorption. SYN parathormone, parathyrin.

pituitary gonadotropic h., SYN anterior pituitary *gonadotropin.*

pituitary growth h., SYN somatotropin.

placental growth h., SYN human placental *lactogen.*

pregnancy h., SYN progesterone.

progestational h., SYN progesterone.

prolactin-inhibiting h. (PIH), SYN prolactostatin.

prolactin-releasing h., SYN prolactoliberin.

proparathyroid h., the immediate precursor of parathyroid h.; proparathyroid differs from parathyroid h. by an N-terminal hexapeptide extension.

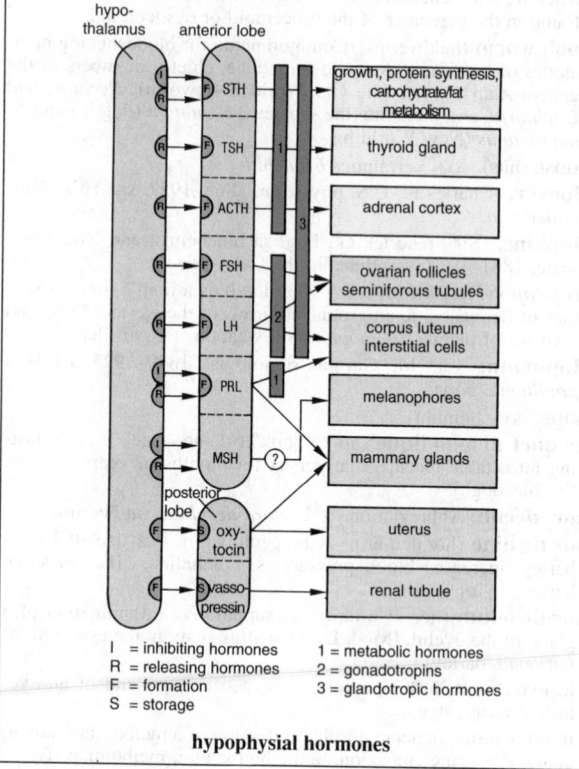

I = inhibiting hormones
R = releasing hormones
F = formation
S = storage

1 = metabolic hormones
2 = gonadotropins
3 = glandotropic hormones

hypophysial hormones

releasing h. (RH), SYN releasing *factors.*

salivary gland h., SYN parotin.

sex h.'s, a general term covering those steroid h.'s that are formed by testicular, ovarian, and adrenocortical tissues, and that are androgens or estrogens. SYN gonadal h.'s.

somatotropic h. (STH), SYN somatotropin.

somatotropin release-inhibiting h. (SIH), SYN somatostatin.

somatotropin-releasing h. (SRH), SYN somatoliberin.

steroid h.'s, those h.'s possessing the steroid ring system; *e.g.,* androgens, estrogens, adrenocortical h.'s.

sympathetic h., SYN sympathin.

thyroid-stimulating h. (TSH), SYN thyrotropin.

thyrotropic h., SYN thyrotropin.

thyrotropin-releasing h. (TRH), SYN thyroliberin.

tissue h.'s, h.'s synthesized by cells other than those in the endocrine system. Cf. endocrine h.'s.

tropic h.'s, trophic h.'s, those h.'s of the anterior lobe of the pituitary that affect the growth, nutrition, or function of other endocrine glands.

vertebrate h.'s, h.'s synthesized in vertebrates.

hor·mo·no·gen·e·sis (hōr′mō-nō-jen′ĕ-sis). The formation of hormones. SYN hormonopoiesis.

hor·mo·no·gen·ic (hōr′mō-nō-jen′ik). Pertaining to the formation of a hormone. SYN hormonopoietic.

hor·mo·no·poi·e·sis (hōr′mō-nō-poy-ē′sis). SYN hormonogenesis. [hormone + G. *poiēsis,* production]

hor·mo·no·poi·et·ic (hōr′mō-nō-poy-et′ik). SYN hormonogenic.

hor·mo·no·priv·ia (hōr′mō-nō-priv′ē-ă). Obsolete term meaning partial or total deprivation of hormones. [hormone + G. *privus,* deprived of]

hor·mo·no·ther·a·py (hōr′mō-nō-thār′ă-pē). Treatment with hormones.

horn (hōrn). Any structure resembling a horn in shape. SYN cornu (1). [A.S.]

Ammon's h., one of the two interlocking gyri composing the hippocampus, the other being the dentate gyrus. SYN cornu ammonis. [G. *Ammōn*, the Egyptian deity *Amūn*]

anterior h., (1) the anterior or frontal division of the lateral ventricle of the brain, extending forward from Monro's interventricular foramen; SEE lateral *ventricle*. **(2)** the anterior or ventral gray column of the spinal cord as appearing in cross section. SEE ALSO anterior *column*, gray *columns*, under *column*. SYN cornu anterius [NA], ventral h.

cicatricial h., a keratinous h. projecting outward from a scar.

coccygeal h., SYN coccygeal *cornua*, under *cornu*.

cutaneous h., a protruding keratotic growth of the skin; the base may show changes of actinic keratosis or carcinoma. SYN cornu cutaneum, warty h.

frontal h., SEE inferior h. of lateral ventricle, inferior h.

greater h. of hyoid bone, the larger and more lateral of the two processes on either side of the hyoid bone. SYN cornu majus ossis hyoidei [NA].

h.'s of hyoid bone, SEE greater h. of hyoid bone, lesser h. of hyoid bone.

iliac h., bony spur of posterior part of ilium, often found in nail-patella syndrome.

inferior h., a lower or downward prolongation of a part or structure of the body. SYN cornu inferius [NA].

inferior h. of falciform margin of saphenous opening, the lower part of the falciform margin of the opening in the fascia lata through which the greater saphenous vein passes. SYN cornu inferius marginalis falciformis hiatus sapheni [NA].

inferior h. of lateral ventricle, the part of the lateral ventricle extending downward and forward into the medial part of the temporal lobe. SEE lateral *ventricle*. SYN cornu inferius ventriculi lateralis [NA], temporal h.

inferior h. of thyroid cartilage, one of the pair of downward prolongations at the back of the thyroid cartilage; it articulates on each side with the cricoid cartilage. SYN cornu inferius cartilaginis thyroideae [NA].

lateral h., the small lateral gray column of the spinal cord as appearing in transverse section containing the interomedial cell column. SEE ALSO gray *columns*, under *column*. SYN cornu laterale [NA].

lesser h. of hyoid bone, the shorter and more medial of the two processes on either side of the hyoid bone. SYN cornu minus ossis hyoidei [NA], styloid cornu.

nail h., obsolete term for overgrown nail.

occipital h., SYN posterior h.

posterior h., the posterior or occipital division of the lateral ventricle of the brain, extending backward into the occipital lobe; the posterior gray column of the spinal cord as appearing in cross section. SYN cornu posterius ventriculi lateralis [NA], cornu posterius, cornua of spinal cord, occipital h.

pulp h., a prolongation of the pulp extending toward the cusp of a tooth.

sacral h.'s, SYN sacral *cornua*, under *cornu*.

h.'s of saphenous opening, SEE inferior h. of falciform margin of saphenous opening, superior h. of falciform margin of saphenous opening.

sebaceous h., a solid outgrowth from a sebaceous cyst.

superior h. of falciform margin of saphenous opening, the upper part of the falciform margin of the opening in the fascia lata through which the greater saphenous vein passes. SYN cornu superius marginalis falciformis [NA], Burns' falciform process, Burns' ligament, Hey's ligament.

superior h. of thyroid cartilage, one of the pair of upward prolongations from the thyroid cartilage to which the lateral hyothyroid ligament attaches. SYN cornu superius cartilaginis thyroideae [NA].

temporal h., SYN inferior h. of lateral ventricle.

h.'s of thyroid cartilage, SEE inferior h. of thyroid cartilage, superior h. of thyroid cartilage.

uterine h., h. of uterus, SYN *cornu* uteri.

ventral h., SYN anterior h.

warty h., SYN cutaneous h.

Horner, Johann F., Swiss ophthalmologist, 1831–1886. SEE H.'s *syndrome, pupil;* Bernard-H. *syndrome;* H.-Trantas *dots,* under *dot.*

Horner, William E., U.S. anatomist, 1793–1853. SEE H.'s *muscle, teeth,* under *tooth.*

hor·ni·fi·ca·tion (hŏr′ni-fi-kā′shŭn). SYN keratinization.

horny (hōrn′ē). Of the nature or structure of horn. SYN corneous, keratic, keratinous (2), keratoid (1), keroid.

ho·rop·ter (hō-rop′ter). The sum of the points in space, the images of which for a given fixation point fall on corresponding retinal points. If the fixation point is 2 meters, the horopter is a straight line; if less, a curve concave to the face; if more, a convex curve. [G. *horos,* limit, + *optēr,* spy, scout, fr. *oraō,* fut. *opsomai,* to see]

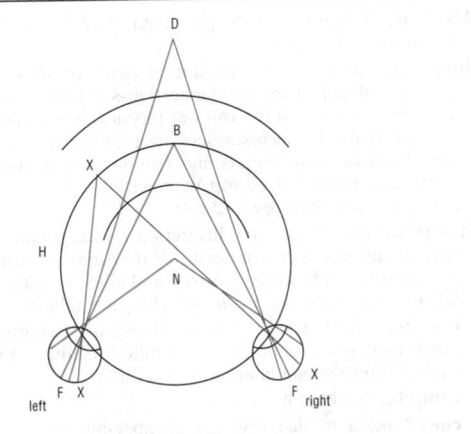

horopter plane

one fixation point (B) is imaged in the fovea (F), while the other fixation point (X) is imaged at the same distance from the fovea in both eyes. Objects outside the horopter plane (D) show a nasal disparity, while those inside it (N) show a temporal disparity

hor·rip·i·la·tion (ho-rip-i-lā′shŭn). Erection of the fine hairs on contraction of the arrectores pilorum. [L. *horreo,* to bristle, + *pilus,* hair]

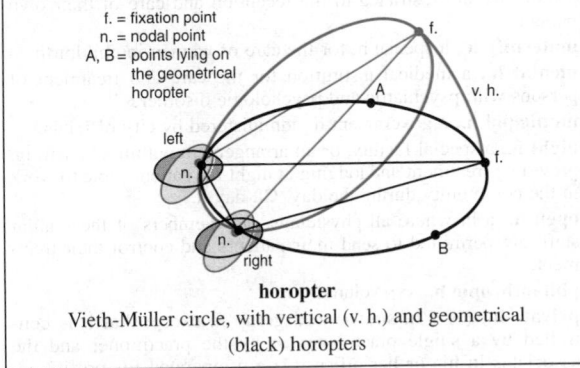

horopter
Vieth-Müller circle, with vertical (v. h.) and geometrical (black) horopters

hor·ror (hor′er). Dread; fear. [L.]

h. autotox′icus, a term introduced by Ehrlich, meaning that immunity is directed against foreign materials but not against the constituents of one's own body; exceptions to this concept are the autoallergic reactions and diseases. [L., dread of self-poisoning]

h. fusio′nis, simultaneous projection into consciousness of retinal images so different that fusion is impossible. SYN macular evasion. [L., dread of intermingling]

horse·fly (hōrs′flī). SEE *Tabanus, Anthomyia canicularis.*

horse·pow·er (hōrs′pow-er). A unit of power, 550 foot-pounds per second, or 745.700 watts.

horse·pox (hōrs′poks). A disease, now rare, that usually appears as typical eruptions, first papular, then vesicular, in the mouth or on the lips and buccal mucosa, sometimes on the skin of the fetlocks; caused by the horsepox virus, a member of the family Poxviridae.

Horsfall, Frank L., Jr., U.S. physician, 1906–1971. SEE Tamm-H. *mucoprotein, protein.*

Horsley, Sir Victor A.H., English surgeon, 1857–1916. SEE H.'s bone *wax.*

hor. som. Abbreviation for L. *hora somni,* before sleep, at bedtime.

Hortega, Pio del Rio, Spanish neurohistologist in South America, 1882–1945. SEE H. *cells,* under *cell;* H.'s neuroglia *stain.*

Horton, Bayard T., U.S. physician, *1895. SEE H.'s *arteritis, cephalalgia, headache.*

hos·pice (hos′pis). An institution that provides a centralized program of palliative and supportive services to dying persons and their families, in the form of physical, psychological, social, and spiritual care; such services are provided by an interdisciplinary team of professionals and volunteers who are available at home and in specialized inpatient settings. [L. *hospitium,* hospitality, lodging, fr. *hospes,* guest]

hos·pi·tal (hos′pi-tăl). An institution for the treatment, care, and cure of the sick and wounded, for the study of disease, and for the training of physicians, nurses, and allied health personnel. [L. *hospitalis,* for a guest, fr. *hospes* (*hospit-*), a host, a guest]
base h., a h. unit located in a military or recreational encampment; usually of small size and limited facilities, for immediate care of illnesses and injuries. SYN camp h.
camp h., SYN base h.
closed h., a h. that restricts membership on its attending or consulting staff, and thereby limits who may admit and treat patients.
day h., a special facility, or an arrangement within a h. setting, that enables the patient to come to the h. for treatment during the day and return home or to another facility at night. Cf. night h.
general h., any large civilian h. that is equipped to care for medical, surgical, maternity, and psychiatric cases, and usually has a resident medical staff.
government h., a h. administered by officials of the city, county, state, or nation. SYN public h.
group h., a private h. organized and controlled by a group of physicians and restricted to the reception and care of their own patients.
maternity h., a special h. for the care of women in childbirth.
mental h., a medical institution for the care and treatment of persons with psychiatric and psychologic disorders.
municipal h., a government h. administered by city officials.
night h., a special facility, or an arrangement within a h. setting, providing treatment and lodging at night for patients able to work in the community during the day. Cf. day h.
open h., a h. where all physicians, not members of the regular staff, are permitted to send their patients and control their treatment.
philanthropic h., SYN voluntary h.
private h., (1) a h. similar to a group h. except that it is controlled by a single practitioner or by the practitioner and the associates in his or her office; (2) a h. operated for profit. SYN proprietary h.
proprietary h., SYN private h.
public h., SYN government h.
special h., a h. for the medical and surgical care of patients with specific types of diseases, as of the ear, nose, and throat, eyes, or mental illness.
state h., a h. supported in part by taxpayers and administered by state government officials.
teaching h., a h. that also functions as a formal center of learning for the training of physicians, nurses, and allied health personnel.
Veterans Administration h., a h. operated at federal government expense and administered by the Veterans Administration for care of veterans of U.S. wars and retired military personnel.
voluntary h., a h. supported in part by voluntary contributions and under the control of a local, usually self-appointed, board of managers; a non-profit h. SYN philanthropic h.
weekend h., a special facility, or an arrangement within a h. setting, which enables a patient to work in the community during the work week and receive treatment in the hospital during the weekend.

hos·pi·tal·ism (hos′pi-tăl-izm). The second stage of a depression observed in the first year of human life, following anaclitic depression, characterized by stupor and a wasting away; usually caused by prolonged hospitalization in which an infant is separated from his or her mother or a mothering influence. SEE anaclitic, anaclitic *depression.*

hos·pi·tal·i·za·tion (hos′pi-tăl-i-zā′shŭn). Confinement in a hospital as a patient for diagnostic study and treatment.

host. The organism in or on which a parasite lives, deriving its body substance or energy from the h. [L. *hospes,* a host]
accidental h., one that harbors an organism which usually does not infect it.
amplifier h., a h. in which infectious agents multiply rapidly to high levels, providing an important source of infection for vectors in vector-borne diseases.
dead-end h., a h. from which infectious agents are not transmitted to other susceptible h.'s.
definitive h., one in which a parasite reaches the adult or sexually mature stage. SYN final h.
final h., SYN definitive h.
intermediate h., intermediary h., (1) one in which larval or developmental stages occur; (2) a host through which a microorganism can pass or which contains an asexual stage of a parasite. SYN secondary h.
paratenic h., an intermediate h. in which no development of the parasite occurs, although its presence may be required as an essential link in the completion of the parasite's life cycle; *e.g.,* the successive fish h.'s that carry the plerocercoid of *Diphyllobothrium latum,* the broad fish tapeworm, to larger food fish eventually eaten by man or other final h.'s. SYN transport h.
reservoir h., the h. of an infection in which the infectious agent multiplies and/or develops, and upon which the agent is dependent for survival in nature; the h. essential for the maintenance of the infection during times when active transmission is not occurring.
secondary h., SYN intermediate h.
transport h., SYN paratenic h.

hot·foot. SYN ignipedites.

hot·ten·tot·ism (hot′en-tot′izm). A form of stammering. [D. fr. Hottentot, (D. *hateren* to stammer, *tateren* to stutter), a people in South Africa named by the Dutch for the sounds of their speech]

Hounsfield, Godfrey N., British electronics engineer, *1919. Developed first practical computed tomography device, the EMI scanner; received the Nobel prize in Medicine in 1979 jointly with physicist A. M. Cormack. SEE H. *unit, number.*

house·fly (hows′flī). SEE *Musca, Fannia.*

house of·fi·cer. An intern or resident employed by a hospital to provide service to patients while receiving training in a medical specialty.

Houssay, Bernardo A., Argentinian physiologist and Nobel laureate, 1887–1971. SEE H. *animal, phenomenon, syndrome.*

Houston, John, Irish physician, 1802–1845. SEE H.'s *folds,* under *fold, muscle, valves,* under *valve.*

Hovius, Jacob, Dutch ophthalmologist, 1710–1786. SEE *canal* of H.

Howard, John Eager, U.S. internist and endocrinologist, 1902–1985. SEE H. *test;* Ellsworth-H. *test.*

Howell, William, U.S. physiologist, 1860–1945. SEE H. *unit;* H.-Jolly *bodies,* under *body.*

Howship, John, British surgeon, 1781–1841. SEE H.'s *lacunae,* under *lacuna;* Romberg-H. *symptom.*

Hoyer, Heinrich F., Polish anatomist and histologist, 1834–

1907. SEE H.'s *anastomoses*, under *anastomosis*, canals, under *canal*; Sucquet-H. *canals*, under *canal*.

HP Abbreviation for haptoglobin.

HPL Abbreviation for human placental *lactogen*.

HPLC Abbreviation for high-pressure liquid chromatography; high-performance liquid *chromatography*.

HPV Abbreviation for human papilloma *virus*.

H₂Q Symbol for ubiquinol.

HRCT Abbreviation for high resolution computed *tomography*.

h.s. Abbreviation for L. *hora somni*, before sleep, at bedtime.

hsp Abbreviation for heat shock *proteins*, under *protein*.

HSV Abbreviation for herpes simplex *virus*.

5-HT Abbreviation for 5-hydroxytryptamine.

Ht Abbreviation for total *hyperopia*.

H-tet·a·nase (tet′ă-nās). Behring's term for the hemolytic constituent of tetanus toxin.

HTLV. Abbreviation for human T-cell lymphoma/leukemia *virus*.

HTLV-I Abbreviation for T-cell lymphotrophic virus type I; human lymphotropic virus, type 1.

HTLV-II Abbreviation for T-cell lymphotrophic virus type II; human lymphotropic virus, type 2.

HTLV-III Abbreviation for human T-cell lymphotropic virus type III. SEE human immunodeficiency *virus*.

hU, hu Abbreviation for dihydrouridine.

Hubrecht, Ambrosius A.W., Dutch zoologist and comparative anatomist, 1853–1915. SEE H.'s protochordal *knot*.

Hucker-Conn stain. See under stain.

Hudson, Arthur Cyril, British ophthalmologist, 1875–1962. SEE H.-Stähli *line*.

hue (hū). One of the three qualities of color; that property by which colors of the spectrum are distinguished from each other and from grays or similar brightness; determined by the wavelength or a combination of wavelengths of light.

Hueck, Alexander F., German anatomist, 1802–1842. SEE H.'s *ligament*.

Huët, G.J., Dutch physician, *1879. SEE Pelger-Huët nuclear *anomaly*.

Hueter, Karl, German surgeon, 1838–1882. SEE H.'s *maneuver*, *sign*.

Hüfner, Carl Gustav von, German physician, 1840–1908. SEE H.'s *equation*.

Huggins, Charles B., Canadian-U.S. surgeon and Nobel laureate, 1901–1994. SEE H.'s *operation*.

Huguier, Pierre C., French surgeon, 1804–1873. SEE H.'s *canal*, *circle, sinus*.

Huhner, Max, U.S. urologist, 1873–1947. SEE H. *test*.

Hull, Edgar, 20th century U.S. cardiologist.

hum (hŭm). A low continuous murmur. [echoic]
  venous h., brief or continuous noise originating from the neck veins that may be confused with cardiac murmurs, particularly with the continuous murmur of patent ductus arteriosus. SYN bruit de diable, nun's murmur.

Human Genome Initiative. SYN Human Genome Project.

Human Genome Project. a comprehensive effort by molecular biologists worldwide to map the human genome, which consists of about 100,000 genes, or 3 billion DNA base pairs. SYN Human Genome Initiative.

    This is a comprehensive effort by molecular biologists worldwide to map the human genome, which consists of about 100,000 genes, or 3 billion DNA base pairs. Sequencing the DNA in all 46 chromosomes is expected to take some 15 years and cost at least $3 billion. Initially, a map of DNA markers will be produced; in 1992 a French laboratory announced it had already carried out this process for 28% of the human genome. The regions between the markers will then be filled in. Supporters of the controversial project argue that mapping the genome will not only further basic understanding of human genetics, but also provide information that will contribute to prevention of inherited disease and perhaps, through gene therapy, lead to treatment of genetic ailments. Critics have countered that DNA sequencing is only a first step to understanding the role of genes in health, mentality, and behavior. Furthermore, the supposedly comprehensive map will be a highly idealized version of the human genome, which varies considerably across populations and among individuals. The wholesale sequencing of the genome would not be possible without the automated method of gene sequencing, invented by Leroy Hood.

hu·mec·tant (hyū-mek′tănt). 1. Moistening. 2. A substance used to obtain a moistening effect (*e.g.,* glycerin solution).

hu·mec·ta·tion (hyū-mek-tā′shŭn). 1. Therapeutic application of moisture. 2. Serous infiltration of the tissues. 3. Soaking of a crude drug in water preparatory to the making of an extract. [L. *humecto,* pp. *-mectus,* to moisten, fr. *humeo,* to be damp]

hu·mer·al (hyū′mer-ăl). Relating to the humerus.

hu·mer·o·ra·di·al (hyū′mer-ō-rā′dē-ăl). Relating to both humerus and radius; denoting especially the ratio of length of one to the other.

hu·mer·o·scap·u·lar (hyū′mer-ō-skap′yū-lăr). Relating to both humerus and scapula.

hu·mer·o·ul·nar (hyū′mer-ō-ŭl′năr). Relating to both humerus and ulna; denoting especially the ratio of length of one to the other.

hu·mer·us, gen. and pl. **hu·meri** (hyū′mer-ŭs, -ī) [NA]. The bone of the arm, articulating with the scapula above and the radius and ulna below. [L. shoulder]

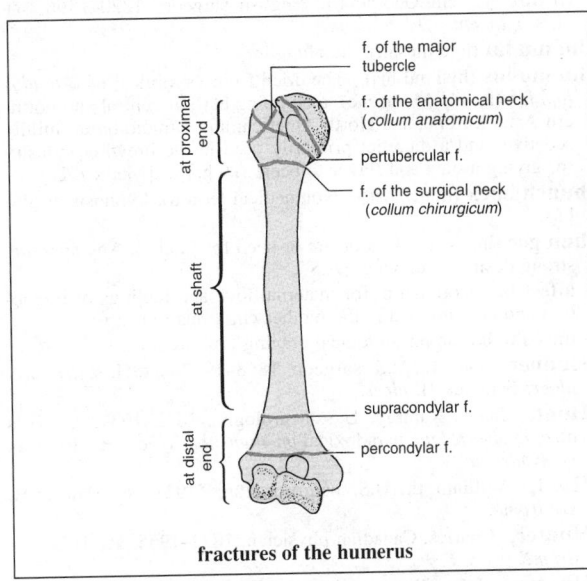

f. of the major tubercle
f. of the anatomical neck (*collum anatomicum*)
pertubercular f.
f. of the surgical neck (*collum chirurgicum*)
at proximal end
at shaft
at distal end
supracondylar f.
percondylar f.

fractures of the humerus

hu·mid·i·ty (hyū-mid′i-tē). Moisture or dampness, as of the air. [L. *humiditas,* dampness]
  absolute h., the mass of water vapor actually present per unit volume of gas or air.
  relative h., the actual amount of water vapor present in the air or in a gas, divided by the amount necessary for saturation at the same temperature and pressure; expressed as a percentage.

hu·min (hyū′min). An insoluble brownish residue obtained upon acid hydrolysis of protein.

Hummelsheim, Eduard K.M.J., German ophthalmologist, 1868–1952. SEE H.'s *operation*.

hu·mor, gen. **hu·mor·is** (hyū′mer, hyū-mōr′is). 1 [NA]. Any clear fluid or semifluid hyaline anatomical substance. 2. One of the elemental body fluids that were the basis of the physiologic and pathologic teachings of the hippocratic school: blood, yellow

hu

bile, black bile, and phlegm. SEE ALSO humoral *doctrine.* [L. correctly, *umor,* liquid]

aqueous h., the watery fluid that fills the anterior and posterior chambers of the eye. It is secreted by the ciliary processes within the posterior chambers and passes through the the pupil into the anterior chamber where it filters through the trabecular meshwork and is reabsorbed into the venous system at the iridocorneal angle by way of the sinus venosus of the sclera; SYN h. aquosus [NA], intraocular fluid.

h. aquo′sus [NA], SYN aqueous h.

Morgagni's h., SYN Morgagni's *liquor.*

ocular h., one of the two h.'s of the eye: aqueous and vitreous.

peccant humors, based on the historic humoral theory of disease, such h.'s or deranged fluids in the body were regarded as the direct causes of various illnesses.

vitreous h., the fluid component of the vitreous body, with which it is often erroneously equated. SYN h. vitreus [NA].

h. vit′reus [NA], SYN vitreous h.

hu·mor·al (hyū′mōr-ăl). Relating to a humor in any sense.

hu·mor·al·ism, hu·mor·ism (hyū′mŏr-ăl-izm, -mŏr-izm). SYN humoral *doctrine.* [L. *umor, humor,* moisture]

hump (hŭmp). A rounded protuberance or bulge.

buffalo h., SYN buffalo *type.*

dowager's h., postmenopausal cervical kyphosis of older women.

Hampton's h., a juxtapleural pulmonary soft tissue density on a chest radiograph, convex toward the hilum, usually at the costophrenic angle; described as a manifestation of pulmonary infarction.

hump·back (hŭmp′bak). Nonmedical term for kyphosis or gibbus.

Humphry, Sir George M., English surgeon, 1820–1896. SEE H.'s *ligament.*

hu·mu·lin (hyū′mū-lin). SYN lupulin.

hu·mu·lus (hyū′mū-lŭs). The dried fruits (strobiles) of *Humulus lupulus* (family Moraceae), a climbing herb of central and northern Asia, Europe, and North America; an aromatic bitter, mildly sedative, and a diuretic; primarily used in the brewing industry for giving aroma and flavor to beer. SYN hops. [Mediev. L.]

hunch·back (hŭnch′bak). Nonmedical term for kyphosis or gibbus.

hun·ger (hŭn′ger). **1.** A desire or need for food. **2.** Any appetite, strong desire, or craving. [A.S.]

affect h., emotional h. for maternal love and feelings of protection and care implied in the mother-child relationship.

narcotic h., the physiological craving for narcotics.

Hunner, Guy L., U.S. surgeon, 1868–1957. SEE H.'s *stricture, ulcer;* Fenwick-H. *ulcer.*

Hunt, James Ramsay, U.S. neurologist, 1872–1937. SEE H.'s *atrophy, neuralgia,* paradoxical *phenomenon, syndrome;* Ramsay H. *syndrome.*

Hunt, William E., U.S. neurosurgeon, *1921. SEE Tolosa-H. *syndrome.*

Hunter, Charles, Canadian physician, 1872–1955. SEE H.'s *syndrome.*

Hunter, John, Scottish surgeon, anatomist, physiologist and pathologist, 1728–1793. SEE H.'s *canal, gubernaculum, operation;* H.-Schreger *bands,* under *line, band, lines,* under *line.*

Hunter, William, Scottish anatomist and obstetrician, 1718–1783. SEE H.'s *ligament, line, membrane.*

Hunter, William, English pathologist, 1861–1937. SEE H.'s *glossitis.*

hunt·ing (hŭnt′ing). The oscillation of a controlled variable, such as the temperature of a thermostat, around its set point. SEE hunting *reaction.*

Huntington, George, U.S. physician, 1850–1916. SEE H.'s *chorea, disease.*

Hurler, Gertrud, Austrian pediatrician, 1889–1965. SEE H.'s *disease, syndrome;* Pfaundler-H. *syndrome.*

Hurst, Arthur Frederick (born Hertz), English physician, 1879–1944.

Hürthle, Karl W., German histologist, 1860–1945. SEE H. *cell,* cell *adenoma,* cell *carcinoma,* cell *tumor.*

Huschke, Emil, German anatomist, 1797–1858. SEE H.'s *cartilages,* under *cartilage, foramen,* auditory *teeth,* under *tooth, valve.*

husk. SYN verminous *bronchitis.*

psyllium husk, the husk of the dried ripe seeds of *Plantago psyllium, P. indica, P. ovata,* and *P. arenaria* (family Plantaginaceae). The husks swell on exposure to water and provide an indigestible mucilaginous mass in the intestines. Used as a bulk laxative and lubricant.

Hutchinson, Sir Jonathan, British surgeon, 1828–1913. SEE H.'s *facies, freckle, mask,* crescentic *notch, patch, pupil, teeth,* under *tooth, triad;* H.-Gilford *disease, syndrome.*

Hutchison, Sir Robert, English pediatrician, 1871–1960. SEE H. *syndrome.*

Huxley, Thomas, English biologist, physiologist, and comparative anatomist, 1825–1895. SEE H.'s *layer, membrane, sheath.*

Huygens, Christian, Dutch physicist, 1629–1695. SEE H.'s *ocular, principle.*

HV Abbreviation for half-value.

HVA Abbreviation for homovanillic acid.

HVL Abbreviation for half-value *layer.*

△**hyal-.** SEE hyalo-.

hy·a·lin (hī′ă-lin). A clear, eosinophilic, homogeneous substance occurring in degeneration; *e.g.,* in arteriolar walls in arteriolar sclerosis and in glomerular tufts in diabetic glomerulosclerosis. [G. *hyalos,* glass]

alcoholic h., SYN Mallory *bodies,* under *body.*

hy·a·li·na·sis cu·tis et mu·co·sae. SYN lipoid *proteinosis.*

hy·a·line (hī′ă-lin, -lēn). Relating to transparent or colorless hyphae or other fungal structures. SYN hyaloid. [G. *hyalos,* glass]

hy·a·lin·i·za·tion (hī′ă-lin-i-zā′shŭn). The formation of hyalin.

hy·a·li·no·sis (hī′ă-li-nō′sis). hyaline *degeneration,* especially that of relatively extensive degree.

systemic h., SYN juvenile hyalin *fibromatosis.*

hy·a·li·nu·ria (hī′ă-li-nū′rē-ă). The excretion of hyalin or casts of hyaline material in the urine. [hyalin + G. *ouron,* urine]

hy·a·li·tis (hī′ă-lī′tis). SYN vitreitis.

suppurative h., purulent vitreous humor due to exudation from adjacent structures, as in panophthalmitis.

△**hyalo-, hyal-.** Glassy, hyalin; vitreous. Cf. vitreo-. [G. *hyalos,* glass]

hy·a·lo·bi·u·ron·ic ac·id (hī′ă-lō-bī-yūr-on′ik). A disaccharide made up of D-glucuronic acid and *N*-acetyl-D-glucosamine in a β1,3 linkage; occurs in hyaluronic acid as the repeating unit. See figure under hyaluronic acid.

hy·a·lo·cyte (hī′ă-lō-sīt). SYN vitreous *cell.* [hyalo- + G. *kytos,* cell]

hy·al·o·gens (hī-al′ō-jenz). Substances similar to mucoids that are found in many animal structures (*e.g.,* cartilage, vitreous humor, hydatid cysts) and yield sugars on hydrolysis.

hy·a·lo·hy·pho·my·co·sis (hī′ă-lō-hī′fō-mī-kō′sis). An infection caused by a fungus with hyaline (colorless) mycelium in tissue, *e.g.,* species of *Fusarium, Penicillium,* and *Scopulariopsis;* circumstances for infections usually involve a decrease in body resistance due to surgery, indwelling catheters, steroid therapy, or immunosuppressive drugs or cytotoxins. [hyalo- + G. *hyphe,* web, + *mykēs,* fungus, + *-osis,* condition]

hy·a·loid (hī′ă-loyd). SYN hyaline. [hyalo- + G. *eidos,* resemblance]

hy·al·o·mere (hī′ă-lō-mēr). The clear periphery of a blood platelet. [hyalo- + G. *meros,* part]

Hy·a·lom·ma (hī-ă-lom′ă). An Old World genus (about 21 species) of large ixodid ticks with submarginal eyes, coalesced festoons, an ornate scutum, and a long rostrum. Adults parasitize all domestic animals and a wide variety of wild animals; larvae or nymphs may parasitize small mammals, birds, and reptiles. Species harbor a great variety of pathogens of humans and animals, and also cause considerable mechanical injury. [hyalo- + G. *omma*, eye]

H. anato'licum, former name for *H. anatolicum anatolicum.*

H. anato'licum anato'licum, a subspecies infesting cattle, camels and horses in Asia, the Near and Middle East, southeastern Europe, and North Africa; it is a vector of bovine tropical theileriosis, of equine babesiosis, and of human Crimean-Congo hemorrhagic fever.

H. margina'tum, a particularly common species of tick carried by birds migrating between Europe and Asia and Africa, and the probable vector of the virus of Crimean hemorrhagic fever.

H. truncat'um, a species causing sweating sickness in cattle in Africa.

H. variega'tum, species of tick that is the vector of the viral agent of lymphocytic choriomeningitis in Ethiopia.

hy·a·lo·pha·gia, hy·a·loph·a·gy (hī′ă-lō-fā′jē-ă, hī-ă-lof′ă-jē). The eating or chewing of glass. [hyalo- + G. *phagō,* to eat]

hy·a·lo·pho·bia (hī′ă-lō-fō′bē-ă). Morbid fear of glass objects. SYN crystallophobia. [hyalo- + G. *phobos,* fear]

hy·al·o·plasm, hy·a·lo·plas·ma (hī′ă-lō-plazm, -plaz′mă). The protoplasmic fluid substance of a cell. [hyalo- + G. *plasma,* thing formed]

nuclear h., SYN karyolymph.

hy·a·lo·se·ro·si·tis (hī′ă-lō-ser-ō-sī′tis). Inflammation of a serous membrane with a fibrinous exudate that eventually becomes hyalinized, resulting in a relatively thick, dense, opaque, glistening, white or gray-white coating; when the process involves the visceral serous membranes of various organs, the grossly apparent condition is sometimes colloquially termed icing liver, sugarcoated spleen, frosted heart, and so on, depending on the site. [hyalo- + Mod. L. *serosa,* serous membrane, + *-itis,* inflammation]

hy·a·lo·sis (hī-ă-lō′sis). Degenerative changes in the vitreous body. [hyalo- + G. *-osis,* condition]

asteroid h., numerous small spherical bodies ("snowball" opacities) in the corpus vitreum, visible ophthalmoscopically; an age change, usually unilateral, and not affecting vision.

punctate h., a condition marked by minute opacities in the vitreous.

hy·al·o·some (hī-al′ō-sōm). An oval or round structure within a cell nucleus that stains faintly but otherwise resembles a nucleolus. [hyalo- + G. *sōma,* body]

hy·a·lu·rate (hī-ă-lū′rāt). SYN hyaluronate.

hy·al·u·ro·nate (hī-ă-lū′ron-āt). A salt or ester of hyaluronic acid. SYN hyalurate.

h. lyase, a lyase cleaving hyaluronic acids, producing hyalobiuronic acid. SEE ALSO hyaluronidase (1), hyaluronoglucosaminidase. SYN hyaluronic lyase.

hy·al·u·ron·ic ac·id (hī′ă-lū-ron′ik). A mucopolysaccharide made up of alternating β1,4-linked residues of hyalobiuronic acid, forming a gelatinous material in the tissue spaces and acting as a lubricant and shock absorbant generally throughout the body; it is hydrolyzed to disaccharide or tetrasaccharide units by hyaluronidase.

hy·al·u·ron·ic ly·ase. SYN *hyaluronate* lyase.

hy·al·u·ron·i·dase (hī′ă-lū-ron′i-dās). **1.** Term used loosely for hyaluronate lyase, hyaluronoglucosaminidase, and hyaluronoglucuronidase, one or more of which are present in testis, sperm, other organs, bee and snake venoms, type II pneumonococci, certain hemolytic streptococci, etc. SYN diffusing factor, Duran-Reynals permeability factor, Duran-Reynals spreading factor, invasin, spreading factor. **2.** A soluble enzyme product prepared from mammalian testes; it is used to increase the effect of local anesthetics and to permit wider infiltration of subcutaneously administered fluids, is suggested in the treatment of certain forms of arthritis to promote resolution of redundant tissue, is used to speed the resorption of traumatic or postoperative edema and hematoma, is used in combination with collagenase to dissociate organs such as liver and heart into viable cell suspensions, and in histochemistry is used on tissue secretions to verify the presence of hyaluronic acid or chondroitin sulfates.

hy·al·u·ron·o·glu·cos·a·min·i·dase (hī-ă-lū′ron-ō-glū′kō-să-

min′i-dās). An enzyme hydrolyzing β1,4 linkages in hyaluronates. SEE ALSO hyaluronidase (1), *hyaluronate* lyase.

hy·al·u·ron·o·glu·cu·ron·i·dase (hī-ă-lū′ron-ō-glū-kur-on′i-dās). An enzyme hydrolyzing β1,3 linkages in hyaluronates. SEE ALSO hyaluronidase (1).

hy·bar·ox·ia (hī-bă-rok′sē-ă). Oxygen therapy with pressures greater than 1 atmosphere or ambient oxygen pressure applied to the entire body in a chamber or room. [G. *hyper,* above, + *baros,* pressure, + *oxys,* acute]

hy·ben·zate (hī-ben′zāt). USAN-approved contraction for *o*-(4-hydroxybenzoyl)benzoate.

hy·brid (hī′brid). **1.** An individual (plant or animal) whose parents are different varieties of the same species or belong to different but closely allied species. **2.** Fused tissue culture cells, as in a hybridoma. SYN crossbreed (1). [L. *hybrida,* offspring of a tame sow and a wild boar, fr. G. *hybris,* violation, wantonness]

DNA-RNA h., double-stranded polynucleic acids in which one strand is DNA and the other strand is the complementary RNA; formed during transcription and during multiplication of oncogenic RNA viruses.

SV40-adenovirus h., a virion consisting of SV40 genetic material encased in an adenovirus capsid.

hy·brid·ism (hī′brid-izm). The state of being hybrid.

hy·brid·i·za·tion (hī′brid-i-zā′shŭn). **1.** The process of breeding a hybrid. **2.** Crossing over between related but nonallelic genes. **3.** The specific reassociation of complementary strands of polynucleic acids; *e.g.,* the formation of a DNA-RNA hybrid. SYN crossbreeding.

cell h., fusion of two or more dissimilar cells, leading to formation of a synkaryon.

cross h., annealing of a DNA probe to an imperfectly matching DNA molecule.

DNA h., a technique used to determine the relatedness of microorganisms by the speed and efficiency of the reassociation of single-stranded DNA to form double-stranded DNA when one of the strands originates from one organism and the other strand from another organism; occurs when the base sequences are complementary or nearly so.

nucleic acid h., SYN anneal (5).

overlap h., SYN chromosome *walking.*

in situ h., a technique developed in 1969 for annealing nucleic acid probes to cellular DNA for detection by autoradiography. Under proper laboratory conditions, the binding process occurs spontaneously. In situ h. constitutes a key step in DNA fingerprinting. SYN in situ nucleic acid h.

in situ nucleic acid h., SYN in situ h.

somatic cell h., production of a heterokaryon.

hy·brid·o·ma (hī-brid-ō′mă). A tumor of hybrid cells used in the *in vitro* production of specific monoclonal antibodies; produced by fusion of an established tissue culture line of lymphocyte tumor cells (*e.g.,* mouse plasmacytoma cells) and specific antibody-producing cells (*e.g.,* splenocytes from specifically immunized mice); fusions are accomplished by use of polyethylene glycol or other methods. [G. *hybris,* violation, wantonness, + *-ōma,* tumor]

hy·can·thone (hī-kan′thōn). 1-[[2-(Diethylamino)ethyl]amino]-4-(hydroxymethyl)thioxan then-9-one; an antischistosomal drug.

hy·clate (hī′klāt). USAN-approved contraction for monohydrochloride hemiethanolate hemihydrate, HCl·½C₂H₅OH·½H₂O.

hy·dan·to·in (hī-dan′tō-in). 2,4-Imidazolidinedione; derived from urea or from allantoin; the NH–CH₂–CO group is prototypical of α-amino acids. SYN glycolylurea.

hy·dan·to·in·ate (hī-dan-tō′in-āt). A salt of hydantoin.

hy·da·tid (hī′da-tid). **1.** SYN hydatid *cyst.* **2.** A vesicular structure resembling an *Echinococcus* cyst. [G. *hydatis,* a drop of water, a hyatid]

Morgagni's h., SYN vesicular *appendices* of uterine tube, under *appendix.*

nonpedunculated h., SYN testicular *appendage.*

pedunculated h., SYN *appendix* of epididymidis.

sessile h., SYN testicular *appendage.*

hy

stalked h., SYN vesicular *appendices* of uterine tube, under *appendix.*

hy·da·tid·i·form (hī-da-tid′i-form). Having the form or appearance of a hydatid.

hy·da·tid·o·cele (hī-da-tid′ō-sēl). A cystic mass composed of one or more hydatids formed in the scrotum. [hydatid + G. *kēlē,* tumor]

hy·da·ti·do·ma (hī′da-ti-dō′mă). A benign neoplasm in which there is prominent formation of hydatids. [hydatid + G. *-oma,* tumor]

hy·da·tid·o·sis (hī′da-ti-dō′sis). The morbid state caused by the presence of hydatid cysts.

hy·da·ti·dos·to·my (hī′da-ti-dos′tō-mē). Surgical evacuation of a hydatid cyst. [hydatid + G. *stoma,* mouth]

Hy·da·tig·e·ra tae·ni·ae·for·mis (hī-da-tij′er-ă tē-ni-ē-fōr′mis). SYN *Taenia taeniaeformis.*

hy·da·toid (hī′da-toyd). **1.** The aqueous humor. **2.** The hyaloid membrane. **3.** Relating to the aqueous humor. **4.** Watery or resembling water. [G. *hydōr* (hydat-), water, + *eidos,* resemblance]

Hyde, James N., U.S. dermatologist, 1840–1910. SEE H.'s *disease.*

hyd·no·car·pus oil (hid-nō-kar′pŭs). SYN chaulmoogra oil.

△**hydr-.** SEE hydro-.

hy·drac·e·tin (hī-dras′ĕ-tin). Pure form of acetylphenylhydrazine.

hy·drad·e·ni·tis (hī′drad-ĕ-nī′tis). SYN hidradenitis.

hy·drad·e·no·ma (hī′drad-ĕ-nō′mă). SYN hidradenoma.

hy·dra·gogue (hī′dră-gog). Producing a discharge of watery fluid; denoting a class of cathartics that retain fluids in the intestine and aid in the removal of edematous fluids, *e.g.,* saline cathartics. [hydr- + G. *agōgos,* drawing forth]

hy·dral·a·zine hy·dro·chlo·ride (hī-dral′ă-zēn). 1-Hydrazinophthalazine hydrochloride; a vasodilating antihypertensive agent.

hy·dral·lo·stane (hī-dral′ō-stān). 11β,17α,21-Trihydroxy-5β-pregnane-3,20-dio ne; a metabolite of cortisole, reduced at the 4,5 double bond. SYN 4,5α-dihydrocortisol.

hy·dra·mi·tra·zine tar·trate (hī-dră-mī′tră-zēn). 2,4-Bis-(Diethylamino)-6-hydrazino-*s*-triazine tartrate; an intestinal antispasmodic.

hy·dram·ni·on, hy·dram·ni·os (hī-dram′nē-on, -nē-os). Presence of an excessive amount of amniotic fluid. [G. *hydōr,* water, + amnion]

hy·dran·en·ceph·a·ly (hī′dran-en-sef′ă-lē). Absence of cerebereal hemispheres, which have been replaced by fluid-filled sacs, lined by leptomeninges. The skull and its brain cavities are normal. [hydr- + G. *an-* priv. + *enkephalos,* brain]

hy·drar·gyr·ia, hy·drar·gy·rism (hī-drar-jir′ē-ă, hī-drar′jir-izm). SYN mercury *poisoning.* [L. *hydrargyrum,* mercury]

hy·drar·gy·rum (hī-drar′ji-rŭm). SYN mercury. [G. *hydrargyros,* quicksilver, fr. *hydōr,* water, + *argyros,* silver]

hy·drar·thro·di·al (hī-drar-thrō′dē-ăl). Relating to hydrarthrosis.

hy·drar·thron (hī-drar′thron). SYN hydrarthrosis.

hy·drar·thro·sis (hī-drar-thrō′sis). Effusion of a serous fluid into a joint cavity. SYN hydrarthron, hydrarthrus, hydrops articuli. [hydr- + G. *arthron,* joint]

intermittent h., a disorder characterized by a periodically recurring serous effusion into the cavity of a joint; the articulation may be the seat of a chronic arthritis or may apparently be normal in the intervals of the attacks.

hy·drar·thrus (hī-drar′thrŭs). SYN hydrarthrosis.

hy·drase (hī′drās). Former name for hydratase.

hy·dras·tine (hī-dras′tēn). An alkaloid of hydrastis; an isoquinoline chemically related to narcotine. As the hydrochloride, was used locally in the treatment of catarrhal inflammation of the mucous membranes, and internally in the treatment of gastric inflammation, as a uterine stimulant, and to check uterine hemorrhage.

hy·dras·ti·nine (hī-dras′ti-nēn). A semisynthetic alkaloid pre-

pared from hydrastine; the hydrochloride has been used in uterine hemorrhage and as an oxytocic; in large doses, it is a powerful depressant of the entire motor tract (motor cortex, nerve, and muscle).

hy·dras·tis (hī-dras′tis). The dried rhizome of *Hydrastis canadensis* (family Ranunculaceae), a native of the eastern U.S.; formerly used in the treatment of chronic catarrhal states of the mucous membranes and in metrorrhagia. SYN golden seal, jaundice root, yellow root. [Mod. L. fr. G. *hydōr* (hydro-), water, + *draō,* to accomplish]

hy·dra·tase (hī′dră-tās). Trivial name applied, together with dehydratase, to certain hydro-lyases (EC class 4.2.1) catalyzing hydration-dehydration; *e.g.,* fumarate-malate interconversion by fumarate hydratase.

hy·drate (hī′drāt). An aqueous solvate (in older terminology, a hydroxide); a compound crystallizing with one or more molecules of water; *e.g.,* $CuSO_4 \cdot 5H_2O$.

hy·drat·ed (hī′drāt-ed). Combined with water, forming a hydrate. SYN hydrous.

hy·dra·tion (hī-drā′shŭn). **1.** Chemically, the addition of water; differentiated from hydrolysis, where the union with water is accompanied by a splitting of the original molecule and the water molecule. SEE ALSO solvation. **2.** Clinically, the taking in of water; used commonly in the sense of reduced h. or dehydration.

absolute h., actual water excess as measured by a difference from the normal or from a given water content.

hy·dra·zide (hī′dră-zīd). An organic compound of the general formula RCO–NHNH₂; an acyl derivative of hydrazine.

hy·dra·zine (hī′dră-zēn). H₂N–NH₂, from which phenylhydrazine and similar products are derived.

hy·dra·zine yel·low. SYN tartrazine.

hy·dra·zi·nol·y·sis (hī′dră-zi-nol′i-sis). Cleavage of chemical bonds by hydrazine (NH₂–NH₂); applied in protein and nucleic acid degradations.

hy·dra·zone (hī′dră-zōn). A substance derived from aldehydes and ketones by reaction with hydrazine or a hydrazine derivative to give the grouping =C=N–NH₂.

hy·dre·mia (hī-drē′mē-ă). A condition in which the blood volume is increased as a result of an increase in the water content of plasma, with or without a reduction in the concentration of protein; there is an excess of plasma in proportion to the cellular elements and a corresponding decrease in hematocrit. SYN dilution anemia, polyplasmia. [hydr- + G. *haima,* blood]

hy·dren·ceph·a·lo·cele (hī-dren-sef′ă-lō-sēl). Protrusion, through a cleft in the skull, of brain substance expanded into a sac containing fluid. SYN encephalocystocele, hydrocephalocele, hydroencephalocele. [hydr- + G. *enkephalos,* brain, + *kēlē,* tumor]

hy·dren·ceph·a·lo·me·nin·go·cele (hī′dren-sef′ă-lō-me-ning′gō-sēl). Protrusion, through a defect in the skull, of a sac containing meninges, brain substance, and cerebrospinal fluid.

hy·dren·ceph·a·lus (hī-dren-sef′ă-lŭs). Rarely used term for internal *hydrocephalus.* [hydr- + G. *enkephalos,* brain]

hy·dri·at·ric, hy·dri·a·tic (hī-drē-at′rik, -at′ik). Relating to the obsolete use of water to treat or cure disease. SYN hydrotherapeutic. [hydr- + G. *iatrikos,* relating to medicine]

hy·dric (hī′drik). Relating to hydrogen in chemical combination.

hy·dride (hī′drīd). A negatively charged hydrogen (*i.e.,* H:⁻) or a compound of hydrogen in which it assumes a formal negative charge, *e.g.,* sodium borohydride (NaBH₄).

hy·drin·dan·tin (hī-drin-dan′tin). The reduced form of ninhydrin.

△**hydro-, hydr-.** **1.** Water, watery. **2.** Containing or combined with hydrogen. **3.** A hydatid. [G. *hydōr,* water]

hy·droa (hī-drō′ă). Any bullous eruption. SYN hidroa. [hydro + G. *ōon,* egg]

h. aestiva′le, SYN h. vacciniforme.

h. fe′brile, SYN *herpes* simplex.

h. gestatio′nis, SYN *herpes* gestationis.

h. herpetifor′me, SYN *dermatitis* herpetiformis.

h. puero′rum, SYN h. vacciniforme.

h. vaccinifor′me, a recurrent eruption of erythema evolving to umbilicated bullae, occurring on exposure to the sun and affecting chiefly male children with resolution before adult life. SYN h. aestivale, h. puerorum.

h. vesiculo′sum, obsolete term for erythema multiforme with iris or vesicular lesions.

hy·dro·a·dip·sia (hī′drō-ă-dip′sē-ă). Absence of thirst for water. [hydro- + G. *a*- priv. + *dipsa*, thirst]

hy·dro·ap·pen·dix (hī′drō-ă-pen′diks). Distention of the vermiform appendix with a serous fluid.

hy·dro·bil·i·ru·bin (hī′drō-bil-i-rū′bin). A dark brown-red pigment that may be formed when bilirubin is reduced.

hy·dro·bro·mate (hī-drō-brō′māt). A salt of hydrobromic acid.

hy·dro·bro·mic ac·id (hī-drō-brō′mik). An aqueous solution of hydrogen bromide; its salts are bromides.

hy·dro·cal·y·co·sis (hī′drō-kal-i-kō′sis). A usually symptomless anomaly of the renal calix that is dilated from obstruction of the infundibulum; usually discovered incidentally at pyelography or autopsy; may become infected. [hydro- + G. *kalyx*, cup of a flower]

hy·dro·car·bon (hī-drō-kar′bŏn). A compound containing only hydrogen and carbon.

Diels h., a phenanthrene derivative obtained by the dehydrogenation of various steroids.

saturated h., a h. that contains the greatest possible number of hydrogen atoms, so that the molecule contains neither rings nor multiple bonds.

hy·dro·cele (hī′drō-sēl). A collection of serous fluid in a sacculated cavity; specifically, such a collection in the tunica vaginalis testis, or in a separate pocket along the spermatic cord. [hydro- + G. *kēlē*, hernia]

cervical h., a cyst formed by secretion into a persistent duct or fissure of the neck; when it involves lymph channels, it is usually a lymphangioma. SYN h. colli.

h. col′li, SYN cervical h.

communicating h., associated with patent processus vaginalis.

congenital h., a collection of fluid in the unobliterated processus vaginalis leading from the abdominal cavity to the investing sac of the testis.

cord h., isolated h. of spermatic cord.

Dupuytren's h., bilocular h. in which the sac fills the scrotum and also extends into the abdominal cavity beneath the peritoneum.

h. fem′inae, accumulation of serous fluid in the labium majus or in Nuck's canal. SYN h. muliebris, Nuck's h.

filarial h., h. due to microfilaria (chiefly of *Wuchereria bancrofti*) in the tunica vaginalis.

funicular h., fluid in a portion of the tunica vaginalis shut off from both testis and abdominal cavity.

h. mulie′bris, SYN h. feminae.

noncommunicating h., obliterated patent processus vaginalis; and isolated h.

Nuck's h., SYN h. feminae.

h. spina′lis, SYN *spina bifida.*

hy·dro·ce·lec·to·my (hī′drō-sē-lek′tō-mē). Excision of a hydrocele. [hydrocele + G. *ektomē*, excision]

hy·dro·ce·phal·ic (hī′drō-se-fal′ik). Relating to or suffering from hydrocephalus.

hy·dro·ceph·a·lo·cele (hī-drō-sef′ă-lō-sēl). SYN hydrencephalocele.

hy·dro·ceph·a·loid (hī-drō-sef′ă-loyd). **1.** Resembling hydrocephalus. **2.** A condition in infants suffering from diarrhea or other debilitating disease, in which there is dehydration and general symptoms resembling those of hydrocephalus without, however, any abnormal accumulation of cerebrospinal fluid.

hy·dro·ceph·a·lus (hī-drō-sef′ă-lŭs). A condition marked by an excessive accumulation of fluid resulting in dilation of the cerebral ventricles and raised intracranial pressure; may also result in enlargement of the cranium and atrophy of the brain. SYN hydrocephaly. [hydro- + G. *kephalē*, head]

communicating h., type of h. in which there is an abnormality in

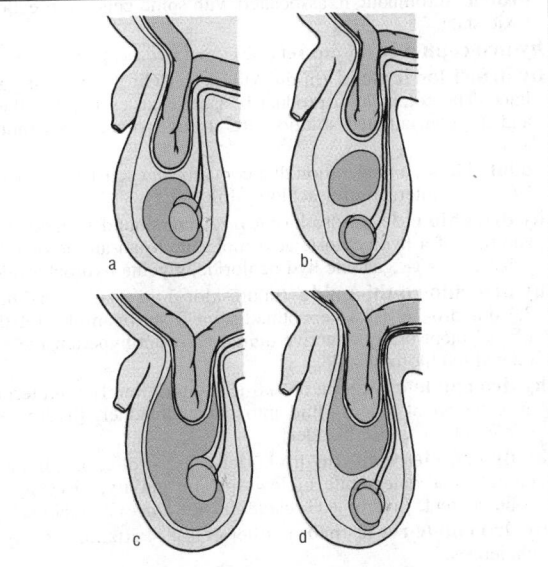

hydrocele (blue) with hernia

a) hernia with hydrocele testis; b) hernia with hydrocele funiculi; c) hernia encystica in open processus vaginalis peritonei; d) hernia encystica with partially obliterated processus vaginalis peritonei

cerebrospinal fluid absorption; there is no obstruction to cerebrospinal fluid flow in the ventricular system or where the cerebrospinal fluid passes into the spinal canal.

congenital h., h. due to a developmental defect of the brain. SYN primary h.

double compartment h., independent supra- and infra-tentorial h. usually due to a veil occlusion of the aqueduct of Sylvius.

external h., (1) accumulation of fluid in the subarachnoid spaces of the brain; **(2)** accumulation of fluid in the subdural space owing to a persistent communication between the subarachnoid and subdural spaces.

h. ex vac′uo, h. due to loss or atrophy of brain tissue; less commonly associated with raised intracranial pressure.

internal h., h. in which the accumulation of fluid is confined to the ventricles; also occurs as an autosomal recessive condition in the Hereford and Holstein breeds of cattle.

noncommunicating h., SYN obstructive h.

normal pressure h., a type of h. developing usually in older people, due to failure of cerebrospinal fluid to be absorbed by the pacchionian granulations, and characterized clinically by progressive dementia, unsteady gait, urinary incontinence, and usually, a normal spinal fluid pressure. SYN occult h.

obstructive h., h. secondary to a block in cerebrospinal fluid flow in the ventricular system or between the ventricular system and spinal canal. SYN noncommunicating h.

occult h., SYN normal pressure h.

otitic h., a form of thrombotic h. associated with otitis media and thrombosis of one or both transverse sinuses of the dura.

postmeningitic h., ventricular dilation following meningitis and secondary to obstruction of cerebrospinal fluid pathways.

posttraumatic h., ventricular dilation following injury, due either to impaired circulation and/or absorption of cerebrospinal fluid or due to loss of brain substance (h. ex vacuo).

primary h., SYN congenital h.

secondary h., an accumulation of fluid in the cranial cavity, due to meningitis or obstruction to the venous flow.

thrombotic h., increase in cerebrospinal fluid and of intracranial pressure following thrombosis of the cerebral veins or sinuses; caused by septic infection, dehydration, tuberculosis, typhoid, leukemia, and other conditions.

hy

toxic h., thrombotic h. associated with some general infection or toxic state.

hy·dro·ceph·a·ly (hī-drō-sef′ă-lē). SYN hydrocephalus.

hy·dro·chlo·ric ac·id (hī-drō-klōr′ik). HCl; the acid of gastric juice. The commercial product is used as an escharotic; the gas and the concentrated solution are strong irritants. SYN muriatic acid.

diluted h. a., a preparation that contains, in each 100 ml, 10 g of HCl; used internally for achlorhydria.

hy·dro·chlo·ride (hī-drō-klōr′īd). A compound formed by the addition of a hydrochloric acid molecule to an amine or related substance; *e.g.,* guanine hydrochloride, glycine hydrochloride.

hy·dro·chlo·ro·thi·a·zide (hī′drō-klōr-ō-thī′ă-zīd). 6-Chloro-3,4-dihydro-2*H*-1,2,4-benzothiadiazine-7-sulfonamide 1,1-dioxide; a potent orally effective diuretic and antihypertensive agent related to chlorothiazide.

hy·dro·cho·le·cys·tis (hī′drō-kō-lē-sis′tis). Rarely used term for an effusion of serous fluid into the gallbladder. [hydro- + G. *cholē*, bile, + *kystis,* bladder]

hy·dro·cho·le·re·sis (hī′drō-kō-ler-ē′sis, -kol-er-). Increased output of a watery bile of low specific gravity, viscosity, and solid content. [hydro- + G. *cholē*, bile, + *hairesis,* a taking]

hy·dro·cho·le·ret·ic (hī′drō-kō-ler-et′ik). Pertaining to hydrocholeresis.

hy·dro·co·done (hī-drō-kō′dōn). A potent analgesic derivative of codeine used as an antitussive and analgesic. SYN dihydrocodeinone.

hy·dro·col·loid (hī-drō-kol′oyd). A gelatinous colloid in unstable equilibrium with its contained water, useful in dentistry for impressions because of its dimensional stability under controlled conditions.

irreversible h., a h. whose physical state is changed by an irreversible chemical reaction when water is added to a powder and an insoluble substance is formed.

reversible h., a h. composed of a base substance whose physical state may be changed to that of a liquid by the application of heat and then changed to that of an elastic gel by cooling.

hy·dro·col·po·cele, hy·dro·col·pos (hī-drō-kol′pō-sēl, -kol′pos). Accumulation of mucus or other nonsanguineous fluid in the vagina. [hydro- + G. *kolpos,* bosom (vagina)]

hy·dro·cor·ta·mate hy·dro·chlo·ride (hī-drō-kōr′tă-māt). 17-Hydroxycorticosterone-21-diethylaminoacetate hydrochloride; cortisol 21-(*N,N*-diethyl)glycinate hydrochloride; an ester-salt of hydrocortisone, used topically in the treatment of acute and chronic dermatoses.

hy·dro·cor·ti·sone (hī-drō-kōr′ti-sōn). 17α-Hydroxycorticosterone, 11β,17α,21-trihydroxy-4-pregnene-3,20-dione; a reduction product (at C-11) of cortisone; a steroid hormone secreted by the adrenal cortex (the active hormone secreted in the greatest quantity by the adrenals) and the most potent of the naturally occurring glucocorticoids in humans. SYN cortisol.

h. acetate, hydrocortisone 21-acetate; similar actions and uses as h. SYN cortisol acetate.

h. cyclopentylpropionate, an ester of h.

h. cypionate, the cyclopentanepropionic ester of cortisone, for oral administration.

h. hydrogen succinate, a form of h. administered intravenously.

h. sodium phosphate, hydrocortisone 21-(disodium phosphate); an anti-inflammatory agent for intravenous or intramuscular administration.

h. sodium succinate, a very soluble ester salt of h. (cortisol), used parenterally in the management of emergencies resulting from acute adrenal insufficiency.

hy·dro·co·tar·nine (hī′drō-kō-tar′nēn). 5,6,7,8-Tetrahydro-4-methoxy-6-methyl-1,3-dioxolo[4,5-*g*]isoquinoline; an alkaloidal principle derived from cotarnine; it is the basic hydrolytic product of narcotine; also obtained from the mother liquors of thebaine.

hy·dro·cu·pre·ine (hī-drō-kū′prē-ēn). 10,11-Dihydro-6′-hydroxycinchonan-9-ol; its 6′ ethers are used as antiseptics, *e.g.,* euprocin hydrochloride.

hy·dro·cy·an·ic ac·id (hī-drō-sī-an′ik). HCN; a colorless, very toxic liquid, with the odor of bitter almonds, present in bitter almonds (amygdalin), the stones of peaches, plums and other fruits, and laurel leaves; inhalation of 300 p.p.m. causes death. SYN hydrogen cyanide, prussic acid.

hy·dro·cy·an·ism (hī-drō-sī′an-izm). Poisoning with hydrocyanic acid.

hy·dro·cyst (hī′drō-sist). A cyst with clear, watery contents. [hydro- + G. *kystis,* bladder]

hy·dro·cys·to·ma (hī′drō-sis-tō′mă). **1.** An eruption of deeply seated vesicles, due to retention of fluid in the sweat follicles. **2.** SYN hidrocystoma. [hydro- + G. *kystis,* bladder, + *-ōma,* tumor]

hy·dro·dip·sia (hī-drō-dip′sē-ă). Water thirst, a characteristic of animals that ordinarily drink water. [hydro- + G. *dipsa,* thirst]

hy·dro·dip·so·ma·nia (hī′drō-dip′sō-mā′nē-ă). Periodic episodes of uncontrollable thirst, occasionally found in epileptic patients. [hydro- + G. *dipsa,* thirst, + *mania,* frenzy]

hy·dro·di·u·re·sis (hī′drō-dī-yū-rē′sis). Diuresis effected by water.

hy·dro·dy·nam·ics (hī′drō-dī-nam′iks). The branch of physics concerned with the flow of liquids. [hydro- + G. *dynamis,* force]

hy·dro·en·ceph·a·lo·cele (hī′drō-en-sef′ă-lō-sēl). SYN hydrencephalocele.

hy·dro·flu·me·thi·a·zide (hī′drō-flū-mě-thī′ă-zīd). 3,4-Dihydro-6-(trifluoromethyl)-2*H*-1,2,4-benzothiadiazine-7-sulfonamide 1,1-dioxide; a diuretic and antihypertensive agent of the thiazide group.

hy·dro·flu·o·ric ac·id (hī-drō-flūr′ik). A solution of hydrogen fluoride gas in water; a poisonous, caustic, foaming liquid that is used to clean metals; extremely irritating to skin and lungs.

hy·dro·gel (hī′drō-jel). A colloid in which the particles are in the external or dispersion phase and water in the internal or dispersed phase. Cf. hydrosol.

hy·dro·gen (H) (hī′drō-jen). **1.** A gaseous element, atomic no. 1, atomic wt. 1.00794. **2.** The molecular form of the element, H_2. [hydro- + G. *-gen,* producing]

activated h., h. removed by a dehydrogenase, *e.g.,* a flavoprotein, from a metabolite for transference to another substance with which it combines.

arseniureted h., SYN arsine.

h. bromide, HBr; a colorless gas that has a very irritating odor and fumes in moist air; in aqueous solution, it is hydrobromic acid.

h. chloride, HCl; a very soluble gas which, in solution, forms hydrochloric acid.

h. cyanide, SYN hydrocyanic acid.

h. dehydrogenase, a hydrogenase enzyme catalyzing the conversion of NAD^+ to NADH by molecular hydrogen (H_2); *i.e.,* H_2 + $NAD^+ \rightarrow H^+$ + NADH.

h. dioxide, SYN h. peroxide.

heavy h., SYN hydrogen-2.

h. peroxide, H_2O_2; an unstable compound readily broken down to water and oxygen, a reaction catalyzed by various powdered metals and by the enzyme, catalase; a 3% solution is used as a mild antiseptic for skin and mucous membranes. SYN h. dioxide, hydroperoxide.

h. phosphide, SYN phosphine.

phosphureted h., SYN phosphine.

h. sulfide, H_2S; a colorless, flammable, toxic gas with a familiar "rotten egg" odor, formed in the decomposition of organic matter containing sulfur; used as a reagent, and in the manufacture of chemicals. SYN sulfureted h.

sulfureted h., SYN h. sulfide.

hy·dro·gen-1 (¹H). The common h. isotope, making up 99.985% of the h. atoms occurring in nature. SYN protium.

hy·dro·gen-2 (²H). The isotope of h. of atomic weight 2; the less common stable isotope of h. making up 0.015% of the h. atoms occurring in nature. SYN deuterium, heavy hydrogen.

hy·dro·gen-3 (³H). A hydrogen isotope of atomic weight 3; weakly radioactive, emitting beta particles to become the stable helium-3; half-life, 12.32 years. SYN tritium.

hy·dro·gen·ase (hī′drō-je-nās, hī-droj′ě-nās). Any enzyme that removes a hydride ion (or H:⁻) from NADH (or NADPH) or adds hydrogen to ferricytochrome or to ferredoxin. SYN hydrogenlyase.

hy·dro·gen·a·tion (hī′drō-jĕ-nā′shŭn, hī-droj′ĕ-nā-shŭn). Addition of hydrogen to a compound, especially to an unsaturated fat or fatty acid; thus, soft fats or oils are solidified or "hardened."

hy·dro·gen ex·po·nent. The logarithm of the hydrogen ion concentration in blood or other fluid; its negative is the pH of that fluid.

hy·dro·gen·ly·ase (hī′drō-gen-lī′ās). SYN hydrogenase.

hy·dro·ki·net·ic (hī′drō-ki-net′ik). Pertaining to the motion of fluids and the forces giving rise to such motion.

hy·dro·ki·net·ics (hī′drō-ki-net′iks). That branch of kinetics concerned with fluids in motion.

hy·dro·la·bile (hī-drō-lā′bil). Unstable in the presence of water.

hy·dro·la·bil·i·ty (hī′drō-lă-bil′i-tē). A state in which the fluid in the tissues readily changes in amount.

hy·dro·las·es (hī′drō-lās-ez). Enzymes (EC class 3) cleaving substrates with addition of H_2O at the point of cleavage; *e.g.*, esterases, phosphatases, nucleases, peptidases. SYN hydrolyzing enzymes.

  cysteine h., h. that utilize an active site cysteinyl residue for the catalytic event.

  serine h., h. that utilize an active site seryl residue for the catalytic event.

hy·dro·ly·as·es (hī-drō-lī′ās-ĕz). A class of lyases (EC class 4.2.1) comprising enzymes removing H and OH as water, leading to formation of new double bonds within the affected molecule; the trivial names usually contain dehydratase or hydratase.

hy·dro·lymph (hī′drō-limf). The circulating fluid in many of the invertebrates.

hy·drol·y·sate (hī-drol′i-sāt). A solution containing the products of hydrolysis.

hy·drol·y·sis (hī-drol′i-sis). A chemical process whereby a compound is cleaved into two or more simpler compounds with the uptake of the H and OH parts of a water molecule on either side of the chemical bond cleaved; h. is effected by the action of acids, alkalies, or enzymes. Cf. hydration. SYN hydrolytic cleavage. [hydro- + G. *lysis*, dissolution]

hy·dro·lyt·ic (hī-drō-lit′ik). Referring to or causing hydrolysis.

hy·dro·lyze (hī′drō-līz). To subject to hydrolysis.

hy·dro·ma (hī-drō′mă). SYN hygroma.

hy·dro·mas·sage (hī′drō-mă-sahzh). Massage produced by streams of water.

hy·dro·me·nin·go·cele (hī′drō-men-ing′gō-sēl). Protrusion of the meninges of brain or spinal cord through a defect in the bony wall, the sac so formed containing cerebrospinal fluid. [hydro- + G. *mēninx*, membrane, + *kēlē*, hernia]

hy·drom·e·ter (hī-drom′ĕ-ter). An instrument for determining the specific gravity of a liquid. SYN areometer, gravimeter. [hydro- + G. *meron*, measure]

hy·dro·me·tra (hī-drō-mē′tră). Accumulation of thin mucus or other watery fluid in the cavity of the uterus. [hydro- + G. *metra*, uterus]

hy·dro·met·ric (hī-drō-met′rik). Relating to hydrometry or the hydrometer.

hy·dro·me·tro·col·pos (hī′drō-mē-trō-kol′pos). Distention of uterus and vagina by fluid other than blood or pus. [hydro- + G. *metra*, uterus, + *kolpos*, bosom (vagina)]

hy·drom·e·try (hī-drom′ĕ-trē). Determination of the specific gravity of a fluid by means of a hydrometer.

hy·dro·mi·cro·ceph·a·ly (hī′drō-mī-krō-sef′ă-lē). Microcephaly associated with an increased amount of cerebrospinal fluid.

hy·dro·mor·phone hy·dro·chlo·ride (hī-drō-mōr′fōn). A synthetic derivative of morphine, with analgesic potency about 10 times that of morphine. SYN dihydromorphinone hydrochloride.

hy·drom·pha·lus (hī-drom′fă-lŭs). A cystic tumor at the umbilicus, most commonly a vitellointestinal cyst. [hydro- + G. *omphalos*, umbilicus]

hy·dro·my·e·lia (hī-drō-mī-ē′lē-ă). An increase of fluid in the dilated central canal of the spinal cord, or in congenital cavities elsewhere in the cord substance. [hydro- + G. *myelos*, marrow]

hy·dro·my·e·lo·cele (hī-drō-mī′ĕ-lō-sēl). Protrusion of a portion of cord, thinned out into a sac distended with cerebrospinal fluid, through a spina bifida. [hydro- + G. *myelos*, marrow, + *kēlē*, tumor, hernia]

hy·dro·my·o·ma (hī-drō-mī-ō′mă). A leiomyoma that contains cystlike foci of proteinaceous fluid; h.'s occur more frequently in leiomyomas of the uterus, as a result of degenerative changes. [hydro- + G. *mys*, muscle, + *-oma*, tumor]

hy·dro·ne·phro·sis (hī′drō-ne-frō′sis). Dilation of the pelvis and calices of one or both kidneys resulting from obstruction to the flow of urine. SYN nephrohydrosis, uronephrosis. [hydro- + G. *nephros*, kidney, + *-osis*, condition]

---

hydronephrosis (causes)

I. mechanical obstruction of urinary tract

  a) changes inside the tract

    1. hyperplasia and carcinoma of the prostate

    2. tumors of the efferent urinary tract

    3. scarring in the ureter or the urethra

    4. formation of stones

    5. congenital or other deformations (nephroptosis)

  b) changes outside the urinary tract

    1. tumors of the pelvis (cervical carcinoma)

    2. tumors and proliferative processes of the retroperitoneum

    3. retroperitoneal fibrosis

    4. pressure from aberrant renal arteries or aneurysms of the renal arteries

    5. pressure from adhesions

II. neuromuscular problems
  spina bifida, paraplegia, tabes dorsalis, multiple sclerosis

III. pregnancy

IV. unknown causes
  functional narrowing of the ureter, at the passage from the renal pelvis: megaloureter-megacystis syndrome

---

hy·dro·ne·phrot·ic (hī′drō-ne-frot′ik). Relating to hydronephrosis.

hy·dro·ni·um (hī-drō′nē-um). SEE hydronium *ion*.

hy·dro·par·a·sal·pinx (hī′drō-par-ă-sal′pinks). Accumulation of serous fluid in the accessory tubes of the oviduct. [hydro- + G. *para*, beside, + *salpinx*, trumpet]

hy·dro·path·ic (hī-drō-path′ik). Relating to hydropathy.

hy·drop·a·thy (hī-drop′ă-thē). The obsolete use of water to treat and cure disease.

hy·dro·pe·nia (hī-drō-pē′nē-ă). Reduction or deprivation of water. [hydro- + G. *penia*, poverty]

hy·dro·pe·nic (hī-drō-pē′nik). Pertaining to or characterized by hydropenia.

hy·dro·per·i·car·di·tis (hī′drō-pār-i-kar-dī′tis). Pericarditis with a large serous effusion.

hy·dro·per·i·car·di·um (hī′drō-pār-i-kar′dē-ŭm). A noninflammatory accumulation of fluid in the pericardial sac.

hy·dro·per·i·to·ne·um, hy·dro·per·i·to·nia (hī′drō-pār-i-tō-nē′ŭm, -tō′nē-ă). SYN ascites. [hydro- + peritoneum]

hy·dro·per·ox·i·das·es (hī′drō-per-oks′i-dā-sez). Those oxidoreductases that require H_2O_2 as hydrogen acceptors; *e.g.*, peroxidases, catalase.

hy·dro·per·ox·ide (hī′drō-per-ok′sīd). SYN hydrogen peroxide.

hy·dro·phil, hy·dro·phile (hī′drō-fil, -fīl). A substance that is hydrophilic.

hy·dro·phil·ia (hī-drō-fil′ē-ă). A tendency of the blood and tissues to absorb fluid. [hydro- + G. *philos*, fond]

hy·dro·phil·ic (hī-drō-fil′ik). Denoting the property of attracting or associating with water molecules, possessed by polar radicals or ions, as opposed to hydrophobic (2). SYN hydrophilous.

hy·droph·i·lous (hī-drof′i-lŭs). SYN hydrophilic.

hy·dro·pho·bia (hī-drō-fō′bē-ă). SYN rabies. [hydro- + G. *phobos*, fear]

hy·dro·pho·bic (hī-drō-fōb′ik). **1.** Relating to or suffering from hydrophobia. **2.** Lacking an affinity for water molecules, as opposed to hydrophilic. SYN apolar (2).

hy·dro·pho·ro·graph (hī′drō-fōr′ō-graf). Obsolete term for an instrument for recording the flow or pressure of a fluid; *e.g.*, the flow of urine or the pressure of spinal fluid. [G. *hydrophoros*, carrying water, + *graphō*, to record]

hy·droph·thal·mia, hy·droph·thal·mos, hy·droph·thal·mus (hī′drof-thal′mē-ă, -thal′mos). SYN buphthalmia. [hydro- + G. *ophthalmos*, eye]

Hy·dro·phy·i·dae (hī-drō-fī′i-de). A family of snakes, the true sea snakes, characterized by a vertically compressed tail, giving it a paddle- or oar-like appearance; their fangs, like those of cobras, are small, grooved, and permanently erect. They are common in shallow waters along coastal margins in many regions of the Pacific basin and are important medically in western Malaysia and coastal Vietnam. There are numerous species, all venomous, but few bite humans.

hy·drop·ic (hī-drop′ik). Containing an excess of water or of watery fluid. SYN dropsical.

hy·dro·pneu·ma·to·sis (hī-drō-nū-mă-tō′sis). Combined emphysema and edema; the presence of liquid and gas in tissues. [hydro- + G. *pneuma*, breath, spirit]

hy·dro·pneu·mo·go·ny (hī′drō-nū-mō′gō-nē). Injection of air into a joint to determine the amount of effusion. [hydro- + G. *pneuma*, air, + *gony*, knee]

hy·dro·pneu·mo·per·i·car·di·um (hī-drō-nū′mō-per-i-kar′dē-ŭm). The presence of a serous effusion and of gas in the pericardial sac. SYN pneumohydropericardium. [hydro- + G. *pneuma*, air, + pericardium]

hy·dro·pneu·mo·per·i·to·ne·um (hī-drō-nū′mō-pār-i-tō-nē′ŭm). The presence of gas and serous fluid in the peritoneal cavity. SYN pneumohydroperitoneum. [hydro- + G. *pneuma*, air, + peritoneum]

hy·dro·pneu·mo·tho·rax (hī′drō-nū-mō-thōr′aks). The presence of both gas and fluids in the pleural cavity. SYN pneumohydrothorax, pneumoserothorax. [hydro- + G. *pneuma*, air, + thorax]

hy·dro·po·sia (hī-drō-pō′zē-ă). Water-drinking, a characteristic of animals that ordinarily drink water. [hydro- + G. *posis*, drinking]

hy·drops (hī′drops). An excessive accumulation of clear, watery fluid in any of the tissues or cavities of the body; synonymous, according to its character and location, with ascites, anasarca, edema, etc. [G. *hydrōps*]

h. artic′uli, SYN hydrarthrosis.

endolymphatic h., SYN Ménière's *disease*.

fetal h., h. fetal′is, abnormal accumulation of serous fluid in the fetal tissues, as in erythroblastosis fetalis.

h. follic′uli, accumulation of fluid in a graafian follicle.

h. of gallbladder, accumulation of clear watery fluid in the gallbladder as a result of long-standing cystic duct obstruction.

immune fetal h., fetal edema and ascites secondary to maternal/fetal blood group incompatibility.

nonimmune fetal h., fetal edema and ascites unrelated to maternal/fetal blood group incompatibilities; multiple etiologies include fetal cardiac disease, fetal viral disease, and fetal structural anomalies.

h. ova′rii, SYN hydrovarium.

h. tu′bae, SYN hydrosalpinx.

h. tu′bae pro′fluens, SYN intermittent *hydrosalpinx*.

hy·dro·py·o·ne·phro·sis (hī′drō-pī′ō-ne-frō′sis). Presence of

purulent urine in the pelvis and calices of the kidney following obstruction of the ureter. [hydro- + G. *pyon*, pus, + nephrosis]

hy·dro·quin·ol (hī-drō-kwin′ol). SYN hydroquinone.

hy·dro·qui·none (hī-drō-kwin′ōn). 1,4-Benzenediol; *p*-dihydroxybenzene; an antioxidant used in ointment. SYN hydroquinol, quinol.

hy·dror·chis (hī-drōr′kis). A collection of water (hydrocele) in the testis, as in the tunica vaginalis or along the spermatic cord. [hydro- + G. *orchis*, testicle]

hy·dro·rhe·o·stat (hī-drō-rē′ō-stat). A rheostat in which resistance to the flow of electric current is provided by water.

hy·dror·rhea (hī-drō-rē′ă). A profuse discharge of watery fluid from any part of the body. [hydro- + G. *rhoia*, flow]

h. grav′idae, h. gravida′rum, discharge of a watery fluid from the vagina during pregnancy.

hy·dro·sal·pinx (hī-drō-sal′pinks). Accumulation of serous fluid in the fallopian tube, often an end result of pyosalpinx. SYN hydrops tubae. [hydro- + G. *salpinx*, trumpet]

intermittent h., intermittent discharge of watery fluid from the oviduct. SYN hydrops tubae profluens.

hy·dro·sar·ca (hī-drō-sar′kă). SYN anasarca. [hydro- + G. *sarx*, flesh]

hy·dro·sar·co·cele (hī-drō-sar′kō-sēl). A chronic swelling of the testis complicated with hydrocele. [hydro- + G. *sarx*, flesh, + *kēlē*, tumor]

hy·dro·sol (hī′dro-sol). A colloid in aqueous solution, the particles being in the dispersed or internal phase and the water in the external or dispersion phase. Cf. hydrogel.

hy·dro·sphyg·mo·graph (hī-drō-sfig′mō-graf). A sphygmograph in which the pulse beat is transmitted to the recorder through a column of water.

hy·dro·stat (hī′drō-stat). A device for regulating water level. [hydro- + G. *statikos*, causing to stand]

hy·dro·stat·ic (hī-drō-stat′ik). Relating to the pressure of fluids or to their properties when in equilibrium.

hy·dro·su·dop·a·thy (hī′drō-sū-dop′ă-thē). SYN hydrosudotherapy. [hydro- + L. *sudor*, sweat, + G. *pathos*, suffering]

hy·dro·su·do·ther·a·py (hī′drō-sū′dō-thār′ă-pē). Hydrotherapy combined with induced sweating, as in the Turkish bath. SYN hydrosudopathy.

hy·dro·sy·rin·go·my·e·lia (hī′drō-sĭ-rin′gō-mī-ē′lē-ă). SYN syringomyelia. [hydro- + G. *hydōr*, water, + *syrinx*, a tube, + *myelos*, marrow]

hy·dro·tax·is (hī-drō-tak′sis). The movement of cells or organisms in relation to water. [hydro- + G. *taxis*, arrangement]

hy·dro·ther·a·peu·tic (hī′drō-thār′ă-pyū′tik). SYN hydriatric.

hy·dro·ther·a·peu·tics (hī′drō-thār′ă-pyū′tiks). SYN hydrotherapy.

hy·dro·ther·a·py (hī′drō-thār′ă-pē). Therapeutic use of water by external application, either for its pressure effect or as a means of applying physical energy to the tissues. SYN hydrotherapeutics. [hydro- + G. *therapeia*, therapy]

hy·dro·ther·mal (hī-drō-ther′măl). Relating to hot water. [hydro- + G. *thermē*, heat]

hy·dro·thi·o·ne·mia (hī′drō-thī-ō-nē′mē-ă). The presence of hydrogen sulfide in the circulating blood. [hydro- + G. *theion*, sulfur, + *haima*, blood]

hy·dro·thi·o·nu·ria (hī′drō-thī-ō-nū′rē-ă). The excretion of hydrogen sulfide in the urine. [hydro- + G. *theion*, sulfur, + *ouron*, urine]

hy·dro·tho·rax (hī-drō-thōr′aks). Presence of fluid in one or both pleural cavities, usually resulting from cardiac failure.

chylous h., SYN chylothorax.

hy·drot·o·my (hī-drot′ō-mē). In histology, tearing apart the tissue elements by injection of water. [hydro- + G. *tomē*, a cutting]

hy·drot·ro·pism (hī-drot′rō-pizm, hī-drō-trō′pizm). The property in growing organisms of turning toward a moist surface (**positive h.**) or away from a moist surface (**negative h.**). [hydro- + G. *tropos*, a turning]

hy·dro·tu·ba·tion (hī′drō-tū-bā′shŭn). Injection of a liquid medication or saline solution through the cervix into the uterine cavity and fallopian tubes for dilation and/or treatment of the tubes.

hy·dro·u·re·ter (hī′drō-yū-rē′ter, -yūr′ē-ter). Distention of the ureter with urine, due to blockage from any cause.

hy·drous (hī′drŭs). SYN hydrated.

hy·dro·va·ri·um (hī-drō-vā′rē-ŭm). A collection of fluid in the ovary. SYN hydrops ovarii.

hy·drox·am·ic ac·ids (hī-drok-sam′ik). R–CO–NH–OH ↔ RC(OH)=N–OH; hydroxylamine derivatives of carboxylic acids, including amino acids, formed by the action of hydroxylamine.

hy·drox·ide (hī-drok′sīd). A compound containing a potentially ionizable hydroxyl group; particularly a compound that liberates OH^- upon dissolving in water.

hy·drox·o·co·bal·a·min (hī-drok′sō-kō-bal′ă-min). Vitamin B_{12b}, differing from cyanocobalamin (vitamin B_{12}) in the presence of a hydroxyl ion in place of the cyanide ion. SEE ALSO *vitamin* B_{12}. SYN hydroxocobemine.

hy·drox·o·co·be·mine (hī-drok′sō-kō-bĕ-mēn). SYN hydroxocobalamin.

⌂**hydroxy-.** Prefix indicating addition or substitution of the –OH group to or in the compound whose name follows. SEE ALSO oxa-, oxo-, oxy-.

hy·drox·y·ace·tic ac·id (hī-drok′sē-a-sē′tik). SYN glycolic acid.

hy·drox·y ac·id (hī-drok′sē). An organic acid containing both OH and COOH groups; *e.g.*, lactic acid.

3-hy·drox·y·ac·yl-CoA de·hy·dro·gen·ase (hī-drok′sē-as′il). β-Hydroxyacyl dehydrogenase; enzyme catalyzing the oxidation of an L-3-hydroxyacyl-CoA to a 3-ketoacyl-CoA with reduction of NAD^+; one of the enzymes of the β oxidation of fatty acids. SYN β-ketohydrogenase, β-ketoreductase.

hy·drox·y·a·cyl·glu·ta·thi·one hy·dro·lase (hī-drok′sē-as′il-glū-tă-thī′ōn). An enzyme with catalytic activity similar to that of lactoylglutathione lyase, but more general; catalyzes the hydrolysis of an S-2-hydroxyacylglutathione, producing glutathione and a 2-hydroxy acid anion. SEE ALSO glyoxalase.

hy·drox·y·am·phet·a·mine hy·dro·bro·mide (hī-drok′sē-am-fet′ă-mēn hī-drō-brō′mīd). α-Methyltyramine hydrobromide; *p*-(2-aminopropyl)phenol hydrobromide; a sympathomimetic, decongestant, and mydriatic.

3-hy·drox·y·anth·ran·il·ic ac·id (hī-drok′sē-anth-ra-nil′ik). A metabolite of tryptophan degradation that can serve as a precursor of NAD^+.

hy·drox·y·ap·a·tite (hī-drok′sē-ap-ă-tīt). $Ca_{10}(PO_4)_6(OH)_2$; a natural mineral structure that the crystal lattice of bones and teeth (*i.e.*, amorphous h.) closely resembles; used in chromatography of nucleic acids; also found in pathologic calcifications (*e.g.*, atherosclerotic aortas). SYN hydroxylapatite.

   amorphous h., containing ion contaminants (*e.g.*, 6-8% CO_3^{2-}, 3-5% Mg^{2+}, F^-, Cl^-, etc.); found in mineralized connective tissue (*e.g.*, bone, dentin, cementum). SYN poorly crystalline h.

   poorly crystalline h., SYN amorphous h.

3-hy·drox·y·bu·ta·no·ic ac·id. SYN 3-hydroxybutyric acid.

β-hy·drox·y·bu·tyr·ic ac·id. SYN 3-hydroxybutyric acid.

3-hy·drox·y·bu·tyr·ic ac·id (hī-drōk′sē-byū-tir′ik). $CH_3CH(OH)CH_2COOH$; the D-stereoisomer is one of the ketone bodies and is formed in ketogenesis; it is an important fuel for extrahepatic tissues; as an acyl derivative it is also an intermediate in fatty acid biosynthesis. The L-isomer is found as a coenzyme A derivative in β oxidation of fatty acids. SYN 3-hydroxybutanoic acid, β-hydroxybutyric acid.

   D-3-h. a. dehydrogenase, an enzyme that reversibly catalyzes the interconversion of the two main ketone bodies, catalyzing acetoacetate + NADH + H^+ ↔ D-3-hydroxybutyrate + NAD^+.

4-hy·drox·y·bu·ty·ric ac·i·du·ria (hī-drok′sē-byū-tir′ik). Elevated levels of 4-hydroxybutyrate in the urine. An inherited disorder that can lead to hypotonia and mental retardation.

hy·drox·y·car·bam·ide (hī-drok′sē-kar′bă-mīd). SYN hydroxyurea.

hy·drox·y·chlo·ro·quine sul·fate (hī-drok′sē-klōr′ō-kwīn). A quinoline derivative; an antimalarial agent whose actions and

uses resemble those of chloroquine phosphate; also used in the treatment of lupus erythematosus and rheumatoid arthritis.

25-hy·drox·y·cho·le·cal·cif·er·ol (HCC) (hī-drok′sē-kō′lē-kal-sif′er-ol). SYN calcidiol.

7α-hy·drox·y·cho·les·ter·ol (hī-droks′ē-kol-es-ter-ol). First intermediate in the conversion of cholesterol to the bile acids; formed in the principal rate-limiting step of bile acid biosynthesis.

hy·drox·y·chro·man (hī-drok-sē-krō′man). SYN chromanol.

hy·drox·y·chro·mene (hī-drok-sē-krō′mēn). SYN chromenol.

hy·drox·y·eph·ed·rine (hī-drok′sē-ĕ-fed′rēn). *p*-Hydroxy-α-[1-(methylamino)ethyl]benzyl alcohol; a sympathomimetic agent for the treatment of shock.

25-hy·drox·y·er·go·cal·cif·er·ol (hī-drok′sēr′gō-kal-sif′er-ol). A biologically active and major circulatory metabolite of vitamin D_2. SYN ercalcidiol.

α-hy·drox·y·eth·yl·thi·a·min py·ro·phos·phate. SYN activated *acetaldehyde*.

hy·drox·y·fat·ty ac·id (hī-drok′sē-fat′te). A fatty acid that has a hydroxyl group covalently attached to it (*e.g.*, in hydroxynervone).

3-hy·drox·y·glu·tar·ic ac·id (hī-drok′sē-glū-tar′ik). $HOOCCH_2CH(OH)CH_2COOH$; accumulates in individuals with glutaric acidemia type I.

hy·drox·y·he·min (hī-drok-sē-hē′min). SYN hematin.

β-hy·drox·y·i·so·bu·tyr·ic ac·id (hī-droks′ē-ī-sō-byu-ter-ik). $HOCH_2CH(CH_3)COOH$; an intermediate in the degradation of L-valine.

3-L-hy·drox·y·ky·nu·ren·ine (hī-drok′sē-ki-nū-rĕ-nēn). An intermediate in the catabolism of L-tryptophan and a precursor of xanthurenate; elevated in cases of a vitamin B_6 deficiency.

hy·drox·y·ky·nu·re·ni·nu·ria (hī-drok′sē-kī-nū′rĕ-ni-nū′rē-ă) [MIM*236800]. An abnormality in tryptophan metabolism, probably due to a defect in kynureninase, characterized by mild mental retardation, migraine-like headaches, and urinary excretion of large amounts of kynurenine, kynurenine-3-monooxygenase, and xanthurenic acid; autosomal recessive inheritance.

hy·drox·yl (hī-drok′sil). The radical, –OH.

hy·drox·yl·a·mine (hī-drok′sil-ă′mēn). NH_2OH; a partially oxidized derivative of ammonia; reacts with carbonyl groups to produce oximes; forms acid salts, *e.g.*, h. hydrochloride ($HONH_2·HCl$ or $HONH_3^+Cl^-$).

   h. reductase, an enzyme catalyzing the reversible reduction of h. to ammonia with a variety of donors (*e.g.*, methylene blue, flavin). SEE ALSO *NADH*-hydroxylamine reductase.

hy·drox·yl·a·mi·no (hī-drok′sil-am-i-nō). The monovalent group, –NH–OH.

hy·drox·yl·ap·a·tite (hī-drok′sil-ap-ă-tīt). SYN hydroxyapatite.

hy·drox·y·las·es (hī-drok′si-lā-sez). Enzymes catalyzing formation of hydroxyl groups by addition of an oxygen atom, hence oxidizing the substrate; most are found in EC subclass 1.14.

hy·drox·yl·a·tion (hī-drok-si-lā′shŭn). Placing of a hydroxyl group on a compound in a position where one did not exist before.

δ-hy·drox·y·ly·sine. SYN 5-hydroxylysine.

5-hy·drox·y·ly·sine (5Hyl). A hydroxylated amino acid found in certain collagens. The decreased ability to form 5-hydroxylysine is associated with Ehlers-Danlos syndrome type VI. SYN δ-hydroxylysine.

p-hy·drox·y·mer·cur·i·ben·zo·ate (hī-drok′sē-mer′kyū-rē-ben′zō-āt). An organic mercurial, $HOHgC_6H_4COO^-$, formed spontaneously by hydrolysis of the *p*-chloro compound. SEE ALSO *p*-mercuribenzoate.

β-hy·drox·y·β-meth·yl·glu·tar·yl-CoA (HMG-CoA). $^-OOCCH_2C(OH)(CH_3)CH_2COS$-CoA; a key intermediate in the synthesis of ketone bodies and of steroids. SYN 3-hydroxy-3-methylglutaryl-CoA.

   β-h.-β-m.-CoA lyase, an enzyme, found primarily in liver and rumen epithelium that catalyzes the formation of acetyl-CoA and acetoacetate from β-h.-β-m.-CoA; a key step in ketogenesis; a deficiency of this enzyme leads to episodes of severe metabolic acidosis without ketosis.

β-h.-β-m.-CoA reductase, an enzyme that catalyzes the rate-limiting step of cholesterol biosynthesis, β-h.-β-m.-CoA + 2NADPH + 2H$^+$ → mevalonate + 2NADP$^+$ + coenzyme A.

β-h.-β-m.-CoA synthase, an enzyme in mitochondria that catalyzes the reaction of acetyl-CoA with acetoacetyl-CoA and water to form β-h.-β-m.-CoA and coenzyme A, a step required for both ketogenesis and steroidogenesis to occur.

3-hy·droxy-3-meth·yl-glu·tar·yl-CoA. SYN β-hydroxy-β-methylglutaryl-CoA.

hy·drox·y·ner·vone (hī-drok-sē-ner′vōn). A cerebroside containing α-hydroxynervonic acid. SYN oxynervone.

hy·drox·y·ner·von·ic ac·id (hī-drok′sē-ner-von′ik). CH$_3$–(CH$_2$)$_7$–CH=CH–(CH$_2$)$_{12}$–CH(OH)COOH; an important constituent of certain cerebrosides.

hy·drox·y·phen·a·mate (hī-drok′sē-fen′ă-māt). 2-Hydroxy-2-phenylbutyl carbamate; a tranquilizer.

***p*-hy·drox·y·phe·nyl·ac·e·tate** (hī-droks-ē-fen′il-as-ē-tāt). A minor side product of L-tyrosine degradation that is elevated in the urine in cases of neonatal tyrosinemia and in Richner-Hanhart syndrome.

***p*-hy·drox·y·phe·nyl·lac·tate** (hī-droks-ē-fen-il-lak-tāt). A metabolite in tyrosine degradation that is elevated in individuals with Richner-Hanhart syndrome.

***p*-hy·drox·y·phe·nyl·py·ru·vate** (hī-droks-ē-fen′il-pī-rū-vāt). A metabolite formed by the transamination of tyrosine; elevated in the urine of individuals with tyrosinemia.

hy·drox·y·phen·yl·u·ria (hī-drok′sē-fen-il-ū′rē-ă). Urinary excretion of tyrosine and phenylalanine, as a result of ascorbic acid deficiency; occurs notably in those premature infants who lack this vitamin.

3α-hy·droxy-5α-preg·nan-20-one. A catabolite of progesterone; found in the urine of pregnant women.

17α-hy·drox·y·pro·ges·ter·one (hī-drok′sē-prō-jes′ter-ōn). 17α-Hydroxy-4-pregnen-3,20-dione; medical use is similar to that of progesterone. The acetate is an orally effective derivative, useful in conditions in which parenterally administered progesterone or the caproate is indicated; it possesses some androgenic potency and may cause virilizing changes in a female fetus. The caproate or hexanoate has essentially the same actions and uses as progesterone, but is more potent and has a longer duration of action. A precursor of the androgens and adrenocortical hormones.

21-hy·drox·y·pro·ges·ter·one. SYN deoxycorticosterone.

3-hy·drox·y·pro·line (3Hyp) (hī-drok′sē-prō′lēn). A derivative of proline found in certain collagens, particularly basement membrane collagen. SYN 3-hydroxy-2-pyrrolidinecarboxylic acid.

4-hy·drox·y·pro·line. 4-Hydroxy-2-pyrrolidinecarboxylic acid; the *trans*-L-isomer is an imino acid found among the hydrolysis products of collagen; not found in proteins other than those of connective tissue. A vitamin C deficiency will result in impaired formation of h.

h. oxidase, (1) a flavoenzyme that catalyzes the conversion of h. to Δ′-pyrroline-3-hydroxy-5-carboxylate using FAD; this enzyme appears to be deficient in individuals with hyperhydroxyprolinemia; **(2)** an enzyme that catalyzes the reaction of h. with NAD$^+$ to form NADH and 4-oxoproline. SYN 4-oxoproline reductase.

hy·drox·y·pro·li·ne·mia (hī-drok′sē-prō-li-nē′mē-ă) [MIM* 236800]. A metabolic disorder characterized by enhanced plasma concentrations and urinary excretion of free hydroxyproline, and associated with severe mental retardation; autosomal recessive inheritance.

β-hy·drox·y·pro·pi·on·ic ac·id (hī-drok′sē-prō′pē-on′ik). A minor intermediate in propionate and methylmalonate metabolism. SEE β-hydroxypropionic aciduria.

β-hy·drox·y·pro·pi·on·ic ac·i·du·ria. Elevated levels of β-hydroxypropionic acid in the urine; seen in defects in methylmalonic acid and propionate metabolism, as well as in ketotic hyperglycinemia syndrome.

15-hy·drox·y·pros·ta·glan·din de·hy·dro·gen·ase (hī-drok′sē-pros-tă-glan′din). An enzyme that catalyzes the oxidation of

prostaglandins, rendering them inactive, by converting the 15-hydroxyl group to a keto group using NAD$^+$.

6-hy·drox·y·pu·rine. SYN hypoxanthine.

3-hy·droxy-2-pyr·ro·li·di·ne·car·box·yl·ic ac·id. SYN 3-hydroxyproline.

8-hy·drox·y·quin·o·line (hī-drok-sē-kwin′ō-lin). A fungistat and chelating agent. SYN quinolinol.

8-hy·drox·y·quin·o·line sul·fate (hī-drok′sē-kwin′ō-lēn). An antiseptic, antiperspirant, and deodorant.

3β-hy·drox·y·ste·roid sul·fate sul·fa·tase (hī-drok′sē-stēr′ōid). An enzyme, found in most mammalian tissues, that is capable of hydrolyzing the sulfate ester bonds of a variety of sulfated sterols; a deficiency of this enzyme will result in X-linked ichthyosis.

hy·drox·y·stil·bam·i·dine is·e·thi·o·nate (hī-drok′sē-stil-bam′i-dēn). 2-Hydroxy-4,4′-stilbenedicarboxamidine di-β-hydroxyethanesulfonate; an antifungal and antiprotozoan agent used in the treatment of the nonprogressive cutaneous form of blastomycosis.

hy·drox·y·to·lu·ic ac·id (hī-drok′sē-tō-lū′ik). SYN mandelic acid.

5-hy·drox·y·tryp·ta·mine (5-HT) (hī-drok-sē-trip′tă-mēn). SYN serotonin.

hy·drox·y·tryp·to·phan de·car·box·yl·ase (hī-drok-sē-trip′tō-fan). SYN aromatic D-amino-acid decarboxylase.

3-hy·drox·y·ty·ra·mine (hī-drok-sē-tī′ră-mēn). SYN dopamine.

hy·drox·y·u·rea (hī-drok′sē-yū-rē′ă). H$_2$NoCONHOH; an oral antineoplastic agent that inhibits DNA synthesis and is used in the treatment in a variety of malignancies including melanoma, chronic myelocytic leukemia, and carcinoma of the ovary. SYN hydroxycarbamide.

hy·drox·y·zine (hī-drok′si-zēn). C$_{21}$H$_{27}$ClN$_2$O$_2$; a mild sedative and minor tranquilizer used in neuroses; available as the hydrochloride and pamoate.

Hy·dro·zoa (hī-drō-zō′ă). A class of coelenterates or jellyfishes, including *Hydra*, a freshwater polyp, *Physalia*, the "Portuguese man-of-war," *Millepora*, a stinging coral, and the sea wasps, *Chironex heckeri* and *Chiropsalmus quadrigatus*, whose stings can cause severe wheals, pain, and skin necrosis, and occasionally rapid death from respiratory and cardiac depression. [hydro- + G. *zōon*, animal]

hy·giei·ol·a·try (hī-jē-yol′ă-trē). Obselete term for an extreme observance of the principles of hygiene. [G. *hygieia*, health, + *latreia*, worship]

hy·giei·ol·o·gy (hī-jē-yol′ō-jē). The science of hygiene and sanitation, and the practice thereof. [G. *hygieia*, health, + *-logia*]

hy·gie·ist (hī′jē-ist). SYN hygienist. [G. *hygieia*, health]

hy·giene (hī′jēn). **1.** The science of health and its maintenance. **2.** Cleanliness that promotes health and well being, especially of a personal nature. [G. *hygieinos*, healthful, fr. *hygiēs*, healthy]

criminal h., obsolete term for the branch of mental h. or penology devoted to the study of the causes and prevention of criminality and the treatment of criminals.

industrial h., practices adopted by an industrial concern to minimize occupation-related disease and/or injury.

mental h., the science and practice of maintaining and restoring mental health; a branch of early twentieth century psychiatry that has become an interdisciplinary field including subspecialties in psychology, nursing, social work, law, and other professions.

oral h., the cleaning of the mouth by means of brushing, flossing, irrigating, massaging, or the use of other devices. SEE ALSO oral *physiotherapy.*

hy·gien·ic (hī-jen′ik, hī-jē-en′ik). Healthful; relating to hygiene; tending to maintain health.

hy·gien·ist (hī-jē′nist, hī′jē-en-ist). One who is skilled in the science of health and its maintenance. SYN hygieist.

dental h., a licensed, professional auxiliary in dentistry who is both an oral health educator and clinician, and who uses preventive, therapeutic, and educational methods for the control of oral diseases.

△**hygr-.** SEE hygro-.

hy·gric (hī′grik). Relating to moisture. [G. *hygros,* moist]

hy·gric ac·id. *N*-Methylproline, the methylbetaine of which is stachydrine.

♻**hygro-, hygr-.** Moisture, humidity; opposite of xero-. [G. *hygros,* moist]

hy·gro·ma (hī-grō′mă). A cystic swelling containing a serous fluid, such as cystic lymphangioma, housemaid's knee, etc. SYN hydroma. [hygro- + G. *-oma,* tumor]

 h. axilla′re, h. of the axillary region.

 cervical h., SYN h. colli cysticum.

 h. col′li cys′ticum, a benign cystic overgrowth of lymphatics of the neck, present at birth, which may form a large tumor-like mass. SYN cervical h.

 cystic h., fetal malformation of fluid accumulations, usually around the neck and shoulders; may be simple or complex; often associated with Turner's syndrome.

 subdural h., accumulation in the subdural space of proteinaceous fluid, usually derived from serum, or of cerebrospinal fluid due to a tear in the arachnoid membrane.

hy·grom·e·ter (hī-grom′ĕ-ter). Any device for measuring the water vapor in the atmosphere, usually indicating relative humidity directly. [hygro- + G. *metron,* measure]

hy·grom·e·try (hī-grom′ĕ-trē). SYN psychrometry.

hy·gro·pho·bia (hī-grō-fō′bē-ă). Morbid fear of dampness or moisture. [hygro- + G. *phobos,* fear]

hy·gro·scop·ic (hī-grō-skop′ik). Denoting a substance capable of readily absorbing and retaining moisture; *e.g.,* NaOH, CaCl₂.

hy·gro·sto·mia (hī′grō-stō′mē-ă). SYN sialism. [hygro- + G. *stoma,* mouth]

Hyl Symbol for hydroxylysine or hydroxylysyl (5Hyl specifically refers to 5-hydroxylysine).

5Hyl Abbreviation for 5-hydroxylysine.

hy·la (hī′lă). A lateral extension of the cerebral (or sylvian) aqueduct. [G. *hylē,* wood]

hy·le·pho·bia (hī-lĕ-fō′bē-ă). Morbid fear of forests. [G. *hylē,* forest, + *phobos,* fear]

hy·lic (hī′lik). Of or pertaining to essential matter; obsolete term denoting the pulp tissue of the embryo. [G. *hylikos* fr. *hylē,* matter]

hy·lo·ma (hī-lō′mă). A neoplasm of pulp tissue, resulting from proliferation of elements derived from the embryonic pulp of epiblastic origin. SYN hylic tumor. [G. *hylē,* stuff, crude matter, + *-oma,* tumor]

 mesenchymal h., a neoplasm of tissue derived from the mesoblastic pulp or mesenchyme.

 mesothelial h., a neoplasm derived from tissue of mesothelial origin.

hy·men (hī′men) [NA]. A thin membranous fold highly variable in appearance which partly occludes the ostium of the vagina prior to its rupture (which may occur for a variety of reasons). It is frequently absent (even in virgins) although remnants are commonly present as hymenal caruncula tags. [G. *hymēn,* membrane]

 h. bifenestra′tus, h. bifo′ris, a h. in which there are two openings separated by a wide septum. Cf. septate h.

 cribriform h., a h. with a number of small perforations.

 denticulate h., a h. with markedly serrated edges.

 imperforate h., a h. in which there is no opening, the membrane completely occluding the vagina.

 infundibuliform h., a projecting, funnel-shaped h. with a central opening with sloping edges.

 h. sculpta′tus, a h. with markedly uneven and ragged edges.

 septate h., a h. in which there are two openings separated by a narrow band of tissue. Cf. h. bifenestratus.

 h. subsep′tus, a h. in which the opening is partly closed by a septum.

 vertical h., a h. in which the opening is perpendicular.

hy·men·al (hī′men-ăl). Relating to the hymen.

hy·me·nec·to·my (hī-me-nek′tō-mē). Excision of the hymen. [G. *hymēn,* membrane, + *ektomē,* excision]

hy·me·ni·tis (hī-me-nī′tis). Inflammation of the hymen.

hy·men·oid (hī′men-oyd). **1.** SYN membranous. **2.** Resembling the hymen.

hy·me·no·le·pi·a·sis (hī-me-nō-lĕ-pī′ă-sis). Illness produced by infection with tapeworms of the genus *Hymenolepis.*

hy·me·no·lep·i·did (hī′men-ō-lep′i-did). Common name for tapeworms of the family Hymenolepididae.

Hy·men·o·lep·i·di·dae (hī′men-ō-lep′i-did-ē). A family of tapeworms (order Cyclophyllidea) that includes the medically important genus *Hymenolepis.* [G. *hymēn,* membrane, + *lepis,* rind]

Hy·me·nol·e·pis (hī-me-nol′ĕ-pis). The largest genus (family Hymenolepididae) of tapeworms in the order Cyclophyllidea; especially common parasites of rodents, shrews, and aquatic birds. [G. *hymēn,* membrane, + *lepis,* rind]

 H. diminu′ta, a tapeworm species of rats and mice, rarely found in man; its cysticercoid larvae are harbored by beetles, fleas, caterpillars, and other insects.

 H. lanceola′ta, a tapeworm of aquatic birds, rarely found in humans.

 H. na′na, the dwarf or dwarf mouse tapeworm; a small tapeworm of man, sometimes found in great numbers in the intestine; the cysticercoid can develop by two pathways: in the final host, with the egg from one human directly infective to another human host, in which both larval and adult stages occur, or through two hosts, an insect (or crustacean) intermediate and a vertebrate final host, the obligate two-host cycle of most cyclophylidean cestodes; in addition, *H. nana* can internally reinfect the same human or rodent host, producing a massive reinfection.

 H. na′na, var. *frater′na,* a race, strain, or subspecies of *H. nana* adapted to mice, although infectivity to humans may remain; the human form, *H. nana,* presumably is derived from the rodent strain.

hy·me·nol·o·gy (hī-mĕ-nol′ō-jē). The branch of anatomy and physiology concerned with the membranes of the body. [G. *hymēn,* membrane, + *logos,* study]

Hy·me·nop·tera (hī-me-nop′ter-ă). An order of insects, including bees, wasps, and ants, characterized by locked pairs of membranous wings and high development of social or colonial behavior. [G. *hymēn,* membrane, + *pteron,* wing]

hy·me·nor·rha·phy (hī-me-nōr′ă-fē). Obsolete term for suture of the hymen in order to close the vagina. [G. *hymēn,* membrane, + *raphē,* a suture]

hy·men·ot·o·my (hī-me-not′ō-mē). Surgical division of a hymen. [G. *hymēn,* membrane, + *tomē,* incision]

Hynes, Wilfred, British plastic surgeon, *1903. SEE Anderson-H. pyeloplasty; H. pharyngoplasty.

♻**hyo-.** U-shaped, hyoid. [G. *hyoeides,* shaped like the letter upsilon, υ]

hy·o·ep·i·glot·tic (hī′ō-ep-i-glot′ik). Relating to the hyoid bone and the epiglottis; denoting the elastic h. ligament connecting the two structures. SYN hyoepiglottidean.

hy·o·ep·i·glot·tid·e·an (hī′ō-ep-i-glo-tid′ē-an). SYN hyoepiglottic.

hy·o·glos·sal (hī′ō-glos′ăl). Relating to the hyoid bone and the tongue. SYN glossohyal.

hy·o·glos·sus (hī′ō-glos′ŭs). SYN hyoglossus *muscle.*

hy·oid (hī′oyd). U-shaped or V-shaped; denoting the *os* hyoideum and the *apparatus* hyoideus. [G. *hyoeidēs,* shaped like the letter upsilon, υ]

hy·o·pha·ryn·ge·us (hī′ō-far′in-jē′ŭs). SEE middle constrictor *muscle* of pharynx.

hy·o·scine (hī′ō-sēn). SYN scopolamine.

h. hydrobromide, SYN *scopolamine* hydrobromide.

hy·o·scy·a·mine (hī-ō-sī′ă-mēn). *l*-Tropine tropate; an alkaloid found in hyoscyamus, belladonna, duboisine, and stramonium; the levorotatory component of the racemic mixture, atropine; used as an antispasmodic, analgesic, and sedative; h. hydrobromide is used for the same purposes. SYN daturine.

h. sulfate, an antispasmodic, hypnotic, and sedative, also used in parkinsonism to relieve tremor, rigidity, and excessive salivation.

dl-**hy·o·scy·a·mine.** SYN atropine.

hy·o·scy·a·mus (hī-ō-sī′ă-mŭs). The leaves and flowering tops of *Hyoscyamus niger* (family Solanaceae); it contains hyoscyamine and hyoscine (scopolamine); an anticholinergic and antispasmodic. SYN henbane. [G. *hyoskyamos,* henbane or hog's bean, fr. *hys,* gen. *hyos,* a hog, + *kyamos,* a bean]

Hy·o·stron·gy·lus ru·bi·dus (hī-ō-stron′ji-lŭs rū′bi-dŭs). The red stomach worm of swine; a small reddish trichostrongyle nematode that burrows into the mucosa of the fundus of the pig stomach and sucks blood; moderate numbers appear to cause little damage unless the animal's resistance is lowered by other factors. [G. *hys,* gen. *hyos,* a hog, + *strongylos,* round]

hy·o·thy·roid (hī′ō-thī′royd). SEE thyrohyoid *membrane.*

Hyp Abbreviation for hypoxanthine; hydroxyproline (3Hyp and 4Hyp specifically refer to 3-hydroxyproline and 4-hydroxyproline, respectively).

3Hyp Abbreviation for 3-hydroxyproline.

△**hyp-.** Variation of the prefix hypo-, often used before a vowel. Cf. sub-.

hyp·a·cu·sia (hī′pă-kū′zē-ă, hip′ă-). SYN hypacusis.

hyp·a·cu·sis (hī′pă-kū′sis, hip′ă-). Hearing impairment of a conductive or neurosensory nature. SYN hypacusia, hypoacusis. [hypo- + G. *akousis,* hearing]

hyp·al·bu·mi·ne·mia (hī′pal-byū-mi-nē′mē-ă, hip′al-). SYN hypoalbuminemia. [G. *hypo,* under, + albuminemia]

hyp·al·ge·sia (hī′pal-jē′zē-ă, hīp′al-). Decreased sensibility to pain. SYN hypalgia, hypoalgesia. [G. *hypo,* under, + *algēsis,* sense of pain]

hyp·al·ge·sic, hyp·al·get·ic (hī′pal-jē′sik, hip′al-; -jet′ik). Relating to hypalgesia; having diminished sensitiveness to pain.

hyp·al·gia (hī-pal′jē-ă, hip-al′). SYN hypalgesia. [G. *hypo,* under, + *algos,* pain]

hyp·am·ni·on, hyp·am·ni·os (hī-pam′nē-on, -nē-os). Presence of an abnormally small amount of amniotic fluid. [G. *hypo,* under, + amnion]

hyp·an·a·ki·ne·sia, hyp·an·a·ki·ne·sis (hī-pan′ă-ki-nē′sē-ă, -kin-ē′sis). Diminution in the normal gastric or intestinal movements. [G. *hypo,* under, + *anakinēsis,* a to-and-fro movement]

hyp·ar·te·ri·al (hī′par-tēr′ē-ăl, hip′ar-). Below or beneath an artery. [G. *hypo,* beneath, + *artēria,* artery]

hyp·ax·i·al (hī-pak′sē-ăl, hip-ak′). Below any axis, such as the spinal axis or the axis of a limb. SEE hypomere. [G. *hypo,* beneath, + axis]

hyp·az·o·tu·ria (hī′paz-ō-tū′rē-ă). SYN hypoazoturia.

hyp·en·ceph·a·lon (hī′pen-sef′ă-lon). The midbrain, pons, and medulla. [G. *hypo,* under, + *enkephalos,* brain]

hyp·en·gy·o·pho·bia (hī-pen′gī-ō-fō′bē-ă). Morbid fear of responsibility. [G. *hypengyos,* responsible, + *phobos,* fear]

△**hyper-.** Excessive, above normal; opposite of hypo-. [G. *hyper,* above, over]

hy·per·ac·an·tho·sis (hī′per-ă-kan-thō′sis). SYN acanthosis.

hy·per·ac·id (hī-per-as′id). Having an excessive concentration of acid.

hy·per·a·cid·i·ty (hī′per-a-sid′i-tē). An abnormally high degree of acidity, as of the gastric juice.

hy·per·ac·tiv·i·ty (hī′per-ak-tiv′i-tē). **1.** SYN superactivity. **2.**

General restlessness or excessive movement such as that characterizing children with attention deficit disorder or hyperkinesis.

hy·per·a·cu·sis, hy·per·a·cu·sia (hī′per-ă-kū′sis, -kū′sē-ă). Abnormal acuteness of hearing due to increased irritability of the sensory neural mechanism. SYN auditory hyperesthesia. [hyper- + G. *akousis,* a hearing]

hy·per·ad·e·no·sis (hī′per-ad-ĕ-nō′sis). Glandular enlargement, especially of the lymphatic glands. [hyper- + G. *adēn,* gland, + *-ōsis,* condition]

hy·per·ad·i·po·sis, hy·per·ad·i·pos·i·ty (hī′per-ad-i-pō′sis, -pos′i-tē). An extreme degree of adiposis or fatness.

hy·per·ad·re·nal·cor·ti·cal·ism (hī′per-ă-drē′năl-kōr′ti-kăl-izm). SYN hypercorticoidism.

hy·per·a·dre·no·cor·ti·cal·ism (hī′per-ă-drē′nō-kōr′ti-kăl-izm). SYN hypercorticoidism.

hy·per·al·a·nine·mia (hī′per-al′ă-nēn-ē′mē-ă). Elevated levels of alanine in the serum.

hy·per·-β-al·a·nine·mia (hī′per-bā′ta-al′ă-nen-ē′mē-a). Elevated levels of β-alanine in the serum; believed to be due to a deficiency of β-alanine:pyruvate aminotransferase; leads to impaired CNS function.

hy·per·al·do·ste·ron·ism (hī′per-al-dos′ter-on-izm). SYN aldosteronism.

hy·per·al·ge·sia (hī-per-al-jē′zē-ă). Extreme sensitiveness to painful stimuli. SYN hyperalgia. [hyper- + G. *algos,* pain]

hy·per·al·ge·sic, hy·per·al·get·ic (hī′per-al-jē′sik, -jet′ik). Relating to hyperalgesia.

hy·per·al·gia (hī′per-al′jē-ă). SYN hyperalgesia.

hy·per·al·i·men·ta·tion (hī′per-al′i-men-tā′shŭn). Administration or consumption of nutrients beyond minimum normal requirements, in an attempt to replace nutritional deficiencies. SYN superalimentation, suralimentation.

parenteral h., h. by intravenous administration of nutrients in greater than normal amounts.

hy·per·al·lan·to·in·u·ria (hī′per-ă-lan′tō-i-nū′rē-ă). Increased excretion of allantoin in the urine.

hy·per·al·pha·lip·o·pro·tei·ne·mia (hi′per-ăl′fa-lip-ō-prō′tēn-ē′mē-ă). An inherited defect that results in elevated levels of high-density lipoproteins in the serum.

hy·per·a·mi·no·ac·i·du·ria (hī′per-am′i-nō-as-i-dū′rē-ă). SYN aminoaciduria.

hy·per·-β-ami·no·iso·bu·ty·ric ac·i·du·ria. Elevated levels of β-aminoisobutyric acid in the urine; believed to be due to a deficiency of liver *R*-β-aminoisobutyrate:pyruvate aminotransferase.

hy·per·am·mo·ne·mia (hī′per-am-ō-nē′mē-ă). SYN ammonemia.

hy·per·am·y·la·se·mia (hī′per-am′i-lā-sē′mē-ă). Elevated serum amylase, usually seen as one of the manifestations of acute pancreatitis. [hyper- + amylase, + G. *haima,* blood]

hy·per·an·a·ci·ne·sia, hy·per·an·a·ci·ne·sis (hī′per-an-ă-si-nē′zē-ă, -nē′sis). SYN hyperanakinesia.

hy·per·an·a·ki·ne·sia, hy·per·an·a·ki·ne·sis (hī′per-an-ă-ki-nē′zē-ă, -ki-nē′sis). Excessive to-and-fro movement, *e.g.,* of the stomach or intestine. SYN hyperanacinesia, hyperanacinesis. [hyper- + G. *anakinēsis,* to-and-fro movement]

hy·per·a·phia (hī′per-ā′fē-ă). Extreme sensitiveness to touch. SYN oxyaphia, tactile hyperesthesia. [hyper- + G. *haphē,* touch]

hy·per·aph·ic (hī-per-af′ik). Marked by hyperaphia.

hy·per·ar·gi·ni·ne·mia (hī′per-ar-jen-in-ē-mē-ă). Elevated levels of arginine in the blood plasma; usually associated with a deficiency of arginase.

hy·per·bar·ic (hī-per-bar′ik). **1.** Pertaining to pressure of ambient gases greater than 1 atmosphere. **2.** Concerning solutions, more dense than the diluent or medium; *e.g.,* in spinal anesthesia, a h. solution has a density greater than that of spinal fluid. [hyper- + G. *baros,* weight]

hy·per·bar·ism (hī-per-bar′izm). Disturbances in the body resulting from the pressure of ambient gases at greater than 1 atmosphere; *e.g.,* nitrogen narcosis, oxygen toxicity, bends, etc. [hyper- + G. *baros,* weight]

hy·per·be·ta·lip·o·pro·tein·e·mia (hī′per-bet-ă-lip′ō-prō-tē-nē′ mē-ă). Enhanced concentration of β-lipoproteins in the blood.
  familial h., SYN type II familial *hyperlipoproteinemia*.
  familial h. and hyperprebetalipoproteinemia, SYN type III familial *hyperlipoproteinemia*.

hy·per·bil·i·ru·bi·ne·mia (hī′per-bil′i-rū-bi-nē′mē-ă). An abnormally large amount of bilirubin in the circulating blood, resulting in clinically apparent icterus or jaundice when the concentration is sufficient.
  neonatal h., serum bilirubin greater than 12.9 mg/dl (220 μol/L) or rising at a rate greater than 5 mg/dl per day; also applied to a nonphysiologic pattern of h., *i.e.,* jaundice in the first 24 hours of life or extending beyond the first week of life in term infants.

hy·per·brach·y·ceph·a·ly (hī′per-brak-ē-sef′ă-lē). An extreme degree of brachycephaly, with a cephalic index of over 85. [hyper- + G. *brachys,* short, + *kephalē,* head]

hy·per·cal·ce·mia (hī′per-kal-sē′mē-ă). An abnormally high concentration of calcium compounds in the circulating blood; commonly used to indicate an elevated concentration of calcium ions in the blood.
  idiopathic h. of infants, persistent h. of unknown cause in very young children, associated with osteosclerosis, renal insufficiency, and sometimes hypertension; also may be associated with supravalvular aortic stenosis, elfin facies, and mental retardation. SYN Williams-Beurer syndrome.

hy·per·cal·ci·nu·ria (hī′per-kal-si-nū′rē-ă). SYN hypercalciuria.

hy·per·cal·ci·u·ria (hī′per-kal-sē-yu′rē-ă). Excretion of abnormally large amounts of calcium in the urine, as in hyperparathyroidism and types of hereditary hypophosphatemic rickets. SYN calcinuric diabetes, hypercalcinuria, hypercalcuria.

hy·per·cal·cu·ria (hī′per-kal-kyū′rē-ă). SYN hypercalciuria.

hy·per·cap·nia (hī-per-kap′nē-ă). Abnormally increased arterial carbon dioxide tension. SYN hypercarbia. [hyper- + G. *kapnos,* smoke, vapor]

hy·per·car·bia (hī-per-kar′bē-ă). SYN hypercapnia.

hy·per·car·dia (hī-per-kar′dē-ă). Hypertrophy of the heart. [hyper- + G. *kardia,* heart]

hy·per·cat·a·bol·ic (hī′-per-kat-ă-bol′ik). Pertaining to hypercatabolism.

hy·per·cat·ab·o·lism (hī′per-kă-tab′ō-lizm). Excessive metabolic breakdown of a specific substance or of body tissue in general, leading to weight loss and wasting.

hy·per·ca·thar·sis (hī′per-kă-thar′sis). Excessive and frequent defecation. [hyper- + G. *katharsis,* a cleansing]

hy·per·ca·thar·tic (hī′per-kă-thar′tik). **1.** Causing excessive purgation. **2.** An agent having an excessive purgative action.

hy·per·ca·thex·is (hī′per-kă-thek′sis). In psychoanalysis, an individual's excessive investment of libido or interest in an object, person, or idea. [hyper- + G. *kathexis,* a holding in, retention]

hy·per·ce·men·to·sis (hī′per-sē-men-tō′sis). Excessive deposition of secondary cementum on the root of a tooth, which may be caused by localized trauma or inflammation, excessive tooth eruption, or osteitis deformans, or may occur idiopathically. SYN cementum hyperplasia. [hyper- + L. *caementum,* a rough quarry stone, + *-osis,* condition]

hy·per·chlor·e·mia (hī′per-klō-rē′mē-ă). An abnormally large amount of chloride ions in the circulating blood. SYN chloremia (2).

hy·per·chlor·hy·dria (hī′per-klōr-hī′drē-ă). Presence of an excessive amount of hydrochloric acid in the stomach. SYN chlorhydria, hyperhydrochloria. [hyper- + chlorhydric (acid)]

hy·per·chlor·u·ria (hī′per-klōr-yū′rē-ă). Increased excretion of chloride ions in the urine.

hy·per·cho·les·ter·e·mia (hī′per-kō-les′ter-ē′mē-ă). SYN hypercholesterolemia.

hy·per·cho·les·ter·in·e·mia (hī′per-kō-les′ter-i-nē′mē-ă). SYN hypercholesterolemia.

hy·per·cho·les·ter·ol·e·mia (hī′per-kō-les′ter-ol-ē′mē-ă). The presence of an abnormally large amount of cholesterol in the cells and plasma of the circulating blood. SYN hypercholesteremia, hypercholesterinemia.

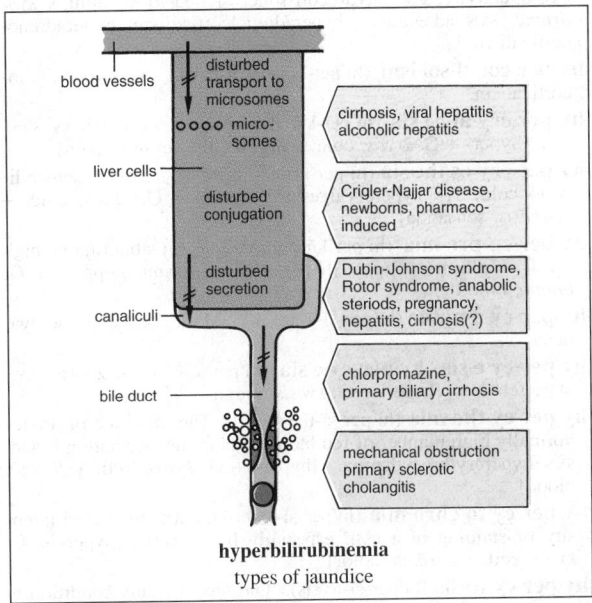

hyperbilirubinemia
types of jaundice

  familial h., SYN type II familial *hyperlipoproteinemia*.
  familial h. with hyperlipemia, SYN type III familial *hyperlipoproteinemia*.

hy·per·cho·les·ter·o·lia (hī′per-kō-les′ter-ō′lē-ă). The presence of an abnormally large quantity of cholesterol in the bile.

hy·per·cho·lia (hī-per-kō′lē-ă). A condition in which an abnormally large amount of bile is formed in the liver. [hyper- + G. *cholē,* bile]

hy·per·chro·maf·fin·ism (hī′-per-krō′maf-in-izm). Presence of a functioning pheochromocytoma.

hy·per·chro·ma·sia (hī′per-krō-mā′zē-ă). SYN hyperchromatism.

hy·per·chro·mat·ic (hī′per-krō-mat′ik). **1.** Abnormally highly colored, excessively stained, or overpigmented. SYN hyperchromic (1). **2.** Showing increased chromatin. [hyper- + G. *chrōma,* color]

hy·per·chro·ma·tism (hī′per-krō′mă-tizm). **1.** Excessive pigmentation. **2.** Increased staining capacity, especially of cell nuclei for hematoxylin. **3.** An increase in chromatin in cell nuclei. SYN hyperchromasia, hyperchromia. [hyper- + G. *chrōma,* color]

hy·per·chro·mia (hī-per-krō′mē-ă). SYN hyperchromatism.
  macrocytic h., hyperchromatic macrocythemia; a misnomer inasmuch as the red blood cells are larger than normal, the total amount of hemoglobin per cell is increased, but the percentage of hemoglobin per cell is usually in the normochromic range.

hy·per·chro·mic (hī-per-krōm′ik). **1.** SYN hyperchromatic (1). **2.** Denoting increased light absorption.

hy·per·chy·lia (hī-per-kī′lē-ă). Excessive secretion of gastric juice. [hyper- + G. *chylos,* juice]

hy·per·chy·lo·mi·cro·ne·mia (hī′per-kī′lō-mī-krō-nē′mē-ă). Increased plasma concentrations of chylomicrons.
  familial h., SYN type I familial *hyperlipoproteinemia*.
  familial h. with hyperprebetalipoproteinemia, SYN type V familial *hyperlipoproteinemia*.

hy·per·ci·ne·sis, hy·per·ci·ne·sia (hī′per-si-nē′sis, -si-nē′zē-ă). SYN hyperkinesis.

hy·per·co·ag·u·la·bil·i·ty (hī′per-kō-ag′ū-lă-bil-i-tē). Abnormally increased coagulability.

hy·per·co·ag·u·la·ble (hī′-per-kō-ag′ū-lă-bl). Characterized by abnormally increased coagulation.

hy·per·cor·ti·coid·ism (hī′per-kōr′ti-koyd-izm). Excessive secretion of one or more steroid hormones of the adrenal cortex; sometimes used also to designate the state produced by therapeutic administration of large quantities of steroids having glucocor-

hy

ticoid activity, *e.g.*, hydrocortisone. SEE ALSO Cushing's *syndrome*. SYN adrenalism, hyperadrenalcorticalism, hyperadrenocorticalism.

hy·per·cor·ti·sol·ism (hī′per-kōr′ti-sol-izm). SEE hyperadrenocorticalism.

hy·per·cry·al·ge·sia (hī′per-krī-al-jē′zē-ă). SYN hypercryesthesia. [hyper- + G. *kryos*, cold, + *algēsis*, the sense of pain]

hy·per·cry·es·the·sia (hī′per-krī-es-thē′zē-ă). Extreme sensibility to cold. SYN hypercryalgesia. [hyper- + G. *kryos*, cold, + *aisthēsis*, sensation]

hy·per·cu·pre·mia (hī′per-kū-prē′mē-ă). An abnormally high level of plasma copper. [hyper- + L. *cuprum*, copper, + G. *haima*, blood]

hy·per·cy·a·not·ic (hī′per-sī-ă-not′ik). Marked by extreme cyanosis.

hy·per·cy·e·sis, hy·per·cy·e·sia (hī′per-sī-ē′sis, -ē′zē-ă). SYN superfetation. [hyper- + G. *kyēsis*, pregnancy]

hy·per·cy·the·mia (hī′per-sī-thē′mē-ă). The presence of an abnormally high number of red blood cells in the circulating blood. SYN hypererythrocythemia. [hyper- + G. *kytos*, cell, + *haima*, blood]

hy·per·cy·to·chro·mia (hī′per-sī-tō-krō′mē-ă). Increased intensity of staining of a cell, especially blood cells. [hyper- + G. *kytos*, cell, + *chrōma*, color]

hy·per·cy·to·sis (hī′per-sī-tō′sis). Old term for any condition in which there is an abnormal increase in the number of cells in the circulating blood or the tissues; frequently used synonymously with leukocytosis.

hy·per·di·crot·ic (hī′per-dī-krot′ik). Pronouncedly dicrotic. SYN superdicrotic.

hy·per·di·cro·tism (hī-per-dik′rō-tizm, -dī′krō-tizm). Extreme dicrotism.

hy·per·dip·loid (hī′per-dip′loid). Having a chromosome number greater than the diploid number.

hy·per·dip·sia (hī-per-dip′sē-ă). Intense thirst that is relatively temporary. [hyper- + G. *dipsa*, thirst]

hy·per·dis·ten·tion (hī′per-dis-ten′shŭn). Extreme distention. SYN superdistention.

hy·per·dy·nam·ia (hī′per-dī-nā′mē-ă, -nam′ē-ă). Extreme violence or muscular restlessness. [hyper- + G. *dynamis*, force]

h. u′teri, excessive uterine contractions in childbirth.

hy·per·dy·nam·ic (hī-per-dī-nam′ik). Marked by hyperdynamia.

hy·per·ech·o·ic (hī′per-ē-kō′ik). **1.** In ultrasonography, pertaining to material that produces echoes of higher amplitude or density than the surrounding medium. **2.** Denoting a region in an ultrasound image in which the echoes are stronger than normal or than surrounding structures.

hy·per·em·e·sis (hī-per-em′ĕ-sis). Excessive vomiting. [hyper- + G. *emesis*, vomiting]

h. gravida′rum, pernicious vomiting in pregnancy.

h. lacten′tium, vomiting by nursing infants with pyloric stenosis.

hy·per·e·met·ic (hī′per-ĕ-met′ik). Marked by excessive vomiting.

hy·per·e·mia (hī-per-ē′mē-ă). The presence of an increased amount of blood in a part or organ. SEE ALSO congestion. [hyper- + G. *haima*, blood]

active h., h. due to an increased afflux of arterial blood into dilated capillaries. SYN arterial h., fluxionary h.

arterial h., SYN active h.

Bier's h., obsolete term for h. produced by Bier's *method* (2).

collateral h., increased blood flow through abundant collateral channels when the circulation through the main artery to a part is arrested, as when the blood supply to one lung or to a portion of it is occluded the blood flow to the other lung or portion of a lung is increased.

constriction h., obsolete term for h. produced by Bier's *method* (2).

fluxionary h., SYN active h.

passive h., h. due to an obstruction in the flow of blood from the affected part, the venous radicles becoming distended. SYN venous h.

peristatic h., SYN peristasis.

reactive h., h. following the arrest and subsequent restoration of the blood supply to a part.

venous h., SYN passive h.

hy·per·e·mic (hī-per-ē′mik). Denoting hyperemia.

hy·per·en·ceph·a·ly (hī′per-en-sef′ă-lē). A fetal developmental deficiency of the vault of the cranium, exposing the poorly formed brain. [hyper- + G. *enkephalos*, brain]

hy·per·e·o·sin·o·phil·ia (hī′per-ē-ō-sin-ō-fil′ē-ă). A greater degree of abnormal increase in the number of eosinophilic granulocytes in the circulating blood or the tissues; *e.g.*, in diseases where the degree of eosinophilia usually ranges from 10 to 30%, an increase to 50 or 60% (or more) might be regarded as h.

hy·per·eph·i·dro·sis (hī′per-ef-i-drō′sis). SYN hyperhidrosis. [hyper- + G. *ephidrōsis*, perspiration]

hy·per·ep·i·thy·mia (hī′per-ep′i-thī′mē-ă). Rarely used term for inordinate desire. [hyper- + G. *epithymia*, yearning]

hy·per·er·ga·sia (hī-per-er-gā′zē-ă). Increased or excessive functional activity. [hyper- + G. *ergasia*, work]

hy·per·er·gia (hī-per-er′jē-ă). An allergic hypersensitivity. SYN hypergia.

hy·per·er·gic (hī-per-er′jik). Relating to hyperergia. SYN hypergic.

hy·per·e·ryth·ro·cy·the·mia (hī′per-ē-rith′rō-sī-thē′mē-ă). SYN hypercythemia.

hy·per·es·o·pho·ria (hī′per-es-ō-fō′rē-ă). A tendency of one eye to deviate upward and inward, prevented by binocular vision. [hyper- + G. *esō*, inward, + *phora*, movement]

hy·per·es·the·sia (hī′per-es-thē′zē-ă). Abnormal acuteness of sensitivity to touch, pain, or other sensory stimuli. SYN oxyesthesia. [hyper- + G. *aisthēsis*, sensation]

auditory h., SYN hyperacusis.

cervical h., the hypersensitivity of teeth in the cervical area due to exposure of the dentin.

gustatory h., SYN hypergeusia.

muscular h., sensitiveness of the muscles to pressure.

olfactory h., h. olfacto′ria, SYN hyperosmia.

h. op′tica, extreme sensitiveness of the eyes to light. SEE photophobia, photosensitivity.

tactile h., SYN hyperaphia.

hy·per·es·thet·ic (hī′per-es-thet′ik). Marked by hyperesthesia.

hy·per·eu·ry·pro·so·pic (hī′per-yū′ri-prō-sop′ik). Pertaining to or characterized by a very low and wide face. [hyper- + G. *eurys*, wide, + *prosōpon*, face]

hy·per·ex·o·pho·ria (hī′per-ek-sō-fō′rē-ă). A tendency of one eye to deviate upward and outward, prevented by binocular vision. [hyper- + G. *exō*, outward, + *phora*, movement]

hy·per·ex·ten·sion (hī′per-eks-ten′shŭn). Extension of a limb or part beyond the normal limit. SYN overextension, superextension.

hy·per·fer·re·mia (hī′per-fer-ē′mē-ă). High serum iron level; found in hemochromatosis.

hy·per·fi·brin·o·ge·ne·mia (hī′per-fī-brin′ō-jĕ-nē′mē-ă). An increased level of fibrinogen in the blood. SYN fibrinogenemia.

hy·per·fi·bri·nol·y·sis (hī′per-fī-brin-ol′i-sis). Markedly increased fibrinolysis, as in subdural hematomas.

hy·per·flex·ion (hī-per-flek′shŭn). Flexion of a limb or part beyond the normal limit. SYN superflexion.

hy·per·fol·lic·u·loid·ism (hī-per-fŏ-lik′yū-loyd-izm). Obsolete term for excessive production of estradiol, as seen in new growths derived from the graafian follicles; a cause of abnormal uterine bleeding, *e.g.*, metropathia hemorrhagica.

hy·per·fruc·to·se·mia (hī′per-frŭk-tō-sē-mē-ă). Elevated serum fructose levels.

hy·per·gal·ac·to·sis (hī′per-ga-lak-tō′sis). Excessive secretion of milk. [hyper- + G. *gala*, milk, + *-ōsis*, condition]

hy·per·gam·ma·glob·u·lin·e·mia (hī′per-gam-ă-glob′yū-li-nē′mē-ă). An increased amount of the γ-globulins in the plasma, such as that frequently observed in chronic infectious diseases.

hy·per·gan·gli·on·o·sis (hī-per-ga'ng-glē-ō-nō'sis). SYN neuronal *hyperplasia.*

hy·per·ga·sia (hī'per-gā'zē-ă). Diminished functional activity. [G. *hypo* (hyp-), under, + *ergasia,* work]

hy·per·gen·e·sis (hī-per-jen'ĕ-sis). Excessive development or redundant production of parts or organs of the body. [hyper- + G. *genesis,* production]

hy·per·ge·net·ic (hī-per-jĕ-net'ik). Relating to hypergenesis.

hy·per·gen·i·tal·ism (hī-per-jen'i-tăl-izm). Abnormally overdeveloped genitalia in adults or for the individual's age.

hy·per·geu·sia (hī-per-gū'sē-ă, -jū'sē-ă). Abnormal acuteness of the sense of taste. SYN gustatory hyperesthesia, oxygeusia. [hyper- + G. *geusis,* taste]

hy·per·gia (hī-per'jē-ă). SYN hyperergia.

hy·per·gic (hī-per'jik). SYN hyperergic.

hy·per·glan·du·lar (hī-per-glan'dyŭ-lăr). Characterized by overactivity or increased size of a gland.

hy·per·glob·u·lia, hy·per·glob·u·lism (hī'per-glob-yū'lē-ă, -glob'yū-lizm). Old term for polycythemia. [hyper- + L. *globulus,* globule]

hy·per·glob·u·lin·e·mia (hī'per-glob'yū-lin-ē'mē-ă). An abnormally large amount of globulins in the circulating blood plasma.

hy·per·gly·ce·mia (hī'per-glī-sē'mē-ă). An abnormally high concentration of glucose in the circulating blood, seen especially in patients with diabetes mellitus. SYN hyperglycosemia. [hyper- + G. *glykys,* sweet, + *haima,* blood]

ketotic h., an inborn error of glycine metabolism characterized by lethargy, vomiting, convulsions, hypertonia, and difficulty breathing; milk protein and casein induce attacks; autosomal recessive inheritance.

nonketotic h., SYN hyperosmolar (hyperglycemic) nonketotic *coma.*

posthypoglycemic h., SYN Somogyi *phenomenon.*

hy·per·glyc·er·i·de·mia (hī'per-glis'er-i-dē'mē-ă). Elevated plasma concentration of glycerides, which usually are present within chylomicrons; normal if transiently present after absorption of a meal containing lipids, abnormal if a persistent state.

endogenous h., type IV familial hyperlipoproteinemia or, more commonly, a nonfamilial sporadic variety.

exogenous h., persistent h. due to retarded rate of removal from plasma of chylomicrons of dietary origin; occurs in alcoholism, hypothyroidism, insulinopenic diabetes mellitus, types I and V hyperlipoproteinemia, and during acute pancreatitis.

hy·per·gly·ci·ne·mia (hī'per-glī-si-nē'mē-ă). Elevated plasma glycine concentration.

ketotic h., an inherited metabolic defect which results from a deficiency of propionyl Coenzyme A carboxylase, the enzyme that converts propionate to methylmalonate; the enzyme requires biotin as a cofactor; clinically, affected infants have overwhelming illness, with lethargy, metabolic acidosis with ketosis, hypotonia; coma and seizures typically develop with early death; propionic acid is markedly elevated in plasma and urine; there is also hyperammonemia, and elevated levels of other metabolites as well, include glycine, hence the original name for the syndrome. SYN methylmalonic acidemia, propionic acidemia.

nonketotic h. [MIM*238300], an inborn error of glycine metabolism, resulting from a defect in the glycine cleavage enzyme system; characteristically overwhelming disease in the newborn period, with coma, seizures and death, or, less often, gradual onset with failure to thrive, focal seizures, and mental retardation; there is massive elevation of plasma glycine, with increased levels in cerebrospinal fluid and urine, plasma hyperosmolality, severe dehydration occur without ketoacidosis; autosomal recessive inheritance.

hy·per·gly·ci·nu·ria (hī'per-glī-si-nū'rē-ă). Enhanced urinary excretion of glycine.

hy·per·gly·co·gen·ol·y·sis (hī'per-glī'kō-jĕ-nol'i-sis). Excessive glycogenolysis. [hyper- + glycogen + G. *lysis,* loosening]

hy·per·gly·cor·rha·chia (hī'per-glī-kō-rak'ē-ă). Excessive sugar in the cerebrospinal fluid. [hyper- + G. *glykys,* sweet, + *rhachis,* spine]

hy·per·gly·co·se·mia (hī'per-glī-kō-sē'mē-ă). SYN hyperglycemia.

hy·per·gly·co·su·ria (hī'per-glī-kō-sū'rē-ă). Persistent excretion of unusually large amounts of glucose in the urine; *i.e.,* an extreme degree of glucosuria.

hy·per·gly·ox·yl·e·mia (hī'per-glī-ok'si-lē'mē-ă). Enhanced plasma (and possibly tissue) concentrations of glyoxylate; may develop during thiamine deficiency.

hy·per·gno·sis (hī-per-nō'sis). **1.** Projection of inner conflicts into the environment. **2.** Exaggerated perception, such as the expansion of an isolated thought. [hyper- + G. *gnōsis,* knowledge]

hy·per·go·nad·ism (hī-per-gō'nad-izm). A clinical state resulting from enhanced secretion of gonadal hormones.

hy·per·go·nad·o·tro·pic (hī'per-gō'nă-dō-trop'ik). Indicating an increased production or excretion of gonadotropic hormones.

hy·per·gran·u·lo·sis (hī'per-gran-yū-lō'sis). Increased thickness of the granular layer of the epidermis, associated with hyperkeratosis. [hyper- + (stratum) granulosum + -*osis,* condition]

hy·per·guan·i·di·ne·mia (hī'per-gwan'i-di-nē'mē-ă). A condition in which there is an abnormally large amount of guanidine in the circulating blood.

hy·per·gy·ne·cos·mia (hī'per-gī-nĕ-koz'mē-ă). Overdevelopment of secondary sex characteristics of the mature female or their precocious development in the young girl. [hyper- + G. *gyne,* woman, + *kosmeō,* to decorate]

hy·per·he·do·nia, hy·per·he·do·nism (hī'per-hē-dō'nē-ă, -hē'don-izm). **1.** The feeling of an abnormally great pleasure in any act or from any happening. **2.** Sexual erethism. [hyper- + G. *hēdonē,* pleasure]

hy·per·he·mo·glo·bi·ne·mia (hī'per-hē'mō-glō-bi-nē'mē-ă). An unusually large amount of hemoglobin in the circulating blood plasma; *i.e.,* much more than that ordinarily observed in most examples of hemoglobinemia.

hy·per·hep·a·ri·ne·mia (hī'per-hep'ar-in-ē'mē-ă) [MIM* 144050]. Elevated plasma concentrations of heparin; believed to be the cause of a heritable bleeding tendency. Genetic evidence of autosomal inheritance is slender.

hy·per·hi·dro·sis (hī'per-hī-drō'sis). Excessive or profuse sweating. SYN hyperephidrosis, hyperidrosis, polyhidrosis, polyidrosis, sudorrhea. [hyper- + hidrosis]

gustatory h., excessive sweating of the lips, nose, and forehead after eating certain foods; it is physiologic in many persons, but sometimes occurs after parotid surgery or as a result of damage to the parasympathetic or sympathetic nerves of the head and neck.

h. oleo'sa, SYN *seborrhea* oleosa.

hy·per·hy·dra·tion (hī'per-hī-drā'shŭn). Excess water content of the body; may result from the intravenous administration of unduly large amounts of glucose solution. SYN overhydration.

hy·per·hy·dro·chlo·ria (hī'per-hī-drō-klōr'ē-ă). SYN hyperchlorhydria.

hy·per·hy·dro·chlor·id·i·a (hī'-per-hī'-drō-chlōr-id-ē-ă). Excessive acid secretion by the stomach; associated with peptic ulcer disease. [hyper + *hydrochloric,* acid + -ia]

hy·per·hy·dro·pexy, hy·per·hy·dro·pex·is (hī-per-hī'drō-pek-sē, hī'per-hī-drō-pek'sis). Increased fixation of water in tissues. [hyper- + G. *hydōr,* water, + *pēgnymi,* to fasten]

hy·per·hy·drox·y·pro·line·mia (hī'per-hī-drok'sē-prō-lēn-ē-mē-a). SEE hydroxyprolinemia.

hy·per·i·cin (hī-per'i-sin). A photosensitizing substance present in *Hypericum perforatum,* St. John's wart, which can cause a photosensitivity similar to fagopyrism in grazing animals.

hy·per·i·dro·sis (hī'per-i-drō'sis). SYN hyperhidrosis.

hy·per·im·i·do·di·pep·ti·du·ria (hī'per-im'i-dō-dī-pep'tīd-ūr-ē-ă). Elevated levels of imidodipeptides (*e.g.,* Xaa-Pro) in the urine; due to a deficiency of prolidase.

hy·per·im·mune (hī'per-im-mum'). Having large quantities of specific antibodies in the serum from repeated immunizations or infections.

hy·per·im·mu·ni·ty (hī'per-i-mu'-ni-tē). A high degree of immunity.

hy·per·im·mu·ni·za·tion (hī'per-im-ū-nī-zāshŭn). **1.** The induction of a heightened state of immunity by the administration of repeated doses of antigen, often used in allergy desensitization. **2.** Passively acquired immunity by the injection of hyperimmune gamma globulin.

hy·per·in·di·can·e·mia (hī'per-in'di-kan-ē'mē-ă). An unusually large amount of indican in the circulating blood; *i.e.,* greater than that observed in most instances of indicanemia.

hy·per·in·fec·tion (hī'per-in-fek'shŭn). Infection by very large numbers of organisms as a result of immunologic deficiency.

hy·per·i·no·se·mia (hī'per-i'nō-sē'mē-ă, hī'per-in'ō-). A greatly increased quantity of fibrinogen in the circulating blood; under certain conditions, unusually large amounts of fibrin may be formed, thereby resulting in a greater degree of coagulability of the blood. SYN hyperinosis. [hyper- + G. *is* (*in*-), fiber, + *haima,* blood]

hy·per·i·no·sis (hī-per-i-nō'sis). SYN hyperinosemia.

hy·per·in·su·li·ne·mia (hī'per-in'sū-lin-ē'mē-ă). SYN hyperinsulinism.

hy·per·in·su·lin·ism (hī'per-in'sū-lin-izm). Increased levels of insulin in the plasma due to increased secretion of insulin by the beta cells of the pancreatic islets; decreased hepatic removal of insulin is a cause in some patients, although h. usually is associated with insulin resistance and is commonly found in obesity in association with varying degrees of hyperglycemia. SYN hyperinsulinemia.
alimentary h., elevated levels of insulin in the plasma following ingestion of meals by individuals with abnormally rapid gastric emptying (*e.g.,* following gastroenterostomy or vagotomy); rapid glucose absorption leads to excessive insulin release which in turn can lead to a marked fall in blood glucose to hypoglycemic levels.

hy·per·in·vo·lu·tion (hī'per-in'vō-lū'shŭn). SYN superinvolution.

hy·per·i·so·ton·ic (hī'per-ī-sō-ton'ik). SYN hypertonic.

hy·per·ka·le·mia (hī'per-kă-lē'mē-ă). A greater than normal concentration of potassium ions in the circulating blood. SYN hyperkaliemia, hyperpotassemia. [hyper- + Mod. L. *kalium,* potash, + G. *haima,* blood]

hy·per·kal·i·e·mia (hī'per-kal-i-ē'mē-ă). SYN hyperkalemia.

hy·per·kal·u·re·sis (hī'per-kal-yū-rē'sis). Excessive urinary excretion of potassium. [hyper- + Mod. L. *kalium,* potassium, + G. *oureō,* to urinate]

hy·per·ker·a·tin·i·za·tion (hī'per-ker'at-i-ni-zā'shŭn). SYN hyperkeratosis.

hy·per·ker·a·to·my·co·sis (hī'per-ker'ă-tō-mī-kō'sis). Thickening of the horny layer of the skin due to mycotic infection.

hy·per·ker·a·to·sis (hī'per-ker-ă-tō'sis). Thickening of the horny layer of the epidermis or mucous membrane. SEE ALSO keratoderma, keratosis. SYN hyperkeratinization.
bovine h., a specific disease characterized by thickening and hardening of the skin and proliferation of the epithelium of some of the mucous membranes; caused by poisoning (*e.g.,* from processed feed grains contaminated with certain highly chlorinated naphthalenes used as wood preservatives and constituents of lubricating greases). SYN X disease of cattle.
h. congen'ita, SYN *ichthyosis* vulgaris.
h. eccen'trica, SYN porokeratosis.
epidermolytic h. [MIM*144200], hyperkeratosis, hypergranulosis, and reticular degeneration in the upper epidermis. Generalized epidermolytic h. is present in bullous congenital ichthyosiform erythroderma. Localized epidermolytic h. may be found in epidermal nevi and benign keratoses. SYN porcupine skin.
h. figura'ta centrif'uga atroph'ica, SYN porokeratosis.
h. follicula'ris et parafollicula'ris, discrete and confluent horny follicular plugs on a crateriform base, often occurring on the arms and legs in diabetics with renal failure; possibly a severe form of perforating folliculitis. SYN h. penetrans, Kyrle's disease.
generalized epidermolytic h., SYN bullous congenital ichthyosiform *erythroderma.*

h. lenticula'ris per'stans [MIM*144150], small keratotic papules on the dorsa of the feet and legs, and occasionally elsewhere, with pinpoint keratotic papules of the palms and soles; onset in the fourth and fifth decades; possibly an autosomal dominant trait. SYN Flegel's disease.
h. pen'etrans, SYN h. follicularis et parafollicularis.
h. subungua'lis, h. affecting the nailbeds of the fingers or toes.

hy·per·ke·to·ne·mia (hī'per-kē'tō-nē'mē-ă). Elevated concentrations of ketone bodies in the blood.

hy·per·ke·ton·u·ria (hī'per-kē'tō-nū'rē-ă). Increased urinary excretion of ketonic compounds.

hy·per·ki·ne·mia (hī'per-ki-nē'mē-ă). Increased circulation rate; increased volume flow through the circulation; supernormal cardiac output. [hyper- + G. *kineō,* to move, + *haima,* blood]

hy·per·ki·ne·sis, hy·per·ki·ne·sia (hī'per-ki-nē'sis, -nē'zē-ă). **1.** Excessive motility. **2.** Excessive muscular activity. SYN hypercinesis, hypercinesia, supermotility. [hyper- + G. *kinēsis,* motion]

hy·per·ki·net·ic (hī'per-ki-net'ik). Pertaining to or characterized by hyperkinesia.

hy·per·lac·ta·tion (hī'per-lak-tā'shŭn). SYN superlactation.

hy·per·leu·ko·cy·to·sis (hī'per-lū'kō-sī-tō'sis). An unusually great increase in the number and proportion of leukocytes in the circulating blood or the tissues; *i.e.,* much more than that ordinarily observed in most instances of leukocytosis.

hy·per·lex·ia (hī-per-lek'sē-ă). In retarded children, the presence of relatively advanced reading ability. [hyper- + G. *lexis,* word, phrase]

hy·per·li·pe·mia (hī'per-li-pē'mē-ă). H. is associated with a deficiency of δ-aminoadipic semialdehyde synthase. SEE ALSO lipemia. [hyper- + G. *lipos,* fat, + *haima,* blood]
carbohydrate-induced h., SYN type III familial *hyperlipoproteinemia,* type IV familial *hyperlipoproteinemia.*
combined fat- and carbohydrate-induced h., SYN type V familial *hyperlipoproteinemia.*
familial combined h., SEE familial *hyperlipoproteinemia.*
familial fat-induced h., SYN type I familial *hyperlipoproteinemia.*
idiopathic h., SYN type I familial *hyperlipoproteinemia.*
mixed h., SYN type V familial *hyperlipoproteinemia.*

hy·per·lip·id·e·mia (hī'per-lip-i-dē'mē-ă). SYN lipemia.
mixed h., SYN mixed hyperlipoproteinemia familial, type 5 h.
mixed hyperlipoproteinemia familial, type 5 h., elevations of VLDL and chylomicrons found in plasma. SYN mixed h.

hy·per·lip·oi·de·mia (hī'per-lip-oy-dē'mē-ă). SYN lipemia.

hy·per·lip·o·pro·tein·e·mia (hī'per-lip'ō-prō'tē-in-ē'mē-ă, -prō'tēn-). An increase in the lipoprotein concentration of the blood.
acquired h., nonfamilial h. that develops as a consequence of some primary disease, such as thyroid deficiency.
familial h., a group of diseases characterized by changes in concentration of β-lipoproteins and pre-β-lipoproteins and the lipids associated with them. SEE type I familial h., type II familial h., type III familial h., type IV familial h., type V familial h.
lipoprotein(a) h., elevated levels of lipoprotein(a) in the serum; associated with an increased risk of coronary disease.
type I familial h. [MIM*238600], h. characterized by the presence of large amounts of chylomicrons and triglycerides in the plasma when the patient has a normal diet, and their disappearance on a fat-free diet; low α- and β-lipoproteins on a normal diet, with increase on fat-free diet; decreased plasma postheparin lipolytic activity; and low tissue lipoprotein lipase activity. It is accompanied by bouts of abdominal pain, hepatosplenomegaly, pancreatitis, and eruptive xanthomas; autosomal recessive inheritance. SEE ALSO familial lipoprotein lipase *inhibitor.* SYN Bürger-Grütz syndrome, familial fat-induced hyperlipemia, familial hyperchylomicronemia, familial hypertriglyceridemia (1), idiopathic hyperlipemia.
type II familial h. [MIM*144400], h. characterized by increased plasma levels of β-lipoproteins, cholesterol, and phospholipids, but normal triglycerides; heterozygotes have mild lipid changes and are susceptible to atherosclerosis in middle age, but homozy-

gotes have severe changes often with generalized xanthomatosis and xanthelasma, and frank clinical atherosclerosis as young adults. The primary defect is a deficiency of apoprotein of VLDL, and the disorder is divided into two classes: 1) type IIA, which has elevated LDL due to a deficiency of the receptor or a modified apolipoprotein B-100; 2) type IIB, which has elevated LDL and triglycerides; autosomal dominant inheritance. SYN familial hyperbetalipoproteinemia, familial hypercholesteremic xanthomatosis, familial hypercholesterolemia.

type III familial h. [MIM*107741], h. characterized by increased plasma levels of LDL, β-lipoproteins, pre-β-lipoproteins, cholesterol, phospholipids, and triglycerides; hypertriglyceridemia induced by a high carbohydrate diet, and glucose tolerance is abnormal; frequent eruptive xanthomas and atheromatosis, particularly coronary artery disease; biochemical defect lies in apolipoproteins; there are many varieties. SYN carbohydrate-induced hyperlipemia, dysbetalipoproteinemia, familial hyperbetalipoproteinemia and hyperprebetalipoproteinemia, familial hypercholesterolemia with hyperlipemia.

type IV familial h. [MIM*144600], plasma levels of VLDL, pre-β-lipoproteins and triglycerides are increased on a normal diet, but β-lipoproteins, cholesterol, and phospholipids are normal; hypertriglyceridemia is induced by a high carbohydrate diet; may be accompanied by abnormal glucose tolerance and susceptibility to ischemic heart disease; probably autosomal recessive inheritance. SYN carbohydrate-induced hyperlipemia, familial hyperprebetalipoproteinemia, familial hypertriglyceridemia (2).

type V familial h. [MIM*144650], h. characterized by increased plasma levels of chylomicrons, VLDL, pre-β-lipoproteins, and triglycerides, and slight rise of cholesterol on a normal diet, with β-lipoproteins normal; may be accompanied by bouts of abdominal pain, hepatosplenomegaly, susceptibility to atherosclerosis, and abnormal glucose tolerance; probably autosomal recessive inheritance. SYN combined fat- and carbohydrate-induced hyperlipemia, familial hyperchylomicronemia with hyperprebetalipoproteinemia, mixed hyperlipemia.

hy·per·li·po·sis (hī′per-li-pō′sis). **1.** Excessive adiposity. **2.** An extreme degree of fatty degeneration. [hyper- + G. *lipos*, fat]

hy·per·li·thu·ria (hī′per-li-thu′rē-ă). An excessive excretion of uric (lithic) acid in the urine.

hy·per·lo·gia (hī-per-lō′jē-ă). Morbid verbosity or loquacity. SEE logorrhea. [hyper- + G. *logios*, eloquent]

hy·per·lor·do·sis (hī′per-lōr-dō′sis). Extreme lordosis.

hy·per·lu·cent (hī′-per-lū′sent). A region on a chest film showing greater than normal film blackening from increased transmission of x-rays. SEE unilateral hyperlucent *lung*. [hyper- + L. *lucens*, shining, fr. *luceo*, to shine]

hy·per·ly·si·ne·mia (hī′per-lī-si-nē′mē-ă). Abnormal increase of the amino acid lysine in the circulating blood; associated with mental retardation, convulsions, anemia, and asthenia; autosomal recessive inheritance [MIM*238700]. A rare form [MIM*238759] has an accompanying hyperammonemia. Another variant [MIM*238710] is thought to be a mitochondrial defect; associated with a deficiency of α-aminoadipic semialdehyde synthase.

hy·per·ly·si·nu·ria (hī′per-lī-si-nū′rē-ă). The presence of abnormally high concentrations of lysine in the urine; a form of aminoaciduria that occurs in cystinuria, hepatolenticular degeneration, and the Fanconi syndrome.

hy·per·mag·ne·se·mia (hī′per-mag-nĕ-sē′mē-ă). An abnormally large concentration of magnesium in the blood serum.

hy·per·mas·tia (hī-per-mas′tē-ă). **1.** SYN polymastia. **2.** Excessively large mammary glands. [hyper- + G. *mastos*, breast]

hy·per·men·or·rhea (hī′per-men-ō-rē′ă). Excessively prolonged or profuse menses. SYN menorrhagia, menostaxis. [hyper- + G. *mēn*, month, + *rhoia*, flow]

hy·per·me·tab·o·lism (hī′per-me-tab′ŏ-lizm). Heat production by the body above normal, as in thyrotoxicosis.

extrathyroidal h., a state of increased metabolic rate with normal levels of thyroid hormone production.

hy·per·met·a·mor·pho·sis (hī′per-met-ă-mōr′fŏ-sis). Excessive and rapid change of ideas occurring in a mental disorder. SEE

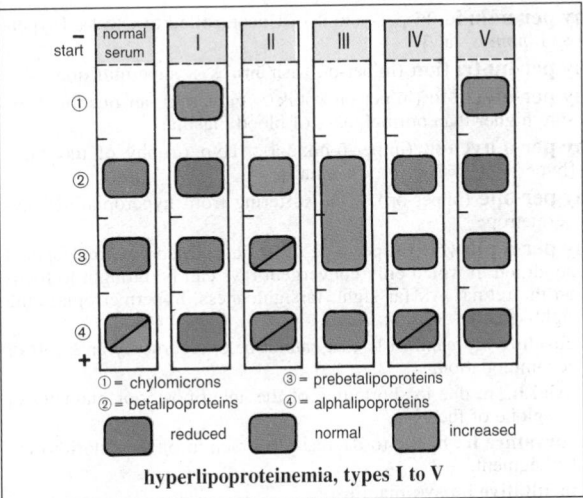

hyperlipoproteinemia, types I to V

① = chylomicrons ③ = prebetalipoproteins
② = betalipoproteins ④ = alphalipoproteins

reduced normal increased

mania, manic-depressive, manic *excitement*. [hyper- + G. *metamorphōsis,* transformation]

hy·per·me·thi·o·nine·mia (hī-per-meth-ī-ō-mēn-ē-mē-ă). Elevated levels of methionine in the sera.

hy·per·me·tria (hī-per-mē′trē-ă). Ataxia characterized by overreaching a desired object or goal; usually seen with cerebellar disorders. Cf. hypometria. [hyper- + G. *metron,* measure]

hy·per·met·rope (hī-per-met′rōp). SYN hyperope.

hy·per·me·tro·pia (hī′per-me-trō′pē-ă). SYN hyperopia. [hyper- + G. *metron,* measure, + *ōps,* eye]

index h., h. arising from decreased refractivity of the lens.

hy·perm·ne·sia (hī-perm-nē′zē-ă). **1.** Extreme power of memory. **2.** A capacity under hypnosis for immediate registration and precise recall of many more individual items than is thought possible under ordinary circumstances. Cf. hypomnesia. [hyper- + G. *mnēmē,* memory]

hy·per·mo·bil·i·ty (hī′per-mō-bil′i-tē). Increased range of movement of joints, joint laxity, occurring normally in young children or as a result of disease, *e.g.,* Marfan's or Ehlers-Danlos syndrome; h. may result in degenerative joint disease.

hy·per·morph (hī′per-mōrf). **1.** Person whose sitting height is low in proportion to the standing height, owing to excessive length of limb. Cf. hypomorph, ectomorph. **2.** A mutant gene that causes an increase in the activity controlled by the gene. Cf. hypomorph. [hyper- + G. *morphē,* form]

hy·per·my·o·to·nia (hī′per-mī-ō-tō′nē-ă). Extreme muscular tonus. [hyper- + G. *mys,* muscle, + *tonos,* tension]

hy·per·my·ot·ro·phy (hī′per-mī-ot′rō-fē). Muscular hypertrophy. [hyper- + G. *mys,* muscle, + *trophē,* nourishment]

hy·per·na·tre·mia (hī′per-nă-trē′mē-ă). An abnormally high plasma concentration of sodium ions. [hyper- + natrium, + G. *haima,* blood]

hy·per·ne·o·cy·to·sis (hī′per-nē′ō-sī-tō′sis). Hyperleukocytosis in which there are considerable numbers of immature and young cells (especially in the granulocytic series); *i.e.,* a "shift to the left" in the hemogram. SYN hyperskeocytosis. [hyper- + G. *neos,* new, + *kytos,* cell, + *-osis,* condition]

hy·per·neph·roid (hī-per-nef′royd). Resembling or of the type of the adrenal gland. [hyper- + G. *nephros,* kidney, + *eidos,* appearance]

hy·per·ne·phro·ma (hī′per-ne-frō′mă). SYN renal *adenocarcinoma.* [hyper- + G. *nephros,* kidney, + *-oma,* tumor]

hy·per·neph·ro·nia (hī′per-ne-frōn-ē-ă). SYN renal *adenocarcinoma.*

hy·per·noia (hī-per-noy′ă). **1.** Great rapidity of thought. **2.** Excessive mental activity or imagination of the type seen in the manic phase of manic depression. SEE depression, hyperpragia. [hyper- + G. *noeō,* to think]

hy

hy·per·nom·ic (hī-per-nom′ik).   Uncontrolled to excess. [hyper- + G. *nomos,* law]

hy·per·nu·tri·tion (hī′per-nū-trish′ŭn).   SYN supernutrition.

hy·per·on·cot·ic (hī′per-on-kot′ik).   Indicating an oncotic pressure higher than normal, *e.g.,* of blood plasma.

hy·per·o·nych·ia (hī′per-ō-nik′ē-ă).   Hypertrophy of the nails. [hyper- + G. *onyx, (onych-),* nail]

hy·per·ope (hī′per-ōp).   One suffering from hyperopia. SYN hypermetrope.

hy·per·o·pia (H) (hī-per-ō′pē-ă).   Longsightedness; that optical condition in which only convergent rays can be brought to focus on the retina. SYN far sight, farsightedness, hypermetropia, long sight. [hyper- + G. *ōps,* eye]

absolute h., manifest h. that cannot be overcome by an effort of accommodation.

axial h., h. due to shortening of the anteroposterior diameter of the globe of the eye.

curvature h., h. due to decreased refraction of the anterior ocular segment.

facultative h., SYN manifest h.

latent h., the difference between total and manifest h.

manifest h., h. that can be compensated by accommodation. SYN facultative h.

total h. (Ht), that which can be determined after complete paralysis of accommodation by means of a cycloplegic.

hy·per·o·pic (H) (hī-per-ō′pik).   Pertaining to hyperopia.

hy·per·o·ral·i·ty (hī′per-ō-ral′i-tē).   A condition in which inappropriate objects are placed in the mouth. [hyper- + L. *os (or-),* mouth]

hy·per·or·chi·dism (hī-per-ōr′ki-dizm).   Obsolete term for increased size or functioning of the testes. [hyper- + G. *orchis,* testis]

hy·per·o·rex·ia (hī′per-ō-rek′sē-ă).   SYN *bulimia* nervosa. [hyper- + G. *orexis,* appetite]

hy·per·or·ni·thi·ne·mia (hī′per-ōrn′a-thēn-ē-mē-ă).   Elevated levels of ornithine in the serum; sometimes associated with hyperammonemia and homocitrullinuria.

hy·per·or·tho·cy·to·sis (hī′per-ōr′thō-sī-tō′sis).   Hyperleukocytosis in which the relative percentages of the various types of white blood cells are within the normal range and immature forms are not observed. [hyper- + G. *orthos,* correct, + *kytos,* cell, + *-osis,* condition]

hy·per·os·mia (hī-per-oz′mē-ă).   An exaggerated or abnormally acute sense of smell. SYN hyperosphresia, hyperosphresis, olfactory hyperesthesia, hyperesthesia olfactoria, oxyosmia, oxyosphresia. [hyper- + G. *osmē,* sense of smell]

hy·per·os·mo·lal·i·ty (hī′per-oz-mō-lal′i-tē).   Increased concentration of a solution expressed as osmoles of solute per kilogram of serum water.

hy·per·os·mo·lar·i·ty (hī′per-oz-mō-lar′i-tē).   An increase in the osmotic concentration of a solution expressed as osmoles of solute per liter of solution.

hy·per·os·mot·ic (hī′per-oz-mot′ik).   **1.** Having an osmolality greater than another fluid, ordinarily assumed to be plasma or extracellular fluid. **2.** Relating to increased osmosis.

hy·per·os·phre·sia, hy·per·os·phre·sis (hī′per-os-frē′sē-ă, hī′per-os-frē′sis).   SYN hyperosmia. [hyper- + G. *osphrēsis,* smell]

hy·per·os·te·oi·do·sis (hī′per-os-tē-oy-dō′sis).   Excessive formation of osteoid, as seen in rickets and osteomalacia.

hy·per·os·to·sis (hī′per-os-tō′sis).   **1.** Hypertrophy of bone. **2.** SYN exostosis. [hyper- + G. *osteon,* bone, + *-ōsis,* condition]

ankylosing h., SYN diffuse idiopathic skeletal h.

h. cortica′lis defor′mans [MIM*239000], marked irregular thickening of the skull and bone cortex, with thickening and widening of the shafts of long bones and high serum alkaline phosphatase; autosomal recessive inheritance.

diffuse idiopathic skeletal h. (DISH), a generalized spinal and extraspinal articular disorder characterized by calcification and ossification of ligaments, particularly of the anterior longitudinal ligament; distinct from ankylosing spondylitis or degenerative joint disease. SYN ankylosing h., Forestier's disease, hyperostotic spondylosis.

flowing h., SYN rheostosis.

h. fronta′lis inter′na, abnormal deposition of bone on the inner aspect of the os frontale, visible by x-ray; may be a part of Morgagni's syndrome.

generalized cortical h., SYN van Buchem's *syndrome.*

infantile cortical h. [MIM*114000], neonatal subperiosteal bone formation over many bones, especially the mandible and clavicles and the shafts of long bones; it follows fever, usually appearing before 6 months of age and disappearing during childhood. SYN Caffey's disease, Caffey's syndrome, Caffey-Silverman syndrome.

streak h., SYN rheostosis.

hy·per·o·var·i·an·ism (hī′per-ō-vā′rē-an-izm).   Sexual precocity in young girls due to premature development of ovaries accompanied by the secretion of ovarian hormones.

hy·per·ox·al·u·ria (hī′per-ok-să-lū′rē-ă).   Presence of an unusually large amount of oxalic acid or oxalates in the urine. SYN oxaluria.

primary h. and oxalosis [MIM*259900 & MIM*260600], a metabolic disorder characterized by calcium oxalate nephrocalcinosis and nephrolithiasis, extrarenal oxalosis, and increased urinary output of oxalic and glycolic acids; usually evident clinically in the first decade of life, with progressive renal failure and uremia; autosomal recessive inheritance. Type I is due to an alteration in alanine:glyoxylate aminotransferase; type II is due to an alteration in D-glycerate dehydrogenase.

hy·per·ox·ia (hī-per-ok′sē-ă).   **1.** An increased amount of oxygen in tissues and organs. **2.** A greater oxygen tension than normal, such as that produced by breathing air or oxygen at pressures greater than 1 atmosphere.

hy·per·ox·i·da·tion (hī′per-oks-i-dā′shŭn).   Excessive oxidation.

hy·per·pan·cre·a·tism (hī′per-pan′krē-ă-tizm).   A condition of increased activity of the pancreas, trypsin being in excess among the enzymes.

hy·per·par·a·site (hī-per-par′ă-sīt).   A secondary parasite capable of development within a previously existing parasite.

hy·per·par·a·sit·ism (hī-per-par′ă-sīt-izm).   A condition in which a secondary parasite develops within a previously existing parasite. SYN biparasitism.

hy·per·par·a·thy·roid·ism (hī′per-par-ă-thī′royd-izm).   A condition due to an increase in the secretion of the parathyroids, causing elevated serum calcium, decreased serum phosphorus, and increased excretion of both calcium and phosphorus, calcium stones and sometimes generalized osteitis fibrosa cystica.

primary h., h. due to neoplasms or idiopathic hyperplasia of the parathyroid glands.

secondary h., h. that arises as a result of disordered metabolism producing hypocalcemia, as in chronic uremia due to renal disease, malabsorption, rickets, or osteomalacia; associated with hyperplasia of the parathyroid glands.

hy·per·pa·rot·i·dism (hī′per-pa-rot′i-dizm).   Increased activity of the parotid glands.

hy·per·path·ia (hī-per-path′ē-ă).   Exaggerated subjective response to painful stimuli, with a continuing sensation of pain after the stimulation has ceased. [hyper- + G. *pathos,* suffering]

hy·per·pep·sia (hī-per-pep′sē-ă).   **1.** Abnormally rapid digestion. **2.** Impaired digestion with hyperchlorhydria. [hyper- + G. *pepsis,* digestion]

hy·per·pep·sin·ia (hī′per-pep-sin′ē-ă).   An excess of pepsin in the gastric juice.

hy·per·per·i·stal·sis (hī′per-per-i-stal′sis).   Excessive rapidity of the passage of food through the stomach and intestine.

hy·per·pha·gia (hī-per-fā′jē-ă).   Gluttony; overeating. [hyper- + G. *phagein,* to eat]

hy·per·pha·lan·gism (hī′per-fă-lan′jizm).   Presence of a supernumerary phalanx in a finger or toe. SYN polyphalangism.

hy·per·phen·yl·a·ni·ne·mia (hī′per-fen′il-al-ă-ni-nē′mē-ă).   The presence of abnormally high blood levels of phenylalanine, which may or may not be associated with elevated tyrosine levels, in newborn infants (premature and full-term), associated with the heterozygous state of phenylketonuria, maternal phenyl-ketonuria, or transient deficiency of phenylalanine hydroxylase or *p*-hydroxyphenylpyruvic acid oxidase.

malignant h., (1) DHPR-deficient form; an inherited disorder in which there is an absence or deficiency of dihydropteridine reductase (DHPR); this results in impaired regeneration of tetrahydrobiopterin, causing an elevation in phenylalanine levels; **(2)** GTP-CH form; an inherited disorder in which there is a deficiency of guanosine triphosphate cyclohydrolase, an enzyme used in the biosynthesis of tetrahydrobiopterin; **(3)** 6-PTS form; an inherited disorder in which there is a deficiency of 6-pyruvoyl tetrahydropterin synthase, an enzyme that participates in the biosynthesis of tetrahydrobiopterin. SYN nonclassical phenylketonuria.

non-PKU h., a benign phenotype in which phenylalanine monooxygenase is deficient but is greater than 1% of normal levels.

hy·per·pho·ne·sis (hī′per-fō-nē′sis). An increase in the percussion sound or of the voice sound in auscultation. [hyper- + G. *phōnēsis,* a sounding]

hy·per·pho·nia (hī′per-fō′nē-ă). Overuse of the voice, as by excessive loudness or tension of the vocal muscles. [hyper- + G. *phōnē,* sound, voice]

hy·per·pho·ria (hī-per-fō′rē-ă). A tendency of the visual axis of one eye to deviate upward, prevented by binocular vision. [hyper- + G. *phora,* motion]

hy·per·phos·pha·ta·se·mia (hī′per-fos′fă-tă-sē′mē-ă). Abnormally high content of alkaline phosphatase in the circulating blood. SEE ALSO hyperphosphatasia.

hy·per·phos·pha·ta·sia (hī′per-fos-fă-tā′zē-ă) [MIM*239300]. Raised alkaline phosphatase, with dwarfism, macrocranium, blue sclerae, and expansion of the diaphyses of tubular bones with multiple fractures; autosomal recessive inheritance. There is also a more of less distinctive dominant type [MIM*146300].

hy·per·phos·pha·te·mia (hī′per-fos-fă-tē′mē-ă). Abnormally high concentration of phosphates in the circulating blood.

hy·per·phos·pha·tu·ria (hī′per-fos-fă-tū′rē-ă). An increased excretion of phosphates in the urine.

hy·per·phre·nia (hī-per-frē′nē-ă). Rarely used term for an excessive degree of intellectual activity; a form of mania. [hyper- + G. *phrēn,* mind]

hy·per·pi·e·sis, hy·per·pi·e·sia (hī′per-pī-ē′sis, -pī-ē′zē-ă). SYN hypertension. [hyper- + G. *piesis,* pressure]

hy·per·pi·et·ic (hī-per-pī-et′ik). Relating to or marked by high blood pressure.

hy·per·pig·men·ta·tion (hī′per-pig-men-tā′shŭn). An excess of pigment in a tissue or part. SYN superpigmentation.

hy·per·pip·e·co·la·te·mia (hī-per-pip′ě-kō-lă-tē′mē-ă). A metabolic disorder in which serum concentrations of pipecolic acid are greatly increased; characterized by hepatomegaly and progressive, generalized demyelination of the nervous system. SYN hyperpipecolic acidemia.

hy·per·pip·e·co·lic ac·i·de·mia (hī′per-pī′pē-ko-lik). SYN hyperpipecolatemia.

hy·per·pi·tu·i·ta·rism (hī′per-pi-tū′i-tă-rizm). Excessive production of anterior pituitary hormones, especially growth hormone; may result in gigantism or acromegaly.

hy·per·pla·sia (hī-per-plā′zē-ă). An increase in number of cells in a tissue or organ, excluding tumor formation, whereby the bulk of the part or organ may be increased. SEE ALSO hypertrophy. SYN numerical hypertrophy, quantitative hypertrophy. [hyper- + G. *plasis,* a molding]

angiofollicular mediastinal lymph node h., SYN benign giant lymph node h.

angiolymphoid h. with eosinophilia, solitary or multiple small benign cutaneous erythematous nodules, occurring mainly on the head and neck in young adults, characterized by dermal proliferation of blood vessels with vacuolated histiocytoid endothelial cells and with a varied infiltrate of eosinophiles, lymphocytes which may form follicles, and histiocytes. SYN Kimura's disease.

atypical melanocytic h., proliferation of melanocytes showing nuclear atypicality, especially as scattered single cells high in the epidermis; interpreted by some pathologists as malignant melanoma in situ.

basal cell h., increase in the number of cells in an epithelium resembling the basal cells.

benign giant lymph node h., solitary masses of lymphoid tissue containing concentric perivascular aggregates of lymphocytes, occurring usually in the mediastinum or hilar region of young adults; similar changes have been reported outside the mediastinum and, if associated with interfollicular sheets of plasma cells, may progress to lymphoma or plasmacytoma. SYN angiofollicular mediastinal lymph node h., Castleman's disease.

cementum h., SYN hypercementosis.

congenital adrenal h., a group of diseases arising from specific enzymatic defects in corticosteroid biosynthesis; adrenal h. with excessive secretion of adrenal androgens develops as a result of these defects. There are four major types, with clinical similarities but distinct genetic and biochemical differences: 1) simple virilizing form [MIM*201710 and *202010]; 2) sodium-losing form [MIM*201810]; 3) hypertensive form [MIM*202010]; 4) pseudohermaphroditic type [MIM*202110]; all autosomal recessive inheritance.

congenital sebaceous h., misnomer for *nevus* sebaceus.

congenital virilizing adrenal h., a series of inherited inborn errors of metabolism with h. of the adrenal cortex and overproduction of virilizing hormones. Most common forms are due to partial or complete 21-hydroxylase deficiency, leading to increased ACTH production by the pituitary, stimulating adrenal growth and function. Severe form is characterized by salt-losing state.

cystic h., formation of multiple retention cysts from obstruction of ducts or glands by h. of the lining epithelium, as in fibrocystic disease of the breast and metropathia hemorrhagica.

cystic h. of the breast, SYN fibrocystic *condition* of the breast.

denture h., SYN inflammatory fibrous h.

ductal h., h. characterized by intraductal proliferation of epithelial cells, *e.g.,* in the breast.

fibromuscular h., thickening of arterial media by fibrosis and muscular h., usually involving the renal arteries and causing multifocal stenosis and hypertension; a variety of fibromuscular dysplasia.

focal epithelial h., multiple soft nodular lesions of the lips, buccal mucosa, tongue, and other oral sites in children and adolescents; lesions spontaneously regress after a period of several months, and have been attributed etiologically to some papovaviruses. SYN Heck's disease.

gingival h., gingival enlargement due to proliferation of fibrous connective tissue. SYN gingival proliferation.

inflammatory fibrous h., overgrowth of tissue in the mucobuccal or labial fold, induced by chronic trauma from ill-fitting dentures. SYN denture h., epulis fissuratum.

inflammatory papillary h., closely arranged papules of the palatal mucosa underlying an ill-fitting denture. SYN palatal papillomatosis.

intravascular papillary endothelial h., a benign florid papillary endothelial proliferation within the veins of the skin or subcutis, less often in visceral blood vessels. SYN Masson's pseudoangiosarcoma.

neuronal h., increased numbers of ganglion cells with myenteric plexus h. and increased acetylcholinesterase activity in nerves of the mucosa and submucosa. Clinically, neuronal h. mimics Hirschprung's disease. Similar findings are seen in patients with multiple endocrine neoplasia syndrome, type IIB, and in neurofibromatosis. SYN hyperganglionosis, neuronal intestinal dysplasia.

nodular h. of prostate, glandular and stromal h. occurring very commonly in the middle and lateral lobes of older men, forming nodules that may increasingly obstruct the urethra. SYN benign prostatic hypertrophy.

nodular regenerative h., SYN nodular *transformation* of the liver.

pseudoepitheliomatous h., pseudocarcinomatous h., a benign marked increase and downgrowth of epidermal cells, observed in chronic inflammatory dermatoses; microscopically, it resembles well-differentiated squamous cell carcinoma.

hy

senile sebaceous h., h. of mature sebaceous glands, forming a nodule on the skin of the face or forehead in elderly persons.

squamous cell h., Increase in the number of cells in a squamous epithelium. SYN hypertrophic dystrophy.

transmissible murine colonic h., a disease of young mice caused by the bacterium *Citrobacter freundii* and characterized by diarrhea and mucosal h. of the descending colon.

verrucous h., a non-invasive precursor of verrucous or squamous carcinoma of the oral mucosa, occurring in the elderly, characterized by sharp or blunt upward papillary projections of squamous epithelium.

hy·per·plas·tic (hī-per-plas′tik). Relating to hyperplasia.

hy·per·pnea (hī-per-nē′ă, hī-perp′nē-ă). Breathing that is deeper and more rapid than is normal at rest. [hyper- + G. *pnoē,* breathing]

hy·per·po·lar·i·za·tion (hī′per-pō′lăr-i-zā′shŭn). An increase in polarization of membranes of nerves or muscle cells; the reverse change from that associated with excitatory action.

hy·per·po·ne·sis (hī′per-pō-nē′sis). Exaggerated activity within the motor portion of the nervous system. [hyper- + G. *ponos,* toil]

hy·per·po·tas·se·mia (hī′per-pō-tas-ē′mē-ă). SYN hyperkalemia.

hy·per·pra·gia (hī-per-prā′jē-ă). Rarely used term for excessive mental activity, as in the manic phase of bipolar disorder. [hyper- + G. *prassō,* to do]

hy·per·prax·ia (hī-per-prak′sē-ă). Rarely used term for excessive activity. [hyper- + G. *praxis,* action]

hy·per·pre·be·ta·lip·o·pro·tein·e·mia (hī′per-prē-bā′tă-lip-ō-prō′tē-in-ē′mē-ă, -prō′tēn-). Increased concentrations of pre-β-lipoproteins in the blood.

  familial h., SYN type IV familial *hyperlipoproteinemia.*

hy·per·pro·chor·e·sis (hī′per-prō-kōr-ē′sis). Rarely used term for hyperperistalsis. [hyper- + G. *pro-chōreō,* to go forward]

hy·per·pro·in·su·li·ne·mia (hī′per-prō-in′sŭl-i-nē′mē-ă). Elevated plasma levels of proinsulin or proinsulin-like material.

hy·per·pro·lac·ti·ne·mia (hī′per-prō-lak-ti-nē′mē-ă). Elevated levels of prolactin in the blood, which is a normal physiological reaction during lactation, but pathological otherwise; prolactin may also be elevated in cases of certain pituitary tumors, and amenorrhea is often present.

hy·per·pro·li·ne·mia (hī′per-prō-li-nē′mē-ă) [MIM*239500 & MIM*239510]. A metabolic disorder characterized by enhanced plasma proline concentrations and urinary excretion of proline, hydroxyproline, and glycine; autosomal recessive inheritance. Type I h. is associated with a deficiency of proline oxidase and renal disease; Type II h. is associated with a deficiency of Δ-pyrroline-5-carboxylate dehydrogenae and mental retardation.

hy·per·pro·sex·ia (hī′per-prō-sek′sē-ă). Fixation of the mind on one idea. [hyper- + G. *prosexis,* attention]

hy·per·pro·tein·e·mia (hī′per-prō′tē-in-ē′mē-ă, -prō′tēn-). An abnormally large concentration of protein in plasma.

hy·per·pro·te·o·sis (hī′per-prō-tē-ō′sis). The condition due to an excessive amount of protein in the diet.

hy·per·py·ret·ic (hī′per-pī-ret′ik). Relating to hyperpyrexia. SYN hyperpyrexial.

hy·per·py·rex·ia (hī′per-pī-rek′sē-ă). Extremely high fever. [hyper- + G. *pyrexis,* feverishness]

  fulminant h., SYN malignant *hyperthermia.*

  heat h., SYN heatstroke.

  malignant h., SYN heatstroke.

hy·per·py·rex·i·al (hī′per-pī-rek′sē-ăl). SYN hyperpyretic.

hy·per·re·flex·ia (hī′per-rē-flek′sē-ă). A condition in which the deep tendon reflexes are exaggerated.

  detrusor h., SYN detrusor *instability.*

hy·per·res·o·nance (hī-per-rez′ō-nans). **1.** An extreme degree of resonance. **2.** Resonance increased above the normal, and often of lower pitch, on percussion of an area of the body; occurs in the chest due to overinflation of the lung as in emphysema or pneumothorax and in the abdomen over a distended bowel.

hy·per·sal·e·mia (hī′per-sal-ē′mē-ă). An increase in the salt content of the circulating blood.

hy·per·sa·line (hī-per-sā′lēn, -sā′līn). Marked by increased salt in a saline solution.

hy·per·sal·i·va·tion (hī′per-sal-i-vā′shŭn). Increased salivation.

hy·per·sar·co·si·ne·mia (hī′per-sar-kō-si-nē′mē-ă). SYN sarcosinemia.

hy·per·sen·si·tive·ness (hī-per-sen′si-tiv-nes). SYN hypersensitivity.

hy·per·sen·si·tiv·i·ty (hī′per-sen-si-tiv′i-tē). Abnormal sensitivity, a condition in which there is an exaggerated response by the body to the stimulus of a foreign agent. SEE allergy. SYN hypersensitiveness.

  contact h., **(1)** SYN contact *dermatitis.* **(2)** SYN delayed *reaction.*

  delayed h., **(1)** SYN cell-mediated *immunity.* **(2)** SYN delayed *reaction.* **(3)** a cell-mediated response which occurs in immune individuals peaking at 24–48 hours after challenge with the same antigen used in an initial challenge. The interaction of T lymphocytes with MHC class II positive antigen- presenting cells initiates the response.

  immediate h., an exaggerated immune response mediated by antibodies, in particular IgE. SEE allergy.

  tuberculin-type h., SYN delayed *reaction.*

hy·per·sen·si·ti·za·tion (hī′per-sen′si-ti-zā′shŭn). The immunological process by which hypersensitivity is induced.

hy·per·se·ro·to·ne·mia (hī′per-sēr′ō-tō-nē′mē-ă). Unusually large amounts of serotonin in the circulating blood; probable cause of some of the symptoms and signs in the carcinoid syndrome.

hy·per·ske·o·cy·to·sis (hī′per-skē′ō-sī-tō′sis). SYN hyperneocytosis. [G. *skaios,* left, + *kytos,* cell, + *-osis,* condition]

hy·per·so·ma·to·tro·pism (hī′per-sō′mă-tō-trō′pizm). A state characterized by abnormally enhanced secretion of pituitary growth hormone (somatotropin).

hy·per·som·nia (hī-per-som′nē-ă). A condition in which sleep periods are excessively long, but the person responds normally in the intervals; distinguished from somnolence. [hyper- + L. *somnus,* sleep]

hy·per·son·ic (hī-per-son′ik). Pertaining to or characterized by supersonic speeds of Mach 5 or greater. While any speed above the speed of sound may be referred to as supersonic, speeds of Mach 5 or greater are specifically referred to as h. [hyper- + L. *sonus,* sound]

hy·per·sphyx·ia (hī-per-sfik′sē-ă). A condition of high blood pressure and increased circulatory activity. [hyper- + G. *sphyxis,* pulse]

hy·per·splen·ism (hī-per-splēn′izm). Any of a group of conditions in which the cellular components of the blood or platelets are removed at an abnormally high rate by the spleen, resulting in low circulating levels.

hy·per·ste·a·to·sis (hī′per-stē-ă-tō′sis). Excessive sebaceous secretion.

hy·per·sthe·nia (hī-per-sthē′nē-ă). Excessive tension or strength. [hyper- + G. *sthenos,* strength]

hy·per·sthen·ic (hī-per-sthen′ik). Pertaining to or marked by hypersthenia.

hy·per·sthen·u·ria (hī′per-sthen-yū′rē-ă). Excretion of urine of unusually high specific gravity and concentration of solutes, resulting usually from loss or deprivation of water. [hyper- + G. *sthenos,* strength, + *ouron,* urine]

hy·per·sus·cep·ti·bil·i·ty (hī′per-sŭ-sep-ti-bil′i-tē). Increased susceptibility or response to an infective, chemical, or other agent.

hy·per·sys·to·le (hī-per-sis′tō-lē). Abnormal force or duration of the cardiac systole.

hy·per·sys·tol·ic (hī′per-sis-tol′ik). Relating to or marked by hypersystole.

hy·per·tel·or·ism (hī-per-tel′ōr-izm). Abnormal distance between two paired organs. [hyper- + G. *tēle,* far off, + *horizō,* to separate, fr. *horos,* a boundary]

  Bixler type h., accompanying features are microtia and clefting of the lip, palate, and nose, mental deficiency, atresia of the auditory canals, ectopic kidneys, and thenar hypoplasia; autosomal recessive inheritance

canthal h., SYN telecanthus.

ocular h. [MIM*145400], increased width between the eyes due to an enlarged sphenoid bone; other congenital deformities and mental retardation may be associated. An apparently distinct form [MIM*145410] shows many other congenital defects. SEE ALSO faciodigitogenital *dysplasia.* SYN Greig's syndrome.

hy·per·ten·sin (hī-per-ten'sin). Former name for angiotensin.

hy·per·ten·sin·o·gen (hī′per-ten-sin′ō-jen). Former name for angiotensinogen.

hy·per·ten·sion (hī′per-ten′shŭn). High blood pressure. Despite many discrete and inherited but rare forms that have been identified, the evidence is that for the most part blood pressure is a multifactorial, perhaps galtonian trait. Its strong cybernetic properties may also be largely inherited but would not be reflected in measurements of heritability. The definition of what is "high" or "low" blood pressure is then entirely arbitrary, but extreme cases are undoubtedly dysgenic. SYN hyperpiesis, hyperpiesia. [hyper- + L. *tensio,* tension]

accelerated h., h. advancing rapidly with increasing blood pressure and associated with acute and rapidly worsening signs and symptoms.

adrenal h., h. due to an adrenal medullary pheochromocytoma or to hyperactivity or functioning tumor of the adrenal cortex.

benign h., h. that runs a relatively long and symptomless course.

borderline h., by consensus, that blood pressure zone between highest acceptable "normal" blood pressure and hypertensive blood pressure. The Framingham Heart Study defines this as pressures between 140 and 160 mm Hg systolic and 90 and 95 mm Hg diastolic.

essential h., h. without known cause. SYN idiopathic h., primary h.

Goldblatt h., increased blood pressure following obstruction of blood flow to one kidney. SYN Goldblatt phenomenon.

idiopathic h., SYN essential h.

labile h., frequently changing levels of elevated blood pressure.

malignant h., severe h. that runs a rapid course, causing necrosis of arteriolar walls in kidney, retina, etc.; hemorrhages occur, and death most frequently is caused by uremia or rupture of a cerebral vessel.

pale h., h. with pallor of the skin, a severe form with pronounced constriction of peripheral vessels.

portal h., h. in the portal system as seen in cirrhosis of the liver and other conditions causing obstruction to the portal vein.

postpartum h., increased blood pressure immediately following the completion of labor.

primary h., SYN essential h.

pulmonary h., h. in the pulmonary circuit; may be primary, or secondary to pulmonary or cardiac disease, *e.g.,* fibrosis of the lung or mitral stenosis.

renal h., h. secondary to renal disease.

renovascular h., h. produced by renal arterial obstruction.

secondary h., arterial h. produced by a known cause, *e.g.,* hyperthyroidism, kidney disease, etc., in contrast to primary h. that is of unknown cause.

systemic venous h., increased pressure in the veins ultimately leading to the right atrium nearly always due to disease of the right heart but occasionally due to blockade of one or both venae cavae.

hy·per·ten·sive (hī-per-ten'siv). **1.** Marked by an increased blood pressure. **2.** Denoting a person suffering from high blood pressure.

hy·per·ten·sor (hī-per-ten'ser, -sōr). SYN pressor.

hy·per·tes·toid·ism (hī-per-tes'toyd-izm). Hypergonadism in the male, characterized by proliferation of Leydig cells with excessive production of testosterone.

hy·per·the·co·sis (hī′per-thē-kō′sis). Diffuse hyperplasia of the theca cells of the graafian follicles.

stromal h., condition in which luteinized cells are present in ovarian stroma at a distance from follicular structures.

testoid h., hyperplasia of Leydig cells of the testis.

hy·per·the·lia (hī-per-thē′lē-ă). SYN polythelia. [hyper- + G. *thēlē,* nipple]

hy·per·ther·mal·ge·sia (hī′per-ther-măl-jē′zē-ă). Extreme sensitiveness to heat. [hyper- + G. *thermē,* heat, + *algēsis,* pain]

hy·per·ther·mia (hī-per-ther′mē-ă). Therapeutically induced hyperpyrexia. [hyper- + G. *thermē,* heat]

malignant h., rapid onset of extremely high fever with muscle rigidity, precipitated by exogenous agents in genetically susceptible persons, especially by halothane or succinylcholine. Cf. futile *cycle.* SYN fulminant hyperpyrexia, porcine stress syndrome.

hy·per·ther·mo·es·the·sia (hī-per-ther′mō-es-thē′zē-ă). Extreme sensitiveness to heat. [hyper- + G. *thermē,* heat, + *aisthēsis,* feeling]

hy·per·throm·bi·ne·mia (hī′per-throm-bi-nē′mē-ă). An abnormal increase of thrombin in the blood, frequently resulting in a tendency to intravascular coagulation.

hy·per·thy·mia (hī-per-thī′mē-ă). State of overactivity, greater than average and less than the overactivity of the manic state of manic-depressive disorder. [hyper- + G. *thymos,* soul, thought]

hy·per·thy·mic (hī-per-thī′mik). **1.** Pertaining to hyperthymia. **2.** Pertaining to hyperthymism.

hy·per·thy·mism (hī-per-thī′mizm). Excessive activity of the thymus gland; formerly postulated to be a causal factor in certain instances of unexpected and sudden death, such as status thymicolymphaticus. SYN hyperthymization.

hy·per·thy·mi·za·tion (hī′per-thī-mi-zā′shŭn). SYN hyperthymism.

hy·per·thy·rea (hī′per-thī-rē-ă). SYN hyperthyroidism.

hy·per·thy·roid·ism (hī-per-thī′royd-izm). An abnormality of the thyroid gland in which secretion of thyroid hormone is usually increased and is no longer under regulatory control of hypothalamic-pituitary centers; characterized by a hypermetabolic state, usually with weight loss, tremulousness, elevated plasma levels of thyroxin and/or triiodothyronine, and sometimes exophthalmos; may progress to severe weakness, wasting, hyperpyrexia, and other manifestations of thyroid storm; often associated with exophthalmos (Graves' disease). SYN hyperthyrea, thyroidism (1), thyrointoxication.

hereditary h., a rare inherited (autosomal dominant) disorder with constitutive stimulation of the thyrocytes.

iodine-induced h., SYN Jod-Basedow *phenomenon.*

masked h., h. occurring without the usual manifestations, especially lack of hyperactivity and eye findings, often with hypoactivity, even somnolence. Manifestation can be limited to heart failure.

ophthalmic h., SYN Graves' *disease.*

primary h., h. due to a disorder originating within the thyroid gland, in contrast to one of pituitary origin; may be due to generalized overactivity of the gland, to a localized hyperactive nodule, or to circulating antibody, which stimulates the gland (long-acting thyroid *stimulator*).

secondary h., h. due to stimulation of the thyroid gland by an excess of thyrotrophin secreted by the pituitary gland.

hy·per·thy·rox·i·ne·mia (hī′per-thī-rok-si-nē′mē-ă). An elevated thyroxine concentration in the blood.

hy·per·to·nia (hī-per-tō′nē-ă). Extreme tension of the muscles or arteries. SYN hypertonicity (1). [hyper- + G. *tonos,* tension]

h. polycythe′mica, a form of polycythemia without a prominent degree of splenomegaly, but with increased blood pressure.

sympathetic h., overfunction of the sympathetic nervous system, often experienced as anxiety.

hy·per·ton·ic (hī-per-ton′ik). **1.** Having a greater degree of tension. SYN spastic (1). **2.** Having a greater osmotic pressure than a reference solution, which is ordinarily assumed to be blood plasma or interstitial fluid; more specifically, refers to a fluid in which cells shrink. SYN hyperisotonic.

hy·per·to·nic·i·ty (hī′per-tō-nis′i-tē). **1.** SYN hypertonia. **2.** An increased effective osmotic pressure of body fluids.

hy·per·tri·chi·a·sis (hī′per-tri-kī′ă-sis). SYN hypertrichosis.

hy

hy·per·trich·o·phry·dia (hī′per-trik-ō-fri′dē-ă). Excessively thick eyebrows. [hyper- + G. *thrix*, hair, + *ophrys*, eyebrow]

hy·per·tri·cho·sis (hī′per-tri-kō′sis). Growth of hair in excess of the normal. SEE ALSO hirsutism. SYN hypertrichiasis. [hyper- + G. *trichōsis*, being hairy]

h. lanugino′sa, excessive growth of lanugo hair associated with internal malignancy.

nevoid h., congenital growth of hair abnormal for its site, texture, color, or length; often associated with other nevoid abnormalities.

h. partia′lis, abnormally excessive hair growth in patches in unusual areas.

h. universa′lis, generalized excessive hair growth.

hy·per·tri·glyc·er·i·de·mia (hī′per-trī-glis′er-i-dē′mē-ă). Elevated triglyceride concentration in the blood.

familial h., (1) SYN type I familial *hyperlipoproteinemia*. **(2)** SYN type IV familial *hyperlipoproteinemia*.

hy·per·troph (hī′per-trof). A microorganism that requires living cells to supply the enzyme systems necessary for growth and reproduction.

hy·per·tro·phia (hī-per-trō′fē-ă). SYN hypertrophy.

hy·per·tro·phic (hī-per-trof′ik). Relating to or characterized by hypertrophy.

hy·per·tro·phy (hī-per′trō-fē). General increase in bulk of a part or organ, not due to tumor formation. Use of the term may be restricted to denote greater bulk through increase in size, but not in number, of the individual tissue elements. SEE ALSO hyperplasia. SYN hypertrophia. [hyper- + G. *trophē*, nourishment]

adaptive h., thickening of the walls of a hollow organ, like the urinary bladder, when there is obstruction to outflow.

benign prostatic h., SYN nodular *hyperplasia* of prostate.

compensatory h., increase in size of an organ or part of an organ or tissue, when called upon to do additional work or perform the work of destroyed tissue or of a paired organ.

compensatory h. of the heart, thickening of the walls of the heart in response to vascular, valvular, other heart disease, or athletic conditioning.

complementary h., increase in size or expansion of part of an organ or tissue to fill the space left by the destruction of another portion of the same organ or tissue.

concentric h., thickening of the walls of the heart or any cavity with apparent diminution of the capacity of the cavity.

eccentric h., thickening of the wall of the heart or other cavity, with dilation.

endemic h., enlargement of the calcaneus preceded by fever and pain in the heel, reported from the Gold Coast (now Ghana) and in Taiwan among the indigenous population.

false h., SYN pseudohypertrophy.

functional h., SYN physiologic h.

giant h. of gastric mucosa, SYN Ménétrier's *disease*.

hemangiectatic h., SYN Klippel-Trenaunay-Weber *syndrome*.

lipomatous h., SYN lipomatous *infiltration*.

numerical h., SYN hyperplasia.

physiologic h., temporary increase in size of an organ or part to provide for a natural increase of function, such as the kind that occurs in the walls of the uterus and in the mammae during pregnancy. SYN functional h.

quantitative h., SYN hyperplasia.

simple h., increase in size of cells.

simulated h., increased size of a part due to continued growth unrestrained by attritions, as is seen in the case of the teeth of certain animals when the opposing teeth have been destroyed.

true h., an increase in size involving all the different tissues composing the part.

vicarious h., h. of an organ following failure of another organ because of a functional relationship between them; *e.g.,* enlargement of the pituitary gland, after destruction of the thyroid.

hy·per·tro·pia (hī′per-trō′pē-ă). An ocular deviation with one eye higher than the other. [hyper- + G. *trope*, a turn]

hy·per·ty·ro·si·ne·mia (hī′per-tī′rō-si-nē′mē-ă). SYN tyrosinemia.

hy·per·ura·cil thy·mi·nu·ria (hī′per-ūr′a-sil). An inherited disorder in which there are elevated levels of uracil and thymine in the urine; associated with a deficiency of dihydropyrimidine dehydrogenase and resultant impaired CNS function.

hy·per·u·re·sis (hī′per-yū-rē′sis). Obsolete term for polyuria. [hyper- + G. *oureō*, to urinate]

hy·per·u·ri·ce·mia (hī′per-yū-rē-sē′mē-ă). Enhanced blood concentrations of uric acid.

hy·per·u·ri·ce·mic (hī′per-yū-ri-sē′mik). Relating to or characterized by hyperuricemia.

hy·per·u·ri·cu·ria (hī′per-yū-ri-kyū′rē-ă). Increased urinary excretion of uric acid.

hy·per·vac·ci·na·tion (hī′per-vak-si-nā′shŭn). Repeated inoculation of an individual already immunized; used as a means of preparing a highly potent antiserum.

hy·per·val·i·ne·mia (hī′per-val-i-nē′mē-ă). Abnormally high plasma concentrations of valine, a common finding in maple syrup urine disease.

hy·per·vas·cu·lar (hī′per-vas′kyū-ler). Abnormally vascular; containing an excessive number of blood vessels. [hyper- + L. *vas*, a vessel]

hy·per·ven·ti·la·tion (hī′per-ven-ti-lā′shŭn). Increased alveolar ventilation relative to metabolic carbon dioxide production, so that alveolar carbon dioxide pressure decreases to below normal. SYN overventilation.

hy·per·vi·ta·min·o·sis (hī′per-vī′tă-mi-nō′sis). A condition resulting from the ingestion of an excessive amount of a vitamin preparation, symptoms varying according to the particular vitamin implicated; serious effects may be caused by overdosage with fat-soluble vitamins, especially A or D, and rarely with water-soluble vitamins.

hy·per·vo·le·mia (hī′per-vō-lē′mē-ă). Abnormally increased volume of blood. SYN plethora (1), repletion (1). [hyper- + L. *volumen*, volume, + G. *haima*, blood]

hy·per·vo·le·mic (hī′per-vō-lē′mik). Pertaining to or characterized by hypervolemia.

hy·per·vo·lia (hī-per-vō′lē-ă). Augmented water content or volume of a given compartment; *e.g.,* cellular h.

hyp·es·the·sia (hī-pes-thē′zē-ă). Diminished sensitivity to stimulation. SYN hypoesthesia. [G. *hypo*, under, + *aisthēsis*, feeling]

olfactory h., SYN hyposmia.

hy·pha, pl. **hy·phae** (hī′fă, hī′fē). A branching tubular cell characteristic of the filamentous fungi (molds). In most species the hyphae are divided by cross-walls (septa) into multicellular hyphae; intercommunicating hyphae constitute a mycelium, the visible colony on natural substrates or artificial laboratory media. The terms hypha and mycelium often are used interchangeably. [G. *hyphē*, a web]

racquet h., a vegetative h. with distal ends of successive cells inflated, resembling a string of elongated snowshoes or tennis racquets; seen in many mycelial fungi, *e.g.,* many dermatophyte species in culture.

spiral hyphae, hyphae that end in a flat or helical coil, as in laboratory colonies of *Trichophyton mentagrophytes*.

hyp·he·do·nia (hīp-hē-dō′nē-ă). A habitually lessened or attenuated degree of pleasure from that which should normally give great pleasure. [G. *hypo*, under, + *hēdonē*, pleasure]

hy·phe·ma (hī-fē′mă). Blood in the anterior chamber of the eye. [G. *hyphaimos*, suffused with blood]

hy·phe·mia (hī-fē′mē-ă). SYN hypovolemia. [hypo- + G. *haima*, blood]

intertropical h., tropical h., SYN ancylostomiasis.

Hy·pho·my·ces des·tru·ens (hī-fō-mī′sēs des′trū-enz). SYN *Pythium insidiosum*.

Hy·pho·my·ce·tes (hī′fō-mī-sē′tēs). A class of fungi that includes all of the filamentous members of the Fungi Imperfecti which form neither acervuli nor pycnidia. No sexual reproduction occurs; most members of this group produce asexual spores. [G. *hyphe*, web, + *mykēs*, fungus]

hy·pho·my·co·sis (hī′fō-mī-kō′sis). A disease of horses and mules (rarely of man) caused by the fungus *Pythium insidiosum*

(*Hyphomyces destruens*), characterized by granulomatous and necrotic lesions that appear on the head and lower legs, ulcerate, and enlarge by subcutaneous extension.

hypn-. SEE hypno-.

hyp·na·gog·ic (hip-nă-goj′ik). Denoting a transitional state, related to the hypnoidal, preceding sleep; applied also to various hallucinations that may manifest themselves at that time. SEE hypnoidal. [hypno- + G. *agōgos*, leading]

hyp·na·gogue (hip′nă-gog). An agent that induces sleep. [hypno- + G. *agōgos*, leading]

hyp·nal·gia (hip-nal′jē-ă). Pain occurring during sleep. SYN dream pain. [hypno- + G. *algos*, pain]

hyp·nap·a·gog·ic (hip-nap-ă-goj′ik). Denoting a state similar to the hypnagogic, through which the mind passes in coming out of sleep; denoting also hallucinations experienced at such time. [hypno- + G. *apo*, from, + *agōgos*, leading]

hyp·nes·the·sia (hip-nes-thē′zē-ă). SYN drowsiness. [hypno- + G. *aisthēsis*, sensation]

hyp·nic (hip′nik). Relating to or causing sleep. [G. *hypnikos*, relating to sleep]

hypno-, hypn-. Sleep, hypnosis. [G. *hypnos*,]

hyp·no·a·nal·y·sis (hip′nō-ă-nal′i-sis). Psychoanalysis or other psychotherapy which employs hypnosis as an adjunctive technique.

hyp·no·an·a·lyt·ic (hip′nō-an-ă-lit′ik). Pertaining to hypnoanalysis.

hyp·no·ca·thar·sis (hip′nō-kă-thar′sis). Ventilation of suppressed or repressed emotional tension, conflicts, and anxiety under hypnosis. [hypno- + G. *katharsis*, purification]

hyp·no·cin·e·mat·o·graph (hip′nō-sin-ĕ-mat′ō-graf). Obsolete term for somnocinematograph. [hypno- + G. *kinēma*, movement, + *graphē*, a record]

hyp·no·cyst (hip′nō-sist). A quiescent or "sleeping" cyst; an encysted protozoon, the reproductive activity of which is in abeyance. [hypno- + G. *kystis*, bladder (cyst)]

hyp·no·don·tics (hip-nō-don′tiks). Hypnosis as applied to the practice of dentistry. [hypno- + G. *odous*, tooth]

hyp·no·gen·e·sis (hip-nō-jen′ĕ-sis). The induction of sleep or of the hypnotic state. [hypno- + G. *genesis*, production]

hyp·no·gen·ic, hyp·nog·e·nous (hip-nō-jen′ik, -noj′ĕ-nŭs). **1.** Relating to hypnogenesis. **2.** An agent capable of inducing a hypnotic state. SEE hypnosis.

hyp·noi·dal (hip-noy′dăl). Resembling hypnosis; denoting the subwaking state, a mental condition intermediate between sleeping and waking. SEE hypnagogic. [hypno- + G. *eidos*, resemblance]

hyp·nol·o·gist (hip-nol′ō-jist). **1.** A student of sleep or hypnosis who studies hypnology. **2.** SYN hypnotist.

hyp·nol·o·gy (hip-nol′ō-jē). The branch of scientific inquiry regarding sleep or hypnosis and its phenomena. [hypno- + G. *logos*, study]

hyp·no·pho·bia (hip-nō-fō′bē-ă). Morbid fear of falling asleep. [hypno- + G. *phobos*, fear]

hyp·no·pom·pic (hip-nō-pom′pik). Denoting the occurrence of visions or dreams during the drowsy state following sleep. [hypno- + G. *pompē*, procession]

hyp·no·sis (hip-nō′sis). An artificially induced trancelike state, resembling somnambulism, in which the subject is highly susceptible to suggestion, oblivious to all else, and responds readily to the commands of the hypnotist; its popularity and scientific validity has been accepted and rejected through several cycles during the past two centuries. SEE mesmerism. SYN hypnotic sleep, hypnotic state. [G. *hypnos*, sleep, + *-osis*, condition]

lethargic h., the deep sleep following major h. SYN trance coma.

major h., a state of extreme suggestibility in h. in which the subject is insensible to all outside impressions except the commands of the hypnotist.

minor h., an induced state resembling normal sleep in which the subject is susceptible to suggestion, though not to the extent of catalepsy or somnambulism.

hyp·no·ther·a·py (hip-nō-thār′ă-pē). **1.** Psychotherapeutic treat-

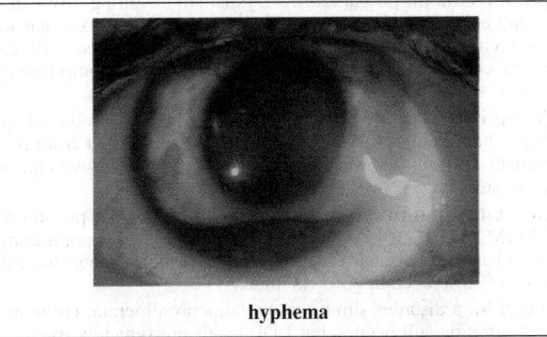

hyphema

ment by means of hypnotism. **2.** Treatment of disease by inducing a trance-like sleep.

hyp·not·ic (hip-not′ik). **1.** Causing sleep. **2.** An agent that promotes sleep. **3.** Relating to hypnotism. [G. *hypnōtikos*, causing one to sleep]

h. suggestion, SEE minor *hypnosis*.

hyp·no·tism (hip′nō-tizm). **1.** The process or act of inducing hypnosis. SYN somnipathy (2), somnolism. **2.** The practice or study of hypnosis. SEE mesmerism. [G. *hypnos*, sleep]

hyp·no·tist (hip′nō-tist). One who practices hypnotism. SYN hypnologist (2).

hyp·no·tize (hip′nō-tīz). To induct one into hypnosis.

hyp·no·toid (hip′nō-toyd). Resembling hypnosis.

hyp·no·zo·ite (hip-nō-zō′īt). Exoerythrocytic schizozoite of *Plasmodium vivax* or *P. ovale* in the human liver, characterized by delayed primary development; thought to be responsible for malarial relapse.

hypo-. **1.** Prefix denoting deficient, below normal. SEE ALSO hyp-. Cf. sub-. **2.** In chemistry, denoting the lowest, or least rich in oxygen, of a series of chemical compounds. [G. *hypo*, under]

hy·po·a·cid·i·ty (hī′pō-a-sid′i-tē). A lower than normal degree of acidity, as of the gastric juice.

hy·po·a·cu·sis (hī′pō-ă-kū′sis). SYN hypacusis.

hy·po·a·de·nia (hī-pō-ă-dē′nē-ă). Any deficiency in the function of a glandular organ or tissue. [hypo- + G. *adēn*, gland]

hy·po·a·dre·nal·ism (hī′pō-ă-drē′năl-izm). Reduced adrenocortical function.

hy·po·al·bu·mi·ne·mia (hī′pō-al-bū-mi-nē′mē-ă). An abnormally low concentration of albumin in the blood. SYN hypalbuminemia.

hy·po·al·dos·ter·on·ism (hī′pō-al-dos′ter-on-izm). A condition due to deficient secretion of aldosterone; can occur in two forms: 1) as part of generalized adrenocortical insufficiency; 2) as a selective deficiency caused by a primary defect of the adrenal gland or a defect in control of aldosterone secretion.

hyporeninemic h., selective aldosterone deficiency resulting from low renin production.

selective h., isolated h., aldosterone deficiency without a concomitant deficiency of glucocorticoid hormones.

hy·po·al·do·ster·on·u·ria (hī′pō-al-dos′ter-on-ū′rē-ă). Abnormally low levels of aldosterone in the urine.

hy·po·al·ge·sia (hī-pō-al-jē′zē-ă). SYN hypalgesia. [hypo- + G. *algēsis*, a sense of pain]

hy·po·al·i·men·ta·tion (hī′pō-al-i-men-tā′shŭn). SYN subalimentation.

hy·po·az·o·tu·ria (hī′pō-az-ō-tū′rē-ă). Excretion of abnormally small quantities of nonprotein nitrogenous material (especially urea) in the urine. SYN hypazoturia. [hypo- + Fr. *azote*, nitrogen, + G. *ouron*, urine]

hy·po·bar·ia (hī-pō-bar′ē-ă). SYN hypobarism.

hy·po·bar·ic (hī-pō-bar′ik). **1.** Pertaining to pressure of ambient gases below 1 atmosphere. **2.** With respect to solutions, less dense than the diluent or medium; *e.g.*, in spinal anesthesia, a h. solution has a density lower than that of spinal fluid. [hypo- + G. *baros*, weight]

hy

hy·po·bar·ism (hī-pō-bar′izm). Dysbarism resulting from decreasing barometric pressure on the body without hypoxia; gas in body cavities tends to expand, and gases dissolved in body fluids tend to come out of solution as bubbles. Cf. decompression *sickness*. SYN hypobaria.

hy·po·ba·rop·a·thy (hī′pō-ba-rop′ă-thē). Sickness produced by reduced barometric pressure; not always distinguished from hypobarism and altitude sickness. [hypo- + G. *baros*, weight, + *pathos*, suffering]

hy·po·be·ta·lip·o·pro·tein·e·mia (hī′pō-bā′tă-lip′ō-prō′tēn-ē′mē-ă) [MIM*107730]. Abnormally low levels of β-lipoproteins in the plasma occasionally with acanthocytosis and neurological signs. SEE ALSO abetalipoproteinemia.

familial h., a disorder similar to abetalipoproteinemia; chylomicron formation still occurs, but LDL levels are typically low.

h. with apo B-37, a disorder in which LDL levels are very low, there is a mild fat malabsorption, and a truncated apolipoprotein B-37 is formed.

hy·po·blast (hī′pō-blast). SYN endoderm. [hypo- + G. *blastos*, germ]

hy·po·blas·tic (hī-pō-blas′tik). Relating to or derived from the hypoblast.

hy·po·bran·chi·al (hī-pō-brang′kē-ăl). Located beneath the branchial apparatus.

hy·po·bro·mite (hī-pō-brō′mīt). A salt of hypobromous acid.

hy·po·bro·mous ac·id (hī-pō-brō′mŭs). An acid, HOBr, the aqueous solution of which possesses oxidizing and bleaching properties.

hy·po·cal·ce·mia (hī′pō-kal-sē′mē-ă). Abnormally low levels of calcium in the circulating blood; commonly denotes subnormal concentrations of calcium ions.

hy·po·cal·ci·fi·ca·tion (hī′pō-kal-si-fi-kā′shŭn). Deficient calcification of bone or teeth.

enamel h. [MIM*104500], a defect of enamel maturation, exacerbated by local, systemic, or hereditary factors, and characterized by low mineral content. A variety of amelogenesis imperfecta.

hy·po·cap·nia (hī-pō-kap′nē-ă). Abnormally decreased arterial carbon dioxide tension. SYN hypocarbia. [hypo- + G. *kapnos*, smoke, vapor]

hy·po·car·bia (hī-pō-kar′bē-ă). SYN hypocapnia.

hy·po·ce·lom (hī-pō-sē′lom). Rarely used term for the ventral portion of the celom, or body cavity, of the embryo. [hypo- + G. *koilos*, hollow]

hy·po·chlor·e·mia (hī′pō-klō-rē′mē-ă). An abnormally low level of chloride ions in the circulating blood.

hy·po·chlor·e·mic (hī′pō-klō-rē′mik). Pertaining to or characterized by hypochloremia.

hy·po·chlor·hy·dria (hī′pō-klōr-hī′drē-ă, -hid′rĭ-ah). Presence of an abnormally small amount of hydrochloric acid in the stomach. SYN hypohydrochloria.

hy·po·chlo·rite (hī-pō-klōr′īt). A salt of hypochlorous acid.

hy·po·chlo·rous ac·id (hī-pō-klōr′ŭs). An acid, HOCl, having oxidizing and bleaching properties.

hy·po·chlor·u·ria (hī′pō-klōr-yū′rē-ă). Excretion of abnormally small quantities of chloride ions in the urine.

hy·po·cho·les·ter·e·mia (hī′pō-kō-les-tĕ-rē′mē-ă). SYN hypocholesterolemia.

hy·po·cho·les·ter·in·e·mia (hī′pō-kō-les′tĕ-ri-nē′mē-ă). SYN hypocholesterolemia.

hy·po·cho·les·ter·ol·e·mia (hī′pō-kō-les′ter-ol-ē′mē-ă). The presence of abnormally small amounts of cholesterol in the circulating blood. SYN hypocholesteremia, hypocholesterinemia.

hy·po·cho·lia (hī-pō-kō′lē-ă). Rarely used term for oligocholia.

hy·po·chon·dria (hī-pō-kon′drē-ă). SYN hypochondriasis.

hy·po·chon·dri·ac (hī-pō-kon′drē-ak). **1.** A person with a somatic overconcern, including morbid attention to the details of bodily functioning and exaggeration of any symptoms no matter how insignificant. **2.** A person manifesting hypochondriasis. **3.** Beneath the ribs; relating to the hypochondrium.

hy·po·chon·dri·a·cal (hī′pō-kon-drī′ă-kăl). Relating to or suffering from hypochondriasis.

hy·po·chon·dri·a·sis (hī′pō-kon-drī′ă-sis). A morbid concern about one's own health and exaggerated attention to any unusual bodily or mental sensations; a delusion that one is suffering from some disease for which no physical basis is evident. SYN hypochondria, hypochondriacal neurosis. [fr. hypochondrium, regarded as the site of hypochondria, + G. *-iasis,* condition]

hy·po·chon·dri·um, pl. **hy·po·chon·dria** (hī-pō-kon′drē-ŭm, -ă). SYN hypochondriac *region*. [L. fr. G. *hypochondrion*, abdomen, belly, from *hypo,* under, + *chondros,* cartilage (of ribs)]

hy·po·chon·dro·pla·sia (hī′pō-kon-drō-plā′zē-ă) [MIM* 146000]. Dwarfism similar to but milder than achondroplasia and neither seen with achondroplasia in the same families nor evident until mid-childhood; the skull and facies are normal; autosomal dominant inheritance. [hypo- + G. *chondros,* cartilage, + *plasis,* a molding]

hy·po·chord·al (hī-pō-kōr′dăl). On the ventral side of the spinal cord. [hypo- + G. *chordē,* cord]

hy·po·chro·ma·sia (hī′pō-krō-mā′zē-ă). SYN hypochromia.

hy·po·chro·mat·ic (hī′-pō-krō-mat′ik). Containing a small amount of pigment, or less than the normal amount for the individual tissue. SYN hypochromic (1). [hypo- + G. *chrōma,* color]

hy·po·chro·ma·tism (hī-pō-krō′mă-tizm). **1.** The condition of being hypochromatic. **2.** SYN hypochromia.

hy·po·chro·mia (hī-pō-krō′mē-ă). An anemic condition in which the percentage of hemoglobin in the red blood cells is less than the normal range. SYN hypochromasia, hypochromatism (2), hypochrosis. [hypo- + G. *chrōma,* color]

hy·po·chro·mic (hī-pō-krō′mik). **1.** SYN hypochromatic. **2.** Denoting decrease in light absorption with a shift in λinferior to a lower wavelength.

hy·po·chro·sis (hī-pō-krō′sis). SYN hypochromia. [hypo- + G. *chrōsis,* a tinting]

hy·po·chy·lia (hī-pō-kī′lē-ă). Rarely used term for oligochylia. [hypo- + G. *chylos,* juice]

hy·po·ci·ne·sis, hy·po·ci·ne·sia (hī′pō-si-nē′sis, -nē′zē-ă). SYN hypokinesis.

hy·po·cit·ra·tur·ia (hī′pō-si-trā-tūr′ē-ă). Abnormally low concentration of citrate in the urine.

hy·po·com·ple·men·te·mia (hī′pō-kom′plĕ-men-tē′mē-ă). A condition in which one or another component of complement is lacking or reduced in amount; associated with immune complex diseases and cases of membranoproliferative glomerulonephritis in which nephritic factor is present. Various autosomal forms are known, dominant [MIM*120550-120980] and recessive [MIM*216950-217070].

hy·po·cone (hī′pō-kōn). The distolingual cusp of an upper molar tooth. [hypo- + G. *kōnos,* pine cone]

hy·po·con·id (hī-pō-kon′id). The distobuccal cusp of a lower molar tooth.

hy·po·con·ule (hī-pō-kon′yūl). The distal, or fifth, cusp of an upper molar tooth. [hypo- + Mod. L. dim. of L. *conus,* cone]

hy·po·con·u·lid (hī-pō-kon′yū-lid). The distal, or fifth, cusp of a lower molar tooth. [hypo- + Mod. L. dim. of L. *conus,* cone]

hy·po·cor·ti·coid·ism (hī-pō-kōr′ti-koyd-izm). SYN adrenocortical *insufficiency*.

hy·po·cu·pre·mia (hī′pō-kū-prē′mē-ă). Reduced copper content of the blood; found in Wilson's disease because ceruloplasmin is depressed, even though serum albumin-attached copper is increased. [hypo- + L. *cuprum,* copper, + G. *haima,* blood]

hy·po·cy·cloi·dal (hī′-pō-sī-kloy′dăl). A tricyclic motion used by mechanical tomography units to optimize blurring and reduce artifacts. [hypo- + G. *kuklos,* circle, + *-oeidēs,* appearance]

hy·po·cys·tot·o·my (hī′pō-sis-tot′ō-mē). Perineal cystotomy.

hy·po·cy·the·mia (hī′pō-sī-thē′mē-ă). Hypocytosis of the circulating blood, such as that observed in aplastic anemia. [hypo- + G. *kytos,* cell, + *haima,* blood]

hy·po·cy·to·sis (hī′pō-sī-tō′sis). Varying degrees of abnormally low numbers of red and white cells and other formed elements of the blood; in some instances, the term is also used to indicate a paucity of component cells of any tissue. SEE ALSO cytopenia, pancytopenia. [hypo- + G. *kytos,* cell, + *-osis,* condition]

hy·po·dac·ty·ly, hy·po·dac·tyl·ia, hy·po·dac·tyl·ism (hī'pō-dak'ti-lē, -dak-til'ē-ă, -dak'til-izm). Less than the full normal complement of digits. [hypo- + G. *daktylos,* finger]

hy·po·derm (hī'pō-derm). SYN superficial *fascia.* [hypo- + G. *derma,* skin]

Hy·po·der·ma (hī-pō-der'mă). A genus of botflies whose larvae are the cause of a tropical form of myiasis linearis (cutaneous larva migrans) of man; occasionally they invade the interior of the eye. Two species, *H. bovis* and *H. lineatum,* are botflies of cattle. The ova of *H. bovis* are deposited on hairs of the legs, and the larvae penetrate the skin and migrate through the tissues to the skin of the back, where they appear during late winter as the common warbles; these ulcerate to the surface and mature larvae escape in early summer, fall to the ground, pupate, and give rise to a new generation of flies. [hypo- + G. *derma,* skin]

hy·po·der·mat·ic (hī'pō-der-mat'ik). Rarely used term for subcutaneous.

hy·po·der·mat·oc·ly·sis (hī'pō-der-mă-tok'li-sis). Rarely used spelling of hypodermoclysis.

hy·po·der·mat·o·my (hī'pō-der-mat'ō-mē). Subcutaneous division of a structure. [hypo- + G. *derma,* skin, + *tomē,* incision]

hy·po·der·ma·to·sis (hī'pō-der-mă-tō'sis). Infection of herbivores and man with larvae of flies of the genus *Hypoderma.*

hy·po·der·mic (hī'pō-der'mik). **1.** SYN subcutaneous. **2.** SYN hypodermic *injection.* **3.** SYN hypodermic *syringe.*

hy·po·der·mis (hī-pō-der'mis). SYN superficial *fascia.*

hy·po·der·moc·ly·sis (hī'pō-der-mok'li-sis). Subcutaneous injection of a saline or other solution. [hypo- + G. *derma,* skin, + *klysis,* a washing out]

hy·po·der·mo·li·thi·a·sis (hī'pō-der'mō-li-thī'ă-sis). Subcutaneous deposits of calcium. SEE ALSO *calcinosis* cutis. [hypo- + G. *derma,* skin, + lithiasis]

hy·po·dip·loid (hī'-pō-dip'loid). Having a chromosome number less than the diploid number.

hy·po·dip·sia (hī-pō-dip'sē-ă). A physiologic condition, perhaps caused by hypertonicity of body fluids, insufficient to initiate drinking but at times sufficient to sustain drinking when started; loosely, oligodipsia. SYN insensible thirst, subliminal thirst. [hypo- + G. *dipsa,* thirst]

hy·po·don·tia (hī-pō-don'shē-ă). A condition of having fewer than the normal complement of teeth, either congenital or acquired. SYN oligodontia, partial anodontia. [hypo- + G. *odous,* tooth]

hy·po·dy·nam·ia (hī'pō-dī-nā'mē-ă, -dī-nam'ē-ă). Diminished power. [hypo- + G. *dynamis,* force]

h. cor'dis, diminished force of cardiac contraction.

hy·po·dy·nam·ic (hī'pō-dī-nam'ik). Possessing or exhibiting subnormal power or force.

hy·po·ec·cri·sis (hī'pō-ek'ri-sis). Reduced excretion of waste matter. [hypo- + G. *eccrisis,* separation]

hy·po·ec·crit·ic (hī'pō-ĕ-krit'ik). Characterized by hypoeccrisis.

hy·po·ech·o·ic (hī'pō-ē-kō'ik). A region in an ultrasound image in which the echoes are weaker or fewer than normal or in the surrounding regions. [hypo- + echo + -ic]

hy·po·e·o·sin·o·phil·ia (hī'pō-ē'ō-sin-ō-fil'ē-ă). SYN eosinopenia.

hy·po·es·o·pho·ria (hī'pō-es-ō-fō'rē-ă). A tendency of the visual axis of one eye to deviate downward and inward, prevented by binocular vision. [hypo- + G. *esō,* within, + *phoros,* bearing]

hy·po·es·the·sia (hī'pō-es-thē'zē-ă). SYN hypesthesia.

hy·po·ex·o·pho·ria (hī'pō-ek-sō-fō'rē-ă). A tendency of the visual axis of one eye to deviate downward and outward, prevented by binocular vision. [hypo- + G. *exō,* without, + *phoros,* bearing]

hy·po·fer·re·mia (hī'pō-fer-ē'mē-ă). A deficiency of iron in the circulating blood.

hy·po·fi·brin·o·ge·ne·mia (hī'pō-fī-brin'ō-jĕ-nē'mē-ă). Abnormally low concentration of fibrinogen in the circulating blood plasma.

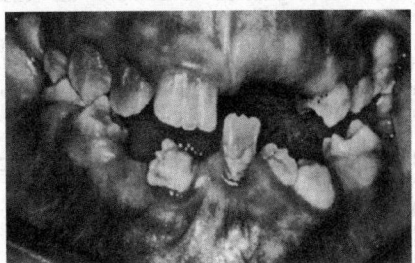
hypodontia (in dentinogenesis imperfecta)

hy·po·func·tion (hī'pō-fŭnk-shŭn). Reduced, low, or inadequate function.

hy·po·ga·lac·tia (hī'pō-ga-lak'shē-ă). Less than normal milk secretion. [hypo- + G. *gala,* milk]

hy·po·ga·lac·tous (hī'pō-ga-lak'tŭs). Producing or secreting a less than normal amount of milk.

hy·po·gam·ma·glo·bi·ne·mia (hī'pō-gam'ă-glō'bi-nē'mē-ă). SYN hypogammaglobulinemia.

hy·po·gam·ma·glob·u·lin·e·mia (hī'pō-gam'ă-glob'yū-li-nē'mē-ă). Decreased quantity of the gamma fraction of serum globulin; sometimes used loosely to denote decreased quantity of immunoglobulins in general; associated with increased susceptibility to pyogenic infections; also observed in type III isolated growth hormone deficiency. SYN hypogammaglobinemia.

acquired h., SYN common variable *immunodeficiency.*

primary h., h. due to a primary immunodeficiency of immunoglobulin-forming cells (B-lymphocytes).

secondary h., SYN secondary *immunodeficiency.*

transient h. of infancy, a type of primary immunodeficiency that occurs in infants of both sexes, usually before the sixth month of life, probably resulting from immaturity of lymphoid tissue. SYN transient agammaglobulinemia.

X-linked h., X-linked infantile h. [MIM*300300], a congenital, X-linked recessive, primary immunodeficiency characterized by decreased numbers (or absence) of circulating B-lymphocytes with corresponding decrease in immunoglobulins of the five classes; associated with marked susceptibility to infection by pyogenic bacteria (notably, pneumococci and *Haemophilus influenzae*) beginning after loss of maternal antibodies.

X-linked h. with growth hormone deficiency, h. combined with a reduced number of B cells; characterized by short stature, delayed puberty, and recurrent infections.

hy·po·gan·gli·o·no·sis (hī'pō-gang-lē-on-ō'sis). A reduction in the number of ganglionic nerve cells.

hy·po·gas·tric (hī-pō-gas'trik). Relating to the hypogastrium.

hy·po·gas·tri·um (hī'pō-gas'trē-ŭm) [NA]. SYN pubic *region,* pubic *region.* [G. *hypogastrion,* lower belly, fr. *hypo,* under, + *gastēr,* belly]

hy·po·gas·tro·cele (hī'pō-gas'trō-sēl). Hernia of the lower part of the abdomen. [hypogastrium + G. *kēlē,* hernia]

hy·po·gas·trop·a·gus (hī'pō-gas-trop'ă-gŭs). Twins joined at the hypogastrium. SEE conjoined *twins,* under *twin.* [hypogastrium + G. *pagos,* fr. *pēgnynai,* to fasten]

hy·po·gas·tros·chi·sis (hī'pō-gas-tros'ki-sis). Congenital fissure of the abdominal wall in the hypogastric region. [hypogastrium + G. *schisis,* cleaving]

hy·po·gen·e·sis (hī'pō-jen'ĕ-sis). Congenital defect of growth with underdevelopment of parts or organs of the body. [hypo- + G. *genesis,* origin]

polar h., a less than normal degree of development at the cephalic or caudal extremity of the embryo.

hy·po·ge·net·ic (hī'pō-jĕ-net'ik). Relating to hypogenesis.

hy·po·gen·i·tal·ism (hī-pō-jen'i-tăl-izm). Partial or complete failure of maturation of the genitalia; commonly, a consequence of hypogonadism.

hy·po·geu·sia (hī-pō-gū′sē-ă). Blunting of the sense of taste. [hypo- + G. *geusis*, taste]

hy·po·glob·u·lia (hī′pō-glo-byū′lē-ă). Old term for abnormally low numbers of red blood cells in the circulating blood; also used infrequently with reference to abnormally decreased proportions of erythroid elements in the bone marrow. [hypo- + G. *globulus*, globule]

hy·po·glos·sal (hī-pō-glos′ăl). 1. Below the tongue. 2. Relating to the twelfth cranial nerve, nervus hypoglossus. SYN hypoglossus [NA]. [L. *hypoglossus* fr. hypo- + *glossus*, tongue]

hy·po·glos·sis (hī-pō-glos′is). SYN hypoglottis.

hy·po·glos·sus (hī′pō-glos′ŭs) [NA]. SYN hypoglossal, hypoglossal. [L.]

hy·po·glot·tis (hī′pō-glot′is). The undersurface of the tongue. SYN hypoglossis. [G. *hypoglōssis*, or -*glōttis*, undersurface of tongue, fr. *hypo*, under, + *glōssa*, tongue]

hy·po·gly·ce·mia (hī′pō-glī-sē′mē-ă). An abnormally small concentration of glucose in the circulating blood, *i.e.*, less than the minimum of the normal range. SYN glucopenia.

    fasting h., excessively low blood glucose in association with fasting; can be seen in patients with hyperinsulinism but also occurs without definable disease.

    leucine h., reduction in blood glucose concentration produced by administration of leucine; believed to reflect the ability of this amino acid to stimulate insulin secretion.

    leucine-induced h., rare cause of h. occurring following ingestion of leucine. Seen especially in infants.

    mixed h., h. due to more than one cause.

    neonatal h. [MIM*240900], familial onset of symptomatic h. during infancy, with persistently low blood glucose; a variant form [MIM*240800] is leucine-induced with hyperinsulinism and variable mental retardation.

hy·po·gly·ce·mic (hī′pō-glī-sē′mik). Pertaining to or characterized by hypoglycemia.

hy·po·gly·co·gen·ol·y·sis (hī′pō-glī′kō-jĕ-nol′i-sis). Deficient glycogenolysis.

hy·po·gly·cor·rha·chia (hī-pō-glī-kō-rak′ē-ă). Depressed concentration of glucose in the cerebrospinal fluid; a characteristic of bacterial, fungal, and tuberculous meningitis. [hypo- + G. *glykys*, sweet, + *rhachis*, spine]

hy·pog·na·thous (hī′pō-nath′ŭs, hī-pog′na-thŭs). Having a congenitally defectively developed lower jaw. [hypo- + G. *gnathos*, jaw]

hy·pog·na·thus (hī′pō-nath′ŭs, hī-pog′na-thŭs). Unequal conjoined twins in which the rudimentary parasite is attached to the mandible of the autosite. SEE conjoined *twins*, under *twin*. [hypo- + G. *gnathos*, jaw]

hy·po·go·nad·ism (hī′pō-gō′nad-izm). Inadequate gonadal function, as manifested by deficiencies in gametogenesis and/or the secretion of gonadal hormones; results in atrophy or deficient development of secondary sexual characteristics and, when occurring in prepubertal males, in altered body habitus characterized by a short trunk and long limbs.

    familial hypogonadotropic h. [MIM*312100 & MIM*307300], a group of disorders characterized by failure of sexual development, owing to inadequate secretion of pituitary gonadotropins; perhaps X-linked or autosomal recessive inheritance.

    hypergonadotropic h., defective gonadal development or function of the gonads, resulting from elevated levels of gonadotropins.

    hypogonadotropic h., defective gonadal development or function, or both, resulting from inadequate secretion of pituitary gonadotropins. SYN hypogonadotropic eunuchoidism, secondary h.

    male h., SYN eunuchoidism.

    primary h., defective gonadal development or function, or both, due to abnormality or loss of the gonad itself.

    secondary h., SYN hypogonadotropic h.

    h. with anosmia [MIM*308700], failure of sexual development secondary to inadequate secretion of pituitary gonadotropins, associated with anosmia due to agenesis of the olfactory lobes of the brain; probably X-linked inheritance. SYN Kallmann's syndrome.

hy·po·go·nad·o·tro·pic (hī′pō-gon′ă-dō-trop′ik). Indicating inadequate secretion of gonadotropins and its consequences.

hy·po·gran·u·lo·cy·to·sis (hī′pō-gran′yū-lō-sī-tō′sis). SYN granulocytopenia.

hy·po·he·pat·ia (hī′pō-hĕ-pat′ē-ă). Rarely used term for underfunctioning of the liver. [hypo- + G. *hēpar*, liver]

hy·po·hi·dro·sis (hī′pō-hī-drō′sis). Diminished perspiration.

hy·po·hi·drot·ic (hī′pō-hi-drot′ik). Characterized by diminished sweating.

hy·po·hy·dre·mia (hī′pō-hī-drē′mē-ă). Any deficiency in the amount of fluid in the blood. [hypo- + G. *hydōr*, water, + *haima*, blood]

hy·po·hy·dro·chlo·ria (hī′pō-hī-drō-klōr′ē-ă). SYN hypochlorhydria.

hy·po·hy·lo·ma (hī′pō-hī-lō′mă). A neoplasm resulting from abnormal proliferation of tissue derived from the embryonic pulp of hypoblastic origin. [hypo- + G. *hylē*, substance, + *-oma*, tumor]

hy·po·hyp·not·ic (hī′pō-hip-not′ik). Denoting incomplete or light slumber. [hypo- + G. *hypnos*, sleep]

hy·po·i·so·ton·ic (hī′pō-ī-sō-ton′ik). SYN hypotonic.

hy·po·ka·le·mia (hī′pō-ka-lē′mē-ă). The presence of an abnormally small concentration of potassium ions in the circulating blood; occurs in familial periodic paralysis and in potassium depletion due to excessive loss from the gastrointestinal tract or kidneys. The changes of h. may include vacuolation of renal tubular epithelial cytoplasm with impairment of urinary concentrating power and acidification, flattening of the T wave of the electrocardiogram, and muscle weakness. SYN hypopotassemia. [hypo- + Mod. L. *kalium*, potassium, + G. *haima*, blood]

hy·po·ki·ne·mia (hī′pō-ki-nē′mē-ă). Reduced circulation rate; reduced volume flow through the circulation; subnormal cardiac output. [hypo- + G. *kineo*, to move, + *haima*, blood]

hy·po·ki·ne·sis, hy·po·ki·ne·sia (hī′pō-ki-nē′sis, -nē′zē-ă). Diminished or slow movement. SYN hypocinesis, hypocinesia, hypomotility. [hypo- + G. *kinēsis*, movement]

hy·po·ki·net·ic (hī′pō-ki-net′ik). Relating to or characterized by hypokinesis.

hy·po·lep·i·do·ma (hī′pō-lep-i-dō′mă). A neoplasm resulting from abnormal proliferation of one of the tissues derived from the hypoblast. [hypo- + G. *lepis*, rind, + *-oma*, tumor]

hy·po·leu·ke·mia (hī′pō-lū-kē′mē-ă). SYN subleukemic *leukemia*.

hy·po·ley·dig·ism (hī-pō-lī′dig-izm). Subnormal secretion of androgens by the interstitial (Leydig's) cells of the testes.

hy·po·lip·o·pro·teine·mia (hī′pō-lip′ō-prō-tēn-ē-mē-ă). Decreased levels of a lipoprotein in the serum.

hy·po·li·po·sis (hī′pō-li-pō′sis). Presence of an abnormally small amount of fat in the tissues.

hy·po·lo·gia (hī′pō-lō′jē-ă). Lack of ability for speech. [hypo- + G. *logos*, word]

hy·po·lym·phe·mia (hī′pō-lim-fē′mē-ă). Abnormally small numbers of lymphocytes in the circulating blood.

hy·po·mag·ne·se·mia (hī′pō-mag-nē-sē′mē-ă). Subnormal blood serum concentration of magnesium; may cause convulsions and concurrent hypocalcemia.

hy·po·ma·nia (hī′pō-mā′nē-ă). A mild degree of mania.

hy·po·mas·tia (hī′pō-mas′tē-ă). Atrophy or congenital smallness of the breasts. SYN hypomazia. [hypo- + G. *mastos*, breast]

hy·po·ma·zia (hī-pō-mā′zē-ă). SYN hypomastia.

hy·po·mel·an·cho·lia (hī′pō-mel-an-kō′lē-ă). A mild degree of mental depression.

hy·po·mel·a·no·sis (hī′pō-mel-ă-nō′sis). SYN leukoderma.

    h. of Ito, SYN *incontinentia* pigmenti achromians.

hy·po·me·lia (hī-pō-mē′lē-ă). General term for hypoplasia of some or all parts of one or more limbs. [hypo- + G. *melos*, limb]

hy·po·men·or·rhea (hī′pō-men-ō-rē′ă). Diminution of the flow or a shortening of the duration of menstruation. [hypo- + G. *mēn,* month, + *rhoia,* flow]

hy·po·mere (hī′pō-mēr). **1.** The portion of the myotome that extends ventrolaterally to form body-wall muscle, innervated by the primary ventral ramus of a spinal nerve. SEE hypaxial. **2.** Less commonly, the somatic and splanchnic layers of the lateral mesoderm which give rise to the lining of the celom. [hypo- + G. *meros,* part]

hy·po·me·tab·o·lism (hī′pō-me-tab′ō-lizm). Reduced metabolism. SEE ALSO hypometabolic *state.*

euthyroid h., an unusual condition resembling myxedema but with an apparently normal thyroid gland.

hy·po·met·ria (hī′pō-mē′trē-ă). Ataxia characterized by underreaching an object or goal; seen with cerebellar disease. Cf. hypermetria. [hypo- + G. *metron,* measure]

hy·pom·ne·sia (hī-pō-nē′zē-ă). Impaired memory. Cf. hypermnesia. [hypo- + G. *mnēmē,* memory]

hy·po·morph (hī′pō-mōrf). **1.** A person whose standing height is short in proportion to the sitting height, owing to shortness of the limbs. Cf. hypermorph, endomorph. **2.** A mutant gene that causes a partial decrease in the activity controlled by the gene. Cf. hypermorph. [hypo- + G. *morphē,* form]

hy·po·mo·til·i·ty (hī′pō-mō-til′i-tē). SYN hypokinesis.

hy·po·my·e·li·na·tion, hy·po·my·e·lin·o·gen·e·sis (hī′pō-mī′ĕ-lin-ā-shun, -ō-jen′ĕ-sis). Defective formation of myelin in the spinal cord and brain; the basis for a number of demyelinating diseases.

hy·po·my·o·to·nia (hī′pō-mī-ō-tō′nē-ă). A condition of diminished muscular tonus. [hypo- + G. *mys (myo-)* muscle, + *tonos,* tension]

hy·po·myx·ia (hī′pō-mik′sē-ă). A condition in which the secretion of mucus is diminished. [hypo- + G. *myxa,* mucus]

hy·po·na·tre·mia (hī′pō-nă-trē′mē-ă). Abnormally low concentrations of sodium ions in the circulating blood. [hypo- + natrium, + G. *haima,* blood]

depletional h., decreased serum sodium concentration associated with loss of sodium from the circulating blood via the GI tract, kidney, skin, or into "third space." Accompanied by hypovolemic and hypotonic state.

hy·po·ne·o·cy·to·sis (hī′pō-nē′ō-sī-tō′sis). Leukopenia associated with the presence of immature and young leukocytes (especially in the granulocytic series), *i.e.,* a "shift to the left" in the hemogram. SYN hyposkeocytosis. [hypo- + G. *neos,* new, + *kytos,* cell, + *-osis,* condition]

hy·po·noia (hī′pō-noy′-ă). Deficient or sluggish mental activity or imagination. [hypo- + G. *noeō,* to think]

hy·po·nych·i·al (hī′pō-nik′ē-ăl). **1.** SYN subungual. **2.** Relating to the hyponychium.

hy·po·nych·i·um (hī′pō-nik′ē-ŭm) [NA]. The epithelium of the nail bed, particularly its proximal part in the region of the nailroot and lunula, forming the nail matrix. [hypo- + G. *onyx,* nail]

hy·pon·y·chon (hī-pon′i-kon). An ecchymosis beneath a fingernail or toenail. [hypo- + G. *onyx,* nail]

hy·po·on·cot·ic (hī′pō-on-kot′ik). Indicating an oncotic pressure less than normal, *e.g.,* of blood plasma.

hy·po·or·tho·cy·to·sis (hī′pō-ōr′thō-sī-tō′sis). Leukopenia in which the relative numbers of the various types of white blood cells are within the normal range, and no immature cells are found in the circulating blood. [hypo- + G. *orthos,* correct, + *kytos,* cell, + *-osis,* condition]

hy·po·o·var·i·an·ism (hī′pō-ō-vā′rē-an-izm). Inadequate ovarian function, commonly referring to reduced secretion of ovarian hormones. SYN hypovarianism.

hy·po·pan·cre·a·tism (hī′pō-pan′krē-ă-tizm). A condition of diminished activity of digestive enzyme secretion by the pancreas.

hy·po·pan·cre·or·rhea (hī′pō-pan′krē-ō-rē′ă). Reduced delivery of pancreatic digestive enzyme secretions. [hypo- + pancreas + G. *rhoia,* flow]

hy·po·par·a·thy·roid·ism (hī′pō-par-ă-thī′royd-izm). A condition due to diminution or absence of the secretion of the parathy-

roid hormones, with low serum calcium and tetany, and sometimes with increased bone density. SEE ALSO pseudohypoparathyroidism. SYN parathyroid insufficiency.

familial h., idiopathic h. in members of the same family with low serum calcium and tetany, and sometimes with increased bone density; all three mendelian forms of inheritance are known [MIM*146200, *241400, *307700].

hy·po·pep·sia (hī-pō-pep′sē-ă). Impaired digestion, especially that due to a deficiency of pepsin. SYN oligopepsia. [hypo- + G. *pepsis,* digestion]

hy·po·per·i·stal·sis (hī′pō-per-i-stal′sis). Reduced or inadequate peristalsis.

hy·po·pha·lan·gism (hī′pō-fă-lan′jizm). Congenital absence of one or more of the phalanges of a finger or toe.

hy·po·phar·ynx (hī′pō-far′inks). SYN laryngopharynx.

hy·po·pho·ne·sis (hī′pō-fō-nē′sis). In percussion or auscultation, a sound that is diminished or fainter than usual. [hypo- + G. *phōnēsis,* a sounding]

hy·po·pho·nia (hī′pō-fō′nē-ă). An abnormally weak voice due to incoordination of the muscles concerned in vocalization. SYN leptophonia, microphonia, microphony. [hypo- + G. *phōnē,* voice]

hy·po·pho·ria (hī′pō-fō′rē-ă). A tendency of the visual axis of one eye to deviate downward, prevented by binocular vision. [hypo- + G. *phora,* motion]

hy·po·phos·pha·ta·se·mia (hī′pō-fos′fă-tă-sē′mē-ă). SYN hypophosphatasia.

hy·po·phos·pha·ta·sia (hī′pō-fos′fă-tā′zē-ă). An abnormally low content of alkaline phosphatase in the circulating blood. SYN hypophosphatasemia.

adult h., an autosomal dominant trait with early loss of teeth, bowing, and beaten-copper skull; there is evidence that the basic defect is in liver alkaline phosphatase.

childhood h., a relatively mild autosomal recessive form of h.; it may be allelic with congenital h.

congenital h. [MIM*241500], a rare disorder associated with a low level of serum alkaline phosphatase, hyperphosphaturia, hypercalcemia, skeletal abnormalities, pathologic fractures, craniostenosis, and often early death; eyes may show blue sclerae, lid retraction, band-shaped keratopathy, cataracts, papilledema, and optic atrophy.

hy·po·phos·pha·te·mia (hī′pō-fos-fă-tē′mē-ă). Abnormally low concentrations of phosphates in the circulating blood. See also entries under rickets.

hy·po·phos·pha·tu·ria (hī′pō-fos′fă-tū′rē-ă). Reduced urinary excretion of phosphates.

hy·po·phos·pho·rous ac·id (hī-pō-fos′fō-rŭs). An aqueous solution containing 31% HPH_2O_2; used as a stabilizing reducing agent in pharmaceutical preparations.

hy·po·phra·sia (hī′pō-frā′zē-ă). Slowness or lack of speech associated with a psychosis or brain injury. [hypo- + G. *phrasis,* speaking]

hy·po·phy·se·al (hī′pō-fiz′ē-ăl). SYN hypophysial.

hy·po·phy·sec·to·mize (hī′pof-i-sek′tō-mīz). To remove the pituitary gland.

hy·poph·y·sec·to·my (hī′pof-i-sek′tō-mē). Surgical removal of the hypophysis or pituitary gland.

hy·po·phys·e·o·priv·ic (hī′pō-fiz′ē-ō-priv′ik). SYN hypophysioprivic.

hy·po·phys·e·o·tro·pic (hī′pō-fiz′ē-ō-trop′ik). SYN hypophysiotropic.

hy·po·phy·si·al (hī′pō-fiz′ē-ăl). Relating to a hypophysis. SYN hypophyseal.

hy·poph·y·sin (hī-pof′i-sin). An aqueous extract of the posterior lobe of the fresh hypophysis of cattle; contains oxytocin and vasopressin.

hy·po·phys·i·o·priv·ic (hī′pō-fiz′ē-ō-priv′ik). Denoting the condition in which the pituitary gland may be functionally inactive or may be absent, as after hypophysectomy. SYN hypophyseoprivic. [hypophysis + L. *privus,* deprived of]

hy·po·phys·i·o·tro·pic (hī′pō-fiz′ē-ō-trop′ik). Denoting a stimu-

hy

latory hormone that acts on the pituitary gland (hypophysis). SYN hypophyseotropic.

hy·poph·y·sis (hī-pof′i-sis) [NA]. An unpaired compound gland suspended from the base of the hypothalamus by a short extension of the infundibulum, the infundibular or pituitary stalk. The h. consists of two major subdivisions: 1) the neurohypophysis, comprising the infundibulum and its bulbous termination, the neural part or infundibular process (posterior lobe), which is composed of neuroglia-like pituicytes, blood vessels, and unmyelinated nerve fibers of the hypothalamohypophyseal tract whose cell bodies reside in the supraoptic and paraventricular nuclei of the hypothalamus, and convey to the lobe for storage and release the neurosecretory hormones oxytocin and antidiuretic hormone; 2) the adenohypophysis, comprising the larger distal part, a sleeve-like extension of this lobe (infundibular part) which invests the infundibular stalk, and a thin intermediate part (poorly developed in humans) between the anterior and posterior lobes; the anterior lobe consists of cords of cells of several different types interspersed with capillaries of the hypothalamohypophysial portal system; secretion of somatotropins, prolactin, thyroid-stimulating hormone, gonadotropins, adrenal corticotropin, and other related peptides in the adenohypophysis is regulated by releasing and inhibiting factors elaborated by neurons in the hypothalamus which are taken up by a primary plexus of capillaries in the median eminence and transported via portal vessels in the infundibular part and infundibular stem to a secondary plexus of capillaries in the distal part. SEE ALSO hypothalamus. SYN glandula pituitaria [NA], basal gland, glandula basilaris, h. cerebri, master gland, pituitary gland. [G. an undergrowth]

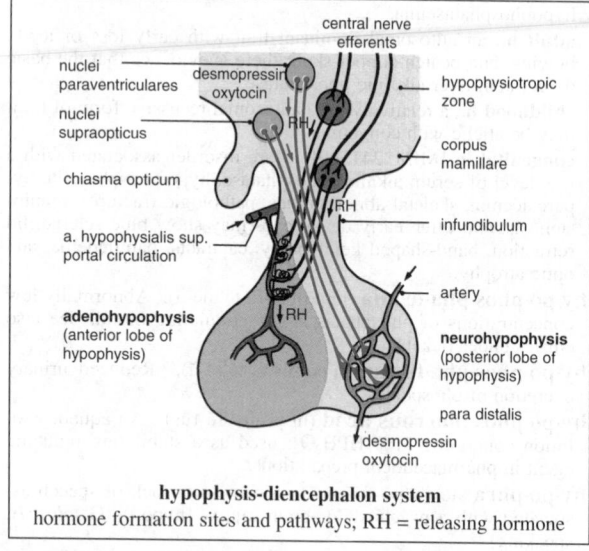

nuclei paraventriculares
desmopressin oxytocin
central nerve efferents
hypophysiotropic zone
nuclei supraopticus
corpus mamillare
chiasma opticum
RH
RH
infundibulum
a. hypophysialis sup. portal circulation
artery
adenohypophysis (anterior lobe of hypophysis)
RH
neurohypophysis (posterior lobe of hypophysis)
para distalis
desmopressin oxytocin

hypophysis-diencephalon system
hormone formation sites and pathways; RH = releasing hormone

h. cere′bri, SYN hypophysis.

pharyngeal h., residual tissue derived from the hypophysial diverticulum that lies in the lamina propria of the nasopharynx; its cells and their arrangement are identical with those of the pars distalis. SYN pars pharyngea hypophyseos.

h. sic′ca, SYN posterior *pituitary.*

hy·poph·y·si·tis (hī-pof-i-sī′tis). Inflammation of the hypophysis.

lymphocytic h., an acute anterior pituitary lymphocytic reaction characterized clinically by signs and symptoms of anterior pituitary insufficiency; probably an autoimmune disorder because antipituitary antibodies are present in the serum. SYN lymphoid h.

lymphoid h., SYN lymphocytic h.

hy·po·pi·e·sis (hī′pō-pī-ē′sis). SYN hypotension (1). [hypo- + G. *piesis,* pressure]

orthostatic h., SYN orthostatic *hypotension.*

hy·po·pi·tu·i·ta·rism (hī′pō-pi-tū′i-tă-rizm). A condition due to diminished activity of the anterior lobe of the hypophysis, with inadequate secretion, to varying degrees, of one or more anterior pituitary hormones.

hy·po·pla·sia (hī′pō-plā′zē-ă). **1.** Underdevelopment of a tissue or organ, usually due to a decrease in the number of cells. **2.** Atrophy due to destruction of some of the elements and not merely to their general reduction in size. [hypo- + G. *plasis,* a molding]

cartilage-hair h. [MIM*250250 & MIM*250460], an autosomal recessive form of dwarfism characterized by shortness of the extremities without skull defects, and with sparse, brittle hair of light color. There is a peculiar, not adequately explained severity in the clinical course of varicella and herpes in such patients.

enamel h., a developmental disturbance of teeth characterized by deficient or defective enamel matrix formation; may be hereditary, as in amelogenesis imperfecta, or acquired, as encountered in dental fluorosis, local infection, childhood fevers, and congenital syphilis.

focal dermal h. [MIM*305600], widely distributed linear areas of dermal hypoplasia resembling striae distensae, with soft yellow nodules of fat herniation usually in females, probably an X-linked dominant trait with high intrauterine homozygous male mortality. SYN Goltz syndrome.

optic nerve h., congenitally small optic disk resulting from failure of development of retinal ganglion cells, with a reduced number of axons; visual impairment may be marked. SEE de Morsier's *syndrome.*

renal h., an abnormally small kidney that is morphologically normal but has either a reduced number of nephrons or smaller nephrons.

h. of right ventricle, failure of development of the right ventricle resulting in its having little muscle and much connective tissue instead of the reverse.

right ventricular h., SYN parchment *heart.*

thymic h., SYN *immunodeficiency* with hypoparathyroidism.

hy·po·plas·tic (hī′pō-plas′tik). Pertaining to or characterized by hypoplasia.

hy·po·pnea (hī-pop′nē-ă). Breathing that is shallower, and/or slower, than normal. SYN oligopnea. [hypo- + G. *pnoē,* breathing]

hy·po·po·sia (hī′pō-pō′sē-ă). Hypodipsia, with emphasis on reduced tendency to drink rather than on the reduced sensation of thirst. [hypo- + G. *posis,* drinking]

hy·po·po·tas·se·mia (hī′pō-pō-ta-sē′mē-ă). SYN hypokalemia.

hy·po·prax·ia (hī-pō-prak′sē-ă). Deficient activity. [hypo- + G. *praxis,* action, + *-ia,* condition]

hy·po·pro·ac·cel·er·i·ne·mia (hī′pō-prō-ak-sel′er-i-nē′mē-ă). Abnormally low concentration of blood-clotting factor V, *i.e.,* proaccelerin, in the circulating blood.

hy·po·pro·con·ver·ti·ne·mia (hī′pō-prō-kon-ver′ti-nē′mē-ă). Abnormally low concentration of blood-clotting factor VII, *i.e.,* proconvertin, in the circulating blood; a deficiency causes a quantitative prolongation of the prothrombin time.

hy·po·pro·tein·e·mia (hī′pō-prō′tē-in-ē′mē-ă, -prō′tēn-). Abnormally small amounts of total protein in the circulating blood plasma.

hy·po·pro·tein·o·sis (hī′pō-prō′tē-in-o′sis, -prō′tēn-). A condition, especially in children, due to a dietary deficiency of protein; characterized by anorexia, vomiting, retardation of growth, anemia, and increased susceptibility to infections.

hy·po·pro·throm·bin·e·mia (hī′pō-prō-throm′bin-ē′mē-ă). Abnormally small amounts of prothrombin in the circulating blood. SYN prothrombinopenia.

hy·pop·ty·a·lism (hī′pō-tī′ă-lizm). SYN hyposalivation. [hypo- + G. *ptyalon,* saliva]

hy·po·py·on (hī-pō′pi-on). The presence of leukocytes in the anterior chamber of the eye. [hypo- + G. *pyon,* pus]

recurrent h., SYN Behçet's *syndrome.*

hy·po·re·flex·ia (hī′pō-rē-flek′sē-ă). A condition in which the reflexes are weakened.

hy·po·ren·i·ne·mia (hī′pō-ren-i-nē′mē-ă). Low levels of renin in the circulating blood.

hy·po·ren·i·nem·ic (hī′pō-ren-i-nē′mik). Denoting or characterized by hyporeninemia.

hy·po·ri·bo·fla·vin·o·sis (hī′pō-rī′bō-flā-vi-nō′sis). A more correct term than the more commonly used ariboflavinosis (*q.v.,*)

hy·po·sal·e·mi·a (hī-pō-să-lē′mē-ă). Obsolete term meaning abnormally small amounts of various salts in the circulating blood; sometimes was used as a synonym for hypochloremia. [hypo- + L. *sal,* salt, + G. *haima,* blood]

hy·po·sal·i·va·tion (hī′pō-sal′i-vā′shŭn). Reduced salivation. SYN hypoptyalism.

hy·po·sar·ca (hī′pō-sar′kă). Extreme anasarca of the subcutaneous connective tissue. [hypo- + G. *sarx* (sark-), flesh]

hy·pos·che·ot·o·my (hī-pos-kē-ot′ō-mē). Incision or puncture into a hydrocele at its most dependent point. [hypo- + G. *oscheon,* scrotum, + *tomē,* incision]

hy·po·scle·ral (hī-pō-sklēr′ăl). Beneath the sclerotic coat of the eyeball.

hy·po·sen·si·tiv·i·ty (hī′pō-sen-si-tiv′i-tē). A condition of subnormal sensitivity, in which the response to a stimulus is unusually delayed or lessened in degree.

hy·po·sen·si·ti·za·tion. SYN desensitization.

hy·po·ske·o·cy·to·sis (hī′pō-skē′ō-sī-tō′sis). SYN hyponeocytosis. [hypo- + *skaios,* left, + *kytos,* cell, + *-osis,* condition]

hy·pos·mia (hī-poz′mē-ă). Diminished sense of smell. SYN hyposphresia, olfactory hypesthesia. [hypo- + G. *osmē,* smell]

hy·pos·mo·sis (hī-pos-mō′sis). A reduction in the rapidity of osmosis.

hy·pos·mot·ic (hī-pos-mot′ik). Having an osmolality less than another fluid, ordinarily assumed to be plasma or extracellular fluid.

hy·po·so·ma·to·tro·pism (hī′pō-sō′mă-tō-trō′pizm). A state characterized by deficient secretion of pituitary growth hormone (somatotropin).

hy·po·so·mia (hī′pō-sō′mē-ă). Inadequate development of the body. [hypo- + G. *sōma,* body]

hy·po·som·ni·ac (hī′pō-som′nē-ak). Pertaining to reduction in time of sleeping. [hypo- + L. *somnus,* sleep]

hy·po·spa·di·ac (hī′pō-spā′dē-ak). Relating to hypospadias.

hy·po·spa·di·as (hī′pō-spā′dē-ăs). A developmental anomaly characterized by a defect on the ventrum of the penis so that the urethral meatus is more proximal than its normal glandular location; may be associated with chordee; also a similar defect in the female in which the urethra opens into the vagina. Cf. epispadias. [G. one having the orifice of the penis too low, fr. *hypospaō,* to draw away from under]

balanic h., SYN glanular h.

coronal h., ventral and proximal malposition of meatus in the coronal sulcus.

glanular h., ventral and proximal glanular malposition of urethral meatus in a male. SYN balanic h.

penile h., ventral and proximal malposition of urethral meatus on penile shaft.

penoscrotal h., h. with the urethral opening at the junction of the penis and scrotum.

perineal h., h. in which the urethral defect continues along the perineum to near the anus; the scrotum is usually cleft, the testes undescended, and the penis rudimentary.

subcoronal h., ventral and proximal malposition of coronal meatus just proximal to coronal sulcus.

hy·pos·phre·sia (hī′pos-frē′zē-ă). SYN hyposmia. [hypo- + G. *osphrēsis,* smell]

hy·po·sphyx·ia (hī′pō-sfik′sē-ă). Abnormally low blood pressure with sluggishness of the circulation. [hypo- + G. *sphyxis,* pulse]

hy·po·splen·ism (hī′pō-splēn′izm). Absent or reduced splenic function, usually due to surgical removal, congenital aplasia, tumor replacement, or splenic vascular accident. Red cell abnormalities, including the presence of inclusions, nucleated erythrocytes, and target cells, are commonly present. Patients with h. are at increased risk of bacterial sepsis, especially due to pneumococcus.

hy·pos·ta·sis (hi-pos′tă-sis). **1.** Formation of a sediment at the bottom of a liquid. **2.** SYN hypostatic *congestion.* **3.** The phenomenon whereby the phenotype that would ordinarily be manifested at one locus is obscured by the genotype at another epistatic locus; *e.g.,* in humans, the phenotype for the ABO blood group locus can be expressed only in the presence of its precursor, H substance. The Bombay factor in the homozygous state blocks H formation and obscures the ABO phenotype. [G. *hypo-stasis,* a standing under, sediment]

postmortem h., SYN postmortem *livedo.*

pulmonary h., hydrostatic congestion of the lung.

hy·po·stat·ic (hī-pō-stat′ik). **1.** Sedimentary; resulting from a dependent position. **2.** Relating to hypostasis.

hy·po·sthe·nia (hī′pō-thē′nē-ă). Weakness. SEE asthenia. [hypo- + G. *sthenos,* strength]

hy·pos·the·ni·ant (hī′pos-thē′nē-ant). **1.** Weakening. **2.** An agent that reduces strength.

hy·po·sthen·ic (hī-pos-then′ik). Weak.

hy·pos·the·nu·ria (hī′pos-thĕ-nū′rē-ă). Secretion of urine of low specific gravity, due to inability of the tubules of the kidneys to produce a concentrated urine; also occurs following excessive water ingestion in diabetes insipidus. [hypo- + G. *sthenos,* strength, + *ouron,* urine]

hy·po·stome (hī′pō-stōm). The central unpaired holdfast organ of the tick capitulum; the h. is covered with recurved spines that enable it to serve as an anchoring device while the tick feeds. [hypo- + G. *stoma,* mouth]

hy·po·sto·mia (hī′pō-stō′mē-ă). A form of microstomia in which the oral opening is a small vertical slit. [hypo- + G. *stoma,* mouth]

hyp·os·to·sis (hīp-os-tō′sis). Deficient development of bone. [hypo- + G. *osteon,* bone, + *-osis,* condition]

hy·po·styp·sis (hī′pō-stip′sis). A state of mild astringence. [hypo- + G. *stypsis,* astringence]

hy·po·styp·tic (hī′pō-stip′tik). Mildly styptic or astringent.

hy·po·supra·dren·al·ism (hī′pō-sū′pră-ă-drē′nal- izm). SYN chronic adrenocortical *insufficiency.*

hy·po·sys·to·le (hī′pō-sis′tō-lē). A weak or incomplete cardiac systole.

hy·po·tax·ia (hī′pō-tak′sē-ă). A condition of weak or imperfect coordination. [hypo- + G. *taxis,* order]

hy·po·tel·or·ism (hī-pō-tel′ōr-izm). Abnormal closeness of eyes. [hypo- + G. *tēle,* far off, + *horizō,* to separate, fr. *horos,* boundary]

hy·po·ten·sion (hī′pō-ten′shŭn). **1.** Subnormal arterial blood pressure. SYN hypopiesis. **2.** Reduced pressure or tension of any kind. [hypo- + L. *tensio,* a stretching]

arterial h., SEE hypotension (1).

idiopathic orthostatic h., the tendency for blood pressure to drop for unknown reasons on assuming upright posture.

induced h., controlled h., deliberate acute reduction of arterial blood pressure to reduce operative blood loss by pharmacologic means during anesthesia and surgery.

intracranial h., subnormal pressure of cerebrospinal fluid; most commonly following lumbar puncture and associated with headache, nausea, vomiting, stiffness of the neck, and sometimes fever; may also result from dehydration.

orthostatic h., a form of low blood pressure that occurs in a standing posture. SYN orthostatic hypopiesis, postural h.

postural h., SYN orthostatic h.

hy·po·ten·sive (hī′pō-ten′siv). Characterized by low blood pressure or causing reduction in blood pressure.

hy·po·ten·sor (hī-pō-ten′ser, -sōr). SYN depressor (4).

hy·po·thal·a·mo·hy·po·phy·si·al (hī′pō-thal′ă-mō-hī′pō-fiz′ē-ăl). Relating to both the hypothalamus and the hypophysis.

hy·po·thal·a·mus (hī′pō-thal′ă-mŭs) [NA]. The ventral and medial region of the diencephalon forming the walls of the ventral half of the third ventricle; it is delineated from the thalamus by the hypothalamic sulcus, lying medial to the internal capsule and subthalamus, continuous with the precommissural septum anteriorly and with the mesencephalic tegmentum and central gray

hy

substance posteriorly. Its ventral surface is marked by, from before backward, the optic chiasma, the unpaired infundibulum that extends by way of the infundibular stalk into the posterior lobe of the hypophysis, and the paired mamillary bodies. The nerve cells of the h. are grouped into the supraoptic paraventricular, lateral preoptic, lateral hypothalamic, tuberal, anterior hypothalamic, ventromedial, dorsomedial, arcuate, posterior hypothalamic, and premamillary nuclei and the mamillary body. It has afferent fiber connections with the mesencephalon, limbic system, cerebellum, and efferent fiber connections with the same structures and with the posterior lobe of the hypophysis; its functional connection with the anterior lobe of the hypophysis is established by the hypothalamohypophysial portal system. The h. is prominently involved in the functions of the autonomic nervous system and, through its vascular link with the anterior lobe of the hypophysis, in endocrine mechanisms; it also appears to play a role in neural mechanisms underlying moods and motivational states. SEE ALSO hypophysis. [hypo- + thalamus]

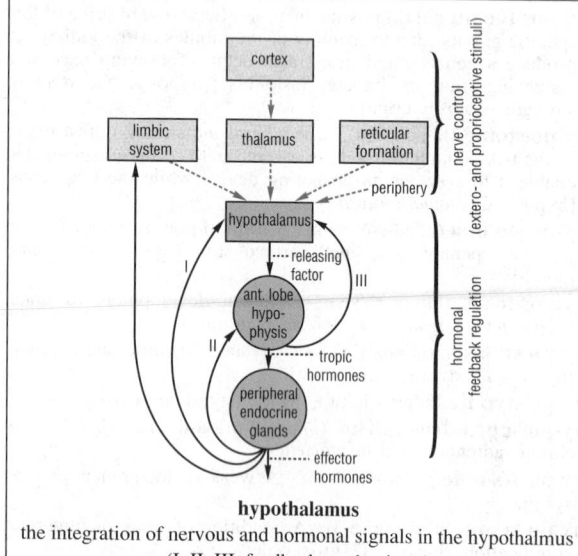

hypothalamus
the integration of nervous and hormonal signals in the hypothalmus
(I, II, III, feedback mechanisms)

hy·po·the·nar (hī'pō-thē'nar, hī-poth'ĕ-nar). **1** [NA]. SYN hypothenar *eminence.* **2.** Denoting any structure in relation with the hypothenar eminence or its underlying collective components. [hypo- + G. *thenar,* the palm]

hy·po·ther·mal (hī-pō-ther'măl). Denoting hypothermia.

hy·po·ther·mia (hī'pō-ther'mē-ă). A body temperature significantly below 98.6°F (37°C). [hypo- + G. *thermē,* heat]

accidental h., unintentional decrease in body temperature, especially in the newborn, infants, and elderly, particularly during operations.

moderate h., a body temperature of 23–32°C. induced by surface cooling.

profound h., a body temperature of 12–20°C.

regional h., reduction of the temperature of an extremity or organ by external cold or perfusion with cold blood or solutions.

total body h., the deliberate reduction of total body temperature, in order to reduce tissue metabolism.

hy·poth·e·sis (hī-poth'ĕ-sis). A conjecture advanced for heuristic purposes, cast in a form that is amenable to confirmation or refutation by the conductance of definable experiments and the critical assembly of empirical data; not to be confused with assumption, postulation, or unfocused speculation. SEE ALSO postulate, theory. [G. foundation, assumption fr. *hypotithenai,* to lay down]

adaptor h., a h., proposed by F.H.C. Crick, that an adaptor molecule must be present between the information-containing DNA and the protein being synthesized.

alternative h., in Neyman-Pearson testing of a h., the h. or family of hypotheses about the numerical value of a parameter if and only if the null h. is rejected as untenable.

autocrine h., that tumor cells containing viral oncogenes may have encoded a growth factor, normally produced by other cell types, and thereby produce the factor autonomously, leading to uncontrolled proliferation.

Avogadro's h., SYN Avogadro's *law.*

Bayesian h., an array of surmised values of a parameter to be severally explored in the light of a current set of data, with logical symmetry being preserved among all. The merits of each h. entertained are based on quantity, the prior probability. The probability of the data conditional on the h. is computed as the conditional probability for each; the product of the two for each h. is the joint probability, and the ratio of each joint probability to the sum of all the joint probabilities is the posterior probability for that h. Unlike the Neyman-Pearson test of hypotheses, the answer is a statement about the h., not about the sample conditional on the h. No h. is preferred or prevails by default. The procedure may be applied recursively any number of times, as the data becomes available.

frustration-aggression h., the theory that frustration may lead to aggression, but that aggression is always the result of some form of frustration.

gate-control h., SYN gate-control *theory.*

Gompertz' h., a theory that the force of mortality increases in geometrical progression, being based on the assumption that the average exhaustion of a person's power to avoid death is such that at the end of equal infinitely small intervals of time he loses equal proportions of the power to oppose destruction which he had at the commencement of each of these intervals.

insular h., obsolete theory of the origin of diabetes mellitus from destruction or loss of function of the islets of Langerhans in the pancreas.

Lyon h., SYN lyonization.

Makeham's h., a development of Gompertz' h. as to the force of mortality following some mathematical law. Makeham assumed that death was the consequence of two generally coexisting causes: 1) chance; 2) a deterioration or increased inability to withstand destruction. The first of these is constant, the second is an increasing geometrical progression.

Michaelis-Menten h., that a complex is formed between an enzyme and its substrate (the O'Sullivan-Tompson h.), which complex then decomposes to yield free enzyme and the reaction products (Brown h.), the latter rate determining the overall rate of substrate-product conversion. SEE ALSO Michaelis-Menten *constant,* Michaelis-Menten *equation.*

mnemic h., the theory that stimuli or irritants leave definite traces (engrams) on the protoplasm of the animal or plant, and when these stimuli are regularly repeated they induce a habit which persists after the stimuli cease; assuming that the germ cells share with the nerve cells in the possession of engrams, acquired habits may thus be transmitted to the descendants. SYN mnemic theory, mnemism, Semon-Hering theory.

Neyman-Pearson statistical h., a formal conjecture about the numerical value of a parameter to be tested exclusively in the light of an immediate set of data without attention to prior knowledge or convictions and ignoring other sets of evidence treated in a similar fashion. The answer is a statement about whether the h. is true but whether it is an acceptable explanation of the data or should be rejected in favor of another h.

null h., the statistical hypothesis that one variable has no association with another variable or set of variables, or that two or more populations do not differ from each other; the statement that results do not differ from those that might be expected by the operation of chance alone; if rejected, it increases confidence in the h.

sequence h., that the amino acid sequence of a protein is determined by a particular sequence of nucleotides (the cistron) in the DNA of the organism producing the protein.

sliding filament h., the theory that the contracting muscle shortens because two sets of filaments slide past each other.

Starling's h., the principle that net filtration through capillary membranes is proportional to the transmembrane hydrostatic pressure difference minus the transmembrane oncotic pressure difference; although well established, it is called Starling's h. to distinguish it from Starling's law of the heart.

wobble h., SEE wobble *base*, wobble.

zwitter h., that an amphoteric molecule (*e.g.*, an amino acid) has, at its isoelectric point, equal numbers of positive and negative charges, thus becoming a zwitterion.

hy·po·throm·bi·ne·mia (hī′pō-throm-bin-ē′mē-ă). Abnormally small amounts of thrombin in the circulating blood, thereby resulting in bleeding tendency.

hy·po·throm·bo·plas·ti·ne·mia (hī′pō-throm′bō-plas-ti-nē′mē-ă). Abnormally small amounts of thromboplastin in the blood, as a result of deficient quantities being released from the tissues.

hy·po·thy·mia (hī′pō-thī′mē-ă). Depression of spirits; the "blues." [hypo- + G. *thymos*, mind, soul]

hy·po·thy·mic (hī′pō-thī′mik). **1.** Obsolete term denoting or characteristic of hypothymia. **2.** Obsolete term pertaining to hypothymism.

hy·po·thy·mism (hī′pō-thī′mizm). Obsolete term for inadequate function of the thymus.

hy·po·thy·roid (hī′pō-thī′royd). Marked by reduced thyroid function.

hy·po·thy·roid·ism (hī′pō-thī′royd-izm). Diminished production of thyroid hormone, leading to clinical manifestations of thyroid insufficiency, including low metabolic rate, tendency to weight gain, somnolence and sometimes myxedema. SYN athyrea (1). [hypo- + G. *thyreoeidēs*, thyroid]

congenital h., lack of thyroid secretion. SEE infantile h.

infantile h., can be due to endemic congenital goiter, nonendemic cases are usually due to defective thyroidal embryogenesis, defective hypothalamic-pituitary function, congenital defects in thyroid hormone synthesis or action, or intrauterine exposure to goitrogenic agents. SYN Brissaud's infantilism, congenital myxedema, dysthyroidal infantilism, hypothyroid dwarfism, hypothyroid infantilism, infantile myxedema, myxedematous infantilism.

secondary h., h. that arises as a consequence of inadequate thyrotropin secretion by the anterior pituitary gland.

hy·po·thy·rox·i·ne·mia (hī′pō-thī-rok-sin-ē′mē-ă). A subnormal thyroxine concentration in the blood.

hy·po·to·nia (hī′pō-tō′nē-ă). **1.** Reduced tension in any part, as in the eyeball. **2.** Relaxation of the arteries. **3.** A condition in which there is a diminution or loss of muscular tonicity, in consequence of which the muscles may be stretched beyond their normal limits. SYN hypotonicity (1), hypotonus, hypotony. [hypo- + G. *tonos*, tone]

hy·po·ton·ic (hī′pō-ton′ik). **1.** Having a lesser degree of tension. **2.** Having a lesser osmotic pressure than a reference solution, which is ordinarily assumed to be blood plasma or interstitial fluid; more specifically, refers to a fluid in which cells would swell. SYN hypoisotonic.

hy·po·to·nic·i·ty (hī′pō-tō-nis′i-tē). **1.** SYN hypotonia. **2.** A decreased effective osmotic pressure.

hy·po·to·nus, hy·pot·o·ny (hī′pō-tō′nŭs, hī-pot′ō-nē). SYN hypotonia.

hy·po·tox·ic·i·ty (hī′pō-toks-is′i-tē). Reduced toxicity; the quality of being only slightly poisonous.

hy·po·tri·chi·a·sis (hī′pō-tri-kī′ă-sis). **1.** SYN hypotrichosis. **2.** SYN *alopecia* congenitalis. [hypo- + G. *trichiasis*, hairiness]

hy·po·tri·cho·sis (hī′pō-tri-kō′sis). A less than normal amount of hair on the head and/or body. SYN hypotrichiasis (1), oligotrichia, oligotrichosis. [hypo- + G. *trichōsis*, hairiness]

h. congen′ita, autosomal recessive condition seen in Guernsey and Holstein cattle.

hy·po·tro·pia (hī′pō-trō′pē-ă). An ocular deviation with one eye lower than the other. [hypo- + G. *trope*, turn]

hy·po·tym·pa·not·o·my (hī′pō-tim-pă-not′ō-mē). Operative procedure for the complete surgical extirpation, without sacrifice of hearing, of small tumors confined to the lower tympanic cavity. [hypo- + G. *tympanon*, tympanum, + *tome*, incision]

hy·po·tym·pa·num (hī′pō-tim′pă-nŭm). The lower part of the tympanic cavity. It is separated by a bony wall from the jugular bulb.

hy·po·u·re·sis (hī′pō-yū-rē′sis). Reduced flow of urine.

hy·po·u·ri·ce·mia (hī′pō-yū-ri-sē′mē-ă). Reduced blood concentration of uric acid.

hy·po·u·ri·cu·ria (hī′pō-yū′ri-kyū′rē-ă). Reduced excretion of uric acid in the urine.

hereditary renal h., an autosomal recessive disorder caused by defective reabsorption of urate in the renal proximal tubule.

hy·po·var·i·an·ism (hī′pō-vā′rē-an-izm). SYN hypoovarianism.

hy·po·ven·ti·la·tion (hī′pō-ven-ti-lā′shŭn). Reduced alveolar ventilation relative to metabolic carbon dioxide production, so that alveolar carbon dioxide pressure increases above normal. SYN underventilation.

hy·po·vi·ta·min·o·sis (hī′pō-vī′tă-min-ō′sis). A nutritional deficiency state characterized by relative insufficiency of one or more vitamins in the diet; manifested first by depletion of tissue levels, then by functional changes, and finally by appearance of morphologic lesions. Cf. avitaminosis.

hy·po·vo·le·mia (hī′pō-vō-lē′mē-ă). A decreased amount of blood in the body. SYN hyphemia. [hypo- + L. *volumen*, volume, + G. *haima*, blood]

hy·po·vo·le·mic (hī′pō-vō-lē′mik). Pertaining to or characterized by hypovolemia.

hy·po·vo·lia (hī-pō-vō′lē-ă). Diminished water content or volume of a given compartment; *e.g.*, extracellular h. [hypo- + L. *volumen*, volume]

hy·po·xan·thine (Hyp) (hī-pō-zan′thin). 6-Oxypurine; purin-6(1*H*)-one; a purine present in the muscles and other tissues, formed during purine catabolism by deamination of adenine; elevated in molybdenum-cofactor deficiency. SYN 6-hydroxypurine.

h. guanine phosphoribosyltransferase (HGPRT), SYN h. phosphoribosyltransferase.

h. oxidase, SYN *xanthine* oxidase.

h. phosphoribosyltransferase, an enzyme present in human tissue that converts h. and guanine to their respective 5′ nucleotides, with 5-phosphoribose 1-diphosphate as the ribose-phosphate donor; a partial deficiency of this enzyme can result in elevated purine biosynthesis resulting in gout; another level of deficiency is associated with Lesch-Nyhan syndrome. SYN h. guanine phosphoribosyltransferase.

hy·po·xan·thin·o·sine (hī′pō-zan-thēn′ō-sēn). SYN inosine.

hy·pox·e·mia (hī-pok-sē′mē-ă). Subnormal oxygenation of arterial blood, short of anoxia. [hypo- + oxygen, + G. *haima*, blood]

hy·pox·ia (hī-pok′sē-ă). Decrease below normal levels of oxygen in inspired gases, arterial blood, or tissue, short of anoxia. [hypo- + oxygen]

anemic h., h. resulting from a decreased concentration of functional hemoglobin or a reduced number of erythrocytes; it is caused by hemorrhage or anemia of various types, or by poisoning with CO_2, nitrites, or chlorates.

diffusion h., abrupt transient decrease in alveolar oxygen tension when room air is inhaled at the conclusion of a nitrous oxide anesthesia, because nitrous oxide diffusing out of the blood dilutes the alveolar oxygen.

hypoxic h., h. resulting from a defective mechanism of oxygena-

---

⚠ **Combining forms**	**[NA] Nomina Anatomica**
Word*Finder*	**[MIM] Mendelian**
Multi-term entry finder	**Inheritance in Man**
Preceding letter A	
	☆ **Official alternate term**
A.D.A.M. Anatomy Plates	
Between letters L and M	☆**[NA] Official alternate**
	Nomina Anatomica term
Appendices:	
Following letter Z	
	High Profile Term
SYN Synonym; Cf., compare	

symptoms of general hypoxia			
organ/function	light	medium	severe
mind or brain	euphoria, loss of orientation	vision difficulties, anxiety	dizziness, delirium, coma
gastro-intestinal tract	nausea	desire to vomit	vomiting
neurosensory tract	headache	chest pains	depression, irregular Cheyne-Stokes respiration, cessation
breathing	faster and deeper	apnea, after O_2 intake	abrupt drop
arterial blood pressure	slightly increased (systolic and diastolic)	high	very weak, arrhythmic, vanishing
pulse	faster, sometimes irregular	slower, strained, irregular	relaxation, paralysis
muscles	lack of coordination	spasms, rigidity, convulsions	dark blue, blue-gray, then clammy
skin			
with normal Hb	lightly cyanotic (acc. to Hb content) warm, moist	blue-red deep cyanotic warm and moist	gray, clammy
with anemia	bluish, relatively dry	blue-gray, moist, sometimes heavy sweating	
pupils	irregular	alternating wideness	extremely dilated, rigid
venous pressure	somewhat higher	much increased	falling

tion in the lungs; may be caused by a low tension of oxygen, abnormal pulmonary function or respiratory obstruction, or a right-to-left shunt in the heart.

ischemic h., tissue h. characterized by tissue oligemia and caused by arterial or arteriolar obstruction or vasoconstriction.

oxygen affinity h., h. due to reduced ability of hemoglobin to release oxygen.

stagnant h., tissue h. characterized not by tissue oligemia (tissue blood volume being normal or even increased), but by intravascular stasis due to impairment of venous outflow or (in some instances) to decreased arterial inflow.

hy·pox·ic (hī-pok′sik). Denoting or characterized by hypoxia.

hyp·sa·rhyth·mia, hyp·sar·rhyth·mia (hip′să-rith′mē-ă). The abnormal and characteristically chaotic electroencephalogram commonly found in patients with infantile spasms. [G. *hypsi*, high, + *a*- priv. + *rhythmos*, rhythm]

△**hypsi-, hypso-.** High, height. [G. *hypsos*, height]

hyp·si·brach·y·ce·phal·ic (hip-sē-brak′e-sĕ-fal′ik). Having a high broad head. [hypsi- + G. *brachys*, broad, + *kephalē*, head]

hyp·si·ceph·a·ly (hip-si-sef′ă-lē). SYN oxycephaly. [hypsi- + G. *kephalē*, head]

hyp·si·con·chous (hip-si-kon′kŭs). Having a high orbit, with an orbital index above 85. [hypsi- + G. *konchos*, a shell, the upper part of the skull]

hyp·si·loid (hip′si-loyd). Y-shaped; U-shaped. SYN upsiloid, ypsiliform. [G. *upsilon (ypsilon)*]

hyp·si·sta·phyl·ia (hip′si-stă-fil′ē-ă). A condition in which the palate is high and narrow. [hypsi- + G. *staphylē*, uvula]

hyp·si·sten·o·ce·phal·ic (hip-si-sten′ō-sĕ-fal′ik). Having a high, narrow head. [hypsi- + G. *stenos*, narrow, + *kephalē*, head]

△**hypso-.** SEE hypsi-.

hyp·so·ceph·a·ly (hip-sō-sef′ă-lē). SYN oxycephaly. [hypso- + G. *kephalē*, head]

hyp·so·chro·mic (hip-sō-krōm′ik). Denoting the shift of an absorption spectrum maximum to a shorter wavelength (greater energy). [hypso- + G. *chroma*, color]

hyp·so·dont (hip′sō-dont). Having long teeth. [hypso- + G. *odous*, tooth]

hy·pur·gia (hī-per′jē-ă). A rarely used term for any minor factor(s) modifying the course of a disease for good or for ill, especially the former. [G. *hypourgia*, help, service, fr. *hypo*, + *ergon*, work]

Hyrtl, Joseph, Austrian anatomist, 1810–1894. SEE H.'s *anastomosis, foramen, loop,* epitympanic *recess, sphincter.*

△**hyster-.** SEE hystero-.

hys·ter·al·gia (his′ter-al′jē-ă). Pain in the uterus. SYN hysterodynia, metrodynia. [hystero- + G. *algos*, pain]

hys·ter·a·tre·sia (his′ter-ă-trē′zē-ă). Atresia of the uterine cavity, usually resulting from inflammatory endocervical adhesions.

hys·ter·ec·to·my (his-ter-ek′tō-mē). Removal of the uterus; unless otherwise specified, usually denotes complete removal of the uterus (corpus and cervix). SYN uterectomy. [hystero- + G. *ektomē*, excision]

abdominal h., removal of the uterus through an incision in the abdominal wall. SYN abdominohysterectomy, celiohysterectomy, laparohysterectomy.

abdominovaginal h., a combined vaginal and abdominal surgical approach that allows partial or complete removal of vagina, vulva, rectum, and perineum (abdominoperineal approach), as well as pelvic organs; usually done in cases of advanced pelvic cancer.

cesarean h., cesarean section followed by h. SYN Porro h., Porro operation.

modified radical h., an extended h. in which a portion of the upper vagina is removed; the ureters are exposed and pulled back laterally without dissection from the ureteral bed. SYN TeLinde operation.

paravaginal h., obsolete term for removal of the uterus through a perineal incision involving only the lower two-thirds of the vaginal wall.

Porro h., SYN cesarean h.

radical h., complete removal of the uterus, upper vagina, and parametrium.

subtotal h., SYN supracervical h.

supracervical h., removal of the fundus of the uterus, leaving the cervix *in situ.* SYN subtotal h.

vaginal h., removal of the uterus through the vagina without incising the wall of the abdomen. SYN colpohysterectomy, vaginohysterectomy.

hys·ter·e·sis (his-ter-ē′sis). **1.** Failure of either one of two related phenomena to keep pace with the other; or any situation in which the value of one depends upon whether the other has been increasing or decreasing. Cf. allosterism, cooperativity. **2.** The lag of a magnetic effect behind its cause. SYN magnetic inertia. **3.** The temperature differential that exists when a substance, such as reversible hydrocolloid, melts at one temperature and solidifies at another. **4.** The basis of a type of cooperativity observed in many enzyme-catalyzed reactions in which the degree of cooperativity is associated with a slow conformational change of the enzyme. Cf. allosterism, cooperativity. [G. *hysterēsis*, a coming later]

static h., the difference in the value reached by a dependent variable at a particular constant value of the independent variable, depending on whether the latter value had been approached from above or below; *e.g.*, in measuring the pressure volume relations of the lungs, if one completely expires and then inspires to a particular volume and holds it constant, the transpulmonary pressure required to maintain that lung volume is greater than if one had completely inspired and then expired to the same volume and held it constant.

hys·ter·eu·ry·sis (his-ter-yū′rē-sis). Dilation of the lower segment and cervical canal of the uterus. [hystero- + G. *eurynō*, to dilate, fr. *eurys*, wide]

hys·te·ria (his-ter′ē-ă, his-tēr′). A somatoform (psychoneurotic or psychosomatic) disorder in which there is an alteration or loss of physical functioning that suggests a physical disorder such as paralysis of an arm or disturbance of vision, but that is instead apparently an expression of a psychological conflict or need; a diagnostic term, referable to a wide variety of psychogenic symptoms involving disorder of function, which may be mental, sensory, motor, or visceral. SEE somatoform *disorder.* [G. *hystera,* womb, from the original notion of womb-related disturbances in women]

anxiety h., h. characterized by manifest anxiety.

canine h., syndrome in dogs caused in ingestion of nitrogen trichloride, formerly in common use as a bleaching agent for flour.

conversion h., h. characterized by the substitution, through psychic transformation, of physical signs or symptoms for anxiety; generally restricted to such major symptoms as blindness, deafness, and paralysis, or lesser ones such as blurred vision and numbness. SYN conversion hysteria neurosis, conversion neurosis, conversion reaction.

dissociative h., an unconscious process sometimes seen in patients with multiple personalities, or in h., in which a group of mental processes is separated from the rest of the thinking processes, resulting in an independent functioning of these processes and a loss of the usual relationships among them.

epidemic h., SYN mass h.

major h., a syndrome, now rarely seen, described by Charcot and characterized by a first stage of aura, a second stage of epileptoid convulsions, a third stage of tonic and clonic spasms, a fourth stage of dramatic behavior, and a fifth stage of delirium; the entire attack may last from a few minutes to half an hour. Sometimes used as a synonym for hysteroepilepsy.

mass h., (1) spontaneous, en masse development of identical physical and/or emotional symptoms among a group of individuals, as seen in a classroom of schoolchildren; (2) a socially contagious frenzy of irrational behavior in a group of people as a reaction to an event. SYN epidemic h.

minor h., a mild form of h. characterized chiefly by subjective pains, nervousness, undue sensitiveness, and sometimes episodes of emotional excitement, but without paralysis or other such symptoms.

hys·ter·i·cal, hys·ter·ic (his-ter′ē-kăl, -ter′ik). Relating to or characterized by hysteria.

hys·ter·i·co·neu·ral·gic (his-ter′i-kō-nū-ral′jik). Relating to neuralgic pains of hysterical origin.

hys·ter·ics (his-ter′iks). An expression of emotion accompanied often by crying, laughing, and screaming.

△**hystero-, hyster-.** **1.** The uterus. SEE ALSO metr-, utero-. [G. *hystera,* womb (uterus)] **2.** Hysteria. [G. *hystera,* womb (uterus)] **3.** Later, following. [G. *hysteros,* later]

hys·ter·o·cat·a·lep·sy (his′ter-ō-kat′ă-lep-sē). Hysteria with cataleptic manifestations.

hys·ter·o·cele (his′ter-ō-sēl). **1.** An abdominal or perineal hernia containing part or all of the uterus. **2.** Protrusion of uterine contents into a weakened, bulging area of uterine wall. [hystero- + G. *kēlē,* hernia]

hys·ter·o·clei·sis (his′ter-ō-klī′sis). Operative occlusion of the uterus. [hystero- + G. *kleisis,* closure]

hys·ter·o·col·po·scope (his′ter-ō-kol′pō-skōp). Instrument for

inspection of the uterine cavity and vagina. [hystero- + G. *kolpos,* vagina, + *skopeō,* to view]

hys·ter·o·cys·to·pexy (his′ter-ō-sis′tō-pek-sē). Attachment of both uterus and bladder to the abdominal wall to correct prolapse. [hystero- + G. *kystis,* bladder, + *pēxis,* fixation]

hys·ter·o·dyn·ia (his′ter-ō-din′ē-ă). SYN hysteralgia. [hystero- + G. *odynē,* pain]

hys·ter·o·ep·i·lep·sy (his′ter-ō-ep′i-lep-sē). Hysterical convulsions. SEE major *hysteria.*

hys·ter·o·gen·ic, hys·ter·og·en·ous (his′ter-ō-jen′ik, his-ter-oj′ ĕ-nŭs). Causing hysterical symptoms or reactions. [hysteria + G. -*gen,* producing]

hys·ter·o·gram (his′ter-ō-gram). **1.** X-ray examination of the uterus, usually using a contrast medium. **2.** A recording of the strength of uterine contractions.

hys·ter·o·graph (his′ter-ō-graf). Apparatus for recording the strength of uterine contractions.

hys·ter·og·ra·phy (his′ter-og′ră-fē). **1.** Radiographic examination of the uterine cavity filled with a contrast medium. **2.** Graphic procedure used to record uterine contractions. SYN metrography. [hystero- + G. *graphō,* to write]

hys·ter·oid (his′ter-oyd). Resembling or simulating hysteria. [hystero- + G. *eidos,* resemblance]

hys·ter·o·lith (his′ter-ō-lith). SYN uterine *calculus.* [hystero- + G. *lithos,* stone]

hys·ter·ol·y·sis (his-ter-ol′i-sis). Breaking up of adhesions between the uterus and neighboring parts. [hystero- + G. *lysis,* dissolution]

hys·ter·om·e·ter (his-ter-om′ĕ-ter). A graduated sound for measuring the depth of the uterine cavity. SYN uterometer. [hystero- + G. *metron,* measure]

hys·ter·o·my·o·ma (his′ter-ō-mī-ō′mă). A myoma of the uterus. [hystero- + G. *mys,* muscle, + -*oma,* tumor]

hys·ter·o·my·o·mec·to·my (his′ter-ō-mī-ō-mek′tō-mē). Operative removal of a uterine myoma. [hysteromyoma + G. *ektomē,* excision]

hys·ter·o·my·ot·o·my (his′ter-ō-mī-ot′ō-mē). Incision into the muscles of the uterus. [hystero- + G. *mys,* muscle, + *tomē,* incision]

hys·ter·o·nar·co·lep·sy (his′ter-ō-nar′kō-lep-sē). Narcolepsy of emotional origin.

hys·ter·o·oo·pho·rec·to·my (his′ter-ō-ō′of-ō-rek′tō-mē). Surgical removal of the uterus and ovaries. [hystero- + G. *ōon,* egg, + *phoros,* bearing, + *ektomē,* excision]

hys·ter·op·a·thy (his-ter-op′ă-thē). Any disease of the uterus. [hystero- + G. *pathos,* suffering]

hys·ter·o·pex·y (his′ter-ō-pek-sē). Fixation of a misplaced or abnormally movable uterus. SYN uterofixation, uteropexy. [hystero- + G. *pēxis,* fixation]

abdominal h., attachment of the uterus to the anterior abdominal wall. SYN laparohysteropexy.

hys·ter·o·phore (his′ter-ō-fōr). A pessary or other support for a prolapsed or displaced uterus. [hystero- + G. *phoros,* bearing]

hys·ter·o·plas·ty (his′ter-ō-plas-tē). SYN uteroplasty.

hys·ter·or·rha·phy (his-ter-ōr′ă-fē). Sutural repair of a lacerated uterus. [hystero- + G. *rhaphē,* suture]

hys·ter·or·rhex·is (his′ter-ō-rek′sis). Rupture of the uterus. SYN metrorrhexis. [hystero- + G. *rhēxis,* rupture]

hys·ter·o·sal·pin·gec·to·my (his′ter-ō-sal-pin-jek′tō-mē). Operation for the removal of the uterus and one or both uterine tubes. [hystero- + G. *salpinx,* a trumpet, + *ektomē,* excision]

hys·ter·o·sal·pin·gog·ra·phy (his′ter-ō-sal-ping-gog′ră-fē). Radiography of the uterus and fallopian tubes after the injection of radiopaque material. SYN gynecography, hysterotubography, metrosalpingography, uterosalpingography, uterotubography. [hystero- + G. *salpinx,* a trumpet, + *graphō,* to write]

hys·ter·o·sal·pin·go·oo·pho·rec·to·my (his′ter-ō-sal-ping′gō-ō-of-ō-rek′tō-mē). Excision of the uterus, oviducts, and ovaries. [hystero- + G. *salpinx,* trumpet, + *ōon,* egg, + *phoros,* bearing, + *ektomē,* excision]

hys·ter·o·sal·pin·gos·to·my (his′ter-ō-sal-ping-gos′tō-mē). Op-

hy

eration to restore patency of a uterine tube. [hystero- + G. *salpinx*, trumpet, + *stoma*, mouth]

hys·ter·o·scope (his′ter-ō-skōp). An endoscope used in direct visual examination of the uterine cavity. SYN metroscope, uteroscope. [hystero- + G. *skopeō*, to view]

hys·ter·os·co·py (his-ter-os′kŏ-pē). Visual instrumental inspection of the uterine cavity. SYN uteroscopy.

laparoscopic-assisted vaginal h. (LAVH), a procedure for viewing the interior of the uterus.

Carbon dioxide or sugar water is injected through the cervix to inflate the uterus; then a hysteroscope is threaded in under local anesthesia. As in standard laparoscopy, the hysteroscope may be fitted with tools to enable minor surgery.

hys·ter·o·spasm (his′ter-ō-spazm). Spasm of the uterus.

hys·ter·o·sys·to·le (his-ter-ō-sis′tō-lē). A delayed contraction of the heart; opposed to premature contraction or extrasystole. [G. *hysteros*, following, after, + *systolē*, a contracting]

hys·ter·o·ther·mom·e·try (his′ter-ō-ther-mom′ě-trē). Measurement of uterine temperature.

hys·ter·ot·o·my (his-ter-ot′ō-mē). Incision of the uterus. SYN metrotomy, uterotomy. [hystero- + G. *tomē*, incision]

abdominal h., transabdominal incision into the uterus. Also variously called abdominohysterotomy; celiohysterotomy; laparohysterotomy; laparouterotomy. SYN abdominohysterotomy, celiohysterotomy, laparohysterotomy, laparouterotomy.

vaginal h., incision into the uterus via the vagina. SYN colpohysterotomy.

hys·ter·o·to·nin (his′ter-ō-tō′nin). Obsolete term for pressor substance found in decidua and amniotic fluid of patients with toxemia of pregnancy. [hystero- + G. *tonos*, tension]

hys·ter·o·trach·e·lec·to·my (his′ter-ō-trak-el-ek′tō-mē). Removal of the cervix uteri. [hystero- + G. *trachēlos*, neck, + *ektomē*, excision]

hys·ter·o·trach·e·lo·plas·ty (his′ter-ō-trak′ě-lō-plas-tē). Plastic surgery of the cervix uteri. [hystero- + G. *trachēlos*, neck, + *plastos*, formed, shaped]

hys·ter·o·tra·che·lor·rha·phy (his′ter-ō-trak-ě-lōr′ă-fē). Sutural repair of a lacerated cervix uteri. [hystero- + G. *trachēlos*, neck, + *rhaphē*, a seam]

hys·ter·o·trach·e·lot·o·my (his′ter-ō-trak-ě-lot′ō-mē). Incision of the cervix uteri. [hystero- + G. *trachēlos*, neck, + *tomē*, incision]

hys·ter·o·tris·mus (his′ter-ō-tris′mŭs). Symptoms of lockjaw with a psychologic, functional basis.

hys·ter·o·tu·bog·ra·phy (his′ter-ō-tū-bog′ră-fē). SYN hysterosalpingography.

Hz Abbreviation for hertz.

I

ι Abbreviation for iota, the 9th letter in the Greek alphabet.

I 1. Symbol for iodine; luminous *intensity* or radiant *intensity*; ionic *strength* (in mol/L); isoleucine; inosine. **2.** Abbreviation for intensity of electrical current, expressed in amperes. **3.** As a subscript, symbol for inspired *gas*. **4.** Designation for I blood group (see Blood Groups appendix).

¹²³I. Symbol for iodine-123.

¹²⁵I. Symbol for iodine-125.

¹²⁷I Symbol for iodine-127.

¹³¹I. Symbol for iodine-131.

¹³²I. Symbol for iodine-132.

-ia. Condition, used in formation of names of many diseases. Cf. -ism. [G. *-ia,* an ancient noun-forming suffix]

IANC Abbreviation for International Anatomical Nomenclature Committee. SEE Nomina Anatomica.

IAP Abbreviation for intermittent acute *porphyria.*

-iasis. A condition or state, especially an unhealthy one; in medical neologisms it has the same value as, and is sometimes interchangeable with, G. *-osis.* [G. suffix forming nouns from verbs]

ia·tra·lip·tic (ī′ă-tră-lip′tik). Obsolete term denoting treatment by inunction. [G. *iatros,* physician, + *aleiptēs,* an anointer]

ia·tra·lip·tics (ī′ă-tră-lip′tiks). Method of treatment by inunction.

iat·ric (ī-at′rik). Pertaining to medicine or to a physician or healer. [G. *iatros,* physician]

iatro-. Physicians, medicine, treatment. Cf. medico-. [G. *iatros,* physician]

iat·ro·chem·i·cal (ī-at-rō-kem′i-kăl). Denoting a school of medicine practicing iatrochemistry.

iat·ro·chem·ist (ī-at-rō-kem′ist). A member of the iatrochemical school.

iat·ro·chem·is·try (ī-at-rō-kem′is-trē). The study of chemistry in relation to physiologic and pathologic processes, and the treatment of disease by chemical substance as practiced by a school of medical thought in the 17th century. SYN chemiatry.

iat·ro·gen·ic (ī-at-rō-jen′ik). Denoting response to medical or surgical treatment, induced by the treatment itself; usually used for unfavorable responses. [iatro- + G. *-gen,* producing]

ia·trol·o·gy (ī-a-trol′ō-jē). Rarely used term for medical science. [iatro- + G. *logos,* study]

iat·ro·math·e·mat·i·cal (ī-at′rō-math-ĕ-mat′i-kăl). SYN iatrophysical.

iat·ro·me·chan·i·cal (ī-at′rō-mĕ-kan′i-kăl). SYN iatrophysical.

iat·ro·phys·i·cal (ī-at′rō-fiz′i-kăl). Denoting a school of medical thought in the 17th century which explained all physiologic and pathologic phenomena by the laws of physics. SYN iatromathematical, iatromechanical.

iat·ro·phys·i·cist (ī-at′rō-fiz′-i-sist). A member of the iatrophysical school.

iat·ro·phys·ics (ī-at′rō-fiz′iks). Physics as applied to medicine.

iat·ro·tech·nique (ī-at′rō-tek-nēk′). Rarely used term for the art of medicine and surgery; the technique or mode of application of medical science. [iatro- + G. *technē,* art]

IBC Abbreviation for iron-binding *capacity.*

ibo·ga·ine (ī′bō-gān). Indole alkaloid of the *iboga* group. Obtained from several parts of the African shrub *Tabernanthe iboga* (family Apocynaceae). Used by African hunters to arrest movement of the hunter; hallucinogenic, antidepressant, and euphoric.

ibo·ten·ic ac·id (ī′bō-ten-ik). Chemical similar to kainic acid extracted from poisonous mushroom species *Amanita muscaria* and *A. pantherina* (family Agaricaceae). Exhibits substantial neuroexcitatory properties. Used in neuropharmacologic research.

IBR Abbreviation for infectious bovine *rhinotracheitis.*

ibu·pro·fen (ī-bū′prō-fen). *dl-p*-Isobutylhydratropic acid; an anti-inflammatory agent.

IBV Abbreviation for infectious bronchitis *virus.*

-ic. 1. Suffix denoting of, pertaining to. **2.** Chemical suffix denoting an element in a compound in one of its highest valencies. Cf. -ous (1). **3.** Suffix indicating an acid. [L. *-icus,* fr. G. *-ikos*]

ICAM-1 Abbreviation for intercellular adhesion *molecule*-1.

ICD Abbreviation for *International Classification of Diseases of the World Health Organization.*

ICDA Abbreviation for *International Classification of Diseases, Adapted for Use in the United States;* includes a classification of surgical operations and other therapeutic and diagnostic procedures.

ice pack. A cold local application to limit or reduce swelling in recently traumatized tissues; usually in the form of a water-impervious container for ice. Improvised means for containing ice (plastic bags, towels, etc.) are often employed, as are chemical sacks that when struck allow the commingling of chemicals that react endothermically.

ICF Abbreviation for intracellular *fluid.*

ich·no·gram (ik′nō-gram). Imprint of the soles of the feet, taken standing. [G. *ichnos,* footstep, + *gramma,* a drawing, fr. *graphō,* to write]

ichor (ī′kōr). Rarely used term for a thin watery discharge from an ulcer or unhealthy wound. [G. *ichōr,* serum]

icho·re·mia (ī-kō-rē′mē-ă). SYN ichorrhemia.

icho·roid (ī′kō-royd). Denoting a thin purulent discharge. [G. *ichōr,* serum, + *eidos,* resemblance]

ichor·ous (ī′kōr-ŭs). Relating to or resembling ichor.

ichor·rhea (ī′kō-rē′ă). A profuse ichorous discharge. [G. *ichōr,* serum, + *rhoia,* a flow]

ichor·rhe·mia (ī-kō-rē′mē-ă). Sepsis resulting from infection accompanied by an ichorous discharge. SYN ichoremia. [G. *ichōr,* serum, + *rhoia,* a flow, + *haima,* blood]

ICHPPC Abbreviation for International Classification of Health Problems in Primary Care.

ich·tham·mol (ik′tham-mol). Sulfonated bitumen; ammonium sulfoichthyolate; a viscous fluid, reddish brown to brownish black in color, with a strong, characteristic, empyreumatic odor, soluble in water and in glycerin; obtained by the destructive distillation of certain bituminous schists, sulfonating the distillate and neutralizing the product with ammonia. It is used in skin disorders; its beneficial effect is due to its mild irritant, stimulant, antiseptic, and analgesic action; has been used in 10 and 20 percent concentration in an ointment ("drawing salve"). SYN ammonium ichthosulfonate.

ich·thy·ism (ik′thi-izm). Poisoning by eating stale or otherwise unfit fish. SYN ichthyismus. [G. *ichthys,* fish]

ich·thy·is·mus (ik-thi-iz′mŭs). SYN ichthyism. [G. *ichthys,* fish]
  i. exanthemat′icus, toxic erythematous eruption due to ingestion of spoiled fish.
  i. hys′trix, SYN bullous congenital ichthyosiform *erythroderma.*

ichthyo-. Fish. [G. *ichthys*]

ich·thy·o·a·can·tho·tox·ism (ik′thi-ō-ă-kan′thō-tok′sizm). Poisoning from the stings or spines of venomous fishes. [ichthyo- + G. *akantha,* thorn, + *toxikon,* poison]

ich·thy·o·col·la (ik-thē-ō-kol′ă). Fish gelatin obtained from sounds or swim bladders of fish such as the hake, cod, and sturgeon; used as a glue, a food substitute, and a clarifying agent. SYN isinglass. [ichthyo- + G. *kolla,* glue]

ich·thy·o·he·mo·tox·in (ik′thē-ō-hē′mō-tok′sin). The toxic substance in the blood of certain fishes. [ichthyo- + G. *haima,* blood, + *toxikon,* poison]

ich·thy·o·he·mo·tox·ism (ik′thē-ō-hē′mō-tok′sizm). Poisoning resulting from the ingestion of fish containing the toxic substance, ichthyohemotoxin.

ic

ich·thy·oid (ik′thē-oyd). Fish-shaped. [ichthyo- + G. *eidos*, resemblance]

ich·thy·o·o·tox·in (ik′thē-ō-ō-tok′sin). Toxic substance restricted to the roe of fishes. [ichthyo- + G. *ōon*, egg, + *toxikon*, poison]

ich·thy·oph·a·gous (ik-thē-of′ă-gŭs). Fish-eating; subsisting on fish. [ichthyo- + G. *phagō*, to eat]

ich·thy·o·pho·bia (ik′thē-ō-fō′bē-ă). Morbid fear of fish. [ichthyo- + G. *phobos*, fear]

ich·thy·o·sar·co·tox·in (ik′thē-ō-sar′kō-tok′sin). Toxic substance found in the flesh or organs of fishes. [ichthyo- + G. *sarx*, flesh, + *toxikon*, poison]

ich·thy·o·sar·co·tox·ism (ik′thē-ō-sar′kō-tok′sizm). Poisoning caused by the toxic substance (ichthyosarcotoxin) in the flesh or organs of fish. [ichthyo- + G. *sarx*, flesh, + *toxikon*, poison]

ich·thy·o·sis (ik-thē-ō′sis). Congenital disorders of keratinization characterized by noninflammatory dryness and scaling of the skin, often associated with other defects and with abnormalities of lipid metabolism; distinguishable genetically, clinically, microscopically, and by epidermal cell kinetics. SYN alligator skin, fish skin, sauriasis, sauriderma, sauriosis, sauroderma. [ichthyo- + G. *-osis*, condition]

acquired i., a thickening and scaling of the skin associated with some malignant diseases (*e.g.,* Hodgkin's disease, lymphosarcoma), leprosy, and severe nutritional deficiencies.

i. congen′ita neonato′rum, generalized i. with parchment-like skin seen in premature babies.

i. cor′neae, an ocular complication of a congenital abnormality of the skin with corneal keratinization, dryness, and scaling.

i. feta′lis, (1) SYN harlequin *fetus*. **(2)** recessive condition in Holstein and Norwegian red poll cattle resembling harlequin fetus in humans.

i. follicula′ris, a form of autosomal dominant type of i., with horny follicular plugging of the extensor surfaces of the extremities; onset in early childhood.

harlequin i., fetal form of i. distinct from lamellar i. in its patchy character and the poor prospect of the patient surviving the neonatal period.

i. hys′trix, SYN bullous congenital ichthyosiform *erythroderma*. [G. *hystrix*, hedgehog]

i. intrauteri′na, SYN i. vulgaris.

lamellar i. [MIM*262300], a dry form of congenital ichthyosiform erythroderma, an autosomal recessive trait present at birth; characterized by large, coarse scales over most of the body with thickened palms and soles, and associated with ectropion; histologically, there is hyperkeratosis, a prominent granular layer in the epidermis, slight acanthosis, many mitotic figures, and normal or reduced epidermal cell turnover. SEE ALSO collodion *baby*, harlequin *fetus*.

i. linea′ris circumflex′a [MIM*256500], congenital or infantile migratory polycyclic erythema and scaling that shows a peripheral double margin; persists throughout life and may be associated with trichorrhexis invaginata in Netherton's syndrome; autosomal recessive inheritance.

nacreous i., a variant of i. characterized by dry pearly scales.

i. palma′ris et planta′ris, SYN palmoplantar *keratoderma*.

i. scutula′ta, i. marked by diamond-shaped or shield-shaped lesions.

i. seba′cea, the presence of an unusual amount of vernix caseosa.

i. seba′cea cor′nea, a type of i. with vernix caseosa as seen in the newborn.

i. sim′plex, SYN i. vulgaris.

i. spino′sa, SYN congenital ichthyosiform *erythroderma*.

i. u′teri, transformation of the columnar epithelium of the endometrium into stratified squamous epithelium.

i. vulga′ris [MIM*146700], an autosomal dominant trait, with onset in childhood of scales on the trunk and extremities but not on the flexural areas, and associated with atopy and prominent palmar and plantar markings; histologically, there is hyperkeratosis, absence of a granular layer in the epidermis, and normal epidermal cell turnover. SYN hyperkeratosis congenita, i. intrauterina, i. simplex, keratosis diffusa fetalis.

X-linked i. [MIM*308100], a form of i., due to 3-β-hydroxysteroidsulfate sulfatase deficiency, that appears at birth or in early infancy and affects males; characterized by scaling predominantly on the neck and trunk but not on the palms and soles; histologically, there is hyperkeratosis, a granular layer in the epidermis, and normal epidermal cell turnover. SYN steroid sulfatase deficiency.

ich·thy·ot·ic (ik-thē-ot′ik). Relating to ichthyosis.

ich·thy·o·tox·i·col·o·gy (ik′thē-ō-tok-si-kol′ō-jē). The study of the poisons produced by fishes, and their recognition, effects, and antidotes. [ichthyo- + G. *toxikon*, poison, + *logos*, study]

ich·thy·o·tox·i·con (ik-thē-ō-tok′si-kon). A toxic principle in certain fishes. SYN fish poison (1). [ichthyo- + G. *toxikon*, poison]

ich·thy·o·tox·in (ik′thē-ō-tok′sin). The hemolytic active principle of eel serum. [ichthyo- + G. *toxicon*, poison]

ich·thy·o·tox·ism (ik′thē-ō-tok′sizm). Poisoning by fish. [ichthyo- + G. *toxikon*, poison]

ICIDH Abbreviation for International Classification of Impairments, Disabilities and Handicaps.

icon·o·ma·nia (ī′kon-ō-mā′nē-ă). Rarely used term for a morbid impulse to worship images. [G. *eikōn*, image, + *mania*, insanity]

ico·sa·he·dral (ī′kō-să-hē′drăl). Having 20 equilateral triangular surfaces and 12 vertices, as do most viruses with cubic symmetry. [G. *eikosi*, twenty, + *-edros*, having sides or bases]

n-**ico·sa·no·ic ac·id** (ī′kō-să-nō′ik). SYN arachidic acid.

ICP Abbreviation for intracranial *pressure*.

ICRP Abbreviation for International Commission on Radiological Protection.

△-**ics.** Organized knowledge, practice, treatment. [-ic + -s]

ICSH Abbreviation of interstitial cell-stimulating hormone.

ic·tal (ik′tăl). Relating to or caused by a stroke or seizure. [L. *ictus*, a stroke]

ic·ter·ic (ik-ter′ik). Relating to or marked by jaundice. [G. *ikterikos*, jaundiced]

△**ictero-.** Icterus. [G. *ikteros*, jaundice]

ic·ter·o·a·ne·mia (ik′ter-ō-ă-nē′mē-ă). SYN acquired hemolytic *icterus*.

swine i., an infectious disease of swine manifested by icterus, anemia, and emaciation; caused by *Eperythrozoon suis*.

ic·ter·o·gen·ic (ik′ter-ō-jen′ik). Causing jaundice. [ictero- + G. *-gen*, producing]

ic·ter·o·he·ma·tu·ric (ik′ter-ō-hē′mă-tū′rik). Denoting jaundice with the passage of blood in the urine. [ictero- + G. *haima*, blood, + *ouron*, urine]

ic·ter·o·he·mo·glo·bi·nu·ria (ik′ter-ō-hē′mō-glō-bi-nū′rē-ă). Jaundice with hemoglobin in the urine.

ic·ter·o·hep·a·ti·tis (ik′ter-ō-hep-ă-tī′tis). Inflammation of the liver with jaundice as a prominent symptom. [ictero- + G. *hēpar*, liver, + *-itis*, inflammation]

ic·ter·oid (ik′ter-oyd). Yellow-hued, or seemingly jaundiced. [ictero- + G. *eidos*, resemblance]

ic·ter·us (ik′ter-ŭs). SYN jaundice. [G. *ikteros*]

acquired hemolytic i., i. and anemia occuring in association with a moderate degree of splenomegaly, increased fragility of red blood cells, and increased amounts of urobilin in the urine. SYN icteroanemia.

benign familial i., SYN familial nonhemolytic *jaundice*.

chronic familial i., SYN hereditary *spherocytosis*.

congenital hemolytic i., SYN hereditary *spherocytosis*.

cythemolytic i., i. caused by absorption of bile produced in excess through stimulation by free hemoglobin caused by the destruction of red blood corpuscles.

i. gra′vis, jaundice associated with high fever and delirium; seen in severe hepatitis and other diseases of the liver with severe functional failure. SYN malignant jaundice.

infectious i., SYN Weil's *disease*.

i. mel′as, a form in which the skin assumes a dirty dark brown color.

i. neonato′rum, i. which can be accentuated by many factors including excessive hemolysis, sepsis, neonatal hepatitis or congenital atresia of the biliary system. SYN physiologic i. SYN jaundice of the newborn, neonatal jaundice, physiologic jaundice.

physiologic i., SYN i. neonatorum.

i. prae′cox, a relatively innocent but rapidly developing type of jaundice with mild anemia in the newborn, most frequently caused by ABO incompatibility between mother and fetus.

ic·tom·e·ter (ik-tom′ĕ-ter). An apparatus for determining the force of the apex beat of the heart. [L. *ictus,* stroke, + G. *metron,* measure]

ic·tus (ik′tŭs). **1.** A stroke or attack. **2.** A beat. [L.]

i. cor′dis, SYN heart *beat.*

i. epilep′ticus, an epileptic convulsion.

i. paralyt′icus, a paralytic stroke.

i. so′lis, SYN sunstroke.

ICU Abbreviation for intensive care *unit.*

I.D. Abbreviation for infecting dose. SEE minimal infecting *dose.*

id. 1. In psychoanalysis, one of three components of the psychic apparatus in the freudian structural framework, the other two being the ego and superego. It is completely in the unconscious realm, is unorganized, is the reservoir of psychic energy or libido, and is under the influence of the primary processes. **2.** The total of all psychic energy available from the innate biologic hungers, appetites, bodily needs, drives and impulses, in a newborn infant; through socialization this diffuse undirected energy becomes channeled in less egocentric and more socially responsive directions (development of the ego from the id). [L. *id,* that]

-id. 1. A state of sensitivity of the skin in which a part remote from the primary lesion reacts ("-id reaction") to substances of the pathogen, giving rise to a secondary inflammatory lesion; the lesion manifesting the reaction is designated by the use of -id as a suffix. [G. *-eidēs,* resembling, through Fr. *-id*] **2.** Small, young specimen. [G. *-idion,* a diminutive ending]

IDA Abbreviation for iminodiacetate, whose derivatives are used in radiopharmaceuticals with a ^{99m}Tc label. SEE HIDA. SEE ALSO DISIDA.

IDDM Abbreviation for insulin-dependent *diabetes* mellitus.

-ide. 1. Suffix denoting the more electronegative element in a binary chemical compound; formerly denoted by the qualification, -ureted; *e.g.,* hydrogen sulfide was sulfureted hydrogen. **2.** Suffix (in a sugar name) indicating substitution for the H of the hemiacetal OH; *e.g.,* glycoside.

idea (ī-dē′ă). Any mental image or concept. [G. semblance]

autochthonous i.'s, thoughts that suddenly burst into awareness as if they are vitally important, often as if they have come from an outside source.

compulsive i., a fixed and repetitively recurring i.

dominant i., an i. that governs all one's actions and thoughts.

fixed i., (1) an exaggerated notion, belief, or delusion that persists, despite evidence to the contrary, and controls the mind; **(2)** the obstinate conviction of a psychotic person regarding the correctness of his delusion. SYN idée fixe, overvalued i., permanent dominant i.

flight of i.'s, an uncontrollable symptom of the manic phase of a bipolar depressive disorder in which streams of unrelated words and i.'s occur to the patient at a rate that is impossible to vocalize despite a marked increase in the individual's overall output of words. SEE ALSO mania.

hyperquantivalent i., an i. that dominates all thought and cannot easily be changed.

overvalued i., SYN fixed i.

permanent dominant i., SYN fixed i.

i. of reference, the misinterpretation that other people's statements or acts or neutral objects in the environment are directed toward one's self when, in fact, they are not.

ide·al (ī-dēl′). A standard of perfection.

ego i., the part of the personality that comprises the goals, aspirations, and aims of the self, usually growing out of the emulation of a significant person with whom one has identified.

ide·a·tion (ī-dē-ā′shŭn). The formation of ideas or thoughts.

ide·a·tion·al (ī-dē-ā′shŭn-ăl). Relating to ideation.

idée fixe (ē-dā′fēks′). SYN fixed *idea.* [Fr. obsession]

iden·ti·fi·ca·tion (ī-den′ti-fi-kā′shŭn). A sense of oneness, or psychic continuity with another person or group; one of the freudian defense mechanisms common to everyone whereby anxiety regarding one's personal identity or worth is dissipated via the mechanism of perceiving oneself as having characteristics in common with a person in the public eye, or in childhood identifying with a more powerful person such as a parent. SYN incorporation. [Mediev. L. *identicus,* fr. L. *idem,* the same, + *facio,* to make]

iden·ti·ty (ī-den′ti-tē). The social role of the person and his or her perception of it.

ego i., the ego's sense of its own identity.

gender i., the sex role adopted by an individual; the degree to which an individual acts out a stereotypical masculine or feminine role in everyday behavior. Cf. gender *role,* sex *role.*

sense of i., one's sense of his or her own identity or psychological selfhood.

ideo-. Ideas; ideation Cf. idio-. [G. *idea,* form, notion]

ide·o·ki·net·ic (ī′dē-ō-ki-net′ik). SYN ideomotor.

ide·ol·o·gy (ī-dē-ol′ō-jē, id-ē-). The composite system of ideas, beliefs, and attitudes that constitutes an individual's or group's organized view of others. [ideo- + G. *logos,* study]

ide·o·mo·tion (ī-dē-ō-mō′shŭn). Muscular movement executed under the influence of a dominant idea, being practically automatic and not volitional.

ide·o·mo·tor (ī′dē-ō-mō′ter). Relating to ideomotion. SYN ideokinetic.

ide·o·pho·bia (ī′dē-ō-fō′bē-ă). Morbid fear of new or different ideas.

ide·o·plas·tia (ī′dē-ō-plas′tē-ă). Rarely used term for the receptive condition in a hypnotized person in which he or she is thought to be completely open to suggestion. [ideo- + G. *plassō,* to form]

idio-. Private, distinctive, peculiar to. Cf. ideo-. [G. *idios,* one's own]

id·i·o·ag·glu·ti·nin (id′ē-ō-ă-glū′tin-in). An agglutinin that occurs naturally in the blood of a person or an animal, without the injection of a stimulating antigen or the passive transfer of antibody.

id·i·o·dy·nam·ic (id′ē-ō-dī-nam′ik). Independently active.

id·i·og·a·mist (id′ē-og′ă-mist). Rarely used term for one who is capable of sexual union with only one or a few individuals of the opposite sex, being impotent in the presence of any others. [idio- + G. *gamos,* marriage]

id·i·o·gen·e·sis (id′ē-ō-jen′ĕ-sis). Origin without evident cause; denoting especially that of an idiopathic disease. [idio- + G. *genesis,* production]

id·i·o·glos·sia (id′ē-ō-glos′ē-ă). An extreme form of lalling or vowel or consonant substitution, by which the speech of a child may be made unintelligible and appear to be another language to one who does not have the key to the literal changes. [idio- + G. *glōssa,* tongue, speech]

id·i·o·glot·tic (id′ē-ō-glot′ik). Relating to idioglossia.

id·i·o·gram (id′ē-ō-gram). **1.** SYN karyotype. **2.** Diagrammatic representation of chromosome morphology characteristic of a species or population. [idio- + G. *gramma,* something written]

id·i·o·graph·ic (id′ē-ō-graf′ik). Pertaining to the characteristics or behavior of a particular individual as an individual, as opposed to nomothetic. [idio- + G. *graphō,* to write]

id·i·o·het·er·o·ag·glu·ti·nin (id′ē-ō-het′er-ō-ă-glū′tin-in). An idioagglutinin occurring in the blood of one animal, but capable of combining with the antigenic material from another species. [idio- + G. *heteros,* another, + agglutinin]

id·i·o·het·er·o·ly·sin (id′ē-ō-het-er-ol′i-sin). An idiolysin occurring in the blood of an animal of one species, but capable of combining with the red blood cells of another species, thereby causing hemolysis when complement is present.

id·i·o·hyp·no·tism (id′ē-ō-hip′nō-tizm). SYN autohypnosis.

id·i·o·i·so·ag·glu·ti·nin (id′ē-ō-ī′sō-ă-glū′tin-in). An idioagglu-

id

tinin occurring in the blood of an animal of a certain species, capable of agglutinating the cells from animals of the same species. [idio- + G. *isos*, equal, + agglutinin]

id·i·o·i·sol·y·sin (id′ē-ō-ī-sol′i-sin). An idiolysin occurring in the blood of an animal of a certain species, capable of combining with the red blood cells from animals of the same species, thereby causing hemolysis when complement is present.

id·i·o·la·lia (id′ē-ō-lā′lē-ă). Use of a language invented by the person himself. [idio- + G. *lalia*, talk]

id·i·ol·y·sin (id-ē-ol′i-sin). A lysin that occurs naturally in the blood of a person or an animal, without the injection of a stimulating antigen or the passive transfer of antibody.

id·i·o·mus·cu·lar (id′ē-ō-mŭs′kyū-lăr). Relating to the muscles alone, independent of the nervous control.

id·i·o·nod·al (id′ē-ō-nō′dăl). Arising from the A-V node itself; applied to the ventricular rhythm in complete S-A or A-V block, or in other forms of A-V dissociation, when the A-V node rather than an ectopic ventricular focus controls the ventricles. More accurately idiojunctional, since it is usually impossible to more accurately locate an "A-V nodal" rhythm; the A-V node is part of the A-V junction. SEE ALSO idioventricular.

id·i·o·pa·thet·ic (id′ē-ō-pă-thet′ik). Rarely used term for idiopathic.

id·i·o·path·ic (id′ē-ō-path′ik). Denoting a disease of unknown cause. SYN agnogenic. [idio- + G. *pathos*, suffering]

id·i·op·a·thy (id-ē-op′ă-thē). An idiopathic disease. [idio- + G. *pathos*, suffering]

id·i·o·phren·ic (id′ē-ō-fren′ik). Relating to, or originating in, the mind or brain alone, not reflex or secondary. [idio- + G. *phrēn*, mind]

id·i·o·psy·cho·log·ic (id′ē-ō-sī-kō-loj′ik). Relating to ideas developed within one's own mind, independent of suggestion from without.

id·i·o·re·flex (id-ē-ō-rē′fleks). A reflex due to a stimulus or irritation originating in the organ or part in which the reflex occurs.

id·i·o·some (id′ē-ō-sōm). The centrosome of a spermatid or of an oocyte. [idio- + G. *sōma*, body]

id·i·o·spasm (id′ē-ō-spazm). A localized spasm.

id·i·o·syn·cra·sy (id′ē-ō-sin′kră-sē). **1.** An individual mental, behavioral, or physical characteristic or peculiarity. **2.** In pharmacology, an abnormal reaction to a drug, sometimes specified as genetically determined. [G. *idiosynkrasia*, fr. *idios*, one's own, + *synkrasis*, a mixing together]

id·i·o·syn·crat·ic (id′ē-ō-sin-krat′ik). Relating to or marked by an idiosyncrasy.

id·i·o·tope (id′ē-ō-tōp). Antigenic determinant of an idiotype. SEE ALSO idiotypic antigenic *determinant*. [idio- + -tope]

id·i·ot-prod·i·gy (id′ē-ŏt prod′i-jē). SYN idiot-savant.

id·i·o·tro·phic (id′ē-ō-trof′ik). Capable of choosing its own food. [idio- + G. *trophē*, food]

id·i·o·tro·pic (id′ē-ō-trop′ik). Turning inward upon one's self. [idio- + G. *tropē*, a turning]

id·i·ot-sa·vant (ē-dē-ō′ sah-vahn′). A person of low general intelligence who possesses an unusual faculty in performing certain mental tasks of which most normal persons are incapable. SYN idiot-prodigy. [Fr.]

id·i·o·type (id′ē-ō-tīp). A determinant that confers on an immunoglobulin molecule an antigenic "individuality" and is frequently a unique attribute of a given antibody in a given animal. It is the product of a limited number of B lymphocyte clones. Collection of idiotopes located within the variable region of an antibody molecule or the T-cell receptor. SEE idiotope. SYN idiotypic antigenic determinant. [idio- + G. *typos*, model]

set of i.'s, (antigenic determinants) of either the immunoglobulin or T cell receptor variable regions.

id·i·o·ven·tric·u·lar (id-ē-ō-ven-trik′yū-lăr). Pertaining to or associated with the cardiac ventricles alone.

id·i·tol (ī′di-tol). Reduction product of the hexose idose.

IDL Abbreviation for intermediate density *lipoprotein*.

id·ose (ī′dōs). One of the aldohexoses, isomeric with galactose; L-i. is epimeric with D-glucose. SEE sugar.

idox·ur·i·dine (IDU) (ī-doks-yū′ri-dēn). 2′-Deoxy-5-iodouridine; 5-iododeoxyuridine; a pyrimidine analogue that produces both antiviral and anticancer effects by interference with DNA synthesis; used locally in the eye for the treatment of keratitis from herpes simplex or vaccinia.

IDP Abbreviation for inosine 5′-diphosphate.

idro·sis (ī-drō′sis). SYN hidrosis. [G. *hidrōs*, sweat]

IDU Abbreviation for idoxuridine.

id·ur·o·nate (ī-dūr-on′āt). The salt or ester of iduronic acid.

i. sulfatase, an enzyme required for the desulfation of 2-sulfate i. residues in heparan sulfate. It is also required in dermatan sulfate degradation; Hunter's syndrome is associated with a deficiency of this enzyme.

idur·on·ic ac·id (ī-dūr-on′ik). The uronic acid of idose; a constituent of dermatan sulfate.

α-L-id·ur·on·id·ase (ī-dūr-on′i-dās). An enzyme that hydrolyzes terminal desulfated α-L-iduronic acid residues of dermatan sulfate and of heparan sulfate; a deficiency of this enzyme is associated with Hurler syndrome and Scheie syndrome.

IEP Abbreviation for isoelectric *point*.

IF Abbreviation for initiation *factor*; intrinsic *factor*.

IFN Abbreviation for interferon.

IFN-α Abbreviation for *interferon* alpha.

IFN-β Abbreviation for *interferon* beta.

IFN-γ Abbreviation for *interferon* gamma.

Ig Abbreviation for immunoglobulin.

IgA Abbreviation for immunoglobulin A.

IgD Abbreviation for immunoglobulin D.

IgE Abbreviation for immunoglobulin E.

IGF Abbreviation for insulin-like growth *factors*, under *factor*.

IgG Abbreviation for immunoglobulin G.

IgM Abbreviation for immunoglobulin M.

ig·na·tia (ig-nā′shē-ă). The dried ripe seed of *Strychnos ignatii* (family Loganiaceae). It is similar in its properties to nux vomica and is a source of strychnine. [St. Ignatius]

ig·ni·pe·di·tes (ig′ni-pe-dī′tēz). Burning pain in the soles of the feet, in multiple neuritis. SYN hotfoot. [L. *ignis*, fire, + *pes* (*ped*-), foot, + G. *itēs*]

ig·ni·punc·ture (ig′ni-pŭngk-chūr). The original procedure of closing a retinal separation by transfixation of the break with cautery. [L. *ignis*, fire, + puncture]

ig·no·tine (ig′nō-tēn). SYN carnosine.

IH Abbreviation for infectious *hepatitis*.

IJP Abbreviation for inhibitory junction *potential*.

iko·ta (ī-kō′tă). A neurosis, similar to latah, affecting married women among the Samoyeds of Siberia.

IL-1 Abbreviation for interleukin-1.

IL-2 Abbreviation for interleukin-2.

IL-3 Abbreviation for interleukin-3.

IL-4 Abbreviation for interleukin-4.

IL-5 Abbreviation for interleukin-5.

IL-6 Abbreviation for interleukin-6.

IL-7 Abbreviation for interleukin-7.

IL-8 Abbreviation for interleukin-8.

IL-9 Abbreviation for interleukin-9.

IL-10 Abbreviation for interleukin-10.

IL-11 Abbreviation for interleukin-11.

IL-12 Abbreviation for interleukin-12.

IL-13 Abbreviation for interleukin-13.

ILA Abbreviation for insulin-like *activity*.

il·e·ac (il′ē-ak). **1.** Relating to the ileus. **2.** Relating to the ileum.

il·e·a·del·phus (il′ē-ă-del′fŭs). SYN *duplicitas* posterior.

il·e·al (il′ē-ăl). Of or pertaining to the ileum.

il·e·ec·to·my (il-ē-ek′tō-mē). Removal of the ileum. [ileum + G. *ektomē*, excision]

il·e·i·tis (il-ē-ī′tis). Inflammation of the ileum.

backwash i., involvement of the terminal ileum by the inflammatory and ulcerative changes seen in chronic ulcerative colitis; distinguished from involvement of ileum and proximal colon by regional (granulomatous) enteritis (*e.g.,* Crohn's disease of terminal ileum and proximal colon).

distal i., regional i., terminal i., SYN regional *enteritis.*

△**ileo-.** The ileum; bottom of the small intestine. [New L. *ileum,* groin]

il·e·o·ce·cal (il′ē-ō-sē′kăl). Relating to both ileum and cecum.

il·e·o·ce·co·cys·to·plas·ty (il′ē-ō-sē′kō-sis′tō-plas-tē). Bladder reconstruction and augmentation with a piece of ileocecum. [ileo- + ceco- + G. *kystis,* bladder, + *plastos,* formed]

il·e·o·ce·cos·to·my (il′ē-ō-sē-kos′tō′mē). Anastomosis of the ileum to the cecum. SYN cecoileostomy.

il·e·o·ce·cum (il-ē-ō-sē′kŭm). The combined ileum and cecum.

il·e·o·co·lic (il′ē-ō-kol′ik). Relating to the ileum and the colon. SYN ileocolonic.

il·e·o·co·li·tis (il′ē-ō-kō-lī′tis). Inflammation to a varying extent of the mucous membrane of both ileum and colon.

il·e·o·co·lon·ic (il′ē-ō-kō-lon′ik). SYN ileocolic.

il·e·o·co·los·to·my (il′ē-ō-kō-los′tō-mē). Establishment of a new communication between the ileum and the colon. [ileo- + colostomy]

il·e·o·cys·to·plas·ty (il′ē-ō-sis′tō-plas-tē). Surgical reconstruction of the bladder involving the use of an isolated intestinal segment to augment bladder capacity. [ileo- + G. *kystis,* bladder, + *plastos,* formed]

il·e·o·en·tec·tro·py (il′ē-ō-en-tek′trō-pē). Rarely used term for eversion of a segment of the ileum. [ileo- + G. *entos,* within, + *ek,* out, + *tropē,* a turning]

il·e·o·il·e·os·to·my (il′ē-ō-il-ē-os′tō-mē). **1.** Establishment of a communication between two segments of the ileum. **2.** The opening so established. [ileum + ileum + G. *stoma,* mouth]

il·e·o·je·ju·ni·tis (il′ē-ō-je-jū-nī′tis). A chronic inflammatory condition involving the jejunum and parts or most of the ileum; occurs in different forms: a granulomatous state resembling regional ileitis, pseudodiverticula, or cicatricial stenosis of the bowel.

il·e·o·pexy (il′ē-ō-pek′sē). Surgical fixation of ileum. [ileo- + G. *pēxis,* fixation]

il·e·o·proc·tos·to·my (il′ē-ō-prok-tos′tō-mē). Establishment of a communication between the ileum and the rectum. SYN ileorectostomy. [ileo- + G. *prōktos,* anus (rectum), + *stoma,* mouth]

il·e·o·rec·tos·to·my (il′ē-ō-rek-tos′tō-mē). SYN ileoproctostomy. [ileum + rectum + G. *stoma,* mouth]

il·e·or·rha·phy (il′ē-ō-ōr′ă-fē). Suturing the ileum. [ileo- + G. *rhaphē,* suture]

il·e·o·sig·moid·os·to·my (il′ē-ō-sig′moyd-os′tō-mē). Establishment of a communication between the ileum and the sigmoid colon. [ileo- + sigmoid, + G. *stoma,* mouth]

il·e·os·to·my (il′ē-os′tō-mē). Establishment of a fistula through which the ileum discharges directly to the outside of the body. [ileo- + G. *stoma,* mouth]

Brooke i., i. in which the divided proximal ileum, brought through the abdominal wall, is evaginated and its edge is sutured to the dermis; a 2 cm protrusion is maintained by additional suturing.

Kock i., SYN Kock *pouch.*

il·e·ot·o·my (il′ē-ot′ō-mē). Incision into the ileum. [ileo- + G. *tomē,* incision]

il·e·o·trans·ver·sos·to·my (il′ē-ō-tranz-vers-os′tō-me). Anastomosis of the ileum to the transverse colon. [ileum + transverse colon, + G. *stoma,* mouth]

il·e·um (il′ē-ŭm) [NA]. The third portion of the small intestine, about 12 feet in length, extending from the junction with the jejunum to the ileocecal opening. It is distinct from jejunum in being typically smaller in diameter with thinner walls, having smaller and less complex plicae circulares, its mesentery having more fat and its arteries (ileal arteries) forming more tiers of

arterial arcades with shorter vasa recta. [L. fr. G. *eileō,* to roll up, twist]

i. du′plex, tubular or cystic segmental duplications of alimentary tract.

il·e·us (il′ē-ŭs). Mechanical, dynamic, or adynamic obstruction of the bowel; may be accompanied by severe colicky pain, abdominal distention, vomiting, absence of passage of stool, and often fever and dehydration. [G. *eileos,* intestinal colic, from *eilō,* to roll up tight]

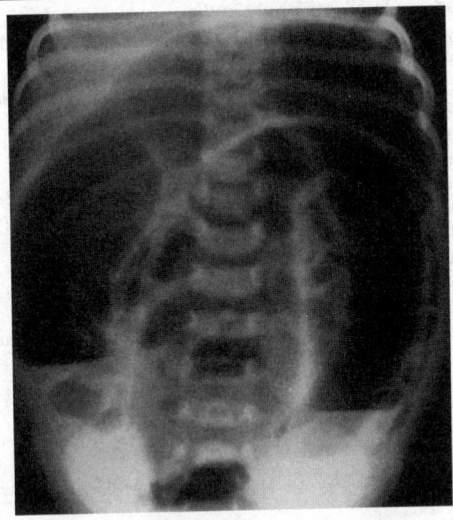

ileus
with expansion of the intestinal coils and mirror-formation of the lower small intestine and large intestine

adynamic i., obstruction of the bowel due to paralysis of the bowel wall, usually as a result of localized or generalized peritonitis or shock. SYN paralytic i.

dynamic i., intestinal obstruction due to spastic contraction of a segment of the bowel. SYN spastic i.

gallstone i., obstruction of the small intestine produced by passage of a gallstone from the biliary tract (usually the gallbladder as a result of cholecystitis) into the intestinal tract (usually by means of a fistulous connection between the gallbladder and the small intestine); occurrence and site of obstruction depend upon size of the stone, but the usual location is at or near the ileocecal junction.

mechanical i., obstruction of the bowel due to some mechanical cause, *e.g.,* volvulus, gallstone, adhesions.

meconium i., intestinal obstruction in the fetus and newborn following inspissation of meconium and caused by lack of trypsin; associated with cystic fibrosis.

occlusive i., complete mechanical blocking of the intestinal lumen.

paralytic i., SYN adynamic i.

spastic i., SYN dynamic i.

i. subpar′ta, obstruction of the large bowel by pressure of the pregnant uterus.

terminal i., obstruction of the lower part of the small bowel.

verminous i., obstruction due to masses of intestinal parasites.

il·i·ac (il′ē-ak). Relating to the ilium.

il·i·a·cus (il-ī′ă-kŭs). SEE iliacus *muscle.*

il·i·a·del·phus (il′ē-ă-del′fŭs). SYN *duplicitas* posterior. [L. *ilium* + G. *adelphos,* brother]

△**ilio-.** The ilium; top of hip bone. [L. *ilium*]

il·i·o·coc·cyg·e·al (il′ē-ō-kok-sij′ē-ăl). Relating to the ilium and the coccyx.

il·i·o·co·lot·o·my (il′ē-ō-kō-lot′ō-mē). The operation of opening

il

into the colon in the inguinal (iliac) region. [ilio- + G. *kolon*, colon, + *tomē*, incision]

il·i·o·cos·tal (il′ē-ō-kos′tăl). Relating to the ilium and the ribs; denoting muscles passing between the two parts.

il·i·o·cos·ta·lis (il′ē-ō-kos-tā′lis). SEE iliocostalis *muscle*.

il·i·o·fem·o·ral (il′ē-ō-fem′ŏ-răl). Relating to the ilium and the femur.

il·i·o·fem·o·ro·plas·ty (il-ē-o-fem′ŏr-ō-plas-tē). An obsolete method of securing a hip fusion by an extra-articular technique (a joint bypass procedure) in which a turned down bone flap from the ilium is placed into a split in the greater trochanter.

il·i·o·hy·po·gas·tric (il′ē-ō-hī-pō-gas′trik). Relating to the iliac and the hypogastric regions.

il·i·o·in·gui·nal (il′ē-ō-ing′gwi-năl). Relating to the iliac region and the groin.

il·i·o·lum·bar (il-ē-ō-lŭm′băr). Relating to the iliac and the lumbar regions.

il·i·om·e·ter (il-ē-om′ĕ-ter). An instrument for measuring exact position of iliac spines and lower vertebrae. [ilio- + G. *metron*, measure]

il·i·op·a·gus (il-ē-op′ă-gŭs). Conjoined twins in which the fusion is restricted to the iliac region. SEE conjoined *twins*, under *twin*. [ilio- + G. *pagos*, something fixed]

il·i·o·pec·tin·e·al (il′ē-ō-pek-tin′ē-ăl). Relating to the ilium and the pubis.

il·i·o·pel·vic (il′ē-ō-pel′vik). Relating to the iliac region and the cavity of the pelvis.

il·i·o·sa·cral (il′ē-ō-sā′krăl). Relating to the ilium and the sacrum.

il·i·o·sci·at·ic (il′ē-ō-sī-at′ik). Relating to the ilium and the ischium.

il·i·o·spi·nal (il′ē-ō-spī′năl). Relating to the ilium and the spinal column.

il·i·o·tho·ra·cop·a·gus (il′ē-ō-thōr-ă-kop′ă-gŭs). Conjoined twins in which union occurs through the ilia and extends to involve the thoraces. SEE conjoined *twins*, under *twin*. SYN ischiothoracopagus. [ilio- + G. *thorax*, chest, + *pagos*, fixed]

il·i·o·tib·i·al (il′ē-ō-tib′ē-ăl). Relating to the ilium and the tibia.

il·i·o·tro·chan·ter·ic (il′ē-ō-trō-kan-ter′ik). Relating to the ilium and the great trochanter of the femur.

il·i·o·xi·phop·a·gus (il′ē-ō-zī-fop′ă-gŭs). Conjoined twins in which the fusion extends from the xiphoid to the iliac region. SEE conjoined *twins*, under *twin*. [ilio- + xiphoid, + G. *pagos*, fixed]

il·i·um, pl. **il·i·a** (il′ē-ŭm, il′ē-ă). The broad, flaring portion of the hip bone, distinct at birth but later becoming fused with the ischium and pubis; it consists of a body, which joins the pubis and ischium to form the acetabulum and a broad thin portion, called the ala or wing. SYN os ilium [NA], os iliacum★, flank bone, iliac bone. [L. groin, flank]

ill. In veterinary medicine, a term used in the common names of several diseases.

joint i., a chronic suppurative inflammation of the joints of foals and other newly born animals, due to umbilical infection with pyogenic bacteria, one of the most common being *Actinobacillus equuli*. SYN joint evil.

louping i., a highly virulent viral encephalomyelitis of sheep in Great Britain and the Iberian peninsula characterized by cerebellar ataxia; caused by a flavivirus (louping-ill virus) and transmitted by the tick, *Ixodes ricinus*.

navel i., a term applied to any kind of acute generalized infections of young mammals having their origin in a wound infection occurring in the stump of the umbilical cord; these infections generally are pyemic, and liver and lung abscesses and multiple acute arthritis are characteristic.

il·lic·i·um (il-lis′ē-ŭm). Chinese or star anise, the dried fruit of *Illhicium verum* (family Magnoliaceae), an evergreen shrub or small tree of southern China; used as a stimulating carminative. [L. an allurement, fr. *il-licio*, to allure]

il·lin·i·tion (il-in-ish′ŭn). The friction of a surface to facilitate absorption of an ointment. [L. *il-lino*, pp. -*litus*, to smear on (*in* + *lino*)]

ill·ness (il′nes). SYN disease (1).

functional i., SYN functional *disorder*.

manic-depressive i., an obsolete term for one of the mood disorders previously called manic-depressive *disorder*.

mental i., (1) a broadly inclusive term, generally denoting one or all of the following: 1) a disease of the brain, with predominant behavioral symptoms, as in paresis or acute alcoholism; 2) a disease of the "mind" or personality, evidenced by abnormal behavior, as in hysteria or schizophrenia; also called mental or emotional disease, disturbance, or disorder, or behavior disorder; (2) any psychiatric illness listed in *Current Medical Information and Terminology* of the American Medical Association or in the *Diagnostic and Statistical Manual for Mental Disorders* of the American Psychiatric Association. SEE ALSO behavior *disorder*.

il·lu·mi·na·tion (i-lū′mi-nā′shŭn). **1.** Throwing light on the body or a part or into a cavity for diagnostic purposes. **2.** Lighting an object under a microscope. [L. *il-lumino*, pp. -atus, to light up]

axial i., the transmission or reflection of light in the direction of the axis of an optical system. SYN central i.

central i., SYN axial i.

contact i., i. of the eye by means of an instrument in contact with the cornea or bulbar conjunctiva.

critical i., the precise focusing of the light source directly upon the object being examined.

dark-field i., a procedure in which a black circular shield is used to block the majority of the vertically directed rays of light (*e.g.,* the field is dark), and a circumferential, suitably angled, mirrored surface is used to direct the peripheral rays horizontally against the object, thereby reflecting the light vertically through the objective lens and along the optical axis; thus, the object is well illuminated in a contrasting dark background. SYN dark-ground i.

dark-ground i., SYN dark-field i.

direct i., an i. in which the rays of light are directed downward, almost perpendicularly onto the upper surface of the object, which reflects the rays upward into the optical system. SYN erect i., vertical i.

erect i., SYN direct i.

focal i., i. in which a beam of light is directed diagonally to an object so that it is brilliantly illuminated while the surrounding area is in shadow. SYN lateral i., oblique i.

Köhler i., a method of i. of microscopic objects in which the image of the light source is focused on the substage condenser diaphragm and the diaphragm of the light source is focused in the same plane with the object to be observed; maximizes both the brightness and uniformity of the illuminated field.

lateral i., SYN focal i.

oblique i., SYN focal i.

vertical i., SYN direct i.

il·lu·mi·nism (i-lū′mi-nizm). A psychotic state of exaltation in which one has delusions and hallucinations of communion with supernatural or exalted beings.

il·lu·sion (i-lū′zhŭn). A false perception; the mistaking of something for what it is not. [L. *illusio*, fr. *il- ludo*, pp. -*lusus*, to play at, mock]

i. of doubles, SYN Capgras' *syndrome*.

i. of movement, successive stimulation of neighboring retinal points which causes the sensation of movement.

oculogravic i., apparent movement of the visual field when the body is subjected to acceleration; due to gravity.

oculogyral i., an i. occurring in angular acceleration in which the position of fixed light appears to drift.

optical i., a false interpretation of the color, form, size, or movement of a visual sensation.

il·lu·sion·al (i-lū′zhŭn-ăl). Relating to or of the nature of an illusion.

ILO Abbreviation for International Labour Organization.

Ilosvay, Lajos de, Hungarian chemist, *1851. SEE I. *reagent*.

IM Abbreviation for internal *medicine*.

I.M., i.m. Abbreviation for intramuscular, or intramuscularly.

ima (ī′mă). Lowest. SEE ALSO imus. [L.]

im·age (im′ij). **1.** Representation of an object made by the rays of light emanating or reflected from it. **2.** Representation produced by x-rays, ultrasound, tomography, thermography, radioisotopes, etc.; as a verb, to produce such representations. [L. *imago,* likeness]

accidental i., SYN afterimage.

body i., (1) the cerebral representation of all body sensation organized in the parietal cortex; **(2)** personal conception of one's own body as distinct from one's actual anatomic body or the conception other persons have of it. SYN body schema.

catatropic i., SYN Purkinje-Sanson i.'s.

direct i., SYN virtual i.

eidetic i., vivid mental i. in the form of a dream, fantasy, or an unusual power of memory and visualization of objects previously seen or imagined.

false i., the i. in the deviating eye in strabismus.

heteronymous i., a double i. in physiological diplopia, when fixation is directed beyond an object; the right i. arises from the left eye, while the left i. arises from the right eye; *i.e.,* there is a crossed diplopia.

homonymous i.'s, double i.'s produced by stimuli arising from points proximal to the horopter. SYN homonymous diplopia, simple diplopia, uncrossed diplopia.

hypnagogic i., imagery occurring between wakefulness and sleep.

hypnopompic i., imagery occurring after the sleeping state and before complete wakefulness; similar to hypnagogic imagery except for the time of occurrence.

inverted i., SYN real i.

mental i., a picture of an object not present, produced in the mind by memory or imagination.

mirror i., a representation of an object or part thereof as its reflected i. in a glass mirror.

motor i., the i. of body movements.

negative i., SYN afterimage.

optical i., an i. formed by the refraction or reflection of light.

phase i., a magnetic resonance i. showing only phase shift information, to detect motion.

Purkinje i.'s, SYN Purkinje-Sanson i.'s.

Purkinje-Sanson i.'s, the two images formed by the anterior and posterior surfaces of the cornea and the two images formed by the anterior and posterior surfaces of the lens. SYN catatropic i., Purkinje i.'s, Sanson's i.'s.

real i., an i. formed by the convergence of the actual rays of light from an object. SYN inverted i.

retinal i., a real i. formed on the retina.

Sanson's i.'s, SYN Purkinje-Sanson i.'s.

sensory i., an i. based on one or more types of sensation.

specular i., the i. of a source of light made visible by the reflection from a mirror.

tactile i., an i. of an object as perceived by the sense of touch.

unequal retinal i., SYN aniseikonia.

virtual i., an erect i. formed by projection of divergent rays from an optical system. SYN direct i.

visual i., a collection of foci corresponding to all the luminous points of an object.

im·age in·ten·si·fi·er. SYN image *amplifier.*

im·ag·e·ry (im′ij-rē). A technique in behavior therapy in which the client or patient is conditioned to substitute pleasant fantasies to counter the unpleasant feelings associated with anxiety.

imag·i·nal (ĭ-maj′i-năl). Relating to an image or to the process of imagining.

imag·ing (im′ă-jing). Radiological production of a clinical image using x-rays, ultrasound, computed tomography, magnetic resonance, radionuclide scanning, thermography, etc.; especially, cross-sectional imaging, such as ultrasonography, CT, or MRI. [see image]

blood pool i., nuclear medicine study using a radionuclide that is confined to the vascular compartment.

exercise i., SEE stress *test.*

magnetic resonance i. (MRI), a diagnostic radiological modali-

ty, using nuclear magnetic resonance technology, in which the magnetic nuclei (especially protons) of a patient are aligned in a strong, uniform magnetic field, absorb energy from tuned radiofrequency pulses, and emit radiofrequency signals as their excitation decays. These signals, which vary in intensity according to nuclear abundance and molecular chemical environment, are converted into sets of tomographic images by using field gradients in the magnetic field, which permits 3-dimensional localization of the point sources of the signals. SYN nuclear magnetic resonance i., NMR i., nuclear magnetic resonance tomography.

The basic idea of MRI was conceived in 1948 but could not be implemented until the advent of computers and the mathematical technique known as algebraic reconstruction. Unlike conventional radiography or CT, MRI does not expose patients to ionizing radiation. In addition, it provides superior 3-D images of the body's interior, delineating muscle, bone, blood vessel, nerve, organ, and tumor tissue.

nuclear magnetic resonance i., NMR i., SYN magnetic resonance i.

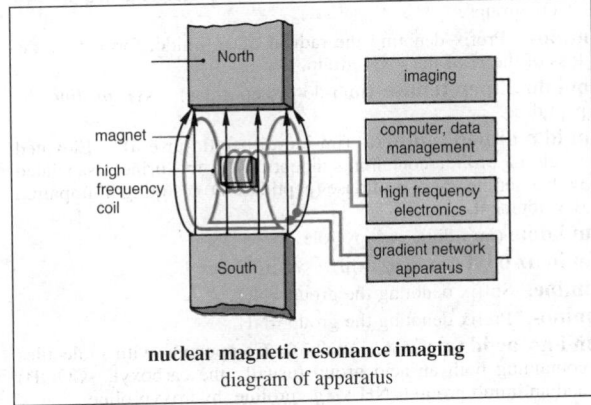

nuclear magnetic resonance imaging
diagram of apparatus

pharmacologic stress i., SEE stress *test.*

through transfer i., SYN transfer i.

transfer i., the production of an ultrasound image by detection and analysis of sound on the opposite side of the body from the emitting transducer. SYN through transfer i.

imag·ing de·part·ment. the diagnostic radiology department. SEE imaging, radiology.

ima·go, pl. **imag·ines** (i-mā′gō, i-maj′i-nēz). **1.** The last stage of an insect after it has completed all its metamorphoses through the egg, larva, and pupa; the adult insect form. **2.** SYN archetype (2). [L. image]

im·bal·ance (im-bal′ans). **1.** Lack of equality between opposing forces. **2.** Lack of equality in some aspect of binocular vision, such as muscle balance, image size, and/or image shape. [L. *in-* neg. + *bi-lanx* (*-lanc-*), having two scales, fr. *bis,* twice, + *lanx,* dish, scale of a balance]

autonomic i., a lack of balance between sympathetic and parasympathetic nervous systems, especially in relation to the vasomotor disturbances. SYN vasomotor i.

occlusal i., an inharmonious relationship between the teeth of the maxilla and mandible during closing or functional movements of the jaw.

sex chromosome i., any abnormal pattern of sex chromosomes; *e.g.,* XXY in men with seminiferous tubule dysgenesis, XO in women with Turner's syndrome; rarer patterns of i. are XXX, XXXY, and XYY. SEE ALSO isochromosome.

sympathetic i., SYN vagotonia.

vasomotor i., SYN autonomic i.

im·be·cile (im′bĕ-sil). An obsolete term for a subclass of mental *retardation* or the individual classified therein. [L. *imbecillus,* weak, silly]

im·bed. SYN embed.

im·bi·bi·tion (im-bi-bish'ŭn). **1.** Absorption of fluid by a solid body without resultant chemical change in either. **2.** Taking up of water by a gel, thereby increasing its size. [L. *im-bibo,* to drink in (*in + bibo*)]

im·bri·cate, im·bri·cat·ed (im'bri-kāt, im'bri-kā-ted). Overlapping like shingles. [L. *imbricatus,* covered with tiles]

im·bri·ca·tion (im'bri-kā'shŭn). The operative overlapping of layers of tissue in the closure of wounds or the repair of defects. [see imbricate]

im·id·a·zole (im-id-az'ōl). 1,3-Diazole; 1,3-diaza-2,4-cyclopentadiene; a five-membered heterocyclic compound occurring in L-histidine and other biologically important compounds.

    i. alkaloids, alkaloids containing one or more i. moieties as part of its structure (*e.g.,* pilocarpine).

4-im·id·a·zo·lone-5-pro·pi·on·ate (im-id-a-zō'lōn). An intermediate in histidine degradation; seen in reduced levels in urocanic aciduria.

im·id·az·o·lyl (im-id-az'ō-lil). The radical of imidazole. SYN iminazolyl.

im·ide (im'īd). The radical or group, =NH, attached to two –CO– groups.

△**imido-.** Prefix denoting the radical of an imide, formed by the loss of the H of the =NH group.

im·i·do·di·pep·ti·dase (im'i-dō-dī-pep'ti-dās). SYN *proline* dipeptidase.

im·id·o·di·pep·ti·du·ria (im-idō-dī-pep'tīd-ūr-ē-ă). Elevated levels of proline-containing dipeptides in the urine; associated with a deficiency of prolidase (peptidase D) resulting in impaired development.

im·i·dole (im'i-dōl). SYN pyrrole.

im·in·az·o·lyl (im-in-az'ō-lil). SYN imidazolyl.

△**-imine.** Suffix denoting the group =NH.

△**imino-.** Prefix denoting the group =NH.

im·i·no ac·ids (im'i-nō, i-mē'nō). Compounds with molecules containing both an acid group (usually the carboxyl, –COOH) and an imino group (=NH); *e.g.,* proline, hydroxyproline.

im·i·no·car·bon·yl (im'i-nō-kar'bon-il). SEE carboxamide.

im·i·no·di·pep·ti·dase (im'i-nō-dī-pep'ti-dās). SYN *prolyl* dipeptidase.

im·i·no·gly·ci·nu·ria (im'i-nō-glī-si-nū'rē-ă) [MIM*242600]. A benign inborn error of amino acid transport in renal tubule and intestine; glycine, proline, and hydroxyproline are excreted in the urine.

im·i·no·hy·dro·las·es (im'i-nō-hī'drō-lās-ez) [EC class 3.5.3]. Enzymes that hydrolyze imino groups; *e.g.,* arginine deiminase. SYN deiminases.

im·in·os·til·benes (im'i-nō-stil'bēnz). A chemical class of agents of which carbamazepine, an antiepileptic drug, is the most prominent.

im·i·pen·em (im-i-pen'em). $C_{12}H_{17}N_3O_4S \cdot H_2O$; a thienamycin antibiotic with broad spectrum activity used, in combination with cilastin, to treat a variety of infections.

imip·ra·mine hy·dro·chlo·ride (im-ip'ră-mēn). 5-(3-Dimethylaminopropyl)-10,11-dihydro-5*H*-dibenz(*b,f*)azepine hydrochloride; a tricyclic antidepressant.

IML. Abbreviation for intermediolateral cell column of the spinal cord gray matter.

Imlach, Francis, Scottish anatomist and surgeon, 1819–1891. SEE I.'s *fat-pad, ring.*

im·me·di·ca·ble (im-med'i-kă-bl). Obsolete term meaning not curable by medicinal remedies. [L. *in-* neg. + *medicabilis,* curable]

im·mer·sion (i-mer'zhŭn). **1.** The placing of a body under water or other liquid. **2.** In microscopy, filling the space between the objective lens and the top of the cover glass with a fluid, such as water or oil, to reduce spherical aberration and increase effective numerical aperture by elimination of refractive effects that result from an air-glass interface; the best resolution is achieved when the space between the condenser lens and the specimen slide is also filled with the fluid. [L. *im-mergo,* pp. *-mersus,* to dip in (*in + mergo*)]

    homogeneous i., in i. microscopy, use of a fluid, such as oil, that has a refractive index virtually identical to that of glass, providing the highest possible numerical aperture.

    oil i., water i., SEE immersion (2).

im·mis·ci·ble (i-mis'i-bl). Incapable of mutual solution; *e.g.,* oil and water. [L. *im-misceo,* to mix in (*in + misceo*)]

im·mit·tance (i-mit'ans). In audiology, a general term describing measurements made of tympanic membrane impedance, compliance, or admittance. [L. *immitto,* to send in]

im·mo·bi·li·za·tion (i-mo'bi-li-zā'shŭn). The act of making immovable. [see immobilize]

im·mo·bi·lize (i-mō'bi-līz). To render fixed or incapable of moving. [L. *in-* neg. + *mobilis,* movable]

im·mor·tal·i·za·tion (i-mŏr'tăl-i-zā'shŭn). Conferring on normal cells cultured *in vitro* the property of an infinite lifespan, as from spontaneous mutation, by exposure to chemical carcinogens, or by viral infection. I. of primary cells in culture is the first of several steps in the expression of transforming genes of DNA tumor viruses, of retrovirus oncogenes, and cellular oncogenes derived from human cancer cells.

im·mune (i-myūn'). **1.** Free from the possibility of acquiring a given infectious disease; resistant to an infectious disease. **2.** Pertaining to the mechanism of sensitization in which the reactivity is so altered by previous contact with an antigen that the responsive tissues respond quickly upon subsequent contact, or to *in vitro* reactions with antibody-containing serum from such sensitized individuals. [L. *immunis,* free from service, fr. *in,* neg., + *munus* (*muner-*), service]

im·mu·ni·fa·cient (im'yū-ni-fā'shent). Making immune after a specific disease. [L. *immunis,* exempt, + *faciens,* making, pr. part. of *facio*]

im·mu·ni·ty (i-myū'ni-tē). The status or quality of being immune (1). SYN insusceptibility. [L. *immunitas* (see immune)]

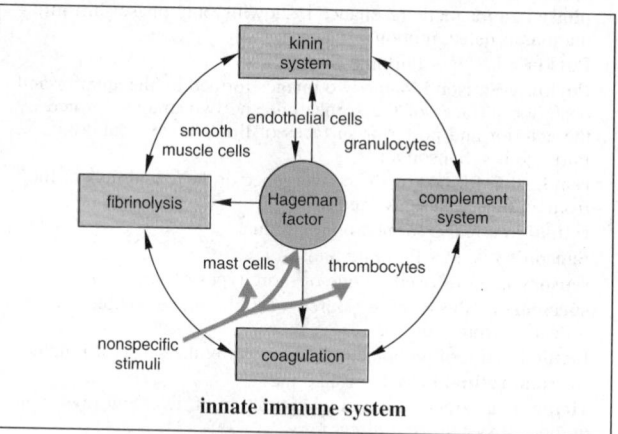

innate immune system

acquired i., resistance resulting from previous exposure of the individual in question to an infectious agent or antigen; it may be *active* and *specific,* as a result of naturally acquired (apparent or inapparent) infection or intentional vaccination (artificial active i.); or it may be *passive,* being acquired from transfer of antibodies from another person or from an animal, either naturally, as from mother to fetus, or by intentional inoculation (artificial passive i.), and, with respect to the particular antibodies transferred, it is *specific.* Passive, cell-mediated i. produced by the transfer of living lymphoid cells from an immune (allergic or sensitive) animal to a normal one is sometimes referred to as adoptive i.

active i., SEE acquired i.

adoptive i., SEE acquired i.

antiviral i., i. resulting from virus infection, either naturally acquired or produced by intentional vaccination; compared to some bacterial i.'s, it is of relatively long duration, but this may be the result of infection-immunity rather than being peculiar to virus infection per se, since it occurs also in bacterial i. after infections such as typhoid fever.

artificial active i., SEE acquired i.

artificial passive i., SEE acquired i.

bacteriophage i., the state induced in a bacterium by lysogenization, the lysogenic bacterium being insusceptible to further lysogenization or to a lytic cycle by a superinfecting bacteriophage, in contradistinction to bacteriophage resistance.

cell-mediated i. (CMI), cellular i., immune responses which are initiated by T lymphocytes and mediated by T lymphocytes, macrophages, or both (*e.g.,* graft rejection, delayed-type hypersensitivity). SYN delayed hypersensitivity (1).

concomitant i., SYN infection i.

general i., i. associated with widely diffused mechanisms that tend to protect the body as a whole, as compared with local i.

group i., SYN herd i.

herd i., the resistance to invasion and spread of an infectious agent in a group or community, based on the resistance to infection of a high proportion of individual members of the group; resistance is a product of the number susceptible and the probability that susceptibles will come into contact with an infected person. SYN group i.

humoral i., i. associated with circulating antibodies, in contradistinction to cellular i.

infection i., the paradoxical immune status in which resistance to reinfection coincides with the persistence of the original infection. SYN concomitant i.

innate i., resistance manifested by a species (or by races, families, and individuals in a species) that has not been immunized (sensitized, allergized) by previous infection or vaccination; much of it results from body mechanisms that are poorly understood, but are different from those responsible for the altered reactivity associated with the specific nature of acquired i.; in general, innate i. is nonspecific and is not stimulated by specific antigens. SEE ALSO self. SYN natural i., nonspecific i.

local i., a natural or acquired i. to certain infectious agents, as manifested by an organ or a tissue, as a whole or in part.

maternal i., i. acquired by a fetus because of the presence of maternal IgG that passes through the placenta.

natural i., nonspecific i., SYN innate i.

passive i., SEE acquired i.

relative i., a modified, not completely effective resistance that results when there is a sort of "fluctuating equilibrium" between the defense mechanisms of the host and the infective agent.

specific i., the immune status in which there is an altered reactivity directed solely against the antigenic determinants (infectious agent or other) that stimulated it. SEE acquired i.

specific active i., SEE acquired i.

specific passive i., SEE acquired i.

stress i., insusceptibility or resistance to the effects of emotional strain.

im·mu·ni·za·tion. Protection of susceptible individuals from communicable diseases by administration of a living modified agent (*e.g.,* yellow fever vaccine), a suspension of killed organisms (*e.g.,* pertussis vaccine), or an inactivated toxin (*e.g.,* tetanus). SEE ALSO vaccination, allergization.

active i., the production of active immunity.

passive i., the production of passive immunity.

im·mu·nize (im′yū-nīz). To render immune.

immuno-. Immune, immunity. [L. *immunis,* immune]

im·mu·no·ad·ju·vant (im′yū-nō-ad′jū-vant). SEE adjuvant (2).

im·mu·no·ag·glu·ti·na·tion (im′yū-nō-ă-glū-ti-nā′shŭn). Specific agglutination effected by antibody.

im·mu·no·as·say (im′yū-nō-as′ā). Detection and assay of substances by serological (immunological) methods; in most applications the substance in question serves as antigen, both in antibody production and in measurement of antibody by the test substance. SEE ALSO radioimmunoassay, radioimmunoelectrophoresis, immunologic pregnancy *test.* SYN immunochemical assay.

double antibody i., SYN double antibody *precipitation.*

enzyme i., any of several i. methods that use an enzyme covalently linked to an antigen or antibody as a label; the most

common types are enzyme-linked immunosorbent assay (ELISA) and enzyme-multiplied immunoassay technique (EMIT). SEE ALSO enzyme-linked immunosorbent *assay,* enzyme-multiplied i. technique.

enzyme-multiplied i. technique (EMIT), a type of i. in which the ligand is labeled with an enzyme, and the enzyme-ligand-antibody complex is enzymatically inactive, allowing quantitation of unlabeled ligand. SEE ALSO competitive binding *assay,* enzyme-linked immunosorbent *assay.*

solid phase i., i. in which the antigen or serum is bound to a solid surface, such as a microplate wall or the sides of a tube, the other reactants being free in solution.

thin-layer i., a method for detection of antigen-antibody reactions, applicable to detection of either antigen or antibody, based on the fact that either reactant, when added to a polystyrene surface (such as a well in a polystyrene plate) is adsorbed as a thin layer and acts as an immunosorbent capable of binding with the second reactant.

im·mun·o·bi·ol·o·gy (im′ū-nō-bī-ōl-ō-ijē). The study of the immune factors that affect the growth, development, and health of biological organisms.

im·mu·no·blast (im′yū-nō-blast). An antigenically stimulated lymphocyte; a large cell with well-defined basophilic cytoplasm, a large nucleus with prominent nuclear membrane, distinct nucleoli, and clumped chromatin. SEE ALSO lymphocyte *transformation.* [immuno- + G. *blastos,* germ]

im·mu·no·blot, im·mu·no·blot·ting. Process by which antigens can be separated by electrophoresis and allowed to adhere onto nitrocellulose sheets where they bind nonspecifically and then are subsequently identified by staining with appropriately labeled antibodies. SEE ALSO Western blot *analysis.*

im·mu·no·blot·ting. SEE immunoblot.

im·mu·no·chem·is·try (im′yū-nō-kem′is-trē). The field of chemistry concerned with chemical aspects of immunologic phenomena, *e.g.,* chemical reactions related to antigen stimulation of tissues, chemical studies of antigens and antibody. SYN chemoimmunology.

im·mu·no·com·pe·tence (im′yū-nō-kom′pě-tens). The ability to produce a normal immune response. SYN immunological competence.

im·mu·no·com·pe·tent (im′yū-nō-kom′pě-tent). Possessing the ability to mount a normal immune response.

im·mu·no·com·plex. Complexes of antibody and antigen. SEE immune *complex.*

im·mu·no·com·pro·mised (im′yū-nō-kom′pro-mīzd). Denoting an individual whose immunologic mechanism is deficient either because of an immunodeficiency disorder or because it has been rendered so by immunosuppressive agents.

im·mu·no·con·glu·ti·nin (im′yū-nō-kon-glū′ti-nin). An autoantibody-like immunoglobulin (IgM) formed in animals (or man) against their own complement following injection of complement-containing complexes or sensitized bacteria.

im·mu·no·cyte (im′yū-nō-sīt). An immunologically competent leukocyte capable, actively or potentially, of producing antibodies or reacting in cell-mediated immunity reactions. SEE ALSO I cell. [immuno- + G. *kytos,* cell]

im·mu·no·cy·to·ad·her·ence (im′ū-nō-sī′tō-ad-her′ens). A method for determining cell surface properties, in which immunoglobulin or receptors on the surface of one cell population cause cells with corresponding molecular configurations on their surface to adhere in rosettes around the cells.

im·mu·no·cy·to·chem·is·try (im′yū-nō-sī-tō-kem′is-trē). The study of cell constituents by immunologic methods, such as the use of fluorescent antibodies.

im·mu·no·de·fi·cien·cy (im′yū-nō-dē-fish′en-sē). A condition resulting from a defective immune mechanism; may be *primary* (due to a defect in the immune mechanism itself) or *secondary* (dependent upon another disease process), *specific* (due to a defect in either the B-lymphocyte or the T-lymphocyte system, or both), or *nonspecific* (due to a defect in one or another component of the nonspecific immune mechanism: the complement, properdin, or phagocytic system). SYN immune deficiency, immunity deficiency, immunological deficiency.

im

congenital immunodeficiency disorders				
defects of the B-cell series	defects of the T-cell series	combined T- and B-cell defects	phagocytosis problems	defects of complement
congenital sex-linked agammaglobulinemia (Bruton type) selective IgA deficiency transitory hypogamma-globulinemia of infants and small children dysimmunoglobulinemias	DiGeorge syndrome Nezelof syndrome chronic mycocutaneous candidiasis	reticular dysgenesis agammaglobulinemia–"Swiss" type immunodeficiency with disproportionate dwarfism Louis-Bar syndrome Wiskott-Aldrich syndrome episodic lymphopenia with lymphocytotoxin variable, not yet classified immunodeficiencies	progressive septic granulomatosis myeloperoxydase-defect Chédiak-Higashi syndrome Job syndrome lazy leukocyte syndrome	C1q defect C1r defect C1s defect in combination with C1r defect C1s inhibitor defect (hereditary angioedema) C2 defect homozygotic C3 defect C3b inactivator-defect C5 dysfunction C6 defect C7 defect C8 defect

cellular i. with abnormal immunoglobulin synthesis, an ill-defined group of sporadic disorders of unknown cause, occurring in both males and females and associated with recurrent bacterial, fungal, protozoal, and viral infections; there is thymic hypoplasia with depressed cellular (T-lymphocyte) immunity combined with defective humoral (B-lymphocyte) immunity, although immunoglobulin levels may be normal. SYN Nezelof syndrome, Nezelof type of thymic alymphoplasia.

combined i., i. of both the B-lymphocytes and T-lymphocytes.

common variable i. [MIM*240500], i. of unknown cause, and usually unclassifiable; usually occurs after age 15 years but may occur at any age in either sex; the total quantity of immunoglobulin is commonly less than 300 mg/dl; the number of B-lymphocytes is often within normal limits but there is a lack of plasma cells in lymphoid tissue; cellular (T-lymphocyte) immunity is usually intact; there is an increased susceptibility to pyogenic infection and often autoimmune disease. SYN acquired agammaglobulinemia, acquired hypogammaglobulinemia.

phagocytic dysfunction i., suppression in number or function of phagocytic cells such as in chronic granulomatous disease. SYN phagocytic dysfunction disorders i.

phagocytic dysfunction disorders i., SYN phagocytic dysfunction i.

secondary i., i. in which there is no evident defect in the lymphoid tissues, but rather hypercatabolism or loss of immunoglobulins such as occurs in familial idiopathic hypercatabolic hypoproteinemia or in defects associated with the nephrotic syndrome. SYN secondary agammaglobulinemia, secondary antibody deficiency, secondary hypogammaglobulinemia.

severe combined i. (SCID) [MIM*202500 & MIM*300400], **(1)** absence of both humoral (antibody) and cellular immunity with alymphoplasia or lymphopenia (both B-type and T-type lymphocytes), associated with marked susceptibility to infection by bacteria, fungi, protozoa, and viruses, and to progressive disease from live vaccines; death occurs usually before the end of the first year of life, although bone marrow transplants have been effective; both X-linked recessive and autosomal recessive forms occur; autosomal recessive mutation that results in a severe i. SCID can be inherited as either an X-linked recessive or autosomal recessive. About one-half of those with autosomal recessive SCID have adenosine deaminase deficiency. i.'s disease individuals have a deficiency of adenosine deaminase; there is also an X-linked severe combined i. with a major histocompatability class I and/or class II deficiency; **(2)** SCID mice lack mature T- and B- cells and are therefore used for transplantation and study of human lymphoid tissues resulting in a SCID-human mouse chimera. SYN Swiss type agammaglobulinemia.

i. with elevated IgM, i. with reduced IgG and IgA-bearing cells; there is recurrent pyogenic infection; X-linked in some families.

i. with hypoparathyroidism, SYN DiGeorge *syndrome*. SYN thymic hypoplasia.

im·mu·no·de·fi·cient (im′yū-nō-dē-fish′ent). Lacking in some essential function of the immune system.

im·mu·no·de·pres·sant (im′yū-nō-dē-pres′ănt). SYN immuno-suppressant.

im·mu·no·de·pres·sor (im′yū-nō-dē-pres′ŏr, -ōr). SYN immuno-suppressant.

im·mu·no·di·ag·no·sis (im′yū-nō-dī-ag-nō′sis). The process of determining specified immunologic characteristics of individuals or of cells, serum, or other biologic specimens.

im·mu·no·dif·fu·sion (im′yū-nō-di-fyū′zhŭn, i-myū′nō-). A technique of study of antigen-antibody reactions by observing precipitates formed by combination of specific antigen and antibodies which have diffused in a gel in which they have been separately placed.

double i., SEE gel diffusion precipitin *tests* in two dimensions, under *test*.

radial i. (RID), SEE gel diffusion precipitin *tests* in two dimensions, under *test*.

single i., SEE gel diffusion precipitin *tests* in one dimension, under *test*, gel diffusion precipitin *tests* in two dimensions, under *test*.

im·mu·no·e·lec·tro·pho·re·sis (im′yū-nō-ē-lek′trō-fō-rē′sis). A kind of precipitin test in which the components of one group of immunological reactants (usually a mixture of antigens) are first separated on the basis of electrophoretic mobility in agar or other medium, the separated components then being identified, by means of the technique of double diffusion, on the basis of precipitates formed by reaction with components of the other group of reactants (antibodies).

crossed i., SYN two-dimensional i.

rocket i., a quantitative method for serum proteins which involves electrophoresis of antigen into a gel containing antibody; the technique is restricted to detection of antigens that move to the positive pole on electrophoresis. SEE electroimmunodiffusion.

two-dimensional i., a combination of conventional electrophoretic separation and electroimmunodiffusion; electrophoresis is first carried out, then the electrophoretic strip is placed on a second slide and an antibody-containing agarose solution is allowed to solidify adjacent to it; electrophoresis is then performed at right angles to the original separation. SYN crossed i.

im·mu·no·en·hance·ment (im′yū-nō-en-hans′ment). In immunology, the potentiating effect of specific antibody in establishing and in delaying rejection of a tumor allograft; aside from antibody, nonspecific substances may also act to enhance immune response. SYN immunological enhancement.

im·mu·no·en·hanc·er (im′yū-nō-en-hans′er). Any specific or nonspecific substance that increases the degree of the immune response.

im·mu·no·fer·ri·tin (im′yū-nō-fer′i-tin). Antibody-ferritin conjugate used to identify specific antigen by electron microscopy.

im·mu·no·flu·o·res·cence (im′yū-nō-flūr-es′ens, i-myū′nō-). An immunohistochemical technique using labeling of antibodies by fluorescein, or rhodamine, isothiocyanates to identify bacterial, viral, or other antigenic material specific for the labeled antibody; the specific binding of antibody can be determined microscopically through the production of a characteristic visible light by the application of ultraviolet rays to the preparation. SEE ALSO fluorescent antibody *technique*.

im·mu·no·gen (i-myū′nō-jen). SYN antigen.

behavioral i., not smoking, regular exercise, and related health-enhancing personal habits and lifestyle of an individual which are associated with a decreased risk of physical illness and dysfunction, and with greater longevity.

im·mu·no·ge·net·ics (im′yū-nō-jĕ-net′iks). The study of the genetics of transplantation and tissue rejection, histochemical loci, immunologic response, immunoglobulin structure, and immunosuppression.

im·mu·no·gen·ic (im′yū-nō-jen′ik). SYN antigenic.

im·mu·no·ge·nic·i·ty (im′yū-nō-jĕ-nis′i-tē). SYN antigenicity.

im·mu·no·glob·u·lin (Ig) (im′yū-nō-glob′yū-lin) [MIM* 146880-146910]. One of a class of structurally related proteins, each consisting of two pairs of polypeptide chains, one pair of light (L) [low molecular weight] chains (κ or λ), and one pair of heavy (H) chains (γ, α, δ, and ε), all four linked together by disulfide bonds. On the basis of the structural and antigenic properties of the H chains, Ig's are classified (in order of relative amounts present in normal human serum) as IgG (7 S in size, 80%), IgA (10 to 15%), IgM (19 S, a pentamer of the basic unit, 5 to 10%), IgD (less than 0.1%), and IgE (less than 0.01%). All of these classes are homogeneous and susceptible to amino acid sequence analysis. Each class of H chain can associate with either κ or λ L chains. Subclasses of Ig's, based on differences in the H chains, are referred to as IgG1, etc.

When split by papain, IgG yields three pieces: the Fc piece, consisting of the C-terminal portion of the H chains, with no antibody activity but capable of fixing complement, and crystallizable; and two identical Fab pieces, carrying the antigen-binding sites and each consisting of an L chain bound to the remainder of an H chain.

Antibodies are Ig's, and all Ig's probably function as antibodies. However, Ig refers not only to the usual antibodies, but also to a great number of pathological proteins classified as myeloma proteins, which appear in multiple myeloma along with Bence Jones proteins, myeloma globulins, and Ig fragments.

From the amino acid sequences of Bence Jones proteins, it is known that all L chains are divided into a region of variable sequence (V_L) and one of constant sequence (C_L), each comprising about half the length of the L chain. The constant regions of all human L chains of the same type (κ or λ) are identical except for a single amino acid substitution, under genetic controls. H chains are similarly divided, although the V_H region, while similar in length to the V_L region, is only one-third or one-fourth the length of the C_H region. Binding sites are a combination of V_L and V_H protein regions. The large number of possible combinations of L and H chains make up the "libraries" of antibodies of each individual.

anti-D i., SYN RH₀(D) immune *globulin*.

chickenpox i., SYN chickenpox immune *globulin* (human).

i. domains, structural units of i. heavy or light chains that are composed of approximately 110 amino acids. Light chains of an i. are composed of one constant domain and one variable domain. Heavy chains are composed of either three or four constant domains and one variable domain.

i. G subclass deficiency, a rare inherited disorder in which there are reduced levels of one or more IgG subclasses resulting from

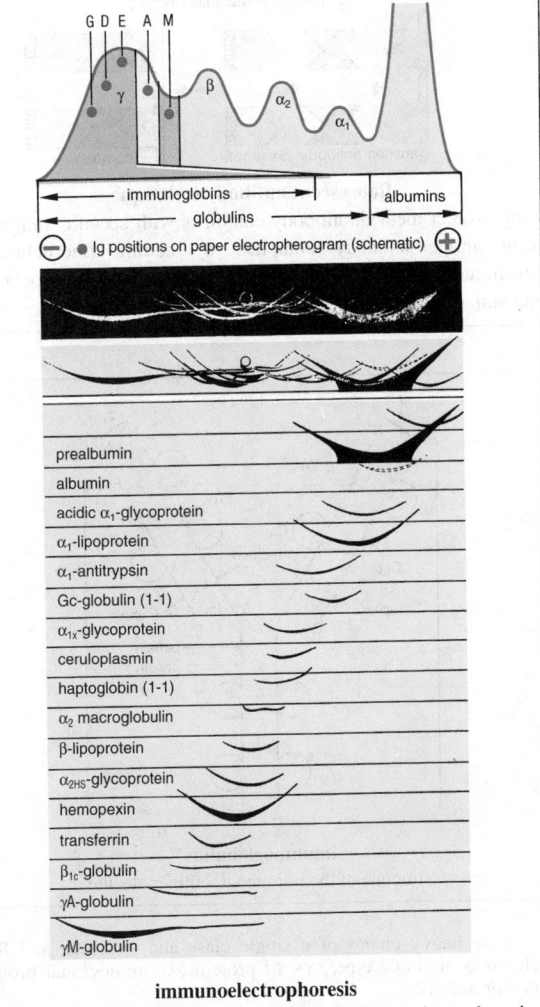

immunoelectrophoresis
(above) distribution of plasma protein; (below) immunoelectrophoresis diagram

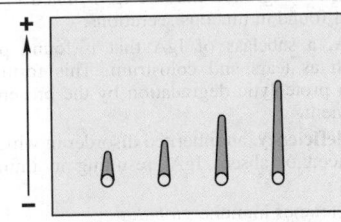

rocket immunoelectrophoresis
schematic view of electrophoresis of antigen in a gel containing antibody; the greater the concentration of antigen, the greater the movement to the positive pole

defective heavy chain genes or an abnormality in the regulation of i. isotype switching.

human normal i., SYN human gamma *globulin*.

measles i., SYN measles immune *globulin* (human).

monoclonal i., a homogenous i. resulting from the proliferation of a single clone of plasma cells and which, during electrophoresis of serum, appears as a narrow band or "spike"; it is character-

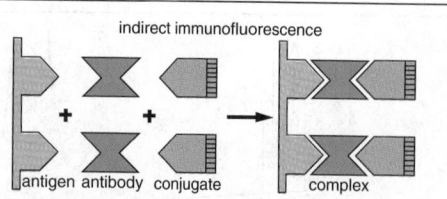

fluorescent antibody technique

with indirect method, antibody combines with specific antigen to form antigen-antibody complex; by adding fluorochromed anti-immunoglobulin serum with conjugates from fluorochrome and antiantibody, complex becomes indirectly visible

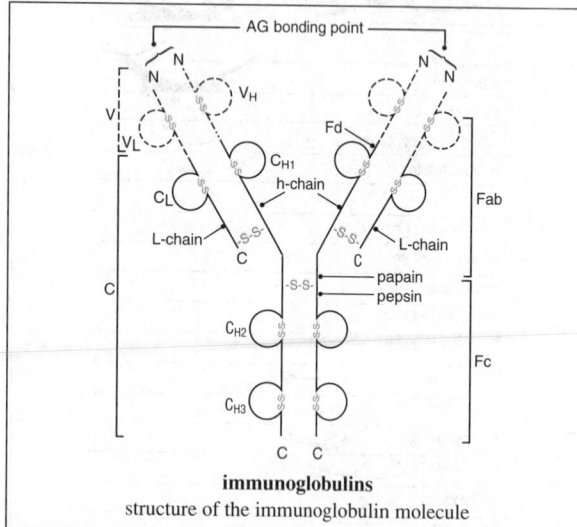

immunoglobulins
structure of the immunoglobulin molecule

ized by heavy chains of a single class and subclass, and light chains of a single type. SYN M protein (2), monoclonal protein, paraprotein (2).

pertussis i., SYN pertussis immune *globulin*.

poliomyelitis i., SYN poliomyelitis immune *globulin* (human).

rabies i., SYN rabies immune *globulin* (human).

Rh₀(D) i., SYN RH₀(D) immune *globulin*.

secretory i., usually IgA but may be IgM linked to a secretory component and found in mucous secretions.

secretory i. A, a subclass of IgA that is found primarily in secretions such as tears and colostrum. This form of IgA is protected from proteolytic degradation by the presence of a secretory component.

selective i. A deficiency, an inherited disorder in which there is a markedly reduced or absent IgA, resulting in immature IgA-bearing B cells.

tetanus i., SYN tetanus immune *globulin*.

thyroid-stimulating i.'s (TSI), in Graves' disease, the antibodies to TSH receptors in the thyroid gland. These antibodies are produced by B-lymphocytes and stimulate the receptors, causing hyperthyroidism. Formerly known as LATS (long-acting thyroid *stimulator*).

im·mu·no·he·ma·tol·o·gy (im′yū-nō-hē-mă-tol′ō-jē, i-myū′nō-). That division of hematology concerned with immune, or antigen-antibody reactions and with related changes in the blood.

im·mu·no·his·to·chem·is·try (im′yū-nō-his′tō-kem′is-trē). Demonstration of specific antigens in tissues by the use of markers that are either fluorescent dyes or enzymes such as horseradish peroxidase.

im·mu·no·lo·cal·i·za·tion (im′ū-nō-lō′cal-ī-zā-shŭn). Refers to use of immunological techniques, including specific antibody, to identify the location of molecules or structures within cells or tissues.

im·mu·nol·o·gist (im-yū-nol′ō-jist). A specialist in the science of immunology.

im·mu·nol·o·gy (im′yū-nol′ō-jē). **1.** The science concerned with the various phenomena of immunity, induced sensitivity, and allergy. **2.** Study of the structure and function of the immune system. [immuno- + G. *logos,* study]

im·mu·no·mod·u·la·to·ry (im′yū-nō-mod′ū-la-to-rē). **1.** Capable of modifying or regulating one or more immune functions. **2.** An immunological adjustment, regulation, or potentiation.

im·mu·no·pa·thol·o·gy (im′yū-nō-pă-thol′ō-jē, i-myū′nō-). The study of diseases or conditions resulting from immune reactions.

im·mu·no·po·ten·ti·a·tion (im′yū-nō-pō-ten-shē-ā′shŭn). Enhancement of the immune response by increasing its rate or prolonging its duration.

im·mu·no·po·ten·ti·a·tor (im′yū-nō-pō-ten′shē-ā-tŏr). Any of a wide variety of specific or nonspecific substances which on inoculation enhances or augments an immune response.

im·mu·no·pre·cip·i·ta·tion (im′yū-nō-prē-sip-i-tā′shŭn). The phenomenon of aggregation of sensitized antigen upon addition of specific antibody (precipitin) to antigen in solution. SYN immune precipitation.

im·mu·no·re·ac·tion (im′yū-nō-rē-ak′shŭn). An immunologic reaction, especially *in vitro* between antigen and antibody.

im·mu·no·re·ac·tive (im′yū-nō-rē-ak′tiv). Denoting or exhibiting immunoreaction.

im·mu·no·se·lec·tion (im′yū-nō-se-lek′shŭn). **1.** Selective death or survival of fetuses of different genotypes depending on immunologic incompatibility with the mother. **2.** The survival of certain cells depending on their surface antigenicity.

im·mu·no·sor·bent (im′yū-nō-sōr′bent). An antibody (or antigen) used to remove specific antigen (or antibody) from solution or suspension; commonly used with reference to antibody bound to a particulate substance such as a dextran polymer used to remove soluble antigen (*e.g.,* insulin) from solution.

im·mu·no·sup·pres·sant (im′yū-nō-sŭ-pres′ant). An agent that induces immunosuppression. SYN immunodepressant, immunodepressor, immunosuppressive (2).

im·mu·no·sup·pres·sion (im′yū-nō-sŭ-presh′ŭn). Prevention or interference with the development of immunologic response; may reflect natural immunologic unresponsiveness (tolerance), may be artificially induced by chemical, biological, or physical agents, or may be caused by disease.

im·mu·no·sup·pres·sive (im′yū-nō-sŭ-pres′iv). **1.** Denoting or inducing immunosuppression. **2.** SYN immunosuppressant.

im·mu·no·sur·veil·lance. Theory that holds that the immune system eliminates tumor cells that arise spontaneously.

im·mu·no·sym·pa·thec·to·my (im′yū-nō-sim′pă-thek′tō-mē). Inhibition of development of sympathetic ganglia induced in newborn animals by injection of antiserum specific for the protein which selectively enhances growth of sympathetic neurons.

im·mu·no·ther·a·py (im′yū-nō-thār′ă-pē). Originally, therapeutic administration of serum or gamma globulin containing preformed antibodies produced by another individual; currently, i. includes nonspecific systemic stimulation, adjuvants, active specific i., and adoptive i. New forms of immunotherapy include the use of monoclonal antibodies. SYN biological i.

This approach has been widely adopted by cancer specialists, often in cases which fail to respond to other treatment. Immunotherapy aims to boost immune system function, as with the administration of interferons and interleukin-2, or to attack cancerous cells directly, as with the injection of monoclonal antibodies. Various immunotherapeutic techniques have also been employed among AIDS patients. In addition, a number of alternative medical practices are claimed to enhance immune function, and various over-the-counter substances (*e.g.,* goldenseal, lysine have gained popularity for this supposed property.

two-phase mechanism of immunoreaction

		initial phase		effectual phase		
		immunologically specific, clinically nonapparent		immunologically nonspecific, clinically apparent		
	mediator	characteristics	reaction with antigen	primary effect	secondary effect	tertiary effect
type I anaphylactic reaction	IgE (IgG)	fixed on mast cells nonprecipitating, noncomplement-activating, heat-labile	on mast cell surface	→ release of H-substances	→ vasodilation, increase of permeability, contraction of smooth muscle	→ return to normal; no tissue damage
type II cytotoxic reaction	IgG (IgM)	circulates with serum	on cell surface (sometimes only absorption after reaction)	→ activation of complement	→ injury to cell membrane	→ cytolysis
type III Arthus reaction	IgG (IgM)	circulates with serum; precipitating, complement activating, heat-stable	near vessels	→ activation of complement	→ chemotaxis (segmented neutrophilic), phagocytosis, leucocytosis	→ enzyme release, tissue damage
type IV cell-mediated reaction	"sensitized" lymphocytes	circulates through tissue: complement-independent, long-lived	in periphery of tissue	→ synthesis and secretion of lymphokines	→ chemotaxis (mononuclear), migration inhibiting, mitogenic stimulation, activation of macrophages	→ enzyme release, cytotoxicity, tissue damage

adoptive i., passive transfer of immunity from an immune donor through inoculation of sensitized lymphocytes, transfer factor, immune RNA, or antibodies in serum or gamma globulin.

biological i., SYN immunotherapy.

im·mu·no·tol·er·ance (im'yū-nō-tol'er-ăns). SYN immunologic tolerance.

im·mu·no·trans·fu·sion (im'yū-nō-trans-fyū'zhŭn, i-myū'nō-). An indirect transfusion in which the donor is first immunized by means of injections of an antigen prepared from microorganisms isolated from the recipient; later, the donor's blood is collected, defibrinated, and then administered to the patient; the latter is then presumably passively immunized by means of antibody formed in the donor, e.g., antibody that reacts with the microorganisms in the patient.

imol·a·mine (i-mol'ă-mēn). 4-[2-(Diethylamino)ethyl]-5-imino-3-phenyl-Δ²-1,2,4-oxadiazoline; used for relief of angina pectoris.

IMP Abbreviation for inosine 5'-monophosphate.

im·pact. **1** (im'pakt). The forcible striking of one body against another. **2** (im-pakt'). To press closely together so as to render immovable. [L. *impingo*, pp. *-pactus*, to strike at (*in* + *pango*), fasten, drive in]

im·pact·ed (im-pak'ted). Wedged or pressed closely so as to be immovable.

im·pac·tion (im-pak'shŭn). The process or condition of being impacted.

dental i., confinement of a tooth in the alveolus and prevention of its eruption into normal position. SEE ALSO impacted *tooth*.

fecal i., an immovable collection of compressed or hardened feces in the colon or rectum.

food i., the forcible wedging of food between adjacent teeth during mastication, producing gingival recession and pocket formation.

mucus i., filling of the proximal bronchi, and also the bronchioles, with mucus.

im·pair·ment (im-pār'ment). A physical or mental defect at the level of a body system or organ. The official WHO definition is: any loss or abnormality of psychological, physiological or anatomical structure or function.

mental i., a disorder characterized by the display of an intellectual defect, as manifested by diminished cognitive, interpersonal, social, and vocational effectiveness and quantitatively evaluated by psychological examination and assessment.

im·par·i·dig·i·tate (im-par-i-dij'i-tāt). SYN perissodactyl (1). [L. *impar*, unequal, + *digitus*, digit]

IMP-as·par·tate li·gase. SYN adenylosuccinate synthase.

im·pat·ent (im-pat'ent, im-pā'tent). Not patent; closed.

im·ped·ance (im-pē'dăns). **1.** Total opposition to flow. When flow is steady, i. is simply the resistance, e.g., the driving pressure per unit flow; when flow is changing, i. also includes the factors that oppose changes in flow. Thus, deviations of i., from simple ohmic resistance because of the effects of capacitance and inductance, become more important in alternating current as the frequency of oscillations increases. In fluid analogies (e.g., pulsatile flow of blood, to-and-fro flow of respiratory gas), i. depends not only on viscous resistance but also upon compressibility, compliance, inertance, and the frequency of imposed oscillations. **2.** Resistance of an acoustic system to being set in motion.

acoustic i., the resistance that a material offers to the passage of a sound wave (colloquial); a property of a medium computed as the product of density and sound propagation speed (characteristic acoustic i.). Discontinuities in acoustic i. are responsible for the echoes on which ultrasound imaging is based. Unit: the rayl.

im·per·cep·tion (im-per-sep'shŭn). Inability to form a mental image of an object by combining the sensory data obtained therefrom. [L. *in-*, not, + *per-cipio*, pp. *-ceptus*, to perceive]

im·per·fo·rate (im-per'fōr-āt). SYN atretic.

im·per·fo·ra·tion (im-per-fōr-ā'shŭn). Condition of being atretic, occluded, or closed; indicated in compound words by the prefix *atreto-* or the suffix *-atresia*. [L. *im-* neg. + *per-foro*, pp. *-atus*, to bore through]

im·per·me·a·ble (im-per'mē-ă-bl). Not permeable; not permitting the passage of substances (e.g., liquids, gases) or heat through a membrane or other structure. SYN impervious. [L. *impermeabilis*, not to be passed through]

im·per·me·ant (im-per'mē-ant). Unable to pass through a particular semipermeable membrane. [L. *im-*, neg., + *permano*, to penetrate]

im·per·sis·tence (im-per-sis'tens). A transitory existence or occurrence, lasting only a short time. [L. *im-*, neg. + *persisto*, to persist]

motor i., inability to sustain a movement.

im·per·vi·ous (im-per'vē-ŭs). SYN impermeable.

im·pe·tig·i·ni·za·tion (im'pe-tij'i-ni-zā'shŭn). The occurrence of impetigo in an area of preexisting dermatosis.

im·pe·tig·i·nous (im-pe-tij'i-nŭs). Relating to impetigo.

im·pe·ti·go (im-pe-tī'gō). A contagious superficial pyoderma, caused by *Staphylococcus aureus* or Group A streptococci, that begins with a superficial flaccid vesicle which ruptures and forms a thick yellowish crust, most commonly occurring on the face of children. SYN crusted tetter, i. contagiosa, i. vulgaris. [L. a scabby eruption, fr. *im-peto* (*inp-*), to rush upon, attack]

Bockhart's i., SYN follicular i.

i. bullo′sa, i. with lesions of large size, forming bullae.

bullous i. of newborn, usually, widely disseminated bullous lesions appearing soon after birth, caused by infection with *Staphylococcus aureus*. SYN i. neonatorum (2), pemphigus gangrenosus (2).

i. circina′ta, a ringlike configuration of bullous lesions of i. formed by confluence of several bullae or by the rupture of a single lesion with crusting of the periphery.

i. contagio′sa, SYN impetigo.

i. contagiosa bullosa, discrete purulent skin lesions occasionally seen with streptococcal pyoderma.

i. eczemato′des, SYN *eczema* pustulosum.

follicular i., a superficial follicular pustular eruption involving the scalp or other hairy area. SYN Bockhart's i., superficial pustular perifolliculitis.

i. herpetifor′mis, a rare pyoderma, occurring most commonly in pregnant women in the third trimester, as an eruption of small closely aggregated pustules developing upon an inflammatory base and accompanied by severe constitutional symptoms and fetal death.

i. neonato′rum, (1) SYN *dermatitis* exfoliativa infantum. (2) SYN bullous i. of newborn.

i. vulga′ris, SYN impetigo.

im·pe·tus (im'pe-tŭs). In psychoanalysis, the motor element of an instinct; the amount of force of the individual's energy which the instinctive impulse demands. [L. an onset, fr. *im-peto*, to attack]

im·plant. 1 (im-plant′). To graft or insert. 2 (im′plant). Material inserted or grafted into tissues. SEE ALSO graft, transplant. 3. In dentistry, a graft or insert set in or onto the alveolar recess prepared for its insertion. SEE ALSO implant *denture*. 4. In orthopaedics, a metallic or plastic device employed in joint reconstruction. [L. *im-*, in, + *planto*, pp. *-atus*, to plant, fr. *planta*, a sprout, shoot]

bag-gel i., an i. composed of a silicone rubber bag containing a silicone gel; used in augmentation mammaplasty.

carcinomatous i.'s, transference of carcinoma cells from a primary tumor to adjacent tissues where growth continues.

cochlear i., an electronic device implanted under the skin with electrodes in the middle ear on the promontory or cochlear window or in the inner ear in the cochlea to create sound sensation in total sensory deafness. SYN cochlear prosthesis.

A microphone behind the ear feeds sound waves into a microprocessor carried on the body, which analyzes the data and sends information back to a radio transmitter that triggers the electrodes in the middle or inner ear to produce the appropriate electrical pulses. This does not enable the patient actually to hear, but rather to distinguish different sounds according to the neural sensation they produce. The first successful cochlear implant was performed in 1978 in Melbourne, Australia. Such devices are among many implanted aids which have been made possible by the advent of microchip technology.

dental i.'s, crowns, bridges, or dentures attached permanently to the jaw by means of metal anchors, most frequently titanium posts.

The implant technique was developed in the 1950s but not widely adopted until 30 years later. Since 1986, when dentists performed 115,000 implant procedures, demand has risen. In 1990, 435,000 implants were done. The most common approach takes up to 8 months. First, the teeth to be replaced are removed. After as long as 2 months for healing, holes are drilled in the jawbone under local anesthetic and cylindrical titanium implants are screwed into them. Within 3 to 6 months, bone fuses around the implants, creating a solid base to which crowns, bridges, or dentures are permanently attached. In a few cases (about 1 in 1,000 according to one study), the bone fails to fuse properly. Also, early implant patients reported chronic infections. Costs remain substantially higher than for conventional dentures.

endometrial i.'s, fragments of endometrial mucosa implanted on pelvic structure following retrograde transference through the oviducts.

endo-osseous i., an i. into alveolar bone inserted through the prepared root canal of a tooth in order to increase effective root length.

endosteal i., an i. that is inserted into the alveolar and/or basal bone and protrudes through the mucoperiosteum.

inflatable i., an i. consisting of an empty silicone rubber bag with an inlet tube and a valve; after insertion into or behind the breast, the bag is inflated with a liquid to the desired size; used in augmentation mammaplasty.

intraocular i., a plastic lens placed in the anterior or posterior chamber of the eye to substitute for the lens removed in cataract extraction.

magnetic i., a tissue-tolerated, magnetized metal placed within the bone to aid in denture retention; a similar magnet is placed in the overlying denture to complete the field.

orbital i., the glass, plastic, or metal device placed in the muscle cone after enucleation of an eye.

penile i., a rigid, flexible, or inflatable device surgically placed in the corpora cavernosa to produce an erection.

pin i., a type of i. usually rod-shaped, used in the area of the maxillary sinuses.

post i., that portion of an i. substructure that protrudes through the mucosa to connect with the restoration.

silicone i., i. composed of silicone; common form of breast i. for augmentation.

submucosal i., an i. resting beneath the mucosa. SEE ALSO implant *denture*.

subperiosteal i., an artificial metal appliance made to conform to the shape of a bone and placed on its surface beneath the periosteum. SEE implant denture *substructure*.

supraperiosteal i., an alloplastic graft inserted superficial to the periosteum to change the contour of an area.

testicular i., a device placed surgically in the scrotum in males with absence or severe hypoplasia of the testis. SYN testicular prosthesis.

triplant i., a combination of three pin i.'s to form a single abutment to support or retain a dental prosthesis.

im·plan·ta·tion (im-plan-tā'shŭn). 1. Attachment of the fertilized ovum (blastocyst) to the endometrium, and its subsequent embedding in the compact layer, occurring 6 or 7 days after fertilization of the ovum. 2. Insertion of a natural tooth into an artificially constructed alveolus. 3. Tissue grafting. SEE ALSO transplantation.

central i., i. in which the blastocyst remains in the uterine cavity, as in carnivores, rhesus monkeys, and rabbits. SYN circumferential i., superficial i.

circumferential i., SYN central i.

cortical i., i. of blastocyst in the ovarian cortex, causing an ovarian pregnancy. SEE ectopic *pregnancy*.

delayed i., a phenomenon characterized by an interval ranging from a few weeks to approximately 6 months between the time an ovum is fertilized and subsequent i. of the zygote, as in the marten and the armadillo.

eccentric i., i. in which the blastocyst lies in a uterine crypt, as in the mouse, rat, and hamster.

interstitial i., i. in which the blastocyst lies within the substance of the endometrium, as in humans and guinea pigs.

nerve i., planting one nerve into the sheath of another nerve.

pellet i., intramuscular or subcutaneous insertion of an active therapeutic agent in pellet form to provide protracted absorption at a rate slower than subcutaneous or intramuscular injection and as a means of providing a sustained therapeutic effect without repeated administration.

periosteal i., insertion of a normal tendon into a periosteum as part of a tendon transplantation operation.

subcutaneous i., insertion of material under the skin.

superficial i., SYN central i.

im·plo·sion (im-plō'shŭn). **1.** A sudden collapse, as of an evacuated vessel, in which there is a bursting inward rather than outward as in explosion. **2.** A type of behavior therapy, similar to flooding, during which the patient is given massive exposure to extreme anxiety-arousing stimuli by being asked to describe, and thus relive in his imagination, those life events or situations typically producing these overwhelming emotional reactions. As the patient does so, the therapist attempts to extinguish the future influence of such unconscious material over the patient's behavior and feelings, and previous avoidance responses to the stimuli are replaced by more appropriate responses.

im·po·tence, im·po·ten·cy (im'pŏ-tens, -ten-sē). **1.** Weakness; lack of power. **2.** Specifically, inability of the male to achieve and/or maintain penile erection and thus engage in copulation; a manifestation of neurological, vascular, or psychological dysfunction. [L. *impotentia,* inability, fr. *in-* neg. + *potentia,* power]

paretic i., i. caused by a lesion of the nervous system.

psychic i., that caused by psychologic factors.

symptomatic i., i. caused by disturbance of the sensory perineal reflexes.

vasculogenic i., i. due to alterations in the flow of blood to and from the penis.

im·preg·nate (im-preg'nāt). **1.** To fecundate; to cause to conceive. **2.** To diffuse or permeate with another substance. SEE ALSO saturate. [L. *im-,* in, + *praegnans,* with child]

im·preg·na·tion (im-preg-nā'shŭn). **1.** The act of making pregnant. **2.** The process of diffusing or permeating with another substance, as in metallic i. of tissue components with silver nitrate or ammoniacal silver. SEE ALSO saturation.

im·pres·sio, pl. **im·pres·si·o·nes** (im-pres'ē-ō, im-pres-ē-ō'nēz) [NA]. SYN impression. [L.]

i. cardi'aca hep'atis [NA], SYN cardiac *impression* of liver.

i. cardi'aca pulmo'nis [NA], SYN cardiac *impression* of lung.

i. col'ica [NA], SYN colic *impression.*

impressio'nes digita'tae [NA], SYN *impressions* for cerebral gyri.

i. duodena'lis [NA], SYN duodenal *impression.*

i. esopha'gea [NA], SYN esophageal *impression.*

i. gas'trica [NA], SYN gastric *impression.*

i. ligamen'ti costoclavicula'ris [NA], SYN *impression* for costoclavicular ligament.

i. petro'sa pal'lii, SYN petrosal *impression* of the pallium.

i. rena'lis [NA], SYN renal *impression.*

i. suprarena'lis [NA], SYN suprarenal *impression.*

i. trigemina'lis [NA], SYN trigeminal *impression.*

im·pres·sion (im-presh'ŭn). **1.** A mark seemingly made by pressure of one structure or organ on another. See also *groove* for the various impressions of the lungs, *e.g.,* descending aorta, subclavian artery and vena cavae. **2.** An effect produced upon the mind by some external object acting through the organs of sense. SYN mental i. **3.** An imprint or negative likeness; especially, the negative form of the teeth and/or other tissues of the oral cavity, made in a plastic material which becomes relatively hard or set while in contact with these tissues, made in order to reproduce a positive form or cast of the recorded tissues; classified, according

to the materials of which they are made, as reversible and irreversible hydrocolloid i., modeling plastic i., plaster i., and wax i. SYN impressio [NA]. [L. *impressio,* fr. *im- primo,* pp. *-pressus,* to press upon]

basilar i., an invagination of the base of the skull into the posterior fossa with compression of the brainstem and cerebellar structures into the foramen magnum. Cf. platybasia.

cardiac i. of liver, a depression on the superior area of the diaphragmatic surface of the liver corresponding to the position of the heart. SYN impressio cardiaca hepatis [NA].

cardiac i. of lung, the depression on the medial surface of each lung produced by the presence of the heart. It is more pronounced on the left lung. SYN impressio cardiaca pulmonis [NA].

i. for cerebral gyri, the depressions on the inner surface of the skull which correspond to the convolutions of the brain. SYN impressiones digitatae [NA], digitate i.'s.

colic i., a hollow on the visceral surface of the right lobe of the liver anteriorly, corresponding to the situation of the right flexure and beginning of the transverse colon. SYN impressio colica [NA].

complete denture i., (**1**) an i. of an edentulous arch made for the purpose of constructing a complete denture; (**2**) a negative registration of the entire denture-bearing, stabilizing area of either the maxillae or mandible; (**3**) a negative registration of the entire denture foundation and border seal areas present in the edentulous mouth.

i. for costoclavicular ligament, an irregular pitted area on the inferior surface of the clavicle at its sternal end, giving attachment to the costoclavicular ligament. SYN impressio ligamenti costoclavicularis [NA], costal tuberosity, rhomboid i., tuberositas costalis.

deltoid i., SYN deltoid *tuberosity.*

digitate i.'s, SYN i. for cerebral gyri.

direct bone i., an i. of denuded bone, used in the construction of subperiosteal denture implants.

duodenal i., a hollow on the visceral surface of the right lobe of the liver alongside the gallbladder, marking the situation of the duodenum. SYN impressio duodenalis [NA].

esophageal i., the marking of the esophagus on the back of the left lobe of the liver. SYN impressio esophagea [NA].

i.'s of esophagus, SYN esophageal *constrictions,* under *constriction.*

final i., in dentistry, the i. that is used to make the master cast.

gastric i., a hollow on the visceral surface of the left lobe of the liver corresponding to the location of the stomach. SYN impressio gastrica [NA].

mental i., SYN impression (2).

partial denture i., an i. or negative copy of all or a part of the partially edentulous dental arch or area, made for the purpose of designing or constructing a partial denture.

petrosal i. of the pallium, a shallow impression on the inferior surface of the cerebral hemisphere made by the superior margin of the petrous part of the temporal bone. SYN impressio petrosa pallii.

preliminary i., primary i., in dentistry, one made for the purpose of diagnosis or the construction of a tray.

renal i., a hollow on the visceral surface of the right lobe of the liver, in which lies the right kidney. SYN impressio renalis [NA].

rhomboid i., SYN i. for costoclavicular ligament.

sectional i., an i. that is made in sections.

suprarenal i., a hollow on the visceral surface of the right lobe of the liver, adjoining the groove for inferior venae cava, in which lies the right suprarenal gland. SYN impressio suprarenalis [NA].

trigeminal i., a depression on the anterior surface of the petrous portion of the temporal bone, near the apex, lodging the trigeminal ganglion. SYN impressio trigeminalis [NA].

im·print·ing. A particular kind of learning characterized by its occurrence in the first few hours of life, and which determines species-recognition behavior.

im·pro·mi·dine (im'prō-mĭ-dēn). An agent which is an agonist at H_2-type histamine receptors. Causes gastric acid secretion and

im

tachycardia. Actions can be blocked by agents such as cimetidine and ranitidine.

im·pulse (im'pŭls). **1.** A sudden pushing or driving force. **2.** A sudden, often unreasoning, determination to perform some act. **3.** The action potential of a nerve fiber. [L. *im-pello,* pp. *-pulsus,* to push against, impel (*inp-*)]

apex i., conventionally the lowermost, leftmost area of cardiac pulsation that is usually palpable.

cardiac i., movement of the chest wall produced by cardiac contraction.

ectopic i., an electrical i. from an area of the heart other than the sinus node.

escape i., one or more i.'s (atrial, junctional, or ventricular) arising as a result of delay in the formation or arrival of impulses from the prevailing pacemaker.

irresistible i., a compulsion to act such that one feels or claims it cannot be resisted.

morbid i., an i. that drives one to commit some act, usually of a deviant or forbidden nature, notwithstanding efforts to restrain oneself.

right parasternal i.'s, cardiac activity as palpable or recordable just to the right of the sternum.

im·pul·sion (im-pŭl'shŭn). An abnormal urge to perform a certain activity.

im·pul·sive (im-pŭl'siv). Relating to or actuated by an impulse, rather than controlled by reason or careful deliberation.

imus (ī'mŭs). Lowest; the most inferior or caudal of several similar structures. [L.]

IMV Abbreviation for intermittent mandatory *ventilation.*

IMViC Acronym for *i*ndole production, *m*ethyl red, *V*oges-Proskauer reaction, and ability to use *c*itrate as a sole source of carbon (*i* inserted for euphony); used primarily to differentiate *Escherichia coli* from *Enterobacter aerogenes* and related organisms.

In Symbol for indium; inulin.

¹¹¹In Symbol for indium-111.

¹¹³ᵐIn Abbreviation for indium-113m.

⌂**in-.** **1.** Not, akin to G. *a-, an-* or Eng. *un-.* **2.** In, within, inside. **3.** Very; appears as im- before b, p, or m. [L.]

in·ac·tion (in-ak'shŭn). Inactivity, rest, or lack of response to a stimulus.

in·ac·ti·vate (in-ak'ti-vāt). To destroy the biological activity or the effects of an agent or substance, as the activity of complement is destroyed when serum is heated.

in·ac·ti·va·tion (in-ak-ti-vā'shŭn). The process of destroying or removing the activity or the effects of an agent or substance; *e.g.,* the complementary effect of a serum may be destroyed by means of i. at 56°C for 30 min.

insertional i., a technique of recombinant DNA technology used to select bacteria that carry recombinant plasmids; a fragment of foreign DNA is inserted into a restriction site within a gene for antibiotic resistance, thus causing that gene to become nonfunctional.

X i., SEE lyonization.

in·an·i·mate (in-an'i-māt). Not alive. [L. *in-* neg. + *anima,* breath, soul]

in·a·ni·tion (in'ă-nish'ŭn). Severe weakness and wasting as occurs from lack of food, defect in assimilation, or neoplastic disease. [L. *inanis,* empty]

in·ap·par·ent (in'ă-pār'ent). Not apparent; beneath the threshold of clinical recognition, as an inapparent infection.

in·ap·pe·tence (in-ap'ĕ-tens). Lack of desire or of craving. [L. *in-* neg. + *ap-peto,* pp. *-petitus,* to strive after, long for (*adp-*)]

in·ar·tic·u·late (in-ar-tik'yū-lit). **1.** Not articulate in the form of intelligible speech. **2.** Unable to satisfactorily express oneself in words.

in·as·sim·i·la·ble (in-ă-sim'il-ă-bl). Not assimilable; not capable of undergoing assimilation. SEE assimilation.

in·at·ten·tion (in-ă-ten'shŭn). Lack of attention; negligence.

selective i., an aspect of attentiveness in which a person attempts to ignore or avoid perceiving that which generates anxiety.

sensory i., the inability to feel a tactile stimulus when a similar stimulus, presented simultaneously in a homologous area of the body, is perceived.

visual i., the inability to perceive a photic stimulus in a visual field when a similar but perceived stimulus is presented simultaneously in the homologous field.

in·born (in'bōrn). Implanted during development *in utero.* In the specific context of i. error of metabolism, it connotes a genetic disruption of an enzyme. SEE inborn *errors* of metabolism, under *error.* SYN innate.

in·bred. Denoting populations (groups, genetic lines, etc.) descended over several generations almost exclusively from a small set of ancestors, and hence having a high rate of consanguinity, often occult.

in·breed·ing (in'brēd-ing). **1.** Mating between organisms that are genetically more closely related than organisms selected at random from the population. **2.** A practice of mating animals that are closely related. The term is clearly relative to how the population is defined; the higher the i. in the population, the less it will lie in the individual mating.

in·car·cer·at·ed (in-kar'ser-ā-ted). Confined; imprisoned; trapped. [L. *in,* in, + *carcero,* pp. *-atus,* to imprison, fr. *carcer,* prison]

in·car·nant (in-kar'nant). Promoting or accelerating the granulation of a wound. SYN incarnative. [L. *incarno,* fr. *in* + *caro* (*carn-*), flesh]

in·car·na·tive (in-kar'nă-tiv). SYN incarnant.

in·cen·di·a·rism (in-sen'di-ă-rizm). SYN pyromania. [L. *incendiarius,* causing a conflagration]

in·cen·tive (in-sen'tiv). In experimental psychology, an object or goal of motivated behavior. [LL. *incentivus,* provocative]

in·cer·tae se·dis (in-ser'tē sē'dis). Of uncertain or doubtful affiliation or doubtful position, said of organisms in taxonomic classifications. [L.]

in·cest (in'sest). **1.** Sexual relations between persons closely related by blood, especially between parents and children, brother and sister. **2.** The crime of sexual relations between persons related by blood, where such cohabitation is prohibited by law. [L. *incestus,* unchaste, fr. *in-,* not, + *castus,* chaste]

in·ces·tu·ous (in-ses'chū-ŭs). **1.** Pertaining to incest. **2.** Guilty of incest.

in·ci·dence (in'si-dens). **1.** The number of specified new events, *e.g.,* persons falling ill with a specified disease, during a specified period in a specified population. **2.** In optics, intersection of a ray of light with a surface. [L. *incido,* to fall into or upon, to happen]

in·ci·dent (in'si-dent). Going toward; impinging upon, as incident rays. [L. *incido,* pp. *-casus,* to fall into, to meet with]

in·ci·dent·a·lo·ma (in'sĭ-den-tă-lō'-mă). Mass lesion, usually of the adrenal gland, serendipitously noted during computerized tomographic examinations performed for other reasons. [incidental + *-oma,* tumor]

in·ci·sal (in-sī'zăl). Cutting; relating to the cutting edges of the incisor and cuspid teeth. [L. *incido,* pp. *-cisus,* to cut into]

in·cise (in-sīz'). To cut with a knife.

in·ci·sion (in-sizh'ŭn). A cut; a surgical wound; a division of the soft parts made with a knife. [L. *incisio*]

bucket-handle i., a bilateral subcostal abdominal i.

celiotomy i., an i. through the abdominal wall.

chevron i., a bilateral subcostal i. in the abdomen, in the shape of an inverted "V"; used in upper gastrointestinal, renal, or adrenal surgery.

collar i., a cervical incision, placed one to two fingerbreadths above the sternal notch, that is frequently used for thyroid or parathyroid surgery.

Deaver's i., an i. in the right lower abdominal quadrant, with medial displacement of the rectus muscle.

Dührssen's i.'s, three surgical i.'s of an incompletely dilated cervix, corresponding roughly to 2, 6, and 10 o'clock, used as a means of effecting immediate delivery of the fetus.

endaural i., i. through the external auditory canal to permit mastoid surgery.

Fergusson's i., an i. used in maxillectomy, along the junction of cheek and nose, to bisect the upper lip.

flank i., an i. usually made near and parallel to the twelfth rib between the iliac crest on the lower side and the ribs on the upper.

Kocher's i., an i. parallel with right costal margin.

McBurney's i., an i. parallel with the course of the external oblique muscle, one or two inches cephalad to the anterior superior spine of the ilium.

midline i., a vertical abdominal i. placed in the midline aponeurosis between the two sheaths of the rectus muscles of the abdomen.

paramedian i., an i. lateral to the midline.

Pfannenstiel's i., an i. made transversely, and through the external sheath of the recti muscles, about an inch above the pubes, the muscles being split or separated in the direction of their fibers.

transverse abdominal i., an abdominal i. that is placed perpendicular to the axis of the rectus muscles of the abdomen.

in·ci·sive (in-sī′siv). **1.** Cutting; having the power to cut. **2.** Relating to the incisor teeth.

in·ci·sor (in-sī′zŏr). One of the cutting teeth, i. teeth, four in number in each jaw at the apex of the dental arch. [L. *incido*, to cut into]

central i., the first tooth in the maxilla and mandible on either side of the midsagittal plane of the head.

lateral i., SYN second i.

scalpriform i.'s, the cutting or gnawing i.'s of a rodent.

second i., second maxillary or mandibular permanent or deciduous tooth on either side of the midsagittal plane of the head. SYN lateral i.

INCISURA

in·ci·su·ra, pl. **in·ci·su·rae** (in′sī-sū′ră, in′si-sū′rē) [NA]. SYN notch. [L. a cutting into]

i. acetab′uli [NA], SYN acetabular *notch*.

i. angula′ris [NA], SYN angular *notch*.

i. ante′rior au′ris [NA], SYN anterior *notch* of ear.

i. ap′icis cor′dis [NA], SYN *notch* of apex of heart.

i. cardi′aca [NA], SYN cardiac *notch*.

i. cardi′aca pulmo′nis sinis′tri [NA], SYN cardiac *notch* of left lung.

incisurae cartilag′inis mea′tus acus′tici exter′ni [NA], SYN *notches* in cartilage of external acoustic meatus, under *notch*.

i. cerebel′li ante′rior, SYN anterior cerebellar *notch*.

i. cerebel′li poste′rior, SYN posterior cerebellar *notch*.

i. clavicula′ris [NA], SYN clavicular *notch* of sternum.

i. costa′lis [NA], SYN costal *notch*.

i. ethmoida′lis [NA], SYN ethmoidal *notch*.

i. fibula′ris [NA], SYN fibular *notch*.

i. fronta′lis [NA], SYN frontal *notch*.

i. interarytenoi′dea [NA], SYN interarytenoid *notch*.

i. intertrag′ica [NA], SYN intertragic *notch*.

i. ischiad′ica ma′jor [NA], SYN greater sciatic *notch*.

i. ischiad′ica mi′nor [NA], SYN lesser sciatic *notch*.

i. jugula′ris os′sis occipita′lis [NA], SYN jugular *notch* of occipital bone.

i. jugula′ris os′sis tempora′lis [NA], SYN jugular *notch* of temporal bone.

i. jugula′ris sterna′lis [NA], SYN suprasternal *notch*.

i. lacrima′lis [NA], SYN lacrimal *notch*.

i. ligamen′ti tere′tis hep′atis [NA], SYN *notch* for round ligament of liver.

i. mandib′ulae [NA], SYN mandibular *notch*.

i. mastoi′dea [NA], SYN mastoid *groove*.

i. nasa′lis [NA], SYN nasal *notch*.

i. pancrea′tis [NA], SYN pancreatic *notch*.

i. parieta′lis [NA], SYN parietal *notch*.

i. preoccipita′lis [NA], SYN preoccipital *notch*.

i. pterygoi′dea [NA], SYN pterygoid *fissure*.

i. radia′lis [NA], SYN radial *notch*.

i. rivi′ni, SYN tympanic *notch*.

incisurae santori′ni, SYN *notches* in cartilage of external acoustic meatus, under *notch*.

i. scap′ulae [NA], SYN scapular *notch*.

i. semiluna′ris ul′nae, SYN trochlear *notch*.

i. sphenopalati′na [NA], SYN sphenopalatine *notch*.

i. supraorbita′lis [NA], SYN supraorbital *notch*. SEE ALSO supraorbital *foramen*.

i. tento′rii [NA], SYN tentorial *notch*.

i. termina′lis au′ris [NA], SYN terminal *notch* of auricle.

i. thyroi′dea infe′rior [NA], SYN inferior thyroid *notch*.

i. thyroi′dea supe′rior [NA], SYN superior thyroid *notch*.

i. trag′ica, SYN intertragic *notch*.

i. trochlea′ris [NA], SYN trochlear *notch*.

i. tympan′ica [NA], SYN tympanic *notch*.

i. ulna′ris [NA], SYN ulnar *notch*.

i. umbilica′lis, SYN *notch* for round ligament of liver.

i. vertebra′lis [NA], SYN vertebral *notch*.

in·ci·sure (in-sī′zhūr). SYN notch. [L. *incisura*]

Lanterman's i.'s, SYN Schmidt-Lanterman i.'s.

Rivinus' i., SYN tympanic *notch*.

Santorini's i.'s, SYN *notches* in cartilage of external acoustic meatus, under *notch*.

Schmidt-Lanterman i.'s, funnel-shaped interruptions in the regular structure of the myelin sheath of nerve fibers, formerly interpreted as actual breaks in the sheath but shown by electron microscopy to correspond each to a strand of cytoplasm locally separating the two otherwise fused oligodendroglial (or, in peripheral nerves, Schwann cell) membranes composing the myelin sheath. SYN Lanterman's i.'s, Schmidt-Lanterman clefts.

tympanic i., SYN tympanic *notch*.

in·cli·na·tio, pl. **in·cli·na·ti·o·nes** (in′kli-nā′shē-ō, -nā-shē-ō′nēz). SYN inclination. [L.]

i. pel′vis [NA], SYN *inclination* of pelvis.

in·cli·na·tion (in-kli-nā′shŭn). **1.** A leaning or sloping. **2.** In dentistry, deviation of the long axis of a tooth from the perpendicular. SYN inclinatio, version (3). [L. *inclinatio*, a leaning]

condylar guidance i., the angle of i. of the condylar guidance to an accepted horizontal plane.

enamel rod i., the direction of the enamel rods with reference to the outer surface of the enamel of a tooth.

lateral condylar i., the direction of the lateral condyle path.

i. of pelvis, the angle which the plane of the superior pelvic aperture makes with the horizontal plane. SYN inclinatio pelvis [NA].

in·cli·nom·e·ter (in′kli-nom′ĕ-ter). Obsolete instrument for de-

♻ **Combining forms**	**[NA] Nomina Anatomica**
Word*Finder* Multi-term entry finder Preceding letter A	**[MIM] Mendelian Inheritance in Man**
A.D.A.M. Anatomy Plates Between letters L and M	☆ **Official alternate term**
Appendices: Following letter Z	☆[NA] **Official alternate Nomina Anatomica term**
SYN Synonym; Cf., compare	**High Profile Term**

in

termining the direction of the ocular axes in astigmatism. [L. *in-clino,* to incline, + G. *metron,* measure]

in·clu·sion (in-klū′zhŭn). **1.** Any foreign or heterogenous substance contained in a cell or in any tissue or organ, not introduced as a result of trauma. **2.** The process by which a foreign or heterogenous structure is misplaced in another tissue. [L. *in-clusio,* a shutting in, fr. *in-cludo,* pp. *-clusis,* to close in]

cell i.'s, (1) the residual elements of the cytoplasm that are metabolic products of the cell, *e.g.,* pigment granules or crystals; SYN metaplasm. **(2)** storage materials such as glycogen or fat; **(3)** engulfed material such as carbon or other foreign substances. SEE ALSO inclusion *bodies,* under *body.*

Döhle i.'s, SYN Döhle *bodies,* under *body.*

fetal i., unequal conjoined twins in which the incompletely developed parasite is wholly enclosed in the autosite.

leukocyte i.'s, SYN Döhle *bodies,* under *body.*

in·co·her·ent (in-kō-hēr′ent). Not coherent; disjointed; confused; denoting a lack of connectedness or organization of parts during verbal expression. [L. *in-* neg. + *co-haereo,* pp. *-haesus,* to cling together, fr. *haereo,* to stick]

in·com·pat·i·bil·i·ty (in′kom-pat-i-bil′i-tē). The quality of being incompatible.

physiologic i., a form of i. in which the substances in a mixture exert opposing physiologic actions. SYN therapeutic i.

therapeutic i., SYN physiologic i.

in·com·pat·i·ble (in-kom-pat′i-bl). **1.** Not of suitable composition to be combined or mixed with another agent or substance, without resulting in an undesirable reaction (including chemical alteration or destruction or pharmacological effect). **2.** Denoting persons who are unable to associate with one another without resulting anxiety and conflict. **3.** Having genotypes that put progeny at high risk of severe recessive disorders or that promote harmful maternal-fetal reaction (*e.g.,* erythroblastosis fetalis is Rh i.). [L. *in-* neg., + *con-,* with, + *patior,* pp. *passus,* to suffer, tolerate]

in·com·pe·tence, in·com·pe·ten·cy (in-kom′pe-tens, in-kom′pĕ-ten-sē). **1.** The quality of being incompetent or incapable of performing the allotted function, especially failure of cardiac or venous valves to close completely. SYN insufficiency (2). **2.** In forensic psychiatry, the inability to distinguish right from wrong or to manage one's affairs. [L. *in-,* neg. + *com-peto,* strive after together]

aortic i., defective closure of the aortic valve permitting regurgitation into the left ventricle during diastole.

cardiac i., inability of the ventricles to pump out the blood returning to the atria fast enough to prevent an abnormal rise in atrial pressure or to pump sufficient blood to maintain normal circulatory function.

cardiac valvular i., failure of a valve to perform its fundamental function: insurance of one-way flow; manifested by regurgitation of blood in the opposite direction when the valve is supposed to be closed.

mitral i., defective closure of the mitral valve permitting regurgitation into the left atrium during systole.

muscular i., imperfect closure of an anatomically normal cardiac valve, in consequence of defective action of its papillary muscles.

pulmonary i., pulmonic i., defective closure of the pulmonic valve permitting regurgitation into the right ventricle during diastole.

pyloric i., a patulous state or want of tone of the pylorus that allows the passage of food into the intestine before gastric digestion is completed.

relative i., imperfect closure of a cardiac valve, in consequence of excessive dilation of the corresponding cavity of the heart.

tricuspid i., defective closure of the tricuspid valve permitting regurgitation into the right atrium during systole.

valvular i., SYN valvular *regurgitation.*

in·con·stant (in-kon′stant). **1.** Irregular. **2.** In anatomy, denoting a structure, such as an artery, nerve, etc., that may or may not be present.

in·con·ti·nence (in-kon′ti-nens). **1.** Inability to prevent the dis-

charge of any of the excretions, especially of urine or feces. **2.** Lack of restraint of the appetites, especially sexual. Cf. intemperance. SYN incontinentia. [L. *in-continentia,* fr. *in-* neg. + *con-tineo,* to hold together, fr. *teneo,* to hold]

fecal i., SYN i. of feces.

i. of feces, the involuntary voiding of feces into clothing or bedclothes, usually due to pathology affecting sphincter control or loss of cognitive functions. SYN fecal i.

i. of milk, SYN galactorrhea.

overflow i., involuntary loss of urine associated with overdistention of the bladder, with or without a detrusor contraction. SYN paradoxical i.

paradoxical i., SYN overflow i.

passive i., dribbling of urine by reason of inability of the bladder to empty itself and of consequent overdistention. SEE ALSO overflow i.

i. of pigment, loss of melanin from the epidermis, and accumulation in melanophages in the upper dermis; seen in several inflammatory diseases of the skin and in incontinentia pigmenti.

reflex i., in neurogenic disorders, loss of urine due to detrusor hyperreflexia and/or involuntary urethral relaxation in the absence of the desire to void.

stress urinary i. (SUI), leakage of urine as a result of coughing, straining, or some sudden voluntary movement, due to weakness of the fascia muscles and at the neck of the bladder. SYN urinary exertional i.

urge i., urgency i., leakage of urine during a strong desire to void.

urinary exertional i., SYN stress urinary i.

i. of urine, the involuntary voiding of urine into clothing or bedclothes. A common problem in elderly populations, especially those in nursing homes, it may be due to neurologic abnormalities, loss of sphincter function (especially common in multiparous women), chronic bladder outlet obstruction, or loss of cognitive functions.

in·con·ti·nent (in-kon′ti-nent). Denoting incontinence.

in·con·ti·nen·tia (in-kon′ti-nen′shē-ă). SYN incontinence. [L.]

i. pigmen′ti [MIM*308300 & MIM*308310], genodermatosis that may also involve other structures; characterized by pigmented lesions in linear, zebra-stripe, and other bizarre configurations, sometimes preceded by vesicles and bullae containing eosinophils, and often followed by verrucous lesions; occasionally accompanied by other developmental abnormalities; the disorder is X-linked and a genetic lethal in males. Cf. Naegeli *syndrome.* SYN Bloch-Sulzberger disease, Bloch-Sulzberger syndrome.

i. pigmen′ti achro′mians [MIM*146150], inherited hypopigmented macules in a "marble-cake" pattern, variably associated with epidermal nevi, alopecia, and ocular, skeletal, and neural abnormalities. SYN hypomelanosis of Ito.

in·co·or·di·na·tion (in-kō-ōr-di-nā′shŭn). SYN ataxia. [L. *in-* neg. + coordination]

in·cor·po·ra·tion (in-kōr-pŏ-rā′shŭn). SYN identification. [L. *in-,* in, + *corporare,* pp. *corporatus,* to make into a body]

in·crease (in′krēs). Any growth in quantity.

absolute cell i., an actual i. in one of the types of leukocytes, the absolute number of leukocytes in 1 cu mm of blood being obtained by multiplying the total leukocyte count by the percentage of the cell types in question.

in·cre·ment (in′kre-ment). A change in the value of a variable; usually an increase, with "decrement" applied to a decrease, though "increment" can also correctly be applied to both. [L. *incrementum,* increase]

in·cre·tion (in-krē′shŭn). The functional activity of an endocrine gland. [in- + secretion]

in·crus·ta·tion (in′krŭs-tā′shŭn). **1.** Formation of a crust or a scab. **2.** A coating of some adventitious material or an exudate; a scab. [L. *in-crusto,* pp. *-atus,* to incrust, fr. *crusta,* crust]

in·cu·ba·tion (in′kyū-bā′shŭn). **1.** Act of maintaining controlled environmental conditions for the purpose of favoring growth or development of microbial or tissue cultures. **2.** Maintenance of an artificial environment for an infant, usually a premature or hypoxic one, by providing proper temperature, humidity, and, usually, oxygen. **3.** The development, without sign or symptom, of an infection from the time the infectious agent gains entry until the appearance of the first signs or symptoms. [L. *incubo*, to lie on]

in·cu·ba·tor (in'kyū-bā'tōr). **1.** A container in which controlled environmental conditions may be maintained; *e.g.*, for culturing microorganisms. **2.** An apparatus for maintaining an infant (usually premature) in an environment of proper oxygenation, humidity, and temperature.

in·cu·bus (in'kū-bŭs). **1.** Originally, an evil spirit which lay upon and oppressed sleeping persons; especially, a male spirit which copulated with sleeping women. Cf. succubus. **2.** SYN nightmare. [L. fr. *incubo*, to lie on]

in·cu·dal (in'kū-dăl). Relating to the incus.

in·cu·dec·to·my (in-kū-dek'tō-mē). Removal of the incus of the tympanum. [incus + G. *ektomē*, excision]

in·cu·des (in-kū'dēz). Plural of incus. [L.]

in·cu·di·form (in-kū'di-fōrm). Shaped like an anvil. [L. *incus (incud-)*, anvil]

in·cu·do·mal·le·al·ar (in-kū'dō-mal'lē-ăl). Relating to the incus and the malleus; denoting the articulation between the incus and the malleus in the middle ear. SYN ambomalleal.

in·cu·do·sta·pe·di·al (in-kū'dō-stā-pē'dē-ăl). Relating to the incus and the stapes; denoting the articulation between the incus and the stapes in the middle ear.

in·cur·a·ble (in-kyūr'ă-bl). Denoting a disease or morbid process that is unresponsive to medical or surgical treatment.

in·cur·va·tion (in'ker-vā'shŭn). An inward curvature; a bending inward.

in·cus, gen. **in·cu·dis**, pl. **in·cu·des** (ing'kŭs, in-kū'dis, in-kū'dēz) [NA]. The middle of the three ossicles in the middle ear; it has a body and two limbs or processes (long crus of incus and short crus of incus); at the tip of the long crus is a small knob, the lenticular process which articulates with the head of the stapes. SYN anvil. [L. anvil]

in·cy·clo·duc·tion (in-sī-klō-dŭk'shŭn). A cycloduction in which the upper pole of the cornea is rotated inward (medially). [in- + cyclo- + L. *duco*, pp. *ductus*, to lead]

in·cy·clo·pho·ria (in-sī'klō-fō'rē-ă). A cyclophoria in which the 12 o'clock position in the iris tends to twist medially. [L. in- + cyclo- + G. *phora*, a carrying]

in·cy·clo·tro·pia (in-sī-klō-trō'pē-ă). A cyclotropia in which the upper poles of the corneas are rotated inward (medially) to each other. [in- + cyclo- + G. *trope*, a turning]

in d. Abbreviation for L. *in dies*, daily.

in·dan·e·di·one de·riv·a·tives. Anticoagulants similar to warfarin in action. Anisindione and phenindione are clinically used; diphenadione is very long acting and used as a rodenticide.

in·dan·e·di·ones (in-dān'ĕ-dī-ōnēz). A class of orally effective indirect-acting anticoagulants of which phenindione is representative.

in·dap·a·mide (in-dap'ă-mīd). 4-Chloro-*N*-(2-methyl-1-indolinyl)-3-sulfamoylbenzamide; an antihypertensive loop diuretic used to treat edema associated with congestive heart failure, hepatic cirrhosis, and renal disease.

in·dec·ain·ide (in-dē-kān'īd). A cardiac depressant used as an antiarrhythmic agent.

in·de·cid·u·ate (in-dē-sid'yū-āt). Relating to the mammals (Indecidua) that do not shed any maternal uterine tissue when expelling the placenta at birth (*e.g.*, horse, pig), in contrast to deciduate mammals (*e.g.*, human, dog, rodent).

in·den·i·za·tion (in-den-i-zā'shŭn). SYN innidiation. [in- + denizen]

in·den·ta·tion (in-den-tā'shun). **1.** The act of notching or pitting. **2.** A notch. **3.** A state of being notched. [Mediev. L. *in-dento*, pp. -*atus*, to make notches like teeth, fr. L. *dens (dent-)*, tooth]

in·de·pen·dence. **1.** The relationship between two or more events in which no information about any combination of some of them contains any information about any combination of the others. **2.** The state of mutual detachment between or among autonomous units.

causal i., the state of systems that share no causes or effects.

stochastic i., i. of two or more events or variables; the state in which their joint probability or distribution is equal to the product of their marginal probabilities or distributions.

INDEX

in·dex, gen. **in·di·cis**, pl. **in·di·ces**, **in·dex·es** (in'deks, -di-sis, -di-sēz, -dek-sĕz). **1** [NA]. SYN index *finger*. **2.** A guide, standard, indicator, symbol, or number denoting the relation in respect to size, capacity, or function, of one part or thing to another. SEE ALSO quotient, ratio. **3.** A core or mold used to record or maintain the relative position of a tooth or teeth to one another and/or to a cast. **4.** A guide, usually made of plaster, used to reposition teeth, casts, or parts. **5.** In epidemiology, a rating scale. [L. one that points out, an informer, the forefinger, an index, fr. *in-dico*, pp. -*atus*, to declare]

absorbancy i., (1) SYN specific absorption *coefficient*. (2) SYN molar absorption *coefficient*.

alveolar i., (1) SYN gnathic i. (2) SYN basilar i.

anesthetic i., ratio of the number of units of anesthetic required for anesthesia to the number of units of anesthetic required to produce respiratory or cardiovascular failure.

antitryptic i., an obsolete term for the relative retardation in loss of viscosity of a solution of casein incubated with trypsin, to which a drop of abnormal blood serum (as from a cancerous patient) has been added, compared with that in a similar solution to which normal serum has been added; if the former drips through the tube of the viscosimeter in 100 seconds, and the latter in 104 seconds, the antitryptic i. is 4.

Arneth i., an expression based on adding the percentages of polymorphonuclear neutrophils with 1 or 2 lobes in their nuclei, plus one-half the percentage with 3 lobes; the normal value is 60%. SEE ALSO Arneth *formula*, Arneth *count*.

auricular i., relation of the width to the height of the auricle or pinna: (width of pinna × 100)/length of pinna.

Ayala's i., the cerebrospinal i. when 10 ml of cerebrospinal fluid have been removed. SYN Ayala's quotient, spinal quotient.

basilar i., ratio between the basialveolar line and the maximum length of the cranium, according to the formula: (basialveolar line × 100)/length of cranium. SYN alveolar i. (2).

Bödecker i., a modification of the DMF caries i.

body mass i., an anthropometric measure of body mass, defined as weight in kilograms divided by height in meters squared; a method of determining caloric nutritional status.

buffer i., SYN buffer *value*.

cardiac i., the amount of blood ejected by the heart in a unit of time divided by the body surface area; usually expressed in liters per minute per square meter.

centromeric i., the ratio of the length of the short arm of the chromosome to that of the total chromosome; ordinarily expressed as a percentage.

cephalic i., the ratio of the maximal breadth to the maximal length of the head, obtained by the formula: (breadth × 100)/length. SYN length-breadth i.

cephalo-orbital i., the ratio of the cubic content of the two orbits to that of the cranial cavity multiplied by 100.

cephalorrhachidian i., SYN cerebrospinal i.

cerebral i., the ratio of the transverse to the anteroposterior diameter of the cranial cavity multiplied by 100.

cerebrospinal i., the figure obtained by multiplying the pressure of the cerebrospinal fluid, after fluid has been withdrawn by spinal puncture, by the quantity of fluid withdrawn and then dividing by the original pressure. SYN cephalorrhachidian i.

chemotherapeutic i., the ratio of the minimal effective dose of a chemotherapeutic agent to the maximal tolerated dose. Originally used by Ehrlich to express the relative toxicity of a chemotherapeutic agent to a parasite and to its host.

chest i., SYN thoracic i.

cranial i., the ratio of the maximal breadth to the maximal length of the skull, obtained by the formula: (breadth × 100)/length.

Cumulative I. Medicus, collection of medical literature, published annually, which began in the US Army Surgeon General's office in the last century. It has been taken over by the National Library of Medicine and has evolved into a database called MEDLINE.

Dean's fluorosis i., an i. that measures the degree of mottled enamel (fluorosis) in teeth; used most often in epidemiological field studies.

def caries i., DEF caries i., an i. of past caries experience based upon the number of decayed, extracted, and filled deciduous (indicated by lower case letters) or permanent (indicated by capital letters) teeth.

degenerative i., the percentage of granulocytes that contain toxic granules in the cytoplasm, as compared with the total percentage of granulocytes.

dental i. (DI), (1) relation of the dental length (distance from the mesial surface of the first premolar to the distal surface of the third molar) to the basinasal (basion to nasion) length: (dental length ×100)/basinasal length; **(2)** a system of numbers for indicating comparative size of the teeth. SYN Flower's dental i.

df caries i., DF caries i., an i. of past caries experience based upon the number of decayed and filled deciduous (indicated by lower case letters) or permanent (indicated by capital letters) teeth. SYN df, DF.

dmfs caries i., DMFS caries i., an i. of past caries experience based upon the number of decayed, missing, and filled surfaces of deciduous (indicated by lower case letters) or permanent (indicated by capital letters) teeth.

effective temperature i., a composite i. of environmental comfort which is compared after exposure to different combinations of air temperature, humidity, and movement.

empathic i., the degree of emotional understanding or empathy experienced by a health services provider or other person concerning another person, more particularly of a sufferer from some emotional or somatic condition.

endemic i., the percentage of children infected with malaria or other endemic disease, in any given locality.

erythrocyte indices, calculations for determining the average size, hemoglobin content, and concentration of hemoglobin in red blood cells, specifically mean cell volume, mean cell hemoglobin, and mean cell hemoglobin concentration.

facial i., relation of the length of the face to its maximal width between the zygomatic prominences; to get **superior facial i.,** the length of the face is measured from the nasion to the alveolar point: (nasialveolar length × 100)/bizygomatic width; for **total facial i.,** length is measured from the nasion to the mental tubercle: (nasimental length × 100)/bizygomatic width.

Flower's dental i., SYN dental i.

free thyroxine i. (FTI), an arbitrary value obtained by multiplying the triiodothyronine uptake by the serum thyroxine concentration; it largely corrects for variations in thyroid-bound globulin concentration by providing a clinically valid estimate of the physiologically active free thyroxine; direct assay or laboratory measurement of free serum thyroxine yields a more accurate value.

gnathic i., relation between the basialveolar (basion to alveolar point) and basinasal (basion to nasion) lengths: (basialveolar length × 100)/basinasal length; the result indicates the degree of projection of the maxilla or upper jaw. SYN alveolar i. (1).

health status i., set of measurements designed to detect short-term fluctuations in health of members of a population; the measurements usually include physical function, emotional well-being, activities of daily living, feelings, etc.

height-length i., SYN vertical i.

icteric i., SEE icterus i.

icterus i., the value that indicates the relative level of bilirubin in serum or plasma; calculated by comparing (in a colorimeter) the intensity of the color of the specimen with that of a standard solution (potassium dichromate, 0.05 g, in 500 ml of water, plus 0.2 ml of sulfuric acid); the normal range is 3 to 5, and values greater than 15 are usually associated with clinically apparent jaundice; an i. less than 3 is observed in various examples of secondary anemia, aplastic anemia, and chlorosis. Sometimes erroneously called icteric i.: it is an i. of jaundice, not a jaundiced i.

iron i., an obsolete i. of iron obtained by dividing the figure for the average content of iron in normal blood (42.74 mg) by the red cell count in millions; it normally varies between 8 and 9; in pernicious anemia, the i. is usually greater than 10, but it tends to be normal in chronic secondary anemia.

karyopyknotic i., an i. used to monitor the hormonal status of the patient as reflected by exfoliated vaginal cells and their morphology; an expression of the percentage of intermediate and superficial cells from squamous cells of vaginal epithelium which have pyknotic nuclei.

length-breadth i., SYN cephalic i.

length-height i., SYN vertical i.

leukopenic i., a significant decrease in the white blood count after ingestion of food to which a patient is hypersensitive, a count made during the normal fasting state being used as the basis for evaluation of the postprandial count.

maturation i., an i. indicating the degree of maturation attained by the vaginal epithelium as adjudged by the cell types being exfoliated; serves as an objective means of evaluating hormonal secretion or response; represents the percentage of parabasal cells/intermediate cells/superficials, in that order; "shift to the left" indicates more immature cells on the surface (atrophy), while "shift to the right" indicates more mature epithelium.

metacarpal i., the average ratio of length to breadth of metacarpals II to V; this ratio is increased in the Marfan syndrome.

mitotic i., the ratio of cells in a tissue that are undergoing mitosis, often expressed as either the number of cells in a specified area of tissue section or as a percentage of the total cell sample.

molar absorbancy i., SYN molar absorption *coefficient*.

nasal i., relation of the greatest width of the nasal aperture to the length of a line from the nasion to the lower border of the nasal aperture: (nasal width × 100)/nasal height.

nucleoplasmic i., the quotient of the nuclear volume divided by the cytoplasmic volume.

obesity i., body weight divided by body volume.

opsonic i., a value that indicates the relative content of opsonin in the blood of a person with an infectious disease, as evaluated *in vitro* in comparison with presumably normal blood; the opsonic i. is calculated from the following equation: phagocytic i. of normal serum ÷ phagocytic i. of test serum = $1 \div x$, where x represents the opsonic i.

orbital i., relation of the height of the orbit to its width: (orbital height × 100)/orbital width.

orbitonasal i., the ratio of the width between the lateral angles of the eyes, measured with a tape measure passing over the root of the nose times 100, to the width between the lateral angles of the eyes measured with a caliper.

palatal i., palatine i., SYN palatomaxillary i.

palatomaxillary i., relation of the palatomaxillary width, measured between the outer borders of the alveolar arch just above the middle of the second molar tooth, and the palatomaxillary length, measured from the alveolar point to the middle of a transverse line touching the posterior borders of the two maxillae: (palatomaxillary width × 100)/palatomaxillary length; it notes the varying forms of the dental arcade and palate. SYN palatal i., palatine i.

pelvic i., the ratio of the conjugate of the pelvic inlet to the transverse diameters of the pelvis: (conjugate of pelvic inlet × 100)/transverse diameter.

phagocytic i., the average number of bacteria observed in the cytoplasm of polymorphonuclear leukocytes after mixing and incubating, at 37°C, 1) a suspension of washed, presumably normal leukocytes, 2) the serum to be tested for opsonin, and 3) a young culture of microorganisms that are causing disease in the patient.

Pirquet's i., an obsolete method of establishing the presence of malnutrition by dividing the weight (grams/10) by the sitting height (in cm); the cube root of the quotient if < 0.945 was considered as indicating malnutrition.

PMA i., an i. which measures the presence or absence of gingival inflammation as occurring on the papillae or the marginal or attached gingivae.

ponderal i., cube root of body weight times 100 divided by height in cm.

pressure-volume i., method of evaluating the cerebrospinal fluid hydrodynamics.

pulsatility i., calculation of Doppler measurements of systolic and diastolic velocities in the uterine, umbilical, or fetal circulations.

refractive i. (n), the relative velocity of light in another medium compared to the velocity in air; *e.g.,* in the case of air to crown glass, $n = 1.52$; in the case of air to water, $n = 1.33$. SEE ALSO *law of refraction.*

Robinson i., an i. used to calculate heart work load. SEE *double product.*

Röhrer's i., body weight in grams times 100 divided by the cube of height in centimeters.

root caries i., the ratio of the number of teeth with carious lesions of the root, and/or restorations of the root, to the number of teeth with exposed root surfaces.

sacral i., a ratio obtained by multiplying the greatest breadth of the sacrum by 100 and dividing by the length.

saturation i., an indication of the relative concentration of hemoglobin in the red blood cells, calculated as: grams of hemoglobin per 100 ml (expressed as percent of normal) ÷ hematocrit value (expressed as percent of normal) = saturation i. The normal i. for adults and infants is 0.97 to 1.02; in primary and secondary anemia, the i. is usually considerably less than 0.97.

Schilling's i., SYN Schilling's *blood count.*

shock i., the quotient of the cardiac rate divided by the systolic blood pressure; normally approximately 0.5, but in shock (*e.g.,* rising pulse rate with falling blood pressure), the i. may reach 1.0.

small increment sensitivity i., SEE SISI *test.*

spiro-i., SEE spiro-index.

splenic i., a rough indication of the salubrity, or the reverse, in regard to malaria of a particular district, judged by the relative absence or prevalence of enlarged spleens among the population.

staphylo-opsonic i., the opsonic i. calculated in relation to a staphylococcal infection, with a young culture of *Staphylococcus aureus* or the strain of staphylococcus from the patient being used in the test.

stroke work i., a measure of the work done by the heart with each contraction, adjusted for body surface area; equal to the stroke volume of the heart multiplied by the arterial pressure and divided by body surface area; the normal stroke work i. does not exceed 40 gram-meters per square meter.

therapeutic i., the ratio of LD_{50} to ED_{50}, used in quantitative comparison of drugs.

thoracic i., anteroposterior diameter of the thorax times 100 divided by the transverse diameter of the thorax. SYN chest i.

tibiofemoral i., the ratio obtained by multiplying the length of the tibia by 100 and dividing by the length of the femur.

transversovertical i., SYN vertical i.

tuberculo-opsonic i., the opsonic i. calculated in relation to tuberculous infection, with an actively growing culture of *Mycobacterium tuberculosis* or the strain of tubercle bacillus from the patient being used in the test.

uricolytic i., the percentage of uric acid oxidized to allantoin before being secreted.

vertical i., the relation of the height to the length of the skull: (height × 100)/length. SYN height-length i., length-height i., transversovertical i.

vital i., the ratio of births to deaths within a population during a given time.

Volpe-Manhold i. (V-MI), An index for comparing the amount of dental calculus in individuals.

volume i., an indication of the relative size (*e.g.,* volume) of erythrocytes, calculated as follows: hematocrit value, expressed as per cent of normal ÷ red blood cell count, expressed as per cent of normal = volume i.

zygomaticoauricular i., the ratio between the zygomatic and the auricular diameters of the skull or head.

in·di·can (in'di-kan). **1.** Indoxyl β-D-glucoside from *Indigofera* species; a source of indigo. SYN plant i. **2.** 3-Indoxylsulfuric acid, a substance found (as its salts) in sweat and in variable amounts in urine; indicative, when in quantity, of protein putrefaction in the intestine (indicanuria). SYN metabolic i., uroxanthin.

metabolic i., SYN indican (2).

plant i., SYN indican (1).

in·di·can·i·dro·sis (in'di-kan-i-drō'sis). Excretion of indican in the sweat. [indican + G. *hidrōs,* sweat]

in·di·cant (in'di-kant). **1.** Pointing out; indicating. **2.** An indication; especially a symptom indicating the proper line of treatment. [L. *in-dico,* pres. p. *-ans* (*-ant*), to point out]

in·di·can·u·ria (in'di-kan-yū'rē-ă). An increased urinary excretion of indican, a derivative of indol formed chiefly in the intestine when protein is putrefied; indol is also formed during the putrefaction of protein in other sites.

in·di·ca·tion (in-di-kā'shŭn). The basis for initiation of a treatment for a disease or of a diagnostic test; may be furnished by a knowledge of the cause (**causal i.**), by the symptoms present (**symptomatic i.**), or by the nature of the disease (**specific i.**). [L. fr. *in-dico,* pp. *-atus,* to point out, fr. *dico,* to proclaim]

in·di·ca·tor (in'di-kā-ter, -tōr). In chemical analysis, a substance that changes color within a certain definite range of pH or oxidation potential, or in any way renders visible the completion of a chemical reaction; *e.g.,* litmus, phenolsulfonphthalein. [L. one that points out]

alizarin i., a solution consisting of 1 g sodium alizarin sulfonate dissolved in 100 cc distilled water; used as an i. for free acidity in gastric contents.

health i., variable, susceptible to direct measurement, that reflects the state of health of persons in a community.

oxidation-reduction i., a substance that undergoes a definite color change at a specific oxidation potential. SYN redox i.

redox i., SYN oxidation-reduction i.

in·di·ces (in'di-sēz). Alternative plural of index.

In·di·el·la (in-dē-el'ă). Old name for *Madurella.*

in·dig·e·nous (in-dij'ĕ-nŭs). Native; natural to the country where found. [L. *indigenus,* born in fr. *indu,* within (old form of *in*), + G. *-gen,* producing]

in·di·ges·tion (in-di-jes'chŭn). Nonspecific term for a variety of symptoms resulting from a failure of proper digestion and absorption of food in the alimentary tract.

acid i., i. resulting from hyperchlorhydria; often used by the laity as a synonym for pyrosis.

fat i., SYN steatorrhea.

gastric i., SYN dyspepsia.

nervous i., i. caused by emotional upsets or stress.

in·di·go (in'dĭ-gō) [C.I. 73000]. $C_{16}H_{10}N_2O_2$; ($\Delta^{2,2'}$-biindoline)-3,3'-dione; a blue dyestuff obtained from *Indigofera tinctoria,* and other species of *Indigofera* (family Leguminosae); also made synthetically. SYN indigo blue, indigotin. [L. *indicum,* fr. G. *indikon,* indigo, ntr. of *Indikos,* Indian]

in·di·go blue. SYN indigo.

in·di·go car·mine [C.I. 73015]. $C_{16}H_8N_2Na_2O_8S_2$; sodium indigotin 5,5'-disulfonate; a blue dye used for measurement of kidney function and as a special stain for Negri bodies. SYN sodium indigotin disulfonate.

in·dig·o·tin (in-dig'ō-tin, in-di-gō'-tin). SYN indigo.

in·di·go·u·ria, in·di·gu·ria (in'dĭ-gō-yū'rē-ă, in-di-gū'rē-ă). The excretion of indigo in the urine.

in·dis·po·si·tion (in-dis-pō-zish'ŭn). Illness, usually slight; malaise. [L. *in* neg. + *dispositio,* an arrangement, fr. *dis-pono,* pp. *-positus,* to place apart]

in·di·um (In) (in'dē-ŭm). A metallic element, atomic no. 49,

in

atomic wt. 114.82. [*indigo*, because of its blue line in the spectrum]

in·di·um-111 (**¹¹¹In**). A cyclotron-produced radionuclide with a half-life of 2.8049 days and with gamma ray emissions of 171.2 and 245.3 kiloelectron volts. In a chloride form, it is used as a bone marrow and tumor-localizing tracer; in a chelate form, as a cerebrospinal fluid tracer.

i. chloride, i. trichloride, Cl_3In; used in electron microscopy to stain nucleic acids in thin tissue sections.

in·di·um-113m (**¹¹³ᵐIn**). A radioactive isomer of ¹¹³In; it has a half-life of 1.658 hours; it has been used in cisternography and as a diagnostic aid in cardiac output.

in·di·vid·u·a·tion (in′di-vid-yū-ā′shŭn). **1.** Development of the individual from the specific. **2.** In jungian psychology, the process by which one's personality is differentiated, developed, and expressed. **3.** Regional activity in an embryo as a response to an organizer.

in·do·cy·a·nine green (in-dō-sī′ă-nēn). A tricarbocyanine dye that binds to serum albumin and is used in blood volume determinations and in liver function tests.

in·do·cy·bin (in-dō-sī′bin). SYN psilocybin.

in·dol·ac·e·tu·ria (in′dōl-as-ĕ-tū′rē-ă). Excretion of an appreciable amount of indoleacetic acid in the urine; a manifestation of Hartnup disease.

in·dol·a·mine (in-dol′ă-mēn). General term for an indole or indole derivative containing a primary, secondary, or tertiary amine group (*e.g.,* serotonin).

in·dole (in′dōl). **1.** 2,3-Benzopyrrole; basis of many biologically active substances (*e.g.,* serotonin, tryptophan); formed in degradation of tryptophan. SYN ketole. **2.** Any of many alkaloids containing the i. (1) structure.

in·do·lent (in′dō-lent). Inactive; sluggish; painless or nearly so, said of a morbid process. [L. *in-* neg. + *doleo,* pr. p. *dolens* (*-ent-*), to feel pain]

in·dol·ic ac·ids (in-dōl′ik). Metabolites of L-tryptophan formed within the body or by intestinal microorganisms; the principal i. a. encountered in urine are indoleacetic acid, indoleacetylglutamine, 5-hydroxyindoleacetic acid, and indolelactic acid.

in·do·log·e·nous (in′dō-loj′ĕ-nŭs). Producing or causing the production of indole.

in·do·lu·ria (in-dō-lū′rē-ă). Excretion of indole in the urine; actual reference commonly is to indolic acids and indoxyl, as indole itself rarely appears in the urine.

in·do·lyl (in′dō-lil). The radical of indole.

in·do·meth·a·cin (in-dō-meth′ă-sin). 1-(*p*-Chlorobenzoyl)-5-methoxy-2-methylindole-3-acetic acid; an analgesic, antipyretic, and anti-inflammatory nonsteroidal agent used in the management of rheumatoid arthritis and in the treatment of osteoarthritis, ankylosing spondylitis, and gout.

in·do·phe·nol·ase (in-dō-fē′nol-ās). SYN cytochrome *c* oxidase.

in·do·phe·nol ox·i·dase (in-dō-fē′nol). SYN cytochrome *c* oxidase.

in·do·pro·fen (in-do-prō′fen). *p*-(1-Oxo-2-isoindolinyl)-hydratropic acid; a nonsteroidal anti-inflammatory agent with analgesic and antipyretic properties.

in·dor·a·min (in-dor′ă-min). A selective competitive α_1-antagonist that has been used for the treatment of hypertension; also an antagonist at H_1-histamine receptors and 5-HT receptors.

in·dox·yl (in-dok′sil). The radical of 3-hydroxyindole; a product of intestinal bacterial degradation of indoleacetic acid, excreted in the urine as indoleaceturic acid (conjugated with glycine), as a sulfate (urinary indican), or as a glucuronide (glucosiduronate); increased amounts are excreted in phenylketonuria.

in·dox·yl·u·ria (in-dok-sil-yū′rē-ă). The excretion of indoxyl, especially indoxyl sulfate, in the urine; i. may be associated with indicanuria, inasmuch as hydrolysis of indican results in formation of indoxyl.

in·duce (in-dūs′). To cause or bring about. SEE induction.

in·duc·er (in-dūs′er). A molecule, usually a substrate of a specific enzyme pathway, that combines with and deactivates an active repressor (produced by a regulator gene); this allows an operator

gene previously repressed to activate the structural genes controlled by it to result in enzyme production; a homeostatic mechanism for regulating enzyme production in an inducible enzyme system.

embryonal i., any compound that will effect differentiation in the early stages of development.

gratuitous i., an analog of a natural i. that is capable of inducing an operon while not serving as a substrate for the enzyme being induced.

in·duc·tance (L) (in-dŭk′tans). The coefficient of electromagnetic induction; the unit of inductance is the henry. [see induction]

in·duc·tion (in-dŭk′shŭn). **1.** Production or causation. **2.** Production of an electric current or magnetic state in a body by electricity or magnetism in another body close to the first body. **3.** The period from the start of anesthesia to the establishment of a depth of anesthesia adequate for a surgical procedure. **4.** In embryology, the influence exerted by an organizer or evocator on the differentiation of adjacent cells or on the development of an embryonic structure. **5.** A modification imposed on the offspring by the action of environment on the germ cells of one or both parents. **6.** In microbiology, the change from probacteriophage to vegetative phage that may occur spontaneously or after stimulation by certain physical and chemical agents. **7.** In enzymology, the process of increasing the amount or the activity of a protein. SEE ALSO inducer. **8.** A stage in the process of hypnosis. **9.** Causal analysis; a method of reasoning in which an inference is made from one or more specific observations to a more general statement. Cf. deduction. [L. *inductio,* a leading in]

electromagnetic i., electromagnetic waves propagated by i. in an electromagnetic field.

lysogenic i., i. that occurs when prophage is transferred to a nonlysogenic bacterium by conjugation or by transduction.

spinal i., the manner in which one sensory stimulus lowers the threshold for another.

in·duc·tor (in-dŭk′ter, -tōr). **1.** That which brings about induction. **2.** In embryology, an evocator or an organizer.

in·duc·to·ri·um (in-dŭk-tō′rē-ŭm). An instrument formerly used in physiologic experiments to generate pulses of induced electricity for stimulating nerve or muscle.

in·duc·to·therm (in-dŭk′tō-therm). The apparatus used in inductothermy.

in·duc·to·ther·my (in-dŭk′tō-ther-mē). Artificial fever production by means of electromagnetic induction. [induction + G. *thermē,* heat]

in·du·lin (in′dū-lin) [C.I. 50400-50415]. A blue quinone-imine dye related to nigrosin; occasionally used as a stain in histology and bacteriology.

in·du·lin·o·phil, in·du·lin·o·phile (in-dū-lin′ō-fil, -fīl). Taking an indulin stain readily. [indulin + G. *philos,* fond]

in·du·rat·ed (in′dū-rāt-ed). Hardened, usually used with reference to soft tissues becoming extremely firm but not as hard as bone. [L. *in-duro,* pp. *-duratus,* to harden, fr. *durus,* hard]

in·du·ra·tion (in-dū-rā′shŭn). **1.** The process of becoming extremely firm or hard, or having such physical features. **2.** A focus or region of indurated tissue. SYN sclerosis (1). [L. *induratio* (see indurated)]

brown i. of the lung, a condition characterized by firmness of the lungs, and a brown color associated with hemosiderin-pigmented macrophages in alveoli, consequent upon long-continued congestion due to heart disease. SYN pigment i. of the lung.

cyanotic i., i. related to persistent, chronic venous congestion in an organ or tissue, frequently resulting in fibrous thickening of the walls of the veins and eventual fibrosis of adjacent tissue; the affected tissue becomes firmer than normal, and tends to have an unusual, red-blue color.

Froriep's i., SYN *myositis* fibrosa.

gray i., a condition occurring in lungs during and after pneumonic processes in which there is failure of resolution; there is a conspicuous increase in fibrous connective tissue in the walls of the alveoli, and also within the alveoli (*e.g.,* fibrous organization of exudate); in contrast to brown i., there is usually not a prominent degree of pigmentation, unless chronic passive congestion is also present.

pigment i. of the lung, SYN brown i. of the lung.

plastic i., sclerosis of corpus cavernosum of penis.

red i., a condition observed in lungs in which there is an advanced degree of acute passive congestion, or acute pneumonitis (sometimes termed interstitial pneumonia), or a similar pathologic process.

in·du·ra·tive (in′dū-ră-tiv). Pertaining to, causing, or characterized by induration.

in·du·si·um, pl. **in·du·sia** (in-dū′zē-ŭm, -zē-ă). **1.** A membranous layer or covering. **2.** The amnion. [L. a woman's undergarment, fr. *induo,* to put on]

i. gris′eum [NA], a thin layer of gray matter on the dorsal surface of the corpus callosum in which the medial and lateral longitudinal stria lie embedded. The i. griseum is a rudimentary component of the hippocampus, continuous caudally around the splenium of the corpus callosum with the fasciolar gyrus, a slender convolution in turn continuous with the dentate gyrus of the hippocampus; rostrally the i. griseum curves around the genu and rostrum of corpus callosum and extends ventralward to the olfactory trigone as the tenia tecta or rudimentum hippocampi, hidden in the depth of the posterior parolfactory sulcus that marks the anterior border of the subcallosal gyrus or precommissural septum. SYN supracallosal gyrus.

in·e·bri·ant (in-ē′brē-ant). **1.** Making drunk; intoxicating. **2.** An intoxicant, such as alcohol. [see inebriety]

in·e·bri·a·tion (in-ē-brē-ā′shŭn). Intoxication, especially by alcohol. [see inebriety]

in·e·bri·e·ty (in-ē-brī′ĕ-tē). Habitual indulgence in alcoholic beverages in excessive amounts. [L. *in-* intensive + *ebrietas,* drunkenness]

in·ert (in-ert′). **1.** Slow in action; sluggish; inactive. **2.** Devoid of active chemical properties, as the inert gases. **3.** Denoting a drug or agent having no pharmacologic or therapeutic action. [L. *iners,* unskillful, sluggish, fr. *in,* neg. + *ars,* art]

in·er·tia (in-er′shē-ă, in-er′shăh). **1.** The tendency of a physical body to oppose any force tending to move it from a position of rest or to change its uniform motion. **2.** Denoting inactivity or lack of force, lack of mental or physical vigor, or sluggishness of thought or action. [L. want of skill, laziness]

magnetic i., SYN hysteresis (2).

psychic i., a psychiatric term denoting resistance to any change in ideas or to progress; fixation of an idea.

uterine i., absence of effective uterine contractions during labor; **primary uterine i., true uterine i.,** uterine i. that occurs when the uterus fails to contract with sufficient force to effect continuous dilation or effacement of the cervix or descent or rotation of the fetal head, and when the uterus is easily indentable at the acme of contraction; **secondary uterine i.,** uterine i. that occurs when the uterine contractions are vigorous but, as a result of the exhaustion or dehydration of the patient, decrease in vigor, and the progress of labor ceases.

in ex·tre·mis (in eks-trē′mis). At the point of death. [L. *extremus,* last]

in·fan·cy (in′fan-sē). Babyhood; the earliest period of extrauterine life; roughly, the first year of life.

in·fant. A child under the age of 1 year; more specifically, a newborn baby. [L. *infans,* not speaking]

i. Hercules, term applied to young children with precocious sexual and muscular development due to a virilizing adrenocortical disorder.

liveborn i., the product of a livebirth; an i. who shows evidence of life after birth; life is considered to be present after birth if any one of the following is observed: 1) if the infant breathes; 2) if the infant shows beating of the heart; 3) if pulsation of the umbilical cord occurs; or 4) if there is definite movement of voluntary muscles.

postmature i., a baby born after over 42 weeks of gestation, which puts the child at risk because of inadequate placental function. The infant usually shows wrinkled skin, sometimes more serious abnormalities.

post-term i., an i. with a gestational age of 42 completed weeks or more (294 days or more).

preterm i., an i. with gestational age of less than 37 completed weeks (259 completed days).

stillborn i., an i. who shows no evidence of life after birth. Cf. liveborn i.

term i., an i. with gestational age between 37 completed weeks (259 completed days) and 42 completed weeks (294 completed days).

in·fan·ti·cide (in-fan′ti-sīd). **1.** The killing of an infant. **2.** One who murders an infant. [infant + L. *caedo,* to kill]

in·fan·tile (in′făn-tīl). **1.** Relating to, or characteristic of, infants or infancy. **2.** Denoting childish behavior.

in·fan·ti·lism (in-fan′ti-lizm). **1.** A state marked by slow development of mind and body. SYN infantile dwarfism. **2.** Childishness, as characterized by a temper tantrum of an adolescent or adult. **3.** Underdevelopment of the sexual organs.

Brissaud's i., SYN infantile *hypothyroidism.*

dysthyroidal i., SYN infantile *hypothyroidism.*

hepatic i., delayed development as a result of liver disease.

hypophysial i., growth hormone deficiency due to failure of hypothalamic growth hormone-releasing hormone (also known as somatocrinin.)

hypothyroid i., SYN infantile *hypothyroidism.*

idiopathic i., dwarfism generally associated with hypogonadism; may be caused by deficient secretion of anterior pituitary hormones. SYN Lorain's disease, proportionate i., universal i.

Lorain-Lévi i., SYN pituitary *dwarfism.*

myxedematous i., SYN infantile *hypothyroidism.*

pancreatic i., i. associated with deficiency or absence of pancreatic secretion.

pituitary i., SYN pituitary *dwarfism.*

proportionate i., SYN idiopathic i.

renal i., SYN renal *rickets.*

sexual i., failure to develop secondary sexual characteristics after the normal time of puberty.

static i., a condition observed in young children resembling spastic spinal paralysis; it is marked by hypotonia of the muscles of the trunk and hypertonia of the muscles of the extremities.

tubal i., a term descriptive of a corkscrew-like fallopian tube as seen in fetal life.

universal i., SYN idiopathic i.

in·farct (in′farkt). An area of necrosis resulting from a sudden insufficiency of arterial or venous blood supply. SYN infarction (2). [L. *in-farcio,* pp. *-fartus* (*-ctus,* an incorrect form), to stuff into]

anemic i., an i. in which little or no bleeding into tissue spaces occurs when the blood supply is obstructed. SYN pale i., white i. (1).

bland i., an uninfected i.

bone i., an area of bone tissue that has become necrotic as a result of loss of its arterial blood supply.

Brewer's i.'s, dark-red, wedge-shaped areas resembling i.'s, seen on section of a kidney in pyelonephritis.

embolic i., an i. caused by an embolus.

hemorrhagic i., an i. red in color from infiltration of blood from collateral vessels into the necrotic area. SYN hemorrhagic gangrene (1), red i.

pale i., SYN anemic i.

red i., SYN hemorrhagic i.

Roesler-Bressler i., SYN myocardial *infarction* in dumbbell form.

septic i., an area of necrosis resulting from vascular obstruction due to emboli comprised of clumps of bacteria or infected material.

thrombotic i., an i. caused by a thrombus.

uric acid i., precipitates of uric acid distending renal collecting tubules in the newborn; since there is no necrosis, the term infarct is a misnomer.

white i., (1) SYN anemic i. **(2)** in the placenta, intervillous fibrin with ischemic necrosis of villi.

Zahn's i., a pseudoinfarct of the liver, consisting of an area of

in

congestion with parenchymal atrophy but no necrosis; due to obstruction of a branch of the portal vein.

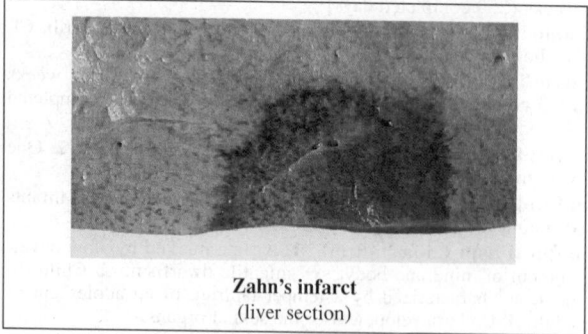

Zahn's infarct
(liver section)

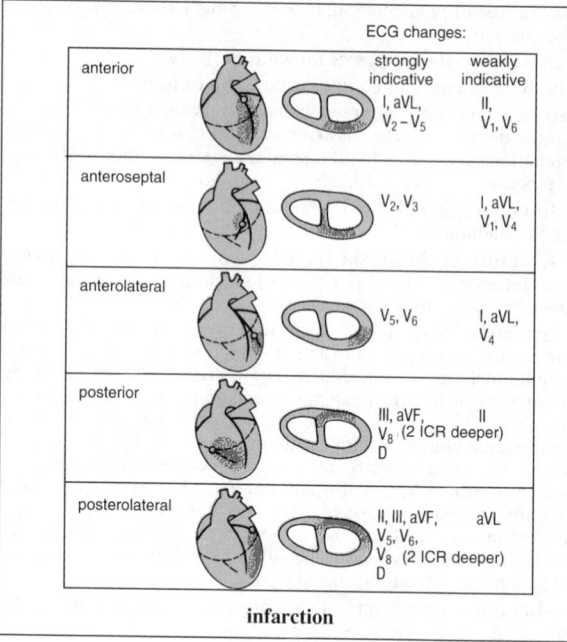

ECG changes:

infarction

in·farc·tion (in-fark'shŭn). **1.** Sudden insufficiency of arterial or venous blood supply due to emboli, thrombi, vascular torsion, or pressure that produces a macroscopic area of necrosis; the heart, brain, spleen, kidney, intestine, lung, and testes are likely to be affected, as are tumors, especially of the ovary or uterus. **2.** SYN infarct.

anterior myocardial i., i. involving the anterior wall of the heart, and producing indicative electrocardiographic changes in the anterior chest leads and often in limb lead I.

anteroinferior myocardial i., i. involving both anterior and inferior walls of the heart simultaneously.

anterolateral myocardial i., extensive anterior i. producing indicative changes across the precordium as well as in leads I and aVL.

anteroseptal myocardial i., an anterior i. in which indicative electrocardiographic changes are confined to the medial chest leads (V_1-V_4).

cardiac i., SYN myocardial i.

diaphragmatic myocardial i., SYN inferior myocardial i.

inferior myocardial i., i. in which the inferior or diaphragmatic wall of the heart is involved, producing indicative changes in leads II, III, and aVF in the electrocardiogram. SYN diaphragmatic myocardial i.

inferolateral myocardial i., i. involving the inferior and lateral surfaces of the heart and producing indicative changes in the electrocardiogram in leads II, III, aVF, V5, and V6.

lateral myocardial i., i. involving only the lateral wall of the heart, producing indicative electrocardiographic changes confined to leads I, aVL, V5, and V6.

myocardial i. (MI), i. of an area of the heart muscle, usually as a result of occlusion of a coronary artery. SYN cardiac i.

myocardial i. in dumbbell form, i. involving the septum along with both inferior and anterior walls to make an H- or dumbbell-shaped configuration. SYN Roesler-Bressler infarct.

nontransmural myocardial i. (NTMI), necrosis of heart muscle that fails to extend from the endocardium to the epicardium, often erroneously considered relatively benign.

posterior myocardial i., i. involving the posterior wall of the heart; also formerly used erroneously of i.'s involving the inferior or diaphragmatic surface of the heart.

silent myocardial i., i. that produces none of the characteristic symptoms and signs of myocardial i.

subendocardial myocardial i., i. that involves only the layer of muscle subjacent to the endocardium.

through-and-through myocardial i., SYN transmural myocardial i.

transmural myocardial i., i. that involves the whole thickness of the heart muscle from endocardium to epicardium. SYN through-and-through myocardial i.

watershed i., cortical i. in an area where the distribution of major cerebral arteries meet or overlap.

in·fect (in-fekt'). **1.** To enter, invade, or inhabit another organism, causing infection or contamination. **2.** To dwell internally, endoparasitically, as opposed to externally (infest). [L. *in-ficio,* pp. *-fectus,* to dip into, dye, corrupt, infect, fr. *in + facio,* to make]

in·fec·tion (in-fek'shŭn). Multiplication of parasitic organisms within the body; multiplication of usual bacterial flora of the intestinal tract is not usually viewed as i.

agonal i., SYN terminal i.

airborne i., a mechanism of transmission of an infectious agent by particles, dust, or droplet nuclei suspended in the air.

apical i., implantation of microorganisms at the apex of a tooth, usually the result of the migration of microorganisms from the pulp canal through the apical foramen.

cross i., i. spread from one source to another, person to person, animal to person, person to animal, animal to animal.

cryptogenic i., bacterial, viral, or other i., the source of which is unknown.

disseminated gonococcal i., i. from *Neisseria gonorrhea* which is spread to distant parts of the body beyond the original portal of entry (usually the lower genital tract). Usually manifest by rash and arthritis.

droplet i., i. acquired through the inhalation of droplets or aerosols of saliva or sputum containing virus or other microorganisms expelled by another person during sneezing, coughing, laughing, or talking.

endogenous i., i. caused by an infectious agent already present in the body, the previous i. having been inapparent.

focal i., an old term which distinguishes local i.'s (focal) from generalized i.'s (sepsis).

inapparent i., presence of i. in a host without the occurrence of recognizable symptoms or signs.

latent i., an asymptomatic i. capable of manifesting symptoms under particular circumstances or if activated.

mass i., i. resulting from the entrance of a large number of pathogens into the circulation or tissues.

mixed i., i. by more than one variety of pathogenic microorganisms.

pyogenic i., i. characterized by severe local inflammation, usually with pus formation, generally caused by one of the pyogenic bacteria.

Salinem i., SYN Salinem *fever.*

scalp i., an i. external to the galea; *e.g.,* folliculitis or cellulitis.

secondary i., an i., usually septic, occurring in a person or animal already suffering from an i. of another nature.

terminal i., an acute i., commonly pneumonic or septic, occurring toward the end of any disease and often the cause of death. SYN agonal i.

urinary tract i. (UTI), microbial i., usually bacterial, of any part of the urinary tract; can involve the parenchyma of the kidney, the renal pelvis, the ureter, the bladder, the urethra or combinations of these organs; often the entire urinary tract is affected; the most common organism causing such infection is *Escherichia coli.*

Vincent's i., SYN necrotizing ulcerative *gingivitis.*

zoonotic i., an i. shared in nature by man with other species of vertebrate animals.

in·fec·tion-im·mu·ni·ty. SEE infection *immunity.*

in·fec·ti·os·i·ty (in-fek-shē-os'i-tē). SYN infectiousness.

in·fec·tious (in-fek'shŭs). **1.** Capable of being transmitted by infection, with or without actual contact. **2.** SYN infective. **3.** Denoting a disease due to the action of a microorganism.

in·fec·tious·ness (in-fek'shŭs-nes). The state or quality of being infectious. SYN infectiosity.

in·fec·tive (in-fek'tiv). Capable of transmitting an infection. SYN infectious (2).

in·fec·tiv·i·ty (in-fek-tiv'i-tē). **1.** The characteristic of a disease agent that embodies capability of entering, surviving in, and multiplying in a susceptible host. **2.** The proportion of exposures in defined circumstances that result in infection.

in·fe·cun·di·ty (in-fē-kŭn'di-tē). SYN female *sterility.* [L. *infecunditas,* barrenness]

in·fer·ence (in'-fer-ens). The logical process of passing from observations and axioms to generalizations; in statistics, the development of generalizations from sample data, usually with calculated degrees of uncertainty.

in·fe·ri·or (in-fē'rē-ōr). **1.** Situated below or directed downward. **2** [NA]. In human anatomy, situated nearer the soles of the feet in relation to a specific reference point; opposite of superior. **3.** Less useful or of poorer quality. [L. lower]

in·fe·ri·or·i·ty (in-fēr-ē-ōr'i-tē). The condition or state of being or feeling inadequate or inferior, especially relative to one's peers or to others similarly situated.

in·fer·til·i·ty (in-fer-til'i-tē). Diminished or absent ability to produce offspring; does not imply (either in the male or the female) the existence of as positive or irreversible a condition as sterility. [L. *in-* neg. + *fertilis,* fruitful]

in·fest (in-fest'). To occupy a site and dwell ectoparasitically on external surface tissue, as opposed to internally (infect). [L. *infesto,* pp. *-atus,* to attack]

in·fes·ta·tion. Development on (rather than in) the body of a pathogenic agent, *e.g.,* body lice. SYN ectoparasitism.

in·fil·trate (in-fil'trāt). **1.** To perform or undergo infiltration. **2.** SYN infiltration (2). **3.** The description of a cellular infiltration (1) in the lung as inferred from appearance of a localized, ill-defined opacity on a chest radiograph; commonly used improperly to describe the shadow on the radiograph. [L. *in* + Mediev. L. *filtro,* pp. *-atus,* to strain through felt, fr. *filtrum,* felt]

Assmann's tuberculous i., SYN infraclavicular i.

infraclavicular i., an incipient lesion of tuberculous infection. SYN Assmann's tuberculous i.

in·fil·tra·tion (in'fil-trā'shŭn). **1.** The act of permeating or penetrating into a substance, cell, or tissue; said of gases, fluids, or matter held in solution. **2.** The gas, fluid, or dissolved matter that has entered any substance, cell, or tissue. SYN infiltrate (2). **3.** Injection of solution into tissues, as in infiltration anesthesia. **4.** Extravasation of solutions intended for intravascular injection.

adipose i., growth of normal adult fat cells in sites where they are not usually present.

calcareous i., SYN calcification.

cellular i., migration of cells from their sources of origin, or direct extension of cells as a result of unusual growth and multiplication, thereby resulting in fairly well-defined foci, irregular accumulations, or diffusely distributed individual cells in the connective tissue and interstices of various organs and tissues; used especially with reference to such changes associated with inflammations and certain types of malignant neoplasms.

epituberculous i., an i. superimposed upon a tuberculous lesion.

fatty i., abnormal accumulation of fat droplets in the cytoplasm of cells, particularly of fat derived from outside the cells. SEE ALSO fatty *degeneration.*

gelatinous i., SYN gray i.

gray i., a term sometimes used for the relatively rapidly formed, semisolid, gray or gray-white exudate (chiefly necrotic cells and remnants of tissue, and macrophages) resulting from unusually acute, overwhelming, diffuse tuberculous infection in the lung. SYN gelatinous i.

lipomatous i., nonencapsulated adipose tissue forming a lipoma-like mass, usually in the cardiac interatrial septum where it may cause arrhythmia and sudden death. SYN lipomatous hypertrophy.

paraneural i., i. adjacent to or along a nerve.

perineural i., i. about a nerve.

in·fin·i·ty (in-fin'i-tē). SYN infinite *distance.*

in·firm (in-ferm'). Weak or feeble because of old age or disease. [L. *in-firmus,* fr. *in-* neg. + *firmus,* strong]

in·fir·ma·ry (in-fer'mă-rē). A clinic or small hospital, especially in a school or college. [L. *infirmarium;* see infirm]

in·fir·mi·ty (in-fer'mi-tē). A weakness; an abnormal, more or less disabling, condition of mind or body. [see infirm]

in·flam·ma·ble (in-flam'ă-bl). SYN flammable. [L. *in-,* intensive, + *flamma,* flame]

in·flam·ma·tion (in-flă-mā'shŭn). A fundamental pathologic process consisting of a dynamic complex of cytologic and chemical reactions that occur in the affected blood vessels and adjacent tissues in response to an injury or abnormal stimulation caused by a physical, chemical, or biologic agent, including: 1) the local reactions and resulting morphologic changes, 2) the destruction or removal of the injurious material, 3) the responses that lead to repair and healing. The so-called "cardinal signs" of i. are: *rubor,* redness; *calor,* heat (or warmth); *tumor,* swelling; and *dolor,* pain; a fifth sign, *functio laesa,* inhibited or lost function, is sometimes added. All of the signs may be observed in certain instances, but no one of them is necessarily always present. [L. *inflammo,* pp. *-atus,* fr. *in,* in, + *flamma,* flame]

active i., SYN acute i.

acute i., any i. that has a fairly rapid onset, quickly becomes severe, usually manifested for only a few days, but may persist for several days or even a few weeks. SYN active i.

adhesive i., i. in which the amount of fibrin in the exudate is sufficient to result in a slight or moderate degree of adherence of adjacent tissues, as in healing by first intention.

allergic i., SEE allergic *reaction.*

alterative i., a local reaction to injury, occasionally observed in the walls of blood vessels and in parenchymal cells of various organs in reacting to certain chemicals, viruses, and other intracellular agents; the response is characterized by degenerative changes in the cytoplasm and nucleus, frequently resulting in necrosis, but exudation (if any) is ordinarily observed only in the wall of the affected vessel, or in the interstices immediately adjacent to the affected vessel or parenchymal cells. SYN degenerative i.

atrophic i., a form of chronic i. or repeated episodes of acute i. in which the continued or recurrent proliferation of fibroblasts results in the formation of fibrous tissue that eventually contracts and leads to compression and atrophy of parenchymal tissue. SYN fibroid i.

catarrhal i., an inflammatory process that is most frequent in the respiratory tract, but may occur in any mucous membrane, and is characterized by hyperemia of the mucosal vessels, edema of the interstitial tissue, enlargement of the secretory epithelial cells (which proliferate and form conspicuous globules of mucus), and an irregular layer of viscous, mucinous material on the surface; as exudation progresses, variable numbers of neutrophils migrate into the affected tissue and are included in the exudate, along with fragments of degenerated and necrotic epithelial cells; such an i. may frequently become mucopurulent.

chronic i., an i. that may begin with a relatively rapid onset or in a slow, insidious, and even unnoticed manner, tends to persist for several weeks, months, or years and has a vague and indefinite termination; results when the injuring agent (or products resulting from its presence) persists in the lesion, and the host's tissues

in

respond in a manner (or to a degree) that is not sufficient to overcome completely the continuing effects of the injuring agent.

chronic active i., the coexistence of chronic i. and superimposed acute i.

degenerative i., SYN alterative i.

exudative i., i. in which the conspicuous or distinguishing feature is an exudate, which may be chiefly serous, serofibrinous, fibrinous, or mucous (*e.g.,* relatively few cells are present), or may be characterized by relatively large numbers of neutrophils, eosinophils, lymphocytes, monocytes, or plasma cells, frequently with one or two types being predominant; it occurs not only as a separate and distinct pathologic process, but also frequently as a part of certain granulomatous i.'s.

fibrinopurulent i., a purulent i. in which the exudate contains an unusually large amount of fibrin; also, a fibrinous or serofibrinous i. in which the accumulation of large numbers of polymorphonuclear leukocytes results in liquefactive necrosis of tissue and the formation of pus with a relatively large quantity of fibrin.

fibrinous i., an exudative i. in which there is a disproportionately large amount of fibrin.

fibroid i., SYN atrophic i.

granulomatous i., a form of proliferative i. SEE ALSO granuloma.

hyperplastic i., SYN proliferative i.

immune i., SEE allergic *reaction.*

interstitial i., i. in which the inflammatory reaction occurs chiefly in the supportive fibrous connective tissue or stroma of an organ.

necrotic i., necrotizing i., usually an acute inflammatory reaction in which the predominant histologic change is fairly rapid necrosis that occurs diffusely or extensively in relatively large foci throughout the affected tissue, frequently with only little or no evidence of cells in the exudate.

productive i., a vague term ordinarily used with reference to proliferative i., with or without an exudate; also sometimes used to indicate any i. in which grossly visible exudate is formed.

proliferative i., an inflammatory reaction in which the distinguishing feature is an actual increase in the number of tissue cells, especially the reticuloendothelial macrophages, in contrast to cells exuded from blood vessels; in addition, exudates of various types are likely to be observed in granulomas and other forms of proliferative i., but the latter may occur without an exudate being formed (as in certain infections caused by virus). SYN hyperplastic i.

pseudomembranous i., a form of exudative i. that involves mucous and serous membranes; relatively large quantities of fibrin in the exudate result in a rather tenacious membrane-like covering that is fairly adherent to the underlying acutely inflamed tissue; the pseudomembrane usually contains (in addition to the dense network of fibrin) varying quantities of plasma protein, degenerated and necrotic elements from the affected tissue, polymorphonuclear leukocytes, bacteria, etc.

purulent i., an acute exudative i. in which the accumulation of polymorphonuclear leukocytes is sufficiently great that their enzymes cause liquefaction of the affected tissues, focally or diffusely; the purulent exudate is frequently termed pus, and consists of plasma and its constituents, end products of the enzymatic digestion of tissue, degenerated and necrotic cells and their debris, polymorphonuclear leukocytes and other white blood cells, the causal agent of the i., etc. SYN suppurative i.

sclerosing i., i. leading to extensive formation of fibrous and scar tissue.

serofibrinous i., i. in which the exudate consists chiefly of serous fluid with an unusually large proportion of fibrin.

serous i., an exudative i. in which the exudate is predominantly fluid (*e.g.,* exuded from the blood vessels), with the protein, electrolytes, and other material contained therein; relatively few (if any) cells are observed.

subacute i., an i. that is intermediate in duration between that of an acute i. and that of a chronic i., usually persisting longer than 3 or 4 weeks.

suppurative i., SYN purulent i.

in·flam·ma·to·ry (in-flam'ă-tōr-ē). Pertaining to, characterized by, causing, resulting from, or becoming affected by inflammation.

in·fla·tion (in-flā'shŭn). Distention by a fluid or gas. SYN vesiculation (2). [L. *inflatio,* fr. *in-flo,* pp. *-flatus,* to blow into, inflate]

in·fla·tor (in-flā'ter, -tŏr). An instrument for injecting air.

in·flec·tion, in·flex·ion (in-flek'shŭn). **1.** An inward bending. **2.** Obsolete term for diffraction. [L. *in-flecto,* pp. *-flexus,* to bend]

in·flu·en·za (in-flū-en'ză). An acute infectious respiratory disease, caused by influenza viruses, which are found in the family Orthomyxoviridae, in which the inhaled virus attacks the respiratory epithelial cells of susceptible persons and produces a catarrhal inflammation; characterized by sudden onset, chills, fever of short duration (3 days), severe prostration, headache, muscle aches, and a cough that usually is dry until secondary infection occurs. The disease commonly occurs in epidemics, sometimes in pandemics, which develop quickly and spread rapidly; mortality rate is usually low, but may be high in cases with secondary bacterial pneumonia, particularly in the elderly and those with underlying debilitating diseases; strain-specific immunity develops, but mutations in the virus are frequent, and the immunity usually does not affect new, antigenically different strains. SYN flu, grip (1), grippe. [It. influence (of planets or stars), fr. L. *influentia,* fr. *in-fluo,* to flow in]

i. A, i. caused by strains of influenza virus type A. These strains have a high propensity for antigenic change. The infections occur in epidemics, which vary in size and severity; perhaps the most important of the three types of i. (A, B, and C).

Asian i., a worldwide i., apparently originating in China in the summer of 1957, which produces a milder disease than that of the pandemic of 1917–1919.

avian i., SYN fowl *plague.*

i. B, i. caused by strains of influenza virus type B; outbreaks are usually more limited than those due to influenza virus type A, although infections by the two types are clinically indistinguishable; occasionally associated with Reye's syndrome.

i. C, i. caused by strains of type C influenza virus; the disease is milder than that caused by types A and B and has become uncommon in recent years.

endemic i., i., usually of a less severe type, occurring with some degree of regularity during the winter season, especially in the larger cities of the world. SYN i. nostras.

equine i., a highly contagious upper respiratory infection of horses and other equids caused by equine strains of influenza virus type A; characterized by fever and respiratory signs similar to but more severe than those of equine rhinopneumonitis; edema of the lower trunk and limbs (epizootic cellulitis) may occur; the disease is frequently fatal when secondary bacterial pneumonia intervenes.

Hong Kong i., influenza caused by a serotype of influenza virus type A and first identified in Hong Kong.

i. nos'tras, SYN endemic i.

Russian i., a pandemic of a strain i. A virus thought to have originated in Russia; occurred in 1978.

Spanish i., i. that caused several waves of pandemic in 1918–1919, resulting in more than 20 million deaths worldwide; it was particularly severe in Spain (hence the name), but now is thought to have originated in the U.S. as a form of swine i.

swine i., an acute respiratory disease of swine caused by strains of influenza virus type A; it is believed to have become adapted to swine in the United States during the great human pandemic in 1918; fatal cases, as in such cases of pandemic i. in man, are commonly associated with secondary bacterial pneumonia.

in·flu·en·zal (in-flū-en'zăl). Relating to, marked by, or resulting from influenza.

In·flu·en·za·vi·rus (in-flū-en'ză-vī-rŭs). The genus of Orthomyxoviridae that comprises the influenza viruses types A and B. Each type of virus has a stable nucleoprotein group antigen common to all strains of the type, but distinct from that of the other type; each also has a mosaic of surface antigens (hemagglutinin and neuraminidase) which characterize the strains and which are subject to variations of two kinds: 1) a rather continual drift that occurs independently within the hemagglutinin and neuraminidase antigens; 2) after a period of years, a sudden shift (notably in type A virus of human origin) to a different hemagglutinin or neuraminidase antigen. The sudden major shifts are the basis of subdivisions of type A virus of human origin. Strain notations indicate type, geographic origin, year of isolation, and, in the case of type A strains, the characterizing subtypes of hemagglutinin and neuraminidase antigens (*e.g.,* A/Hong Kong/1/68 ($H_3 N_2$); B/Hong Kong/5/72).

in·fold (in-fōld′). To inclose within a fold, as in "infolding" an ulcer of the stomach, in which the walls on either side of the lesion are brought together and sutured.

in·formed con·sent. voluntary consent given by a person or a responsible proxy (*e.g.,* a parent) for participation in a study, immunization program, treatment regimen, etc., after being informed of the purpose, methods, procedures, benefits, and risks. The essential criteria of i. c. are that the subject has both knowledge and comprehension, that consent is freely given without duress or undue influence, and that the right of withdrawal at any time is clearly communicated to the subject. Other aspects of i. c. in the context of epidemiologic and biomedical research, and criteria to be met in obtaining it, are specified in *International Guidelines for Ethical Review of Epidemiologic Studies* (Geneva: CIOMS/WHO 1991) and *International Ethical Guidelines for Biomedical Research Involving Human Subjects* (Geneva: CIOMS/WHO 1993).

in·for·mo·fers (in-fōr′mō-fers). Name suggested for the protein particles that appear when RNA is removed from nucleoprotein particles. [information + -fer]

in·for·mo·somes (in-fōr′mō-sōmz). Name suggested for the bodies composed of messenger (informational) RNA and protein that are found in the cytoplasm of animal cells. [*inform*ation + G. *sōma,* body]

△**infra-.** A position below the part denoted by the word to which it is joined. [L. below]

in·fra·ax·il·lary (in′fră-ak′si-lār-ē). SYN subaxillary.

in·fra·bulge (in′fră-bŭlj). **1.** That portion of the crown of a tooth gingival to the height of contour. **2.** That area of a tooth where the retentive portion of a clasp of a removable partial denture is placed.

in·fra·car·di·ac (in′fră-kar′dē-ak). Beneath the heart; below the level of the heart.

in·fra·ce·re·bral (in′fră-ser′e-brăl). Pertaining to that portion of the nervous system below the level of the cerebrum.

in·fra·cla·vic·u·lar (in′fră-kla-vik′yū-lăr). SYN subclavian (1).

in·fra·clu·sion (in-fră-klū′zhŭn). The state wherein a tooth has failed to erupt to the maxillomandibular plane of interdigitation. SYN infraocclusion, infraversion (3).

in·fra·cor·ti·cal (in′fră-kōr′ti-kăl). Beneath the cortex of an organ, mainly the brain or kidney. SEE subcortical.

in·fra·cos·tal (in-fră-kos′tăl). SYN subcostal (1).

in·fra·cot·y·loid (in-fră-kot′i-loyd). Below the acetabulum or cotyloid cavity.

in·fra·cris·tal (in-fră-kris′tăl). Below the supraventricular crest; usually used in reference to ventricular septal defect. [infra- + L. *crista,* crest]

in·frac·tion (in-frak′shŭn). A fracture; especially one without displacement. SYN infracture. [L. *infractio,* a breaking, fr. *infringere,* to break]

in·frac·ture (in-frak′chūr). SYN infraction.

in·fra·den·ta·le (in′fră-den-tā′lē). In craniometrics, the apex of the septum between the mandibular central incisors. SYN lower alveolar point.

in·fra·di·an (in-frā′dē-ăn). Relating to biologic variations or rhythms occurring in cycles less frequent than every 24 hours. Cf. circadian, ultradian. [infra- + L. *dies,* day]

in·fra·di·a·phrag·mat·ic (in′fră-dī′ă-frag-mat′ik). SYN subdiaphragmatic.

in·fra·duc·tion (in-fră-dŭk′shŭn). SYN deorsumduction.

in·fra·gle·noid (in′fră-glē′noyd). Inferior to the glenoid cavity of the scapula. SYN subglenoid.

in·fra·glot·tic (in-fră-glot′ik). Inferior to the glottis. SYN subglottic.

in·fra·he·pa·tic (in-fră-he-pat′ik). SYN subhepatic.

in·fra·hy·oid (in′fră-hī′oyd). Below the hyoid bone; denoting especially a group of muscles: the sternohyoideus, sternothyroideus, thyrohyoideus, and omohyoideus. SYN subhyoid, subhyoidean.

in·fra·mam·il·lary (in-fră-mam′ĭ-lār-ē). Relating to that which is situated below a nipple.

in·fra·mam·ma·ry (in-fră-mam′ă-rē). Inferior to the mammary gland. SYN submammary (2).

in·fra·man·dib·u·lar (in-fră-man-dib′yū-lăr). SYN submandibular.

in·fra·mar·gin·al (in-fră-mar′ji-năl). Below any margin or edge.

in·fra·max·il·lary (in-fră-mak′si-lā-rē). SYN mandibular.

in·fra·na·tant (in′fră-nā′tănt). SEE infranatant *fluid.* [infra- + L. *natare,* to swim]

in·fra·oc·clu·sion (in′fră-ŏ-klū′zhun). SYN infraclusion.

in·fra·or·bit·al (in′fră-ōr′bi-tăl). Below or beneath the orbit. SYN suborbital.

in·fra·pa·tel·lar (in-fră-pa-tel′ăr). Inferior to the patella; denoting especially a bursa, a pad of fat, or a synovial fold. SYN subpatellar (2).

in·fra·psy·chic (in-fră-sī′kik). Denoting ideas or actions originating below the level of consciousness.

in·fra·red (in′fră-red). That portion of the electromagnetic spectrum with wavelengths between 770 and 1000 nm.

in·fra·scap·u·lar (in-fră-skap′yū-lăr). Inferior to the scapula. SYN subscapular (2).

in·fra·son·ic (in′fră-son′ik). Denoting those frequencies that lie below the range of human hearing. [infra- + L. *sonus,* sound]

in·fra·spi·na·tus (in-fră-spī-nā′tŭs). SEE infraspinatus *muscle.*

in·fra·spi·nous (in-fră-spī′nŭs). Below a spine or spinous process; specifically, the fossa infraspinata. SYN subspinous (1).

in·fra·splen·ic (in′fră-splen′ik, -sple′nik). Beneath or below the spleen.

in·fra·ster·nal (in-fră-ster′năl). Inferior to the sternum. SYN substernal (2).

in·fra·sub·spe·cif·ic (in′fră-sŭb-spe-si′fik). Denoting a category of organisms of rank lower than subspecies.

in·fra·tem·po·ral (in-fră-tem′pŏ-răl). Below the temporal fossa.

in·fra·tho·rac·ic (in′fră-thō-ras′ik). Below or at the lower portion of the thorax.

in·fra·ton·sil·lar (in-fră-ton′si-lăr). Below the palatine tonsil or cerebellar tonsil.

in·fra·troch·le·ar (in′fră-trok′lē-ăr). Inferior to the trochlea or pulley of the superior oblique muscle of the eye.

in·fra·um·bil·i·cal (in′fră-ŭm-bil′i-kăl). Inferior to the umbilicus. SYN subumbilical.

in·fra·ver·sion (in′fră-ver′shŭn). **1.** A turning (version) downward. **2.** In physiological optics, rotation of both eyes downward. **3.** SYN infraclusion.

in·fric·tion (in-frik′shŭn). The application of liniments or ointments combined with friction. [L. *in,* on, + *frictio,* a rubbing]

in·fun·dib·u·la (in-fŭn-dib′yū-lă). Plural of infundibulum.

in·fun·dib·u·lar (in-fŭn-dib′yū-lăr). Relating to an infundibulum.

in·fun·dib·u·lec·to·my (in′fŭn-dib′yū-lek′tō-mē). Excision of the infundibulum, especially of hypertrophied ventricular septal myocardium encroaching on the superior ventricular outflow tract. [infundibulum + G. *ektomē,* excision]

in·fun·dib·u·li·form (in-fŭn-dib′yū-li-fōrm). SYN choanoid. [L. *infundibulum,* funnel, + *forma,* form]

in·fun·dib·u·lin (in-fŭn-dib′yū-lin). A 20% solution of an extract of the posterior lobe of the hypophysis cerebri.

in·fun·dib·u·lo·fol·lic·u·li·tis (in-fŭn-dib′yū-lō-fo-lik′yū-lī′tis). Inflammation of the follicular infundibulum, the superficial part of the hair follicle above the opening of the sebaceous gland.

    disseminated recurrent i., a pruritic papular follicular eczema of the trunk and proximal extremities; usually occurs in blacks.

in·fun·dib·u·lo·ma (in-fŭn-dib′yū-lō′mă). A pilocytic astrocytoma arising in the neurohypophysis of the pituitary. [infundibulum + G. -*oma*, tumor]

in·fun·dib·u·lo-ovar·i·an (in-fŭn-dib′yū-lō-ō-vā′rē-an). Relating to the fimbriated extremity of a uterine tube and the ovary.

in·fun·dib·u·lo·pel·vic (in-fŭn-dib′yū-lō-pel′vik). Relating to any two structures called infundibulum and pelvis, such as the expanded portion of a calyx and the pelvis of the kidney, or the fimbriated extremity of the uterine tube and the pelvis.

in·fun·dib·u·lum, pl. **in·fun·dib·u·la** (in-fŭn-dib′yū-lŭm, -yū-lă). **1** [NA]. A funnel or funnel-shaped structure or passage. **2.** SYN i. of uterine tube. **3.** The expanding portion of a calix as it opens into the pelvis of the kidney. **4** [NA]. ☆official alternate term for arterial *cone*. **5.** Termination of a bronchiole in the alveolus. **6.** Termination of the cochlear canal beneath the cupola. **7** [NA]. The funnel-shaped, unpaired prominence of the base of the hypothalamus behind the optic chiasm, enclosing the infundibular recess of the third ventricle and continuous below with the stalk of the hypophysis. **8.** The contact surface indentation in the incisor and cheek teeth of a horse. SYN i. of teeth, mark (2). [L. a funnel]

ethmoid i., SYN ethmoidal i.

ethmoidal i., a passage from the middle meatus of the nose communicating with the anterior ethmoidal cells and frontal sinus. SYN i. ethmoidale [NA], ethmoid i.

i. ethmoida′le [NA], SYN ethmoidal i.

i. hypothal′ami [NA], SYN hypothalamic i.

hypothalamic i., the apical portion of the tuber cinereum extending into the stalk of the hypophysis. SYN i. hypothalami [NA].

i. of lungs, in the embryo, one of the expanded extremities of the subdivisions of the lung buds; in later development minute pouches (the air sacs) appear in its wall.

i. of teeth, SYN infundibulum (8).

i. tu′bae uteri′nae [NA], SYN i. of uterine tube.

i. of uterine tube, the funnel-like expansion of the abdominal extremity of the uterine (fallopian) tube. SYN i. tubae uterinae [NA], infundibulum (2).

in·fu·si·ble (in-fū′zi-bl). **1.** Incapable of being melted or fused. **2.** Capable of being made into an infusion.

in·fu·sion (in-fyū′zhŭn). **1.** The process of steeping a substance in water, either cold or hot (below the boiling point), in order to extract its soluble principles. **2.** A medicinal preparation obtained by steeping the crude drug in water. **3.** The introduction of fluid other than blood, *e.g.,* saline solution, into a vein. [L. *infusio,* fr. *in-fundo,* pp. -*fusus,* to pour in]

in·fu·so·de·coc·tion (in-fyū′zō-dē-kok′shŭn). Rarely used term for: **1.** Infusion followed by decoction. **2.** A medicinal preparation made by steeping the crude drug first in cold water and then in boiling water.

In·fu·so·ria (in-fyūsō′rē-ă). Archaic term for Ciliophora. [Mod. L. pertaining to or found in an infusion, fr. *in-fundo,* pp. *in-fusus,* to pour in]

in·fu·so·ri·an (in-fyū-sō′rē-an). Archaic term for a member of the class Infusoria, now the phylum Ciliophora.

in·ges·ta (in-jes′tă). Solid or liquid nutrients taken into the body. [pl. of L. *ingestum,* ntr. pp. of *in-gero, -gestus,* to carry in]

in·ges·tion (in-jes′chŭn). **1.** Introduction of food and drink into the stomach. **2.** Incorporation of particles into the cytoplasm of a phagocytic cell by invagination of a portion of the cell membrane as a vacuole. [L. *in-gero,* to carry in]

in·ges·tive (in-jes′tiv). Relating to ingestion.

Ingrassia, Giovanni F., Italian anatomist, 1510–1580. SEE I.'s *apophysis, wing.*

in·gra·ves·cent (in-gră-ves′ent). Increasing in severity. [L. *in-gravesco,* to grow heavier, fr. *gravis,* heavy]

in·guen (ing′gwen). SYN inguinal *region.* [L.]

in·gui·nal (ing′gwi-năl). Relating to the groin.

in·gui·no·cru·ral (ing′gwi-nō-krū′răl). Relating to the groin and the thigh.

in·gui·no·dyn·ia (ing′gwi-nō-din′ē-ă). Rarely used term for pain in the groin. [L. *inguen* (*inguin-*), groin, + G. *odynē,* pain]

in·gui·no·la·bi·al (ing′gwi-nō-lā′bē-ăl). Relating to the groin and the labium.

in·gui·no·per·i·to·ne·al (ing′gwi-nō-per′i-tō-nē′ăl). Relating to the groin and the peritoneum.

in·gui·no·scro·tal (ing′gwi-nō-skrō′tăl). Relating to the groin and the scrotum.

INH Abbreviation for isonicotinic acid hydrazide.

in·hal·ant (in-hā′lant). **1.** That which is inhaled; a remedy given by inhalation. **2.** A drug (or combination of drugs) with high vapor pressure, carried by an air current into the nasal passage, where it produces its effect. **3.** Group of products consisting of finely powdered or liquid drugs that are carried to the respiratory passages by the use of special devices such as low pressure aerosol containers. SYN insufflation (2). SEE ALSO inhalation, aerosol. [see inhalation]

in·ha·la·tion (in-hă-lā′shŭn). **1.** The act of drawing in the breath. SYN inspiration. **2.** Drawing a medicated vapor with the breath. **3.** A solution of a drug or combination of drugs for administration as a nebulized mist intended to reach the respiratory tree. [L. *in-halo,* pp. -*halatus,* to breathe at or in]

solvent i., i. of volatile organic solvents used in glue, nail polish remover, lacquer thinners, cleaning fluid, lighter fluid, and gasoline, for the purpose of self-intoxication. SEE ALSO glue-sniffing.

in·hale (in-hāl′). To draw in the breath. SYN inspire.

in·hal·er (in-hāl′er). **1.** SYN respirator (1). **2.** An apparatus for administering pharmacologically active agents by inhalation.

in·her·ent (in-her′ent). Occurring as a natural part or consequence; latent imminent; intrinsic. [L. *inhaerens,* sticking to, adhering]

in·her·i·tance (in-her′i-tans). **1.** Characters or qualities that are transmitted from parent to offspring by coded cytological data; that which is inherited. **2.** Cultural or legal endowment. **3.** The act of inheriting. [L. *heredito,* inherit, fr. *heres* (*hered-*), an heir]

alternative i., (1) SYN mendelian i. **(2)** Galton's term for an assumed form in which all the characters are derived from one parent.

blending i., Galton's term for i. in which no component is conspicuous or obtrusive.

codominant i., i. in which two alleles are individually expressed in the presence of each other; there may be other alleles available at the locus that may or may not exhibit codominance.

collateral i., the appearance of characters in collateral members of a family group, as when an uncle and a niece show the same character inherited from a common ancestor; in recessive characters it may appear irregularly, in contrast to dominant characters transmitted directly from one generation to the next.

cytoplasmic i., transmission of characters dependent on self-perpetuating elements not nuclear in origin (*e.g.,* mitochondrial DNA). SYN extranuclear i.

dominant i., SEE *dominance* of traits.

extrachromosomal i., transmission of characters dependent on some factor not connected with the chromosomes.

extranuclear i., SYN cytoplasmic i.

galtonian i., i. in which a measurable phenotype is generated by many loci, the contributions of which are statistically independent, additive, and of about equal value. (The latter are in accordance with the classical central limit therein and justify the use of the multivariate normal distribution in galtonian genetics). SYN polygenic i.

holandric i., SYN Y-linked i.

hologynic i., transmission of a trait from mother to her daughters but to no sons, attributed to attached (partially fused) X chromosomes, to cytoplasmic i., or to sex limitation with abnormal segregation, *e.g.,* hematocolpos.

maternal i., transmission of characters that are dependent on peculiarities of the egg cytoplasm produced, in turn, by nuclear genes.

mendelian i., i. in which stable and undecomposable characters controlled entirely or overwhelmingly by a single genetic locus are transmitted over many generations. SEE Mendel's first *law, law* of segregation, *law* of independent assortment. SYN alternative i. (1).

mosaic i., i. in which the paternal influence is dominant in one group of cells and the maternal in another. Cf. lyonization.

multifactorial i., i. involving many factors, of which at least one is genetic but none is of overwhelming importance, as in the causation of a disease by multiple genetic and environmental factors. Cf. galtonian i.

polygenic i., SYN galtonian i.

recessive i., SEE *dominance* of traits.

sex-influenced i., i. that is autosomal but has a different intensity of expression in the two sexes, *e.g.,* male pattern baldness.

sex-limited i., of a trait that can be expressed in one sex only, *e.g.,* testicular feminization.

sex-linked i., the pattern of inheritance that may result from a mutant gene located on either the X or Y chromosome.

X-linked i., the pattern of i. that may result from a mutant gene on an X chromosome.

Y-linked i., the pattern of i. that may result from a mutant gene located on a Y chromosome. SYN holandric i.

in·her·it·ed (in-her′it-ed). Derived from a preformed genetic code present in the parents. Contrast with acquired.

in·hib·in (in-hib′in). Two glycoproteins, i. A and i. B, secreted by Sertoli cells in the testis and granulosa cells in the ovary, which inhibit FSH secretion by direct action on the pituitary. [inhibit + -in]

in·hib·it (in-hib′it). To curb or restrain.

in·hib·i·tine (in-hib′i-tēn). SYN carnosine.

in·hi·bi·tion (in-hi-bish′ŭn). **1.** Depression or arrest of a function. SEE ALSO inhibitor. **2.** In psychoanalysis, the restraining of instinctual or unconscious drives or tendencies, especially if they conflict with one's conscience or with societal demands. **3.** In psychology, a generic term for a variety of processes associated with the gradual attenuation, masking, and extinction of a previously conditioned response. [L. *in-hibeo,* pp. *-hibitus,* to keep back, fr. *habeo,* to have]

allogeneic i., i. or injury to allogeneic cells that occurs when lymphocytes are mixed and cultured with other cells of different genotypes *in vitro.*

central i., suppression or diminution of outgoing impulses from a reflex center.

competitive i., blocking of the action of an enzyme by a compound that binds to the free enzyme, preventing the substrate from binding and thus prevents the enzyme from acting on that substrate. The competitive inhibitor is often a substrate analog and binds at the active site; however, this is not an absolute requirement for competitive i. Saturating levels of substrate can remove the inhibition. Cf. isostery. SYN selective i.

contact i., cessation of replication of dividing cells that come into contact, as in the center of a healing wound.

end product i., SYN feedback i.

feedback i., i. of activity by an end product of the pathway of which that activity is a part; *e.g.,* thyroliberin stimulates thyroglobulin production, and thyroglobulin decreases thyrotropin formation. SYN end product i., retroinhibition.

hapten i. of precipitation, i. of precipitation that occurs when the precipitin has combined with hapten of the same specificity as the subsequently added antigen.

hemagglutination i., i. of nonimmune hemagglutination by antibody specific for the hemagglutinin; *e.g.,* viral hemagglutination will not occur if antibody specific for the virus is added before addition of red blood cells. The i. is specific and is widely used for virus identification and for antibody determination.

noncompetitive i., a type of enzyme i. in which the inhibiting compound does not compete with the natural substrate for the active site on the enzyme, but inhibits the reaction by combining with the enzyme-substrate complex, once the latter has been formed, and with the free enzyme.

potassium i., arrest of the heart in the fully relaxed state as a result of potassium intoxication.

proactive i., a type of interference or negative transfer, observed in memory experiments and other learning situations, when something learned previously interferes with present learning or recall. Cf. retroactive i.

product i., i. of an enzyme activity by a product of the reaction catalyzed by that enzyme.

reciprocal i., **(1)** SYN reciprocal *innervation.* **(2)** SYN systematic *desensitization.*

reflex i., a situation in which sensory stimuli decrease reflex activity.

residual i., the i. or suppression of tinnitus by use of a sound-generating device (residual inhibitor) which masks the sounds of tinnitus and produces a residual sound-inhibiting effect when the device is turned off.

retroactive i., the partial or complete obliteration of memory by a more recent event, particularly new learning. Cf. proactive i.

selective i., SYN competitive i.

substrate i., i. of an enzyme activity by a substrate of the reaction catalyzed by that enzyme; often, this type of i. occurs at elevated substrate levels in which the substrate is binding to a second, non-active site on the enzyme.

uncompetitive i., an inhibitory effect on a metabolic function, such as an enzyme, not based on competition for the binding site of the naturally occurring substrate, but on a different effect on the molecule whose function is being inhibited.

Wedensky i., i. of muscle response resulting from application of a series of rapidly repeated stimuli to the motor nerve where slower frequency of stimulation results in muscle response.

in·hib·i·tor (in-hib′i-ter, -tōr). **1.** An agent that restrains or retards physiologic, chemical, or enzymatic action. **2.** A nerve, stimulation of which represses activity. SEE ALSO inhibition.

angiotensin-converting enzyme i.'s (ACEI), a class of drugs used in the treatment of hypertension; they produce a reduction of peripheral arterial resistance, although the exact mechanism of action has not been fully determined; they block the conversion of angiotensin I to angiotensin II, a powerful vasoconstrictor.

aromatase i.'s, drugs, such as aminoglutethimide, that inhibit aromatase, an enzyme used in the synthesis of estrogens.

Bowman-Birk i., a polypeptide that will inhibit both trypsin and chymotrypsin.

carbonate dehydratase i., an agent, usually chemically related to the sulfonamides, that inhibits the activity of carbonate dehydratase, producing a general decrease in the formation of H_2CO_3 in the tissues. SEE ALSO acetazolamide, dichlorphenamide. SYN carbonic anhydrase i.

carbonic anhydrase i., SYN carbonate dehydratase i.

C1 esterase i., an α_2-neuraminoglycoprotein that inhibits the enzymatic activity of C1 esterase, the activated first component of complement. A deficiency of this i. results in a lack of inhibition of C1r and C1s leading to uncontrolled activation of the complement cascade and edema.

cholinesterase i., a drug, such as neostigmine, which, by inhibiting biodegradation of acetylcholine, restores myoneural function in myasthenia gravis or after nondepolarizing neuromuscular relaxants have been administered.

familial lipoprotein lipase i., an i. found in certain individuals that inhibits lipoprotein lipase resulting in accumulation of chylomicrons, VLDL, and triacylglycerols; similar in symptoms to familial lipoprotein lipase deficiency.

glucosidase i.'s, agents such as acarbose which reduce gastrointestinal absorption of carbohydrates. This group of drugs has been known popularly as "starch blockers". They lower plasma glucose levels and tend to cause weight loss. A limiting side effect is flatulence.

HMG CoA reductase i.'s, drugs, such as lovastatin and pravastatin, which interfere with the biosynthesis of cholesterol; used to treat hyperlipidemia.

human α_1-proteinase i. (α_1PI), SYN α_1-antitrypsin.

β-lactamase i.'s, drugs such as clavulanic acid, which are used to inhibit bacterial β-lactamases; often used with a penicillin or cephalosporin to overcome drug resistance.

lipoprotein-associated coagulation i. (LACI), formerly known as anticonvertin; a protein that inhibits the extrinsic pathway of coagulation by binding to the tissue factor III-factor VII-Ca^{2+}-factor Xa complex.

mechanism-based i., SYN suicide *substrate.*

in

monoamine oxidase i. (MAOI), any of the hydrazine ($-NHNH_2$) and hydrazide ($-CONHNH_2$) derivatives that inhibit several enzymes and raise the brain norepinephrine and 5-hydroxytryptamine levels; used as antidepressant and hypotensive agents.

ovulation i., a compound that inhibits ovulation; often found in oral contraceptives.

residual i., a sound-generating device, worn in the ear, which inhibits or suppresses the sounds of tinnitus by masking, with a residual inhibitory effect when the device is turned off.

respiratory i., a compound that inhibits the respiratory chain. SYN respiratory poison.

serine protease i.'s, a class of highly polymorphic inhibitors of trypsin, elastase, and certain other proteases synthesized by hepatocytes and macrophages SEE ALSO α_1-antitrypsin. SYN serpins.

trypsin i., **(1)** a peptide hydrolyzed off trypsinogen under the catalytic influence of enteropeptidase, with trypsin produced as a result; so called because the peptide masks or inhibits the active site of the trypsin molecule; **(2)** one of the polypeptides, from various sources (*e.g.*, human and bovine colostrum, soybeans, egg white), that inhibit the action of trypsin. Cf. Bowman-Birk i. α_1**-trypsin i.,** SYN α_1-antitrypsin.

in·hib·i·to·ry (in-hib'i-tōr-ē). Restraining; tending to inhibit.

in·i·ac (in'ē-ak). Relating to the inion. SYN inial.

in·i·ad (in'ē-ad). In a direction toward the inion. [L. *ad*, to]

in·i·al (in'ē-ăl). SYN iniac.

in·i·en·ceph·a·ly (in'ē-en-sef'ă-lē). Malformation consisting of a cranial defect at the occiput, with the brain exposed; often in combination with a cervical rachischisis and retroflexion. [G. *inion*, back of the head, + *enkephalos*, brain]

in·i·on (in'ē-on) [NA]. A point located on the external occipital protuberance at the intersection of the midline with a line drawn tangent to the uppermost convexity of the right and left superior nuchal lines. [G. nape of the neck]

in·i·op·a·gus (in'ē-op'ă-gŭs). SYN *craniopagus* occipitalis. [inion + G. *pagos*, fixed]

in·i·ops (in'ē-ops). SYN *janiceps* asymmetrus. [inion + G. *ōps*, eye, face]

in·i·ti·a·tion (i-ni-shē-ā'shŭn). **1.** The first stage of tumor induction by a carcinogen; subtle alteration of cells by exposure to a carcinogenic agent so that they are likely to form a tumor upon subsequent exposure to a promoting agent (promotion). **2.** Starting point of replication or translation in macromolecule biosynthesis. **3.** Start of chemical or enzymatic reaction.

in·i·tis (in-ī'tis). **1.** Inflammation of fibrous tissue. **2.** SYN myositis. [G. *is* (*in-*), fiber, + *-itis*, inflammation]

in·ject (in-jekt'). To introduce into the body; denoting a fluid forced beneath the skin or into a blood vessel. SEE ALSO injection. [L. *injicio*, to throw in]

in·ject·a·ble (in-jek'tă-bl). **1.** Capable of being injected into anything. **2.** Capable of receiving an injection.

in·ject·ed (in-jek'ted). **1.** Denoting a fluid introduced into the body. **2.** Denoting blood vessels visibly distended with blood.

in·jec·tion (in-jek'shŭn). **1.** Introduction of a medicinal substance or nutrient material into the subcutaneous tissue (subcutaneous or hypodermic i.), the muscular tissue (intramuscular i.), a vein (intravenous i.), an artery (intraarterial i.), the rectum (rectal i. or enema), the vagina (vaginal i. or douche), the urethra, or other canals or cavities of the body. **2.** An injectable pharmaceutical preparation. **3.** Congestion or hyperemia. [L. *injectio*, a throwing in, fr. *in-jicio*, to throw in]

adrenal cortex i., obsolete treatment involving the parenteral administration of extract of the adrenal cortex; formerly used in treatment of Addison's *disease*.

collagen i., correction of superficial soft tissue deformities, acne scars, or age-related skin changes by i. (implantation) of collagen; bovine collagen preparations are commonly used. Prior intradermal testing is necessay to exclude hypersensitivity.

depot i., an i. of a substance in a vehicle that tends to keep it at the site of i. so that absorption occurs over a prolonged period.

hypodermic i., the administration of a remedy in liquid form by i. into the subcutaneous tissues. SYN hypodermic (2).

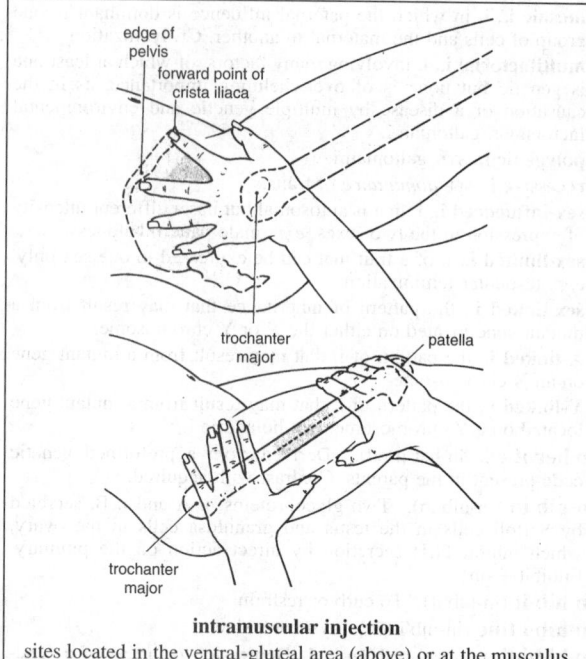

intramuscular injection
sites located in the ventral-gluteal area (above) or at the musculus vastus lateralis (below)

insulin i., a preparation that may contain 20, 40, 80, 100, or 500 USP insulin units per ml, although the trend is toward standardizing all insulin preparations at 100 units per ml; it is administered subcutaneously, occasionally intravenously, and has a rapid onset of action, has a brief duration (5 to 7 hours), and is compatible for mixing with long-acting insulin preparations; used in the treatment of diabetic acidosis and insulin coma. SYN regular insulin i.

intrathecal i., introduction of material for diffusion throughout the subarachnoid space by means of lumbar puncture.

intraventricular i., the introduction of materials for diffusion throughout the ventricular and subarachnoid space by means of ventricular puncture.

jet i., hypodermic i. of drugs by a jet injector.

lactated Ringer's i., a sterile solution of calcium chloride, potassium chloride, sodium chloride, and sodium lactate in water for injection; used intravenously as a systemic alkalizer and a fluid and electrolyte replenisher.

regular insulin i., SYN insulin i.

Ringer's i., a sterile solution of sodium chloride, potassium chloride, and calcium chloride, containing in each 100 ml between 820 and 900 mg of sodium chloride, between 25 and 35 mg of potassium chloride, and between 30 and 37 mg of calcium chloride; used intravenously as a fluid and electrolyte replenisher.

selective i., i. of contrast medium following selective catheterization of a branch artery or vein for angiography.

sensitizing i., an i. that sensitizes a person so that subsequent exposure to the antigen (allergen) evokes an allergic response.

test i., intravenous i. of a few milliliters of radiographic contrast medium to screen for allergic or idiosyncratic responses.

Z-tract i., a technique in which the skin and subcutaneous tissue are displaced laterally before inserting the needle intramuscularly; used to prevent leakage along the track of the needle and consequent tissue irritation.

in·jec·tor (in-jek'ter). A device for making injections.

jet i., an i. that uses high pressure to force a liquid through a small orifice at a velocity sufficient to penetrate skin or mucous membrane without the use of a needle.

power i., an i. for rapid contrast medium injection in angiography or computed tomography.

in·jure (in'jer). To wound, hurt, or harm.

in·ju·ry (in'jer-ē). The damage or wound of trauma. [L. *injuria,* fr. *in-* neg. + *jus (jur-),* right]

blast i., tearing of lung tissue or rupture of abdominal viscera without external i., as by the force of an explosion.

closed head i., a head i. in which continuity of the scalp and mucous membranes is maintained.

contrecoup i. of brain, an i. occurring beneath the skull opposite to the area of impact.

coup i. of brain, an i. occurring directly beneath the skull at the area of impact.

current of i., SEE *current* of injury.

degloving i., avulsion of the skin of the hand (or foot) in which the part is skeletonized by removal of most or all of the skin and subcutaneous tissue.

egg-white i., SYN egg-white *syndrome.*

hyperextension-hyperflexion i., violence to the body causing the unsupported head to hyperextend and hyperflex the neck rapidly; does not imply any specific resultant trauma or pathology.

i. of intervertebral disk, SEE traumatic cervical *discopathy.*

open head i., a head i. in which there is a loss of continuity of scalp or mucous membranes; the term is sometimes used to indicate a communication between the exterior and the intracranial cavity. SEE ALSO penetrating *wound.*

pneumatic tire i., separation of the skin and subcutaneous tissue from the underlying fascia, classically occurring when an extremity is crushed and rolled over by the tire of a vehicle but may be incurred through other mechanisms that produce shear forces; may occur particularly in cases of obesity.

reperfusion i., myocardial impairment, usually with arrhythmia, following the opening of arterial blockage and considered to be due to oxygen-derived free radicals.

steering wheel i., trauma to the anterior chest wall caused by impact with the steering wheel during an automobile accident; can include fractured sternum and ribs, cardiac contusion, tear of the aorta or other great vessels, as well as lung injuries.

whiplash i., popular term for hyperextension-hyperflexion i.

in·lay (in'lā). **1.** In dentistry, a prefabricated restoration sealed in the cavity with cement. **2.** A graft of bone into a bone cavity. **3.** A graft of skin into a wound cavity for epithelialization. **4.** In orthopaedics, an orthomechanical device inserted into a shoe; commonly called an "arch support."

epithelial i., SYN inlay *graft.*

gold i., a gold restoration fabricated by casting in a mold made from a wax pattern; the restoration is sealed in the prepared cavity with dental cement.

porcelain i., a fused porcelain restoration luted in a cavity prepared in a tooth.

in·let. A passage leading into a cavity. SYN aditus [NA].

i. of larynx, the aperture between the pharynx and larynx, bounded by the superior edges of the epiglottis (anteriorly), the aryepiglottic folds (laterally), and the mucosa between the arytenoids (posteriorly). SYN aditus laryngis [NA], laryngeal aperture.

pelvic i., SYN superior pelvic *aperture.*

in·nate (i'nāt, i-nāt'). SYN inborn. [L. *in-nascor,* pp. *-natus,* to be born in, pp. as adj. inborn, innate]

in·ner·va·tion (in'er-vā'shŭn). The supply of nerve fibers functionally connected with a part. [L. *in,* in, + *nervus,* nerve]

reciprocal i., contraction in a muscle is accompanied by a loss of tone or by relaxation in the antagonistic muscle. SYN reciprocal inhibition (1).

in·nid·i·a·tion (i-nid-ē-ā'shŭn). The growth and multiplication of abnormal cells in another location to which they have been transported by means of lymph or the blood stream, or both. SEE ALSO metastasis. SYN colonization (1), indenization. [L. *in,* in, + *nidus,* nest]

in·no·cent (in'ō-sent). **1.** Not apparently harmful. **2.** Free from moral wrong. [L. *innocens (-ent-),* fr. *in,* neg., + *noceo,* to injure]

in·noc·u·ous (i-nok'yū-ŭs). Harmless. SYN innoxious. [L. *in-nocuus*]

in·nom·i·na·tal (i-nom'i-nā-tăl). Relating to the hip bone.

in·nom·i·nate (i-nom'i-nāt). SYN anonyma. [L. *innominatus,* fr. *in-* neg. + *nomen (nomin-),* name]

in·nox·ious (i-nok'shŭs). SYN innocuous. [L. *in-noxius,* fr. *in,* neg. + *noceo,* to injure]

Ino Symbol for inosine.

△**ino-, in-.** Obsolete prefix for fiber, fibrous; replaced in most terms by fibro-. [G. *is (in-),* fiber]

in·oc·u·la·bil·i·ty (i-nok'yū-lă-bil'i-tē). The quality of being inoculable.

in·oc·u·la·ble (i-nok'yū-lă-bl). **1.** Transmissible by inoculation. **2.** Susceptible to a disease transmissible by inoculation.

in·oc·u·late (i-nok'yū-lāt). **1.** To introduce the agent of a disease or other antigenic material into the subcutaneous tissue or a blood vessel, or through an abraded or absorbing surface for preventive, curative, or experimental purposes. **2.** To implant microorganisms or infectious material into or upon culture media. **3.** To communicate a disease by transferring its virus. [L. *inoculo,* pp. *-atus,* to ingraft]

in·oc·u·la·tion (i-nok-yū-lā'shŭn). Introduction into the body of the causative organism of a disease.

stress i., in clinical psychology, an approach intended to provide patients with cognitive and attitudinal skills that they can use to cope with stress.

in·oc·u·lum (i-nok'yū-lŭm). The microorganism or other material introduced by inoculation.

In·o·cy·be (i-nō'sī-bē). A genus of mushrooms containing several species that have a high yield of muscarine.

in·o·pec·tic (in-ō-pek'tik). Relating to inopexia.

in·op·er·a·ble (in-op'er-ă-bl). Denoting that which cannot be operated upon, or cannot be corrected or removed by an operation.

in·o·pex·ia (in'ō-peksē-ă). A tendency toward spontaneous coagulation of the blood. [ino + G. *pexis,* fixation, + -ia]

in·or·gan·ic (in-ōr-gan'ik). **1.** Not organic; not formed by living organisms. **2.** SEE inorganic *compound.* **3.** Not containing carbon.

in·os·a·mine (in-ōs'ă-mēn). An inositol in which an –OH group is replaced by an –NH$_2$ group.

in·os·co·py (in-os'kŏ-pē). The microscopic examination of biologic materials (*e.g.,* tissue, sputum, clotted blood) after dissecting or chemically digesting the fibrillary elements and strands of fibrin. [ino- + G. *skopeō,* to look at]

in·ose (in'ōs). SYN inositol.

in·o·se·mia (in-ō-sē'mē-ă). **1.** The presence of inositol in the circulating blood. **2.** SYN fibremia. [inose + G. *haima,* blood]

in·o·si·nate (in-ō'si-nāt). A salt or ester of inosinic acid.

in·o·sine (I, Ino) (in'ō-sēn). 9-β-D-Ribosylhypoxanthine; a nucleoside formed by the deamination of adenosine. SYN hypoxanthinosine.

in·o·sine 5'-di·phos·phate (IDP). Inosine esterified at its 5' position with diphosphoric acid.

in·o·sine 5'-mon·o·phos·phate (IMP). SYN inosinic acid.

IMP dehydrogenase, an enzyme that catalyzes the reaction of IMP, water, and NAD$^+$ to form NADH and xanthosine 5'-monophosphate (XMP), the immediate precursor of GMP.

in·o·sine pran·o·bex (in'ō-sēn pran'ō-beks). A 1:3 molar complex of 1-dimethylaminopropan-2-ol-4-acetamidobenzoate and inosine, used as an antiviral agent.

in·o·sine 5'-tri·phos·phate (ITP). (in'ō-sēn). Inosine with triphosphoric acid esterified at its 5' position; participates in a number of enzyme-catalyzed reactions.

in·o·sin·ic ac·id (in-ō-sin'ik). A mononucleotide found in muscle and other tissues; a key intermediate in purine biosynthesis; also produced in relatively high levels in muscle. SYN inosine 5'-monophosphate.

in·o·sin·i·case (in-o-sin'-a-kās). An enzyme that functions in purine biosynthesis and catalyzes the ring closure reaction that produces inosinic acid from 5'-phosphoribosyl 5-formamidoimidazole-4-carboxamide.

in·o·sin·yl (in-ō'si-nil). The radical of inosinic acid.

in·o·site (in′ō-sīt). SYN inositol.

in·o·si·tide (in-ō′si-tīd). Term used for phosphatidylinositol or any inositol-containing phospholipid.

in·o·si·tol (in-ō′si-tōl, -tol). 1,2,3,4,5,6-Hexahydroxycyclohexane; a member of the vitamin B complex necessary for growth of yeast and of mice; absence from the diet causes alopecia and dermatitis in mice and "spectacle eyes" in rats. It occurs in a number of stereoisomeric forms: *cis-*, *epi-*, *allo-*, *neo-*, *myo-*, *muco-*, *chiro-*, and *scyllo-*inositols; the most abundant naturally occurring one is *myo-*inositol (usually meant when "inositol" occurs alone). SYN antialopecia factor, cyclohexitol, inose, inosite, liposital, mouse antialopecia factor.

i. niacinate, hexanicotinoyl inositol; a peripheral vasodilator.

i. 1,3,4,5-tetraphosphate, a phosphorylated derivative of i. formed from inositol 1,4,5-trisphosphate that causes Ca^{2+} entry into the cytosol from the extracellular medium; inactivated by hydrolysis to form inositol 1,3,4-trisphosphate.

i. 1,4,5-trisphosphate (IP₃), a second messenger formed from phosphatidylinositol 4,5-bisphosphate; triggers the release of calcium ions from special vesicles of the endoplasmic reticulum; has a role in the activation of neutrophils.

meso-in·o·si·tol. 1. Generic term for any isomer of *meso-*inositol in which the hydroxyl groups are so arranged that the molecule as a whole possesses a plane of symmetry and is optically inactive. 2. Former name for *myo-*inositol.

myo-in·o·si·tol. 1,2,3,5/4,6-Inositol; a constituent of various phosphatidylinositols and the most widely distributed form of inositol found in microorganisms, higher plants, and animals. In plants, it is found as phytic acid and as phytin; partially phosphorylated and free forms occur throughout nature, and in many tissues.

in·o·si·tu·ria (in′ō-sī-tū′rē-ă). The excretion of inositol in the urine. SYN inosuria (1). [inositol + G. *ouron,* urine]

in·o·su·ria (in-ō-sū′rē-a). 1. SYN inosituria. 2. The occurrence of fibrin in the urine.

in·o·tro·pic (in-ō-trop′ik). Influencing the contractility of muscular tissue. [ino- + G. *tropos,* a turning]

negatively i., weakening muscular action.

positively i., strengthening muscular action.

Ino·vir·i·dae (i-nō-vir′i-dē). Provisional name for a family of filamentous bacterial viruses with a genome of single-stranded DNA (molecular weight 1.9 to 2.7×10^6). Coliphage fd, the type species of the fd phage group genus, adsorbs to the tips of pili of male enterobacteria and, after multiplication, particles are released without causing lysis of the host bacterium. [ino- + virus]

in phase. Moving in the same direction at the same time; a possible characteristic of two simultaneous oscillations of similar frequency.

in·quest (in′kwest). A legal inquiry into the cause of sudden, violent, or mysterious death. [L. *in,* in, + *quaero,* pp. *quaesitus,* to seek]

in·qui·line (in′kwi-līn, -lin). An animal that lives habitually in the abode of some other species (an oyster crab within the shell of an oyster) causing little or no inconvenience to the host. SEE ALSO commensal. [L. *inquilinus,* an inhabitant of a place that is not his own, fr. *in,* in, + *colo,* to inhabit]

in·sa·lu·bri·ous (in-să-lū′brē-ŭs). Unwholesome; unhealthful; usually in reference to climate. [L. *in-salubris,* unwholesome]

in·sane (in-sān′). 1. Of unsound mind; severely mentally impaired; deranged; crazy. 2. Relating to insanity. [L. *in-* neg. + *sanus,* sound, sane]

in·san·i·tary (in-san′i-tār-ē). Injurious to health, usually in reference to an unclean or contaminated environment. SYN unsanitary. [L. *in-* neg. + *sanus,* sound]

in·san·i·ty (in-san′i-tē). 1. An outmoded term referring to severe mental illness or psychosis. 2. In law, that degree of mental illness which negates the individual's legal responsibility or capacity. [L. *in-* neg. + *sanus,* sound]

criminal i., in forensic psychiatry, a term that describes the degree of mental competence and that is defined by such currently applicable legal precedents as the American Law Institute

rule, Durham rule, M'Naghten rule, and the New Hampshire rule.

i. defense, in forensic psychiatry, the use in the courtroom of i. as a mitigating factor in the defense of an individual on trial for a serious criminal offense. SEE criminal i.

in·scrip·tio (in-skrip′shē-ō). SYN inscription. [L. fr. *in-scribo,* pp. *-scriptus,* to write on]

i. tendin′ea, SYN tendinous *intersection.*

in·scrip·tion (in-skrip′shŭn). 1. The main part of a prescription; that which indicates the drugs and the quantity of each to be used in the mixture. 2. A mark, band, or line. SYN inscriptio. [L. *inscriptio*]

tendinous i., SYN tendinous *intersection.*

In·sec·ta (in-sek′tă). The insects, the largest class of the phylum Arthropoda and the largest major grouping of living things, chiefly characterized by flight, great adaptability, vast speciation in terrestrial and freshwater environments, and possession of three pairs of jointed legs and, usually, two pairs of wings. Some are parasitic, others serve as intermediate hosts for parasites, including those that cause many human diseases. Some are wingless; others, such as the Diptera, have only one pair of wings. Respiration is by tracheoles, cuticle-lined air tubes that pass air directly to the tissues. Development in higher forms is holometabolous and passes through distinctive egg, larval, pupal, and adult stages. SYN Hexapoda. [L. pl. of *insectus,* insect, fr. *in-seco,* pp. *-sectus,* to cut into]

in·sec·tar·i·um (in-sek-tā′rē-ŭm). Place for keeping and breeding insects for scientific purposes. [L.]

in·sec·ti·cide (in-sek′ti-sīd). An agent that kills insects. [insect + L. *caedō,* to kill]

in·sec·ti·fuge (in-sek′ti-fūj). A substance that drives off insects. [insect + L. *fugo,* to put to flight]

In·sec·tiv·o·ra (in-sek-tiv′ō-ră). An order of small, plantigrade, placental mammals that are extremely active and often highly predaceous; they feed mostly on insects and small rodents, although the jes or potomogale of Africa feeds on fish. Eight living families include the solenodons of Cuba and Haiti, tenrecs of Madagascar, hedgehog of Europe and Asia, and shrews and moles of the U.S., Africa, and Asia. [insect + L. *voro,* to devour]

in·sec·tiv·o·rous (in-sek-tiv′ŏ-rŭs). Insect-eating. [insect + L. *voro,* to devour]

in·se·cu·ri·ty (in-sē-kyūr′i-tē). A feeling of unprotectedness and helplessness.

in·sem·i·na·tion (in-sem-i-nā′shŭn). Deposit of seminal fluid within the vagina, normally during coitus. SYN semination. [L. *in-semino,* pp. *-atus,* to sow or plant in, fr. *semen,* seed]

artificial i., the introduction of semen into the vagina other than by coitus.

donor i., SYN heterologous i.

heterologous i., artificial i. with semen from a donor who is not the woman's husband. SYN donor i.

homologous i., artificial i. with the husband's semen.

in·se·nes·cence (in-sē-nes′ens). The process of growing old. [L. *insenesco,* to begin to grow old]

in·sen·si·ble (in-sen′si-bl). 1. SYN unconscious. 2. Not appreciable by the senses. [L. *in-sensibilis,* fr. *in,* neg. + *sentio,* pp. *sensus,* to feel]

in·sert (in′sert). 1. An additional length of base pairs in DNA that has been introduced into that DNA. 2. An additional length of bases that has been introduced into RNA. 3. An additional length of amino acids that has been introduced into a protein.

in·ser·tion (in-ser′shŭn). 1. A putting in. 2. The attachment of a muscle to the more movable part of the skeleton, as distinguished from origin. 3. In dentistry, the intraoral placing of a dental prosthesis. 4. Intrusion of fragments of any size from molecular to cytogenetic into the normal genome. [L. *insertio,* a planting in, fr. *inserto, -sertus,* to plant in]

parasol i., SYN velamentous i.

velamentous i., a form of i. of the fetal blood vessels into the placenta, in which the vessels separate before reaching the placenta and develop toward it in a fold of amnion, somewhat like the ribs of an open parasol. SYN parasol i.

in·sheathed (in-shēthd′). Enclosed in a sheath or capsule.

in·sid·i·ous (in-sid′ē-ŭs). Treacherous; stealthy; denoting a disease that progresses gradually with inapparent symptoms. [L. *insidiosus,* cunning, fr. *insidiae* (pl.), an ambush]

in·sight (in′sīt). Self-understanding as to the motives and reasons behind one's own actions or those of another's.

in si·tu (in sī′tū). In position, not extending beyond the focus or level of origin. [L. *in,* in, + *situs,* site]

in·so·la·tion (in-sō-lā′shŭn). **1.** Exposure to the sun's rays. **2.** SYN sunstroke. [L. *insolare,* to place in the sun]

in·sol·u·ble (in-sol′yū-bl). Not soluble.

in·som·nia (in-som′nē-ă). Inability to sleep, in the absence of external impediments, such as noise, a bright light, etc., during the period when sleep should normally occur; may vary in degree from restlessness or disturbed slumber to a curtailment of the normal length of sleep or to absolute wakefulness. SYN sleeplessness. [L. fr. *in-* priv. + *somnus,* sleep]

conditioned i., a form of insomnia resulting from conditioned behaviors that are incompatible with sleep, *e.g.,* each time a person walks into his bedroom, his first thought is that he is not going to be able to sleep.

subjective i., a condition characterized by the subjective experience of greatly reduced sleep, in the context of relatively normal physiologic measures of sleep.

in·som·ni·ac (in-som′nē-ak). **1.** A sufferer from insomnia. **2.** Exhibiting, tending toward, or producing insomnia.

in·sorp·tion (in-sōrp′shŭn). Movement of substances from the lumen of the gut into the blood. [L. *in,* in, + *sorbēre,* to suck]

in·spec·tion·ism (in-spek′shŭn-izm). Sexual pleasure from looking at genitals.

in·sper·sion (in-sper′shŭn, -zhŭn). Sprinkling with a fluid or a powder. [L. *inspersio,* fr. *in-spergo,* pp. *-spersus,* to scatter upon, fr. *spargo,* to scatter]

in·spi·ra·tion (in-spi-rā′shŭn). SYN inhalation (1). [L. *inspiratio,* fr. *in-spiro,* pp. *-atus,* to breathe in]

crowing i., noisy breathing associated with respiratory obstruction, usually at the larynx.

in·spi·ra·to·ry (in-spī′ră-tō-rē). Relating to or timed during inhalation.

in·spire (in-spīr′). SYN inhale.

in·spi·rom·e·ter (in-spī-rom′ĕ-ter). An instrument for measuring the force, frequency, or volume of inspirations. [L. *in-spiro,* to breathe in, + G. *metron,* measure]

in·spis·sate (in-spis′āt). To perform or undergo inspissation.

in·spis·sa·tion (in-spi-sā′shŭn). **1.** The act of thickening or condensing, as by evaporation or absorption of fluid. **2.** An increased thickening or diminished fluidity. [L. *in,* intensive, + *spisso,* pp. *-atus,* to thicken]

in·spis·sa·tor (in-spis′ă-tŏr). An apparatus for evaporating fluids.

in·sta·bil·i·ty (in-stă-bil′i-tē). The state of being unstable, or lacking stability.

detrusor i., a bladder that has detrusor contractions that occur inappropriately, either at inappropriately low volumes or involuntarily. SYN detrusor hyperreflexia.

spinal i., the inability of the spinal column, under physiologic loads, to maintain its normal configuration; may result in damage to the spinal cord or nerve roots or lead to the development of a painful spinal deformity.

in·star (in′stahr). Any of the successive nymphal stages in the metamorphosis of hemimetabolous insects (simple or incomplete metamorphosis), or the stages of larval change by successive molts that characterize the holometabolous insects (complex or complete metamorphosis). [L. *form*]

in·step. The arch, or highest part of the dorsum of the foot. SEE ALSO tarsus.

in·stil·la·tion (in-sti-lā′shŭn). Dropping of a liquid on or into a part. [L. *instillatio,* fr. *in-stillo,* pp. *-atus,* to pour in by drops, fr. *stilla,* a drop]

in·stil·la·tor (in′sti-lā-ter). A device for performing instillation. SYN dropper.

in·stinct (in′stinkt). **1.** An enduring disposition or tendency of an organism to act in an organized and biologically adaptive manner characteristic of its species. **2.** The unreasoning impulse to perform some purposive action without an immediate consciousness of the end to which that action may lead. **3.** In psychoanalytic theory, the forces assumed to exist behind the tension caused by the needs of the id. [L. *instinctus,* impulse]

aggressive i., SYN death i.

death i., the i. of all living creatures toward self-destruction, death, or a return to the inorganic lifelessness from which they arose. SYN aggressive i.

ego i.'s, self-preservative needs and self-love, as opposed to object love; drives that are primarily erotic.

herd i., tendency or inclination to band together with and share the customs of others of a group, and to conform to the opinions and adopt the views of the group. SYN social i.

life i., the i. of self-preservation and sexual procreation; the basic urge toward preservation of the species. SYN sexual i.

sexual i., SYN life i.

social i., SYN herd i.

in·stinc·tive, in·stinc·tu·al (in-stink′tiv, -stink′chū-ăl). Relating to instinct.

in·stru·ment (in′strū-ment). A tool or implement. [L. *instrumentum*]

diamond cutting i.'s, in dentistry, cylinders, disks, and other cutting i.'s to which numerous small diamond pyramids have been attached by a plating of metal.

Krueger i. stop, a mechanical device limiting the insertion of a root canal i. into a canal.

plugging i., SYN plugger.

purse-string i., an intestinal clamp with jaws at an angle to the handle; when closed across the bowel, large grooved interdigitating serrations allow passage of a straight needle and suture through each side to form a purse-string suture, after which the clamp is removed.

Sabouraud-Noiré i., an obsolete device for measuring the quantity of x-rays by means of the change in color of a disk of barium platinocyanide which exposure to them produces; the unit used in this method is called tint B = erythema dose.

stereotactic i., stereotaxic i., an apparatus attached to the head, used to localize precisely an area in the brain by means of coordinates related to intracerebral structures.

test handle i., a root canal i. the handle of which is similar to a collet chuck and which can be secured in position on the root canal i. to adjust its effective length.

in·stru·men·tar·i·um (in′strū-men-tār′ē-ŭm). A collection of instruments and other equipment for an operation or for a medical procedure.

in·stru·men·ta·tion (in′strū-men-tā′shŭn). **1.** The use of instruments. **2.** In dentistry, the application of armamentarium in a restorative procedure.

in·suc·ca·tion (in′sŭ-kā′shŭn). Maceration or soaking, especially of a crude drug to prepare it for further pharmaceutical operation. [L. *insuco,* pp. *-atus,* to soak in, fr. *in,* in, + *sucus,* juice, sap (improp. *succ-*)]

in·su·date (in′sū-dāt). Fluid swelling within an arterial wall (ordinarily serous), differing from an exudate in that it does not come to lie extramurally. [L. *in,* in, + *sudo,* pp. *-atus,* to sweat]

in·suf·fi·cien·cy (in-sŭ-fish′en-sē). **1.** Lack of completeness of function or power. **2.** SYN incompetence (1). [L. *in-,* neg. + *sufficientia,* fr. *sufficio* to suffice]

acute adrenocortical i., severe adrenocortical i. when an intercurrent illness or trauma causes an increased demand for adrenocortical hormones in a patient with adrenal insufficiency due to disease or use of relatively large amounts of similar hormones as therapy; characterized by nausea, vomiting, hypotension, and frequently hyperthemia, hyponatremia, hyperkalemia, and hypoglycemia; can be fatal if untreated. SYN addisonian crisis, adrenal crisis, Bernard-Sergent syndrome.

adrenocortical i., loss, to varying degrees, of adrenocortical function. SYN hypocorticoidism.

aortic i., SEE valvular i.

in

cardiac i., SYN heart *failure* (1).

chronic adrenocortical i., adrenocortical i. usually as the result of idiopathic atrophy or destruction of both adrenal glands by tuberculosis, an autoimmune process, or other diseases; characterized by fatigue, decreased blood pressure, weight loss, increased melanin pigmentation of the skin and mucous membranes, anorexia, and nausea or vomiting; without appropriate replacement therapy, it can progress to acute adrenocortical i. SYN Addison's disease, addisonian syndrome, hyposupradrenalism, morbus Addisonii.

convergence i., that condition in which an esophoria or esotropia is more marked for far vision than for near vision.

coronary i., inadequate coronary circulation leading to anginal pain. SYN coronarism (1).

divergence i., that condition in which an exophoria or exotropia is more marked for near vision than for far vision.

exocrine pancreatic i., lack of exocrine secretions of pancreas, due to destruction of acini, usually by chronic pancreatitis; lack of digestive enzymes from pancreas results in diarrhea, usually fatty (steatorrhea) because of lack of pancreatic enzymes.

hepatic i., defective functional activity of the liver cells.

latent adrenocortical i., adrenocortical i. not clinically evident but which can become severe if a sudden stress, such as an intercurrent acute illness, develops.

mitral i., SEE valvular i.

muscular i., failure of any muscle to contract with its normal force, especially such failure of any of the eye muscles.

myocardial i., SYN heart *failure* (1).

parathyroid i., SYN hypoparathyroidism.

partial adrenocortical i., normal basal adrenocortical function with failure of adrenocortical reserve to respond to ACTH stimulation.

primary adrenocortical i., adrenocortical i. caused by disease, destruction, or surgical removal of the adrenal cortices.

pulmonary i., SEE valvular i.

pyloric i., patulousness of the pyloric outlet of the stomach, allowing regurgitation of duodenal contents into the stomach.

renal i., defective function of the kidneys, with accumulation of waste products (particularly nitrogenous) in the blood.

respiratory i., failure to adequately provide oxygen to the cells of the body and to remove excess carbon dioxide from them.

secondary adrenocortical i., adrenocortical i. caused by failure of ACTH secretion resulting from anterior pituitary disease or inhibition of ACTH production resulting from exogenous steroid therapy.

thyroid i., subnormal secretion of hormones by the thyroid gland. SEE ALSO hypothyroidism.

tricuspid i., SEE valvular i.

uterine i., atony of the uterine musculature.

valvular i., SYN valvular *regurgitation.*

velopharyngeal i., anatomical or functional deficiency in the soft palate or superior constrictor muscle, resulting in the inability to achieve velopharyngeal closure.

venous i., inadequate drainage of venous blood from a part, resulting in edema or dermatosis.

in·suf·flate (in-sŭf'lāt). May involve injection of carbon dioxide into the peritoneum to achieve pneumoperitoneum during laparoscopy and laparoscopic surgery. [L. *in-sufflo,* to blow on or into]

in·suf·fla·tion (in-sŭf-lā'shŭn). 1. The act or process of insufflating. 2. SYN inhalant (3).

perirenal i., an obsolete technique involving injection of air or carbon dioxide about the kidneys for radiography of the adrenal glands.

in·suf·fla·tor (in'sŭf-lā-ter). An instrument used in insufflation.

in·su·la, gen. and pl. **in·su·lae** (in'sū-lă, -lē). 1 [NA]. An oval region of the cerebral cortex overlying the extreme capsule, lateral to the lenticular nucleus, buried in the depth of the fissura lateralis cerebri (sylvian fissure). SYN insular area, insular cortex, island of Reil. 2. SYN island. 3. Any circumscribed body or patch on the skin. [L. island]

Haller's i., a doubling of the thoracic duct for part of its course through the thorax. SYN Haller's annulus.

in·su·lar (in'sū-lăr). Relating to any insula, especially the island of Reil.

in·su·late (in'sŭ-lāt). To prevent the passage of electric or radiant energy by the interposition of a nonconducting substance. [L. *insulatus,* made like an island]

in·su·la·tion (in-sŭ-lā'shŭn). 1. The act of insulating. 2. The nonconducting substance so used. 3. The state of being insulated.

in·su·la·tor (in'sŭ-lā-ter). A nonconducting substance used as insulation.

in·su·lin (in'sŭ-lin). A polypeptide hormone, secreted by beta cells in the islets of Langerhans, that promotes glucose utilization, protein synthesis, and the formation and storage of neutral lipids; obtained from various animals and available in a variety of preparations, i. is used parenterally in the treatment of diabetes mellitus. [L. *insula,* island, + -in]

biphasic i., the specific antidiabetic principle of the pancreas of the ox in a solution of that from the pancreas of the pig.

globin i., SYN regular i.

globin zinc i., a sterile solution of i. modified by the addition of zinc chloride and globin; it contains 40 or 80 units per ml; duration of action is about 18 hours.

human i., a protein that has the normal structure of i. produced by the human pancreas, prepared by recombinant DNA techniques or by semisynthetic processes.

immunoreactive i. (IRI), that portion of i. in blood measured by immunochemical methods for the hormone; presumed to represent the free (unbound) and biologically active fraction of total blood i.

isophane i., a modified form of i. composed of i., protamine, and zinc; an intermediately acting preparation used for the treatment of diabetes mellitus. SYN NPH i.

lente i., SYN insulin zinc *suspension.*

NPH i., SYN isophane i. [*N*eutral *P*rotamine *H*agedorn]

protamine zinc i., i. modified by the addition of protamine and zinc chloride; it contains 40 or 80 units per ml.

regular i., a rapidly acting form of i. which is a clear solution and may be administered intravenously as well as subcutaneously; may be mixed with longer acting forms of i. to extend the duration of effect. Onset of effect occurs in ½ to 1 hour, peak effects are observed in 2 to 3 hours, and the duration of effect is about 5 to 7 hours. SYN globin i.

semilente i., SYN prompt insulin zinc *suspension.*

ultralente i., a form of zinc precipitated i. in suspension in which the particle size is large, and thus release into the bloodstream after subcutaneous injection is slow; it can be mixed with other i.'s having different particle sizes to achieve different durations of activity. Can be derived from porcine, bovine, or genetically engineered human type.

in·su·li·ne·mia (in'sŭ-li-nē'mē-ă). Literally, insulin in the circulating blood; usually connotes abnormally large concentrations of insulin in the circulating blood. [insulin + G. *haima,* blood]

in·su·lin·o·gen·e·sis (in'sŭ-lin-ō-jen'ĕ-sis). Production of insulin. [insulin + G. *genesis,* production]

in·su·lin·o·gen·ic, in·su·lo·gen·ic (in'sŭ-lin-ō-jen'ik, in'sŭ-lō-jen'ik). Relating to insulinogenesis.

in·su·li·no·ma (in'sŭ-li-nō'mă). An islet cell adenoma that secretes insulin. SYN insuloma.

in·su·li·tis (in'sŭ-lī'tis). Inflammation of the islands of Langerhans, with lymphocytic infiltration which may result from viral infection and be the initial lesion of insulin-dependent diabetes mellitus. [L. *insula,* island, + *-itis,* inflammation]

in·su·lo·ma (in-sŭ-lō'mă). SYN insulinoma. [L. *insula,* island, + *-oma,* tumor]

in·sult (in'sŭlt). An injury, attack, or trauma. [LL. *insultus,* fr L. *insulto,* to spring upon]

in·sus·cep·ti·bil·i·ty (in'sŭ-sep'ti-bil'i-tē). SYN immunity. [L. *suscipio,* pp. *-ceptus,* to take upon one, fr. *sub,* under, + *capio,* to take]

int. cib. Abbreviation for L. *inter cibos,* between meals.

in·te·gral (int′ē-gral). **1.** Constituent. **2.** Integrated. **3.** SEE integration (3).

in·te·gra·tion (in-tĕ-grā′shŭn). **1.** The state of being combined, or the process of combining, into a complete and harmonious whole. **2.** In physiology, the process of building up, as by accretion, anabolism, etc. **3.** In mathematics, the process of ascertaining a function from its differential. **4.** In molecular biology, a recombination event in which a genetic element is inserted. [L. *integro*, pp. *-atus*, to make whole, fr. *integer*, whole]

personality i., the effective organization of old and new experience, data, and emotional capacities into the personality; the harmonious organization of the personality.

in·te·grins (in-te′grinz). A class of proteins that link the outside of cells with their interior, thus integrating response, *e.g.*, the mediation of adhesion of neutrophils to endothelial cells. [L. *integer*, whole, intact, fr. *in-* + *tango*, to touch + *-in*]

in·teg·ri·ty (in-teg′ri-tē). Soundness or completeness of structure; a sound or unimpaired condition.

marginal i. of amalgam, the ability of a dental amalgam restoration to maintain its original marginal form at the cavosurface margins.

in·teg·u·ment (in-teg′yū-ment). **1.** The enveloping membrane of the body; includes, in addition to the epidermis and dermis, all of the derivatives of the epidermis, *e.g.*, hairs, nails, sudoriferous and sebaceous glands, and mammary glands. **2.** The rind, capsule, or covering of any body or part. SYN tegument (2). SYN integumentum commune [NA], tegument (1). [L. *integumentum*, a covering, fr. *in-tego*, to cover]

in·teg·u·men·ta·ry (in-teg-yū-men′tă-rē). Relating to the integument. SEE ALSO cutaneous, dermal.

in·teg·u·men·tum com·mune (in-teg-yū-men′tŭm ko-myūn′) [NA]. SYN integument.

in·tel·lec·tu·al·i·za·tion (in-te-lek′chū-ăl-i-zā′shŭn). An unconscious defense mechanism in which reasoning, logic, or focusing on and verbalizing intellectual minutiae is used in an attempt to avoid confrontation with an objectionable impulse, affect, or interpersonal situation. [L. *intellectus*, perception, discernment]

in·tel·li·gence (in-tel′i-jens). **1.** An individual's aggregate capacity to act purposefully, think rationally, and deal effectively with the environment, especially in relation to the extent of one's perceived effectiveness in meeting challenges. **2.** In psychology, an individual's relative standing on two quantitative indices, measured i. and effectiveness of adaptive behavior; a quantitative score or similar index on both indices constitutes the operational definition of i. [L. *intelligentia*]

abstract i., the capacity to understand and manage abstract ideas and symbols.

artificial i., (1) a branch of computer science in which attempts are made to replicate human intellectual functions. One application is the development of computer programs for diagnosis. Such programs are often based on epidemiologic analysis of data in large numbers of medical records; **(2)** a machine that replicates human intellectual functions, although no machine (*i.e.,* computer) can do this yet.

measured i., that i. which can be ranked relative to an age or peer group quantitative index by use of scores on i. tests.

mechanical i., the capacity to understand and manage technical mechanisms.

social i., the capacity to understand and manage one's human relations and social affairs.

in·tem·per·ance (in-tem′per-ăns). Lack of proper self-control, usually in reference to the use of alcoholic beverages. Cf. incontinence (2). [L. *intemperantia*, fr. *in-*, neg. + *temperantia*, moderation]

in·ten·si·ty (in-ten′si-tē). Marked tension; great activity; often used simply to denote a measure of the degree or amount of some quality. [L. *in- tendo*, pp. *-tensus*, to stretch out]

luminous i. (I), the luminous flux per unit solid angle in a given direction. SYN candle-power, radiant i.

radiant i. (I), SYN luminous i.

i. of sound, the objective measurement of the amplitude of vibration of a sound wave.

insulin (metabolic effects)			
metabolic change	effect	mechanism	main organ
1. glucose transport	+	unknown	muscles, fatty tissue
2. amino acid transport	+	unknown	muscles, fatty tissue
3. potassium transport	+	unknown; sometimes in connection with glucose transport	liver muscles
4. glucose oxidation	+	increased glucose production in the cell	muscles, fatty tissue
5. glycogen synthesis	+	increased glucose production in the cell; activation of glycogensynthetase through dephosphorylation of the enzyme	muscles, liver
6. fatty acid synthesis	+	as in 4; plus reduction of acyl-CoA, increased acetyl-CoA from glucose resulting from activation of pyruvate dehydrogenase; release of acetyl-CoA-carboxylase	fatty tissue, liver
7. lipid synthesis	+	as in 4; plus production of α–glycerophosphate from glucose	fatty tissue, liver, muscles
8. protein synthesis	+	activation of ribosomes (translation of messenger RNA)	muscles, fibro-blasts
9. lipolysis	−	antagonistic to lypolytic hormones; inhibition of adenylatcyclase	fatty tissue, liver
10. keto-genesis	−	inhibition of fatty acid production through antilipolysis (see 9)	liver
11. gluco-neogene-sis and glyco-genolysis	−	inhibition of glucagon-stimulated glucose release; inhibition of adenylatcyclase	liver
12. proteo-lysis	−	unknown; inhibition of urea production in the liver, through reduced production of amino acids	liver, muscle

in·ten·sive (in-ten′siv). Relating to or marked by intensity; denoting a form of treatment by means of very large doses or of substances possessing great strength or activity.

in·ten·tion (in-ten′shŭn). **1.** An objective. **2.** In surgery, a process or operation. [L. *intentio*, a stretching out; intention]

△**inter-.** Among, between. [L. *inter*, between]

in

in·ter·ac·i·nar (in-ter-as′i-nar). SYN interacinous.

in·ter·ac·i·nous (in-ter-as′i-nŭs). Between the acini of a gland. SYN interacinar.

in·ter·ac·tion (int′er-ak′shŭn). **1.** The reciprocal action between two entities in a common environment as in chemical i., ecological i., social i., etc. **2.** The effects when two entities concur that would not be observed with either in isolation. **3.** In statistics, pharmacology, and quantitative genetics, the phenomenon that the combined effects of two causes differ from the sum of the effects separately (as in synergism and antagonism). **4.** Independent operation of two or more causes to produce or prevent an effect. **5.** In statistics, the necessity for a product term in a linear model.

apolar i., SYN hydrophobic i.

hydrophobic i., i. between uncharged substituents on different molecules without a sharing of electrons or protons; entropy-driven i. SYN apolar i.

in·ter·al·ve·o·lar (in′ter-al-vē′ō-lăr). Between any alveoli, especially the alveoli of the lungs.

in·ter·an·nu·lar (in-ter-an′yū-lăr). Between any two ringlike structures or constrictions. [inter- + L. *anulus,* ring]

in·ter·arch (in′ter-arch). SEE interarch *distance.*

in·ter·ar·tic·u·lar (in-ter-ar-tik′yū-lăr). **1.** Between two joints. **2.** Between two joint surfaces. [inter- + L. *articulus,* joint]

in·ter·ar·y·te·noid (in′ter-ăr′i-tē′noyd). Between the arytenoid cartilages.

in·ter·as·ter·ic (in-ter-ă-stē′rik). Between the two asteria. SEE asterion.

in·ter·a·tri·al (in-ter-ā′trē-ăl). Between the atria of the heart. SYN interauricular (1).

in·ter·au·ric·u·lar (in′ter-aw-rik′yū-lăr). **1.** SYN interatrial. **2.** Between the auricles or pinnae.

in·ter·body (in′ter-bod′ē). Between the bodies of two adjacent vertebrae.

in·ter·ca·dence (in-ter-kā′dens). The occurrence of an extra beat between the two regular pulse beats. [inter- + L. *cado,* pr. p. *cadens* (-*ent*-), to fall]

in·ter·ca·dent (in-ter-kā′dent). Irregular in rhythm; characterized by intercadence.

in·ter·ca·lary (in-ter′kă-ler-ē, in-ter-kal′er-ē). **1.** Occurring between two others; as in a pulse tracing, an upstroke interposed between two normal pulse beats. **2.** In fungi, located in a hypha or between hyphal segments, not at a hyphal terminus. [L. *intercalarius,* concerning an insertion]

in·ter·ca·lat·ed (in-ter′kă-lā-ted). Interposed; inserted between two others. [L. *intercalatus*]

in·ter·ca·la·tion (in′ter-kă′lā-shun). The process of insertion between two other entities; *e.g.,* insertion of a dye or drug between stacked bases in DNA.

in·ter·can·a·lic·u·lar (in-ter-kan-ă-lik′yū-lăr). Between canaliculi.

in·ter·cap·il·lary (in-ter-kap′i-lā-rē). Between or among capillary vessels.

in·ter·ca·rot·ic, in·ter·ca·rot·id (in-ter-ka-rot′ik, -id). Between the internal and external carotid arteries.

in·ter·car·pal (in-ter-kar′păl). Between the carpal bones.

in·ter·car·ti·lag·i·nous (in′ter-kar-ti-laj′i-nŭs). Between or connecting cartilages. SYN interchondral.

in·ter·cav·ern·ous (in′ter-kav′er-nŭs). Between two cavities.

in·ter·cel·lu·lar (in-ter-sel′yū-lăr). Between or among cells.

in·ter·cen·tral (in-ter-sen′trăl). Connecting or lying between two or more centers.

in·ter·cen·trum, pl. **in·ter·cen·tra** (in-ter-sen′trŭm, -tră). In veterinary anatomy, an intervertebral disc between vertebrae, and the hemal arch beneath vertebrae of some reptiles, birds, and mammals. SEE ALSO hemal *arches,* under *arch.*

in·ter·ce·re·bral (in′ter-ser′ē-brăl). Between the cerebral hemispheres.

in·ter·chon·dral (in-ter-kon′drăl). SYN intercartilaginous. [inter- + L. *chondros,* cartilage]

in·ter·cil·i·um (in-ter-sil′ē-ŭm). SYN glabella. [inter- + L. *cilium,* eyelid]

in·ter·cla·vic·u·lar (in-ter-kla-vik′yū-lăr). Between or connecting the clavicles.

in·ter·coc·cyg·e·al (in′ter-kok-sij′ē-ăl). Situated between unfused segments of the coccyx.

in·ter·co·lum·nar (in-ter-kŏ-lŭm′nar). Between any two columns, as the columns or crura of the superficial inguinal ring.

in·ter·con·dy·lar, in·ter·con·dyl·ic, in·ter·con·dy·loid (in-ter-kon′di-lăr, -kon-dil′ik, -kon′di-loyd). Between two condyles.

in·ter·con·ver·sion (in-ter-kon-ver′shun). A mutual alteration of the physical or chemical nature of a substance or entity; *e.g.,* i. of chemical compounds or of foodstuffs.

enzyme i., the reversible transformation of one enzyme form into another, typically with an alteration in the enzyme activity or regulation, *e.g.,* phosphorylation of a glycogen phosphorylase.

in·ter·cos·tal (in-ter-kos′tăl). Between the ribs. [inter- + L. *costa,* rib]

in·ter·cos·to·hu·mer·al (in′ter-kos′tō-hyū′mer-ăl). Relating to an intercostal space and the arm. SEE intercostobrachial *nerves,* under *nerve.*

in·ter·cos·to·hu·me·ra·lis (in-ter-kos′tō-hyū-mer-ā′lis). SEE intercostobrachial *nerves,* under *nerve.*

in·ter·course (in′ter-kōrs). Communication or dealings between or among people. [L. *intercursus,* a running between]

sexual i., SYN coitus.

in·ter·cri·co·thy·rot·o·my (in-ter-krī′kō-thī-rot′ō-mē). SYN cricothyrotomy.

in·ter·cris·tal (in-ter-kris′tăl). Between two crests, as between the crests of the ilia, applied to one of the pelvic measurements.

in·ter·cross (in′ter-kros). A mating between two individuals both heterozygous at a specified locus or loci.

in·ter·cru·ral (in-ter-krū′răl). Between two crura; *e.g.,* the cerebral peduncles of the brain, etc .

in·ter·cur·rent (in-ter-ker′ent). Intervening; said of a disease attacking a person already ill of another malady. [inter- + L. *curro,* pr. p. *currens* (-*ent*-), to run]

in·ter·cus·pa·tion (in′ter-kŭs-pā′shun). **1.** The cusp-to-fossa relation of the maxillary and mandibular posterior teeth to each other. **2.** The interlocking or fitting together of the cusps of opposing teeth. SYN interdigitation (4). SYN intercusping.

in·ter·cusp·ing (in-ter-kŭs′ping). SYN intercuspation. [L. *inter,* among, mutually, + cusp]

in·ter·cu·ta·ne·o·mu·cous (in′ter-kyū-tā′nē-ō-mŭ′kŭs). Between skin and mucous membrane, as in the cheek or lip or at the mucocutaneous border of the lips or anus.

in·ter·de·fer·en·tial (in-ter-def-er-en′shăl). Between the deferent ducts.

in·ter·den·tal (in-ter-den′tăl). **1.** Between the teeth. **2.** Denoting the relationship between the proximal surfaces of the teeth of the same arch. [inter- + L. *dens,* tooth]

in·ter·den·ti·um (in-ter-den′shē-ŭm). The interval between any two contiguous teeth.

in·ter·dig·it (in-ter-dij′it). That part of the hand or foot lying between any two adjacent fingers or toes.

in·ter·dig·i·tal (in-ter-dij′i-tăl). Between the fingers or toes.

in·ter·dig·i·ta·tion (in′ter-dij-i-tā′shŭn). **1.** The mutual interlocking of toothed or tonguelike processes. **2.** The processes thus interlocked. **3.** Infoldings or plicae of adjacent cell or plasma membranes. **4.** SYN intercuspation (2). [inter- + L. *digitus,* finger]

in·ter·dis·ci·pli·nary (in-ter-dis′i-pli-nār-ē). Denoting the overlapping interests of different fields of medicine and science. [inter- + L. *disciplina,* knowledge]

in·ter·face (in′ter-fās). **1.** A surface that forms a common boundary of two bodies. **2.** The boundary between regions of different radiopacity, acoustic, or magnetic resonance properties; the projection of the i. between tissues of different such properties on an image.

crystalline i., in dentistry, a boundary between adjacent crystals.

dermoepidermal i., the line of meeting of the dermis and epidermis.

metal i., in dentistry, a boundary between metal and nonsolvent solder, or between metal and surface oxide.

structural i., in dentistry, a boundary between tooth and restorative material.

in·ter·fa·cial (in-ter-fā′shăl). Relating to an interface.

in·ter·fas·cic·u·lar (in′ter-fă-sik′yū-lăr). Between fasciculi.

in·ter·fem·o·ral (in-ter-fem′ŏ-răl). Between the thighs.

in·ter·fer·ence (in-ter-fēr′ens). **1.** The coming together of waves in various media in such a way that the crests of one series correspond to the hollows of the other, the two thus neutralizing each other; or so that the crests of the two series correspond, thus increasing the excursions of the waves. **2.** Collision within the myocardium of two waves of excitation at the junction of territories controlled by each, as is seen in A-V dissociation. **3.** Also, in A-V dissociation, the disturbance of the regular rhythm of the ventricles by a conducted impulse from the atria, *e.g.,* by a ventricular capture (interference beat). **4.** The condition in which infection of a cell by one virus prevents superinfection by another virus, or in which superinfection prevents effects which would result from infection by either virus alone, even though both viruses persist. [inter- + L. *ferio,* to strike]

bacterial i., the condition in which colonization by one bacterial strain prevents colonization by another strain.

cuspal i., SYN deflective occlusal *contact.*

in·ter·fer·om·e·ter (in′ter-fe-rom′ĕ-ter). An instrument for measuring minute distances or movements through the interference of light waves thereby produced. [interfere + G. *metron,* measure]

electron i., an i. that employs an electron beam in place of a light beam.

in·ter·fer·o·me·try (in′ter-fe-rom′ĕ-trē). Measurement of minute distances or movements by interaction of waves of electromagnetic energy.

electron i., i. in which a beam of electrons is used instead of a beam of light.

in·ter·fer·on (IFN) (in-ter-fēr′on). A class of small (MW 26,000–38,000) glycoproteins that exert antiviral activity at least in homologous cells through cellular metabolic processes involving synthesis of double-stranded RNA, which is an intermediate in replication of RNA viruses. Antiviral mechanisms include the effect on viral translation. These substances also have numerous non-antiviral actions, and can regulate many cell properties and functions. IFN's are classified into three major groups, alpha, beta, and gamma, based on their reactivities with antibodies as well as their physico-chemical properties and their cells of origin and method of induction; Arabic numerals and letters are appended to the Greek letter to delineate subcategories. [interfere + -on]

i. alpha (IFN-α), a number of different subtypes exist that are elaborated by leukocytes in response to viral infection and stimulation with double-stranded RNA; IFN-α-2A and -2B are protein products made by recombinant DNA techniques and are used as antineoplastic agents. SYN leukocyte i.

antigen i., SYN i. gamma.

i. beta (IFN-β), i. elaborated by fibroblasts in response to the same stimuli as i. alpha. SYN fibroblast i.

fibroblast i., SYN i. beta.

i. gamma (IFN-γ), i. elaborated by T lymphocytes in response to either specific antigen or mitogenic stimulation. SYN antigen i., immune i.

immune i., SYN i. gamma.

leukocyte i., SYN i. alpha.

in·ter·fer·on-β2. SYN interleukin-6.

in·ter·fi·bril·lar, in·ter·fi·bril·lary (in′ter-fī′bri-lăr, -fī′bri-lār-ē; -fī-bril′ăr). Between fibrils.

in·ter·fi·brous (in-ter-fī′brŭs). Between fibers.

in·ter·fil·a·men·tous (in′ter-fil-ă-men′tŭs). Between filaments.

in·ter·fron·tal (in-ter-fron′tăl). Between the unfused halves of the frontal bone; denoting a persistent suture there present. (anomalous)

interferons (clinical experience)	
herpes keratitis (HSV 1)	successful treatment (since 1978)
herpes zoster (VZV)	reduction, side effects
herpes simplex infections	not yet determined
condyloma (condyloma acuminatum)	good clinical effect
cytomegalovirus (CMV) (chronic active infection)	meager improvement side effects
hepatitis-B virus (chronic active infection)	permanent reduction and disappearance of Dane particles, etc.
viral infection of the respiratory tract (influenza, rhinovirus)	no convincing effect
other viral illnesses	varying
metastatizing illnesses osteosarcoma	apparent success, in combination with chemotherapy
chronic myeloic leukemia and hairy cell leukemia	proven therapeutic activity
multiple myeloma	very good reaction
breast cancer	not complete; improvement
Hodgkin's disease	variable remission
melanoma	disappearance of tumor

in·ter·gan·gli·on·ic (in′ter-gang′lē-on′ik). Between or among or connecting ganglia.

in·ter·gem·mal (in′ter-jem′ăl). Between any two or more bud-like or bulblike bodies such as the taste buds; denoting especially a nerve termination between two end bulbs. [inter- + L. *gemma,* bud]

in·ter·ge·nal (in-ter-jēn′al). Between different genes.

in·ter·glob·u·lar (in-ter-glob′yū-lăr). Between globules.

in·ter·glu·te·al (in-ter-glū′tē-ăl). Between the buttocks. [inter- + G. *gloutos,* buttock]

in·ter·go·ni·al (in-ter-gō′nē-ăl). Between the two gonia. SEE gonion. [inter- + G. *gōnia,* angle]

in·ter·gy·ral (in-ter-jī′răl). Between the gyri or convolutions of the brain.

in·ter·hem·i·ce·re·bral (in′ter-hem′ē-ser′ē-brăl). Between the cerebral hemispheres.

in·ter·ic·tal (in-ter-ik′tăl). The period between convulsions. [inter- + L. *ictus,* stroke]

in·te·ri·or (in-tēr′ē-ōr). Relating to the inside; situated within.

in·ter·is·chi·ad·ic (in-ter-is-kē-ad′ik). Between the two ischia;

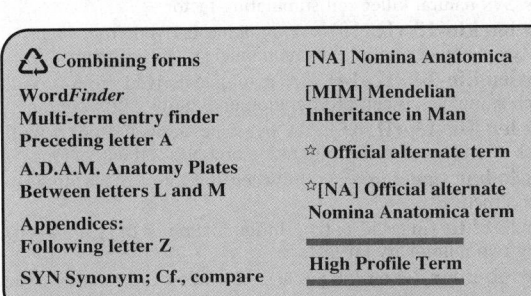

♻ **Combining forms**	**[NA] Nomina Anatomica**
WordFinder Multi-term entry finder Preceding letter A	**[MIM] Mendelian Inheritance in Man**
A.D.A.M. Anatomy Plates Between letters L and M	☆ **Official alternate term**
Appendices: Following letter Z	☆**[NA] Official alternate Nomina Anatomica term**
SYN Synonym; Cf., compare	**High Profile Term**

in

especially, between the two tuberosities of the ischia. SYN intersciatic.

in·ter·ki·ne·sis (in′ter-ki-nē′sis). Period between the first and second divisions of meiosis; comparable to interphase of mitosis. [inter- + G. *kinēsis,* movement]

in·ter·la·mel·lar (in′ter-lă-mel′ăr, -lam′ĕ- lăr). Between lamellae.

in·ter·leukin. The name given to cytokines once their amino acid structure is known. SEE lymphokines, cytokine. [inter- + *leuk*ocyte + -in]

in·ter·leu·kin-1 (IL-1) (in-ter-lū′kin). A cytokine, derived primarily from mononuclear phagocytes, which enhances the proliferation of T helper cells and growth and differentiation of B cells. When secreted in larger quantities, IL-1 enters the bloodstream and can cause fever, induce synthesis of acute phase proteins, and initiate metabolic wasting. There are two distinct forms of IL-1: alpha and beta, both of which perform the same functions, but represent different proteins.

in·ter·leu·kin-2 (IL-2). A cytokine derived from T helper lymphocytes that causes proliferation of T lymphocytes and activated B lymphocytes. SYN T-cell growth factor-1, T-cell growth factor.

in·ter·leu·kin-3 (IL-3). A cytokine derived from monocytes, fibroblasts, and endothelial cells that increases production of monocytes. SYN multi-colony-stimulating factor.

in·ter·leu·kin-4 (IL-4). A cytokine derived from T4 lymphocytes that causes differentiation of B lymphocytes. SYN B-cell differentiating factor, T-cell growth factor-2.

in·ter·leu·kin-5 (IL-5). A cytokine derived from T lymphocytes that causes activation of B lymphocytes and differentiation of eosinophils.

in·ter·leu·kin-6 (IL-6). A cytokine derived from fibroblasts, macrophages, and tumor cells that increases synthesis and secretion of immunoglobulins by B lymphocytes. SYN B-cell stimulatory factor 2, interferon-β2.

in·ter·leu·kin-7 (IL-7). A cytokine derived from bone marrow cells that causes proliferation of B and T lymphocytes.

in·ter·leu·kin-8 (IL-8). A cytokine derived from endothelial cells, fibroblasts, keratinocytes, macrophages, and monocytes which causes chemotaxis of neutrophils and T cell lymphocytes. SYN anionic neutrophil activating peptide, monocyte derived neutrophil chemotactic factor, neutrophil activating factor, neutrophil activating protein, neutrophil chemotactant factor.

in·ter·leu·kin-9 (IL-9). A cytokine derived from T cells which causes growth and proliferation of T cells.

in·ter·leu·kin-10 (IL-10). A cytokine derived from helper T cell lymphocytes, B cell lymphocytes, and monocytes that inhibits gamma-interferon (IFNγ) secretion by T cell lymphocytes and it inhibits mononuclear cell inflammation.

in·ter·leu·kin-11 (IL-11). A cytokine derived from bone marrow stromal cells (endothelial cells, macrophages, and preadipocytes) which stimulates increased plasma concentrations of acute phase proteins (C-reactive protein (CRP), mannose-binding protein, serum amyloid P component, α_1-antitrypsin, fibrinogen, ceruloplasmin, and complement components C9 and factor B).

in·ter·leu·kin-12 (IL-12). A cytokine derived from B lymphocytes, T lymphocytes, and macrophages that induces gamma-interferon (IFNγ) gene expression in T lymphocytes and NK cells. SYN natural killer cell stimulating factor.

in·ter·leu·kin-13 (IL-13). A cytokine derived from helper T cell lymphocytes that inhibits mononuclear cell inflammation.

in·ter·leu·kin-14 (IL-14). A cytokine derived from T cells which stimulates B cell proliferation and inhibits Ig secretion.

in·ter·leu·kin-15 (IL-15). A cytokine derived from T cells which stimulates T cell proliferation and NK cell activation.

in·ter·lo·bar (in-ter-lō′bar). Between the lobes of an organ or other structure.

in·ter·lo·bi·tis (in′ter-lō-bī′tis). Inflammation of the pleura separating two pulmonary lobes.

in·ter·lob·u·lar (in-ter-lob′yū-lăr). Between the lobules of an organ.

in·ter·mal·le·o·lar (in-ter-mal-ē′ō-lăr). Between the malleoli.

in·ter·mam·ma·ry (in-ter-mam′ă-rē). Between the breasts. [inter- + L. *mamma,* breast]

in·ter·mam·mil·lary (in-ter-mam′i-lā-rē). Between the breasts; between the nipples; denoting a line drawn between the two nipples. [inter- + L. *mammilla,* breast, nipple]

in·ter·mar·riage (in-ter-mar′ij). **1.** Marriage of relatives. **2.** Marriage of persons of different races or cultures.

in·ter·max·il·la (in-ter-maks-il′ă). SYN os incisivum.

in·ter·max·il·lary (in-ter-mak′si-lā-rē). Between the maxillae, or upper jaw bones.

in·ter·me·di·ary (in′ter-mē′dē-ār-ē). Occurring between. [L. *intermedius,* lying between, fr. *medius,* middle]

in·ter·me·di·ate (in′ter-mē′dē-it). **1.** Between two extremes; interposed; intervening. **2.** A substance formed in the course of chemical reactions that then proceeds to participate rapidly in further reactions, so that at any given moment it is present in minute concentrations only; such substances, when appearing in the course of the reactions involved in metabolism, are metabolic i.'s. **3.** In dentistry, a cement base. **4.** An element or organ between right and left (or lateral and medial) structures. SYN intermedius [NA].

replicative i., during the copying of the viral RNA of an RNA virus, the opposite sense strand that serves as a template for positive strand production.

in·ter·me·din (in-ter-mē′din). SYN melanotropin.

in·ter·me·di·o·lat·er·al (in-ter-mē′dē-ō-lat′er-ăl). Intermediate, and to one side, not central. Used especially to denote the intermediolateral cell column of spinal cord gray mattter, abbreviated IML, the location of all presynaptic sympathetic nerve cell bodies.

in·ter·me·di·us (in-ter-mē′dē-ŭs) [NA]. SYN intermediate. [L.]

in·ter·mem·bra·nous (in-ter-mem′bră-nŭs). Between membranes.

in·ter·me·nin·ge·al (in′ter-me-nin′jē-ăl). Between the meninges.

in·ter·men·stru·al (in-ter-men′strū-ăl). Between two consecutive menstrual periods.

in·ter·met·a·car·pal (in-ter-met′ă-kar′păl). Between the metacarpal bones.

in·ter·met·a·mer·ic (in′ter-met′ă-mer′ik). Between two metameres; denoting especially the intervertebral disks.

in·ter·met·a·tar·sal (in-ter-met′ă-tar′săl). Between the metatarsal bones.

in·ter·met·a·tar·se·um (in-ter-met′ă-tar′sē-ŭm). SYN os intermetatarseum.

in·ter·mis·sion (in-ter-mish′ŭn). **1.** A temporary cessation of symptoms or of any action. **2.** An interval between two paroxysms of a disease, such as malaria. [L. *intermissio,* fr. *intermitto,* to leave off, intermit, fr. *mitto,* to send]

in·ter·mit. To cease for a time.

in·ter·mit·tence, in·ter·mit·ten·cy (in-ter-mit′ens, -en-sē). **1.** A condition marked by intermissions or interruptions in the course of a disease or other process or state or in any continued action; denoting especially a loss of one or more pulse beats. **2.** Complete cessation of symptoms between two periods of activity of a disease.

in·ter·mit·tent (in-ter-mit′ent). Marked by intervals of complete quietude between two periods of activity.

in·ter·mus·cu·lar (in-ter-mŭs′kyū-lăr). Between the muscles.

in·tern. An advanced student or recent graduate undertaking further education by assisting in the medical or surgical care of hospital patients, with supervision and instruction; formerly, one who resided within the institution. [F. *interne,* inside]

in·ter·nal (in-ter′năl). Away from the surface; often incorrectly used to mean medial. SYN internus [NA]. [L. *internus*]

in·ter·nal·i·za·tion (in-ter′năl-i-zā′shŭn). Adopting as one's own the standards and values of another person or society.

in·ter·na·ri·al (in-ter-nā′rē-ăl). Between the nares or nostrils. SYN internasal.

in·ter·na·sal (in-ter-nā′săl). SYN internarial.

In·ter·na·tion·al Clas·si·fi·ca·tion of Dis·ease (ICD). The classification of specific conditions and groups of conditions determined by an internationally representative expert committee that advises the World Health Organization, which publishes the complete list in a periodically revised book, the *Manual of the International Statistical Classification of Diseases, Injuries and Causes of Death.* The Tenth Revision (ICD) came into use in 1992; it has 20 chapters, each with a hierarchical arrangement of subdivisions (rubrics); some chapters are etiological, more relate to body systems, some to classes of conditions, some to procedures.

In·ter·na·tion·al Clas·si·fi·ca·tion of Health Prob·lems in Pri·ma·ry Care. A classification of diseases, conditions and problems arranged for use in primary care where diagnostic precision is seldom possible.

In·ter·na·tion·al Clas·si·fi·ca·tion of Im·pair·ments, Dis·a·bil·i·ties and Hand·i·caps. A WHO-sponsored numerical taxonomy of the impairments, disabilities and handicaps consequent upon injury and disease.

In·ter·na·tion·al Com·mit·tee of the Red Cross. A neutral Swiss organization serving as an intermediary between contending forces in armed conflict, in civil war, or internal strife, to help victims receive protection and other humanitarian assistance under the Geneva Conventions in accordance with the fundamental principles of the Red Cross.

In·ter·na·tion·al Sys·tem of Units (SI). A system of measurements, based on the metric system, adopted at the 11th General Conference on Weights and Measures of the International Organization for Standardization (1960) to cover both the coherent units (basic, supplementary, and derived units) and the decimal multiples and submultiples of these units formed by use of prefixes proposed for general international scientific and technological use. SI proposes seven basic units: meter (m), kilogram (kg), second (s), ampere (A), Kelvin (K), candela (cd), and mole (mol) for the basic quantities of length, mass, time, electric current, temperature, luminous intensity, and amount of substance; supplementary units proposed include the radian (rad) for plane angle and steradian (sr) for solid angle; derived units (*e.g.,* force, power, frequency) are stated in terms of the basic units (*e.g.,* velocity is in meters per second, m/s^{-1}). Multiples (prefixes) in descending order are: exa- (E, 10^{18}), peta- (P, 10^{15}), tera- (T, 10^{12}), giga- (G, 10^9), mega- (M, 10^6), kilo- (k, 10^3), hecto- (h, 10^2), deca- (da, 10^1), deci- (d, 10^{-1}), centi- (c, 10^{-2}), milli- (m, 10^{-3}), micro- (μ, 10^{-6}), nano- (n, 10^{-9}), pico- (p, 10^{-12}), femto- (f, 10^{-15}), atto- (a, 10^{-18}). The prefix zepto (z) has been proposed for 10^{-21}. Those involving a multiple of 10^3 are recommended; compounds of these are not recommended (*e.g.,* mμ for n). [Fr. *Système International d'Unités*]

in·terne. Intern.

in·ter·neu·ro·mer·ic (in'ter-nūr-ō-mer'ik). Between the neuromeres.

in·ter·neu·rons (in'ter-nū'ronz). Combinations or groups of neurons between sensory and motor neurons that govern coordinated activity.

in·tern·ist (in-ter'nist, in'ter-nist). A physician trained in internal medicine.

in·ter·nod·al (in-ter-nō'dăl). Between two nodes; relating to an internode.

in·ter·node (in'ter-nōd). SYN internodal *segment.*

in·ter·nu·cle·ar (in-ter-nū'klē-ăr). Between nerve cell groups in the brain or retina.

in·ter·nun·ci·al (in-ter-nun'sē-ăl). **1.** Indicating a neuron functionally interposed between two or more other neurons. **2.** Acting as a medium of communication between two organs. [L. *internuntius* (or *-nuncius*), a messenger between two parties, fr. *inter,* between, + *nuncius,* a messenger]

in·ter·nus (in-ter'nŭs) [NA]. SYN internal. [L.]

in·ter·oc·clu·sal (in'ter-ŏ-klū'săl). Between the occlusal surfaces of opposing teeth.

in·ter·o·cep·tive (in'ter-ō-sep'tiv). Relating to the sensory nerve cells innervating the viscera (thoracic, abdominal and pelvic organs, and the cardiovascular system), their sensory end organs, or the information they convey to the spinal cord and the brain. [inter- + L. *capio,* to take]

in·ter·o·cep·tor (in'ter-ō-sep'ter). One of the various forms of small sensory end organs (receptors) situated within the walls of the respiratory and gastrointestinal tracts or in other viscera. [inter- + L. *capio,* to take]

in·ter·ol·i·vary (in-ter-ol'i-vār-ē). Between the left and right inferior olive of the medulla oblongata.

in·ter·or·bit·al (in-ter-ōr'bi-tăl). Between the orbits.

in·ter·os·se·al (in-ter-os'ē-ăl). SYN interosseous.

in·ter·os·sei (in-ter-os'ē-ī). Plural of interosseus.

in·ter·os·se·ous (in'ter-os'ē-ŭs). Lying between or connecting bones; denoting certain muscles and ligaments. SYN interosseal. [inter- + L. *os,* bone]

in·ter·os·se·us, pl. **in·ter·os·sei** (in'ter-os'ē-ŭs, -os'e-ī). SEE muscle.

in·ter·pal·pe·bral (in-ter-pal'pe-brăl). Between the eyelids.

in·ter·pa·ri·e·tal (in'ter-pă-rī'ĕ-tăl). Between the walls of a part, or between the parietal bones. [inter- + L. *paries,* wall]

in·ter·par·ox·ys·mal (in-ter-par-ok-siz'măl). Occurring between successive paroxysms of a disease.

in·ter·pe·dic·u·late (in-ter-pe-dik'yū-lāt). Between vertebral pedicles.

in·ter·pe·dun·cu·lar (in-ter-pe-dŭnk'yū-lăr). Between any two peduncles.

in·ter·per·son·al (in-ter-per'sŏn-ăl). Pertaining to relations and social exchanges between persons.

in·ter·pha·lan·ge·al (in'ter-fă-lan'jē-ăl). Between two phalanges; denoting the finger or toe joints.

in·ter·phase (in'ter-fāz). The stage between two successive divisions of a cell nucleus in which the biochemical and physiologic functions of the cell are performed and replication of chromatin occurs. SYN karyostasis.

in·ter·phy·let·ic (in'ter-fī-let'ik). Denoting the transitional forms between two kinds of cells during the course of metaplasia. [inter- + G. *phylē,* tribe]

in·ter·plant. The material transferred from donor to host in interplanting.

in·ter·plant·ing. In experimental embryology, the transferring of a primordial cell mass from one embryo to an indifferent environment in another embryo, as in chorioallantoic grafts or intraocular transplants.

in·ter·pre·ta·tion (in-ter-pre-tā'shŭn). **1.** In psychoanalysis, the characteristic therapeutic intervention of the analyst. **2.** In clinical psychology, drawing inferences and formulating the meaning in terms of the psychological dynamics inherent in an individual's responses to psychological tests or during psychotherapy.

in·ter·prox·i·mal (in-ter-prok'si-măl). Between adjoining surfaces.

in·ter·pu·bic (in-ter-pyū'bik). Between the two pubic bones.

in·ter·pu·pil·lary (in-ter-pyū'pi-lār-ē). Between the pupils.

in·ter·ra·di·al (in-ter-rā'dē-ăl). Situated between radii or rays.

in·ter·re·nal (in-ter-rē'năl). Between the two kidneys.

in·ter·scap·u·lar (in-ter-skap'yū-lăr). Between the scapulae.

in·ter·scap·u·lum (in-ter-skap'yū-lŭm). The part of the back between the shoulders, or that between the scapulae.

in·ter·sci·at·ic (in-ter-sī-at'ik). SYN interischiadic.

in·ter·sec·tio, pl. **in·ter·sec·ti·o·nes** (in'ter-sek'shē-ō, -sek-shē-ō'nēz) [NA]. SYN intersection. [L.]

   i. tendin'ea [NA], SYN tendinous *intersection.*

in·ter·sec·tion (in'ter-sek-shŭn). The site of crossing of two structures. SYN intersectio [NA].

   tendinous i., a tendinous band or partition running across a muscle. SYN intersectio tendinea [NA], inscriptio tendinea, tendinous inscription.

in·ter·sec·ti·o·nes (in-ter-sek-shē-ō'nēz). Plural of intersectio.

in·ter·seg·men·tal (in-ter-seg-men'tăl). Between two segments, such as metameres or myotomes.

in·ter·sep·tal (in-ter-sep'tăl). Lying between two septa.

in

in·ter·sep·to·val·vu·lar (in'ter-sep-tō-val'vyū-lăr). Between the embryonic septum primum and septum spurium.

in·ter·sep·tum (in-ter-sep'tŭm). SYN diaphragm (1). [L]

in·ter·sex·u·al (in-ter-seks'yū-ăl). Relating to or characterized by intersexuality.

in·ter·sex·u·al·i·ty (in'ter-seks-yū-al'i-tē). The condition of having both male and female characteristics; being intermediate between the sexes.

in·ter·space (in'ter-spās). Any space between two similar objects, such as a costal i. or interval between two ribs.

in·ter·spi·nal (in-ter-spī'năl). Between two spines, such as the spinous processes of the vertebrae. SYN interspinous.

in·ter·spi·na·lis (in-ter-spī-nā'lis). SEE interspinales *muscles*, under *muscle*.

in·ter·spi·nous (in-ter-spī'nŭs). SYN interspinal.

in·ter·stice, pl. **in·ter·stic·es** (in-ter'stis, -sti-sēz). SYN interstitium. [L. *interstitium*, fr. *sisto*, to stand]

in·ter·sti·tial (in-ter-stish'ăl). **1.** Relating to spaces or interstices in any structure. **2.** Relating to spaces within a tissue or organ, but excluding such spaces as body cavities or potential space. Cf. intracavitary.

in·ter·stit·i·um (in-ter-stish'ē-ŭm). A small area, space, or gap in the substance of an organ or tissue. SEE ALSO connective *tissue*. SYN interstice. [L.]

in·ter·sys·to·le (in'ter-sis'tō-lē). The period intervening between the systole of the atrium and that of the ventricle of the heart.

in·ter·tar·sal (in-ter-tar'săl). Denoting the articulations of the tarsal bones with each other. SYN tarsotarsal.

in·ter·tha·lam·ic (in-ter-thal'ă-mik). Between the thalami.

in·ter·trans·ver·sa·lis (in-ter-trans-ver-sā'lis). Intertransversarius. SEE muscle.

in·ter·trans·verse (in'ter-trans'vers). Between the transverse processes of the vertebrae.

in·ter·trig·i·nous (in-ter-trij'i-nŭs). Characterized by or related to intertrigo.

in·ter·tri·go (in-ter-trī'gō). Irritant dermatitis occurring between folds or juxtaposed surfaces of the skin, as between the buttocks, between the scrotum and the thigh, beneath pendulous breasts, etc.; caused by friction, sweat retention, moisture, warmth, and concomitant overgrowth of resident microorganisms; occurring in young children and obese adults. [L. a galling of the skin, fr. *inter*, between, + *tero*, to rub]

in·ter·tro·chan·ter·ic (in'ter-trō-kan-tăr'ik). Between the two trochanters of the femur.

in·ter·tu·bu·lar (in-ter-tū'byū-lăr). Between or among tubules.

in·ter·u·re·ter·al (in'ter-yū-rē'ter-ăl). Between the two ureters. SYN interureteric.

in·ter·u·re·ter·ic (in-ter-yū-rē-tăr'ik). SYN interureteral.

in·ter·val (in'ter-văl). A time or space between two periods or objects; a break in continuity. [L. *inter-vallum*, space between breastworks in a camp, an interval, fr. *vallum*, a rampart, wall]

A-H i., the time from the initial rapid deflection of the atrial wave to the initial rapid deflection of the His bundle (H) potential; it approximates the conduction time through the A-V node (normally 50-120 msec).

A-N i., the time between onset of the atrial deflection and the nodal potential (normally 40-100 msec).

atriocarotid i., a-c i., obsolete term for the time between the beginning of the atrial and that of the carotid waves in a tracing of the jugular pulse.

atrioventricular i., SYN auriculoventricular i.

auriculoventricular i., the time between depolarization of the atria and of the ventricle. SYN atrioventricular i.

A-V i., the time from the beginning of atrial systole to the beginning of ventricular systole as measured from pressure pulses or cardiac volume curves in animals, or from the electrocardiogram in humans.

BH i., the duration of the His bundle deflections (normally 15-20 msec).

cardioarterial i., c-a i., the time between the apex beat of the heart and the radial pulse beat.

confidence i., a range of values for a variable of interest, constructed so that this range has a specified probability of including the true value of the variable.

coupling i., the i., usually expressed in hundredths of a second, between a normal sinus beat and the ensuing premature beat.

escape i., the time between the last beat of the patient's basic rhythm (ectopic or sinus beat) and a beat from a spontaneous escape focus or the initial electronic pacemaker impulse (a preset i. in the circuitry); it may be either a shorter or a longer time period than the pulse i.

focal i., the distance between the anterior and posterior focal points of the eye.

H-V i., the time from the initial deflection of the His bundle (H) potential and the onset of ventricular activity (normally 35-45 msec).

interectopic i., the distance between consecutive ectopic complexes in the electrocardiogram.

isovolumic i., time during which both an A-V and a semilunar valve are closed.

lucid i., in psychoses or delirium, a rational period appearing in the course of the mental disorder.

P-A i., the time from onset of the P wave to the initial rapid deflection of the A wave in the His bundle electrogram (normally 25-45 msec); it represents the intra-atrial conduction time.

P-J i., the time elapsing from the beginning of the P wave to the end of the QRS complex (J for junction between QRS and S-T segment) in the electrocardiogram.

P-P i., the distance between consecutive P waves in the electrocardiogram.

P-Q i., SYN P-R i.

P-R i., in the electrocardiogram, the time elapsing between the beginning of the P wave and the beginning of the next QRS complex; it corresponds to the a-c i. of the venous pulse and is normally 0.12-0.20 sec. SYN P-Q i.

Q-R i., the time elapsing from the onset of the QRS complex to the peak of the R wave; measures the time of onset of the intrinsicoid deflection if determined in an appropriate unipolar lead tracing.

Q-RB i., the time between the onset of the Q wave of the QRS complex and the right bundle-branch potential (normally 15-20 msec).

QRS i., the duration of the QRS complex in the electrocardiogram.

Q-S$_2$ i., SYN electromechanical *systole*.

Q-T i., time from electrocardiogram Q wave to the end of the T wave corresponding to electrical systole.

R-R i., the time elapsing between two consecutive R waves in the electrocardiogram.

sphygmic i., the period in the cardiac cycle when the semilunar valves are open and blood is being ejected from the ventricles into the arterial system. SYN ejection period.

Sturm's i., the distance between the anterior and posterior focal lines in a spherocylindrical lens combination.

systolic time i.'s, SEE electromechanical *systole*, left ventricular ejection *time*, preejection *period*.

in·ter·vas·cu·lar (in-ter-vas'kyū-lăr). Between blood or lymph vessels.

in·ter·ven·tion (in-ter-ven'shŭn). An action or ministration that produces an effect or that is intended to alter the course of a pathologic process. [L. *inter-ventio*, a coming between, fr *intervenio*, to come between]

crisis i., a psychotherapeutic technique directed at counseling at the time of an acute life crisis and limited in aim to helping resolve the crisis.

in·ter·ven·tric·u·lar (in-ter-ven-trik'yū-lăr). Between the ventricles.

in·ter·ver·te·bral (in-ter-ver'te-brăl). Between two vertebrae.

in·ter·vil·lous (in-ter-vil'ŭs). Between or among villi.

in·tes·ti·nal (in-tes'ti-năl). Relating to the intestine.

i. pseudo-obstruction, clinical manifestations falsely suggesting obstruction of the small intestine, usually occurring in patients with multiple jejunal diverticula.

in·tes·tine (in-tes′tin). SYN intestinum (1). [L. *intestinum*]

large i., the portion of the digestive tube extending from the ileocecal valve to the anus; it comprises the cecum, colon, rectum, and anal canal. SYN intestinum crassum [NA].

small i., the portion of the digestive tube between the stomach and the cecum or beginning of the large intestine; it consists of three portions: duodenum, jejunum, and ileum. SYN intestinum tenue [NA].

in·tes·ti·no·tox·in (in-tes′ti-nō-tok′sin). SYN enterotoxin.

in·tes·ti·num, pl. **in·tes·ti·na** (in-tes-tī′nŭm, -nă). **1** [NA]. The digestive tube passing from the stomach to the anus. It is divided primarily into the i. tenue (small intestine) and the i. crassum (large intestine). SYN bowel, intestine. **2.** Inward; inner. [neuter of *intestinus*] SYN gut (1). [L. *intestinus*, internal, ntr. as noun, the entrails, fr. *intus*, within]

i. ce′cum, SYN cecum (1).

i. cras′sum [NA], SYN large *intestine*.

i. il′eum, twisted intestine. SEE ileum.

i. jeju′num, empty intestine. SEE jejunum.

i. rec′tum, straight intestine. SEE rectum.

i. ten′ue [NA], SYN small *intestine*.

i. ten′ue mesenteria′le, the freely movable portion of the small intestine supplied with a mesentery, comprising the jejunum and ileum. SYN mesenteric portion of small intestine.

in·ti·ma (in′ti-mă). Innermost. SEE *tunica* intima. [L. fem. of *intimus*, inmost]

in·ti·mal (in′ti-măl). Relating to the intima or inner coat of a vessel.

in·ti·mi·tis (in-ti-mī′tis). Inflammation of an intima, as in endangiitis. [intima + G. *-itis*, inflammation]

proliferative i., eruption characterized by dusky erythema and small ulcers due to proliferative changes in capillary bed.

in·toe (in′tō). Medial deviation of the axis of the foot. SYN *metatarsus* varus.

in·tol·er·ance (in-tol′er-ăns). Abnormal metabolism, excretion, or other disposition of a given substance; term often used to indicate impaired utilization or disposal of dietary constituents.

hereditary fructose i. [MIM*229600], a metabolic error due to deficiency of hepatic fructose 1,6-bisphosphate aldolase B (which also acts on fructose 1-phosphate); the second enzyme in the specific fructose pathway; vomiting and hypoglycemia follow ingestion of fructose; prolonged fructose ingestion in young children results in failure to thrive and in jaundice, hepatomegaly, albuminuria, aminoaciduria, and sometimes cachexia and death; autosomal recessive inheritance in most families.

lactose i., a disorder characterized by abdominal cramps and diarrhea after consumption of food containing lactose (*e.g.,* milk, ice cream); believed to reflect a deficiency of intestinal lactase and may appear first in young adults who had tolerated milk well as infants.

lysinuric protein i., an autosomal recessive disorder characterized by elevated levels of dibasic amino acids (*e.g.,* L-lysine, L-arginine, and L-ornithine) in the urine; apparently due to a defect in dibasic amino acid transport.

in·tor·sion (in-tōr′shŭn). Conjugate rotation of the upper poles of each cornea inward. [L. *in-torqueo,* pp. *tortus,* to twist]

in·tor·tor (in-tōr′tōr). A muscle that turns a part medialward. SEE ALSO invertor. SYN medial rotator.

in·tox·a·tion (in-tok-sā′shŭn). Poisoning, especially by the toxic products of bacteria or poisonous animals, other than alcohol. [see intoxication]

in·tox·i·cant (in-tok′si-kant). **1.** Having the power to intoxicate. **2.** An intoxicating agent, such as alcohol.

in·tox·i·ca·tion (in-tok-si-kā′shŭn). **1.** SYN poisoning. **2.** SYN acute *alcoholism*. [L. *in,* in, + G. *toxikon,* poison]

acid i., poisoning by acid products (β-oxybutyric acid, diacetic acid, or acetone) formed as a result of faulty metabolism (*e.g.,* uncontrolled diabetes mellitus) or by acids introduced from with-

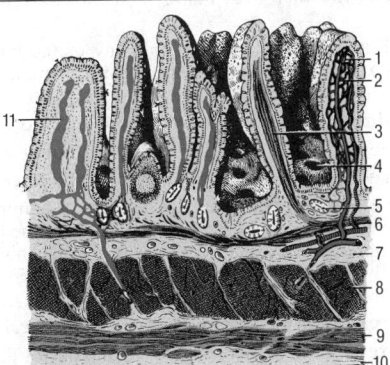

small intestine wall structure
1) arteriole; 2) capillary network to the villi; 3) smooth muscle cells; 4) entrance to crypt; 5) Lieberkühn's crypt; 6) muscular mucosa; 7) tunica submucosa; 8) ring muscle; 9) longitudinal muscle; 10) serosa; 11) central chyle vessel

out; marked by epigastric pain, headache, loss of appetite, constipation, restlessness, and an odor of acetone in the breath, followed by air hunger, coma, and collapse.

anaphylactic i., i. following an anaphylactic reaction.

citrate i., a toxic condition that may develop during massive replacement therapy with transfused blood that contains citrate as an anticoagulant; the citrate combines with calcium ions and may result in tetany.

intestinal i., SYN autointoxication.

septic i., SYN septicemia.

water i., a metabolic encephalopathy resulting from severe overhydration.

intra-. Inside, within; opposite of extra-. SEE ALSO endo-, ento-. [L. within]

in·tra·ab·dom·i·nal (in′tră-ab-dom′i-năl). Within the abdomen.

in·tra·ac·i·nous (in-tră-as′i-nŭs). Within an acinus.

in·tra·ad·e·noi·dal (in′tră-ad-ĕ-noy′dăl). Within the adenoids.

in·tra·ar·te·ri·al (in′tră-ar-tēr′ē-ăl). Within an artery or the arteries.

in·tra·ar·tic·u·lar (in′tră-ar-tik′yūlăr). Within the cavity of a joint. [intra- + L. *articulus,* joint]

in·tra·a·tri·al (in′tră-ā-trē-ăl). Within one or both of the atria of the heart.

in·tra·au·ral (in′tră-aw′răl). Within the ear. [intra- + L. *auris,* ear]

in·tra·au·ric·u·lar (in′tră-aw-rik′yū-lăr). **1.** Within an auricle (*e.g.,* of the ear). **2.** Obsolete term for intra-atrial.

in·tra·bron·chi·al (in-tră-brong′kē-ăl). Within the bronchi or bronchial tubes. SYN endobronchial.

in·tra·buc·cal (in′tră-bŭk′ăl). **1.** Within the mouth. **2.** Within the substance of the cheek. [intra- + L. *bucca,* cheek]

in·tra·can·a·lic·u·lar (in′tră-kan-ă-lik′yū-lăr). Within a canaliculus or canaliculi.

in·tra·cap·su·lar (in′tră-kap′sū-lăr). Within a capsule, especially the capsule of a joint.

in·tra·car·di·ac (in′tră-kar′dē-ak). Within one of the chambers of the heart. SYN endocardiac (1), endocardial, intracordal. [intra- + G. *kardia,* heart]

in·tra·car·pal (in-tră-kar′păl). Within the carpus; among the carpal bones.

in·tra·car·ti·lag·i·nous (in′tră-kar-ti-laj′i-nŭs). Within a cartilage or cartilaginous tissue. SYN enchondral, endochondral.

in·tra·cath·e·ter (in′tră-kath′e-ter). A plastic tube, usually attached to the puncturing needle, inserted into a blood vessel for infusion, injection, or pressure monitoring.

in

in·tra·cav·i·tary (in′tră-cav′i-tār-ē). Within an organ or body cavity.

in·tra·ce·li·al (in′tră-sē′lē-ăl). Within any of the body cavities, especially within one of the ventricles of the brain. [intra- + G. *koilia*, cavity]

in·tra·cel·lu·lar (in-tră-sel′yū-lăr). Within a cell or cells.

in·tra·cer·e·bel·lar (in′tră-ser-ĕ-bel′ăr). Within the cerebellum.

in·tra·ce·re·bral (in′tră-ser′ē-brăl). Within the cerebrum.

in·tra·cer·e·bro·ven·tric·u·lar. The locus of administration of drugs or chemicals into the ventricular system of the brain. Often used in animal studies and occasionally for the introduction of anti-infectives that do not penetrate the blood-brain barrier into the brain in humans.

in·tra·cer·vi·cal (in′tră-ser′vi-kăl). SYN endocervical (1).

in·tra·cis·ter·nal (in′tră-sis-ter′năl). Within one of the subarachnoid cisternae; usually refers to the introduction of a cannula into the cerebellomedullary cistern for aspiration of cerebrospinal fluid or the injection of air into the ventricles of the brain.

in·tra·co·lic (in′tră-kol′ik). Within the colon.

in·tra·cor·dal (in′tră-kōr′dăl). SYN intracardiac. [intra- + L. *cor*, heart]

in·tra·cor·o·nal (in′tră-kōr′ŏ-năl). Within the crown portion of a tooth.

in·tra·cor·po·re·al (in′tră-kōr-po′rē-ăl). 1. Within the body. 2. Within any structure anatomically styled a corpus. [intra- + L. *corpus*, body]

in·tra·cor·pus·cu·lar (in′tră-kōr-pŭs′kyū-lăr). Within a corpuscle, especially a red blood corpuscle. SYN intraglobular (2).

in·tra·cos·tal (in′tră-kos′tăl). On the inner surface of the ribs.

in·tra·cra·ni·al (in′tră-krā′nē-ăl). Within the skull.

in·trac·ta·ble (in′trak′tă-bl). 1. SYN refractory (1). 2. SYN obstinate (1). [L. *in-tractabilis*, fr. *in-* neg. + *tracto*, to draw, haul]

in·tra·cu·ta·ne·ous (in′tră-kū-tā′nē-ŭs). Within the substance of the skin, particularly the dermis. SYN intradermal, intradermic. [intra- + L. *cutis*, skin]

in·tra·cys·tic (in′tră-sis′tik). Within a cyst or the urinary bladder.

in·trad. Toward the inner part.

in·tra·der·mal, in·tra·der·mic (in′tră-der′măl, -der′mik). SYN intracutaneous. [intra- + G. *derma*, skin]

in·tra·duct (in′tră-dŭkt). Within the duct or ducts of a gland.

in·tra·du·ral (in′tră-dū′răl). Within or enclosed by the dura mater.

in·tra·em·bry·on·ic (in′tră-em-brē-on′ik). Within the embryonic body, *e.g.*, the portion of the umbilical vein within the embryo (in contrast to the portion in the umbilical cord which is discarded at birth). Cf. extraembryonic.

in·tra·ep·i·der·mal (in′tră-ep-i-der′măl). Within the epidermis.

in·tra·ep·i·phys·i·al (in′tră-ep-i-fiz′ē-ăl). Within the epiphysis of a long bone.

in·tra·ep·i·the·li·al (in′tră-ep-i-thē′lē-ăl). Within or among the epithelial cells.

in·tra·far·a·di·za·tion (in′tră-fa-ră-di-zā′shŭn). Application of a faradic cauterizing current to the inner surface of a cavity or hollow organ.

in·tra·fas·cic·u·lar (in′tră-fă-sik′yū-lăr). Within the fasciculi of a tissue or structure (*e.g.*, fasciculus intrafasciculus).

in·tra·fe·brile (in′tră-fē′bril, -feb′ril). Occurring during the febrile stage of a disease. SYN intrapyretic.

in·tra·fi·lar (in′tră-fī′lăr). Lying within the meshes of a network. [intra- + L. *filum*, thread]

in·tra·fu·sal (in′tră-fyū′săl). Applied to structures within the muscle spindle.

in·tra·gal·va·ni·za·tion (in′tră-gal-van-i-zā′shŭn). Application of a galvanic cauterizing current to the interior of a cavity or hollow organ.

in·tra·gas·tric (in′tră-gas′trik). Within the stomach.

in·tra·gem·mal (in′tră-jem′ăl). Within any budlike or bulblike body; denoting especially a nerve termination within an end bulb or taste bud. [intra- + L. *gemma*, bud]

in·tra·ge·nal (in′tră-jēn′al). Within a gene.

in·tra·glan·du·lar (in′tră-glan′dū-lăr). Within a gland or glandular tissue.

in·tra·glob·u·lar (in′tră-glob′yū-lăr). 1. Within a globule in any sense. 2. SYN intracorpuscular.

in·tra·gy·ral (in′tră-jī′răl). Within a gyrus or convolution of the brain.

in·tra·he·pat·ic (in′tră-he-pat′ik). Within the liver.

in·tra·hy·oid (in′tră-hī′oyd). Within the hyoid bone; denoting certain accessory thyroid glands that lie in the hollow or within the substance of the hyoid bone.

in·tra·la·ryn·ge·al (in′tră-lă-rin′je-ăl). Within the larynx.

in·tra·lig·a·men·tous (in′tră-lig-ă-men′tŭs). Within a ligament, especially the broad ligament of the uterus.

in·tra·lo·bar (in′tră-lō′bar). Within a lobe of any organ or other structure.

in·tra·lob·u·lar (in′tră-lob′yū-lăr). Within a lobule.

in·tra·loc·u·lar (in-tră-lok′yū-lăr). Within the loculi of any structure or part.

in·tra·lu·mi·nal (in-tră-lū′mi-năl). SYN intratubal.

in·tra·med·ul·lary (in′tră-med′yū-lār-ē). 1. Within the bone marrow. 2. Within the spinal cord. 3. Within the medulla oblongata.

in·tra·mem·bra·nous (in′tră-mem′brā-nŭs). 1. Within, or between the layers of, a membrane. 2. Denoting a method of bone formation directly from mesenchymal cells without an intervening cartilage stage (occurring, for example, in the calvaria), as distinguished from intracartilaginous bone formation.

in·tra·me·nin·ge·al (in′tră-mĕ-nin′jē-ăl). Within or enclosed by the meninges of the brain or spinal cord.

in·tra·mi·to·chon·dri·al (in′tră-mī-tō-kon′drē-al). Within the mitochondria.

in·tra·mo·lec·u·lar (in′tră-mŏ-lek′yū-lăr). Referring to situations and events within a molecule.

in·tra·mu·ral (in′tră-myū′răl). Within the substance of the wall of any cavity or hollow organ. SYN intraparietal (1).

in·tra·mus·cu·lar (I.M., i.m.) (in′tră-mŭs′kyū-lăr). Within the substance of a muscle.

in·tra·my·o·car·di·al (in′tră-mī′ō-kar′dē-ăl). Within the myocardium.

in·tra·my·o·me·tri·al (in′tră-mī′ō-mē′trē-ăl). Within the muscular coat of the uterus.

in·tra·na·sal (in′tră-nā′săl). Within the nasal cavity.

in·tra·na·tal (in′tră-nā′tăl). During or at the time of birth. [intra- + L. *natalis*, relating to birth]

in·tra·neu·ral (in′tră-nū′răl). Within a nerve. [intra- + G. *neuron*, nerve]

in·tra·nu·cle·ar (in′tră-nū′klē-ăr). Within the nucleus of a cell.

in·tra·oc·u·lar (in′tră-ok′yū-lăr). Within the eyeball.

in·tra·o·ral (in′tră-ō′răl). Within the mouth. [intra- + L. *os*, mouth]

in·tra·or·bit·al (in′tră-ōr′bi-tăl). Within the orbit.

in·tra·os·se·ous (in′tră-os′ē-ŭs). Within bone. SYN intraosteal. [intra- + L. *os*, bone]

in·tra·os·te·al (in′tră-os′tēăl). SYN intraosseous.

in·tra·o·var·i·an (in′tră-ō-vā′rē-an). Within the ovary.

in·tra·ov·u·lar (in′tră-ov′yū-lăr). Within the ovum.

in·tra·pa·ri·e·tal (in′tră-pă-rī′ĕ-tăl). 1. SYN intramural. 2. Denoting the intraparietal sulcus.

in·tra·par·tum (in′tră-par′tŭm). During labor and delivery or childbirth. Cf. antepartum, postpartum. [intra- + L. *partus*, childbirth]

in·tra·pel·vic (in′tră-pel′vik). Within the pelvis.

in·tra·per·i·car·di·ac, in·tra·per·i·car·di·al (in′tră-per′ē-kar′dē-ak, -kar′dē-ăl). Within the pericardial cavity. SYN endopericardiac.

in·tra·per·i·to·ne·al (I.P., i.p.) (in′tră-per′i-tō-nē′ăl). Within the peritoneal cavity.

in·tra·per·son·al (in′tră-per′sŏn-ăl). SYN intrapsychic.

in·tra·pi·al (in′tră-pī′ăl). Within the pia mater.

in·tra·pleu·ral (in′tră-plū′răl). Within the pleura or the pleural cavity.

in·tra·pon·tine (in′tră-pon′tīn). Within the pons of the brainstem.

in·tra·pros·tat·ic (in′tră-pros-tat′ik). Within the prostate gland.

in·tra·pro·to·plas·mic (in′tră-prō-tō-plas′mik). Within the protoplasm of a cell.

in·tra·psy·chic (in′tră-sī′kik). Denoting the psychological dynamics that occur inside the mind without reference to the individual's exchanges with other persons or events. SYN intrapersonal.

in·tra·pul·mo·nary (in′tră-pul′mo-nār-ē). Within the lungs.

in·tra·py·ret·ic (in′tră-pī-ret′ik). SYN intrafebrile. [intra- + L. *pyretos,* fever]

in·tra·rec·tal (in′tră-rek′tăl). Within the rectum.

in·tra·re·nal (in′tră-rē′năl). Within the kidney. [intra- + L. *ren,* kidney]

in·tra·ret·i·nal (in′tră-ret′i-năl). Within the retina.

in·trar·rha·chid·i·an, in·tra·ra·chid·i·an (in′tră-ră-kid′ē-an). SYN intraspinal. [intra- + G. *rachis,* spine]

in·tra·scro·tal (in′tră-skrō′tăl). Within the scrotum.

in·tra·spi·nal (in′tră-spī′năl). Within the vertebral canal or spinal cord. SYN intrarrhachidian, intrarachidian.

in·tra·splen·ic (in′tră-splen′ik). Within the spleen.

in·tra·stro·mal (in′tră-strō′măl). Within the stroma or foundation substance of any organ or part.

in·tra·syn·ov·i·al (in′tră-si-nō′vē-ăl). Within the synovial sac of a joint or a synovial tendon sheath.

in·tra·tar·sal (in′tră-tar′săl). Within the tarsus; among the tarsal bones.

in·tra·the·cal (in′tră-thē′kăl). **1.** Within a sheath. **2.** Within either the subarachnoid or the subdural space.

in·tra·tho·rac·ic (in′tră-thō-ras′ik). Within the cavity of the chest.

in·tra·ton·sil·lar (in′tră-ton-si-lăr). Within the substance of a tonsil.

in·tra·tub·al (in′tră-tū′băl). Within any tube. SYN intraluminal.

in·tra·tu·bu·lar (in′tră-tū′byū-lăr). Within any tubule.

in·tra·tym·pan·ic (in′tră-tim-pan′ik). Within the middle ear or tympanic cavity.

in·tra·u·ter·ine (in′tră-yū′ter-in). Within the uterus.

in·tra·vas·cu·lar (in′tră-vas′kyū-lăr). Within the blood vessels or lymphatics.

in·tra·ve·nous (I.V., i.v.) (in′tră-vē′nŭs). Within a vein or veins. SYN endovenous.

in·tra·ven·tric·u·lar (I-V) (in′tră-ven-trik′yū-lăr). Within a ventricle of the brain or heart.

in·tra·ves·i·cal (in′tră-ves′i-kăl). Within a bladder, especially the urinary bladder.

in·tra vi·tam (in′tră vī′tăm). During life. [L. *vita,* life]

in·tra·vi·tel·line (in′tră-vi-tel′in, -ēn). Within the vitellus or yolk.

in·tra·vit·re·ous (in′tră-vit′rē-ŭs). Within the vitreous body.

in·trin·sic (in-trin′sik). **1.** Belonging entirely to a part. **2.** In anatomy, denoting those muscles whose origin and insertion are both within the structure under consideration, distinguished from the extrinsic muscles which have their origin outside of the structure under consideration; applied especially to the limbs but also to the ciliary muscle as distinguished from the recti and other orbital muscles which are outside the eyeball. SYN essential (6). [L. *intrinsecus,* on the inside]

△**intro-.** Inwardly, into; opposite of extra-. Cf. intra-. [L. *intro,* into]

in·tro·duc·er (in-trō-dūs′er). An instrument, such as a catheter,

needle, or endotracheal tube, for introduction of a flexible device. SYN intubator. [L. *intro-duco,* to lead into, introduce]

in·tro·flec·tion, in·tro·flex·ion (in′trō-flek′shŭn). A bending inward. [intro- + L. *flecto,* pp. *flectus,* to bend]

in·tro·gas·tric (in-trō-gas′trik). Leading or passed into the stomach. [intro- + G. *gastēr,* belly, stomach]

in·tro·i·tus (in-trō′i-tŭs). The entrance into a canal or hollow organ, as the vagina. [L. entrance, fr. *intro-eo,* to go into]

i. cana′lis, SYN i. of facial canal.

i. of facial canal, entrance to facial canal, through which the facial nerve passes, at end of internal acoustic meatus. SYN i. canalis.

vaginal i., SYN *vestibule* of vagina.

in·tro·jec·tion (in-trō-jek′shŭn). A psychological defense mechanism involving appropriation of an external happening and its assimilation by the personality, making it a part of the self. [intro- + L. *jacto,* to throw]

in·tro·mis·sion (in-trō-mish′ŭn). The insertion or introduction of one part into another. [intro- + L. *mitto,* to send]

in·tro·mit·tent (in-trō-mit′ent). Conveying or sending into a body or cavity.

in·tron (in′tron). A portion of DNA that lies between two exons, is transcribed into RNA, but does not appear in that RNA after maturation, and so is not expressed (as protein) in protein synthesis. SYN intervening sequence. [inter- + -on]

in·tro·spec·tion (in-trō-spek′shŭn). Looking inward; self-scrutinizing; contemplating one's own mental processes. [intro- + L. *specto,* to look at, inspect]

in·tro·spec·tive (in-trō-spek′tiv). Relating to introspection.

in·tro·sus·cep·tion (in′trō-sŭs-sep′shŭn). SYN intussusception.

in·tro·ver·sion (in-trō-ver′zhŭn). **1.** The turning of a structure into itself. SEE ALSO intussusception, invagination. **2.** A trait of preoccupation with oneself, as practiced by an introvert. Cf. extraversion. [intro- + L. *verto,* pp. *versus,* to turn]

in·tro·vert. 1 (in′trō-vert). One who tends to be unusually shy, introspective, self-centered, and avoids becoming concerned with or involved in the affairs of others. Cf. extrovert. **2** (in-trō-vert′). To turn a structure into itself.

in·tu·bate (in′tū-bāt). To perform intubation.

in·tu·ba·tion (in-tū-bā′shŭn). Insertion of a tubular device into a canal, hollow organ, or cavity; specifically, passage of an oro- or nasotracheal tube for anesthesia or for control of pulmonary ventilation. [L. *in,* in, + *tuba,* tube]

altercursive i., rarely used term for diversion of secretion intermittently to the exterior from its normal destination, *e.g.,* of the bile from the intestine.

aqueductal i., insertion of a tube in the sylvian aqueduct to relieve atresia or narrowing of the aqueduct.

blind nasotracheal i., passage of a tracheal tube through the nose and into the trachea without using a laryngoscope.

endotracheal i., passage of a tube through the nose or mouth into the trachea for maintenance of the airway during anesthesia or for maintenance of an imperiled airway. SYN intratracheal i.

intratracheal i., SYN endotracheal i.

nasotracheal i., tracheal i. through the nose.

orotracheal i., tracheal i. through the mouth.

tracheal i., passage of a tube through the nose, mouth, or a tracheotomy into the trachea for maintenance of patency of the airway.

in·tu·ba·tor (in′tū-bā-tŏr). SYN introducer.

in·tu·mesce (in-tū-mes′). To swell up; to enlarge. [L. *in-tumesco,* to swell up, fr. *tumeo,* to swell]

in·tu·mes·cence (in-tū-mes′ens). **1.** SYN enlargement. **2.** The process of enlarging or swelling; used to describe the spinal enlargements.

tympanic i., SYN tympanic *enlargement.*

in·tu·mes·cent (in-tū-mes′ent). Enlarging; becoming enlarged or swollen.

in·tu·mes·cen·tia (in-tū-mes-sen′shē-ă) [NA]. SYN enlargement. [Mod. L.]

i. cervica′lis [NA], SYN cervical *enlargement.*

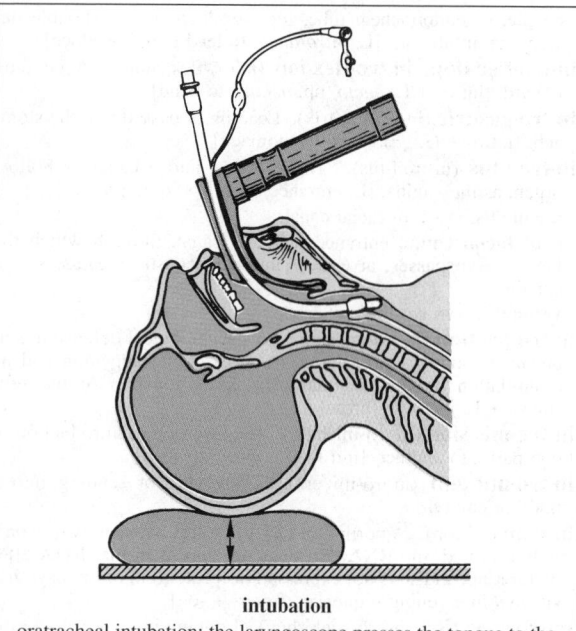

intubation

oratracheal intubation: the laryngoscope presses the tongue to the floor of the mouth

i. gangliofor′mis, SYN geniculate *ganglion.*

i. lumba′lis [NA], SYN lumbar *enlargement.*

i. tympan′ica, SYN tympanic *enlargement.*

in·tus·sus·cep·tion (in′tŭs-sŭ-sep′shŭn). **1.** The taking up or receiving of one part within another, especially the enfolding of one segment of the intestine within another. SEE ALSO introversion, invagination. **2.** Often, specifically, the process of incorporation of new material in the growth of the cell wall. SYN introsusception. [L. *intus,* within, + *sus-cipio,* to take up, fr. *sub* + *capio,* to take]

colic i., the ensheathing of one portion of the colon into another.

double i., a second i. that involves the bowel above the first; the first i. is followed by contraction of the bowel wall around it, and the solid mass so formed is enveloped by the proximal portion of the bowel and is thus the cause of the second i.

ileal i., i. in which one portion of the ileum is ensheathed in another portion of the same division of the bowel.

ileocecal i., i. in which the lower segment of the ileum passes through the valve of the colon into the cecum.

ileocolic i., i. in which the lower portion of the ileum with the valve of the cecum passes into the ascending colon.

jejunogastric i., a rare complication following gastrojejunostomy in which the afferent or the efferent loop of bowel invaginates into the stomach.

retrograde i., the invagination of a lower segment of the bowel into one just above.

in·tus·sus·cep·tive (in′tŭs-sŭ-sep′tiv). Relating to or characterized by intussusception.

in·tus·sus·cep·tum (in′tŭs-sŭ-sep′tŭm). The inner segment in an intussusception; that part of the bowel which is received within the other part.

in·tus·sus·cip·i·ens (in′tŭs-sŭ-sip′ē-enz). The portion of the bowel, in intussusception, which receives the other portion. [L. *intus,* within, + *suscipiens,* pr. p. of *suscipio,* to take up]

in·u·lase (in′yū-lās). SYN inulinase.

in·u·lin (In) (in′yū-lin). A fructose polysaccharide from the rhizome of *Inula helenium* or *elecampane* (family Compositae) and other plants; a hygroscopic powder used by intravenous injection to determine the rate of glomerular filtration. Also used in bread for diabetics. Cf. inulin *clearance.* SYN alant starch, alantin, dahlin.

in·u·lin·ase (in′yū-lin-ās). An enzyme acting upon 2,1-β-D-fructoside links in inulin, releasing D-fructose. SYN inulase.

in·u·lol (in′yū-lol). SYN alantol.

in·unc·tion (in-ŭngk′shŭn). Administration of a drug in ointment form by rubbing to cause absorption of the active ingredient. [L. *inunctio,* an anointing, fr. *inunguo,* pp. *-unctus,* to smear on]

in·vac·ci·na·tion (in-vak-si-nā′shŭn). Accidental inoculation of some disease, *e.g.,* syphilis, during vaccination.

in·vag·i·nate (in-vaj′i-nāt). To ensheathe, infold, or insert a structure within itself or another. [L. *in,* in, + *vagina,* a sheath]

in·vag·i·na·tion (in-vaj′i-nā′shŭn). **1.** The ensheathing, enfolding, or insertion of a structure within itself or another. **2.** The state of being invaginated. SEE ALSO introversion, intussusception.

basilar i., SYN platybasia.

in·vag·i·na·tor (in-vag′i-nā-ter, -tōr). An instrument for pushing inward any tissue.

in·va·lid (in′vă-lid). **1.** Weak; sick. **2.** A person partially or completely disabled. [L. *in-* neg. + *validus,* strong]

in·va·lid·ism (in′vă-lid-izm). The condition of being an invalid.

in·va·sin (in-vā′sin). SYN hyaluronidase (1).

in·va·sion (in-vā′zhŭn). **1.** The beginning or incursion of a disease. **2.** Local spread of a malignant neoplasm by infiltration or destruction of adjacent tissue; for epithelial neoplasms, i. signifies infiltration beneath the epithelial basement membrane. **3.** Entrance of foreign cells into a tissue, such as polymorphonuclear leukocytes in inflammation. [L. *invasio,* fr. *in-vado,* pp. *-vasus,* to go into, attack]

in·va·sive (in-vā′siv). **1.** Denoting or characterized by invasion. **2.** Denoting a procedure requiring insertion of an instrument or device into the body through the skin or a body orifice for diagnosis or treatment.

in·ven·to·ry (in′ven-tōr-ē). A detailed, often descriptive, list of items.

Millon clinical multiaxial i. (MCMI), SYN Millon Clinical Multiaxial Inventory *test.*

Minnesota Multiphasic Personality i., SYN Minnesota multiphasic personality inventory *test.*

personality i., a psychological test for evaluation of habitual modes of behavior, thinking, and feeling based on the comparable characteristics of individuals in one's peer group.

in·ver·mi·na·tion (in-ver-mi-nā′shŭn). SYN helminthiasis. [L. *in,* in, + *vermis* (*vermin-*), worm]

in·ver·sion (in-ver′zhŭn). **1.** A turning inward, upside down, or in any direction contrary to the existing one. **2.** Conversion of a disaccharide or polysaccharide by hydrolysis into a monosaccharide; specifically, the hydrolysis of sucrose to D-glucose and D-fructose; so called because of the change in optical rotation. **3.** Alteration of a DNA molecule made by removing a fragment, reversing its orientation, and putting it back into place. **4.** Heat-induced transition of silica, in which the quartz tridymite or cristobalite changes its physical properties as to thermal expansion. [L. *inverto,* pp. *-versus,* to turn upside down, to turn about]

i. of chromosomes, a chromosome aberration resulting from a double break in a segment of the chromosome, with end for end rotation of the fragment between the fracture lines, and refusion of the fragments; this results in reversal of the order of genes in that segment.

paracentric i., i. in a chromosome of a single segment in which the centromere is not included.

pericentric i., i. in a chromosome of a single segment that includes the centromere.

i. of the uterus, a turning of the uterus inside out, usually following childbirth.

visceral i., SYN *situs* inversus viscerum.

in·vert (in′vert). **1.** In chemistry, subjected to inversion, *e.g.,* invert sugar. **2.** Rarely used term for a homosexual. [see inversion]

in·vert·ase (in′ver-tās). SYN β-fructofuranosidase.

In·ver·te·bra·ta (in-ver-tĕ-brā′tă). A general category of the kingdom Animalia (multicellular animals) including those phyla whose members lack a notochord; *i.e.*, all animals except vertebrates in the phylum Chordata.

in·ver·te·brate (in-ver′tĕ-brāt). **1.** Not possessed of a spinal or vertebral column. **2.** Any animal that has no spinal column.

in·vert·ed re·peat. A sequence of nucleotides that is repeated nearly without change except in the opposite direction, usually at some point distant from the original sequence; often associated with gene insertion.

in·ver·tin (in′ver-tin). SYN β-fructofuranosidase.

in·ver·tor (in-ver′ter, -tōr). A muscle that inverts or causes inversion or turns a part, such as the foot, inward. [see inversion]

in·vest·ing. 1. In dentistry, covering or enveloping wholly or in part an object such as a denture, tooth, wax form, crown, etc., with a refractory investment material before curing, soldering, or casting. **2.** In psychoanalysis, allocating to or charging an object with psychic energy or cathexis.
vacuum i., the i. of a pattern within a vacuum.

in·vest·ment. 1. In dentistry, any material used in investing. **2.** In psychoanalysis, the psychic charge or cathexis invested in an object.
refractory i., an i. material which can withstand the high temperatures used in soldering or casting.

in·vet·er·ate (in-vet′er-āt). Long seated; firmly established; said of a disease or of confirmed habits. [L. *in-vetero*, pp. *-atus*, to render old, fr. *vetus*, old]

in·vis·ca·tion (in-vis-kā′shŭn). **1.** Smearing with mucilaginous matter. **2.** The mixing of the food, during mastication, with the buccal secretions. [L. *in*, in, on, + *viscum*, birdlime]

in vit·ro (in vē′trō). In an artificial environment, referring to a process or reaction occurring therein, as in a test tube or culture media. Cf. *in vivo*. [L. in glass]

in·vo·lu·cre (in′vō-lū-ker). SYN involucrum.

in·vo·lu·crin (in-vō-lū′krin). A non-keratin soluble precursor of the highly cross-linked protein known as the corneocyte envelope. [fr. L. *involucrum*, a wrapper]

in·vo·lu·crum, pl. **in·vo·lu·cra** (in-vō-lū′krŭm, -lū′kră). **1.** An enveloping membrane, *e.g.*, a sheath or sac. **2.** The sheath of new bone that forms around a sequestrum. SYN involucre. [L. a wrapper, fr. *in-volvo*, to roll up]

in·vol·un·tary (in-vol′ŭn-tār-ē). **1.** Independent of the will; not volitional. **2.** Contrary to the will. [L. *in-* neg. + *voluntarius*, willing, fr. *volo*, to wish]

in·vo·lu·tion (in-vō-lū′shŭn). **1.** Return of an enlarged organ to normal size. **2.** Turning inward of the edges of a part. **3.** In psychiatry, mental decline associated with advanced age. SYN catagenesis. [L. *in-volvo*, pp. *-volutus*, to roll up]
senile i., the retrogression of vital organs and psychological processes incident to aging.
i. of the uterus, the process of reduction of the uterus to its normal nonpregnant size and state following childbirth.

in·vo·lu·tion·al (in-vō-lū′shŭn-ăl). Relating to involution.

io·ben·zam·ic ac·id (ī-ō-ben-zam′ik). *N*-(3-Amino-2,4,6-triiodobenzoyl)-*N*-phenyl-β-alanine; a radiographic contrast medium for oral cholecystography.

io·ce·tam·ic ac·id (ī′ō-sē-tam′ik). *N*-Acetyl-*N*-(3-amino-2,4,6-triiodophenyl)-2-methyl-β-alanine; a radiographic contrast medium for oral cholecystography.

io·da·mide (ī-ō′dă-mīd). α,5-Diacetamide-2,4,6-triiodo-*m*-toluic acid; a radiographic contrast medium formerly used for oral cholecystography. SYN ametriodinic acid.

Iod·a·moe·ba (ī-od-ă-mē′bă). A genus of parasitic amebae in the superclass Rhizopoda, order Amoebida.
I. bütsch′lii, a parasitic ameba in the large intestine of man; trophozoites are usually 9 to 14 μm in diameter; the cysts are usually 8 to 10 μm in diameter, uninucleate and somewhat irregular in shape, with a thick wall and a large compact mass of glycogen that stains deeply with a solution of iodine; clinically recognizable amebiasis caused by this organism is rare, with symptoms resembling those of chronic disease caused by *Entamoeba histolytica;* it is also found in other primates and is the commonest ameba of pigs.

io·date (ī′ō-dāt). A salt of iodic acid.

iod·ic (ī-od′ik). **1.** Relating to, or caused by, iodine or an iodide. **2.** Denoting a compound of iodine in its pentavalent state.

iod·ic ac·id. HIO_3; crystalline powder, soluble in water; used as an astringent, caustic, disinfectant, deodorant, and intestinal antiseptic.

io·dide (ī′ō-dīd). The negative ion of iodine, I^-.
i. peroxidase, an oxidoreductase catalyzing reactions between iodine and water to yield iodide and H_2O_2; also catalyzes iodination and deiodination of tyrosine compounds; a deficiency of this enzyme leads to a loss of the iodotyrosine derivatives and iodine from the thyroid and results in goiter. SYN iodinase, iodotyrosine deiodase.
sodium i. iodine-131, prepared from radioactive iodine (^{131}I); practically carrier-free, with a half-life of 8.0 days; used as a diagnostic agent in suspected thyroid disease and in the treatment of selected thyroid diseases.

io·dim·e·try (ī-ō-dim′ĕ-trē). SYN iodometry. [iodine + G. *metron,* measure]

io·di·nase (ī′ō-din-ās). SYN *iodide* peroxidase.

io·di·nate (ī′ō-di-nāt). To treat or combine with iodine.

io·dine (I) (ī′ō-dīn, -dēn). A nonmetallic chemical element, atomic no. 53, atomic wt. 126.90447; used in the manufacture of i. compounds and as a catalyst, reagent, tracer, constituent of radiographic contrast media, topical antiseptic, therapy in thyroid disease, antidote for alkaloidal poisons, and in certain stains and solutions. [G. *iōdēs,* violet-like, fr. *ion,* a violet, + *eidos,* form]
butanol-extractable i. (BEI), i. that can be separated from plasma proteins by butanol or other extractable solvents; used to measure thyroid function.
Gram's i., a solution containing i. and potassium iodide, used in Gram's stain.
povidone i., a water soluble complex of i. with polyvinylpyrrolidone. Applied as an antiseptic in the form of solutions or ointments, it releases i. Used in cleansing and disinfecting the skin, preparing the skin preoperatively, and treating infections susceptible to i. SYN polyvinylpyrrolidone-iodine complex, povidone-iodine.
protein-bound i. (PBI), thyroid hormone in its circulating form, consisting of one or more of the iodothyronines bound to one or more of the serum proteins.
radioactive i., the i. radioisotopes ^{131}I, ^{125}I, or ^{123}I used as tracers in biology and medicine.
tamed i., SYN iodophor.
i. tincture, a hydroalcoholic solution containing 2% elemental i. and 2.4% potassium iodide to facilitate dissolution and 47% alcohol; used as an antiseptic/germicide on the skin surface for cuts and scratches. Has been used as a skin disinfectant before surgery but is now largely replaced by organic forms of i.

io·dine-123 (^{123}I). A radioisotope of iodine with a 159 keV gamma emission and a physical half-life of 13.2 hr, frequently used for studies of thyroid disease and of renal function.

io·dine-125 (^{125}I). Radioactive iodine isotope that decays by K-capture (internal conversion) with a half-life of 59.4 days; used as a tracer in thyroid studies and as a label in immunoassay and in imaging.

io·dine-127 (^{127}I, ^{127}I). Stable, nonradioactive iodine, the most abundant iodide isotope found in nature; dietary deficiency causes simple goiter; used to block thyroid uptake of radioactive iodine released from nuclear accidents.

io·dine-131 (^{131}I). A radioactive iodine isotope; beta and gamma emitter with a half-life of 8 days; used as a tracer in thyroid studies, as therapy in hyperthyroidism, thyroid cancer, and heart disease, and as a label in immunoassay and imaging.

io·dine-132 (^{132}I). A beta- and gamma-emitting radioisotope of iodine with a physical half-life of 2.28 hr, usually obtained from a tellurium-132 radionuclide generator; its clinical use has been supplanted by ^{131}I and ^{123}I.

io·dine-fast. Denoting hyperthyroidism unresponsive to iodine therapy, which develops frequently in most cases so treated.

io·din·o·phil, io·din·o·phile (ī-ō-din′ō-fil, -fīl). **1.** Staining

io

readily with iodine. SYN iodinophilous. **2.** Any histologic element that stains readily with iodine. [iodine + G. *philos*, fond]

io·din·oph·i·lous (ī-ō-din-of'i-lŭs). SYN iodinophil (1).

io·dip·a·mide (ī-ō-dip'ă-mīd). N,N'-Adipylbis(3-amino-2,4,6-triiodobenzoic acid); an ionic, dimeric, water-soluble radiographic contrast medium for intravenous cholangiography; used as the sodium or methylglucamine salt. SYN Adipiodone.

methylglucamine i., bis-N-methylglucamine salt of iodipamide; a water-soluble organic iodine compound used for intravenous cholangiography and cholecystography.

io·dism (ī'ō-dizm). Poisoning by iodine, a condition marked by severe coryza, an acneform eruption, weakness, salivation, and foul breath; caused by the continuous administration of iodine or one of the iodides.

io·dix·an·ol (ī-ō-diks'ă-nol). 5,5'-[(2-Hydroxy-1,3-propane)bis-(acetylamino)]bis[N,N'-bis(2,3- dihydroxypropyl)-2,4,6- triiodo-1,3-benzenedicarboxamide]; a dimeric, nonionic, low osmolar, water-soluble radiographic contrast medium for intravascular use.

io·dize (ī'ō-dīz). To treat or impregnate with iodine.

i·o·dized oil (ī'ō-dīzd). An iodine addition product of vegetable oils, containing not less than 38% and not more than 42% of organically combined iodine; a radiopaque medium.

io·do·a·cet·a·mide (ī-ō'dō-ă-sē'tă-mīd). ICH_2–$CONH_2$; a chemical reacting readily with sulfhydryl groups and therefore a strong inhibitor of many enzymes.

io·do·al·phi·on·ic ac·id (ī-ō'dō-al-fē-on'ik). β-(4-Hydroxy-3,5-diiodophenyl)-α-phenylpropionic acid; a formerly used radiographic contrast medium for cholecystography.

io·do·ca·sein (ī-ō-dō-kā'sēn). A compound of iodine with casein, in which the iodine is attached to tyrosine molecules; possesses thyroxine activity.

io·do·chlor·hy·drox·y·quin, io·do·chlo·ro·hy·drox·y·quin-o·line (ī'ō-dō-klōr'hī-drok'si-kwin, -klōr'ō-hī-drok'si-kwin'ō-lēn). 5-Chloro-7-iodo-8-quinolinol; 5-chloro-8-hydroxy-7-iodo-quinoline; used topically as a local anti-infective and in a wide range of dermatoses, intravaginally in *Trichomonas vaginalis* vaginitis, and internally for the treatment of mild or asymptomatic intestinal amebiasis. SYN chloriodoquin, clioquinol.

io·do·chlo·rol (ī'ō-dō-klōr'ol). SYN chloriodized oil.

io·do·der·ma (ī-ō'dō-der'mă). An eruption of follicular papules and pustules, or a granulomatous lesion, caused by iodine toxicity or sensitivity.

io·do·form (ī-ō'dō-fōrm). CHI_3; a topical antiseptic. SYN triiodomethane.

io·do·glob·u·lin (ī-ō'dō-glob'yū-lin). SYN thyroglobulin (1).

io·do·gor·go·ic ac·id (ī-ō'dō-gōr-gō'ik). 3,5-Diiodotyrosine; a precursor of thyroxine.

io·do·hip·pu·rate so·di·um (ī-ō'dō-hip'pū-rāt). Sodium *o*-iodo-hippurate; a radiopaque compound formerly used intravenously, orally, or for retrograde urography. When tagged with iodine-131, it was used to measure effective renal plasma flow and to image the kidneys for radioisotopic renography.

io·do·meth·a·mate so·di·um (ī-ō'dō-meth'ă-māt). N-Methyl-3,5-diiodo-4-pyridone-2,6-dicarboxylate; a high osmolar, ionic, water-soluble, radiographic contrast medium formerly used widely as the disodium salt for intravenous urography.

io·do·met·ric (ī-ō'dō-met'rik). Relating to iodometry.

io·dom·e·try (ī-ō-dom'ĕ-trē). Analytical techniques involving titrations in which iodine is either formed or consumed, the sudden appearance or disappearance of iodine marking the end point. SYN iodimetry. [iodine + G. *metron*, measure]

io·do·pa·no·ic ac·id (ī-ō'dō-pa-nō'ik). SYN iopanoic acid.

io·do·phen·dyl·ate (ī-ō'dō-fen'dil-āt). SYN iophendylate.

io·do·phil·ia (ī-ō'dō-fil'ē-ă). An affinity for iodine, as manifested by some leukocytes in certain conditions. When treated with a solution of iodine and potassium iodide, normal polymorphonuclear leukocytes stain a fairly bright yellow; in certain pathologic conditions, the polymorphonuclear leukocytes frequently stain diffusely brown or yellow-brown; the reaction may be intracellular (as described) or extracellular, affecting the particles in the

immediate vicinity of the leukocytes. [iodine + G. *phileō*, to love]

io·do·phor (ī-ō'dō-fōr). A combination of iodine with a surfactant carrier, usually polyvinylpyrrolidone. Commercial preparations generally contain 1% "available" iodine, which is slowly released to take effect against microorganisms; used as skin disinfectants, particularly for surgical scrubs. SYN tamed iodine. [iodine + G. *phora*, a carrying]

io·do·phtha·lein (ī-ō'dō-thal'ēn, -dof-thal'e-in). A radiographic contrast medium. The disodium salt was once used in radiography of the gallbladder. SYN tetraiodophenolphthalein sodium.

3-io·do-1,2-pro·pane·di·ol. SYN glyceryl iodide.

γ-io·do·pro·py·lene·gly·col. SYN glyceryl iodide.

io·do·pro·pyl·i·dene glyc·er·ol. SYN iodinated *glycerol*.

io·do·pro·teins (ī-ō'dō-prō'tēnz). Proteins containing iodine bound to tyrosine groups.

io·dop·sin (ī-ō-dop'sin). A visual pigment, composed of 11-*cis*-retinal bound to an opsin, found in the cones of the retina. SYN visual violet. [G. *ion*, violet, + *ōps*, eye, + -in]

io·do·py·ra·cet (ī-ō'dō-pī'ră-set). 3,5-Diiodo-4-pyridone-N-acetate; a radiographic contrast medium used for intravenous urography; also used to determine the renal plasma flow and the renal tubular excretory mass. SYN diodone.

io·do·qui·nol (ī-ō'dō-kwin'ol). Drug used as an amebicide prepared by the action of iodine monochloride on 8-hydroxyquinoline.

io·do·ther·a·py (ī'ō-dō-thār'ă-pē). Treatment with iodine.

io·do·thy·ro·nines (ī-ō'dō-thī'rō-nēnz). Iodinated derivatives of thyronine.

io·do·ty·ro·sine (ī-ō'dō-tī'rō-sēn). An iodinated tyrosine.

i. deiodase, SYN *iodide* peroxidase.

io·dox·a·mate meg·lu·mine (ī-ō-doks'ă-māt). 3,3'-[Ethylenebis(oxyethylene-oxyethylenecar bonylimino)]bis-[2,4,6-triiodobenzoic acid] compound with 1-deoxy-1-(methyla-mino)-D-glucitol (1:2); the methylglucamine salt of an ionic, water-soluble, dimeric, radiographic contrast medium; formerly used primarily for intravenous cholangiography.

io·du·ria (ī-ō-dū'rē-ă). Urinary excretion of iodine.

io·gly·cam·ic ac·id (ī'ō-glī-kam'ik). An ionic, water-soluble, dimeric, radiographic contrast medium, formerly used for intravenous cholangiography.

io·hex·ol (ī'ō-heks'ol). $C_{19}H_{26}I_3N_3O_9$; N,N'-Bis(2,3-dihydrox-ypropyl)-5-[(N-2,3-dihydroxypropyl)acetamido]-2,4,6-triiodo-isophthalamide; a monomeric, nonionic, water-soluble, low osmolar radiographic contrast medium for urography or angiography. Used intrathecally and intravascularly.

iom·e·ter (ī-om'ĕ-ter). An apparatus for measuring ionization. [ion + G. *metron*, measure]

ion (ī'on). An atom or group of atoms carrying an electric charge by virtue of having gained or lost one or more electrons. I.'s charged with negative electricity (anions) travel toward a positive pole (anode); those charged with positive electricity (cations) travel toward a negative pole (cathode). I.'s may exist in solid, liquid, or gaseous environments, although those in liquid (electrolytes) are more common and familiar. [G. *iōn*, going]

aquo-i., SEE aquo-ion.

dipolar i.'s, i.'s possessing both a negative charge and a positive charge, each localized at a different point in the molecule, which thus has both positive and negative "poles"; amino acids are the most notable dipolar i.'s, containing a positively charged NH_3^+ group and a negatively charged COO^- group at neutral pH. SYN amphions, zwitterions.

gram-i., SEE gram-ion.

hydride i., the H^- i., transferred to acceptor molecules in some biological oxidations.

hydrogen i. (H^+), a hydrogen atom minus its electron and therefore carrying a unit positive charge (*i.e.,* a proton); in water, it combines with a water molecule to form hydronium i., H_3O^+.

hydronium i., the hydrated proton, H_3O^+, a form in which hydrogen i. exists in aqueous solutions; also, $H_3O^+ \cdot H_2O$, $H_3O^+ \cdot 2H_2O$, etc. SYN oxonium i.

oxonium i., SYN hydronium i.

sulfonium i., a compound in which a sulfur atom has three single covalent bonds and therefore has a positive charge analogous to the nitrogen of an ammonium compound; *e.g.,* S-adenosyl-L-methionine.

Ionescu. SEE Jonnesco.

ion ex·change (ī'on eks-chanj'). SEE anion exchange, cation exchange, ion exchange *chromatography.*

ion ex·chang·er (ī'on eks-chanj'er). SEE anion exchanger, cation exchanger.

ion·ic (ī-on'ik). Relating to an ion.

io·ni·um (ī-ō'nē-ŭm). Former term for thorium-230. [G. *iōn,* going]

ion·i·za·tion (ī'on-i-zā'shŭn). **1.** Dissociation into ions, occurring when an electrolyte is dissolved in water or certain liquids or when molecules are subjected to electrical discharge or ionizing radiation. **2.** Production of ions as a result of interaction of radiation with matter. **3.** SYN iontophoresis.

ion·ize (ī'on-īz). To separate into ions; to dissociate atoms or molecules into electrically charged atoms or radicals.

ion·o·gram (ī'on-ō-gram). SYN electropherogram.

io·none (ī'ō-nōn). A cyclic ketone with an odor of violets or cedar wood, the α and β varieties of which differ in the location of the double bond in the ring: provitamins A and vitamin A have i. configuration in the ring portion; α-carotene contains one α- and one β-ionone moieties, β-carotene contains two β-ionone moieties, and γ-carotene contains one β-ionone moiety.

ion·o·pher·o·gram (ī'on-ō-fer'ō-gram). SYN electropherogram.

ion·o·phore (ī-on'ō-fōr). A compound or substance that forms a complex with an ion and transports it across a membrane. [ion + G. *phore,* a bearer]

ion·o·pho·re·sis (ī-on'ō-fōr-ē'sis). SYN electrophoresis. [ion + G. *phorēsis,* a carrying]

ion·o·pho·ret·ic (ī-on'ō-fōr-et'ik). SYN electrophoretic.

ion·to·pho·re·sis (ī-on'tō-fōr-ē'sis). The introduction into the tissues, by means of an electric current, of the ions of a chosen medicament. SYN ionic medication, ionization (3), iontotherapy. [ion + G. *phorēsis,* a carrying]

ion·to·pho·ret·ic (ī-on'tō-fōr-et'ik). Relating to iontophoresis.

ion·to·ther·a·py (ī-on'tō-thār'ă-pē). SYN iontophoresis.

io·pam·i·dol (ī'ō-pam'i-dol). (S)-5-Lactamido-2,4,6-triiodo-N,N′-bis(1,3)dihydroxypropyl)isophthalamide; a monomeric, nonionic, water-soluble, low osmolar radiographic contrast medium for urography or angiography.

io·pa·no·ic ac·id (ī'ō-pa-nō'ik). 3-(3-Amino-2,4,6-triiodophenyl)-2-ethylpropionic acid; a water-insoluble radiographic contrast medium, once used widely for oral cholecystography. SYN iodopanoic acid.

io·pen·tol (ī'ō-pen'tol). N,N′-Bis(2,3-dihydroxypropyl)-5-[N-(2-hydroxy-3-methoxypropyl) acetamido]-2,4,6-triiodoisophthalamide; a nonionic, monomeric, low osmolar radiographic contrast medium for intravenous urography or angiography.

io·phen·dyl·ate (ī-ō-fen'dil-āt). Ethyl 10-(p-iodophenyl)-undecylate; a mixture of isomers of ethyl iodophenylundecylate, an iodized fatty acid of low viscosity; used for radiography of the spinal canal. SYN iodophendylate.

io·phe·no·ic ac·id (ī'ō-fen-ō-ik). SYN iophenoxic acid.

io·phen·ox·ic ac·id (ī'ō-fen-oks'ik). α-Ethyl-3-hydroxy-2,4,6-triiodohydrocinnamic acid; a radiographic contrast medium; formerly used for oral cholecystography. SYN iophenoic acid.

io·pho·bia (ī-ō-fō'bē-ă). Morbid fear of poisons. [G. *ios,* poison, + *phobos,* fear]

io·pro·mide (ī-ō'prō-mid). A monomeric, nonionic, water-soluble, low osmolar radiographic contrast medium for intravenous urography or angiography.

i·o·ta (ι) (ī-ōt'a). The ninth letter in the Greek alphabet. **2.** In chemistry, denotes the ninth in a series, or the ninth atom from a carboxyl group or other functional group. **3.** A tiny or minute amount.

io·ta·cism (ī-ō'tă-sizm). A speech defect marked by the frequent substitution of a long *e* sound (that of the Greek iota) for other vowels. [G. *iōta,* the letter ι]

io·tha·lam·ic ac·id (ī'ō-thă-lam'ik). 5-Acetamido-2,4,6-triiodo-N-methylisophthalamic acid; an ionic, monomeric, water-soluble radiographic contrast medium, widely used as the sodium or methylglucamine salt (iothalamate) for intravenous urography and angiography.

io·thi·o·u·ra·cil so·di·um (ī'ō-thī-ō-yūr'ă-sil). The sodium salt of 5-iodo-2-thiouracil; an organic iodine derivative of thiouracil with the thyroid-involuting action of iodine and the capability of inhibiting thyroxine production.

io·trol (ī'ō-trol). SYN iotrolan.

io·tro·lan (ī-ō'trō-lan). 5,5′-[Malonylbis(methylimino)]bis[N, N′-bis[2,3-dihydroxy-1-(hydroxymethyl)propyl]-2,4,6-triiodoisophthalamide]; a dimeric, nonionic, water-soluble, low osmolar radiographic contrast medium, used for myelography and other nonvascular applications. SYN iotrol.

io·ver·sol (ī-ō-ver'sol). N,N′-Bis(2,3-dihydroxypropyl)-5-[N-[2-hydroxyethyl)glycolamido]-2,4,6-triiodoisophthalamide; a water-soluble, nonionic, low osmolar, radiographic contrast medium.

iox·ag·late (ī-oks-ag'lāt). A diagnostic radiopaque medium, usually a combination of i. meglumine ($C_{24}H_{21}I_6N_5O_8 \cdot C_7H_{17}NO_5$), and i. sodium ($C_{24}H_{20}I_6N_5NaO_8$); used in angiography, aortography, arteriography, venography, and urography.

iox·i·lan (ī-oks'ī-lan). A monomeric, nonionic, water-soluble, low osmolar radiographic contrast medium for urography or angiography.

iox·i·thal·a·mate (ī-oks-ī-thal'ă-māt). 5-Acetamido-2,4,6-triiodo-N-(2-hydroxyethyl)isophthalamic acid; an ionic, monomeric, water-soluble radiographic contrast medium for urography and angiography.

I.P., i.p. Abbreviation for intraperitoneal or intraperitoneally; isoelectric *point.*

IP₃ Abbreviation for *inositol* 1,4,5-trisphosphate.

ip·e·cac (ip'ē-kak). SYN ipecacuanha.

powdered i., a form of i. used in the preparation of ipecac syrup.

ip·e·cac·u·a·nha (ip-ē-kak-yū-an'ă). The dried root of *Uragoga (Cephaelis) ipecacuanha* (family Rubiaceae), a shrub of Brazil and other parts of South America; contains emetine, cephaeline, emetamine, ipecacuanhic acid, psychotrine, and methylpsychotrine; has expectorant, emetic, and antidysenteric properties. SYN ipecac. [native Brazilian word]

de-emetinized i., i. from which the emetic principle has been extracted; has been used as an antidysenteric agent.

prepared i., a fine powder to contain 2% of the total alkaloids of i., calculated as emetine.

IPF Abbreviation for idiopathic pulmonary *fibrosis* or interstitial pulmonary *fibrosis.*

ipo·date. 3-[(Dimethylaminomethylene)amino]-2,4,6-triiodohydrocinnamic acid; a radiographic contrast medium, given orally as the sodium or, more often, the calcium salt, for opacification of the gallbladder and central biliary tree.

ipo·date so·di·um (ī'pō-dāt). Sodium 3-[(dimethylaminomethylene)amino]-2,4,6- triiodohydrocinnamate; a radiopaque medium.

ip·o·mea (ī-pō-mē'ă). The dried root of *Ipomoea orizabensis* (family Convolvulaceae). SEE ALSO ipomea *resin.* SYN orizaba jalap root. [G. *ips* (*ip-*), a worm, + *homoios,* like]

Ip·o·moea (ī-pō-mē'ă). A plant genus of the family Convolvulaceae. [L. ipomea]

I. rubrocoeru'lea var. *prae'cox,* the seeds contain lysergic acid amide, isolysergic acid amide, chanoclavine, elymoclavine, and other ergot (indole) alkaloids; ingestion of the seeds produces hallucinatory and euphoric effects. SYN morning glory (1).

I. versico'lor, a species whose seeds contain hallucinogenic ergot (indole) alkaloids.

IPPB Abbreviation for intermittent positive pressure *breathing.*

IPPV Abbreviation for intermittent positive pressure *ventilation.*

ipra·tro·pi·um (i-pră-trō'pē-ŭm). (8r)-3α-Hydroxy-8-isopropyl-1α H,5αH-tropanium bromide (±)-tropate monohydrate; a synthetic quaternary ammonium compound, chemically related to

ip

atropine, that has anticholinergic activity and is used as an inhalant in the treatment of bronchospasm.

ip·rin·dole (ĭ-prin′dōl). An antidepressant containing a three-ring structure of which the center ring consists of an indole nucleus.

ipro·ni·a·zid (ī-prō-nī′ă-zid). 1-Isonicotinoyl-2-isopropylhydrazine; an antituberculous and antidepressant agent similar to isoniazid, but more toxic and rarely used; it inhibits monoamine oxidase. The first antidepressant agent.

ipro·ni·da·zole (ī-prō-nī′dă-zōl). 2-Isopropyl-1-methyl-5-nitroimidazole; an antiprotozoal agent.

ipro·ver·a·tril (ī-prō-ver′ă-tril). SYN verapamil.

iPrSGal Abbreviation for isopropylthiogalactoside.

Ips Abbreviation for pipsyl.

ip·se·fact (ip′se-fakt). All parts or aspects of the environment that an individual, colony, population, or species of animal has modified chemically or physically by its own behavior (*e.g.*, a nest or home, rodent or deer runs, excrement, pheromones). [L. *ipse*, self, + *factum*, a thing done]

ip·si·lat·er·al (ip-si-lat′er-ăl). On the same side, with reference to a given point, *e.g.*, a dilated pupil on the same side as an extradural hematoma with contralateral limbs being paretic. SYN homolateral. [L. *ipse*, same, + *latus* (*later*-), side]

IPSP Abbreviation for inhibitory postsynaptic *potential*.

IPTG Abbreviation for isopropylthiogalactoside.

IPV Abbreviation for inactivated poliovirus *vaccine*. SEE poliovirus *vaccines*, under *vaccine*.

IQ Abbreviation for intelligence *quotient*.

IR Abbreviation for infrared.

Ir Symbol for iridium.

IRI Abbreviation for immunoreactive *insulin*.

△**irid-.** SEE irido-.

ir·i·dal (ī′ri-dăl, ir′i-dăl). Relating to the iris. SYN iridial, iridian, iridic.

ir·i·dec·to·my (ir′i-dek′tō-mē). 1. Excision of a portion of the iris. 2. The hole in the iris produced by a surgical iridectomy. [irido- + G. *ektomē*, excision]

buttonhole i., SYN peripheral i.

optical i., i. performed for the purpose of improving vision by making an artificial pupil.

peripheral i., in narrow-angle glaucoma, the surgical removal of a minute portion of the iris at its root; in intracapsular extraction of cataract, removal of one or more minute sections near the peripheral border, leaving the pupillary margin intact. SYN buttonhole i., stenopeic i.

sector i., an i. in which a portion of the pupillary margin is excised.

stenopeic i., SYN peripheral i.

therapeutic i., an i. performed for the prevention or cure of disease, *e.g.*, angle-closure glaucoma.

ir·i·den·clei·sis (ir′i-den-klī′sis). The incarceration of a portion of the iris by corneoscleral incision in glaucoma to effect filtration between the anterior chamber and subconjunctival space. [irido- + G. *enkleiō*, to shut in]

ir·i·der·e·mia (ir′i-der-ē′mē′ă, ī′rid-). Condition wherein the iris is so rudimentary as to appear to be absent. Cf. aniridia. [irido- + G. *erēmia*, absence]

ir·i·des (ir′i-dēz). Plural of iris. [G.]

ir·i·des·cent (ir-i-des′ent). Presenting multiple bright refractile colors, typically as a result of optical interference when incident white light is broken into its spectral components when reflected back through several thin-layered films. [G. *iris*, rainbow]

irid·e·sis (i-rid′ĕ-sis, ī-ri-dē′sis). Ligature of a portion of the iris brought out through an incision in the cornea. [irido- + G. *desis*, a binding together]

irid·i·al, irid·i·an, irid·ic (ī-rid′ē-al; ī-rid′ē-an; ī-rid′ik, i-rid′-). SYN iridal.

ir·i·din (ir′i-din). 1. Irigenin 7-glucoside from orris root, *Iris florentina*. 2. A resinoid from blue flag, *Iris versicolor;* used as a cholagogue and cathartic. SYN irisin.

irid·i·um (Ir) (i-rid′ē-ŭm). A white, silvery metallic element, atomic no. 77, atomic wt. 192.22; ^{192}Ir is a radioisotope (half-life of 73.83 days) that has been used in the interstitial treatment of certain tumors. [L. *iris*, rainbow]

△**irido-, irid-.** The iris. [G. *iris* (*irid*-), rainbow]

ir·i·do·a·vul·sion (ir′i-dō-ă-vŭl′shŭn). Avulsion, or tearing away, of the iris.

ir·i·do·cele (ir′i-dō-sēl). Herniation of a portion of the iris through a corneal defect. [irido- + G. *kēlē*, hernia]

ir·i·do·cho·roid·i·tis (ir′i-dō-kō-roy-dī′tis). Inflammation of both iris and choroid.

ir·i·do·col·o·bo·ma (ir′i-dō-ko-lō-bō′mă). A coloboma or congenital defect of the iris. [irido- + G. *kolobōma*, coloboma]

ir·i·do·cor·ne·al (ir′i-dō-kōr′nē-ăl). Relating to the iris and the cornea.

ir·i·do·cy·clec·to·my (ir′i-dō-sī-klek′tō-mē). Removal of the iris and ciliary body for excision of a tumor. [irido- + G. *kyklos*, circle (ciliary body), + *ektomē*, excision]

ir·i·do·cy·cli·tis (ir′i-dō-sī-klī′tis). Inflammation of both iris and ciliary body. SEE ALSO iritis, uveitis. [irido- + G. *kyklos*, circle (ciliary body), + *-itis*, inflammation]

i. sep′tica, SYN Behçet's *syndrome*.

ir·i·do·cy·clo·cho·roid·i·tis (ir′i-dō-sī′klō-kō-royd-ī′tis). Inflammation of the iris, involving the ciliary body and the choroid.

ir·i·do·cys·tec·to·my (ir′i-dō-sis-tek′tō-mē). An operation for making an artificial pupil when posterior synechiae follow extracapsular extraction of cataract; the border of the iris and a portion of the capsule of the lens are drawn out through an incision in the cornea and cut off. [irido- + G. *kystis*, bladder (capsule), + *ektomē*, excision]

ir·i·do·di·ag·no·sis (ir′i-dō-dī-ag-nō′sis). Diagnosis of systemic diseases by observation of changes in form and color of the iris.

ir·i·do·di·al·y·sis (ir′i-dō-dī-al′i-sis). A colobomatous defect of the iris caused by its separation from the scleral spur. [irido- + G. *dialysis*, loosening]

ir·i·do·di·la·tor (ir′i-dō-dī-lā′ter). Causing dilation of the pupil; applied to the musculus dilator pupillae.

ir·i·do·do·ne·sis (ir′i-dō-dō-nē′sis). Agitated motion of the iris. SYN tremulous iris. [irido- + G. *doneō*, to shake to and fro]

ir·i·do·ki·net·ic (ir′i-dō-ki-net′ik). Relating to the movements of the iris. SYN iridomotor.

ir·i·dol·o·gy (ir-i-dol′ō-jē). A system of medicine based on an examination of the iris, using a chart on which certain areas of the iris are diagnostically specific for particular organs, systems, and structures. [irido- + G. *logos*, study]

ir·i·do·ma·la·cia (ir′i-dō-mă-lā′shē-ă). Degenerative softening of the iris. [irido- + G. *malakia*, softness]

ir·i·do·mes·o·di·al·y·sis (ir′i-dō-mes′ō-dī-al′i-sis). Separation of adhesions around the inner margin of the iris. [irido- + G. *mesos*, middle, + *dialysis*, loosening]

ir·i·do·mo·tor (ir′i-dō-mō′tŏr). SYN iridokinetic, pupillomotor.

ir·i·do·pa·ral·y·sis (ir′i-dō-pă-ral′i-sis). SYN iridoplegia.

ir·i·dop·a·thy (ir-i-dop′ă-thē). Pathologic lesions in the iris.

ir·i·do·ple·gia (ir′i-dō-plē′jē-ă). Paralysis of the musculus sphincter iridis. SYN iridoparalysis. [irido- + G. *plēgē*, stroke]

complete i., paralysis of both the dilator and sphincter muscles of the iris.

reflex i., absence of the pupillary light reflex, as in the Argyll Robertson pupil.

sympathetic i., i. due to the paralysis of the sympathetically innervated dilator pupillae muscle.

ir·i·dop·to·sis (ir′i-dop-tō′sis). Prolapse of the iris. [irido- + G. *ptōsis*, a falling]

ir·i·dor·rhex·is (ir′i-dō-rek′sis). Deliberate, surgical tearing of the iris from the scleral spur in order to increase the breadth of a coloboma. [irido- + G. *rhēxis*, rupture]

ir·i·dos·chi·sis (ir-i-dos′ki-sis). Separation of the anterior layer of the iris from the posterior layer; ruptured anterior fibers float in the aqueous humor. [irido- + G. *schisma*, cleft]

ir·i·do·scle·rot·o·my (ir′i-dō-skle-rot′ō-mē). An incision involving both sclera and iris. [irido- + sclera, + G. *tomē*, incision]

ir·i·dot·o·my (ir-i-dot′ō-mē). Transverse division of some of the fibers of the iris, forming an artificial pupil. [irido- + G. *tomē*, incision]

laser i., peripheral iridectomy as performed by laser.

> This is a refinement of the surgical technique devised in 1858 by von Graefe. In acute glaucoma the aqueous humor cannot flow freely around the lens and through the pupil to be absorbed in the angle of the anterior chamber. Laser peripheral iridectomy corrects this problem by producing a small hole in the iris to permit aqueous flow. The procedure takes only a few seconds and employs a laser attached to a slit lamp.

Ir·i·do·vir·i·dae (ir′i-do-vir′i-dē). A family of viruses including iridescent viruses of insects (*Iridovirus*), the virions of which are nonenveloped, and, probably, also viruses of vertebrates (perhaps including African swine fever virus), the virions of which have envelopes containing 15% lipid. In general, the virus has large icosahedral virions (130 to 300 nm in diameter), the capsids of which contain about 1500 capsomeres. The genome is a single molecule of double stranded DNA with molecular weight of 130 to 160×10^6.

Ir·i·do·vi·rus (ir′i-dō-vī′rŭs). A genus of viruses (family Iridoviridae) comprised of the iridescent insect viruses of which the type species is the tipula iridescent virus.

iri·gen·in (i-ri-jen′in). A trihydroxy trimethoxy isoflavone component of iridin.

iris, pl. **ir·i·des** (ī′ris, ir′i-dēz) [NA]. The anterior division of the vascular tunic of the eye, a diaphragm, perforated in the center (the pupil), attached peripherally to the scleral spur; it is composed of stroma and a double layer of pigmented retinal epithelium from which are derived the sphincter and dilator muscles of the pupil. SYN orris. [G. rainbow, the iris of the eye]

i. bicolor, a variegated or two-colored i. SYN monocular heterochromia.

i. bombé, a condition occurring in posterior annular synechia, in which an increase of fluid in the posterior chamber causes a forward bulging of the peripheral i.

plateau i., in angle-closure glaucoma, a flat appearance of the i. rather than a forward convexity.

tremulous i., SYN iridodonesis.

iris frill. SYN collarette.

iri·sin (ī′ri-sin). SYN iridin (2).

irit·ic (ī-rit′ik). Relating to iritis.

iri·tis (ī-rī′tis). Inflammation of the iris. SEE ALSO iridocyclitis, uveitis.

fibrinous i., acute inflammation of the iris, with profuse exudate; occurs in uveitis of tertiary syphilis.

follicular i., rarely used term for chronic i. with glassy nodules situated deep down between the anterior and posterior layers of the iris.

i. glaucomato′sa, an outpouring of exudate and cells after control of angle-closure glaucoma.

hemorrhagic i., i. with such severe hyperemia that hyphema occurs.

nodular i., i. with aggregations of round cells in the iris.

plastic i., i. with a fibrinous exudation.

quiet i., i. without inflammatory signs such as redness or edema of the cornea.

serous i., inflammation of the iris, with a serous exudate in the anterior chamber.

sympathetic i., i. consecutive to a similar condition in the other eye.

iron (Fe) (ī′ern, ī′rŭn). A metallic element, atomic no. 26, atomic wt. 55.847, that occurs in the heme of hemoglobin, myoglobin, transferrin, ferritin, and iron-containing porphyrins, and is an essential component of enzymes such as catalase, peroxidase, and the various cytochromes; its salts are used medicinally. For individual salts not listed below, see ferric and ferrous entries. [A.S. *iren*]

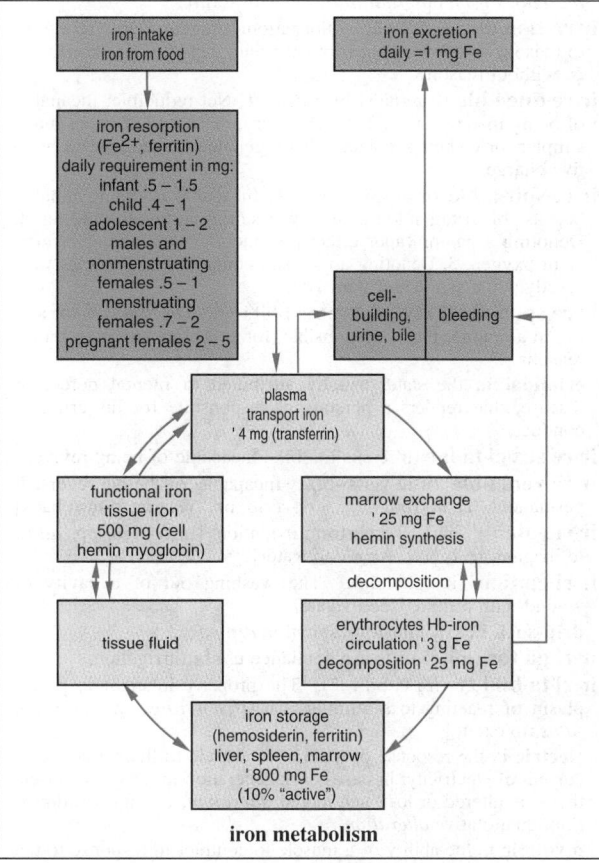

iron metabolism

albuminized i., i. albuminate, a compound of i. oxide and albumin; rendered soluble by the presence of sodium citrate; occurs as reddish brown, lustrous granules, odorless or nearly so; used in anemia.

i. alum, SYN ferric ammonium sulfate.

i. dextrin, a complex of dextrin with ferric hydroxide; used intravenously in the treatment of iron deficiency.

peptonized i., a compound of i. oxide and peptone, rendered soluble by the presence of sodium citrate; used in the treatment of iron deficiency anemia.

i. protoporphyrin, a protoporphyrin to which an i. atom is complexed; *e.g.,* heme.

i. pyri′tes, native sulfide of i.

i. sorbitex, a complex of iron, sorbitol, and citric acid in stable solution for intramuscular administration in the treatment of iron deficiency anemia in patients who are unable to take sufficient amounts of iron by the oral route. SYN i. sorbitol.

i. sorbitol, SYN i. sorbitex.

iron-52 (^{52}**Fe**). A radioactive iron isotope; a cyclotron-produced positron emitter with a half-life of 8.28 hr, used to study iron metabolism.

iron-55 (^{55}**Fe**). An iron isotope; a positron emitter with a half-life of 2.73 years; used (less often than ^{59}Fe) as a tracer in study of iron metabolism and in blood perfusion studies.

iron-59 (^{59}**Fe**). An iron isotope; a gamma and beta emitter with a half-life of 44.51 days; used as tracer in study of iron metabolism, determination of blood volume, and in blood transfusion studies.

ir·ra·di·ate (i-rā′dē-āt). To apply radiation from a source to a structure or organism. [see irradiation]

ir·ra·di·a·tion (i-rā-dē-ā′shŭn). **1.** The subjective enlargement of a bright object seen against a dark background. **2.** Exposure to the action of electromagnetic radiation (*e.g.,* heat, light, x-rays).

3. The spreading of nervous impulses from one area in the brain or cord, or from a tract, to another tract. SEE ALSO radiation. [L. *ir-radio,* (*in-r*), pp. *-radi-atus,* to beam forth]

ir·ra·tion·al (i-rash'ŭn-ăl). Not rational; unreasonable (contrary to reason) or unreasoning (not exercising reason). [L. *irrational-is,* without reason]

ir·re·duc·i·ble (ir-rē-dū'si-bl, i-rē-). **1.** Not reducible; incapable of being made smaller. **2.** In chemistry, incapable of being made simpler, or of being replaced, hydrogenated, or reduced in positive charge.

ir·re·spir·a·ble (ir-rē-spīr'ă-bl). **1.** Incapable of being inhaled because of irritation to the airway, resulting in breath-holding. **2.** Denoting a gas or vapor either poisonous or containing insufficient oxygen. **3.** Denoting an aerosol composed of particles with aerodynamic size larger than 10 μ.

ir·re·spon·si·bil·i·ty (ir'rē-spons-i-bil'i-tē). The state of not acting in a manner that is responsible, for conscious or unconscious reasons.

criminal i., the state, usually attributed to mental defect or disease, that renders a person not responsbile for his criminal conduct.

ir·re·sus·ci·ta·ble (ir'rē-sŭs'i-tă-bl). Incapable of being revived.

ir·re·vers·i·ble (ir-rē-ver'si-bl). Incapable of being reversed; permanent. [L. *in-* (*ir-*) neg. + *re-verto,* pp. *-versus,* to turn back]

ir·ri·gate (ir'i-gāt). To perform irrigation. [L. *ir-rigo,* pp. *-atus,* to irrigate, fr. *in,* on, + *rigo,* to water]

ir·ri·ga·tion (ir-i-gā'shŭn). The washing out of a cavity or wound with a fluid. [see irrigate]

drip-suck i., SYN infusion-aspiration *drainage.*

ir·ri·ga·tor (ir'i-gā-ter). An appliance used in irrigation.

ir·ri·ta·bil·i·ty (ir'i-tă-bil'i-tē). The property inherent in protoplasm of reacting to a stimulus. [L. *irritabilitas,* fr. *irrito,* pp. *-atus,* to excite]

electric i., the response of a nerve or muscle to the passage of a current of electricity; in cases of degeneration in nerve or muscle this i. is altered or lost. SEE modal *alteration,* qualitative *alteration,* quantitative *alteration.*

myotatic i., the ability of a muscle to contract in response to the stimulus produced by a sudden stretching.

ir·ri·ta·ble (ir'i-tă-bl). **1.** Capable of reacting to a stimulus. **2.** Tending to react immoderately to a stimulus. Cf. excitable.

ir·ri·tant (ir'i-tant). **1.** Irritating; causing irritation. **2.** Any agent with this action.

primary i., a substance that causes inflammation and other evidence of irritation, particularly of the skin, on first contact or exposure; a reaction of irritation not dependent on a mechanism of sensitization.

ir·ri·ta·tion (ir-i-tā'shŭn). **1.** Extreme incipient inflammatory reaction of the tissues to an injury. **2.** The normal response of nerve or muscle to a stimulus. **3.** The evocation of a normal or exaggerated reaction in the tissues by the application of a stimulus. [L. *irritatio*]

ir·ri·ta·tive (ir-i-tā'tiv). Causing irritation.

ir·ru·ma·tion (ir'ū-mā'shŭn). SYN fellatio. [L. *irrumo,* pp. *-atus,* to give suck]

ir·rup·tion (i-rŭp'shŭn). Act or process of breaking through to a surface. [L. *irruptio,* fr. *irrumpo,* to break in]

ir·rup·tive (i-rŭp'tiv). Relating to or characterized by irruption.

IRV Abbreviation for inspiratory reserve *volume.*

Irvine, A. Ray, Jr., U.S. ophthalmologist, *1917. SEE I.-Gass *syndrome.*

ISA Abbreviation for intrinsic sympathomimetic *activity.*

Is·a·mine blue (is'ă-mēn, ī'să-). SYN pyrrol blue.

is·aux·e·sis (ī-sawk-zē'sis). Growth of parts at the same rate as growth of the whole. [G. *isos,* even, + *auxēsis,* increase]

is·che·mia (is-kē'mē-ă). Local anemia due to mechanical obstruction (mainly arterial narrowing) of the blood supply. [G. *ischō,* to keep back, + *haima,* blood]

myocardial i., inadequate circulation of blood to the myocardium, usually as a result of coronary artery disease. SEE ALSO *angina* pectoris, myocardial *infarction.*

postural i., the reduced blood pressure and flow induced in a part, *e.g.,* the leg or foot, by raising it above the heart level; used to reduce bleeding during surgical operations on the extremities.

i. ret'inae, diminished blood supply in the retina due to failure of the arterial circulation; it may occur as a result of arterial embolism or spasm; poisoning, as by quinine; or exsanguination from recurring profuse hemorrhages (*e.g.,* in parturition, gastric and duodenal ulcers, and pulmonary tuberculosis); bilateral transitory or permanent blindness may result.

silent i., myocardial i. without accompanying signs or symptoms of angina pectoris; can be detected by EKG and other lab techniques. SEE ALSO silent myocardial *infarction.*

is·che·mic (is-kē'mik). Relating to or affected by ischemia.

is·che·sis (is-kē'sis). Suppression of any discharge, especially of a normal one. [G. *ischō,* to hold back]

is·chia (is'kē-ă). Plural of ischium.

is·chi·ad·ic (is-kē-ad'ik). SYN sciatic (1).

is·chi·a·di·cus (is-kē-ad'i-kŭs) [NA]. SYN sciatic. [L.]

is·chi·al (is'kē-ăl). SYN sciatic (1).

is·chi·al·gia (is-kē-al'jē-ă). **1.** Pain in the hip; specifically, the ischium. SYN ischiodynia. **2.** Rarely used term for sciatica. SYN ischioneuralgia. [G. *ischion,* hip, + *algos,* pain]

is·chi·at·ic (is-kē-at'ik). SYN sciatic (1).

is·chi·dro·sis (is-ki-drō'sis). Obsolete term for anhidrosis. [G. *ischō,* to hold back, + *hidrōsis,* perspiration]

△**ischio-.** The ischium. [G. *ischion,* hip joint, haunch (ischium)]

is·chi·o·a·nal (is-kē-ō-ā'năl). Relating to the ischium and the anus.

is·chi·o·bul·bar (is-kē-ō-bŭl'bar). Relating to the ischium and the bulb of the penis.

is·chi·o·cap·su·lar (is-kē-ō-kap'sū-lăr). Relating to the ischium and the capsule of the hip joint; denoting that part of the capsule which is attached to the ischium.

is·chi·o·cav·er·no·sus. SEE ischiocavernous *muscle.*

is·chi·o·cav·ern·ous (is-kē-ō-kav'er-nŭs). Relating to the ischium and the corpus cavernosum.

is·chi·o·cele (is'kē-ō-sēl). SYN sciatic *hernia.* [ischio- + G. *kēlē,* hernia]

is·chi·o·coc·cyg·e·al (is-kē-ō-kok-sij'ē-ăl). Relating to the ischium and the coccyx.

is·chi·o·coc·cyg·e·us (is-kē-ō-kok-sij'ē-ŭs). SEE muscle.

is·chi·o·dyn·ia (is'kē-ō-din'ē-ă). SYN ischialgia (1). [ischio- + G. *odynē,* pain]

is·chi·o·fem·o·ral (is-kē-ō-fem'ŏ-răl). Relating to the ischium, or hip bone, and the femur, or thigh bone.

is·chi·o·fib·u·lar (is'kē-ō-fib'yū-lăr). Relating to or connecting the ischium and the fibula.

is·chi·o·me·lus (is-ki-om'ē-lŭs). Unequal conjoined twins in which the parasite, often only an arm or a leg, arises from the pelvic region of the autosite. SEE conjoined *twins,* under *twin.* [ischio- + G. *melos,* limb]

is·chi·o·neu·ral·gia (is-kē-ō-nū-ral'jē-ă). SYN ischialgia.

is·chi·o·ni·tis (is'kē-ō-nī'tis). Inflammation of the ischium.

is·chi·op·a·gus (is-kē-op'ă-gŭs). Conjoined twins united in their ischial region. SEE conjoined *twins,* under *twin.* [ischio- + G. *pagos,* fixed]

is·chi·o·per·i·ne·al (is'kē-ō-per-i-nē'ăl). Relating to the ischium and the perineum.

is·chi·o·pu·bic (is'kē-ō-pū'bik). Relating to both ischium and pubis.

is·chi·o·rec·tal (is'kē-ō-rek'tăl). Relating to the ischium and the rectum.

is·chi·o·sa·cral (is-kē-ō-sā'krăl). Relating to the ischium and the sacrum.

is·chi·o·tho·ra·cop·a·gus (is'kē-ō-thōr-ă-kop'ă-gŭs). SYN ilio-thoracopagus.

is·chi·o·tib·i·al (is'kē-ō-tib'ē-ăl). Relating to or connecting the ischium and the tibia.

is·chi·o·vag·i·nal (is-kē-ō-vaj′i-năl). Relating to the ischium and the vagina.

is·chi·o·ver·te·bral (is-kē-ō-ver′tĕ-brăl). Relating to the ischium and the vertebral column.

is·chi·um, gen. **is·chii**, pl. **is·chia** (is′kē-ŭm, is′kē-ă). The lower and posterior part of the hip bone, distinct at birth but later becoming fused with the ilium and pubis; it consists of a body, where it joins the ilium and superior ramus of the pubis to form the acetabulum, and a ramus joining the inferior ramus of the pubis. SYN os ischii [NA], ischial bone. [Mod. L. fr. G. *ischion,* hip]

is·cho·chy·mia (is-kō-kī′mē-ă). Retention of food in the stomach due to dilation of that organ. [G. *ischō,* to keep back, + *chymos,* juice]

is·chu·ret·ic (is-kū-ret′ik). **1.** Relating to or relieving ischuria. **2.** An agent that relieves retention or suppression of urine.

is·chu·ria (is-kū′rē-ă). Retention or suppression of urine. [G. *ischō,* to keep back, + *ouron,* urine]

is·e·thi·o·nate (ī-sĕ-thī′ō-nāt). A salt or ester of isethionic acid.

is·e·thi·on·ic ac·id (ī′sĕ-thī-on′ik). HOCH₂CH₂SO₃H; 2-hydroxyethanesulfonic acid; a colorless viscous liquid, miscible with water and alcohols, that forms crystalline salts with organic acids.

Ishak. SEE Luna-Ishak *stain.*

Ishihara, Shinobu, Japanese ophthalmologist, 1879–1963. SEE I. *test.*

isin·glass (ī′zing-glas). SYN ichthyocolla. [Old Ger. *huysenblas,* sturgeon's bladder]

is·land (ī′land). In anatomy, any isolated part, separated from the surrounding tissues by a groove, or marked by a difference in structure. SYN insula (2). [A.S. *īgland*]

blood i., an aggregation of splanchnic mesodermal cells on the embryonic yolk sac, with the potentiality of forming vascular endothelium and primitive blood cells. SYN blood islet.

bone i., a macroscopic focus of cortical bone within medullary bone, commonly seen as a dense round or oval opacity on radiographs of the pelvis, femoral head, humerus, or ribs.

i.'s of Calleja, dense clusters of very small nerve cells (granule cells) characteristic of the olfactory tubercle at the base of the forebrain.

epimyoepithelial i.'s (ep′ē-mī-ō-ep′ē-thē′lī-al), proliferation of salivary gland ductal epithelium and myoepithelium. Characteristic of benign lymphoepithelial lesions and Sjögren's syndrome.

Langerhans' i.'s, SYN *islets* of Langerhans, under *islet.*

pancreatic i.'s, SYN *islets* of Langerhans, under *islet.*

i. of Reil, SYN insula (1).

is·let (ī′let). A small island.

blood i., SYN blood *island.*

i.'s of Langerhans, cellular masses varying from a few to hundreds of cells lying in the interstitial tissue of the pancreas; they are composed of different cell types that comprise the endocrine portion of the pancreas and are the source of insulin and glucagon. SYN islet tissue, Langerhans' islands, pancreatic islands, pancreatic i.'s.

pancreatic i.'s, SYN i.'s of Langerhans.

principal i.'s, separate globular aggregates made up mostly of endocrine pancreatic tissue; present in some fishes and snakes.

△**-ism. 1.** A medical condition or a disease resulting from or involving some specified thing. **2.** A practice, doctrine. Cf. -ia, -ismus. [G. *-isma, -ismos,* noun-forming suffix]

△**-ismus.** L. for -ism; customarily used to imply spasm, contraction. [L. fr. G. *-ismos,* suffix forming nouns of action]

△**iso-. 1.** Prefix meaning equal, like. **2.** In chemistry, prefix indicating "isomer of" (isomerism); *e.g.,* isocyanate vs. cyanate. **3.** In immunology, prefix designating sameness with respect to species; in recent years, the meaning has shifted to sameness with respect to genetic constitution of individuals. [G. *isos,* equal]

iso·ac·cept·or tRNA (ī′sō-ak′sep-tor). Different tRNA species that bind to alternate codons for the same amino acid residue; can be one tRNA that recognizes the various codons that signify those for the particular amino acid residue.

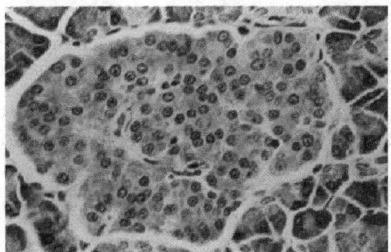
islets of Langerhans

iso·ag·glu·ti·na·tion (ī′sō-ă-glū-ti-nā′shŭn). Agglutination of red blood cells as a result of the reaction between an isoagglutinin and specific antigen in or on the cells. SYN isohemagglutination. [iso- + L. *ad,* to, + *gluten,* glue]

iso·ag·glu·ti·nin (ī′sō-ă-glū′ti-nin). An isoantibody that causes agglutination of cells of genetically different members of the same species. SYN isohemagglutinin.

iso·ag·glu·tin·o·gen (ī′sō-ă-glū-tin′ō-jen). An isoantigen that induces agglutination of the cells to which it is attached upon exposure to its specific isoantibody.

iso·al·lele (ī′sō-ă-lēl′). One of a number of alleles that can be distinguished only by special analyses.

iso·al·lox·a·zine (ī′sō-ă-loks′ă-zēn). The heterocyclic compound of riboflavin and other flavins.

iso·am·i·nile (ī-sō-am′i-nīl). 4-(Dimethylamino)-2-isopropyl-2-phenylvaleronitrile; an antitussive agent.

iso·am·yl (ī-sō-am′il). SEE amyl.

iso·am·y·lase (ī-sō-am′il-ās). A hydrolase that cleaves 1,6-α-D-glucosidic branch linkages in glycogen, amylopectin, and their β-limit dextrins; part of the complex known as debranching enzyme; similar to α-dextrin endo-1,6-α-glucosidase but unable to act on pullulan.

iso·an·dros·ter·one (ī′sō-an-dros′ter-ōn). SYN epiandrosterone.

iso·an·ti·body (ī′sō-an′ti-bod-ē). **1.** An antibody that occurs only in some individuals of a species and reacts specifically with a particular foreign isoantigen. For specific i.'s of blood groups, see the Blood Groups appendix. **2.** Sometimes used as a synonym of alloantibody. [G. *isos,* equal]

iso·an·ti·gen (ī′sō-an′ti-jen). **1.** An antigenic substance that occurs only in some individuals of a species, such as the blood group antigens of humans. For specific i.'s of blood groups, see the Blood Groups appendix. **2.** Sometimes used as a synonym of alloantigen.

iso·bar (ī′sō-bar). **1.** One of two or more nuclides having the same total number of protons plus neutrons, but with different distribution; *e.g.,* argon-40 with 18 protons and 22 neutrons, potassium-40 with 19 protons and 21 neutrons, calcium-40 with 20 protons and 20 neutrons. The product of a β-disintegration is an i. of its parent. **2.** The line on a map connecting points of equal barometric pressure. [iso- + G. *baros,* weight]

iso·bar·ic (ī-sō-bar′ik). **1.** Having equal weights or pressures. **2.** With respect to solutions, having the same density as the diluent or medium; *e.g.,* in spinal anesthesia, an i. solution has the same specific gravity as has spinal fluid.

iso·bes·tic (ī-sō-bes′tik). Erroneous spelling of isosbestic.

iso·bor·nyl thi·o·cy·a·no·ac·e·tate (ī-sō-bōr′nil thī-ō-sī′ă-nō-as′ĕ-tāt). C₁₃H₁₉NO₂S; a pediculicide.

iso·bu·tane (ī′sō-byū′tān). SEE butane.

iso·bu·te·ine (ī-sō-byū-tē-ēn). *S*-(2-Carboxypropyl)cysteine; a sulfur-containing compound in urine.

iso·bu·tyl al·co·hol (ī-sō-byū′til). SEE *butyl* alcohol.

iso·bu·tyl ni·trite. A liquid present in commercial amyl nitrite, with similar antispasmodic and vasodilator properties.

iso·bu·tyr·ic ac·id (ī′sō-byū-tir′ik). SEE butyric acid.

iso·bu·zole (ī-sō-byū′zōl). *N*-(5-Isobutyl-1,3,4-thiadiazol-2-yl)-

p-methoxybenzenesulfonamide; an oral hypoglycemic agent for the treatment of diabetes mellitus. SYN glysobuzole.

iso·cap·nia (ī-sō-kap′nē-ă). A state in which the arterial carbon dioxide pressure remains constant or unchanged. [iso- + G. *kapnos,* vapor]

iso·car·box·az·id (ī′sō-kar-bok′să-zid). 1-Benzyl-2-(5-methyl-3-isoxazolylcarbonyl)hydrazine; a monoamine oxidase inhibitor used in the treatment of depressive disorders.

iso·cel·lu·lar (ī′sō-sel′yū-lăr). Composed of cells of equal size or of similar character. [iso- + L. *cellula,* dim. of *cella,* a storeroom]

iso·chor·ic (ī′sō-kōr′ik). SYN isovolumic. [iso- + G. *chōra,* space]

iso·chro·mat·ic (ī-sō-krō-mat′ik). **1.** Of uniform color. SYN isochrous. **2.** Denoting two objects of the same color. [iso- + G. *chrōma,* color]

iso·chro·mat·o·phil, iso·chro·mat·o·phile (ī′sō-krō-mat′ō-fil, fīl). Having an equal affinity for the same dye; said of cells or tissues. [iso- + G. *chrōma,* color, + *philos,* fond]

iso·chro·mo·some (ī′sō-krō′mō-sōm). A chromosomal aberration that arises as a result of transverse rather than longitudinal division of the centromere during meiosis; two daughter chromosomes are formed, each lacking one chromosome arm but with the other doubled.

iso·chro·nia (ī-sō-krō′nē-ă). **1.** The state of having the same chronaxie. **2.** Agreement, with respect to time, rate, or frequency, between processes. [iso- + G. *chronos,* time]

isoch·ro·nous (ī-sok′rŏ-nŭs). Occurring during the same time.

isoch·ro·ous (ī-sok′rŏ-ŭs). SYN isochromatic (1).

iso·cit·rase, iso·cit·ra·tase (ī-sō-sit′rās, -sit′ră-tās). SYN *isocitrate* lyase.

iso·ci·trate. (ī-sŝit′rāt) A salt or ester of isocitric acid.
i. dehydrogenase, one of two enzymes that catalyze the conversion of *threo*-Dₛ-isocitrate, the product of the action of both aconitase and isocitrate lyase, to α-ketoglutarate (2-oxoglutarate) and CO_2; one of the isozymes uses NAD^+ (participating in the tricarboxylic acid cycle) while the other uses $NADP^+$. SYN isocitric acid dehydrogenase, oxalosuccinic carboxylase.
i. lyase, an enzyme that catalyzes the reversible aldol condensation of glyoxylate and succinate, forming *threo*-Dₛ-isocitrate; participates in the glyoxylate cycle. SYN isocitrase, isocitratase, isocitritase.

iso·cit·ric ac·id (ī-sō-sit′rik). $HOOCCH_2CH(COOH)CH(OH)COOH$; an intermediate in the tricarboxylic acid cycle.
i. a. dehydrogenase, SYN *isocitrate* dehydrogenase.

iso·cit·ri·tase (ī-sō-sit′ri-tās). SYN *isocitrate* lyase.

iso·cline (ī′sō-klīn). A line in a geographical region that joins all points at which in a population there is the same average frequency for the various alleles at a genetic locus. SEE ALSO cline. [iso- + G. *klinō,* to slope]

iso·con·a·zole (ī′sō-kō′nă-zōl). Antibacterial and antifungal agent related to ketoconazole and oxiconazole.

iso·co·ria (ī-sō-kō′rē-ă). Equality in the size of the two pupils. [iso- + G. *korē,* pupil]

iso·cor·tex (ī-sō-kōr′teks). O. and C. Vogt's term for the larger part of the mammalian cerebral cortex, distinguished from the allocortex by being composed of a larger number of nerve cells arranged in six layers. SEE ALSO cerebral *cortex.* SYN homotypic cortex, neocortex, neopallium.

iso·cy·a·nate (ī-sō-sī′ă-nāt). The radical –N=C=O from isocyanic acid.

iso·cy·an·ic ac·id (ī-sō-sī′ă-nik). HNCO; a highly reactive chemical.

iso·cy·a·nide (ī-sō-sī′ă-nīd). The radical –NC; organic i.'s are called isonitriles.

iso·cy·tol·y·sin (ī′sō-sī-tol′i-sin). A cytolysin that reacts with the cells of certain other animals of the same species, but not with the cells of the individual that formed the i.

iso·dac·tyl·ism (ī-sō-dak′ti-lizm). Condition in which the fingers or toes are all approximately of equal length. [iso- + G. *daktylos,* finger]

iso·dense (ī′sō-dens). Denoting a tissue having a radiopacity (radiodensity) similar to that of another or adjacent tissue.

iso·des·mo·sine (ī-sō-des′mō-sēn). A cross-linking amino acid formed from lysyl residues; found in elastin.

iso·dul·cit (ī-sō-dŭl′sit). SYN L-rhamnose.

iso·dy·nam·ic (ī′sō-dī-nam′ik). **1.** Of equal force or strength. **2.** Relating to foods or other materials that liberate the same amount of energy on combustion. [iso- + G. *dynamis,* force]

iso·dy·na·mo·gen·ic (ī′sō-dī-nă-mō-jen′ik, -dī-nam′ō-). **1.** SYN isoenergetic. **2.** Producing equal nerve force. [iso- + G. *dynamis,* force, + *-gen,* producing]

iso·e·lec·tric (ī′sō-ē-lek′trik). Of equal electrical potential. Cf. isoelectric *point.* SYN isopotential.
i. focusing, electrophoresis of small molecules or macromolecules in a pH gradient.

iso·en·er·get·ic (ī′sō-en-er-jet′ik). Exerting equal force; equally active. SYN isodynamogenic (1).

iso·en·zyme (ī-sō-en′zīm). One of a group of enzymes that catalyze the same reaction but may be differentiated by variations in physical properties, such as isoelectric point, electrophoretic mobility, kinetic parameters, or modes of regulation; *e.g.,* lactate dehydrogenase, a tetramer composed of varying amounts of α and β subunits (*i.e.,* 4α; 3α + 1β; 2α + 2β; 1α + 3β; and 4β). SYN isozyme.
creatine kinase i.'s, the isoenzymes of creatine kinase. Creatine kinase is a dimer with M (muscle) and/or B (brain) subunits; it exists in three isoenzyme forms: CK-MM, the predominant form, found primarily in skeletal muscle; CK-MB, found in cardiac muscle, tongue, diaphragm, and in small amounts in skeletal muscle; and CK-BB found in the brain, smooth muscle, thyroid, lungs, and prostate. Elevations detected by electrophoresis or other methodologies can be used to help in the differential diagnosis of a variety of disease states, with CK-MB elevations as an important marker following myocardial infarctions, elevations in CK-MM an indicator of muscle disease, and increases in CK-BB an occasional finding following brain infarcts, bowel infarcts, or in the presence of certain malignancies.

iso·e·ryth·rol·y·sis (ī′sō-ĕ-rith-rol′i-sis). Destruction of erythrocytes by isoantibodies. [iso- + erythrocyte = G. *lysis,* dissolution]
neonatal i., (1) i. in the newborn animal; **(2)** hemolytic icterus of the newborn.

iso·eth·a·rine (ī-sō-eth′ă-rēn). α-(1-Isopropylaminopropyl)-protocatechuyl alcohol; a bronchodilator for the treatment of bronchial asthma; it possesses actions similar to metaproterenol.

iso·flu·or·phate (ī-sō-flūr′fāt). $[(CH_3)_2CH–O]_2P(O)F$; a toxic cholinergic agent that acts by irreversible inhibition of cholinesterase; an ophthalmic cholinergic agent; also used in biochemical research as an enzyme inhibitor. SYN diisopropyl fluorophosphate.

iso·flu·rane (ī-sō-flūr′ān). 1-Chloro-2,2,2-trifluoroethyl difluoromethyl ether; a nonflammable, nonexplosive, halogenated ether with potent anesthetic action; an isomer of enflurane.

iso·ga·mete (ī-sō-gam′ēt). **1.** One of two or more similar cells that conjugate or fuse and subsequently divide, resulting in reproduction. **2.** A gamete of the same size as the gamete with which it unites. [iso- + G. *gametēs* or *gametē,* husband or wife]

isog·a·my (ī-sog′ă-mē). Conjugation between two equal gametes or two individual cells alike in all respects. [iso- + G. *gamos,* marriage]

iso·ge·ne·ic, iso·gen·ic (ī′sō-jĕ-nē′ik, -jen′ik). SYN syngeneic.

isog·e·nous (ī-soj′ĕ-nŭs). Of the same origin, as in development from the same tissue or cell. [iso- + G. *genos,* family, kind]

iso·gen·ti·o·bi·ose (ī′sō-jen-shi-ō-bī′ōs). SYN isomaltose.

iso·glu·ta·mine (ī-sō-glū′tă-mēn). $H_2NCO–CH(NH_3^+)-CH_2CH_2COO^-$; a glutamic amide.

iso·gna·thous (ī-sog′nā-thŭs). Having jaws of approximately the same width. [iso- + G. *gnathos,* jaw]

iso·graft (ī′sō-graft). SYN syngraft.

iso·he·mag·glu·ti·na·tion (ī′sō-hē′mă-glū′ti-nā′shŭn). SYN isoagglutination. [iso- + G. *haima,* blood, + L. *ad,* to, + *gluten,* glue]

iso·he·mag·glu·ti·nin (ī′sō-hē′mă-glū′ti-nin). SYN isoagglutinin.

iso·he·mo·ly·sin (ī′sō-hē-mol′i-sin). An isolysin that reacts with red blood cells.

iso·he·mol·y·sis (ī′sō-hē-mol′i-sis). A form of isolysis in which there is dissolution of red blood cells as a result of the reaction between an isolysin (isohemolysin) and specific antigen in or on the cells. [iso- + G. *haima,* blood, + *lysis,* dissolution]

iso·hy·dric (ī-sō-hī′drik). Denoting two substances possessing the same pH.

iso·hy·dru·ria (ī′sō-hī-drū′rē-ă). Fixation of the pH of the urine without the usual variation. [iso- + G. *hydor,* water, + *ouron,* urine, + -ia]

iso·hy·per·cy·to·sis (ī′sō-hī-per-sī-tō′sis). Obsolete term for a condition in which the number of leukocytes in the circulating blood is increased, but the relative proportions of the various types (especially the granulocytes) are within the usual range. [iso- + G. *hyper,* above, + *kytos,* cell, + -*osis,* condition]

iso·hy·po·cy·to·sis (ī′sō-hī-pō-sī-tō′sis). Obsolete term for a condition in which there is an abnormally small number of leukocytes in the circulating blood, but the relative proportions of the various types (especially the granulocytes) are within the usual range. [iso- + G. *hypo,* below, + *kytos,* cell, + -*osis,* condition]

iso·im·mu·ni·za·tion (ī′sō-im′yū-nī-zā′shŭn). Development of a significant titer of specific antibody as a result of antigenic stimulation with material contained on or in the red blood cells of another individual of the same species; *e.g.,* i. is likely to occur when an Rh-negative person is treated with a transfusion of Rh-positive blood from another human being, or an Rh-negative woman has a pregnancy in which the fetus inherits Rh-positive red blood cells.

iso·late (ī′sō-lāt). **1.** To separate, to set apart others; that which is so treated. **2.** To free of chemical contaminants. **3.** In psychoanalysis, to separate experiences or memories from the affects pertaining to them. **4.** In group psychotherapy an individual who is not responded to by others in the group. **5.** Viable organisms separated on a single occasion from a field sample in experimental hosts, culture systems, or stabilates. **6.** A population that for geographic, linguistic, cultural, social, religious, or other reasons is subject to little or no gene flow. SYN genetic i. [It. *isolare;* Mediev. L. *insulo,* pp. -*atus,* to insulate, fr. L. *insula,* island]

genetic i., SYN isolate (6).

mating i., a population separated from its neighbors by any means so that all or most matings occur within the population group.

iso·la·tion. 1. In microbiology, separation of an organism from others, usually by making serial cultures. **2.** Separation for the period of communicability of infected persons or animals from others, so as to prevent or limit the direct or indirect transmission of the infectious agent from those who are infected to those who are susceptible.

iso·lec·i·thal (ī-sō-les′i-thăl). Denoting an ovum in which there is a moderate amount of uniformly distributed yolk.

iso·leu·cine (I) (ī-sō-lū′sēn). $CH_3CH_2CH(CH_3)CH-$ (NH_3^+) COO^-; 2-amino-3-methylvaleric acid; the L-amino acid found in almost all proteins; an isomer of leucine and, like it, a dietary essential amino acid.

iso·leu·cyl (ī-sō-lū′sil). The acyl radical of isoleucine.

iso·leu·ko·ag·glu·ti·nin (ī′sō-lū′kō-ă-glū′ti-nin). Naturally occurring abnormal antibody in the blood of some persons with certain conditions, capable of agglutinating human leukocytes.

isol·o·gous (ī-sol′ō-gŭs). SYN syngeneic. [iso- + G. *logos,* ratio]

isol·y·sin (ī-sol′i-sin). An antibody that combines with, sensitizes, and results in complement-fixation and dissolution of cells that contain the specific isoantigen; i.'s occur in the blood of some members of a species and they react with the cells of that species, but not with the cells of the individual (or the same type) in which the i.'s are naturally formed.

isol·y·sis (ī-sol′i-sis). Lysis or dissolution of cells as a result of the reaction between an isolysin and specific antigen in or on the cells. SEE ALSO isohemolysis. [iso- + G. *lysis,* dissolution]

iso·lyt·ic (ī-sō-lit′ik). Pertaining to, characterized by, or causing isolysis.

iso·malt·ase (ī-sō-mal′tās). SYN oligo-α1,6-glucosidase. SEE ALSO sucrose α-D-glucohydrolase.

iso·malt·ose (ī-sō-mal′tōs). A disaccharide in which two glucose molecules are attached by an α1,6 link, rather than an α1,4 link as in maltose. SYN isogentiobiose.

iso·mas·ti·gote (ī-sō-mas′ti-gōt). Denoting a protozoan having two or four flagella of equal length at one extremity. [iso- + G. *mastix,* whip]

iso·mer (ī′sō-mer). **1.** One of two or more substances displaying isomerism; *e.g.,* L-glucose and D-glucose or citrate and isocitrate. Cf. stereoisomer. **2.** One of two or more nuclides having the same atomic and mass numbers but differing in energy states for a finite period of time; *e.g.,* ^{99m}Tc and ^{99}Tc. [iso- + G. *meros,* part]

geometric i., SEE geometric *isomerism.*

isom·er·ase (ī-som′er-ās). A class of enzymes (EC class 5) catalyzing the conversion of a substance to an isomeric form; *e.g.,* glucosephosphate isomerase.

iso·mer·ic (ī-sō-mār′ik). Relating to or characterized by isomerism. SYN isomerous.

isom·er·ism (ī-som′er-izm). The existence of a chemical compound in two or more forms that are identical with respect to percentage composition but differ as to the positions of one or more atoms within the molecules, and also in physical and chemical properties.

geometric i., a form of i. displayed by unsaturated or ring compounds where free rotation about a bond (usually a carbon-carbon bond) is restricted; *e.g.,* the i. of a *cis-* or *trans-* compound as in oleic acid and elaidic acid. Cf. cis-, entgegen, trans-, zusammen.

optical i., stereoisomerism involving the arrangement of substituents about an asymmetric atom or atoms (usually carbon) so that there is a difference in the behavior of the various isomers with regard to the extent of their rotation of the plane of polarized light. Cf. stereoisomerism.

stereochemical i., SYN stereoisomerism.

structural i., i. involving the same atoms in different arrangements; *e.g.,* butyric acids, leucine and isoleucine, glucose and fructose.

isom·er·i·za·tion (ī-som′er-ī-zā′shŭn). A process in which one isomer is formed from another, as in the action of isomerases.

enzyme i., reversible changes in enzyme conformation.

isom·er·ous (ī-som′er-ŭs). SYN isomeric.

iso·meth·a·done (ī-sō-meth′ă-dōn). 6-(Dimethylamino)-5-methyl-4,4-diphenyl-3-hexanone; a narcotic analgesic.

iso·meth·ep·tene (ī′sō-meth-ep′ten). *N,*1,5-Trimethyl-4-hexenylamine; an unsaturated aliphatic sympathomimetic amine with antispasmodic and vasoconstrictor actions.

iso·met·ric (ī-sō-met′rik). **1.** Of equal dimensions. **2.** In physiology, denoting the condition when the ends of a contracting muscle are held fixed so that contraction produces increased tension at a constant overall length. Cf. auxotonic, isotonic (3), isovolumic. [iso- + G. *metron,* measure]

iso·me·tro·pia (ī′sō-me-trō′pē-ă). Equality in refraction in the two eyes. [iso- + G. *metron,* measure, + *ōps* (*ōp-*), eye]

iso·mor·phic (ī-sō-mōr′fik). SYN isomorphous.

iso·mor·phism (ī-sō-mōr′fizm). Similarity of form between two or more organisms or between parts of the body. [iso- + G. *morphē,* shape]

iso·mor·phous (ī-sō-mōr′fŭs). Having the same form or shape, or being morphologically equal. SYN isomorphic.

iso·naph·thol (ī-sō-naf′thol). SEE naphthol.

ison·cot·ic (ī-son-kot′ik). Of equal oncotic pressure.

iso·ni·a·zid (ī-sō-nī′ă-zid). $C_6H_7N_3O$; isonicotinic acid hydrazide; a compound effective in the treatment of tuberculosis.

iso·nic·o·tin·ic ac·id (ī-sō-nik-ō-tin′ik). 4-Pyridinecarboxylic acid; its hydrazide is isoniazid.

iso·ni·trile (ī-sō-nī′tril). An organic isocyanide.

iso·ni·tro·so·ac·e·tone (ī′sō-nī-trō-sō-as′ĕ-tōn). $CH_3CO-CH=$

NOH; propanone 1-oxine; a cholinesterase reactivator that can penetrate the blood-brain barrier readily and cause significant reactivation of phosphorylated acetylcholinesterase in the central nervous system; used to protect human beings and animals against otherwise lethal poisoning with organophosphorous anticholinesterase agents. SYN monoisonitrosoacetone, pyruvaldoxine.

iso·nor·mo·cy·to·sis (ī′sō-nōr-mō-sī-tō′sis). Obsolete term for a condition in which the actual number and the relative proportions of the various types of leukocytes in the circulating blood are within normal range. [iso- + L. *norma*, rule, + G. *kytos*, cell, + *-osis*, condition]

iso-os·mot·ic (ī′sō-os-mot′ik). SYN isosmotic.

isop·a·thy (ī-sop′ă-thē). Treatment of disease by means of the causal agent or a product of the same disease; or treatment of a diseased organ by an extract of a similar organ from a healthy animal. SEE ALSO homeopathy. [iso- + G. *pathos*, suffering]

iso·pen·ten·yl·py·ro·phos·phate (ī-sō-pen-tēn-il′pī-rō-fos′fāt). H₂C=C(CH₃)CH₂CH₂OP₂O₆²⁻; an intermediate in the biosynthesis of steroids, terpenes, dolichol, and prenylated proteins.

iso·pen·tyl (ī-sō-pen′til). SEE amyl.

iso·pep·tide (ī-sō-pep′tīd). SEE isopeptide *bond*.

isoph·a·gy (ī-sof′ă-jē). SYN autolysis. [iso- + G. *phagō*, to eat]

iso·plas·sonts (ī-sō-plas′onts). Like-formed entities having certain features in common. [iso- + G. *plassō*, to form]

iso·plas·tic (ī-sō-plas′tik). SYN syngeneic. [iso- + G. *plassō*, to form]

iso·pleth (ī′sō-pleth). A line on a Cartesian nomogram consisting of all points that represent a particular value of a variable; *e.g.*, an isobar is an i. for a particular pressure.

iso·po·ten·tial (ī′sō-pō-ten′chŭl). SYN isoelectric.

iso·pre·cip·i·tin (ī′sō-prē-sip′i-tin). An antibody that combines with and precipitates soluble antigenic material in the plasma or serum, or in an extract of the cells, from another member, but not all members, of the same species. [iso- + precipitin]

iso·pren·a·line hy·dro·chlo·ride (ī-sō-pren′ă-lēn). SYN isoproterenol hydrochloride.

iso·pren·a·line sul·fate. SYN isoproterenol sulfate.

iso·prene (ī′sō-prēn). CH₂=CH–C(CH₃)=CH₂; 2-methyl-1,3-butadiene; an unsaturated five-carbon hydrocarbon with a branched chain, which in the plant and animal kingdom is used as the basis for the formation of isoprenoids; *e.g.*, terpenes, carotenoids and related pigments, rubber. Fat-soluble vitamins either are isoprenoid or have isoprenoid side chains; steroids are synthesized via isoprenoid intermediates as are ubiquinone, dolichol, and prenylated proteins.

iso·pre·noids (ī-sō-prēn′oydz). Polymers whose carbon skeletons consist in whole or in large part of isoprene units joined end to end; *e.g.*, carotene, lycopene, vitamin A. Vitamins K and E and the coenzymes Q have isoprenoid side chains.

iso·pre·nyla·tion (ī-sō-pren′il-ā′shun). SYN prenylation. SEE prenylation.

iso·pro·pa·mide io·dide (ī-sō-prō′pă-mīd). (3-Carbamoyl-3,3-diphenylpropyl)diisopropylmethylammonium iodide; an anticholinergic agent.

iso·pro·pa·nol (ī-sō-prō′pă-nol). SYN isopropyl alcohol.

iso·pro·phen·a·mine hy·dro·chlo·ride (ī′sō-prō-fen′ă-mēn). SYN clorprenaline hydrochloride.

iso·pro·pyl al·co·hol (ī-sō-prō′pil). (CH₃)₂CHOH; an isomer of propyl alcohol and a homologue of ethyl alcohol, similar in its properties, when used externally, to the latter, but more toxic when taken internally; used as an ingredient of various cosmetics and of medicinal preparations for external use; also available as isopropyl rubbing alcohol, which contains 68 to 72% of isopropyl alcohol (by volume) in water; used as a rubefacient. SYN dimethylcarbinol, isopropanol.

iso·pro·pyl·ar·te·re·nol hy·dro·chlo·ride (ī-sō-prō′pil-ar-ter′ĕ-nol). SYN isoproterenol hydrochloride.

iso·pro·pyl·car·bi·nol (ī′sō-prō-pil-kar′bin-ol). SEE butyl alcohol.

iso·pro·pyl myr·is·tate (ī-sō-prō′pil). A pharmaceutic aid used

in topical medicinal preparations to promote absorption through the skin.

iso·pro·pyl·thi·o·ga·lac·to·side (iPrSGal, IPTG) (ī-sō-pro′pil-thī′ō-gă-lak′tō-sīd). An artificial galactoside capable of inducing β-galactosidase in *Escherichia coli* without being split, as are the natural substrates such as lactose.

iso·pro·te·re·nol hy·dro·chlo·ride (ī′sō-prō-ter′ĕ-nol). 3,4-Dihydroxy-α-[(isopropylamino)methyl]benzyl alcohol hydrochloride; a sympathomimetic β-receptor stimulant possessing the cardiac excitatory, but not the vasoconstrictor, actions of epinephrine. Chemically it differs from epinephrine in having an isopropyl group replacing the methyl group attached to the nitrogen atom; used in the treatment of bronchial asthma and heart block, including Adams-Stokes attacks. SYN isoprenaline hydrochloride, isopropylarterenol hydrochloride.

iso·pro·te·re·nol sul·fate. Used for inhalation as an aerosol in the treatment of acute asthmatic attacks and chronic pulmonary emphysema. SYN isoprenaline sulfate.

isop·ter (ī-sop′ter). A line of equal retinal sensitivity in the visual field. [iso- + G. *optēr*, observer]

iso·pyk·nic (ī-sō-pik′nik). Having the same density. [iso- + G. *phknos*, thick, dense, + -ic]

iso·py·ro·cal·cif·er·ol (ī-sō-pī′rō-cal-sif′er-ol). 9β-Ergosterol; a thermal decomposition product of calciferol; a stereoisomer of pyrocalciferol and ergosterol.

iso·quin·o·line (ī-sō-kwin′ō-lēn). **1.** Benzo[*c*]pyridine; ring structure is characteristic of the group of opium alkaloids represented by papaverine. **2.** A class of alkaloids containing the i. (1) ring structure.

iso·ri·bo·fla·vin (ī′sō-rī′bō-flā-vin). 8-Demethyl-6-methylriboflavin; a riboflavin antimetabolite, differing from riboflavin in that the methyl groups on the isoalloxazine nucleus are in the 6,7 positions rather than the 7,8.

isor·rhea (ī-sō-rē′ă). Equality of intake and output of water; maintenance of water equilibrium. [iso- + G. *rhoia*, a flow]

isos·best·ic (ī-sos-bes′tik). Denoting the wavelength of light at which two related compounds have identical extinction coefficients; *e.g.*, the wavelength at which the absorption spectra of hemoglobin and oxyhemoglobin cross is their i. point. Spectrophotometry at that wavelength measures total concentration of hemoglobin, regardless of the extent to which it might be oxygenated. [Ger. *isosbestisch*, fr. G. *isos*, equal, + *sbestos*, extinguished]

iso·schiz·o·mer (ī-sō′-skiz′ō-mer). A restriction endonuclease from different organisms that recognizes and hydrolyzes at the same DNA sequence. [jiso- + G. *schizō* to split, + -mer]

iso·sen·si·tize (ī-sō-sen′si-tīz). SYN autosensitize.

iso·sex·u·al (ī-sō-sek′shū-ăl). **1.** Relating to the existence of characteristics or feelings of both sexes in one person. **2.** Descriptive of an individual's somatic characteristics, or of processes occurring within, that are consonant with the sex of that individual.

is·os·mot·ic (ī′sos-mot′ik). Having the same total osmotic pressure or osmolality as another fluid (ordinarily intracellular fluid); such a fluid is not isosmotic if it includes solutes that freely permeate cell membranes. SYN iso-osmotic.

iso·sor·bide. A compound with diuretic properties prepared by acid dehydration of D-glucitol.

iso·sor·bide di·ni·trate (ī-sō-sōr′bīd dī-nī′trāt). 1,4:3,6-Dianhydro-D-glucitol dinitrate; a coronary vasodilator; large doses may produce headache, flushing of the face, fainting, and methemoglobinemia.

Isos·po·ra (ī-sos′pō-ră). A genus of coccidia (family Eimeriidae, class Sporozoea), with species chiefly in mammals; the ripe oocysts contain two sporocysts, each of which contains four sporozoites. This genus is now known to be closely related to *Toxoplasma* and *Sarcocystis*, with a similar sexual phase in the life cycle and a similar apical complex. [iso- + G. *sporos*, seed]

I. bel′li, a relatively rare species occurring in the small intestine of man, most common in the tropics but probably of worldwide distribution; most infections are subclinical, but sometimes they may cause mucous diarrhea.

I. bigem'ina, a species that occurs in the small intestine of the dog, cat, fox, mink, and possibly other carnivores; the most pathogenic coccidium in dogs and cats, causing enteritis and diarrhea; the oocysts are usually sporulated when passed in the feces, but are indistinguishable from those of *Toxoplasma gondii,* so considerable question remains as to the status of these parasites.

I. ca'nis, a species of worldwide distribution that is mildly pathogenic in dogs and is not infective in cats.

I. fe'lis, a species found in the small intestine and sometimes the cecum and colon of cats, lions, and other felids; it is only slightly, if at all, pathogenic in cats and is not infective in dogs.

I. rivol'ta, a species that occurs in the small intestine of dogs, cats, dingos, and probably other wild carnivores; pathogenic capabilities are similar to those of *I. bigemina.*

I. su'is, a species that affects the small intestine of the pig, producing mild diarrhea.

isos·po·ri·a·sis (ī-sos-pō-rī′ă-sis). Disease caused by infection with a species of *Isospora,* such as *I. belli* of humans; human disease usually is mild except in cases of immunosuppression, as in AIDS, where it may cause an intractable diarrhea.

iso·stere (ī′sō-stēr). One of two or more atoms or molecules having the same electron arrangement; *e.g.,* N_2 and CO. [iso- + G. *stereos,* solid]

iso·stery (ī-sō-stēr′ē). Physiological enzyme or metabolic regulation via competitive inhibition by structural analogs of natural substrates.

isos·the·nu·ria (ī-sos′thē-nū′rē-ă, ī′sō-sthē-). A state in chronic renal disease in which the kidney cannot form urine with a higher or a lower specific gravity than that of protein-free plasma; specific gravity of the urine becomes fixed around 1.010, irrespective of the fluid intake. [iso- + G. *sthenos,* strength, + *ouron,* urine]

iso·suc·cin·ic ac·id (ī′sō-sŭk-sin′ik). SYN methylmalonic acid.

iso·sul·fa·mer·a·zine (ī′sō-sŭl-fă-mer′ă-zēn). SYN sulfaperin.

iso·sul·fan blue (ī-sō-sŭl′fan). $C_{27}H_{31}N_2NaO_6S_2$; a dye used as a radiographic adjunct to mark lymphatic vessels during lymphography.

iso·ther·mal (ī-sō-ther′măl). Having the same temperature. [iso- + G. *thermē,* heat]

iso·thi·o·cy·a·nate (ī′sō-thī-ō-sī′ă-nāt). The radical of isothiocyanic acid, –N=C=S.

iso·thi·pen·dyl (ī′sō-thī-pen′dil). 10-(2-Dimethylamino-2-methylethyl)-10*H*-pyrido[3,2-*b*][1,4]benzothiazine; an antihistaminic.

iso·tone (ī′sō-tōn). One of several nuclides having the same number of neutrons in their nuclei; *e.g.,* $^{39}_{19}K$ and $^{40}_{20}Ca$ with 20 each, $^{56}_{26}Fe$ and $^{58}_{28}Ni$ with 30 each. [iso- + G. *tonos,* stretching, tension]

iso·to·nia (ī-sō-tō′nē-ă). A condition of tonic equality in which tension or osmotic pressure in two substances or solutions is the same. [iso- + G. *tonos,* tension]

iso·ton·ic (ī-sō-ton′ik). **1.** Relating to isotonicity or isotonia. **2.** Having equal tension; denoting solutions possessing the same osmotic pressure; more specifically, limited to solutions in which cells neither swell nor shrink. Thus, a solution that is isosmotic with intracellular fluid will not be i. if it includes solute, such as urea, that freely permeates cell membranes. **3.** In physiology, denoting the condition when a contracting muscle shortens against a constant load, as when lifting a weight. Cf. auxotonic, isometric (2).

iso·to·nic·i·ty (ī-sō-tō-nis′i-tē). **1.** The quality of possessing and maintaining a uniform tone or tension. **2.** The property of a solution in being isotonic.

iso·tope (ī′sō-tōp). One of two or more nuclides that are chemically identical, having the same number of protons, yet differ in mass number, since their nuclei contain different numbers of neutrons; individual i.'s are named with the inclusion of their mass number in the superior position (^{12}C) and the atomic number (nuclear protons) in the inferior position ($_6C$). In former usage, the mass numbers follow the chemical symbol (C-12). [iso- + G. *topos,* part, place]

daughter i., an element produced by radioactive decay of another. SEE radionuclide *generator,* cow.

radioactive i., an i. with an unstable nuclear composition; such nuclei decompose spontaneously by emission of a nuclear electron (β particle) or helium nucleus (α particle) and radiation (γ rays), thus achieving a stable nuclear composition; used as tracers, and as radiation and energy sources. SEE half-life.

stable i., a nonradioactive nuclide; an i. that shows no tendency to undergo radioactive decomposition.

iso·to·pic (ī-sō-top′ik). Of identical chemical composition but differing in some physical property, such as atomic weight.

iso·trans·plan·ta·tion (ī′sō-tranz-plan-tā′shŭn). Transfer of an isograft (syngraft).

iso·tret·i·noin (ī-sō-tret′i-noyn). 13-*cis*-Retinoic acid; a retinoid used for treatment of severe recalcitrant cystic acne; a known human teratogen.

iso·tro·pic, isot·ro·pous (ī-sō-trop′ik, ī-sot′rō-pŭs). Having properties which are the same in all directions. [iso- + G. *tropē,* a turn]

iso·type (ī′sō-tīp). An antigenic determinant (marker) that occurs in all members of a subclass of an immunoglobulin class. Whereas a given allotypic marker or determinant is thought to occur in only one subclass, an antigenic marker that is isotypic in one subclass may also occur as an allotypic marker in another subclass. [iso- + G. *typos,* model]

»nuclide chart«

isotopes

iso·typ·ic (ī-sō-tip′ik). Pertaining to an isotype.

iso·va·ler·ic ac·id (ī′so-vă-lār′ik, -lēr′ik). $(CH_3)_2CHCH_2COOH$; 3-Methylbutyric acid; a metabolic intermediate in oxidative processes; elevated in cases of isovaleric acidemia.

iso·va·ler·ic ac·i·de·mia [MIM*243500]. A disorder of leucine metabolism characterized by the excessive production of isovaleric acid upon protein ingestion or during infectious episodes; severe metabolic acidosis results from the large quantities of acid formed; autosomal recessive inheritance; due to a deficiency of isovaleryl-CoA dehydrogenase. SYN sweaty feet syndrome.

iso·va·ler·yl-CoA (ī-sō-văl′er-il). The condensation product of isovaleric acid and coenzyme A; an intermediate in the catabolism of L-leucine. SYN isovalerylcoenzyme A.

i.-CoA dehydrogenase, an enzyme that participates in the catabolism of L-leucine; it converts i.-CoA to 3-methylcrotonyl-CoA using FAD; a deficiency in this enzyme will result in isovaleric acidemia.

iso·va·ler·yl·co·en·zyme A. SYN isovaleryl-CoA.

iso·val·thine (ī-sō-val′thēn). $(CH_3)_2CHCH(COOH)–S–CH_2CH(NH_2)COOH$; *S*-(1-carboxy-2-methylpropyl)-L-cysteine; a sulfur-containing compound found in urine.

iso·vol·ume (ī-sō-vol′yūm). At the same or equal volume. SEE ALSO isovolumic.

iso·vol·u·met·ric (ī′sō-vol-yū-met′rik). SYN isovolumic.

iso·vol·u·mic (ī′sō-vol-yū′mik). Occurring without an associated alteration in volume, as when, in early ventricular systole, the muscle fibers initially increase their tension without shortening so that ventricular volume remains unaltered. SEE ALSO isometric. SYN isochoric, isovolumetric.

iso·xi·cam (ī-soks′i-kam). Nonsteroidal anti-inflammatory drug with antipyretic and analgesic properties; resembles piroxicam.

is

isox·sup·rine hy·dro·chlo·ride (ī-soks'sū-prēn). 1-(*p*-Hydrox-yphenyl)-2-[(1'-methyl- 2'-phenoxy)ethylamino]-1-propanol hy-drochloride; sympathomimetic amine with potent inhibitory effects on vascular, uterine, and other smooth muscles; used as a vasodilator in various vascular diseases and as a uterine relaxant.

iso·zyme (ī'sō-zīm). SYN isoenzyme.

is·sue (ish'ū). Archaic term for a discharge of pus, blood, or other matter. [Fr. a going out]

nature-nurture i., a controversy concerning the relative importance of heredity (nature) and environment (nurture) in various aspects of individual development, such as intelligence, personality, or mental illness.

isth·mec·to·my (is-mek'tō-mē). Excision of the midportion of the thyroid. [G. *isthmos*, isthmus, + *ektomē*, excision]

isth·mic, isth·mi·an (is'mik, is'mē-an). Denoting an anatomical isthmus.

isth·mo·pa·ral·y·sis (is'mō-pă-ral'i-sis). Paralysis of the velum pendulum palati and the muscles forming the anterior pillars of the fauces. SYN faucial paralysis, isthmoplegia. [G. *isthmos*, isthmus, + paralysis]

isth·mo·ple·gia (is'mō-plē'jē-ă). SYN isthmoparalysis. [G. *isthmos*, isthmus, + *plēgē*, stroke]

isth·mus, pl. **isth·mi, isth·mus·es** (is'mŭs, -mī, -mŭs-ez). **1.** A constriction connecting two larger parts of an organ or other anatomical structure. **2.** A narrow passage connecting two larger cavities. **3.** The narrowest portion of the brainstem at the junction between midbrain and hindbrain. [G. *isthmos*]

i. of aorta, a slight constriction of the aorta immediately distal to the left subclavian artery at the point of attachment of the ductus arteriosus. SYN i. aortae [NA].

i. aor'tae [NA], SYN i. of aorta.

i. of auditory tube, the narrowest portion of the auditory tube at the junction of the cartilaginous and bony portions. SYN i. tubae auditivae [NA], i. of eustachian tube.

i. of cartilage of ear, a narrow bridge connecting the cartilage of the external acoustic meatus and the lamina of the tragus with the main portion of the cartilage of the auricle. SYN i. cartilaginis auris [NA].

i. cartilag'inis au'ris [NA], SYN i. of cartilage of ear.

i. of cingulate gyrus, the narrowing of the cingulate gyrus, at its transition with the hippocampal gyrus behind and below the splenium of the corpus callosum, caused by the anterior extension of the conjoined parieto-occipital and calcarine sulci. SYN i. gyri cinguli [NA], i. of gyrus fornicatus, i. of limbic lobe.

i. of eustachian tube, SYN i. of auditory tube.

i. of external acoustic meatus, the narrowest portion of this canal in the bony part near its deep termination. SYN i. meatus acustici externi.

i. of fauces, the constricted and short space which establishes the connection between the cavity of the mouth and the oro-pharynx, bounded anteriorly by the palatoglossal folds and posteriorly by the palatopharyngeal folds; the lateral well is the tonsillar fossa. SYN i. faucium [NA].

i. fau'cium [NA], SYN i. of fauces.

i. glan'dulae thyroid'eae [NA], SYN i. of thyroid.

Guyon's i., SYN i. of uterus.

i. gy'ri cin'guli [NA], SYN i. of cingulate gyrus.

i. of gy'rus fornica'tus, SYN i. of cingulate gyrus.

i. of His, SYN rhombencephalic i.

Krönig's i., the narrow straplike portion of the resonant field that extends over the shoulder, connecting the larger areas of resonance over the pulmonary apex in front and behind.

i. of limbic lobe, SYN i. of cingulate gyrus.

i. mea'tus acus'tici exter'ni, SYN i. of external acoustic meatus.

pharyngeal i., communicating space between nasopharynx and oropharynx, sealed off by elevation of the soft palate and contraction of portions of the superior pharyngeal constrictor (palatopharyngal sphincter) during swallowing.

i. pharyngonasa'lis, SYN choana.

i. pros'tatae [NA], SYN i. of prostate.

i. of prostate, the narrow middle part of the prostate anterior to the urethra. SYN i. prostatae [NA].

i. rhombenceph'ali [NA], SYN rhombencephalic i.

rhombencephalic i., (1) a constriction in the embryonic neural tube delineating the mesencephalon from the rhombencephalon; **(2)** the anterior portion of the rhombencephalon connecting with the mesencephalon. SYN i. rhombencephali [NA], i. of His.

i. of thyroid, the central part of the thyroid gland joining the two lateral lobes. SYN i. glandulae thyroideae [NA].

i. tu'bae auditi'vae [NA], SYN i. of auditory tube.

i. tu'bae uteri'nae [NA], SYN i. of uterine tube.

i. u'teri [NA], SYN i. of uterus.

i. of uterine tube, the narrow portion of the uterine tube adjoining the uterus. SYN i. tubae uterinae [NA].

i. of uterus, an elongated constriction at the junction of the body and cervix of the uterus. SYN i. uteri [NA], Guyon's i., orificium internum uteri, os uteri internum, ostium uteri internum.

Vieussens' i., SYN *limbus* fossae ovalis.

it·a·con·ic ac·id (it'ă-kon'ik). $CH_2=C(COOH)CH_2COOH$; the decarboxylation product of *cis*-aconitic acid. SYN methylenesuccinic acid.

itch. 1. A peculiar irritating sensation in the skin that arouses the desire to scratch. **2.** Common name for scabies. **3.** SYN pruritus (2). SYN pruritus (2). [A.S. *gikkan*]

azo i., itching that occurs among workers in azo dyes.

baker's i., an eruption on the hands and arms of bakers due to an allergic reaction to flour or other substances handled, or to the grain itch mite.

barber's i., SYN *tinea* barbae.

bath i., SYN bath *pruritus*.

coolie i., SYN cutaneous *ancylostomiasis*.

copra i., a dermatitis occurring in workers in copra mills, caused by the presence of a mite, *Tyrophagus putrescentiae*.

Cuban i., SYN alastrim.

dew i., SYN cutaneous *ancylostomiasis*.

dhobie i., SYN *tinea* cruris.

frost i., SYN *dermatitis* hiemalis.

grain i., a cutaneous eruption occasionally noted in farmers and grain handlers, caused by the action of the mite *Pyemotes ventricosus*.

grocer's i., a vesicular dermatitis seen in grocers and bakers who handle sugar or flour; caused by a mite of the genus *Glycophagus*.

ground i., SYN cutaneous *ancylostomiasis*.

jock i., SYN *tinea* cruris.

kabure i., SYN *schistosomiasis* japonica.

lumberman's i., SYN *dermatitis* hiemalis.

mad i., SYN pseudorabies.

Malabar i., SYN *tinea* imbricata.

Norway i., SYN Norwegian *scabies*.

poultryman's i., eruption due to infestation with the mite, *Dermanyssus gallinae*.

prairie i., pruritus of varied origin, affecting farm laborers.

rice i., SYN *schistosomiasis* japonica.

Saint Ignatius' i., SYN pellagra.

straw i., straw-bed i., an urticarial eruption caused by the mite, *Pyemotes ventricosus*, which can infest straw used in mattresses. SYN dermatitis pediculoides ventricosus.

summer i., SYN *pruritus* aestivalis.

swamp i., SYN cutaneous *ancylostomiasis*.

sweet i., a pruritic dermatosis of horses caused by an allergic reaction to midges of the genus *Culicoides*.

swimmer's i., (1) SYN cutaneous *ancylostomiasis*. **(2)** SYN schistosomal *dermatitis*.

toe i., SYN cutaneous *ancylostomiasis*.

warehouseman's i., eczema of the hands from handling irritating substances.

washerwoman's i., an eczematous eruption of the hands and arms of washerwomen, dishwashers, and others whose hands are excessively immersed in water.

water i., (1) SYN cutaneous *ancylostomiasis.* **(2)** SYN schistosomal *dermatitis.*

winter i., SYN *dermatitis* hiemalis.

itch·ing. An uncomfortable sensation of irritation of the skin or mucous membranes which causes scratching or rubbing of the affected parts. SYN pruritus (1).

-ite. 1. Of the nature of, resembling. **2.** A salt of an acid that has the termination -ous. **3.** In comparative anatomy, a suffix denoting an essential portion of the part to the name of which it is attached. SEE ALSO -ites. [G. *-itēs,* fem. *-itis*]

iter (ī′ter). A passage leading from one anatomical part to another. SEE ALSO canaliculus. [L. *iter (itiner-),* a way, journey]

i. chor′dae ante′rius, SYN anterior *canaliculus* of chorda tympani.

i. chor′dae poste′rius, SYN posterior *canaliculus* of chorda tympani.

i. den′tis, the route or routes by which one or more teeth erupt. SYN iter dentium.

i. a ter′tio ad quar′tum ventric′ulum, SYN cerebral *aqueduct.* [L. path from the third to the fourth ventricle]

iter·al (ī′ter-ăl). Relating to an iter.

-ites. Adjectival suffix to nouns, corresponding to L. *-alis, -ale,* or *-inus, -inum,* or Eng. -y, -like, or the hyphenated nouns; the adjective so formed is used without the qualified noun. The feminine form, *-itis* (agreeing with *nosos,* disease), is so often associated with inflammatory disease that it has acquired in most cases the significance of inflammation. Thus, tympanites is *ho tympanitēs hydrōps,* the drumlike swelling of the abdomen, but tympanitis is *hē tympanitis nosos,* the inflammation of the tympanum. SEE ALSO -ite. [G. *itēs,* m., or *-ites,* n.]

ith·y·ky·pho·sis, ith·y·cy·pho·sis (ith′ĭ-kī-fō′sis, ith′ĭ-sī-). Obsolete term for pure kyphosis without lateral displacement of the spine. [G. *ithys,* straight, + *kyphos,* a hump]

ith·y·lor·do·sis (ith′ē-lōr-dō′sis). Obsolete term for a pure lordosis without lateral curvature of the spine. [G. *ithys,* straight, + *lordōsis,* a forward curvature of the spine, fr. *lordos,* bent backward (opp. of *kyphos,* humped]

-itides. Plural of -itis.

-itis. SEE -ites. [G. fem. of *-ites*]

Ito, Hayozo, 19th century Japanese physician, *1865. SEE Ito-Reenstierna *test.*

Ito, Minor, 20th century Japanese dermatologist. SEE Ito's *nevus; hypomelanosis* of I.

Ito, T., 20th century Japanese physician. SEE I. *cells,* under *cell.*

ITP Abbreviation for idiopathic thrombocytopenic *purpura;* inosine 5′-triphosphate.

itra·min tos·yl·ate (ī′tră-min). 2-Aminoethyl nitrate *p*-toluenesulfonate; a vasodilator.

IU Abbreviation for international *unit.*

IUB Abbreviation for International Union of Biochemistry.

IUCD Abbreviation for intrauterine contraceptive *devices.*

IUD Abbreviation for intrauterine *devices,* under *device.*

IUPAC Abbreviation for International Union of Pure and Applied Chemistry.

I-V Abbreviation for intraventricular.

I.V., i.v. Abbreviation for intravenous, or intravenously.

IVB Abbreviation for intraventricular *block.*

IVC Abbreviation for inferior *vena* cava.

Ivemark, Björn, Swedish pathologist, *1925. SEE I.'s *syndrome.*

iver·mec·tin (ī-ver-mek′tin). A semisynthetic macrolide antibiotic effective in the treatment of filariasis. The drug destroys *Onchocerca microfilaria* and *Filaria bancrofti.*

IVF Abbreviation for *in vitro fertilization.*

IVF-ET. Abbreviation for *in vitro* fertilization and *in vivo* transfer of the embryo to the uterus, Fallopian tube, or the peritoneal cavity.

ivo·ry (ī′vŏ-rē). A term applied to the tusks of the elephant, walrus, narwhal, hippopotamus, and warthog, and to all of the teeth of the sperm whale; the material is dentinum, the inner layer of the tooth derived from the mesoderm. In all of these animals, as well as in several others, the hard enamel layer fails to develop, or develops incompletely, leaving the softer dentinum core exposed. [L. *ebur*]

IVP Abbreviation for intravenous *pyelography* or pyelogram.

IVU Abbreviation for intravenous urogram; preferred to IVP. SEE intravenous *urography.*

Ivy, Robert H., U.S. oral and plastic surgeon, 1881–1974. SEE I. loop *wiring,* bleeding time *test.*

Ix·o·des (ik-sō′dēz). A genus of hard ticks (family Ixodidae), many species of which are parasitic on man and animals; severe reactions frequently follow their bites; they are characterized by an anal groove surrounding the anus anteriorly, absence of eyes and festoons, and marked sexual dimorphism; about 40 species have been described from North America. [G. *ixōdēs,* sticky, like bird-lime, fr. *ixos,* mistletoe, + *eidos,* form]

I. bicor′nis, a species, found in Mexico, whose bite causes fever and extreme malaise.

I. cook′ei, a species that is a vector of Powassan virus in Canada.

I. damm′ini, a species that is a vector of Lyme disease (*Borrelia burgdorferi*) and human babesiosis (*Babesia microti*) in the U.S. Bites causing Lyme disease in humans are from nymphal ticks about the size of a pencil point, infected with *B. burgdorferi* from white-footed field mice. Adult ticks complete their two-year life cycle feeding on deer.

I. holocyc′lus, a species in Australia that infests the kangaroo and transmits a paralytic disease to young cattle.

I. pacif′icus, the California black-legged tick, a species that is the vector of Lyme disease in the western U.S.

I. persulca′tus, a Eurasian species that is a vector for Russian spring-summer encephalitis and Lyme disease, and is associated with the taiga forest of the area formerly known as the USSR.

I. pilo′sus, the paralysis tick, a species that infests sheep in South Africa and causes paralysis.

I. rici′nus, the castor bean tick, a Euroasian species that infests cattle, sheep, and wild animals, and transmits the virus of louping ill, the piroplasm *Babesia divergens,* the central European tick-borne encephalitis virus, and the Lyme disease bacterium.

I. scapula′ris, the black-legged or shoulder tick, a species found on animals in the southern and eastern U.S.; capable of inflicting a painful bite to humans, and of being a vector of Lyme disease.

I. spinipal′pis, a species parasitic on wild rodents in British Columbia and the vector of Powassan virus in mice of the genus *Peromyscus.*

ix·o·di·a·sis (ik-sō-dī′ă-sis). Skin lesions caused by the bites of certain ixodid ticks. In some cases the tick burrows under the skin, causing some degree of irritation, but in most cases an urticarioid eruption is the only result.

ix·od·ic (ik-sod′ik). Relating to or caused by ticks.

ix·o·did (ik′sō-did). Common name for members of the family Ixodidae.

ix

Ix·od·i·dae (ik-sod′i-dē). A family of ticks (order Acarina, suborder Ixodides), the so-called "hard" ticks, characterized by rigid body form, presence of a dorsal shield, and an anteriorly projecting capitulum. It includes the genera *Ixodes, Hyalomma, Amblyomma, Boophilus, Margaropus, Dermacentor, Haemaphysalis,* and *Rhipicephalus,* species of which transmit many important human and animal diseases and cause tick paralysis; they occasionally attack man, a few habitually so. [G. *ixōdēs,* sticky]

Ix·o·doi·dea (ik′sō-dō-id′ē-ă). Superfamily of the order Acarina that includes the families Ixodidae and Argasidae. [G. *ixōdēs,* sticky]

J Symbol for joule; Joule's *equivalent*; electric current density.

J Symbol for flux (4).

jaag·siek·te (yahg′zēk-tē). SYN pulmonary *adenomatosis* of sheep. [Afrikaans, drive sickness]

Ja·bo·ran·di. SYN pilocarpus.

Jaboulay, Mathieu, French surgeon, 1860–1913. SEE J. *pyloroplasty;* J.'s *amputation.*

Jaccoud, François Sigismond, French physician, 1830–1913. SEE J.'s *arthritis, arthropathy.*

jack·et (jak′et). **1.** A fixed bandage applied around the body in order to immobilize the spine. **2.** In dentistry, a term commonly used in reference to an artificial crown composed of fired porcelain or acrylic resin. [M.E., fr. O.Fr. *jaquet,* dim. of *jaque,* tunic, fr. *Jacques,* nickname of Fr. peasants.]

Minerva j., a plaster of Paris body cast incorporating the head and trunk, usually for fracture of the cervical spine.

Sayre's j., a plaster of Paris j. applied while the patient is suspended by the head and axillae.

straight j., SEE straight j.

jack·screw (jak′skrū). A threaded device used in appliances for the separation of approximated teeth or jaws.

Jackson, Jabez N., U.S. surgeon, 1868–1935. SEE J.'s *membrane, veil.*

Jackson, John Hughlings, English neurologist, 1835–1911. SEE jacksonian *epilepsy;* J.'s *law, rule, sign.*

jack·so·ni·an (jak-sō′nē-an). Described by John Hughlings Jackson. SEE jacksonian *epilepsy,* Jacksonian *seizure.*

Jacobaeus, Hans C., Swedish surgeon, 1879–1937. SEE J. *operation.*

Jacobson, Ludwig L., Danish anatomist, 1783–1843. SEE J.'s *anastomosis, canal, cartilage, nerve, organ, plexus, reflex.*

Jacquart, Henri, 19th century French physician. SEE J.'s *facial angle.*

Jacquemet, Marcel, French anatomist, 1872–1908. SEE J.'s *recess.*

Jacquemin, Emile, 19th century French chemist. SEE Jacquemin's *test.*

Jacques, Paul, 19th century French physician. SEE J.'s *plexus.*

Jacquet, Leonard L., French dermatologist, 1860–1914. SEE J.'s *erythema.*

jac·ti·ta·tion (jak-ti-tā′shŭn). Rarely used term for extreme restlessness or tossing about from side to side. [L. *jactatio,* a tossing, fr. *jacto,* pp. *-atus,* to throw]

Jadassohn, Josef, German dermatologist in Switzerland, 1863–1936; introduced the patch *test* for contact dermatitis. SEE J.'s *nevus;* Borst-J. type intraepidermal *epithelioma;* J.-Pellizzari *anetoderma;* J.-Tièche *nevus;* Franceschetti-J. *syndrome;* J.-Lewandowski *syndrome.*

Jaeger, Eduard, Ritter von Jaxthal, Austrian ophthalmologist, 1818–1884. SEE J.'s *test types.*

Jaffe, Henry L., U.S. pathologist, 1896–1979 SEE J.-Lichtenstein *disease.*

Jaffe, Max, German biochemist, 1841–1911. SEE J. *reaction;* J.'s *test.*

Jahnke's syn·drome. See under syndrome.

Jakob, Alfons M., German neuropsychiatrist, 1884–1931. SEE Creutzfeldt-J. *disease;* J.-Creutzfeldt *disease.*

jal·ap. The dried tuberous root of *Exogonium purga, Exogonium jalapa,* or *Ipomoea purga* (family Convolvulaceae); used as a cathartic. [*Jalapa* or *Xalapa,* a Mexican city whence the drug was exported]

James, George C.W., 20th century U.S. radiologist. SEE Swyer-J. *syndrome;* Swyer-J.-MacLeod *syndrome.*

James, Thomas N., U.S. cardiologist and physiologist, *1925. SEE J. *fibers,* under *fiber, tracts,* under *tract.*

James, William, U.S. psychologist, 1842–1910. SEE J.-Lange *theory.*

James·town weed. SYN *Datura stramonium.*

Janet, Pierre M.F., French neurologist, 1859–1947. SEE J.'s *test.*

Janeway, Edward G., U.S. physician, 1841–1911. SEE J. *lesion.*

jan·i·ceps (jan′i-seps). Conjoined twins having their two heads fused together, with the faces looking in opposite directions. SEE conjoined *twins,* under *twin.* SEE ALSO craniopagus, syncephalus. [L. *Janus,* a Roman diety having two faces, + *caput,* head]

j. asym′metrus, a j. with one very small and imperfectly developed face. SYN iniops, syncephalus asymmetros.

j. parasit′icus, a j. in which one of the twins is a small and incompletely formed parasite attached to the more fully formed autosite.

Jansen, Albert, German otologist, 1859–1933. SEE J.'s *operation.*

Jansky, Jan, Czech physician, 1873–1921. SEE J.-Bielschowsky *disease;* J.'s *classification.*

Janus green B [C.I. 11050]. $C_{30}H_{31}N_6Cl$; diethylsafraninazodimethylaniline chloride; a basic dye used in histology and to stain mitochondria supravitally.

jar. **1.** To jolt or shake. **2.** A jolting or shaking.

heel j., the patient standing on tiptoe feels pain on suddenly bringing the heels to the ground: **(1)** in the spine in Pott's disease or disk space infection; **(2)** in one lumbar region in renal calculus.

jar·gon (jar′gŏn). **1.** Language or terminology peculiar to a specific field, profession, or group. **2.** SYN paraphasia. [Fr. gibberish]

Jarisch, Adolf, Austrian dermatologist, 1850–1902. SEE J.-Herxheimer *reaction;* Bezold-J. *reflex.*

Jarjavay, Jean F., French anatomist and surgeon, 1815–1868. SEE J.'s *ligament.*

Jar·vik. Robert Koffler, U.S. cardiologist. SEE Jarvik artificial *heart.*

Ja·tro·pha (jat′rō-fă). A genus of plants of the family Euphorbiaceae; a poisonous plant found in eastern Africa and the West Indies. [G. *iatros,* physician, + *trophē,* nourishment]

J. cur′cas, Barbados nut or physic-nut, the seed of which furnishes a purgative oil similar to croton oil. SYN *J. glandulifera.*

J. glandulif′era, SYN *J. curcas.*

J. u′rens, a species of South America; the macerated fresh leaves are used as a rubefacient and stimulating poultice; the seeds furnish a purgative oil.

jaun·dice (jawn′dis). A yellowish staining of the integument, sclerae, and deeper tissues and the excretions with bile pigments, which are increased in the plasma. SYN icterus. [Fr. *jaune,* yellow]

acholuric j., j. with excessive amounts of unconjugated bilirubin in the plasma and without bile pigments in the urine.

anhepatic j., j. due to hemolysis, with normal function of the liver and biliary tract. SYN anhepatogenous j.

anhepatogenous j., SYN anhepatic j.

catarrhal j., obsolete term for viral *hepatitis* type A.

choleric j., j. with the presence of biliary derivatives in the urine; occurs in regurgitation hyperbilirubinemia.

cholestatic j., j. produced by inspissated bile or bile plugs in small biliary passages in the liver.

chronic acholuric j., SYN hereditary *spherocytosis.*

chronic familial j., SYN hereditary *spherocytosis.*

chronic idiopathic j., SYN Dubin-Johnson *syndrome.*

congenital hemolytic j., SYN hereditary *spherocytosis.*

familial nonhemolytic j. [MIM*143500], mild j. due to increased amounts of unconjugated bilirubin in the plasma without evidence of liver damage, biliary obstruction, or hemolysis; thought to be due to an inborn error of metabolism in which the excretion of bilirubin by the liver is defective, ascribed to de-

ja

creased conjugation of bilirubin as a glucuronide or impaired uptake of hepatic bilirubin. SYN benign familial icterus, constitutional hepatic dysfunction, Gilbert's disease, Gilbert's syndrome, Hebra's disease (2).

hematogenous j., SYN hemolytic j.

hemolytic j., j. resulting from increased production of bilirubin from hemoglobin as a result of any process (toxic, genetic, or immune) causing increased destruction of erythrocytes. SYN hematogenous j., toxemic j.

hepatocellular j., j. resulting from diffuse injury or inflammation or failure of function of the liver cells, usually referring to viral or toxic hepatitis.

hepatogenous j., j. resulting from disease of the liver, as distinguished from that due to blood changes.

homologous serum j., obsolete term for viral *hepatitis* type B.

human serum j., obsolete name for hepatitis transmitted parenterally, usually by blood or blood products; usually due to hepatitis B.

infectious j., (1) SYN Weil's *disease.* (2) sometimes used in referring to viral *hepatitis* type A.

infective j., acute onset of malaise, fever, myalgia, nausea, anorexia, abdominal pain, and icterus caused by members of the genus *Leptospira.*

leptospiral j., j. associated with infection by various species of *Leptospira.*

malignant j., SYN *icterus* gravis.

mechanical j., SYN obstructive j.

neonatal j., SYN *icterus* neonatorum.

j. of the newborn, SYN *icterus* neonatorum.

nonobstructive j., any j. in which the main biliary passages are not obstructed, *e.g.,* hemolytic j. or j. due to hepatitis.

nuclear j., SYN kernicterus.

obstructive j., j. resulting from obstruction to the flow of bile into the duodenum, whether intra- or extrahepatic. SYN mechanical j.

painless j., j. not associated with abdominal pain; usually used for obstructive j. resulting from obstruction of the common bile duct at the head of the pancreas by a tumor or impaction of a stone.

physiologic j., SYN *icterus* neonatorum.

postarsphenamine j., liver toxicity, causing j., in a patient who has received arsphenamine.

regurgitation j., j. due to biliary obstruction, the bile pigment having been conjugated and secreted by the hepatic cells and then reabsorbed into the bloodstream.

retention j., j. due to insufficiency of liver function or to an excess of bile pigment production; the bilirubin is unconjugated because it has not passed through the liver cells; van den Bergh test is indirect.

Schmorl's j., kernicterus.

spherocytic j., hemolytic j. associated with spherocytosis.

spirochetal j., j. caused by infection with *Leptospira* species, usually *Leptospira icterohemorrhagica.*

toxemic j., SYN hemolytic j.

jaun·dice root. SYN hydrastis.

jaw. 1. One of the two bony structures, in which the teeth are set, forming the framework of the mouth. **2.** Common name for either the maxillae or the mandible. [A.S. *ceōwan,* to chew]

crackling j., chronic subluxation with clicking on motion.

Hapsburg j., prognathism and pouting lower lip, characteristic of the Hispano-Austrian imperial dynasty.

jaw winking, a paradoxical movement of eyelids associated with movements of the jaw.

lock-j., SYN trismus.

lower j., SYN mandible.

lumpy j., SYN actinomycosis.

parrot j., a condition caused by protrusion of incisor teeth.

upper j., SYN maxilla.

Jaworski, Walery, Polish physician, 1849–1924. SEE J.'s *bodies,* under *body.*

Jeanselme, A. Edouard, French dermatologist, 1858–1935. SEE J.'s *nodules,* under *nodule.*

Jeghers, Harold, U.S. physician, *1904. SEE Peutz-J. *syndrome;* J.-Peutz *syndrome.*

jejun-. SEE jejuno-.

je·ju·nal (je-jū′năl). Relating to the jejunum.

je·ju·nec·to·my (je-jū-nek′tō-mē). Excision of all or a part of the jejunum. [jejunum + G. *ektomē,* excision]

je·ju·ni·tis (je-jū-nī′tis). Inflammation of the jejunum.

jejuno-, jejun-. The jejunum, jejunal. [L. *jejunus,* empty]

je·ju·no·co·los·to·my (je-jū-nō-kō-los′tō-mē). Establishment of a communication between the jejunum and the colon. [jejuno- + colon + G. *stoma,* mouth]

je·ju·no·il·e·al (je-jū′nō-il′ē-ăl). Relating to the jejunum and the ileum.

je·ju·no·il·e·i·tis (je-jū′nō-il-ē-ī′tis). Inflammation of the jejunum and ileum.

je·ju·no·il·e·os·to·my (je-jū′nō-il-ē-os′tō-mē). Establishment of a new communication between the jejunum and the ileum. [jejuno- + ileum + G. *stoma,* mouth]

jejunocecostomy	Payne et al. Shibata et al.	1961 1967	
jejunoileostomy	Buchwald Jensen Payne Salmon Scott	1971 1969 1970 1971 1970	
jejunoileostomy with fistula	Bünte	1973	entrance

jejunoileostomy
modifications of partial removal of ileum

je·ju·no·je·ju·nos·to·my (je-jū′nō-jĕ-jū-nos′tō-mē). An anastomosis between two portions of jejunum. [jejuno- + jejuno- + G. *stoma,* mouth]

je·ju·no·plas·ty (je-jū′nō-plas-tē). A corrective surgical procedure on the jejunum. [jejuno- + G. *plastos,* molded]

je·ju·nos·to·my (je-jū-nos′tō-mē). Operative establishment of an opening from the abdominal wall into the jejunum, usually with creation of a stoma on the abdominal wall. [jejuno- + G. *stoma,* mouth]

je·ju·not·o·my (je-jū-not′ō-mē). Incision into the jejunum. [jejuno- + G. *tomē,* incision]

je·ju·num (jĕ-jū′nŭm) [NA]. The portion of small intestine, about 8 feet in length, between the duodenum and the ileum. The jejunum is distinct from the ileum in being more proximal, of larger diameter with a thicker wall, having larger, more highly developed plicae circulares, being more vasculer (redder in appearance) with the jejunal arteries forming fewer tiers of arterial arcades and longer vasa recti. [L. *jejunus,* empty]

Jellinek, Edward J., British physician specializing in alcohol-related disorders, 1890–1963. SEE Jellinek *formula.*

jel·ly (jel′ē). A semisolid tremulous compound usually containing some form of gelatin in aqueous solution. [L. *gelo,* to freeze]

cardiac j., term introduced by C.L. Davis for the gelatinous, noncellular material between the endothelial lining and the myocardial layer of the heart in very young embryos; later in development it serves as a substratum for cardiac mesenchyme.

interlaminar j., term introduced by B.M. Patten for the gelatinous material between ectoderm and endoderm that serves as the substrate on which mesenchymal cells migrate.

Wharton's j., the mucous connective tissue of the umbilical cord.

jel·ly·fish (jel′ē-fish). Marine coelenterates (class Hydrozoa) including some poisonous species, notably *Physalia*, the Portuguese man-of-war; toxin is injected into the skin by nematocysts on the tentacles, causing linear wheals.

Jendrassik, Ernö, Hungarian physician, 1858–1921. SEE J.'s *maneuver.*

Jenner, Edward, 1749–1823; English physician and naturalist who discovered the method of vaccinating against smallpox by inoculating susceptible persons with cowpox (vaccinia); Jenner's method led directly to the eradication of smallpox worldwide in 1977, the greatest public health achievement ever.

Jenner, Harley D., Canadian physician, *1907. SEE J.-Kay *unit.*

Jenner, Louis, English physician, 1866–1904. SEE J.'s *stain.*

Jensen, Carl O., Danish veterinary surgeon and pathologist, 1864–1934. SEE J.'s *sarcoma.*

Jensen, Edmund Z., Danish ophthalmologist, 1861–1950. SEE J.'s *disease.*

jerk. **1.** A sudden pull. **2.** SYN deep *reflex.*
 ankle j., SYN Achilles *reflex.*
 chin j., SYN jaw *reflex.*
 crossed j., SYN crossed *reflex.*
 crossed adductor j., SYN crossed adductor *reflex.*
 crossed knee j., SYN crossed knee *reflex.*
 elbow j., SYN triceps *reflex.*
 jaw j., SYN jaw *reflex.*
 knee j., SYN patellar *reflex.*
 supinator j., SYN brachioradial *reflex.*

jerks (pl.). Chorea or any form of tic.

Jervell, Anton, 20th century Norwegian cardiologist. SEE J. and Lange-Nielsen *syndrome.*

Jes·u·its′ bark. SYN cinchona.

jet. A region of very high blood velocity just downstream of a vessel stenosis.

jet lag. An imbalance of the normal circadian rhythm resulting from subsonic or supersonic travel through a varied number of time zones and leading to fatigue, irritability, and various functional disturbances.

Jeune, M., 20th century French pediatrician. SEE J.'s *syndrome.*

Jewett, Hugh, U.S. urologist, 1903–1990. SEE J. *sound,* and Strong *staging.*

jig·ger. Common name for *Tunga penetrans.* SEE ALSO chigoe.

jim·son weed. SYN *Datura stramonium.*

jird (jerd). A rodent of the genus *Meriones;* distinct from the gerbil, with which it is frequently confused.

Jk blood group. See Kidd blood group, Blood Groups appendix.

JNA Abbreviation for *Jena Nomina Anatomica,* 1935. SEE Nomina Anatomica.

Jobert de Lamballe, Antoine, French surgeon, 1799–1867. SEE J. de L.'s *fossa, suture.*

Jod-Basedow, jod·bas·e·dow (yod-bas′ĕ-dō). SEE Jod-Basedow *phenomenon.* [Ger. *Jod,* iodine, + K.A. von *Basedow*]

Joest, Ernst, German veterinary pathologist, 1873–1926. SEE J. *bodies,* under *body.*

Joffroy, Alexis, French physician, 1844–1908. SEE J.'s *reflex, sign.*

Johne, H. Albert, German physician, 1839–1910. SEE johnin; J.'s *bacillus, disease.*

joh·nin (yō′nin). A product used as a diagnostic agent, analogous to tuberculin but made from *Mycobacterium paratuberculosis* (the causative organism of Johne's disease) grown in a broth medium containing *Mycobacterium phlei* (timothy hay bacillus); used as an allergen to provoke reactions in infected animals. [A. *Johne*]

Johnson, Frank B., U.S. pathologist, *1919. SEE Dubin-J. *syndrome.*

Johnson, Frank C., U.S. pediatrician, 1894–1934. SEE Stevens-J. *syndrome.*

Johnson, Harry B., U.S. dentist. SEE J.'s *method.*

Johnson, Treat Baldwin, U.S. chemist, 1875–1947. SEE Wheeler-J. *test.*

JOINT

joint (joynt). In anatomy, the place of union, usually more or less movable, between two or more bones. J.'s between skeletal elements exhibit a great variety of form and function, and are classified into three general morphological types: fibrous j.'s; cartilaginous j.'s; and synovial j.'s. SYN articulatio [NA], arthrosis (1), articulation (1), articulus, junctura (1). [L. *junctura;* fr. *jungo,* pp. *junctus,* to join]

acromioclavicular j., a plane synovial joint between the acromial end of the clavicle and the medial margin of the acromion. SYN articulatio acromioclavicularis [NA].

ankle j., a hinge synovial joint between the tibia and fibula above and the talus below. SYN articulatio talocruralis [NA], ankle (1), mortise j., talocrural articulation, talocrural j.

anterior intraoccipital j., SYN anterior intraoccipital *synchondrosis.*

arthrodial j., SYN plane j.

atlantoaxial j., compound j. between first and second cervical vertebrae.

atlanto-occipital j., a condylar synovial joint between the superior articular facets of the atlas and the condyles of the occipital bone. SYN articulatio atlanto-occipitalis [NA], atlanto-occipital articulation.

j.'s of auditory ossicles, the joints of the ossicular chain consisting of incudomallear j., incudostapedeal j., and the tympanostapedeal syndesmosis. SYN articulationes ossiculorum auditus [NA], j.'s of ear bones.

ball-and-socket j., a multiaxial synovial joint in which a more or less extensive sphere on the head of one bone fits into a rounded cavity in the other bone, as in the hip joint. SYN articulatio spheroidea [NA], articulatio cotylica* [NA], cotyloid j., enarthrodial j., enarthrosis, socket j., spheroid articulation, spheroid j.

biaxial j., one in which there are two principal axes of movement situated at right angles to each other; *e.g.,* saddle j.'s.

bicondylar j., a synovial joint in which two more or less distinct, rounded surfaces of one bone articulate with shallow depressions on another bone. SYN articulatio bicondylaris [NA], bicondylar articulation.

bilocular j., one in which the intra-articular disk is complete, dividing the j. into two distinct cavities.

Budin's obstetrical j., SYN posterior intraoccipital *synchondrosis.*

calcaneocuboid j., a somewhat saddle-shaped synovial joint between the anterior surface of the calcaneus and the posterior surface of the cuboid. This is the lateral element of the compound transverse tarsal joint. SYN articulatio calcaneocuboidea [NA].

capitular j., SYN j. of head of rib.

carpal j.'s, **(1)** SYN intercarpal j.'s. **(2)** SYN wrist j.

carpometacarpal j.'s, the synovial joints between the carpal and metacarpal bones; these are all plane joints except that of the thumb, which is saddle-shaped. SYN articulationes carpometacarpeae [NA].

carpometacarpal j. of thumb, the saddle-shaped synovial articulation between the trapezium and the base of the first metacarpal bone. SYN articulatio carpometacarpea pollicis [NA].

cartilaginous j., a joint in which the apposed bony surfaces are united by cartilage; they are divided into synchondroses and symphyses; in synchondroses, the cartilage connecting the apposed surfaces is, as a rule, ultimately converted to bone, as between epiphyses and diaphyses of long bones; exceptions are the sternal synchondroses and the cartilaginous union of the first rib and the manubrium of the sternum; in symphyses the bones are connected by a flat disk of fibrocartilage which remains unossified throughout life; *e.g.,* the intervertebral disk and the

jo

symphysis pubis. SYN articulatio cartilaginis [NA], cartilaginous articulation, junctura cartilaginea, synarthrodial j. (2).

Charcot's j., SYN tabetic *arthropathy.*

Chopart's j., SYN transverse tarsal j.

Clutton's j.'s, symmetrical arthrosis, especially of the knee joints, in cases of congenital syphilis.

coccygeal j., SYN sacrococcygeal j.

cochlear j., a variety of hinge j. in which the elevation and depression, respectively, on the opposing articular surfaces form part of a spiral, flexion being then accompanied by a certain amount of lateral deviation. SYN screw j., spiral j.

coffin j., the distal interphalangeal articulation of the horse, a compound synovial j. between the middle and distal phalanges and also with the distal sesamoid or navicular bone on the caudal side.

composite j., SYN compound j.

compound j., a joint composed of three or more skeletal elements, or in which two anatomically separate joints function as a unit. For example, the telonavicular and calcaneocuboid joints act together as the compound transverse tarsal joint. SYN articulatio complexa [NA], articulatio composita [NA], composite j., compound articulation.

condylar j., SYN ellipsoidal j.

costochondral j., the cartilaginous joint between the sternal end of a rib and the lateral end of a costal cartilage. SYN articulatio costochondralis [NA], costochondral junction.

costotransverse j., the synovial articulation between the neck and tubercle of a rib and the transverse process of a vertebra. SYN articulatio costotransversaria [NA].

costovertebral j.'s, the synovial joints uniting ribs and vertebrae; they consist of the j. capitis costae and the j. costotransversaria. SYN articulationes costovertebrales [NA].

cotyloid j., SYN ball-and-socket j.

cricoarytenoid j., the synovial joint between the base of each arytenoid cartilage and the upper border of the lamina of the cricoid cartilage. SYN articulatio cricoarytenoidea [NA], cricoarytenoid articulation.

cricothyroid j., the synovial articulation between the inferior horn of the thyroid cartilage and the side of the cricoid cartilage. SYN articulatio cricothyroidea [NA], cricothyroid articulation.

Cruveilhier's j., SYN median atlantoaxial j.

cubital j., SYN elbow j.

cuboideonavicular j., a fibrous j. between adjacent parts of the cuboid and navicular bones; occasionally a synovial cavity is found here as an extension of the cuneonavicular j.

cuneocuboid j., the synovial articulation between the lateral surface of the lateral cuneiform and the anterior two-thirds of the medial surface of the cuboid.

cuneometatarsal j.'s, SYN tarsometatarsal j.'s.

cuneonavicular j., the synovial joint between the anterior surface of the navicular and the posterior surfaces of the three cuneiform bones. SYN articulatio cuneonavicularis [NA], cuneonavicular articulation.

dentoalveolar j., SYN gomphosis.

diarthrodial j., SYN synovial j.

digital j.'s, SYN interphalangeal j.'s of hand.

DIP j.'s, SYN distal interphalangeal j.'s.

distal interphalangeal j.'s, the synovial j.'s between the middle and distal phalanges of the fingers and of the toes. SYN DIP j.'s.

distal radioulnar j., the pivot synovial joint between the head of the ulna and the ulnar notch on the radius; an articular disk passes across the distal part of the joint. SYN articulatio radioulnaris distalis [NA], distal radioulnar articulation, inferior radioulnar j.

distal tibiofibular j., SYN tibiofibular *syndesmosis.*

j.'s of ear bones, SYN j.'s of auditory ossicles.

elbow j., a compound hinge synovial joint between the humerus and the bones of the forearm; it consists of the j. humeroradialis and the j. humeroulnaris. SYN articulatio cubiti [NA], cubital j.

ellipsoidal j., a modified ball-and-socket synovial joint in which the joint surfaces are elongated or ellipsoidal; it is a biaxial joint, *i.e.,* two axes of motion at right angles to each other, the radio-

carpal being an example. SYN articulatio ellipsoidea [NA], articulatio condylaris★ [NA], condylar articulation, condylar j.

enarthrodial j., SYN ball-and-socket j.

facet j.'s, SYN zygapophyseal j.'s.

false j., SYN pseudarthrosis.

femoropatellar j., the articulation of the facets on the articular surface of the patella with corresponding surfaces on the femoral condyles.

fibrous j., a union of two bones by fibrous tissue such that there is no joint cavity and almost no motion possible; the types of fibrous joints are sutures, syndesmoses, and gomphoses. SYN articulatio fibrosa [NA], immovable j., junctura fibrosa, synarthrodia, synarthrodial j. (1).

flail j., a j. with loss of function caused by loss of ability to stabilize the j. in any plane within its normal range of motion.

j.'s of foot, j.'s including the talocrural, intertarsal, tarsometatarsal, intermetatarsal, metatarsophalangeal and interphalangeal joints. SYN articulationes pedis [NA], articulations of foot.

j.'s of free inferior limb, SYN j.'s of free lower limb.

j.'s of free lower limb, the joints uniting the bones of the free inferior limb to one another and to the pelvic girdle; they are the hip joint, knee joint, tibiofibular joint, and the joints of the ankle and foot. SYN articulationes membri inferioris liberi [NA], j.'s of free inferior limb, juncturae membri inferioris liberi.

j.'s of free superior limb, SYN j.'s of free upper limb.

j.'s of free upper limb, the joints uniting the bones of the free superior limb girdle; they are the shoulder joint, elbow joint, radioulnar joints, and joints of the wrist and hand. SYN articulationes membri superioris liberi [NA], j.'s of free superior limb, juncturae membri superioris liberi.

ginglymoid j., SYN hinge j.

gliding j., SYN plane j.

gomphilic j., SYN gomphosis.

j.'s of hand, these joints include the radiocarpal or wrist joint; intercarpal, carpometacarpal, intermetacarpal; metacarpophalangeal and interphalangeal joints. SYN articulationes manus [NA], articulations of hand.

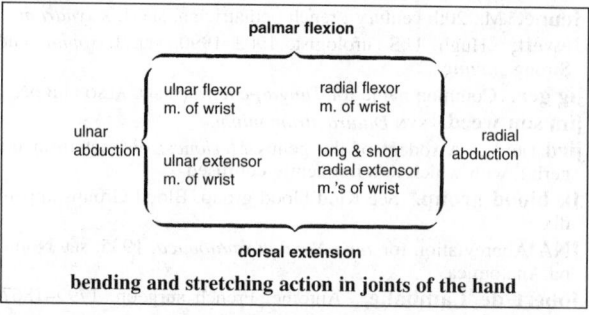

bending and stretching action in joints of the hand

j. of head of rib, the synovial joint between a rib and bodies of two adjacent vertebrae; the joint cavity is divided by an intra-articular ligament which attaches to the intervertebral disk; the first, tenth, eleventh, and twelfth ribs articulate with only one vertebra. SYN articulatio capitis costae [NA], capitular j.

hemophilic j., chronic arthroplasty due to repeated hemarthrosis in a hemophiliac.

hinge j., a uniaxial joint in which a broad, transversely cylindrical convexity on one bone fits into a corresponding concavity on the other, allowing of motion in one plane only, as in the elbow. SYN ginglymus [NA], ginglymoid j.

hip j., the ball-and-socket synovial joint between the head of the femur and the acetabulum. SYN articulatio coxae [NA], coxa (2), thigh j.

humeroradial j., the portion of the elbow joint between the capitulum of the humerus and the head of the radius. SYN articulatio humeroradialis [NA], humeroradial articulation.

humeroulnar j., the portion of the elbow joint between the trochlea of the humerus and the trochlear notch of the ulna. SYN articulatio humeroulnaris [NA].

hysterical j., a simulation of j. disease, with symptoms of pain, possibly swelling, and impairment of motion.

immovable j., SYN fibrous j.

incudomalleolar j., the saddle synovial joint between the incus and the malleus. SYN articulatio incudomallearis [NA], incudomalleolar articulation.

incudostapedial j., the synovial joint between the lenticular process on the long crus of the incus and the head of the stapes. SYN articulatio incudostapedia [NA], incudostapedial articulation.

j.'s of inferior limb girdle, SYN j.'s of pelvic girdle.

inferior radioulnar j., SYN distal radioulnar j.

inferior tibiofibular j., SYN tibiofibular *syndesmosis*.

interarticular j.'s, SYN zygapophyseal j.'s.

intercarpal j.'s, the synovial joints between the carpal bones. SYN articulationes intercarpeae [NA], carpal j.'s (1).

interchondral j.'s, the synovial joints between the contiguous surfaces of the fifth, sixth, seventh, eighth, ninth, and tenth costal cartilages, forming the costal arch. SYN articulationes interchondrales [NA], interchondral articulations.

intercuneiform j.'s, the articulations between contiguous surfaces of the cuneiform bones.

intermetacarpal j.'s, the synovial joints between the bases of the second, third, fourth, and fifth metacarpal bones. SYN articulationes intermetacarpeae [NA].

intermetatarsal j.'s, the synovial joints between the bases of the five metatarsal bones. SYN articulationes intermetatarseae [NA], intermetatarsal articulations.

interphalangeal j.'s of hand, the hinge synovial j.'s between the phalanges of the fingers. SYN articulationes interphalangeae manus [NA], digital j.'s, interphalangeal articulations, phalangeal j.'s.

interphalangeal j.'s of foot, the hinge synovial j.'s between the phalanges of the toes. SYN articulationes interphalangeae pedis [NA].

intersternebral j.'s, SYN *synchondroses* intersternebrales, under *synchondrosis*.

intertarsal j.'s, the synovial joints which unite the tarsal bones. SYN articulationes intertarseae [NA], intertarsal articulations, tarsal j.'s.

jaw j., SYN temporomandibular j.

knee j., a compound condylar synovial joint consisting of the joint between the condyles of the femur and the condyles of the tibia, articular menisci (semilunar cartilages) being interposed, and the articulation between femur and patella. SYN articulatio genus [NA].

lateral atlantoaxial j., a condylar synovial joint between the inferior articular facets of the atlas and the superior articular facets of the axis. SYN articulatio atlantoaxialis lateralis [NA], lateral atlantoepistrophic j.

lateral atlantoepistrophic j., SYN lateral atlantoaxial j.

Lisfranc's j.'s, SYN tarsometatarsal j.'s.

lumbosacral j., the articulation of the fifth lumbar vertebra with the sacrum. SYN articulatio lumbosacralis [NA], junctura lumbosacralis.

Luschka's j.'s, SYN uncovertebral j.'s.

mandibular j., SYN temporomandibular j.

manubriosternal j., the early union, by hyaline cartilage, of the manubrium and the body of the sternum, which later becomes a symphysial type of joint. SYN synchondrosis manubriosternalis [NA].

median atlantoaxial j., a pivot synovial joint between the dens of the axis and the ring formed by the anterior arch and the transverse ligament of the atlas. SYN articulatio atlantoaxialis mediana [NA], Cruveilhier's j., middle atlantoepistrophic j.

metacarpophalangeal j.'s, the spheroid synovial joints between the heads of the metacarpals and the bases of the proximal phalanges. SYN articulationes metacarpophalangeae [NA], metacarpophalangeal articulations, MP j.'s (1).

metatarsophalangeal j.'s, the spheroid synovial joints between the heads of the metatarsals and the bases of the proximal phalanges of the toes. SYN articulationes metatarsophalangeae [NA], metatarsophalangeal articulations, MP j.'s (2).

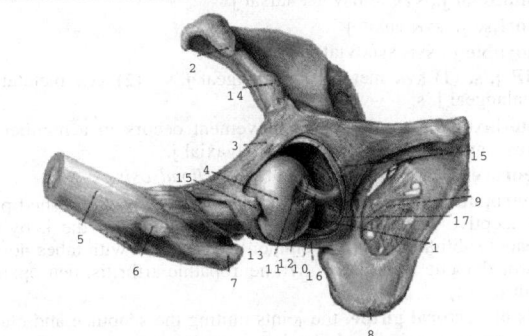

hip joint (articulatio coxae)
1) acetabulum, 2) spina iliaca anterior superior, 3) lig. iliofemorale, 4) caput femoris, 5) corpus femoris, 6) trochanter minor, 7) trochanter major, 8) tuber ischiadicum (ischiale), 9) membrana obturatoria, 10) lig. capitis femoris, 11) fovea capitis femoris, 12) labrum acetabulare, 13) zona orbicularis, 14) spina iliaca anterior inferior, 15) lig. pubofemorale, 16) lig. ischiofemorale, 17) capsula articularis

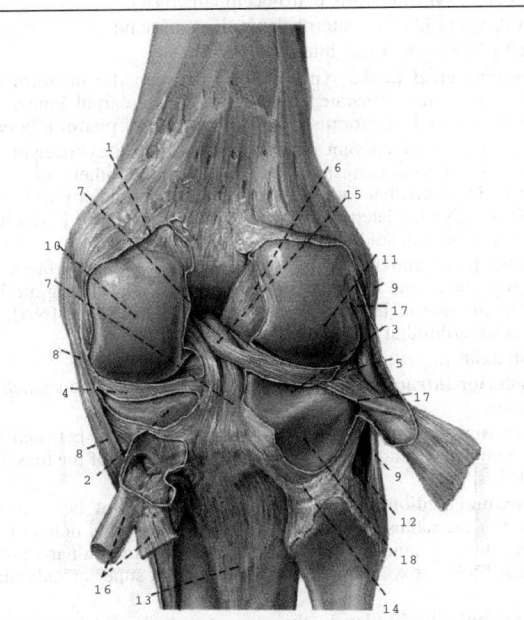

knee joint
1) capsula articularis, 2) condylus medialis (tibiae), 3) condylus lateralis (tibiae), 4) meniscus medialis, 5) meniscus lateralis, 6) lig. cruciatum anterius, 7) lig. cruciatum posterius, 8) lig. collaterale tibiale, 9) lig. collaterale fibulare, 10) condylus medialis (femoris), 11) condylus lateralis (femoris), 12) caput fibulae (fibulare), 13) tibia, 14) articulatio tibiofibularis, 15) lig. meniscofemorale posterius, 16) m. semimembranosus, 17) m. popliteus, 18) recessus subpopliteus

midcarpal j., the synovial joint between the proximal and distal rows of carpal bones. SYN articulatio mediocarpea [NA], middle carpal j.

middle atlantoepistrophic j., SYN median atlantoaxial j.

middle carpal j., SYN midcarpal j.

middle radioulnar j., SYN radioulnar *syndesmosis*.

jo

midtarsal j., SYN transverse tarsal j.

mortise j., SYN ankle j.

movable j., SYN synovial j.

MP j.'s, (1) SYN metacarpophalangeal j.'s. **(2)** SYN metatarsophalangeal j.'s.

multiaxial j., one in which movement occurs in a number of axes. SEE ball-and-socket j. SYN polyaxial j.

neurocentral j., SYN neurocentral *synchondrosis.*

neuropathic j., destructive j. disease caused by diminished proprioceptive sensation, with gradual destruction of the j. by repeated subliminal injury, commonly associated with tabes dorsalis or diabetic neuropathy. SYN neuropathic arthritis, neuropathic arthropathy.

j.'s of pectoral girdle, the joints uniting the scapulae and clavicles to each other and the latter to the sternum forming the superior limb girdle; these are the acromioclavicular and the sternoclavicular joints. SYN articulationes cinguli membri superioris [NA], j.'s of superior limb girdle, juncturae cinguli membri superioris.

peg-and-socket j., SYN gomphosis.

j.'s of pelvic girdle, the j.'s that unite the sacrum and the two hip bones to form the pelvic girdle; these are the sacroiliac j.'s, the pubic symphysis, the sacrotuberal and sacrospinal ligaments, and the obturator membrane. SYN articulationes cinguli membri inferioris [NA], j.'s of inferior limb girdle.

petro-occipital j., fibrocartilage filling the petro-occipital fissure. SYN synchondrosis petro-occipitalis [NA].

phalangeal j.'s, SYN interphalangeal j.'s of hand.

PIP j.'s, SYN proximal interphalangeal j.'s.

pisotriquetral j., the synovial joint between the pisiform and triquetrum; it is separate from the other intercarpal joints. SYN articulatio ossis pisiformis [NA], articulation of pisiform bone.

pivot j., a synovial joint in which a section of a cylinder of one bone fits into a corresponding cavity on the other, as in the proximal radioulnar joint. SYN articulatio trochoidea [NA], helicoid ginglymus, lateral ginglymus, rotary j., rotatory j., trochoid articulation, trochoid j.

plane j., a synovial joint in which the opposing surfaces are nearly planes and in which there is only a slight, gliding motion, as in the intermetacarpal joints. SYN articulatio plana [NA], arthrodia, arthrodial articulation, arthrodial j., gliding j.

polyaxial j., SYN multiaxial j.

posterior intraoccipital j., SYN posterior intraoccipital *synchondrosis.*

proximal interphalangeal j.'s, the synovial j.'s between the proximal and middle phalanges of the fingers and of the toes. SYN PIP j.'s.

proximal radioulnar j., the pivot synovial joint between the head of the radius and the ring formed by the radial notch of the ulna and the annular ligament. SYN articulatio radioulnaris proximalis [NA], proximal radioulnar articulation, superior radioulnar j.

proximal tibiofibular j., the plane synovial joint between the lateral condyle of the tibia and the head of the fibula. SYN articulatio tibiofibularis [NA], superior tibial articulation, superior tibiofibular articulation (1).

radiocarpal j., SYN wrist j.

rotary j., rotatory j., SYN pivot j.

sacrococcygeal j., the cartilaginous articulation of the coccyx with the sacrum. SYN articulatio sacrococcygea [NA], coccygeal j., junctura sacrococcygea, sacrococcygeal junction, symphysis sacrococcygea.

sacroiliac j., the synovial joint on either side between the auricular surface of the sacrum and that of the ilium. SYN articulatio sacroiliaca [NA], sacroiliac articulation.

saddle j., a biaxial synovial joint in which the double motion is effected by the opposition of two surfaces, each of which is concave in one direction and convex in the other; as in the carpometacarpal joint of the thumb. SYN articulatio sellaris [NA], articulatio ovoidalis.

schindyletic j., SYN wedge-and-groove j.

screw j., SYN cochlear j.

shoulder j., a ball-and-socket synovial joint between the head of the humerus and the glenoid cavity of the scapula. SYN articulatio humeri [NA], glenohumeral articulation, humeral articulation.

simple j., one composed of two bones only. SYN articulatio simplex [NA].

socket j., SYN ball-and-socket j.

spheno-occipital j., SYN spheno-occipital *synchondrosis.*

spheroid j., SYN ball-and-socket j.

spiral j., SYN cochlear j.

sternal j.'s, SYN sternal *synchondroses,* under *synchondrosis.*

sternoclavicular j., the synovial articulation between the medial end of the clavicle and the manubrium of the sternum and cartilage of the first rib; an articular disk subdivides the joint into two cavities. SYN articulatio sternoclavicularis [NA].

sternocostal j.'s, the joints between the cartilages of the first seven ribs and the sternum; synovial cavities are variable in occurrence in these joints. SYN articulationes sternocostales [NA], sternocostal articulations.

stifle j., the femorotibial articulation in the hind leg of the horse and other quadrupeds; it corresponds to the knee in humans. SYN stifle.

subtalar j., a plane synovial joint between the inferior surface of the talus and the posterior articular surface of the calcaneus. The term is also used clinically to refer to the compound joint formed by the talocalcaneal and talocalcaneonavicular joints. SYN articulatio subtalaris [NA], talocalcaneal j.

j.'s of superior limb girdle, SYN j.'s of pectoral girdle.

superior radioulnar j., SYN proximal radioulnar j.

superior tibiofibular j., SYN proximal tibiofibular j.

suture j., SYN suture.

synarthrodial j., (1) SYN fibrous j. **(2)** SYN cartilaginous j.

synchondrodial j., SYN synchondrosis.

syndesmodial j., syndesmotic j., SYN syndesmosis.

synovial j., a joint in which the opposing bony surfaces are covered with a layer of hyaline cartilage or fibrocartilage, there is a joint cavity containing synovial fluid, lined with synovial membrane and reinforced by a fibrous capsule and ligaments, and there is some degree of free movement possible. SYN articulatio synovialis [NA], diarthrodial j., diarthrosis, junctura synovialis, movable j., perarticulation.

talocalcaneal j., SYN subtalar j.

talocalcaneonavicular j., a ball-and-socket synovial joint, part of which participates in the transverse tarsal joint, formed by the head of the talus articulating with the navicular bone and the anterior part of the calcaneus. SYN articulatio talocalcaneonavicularis [NA].

talocrural j., SYN ankle j.

talonavicular j., the part of the talocalcaneonavicular j. which forms the medial element of the compound transverse tarsal j.

tarsal j.'s, SYN intertarsal j.'s.

tarsometatarsal j.'s, the three synovial joints between the tarsal and metatarsal bones, consisting of a medial joint between the first cuneiform and first metatarsal, an intermediate joint between the second and third cuneiforms and corresponding metatarsals, and a lateral joint between the cuboid and fourth and fifth metatarsals. SYN articulationes tarsometatarseae [NA], cuneometatarsal j.'s, Lisfranc's j.'s.

temporomandibular j., the synovial articulation between the head of the mandible and the mandibular fossa and articular tubercle of the temporal bone; a fibrocartilaginous articular disk divides the joint into two cavities. SYN articulatio temporomandibularis [NA], articulatio mandibularis, jaw j., mandibular j., temporomandibular articulation.

thigh j., SYN hip j.

transverse tarsal j., the synovial joints between the talus and navicular bone medially and the calcaneus and navicular bones laterally which act as a unit in allowing the front of the foot to pivot relative to the back of the foot about the longitudinal axis of the foot, contributing to the total inversion and eversion movements. SYN articulatio tarsi transversa [NA], Chopart's j., midtarsal j., transverse tarsal articulation.

trochoid j., SYN pivot j.

uncovertebral j.'s, small synovial j.'s between adjacent lateral lips of the bodies of the lower cervical vertebrae. SYN Luschka's j.'s.

uniaxial j., one in which movement is around one axis only.

unilocular j., one in which an intra-articular disk is incomplete or absent, the j. having but a single cavity.

wedge-and-groove j., a form of fibrous joint in which the sharp edge of one bone is received in a cleft in the edge of the other, as in the articulation of the vomer with the rostrum of the sphenoid. SYN schindylesis [NA], schindyletic j., wedge-and-groove suture.

wrist j., the synovial joint between the distal end of the radius and its articular disk and the proximal row of carpal bones with the exception of the pisiform bone. SYN articulatio radiocarpea [NA], carpal articulation, carpal j.'s (2), radiocarpal articulation, radiocarpal j.

xiphisternal j., the cartilaginous union between the xiphoid process and the body of the sternum. SYN synchondrosis xiphosternalis [NA].

zygapophyseal j.'s, the synovial joints between zygapophyses or articular processes of the vertebrae. SYN articulationes zygapophyseales [NA], facet j.'s, interarticular j.'s, juncturae zygapophyseales.

---

joint mice. Small fibrous, cartilaginous, or bony loose bodies in the synovial cavity of a joint.

Jolles, Adolf, Austrian chemist, 1863–1944. SEE J.'s *test.*

Jolly, Friedrich, German neurologist, 1844–1904. SEE J.'s *reaction.*

Jolly, Justin, French histologist, 1870–1953. SEE J. *bodies,* under *body;* Howell-J. *bodies,* under *body.*

Jones, Ernest, British psychiatrist, 1879–1958. SEE Ross-J. *test.*

Jones, Henry Bence. SEE Bence J.

Jonnesco (Ionescu), Thomas, Roumanian surgeon, 1860–1926. SEE J.'s *fossa.*

Jonston, Johns, Scottish physician in Poland, 1603–1675. SEE J.'s *alopecia, area.*

Joseph, Jacques, German surgeon, 1865–1934. SEE J. *rhinoplasty, knife.*

Joubert, Marie, 20th century Canadian neurologist. SEE J.'s *syndrome.*

Joule, James P., British physicist, 1818–1889. SEE joule; J.'s *equivalent.*

joule (J) (jūl, jowl). A unit of energy; the heat generated, or energy expended, by an ampere flowing through an ohm for 1 second; equal to 10^7 ergs and to a newton-meter. It is an approved multiple of the SI fundamental unit of energy, the erg, and is intended to replace the calorie (4.184 J). SYN unit of heat (3). [J.P. *Joule*]

juc·cu·ya (ŭ-kū′yă). SYN cutaneous *leishmaniasis.*

Judkins, Melvin P., U.S. radiologist, 1922–1985; pioneer in coronary angiography and angioplasty. SEE J. *technique.*

ju·ga (jū′gă). Plural of jugum.

ju·gal (jū′găl). **1.** Connecting; yoked. **2.** Relating to the zygomatic bone. [L. *jugalis,* yoked together, fr. *jugum,* a yoke]

ju·ga·le (jū-gā′lē). A craniometric point at the union of the temporal and frontal processes of the zygomatic bone. SYN jugal point.

ju·go·max·il·lary (jū′gō-mak′si-lār-ē). Relating to the zygomatic bone and the maxilla.

jug·u·lar (jŭg′yū-lar). **1.** Relating to the throat or neck. **2.** Relating to the j. veins. **3.** A j. vein. [L. *jugulum,* throat]

jug·u·lum (jŭg′yū-lŭm). SYN throat (2).

ju·gum, pl. **ju·ga** (jū′gŭm, -gă). **1.** A ridge or furrow connecting two points. SYN yoke. **2.** A type of forceps. [L. a yoke]

j. alveola′re, pl. **ju′ga alveola′ria** [NA], one of the eminences on the outer surface of the alveolar process of the maxilla or mandible, formed by the roots of the incisor teeth. SYN alveolar yoke.

j. sphenoida′le [NA], a plane surface on the sphenoid bone, in front of the sella turcica, connecting the two lesser wings, and forming part of the anterior cranial fossa and especially later in life, the roof of the anteriormost portion of the sphenoidal sinus. SYN planum sphenoidale.

juice (jūs). **1.** The interstitial fluid of a plant or animal. **2.** A digestive secretion. [L. *jus,* broth]

appetite j., gastric j. secreted upon the sight or smell of food and at the time of eating, influenced by the attractiveness of the food and delight in the food ingested; a conditioned reflex.

cancer j., turbid, white to yellow-white or gray-white fluid (chiefly plasma) that may be expressed from certain forms of malignant neoplastic tissue, and is likely to contain neoplastic cells and debris; formed especially in relatively large, degenerating, partly necrotic foci of rapidly growing neoplastic tissue.

gastric j., the digestive fluid secreted by the glands of the stomach; a thin colorless liquid of acid reaction containing primarily hydrochloric acid, chymosin, pepsinogen, and intrinsic factor plus mucus.

intestinal j., an alkaline straw-colored fluid secreted by the intestinal glands; its enzymes (peptidases, saccharases, nucleases, lecithinases, phosphatases, lipases) complete the hydrolysis of carbohydrates, proteins, and lipids.

pancreatic j., the external secretion of the pancreas; a clear alkaline fluid containing several enzymes: α-amylase, nucleases, trypsinogen, chymotrypsinogen, and triacylglycerol lipase.

Jukes (jūks). The pseudonym for a celebrated family, most of whose members were social misfits, feebleminded, and degenerate. SEE ALSO Kallikak.

junc·tion (jŭngk′shŭn). SYN junctura (2).

amelodental j., amelodentinal j., rarely used terms for dentino-enamel j.

amnioembryonic j., the line of amniotic attachment to the periphery of the embryonic disk.

anorectal j., transition from rectum to anal canal; corresponds to the perineal flexure, or the level at which the gut perforates the pelvic diaphragm; here the rectal ampulla narrows abruptly into a narrow slip.

A-V j., imprecisely defined zone surrounding and including the A-V node and the adjacent atrial and ventricular myocardium.

cardioesophageal j., the abrupt transition from esophageal mucosa to that of the cardiac portion of stomach, demarcated internally in the living by the z-line, and approximated externally by the cardiac notch.

cementodentinal j., the surface at which the cementum and dentin of the root of a tooth are joined. SYN dentinocemental j.

cementoenamel j., the surface at which the enamel of the crown and the cementum of the root of a tooth are joined. SEE ALSO cervical *line.*

choledochoduodenal j., that part of the duodenal wall traversed by the ductus choledochus, ductus pancreaticus, and ampulla.

costochondral j., SYN costochondral *joint.*

dentinocemental j., SYN cementodentinal j.

dentinoenamel j., the surface at which the enamel and the dentin of the crown of a tooth are joined.

duodenojejunal j., point along the course of the gastrointestinal tract where the duodenum ends and the jejunum begins; occurs approximately at the level of the L2 vertebra, 2–3 cm to the left of the midline; usually takes the form of an acute angle, the duodenojejunal flexure, and is supported by the attachment of the suspensory muscle (ligament) of the duodenum.

electrotonic j., SYN gap j.

esophagogastric j., terminal end of esophagus and beginning of stomach at the cardiac orifice; site of the physiologic inferior esophageal sphincter.

gap j., (1) an intercellular j. formerly considered to be a tight, membrane-to-membrane j. (macula occludens) but now shown to have a 2-nm gap between apposed cell membranes; the gap is not void but contains subunits in the form of polygonal lattices; it occurs in epithelia, between certain nerve cells, and in smooth and cardiac muscle; it is believed to mediate electrotonic coupling which allows ionic currents to pass from one cell to another. SEE ALSO synapse. (2) areas of increased electrochemical communication between myometrial cells which aid in the propagation of the contractions of labor. SYN electrotonic j., electrotonic synapse, macula communicans, nexus.

ju

Holliday j., the cross-strand structure formed when two DNA duplexes cross in a recombination event. SYN Holliday structure.

ileocecal j., point along the course of the gastrointestinal tract where the small intestine (ileum) ends as it opens into the cecal portion of the large intestine; occurs usually within the iliac fossa, demarcated internally as the ileocecal orifice.

intercellular j.'s, specializations of the cellular margins that contribute to the adhesion or allow for communication between cells; they include the macula adherens (desmosome), zonula adherens, zonula occludens, and nexus (gap junction).

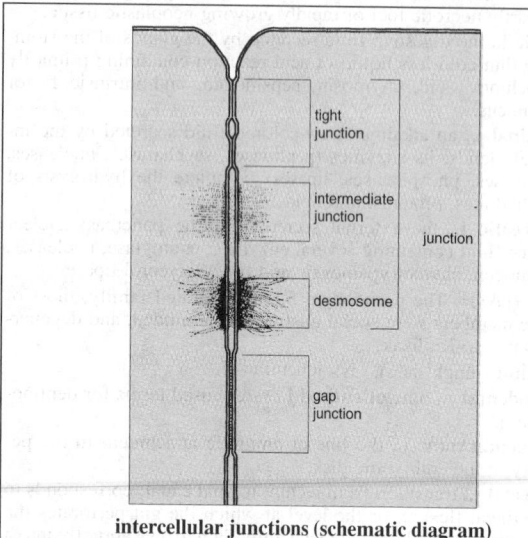

intercellular junctions (schematic diagram)

intermediate j., SYN *zonula* adherens.

j. of lips, SYN *commissure* of lips.

manubriosternal j., SYN sternal *angle.*

mucocutaneous j., the site of transition from epidermis to the epithelium of a mucous membrane.

muscle-tendon j., SYN muscle-tendon *attachment.*

myoneural j., the synaptic connection of the axon of the motor neuron with a muscle fiber. SEE motor *endplate.* SYN neuromuscular j.

neuroectodermal j., the margin of the embryonic neural plate separating it from the embryonic ectoderm; cells from this region form the neural crest. SYN neurosomatic j.

neuromuscular j., SYN myoneural j.

neurosomatic j., SYN neuroectodermal j.

rectosigmoid j., the site where the sigmoid colon becomes the rectum; usually takes the form of an acute angle, demarcated externally by a discontinuation of appendices epiploicae, a spreading out of the teniae coli to completely encircle the rectum, and consequently, termination of the sacculations (haustrae) between the teniae.

right splicing j., boundary between the right end of an intron and the left end of the adjacent exon. SYN acceptor splicing site.

sacrococcygeal j., SYN sacrococcygeal *joint.*

sclerocorneal j., SYN *limbus* of cornea.

squamocolumnar j., the site of transition from stratified squamous epithelium to columnar epithelium, usually characterized by stratified columnar epithelium.

ST j., SYN J *point.*

sternomanubrial j., SYN manubriosternal *symphysis.*

tight j., an intercellular j. between epithelial cells in which the outer leaflets of lateral cell membranes fuse to form a variable number of parallel interweaving strands that greatly reduce transepithelial permeability to macromolecules, solutes, and water via the paracellular route.

tympanostapedial j., the connection of the base or foot-plate of the stapes with the vestibular (oval) window. SYN syndesmosis tympanostapedia [NA].

ureteropelvic j. (UPJ), site of origin of the ureter from the renal pelvis, a common location for congenital or acquired obstruction.

junc·tu·ra, pl. **junc·tu·rae** (jŭngk-tū'ră, -rē). **1.** SYN joint. **2.** The point, line, or surface of union of two parts, mainly bones or cartilages. SYN junction, juncture. [L. a joining]

j. cartilagi'nea, SYN cartilaginous *joint.*

junctu'rae cin'guli mem'bri superio'ris, SYN *joints* of pectoral girdle, under *joint.*

j. fibro'sa, SYN fibrous *joint.*

j. lumbosacra'lis, SYN lumbosacral *joint.*

junctu'rae mem'bri inferio'ris li'beri, SYN *joints* of free lower limb, under *joint.*

junctu'rae mem'bri superio'ris li'beri, SYN *joints* of free upper limb, under *joint.*

junctu'rae os'sium, alternative name for articulationes. SEE articulatio.

j. sacrococcy'gea, SYN sacrococcygeal *joint.*

j. synovia'lis, SYN synovial *joint.*

junctu'rae ten'dinum, SYN intertendinous *connections,* under *connection.*

junctu'rae zygapophysea'les, SYN zygapophyseal *joints,* under *joint.*

junc·ture (jŭngk'chūr). SYN junctura (2).

Jung, Carl Gustav, Swiss psychiatrist and psychologist, 1875–1961. SEE jungian *psychoanalysis.*

Jung, Karl G., Swiss anatomist, 1793–1864. SEE J.'s *muscle.*

jung·i·an (yung'ē-an). The psychological system or the psychoanalytic form of treatment deriving from it; developed by Carl Gustav Jung.

Jüngling, Adolph O., German surgeon, 1884–1944. SEE J.'s *disease.*

ju·ni·per (jū'ni-per). The dried ripe fruit of *Juniperus communis* (family Pinaceae). [L. the juniper tree]

j. berry oil, SYN *oil* of juniper.

j. tar, the empyreumatic volatile oil obtained from the woody portion of *Juniperus oxycedrus;* used externally for skin diseases. SYN cade oil.

Junius, Paul, German ophthalmologist, *1871. SEE Kuhnt-J. *degeneration, disease.*

Junod, Victor T., French physician, 1809–1881. SEE J.'s *boot.*

jur·is·pru·dence (jūr-is-prū'dens). The science of law, its principles and concepts. [L. *juris prudentia,* knowledge of law]

dental j., SYN forensic *dentistry.*

medical j., SYN forensic *medicine.*

jus·tice. The ethical principle that persons who have similar circumstances and conditions should be treated alike; sometimes known as distributive justice. [L. *justitia,* fr. *jus,* right, law]

jus·to ma·jor (jus'tō mā'jer). SEE *pelvis* justo major.

jus·to mi·nor (jus'tō mī'ner). SEE *pelvis* justo minor.

ju·ve·nile de·lin·quent. A minor who cannot be controlled by parental authority and commits antisocial or criminal acts, such as vandalism, violence, or robbery.

jux·ta·crine (juks'tă-krin). A mode of hormone action that requires the cell producing the effector to be in direct contact with the cell containing the appropriate receptor. [L. *juxta,* close to, + G. *krinō,* to separate]

jux·ta·ep·i·phys·i·al (juks'tă-ep-i-fiz'ē-ăl). Close to or adjoining an epiphysis.

jux·ta·glo·mer·u·lar (juks'tă-glō-mer'yū-lăr). Close to or adjoining a renal glomerulus.

jux·tal·lo·cor·tex (juks'tă-lō-kōr'teks). O. Vogt's collective term for several regions of the cerebral cortex which occupy an intermediate position between the isocortex and the allocortex.

jux·ta·med·ul·lary (juks'tă-med'ŭ-lăr-ē). Close to or adjoining the medullary border.

jux·ta·po·si·tion (juks'tă-pō-zish'ŭn). A position side by side. SEE ALSO apposition, contiguity. [L. *juxta,* near to, + *positio,* a placing, fr. *pono,* pp. *positus,* to place]

K

κ Symbol for kappa, the tenth letter in the Greek alphabet.

K 1. Symbol for potassium; kalium; phylloquinone; kelvin; lysine. **2.** In optics, the coefficient of scleral rigidity. **3.** In contact lens fitting, the radius of curvature of the flattest meridian of the apical cornea.

^{40}**K** Symbol for potassium-40.

^{42}**K** Symbol for potassium-42.

^{43}**K** Symbol for potassium-43.

K Symbol for dissociation *constant.* SEE K_d.

K_a Symbol for dissociation *constant* of an acid; association *constant* (2) (often used with gases).

K_b Symbol for dissociation *constant* of a base.

K_d Symbol for dissociation *constant.*

K_{eq} Symbol for equilibrium *constant.*

K_i Symbol for the dissociation constant of an inhibitor; in enzyme kinetics, K_{ii} reflects the values of K_i that affect the intercept of a double-reciprocal plot while K_{is} reflects the values of K_i that affect the slope of the same plot.

K_m. Symbol for Michaelis *constant*; Michaelis-Menten *constant.*

K_w Symbol for dissociation *constant* of water.

k Symbol for kilo-.

k Symbol for rate *constants,* under *constant* or velocity *constants,* under *constant.*

k_{cat} The overall catalytic rate of an enzyme; symbol for turnover *number;* V_{max} divided by the total enzyme concentration.

Ka Abbreviation for kathode or kathodal.

ka·bu·re (kah-bū′rē). SYN *schistosomiasis* japonica.

Kaes, Theodor, German neurologist, 1852–1913. SEE *line* of K.; *band* of K.-Bechterew.

ka·fin·do (kă-fin′dō). SYN onyalai.

kai·nic ac·id (kā′in-ik). 2-Carboxy-4-(1-methylethenyl)-3-pyrrolidineacetic acid; a glutamate analog that exhibits powerful and long-acting excitatory and toxic activity on neurons; used as a research tool in neurobiology to destroy neurons and as an activator of glutamate receptors. Has been used as an anthelmintic against nematodes.

kai·ro·mones (kī′rō-mōn). A flower scent used to attract or repel other species. Cf. pheromones, allomones.

Kaiserling, Karl, German pathologist, 1869–1942. SEE K.'s *fixative.*

△**kak-, kako-.** SEE caco-.

kak·ké (kahk′kā). SYN beriberi. [Jap.]

△**kal-, kali-.** Potassium; sometimes improperly written as *kalio-*. [L. *kalium,* potassium]

ka·la azar (kah′lah ah-zahr′). SYN visceral *leishmaniasis.* [Hind. *kala,* black, + *azar,* poison]

ka·le·mia (kă-lē′mē-ă). The presence of potassium in the blood.

ka·li·o·pe·nia (kā′lē-ō-pē′nē-ă). Insufficiency of potassium in the body. [Mod. L. *kalium,* potassium, + G. *penia,* poverty]

ka·li·o·pe·nic (kā′lē-ō-pē′nik). Relating to kaliopenia.

Kalischer, Siegfried, German physician, *1862. SEE Sturge-K.-Weber *syndrome.*

ka·li·um (K) (kā′lē-ŭm). SYN potassium. [Mod. L. fr. Ar. *quali,* potash]

ka·li·u·re·sis (kā′lē-yū-rē′sis). SYN kaluresis.

ka·li·u·ret·ic (kā′lē-yū-ret′ik). SYN kaluretic.

kal·lak (kah-lak′). A pustular dermatitis observed among Eskimos. [Eskimo word meaning skin disease]

kal·li·din (kal′i-din). Bradykinin with a lysyl group attached to the amino terminus; this group can be removed by an aminopeptidase in the blood to yield bradykinin; a decapeptide vasodilator. SYN bradykininogen, k. 10, k. II, lysyl-bradykinin.

k. 9, SYN bradykinin.

k. 10, SYN kallidin.

k. I, SYN bradykinin.

k. II, SYN kallidin.

Kal·li·kak (kal′ĭ-kak). The pseudonym for a celebrated family with two lines of descendants, one of respectable citizens, the other of social misfits and criminals. SEE ALSO Jukes.

kal·li·kre·in (kal-i-krē′in). A group of enzymes (*e.g.,* plasma, tissue, pancreatic, urinary, submandibular k.) that can convert kininogen by proteolysis to bradykinin or kallidin; trypsin and plasmin can also effect the conversion; plasma k. activates the Hageman factor and acts on kininogen. SYN kininogenase, kininogenin.

Kallmann, Franz Josef, U.S. medical geneticist and psychiatrist, 1897–1965. SEE K.'s *syndrome.*

kal·u·re·sis (kal-yū-rē′sis). The increased urinary excretion of potassium. SYN kaliuresis. [Mod. L. *kalium,* potassium, + G. *ourēsis,* urination]

kal·u·ret·ic (kal-yū-ret′ik). Relating to, causing, or characterized by kaluresis. SYN kaliuretic.

ka·na·my·cin sul·fate (kan-ă-mī′sin). An aminoglycoside antibiotic substance derived from strains of *Streptomyces kanamycetius;* a thermostable, water-soluble, polybasic substance consisting of two amino sugars glycosidally linked to deoxystreptamine. The antibacterial activity *in vitro* is nearly identical with that of neomycin and is active against many aerobic Gram-positive and Gram-negative bacteria (*Aerobacter, Escherichia coli, Proteus, Klebsiella, Neisseria, Shigella,* and *Salmonella*). Excessive doses and prolonged administration may result in irreversible damage to the auditory portion and/or vesitibular portion of the eighth cranial nerve.

Kandori, Fumio, Japanese ophthalmologist, *1904. SEE fleck *retina* of Kandori.

Kanner, Leo, Austrian psychiatrist in U.S., *1894. SEE K.'s *syndrome.*

kan·yem·ba (kan-yem′bă). SYN chiufa.

ka·od·ze·ra (kah′od-ze′rā). A disease prevalent in Zimbabwe (formerly Rhodesia), similar to sleeping sickness, caused by *Trypanosoma rhodesiense.* SEE ALSO Rhodesian *trypanosomiasis.*

ka·o·lin (kā′ō-lin). when powdered and freed from gritty particles by elutriation, k. is used as a demulcent and adsorbent; in dentistry, it is used to add toughness and opacity to porcelain teeth. SYN aluminum silicate. [Ch. *kao lin,* High Ridge, name of a locality in China where the substance is found in abundance]

ka·o·lin·o·sis (kā′ō-lin-ō′sis). Pneumonoconiosis caused by the inhalation of clay dust.

Kaposi, Moritz, (born Moritz Kohn), Hungarian dermatologist in Austria, 1837–1902. SEE K.'s varicelliform *eruption, sarcoma.*

kap·pa (κ) (kap′a). **1.** The tenth letter in the Greek alphabet. **2.** In chemistry, denotes the position of a substituent located on the tenth atom from the carboxyl or other functional group. **3.** A measure of the degree of nonrandom agreement between observers or measurements of the same categorical variable.

kap·pa·cism (kap′ă-sizm). Faulty pronunciation of the "k" sound. [G. *kappa,* the letter κ]

Karman can·nu·la. See under cannula.

Karmen, Albert, U.S. internist and clinical pathologist, *1930. SEE K. *unit.*

Karnofsky, D.A., 20th century U.S. physician. SEE K. *scale.*

Kartagener, Manes, Swiss physician, 1897–1975. SEE K.'s *syndrome, triad.*

△**karyo-.** Nucleus. Cf. nucleo-. [G. *karyon,* nucleus]

kar·y·o·chrome (kar′ē-ō-krōm). A nerve cell body having little or no Nissl substance visible but a nucleus that stains intensely. [karyo- + G. *chroma,* color]

kar·y·oc·la·sis (kar-ē-ok′lă-sis). SYN karyorrhexis. [karyo- + G. *klasis,* a breaking]

kar·y·o·cyte (kar′ē-ō-sīt). A young, immature normoblast. [karyo- + G. *kytos,* cell]

ka

kar·y·o·gam·ic (kar-ē-ō-gam′ik). Relating to or marked by karyogamy.

kar·y·og·a·my (kar-ē-og′ă-mē). Fusion of the nuclei of two cells, as occurs in fertilization or true conjugation. [karyo- + G. *gamos,* marriage]

kar·y·o·gen·e·sis (kar-ē-ō-jen′ĕ-sis). Formation of the nucleus of a cell. [karyo- + G. *genesis,* production]

kar·y·o·gen·ic (kar-ē-ō-jen′ik). Relating to karyogenesis; forming the nucleus.

kar·y·o·go·nad (kar′ē-ō-gō′nad). SYN micronucleus (2). [karyo- + G. *gonē,* generation, descent]

kar·y·o·gram (kar′ē-ō-gram). SYN karyotype.

kar·y·ol·o·gy (kar-ē-ol′o-jē). The branch of cytology that deals with the study of the cell nucleus, its organelles, structures, and functions. [karyo- + -logy]

kar·y·o·lymph (kar′ē-ō-limf). The presumably fluid substance or gel of the nucleus in which stainable elements were believed to be suspended; much that was formerly considered to be k. is now known to be euchromatin. SYN nuclear hyaloplasm, nuclear sap, nucleochylema, nucleochyme. [karyo- + L. *lympha,* clear water]

kar·y·ol·y·sis (kar-ē-ol′i-sis). Apparent destruction of the nucleus of a cell by swelling and the loss of affinity of its chromatin for basic dyes. [karyo- + G. *lysis,* dissolution]

kar·y·o·lyt·ic (kar′ē-ō-lit′ik). Relating to karyolysis.

kar·y·o·mere (kar′ē-ō-mer′). A vesicle containing only a small part of the typical nucleus, usually following an abnormal mitosis. [karyo- + G. *meros,* part]

kar·y·o·mi·cro·some (kar-ē-ō-mī′krō-sōm). One of the minute particles or granules making up the substance of the cell nucleus. SYN nucleomicrosome. [karyo- + G. *mikros,* small, + *soma,* body]

kar·y·o·mi·to·me (kar′-ē-ōm-ī-tom). The nuclear chromatin network. [karyo- + mitosis + -ome]

kar·y·o·mor·phism (kar′ē-ō-mōr′fizm). **1.** Development of the nucleus of a cell. **2.** Denoting the nuclear shapes of cells, especially leukocytes. [karyo- + G. *morphē,* form]

kar·y·on (kar′ē-on). SYN nucleus (1). [G. *karyon,* a nut, kernel]

kar·y·o·phage (kar′ē-ō-fāj). An intracellular parasite that feeds on the host nucleus. [karyo- + G. *phagō,* to devour]

kar·y·o·plasm (kar′ē-ō-plazm). Rarely used term for nucleoplasm.

kar·y·o·plas·mol·y·sis (kar′ē-ō-plaz-mol′i-sis). SYN achromatolysis.

kar·y·o·plast (kar′ē-ō-plast). A cell nucleus surrounded by a narrow band of cytoplasm and a plasma membrane. [karyo- + G. *plastos,* formed]

kar·y·o·plas·tin (kar′ē-ō-plas′tin). The achromatic nuclear material that forms the spindle apparatus.

kar·y·o·pyk·no·sis (kar′ē-ō-pik-nō′sis). Cytologic characteristics of the superficial or cornified cells of stratified squamous epithelium in which there is shrinkage of the nuclei and condensation of the chromatin into structureless masses. [karyo- + G. *pyknos,* thick, crowded, + *-osis,* condition]

kar·y·o·pyk·not·ic (kar′ē-ō-pik-not′ik). Pertaining to or causing karyopyknosis.

kar·y·or·rhex·is (kar-ē-ō-rak′sis). Fragmentation of the nucleus whereby its chromatin is distributed irregularly throughout the cytoplasm; a stage of necrosis usually followed by karyolysis. SYN karyoclasis. [karyo- + G. *rhexis,* rupture]

kar·y·o·some (kar′ē-ō-sōm). A mass of chromatin often found in the interphase cell nucleus representing a more condensed zone of chromatin filaments. SYN chromatin nucleolus, chromocenter, false nucleolus, net knot. [karyo- + G. *sōma,* body]

kar·y·os·ta·sis (kar-ē-os′tă-sis). SYN interphase. [karyo- + G. *stasis,* a standing still]

kar·y·o·the·ca (kar′ē-ō-thē′kă). SYN nuclear *envelope.* [karyo- + G. *thēkē,* box, sheath]

kar·y·o·type (kar′ē-ō-tīp). The chromosome characteristics of an individual cell or of a cell line, usually presented as a systematized array of metaphase chromosomes from a photomicrograph

of a single cell nucleus arranged in pairs in descending order of size and according to the position of the centromere. SYN idiogram (1), karyogram. [karyo- + G. *typos,* model]

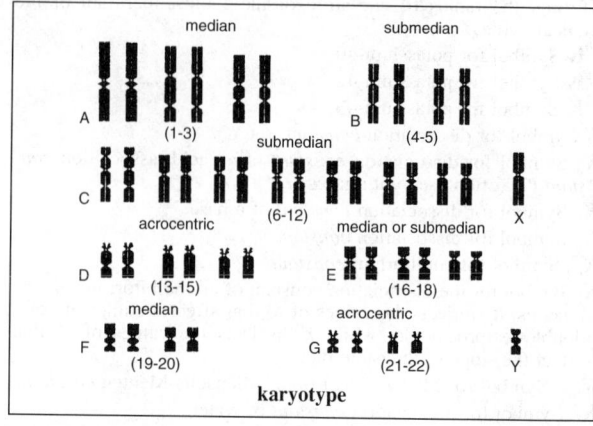

karyotype

kar·y·o·zo·ic (kar′ē-ō-zō′ik). Denoting a parasite inhabiting the cell nucleus of its host. [karyo- + G. *zōon,* animal]

Kasabach, Haig H., U.S. physician, 1898–1943. SEE K.-Merritt *syndrome.*

Kasai, Morio, 20th century Japanese surgeon. SEE K. *operation.*

ka·sai (kă-sī′). A form of anemia occurring in natives of Zaire (formerly the Belgian Congo), with associated edema of subcutaneous tissues, depigmented regions in the skin, and various gastrointestinal disturbances; thought to result from deficiencies in nutrition. SYN Belgian Congo anemia.

Kashin, Nikolai I., Russian orthopedist, 1825–1872. SEE K.-Bek *disease.*

Kasten, Frederick H., U.S. histochemist and cell biologist, *1927. SEE K.'s fluorescent Schiff *reagents,* under *reagent,* fluorescent Feulgen *stain,* fluorescent PAS *stain.*

kat Abbreviation for katal.

△**kata-.** Alternative spelling for cata-; down. [G. *kata,* down]

kat·al (kat) (kat′ăl). Unit of catalytic activity equal to one mole of product formed (or substrate consumed) per second, as of the amount of enzyme that catalyzes transformation of one mole of substrate per second.

kat·a·ther·mom·e·ter (kat′ă-ther-mom′ĕ-ter). An alcohol-filled thermometer of specified design that is heated above ambient temperature and then allowed to cool; the time taken to cool between specified temperatures is a measure of the heat content of the environment that takes into account air movement as well as temperature. The bulb may be silvered to minimize radiation effects or blackened to maximize them.

Katayama, Kunika, Japanese physician, 1856–1931. SEE K.'s *test.*

kath·o·dal (Ka), kath·ode (kath′ō-dăl, kath′ōd). Obsolete spelling of cathodal, cathode.

kat·i·on (kat′ī-on). Obsolete spelling of cation.

Katz, Sir Bernard, German-British neurophysiologist and Nobel laureate, *1911. SEE Goldman-Hodgkin-K. *equation.*

ka·va (kah′vah). **1.** SYN methysticum. **2.** SYN yaqona. [Tongan and Marquesan, Litter]

Kawasaki, Tomisaku, 20th century Japanese pediatrician. SEE K.'s *disease, syndrome.*

Kay, Herbert D., British biochemist, *1893. SEE Jenner-K. *unit.*

Kayser, Bernhard, German physician, 1869–1954. SEE K.-Fleischer *ring.*

Kazanjian, Varaztad H., Armenian otorhinolaryngologist in the U.S., 1879–1974. SEE K.'s *operation.*

kb Abbreviation for kilobase.

K blood group, k blood group. See Kell blood group, Blood Groups appendix.

kc Abbreviation for kilocycle.

kcal Abbreviation for kilogram *calorie*; kilocalorie.

Kearns, Thomas P., U.S. ophthalmologist, *1922. SEE K.-Sayre *syndrome.*

Keating-Hart, Walter V., French physician, 1870–1922. SEE Keating-Hart's *method.*

ked. SYN *Melophagus ovinus.*

keel (kēl). Paratyphoid or salmonellosis of ducklings.

Keen, William W., U.S. surgeon, 1837–1932. SEE K.'s *operation, sign.*

Kegel, A.H., 20th century U.S. gynecologist. SEE K.'s *exercises,* under *exercise.*

Kehr, Hans, German surgeon, 1862–1916. SEE K.'s *sign.*

kei·ro·spasm (kī'rō-spazm). SYN shaving *cramp.* [G. *keirō,* to shear]

Keith, Sir Arthur, Scottish anatomist, 1866–1955. SEE K.'s *bundle, node;* K. and Flack *node.*

ke·lec·tome (kē'lek-tōm). An instrument used, like the harpoon, to remove a specimen of tumor substance for examination. [G. *kēlē,* tumor, + *ektomē,* excision]

Kell blood group. See Blood Groups appendix.

Keller, William Lordan, U.S. surgeon, 1874–1959. SEE K. *bunionectomy.*

Kellie, George, 18th century Scottish anatomist. SEE Monro-K. *doctrine.*

Kelly, Adam B., British otolaryngologist, 1865–1941. SEE Paterson-K. *syndrome;* Paterson-Brown-K. *syndrome.*

Kelly, Howard A., U.S. gynecologist, 1858–1943. SEE K. *clamp;* K.'s *operation,* rectal *speculum.*

ke·loid (kē'loyd). A nodular, firm, movable, nonencapsulated, often linear mass of hyperplastic scar tissue, tender and frequently painful, consisting of wide irregularly distributed bands of collagen; occurs in the dermis and adjacent subcutaneous tissue, usually after trauma, surgery, a burn, or severe cutaneous disease such as cystic acne, and is more common in blacks. SYN cheloid. [G. *kēlē,* a tumor (or *kēlis,* a spot), + *eidos,* appearance]
acne k., a chronic eruption of fibrous papules which develop at the site of follicular lesions, usually on the back of the neck at the hairline. SYN dermatitis papillaris capillitii, folliculitis keloidalis, sycosis frambesiformis.

ke·loi·do·sis (kē'loy-dō'sis). Multiple keloids.

ke·lo·plas·ty (kē'lō-plas-tē). Operative removal of a scar or keloid. [keloid + G. *plastos,* formed]

ke·lo·so·mia (kē-lō-sō'mē-ă). SYN celosomia.

Kelvin, Lord William Thomson, Scottish physicist, 1824–1907. SEE kelvin; K. *scale.*

kel·vin (K). A unit of thermodynamic temperature equal to $^{1}/_{273.16}$ of the thermodynamic temperature of the triple point of water. SEE Kelvin scale. [Lord *Kelvin*]

Kendall. SEE Abell-Kendall *method.*

Kennedy, Edward, U.S. dentist, *1883. SEE K. *classification.*

Kennedy, Robert Foster, U.S. neurologist, 1884–1952. SEE K.'s *syndrome;* Foster K. *syndrome.*

Kennedy, William, U.S. neurologist. SEE Kennedy's *disease.*

Kenny, Elizabeth, Australian nurse, 1886–1952. SEE K.'s *treatment.*

△**keno-.** SEE ceno- (3). [G. *kenos,* empty]

Kent, Albert F.S., English physiologist, 1863–1958. SEE K.'s *bundle;* K.-His *bundle.*

keph·a·lin (kef'ă-lin). SYN cephalin.

kep·one (kē-pōn'). An insecticide consisting of a cage structure; neurotoxic chemical.

Kerandel, Jean F., French physician, 1873–1934. SEE K.'s *symptom.*

ker·a·phyl·lo·cele (ker-ă-fil'ō-sēl). A horny tumor on the internal face of the wall of a horse's foot. [G. *keras,* horn, + *phyllon,* leaf, + *kēlē,* hernia, tumor]

ker·a·sin (ker'ă-sin). Obsolete term for glucocerebroside. SYN cerasin.

△**kerat-.** SEE kerato-.

ker·a·tan sul·fate (ker'ă-tan). A type of sulfated mucopolysaccharide containing D-galactose in place of the uronic acid of hyaluronic acid or chondroitin; also containing unsulfated and 6-sulfated N-acetyl-D-glucosamine; found in cartilage, bone, connective tissue, the cornea, aorta, and in the intervertebral discs; accumulates in Morquio syndrome; k. s. I is abundant in cornea and is attached to a protein via an asparaginyl residue; k. s. II is found in loose connective tissue and is linked to a seryl or threonyl residue. SYN keratosulfate.

ker·a·tec·ta·sia (ker-ă-tek-tā'zē-ă). SYN keratoectasia. [kerato- + G. *ektasis,* extrusion]

ker·a·tec·to·my (ker-ă-tek'tō-mē). An operation done to change the refraction of the cornea; a crescentic piece of corneal stroma is removed and the resultant corneal wound is sutured. This steepens the cornea and increases its power in that axis. [kerato- + G. *ektomē,* excision]
photorefractive k., removal of part of the cornea with a laser to change its shape, and thus to modify the refractive error of the eye (reduce its myopia, for example).

ker·a·te·in (ker'ă-tē-in). The easily digested reduction product of keratin, in which the disulfide links are reduced to SH groups, the individual peptide chains being separated.

ker·a·ti·a·sis (ker-ă-tī'ă-sis). SYN keratosis.

ke·rat·ic (ke-rat'ik). SYN horny. [G. *keras (kerat-),* horn]

ker·a·tin (ker'ă-tin). A scleroprotein or albuminoid present largely in cuticular structures (*e.g.,* hair, nails, horns); it contains a relatively large amount of sulfur, is insoluble in the gastric juices, and is sometimes used for coating enteric pills that are intended to be dissolved only in the intestine. There are at least eleven k.'s. α-Keratin has a folded configuration; β-keratin has an extended configuration. SYN ceratin. [G. *keras (kerat-),* horn, + -in]

ker·a·tin·as·es (ker'ă-tin-ās-ez). Hydrolases catalyzing the hydrolysis of keratin; each having slightly different specificities.

ker·a·tin·i·za·tion (ker'ă-tin-i-zā'shŭn). Keratin formation or development of a horny layer; may also apply to premature formation of keratin. SYN cornification, hornification.

ker·a·tin·ized (ker'ă-ti-nīzd). Having become horny. SYN cornified.

ke·rat·i·no·cyte (ke-rat'i-nō-sīt). A cell of the living epidermis and certain oral epithelium that produces keratin in the process of differentiating into the dead and fully keratinized cells of the stratum corneum.

ke·rat·i·no·phil·ic (ke-rat'i-nō-fil'ik). Denoting fungi that use keratin as a substrata, *e.g.,* dermatophytes. [keratin + Gr. *philos,* love, attraction, + -ic]

ke·rat·i·no·some (ke-rat'i-nō-sōm). A membrane-bound granule, 100 to 500 nm in diameter, located in the upper layers of the stratum spinosum of certain stratified squamous epithelia. SYN lamellar granule, membrane-coating granule, Odland body.

ke·rat·i·nous (ke-rat'i-nŭs). 1. Relating to keratin. 2. SYN horny.

ker·a·ti·tis (ker-ă-tī'tis). Inflammation of the cornea. SEE ALSO keratopathy. [kerato- + G. *-itis,* inflammation]
actinic k., a reaction of the cornea to ultraviolet light.
deep punctate k., sharply defined opacities in an otherwise clear cornea, occurring in syphilitic iritis.
dendriform k., dendritic k., a form of herpetic k.
diffuse deep k., SYN k. profunda.
Dimmer's k., SYN k. nummularis.
disciform k., large disk-shaped infiltration of the central or paracentral corneal stroma. This lesion is deep and nonsuppurative and is seen in virus infections, particularly herpetic. SYN k. disciformis.
k. discifor'mis, SYN disciform k.
exposure k., inflammation of the cornea resulting from irritation caused by inability to close the eyelids. SYN lagophthalmic k.
fascicular k., a phlyctenular k. followed by the formation of a band or fascicle of blood vessels extending from the margin toward the center.
filamentary k., a condition characterized by the formation of epithelial filaments of varying size and length on the corneal surface. SYN k. filamentosa.

ke

k. filamento′sa, SYN filamentary k.

geographic k., k. with coalescence of superficial lesions in herpes keratitis.

herpetic k., inflammation of the cornea (or cornea and conjunctiva) due to herpes simplex virus. SYN herpes corneae, herpetic keratoconjunctivitis.

infectious bovine k., a highly contagious keratoconjunctivitis that occurs in range or pastured cattle during the summer months, is transmitted most commonly by contact with infectious discharges, and is caused by *Moraxella bovis.*

interstitial k., an inflammation of the corneal stroma, often with neovascularization.

lagophthalmic k., SYN exposure k.

k. linea′ris mi′grans, a deep, linear corneal opacity stretching from limbus to limbus; associated with congenital syphilis.

marginal k., a corneal inflammation at the limbus.

metaherpetic k., a postinfectious corneal inflammation in herpetic k. leading to epithelial erosion; not due to virus replication.

mycotic k., an infection of the cornea of the eye caused by a fungus.

neuroparalytic k., SYN neurotrophic *keratitis.*

neurotrophic k., inflammation of the cornea after corneal anesthesia.

k. nummula′ris, coin-shaped or round, discrete, grayish areas 0.5 to 1.5 mm in diameter scattered throughout the various layers of the cornea. SYN Dimmer's k.

phlyctenular k., an inflammation of the corneal conjunctiva with the formation of small red nodules of lymphoid tissue (phlyctenulae) near the corneoscleral limbus. SYN scrofulous k.

pneumococcal/suppurative k., SYN serpiginous k.

polymorphic superficial k., epithelial degeneration occurring in starvation.

k. profun′da, an inflammation of the posterior corneal stroma. SYN diffuse deep k.

punctate k., k. puncta′ta, SYN keratic *precipitates,* under *precipitate.*

sclerosing k., inflammation of the cornea complicating scleritis; characterized by opacification of the corneal stroma.

scrofulous k., SYN phlyctenular k.

serpiginous k., a severe, creeping, central, suppurative ulcer often due to pneumococci. SYN pneumococcal/suppurative k., serpent ulcer of cornea.

k. sic′ca, SYN *keratoconjunctivitis* sicca.

superficial linear k., spontaneous, painful k. with epithelial erosion and folds in Bowman's membrane.

superficial punctate k., epithelial punctate k. associated with viral conjunctivitis. SYN Thygeson's disease.

trachomatous k., SEE pannus, corneal *pannus.*

vascular k., superficial cellular infiltration of the cornea and neovascularization between Bowman's membrane and the epithelium.

vesicular k., k. with coalescence of areas of epithelial corneal edema.

xerotic k., SYN keratomalacia.

△**kerato-, kerat-. 1.** The cornea. **2.** Horny tissue or cells. SEE ALSO cerat-, cerato-. [G. *keras,* horn]

ker·a·to·ac·an·tho·ma (ker′ă-tō-ak′an-thō′mă). A rapidly growing tumor which may be umbilicated, usually occurring on exposed areas of the skin, which invades the dermis but remains localized and usually resolves spontaneously if untreated; microscopically, the nodule is composed of well-differentiated squamous epithelium with a central keratin mass that opens on the skin surface. [kerato- + G. *akantha,* thorn, +-*oma,* tumor]

ker·a·to·an·gi·o·ma (ker′ă-tō-an-jē-ō′mă). SYN angiokeratoma.

ker·a·to·at·ro·pho·der·ma (ker′ă-tō-at′rō-fō-der′mă). SYN porokeratosis. [kerato- + G. *atrophia,* atrophy, + *derma,* skin]

ker·a·to·cele (ker′ă-tō-sēl). Hernia of Descemet's membrane through a defect in the outer layers of the cornea. [kerato- + G. *kēlē,* hernia]

ker·a·to·con·junc·ti·vi·tis (ker′ă-tō-kon-jŭngk′ti-vī′tis). Inflammation of the conjunctiva and of the cornea.

atopic k., a chronic papillary inflammation, of the conjunctiva showing Trantas dots in a patient with a history of hypersensitivity.

epidemic k., follicular conjunctivitis followed by subepithelial corneal infiltrates; often caused by adenovirus type 8, less commonly by other types. SYN virus k.

flash k., SYN ultraviolet k.

herpetic k., SYN herpetic *keratitis.*

infectious bovine k., a disease of cattle caused by the bacterium *Moraxella bovis* and characterized by blepharospasm, conjunctivitis, lacrimation, and corneal opacity and ulceration. SYN infectious ophthalmia, pinkeye (2).

microsporidian k., a form of k. often associated with immunosuppressed persons, such as those suffering from AIDS.

k. sic′ca, k. associated with decreased tears. SEE ALSO Sjögren's *syndrome.* SYN dry eye syndrome, keratitis sicca.

superior limbic k., inflammatory edema of the superior corneoscleral limbus.

ultraviolet k., acute k. resulting from exposure to intense ultraviolet irradiation. SYN actinic conjunctivitis, arc-flash conjunctivitis, flash k., ophthalmia nivalis, snow conjunctivitis, welder's conjunctivitis.

vernal k., SYN vernal *conjunctivitis.*

virus k., SYN epidemic k.

ker·a·to·co·nus (ker′ă-tō-kō′nŭs). A conical protrusion of the cornea caused by thinning of the stroma; usually bilateral. SEE ALSO Fleischer's *ring,* Munson's *sign.* SYN conical cornea. [kerato- + G. *kōnos,* cone]

ker·a·to·cri·coid (ker′ă-tō-krī′koyd). SYN ceratocricoid.

ker·a·to·cyst (ker′ă-tō-sist). Odontogenic cyst derived from remnants of the dental lamina and appearing as a unilocular or multilocular radiolucency which may produce jaw expansion; epithelial lining is characterized microscopically by a uniform thickness, a corrugated superficial layer of parakeratin, and a prominent basal layer composed of palisaded columnar cells; associated with the bifid rib basal cell nevus syndrome.

odontogenic k. (ke-rā′tō-sist), a cyst of dental lamina origin with a high recurrence rate and well-defined histologic criteria of a corrugated parakeratin surface, uniformly thin epithelium, and a palisaded basal layer. One manifestation of the basal cell nevus syndrome.

ker·a·to·cyte (ker′ă-tō-sīt). The fibroblastic stromal cell of the cornea.

ker·a·to·der·ma (ker′ă-tō-der′mă). **1.** Any horny superficial growth. **2.** A generalized thickening of the horny layer of the epidermis. [kerato- + G. *derma,* skin]

k. blennorrhag′ica, SYN *keratosis* blennorrhagica.

k. blennorrhagicum (blen-ō-raj′ĭ-kŭm), the scattered, thickened, hyperkeratotic skin lesions seen in Reiter's syndrome.

k. eccen′trica, SYN porokeratosis.

lymphedematous k., SYN mossy *foot.*

mutilating k. [MIM*124500], diffuse k. of the extremities, with the development during childhood of constricting fibrous bands around the middle phalanx of the fingers or toes which may lead to spontaneous amputation; autosomal dominant inheritance. SYN keratoma hereditarium mutilans, Vohwinkel syndrome.

k. palma′ris et planta′ris, SYN palmoplantar k.

palmoplantar k. [MIM*148600 & MIM*244850], the occurrence of symmetrical diffuse or patchy areas of hypertrophy of the horny layer of the epidermis on the palms and soles; a group of ectodermal dysplasias of considerable variety, and either autosomal dominant or recessive inheritance. SYN ichthyosis palmaris et plantaris, k. palmaris et plantaris, k. symmetrica, keratoma plantare sulcatum, keratosis palmaris et plantaris, tylosis palmaris et plantaris.

k. planta′re sulca′tum, hyperkeratosis and fissure formation on the soles. SYN cracked heel.

punctate k., horny papules over the palms, soles, and digits that develop central plugs; seen commonly in blacks. SYN keratoma disseminatum, keratosis punctata.

senile k., SYN actinic *keratosis.*

k. symmet′rica, SYN palmoplantar k.

ker·a·to·der·ma·ti·tis (ker'ă-tō-der-mă-tī'tis). Inflammation with proliferation of the horny layer of the skin. [kerato- + G. *derma*, skin, + -*itis*, inflammation]

ker·a·to·ec·ta·sia (ker'ă-tō-ek-tā'zē-ă). A bulging forward of the cornea. SYN corneal ectasia, keratectasia.

ker·a·to·elas·toid·o·sis (ker'ă-tō-ă-las'toy-dō-sis). Hyperkeratosis and degeneration of dermal elastic tissue. SEE ALSO acrokeratoelastoidosis. [kerato- + Mod. L. *elasticus*, elastic, fr. G. *elastikos*, propulsive, fr. *elaunō*, to drive + *eidos*, resemblance, + suffix -*ōsis*, condition]

k. marginalis (mar-gin-āl'is), hyperkeratosis and solar elastosis presenting as linear papules along the junction of the palms and dorsal surface of the hands in the elderly. [L. marginal]

ker·a·to·ep·i·the·li·o·plas·ty (ker'ă-tō-ep-i-thē'lē-ō-plas-tē). A surgical procedure for the repair of persistent corneal epithelial defects. All the corneal epithelium is removed from the recipient cornea, and small pieces of donor cornea, with epithelium attached, are placed at the corneoscleral limbus. The donor corneal epithelium grows and spreads out to cover the recipient cornea. [kerato- + epithelio- + G. *plastos*, formed]

ker·a·to·gen·e·sis (ker'ă-tō-jen'ĕ-sis). Production or origin of horny cells or tissue. [kerato- + G. *genesis*, production]

ker·a·to·ge·net·ic (ker'ă-tō-jĕ-net'ik). Relating to keratogenesis.

ker·a·tog·e·nous (ker-ă-toj'ĕ-nŭs). Causing a growth of cells that produce keratin and result in the formation of horny tissue, such as fingernails, scales, feathers, etc.

ker·a·to·glo·bus (ker-ă-tō-glō'bŭs). Congenital anomaly consisting of an enlarged anterior segment of the eye. SYN anterior megalophthalmos, megalocornea. [kerato- + L. *globus*, ball]

ker·a·to·glos·sus (ker'ă-tō-glos'sŭs). SYN chondroglossus *muscle*.

ker·a·tog·ra·phy (ker'ah-tog'ra-fē). A record or portrayal of the cornea. SEE photokeratoscope, videokeratoscope. [kerato- + G. *graphō*, to write]

ker·a·to·hy·al (ker'ă-tō-hī'ăl). SYN ceratohyal.

ker·a·to·hy·a·lin (ker'ă-tō-hī'ă-lin). The substance in the large basophilic granules of the stratum granulosum of the epidermis. [kerato- + hyalin]

ker·a·toid (ker'ă-toyd). 1. SYN horny. 2. Resembling corneal tissue. [kerato- + G. *eidos*, resemblance]

ker·a·to·lep·tyn·sis (ker'ă-tō-lep-tin'sis). 1. SYN gutter *dystrophy* of cornea. 2. An operation for removing the surface of the cornea and replacement by bulbar conjunctiva for cosmetic reasons. [kerato- + G. *leptynsis*, a making thin]

ker·a·to·leu·ko·ma (ker'ă-tō-lū-kō'mă). A white corneal opacity. [kerato- + G. *leukos*, white, + -*ōma*, growth]

ker·a·tol·y·sis (ker-ă-tol'i-sis). 1. Separation or loosening of the horny layer of the epidermis. 2. Specifically, a disease characterized by a shedding of the epidermis recurring at more or less regular intervals. SYN deciduous skin. [kerato- + G. *lysis*, loosening]

k. exfoliati'va [MIM*270300], familial continual skin peeling characterized by a separation of stratum corneum in leaflike flakes occurring everywhere except on the palms and soles; the cause is unknown. SYN erythema exfoliativa, erythroderma exfoliativa.

pitted k., noninflammatory Gram-positive bacterial infection of the plantar surfaces producing small depressions in the stratum corneum, associated frequently with humidity and hyperhidrosis. SYN k. plantare sulcatum.

k. planta're sulca'tum, SYN pitted k.

ker·a·to·lyt·ic (ker'ă-tō-lit'ik). Relating to keratolysis.

ker·a·to·ma (ker-ă-tō'mă). 1. SYN callosity. 2. A horny tumor. [kerato- + G. -*oma*, tumor]

k. dissemina'tum, SYN punctate *keratoderma*.

k. heredita'rium mu'tilans, SYN mutilating *keratoderma*.

k. malig'num, SYN congenital ichthyosiform *erythroderma*.

k. planta're sulca'tum, SYN palmoplantar *keratoderma*.

senile k., SYN actinic *keratosis*.

ker·a·to·ma·la·cia (ker'ă-tō-mă-lā'shē-ă). Dryness with ulceration and perforation of the cornea, with absence of inflammatory

reactions, occurring in cachectic children; results from severe vitamin A deficiency. SYN xerotic keratitis. [kerato- + G. *malakia*, softness]

ker·a·tome (ker'ă-tōm). A knife used for incising the cornea. SYN keratotome.

ker·a·tom·e·ter (ker-ă-tom'ĕ-ter). An instrument for measuring the curvature of the anterior corneal surface. SYN ophthalmometer. [kerato- + G. *metron*, measure]

ker·a·tom·e·try (ker-ă-tom'ĕ-trē). Measurement of the radii of corneal curvature.

ker·a·to·mi·leu·sis (ker'ă-tō-mī-lū'sis). Surgical alteration of refractive error by changing the shape of a deep layer of the cornea: the anterior lamella is peeled back, frozen, and recarved on its back surface on a lathe; or, some of the corneal stroma can be removed from the bed with a laser or a knife. [coinage, prob. fr. G. *keras* (*kerat-*), horn, cornea, + *smileusis*, carving]

ker·a·to·my·co·sis (ker-ă-tō-mī-kō'sis). Fungal infection of the cornea.

ker·a·to·no·sis (ker'ă-tō-nō'sis). Any abnormal noninflammatory, usually hypertrophic, affection of the horny layer of the skin. [kerato- + G. -*osis*, condition]

ker·a·to·pach·y·der·ma (ker'ă-tō-pak-i-der'mă). A syndrome of congenital deafness with development of hyperkeratosis of the skin of the palms, soles, elbows, and knees in childhood, and with bandlike constrictions of the fingers. [kerato- + G. *pachys*, thick, + *derma*, skin]

ker·a·top·a·thy (ker-ă-top'ă-thē). Any corneal disease, damage, dysfunction, or abnormality. [kerato- + G. *pathos*, suffering, disease]

band-shaped k., a horizontal, gray, interpalpebral opacity of the cornea that begins at the periphery and progresses centrally; occurs in hypercalcemia, chronic iridocyclitis, and Still's disease.

bullous k., edema of the corneal stroma and epithelium; occurs in Fuchs' epithelial dystrophy, advanced glaucoma and iridocyclitis, and sometimes after intraocular lens implantation.

climatic k., a bilateral, symmetrical corneal dystrophy caused by prolonged exposure to extremes of heat or cold; nodular opacities are limited to the interpalpebral area and vision is only mildly affected. SYN Labrador k.

filamentary k., formation of fine elongations of corneal epithelium in inflammation, edema, and degenerative states.

Labrador k., SYN climatic k.

lipid k., occurrence of fats in an area of corneal vascularization.

neuroparalytic k., corneal inflammation or ulceration associated with dysfunction of the ophthalmic branch of the trigeminal nerve.

striate k., corneal stromal edema with formation of criss-cross tracts.

vesicular k., corneal epithelial edema with formation of vacuoles.

ker·a·to·pha·kia (ker'ă-tō-fak'ē-ă). Implantation of a donor cornea or plastic lens within the corneal stroma to modify refractive error. SYN keratophakic keratoplasty. [kerato- + G. *phakos*, lens]

ker·a·to·plas·ia (ker'ă-tō-plā'zē-ă). The formation or renewal of a horny layer. [kerato- + G. *plassō*; to fashion]

ker·a·to·plas·ty (ker'ă-tō-plas-tē). Any surgical modification of the cornea; the removal of a portion of the cornea containing an opacity and the insertion in its place of a piece of cornea of the same size and shape removed from elsewhere. SYN corneal graft, corneal transplantation, corneal trepanation, trepanation of cornea, transplantation of cornea. [kerato- + G. *plassō*, to form]

allopathic k., corneal transplant with donor material of glass, plastic, or other inert material.

autogenous k., corneal transplant with donor material from the same individual.

epikeratophakic k., SYN epikeratophakia.

heterogenous k., corneal transplant with donor material from another species.

homogenous k., corneal transplant with donor material from another individual of the same species.

keratophakic k., SYN keratophakia.

lamellar k., layered k., SYN nonpenetrating k.

ke

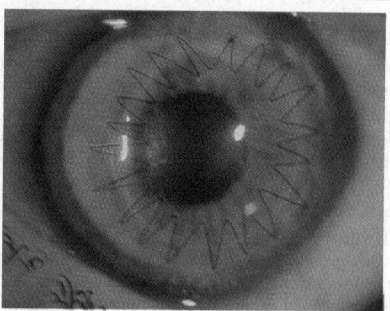

keratoplasty
in this corneal graft, nylon thread is used as suture material

nonpenetrating k., k. in which only the anterior layer of the cornea is used (not a tectonic k.). SYN lamellar k., layered k.

optical k., transplantation of transparent corneal tissue to replace a leukoma or scar that impairs vision.

penetrating k., corneal transplant with replacement of all layers of the cornea, but retaining the peripheral cornea. SYN perforating k.

perforating k., SYN penetrating k.

refractive k., any procedure in which the shape of the cornea is modified, with the intent of changing the refractive error of the eye; for example, if the cornea is flattened, the eye becomes less myopic. SEE photorefractive *keratectomy*, keratophakia, lamellar k., thermokeratoplasty, keratomileusis, radial *keratotomy*. SYN keratorefractive surgery.

tectonic k., grafting to replace lost corneal tissue.

total k., corneal transplant in which the entire cornea is removed and replaced.

ker·a·to·pros·the·sis (ker'ă-tō-pros-thē'sis). Replacement of the central area of an opacified cornea by plastic. [kerato- + G. *prosthesis*, addition]

ker·a·to·rhex·is, ker·a·tor·rhex·is (ker'ă-tō-rek'sis). Rupture of the cornea, due to trauma or perforating ulcer. [kerato- + G. *rhēxis*, a bursting]

ker·a·to·rus (ker-a-tō'rŭs). Vault-like corneal herniation with severe regular myopic astigmatism. [kerat- + L. *torus*, swelling, knot, bulge]

ker·a·to·scle·ri·tis (ker'ă-tō-skle-rī'tis). Inflammation of both cornea and sclera.

ker·a·to·scope (ker'ă-tō-skōp). An instrument marked with lines or circles by means of which the corneal reflex can be observed. SYN Placido da Costa's disk. [kerato- + G. *skopeō*, to examine]

ker·a·tos·co·py (ker-a-tos'kŏ-pē). 1. Examination of the reflections from the anterior surface of the cornea in order to determine the character and amount of corneal astigmatism. 2. A term first applied by Cuignet to his method of retinoscopy. [kerato- + G. *skopeō*, to examine]

ker·a·tose (ker'ă-tōs). Keratotic, relating to or marked by keratosis.

ker·a·to·sis, pl. **ker·a·to·ses** (ker-ă-tō'sis, -sēz). Any lesion on the epidermis marked by the presence of circumscribed overgrowths of the horny layer. SYN keratiasis. [kerato- + G. *-osis*, condition]

actinic k., a premalignant warty lesion occurring on the sun-exposed skin of the face or hands in aged light-skinned persons; hyperkeratosis may form a cutaneous horn, and squamous cell carcinoma of low-grade malignancy may develop in a small proportion of untreated patients. SYN senile keratoderma, senile keratoma, senile k., k. senilis, senile wart, solar k., verruca plana senilis, verruca senilis.

arsenical k., multiple keratoses, most commonly of the palms and soles but also of the fingers and proximal portions of the extremities, resulting from long-term arsenic ingestion; they resemble Bowen's disease microscopically and may become malignant.

k. blennorrhag'ica, pustules and crusts associated with Reiter's disease. SYN keratoderma blennorrhagica.

k. diffu'sa feta'lis, SYN *ichthyosis* vulgaris.

k. follicula'ris [MIM*124200], a familial, autosomal dominant eruption, beginning usually in childhood, in which keratotic papules originating from both follicles and interfollicular epidermis of the trunk, face, scalp, and axillae become crusted and verrucous; the papules are often intensely pruritic. Microscopically, dyskeratotic cells termed corps ronds are seen in the epidermis. SYN Darier's disease, k. vegetans.

k. follicula'ris contagio'sa, a rare condition simulating k. follicularis. SYN Brooke's disease (2).

inverted follicular k., a solitary benign epithelial tumor of infundibular hair follicle origin occurring on the face, consisting of a lobulated epidermal downgrowth of keratinizing squamous cells with a pattern of eddies or whorls.

k. labia'lis, thickening of stratum corneum on the lips.

lichenoid k., a solitary benign papule or plaque, with microscopic features resembling lichen planus, occurring on sun-exposed or unexposed skin. SYN lichen planus-like k.

lichen planus-like k., SYN lichenoid k.

k. ni'gricans, SYN *acanthosis* nigricans.

k. obtu'rans, an accretion of epithelia in the external auditory canal. SYN laminated epithelial plug.

k. palma'ris et planta'ris, SYN palmoplantar *keratoderma*.

k. pila'ris atroph'icans facie'i, erythema and horny plugs of outer portions of the eyebrows with destruction of follicles; onset in early infancy.

k. puncta'ta, SYN punctate *keratoderma*.

k. ru'bra figura'ta, SYN *erythrokeratoderma* variabilis.

seborrheic k., k. seborrhe'ica, superficial, benign, verrucous, often pigmented, greasy lesions consisting of proliferating epidermal cells, resembling basal cells, enclosing horn cysts; they usually occur after the third decade. SYN basal cell papilloma, seborrheic verruca, seborrheic wart.

senile k., k. seni'lis, SYN actinic k.

solar k., SYN actinic k.

tar k., warty lesions of the face and hands resulting from repeated, prolonged exposure to tar and pitch; also occurs as keratoacanthoma-like lesions that can become malignant, particularly on the scrotum.

k. veg'etans, SYN k. follicularis.

ker·a·to·sul·fate (ker'ă-tō-sŭl-fāt). SYN keratan sulfate.

ker·a·to·tome (ker'ă-tō-tōm). SYN keratome.

ker·a·tot·o·my (ker'ă-tot'ō-mē). 1. Any incision through the cornea. 2. An operation making a partial thickness incision into the cornea to flatten it and reduce its refractive power in that meridian. [kerato- + G. *tomē*, incision]

delimiting k., incision in the cornea along the margin of an advancing ulcer.

radial k., a k. with radial incisions around a clear central zone. A form of refractive keratoplasty used in the treatment of myopia.

refractive k., modification of corneal curvature by means of corneal incisions to minimize hyperopia, myopia, or astigmatism.

> In this type of radial keratotomy surgery, performed by excimer laser, pie-shaped pieces of cornea are removed under local anesthetic. The resulting scar tissue formation reshapes the cornea. This class of surgery is somewhat unpredictable, and its long-term effects are still unknown.

ke·rau·no·pho·bia (kě-raw'nō-fō'bē-ă). Morbid fear of thunder and lightning. [G. *keraunos*, thunderbolt, + *phobos*, fear]

Kerckring (Kerckringius). Theodor, Dutch anatomist, 1640–1693. SEE Kerckring's *center*, Kerckring's *folds*, under *fold*, ossicle, Kerckring's *valves*, under *valve*.

ke·ri·on (kē'rē-on). A granulomatous secondarily infected lesion complicating fungal infection of the hair; typically, a raised boggy lesion. [G. *kērion*, honeycomb; a skin disease, fr. *kēros*, beeswax]

Celsus k., SYN *tinea* kerion.

Kerley, Peter J., English radiologist, *1900. SEE K. B *lines,* under *line.*

ker·nel (ker′nĕl). The central portion of the software expression of a mathematical algorithm, as in computed tomography. [O.E. *cyrnel,* a little corn]

ker·nic·ter·us (ker-nik′ter-ŭs). Associated with high levels of unconjugated bilirubin, or, in small premature infants with more modest degrees of bilirubinemia; yellow staining and degenerative lesions are found chiefly in basal ganglia including in the lenticular nucleus, subthalamus, Ammon's horn, and other areas; may occur with hemolytic disorder such as Rh or ABO erythroblastosis or G6PD deficiency as well as with neonatal sepsis or Crigler-Najjas syndrome; characterized early clinically by opisthotonus, high-pitched cry, lethargy, and poor sucking, as well as abnormal or absent Moro reflex, and loss of upward gaze; later consequences include deafness, cerebral palsy, other sensineural deficits, and mental retardation. SYN bilirubin encephalopathy, nuclear jaundice. [Ger. *Kern,* kernel (nucleus), + *Ikterus,* jaundice]

Kernig, Vladimir, Russian physician, 1840–1917. SEE K.'s *sign.*

Kernohan, J.W., U.S. pathologist, *1897. SEE K.'s *notch.*

ker·oid (ker′oyd). SYN horny. [G. *keroeidēs,* horn-like]

ker·o·sene (ker′ō-sēn). A mixture of petroleum hydrocarbons, chiefly of the methane series; the fifth fraction in the distillation of petroleum, used as fuel for lamps and stoves, as a degreaser and cleaner, and in insecticides. Contact on human skin can lead to irritation and infection; inhalation may cause headache, drowsiness, coma; swallowing causes irritation, vomiting, and diarrhea. Vomiting should not be induced, as aspiration of vomitus causes pneumonitis. [G. *kēros,* wax, + -ene]

ker·o·ther·a·py (ker-ō-thăr′ă-pē). Treatment of burns and denuded surfaces with wax or paraffin preparations. [G. *kēros,* wax, + *therapeia,* treatment]

Kerr, Harry Hyland, U.S. surgeon, 1881–1963. SEE Parker-K. *suture.*

Kestenbaum, U.S. ophthalmologist, 1890–1961. SEE Kestenbaum's *sign,* Kestenbaum's *number.*

Kestenbaum's sign. See under sign.

ke·tal (kē′tăl). RC(OR′)(R″)OR‴; a hydrated ketone in which both hydroxyl groups are esterified with alcohols.

ket·a·mine (kēt′ă-mēn). DL-2-(*o*-Chlorophenyl)-2-(methylamino)cyclohexanone; a parenterally administered anesthetic that produces catatonia, profound analgesia, increased sympathetic activity, and little relaxation of skeletal muscles; side effects include sialorrhea and occasional pronounced dysphoria, especially in adults; chemically related to phencyclidine (PCP), it can produce hallucinations.

ke·tan·ser·in (kēt-an′ser-in). Specific serotonin 5HT₂-receptor antagonist with antihypertensive properties; the drug also reduces platelet aggregation produced by serotonin.

ke·tene (kē′tēn). CH₂=C=O; a very reactive acetylating agent, used in chemical syntheses.

ket·i·mine (kē′ta-mēn). R–N=C(R′)(R″); a tautomer of an aldimine, formed in many enzyme-catalyze reactions; *e.g.,* aminotransferases.

keto-. Combining form denoting a compound containing a ketone group; replaced by oxo- in systematic nomenclature. [Ger.]

ke·to ac·id (kē′tō). An acid containing a ketone group (–CO–) in addition to the acid group(s); α-k. a. refers to a 2-oxo acid (*e.g.,* pyruvic acid); β-k. a. refers to a 3-oxo acid (*e.g.,* acetoacetic acid), etc. SYN oxo acid.

α-k. a. dehydrogenase, one of several distinct multienzyme complexes that catalyzes the formation of an acyl-CoA derivative, CO₂, and NADH from an α-keto acid, NAD⁺, and coenzyme A; maple syrup urine disease results from several different inherited defects in the mitochondrial branched chain α-keto acid dehydrogenase complex.

3-ke·to·ac·id-CoA trans·fer·ase. SYN 3-oxoacid-CoA transferase.

ke·to·ac·id·e·mia (kē′tō-as-id-ē′mē-ă). SYN maple syrup urine *disease.*

ke·to·ac·i·do·sis (kē′tō-as-i-dō′sis). Acidosis, as in diabetes or starvation, caused by the enhanced production of ketone bodies.

ke·to·ac·i·du·ria (kē′tō-as-i-dū′rē-ă). Excretion of urine having an elevated content of ketonic acids.

branched chain k., SYN maple syrup urine *disease.*

β-ke·to·ac·yl-ACP re·duc·tase (kē-tō-as′il). SYN 3-oxoacyl-ACP reductase.

β-ke·to·ac·yl-ACP syn·thase. SYN 3-oxoacyl-ACP synthase.

3-ke·to·ac·yl-CoA thi·o·lase. SYN *acetyl-CoA* acyltransferase.

2-ke·to·a·dip·ic ac·id (kē′tō-a-dip′ik). HOOCCH₂CH₂CH₂COCOOH; an intermediate in L-tryptophan and L-lysine catabolism; 2-k. a. accumulates in certain inherited disorders, probably due to a deficiency of one of the proteins in the α-ketoadipate dehydrogenase complex.

2-k. a. dehydrogenase complex, the multienzyme complex that reacts 2-k. a. with coenzyme A and NAD⁺ to produce glutaryl-CoA, CO₂, and NADH + H⁺ in L-lysine and L-tryptophan catabolism; a deficiency of one of the proteins in this complex results in 2-ketoadipic acidemia.

2-ke·to·a·dip·ic ac·i·de·mia (ē′tō-a-dip′ik). Elevated levels of 2-ketoadipic acid in the serum.

ke·to·con·a·zole (kē-tō-kō′nă-zōl). *cis*-1-Acetyl-4-[4-[[2-(2,4-dichlorophenyl-2-(imidazol-1-ylmethyl)1,3-dioxolan-4-yl]methoxy]phenyl]piperazine; a broad spectrum antifungal agent used to treat systemic and topical fungal infections.

α-ke·to·de·car·box·y·lase (kē′tō-dē-kar-boks′i-lās). Formerly, the enzyme system converting pyruvate (a 2-oxoacid) to acetyl-CoA and CO₂, with reduction of NAD⁺ to NADH and the participation of lipoamide and thiamin pyrophosphate; now known to involve at least three enzymes in succession: pyruvate dehydrogenase, dihydrolipoamide acetyltransferase, and dihydrolipoamide dehydrogenase. Cf. *pyruvate* dehydrogenase (lipoamide).

ke·to·gen·e·sis (kē-tō-jen′ě-sis). Metabolic production of ketones or ketone bodies.

ke·to·gen·ic (kē-tō-jen′ik). Giving rise to ketone bodies in metabolism.

α-ke·to·glu·tar·am·ic ac·id (kē′tō-glū-tār-ik). H₂N–COCH₂CH₂COCOOH; a metabolite of glutamine formed by the action of glutamine aminotransferase; elevated in certain cases of hepatocoma. SYN 2-oxoglutaric acid.

α-ke·to·glu·tar·ate. A salt or ester of α-ketoglutaric acid.

α-k. dehydrogenase, an enzyme that catalyzes the oxidative decarboxylation of 2-ketoglutaric acid to succinyldihydrolipoate; the succinyl group is later transferred to CoA and the reduced lipoate is oxidized by NAD⁺; a complex that is a part of the tricarboxylic acid cycle. SYN 2-oxoglutarate dehydrogenase, α-ketoglutarate dehydrogenase complex.

ke·to·hep·tose (kē-tō-hep′tōs). A seven-carbon sugar possessing a ketone group. SYN heptulose.

ke·to·hex·ose (kē-tō-heks′ōs). A six-carbon sugar possessing a ketone group; *e.g.,* fructose. SYN hexulose.

β-ke·to·hy·dro·gen·ase (kē-tō-hī′drō-jen-ās). SYN 3-hydroxyacyl-CoA dehydrogenase.

ke·to·hy·drox·y·es·trin (kē′tō-hī-drok-sē-es′trin). SYN estrone.

ke·tol (kē′tol). A ketone that has an OH group near the CO group. In an α-k., the OH is attached to a carbon atom that is attached to the CO carbon atom; in a β-k., one carbon atom intervenes.

ke·tole (kē′tōl). SYN indole (1).

ke·tole group. Carbons 1 and 2 of a 2-ketose (HOCH₂CO–); *trans*-ketolation from D-xylose 5-phosphate to C-1 of aldoses is important in various metabolic pathways involving carbohydrates (*e.g.,* photosynthesis, Dickens shunt); the two-carbon unit is transferred as α,β-dihydroxyethyl thiamin pyrophosphate.

ke·to·lyt·ic (kē-tō-lit′ik). Causing the dissolution of ketone or acetone substances, referring usually to oxidation products of glucose and allied substances.

ke·tone (kē′tōn). A substance with the carbonyl group

$$\underset{\displaystyle -CO-}{\overset{\displaystyle O}{\|}}$$

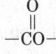
ke

linking two carbon atoms; the most important in medicine and the simplest in chemistry is dimethyl k. (acetone).

ke·tone al·co·hol. A compound containing a carbonyl or ketone group as well as a hydroxyl group; *e.g.,* dihydroxyacetone.

ke·tone-al·de·hyde mu·tase. SYN lactoylglutathione lyase.

ke·to·ne·mia (kē-tō-nē′mē-ă). The presence of recognizable concentrations of ketone bodies in the plasma. [ketone + G. *haima,* blood]

ke·ton·ic (kē-tōn′ik). Pertaining to, or possessing the characteristics of, a ketone.

ke·to·ni·za·tion (kē-tō-ni-zā′shŭn). Conversion into a ketone.

ke·ton·u·ria (kē-tō-nū′rē-ă). Enhanced urinary excretion of ketone bodies.

branched chain k., SYN maple syrup urine *disease.*

ke·to·pan·to·ic ac·id (kē′tō-pan-tō′ik). Oxidized precursor of pantoic acid, intermediate on the synthetic pathway between α-ketoisovaleric acid and pantothenic acid.

ke·to·pen·tose (kē-tō-pen′tōs). A five-carbon sugar in which carbons 2, 3, or 4 make up part of a carbonyl group; *e.g.,* ribulose.

ke·to·pro·fen (kē-tō-prō′fen). *m*-Benzoylhydratropic acid; a nonsteroidal anti-inflammatory drug chemically related to fenoprofen and ibuprofen; useful in inflammatory disorders such as rheumatoid arthritis and osteoarthritis. Also has analgesic properties.

β-ke·to·re·duc·tase (kē′tō-rē-dŭk′tās). SYN 3-hydroxyacyl-CoA dehydrogenase.

ket·or·o·lac. A pyrrolo-pyrrole nonsteroidal anti-inflammatory agent with antipyretic and analgesic properties; similar in actions to ibuprofen but substantially more potent and capable of relieving severe pain. Often used by injection.

ke·tose (kē′tōs). A carbohydrate containing the characteristic carbonyl group of the ketones; *i.e.,* a polyhydroxyketone; *e.g.,* fructose, ribulose, sedoheptulose; the majority of the naturally occurring k.'s have the carbonyl on the second carbon.

ke·tose-1-phos·phate al·dol·ase. Fructose bisphosphate aldolase.

ke·tose re·duc·tase. SYN D-sorbitol-6-phosphate dehydrogenase.

ke·to·sis (kē-tō′sis). A condition characterized by the enhanced production of ketone bodies, as in diabetes mellitus or starvation. [ketone + *-osis,* condition]

bovine k., a common metabolic disease of cows which appears as a rule within a few weeks after parturition; characterized by hypoglycemia, ketonuria, loss of appetite, lethargy, loss of milk production, and rapid emaciation. SYN bovine acetonemia.

17-ke·to·ste·roids (17-KS) (kē-tō-stēr′oydz). Nominally, any steroid with a ketone group on C-17; commonly used to designate urinary C_{19} steroidal metabolites of androgenic and adrenocortical hormones that possess this structural feature. SYN 17-oxosteroids.

α-ke·to·suc·ci·nam·ic ac·id (kē′tō-sŭk-si-nam′ik). NH_2-CO-CH_2-CO-COOH; the transamination product of asparagine; acted upon by ω-amidase.

ke·to·suc·ci·nic ac·id (kē-tō-sŭk′si-nik). SYN oxaloacetic acid.

ke·to·su·ria (kē′tō-su′rē-ă′). The presence of ketones in the urine.

ke·to·tet·rose (kē′tō-tet′rōs). A four-carbon sugar possessing a ketone group; *e.g.,* erythrulose.

β-ke·to·thi·o·lase (kē-tō-thī′ō-lās). SYN *acetyl-CoA* acyltransferase.

ke·to·tic (kē′tot-ik). Pertaining to ketone bodies; presence of acidosis due to excess ketone body production such as occurs in uncontrolled insulin-dependent diabetes.

ke·to·tri·ose (kē′tō-trī′ōs). A three-carbon sugar possessing a ketone group; *i.e.,* dihydroxyacetone.

keV. Abbreviation for kiloelectron volts, a unit of effective mean x-ray tube voltage in diagnostic radiography.

Key, Charles Alston, English physician, 1793–1849.

Key, Ernst A.H., Swedish anatomist and physician, 1832–1901.

SEE K.-Retzius *corpuscles,* under *corpuscle; foramen* of K.; *sheath* of K. and Retzius.

key·way (kē′wā). The female portion of a precision attachment.

kg Abbreviation for kilogram.

khat (kot). The tender fresh parts of *Catha edulis.*

khel·lin (kel′in). Dimethoxymethylfuranochromone; the active principle in extracts of *Ammi visnaga,* an umbelliferous plant growing in the Near East; used in angina pectoris and asthma. [Ar. *khella*]

KHN Abbreviation for Knoop hardness *number.*

kick (kik). A brisk mechanical stimulus.

atrial k., the priming force contributed by atrial contraction immediately before ventricular systole to increase the efficiency of ventricular ejection due to increased preload.

idioventricular k., the increased contractility of the initially contracting ventricular fibers which, by stretching the later contracting fibers, increases their force of contraction.

Kidd blood group. See Blood Groups appendix.

kid·ney (kid′nē). One of the two organs that excrete the urine. The k.'s are bean-shaped organs (about 11 cm long, 5 cm wide, and 3 cm thick) lying on either side of the vertebral column, posterior to the peritoneum, about opposite the twelfth thoracic and first three lumbar vertebrae. SYN ren [NA], nephros[*]. [A.S. *cwith,* womb, belly, + *neere,* kidney (L. *ren,* G. *nephros*)]

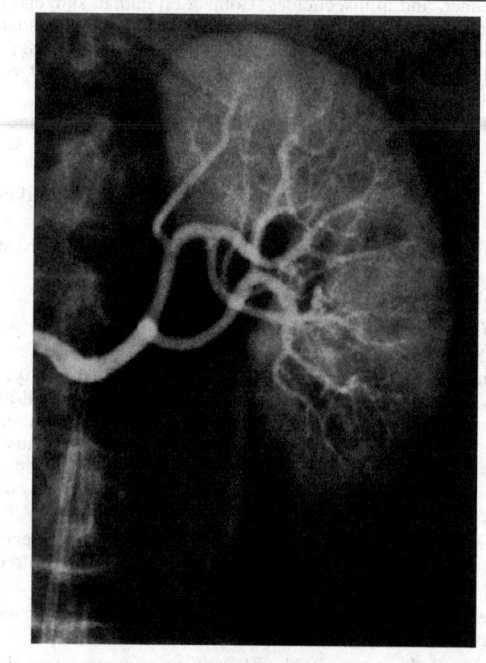

renal angiography

amyloid k., a k. in which amyloidosis has occurred, usually in association with some chronic illness such as multiple myeloma, tuberculosis, osteomyelitis, or other chronic suppurative inflammation; such k.'s are moderately enlarged and grossly manifest a waxy appearance, with amyloid deposited beneath the endothelium in the glomerular loops and in the arterioles, apparently beginning as foci of thickening of the basement membranes. SYN waxy k.

Armanni-Ebstein k., glycogen vacuolization of the loops of Henle, seen in diabetics before the introduction of insulin. SYN Armanni-Ebstein change.

arteriolosclerotic k., a k. in which there is sclerosis of the arterioles, *i.e.,* arteriolar nephrosclerosis resulting from long-standing benign hypertension. Such k.'s tend to be pale red-brown or relatively gray, moderately reduced in size, and firmer than normal organs; the capsular surfaces are uniformly finely granular. Most of the arterioles are thickened and hyalinized, thereby resulting in varying degrees of narrowing of the lumens, ischemia, and fibrosis in the interstitial tissue, leading to uniform contraction of the cortex.

arteriosclerotic k., a k. in which there is sclerosis of arterial vessels larger than arterioles. Such k.'s are usually not significantly reduced in size, but are likely to be paler than usual; the capsular surface may be marked by a few, possibly several, conical, relatively deep V-shaped scars that result from fibrosis and ischemic atrophy of the region supplied by the affected vessel.

artificial k., SYN hemodialyzer.

Ask-Upmark k., true renal hypoplasia with decreased lobules and deep transverse grooving of the cortical surfaces of the kidney.

atrophic k., a k. that is diminished in size because of inadequate circulation and/or loss of nephrons.

cake k., a solid, irregularly lobed organ of bizarre shape, usually situated in the pelvis toward the midline, produced by fusion of the renal anlagen.

contracted k., a diffusely scarred k. in which the relatively large amount of abnormal fibrous tissue and ischemic atrophy leads to a moderate or great reduction in the size of the organ, as in arteriolar nephrosclerosis and chronic glomerulonephritis.

cow k., a k. containing an abnormally large number of minor calices, resembling normal bovine renal anatomy.

crush k., acute oliguric renal failure following crushing injuries of muscle; k.'s show the changes of hypoxic tubular damage, plus pigment casts in renal tubules that contain myoglobin.

cystic k., a general term used to indicate a k. that contains one or more cysts, including polycystic disease, solitary cyst, multiple simple cysts, and retention cysts (associated with parenchymal scarring).

disk k., SYN pancake k.

duplex k., a k. in which two pelviocaliceal systems are present.

fatty k., a k. in which there is fatty metamorphosis of the parenchymal cells, especially fatty degeneration.

flea-bitten k., the k. seen at autopsy in some cases of bacterial endocarditis, the appearance being caused by diffuse petechial hemorrhages resulting from focal glomerulonephritis.

floating k., the abnormally mobile k. in nephroptosis. SYN movable k., wandering k.

Formad's k., an enlarged and deformed k. sometimes seen in chronic alcoholism.

fused k., a single, anomalous organ produced by fusion of the renal anlagen.

Goldblatt k., a k. whose arterial blood supply has been compromised, as a consequence of which arterial (renovascular) hypertension develops.

granular k., a k. in which fairly uniform, diffusely and evenly situated foci of scarring of the interstitial tissue of the cortex (and sometimes scarring of glomeruli), and the associated slight degree of bulging of groups of dilated tubules, leads to the development of a minutely bosselated surface; such k.'s are seen in arteriolar nephrosclerosis or chronic glomerulonephritis. SYN sclerotic k.

head k., SYN pronephros (1).

hind k., SYN metanephros.

horseshoe k., union of the lower or occasionally the upper extremities of the two k.'s by a band of tissue extending across the vertebral column.

medullary sponge k., cystic disease of the renal pyramids associated with calculus formation and hematuria; differs from cystic disease of the renal medulla in that renal failure does not usually develop.

middle k., SYN mesonephros.

mortar k., SYN putty k.

movable k., SYN floating k.

pancake k., a disk-shaped organ produced by fusion of both poles of the contralateral k. anlagen. SYN disk k.

pelvic k., k. that has been displaced into the pelvis.

polycystic k., a progressive disease characterized by formation

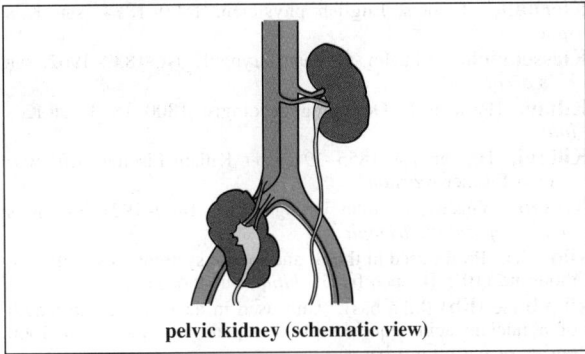

pelvic kidney (schematic view)

of multiple cysts of varying size scattered diffusely throughout both k.'s, resulting in compression and destruction of k. parenchyma, usually with hypertension, gross hematuria, and uremia; there are two major types: 1) with onset in infancy or early childhood, usually with autosomal recessive inheritance [MIM*263200]; 2) with onset in adulthood, with autosomal dominant inheritance [MIM*174000]. SYN polycystic disease of kidneys.

primordial k., SYN pronephros.

putty k., a k. containing caseous material trapped by stricture of the ureter due to tuberculous granulations in renal tuberculosis. SYN mortar k.

pyelonephritic k., a k. deformed by multiple scars as a result of chronic or recurrent renal infection.

Rose-Bradford k., a form of fibrotic k. of inflammatory origin found in young persons.

sclerotic k., SYN granular k.

sigmoid k., upper pole of one k. fused with the lower pole of the other.

supernumerary k., a k., in addition to the two usually present, developed from the splitting of the nephrogenic blastema or from a separate metanephric blastema, into which a partial or complete reduplication of the ureteral stalk enters to form a separate, capsulated k.; in some cases, the separation of the reduplicated organ is incomplete.

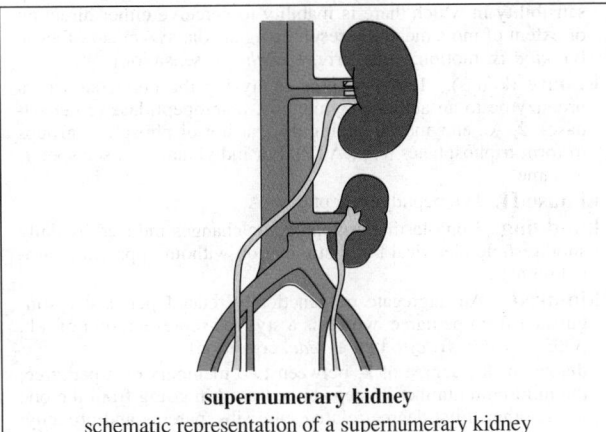

supernumerary kidney
schematic representation of a supernumerary kidney

thoracic k., ectopic k. that partially lies above the diaphragm in the posterior mediastinum.

wandering k., SYN floating k.

waxy k., SYN amyloid k.

Kiel clas·si·fi·ca·tion. See under classification.

Kielland. SEE Kjelland.

Kien, Alphonse M.J., 19th century German physician. SEE Kussmaul-K. *respiration.*

Kienböck, Robert, Austrian roentgenologist, 1871–1953. SEE K.'s atrophy, *disease, dislocation, unit.*

Kiernan, Francis, English physician, 1800–1874. SEE K.'s *space*.

Kiesselbach, Wilhelm, German laryngologist, 1839–1902. SEE K.'s *area*.

Kilian, Hermann F., German gynecologist, 1800–1863. SEE K.'s *line*.

Kiliani, H., chemist, 1855–1945. SEE Kiliani-Fischer *synthesis;* Kiliani-Fischer *reaction*.

Killian, Gustav, German laryngologist, 1860–1921. SEE K.'s *bundle, operation, triangle*.

kilo- (k). Prefix used in the SI and metric systems to signify one thousand (10^3). [French fr. G. *chilioi,* one thousand]

kil·o·base (kb) (kil′ō-bās). Unit used in designating the length of a nucleic acid sequence; 1 kb equals a sequence of 1000 purine or pyrimidine bases.

kil·o·cal·o·rie (kcal) (kil′ō-kal-ō-rē). SYN large *calorie*.

kil·o·cy·cle (kc) (kil′ō-sī-kl). One thousand cycles per second.

kil·o·gram (kg) (kil′ō-gram). The SI unit of mass, 1000 g; equivalent to 15,432.358 gr, 2.2046226 lb. avoirdupois, or 2.6792289 lb. troy.

kil·o·gram-me·ter. The energy exerted, or work done, when a mass of 1 kg is raised a height of 1 m; equal to 9.80665 J in the SI system.

kil·o·hertz. A unit of frequency equal to 10^3 hertz.

kil·ohm. A unit of electrical resistance equal to 10^3 ohms. [kilo + ohm]

kil·o·joule. A unit of energy, work, or quantity of heat equal to 10^3 joules. [kilo + joule]

kil·o·roent·gen (kil-ō-rent′gen). Term used to denote an exposure of 10^3 roentgens.

kil·o·volt (kv) (kil′ō-vōlt). A unit of electrical potential, potential difference, or electromotive force, equal to 10^3 volts. [kilo + volt]

kil·o·volt·me·ter (kil′ō-vōlt-mē′ter). An instrument designed to measure electromotive force in kilovolts.

Kimmelstiel, Paul, German pathologist in the U.S., 1900–1970. SEE K.-Wilson *disease, syndrome*.

Kimura, T., 20th century Japanese pathologist. SEE K.'s *disease*.

kin-, kine-. Movement, motion. SEE ALSO cine-. [G. *kinēsis*]

kin·an·es·the·sia (kin-an-es-thē′zē-ă). A disturbance of deep sensibility in which there is inability to perceive either direction or extent of movement, the result being ataxia. SYN cinanesthesia. [G. *kinēsis,* motion, + *an*- priv. + *aisthēsis,* sensation]

ki·nase (kī′nās). **1.** An enzyme catalyzing the conversion of a proenzyme to an active enzyme; *e.g.,* enteropeptidase (enterokinase). **2.** An enzyme catalyzing the transfer of phosphate groups to form triphosphates (*e.g.,* ATP). For individual k.'s, see specific name.

ki·nase II. SYN peptidyl dipeptidase A.

kin·d·ling. Long-lasting epileptogenic changes induced by daily subthreshold electrical brain stimulation without apparent neuronal damage.

kin·dred. An aggregate of genetically related persons; distinguished from pedigree, which is a stylized representation of a k. [O.E. *kynrēde,* fr. *cyn,* kin, + *rēde,* condition]

degree of k., degree of k. between two members of a pedigree, the minimum number of steps to be traced in going from the one to the other. First degree relatives are sibs, parents and progeny; second degree are uncles, aunts, nephews, and nieces and so forth. The term is defined for legal purposes *e.g.,* consanguineous marriages, and may be misleading in genetics. Use of groups constituted by lumping together "first degree relatives" regardless of sex or the mode of inheritance in question and that fails to distinguish progeny from sibs is to be deplored.

kin·e·mat·ics (kin-ĕ-mat′iks). In physiology, the science concerned with movements of the parts of the body. SYN cinematics. [G. *kinēmatica,* things that move]

kin·e·mom·e·ter (kin-ĕ-mom′ĕ-ter). An electromagnetic device, similar in principle to the velocity ballistocardiograph, used to measure the contraction and relaxation elicited in a tendon reflex. [G. *kinēsis,* movement, + *metron,* measure]

kin·e·plas·tics (kin′ĕ-plas-tiks). SYN cineplastic *amputation*.

kin·e·sal·gia (kin-ĕ-sal′jē-ă). Pain caused by muscular movement. SYN kinesialgia. [G. *kinēsis,* motion, + *algos,* pain]

kin·e·scope (kin′ĕ-skōp). Obsolete instrument for determining the refraction of the eyes; the subject observes the apparent "with" or "against" movement of the test object through a stenopeic slit moved across the front of the eye. [G. *kinēsis,* motion, + *skopeō,* to examine]

kinesi-, kinesio-, kineso-. Motion. [G. *kinēsis*]

ki·ne·sia (ki-nē′sē-ă, -nē′zē-). SYN motion *sickness*. [G. *kinēsis,* movement]

ki·ne·si·al·gia (ki-nē-sē-al′jē-ă). SYN kinesalgia.

ki·ne·si·at·rics (ki-nē′sē-at′riks). SYN kinesitherapy. [G. *kinēsis,* movement, + *iatrikos,* relating to medicine]

ki·ne·sics (ki-nē′siks). The study of nonverbal, bodily motion in communication. SEE body *language*.

kin·e·sim·e·ter (kin-ĕ-sim′ĕ-ter). An instrument for measuring the extent of a movement. SYN kinesiometer. [G. *kinēsis,* movement, + *metron,* measure]

ki·ne·sin (ki-nē′sin). A motor protein associated with microtubules; participates in the transport of vesicles and other entities; directs anterograde axonal transport.

kinesio-. SEE kinesi-.

ki·ne·si·ol·o·gy (ki-nē-sē-ol′ō-jē). The science or the study of movement, and the active and passive structures involved. [G. *kinēsis,* movement, + *-logos,* study]

ki·ne·si·om·e·ter (ki-nē-sē-om′ĕ-ter). SYN kinesimeter.

ki·ne·si·o·neu·ro·sis (ki-nē′sē-ō-nū-rō′sis). Rarely used term for a neurosis, or functional nervous disease, marked by tics, spasms, or other motor disorders. [G. *kinēsis,* movement]

kin·e·sip·a·thist (kin-ĕ-sip′ă-thist). A nonmedical person who treats disease by movements of various kinds.

kin·e·sip·a·thy (kin-ĕ-sip′ă-thē). **1.** An affection marked by motor disturbances. **2.** SYN kinesitherapy. [G. *kinēsis,* movement, + *pathos,* suffering]

ki·ne·sis (ki-nē′sis). Motion. As a termination, used to denote movement or activation, particularly the kind induced by a stimulus. [G.]

ki·ne·si·ther·a·py (ki-nē-si-thār′ă-pē). Physical therapy involving motion and range of motion exercises. SEE movement. SYN kinesiatrics, kinesipathy (2).

kineso-. SEE kinesi-.

ki·ne·so·pho·bia (ki-nē-sō-fō′bē-ă). Morbid fear of movement. [G. *kinēsis,* movement, + *phobos,* fear]

kin·es·the·sia (kin′es-thē′zē-ă). **1.** The sense perception of movement; the muscular sense. **2.** An illusion of moving in space. [G. *kinēsis,* motion, + *aisthēsis,* sensation]

kinesthesia k., the sense of movement of one or more muscles, when no movement is taking place.

kin·es·the·si·om·e·ter (kin′es-thē′zē-om′ĕ-ter). An instrument for determining the degree of muscular sensation. [kinesthesia, + G. *metron,* measure]

kin·es·the·sis (kin′es-thē-sēz). SEE kinesthesia.

kin·es·thet·ic (kin-es-thet′ik). Relating to kinesthesia.

ki·net·ic (ki-net′ik). Relating to motion or movement. [G. *kinētikos,* of motion, fr. *kinētos,* moving]

ki·net·ics (ki-net′iks). The study of motion, acceleration, or rate of change.

chemical k., the study of the rates of chemical reactions.

enzyme k., the study of the rates, and alterations in those rates, of enzyme-catalyzed reactions; includes the reactions catalyzed by synzymes, abzymes, and ribozymes.

kineto-. Motion. [G. *kinētos,* moving, movable]

ki·ne·to·car·di·o·gram (ki-nē′tō-kar′dē-ō-gram, ki-net′ō-). One type of graphic recording of the vibrations of the chest wall produced by cardiac activity.

ki·ne·to·car·di·o·graph (ki-nē′tō-kar′dē-ō-graf, ki-net′ō-). A device for recording precordial impulses due to cardiac movement; the absolute displacement of a point on the chest wall is recorded relative to a fixed reference point above the recumbent patient.

ki·ne·to·chore (ki-nē'tō-kōr, ki-net'ō-). The structural portion of the chromosome to which microtubules attach. Cf. centromere. [kineto- + G. *chōra*, space]

ki·ne·to·chores (ki-nē'tō-korz). The protein-bound region of the centromere.

ki·ne·to·gen·ic (ki-nē-tō-jen'ik, ki-net-ō-). Causing or producing motion.

ki·ne·to·plasm (ki-nē'tō-plazm). **1.** The most contractile part of a cell. **2.** The cytoplasm of the droplet that covers the sperm head during maturation. SYN cinetoplasm, cinetoplasma, kinoplasm. [kineto- + G. *plasma*, a thing formed]

ki·ne·to·plast (ki-nē'tō-plast, ki-net'ō-). An intensely staining rod-, disc-, or spherical-shaped extranuclear DNA structure found in parasitic flagellates (family Trypanosomatidae) near the base of the flagellum, posterior to the blepharoplast, and often at right angles to the nucleus. Electron micrographs show it to be part of a single giant mitochondrion filling most of the cytoplasm of amastigote flagellates, the k. portion being visible by light microscopy. DNA of the k. is termed kDNA to distinguish it from nuclear DNA, or nDNA. The k. divides independently, along with the basal body, prior to nuclear division. The term k. formerly included parabasal body and blepharoplast in a locomotory apparatus, but is now recognized as a distinct organelle of most trypanosomatids. SEE ALSO parabasal *body*. [kineto- + G. *plastos*, formed]

ki·ne·to·scope (ki-ne'to-skōp). An apparatus for taking serial photographs to record movement. [kineto- + G. *skopeō*, to examine]

ki·net·o·some (ki-nē'tō-sōm, ki-net'ō-). SYN basal *body*. [kineto- + G. *sōma*, body]

King, Earl J., Canadian biochemist, 1901–1962. SEE K. *unit;* K.-Armstrong *unit.*

king·dom (king'dum). One of the three categories into which natural objects are usually classified: the animal kingdom, including all animals; the plant kingdom, including all plants; and the mineral kingdom, including all objects and substances without life. [A.S. *cyningdōm*, fr. *cyning*, king, + *-dom*, state, condition]

Kin·gel·la (kin-jel'ah). Newly recognized member of the family Neisseriaceae; a Gram-negative cocci with a requirement of enhanced carbon dioxide for recovery in culture.

K. indolog'enes, a species that causes eye infections or endocarditis (when prosthetic heart valves are present) in humans.

K. kin'gae, a species that causes endocarditis in humans; formerly *Moraxella kingae.* SEE HACEK *group.* SYN *Moraxella kingae.*

Kingsley, N.W., U.S. dentist, 1829–1913. SEE K. *splint.*

kin·ic ac·id (kin'ik). SYN quinic acid.

ki·nin (ki'nin). One of a number of widely differing substances having pronounced and dramatic physiological effects. Some (*e.g.,* kallidin and bradykinin) are polypeptides, formed in blood by proteolysis secondary to some pathological process, that stimulate visceral smooth muscle but relax vascular smooth muscle, thus producing vasodilation; others (*e.g.,* kinetin) are plant growth regulators. [G. *kineō,* to move, + *-in*]

k. 9, SYN bradykinin.

ki·nin·o·gen (ki-nin'ō-jen). The globulin precursor of a (plasma) kinin.

high molecular weight k., a plasma protein of 110,000 molecular weight that normally exists in plasma in a 1:1 complex with prekallikrein. The complex is a cofactor in the activation of coagulation factor XII. The product of this reaction, XIIa, in turn activates prekallikrein to kallikrein. SYN Fitzgerald *factor,* Flaujeac *factor,* Williams *factor.*

low molecular weight k., a protein of 50,000 molecular weight that occurs in various normal tissues and which, upon cleavage by kallikrein or other k.'s, forms kallidin. Kallidin, in turn, is converted into bradykinin.

ki·nin·o·ge·nase (ki-nin'ō-jĕ-nās). SYN kallikrein.

ki·nin·o·gen·in (ki-nin'ō-jen-in). SYN kallikrein.

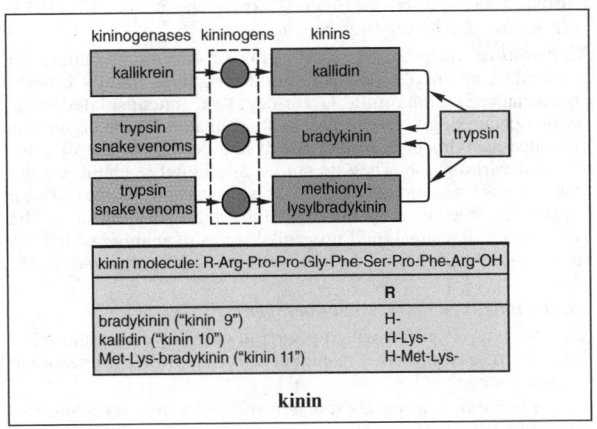

kinin

kink. An angulation, bend, or twist.

Lane's k., SYN Lane's *band.*

△**kino-.** Movement. [G. *kineō,* to move]

kin·o·cen·trum (kin-ō-sen'trŭm). SYN cytocentrum. [kino- + G. *kentron,* center]

ki·no·cil·i·um (kī-nō-sil'ē-ŭm). A cilium, usually motile, having nine peripheral double microtubules and two single central ones. [kino- + cilium]

kin·o·hapt (kin'ō-hapt). An esthesiometer for applying several stimuli to the skin at different distances and frequencies. [kino- + G. *haptō,* to touch]

kin·o·mom·e·ter (kin-ō-mom'ĕ-ter). An instrument for measuring degree of motion. [kino- + G. *metron,* measure]

kin·o·plasm (kin'ō-plazm, kī'nō). SYN kinetoplasm.

kin·o·plas·mic (kin-ō-plas'mik, kī-nō-). Relating to kinoplasm (kinetoplasm).

kin·ship. The state of being genetically related.

Kinyoun, Joseph J., U.S. physician, 1860–1919. SEE K. *stain.*

ki·on (kī'on). Obsolete term for uvula. See entries under cion- as a combining form of uvula. [G. *kiōn,* pillar, the uvula]

△**kion-, kiono-.** Obsolete combining form relating to the uvula. SEE uvulo-, uvul-. [G. *kiōn,* uvula]

Kirk, Norman Thomas, U.S. Army surgeon, 1888–1960. SEE K.'s *amputation.*

Kirkland, Olin, U.S. periodontist, 1876–1969. SEE K. *knife.*

Kirschner, Martin, German surgeon, 1879–1942. SEE K.'s *apparatus,* wire.

Kisch, Bruno, German physiologist, 1890–1966. SEE K.'s *reflex.*

Kitasato, Shibasaburo, Baron, Japanese bacteriologist, 1856–1931. SEE K.'s *bacillus.*

Kjeldahl, Johan G.C., Danish chemist, 1849–1900. SEE K. *apparatus,* method; macro-K. *method;* micro-K. *method.*

Kjelland (Kielland), Christian, Norwegian obstetrician, 1871–1941. SEE K.'s *forceps.*

Klapp, Rudolph, German surgeon, 1873–1949. SEE K.'s *method.*

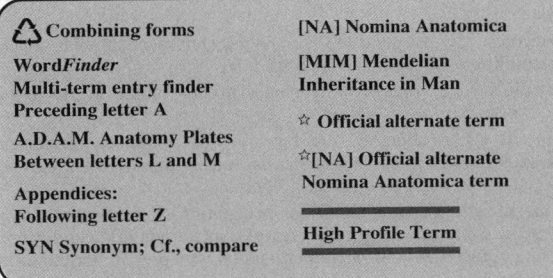
Kl

Klebs, Theodor Albrecht Edwin, German physician, 1834–1913. SEE *Klebsiella;* K.-Loeffler *bacillus.*

Kleb·si·el·la (kleb-sē-el′ă). A genus of aerobic, facultatively anaerobic, nonmotile, nonsporeforming bacteria (family Enterobacteriaceae) containing Gram-negative, encapsulated rods which occur singly, in pairs, or in short chains. These organisms produce acetylmethylcarbinol and lysine decarboxylase or ornithine decarboxylase. They do not usually liquefy gelatin. Citrate and glucose are ordinarily used as sole carbon sources. These organisms may or may not be pathogenic. They occur in the respiratory, intestinal, and urogenital tracts of man as well as in soil, water, and grain. The type species is *K. pneumoniae.* [E. *Klebs*]

K. mo′bilis, SYN *Enterobacter aerogenes.*

K. ozae′nae, a species which occurs in cases of ozena and other chronic diseases of the respiratory tract. SYN *K. pneumoniae* subsp. *ozaenae.*

K. pneumo′niae, a species found in soil and water, on grain, and in the intestinal tract of humans and other animals; it also occurs in association with several pathologic conditions, urinary tract infections, sputum, feces, and metritis in mares; capsular types 1, 2, and 3 of this organism may be causative agents in pneumonia; organisms previously identified as nonmotile strains of *Aerobacter aerogenes* are now placed in this species; it is the type species of *K.* SYN Friedländer's bacillus, pneumobacillus.

K. pneumo′niae subsp. *ozae′nae,* SYN *K. ozaenae.*

K. rhinosclero′matis, a species found in cases of rhinoscleroma.

klee·blatt·schä·del (klā-blat-she′dl). SEE cloverleaf skull *syndrome.* [Ger. cloverleaf skull]

Kleffner. SEE Landau-Kleffner *syndrome.*

Kleihauer. SEE Kleihauer's *stain,* Betke-Kleihauer *test.*

Klein, Edward E., Hungarian histologist, 1844–1925. SEE K.'s *muscle;* K.-Gumprecht shadow *nuclei,* under *nucleus.*

Kleine, Willi, 20th century German neuropsychiatrist. SEE K.-Levin *syndrome.*

klep·to·lag·nia (klep-tō-lag′nē-ă). Erotic feelings induced by stealing. [G. *kleptō,* to steal, + *lagneia,* lust, coition]

klep·to·ma·nia (klep-tō-mā′nē-ă). A disorder of impulse control characterized by a morbid tendency to steal. [G. *kleptō,* to steal, + *mania,* insanity]

klep·to·ma·ni·ac (klep-tō-mā′nē-ak). A person exhibiting kleptomania.

klep·to·pho·bia (klep-tō-fō′bē-ă). Morbid fear of stealing or of becoming a thief. [G. *kleptō,* to steal, + *phobos,* fear]

Klinefelter, Harry F., Jr., U.S. physician, *1912. SEE K.'s *syndrome.*

Klinger-Ludwig ac·id-thi·o·nin stain for sex chro·ma·tin. See under stain.

Klippel, Maurice, French neurologist, 1858–1942. SEE K.-Feil *syndrome;* K.-Trenaunay-Weber *syndrome.*

Klumpke. SEE Dejerine-Klumpke.

Klüver, Heinrich, German-born U.S. neurologist, *1897. SEE K.-Barrera Luxol fast blue *stain;* K.-Bucy *syndrome.*

Kluy·ve·ra (klooy-ver′ah). Newly named genus of Enterobacteriaceae.

Knapp, Herman J., U.S. ophthalmologist, 1832–1911. SEE K.'s *streaks,* under *streak, striae,* under *stria.*

Knaus, Hermann, Austrian gynecologist, *1892. SEE Ogino-K. *rule.*

knee (nē). **1.** SYN genu (1). **2.** Any structure of angular shape resembling a flexed knee. [A.S. *cneōw*]

Brodie's k., chronic hypertrophic synovitis of the k. SYN Brodie's disease (1).

capped k., swelling of the bursa of the extensor metacarpi magnus muscle in cattle, usually caused by injury to the carpus in getting up and down on hard floors.

housemaid's k., an adventitious occupational bursitis occurring over the tibial tuberosity, the area of contact when kneeling; not to be confused with infrapatellar bursitis. SYN prepatellar bursitis.

locked k., a condition in which the k. lacks full extension and

flexion because of internal derangement, usually the result of a torn medial meniscus.

knee·cap (nē′kap). SYN patella.

Kne·mi·do·kop·tes (nē′mi-dō-kop′tēz). A genus of microscopic burrowing sarcoptid mites that infect fowl and caged birds; species include *K. laevis* var. *gallinae,* the depluming mite, and *K. mutans,* the scaly leg mite. [G. *knēmē,* leg, + *koptō,* to cut]

KNF mod·el Abbreviation for Koshland-Némethy-Filmer *model.*

Kniest, Wilhelm, 20th century German pediatrician. SEE K. *syndrome.*

knife, pl. **knives** (nīf, nīvz). A cutting instrument used in surgery and dissection. [M.E. *knif,* fr. A.S. *cnif,* fr. O. Norse *knīfr*]

amputation k., a broad-bladed k. used primarily for transecting large muscles during major amputations.

Beer's k., a triangular k. with a sharp point and one sharp edge, formerly used for incision for cataract.

cartilage k., SYN chondrotome.

cautery k., a k. that sears while cutting, to diminish bleeding.

chemical k., term sometimes used for restriction *endonuclease.*

electrode k., a blade-shaped electrical instrument used to cut tissues by means of a high-frequency electrical current.

fistula k., SYN fistulatome.

free-hand k., a manually operated k. or blade usually used to take split-thickness skin grafts; *e.g.,* Blair-Brown k., Humby k., Theirsh k.

gamma ray k., a beam of high energy x-rays. SEE radiosurgery.

Goldman-Fox knives, a set of knives used in periodontal surgery.

Graefe's k., a narrow-bladed k. used in making a section of the cornea.

hernia k., a slender bladed k., with short cutting edge, for dividing the constricting tissues at the mouth of the hernial sac. SYN herniotome.

Humby k., a k. with a roller and a calibration device to cut skin grafts of different thickness.

Joseph k., a k. for use in rhinoplasty to separate the overlying skin from the nasal dorsum.

Kirkland k., a heart-shaped k. used in gingival surgery.

lenticular k., a scraper resembling a sharp spoon.

Liston's knives, long-bladed knives of various sizes used in amputations.

Merrifield k., a long, narrow, triangularly shaped k. used in gingival surgery.

valvotomy k., a k. used in mitral or venous valvular surgery; also called valvulotome.

knis·mo·gen·ic (nis′mō-jen′ik). Causing a tickling sensation. [G. *knismos,* tickling, + *-gen,* production]

knis·mo·lag·nia (nis-mō-lag′nē-ă). Sexual gratification from the act of tickling. [G. *knismos,* tickling, + *lagneia,* lust]

knit·ting (nit′ing). Nonmedical term denoting the process of union of the fragments of a broken bone or of the edges of a wound. [M.E., *knitten,* to knot, fr. A.S. *cnyttan*]

knob (nob). A protuberance; a mass; a nodule.

aortic k., the prominent shadow of the aortic arch on a frontal chest radiograph.

Engelmann's basal k.'s, obsolete eponym for blepharoplast.

malarial k.'s, rounded protrusions of a red blood cell infected with *Plasmodium falciparum,* responsible for the adhesion of infected red cells to one another and to the endothelium of the blood vessels containing these infected cells; results in capillary blockage responsible for much of the pathology of malignant tertian malaria.

knock (nok). **1.** Colloquialism for a blow, especially a blow to the head. **2.** A sound simulating that of a blow or rap.

pericardial k., an early diastolic sound analogous to the normal third heart sound, but occurring somewhat earlier, due to rapid ventricular filling being abruptly halted by the restricting pericardium; a truly "knocking" quality is uncommon.

knock-knee (nok′nē). SYN genu valgum.

Knoll, Philipp, Bohemian physiologist, 1841–1900. SEE K.'s *glands,* under *gland.*

Knoop, Hedwig, German physician, *1908. SEE K.'s *theory.*

Knoop hard·ness num·ber (KHN). See under number.

knot (not). **1.** An intertwining of the ends of two cords, tapes, sutures, etc. in such a way that they cannot spontaneously become separated; or a similar twining or infolding of a cord in its continuity. **2.** In anatomy or pathology, a node, ganglion, or circumscribed swelling suggestive of a k. [A.S. *cnotta*]

false k.'s, false k.'s of umbilical cord, local increases in length or varicosity of the umbilical vein, causing markedly apparent twisting of the cord.

granny k., a double k. in which the free ends of the second loop are asymmetric and not in the same plane as the free ends of the first loop.

Hensen's k., SYN primitive *node.*

Hubrecht's protochordal k., SYN primitive *node.*

laparoscopic k., a k. placed intracorporally through a laparoscopic instrument. The k. itself may be tied extracorporally and passed into the body through a cannula or the k. may be both placed and tied intracorporally.

net k., SYN karyosome.

primitive k., SYN primitive *node.*

protochordal k., SYN primitive *node.*

surgeon's k., the first loop of the k. has two throws rather than a single throw. The second loop has only one throw and that is placed in a square knot fashion leaving the free ends in the same plane as the first loop.

syncytial k., a localized aggregation of syncytiotrophoblastic nuclei in the villi of the placenta during early pregnancy. SYN syncytial bud, syncytial sprout.

true k., true k. of umbilical cord, actual intertwining of a segment of umbilical cord; circulation is usually not obstructed.

vital k., SYN noeud vital.

knuck·le (nŭk′l). **1.** A joint of a finger when the fist is closed, especially a metacarpophalangeal joint. **2.** A kink or loop of intestine, as in a hernia. [M.E. *knokel*]

aortic k., the contour of the aortic arch protruding from the mediastinal silhouette in an anteroposterior (AP) radiograph of the chest.

cervical aortic k., an anomalous aortic arch in which the aorta extends into the neck and forms an anteroposterior arch, which may be as high as the hyoid bone; the common carotid artery of one side is given off from the summit of the arch, and the common carotid of the other side arises from the more proximal part of the aorta; the pulsating arch may be mistaken for an aneurysm, but the radial pulses are equal.

knuck·ling (nŭk′ling). Talipes in the horse, caused by a contraction of the posterior fetlock tendons.

Kobelt, Georg L., German physician, 1804–1857. SEE K.'s *tubules,* under *tubule.*

Kober, Philip A., U.S. chemist, *1884. SEE K. *test.*

Kober test. See under test.

Köbner, H., German dermatologist, 1838–1904. SEE K.'s *phenomenon.*

Koch, Robert, German bacteriologist and Nobel laureate, 1843–1910. SEE K.'s *bacillus,* blue *bodies,* under *body, law,* old *tuberculin,* original *tuberculin, phenomenon, postulates,* under *postulate;* K.-Weeks *bacillus.*

Koch, Walter, German surgeon, *1880. SEE K.'s *node, triangle.*

Kocher, E. Theodor, Swiss surgeon and Nobel laureate, 1841–1917. SEE K. *clamp;* K.'s *incision, sign;* K.-Debré-Sémélaigne *syndrome.*

Kock, Nils G., 20th century Swedish surgeon. SEE K. *pouch.*

Koenen's tu·mor. See under tumor.

Koenig, Franz, German surgeon, 1832–1910. SEE K.'s *syndrome.*

Koerber, H., 20th century German ophthalmologist.

Koerber-Salus-Elschnig syn·drome. See under syndrome.

Koerte, Werner, German surgeon, 1853–1937. SEE K.-Ballance *operation.*

Koettstorfer, J., 19th century German chemist. SEE K. *number.*

Koettstorfer num·ber. See under number.

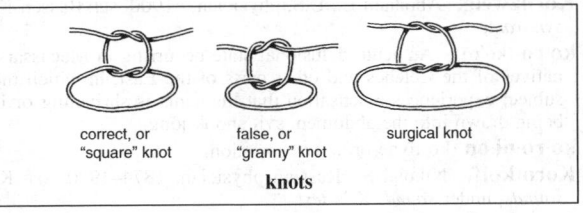

correct, or "square" knot   false, or "granny" knot   surgical knot

knots

Kogoj, Franz, Yugoslavian physician, *1894. SEE spongiform *pustule* of K.

Köhler, Alban, German roentgenologist, 1874–1947. SEE K.'s *disease.*

Köhler, August, German microscopist, 1866–1948. SEE K. *illumination.*

Kohlrausch, Otto L.B., German physician, 1811–1854. SEE K.'s *muscle, valves,* under *valve.*

Kohn, Hans N., German pathologist, *1866. SEE K.'s *pores,* under *pore.*

Kohnstamm, Oskar, German physician, 1871–1917. SEE K.'s *phenomenon.*

koi·lo·cyte (koy′lō-sīt). A squamous cell, often binucleated, showing a perinuclear halo; characteristic of condyloma acuminatum. [G. *koilos,* hollow, + *kytos,* cell]

koi·lo·cy·to·sis (koy′lō-sī-tō′sis). Perinuclear vacuolation. SEE ALSO koilocyte. [G. *koilos,* hollow, + *kytos,* cell, + *-osis,* condition]

koi·lo·nych·ia (koy-lō-nik′ē-ă). A malformation of the nails in which the outer surface is concave; often associated with iron deficiency or softening by occupational contact with oils. SYN celonychia, spoon nail. [G. *koilos,* hollow, + *onyx (onych-),* nail]

koil·o·ster·nia (koy-lō-ster′nē-ă). SYN *pectus* excavatum. [G. *koilos,* hollow, + *sternon,* chest (sternum)]

Kojewnikoff (Kozhevnikov), Aleksei Y., Russian neurologist, 1836–1902. SEE K.'s *epilepsy.*

ko·jic ac·id (kō′jik). 5-Hydroxy-2-(hydroxymethyl)-4-pyranone; an antibiotic product of D-glucose catabolism in some molds; can be converted into flavor enhancers.

ko·la (kō′lă). The dried cotyledons of *Cola nitida* or other species of *Cola* (family Sterculiaceae) which contains caffeine, theobromine, and a soluble principle, colatin; used as a cardiac and central nervous system stimulant. SYN cola (1).

Kölliker, Rudolph A. von, Swiss histologist, 1817–1905. SEE K.'s *layer, reticulum.*

Kollmann, Arthur, 19th century German urologist. SEE K.'s *dilator.*

Kolmer, John A., U.S. pathologist, 1886–1962. SEE K. *test.*

Kolopp, P., 20th century French dermatologist. SEE Woringer-K. *disease.*

△**kolp-.** SEE colpo-.

ko·lyt·ic (kō-lit′ik). Denoting an inhibitory action. [G. *kolyō,* to hinder]

Kondoleon, Emmanuel, Greek surgeon, 1879–1939. SEE K. *operation.*

ko·ni·o·cor·tex (kō′nē-ō-kōr′teks). Regions of the cerebral cortex characterized by a particularly well developed inner granular layer (layer 4); this type of cerebral cortex is represented by the primary sensory area 17 of the visual cortex, areas 1 to 3 of the somatic sensory cortex, and area 41 of the auditory cortex. SEE ALSO cerebral *cortex.* [G. *konis,* dust, + L. *cortex,* bark]

Koplik, Henry, U.S. physician, 1858–1927. SEE K.'s *spots,* under *spot.*

kop·o·pho·bia (kop-ō-fō′bē-ă). Morbid fear of fatigue. [G. *kopos,* fatigue, + *phobos,* fear]

△**kopro-.** SEE copro-.

Korff, Karl von, 20th century German anatomist and histologist. SEE K.'s *fibers,* under *fiber.*

Kornberg, A., U.S. biochemist and Nobel laureate, *1918. SEE K. *enzyme.*

Kornzweig, Abraham L., U.S. physician, *1900. SEE Bassen-K. *syndrome.*

ko·ro (kō'rō). An acute delusional state occurring in Macassars, natives of the Celebes and other parts of the East, in which the subject experiences a sensation that his penis is shriveling or is being drawn into the abdomen. SYN shook jong.

ko·ro·ni·on (kŏ-rō'nē-on). SYN coronion.

Korotkoff, Nikolai S., Russian physician, 1874–1920. SEE K. *sounds,* under *sound;* K.'s *test.*

Korsakoff, Sergei S., Russian neurologist, 1853–1900. SEE K.'s *psychosis, syndrome;* Wernicke-K. *encephalopathy, syndrome.*

Koshland, Daniel E., U.S. biochemist, *1920. SEE Adair-K.-Némethy-Filmer *model;* K.-Némethy-Filmer *model.*

Kossa, SEE von Kossa.

Koyanagi, Yosizo, Japanese ophthalmologist, 1880–1954. SEE Vogt-K. *syndrome.*

Koyter. SEE Coiter.

Kr Symbol for krypton.

Krabbe, Knud H., Danish neurologist, 1885–1961. SEE K.'s *disease;* Christensen-K. *disease.*

krait (krīt). Elapid snakes of the genus *Bungaris,* found in northern India, whose bite is associated with generalized anesthetic and paralytic effects, as opposed to local pain, discoloration, or edema; neurotoxic symptoms are similar to those induced by cobra venom. [Hindi *karait*]

kra-kra. SYN craw-craw.

Krantz, Kermit E., U.S. obstetrician-gynecologist, *1923. SEE Marshall-Marchetti-K. *operation.*

Kraske, Paul, German surgeon, 1851–1930. SEE K.'s *operation.*

krau·ro·sis vul·vae (kraw-rō'sis vŭl've). Atrophy and shrinkage of the epithelium of the vagina and vulva, often accompanied by a chronic inflammatory reaction in the deeper tissues, as in lichen sclerosus. SYN leukokraurosis. [G. *krauros,* dry, brittle]

Krause, Fedor, German surgeon, 1857–1937. SEE K. *graft;* K.'s *method;* Wolfe-K. *graft.*

Krause, Karl F.T., German anatomist, 1797–1868. SEE K.'s *glands,* under *gland, ligament, muscle.*

Krause, Wilhelm J.F., German anatomist, 1833–1910. SEE K.'s *bone,* end *bulbs,* under *bulb,* respiratory *bundle, valve.*

kreb·i·o·zen (krē'bē-oz'en). An extract from peach kernels, the composition of which has not been fully described but which gained notoriety in the 1960's and 1970's as a dubious but exploited remedy for cancer; currently not regarded as effective. [Ger. *Krebs,* crab, cancer]

Krebs, Sir Hans Adolph, German biochemist in England and Nobel laureate, 1900–1981. SEE K. *cycle;* K.-Henseleit *cycle;* K.-Ringer *solution.*

Kretschmann, Friederich, German otologist, 1858–1934. SEE K.'s *space.*

Kreysig, Friedrich L., German physician, 1770–1839. SEE K.'s *sign;* Heim-K. *sign.*

krin·gle (krin'gle). A structural motif or domain seen in certain proteins in which a fold of large loops is stabilized by disulfide bonds; an important structural feature in blood coagulation factors. [Ger. *Kringel,* curl]

Krogh, August, Danish physiologist and Nobel laureate, 1874–1949. SEE K. *spirometer.*

Kromayer, Ernst L.F., German dermatologist, 1862–1933. SEE K.'s *lamp.*

Kronecker, Karl H., Swiss physiologist, 1839–1914. SEE K.'s *stain.*

Krönig, Georg, German physician, 1856–1911. SEE K.'s *isthmus, steps,* under *step.*

Krönlein, Rudolph U., Swiss surgeon, 1847–1910. SEE K. *operation;* K.'s *hernia.*

Krueger in·stru·ment stop. See under instrument.

Krukenberg, Adolph, German anatomist, 1816–1877. SEE K.'s *veins,* under *vein.*

Krukenberg, Friedrich, German pathologist, 1871–1946. SEE K.'s *amputation, spindle, tumor.*

Kruse, Walther, German bacteriologist, 1864–1943. SEE K.'s *brush;* Shiga-Kruse *bacillus.*

△**krymo-, kryo-.** SEE crymo-, cryo-.

kryp·ton (Kr) (krip'ton). One of the inert gases, present in small amounts in the atmosphere (1.14 ppm by dry volume); atomic no. 36, atomic wt. 83.80; ^{85}Kr (half-life of 10.73 years) has been used in studies of cardiac abnormalities. [G. *kryptos,* concealed]

17-KS Abbreviation for 17-ketosteroids.

KUB. Abbreviation for kidneys, ureters, bladder; archaic term for a plain frontal supine radiograph of the abdomen.

ku·bi·sa·ga·ri, ku·bi·sa·ga·ru (kū-bi-sah-gah're, kū-bi-sah-gah'rū). SYN vestibular *neuronitis.* [Jap. *kubi,* head, neck, + *sagaru,* to hang down]

Kufs, H., German psychiatrist, 1871–1955. SEE K. *disease.*

Kugelberg, Eric, Swedish neurologist, 1913–1983. SEE K.-Welander *disease;* Wohlfart-K.-Welander *disease.*

Kugel's anastomotic ar·tery. See under artery.

Kühne, Wilhelm (Willy) F., German physiologist and histologist, 1837–1900. SEE K.'s *fiber, methylene blue, phenomenon, plate, spindle.*

Kuhnt, Hermann, German ophthalmologist, 1850–1925. SEE K.'s *spaces,* under *space;* K.-Junius *degeneration, disease.*

Kulchitsky, Nicholas, Russian histologist, 1856–1925. SEE K. *cells,* under *cell.*

Külz, Rudolph E., German physician, 1845–1895. SEE K.'s *cylinder.*

Kümmell, Hermann, German surgeon, 1852–1937. SEE K.'s *spondylitis.*

Küntscher, Gerhard, German surgeon, 1902–1972. SEE K. *nail.*

Kupffer, Karl W. von, German anatomist, 1829–1902. SEE K. *cells,* under *cell.*

kur·chi bark (ker'chē). SYN conessi.

Kurloff, Mikhail G., Russian physician, 1859–1932. SEE K.'s *bodies,* under *body.*

Kürsteiner (Kuersteiner), W., 19th century German anatomist. SEE K.'s *canals,* under *canal.*

kur·to·sis (kur-tō'sis). The extent to which a unimodal distribution is peaked. [G., an arching]

ku·ru (kū'rū). A progressive, fatal form of spongiform encephalopathy endemic to certain Melanesian tribes in the highlands of New Guinea, initially attributed to a "slow virus" infection, but now known to be caused by prions. Transmission is believed to be effected by contamination and ingestion during ritual cannabalism. SEE prion. [native dialect, to shiver from fear or cold]

Kurzrok-Ratner test. See under test.

Kussmaul, Adolph, German physician, 1822–1902. SEE K. *respiration;* K.'s *aphasia, coma, disease,* paradoxical *pulse, sign, symptom;* K.-Kien *respiration;* K.'s *pulse.*

Küster, Herman, early 20th century German gynecologist. SEE Mayer-Rokitansky-K.-Hauser *syndrome;* Rokitansky-K.-Hauser *syndrome.*

Küstner, Heinz, German gynecologist, *1897. SEE Prausnitz-K. *antibody, reaction;* reversed K. *reaction.*

kv Abbreviation for kilovolt.

Kveim, Morton A., Norwegian physician, *1892. SEE K. *antigen, test;* K.-Stilzbach *antigen, test;* Nickerson-K. *test.*

kVp Abbreviation for kilovolts peak, the highest instantaneous energy across an x-ray tube, corresponding to the highest energy x-rays emitted.

kwa·shi·or·kor (kwah-shē-ōr'kōr). A disease seen originally in African natives, particularly children one to three years old, due to dietary deficiency, particularly of protein; characterized by marked hypoalbuminemia, anemia, edema, pot belly, depigmentation of the skin, loss of hair or change in hair color to red, and bulky stools containing undigested food; fatty changes in the cells of the liver, atrophy of the acinar cells of the pancreas, and hyalinization of the renal glomeruli are found postmortem. SYN infantile pellagra, malignant malnutrition. [Native, red boy or displaced child]

marasmic k., severe protein-calorie malnutrition characterized by extreme weight loss, weakness, and features of k.

⟁**ky-.** For words beginning thus and not found below, see cy-.

kyl·lo·sis (kil-ō′sis). Obsolete term for talipes. [G. *kyllōsis,* a crippling]

ky·ma·tism (kī′mă-tizm). SYN myokymia. [G. *kyma,* wave]

ky·mo·gram (kī′mō-gram). The graphic curve made by a kymograph.

ky·mo·graph (kī′mō-graf). An instrument for recording wave-like motions or modulation, especially for recording variations in blood pressure; it consists of a drum usually revolved by clockwork and covered with smoked paper upon which the curve is inscribed by a stylet or other writing point. [G. *kyma,* wave, + *graphō,* to record]

ky·mog·ra·phy (kī-mog′ră-fē). Use of the kymograph.

ky·mo·scope (kī′mō-skōp). An apparatus once used for measuring the pulse waves, or the variation in blood pressure. [G. *kyma,* wave, + *skopeō,* to regard]

kyn·u·ren·ic ac·id (kin-yū-rē′nik, -ren′ik). 4-Hydroxyquinoline-2-carboxylic acid; a product of the metabolism of L-tryptophan; appears in human urine in states of marked pyridoxine deficiency.

kyn·u·ren·i·nase (kī-nū-ren′i-nās). A liver enzyme catalyzing the hydrolysis of the L-kynurenine side chain, with the formation of anthranilic acid and L-alanine, in L-tryptophan metabolism.

kyn·u·ren·ine (kī-nū′rĕ-nēn, -nin). 3-Anthraniloylalanine; a product of the metabolism of L-tryptophan, excreted in the urine in small amounts.

  k. formamidase, SYN formamidase.

  k. 3-hydroxylase, SYN k. 3-monooxygenase.

  k. 3-monooxygenase, an enzyme catalyzing addition of a 3-OH to L-kynurenine, with the aid of NADPH and O_2, producing 3-hydroxy-L-kynurenine, $NADP^+$, and water; a step in the catabolism of L-tryptophan. SYN k. 3-hydroxylase.

ky·phos (kī′fos). A hump, the convex prominence in kyphosis. [G.]

ky·pho·sco·li·o·sis (kī′fō-skō-lē-ō′sis). Kyphosis combined with scoliosis; severe congestive heart failure is not infrequently a late complication.

ky·pho·sis (kī-fō′sis). A deformity of the spine characterized by extensive flexion. [G. *kyphōsis,* hump-back, fr. *kyphos,* bent, hump-backed]

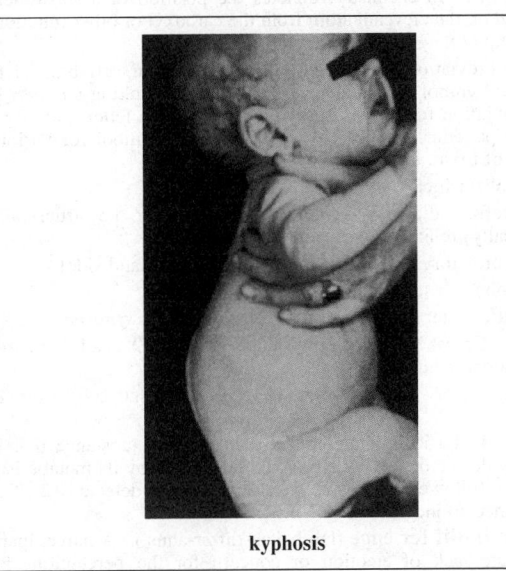

kyphosis

  juvenile k., SYN Scheuermann's *disease.*

ky·phot·ic (kī-fot′ik). Relating to or suffering from kyphosis.

ky·pho·tone (kī′fō-tōn). A brace for use in tuberculosis of the spine. [G. *kyphos,* hump, + *tonos,* brace]

Kyrle, J., German dermatologist, 1880–1926. SEE K.'s *disease.*

⟁**kyto-.** SEE cyto-.

ky

λ SEE Λ.

Λ, λ **1.** The 11th letter of the Greek alphabet, lambda. **2.** Symbol (λ) for Avogadro's *number*; wavelength; radioactive *constant*; Ostwald's solubility *coefficient*; molar conductivity of an electrolyte (Λ). **3.** In chemistry, denotes the position of a substituent located on the eleventh atom from the carboxyl or other functional group (λ).

L 1. Abbreviation for left (*e.g.*, left eye); lumbar vertebra (L1 to L5). **2.** Symbol for inductance; liter; linking *number*. **3.** Abbreviation for limes; used with a lower case letter, plus sign, subscript letter, or subscript plus sign as a symbol for various doses of toxin. SEE dose.

l Symbol for liter.

△**L-.** Prefix indicating a chemical compound to be structurally (sterically) related to L-glyceraldehyde. Cf. D-.

△**l-.** Levorotatory. Cf. *d-*. [L. *laevus*, on the left-hand side]

La Symbol for lanthanum.

Laband, Peter F., U.S. dentist, *1900. SEE L.'s *syndrome*.

Labbé, Ernest M., French physician, 1870–1939. SEE L.'s neurocirculatory *syndrome*.

Labbé, Leon, French surgeon, 1832–1916. SEE L.'s *triangle, vein*.

la·bel. 1. To incorporate into a compound a substance that is readily detected, such as a radionuclide, whereby its metabolism can be followed or its physical distribution detected. **2.** The substance so incorporated.

la belle in·dif·fér·ence (lah bel an-dif-er-ahns'). A naive, inappropriate lack of emotion or concern for the perceptions by others of one's disability, typically seen in persons with conversion hysteria. [Fr.]

la·bet·a·lol hy·dro·chlo·ride (la-bet'ă-lol). 5-[1-Hydroxy-2-[(1-methyl-3-phenylpropyl)amino]ethyl]salicyamide monohydrochloride; an α-adrenergic and β-adrenergic blocking agent used in the treatment of hypertension.

la·bia (lā'bē-ă). Plural of labium.

la·bi·al (lā'bē-ăl). **1.** Relating to the lips or any labium. **2.** Toward a lip. **3.** One of the letters formed by means of the lips. [L. *labium*, lip]

la·bi·al·ism (lā'bē-ăl-izm). A form of stammering in which there is confusion in the use of the labial consonants.

la·bi·al·ly (lā'bē-ăl-ē). Toward the lips.

la·bile (lā'bīl, -bil). Unstable; unsteady, not fixed; denoting: **1.** An adaptability to alteration or modification, *i.e.*, relatively easily changed or rearranged. **2.** Certain constituents of serum affected by increases in heat. **3.** An electrode that is kept moving over the surface during the passage of an electric current. **4.** In psychology or psychiatry, denoting free and uncontrolled mood or behavioral expression of the emotions. **5.** Easily removable; *e.g.*, a l. hydrogen. [L. *labilis*, liable to slip, fr. *labor*, pp. *lapsus*, to slip]

la·bil·i·ty (lă-bil'i-tē). The state of being labile.

△**labio-.** The lips. SEE ALSO cheilo-. [L. *labium*, lip]

la·bi·o·cer·vi·cal (lā'bē-ō-ser'vi-kăl). Relating to a lip and a neck; specifically, to the labial or buccal surface of the neck of a tooth. [labio- + L. *cervix*, neck]

la·bi·o·cho·rea (lā-bē-ō-kōr-ē'ă). A chronic spasm of the lips, interfering with speech. [labio- + G. *choreia*, dance]

la·bi·o·cli·na·tion (lā'bē-ō-kli-nā'shŭn). Inclination of position more toward the lips than is normal; said of a tooth.

la·bi·o·den·tal (lā-bē-ō-den'tăl). Relating to the lips and the teeth; denoting certain letters the sound of which is formed by both lips and teeth. [labio- + L. *dens*, tooth]

la·bi·o·gin·gi·val (lā'bē-ō-jin'ji-văl). Relating to the point of junction of the labial border and the gingival line on the distal or mesial surface of an incisor tooth.

la·bi·o·glos·so·la·ryn·ge·al (lā'bē-ō-glos'ō-lă-rin'jē-ăl). Relating to the lips, tongue, and larynx; describing bulbar paralysis in which these parts are involved. [labio- + G. *glōssa*, tongue, + larynx]

la·bi·o·glos·so·pha·ryn·ge·al (lā'bē-ō-glos'ō-fă-rin'jē-ăl). Relating to the lips, tongue, and pharynx; describing bulbar paralysis involving these parts. [labio- + G. *glōssa*, tongue, + pharynx]

la·bi·o·graph (lā'bē-ō-graf). An instrument for recording the movements of the lips in speaking. [labio- + G. *graphō*, to record]

la·bi·o·men·tal (lā'bē-ō-men'tăl). Relating to the lower lip and the chin. [labio- + L. *mentum*, chin]

la·bi·o·na·sal (lā'bē-ō-nā'săl). **1.** Relating to the upper lip and the nose, or to both lips and the nose. **2.** Denoting a letter which is both labial and nasal in the production of its sound.

la·bi·o·pal·a·tine (lā'bē-ō-pal'ă-tīn). Relating to the lips and the palate.

la·bi·o·place·ment (lā'bē-ō-plās'ment). Positioning (*e.g.*, of a tooth) more toward the lips than normal.

la·bi·o·plas·ty (lā'bē-ō-plas-tē). Plastic surgery of a lip. [labio- + G. *plastos*, formed]

la·bi·o·ver·sion (lā'bē-ō-ver-zhŭn). Malposition of an anterior tooth from the normal line of occlusion toward the lips.

lab·i·tome (lab'i-tōm). A forceps with sharp blades. SYN cutting forceps. [G. *labis*, pincers, + *tomē*, an incision]

la·bi·um, gen. **la·bii,** pl. **la·bia** (lā'bē-ŭm, -bē-ē, -bē-ă) [NA]. SYN lip. **2.** Any lip-shaped structure. [L.]

l. ante'rius ostii uteri [NA], SYN anterior *lip* of uterine os.

l. exter'num cris'tae ili'acae [NA], SYN external *lip* of iliac crest.

l. infe'rius o'ris [NA], SYN lower *lip*.

l. inter'num cris'tae ili'acae [NA], SYN internal *lip* of iliac crest.

l. latera'le lin'eae as'perae [NA], SYN lateral *lip* of linea aspera.

l. lim'bi tympan'icum laminae spiralis [NA], SYN tympanic l. of limbus of spiral lamina.

l. lim'bi vestibula're laminae spiralis [NA], SYN vestibular l. of limbus of spiral lamina.

l. majus, one of two rounded folds of integument forming the lateral boundaries of the pudendal cleft. The labia majora are the female homolog of the scrotum. SYN l. majus pudendi [NA], large pudendal lip.

l. ma'jus puden'di, pl. **la'bia majo'ra** [NA], SYN l. majus.

l. media'le lin'eae as'perae [NA], SYN medial *lip* of linea aspera.

l. minus, one of two narrow longitudinal folds of mucous membrane enclosed in the pudendal cleft within the labia majora; posteriorly, they gradually merge into the labia majora and join to form the frenulum labiorum pudendi (fourchette); anteriorly, each l. divides into two portions which unite with those of the opposite side in front of the glans clitoridis to form the prepuce. SYN l. minus pudendi [NA], small pudendal lip.

l. mi'nus puden'di, pl. **la'bia mino'ra** [NA], SYN l. minus.

la'bia o'ris [NA], SYN lips of mouth, under *lip*. SEE lip (1).

l. poste'rius ostii uteri [NA], SYN posterior *lip* of uterine os.

l. supe'rius o'ris [NA], SYN upper *lip*.

tympanic l. of limbus of spiral lamina, the lower, long periosteal extension of the limbus laminae spiralis osseae that rests on the basilar lamina of the spiral organ (of Corti). SYN l. limbi tympanicum laminae spiralis [NA], tympanic lip of limbus of spiral lamina.

l. ure'thrae, one of the two lateral margins of the external urethral orifice of the female.

la'bia u'teri, SEE anterior *lip* of uterine os, posterior *lip* of uterine os.

vestibular l. of limbus of spiral lamina, the upper, short periosteal extension of the limbus laminae spiralis osseae which provides the central attachment for the tectorial membrane. SYN l. limbi vestibulare laminae spiralis [NA], lamina dentata, vestibular lip of limbus of spiral lamina.

l. voca'le, pl. **la'bia voca'lia,** SYN vocal *fold*.

la·bor (lā'bŏr). The process of expulsion of the fetus and the placenta from the uterus. The **stages of l.** include: **first stage**, beginning with the onset of uterine contractions through the period of dilation of the os uteri; **second stage**, the period of expulsive effort, beginning with complete dilation of the cervix and ending with expulsion of the infant; **third s.** or **placental stage**, the period beginning at the expulsion of the infant and ending with the completed expulsion of the placenta and membranes. [L. toil, suffering]

active l., contractions resulting in progressive effacement and dilation of the cervix.

dry l., obsolete term for l. after spontaneous loss of the amniotic fluid.

false l., contractions which do not produce cervical dilation or effacement.

missed l., brief uterine contractions which do not lead to labor and expulsion of the infant, but which cease, resulting in the indefinite retention of the fetus (usually lifeless) either *in utero* or extrauterine, *e.g.,* in the abdominal cavity.

precipitate l., very rapid l. ending in delivery of the fetus.

premature l., onset of labor before the 37th completed week of pregnancy dated from the last normal menstrual period.

lab·o·ra·to·ri·an (lab'ŏ-ră-tōr'ē-an). One who works in a laboratory; in the medical and allied health professions, one who examines or performs tests (or supervises such procedures) with various types of chemical and biologic materials, chiefly as an aid in the diagnosis, treatment, and control of disease, or as a basis for health and sanitation practices.

lab·o·ra·tory (lab'ŏ-ră-tō-rē, lab'ră-). A place equipped for the performance of tests, experiments, and investigative procedures and for the preparation of reagents, therapeutic chemical materials, and so on. [Mediev. L. *laboratorium,* a workplace, fr. L. *laboro,* pp. *-atus,* to labor]

personal growth l., a sensitivity training setting in which the primary emphasis is on each participant's potentialities for creativity, empathy, and leadership. SEE ALSO sensitivity training *group.*

la·bra (lā'bră). Plural of labrum. [L.]

la·bra·le in·fe·ri·us (lă-brā'lē in-fē'rē-ŭs). A point where the boundary of the vermilion border of the lower lip and the skin is intersected by the median plane.

la·bra·le su·pe·ri·us (lă-brā'lē sū-pē'rē-ŭs). The point on the upper lip lying in the median sagittal plane on a line drawn across the boundary of the vermilion border and skin.

lab·ro·cyte (lab'rō-sīt). SYN mast *cell.*

la·brum, pl. **la·bra** (lā'brŭm, lā'bră) [NA]. **1.** A lip. **2.** A lip-shaped structure. [L.]

acetabular l., a fibrocartilaginous rim attached to the margin of the acetabulum of the hip bone. SYN l. acetabulare [NA], acetabular lip, circumferential cartilage (1), cotyloid ligament, ligamentum cotyloideum.

l. acetabula're [NA], SYN acetabular l.

articular l., a fibrocartilaginous lip around the margin of the concave portion of some joints. SYN l. articulare [NA], articular lip.

l. articula're [NA], SYN articular l. SEE acetabular l., glenoid l.

glenoid l., a ring of fibrocartilage attached to the margin of the glenoid cavity of the scapula to increase its depth. SYN l. glenoidale [NA], articular margin, circumferential cartilage (2), glenoid ligament (1), glenoidal lip, ligamentum glenoidale.

l. glenoida'le [NA], SYN glenoid l.

lab·y·rinth (lab'i-rinth). Any of several anatomical structures with numerous intercommunicating cells or canals. **1.** The internal or inner ear, composed of the semicircular ducts, vestibule, and cochlea. **2.** Any group of communicating cavities, as in each lateral mass of the ethmoid bone. **3.** SYN convoluted *part* of kidney lobule. **4.** A group of upright test tubes terminating below in a base of communicating, alternately ∪-shaped and ∩-shaped tubes, used for isolating motile from nonmotile organisms in culture, or a motile from a less motile organism (as the typhoid from the colon bacillus), the former traveling faster and farther through the tubes than the latter.

bony l., a series of cavities (cochlea, vestibule, and semicircular

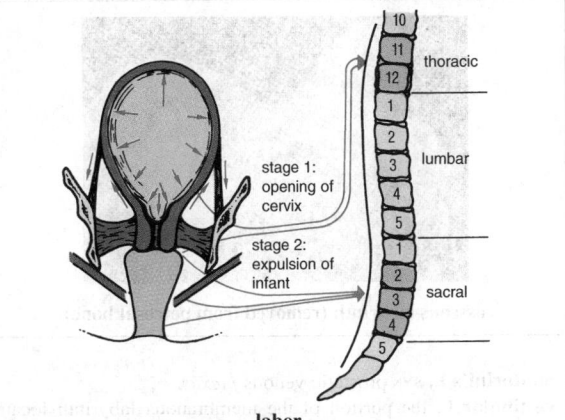

labor

pathways of labor pains and effect of labor on the opening of the cervical canal (first stage) and on the infant in the uterus (second stage); contractions of the uterus move in the direction of the pelvis because the neck of the uterus is fixed inside the pelvis by parametrial connective tissue, and the fundus of the uterus is anchored to the pelvic ring by uteroinguinal chords and is in an upright position by its proximity to the anterior abdominal wall

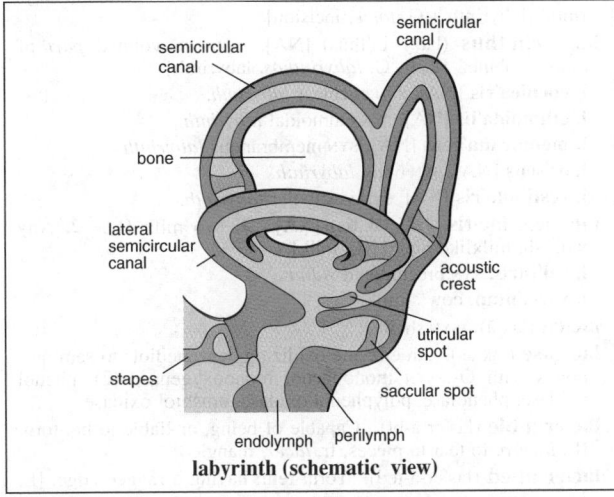

labyrinth (schematic view)

canals) contained within the otic capsule of the petrous portion of the temporal bone; the bony labyrinth is filled with perilymph, in which the delicate, endolymph-filled membranous labyrinth is suspended. SYN labyrinthus osseus [NA], osseous l.

cochlear l., the content of the cochlea including the portion of the membranous labyrinth containing the spiral organ (cochlear duct) and the perilymphatic channels (scalae) which lie on either side. SYN labyrinthus cochlearis [NA], organ of hearing.

ethmoidal l., a mass of air cells with thin bony walls forming part of the lateral wall of the nasal cavity; the cells are arranged in three groups, anterior, middle, and posterior, and are closed laterally by the orbital plate which forms part of the wall of the orbit. SYN labyrinthus ethmoidalis [NA], ectethmoid, ectoethmoid, lateral mass of ethmoid bone.

Ludwig's l., SYN convoluted *part* of kidney lobule.

membranous l., a complex arrangement of communicating membranous canaliculi and sacs, filled with endolymph and surrounded by perilymph, suspended within the cavity of the bony labyrinth; its chief divisions are the cochlear labyrinth and the vestibular labyrinth. SYN labyrinthus membranaceus [NA].

osseous l., SYN bony l.

renal l., SYN convoluted *part* of kidney lobule.

la

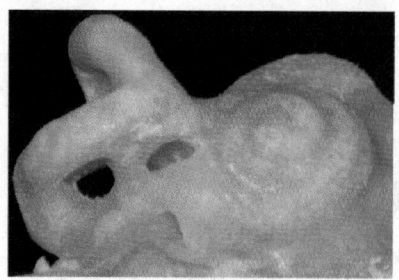

osseous labyrinth (removed from petrosal bone)

Santorini's l., SYN prostatic venous *plexus.*

vestibular l., the portion of the membranous labyrinth located within the semicircular canals and the vestibule of the osseous labyrinth. It is surrounded with perilymph and involved with vestibular functions. SYN labyrinthus vestibularis [NA].

lab·y·rin·thec·to·my (lab-ĭ-rin-thek'tō-mē). Excision of the labyrinth; a destructive operation to destroy labyrinthine function. [labyrinth + G. *ektomē,* excision]

lab·y·rin·thine (lab-ĭ-rin'thin). Relating to any labyrinth.

lab·y·rin·thi·tis (lab'ĭ-rin-thī'tis). Inflammation of the labyrinth (the internal ear), sometimes accompanied by vertigo and deafness. SYN otitis interna.

lab·y·rin·thot·o·my (lab-ĭ-rin-thot'ō-mē). Incision into the labyrinth. [labyrinth + G. *tomē,* incision]

lab·y·rin·thus (lab-i-rin'thŭs) [NA]. SYN convoluted *part* of kidney lobule. [L. fr. G. *labyrinthos,* labyrinth]

l. cochlea'ris [NA], SYN cochlear *labyrinth.*

l. ethmoida'lis [NA], SYN ethmoidal *labyrinth.*

l. membrana'ceus [NA], SYN membranous *labyrinth.*

l. os'seus [NA], SYN bony *labyrinth.*

l. vestibula'ris [NA], SYN vestibular *labyrinth.*

lac, gen. **lac·tis** (lak, lak'tis) [NA]. **1.** SYN milk (1). **2.** Any whitish, milklike liquid. [L. milk]

l. sul'furis, SYN precipitated *sulfur.*

l. vacci'num, cow's milk.

lac·ca (lak'ă). SYN shellac.

lac·case (lak'ās). An enzyme oxidizing benzenediols to semiquinones with O_2. SYN monophenol monooxygenase (2), phenol oxidase, phenolase, polyphenol oxidase, urushiol oxidase.

lac·er·a·ble (las'er-ă-bl). Capable of being, or liable to be, torn. [L. *lacero,* to tear to pieces, fr. *lacer,* mangled]

lac·er·at·ed (las'er-ā-ted). Torn; rent; having a ragged edge. [L. *lacero,* pp. *-atus,* to tear to pieces]

lac·er·a·tion (las-er-ā'shŭn). **1.** A torn or jagged wound, or an accidental cut wound. **2.** The process or act of tearing the tissues. [L. *lacero,* pp. *-atus,* to tear to pieces]

brain l., gross tearing of neural tissue.

scalp l., a tear of the dermis or underlying tissues and galea aponeurotica of the scalp.

through-and-through laceration, a l. that penetrates two surfaces of a structure, generally restricted to skin or mucosal surfaces, such as the cheek, lip, ala nasi, pinna, etc.

vaginal l., SYN colporrhexis.

la·cer·tus (lă-ser'tŭs). **1.** Originally the muscular part of the upper limb from shoulder to elbow. **2** [NA]. A fibrous band, bundle, or slip related to a muscle. [L.]

l. cor'dis, one of the trabeculae carneae.

l. fibro'sus, SYN bicipital *aponeurosis.*

l. of lateral rectus muscle, the part of the tendon of origin of the lateral rectus muscle attaching to the greater wing of the sphenoid bone, lateral to the common tendinous ring; often incorrectly equated to the lateral check ligament of the eyeball. SYN l. musculi recti lateralis [NA].

l. me'dius, SYN anterior longitudinal *ligament.*

l. mus'culi rec'ti latera'lis [NA], SYN l. of lateral rectus muscle.

lach·ry·mal (lak'ri-măl). SYN lacrimal.

LACI Abbreviation for lipoprotein-associated coagulation *inhibitor.*

la·cin·i·ae tu·bae (la-sin'ē-ē tū'bē). SYN *fimbriae* of uterine tube, under *fimbria.* [L. *lacinia,* fringe]

lac·ri·mal (lak'ri-măl). Relating to the tears, their secretion, the secretory glands, and the drainage apparatus. SYN lachrymal. [L. *lacrima,* a tear]

lac·ri·ma·tion (lak'ri-mā'shŭn). The secretion of tears, especially in excess. [L. *lacrimatio*]

lac·ri·ma·tor (lak'ri-mā-ter). An agent (such as tear gas) that irritates the eyes and produces tears. [L. *lacrima,* tear]

lac·ri·ma·to·ry (lak'ri-mă-tō-rē). Causing lacrimation.

lac·ri·mot·o·my (lak-ri-mot'ō-mē). The operation of incising the lacrimal duct or sac. [L. *lacrima,* tear, + G. *tomē,* incision]

△**lact-, lacti-, lacto-.** Milk. SEE ALSO galacto-. [L. *lac, lactis*]

lac·tac·i·de·mia (lak-tas-i-dē'mē-ă). SYN lactic acidemia.

lac·tac·i·do·sis (lak-tas-i-dō'sis). Acidosis due to increased lactic acid.

lac·tal·bu·min (lak-tal-byū'min). The albumin fraction of milk. It contains two proteins: α- and β-l.; the former, minor l., interacts with galactosyl transferase to form lactose synthase which synthesizes lactose from D-glucose and UDP-galactose in milk production; β-l. is the chief whey protein in bovine milk; α-l. is the most heat-stable of the whey proteins.

lac·tam, lac·tim (lak'tam, -tim). Contractions of "lactoneamine" and "lactoneimine," and applied to the tautomeric forms –NH–CO– and –N=C(OH)–, respectively, observed in many purines, pyrimidines, and other substances; the latter form accounts for the acidic properties of uric acid.

β-lac·tam. A class of broad spectrum antibiotics that are structurally and pharmacologically related to the penicillins and cephalosporins.

β-lac·ta·mase (lak'tă-mās). An enzyme that brings about the hydrolysis of a β-lactam (as penicillin to penicilloic acid); found in most staphylococcus strains that are naturally resistant to penicillin. SYN cephalosporinase, penicillinase (1).

lac·tase (lak'tās). SYN β-D-galactosidase.

lac·tate (lak'tāt). **1.** A salt or ester of lactic acid. **2.** To produce milk in the mammary glands.

l. dehydrogenase (LDH), name for four enzymes: L-l. dehydrogenase (cytochrome), D-l. dehydrogenase (cytochrome), L-l. dehydrogenase, and D-l. dehydrogenase. The first two enzymes transfer H to ferricytochrome *c* (EC 1.1.2.3 is cytochrome b_2), the last two enzymes transfer it to NAD^+, in catalyzing the oxidation of lactate to pyruvate; the isozyme distribution of heart and muscle l. dehydrogenase is of significant use in cases of myocardial infarction; a deficiency of a subunit will result in myoglobinuria after intense exercise. SYN lactic acid dehydrogenase.

excess l., the increase in l. concentration beyond what would be expected from the increase in pyruvate concentration resulting from a change in redox potential; used as an index of anaerobic carbohydrate metabolism.

lac·tate 2-mon·o·ox·y·gen·ase. A flavoprotein oxidoreductase catalyzing oxidation (with O_2) of L-lactate to acetate plus CO_2 and water. SYN lactic acid oxidative decarboxylase.

lac·ta·tion (lak-tā'shŭn). **1.** Production of milk. **2.** Period following birth during which milk is secreted in the breasts. [L. *lactatio,* suckle]

lac·ta·tion·al (lak-tā'shŭn-ăl). Relating to lactation.

lac·te·al (lak'tē-ăl). **1.** Relating to or resembling milk; milky. **2.** A lymphatic vessel that conveys chyle from the intestine. SYN chyle vessel, lacteal vessel.

central l., the blindly ending lymphatic capillary in the center of an intestinal villus.

lac·te·nin (lak'tĕ-nin). An antibacterial agent active against streptococci isolated from cow's milk.

lac·tes·cent (lak-tes'ent). Resembling milk; milky.

△**lacti-.** SEE lact-.

lac·tic (lak'tik). Relating to milk. [L. *lac* (*lact-*), milk]

lac·tic ac·id. CH₃–CHOH–COOH; 2-hydroxypropionic acid; a normal intermediate in the fermentation (oxidation, metabolism) of sugar. In pure form, a syrupy, odorless, and colorless liquid obtained by the action of the l. a. bacillus on milk or milk sugar; in concentrated form, a caustic used internally to prevent gastrointestinal fermentation. A culture of the bacillus, or milk containing it, is usually given in place of the acid. L-L. a. is also known as sarcolactic acid.

lac·tic ac·id de·hy·dro·gen·ase. SYN *lactate* dehydrogenase.

lac·tic ac·i·de·mia (lak'tik-as-i-dē'mē-ă). The presence of dextrorotatory lactic acid in the circulating blood. SYN lactacidemia. [lactic acid + G. *haima*, blood]

lac·tic ac·id ox·i·da·tive de·car·box·yl·ase. SYN lactate 2-mono-oxygenase.

lac·tif·er·ous (lak-tif'er-ŭs). Yielding milk. SYN lactigerous. [lacti- + L. *fero*, to bear]

lac·tif·u·gal (lak-tif'yū-găl). SYN lactifuge (1).

lac·ti·fuge (lak'ti-fyūj). **1.** Causing arrest of the secretion of milk. SYN lactifugal. **2.** An agent having such an effect. SYN phygogalactic. [lacti- + L. *fugo*, to drive away]

lac·tig·e·nous (lak-tij'ĕ-nŭs). Producing milk. [lacti- + -gen, producing]

lac·tig·er·ous (lak-tij'er-ŭs). SYN lactiferous. [lacti- + L. *gero*, to carry]

lac·tim (-tim). SEE lactam.

lac·ti·mor·bus (lak-ti-mōr'bŭs). SYN milk *sickness*. [lacti- + L. *morbus*, disease]

lac·ti·nat·ed (lak'ti-nā-ted). Prepared with or containing milk sugar.

△**lacto-.** SEE lact-.

Lac·to·bac·il·la·ce·ae (lak'tō-bas'i-lā'sē-ē). A family of anaerobic to facultatively anaerobic, ordinarily nonmotile bacteria (order Eubacteriales) containing straight or curved, Gram-positive rods which usually occur singly or in chains; motile cells are peritrichous. These organisms have complex organic nutritional requirements; they produce lactic acid from carbohydrates. They are found in fermenting animal and plant products where carbohydrates are available; they are also found in the mouth, vagina, and intestinal tract of various warm-blooded animals, including humans. Only a few species are pathogenic. The type genus is *Lactobacillus*.

lac·to·ba·cil·li (lak-tō-bă-sil'ī). Plural of lactobacillus.

lac·to·ba·cil·lic ac·id (lak'tō-bă-sil'ik). CH₃(CH₂)₄CH₂–CH–CH–(CH₂)₉COOH; (1*R-cis*)-2-hexycyclopropanedecanoic acid; a major constituent of the lipids of lactobacilli; notable for the presence of a cyclopropane ring in the molecule.

Lac·to·ba·cil·lus (lak-tō-bă-sil'ŭs). A genus of microaerophilic or anaerobic, nonsporeforming, ordinarily nonmotile bacteria (family Lactobacillaceae) containing Gram-positive rods which vary from long and slender cells to short coccobacilli; chains are commonly produced, especially in the later part of the logarithmic phase of growth. These organisms possess complex nutritional requirements, generally characteristic for each species; metabolism is fermentative and at least half of the end product is lactic acid. They are found in dairy products and effluents to grain and meat products, water, sewage, beer, wine, fruits and fruit juices, pickled vegetables, and in sour dough and mash, and are part of the normal flora of the mouth, intestinal tract, and vagina of many warm-blooded animals, including humans; rarely are they pathogenic. The type species is *L. delbrueckii*. [lacto- + bacillus]

L. acidoph'ilus, a species found in the feces of milk-fed infants and also in the feces of older persons on a high milk-, lactose-, or dextrin-containing diet.

L. bi'fidus, former name for *Bifidobacterium bifidum*.

L. bi'fidus subsp. *pennsylva'nicus*, former name for *Bifidobacterium bifidum*.

L. bre'vis, a species widely distributed in nature, especially in plant and animal products; it is also found in the mouth and intestinal tract of humans and rats.

L. buch'neri, a species widely distributed in fermenting substances.

L. bulgar'icus, a species used in the production of yogurt.

L. ca'sei, a species found in milk and cheese.

L. catenafor'mis, an anaerobic species found in the intestines and pulmonary cavities of humans.

L. cellobio'sus, SYN *L. fermentum*.

L. confu'sus, a species found in cow dung.

L. coproph'ilus, former name for *Lactobacillus confusus*.

L. corynifor'mis, a species found primarily in silage but also in cow dung and dairy barn air.

L. crispa'tus, a species found in pus from a dental abscess.

L. curva'tus, a species found in cow dung, dairy barn air, silage, milk, and in a case of endocarditis.

L. delbrueck'ii, a species found in fermenting vegetables and grain mashes; it is the type species of the genus *L.*

L. fermen'tum, a species found widely distributed in nature, especially in fermenting plant and animal products. Also found in the mouth of human beings. SYN *L. cellobiosus*.

L. fructiv'orans, a species isolated from spoiled mayonnaise and salad dressings.

L. helvet'icus, a species found in sour milk and Swiss cheese.

L. heterohio'chi, a species found in spoiled sake.

L. hilgar'dii, a species isolated from California table wines.

L. homohio'chii, a species found in spoiled sake.

L. jensen'ii, a species isolated from human sources such as vaginal discharge and blood clot.

L. lac'tis, a species found in milk and cheese; not pathogenic.

L. leichman'nii, a species found in dairy and plant products.

L. planta'rum, a species found in dairy products and environments, fermenting plants, silage, sauerkraut, pickled vegetables, spoiled tomato products, sour dough, cow dung, and the human mouth, intestinal tract, and stools.

L. saliva'rius, a species found in the mouth and intestinal tract of the hamster, the mouth of humans, and the intestinal tract of the hen.

L. tricho'des, a species found in wines containing 20% ethanol and in lees in California, Australia, France, and Spain; in California this organism is commonly referred to as the hair bacillus, cottony bacillus, cottony mold, or Fresno mold.

L. virides'cens, a species found in discolored cured meat products such as sausage and bologna.

lac·to·ba·cil·lus (lak-tō-bă-sil'ŭs). A vernacular term used to refer to any member of the genus *Lactobacillus*.

lac·to·bu·ty·rom·e·ter (lak'tō-byū-ti-rom'ĕ-ter). A type of lactocrit. [lacto- + G. *boutyron*, butter, + *metron*, measure]

lac·to·cele (lak'tō-sēl). SYN galactocele. [lacto- + G. *kēlē*, tumor]

lac·to·chrome (lak'tō-krōm). SYN lactoflavin (1).

lac·to·crit (lak'tō-krit). An instrument used to estimate the amount of butterfat in milk. [lacto- + G. *krinō*, to separate]

lac·to·den·sim·e·ter (lak'tō-den-sim'ĕ-ter). A type of galactometer. [lacto- + L. *densus*, thick, + G. *metron*, measure]

lac·to·fer·rin (lak'tō-fār-in). A transferrin found in the milk of several mammalian species and thought to be involved in the transport of iron to erythrocytes; relatively high concentrations in human milk.

lac·to·fla·vin (lak'tō-flā-vin). **1.** The flavin in milk. SYN lactochrome. **2.** SYN riboflavin.

lac·to·gen (lak'tō-jen). An agent that stimulates milk production or secretion. [lacto- + G. *-gen*, producing]

human placental l. (HPL), l. isolated from human placentas and structurally similar to somatotropin; its biological activity weakly mimics that of somatotropin and prolactin; secreted into maternal circulation; a deficiency of HPL during pregnancy leads to children having abnormal intrauterine and postnatal growth. SYN choriomammotropin, chorionic "growth hormone-prolactin", human chorionic somatomammotropic hormone, human chorionic somatomammotropin, placenta protein, placental growth hormone, purified placental protein.

lac·to·gen·e·sis (lak-tō-jen'ĕ-sis). Milk production. [lacto- + G. *genesis*, production]

la

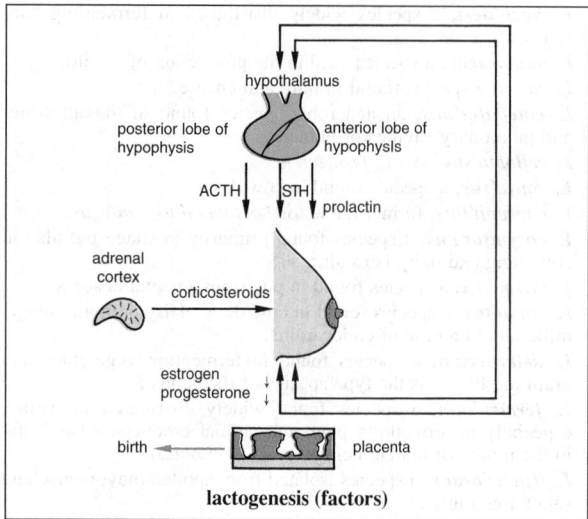

lactogenesis (factors)

lac·to·gen·ic (lak-tō-jen'ik). Pertaining to lactogenesis.

lac·to·glob·u·lin (lak-tō-glob'yū-lin). The globulin present in milk, comprising 50 to 60% of bovine whey protein.

lac·tom·e·ter (lak-tom'ĕ-ter). SYN galactometer. [lacto- + G. *metron*, measure]

lac·to·nase (lak'tō-nās). SYN gluconolactonase.

lac·tone (lak'tōn). An intramolecular organic anhydride formed from a hydroxyacid by the loss of water between an –OH and a –COOH group; a cyclic ester.

lac·to·per·ox·i·dase (lak'tō-per-oks'i-dās). A peroxidase obtained from milk.

lac·to·pro·tein (lak-tō-prō'tēn). Any protein normally present in milk.

lac·tor·rhea (lak-tō-rē'ă). SYN galactorrhea. [lacto- + G. *rhoia*, a flow]

lac·to·scope (lak'tō-skōp). SYN galactoscope. [lacto- + G. *skopeō*, to view]

lac·tose (lak'tōs). 4-(β-D-Galactosido)-D-glucose; a disaccharide present in mammalian milk, occurring naturally as α- and β-l.; obtained from cow's milk and used in modified milk preparations, in food for infants and convalescents, and in pharmaceutical preparations; large doses act as an osmotic diuretic and as a laxative. SYN milk sugar, saccharum lactis.
l. synthase, the enzyme responsible for the synthesis of l., catalyzing the reaction between UDP-galactose and D-glucose to l. and UDP.

lac·tos·u·ria (lak'tō-sū'rē-ă). Excretion of lactose (milk sugar) in the urine; a common finding during pregnancy and lactation, and in the newborn, especially premature babies. [lactose + G. *ouron*, urine, + -ia]

lac·to·ther·a·py (lak-tō-thār'ă-pē). SYN galactotherapy.

lac·to·tro·pin (lak-tō-trō'pin). SYN prolactin.

lac·to·veg·e·tar·i·an (lak'tō-vej-ĕ-tā'rē-ăn). One who lives on a mixed diet of milk and milk products, eggs, and vegetables, but eschews meat.

lac·to·yl·glu·ta·thi·one ly·ase (lak'tō-il-glū-tă-thī'ōn). Glyoxalase I; a lyase cleaving *S*-D-lactoylglutathione to glutathione and methylglyoxal. SYN aldoketomutase, ketone-aldehyde mutase, methylglyoxalase.

lac·tu·lose (lak'tū-lōs). 4-*O*-β-D-Galactopyranosyl-D-fructose; a synthetic disaccharide used to treat hepatic encephalopathy and chronic constipation.

α-lac·tyl-·thi·am·in py·ro·phos·phate. SYN active *pyruvate*.

la·cu·na, pl. **la·cu·nae** (lă-kū'nă, -kū'nē). **1** [NA]. A small space, cavity, or depression. **2.** A gap or defect. **3.** An abnormal space between strata or between the cellular elements of the

epidermis. **4.** SYN corneal *space*. [L. a pit, dim. of *lacus*, a hollow, a lake]

cartilage l., a cavity within the matrix of cartilage, occupied by a chondrocyte. SYN cartilage space.

cerebral l., a small circumscribed loss of brain tissue caused by occlusion of one of the small penetrating arteries. SYN l. cerebri.
l. cer'ebri, SYN cerebral l.

Howship's lacunae, tiny depressions, pits, or irregular grooves in bone that is being resorbed by osteoclasts. SYN resorption lacunae.

intervillous l., one of the blood spaces in the placenta into which the chorionic villi project.

lateral lacunae, SYN lateral venous lacunae.

lacunae latera'les [NA], SYN lateral venous lacunae.

lateral venous lacunae, lateral expansions of the superior sagittal sinus of the dura mater, often increasing in width with advancing age until, in the very old, they may extend two centimeters lateral to the midline; the endothelium-lined lumen of the lacunae are usually reduced to a spongelike labyrinth by numerous arachnoid granulations and dural trabeculae. SYN lacunae laterales [NA], lateral lacunae, lateral lakes, parasinoidal sinuses.

l. mag'na, a recess on the roof of the fossa navicularis of the penis, formed by a fold of mucous membrane, the valve of the navicular fossa.

Morgagni's l., SYN urethral l.

muscular l., the lateral compartment beneath the inguinal (Poupart's) ligament, for the passage of the iliopsoas muscle and femoral nerve; it is separated by the iliopectineal arch from the vascular lacuna. SYN l. musculorum [NA].

l. musculo'rum [NA], SYN muscular l.

osseous l., a cavity in bony tissue occupied by an osteocyte.

l. pharyn'gis, a depression near the pharyngeal opening of the auditory (eustachian) tube.

resorption lacunae, SYN Howship's lacunae.

trophoblastic l., one of the spaces in the early syncytiotrophoblastic layer of the chorion before the formation of villi; in human embryos maternal blood enters these spaces by the 10th day; with the differentiation of the chorionic villi they become intervillous spaces, sometimes called intervillous lacunae.

urethral l., one of a number of little recesses in the mucous membrane of the spongy urethra into which empty the ducts of the urethral glands. SYN l. urethralis [NA], Morgagni's l.

l. urethra'lis, pl. **lacu'nae urethra'les** [NA], SYN urethral l.

vascular l., the medial compartment beneath the inguinal ligament, for the passage to the femoral vessels; it is separated from the muscular l. by the iliopectineal arch. SYN l. vasorum [NA].

l. vaso'rum [NA], SYN vascular l.

la·cu·nar (lă-kū'năr). Relating to a lacuna.

la·cu·nule (lă-kū'nūl). A very small lacuna. [Mod. L. *lacunula*, dim. of L. *lacuna*]

la·cus, pl. **la·cus** (lā'kŭs). A small collection of fluid. SYN lake (1). [L. lake]

l. lacrima'lis [NA], SYN lacrimal *lake*.

l. semina'lis, the vault of the vagina after insemination. SYN seminal lake.

LAD Abbreviation for *leukocyte* adhesion deficiency.

Ladd, William E., U.S. pediatric surgeon, 1880–1967. SEE L.'s *band, operation.*

Ladd-Franklin, Christine, U.S. psychologist, 1847–1930. SEE Ladd-Franklin *theory.*

Lae·laps echid·ni·nus (lē'laps ē-kid-nī'nŭs). The spiny rat mite, a common worldwide ectoparasite of the wild Norway rat and occasionally found on the house mouse, cotton rat, and other rodents; it is the natural vector of *Hepatozoon muris* and can transmit the agent of tularemia experimentally. Junin virus has been isolated from this species in South America.

Laënnec, René T.H., French physician, 1781–1826. SEE L.'s *cirrhosis, pearls,* under *pearl.*

la·e·trile (lā'ĕ-tril). An allegedly antineoplastic drug consisting chiefly of amygdalin derived from apricot pits; its antitumor effect is unproven.

△**laev-.** SEE levo-.

Lafora, Gonzalo Rodriguez, Spanish neurologist, 1887–1971. SEE L. *body,* body *disease;* L.'s *disease.*

lag. 1. To move or progress more slowly than normal; to fall behind. **2.** The act or condition of falling behind. **3.** The time interval between a change in one variable and a consequent change in another variable.

anaphase l., slowing or arrest in the normal migration of chromosomes during anaphase, resulting in such chromosomes being excluded from one of the daughter cells.

homeostatic l., the interval in a homeostatic process between a change of the trait controlled and the appropriate response, due to afferent, efferent, and central components. The l. may be a pure random variable, *e.g.,* the waiting time of an exponential process or the sum of several such processes taking any value greater than zero but with a mean considerably greater than zero; sometimes it may be deterministic or almost so and with a minimum sharply defined and greater than zero for anatomical reasons. For instance, the partial pressures of oxygen and carbon dioxide are controlled in the lungs but based on afferent information obtained from the carotid body that is already dated because of the circulation time of ten seconds or so between the two sites.

la·ge·na, pl. **la·ge·nae** (lă-jē'nă, -jē-nē). **1.** SYN cupular *cecum* of the cochlear duct. **2.** One of the three parts of the membranous labyrinth of the inner ear of lower vertebrates; in mammals, the l. becomes the cochlea. [L. flask]

lag·ging. Retarded or diminished ventilatory movement of the affected side of the chest due to pleural disease with muscle splinting or collapse of a lung.

lag·o·morph (lā'gō-mōrf). A member of the order Lagomorpha.

Lag·o·mor·pha (lā-gō-mōr'fă). An order of herbivorous mammals (class Eutheria) resembling rodents (order Rodentia) but having two pairs of upper incisors one behind the other; it includes the rabbits, hares, and pikas. [G. *lagōs,* hare, + *morphē,* form]

lag·oph·thal·mia (lag-of-thal'mē-ă). SEE lagophthalmos.

lag·oph·thal·mos, lag·oph·thal·mia (lag-of-thal'mŏs, lag-of-thal'mē-ă). A condition in which a complete closure of the eyelids over the eyeball is difficult or impossible. [G. *lagōs,* hare + *ophthalmos,* eye]

Lagrange, Pierre F., French ophthalmologist, 1857–1928.

Lahey, Frank H., U.S. surgeon, 1880–1935. SEE L. *forceps.*

LAK Abbreviation for lymphokine activated killer cells.

lake (lāk). **1.** SYN lacus. **2.** To cause blood plasma to become red as a result of the release of hemoglobin from the erythrocytes, as when the latter are suspended in water. SEE ALSO lacuna. [A.S. *lacu,* fr. L. *lacus,* lake]

capillary l., the total mass of blood contained in capillary vessels.

lacrimal l., the small cistern-like area of the conjunctiva at the medial angle of the eye, in which the tears collect after bathing the anterior surface of the eyeball and the conjunctival sac. SYN lacus lacrimalis [NA], lacrimal bay.

lateral l.'s, SYN lateral venous *lacunae,* under *lacuna.*

seminal l., SYN *lacus* seminalis.

subchorial l., SYN subchorial *space.*

venous l.'s, (1) thin-walled collections of blood, resembling blood blisters, found commonly in the ears and less often on the lips and on the face and neck of elderly sun-damaged men; **(2)** discontinuous venous cavities or channels; Cf. marginal *sinuses* of placenta, under *sinus.* **(3)** in skull radiography, round to oval radiolucent foci in the frontal or parietal bones caused by dilated diploic venous channels.

Laki-Lorand fac·tor. See under factor.

laky (lā'kē). Pertaining to the transparent bright red appearance of blood serum or plasma, developing as a result of hemoglobin being released from destroyed red blood cells.

la·li·a·try (lă-lī'ă-trē). The study and treatment of speech disorders. [G. *lalia,* speech, chatter, + *iatria,* cure]

lal·i·o·pho·bia (lal'ē-o-fō'bē-ă). Morbid fear of speaking or stuttering. [G. *lalia,* speech, + *phobos,* fear]

Lallemand, Claude F., French surgeon, 1790–1853. SEE L.'s *bodies,* under *body;* Trousseau-L. *bodies,* under *body.*

lal·ling (lal'ing). A form of stammering in which the speech is almost unintelligible. [G. *laleō,* to chatter]

Lallouette, Pierre, French physician, 1711–1792. SEE L.'s *pyramid.*

lal·o·che·zia (lal-ō-kē'zē-ă). Emotional discharge gained by uttering indecent or filthy words. [G. *lalia,* speech, + *chezō,* to relieve oneself]

lal·og·no·sis (lal'og-nō'sis). Understanding and knowledge of speech. [G. *lalia,* speech, + *gnosis,* knowledge]

la·lo·ple·gia (la-lō-plē'jē-ă). Paralysis of the muscles concerned in the mechanism of speech. [G. *lalia,* speech, + *plēgē,* a stroke]

Lamarck, Jean-Baptiste P.A., French botanist, zoologist, and biological philosopher, 1744–1829. SEE lamarckian *theory.*

Lamaze, Fernand, French obstetrician, 1890–1957. SEE L. *method.*

LAMB Acronym for *l*entigines, *a*trial myxoma, *m*ucocutaneous myxomas, and *b*lue nevi. SEE LAMB *syndrome.*

Lam B. Outer membrane protein of Gram-negative bacteria.

lamb·da (lam'dă). **1.** The 11th letter of the Greek alphabet, λ. **2.** The craniometric point at the junction of the sagittal and lambdoid sutures.

lamb·da·cism (lam'dă-sizm). **1.** Mispronunciation or disarticulation of the letter *l.* **2.** Substitution of the letter *l* for the letter *r.* [G. *lambda,* the letter L]

lamb·doid (lam'doyd). Resembling the Greek letter lambda, as does the lambdoid suture. [lambda + G. *eidos,* resemblance]

Lambert, Edward H., U.S. physician, *1915. SEE L.-Eaton *syndrome;* Eaton-L. *syndrome.*

lam·bert. A unit of brightness; the brightness of a perfectly diffusing surface emitting or reflecting a total luminous flux of 1 lumen per sq cm of surface. [J.H. *Lambert,* German physicist and mathematician, 1728–1777]

Lam·blia in·tes·ti·na·lis (lam'blē-ă in-tes-ti-nā'lis). Old term for *Giardia lamblia,* though still frequently used, especially by protozoologists in the former Soviet Union.

lam·bli·a·sis (lam-blī'ă-sis). SYN giardiasis.

lam·bo lam·bo (lam'bō-lam'bō). SYN *myositis* purulenta tropica.

Lambrinudi, Constantine, British orthopaedic surgeon, 1890–1943. SEE Lambrinudi *operation.*

la·mel·la, pl. **la·mel·lae** (lă-mel'ă, -mel'ē). **1.** A thin sheet or layer, such as occurs in compact bone. **2.** A preparation in the form of a medicated gelatin disc, used as a means of making local applications to the conjunctiva in place of solutions. SYN discus [NA], disc (2), disk (1). [L. dim. of *lamina,* plate, leaf]

annulate lamellae, several pairs of parallel, smooth membranes, each pair containing regularly spaced pores resembling those of the nuclear envelope; they occur in germ cells, embryonic cells, and neoplastic cells.

articular l., the compact layer of bone on its articular surface that is firmly attached to the overlying articular cartilage.

l. of bone, a concentric, circumferential, or interstitial l.

circumferential l., a bony l. that encircles the outer or inner surface of a bone.

concentric l., one of the concentric tubular layers of bone surrounding the central canal in an osteon. SYN haversian l.

cornoid l., a narrow vertical column of parakeratosis in the epidermal stratum corneum; characteristic of porokeratosis.

elastic l., a thin sheet or membrane composed of elastic fibers; distinguished from elastic membrane, which usually refers to a condensed mass of fibers, as in an artery, whereas an elastic l. may be a looser elastic layer such as found in a vein or the respiratory tract.

enamel l., an organic defect in enamel; a thin, leaflike structure that extends from the enamel surface toward the dentinoenamel junction.

glandulopreputial l., a layer of embryonic epithelial tissue that gives rise to the prepuce.

ground l., SYN interstitial l.

haversian l., SYN concentric l.

la

intermediate l., SYN interstitial l.

interstitial l., one of the lamellae of partially resorbed osteons occurring between newer, complete osteons. SYN ground l., intermediary system, intermediate l.

triangular l., SYN choroid *tela* of third ventricle.

vitreous l., SYN *lamina* basalis choroideae.

lam·el·lar (lam′ĕ-lăr, lă-mel′ăr). **1.** Arranged in thin plates or scales. SYN lamellate, lamellated. **2.** Relating to lamellae.

lam·el·late, lam·el·lat·ed (lam′ĕ-lāt, -ed). SYN lamellar (1).

la·mel·li·po·di·um, pl. **la·mel·li·po·dia** (lă-mel-i-pō′dē-ŭm, -ă). A cytoplasmic veil produced on all sides of migrating polymorphonuclear leukocytes.

LAMINA

lam·i·na, pl. **lam·i·nae** (lam′i-nă, lam′i-nē) [NA]. Thin plate or flat layer. SEE ALSO layer, stratum. [L]

l. affix′a [NA], that part of the medial ependymal wall of the lateral ventricle of the embryonic brain that in later development becomes adherent to the superior surface of the thalamus and thus comes to form the floor of the central part of the lateral ventricle; it covers the thalamostriate and choroidal veins.

l. ala′ris [NA], SYN alar l. of neural tube.

alar l. of neural tube, the dorsal division of the lateral walls of the neural tube in the embryo; it gives rise to neurons relaying afferent impulses to higher centers; in the adult such neurons compose the sensory nuclei of the spinal cord and brainstem. SYN l. alaris [NA], alar plate of neural tube, dorsolateral plate of neural tube, l. dorsalis, wing plate.

lam′inae al′bae cerebel′li [NA], layers of white substance seen on section of the cerebellum. SYN laminae medullares cerebelli.

l. ante′rior vagi′nae mus′culi rec′ti abdo′minis [NA], SYN anterior *layer* of rectus abdominis sheath.

l. ar′cus ver′tebrae [NA], SYN l. of vertebral arch.

basal l., (1) an amorphous extracellular layer applied to the basal surface of epithelium and also investing muscle cells, fat cells, and Schwann cells; thought to be a selective filter and to serve both structural and morphogenetic functions. It is comprised of a 20–100 nm network of file filaments called the l. densa which appears dense in the electron microscope, and on either side of this layer is a less dense layer called the l. rarae; SEE ALSO basement *membrane*, l. densa. **(2)** SYN l. densa.

basal l. of choroid, SYN l. basalis choroideae.

basal l. of ciliary body, the inner layer of the ciliary body, continuous with the basal layer of the choroid and supporting the pigment epithelium of the ciliary retina. SYN l. basalis corporis ciliaris [NA], basal layer of ciliary body.

basal l. of cochlear, SYN basilar *membrane*.

l. basa′lis [NA], SYN basal l. of neural tube.

l. basa′lis choroi′deae [NA], the transparent, nearly structureless inner layer of the choroid in contact with the pigmented layer of the retina. SYN basal l. of choroid, basal layer of choroid, Bruch's membrane, Henle's membrane, l. vitrea, vitreous lamella, vitreous membrane (3).

l. basa′lis cor′poris cilia′ris [NA], SYN basal l. of ciliary body.

basal l. of neural tube, the ventral division of the lateral walls of the neural tube in the embryo; it contains neuroblasts giving rise to somatic and visceral motor neurons. SYN l. basalis [NA], basal plate of neural tube, l. ventralis, ventral plate of neural tube.

basal l. of semicircular duct, SYN basal *membrane* of semicircular duct.

basement l., SYN basement *membrane*.

basilar l., SYN basilar *membrane*.

l. basila′ris coch′leae [NA], SYN basilar *membrane*.

boundary l., a basement membrane-like structure that invests muscle cells, fat cells, and Schwann cells. SEE ALSO basement *membrane*, basal l.

l. cartilag′inis cricoi′deae [NA], SYN l. of cricoid cartilage.

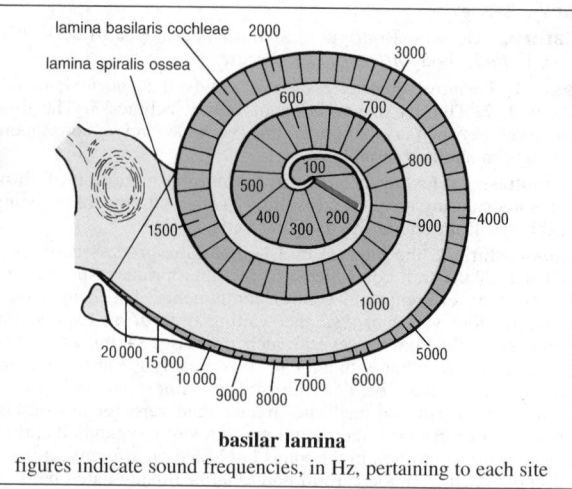

basilar lamina
figures indicate sound frequencies, in Hz, pertaining to each site

l. cartilag′inis latera′lis tubae auditivae [NA], ☆official alternate term for lateral l. of cartilaginous auditory tube.

l. cartilag′inis media′lis tubae auditivae [NA], ☆official alternate term for medial l. of cartilaginous auditory tube, medial l. of cartilaginous auditory tube.

l. cartilag′inis thyroi′deae [NA], SYN l. of thyroid cartilage.

l. choriocapilla′ris, SYN choriocapillary *layer*.

l. choroi′dea, SYN epithelial l.

l. choroi′dea epithelia′lis, SYN epithelial l.

l. choroidocapilla′ris [NA], SYN choriocapillary *layer*.

l. cine′rea, SYN l. terminalis of cerebrum.

l. cribro′sa os′sis ethmoida′lis [NA], SYN cribriform *plate* of ethmoid bone.

l. cribro′sa scle′rae, the portion of the sclera through which pass the fibers of the optic nerve. SYN cribrous l., perforated layer of sclera.

cribrous l., SYN l. cribrosa sclerae.

l. of cricoid cartilage, a quadrate plate forming the posterior part of the cricoid cartilage. It resembles the shield of a signet ring, the arch of the cricoid representing the remainder of the ring. SYN l. cartilaginis cricoideae [NA].

deep l., SYN deep *layer*.

l. den′sa, (1) the electron-dense layer of the basal l. as seen in the electron microscope; SEE ALSO basement *membrane*. **(2)** the extraordinarily thick basal l. of the renal glomerulus. SYN basal l. (2).

dental l., SYN dental *ledge*.

l. denta′ta, SYN vestibular *labium* of limbus of spiral lamina.

dentogingival l., SYN dental *ledge*.

l. dorsa′lis, SYN alar l. of neural tube.

l. du′ra, the hard layer lining the dental alveoli.

l. elas′tica ante′rior, SYN anterior limiting *layer* of cornea.

l. elas′tica poste′rior, SYN posterior limiting *layer* of cornea.

elastic laminae of arteries, 1) external: the layer of elastic connective tissue lying immediately outside the smooth muscle of the tunica media; 2) internal: a fenestrated layer of elastic tissue of the tunica intima. SYN elastic layers of arteries, Henle's fenestrated elastic membrane.

episcleral l., the delicate moveable layer of loose connective tissue between the external surface of the sclera and the fascial sheath of the eyeball. SYN l. episcleralis [NA].

l. episclera′lis [NA], SYN episcleral l.

epithelial l., the layer of modified ependymal cells that forms the inner layer of the tela choroidea, facing the ventricle. SYN l. epithelialis [NA], epithelial choroid layer, l. choroidea epithelialis, l. choroidea.

l. epithelia′lis [NA], SYN epithelial l.

l. exter′na cra′nii [NA], SYN outer *table* of skull.

l. fibrocartilagin′ea interpu′bica, SYN interpubic *disc*.

l. fibroreticula′ris, a layer of the basement membrane in continuity with associated connective tissue; it is often discontinuous and may be lacking entirely in some cases.

l. fusca of sclera, an exceedingly delicate layer of loose, pigmented connective tissue on the inner surface of the sclera, connecting it with the choroid. SYN l. fusca sclerae [NA], brown layer, membrana fusca.

l. fus′ca scle′rae [NA], SYN l. fusca of sclera.

hepatic laminae, the plates of liver cells that radiate from the center of the liver lobule.

l. horizonta′lis os′sis palati′ni [NA], SYN horizontal *plate* of palatine bone.

l. inter′na cra′nii [NA], SYN inner *table* of skull.

internal medullary l., SEE medullary laminae of thalamus.

l. internal ossium cranii, SYN vitreous *table*.

iridopupillary l., embryonic precursor of the anterior stroma of the iris which forms the inner (posterior or deep) wall of the primary anterior chamber of the eye. Its central portion becomes attenuated as the pupillary membrane (membrana pupillaris [NA]).

labiogingival l., a band of ectodermal epithelial cells growing into the mesenchyme of the embryonic jaws between the developing lip and the growing gingival elevation; it later opens to form the labiogingival groove.

lateral l. of cartilaginous auditory tube, the narrow lateral portion of the cartilaginous part of the auditory tube. SYN l. lateralis cartilaginis tubae auditivae [NA], l. cartilaginis lateralis tubae auditivae★ [NA], lateral cartilaginous layer, lateral layer of cartilaginous auditory tube.

l. latera′lis cartilaginis tubae auditivae [NA], SYN lateral l. of cartilaginous auditory tube.

l. latera′lis proces′sus pterygoid′ei [NA], SYN lateral pterygoid *plate.*

lateral medullary l. of corpus striatum, a thin, sharply defined layer of fibers separating the putamen from the globus pallidus. SYN l. medullaris lateralis corporis striati [NA].

l. of lens, one of a series of concentric layers composed of the lens fibers that make up the substance of the lens.

l. lim′itans ante′rior cor′neae [NA], SYN anterior limiting *layer* of cornea.

l. lim′itans poste′rior cor′neae [NA], SYN posterior limiting *layer* of cornea.

l. lu′cida, the lightly staining layer of the basement membrane in contact with the plasmalemma of epithelial cells or other cells having an investment of basement membrane.

medial l. of cartilaginous auditory tube, the broad medial portion of the cartilaginous part of the auditory tube. SYN l. medialis cartilaginis tubae auditivae [NA], l. cartilaginis medialis tubae auditivae★ [NA], medial cartilaginous layer, medial layer of cartilaginous auditory tube.

l. media′lis cartilaginis tubae auditivae [NA], SYN medial l. of cartilaginous auditory tube.

l. media′lis proces′sus pterygoi′dei [NA], SYN medial pterygoid *plate.*

medial medullary l. of corpus striatum, a fiber layer separating the medial and lateral segments of the globus pallidus. SYN l. medullaris medialis corporis striati [NA].

lam′inae medulla′res cerebel′li, SYN laminae albae cerebelli.

lam′inae medulla′res thal′ami [NA], SYN medullary laminae of thalamus.

l. medulla′ris latera′lis cor′poris stria′ti [NA], SYN lateral medullary l. of corpus striatum.

l. medulla′ris media′lis cor′poris stria′ti [NA], SYN medial medullary l. of corpus striatum.

medullary laminae of thalamus, layers of myelinated fibers that appear on transverse sections of the thalamus; the l. medullaris externa marks the ventral and lateral borders of the thalamus and delimits it from the subthalamus and reticular nucleus of thalamus; the l. medullaris interna is interposed between the mediodorsal and ventral nuclei of the thalamus and encloses the intralaminar nuclei (centromedian, paracentral, and central lateral

nuclei). SYN laminae medullares thalami [NA], medullary layers of thalamus.

l. membrana′cea cartilaginis tubae auditivae [NA], SYN membranous l. of cartilaginous auditory tube.

membranous l. of cartilaginous auditory tube, the connective tissue membrane that, with the lateral l., completes the lateral and inferior walls of the cartilaginous part of the auditory tube. SYN l. membranacea cartilaginis tubae auditivae [NA], membranous layer.

l. of mesencephalic tectum, the roofplate of the mesencephalon formed by the quadrigeminal bodies. SYN l. tecti mesencephali [NA], tectum mesencephali [NA], l. quadrigemina, quadrigeminal l., quadrigeminal plate.

l. modi′oli [NA], SYN *plate* of modiolus.

l. muscula′ris muco′sae [NA], SYN *muscularis* mucosae.

nuclear l., a protein-rich layer lining the inner surface of the nuclear membrane in interphase cells.

orbital l. of ethmoid bone, SYN orbital *plate* of ethmoid bone.

l. orbita′lis os′sis ethmoida′lis [NA], SYN orbital *plate* of ethmoid bone.

osseous spiral l., a double plate of bone winding spirally around the modiolus dividing the spiral canal of the cochlea incompletely into two, scala tympani and scala vestibuli; between the two plates of this l. the fibers of the cochlear nerve reach the spiral organ (of Corti). SYN l. spiralis ossea [NA], spiral plate.

l. papyra′cea, SYN orbital *plate* of ethmoid bone.

l. parieta′lis [NA], SYN parietal *layer.*

l. parietalis pericar′dii, SYN parietal *layer* of serous pericardium.

l. parietalis tu′nicae vagina′lis tes′tis, SYN parietal *layer* of tunica vaginalis.

periclaustral l., SYN external *capsule.*

l. perpendicula′ris [NA], SYN perpendicular *plate.*

l. perpendicularis ossis ethmoidalis [NA], SYN perpendicular *plate* of ethmoid bone.

l. perpendicularis ossis palatini [NA], SYN perpendicular *plate* of palatine bone.

l. poste′rior vagi′nae mus′culi rec′ti abdo′minis [NA], SYN posterior *layer* of rectus abdominis sheath.

l. pretrachea′lis [NA], SYN pretracheal *fascia.*

l. prevertebra′lis [NA], SYN prevertebral *fascia.*

primary dental l., SYN dental *ledge.*

l. profun′da [NA], SYN deep *layer.*

l. profunda fas′ciae tempora′lis, SYN deep *layer* of temporalis fascia.

l. profunda mus′culi levato′ris palpe′brae superio′ris, SYN deep *layer* of levator palpebrae superioris muscle.

lamina l., the layer of connective tissue underlying the epithelium of a mucous membrane. SYN l. propria mucosae [NA].

l. pro′pria muco′sae [NA], SYN lamina l.

lamina l. of semicircular duct, the meshwork of connective tissue fibers between the semicircular duct and the bony semicircular canal; it encloses the perilymph in its spaces. SYN membrana propria ductus semicircularis [NA].

pterygoid laminae, SEE lateral pterygoid *plate,* medial pterygoid *plate.*

l. quadrigem′ina, SYN l. of mesencephalic tectum.

quadrigeminal l., SYN l. of mesencephalic tectum.

l. ra′ra, the relatively electron-lucent layer on either side of the l. densa of the basement membrane.

reticular l., a major component of the basement membrane, as seen by light microscopy; it consists largely of reticular fibers and ground substances.

l. of Rexed, a division of the gray matter of the spinal cord into nine laminae (I-IX) and a gray area around the central canal (area X) based on cytoarchitectural features; the dorsal (posterior) horn is composed of laminae I-VI, the intermediate zone of lamina VII, and the ventral horn of laminae VIII and IX; general correlation of laminae with major nuclei: I, posteromarginal nucleus; II, substantia gelatinosa; III, IV, nucleus proprius (posterior); V, VI, nucleus proprius (anterior); VII, Clarke's nucleus, intermediolateral cell column; VIII, commissural nuclei, interneurons; IX, motor nuclei of ventral horn.

la

rostral l., a whitish line appearing on perfectly median sections of the brain as a thin bridge connecting the rostrum of the corpus callosum with the lamina terminalis; the rostral l. contains no commissural fibers; instead, it corresponds to the line along which the pia mater reflects from the medial surface of one hemisphere to that of the other. SYN l. rostralis, rostral layer, teniola corporis callosi.

l. rostra'lis, SYN rostral l.

secondary spiral l., a ridge on the outer wall of the first turn of the cochlea opposite the spiral l. SYN l. spiralis secundaria [NA], secondary spiral plate.

l. sep'ti pellu'cidi [NA], SYN l. of septum pellucidum.

l. of septum pellucidum, one of the two thin layers of the transparent septum, which extend from the corpus callosum to the fornix; often separated from each other by a space, the cavity of septum pellucidum. SYN l. septi pellucidi [NA].

l. spira'lis os'sea [NA], SYN osseous spiral l.

l. spira'lis secunda'ria [NA], SYN secondary spiral l.

substantia l. of cornea, proper substance of cornea, modified transparent connective tissue, between the layers of which are open spaces or lacunae nearly filled with the corneal cells or corpuscles. SYN substantia propria corneae [NA].

superficial l., SYN superficial *layer.*

l. superficia'lis [NA], SYN superficial *layer.*

l. superficialis fas'ciae cervica'lis [NA], SYN investing *layer* of deep cervical fascia.

l. superficialis fas'ciae tempora'lis [NA], SYN superficial *layer* of temporalis fascia.

l. superficialis mus'culi levato'ris pal'pebrae superio'ris [NA], SYN superficial *layer* of the levator palpebrae superioris muscle.

suprachoroid l., a layer of loose, pigmented connective tissue on the outer surface of the choroid, resembling and attached to the l. fusca sclerae. SYN l. suprachoroidea [NA], ectochoroidea, suprachoroid layer, suprachoroidea.

l. suprachoroi'dea [NA], SYN suprachoroid l.

l. supraneuropor'ica, that part of the choroid membrane of the third ventricle that forms the roof of the foramen of Monro.

l. tec'ti mesenceph'ali [NA], SYN l. of mesencephalic tectum.

l. termina'lis cer'ebri [NA], SYN l. terminalis of cerebrum.

l. terminalis of cerebrum, a thin plate passing upward from the optic chiasm and forming the rostral boundary of the third ventricle; membrane closing the rostral neuropore. SYN l. terminalis cerebri [NA], l. cinerea, terminal plate, velum terminale.

l. of thyroid cartilage, one of the paired (dextra et sinistra) thin quadrilateral plates of the thyroid cartilage that are joined anteriorly and form an open angle posteriorly. SYN l. cartilaginis thyroideae [NA].

l. tra'gi [NA], SYN l. of tragus.

l. of tragus, a longitudinal curved plate of cartilage, the beginning of the cartilaginous portion of the external acoustic meatus. SYN l. tragi [NA].

vascular l. of choroid, the outer portion of the choroid of the eye containing the largest blood vessels. SYN l. vasculosa choroideae [NA], Haller's vascular tissue, uvaeformis, vascular layer of choroid coat of eye, vascular l.

l. vasculo'sa choroi'deae [NA], SYN vascular l. of choroid.

l. ventra'lis, SYN basal l. of neural tube.

l. of vertebral arch, the flattened posterior portion of the vertebral arch extending between the pedicles and the midline, forming the dorsal wall of the vertebral foramen, and from the midline junction of which the spinous process extends. SYN l. arcus vertebrae [NA], neurapophysis.

l. viscera'lis [NA], SYN visceral *layer.*

l. visceralis pericar'dii [NA], SYN visceral *layer* of serous pericardium.

l. visceralis tu'nicae vagina'lis tes'tis [NA], SYN visceral *layer* of tunica vaginalis of testis.

l. vit'rea, SYN l. basalis choroideae.

lam·i·na·gram (lam'i-nă-gram). An image made by laminagraphy.

lam·i·na·graph (lam'i-nă-graf). A device for laminagraphy; a laminagram.

lam·i·nag·ra·phy, lami·nog·ra·phy (lam'i-nahg'ră-fē, lam'i-nog-ră-fē). Radiographic technique in which the images of tissues above and below the plane of interest are blurred out by movement of the x-ray tube and film holder, to show a specific area more clearly. SEE ALSO tomography. [lamina + G. *graphē,* a writing]

lam·i·nar (lam'i-nar). **1.** Arranged in plates or laminae. SYN laminated. **2.** Relating to any lamina.

lam·i·nar·ia (lam-i-nā're-ă). Sterile rod made of kelp (genus *Laminaria*) which is hydrophilic, and, when placed in the cervical canal, absorbs moisture, swells, and gradually dilates the cervix. [L. *lamina,* a blade]

lam·i·nar·in (lam-i-nar'in). An algal polysaccharide, made up chiefly of β-D-glucose residues, obtained from *Laminaria* species (family Laminariaceae); variable proportions of the glucose chains contain at the potential reducing end a molecule of mannitol that can be sulfated.

l. sulfate, l. sulfated to varying degrees; two sulfate groups per glucose unit results in maximum stability and anticoagulant activity similar to that of heparin; l. with fewer sulfate groups has only antilipemic activity.

lam·i·nat·ed (lam'i-nāt-ed). SYN laminar (1).

lam·i·na·tion (lam-i-nā'shŭn). **1.** An arrangement in the form of plates or laminae. **2.** Embryotomy by removing the fetal head in slices.

lam·i·nec·to·my (lam-i-nek'tō-mē). Excision of a vertebral lamina; commonly used to denote removal of the posterior arch. SYN rachitomy, spondylotomy. [L. *lamina,* layer, + G. *ektomē,* excision]

lam·i·nin (lam'i-nin). A large multimeric glycoprotein component of the basement membrane; particularly its unstained laminae; a major protein component of the laminae of the renal glomerulus.

lam·i·ni·tis (lam-i-nī'tis). **1.** Inflammation of any lamina. **2.** A painful inflammation of the sensitive lamina to which the hoof of the horse is attached. SYN founder (2).

lami·nog·ra·phy (lam'i-nog-ră-fē). SEE laminagraphy.

lam·i·not·o·my (lam'i-not'ō-mē). An operation on one or more vertebral laminae. SYN rachiotomy. [L. *lamina,* layer, + G. *tomē,* incision]

lam·ins (lam'inz). Fibrous network associated with the inner membranes of cell nuclei, composed of polypeptides of varying molecular weights (60,000–80,000) and classified as A, B, C, etc. on the basis of physical properties; the phosphorylation of l. is associated with mitosis.

lam·o·tri·gine (lă-mō'trī-jēn). New structural class of antiepileptics; an anticonvulsant which appears in preclinical studies to resemble phenytoin.

lamp. Illuminating device; source of light. SEE ALSO light.

annealing l., an alcohol l. with a soot-free flame used in dentistry to drive off the protective NH_3 gas coating from the surface of cohesive gold foil.

Edridge-Green l., a lantern used to test recognition of colored signals; it displays a single light with color filters in rotating disks that can be modified to simulate conditions of weather and atmosphere. This test for color blindness was officially adopted in Great Britain in 1915 in place of the Holmgren wool test, but is now seldom used.

heat l., a l. that emits infrared light and produces heat; used to apply topical heat to the skin. SYN thermolamp.

Kromayer's l., a U-shaped quartz l. of mercury vapor, giving out actinic rays; used in the treatment of skin diseases.

mercury vapor l., a l. in which the electric arc is in an ionized mercury vapor atmosphere; it produces ultraviolet light that can be used therapeutically or in diagnostic photometry.

mignon l., a minute electric light used in various endoscopic instruments.

slit l., a combination of a microscope and a narrow beam of collimated light, used to examine the eye.

spirit l., a l., used mainly for heating in laboratory work, in which alcohol is burned.

tungsten arc l., a l. having highly compressed tungsten elements.

ultraviolet l., a l. that emits rays in the ultraviolet band of the spectrum. SEE ALSO ultraviolet.

uviol l., an electric l. with uviol glass, furnishing especially violet rays; used in phototherapy.

Wood's l., an ultraviolet l. with a nickel oxide filter that only passes light with a maximal wavelength of about 3660 Å; used to detect by fluorescence hairs infected with species *M. audouinii,* *M. canis,* var. *distortum,* or *M. ferrugineum,* producing greenish-yellow fluorescence.

Lamy, Maurice, French physician, 1895–1975. SEE Maroteaux-L. *syndrome.*

la·na, gen. and pl. **la·nae** (lan'ă, lan'ē). SYN wool. [L.]

la·nat·o·side D (lă-nat'ō-sīd). A digitales glycoside from the leaves of *Digitalis lanata,* yielding the genin diginatigenin (12-hydroxygitoxigenin; 16-hydroxydigoxigenin).

la·nat·o·sides A, B, and C (lă-nat'ō-sīdz). Digilanides A, B, and C; the cardioactive precursor glycosides obtained from *Digitalis lanata.* Removal of the acetyl group yields desacetyllanatosides A, B, and C (purpurea glycosides A, B, and C, respectively); removal of the glucose from lanatosides A, B, and C yields acetyldigitoxin, acetylgitoxin, and acetyldigoxin, respectively; removal of glucose and the acetyl group yields digitoxin, gitoxin, and digoxin, respectively. SEE ALSO purpurea glycosides A.

lance (lans). **1.** To incise a part, as an abscess or boil. **2.** A lancet. [L. *lancea,* a slender spear]

Lancefield, Rebecca Craighill, U.S. bacteriologist, *1895. SEE L. *classification.*

lan·cet (lan'set). A surgical knife with a short, wide, sharp-pointed, two-edged blade. [Fr. *lancette*]

gum l., a l. used for incising the gum over the crown of an erupting tooth.

spring l., a l. with a handle containing a blade that is activated by a spring.

thumb l., a l. with short flat blade which folds back, when closed, between two plates of the handle.

lan·ci·nat·ing (lan'si-nāt'ing). Denoting a sharp cutting or tearing pain. [L. *lancino,* pp. *-atus,* to tear]

Lancisi, Giovanni M., Italian physician, 1654–1720. SEE L.'s *sign;* striae lancisi, under *stria.*

Landau-Kleffner syn·drome. See under syndrome.

Landolfi's sign. See under sign.

Landolt, Edmund, French ophthalmologist, 1846–1926. SEE L.'s *bodies,* under *body.*

Landouzy, Louis T.J., French neurologist, 1845–1917. SEE L.-Dejerine *dystrophy;* L.-Grasset *law.*

Landry, Jean B.O., French physician, 1826–1865. SEE L.'s *paralysis;* L. *syndrome;* L.-Guillain-Barré *syndrome.*

Landschutz tu·mor. See under tumor.

Landsteiner, Karl, Austrian-U.S. pathologist and Nobel laureate, 1868–1943. SEE L.-Donath *test;* Donath-L. cold *autoantibody, phenomenon.*

Landström, John, Swedish surgeon, 1869–1910. SEE L.'s *muscle.*

Landzert, T., 19th century German anatomist. SEE L.'s *fossa;* Gruber-L. *fossa.*

Lane, Sir W. Arbuthnot, English surgeon, 1856–1943. SEE L.'s *band, disease, plates,* under *plate.*

Lang, Basil T., English ophthalmologist, 1880–1928.

Lange, Carl F.A., German biochemist, *1883. SEE L.'s *solution, test.*

Lange, Carl G., Danish psychologist, 1834–1900. SEE James-L. *theory.*

Lange, Cornelia de. See under de Lange.

Langenbeck, Bernhard R.K. von, German surgeon, 1810–1887. SEE L.'s *triangle.*

Langendorff, Oscar, German physiologist, 1853–1908. SEE L.'s *method.*

Lange-Nielsen, F., 20th century Norwegian cardiologist. SEE Jervell and Lange-Nielsen *syndrome.*

Langer, Carl (Ritter von Edenberg), Austrian anatomist, 1819–1887. SEE L.'s *arch, lines,* under *line, muscle.*

Langerhans, Paul, German anatomist, 1847–1888. SEE L.'s *cells,* under *cell, granule, islands,* under *island; islets* of L., under *islet.*

Langhans, Theodor, German pathologist, 1839–1915. SEE L.'s *cells,* under *cell;* L.'s-type giant *cells,* under *cell;* L.'s *layer, stria.*

Langley, John N., English physiologist, 1852–1925. SEE L.'s *granules,* under *granule.*

Langmuir, Irving, U.S. chemist and Nobel laureate, 1881–1957. SEE L. *trough.*

lan·guage (lang'gwij). Any means or form, vocal or other, of expression or communication. [L. *lingua*]

body l., (1) the expression of thoughts and feelings by means of nonverbal bodily movements, *e.g.,* gestures, or via the symptoms of hysterical conversion; SEE kinesics. **(2)** communication by means of bodily signs.

lan·i·ary (lan'i-ār-ē). Adapted for tearing; in anatomy, sometimes applied to canine teeth, as l. teeth. [L. *laniarius,* to tear to pieces]

lan·ka·my·cin (lān'kă-mī-sin). Macrolide antibiotic produced by *Streptomyces violaceoniger* from the soil of Ceylon.

Lannelongue, Odilon M., French surgeon and pathologist, 1840–1911. SEE L.'s *foramina,* under *foramen, ligaments,* under *ligament.*

lan·o·lin (lan'ō-lin). SYN adeps lanae. SYN wool fat. [L. *lana,* wool, + *oleum,* oil]

anhydrous l., l. that contains not more than 0.25% of water; used as a water-adsorbable ointment base.

la·nos·ter·ol (lan-ō'stēr-ol). 5α-Lanosta-8(9),24-dien-3β-ol; a zoosterol synthesized from squalene and a precursor to cholesterol.

Lanterman, A.J., 19th century U.S. anatomist in Strasbourg. SEE L.'s *incisures,* under *incisure, segments,* under *segment;* Schmidt-L. *clefts,* under *cleft, incisures,* under *incisure.*

lan·tha·nic (lan'thă-nik). Rarely used term denoting a disease process that produces no symptoms or clinical evidence of illness. [G. *lanthanō,* to lie hidden]

lan·tha·nides (lan'thă-nīdz). Those elements with atomic numbers 57–71 which closely resemble one another chemically and were once difficult to separate from one another. SYN rare earth elements. [*lanthanum,* first element of the series]

lan·tha·num (La) (lan'thă-nŭm). A metallic element, atomic no. 57, atomic wt. 138.9055; first of the rare earth elements (lanthanides). [G. *lanthanein,* to lie hidden]

l. nitrate, La(NO$_3$)$_3$; used in electron microscopy as a stain for extracellular mucopolysaccharides.

lan·thi·o·nine (lan-thī'ō-nēn). S(CH$_2$–CH(NH$_3$)$^+$–COO$^-$)$_2$; 3,3'-thiodialanine; an amino acid obtained from wood which resembles cystine but has only one sulfur atom in the molecule rather than two; *i.e.,* a sulfide rather than a disulfide.

la·nu·gi·nous (lă-nū'ji-nŭs). Covered with lanugo.

la·nu·go (lă-nū'gō) [NA]. Fine, soft, lightly pigmented fetal hair with minute shafts and large papillae; it appears toward the end of the third month of gestation. SYN lanugo hair. [L. down, wooliness, from *lana,* wool]

Lanz, Otto, Swiss surgeon in Amsterdam, 1865–1935. SEE L.'s *line.*

LAO Abbreviation for left anterior oblique projection, used in chest radiography, especially to assess the size of the left atrium and ventricle.

LAP Abbreviation for leukocyte alkaline phosphatase. SEE alkaline *phosphatase.*

lap·a·rec·to·my (lap'ă-rek'tō-mē). Excision of strips or gores from the abdominal wall and suture of the edges of the wounds,

la

in cases of abnormal laxity of the abdominal muscles. [laparo- + G. *ektomē,* excision]

△**laparo-.** The loins (less properly, the abdomen in general). [G. *lapara,* flank, loins]

lap·a·ro·cele (lap′ă-rō-sēl). SYN abdominal *hernia.* [laparo- + G. *kēlē,* hernia]

lap·a·ro·gas·tros·co·py (lap′ă-rō-gas-tros′kŏ-pē). Inspection of interior of the stomach after a gastrotomy. [laparo- + G. *gastēr,* stomach, + *skopeō,* to view]

lap·a·ro·hys·ter·ec·to·my (lap′ă-rō-his-ter-ek′tō-mē). SYN abdominal *hysterectomy.*

lap·a·ro·hys·tero-o·o·pho·rec·to·my (lap′ă-rō-his′ter-ō-ō-of′ō-rek′tō-mē). Removal of the uterus and ovaries through an incision in the abdominal wall. [laparo- + G. *hystera,* uterus, + oophorectomy]

lap·a·ro·hys·ter·o·pexy (lap′ă-rō-his′ter-ō-pek-sē). SYN abdominal *hysteropexy.* [laparo- + G. *hystera,* uterus, + *pēxis,* fixation]

lap·a·ro·hys·ter·o·sal·pin·go-o·o·pho·rec·to·my (lap′ă-rō-his′ter-ō-sal′pin-gō-ō′of-ōr-ek′tō-mē). Removal of uterus and adnexa (tubes and ovaries) through an abdominal incision.

lap·a·ro·hys·ter·ot·o·my (lap′ă-rō-his-te-rot′ō-mē). SYN abdominal *hysterotomy.* [laparo- + G. *hystera,* uterus, + *tomē,* incision]

lap·a·ro·my·o·mec·to·my (lap′ă-rō-mī-ō-mek′tō-mē). SYN abdominal *myomectomy.*

lap·a·ro·my·o·si·tis (lap′ă-rō-mī′ō-sī′tis). Inflammation of the lateral abdominal muscles. [laparo- + G. *mys,* muscle, + *-itis,* inflammation]

lap·a·ror·rha·phy (lap′ă-rōr′ă-fē). SYN celiorrhaphy.

lap·a·ro·sal·pin·gec·to·my (lap′ă-rō-sal-pin-jek′tō-mē). SYN abdominal *salpingectomy.*

lap·a·ro·sal·pin·go-o·o·pho·rec·to·my (lap′ă-rō-sal′ping-gō-ō-of′ō-rek′tō-mē). Removal of the fallopian tube and ovary through an abdominal incision. SYN abdominal salpingo-oophorectomy.

lap·a·ro·sal·pin·got·o·my (lap′ă-rō-sal-ping-got′ō-mē). SYN abdominal *salpingotomy.*

lap·a·ro·scope (lap′ă-rō-skōp). An endoscope for examining the peritoneal cavity. SYN peritoneoscope. [laparo- + G. *skopeō,* to view]

lap·a·ros·co·py (lap-ă-ros′kŏ-pē). Examination of the contents of the peritoneum with a laparoscope passed through the abdominal wall. SEE peritoneoscopy.

The laparoscope is a type of endoscope, the earliest of which, dating from 150 years ago, was a crude tube down which lamplight was reflected. With the advent of fiberoptics in the 1960s and of high-intensity, low-heat, halogen bulbs in the 1970s, endoscopy became clinically practical. Typically, in laparoscopy, the abdomen is first inflated with carbon dioxide, and the laparoscope passed through a small incision in the abdominal wall. The device is frequently used to view the female reproductive organs, in particular where endometriosis or pelvic inflammatory disease is thought to be present, or infertility is suspected because of obstruction of the fallopian tubes by scarring (adhesions). Fitted with grasping and cutting tools, the laparoscope can perform minor surgery, take tissue samples for biopsy, and remove eggs from the ovaries (as in gamete intrafallopian transfer). Often done on an ambulatory basis, laparoscopy is among the new techniques that have revolutionized modern surgery.

closed l., l. performed after insufflation of the abdominal cavity using a percutaneously placed needle.

open l., l. performed after insufflation of the abdomen using a trocar placed under direct vision after making a small celiotomy incision.

lap·a·rot·o·my (lap′ă-rot′ō-mē). **1.** Incision into the loin. **2.** SYN celiotomy. [laparo- + G. *tomē,* incision]

lap·a·ro·trach·e·lot·o·my (lap′ă-rō-trak-ĕ-lot′ō-mē). A low cervical cesarean section. [laparo- + G. *trachēlos,* neck, + *tomē,* incision]

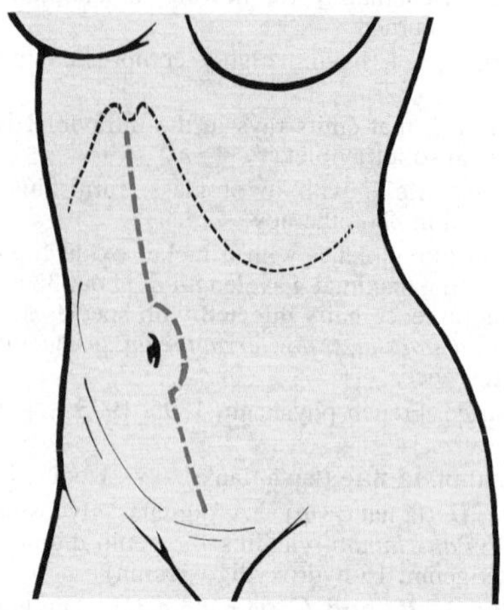

laparotomy (typical abdominal incision)

lap·a·ro·u·ter·ot·o·my (lap′ă-rō-yū-ter-ot′ō-mē). SYN abdominal *hysterotomy.* [laparo- + uterus + G. *tomē,* incision]

Lapicque, Louis, French physiologist, 1866–1952. SEE L.'s *law.*

lap·i·ni·za·tion (lap′i-ni-zā′shŭn). Serial passage of a virus or vaccine in rabbits. [Fr. *lapin,* rabbit]

lap·i·nized (lap′i-nīzd). Denoting viruses which have been adapted to develop in rabbits by serial transfers in this species. [Fr. *lapin,* rabbit]

Laplace, Ernest, U.S. surgeon, 1861–1924. SEE L.'s *forceps.*

Laplace, Pierre S. de, French mathematician, 1749–1827. SEE L.'s *law.*

Laquer, Ernst, German physiologist, *1910. SEE L.'s *stain* for alcoholic hyalin.

lar·bish. A form of creeping eruption observed in Senegal.

lard. SYN adeps (2). [L. *lardum*]

benzoinated l., used as a lubricant, in the manufacture of soap, for oiling wool, and as an illuminant. Formerly used as an ointment base.

lark·spur (lark′sper). SYN *Delphinium ajacis.*

Laron, Zvi, Israeli pediatric endocrinologist, *1927. SEE L. type *dwarfism.*

Laroyenne, Lucien, French surgeon, 1831–1902. SEE L.'s *operation.*

Larrey, Baron Dominique Jean de, French surgeon, 1766–1842. SEE L.'s *amputation, cleft;* L.-Weil *disease.*

Larsen, Loren J., U.S. orthopedic surgeon, *1914. SEE L.'s *syndrome.*

Larsson, Tage Konrad Leopold, Swedish scientist, *1905. SEE Sjögren-L. *syndrome.*

lar·va, pl. **lar·vae** (lar′vă, lar′vē). **1.** The wormlike developmental stage or stages of an insect or helminth that are markedly different from the adult and undergo subsequent metamorphosis; a grub, maggot, or caterpillar. **2.** The second stage in the life cycle of a tick; the stage which hatches from the egg and, following engorgement, molts in the nymph. **3.** The young of fishes or amphibians which often differ in appearance from the adult. [L. a mask]

filariform l., infective third-stage l. of the hookworm, *Ascaris,* and other nematodes with penetrating larvae or with larvae that migrate through the body to reach the intestine.

rhabditiform l., early developmental larval stages (first and second) of soil-borne nematodes such as *Necator, Ancylostoma,* and *Strongyloides,* which precede the infectious third-stage filariform l.

lar·va·ceous (lar-vā′shŭs). SYN larvate.

lar·va cur·rens (lar′vă kŭr′enz). Cutaneous larva migrans caused by rapidly moving larvae of *Strongyloides stercoralis* (up to 10 cm/hr), typically extending from the anal area down the upper thighs and observed as a rapidly progressing linear urticarial trail; may also be caused by zoonotic species of *Strongyloides*. [L. *larva*, mask + *currens*, racing]

lar·val (lar′văl). 1. Relating to larvae. 2. SYN larvate.

lar·va mi·grans (lar′vă mī′granz). A larval worm, typically a nematode, that wanders for a period in the host tissues but does not develop to the adult stage; this usually occurs in abnormal hosts that inhibit normal development of the parasite. [L. *larva*, mask, + *migro*, to transfer, migrate]

  cutaneous l. m., an advancing serpiginous or netlike tunneling in the skin, with marked pruritus, caused by wandering hookworm larvae not adapted to intestinal maturation in man; especially common in the eastern and southern coastal U.S. and other tropical and subtropical coastal areas; various hookworms of dogs and cats have been implicated, chiefly *Ancylostoma braziliense* in the U.S., but also *Ancylostoma caninum* of dogs, *Uncinaria stenocephala*, the European dog hookworm, and *Bunostomum phlebotomum*, the cattle hookworm; *Strongyloides* species of animal origin may also contribute to human cutaneous l. m. SYN creeping eruption.

  ocular l. m., visceral l. m. involving the eyes, primarily of older children; clinical symptoms include decreased visual acuity and strabismus.

  spiruroid l. m., extraintestinal migration by nematode larvae of the order Spiruroidea, not adapted to maturation in the human intestine; caused chiefly by species of *Gnathostoma spinigerum* and *G. hispidum* in Japan and Thailand, following ingestion of uncooked fish infected with encapsulated third-stage infective larvae, and possibly by ingestion of infected copepods (the first intermediate host) in contaminated drinking water; the anteriorly spined larvae produce serpiginous tunnels in the skin or may cause subcutaneous or pulmonary abscess, or may invade the eye or brain.

  visceral l. m., a disease, chiefly of children, caused by ingestion of infective ova of *Toxocara canis*, less commonly by other ascarid nematodes not adapted to humans, whose larvae hatch in the intestine, penetrate the gut wall, and wander in the viscera (chiefly the liver) for periods of up to 18 or 24 months; may be asymptomatic or may be marked by hepatomegaly (with granulomatous lesions caused by encapsulated larvae in the enlarged liver), pulmonary infiltration, fever, cough, hyperglobulinemia, and sustained high eosinophilia.

lar·vate (lar′vāt). Masked or concealed; applied to a disease with undeveloped, absent, or atypical symptoms. SYN larvaceous, larval (2). [L. *larva*, mask]

lar·vi·cid·al (lar-vi-sī′dăl). Destructive to larvae.

lar·vi·cide (lar′vi-sīd). An agent that kills larvae. [larva + L. *caedo*, to kill]

lar·vip·a·rous (lar-vip′ă-rŭs). Larvae-bearing; denoting passage of larvae, rather than eggs, from the body of the female, as in certain nematodes and insects. [larva + L. *pario*, to bear]

lar·vi·phag·ic (lar′vi-fā′jik). Consuming larvae; certain l. fish are used in mosquito control. [larva + G. *phagō*, to eat]

△**laryng-.** SEE laryngo-.

la·ryn·ge·al (lă-rin′jē-ăl). Relating in any way to the larynx.

la·ryn·gec·to·my (lar′in-jek′tō-mē). Excision of the larynx. [laryngo- + G. *ektomē*, excision]

la·ryn·ges (lă-rin′jēz). Plural of larynx. [L.]

lar·yn·gis·mus (lar-in-jiz′mŭs). A spasmodic narrowing or closure of the rima glottidis. [L. fr. G. *larynx*, + -*ismos*, -ism]

  l. strid′ulus, a spasmodic closure of the glottis, lasting a few seconds, followed by a noisy inspiration. Cf. *laryngitis* stridulosa. SYN pseudocroup, spasmus glottidis.

lar·yn·git·ic (lar-in-jit′ik). Relating to or caused by laryngitis.

lar·yn·gi·tis (lar-in-jī′tis). Inflammation of the mucous membrane of the larynx. [laryngo- + G. -*itis*, inflammation]

  chronic subglottic l., SYN *chorditis* vocalis inferior.

  croupous l., inflammation of the subglottic larynx associated with respiratory infection and croupy or noisy breathing.

  membranous l., a form in which there is a pseudomembranous exudate on the vocal cords.

  spasmodic l., SYN l. stridulosa.

  l. stridulo′sa, catarrhal inflammation of the larynx in children, accompanied by night attacks of spasmodic closure of the glottis, causing inspiratory stridor. SYN spasmodic l.

△**laryngo-, laryng-.** The larynx. [G. *larynx*]

la·ryn·go·cele (lă-ring′gō-sēl). An air sac communicating with the larynx through the ventricle, often bulging outward into the tissue of the neck, especially during coughing. [laryngo- + G. *kēlē*, hernia]

la·ryn·go·fis·sure (lă-ring′gō-fish′er). Operative opening into the larynx, generally through the midline, commonly done for the excision of early carcinoma or the correction of laryngostenosis. SYN median laryngotomy, thyrofissure, thyroidotomy, thyrotomy (2).

la·ryn·go·graph (lă-ring′gō-graf). An instrument for making a tracing of the movements of the vocal folds. [laryngo- + G. *graphō*, to write]

la·ryn·gog·ra·phy (lă-ring-og′-ră-fē). Radiography of the larynx after coating mucosal surfaces with contrast material.

lar·yn·gol·o·gy (lar′ing-gol′ō-jē). The branch of medical science concerned with the larynx; the specialty of diseases of the larynx. [laryngo- + G. *logos*, study]

la·ryn·go·ma·la·cia (lă-ring′gō-mă-lā′shē-ă). SYN *chondromalacia* of larynx. [laryngo- + G. *malakia*, a softness]

la·ryn·go·pa·ral·y·sis (lă-ring′gō-pă-ral′i-sis). Paralysis of the laryngeal muscles. SYN laryngoplegia.

la·ryn·go·pha·ryn·ge·al (lă-ring′gō-fă-rin′jē-ăl). Relating to both larynx and pharynx or to the laryngopharynx.

la·ryn·go·phar·yn·gec·to·my (lă-ring′gō-far′in-jek′tō-mē). Resection or excision of both larynx and pharynx.

la·ryn·go·pha·ryn·ge·us (lă-ring′gō-făr′in-jē′ŭs). SYN inferior constrictor *muscle* of pharynx. [L.]

la·ryn·go·phar·yn·gi·tis (lă-ring′gō-far-in-jī′tis). Inflammation of the larynx and pharynx.

la·ryn·go·phar·ynx (lă-ring′gō-far-ingks). The part of the pharynx lying below the aperture of the larynx and behind the larynx; it extends from the vestibule of the larynx to the esophagus at the level of the inferior border of the cricoid cartilage. SYN pars laryngea pharyngis [NA], hypopharynx, laryngeal part of pharynx, laryngeal pharynx.

la·ryn·go·phthi·sis (lă-ring′gō-thī′sis). Tuberculosis of the larynx. [laryngo- + G. *phthisis*, a wasting]

la·ryn·go·plas·ty (lă-ring′gō-plas-tē). Reparative or plastic surgery of the larynx. [laryngo- + G. *plassō*, to form]

la·ryn·go·ple·gia (lă-ring′gō-plē′jē-ă). SYN laryngoparalysis. [laryngo- + G. *plēgē*, stroke]

la·ryn·go·pto·sis (lă-ring-gō-tō′sis). An abnormally low position of the larynx at birth, which may be congenital or acquired; does not impair the health of the neonate. Some degree of l. occurs with aging. [laryngo- + G. *ptōsis*, a falling]

la·ryn·go·scope (lă-ring′gō-skōp). Any of several types of hollow tubes, equipped with electrical lighting, used in examining or operating upon the interior of the larynx through the mouth. [laryngo- + G. *skopeō*, to inspect]

la·ryn·go·scop·ic (lă-ring′gō-skop′ik). Relating to laryngoscopy.

lar·yn·gos·co·pist (lar′ing-gos′kŏ-pist). A person skilled in the use of the laryngoscope.

lar·yn·gos·co·py (lar′ing-gos′kŏ-pē). Inspection of the larynx by means of the laryngoscope.

  direct l., inspection of the larynx by means of either a rigid, hollow instrument or a fiberoptic cable.

  indirect l., inspection of the larynx by means of a reflected image on a mirror.

  suspension l., support of the laryngoscope by leverage from the anterior chest wall or other supportive structure to provide maximum exposure of the pharyngeal cavity and larynx.

la·ryn·go·spasm (lă-ring′gō-spazm). Spasmodic closure of the glottic aperture. SYN glottidospasm, laryngospastic reflex.

la

la·ryn·go·ste·no·sis (lă-ring′gō-stĕ-nō′sis). Stricture or narrowing of the lumen of the larynx. [laryngo- + G. *stenōsis*, a narrowing]

lar·yn·gos·to·my (lar′ing-gos′tō-me). The establishment of a permanent opening from the neck into the larynx. [laryngo- + G. *stoma*, mouth]

la·ryn·go·stro·bo·scope (lă-ring′gō-strō′bō-skōp, -strob′ō-skōp). Stroboscopic apparatus for observing the motion of the vocal folds during phonation.

lar·yn·got·o·my (lar-ing-got′ō-me). A surgical incision of the larynx. [laryngo- + G. *tomē*, incision]

inferior l., SYN cricothyrotomy.

median l., SYN laryngofissure.

superior l., incision through the thyrohyoid membrane.

la·ryn·go·tra·che·al (lă-ring′gō-trā′ke-ăl). Relating to both larynx and trachea.

la·ryn·go·tra·che·i·tis (lă-ring′gō-trā-ke-ī′tis). Inflammation of both larynx and trachea.

avian infectious l., a severe, specific, infectious disease of chickens and other birds, caused by avian herpesvirus 1; manifested by severe hemorrhagic inflammation of the trachea and upper air passages.

la·ryn·go·tra·che·o·bron·chi·tis (lă-ring′gō-trā′ke-ō-brong-kī′tis). An acute respiratory infection involving the larynx, trachea, and bronchi. SEE croup.

lar·ynx, pl. **la·ryn·ges** (lar′ingks, lă-rin′jēz) [NA]. The organ of voice production; the part of the respiratory tract between the pharynx and the trachea; it consists of a framework of cartilages and elastic membranes housing the vocal folds and the muscles which control the position and tension of these elements. [Mod. L. fr. G.]

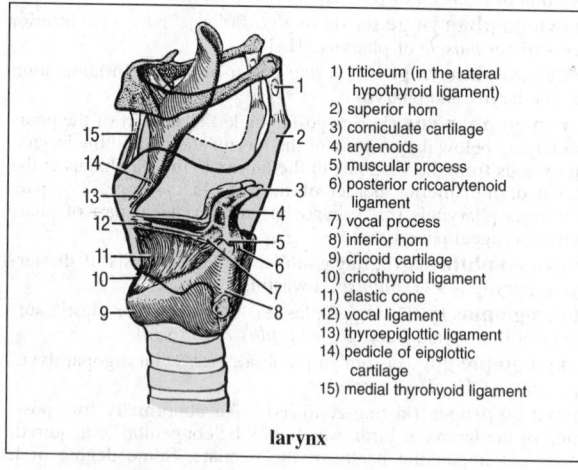

1) triticeum (in the lateral hypothyroid ligament)
2) superior horn
3) corniculate cartilage
4) arytenoids
5) muscular process
6) posterior cricoarytenoid ligament
7) vocal process
8) inferior horn
9) cricoid cartilage
10) cricothyroid ligament
11) elastic cone
12) vocal ligament
13) thyroepiglottic ligament
14) pedicle of eipglottic cartilage
15) medial thyrohyoid ligament

larynx

lase (lāz). To cut, divide, or dissolve a substance, or to treat an anatomical structure, with a laser beam.

Lasègue, Ernest C., French physician, 1816–1883. SEE L.'s *disease, sign, syndrome.*

la·ser (lā′zer). **1.** (noun) A device that concentrates high energies into an intense narrow beam of nondivergent monochromatic electromagnetic radiation; used in microsurgery, cauterization, and for a variety of diagnostic purposes. L.'s using ruby, argon, krypton, neodymium, helium-neon, or carbon dioxide are available. L.'s are widely used in printers of text or x-ray images. **2.** (verb) To treat a structure with a laser beam. [acronym coined from *l*ight *a*mplification by *s*timulated *e*mission of *r*adiation]

pulsed dye l., extremely short bursts of focused yellow light absorbed by hemoglobin, used to treat hemangiomas without anesthesia in young children.

la·ser·ing (lā′zing). The use of a laser beam to cut, divide, or dissolve a substance, or to treat an anatomical structure.

Lash, Abraham Fae, U.S. obstetrician-gynecologist, *1898. SEE L.'s *operation.*

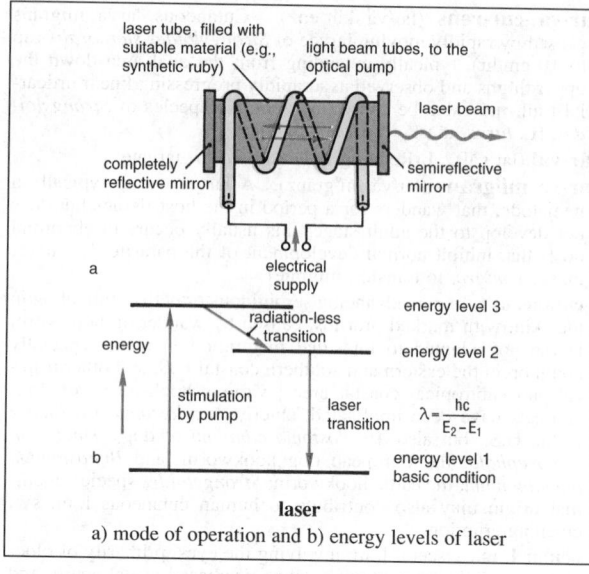

laser tube, filled with suitable material (e.g., synthetic ruby)

light beam tubes, to the optical pump

laser beam

completely reflective mirror

semireflective mirror

electrical supply

a

energy

radiation-less transition

energy level 3

energy level 2

stimulation by pump

laser transition

$\lambda = \dfrac{hc}{E_2 - E_1}$

energy level 1 basic condition

b

laser

a) mode of operation and b) energy levels of laser

lash. An eyelash.

La·si·o·he·lea (las′ē-ō-hē′le-ă). A genus of small bloodsucking gnats.

las·si·tude (las′i-tūd). A sense of weariness. [L. *lassitudo,* fr. *lassus,* weary]

la·tah (lah′tah). One of the pathological startle syndromes. A culture bound disorder characterized by an exaggerated physical response to being startled or to unexpected suggestion, the subjects involuntarily uttering cries or executing movements in response to command or in imitation of what they hear or see in others. SEE ALSO jumping *disease.* [Malay, ticklish]

Latarget, André, French anatomist, 1877–1947. SEE L.'s *nerve, vein.*

lat·e·bra (lat′ē-bră). A flask-shaped region in large-yolked eggs extending from the animal pole to a dilated terminal portion near the center of the yolk; it contains the main bulk of the white yolk. [L. hiding place]

la·ten·cy (lā′ten-sē). **1.** The state of being latent. **2.** In conditioning, or other behavioral experiments, the period of apparent inactivity between the time the stimulus is presented and the moment a response occurs. **3.** In psychoanalysis, the period of time from approximately age five to puberty.

la·tent (lā′tent). Not manifest, dormant, but potentially discernible. [L. *lateo,* pres. p. *latens* (-*ent*-), to lie hidden]

lat·er·ad (lat′er-ad). Toward the side. [L. *latus,* side, + *ad,* to]

lat·er·al (lat′er-ăl). **1.** On the side. SYN lateralis [NA]. **2.** Farther from the median or midsagittal plane. SYN lateralis [NA]. **3.** In dentistry, a position either right or left of the midsagittal plane. **4.** A radiographic projection made with the film in the sagittal plane; especially, the second view of a chest series. SYN lateralis [NA]. [L. *lateralis,* lateral, fr. *latus,* side]

la·te·ra·lis (lat-er-ā′lis) [NA]. SYN lateral (1), lateral (2), lateral. [L.]

lat·er·al·i·ty (lat-er-al′i-tē). Referring to a side of the body or of a structure; specifically, the dominance of one side of the brain or the body.

crossed l., right dominance of some members, *e.g.,* arm or leg, and left dominance of other members.

lat·er·al·i·za·tion (lat′er-al-ī-zā′shŭn). The process whereby certain embryological asymmetries of structure (such as the right-side location of the liver and the structure of the great vessels) and function (handedness) are ordained phylogenetically, coded genetically, and realized ontogenetically.

lat·er·i·flex·ion, lat·er·i·flec·tion (lat-er-i-flek′shŭn). SYN lateroflexion.

△**latero-.** Lateral, to one side. [L. *lateralis,* lateral, fr. *latus,* side]

lat·er·o·ab·dom·i·nal (lat′er-ō-ab-dom′i-năl). Relating to the sides of the abdomen, to the loins or flanks.

lat·er·o·de·vi·a·tion (lat′er-ō-dē-vē-ā′shŭn). A bending or a displacement to one side. [latero- + L. *devio,* to turn aside, fr. *via,* a way]

lat·er·o·duc·tion (lat′er-ō-dŭk′shŭn). A drawing to one side; denoting a movement of a limb or turning of the eyeball away form the midline. SYN exduction. [latero- + L. *duco,* pp. *ductus,* to lead]

lat·er·o·flex·ion, lat·er·o·flec·tion (lat′er-ō-flek′shŭn). A bending or curvature to one side. SYN lateriflexion, lateriflection. [latero- + L. *flecto,* pp. *flexus,* to bend]

lat·er·o·po·si·tion (lat′er-ō-pō-zish′ŭn). A shift to one side.

lat·er·o·pul·sion (lat′er-ō-pŭl′shŭn). An involuntary sidewise movement occurring in certain nervous affections. [latero- + L. *pello,* pp. *pulsus,* to push, drive]

lat·er·o·tor·sion (lat′er-ō-tōr′shŭn). A twisting to one side; denoting rotation of the eyeball around its anteroposterior axis, so that the top part of the cornea turns away from the sagittal plane. [latero- + L. *torsio,* a twisting]

lat·er·o·tru·sion (lat′er-ō-trū′zhŭn). The outward thrust given by the muscles of mastication to the rotating mandibular condyle during movement of the mandible. [latero- + L. *trudo,* pp. *trusus,* to thrust]

lat·er·o·ver·sion (lat′er-ō-ver′shŭn). Version to one side or the other, denoting especially a malposition of the uterus. [latero- + L. *verto,* pp. *versus,* to turn]

la·tex (lā′teks). **1.** An emulsion or suspension produced by some seed plants; it contains suspended microscopic globules of natural rubber. **2.** Similar synthetic materials such as polystyrene, polyvinyl chloride, etc. [L. liquid]

lathe (lādh). A motor-driven machine with a rotating shaft that can be fitted with various types of cutting instruments, grinding stones and polishing wheels; used in finishing and polishing dental appliances.

lath·y·rism (lath′i-rizm). **1.** A disease occurring in Ethiopia, Algeria, and India, characterized by various nervous manifestations, tremors, spastic paraplegia, and paresthesias; prevalent in districts where vetches, khasari (*Lathyrus sativus*), and allied species form the main food. **2.** Poisoning of horses from eating certain varieties of peas, particularly *L. sativus,* a plant introduced into Europe from India; manifested by paralytic symptoms. SEE ALSO githagism. **3.** Experimentally, a form of bone disease induced in laboratory animals by feeding *L. sativus* peas, or a principle derived from them, especially β-aminoproprionitrile. SYN lupinosis. [L. *lathyrus,* vetch]

lath·y·ro·gen (lath′i-rō-jen). An agent or drug, occurring naturally or used experimentally, that induces lathyrism.

La·tin square. A statistical design for experiments that removes from experimental error the variation from two sources that may be identified with the rows and columns of a square. The allocation of experimental treatments is such that each treatment occurs exactly once in each row and column. For example, a design for a 5 × 5 square is as follows:

A	B	C	D	E
B	A	E	C	D
C	D	A	E	B
D	E	B	A	C
E	C	D	B	A

lat·i·tude (la′ti-tūd). The range of light or x-ray exposure acceptable with a given photographic emulsion. SEE latitude *film.* SYN digital gray scale, gray scale. [L. *latitudo,* width, fr. *latus,* wide]

La·tro·dec·tus (lat-rō-dek′tŭs). A genus of relatively small spiders, the widow spiders, capable of inflicting highly poisonous, neurotoxic, painful bites; they are responsible, along with *Loxosceles* (the brown spider), for most of the severe reactions from spider envenomation. Medically important species are known from Australia, North and South America, South Africa, and New Zealand. Some venomous species, in addition to *L. mactans*

(the black widow spider), are *L. bishopi* (the red-legged widow spider), *L. euracaviensis, L. geometricus,* and *L. tredecimguttatus.* [L. *latro,* servant, robber, + G. *dēktēs,* a biter]

L. mac′tans, the black widow spider, a venomous jet-black spider found in protected dark places; it is especially common in the southern U.S.; the full mature female (slightly more than 1 cm long) has a brilliant red dumbbell- or hourglass-shaped mark on the ventral aspect of the abdomen, and her bite may be extremely painful, producing a syndrome mimicking an acute abdominal crisis; some deaths, though rare, have been reported, particularly in small children; the male spider lacks the hourglass mark and is not venomous.

LATS Abbreviation for long-acting thyroid *stimulator.*

lat·tice (lat′is). A regular arrangement of units into an array such that a plane passing through two units of a particular type or in a particular interrelationship will pass through an indefinite number of such units; *e.g.,* the atom arrangement in a crystal.

la·tus, gen. **la·te·ris,** pl. **la·te·ra** (lā′tŭs, lat′er-is, lat′er-ă). The side of the body between the pelvis and the ribs. SYN flank. [L. broad]

Latzko, Wilhelm, Austrian obstetrician, 1863–1945. SEE L.'s cesarean *section.*

laud·a·ble (law′dă-bl). A term formerly used to describe a quality of pus that was thick and creamy and not indicating an infection that would spread, leading to blood poisoining and death. [L. *laudabilis,* praiseworthy]

lau·da·nine (law′dă-nēn). $C_{20}H_{25}NO_4$; an isoquinoline alkaloid derived from the mother liquor of morphine; it causes tetanoid convulsions, with action similar to that of strychnine.

lau·da·no·sine (law′dă-nō-sēn). $C_{21}H_{27}NO_4$; an isoquinoline alkaloid obtained from the mother liquor of morphine; it causes tetanic convulsions.

lau·da·num (law′dă-nŭm). A tincture containing opium. [G. *lēdanon,* a resinous gum]

Laugier, Stanislas, French surgeon, 1799–1872. SEE L.'s *hernia, sign.*

Laumonier, Jean B.P.N.R., French surgeon, 1749–1818. SEE L.'s *ganglion.*

Launois, Pierre E., French physician, 1856–1914. SEE L.-Cléret *syndrome;* L.-Bensaude *syndrome.*

Laurence, John Zachariah, British ophthalmologist, 1830–1874. SEE L.-Moon-Biedl *syndrome.*

Laurer, Johann F., German pharmacologist, 1798–1873. SEE L.'s *canal.*

lau·ric ac·id (law′rik). $CH_3(CH_2)_{10}COOH$; a fatty acid occurring in spermaceti, in milk, and in laurel, coconut, and palm oils as well as waxes and marine fats. SYN *n*-dodecanoic acid.

Lauth, Charles, English chemist, 1836–1913. SEE L.'s *violet.*

Lauth, Ernst A., German physician, 1803–1837. SEE L.'s *canal.*

Lauth, Thomas, German anatomist and surgeon, 1758–1826. SEE L.'s *ligament.*

Lauth's vi·o·let. SYN thionine.

LAV Abbreviation for lymphadenopathy-associated *virus.*

la·vage (lă-vahzh′). The washing out of a hollow cavity or organ by copious injections and rejections of fluid. [Fr. from L. *lavo,* to wash]

Lavdovsky, Michail D., Russian histologist, 1846–1902. SEE L.'s *nucleoid.*

La·ver·an·ia (lav-er-ā′nē-ă). Old generic name for malaria-causing and other hematozoan protozoa. *L. falciparum* is a distinctive generic name for *Plasmodium falciparum,* and is preferred by some who believe that crescentic gametocytes should be the basis for classifying the causal agent of falciparum malaria in a separate genus. SEE *Plasmodium, Haemoproteus.* [C. Laveran, Fr. protozoologist and Nobel laureate, 1845–1922]

la·veur (lă-vŭr′). An instrument for irrigation or lavage. [Fr.]

LAVH. Abbreviation for laparoscopic-assisted vaginal *hysteroscopy.*

LA

LAW

law. 1. A principle or rule. 2. A statement of a sequence or relation of phenomena that is invariable under the given conditions. SEE ALSO principle, rule, theorem. [A.S. *lagu*]

all or none l., SYN Bowditch's l.

Ambard's l.'s, obsolete l.'s for output of urea: 1) with the urinary urea concentration constant, urea output varies directly as the square of the concentration of the blood urea; 2) with the blood urea concentration constant, urea output varies inversely as the square root of its urinary concentration.

Ångström's l., a substance absorbs light of the same wavelength as it emits when luminous.

Arndt's l., obsolete l. stating that weak stimuli excite physiologic activity, moderately strong ones favor it, strong ones retard it, and very strong ones arrest it.

Arrhenius l., SYN Arrhenius *doctrine*.

l.'s of association, principles formulated by Aristotle to account for the functional relationships between ideas; the l. of contiguity (association) proved most useful to experimental psychologists, culminating in modern studies of respondent conditioning.

l. of average localization, visceral pain is most accurately localized in the least mobile viscera and least accurately in the most mobile.

Avogadro's l., equal volumes of gases contain equal numbers of molecules, the conditions of pressure and temperature being the same. SYN Ampère's postulate, Avogadro's hypothesis, Avogadro's postulate.

Baer's l., the general organ characteristics found in all members of a group appear earlier in embryogenesis than the special organ characteristics that distinguish specific members of the group; this law is the predecessor of the recapitulation theory.

Baruch's l., the effect of any hydriatric procedure is in direct proportion to the difference between the temperature of the water and that of the skin; when the temperature of the water is above or below that of the skin the effect is stimulating; when the two temperatures are the same the effect is sedative.

Beer-Lambert l., the absorbance of light is directly proportional to the thickness of the ligand through which the light is being transmitted multiplied by the concentration of absorbing chromophore; *i.e.,* $A = \varepsilon bc$ where A is the absorbance, ε is the molar extinction coefficient, b is the thickness of the solution, and c is the concentration.

Beer's l., the intensity of a color or of a light ray is inversely proportional to the depth of liquid through which it is transmitted; it is concluded that the absorption is dependent upon the number of molecules in the path of the ray. Cf. Beer-Lambert l.

Behring's l., parenteral administration of serum from an immunized person provides a relative, passive immunity to that disease (*i.e.,* prevents it, or favorably modifies its course) in a previously susceptible person.

Bell-Magendie l., SYN Bell's l.

Bell's l., the ventral spinal roots are motor, the dorsal are sensory. SYN Bell-Magendie l., Magendie's l.

Bernoulli's l., when friction is negligible, the velocity of flow of a gas or fluid through a tube is inversely related to its pressure against the side of the tube; *i.e.,* velocity is greatest and pressure lowest at a point of constriction. SYN Bernoulli's principle, Bernoulli's theorem.

Berthollet's l., salts in solution will always react with each other so as to form a less soluble salt, if possible.

biogenetic l., l. of biogenesis, SYN recapitulation *theory*.

Blagden's l., the depression of the freezing point of dilute solutions is proportional to the amount of the dissolved substance.

Bowditch's l., consistently total response to any effective stimulus. SYN all or none l.

Boyle's l., at constant temperature, the volume of a given quantity of gas varies inversely with its absolute pressure. SYN Mariotte's l.

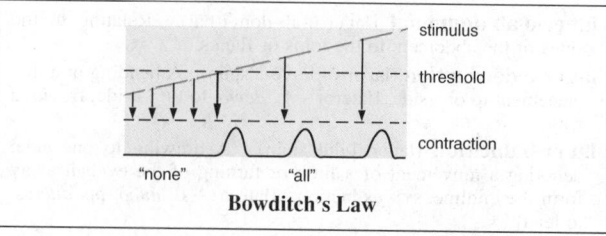

Bowditch's Law

Broadbent's l., lesions of the upper segment of the motor tract cause less marked paralysis of muscles that habitually produce bilateral movements than of those that commonly act independently of the opposite side.

Bunsen-Roscoe l., in two photochemical reactions, *e.g.,* the darkening of a photographic plate or film, if the product of the intensity of illumination and the time of exposure are equal, the quantities of chemical material undergoing change will be equal; the retina for short periods of exposure obeys this l. SYN reciprocity l., Roscoe-Bunsen l.

Charles l., all gases expand equally on heating, namely, $\frac{1}{273.16}$ of their volume at 0°C for every degree Celsius. SYN Gay-Lussac's l.

l. of constant numbers in ovulation, the number of ova discharged at each ovulation is nearly constant for any given species.

l. of contiguity, when two ideas or psychologically perceived events have once occurred in close association they are likely to so occur again, the subsequent occurrence of one tending to elicit the other; this l. figures prominently in modern theories of conditioning and learning.

l. of contrary innervation, SYN Meltzer's l.

Coppet's l., solutions having the same freezing point have equal concentrations of dissolved substances.

Courvoisier's l., enlargement of the gallbladder with jaundice is likely to result from carcinoma of the head of the pancreas and not from a stone in the common duct, because in the latter the gallbladder is usually scarred from infection and does not distend. SYN Courvoisier's sign.

Dale-Feldberg l., an identical chemical transmitter is liberated at all the functional terminals of a single neuron.

Dalton-Henry l., in dissolving a mixture of gases, a liquid will absorb as much of each gas in the mixture as if that were the only gas dissolved.

Dalton's l., each gas in a mixture of gases exerts a pressure proportionate to the percentage of the gas and independent of the presence of the other gases present. SYN l. of partial pressures.

l. of definite proportions, the relative weights of the several elements forming a chemical compound are invariable. SYN Proust's l.

l. of denervation, when a structure is denervated, its irritability to certain chemical agents is increased; *e.g.,* the greater sensitivity of the pupil to acetylcholine after section and degeneration of the third nerve, and of the nictitating membrane to adrenaline after excision of the superior cervical ganglion.

Descartes' l., SYN l. of refraction.

Donders' l., the rotation of the eyeball is determined by the distance of the object from the median plane and the line of the horizon.

Draper's l., a chemical change is produced in a photochemical substance only by those light rays that are absorbed by that substance.

Du Bois-Reymond's l., SYN l. of excitation.

Dulong-Petit l., the specific heats of many solid elements are inversely proportional to their atomic weights.

Einthoven's l., in the electrocardiogram the potential of any wave or complex in lead II is equal to the sum of the potentials of leads I and III. SYN Einthoven's equation.

Elliott's l., adrenaline acts upon those structures innervated by sympathetic nerve fibers.

l. of excitation, a motor nerve responds, not to the absolute value, but to the alteration of value from moment to moment, of the electric current; *i.e.,* rate of change of intensity of the current is a factor in determining its effectiveness. SYN Du Bois-Reymond's l.

Faraday's l.'s, (1) the amount of an electrolyte decomposed by an electric current is proportional to the amount of the current; **(2)** when the same current is passed through several electrolytes, the amounts of the different substances decomposed are proportional to their chemical equivalents.

Farr's l., the curve of cases of an epidemic rises rapidly at first, then climbs slowly to a peak from which the fall is steeper than the previous rise.

Fechner-Weber l., SYN Weber-Fechner l.

Ferry-Porter l., the critical fusion is directly proportional to the logarithm of the light intensity.

Fick's l.'s of diffusion, (1) the direction of movement of solutes by diffusion is always from a higher to a lower concentration and the diffusive flux J_A of solute A across a plane at x is proportional to the concentration gradient of A at x; *i.e.,* $J_A = -D(C_A/x)$; **(2)** the increase of concentration of solute A with time, C_A/t, is directly proportional to the change in the concentration gradient, *i.e.,* $C_A/t = D(fl^2/x^2)$.

Flatau's l., a l. concerning the excentric position of the long spinal tracts; the greater the distance the nerve fibers run lengthwise in the cord, the more they tend to be situated toward its periphery.

Galton's l., in a population mating at random, the progeny of a parent with an extreme value for a measurable phenotype will tend on average to have values nearer the population mean than in the extreme parent. SEE ALSO l. of regression to mean. SYN l. of regression to mean.

Gay-Lussac's l., SYN Charles l.

Gerhardt-Semon l., obsolete l. formerly used to account for the position of an affected vocal cord or cords after injury to the recurrent laryngeal nerve or nerves.

Godélier's l., tuberculosis of the peritoneum is always associated with tuberculosis of the pleura on one or both sides.

Gompertz' l., the proportional relationship of mortality to age; after age 35–40, the increase in mortality with age tends to be logarithmic.

Graham's l., the relative rapidity of diffusion of two gases varies inversely as the square root of their densities, *i.e.,* their molecular weights.

Grasset's l., SYN Landouzy-Grasset l.

l. of gravitation, SYN Newton's l.

Guldberg-Waage l., SYN l. of mass action.

Haeckel's l., SYN recapitulation *theory.*

Halsted's l., transplanted tissue will grow only if there is a lack of that tissue in the host.

Hamburger's l., albumins and phosphates pass from red corpuscles to serum and chlorides pass from serum to cells when blood is acid; the reverse occurs when blood is alkaline.

Hardy-Weinberg l., if mating occurs at random with respect to any one autosomal locus in a population in which the gene frequencies are equal in the two sexes, and the factors tending to change gene frequencies (mutation, differential selection, migration) are either absent or negligible, then in one generation the probabilities of all possible genotypes will on average equal the same proportions as if the genes were assembled at random. The l. does not apply to two or more loci jointly, nor to X-linked traits where the initial gene frequencies differ in the two sexes.

l. of the heart, the energy liberated by the heart when it contracts is a function of the length of its muscle fibers at the end of diastole. SYN Starling's l.

Heidenhain's l., glandular secretion is always accompanied by an alteration in the structure of the gland.

Hellin's l., twins occur once in 89 births, triplets once in 89^2, and quadruplets once in 89^3. If the frequency of twins in a population is *p*, the frequency of triplets is p^2, and the frequency of quadruplets is p^3.

Henry's l., at equilibrium, at a given temperature, the amount of gas dissolved in a given volume of liquid is directly proportional to the partial pressure of that gas in the gas phase (this only holds for gases that do not react chemically with the solvent).

Hess' l., the amount of heat generated by a reaction is the same whether the reaction takes place in one step or several steps; *i.e.,* ΔH values (and thus ΔG values) are additive.

Hilton's l., the nerve supplying a joint supplies also the muscles which move the joint and the skin covering the articular insertion of those muscles.

Hooke's l., the stress applied to stretch or compress a body is proportional to the strain, or change in length thus produced, so long as the limit of elasticity of the body is not exceeded.

l. of independent assortment, different hereditary factors assort independently when the gametes are formed; traits at linked loci are an exception. SYN Mendel's second l.

l. of initial value, SYN Wilder's l. of initial value.

l. of intestine, SYN myenteric *reflex.*

inverse square l., as applied to point sources, the intensity of radiation diminishes in proportion to the square of the distance from the source.

l. of isochronism, a nerve and the muscle which it innervates have the same chronaxie values.

isodynamic l., for energy purposes, the different foodstuffs may replace one another in accordance with their caloric values when burned in a calorimeter.

Jackson's l., loss of mental functions due to disease retraces in reverse order its evolutionary development.

Koch's l., SYN Koch's *postulates,* under *postulate.*

Lambert's l., (1) each layer of equal thickness absorbs an equal fraction of the light that traverses it; Cf. Beer-Lambert l. **(2)** the illumination of a surface on which the light falls normally from a point source is inversely proportional to the square of the distance from the source.

Landouzy-Grasset l., in lesions of one hemisphere, the patient's head is turned to the side of the affected muscles if there is spasticity and to that of the cerebral lesion if there is paralysis. SYN Grasset's l.

Lapicque's l., the chronaxie is inversely proportional to the diameter of an axon.

Laplace's l., the equilibrium relationship between transmural pressure difference (ΔP), wall tension (T), and radius of curvature (R) in a concave surface; for a sphere: $\Delta P = 2T/R$; for a cylinder: $\Delta P = T/R$.

Le Chatelier's l., if external factors such as temperature and pressure disturb a system in equilibrium, adjustment occurs in such a way that the effect of the disturbing factors is reduced to a minimum. SYN Le Chatelier's principle.

Listing's l., when the eye leaves one object and fixes upon another, it revolves about an axis perpendicular to a plane cutting both the former and the present lines of vision.

Louis' l., tuberculosis in any organ is associated with tuberculosis in the lung.

Magendie's l., SYN Bell's l.

Marey's l., the pulse rate varies inversely with the blood pressure; *i.e.,* the pulse is slow when the pressure is high; an expression of baroreceptor reflex influences on heart rate.

Marfan's l., the healing of localized tuberculosis protects against subsequent development of pulmonary tuberculosis.

Mariotte's l., SYN Boyle's l.

mass l., SYN l. of mass action.

l. of mass action, the rate of a chemical reaction is proportional

♻ **Combining forms**	**[NA]** Nomina Anatomica
Word*Finder*	**[MIM]** Mendelian
Multi-term entry finder	**Inheritance in Man**
Preceding letter A	
	☆ **Official alternate term**
A.D.A.M. Anatomy Plates	
Between letters L and M	☆**[NA]** Official alternate
	Nomina Anatomica term
Appendices:	
Following letter Z	▬▬▬▬▬
SYN Synonym; Cf., compare	**High Profile Term**

la

to the concentrations of the reacting substances; when the forward reaction rate equals the reverse reaction rate (*i.e.*, at equilibrium) then, at constant temperature, the product of the concentrations of all the products divided by the product of the concentrations of all the reactants is itself a constant (K_{eq}). SYN Guldberg-Waage l., mass l.

Meltzer's l., "all living functions are continually controlled by two opposite forces: augmentation or action on the one hand, and inhibition on the other." SYN l. of contrary innervation.

Mendeléeff's l., the properties of elements are periodical functions of their atomic weights; *i.e.,* if the elements are arranged in the order of their atomic weights, every element in the series will be related in respect to its properties to the eighth in order before or after it. SYN periodic l.

Mendel's first l., SYN l. of segregation.

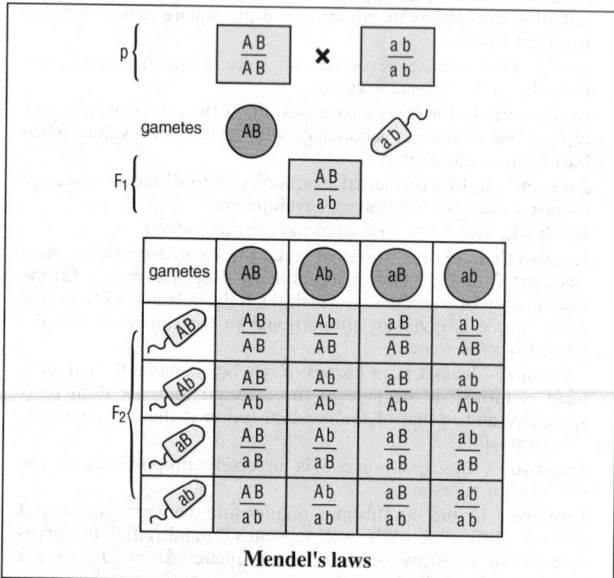

Mendel's laws

Mendel's second l., SYN l. of independent assortment.

l. of the minimum, growth and development of plants and animals are determined by the availability of that essential nutrient which is present in the smallest amount.

Müller's l., each type of sensory nerve ending, however stimulated (electrically, mechanically, etc.), gives rise to its own specific sensation; moreover, each type of sensation depends not upon any special character of the different nerves but upon the part of the brain in which their fibers terminate. SYN l. of specific nerve energies.

l. of multiple proportions, SYN l. of reciprocal proportions.

Nasse's l., an early statement of the pattern of X-linked recessive inheritance: hemophilia affects only boys but is transmitted through mothers and sisters.

Neumann's l., in compounds of analogous chemical constitution, the molecular heat, or the product of the specific heat by the atomic weight, is always the same.

Newton's l., the attractive force between any two bodies is proportional to the product of their masses, and inversely proportional to the square of the distance between their centers. SYN l. of gravitation.

Nysten's l., rigor mortis affects first the muscles of the head and spreads toward the feet.

Ochoa's l., the content of the X-chromosome tends to be phylogenetically conserved.

Ohm's l., in an electric current passing through a wire, the intensity of the current (I) in amperes equals the electromotive force (E) in volts divided by the resistance (R) in ohms: $I = E/R$.

l. of partial pressures, SYN Dalton's l.

Pascal's l., fluids at rest transmit pressure equally in every direction.

periodic l., SYN Mendeléeff's l.

Pflüger's l., SYN l. of polar excitation.

Plateau-Talbot l., when successive light stimuli follow each other sufficiently rapidly to become fused, their apparent brightness is diminished.

Poiseuille's l., in laminar flow, the volume of a homogeneous fluid passing per unit time through a capillary tube is directly proportional to the pressure difference between its ends and to the fourth power of its internal radius, and inversely proportional to its length and to the viscosity of the fluid.

l. of polar excitation, a given segment of a nerve is irritated by the development of catelectrotonus and the disappearance of anelectrotonus, but the reverse does not hold; *i.e.,* excitation occurs at the cathode when the circuit is closed and at the anode when it is opened. SYN Pflüger's l.

l. of priority, use of the earliest published name (senior synonym) of two or more names of an organism as the correct name.

Profeta's l., the subject of congenital syphilis is immune against the acquired disease.

Proust's l., SYN l. of definite proportions.

Raoult's l., the vapor pressure of a solution of a nonvolatile nonelectrolyte is that of the pure solvent multiplied by the mole-fraction of the solvent in the solution.

l. of recapitulation, SYN recapitulation *theory.*

l. of reciprocal proportions, the relative weights in which two substances form a chemical union singly with a third are the same as, or simple multiples of, those in which they unite with each other; a corollary of the law of definite proportions. SYN l. of multiple proportions.

reciprocity l., SYN Bunsen-Roscoe l.

l. of referred pain, pain arises only from irritation of nerves which are sensitive to those stimuli that produce pain when applied to the surface of the body.

l. of refraction, for two given media, the sine of the angle of incidence bears a constant relation to the sine of the angle of refraction. SYN Descartes' l., Snell's l.

l. of regression to mean, SYN Galton's l.

Riccò's l., for small images, light intensity × area = constant for the threshold.

Ritter's l., a nerve is stimulated at both the opening and the closing of an electrical current. SEE l. of polar excitation.

Roscoe-Bunsen l., SYN Bunsen-Roscoe l.

Rosenbach's l., (1) in affections of the nerve trunks or nerve centers, paralysis of the flexor muscles appears later than that of the extensors; (2) in cases of abnormal stimulation of organs with rhythmical functional periodicity, there is often a grouping of the individual acts with corresponding lengthening of the pauses, in such a way that the proportion of total rest and activity remains nearly the same.

Rubner's l.'s of growth, (1) the l. of constant energy consumption: the rapidity of growth is proportional to the intensity of the metabolic processes; (2) the l. of the constant growth quotient: in most young mammals, 24% of the entire food energy, or calories, is utilized for growth; in humans only 5% is utilized.

Schütz' l., SYN Schütz *rule.*

second l. of thermodynamics, the entropy of the universe moves toward a maximum; similarly, the entropy of any isolated microcosm (*e.g.,* a chemical reaction) proceeds spontaneously only in that direction that yields an increase in entropy, entropy being maximal at equilibrium. To quote G.N. Lewis, ";Every process that occurs spontaneously is capable of doing work; to reverse any such process requires the expenditure of work from the outside."

l. of segregation, factors that affect development retain their individuality from generation to generation, do not become contaminated when mixed in a hybrid, and become sorted out from one another when the next generation of gametes is formed. SYN Mendel's first l.

Semon's l., an obsolete l. stating that injury to the recurrent laryngeal nerve results in paralysis of the abductor muscle of the vocal cords before paralysis of the adductor muscles.

Sherrington's l., every dorsal spinal nerve root supplies a particular area of the skin, the dermatome (3), which is, however, invaded above and below by fibers from the adjacent spinal segments.

l. of similars, SEE similia similibus curantur.

Snell's l., SYN l. of refraction.

Spallanzani's l., the younger the individual the greater is the regenerative power of its cells.

l. of specific nerve energies, SYN Müller's l.

Starling's l., SYN l. of the heart.

Stokes' l., (1) a muscle lying above an inflamed mucous or serous membrane is frequently the seat of paralysis; **(2)** a relationship of the rate of fall of a small sphere in a viscous fluid; applicable to centrifugation of macromolecules; **(3)** the wavelength of light emitted by a fluorescent material is longer than that of the radiation used to excite the fluorescence.

Tait's l., an obsolete dictum that an exploratory laparotomy should be performed in every case of obscure pelvic or abdominal disease that threatens health or life.

Thoma's l.'s, the development of blood vessels is governed by dynamic forces acting on their walls as follows: an increase in velocity of blood flow causes dilation of the lumen; an increase in lateral pressure on the vessel wall causes it to thicken; an increase in end-pressure causes the formation of new capillaries.

van der Kolk's l., in a mixed nerve, the sensory fibers are distributed to the parts moved by the muscles controlled by the motor fibers.

van't Hoff's l., (1) in stereochemistry, all optically active substances have one or more multivalent atoms united to four different atoms or radicals so as to form in space an unsymmetrical arrangement; **(2)** the osmotic pressure exerted by any substance in very dilute solution is the same that it would exert if present as gas in the same volume as that of the solution; or, at constant temperature, the osmotic pressure of dilute solutions is proportional to the concentration (number of molecules) of the dissolved substance; *i.e.,* the osmotic pressure, Π, in dilute solutions is $\pi = RT\Sigma c_i$, where R is the universal gas constant, T is the absolute temperature, and c_i is the molar concentration of solute i; **(3)** the rate of chemical reactions increases between two- and three-fold for each 10°C rise in temperature.

Virchow's l., there is no special or distinctive neoplastic cell, inasmuch as the component cells of neoplasms originate from preexisting forms.

Vogel's l., when a phenotype may be transmitted by various modes of mendelian inheritance, the dominant will have the least deleterious phenotype, the recessive the most, and the X-linked intermediate between the two.

wallerian l., after section of the posterior root of a spinal nerve between the root ganglion and the spinal cord, the central portion degenerates; after division of the anterior root, the peripheral portion degenerates; the trophic center of the posterior root is therefore the ganglion, that of the anterior root the spinal cord.

Weber-Fechner l., the intensity of a sensation varies by a series of equal increments (arithmetically) as the strength of the stimulus is increased geometrically; if a series of stimuli is applied and so adjusted in strength that each stimulus causes a just perceptible change in intensity of the sensation, then the strength of each stimulus differs from the preceding one by a constant fraction; thus, if a just perceptible change in a visual sensation is produced by the addition of 1 candle to an original illumination of 100 candles, 10 candles will be required to produce any change in sensation when the original illumination was one of 1000 candles. SYN Fechner-Weber l., Weber's l.

Weber's l., SYN Weber-Fechner l.

Weigert's l., the loss or destruction of a part or element in the organic world is likely to result in compensatory replacement and overproduction of tissue during the process of regeneration or repair (or both), as in the formation of callus when a fractured bone heals. SYN overproduction theory.

Wilder's l. of initial value, the direction of response of a body function to any agent depends to a large degree on the initial level of that function. SYN l. of initial value.

Williston's l., as the vertebrate scale is ascended, the number of bones in the skull is reduced.

Wolff's l., every change in the form and the function of a bone,

or in its function alone, is followed by certain definite changes in its internal architecture and secondary alterations in its external conformation.

Lawrence, R.D., 20th century English physician. SEE L.-Seip *syndrome.*

law·ren·ci·um (Lr) (law-ren′sē-ŭm). An artificial transplutonium element; atomic no. 103; atomic wt. 262.11. [E.O. *Lawrence,* U.S. physicist and Nobel laureate, 1901–1958]

lax·a·tion (lak-sā′shŭn). Bowel movement, with or without laxatives. [see laxative]

lax·a·tive (lak′să-tiv). **1.** Mildly cathartic; having the action of loosening the bowels. **2.** A mild cathartic; a remedy that moves the bowels slightly without pain or violent action. [L. *laxativus,* fr. *laxo,* pp. *-atus,* to slacken, relax]

diphenylmethane l.'s, members of a chemical class of l. agents including phenolphthalein and bisacodyl.

la·xa·tor tym·pa·ni (lak-sā′tor tim′pan-ī). One of two supposed muscles, probably ligaments of the malleus. [Mod. L.]

LAYER

lay·er (lā′er). A sheet of one substance lying on another and distinguished from it by a difference in texture or color or by not being continuous with it. SEE ALSO stratum, lamina.

ameloblastic l., the internal l. of the enamel organ. SYN enamel l.

anterior elastic l., SYN anterior limiting l. of cornea.

anterior limiting l. of cornea, a transparent homogeneous acellular layer, 6 to 9 μm thick, lying between the basal l. of the outer layer of stratified epithelium and the substantia propria of the cornea; considered to be a basement membrane. SYN lamina limitans anterior corneae [NA], anterior elastic l., Bowman's membrane, lamina elastica anterior, limiting l.'s of cornea.

anterior l. of rectus abdominis sheath, the portion of the rectus sheath that lies anterior to the muscle, consisting in its upper two-thirds of contributions from the aponeuroses of the external and internal oblique muscles, and in its lower third (below the arcuralt line) of contributions from the aponeuroses of all three muscles of the anterolateral abdominal wall. SYN lamina anterior vaginae musculi recti abdominis [NA].

bacillary l., SYN l. of rods and cones.

basal l., SYN *stratum* basale (1).

basal cell l., SYN *stratum* basale epidermidis.

basal l. of choroid, SYN *lamina* basalis choroideae.

basal l. of ciliary body, SYN basal *lamina* of ciliary body.

l. of Bechterew, SYN *band* of Kaes-Bechterew.

blastodermic l.'s, the primordial cell l.'s on the yolk surface of a telolecithal egg; in the earliest stages they consist of protoderm, and they later differentiate into ectoderm, endoderm, and mesoderm.

brown l., SYN *lamina* fusca of sclera.

cambium l., (1) the inner osteogenic l. of the periosteum; **(2)** a highly cellular zone immediately beneath the epithelium covering a botryoid sarcoma.

l.'s of cerebellar cortex, SEE cerebellar *cortex.*

l.'s of cerebral cortex, SEE cerebral *cortex.*

cerebral l. of retina, the internal l. of the retina containing the neural elements, as distinguished from the outer leaf of the retina, or pigmented layer. SYN pars optica retinae [NA], neural l. of retina, optic part of retina, stratum cerebrale retinae.

Chievitz' l., in the developing retina of an embryo, a transitory zone between the inner and outer neuroblastic l.'s that is devoid of nuclei.

choriocapillary l., the internal layer of the choroidea of the eye, composed of a very close capillary network. SYN lamina choroidocapillaris [NA], choriocapillaris, entochoroidea, lamina choriocapillaris, membrana choriocapillaris, Ruysch's membrane.

la

circular l. of muscular coat, the inner, circular l. of the smooth muscle of the muscular coat. Nomina Anatomica lists circular l.'s of muscular coats (stratum circulare tunicae muscularis ...) of the following: 1) colon (... coli [NA]); 2) rectum (... recti [NA]); 3) small intestine (... intestini tenuis [NA]); 4) stomach (... gastrici [NA]). SYN stratum circulare tunicae muscularis gastricae [NA], stratum circulare tunicae [NA].

circular l.'s of muscular tunics, SEE circular l. of muscular coat.

circular l. of tympanic membrane, SYN *stratum* circulare membranae tympani.

claustral l., the l. of subcortical gray matter between the external capsule and the white matter of the insula or extreme capsule.

clear l. of epidermis, SYN *stratum* lucidum.

columnar l., SYN *stratum* basale epidermidis.

conjunctival l. of bulb, SYN bulbar *conjunctiva*.

conjunctival l. of eyelids, SYN palpebral *conjunctiva*.

corneal l. of epidermis, SYN *stratum* corneum epidermidis.

cornified l. of nail, SYN *stratum* corneum unguis.

cutaneous l. of tympanic membrane, SYN *stratum* cutaneum membranae tympani.

deep l., in a stratified structure, the stratum which lies beneath all others, furthest from the surface. SEE deep l. of levator palpebrae superioris muscle, deep l. of temporalis fascia. SYN lamina profunda [NA], deep lamina.

deep gray l. of superior colliculus, a l. of myelinated fibers, the deepest layer of the colliculus superior, delimiting the latter from the central gray substance surrounding the cerebral aqueduct. SYN stratum album profundum.

deep l. of levator palpebrae superioris muscle, the deeper fibers of the levator muscle of the superior eyelid which are inserted into the superior tarsal plate. SYN lamina profunda musculi levatoris palpebrae superioris.

deep l. of temporalis fascia, the deep part of the temporal fascia attaching to the medial surface of the zygomatic arch; SYN lamina profunda fasciae temporalis.

deep white l. of superior colliculus, SEE gray l. of superior colliculus.

elastic l.'s of arteries, SYN elastic *laminae* of arteries, under *lamina*.

elastic l.'s of cornea, SEE anterior limiting l. of cornea, posterior limiting l. of cornea.

enamel l., SYN ameloblastic l.

ependymal l., an inner epithelial l. of cells bordering the lumen of the embryonic neural tube and brain, formed during the latter's stratification, and persisting in modified form throughout life. SYN ependymal zone, ventricular l.

epithelial l.'s, SEE epithelium.

epithelial choroid l., SYN epithelial *lamina*.

epitrichial l., the superficial flattened-cell l. of the epidermis of a young embryo before the definitive stratification has developed.

external nuclear l. of retina, SYN neuroepithelial l. of retina.

fatty l. of superficial fascia, SYN Camper's *fascia*.

fibrous l., the outer dense connective tissue l. of the periosteum.

fillet l., SYN *stratum* lemnisci.

fusiform l., l. 6 of the cortex cerebri. SYN multiform l., polymorphous l., spindle-celled l.

ganglionic l. of cerebellar cortex, SYN piriform neuron l.

ganglionic l. of cerebral cortex, l. 5 of the cortex cerebri.

ganglionic l. of optic nerve, the inner l. of multipolar neurons in the retina consisting of the relatively large neurons that give rise to the fibers of the optic nerve. SYN stratum ganglionare nervi optici.

ganglionic l. of retina, the intermediate l. of neurons in the retina composed largely of bipolar cells. SYN internal nuclear l. of retina, stratum ganglionare retinae, stratum nucleare internum retinae.

germ l., one of the three primordial cell l.'s (ectoderm, endoderm, mesoderm) established in an embryo during gastrulation and the immediately following stages.

germinative l., SYN *stratum* basale epidermidis.

germinative l. of nail, SYN *stratum* germinativum unguis.

glomerular l. of olfactory bulb, a l. composed of spherical bodies, called glomeruli, formed by the synapses of mitral cells with the olfactory nerve fibers derived from the cells of the olfactory epithelium.

granular l. of cerebellar cortex, SYN granular l. of cerebellum.

granular l. of cerebellum, the deepest of the three l.'s of the cortex; it contains large numbers of granule cells, the dendrites of which synapse with incoming mossy fibers in cerebellar glomeruli. Thin, unmyelinated axons of granule cells ascend perpendicularly into the molecular l. in which they bifurcate into fibers coursing parallel to the long axis of the cerebellar folia. Parallel fibers form numerous synapses with the dendrites of Purkinje cells, basket cells, and stellate cells. SYN stratum granulosum cerebelli [NA], granular l. of cerebellar cortex.

granular l.'s of cerebral cortex, l.'s 2 (outer) and 4 (inner) of the cortex cerebri.

granular l. of epidermis, a l. of somewhat flattened cells containing basophilic granules of keratohyalin and lying just above the stratum spinosum and deeply to the stratum corneum. SYN stratum granulosum epidermidis [NA].

granular l.'s of retina, SYN nuclear l.'s of retina.

granular l. of a vesicular ovarian follicle, SYN *stratum* granulosum folliculi ovarici vesiculosi.

gray l. of superior colliculus, term applied to any one of the three major l.'s of gray matter of the superior colliculus that alternate with l.'s composed chiefly of nerve fibers: 1) the superficial gray l. of superior colliculus, above the largely white layer of the incoming fibers of the optic tract (optic l.); 2) the middle gray l. of superior colliculus, placed between the optic l. and a more deeply located l. of fibers, the l. lemnisci; 3) the deep gray layer of superior colliculus, between the l. lemnisci and the central gray substance surrounding the cerebral aqueduct, and containing the large nerve cells from which most of the colliculus descending connections (tectobulbar, tectopontine, and tectospinal tract) originate. SYN stratum griseum colliculi superioris [NA], stratum cinereum colliculi superioris.

half-value l. (HVL), the thickness of a specific absorber (*e.g.,* Al) that will reduce the intensity of a beam of radiation to one-half its initial value.

Henle's l., the outer l. cells of the inner root sheath of the hair follicle.

Henle's fiber l., the l. of inner cone fibers in the central area of the retina.

Henle's nervous l., SYN entoretina.

horny l. of epidermis, SYN *stratum* corneum epidermidis.

horny l. of nail, SYN *stratum* corneum unguis.

Huxley's l., a l. of cells interposed between Henle's l. and the cuticle of the inner root sheath of the hair follicle. SYN Huxley's membrane, Huxley's sheath.

infragranular l., the cellular band deep to the inner granular l. of the developing human cerebral cortex, which differentiates into the ganglionic l. and multiform l. by the sixth fetal month.

intermediate l., SYN mantle l.

internal nuclear l. of retina, SYN ganglionic l. of retina.

investing l. of deep cervical fascia, the part of the cervical fascia investing the sternocleidomastoid and trapezius muscles and completely encircling the neck. SYN lamina superficialis fasciae cervicalis [NA], investing fascia, superficial l. of deep cervical fascia.

Kölliker's l., the l. of connective tissue in the iris.

Langhans' l., SYN cytotrophoblast.

lateral cartilaginous l., SYN lateral *lamina* of cartilaginous auditory tube.

lateral l. of cartilaginous auditory tube, SYN lateral *lamina* of cartilaginous auditory tube.

latticed l., a cortical cell l. in the hippocampus.

limiting l.'s of cornea, SYN anterior limiting l. of cornea, posterior limiting l. of cornea.

longitudinal l. of muscular coat, the outer, longitudinal l. of the smooth muscle of the muscular coat. Nomina Anatomica lists longitudinal l.'s of muscular coats (stratum longitudinale tunicae muscularis ...) of the following: 1) colon (... coli [NA]); 2) rectum (... recti [NA]); 3) small intestine (... intestini tenuis [NA]); 4) stomach (... gastrici [NA]). SYN stratum longitudinale tunicae muscularis gastricae [NA], stratum longitudinale tunicae muscularis [NA].

longitudinal l.'s of muscular tunics, SEE longitudinal l. of muscular coat.

malpighian l., SYN malpighian *stratum*.

mantle l., the nuclear zone of the developing neural tube between the marginal l. and the ependymal l.; forms the gray matter of the central nervous system. SYN intermediate l., mantle zone (1).

marginal l., the outer, nonnuclear l. of the embryonic neural tube; into its fibrous network grow the longitudinal nerve fibers which eventually become the white matter of the cord and brain stem. SYN marginal zone.

medial cartilaginous l., SYN medial *lamina* of cartilaginous auditory tube.

medial l. of cartilaginous auditory tube, SYN medial *lamina* of cartilaginous auditory tube.

medullary l.'s of thalamus, SYN medullary *laminae* of thalamus, under *lamina*.

membranous l., SYN membranous *lamina* of cartilaginous auditory tube.

membranous l. of superficial fascia, (1) SYN superficial *fascia* of perineum. **(2)** SYN Scarpa's *fascia*.

meningeal l. of dura mater, SEE *dura mater* of brain.

Meynert's l., SYN pyramidal cell l.

middle gray l. of superior colliculus, SEE gray l. of superior colliculus.

molecular l., term applied to any l. of brain tissue that contains few nerve-cell bodies and is composed largely of terminal arborizations of dendrites and axons; notable examples are the superficial l. (first l.) of the cerebral cortex and the molecular l. of cerebellum. SYN plexiform l., stratum moleculare.

molecular l. of cerebellar cortex, SYN molecular l. of cerebellum.

molecular l. of cerebellum, the outer lamina of the cortex, containing the cell bodies and dendrites of Purkinje cells, the axons of the granule cells, and the cell bodies, dendrites, and axons of basket cells. SYN stratum moleculare cerebelli [NA], molecular l. of cerebellar cortex.

molecular l. of cerebral cortex, l. 1 of the cortex cerebri. SYN plexiform l. of cerebral cortex.

molecular l.'s of olfactory bulb, the l.'s, composed mainly of nerve fibers, on the outer and inner sides of the l. of mitral cells of the bulb.

molecular l. of retina, name applied to each of the plexiform l.'s of the retina. SYN stratum moleculare retinae.

multiform l., SYN fusiform l.

muscular l. of mucosa, SYN *muscularis* mucosae.

neural l. of optic retina, SEE retina.

neural l. of retina, SYN cerebral l. of retina.

neuroepithelial l. of retina, the outermost l. of the cerebral l. of retina, composed of the primary receptor cells of the retina; the stratum consists of two sublayers: 1) an external l. made up of the rods and cones, the photosensitive processes of the receptor cells, and 2) the external nuclear l. containing the cell bodies of these cells; the external limiting membrane forms a perforated supporting plate between the two sublayers; the name refers to the fact that the retinal receptor cells are a specialized form of (epithelial) ependyma cell and thus, in a sense, are comparable to the neuroepithelial cells (*e.g.,* hair cells) of other sense organs. SYN external nuclear l. of retina, stratum neuroepitheliale retinae, stratum nucleare externum retinae.

Nitabuch's l., SYN Nitabuch's *membrane*.

nuclear l.'s of retina, the outer nuclear l., l. 4, of the retina, neuroepithelial l. of retina, and the inner l., l. 6, of the retina, ganglionic l. of retina. SYN granular l.'s of retina, stratum nucleare externum et internum retinae.

odontoblastic l., a l. of connective tissue cells at the periphery of the dental pulp of the tooth.

optic l., (1) a layer of white matter interspersed with nerve-cell bodies, immediately below the superficial gray l. of the superior colliculus, composed of myelinated fibers originating in the retina and striate cortex; **(2)** the inner l. of the retina, consisting of the fibers originating from the cells of the ganglionic l. of optic nerve; in their further course these fibers combine to form the optic nerve or optic tract. SYN stratum opticum.

orbital l. of ethmoid bone, SYN orbital *plate* of ethmoid bone.

osteogenetic l., the inner bone-forming l. of the periosteum.

palisade l., SYN *stratum* basale epidermidis.

papillary l., SYN *stratum* papillare corii.

parietal l., the outer l. of an enveloping sac or bursa, usually lining the walls of the cavity or space occupied by the enveloped structure, the structure itself being covered with the inner or visceral layer of the enveloping sac; an actual or potential space is enclosed by the two layers and intervenes between parietal and visceral layers. The parietal l. is usually the more substantial l. SYN lamina parietalis [NA].

parietal l. of leptomeninges, SYN arachnoid.

parietal l. of serous pericardium, the outer part of the serous pericardium suported by the fibrous pericardium. SYN lamina parietalis pericardii.

parietal l. of tunica vaginalis, the outer part of the tunica vaginalis testis supported by the internal spermatic fascia. SYN lamina parietalis tunicae vaginalis testis.

perforated l. of sclera, SYN *lamina* cribrosa sclerae.

periosteal l. of dura mater, SEE *dura mater* of brain.

pigmented l. of ciliary body, SYN *stratum* pigmenti corporis ciliaris.

pigmented l. of iris, SYN *stratum* pigmenti iridis.

pigmented l. of retina, the outer l. of the retina, consisting of pigmented epithelium. SYN ectoretina, stratum pigmenti bulbi, stratum pigmenti retinae, tapetum nigrum, tapetum oculi.

piriform neuron l., the layer of Purkinje cells between the molecular and granular layers of the cerebellar cortex. SYN stratum neuronorum piriformium [NA], ganglionic l. of cerebellar cortex, l. of piriform neurons, Purkinje's l., stratum gangliosum cerebelli.

l. of piriform neurons, SYN piriform neuron l.

plasma l., SYN still l.

plexiform l., SYN molecular l.

plexiform l. of cerebral cortex, SYN molecular l. of cerebral cortex.

plexiform l.'s of retina, l.'s of the retina where synapses occur; in the external l., processes of rods and cones synapse with bipolar neuron dendrites; in the internal l., axon terminals of bipolar cells synapse with ganglion cell dendrites. SEE retina. SYN stratum plexiforme externum et internum retinae.

polymorphous l., SYN fusiform l.

posterior elastic l., SYN posterior limiting l. of cornea.

posterior limiting l. of cornea, a transparent homogeneous acellular layer between the substantia propria and the endothelial layer of the cornea; considered to be a highly developed basement membrane. SYN lamina limitans posterior corneae [NA], membrana vitrea [NA], Descemet's membrane, Duddell's membrane, entocornea, hyaloid membrane, lamina elastica posterior, limiting l.'s of cornea, membrana hyaloidea, posterior elastic l., tunica vitrea, vitreous membrane (1).

posterior l. of rectus abdominis sheath, the portion of the sheath of the rectus abdominis muscle that lies posterior to the muscle covering only its upper two-thirds; it is formed by contributions from the aponeuroses of the internal oblique and transversus abdominis muscles; its free inferior margin forms the arcuate line; it is deficient below this, the posterior aspect of the muscle being covered only by transversalis fascia and peritoneum. SYN lamina posterior vaginae musculi recti abdominis [NA].

pretracheal l., SYN pretracheal *fascia*.

prevertebral l., SYN prevertebral *fascia*.

prickle cell l., SYN *stratum* spinosum epidermidis.

Purkinje's l., SYN piriform neuron l.

pyramidal cell l., l. 3 of the cortex cerebri. SYN Meynert's l.

radiate l. of tympanic membrane, SYN *stratum* radiatum membranae tympani.

la

Rauber's l., (1) the thinned-out trophoblastic membrane over the embryonic disk in developing carnivores and ungulates; **(2)** outermost cell layer which helps form the blastodisk; called blastodermic or primitive ectoderm.

reticular l. of corium, SYN *stratum* reticulare corii.

l.'s of retina, SEE retina.

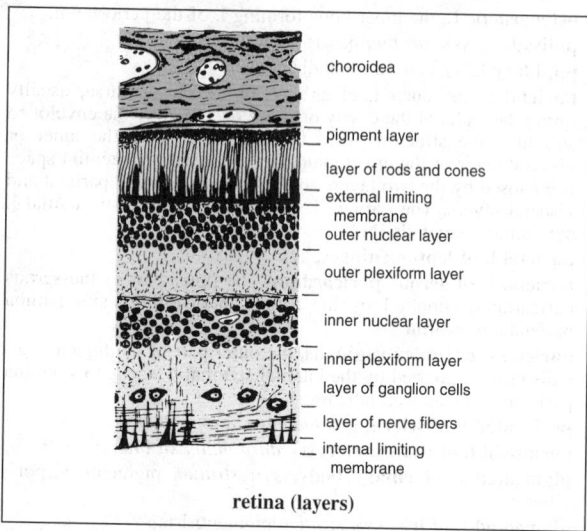

choroidea

pigment layer

layer of rods and cones

external limiting membrane

outer nuclear layer

outer plexiform layer

inner nuclear layer

inner plexiform layer

layer of ganglion cells

layer of nerve fibers

internal limiting membrane

retina (layers)

l. of rods and cones, the l. of the retina next to the pigment l. and containing the visual receptors. SEE ALSO retina, granular l.'s of retina, neuroepithelial l. of retina. SYN bacillary l.

rostral l., SYN rostral *lamina*.

Sattler's elastic l., the middle l. of the choroid.

serous l. of peritoneum, simple squamous epithelium that forms the glistening surface of the parietal and visceral layers of peritoneum. SYN tunica serosa peritonei [NA].

l.'s of skin, SEE epidermis, dermis.

sluggish l., SYN still l.

somatic l., the external l. of the lateral mesoderm of the embryo, lying adjacent to the ectoderm and together with it constituting the somatopleure.

spindle-celled l., SYN fusiform l.

spinous l., SYN *stratum* spinosum epidermidis.

splanchnic l., the internal l. of the lateral mesoderm, lying adjacent to the endoderm and together with it forming the splanchnopleure.

still l., the l. of the bloodstream in the capillary vessels, next to the wall of the vessel, that flows slowly and transports the white blood cells along the l. wall, while in the center the flow is rapid and transports the red blood cells. SYN plasma l., Poiseuille's space, sluggish l.

subendocardial l., the loose connective tissue l. that joins the endocardium and myocardium; in the ventricles, it contains branches of the conducting system of the heart.

subendothelial l., the thin l. of connective tissue lying between the endothelium and elastic lamina in the intima of blood vessels.

subpapillary l., the vascular l. of the corium.

subserous l., the layer of connective tissue beneath a serous membrane such as that of the periconeum or pericardium. SYN tela subserosa [NA].

superficial l., in a stratified structure, the outermost or topmost of the strata; the stratum nearest the surface. SEE superficial l. of deep cervical fascia, superficial l. of the levator palpebrae superioris muscle, superficial l. of temporalis fascia. SYN lamina superficialis [NA], superficial lamina.

superficial l. of deep cervical fascia, SYN investing l. of deep cervical fascia.

superficial gray l. of superior colliculus, SEE gray l. of superior colliculus.

superficial l. of the levator palpebrae superioris muscle, the superficial fibers of the levator muscle of the superior eyelid which are inserted into the skin of the superior eyelid. SYN lamina superficialis musculi levatoris palpebrae superioris [NA].

superficial l. of temporalis fascia, the superficial part of the temporal fascia attaching to the lateral surface of the zygomatic arch. SYN lamina superficialis fasciae temporalis [NA].

suprachoroid l., SYN suprachoroid *lamina*.

Tomes' granular l., a thin l. of dentin adjacent to the cementum, appearing granular in ground sections; the granules are small uncalcified spaces.

vascular l., SYN vascular *lamina* of choroid.

vascular l. of choroid coat of eye, SYN vascular *lamina* of choroid.

ventricular l., SYN ependymal l.

visceral l., the inner l. of an enveloping sac or bursa which lines the outer surface of the enveloped structure, as opposed to the parietal layer which lines the walls of the occupied space or cavity. The visceral l. is usually thin, delicate and not apparent as being separate, but rather appears to be the outer surface of the structure itself. SYN lamina visceralis [NA].

visceral l. of serous pericardium, the inner part of the serous pericardium applied directly on the heart. SYN epicardium [NA], lamina visceralis pericardii [NA].

visceral l. of tunica vaginalis of testis, the inner part of the tunica vaginalis testis applied directly to the testis and epididymis. SYN lamina visceralis tunicae vaginalis testis [NA].

Waldeyer's zonal l., SYN dorsolateral *fasciculus*.

Weil's basal l., the l. beneath the odontoblasts of the tooth; it contains reticular fibers but few if any cells. SYN Weil's basal zone.

zonular l., (1) a thin l. of white substance covering the upper surface of the thalamus and forming part of the floor of the body of the lateral ventricle; **(2)** a l. of white substance on the surface of the superior colliculus. SYN stratum zonale [NA].

laz·a·ret, laz·a·ret·to (laz′ă-ret, -ret′ō). Obsolete term for: **1.** SYN leprosarium. **2.** A hospital for the treatment of contagious diseases. **3.** A place of detention for persons in quarantine. [It. *lazzaretto,* fr. *lazzaro,* a leper]

lb. Abbreviation for pound.

LBF Abbreviation for *Lactobacillus bulgaricus factor.*

LCAT Abbreviation for lecithin:cholesterol acyltransferase.

l-cone. Long wavelength sensitive cone (red cone).

LD Abbreviation for lethal *dose.*

LDH Abbreviation for *lactate* dehydrogenase.

LDL Abbreviation for low density lipoprotein. See lipoprotein.

LE, L.E. Abbreviation for left eye; *lupus* erythematosus.

leach·ing (lēch′ing). Removal of the soluble constituents of a substance by running water through it. SYN lixiviation. [A.S. *leccan,* to wet]

lead (Pb) (led). A metallic element, atomic no. 82, atomic wt. 207.2; occurs in nature as an oxide or one of the salts, but chiefly as the sulfide, or galena; ^{210}Pb (half-life equal to 22.6 years) has been used in the treatment of certain eye conditions. SYN plumbum.

l. acetate, has been used as an astringent in diarrhea, and in aqueous solution as a wet dressing in certain dermatoses. SYN sugar of lead.

black l., SYN graphite.

l. carbonate, a heavy white powder that is insoluble in water; occasionally, it is used to relieve irritation in dermatitis, but it is used largely in the manufacture of paint and in the arts and is thus productive of l. poisoning. SYN ceruse, white l.

l. chromate, SYN chrome yellow.

l. monoxide, has been used as an ingredient in external applications such as l. plaster. SYN l. oxide (yellow), litharge, massicot.

l. oxide (yellow), SYN l. monoxide.

red l., SYN l. tetroxide.

red oxide of l., SYN l. tetroxide.

l. sulfide, PbS; the native form in which l. is chiefly found. SYN galena.

l. tetraethyl, SYN tetraethyllead.

l. tetroxide, a bright orange-red powder that turns black when heated; used in ointments and plasters. SYN red l., red oxide of l.

white l., SYN l. carbonate.

lead (lēd). An electrocardiographic cable with connections within the electronics of the machine designated for an electrode placed at a particular point on the body surface.

ABC l.'s, the l.'s for recording one kind of vectorcardiogram utilizing the Arrighi triangle; supplanted by XYZ l.'s.

augmented l., electrocardiogram recorded between one limb and two other limbs. The augmented l. are designated aVF, aVL, and aVR for recordings made between the foot (left), left arm, and right arm, respectively, and the other two limbs.

bipolar l., a record obtained with two electrodes placed on different regions of the body, each electrode contributing significantly to the record; e.g., a standard limb l.

CB l., a bipolar chest l. with the negative electrode placed upon the subject's back.

CF l., a bipolar chest l. with the negative electrode placed on the subject's left leg.

chest l.'s, those in which the exploring electrode is on the chest overlying the heart or its vicinity. SYN precordial l.'s, semidirect l.'s.

CL l., a bipolar chest l. with the negative electrode placed on the subject's left arm.

CR l., a bipolar chest l. with the negative electrode placed on the subject's right arm.

direct l., in electrocardiography, a unipolar l. recorded with the exploring electrode placed directly on the surface of the exposed heart.

esophageal l., an electrocardiographic l. passed down the throat into the esophagus to record the electrocardiogram at various levels of the esophagus; especially useful for certain types of arrhythmias. Similarly, a transducer for echocardiography can be passed into the esophagus.

indirect l., SYN standard limb l.

intracardiac l., the record obtained when the exploring electrode is placed within one of the heart's chambers, usually by means of cardiac catheterization.

limb l., one of the three standard l.'s (l.'s I, II, III) or one of the unipolar limb l.'s (aVR, aVL, aVF).

precordial l.'s, SYN chest l.'s.

semidirect l.'s, SYN chest l.'s.

standard limb l., one of the three original bipolar limb l.'s of the clinical electrocardiogram, designated I, II and III: l. I records the potential difference between the right and left arms; l. II the difference between right arm and left leg; and l. III the difference between left arm and left leg. SYN indirect l.

unipolar l.'s, those in which the exploring electrode is on the chest in the vicinity of the heart or on one of the limbs, while the other or indifferent electrode is the central terminal.

V l., a unipolar l. with the central terminal as the indifferent electrode; V is the symbol for unipolar (Latin "U").

leaf·let (lēf′let). A layer of phospholipid; thus, a bilayer has two leaflets.

League of Red Cross So·ci·e·ties. The international federation of national Red Cross and similar societies.

learned help·less·ness. A laboratory model of depression involving both classical (respondent) and instrumental (operant) conditioning techniques; application of unavoidable shock is followed by failure to cope in situations where coping might otherwise be possible.

learn·ing (lern′ing). Generic term for the relatively permanent change in behavior that occurs as a result of practice. SEE ALSO conditioning, forgetting, memory.

incidental l., l. without a direct attempt. SYN passive l.

insight l., the grasp of the solution to a problem without the intervening series of the trial and error steps that are associated with most types of learning (e.g., a monkey housed behind the bars of a cage who, without proceeding through countless hours of futile attempts with one stick or the other, fits two sticks together to retrieve a banana outside the distance measured by either stick alone).

latent l., that l. which is not evident to the observer at the time it occurs, but which is inferred from later performance in which l. is more rapid than would be expected without the earlier experience.

passive l., SYN incidental l.

rote l., the l. of arbitrary relationships, usually by repetition of the l. procedure through memorization and without an understanding of the relationships.

state-dependent l., l. during a specific state of sleep or wakefulness, or during a chemically altered state, where retrieval of learned information (e.g., as measured by performance of a learned response) cannot be demonstrated unless the subject is restored to the state that originally existed during l.

least squares. A principle of estimation invented by Gauss in which the estimates of a set of parameters in a statistical model are the quantities that minimize the sum of squared differences between the observed values of the dependent variable and the values predicted by the model.

Le Bel, Joseph Achille, French chemist, 1847–1930. SEE Le B.-van't Hoff *rule.*

Leber, Theodor, German ophthalmologist, 1840–1917. SEE L.'s idiopathic stellate *neuroretinitis,* hereditary optic *atrophy, plexus; amaurosis* congenita of L.

Le Chatelier, Henri, French physical chemist, 1850–1936. SEE Le C.'s *law, principle.*

lec·i·thal (les′i-thăl). Having a yolk or pertaining to the yolk of any egg; used especially as a suffix. [G. *lekithos,* egg yolk]

lec·i·thin (les′i-thin). Traditional term for 1,2-diacyl-*sn*-glycero-3-phosphocholines or 3-*sn*-phosphatidylcholines, phospholipids that on hydrolysis yield two fatty acid molecules and a molecule each of glycerophosphoric acid and choline. In some varieties of l., both fatty acids are saturated, others contain only unsaturated acids (e.g., oleic, linoleic, or arachidonic acid); in others again, one fatty acid is saturated, the other unsaturated. L.'s are yellowish or brown waxy substances, readily miscible in water in which they appear under the microscope as irregular elongated particles known as "myelin forms," and are found in nervous tissue, especially in the myelin sheaths, in egg yolk, and as essential constituents of animal and vegetable cells. [G. *lekithos,* egg yolk]

l. acyltransferase, SYN lecithin-cholesterol acyltransferase.

l.-cholesterol l., a plasma enzyme that catalyzes the uptake of cholesterol esters by intermediate-density lipoproteins formed by high density lipoproteins.

lec·i·thi·nase (les′i-thi-nās). SYN phospholipase.

l. A, SYN *phospholipase* A$_2$.

l. B, SYN lysophospholipase.

l. C, SYN *phospholipase* C.

l. D, SYN *phospholipase* D.

lec·i·thin-cho·les·ter·ol ac·yl·trans·fer·ase (LCAT). An enzyme that reversibly transfers an acyl residue from a lecithin to cholesterol, forming a 1-acylglycerophosphocholine (a lysolecithin) and a cholesterol ester; a deficiency of this enzyme leads to an accumulation of unesterified cholesterol in plasma resulting in anemia, proteinuria, renal failure, and corneal opacities; LCAT is also low in individuals with fish-eye disease. SYN lecithin acyltransferase.

lec·i·tho·blast (les′i-thō-blast). One of the cells proliferating to form the yolk-sac endoderm. [G. *lekithos,* egg yolk, + *blastos,* germ]

lec·i·tho·pro·tein (les′i-thō-prō′tēn). A conjugated protein, with lecithin as the prosthetic group.

Leclef. SEE Denys-Leclef *phenomenon.*

lec·tin (lek′tin). A protein of primarily plant (usually seed) origin that binds to glycoproteins on the surface of cells causing agglutination, precipitation, or other phenomena resembling the action of specific antibody; l.'s include plant agglutinins (phytoagglutinins, phytohemagglutinins), plant precipitins, and perhaps certain animal proteins; some have mitogenic properties. [L. *lego,* pp. *lectum,* to select, + -in]

le

mitogenic l., a l. that induces the replication of polynucleic acids and the proliferation of lymphocytes.

Lederer, Max, U.S. pathologist, 1885–1952. SEE L.'s *anemia.*

Ledermann, Sully, French psychiatrist. SEE Ledermann *formula.*

ledge (lej). In anatomy, a structure resembling a ledge. SEE ALSO shelf, lamina.

dental l., a band of ectodermal cells growing from the epithelium of the embryonic jaws into the underlying mesenchyme; local buds from the l. give rise to the primordia of the enamel organs of the teeth. SYN dental lamina, dental shelf, dentogingival lamina, enamel l., primary dental lamina.

enamel l., SYN dental l.

Lee, Robert, English physician, 1793–1877. SEE L.'s *ganglion.*

Lee, Roger I., U.S. physician, *1881. SEE L.-White *method.*

leech (lēch). **1.** A bloodsucking aquatic annelid worm (genus *Hirudo,* class Hirudinea) formerly used in medicine for local withdrawal of blood. For various *l.* species, see *Hirudo.* **2.** To treat medically by applying leeches. [A.S. *laece,* a physician; a leech, because of its therapeutic use]

leech·ing (lēch'ing). The former practice of applying leeches to the body to draw blood for therapeutic purposes.

Leede, Carl S., U.S. physician, *1882. SEE Rumpel-L. *sign, test;* L.-Rumpel *phenomenon.*

LEEP Abbreviation for loop electrocautery excision *procedure.*

Leeuwenhoek, Anton van, Dutch microscopist, 1632–1723. SEE L.'s *canals,* under *canal.*

Lefèvre, Paul, 20th century French dermatologist. SEE Papillon-L. *syndrome.*

Le Fort, Léon C., French surgeon and gynecologist, 1829–1893. SEE Le F. I *fracture,* II *fracture,* III *fracture, sound;* Le F.'s *amputation.*

left-foot·ed. SYN sinistropedal.

left-hand·ed. Denoting the habitual or more skillful use of the left hand for writing and for most manual operations. SYN sinistromanual.

left-sid·ed·ness. The normal left-sided location of certain unpaired organs, such as the spleen and most of the stomach.

bilateral l.-s., a syndrome in which normally unpaired organs develop more symmetrically in mirror image; two spleens, one on each side, are usually present, and cardiovascular anomalies are common. SYN polysplenia syndrome.

leg. 1. The segment of the inferior limb between the knee and the ankle; commonly used to mean the entire inferior limb. **2.** A structure resembling a leg. SYN crus (1) [NA].

l. of antihelix, SYN *crus* of antihelix.

Barbados l., SYN elephantiasis.

bow-l., SEE *genu* varum.

elephant l., SYN elephantiasis.

milk l., SYN *phlegmasia* alba dolens.

restless l.'s, SYN restless legs *syndrome.*

rider's l., a strain of the adductor muscles of the thigh.

scaly l., a thickened, encrusted condition of the legs of fowls caused by the mite, *Knemidokoptes mutans.*

tennis l., a rupture of the gastrocnemius muscle at the musculotendinous junction, resulting from forcible contractions of the calf muscles; commonly seen in tennis players.

white l., SYN *phlegmasia* alba dolens.

Legal, Emmo, German physician, 1859–1922. SEE L.'s *test.*

Legendre, Gaston J., French physician, *1887. SEE L.'s *sign.*

Legg, Arthur T., U.S. surgeon, 1874–1939. SEE L.-Calvé-Perthes *disease.*

-legia. Reading, as distinguished from the G. derivatives, *-lexis* and *-lexy,* which signify speech. from G. *legō,* to say. [L. *lego,* to read]

Le·gion·el·la (lē-jŭ-nel'lă). A genus of aerobic, motile, non-acid-fast, non-encapsulated, Gram-negative bacilli (family Legionellaceae) that have a nonfermentative metabolism and require L-cysteine HCl and iron salts for growth; they are water-dwelling

and airborne-spread, and are pathogenic for humans. The type species is *L. pneumophila.*

L. bozeman'ii, a species that causes human pneumonia.

L. dumoffii, a species implicated in pneumonia.

L. feeleii, a species implicated in pneumonia.

L. gormanii, a species implicated in pneumonia.

L. longbeachae, a species implicated in pneumonia.

L. micda'dei, a species that causes Pittsburgh pneumonia, a variant of Legionnaires' disease. Accounts for approximately 60% of *Legionella* pneumonias other than those caused by *L..* SYN Pittsburgh pneumonia agent.

L. pneumo'phila, a species that is the etiologic agent of Legionnaires' disease; believed to grow in plumbing systems or in standing water in ventilation systems. The type species of the genus *L.*

L. wadsworthii, a species implicated in pneumonia.

le·gi·o·nel·lo·sis (lē-jŭ-nel-ō'sis). SYN Legionnaire's *disease.*

le·gu·min (lĕ-gū'min, leg'ū-min). SYN avenin.

le·gu·mi·niv·o·rous (le-gū-mi-niv'ō-rŭs). Feeding on beans, peas, and other legumes.

Lehmann, J.O. Orla, Swedish physician, *1927. SEE Börjeson-Forssman-L. *syndrome.*

Leichtenstern, Otto, German physician, 1845–1900. SEE L.'s *phenomenon, sign.*

Leigh, Denis, British psychiatrist, *1915. SEE L.'s *disease.*

Leiner, Karl, Austrian pediatrician, 1871–1930. SEE L.'s *disease.*

leio-. Smooth. [G. *leios*]

lei·o·der·mia (lī-ō-der'mē-ă). Smooth, glossy skin. [leio- + G. *derma,* skin]

lei·o·my·o·fi·bro·ma (lī-ō-mī'ō-fī-brō'mă). SYN fibroleiomyoma.

lei·o·my·o·ma (lī'ō-mī-ō'mă). A benign neoplasm derived from smooth (nonstriated) muscle. [leio- + G. *mys,* muscle, + *-oma,* tumor]

l. cu'tis, cutaneous eruption of multiple small painful nodules composed of smooth muscle fibers; derived from arrector muscles of hair. SYN dermatomyoma.

parasitic l., a uterine l. which has become detached from the uterus and adherent to another peritoneal surface from which it derives a blood supply.

vascular l., a markedly vascular l., apparently arising from the smooth muscle of blood vessels. SYN angioleiomyoma, angiomyofibroma, angiomyoma.

lei·o·my·o·ma·to·sis (lī'ō-mī-ō-mă-tō'sis). The state of having multiple leiomyomas throughout the body.

lei·o·my·o·mec·to·my (lī'ō-mī-ō-mek'tō-mē). Surgical resection of a leiomyoma, usually of the uterus.

lei·o·my·o·sar·co·ma (lī'ō-mī'ō-sar-kō'mă). A malignant neoplasm derived from smooth (nonstriated) muscle. [leio- + myosarcoma]

lei·ot·ri·chous (lī-ot'ri-kŭs). Having straight hair. [leio- + G. *thrix,* hair]

leipo-. SEE lipo-.

Leipzig yel·low [C.I. 77600]. SYN chrome yellow.

Leishman, Sir William B., Scottish surgeon, 1865–1926. SEE *Leishmania;* L.'s chrome *cells,* under *cell, stain;* L.-Donovan *body.*

Leish·man·ia (lēsh-man'ē-ă). A genus of digenetic, asexual, protozoan flagellates (family Trypanosomatidae) that occur as amastigotes in the macrophages of vertebrate hosts, and as promastigotes in invertebrate hosts and in cultures. Species are largely indistinguishable morphologically, but may be separated by clinical manifestations, geographic distribution and epidemiology, developmental patterns of promastigotes in their sandfly hosts, virulence testing of clones *in vivo,* the effect of test sera on growth in culture, cross-immunity tests, and serotyping with promastigote excreted factors; strains also can be distinguished by various biochemical analyses. Such procedures have identified all of the recognized groups and confirmed the separation of New World leishmaniasis agents into two species complexes, *L. mexicana* and *L. braziliensis.* [W. B. *Leishman*]

L. aethio'pica, an African species of *L.* responsible for human cutaneous leishmaniasis in Ethiopia, with a reservoir of human infection in the rock hyraxes, *Procavia capensis* and *Heterohyrax brucei,* and in Kenya, with reservoirs in the tree hyrax, *Dendrohyrax arboreus,* and the giant rat, *Cricetomys gambianus;* vectors are the sandflies *Phlebotomus longpipes* and *P. pedifer.* It causes a cutaneous leishmaniasis of three types: classical oriental sore, mucocutaneous leishmaniasis, and diffuse cutaneous leishmaniasis; ulceration is late or absent and healing takes one to three years.

L. brazilien'sis, a species that is the causal agent of mucocutaneous leishmaniasis, endemic in southern Mexico and Central and South America, and transmitted by various species of *Lutzomyia* (New World sandflies); forest rodents and other neotropical arboreal animals serve as reservoir hosts. *L. braziliensis* is currently divided into three clinically, epidemiologically, and biochemically distinct strains or subspecies: *L. b. braziliensis, L. b. guyanensis,* and *L. b. panamensis.*

L. brazilien'sis brazilien'sis, the type subspecies of *L. braziliensis* and the agent of mucocutaneous leishmaniasis. A natural reservoir of infection remains unknown, but the proven vector in Brazil is *Lutzomyia (Psychodopygus) wellcomei;* other sandflies may also transmit the infection.

L. brazilien'sis guyanen'sis, a subspecies within the *L. braziliensis* complex from Brazil and Guyana, and the cause of the cutaneous leishmaniasis condition locally known as "pian bois"; the reservoir host in Brazil is the sloth *Choloepus hoffmani* and the vector is the sandfly *Lutzomyia umbratilis.*

L. brazilien'sis panamen'sis, a subspecies of *L. braziliensis* found in Panama, Colombia, and neighboring regions; it causes ulcerating lesions of cutaneous leishmaniasis which do not heal spontaneously and often involve nearby lymphatic tissues, but nasopharyngeal involvement is rare. The sloth *Choloepus hoffmani* is the reservoir in Panama and Costa Rica; the sandfly *Lutzomyia trapidoi* has been proven to be a vector.

L. donova'ni, a species that is the causal agent of visceral leishmaniasis in Mediterranean and adjacent countries, the south central section of the area formerly known as the USSR, eastern India, northern China, Kenya, Ethiopia, and the Sudan; also found in Brazil, Argentina, Colombia, and Venezuela; in the Old World, it is transmitted by various species of *Phlebotomus;* New World vectors are species of *Lutzomyia;* dogs and other carnivores are known as reservoir hosts in some areas. The intracellular amastigote form multiplies in macrophages and produces a reticuloendothelial hyperplasia grossly affecting the spleen and liver, with other lymphoid tissues being involved as well, resulting in severe hepatosplenomegaly which usually is fatal if untreated.

L. donova'ni archibal'di, SEE *L. donovani donovani.*

L. donova'ni chaga'si, a subspecies of *L.* found in South America, chiefly in Brazil, producing visceral leishmaniasis; infections have been found in domestic dogs and in foxes, though the primary reservoir host is unclear. The vector remains undiscovered, and the taxonomic status of this subspecies is uncertain.

L. donova'ni donova'ni, the type subspecies and agent of visceral leishmaniasis in Asia, Africa, and the Indian subcontinent; a few cases occur in the south central section of the area known as the former USSR, and in Iran, Iraq, and possibly Yemen; the dog and jackal are animal reservoirs. The form in Africa may be this subspecies, though the name *L. donovani archibaldi* is also used.

L. donova'ni infan'tum, a strain or subspecies of *L. donovani* that causes visceral leishmaniasis in young children in Mediterranean countries; the reservoir is the domestic dog.

L. furunculo'sa, former name for *L. tropica.*

L. ma'jor, a species responsible for zoonotic cutaneous leishmaniasis in a large area of the Mediterranean region and Asia Minor. The animal reservoirs are usually ground squirrels, such as *Rhombomys opimus* in the area formerly known as the USSR and elsewhere in south central Asia, and other rodents in northwest India, the Middle East, and northern Africa; proven sandfly vectors include *Phlebotomus papatasi, P. duboscqi,* and *P. salehi.* SYN *L. tropica major.*

L. mexica'na, the agent of many forms of cutaneous leishmaniasis, now considered a complex of several subspecies or possibly species, each with distinctive DNA and enzyme characteristics, distribution, and vector-reservoir host association, resulting in distinct manifestations of human leishmaniasis; reservoir hosts are extremely diverse and include a wide array of arboreal rodents as well as marsupials, primates, and small carnivores. Typical disease forms caused by this species are chiclero's ulcer and diffuse cutaneous leishmaniasis, in contrast with mucocutaneous leishmaniasis, more characteristic of *L. braziliensis* infection. SYN *L. tropica mexicana.*

L. mexica'na amazonen'sis, a particularly widespread form of *L. mexicana* in the Amazon basin (Bolivia, Brazil, Colombia, Ecuador, and southern Venezuela), where it infects a variety of forest rodents, the reservoirs of human infection. The disease is rare in humans, but the single or multiple lesions, when induced, rarely heal spontaneously; the disseminated form is common, but nasopharyngeal involvement does not occur. The vector is the sandfly *Lutzomyia flaviscutellata.*

L. mexica'na garnha'mi, a subspecies of *L. mexicana,* found in western Venezuela, causing single or multiple lesions in humans that heal spontaneously in about six months; the probable sandfly vector is *Lutzomyia townsendi.*

L. mexica'na mexica'na, a species described from Mexico, Guatemala, and Belize; agent of a form of New World cutaneous leishmaniasis called chiclero's ulcer, associated with chicle gum and mahogany forest workers. The New World sandfly, *Lutzomyia olmeca,* is a proven vector of this subspecies.

L. mexica'na pifa'noi, a strain of *L. mexicana* accorded species status by those who consider it responsible for the diffuse or disseminated form of cutaneous leishmaniasis. It is responsible for this condition in Venezuela, where it was described, but it is now recognized that several species and subspecies of *L.* cause similar disseminated forms of leishmaniasis in widely separated regions (*L. mexicana amazonensis, L. aethiopica*); absence or suppression of the cell-mediated immune response in the host is also an important factor in induction of diffuse cutaneous leishmaniasis. SYN *L. pifanoi.*

L. mexica'na venezuelen'sis, a recently described subspecies of *L. mexicana* from Venezuela that causes indolent, nodular, single lesions of cutaneous leishmaniasis to develop, sometimes with curable disseminated cutaneous leishmaniasis; infection has also been found in equines.

L. peruvia'na, species of *L.* found infecting humans in the high Andean valleys of Peru and Bolivia; cause of a distinct form of New World cutaneous leishmaniasis called uta.

L. pifa'noi, SYN *L. mexicana pifanoi.*

L. trop'ica, species that is the causal agent of anthroponotic cutaneous leishmaniasis; formerly endemic throughout the Mediterranean basin, the Middle East, parts of the southern section of the area formerly known as the USSR and elsewhere in Asia, and also reported from western Africa; it is transmitted by *Phlebotomus papatasi, P. sergenti,* and related species of sandflies; small rodents such as various ground squirrels serve as reservoir hosts.

L. trop'ica ma'jor, SYN *L. major.*

L. trop'ica mexica'na, SYN *L. mexicana.*

---

leish·man·i·a·sis (lēsh'mă-nī'ă-sis). Infection with a species of *Leishmania* resulting in a clinically ill-defined group of diseases traditionally divided into four major types: 1) visceral l. (kala azar); 2) Old World cutaneous l.; 3) New World cutaneous l.; 4) mucocutaneous l. Each is clinically and geographically distinct and each has in recent years been subdivided further into clinical and epidemiological categories. Transmission is by various sandfly species of the genus *Phlebotomus* or *Lutzomyia.* SEE tropical *diseases,* under *disease.* SYN leishmaniosis.

acute cutaneous l., SYN zoonotic cutaneous l.

American l., l. america'na, SYN mucocutaneous l.

anergic l., SYN diffuse cutaneous l.

anthroponotic cutaneous l., a form of Old World cutaneous l., usually with a prolonged incubation period and confined to urban areas. SYN chronic cutaneous l., dry cutaneous l., urban cutaneous l.

canine l., a mild infection of dogs, usually confined to the

le

muzzle or ears, produced by human disease-causing species of *Leishmania;* dogs therefore are important reservoirs of human infection, such as with visceral l. in the Mediterranean region.

chronic cutaneous l., SYN anthroponotic cutaneous l.

cutaneous l., infection with promastigotes (leptomonads) of *Leishmania tropica* and of *L. major* inoculated into the skin by the bite of an infected sandfly, *Phlebotomus* (commonly *P. papatasi*); it is endemic in parts of Asia Minor, northern Africa, and India, and is known by innumerable names, each indicating its locality (*e.g.,* Aleppo, Baghdad, Delhi, or Jericho boil; Aden ulcer; Biskra button); the ulcer begins as a papule that enlarges to a nodule and then breaks down into an ulcer. Two distinctive clinical and epidemiological diseases are recognized, the more common and widespread zoonotic rural disease with a moist acute form, caused by *L. major,* with reservoir rodent hosts; and an urban, anthroponotic, dry, chronic form of l. caused by *L. tropica,* without a reservoir host, and now largely controlled. SEE zoonotic cutaneous l., anthroponotic cutaneous l. SYN juccuya, Old World l., tropical sore.

diffuse l., SYN diffuse cutaneous l.

diffuse cutaneous l., l. caused by several New and Old World species and strains of *Leishmania* (*L. mexicana amazonensis, L. m. pifanoi,* possibly *L. m. garnhami* and *L. m. venezuelensis;* in Ethiopia, *L. aethiopica,* and unidentified leishmanial agents in Namibia and Tanzania). The condition is associated with a suppressed cell-mediated immune response, so that the non-ulcerating, non-necrotizing cutaneous lesions can spread widely over the body; great numbers of parasite-filled macrophages are found in the dermal lesions. Healing does not appear to occur unless an acquired cellular hypersensitivity can develop. SYN anergic l., diffuse l., disseminated cutaneous l., l. tegumentaria diffusa, pseudolepromatous l.

disseminated cutaneous l., SYN diffuse cutaneous l.

dry cutaneous l., SYN anthroponotic cutaneous l.

infantile l., visceral l. in infants, from *Leishmania donovani infantum.*

lupoid l., SYN l. recidivans.

mucocutaneous l., a grave disease caused by *Leishmania braziliensis braziliensis,* endemic in southern Mexico and Central and South America, except for the equatorial region of Chile; the organism does not invade the viscera, and the disease is limited to the skin and mucous membranes, the lesions resembling the sores of cutaneous l. caused by *L. mexicana* or *L. tropica;* the chancrous sores heal after a time, but some months or years later, fungating and eroding forms of ulceration may appear on the tongue and buccal or nasal mucosa; many variants of the disease exist, marked by differences in distribution, vector, epidemiology, and pathology, which suggest that it may in fact be caused by a number of closely related etiological agents. SEE ALSO espundia. SYN American l., l. americana, nasopharyngeal l., New World l.

nasopharyngeal l., SYN mucocutaneous l.

New World l., SYN mucocutaneous l.

Old World l., SYN cutaneous l.

pseudolepromatous l., SYN diffuse cutaneous l.

l. recid'ivans, a partially healing leishmanial lesion caused by *Leishmania tropica* and characterized by an extreme form of cellular immune response, intense granuloma production, fibrinoid necrosis without caseation, and frequent development of satellite lesions that continue the production of granulomatous tissue without healing, sometimes over a period of many years; organisms are difficult to demonstrate but can be cultured. SYN lupoid l.

rural cutaneous l., SYN zoonotic cutaneous l.

l. tegumenta'ria diffu'sa, SYN diffuse cutaneous l.

urban cutaneous l., SYN anthroponotic cutaneous l.

visceral l., a chronic disease, occurring in India, Assam, China, the area formerly known as the Mediterranean littoral areas, the Middle East, India, Pakistan, China, South and Central America, Asia, Africa caused by *Leishmania donovani* and transmitted by the bite of an appropriate species of sandfly of the genus *Phlebotomus* or *Lutzomyia;* the organisms grow and multiply in macrophages, eventually causing them to burst and liberate amastigote parasites which then invade other macrophages; prolifera-

tion of macrophages in the bone marrow causes crowding out of erythroid and myeloid elements, resulting in leukopenia, and anemia, splenomegaly, and hepatomegaly which are characteristic, along with enlargement of lymph nodes; fever, fatigue, malaise, and secondary infections also occur; different strains of *L. donovani* occur; *L. infantum* in Eurasia, *L. chagasi* in Latin America. SYN Assam fever, black sickness, Burdwan fever, cachectic fever, Dumdum fever, kala azar, tropical splenomegaly.

visceral l., Visceral l. caused by *Leishmania tropica,* cultured from bone marrow aspirates of military patients following Operation Desert Storm.

wet cutaneous l., SYN zoonotic cutaneous l.

zoonotic cutaneous l., a form of cutaneous l. characterized by rural distribution of human cases near infected rodents, particularly communal ground squirrels; characterized by acute rapidly developing dermal lesions that become severely inflamed, with moist necrotizing sores or ulcers that heal in two to eight months after a two to four month incubation period; among nonimmune immigrants, multiple lesions may develop, which heal more slowly and leave disabling or disfiguring scars. A strong delayed hypersensitivity and involvement of immune complexes play a role in necrosis, which is part of the healing process and of the strong specific immunity that follows. SYN acute cutaneous l., rural cutaneous l., wet cutaneous l.

leish·man·i·o·sis (lēsh'man-ē-ō'sis). SYN leishmaniasis.

leish·man·oid (lēsh'mă-noyd). A condition resembling leishmaniasis.

dermal l., SYN post-kala azar dermal l.

post-kala azar dermal l., a chronic, progressive, granulomatous, nonulcerating hypopigmented nodular cutaneous outbreak that may appear 6 months to 5 years after spontaneous or drug cure of visceral leishmaniasis (kala azar); this condition was first described in India and is most characteristic of kala azar in that country. SYN dermal l.

Leiter, Russell G., U.S. psychologist, *1901. SEE L. International Performance *Scale.*

Lejeune, Jerôme J.L.M., French cytogeneticist, *1926. SEE L. *syndrome.*

Lembert, Antoine, French surgeon, 1802–1851. SEE L. *suture;* Czerny-L. *suture.*

le·mic (lē'mik). Relating to plague or any epidemic disease. [G. *loimos,* plague]

Lemli, Luc, 20th century U.S. pediatrician. SEE Smith-L.-Opitz *syndrome.*

lem·mo·blast (lem'ō-blast). In an embryo, a cell of neural crest origin capable of forming a cell of the neurilemma sheath. [G. *lemma,* husk, + *blastos,* germ]

lem·mo·cyte (lem'ō-sīt). One of the cells of the neurolemma. [G. *lemma,* husk, + *kytos,* cell]

lem·nis·cus, pl. **lem·nis·ci** (lem-nis'kŭs, -nis'ī) [NA]. A bundle of nerve fibers ascending from sensory relay nuclei to the thalamus. SYN fillet (1). [L. from G. *lēmniskos,* ribbon or fillet]

acoustic l., SYN lateral l.

auditory l., SYN lateral l.

gustatory l., the uncrossed secondary-sensory fiber system ascending from the rhombencephalic gustatory nucleus to the parabrachial nuclei (rostral pontine level) and directly to the thalamic gustatory nucleus (ventral postero-medial nucleus, pars parvicellularis).

lateral l., a bundle of ascending fibers that originate from the cochlear and auditory relay nuclei of the rhombencephalon, enter the trapezoid body, a transverse fiber stratum in which about half their number decussate, and from here turn rostrally along the lateral side of the spinothalamic tract; in the midbrain, it arches dorsally and enters the inferior colliculus in which all of its fibers terminate; the auditory pathway is transsynaptically extended from here by the brachium of the inferior colliculus to the medial geniculate body of the thalamus, from which in turn the auditory radiation leads to the auditory cortex; intercalated in the trapezoid body and along the ascending trajectory of the l. are several cell groups in which part of the fibers synapse. SYN l. lateralis [NA], acoustic l., auditory l., auditory tract, lateral fillet.

l. latera'lis [NA], SYN lateral l.

medial l., a band of white fibers originating from the gracile and cuneate nuclei and decussating in the lower medulla; thence it passes upward through the center of the medulla oblongata, close to the median raphe; on entering the pons it spreads out laterally to form a flat band ascending over the dorsal border of the pontine nuclei; in the mesencephalon it passes over the dorsal border of the substantia nigra and is displaced laterally by the red nucleus; passing medial to the medial geniculate body, the bundle enters and terminates in the ventral posterior nucleus of the thalamus. Throughout their course, the fibers retain a somatotopic order such that those originating from the gracile nucleus and representing the lower extremity lie lateral to those originating in the cuneate nucleus and representing the arm. The medial l. conveys somatic-sensory information involved in tactile discrimination (two-point discrimination), position sense, and vibration sense. SYN l. medialis [NA], medial fillet, Reil's band (2), Reil's ribbon.

l. media′lis [NA], SYN medial l.

spinal l., SYN spinothalamic *tract*.

l. spina′lis [NA], SYN spinothalamic *tract*.

trigeminal l., collective term denoting the fibers ascending from the sensory nucleus of the trigeminus; one such fiber system originates from the main sensory nucleus, largely decussates, and ascends as the ventral trigeminal l. to join the medial l. with which it enters the ventral posterior nucleus of thalamus, terminating in the mediodorsal region of that nucleus; a second, uncrossed, fiber group follows an ascending course through central parts of the mesencephalic tegmentum ("dorsal trigeminal l."). The trigeminal l. conveys tactile, pain, and temperature impulses from the skin of the face, the mucous membranes of the nasal and oral cavities, and the eye, as well as proprioceptive information from the facial and masticatory muscles. SYN l. trigeminalis [NA].

l. trigemina′lis [NA], SYN trigeminal l.

lem·on (lem′ŏn). The fruit of *Citrus limon* (family Rutaceae); a source of citric and ascorbic acid; the freshly expressed juice of the ripe fruit is used as a refrigerant diuretic in fever, in the form of lemonade. SYN limon. [L. *limon*]

lem·on yel·low. SYN chrome yellow.

Lendrum, A.C., 20th century Scottish pathologist. SEE L.'s phloxine-tartrazine *stain;* Fraser-L. *stain* for fibrin.

Lenègre, Jean, 20th century French cardiologist. SEE L.'s *disease, syndrome.*

length. Linear distance between two points.

arch l., the amount of space required for the permanent teeth as measured from the mesial aspect of the first molar on one side to the mesial aspect of the first molar on the opposite side, as measured through the contact points along an imaginary line of the dental arch.

available arch l., the amount of space available for the permanent teeth around the dental arch from first permanent molar to first permanent molar.

crown-heel l. (CH), l. of an outstretched embryo or fetus from skull vertex to heel. SEE Streeter's developmental horizon(s).

crown-rump l. (CR, CRL), a measurement from the skull vertex to the midpoint between the apices of the buttocks of an embryo or fetus, that permits approximation of embryonic or fetal age.

greatest l., measurement from the cranial to caudal end of the embryo prior to folding.

required arch l., the sum of the mesiodistal widths of the permanent teeth from first permanent molar to first permanent molar.

resting l., the length at rest from which a muscle develops maximum isometric tension.

spinal l. (SL), a measurement from the distal surface of the embryo where the plane passes through the developing eye (this is the cranial limit of the spinal cord) down to the rump.

Lenhossék, Michael (Mihály) von, Hungarian anatomist, 1863–1937. SEE L.'s *processes,* under *process.*

len·i·tive (len′i-tiv). **1.** Soothing; relieving discomfort or pain. **2.** Rarely used term for a demulcent. [L. *lenio,* pp. *lenitus,* to soften, fr. *lenis,* mild]

Lennert, K. SEE L.'s *lymphoma; L. classification.*

Lennox, William G., U.S. neurologist, 1884–1960. SEE L. *syndrome;* L.-Gastaut *syndrome.*

Lenoir, Camille A.H., French anatomist, *1867. SEE L.'s *facet.*

lens (lenz). **1.** A transparent material with one or both surfaces having a concave or convex curve; acts upon electromagnetic energy to cause convergence or divergence of light rays. **2** [NA]. The transparent biconvex cellular refractive structure lying between the iris and the vitreous humor, consisting of a soft outer part (cortex) with a denser part (nucleus), and surrounded by a basement membrane (capsule); the anterior surface has a cuboidal epithelium, and at the equator the cells elongate to become lens fibers. SYN crystalline l. [L. a lentil]

achromatic l., a compound l. made of two or more l.'s having different indices of refraction, so correlated as to minimize chromatic aberration.

acoustic l., in ultrasonography, a l. used to focus or diverge a sound beam; may be simulated by electronic manipulation of signals.

aplanatic l., a l. designed to correct spherical aberration and coma (*q.v.*). SYN periscopic meniscus.

apochromatic l., a compound l. designed to correct both spherical and chromatic aberrations.

aspheric l., a l. with a paraboloidal surface that eliminates spherical aberration.

astigmatic l., SYN cylindrical l.

biconcave l., a l. that is concave on two opposing surfaces. SYN concavoconcave l., double concave l.

biconvex l., a l. with both surfaces convex. SYN convexoconvex l., double convex l.

bifocal l., a l. used in cases of presbyopia, in which one portion is suited for distant vision, the other for reading and close work in general; the reading addition may be cemented to the l., fused to the front surface, or ground in one-piece form; other bifocal l.'s are the flat-top Franklin type, or blended invisible.

cataract l., any l. prescribed for aphakia.

compound l., an optical system of two or more lenses.

concave l., a diverging minus power lens. SYN minus l.

concavoconcave l., SYN biconcave l.

concavoconvex l., a converging meniscus l. that is concave on one surface and convex on the opposite surface.

contact l., a l. that fits over the cornea and sclera or cornea only; used to correct refractive errors.

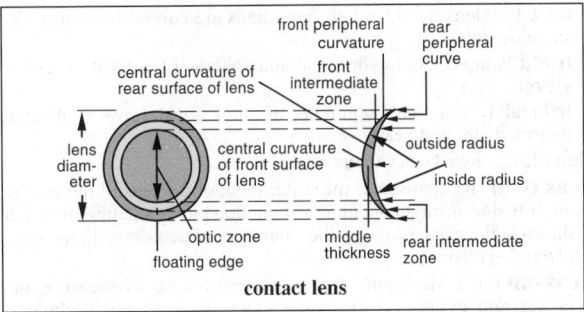

contact lens

convex l., a converging l. SYN plus l.

convexoconcave l., a minus power l. having one surface convex and the opposite surface concave, with the latter having the greater curvature.

convexoconvex l., SYN biconvex l.

corneal l., contact l. of plastic without scleral portions.

crystalline l., SYN lens (2).

cylindrical l. (cyl., C), a l. in which one of the surfaces is curved in one meridian and less curved in the opposite meridian; *e.g.,* a teaspoon or a football. SYN astigmatic l.

decentered l., a l. so mounted that the visual axis does not pass through the axis of the l.

dislocation of l., SYN *ectopia* lentis.

double concave l., SYN biconcave l.

double convex l., SYN biconvex l.

eye l., the upper of the two planoconvex l.'s of Huygens' ocular. SYN ocular l.

field l., the lower of the two planoconvex l.'s of Huygens' ocular.

Fresnel l., a l. with a surface consisting of a concentric series of zones that duplicate the power of a l. or prism but with less thickness. SYN lighthouse l.

immersion l., an objective (for a microscope) constructed in such a manner that the lower l. may be moved downward into direct contact with a fluid which is placed on the object being examined; by using a fluid with a refractive index closely similar to that of glass, the loss of light is minimized.

lighthouse l., SYN Fresnel l.

meniscus l., a l. having a spherical concave curve on one side and a spherical convex curve on the other. SYN meniscus (1).

minus l., SYN concave l.

multifocal l., a l. with segments providing two or more powers; commonly, a trifocal l.

ocular l., SYN eye l.

omnifocal l., a l. for near and distant vision in which the reading portion is a continuously variable curve.

orthoscopic l., a spectacle l. corrected for distortion and curvature of the periphery.

periscopic l., a lens with 1.25 D base curve.

photochromic l., a light-sensitive spectacle l. that reduces light transmission in sunlight and increases transmission in reduced light.

planoconcave l., a l. that is flat on one side and concave on the other.

planoconvex l., a l. that is flat on one side and convex on the other.

plus l., SYN convex l.

safety l., a l. that meets government specifications of impact resistance; the increased impact resistance required for safety l.'s is obtained by tempering, by an ion-exchange process, or by using laminated or plastic lenses.

slab-off l., a spectacle l. with a base-up prism below; used in unequal myopia to equalize image displacement when reading.

spherical l. (S, sph.), a l. in which all refracting surfaces are spherical.

spherocylindrical l., a combined spherical and cylindrical l., one surface being spherical, the other cylindrical. SYN spherocylinder.

toric l., a lens in which both meridians are curved but not to the same degree.

trial l.'s, a series of cylindrical and spherical l.'s used in testing vision.

trifocal l., a l. with segments of three focal powers: distant, intermediate, and near.

lens l. c., SYN Geneva lens measure.

lens·ec·to·my (len-sek'tō-mē). Removal of the lens of the eye by an infusion-aspiration cutter; often done by puncture incision through the pars plana in the course of vitrectomy. [lens + G. *ektomē*, excision]

lens·om·e·ter (len-zom'ĕ-ter). An instrument to measure the power and cylindrical axis of a spectacle lens. SYN focimeter, vertometer. [lens + G. *metron*, measure]

lens·op·a·thy (lenz-op'ă-thē). The process by which tear proteins are deposited on a contact lens. [lens + G. *pathos*, suffering]

len·ti·co·nus (len-ti-kō'nŭs). Conical projection of the anterior or posterior surface of the lens of the eye, occurring as a developmental anomaly. [lens + L. *conus*, cone]

len·tic·u·la (len-tik'yū-lă). **1.** SYN lenticular *nucleus.* **2.** SYN lentigo. [L. dim. of *lens*]

len·tic·u·lar (len-tik'yū-lăr). **1.** Relating to or resembling a lens of any kind. **2.** Of the shape of a lentil. [L. *lenticula*, a lentil]

len·tic·u·lo-op·tic (len-tik'yū-lō-op'tik). Relating to the lentiform nucleus and the optic tract; specifically refers to branches of the middle cerebral artery considered to supply these structures.

len·tic·u·lo-pap·u·lar (len-tik'yū-lō-pap'yū-lăr). Indicating an eruption with dome-shaped or lens-shaped papules.

len·tic·u·lo·stri·ate (len-tik'yū-lō-strī'āt). Relating to the lenticular nucleus and the caudate nucleus; specifically refers to branches of the middle cerebral artery supplying these gray masses.

len·tic·u·lo·tha·lam·ic (len-tik'yū-lō-tha-lam'ik). Pertaining to the lentiform (lenticular) nucleus and the thalamus.

len·tic·u·lus, pl. **len·tic·u·li** (len-tik'yū-lŭs, -lī). Seldom-used term for an intraocular lens prosthesis placed in the anterior or posterior chamber of the eye, or attached to the iris after cataract extraction. SYN prosthetophacos, pseudophacos. [L. dim. of *lens, lentis,* a little lens]

len·ti·form (len'ti-fōrm). Lens-shaped.

len·tig·i·nes (len-tij'i-nēz). Plural of lentigo. [L.]

len·tig·i·no·sis (len-tij-i-nō'sis). Presence of lentigenes in very large numbers or in a distinctive configuration.

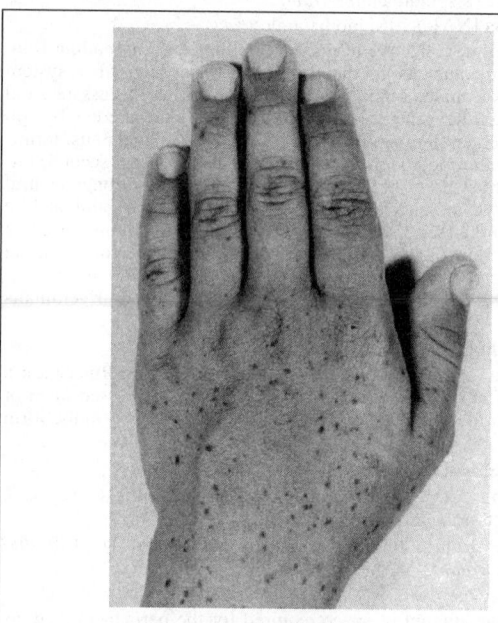

lentiginosis

centrofacial l. [MIM*151000 & MIM*151001], uncommon autosomal dominant syndrome of small hyperpigmented macules in a horizontal band across the center of the face at one year, increasing in number up to ten years, and associated with skeletal and neural defects.

generalized l., lentigines occurring singly or in groups from infancy onward.

len·ti·glo·bus (len-ti-glō'bŭs). Rare congenital anomaly with a spheroid elevation on the posterior surface of the lens of the eye. [lens + L. *globus*, sphere]

len·ti·go, pl. **len·tig·i·nes** (len-tī'gō, len-tij'i-nēz). A brown macule resembling a freckle except that the border is usually regular, and microscopic proliferation of rete ridges is present; scattered melanocytes are seen in the basal cell layer. SEE ALSO junction *nevus.* SYN lenticula (2). [L. fr. *lens (lent-),* a lentil]

l. maligna, a brown or black mottled, irregularly outlined, slowly enlarging lesion resembling a l. in which there are increased numbers of scattered atypical melanocytes in the epidermis, usually occurring on the face of older persons; after many years the dermis may be invaded and the lesion is then termed l. maligna melanoma. SYN Hutchinson's freckle, melanotic freckle.

senile l., a variably pigmented l. occurring on exposed skin of older Caucasians. SYN liver spot, solar l.

solar l., SYN senile l.

Len·ti·vir·i·nae (len'ti-vir'i-nē). A subfamily of viruses (family

Retroviridae) that includes the slow viruses of sheep (visna virus and maedi virus) and human T-cell lymphotropic viruses, including human immunodeficiency viruses 1 and 2. The viruses resemble the C-type RNA tumor viruses (Oncovirinae) in many ways, including production of reverse transcriptase. [L. *lentus,* sluggish, slow]

len·ti·vi·rus (len'ti-vī-rŭs). Any virus of the subfamily Lentivirinae.

len·to·gen·ic (len-tō-jen'ik). Denoting the virulence of a virus capable of inducing lethal infection in embryonic hosts after a long incubation period and an inapparent infection in immature and adult hosts; the term is used in characterizing Newcastle disease virus, particularly strains used as vaccines administered in water or as sprays. [L. *lentus,* sluggish, inactive, + G. *-gen,* producing]

len·tu·la, len·tu·lo (len'tyū-lă, -lō). A motorized, flexible, spiral wire instrument used in dentistry to apply paste filling material into the root canal(s) of a tooth. [L. *lentus,* pliant, flexible]

le·on·ti·a·sis (lē-on-tī'ă-sis). The ridges and furrows on the forehead and cheeks of patients with advanced lepromatous leprosy, giving a leonine appearance. SYN leonine facies. [G. *leōn (leont-),* lion]

l. os'sea, SYN megacephaly.

LEOPARD [MIM*151101] Acronym for *l*entigines (multiple), *e*lectrocardiographic abnormalities, *o*cular hypertelorism, *p*ulmonary stenosis, *a*bnormalities of genitalia, *r*etardation of growth, and *d*eafness (sensorineural).

leop·ard's bane. SYN arnica.

Leopold, Christian G., German physician, 1846–1911. SEE L.'s *maneuvers,* under *maneuver.*

Lepehne, Georg, German physician, *1887. SEE L.-Pickworth *stain.*

lep·er (lep'er). A person who has leprosy. [G. *lepra*]

le·pid·ic (lě-pid'ik). Relating to scales or a scaly covering layer. [G. *lepis (lepid-),* scale, rind]

Lep·i·dop·tera (lep-i-dop'ter-ă). An order of insects comprised of the moths and butterflies, characterized by wings covered with delicate scales. [G. *lepis,* scale, + *pteron,* wing]

lep·i·do·sis (lep-i-dō'sis). Any scaly or desquamating eruption. [G. *lepis,* scale, rind, + *-osis,* condition]

Lep·or·i·pox·vi·rus (lep'ō-ri-poks'vī-rŭs). The genus of viruses (family Poxviridae) that comprises the fibroma and myxoma viruses of rabbits; unlike the orthopoxviruses, they are ether-sensitive. [L. *leporis,* gen. of *lepus,* a hare, + virus]

lep·o·thrix (lep'ō-thriks). SYN *trichomycosis* axillaris. [G. *lepos,* rind, husk, + *thrix,* hair]

lep·ra (lep'ră). Obsolete term for leprosy. [G. leprosy]

lep·re·chaun·ism (lep'rě-kawn-izm) [MIM*246200]. A congenital form of dwarfism characterized by extreme growth retardation, endocrine disorders, and emaciation, with elfin facies and large low-set ears; autosomal recessive inheritance. SYN Donohue's disease, Donohue's syndrome. [Irish *leprechaun,* elf]

lep·rid. Early cutaneous lesion of leprosy. [G. *lepra,* leprosy, + *-id* (1)]

le·prol·o·gist (lě-prol'ŏ-jist). A physician who specializes in the study of leprosy.

le·prol·o·gy (lě-prol'ŏ-jē). The science and study of leprosy. [G. *lepra,* leprosy, + *logos,* study]

le·pro·ma (lě-prō'mă). A fairly well-circumscribed discrete focus of granulomatous inflammation, caused by *Mycobacterium leprae,* which consists chiefly of an accumulation of large mononuclear phagocytic cells in which the cytoplasm seems finely vacuolated (*i.e.,* foam cells); the foamlike character of the macrophages is related to the engulfing of numerous acid-fast organisms. [G. *lepros,* scaly, + *-oma,* tumor]

lep·rom·a·tous (lep-rō'mă-tŭs). Pertaining to, or characterized by, the features of a leproma.

lep·ro·min (lep'rō-min). An extract of tissue infected with *Mycobacterium leprae* used in skin tests to classify the stage of leprosy. SEE ALSO lepromin *reaction,* test.

lep·ro·sar·i·um (lep'rō-sar'ē-ŭm). A hospital especially designed for the care of those suffering from leprosy, especially those who need expert care. SYN lazaret (1), lazaretto.

lep·rose (lep'rōs). SYN leprous.

lep·ro·sery (lep'rō-ser-ē). A leper home or colony.

lep·ro·stat·ic (lep-rō-stat'ik). **1.** Inhibiting to the growth of *Mycobacterium leprae.* **2.** An agent having this action.

lep·ro·sy (lep'rō-sē). **1.** A name used in the Bible to describe various cutaneous diseases, especially those of a chronic or contagious nature, which probably included psoriasis and leukoderma. **2.** Chronic granulomatous infection caused by *Mycobacterium leprae* (Hansen's bacillus) and affecting various parts of the body including the skin. SYN Hansen's disease. [G. *lepra,* from *lepros,* scaly]

anesthetic l., a form of l. chiefly affecting the nerves, marked by hyperesthesia succeeded by anesthesia, and by paralysis, ulceration, and various trophic disturbances, terminating in gangrene and mutilation. SYN Danielssen's disease, Danielssen-Boeck disease, dry l., trophoneurotic l.

articular l., a late stage of anesthetic l. SYN mutilating l.

borderline l., a form of l. that is very unstable immunologically; the cutaneous nerves frequently present bacilli, but the lepromin test is usually negative; cutaneous lesions are comprised of flat bands or plaques. SYN dimorphous l.

dimorphous l., SYN borderline l.

dry l., SYN anesthetic l.

histoid l., a form of lepromatous l. with lesions microscopically resembling dermatofibromas or other spindle-celled tumors.

indeterminate l., a transitory form of l. in which the immunologic status is not yet formed, and the histologic and clinical features are not yet characteristic of any of the major types of l.

lazarine l., SYN Lucio's l. [*Lazarus,* Biblical character]

lepromatous l., a form of l. in which nodular cutaneous lesions are infiltrated, have ill-defined borders, and are bacteriologically positive; the lepromin test is negative, *i.e.,* the immunologic mechanism of the patient is not responsive to the *Mycobacterium leprae* infection.

Lucio's l., an acute form occurring in pure diffuse lepromatous l. presenting irregularly shaped, intensely erythematous, tender plaques, especially of the legs, with tendency to ulceration and scarring. SYN lazarine l., Lucio's leprosy phenomenon.

macular l., a form of tuberculoid l. in which the lesions are small, hairless, and dry, and are erythematous in light skin and hypopigmented or copper-colored in dark skin.

Malabar l., SYN elephantiasis.

mouse l., murine l., SYN rat l.

mutilating l., SYN articular l.

nodular l., SYN tuberculoid l.

rat l., a slowly but progressively fatal form of l. occurring in rats, caused by *Mycobacterium lepraemurium;* it appears in two forms, glandular and musculocutaneous; causes induration, alopecia, and eventually ulceration. SYN mouse l., murine l.

smooth l., SYN tuberculoid l.

trophoneurotic l., SYN anesthetic l.

tuberculoid l., a benign, stable, and resistant form of the disease in which the lepromin reaction is strongly positive and in which the lesions are erythematous, insensitive, infiltrated plaques with clear-cut edges. SYN nodular l., smooth l.

lep·rot·ic (lep-rot'ik). SYN leprous.

lep·rous (lep'rŭs). Relating to or suffering from leprosy. SYN leprose, leprotic.

⊘-lepsis, -lepsy. A seizure. [G. *lēpsis*]

lep·tan·dra (lep-tān'dră). Dried rhizome and roots of *Veronicastrum virginicum* (family Serophulariaceae). Indigenous to North America. Formerly used as a cathartic. SYN black root, Culver's root.

⊘lepto-. Light, thin, frail. [G. *leptos,* slender, delicate, weak]

lep·to·ceph·a·lous (lep-tō-sef'ă-lŭs). Having an abnormally tall, narrow cranium. [lepto- + G. *kephalē,* head]

lep·to·ceph·a·ly (lep-tō-sef'ă-lē). A malformation characterized by an abnormally tall, narrow cranium. [lepto- + G. *kephalē,* head]

lep·to·chroa (lep-tō-krō′ă). Abnormally delicate skin. [lepto- + G. *chrōa*, skin]

lep·to·chro·mat·ic (lep′tō-krō-mat′ik). Having a very fine chromatin network.

lep·to·cyte (lep′tō-sīt). A target or Mexican hat cell, *i.e.*, an unusually thin or flattened red blood cell in which there is a central rounded area of pigmented material, a middle clear zone that contains no pigment, and an outer pigmented rim at the edge of the cell. L.'s are thought to be erythrocytes in which the cellular envelope or membrane is unusually large in proportion to its contents. [lepto- + G. *kytos*, cell]

lep·to·cy·to·sis (lep′tō-sī-tō′sis). The presence of leptocytes in the circulating blood, as in thalassemia, some instances of jaundice (even in the absence of anemia), occasional examples of hepatic disease (in the absence of jaundice), and some patients who have had the spleen removed.

lep·to·dac·ty·lous (lep-tō-dak′ti-lŭs). Having slender fingers. [lepto- + G. *daktylos*, finger]

lep·to·der·mic (lep-tō-der′mik). Thin-skinned. [lepto- + G. *derma*, skin]

lep·to·me·nin·ge·al (lep′tō-me-nin′jē-ăl). Pertaining to the leptomeninges.

lep·to·me·nin·ges, lep·to·me·ninx, sing. **lep·to·me·ninx** (lep-tō-me-nin′jēz, lep′tō-mē′ninks, lep′tō-mē′ninks). The two delicate layers of the meninges, the arachnoid mater and pia mater (vs. the tough pachymeninx or dura mater), considered together; by this concept, the arachnoid and pia are two parts of a single layer, much like the parietal and visceral layers of a serous membrane or bursa; although separated by the subarachnoid space they are connected via the arachnoid trabeculae and become continuous where the nerves and filum terminale exit the subarachnoid space (the cerebrospinal fluid-filled space bounded by the leptomeninges). SEE ALSO arachnoid, pia mater. SYN meninx tenuis, pia-arachnoid, piarachnoid. [lepto- + G. *mēninx*, pl. *mēninges*, membrane]

lep·to·men·in·gi·tis (lep′tō-men-in-jī′tis). Inflammation of leptomeninges. SEE ALSO arachnoiditis. SYN pia-arachnitis.

basilar l., inflammation of the arachnoid at the base of the brain; often found in chronic meningitis of tuberculous, luetic, or mycotic origin.

lep·to·mere (lep′tō-mēr). A very minute particle of living matter; Asclepiades believed the body was composed of an aggregation of vast numbers of l.'s. [lepto- + G. *meros*, part]

lep·to·mo·nad (lep′tō-mō′nad, lep-tom′ŏ-nad). **1.** Common name for a member of the genus *Leptomonas*. **2.** SEE promastigote.

Lep·tom·o·nas (lep′tō-mō′nas, lep-tom′ŏ-nŭs). A genus of asexual, monogenetic, parasitic flagellates (family Trypanosomatidae) commonly found in the hindgut of insects. [lepto- + G. *monas*, unit]

lep·to·ne·ma (lep-tō-nē′mă). SYN leptotene. [lepto- + G. *nēma*, thread]

lep·to·pho·nia (lep′tō-fō′nē-ă). SYN hypophonia. [lepto- + G. *phōnē*, sound, voice]

lep·to·phon·ic (lep′tō-fon′ik). Weak-voiced.

lep·to·po·dia (lep-tō-pō′dē-ă). The condition of having slender feet. [lepto- + G. *pous*, foot]

lep·to·pro·so·pia (lep′tō-prō-sō′pē-ă). Narrowness of the face. [lepto- + G. *prosōpon*, face]

lep·to·pro·so·pic (lep′tō-prō-sō′pik). Having a thin, narrow face. Cf. leptosomatic.

lep·tor·rhine (lep′tō-rīn). Having a thin nose. Applied to a skull with a nasal index below 47 (Frankfort agreement) or 48 (Broca). [lepto- + G. *rhis*, nose]

lep·to·scope (lep′tō-skōp). An apparatus for measuring cell membranes.

lep·to·so·mat·ic, lep·to·som·ic (lep′tō-sō-mat′ik, -tō-sō′mik). Having a slender, light, or thin body. [lepto- + G. *sōma*, body]

Lep·to·spi·ra (lep′tō-spī′ră). A genus of aerobic bacteria (order Spirochaetales) containing thin, tightly coiled organisms 6 to 20 μm in length. They possess an axial filament, and one or both

ends may be bent into a semicircular hook. They stain with difficulty except with Giemsa's stain or silver impregnation. Associated with icterohemorrhagic fever. The type species is *L. interrogans*. [lepto- + G. *speira*, a coil]

L. inter′rogans, a species containing more than 170 named parasitic or pathogenic serovars, including *L. interrogans serovar- canicola, -grippotyphosa, -pomona, -icterohaemorrhagiae, - autumnalis* (implicated in Fort Bragg fever), *-ballum,*, and *- australis*. Causative agent of leptospirosis. It is the type species of the genus *L.*

lep·to·spire (lep′tō-spīr). Common name for any organism belonging to the genus *Leptospira*.

lep·to·spi·ro·sis (lep′tō-spī-rō′sis). Infection with *Leptospira interrogans*.

anicteric l., infection with one of the species of the *Leptospira* group, usually mild, with limited liver and kidney involvement, as opposed to Weil's *disease*.

l. icterohemorrhagica (ik′ter-ō-hem-ōr-aj′ĭ-kă), SYN icterohemorrhagic *fever*.

lep·to·spi·ru·ria (lep′tō-spī-rū′rē-ă). Presence of species of the genus *Leptospira* in the urine, as a result of leptospirosis in the renal tubules.

lep·to·tene (lep′tō-tēn). Early stage of prophase in meiosis in which the chromosomes contract and become visible as long filaments well separated from each other. SYN leptonema. [lepto- + G. *tainia*, band, tape]

lep·to·thri·co·sis (lep′tō-thri-kō′sis). Obsolete term for any disease caused by the now invalid genus *Leptothrix*.

Lep·to·thrix (lep′tō-thriks). Invalid name for a genus of organisms that would probably now be classified as actinomycetes, nocardiae, or corynebacteria.

Lep·to·trich·ia (lep-tō-trik′ē-ă). A genus of anaerobic, nonmotile bacteria containing Gram-negative, straight or slightly curved rods, 5 to 15 μm in length, with one or both ends rounded, often pointed. Granules are distributed evenly along the long axis, and one or more large granules may localize near the end of the cell. Branched or clubbed forms do not occur. Two or more cells join together and form septate filaments of varying length; in older cultures, filaments up to 200 μm may form and twist around each other; large, coccoid bodies may be found within a filament as a cell lyses. Carbon dioxide is essential for optimal growth. Lactic acid is produced from glucose. These organisms occur in the oral cavity of humans. The type species is *L. buccalis*. [lepto- + G. *thrix*, hair]

L. bucca′lis, a species found in the human mouth; it is the type species of the genus *L.*

Lep·to·trom·bid·i·um (lep′tō-trom-bid′ē-ŭm). An important genus of trombiculid mites, formerly considered a subgenus of the genus *Trombicula*, which includes all of the vectors of scrub typhus (tsutsugamushi disease). Members of *L.* that serve as vectors of scrub typhus are within the *L. deliense* group: *L. akamushi* is the classical vector in Japan; *L. deliense* is the primary vector, extending from New Guinea, Australia, the Philippines, China, and Southeast Asia to western Pakistan; *L. fletcheri* is found in Malaysia, New Guinea, and the Philippines. Some eight other species have also been implicated in scrub typhus transmission in more limited areas.

L. akamu′shi, one of two species, the other being *L. deliensis* (*T. deliensis*), implicated in the transmission of *Rickettsia tsutsugamushi*, agent of tsutsugamushi disease in Japan and elsewhere in the Orient; the larvae of these species are characteristic parasites of rodents, which therefore are reservoirs of human infections, although the mites themselves are also reservoirs, as the rickettsial parasites are transovarially transmitted from generation to generation (a requirement for transmission to humans as only larval mites feed parasitically and then only once in their lifetimes). SYN *Trombicula akamushi*.

ler·go·trile (ler′gō-trīl). A derivative of ergot which exerts agonistic properties on dopamine receptors; similar to bromocriptine and lisuride.

Leri, André, French orthopedic surgeon, 1875–1930. SEE L.'s *pleonosteosis, sign*; L.-Weill *disease, syndrome*.

Leriche, René, French surgeon, 1879–1955. SEE L.'s *operation, syndrome.*

Lermoyez, Marcel, French otolaryngologist, 1858–1929. SEE L.'s *syndrome.*

Lerner, I.M., U.S. population geneticist, 1910–1967. SEE L. *homeostasis.*

Leroy, Edgar August, French physician, *1883. SEE Fiessinger-L.-Reiter *syndrome.*

LES Acronym for lower esophageal *sphincter;* Lambert-Eaton *syndrome.*

les·bi·an (lez′bē-ăn). **1.** A female homosexual or a female homosexual lifestyle. **2.** One who practices lesbianism. SEE gay.

les·bi·an·ism (lez′bē-ăn-izm). Homosexuality between women. SYN sapphism. [G. *lesbios,* relating to the island of Lesbos]

Lesch, Michael, U.S. pediatrician, *1939. SEE L.-Nyhan *syndrome.*

Leser, Edmund, German surgeon, 1828–1916. SEE L.-Trélat *sign.*

le·sion (lē′zhŭn). **1.** A wound or injury. **2.** A pathologic change in the tissues. **3.** One of the individual points or patches of a multifocal disease. [L. *laedo,* pp. *laesus,* to injure]

Baehr-Lohlein l., SYN Lohlein-Baehr l.

benign lymphoepithelial l., benign tumor-like masses of lymphoid tissue in the parotid gland, containing scattered small, mainly solid islands of epithelial cells. SYN Godwin tumor.

Bracht-Wachter l., a focal collection of lymphocytes and mononuclear cells within the myocardium in bacterial endocarditis.

caviar l., a dilated vein or varicule existing in the venous collecting system under the tongue.

coin l. of lungs, SYN nodular *opacity.*

Councilman's l., SYN Councilman *body.*

Dreulofoy's l., an abnormally large submucosal artery located in the proximal stomach that may be the site of acute and recurrent episodes of massive hemorrhage.

Duret's l., small hemorrhage(s) in the floor of the fourth ventricle or beneath the aqueduct of Sylvius.

Ghon's primary l., SYN Ghon's *tubercle.*

gross l., a l. plainly visible to the naked eye.

Hill-Sachs l., an irregularity seen in the head of the humerus following dislocation of the shoulder; caused by impaction of the head of the humerus against the edge of the glenoid.

Janeway l., one of the stigmata of infectious endocarditis: irregular, erythematous, flat, painless macules on the palms, soles, thenar and hypothenar eminences of the hands, tips of the fingers, and plantar surfaces of the toes; rarely a diffuse rash. In acute endocarditis the lesions may be hemorrhagic or purple.

Lennert's l., SYN Lennert's *lymphoma.*

Lohlein-Baehr l., focal embolic glomerulonephritis occurring in bacterial endocarditis. SYN Baehr-Lohlein l.

lower motor neuron l., injury to motor cells in the brainstem or spinal cord, or of the axons derived from them.

Mallory-Weiss l., laceration of the gastric cardia, as seen in the Mallory-Weiss syndrome. SYN Mallory-Weiss tear.

precancerous l., a noninvasive l. with a predictable likelihood of becoming malignant; *e.g.,* actinic keratosis.

radial sclerosing l., a variant of sclerosing adenosis of the breast with central scar formation and radiating hyperplastic ducts. SYN radial scar.

ring-wall l., a small ring hemorrhage in the brain that stimulates proliferation of a glial ring.

supranuclear l., injury to cerebral descending (corticonuclear) fibers above the brainstem or spinal motor nerve nucleus. SYN upper motor neuron l.

upper motor neuron l., SYN supranuclear l.

wire-loop l., thickening of the basement membrane, with fibrinoid staining, of scattered peripheral capillaries in renal glomeruli; characteristic of renal involvement in systemic lupus erythematosus; the appearance of an affected capillary wall resembles a loop used in microbiology.

Lesser, Ladislaus Leo, German surgeon born in Poland, 1846–1925.

Lesser's tri·an·gle. See under triangle.

Lesshaft, Pjotr F., Russian physician, 1836–1909. SEE L.'s *triangle.*

LET Abbreviation for linear energy *transfer.*

le·thal (lē′thăl). Pertaining to or causing death; denoting especially the causal agent. [L. *letalis,* fr. *letum,* death]

clinical l., a disorder that culminates in premature death.

l. equivalent, expression used of the genetic load of recessive genes in heterozygous state that if in homozygous state would cause death or carry a risk of death. The expected number of deaths from all such genes is expressed in l. equivalent.

genetic l., a disorder that prevents effective reproduction by those affected; *e.g.,* Klinefelter syndrome.

le·thal·i·ty (lē-thal′i-tē). The quality or state of being lethal.

leth·ar·gy (leth′ar-jē). A state of deep and prolonged unconsciousness, resembling profound slumber, from which one can be aroused but into which one immediately relapses. [G. *lēthargis,* drowsiness]

LETS Acronym for *large, external transformation-sensitive* fibronectin. SEE fibronectins.

Letterer, Erich, German pathologist, *1895. SEE L.-Siwe *disease.*

Leu Symbol for leucine radical.

△**leuc-, leuco-.** White; white blood cell. SEE leuko-, leuk-. [G. *leukos,* white]

leu·cin (lū′sin). SYN leukin.

leu·cine (Leu, L) (lū′sēn). (CH₃)₂CHCH₂CH(N₃⁺)COO⁻; 2-Amino-4-methylvaleric acid; the L-isomer is one of the amino acids of proteins; a nutritionally essential amino acid.

l. aminopeptidase, aminopeptidase (cytosol).

l. dehydrogenase, an enzyme that catalyzes the reaction of L-l., water, and NAD⁺ to produce NADH, ammonia, and 4-methyl-2-oxopentanoate; used in the treatment of certain tumors.

l. zipper, a structural motif found in a number of proteins (*e.g.,* some of the DNA-binding regulatory proteins) in which leucyl residues align along one edge of the helix and can interdigitate with a similar structure on another protein molecule. [Zipper, orig. a trademark for a fastening device with two rows of interlocking teeth]

leu·ci·no·sis (lū′si-nō′sis). A condition in which there is an abnormally large proportion of leucine in the tissues and body fluids.

leu·cin·u·ria (lū-si-nū′rē-ă). The excretion of leucine in the urine.

Leu·co·cy·to·zo·on (lū′kō-sī-tō-zō′on). A genus of sporozoan parasites (family Plasmodiidae, suborder Haemosporina) that attack the immature red blood cells of birds and are capable of causing acute outbreaks of disease, particularly in turkeys and ducks; vectors are black flies, *Simulium* species, and the blood-sucking gnat *Culicoides.* SYN *Leukocytozoon.* [G. *leukos,* white, + *kytos,* cell, + *zōon,* animal]

L. marchou′xi, a species of unknown pathogenicity, but fairly common in wild doves and pigeons.

L. sabraze′si, a species that is a cause of leucocytozoonosis of chickens, particularly in Indochina, Malaysia, India, Sumatra, and Java.

L. simon′di, a species that causes disease in domestic and wild ducks, geese, and related waterfowl in the northern U.S. and Canada; it is severely pathogenic, especially in young birds.

L. smith′i, a species that causes disease in domestic turkeys.

leu·co·cy·to·zo·o·no·sis (lū′kō-sī′tō-zo-ō-nō′sis). Infection of ducks, turkeys, chickens, pigeons, and doves with species of the protozoan genus *Leucocytozoon.* The disease is most acute and damaging in young turkeys and ducks, and is characterized by enlargement of the spleen and liver, anemia, listlessness, weakness, and frequently death. SYN leukocytozoonosis.

leu·co·har·mine (lū-kō-har′mēn). SYN harmine.

leu·co·line (lū′kō-lēn). SYN quinoline (1).

leu·co·meth·yl·ene blue (lu′kō-meth′i-lēn). The reduced and colorless form of methylene blue. SYN methylene white.

Leu·co·nos·toc (lū-kō-nos′tok). A genus of microaerophilic to facultatively anaerobic bacteria (family Lactobacillaceae) con-

le

taining Gram-positive, spherical cells which may, under certain conditions, lengthen and become pointed and even form rods. Lactic and acetic acids are produced by these organisms. They are found in plant juices and in milk. The type species is *L. mesenteroides.* [G. *leukos,* white, + *nostoc,* a genus of algae (a word coined by Paracelsus)]

L. mesenteroi′des, a species found in fermenting vegetables and other plant materials and in prepared meat products; it is an active slime (dextran) producer, the dextran commonly used as a plasma expander; it is the type species of the genus *L.*

leu·co pa·tent blue (lū′kō pat′ent) [C.I. 42051]. A sulfonated triphenylmethane dye reduced and decolorized with zinc and acetic acid to produce a stable solution; used to demonstrate hemoglobin peroxidase. SYN patent blue V.

leu·co·vo·rin (lū′kō-vōr-in). SYN folinic acid.

l. calcium, the calcium salt of leucovorin (folinic acid); used to counteract toxic effects of folic acid antagonists, for the treatment of megaloblastic anemias, and as an adjunct to cyanocobalamin in pernicious anemia. SYN calcium folinate.

Leudet, Théodor E., French physician, 1825–1887. SEE L.'s *tinnitus.*

leu·en·keph·a·lin (lū-en-kef′ă-lin). SEE enkephalins.

△**leuk-.** SEE leuko-.

leuk·a·ne·mia (lū-kă-nē′mē-ă). Former term for erythroleukemia. [leukemia + anemia]

leuk·a·phe·re·sis (lū′kă-fĕ-rē′sis). A procedure, analogous to plasmapheresis, in which leukocytes are removed from the withdrawn blood and the remainder of the blood is retransfused into the donor. [leuko- + G. *aphairesis,* a withdrawal]

leu·kas·mus (lū-kaz′mŭs). SYN vitiligo. [G. *leukasmos,* a growing white]

leu·ke·mia (lū-kē′mē-ă). Progressive proliferation of abnormal leukocytes found in hemopoietic tissues, other organs, and usually in the blood in increased numbers. L. is classified by the dominant cell type, and by duration from onset to death. This occurs in *acute l.* within a few months in most cases, and is associated with acute symptoms including severe anemia, hemorrhages, and slight enlargement of lymph nodes or the spleen. The duration of *chronic l.* exceeds one year, with a gradual onset of symptoms of anemia or marked enlargement of spleen, liver, or lymph nodes. SYN leukocytic sarcoma. [leuko- + G. *haima,* blood]

acute lymphocytic leukemia (ALL), SEE lymphocytic l.

acute promyelocytic l., l. presenting as a severe bleeding disorder, with infiltration of the bone marrow by abnormal promyelocytes and myelocytes, a low plasma fibrinogen, and defective coagulation.

adult T-cell l. (ATL), SYN adult T-cell *lymphoma.*

aleukemic l., l. in which abnormal (or leukemic) cells are absent in the peripheral blood.

basophilic l., basophilocytic l., a form of granulocytic l. in which there are unusually great numbers of basophilic granulocytes in the tissues and circulating blood; in some instances, the immature and mature basophilic forms may represent from 40 to 80% of the total numbers of white blood cells. SYN mast cell l.

bovine l., SYN enzootic bovine *leukosis.*

l. cu′tis, yellow-brown, red, blue-red, or purple, sometimes nodular lesions associated with diffuse infiltration of leukemic cells in the skin; the involvement may be diffuse and generalized, *i.e.,* so-called universal l. cutis, or it may be localized.

embryonal l., SYN stem cell l.

eosinophilic l., eosinophilocytic l., a form of granulocytic l. in which there are conspicuous numbers of eosinophilic granulocytes in the tissues and circulating blood, or in which such cells are predominant; in chronic disease of this type, the total white blood cell count may be as high as 200,000 to 250,000 per cu mm, with as many as 80 or 90% being eosinophils, chiefly adult forms.

feline l., a leukemic disorder of cats caused by feline l. virus, a member of the family Retroviridae, and characterized by depression and mild fever, and by the presence of tumors in the mediastinal and mesenteric lymph nodes, followed by multiple tumor

formation throughout the body; during the terminal stages of the disease lymphoblasts may appear in the peripheral blood.

l. of fowls, SYN avian *leukosis.*

granulocytic l., a form of l. characterized by an uncontrolled proliferation of myelopoietic cells in the bone marrow and in extramedullary sites, and the presence of large numbers of immature and mature granulocytic forms in various tissues (and organs) and in the circulating blood; the total count may range from 1000 (aleukemic variety) to several hundred thousand per cu mm. The predominant cell is usually of the neutrophilic series, but, in a few instances, eosinophilic or basophilic granulocytes, or even megakaryocytes, may represent the chief form; early in granulocytic l., the circulating blood may contain excessive numbers of all of the granulocytic forms. SYN leukemic myelosis (1), myelocytic l., myelogenic l., myelogenous l., myeloid l.

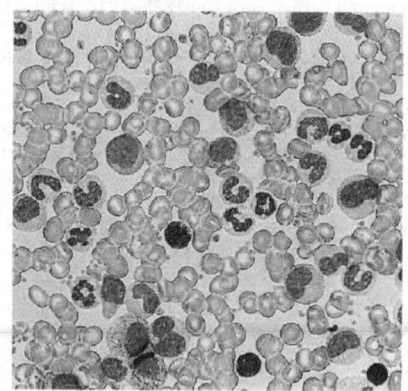

granulocytic leukemia (blood smear)
high leukocyte count, with myeloblasts

hairy cell l., a rare, usually chronic disorder characterized by proliferation of hairy cells in reticuloendothelial organs and blood.

leukemic l., a redundant term sometimes used to emphasize the occurrence of abundant numbers of leukemic cells in the circulating blood; this classic form of l. is usually termed simply *leukemia.*

leukopenic l., a form of lymphocytic, granulocytic, or monocytic l. in which the total number of white blood cells in the circulating blood is in the normal range, or may be diminished to various levels that are significantly less than normal.

lymphatic l., SYN lymphocytic l.

lymphoblastic l., acute lymphocytic l. in which the abnormal cells are chiefly (or almost totally) blast forms of the lymphocytic series, or in which unusually large numbers of the immature forms occur in association with adult lymphocytes.

lymphocytic l., a variety of l. characterized by an uncontrolled proliferation and conspicuous enlargement of lymphoid tissue in various sites (*e.g.,* lymph nodes, spleen, bone marrow, lungs), and the occurrence of increased numbers of cells of the lymphocytic series in the circulating blood and in various tissues and organs; in chronic disease, the cells are adult lymphocytes, whereas conspicuous numbers of lymphoblasts are observed in the more acute syndromes. SYN lymphatic l., lymphoid l.

lymphoid l., SYN lymphocytic l.

mast cell l., SYN basophilic l.

mature cell l., chronic granulocytic l.

megakaryocytic l., an unusual form of myelopoietic disease that is characterized by a seemingly uncontrolled proliferation of megakaryocytes in the bone marrow, and sometimes by the presence of a considerable number of megakaryocytes in the circulating blood. When bone marrow is examined at various intervals in some instances of chronic myelocytic l., the proliferation of megakaryocytes is more prominent than that of the granulocytes; at such times, the circulating blood may contain megakaryocytes or fragments of megakaryocytic nuclei and cytoplasm, or both, amounting to as much as 5 or 6% of the total number of leukocytes.

meningeal l., infiltration of the meninges by leukemic cells, a common occurrence in relapse following systemic administration of chemotherapeutic agents to leukemia patients.

micromyeloblastic l., a form of myelocytic l. in which relatively large proportions of micromyeloblasts are found in the circulating blood and in bone marrow and other tissues.

mixed l., mixed cell l., term infrequently used as a designation for granulocytic l., thereby emphasizing the occurrence of different types of cells in the myeloid series (*i.e.,* neutrophilic, eosinophilic, and basophilic granulocytes), in contrast to the comparatively monotonous pattern observed in lymphocytic and monocytic l.

monocytic l., a form of l. characterized by large numbers of cells that can be definitely identified as monocytes, in addition to larger, apparently related cells formed from the uncontrolled proliferation of the reticuloendothelial tissue; l. in which these two types of cells seem to "overrun" the usual sites of the reticuloendothelial system, and occur in conspicuous numbers in the circulating blood, is frequently referred to as the Schilling type of monocytic l., or sometimes as true monocytic l. The disease runs an acute or subacute course in older persons, and is characterized by swelling of gums, oral ulceration, bleeding in skin or mucous membranes, secondary infection, and splenomegaly. SYN leukemic reticulosis.

murine l., a leukemic disorder of mice caused by a number of different type C retroviruses.

myeloblastic l., a form of granulocytic l. in which there are large numbers of myeloblasts in various tissues (and organs) and in the circulating blood; the immature forms may amount to 30 to 60% (or even a greater proportion) of the increased total number of white blood cells. Used synonymously for acute granulocytic l. SYN leukemic myelosis (2).

myelocytic l., myelogenic l., myelogenous l., myeloid l., SYN granulocytic l.

myelomonocytic l., a variant of granulocytic l. with monocytosis in the peripheral blood. SYN Naegeli type of monocytic l.

Naegeli type of monocytic l., SYN myelomonocytic l.

neutrophilic l., an unusual form of chronic granulocytic l. in which the greatly increased number of leukocytes in the circulating blood are mature polymorphonuclear neutrophils, with virtually no young or immature granulocytes being observed.

plasma cell l., an unusual disease characterized by leukocytosis and other signs and symptoms that are suggestive of l., in association with diffuse infiltrations and aggregates of plasma cells in the spleen, liver, bone marrow, and lymph nodes, and the presence of considerable numbers of plasma cells in the circulating blood; the total number of leukocytes in the latter may range from normal levels to 80,000 or 90,000 per cu mm, and 5 to 90% may be plasma cells; multiple myelomas are observed in some examples of plasma cell l., but discrete nodules are not formed in bone. Although there are other clinicopathologic differences in the two conditions, they may be phases of the same basic process.

polymorphocytic l., granulocytic l., especially any variety in which the predominant cells are mature, segmented granulocytes.

Rieder cell l., a special form of acute granulocytic l. in which the affected tissues and the circulating blood contain relatively large numbers of atypical myeloblasts (*i.e.,* Rieder cells) that have the usual, faintly granular, immature type of cytoplasm, and a bizarre, comparatively mature nucleus with several wide and deep indentations (suggestive of lobulation).

Schilling type of monocytic l., SEE monocytic l.

splenic l., a form of l. in which there is an unusually great degree of enlargement of the spleen, as observed frequently in chronic granulocytic l.

stem cell l., a form of l. in which the abnormal cells are thought to be the precursors of lymphoblasts, myeloblasts, or monoblasts. SYN embryonal l.

subleukemic l., a form of l. in which abnormal cells are present in the peripheral blood, but the total leukocyte count is not elevated. SYN hypoleukemia, leukopenic myelosis, subleukemic myelosis, subleukemia.

leu·ke·mic (lū-kē′mik). Pertaining to, or having the characteristics of, any form of leukemia.

leu·ke·mid (lū-kem′id). Any nonspecific type of cutaneous lesion that is frequently associated with leukemia (as a feature of the syndrome), but is not a localized accumulation of leukemic cells; *e.g.,* petechiae, vesicles, wheals, bullae, hematomas, and the lesions of exfoliative dermatitis and herpes zoster. [leuko- + G. *haima,* blood, + *id* (1)]

leu·ke·mo·gen (lū-kē′mō-jen). Any substance or entity (*e.g.,* benzene, ionizing radiation) considered to be a causal factor in the occurrence of leukemia.

leu·ke·mo·gen·e·sis (lū-kē-mō-jen′ĕ-sis). The causation (or induction), development, and progression of a leukemic disease. [leukemia + G. *genesis,* production]

leu·ke·mo·gen·ic (lū-kē-mō-jen′ik). Pertaining to the causation, induction, and development of leukemia; manifesting the ability to cause leukemia.

leu·ke·moid (lū-kē′moyd). Resembling leukemia in various signs and symptoms, especially with reference to changes in the circulating blood. SEE ALSO leukemoid reaction. [leukemia + G. *eidos,* resemblance]

leu·ke·moid re·ac·tion. A moderate, advanced, or sometimes extreme degree of leukocytosis in the circulating blood, similar to that occurring in various forms of leukemia, but not the result of leukemic disease; usually, there is a disproportionate increase in the number of forms (including immature stages) in one series of leukocytes, and various examples of myelocytic, lymphocytic, monocytic, or plasmocytic l. r. may be also indistinguishable from leukocytosis that is associated with certain forms of leukemia. l. r.'s are sometimes observed as a feature of: 1) infectious disease caused by certain bacteria and other biologic agents, *e.g.,* tuberculosis, diphtheria, chickenpox, and others; 2) intoxication of various types, *e.g.,* eclampsia, serious burns, mustard gas poisoning, and others; 3) malignant neoplasms, *e.g.,* carcinoma of the colon, of the lung, of the kidney, or of other organs; 4) acute hemorrhage or hemolysis.

lymphocytic l. r., leukocytosis of varying degree, with adult lymphocytes and immature forms amounting to 40% (or more) of the total number of white blood cells in the circulating blood; may be observed in association with pertussis, infectious mononucleosis, gonorrhea, chickenpox, and sarcoidosis.

monocytic l. r., leukocytosis of varying degree, *e.g.,* 30,000 to 40,000 per cu mm, with adult monocytes and immature forms amounting to 30% (or more) of the total number of white blood cells in the circulating blood; may be observed in association with tuberculosis, especially the first infection, miliary type.

myelocytic l. r., leukocytosis of at least moderate degree, *e.g.,* 50,000 or more per cu mm, with a few immature forms, *e.g.,* 1 or 2% myelocytes, but chiefly mature polymorphonuclear leukocytes in the circulating blood; may be observed in association with tuberculosis, chronic osteomyelitis, various types of empyema, malaria, pneumococcal pneumonia, meningococcal meningitis, Hodgkin's disease, and metastases of carcinoma in the bone marrow.

plasmocytic l. r., the presence of unusual numbers of plasma cells, *i.e.,* plasmocytosis, in the bone marrow; may be observed in association with sarcoidosis, rheumatoid arthritis, cirrhosis, Hodgkin's disease, and certain of the so-called collagen diseases.

leu·kin (lū′kin). A thermostable bactericidal substance extracted from leukocytes. SYN leucin. [*leuko*cyte + *-in*]

⚠**leuko-, leuk-.** White; white blood cells. For some words beginning thus, see leuc- and leuco-. [G. *leukos,* white]

leu·ko·ag·glu·ti·nin (lū′kō-ă-glū′ti-nin). An antibody that agglutinates white blood cells.

leu·ko·bil·in (lū-kō-bil′in). SYN white *bile.* [leuko- + L. *bilis,* bile]

leu·ko·blast (lū′kō-blast). An immature white blood cell that is transitional between the lymphoidocyte (or the myeloblast of Naegeli and Downey) and the promyelocyte; the cytoplasm is polychromatophilic or slightly acidophilic and, as compared with the lymphoidocyte, the nuclear network of chromatin is thicker

le

and the nucleoli less distinct. SYN proleukocyte. [leuko- + G. *blastos*, germ]

granular l., obsolete term for promyelocyte.

leu·ko·blas·to·sis (lū′kō-blas-tō′sis). A general term for the abnormal proliferation of leukocytes, especially that occurring in myelocytic and lymphocytic leukemia.

leu·ko·chlo·ro·ma (lū′kō-klō-rō′mă). SYN myelocytomatosis (1). [leuko- + G. *chlorōs*, green, + *-oma*, tumor]

leu·ko·ci·din (lū-kos′i-din, lū-kō-sī′din). A heat-labile substance that is elaborated by many strains of *Staphylococcus aureus*, *Streptococcus pyogenes*, and pneumococci and manifests a destructive action on leukocytes, with or without lysis of the cells. [leukocyte + L. *caedo*, to kill]

leu·ko·co·ria, leu·ko·ko·ria (lū-kō-kō′rē-ă, lū-kō-kō′rē-ă). Reflection from a white mass within the eye giving the appearance of a white pupil. SYN leukokoria, white pupillary *reflex.* [*leuko-* white, + G. *korē*, pupil]

leu·ko·cy·tac·tic (lū′kō-sī-tak′tik). SYN leukocytotactic.

leu·ko·cy·tal (lū-kō-sī′tăl). SYN leukocytic.

leu·ko·cy·tax·ia, leu·ko·cy·tax·is (lū′kō-sī-tak′sē-ă, -tak′sis). SYN leukocytotaxia.

leu·ko·cyte (lū′kō-sīt). A type of cell formed in the myelopoietic, lymphoid, and reticular portions of the reticuloendothelial system in various parts of the body, and normally present in those sites and in the circulating blood (rarely in other tissues). Under various abnormal conditions, the total numbers or proportions, or both, may be characteristically increased, decreased, or not altered, and they may be present in other tissues and organs. L.'s represent three lines of development from primitive elements: myeloid, lymphoid, and monocytic series. On the basis of features observed with various methods of staining with polychromatic dyes (*e.g.,* Wright's stain, and others), cells of the myeloid series are frequently termed granular l.'s, or granulocytes; cells of the lymphoid and monocytic series also have granules in the cytoplasm but, owing to their tiny, inconspicuous size and different properties (frequently not clearly visualized with routine methods), lymphocytes and monocytes are sometimes termed nongranular or agranular l.'s. Granulocytes are commonly known as polymorphonuclear l.'s (also polynuclear or multinuclear l.'s), inasmuch as the mature nucleus is divided into two to five rounded or ovoid lobes that are connected with thin strands or small bands of chromatin; they consist of three distinct types: neutrophils, eosinophils, and basophils, named on the basis of the staining reactions of the cytoplasmic granules. Cells of the lymphocytic series occur as two, somewhat arbitrary, normal varieties: small and large lymphocytes; the former represent the ordinary forms and are conspicuously more numerous in the circulating blood and normal lymphoid tissue; the latter may be found in normal circulating blood, but are more easily observed in lymphoid tissue. The small lymphocytes have nuclei that are deeply or densely stained (the chromatin is coarse and bulky) and almost fill the cells, with only a slight rim of cytoplasm around the nuclei; the large lymphocytes have nuclei that are approximately the same size as, or only slightly larger than, those of the small forms, but there is a broader, easily visualized band of cytoplasm around the nuclei. Cells of the monocytic series are usually larger than the other l.'s, and are characterized by a relatively abundant, slightly opaque, pale blue or blue-gray cytoplasm that contains myriads of extremely fine reddish-blue granules. Monocytes are usually indented, reniform, or shaped similarly to a horseshoe, but are sometimes rounded or ovoid; their nuclei are usually large and centrally placed and, even when eccentrically located, are completely surrounded by at least a small band of cytoplasm. SYN white blood cell. [leuko- + G. *kytos,* cell]

acidophilic l., SYN eosinophilic l.

agranular l., SYN nongranular l.

basophilic l., a polymorphonuclear l. characterized by many large, coarse, metachromatic granules (dark purple or blue-black when treated with Wright's or similar stains) that usually fill the cytoplasm and may almost mask the nucleus; these l.'s are unique in that they usually do not occur in increased numbers as the result of acute infectious disease, and their phagocytic qualities are probably not significant; the granules, which contain heparin and histamine, may degranulate in response to hypersensitivity reactions and can be of significance in general inflammation. SYN basocyte, basophilocyte, mast l.

cystinotic l., a l. having an enhanced content of cystine, found in patients with disorders characterized by the storage of cystine; within the l., the cystine, largely in noncrystalline form, is associated with dense lysosomal particles.

endothelial l., old term for a monocyte, a type of l. thought to be derived from reticuloendothelial tissue.

eosinophilic l., a polymorphonuclear l. characterized by many large or prominent, refractile, cytoplasmic granules that are fairly uniform in size and bright yellow-red or orange when treated with Wright's or similar stains; the nuclei are usually larger than those of neutrophils, do not stain as deeply, and characteristically have two lobes (a third lobe is sometimes interposed on the connecting strand of chromatin); these l.'s are motile phagocytes with distinctive antiparasitic functions. SYN acidophilic l., eosinocyte, eosinophil, eosinophile, oxyphil (2), oxyphile, oxyphilic l.

filament polymorphonuclear l., any mature polymorphonuclear l., especially a neutrophilic l., in which the lobes of the nucleus are interconnected with a thin strand or filament of chromatin.

globular l., a type of wandering cell with a small, round nucleus found in the epithelium and lamina propria of the intestinal mucosa of many animals; its cytoplasm contains large eosinophilic globules or droplets.

granular l., any one of the polymorphonuclear l.'s, especially a neutrophilic l. SEE ALSO granulocyte, basophilic l., eosinophilic l.

hyaline l., old term for a monocyte, and for a mononuclear macrophage in various lesions.

mast l., SYN basophilic l.

motile l., any l. that manifests active ameboid movement, especially a mature granulocytic l. (eosinophils are less motile than neutrophils or basophils); monocytes manifest a slow, but persistent, wavelike movement.

multinuclear l., SYN polymorphonuclear l.

neutrophilic l., a neutrophilic granulocyte, the most frequent of the polymorphonuclear l.'s, and also the most active phagocyte among the various types of white blood cells; when treated with Wright's stain (or similar preparations), the fairly abundant cytoplasm is faintly pink, and numerous tiny, slightly refractile, relatively bright pink or violet-pink, diffusely scattered granules are recognizable in the cytoplasm; the deeply stained blue or purple-blue nucleus is sharply distinguished from the cytoplasm and is distinctly lobated, with thin strands of chromatin connecting the three to five lobes.

nonfilament polymorphonuclear l., a neutrophil, basophil, or eosinophil that is not completely matured, *i.e.,* the lobes of the nuclei remain connected with bands of chromatin, in contrast to the thin strands observed in mature cells.

nongranular l., a general, nonspecific term frequently used with reference to lymphocytes, monocytes, and plasma cells; although the cytoplasm of a lymphocyte or monocyte contains tiny granules, it is "nongranular" in comparison with that of a neutrophil, basophil, or eosinophil. SEE ALSO leukocyte. SYN agranular l.

nonmotile l., a term sometimes used with reference to lymphocytes, monocytes, and plasma cells; although such forms actually have some degree of motility, they are "nonmotile" in comparison with the actively ameboid, neutrophilic, basophilic, and eosinophilic l.'s.

oxyphilic l., SYN eosinophilic l.

polymorphonuclear l., polynuclear l., common term for granulocyte or granulocytic l.; the term includes basophilic, eosinophilic, and neutrophilic l.'s, but is usually used especially with reference to the neutrophilic l.'s. SYN multinuclear l.

segmented l., any mature polymorphonuclear l., especially a neutrophilic l.

transitional l., old term for a monocyte.

Türk's l., SYN Türk *cell.*

leu·ko·cy·the·mia (lū′kō-sī-thē′mē-ă). A seldom used term for leukemia. [leukocyte + G. *haima,* blood]

leu·ko·cyt·ic (lū-kō-sit′ik). Pertaining to or characterized by leukocytes. SYN leukocytal.

leu·ko·cy·to·blast (lū-kō-sī′tō-blast). A nonspecific term for any immature cell from which a leukocyte develops, including lymphoblast, myeloblast, and the like. [leukocyte + G. *blastos,* germ]

leu·ko·cy·toc·la·sis (lū′kō-sī-tok′lă-sis). Karyorrhexis of leukocytes. [leuko- + G. *kytos,* cell, + *klasia,* a breaking]

leu·ko·cy·to·gen·e·sis (lū′kō-sī-tō-jen′ĕ-sis). The formation and development of leukocytes. [leukocyte + G. *genesis,* production]

leu·ko·cy·toid (lū′kō-sī-toyd). Resembling a leukocyte. [leukocyte + G. *eidos,* resemblance]

leu·ko·cy·tol·y·sin (lū′kō-sī-tol′i-sin). Any substance (including lytic antibody) that causes dissolution of leukocytes. SYN leukolysin.

leu·ko·cy·tol·y·sis (lū′kō-sī-tol′i-sis). Dissolution or lysis of leukocytes. SYN leukolysis. [leukocyte + G. *lysis,* dissolution]

leu·ko·cy·to·lyt·ic (lū′kō-sī-tō-lit′ik). Pertaining to, causing, or manifesting leukocytolysis. SYN leukolytic.

leu·ko·cy·to·ma (lū′kō-sī-tō′mă). A fairly well circumscribed, nodular, dense accumulation of leukocytes. [leukocyte + G. *-oma,* tumor]

leu·ko·cy·tom·e·ter (lū′kō-sī-tom′ĕ-ter). A standarized glass slide that is suitably ruled for counting the leukocytes in a measured volume of accurately diluted blood (or other specimens). [leukocyte + G. *metron,* measure]

leu·ko·cy·to·pe·nia (lū′kō-sī-tō-pē′nē-ă). SYN leukopenia.

leu·ko·cy·to·pla·nia (lū′kō-sī-tō-plā′nē-ă). Movement of leukocytes from the lumens of blood vessels, through serous membranes, or in the tissues. [leukocyte + G. *planē,* a wandering]

leu·ko·cy·to·poi·e·sis (lū′kō-sī-tō-poy-ē′sis). SYN leukopoiesis. [leukocyte + G. *poiēsis,* a making]

leu·ko·cy·to·sis (lū′kō-sī-tō′sis). An abnormally large number of leukocytes, as observed in acute infections. A white blood cell count of 10,000 or more per cu mm usually indicates l. Most examples of l. represent a disproportionate increase in the number of cells in the neutrophilic series, and the term is frequently used synonymously with the designation neutrophilia. L. of 15,000 to 25,000 per cu mm is frequently observed in various pathologic conditions, and values as high as 40,000 are not unusual; occasionally, as in some examples of leukemoid reactions, white blood cell counts may range up to 100,000 per cu mm. [leukocyte + G. *-osis,* condition]

absolute l., an actual increase in the total number of leukocytes in the circulating blood, as distinguished from a relative increase (such as that observed in dehydration).

agonal l., SYN terminal l.

basophilic l., the presence of an abnormally large number of basophilic granulocytes in the blood. SYN basocytosis.

digestive l., l. occurring normally after ingestion of food.

distribution l., an abnormally large proportion of one or more types of leukocytes.

emotional l., an abnormally high white blood cell count that is thought to be related only to an emotional disturbance.

eosinophilic l., a form of relative l. in which the greatest proportionate increase is in the eosinophils. SYN eosinophilia.

lymphocytic l., SYN lymphocytosis.

monocytic l., SYN monocytosis.

neutrophilic l., SYN neutrophilia.

l. of the newborn, an apparently "physiologic" l. usually observed in newborn infants, in whom the white blood cell counts are usually greater than 10,000 per cu mm, and sometimes range to 45,000 per cu mm, resulting chiefly from increased numbers of neutrophils (especially single and bilobed forms). On the third or fourth day of life, the count generally decreases rapidly, and then fluctuates for several days; beginning about the fourth week of life, a relative lymphocytosis is observed, and this normally continues for a few years.

physiologic l., any form of l. that is associated with apparently normal situations and that is not directly related to a pathologic condition; *e.g.,* the temporary increase in the total number of white blood cells that may occur during a single day, or from day to day, as well as in the newborn period, during childhood, after strenuous exercise, during attacks of paroxysmal tachycardia, and in association with various other situations.

relative l., an increased proportion of one or more types of leukocytes in the circulating blood, without an actual increase in the total number of white blood cells.

terminal l., one that occurs in a person just prior to death, especially in one who has a "slow death." SYN agonal l.

leu·ko·cy·to·tac·tic (lū′kō-sī-tō-tak′tik). Pertaining to, characterized by, or causing leukocytotaxia. SYN leukocytactic, leukotactic.

leu·ko·cy·to·tax·ia (lū′kō-sī-tō-tak′sē-ă). 1. The active ameboid movement of leukocytes, especially the neutrophilic granulocytes, either toward (**positive l.**) or away from (**negative l.**) certain microorganisms as well as various substances frequently formed in inflamed tissue. 2. The property of attracting or repelling leukocytes. SYN leukocytaxia, leukocytaxis, leukotaxia, leukotaxis. [leukocyte + G. *taxis,* arrangement]

leu·ko·cy·to·tox·in (lū′kō-sī-tō-tok′sin). Any substance that causes degeneration and necrosis of leukocytes, including leukolysin and leukocidin. SYN leukotoxin. [leukocyte + G. *toxikon,* poison]

Leu·ko·cy·to·zo·on (lū′kō-sī-tō-zō′on). SYN *Leucocytozoon.*

leu·ko·cy·to·zo·o·no·sis (lū′kō-sī′tō-zō-ō-nō′sis). SYN leucocytozoonosis.

leu·ko·cy·tu·ria (lū′kō-sī-tū′rē-ă). The presence of leukocytes in urine that is recently voided or collected by means of a catheter. [leukocyte + G. *ouron,* urine]

leu·ko·der·ma (lū-kō-der′mă). An absence of pigment, partial or total, in the skin. SYN achromoderma, hypomelanosis, leukopathia, leukopathy. [leuko- + G. *derma,* skin]

acquired l., SYN vitiligo.

l. acquisi′tum centrifu′gum, SYN halo *nevus.*

l. col′li, SYN syphilitic l.

syphilitic l., a fading of the roseola of secondary syphilis, leaving reticulated depigmented and hyperpigmented areas located chiefly on the sides of the neck. SYN l. colli, melanoleukoderma colli.

leu·ko·der·ma·tous (lū-kō-der′mă-tŭs). Relating to or resembling leukoderma.

leu·ko·don·tia (lū-kō-don′shē-ă). The condition of having white teeth. [leuko- + G. *odous,* tooth]

leu·ko·dys·tro·phia (lū-kō-dis-trō′fē-ă). SYN leukodystrophy.

l. cer′ebri progres′siva, SYN leukodystrophy.

leu·ko·dys·tro·phy (lū-kō-dis′trō-fē). Term for a group of white matter diseases, some familial, characterized by progressive cerebral deterioration usually in early life, and pathologically by primary absence or degeneration of the myelin of the central and peripheral nervous systems with glial reaction; probably related to a defect in lipid metabolism; the adult type of Pelizaeus-Merzbacher *disease* is inherited as an autosomal dominant trait [MIM*169500]. SEE ALSO Canavan's *disease.* SYN leukodystrophia cerebri progressiva, leukodystrophia, sclerosis of white matter. [leuko- + G. *dys,* bad, + *trophē,* nourishment]

adrenal l., sudanophilic leukodystrophy with bronzing of skin and adrenal atrophy. A metabolic disorder of young males, characterized by widespread myelin degeneration and associated adrenal insufficiency. The myelin degeneration is massive in various portions of the brain and sometimes the spinal cord, with the accumulation of degradation products of myelin in macrophages: sudanophilic demyelination; atrophy is present in the adrenal glands and testes, and markedly increased amounts of very long-chain fatty acid are present in both the brain and adrenal glands. Symptoms include bronzing of the skin, dysarthria, cortical blindness, bilateral hemiplegia, pseudobulbar paralysis, and progressive dementia. Probably sex-linked recessive inheritance.

l. with diffuse Rosenthal fiber formation, a metabolic disorder whose onset can be in infancy, adolescence, or adulthood; characterized pathologically by widespread cerebral demyelination with astrocyte and primitive oligodendroglial cell proliferation; refractile Rosenthal fibers result from the degeneration of these proliferating cells; etiology unknown, but possibly due to a metabolic defect of astrocytes; sex-linked recessive disorder.

globoid cell l. [MIM*245200], a metabolic disorder of infancy with rapidly progressive cerebral degeneration, massive loss of myelin, severe astrocytic gliosis, and infiltration of the white matter with characteristic multinucleate globoid cells; metabolically there is gross deficiency of lysosomal cerebrosidase (galactosylceramide β-galactosidase); autosomal recessive inheritance. SYN diffuse infantile familial sclerosis, galactosylceramide lipoidosis, Krabbe's disease.

metachromatic l., a metabolic disorder, usually of infancy, characterized by myelin loss, accumulation of metachromatic lipids (galactosyl sulfatidates) in the white matter of the central and peripheral nervous systems, progressive paralysis, and mental retardation; psychosis and dementia are seen in adults; autosomal recessive inheritance; autosomal dominant [MIM*156310, *176801] and recessive [MIM*250100] inheritance; a deficiency of arylsulfatase A. SYN sulfatide lipidosis.

leu·ko·e·de·ma (lū′kō-e-dē′mă). A bluish-white opalescence of the buccal mucosa which becomes the normal mucosal color on stretching the tissue; most commonly observed in blacks and may be considered a normal anatomic variation.

leu·ko·en·ceph·a·li·tis (lū′kō-en-sef-ă-lī′tis). Encephalitis restricted to the white matter.

acute epidemic l., a disease characterized by acute onset of fever, followed by convulsions, delirium, and coma, and associated with perivascular demyelination and hemorrhagic foci in the central nervous system. SYN acute primary hemorrhagic meningoencephalitis, Strümpell's disease (2).

acute hemorrhagic l., SYN acute necrotizing hemorrhagic *encephalomyelitis*.

acute necrotizing hemorrhagic l., SYN acute necrotizing hemorrhagic *encephalomyelitis*.

sclerosing l., SYN subacute sclerosing *panencephalitis*.

subacute sclerosing l., SYN subacute sclerosing *panencephalitis*.

leu·ko·en·ceph·a·lop·a·thy (lū′kō-en-sef-ă-lop′ă-thē). White matter changes first described in children with leukemia, associated with radiation and chemotherapy injury, often associated with methotrexate; pathologically characterized by diffuse reactive astrocytosis with multiple areas of necrotic foci without inflammation. [leuko- + G. *enkephalos,* brain, + *pathos,* suffering]

progressive multifocal l. (PML), a rare, subacute, afebrile disease characterized by areas of demyelinization surrounded by markedly altered neuroglia, including inclusion bodies in glial cells; it occurs usually in individuals with AIDS, leukemia, lymphoma, or other debilitating diseases, or in those who have been receiving immunosuppressive treatment. Caused by JC virus, a human polyoma virus. SYN progressive subcortical encephalopathy.

leu·ko·e·ryth·ro·blas·to·sis (lū′kō-ĕ-rith′rō-blas-tō′sis). Any anemic condition resulting from space-occupying lesions in the bone marrow; the circulating blood contains immature cells of the granulocytic series and nucleated red blood cells, frequently in numbers that are disproportionately large in relation to the degree of anemia. SYN leukoerythroblastic anemia, myelophthisic anemia, myelopathic anemia.

leu·ko·ker·a·to·sis (lū′kō-ker-ă-tō′sis). Rarely used term for leukoplakia.

leu·ko·ki·net·ic (lū′kō-ki-net′ik). Pertaining to leukokinetics. [leukocyte + G. *kinētikos,* of motion, fr. *kineō,* to move]

leu·ko·ki·net·ics (lū′kō-ki-net′iks). The study of the formation, circulation, and fate of leukocyte, usually by use of a radioactive tracer. [leukocyte + G. *kinetikos,* of or for putting in motion]

leu·ko·ko·ria (lū-kō-kō′rē-ă). SEE leukocoria.

leu·ko·krau·ro·sis (lū′kō-kraw-rō′sis). SYN kraurosis vulvae.

leu·ko·lymph·o·sar·co·ma (lū′kō-lim′fō-sar-kō′mă). Obsolete term for malignant *lymphoma*.

leu·kol·y·sin (lū-kol′i-sin). SYN leukocytolysin.

leu·kol·y·sis (lū-kol′i-sis). SYN leukocytolysis.

leu·ko·lyt·ic (lū-kō-lit′ik). SYN leukocytolytic.

leu·ko·ma (lū-kō′mă). A dense, opaque, white opacity of the cornea. [G. whiteness, a white spot in the eye, fr. *leukos,* white]

adherent l., a cicatrix of the cornea to which a portion of the iris is attached.

leu·ko·ma·tous (lū-kō′mă-tŭs). Denoting leukoma.

leu·ko·mye·li·tis (loo′kō-mī-e-lī′tis). An inflammatory process involving the white matter of the spinal cord.

necrotizing hemorrhage l., the pathological substrate responsible for the clinical disorder of acute necrotizing *myelitis*.

leu·ko·my·e·lop·a·thy (lū′kō-mī′ĕ-lop′ă-thē). Any systemic disease involving the white matter or the conducting tracts of the spinal cord. [leuko- + G. *myelos,* marrow, + *pathos,* suffering]

leu·kon (lū′kon). The total mass of circulating leukocytes as well as the cells and leukopoietic cells from which it originates.

leu·ko·ne·cro·sis (lū′kō-ne-krō′sis). SYN white *gangrene.* [leuko- + G. *nekrōsis,* deadness]

leu·ko·nych·ia (lū-kō-nik′ē-ă). The occurrence of white spots or patches under the nails, due to the presence of air bubbles between the nail and its bed; the decoloration may be total or in the form of lines (striate l.) or dots (punctate l.). SYN achromia unguium, canities unguium, leukopathia unguis. [leuko- + G. *onyx (onych-),* nail]

apparent l., pallor of the nail not due to subungual air bubbles.

leu·ko·path·ia, leu·kop·a·thy (lū-kō-path′ē-ă, lū-kop′ă-thē). SYN leukoderma. [leuko- + G. *pathos,* disease]

acquired l., SYN vitiligo.

l. un′guis, SYN leukonychia.

leu·ko·pe·de·sis (lū′kō-pē-dē′sis). The movement of white blood cells (especially polymorphonuclear leukocytes) through the walls of capillaries and into the tissues. [leuko- + G. *pēdēsis,* a leaping]

leu·ko·pe·nia (lū-kō-pē′nē-ă). The antithesis of leukocytosis; any situation in which the total number of leukocytes in the circulating blood is less than normal, the lower limit of which is generally regarded as 4000–5000 per cu mm. SYN leukocytopenia. [leuko(cyte) + G. *penia,* poverty]

basophilic l., a decrease in the number of basophilic granulocytes normally present in the circulating blood (difficult to evaluate, owing to the small and variable number normally present). SYN basocytopenia, basopenia.

eosinophilic l., a decrease in the number of eosinophilic granulocytes normally present in the circulating blood.

lymphocytic l., SYN lymphopenia.

monocytic l., SYN monocytopenia.

neutrophilic l., SYN neutropenia.

leu·ko·pe·nic (lū-kō-pē′nik). Pertaining to leukopenia.

leu·ko·phleg·ma·sia (lū-kō-fleg-mā′zē-ă). SYN lymphatic *edema.* [leuko- + phlegmasia]

l. do′lens, SYN *phlegmasia* alba dolens.

leu·ko·pla·kia (lū-kō-plā′kē-ă). A white patch of oral mucous membrane which cannot be wiped off and cannot be diagnosed clinically as any specific disease entity; in current usage, a clinical term without histologic or premalignant connotation. [leuko- + G. *plax,* plate]

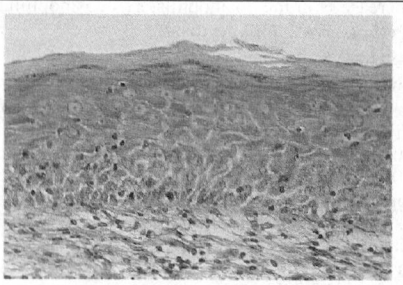

leukoplakia (of the oral mucosa)

hairy l., a white lesion appearing on the tongue, occasionally on the buccal mucosa, of patients with AIDS; the lesion appears raised, with a corrugated or "hairy" surface due to keratin projections.

Appearing in otherwise healthy individuals, hairy leukoplakia, caused by the Epstein-Barr virus, rarely becomes cancerous (in an estimated 5% of cases, over a 20-year period after first appearance). However, among those with AIDS, the risk is elevated. As with oral candidiasis, this is frequently among the first symptoms to arise in HIV-positive persons. Perhaps 20% of those with hairy leukoplakia are HIV positive. When the lesion does not spontaneously regress, it is sometimes treated with antiviral drugs (*e.g.,* acyclovir, zidovudine).

l. vul'vae, a clinical term for hyperkeratotic white patches of the vulvar epithelium; biopsy is necessary for specific diagnosis. SYN leukoplakic vulvitis.

leu·ko·poi·e·sis (lū′kō-poy-ē′sis). Formation and development of the various types of white blood cells. SYN leukocytopoiesis. [leuko- + G. *poiēsis,* a making]

leu·ko·poi·et·ic (lū′kō-poy-et′ik). Pertaining to or characterized by leukopoiesis, as manifested by portions of the bone marrow and reticuloendothelial and lymphoid tissues, which form (respectively) the granulocytes, monocytes, and lymphocytes.

leu·ko·pro·te·ase (lū-kō-prō′tē-ās). An ill-defined proteolytic enzyme product of polynuclear leukocytes, formed in an area of inflammation, that causes liquefaction of dead tissue.

leu·ko·ri·bo·fla·vin (lū-kō-rī′bō-flā-vin). The colorless nonfluorescing dihydro compound formed by the reduction of riboflavin.

leu·kor·rha·gia (lū-kō-rā′jē-ă). SYN leukorrhea. [leuko- + G. *rhēgnymi,* to burst forth]

leu·kor·rhea (lū-kō-rē′ă). Discharge from the vagina of a white or yellowish viscid fluid containing mucus and pus cells. SYN leukorrhagia. [leuko- + G. *rhoia,* flow]

menstrual l., intermittent l. recurring at or just before each menstrual period.

leu·kor·rhe·al (lū-kō-rē′ăl). Relating to or characterized by leukorrhea.

leu·ko·sar·co·ma (lū′kō-sar-kō′mă). Obsolete term for malignant *lymphoma.*

leu·ko·sar·co·ma·to·sis (lū′kō-sar-kō-mă-tō′sis). Obsolete term for a condition characterized initially by numerous widespread nodules or masses of lymphosarcoma, and the subsequent presence of similar cells in the circulating blood as in leukosarcoma.

leu·ko·sis (lū-kō′sis). Abnormal proliferation of one or more of the leukopoietic tissues; the term includes myelosis, certain forms of reticuloendotheliosis, and lymphadenosis.

avian l., a group of conditions (*e.g.,* lymphoid, erythroid, or myeloid l.) that occur chiefly in chickens and are characterized by an abnormal proliferation of myelopoietic, erythropoietic, or lymphoid tissues; etiologic agents are a group of closely related viruses in the family Retroviridae, and the conditions are transmissible. SEE ALSO avian leukosis-sarcoma *complex.* SYN fowl l., leukemia of fowls.

enzootic bovine l., a fatal infectious disease of cattle older than 3 years caused by the bovine leukemia virus in the family Retroviridae; characterized clinically by enlargement of peripheral lymph nodes, anorexia, weight loss, and decreased milk production, and pathologically by development of lymphosarcoma in various tissues and organs. SYN bovine leukemia.

fowl l., SYN avian l.

sporadic bovine l., a rare disease of cattle less than 3 years of age, of unknown cause, characterized by the development of lymphosarcoma; three clinicopathological forms are recognized: calf or juvenile form, thymic form, and cutaneous form.

leu·ko·tac·tic (lū-kō-tak′tik). SYN leukocytotactic.

leu·ko·tax·ia (lū-kō-tak′sē-ă). SYN leukocytotaxia.

leu·ko·tax·ine (lū-kō-tak′sēn). A cell-free nitrogenous material prepared from injured, acutely degenerating tissue and from inflammatory exudates.

leu·ko·tax·is (lū-kō-tak′sis). SYN leukocytotaxia.

leu·kot·ic (lū-kot′ik). Pertaining to, characterized by, or manifesting leukosis.

leu·ko·tome (lū′kō-tōm). An instrument for performing leukotomy.

leu·kot·o·my (lū-kot′ō-mē). Incision into the white matter of the frontal lobe of the brain. [leuko- + G. *tomē,* a cutting]

prefrontal l., SYN prefrontal *lobotomy.*

transorbital l., SYN transorbital *lobotomy.*

leu·ko·tox·in (lū-kō-tok′sin). SYN leukocytotoxin.

leu·ko·trich·ia (lū-kō-trik′ē-ă). Whiteness of the hair. [leuko- + G. *thrix,* hair]

l. annula'ris, SYN ringed *hair.*

leu·kot·ri·chous (lū-kot′ri-kŭs). Having white hair.

leu·ko·tri·enes (LT) (lū-kō-trī′ēnz). Products of eicosanoid metabolism (usually, arachidonic acid) with postulated physiologic activity such as mediators of inflammation and roles in allergic reactions; differ from the related prostaglandins and thromboxanes by not having a central ring; so named because discovered in association with leukocytes and of three conjugated double bonds; letters A through F identify the six metabolites thus far isolated, with subscript numbers to indicate the number of double bonds (*e.g.,* leukotriene C_4).

peptidyl l., l. having amino acids present (even single amino acids) although not true peptides; *e.g.,* LTC_4 is an *S*-substituted glutathione, LTD_4 is an *S*-substituted cysteinylglycine, LTE_4 is an *S*-substituted cysteine, and LTF_4 (also known as γ-glutamyl-LTE_4) is an *S*-substituted γ-glutamylcysteine.

Leu·ko·vi·rus (lū′kō-vī′rŭs). A former genus composed of the RNA tumor viruses now included in the family Retroviridae.

leu·pep·tin (lū-pep′tin). A peptide (*N*-acetylleucylleucylarginyl) from *Streptomyces* species that inhibits cathepsin B, papain, trypsin, plasmin, and cathepsin D.

leu·pro·lide ac·e·tate (lū′prō-līd). A synthetic nonapeptide analog of naturally occurring gonadotropin-releasing hormone; used in the palliative treatment of advanced prostatic cancer.

leu·ro·cris·tine (lū′rō-kris′tin). SYN vincristine sulfate.

Lev, Maurice, U.S. pathologist, *1908. SEE L.'s *disease,* syndrome.

Levaditi, Constantin, Roumanian bacteriologist in Paris, 1874–1928. SEE L. *stain.*

lev·al·lor·phan tar·trate (lev-ă-lōr′fan). 1-*N*-Allyl-3-hydroxymorphinan tartrate; the *N*-allyl analog of levorphanol, antagonistic to the actions of narcotic analgesics; used in the treatment of respiratory depression due to overdosage of narcotics.

lev·am·iso·le (lē-vam′ĭ-sōl). Formerly used as an anthelmintic; increases immune responses and is used adjunctively with antineoplastic agents to improve response and suppress recurrence.

lev·an. SYN fructosan.

lev·an·su·crase (lev-an-sū′krās). An enzyme catalyzing transfer of the fructose moiety of sucrose to polyfructose (a levan), releasing D-glucose.

lev·ar·te·re·nol (lev-ar-tēr′ĕ-nol). SYN norepinephrine.

l. bitartrate, SYN *norepinephrine* bitartrate.

le·va·tor (le-vā′ter, tōr). **1.** A surgical instrument for prying up the depressed part in a fracture of the skull. **2.** One of several muscles whose action is to raise the part into which it is inserted. [L. a lifter, fr. *levo,* pp. -*atus,* to lift, fr. *levis,* light]

LeVeen, Harry H., U.S. surgeon, *1914. SEE LeV. *shunt.*

lev·el. Any rank, position, or status in a graded scale of values.

acoustic reference l., the biological reference l. for sound mea-

---

♻ **Combining forms**	**[NA]** Nomina Anatomica
Word*Finder*	**[MIM]** Mendelian
Multi-term entry finder	**Inheritance in Man**
Preceding letter A	
A.D.A.M. Anatomy Plates	☆ **Official alternate term**
Between letters L and M	
Appendices:	☆**[NA]** Official alternate
Following letter Z	**Nomina Anatomica term**
SYN Synonym; **Cf.,** compare	**High Profile Term**

le

surements. When the term decibel is used to indicate the noise l., a reference quantity is implied; this reference value is usually expressed as a sound pressure of 20 micronewtons per square meter. The reference l. is referred to as 0 decibels, the baseline of the scale of noise l.'s; this baseline is considered the weakest sound that can be heard by a person with very good hearing in an extremely quiet location. Other equivalent reference l.'s still being used include 0.0002 microbar and 0.0002 dyne per square centimeter.

l. of aspiration, in clinical psychology, the degree or quality of performance (exhibited in a testing situation) which an individual desires to attain or feels he can achieve.

background l., the concentration (usually low) at which a substance or agent is present or occurs at a particular time and place in the absence of a specific hazard under investigation; an example is the background level of ionizing radiation.

Clark's l., the l. of invasion of primary malignant melanoma of the skin; limited to the epidermis, I; into the underlying papillary dermis, II; to the junction of the papillary and reticular dermis, III; into the reticular dermis, IV; into the subcutaneous fat, V. The prognosis is worse with each successive deeper l. of invasion.

hearing l., the measure of the status of hearing as read directly on the hearing loss scale of an audiometer; described in decibels as a deviation from a standard value for zero on the audiometer.

sound pressure l. (SPL), a measure of sound energy relative to 0.0002 dynes/cm^2, expressed in decibels.

window l., the CT number setting in Hounsfield units of the midpoint of the window width, which is the gray scale of the image; a typical window l. for imaging the lungs if −500; for the abdomen, 0.

Leventhal, Michael L., U.S. obstetrician-gynecologist, 1901–1971. SEE Stein-L. *syndrome.*

le·ver (lev′er, lē′ver). An instrument used to lift or pry. [Fr. *lever,* to lift]

dental l., SYN elevator (2).

le·ver·age (lē′ver-ij). **1.** The actual lift or elevating direction of a lever or elevator. **2.** The mechanical advantage gained thereby.

Lévi, E. Leopold, French endocrinologist, 1868–1933. SEE dominantly inherited L.'s *disease;* Lorain-L. *dwarfism, infantilism, syndrome.*

Levin, Abraham, U.S. physician, 1880–1940. SEE L. *tube.*

Levin, Max, U.S. neurologist, *1901. SEE Kleine-L. *syndrome.*

Levine, Samuel A., U.S. cardiologist, 1891–1966. SEE Lown-Ganong-L. *syndrome.*

Le·vin·ea (lĕ-vin′ē-ă). A former genus of bacteria (of the family Enterobacteriaceae) whose species are now assigned to the genus *Citrobacter.* [Max *Levine,* U.S. bacteriologist, *1889]

L. amalona′tica, SYN *Citrobacter amalonatica.*

L. diversus, SYN *Citrobacter diversus.*

L. malona′tica, SYN *Citrobacter diversus.*

lev·i·ta·tion (lev-i-tā′shŭn). Support of the patient on a cushion of air. [L. *levitas,* lightness]

Le·vi·vir·i·dae (lĕ-vi-vir′i-dē). Provisional name for a family of small, nonenveloped, isometric bacterial viruses with genomes of single-stranded RNA (MW 1×10^6). Virions adsorb to the sides of bacterial pili, and crystalline arrays are formed in infected bacteria. The type species is coliphage R17. [L. *levis,* light (not heavy)]

△**levo-.** Left, toward or on the left side. [L. *laevus*]

le·vo·bu·no·lol hy·dro·chlo·ride (lē-vō-byū′nō-lol). (−)-5-[3-(*tert*-Butylamino)-2-hydroxypropoxy]-3,4-dihydro-1(2*H*)-naphthalenonehydrochloride; a β-adrenergic blocking agent used primarily as an eye drop in the treatment of chronic open-angle glaucoma and ocular hypertension.

le·vo·car·dia (lē-vō-kar′dē-ă). Situs inversus of the other viscera but with the heart normally situated on the left; congenital cardiac lesions are commonly associated. [levo- + G. *kardia,* heart]

le·vo·car·di·o·gram (lē-vō-kar′dē-ō-gram). That part of the bi-cardiogram, or normal curve, that is the effect of the left ventricle.

levo·car·ni·tine (lē′vō-kar′nĭ-tēn). Used as a supplement for carnitine deficiency.

le·vo·cli·na·tion (lē′vō-kli-nā′shŭn). SYN levotorsion (2). [levo- + L. *clino,* pp. -*atus,* to bend]

levocycleduction. SYN levotorsion.

le·vo·cy·clo·duc·tion (lē′vō-sī-klō-dŭk′shŭn). levotorsion of one eye. [levo- + cyclo- + L. *duco,* pp. *ductus,* to lead]

le·vo·do·pa (lē-vō-dō′pă). The biologically active form of dopa; an antiparkinsonian agent that is converted to dopamine. SYN L-dopa.

le·vo·duc·tion (lē-vō-dŭk′shŭn). Turning of one eye to the left; exduction of left eye or euduction of right eye. [levo- + L. *duco,* pp. *ductus,* to lead]

le·vo·form (lē′vō-fōrm). Denoting the structure of a substance that rotates the plane of polarized light counterclockwise (left).

le·vo·glu·cose (lē-vō-glū′kōs). D-Fructose. SEE fructose.

le·vo·gram (lē′vō-gram). Electrocardiographic record in an experimental animal representing spread of impulse through the left ventricle alone.

le·vo·gy·rate, le·vo·gy·rous (lē-vō-jī′rāt, -jī′rŭs). SYN levorotatory. [levo- + L. *gyro,* to turn in a circle]

le·vo·nor·def·rin (lē′vō-nōr-def′rin). α-(1-Aminoethyl)-3,4-dihydroxybenzyl alcohol; used as a nasal decongestant and as a vasoconstrictor given with infiltration anesthetics.

le·vo·pha·ce·top·er·ane (lē′vō-fa-sĕ-top′er′ān). α-Phenyl-2-piperidinemethanol acetate; an antidepressant with anorexigenic properties.

le·vo·pho·bia (lev′ō-fō′bē-ă). Fear of objects to the left.

le·vo·pro·pox·y·phene nap·syl·ate (lē′vō-prō-pok′si-fēn). α-4-(Dimethylamino)-3-methyl-1,2-diphenyl-2-butanol propionate 2-naphthalenesulfonate; an antitussive.

le·vo·ro·ta·tion (lē-vō-rō-tā′shŭn). **1.** A turning or twisting to the left; in particular, the counterclockwise twist given the plane of plane-polarized light by solutions of certain optically active substances. Cf. dextrorotation. **2.** SYN sinistrotorsion. [levo- + L. *roto,* to turn]

le·vo·ro·ta·to·ry (lē-vō-rō′tă-tōr-ē). Denoting levorotation, or certain crystals or solutions capable of doing so; as a chemical prefix, usually abbreviated *l-* or (−). Cf. dextrorotatory. SYN levogyrate, levogyrous.

lev·or·pha·nol tar·trate (lev-ōrf′ă-nol). L-3-Hydroxy-*N*-methylmorphinan tartrate dihydrate; an analgesic similar in action to morphine.

le·vo·tor·sion (lē-vō-tōr′shŭn). **1.** SYN sinistrotorsion. **2.** Rotation of the upper pole of the cornea of one or both eyes to the left. SYN levoclination. SYN levocycleduction. [levo- + L. *torsio,* a twisting]

le·vo·ver·sion (lē′vō-ver′zhŭn). **1.** Version toward the left. **2.** Conjugate turning of both eyes to the left. [levo- + L. *verto,* pp. *versus,* to turn]

Levret, André, French obstetrician, 1703–1780. SEE L.'s *forceps;* Mauriceau-L. *maneuver.*

lev·u·lan (lev′yū-lan). SYN fructosan.

lev·u·lic ac·id (lev′yū-lik). SYN levulinic acid.

lev·u·lin (lev′yū-lin). SYN fructosan.

lev·u·li·nate (lev′yū-lin-āt). A salt or ester of levulinic acid.

lev·u·lin·ic ac·id (lev-yū-lin′ik). 4-Oxopentanoic acid; $CH_3COCH_2CH_2COOH$, formed by the action of hot, strong acids on hexoses. SEE ALSO δ-aminolevulinic acid. SYN levulic acid.

lev·u·lo·san (lev′yū-lō-san). SYN fructosan.

lev·u·lose (lev′yū-lōs). D-Fructose. SEE fructose.

lev·u·lo·se·mia (lev′yū-lō-sē′mē-ă). SYN fructosemia.

lev·u·lo·su·ria (lev′yū-lō-sū′rē-ă). SYN fructosuria.

Lévy, Gabrielle, French neurologist, 1886–1935. SEE Roussy-L. *disease, syndrome.*

Lewandowski, Felix, German dermatologist, 1879–1921. SEE Jadassohn-L. *syndrome; nevus* elasticus of L.

Lewis, Gilbert N., U.S. chemist, 1875–1946. SEE ALSO L. *acid, base;* second *law* of thermodynamics.

Lewis Blood Group, Le Blood Group. See Blood Groups Appendix.

lew·is·ite (lū′i-sīt). $C_2H_2AsCl_3$; dichloro(2-chlorovinyl)arsine; a war gas. It is a vesicant, a lung irritant like mustard gas, a systemic poison entering the circulation through the lungs or skin, and a mitotic poison arresting mitosis in the metaphase; dimercaprol is the antidote. SYN β-chlorovinyldichloroarsine. [W. Lee *Lewis,* U.S. chemist 1898–1943]

Lewy (Lewey), Frederic H., German neurologist in the U.S., 1885–1950. SEE L. *bodies,* under *body.*

-lexis, -lexy. Suffixes that properly relate to speech, although often confused with -legia (Latin *-legis*) and thus erroneously employed to relate to reading. [G. *lexis,* word, speech, from *legō,* to say]

Leyden, Ernst V. von, German physician, 1832–1910. SEE L.'s *ataxia, crystals,* under *crystal, neuritis;* L.-Möbius muscular *dystrophy.*

Leydig, Franz von, German anatomist, 1821–1908. SEE L.'s *cells,* under *cell;* L. cell *adenoma.*

ley·dig·ar·che (lī′dig-ar-kē). Obsolete term for the beginning of gonadal function in the male, *e.g.,* male puberty. [Leydig (see Leydig cells), + G. *arche,* beginning]

Lf, L$_f$. SEE dose.

LFA Abbreviation for left frontoanterior position; lymphocyte function associated *antigen.*

LFP Abbreviation for left frontoposterior position.

LFT Abbreviation for left frontotransverse position.

LH Abbreviation for luteinizing *hormone.*

Lhermitte, Jean, French neurologist, 1877–1959. SEE L.'s *sign.*

LH/FSH-RF Abbreviation for luteinizing hormone/follicle-stimulating hormone-releasing *factor.*

LH-RF Abbreviation for luteinizing hormone-releasing *factor.*

LH-RH Abbreviation for luteinizing *hormone*-releasing *hormone.*

Li, Frederick P., 20th century epidemiologist. SEE L.-Fraumeni cancer *syndrome.*

Li Symbol for lithium.

lib·er·a·tor (lib′er-ā-ter, -tōr). An agent that stimulates or activates a physiological chemical or an enzymatic action.

    histamine l.'s, substances that cause the release of histamine from mast cells or basophils.

li·ber·ins (lib′er-ins). SYN releasing *factors.* [L. *libero,* to free, + -in]

lib·er·o·mo·tor (lib′er-ō-mō′ter). Relating to voluntary movements. [L. *liber,* free, + *motor,* mover]

li·bid·i·ni·za·tion (li-bid′i-ni-zā′shŭn). SYN erotization.

li·bid·i·nous (li-bid′i-nŭs). Lascivious; invested with or arousing sexual desire or energy. [L. *libidinosus,* fr. *libido* (*libidin-*), pleasure, desire]

li·bi·do (li-bē′dō, -bī′dō). **1.** Conscious or unconscious sexual desire. **2.** Any passionate interest or form of life force. **3.** In jungian psychology, synonymous with psychic *energy.* [L. lust]

    object l., l. invested in the object, in contradistinction to that invested in the ego.

Libman, Emanuel, U.S. physician, 1872–1946. SEE L.-Sacks *endocarditis, syndrome.*

Liborius, Paul, 19th century Russian bacteriologist. SEE L.'s *method.*

li·brary (lī′brār-ē). A collection of cloned fragments that represent the entire genome.

    cDNA l., a collection of copy (cDNA) fragments that have been made by reverse transcriptase from the mRNA of a particular cell, organ, or organism.

    genomic l., l. in which both introns and exons are represented.

    l. screening, the process of selection of a desired clone from the collection.

lice (līs). Plural of louse.

li·chen (lī′ken). A discrete flat papule or an aggregate of papules giving a patterned configuration resembling lichens growing on rocks. [G. *leichēn,* lichen; a lichen-like eruption]

l. acumina′tus, SYN l. planus.

l. a′grius, acute papular eczema of severe type. SYN Celsus' papules.

l. al′bus, chronic lichenoid dermatitis with depigmentation.

l. annula′ris, SYN *granuloma* annulare.

l. hemorrhag′icus, a papular eruption due to hemorrhage into the hair follicles.

l. infan′tum, SYN *miliaria* rubra.

l. i′ris, ringworm with concentric rings of erythematous papules.

l. myxedemato′sus, a lichenoid eruption of papules or plaques of mucinous edema due to deposit of glycosaminoglycans in the skin and fibroblast proliferation, in the absence of endocrine disease. SEE ALSO scleromyxedema. SYN papular mucinosis.

l. niti′dus, minute asymptomatic whitish or pinkish papules; lesions, which are flat-topped, rarely may coexist with l. planus and may involve male genitalia.

l. nu′chae, l. simplex of the neck, usually in women.

l. obtu′sus, a form in which the papules are large and rounded instead of flattened.

oral (erosive) l. planus, oral manifestations of l. planus characterized by white striae (Wickham's striae) of the oral mucous membrane and sometimes associated with ulceration; patients may or may not exhibit a history of cutaneous l. planus.

l. planopila′ris, follicular hyperkeratosis of the scalp with lymphocytic perifolliculitis and l. planus elsewhere. SYN Graham Little syndrome, l. planus et acuminatus atrophicans.

l. pla′nus, eruption of flat-topped, shiny, violaceous papules on flexor surfaces, male genitalia, and buccal mucosa of unknown cause; may form linear groups; microscopically characterized by a bead-like subepidermal lymphocytic infiltrate. Spontaneous resolution is common after months to years. SYN l. acuminatus, l. ruber planus, Wilson's l.

l. pla′nus et acumina′tus atro′phicans, SYN l. planopilaris.

l. pla′nus annula′ris, a form in which the papules are grouped in ring figures.

l. pla′nus follicula′ris, l. planus of the hair follicles, usually of the scalp.

l. pla′nus hypertro′phicus, verrucoid or warty lesions occurring on legs and thighs in association with l. planus elsewhere. SYN l. planus verrucosus, l. ruber verrucosus.

l. pla′nus verruco′sus, SYN l. planus hypertrophicus.

l. ru′ber, obsolete term for l. planus.

l. ru′ber monilifor′mis, a rare dermatosis consisting of small reddish papules arranged in narrow beaded bands and covering large areas of the body.

l. ru′ber pla′nus, SYN l. planus.

l. ru′ber verruco′sus, SYN l. planus hypertrophicus.

l. sclero′sus et atro′phicus, an eruption consisting of white atrophic papules which may be discrete or confluent and may contain a central depression or a black keratotic plug microscopically showing epidermal hyperkeratosis and atrophy, superficial dermal edema and homogenization, and mid-dermal inflammation; vulval involvement was formerly called kraurosis vulvae.

l. scrofuloso′rum, small asymptomatic l. papules on the trunk of children with tuberculosis; acid-fast bacilli are not seen in the dermal granulomas. SYN acne scrofulosorum, papular scrofuloderma, papular tuberculid.

l. sim′plex chronicus, a thickened area of itching skin resulting from rubbing and scratching.

l. spinulo′sus, eruption of conical papules, of unknown cause, which have an adherent scaly surface; may be related to l. planus.

l. stria′tus, a self-limited papular eruption occurring primarily in children (more commonly in females); the lesions are arranged in linear groups and usually occur on one extremity.

l. strophulo′sus, SYN *miliaria* rubra.

l. syphilit′icus, SYN follicular *syphilid.*

tropical l., l. trop′icus, SYN *miliaria* rubra.

l. urtica′tus, SYN papular *urticaria.*

Wilson's l., SYN l. planus.

li·chen·i·fi·ca·tion (lī′ken-i-fi-kā′shŭn). Leathery induration and

li

thickening of the skin with hyperkeratosis, caused by scratching in atopic or chronic contact dermatitis. SYN lichenization. [lichen + L. *facio,* to make]

li·chen·in (lī'ken-in). A variety of polysaccharide obtained from Iceland moss; used as a demulcent. SYN moss starch.

li·chen·i·za·tion (lī'ken-i-zā'shŭn). SYN lichenification.

li·chen·oid (lī'kĕ-noyd). **1.** Resembling lichen. **2.** Accentuation of normal skin markings observed in cases of chronic eczema. **3.** Microscopically resembling lichen planus.

Lichtenstein, Louis, U.S. physician, 1906–1977. SEE Jaffe-L. *disease.*

Lichtheim, Ludwig, German physician, 1845–1928. SEE L.'s *sign;* Dejerine-Lichtheim *phenomenon.*

lic·o·rice (lik'ŏ-ris). SYN glycyrrhiza.

lid. SYN eyelid. [A.S. *hlid*]

granular l.'s, SYN trachoma.

lower l., SYN lower *eyelid.*

Liddell, Edward G.T., English neurophysiologist, 1895–1981. SEE L.-Sherrington *reflex.*

li·do·caine hy·dro·chlo·ride (lī'dō-kān). Diethylamino-2,6-acetoxylidide hydrochloride; a local anesthetic with antiarrhythmic and anticonvulsant properties.

li·do·fla·zine (lī-dō-flā'zēn). 4-[4,4-Bis(*p*-fluorophenyl)butyl]-1-piperazineaceto-2′,6′-xylidide; a coronary vasodilator.

lie (lī). Relationship of the long axis of the fetus to that of the mother.

longitudinal l., that relationship in which the long axis of the fetus is longitudinal and roughly parallel to the long axis of the mother; the presenting part may be either the head or the breech.

oblique l., that relationship in which the long axis of the fetus crosses the maternal axis at an angle other than a right angle.

transverse l., that relationship in which the long axis of the fetus is transverse or at right angles to that of the mother.

Lieberkühn, Johann N., German anatomist, 1711–1756. SEE L.'s *crypts,* under *crypt, follicles,* under *follicle, glands,* under *gland.*

lie·ber·kühn (lē'ber-kūn). A concave reflector around the objective of a microscope, for the purpose of directing a concentrated beam of light on the material being examined. [J.N. *Lieberkühn*]

Liebermann, Leo von S., Hungarian physician, 1852–1926. SEE Burchard-L. *reaction;* L.-Burchard *test.*

Liebermeister, Carl von, German physician, 1833–1901. SEE L.'s *rule.*

Liebig, Baron Justus von, German chemist, 1803–1873. SEE L.'s *theory.*

Liebow (lē'-bō), Averill A., Austrian-U.S. pulmonary pathologist, 1911–1978. SEE usual interstitial *pneumonia* of Liebow.

lie de·tec·tor. SYN polygraph (2).

li·en (lī'en) [NA]. ✗official alternate term for spleen. [L.]

l. accesso′rius, SYN accessory *spleen.*

l. mo′bilis, SYN floating *spleen.*

l. succenturia′tus, SYN accessory *spleen.*

△**lien-, lieno-.** The spleen; most terms beginning thus are obsolete or obsolescent. SEE spleno-. [L. *lien*]

li·e·nal (lī'ĕ-năl). SYN splenic.

li·en·cu·lus (lī-en'kyū-lŭs). SYN accessory *spleen.* [Mod. L. dim. of L. *lien,* spleen]

li·e·nec·to·my (lī'ĕ-nek'tō-mē). Obsolete term for splenectomy.

li·e·no·med·ul·lary (lī'ĕ-nō-med'yū-lār-ē). SYN splenomyelogenous. [lieno- + G. *medulla,* marrow]

li·e·no·my·e·log·e·nous (lī'ĕ-nō-mī-ĕ-loj'ĕ-nŭs). SYN splenomyelogenous.

li·e·no·pan·cre·at·ic (lī'ĕ-nō-pan'krē-at'ik). SYN splenopancreatic.

li·e·no·re·nal (lī'ĕ-nō-rē'năl). SYN splenorenal. [lieno- + L. *ren,* kidney]

li·en·ter·ic (lī-en-ter'ik). Relating to, or marked by, lientery.

li·en·tery (lī'en-ter-ē). Passage of undigested food in the stools. [G. *leienteria,* fr. *leios,* smooth, + *enteron,* intestine]

li·en·un·cu·lus (lī'ĕ-nun'kyū-lŭs). SYN accessory *spleen.* [Mod. L. dim. of L. *lien,* spleen]

Liesegang, Ralph E., German chemist, 1869–1947. SEE L. *rings,* under *ring.*

Lieutaud, Joseph, French anatomist and pathologist, 1703–1780. SEE L.'s *body, triangle, trigone, uvula.*

life (līf). **1.** Vitality, the essential condition of being alive; the state of existence characterized by such functions as metabolism, growth, reproduction, adaptation, and response to stimuli. **2.** Living organisms such as animals and plants. [A.S. *lif*]

half-l., SEE half-life.

postnatal l., that interval of l. after birth; in man, usually divided into periods: neonatal, infancy, childhood, adolescence, and adulthood.

prenatal l., that interval of l. between conception and birth; in humans, usually divided into embryonic and fetal periods.

sexual l., in psychiatry and psychoanalysis, the specifically erotic or sexual interests, fantasies, inclinations, and conduct of the patient.

vegetative l., the simple metabolic and reproductive activity of humans or animals, apart from the exercise of conscious mental or psychic processes.

life e·vents. Occurrences in one's daily life, some of which act as stressors.

life·span. 1. The duration of life of an individual. **2.** The normal or average duration of life of members of a given species. SEE ALSO longevity.

life-style. The set of habits and customs that is influenced by the lifelong process of socialization, including social use of substances such as alcohol and tobacco, dietary habits, exercise, etc., all of which have important implications for health.

LIGAMENT

lig·a·ment (lig'ă-ment). **1.** A band or sheet of fibrous tissue connecting two or more bones, cartilages, or other structures, or serving as support for fasciae or muscles. **2.** A fold of peritoneum supporting any of the abdominal viscera. **3.** Any structure resembling a l. though not performing the function of such. **4.** The cordlike remains of a fetal vessel or other structure that has lost its original lumen. SYN ligamentum [NA]. [L. *ligamentum,* a band, bandage]

accessory l.'s, l.'s about a joint that are in addition to the articular capsule. They may lie within, or on the outside of the latter.

accessory plantar l.'s, SYN plantar l.'s.

accessory volar l.'s, SYN palmar l.'s.

acromioclavicular l., a fibrous band extending from the acromion of the scapula to the clavicle. SYN ligamentum acromioclaviculare [NA].

alar l.'s, (1) one of a pair of short stout bands that extends from the side of the dens of the axis to the tubercle on the medial aspect of the occipital condyle; SYN check l.'s of odontoid. **(2)** SYN alar *folds,* under *fold.*

alveolodental l., SYN periodontal l.

annular l., one of a number of l.'s encircling various parts; the principal annular l.'s are those of the stapes, radius, and trachea. SEE annular l. of the radius, annular l. of the stapes, annular l.'s of the trachea. SYN ligamentum annulare, orbicular l.

annular l. of the radius, the l. that encircles and holds the head of the radius in the radial notch of the ulna, forming the proximal radioulnar joint and enabling pronation/supination of forearm; receives the radial collateral l. of the elbow. SYN ligamentum annulare radii [NA], ligamentum orbiculare radii, orbicular l. of radius.

annular l. of the stapes, a ring of elastic fibers that attaches the base of the stapes to the margin of the fenestra vestibuli. SYN ligamentum annulare stapedis [NA].

annular l.'s of the trachea, the fibrous membranes that connect adjacent tracheal cartilages. SYN ligamenta annularia trachealia [NA], ligamenta trachealia [NA].

anococcygeal l., a musculofibrous band that passes between the anus and the coccyx. SYN ligamentum anococcygeum [NA], anococcygeal body, raphe anococcygea, Symington's anococcygeal body.

anterior costotransverse l., SYN superior costotransverse l.

anterior cruciate l., the l. that extends from the anterior intercondylar area of the tibia to the posterior part of the medial surface of the lateral condyle of the femur. SYN ligamentum cruciatum anterius [NA].

anterior l. of head of fibula, a l. uniting the anterior part of the head of the fibula to the tibia. SYN ligamentum capitis fibulae anterius.

anterior l. of Helmholtz, SEE anterior l. of malleus.

anterior longitudinal l., the wide fibrous band interconnecting the anterior surfaces of the vertebral bodies. SYN lacertus medius, ligamentum longitudinale anterius.

anterior l. of malleus, consists of two portions: Meckel's band, passing from the base of the anterior process to the spine of the sphenoid through the petrotympanic fissure; and the anterior l. of Helmholtz, extending from the anterior aspect of the neck of the malleus to the anterior boundary of the tympanic notch. SYN ligamentum mallei anterius [NA].

anterior meniscofemoral l., the ligamentous band that passes anterior to the posterior cruciate l., extending between the posterior portion of the lateral meniscus and the upper end of the anterior cruciate l. SYN ligamentum meniscofemorale anterius [NA], Humphry's l.

anterior sacrococcygeal l., SYN ventral sacrococcygeal l.

anterior sacroiliac l.'s, the strong fibrous bands that reinforce the sacroiliac joint anteriorly. SYN ligamenta sacroiliaca anteriora [NA], ventral sacroiliac l.'s.

anterior sacrosciatic l., SYN sacrospinous l.

anterior sternoclavicular l., a fibrous band that reinforces the sternoclavicular anteriorly. SYN ligamentum sternoclaviculare anterius [NA].

anterior talofibular l., the band of fibers that extends from the lateral malleolus to the neck of the talus. SYN ligamentum talofibulare anterius [NA].

anterior talotibial l., SYN anterior tibiotalar l. SEE ALSO deltoid l.

anterior tibiofibular l., the l. that binds the anterior aspect of the tibiofibular syndesmosis. SYN ligamentum tibiofibulare anterius [NA].

anterior tibiotalar l., the part of the medial or deltoid l. that extends from the medial malleolus to the neck of the talus. SYN pars tibiotalaris anterior ligamenti medialis [NA], anterior talotibial l., anterior tibiotalar part of deltoid ligament, ligamenti medialis, ligamentum talotibiale anterius.

apical l. of dens, a l. that extends from the apex of the dens of the axis to the anterior margin of the foramen magnum; includes vestiges of notochord. SYN ligamentum apicis dentis [NA].

Arantius' l., SYN *ligamentum* venosum.

arcuate popliteal l., a broad fibrous band attached above to the lateral condyle of the femur and passing medially and downward, blending with the posterior part of the fibrous capsule of the knee joint, arching over the tendon of the popliteus muscle. SYN ligamentum popliteum arcuatum [NA], popliteal arch, posterior l. of knee.

arcuate pubic l., the l. that arches across the inferior aspect of the pubic symphysis. SYN ligamentum arcuatum pubis [NA], inferior pubic l.

arterial l., SYN *ligamentum* arteriosum.

l.'s of auditory ossicles, the l.'s connecting the ear bones with one another and with the walls of the tympanic cavity. SYN ligamenta ossiculorum auditus [NA].

auricular l.'s, the three l.'s that attach the auricle to the side of the head: anterior auricular l. (*ligamentum* auriculare anterius), which extends from the root of the zygomatic process to the spine of the helix; posterior auricular l. (*ligamentum* auriculare posterius), which extends from the mastoid process to the conchal eminence; superior auricular l. (*ligamentum* auriculare superius), which extends from the superior margin of the osseous

external acoustic meatus to the spine of the helix. SYN ligamenta auricularia [NA], Valsalva's l.'s.

axis l. of malleus, SYN Helmholtz' axis l.

Bardinet's l., the posterior band of the ulnar collateral l. of the elbow.

Barkow's l.'s, the anterior and posterior portions of the fibrous capsule of the elbow joint.

Bellini's l., a fasciculus from the ischiofemoral portion of the articular fibrous capsule of the hip which extends to the great trochanter.

Berry's l.'s, SYN lateral thyrohyoid l.

Bertin's l., SYN iliofemoral l.

Bichat's l., the lower fasciculus of the posterior sacroiliac l.

bifurcate l., a strong V-shaped l. on the dorsum of the foot that passes from the calcaneus distal to the tarsal sinus and attaches to cuboid and navicular bones; it is divided into the dorsal calcaneocuboid l. and the calcaneonavicular l. SYN ligamentum bifurcatum [NA], bifurcated l.

bifurcated l., SYN bifurcate l.

Bigelow's l., SYN iliofemoral l.

Botallo's l., SYN *ligamentum* arteriosum.

Bourgery's l., SYN oblique popliteal l.

broad l. of the uterus, the peritoneal fold passing from the lateral margin of the uterus to the wall of the pelvis on either side, and in so doing also ensheathing the ovaries and uterine tubes. SYN ligamentum latum uteri [NA].

Brodie's l., SYN transverse humeral l.

Burns' l., SYN superior *horn* of falciform margin of saphenous opening.

calcaneocuboid l., the lateral part of the bifurcate l. SYN ligamentum calcaneocuboideum [NA].

calcaneofibular l., the middle of the three fascicles that form the lateral collateral l. of the ankle joint, reinforcing the lateral side of the ankle joint; the remaining two l.'s of the lateral collateral l.'s are the anterior and posterior talofibular l.'s. SYN ligamentum calcaneofibulare [NA].

calcaneonavicular l., the medial part of the l. bifurcatum. SYN ligamentum calcaneonaviculare [NA].

calcaneotibial l., SYN tibiocalcaneal l. SEE ALSO deltoid l.

Caldani's l., SYN coracoclavicular l.

Campbell's l., SYN suspensory l. of axilla.

Camper's l., SYN inferior *fascia* of urogenital diaphragm.

capsular l., thickened portions of the fibrous membrane of an articular capsule. SYN ligamentum capsulare.

cardinal l., a fibrous band attached to the uterine cervix and the vault of the lateral fornix of the vagina; continuous with the tissue ensheathing the pelvic vessels. SYN cervical l. of uterus, ligamentum transversale colli, Mackenrodt's l.

caroticoclinoid l., the l. that connects the anterior to the middle clinoid process of the sphenoid bone.

carpometacarpal l.'s, the l.'s uniting the metacarpal and carpal bones. SYN ligamenta carpometacarpalia [NA].

caudal l., SYN caudal *retinaculum*.

ceratocricoid l., SYN *ligamentum* ceratocricoideum.

cervical l. of uterus, SYN cardinal l.

check l.'s of eyeball, medial and lateral, expansions of the sheaths of the medial and lateral rectus muscles of the eyeball which are attached, respectively, to the lacrimal bone and to the orbital tubercle of the zygomatic bone; they serve to prevent overaction of these muscles.

check l.'s of odontoid, SYN alar l.'s (1).

chondroxiphoid l., SYN costoxiphoid l.

ciliary l., SYN ciliary *muscle*.

Civinini's l., SYN pterygospinous l.

Clado's l., a mesenteric fold running from the broad l. on the right side to the appendix.

collateral l., one of a number of l.'s on either side of, and serving as a radius of movement of, a joint having a hingelike movement; they occur at the following joints: elbow, knee, wrist, and the metacarpo- or metatarsophalangeal, proximal interpha-

li

langeal, and distal interphalangeal joints of the hands and feet. SYN ligamentum collaterale [NA].

Colles' l., SYN reflected inguinal l.

conjugate l., a l. in some mammals which is the homologue of the intra-articular l. present in the joints between the heads of the ribs and the vertebrae. SYN ligamentum conjugale.

conoid l., the medial part of the coracoclavicular l. that attaches to the conoid tubercle of the clavicle. SYN ligamentum conoideum [NA].

Cooper's l.'s, (1) SYN suspensory l.'s of breast. **(2)** SYN pectineal l. **(3)** SYN transverse l. of elbow.

coracoacromial l., the heavy arched fibrous band that passes between the coracoid process and the acromion above the shoulder joint; the osseofibrous arch thus formed prevents upward dislocation of the shoulder (glanohumeral) joint. SYN ligamentum coracoacromiale [NA].

coracoclavicular l., the strong l. that unites the clavicle to the coracoid process; it is subdivided into the conoid ligamentum and the trapezoid ligamentum. The free upper limb is passively suspended from the clavicular "strut" by the coracoclavicular l.; the l. also plays an important role in preventing dislocation of the acromioclavicular joint. SYN ligamentum coracoclaviculare [NA], Caldani's l.

coracohumeral l., the l. that passes from the base of the coracoid process to the greater tubercle of the humerus. SYN ligamentum coracohumerale [NA].

corniculopharyngeal l., SYN cricopharyngeal l.

coronary l. of knee, portions of the articular capsule of the knee joint which connect the circumference of the menisci with the margins of the condyles of the tibia.

coronary l. of liver, peritoneal reflections from the liver to the diaphragm at the margins of the bare area of the liver. SYN ligamentum coronarium hepatis [NA].

costoclavicular l., the l. that connects the first rib and the clavicle near its sternal end; limits elevation of shoulder (at sternoclavicular joint). SYN ligamentum costoclaviculare [NA], rhomboid l.

costocolic l., SYN phrenicocolic l.

costotransverse l., the l. that connects the dorsal aspect of the neck of a rib to the ventral aspect of the corresponding transverse process. SYN ligamentum costotransversarium [NA], ligamentum colli costae, middle costotransverse l.

costoxiphoid l., the l. that connects the xiphoid process to the seventh, and often to the sixth, costal cartilages. SYN ligamentum costoxiphoideum [NA], chondroxiphoid l.

cotyloid l., SYN acetabular *labrum*.

Cowper's l., the part of the fascia lata which is anterior to and provides origin for fibers of the pectineus muscle.

cricopharyngeal l., an elastic band connecting the tip of the corniculate (Santorini's) cartilage and the lamina of the cricoid cartilage and continuing into the pharyngeal mucosa covering the cricoid lamina. SYN ligamentum cricopharyngeum [NA], corniculopharyngeal l., cricosantorinian l., jugal l., ligamentum corniculopharyngeum, ligamentum jugale.

cricosantorinian l., SYN cricopharyngeal l.

cricothyroid l., the strong band that connects the cricoid and thyroid cartilages in the midline anteriorly; it is continuous posteriorly with the conus elasticus. SYN conus elasticus (2) [NA], ligamentum cricothyroideum [NA].

cricotracheal l., a midline fibrous band connecting the cricoid cartilage with the first ring of the trachea. SYN ligamentum cricotracheale [NA], cricotracheal membrane.

crucial l., (1) SEE inferior extensor *retinaculum*, superior extensor *retinaculum*. **(2)** SYN cruciate l.'s of knee. **(3)** SYN cruciform l. of atlas. **(4)** SYN cruciform *part* of fibrous digital sheath.

cruciate l. of the atlas, SYN cruciform l. of atlas.

cruciate l.'s of knee, the two l.'s which pass from the intercondylar area of the tibia to the intercondylar fossa of the femur. SEE anterior cruciate l., posterior cruciate l. SYN ligamenta cruciata genus [NA], crucial l. (2).

cruciate l. of leg, SYN inferior extensor *retinaculum*.

cruciform l. of atlas, the strong l. that lies posterior to the dens of the axis holding it against the anterior arch of the atlas; it consists primarily of the transverse l. of the atlas that forms the cross-bar of the cross and is most important functionally, and longitudinal bands of the cruciform l., forming the upright or vertical beams of the cross. SYN ligamentum cruciforme atlantis [NA], crucial l. (3), cruciate l. of the atlas, ligamentum cruciatum atlantis.

Cruveilhier's l.'s, SYN plantar l.'s.

cuboideonavicular l.'s, l. uniting the cuboid bone with the navicular bone. SEE dorsal cuboideonavicular l., plantar cuboideonavicular l. SYN ligamentum cuboideonaviculare [NA].

cuneocuboid l.'s, ligament uniting the lateral cuneiform bone with the cuboid bone. SEE dorsal cuneocuboid l., interosseous cuneocuboid l., plantar cuneocuboid l. SYN ligamentum cuneocuboideum [NA].

cuneonavicular l.'s, SEE dorsal cuneonavicular l.'s, plantar cuneonavicular l.'s.

cystoduodenal l., a peritoneal fold that sometimes passes from the gallbladder to the first part of the duodenum.

deep dorsal sacrococcygeal l., the continuation of the posterior longitudinal l. uniting the sacrum and coccyx. SYN ligamentum sacrococcygeum posterius profundum [NA], deep posterior sacrococcygeal l.

deep posterior sacrococcygeal l., SYN deep dorsal sacrococcygeal l.

deep transverse metacarpal l., the l. that interconnects the palmar surface of the heads of the second to fifth metacarpals, being continuous with the palmar l.'s on palmar plates; it lies in the plane of the palmar interosseous fascia. SYN ligamentum metacarpale transversum profundum [NA], transverse metacarpal l.

deep transverse metatarsal l., the l. that interconnects the plantar surface of the heads of the metatarsals, being continuous with the plantar l.'s. SYN ligamentum metatarsale transversum profundum [NA], transverse metatarsal l.

deltoid l., compound l. consisting of four component l.'s which pass downward from the medial malleolus of the tibia to the tarsal bones: 1) tibionavicular l. (pars tibionavicularis [NA]), 2) tibiocalcaneal l. (pars tibiocalcanea [NA]), 3) anterior tibiotalar l. (pars tibiotalaris anterior [NA]), and 4) posterior tibiotalar l. (pars tibiotalaris posterior [NA]). SYN ligamentum mediale articulationis talocruralis [NA], ligamentum deltoideum✩, medial l. of talocrural joint.

Denonvilliers' l., SYN puboprostatic l.

dentate l. of spinal cord, rarely used variation on the spelling of denticulate l.

denticulate l., a serrated, shelflike extension of the spinal pia mater projecting in a frontal plane from either side of the cervical and thoracic spinal cord; its 21 pointed processes fuse laterally with the arachnoid and dura mater midway between the exits of the roots of adjacent spinal nerves. SYN ligamentum denticulatum [NA].

Denucé's l., SYN quadrate l.

diaphragmatic l. of the mesonephros, the segment of the urogenital ridge that extends from the mesonephros to the diaphragm; becomes the suspensory l. of the ovary. SYN urogenital mesentery.

dorsal calcaneocuboid l., SEE bifurcate l.

dorsal carpal l., SYN extensor *retinaculum*.

dorsal carpometacarpal l.'s, fibrous bands that connect the dorsal surfaces of the carpal and metacarpal bones. SYN ligamentum carpometacarpalia dorsalia.

dorsal cuboideonavicular l., the l. that unites the dorsal surfaces of the cuboid and navicular bones of the tarsus. SYN ligamentum cuboideonaviculare dorsale [NA].

dorsal cuneocuboid l., the fibrous band that unites the dorsal margins of the lateral cuneiform and cuboid bones. SYN ligamentum cuneocuboideum dorsale [NA].

dorsal cuneonavicular l.'s, several l.'s connecting the dorsal surface of the navicular with the three cuneiform bones. SYN ligamenta cuneonavicularia dorsalia.

dorsal metacarpal l.'s, fibrous bands connecting the dorsal aspects of the bases of metacarpals two to five. SYN ligamenta metacarpalia dorsalia.

dorsal metatarsal l.'s, fibrous bands that connect the dorsal aspects of the bases of the metatarsals. SYN ligamenta metatarsalia dorsalia.

dorsal radiocarpal l., the l. that extends from the distal end of the radius posteriorly to the proximal row of carpal bones. SYN ligamentum radiocarpale dorsale [NA].

dorsal sacroiliac l.'s, SYN posterior sacroiliac l.'s.

dorsal talonavicular l., the broad band that passes from the dorsal side of the neck of the talus to the dorsal surface of the navicular bone. SYN ligamentum talonaviculare [NA], talonavicular l.

duodenorenal l., a fold of peritoneum occasionally passing from the termination of the hepatoduodenal l. to the front of the right kidney. SYN ligamentum duodenorenale.

l. of epididymis, one of two folds (superior and inferior) of the tunica vaginalis between the epididymis and the testis. SYN ligamentum epididymidis [NA].

epihyal l., SYN stylohyoid l.

external collateral l. of wrist, SYN radial collateral l. of wrist.

extracapsular l.'s, l.'s associated with a synovial joint but separate from and external to its articular capsule. SYN ligamenta extracapsularia [NA].

falciform l., SYN falciform *process*.

falciform l. of liver, a crescentic fold of peritoneum extending to the surface of the liver from the diaphragm and anterior abdominal wall; the round ligament lies in its free inferior border, derivative of embryonic ventral mesogastrium. SYN ligamentum falciforme hepatis [NA].

fallopian l., SYN inguinal l.

Ferrein's l., SYN lateral temporomandibular l.

fibular collateral l., the cordlike l. that passes from the lateral epicondyle of the femur to the head of the fibula. SYN ligamentum collaterale fibulare [NA], lateral l. of knee, Winslow's l.

fibular collateral l. of ankle, SYN lateral collateral l. of ankle.

Flood's l., a band of the coracohumeral ligament, attached to the lower part of the lesser tuberosity of the humerus.

fundiform l. of foot, SYN Retzius' l.

fundiform l. of penis, a band of elastic fibers of the superficial fascial layer that extends from the linea alba above the pubic symphysis splitting to surround the penis before attaching to the fascia of the penis. SYN ligamentum fundiforme penis [NA].

gastrocolic l., the major, apron-like portion of the greater omentum that extends between the stomach and the transverse colon. SYN ligamentum gastrocolicum [NA].

gastrodiaphragmatic l., SYN gastrophrenic l.

gastrolienal l., SYN gastrosplenic l.

gastrophrenic l., the portion of the greater omentum that extends from the greater curvature of the stomach to the inferior surface of the diaphragm. SYN ligamentum gastrophrenicum [NA], gastrodiaphragmatic l., phrenogastric l.

gastrosplenic l., the portion of the greater omentum that lies between the greater curvature of the stomach and the hilum of the spleen. SYN ligamentum gastrosplenicum [NA], ligamentum gastrolienale☆ [NA], gastrolienal l., gastrosplenic omentum.

genital l., an embryonic mesenchymatous band providing support for the internal genitalia. SYN suspensory l. of gonad.

genitoinguinal l., in the fetus, a fold of the mesorchium containing the gubernaculum testis. SYN ligamentum genitoinguinale [NA], plica gubernatrix.

Gerdy's l., SYN suspensory l. of axilla.

Gillette's suspensory l., SYN cricoesophageal *tendon*.

Gimbernat's l., SYN lacunar l.

gingivodental l., SYN periodontal l.

glenohumeral l.'s, three fibrous bands that reinforce the anterior part of the articular capsule of the shoulder joint; they are in continuity with the glenoid labrum at the supraglenoid tubercle of the scapula and blend with the fibrous capsule as it attaches to the anatomic neck of the humerus. SYN ligamenta glenohumeralia [NA].

glenoid l., (1) SYN glenoid *labrum*. (2) SYN plantar l.'s.

glossoepiglottic l., an elastic ligamentous band passing from the base of the tongue to the epiglottis in the middle glossoepiglottic fold.

Günz' l., a portion of the superficial layer of the obturator membrane.

hammock l., the part of the periodontium below the growing end of the root of the tooth.

l. of head of femur, a flattened l. that passes from the fovea in the head of the femur to the borders of the acetabular notch (transverse acetabular l.); developmentally, an artery passes to the head of the femur with the l. which may or may not persist into adulthood; the l. does not contribute to the integrity of the joint or control movements there. SYN ligamentum capitis femoris [NA], ligamentum teres femoris, round l. of femur.

Helmholtz' axis l., a l. forming the axis about which the malleus rotates; it consists of two portions extending from the anterior and the posterior border, respectively, of the tympanic notch to the malleus. SYN axis l. of malleus.

Hensing's l., the left superior colic l.; a small serous horizontal or oblique fold sometimes found extending between the upper end of the descending colon and the abdominal wall. SEE phrenicocolic l.

hepatocolic l., an inconstant extension of the hepatoduodenal l. to the transverse colon. SYN ligamentum hepatocolicum [NA].

hepatoduodenal l., the portion of the lesser omentum that connects the liver and duodenum. SYN ligamentum hepatoduodenale [NA].

hepatoesophageal l., the part of the lesser omentum that extends between the liver and the abdominal part of the esophagus. SYN ligamentum hepatoesophageum.

hepatogastric l., the part of the lesser omentum that extends between the liver and lesser curvature of the stomach. SYN ligamentum hepatogastricum [NA].

hepatorenal l., a prolongation of the coronary l. downward over the right kidney. SYN ligamentum hepatorenale [NA].

Hesselbach's l., SYN interfoveolar l.

Hey's ligament, SYN superior *horn* of falciform margin of saphenous opening.

Holl's l., l. joining the corpora cavernosa clitoridis in front of the urinary meatus.

Hueck's l., SYN trabecular *reticulum*.

Humphry's l., SYN anterior meniscofemoral l.

Hunter's l., SYN round l. of uterus.

hyalocapsular l., attachment of the vitreous body to the posterior surface of the lens of the eye. SYN ligamentum hyaloideo-capsulario.

hyoepiglottic l., a short elastic band that unites the epiglottis to the upper border of the hyoid bone. SYN ligamentum hyoepiglotticum [NA].

hypsiloid l., SYN iliofemoral l.

iliofemoral l., a triangular l. attached by its apex to the anterior inferior spine of the ilium and rim of the acetabulum, and by its base to the anterior intertrochanteric line of the femur; the strong medial band is attached to the lower part of the intertrochanteric line; the strong lateral part is fixed to the tubercle at the upper part of this line; the bands diverge, forming a Y-like figure with a weak area between; among the strongest of the body's l.'s, it limits extension at the hip joint. SYN ligamentum iliofemorale [NA], Bertin's l., Bigelow's l., hypsiloid l., Y-shaped l.

iliolumbar l., the strong l. that connects the fourth and fifth lumbar vertebrae with the ilium, spanning the "notch" between the vertebral column and the wing of the ileum. SYN ligamentum iliolumbale [NA].

iliopectineal l., SYN iliopectineal *arch*.

iliotrochanteric l., the lateral strong band of the Y-shaped iliofemoral l.; it is attached below to the tubercle at the upper part of the intertrochanteric line.

inferior calcaneonavicular l., SYN plantar calcaneonavicular l.

inferior l. of epididymis, the lower of the folds of the tunica vaginalis between the body of the epididymis and the testis. SYN ligamentum epididymidis inferius.

inferior pubic l., SYN arcuate pubic l.

inferior transverse scapular l., an inconstant fibrous band that

li

passes from the lateral border of the spine of the scapula to the posterior margin of the glenoid cavity. SYN ligamentum transversum scapulae inferius [NA], spinoglenoid l.

infundibulo-ovarian l., SYN ovarian *fimbria.*

infundibulopelvic l., SYN suspensory l. of ovary.

inguinal l., a fibrous band formed by the thickened inferior border of the aponeurosis of the external oblique that extends from the anterior superior spine of the ilium to the pubic tubercle bridging, muscular and vascular lacunae;forms the floor of the inguinal canal; gives origin to the lowermost fibers of internal oblique and transversus abdominis muscles. SEE ALSO *aponeurosis* of external abdominal oblique muscle. SYN ligamentum inguinale [NA], arcus inguinalis⋆ [NA], crural arch, fallopian arch, fallopian l., femoral arch, Poupart's l.

inguinal l. of the kidney, the segment of the mesonephros extending to the inguinal region.

intercapital l., SYN *ligamentum* intercapitale.

intercarpal l.'s, three sets of short fibrous bands that bind together the two rows of carpal bones; according to their location they are named dorsal intercarpal l. (ligamentum intercarpalia dorsalia), interosseous intercarpal l. (ligamentum intercarpalia interossea), and palmar intercarpal l. (ligamentum intercarpalia palmaria). SYN ligamenta intercarpalia [NA].

interclavicular l., a strong l. that connects the two sternoclavicular joints across the upper border of the manubrium. SYN ligamentum interclaviculare [NA].

interclinoid l., a band of dura mater connecting the anterior and posterior clinoid processes of the sphenoid bone; may become ossified.

intercornual l., SYN lateral sacrococcygeal l.

intercostal l.'s, SYN intercostal *membranes,* under *membrane.*

intercuneiform l.'s, fibrous bands that unite the cuneiform bones; they are arranged in three sets: dorsal intercuneiform l. (ligamentum intercuneiformia dorsalia), interosseous intercuneiform l. (ligamentum intercuneiformia interossea), and plantar intercuneiform l. (ligamentum intercuneiformia plantaria). SYN ligamenta intercuneiformia [NA].

interfoveolar l., fibrous or muscular strands that lie medial to the deep inguinal ring, extending from the lower border of the transversus muscle to the lacunar l. and pectineal fascia. SYN ligamentum interfoveolare [NA], Hesselbach's l.

internal collateral l. of the wrist, SYN ulnar collateral l. of wrist.

interosseous cuneocuboid l., the fibrous band that unites adjacent margins of the distal end of the lateral cuneiform and cuboid bones. SYN ligamentum cuneocuboideum interosseum [NA].

interosseous cuneometatarsal l.'s, l.'s that pass from the cuneiform bones to the metatarsals, the one from the first cuneiform to the second metatarsal being the strongest. SYN ligamenta cuneometatarsalia interossea [NA], Lisfranc's l.'s.

interosseous metacarpal l.'s, fibrous bands connecting the bases of metacarpals two to five; they extend between the dorsal and palmar metacarpal ligaments. SYN ligamenta metacarpalia interossea.

interosseous metatarsal l.'s, fibrous bands that connect the bases of the metatarsals; they extend between the dorsal and plantar metatarsal ligaments. SYN ligamenta metatarsalia interossea.

interosseous sacroiliac l.'s, short obliquely directed fibrous bands that pass between the sacrum and ilium in the narrow cleft behind the auricular surfaces of these bones. SYN ligamenta sacroiliaca interossea [NA].

interosseous talocalcaneal l., a strong fibrous band occupying the tarsal sinus. SYN ligamentum talocalcaneare interosseum.

interosseous tibiofibular l., SYN transverse tibiofibular l.

interspinous l., bands of fibrous tissue that connect the spinous processes of adjacent vertebrae. SYN ligamentum interspinale [NA].

intertransverse l., one of the ligaments that connect the transverse processes of adjacent vertebrae. SYN ligamentum intertransversarium [NA].

intra-articular l. of costal head, transverse fibers extending within the capsule from the ridge between the two facets on the head of the rib to the intervertebral disk. SYN ligamentum capitis costae intra-articulare [NA].

intra-articular sternocostal l., a l. within the articular capsule between a costal cartilage and the sternum; especially well developed at second costal cartilage. SYN ligamentum sternocostale intra-articulare [NA].

intracapsular l.'s, ligaments located within and separate from the articular capsule of a synovial joint. SYN ligamenta intracapsularia [NA].

ischiocapsular l., SYN ischiofemoral l.

ischiofemoral l., the thickened part of the capsule of the hip joint that passes from the ischium upward and laterally over the femoral neck; some of its fibers continue into the zona orbicularis. SYN ligamentum ischiofemorale [NA], ischiocapsular l., ligamentum ischiocapsulare.

Jarjavay's l., SYN sacrouterine *fold.*

jugal l., SYN cricopharyngeal l.

Krause's l., SYN transverse perineal l.

laciniate l., SYN flexor *retinaculum* of lower limb.

lacunar l., a curved fibrous band that passes horizontally backward from the medial end of the inguinal l. to the pectineal line; it forms the medial boundary of the femoral ring. SEE ALSO *aponeurosis* of external abdominal oblique muscle. SYN ligamentum lacunare [NA], Gimbernat's l.

Lannelongue's l.'s, SYN sternopericardial l.

lateral arcuate l., one of Haller's arches; a thickening of the fascia of the quadratus lumborum muscle between the transverse process of the first lumbar vertebra and the twelfth rib on either side that gives attachment to a portion of the diaphragm. SYN ligamentum arcuatum laterale [NA], arcus lumbocostalis lateralis, lateral lumbocostal arch.

lateral l.'s of the bladder, condensations of fibroareolar tissue which pass one from each side of the bladder to blend with the pelvic fascia; smooth muscle is usually present in this tissue and is referred to as the musculus rectovesicalis.

lateral collateral l. of ankle, the calcaneofibular l., anterior talofibular l., and posterior talofibular l. together maintaining the integrity of the lateral aspect of the talocrural joint. SYN fibular collateral l. of ankle.

lateral costotransverse l., the short quadrangular l., actually a thickening of the posterior aspect of the costotransverse joint, extending from the tip of the transverse process to the posterior surface of the neck of the rib. SYN ligamentum costotransversarium laterale [NA], ligamentum costotransversarium posterius, ligamentum tuberculi costae, posterior costotransverse l.

lateral l. of elbow, SYN radial collateral l. of elbow.

lateral l. of knee, SYN fibular collateral l.

lateral malleolar l., SEE anterior tibiofibular l., posterior tibiofibular l.

lateral l. of malleus, a short fan-shaped l. converging from the posterior half of the tympanic notch to the neck of the malleus. SYN ligamentum mallei laterale [NA].

lateral palpebral l., the band that attaches the tarsal plates to the orbital eminence of the zygomatic bone. SYN ligamentum palpebrale laterale [NA], ligamentum palpebrale externum, ligamentum tarsale externum.

lateral puboprostatic l., SYN *ligamentum* puboprostaticum laterale. SEE puboprostatic l.

lateral sacrococcygeal l., a l. that extends from the lateral inferior margin of the sacrum to the transverse process of the first coccygeal vertebra. SYN ligamentum sacrococcygeum laterale [NA], intercornual l.

lateral talocalcaneal l., a l. extending from the trochlea of the talus to the lateral surface of the calcaneus. SYN ligamentum talocalcaneare laterale.

lateral temporomandibular l., the capsular l. that passes obliquely down and backward across the lateral surface of the temporomandibular joint. SYN ligamentum laterale articulationis temporomandibularis [NA], Ferrein's l., lateral l. of temporomandibular joint, ligamentum temporomandibulare, temporomandibular l.

lateral l. of temporomandibular joint, SYN lateral temporomandibular l.

lateral thyrohyoid l., thickened elastic bundle connecting the superior horn of the thyroid cartilage to the tip of the greater horn of the hyoid cartilage; forms the posterior border of the thyrohyoid membrane. SYN ligamentum thyrohyoideum laterale [NA], Berry's l.'s, ligamentum hyothyroideum laterale.

lateral umbilical l., SYN *ligamentum* umbilicale laterale.

lateral l. of wrist, SYN radial collateral l. of wrist.

Lauth's l., SYN transverse l. of the atlas.

l. of left superior vena cava, the obliterated left common cardinal vein that extends from the left brachiocephalic vein to the oblique vein of the left atrium.

left triangular l., a triangular fold of fibrous connective tissue and peritoneum that extends from the left lobe of the liver to the diaphragm. SYN ligamentum triangulare sinistrum [NA].

l. of left vena cava, the obliterated left common cardinal vein; it extends from the left brachiocephalic vein to the oblique vein of the left atrium. SYN ligamentum venae cavae sinistrae.

lienophrenic l., SYN splenorenal l.

lienorenal l., SYN splenorenal l.

Lisfranc's l.'s, SYN interosseous cuneometatarsal l.'s.

Lockwood's l., SYN suspensory l. of eyeball.

longitudinal l., one of two extensive fibrous bands running the length of the vertebral column: the anterior longitudinal l. and the posterior longitudinal l. SYN ligamentum longitudinale [NA].

long plantar l., a strong l. that extends from the calcaneus to the cuboid and lateral metatarsals on the plantar aspect of the foot; part of the passive support system for maintaining the longitudinal arch of the foot. SYN ligamentum plantare longum [NA].

lumbocostal l., a strong band that unites the twelfth rib with the tips of the transverse processes of the first and second lumbar vertebrae. SYN ligamentum lumbocostale [NA].

Luschka's l.'s, SYN sternopericardial l.

Mackenrodt's l., SYN cardinal l.

l.'s of malleus, SEE anterior l. of malleus, lateral l. of malleus, superior l. of malleus.

Mauchart's l.'s, SEE alar l.'s.

Meckel's l., SYN Meckel's *band*.

medial l., the bundle of fibers strengthening the medial part of the articular capsule of the temporomandibular joint. SYN ligamentum mediale articulationis temporomandibularis [NA].

medial arcuate l., one of Haller's arches; a tendinous thickening of the psoas fascia that extends from the body of the first lumbar vertebra to its transverse process on either side. A portion of the diaphragm arises from it. SYN ligamentum arcuatum mediale [NA], arcus lumbocostalis medialis, medial lumbocostal arch.

medial collateral l. of elbow, SYN ulnar collateral l. of elbow.

medial l. of knee, SYN tibial collateral l.

medial palpebral l., the fibrous band that attaches the medial ends of the tarsal plates to the maxilla at the medial orbital margin. SYN ligamentum palpebrale mediale [NA], ligamentum tarsale internum, tendo oculi, tendo palpebrarum.

medial puboprostatic l., SYN *ligamentum* puboprostaticum mediale. SEE puboprostatic l.

medial talocalcaneal l., a l. extending from the medial tuberosity of the posterior talar process and the sustentaculum tali. SYN ligamentum talocalcaneare mediale.

medial l. of talocrural joint, SYN deltoid l.

medial umbilical l., the obliterated umbilical artery that persists as a fibrous cord passing upward alongside the bladder to the umbilicus. SYN ligamentum umbilicale mediale [NA].

medial l. of wrist, SYN ulnar collateral l. of wrist.

median arcuate l., a tendinous connection between the crura of the diaphragm that arches over the aorta, forming the anterosuperior margin of the aortic hiatus. SYN ligamentum arcuatum medianum [NA].

median thyrohyoid l., the central thickened portion of the thyrohyoid membrane. SYN ligamentum thyrohyoideum medianum [NA], ligamentum hyothyroideum medium.

median umbilical l., the remnant of the urachus, contained in the median umbilical fold; it persists as a midline fibrous cord between the apex of the bladder and the umbilicus. SYN ligamentum umbilicale medianum [NA], middle umbilical l., urachal l.

meniscofemoral l.'s, one of two l.'s that extend from the posterior part of the lateral meniscus to the lateral surface of the medial meniscus: anterior meniscofemoral l. and posterior meniscofemoral l. SYN ligamenta meniscofemorale [NA].

middle costotransverse l., SYN costotransverse l.

middle umbilical l., SYN median umbilical l.

nuchal l., SYN *ligamentum* nuchae.

oblique l. of elbow joint, a slender band extending from the lateral part of the coronoid process of the ulna distad and laterad to the radius immediately distal to the bicipital tuberosity. SYN chorda obliqua [NA], oblique cord, round l. of elbow joint, Weitbrecht's cord, Weitbrecht's l.

oblique popliteal l., reflected tendon of insertion of semimembranous muscle; a fibrous band that extends across the back of the knee from its separation from the direct tendon of insertion on the medial condyle of the tibia to the lateral condyle of the femur. SYN ligamentum popliteum obliquum [NA], Bourgery's l.

occipitoaxial l.'s, l.'s connecting the axis with the occipital bone. SEE alar l.'s, apical l. of dens.

odontoid l., SYN alar *folds*, under *fold*.

orbicular l., SYN annular l.

orbicular l. of radius, SYN annular l. of the radius.

ovarian l., a cordlike bundle of fibers passing to the side of the uterus from the lower end of the ovary, between the folds of the broad l. (mesovarium). SYN ligamentum ovarii proprium [NA], proper l. of ovary.

palmar l.'s, the fibrocartilaginous plates, one located on the anterior aspect of each metacarpophalangeal and interphalangeal joint, that are firmly attached to the bases of the phalanges and the heads of the next proximal bones; they are grooved to accommodate the long flexor tendons. SYN ligamenta palmaria [NA], accessory volar l.'s.

palmar carpal l., SYN antebrachial flexor *retinaculum*.

palmar carpometacarpal l.'s, fibrous bands that connect the palmar surfaces of the carpal and metacarpal bones. SYN ligamentum carpometacarpalia palmaria.

palmar metacarpal l.'s, fibrous bands connecting the palmar aspects of the bases of metacarpals two to five. SYN ligamenta metacarpalia palmaria.

palmar radiocarpal l., a strong l. that passes from the distal end of the radius to the proximal row of carpal bones on the anterior surface of the wrist joint. SYN ligamentum radiocarpale palmare [NA].

palmar ulnocarpal l., the fibrous band that passes from the ulnar styloid process to the carpal bones. SYN ligamentum ulnocarpale palmare [NA].

patellar l., a strong flattened fibrous band passing from the apex and adjoining margins of the patella to the tuberosity of the tibia; considered by some to be part of the tendon of the quadriceps femoris muscle, in which the patella is embedded as a sesamoid bone. SYN ligamentum patellae [NA].

pectinate l.'s of iridocorneal angle, SYN trabecular *reticulum*.

pectinate l.'s of iris, SEE trabecular *reticulum*.

pectineal l., a thick, strong fibrous band that passes laterally from the lacunar l. along the pectineal line of the pubis. SEE ALSO *aponeurosis* of external abdominal oblique muscle. SYN ligamentum pectineale [NA], Cooper's l.'s (2).

peridental l., SYN periodontal l.

periodontal l., the connective tissue that surrounds the tooth root and attaches it to its bony socket; it consists of fibers anchored in the cementum and extending into the alveolar bone; the tissues that surround and support the teeth, including the gingivae, cementum, periodontal l., and alveolar and supporting bone. SYN periodontium [NA], alveolar periosteum, periosteum alveolare, alveolodental l., alveolodental membrane, gingivodental l., paradentium, parodontium, peridental l., peridental membrane, peridentium, periodontal membrane, tapetum alveoli.

Petit's l., SYN sacrouterine *fold*.

phrenicocolic l., a triangular fold of peritoneum attached to the left flexure of the colon and to the diaphragm, on which rests the inferior pole or extremity of the spleen. SYN ligamentum phrenicocolicum [NA], costocolic l.

phrenicolienal l., SYN splenorenal l.

phrenicosplenic l., SYN splenorenal l.

li

phrenogastric l., SYN gastrophrenic l.

phrenosplenic l., SYN splenorenal l.

pisohamate l., a strong fibrous band that extends from the pisiform bone to the hook of the hamate. SYN ligamentum pisohamatum [NA], pisounciform l., pisouncinate l.

pisometacarpal l., a strong fibrous band extending from the pisiform bone to the base of the fifth metacarpal bone; this l., together with the pisohamate l., forms the tendon of insertion of the flexor carpi ulnaris, in which the pisiform bone is like a sesamoid bone. SYN ligamentum pisometacarpeum [NA].

pisounciform l., SYN pisohamate l.

pisouncinate l., SYN pisohamate l.

plantar l.'s, the counterparts in the foot of the palmar l.'s in the hand. SYN ligamenta plantaria [NA], accessory plantar l.'s, Cruveilhier's l.'s, glenoid l. (2).

plantar calcaneocuboid l., a strong band that passes forward and medially from the plantar surface of the calcaneus to the cuboid bone, actually forming a part of the articular "socket." SYN ligamentum calcaneocuboideum plantare [NA].

plantar calcaneonavicular l., a dense fibroelastic l. that extends from the sustentaculum tali to the plantar surface of the navicular bone; it supports the head of the talus. SYN ligamentum calcaneonaviculare plantare [NA], inferior calcaneonavicular l., spring l.

plantar cuboideonavicular l., the l. that unites the plantar surfaces of the cuboid and navicular bones of the tarsus. SYN ligamentum cuboideonaviculare plantare [NA].

plantar cuneocuboid l., the fibrous band that unites the apex of the lateral cuneiform with the medial margin of the plantar suface of the cuboid. SYN ligamentum cuneocuboideum plantare [NA].

plantar cuneonavicular l.'s, l.'s connecting the plantar surface of the navicular with the three cuneiform bones. SYN ligamenta cuneonavicularia plantaria.

plantar metatarsal l.'s, fibrous bands connecting the plantar aspects of the bases of the metatarsals. SYN ligamenta metatarsalia plantaria.

posterior costotransverse l., SYN lateral costotransverse l.

posterior cricoarytenoid l., the l. that passes downward from the posterior border of the arytenoid cartilage to the lamina of the cricoid cartilage. SYN ligamentum cricoarytenoideum posterius [NA].

posterior cruciate l., the strong fibrous cord that extends from the posterior intercondylar area of the tibia to the anterior part of the lateral surface of the medial condyle of the femur. SYN ligamentum cruciatum posterius [NA].

posterior l. of head of fibula, a l. uniting the posterior part of the head of the fibula to the tibia. SYN ligamentum capitis fibulae posterius.

posterior l. of incus, ligamentous band extending from short crus of fincus. SYN ligamentum incudis posterius.

posterior l. of knee, SYN arcuate popliteal l.

posterior longitudinal l., the fibrous band interconnecting the posterior surfaces of the vertebral bodies; it narrows to pass between the pedicles and spreads out to blend with the posterior annulus fibrosus of the intervertebral discs; forms the anterior wall of the vertebral canal. SYN ligamentum longitudinale posterius.

posterior meniscofemoral l., the band that passes posterior to the posterior cruciate l. extending between the medial condyle of the femur and the posterior crus of the lateral meniscus. SYN ligamentum meniscofemorale posterius [NA], ligamentum cruciatum tertium genus, ligamentum menisci lateralis, Wrisberg's l.

posterior occipitoaxial l., SYN tectorial *membrane*.

posterior sacroiliac l.'s, the heavy fibrous bands that pass from the ilium to the sacrum posterior to the sacroiliac joint. SYN ligamenta sacroiliaca posteriora [NA], dorsal sacroiliac l.'s, ligamentum sacroiliacum posterius.

posterior sacrosciatic l., SYN sacrotuberous l.

posterior sternoclavicular l., a fibrous band that reinforces the sternoclavicular joint posteriorly. SYN ligamentum sternoclaviculare posterius [NA].

posterior talofibular l., the nearly horizontal fibrous band that extends from the posterior border of the talus to the malleolar fossa. SYN ligamentum talofibulare posterius [NA].

posterior talotibial l., SYN posterior tibiotalar l. SEE ALSO deltoid l.

posterior tibiofibular l., the fibrous band that horizontally crosses the posterior aspect of the tibiofibular syndesmosis, contributing the posterior "wall" of the "socket" which receives the trochlea of the talus. SYN ligamentum tibiofibulare posterius [NA].

posterior tibiotalar l., the part of the medial or deltoid l. that extends from the medial malleolus to the posterior process of the talus. SYN pars tibiotalaris posterior ligamenti medialis [NA], ligamentum talotibiale posterius, posterior talotibial l., posterior tibiotalar part of deltoid ligament.

Poupart's l., SYN inguinal l.

proper l. of ovary, SYN ovarian l.

pterygomandibular l., SYN pterygomandibular *raphe*.

pterygospinal l., SYN pterygospinous l.

pterygospinous l., a membranous l. extending from the spine of the sphenoid to the upper part of the posterior border of the lateral pterygoid lamina. SYN ligamentum pterygospinale [NA], Civinini's l., pterygospinal l.

pubocapsular l., SYN pubofemoral l.

pubofemoral l., a thickened part of the capsule of the hip joint that extends from the superior ramus of the pubis to the intertrochanteric line of the femur. SYN ligamentum pubofemorale [NA], ligamentum pubocapsulare, pubocapsular l.

puboprostatic l., the localized thickening of the superior fascia of the pelvic diaphragm anteriorly that anchors the prostate and neck of the bladder to the pubis on each side. It is composed of medial and lateral parts (l.'s) and usually contains smooth muscle. SYN ligamentum puboprostaticum [NA], Denonvilliers' l.

pubovesical l., in the female the fascial thickening comparable to the puboprostatic l. SYN ligamentum pubovesicale [NA].

pulmonary l., two-layered fold formed as the pleura of the mediastinum is reflected onto the lung inferior to the root of the lung. SYN ligamentum pulmonale [NA], ligamentum latum pulmonis, Teutleben's l.

quadrate l., fibers that pass from the distal margin of the radial notch of the ulna to the neck of the radius. SYN ligamentum quadratum [NA], Denucé's l.

radial collateral l., SYN radial collateral l. of elbow.

radial collateral l. of elbow, the l. that connects the lateral epicondyle of the humerus with the annular l. of the radius. SYN ligamentum collaterale radiale [NA], lateral l. of elbow, radial collateral l.

radial collateral l. of wrist, the l. that extends distally from the styloid process of the radius to the carpal bones. SYN ligamentum collaterale carpi radiale [NA], external collateral l. of wrist, lateral l. of wrist.

radiate l., SYN radiate l. of head of rib.

radiate l. of head of rib, the radiate, stellate, or anterior costovertebral l. connecting the head of each rib to the bodies of the two vertebrae with which it articulates. SYN ligamentum capitis costae radiatum [NA], ligamentum radiatum, radiate l., stellate l.

radiate sternocostal l.'s, fibers of the articular capsule that radiate from the costal cartilages to the anterior surface of the sternum. SYN ligamenta sternocostalia radiata [NA].

radiate l. of wrist, the ligament that extends from the capitate bone to the scaphoid, lunate, and triquetrum on the palmar side of the wrist. SYN ligamentum carpi radiatum [NA].

reflected inguinal l., a triangular fibrous band extending from the aponeurosis of the external oblique to the pubic tubercle of the opposite side. SEE ALSO *aponeurosis* of external abdominal oblique muscle. SYN ligamentum reflexum [NA], Colles' l., fascia triangularis abdominis, reflex l., triangular fascia.

reflex l., SYN reflected inguinal l.

Retzius' l., the deep attachment of the inferior extensor retinaculum in the tarsal sinus, it acts as a sling for the extensor tendons of the toes. SYN fundiform l. of foot.

rhomboid l., SYN costoclavicular l.

right triangular l., a triangular fold of peritoneum that passes from the right lobe of the liver to the diaphragm; it is a formation of the coronary l., formed as the coronary l. makes an acute angle upon reaching its most lateral point on the right side as it surrounds the bare area of the liver. SYN ligamentum triangulare dextrum [NA].

ring l., SYN *zona* orbicularis.

round l. of elbow joint, SYN oblique l. of elbow joint.

round l. of femur, SYN l. of head of femur.

round l. of liver, the remains of the umbilical vein running within the free edge of the falciform l. from umbilicus to the liver, where it continues within the fissure for the round l. to the origin of the left portal vein within the porta hepatis. SYN ligamentum teres hepatis [NA].

round l. of uterus, a fibromuscular band that is attached to the uterus on either side in front of and below the opening of the uterine tube; it passes through the inguinal canal to the labium majus; corresponds to the spermatic cord of male in that it passes through the inguinal canal and gains similar coverings, but is not homologous. SYN ligamentum teres uteri [NA], Hunter's l.

sacrodural l., a longitudinal bundle of fibrous filaments running from the midline of the inferior part of the dural sac to the posterior longitudinal ligament of the sacrum. SYN ligamentum sacrodurale.

sacrospinous l., the fibrous band that passes from the ischial spine to the sacrum and coccyx. SYN ligamentum sacrospinale [NA], anterior sacrosciatic l., ligamentum sacrospinosum.

sacrotuberous l., the l. that passes from the ischial tuberosity to the ilium, sacrum, and coccyx, transforming the scialic notch to a large scialic foramen, which is then further subdivided by the sacrospinous l. SYN ligamentum sacrotuberale [NA], ligamentum sacrotuberosum, posterior sacrosciatic l.

serous l., one of a number of peritoneal folds attaching certain of the viscera to the abdominal wall or to each other. SYN ligamentum serosum.

sheath l.'s, SEE fibrous digital *sheaths* of hand, under *sheath,* fibrous digital *sheaths* of foot, under *sheath,* fibrous tendon *sheath.*

Simonart's l.'s, SYN amniotic *bands,* under *band.*

Soemmerring's l., small fibers attaching the lacrimal gland to the periorbita.

sphenomandibular l., the fibrous band that passes from the spine of the sphenoid bone to the lingula of the mandible; it is a primary passive support of the mandible serving as a "swinging axis", enabling depression and elevation around a transverse axis passing through the two lingulae, while at the same time enabling protraction and retraction. SYN ligamentum sphenomandibulare [NA].

spinoglenoid l., SYN inferior transverse scapular l.

spiral l. of cochlea, the thickened periosteal lining of the bony cochlea forming the outer wall of the cochlear duct to which the basal lamina attaches. SYN crista spiralis [NA], ligamentum spirale cochleae [NA], spiral crest.

splenorenal l., a peritoneal fold (portion of the greater omentum) which extends from the diaphragm and the anterior aspect of the left kidney to the hilar region of the spleen, conducting the splenic vessels from the posterior body wall to the spleen. SYN ligamentum lienorenale [NA], ligamentum phrenicolienale [NA], ligamentum splenorenale [NA], lienophrenic l., lienorenal l., ligamentum phrenicosplenicum, phrenicolienal l., phrenicosplenic l., phrenosplenic l., sustentaculum lienis.

spring l., SYN plantar calcaneonavicular l.

Stanley's cervical l.'s, fibers of the capsule of the hip joint reflected onto the neck of the femur.

stellate l., SYN radiate l. of head of rib.

sternoclavicular l., l. uniting the clavicle to the manubrium of the sternum. SEE anterior sternoclavicular l., posterior sternoclavicular l. SYN ligamentum sternoclaviculare [NA].

sternopericardial l., fibrous bands that pass from the pericardium to the sternum. SYN ligamenta sternopericardiaca [NA], Lannelongue's l.'s, Luschka's l.'s.

stylohyoid l., a fibrous cord that passes from the tip of the styloid process to the lesser cornu of the hyoid bone; it is occa-

sionally ossified. SYN ligamentum stylohyoideum [NA], epihyal l.

stylomandibular l., a condensation of the deep cervical fascia extending from the tip of the styloid process of the temporal bone to the posterior border of the angle of the jaw; blends with parotid sheath. SYN ligamentum stylomandibulare [NA], stylomaxillary l.

stylomaxillary l., SYN stylomandibular l.

superficial dorsal sacrococcygeal l., the continuation of the supraspinal l. from the sacrum to the coccyx. SYN ligamentum sacrococcygeum posterius superficiale [NA], superficial posterior sacrococcygeal l.

superficial posterior sacrococcygeal l., SYN superficial dorsal sacrococcygeal l.

superficial transverse metacarpal l., a thickening of the deep fascia in the most distal part of the (base) of the triangular palmar aponeurosis. SYN ligamentum metacarpale transversum superficiale [NA], Gerdy's fibers, ligamentum natatorium.

superficial transverse metatarsal l., a thickening of the distal part (base) of the plantar aponeurosis, at the level of the heads of the metatarsal bones. SYN ligamentum metatarsale transversum superficiale [NA].

superior costotransverse l., the fibrous band that extends upward from the neck of a rib to the transverse process of the next higher vertebra. SYN ligamentum costotransversarium superius [NA], anterior costotransverse l., ligamentum costotransversarium anterius.

superior l. of epididymis, the uppermost of the two folds of the tunica vaginalis between the head of the epididymis and the testis. SYN ligamentum epididymidis superius.

superior l. of incus, connects the body of the incus with the roof of the tympanic recess. SYN ligamentum incudis superius.

superior l. of malleus, a l. extending from the head of the malleus to the roof of the epitympanic recess. SYN ligamentum mallei superius [NA].

superior pubic l., fibers that pass transversely above the pubic symphysis. SYN ligamentum pubicum superius [NA].

superior transverse scapular l., the strong fibrous band that bridges the scapular notch creating a foramen that gives passage to the suprascapular nerve, while the suprascapular vessels pass over the l. superiorly. SYN ligamentum transversum scapulae superius [NA], suprascapular l.

suprascapular l., SYN superior transverse scapular l.

supraspinous l., the longitudinal fibrous band attached to the tips of the spinous processes of the vertebrae; in the cervical region it is altered to form the ligamentum nuchae. SYN ligamentum supraspinale [NA].

suspensory l. of axilla, the continuation of the clavipectoral fascia downward to attach to the axillary fascia; it maintains the characteristic hollow of the armpit. SYN Campbell's l., Gerdy's l.

suspensory l.'s of breast, well developed retinacula cutis that extend from the fibrous stroma of the mammary gland to the overlying skin. SYN ligamenta suspensoria mammae [NA], Cooper's l.'s (1), suspensory l.'s of Cooper.

suspensory l. of clitoris, a fibrous band at the deep fascial level that extends from the pubic symphysis to the deep fascia of the clitoris, anchoring the clitoris to the pubic symphysis. SYN ligamentum suspensorium clitoridis [NA].

suspensory l.'s of Cooper, SYN suspensory l.'s of breast.

suspensory l. of esophagus, SYN cricoesophageal *tendon.*

suspensory l. of eyeball, a thickening of the inferior part of the bulbar sheath which supports the eye within the orbit; it extends between the lateral and medial orbital margins and includes the medial and lateral check l.'s. SYN Lockwood's l.

suspensory l. of gonad, SYN genital l.

suspensory l. of lens, SYN ciliary *zonule.*

suspensory l. of ovary, a band of peritoneum that extends upward from the upper pole of the ovary; it contains the ovarian vessels and ovarian plexus of nerves. SYN ligamentum suspensorium ovarii [NA], infundibulopelvic l.

suspensory l. of penis, a fibrous band at the deep fascial layer that extends from the pubic symphysis to the deep fascia of the

li

penis anchoring the roof of the penis. SYN ligamentum suspensorium penis [NA].

suspensory l. of testis, the cranial atrophic portion of the urogenital ridge attached to the cranial pole of the intra-abdominal embryonic testis.

suspensory l. of thyroid gland, one of several fibrous bands which pass from the sheath of the thyroid gland to the thyroid and cricoid cartilages.

sutural l., a delicate membrane binding the bones at the cranial sutures.

synovial l., one of the large synovial folds in a joint.

talocalcaneal l., any of three l.'s uniting the talus and calcaneus: interosseous talocalcaneal l., lateral talocalcaneal l., and medial talocalcaneal l. SYN ligamentum talocalcaneare [NA].

talonavicular l., SYN dorsal talonavicular l.

tarsal l.'s, the l.'s that interconnect the tarsal bones; they are grouped into three sets: dorsal tarsal l.'s, interosseous tarsal l.'s, and plantar tarsal l.'s, and are individually named according to their attachments. SYN ligamenta tarsi [NA].

tarsometatarsal l.'s, the ligaments that unite tarsal and metatarsal bones; they are arranged in dorsal, interosseous, and plantar sets. SYN ligamenta tarsometatarsalia [NA].

temporomandibular l., SYN lateral temporomandibular l.

Teutleben's l., SYN pulmonary l.

Thompson's l., SYN iliopubic *tract.*

thyroepiglottic l., thyroepiglottidean l., an elastic band that connects the petiole of the epiglottis to the interior of the thyroid cartilage near the superior thyroid notch. SYN ligamentum thyroepiglotticum [NA].

tibial collateral l., the broad fibrous band that passes from the medial epicondyle of the femur to the medial margin and medial surface of the tibia; the medial meniscus is attached to its deep surface; it is continuous with (a thickening of) the fibrous capsule of the knee joint. SYN ligamentum collaterale tibiale [NA], medial l. of knee.

tibiocalcaneal l., the part of the medial or deltoid l. that extends from the medial malleolus to the sustentaculum tali of the calcaneus. SYN pars tibiocalcanea ligamenti medialis [NA], calcaneotibial l., ligamentum calcaneotibiale, tibiocalcaneal part of deltoid ligament.

tibiofibular l., SEE anterior tibiofibular l., interosseous *membrane* of leg, posterior tibiofibular l. SEE ALSO tibiofibular *syndesmosis.*

tibionavicular l., the part of the medial or deltoid l. that extends from the medial malleolus to the navicular bone. SEE ALSO deltoid l. SYN pars tibionavicularis ligamenti medialis [NA], ligamentum tibionaviculare, tibionavicular part of deltoid ligament.

transverse l. of acetabulum, portion of the acetabular labrum that passes across the acetabular notch. SYN ligamentum transversum acetabuli [NA].

transverse atlantal l., SYN transverse l. of the atlas.

transverse l. of the atlas, thick, strong, centrally flattened band spanning the vertebral foramen of the atlas as it extends from the medial aspect of one lateral mass to the other, passing dorsal to the dens with which it articulates; it forms the dorsal portion of the opening for the dens, tightly embracing its neck. It forms a part of the "cross-bar" of the cruciform l. of the atlas. SEE ALSO cruciform l. of atlas. SYN ligamentum transversum atlantis [NA], Lauth's l., transverse atlantal l.

transverse carpal l., a strong fibrous band crossing the front of the carpus and binding down the flexor tendons of the digits and the flexor carpi radialis tendon and the median nerve; in so doing it creates the carpal tunnel. SYN retinaculum flexorum [NA], deep part of flexor retinaculum, flexor retinaculum, ligamentum carpi transversum, ligamentum carpi volare, volar carpal l.

transverse crural l., SYN superior extensor *retinaculum.*

transverse l. of elbow, a bundle of fibers running from the olecranon to the coronoid process in association with the ulnar collateral l. SYN Cooper's l.'s (3).

transverse genicular l., SYN transverse l. of knee.

transverse humeral l., a fibrous band running more or less obliquely from the greater to the lesser tuberosity of the humerus, bridging over the bicipital groove. SYN Brodie's l.

transverse l. of knee, a transverse band that passes between the lateral and medial menisci in the anterior part of the knee joint. SYN ligamentum transversum genus [NA], transverse genicular l.

transverse l. of leg, SYN superior extensor *retinaculum.*

transverse metacarpal l., SYN deep transverse metacarpal l.

transverse metatarsal l., SYN deep transverse metatarsal l.

transverse l. of pelvis, SYN transverse perineal l.

transverse perineal l., the thickened anterior border of the urogenital diaphragm, formed by the fusion of its two fascial layers. SYN ligamentum transversum perinei [NA], Krause's l., ligamentum transversum pelvis, transverse l. of pelvis, transverse l. of perineum.

transverse l. of perineum, SYN transverse perineal l.

transverse tibiofibular l., the distal continuation of the interosseous membrane forming a strong l. that unites the distal end of the tibia and fibula; it lies deep to the posterior tibiofibular l. SYN interosseous tibiofibular l.

trapezoid l., the lateral part of the coracoclavicular l. that attaches to the trapezoid line of the clavicle. SYN ligamentum trapezoideum [NA].

Treitz's l., SYN suspensory *muscle* of duodenum.

triangular l., SYN inferior *fascia* of urogenital diaphragm.

triangular l.'s of liver, SEE right triangular l., left triangular l.

ulnar collateral l., SYN ulnar collateral l. of elbow.

ulnar collateral l. of elbow, the triangular l. extending from the medial epicondyle of the humerus to the medial side of the coronoid process and olecranon of the ulna. SYN ligamentum collaterale ulnare [NA], medial collateral l. of elbow, ulnar collateral l.

ulnar collateral l. of wrist, a l. that passes from the styloid process of the ulna to the pisiform and triquetrum. SYN ligamentum collaterale carpi ulnare [NA], internal collateral l. of the wrist, medial l. of wrist.

urachal l., SYN median umbilical l.

uterosacral l., SYN sacrouterine *fold.*

uterovesical l., a peritoneal fold extending from the uterus to the posterior portion of the bladder. SYN plica uterovesicalis, plica vesicouterina, uterovesical fold, vesicouterine l.

Valsalva's l.'s, SYN auricular l.'s.

venous l., SYN *ligamentum* venosum.

ventral sacrococcygeal l., the continuation of the anterior longitudinal l. uniting the sacrum and coccyx. SYN ligamentum sacrococcygeum anterius [NA], anterior sacrococcygeal l.

ventral sacroiliac l.'s, SYN anterior sacroiliac l.'s.

ventricular l., SYN vestibular l.

vertebropelvic l.'s, SEE iliolumbar l., sacrospinous l., sacrotuberous l.

vesicoumbilical l., one of the l.'s between the urinary bladder and the umbilicus. SEE median umbilical l., medial umbilical l.

vesicouterine l., SYN uterovesical l.

vestibular l., the thin fibrous layer that lies in the ventricular fold of the larynx. SYN ligamentum vestibulare [NA], ligamentum ventriculare, ventricular l.

vocal l., the band that extends on either side from the thyroid cartilage to the vocal process of the arytenoid cartilage; it is the thickened, free upper border of the conus elasticus of the larynx. SYN ligamentum vocale [NA].

volar carpal l., SYN transverse carpal l.

Weitbrecht's l., SYN oblique l. of elbow joint.

Winslow's l., SYN fibular collateral l.

Wrisberg's l., SYN posterior meniscofemoral l.

yellow l., SYN *ligamentum* flavum.

Y-shaped l., SYN iliofemoral l.

Zaglas' l., a short thick fibrous band extending from the posterior superior spine of the ilium to the second transverse tubercle of the sacrum.

Zinn's l., SYN common tendinous *ring.*

lig·a·men·ta (lig'ă-men'tă). Plural of ligamentum. [L.]
lig·a·men·to·pex·is, lig·a·men·to·pexy (lig'ă-men-tō-pek'sis,

-pek′sē). Shortening of any ligament of the uterus. [ligament + G. *pēxis*, fixation]

lig·a·men·tous (lig′ă-men′tŭs). Relating to or of the form or structure of a ligament.

LIGAMENTUM

lig·a·men·tum, pl. **lig·a·men·ta** (lig′ă-men′tŭm, -men′tă) [NA]. SYN ligament. [L. a band, tie, fr. *ligo*, to bind]

l. acromioclavicula′re [NA], SYN acromioclavicular *ligament*.

ligamen′ta ala′ria [NA], SYN alar *folds*, under *fold*.

l. annula′re, SYN annular *ligament*.

l. annula′re bul′bi, SYN trabecular *reticulum*.

l. annula′re digito′rum, SYN annular *part* of fibrous digital sheath.

l. annula′re ra′dii [NA], SYN annular *ligament* of the radius.

l. annula′re stape′dis [NA], SYN annular *ligament* of the stapes.

ligamen′ta annula′ria trachea′lia [NA], SYN annular *ligaments* of the trachea, under *ligament*.

l. anococcy′geum [NA], SYN anococcygeal *ligament*.

l. ap′icis den′tis [NA], SYN apical *ligament* of dens.

l. arcua′tum latera′le [NA], SYN lateral arcuate *ligament*.

l. arcua′tum media′le [NA], SYN medial arcuate *ligament*.

l. arcua′tum media′num [NA], SYN median arcuate *ligament*.

l. arcua′tum pu′bis [NA], SYN arcuate pubic *ligament*.

l. arterio′sum [NA], the remains of the ductus arteriosus. SYN arterial ligament, Botallo′s ligament.

ligamen′ta auricula′ria [NA], SYN auricular *ligaments*, under *ligament*.

l. bifurca′tum [NA], SYN bifurcate *ligament*.

l. calcaneocuboi′deum [NA], SYN calcaneocuboid *ligament*.

l. calcaneocuboi′deum planta′re [NA], SYN plantar calcaneocuboid *ligament*.

l. calcaneofibula′re [NA], SYN calcaneofibular *ligament*.

l. calcaneonavicula′re [NA], SYN calcaneonavicular *ligament*.

l. calcaneonavicula′re planta′re [NA], SYN plantar calcaneonavicular *ligament*.

l. calcaneotibia′le, SYN tibiocalcaneal *ligament*. SEE ALSO deltoid *ligament*.

l. cap′itis cos′tae intra-articula′re [NA], SYN intra-articular *ligament* of costal head.

l. cap′itis cos′tae radia′tum [NA], SYN radiate *ligament* of head of rib.

l. cap′itis fem′oris [NA], SYN *ligament* of head of femur.

l. cap′itis fib′ulae ante′rius, SYN anterior *ligament* of head of fibula.

l. cap′itis fib′ulae poste′rius, SYN posterior *ligament* of head of fibula.

ligamen′ta capitulo′rum transver′sa, SEE deep transverse metacarpal *ligament*, deep transverse metatarsal *ligament*.

l. capsula′re, SYN capsular *ligament*.

l. car′pi dorsa′le, SYN extensor *retinaculum*.

l. car′pi radia′tum [NA], SYN radiate *ligament* of wrist.

l. car′pi transver′sum, SYN transverse carpal *ligament*.

l. car′pi vola′re, SYN transverse carpal *ligament*.

ligamen′ta carpometacarpa′lia [NA], SYN carpometacarpal *ligaments*, under *ligament*.

l. carpometacarpa′lia dorsa′lia, SYN dorsal carpometacarpal *ligaments*, under *ligament*.

l. carpometacarpa′lia palma′ria, SYN palmar carpometacarpal *ligaments*, under *ligament*.

l. cauda′le, SYN caudal *retinaculum*.

l. ceratocricoi′deum, one of three ligaments (anterior, posterior, and lateral) reinforcing the capsule of the cricothyroid articulation on either side. SYN ceratocricoid ligament.

l. collatera′le, pl. **ligamen′ta collatera′lia** [NA], SYN collateral *ligament*.

l. collatera′le car′pi radia′le [NA], SYN radial collateral *ligament* of wrist.

l. collatera′le car′pi ulna′re [NA], SYN ulnar collateral *ligament* of wrist.

l. collatera′le fibula′re [NA], SYN fibular collateral *ligament*.

l. collatera′le radia′le [NA], SYN radial collateral *ligament* of elbow.

l. collatera′le tibia′le [NA], SYN tibial collateral *ligament*.

l. collatera′le ulna′re [NA], SYN ulnar collateral *ligament* of elbow.

l. col′li cos′tae, SYN costotransverse *ligament*.

l. conjuga′le, SYN conjugate *ligament*.

l. conoid′eum [NA], SYN conoid *ligament*.

l. coracoacromia′le [NA], SYN coracoacromial *ligament*.

l. coracoclavicula′re [NA], SYN coracoclavicular *ligament*.

l. coracohumera′le [NA], SYN coracohumeral *ligament*.

l. corniculopharynge′um, SYN cricopharyngeal *ligament*.

l. corona′rium hep′atis [NA], SYN coronary *ligament* of liver.

l. costoclavicula′re [NA], SYN costoclavicular *ligament*.

l. costotransversa′rium [NA], SYN costotransverse *ligament*.

l. costotransversa′rium ante′rius, SYN superior costotransverse *ligament*.

l. costotransversa′rium latera′le [NA], SYN lateral costotransverse *ligament*.

l. costotransversa′rium poste′rius, SYN lateral costotransverse *ligament*.

l. costotransversa′rium supe′rius [NA], SYN superior costotransverse *ligament*.

l. costoxiphoi′deum [NA], SYN costoxiphoid *ligament*.

l. cotyloid′eum, SYN acetabular *labrum*.

l. cricoarytenoi′deum poste′rius [NA], SYN posterior cricoarytenoid *ligament*.

l. cricopharyn′geum [NA], SYN cricopharyngeal *ligament*.

l. cricothyroi′deum [NA], SYN cricothyroid *ligament*.

l. cricotrachea′le [NA], SYN cricotracheal *ligament*.

ligamen′ta crucia′ta digito′rum, SYN cruciform *part* of fibrous digital sheath.

ligamen′ta crucia′ta ge′nus [NA], SYN cruciate *ligaments* of knee, under *ligament*.

l. crucia′tum ante′rius [NA], SYN anterior cruciate *ligament*.

l. crucia′tum atlan′tis, SYN cruciform *ligament* of atlas.

l. crucia′tum cru′ris, SYN inferior extensor *retinaculum*.

l. crucia′tum poste′rius [NA], SYN posterior cruciate *ligament*.

l. crucia′tum ter′tium ge′nus, SYN posterior meniscofemoral *ligament*.

l. crucifor′me atlan′tis [NA], SYN cruciform *ligament* of atlas.

l. cuboideonavicular [NA], SYN cuboideonavicular *ligaments*, under *ligament*.

l. cuboideonavicula′re dorsa′le [NA], SYN dorsal cuboideonavicular *ligament*.

l. cuboideonavicula′re planta′re [NA], SYN plantar cuboideonavicular *ligament*.

l. cuneocuboidenum [NA], SYN cuneocuboid *ligaments*, under *ligament*.

l. cuneocuboideum dorsa′le [NA], SYN dorsal cuneocuboid *ligament*.

l. cuneocuboideum interos′seum [NA], SYN interosseous cuneocuboid *ligament*.

l. cuneocuboideum planta′re [NA], SYN plantar cuneocuboid *ligament*.

ligamen′ta cuneometatarsa′lia interos′sea [NA], SYN interosseous cuneometatarsal *ligaments*, under *ligament*.

l. cuneonaviculare planta′re,

ligamen′ta cuneonavicula′ria dorsa′lia, SYN dorsal cuneonavicular *ligaments*, under *ligament*.

l. cuneonavicula′ria planta′ria, SYN plantar cuneonavicular *ligaments*, under *ligament*.

l. deltoi′deum, ☆official alternate term for deltoid *ligament*.

l. denticula′tum [NA], SYN denticulate *ligament.*

l. duc′tus veno′si, SYN l. venosum.

l. duodenorena′le, SYN duodenorenal *ligament.*

l. epididym′idis [NA], SYN *ligament* of epididymis.

l. epididym′idis infe′rius, SYN inferior *ligament* of epididymis.

l. epididym′idis supe′rius, SYN superior *ligament* of epididymis.

ligamen′ta extracapsula′ria [NA], SYN extracapsular *ligaments,* under *ligament.*

l. falcifor′me, SYN falciform *process.*

l. falcifor′me hep′atis [NA], SYN falciform *ligament* of liver.

l. fla′vum [NA], one of the paired ligaments of yellow elastic fibrous tissue, which bind together the laminae of adjoining vertebrae, forming the dorsal wall of the vertebral canal between the vertebra or laminae; penetration of the ligamentum flavum with a trochar during epidural or spinal puncture produces a distinct feel, letting the practitioner know that the tip of the trochar has entered the epidural space. SYN yellow ligament.

l. fundifor′me pe′nis [NA], SYN fundiform *ligament* of penis.

l. gastrocol′icum [NA], SYN gastrocolic *ligament.*

l. gastroliena′le [NA], ✩official alternate term for gastrosplenic *ligament,* gastrosplenic *ligament.*

l. gastrophren′icum [NA], SYN gastrophrenic *ligament.*

l. gastrosple′nicum [NA], SYN gastrosplenic *ligament.*

l. genitoinguina′le [NA], SYN genitoinguinal *ligament.*

ligamen′ta glenohumera′lia [NA], SYN glenohumeral *ligaments,* under *ligament.*

l. glenoida′le, SYN glenoid *labrum.*

l. hepatocol′icum [NA], SYN hepatocolic *ligament.*

l. hepatoduodena′le [NA], SYN hepatoduodenal *ligament.*

l. hepatoesopha′geum, SYN hepatoesophageal *ligament.*

l. hepatogas′tricum [NA], SYN hepatogastric *ligament.*

l. hepatorena′le [NA], SYN hepatorenal *ligament.*

l. hyaloi′deo-capsula′rio, SYN hyalocapsular *ligament.*

l. hyoepiglot′ticum [NA], SYN hyoepiglottic *ligament.*

l. hyothyroi′deum latera′le, SYN lateral thyrohyoid *ligament.*

l. hyothyroi′deum me′dium, SYN median thyrohyoid *ligament.*

l. iliofemora′le [NA], SYN iliofemoral *ligament.*

l. iliolumba′le [NA], SYN iliolumbar *ligament.*

l. iliopectinea′le, SYN iliopectineal *arch.*

l. in′cudis poste′rius, SYN posterior *ligament* of incus.

l. in′cudis supe′rius, SYN superior *ligament* of incus.

l. inguina′le [NA], SYN inguinal *ligament.*

l. intercapita′le, a part of the l. capitis costae intra-articulare; which connects the heads of opposite ribs by passing over the intervertebral fibrocartilage, and thus holds the ribs in their articular sockets; not present in man but well developed in the dog and cat. SYN intercapital ligament.

ligamen′ta intercarpa′lia [NA], SYN intercarpal *ligaments,* under *ligament.*

l. intercarpalia dorsalia, dorsal intercarpal ligament. SEE intercarpal *ligaments,* under *ligament.*

l. intercarpalia interossea, interosseous intercarpal ligament. SEE intercarpal *ligaments,* under *ligament.*

l. intercarpalia palmaria, palmar intercarpal ligament. SEE intercarpal *ligaments,* under *ligament.*

l. interclavicula′re [NA], SYN interclavicular *ligament.*

ligamen′ta intercosta′lia, SYN intercostal *membranes,* under *membrane.*

ligamen′ta intercuneifor′mia [NA], SYN intercuneiform *ligaments,* under *ligament.*

l. intercuneiformia dorsalia, dorsal intercuneiform ligament. SEE intercuneiform *ligaments,* under *ligament.*

l. intercuneiformia interossea, interosseous intercuneiform ligament. SEE intercuneiform *ligaments,* under *ligament.*

l. intercuneiformia plantaria, plantar intercuneiform ligament. SEE intercuneiform *ligaments,* under *ligament.*

l. interfoveola′re [NA], SYN interfoveolar *ligament.*

l. interspina′le [NA], SYN interspinous *ligament.*

l. intertransversa′rium [NA], SYN intertransverse *ligament.*

ligamen′ta intracapsula′ria [NA], SYN intracapsular *ligaments,* under *ligament.*

l. ischiocapsula′re, SYN ischiofemoral *ligament.*

l. ischiofemora′le [NA], SYN ischiofemoral *ligament.*

l. juga′le, SYN cricopharyngeal *ligament.*

l. lacinia′tum, SYN flexor *retinaculum* of lower limb.

l. lacuna′re [NA], SYN lacunar *ligament.*

l. latera′le articulatio′nis temporomandibula′ris [NA], SYN lateral temporomandibular *ligament.*

l. la′tum pulmo′nis, SYN pulmonary *ligament.*

l. la′tum u′teri [NA], SYN broad *ligament* of the uterus.

l. lienorena′le [NA], SYN splenorenal *ligament,* splenorenal *ligament.*

l. longitudin′ale [NA], SYN longitudinal *ligament.*

l. longitudina′le ante′rius, SYN anterior longitudinal *ligament.*

l. longitudina′le poste′rius, SYN posterior longitudinal *ligament.*

l. lumbocosta′le [NA], SYN lumbocostal *ligament.*

l. mal′lei ante′rius [NA], SYN anterior *ligament* of malleus.

l. mal′lei latera′le [NA], SYN lateral *ligament* of malleus.

l. mal′lei supe′rius [NA], SYN superior *ligament* of malleus.

l. malle′oli latera′lis, SEE anterior tibiofibular *ligament,* posterior tibiofibular *ligament.*

l. media′le articulatio′nis talocrura′lis [NA], SYN deltoid *ligament.*

l. media′le articulatio′nis temporomandibula′ris [NA], SYN medial *ligament.*

l. media′lis, SYN anterior tibiotalar *ligament.*

l. menis′ci latera′lis, SYN posterior meniscofemoral *ligament.*

ligamen′ta meniscofemora′le [NA], SYN meniscofemoral *ligaments,* under *ligament.*

l. meniscofemora′le ante′rius [NA], SYN anterior meniscofemoral *ligament.*

l. meniscofemora′le poste′rius [NA], SYN posterior meniscofemoral *ligament.*

l. metacarpa′le transver′sum profun′dum [NA], SYN deep transverse metacarpal *ligament.*

l. metacarpa′le transver′sum superficia′le [NA], SYN superficial transverse metacarpal *ligament.*

ligamen′ta metacarpa′lia dorsa′lia, SYN dorsal metacarpal *ligaments,* under *ligament.*

ligamen′ta metacarpa′lia interos′sea, SYN interosseous metacarpal *ligaments,* under *ligament.*

ligamen′ta metacarpa′lia palma′ria, SYN palmar metacarpal *ligaments,* under *ligament.*

l. metatarsa′le transver′sum profun′dum [NA], SYN deep transverse metatarsal *ligament.*

l. metatarsa′le transver′sum superficia′le [NA], SYN superficial transverse metatarsal *ligament.*

ligamen′ta metatarsa′lia dorsa′lia, SYN dorsal metatarsal *ligaments,* under *ligament.*

ligamen′ta metatarsa′lia interos′sea, SYN interosseous metatarsal *ligaments,* under *ligament.*

ligamen′ta metatarsa′lia planta′ria, SYN plantar metatarsal *ligaments,* under *ligament.*

l. natato′rium, SYN superficial transverse metacarpal *ligament.*

ligamen′ta navicularicuneifor′mia, SEE dorsal cuneonavicular *ligaments,* under *ligament,* plantar cuneonavicular *ligaments,* under *ligament.*

l. nu′chae [NA], a sagittal ligamentous band at the back of the neck, formed of thickened supraspinous ligaments; it extends from the external occipital protuberance to the posterior border of the foramen magnum, cranially, to the seventh cervical spinous process, caudally. SYN apparatus ligamentosus colli, nuchal ligament.

l. orbicula′re ra′dii, SYN annular *ligament* of the radius.

ligamen′ta ossiculo′rum audi′tus [NA], SYN *ligaments* of auditory ossicles, under *ligament.*

l. ova′rii pro′prium [NA], SYN ovarian *ligament.*

ligamen′ta palma′ria [NA], SYN palmar *ligaments,* under *ligament.*

l. **palpebra′le exter′num,** syn lateral palpebral *ligament.*

l. **palpebra′le latera′le** [NA], syn lateral palpebral *ligament.*

l. **palpebra′le media′le** [NA], syn medial palpebral *ligament.*

l. **patel′lae** [NA], syn patellar *ligament.*

l. **pectina′tum** [NA], pectinate ligaments of iridocorneal angle. see trabecular *reticulum.*

l. **pectina′tum an′guli iridocornea′lis,** pectinate ligaments of iridocorneal angle. see trabecular *reticulum.*

l. **pectina′tum ir′idis,** pectinate ligaments of iridocorneal angle. see trabecular *reticulum.*

l. **pectinea′le** [NA], syn pectineal *ligament.*

l. **phrenicocol′icum** [NA], syn phrenicocolic *ligament.*

l. **phrenicoliena′le** [NA], syn splenorenal *ligament.*

l. **phrenicosple′nicum,** [NA] syn splenorenal *ligament.*

l. **pisohama′tum** [NA], syn pisohamate *ligament.*

l. **pisometacarp′eum** [NA], syn pisometacarpal *ligament.*

l. **planta′re lon′gum** [NA], syn long plantar *ligament.*

ligamen′ta **planta′ria** [NA], syn plantar *ligaments,* under *ligament.*

l. **poplit′eum arcua′tum** [NA], syn arcuate popliteal *ligament.*

l. **poplit′eum obli′quum** [NA], syn oblique popliteal *ligament.*

l. **pterygospina′le** [NA], syn pterygospinous *ligament.*

l. **pu′bicum supe′rius** [NA], syn superior pubic *ligament.*

l. **pubocapsula′re,** syn pubofemoral *ligament.*

l. **pubofemora′le** [NA], syn pubofemoral *ligament.*

l. **puboprostat′icum** [NA], syn puboprostatic *ligament.*

l. **puboprostat′icum latera′le,** see puboprostatic *ligament.* syn lateral puboprostatic ligament.

l. **puboprostat′icum media′le,** see puboprostatic *ligament.* syn medial puboprostatic ligament.

l. **pubovesica′le** [NA], syn pubovesical *ligament.*

l. **pulmona′le** [NA], syn pulmonary *ligament.*

l. **quadra′tum** [NA], syn quadrate *ligament.*

l. **radia′tum,** syn radiate *ligament* of head of rib.

l. **radiocarpa′le dorsa′le** [NA], syn dorsal radiocarpal *ligament.*

l. **radiocarpa′le palma′re** [NA], syn palmar radiocarpal *ligament.*

l. **reflex′um** [NA], syn reflected inguinal *ligament.*

l. **sacrococcyg′eum ante′rius** [NA], syn ventral sacrococcygeal *ligament.*

l. **sacrococcyg′eum latera′le** [NA], syn lateral sacrococcygeal *ligament.*

l. **sacrococcyg′eum poste′rius profun′dum** [NA], syn deep dorsal sacrococcygeal *ligament.*

l. **sacrococcyg′eum poste′rius superficia′le** [NA], syn superficial dorsal sacrococcygeal *ligament.*

l. **sacrodura′le,** syn sacrodural *ligament.*

ligamen′ta **sacroili′aca ante′riora** [NA], syn anterior sacroiliac *ligaments,* under *ligament.*

ligamen′ta **sacroili′aca interos′sea** [NA], syn interosseous sacroiliac *ligaments,* under *ligament.*

ligamen′ta **sacroil′iaca poste′riora** [NA], syn posterior sacroiliac *ligaments,* under *ligament.*

l. **sacroili′acum poste′rius,** syn posterior sacroiliac *ligaments,* under *ligament.*

l. **sacrospina′le** [NA], syn sacrospinous *ligament.*

l. **sacrospino′sum,** syn sacrospinous *ligament.*

l. **sacrotubera′le** [NA], syn sacrotuberous *ligament.*

l. **sacrotubero′sum,** syn sacrotuberous *ligament.*

l. **sero′sum,** syn serous *ligament.*

l. **sphenomandibula′re** [NA], syn sphenomandibular *ligament.*

l. **spira′le coch′leae** [NA], ☆official alternate term for spiral *ligament* of cochlea, spiral *ligament* of cochlea.

l. **splenorena′le** [NA], syn splenorenal *ligament.*

l. **sternoclaviculare** [NA], syn sternoclavicular *ligament.*

l. **sternoclavicula′re ante′rius** [NA], syn anterior sternoclavicular *ligament.*

l. **sternoclavicula′re poste′rius** [NA], syn posterior sternoclavicular *ligament.*

l. **sternocosta′le intra-articula′re** [NA], syn intra-articular sternocostal *ligament.*

ligamen′ta **sternocosta′lia radia′ta** [NA], syn radiate sternocostal *ligaments,* under *ligament.*

ligamen′ta **sternoper′icardi′aca** [NA], syn sternopericardial *ligament.*

l. **stylohyoi′deum** [NA], syn stylohyoid *ligament.*

l. **stylomandibula′re** [NA], syn stylomandibular *ligament.*

l. **supraspina′le** [NA], syn supraspinous *ligament.*

ligamen′ta **suspenso′ria mam′mae** [NA], syn suspensory *ligaments* of breast, under *ligament.*

l. **suspenso′rium clitor′idis** [NA], syn suspensory *ligament* of clitoris.

l. **suspenso′rium ova′rii** [NA], syn suspensory *ligament* of ovary.

l. **suspenso′rium pe′nis** [NA], syn suspensory *ligament* of penis.

l. **talocalcanea′re** [NA], syn talocalcaneal *ligament.*

l. **talocalcanea′re interos′seum,** syn interosseous talocalcaneal *ligament.*

l. **talocalcanea′re latera′le,** syn lateral talocalcaneal *ligament.*

l. **talocalcanea′re media′le,** syn medial talocalcaneal *ligament.*

l. **talofibula′re ante′rius** [NA], syn anterior talofibular *ligament.*

l. **talofibula′re poste′rius** [NA], syn posterior talofibular *ligament.*

l. **talonavicula′re** [NA], syn dorsal talonavicular *ligament.*

l. **talotibia′le ante′rius,** syn anterior tibiotalar *ligament.* see also deltoid *ligament.*

l. **talotibia′le poste′rius,** syn posterior tibiotalar *ligament.* see also deltoid *ligament.*

l. **tarsa′le exter′num,** syn lateral palpebral *ligament.*

l. **tarsa′le inter′num,** syn medial palpebral *ligament.*

ligamen′ta **tar′si** [NA], syn tarsal *ligaments,* under *ligament.*

ligamen′ta **tarsometatarsa′lia** [NA], syn tarsometatarsal *ligaments,* under *ligament.*

l. **temporomandibula′re,** syn lateral temporomandibular *ligament.*

l. **te′res fem′oris,** syn *ligament* of head of femur.

l. **te′res hep′atis** [NA], syn round *ligament* of liver.

l. **te′res u′teri** [NA], syn round *ligament* of uterus.

l. **tes′tis,** the caudal portion of the embryonic urogenital ridge; the upper third of the gubernaculum testis.

l. **thyroepiglot′ticum** [NA], syn thyroepiglottic *ligament.*

l. **thyrohyoi′deum latera′le** [NA], syn lateral thyrohyoid *ligament.*

l. **thyrohyoi′deum media′num** [NA], syn median thyrohyoid *ligament.*

l. **tibiofibula′re ante′rius** [NA], syn anterior tibiofibular *ligament.*

l. **tibiofibula′re me′dium,** syn interosseous *membrane* of leg.

l. **tibiofibula′re poste′rius** [NA], syn posterior tibiofibular *ligament.*

l. **tibionavicula′re,** syn tibionavicular *ligament.* see also deltoid *ligament.*

ligamen′ta **trachea′lia** [NA], syn annular *ligaments* of the trachea, under *ligament.*

l. **transversa′le col′li,** syn cardinal *ligament.*

l. **transver′sum acetab′uli** [NA], syn transverse *ligament* of acetabulum.

l. **transver′sum atlan′tis** [NA], syn transverse *ligament* of the atlas.

l. **transver′sum cru′ris,** syn superior extensor *retinaculum.*

l. **transver′sum ge′nus** [NA], syn transverse *ligament* of knee.

l. **transver′sum pel′vis,** syn transverse perineal *ligament.*

l. **transver′sum perine′i** [NA], syn transverse perineal *ligament.*

l. **transver′sum scap′ulae infe′rius** [NA], syn inferior transverse scapular *ligament.*

l. **transver′sum scap′ulae supe′rius** [NA], syn superior transverse scapular *ligament.*

l. **trapezoi′deum** [NA], syn trapezoid *ligament.*

l. **triangula′re,** syn inferior *fascia* of urogenital diaphragm.

li

l. triangula′re dex′trum [NA], SYN right triangular *ligament.*

l. triangula′re sinis′trum [NA], SYN left triangular *ligament.*

l. tuber′culi cos′tae, SYN lateral costotransverse *ligament.*

l. ulnocarpa′le palma′re [NA], SYN palmar ulnocarpal *ligament.*

l. umbilica′le latera′le, an old name for l. umbilicale mediale. SYN lateral umbilical ligament.

l. umbilica′le media′le [NA], SYN medial umbilical *ligament.*

l. umbilica′le media′num [NA], SYN median umbilical *ligament.*

l. ve′nae ca′vae sinis′trae, SYN *ligament* of left vena cava.

l. veno′sum [NA], a thin fibrous cord, lying in the fissure of the ligamentum venosum, the remains of the ductus venosus of the fetus. SYN Arantius' ligament, l. ductus venosi, venous ligament.

l. ventricula′re, SYN vestibular *ligament.*

l. vestibula′re [NA], SYN vestibular *ligament.*

l. voca′le [NA], SYN vocal *ligament.*

---

lig·and (lig′and, lī′gand). **1.** An organic molecule attached to a central metal ion by multiple coordinate bonds; *e.g.,* the porphyrin portion of heme, the corrin nucleus of the B_{12} vitamins. **2.** An organic molecule attached to a tracer element, *e.g.,* a radioisotope. **3.** A molecule that binds to a macromolecule, *e.g.,* a l. binding to a receptor. **4.** The analyte in competitive binding assays, such as radioimmunoassay. [L. *ligo,* to bind]

addressing l.'s, l.'s on cells for specific homing receptors on lymphocytes.

lig·and·in (lī-gan′din). SYN *glutathione S-transferase.*

li·gase (lī′gās). Generic term for enzymes (EC class 6) catalyzing the joining of two molecules coupled with the breakdown of a pyrophosphate bond in ATP or a similar compound. SEE ALSO synthetase.

li·gate (lī′gāt). To apply a ligature. [L. *ligo,* pp. *-atus,* to bind]

li·ga·tion (lī-gā′shŭn). **1.** Application of a ligature. **2.** The act of binding or annealing. [L. *ligatio,* fr. *ligo,* to bind]

blunt-end l., a reaction that joins two DNA duplexes directly at their blunt ends.

enzyme-catalyzed l., an enzyme-mediated joining of phosphodiester linkage of two stretches of DNA or RNA, or of peptide linkage of two polypeptides.

pole l., a l. at the root of an organ to shut off or diminish blood supply.

surgical l., in dentistry, the surgical exposure of an unerupted tooth so that a metal ligature can be placed around its cervix and fastened to an orthodontic appliance to facilitate eruption.

tooth l., the binding together of teeth with wire for stabilization and immobilization following traumatic injury or orthognathic surgery, or during periodontal therapy.

tubal l., interruption of the continuity of the oviducts by cutting, cautery, or by a plastic or metal device to prevent future conception.

li·ga·tor (lī′gā-ter, -tōr). An instrument used in the ligation of vessels in deep and nearly inaccessible parts.

lig·a·ture (lig′ă-chūr). **1.** A thread, wire, fillet, or the like, tied tightly around a blood vessel, the pedicle of a tumor, or other structure to constrict it. **2.** In orthodontics, a wire or other material used to secure an orthodontic attachment or tooth to an archwire. [L. *ligatura,* a band or tie, fr. *ligo,* to tie]

elastic l., (1) a rubber l. that slowly constricts; **(2)** in orthodontics, a stretchable threadlike material that may be tied from a tooth to an archwire or from tooth to tooth to gain movement of these units.

intravascular l., balloon occlusion of the feeding vessels of a cerebral arteriovenous malformation.

nonabsorbable l., a permanent l. of inert material, such as silk, wire, or synthetic fiber, that does not undergo dissolution in human tissues.

occluding l., a l. to shut off completely the distal blood supply.

provisional l., a l. applied to an artery in continuity at the beginning of an operation to prevent hemorrhage, but removed when the operation is completed.

soluble l., a temporary l. of material that can be absorbed by human tissues.

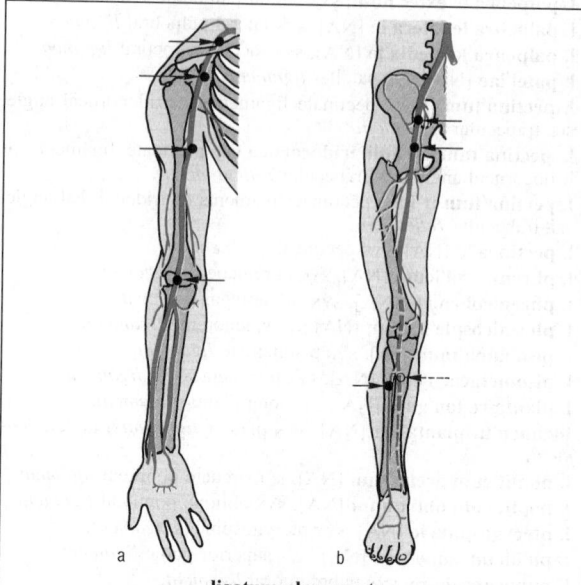

ligature placement
a) on subclavian and brachial arteries; and b) on femoral artery and its major branches

Stannius l., a l. placed either around the junction between the sinus venosus and atrium of the frog or turtle heart (first Stannius l.) or around the atrioventricular junction (second Stannius l.); demonstrates that the cardiac impulse is conducted from sinus venosus to atria to ventricle, but that successive chambers possess automaticity since each may continue to beat, but the atria now have a slower rate than the sinus venosus, and the ventricle either does not contract or beats at a slower rate than the atria.

suboccluding l., a l. to diminish blood supply and encourage collateral circulation.

suture l., a l. applied by passing a needle with attached thread through or around a structure to more firmly secure the l.

light (līt). That portion of electromagnetic radiation to which the retina is sensitive. SEE ALSO lamp. [A.S. *leōht*]

cold l., (1) SYN bioluminescence (1). **(2)** fluorescent l. as opposed to incandescent l.

infrared l., SEE infrared.

invisible l., historic term for x-rays.

minimum l., SEE visual *threshold.*

polarized l., l. in which, as a result of reflection or transmission through certain media, the vibrations are all in one plane, transverse to the ray, instead of in all planes.

reflected l., l. directed backward from a mirror.

refracted l., bent rays of l. changed in passage from one transparent medium to another of unequal density. SEE ALSO refraction.

transmitted l., l. passed through a transparent medium.

Wood's l., ultraviolet l. produced by Wood's lamp.

light·en·ing (līt′en-ing). Sensation of decreased abdominal distention during the later weeks of pregnancy following the descent of the fetal head into the pelvic inlet.

light green SF yel·low·ish [C.I. 42095]. An acid arylmethane dye, used as a cytoplasmic stain in plant and animal histology; fades badly in bright light.

Lignac, G.O.E., Dutch pediatrician, 1891–1954. SEE L.-Fanconi *syndrome.*

lig·ne·ous (lig′nē-us). Woody; having a woody feeling. [L. *ligneus,* wooden, fr. *lignum,* wood]

lig·nin. A polymer of coniferyl alcohol accompanying cellulose and present in vegetable fiber and wood cells; a source of vanillin (by oxidation of l.); l. composition varies with plant species. [L. *lignum,* wood]

lig·no·cer·ic ac·id (lig-nō-sār′ik, -sēr′ik). $CH_3(CH_2)_{22}COOH$; an acid present in one type of sphingolipid and in small amounts in triacylglycerols. SYN *n*-tetracosanoic acid.

lig·no·pha·gia (lig-nō-fāj′ē-a). An abnormal chewing and eating of wood, seen in horses in restrictive quarters. [L. *lignum,* wood, + G. *phagō,* to eat]

like·li·hood. A statement of the chance that an unknown quantity in reality has a particular value based on the readiness with which it would account for a given set of data; in this way the merits of various competing interpretations may be compared.

Likert, Rensis, U.S. social psychologist, *1903. SEE Likert *scale.*

Lillie, Ralph D., U.S. pathologist, 1896–1979. SEE Glenner-L. *stain* for pituitary. See entries under stain.

Lilly, John C., U.S. physiologist, *1915. SEE Silverman-L. *pneumotachograph.*

limb (lim). **1.** An extremity; a member; an arm or leg. **2.** A segment of any jointed structure. SEE ALSO leg. [A.S. *lim*]

   ampullary l.'s of semicircular ducts, SYN ampullary *crura* of semicircular ducts, under *crus.*

   anacrotic l., the ascending l. of an arterial pulse tracing.

   anterior l. of internal capsule, the portion of the internal capsule between the head of the caudate nucleus and the putamen; it lies anterior to the genu of the internal capsule. SYN crus anterius capsulae internae [NA].

   anterior l. of stapes, SYN anterior *crus* of stapes.

   l.'s of bony semicircular canals, SYN *crura* of bony semicircular canals, under *crus.*

   common l. of membranous semicircular ducts, SYN common *crus* of semicircular ducts.

   l. of helix, SYN *crus* of helix.

   inferior l., SYN lower l.

   lateral l., SYN lateral *crus.*

   lower l., the hip, thigh, leg, ankle, and foot. SYN membrum inferius [NA], inferior l., lower extremity, pelvic l.

   medial l., SYN medial *crus.*

   pelvic l., SYN lower l.

   phantom l., the sensation that an amputated l. is still present, often associated with painful paresthesia. SYN pseudesthesia (3), pseudoesthesia (3), stump hallucination.

   posterior l. of internal capsule, that subdivision of the internal capsule caudal to the genu between the thalamus and lentiform nucleus. SYN crus posterius capsulae internae [NA].

   posterior l. of stapes, SYN posterior *crus* of stapes.

   retrolenticular l. of internal capsule, SYN retrolenticular *part* of internal capsule.

   simple membranous l. of semicircular duct, SYN simple *crus* of semicircular duct.

   sublenticular l. of internal capsule, SYN sublenticular *part* of internal capsule.

   superior l., SYN upper l.

   thoracic l., SYN upper l.

   upper l., the shoulder, arm, forearm, wrist, and hand. SYN membrum superius [NA], superior l., thoracic l., upper extremity.

lim·bic (lim′bik). **1.** Relating to a limbus. **2.** Relating to the limbic *system.*

lim·bus, pl. **lim·bi** (lim′bŭs, lim′bī) [NA]. The edge, border, or fringe of a part. [L. a border]

   l. acetab′uli [NA], SYN *margin* of acetabulum.

   l. alveola′ris, (1) SYN alveolar *arch* of mandible. **(2)** SYN alveolar *arch* of maxilla.

   l. of bony spiral lamina, the border of the spiral lamina; the thickened periosteum covering the upper plate of the bony spiral lamina of the cochlea. SYN l. laminae spiralis osseae [NA].

   l. of cornea, the margin of the cornea overlapped by the sclera. SYN l. corneae [NA], corneal margin, sclerocorneal junction.

   l. cor′neae [NA], SYN l. of cornea.

   l. fos′sae ova′lis, a muscular ring surrounding the fossa ovalis in the wall of the right atrium of the heart. SYN annulus

ovalis, margin of fossa ovalis, Vieussens' annulus, Vieussens' isthmus, Vieussens' l., Vieussens' ring.

   l. lam′inae spira′lis os′seae [NA], SYN l. of bony spiral lamina.

   l. membra′nae tym′pani, SYN l. of tympanic membrane.

   lim′bi palpebra′les [NA], SYN *borders* of eyelids, under *border.*

   l. palpebrales anteriores [NA], SYN anterior *border* of eyelids.

   l. penicilla′tus, SYN brush *border.*

   l. stria′tus, SYN striated *border.*

   l. of tympanic membrane, margin of the tympanic membrane attaching to the tympanic sulcus. SYN l. membranae tympani.

   Vieussens' l., SYN l. fossae ovalis.

lime (līm). **1.** CaO; an alkaline earth oxide occurring in grayish white masses (quicklime); on exposure to the atmosphere it becomes converted into calcium hydrate and calcium carbonate (air-slaked l.); direct addition of water to calcium oxide produces calcium hydrate (slaked l.). SYN calcium oxide, calx (1). **2.** Fruit of the l. tree, *Citrus medica* (family Rutaceae), which is a source of ascorbic acid and acts as an antiscorbutic agent. [O.E. *līm,* birdlime]

   air-slaked l., SEE lime (1).

   chlorinated l., SEE chlorinated lime.

   slaked l., SEE lime (1).

   sulfurated l., SYN crude *calcium* sulfide.

li·men, pl. **li·mi·na** (lī′men, lim′i-nă) [NA]. Entrance; the external opening of a canal or space, such as l. insulae. SYN threshold (4). [L.]

   l. in′sulae [NA], the band of transition between the anterior portion of the gray matter of the insula and the anterior perforated substance; it is formed by a narrow strip of olfactory cortex along the lateral side of the lateral olfactory stria. SYN threshold of island of Reil.

   l. na′si [NA], a ridge marking the boundary between the nasal cavity proper and the vestibule. SYN threshold of nose.

lim·er·ence (lim′er-ens). Emotional excitement of being in love.

limes (L) (lī′mēz). A boundary, limit, or threshold. SEE ALSO L *doses,* under *dose.* [L.]

lim·i·nal (lim′i-năl). **1.** Pertaining to a threshold. **2.** Pertaining to a stimulus just strong enough to excite a tissue, *e.g.,* nerve or muscle. [L. *limen* (*limin*-), a threshold]

lim·i·nom·e·ter (lim-i-nom′ĕ-ter). An instrument for measuring the strength of a stimulus which is barely sufficient to produce a reflex response. [L. *limen,* threshold, + G. *metron,* measure]

lim·it. A boundary or end. [L. *limes,* boundary]

   elastic l., the greatest stress to which a material may be subjected and still be capable of returning to its original dimensions when the forces are released.

   Hayflick's l., the l. of human cell division in subcultures; such cells will divide only about 50 times before dying out.

   permissible exposure l., an occupational health standard to safeguard workers against dangerous contaminants in the workplace.

   proportional l., the greatest stress that a material is capable of sustaining without any deviation from proportionality of stress to strain (Hooke's law).

   quantum l., the shortest wavelength found in an x-ray spectrum.

   short-term exposure l. (STEL), the maximum concentration of a chemical to which workers may be exposed continuously for up to 15 minutes without danger to health or work efficiency and safety.

Lim·na·tis ni·lot·i·ca (lim-nā′tis nī-lot′i-kă). The horse leech; a species of land-leech of southern Europe and northern Africa which may infest the nostrils or gullet and, attaching itself to the mucous membrane, may cause hemorrhages and anemia in horses and other animals drinking leech-infested water. [G. *limnē,* pool]

lim·ne·mia (lim-nē′mē-ă). SYN chronic *malaria.* [G. *limnē,* marsh, + *haima,* blood]

lim·ne·mic (lim-nē′mik). Suffering from chronic malaria.

lim·nol·o·gy (lim-nol′ō-jē). Study of the physical, chemical, meteorological, and biological conditions in fresh water; a branch of ecology. [G. *limnē,* pool, + *logos,* study]

li·mon, gen. **li·mo·nis** (lī′mon, li-mō′nis). SYN lemon. [L.]

li·mo·phoi·tas (lī'mō-foy'tas). Rarely used term for a psychosis induced by starvation. [G. *limos,* hunger, + *phoitas,* frenzy]

li·moph·thi·sis (lī-mof'thī-sis). Rarely used term for emaciation from lack of sufficient nourishment. [G. *limos,* hunger, + *phthisis,* wasting]

li·mo·sis (lī-mō'sis). Rarely used term for hunger, especially abnormal or inordinate hunger. [G. *limos,* hunger]

limp. A lame walk with a yielding step; asymmetrical gait. SEE ALSO claudication.

LINAC Abbreviation for linear *accelerator.*

lin·co·my·cin (lin-kō-mī'sin). An antibacterial substance, composed of substituted pyrrolidine and octapyranose moities, produced by *Streptomyces lincolnensis;* active against Gram-positive organisms; used medicinally as l. hydrochloride.

linc·ture, linc·tus (link'chūr, link'tŭs). An electuary or a confection; originally a medical preparation taken by licking. [L. *lingo,* pp. *linctus,* to lick]

lin·dane (lin'dān). 1,2,3,4,5,6-Hexachlorocyclohexane; used as a scabicide, pediculicide, and insecticide (10 times more toxic for house flies than DDT). SEE ALSO gamma benzene *hexachloride.*

Lindau, Arvid, Swedish pathologist, 1892–1958. SEE L.'s *disease, tumor;* von Hippel-L. *syndrome.*

Lindbergh, Charles A., U.S. aviator, 1902–1974. SEE Carrel-L. *pump.*

Lindner, Karl, Austrian ophthalmologist, 1883–1961. SEE L.'s *bodies,* under *body.*

Lindqvist, Johan Torsten, Swedish physician, *1906. SEE Fahraeus-L. *effect.*

LINE

line (līn). **1.** A mark, strip, or streak. In anatomy, a long narrow mark, strip, or streak distinguished from the adjacent tissues by a color, texture, or elevation. SEE ALSO line. **2.** A unit of measurement used by histologists in the 19th century; it varied in different countries from $\frac{1}{10}$ to $\frac{1}{12}$ of an English inch. **3.** A laboratory derivative of a stock of organisms maintained under defined physical conditions. **4.** A section of tubing supplying fluid or conducting impulses for monitoring equipment; *e.g.,* intravenous l., arterial l. SYN linea [NA]. [L. *linea,* a linen thread, a string, line, fr. *linum,* flax]

absorption l.'s, the dark l.'s in the solar spectrum due to absorption by the solar and the earth's atmosphere; the phenomenon occurs because rays passing from an incandescent body through a colder medium are absorbed by elements in that medium.

accretion l.'s, l.'s seen in microscopic sections of the enamel, marking successive layers of added material.

alveolonasal l., a l. connecting the alveolar point and the nasion.

Amberg's lateral sinus l., a l. dividing the angle formed by the anterior edge of the mastoid process and the temporal l.

anocutaneous l., SYN pectinate l.

anterior axillary l., a vertical line extending inferiorly from the anterior axillary fold. SYN linea axillaris anterior [NA], linea preaxillaris ✶ [NA], preaxillary l.

anterior junction l., radiographic projection of the mediastinal tissue septum between the upper lobes behind the sternum.

anterior median l., the line of intersection of the midsagittal plane with the anterior surface of the body. SYN linea mediana anterior [NA].

arcuate l., an arching or bow-shaped l. SEE arcuate l. of ilium, arcuate l. of rectus sheath. SYN linea arcuata [NA].

arcuate l. of ilium, the iliac portion of the linea terminalis of the bony pelvis. SYN linea arcuata ossis ilii [NA].

arcuate l. of rectus sheath, a crescentic line, not always clearly defined, which marks the lower limit of the posterior layer of the sheath of the rectus abdominis muscle. SYN linea arcuata vaginae musculi recti abdominis [NA], Douglas' l., linea semicircularis, semicircular l.

arterial l., an intra-arterial catheter.

axillary l., SEE anterior axillary l., midaxillary l., posterior axillary l.

Baillarger's l.'s, two laminae of white fibers that course parallel to the surface of the cerebral cortex and are visible as outer and inner l.'s in sections cut perpendicular to the surface; the l. of Gennari in the calcarine cortex represents the outer of these lines. SYN Baillarger's bands.

base l., a l. approximating the base of the skull, passing from the infraorbital ridge to the midline of the occiput, intersecting the superior margin of the external auditory meatus; the skull is in the anatomical position when the base line lies in the horizontal plane. SYN orbitomeatal l.

basinasal l., a l. connecting the basion and the nasion. SYN nasobasilar l.

Beau's l.'s, transverse depressions on the fingernails following severe febrile disease, malnutrition, trauma, myocardial infarction, etc.

l. of Bechterew, SYN *band* of Kaes-Bechterew.

bismuth l., a black zone on the free marginal gingiva, often the first sign of poisoning from prolonged parenteral administration of bismuth.

black l., SYN *linea* nigra.

blue l., a bluish l. along the free border of the gingiva, occurring in chronic heavy metal poisoning.

Bolton-nasion l., SYN Bolton *plane.*

Brödel's bloodless l., l. running somewhat posterior to the lateral convex border of the kidney between anterior and posterior renal segments demarcating the areas of distribution of the anterior and posterior branches of the renal artery; it is in fact only relatively avascular.

Burton's l., a bluish l. on the free border of the gingiva, occurring in lead poisoning.

calcification l.'s of Retzius, incremental l.'s of rhythmic deposition of successive layers of enamel matrix during development. SYN l.'s of Retzius.

Camper's l., the l. running from the inferior border of the ala of the nose to the superior border of the tragus of the ear.

cell l., **(1)** in tissue culture, the cells growing in the first or later subculture from a primary culture. SEE ALSO established cell l. **(2)** a clone of cultured cells derived from an identified parental cell type.

cement l., the refractile boundary of an osteon or interstitial lamellar system in compact bone.

cervical l., a continuous anatomical irregular curved l. marking the cervical end of the crown of a tooth and the cementoenamel junction.

Chamberlain's l., a l. drawn from the posterior margin of the hard palate to the dorsum of the foramen magnum; in basilar impression, the odontoid process rises above this l.

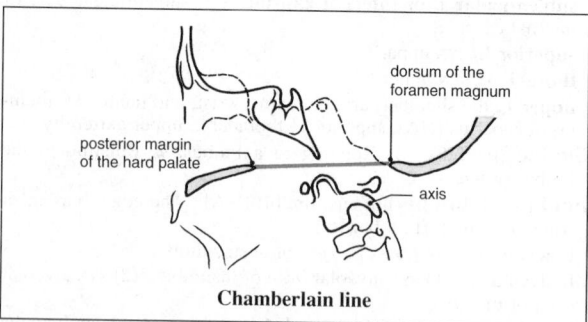

dorsum of the foramen magnum

posterior margin of the hard palate

axis

Chamberlain line

Chaussier's l., the anteroposterior l. of the corpus callosum as appearing on median section of the brain.

Clapton's l., a greenish discoloration of the marginal gingiva in cases of chronic copper poisoning.

cleavage l.'s, lines which can be extrapolated by connecting linear openings made when a round pin is driven into the skin of a cadaver, resulting from the principal axis of orientation of the subcutaneous connective tissue (collagen) fibers of the dermis; they vary in direction with the region of the body surface. SYN Langer's l.'s.

Conradi's l., a l. extending from the base of the ensiform cartilage to the apex beat of the heart, corresponding approximately to the lower edge of the cardiac area.

contour l.'s of Owen, SYN Owen's l.'s.

Correra's l., SYN pleural l.'s.

costoclavicular l., SYN parasternal l.

costophrenic septal l.'s, SYN Kerley B l.'s.

Crampton's l., a l. from the apex of the cartilage of the last rib downward and forward nearly to the crest of the ilium, then forward parallel with it to a little below the anterior superior spine; a guide to the common iliac artery.

Daubenton's l., the l. passing between the opisthion and the basion. SEE ALSO Daubenton's *angle*, Daubenton's *plane*.

l. of demarcation, a zone of inflammatory reaction separating a gangrenous area from healthy tissue.

demarcation l. of retina, junction of avascular and vascular retina in retinopathy of prematurity; line marking the limits of an old retinal detachment.

Dennie's l., an accentuated line or fold below the margin of the lower eyelid; characteristic in atopic dermatitis. SYN Dennie's infraorbital fold.

dentate l., SYN pectinate l.

developmental l.'s, SYN developmental *grooves*, under *groove*.

Douglas' l., SYN arcuate l. of rectus sheath.

Eberth's l.'s, l.'s appearing between the cells of the myocardium when stained with silver nitrate.

Egger's l., seldom-used term for the circular l. of adhesion between the vitreous and posterior lens.

Ehrlich-Türk l., seldom-used term for the vertical, thin deposition of material on the posterior surface of the cornea in uveitis.

epiphysial l., the line of junction of the epiphysis and diaphysis of a long bone where growth in length occurs. SYN linea epiphysialis [NA], synchondrosis epiphyseos.

established cell l., cells that demonstrate the potential for indefinite subculture *in vitro*.

Farre's l., a whitish l. marking the insertion of the mesovarium at the hilum of the ovary.

Feiss l., a l. running from the medial malleolus to the plantar aspect of the first metatarsophalangeal joint.

l. of fixation, a l. joining the object (or point of fixation) with the fovea.

Fleischner l.'s, coarse linear shadows on a chest radiograph, indicating bands of subsegmental atelectasis.

Fraunhofer's l.'s, a number of the most prominent of the absorption l.'s of the solar spectrum.

fulcrum l., an imaginary l. around which a removable partial denture tends to rotate. SYN rotational axis.

Futcher's l., a dorso-ventral line of pigmentation occurring symmetrically and bilaterally for about 10 cm along the lateral edge of the biceps muscle, seen in some blacks. SYN Voigt's l.'s.

l. of Gennari, a prominent white line appearing in perpendicular sections of the visual cortex (Brodmann's area 17) at about mid-thickness of the cortical gray matter, corresponding to the particularly well developed outer line of Baillarger of that cortical area, and composed largely of tangentially disposed intracortical association fibers. SYN Gennari's band, Gennari's stria, stripe of Gennari.

germ l., a collection of haploid cells derived from the specialized cells of the primitive gonad.

gluteal l., one of three rough curved lines on the outer surface of the ala of the ilium: anterior (or middle) gluteal l., inferior gluteal l., and posterior gluteal l.; the two areas bounded by these give attachment to the gluteus minimus muscle below and gluteus medius above. SYN linea glutea [NA].

Granger's l., on lateral skull radiographs, the l. produced by the groove of the optic chiasm or *sulcus* prechiasmatis.

growth arrest l.'s, dense l.'s parallel to the growth plates of long

bones on radiographs, representing temporary slowing or cessation of longitudinal growth. SYN Harris' l.'s.

Gubler's l., the level of the superficial origin of the trigeminus on the pons, a lesion below which causes Gubler's paralysis.

gum l., the position of the margin of the gingiva in relation to the teeth in the dental arch.

Haller's l., SYN *linea* splendens.

Hampton l., a thin radiolucent band across the neck of a contrast-filled benign gastric ulcer, indicating mucosal edema. Cf. Carman's *sign*.

Harris' l.'s, SYN growth arrest l.'s.

Head's l.'s, bands of cutaneous hyperesthesia associated with acute or chronic inflammation of the viscera. SYN Head's zones, tender l.'s, tender zones.

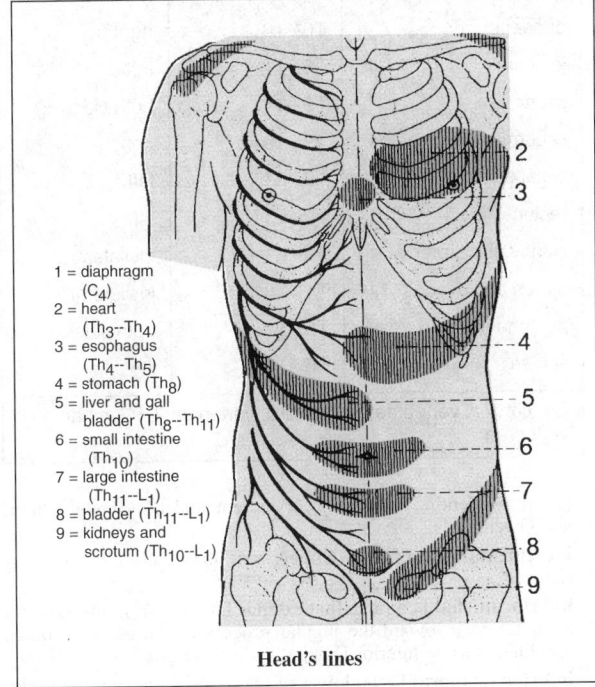

1 = diaphragm (C$_4$)
2 = heart (Th$_3$--Th$_4$)
3 = esophagus (Th$_4$--Th$_5$)
4 = stomach (Th$_8$)
5 = liver and gall bladder (Th$_8$--Th$_{11}$)
6 = small intestine (Th$_{10}$)
7 = large intestine (Th$_{11}$--L$_1$)
8 = bladder (Th$_{11}$--L$_1$)
9 = kidneys and scrotum (Th$_{10}$--L$_1$)

Head's lines

Hensen's l., SYN H *band*.

highest nuchal l., a line above and parallel to the superior nuchal line on the external surface of the occipital bone; it gives attachment to the epicranial aponeurosis and occipitalis muscle. SYN linea nuchae suprema [NA].

high lip l., the greatest height to which the lip is raised in normal function or during the act of smiling broadly.

Hilton's white l., SYN white l. of anal canal.

His' l., a l. extending from the tip of the anterior nasal spine (acanthion) to the hindmost point on the posterior margin of the foramen magnum (opisthion), dividing the face into an upper and a lower, or dental part.

Holden's l., the crease or furrow of the skin of the groin caused by flexion of the thigh.

Hudson-Stähli l., a brown, horizontal l. across the lower third of the cornea, occasionally seen in the aged and also in association with corneal opacities.

Hunter's l., SYN *linea* alba.

Hunter-Schreger l.'s, SYN Hunter-Schreger *bands*, under *band*.

iliopectineal l., SYN *linea* terminalis.

imbrication l.'s of von Ebner, incremental l.'s in the dentin of the tooth that reflect variations in mineralization during dentin formation; the distance between the l.'s corresponds to the daily rate of dentin formation. SYN incremental l.'s of von Ebner.

incremental l.'s, (1) in the enamel, calcification l.'s of Retzius;

li

Head's lines		
organ	dermatomic area	side of body
heart	C3–4–T1–5	right front
thoracic aorta	C3–4–T1–7	both sides
ribs	T2–12	ipsilateral
lungs	C3–4	ipsilateral
esophagus	T1–8	both sides
stomach	T(5) 6–9	left
liver and gall bladder	T(5) 6–9 (10)	right
pancreas	T6–9	left front
duodendum	T6–10	right
jejunum	T8–11	left
ileum	T9–11	both sides
cecum, proximal colon	T9–10–L1	right
distal colon	T9–L1	left
rectum	T9–L1	left
kidney and ureter	T9–L1 (2)	ipsilateral
uterus and ovaries	T12–L1	ipsilateral
peritoneum	T5–12	both sides
spleen	T6–10	left

C = cervical vertebrae; T = thoracic vertebrae; L = lumbar vertebrae

(2) in the dentin, imbrication or incremental l.'s of von Ebner, and Owen's l.'s.

incremental l.'s of von Ebner, SYN imbrication l.'s of von Ebner.

inferior nuchal l., a ridge that extends laterally from the external occipital crest toward the jugular process of the occipital bone. SYN linea nuchae inferior [NA].

inferior temporal l., the lower of two curved lines on the parietal bone; it marks the outer limit of attachment of the temporalis muscle. SYN linea temporalis inferior [NA], temporal ridge.

infracostal l., SYN subcostal *plane.*

intercondylar l. of femur, a faint transverse ridge separating the floor of the intercondylar fossa from the popliteal surface of the femur; it affords attachment to the posterior portion of the articular capsule of the knee. SYN linea intercondylaris femoris [NA].

intermediate l. of iliac crest, the line on the crest of the ilium between the outer and inner lips, for origin of internal oblique muscle. SYN linea intermedia cristae iliacae [NA].

internal oblique l., SYN mylohyoid l.

interspinal l., l. passing through both anterior superior iliac spines indicating the interspinal *plane.* SYN linea interspinalis [NA].

intertrochanteric l., a rough line that separates the neck and shaft of the femur anteriorly; it passes downward and medially from the greater trochanter to the lesser trochanter and continues into the medial lip of the linea aspera. SYN linea intertrochanterica [NA], linea spiralis, spiral l.

intertubercular l., l. passing through tubercles of both iliac crests, indicating the intertubercular *plane.* SYN linea intertubercularis [NA].

isoelectric l., the baseline of the electrocardiogram.

l. of Kaes, SYN *band* of Kaes-Bechterew.

Kerley A l.'s, images of deep interlobular septa; longer, thicker, and more central than Kerley B l.'s; usually in upper lobes.

Kerley B l.'s, fine peripheral septal l.'s. SYN costophrenic septal l.'s.

Kerley C l.'s, a nonspecific fine reticular pattern on chest radiographs.

Kilian's l., a transverse l. marking the promontory of the pelvis.

Langer's l.'s, SYN cleavage l.'s.

Lanz's l., SYN interspinal *plane.*

lateral l., SEE lateral line *system.*

lead l., deposits of lead sulfide in the gingiva in areas of chronic inflammation.

Looser's l.'s, radiolucent bands in the cortex of a bone; usually indicates osteomalacia. SYN Looser's zones.

low lip l., (1) the lowest position of the lower lip during the act of smiling or voluntary retraction; (2) the lowest position of the upper lip at rest.

M l., a fine l. in the center of the A band of the sarcomere of striated muscle myofibrils. SYN M band, mesophragma.

Mach l., the apparent l. of contrasting density bordering a soft tissue shadow on a radiograph; it is an optical illusion constructed by the observer's retina.

mamillary l., a vertical line passing through the nipple on either side. SYN linea mamillaris [NA], nipple l.

mammary l., a transverse l. drawn between the two nipples.

McKee's l., a l. drawn from the tip of the cartilage of the eleventh rib to a point 3.5 cm medial to the anterior superior spine, then curved downward, forward, and inward to just above the deep inguinal ring; a guide to the common iliac artery.

median l., SEE anterior median l., posterior median l.

Mees' l.'s, horizontal white bands of the nails seen in chronic arsenical poisoning, and occasionally in leprosy. SYN Mees' stripes.

mercurial l., a bluish brown pigmentation seen at the gingival margin and associated with mercury poisoning (mercurial stomatitis).

Meyer's l., a l. through the axis of the big toe and passing the midpoint of the heel in a normal foot.

midaxillary l., a vertical line intersecting a point midway between the anterior and posterior axillary folds or lines. SYN linea axillaris media [NA], linea medio-axillaris✩ [NA], middle axillary l.

midclavicular l., a vertical line passing through the midpoint of the clavicle. SYN linea medioclavicularis [NA].

middle axillary l., SYN midaxillary l.

milk l., SYN mammary *ridge.*

Monro-Richter l., a l. passing from the umbilicus to the anterior superior iliac spine. McBurney's point occurs on this line. SYN Monro's l., Richter-Monro l.

Monro's l., SYN Monro-Richter l.

Muehrcke's l.'s, white l.'s, parallel with the lanula and separated from each other by normal pink areas; associated with hypoalbuminemia; the l.'s do not move outward with nail growth, but disappear when the serum albumen returns to normal.

mylohyoid l., a ridge on the inner surface of the mandible running from a point inferior to the mental spine upward and backward to the ramus behind the last molar tooth; it gives attachment to the mylohyoid muscle and the lowermost part of the superior constrictor of the pharynx. SYN linea mylohyoidea [NA], internal oblique l., mylohyoid ridge.

nasobasilar l., SYN basinasal l.

Nélaton's l., a l. drawn from the anterior superior iliac spine to the tuberosity of the ischium; normally the great trochanter lies in this l., but in cases of iliac dislocation of the hip or fracture of the neck of the femur the trochanter is felt above the l. SYN Roser-Nélaton l.

neonatal l., in deciduous teeth, a l. of demarcation between prenatal and postnatal enamel. SYN neonatal ring.

nipple l., SYN mamillary l.

Obersteiner-Redlich l., SYN Obersteiner-Redlich *zone.*

oblique l., a diagonal, sloping or slanting l.; a l. which is neither parallel nor perpendiculr, neither horizontal nor vertical. SEE oblique l. of mandible, oblique l. of thyroid cartilage. SYN linea obliqua [NA].

oblique l. of mandible, the l. on the external surface of the mandible that extends from the mental tubercle to the ramus and separates the alveolar and basilar parts of the bone. SYN linea obliqua mandibulae [NA].

oblique l. of thyroid cartilage, a ridge on the outer surface of the thyroid cartilage that gives attachment to the sternothyroid and thyrohyoid muscles. SYN linea obliqua cartilaginis thyroidea [NA].

l. of occlusion, the alignment of the occluding surfaces of the teeth in the horizontal plane. SEE ALSO occlusal *plane.*

Ogston's l., a l. drawn from the adductor tubercle of the femur to the intercondylar notch; a guide to resection of the medial condyle for knock-knee.

Ohngren's l., a theoretical plane passing between the medial canthus of the eye and the angle of the mandible; used as an arbitrary dividing l. in classifying localized tumors of the maxillary sinus; tumors above the l. invade vital structures early and have a poorer prognosis, whereas those below the l. have a more favorable prognosis.

orbitomeatal l., SYN base l.

Owen's l.'s, accentuated incremental l.'s in the dentin thought to be due to disturbances in the mineralization process. SYN contour l.'s of Owen.

paraspinal l., radiographic image of the interface between the lung and paravertebral soft tissues.

parasternal l., a vertical line equidistant from the sternal and midclavicular lines. SYN linea parasternalis [NA], costoclavicular l.

paravertebral l., a vertical line corresponding to the tips of the transverse processes of the vertebrae. SYN linea paravertebralis [NA].

Paris l., a unit of microscopic measurement as used in Kölliker's *Mikroskopische Anatomie;* it was equal to 0.0888138 of an inch.

Paton's l.'s, fine l.'s on the surface of the retina, concentric to a swollen disc. SYN striae retinae.

pectinate l., the l. between the simple columnar epithelium of the rectum and the stratified epithelium of the anal canal. SYN linea anocutanea [NA], anocutaneous l., dentate l.

pectineal l., a ridge running down the posterior surface of the shaft of the femur from the lesser trochanter to which the pectineus muscle attaches; continuous superiorly with intertrochanteric line and inferiorly with the medial lip of the linea aspera. SYN linea pectinea [NA].

pectineal l. of pubis, SYN *pecten* pubis.

pleural l.'s, on a chest radiograph, the shadow of the soft tissues between the aerated lung and the bones of the thorax. SYN Correra's l.

pleuroesophageal l., on a frontal chest radiograph, the image of the interface between the right lung and esophagus, the boundary of the azygoesophageal recess.

Poirier's l., a l. extending from the nasion to the lambda.

popliteal l., SYN soleal l.

postaxillary l., SYN posterior axillary l.

posterior axillary l., a vertical line extending inferiorly from the posterior axillary fold. SYN linea axillaris posterior [NA], linea postaxillaris ☆ [NA], postaxillary l.

posterior junction l., radiographic image of the mediastinal septum between the upper lobes behind the esophagus, above the aortic arch.

posterior median l., the line of intersection of the midsagittal plane with the posterior surface of the body. SYN linea mediana posterior [NA].

Poupart's l., a vertical l. passing through the center of the inguinal ligament on either side; it marks off the hypochondriac, lumbar, and iliac from the epigastric, umbilical, and hypogastric regions, respectively.

preaxillary l., SYN anterior axillary l.

Reid's base l., a l. drawn from the inferior margin of the orbit to the auricular point (center of the orifice of the external acoustic

meatus) and extending backward to the center of the occipital bone. Used as the zero plane in computed tomography.

retentive fulcrum l., (1) an imaginary l. connecting the retentive points of clasp arms on retaining teeth adjacent to mucosa-borne denture bases; **(2)** an imaginary l. connecting the retentive points of clasp arms, around which l. the denture tends to rotate when subjected to forces such as the pull of sticky foods.

l.'s of Retzius, SYN calcification l.'s of Retzius.

Richter-Monro l., SYN Monro-Richter l.

Roser-Nélaton l., SYN Nélaton's l.

rough l., SYN *linea* aspera.

sagittal l., any l. parallel to the midline, indicating a sagittal *plane.*

Salter's incremental l.'s, transverse l.'s sometimes seen in dentin, due to improper calcification.

S-BP l., a l. connecting the sella with the Bolton point; it indicates the posterior portion of the cranial base in cephalometrics.

scapular l., a vertical line passing through the inferior angle of the scapula. SYN linea scapularis [NA].

Schreger's l.'s, SYN Hunter-Schreger *bands,* under *band.*

semicircular l., SYN arcuate l. of rectus sheath.

semicircular l. of Douglas, a crescent-shaped l. that defines the end of the posterior fascial sheath of the rectus abdominis muscle.

semilunar l., SYN *linea* semilunaris.

septal l.'s, radiographic images of thickened interlobular septa, most often along the lateral border of lung, extending to pleura; Kerley A and B l.'s; usually caused by septal edema and fibrosis, also carcinomatosis.

Sergent's white l., SYN white l. (2).

Shenton's l., a curved l. formed by the top of the obturator foramen and the inner side of the neck of the femur, seen on an anteroposterior frontal radiograph of a normal hip joint; it is disturbed in lesions of the joint such as dislocation or fracture.

S-N l., a l. connecting a point (S) representing the center of the sella turcica with the frontonasal junction (N); it denotes the anterior portion of the cranial base in cephalometrics.

soleal l., a ridge which extends obliquely downward and medially across the back of the tibia from the fibular articular facet; it gives origin to the soleus muscle. SYN linea musculi solei [NA], l. for soleus muscle, linea poplitea, popliteal l.

l. for soleus muscle, SYN soleal l.

Spigelius' l., SYN *linea* semilunaris.

spiral l., SYN intertrochanteric l.

stabilizing fulcrum l., an imaginary l. connecting occlusal rests, around which l. the denture tends to rotate under masticatory force.

sternal l., a vertical line corresponding to the lateral margin of the sternum. SYN linea sternalis [NA].

Stocker's l., a fine l. of pigment in the corneal epithelium near the head of a pterygium.

subcostal l., a transverse l. transecting the inferiormost border of the thoracic cage, indicating the subcostal *plane.* SEE ALSO subcostal *plane.* SYN linea subcostalis [NA].

superior nuchal l., the ridge that extends laterally from the external occipital protuberance toward the lateral angle of the occipital bone; it gives attachment to the trapezius, sternocleido-

---

⟳ **Combining forms**	**[NA] Nomina Anatomica**
Word*Finder* **Multi-term entry finder** **Preceding letter A**	**[MIM] Mendelian** **Inheritance in Man**
A.D.A.M. Anatomy Plates **Between letters L and M**	☆ **Official alternate term**
Appendices: **Following letter Z**	☆**[NA] Official alternate** **Nomina Anatomica term**
SYN Synonym; Cf., compare	**High Profile Term**

li

mastoid, and splenius capitis muscles. SYN linea nuchae superior [NA].

superior temporal l., the upper of two curved lines on the parietal bone; the temporal fascia is attached to it. SYN linea temporalis superior [NA], temporal ridge.

supracrestal l., a transverse l. transecting the high point of both iliac crests, indicating the supracristal *plane*. SEE ALSO supracristal *plane*. SYN linea supracristalis [NA].

survey l., (1) a l. scribed on an abutment tooth of a dental cast by means of a dental surveyor indicating the height of contour of the tooth according to a specific path of insertion; **(2)** a l. which serves as a guide in the proper location of various parts of a clasp assembly for a removable partial denture. SYN clasp guideline, Cummer's guideline.

Sydney l., SYN Sydney *crease*.

sylvian l., the l. of the posterior limb of the lateral sulcus (sylvian fissure) of the cerebral cortex.

temporal l., SEE inferior temporal l., superior temporal l.

tender l.'s, SYN Head's l.'s.

terminal l., SYN *linea* terminalis.

Topinard's l., a l. running between the glabella and the mental point.

tram l.'s, the images of bronchial walls, usually thickened; colloq., British. SYN radiographic parallel line shadows.

transverse l.'s of sacrum, one of four ridges that cross the pelvic surface of the sacrum; these mark the positions of the intervertebral disks between the bodies of the five sacral vertebrae in the immature bone. SYN lineae transversa ossi sacri [NA].

trapezoid l., the area on the inferior surface of the clavicle near its lateral extremity on which the trapezoid ligament attaches. SYN linea trapezoidea [NA], trapezoid ridge.

Ullmann's l., the l. of displacement in spondylolisthesis.

Vesling's l., SYN scrotal *raphe*.

vibrating l., the imaginary l. across the posterior part of the palate, marking the division between the movable and immovable tissues.

l. of vision, SYN visual *axis*.

Voigt's l.'s, SYN Futcher's l.

Wegner's l., a narrow, whitish, slightly curved l. representing an area of preliminary calcification at the junction of the epiphysis and diaphysis of a long bone, related to syphilitic epiphysitis.

white l., (1) SYN *linea* alba. **(2)** a pale streak appearing within 30 to 60 seconds after stroking the skin with a fingernail, and lasting for several minutes; regarded as a sign of diminished arterial tension. SYN Sergent's white l.

white l. of anal canal, a bluish pink, narrow, wavy zone in the mucosa of the anal canal below the pectinate l. at the level of the interval between the subcutaneous part of the external sphincter and the lower border of the internal sphincter, said to be palpable. SYN Hilton's white l.

white l. of Toldt, (1) lateral reflection of posterior parietal pleura of abdomen over the mesentery of the ascending and descending colon. **(2)** junction of parietal peritoneum with Denonvillieri's fascia.

Z l., a cross-striation bisecting the I band of striated muscle myofibrils and serving as the anchoring point of actin filaments at either end of the sarcomere. SYN intermediate disk, Z band, Z disk.

l.'s of Zahn, riblike markings seen by the naked eye on the surface of antemortem thrombi; they consist of a branching framework of platelets and fibrin separating the coagulated blood cells. SYN striae of Zahn.

Zöllner's l.'s, figures devised to show the possibility of optical illusions; a common one consists of two parallel l.'s which are met by numerous short lines obliquely placed; the parallel lines then seeming to converge or diverge.

LINEA

lin·ea, gen. and pl. **lin·e·ae** (lin'ē-ă, -ē-ē) [NA]. SYN line. [L.]

l. al'ba [NA], a fibrous band running vertically the entire length of the center of the anterior abdominal wall, receiving the attachments of the oblique and transverse abdominal muscles. SYN Hunter's line, white line (1).

lin'eae albican'tes, SYN *striae* cutis distensae, under *stria*.

l. anocuta'nea [NA], SYN pectinate *line*.

l. arcua'ta [NA], SYN arcuate *line*.

l. arcua'ta os'sis il'ii [NA], SYN arcuate *line* of ilium.

l. arcua'ta vagi'nae mus'culi rec'ti abdom'inis [NA], SYN arcuate *line* of rectus sheath. SEE ALSO rectus *sheath*, posterior *layer* of rectus abdominis sheath.

l. as'pera [NA], a rough ridge with two pronounced lips running down the posterior surface of the shaft of the femur; the lateral lip of the linea aspera is a continuation of the gluteal tuberosity, the medial lip of the intertrochanteric line; it affords attachment to the vastus medialis, adductor longus, adductor magnus, adductor brevis, the short head of the biceps, and the vastus lateralis muscles as well as to the intermuscular septa of the thigh. SYN rough line.

lin'eae atroph'icae, SYN *striae* cutis distensae, under *stria*.

l. axilla'ris ante'rior [NA], SYN anterior axillary *line*.

l. axilla'ris me'dia [NA], SYN midaxillary *line*.

l. axilla'ris poste'rior [NA], SYN posterior axillary *line*.

l. cor'neae seni'lis, SYN *arcus* cornealis.

l. epiphysia'lis [NA], SYN epiphysial *line*.

l. glu'tea [NA], SYN gluteal *line*.

l. glu'tea ante'rior, anterior gluteal line. SEE gluteal *line*.

l. glutea inferior, inferior gluteal line. SEE gluteal *line*.

l. glutea posterior, posterior gluteal line. SEE gluteal *line*.

l. intercondyla'ris fem'oris [NA], SYN intercondylar *line* of femur.

l. interme'dia cris'tae ili'acae [NA], SYN intermediate *line* of iliac crest.

l. interspina'lis [NA], SYN interspinal *line*. SEE ALSO interspinal *plane*.

l. intertrochanter'ica [NA], SYN intertrochanteric *line*.

l. intertubercula'ris [NA], SYN intertubercular *line*. SEE ALSO intertubercular *plane*.

l. mamilla'ris [NA], SYN mamillary *line*.

l. media'na ante'rior [NA], SYN anterior median *line*.

l. media'na poste'rior [NA], SYN posterior median *line*.

l. medio-axilla'ris [NA], ⭐official alternate term for midaxillary *line*, midaxillary *line*.

l. medioclavicula'ris [NA], SYN midclavicular *line*.

l. mus'culi sol'ei [NA], SYN soleal *line*.

l. mylohyoi'dea [NA], SYN mylohyoid *line*.

l. ni'gra, the l. alba in pregnancy, which then becomes pigmented. SYN black line.

l. nu'chae infe'rior [NA], SYN inferior nuchal *line*.

l. nu'chae media'na, SYN external occipital *crest*.

l. nu'chae supe'rior [NA], SYN superior nuchal *line*.

l. nu'chae supre'ma [NA], SYN highest nuchal *line*.

l. obli'qua [NA], SYN oblique *line*.

l. obliqua cartilag'inis thyroi'dea [NA], SYN oblique *line* of thyroid cartilage.

l. obliqua mandib'ulae [NA], SYN oblique *line* of mandible.

l. parasterna'lis [NA], SYN parasternal *line*.

l. paravertebra'lis [NA], SYN paravertebral *line*.

l. pecti'nea [NA], SYN pectineal *line*.

l. poplit'ea, SYN soleal *line*.

l. postaxilla'ris [NA], ⭐official alternate term for posterior axillary *line*, posterior axillary *line*.

l. preaxilla′ris [NA], ☆official alternate term for anterior axillary *line,* anterior axillary *line.*

l. scapula′ris [NA], SYN scapular *line.*

l. semicircula′ris, SYN arcuate *line* of rectus sheath.

l. semiluna′ris [NA], the slight groove in the external abdominal wall parallel to the lateral edge of the rectus sheath. SYN semilunar line, Spigelius′ line.

l. spira′lis, SYN intertrochanteric *line.*

l. splen′dens, a thickened band of pia mater along the midline of the anterior surface of the spinal cord. SYN Haller′s line.

l. sterna′lis [NA], SYN sternal *line.*

l. subcosta′lis [NA], SYN subcostal *line.* SEE ALSO subcostal *plane.*

l. supracrista′lis [NA], SYN supracrestal *line.* SEE ALSO supracrestal *plane.*

l. tempora′lis infe′rior [NA], SYN inferior temporal *line.*

l. tempora′lis supe′rior [NA], SYN superior temporal *line.*

l. termina′lis [NA], an oblique ridge on the inner surface of the ilium and continued on the pubis, which forms the lower boundary of the iliac fossa; it separates the true from the false pelvis. SYN iliopectineal line, terminal line.

lineae transver′sa ossi sacri [NA], SYN transverse *lines* of sacrum, under *line.*

l. trapezoi′dea [NA], SYN trapezoid *line.*

---

lin·e·age (līn′aj, lin′ē-āj). Descent in a line from a common progenitor or source. [O. Fr. *ligne,* line of descent]

lin·e·ar (lin′ē-ăr). Pertaining to or resembling a line.

line·breed·ing. Practice of successive inbreeding of closely related individuals with the object of concentrating desirable or scientifically interesting genetic characteristics of some individual or group.

li·ner (lī′ner). A layer of protective material.

asbestos l., a layer of asbestos used to line a dental casting ring so that during the heating and expansion of the investment the compression of the l. will free the investment from the restraint of the ring.

cavity l., SYN varnish (dental).

LINES Abbreviation for long interspersed *elements,* under *element.*

Lineweaver, Hans, U.S. physical chemist, *1907. SEE L.-Burk *equation, plot.*

Ling, Per Henrik, Swedish hygienist, 1776–1839. SEE L.′s *method.*

Lin·gel·sheim·ia (lin′jels-hīˑ′mē-ă). SYN *Acinetobacter.* [W. von Lingelsheim]

L. anitra′ta, SYN *Acinetobacter calcoaceticus.*

ling·ism (ling′izm). SYN Ling′s *method.*

lin·gua, gen. and pl. **lin·guae** (ling′gwă, ling′gwē) [NA]. 1. SYN tongue (1). 2. SYN tongue (2). [L. tongue]

l. cerebel′li, SYN *lingula* of cerebellum.

l. dissec′ta, SYN geographic *tongue.*

l. fissura′ta, SYN fissured *tongue.*

l. frena′ta, a tongue with a very short frenum constituting tongue-tie.

l. geograph′ica, SYN geographic *tongue.*

l. ni′gra, SYN black *tongue.*

l. plica′ta, SYN fissured *tongue.*

lin·gual (ling′gwăl). 1. Relating to the tongue or any tongue-like part. SYN glossal. 2. Next to or toward the tongue.

Lin·guat·u·la (ling-gwat′yū-lă). A genus of endoparasitic blood-sucking arthropods (family Linguatulidae, class Pentastomida), commonly known as tongue worms; once thought to be degenerate Acarina, but now generally considered to be a small but distinctive early offshoot of the Arthropoda. Adult worms are found in lungs or air passages of various hosts (*e.g.,* reptiles, birds, carnivores); young worms are found in a great variety of hosts, including humans, but chiefly in animals that serve as prey. [L. *linguatulus,* tongued]

L. rhina′ria, SYN *L. serrata.*

L. serra′ta, a species most common in Europe, but also found in the United States, South America, and probably elsewhere; the adult is a whitish, soft, flattened, annulated worm equipped with hooks by which it attaches itself to the nasal mucosa of dogs and other canids; the larvae develop in the liver and lymph nodes of rodents, swine, cattle, and sometimes man and other primates. SYN *L. rhinaria.*

lin·guat·u·li·a·sis (ling-gwat-yū-lī′ă-sis). Infection with *Linguatula.* SEE ALSO halzoun.

Lin·gua·tu·li·dae (ling-gwat′yū-li-dē). One of the families of Pentastomida of medical interest, the other being the Porocephalidae. L. have flattened bodies; adults inhabit the nasal cavities of various carnivores, such as the dog and cat, and larval forms are found in tissues of rodents, herbivores, and other animals; both larvae and adults have been reported from humans.

lin·gui·form (ling′gwi-fōrm). Tongue-shaped.

lin·gu·la, pl. **lin·gu·lae** (ling′gyū-lă, -lē) [NA]. 1. A term applied to several tongue-shaped processes. 2. When not qualified, the l. of cerebellum. [L. dim. of *lingua,* tongue]

l. cerebel′li [NA], SYN l. of cerebellum.

l. of cerebellum, a tongue-shaped sequence of flattened cerebellar folia forming the anterior (or superior) extreme of the cerebellar vermis, extending forward on the surface of the superior medullary velum between the two emerging superior cerebellar peduncles. SYN l. cerebelli [NA], lingua cerebelli, tongue of cerebellum.

l. of left lung, an inferomedial projection from the anterior aspect of the upper lobe of the left lung which bounds the cardiac notch inferiorly. SYN l. pulmonis sinistri [NA].

l. of mandible, a pointed tongue of bone overlapping the mandibular foramen, giving attachment to the sphenomandibular ligament. SYN l. mandibulae [NA], mandibular tongue, Spix′s spine.

l. mandib′ulae [NA], SYN l. of mandible.

l. pulmo′nis sinis′tri [NA], SYN l. of left lung.

l. sphenoida′lis [NA], a slender process projecting posteriorly between the body and greater wing of the sphenoid bone, on either side, forming the lateral margin of the carotid groove. In the dry skull, it projects into the foramen laccrum.

lin·gu·lar (ling′gyū-lăr). Pertaining to any lingula.

lin·gu·lec·to·my (ling′gyū-lek′tō-mē). 1. SYN glossectomy. 2. Excision of the lingular portion of the left upper lobe of the lung.

△**linguo-.** The tongue. [L. *lingua*]

lin·guo·cli·na·tion (ling′gwō-kli-nā′shŭn). Axial inclination of a tooth when the crown is inclined toward the tongue more than is normal.

lin·guo·clu·sion (ling-gwō-klū′zhŭn). Displacement of a tooth toward the interior of the dental arch, or toward the tongue. SEE ALSO lingual *occlusion* (2). SYN lingual occlusion (1).

lin·guo·dis·tal (ling-gwō-dis′tăl). Relating to the lingual and distal part of the tooth, *e.g.,* the l. cusp. SEE ALSO distolingual.

lin·guo·gin·gi·val (ling-gwō-jin′ji-văl). 1. Relating to the gingival third of the lingual surface of a tooth. 2. Relating to the angle or point of junction of the lingual border and gingival line on the distal or mesial surface of an incisor tooth.

lin·guo·oc·clu·sal (ling′gwō-ŏ-klū′săl). Relating to the line of junction of the lingual and occlusal surfaces of a tooth.

lin·guo·pap·il·li·tis (ling′gwō-pap′i-lī′tis). Small painful ulcers involving the papillae on the tongue margins.

lin·guo·plate (ling′gwō-plāt). A partial denture major connector formed as a lingual bar extended to cover the cingula of the lower anterior teeth. SYN lingual plate.

lin·guo·ver·sion (ling′gwō-ver-zhŭn). Malposition of a tooth lingual to the normal position.

lin·i·ment (lin′i-ment). A liquid preparation for external application or application to the gums; they may be clear dispersions, suspensions, or emulsions, and are frequently applied by friction to the skin; used as counterirritants, rubefacients, anodynes, or cleansing agents. [L., fr. *lino,* to smear]

li·nin (lī′nin). 1. A bitter glycoside obtained from *Linum catharticum* (family Linaceae). 2. A protein in linseed. 3. Obsolete term for the threadlike, nonstaining (achromatic) substance of the cell nucleus, on which chromatin granules were thought to be suspended. [L. *linum,* fr. G. *linon,* flax]

lin·ing (līn′ing). A coating applied to the pulpal wall(s) of a restorative dental preparation to protect the pulp from thermal or chemical irritation; usually a vehicle containing a varnish, resin, and/or calcium hydroxide.

li·ni·tis (li-nī′tis, lī-nī′tis). Inflammation of cellular tissue, specifically of the perivascular tissue of the stomach. [G. *linon,* flax, linen cloth, + *-itis,* inflammation]

l. plas′tica, originally believed to be an inflammatory condition, but now recognized to be due to infiltrating scirrhous carcinoma causing extensive thickening of the wall of the stomach; often called leather-bottle stomach.

link·age (lingk′ij). 1. A chemical covalent bond. 2. The relationship between syntenic loci sufficiently close that the respective alleles are not inherited independently by the offspring; a characteristic of loci, not genes.

genetic l., SEE linkage (2).

medical record l., the assemblage of lifetime or long-term individual medical histories from vital and medical data derived from multiple sources.

record l., a method of assembling the information contained in two or more sets of medical records, or a set of medical records and vital records such as birth or death certificates, and a procedure to ensure that each individual's records are counted only once; facilitated by a unique numbering system such as the Hogben number or soundex code to identify individuals with precision.

sex l., inheritance of a trait or a sex chromosome or gonosome. A man receives all his sex-linked genes from his mother and transmits them all to his daughters but not to his sons; a recessive sex-linked character is much more likely to be expressed in the male. SEE ALSO sex *chromosomes,* under *chromosome.*

link·age map. An abstract mathematical representation of genetic loci that conserves order of loci which are spaced in such a way that the distances are algebraically additive; conventionally, a map is scaled so that as distances between loci become smaller the ratio of the map distance to the value of the recombination fraction approaches 1 and independently assorting loci are infinitely far apart.

linked. Said of two genetic loci that exhibit genetic linkage.

link·er. A fragment of synthetic DNA containing a restriction site that may be used for splicing genes.

link·er scan·ning. A type of deletion mutagenesis where the distance and/or reading frame between potentially important regions is maintained by replacement with a synthetic oligonucleotide of known sequence.

Linné, Carl von, Swedish botanist and physician, 1707-1778. SEE linnaean *system* of nomenclature.

Li·nog·na·thus (li-nog′nă-thŭs). A genus of sucking lice (order Anoplura, family Linognathidae) that includes the species *L. africanus,* the African blue louse of sheep and goats; *L. ovillus,* the sheep body louse; *L. pedalis,* the foot louse of sheep; *L. setosus,* the sucking louse of the dog and other canids; *L. stenopsis,* the sucking louse of goats; and *L. vituli,* the "long-nosed" sucking louse, ox louse, or blue louse of cattle. [G. *linon,* flax, thread, + *gnathos,* jaw]

li·no·le·ate (li-nō′lē-āt). Salt of linoleic acid.

lin·o·le·ic ac·id (lin-ō-lē′ik). $CH_3(CH_2)_3(CH_2CH=CH)_2(CH_2)_7$ COOH; 9,12-octadecadienoic acid; a doubly unsaturated fatty acid, occurring widely in plant glycerides, that is essential in nutrition in mammals. SYN linolic acid. [L. *linum,* flax, + *oleum,* oil]

lin·o·len·ic ac·id (lin-ō-len′ik). $CH_3(CH_2CH=CH)_3(CH_2)_7$ COOH; 9,12,15-cctadecatrienoic acid; an unsaturated fatty acid that is essential in nutrition. γ-l. a. is 6,9,12-octadecatrienoic acid.

linolic acid. SYN linoleic acid.

lin·seed (lin′sēd). The dried ripe seed of *Linum usitatissimum* (family Linaceae), flax, the fiber of which is used in the manufacture of linen; an infusion was used as a demulcent in catarrhal affections of the respiratory and urogenital tracts, and the ground seeds are used in making poultices. SYN flaxseed. [G. *linon,* flax]

l. oil, a fatty oil expressed from the ripe seeds of *Linum usitatissimum;* used in the preparation of lime liniment. SYN flaxseed oil.

lint. A soft, absorbent material used in surgical dressings, usually in the form of a thick, loosely woven material (sheet or patent l.). [O.E. *lin,* flax]

△**lio-.** SEE leio-.

li·o·trix (lī′ō-triks). A mixture of liothyronine sodium and levothyroxine sodium; used as a thyroid hormone.

LIP Acronym for lymphocytic interstitial *pneumonia* or lymphoid interstitial *pneumonia* .

lip. 1. One of the two muscular folds with an outer mucosa having a stratified squamous epithelial surface layer that bound the mouth anteriorly. 2. Any liplike structure bounding a cavity or groove. SEE ALSO labium, labrum. SYN labium (1) [NA]. [A.S. *lippa*]

acetabular l., SYN acetabular *labrum.*

anterior l. of uterine os, the portion of the vaginal part of the uterine cervix that bounds the ostium anteriorly intervening between the ostium and the anterior vaginal fornix. It is slightly shorter than l. posterius. SYN labium anterius ostii uteri [NA].

articular l., SYN articular *labrum.*

cleft l., a congenital facial deformity of the l. (usually the upper l.) due to failure of mesodermal penetration of the ectodermal grooves at the line of fusion of the medial and lateral nasal prominences and maxillary process; frequently but not necessarily associated with cleft alveolus and cleft palate. In many families and in various forms [MIM*119300, *119500, *119530, *119540, and *119550] there seems to be autosomal dominant inheritance; likewise for X-linked inheritance [MIM*303400]. But generally, as with the supposed autosomal dominant recessive forms, the genetics is more confusing and may represent a variable feature of a syndrome. SYN harelip.

double l., congenital or acquired excess tissue on the inner mucosal aspect of the l.; may be a manifestation of Ascher's syndrome.

external l. of iliac crest, the roughened outer margin of the crest that gives attachment to the external oblique and latissimus dorsi muscles above and to the fasciae latae and the tensor fascia lata muscle below. SYN labium externum cristae iliacae [NA].

glenoidal l., SYN glenoid *labrum.*

Hapsburg l., SEE Hapsburg *jaw.*

internal l. of iliac crest, the roughened inner margin of the crest that gives attachment to parts of the transversus abdominis, quadratus lumborum, and erector spinae muscles. SYN labium internum cristae iliacae [NA].

large pudendal l., SYN *labium* majus.

lateral l. of linea aspera, the lateral margin of the linea aspera of the femur that gives attachment to the lateral intermuscular septum and the short head of the biceps femoris muscles. SYN labium laterale lineae asperae [NA].

lower l., the muscular fold bounding the opening of the mouth inferiorly. SYN labium inferius oris [NA].

medial l. of linea aspera, the medial margin of the linea aspera of the femur that provides attachment for part of the vastus medialis muscle. SYN labium mediale lineae asperae [NA].

l.'s of mouth, lips of the mouth. SYN labia oris [NA].

posterior l. of uterine os, the portion of the uterine cervix that bounds the ostium posteriorly. It is slightly longer than l. anterius, intervening between the cervical canal and the posterior fornix of the vagina. SYN labium posterius ostii uteri [NA].

rhombic l., the thickened alar plate of the embryonic rhombencephalon.

small pudendal l., SYN *labium* minus.

tympanic l. of limbus of spiral lamina, SYN tympanic *labium* of limbus of spiral lamina.

upper l., the muscular fold forming the superior border of the mouth. SYN labium superius oris [NA].

vestibular l. of limbus of spiral lamina, SYN vestibular *labium* of limbus of spiral lamina.

△**lip-.** SEE lipo-.

li·pan·cre·a·tin (li-pan'krē-ă-tin, -krē'ă-tin). SYN pancrelipase.

lip·a·ro·cele (lip'ă-rō-sēl). An omental hernia. [G. *liparos*, fatty, + *kēlē*, tumor, hernia]

li·pase (lip'ās). In general, any fat-splitting or lipolytic enzyme; a carboxylesterase; *e.g.*, triacylglycerol lipase, phospholipase A₂, lipoprotein lipase.

lip·ec·to·my (lip-ek'tō-mē). Surgical removal of fatty tissue, as in cases of adiposity. [lipo- + G. *ektomē*, excision]

lip·e·de·ma (lip'e-dē'mă). Chronic swelling, usually of the lower extremities, particularly in middle-aged women, caused by the widespread even distribution of subcutaneous fat and fluid. [lipo- + G. *oidēma*, swelling]

li·pe·mia (lip-ē'mē-ă). The presence of an abnormally large amount of lipids in the circulating blood. SYN hyperlipidemia, hyperlipoidemia, lipidemia, lipoidemia. [lipid + G. *haima*, blood]

    alimentary l., relatively transient l. occurring after the ingestion of foods with a large content of fat. SYN postprandial l.

    diabetic l., development of lactescent plasma upon ingestion of dietary lipids; a rare manifestation of uncontrolled diabetes mellitus caused by defective metabolism of dietary lipids and abolished by the administration of insulin.

    postprandial l., SYN alimentary l.

    l. retina'lis, a creamy appearance of the retinal blood vessels that occurs when the lipids of the blood exceed 5%.

li·pe·mic (li-pē'mik). Relating to lipemia.

lip·id. "Fat-soluble," an operational term describing a solubility characteristic, not a chemical substance, *i.e.*, denoting substances extracted from animal or vegetable cells by nonpolar or "fat" solvents; included in the heterogeneous collection of materials thus extractable are fatty acids, glycerides and glyceryl ethers, phospholipids, sphingolipids, alcohols and waxes, terpenes, steroids, and "fat-soluble" vitamins A, D, and E. [G. *lipos*, fat]

    anisotropic l., a l. in the form of doubly refractive droplets.

    annular l., the layer(s) of l. bound to and/or surrounding an integral membrane protein.

    brain l., impure cephalin possessing marked hemostatic action when locally applied.

    compound l.'s, SYN heterolipids.

    isotropic l., a l. occurring in the form of singly refractive droplets.

    simple l.'s, SYN homolipids.

lip·i·de·mia (lip'i-dē'mē-ă). SYN lipemia.

lip·i·do·ly·tic (lip'ī-dō-lit'ik). Causing breakdown of lipid. [lipid + G. *lysis*, loosening]

lip·i·do·sis, pl. **lip·i·do·ses** (lip-i-dō'sis, -sēz). Hereditary abnormality of lipid metabolism that results in abnormal amounts of lipid deposition; classification is typically based on the responsible enzymatic deficiency and type of lipid involved. Such enzymatic activity takes place in the lysosomes, and the abnormal products appear as lysosomal storage diseases. Sphingolipidoses make up the largest portion of recognized lipidoses, including abnormal metabolism of gangliosides, ceramides, and cerebrosides. [lipid + G. *-ōsis*, condition]

    ceramide lactoside l., an inherited disorder associated with an accumulation of ceramide lactoside due to a deficiency of ceramide lactosidase; results in progressive brain damage with liver and spleen enlargement.

    cerebral l., SYN cerebral *sphingolipidosis*.

    cerebroside l., SYN Gaucher's *disease*.

    ganglioside l., SYN gangliosidosis.

    glycolipid l., SYN Fabry's *disease*.

    sphingomyelin l., SYN Niemann-Pick *disease*.

    sulfatide l., SYN metachromatic *leukodystrophy*.

Lipmann, Fritz A., German-U.S. biochemist in the U.S. and Nobel laureate, 1899–1986. SEE Warburg-L.-Dickens-Horecker *shunt*.

⚭lipo-, lip-. Fatty, lipid. [G. *lipos*, fat]

lip·o·am·ide (lip-ō-am'īd, -am'id). SEE lipoic acid.

lip·o·am·ide de·hy·dro·gen·ase. SYN dihydrolipoamide dehydrogenase.

lip·o·am·ide di·sul·fide. Oxidized lipoic acid in amide combination with the ε-amino group of an L-lysyl group of pyruvic acid dehydrogenase.

lip·o·am·ide re·duc·tase (NADH). SYN dihydrolipoamide dehydrogenase.

lip·o·ar·thri·tis (lip'ō-ar-thrī'tis). Inflammation of the periarticular fatty tissues of the knee. [lipo- + arthritis]

lip·o·ate (lip'ō-āt). A salt or ester of lipoic acid.

lip·o·ate ace·tyl·trans·fer·ase. SYN dihydrolipoamide acetyltransferase.

lip·o·a·tro·phia (lip'ō-ă-trō'fē-ă). SYN lipoatrophy.

    l. annula'ris, a rare condition of unknown cause characterized by localized panatrophy, a depressed area encircling the arm with sclerosis and atrophy of fat.

    l. circumscrip'ta, localized fat atrophy.

lip·o·at·ro·phy (lip-ō-at'rō-fē). Loss of subcutaneous fat, which may be total, congenital, and associated with hepatomegaly, excessive bone growth, and insulin-resistant diabetes. SYN Lawrence-Seip syndrome, lipoatrophia, lipoatrophic diabetes. [G. *lipos*, fat, + *a-*, priv. + *trophē*, nourishment]

    insulin l., SYN insulin *lipodystrophy*.

    partial l., SYN progressive *lipodystrophy*.

lip·o·blast (lip'ō-blast). An embryonic fat cell. [lipo- + G. *blastos*, germ]

lip·o·blas·to·ma (lip'ō-blas-tō'mă). 1. SYN liposarcoma. 2. A benign subcutaneous tumor composed of embryonal fat cells separated into distinct lobules, occurring usually in infants.

lip·o·blas·to·ma·to·sis (lip'ō-blas-tō-mă-tō'sis). A diffuse form of lipoblastoma that infiltrates locally but does not metastasize.

lip·o·car·di·ac (lip'ō-kar'dē-ak). 1. Relating to fatty heart. 2. Denoting a person suffering from fatty degeneration of the heart. [lipo- + G. *kardia*, heart]

lip·o·cat·a·bol·ic (lip'ō-kat-ă-bol'ik). Relating to the breakdown (catabolism) of fat.

lip·o·cer·a·tous (lip-ō-ser'ă-tŭs). SYN adipoceratous.

lip·o·cere (lip'ō-sēr). SYN adipocere. [lipo- + L. *cera*, wax]

lip·o·chon·dria (lip'ō-kon'drē-ă). Temporary storage vacuoles of lipids found in the Golgi apparatus. SEE ALSO phytosterolemia. [lipo- + mitochondria]

lip·o·chon·dro·dys·tro·phy (lip'ō-kon-drō-dis'trō-fē). SYN Hurler's *syndrome*.

lip·o·chrome (lip'ō-krōm). 1. A pigmented lipid, *e.g.*, lutein, carotene. SYN chromolipid. 2. A term sometimes used to designate the wear-and-tear pigments, *e.g.*, lipofuscin, hemofuscin, ceroid. More precisely, l.'s are yellow pigments that seem to be identical to carotene and xanthophyll and are frequently found in the serum, skin, adrenal cortex, corpus luteum, and arteriosclerotic plaques, as well as in the liver, spleen, and adipose tissue; l.'s do not stain with the ordinary dyes for fat. 3. The pigment produced by certain bacteria. [lipo- + G. *chroma*, color]

li·poc·la·sis (li-pok'lă-sis). SYN lipolysis. [lipo- + G. *klasis*, a breaking]

lip·o·clas·tic (lip-ō-klas'tik). SYN lipolytic.

lip·o·crit (lip'ō-krit). An apparatus and procedure for separating and volumetrically analyzing the amount of lipid in blood or other body fluid. [lipo- + G. *krinō*, to separate]

lip·o·cyte (lip'ō-sīt). SYN fat-storing *cell*. [lipo- + G. *kytos*, cell]

lip·o·der·moid (lip-ō-der'moyd). Congenital, yellowish-white, fatty, benign tumor located subconjunctivally. [lipo- + dermoid]

lip·o·di·er·e·sis (lip'ō-dī-er'ĕ-sis). SYN lipolysis. [lipo- + G. *dieresis*, division]

lip·o·dys·tro·phia (lip'ō-dis-trō'fē-ă). SYN lipodystrophy.

    l. intestina'lis, obsolete term for Whipple's *disease*.

    l. progressi'va supe'rior, SYN progressive *lipodystrophy*.

lip·o·dys·tro·phy (lip-ō-dis'trō-fē) [MIM*157660]. Defective metabolism of fat. SYN lipodystrophia. [lipo- + G. *dys-*, bad, difficult, + *trophē*, nourishment]

    congenital total l. [MIM*151680, MIM*151670, MIM*308908], l. characterized by almost complete lack of subcutaneous fat, accelerated rate of growth and skeletal development during the first 3 to 4 years of life, muscular hypertrophy, cardiac enlargement, hepatosplenomegaly, hypertrichosis, renal enlargement, hypertriglyceridemia, and hypermetabolism; both autosomal dominant and X-linked varieties exist.

familial l. [MIM*157680], autosomal dominant; partial lip associated with multifacial hypoplasin, retarded bone age, and hypotichosis.

insulin l., dystrophic atrophy of subcutaneous tissues in diabetics at the site of frequent injections of insulin. SYN insulin lipoatrophy.

intestinal l., obsolete term for Whipple's *disease*.

membranous l., a rare metabolic disease in which bone marrow fat cells are transformed into thick convoluted PAS-staining membranes enclosing weakly osmophilic material; leads to progressive cystic resorption of limb bones and dementia with sudanophilic leukodystrophy.

partial face-sparing l., a syndrome beginning at puberty that resembles total l. but is inherited as an autosomal or X-linked dominant form.

progressive l., a condition characterized by a complete loss of the subcutaneous fat of the upper part of the torso, the arms, neck, and face, sometimes with an increase of fat in the tissues about and below the pelvis. SYN Barraquer's disease, lipodystrophia progessiva superior, partial lipoatrophy, Simons' disease.

lip·o·e·de·ma (lĭp′ō-e-dē′mă). Edema of subcutaneous fat, causing painful swellings, especially of the legs in women. SYN cellulite (2).

lip·o·fec·tin (lĭp′o-fek′tin). A mixture predominantly of phospholipids used for aiding in the transfer of DNA into cells.

lip·o·fec·tion (lĭp′o-fek′shŭn). The process of injecting a lipid-complexed or contained DNA into eucaryotic cells. [lipo- + trans*fection*]

li·pof·er·ous (lip-of′er-ŭs). Transporting fat. [lipo- + L. *fero,* to carry]

lip·o·fi·bro·ma (lĭp′ō-fī-brō′mă). A benign neoplasm of fibrous connective tissue, with conspicuous numbers of adipose cells.

lip·o·fus·cin (lip-ō-fyūs′in). Brown pigment granules representing lipid-containing residues of lysosomal digestion and considered one of the aging or "wear and tear" pigments; found in liver, kidney, heart muscle, adrenal, and ganglion cells.

lip·o·fus·ci·no·sis (lĭp′ō-fyūs-i-nō′sis). Abnormal storage of any one of a group of fatty pigments.

ceroid l., cerebral *sphingolipidosis,* late juvenile type.

neuronal l., a group of diseases characterized by accumulation of abnormal pigments in tissue (previously classified as cerebral sphingolipidoses). Major subtypes include chronic juvenile form (Batten disease), slowly progressive behavior and visual symptoms, autosomal recessive inheritance; acute, late infantile form (Bielschowsky disease); autosomal recessive inheritance; chronic adult form (Kufs disease), variable inheritance; acute infantile form (Santavuori-Haltia disease), fulminating motor and mental deterioration often associated with myoclonic seizures. Minor forms have also been described.

lip·o·gen·e·sis (lip-ō-jen′ĕ-sis). The production of fat, either fatty degeneration or fatty infiltration; also applied to the normal deposition of fat or to the conversion of carbohydrate or protein to fat. SYN adipogenesis. [lipo- + G. *genesis,* production]

lip·o·gen·ic (lip-ō-jen′ik). Relating to lipogenesis. SYN adipogenic, adipogenous, lipogenous.

li·pog·e·nous (li-poj′ĕ-nŭs). SYN lipogenic.

lip·o·gran·u·lo·ma (lĭp′ō-gran-yū-lō′mă). A nodule or focus of granulomatous inflammation (usually of the foreign-body type) in association with lipid material deposited in tissues, *e.g.,* after the injection of certain oils. SEE ALSO paraffinoma. SYN eleoma, oil tumor, oleogranuloma, oleoma.

lip·o·gran·u·lo·ma·to·sis (lĭp′ō-gran′yū-lō-mă-tō′sis). **1.** Presence of lipogranulomas. **2.** Local inflammatory reaction to necrosis of adipose tissue.

disseminated l., a form of mucolipodosis, developing soon after birth because of deficiency of ceramidase; characterized by swollen joints, subcutaneous nodules, lymphadenopathy, and accum-

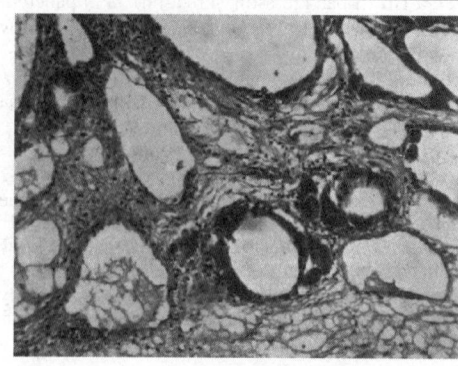

lipogranuloma

ulation in lysosomes of affected cells of PAS-positive lipid consisting of ceramide. SYN Farber's disease, Farber's syndrome.

lip·o·he·mia (lip-ō-hē′mē-ă). Obsolete term for lipemia.

li·po·ic ac·id (li-pō′ik). 6,8-Dimercapto-octanoic acid; functions as the amide (lipoamide) in the oxidized (–S–S–) form in the transfer of "active aldehyde" (acetyl), the two-carbon fragment resulting from decarboxylation of pyruvate, from α-hydroxy-ethylthiamin pyrophosphate to acetyl-CoA, itself being reduced (to the –SH HS– form; *i.e.,* dihydrolipoic acid) in the process; present in yeast and liver extracts, and may be useful in the treatment of mushroom poisoning. SYN acetate replacement factor, ovoprotogen, protogen, protogen A, pyruvate oxidation factor, thioctic acid.

lip·oid (lip′oyd). **1.** Resembling fat. **2.** Former term for lipid. SYN adipoid. [lipo- + G. *eidos,* appearance]

lip·oi·de·mia (lip-oy-dē′mē-ă). SYN lipemia.

lip·oi·do·sis (lip-oy-do′sis). Presence of anisotropic lipoids in the cells.

cerebroside l. (ser-ē′brō-sīd), a group of lysosomal storage diseases characterized by accumulation of lipid in cells of affected tissue and commonly accompanied by a manifest derangement of central nervous system development; *e.g.,* Gaucher's *disease* and Krabbe's *disease.*

l. cor′neae, SYN *arcus* cornealis.

l. cu′tis et muco′sae, SYN lipoid *proteinosis.*

galactosylceramide l., SYN globoid cell *leukodystrophy.*

lip·o·lip·oi·do·sis (lĭp′ō-lip-oy-dō′sis). Fatty infiltration, both neutral fats and anisotropic lipoids being present in the cells. SEE ALSO liposis (2).

li·pol·y·sis (li-pol′i-sis). The splitting up (hydrolysis), or chemical decomposition, of fat. SYN lipoclasis, lipodieresis. [lipo- + G. *lysis,* dissolution]

lip·o·lyt·ic (lip-ō-lit′ik). Relating to or causing lipolysis. SYN lipoclastic.

li·po·ma (li-pō′mă). A benign neoplasm of adipose tissue, comprised of mature fat cells. SYN adipose tumor. [lipo- + G. *-oma,* tumor]

l. annula′re col′li, an encircling growth of l. (or coalescent l.'s) in the neck, resulting in a collar-like enlargement. SEE ALSO Madelung's *neck.*

l. arbores′cens, an irregularly shaped l. involving the synovial membrane of a joint, resulting in fingerlike or treelike hyperplastic folds in the villi.

atypical l., l., occurring primarily in older men on the posterior neck, shoulders, and back, which is benign but microscopically atypical, containing giant cells with multiple overlapping nuclei forming a circle. SYN pleomorphic l.

l. capsula′re, a well-circumscribed mass resulting from a greatly increased amount of adipose tissue adjacent to the breast.

l. caverno′sum, SYN angiolipoma.

l. fibro′sum, SYN fibrolipoma.

infiltrating l., SYN liposarcoma.

lipoblastic l., SYN liposarcoma.

l. myxomatodes, SYN myxolipoma.

l. ossif'icans, a l. in which metaplasia occurs and small foci of bone are formed.

l. petrif'icans, a l. in which degeneration and necrosis results in a considerable amount of dystrophic calcification.

pleomorphic l., SYN atypical l.

l. sarcomato'des, l. sarcomato'sum, SYN liposarcoma.

spindle cell l., a microscopically distinctive form of l. in which adipose tissue is infiltrated by fibroblasts and collagen; usually found in the shoulder or neck of elderly men.

telangiectatic l., SYN angiolipoma.

li·po·ma·toid (li-pō'mă-toyd). Resembling a lipoma, frequently said of accumulations of adipose tissue that is not thought to be neoplastic.

lip·o·ma·to·sis (lip'ō-mă-tō'sis). SYN adiposis.

encephalocraniocutaneous l., a rare syndrome of multiple fibrolipomas or angiofibroma of the face, scalp, and neck present at birth, sometimes with symptomatic intracranial lipomas.

mediastinal l., increased mediastinal fat caused by taking steroids.

multiple symmetric l., accumulation and progressive enlargement of collections of adipose tissue in the subcutaneous tissue of the head, neck, upper trunk, and upper portions of the upper extremities; seen primarily in adult males and of unknown cause. SYN Launois-Bensaude syndrome, Madelung's disease, symmetric adenolipomatosis.

l. neurot'ica, SYN *adiposis* dolorosa.

li·po·ma·tous (li-pō'mă-tŭs). Pertaining to or manifesting the features of lipoma, or characterized by the presence of a lipoma (or lipomas).

lip·o·me·nin·go·cele (lip'ō-mĕ-ning'gō-sēl). An intraspinal cauda equinal lipoma associated with a spina bifida. [lipo- + G. *mēninx,* membrane, + *kēlē,* tumor]

lip·o·mu·co·pol·y·sac·cha·ri·do·sis (lip'ō-myū'ko-pol-ē-sak'ă-ri-dō'sis). SYN *mucolipidosis* I.

lip·o·nu·cle·o·pro·teins (lip'ō-nū'klē-ō-prō'tēnz). Associations or complexes containing lipids, nucleic acids, and proteins.

Lip·o·nys·sus (lip-ō-nis'ŭs). Former name for *Ornithonyssus.* [lipo- + G. *nyssō,* to prick]

lip·o·pe·nia (lip-ō-pē'nē-ă). An abnormally small amount, or a deficiency, of lipids in the body. [lipo- + G. *penia,* poverty]

lip·o·pe·nic (lip-ō-pē'nik). **1.** Relating to or characterized by lipopenia. **2.** An agent or drug that produces a reduction in the concentration of lipids in the blood.

lip·o·pep·tid, lip·o·pep·tide (lip-ō-pep'tid, lip-ō-pep'tīd). A compound or complex of lipid and amino acids.

lip·o·phage (lip'ō-fāj). A cell that ingests fat. [G. *lipos,* fat, + *phagō,* to eat]

lip·o·pha·gia (lip-ō-fā'jē-ă). SYN lipophagy.

l. granulomato'sis, obsolete term for Whipple's *disease.*

lip·o·phag·ic (lip-ō-fā'jik). Relating to lipophagy.

lip·oph·a·gy (lip-of'ă-jē). Ingestion of fat by a lipophage. SYN lipophagia. [lipo- + G. *phagein,* to eat]

lip·o·phan·er·o·sis (lip'ō-fan-er-ō'sis). A change in certain cells whereby previously invisible fat becomes demonstrable as small sudanophilic droplets. SEE fatty *degeneration.* [lipo- + G. *phaneros,* visible, + *-osis,* condition]

lip·o·phil (lip'ō-fil). A substance with lipophilic (hydrophobic) properties. [lipo- + G. *philos,* fond of]

lip·o·phil·ic (lip-ō-fil'ik). Capable of dissolving, of being dissolved in, or of absorbing lipids.

lip·o·phos·pho·di·es·ter·ase I (lip'ō-fos'-fō-dī-es'ter-ās). SYN *phospholipase* C.

lip·o·phos·pho·di·es·ter·ase II. SYN *phospholipase* D.

lip·o·pol·y·sac·cha·ride (LPS) (lip'ō-pol'ē-sak'ă-rīd). A compound or complex of lipid and carbohydrate; the l. (endotoxin) released from the cell walls of Gram-negative organisms that produces septic shock.

lip·o·pro·tein (lip-ō-prō'tēn). Complexes or compounds containing lipid and protein. Almost all the lipids in plasma are present as l.'s and are therefore transported as such. Plasma l.'s migrate electrophoretically with the α- and β-globulins, but are presently characterized by their flotation constants (densities, in g/ml) as follows: chylomicra, <0.93; very low density (VLDL), 0.93-1.006; intermediate density (IDL), 1.006-1.019; low density (LDL), 1.019-1.063; high density (HDL), 1.063-1.21 (divided into two classes: HDL_2 (1.063-1.125) and HDL_3 (1.125-1.21); very high density (VHDL), >1.21. They range in molecular weight from 175,000 to 1×10^9 and from 4 to 98% lipid (the higher the density, the lower the lipid content). The very low- and low-density fractions appear in the β_1-globulin fraction and are particularly rich in triacylglycerols and cholesterol esters, respectively; the high-density and very high-density fractions appear in the α_1-globulin fraction. Levels of l.'s are important in assessing the risk of cardiovascular disease.

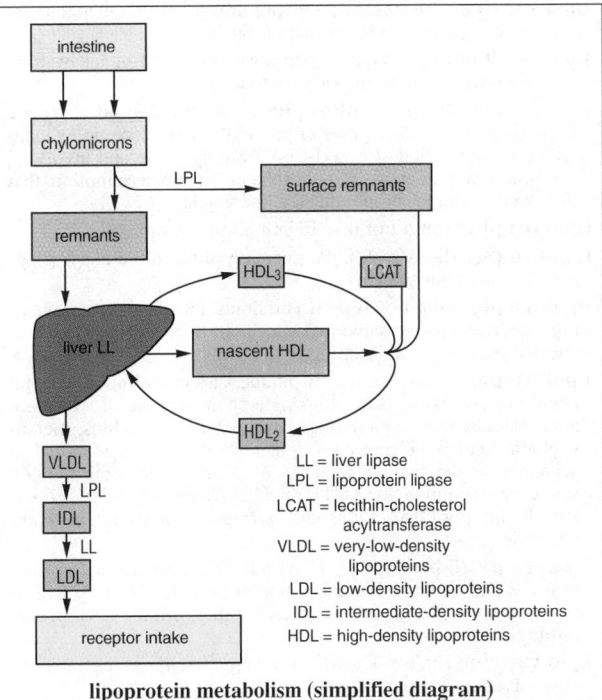

lipoprotein metabolism (simplified diagram)

lipoprotein Lp(a), a l. composed of an LDL particle combined with an additional protein, Lp(a) specific protein; elevated levels have been identified as a risk factor for coronary artery disease.

α_1-**lip·o·pro·tein.** A lipoprotein fraction of relatively low molecular weight, high density, rich in phospholipids, and found in the α_1-globulin fraction of human plasma.

β_1-**lip·o·pro·tein.** A lipoprotein fraction of relatively high molecular weight, low density, rich in cholesterol, and found in the β-globulin fraction of human plasma.

lip·o·pro·tein(a) (lip-ō-prō'tēn). A type of lipoprotein that has been found to be associated with apolipoprotein B and possibly with LDL; it is elevated in certain types of hyperlipoproteinemia and is associated with increased risk of coronary disease.

lip·o·pro·tein li·pase. An enzyme that hydrolyzes one fatty acid from a triacylglycerol; its activity is enhanced by heparin and inactivated by heparinase. It is activated by apolipoprotein C-II; a deficiency of l. l. is associated with familial hyperlipoproteinemia type I. SEE ALSO familial lipoprotein lipase *inhibitor,* clearing *factors,* under *factor.* SYN diacylglycerol lipase, diglyceride lipase.

lip·o·pro·tein-X. An abnormal lipoprotein found in patients with obstructive jaundice.

lip·o·sar·co·ma (lip'ō-sar-kō'mă). A malignant neoplasm of adults that occurs especially in the retroperitoneal tissues and the thigh, usually deep in the intermuscular or periarticular planes; histologically, l.'s are large tumors that may be composed of well-differentiated fat cells or may be dedifferentiated, either myxoid, round celled, or pleomorphic, usually in association with a rich network of capillaries; recurrences are common, and dedifferentiated l.'s metastasize to the lungs or serosal surfaces. SYN infiltrating lipoma, lipoblastic lipoma, lipoblastoma (1), lipoma sarcomatodes, lipoma sarcomatosum. [lipo- + *sarx,* flesh, + *-oma,* tumor]

li·po·sis (li-pō'sis). **1.** SYN adiposis. **2.** Fatty infiltration, neutral fats being present in the cells. SEE ALSO lipolipoidosis. [lipo- + G. *-osis,* condition]

li·pos·i·tol (lip-os'i-tol). SYN inositol.

lip·o·sol·u·ble (lip-ō-sol'yū-bl). Fat-soluble.

lip·o·some (lip'ō-sōm). A spherical particle of lipid substance suspended in an aqueous medium within a tissue. [lipo- + G. *sōma,* body]

lip·o·suc·tion. Method of removing unwanted subcutaneous fat using percutaneously placed suction tubes.

lip·o·suc·tion·ing (lip'ō-sŭk'shŭn-ing). Removal of fat by high vacuum pressure; used in body contouring.

lip·o·thi·am·ide py·ro·phos·phate (lip-ō-thī'am-īd). Name once given to the coenzymes of the multi-enzyme complex catalyzing the formation of acetyl-CoA from pyruvate and involving lipoamide and thiamin pyrophosphate, on the assumption that they were a single compound. SEE lipoic acid.

lip·o·tro·phic (lip-ō-trof'ik). Relating to lipotrophy.

li·pot·ro·phy (li-pot'rō-fē). An increase of fat in the body. [lipo- + G. *trophē,* nourishment]

lip·o·tro·pic (lip-ō-trop'ik). **1.** Pertaining to substances preventing or correcting excessive fat deposits in liver such as occurs in choline deficiency. **2.** Relating to lipotropy.

lip·o·tro·pin (li-pō-trō'pin). A pituitary hormone mobilizing fat from adipose tissue. β-L. is a single-chain peptide of 91 amino acid residues that contains the sequences of endorphins, metenkephalin, and β-melanotropin; γ-l. is shorter and is identical in sequence to the first 58 residues of β-lipotropin; both contain sequences common to ACTH and β-melanotropin. SYN lipid-mobilizing hormone, lipotropic hormone, lipotropic pituitary hormone.

li·pot·ro·py (li-pot'rō-pē). **1.** Affinity of basic dyes for fatty tissue. **2.** Prevention of accumulation of fat in the liver. **3.** Affinity of nonpolar substances for each other. [lipo- + G. *tropē,* turning]

lip·o·vac·cine (lip'ō-vak-sēn). A vaccine having a vegetable oil as a solvent. SEE adjuvant *vaccine.*

lip·o·vi·tel·lin (lip'ō-vi-tel'in). SYN vitellin.

li·pox·e·nous (li-pok'sĕ-nŭs). Pertaining to lipoxeny.

li·pox·e·ny (li-pok'sĕ-nē, lī-). Desertion of the host by a parasite when the development of the latter is complete. [G. *leipō,* to leave, + *xenos,* host]

li·pox·i·dase (li-poks'i-dās). SYN lipoxygenase.

li·pox·y·ge·nase (li-poks'ē-jĕ-nās). An enzyme that catalyzes the oxidation of unsaturated fatty acids with O_2 to yield hydroperoxides of the fatty acids; 5-l. catalyzes the first step in leukotriene biosynthesis, acting on arachidonate. SYN carotene oxidase, lipoxidase.

lip·o·yl (lip'ō-il). The acyl radical of lipoic acid.

lip·o·yl de·hy·dro·gen·ase. SYN dihydrolipoamide dehydrogenase.

lip·ping (lip'ing). The formation of a liplike structure, as at the articular end of a bone in osteoarthritis.

lip·pi·tude, lip·pi·tu·do (lip'i-tūd, lip-i-tū'dō). SYN blear *eye.* [L., fr. *lippus,* blear-eyed]

Lipschütz, Benjamin, Austrian physician, 1878–1931. SEE L. *cell;* L.'s *ulcer.*

li·pu·ria (li-pū'rē-ă). Presence of lipids in the urine. SYN adiposuria. [lipo- + G. *ouron,* urine]

li·pur·ic (li-pū'rik). Pertaining to lipuria.

liq·ue·fa·cient (lik'we-fā'shent). **1.** Making liquid; causing a solid to become liquid. **2.** Denoting a resolvant supposed to cause the resolution of a solid tumor by liquefying its contents. [L.

lique-facio, pres. p. *-faciens,* to make fluid, fr. ligueo, to be liquid]

liq·ue·fac·tion (lik-wĕ-fak'shŭn). The act of becoming liquid; change from a solid to a liquid form. [see liquefacient]

liq·ue·fac·tive (lik-wĕ-fak'tiv). Relating to liquefaction.

li·ques·cent (li-kwes'ent). Becoming or tending to become liquid. [L. *liquesco,* to become liquid]

li·queur (li-ker'). A cordial; a spirit containing sugar and aromatics. [Fr.]

liq·uid (lik'wid). **1.** An inelastic substance, like water, that is neither solid nor gaseous. **2.** Flowing like water. [L. *liquidus*]
Cotunnius' l., SYN perilymph.

li·quor, gen. **li·quor·is,** pl. **li·quo·res** (lik'er, lik'wŏr; -wŏr-is; -wō'rēs). **1.** Any liquid or fluid. **2.** A term used for certain body fluids. **3.** The pharmacopeial term for any aqueous solution (not a decoction or infusion) of a nonvolatile substance and for aqueous solutions of gases. SEE ALSO solution. [L.]

l. am'nii, SYN amniotic *fluid.*

l. cerebrospina'lis [NA], SYN cerebrospinal *fluid.*

l. cotun'nii, SYN perilymph.

l. enter'icus, intestinal secretions.

l. follic'uli, the fluid within the antrum of the ovarian follicle.

malt l., a beverage brewed from malt, such as beer or ale.

Morgagni's l., a fluid found postmortem between the epithelium and the fibers of the lens, resulting from the liquefaction of a semifluid material existing there during life. SYN Morgagni's humor.

mother l., the saturated solution remaining after a crystallization or precipitation.

Scarpa's l., SYN endolymph.

spirituous l., a strong alcoholic l. obtained by distillation, such as whiskey.

vinous l., SYN wine (1).

li·quo·rice (lik'ŏ-ris). SYN glycyrrhiza.

li·quor·rhea (lik-ŏ-rē'ă). The flow of liquid. [L. *liquor,* fluid, + G. *rhoia,* flow]

Lisch, Karl, Austrian ophthalmologist, *1907. SEE L. *nodule.*

Lisfranc (de St. Martin), Jacques, French surgeon, 1790–1847. SEE L.'s *amputation, joints,* under *joint, ligaments,* under *ligament, operation;* scalene *tubercle* of L.

lis·in·o·pril (līs-in'ō-pril). 1-[N^2-[(S)-1-Carboxy- 3-phenylpropyl]-L-lysyl]-L-proline dihydrate; an angiotensin-converting enzyme inhibitor used in the treatment of hypertension.

Lison, Lucien, Belgian scientist, *1907. SEE L.-Dunn *stain.*

lisp·ing. Mispronunciation of the sibilants *s* and *z.* SYN parasigmatism, sigmatism.

lis·sa·mine rho·da·mine B 200 (lis'să-mēn rō'dă-mēn). SYN sulforhodamine B.

Lissauer, Heinrich, German neurologist, 1861–1891. SEE L.'s *bundle, column, fasciculus, tract,* marginal *zone; column* of Spitzka-L.

lis·sen·ce·pha·lia (lis'en-sĕ-fā'lē-ă). SYN agyria. [G. *lissos,* smooth, + *enkephalos,* brain]

lis·sen·ce·phal·ic (lis'en-sĕ-fal'ik). Pertaining to, or characterized by, lissencephalia.

lis·sen·ceph·a·ly (lis-en-sef'ă-lē). SYN agyria. [G. *lissos,* smooth, + *enkephalos,* brain]

lis·sive (lis'iv). Having the property of relieving muscle spasm without causing flaccidity. [G. *lissos,* smooth]

lis·so·sphinc·ter (lis'ō-sfingk'ter). A sphincter of smooth musculature. SYN smooth muscular sphincter. [G. *lissos,* smooth, + sphincter]

lis·so·trich·ic, lis·sot·ri·chous (lis-ō-trik'ik, -trik'ŭs). Having straight hair. [G. *lissos,* smooth, + *thrix (trich-),* hair]

Lister, Joseph (Lord Lister), English surgeon, 1827–1912. SEE *Listerella; Listeria;* listerism; L.'s *dressing, method, tubercle.*

Lis·ter·el·la (lis'ter-el'ă). In bacteriology, a rejected generic name sometimes cited as a synonym of *Listeria.* The type species is *L. hepatolytica.* [Joseph *Lister*]

Lis·te·ria (lis-tēr-ē-ă). A genus of aerobic to microaerophilic, motile, peritrichous bacteria (family Corynebacteriaceae) containing small, coccoid, Gram-positive rods; these organisms tend to produce chains of three to five cells and, in the rough state, elongated and filamentous forms. Cells 18 to 24 hours old may show a palisade arrangement with a few V or Y forms; the bacteria produce acid but no gas from glucose and are found in the feces of humans and other animals, on vegetation, and in silage and are parasitic on poikilothermic and warm-blooded animals, including humans. The type species is *L. monocytogenes.* [Joseph *Lister*]

L. **denitrif·icans,** a species found in cooked blood of beef; pathogenic to rats and mice when injected intraperitoneally.

L. **gra′yi,** a species found in the feces of chinchillas.

L. **monocytog′enes,** a species causing meningitis, encephalitis, septicemia, endocarditis, abortion, abscesses, and local purulent lesions; it is often fatal; it is found in healthy ferrets, insects, and the feces of chinchillas, ruminants, and humans, as well as sewage, decaying vegetation, silage, soil, and fertilizer. Sometimes involved in infections in immunocompromised hosts. A causative agent of perinatal infections, neonatal sepsis and septicemia. Also recently linked to food-borne diseases.

lis·te·ri·o·sis (lis-tēr′ē-ō′sis). A sporadic disease of animals and humans, particularly those who are immunocompromised or pregnant, caused by the bacterium, *Listeria monocytogenes.* The infection in sheep and cattle frequently involves the central nervous system, causing various neurologic signs; in monogastric animals and fowl, the chief manifestations are septicemia and necrosis of the liver. Meningitis, bacteremia, and focal metastatic disease are associated with listeriosis. SYN listeria meningitis. [fr. organism *Listeria*]

lis·ter·ism (lis′ter-izm). SYN Lister's *method.*

Listing, Johann B., German physiologist, 1808–1882. SEE L.'s reduced *eye, law.*

Liston, Robert, English surgeon, 1794–1847. SEE L.'s *knives,* under *knife, shears, splint.*

li·sur·ide (lī′sūr-īd). A soluble ergot derivative with endocrine effects similar to those of bromocriptine; a serotonin inhibitor.

li·ter (L, l) (lē′ter). A measure of capacity of 1000 cubic centimeters or 1 cubic decimeter; equivalent to 1.056688 quarts (U.S., liquid). [Fr., fr. G. *litra,* a pound]

△**lith-.** SEE litho-.

lith·a·gogue (lith′ă-gog). Causing the dislodgment or expulsion of calculi, especially urinary calculi. [litho- + G. *agōgos,* drawing forth]

lith·arge (lith′arj). SYN *lead* monoxide. [litho- + G. *argyros,* silver]

li·thec·to·my (li-thek′tō-mē). SYN lithotomy. [litho- + G. *ektomē,* excision]

li·thi·a·sis (li-thī′ă-sis). Formation of calculi of any kind, especially of biliary or urinary calculi. [litho- + G. *-iasis,* condition]

l. conjuncti′vae, deposits of cellular degeneration into hard masses in Henle's glands.

2,8-dihydroxyalanine l., formation of calculi of 2,8-dihydroxyalanine due to a deficiency or reduced activity of adenine phosphoribosyltransferase.

pancreatic l., the formation of stones in the pancreas, usually associated with chronic inflammation and obstruction of the pancreatic ducts.

lith·ic ac·id (lith′ik). SYN uric acid.

lith·i·um (Li) (lith′ē-ŭm). An element of the alkali metal group, atomic no. 3, atomic wt. 6.941. Many salts have clinical applications. [Mod. L. fr. G. *lithos,* a stone]

l. bromide, LiBr; a white deliquescent powder, used as a sedative and hypnotic.

l. carbonate, Li_2CO_3; an antirheumatic and antilithic agent, also used in the treatment and prophylaxis of depressive, hypomanic, and manic phases of bipolar affective disorders.

l. citrate, $Li_3C_6H_5O_7 \cdot 4H_2O$; a diuretic and antirheumatic, also used in the treatment of manic psychosis.

effervescent l. citrate, a preparation containing l. citrate, sodium bicarbonate, tartaric acid, and citric acid; same use as potassium or sodium citrate.

---

lithiasis
Ultzmann's classification of urinary calculus

combustible	without flame or odor	murexide test: with NH_3, purplish-red with KOH, purplish-violet	uric acid oxalate
		with NH_3, yellow with KOH, orange	xanthine
	light-blue flame, odor of burning fat or flesh		cystine
noncombustible	natural powder, effervesces with HCl		carbonate apatite
	natural powder, does not effervesce	but glows	oxaloacetic chalk
		nor does it glow	earthy (organic) phosphates

---

l. tungstate, used in electron microscopy as a negative stain.

△**litho-, lith-.** A stone, calculus, calcification. [G. *lithos*]

Lith·o·bi·us (li-thō′bē-ŭs). A genus of centipedes characterized by 15 pairs of legs. Species common in the U.S. include *L. multidentatus* and *L. forficatus.* [litho- + G. *bios,* life]

lith·o·cho·lic ac·id (lith-ō-kō′lik). 3α-Hydroxy-5β-cholan-24-oic acid; one of the acids isolated from human bile as well as from cows, rabbits, sheep, and goats.

lith·o·clast (lith′ō-klast). SYN lithotrite. [litho- + G. *klastos,* broken]

lith·o·gen·e·sis, li·thog·e·ny (lith-ō-jen′ĕ-sis, lith-oj′ĕ-nē). Formation of calculi. [litho- + G. *genesis,* production]

lith·o·gen·ic (lith-ō-jen′ik). Promoting the formation of calculi.

lith·og·e·nous (lith-oj′ĕ-nŭs). Calculus-forming.

lith·oid (lith′oyd). Resembling a calculus or stone. [litho- + G. *eidos,* resemblance]

lith·o·kel·y·pho·pe·di·on, lith·o·kel·y·pho·pe·di·um (lith-ō-kel′ĕ-fō-pē′dē-on, -ŭm). A lithopedion in which the fetal parts in contact with the surrounding membranes, as well as the membranes, are calcified. [litho- + G. *kelyphos,* husk, shell, + *paidion,* child]

lith·o·kel·y·phos (lith-ō-kel′ĕ-fos). A type of lithopedion in which the fetal membranes alone undergo calcification. [litho- + G. *kelyphos,* rind, shell]

lith·o·labe (lith′ō-lāb). Obsolete instrument for holding a bladder calculus during its removal. [litho- + G. *lambanō, labein,* to grasp]

li·thol·a·paxy (li-thol′ă-pak-sē). The operation of crushing a stone in the bladder and washing out the fragments through a catheter. [litho- + G. *lapaxis,* an emptying out]

li·thol·y·sis (li-thol′i-sis). The dissolution of urinary calculi. [litho- + G. *lysis,* dissolution]

lith·o·lyte (lith′ō-līt). An instrument for injecting calculary solvents.

lith·o·lyt·ic (li-thō-lit′ik). **1.** Tending to dissolve calculi. **2.** An agent having such properties. [litho- + G. *lysis,* dissolution]

lith·o·myl (lith′ō-mil). An instrument for pulverizing a stone in the bladder. [litho- + G. *mylē,* mill]

lith·o·ne·phri·tis (lith′ō-ne-frī′tis). Interstitial nephritis associated with calculus formation.

lith·o·pe·di·on, lith·o·pe·di·um (lith-ō-pē′dē-on, -ŭm). A retained fetus, usually extrauterine, which has become calcified. [litho- + G. *paidion,* small child]

lith·o·tome (lith′ō-tōm). A knife used in lithotomy.

li·thot·o·mist (li-thot′ō-mist). A person skilled in lithotomy.

li·thot·o·my (li-thot′ō-mē). Cutting for stone; a cutting operation

li

for the removal of a calculus, especially a vesical calculus. SYN lithectomy. [litho- + G. *tomē*, incision]

bilateral l., obsolete term for a l. in which the perineal incision is made transversely across the median raphe.

high l., SYN suprapubic l.

lateral l., l. in which the perineum is incised to one side of the median line.

marian l., SYN median l. [L. *mas* (*mar-*), male]

median l., l. in which the perineal incision is made in the median raphe. SYN marian l.

perineal l., l. in which the bladder is approached by an incision in the perineum.

prerectal l., l. by an incision in the midline of the perineum anterior to anus.

suprapubic l., l. in which the bladder is entered by an incision immediately above the symphysis pubis. SYN high l.

vaginal l., l. in which the bladder is entered through an incision in the vagina.

vesical l., SYN cystolithotomy.

lith·o·tre·sis (lith-ō-trē'sis). The boring of holes in a calculus to facilitate its crushing. [litho- + G. *trēsis,* a boring]

ultrasonic l., the demolition of calculi by high frequency sound waves.

lith·o·trip·sy (lith'ō-trip-sē). The crushing of a stone in the renal pelvis, ureter, or bladder, by mechanical force or sound waves. SYN lithotrity. [litho- + G. *tripsis,* a rubbing]

electrohydraulic shock wave l. (ESWL), destruction of calculi (urinary tract or other) by fragmentation using shock waves sent transcutaneously.

extracorporeal shock wave l. (ESWL) (lith'ō-trip'sē), breaking up of renal or ureteral calculi by focused ultrasound energy.

shock wave l., a method of fragmenting calculi.

lith·o·trip·tic (lith-ō-trip'tik). **1.** Relating to lithotripsy. **2.** An agent that effects the dissolution of a calculus.

lith·o·trip·tor (lith-ō-trip'tŏr). A device used to crush or fragment a calculus in lithotripsy.

lith·o·trip·tos·co·py (lith'ō-trip-tos'kŏ-pē). Crushing of a stone in the bladder under direct vision by use of a lithotriptoscope. [litho- + G. *tribō,* to rub, crush, + *skopeō,* to view]

lith·o·trite (lith'ō-trīt). A mechanical instrument used to crush a urinary calculus in lithotripsy. SYN lithoclast. [litho- + L. *tero,* pp. *tritus,* to rub]

li·thot·ri·ty (li-thot'ri-tē). SYN lithotripsy.

lith·o·troph (lith'ō-trof). An organism whose carbon needs are satisfied by carbon dioxide. Cf. chemoautotroph.

lith·u·re·sis (lith'yū-rē'sis). The passage of gravel in the urine. [litho- + G. *ourēsis,* urination]

li·thu·ria (li-thū'rē-ă). Excretion of uric acid or urates in large amount in the urine. [lithic (acid) + G. *ouron,* urine]

lit·mus (lit'mŭs) [old C.I. 1242]. A blue coloring matter obtained from *Roccella tinctoria* and other species of lichens, the principal component of which is azolitmin; used as an indicator (reddened by acids and turned blue again by alkalies). [a corruption of *lacmus,* fr. deu *lacmus,* fr. Dutch *lakmoes*]

lit·ter (lit'er). **1.** A stretcher or portable couch for moving the sick or injured. **2.** A group of animals of the same parents, born at the same time. SYN brood (1). [Fr. *litière;* fr. *lit,* bed]

Little, James, U.S. surgeon, 1836–1885. SEE L.'s area.

Little, William J., English surgeon, 1810–1894. SEE L.'s disease.

Littré, Alexis, French anatomist, 1658–1726. SEE L.'s glands, under *gland, hernia.*

lit·tri·tis (li-trī'tis). Obsolete term for inflammation of Littré's glands.

Litzmann, Karl K.T., German gynecologist, 1815–1890. SEE L. *obliquity.*

live·birth, live birth (līv'berth). The birth of an infant who shows evidence of life after birth. SEE ALSO liveborn *infant.*

li·ve·do (li-vē'dō). A bluish discoloration of the skin, either in limited patches or general. [L. lividness, fr. *liveo,* to be black and blue]

postmortem l., a purple coloration of dependent parts, except in areas of contact pressure, appearing within one half to two hours after death, as a result of gravitational movement of blood within the vessels. SYN postmortem hypostasis, postmortem lividity, postmortem suggillation.

l. racemo'sa, SYN l. reticularis.

l. reticula'ris, a persistent purplish network-patterned discoloration of the skin caused by dilation of capillaries and venules due to stasis or changes in underlying blood vessels including hyalinization; rarely appears as a developmental defect. SYN angiitis livedo reticularis, dermatopathia pigmentosa reticularis, l. racemosa.

l. reticula'ris idiopath'ica, an extensive and permanent form of l. reticularis; in rare instances associated with central arterial disease.

l. reticula'ris symptomat'ica, a discoloration or mottling of the skin due to some demonstrable cause, such as seen in erythema ab igne, and in certain tuberculids. SEE ALSO *cutis* marmorata.

l. telangiectat'ica, a permanent mottling of the skin due to an anomaly, probably congenital, of the cutaneous capillaries; a form of l. reticularis.

liv·e·doid (liv'ĕ-doyd). Pertaining to or resembling livedo.

liv·er. The largest gland of the body, lying beneath the diaphragm in the right hypochondrium and upper part of the epigastrium; it is of irregular shape and weighs from 1 to 2 kg, or about $\frac{1}{40}$ the weight of the body. It secretes the bile and is also of great importance in both carbohydrate and protein metabolism. SYN hepar [NA]. [A.S. *lifer*]

cardiac l., SYN cardiac *cirrhosis.*

desiccated l., a dried undefatted powder prepared from mammalian l.'s used as human food; contains riboflavin, nicotinic acid, and choline; used in the treatment of macrocytic anemias and as a nutritional supplement.

fatty l., yellow discoloration of the l. due to fatty degeneration of l. parenchymal cells. SYN hepatic steatosis.

frosted l., hyaloserositis of the liver. SYN Curschmann's disease, icing l., sugar-icing l., zuckergussleber.

hobnail l., in Laënnec's cirrhosis, the contraction of scar tissue and hepatic cellular regeneration which causes a nodular appearance of the l.'s surface.

icing l., SYN frosted l.

lardaceous l., SYN waxy l.

nutmeg l., chronic passive congestion of the l., causing accentuation of the lobular pattern with red central and yellow or tan periportal zones.

pigmented l., a l. that contains pigment, such as occurs in Dubin-Johnson *syndrome,* hemochromatosis, long-standing malaria.

polycystic l., gradual cystic dilation of intralobular bile ducts (Meyenburg's complexes) that fail to involute in embryologic development of the l.; frequently associated with bilateral congenital polycystic kidneys and occasionally with cystic involvement of the pancreas, lungs, and other organs. SYN polycystic liver disease.

sugar-icing l., SYN frosted l.

wandering l., SYN hepatoptosis.

waxy l., amyloid degeneration of the l. SYN lardaceous l.

liv·e·tin (liv'ĕ-tin). Any of the three major water-soluble proteins in egg yolk: α-**livetin,** serum albumin; β-**livetin,** α-glycoprotein; γ-**livetin,** serum γ-globulin.

liv·id. Having a black and blue or a leaden or ashy gray color, as in discoloration from a contusion, congestion, or cyanosis. [L. *lividus,* being black and blue]

li·vid·i·ty (li-vid'i-tē). The state of being livid.

postmortem l., SYN postmortem *livedo.*

li·vor (lī'vŏr). The livid discoloration of the skin on the dependent parts of a corpse. [L. a black and blue spot]

lix·iv·i·a·tion (lik-siv-ē-ā'shŭn). SYN leaching. [L. *lixivius,* made into lye, fr. *lix,* lye]

lix·iv·i·um (lik-siv'ē-ŭm). SYN lye. [L. ntr. of *lixivius,* made into lye]

LLAT Abbreviation for *lysolecithin*:lecithin acyltransferase.

LLETZ. Abbreviation for large loop excision of transformation zone of the cervix of the uterus.

LLL Abbreviation for left lower lobe (of lung).

Lloyd, John Uri, U.S. pharmacist, 1849–1936. Noted for investigational work in plant chemistry and phytochemistry as applied to medicines, alkaloids, and glucosides.

Lloyd's re·a·gent. See under reagent.

LLQ Abbreviation for left lower quadrant (of abdomen).

LM Abbreviation for licentiate in midwifery.

lm Abbreviation for lumen (2).

LMA Abbreviation for left mentoanterior position.

LMP Abbreviation for left mentoposterior position.

LMT Abbreviation for left mentotransverse position.

LNPF Abbreviation for lymph node permeability *factor.*

Lo, L₀. SEE Lo *dose.*

LOA Abbreviation for left occipitoanterior position.

load (lōd). A departure from normal body content, as of water, salt, or heat; positive l.'s are quantities in excess of the normal; negative l.'s are quantities in deficit.

    electronic pacemaker l., the impedance to the output, the standard l. being 500 ohms resistance ± 1%.

    genetic l., the aggregate of more or less harmful genes that are carried, mostly hidden, in the genome that may be transmitted to descendants and cause morbidity and disease; in classical genetic dynamics, genetic l. may be seen as undischarged genetic debts that result from previous mutations, each of which is supposed to exact an average number of lethal equivalents dependent only on the pattern of inheritance, regardless of how mild or severe the phenotype may be.

load·ing (lōd'ing). Administration of a substance for the purpose of testing metabolic function.

    carbohydrate l., a procedure popular with long-distance runners and other athletes of filling muscles with a large glycogen pool prior to an athletic event; often, the athlete consumes very few carbohydrates for three days followed by a largely carbohydrate diet for the last three days before the event.

    salt l., the administration of 2 g of sodium chloride (with a regular diet) 3 times a day for 4 days; a diagnostic test in primary aldosteronism, in which the salt l. produces the typical plasma electrolyte pattern.

    soda l., a procedure adopted by a number of athletes of ingesting sodium bicarbonate in an attempt to buffer the production of protons during exercise.

Loa loa (lō'ă lō'ă). The African eye worm, a species of the family Onchocercidae (superfamily Filarioidea) that is indigenous to the western part of equatorial Africa, especially in the region of the Congo River, and is the causal agent of loiasis. Adult worms are white or gray-white, cylindroid, and threadlike, the males averaging 25 to 35 by 0.3 to 0.4 mm (with a curved tail) and the females ranging from 50 to 60 by 0.4 to 0.6 mm; microfilariae are ensheathed, with nuclei extending to the tip of the tail. The life cycle is somewhat similar to that of *Wuchereria* species; humans are the only known definitive host, and parasites are transmitted by *Chrysops* flies (family Tabanidae); infective larvae from the latter require 3 years or more to mature in humans, and the adult forms may persist in man for as long as 17 years. SEE ALSO loiasis.

lo·bar (lō'bar). Relating to any lobe.

    l. nephronia, (1) A focal renal mass related to acute infection. **(2)** Acute focal bacterial nephritis. **(3)** Renal phlegmon (not an abscess; no free pus).

lo·bate (lō'bāt). **1.** Divided into lobes. **2.** Lobe-shaped; denoting a bacterial colony with a deeply undulate margin. SYN lobose, lobous.

lobe (lōb). **1.** One of the subdivisions of an organ or other part, bounded by fissures, connective tissue, septa, or other structural demarcations. **2.** A rounded projecting part, as the l. of the ear. SEE ALSO lobule. **3.** One of the larger divisions of the crown of a tooth, formed from a distinct point of calcification. SYN lobus [NA]. [G. *lobos,* lobe]

anterior l. of hypophysis, ☆official alternate term for adenohypophysis.

    az′ygos l. of lung, a small accessory l. sometimes found on the apex of the right lung; separated from the rest of the upper l. by a deep groove lodging the azygos vein. SYN lobus azygos.

    caudate l., SYN *lobus* caudatus.

    l.'s of cerebrum, SYN *lobi* cerebri, under *lobus.*

    cuneiform l., SYN biventer *lobule.*

    ear l., the lowest part of the auricle; it consists of fat and fibrous tissue not reinforced by the auricular cartilage. SYN lobulus auriculae [NA], lobule of auricle.

    falciform l., SYN cingulate *gyrus.*

    flocculonodular l., the small posterior and inferior subdivision of the cerebellar cortex that borders the line of attachment of the choroid roof of the rhomboid fossa, and consists of the left and right flocculus together with the unpaired nodulus (the most posterior of the folia composing the vermis cerebelli). Its major afferent connections come from the vestibular nuclei and directly from the vestibular nerve; it projects largely to the vestibular nuclei, directly and by way of the fastigial nucleus.

    frontal l., SYN frontal l. of cerebrum.

    frontal l. of cerebrum, the portion of each cerebral hemisphere anterior to the central sulcus. SYN lobus frontalis cerebri [NA], frontal l.

    glandular l. of hypophysis, SYN adenohypophysis.

    Home's l., the enlarged middle l. of the prostate gland.

    inferior l. of lung, it is located below and behind the oblique fissure and contains five bronchopulmonary segments: superior, medial basal, anterior basal, lateral basal, and posterior basal. SYN lobus inferior pulmonis [NA], lower l. of lung.

    left l., the left subdivision of several glands, *e.g.,* prostate, thyroid, thymus. SYN lobus sinister [NA].

    left l. of liver, it is separated from the right lobe above and in front by the falciform ligament, and from the quadrate and caudate lobes by the fissure for the ligamentum teres and the fissure for the ligamentum venosum; the distribution of the portal vein, hepatic artery, and bile ducts does not correspond to the gross lobar divisions of the liver. It contains two segments, superior and inferior. SYN lobus hepatis sinister [NA].

    limbic l., as originally defined by P. Broca: the nearly closed ring of the brain structures surrounding the hilus, or margin, of the cerebral hemisphere of mammals; it is composed of the fornicate gyrus (cingulate gyrus and parahippocampal gyrus), the hippocampus, and the amygdala. SEE limbic *system.*

    lingual l., SYN *cingulum* of tooth.

    lower l. of lung, SYN inferior l. of lung.

    l.'s of mammary gland, the 15 to 20 separate portions of the mammary gland that radiate from the central area deep to the nipple like wheel spokes and comprise the body of the mammary gland; each is drained by a single lactiferous duct. SYN lobi glandulae mammariae [NA].

    middle l. of prostate, the portion of the prostate lying between the urethra and the ejaculatory ducts; indistinct unless hypertrophied. SYN lobus medius prostatae [NA], Morgagni's caruncle.

    middle l. of right lung, it is located anteriorly between the horizontal and oblique fissures and includes lateral and medial bronchopulmonary segments. SYN lobus medius pulmonis dextri [NA].

    nervous l., SYN nervous l. of hypophysis.

    nervous l. of hypophysis, the bulbous part of the neurohypophysis attached to the hypothalamus by the infundibulum. It is composed of pituicytes, blood vessels, and terminals of nerve fibers from the supraoptic and paraventricular nuclei. SYN lobus nervosus, nervous l.

    occipital l., SYN occipital l. of cerebrum.

    occipital l. of cerebrum, the posterior, somewhat pyramid-shaped part of each cerebral hemisphere, demarcated by no distinct surface markings on the lateral convexity of the hemisphere from the parietal and temporal lobes, but sharply delineated from the parietal lobe by the parieto-occipital sulcus on the medial surface. SYN lobus occipitalis cerebri [NA], occipital l.

    parietal l., SYN parietal l. of cerebrum.

lo

parietal l. of cerebrum, the middle portion of each cerebral hemisphere, separated from the frontal lobe by the central sulcus, from the temporal lobe by the lateral sulcus in front and an imaginary line projected posteriorly, and from the occipital lobe only partially by the parieto-occipital sulcus on its medial aspect. SYN lobus parietalis cerebri [NA], parietal l.

placental l.'s, cotyledons of the human placenta, viewed on the maternal surface as irregularly shaped elevations or l.'s.

polyalveolar l., a type of congenital anomaly where a several-fold increase in the total alveolar number leads to congenital lobar emphysema.

posterior l. of hypophysis, SYN neurohypophysis.

l. of prostate, one of the lateral lobes (right or left) or the middle lobe or isthmus of the prostate; in the adult the lobes are ill-defined. SYN lobus prostatae [NA].

pyramidal l. of thyroid gland, an inconstant narrow lobe of the thyroid gland that arises from the upper border of the isthmus and extends upward, sometimes as far as the hyoid bone; it marks the point of continuity with the thyroglossal duct. SYN lobus pyramidalis glandulae thyroideae [NA], Lallouette's pyramid, Morgagni's appendix, pyramid of thyroid.

quadrate l., (1) a lobe on the inferior surface of the liver located between the fossa for the gallbladder and the fissure for the ligamentum teres; **(2)** SYN quadrangular *lobule.* **(3)** SYN precuneus.

renal l., one of the subdivisions of the kidney, consisting of a renal pyramid and the cortical tissue associated with it. SYN lobus renalis [NA].

Riedel's l., an occasional tongue-like process extending downward from the right l. of the liver lateral to the gallbladder; a similar process may, though rarely, extend from the left lobe. SYN lobus appendicularis, lobus linguiformis.

right l., the right subdivision of several glands, *e.g.,* prostate, thyroid, thymus. SYN lobus dexter [NA].

right l. of liver, the largest lobe of the liver, separated from the left lobe above and in front by the falciform ligament and from the caudate and quadrate lobes by the sulcus for the vena cava and the fossa for the gallbladder; it contains two segments, anterior and posterior. SYN lobus hepatis dexter [NA].

Spigelius' l., SYN *lobus* caudatus.

superior l. of lung, the lobe of the right lung that lies above the oblique and horizontal fissures and includes the apical, posterior and anterior bronchopulmonary segments; in the left lung, the lobe lies above the oblique fissure and contains the apicoposterior, anterior, superior lingular and inferior lingular segments. SYN lobus superior pulmonis [NA], upper l. of lung.

supplemental l., in dental anatomy, an extra l.; one that is not included in the typical formation of a tooth.

temporal l., a long l., the lowest of the major subdivisions of the cortical mantle, forming the posterior two-thirds of the ventral surface of the cerebral hemisphere, separated from the frontal and parietal l.'s above it by the lateral sulcus arbitrarily delineated by an imaginary plane from the occipital l. with which it is continuous posteriorly. The temporal l. has a heterogeneous composition: in addition to a large neocortical component consisting of the superior, middle, and inferior temporal gyri and the lateral and medial occipitotemporal gyri, it includes the largely juxtallocortical parahippocampal gyrus with its paleocortical (olfactory) uncus and, beneath the latter, the amygdala. SYN lobus temporalis [NA], temporal cortex.

l.'s of thyroid gland, the two major divisions of the gland lying on the right and left side of the trachea and connected by the isthmus. A smaller pyramidal lobe is frequently present as an upward extension from the isthmus. SYN lobi glandulae thyroideae [NA].

upper l. of lung, SYN superior l. of lung.

lo·bec·to·my (lō-bek'tō-mē). Excision of a lobe of any organ or gland. [G. *lobos,* lobe, + *ektomē,* excision]

lo·be·lia (lō-bē'lē-ă). **1.** The dried leaves and tops of *Lobelia inflata* (family Lobeliaceae); it contains several alkaloids: lobeline, lobelamine, lobelanidine, lobelanine, norlobelanine, norlobelanidine, and isolobelanine. The fluid extract and the tincture have been used as an expectorant in asthma and chronic

bronchitis. **2.** One of a class of alkaloids isolated from l. (1). SYN asthma-weed (1), wild tobacco.

lo·be·line, lo·be·lin (lō'bĕ-lēn, lob'ĕ-lēn, -lin). A piperidylacetophenone; an alkaloid of lobelia with the same actions as nicotine, but with less potency.

l. sulfate, a form of l. occurring in yellow friable masses, soluble in water; used in whooping cough and asthma; it has been suggested as a smoking deterrent.

lo·bi (lō'bī). Plural of lobus. [L.]

lo·bi·tis (lō-bī'tis). Inflammation of a lobe.

Lobo, Jorge, 20th century Brazilian physician. SEE L.'s *disease.*

Lo·boa lo·boi (lō-bō'ă lō-bō'ē). A species of fungus causing lobomycosis. The organism is still classified by some as *Paracoccidioides brasiliensis,* which causes paracoccidioidomycosis.

lo·bo·my·co·sis (lō-bō-mī-kō'sis). A chronic localized mycosis of the skin reported from South America resulting in granulomatous nodules or keloids that contain budding, thick-walled cells about 9 μ in diameter, *i.e.,* the tissue form of *Loboa loboi,* the causative fungus, which has not been cultured. SYN Lobo's disease.

lo·bo·po·di·um, pl. **lo·bo·po·dia** (lō'bō-pō'dē-ŭm, -dē-ă). A thick lobose pseudopodium. [G. *lobos,* lobe, + *pous,* foot]

lo·bose, lo·bous (lō'bōs, lō'bŭs). SYN lobate.

lo·bot·o·my (lō-bot'ō-mē). **1.** Incision into a lobe. **2.** Division of one or more nerve tracts in a lobe of the cerebrum. [G. *lobos,* lobe, + *tomē,* a cutting]

prefrontal l., division of one or more nerve tracts in the prefrontal area of the brain for surgical treatment of pain and emotional disorder. SYN prefrontal leukotomy.

transorbital l., l. by an approach through the roof of the orbit, behind the frontal sinus. SYN transorbital leukotomy.

Lobry de Bruyn, Cornelius A., Dutch chemist, 1857–1904. SEE L. de B.-van Ekenstein *transformation.*

Lobstein, Johann F.G., German pathologist, 1777–1835. SEE L.'s *ganglion.*

lob·u·lar (lob'yū-lăr). Relating to a lobule.

lob·u·late, lob·u·lat·ed (lob'yū-lāt, -ed). Divided into lobules.

lob·ule (lob'yūl). A small lobe or subdivision of a lobe. SYN lobulus [NA].

ala central l., the lateral winglike projection of the central lobule of the cerebellum. SYN ala lobuli centralis [NA], ala cerebelli.

ansiform l., comprises the greater part of the hemisphere of the cerebellum; its superior and inferior surfaces are separated by the horizontal fissure into major parts known as crus I (superior semilunar lobule) and crus II (inferior semilunar lobule).

anterior lunate l., SYN superior semilunar l.

l. of auricle, SYN ear *lobe.*

biventer l., a l. on the undersurface of each cerebellar hemisphere, divided by a curved sulcus into a lateral and medial portion; it corresponds to the pyramid of the vermis. SYN lobulus biventer [NA], biventral l., cuneiform lobe, lobulus biventralis, lobulus cuneiformis.

biventral l., SYN biventer l.

central l., SYN central l. of cerebellum.

central l. of cerebellum, a division of the superior vermis of the cerebellum between the lingula and the monticulus. SYN lobulus centralis cerebelli [NA], central l.

cortical l.'s of kidney, one of the subdivisions of the kidney, consisting of a medullary ray and that portion of the convoluted port (renal corpuscles and convoluted tubules) associated with its collecting duct. SYN lobulus corticalis renalis [NA], renal cortical l., renculus (1), reniculus (1), renunculus (1).

crescentic l.'s of the cerebellum, archaic term designation for *lobulus* semilunaris inferior and *lobulus* semilunaris superior.

l.'s of epididymis, the coiled portion of the efferent ductules that constitute the head of the epididymis; these join the ductus epididymidis. SYN lobuli epididymidis [NA], coni epididymidis [NA], coni vasculosi, Haller's cones, vascular cones.

gracile l., the anterior portion of the posteroinferior lobule of the cerebellum, the posterior portion being the semilunar l. inferior;

the two correspond to the tuber of the vermis. SYN lobulus gracilis, slender l.

hepatic l., the conceptual polygonal histologic unit of the liver consisting of masses of liver cells arranged around a central vein, a terminal branch of one of the hepatic veins; at the periphery are located preterminal and terminal branches of the portal vein, hepatic artery, and bile duct, hepatic lobules have anatomical reality in the pig liver or pathologically in humans, when fibrous septa are present. SYN lobulus hepatis [NA].

inferior parietal l., the area of the parietal lobe of the cerebrum lying below the interparietal sulcus; it contains the angular and the supramarginal gyri. SYN lobulus parietalis inferior [NA], inferior parietal gyrus.

inferior semilunar l., the part of the superior surface of the cerebellar hemisphere lying behind the horizontal fissure. SYN lobulus semilunaris inferior [NA], crus II, posterior lunate l.

l.'s of mammary gland, subdivisions of the lobes of the mammary gland. SYN lobuli glandulae mammariae [NA].

paracentral l., a division of the medial aspect of the cerebral cortex, lying above the singulate sulcus and bounded by the precentral sulcus in front and the marginal part of the cingulate sulcus behind. SYN lobulus paracentralis [NA].

portal l. of liver, a conceptual unit of the liver, emphasizing its exocrine function in bile secretion, which comprises a roughly triangular shaped cross-sectional area with a portal canal at its center and three or more venae centrales hepatis at its periphery.

posterior lunate l., SYN inferior semilunar l.

primary pulmonary l., SYN pulmonary *acinus*.

quadrangular l., the main portion of the superior part of each hemisphere of the cerebellum, corresponding to the monticulus of the vermis; it is divided into two portions, the anterior and the posterior crescentic lobules, corresponding to the culmen and the declive of the vermis. SYN lobulus quadrangularis [NA], lobus quadratus [NA], lobulus quadratus (1), quadrate lobe (2), quadrate l. (1).

quadrate l., **(1)** SYN quadrangular l. **(2)** SYN precuneus.

renal cortical l., SYN cortical l.'s of kidney.

respiratory l., SYN pulmonary *acinus*.

secondary pulmonary l., a pyramidal mass of lung tissue whose sides are bounded by the incomplete interlobular connective tissue septa and whose base, which is 1 to 2 cm in diameter, usually faces the pleural surface of the lung; l.'s that occupy a more central position in the lung are not well defined and are considered to consist of three to five pulmonary acini with proximate terminal bronchioles.

simple l., the smaller anterior part of the posterior lobe of the cerebellum, demarcated by the primary fissure from the anterior lobe rostrally and from the large caudal subdivision of the posterior lobe caudally. SYN lobulus simplex [NA].

slender l., SYN gracile l.

superior parietal l., the area of the convex surface of the parietal lobe of the cerebrum lying between the longitudinal fissure and the interparietal sulcus behind the posterior central gyrus; it is continuous with the precuneus on the medial aspect of the hemisphere. SYN lobulus parietalis superior [NA], superior parietal gyrus.

superior semilunar l., the part of the superior surface of the cerebellar hemisphere lying rostral to the horizontal fissure, and adjoining the folium of the vermis. SYN lobulus semilunaris superior [NA], anterior lunate l., crus I.

l.'s of testis, the subdivisions of the parenchyma of the testis formed by delicate fibrous septa that pass inward from the tunica albuginea to converge at the mediastinum testis. SYN lobuli testis [NA].

l.'s of thymus, areas of thymic tissue 0.5 to 2 mm in diameter with a cortex and medulla. SYN lobuli thymi [NA].

l.'s of thyroid gland, the subdivisions of the lobes, consisting of incompletely separated, irregular groups of thyroid follicles (20 to 40 in number) bound together by delicate connective tissue. SYN lobuli glandulae thyroideae [NA].

lob·u·let, lob·u·lette (lob′yū-let′). A very small lobule or one of the smaller subdivisions of a lobule.

lob·u·lus, gen. and pl. **lob·u·li** (lob′yū-lŭs, yū-lī) [NA]. SYN lobule. [Mod. L. dim. of *lobus,* lobe]

l. auric′ulae [NA], SYN ear *lobe*.

l. biven′ter [NA], SYN biventer *lobule*.

l. biventra′lis, SYN biventer *lobule*.

l. centra′lis cerebel′li [NA], SYN central *lobule* of cerebellum.

l. cli′vi, SYN declive.

l. cortica′lis rena′lis [NA], SYN cortical *lobules* of kidney, under *lobule*.

l. cul′minis, SYN culmen.

l. cune′iform′is, SYN biventer *lobule*.

lob′uli epididym′idis [NA], SYN *lobules* of epididymis, under *lobule*.

l. fo′lii, the part of the superior vermis of the cerebellum lying immediately behind the posterior superior fissure and caudal to the l. clivi.

l. fusifor′mis, SYN fusiform *gyrus*.

lob′uli glan′dulae mamma′riae [NA], SYN *lobules* of mammary gland, under *lobule*.

lob′uli glan′dulae thyroi′deae [NA], SYN *lobules* of thyroid gland, under *lobule*.

l. grac′ilis, SYN gracile *lobule*.

l. hep′atis [NA], SYN hepatic *lobule*.

l. paracentra′lis [NA], SYN paracentral *lobule*.

l. parieta′lis infe′rior [NA], SYN inferior parietal *lobule*.

l. parieta′lis supe′rior [NA], SYN superior parietal *lobule*.

l. quadrangula′ris [NA], SYN quadrangular *lobule*.

l. quadra′tus, (1) SYN quadrangular *lobule*. **(2)** SYN precuneus.

l. semiluna′ris infe′rior [NA], SYN inferior semilunar *lobule*.

l. semiluna′ris supe′rior [NA], SYN superior semilunar *lobule*.

l. sim′plex [NA], SYN simple *lobule*.

lob′uli tes′tis [NA], SYN *lobules* of testis, under *lobule*.

lobuli thy′mi [NA], SYN *lobules* of thymus, under *lobule*.

lo·bus, gen. and pl. **lo·bi** (lō′bŭs, lō′bī) [NA]. SYN lobe. [LL. fr. G. *lobos*]

l. ante′rior hypophys′eos [NA], SYN adenohypophysis.

l. appendicula′ris, SYN Riedel's *lobe*.

l. azygos, SYN azygos *lobe* of lung.

l. cauda′tus [NA], a small lobe of the liver situated posteriorly between the sulcus for the vena cava and the fissure for the ligamentum venosum. SYN caudate lobe, Spigelius' lobe.

lobi cer′ebri [NA], the major divisions of the cerebral hemisphere; they include the frontal, parietal, temporal, and occipital lobes, named for the overlying bones of the skull. SYN lobes of cerebrum.

l. cli′vi, the clivus monticuli and the posterior crescentic lobules of the cerebellum considered as one lobe.

l. dex′ter [NA], SYN right *lobe*.

l. falcifor′mis, SYN cingulate *gyrus*.

l. fronta′lis cer′ebri [NA], SYN frontal *lobe* of cerebrum.

lo′bi glan′dulae mamma′riae [NA], SYN *lobes* of mammary gland, under *lobe*.

lo′bi glan′dulae thyroi′deae [NA], SYN *lobes* of thyroid gland, under *lobe*.

l. glandula′ris hypophys′eos, SYN adenohypophysis.

l. hep′atis dex′ter [NA], SYN right *lobe* of liver.

l. hep′atis sinis′ter [NA], SYN left *lobe* of liver.

l. infe′rior pulmo′nis [NA], SYN inferior *lobe* of lung.

l. linguifor′mis, SYN Riedel's *lobe*.

l. me′dius pro′statae [NA], SYN middle *lobe* of prostate.

l. me′dius pulmo′nis dex′tri [NA], SYN middle *lobe* of right lung.

l. nervo′sus, SYN nervous *lobe* of hypophysis.

l. occipita′lis cer′ebri [NA], SYN occipital *lobe* of cerebrum.

l. parieta′lis cer′ebri [NA], SYN parietal *lobe* of cerebrum.

l. poste′rior hypophys′eos [NA], ✶official alternate term for neurohypophysis. SEE ALSO hypophysis.

l. pro′statae [NA], SYN *lobe* of prostate.

lo

l. pyramida′lis glan′dulae thyroi′deae [NA], SYN pyramidal *lobe* of thyroid gland.

l. quadra′tus [NA], SYN quadrangular *lobule*.

l. rena′lis [NA], SYN renal *lobe*.

l. sinis′ter [NA], SYN left *lobe*.

l. supe′rior pulmo′nis [NA], SYN superior *lobe* of lung.

l. tempora′lis [NA], SYN temporal *lobe*.

LOCA Abbreviation for low osmolar contrast agent.

lo·cal (lō′kăl). Having reference or confined to a limited part; not general or systemic. [L. *localis*, fr. *locus*, place]

lo·cal·i·za·tion (lō′kăl-i-zā′shŭn). **1.** Limitation to a definite area. **2.** The reference of a sensation to its point of origin. **3.** The determination of the location of a morbid process.

auditory l., in sensory psychology, the naming or pointing to directions from which sounds emanate.

cerebral l., the mapping of the cerebral cortex into areas and the correlation of the various areas with cerebral function, or determining the site of a brain lesion, based on the signs and symptoms manifested by the patient or by neuroimaging.

germinal l., determination in very young embryos of the presumptive areas for specific organs or structures. SYN fate map.

radiotherapy l., planning the size and alignment of radiation beams to encompass the neoplasm to be treated.

spatial l., the reference of a visual sensation to a definite locality in space.

stereotaxic l., l. of intracerebral nuclei by coordinates with reference to anatomical landmarks in the brain.

lo·cal·ized (lō′kăl-īzd). Restricted or limited to a definite part.

lo·cant (lō′kant). A number or letter preceding a substituent name in the name of a complex chemical that specifies the position (location) of the substituent on the parent molecule; *e.g.,* 5 in 5-methyluridine, *S* in *S*-adenosylmethionine.

lo·ca·tor (lō′kā-ter, tōr). An instrument or apparatus for finding the position of a foreign object in tissue.

lo·chia (lō′kē-ă). Discharges from the vagina of mucus, blood, and tissue debris, following childbirth. [G. neut. pl. of *lochios*, relating to childbirth, fr. *lochos*, childbirth]

lochia		
name (color)	composition	times (varies for individuals)
lochia rubra (red)	mainly blood, tissue debris, decidua (occasionally vernix caseosa, lanugo, meconium)	1st–3rd day (first week)
lochia fusca (brownish)	increasing hemolysis, less blood; serous secretion (lymph, leukocytes)	3rd–7th day (second week)
lochia serosa (serous)	leukocytes, decidual cells, cervical mucus	7th–14th day
lochia flava (yellowish)	mainly leukocytes, bacteria, detritus (so-called physiological endometritis)	2nd–3rd week
lochia alba (grayish)	decline of weekly flow; endometrial epithelializing; clear mucous secretion of uterine glands	3rd (4th) week

l. al′ba, the last discharge no longer tinged with blood. SYN l. purulenta.

l. cruen′ta, the initial discharge stained with blood. SYN l. rubra.

l. purulen′ta, SYN l. alba.

l. ru′bra, SYN l. cruenta.

l. sanguinolen′ta, thick, dark red vaginal discharge seen a few days after delivery.

l. sero′sa, a thin and watery l.

lo·chi·al (lō′kē-ăl). Relating to the lochia.

lo·chi·o·me·tra (lō-kē-ō-mē′tră). Distention of the uterus with retained lochia. [G. *mētra*, womb]

lo·chi·o·me·tri·tis (lō-kē-ō-mē-trī′tis). Puerperal metritis.

lo·chi·o·per·i·to·ni·tis (lō′kē-ō-per′i-tō-nī′tis). Puerperal peritonitis.

lo·chi·or·rha·gia (lō-kē-ō-rā′jē-ă). SYN lochiorrhea. [lochia + G. *rhēgnymi*, to burst forth]

lo·chi·or·rhea (lō-kē-ō-rē′ă). Profuse flow of the lochia. SYN lochiorrhagia. [lochia + G. *rhoia*, a flow]

lo·ci (lō′sī). Plural of locus.

Locke, Frank S., British physiologist, 1871–1949. SEE L.'s *solutions*, under *solution;* L.-Ringer *solution*.

lock·jaw (lok′jaw). SYN trismus.

Lockwood, Charles B., English anatomist and surgeon, 1858–1914. SEE L.'s *ligament*.

LOCM Abbreviation for low osmolar contrast medium.

lo·co (lō′kō). A disease affecting cattle on the great plains of the western U.S. caused by eating the locoweed; characterized by paresis, incoordination, dullness, and a tendency to become solitary in habit. SYN locoweed disease. [Sp. crack-brained]

lo·co·mo·tive (lō-kō-mō′tiv). SYN locomotor.

lo·co·mo·tor (lō-kō-mō′ter). Relating to locomotion, or movement from one place to another. SYN locomotive, locomotory. [L. *locus*, place, + L. *moveo*, pp. *motus*, to move]

lo·co·mo·to·ri·al (lō-kō-mō-tō′rē-ăl). Relating to the locomotorium.

lo·co·mo·to·ri·um (lō′kō-mō-tō′rē-ŭm). The locomotor apparatus of the body. [L. *locus*, place, + *motorius*, moving]

lo·co·mo·to·ry (lō-kō-mō′tō-rē). SYN locomotor.

loc·u·lar (lok′yū-lăr). Relating to a loculus.

loc·u·late (lok′yū-lāt). Containing numerous loculi.

loc·u·la·tion (lok-yū-lā′shŭn). **1.** A loculate region in an organ or tissue, or a loculate structure formed between surfaces of organs, mucous or serous membranes, and so on. **2.** The process that results in the formation of a loculus or loculi.

loc·u·lus, pl. **loc·u·li** (lok′yū-lŭs, -lī). A small cavity or chamber. [L. dim. of *locus*, place]

lo·cum ten·ant (lō′kum těn′ent). A temporary substitution of one physician by another. SYN locum tenens. [partial anglicization of *locum tenens*]

lo·cum ten·ens (lō′kum těn′ens). SYN locum tenant. [L. one holding a place]

lo·cus, pl. **lo·ci** (lō′kŭs, lō′sī). **1.** A place; usually, a specific site. **2.** The position that a gene occupies on a chromosome lod score. In genetics, the log of the odds ratio of observed to expected distribution of genetic markers. **3.** The position of a point, as defined by the coordinates on a graph. [L.]

l. ceru′leus [NA], a shallow depression, of a blue color in the fresh brain, lying laterally in the most rostral portion of the rhomboidal fossa near the cerebral aqueduct; it lies near the lateral wall of the fourth ventricle and consists of about 20,000 melanin-pigmented neuronal cell bodies whose norepinephrine-containing axons have a remarkably wide distribution in the cerebellum as well as in the hypothalamus and cerebral cortex. SYN substantia ferruginea [NA], l. cinereus, l. ferrugineus.

l. cine′reus, SYN l. ceruleus.

cis-acting l., a section of DNA that affects the activity of DNA sequences on that same molecule of DNA.

complex l., a set of closely linked genetic loci with a common function, as in the major histocompatibility complex l.

l. of control, a theoretical construct designed to assess a person's perceived control over his/her own behavior; classified as *internal* if the person feels in control of events, *external* if others are perceived to have that control.

l. ferrugin′eus, SYN l. ceruleus.

genetic l., the set of homologous parts of a pair of chromosomes that may be occupied by allelic genes. The l. thus comprises a pair of locations (except in the X chromosome in males). The concept of a l. is somewhat idealized, not taking into account accidents that may occur in meiosis such as duplication of loci as a result of unequal crossing-over, translocations, inversions, etc.

marker l., a l. on a chromosome or in a stretch of DNA that can be identified (*e.g.,* a restriction fragment length polymorphism) and can serve in linkage analysis and in the isolation of a disease gene. SEE ALSO linkage *marker.*

l. ni′ger, SYN *substantia* nigra.

l. perfora′tus anti′cus, SYN anterior perforated *substance.*

l. perfora′tus posti′cus, SYN posterior perforated *substance.*

sex-linked l., any l. that in normal karyotypes is borne on a heterosome; commonly but incorrectly applied to an X-linked l.

X-linked l., any l. that in normal karyotypes is borne on the X chromosome.

Y-linked l., any (haploid) l. that in normal karyotypes is borne on the Y chromosome. The known content is so far small.

lod score (lod skōr). A number used in genetic linkage studies; logarithm (base 10) of the odds in favor of genetic linkage. [*logarithm* + *odd*s]

Loeb, Leo, U.S. pathologist, 1869–1959. SEE L.'s *deciduoma.*

Loeffler, Friedrich A.J., German bacteriologist and surgeon, 1852–1915. SEE L.'s *bacillus,* blood culture *medium, stain,* caustic *stain, methylene blue;* Klebs-L. *bacillus.*

Loevit, Moritz, Austrian pathologist, 1851–1918. SEE L.'s *cell.*

Loewenthal, Wilhelm, German physician, 1850–1894. SEE L.'s *bundle, reaction, tract.*

lo·fen·ta·nil (lō-fen′tă-nil). $C_{25}H_{32}N_2O_3$; a potent, long-lasting narcotic and analgesic that is chemically related to fentanyl.

Löffler, Wilhelm, Swiss physician, *1887. SEE L.'s *disease, endocarditis;* Loffler's parietal fibroplastic *endocarditis;* L.'s *syndrome.*

△**log-.** SEE logo-.

log·ag·no·sia (log-ag-nō′sē-ă). SYN aphasia. [logo- + G. *agnosia,* ignorance]

log·a·graph·ia (log-ă-graf′ē-ă). SYN agraphia. [logo- + G. *a*-priv. + *graphō,* to write]

log·am·ne·sia (log-am-nē′zē-ă). SYN aphasia. [logo- + G. *amnēsia,* forgetfulness]

Logan, William H.G., early 20th century U.S. plastic surgeon. SEE L.'s *bow.*

log·a·pha·sia (log-ă-fā′zē-ă). Aphasia of articulation. [logo- + G. *aphasia,* speechlessness]

log·a·rithm (lŏg′ar-ridhm). If a number, *x,* is expressed as a power of another number, *y, i.e.,* if $x = yn$, then n is said to be the logarithm of *x* to base *y.* Common logarithms are to the base 10; natural or Napierian logarithms are to the base e, a mathematical constant. [G. *logos,* word, ratio, + *arithmos,* number]

log·as·the·nia (log-as-thē′nē-ă). SYN aphasia. [logo- + G. *astheneia,* weakness]

lo·get·ro·nog·ra·phy (lo-jê-tron-og′ră-fē). A method of photographic printing in which fine details are emphasized by electronic enhancement of their contrast; formerly used for reproducing radiographic images.

△**-logia.** **1.** The study of the subject noted in the body of the word, or a treatise on the same; the Eng. equivalent is -logy, or, with a connecting vowel, -ology. [G. *logos,* discourse, treatise] **2.** Collecting or picking. [G. *legō,* to collect]

lo·git (lŏg′it). The logarithm of the ratio of frequencies of two different categorical and mutually exclusive outcomes such as healthy and sick.

△**logo-, log-.** Speech, words. [G. *logos,* word, discourse]

log·op·a·thy (log-op′ă-thē). Any speech disorder. [logo- + G. *pathos,* suffering]

log·o·pe·dia (log-ō-pē′dē-ă). SYN logopedics.

log·o·pe·dics (log′ō-pē′diks). A branch of science concerned with the physiology and pathology of the organs of speech and with the correction of speech defects. SYN logopedia. [logo- + G. *pais (paid-),* child]

log·o·ple·gia (log-ō-plē′jē-ă). Paralysis of the organs of speech. [logo- + G. *plēgē,* stroke]

log·or·rhea (log-ō-rē′ă). Rarely used term for abnormal or pathologic talkativeness or garrulousness. [logo- + G. *rhoia,* a flow]

log·o·spasm (log′ō-spazm). **1.** SYN stuttering. **2.** SYN explosive *speech.* [logo- + G. *spasmos,* spasm]

log·o·ther·a·py (log′ō-thār′ă-pē). A form of psychotherapy which places special emphasis on the patient's spiritual life and on the physician as "medical minister." [logo- + G. *therapeia,* cure]

△**-logy.** SEE -logia. [G. *logos,* treatise, discourse]

Lohlein-Baehr le·sion. See under lesion.

lo·i·a·sis (lō-ī′ă-sis). A chronic disease caused by the filarial nematode *Loa loa,* with symptoms and signs first occurring approximately three to four years after a bite by an infected tabanid fly. When the infective larvae mature, the adult worms move about in an irregular course through the connective tissue of the body (as rapidly as 1 cm per minute), frequently becoming visible beneath the skin and mucous membranes; *e.g.,* in the back, scalp, chest, inner surface of the lip, and especially on the conjunctiva. The worms provoke hyperemia and exudation of fluid, often a host response to the worm products, a Calabar or fugitive swelling which causes no serious damage and subsides as the parasites move on; the patient is annoyed by the "creeping" in the tissues and intense itching, as well as occasional pain, especially when the swelling is in the region of tendons and joints. Most patients have an eosinophilia of 10 to 30 or 40% in the circulating blood. SYN Calabar swelling, fugitive swelling.

loin (loyn). The part of the side and back between the ribs and the pelvis. SYN lumbus [NA]. [Fr. *longe;* E. *lumbus*]

Lok, SEE Luer-Lok *syringe.*

lo·li·ism (lō′li-izm). Poisoning by the seeds of a grass, *Lolium temulentum* (in the form of flour made into bread), characterized by giddiness, tremor, green vision, dilated pupils, prostration, and sometimes vomiting. [L. *lolium,* darnel, tares]

Lombard, Etienne, French physician, 1868–1920. SEE L. voice-reflex *test.*

lo·mus·tine (lō-mŭs′tēn). 1-(2-Chloroethyl)-3-cyclohexyl-1-nitrosourea; an antineoplastic agent. SYN CCNU.

London, Fritz, German-U.S. physicist, 1900–1954. SEE L. *forces,* under *force.*

Long, John H., U.S. physician, 1856–1927. SEE L.'s *coefficient, formula.*

long-chain ac·yl-CoA de·hy·dro·gen·ase. SEE *acyl-CoA* dehydrogenase (NADPH⁺).

long-chain fat·ty ac·id-CoA li·gase. Fatty acid thiokinase (long-chain), a ligase forming acyl-CoA, AMP, and pyrophosphate from long-chain fatty acids, ATP, and coenzyme A. SYN acyl-activating enzyme (1), dodecanoyl-CoA synthetase.

lon·gev·i·ty (lon-jev′i-tē). Duration of a particular life beyond the norm for the species. SEE ALSO lifespan. SYN macrobiosis.

lon·gi·tu·di·nal (lon′ji-tū′di-năl). **1.** Running lengthwise; in the direction of the long axis of the body or any of its parts. **2.** Studied over a period of time, diachronic; contrast with cross-sectional or synchronic, which give equivalent results only under certain strict conditions of stability and equilibrium. Strict attention to these conditions is of the greatest importance in the study of survivorship either in demographics or in cell economy (such as the survival pattern of the erythrocytes and platelets). SYN longitudinalis [NA]. [L. *longitudo,* length]

lon·gi·tu·di·na·lis (lon′ji-tū′di-nā′lis) [NA]. SYN longitudinal.

lon·gi·type (lon′ji-tūp). SYN ectomorph.

Longmire, William P., Jr., U.S. surgeon, *1913. SEE L.'s *operation.*

Looney, Joseph M., U.S. biochemist, *1896. SEE Folin-Looney *test.*

loop (lūp). **1.** A sharp curve or complete bend in a vessel, cord, or other cylindrical body, forming an oval or circular ring. SEE ALSO ansa. **2.** A wire (usually of platinum or nichrome) fixed into a

lo

handle at one end and bent into a circle at the other, rendered sterile by flaming, and used to transfer microorganisms. [M.E. *loupe*]

Biebl l., a continuous l. of small intestine brought through the abdominal wall to a subcutaneous location, for observation of motility.

bulboventricular l., the portion of the early-somite embryonic cardiac tube that evolves into the ventricle and bulbus cordis. SYN ventricular l.

capillary l.'s, small blood vessels in the dermal papillae.

cervical l., SYN *ansa* cervicalis.

cruciform l.'s, a secondary structure of DNA formed by the hydrogen bonding of self-complementary regions.

D l., a structure in replicating circular DNA. SYN displacement l.

displacement l., SYN D l.

gamma l., the reflex arc consisting of small anterior horn cells and neuroma, their small fibers projecting to the intrafusal bundle producing its contraction, which initiates the afferent impulses that pass through the posterior root to the anterior horn cells, inducing a stretch reflex. SYN gamma motor neurons, gamma motor system, Granit's l.

Gerdy's interatrial l., a muscular fasciculus in the interatrial septum of the heart, passing backward from the atrioventricular groove.

Granit's l., SYN gamma l.

hairpin l.'s, single-stranded DNA and RNA can fold back on itself under the proper conditions forming irregular double-helical l.'s.

Henle's l., SYN nephronic l.

l. of hypoglossal nerve, SYN *ansa* cervicalis.

Hyrtl's l., a communicating l. between the right and left hypoglossal nerves, lying between the geniohyoid and genioglossus muscles or in the substance of the geniohyoid; it is found in about one in ten persons. SYN Hyrtl's anastomosis.

lenticular l., the pallidal efferent fibers curving around the medial border of the internal capsule. SYN ansa lenticularis [NA], lenticular ansa.

memory l., an electronic device for retrieving data that had been stored and/or displayed upon the oscilloscope at an earlier time; used for reviewing electrical events immediately preceding a specific disturbance.

Meyer-Archambault l., the fibers of the visual radiation that loop around the tip of the temporal horn.

nephronic l., the U-shaped part of the nephron extending from the proximal to the distal convoluted tubules, consisting of descending and ascending limbs, located in the medulla renalis and medullary ray. SYN Henle's ansa, Henle's l.

peduncular l., SYN *ansa* peduncularis.

l.'s of spinal nerves, loops of the spinal nerves, connecting ventral primary rami of the spinal nerves. SYN ansae nervorum spinalium.

subclavian l., SYN *ansa* subclavia.

vector l., an irregular, usually elliptical, curve representing the average direction and magnitude of the heart's action from moment to moment throughout the cardiac cycle. SEE ALSO vector (2), vectorcardiogram.

ventricular l., SYN bulboventricular l.

Vieussens' l., SYN *ansa* subclavia.

loos·en·ing of as·so·ci·a·tion. A manifestation of a severe thought disorder characterized by the lack of an obvious connection between one thought or phrase and the next, or with the response to a question.

Looser, Emil, Swiss physician, 1877–1936. SEE L.'s *zones,* under *zone.*

LOP Abbreviation for left occipitoposterior position.

lop-ear (lop'ēr). Congenital deformity of the external ear, with poor development of helix and anthelix. SYN bat ear.

lo·per·am·ide hy·dro·chlo·ride (lō-per'ă-mīd). 4-(*p*-Chlorophenyl)-4-hydroxy-*N,N*-dimethyl-α,α-diphenyl-1-piperidinebutyramide monohydrochloride; an antiperistaltic agent used to treat diarrhea.

loph·o·dont (lof'ŏ-dont). Having the crowns of the molar teeth formed in transverse or longitudinal crests or ridges, in contrast to bunodont. [G. *lophos,* ridge, + *odous,* tooth]

Lo·phoph·o·ra wil·liam·sii (lō-fof'ŏ-ră wil-yăm'sē-ī). The botanical origin of peyote (mescal button); it contains over a dozen alkaloids, of which mescaline is the most important; others are pellotine, anhalomine, anhalonidine, anhalamine, anhalinine, anhalidine, and lophophorine.

lo·phot·ri·chate (lō-fot'ri-kāt). SYN lophotrichous.

lo·phot·ri·chous (lō-fot'ri-kŭs). Referring to a bacterial cell with two or more flagella at one or both poles. SYN lophotrichate. [G. *lophos,* crest, + *thrix,* hair]

lo·pre·mone (lō'pre-mōn). Former name for protirelin.

Lorain, Paul, French physician, 1827–1875. SEE L.'s *disease;* L.-Lévi *dwarfism, infantilism, syndrome.*

lor·a·ze·pam (lō-ră'zĕ-pam). 7-Chloro-5-(*o*-chlorophenyl)-1,3-dihydro-3-hydroxy-2*H*-1,4-benzodiazepin-2-one; an antianxiety drug of the benzodiazepine group.

lor·cai·nide (lor-kă-nīd). An antiarrhythmic agent used for the treatment of ventricular arrhythmias; much like a cardiac depressant (antiarrhythmic).

lor·do·sco·li·o·sis (lōr'dō-skō-lē-ō'sis). Combined backward and lateral curvature of the spine. [G. *lordos,* bent back, + *skoliōsis,* crookedness, fr. *skolios,* bent, aslant]

lor·do·sis (lōr-dō'sis). An abnormal extension deformity; anteroposterior curvature of the spine, generally lumbar with the convexity looking anteriorly. SYN hollow back, saddle back. [G. *lordōsis,* a bending backward]

lor·dot·ic (lōr-dot'ik). Pertaining to or marked by lordosis.

Lorenz, Adolf, Austrian surgeon, 1854–1946. SEE L.'s *sign.*

Loschmidt, Joseph (Johann), Czech chemist and physicist, 1821–1895. SEE L.'s *number.*

LOT Abbreviation for left occipitotransverse position.

lo·tion (lō'shŭn). A class of pharmacopeial preparations that are liquid suspensions or dispersions intended for external application; some consist of finely powdered, insoluble solids held in more or less permanent suspension by suspending agents or surface-active agents, or both; others are oil-in-water emulsions stabilized by surface-active agents. [L. *lotio,* a washing, fr. *lavo,* to wash]

Louis, Pierre C.A., French physician, 1787–1872. SEE L.'s *angle, law.*

Louis-Bar, Denise, mid-20th century French physician. SEE Louis-Bar *syndrome.*

loupe (lūp). A magnifying lens. [Fr.]

binocular l., a magnifying device, attached to spectacles or a headband, worn as a visual aid when performing operations on small structures.

louse, pl. **lice** (lows, līs). Common name for members of the ectoparasitic insect orders Anoplura (sucking lice) and Mallophaga (biting lice). Important species are *Felicola subrostrata* (cat l.), *Goniocotes gallinae* (fluff l.), *Goniodes dissimilis* (brown chicken l.), *Haemodipsus ventricosus* (rabbit l.), *Lipeurus caponis* (wing l.), *Menacanthus stramineus* (chicken body l.), *Phthirus pubis* (crab or pubic l.), and *Polyplax serratus* (mouse l.). [A.S. *lūs*]

biting l., chewing l., feather l., ectoparasites (order Mallophaga) chiefly found on birds, where they feed on feathers, hair, epidermal debris, and (less commonly) on blood; they possess nipperlike, heavily sclerotized mandibles and a characteristic broad head; many species are host-specific.

sucking l., blood-sucking mammalian ectoparasites (order Anoplura), characterized by a narrow head with piercing and sucking mouthparts that lie in a sac concealed in the head.

lous·i·ness (low'zē-nes). SYN pediculosis.

lousy (low'sē). SYN pediculous.

lo·va·stat·in (lō-vă-stat'in). A cholesterol-lowering agent, isolated from a strain of *Aspergillus terreus,* that reduces both normal and elevated serum cholesterol. SYN mevinolin.

Lovén, Otto C., Swedish physician, 1835–1904. SEE L. *reflex.*

Lovibond, J.L., 20th century English dermatologist.

Lovibond's pro·file sign. See under sign.

Low, George C., English physician, 1872–1952. SEE Castellani-L. *sign.*

Lowe, Charles U., U.S. pediatrician, *1921. SEE L.'s *syndrome;* L.-Terrey-MacLachlan *syndrome.*

Löwenberg, Benjamin B., French laryngologist, 1836–1905. SEE L.'s *canal, forceps, scala.*

Löwenstein, L.W. SEE Buschke-L. *tumor.*

Lower, Richard, English anatomist and physiologist, 1631–1691. SEE L.'s *ring, tubercle.*

Lown, Bernard, U.S. cardiologist, *1921. SEE L.-Ganong-Levine *syndrome.*

Low·ry, Oliver H., U.S. biochemist, *1910. SEE Lowry-Folin *assay;* L. protein *assay.*

Lowry, R. Brian, 20th century Irish medical geneticist in Canada. SEE Coffin-L. *syndrome.*

Lowsley, Oswald S., U.S. urologist, 1884–1955. SEE L. *tractor.*

lox·a·pine (lok'să-pēn). 2-Chloro-11-(4-methyl-1-piperazinyl)-dibenz[*b,f*][1,4]-oxazepine; a neuroleptic antipsychotic agent used as the succinate and hydrochloride salts.

lox·ia (lok'sē-ă). SYN torticollis. [G. *loxos,* oblique, slanting]

Lox·os·ce·les (lok-sos'ĕ-lēz). A genus of venomous spiders, the brown spiders, marked by a fiddle-shaped pattern on the cephalothorax, and found chiefly in South America. They inflict a highly ulcerative, spreading dermal lesion at the site of the bite (loxoscelism). Important species include *L. laeta,* the Chilean brown spider; *L. reclusus,* the brown spider of North America; and *L. rufipes,* the Peruvian brown spider. [G. *loxos,* oblique, + *skelos,* leg]

lox·os·ce·lism (lok-sos'ĕ-lizm). A clinical illness produced by the brown recluse spider, *Loxosceles reclusus,* of North America; characterized by gangrenous slough at the site of the bite, nausea, malaise, fever, hemolysis, and thrombocytopenia.

Lox·o·tre·ma ova·tum (lok-sō-trē'mă ō-vā'tŭm). Former name for *Metagonimus yokogawai.* [G. *loxos,* slanting, + *trēma,* a hole; L. *ovatus,* egg-shaped]

loz·enge (loz'enj). SYN troche. [Fr. *losange,* fr. *lozangé,* rhombic]

LPH Abbreviation for lipotropic *hormone.*

L.P.N. Abbreviation for licensed practical *nurse.*

LPO Abbreviation for left posterior oblique, a radiographic projection.

LPS Abbreviation for lipopolysaccharide.

Lr Symbol for lawrencium.

Lr, L$_r$ SEE Lr *dose.*

L.R.C.P. Abbreviation for Licentiate of the Royal College of Physicians (of England).

L.R.C.P.(E) Abbreviation for Licentiate of the Royal College of Physicians (Edinburgh).

L.R.C.P.(I) Abbreviation for Licentiate of the Royal College of Physicians (Ireland).

L.R.C.S. Abbreviation for Licentiate of the Royal College of Surgeons (of England).

L.R.C.S.(E) Abbreviation for Licentiate of the Royal College of Surgeons (Edinburgh).

L.R.C.S.(I) Abbreviation for Licentiate of the Royal College of Surgeons (Ireland).

LRF Abbreviation for luteinizing hormone-releasing *factor.*

L.R.F.P.S. Abbreviation for Licentiate of the Royal Faculty of Physicians and Surgeons, a Scottish institution.

LRH Abbreviation for luteinizing *hormone*-releasing *hormone.*

LSA Abbreviation for left sacroanterior position.

LSD Abbreviation for *lysergic acid* diethylamide.

LSF Abbreviation for line spread *function.*

LSP Abbreviation for left sacroposterior position.

LST Abbreviation for left sacrotransverse position.

LT Abbreviation for leukotrienes, usually followed by another letter with a subscript number; *e.g.,* LTA$_4$, LTC$_4$.

LTH Abbreviation for luteotropic *hormone.*

LTM Abbreviation for long-term *memory.*

LTR Abbreviation for long terminal repeat *sequences,* under *sequence.*

Lu Symbol for lutetium.

Lubarsch, Otto, German pathologist, 1860–1933. SEE L.'s *crystals,* under *crystal.*

Luc, Henri, French laryngologist, 1855–1925. SEE L.'s *operation;* Caldwell-L. *operation;* Ogston-L. *operation.*

lu·can·thone hy·dro·chlo·ride (lū-kan'thōn). 1,2′-Diethylaminoethylamino-4-methylthiaxanthone hydrochloride; used in the treatment of urinary schistosomiasis (*Schistosoma haematobium*) and intestinal schistosomiasis (*S. mansoni*).

Lucas, Richard C., English anatomist and surgeon, 1846–1915. SEE L.'s *groove.*

lu·cen·so·my·cin (lū-sen-sō-mī'sin). An antibiotic isolated from cultures of *Streptomyces lucensis;* an antifungal agent. SYN lucimycin.

lu·cent (lū'sent). Bright; clear; translucent. [L. *lucere,* to shine]

Lu·ci·bac·te·ri·um (lū'si-bak-tēr-ē-ŭm). A genus of aerobic to facultatively anaerobic, motile, peritrichous bacteria containing Gram-negative rods. Their metabolism is fermentative, and they are usually luminescent. They occur on the surface of dead fish and in sea water. The type species is *L. harveyi.* [L. *luceo,* to shine, + bacterium]
L. harveyi, a species of luminescent bacteria found in sea water; it is the type species of the genus *L.* SYN *Photobacterium harveyi.*

lu·cid (lū'sid). Clear, not obscured or confused, as in a l. moment or l. spoken expression. [L. *lucidus,* clear]

lu·cid·i·fi·ca·tion (lū-sid'i-fi-kā'shŭn). SYN clarification. [L. *lucidus,* clear, + *facio,* to make]

lu·cid·i·ty (lū-sid'i-tē). The quality or state of being lucid.

lu·cif·er·as·es (lū-sif'er-ās-ĕz). Enzymes present in certain luminous organisms that act to bring about the oxidation of luciferins; energy produced in the process is liberated as bioluminescence; such enzymes can be used to detect very low concentrations of metabolites. [L. *lux,* light + *fero,* to bear]

lu·cif·er·ins (lū-sif'er-inz). Chemical substances present in certain luminous organisms that, when acted upon by luciferases, produce bioluminescence.

lu·cif·u·gal (lū-sif'yū-găl). Avoiding light. [L. *lux,* light, + *fugio,* to flee from]

Lu·cil·ia (lū-sil'ē-ă). A genus of scavenging blowflies (family Calliphoridae), commonly called bluebottle or greenbottle flies, whose larvae feed on carrion or excrement; they occasionally cause wound infestation or myiasis.
L. cae'sar, a species whose larvae formerly were used in the treatment of septic wounds. SEE ALSO *Phormia regina.*
L. cupri'na, the most important cause of blowfly strike of sheep in Australia and South Africa.
L. illus'tris, a metallic blue-green blowfly widely distributed in North America; the eggs are deposited chiefly on animal carcasses.
L. serica'ta, SYN *Phaenicia sericata.*

lu·ci·my·cin (lū-si-mī'sin). SYN lucensomycin.

Lucio, R., Mexican physician, 1819–1866. SEE L.'s *leprosy,* leprosy *phenomenon.*

lu·cip·e·tal (lū-sip'i-tăl). Seeking light. [L. *lux,* light, + *peto,* to seek]

Lucké, Balduin, U.S. pathologist, 1889–1954. SEE L. *carcinoma;* L.'s *adenocarcinoma, virus.*

Lücke, George A., German surgeon, 1829–1894. SEE L.'s *test.*

lüc·ken·schä·del (luk-en-shā'dl). Craniolacunia with meningocele or encephalocele. [Ger. *Lücke,* gap + *Schädel,* skull]

lu·co·ther·a·py (lū'kō-thār-ă-pē). SYN phototherapy. [L. *lux,* light, + G. *therapeia,* therapy]

lud·ic (lū'dik). Playlike; playfully pretending. [G. *ludus,* game]

Ludloff, Karl, German surgeon, 1864–1945. SEE L.'s *sign.*

Ludwig, Daniel, German anatomist, 1625–1680. SEE L.'s *angle.*

Ludwig, Karl F.W., German anatomist and physiologist, 1816–1895. SEE depressor *nerve* of L.; L.'s *ganglion, labyrinth, nerve, stromuhr.*

Lu

Ludwig, Kurt, German anatomist, *1922. SEE Klinger-L. acid-thionin *stain* for sex chromatin.

Ludwig, Wilhelm Friedrich von, German surgeon, 1790–1865. SEE L.'s *angina.*

Luebering, J. SEE Rapoport-Luebering *shunt.*

Luer, German instrument maker, †1883. SEE L. *syringe;* L.-Lok *syringe.*

lu·es (lū′ēz). A plague or pestilence; specifically, syphilis. [L. pestilence]

l. vene′rea, SYN syphilis.

lu·et·ic (lū-et′ik). SYN syphilitic.

Luft, John H., U.S. histologist, *1927. SEE L.'s potassium permanganate *fixative.*

Luft, Rolf, 20th century Swedish endocrinologist. SEE L.'s *disease.*

Lugol, Jean G.A., French physician, 1786–1851. SEE Lugol's iodine *solution.*

Lukes-Collins clas·si·fi·ca·tion. See under classification.

LUL Abbreviation for left upper lobe (of lung).

lu·lib·er·in (lū-lib′er-in). A decapeptide hormone from the hypothalamus that stimulates the anterior pituitary to release both follicle-stimulating hormone and luteinizing hormone. SYN luteinizing hormone-releasing hormone. [luteinizing hormone + L. *libero,* to free, + -in]

lum·ba·go (lŭm-bā′gō). Pain in mid and lower back; a descriptive term not specifying cause. SYN lumbar rheumatism. [L. fr. *lumbus,* loin]

ischemic l., an intermittent claudication of the back; a vascular form of backache characterized by a painful cramp of the muscles in the lumbar region excited by the exertion of walking or standing and promptly relieved by rest.

lum·bar (lŭm′bar). Relating to the loins, or the part of the back and sides between the ribs and the pelvis. [L. *lumbus,* a loin]

lum·bar·i·za·tion (lŭm′bar-i-zā′shŭn). A congenital anomaly of the lumbosacral junction characterized by development of the first sacral vertebra as a lumbar vertebra; there are six lumbar vertebrae instead of five.

lum·bi (lŭm′bī). Plural of lumbus. [L.]

lum·bo·ab·dom·i·nal (lŭm′bō-ab-dom′i-năl). Relating to the sides and front of the abdomen.

lum·bo·co·los·to·my (lŭm′bō-kō-los′tō-mē). Obsolete term for formation of a permanent opening into the colon via an incision through the lumbar region. [L. *lumbus,* loin, + G. *kolon,* colon, + *stoma,* mouth]

lum·bo·co·lot·o·my (lŭm′bō-kō-lot′ō-mē). Obsolete term for incision into the colon through the lumbar region. [L. *lumbus,* loin, + G. *kolon,* colon, + *tomē,* incision]

lum·bo·cos·tal (lŭm′bō-kos′tăl). **1.** Relating to the lumbar and the hypochondriac regions. **2.** Relating to the lumbar vertebrae and the ribs; denoting a ligament connecting the first lumbar vertebra with the neck of the twelfth rib. [L. *lumbus,* loin, + *costa,* rib]

lum·bo·il·i·ac (lŭm-bō-il′ē-ak). SYN lumboinguinal.

lum·bo·in·gui·nal (lŭm′bō-ing′gwi-năl). Relating to the lumbar and the inguinal regions. SYN lumboiliac. [L. *lumbus,* loin, + *inguen* (inguin-), groin]

lum·bo·ova·ri·an (lŭm-bō-ō-vā′rē-an). Relating to the ovary and the lumbar regions.

lum·bo·sa·cral (lŭm′bō-sā′krăl). Relating to the lumbar vertebrae and the sacrum. SYN sacrolumbar.

lum·bri·cal (lŭm′bri-kăl). SYN lumbricoid (1). [L. *lumbricus,* earthworm]

lum·bri·ca·lis. SEE lumbrical *muscle* of hand, lumbrical *muscle* of foot.

lum·bri·ci·dal (lŭm-bri-sī′dăl). Destructive to lumbricoid (intestinal) worms.

lum·bri·cide (lŭm′bri-sīd). An agent that kills lumbricoid (intestinal) worms. [L. *lumbricus,* worm, + *caedo,* to kill]

lum·bri·coid (lŭm′bri-koyd). **1.** Denoting or resembling a roundworm, especially *Ascaris lumbricoides.* SYN lumbrical,

lumbricus (1). SEE ALSO scolecoid (2), vermiform. **2.** Obsolete common name for *Ascaris lumbricoides.* [L. *lumbricus,* earthworm, + G. *eidos,* resemblance]

lum·bri·co·sis (lŭm′bri-kō′sis). Infection with round intestinal worms.

lum·bri·cus (lŭm′bri-kŭs). **1.** SYN lumbricoid (1). **2.** Obsolete name for *Ascaris lumbricoides.* [L. earthworm]

lum·bus, gen. and pl. **lum·bi** (lŭm′bŭs, -bī) [NA]. SYN loin. [L.]

lu·men, pl. **lu·mi·na, lu·mens** (lū′men, -min-ă, -menz). **1.** The space in the interior of a tubular structure, such as an artery or the intestine. **2 (lm).** The unit of luminous flux; the luminous flux emitted in a unit solid angle of 1 steradian by a uniform point source of light having a luminous intensity of 1 candela. [L. light, window]

residual l., SYN residual *cleft.*

lu·mi·chrome (lū′mi-krōm). 7,8-Dimethylalloxazine; riboflavin minus its ribityl side chain; produced by ultraviolet irradiation of riboflavin in acid solution.

lu·mi·fla·vin (lū′mi-flā-vin). 7,8,10-Trimethylisoalloxazine; a yellow photoderivative of riboflavin, bearing a methyl group in place of the ribityl; produced by ultraviolet irradiation of riboflavin in alkaline solution.

lu·mi·na (lū′mi-nă). Plural of lumen. [L.]

lu·mi·nal (lū′mi-năl). Relating to the lumen of a blood vessel or other tubular structure.

lu·mi·nance (lū′mi-năns). The brightness of an object, expressed as the luminous flux per unit solid angle per unit projected area, measured in lamberts or in candelas per square meter. [L. *lumino,* to light up, fr. *lumen,* light]

lu·mi·nes·cence (lū-mi-nes′ens). Emission of light from a body as a result of a chemical reaction. SEE bioluminescence. [L. *lumen,* light]

lu·mi·nif·er·ous (lū-mi-nif′er-ŭs). Producing or conveying light. [L. *lumen,* light, + *fero,* to carry]

lu·mi·no·phore (lū′mi-nō-fōr). An atom or atomic grouping in an organic compound that increases its ability to emit light. [L. *lumen,* light, + G. *phoros,* bearing]

lu·mi·nous (lū′mi-nŭs). Emitting light, with or without accompanying heat. [L. *lumen,* light]

lu·mi·rho·dop·sin (lū′mi-rō-dop′sin). An intermediate between rhodopsin and all-*trans*-retinal plus opsin during bleaching of rhodopsin by light; formed from bathorhodopsin and converted to metarhodopsin I with a half-life of about 20 μs. [L. *lumen,* light, + G. *rhodon,* rose, + *opsis,* vision]

lum·is·ter·ol (lūm-ē-stēr′ol). **1.** A by-product in ergocalciferol biosynthesis. **2.** A phosphorylated derivative of ribulose that is an intermediate in the pentose monophosphate shunt.

lump·ec·to·my (lŭm-pek′tō-mē). Removal of either a benign or malignant lesion from the breast with preservation of essential anatomy of the breast. [lump + G. *ektomē,* excision]

Luna, Lee G., 20th century U.S. medical technologist. SEE L.-Ishak *stain.*

lu·na·cy (lū′nă-sē). **1.** An obsolete term for a form of insanity characterized by alternating lucid and insane periods, believed to be influenced by phases of the moon. **2.** Any form of insanity. **3.** Insanity as defined variously by law. [L. *luna,* moon]

lu·nar (lū′ner). **1.** Relating to the moon or to a month. **2.** Resembling the moon in shape, especially a half moon. SYN lunate (1), semilunar. SEE ALSO crescentic. **3.** Relating to silver (the moon was the symbol of silver in alchemy). [L. *luna,* moon]

lunar caustic. SYN toughened *silver* nitrate.

lu·na·re (lū-nā′rē). SYN lunate *bone.*

lu·nate (lū′nāt). **1.** SYN lunar (2). **2.** Relating to the lunate bone.

lu·na·tic (lū′nă-tik). Obsolete term for a mentally ill person. [see lunacy]

lu·na·to·ma·la·cia (lū-nā′tō-mă-lā′shē-ă). SYN Kienböck's *disease.*

lung (lŭng). One of a pair of viscera occupying the pulmonary cavities of the thorax, the organs of respiration in which aeration of the blood takes place. As a rule, the right l. is slightly larger than the left and is divided into three lobes (an upper, a middle,

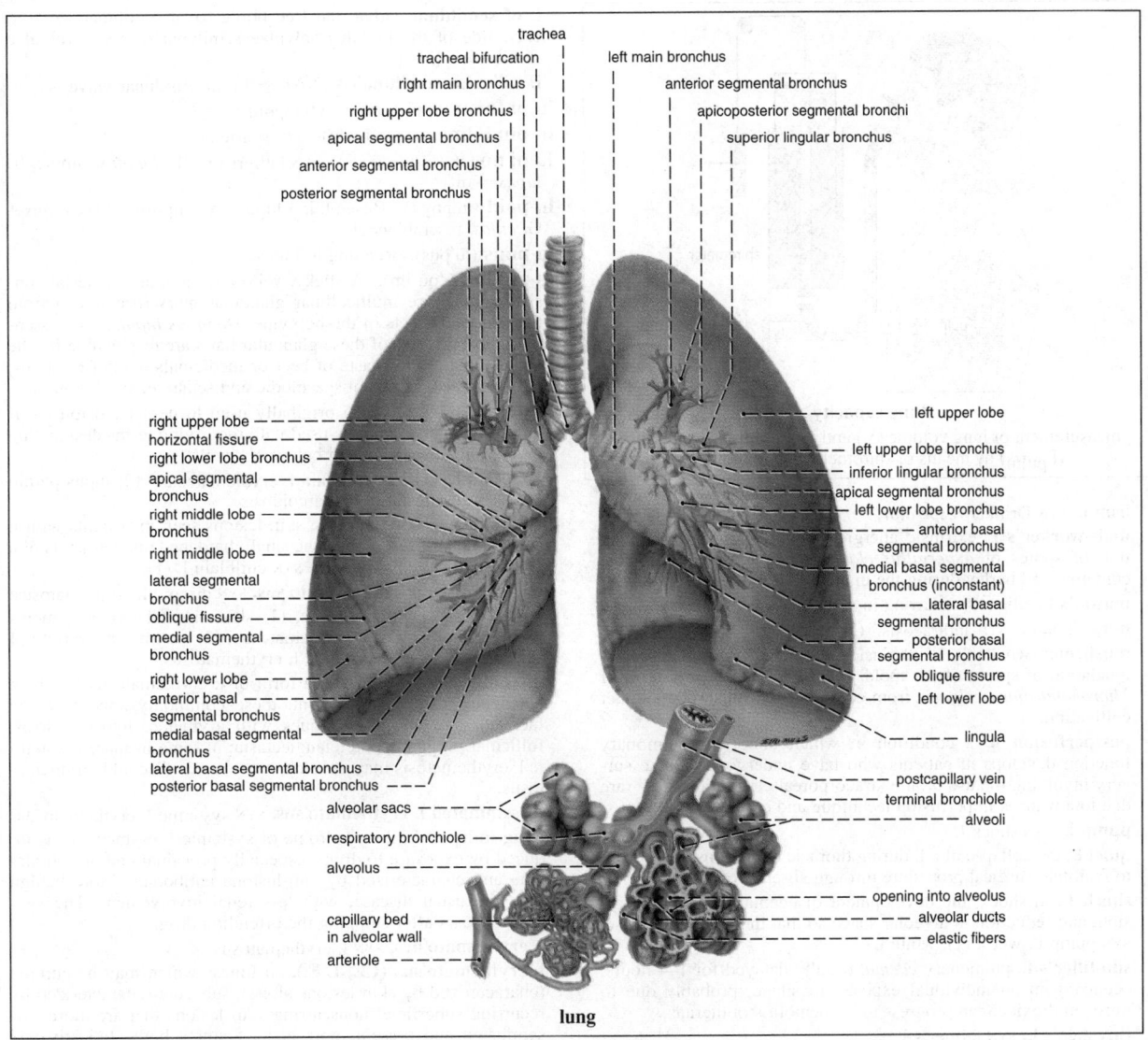

lung

and a lower or basal), while the left has but two lobes (an upper and a lower or basal). Each l. is irregularly conical in shape, presenting a blunt upper extremity (the apex), a concave base following the curve of the diaphragm, an outer convex surface (costal surface), an inner or mediastinal surface (mediastinal surface), a thin and sharp anterior border, and a thick and rounded posterior border. SYN pulmo [NA]. [A.S. *lungen*]

air-conditioner l., an extrinsic allergic alveolitis caused by forced air contaminated by thermophilic actinomycetes and other organisms.

bird-breeder's l., bird-fancier's l., extrinsic allergic alveolitis caused by inhalation of particulate avian emanations; sometimes specified by avian species, *e.g.,* pigeon-breeder's l., budgerigar-breeder's l. SYN bird-breeder's disease.

black l., a form of pneumoconiosis, common in coal miners, characterized by deposit of carbon particles in the l. SYN miner's l. (2).

brown l., obstructive airway disease with asthma produced by exposure to cotton dust, flax or hemp. SEE ALSO byssinosis.

butterfly l., hemorrhagic markings appearing on an animal's l. after inoculation with *Leptospira interrogans* (*L. icterohaemorrhagiae*).

cardiac l., disturbance in pulmonary anatomy and physiology secondary to valvular disease of the heart or to other disturbances of circulation incident to cardiac disease.

cheese worker's l., extrinsic allergic alveolitis caused by inhalation of spores of *Penicillium casei* from moldy cheese.

collier's l., SYN anthracosis.

coptic l., condition caused by the cloth lung.

endstage l., severe diffuse interstitial fibrosis and honeycombing.

farmer's l., a hypersensitivity pneumonitis characterized by fever and dyspnea, caused by inhalation of organic dust from moldy hay containing spores of actinomycetes such as *Micromonospora vulgaris*, *M. faeni*, *Thermopolyspora polyspora*, and certain true fungi, which thrive in the elevated temperatures of hay lofts and silos; repeated exposure may result in alveolar sensitization and, ultimately, granulomatous lung disease with severe l. disability. SYN thresher's l.

fibroid l., chronic interstitial pneumonia in a l.

honeycomb l., the radiological and gross appearance of the l.'s resulting from interstitial fibrosis and cystic dilation of bronchioles and distal air spaces; of unknown cause or a sequel of any of several diseases, including eosinophilic granuloma and sarcoidosis.

hyperlucent l., the radiographic finding that a l. or portion thereof is less dense than normal, as from air trapping by a bronchial foreign body, asymmetric emphysema, or decreasing blood flow. SEE unilateral hyperlucent l.

lu

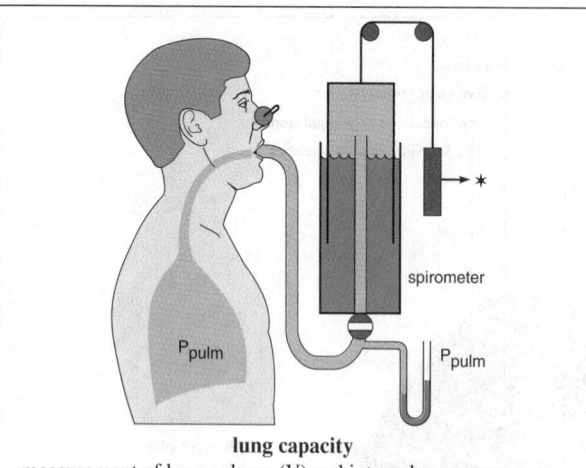

lung capacity
measurement of lung volume (V) and intrapulmonary pressure (P_{pulm}) by means of spirometer and manometer

iron l., SYN Drinker *respirator.*

malt-worker's l., extrinsic allergic alveolitis caused by inhalation of spores of *Aspergillus clavatus* and *A. fumigatus* from contaminated barley during the manufacture of beer.

mason's l., silicosis occurring in stone masons.

miner's l., (1) SYN anthracosis. **(2)** SYN black l.

mushroom-worker's l., extrinsic allergic alveolitis caused by inhalation of spores of the mold *Thermopolyspora polyspora* or *Micromonospora vulgaris* from contaminated mushrooms under cultivation.

postperfusion l., a condition in which abnormal pulmonary function develops in patients who have undergone cardiac surgery involving the use of an extracorporeal circulation; now rare due to advances in perfusion technique and equipment.

pump l., SYN shock l.

quiet l., the collapse of a l. during thoracic operations undertaken to facilitate surgical procedure through absence of l. movement.

shock l., in shock, the development of edema, impaired perfusion, and reduction in alveolar space so that the alveoli collapse. SYN pump l., wet l. (1), white l.

silo-filler's l., pulmonary *edema,* usually delayed for 1–4 hours, occurring in an individual exposed to silage, probably due to nitrogen dioxide; can progress to bronchiolitis obliterans.

thresher's l., SYN farmer's l.

trench l., a psychogenic hyperventilation marked by paroxysmal attacks of rapid breathing, without any signs of organic disease, observed in stressful situations such as battle.

unilateral hyperlucent l., chronic bronchiolitis obliterans predominating on one side. SEE unilateral lobar *emphysema.*

uremic l., perihilar edema of the l. associated with renal failure and hypertension; the peripheral parts of the l. remain clear. SYN uremic pneumonia (1), uremic pneumonitis.

vanishing l., SEE vanishing lung *syndrome.*

welder's l., relatively benign form of pneumoconiosis, associated with welding, resulting from deposit of fine metallic particles in the l.

wet l., white l., (1) SYN shock l. **(2)** SYN adult respiratory distress *syndrome.*

lung·worms (lŭng'wermz). Nematodes that inhabit the air passages of animals, chiefly in the family Metastrongylidae (or Protostrongylidae). SEE *Aelurostrongylus, Crenosoma vulpis, Dictyocaulus, Metastrongylus, Muellerius capillaris, Protostrongylus rufescens.*

lu·nu·la, pl. **lu·nu·lae** (lū'nū-lă, -lē). **1** [NA]. The pale arched area at the proximal portion of the nail plate. SYN arcus unguium, half-moon, selene unguium. **2.** A small semilunar structure. [L. dim. of *luna,* moon]

azure l. of nails, bluish nonblanching discoloration of the lunulae of all the fingernails in hepatolenticular degeneration.

l. of semilunar valve, the free border of a semilunar valve at each side of the nodulus valvulae semilunaris. SYN l. valvulae semilunaris [NA].

l. val'vulae semiluna'ris [NA], SYN l. of semilunar valve.

lu·pi·form (lū'pi-fōrm). SYN lupoid.

lu·pin·i·dine (lū-pin'i-dēn). SYN sparteine.

lu·pi·no·sis (lū-pi-nō'sis). SYN lathyrism. [L. *lupinus,* lupine, fr. *lupus,* wolf]

lu·poid (lū'poyd). Resembling lupus. SYN lupiform. [L. *lupus* + G. *eidos,* resemblance]

lu·pous (lū'pŭs). Relating to lupus.

lu·pu·lin (lū'pū-lin). A sticky, yellowish, granular material consisting of entire multicellular glandular hairs (trichomes) from the fruit and bracts of the hop vine, *Humulus lupulus;* the essential oils and resins of these glandular hairs are responsible for the characteristic bitter taste of beer or medicinals made from hops; has been used as an antispasmodic and sedative. SYN humulin.

lu·pus (lū'pŭs). A term originally used to depict erosion (as if gnawed) of the skin, now used with modifying terms designating the various diseases listed below. [L. wolf]

chilblain l., (1) SYN chilblain l. erythematosus. **(2)** lupus pernio that is a manifestation of sarcoidosis.

chilblain l. erythematosus, skin lesions seen in patients with l. erythematosus, resembling the small, hardened nodular areas of a cold injury called chilblains. SYN chilblain l. (1).

chronic discoid l. erythemato'sus, SYN discoid l. erythematosus.

cutaneous l. erythematosus, (1) skin disease seen in patients with discoid form of l. erythematosus; **(2)** a term for a variety of skin lesions seen in systemic l. erythematosus.

discoid l. erythemato'sus, a form of l. erythematosus in which cutaneous lesions are present; these commonly appear on the face and are atrophic plaques with erythema, hyperkeratosis, follicular plugging, and telangiectasia; in some instances systemic l. erythematosis may develop. SYN chronic discoid l. erythematosus.

disseminated l. erythemato'sus, SYN systemic l. erythematosus.

drug-induced l., the syndrome of systemic l. erythematosus induced by exposure to drugs, especially procainamide or hydralazine and characterized by anti-histone antibodies. More benign than the usual disease, with less renal involvement. The syndrome clears after stopping the offending drug.

l. erythemato'des, SYN l. erythematosus.

l. erythemato'sus (LE, L.E.), an illness which may be chronic (characterized by skin lesions alone), subacute (characterized by recurring superficial nonscarring skin lesions that are more disseminated and present more acute features both clinically and histologically than those seen in the chronic discoid phase), or systemic or disseminated (in which antinuclear antibodies are present and in which there is almost always involvement of vital structures). SEE ALSO discoid l. erythematosus, systemic l. erythematosus. SYN l. erythematodes, l. superficialis.

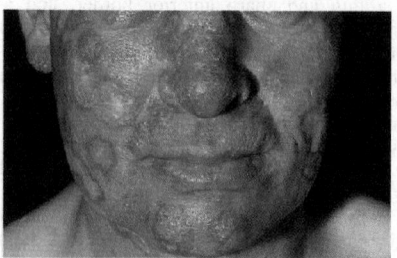

lupus erythematosus
in chronic lupus erythematosus, the lesions are sensitive to touch

l. erythematosus, neonatal, l. erythematosus present at birth as a result of placentally transmitted antibodies from a mother with systemic l. erythematosus; characterized by transient hematopoietic and cutaneous lesions and permanent cardiac abnormalities.

l. erythemato′sus profun′dus, a subcutaneous panniculitis with marked lymphocyte infiltration of fat lobules giving rise to deep-seated, firm, rubbery nodules that sometimes become ulcerated, usually of the face; may occur in systemic and localized l. erythematosus. SYN l. profundus.

l. livi′do, persistent cyanotic lesions on the extremities, associated with the cutaneous manifestations of Raynaud's disease.

l. lymphat′icus, SYN *lymphangioma* circumscriptum.

l. milia′ris dissemina′tus facie′i, a millet-like papular eruption of the face, associated with a (histopathologically) tuberculoid perifollicular infiltration, but probably related to rosacea rather than tuberculous infection.

l. mu′tilans, cutaneous tuberculosis with extensive destruction of tissue.

neonatal l., l. erythematosus occurring in newborn children of mothers who had lupus during pregnancy; anti-SSA antibodies usually should be screened for; 50% have anti-nuclear antibodies. A variety of skin lesions are seen, which can resolve or leave scarring; the syndrome usually resolves; however cardiac manifestations can be fatal. Some children develop systemic lupus later in life.

l. papillomato′sus, SYN *tuberculosis* cutis verrucosa.

l. per′nio, sarcoid lesions, clinically resembling frostbite and microscopically resembling l. vulgaris, involving ears, cheeks, nose, hands, and fingers.

l. profundus (prō-fŭn′dŭs), SYN l. erythematosus profundus. [L. deep]

l. seba′ceus, l. erythematosus with lesions on the face in butterfly areas.

l. serpigino′sus, a cutaneous tuberculous lesion that spreads peripherally, healing centrally with scar formation.

l. superficia′lis, SYN l. erythematosus.

systemic l. erythemato′sus (SLE), an inflammatory connective tissue disease with variable features, frequently including fever, weakness and fatigability, joint pains or arthritis resembling rheumatoid arthritis, diffuse erythematous skin lesions on the face, neck, or upper extremities, with liquefaction degeneration of the basal layer and epidermal atrophy, lymphadenopathy, pleurisy or pericarditis, glomerular lesions, anemia, hyperglobulinemia, and a positive LE cell test, with serum antibodies to double-stranded DNA and acidic nuclear protein (Sm). SYN disseminated l. erythematosus.

l. tuberculo′sus, SYN l. vulgaris.

l. verruco′sus, SYN *tuberculosis* cutis verrucosa.

l. vulga′ris, cutaneous tuberculosis with characteristic nodular lesions on the face, particularly about the nose and ears. SYN l. tuberculosus, tuberculosis cutis luposa.

LUQ Abbreviation for left upper quadrant (of abdomen).

lu·ra (lū′ră). The contracted termination of the infundibulum of the brain. [L. the mouth of a bottle]

lu·ral (lū′răl). Pertaining to the lura.

Luschka, Hubert, German anatomist, 1820–1875. SEE L.'s *bursa, cartilage, ducts,* under *duct, gland, cystic glands,* under *gland, joints,* under *joint, ligaments,* under *ligament, sinus, tonsil; foramen* of L.

Luse, Sarah A., 20th century U.S. physician. SEE L. *bodies,* under *body.*

lute (lūt). To seal or fasten with wax or cement. [L. *lutum,* mud]

lu·te·al (lū′tē-ăl). Relating to the corpus luteum; l. cells, l. hormone, etc. SYN luteus [NA]. [L. *luteus,* saffron-yellow]

lu·te·ci·um (lū-tē′sē-ŭm). SYN lutetium.

lu·te·in (lū′tē-in). **1.** The yellow pigment in the corpus luteum, in the yolk of eggs, or any lipochrome. **2.** SYN xanthophyll. **3.** The dried powdered corpora lutea of the hog, formerly used as a progesterone source. [L. *luteus,* saffron-yellow]

lu·te·in·i·za·tion (lū′tē-in-i-zā′shŭn). Transformation of the mature ovarian follicle and its theca interna into a corpus luteum after ovulation; formation of luteal tissue, which appears yellow in some species.

lu·te·i·nize (lū′tē-ĭ-nīz). To form luteal tissue.

lu·te·i·no·ma (lū′tē-i-nō′mă). SYN luteoma.

Lutembacher, René, French cardiologist, 1884–1916. SEE L.'s *syndrome.*

lu·te·o·gen·ic (lū′tē-ō-jen′ik). Luteinizing; inducing the production or growth of corpora lutea.

lu·te·o·hor·mone (lū′tē-ō-hōr′mōn). SYN progesterone.

lu·te·ol, lu·te·ole (lū′tē-ol, -ōl). SYN xanthophyll.

lu·te·o·lin (lū-tē-ō′lin). 3′,4′,5,7-Tetrahydroxyflavone; the aglycon of galuteolin and cynaroside. SYN cyanidenon.

lu·te·ol·y·sin (lū-tē-ol′i-sin). Any agent, natural or compounded, that destroys the function of the corpus luteum. [L. *luteus,* saffron-yellow, + G. *lysis,* dissolution]

lu·te·ol·y·sis (lū-tē-ol′i-sis). Degeneration or destruction of ovarian luteinized tissue.

lu·te·o·lyt·ic (lū-tē-ō-lit′ik). Promoting or characteristic of luteolysis.

lu·te·o·ma (lū-tē-ō′mă). An ovarian tumor of granulosa or thecalutein cell origin, producing progesterone effects on the uterine mucosa. SYN luteinoma.

pregnancy l., a benign lutein cell tumor of the ovary.

lu·te·o·tro·pic, lu·te·o·tro·phic (lū′tē-ō-trop′ik, -trof′ik). Having a stimulating action on the development and function of the corpus luteum.

lu·te·o·tro·pin (lū′tē-ō-trō′pin). An anterior pituitary hormone whose action maintains the function of the corpus luteum. SYN luteotropic hormone.

lu·te·ti·um (Lu) (lū-tē′shē-ŭm). A rare earth element; atomic no. 71, atomic wt. 174.967. SYN lucecium. [L. *Lutetia,* Paris]

lu·te·us (lū-tē′ŭs) [NA]. SYN luteal, luteal. [L.]

Lu·ther·an Blood Group, Lu Blood Group. See Blood Groups Appendix.

lu·tro·pin (lū′trō-pin). A glycoprotein hormone that stimulates the final ripening of the follicles and the secretion of progesterone by them, their rupture to release the egg, and the conversion of the ruptured follicle into the corpus luteum. SYN interstitial cell-stimulating hormone, luteinizing hormone, luteinizing principle.

lu·tu·trin (lū′tū-trin). A water-soluble protein-like fraction extracted from the corpus luteum of sows' ovaries, resembling relaxin; it causes uterine relaxation and is used in dysmenorrhea.

Lutz, Alfredo, Brazilian physician, 1855–1940. SEE L.-Splendore-Almeida *disease.*

Lutz·o·my·ia (lūt-zō-mī′ă). A genus of New World sandflies or bloodsucking midges (family Psychodidae) that serve as vectors of leishmaniasis and Oroyo fever; formerly combined with the Old World sandfly genus *Phlebotomus.*

L. flaviscutella′ta, a sandfly species that is a vector of *Leishmania mexicana,* the agent of chiclero's ulcer. SYN *Phlebotomus flaviscutellatus.*

L. interme′dius, one of a group of sandfly species that are vectors of *Leishmania braziliensis,* the agent of espundia.

L. longipal′pis, SYN *Phlebotomus longipalpis.*

L. peruen′sis, a sandfly species that is a vector of *Leishmania peruviana,* the agent of uta.

lux (lx) (lŭks). A unit of light or illumination; the reception of a luminous flux of 1 lumen per square meter of surface. SYN candle-meter, meter-candle. [L. light]

lux·a·tio (lŭk-sā′shē-ō). SEE luxation. [L. *luxo,* pp. *-atus,* to dislocate]

l. erec′ta, subglenoid dislocation of the head of the humerus; the arm is raised and abducted and cannot be lowered.

l. perinea′lis, a condition in which the head of the femur is dislocated to the perineum.

lux·a·tion (lŭk-sā′shŭn). **1.** SYN dislocation. **2.** In dentistry, the dislocation or displacement of the condyle in the temporomandibular fossa, or of a tooth from the alveolus. [L. *luxatio*]

Malgaigne's l., SYN nursemaid's *elbow.*

Lux·ol fast blue. Name for a group of closely related copper phthalocyanin dyes used as stains (with PAS, PTAH, hematoxylin, silver nitrate, etc.) for myelin in nerve fibers.

lux·us (lŭks′ŭs). Excess of any sort. [L. extravagance, luxury]

lu

Luys, Jules B., French physician, 1828–1897. SEE L.'s *body;* centre médian de L.; *corpus* luysi; *nucleus* of L.

LVET Abbreviation for left ventricular ejection *time.*

L.V.N. Abbreviation for licensed vocational *nurse.*

Lw Former symbol for lawrencium.

lx Abbreviation for lux.

ly·ase (lī'ās). Class name for those enzymes removing groups nonhydrolytically (EC class 4); prefixes such as "hydro-," "ammonia-," etc., are used to indicate the type of reaction. Trivial names for lyases include synthases, decarboxylases, aldolases, dehydratases. Cf. synthase, synthetase.

ly·can·thro·py (lī-kan'thrō-pē). The morbid delusion that one is a wolf, possibly a mental atavism of the werewolf superstition. [G. *lykos,* wolf, + *anthrōpos,* man]

ly·coc·to·nine (lī-kok'tō-nēn). An alkaloid, $C_{25}H_{41}NO_7$, obtained from *Aconitum lycoctonum,* an exceedingly poisonous species of aconite; it also occurs in other species of *Aconitum* and *Delphinium.*

ly·co·pene (lī'kō-pēn). Ψ,Ψ-Carotene; the red pigment of the tomato that may be considered chemically as the parent substance from which all natural carotenoid pigments are derived; an unsaturated hydrocarbon made up of 8 isoprene units, two of them hydrogenated, with 11 conjugated double bonds.

ly·co·pe·ne·mia (lī'kō-pĕ-nē'mē-ă). A condition in which there is a high concentration of lycopene in the blood, producing carotenoid-like yellowish pigmentation of the skin; found in people who consume excessive amounts of tomatoes or tomato juice, or lycopene-containing fruits and berries. [lycopene + G. *haima,* blood]

Ly·co·per·don (līkō-per'don). A genus of fungi (family Lycoperdaceae), some species of which have been used medicinally, *e.g.,* in folk medicine, by nasal inhalation to treat epistaxis. The spores of *L. bovista* (*L. gemmatum, L. caelatum*) and of *L. pyriforme* may rarely produce lycoperdonosis. SYN puffball. [G. *lykos,* wolf, + *perdomai,* to break wind]

ly·co·per·do·no·sis (lī'kō-per-don-ō'sis). A persisting pneumonitis following inhalation of spores of the puffballs *Lycoperdon pyriforme* and *L. bovista.*

ly·coph·o·ra (lī-kof'ō-ră). The 10-hooked larva of primitive tapeworms of the subclass Cestodaria.

ly·co·po·di·um (lī-kō-pō'dē-ŭm). The spores of *Lycopodium clavatum* (family Lycopodiaceae) and other species of *L.;* a yellow, tasteless, and odorless powder; was used as a dusting powder and in pharmacy to prevent the agglutination of pills in a box. SYN club moss, vegetable sulfur. [G. *lykos,* wolf, + *pous,* foot]

lye (lī). The liquid obtained by leaching wood ashes. SEE *potassium* hydroxide, *sodium* hydroxide. SYN lixivium. [A.S. *leáh*]

Lyell, Aian. SEE L.'s *disease, syndrome.*

ly·go·phil·ia (lī-gō-fil'ē-ă). Morbid preference for dark places. [G. *lygē,* twilight, + *phileō,* to love]

ly·me·cy·cline (lī-mĕ-sī'klēn). Tetracycline-methylene lysine; an antimicrobial agent.

Lym·naea (lim-nē'ă). A genus of snails, species of which are invertebrate hosts for the liver or sheep liver fluke, *Fasciola hepatica,* and other trematodes. [G. *limnē,* marsh]

lymph (limf). A clear, transparent, sometimes faintly yellow and slightly opalescent fluid that is collected from the tissues throughout the body, flows in the lymphatic vessels (through the l. nodes), and is eventually added to the venous blood circulation. L. consists of a clear liquid portion, varying numbers of white blood cells (chiefly lymphocytes), and a few red blood cells. SYN lympha [NA]. [L. *lympha,* clear spring water]

aplastic l., l. containing a relatively large number of leukocytes, but comparatively little fibrinogen; such l. does not form a good clot and manifests only a slight tendency to become organized. SYN corpuscular l.

blood l., l. exuded from the blood vessels and not derived from the fluid in the tissue spaces.

corpuscular l., SYN aplastic l.

croupous l., a form of inflammatory l. with an unusually large content of fibrinogen; as a result of the fibrin that is formed in relatively dense mats, a pseudomembrane is likely to be produced.

dental l., SYN dentinal *fluid.*

euplastic l., l. that contains relatively few leukocytes, but a comparatively high concentration of fibrinogen; such l. clots fairly well and tends to become organized with fibrous tissue.

fibrinous l., a euplastic or croupous l.

inflammatory l., a faintly yellow, usually coagulable fluid (*i.e.,* euplastic l.) that collects on the surface of an acutely inflamed membrane or cutaneous wound.

intercellular l., the fluid in the potential spaces between cells in the various organs and tissues.

intravascular l., l. within the lymphatic vessels, in contrast to intercellular l. and l. that has exuded from the vessels.

plastic l., inflammatory l. that has a tendency to become organized.

tissue l., true l., *i.e.,* l. derived chiefly from fluid in tissue spaces (in contrast to blood l.).

vaccine l., vaccinia l., that collected from the vesicles of vaccinia infection, and used for active immunization against smallpox.

△**lymph-.** SEE lympho-.

lym·pha (lim'fă) [NA]. SYN lymph. [L.]

lym·pha·den (limf'ă-den). SYN lymph node. [lymph- + G. *adēn,* gland]

△**lymphaden-.** SEE lymphadeno-.

lym·phad·e·nec·to·my (lim-fad-ĕ-nek'tō-mē). Excision of lymph nodes. [lymphadeno- + G. *ektomē,* excision]

lym·phad·e·ni·tis (lim'-fad'ĕ-nī'tis). Inflammation of a lymph node or lymph nodes. [lymphadeno- + G. *-itis,* inflammation]

caseous l., a specific disease of sheep caused by *Corynebacterium pseudotuberculosis* and characterized by slowly progressing caseation necrosis of the lymph nodes, particularly those of the thorax.

dermatopathic l., SYN dermatopathic *lymphadenopathy.*

paratuberculous l., old term for chronic inflammation of certain lymph nodes, not specifically tuberculous (*i.e.,* tubercle bacilli are not demonstrable), but associated with proved tuberculous inflammation in another part or organ of the body.

regional l., inflammation of a group of lymph nodes receiving drainage from a site of infection.

regional granulomatous l., SYN cat-scratch *disease.*

streptococcal l., a contagious bacterial disease of pigs caused by a group E streptococcus and characterized by the formation of abscesses in the cervical and/or cephalic lymph nodes.

tuberculosis l., SYN tuberculous l.

tuberculous l., l. resulting from infection by *Mycobacterium tuberculosis;* tuberculosis of the lymph nodes. SYN tuberculosis l.

△**lymphadeno-, lymphaden-.** The lymph nodes. [L. *lympha,* spring water, + G. *adēn,* gland]

lym·phad·e·nog·ra·phy (lim-fad'ĕ-nog'ră-fē). Radiographic visualization of lymph nodes after injection of a contrast medium; lymphography. [lymphadeno- + G. *graphō,* to write]

lym·phad·e·noid (lim-fad'ĕ-noyd). Relating to, or resembling, or derived from a lymph node. [lymphadeno- + G. *eidos,* resemblance]

lym·phad·e·no·ma (lim-fad'ĕ-nō'mă). Obsolete term for: **1.** An enlarged lymph node. **2.** SYN Hodgkin's *disease.* [lymphadeno- + G. *-ōma,* tumor]

lym·phad·e·no·ma·to·sis (lim-fad'ĕ-nō-mă-tō'sis). Obsolete term for a condition characterized by the presence of several to numerous enlarged lymph nodes, as in lymphosarcoma or Hodgkin's disease.

lym·phad·e·nop·a·thy (lim-fad-ĕ-nop'ă-thē). Any disease process affecting a lymph node or lymph nodes. [lymphadeno- + G. *pathos,* suffering]

angioimmunoblastic l. with dysproteinemia (AILD), a lymphoproliferative disorder characterized by generalized l., hepatosplenomegaly, fever, sweats, weight loss, skin lesions, and pruritus with hypergammaglobulinemia; occurs primarily in older adults, often with fatal outcome. Proliferation of B cells, deficiency of T cells has been demonstrated. SYN immunoblastic l.

dermatopathic l., enlargement of lymph nodes, with proliferation of pale-staining interdigitating reticulum cells and macrophages containing fat and melanin; secondary to various forms of dermatitis. SYN dermatopathic lymphadenitis, lipomelanic reticulosis.

immunoblastic l., SYN angioimmunoblastic l. with dysproteinemia.

persistent generalized l., a syndrome characterized by reactive hyperplasia of lymph nodes (of at least one month's duration and at two different body sites, not including the inguinal area) in patients infected with the human immunodeficiency virus. The lymph node lesions progress from benign reactive hyperplasia through a stage of mixed follicular hyperplasia, to follicular involution with lymphocyte depletion. Many go on to a malignant non-Hodgkin's lymphoma.

lym·phad·e·no·sis (lim-fad'ĕ-nō'sis). The basic underlying proliferative process that results in enlargement of lymph nodes, as in lymphocytic leukemia and certain inflammations. [lymphadeno- + G. *-osis,* condition]

benign l., SYN infectious *mononucleosis.*

malignant l., obsolete term for malignant *lymphoma.*

lym·phad·e·no·va·rix (lim-fad'ĕ-nō-vā'riks). Varicose deformity of a lymph node associated with lymphangiectasis. [lymphadeno- + L. *varix*]

lym·pha·gogue (limf'ă-gog). An agent that increases the formation and flow of lymph. [lymph + G. *agōgos,* drawing forth]

lym·phan·ge·i·tis (lim-fan'jē-ī'tis). SYN lymphangitis.

⌂lymphangi-. SEE lymphangio-.

lym·phan·gi·al (lim-fan'jē-ăl). Relating to a lymphatic vessel.

lym·phan·gi·ec·ta·sis, lym·phan·gi·ec·ta·sia (lim-fan'jē-ek'tă-sis, -ek-tā'zē-a). Dilation of the lymphatic vessels, the basic process that may result in the formation of a lymphangioma. SYN lymphectasia, telangiectasia lymphatica. [lymphangio- + G. *ektasis,* a stretching]

cavernous l., SYN *lymphangioma cavernosum.*

cystic l., SYN *lymphangioma cysticum.*

intestinal l. [MIM*152800], familial l. with intestinal loss of lymph causing lymphocytopenia and hypogammaglobulinemia.

simple l., SYN *lymphangioma simplex.*

lym·phan·gi·ec·tat·ic (lim-fan'jē-ek-tat'ik). Relating to or characterized by lymphangiectasis.

lym·phan·gi·ec·to·des (lim-fan'jē-ek-tō'dēz). SYN *lymphangioma* circumscriptum. [lymphangio- + G. *ektasis,* a stretching, + *eidos,* appearance]

lym·phan·gi·ec·to·my (lim-fan'jē-ek'tō-mē). Excision of a lymph channel. [lymphangio- + G. *ektomē,* excision]

lym·phan·gi·i·tis (lim-fan'jē-ī'tis). SYN lymphangitis.

⌂lymphangio-, lymphangi-. The lymphatic vessels. [L. *lympha,* spring water, + G. *angeion,* vessel]

lym·phan·gi·o·en·do·the·li·o·ma (lim-fan'jē-ō-en'dō-thē-lē-ō'mă). A neoplasm consisting of irregular groups or small masses of endothelial cells, as well as congeries of tubate structures that are thought to be derived from lymphatic vessels. [lymphangio- + endothelium + *-oma,* tumor]

lym·phan·gi·og·ra·phy (lim-fan'jē-og'ră-fē). Radiographic demonstration of lymphatics and lymph nodes following the injection of a contrast medium; lymphography. [lymphangio- + G. *graphō,* to write]

lym·phan·gi·ol·o·gy (lim-fan-jē-ol'ō-jē). The branch of medical science concerned with the lymphatic vessels. SYN lymphology. [lymphangio- + G. *logos,* study]

lym·phan·gi·o·ma (lim-fan'jē-ō'mă). A fairly well-circumscribed nodule or mass of lymphatic vessels or channels that vary in size, are usually greatly dilated, and are lined with normal endothelial cells; lymphoid tissue is usually present in the peripheral portions of the lesions, which are present at birth, or shortly thereafter, and probably represent anomalous development of lymphatic vessels (rather than true neoplasms); they occur most frequently in the neck and axilla, but may also devel-

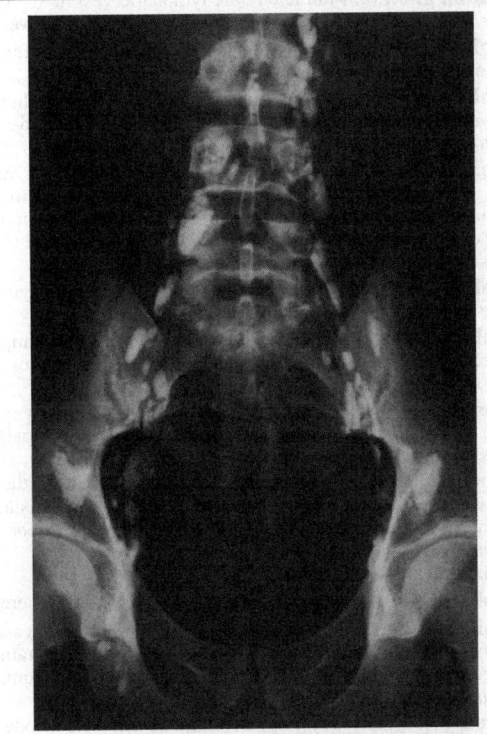

lymphadenography (storage phase)

op in the arm, mesentery, retroperitoneum, and other sites. SYN angioma lymphaticum. [lymphangio- + G. *-oma,* tumor]

l. capilla're varico'sum, SYN l. circumscriptum.

l. caverno'sum, a condition of conspicuous dilation of lymphatic vessels in a fairly circumscribed region, frequently with the formation of cavities or "lakes" filled with lymph. SYN cavernous lymphangiectasis.

l. circumscrip'tum, a congenital nevoid lesion consisting of a circumscribed group of tense lymph vesicles. SYN lupus lymphaticus, lymphangiectodes, l. capillare varicosum, l. superficium simplex.

l. cys'ticum, a condition characterized by a fairly well circumscribed group of several or numerous, cystlike, dilated vessels or spaces lined with endothelium and filled with lymph. SYN cystic lymphangiectasis.

l. sim'plex, a circumscribed region or focus of several to numerous lymphatic vessels that are moderately dilated. SYN simple lymphangiectasis.

l. superfic'ium sim'plex, SYN l. circumscriptum.

l. tubero'sum mul'tiplex, a cutaneous lesion characterized by multiple, slightly red, cystlike nodules (located chiefly on the trunk), resulting from fairly large lymphatic vessels and spaces, and groups of proliferating endothelial cells; the lesion has some gross resemblance to spiradenoma, except for the characteristic location.

l. xanthelasmoid'eum, a capillary l. with colloid degeneration of the elastic tissues of the skin, characterized by yellow-brown or gray-brown plaques that may be only slightly raised above the surface of the skin.

lym·phan·gi·o·ma·tous (lim-fan'jē-ō'mă-tŭs). Pertaining to, characterized by, or containing lymphangioma.

lymph·an·gi·o·my·o·ma·to·sis (lim-fan'gē-ō-mī'ō-ma-tō'sis). A proliferation of abnormal smooth muscle cells, usually occurring in the lung and mediastinum as multiple tumors; often associated with tuberous sclerosis. [lymphangio- + myoma + *-osis,* condition]

ly

lym·phan·gi·on (lim-fan′jē-on). A lymphatic vessel. SEE lymph *vessels*, under *vessel*. [L. *lympha,* lymph, + G. *angeion,* vessel]

lym·phan·gi·o·phle·bi·tis (lim-fan′jē-ō-flĕ-bī′tis). Inflammation of the lymphatic vessels and veins.

lym·phan·gi·o·plas·ty (lim-fan′jē-ō-plas-tē). Surgical alteration of lymphatic vessels. SYN lymphoplasty. [lymphangio- + G. *plastos,* formed]

lym·phan·gi·o·sar·co·ma (lim-fan′jē-ō-sar-kō′mă). A malignant neoplasm derived from vascular tissue, *i.e.,* an angiosarcoma, in which the neoplastic cells originate from the endothelial cells of lymphatic vessels, usually developing in the arm several years after radical mastectomy.

lym·phan·gi·ot·o·my (lim-fan′jē-ot′ō-mē). Incision of lymphatic vessels. [lymphangio- + G. *tomē,* incision]

lym·phan·gi·tis (lim-fan-jī′tis). Inflammation of the lymphatic vessels. SYN lymphangeitis, lymphangiitis. [lymphangio- + G. *-itis,* inflammation]

l. carcinomato′sa, extensive lymphatic permeation by tumor cells, with surrounding fibrosis, producing visible or palpable cords, especially in pleura or skin overlying a carcinoma.

epizootic l., l. primarily involving the lymph channels of the skin of the legs and chest of horses and mules in Europe, Asia, and Africa; the causative agent is *Histoplasma capsulatum* var. *farciminosum.* SYN l. epizootica.

l. epizoot′ica, SYN epizootic l.

lym·pha·phe·re·sis (lim′fă-fĕ-rē′sis). SYN lymphocytapheresis.

lym·phat·ic (lim-fat′ik). **1.** Pertaining to lymph. **2.** A vascular channel that transports lymph. **3.** Sometimes used to pertain to a sluggish or phlegmatic characteristic. SYN vas lymphaticum. [L. *lymphaticus,* frenzied; Mod. L. use, of or for lymph]

afferent l., a l. vessel entering, or bringing lymph to, a node. SYN vas lymphaticum afferens [NA], afferent vessel (3).

efferent l., SYN *vas* efferens (1). SYN vas lymphaticum efferens [NA].

lym·phat·i·cos·to·my (lim-fat-i-kos′tō-mē). Making an opening into a lymphatic duct. [lymphatic + G. *stoma,* mouth]

lymph·at·ics (lim-fat′iks). SYN lymph *vessels,* under *vessel.*

lym·pha·ti·tis (lim-fă-tī′tis). Inflammation of the lymphatic vessels or lymph nodes. [lymphatic + G. *-itis,* inflammation]

lym·pha·tol·o·gy (lim-fă-tol′ō-jē). The study of the lymphatic system. [lymphatic + G. *logos,* study]

lym·pha·tol·y·sis (lim′fă-tol′i-sis). Destruction of the lymphatic vessels or lymphoid tissue, or both. [lymphatic + G. *lysis,* dissolution]

lym·pha·to·lyt·ic (lim′fă-tō-lit′ik). Pertaining to or characterized by lymphatolysis.

lym·phec·ta·sia (lim-fek-tā′zē-ă). SYN lymphangiectasis. [lymph + G. *ektasis,* a stretching]

lymph·e·de·ma (limf′e-dē′mă). Swelling (especially in subcutaneous tissues) as a result of obstruction of lymphatic vessels or lymph nodes and the accumulation of large amounts of lymph in the affected region. [lymph + G. *oidēma,* a swelling]

congenital l., SEE hereditary l.

hereditary l., permanent pitting edema usually confined to the legs; two types, congenital (Milroy's disease [MIM*153100]), or with onset at about the age of puberty (Meige's disease [MIM*153200]); autosomal dominant inheritance.

l. prae′cox, SYN primary l.

primary l., a form of l. observed chiefly in young women and girls, characterized by diffuse swelling of the lower extremities. SYN l. praecox.

lym·phe·mia (lim-fē′mē-ă). The presence of unusually large numbers of lymphocytes or their precursors, or both, in the circulating blood. [lymph(ocyte) + G. *haima,* blood]

lym·phi·za·tion (lim-fi-zā′shŭn). The formation of lymph.

lymph node. One of numerous round, oval, or bean-shaped bodies located along the course of lymphatic vessels, varying greatly in size (1 to 25 mm in diameter) and usually presenting a depressed area, the hilum, on one side through which blood vessels enter and efferent lymphatic vessels emerge. The structure consists of a fibrous capsule and internal trabeculae support-ing lymphoid tissue and lymph sinuses; lymphoid tissue is arranged in nodules in the cortex and cords in the medulla of a node, with afferent vessels entering at many points of the periphery. SYN nodus lymphaticus [NA], lymph gland, lymphaden, lymphoglandula.

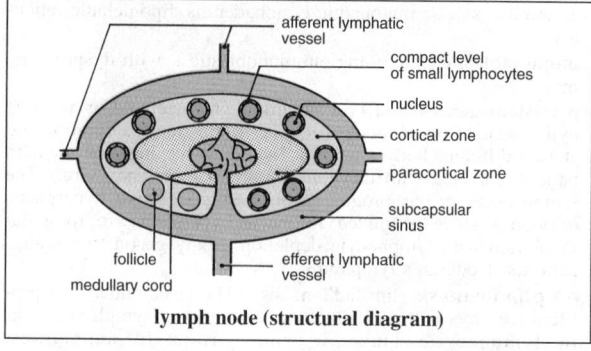

lymph node (structural diagram)

labels: afferent lymphatic vessel; compact level of small lymphocytes; nucleus; cortical zone; paracortical zone; subcapsular sinus; efferent lymphatic vessel; medullary cord; follicle

l. n.'s of abdominal organs, the numerous l. n.'s receiving lymph from abdominal organs located in association with the visceral branches of the aorta. SYN nodi lymphatici abdominis viscerales [NA].

accessory nerve l. n.'s, the nodes of the lateral deep cervical group that are located along the accessory nerve; their efferent vessels pass to the supraclavicular l. n.'s. SYN companion l. n.'s of accessory nerve, nodi lymphatici comitantes nervi accessorii.

anorectal l. n.'s, SYN pararectal l. n.'s.

anterior cervical l. n.'s, the group of l. n.'s located in the anterior region of the neck, divided into superficial and deep groups. SYN nodi lymphatici cervicales anteriores [NA].

anterior deep cervical l. n.'s, the l. n.'s near the larynx, trachea, and thyroid gland. SYN nodi lymphatici cervicales anteriores profundi.

anterior group of axillary l. n.'s, SYN pectoral group of axillary l. n.'s.

anterior jugular l. n.'s, nodes of the lateral deep cervical group located anterior to the internal jugular vein; two nodes are specifically named: the jugulodigastric l. n. and the jugulo-omohyoid l. n. SYN nodi lymphatici jugulares anteriores [NA].

anterior mediastinal l. n.'s, located in the superior mediastinum in relation to the great vessels, these nodes receive lymph from the thymus, pericardium and right side of the heart; their efferent vessels join those of the tracheal nodes to form the bronchomediastinal trunks. SYN nodi lymphatici mediastinales anteriores [NA].

anterior superficial cervical l. n.'s, the l. n.'s in the subcutaneous tissue of the anterior region of the neck. SYN nodi lymphatici cervicales anteriores superficiales.

anterior tibial l. n., a small inconstant l. n. in front of the interosseous membrane along the upper part of the anterior tibial vessels. SYN nodus tibialis anterior [NA], anterior tibial node.

apical group of axillary l. n.'s, the group of l. n.'s located at the apex of the axillary fossa that receive lymphatic drainage from other groups of axillary l. n.'s and then drain in turn into the subclavian lymphatic trunk. SYN nodi lymphatici axillares apicales [NA].

appendicular l. n.'s, nodes along the appendicular vessels in the mesoappendix; they receive afferent vessels from the vermiform appendix and send efferent vessels to the ileocolic l. n.'s. SYN nodi lymphatici appendiculares [NA].

axillary l. n.'s, numerous nodes around the axillary veins which receive the lymphatic drainage from the upper limb, scapular region and pectoral region (including mammary gland); they drain into the subclavian trunk. SYN nodi lymphatici axillares [NA], axillary glands.

l. n. of azygos arch, a l. n. of the posterior mediastinal group located adjacent to the arch of the azygos vein. SYN nodus lymphaticus arcus venae azygos [NA].

bifurcation l. n.'s, SYN inferior tracheobronchial l. n.'s.

brachial l. n.'s, SYN lateral group of axillary l. n.'s.

bronchopulmonary l. n.'s, l. n.'s in the hilum of the lung that receive lymph from the pulmonary l. n.'s, and drain to the tracheobronchial nodes. SYN glandulae bronchiales [NA], bronchial glands (1), hilar l. n.'s, nodi lymphatici bronchopulmonales.

buccal l. n., one of the chain of facial l. n.'s located superficial to the buccinator muscle. SYN nodus buccinatorius [NA], buccinator node, buccal node.

carinal l. n.'s, SYN inferior tracheobronchial l. n.'s.

celiac l. n.'s, nodes located along the celiac trunk which drain lymph from the stomach, duodenum, pancreas, spleen, and biliary tract and drain to the cisterna chyli via the right and left intestinal lymphatic trunks. SYN nodi lymphatici coeliaci [NA], celiac glands.

central group of axillary l. n.'s, nodes located around the midportion of the axillary vein; they receive afferent vessels from the lateral (brachial), pectoral, and subscapular groups of axillary nodes and send efferent vessels to the apical group of axillary l. n.'s;

central mesenteric l. n.'s, SYN middle group of mesenteric l. n.'s. SEE ALSO mesenteric l. n.'s.

colic l. n.'s, SYN nodi lymphatici colici. SEE left colic l. n.'s, middle colic l. n.'s, right colic l. n.'s.

common iliac l. n.'s, nodes located in association with the common iliac vein; they are subdivided into five groups: intermediate (anterior) common iliac l. n.'s, between the common iliac artery and vein; lateral common iliac l. n.'s lateral to the vein; medial common iliac l. n.'s, medial to the vein; promontory common iliac l. n.'s at the sacral promontory; and subaortic common iliac l. n.'s, at the bifurcation of the aorta; they all receive afferent vessels from the external and internal iliac nodes and send efferent vessels to the lumbar nodes. SYN nodi lymphatici iliaci communes [NA].

companion l. n.'s of accessory nerve, SYN accessory nerve l. n.'s.

cubital l. n.'s, two groups of nodes, superficial and deep, lying along the basilic vein above the medial epicondyle; they receive afferents from the ulnar side of the forearm and hand, and send efferents to the brachial nodes. SYN nodi lymphatici cubitales [NA], epitrochlear nodes, l. n.'s of elbow.

cystic l. n., a l. n. at the neck of the gallbladder draining lymph into the hepatic nodes. SYN nodus cysticus [NA], cystic node.

deep inguinal l. n.'s, several small nodes deep to the fascia lata and medial to the femoral vein; they receive lymph from the deep structures of the lower limb, from the glans penis and from superficial inguinal nodes; efferents pass to the external iliac nodes. SYN nodi lymphatici inguinales profundi [NA].

deep parotid l. n.'s, the group of l. n.'s associated with the parotid gland lying deep to the parotid masseteric fascia. SYN nodi lymphatici parotidei profundi [NA].

l. n.'s of elbow, SYN cubital l. n.'s.

external iliac l. n.'s, nodes located in association with the external iliac vein; they are subdivided into three groups: intermediate external iliac l. n.'s, between the vein and the external iliac artery; lateral external iliac l. n.'s, and medial external iliac l. n.'s, medial to the vein; they all receive afferent vessels from the inguinal nodes, lower abdominal wall, and pelvic viscera, and send efferent vessels to the common iliac nodes. SYN nodi lymphatici iliaci externi [NA].

facial l. n.'s, a chain of l. n.'s lying along the facial vein that receive afferent vessels from the eyelids, nose, cheek, lip, and gums, and send efferent vessels to the submandibular nodes. SYN nodi lymphatici faciales [NA].

fibular l. n., a small inconstant l. n. located along the course of the peroneal vein. SYN nodus fibularis [NA], fibular node, peroneal node.

foraminal l. n., one of the hepatic nodes located adjacent to the epiploic foramen. SYN nodus foraminalis [NA], foraminal node.

gastroduodenal l. n.'s, SYN pyloric l. n.'s.

gluteal l. n.'s, nodes of the internal iliac group; they are subdivided into two groups: interior gluteal l. n.'s, located along the inferior gluteal vein; superior gluteal l. n.'s located along the superior gluteal vein. SYN nodi lymphatici gluteales [NA].

hepatic l. n.'s, nodes located along the hepatic artery as far as the porta hepatis; they drain the liver, gallbladder, stomach, duodenum, and pancreas, and send efferents to the celiac nodes. SYN nodi lymphatici hepatici [NA].

hilar l. n.'s, SYN bronchopulmonary l. n.'s.

ileocolic l. n.'s, nodes located along the ileocolic artery that drain lymph from the ascending colon to the superior mesenteric nodes. SYN nodi lymphatici ileocolici [NA].

inferior epigastric l. n.'s, three or four nodes placed along the inferior epigastric vessels; they receive afferents from the lower abdominal wall and empty into the external iliac nodes. SYN nodi lymphatici epigastrici inferiores [NA].

inferior mesenteric l. n.'s >, nodes located along the inferior mesenteric artery and its branches that drain the upper part of the rectum, the sigmoid colon, and descending colon. SYN nodi lymphatici mesenterici inferiores [NA].

inferior phrenic l. n.'s, small l. n.'s associated with the inferior phrenic vessels. SYN nodi lymphatici phrenici inferiores [NA].

inferior tracheobronchial l. n.'s, several large l. n.'s inferior to the tracheal bifurcation; they receive afferents from the bronchopulmonary nodes and the heart, and send efferents to the superior tracheobronchial and tracheal nodes. SYN nodi lymphatici tracheobronchiales inferiores [NA], bifurcation l. n.'s, carinal l. n.'s.

infra-auricular deep parotid l. n.'s, small l. n.'s located deep to the parotid fascia and below the ear. SYN nodi lymphatici parotidei profundi infra-auriculares [NA], infra-auricular subfascial parotid l. n.'s.

infra-auricular subfascial parotid l. n.'s, SYN infra-auricular deep parotid l. n.'s.

intercostal l. n.'s, one or two small nodes located posteriorly in each intercostal space; they receive lymph from the parietal pleura, intercostal space, and posterior body wall; the nodes in the upper spaces empty into the thoracic duct; the nodes in the lower spaces form a descending intercostal trunk that opens into the cisterna chyli. SYN nodi lymphatici intercostales [NA].

interiliac l. n.'s, several l. n.'s located between the external and internal iliac arteries and the obturator artery; these nodes are considered by some to be part of the medial external iliac l. n.'s. SYN nodi lymphatici interiliaci [NA].

intermediate lacunar l. n., a l. n. of the external iliac group located between the external iliac artery and vein at the vascular lacuna. SYN nodus lacunaris intermedius [NA], intermediate lacunar node.

intermediate lumbar l. n.'s, the chain of lymph nodes located between the aorta and the inferior vena cava. SYN nodi lymphatici lumbales intermedii [NA], lumbar l. n.'s.

internal iliac l. n.'s, nodes that lie along the internal iliac artery and its branches; they receive lymph from the pelvic viscera, the gluteal region, and the deep parts of the perineum, and send efferent vessels to the common iliac nodes. SYN nodi lymphatici iliaci interni [NA].

interpectoral l. n.'s, small l. n.'s located between the pectoralis major and minor muscles; they receive lymph from the muscles and the mammary gland, and deliver lymph to the axillary lymphatic plexus. SYN nodi lymphatici interpectorales [NA].

intraglandular deep parotid l. n.'s, small l. n.'s of the deep parotid group lying within the parotid gland. SYN nodi lymphatici parotidei intraglandulares [NA], intraglandular parotid l. n.'s.

intraglandular parotid l. n.'s, SYN intraglandular deep parotid l. n.'s.

jugulo-digastric l. n., a prominent l. n. in the deep lateral cervical group lying below the digastric muscle and anterior to the internal jugular vein; it receives lymphatic drainage from the pharynx, palatine tonsil, and tongue. SYN nodus jugulodigastricus [NA], jugulodigastric node, subdigastric node.

jugulo-omohyoid l. n., a l. n. of the lateral deep cervical group that lies above the intermediate tendon of the omohyoid muscle and anterior to the internal jugular vein; it receives lymphatic drainage from the submental, submandibular, and deep anterior cervical nodes; its efferent vessels go to other deep lateral cervical nodes. SYN nodus jugulo-omohyoideus [NA], jugulo-omohyoid node.

juxta-esophageal pulmonary l. n.'s, **juxta-esophageal l. n.'s,**

several nodes of the posterior mediastinal group located along either side of the esophagus; they receive lymph from both the esophagus and the lungs. SYN nodi lymphatici juxta-esophageales pulmonales [NA].

juxta-intestinal l. n.'s, the mesenteric l. n.'s located in immediate proximity to the jejunum or ileum. SYN nodi lymphatici juxta-intestinales [NA].

lateral deep cervical l. n.'s, the l. n.'s located in the posterior triangle of the neck beneath the deep cervical fascia; they empty into the jugular trunk on the right or left side; the group is subdivided into four smaller chains: anterior jugular l. n.'s, lateral jugular l. n.'s, accessory nerve l. n.'s, and supraclavicular l. n.'s. SYN nodi lymphatici cervicales laterales profundi [NA].

lateral group of axillary l. n.'s, l. n.'s along the brachial vein that receive lymph drainage from most of the free superior limb and send efferent vessels to the central group of axillary l. n.'s. SYN nodi lymphatici brachiales [NA], brachial l. n.'s.

lateral jugular l. n.'s, nodes of the lateral deep cervical group lying lateral to the internal jugular vein; they usually empty into the jugular trunk. SYN nodi lymphatici jugulares laterales [NA].

lateral lacunar l. n., a l. n. of the external iliac group located lateral to the external iliac artery at the vascular lacuna. SYN nodus lacunaris lateralis [NA], lateral lacunar node.

lateral pericardiac l. n.'s, small l. n.'s located along the pericardiacophrenic vessels, they drain the pericardium. SYN nodi lymphatici pericardiales laterales [NA].

lateral superficial cervical l. n.'s, one to four nodes lying along the external jugular vein; they drain the skin and superficial structures over the region of the sternocleidomastoid muscle and send efferent vessels to the deep lateral cervical l. n.'s. SYN nodi lymphatici cervicales laterales superficiales [NA].

left colic l. n.'s, small nodes along the left colic artery and its branches that drain the left flexure and upper part of the descending colon; efferent vessels pass to the inferior mesenteric nodes. SYN nodi lymphatici colici sinistri [NA].

left gastric l. n.'s, nodes located along the left gastric artery and its branches; they are divided into paracardial, upper and lower groups. SYN nodi lymphatici gastrici sinistri [NA], superior gastric l. n.'s.

left gastroepiploic l. n.'s, nodes located in the greater omentum along the left gastroepiploic artery that drain part of the greater curvature of the stomach and greater omentum. SYN nodi lymphatici gastro-omentales sinistri [NA], left gastro-omental nodes.

left lumbar l. n.'s, the chain of l. n.'s associated with the aorta in the abdomen; it is divided into three groups: lateral aortic l. n.'s on the left of the aorta; pre-aortic l. n.'s in front of the aorta; post-aortic l. n.'s, behind the aorta. SYN nodi lymphatici lumbales sinistri [NA], lumbar l. n.'s.

l. n. of ligamentum arteriosum, SYN *node* of ligamentum arteriosum.

lingual l. n.'s, l. n. along the lingual vein receiving drainage from the tongue (except tip); drain to submandibular l. n.'s. SYN nodi lymphatici linguales [NA].

lumbar l. n.'s, SYN right lumbar l. n.'s, intermediate lumbar l. n.'s, left lumbar l. n.'s.

malar l. n., one of the facial l. n.'s located near the zygomatic minor muscle. SYN nodus malaris [NA], malar node.

mandibular l. n., one of the facial l. n.'s located by the facial artery near the point it crosses the mandible. SYN nodus mandibularis [NA], mandibular nodes.

mastoid l. n.'s, SYN retroauricular l. n.'s.

medial lacunar l. n., a l. n. of the external iliac group located medial to the external iliac vein at the vascular lacuna. SYN nodus lacunaris medialis [NA], medial lacunar node.

mesenteric l. n.'s, nodes located in the mesentery; they are of three classes: mesenteric l. n.'s, juxta-intestinal l. n.'s, and the superior middle group of mesenteric l. n.'s. SYN nodi lymphatici mesenterici [NA].

mesocolic l. n.'s, nodes located in the mesocolon; they are of two classes: para-colic l. n.'s, located in immediate proximity to the colon; colic l. n.'s located along the arteries supplying the colon. SYN nodi lymphatici mesocolici [NA], nodi lymphatici paracolici.

middle colic l. n.'s, nodes along the middle colic artery and its branches that drain the right colic flexure and most of the transverse colon. SYN nodi lymphatici colici medii [NA].

middle group of mesenteric l. n.'s, the mesenteric l. n.'s located along the intestinal (jejunal and ileal) branches of the superior mesenteric artery. SYN nodi lymphatici superiores centrales [NA], central mesenteric l. n.'s.

middle rectal l. n., a l. n. along the middle rectal artery that receives afferents from the pararectal nodes and sends efferents to the internal iliac nodes. SYN middle rectal node, nodus rectalis medius.

nasolabial l. n., one of the facial l. n.'s located near the junction of the superior labial and facial arteries. SYN nodus nasolabialis [NA], nasolabial node.

obturator l. n.'s, nodes of the internal iliac group located along the obturator artery. SYN nodi lymphatici obturatorii [NA].

occipital l. n.'s, one or two small nodes along the occipital vessels close to the trapezius muscle that receive afferents from the posterior scalp and drain into the superior deep cervical nodes. SYN nodi lymphatici occipitales [NA].

pancreatic l. n.'s, nodes draining the body and tail of the pancreas; they are subdivided into two groups: inferior pancreatic l. n.'s (nodi lymphatici pancreatici inferiores [NA]), located along the inferior pancreatic artery; superior pancreatic l. n.'s (nodi lymphatici pancreatici superiores [NA]), located along the splenic artery near the origin of its pancreatic branches. SYN nodi lymphatici pancreatici [NA].

pancreaticoduodenal l. n.'s, nodes along the superior and inferior pancreaticoduodenal arteries. SYN nodi lymphatici pancreaticoduodenales [NA].

pancreaticosplenic l. n.'s, l. n.'s of the pancreatic tail and spleen, receiving afferents from both organs plus the greater curvature of the stomach; they drain to the celiac l. n.'s. SYN nodi lymphatici pancreticolienales [NA].

paramammary l. n.'s, several l. n.'s on the lateral side of the mammary gland that receive afferents from the mammary gland and send efferents to the axillary pectoral group of l. n.'s. The paramammary l. n.'s are commonly considered as part of the pectoral group of axillary nodes. SYN nodi lymphatici paramammarii [NA].

pararectal l. n.'s, nodes located on either side of the rectum; they send efferents to the middle rectal and superior rectal nodes. SYN nodi lymphatici pararectales [NA], nodi lymphatici anorectales☆ [NA], anorectal l. n.'s.

parasternal l. n.'s, a number of small nodes that lie along the course of the internal thoracic vessels; lymph enters these nodes from the anterior intercostal spaces, pericardium, diaphragm, liver and medial mammary gland; the efferent vessels pass upward to join the bronchomediastinal trunk of the same side. SYN nodi lymphatici parasternales [NA].

paratracheal l. n., nodes along the sides of the trachea in the neck and in the posterior mediastinum; receive drainage of superior (and inferior) tracheobranchial (nodes, trachea and esophagus); drain to bronchomediastinal lymphatic trunk(s), thoracic duct. SYN nodi lymphatici paratracheales [NA], tracheal l. n.'s.

parauterine l. n.'s, nodes on either side of the uterus draining lymph to the internal iliac nodes and to the lumbar nodes via lymphatic vessels following the ovarian arteries. SYN nodi lymphatici parauterini [NA].

paravaginal l. n.'s, l. n.'s in association with the vagina; they drain to the internal iliac nodes. SYN nodi lymphatici paravaginales [NA].

paravesical l. n.'s, the l. n.'s located around the urinary bladder and, in the male, the prostate; there are three groups: prevesicular l. n.'s, in front of the bladder; lateral vesical l. n.'s, on the right and left sides; postvesicular l. n.'s behind the bladder.

parietal l. n.'s, the l. n.'s draining the walls of the abdomen or of the pelvis. SYN nodi lymphatici parietales [NA], parietal nodes.

pectoral group of axillary l. n.'s, l. n.'s located along the lateral thoracic vein; they receive the drainage of the pectoral region, including most of the drainage of the breast. SYN nodi lymphatici axillaris pectorales [NA], anterior group of axillary l. n.'s.

popliteal l. n.'s, two groups of nodes located in the popliteal fossa: the superficial popliteal l. n.'s, located around the termination of the small saphenous vein, that drain the skin of the back of the leg and lateral side of the foot; and the deep popliteal l. n.'s, located around the popliteal vessels, that drain the superficial group, the deep structures of the leg, and the knee joint. SYN nodi lymphatici popliteales [NA].

posterior group of axillary l. n.'s, SYN subscapular group of axillary l. n.'s.

posterior mediastinal l. n.'s, nodes located along the thoracic aorta; they receive vessels from the esophagus, diaphragm, liver and pericardium and send efferents to the thoracic duct and bronchomediastinal lymphatic trunk(s). SYN nodi lymphatici mediastinales posteriores [NA].

posterior tibial l. n., a small inconstant l. n. located along the course of the posterior tibial artery. SYN nodus tibialis posterior [NA], posterior tibial node.

preauricular deep parotid l. n.'s, SYN *nodi lymphatici parotidei profundi preauriculares,* under *nodus lymphaticus.*

prececal l. n.'s, nodes located in front of the cecum draining lymph to the ileocolic nodes. SYN nodi lymphatici prececales [NA].

prelaryngeal l. n.'s, l. n.'s of the anterior deep cervical group that lie in front of the larynx; they drain into the lateral deep lateral cervical nodes. SYN nodi lymphatici prelaryngeales [NA].

prepericardiac l. n.'s, several small l. n.'s located between the pericardium and the sternum, in the anterior mediastinum. SYN nodi lymphatici prepericardiales [NA].

pretracheal l. n.'s, l. n.'s of the anterior deep cervical group that lie in front of the trachea; they drain into the lateral deep cervical group or into the anterior mediastinal group. SYN nodi lymphatici pretracheales [NA].

prevertebral l. n.'s, l. n.'s posterior to the thoracic aorta. SYN nodi lymphatici prevertebrales [NA].

promontory common iliac l. n.'s, nodes of the common iliac group located at the promontory of the sacrum. SYN nodi lymphatici promontorii [NA], nodi lymphatici iliaci communes promontorii.

pulmonary l. n.'s, small nodes that occur along the bronchi within the lung; they receive the drainage from localized areas of the lung and send efferents to bronchopulmonary nodes. SYN nodi lymphatici pulmonales.

pyloric l. n.'s, group of nodes surrounding the pylorus, draining lymph into the right gastric or the right gastro-omental l. n.'s; it is divided into three smaller groups: suprapyloric l. n.'s, above the pylorus; subpyloric l. n.'s, below the pylorus; and retropyloric l. n.'s, behind the pylorus. SYN nodi lymphatici pylorici [NA], gastroduodenal l. n.'s.

retroauricular l. n.'s, two or three nodes in the region of the mastoid process; they receive afferent lymphatic vessels from the scalp and auricle and send efferent vessels to the superior deep cervical nodes. SYN nodi lymphatici mastoidei [NA], mastoid l. n.'s.

retrocecal l. n.'s, nodes located behind the cecum draining lymph into the ileocolic nodes. SYN nodi lymphatici retrocecales [NA].

retropharyngeal l. n.'s, the three groups of l. n.'s, one median and two lateral, located between the pharynx and the prevertebral fascia; they receive lymph from the nasopharynx, the auditory tube, and the atlanto-occipital and atlantoaxial joints. SYN nodi lymphatici retropharyngeales [NA].

retropyloric l. n.'s, a group of l. n.'s located behind the pylorus. SYN nodi retropylorici [NA], retropyloric nodes.

right colic l. n.'s, nodes located along the right colic artery that drain the upper part of the ascending colon. SYN nodi lymphatici colici dextri [NA].

right gastric l. n.'s, small nodes along the course of the right gastric artery that drain part of the lesser curvature of the stomach. SYN nodi lymphatici gastrici dextri [NA].

right gastroepiploic l. n.'s, nodes located in the greater omentum along the right gastroepiploic artery that drain part of the greater curvature of the stomach and the greater omentum. SYN nodi lymphatici gastro-omentales dextri [NA], right gastro-omental l. n.'s.

right gastro-omental l. n.'s, SYN right gastroepiploic l. n.'s.

right lumbar l. n.'s, the chain of l. n.'s associated with the inferior vena cava; it is divided into three groups: *nodi lymphatici cavales laterales* on the right of the inferior vena cava; *nodi lymphatici precavales,* in front of the inferior vena cava; *nodi lymphatici postcavales,* under *nodus lymphaticus,* behind the inferior vena cava. SYN nodi lymphatici lumbales dextri [NA], lumbar l. n.'s.

sacral l. n.'s, nodes in the concavity of the sacrum that drain the rectum and posterior pelvic wall. SYN nodi lymphatici sacrales [NA].

sigmoid l. n.'s, nodes of the inferior mesenteric group, located along the sigmoid arteries. SYN nodi lymphatici sigmoidei [NA].

splenic l. n.'s, nodes near the hilum of the spleen; they receive afferents from the spleen and stomach, and send efferents to the pancreatic-postsplenic and celiac nodes. SYN nodi lymphatici splenici [NA], nodi lymphatici lienales* [NA].

subaortic l. n.'s, nodes of the common iliac group located at the bifurcation of the aorta. SYN nodi lymphatici subaortici [NA].

submandibular l. n.'s, four or five nodes that lie between the mandible and the submandibular gland; they receive vessels from the face below the eye and from the tongue and drain into the superior deep cervical nodes, particularly the jugulodigastric node. SYN nodi lymphatici submandibulares [NA].

submental l. n.'s, small nodes that lie superficial to the mylohyoid muscle; they receive afferents from the lower lip, chin, and the tip of the tongue, and send efferents to the superior deep cervical nodes. SYN nodi lymphatici submentales [NA].

subpyloric l. n.'s, a group of l. n.'s located below the pylorus. SYN nodi subpylorici [NA], subpyloric node.

subscapular group of axillary l. n.'s, l. n.'s of the axillary region located along the subscapular vein and its tributaries; they receive afferent vessels from the dorsal surface of the thorax and scapular region, and send efferent vessels to the central group of l. n.'s. SYN nodi lymphatici axillares subscapulares [NA], posterior group of axillary l. n.'s.

superficial inguinal l. n.'s, a group of 12 to 20 nodes that lie in the subcutaneous tissue below the inguinal ligament and along the terminal part of the great saphenous vein; they drain the skin and subcutaneous tissue of the lower abdominal wall, perineum, buttock, external genitalia, and lower limb; they are subdivided into three groups: inferior (vertical) group of superficial inguinal l. n.'s, located inferior to the saphenous opening receiving drainage of the lower limb; superolateral (lateral horizontal) superficial inguinal l. n.'s located lateral to the saphenous opening receiving drainage of lateral buttock and lower anterior abdominal wall; and superomedial (medial horizontal) superficial inguinal l. n.'s, located medial to the saphenous opening, receiving drainage of the perineum and external genitalia. SYN nodi lymphatici inguinales superficiales [NA].

superficial parotid l. n.'s, several small l. n.'s located in the subcutaneous tissue in the parotid region. SYN nodi lymphatici parotidei superficiales [NA].

superior gastric l. n.'s, SYN left gastric l. n.'s.

superior mesenteric l. n.'s, the numerous nodes located in the mesentery along the superior mesenteric artery; they receive lymph from the central mesenteric l. n.'s and drain into the intestinal lymph trunk. SYN nodi lymphatici mesenterici superiores [NA], nodi lymphatici centrales.

superior phrenic l. n.'s, three groups of small nodes, anterior, middle, and posterior, on the upper surface of the diaphragm; they receive afferents from the liver, diaphragm, and intercostal spaces and send efferents to parasternal and posterior mediastinal nodes. SYN nodi lymphatici phrenici superiores [NA], diaphragmatic nodes.

superior rectal l. n.'s, nodes of the inferior mesenteric group, located along the superior rectal artery. SYN nodi lymphatici rectales superiores [NA].

superior tracheobronchial l. n.'s, several large lymph nodes of the posterior mediastinal group located superior to the bronchi at their union with the trachea; receives lymph from inferior tracheobronchial lymph nodes and bronchopulmonary nodes; drain to

ly

paratracheal nodes. SYN nodi lymphatici tracheobronchiales superiores [NA].

supraclavicular l. n.'s, the portion of the inferior deep cervical group located between the inferior belly of the omohyoid muscle and the clavicle; afferent vessels come from adjacent regions including the mediastinum; efferent vessels terminate in the subclavian trunk. SYN nodi lymphatici supraclaviculares [NA].

suprapyloric l. n., a l. n. located above the pylorus. SYN nodus suprapyloricus [NA], suprapyloric node.

thyroid l. n.'s, nodes of the anterior deep cervical group located around the thyroid gland; they drain into the lateral deep cervical group. SYN nodi lymphatici thyroidei [NA].

tracheal l. n.'s, SYN paratracheal l. n.

visceral l. n.'s, the l. n.'s draining the viscera of the abdomen or of the pelvis. SYN nodi viscerales [NA], visceral nodes.

△**lympho-, lymph-.** Lymph. [L. *lympha,* spring water]

lym·pho·ad·e·no·ma (lim′fō-adĕ-nō′mǎ). **1.** Obsolete term for an enlarged lymph node. **2.** Obsolete term for Hodgkin's *disease.*

lym·pho·blast (lim′fō-blast). A young immature cell that matures into a lymphocyte and is characterized by more abundant cytoplasm than in a lymphocyte, a nucleus in which the chromatin is finer than in a lymphocyte (but coarser than in a myeloblast), and one or two rather prominent nucleoli. SYN lymphocytoblast. [lympho- + G. *blastos,* germ]

lym·pho·blas·tic (lim-fō-blas′tik). Pertaining to the production of lymphocytes.

lym·pho·blas·to·ma (lim-fō-blas-tō′mǎ). A form of malignant lymphoma in which the chief cells are lymphoblasts. [lymphoblast + G. *-oma,* tumor]

giant follicular l., SYN nodular *lymphoma.*

lym·pho·blas·to·sis (lim′fō-blas-tō′sis). The presence of lymphoblasts in the peripheral blood; sometimes used as a synonym for acute lymphocytic leukemia. [lymphoblast + G. *-osis,* condition]

lym·pho·cele (lim′fō-sēl). A cystic mass that contains lymph, usually from diseased or injured lymphatic channels. SYN lymphocyst. [lympho- + G. *kēlē,* tumor]

lym·pho·cer·as·tism (lim-fō-ser′as-tizm). The process of formation of cells in the lymphocytic series. [lympho- + G. *kerastos,* mixed, mingled]

lym·pho·ci·ne·sis, lym·pho·ci·ne·sia (lim′fō-si-nē′sis, nē-zē-ǎ). SYN lymphokinesis.

lym·pho·cyst (lim′fō-sist). SYN lymphocele. [lympho- + G. *kystis,* bladder]

lym·pho·cy·ta·phe·re·sis (lim′fō-sī-tǎ-fĕ-rē′sis). Separation and removal of lymphocytes from the withdrawn blood, with the remainder of the blood retransfused into the donor. SYN lymphapheresis. [lymphocyte + G. *aphairesis,* a withdrawal]

lym·pho·cyte (lim′fō-sīt). A white blood cell formed in lymphatic tissue throughout the body (*e.g.,* lymph nodes, spleen, thymus, tonsils, Peyer's patches, and sometimes in bone marrow) and in normal adults comprising approximately 22 to 28% of the total number of leukocytes in the circulating blood. L.'s are generally small (7 to 8 μm), but larger forms are frequent (10 to 20 μm); with Wright's (or a similar) stain, the nucleus is deeply colored (purple-blue), and is composed of dense aggregates of chromatin within a sharply defined nuclear membrane; the nucleus is usually round, but may be slightly indented, and is eccentrically situated within a relatively small amount of light blue cytoplasm that ordinarily contains no granules; especially in larger forms, the cytoplasm may be fairly abundant and include several bright red-violet fine granules; in contrast to granules of the myeloid series of cells, those in l.'s do not yield a positive oxidase or peroxidase reaction. SYN lymph cell, lympholeukocyte. [lympho- + G. *kytos,* call]

B l., an immunologically important l. that is not thymus-dependent, is of short life, and resembles the bursa-derived l. of birds in that it is responsible for the production of immunoglobulins, *i.e.,* it is the precursor of the plasma cell and expresses immunoglobulins on its surface but does not release them. It does not play a direct role in cell-mediated immunity. SEE ALSO T l. SYN B cell (2).

lymphocytes		
	T- lymphocytes	B-lymphocytes
place of formation	marrow (from undifferentiated stem cells)	
regulating organ or place of differentiation	thymus	lymphoid tissue of intestine (Peyer's patches); in birds, bursa of Fabricius
function	cell-transmitted immunity	humoral immunity
cell function forms	T-memory, killer, helper, suppressor cells	B-memory, antibody-producing cells (plasma cells)
interactions	see "immunity" (and diagram s.v.)	
surface characteristics of cell membrane	surface structures, distinguished by monoclonal antibodies (see "marker")	
	T-cell (antigen) receptor	receptor for complement factor C3
	receptor for sheep erythrocyte (SRBC [sheep red blood cell] receptor); shown by rosette test	receptor for mouse erythrocyte
transformation (blastogenesis, mitosis) stimulants	antigens (e.g., transplantation or tissue, bacterial antigen), mitogens (e.g., phytohemagglutinin [PHA], concanavalin A [con A])	antigens (indirect) interleukin II, pokeweed mitogen (PWM)
soluble products of activated lymphocytes	lymphokines	immunoglobulins (antibodies)
defects	see "immunodeficiency"	
malignant proliferation	see "lymphoma" (diagram), lymphatic leukemia	

pre-B l., an early B-lymphoid type cell that is recognized by immunofluorescence as a μ-positive, L-chain-negative bone marrow cell.

Rieder's l., an abnormal form of l. that has a greatly indented (or lobed), slightly twisted nucleus; such cells are usually observed in certain examples of chronic lymphocytic leukemia.

T l., a thymocyte-derived l. of immunological importance that is long-lived (months to years) and is responsible for cell-mediated immunity. T l.'s form rosettes with sheep erythrocytes and, in the presence of transforming agents (mitogens), differentiate and divide. These cells have the characteristic T3 surface marker and may be further divided into subsets according to function, such as helper, cytotoxic, etc. SEE ALSO B l. SYN T cell.

transformed l., SEE lymphocyte *transformation.*

tumor-infiltrating l.'s (lim′fō-sītz), l.'s collected from the site of a tumor and exposed to IL-2 *in vitro.* When these cells are injected back into the tumor bearing host, they will specifically kill the tumor from which they originated.

lym·pho·cy·the·mia (lim'fō-sī-thē'mē-ă). SYN lymphocytosis.

lym·pho·cyt·ic (lim-fō-sit'ik). Pertaining to or characterized by lymphocytes.

lym·pho·cy·to·blast (lim-fō-sī'tō-blast). SYN lymphoblast. [lymphocyte + G. *blastos,* germ]

lym·pho·cy·to·ma (lim'fō-sī-tō'mă). A circumscribed nodule or mass of mature lymphocytes, grossly resembling a neoplasm. [lymphocyte + G. *-oma,* tumor]

benign l. cutis, a soft red to violaceous skin nodule often involving the head, caused by dense infiltration of the dermis by lymphocytes and histiocytes, often forming lymphoid follicles, separated from the epidermis by a narrow noninfiltrating layer. SYN Spiegler-Fendt pseudolymphoma, Spiegler-Fendt sarcoid.

lym·pho·cy·to·pe·nia (lim'fō-sī-tō-pē'nē-ă). SYN lymphopenia.

lym·pho·cy·to·poi·e·sis (lim'fō-sī-tō-poy-ē'sis). The formation of lymphocytes. [lymphocyte + G. *poiēsis,* a making]

lym·pho·cy·to·sis (lim'fō-sī-tō'sis). A form of actual or relative leukocytosis in which there is an increase in the number of lymphocytes. SYN lymphocythemia, lymphocytic leukocytosis.

lym·pho·der·ma (lim'fō-der'mă). A condition resulting from any disease of the cutaneous lymphatic vessels. [lympho- + G. *derma,* skin]

lym·pho·duct (lim'fō-dŭkt). A lymphatic vessel. SEE lymph *vessels,* under *vessel.* [lympho- + L. *ductus,* a leading]

lym·pho·ep·i·the·li·o·ma (lim'fō-ep-i-thē-lē-ō'mă). A poorly differentiated radiosensitive squamous cell carcinoma involving lymphoid tissue in the region of the tonsils and nasopharynx; composed of irregular sheets, or small groups, of neoplastic epithelial cells (squamous or undifferentiated), with a slight to moderate amount of fibrous stroma that contains numerous lymphocytes; metastasizes at an early stage to cervical lymph nodes. [lympho- + epithelium + *-oma,* tumor]

lym·pho·gen·e·sis (lim-fō-gen'ĕ-sis). Lymph production. [lympho- + G. *genesis,* production]

lym·pho·gen·ic (lim-fō-jen'ik). SYN lymphogenous (1).

lym·phog·e·nous (lim-foj'ĕ-nŭs). 1. Originating from lymph or the lymphatic system. SYN lymphogenic. 2. Producing lymph.

lym·pho·glan·du·la (lim-fō-glan'dū-lă). SYN lymph node.

lym·pho·gran·u·lo·ma (lim'fō-gran-yū-lō'mă). 1. Old nonspecific term used with reference to a few basically dissimilar diseases in which the pathologic processes result in granulomas or granuloma-like lesions, especially in various groups of lymph nodes (which then become conspicuously enlarged). 2. Old term for Hodgkin's disease.

l. benig'num, old term for sarcoidosis.

l. inguina'le, SYN venereal l.

l. malig'num, old term for Hodgkin's disease.

Schaumann's l., old eponym for sarcoidosis.

venereal l., l. vene'reum, a venereal infection usually caused by *Chlamydia trachomatis,* and characterized by a transient genital ulcer and inguinal adenopathy in the male; in the female, perirectal lymph nodes are involved and rectal stricture is a common occurrence. SYN climatic bubo, l. inguinale, Nicolas-Favre disease, sixth venereal disease, tropical bubo.

lym·pho·gran·u·lo·ma·to·sis (lim-fō-gran'yū-lō-mă-tō'sis). Any condition characterized by the occurrence of multiple and widely distributed lymphogranulomas.

lym·phog·ra·phy (lim-fog'ră-fē). Visualization of lymphatics (lymphangiography), lymph nodes (lymphadenography), or both by radiography following the intra-lymphatic injection of a contrast medium, usually an iodized oil. [lympho- + *graphō,* to write]

lym·pho·his·ti·o·cy·to·sis (lim'fō-his'tē-ō-sī-tō'sis). Proliferation or infiltration of lymphocytes and histiocytes.

lym·phoid (lim'foyd). 1. Resembling lymph or lymphatic tissue, or pertaining to the lymphatic system. 2. SYN adenoid (1). [lympho- + G. *eidos,* appearance]

lym·phoi·dec·to·my (lim-foy-dek'tō-mē). Excision of lymphoid tissue. [lymphoid + G. *ektomē,* excision]

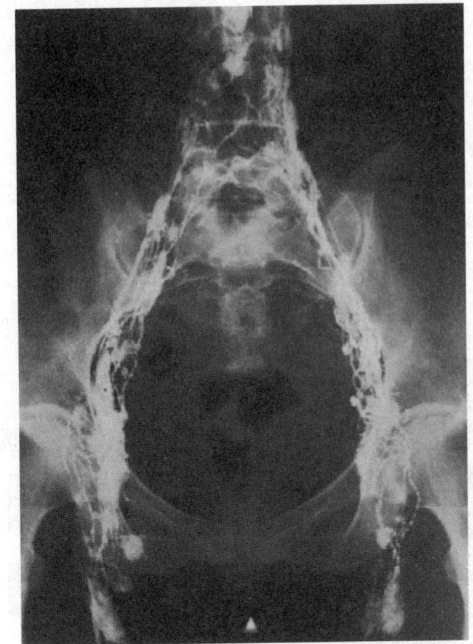

lymphography:
posterior projection of thoracic duct

lym·phoi·do·cyte (lim-foy'dō-sīt). A primitive mesenchymal cell believed to be capable of differentiating into all types of lymphoid cells, including lymphocytes, littoral cells, and reticular cells of lymph nodes.

lym·pho·kines (lim'fō-kīnz). Hormone-like peptides, released by activated lymphocytes that mediate immune responses. [*lympho*cyte + G. *kineō,* to set in motion]

lym·pho·ki·ne·sis (lim'fō-ki-nē'sis). 1. Circulation of lymph in the lymphatic vessels and through the lymph nodes. 2. Movement of endolymph in the semicircular canals of the inner ear. SYN lymphocinesis, lymphocinesia. [lympho- + G. *kinēsis,* movement]

lym·pho·leu·ko·cyte (lim'fō-lū'kō-sīt). SYN lymphocyte.

lym·phol·o·gy (lim-fol'ō-jē). SYN lymphangiology. [lympho- + G. *logos,* study]

lym·pho·ma (lim-fō'mă). Obsolete term for malignant l. [lympho- + G. *-oma,* tumor]

Lymphomas are among the most treatable cancers, with survival rates having steadily climbed from 31% in the 1960s to 50% in the 1990s. Hodgkin's l., which generally strikes between ages 20 and 30, is highly curable, primarily because of therapeutic advances in bone marrow transplants. Non-Hodgkin's types, mainly afflicting those over 50, have proven more difficult. Some ten varieties of l. have been identified, and it represents the third most rapidly increasing form of cancer in the U.S. (affecting about 17 of 100,000 people). Non-Hodgkin's l. and l. of the brain are among the commonest AIDS-related malignancies. Non-Hodgkin's cases among HIV-positive people showed five- to tenfold increases in some locales between the mid-1970s and late 1980s.

adult T-cell l. (ATL), an acute or subacute disease associated with a human T-cell virus, with lymphadenopathy, hepatosplenomegaly, skin lesions, peripheral blood involvement, and hypercalcemia. SYN adult T-cell leukemia.

anaplastic large cell l., a form of lymphoma characterized by

ly

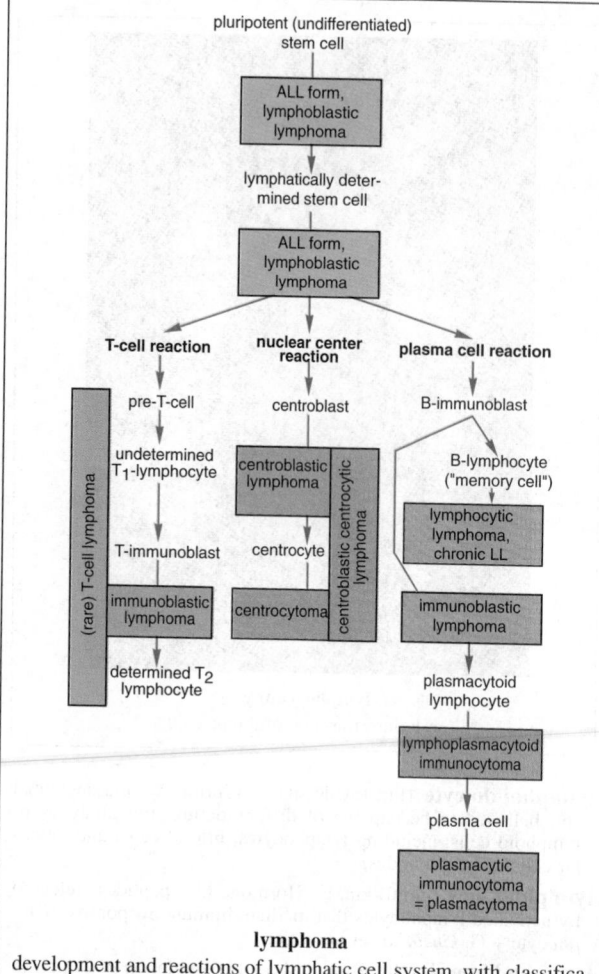

lymphoma

development and reactions of lymphatic cell system, with classification of non-Hodgkin's lymphomas

anaplasia of cells, sinusoidal growth, and immunoreactivity with CD30 (Ki-1 or Ber-H2). SYN Ki-1+ l.

benign l. of the rectum, a rectal polyp composed of lymphoid tissue with follicle formation, covered by mucosa.

Burkitt's l., a form of malignant l. reported in African children, frequently involving facial bones, ovaries, and abdominal lymph nodes, which are infiltrated by undifferentiated stem cells with scattered pale macrophages containing nuclear debris; undifferentiated cells show numerous mitoses from lymphoid germinal center B cells. Geographical distribution of Burkitt's l. suggests that it is found in areas with endemic malaria and caused by Epstein-Barr virus, a member of the family Herpesviridae; occasional cases of l. with similar features have been reported in the United States.

canine malignant l., a progressive fatal disease of dogs characterized by neoplastic transformation and proliferation of lymphoid cells, usually originating in solid lymphoid organs (lymphosarcoma) or bone marrow (lymphocytic leukemia).

diffuse small cleaved cell l., diffuse poorly differentiated lymphocytic l.; follicular center cell l. that lacks a follicular pattern; malignancy is of intermediate grade.

follicular l., SYN nodular l.

follicular predominantly large cell l., a B-cell l. of intermediate malignancy. SYN nodular histiocytic l.

follicular predominantly small cleaved cell l., SYN poorly differentiated lymphocytic l.

histiocytic l., a malignant tumor of reticular tissue composed predominantly of neoplastic histiocytes. SEE ALSO large cell l.

Hodgkin's l., SYN Hodgkin's *disease.*

immunoblastic l., a monomorphous proliferation of immunoblasts involving the lymph nodes; it may develop in some patients with angioimmunoblastic lymphadenopathy.

Ki-1+ l., SYN anaplastic large cell l.

large cell l., l. composed of large mononuclear cells of undetermined type. Many l.'s formerly classified as histiocytic have in recent years been shown to consist of large lymphocytes.

Lennert's l., malignant l. with a high proportion of diffusely scattered epithelioid cells, tonsillar involvement, and an unpredictable course. SYN Lennert's lesion.

lymphoblastic l., a diffuse l. in children, with supradiaphragmatic distribution and T lymphocytes having convoluted nuclei; many patients develop acute lymphoblastic leukemia.

malignant l., general term for ordinarily malignant neoplasms of lymphoid and reticuloendothelial tissues which present as apparently circumscribed solid tumors composed of cells that appear primitive or resemble lymphocytes, plasma cells, or histiocytes. L.'s appear most frequently in lymph nodes, spleen, or other normal sites of lymphoreticular tissue; when disseminated, l.'s, especially of the lymphocytic type, may invade the peripheral blood and manifest as leukemia. L.'s are classified by cell type, degrees of differentiation, and nodular or diffuse pattern; Hodgkin's disease and Burkitt's l. are special forms.

Mediterranean l., SYN immunoproliferative small intestinal *disease.*

nodular l., malignant l. arising from lymphoid follicular B cells which may be small or large, growing in a nodular pattern. SYN follicular l., giant follicular lymphoblastoma.

nodular histiocytic l., SYN follicular predominantly large cell l.

non-Hodgkin's l., a l. other than Hodgkin's disease, classified by Rappaport into a nodular or diffuse tumor pattern and by cell type; a working or international formulation separates such l.'s into low, intermediate, and high grade malignancy and into cytologic subtypes reflecting follicular center cell or other origin.

poorly differentiated lymphocytic l. (PDLL), a B-cell l. with nodular or diffuse lymph node or bone marrow involvement by large lymphoid cells. SYN follicular predominantly small cleaved cell l.

small lymphocytic l., SYN well-differentiated lymphocytic l.

T cell-rich, B cell l., a B cell l. in which more than 90% of the cells are of T cell origin, masking the large cells that form the neoplastic B cell component. SEE ALSO adult T-cell l.

well-differentiated lymphocytic l. (WDLL), essentially the same disease as chronic lymphocytic leukemia, except that lymphocytes are not increased in the peripheral blood; lymph nodes are enlarged and other lymphoid tissue or bone marrow is infiltrated by small lymphocytes. SYN small lymphocytic l.

lym·pho·ma·toid (lim-fō′mă-toyd). Resembling a lymphoma.

lym·pho·ma·to·sis (lim′fō-mă-to′sis). Any condition characterized by the occurrence of multiple, widely distributed sites of involvement with lymphoma.

avian l., a group of virus-induced transmissible diseases of chickens and some other birds in which there is lymphoid cell infiltration or formation of lymphomatous tumors in various tissues and organs; the two principal diseases are: 1) the avian leukosis-sarcoma complex-induced lymphoid leukosis, involving the bursa fabricius and various visceral organs, that is associated with viruses of the family Retroviridae; 2) Marek's disease, caused by avian herpesvirus 2 and involving primarily the peripheral nerves and gonads and, to a lesser and more variable extent, other visceral organs, skin, muscle, and the eye. Variability of lesion site prompted other names for avian l., such as big liver disease, ocular l., visceral l. neurolymphomatosis gallinarum, and fowl paralysis. SYN fowl l.

fowl l., SYN avian l.

ocular l., SEE avian l.

visceral l., SEE avian l.

lym·pho·ma·tous (lim-fō′mă-tŭs). Pertaining to or characterized by lymphoma.

lym·pho·my·e·lo·ma (lim′fō-mī′ĕ-lō′mă). A medullary neoplasm that consists of uninuclear, relatively small cells with morphologic features resembling those of lymphocytic forms. [lympho- + G. *myelos,* marrow, + *-oma,* tumor]

lym·pho·myx·o·ma (lim′fō-mik-sō′mă). A soft nonmalignant neoplasm that contains lymphoid tissue in a matrix of loose, areolar connective tissue. [lympho- + G. *myxa,* mucus, + *-oma,* tumor]

lym·pho·path·ia (lim-fō-path′ē-ă). SYN lymphopathy.
  l. vene′reum, an obsolete term for *lymphogranuloma* venereum.

lym·phop·a·thy (lim-fop′ă-thē). Any disease of the lymphatic vessels or lymph nodes. SYN lymphopathia. [lympho- + G. *pathos,* suffering]

lym·pho·pe·nia (lim-fō-pē′nē-ă). A reduction, relative or absolute, in the number of lymphocytes in the circulating blood. SYN lymphocytic leukopenia, lymphocytopenia. [lympho- + G. *penia,* poverty]

lym·pho·plas·ma·phe·re·sis (lim′fō-plaz′mă-fĕ-rē′sis). Separation and removal of lymphocytes and plasma from the withdrawn blood, with the remainder of the blood retransfused into the donor. [lymphocyte + plasma + G. *aphairesis,* a withdrawal]

lym·pho·plas·ty (lim′fō-plas-tē). SYN lymphangioplasty.

lym·pho·poi·e·sis (lim-fō-poy-ē′sis). The formation of lymphatic tissue. [lympho- + G. *poiēsis,* a making]

lym·pho·poi·et·ic (lim-fō-poy-et′ik). Pertaining to or characterized by lymphopoiesis.

lym·pho·re·tic·u·lo·sis (lim′fō-rĕ-tik-yū-lō′sis). Proliferation of the reticuloendothelial cells (macrophages) of the lymph glands.
  benign inoculation l., SYN cat-scratch *disease.*

lym·phor·rha·gia (lim-fō-rā′jē-ă). SYN lymphorrhea. [lympho- + G. *rhēgnymi,* to burst forth]

lym·phor·rhea (lim-fō-rē′ă). An escape of lymph on the surface from ruptured, torn, or cut lymphatic vessels. SYN lymphorrhagia. [lympho- + G. *rhoia,* a flow]

lym·phor·rhoid (lim′fō-royd). A dilation of a lymph channel, resembling a hemorrhoid. [lymh + *-rrhoid,* tending to leak, on the analogy of *hemorrhoid*]

lym·pho·sar·co·ma (lim′fō-sar-kō′mă). Obsolete term for malignant *lymphoma.* [lympho- + G. *sarkōma,* sarcoma]
  bovine l., a systemic malignancy of the lymphoreticular system of cattle which is seen in two etiologically and clinically distinct forms, enzootic bovine *leukosis* and sporadic bovine *leukosis.*

lym·pho·sar·co·ma·to·sis (lim′fō-sar-kō′mă-tō′sis). Obsolete term for a condition characterized by the presence of multiple, widely distributed masses of lymphosarcoma.

lym·pho·scin·tig·ra·phy (lim′fō-sin-tig′ră-fē). Scintillation scanning of lymphatics or lymph nodes following intralymphatic or subcutaneous injection of a radionuclide.

lym·pho·sis (lim-fō′sis). Rarely used term for lymphocytic *leukemia.*

lym·phos·ta·sis (lim-fos′tă-sis). Obstruction of the normal flow of lymph. [lympho- + G. *stasis,* a standing still]

lym·pho·tax·is (lim-fō-tak′sis). The exertion of an effect that attracts or repels lymphocytes. [lympho- + G. *taxis,* orderly arrangement]

lym·pho·tox·ic·i·ty (lim′fō-tok-sis′i-tē). Toxicity to lymphocytes.

lym·pho·tox·in (lim′fō-tok-sin). A lymphokine that lyses or damages many cell types.

lym·phot·ro·phy (lim-fot′rō-fē). Nourishment of the tissues by lymph in parts devoid of blood vessels. [lympho- + G. *trophē,* nourishment]

lym·phu·ria (lim-fū′rē-ă). Discharge of lymph in the urine. [lympho- + G. *ouron,* urine]

lyn·es·tre·nol (lin-es′tren-ol). 17α-Ethynylestr-4-en-17β-ol; 3-desoxynorlutin; a progestational agent, used with mestranol as an oral contraceptive. SYN ethinylestrenol.

⚠**lyo-.** Dissolution. SEE ALSO lyso-. [G. *lyō,* to loosen, dissolve]

ly·o·en·zyme (lī-ō-en′zīm). SYN extracellular *enzyme.*

ly·ol·y·sis (lī-ol′i-sis). Rarely used term for solvolysis.

Lyon, B. B. Vincent, U.S. physician, 1880–1953. SEE Meltzer-L. *test.*

Lyon, Mary F., English cytogeneticist, *1925. SEE L. *hypothesis;* lyonization.

ly·on·i·za·tion (lī′on-i-zā′shŭn). The normal phenomenon that wherever there are two or more haploid sets of X-linked genes in each cell all but one of the genes is inactivated apparently at random and have no phenotypic expression. L. is usual but not invariable for all loci. Its randomness explains the more variable espressivity of X-linked traits in women than in men. L. occurs in men with the Klinefelter (XXY) karyotype. SEE ALSO gene dosage *compensation.* SYN Lyon hypothesis, X-inactivation. [M. Lyon]

ly·o·phil, ly·o·phile (lī′ō-fil, -fīl). A substance that is lyophilic.

ly·o·phil·ic (lī-ō-fil′ik). In colloid chemistry, denoting a dispersed phase having a pronounced affinity for the dispersion medium; when the dispersed phase is l., the colloid is usually a reversible one. SYN lyotropic. [lyo- + G. *phileō,* to love]

ly·oph·i·li·za·tion (lī-of′i-li-zā′shŭn). The process of isolating a solid substance from solution by freezing the solution and evaporating the ice under vacuum. SYN freeze-drying.

ly·o·phobe (lī′ō-fōb). A substance that is lyophobic.

ly·o·pho·bic (lī-ō-fo′bik). In colloid chemistry, denoting a dispersed phase having but slight affinity for the dispersion medium; when the dispersed phase is l., the colloid is usually an irreversible one. [lyo- + G. *phobos,* fear]

ly·o·sorp·tion (lī-ō-sōrp′shŭn). Adsorption of a liquid on a solid surface.

ly·o·tro·pic (lī-ō-trop′ik). SYN lyophilic. [lyo- + G. *tropē,* a turning]

ly·pres·sin (lī′pres-in). [Lys^8]Vasopressin; vasopressin containing lysine in position 8; an antidiuretic and vasopressor hormone. SYN 8-lysine vasopressin.

ly·ra (lī′ră). A lyre-shaped structure. [L. and G. lyre]
  l. davidis, lyre of David, obsolete terms for *commissura fornicis.*
  l. uteri′na, SYN palmate *folds,* under *fold.*

Lys Symbol for lysine, or its radicals in peptides.

⚠**lys-.** SEE lyso-.

ly·sate (lī′sāt). Material produced by the destructive process of lysis.

lyse (līz). To break up, to disintegrate, to effect lysis. SYN lyze.

ly·se·mia (lī-sē′mē-ă). Disintegration or dissolution of red blood cells and the occurrence of hemoglobin in the circulating plasma and in the urine. [lyso- + G. *haima,* blood]

ly·serg·am·ide (lī-serj′ă-mīd). SYN lysergic acid amide.

ly·ser·gic ac·id (lī-ser′jik). The D-isomer is a cleavage product of alkaline hydrolysis of ergot alkaloids, with mol. wt. 268.315; occurs as shiny crystals, slightly soluble in water; a psychotomimetic.
  l. a. amide, a psychotomimetic agent present in *Rivea corymbosa* and *Ipomoea tricolor;* possesses less hallucinogenic potency than does l. a. diethylamide. SYN ergine, lysergamide.
  l. a. diethylamide (LSD), peripherally, a serotonin antagonist; 1 to 2 μg per kg induces hallucinatory states of a visual rather than auditory nature; its use may precipitate psychoses; it has been occasionally used in the treatment of chronic alcoholism and psychotic disorders. SYN lysergide.
  l. a. monoethylamide, a psychotomimetic agent present in *Rivea corymbosa* and *Ipomoea tricolor;* possesses less hallucinatory potency than does l. a. diethylamide.

ly·ser·gide (lī-ser′jīd). SYN lysergic acid diethylamide.

ly·ser·gol (lī-sŭr-jol). A semisynthetic ergot alkaloid.

ly·sin (lī′sin). **1.** A specific complement-fixing antibody that acts destructively on cells and tissues; the various types are designated in accordance with the form of antigen that stimulates the production of the l., *e.g.,* hemolysin, bacteriolysin. **2.** Any substance that causes lysis.

ly·sine (K, Lys) (lī′sēn). $NH_2(CH_2)_4CH(NH_2)COOH$; 2,6-diaminohexanoic acid; the L-isomer is a nutritionally essential α-amino acid found in many proteins; distinguished by an ε-amino group.
  l. decarboxylase, an enzyme that catalyzes the decarboxylation of L-l., with the production of cadaverine and CO_2.

ly·si·ne·mia (lī-si-nē′mē-ă). SEE hyperlysinemia.

8-ly·sine va·so·pres·sin. SYN lypressin.

ly·sin·i·um (lī-sin'ē-um). The cation form of lysine, either lysinium (+1) or lysinium (+2).

ly·sin·o·gen (lī-sin'ō-jen). An antigen that stimulates the formation of a specific lysin.

ly·si·no·gen·ic (lī'si-nō-jen'ik). Having the property of a lysinogen.

ly·sin·u·ria (lī-si-nū'rē-ă). The presence of lysine in the urine.

ly·sis (lī'sis). **1.** Gradual subsidence of the symptoms of an acute disease, a form of the recovery process, as distinguished from crisis. **2.** Destruction of red blood cells, bacteria, and other structures by a specific lysin, usually referred to by the structure destroyed (*e.g.*, hemolysis, bacteriolysis, nephrolysis); may be due to a direct toxin or an immune mechanism, such as antibody reacting with antigen on the surface of a target cell, usually by binding and activation of a series of proteins in the blood with enzymatic activity (complement system). [G. dissolution or loosening]

△**lyso-, lys-.** Lysis, dissolution. SEE ALSO lyo-. [G. *lysis*, a loosening]

ly·so·ceph·a·lin (lī-sō-sef'ă-lin). A lysophosphatidic acid esterified with serine or ethanolamine, *i.e.*, a lysophosphatidylserine or -ethanolamine; analogous to lysolecithin.

ly·so·gen (lī'sō-jen). **1.** That which is capable of inducing lysis. **2.** A bacterium in the state of lysogeny. [lysin + G. *-gen*, producing]

ly·so·gen·e·sis (lī-sō-jen'ĕ-sis). The production of lysins.

ly·so·gen·ic (lī-sō-jen'ik). **1.** Causing or having the power to cause lysis, as the action of certain antibodies and chemical substances. **2.** Pertaining to bacteria in the state of lysogeny.

ly·so·ge·nic·i·ty (lī'sō-jĕ-nis'i-tē). The property of being lysogenic.

ly·so·ge·ni·za·tion (lī'sō-jĕ-ni-zā'shŭn, lī-soj'ĕ-ni-zā'shŭn). The process by which a bacterium becomes lysogenic.

ly·sog·e·ny (lī-soj'ĕ-nē). The phenomenon by which a bacterium is infected by a temperate bacteriophage whose DNA is integrated into the bacterial genome and replicates along with the bacterial DNA but remains latent or unexpressed; triggering of the lytic cycle may occur spontaneously or by certain agents and will result in the production of bacteriophage and lysis of the bacterial cell.

ly·so·ki·nase (lī-sō-kī'nās). Term proposed for activator agents (*e.g.*, streptokinase, urokinase, staphylokinase) that produce plasmin by indirect or multiple-stage action on plasminogen.

ly·so·lec·i·thin (lī-sō-les'i-thin). A lysophosphatic acid that contains choline; capable of lysing erythrocytes. SYN lysophosphatidylcholine.

l.-lecithin acyltransferase (LLAT), an enzyme that catalyzes the reversible reaction of l. and another phospholipid (*e.g.*, phosphatidylethanolamine) to form lecithin and lysophosphatidylethanolamine; a major route in the restructuring of lecithin.

ly·so·lec·i·thin·ase (lī-sō-les'i-thin-ās). SYN lysophospholipase.

ly·so·phos·pha·tid·ic ac·id (lī'sō-fos'fă-tid'ik). A phosphatidic acid in which only one of the two hydroxyl groups of the glycerophosphate is esterified; most commonly, when carbon-1 of the glycerol moiety is esterified (*e.g.*, 1-acylglycerol-3-phosphate).

l. a. acyltransferase, 1-acylglycerol-3-phosphate acyltransferase, 1-acylglycerol-3-phosphate acyltransferase.

ly·so·phos·pha·ti·dyl·cho·line (lī'sō-fos'fă-tī'dil-kō'lēn). SYN lysolecithin.

ly·so·phos·pha·ti·dyl·ser·ine (lī'sō-fos'fă-tī'dil-ser'ēn). Phos-

phatidylserine from which one fatty acid residue has been removed from the glycerol moiety, typically at carbon-2. Cf. lysophosphatidic acid.

ly·so·phos·pho·li·pase (lī'sō-fos'fō-lip'ās). A hydrolase removing the single acyl group from a lysolecithin, producing glycerophosphocholine and the free fatty acid anion. SYN lecithinase B, lysolecithinase, phospholipase B (1).

ly·so·some (lī'sō-sōm). A cytoplasmic membrane-bound vesicle measuring 5-8 nm (primary l.) and containing a wide variety of glycoprotein hydrolytic enzymes active at an acid pH; serves to digest exogenous material, such as bacteria, as well as effete organelles of the cells. [lyso- + G. *soma*, body]

definitive l.'s, SYN secondary l.'s.

primary l.'s, l.'s produced at the Golgi apparatus where hydrolytic enzymes are incorporated; they fuse with phagosomes or pinosomes to become secondary l.'s.

secondary l.'s, l.'s in which lysis takes place, owing to the activity of hydrolytic enzymes; they are believed to eventually become residual bodies. SYN definitive l.'s, digestive vacuole.

ly·so·staph·in (lī-sō-staf'in). A peptidase enzyme produced by certain strains of *Staphylococcus* microorganisms with antibacterial activity against *Staphylococci*.

ly·so·type (li'sō-typ). A type within a bacterial species determined by its reaction to specific phages. [lyso + type]

ly·so·zyme (lī'sō-zīm). An enzyme hydrolyzing 1,4-β links between *N*-acetylmuramic acid and *N*-acetyl-D-glucosamine, and thus destructive to cell walls of certain bacteria; present in tears and some other body fluids, in egg white, and in some plant tissues; used in the prevention of caries and in the treatment of infant formulas. SYN mucopeptide glycohydrolase, muramidase.

lys·sa (lis'ă). **1.** A cartilage in the tongue of the dog. SYN worm (2). **2.** Old term for rabies. [G. *madness*]

Lys·sa·vi·rus (lis'ă-vī-rŭs). A genus of viruses (family Rhabdoviridae) that includes the rabies virus group.

ly·syl (lī'sil). The univalent radical of lysine.

l. hydroxylase, an enzyme that acts on specific lysyl residues in certain proteins (*e.g.*, collagens) with α-ketoglutarate and O_2 to produce δ-hydroxylysyl residues, succinate, and CO_2; this enzyme, which requires Fe^{2+} and ascorbate, is deficient in Ehlers-Danlos syndrome type VI. SYN l. 2-oxoglutarate dioxygenase.

l. oxidase, an enzyme, which requires Cu^{2+} and O_2, that oxidizes certain lysyl residues in collagen to allysyl residues and hydroxylysyl residues to hydroxyallysyl residues; this is a required step for the cross-linking (via aldol condensations and Amadori rearrangements) of collagen strands; a lower activity of this enzyme is associated with occipital horn syndrome.

l. 2-oxoglutarate dioxygenase, SYN l. hydroxylase.

ly·syl-brad·y·ki·nin (lī'sil-brad-ē-kī'nin). SYN kallidin.

lyt·ic (lit'ik). Pertaining to lysis; used colloq. as an abbreviation for osteolytic.

lyt·ta (lit'ă). Old term for rabies.

lyx·i·tol (lik'si-tol). A pentitol (reduced lyxose) occurring in lyxoflavin.

lyx·o·fla·vin (lik-sō-flā'vin). A compound similar to riboflavin except that D-lyxitol is present in place of the D-ribitol group; present in small quantity in cardiac muscle.

lyx·ose (lik'sōs). An aldopentose; D-l. is epimeric with both D-arabinose and D-xylose; L-l. is epimeric with D-ribose.

lyx·u·lose (liks'yū-lōs). The 2-keto derivative of lyxose.

lyze (līz). SYN lyse.

INDEX TO COLOR ANATOMY

A

Acromion 11-5.
Angle 11-7b.
Angle of mandible 7-22, 8-22.
Angle, left venous 28-17.
Anus 3-23, 4-28.
Aorta, abdominal 23-11.
Apex 1-29.
Apex of bladder 3-6, 4-4.
Aponeurosis of external abdominal oblique muscle 18-13.
Aponeurosis, epicranial 19-1, 20-1.
Appendix, vermiform 2-9e.
Arch, deep palmar 22-21.
Arch, plantar 24-20.
Arch, superficial palmar 22-32.
Arch, zygomatic 8-34, 9-10.
Arteries, common palmar digital 22-33.
Arteries, palmar metacarpal 22-22.
Arteries, perforating (1-3) 23-5, 24-13.
Arteries, plantar digital 24-22.
Arteries, plantar metatarsal 24-21.
Arteries, proper palmar digital 22-24.
Artery, 1st dorsal metatarsal 23-22.
Artery, angular 21-7.
Artery, anterior circumflex humeral 22-7.

Artery, anterior interosseus 22-18.
Artery, anterior tibial 23-7, 24-17.
Artery, anterior ulnar recurrent 22-27.
Artery, arcuate 23-21.
Artery, ascending pharyngeal 21-26.
Artery, axillary 22-4.
Artery, brachial 22-11, and vein 16-6.
Artery, buccal 21-10.
Artery, circumflex scapular, and vein 17-14.
Artery, common carotid 21-31.
Artery, common iliac 23-12.
Artery, common interosseus 22-15.
Artery, deep cervical 21-30.
Artery, deep circumflex iliac 23-2.
Artery, descending genicular 23-17, 24-4.
Artery, dorsalis pedis 23-9.
Artery, external carotid 21-16.
Artery, external iliac 23-1.
Artery, facial 20-31, 21-11.
Artery, femoral 16-14, 23-16, 24-3.
Artery, inferior epigastric 23-14.
Artery, inferior gluteal 24-2.
Artery, inferior labial 21-12, and vein 20-30.
Artery, inferior lateral genicular 24-16.
Artery, inferior medial genicular 24-7.
Artery, inferior ulnar collateral 22-26.
Artery, infraorbital 21-8, and nerve 20-25.
Artery, internal carotid 21-27.
Artery, internal iliac 23-13.
Artery, lateral femoral circumflex 23-3, 24-11.
Artery, lateral malleolar 23-8.
Artery, lateral plantar 24-19.
Artery, lateral thoracic 22-5.
Artery, lingual 21-15.
Artery, maxillary 21-22.
Artery, medial femoral circumflex 23-15.
Artery, medial malleolar 23-20.
Artery, medial plantar 24-9.
Artery, mental 21-13.
Artery, middle collateral 22-13.
Artery, nutrient 14-12.
Artery, occipital 20-8, 21-24.
Artery, opthalmic 21-6.
Artery, peroneal 24-18.
Artery, popliteal 23-18, 24-6.
Artery, posterior auricular 20-5, 21-23.
Artery, posterior circumflex humeral 22-6.
Artery, posterior interosseus 22-17.
Artery, posterior tibial 24-8.
Artery, posterior ulnar recurrent 22-28.
Artery, profunda brachii 22-10.
Artery, profunda femoris 23-4, 24-12.
Artery, radial 15-34, 22-16.
Artery, radial collateral 22-12.
Artery, radial recurrent 22-14.
Artery, radialis indicis 22-23.
Artery, subclavian 22-1.
Artery, submental 21-14.
Artery, subscapular 22-8.
Artery, superficial temporal 21-21, and vein 20-3.
Artery, superior gluteal 24-1.
Artery, superior labial 21-9.
Artery, superior laryngeal 21-17.
Artery, superior lateral genicular 24-15.

Color Anatomy

Color Anatomy

PLATE 1: RESPIRATORY SYSTEM, ANTERIOR VIEW

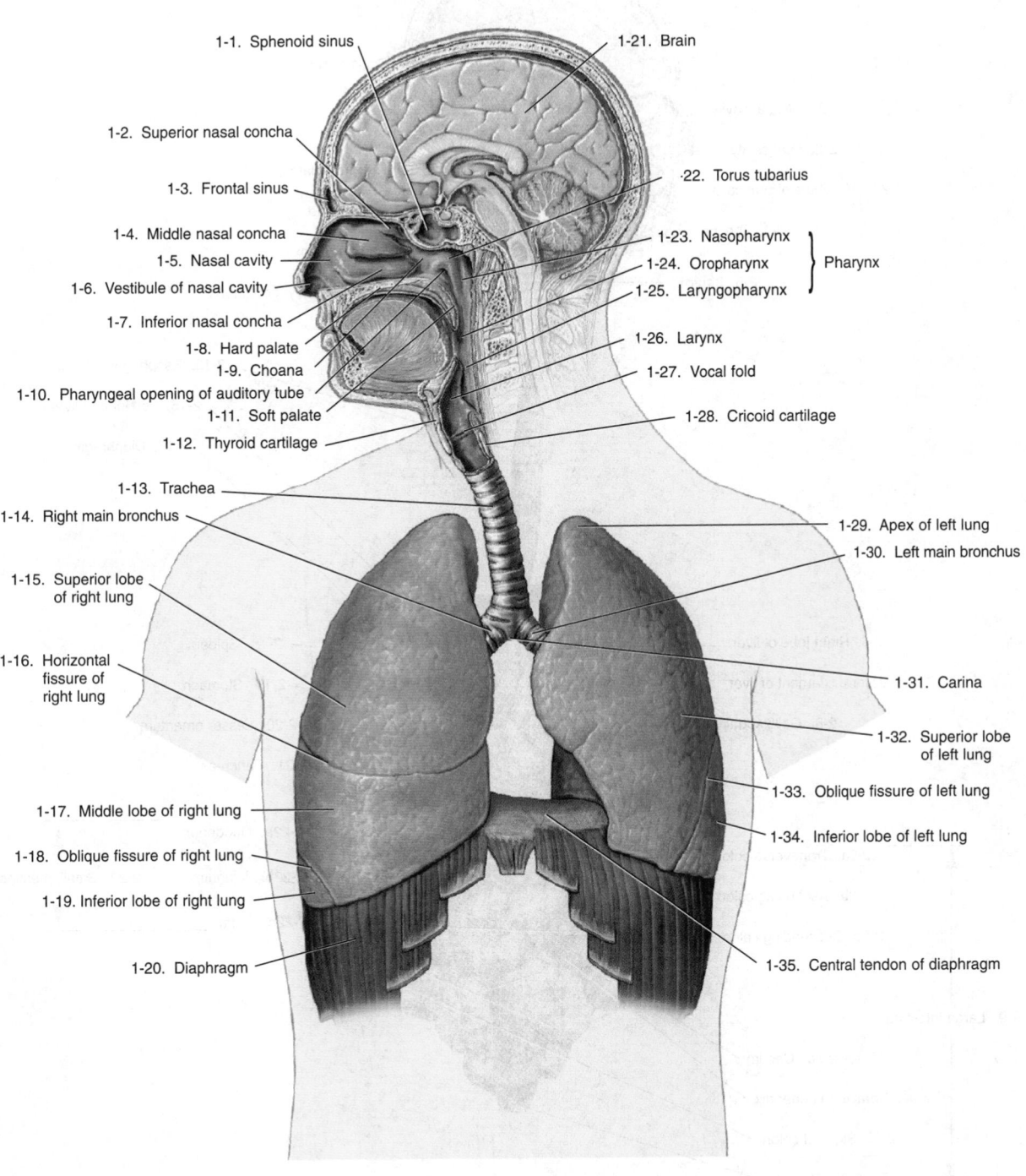

1-1. Sphenoid sinus

1-2. Superior nasal concha

1-3. Frontal sinus

1-4. Middle nasal concha

1-5. Nasal cavity

1-6. Vestibule of nasal cavity

1-7. Inferior nasal concha

1-8. Hard palate

1-9. Choana

1-10. Pharyngeal opening of auditory tube

1-11. Soft palate

1-12. Thyroid cartilage

1-13. Trachea

1-14. Right main bronchus

1-15. Superior lobe of right lung

1-16. Horizontal fissure of right lung

1-17. Middle lobe of right lung

1-18. Oblique fissure of right lung

1-19. Inferior lobe of right lung

1-20. Diaphragm

1-21. Brain

·22. Torus tubarius

1-23. Nasopharynx

1-24. Oropharynx

1-25. Laryngopharynx

} Pharynx

1-26. Larynx

1-27. Vocal fold

1-28. Cricoid cartilage

1-29. Apex of left lung

1-30. Left main bronchus

1-31. Carina

1-32. Superior lobe of left lung

1-33. Oblique fissure of left lung

1-34. Inferior lobe of left lung

1-35. Central tendon of diaphragm

Color Anatomy

PLATE 2: DIGESTIVE SYSTEM, ANTERIOR VIEW

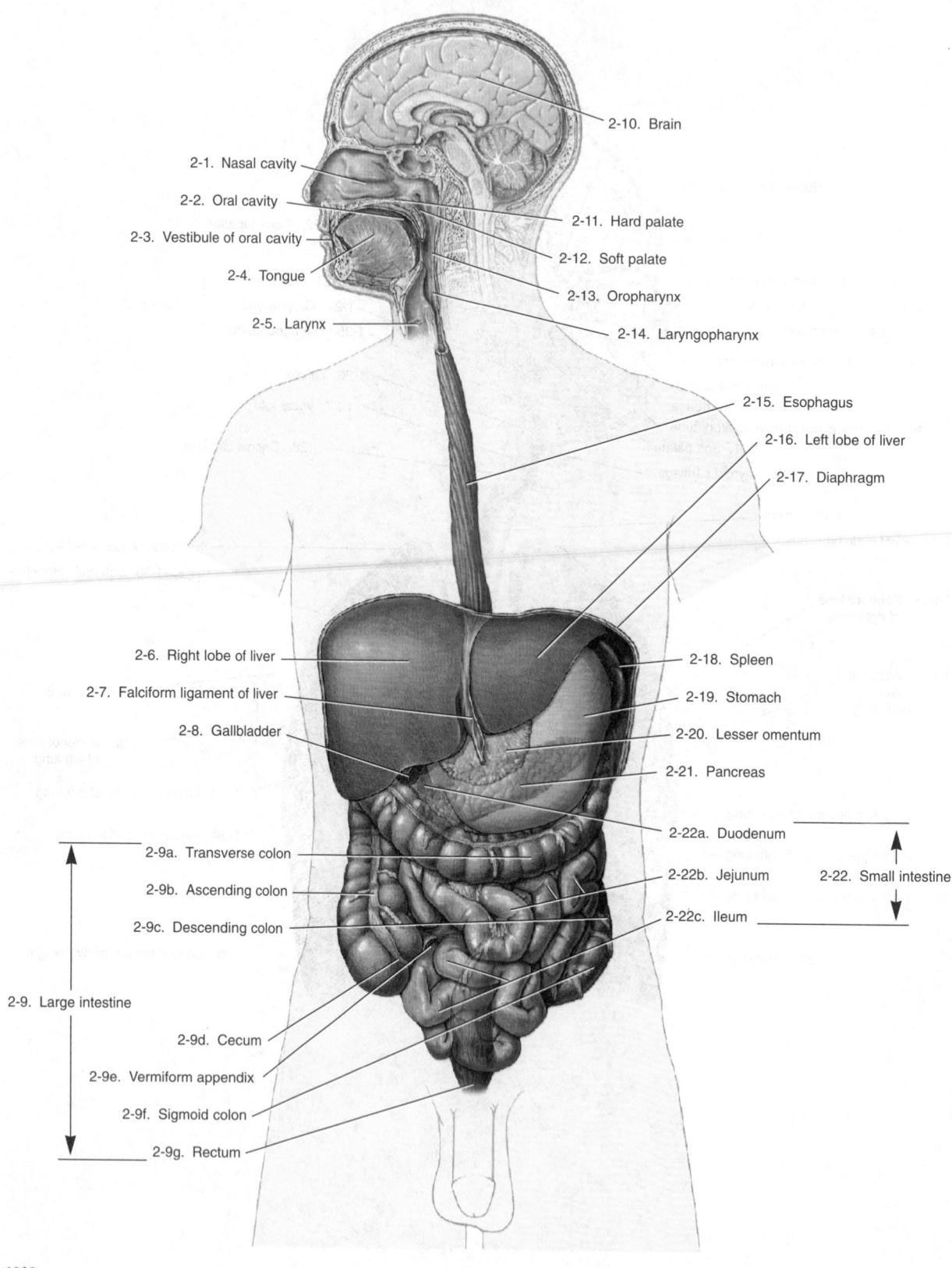

2-10. Brain

2-1. Nasal cavity

2-2. Oral cavity

2-11. Hard palate

2-3. Vestibule of oral cavity

2-12. Soft palate

2-4. Tongue

2-13. Oropharynx

2-5. Larynx

2-14. Laryngopharynx

2-15. Esophagus

2-16. Left lobe of liver

2-17. Diaphragm

2-6. Right lobe of liver

2-18. Spleen

2-7. Falciform ligament of liver

2-19. Stomach

2-8. Gallbladder

2-20. Lesser omentum

2-21. Pancreas

2-22a. Duodenum

2-9a. Transverse colon

2-9b. Ascending colon

2-22b. Jejunum

2-22. Small intestine

2-9c. Descending colon

2-22c. Ileum

2-9. Large intestine

2-9d. Cecum

2-9e. Vermiform appendix

2-9f. Sigmoid colon

2-9g. Rectum

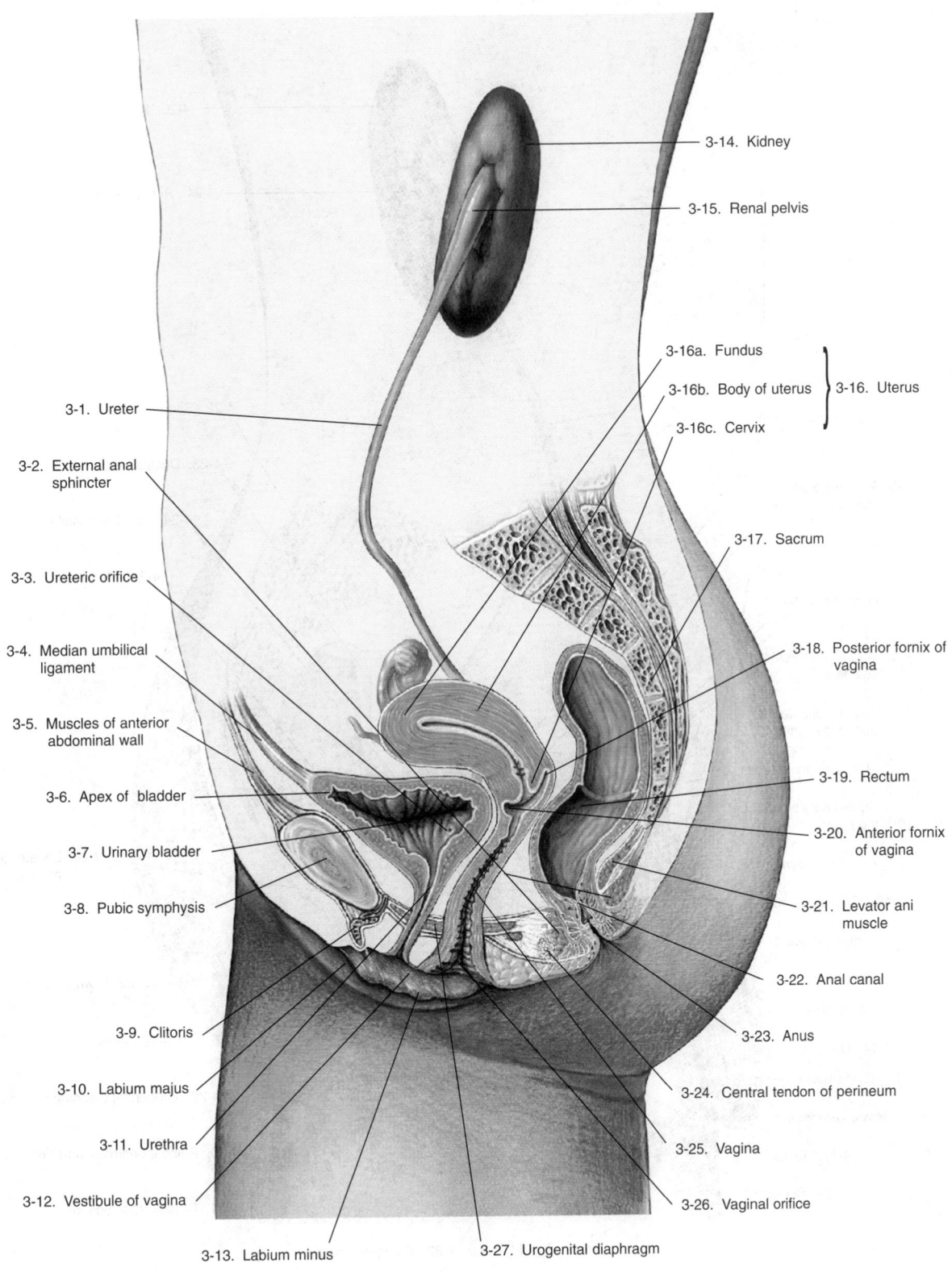

3-14. Kidney

3-15. Renal pelvis

3-16a. Fundus

3-16b. Body of uterus } 3-16. Uterus

3-16c. Cervix

3-1. Ureter

3-2. External anal sphincter

3-17. Sacrum

3-3. Ureteric orifice

3-18. Posterior fornix of vagina

3-4. Median umbilical ligament

3-5. Muscles of anterior abdominal wall

3-19. Rectum

3-6. Apex of bladder

3-20. Anterior fornix of vagina

3-7. Urinary bladder

3-21. Levator ani muscle

3-8. Pubic symphysis

3-22. Anal canal

3-23. Anus

3-9. Clitoris

3-24. Central tendon of perineum

3-10. Labium majus

3-11. Urethra

3-25. Vagina

3-12. Vestibule of vagina

3-26. Vaginal orifice

3-13. Labium minus

3-27. Urogenital diaphragm

Color Anatomy

A.D.A.M. Image

PLATE 4: MALE UROGENITAL SYSTEM, MID-SAGITTAL VIEW FROM LEFT

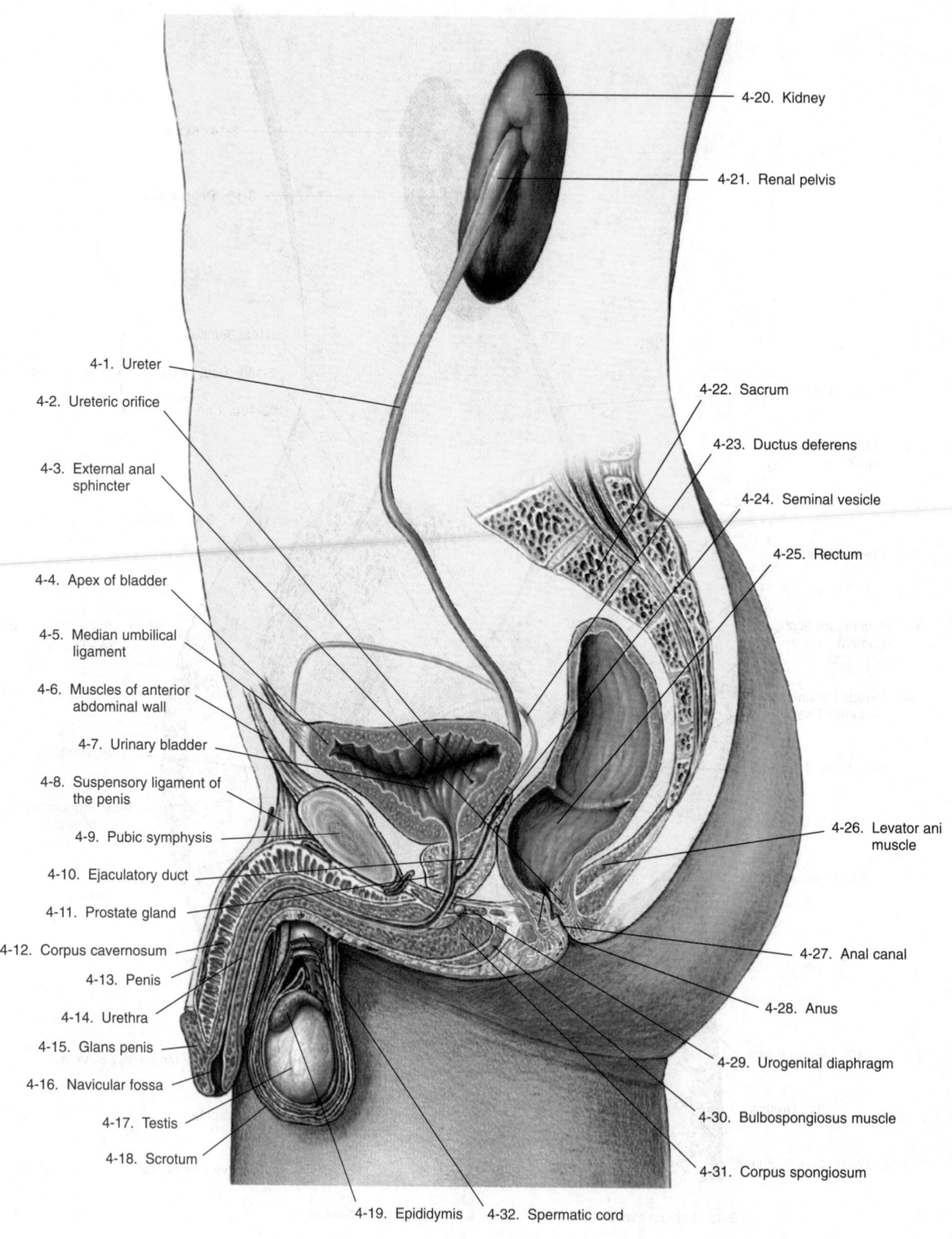

4-20. Kidney

4-21. Renal pelvis

4-1. Ureter

4-2. Ureteric orifice

4-3. External anal sphincter

4-4. Apex of bladder

4-5. Median umbilical ligament

4-6. Muscles of anterior abdominal wall

4-7. Urinary bladder

4-8. Suspensory ligament of the penis

4-9. Pubic symphysis

4-10. Ejaculatory duct

4-11. Prostate gland

4-12. Corpus cavernosum

4-13. Penis

4-14. Urethra

4-15. Glans penis

4-16. Navicular fossa

4-17. Testis

4-18. Scrotum

4-19. Epididymis

4-32. Spermatic cord

4-22. Sacrum

4-23. Ductus deferens

4-24. Seminal vesicle

4-25. Rectum

4-26. Levator ani muscle

4-27. Anal canal

4-28. Anus

4-29. Urogenital diaphragm

4-30. Bulbospongiosus muscle

4-31. Corpus spongiosum

A.D.A.M. Image

PLATE 5: SKELETON, ANTERIOR VIEW

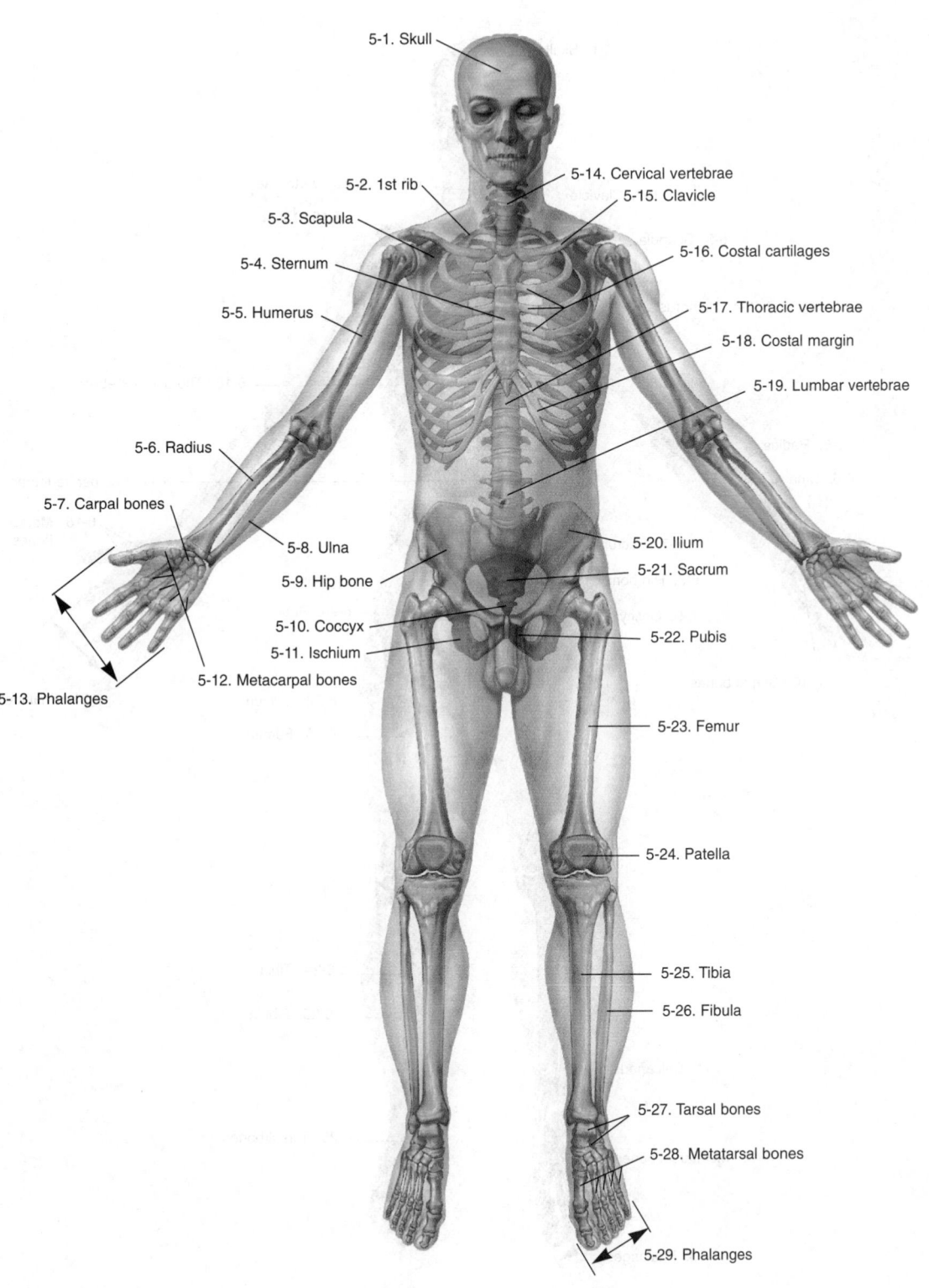

5-1. Skull

5-2. 1st rib

5-3. Scapula

5-4. Sternum

5-5. Humerus

5-6. Radius

5-7. Carpal bones

5-8. Ulna

5-9. Hip bone

5-10. Coccyx

5-11. Ischium

5-12. Metacarpal bones

5-13. Phalanges

5-14. Cervical vertebrae

5-15. Clavicle

5-16. Costal cartilages

5-17. Thoracic vertebrae

5-18. Costal margin

5-19. Lumbar vertebrae

5-20. Ilium

5-21. Sacrum

5-22. Pubis

5-23. Femur

5-24. Patella

5-25. Tibia

5-26. Fibula

5-27. Tarsal bones

5-28. Metatarsal bones

5-29. Phalanges

Color Anatomy

PLATE 6: SKELETON, POSTERIOR VIEW

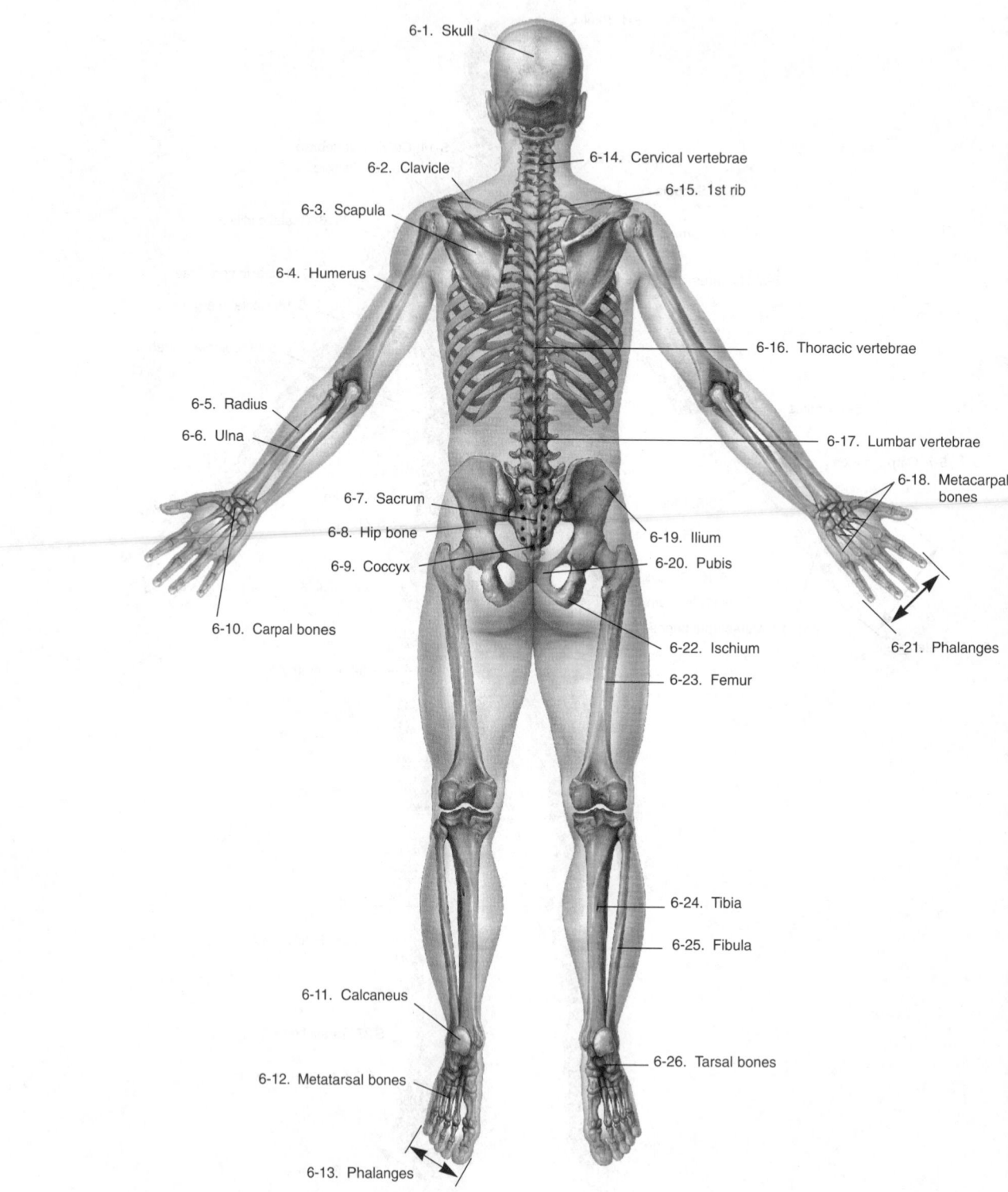

6-1. Skull

6-2. Clavicle

6-3. Scapula

6-4. Humerus

6-5. Radius

6-6. Ulna

6-7. Sacrum

6-8. Hip bone

6-9. Coccyx

6-10. Carpal bones

6-11. Calcaneus

6-12. Metatarsal bones

6-13. Phalanges

6-14. Cervical vertebrae

6-15. 1st rib

6-16. Thoracic vertebrae

6-17. Lumbar vertebrae

6-18. Metacarpal bones

6-19. Ilium

6-20. Pubis

6-21. Phalanges

6-22. Ischium

6-23. Femur

6-24. Tibia

6-25. Fibula

6-26. Tarsal bones

PLATE 7: ANTERIOR VIEW OF SKULL

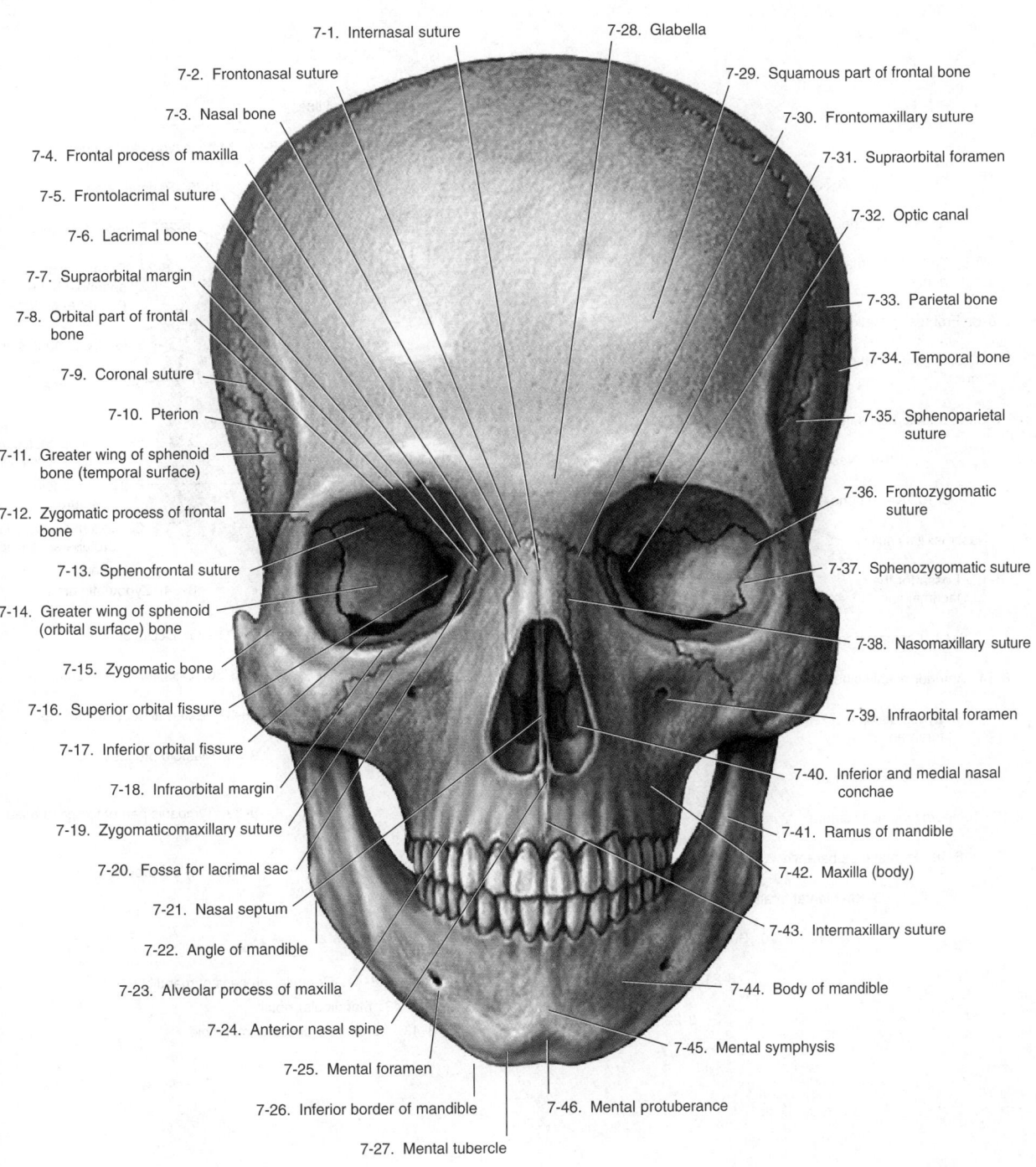

7-1. Internasal suture

7-2. Frontonasal suture

7-3. Nasal bone

7-4. Frontal process of maxilla

7-5. Frontolacrimal suture

7-6. Lacrimal bone

7-7. Supraorbital margin

7-8. Orbital part of frontal bone

7-9. Coronal suture

7-10. Pterion

7-11. Greater wing of sphenoid bone (temporal surface)

7-12. Zygomatic process of frontal bone

7-13. Sphenofrontal suture

7-14. Greater wing of sphenoid (orbital surface) bone

7-15. Zygomatic bone

7-16. Superior orbital fissure

7-17. Inferior orbital fissure

7-18. Infraorbital margin

7-19. Zygomaticomaxillary suture

7-20. Fossa for lacrimal sac

7-21. Nasal septum

7-22. Angle of mandible

7-23. Alveolar process of maxilla

7-24. Anterior nasal spine

7-25. Mental foramen

7-26. Inferior border of mandible

7-27. Mental tubercle

7-28. Glabella

7-29. Squamous part of frontal bone

7-30. Frontomaxillary suture

7-31. Supraorbital foramen

7-32. Optic canal

7-33. Parietal bone

7-34. Temporal bone

7-35. Sphenoparietal suture

7-36. Frontozygomatic suture

7-37. Sphenozygomatic suture

7-38. Nasomaxillary suture

7-39. Infraorbital foramen

7-40. Inferior and medial nasal conchae

7-41. Ramus of mandible

7-42. Maxilla (body)

7-43. Intermaxillary suture

7-44. Body of mandible

7-45. Mental symphysis

7-46. Mental protuberance

Color Anatomy

PLATE 8: LATERAL VIEW OF SKULL

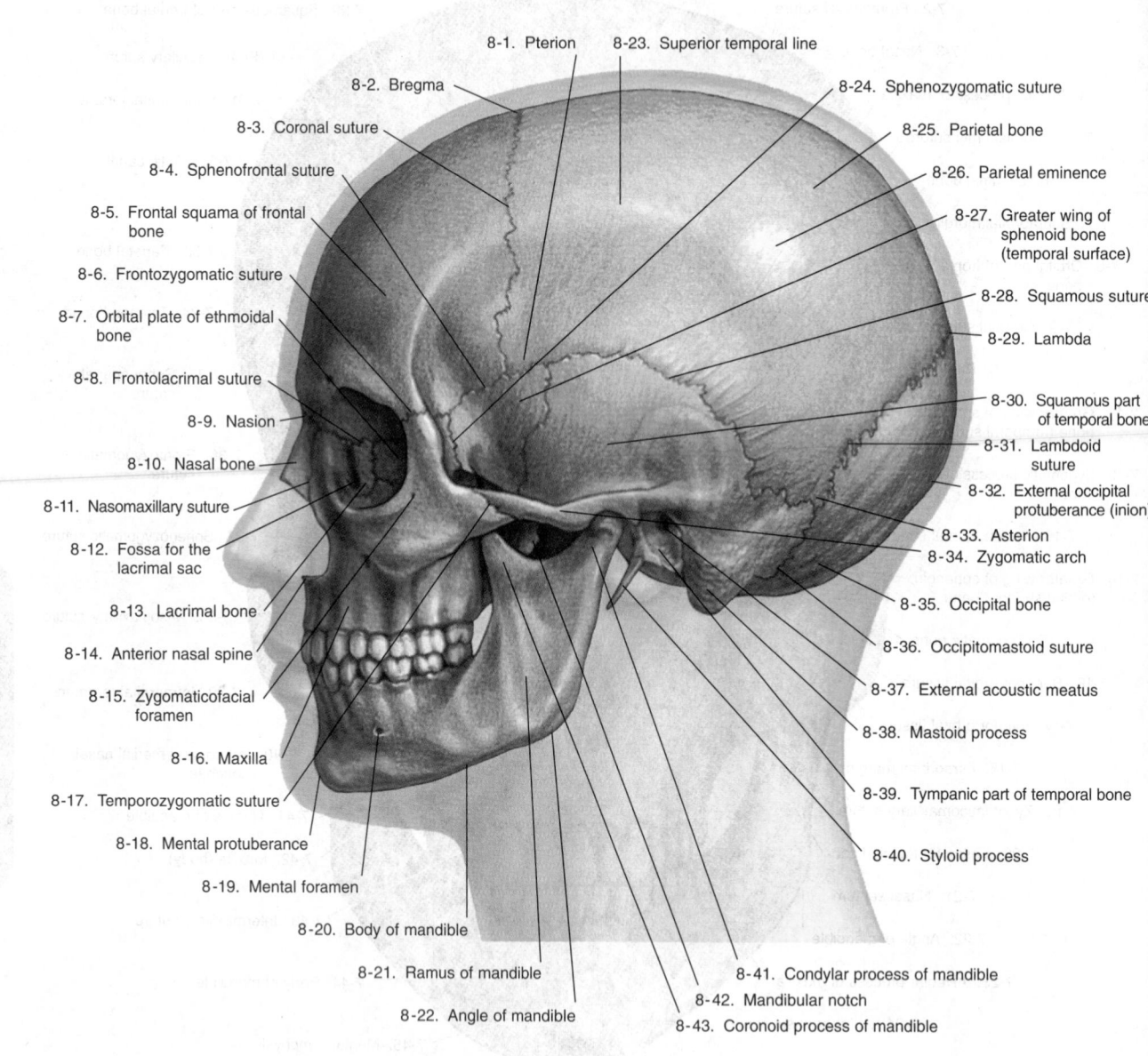

8-1. Pterion

8-2. Bregma

8-3. Coronal suture

8-4. Sphenofrontal suture

8-5. Frontal squama of frontal bone

8-6. Frontozygomatic suture

8-7. Orbital plate of ethmoidal bone

8-8. Frontolacrimal suture

8-9. Nasion

8-10. Nasal bone

8-11. Nasomaxillary suture

8-12. Fossa for the lacrimal sac

8-13. Lacrimal bone

8-14. Anterior nasal spine

8-15. Zygomaticofacial foramen

8-16. Maxilla

8-17. Temporozygomatic suture

8-18. Mental protuberance

8-19. Mental foramen

8-20. Body of mandible

8-21. Ramus of mandible

8-22. Angle of mandible

8-23. Superior temporal line

8-24. Sphenozygomatic suture

8-25. Parietal bone

8-26. Parietal eminence

8-27. Greater wing of sphenoid bone (temporal surface)

8-28. Squamous suture

8-29. Lambda

8-30. Squamous part of temporal bone

8-31. Lambdoid suture

8-32. External occipital protuberance (inion)

8-33. Asterion

8-34. Zygomatic arch

8-35. Occipital bone

8-36. Occipitomastoid suture

8-37. External acoustic meatus

8-38. Mastoid process

8-39. Tympanic part of temporal bone

8-40. Styloid process

8-41. Condylar process of mandible

8-42. Mandibular notch

8-43. Coronoid process of mandible

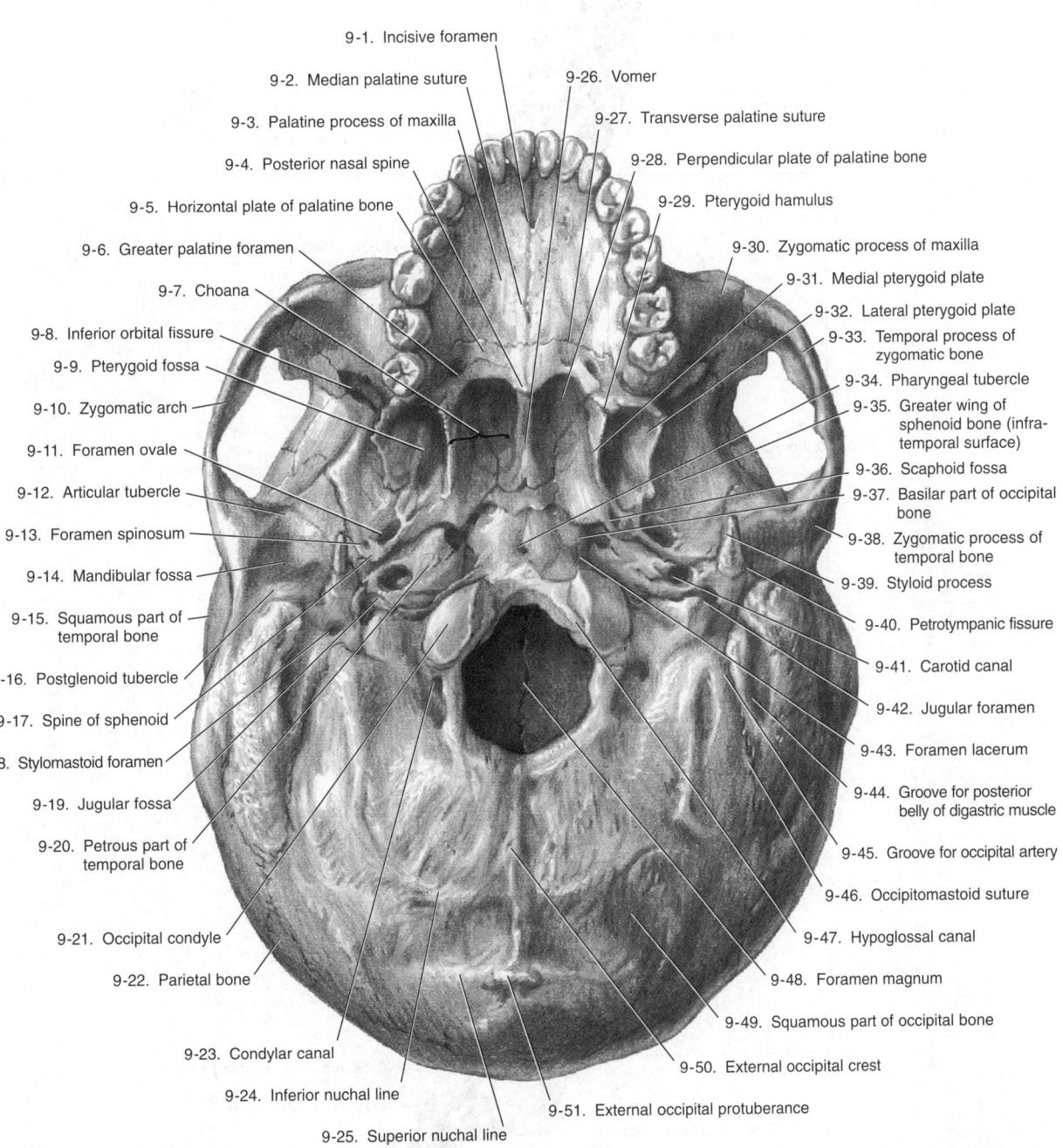

9-1. Incisive foramen

9-2. Median palatine suture

9-3. Palatine process of maxilla

9-4. Posterior nasal spine

9-5. Horizontal plate of palatine bone

9-6. Greater palatine foramen

9-7. Choana

9-8. Inferior orbital fissure

9-9. Pterygoid fossa

9-10. Zygomatic arch

9-11. Foramen ovale

9-12. Articular tubercle

9-13. Foramen spinosum

9-14. Mandibular fossa

9-15. Squamous part of temporal bone

9-16. Postglenoid tubercle

9-17. Spine of sphenoid

9-18. Stylomastoid foramen

9-19. Jugular fossa

9-20. Petrous part of temporal bone

9-21. Occipital condyle

9-22. Parietal bone

9-23. Condylar canal

9-24. Inferior nuchal line

9-25. Superior nuchal line

9-26. Vomer

9-27. Transverse palatine suture

9-28. Perpendicular plate of palatine bone

9-29. Pterygoid hamulus

9-30. Zygomatic process of maxilla

9-31. Medial pterygoid plate

9-32. Lateral pterygoid plate

9-33. Temporal process of zygomatic bone

9-34. Pharyngeal tubercle

9-35. Greater wing of sphenoid bone (infra-temporal surface)

9-36. Scaphoid fossa

9-37. Basilar part of occipital bone

9-38. Zygomatic process of temporal bone

9-39. Styloid process

9-40. Petrotympanic fissure

9-41. Carotid canal

9-42. Jugular foramen

9-43. Foramen lacerum

9-44. Groove for posterior belly of digastric muscle

9-45. Groove for occipital artery

9-46. Occipitomastoid suture

9-47. Hypoglossal canal

9-48. Foramen magnum

9-49. Squamous part of occipital bone

9-50. External occipital crest

9-51. External occipital protuberance

Color Anatomy

PLATE 10: VERTEBRAL COLUMN, LEFT LATERAL VIEW

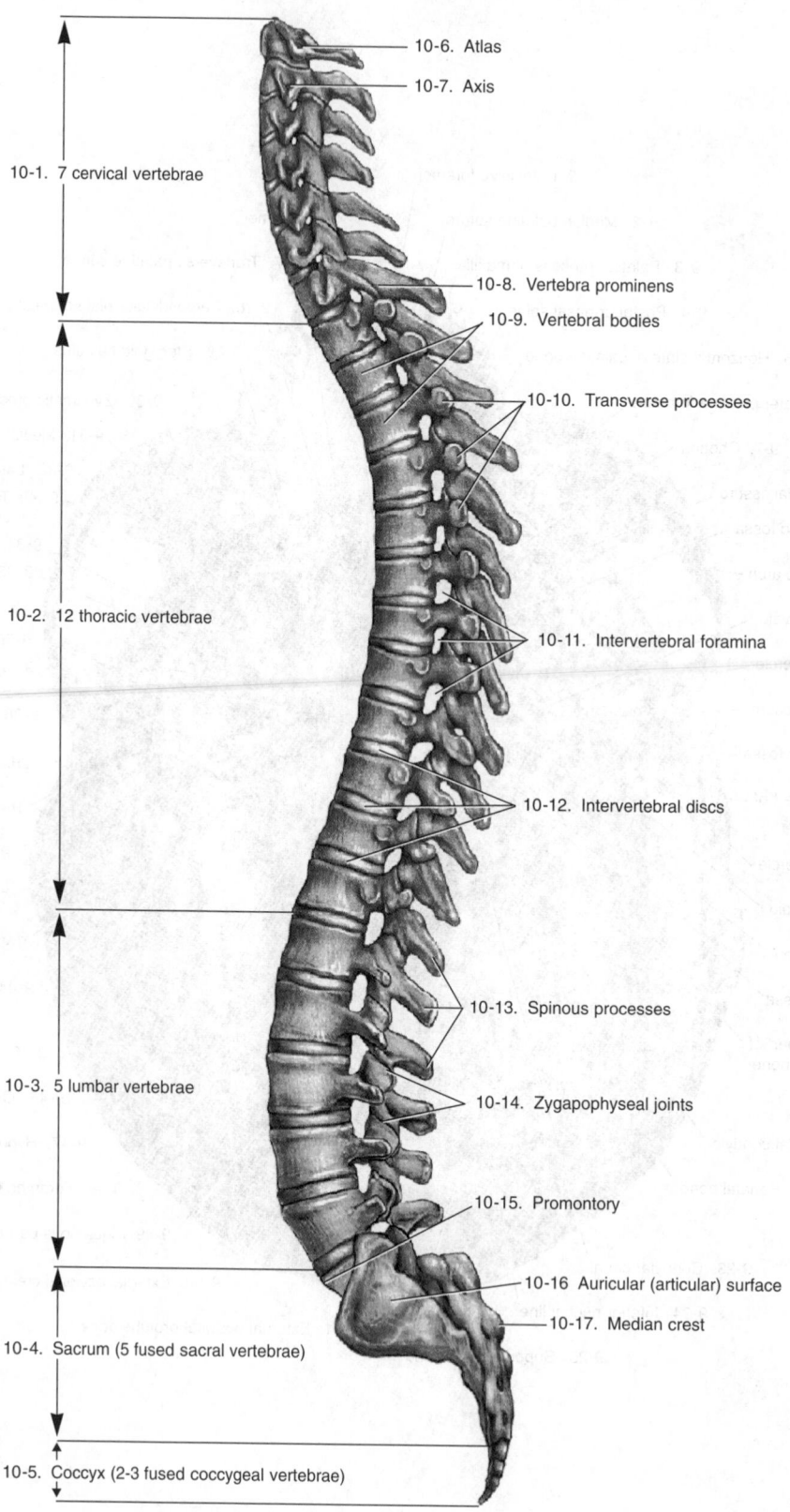

10-6. Atlas

10-7. Axis

10-1. 7 cervical vertebrae

10-8. Vertebra prominens

10-9. Vertebral bodies

10-10. Transverse processes

10-11. Intervertebral foramina

10-2. 12 thoracic vertebrae

10-12. Intervertebral discs

10-13. Spinous processes

10-3. 5 lumbar vertebrae

10-14. Zygapophyseal joints

10-15. Promontory

10-16 Auricular (articular) surface

10-17. Median crest

10-4. Sacrum (5 fused sacral vertebrae)

10-5. Coccyx (2-3 fused coccygeal vertebrae)

A.D.A.M. Image

PLATE 11: SKELETON OF THORAX AND PECTORAL GIRDLE, ANTERIOR VIEW

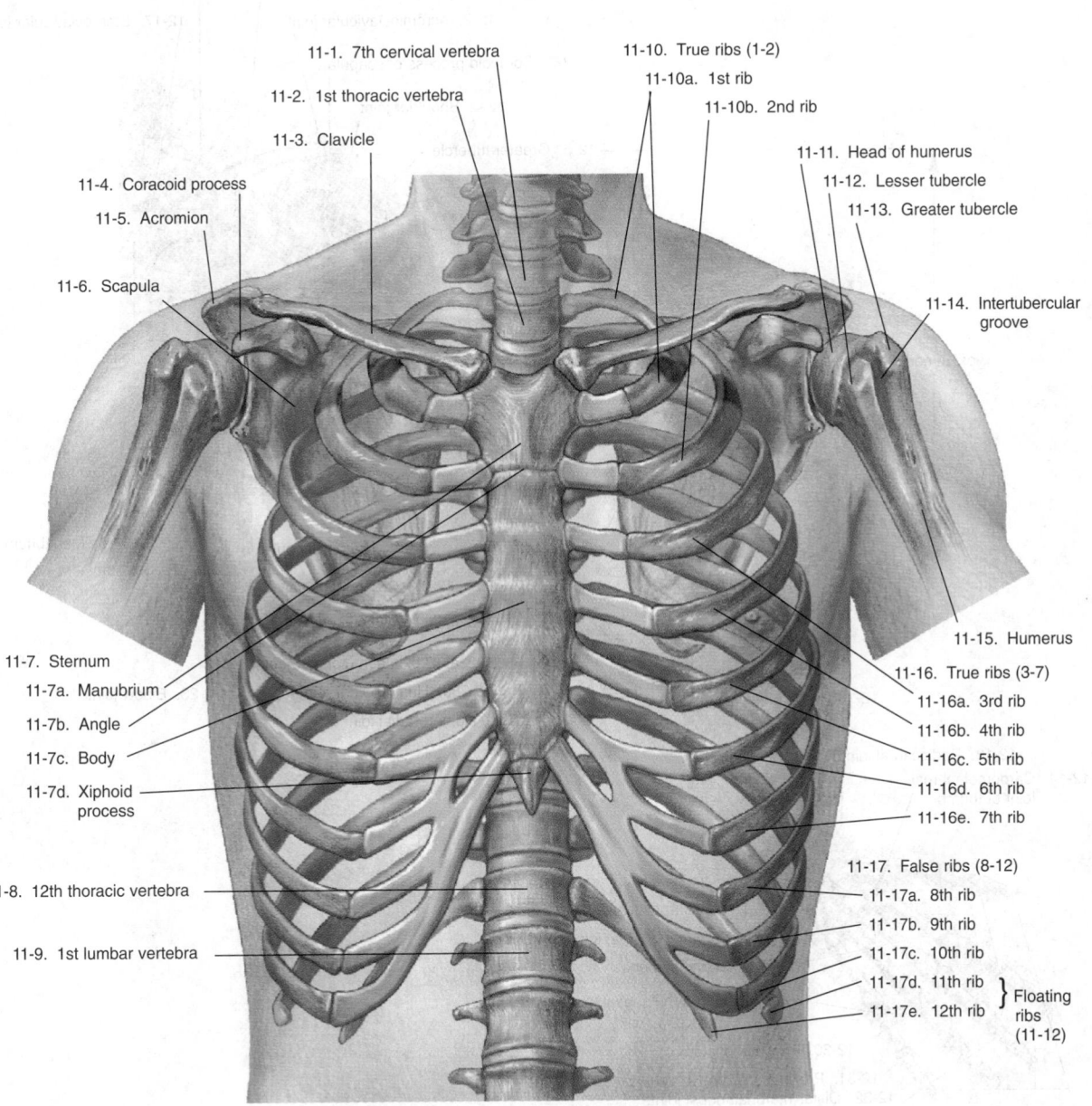

11-1. 7th cervical vertebra

11-2. 1st thoracic vertebra

11-3. Clavicle

11-4. Coracoid process

11-5. Acromion

11-6. Scapula

11-7. Sternum

11-7a. Manubrium

11-7b. Angle

11-7c. Body

11-7d. Xiphoid process

11-8. 12th thoracic vertebra

11-9. 1st lumbar vertebra

11-10. True ribs (1-2)

11-10a. 1st rib

11-10b. 2nd rib

11-11. Head of humerus

11-12. Lesser tubercle

11-13. Greater tubercle

11-14. Intertubercular groove

11-15. Humerus

11-16. True ribs (3-7)

11-16a. 3rd rib

11-16b. 4th rib

11-16c. 5th rib

11-16d. 6th rib

11-16e. 7th rib

11-17. False ribs (8-12)

11-17a. 8th rib

11-17b. 9th rib

11-17c. 10th rib

11-17d. 11th rib

11-17e. 12th rib

} Floating ribs (11-12)

Color Anatomy

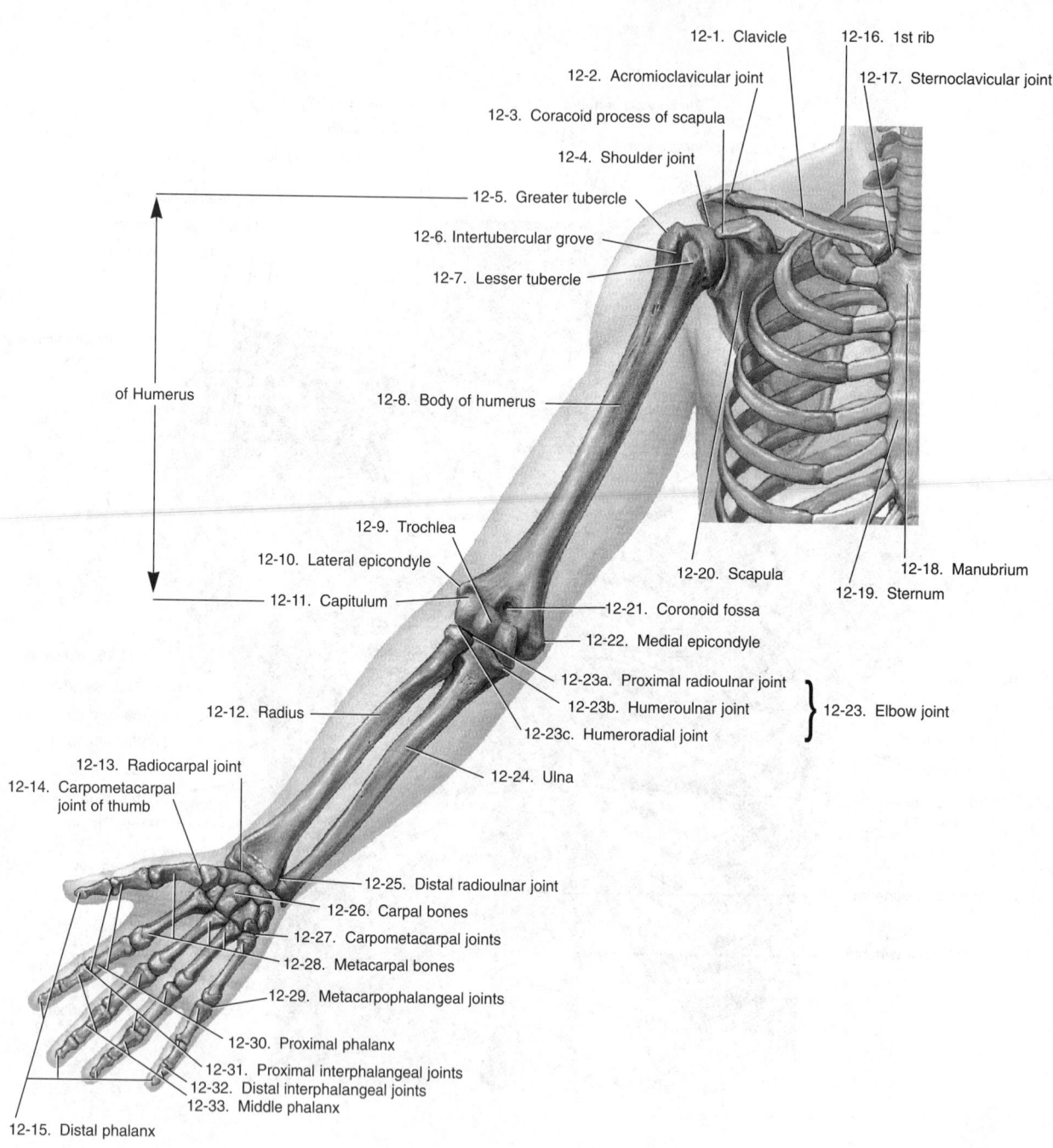

12-1. Clavicle

12-16. 1st rib

12-2. Acromioclavicular joint

12-17. Sternoclavicular joint

12-3. Coracoid process of scapula

12-4. Shoulder joint

12-5. Greater tubercle

12-6. Intertubercular grove

12-7. Lesser tubercle

of Humerus

12-8. Body of humerus

12-9. Trochlea

12-10. Lateral epicondyle

12-11. Capitulum

12-20. Scapula

12-18. Manubrium

12-21. Coronoid fossa

12-22. Medial epicondyle

12-19. Sternum

12-23a. Proximal radioulnar joint

12-23b. Humeroulnar joint

12-23. Elbow joint

12-12. Radius

12-23c. Humeroradial joint

12-24. Ulna

12-13. Radiocarpal joint

12-14. Carpometacarpal joint of thumb

12-25. Distal radioulnar joint

12-26. Carpal bones

12-27. Carpometacarpal joints

12-28. Metacarpal bones

12-29. Metacarpophalangeal joints

12-30. Proximal phalanx

12-31. Proximal interphalangeal joints

12-32. Distal interphalangeal joints

12-33. Middle phalanx

12-15. Distal phalanx

PLATE 13: SKELETON OF LOWER LIMB, ANTERIOR VIEW

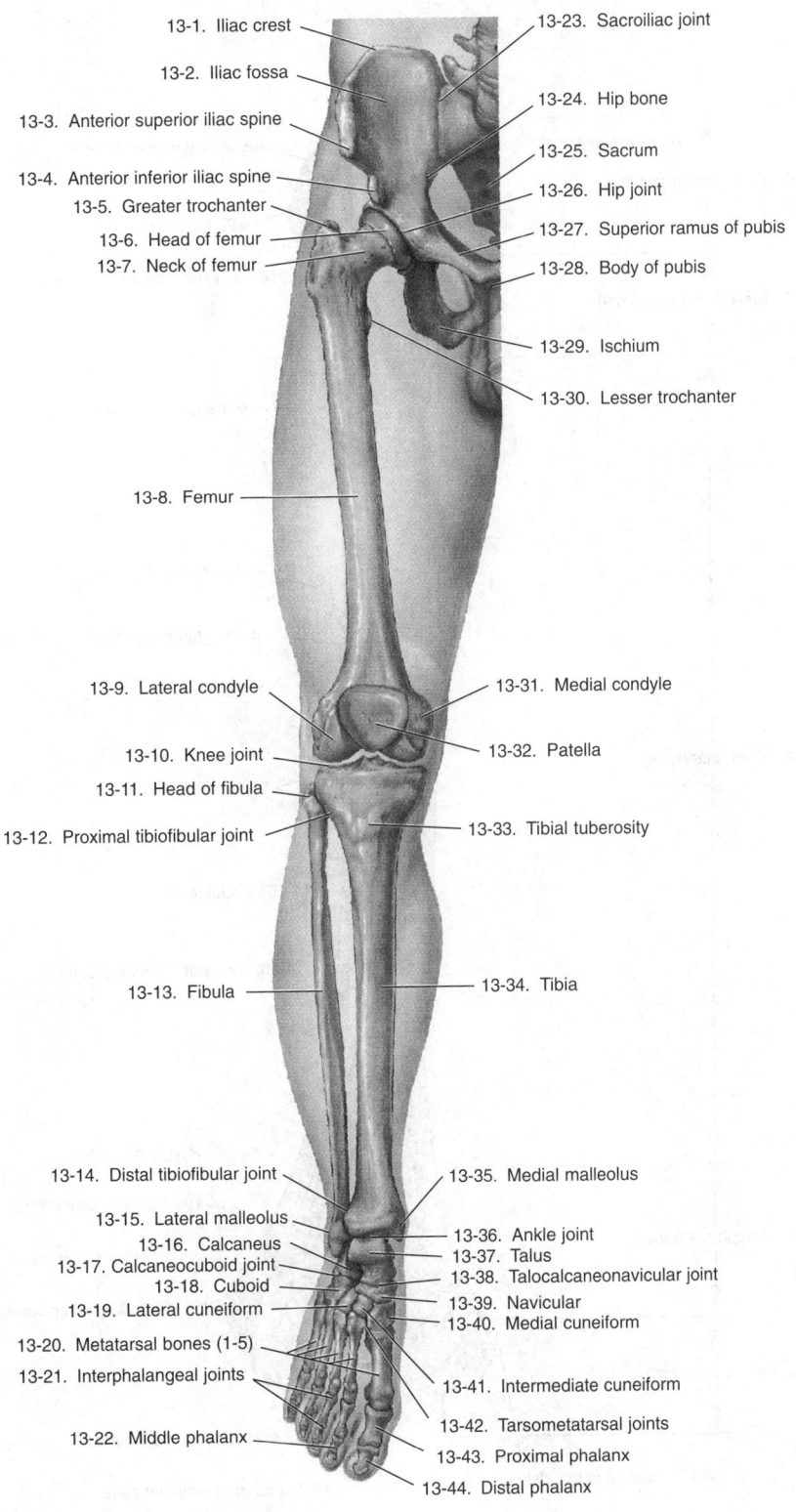

13-1. Iliac crest
13-2. Iliac fossa
13-3. Anterior superior iliac spine
13-4. Anterior inferior iliac spine
13-5. Greater trochanter
13-6. Head of femur
13-7. Neck of femur
13-8. Femur
13-9. Lateral condyle
13-10. Knee joint
13-11. Head of fibula
13-12. Proximal tibiofibular joint
13-13. Fibula
13-14. Distal tibiofibular joint
13-15. Lateral malleolus
13-16. Calcaneus
13-17. Calcaneocuboid joint
13-18. Cuboid
13-19. Lateral cuneiform
13-20. Metatarsal bones (1-5)
13-21. Interphalangeal joints
13-22. Middle phalanx

13-23. Sacroiliac joint
13-24. Hip bone
13-25. Sacrum
13-26. Hip joint
13-27. Superior ramus of pubis
13-28. Body of pubis
13-29. Ischium
13-30. Lesser trochanter
13-31. Medial condyle
13-32. Patella
13-33. Tibial tuberosity
13-34. Tibia
13-35. Medial malleolus
13-36. Ankle joint
13-37. Talus
13-38. Talocalcaneonavicular joint
13-39. Navicular
13-40. Medial cuneiform
13-41. Intermediate cuneiform
13-42. Tarsometatarsal joints
13-43. Proximal phalanx
13-44. Distal phalanx

Color Anatomy

PLATE 14: LONGITUDINALLY SECTIONED LONG BONE (HUMERUS)

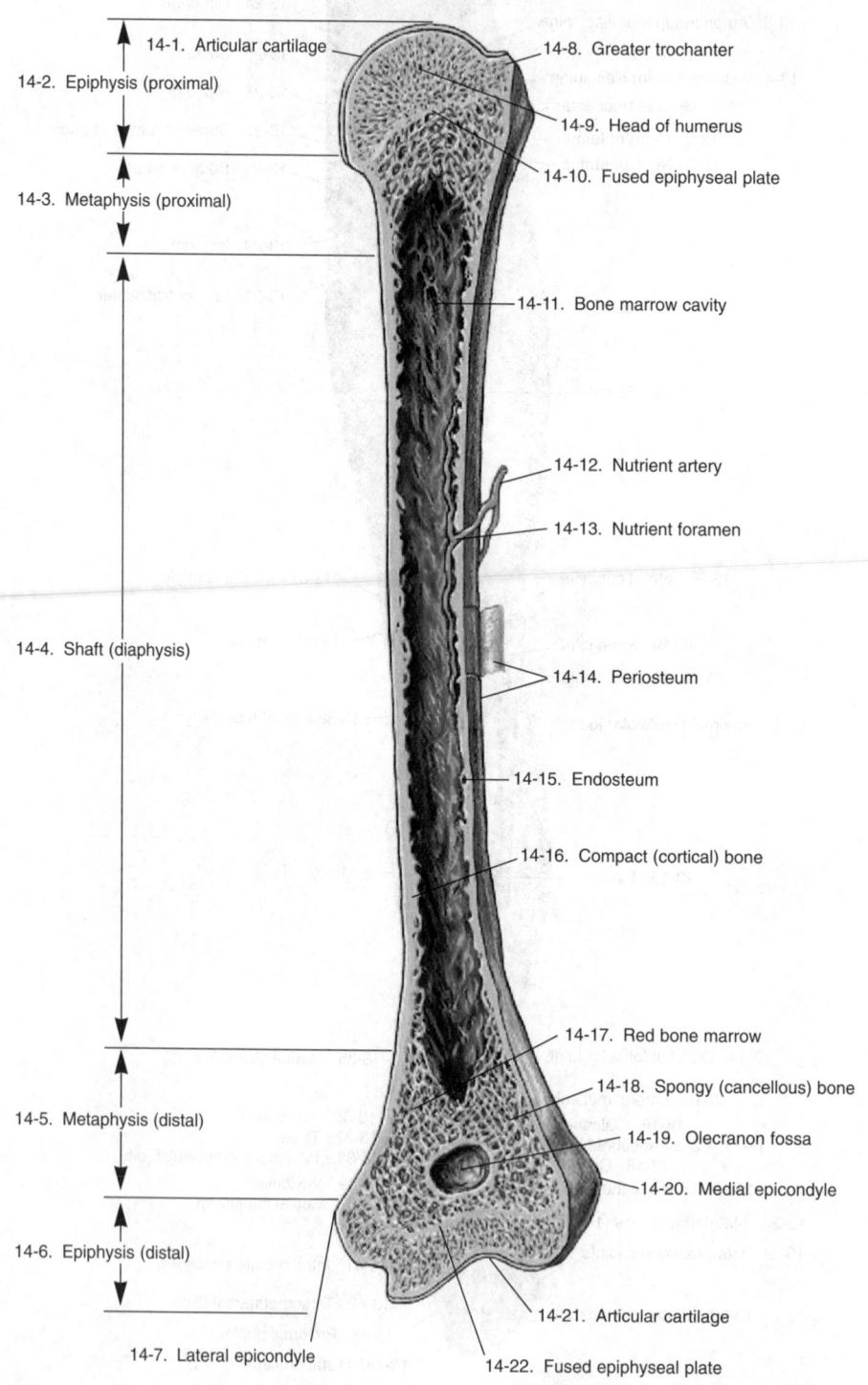

14-1. Articular cartilage

14-2. Epiphysis (proximal)

14-3. Metaphysis (proximal)

14-4. Shaft (diaphysis)

14-5. Metaphysis (distal)

14-6. Epiphysis (distal)

14-7. Lateral epicondyle

14-8. Greater trochanter

14-9. Head of humerus

14-10. Fused epiphyseal plate

14-11. Bone marrow cavity

14-12. Nutrient artery

14-13. Nutrient foramen

14-14. Periosteum

14-15. Endosteum

14-16. Compact (cortical) bone

14-17. Red bone marrow

14-18. Spongy (cancellous) bone

14-19. Olecranon fossa

14-20. Medial epicondyle

14-21. Articular cartilage

14-22. Fused epiphyseal plate

PLATE 15: LATERAL VIEW OF MUSCLES OF THORAX AND UPPER LIMB

15-1. Trapezius muscle

15-2. Acromion process of scapula

15-3. Spine of scapula

15-4. Deltoid muscle

15-5. Infraspinatus muscle

15-6. Teres minor muscle

15-7. Teres major muscle

15-8. Lateral head of triceps brachii muscle

15-9. Lateral intermuscular septum

15-10. Latissimus dorsi muscle

15-11. Olecranon

15-12. Anconeus muscle

15-13. Extensor carpi ulnaris muscle

15-14. Extensor digitorum muscle

15-15. Extensor pollicis longus muscle

15-16. Extensor retinaculum

15-17. 1st dorsal interosseus muscle

15-18. Sternocleidomastoid muscle

15-19. External jugular vein

15-20. Clavicle

15-21. Pectoralis major muscle

15-22. Serratus anterior muscle

15-23. Long head of biceps brachii muscle

15-24. Brachialis muscle

15-25. External abdominal oblique muscle

15-26. Lateral antebrachial cutaneous nerve

15-27. Lateral epicondyle of humerus

15-28. Brachioradialis muscle

15-29. Extensor carpi radialis longus muscle

15-30. Extensor carpi radialis brevis muscle

15-31. Abductor pollicis longus muscle

15-32. Extensor pollicis brevis muscle

15-33. Anatomical snuff box

15-34. Radial artery

15-35. Adductor pollicis muscle

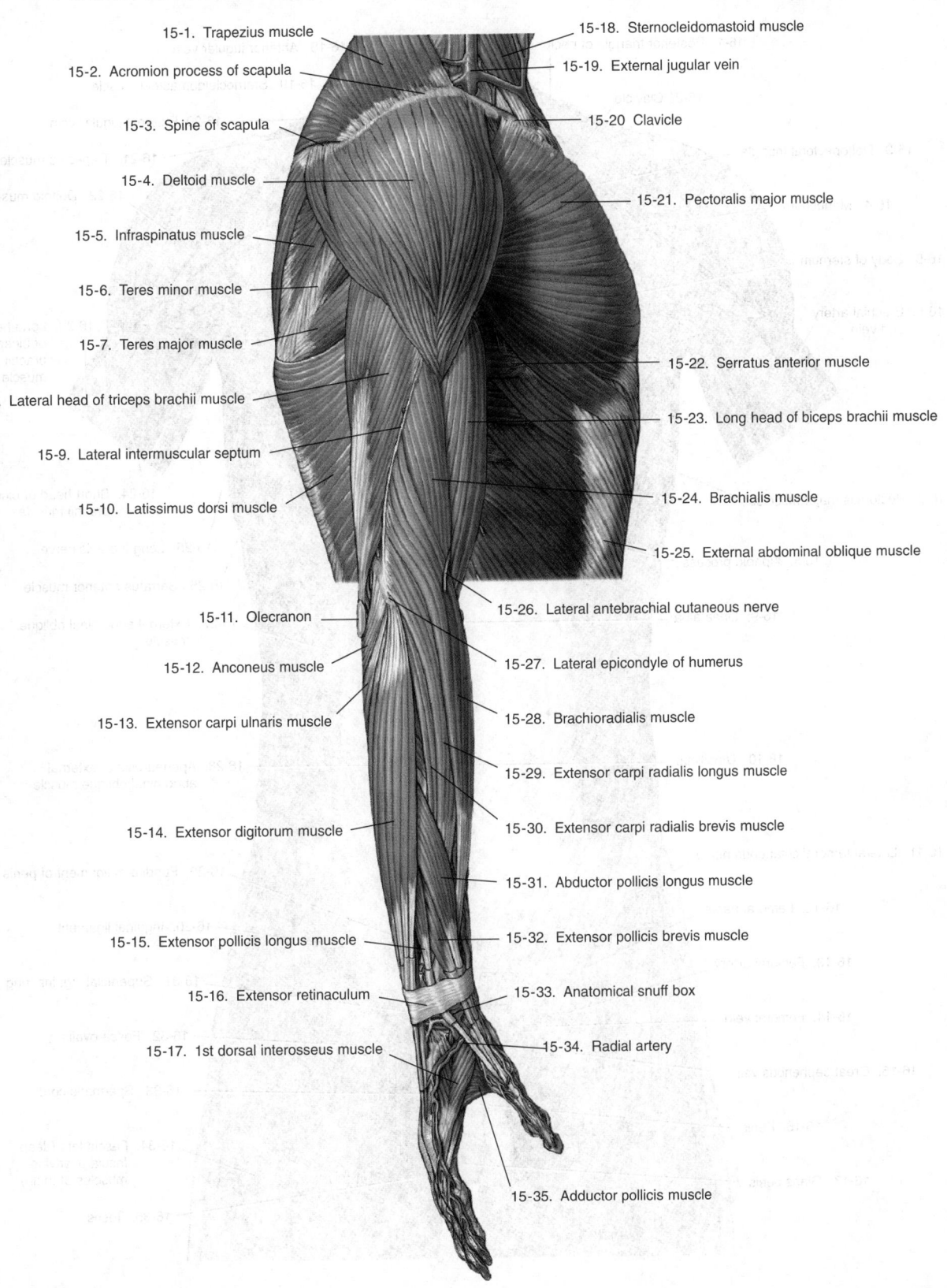

Color Anatomy

A.D.A.M. Image

1033

PLATE 16: ANTERIOR VIEW, MUSCULATURE OF TRUNK AND UPPER THIGH

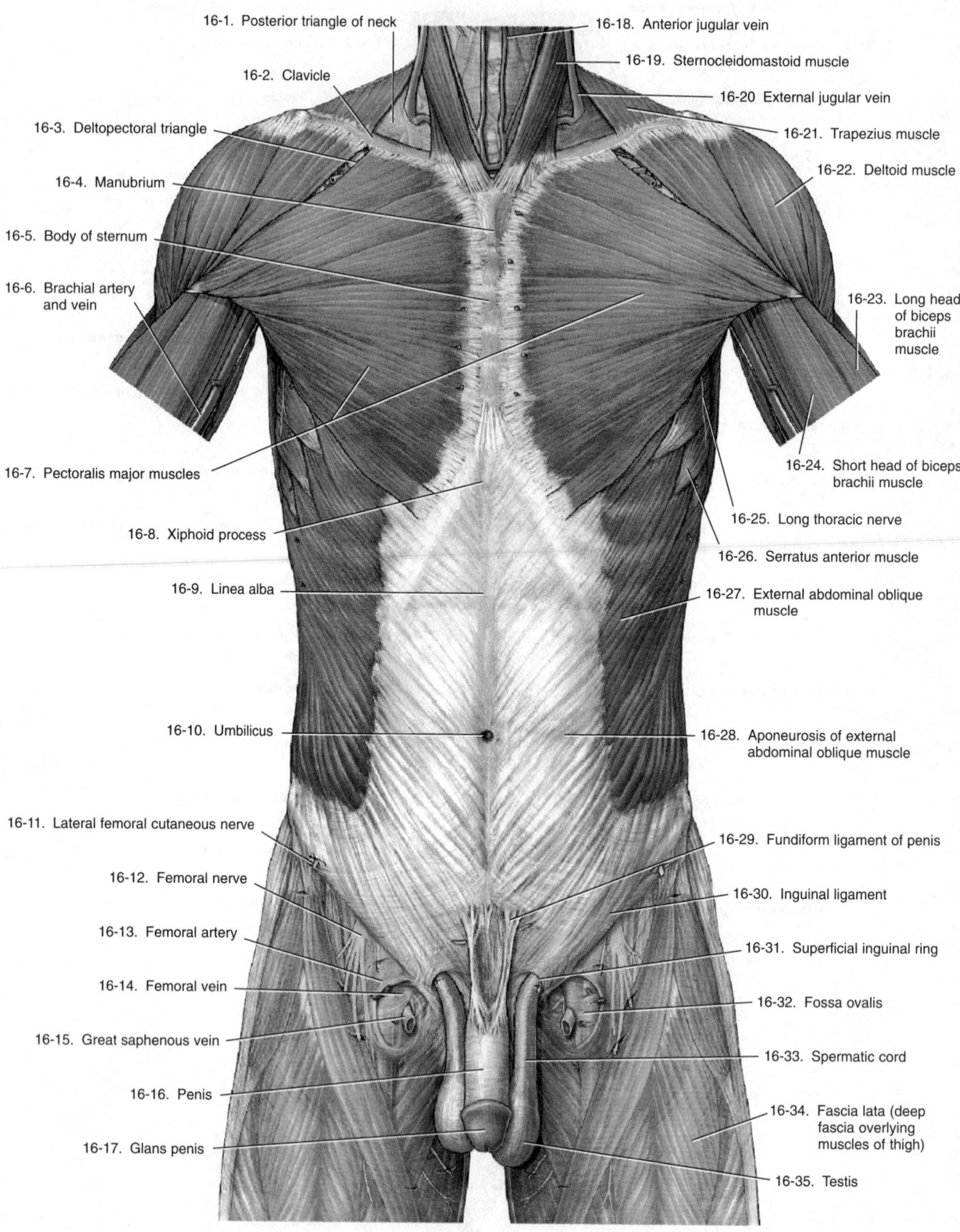

16-1. Posterior triangle of neck

16-2. Clavicle

16-3. Deltopectoral triangle

16-4. Manubrium

16-5. Body of sternum

16-6. Brachial artery and vein

16-7. Pectoralis major muscles

16-8. Xiphoid process

16-9. Linea alba

16-10. Umbilicus

16-11. Lateral femoral cutaneous nerve

16-12. Femoral nerve

16-13. Femoral artery

16-14. Femoral vein

16-15. Great saphenous vein

16-16. Penis

16-17. Glans penis

16-18. Anterior jugular vein

16-19. Sternocleidomastoid muscle

16-20. External jugular vein

16-21. Trapezius muscle

16-22. Deltoid muscle

16-23. Long head of biceps brachii muscle

16-24. Short head of biceps brachii muscle

16-25. Long thoracic nerve

16-26. Serratus anterior muscle

16-27. External abdominal oblique muscle

16-28. Aponeurosis of external abdominal oblique muscle

16-29. Fundiform ligament of penis

16-30. Inguinal ligament

16-31. Superficial inguinal ring

16-32. Fossa ovalis

16-33. Spermatic cord

16-34. Fascia lata (deep fascia overlying muscles of thigh)

16-35. Testis

PLATE 17: POSTERIOR VIEW, SUPERFICIAL MUSCLES OF THE BACK

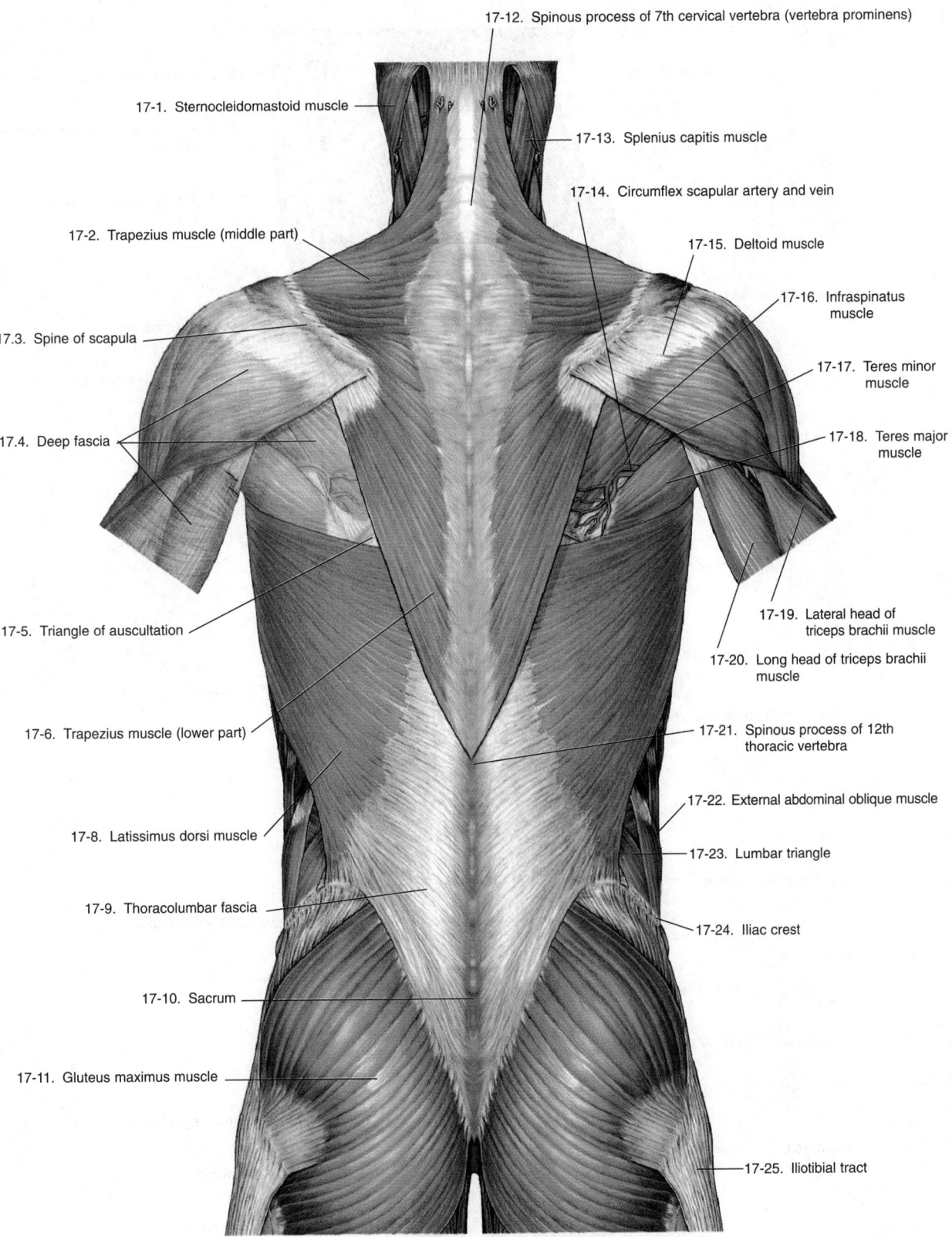

17-12. Spinous process of 7th cervical vertebra (vertebra prominens)

17-1. Sternocleidomastoid muscle

17-13. Splenius capitis muscle

17-14. Circumflex scapular artery and vein

17-2. Trapezius muscle (middle part)

17-15. Deltoid muscle

17-16. Infraspinatus muscle

17-3. Spine of scapula

17-17. Teres minor muscle

17-4. Deep fascia

17-18. Teres major muscle

17-19. Lateral head of triceps brachii muscle

17-5. Triangle of auscultation

17-20. Long head of triceps brachii muscle

17-6. Trapezius muscle (lower part)

17-21. Spinous process of 12th thoracic vertebra

17-22. External abdominal oblique muscle

17-8. Latissimus dorsi muscle

17-23. Lumbar triangle

17-9. Thoracolumbar fascia

17-24. Iliac crest

17-10. Sacrum

17-11. Gluteus maximus muscle

17-25. Iliotibial tract

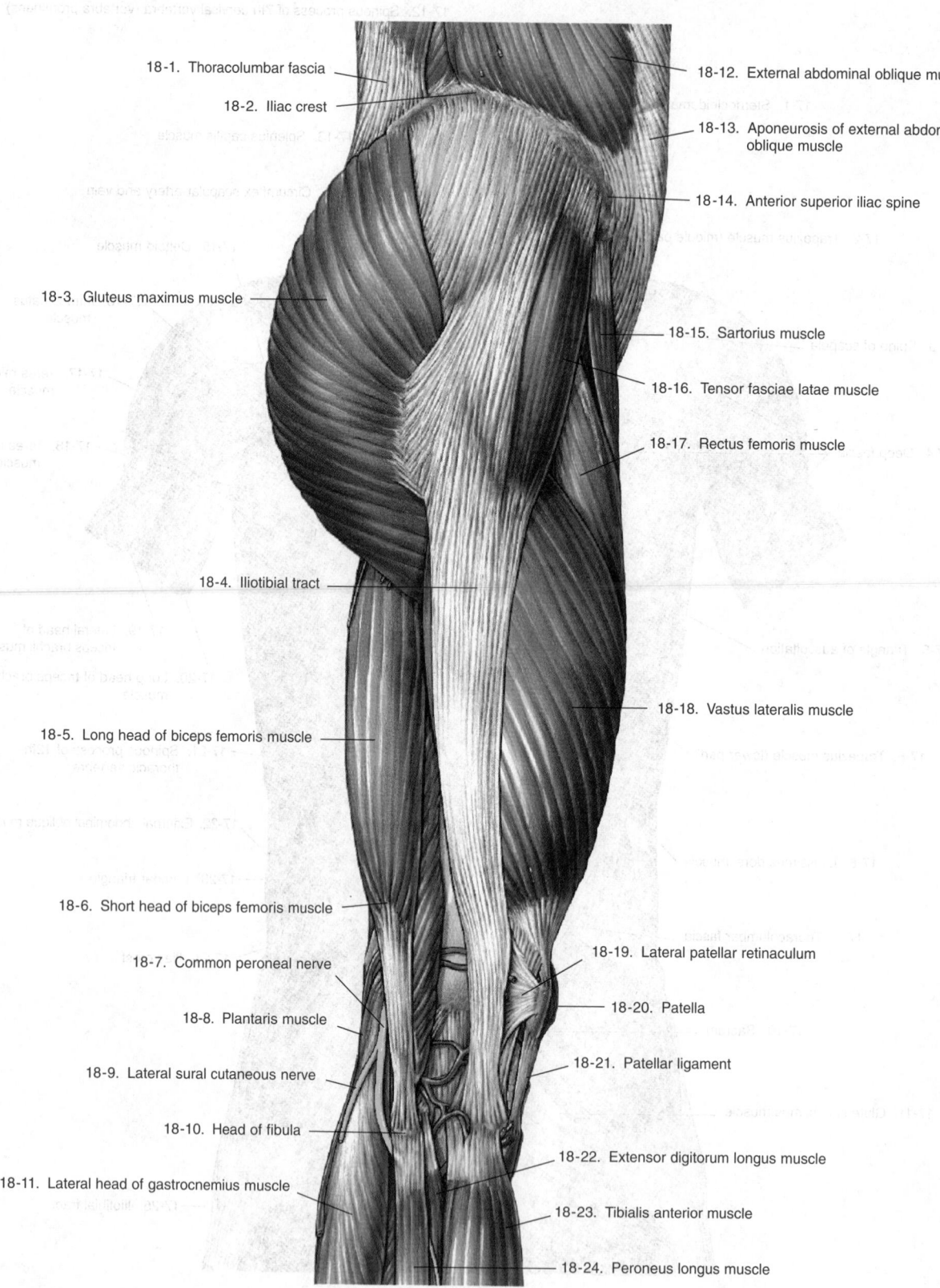

18-1. Thoracolumbar fascia

18-2. Iliac crest

18-3. Gluteus maximus muscle

18-4. Iliotibial tract

18-5. Long head of biceps femoris muscle

18-6. Short head of biceps femoris muscle

18-7. Common peroneal nerve

18-8. Plantaris muscle

18-9. Lateral sural cutaneous nerve

18-10. Head of fibula

18-11. Lateral head of gastrocnemius muscle

18-12. External abdominal oblique muscl

18-13. Aponeurosis of external abdomina oblique muscle

18-14. Anterior superior iliac spine

18-15. Sartorius muscle

18-16. Tensor fasciae latae muscle

18-17. Rectus femoris muscle

18-18. Vastus lateralis muscle

18-19. Lateral patellar retinaculum

18-20. Patella

18-21. Patellar ligament

18-22. Extensor digitorum longus muscle

18-23. Tibialis anterior muscle

18-24. Peroneus longus muscle

PLATE 19: ANTERIOR VIEW OF FACE SHOWING MUSCLES OF FACIAL EXPRESSION

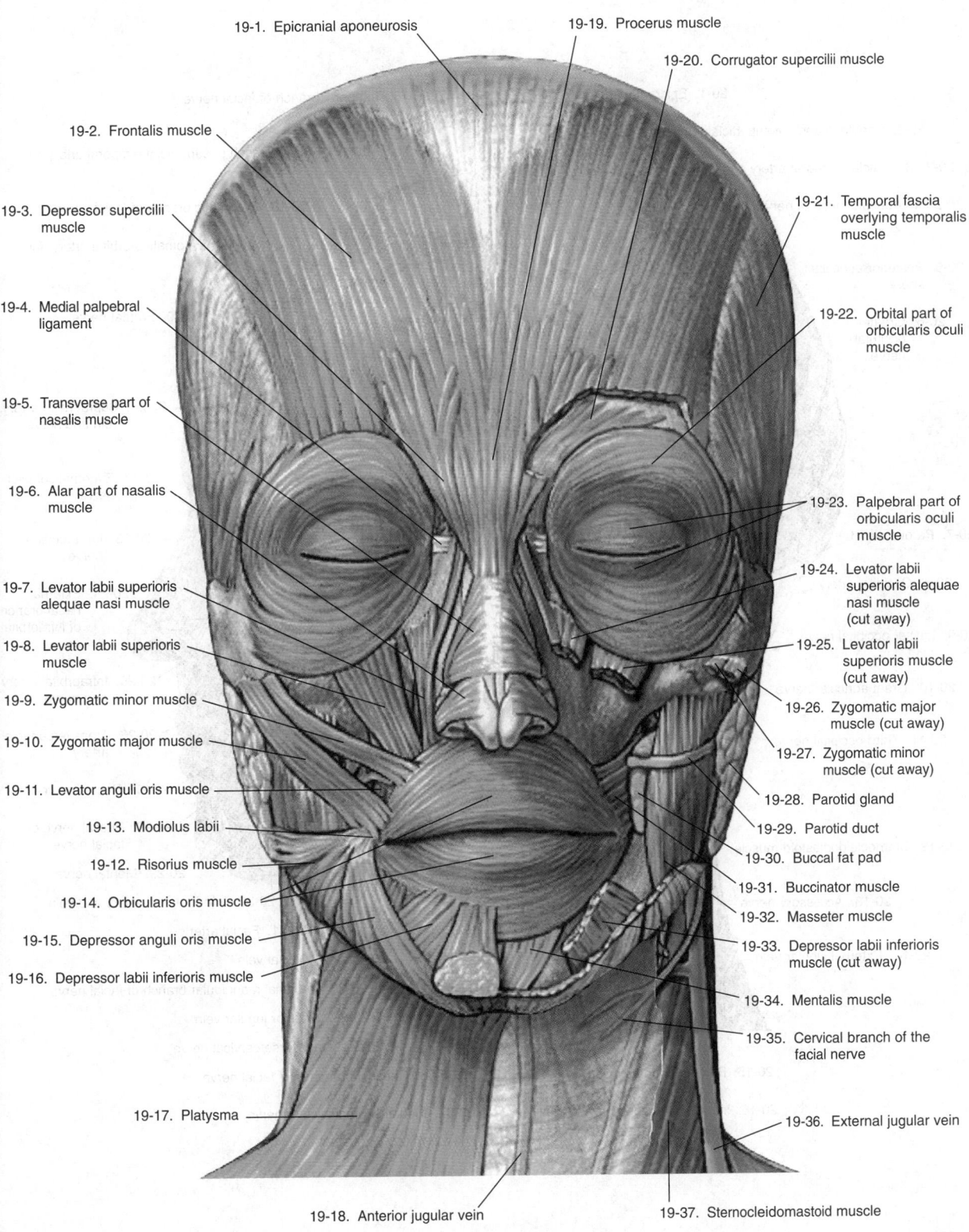

19-1. Epicranial aponeurosis

19-19. Procerus muscle

19-20. Corrugator supercilii muscle

19-2. Frontalis muscle

19-3. Depressor supercilii muscle

19-4. Medial palpebral ligament

19-5. Transverse part of nasalis muscle

19-6. Alar part of nasalis muscle

19-7. Levator labii superioris alequae nasi muscle

19-8. Levator labii superioris muscle

19-9. Zygomatic minor muscle

19-10. Zygomatic major muscle

19-11. Levator anguli oris muscle

19-13. Modiolus labii

19-12. Risorius muscle

19-14. Orbicularis oris muscle

19-15. Depressor anguli oris muscle

19-16. Depressor labii inferioris muscle

19-17. Platysma

19-21. Temporal fascia overlying temporalis muscle

19-22. Orbital part of orbicularis oculi muscle

19-23. Palpebral part of orbicularis oculi muscle

19-24. Levator labii superioris alequae nasi muscle (cut away)

19-25. Levator labii superioris muscle (cut away)

19-26. Zygomatic major muscle (cut away)

19-27. Zygomatic minor muscle (cut away)

19-28. Parotid gland

19-29. Parotid duct

19-30. Buccal fat pad

19-31. Buccinator muscle

19-32. Masseter muscle

19-33. Depressor labii inferioris muscle (cut away)

19-34. Mentalis muscle

19-35. Cervical branch of the facial nerve

19-36. External jugular vein

19-18. Anterior jugular vein

19-37. Sternocleidomastoid muscle

Color Anatomy

A.D.A.M. Image

1037

PLATE 20: SUPERFICIAL ARTERIES AND NERVES OF FACE, LATERAL VIEW

20-1. Epicranial aponeurosis

20-2. Parietal branch of superficial temporal artery

20-3. Superficial temporal artery and vein

20-4. Auriculotemporal nerve

20-5. Posterior auricular artery

20-6. Greater occipital nerve

20-7. Parotid gland

20-8. Occipital artery

20-9. Lesser occipital nerve

20-10. Great auricular nerve

20-11. Third occipital nerve

20-12. Sternocleidomastoid muscle

20-13. Accessory nerve

20-14. External jugular vein

20-15. Posterior supraclavicular nerve

20-16. Intermediate supraclavicular nerve

20-16. Temporal branch of facial nerve

20-17. Frontal branch of superficial temporal artery

20-18. Zygomatic branch of facial nerve

20-19. Zygomatico-orbital artery and vein

20-20. Frontal nerve

20-21. Supraorbital artery, vein and nerve

20-22. Zygomaticofacial nerve

20-23. Infratrochlear nerve

20-24. External nasal branch of infraorbital nerve

20-25. Infraorbital artery and nerve

20-26. Transverse facial artery

20-27. Buccal nerve

20-28. Buccal nerve of facial nerve

20-29. Mental nerve

20-30. Inferior labial artery and vein

20-31. Facial artery

20-32. Facial vein

20-33. Marginal mandibular branch of facial nerve

20-34. Anterior jugular vein

20-35. Transverse cervical nerve

20-36. Cervical branches of facial nerve

20-37. Medial supraclavicular nerve

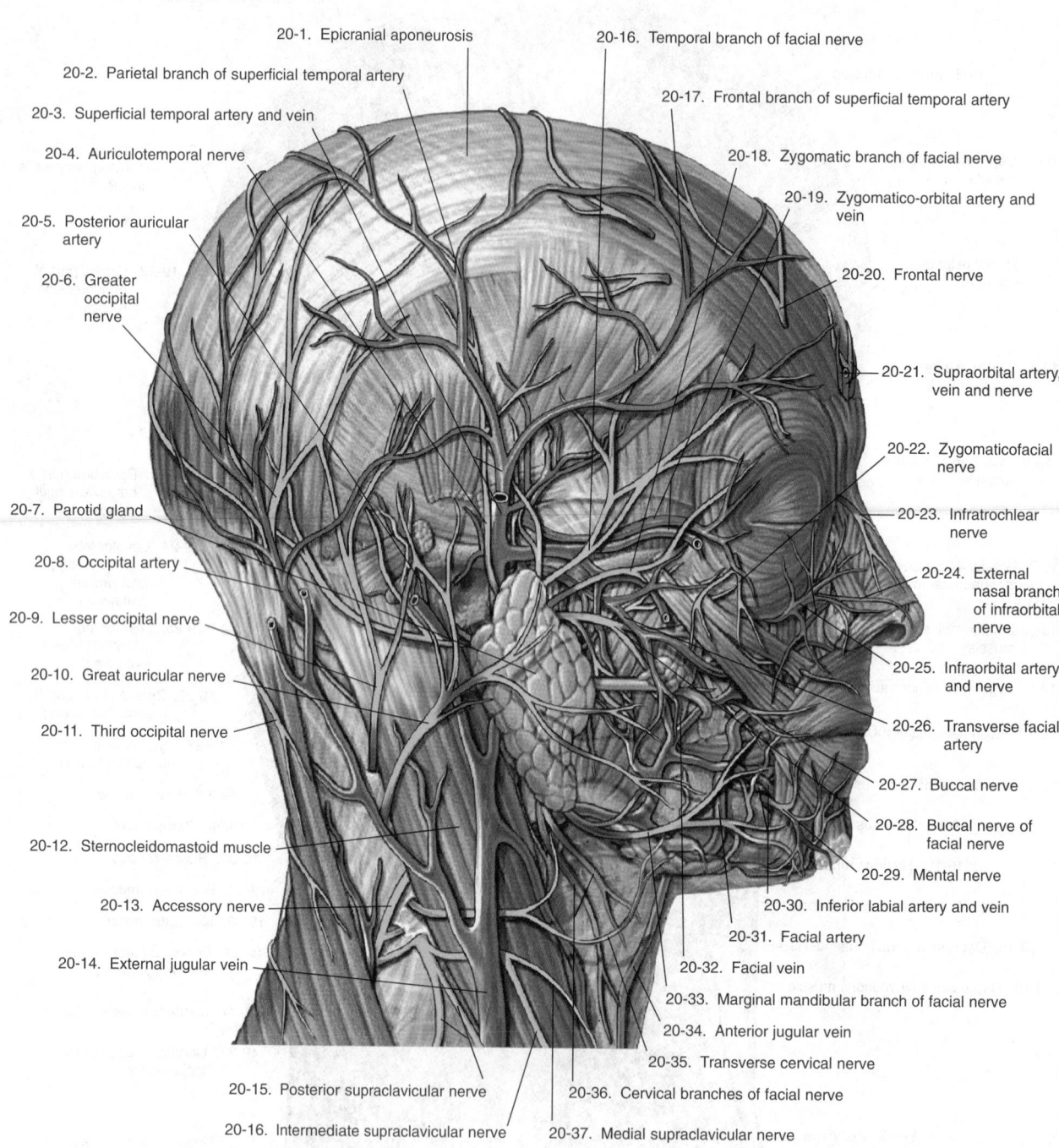

PLATE 21: ARTERIES OF HEAD AND UPPER NECK, LEFT LATERAL VIEW

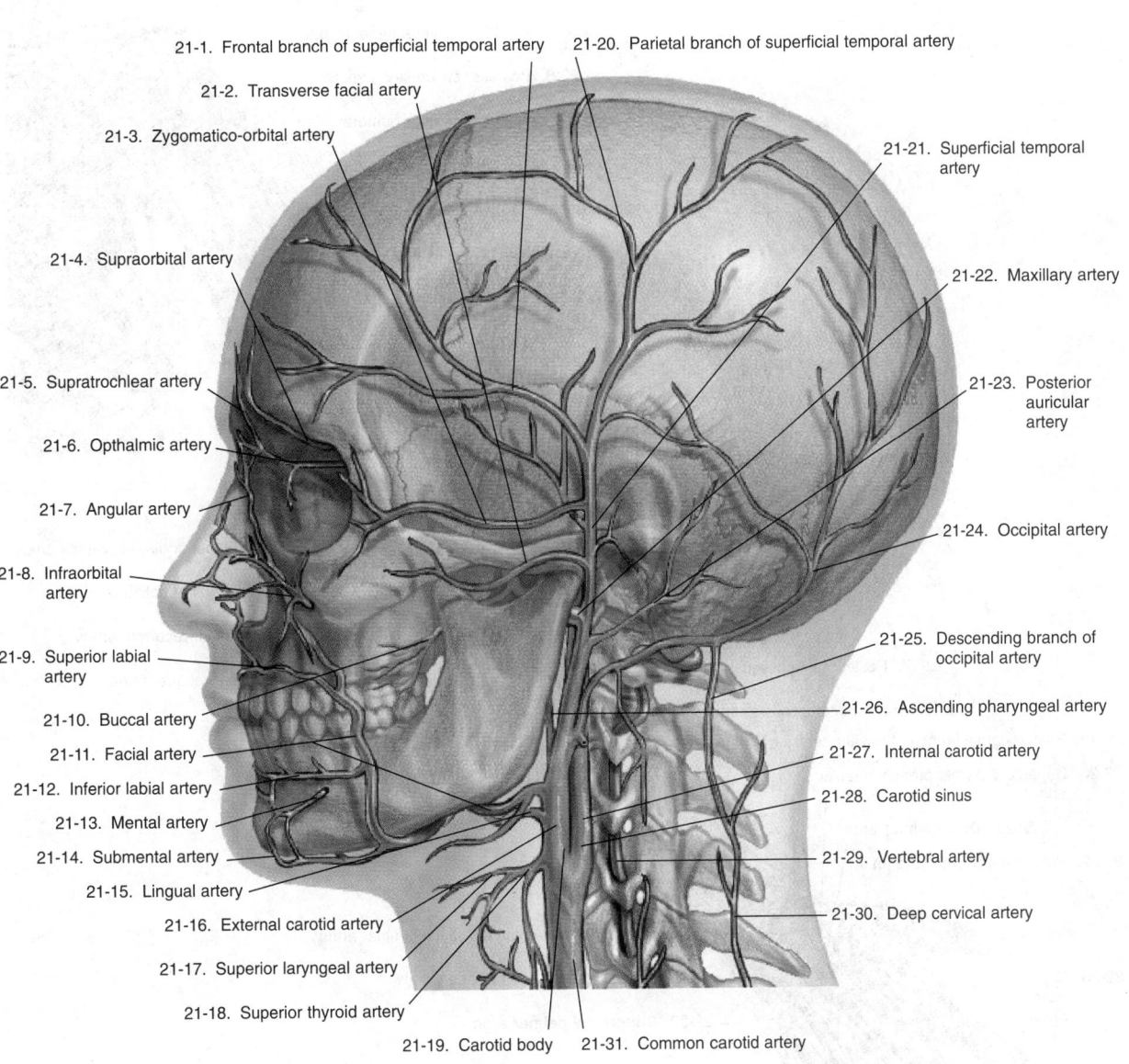

21-1. Frontal branch of superficial temporal artery

21-2. Transverse facial artery

21-3. Zygomatico-orbital artery

21-4. Supraorbital artery

21-5. Supratrochlear artery

21-6. Opthalmic artery

21-7. Angular artery

21-8. Infraorbital artery

21-9. Superior labial artery

21-10. Buccal artery

21-11. Facial artery

21-12. Inferior labial artery

21-13. Mental artery

21-14. Submental artery

21-15. Lingual artery

21-16. External carotid artery

21-17. Superior laryngeal artery

21-18. Superior thyroid artery

21-19. Carotid body

21-20. Parietal branch of superficial temporal artery

21-21. Superficial temporal artery

21-22. Maxillary artery

21-23. Posterior auricular artery

21-24. Occipital artery

21-25. Descending branch of occipital artery

21-26. Ascending pharyngeal artery

21-27. Internal carotid artery

21-28. Carotid sinus

21-29. Vertebral artery

21-30. Deep cervical artery

21-31. Common carotid artery

Color Anatomy

PLATE 22: ARTERIAL SUPPLY OF UPPER LIMB, ANTERIOR VIEW

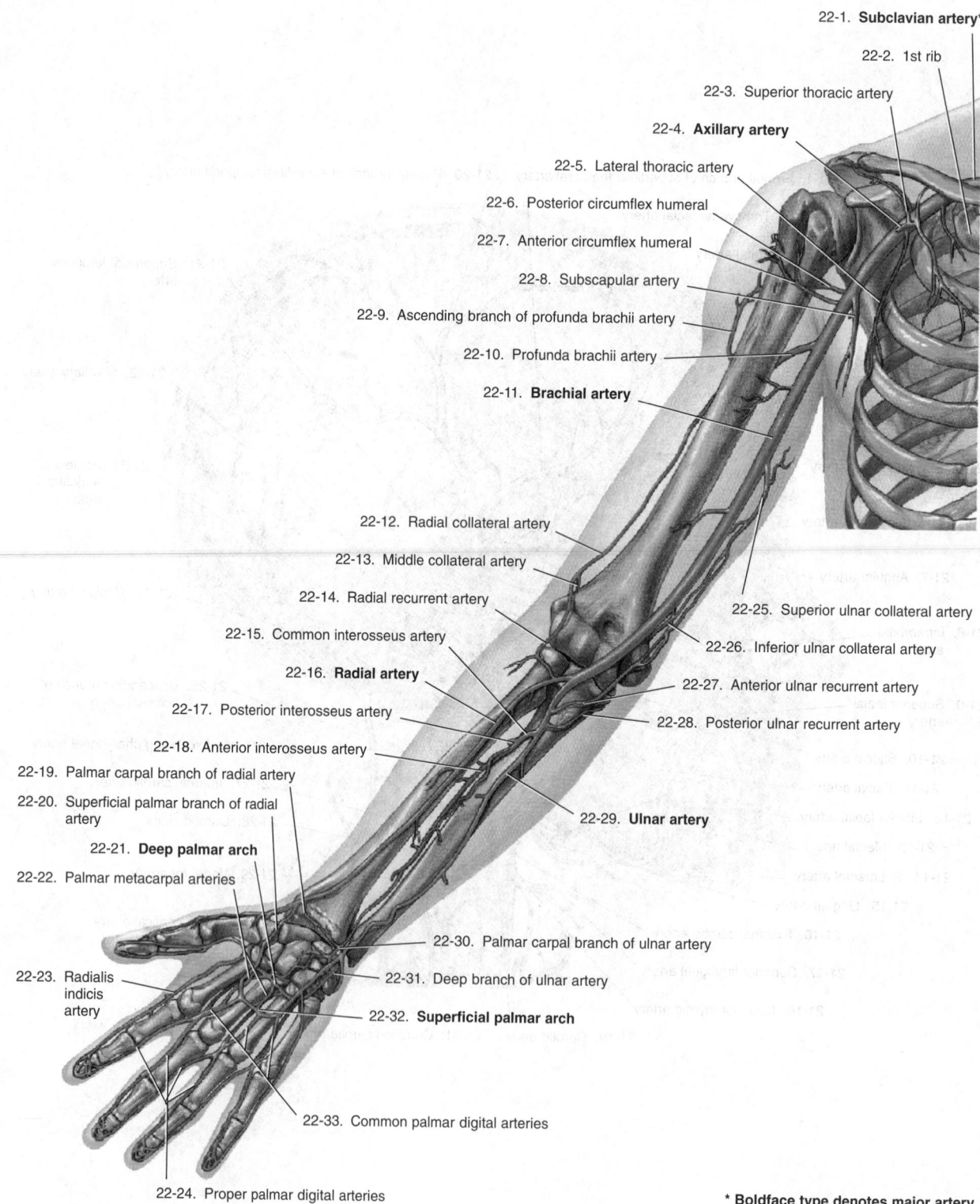

22-1. **Subclavian artery***

22-2. 1st rib

22-3. Superior thoracic artery

22-4. **Axillary artery**

22-5. Lateral thoracic artery

22-6. Posterior circumflex humeral

22-7. Anterior circumflex humeral

22-8. Subscapular artery

22-9. Ascending branch of profunda brachii artery

22-10. Profunda brachii artery

22-11. **Brachial artery**

22-12. Radial collateral artery

22-13. Middle collateral artery

22-14. Radial recurrent artery

22-15. Common interosseus artery

22-16. **Radial artery**

22-17. Posterior interosseus artery

22-18. Anterior interosseus artery

22-19. Palmar carpal branch of radial artery

22-20. Superficial palmar branch of radial artery

22-21. **Deep palmar arch**

22-22. Palmar metacarpal arteries

22-23. Radialis indicis artery

22-24. Proper palmar digital arteries

22-25. Superior ulnar collateral artery

22-26. Inferior ulnar collateral artery

22-27. Anterior ulnar recurrent artery

22-28. Posterior ulnar recurrent artery

22-29. **Ulnar artery**

22-30. Palmar carpal branch of ulnar artery

22-31. Deep branch of ulnar artery

22-32. **Superficial palmar arch**

22-33. Common palmar digital arteries

* **Boldface type denotes major artery**

A.D.A.M. Image

PLATE 23: ARTERIES OF LOWER LIMB, ANTERIOR VIEW

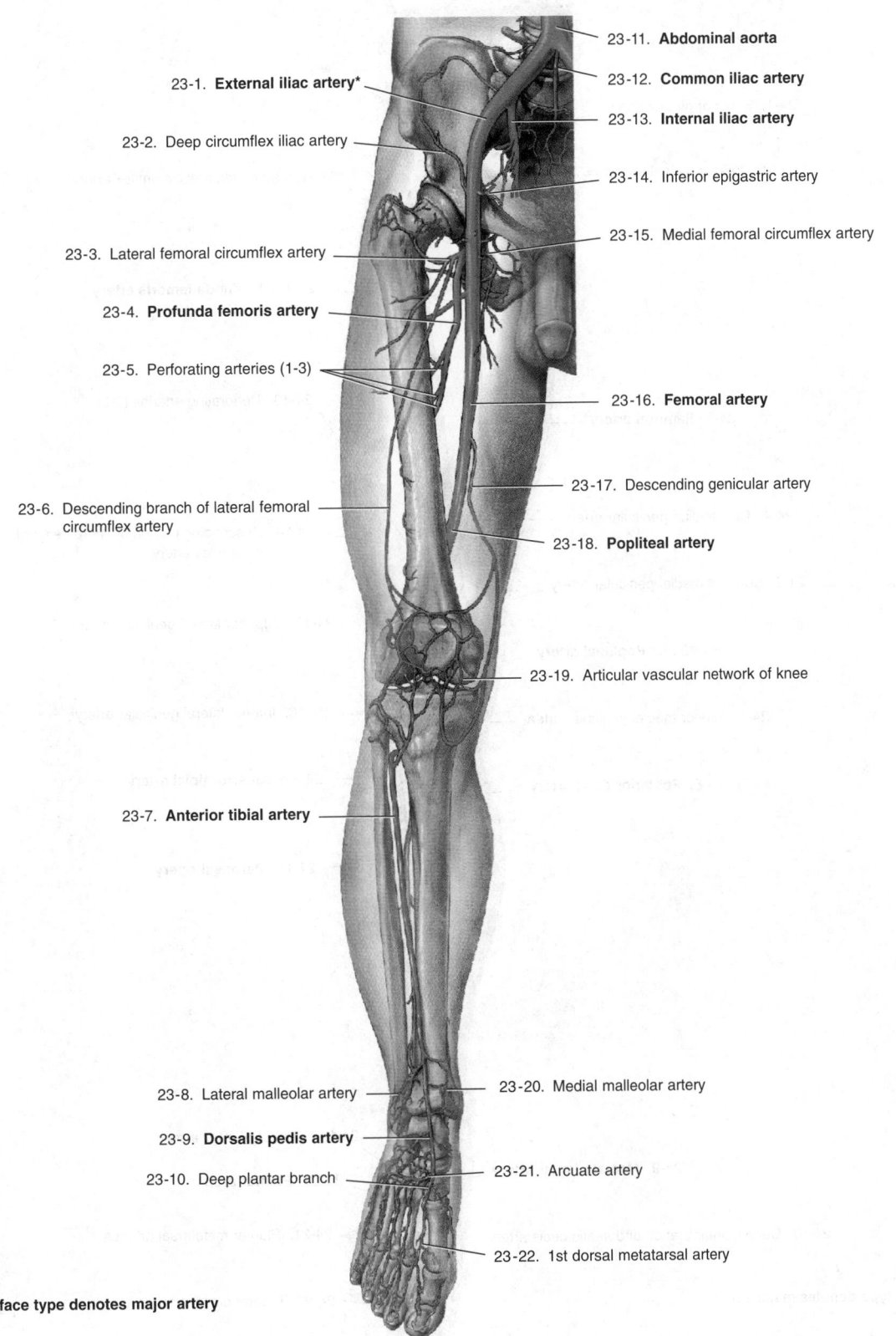

23-1. **External iliac artery***

23-2. Deep circumflex iliac artery

23-3. Lateral femoral circumflex artery

23-4. **Profunda femoris artery**

23-5. Perforating arteries (1-3)

23-6. Descending branch of lateral femoral circumflex artery

23-7. **Anterior tibial artery**

23-8. Lateral malleolar artery

23-9. **Dorsalis pedis artery**

23-10. Deep plantar branch

23-11. **Abdominal aorta**

23-12. **Common iliac artery**

23-13. **Internal iliac artery**

23-14. Inferior epigastric artery

23-15. Medial femoral circumflex artery

23-16. **Femoral artery**

23-17. Descending genicular artery

23-18. **Popliteal artery**

23-19. Articular vascular network of knee

23-20. Medial malleolar artery

23-21. Arcuate artery

23-22. 1st dorsal metatarsal artery

* **Boldface type denotes major artery**

PLATE 24: ARTERIES OF LOWER LIMB, POSTERIOR VIEW

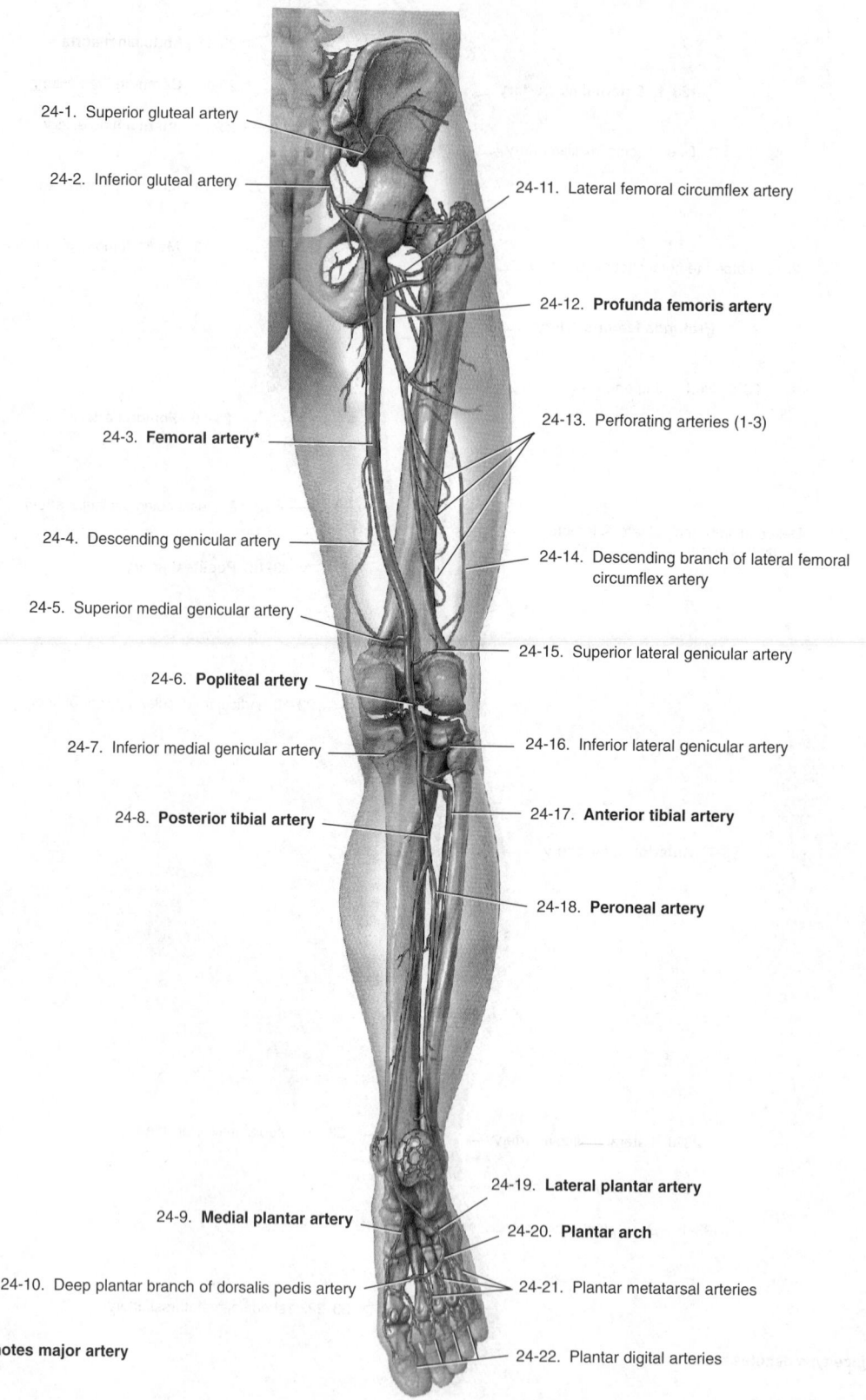

24-1. Superior gluteal artery

24-2. Inferior gluteal artery

24-3. **Femoral artery***

24-4. Descending genicular artery

24-5. Superior medial genicular artery

24-6. **Popliteal artery**

24-7. Inferior medial genicular artery

24-8. **Posterior tibial artery**

24-9. **Medial plantar artery**

24-10. Deep plantar branch of dorsalis pedis artery

* Boldface type denotes major artery

24-11. Lateral femoral circumflex artery

24-12. **Profunda femoris artery**

24-13. Perforating arteries (1-3)

24-14. Descending branch of lateral femoral circumflex artery

24-15. Superior lateral genicular artery

24-16. Inferior lateral genicular artery

24-17. **Anterior tibial artery**

24-18. **Peroneal artery**

24-19. **Lateral plantar artery**

24-20. **Plantar arch**

24-21. Plantar metatarsal arteries

24-22. Plantar digital arteries

A.D.A.M. Image

PLATE 25: NERVES OF ARM, ANTERIOR VIEW

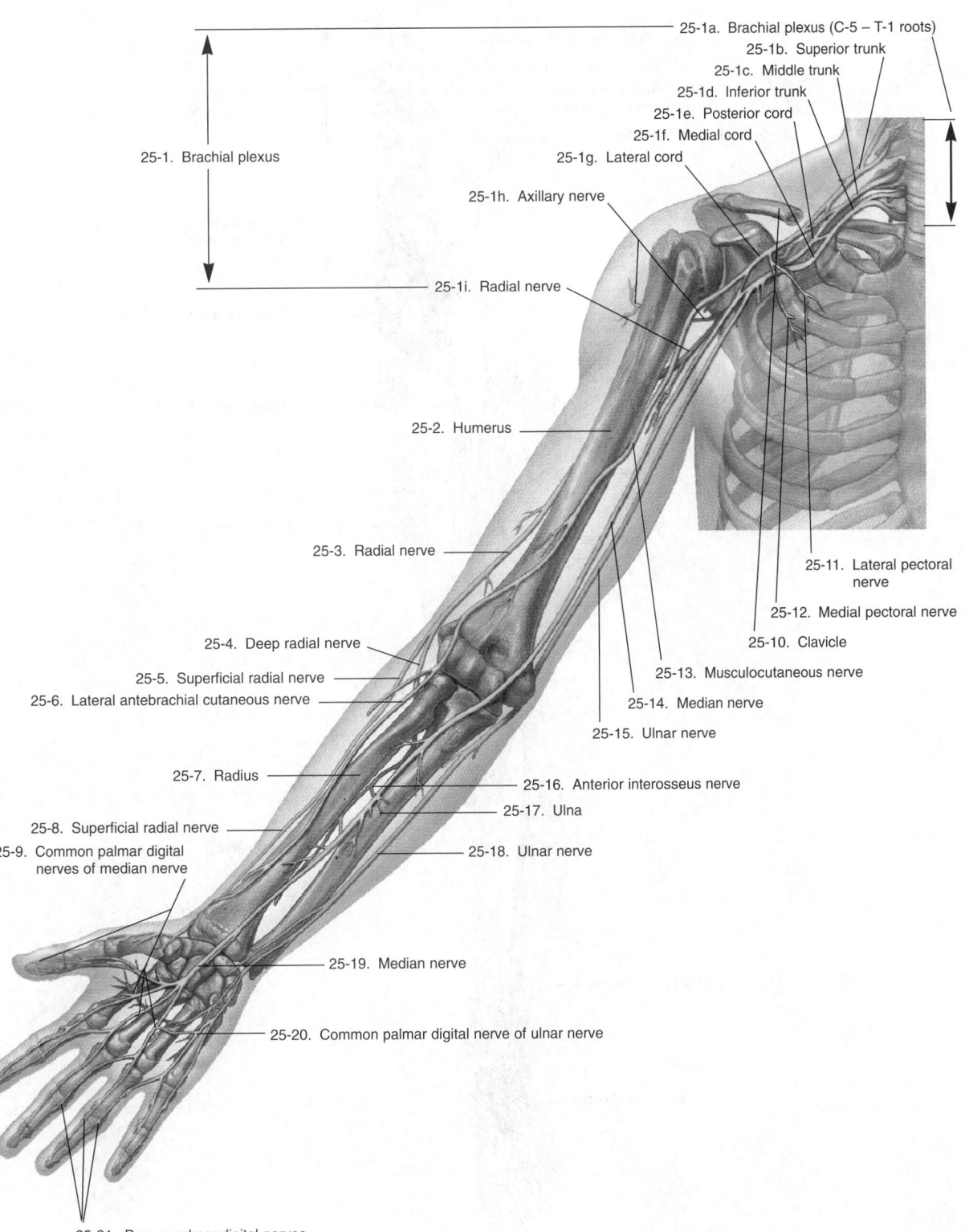

25-1a. Brachial plexus (C-5 – T-1 roots)

25-1b. Superior trunk

25-1c. Middle trunk

25-1d. Inferior trunk

25-1e. Posterior cord

25-1f. Medial cord

25-1g. Lateral cord

25-1. Brachial plexus

25-1h. Axillary nerve

25-1i. Radial nerve

25-2. Humerus

25-3. Radial nerve

25-4. Deep radial nerve

25-5. Superficial radial nerve

25-6. Lateral antebrachial cutaneous nerve

25-7. Radius

25-8. Superficial radial nerve

25-9. Common palmar digital nerves of median nerve

25-11. Lateral pectoral nerve

25-12. Medial pectoral nerve

25-10. Clavicle

25-13. Musculocutaneous nerve

25-14. Median nerve

25-15. Ulnar nerve

25-16. Anterior interosseus nerve

25-17. Ulna

25-18. Ulnar nerve

25-19. Median nerve

25-20. Common palmar digital nerve of ulnar nerve

25-21. Proper palmar digital nerves

Color Anatomy

PLATE 26: NERVES OF LOWER LIMB, ANTERIOR VIEW

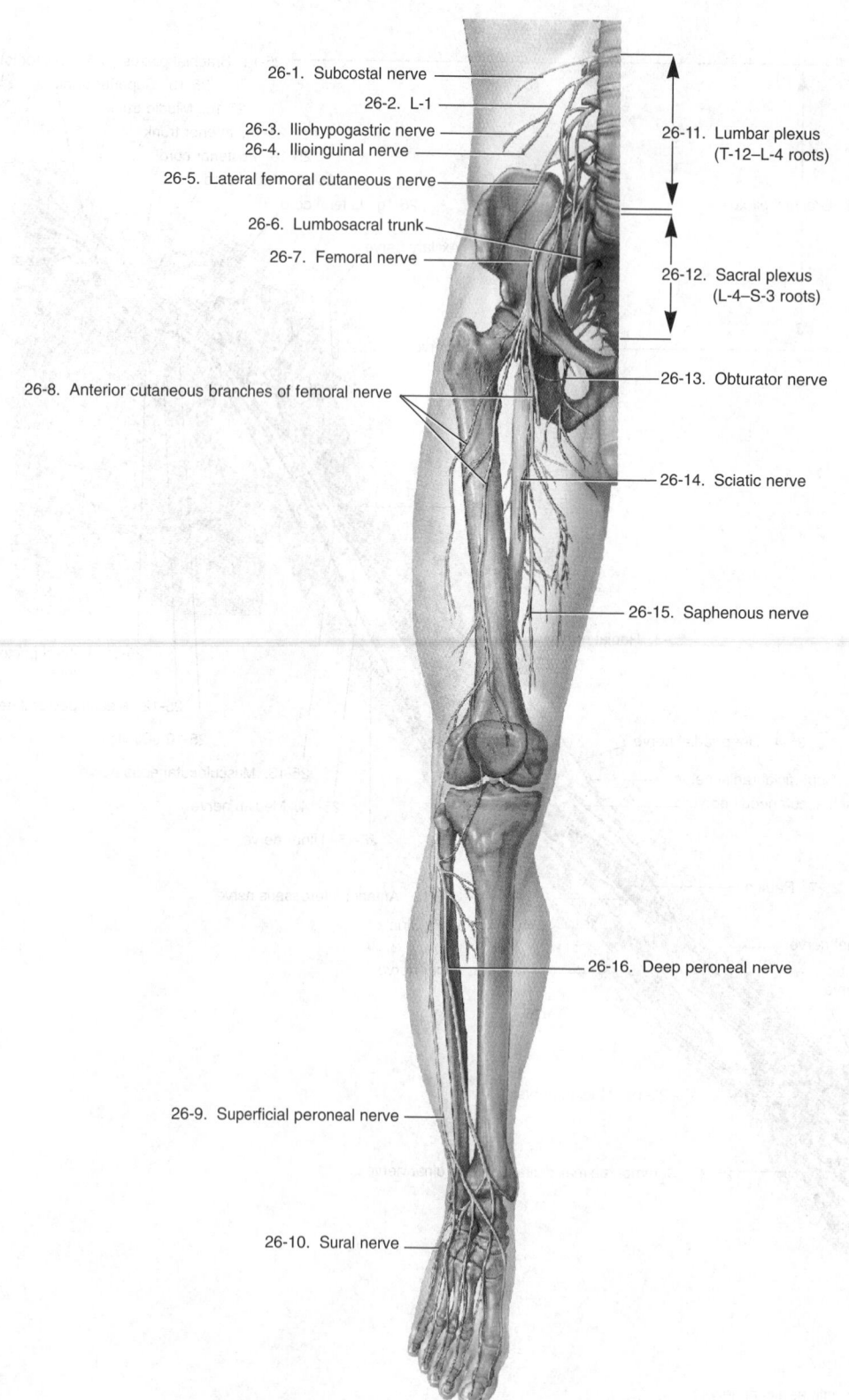

26-1. Subcostal nerve

26-2. L-1

26-3. Iliohypogastric nerve

26-4. Ilioinguinal nerve

26-5. Lateral femoral cutaneous nerve

26-6. Lumbosacral trunk

26-7. Femoral nerve

26-8. Anterior cutaneous branches of femoral nerve

26-9. Superficial peroneal nerve

26-10. Sural nerve

26-11. Lumbar plexus (T-12–L-4 roots)

26-12. Sacral plexus (L-4–S-3 roots)

26-13. Obturator nerve

26-14. Sciatic nerve

26-15. Saphenous nerve

26-16. Deep peroneal nerve

PLATE 27: NERVES OF LOWER LIMB, POSTERIOR VIEW

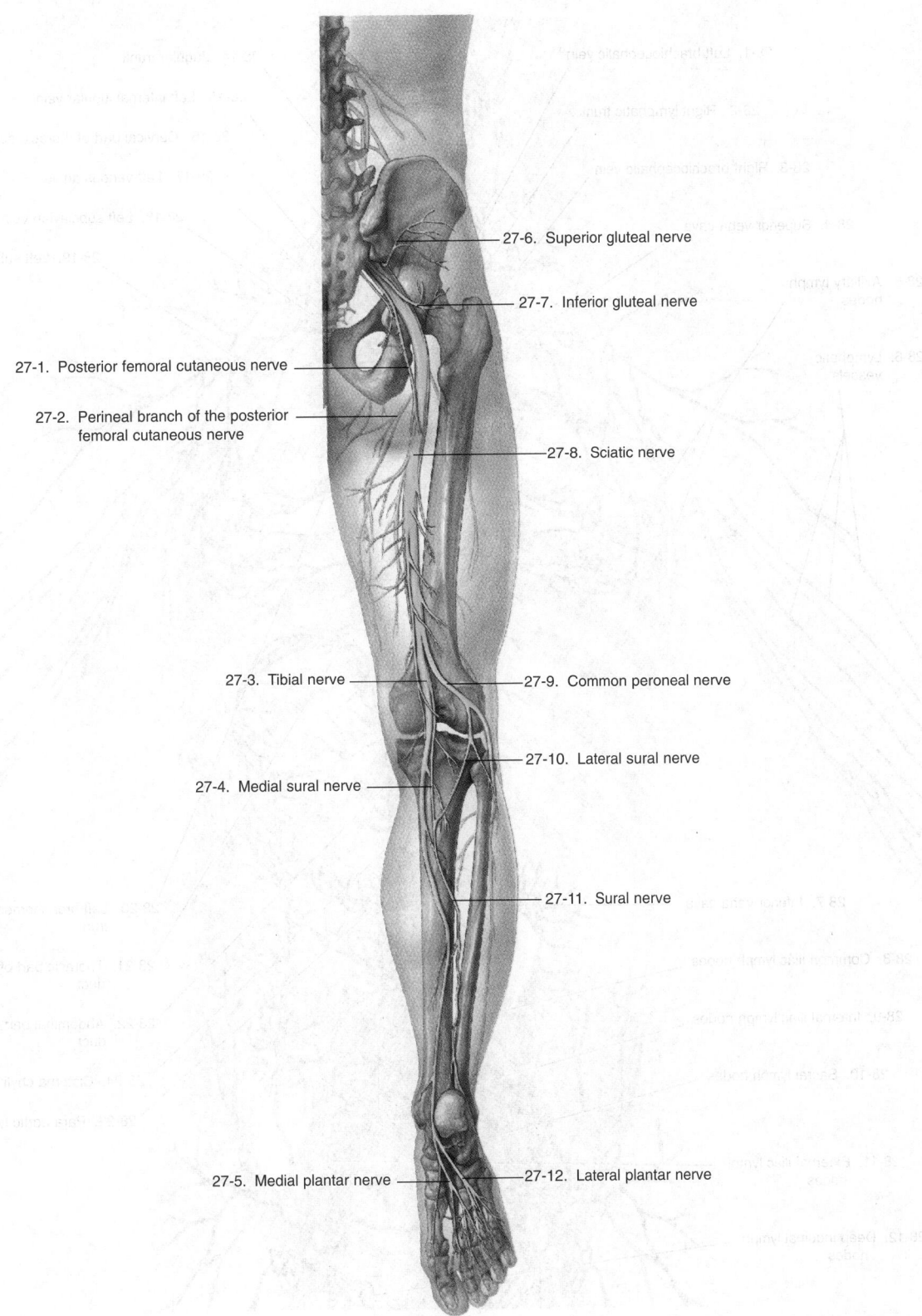

27-6. Superior gluteal nerve

27-7. Inferior gluteal nerve

27-1. Posterior femoral cutaneous nerve

27-2. Perineal branch of the posterior femoral cutaneous nerve

27-8. Sciatic nerve

27-3. Tibial nerve

27-9. Common peroneal nerve

27-10. Lateral sural nerve

27-4. Medial sural nerve

27-11. Sural nerve

27-5. Medial plantar nerve

27-12. Lateral plantar nerve

Color Anatomy

A.D.A.M. Image

PLATE 28: LYMPHATICS OF THE BODY

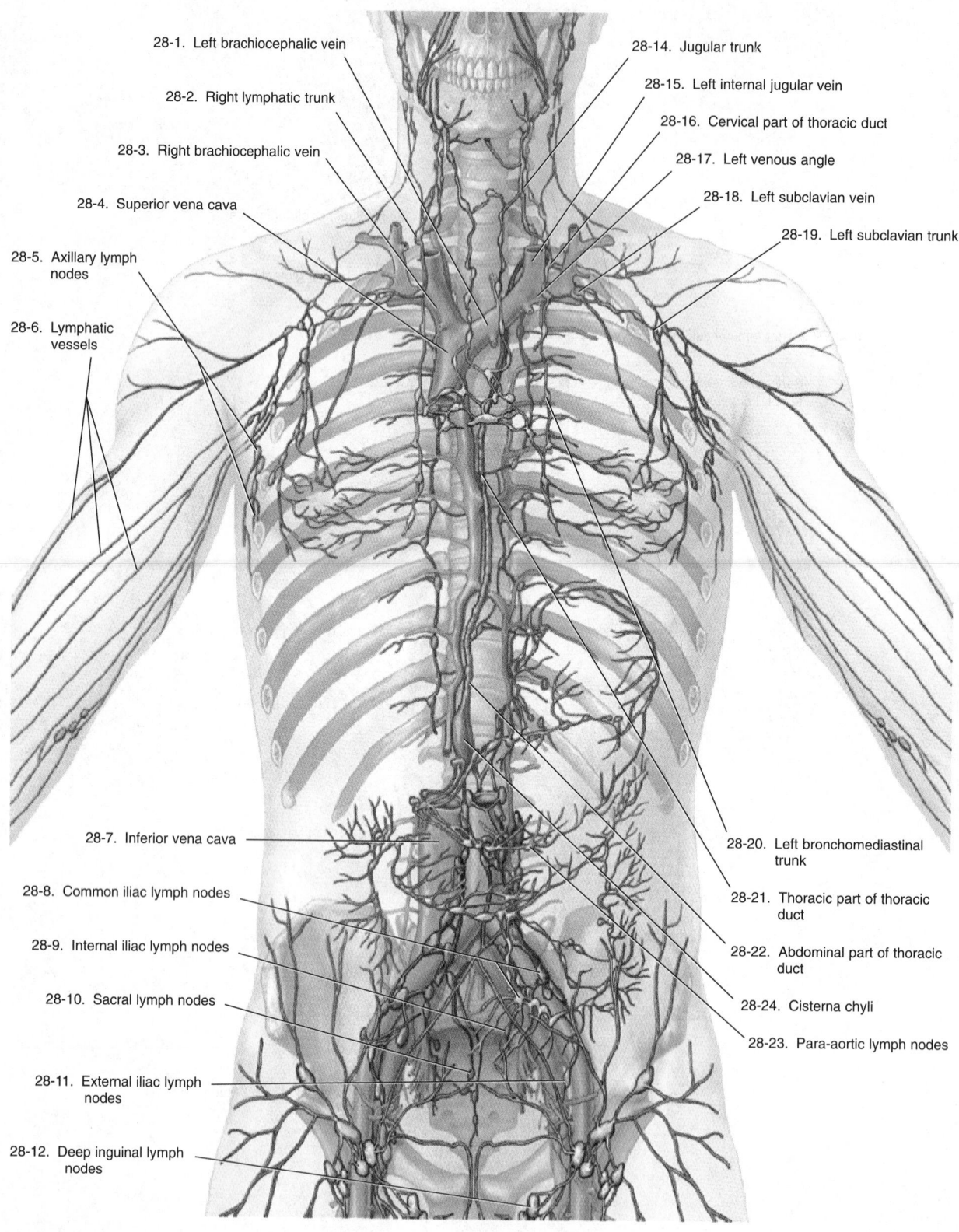

28-1. Left brachiocephalic vein

28-2. Right lymphatic trunk

28-3. Right brachiocephalic vein

28-4. Superior vena cava

28-5. Axillary lymph nodes

28-6. Lymphatic vessels

28-14. Jugular trunk

28-15. Left internal jugular vein

28-16. Cervical part of thoracic duct

28-17. Left venous angle

28-18. Left subclavian vein

28-19. Left subclavian trunk

28-7. Inferior vena cava

28-8. Common iliac lymph nodes

28-9. Internal iliac lymph nodes

28-10. Sacral lymph nodes

28-11. External iliac lymph nodes

28-12. Deep inguinal lymph nodes

28-20. Left bronchomediastinal trunk

28-21. Thoracic part of thoracic duct

28-22. Abdominal part of thoracic duct

28-24. Cisterna chyli

28-23. Para-aortic lymph nodes

PLATE 29: LEFT LATERAL VIEW OF CEREBRUM

29-1. Central sulcus of Rolando
29-2. Precentral sulcus
29-3. Superior frontal gyrus
29-4. Opercular part of inferior frontal gyrus
29-5. Superior frontal sulcus
29-6. Middle frontal gyrus
29-7. Inferior frontal sulcus
29-8. Triangular part of inferior frontal gyrus

29-14. Precentral gyrus
29-15. Postcentral gyrus
29-16. Postcentral sulcus
29-17. Supramarginal gyrus
29-18. Intraparietal sulcus
29-19. Inferior parietal lobule
29-20. Superior parietal lobule
29-21. Angular gyrus
29-22. Transverse occipital sulcus
29-23. Parieto-occipital sulcus

29-9. Frontal pole

29-10. Orbital part of inferior frontal gyrus

29-11. Temporal pole

29-12. Superior temporal gyrus

29-13. Lateral sulcus of Sylvius

29-24. Occipital pole
29-25. Lunate sulcus
29-26. Calcarine sulcus
29-27. Preoccipital notch
29-28. Inferior temporal gyrus
29-29. Inferior temporal sulcus
29-30. Middle temporal gyrus
29-31. Superior temporal sulcus

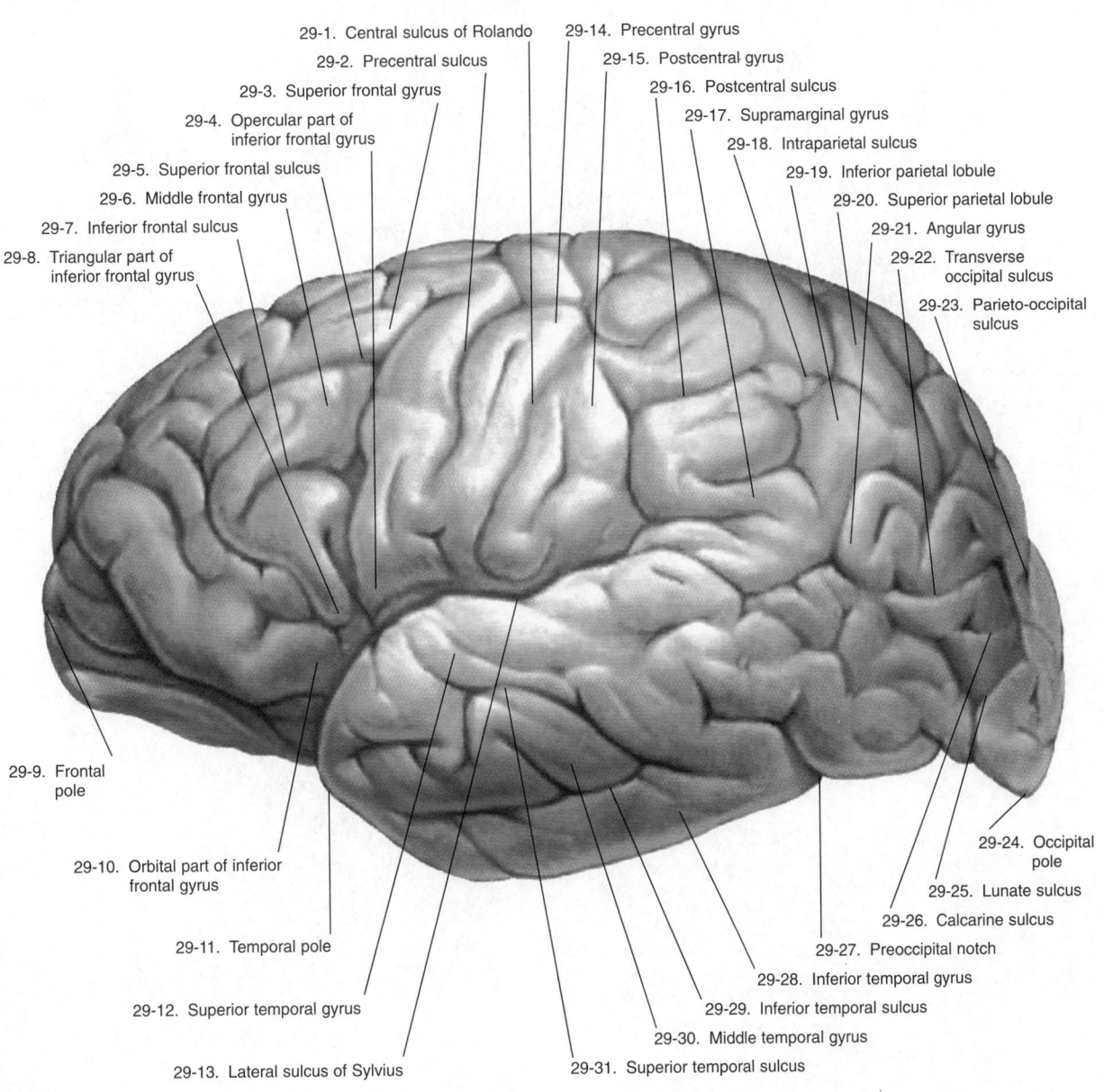

Color Anatomy

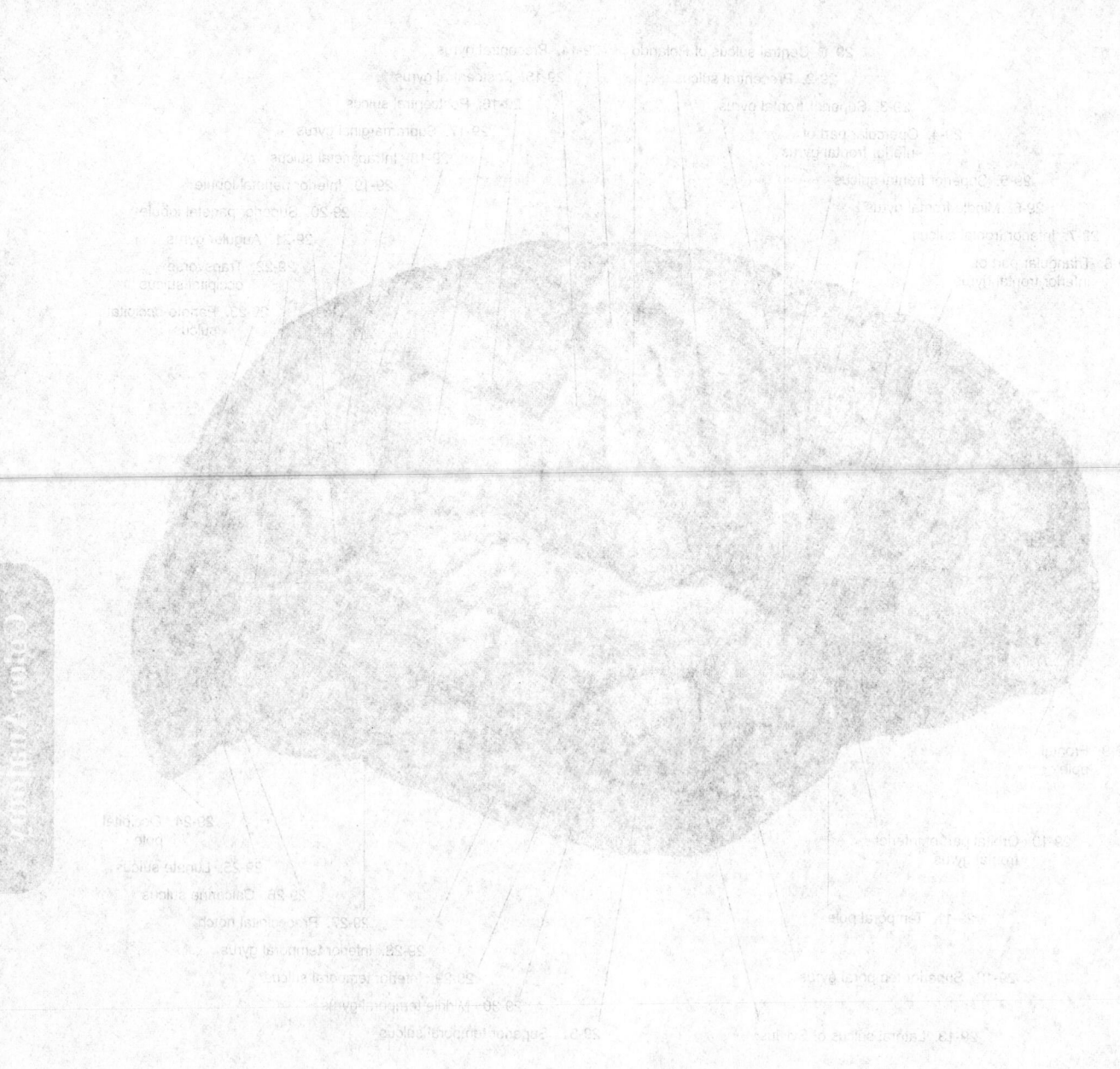

M

μ **1.** 12th Letter of the Greek alphabet. **2.** Symbol for micro- (2); micron; dynamic *viscosity*; magnetic or electric dipole moment of a molecule; chemical *potential*; denotes the position of a substituent located on the 12th atom from the carboxyl or other functional group.

μμ Symbol for micromicro-; micromicron.

μμg Symbol for micromicrogram.

μΩ Symbol for microhm.

μC Symbol for microcoulomb.

μCi Symbol for microcurie.

μg Symbol for microgram.

μl Symbol for microliter.

μM Symbol for micromolar.

μm Symbol for micrometer.

μmol Symbol for micromole.

μV Symbol for microvolt.

M 1. Symbol for mega- (2); morgan; moles per liter (also written *M* or M); myopia or myopic; methionine; 6-mercaptopurine ribonucleoside in a nucleic acid; molarity; L. *misce*, mix. **2.** Symbol for a blood factor. See entries under MNSs blood group, Blood Groups Appendix.

M. Abbreviation for L. *misce*, mix.

M_r Symbol for molecular weight *ratio* or relative molecular *mass*.

m Symbol for meter; milli-; minim; mass; magnetic dipole moment; molality.

mμ Symbol for millimicron.

mM Abbreviation for millimolar (10^{-3} M).

M Symbol for moles per liter (also written M or *M*).

△*m-* Abbreviation for meta- (3).

MA Abbreviation for mental *age*.

ma, mA Abbreviation for milliampere.

MAA Abbreviation for macroaggregated *albumin*.

MAB Abbreviation for monoclonal *antibody*.

MAC 1. Abbreviation for minimal anesthetic *concentration*; minimal alveolar *concentration*; membrane attack *complex*. **2.** Abbreviation for *Mycobacterium avium* complex. SEE *Mycobacterium avium-intracellulare complex*.

△**Mac-.** For proper names beginning thus, see also Mc-.

Ma·ca·ca (mă-kah′kă). A large genus of Old World monkeys (family Cercopithecidae) that includes the macaque and rhesus monkeys, and the Barbary apes. *M. mulatta*, the rhesus monkey, is used as a research animal. [Pg. *macaco,* monkey]

ma·caque (mă-kahk′). SEE *Macaca*. [Fr.]

Macchiavello's stain. See under stain.

MacConkey, Alfred T., British bacteriologist, 1861–1931. SEE MacConkey *agar*.

Mace, MACE Acronym for *m*ethyl*c*hloroform 2-chlor*ace*tophenone (the classical lacrimator) in a light petroleum dispersant and a pressurized propellant.

mac·er·ate (mas′er-āt). To soften by steeping or soaking. [see maceration]

mac·er·a·tion (mas-er-a′shŭn). **1.** Softening by the action of a liquid. **2.** Softening of tissues after death by nonputrefactive (sterile) autolysis; seen especially in the stillborn, with bullous separation of the epidermis. [L. *macero*, pp. *-atus*, to soften by soaking]

Macewen, Sir William, Scottish surgeon, 1848–1924. SEE M.'s *sign, symptom, triangle*.

Mach, Ernst, Austrian scientist, 1838–1916. SEE M.'s *band*; M. *number*.

Machado-Guerreiro test. See under test.

Machado-Joseph. See under disease.

ma·chine (mă-shēn′). Any mechanical apparatus or device. [L. *machina*, contrivance]

anesthesia m., equipment used for inhalation anesthesia, including flowmeters, vaporizers, and sources of compressed gases, but not including the anesthetic circuit or mechanisms for elimination of carbon dioxide.

heart-lung m., a device incorporating a blood pump (artificial heart) and a blood oxygenator (artificial lung) to provide extracorporeal circulation and oxygenation of the blood during cardiac surgery.

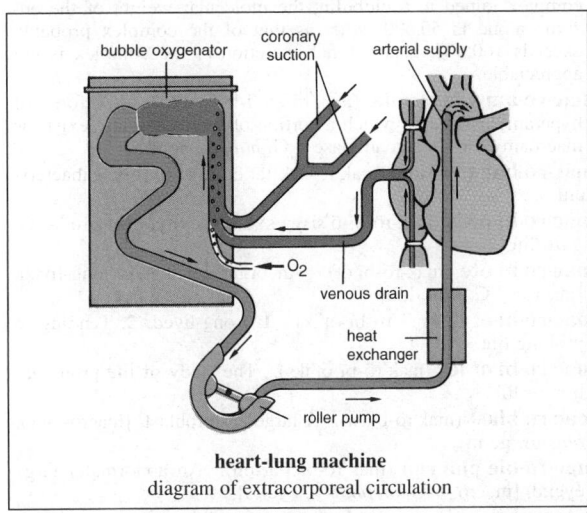

heart-lung machine
diagram of extracorporeal circulation

panoramic rotating m., an x-ray machine using a reciprocating motion of the tube and extraoral film to produce a radiograph of all the teeth and surrounding structures.

Mackay, R. Stuart, U.S. physicist, *1924. SEE M.-Marg *tonometer*.

Mackenrodt, Alwin K., German gynecologist, 1859–1925. SEE M.'s *ligament*.

Mackenzie, Sir James, Scottish physician practicing in London, 1853–1925. SEE M.'s *polygraph*.

Mackenzie, Richard J., Scottish surgeon, 1821–1854. SEE M.'s *amputation*.

MacLachlan, Elsie A., 20th century researcher. SEE Lowe-Terrey-MacL. *syndrome*.

Macleod, Roderick, Scottish physician, 1795–1852. SEE M.'s *rheumatism*.

Macleod, William Mathieson, British physician, 1911–1977. SEE M.'s *syndrome*; Swyer-James-MacLeod *syndrome*.

ma·clur·in (mă-klūr′in) [C.I. 75240]. A natural dye associated with morin and derived from fustic; used to dye fabrics with various metal mordants. It turns deep green on addition of ferric chloride.

MacNeal, Ward J., U.S. bacteriologist, 1881–1946. SEE M.'s tetrachrome blood *stain*; Novy and M. blood *agar*.

△**macr-.** SEE macro-.

Mac·ra·can·tho·rhyn·chus (mak′ră-kan-thō-ring′kŭs). A genus of giant thorny-headed worms (class Acanthocephala). [macro- + G. *akantha*, thorn, + *rhynchos*, snout]

M. hirudina′ceus, the giant thorny-headed worm of the pig, approximately the size of the giant roundworm (*Ascaris*); it inhabits the intestinal tract where nodules develop at the site of penetration of the spiny proboscis of each worm; it has occasionally been reported in man; transmission is by ingestion of infected insects, frequently dung beetles or cockroaches that have fed on feces of infected pigs containing viable eggs and have developed the cystacanth stage infective to the vertebrate host, including humans.

ma

mac·ren·ceph·a·ly, mac·ren·ce·pha·lia (mak′ren-sef′ă-lē, -sĕ-fā′lē-ă). Hypertrophy of the brain; the condition of having a large brain. [macro- + G. *enkephalos,* brain]

⌂**macro-, macr-.** Large, long. SEE ALSO mega-, megalo-. [G. *makros*]

mac·ro·ad·e·no·ma (mak′rō-ad-ĕ-nō′mă). A pituitary adenoma larger than 10 mm in diameter.

mac·ro·am·y·lase (mak-rō-am′i-lās). Descriptive term applied to a form of serum amylase in which the enzyme is present as a complex joined to a globulin; the molecular weight of the enzyme alone is 50,000, whereas that of the complex probably exceeds 160,000; hence, renal excretion of the complex is not appreciable.

mac·ro·am·y·la·se·mia (mak′rō-am′i-lā-sē′mē-ă). A form of hyperamylasemia, in which a portion of serum amylase exists as macroamylase. [macroamylase + G. *haima,* blood]

mac·ro·bac·te·ri·um (mak′rō-bak-tēr′ē-ŭm). SYN megabacterium.

mac·ro·bi·o·sis (mak′rō-bī-ō′sis). SYN longevity. [macro- + G. *bios,* life]

mac·ro·bi·ote (mak-rō-bī′ōt). An organism that is long-lived. [macro- + G. *bios,* life]

mac·ro·bi·ot·ic (mak′rō-bī-ot′ik). **1.** Long-lived. **2.** Tending to prolong life.

mac·ro·bi·ot·ics (mak′rō-bī-ot′iks). The study of the prolongation of life.

mac·ro·blast (mak′rō-blast). A large erythroblast. [macro- + G. *blastos,* germ]

mac·ro·ble·pha·ron (mak′rō-blef′ar-on). An abnormally large eyelid. [macro- + G. *blepharon,* eyelid]

mac·ro·bra·chia (mak-rō-brā′kē-ă). Condition of having abnormally thick or long arms. [macro- + G. *brachiōn,* arm]

mac·ro·car·dia (mak-rō-kar′dē-ă). SYN cardiomegaly.

mac·ro·ce·phal·ic, mac·ro·ceph·a·lous (mak′rō-se-fal′ik, -sef′ă-lŭs). SYN megacephalic. [macro- + G. *kephalē,* head]

mac·ro·ceph·a·ly, mac·ro·ce·pha·lia (mak-rō-sef′ă-lē, -sĕ-fā′lē-ă). SYN megacephaly. [macro- + G. *kephalē,* head]

mac·ro·chei·lia, mac·ro·chi·lia (mak-rō-kī′lē-ă). **1.** Abnormally enlarged lips. SYN macrolabia. **2.** Cavernous lymphangioma of the lip, a condition of permanent swelling of the lip resulting from the presence of greatly distended lymphatic spaces. SYN macrochilia. [macro- + G. *cheilos,* lip]

mac·ro·chei·ria, mac·ro·chi·ria (mak-rō-kī′rē-ă). A condition characterized by abnormally large hands. SYN cheiromegaly, chiromegaly, megalocheiria, megalochiria. [macro- + G. *cheir,* hand]

mac·ro·chem·is·try (mak-rō-kem′is-trē). The use of chemical procedures, the reactions of which (color change, effervescence, etc.) are visible to the unaided eye. Cf. microchemistry.

mac·ro·chi·lia (mak-rō-kī′lē-ă). SYN macrocheilia.

mac·ro·chy·lo·mi·cron (mak′rō-kī-lō-mī′kron). An unusually large chylomicron.

mac·ro·cne·mia (mak-rō-nē′mē-ă). A condition characterized by enlargement of the legs below the knee. [macro- + G. *knēmē,* leg]

mac·ro·coc·cus (mak′rō-kok′ŭs). SYN megacoccus.

mac·ro·co·lon (mak′rō-kō′lon). A sigmoid colon of unusual length; a variety of megacolon.

mac·ro·co·nid·i·um, pl. **mac·ro·co·nid·ia** (mak′rō-kō-nid′ē-ŭm, -ă). **1.** A conidium, or exospore, of large size. **2.** In fungi, the larger of two distinctively different-sized types of conidia in a single species, thick- or thin-walled and composed of 2 to 10 cells; characteristic of most dermatophytes and some other genera e.g., *Histoplasma, Fusarium.* [macro- + Mod. L. dim. fr. G. *konis,* dust]

mac·ro·cor·nea (mak-rō-kōr′nē-ă). An abnormally large cornea.

mac·ro·cra·ni·um (mak-rō-krā′nē-ŭm). An enlarged skull, especially the bones containing the brain, as seen in hydrocephalus; the face appears relatively small in comparison.

mac·ro·cry·o·glob·u·lin (mak-rō-krī-ō-glob′yū-lin). A macroglobulin that has the properties of a cryoglobulin.

mac·ro·cry·o·glob·u·li·ne·mia (mak′rō-krī-ō-glob′yū-lin-ē′mē-ă). The presence of cold-precipitating macroglobulins in the peripheral blood; such macrocryoglobulins are often called cold hemagglutinins.

mac·ro·cyst (mak′rō-sist). A cyst of macroscopic proportions.

mac·ro·cy·tase (mak-rō-sī′tās). According to Metchnikoff, a cytase or complement, formed by the large uninuclear leukocytes, which is effective in the destruction of tissue cells, blood cells, etc.

mac·ro·cyte (mak′rō-sīt). A large erythrocyte, such as those observed in pernicious anemia. SYN macroerythrocyte. [macro- + G. *kytos,* a hollow (cell)]

mac·ro·cy·the·mia (mak′rō-sī-thē′mē-ă). The occurrence of unusually large numbers of macrocytes in the circulating blood. SYN macrocytosis, megalocythemia, megalocytosis. [macrocyte + G. *haima,* blood]

  hyperchromatic m., an inexact term frequently used for macrocytes that contain an unusually large amount of hemoglobin, but are actually normochromic; although the total mass of hemoglobin is greater than normal (owing to the large cells), the percentage of hemoglobin in the cells is not greater than normal.

mac·ro·cy·to·sis (mak′rō-sī-tō′sis). SYN macrocythemia. [macrocyte + G. *-osis,* condition]

mac·ro·dac·tyl·ia, mac·ro·dac·tyl·ism, mac·ro·dac·ty·ly (mak-rō-dak-til′ē-ă, -dak′til-izm, dak′ti-lē). SYN megadactyly.

mac·ro·dont (mak′rō-dont). **1.** A tooth of abnormally large and frequently distorted proportions; the condition may be localized or generalized. **2.** Denoting a skull with a dental index above 44. SYN megadont, megalodont. [macro- + G. *odous* (*odont-*), tooth]

mac·ro·don·tia, mac·ro·don·tism (mak-rō-don′shē-ă, -don′tizm). The state of having abnormally large teeth. SYN megadontism, megalodontia.

mac·ro·dys·tro·phia li·po·ma·to·sa (mak′rō-dis-trō′fē-ă lip-ō-mă-tō′să). A rare nonfamilial disease characterized by enlargement of the fingers by lipomas, with painful degenerative arthropathy of the metacarpophalangeal and interphalangeal joints.

mac·ro·ele·ments (mak′rō-el′ĕ-ments). Inorganic nutrients needed in relatively high daily amounts (*i.e.,* more than 100 mg per day) e.g., calcium, phosphorus, sodium, etc. SYN macrominerals.

mac·ro·en·ceph·a·lon (mak′rō-en-sef′ă-lon). SYN megaloencephalon. [macro- + G. *enkephalos,* brain]

mac·ro·e·ryth·ro·blast (mak′rō-ĕ-rith′rō-blast). A large erythroblast. SYN macronormochromoblast.

mac·ro·e·ryth·ro·cyte (mak′rō-ĕ-rith′rō-sīt). SYN macrocyte.

mac·ro·es·the·sia (mak′rō-es-thē′zē-ă). A subjective sensation that all objects are larger than they are. [macro- + G. *aisthēsis,* sensation]

mac·ro·ga·mete (mak-rō-gam′ēt). The female element in anisogamy; it is the larger of the two sex cells, with more reserve material, and usually nonmotile. SYN megagamete. [macro- + G. *gametē,* wife]

mac·ro·ga·me·to·cyte (mak′rō-gă-mē′tō-sīt). The female gametocyte or mother cell producing the female or macrogamete among fungi or protozoa that undergo anisogamy. SYN macrogamont.

mac·ro·gam·ont (mak-rō-gam′ont). SYN macrogametocyte.

ma·crog·a·my (mă-krog′ă-mē). Conjugation of two adult cells or gametes. [macro- + G. *gamos,* marriage]

mac·ro·gas·tria (mak-rō-gas′trē-ă). SYN megalogastria.

mac·ro·gen·i·to·so·mia (mak′rō-jen′i-tō-sō′mē-ă). Excessive bodily and genital development. [macro- + L. *genitalis,* genital, + G. *sōma,* body]

  m. prae′cox, a disorder in which gonadal maturation (puberty) and the adolescent growth spurt in bodily height occur in the first decade of life; often associated with a pineal tumor or lesions in hypothalamic areas known to regulate gonadotrophin secretion. SYN Pellizzi's syndrome.

  m. prae′cox su′prarena′lis, precocious somatic growth and isosexual maturation of secondary sexual characteristics, resulting from an adrenocortical tumor.

ma·crog·lia (ma-krog'lē-ă). SYN astrocyte. [macro- + G. *glia*, glue]

mac·ro·glob·u·lin·e·mia (mak'rō-glob'yū-li-nē'mē-ă). The presence of increased levels of macroglobulins in the circulating blood.

Waldenström's m., m. occurring in elderly persons, characterized by proliferation of cells resembling lymphocytes or plasma cells in the bone marrow, anemia, increased sedimentation rate, and hyperglobulinemia with a narrow peak in γ-globulin or β₂-globulin at about 19 S units. The spleen, liver, or lymph nodes are often enlarged and there is frequently purpura or mucosal bleeding. SYN hyperglobulinemic purpura, Waldenström's purpura, Waldenström's syndrome.

mac·ro·glob·u·lins (mak-rō-glob'yū-lins). Plasma globulins of unusually large molecular weight, *e.g.,* as much as 1,000,000; α₂-macroglobulin inhibits thrombin and other proteases.

mac·ro·glos·sia (mak-rō-glos'ē-ă). Enlargement of the tongue, either developmental in origin or secondary to a neoplasm or vascular hamartoma. SYN megaloglossia. [macro- + G. *glōssa*, tongue]

mac·ro·gna·thia (mak-rō-nā'thē-ă). Enlargement or elongation of the jaw. SYN megagnathia. [macro- + G. *gnathos,* jaw]

ma·crog·ra·phy (mă-krog'ră-fē). Rarely used term for writing with very large letters. SYN megalographia. [macro- + G. *graphō,* to write]

mac·ro·gy·ria (mak-rō-jī'rē-ă). SYN pachygyria. [macro- + G. *gyros,* circle (gyrus)]

mac·ro·la·bia (mak'rō-lā'bē-ă). SYN macrocheilia (1). [macro- + L. *labium,* lip]

mac·ro·leu·ko·blast (mak-rō-lū'kō-blast). An unusually large leukoblast.

mac·ro·lides (mak'rō-līdz). A class of antibiotics discovered in streptomycetes, characterized by molecules made up of large-ring lactones; *e.g.,* erythromycin; many inhibit protein biosynthesis.

mac·ro·mas·tia, mac·ro·ma·zia (mak-rō-mas'tē-a, -mā'zē-ă). Abnormally large breasts. SEE ALSO hypermastia (2). [macro- + G. *mastos,* breast]

mac·ro·mel·a·no·some (mak-rō-mel'ă-nō-sōm). SYN giant *melanosome.*

mac·ro·me·lia (mak-rō-mē'lē-ă). Abnormal size of one or more of the limbs. SYN megalomelia. [macro- + G. *melos,* limb]

mac·ro·mere. A blastomere of large size, as in amphibians. [macro- + G. *meros,* part]

mac·ro·mer·o·zo·ite (mak'rō-mer-ō-zō'īt). A large merozoite. SYN megamerozoite. [macro- + G. *meros,* part, + *zōon,* animal]

mac·ro·min·er·als (mak-rō-min-er-alz). SYN macroelements.

mac·ro·mol·e·cule (mak-rō-mol'ĕ-kyūl). A molecule of colloidal size; *e.g.,* proteins, polynucleic acids, polysaccharides.

mac·ro·mon·o·cyte (mak-rō-mon'ō-sīt). An unusually large monocyte.

mac·ro·my·e·lo·blast (mak-rō-mī'ĕ-lō-blast). An abnormally large myeloblast.

mac·ro·nor·mo·blast (mak-rō-nōr'mō-blast). 1. A large normoblast. 2. A large, incompletely hemoglobiniferous, nucleated red blood cell with a "cart-wheel" nucleus.

mac·ro·nor·mo·chro·mo·blast (mak'rō-nōr-mō-krō'mō-blast). SYN macroerythroblast.

mac·ro·nu·cle·us (mak-rō-nū'klē-ŭs). 1. A nucleus that occupies a relatively large portion of the cell, or the larger nucleus where two or more are present in a cell. SYN meganucleus. 2. The larger of the two nuclei in ciliates, which governs vegetative metabolic functions and not reproduction. SYN somatic nucleus, trophic nucleus, trophonucleus. SEE ALSO micronucleus (2).

mac·ro·nu·tri·ents (mak-rō-nū'trē-ents). Nutrients required in the greatest amount; *e.g.,* carbohydrates, protein, fats.

mac·ro·nych·ia (mak-rō-nik'ē-ă). Abnormally large fingernails or toenails. SYN megalonychosis. [macro- + G. *onyx,* nail]

mac·ro·or·chid·ism (mak-rō-ōr'kĭ-dizm). Having abnormally large testes; seen in males with fragile X syndrome. [macro- + G. *orchis (orchid-),* testicle]

mac·ro·par·a·site (mak-rō-par'ă-sīt). A parasite, such as a louse or an intestinal worm, that is visible to the naked eye.

mac·ro·pa·thol·o·gy (mak'rō-pa-thol'ŏ-jē). The phase of pathology that pertains to the gross anatomical changes in disease.

mac·ro·pe·nis (mak-rō-pē'nis). An abnormally large penis. SYN macrophallus.

mac·ro·phage (mak'rō-fāj). Any mononuclear, actively phagocytic cell arising from monocytic stem cells in the bone marrow; these cells are widely distributed in the body and vary in morphology and motility, though most are large, long-lived cells with a nearly round nucleus and have abundant endocytic vacuoles, lysosomes, and phagolysosomes. Phagocytic activity is typically mediated by serum recognition factors, including certain immunoglobulins and components of the complement system, but also may be nonspecific for some inert materials and bacteria, as in the case of alveolar m.'s; m.'s also are involved in both the production of antibodies and in cell-mediated immune responses, participate in presenting antigens to lymphocytes, and secrete a variety of immunoregulatory molecules. SYN clasmatocyte, macrophagocyte, rhagiocrine cell. [macro- + G. *phagō,* to eat]

activated m., a mature m., in an active metabolic state, that is cytotoxic to tumor/target cells, usually following exposure to certain cytokines. SYN armed m.

alveolar m., a vigorously phagocytic m. on the epithelial surface of lung alveoli where it ingests inhaled particulate matter. SYN coniophage, dust cell.

armed m., SYN activated m.

associated m., a mature m. in an active metabolic state that is cytotoxic to tumor/target cells, usually following exposure to certain cytokines.

fixed m., a relatively immotile m. found in connective tissue, lymph nodes, spleen, and bone marrow. SYN resting wandering cell.

free m., an actively motile m. typically found in sites of inflammation.

Hansemann m., large histiocytes with abundant cytoplasm that may contain Michaelis-Gutmann bodies and one or several nuclei; described in lesions of malacoplakia.

inflammatory m., a m. found at sites of inflammation.

mac·ro·phag·o·cyte (mak-rō-fag'ō-sīt). SYN macrophage.

mac·ro·phal·lus (mak-rō-fal'lŭs). SYN macropenis. [macro- + G. *phallos,* penis]

mac·roph·thal·mia (mak-rof-thal'mē-ă). SYN megalophthalmos. [macro- + G. *ophthalmos,* eye]

mac·ro·po·dia (mak-rō-pō'dē-ă). Abnormally large feet. SYN megalopodia, pes gigas. [macro- + G. *pous,* foot]

mac·ro·pol·y·cyte (mak-rō-pol'ē-sīt). An unusually large polymorphonuclear neutrophilic leukocyte that contains a multisegmented nucleus (*e.g.,* 8, 10, or more lobes); the arrangement of chromatin is less compact than in the normal neutrophil, and the cytoplasmic granules tend to be larger and more acidophilic. Such changes frequently precede significant alterations in the red blood cells, *e.g.,* as in pernicious anemia and certain other forms of anemia. [macro- + G. *polys,* many, + *kytos,* cell]

mac·ro·pro·my·e·lo·cyte (mak'rō-prō-mī'ĕ-lō-sīt). An unusually large promyelocyte.

mac·ro·pro·so·pia (mak'rō-prō-sō'pē-ă). A condition in which the face is too large in proportion to the size of the cranial vault. SYN megaprosopia. [macro- + G. *prosōpon,* face]

mac·ro·pro·so·pous (mak-rō-prō'sō-pŭs, -prō-sō'pŭs). Relating to or exhibiting macroprosopia. SYN megaprosopous.

ma·crop·sia (mă-krop'sē-ă). Perception of objects as larger than they are. SYN megalopia, megalopsia. [macro- + G. *opsis,* vision]

mac·ro·rhin·ia (mak-rō-rin'ē-ă). Excessive size of the nose, either congenital or pathologic. [macro- + G. *rhis (rhin-),* nose]

mac·ro·sce·lia (mak-rō-sē'lē-ă). Abnormally increased length or thickness of the legs. [macro- + G. *skelos,* leg]

mac·ro·scop·ic (mak-rō-skop'ik). 1. Of a size visible with the naked eye or without the use of a microscope. 2. Relating to macroscopy.

ma

ma·cros·co·py (mă-kros′kŏ-pē). Examination of objects with the naked eye. [macro- + G. *skopeō*, to view]

mac·ro·sig·moid (mak-rō-sig′moyd). Enlargement or dilation of the sigmoid colon. SYN megasigmoid.

ma·cro·sis (mă-krō′sis). Increase in length or volume. [G.]

mac·ros·mat·ic (mak′roz-mat′ik). Denoting an abnormally keen olfactory sense. [macro- + G. *osmē*, smell]

mac·ro·so·mia (mak-rō-sō′mē-ă). Abnormally large size of the body. SYN megasomia. [macro- + G. *sōma*, body]

mac·ro·splanch·nic (mak-rō-splangk′nik). SYN megalosplanchnic.

mac·ro·spore (mak′rō-spōr). The larger of two spore types of certain protozoans or fungi. SYN megalospore, megaspore. [macro- + G. *sporos*, seed]

mac·ro·ster·e·og·no·sis (mak′rō-ster-ē-og-nō′sis). An error of perception in which objects appear larger than they are. [macro- + G. *stereos*, solid, + *gnōsis*, recognition]

mac·ro·sto·mia (mak-rō-stō′mē-ă). Abnormally large size of the mouth resulting from failure of fusion between the maxillary and mandibular processes of the embryonic face. [macro- + G. *stoma*, mouth]

mac·ro·tia (mak-rō′shē-ă). Congenital excessive enlargement of the auricle, particularly the pinna. [macro- + G. *ous*, ear]

mac·ro·tome (mak′rō-tōm). An instrument for making gross anatomical sections. [macro- + G. *tomē*, cutting]

mac·u·la, pl. **mac·u·lae** (mak′yū-lă, -yū-lē). **1** [NA]. A small spot, perceptibly different in color from the surrounding tissue. **2.** A small, discolored patch or spot on the skin, neither elevated above nor depressed below the skin's surface. SEE ALSO spot. SYN macule, spot (1). [L. a spot]

mac′ulae acus′ticae, SEE m. of saccule, m. of utricle.

m. adher′ens, SYN desmosome.

m. al′bida, pl. **mac′ulae al′bidae,** gray-white or white, rounded or irregularly shaped, slightly opaque patches or spots that are sometimes observed postmortem in the epicardium, especially in middle-aged or older persons; they result from fibrous thickening, and sometimes hyalinization, of the epicardium; similar lesions may also occur in the visceral layer of the peritoneum. SYN m. lactea, m. tendinea, tache blanche, tache laiteuse (2), tendinous spot, white spot.

m. atroph′ica, an atrophic glistening white spot on the skin.

m. ceru′lea, a bluish stain on the skin caused by the bites of fleas or lice, especially pediculosis pubis. SYN blue spot (1), tache bleuâtre.

m. commu′nicans, SYN gap junction.

m. commu′nis, the thickened area in the medial wall of the auditory vesicle that later subdivides to form the maculae of the sacculus and utriculus as well as the cristae of the ampullae of the semicircular ducts.

m. cor′neae, a moderately dense opacity of the cornea. SYN corneal spot.

m. cribro′sa, pl. **mac′ulae cribro′sae** [NA], one of three areas on the wall of the vestibule of the labyrinth, marked by numerous foramina giving passage to nerve filaments supplying portions of the membranous labyrinth; **m. cribrosa inferior,** located in the posterior bony ampulla for passage of posterior ampullary nerve fibers; **m. cribrosa media,** area near the base of the cochlea through which the saccular nerve fibers pass; **m. cribrosa superior,** perforated area above the elliptical recess for passage of the utriculoampullary nerve fibers; **m. cribrosa quarta,** a name sometimes applied to the opening for the cochlear nerve.

m. den′sa, a closely packed group of densely staining cells in the distal tubular epithelium of a nephron, in direct apposition to the juxtaglomerular cells; they may function as either chemoreceptors or as baroreceptors feeding information to the juxtaglomerular cells.

false m., an extrafoveal point of fixation.

m. fla′va, a yellowish spot at the anterior extremity of the rima glottidis where the two vocal folds join.

m. germinati′va, archaic term for the nucleolus in the nucleus of an ovum; also refers to any germinal area.

m. gonorrho′ica, a spot of red brighter than the surrounding

membrane, at the congested orifice of the duct of Bartholin's gland, sometimes seen in gonorrhea. SYN Saenger's m.

honeycomb m., edema of the macular region of the retina.

m. lac′tea, SYN m. albida.

m. lu′tea, SYN m. retinae.

mongolian m., SYN mongolian *spot*.

m. pellu′cida, SYN follicular *stigma*.

m. ret′inae [NA], an oval area of the sensory retina, 3 by 5 mm, temporal to the optic disk corresponding to the posterior pole of the eye; at its center is the central fovea, which contains only retinal cones. SYN area centralis, m. lutea, macular area, punctum luteum, Soemmerring's spot, yellow spot.

m. of saccule, the oval neuroepithelial sensory receptor in the anterior wall of the saccule; hair cells of the neuroepithelium support the statoconial membrane and have terminal arborizations of vestibular nerve fibers around their bodies. SYN m. sacculi [NA], saccular spot.

m. sac′culi [NA], SYN m. of saccule.

Saenger's m., SYN m. gonorrhoica.

m. tendin′ea, SYN m. albida.

m. of utricle, the neuroepithelial sensory receptor in the inferolateral wall of the utricle; hair cells of the neuroepithelium support the statoconial membrane and have terminal arborizations of vestibular nerve fibers around their bodies; sensitive to linear acceleration in the longitudinal axis of the body and to gravitational influences. SYN m. utriculi [NA], utricular spot.

m. utric′uli [NA], SYN m. of utricle.

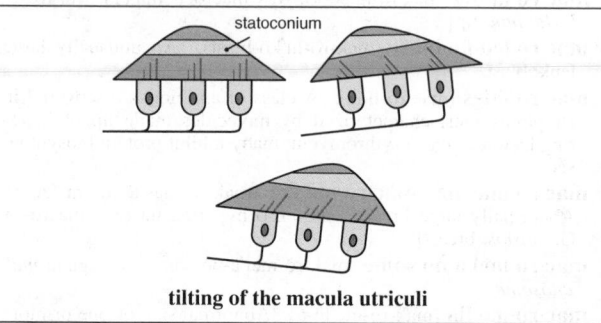

tilting of the macula utriculi

mac·u·lar, mac·u·late (mak′yū-lăr, -lāt). **1.** Relating to or marked by macules. **2.** Denoting the central retina, especially the macula retinae.

mac·u·la·tion (mak-yū-lā′shŭn). The formation or the presence of macules.

mac·ule (mak′yūl). SYN macula. [L. *macula,* spot]

mac·u·lo·ce·re·bral (mak′yū-lō-ser′ĕ-brăl). Relating to the macula lutea and the brain; denoting a type of nervous disease marked by degenerative lesions in both the retina and the brain.

mac·u·lo·er·y·the·ma·tous (mak′yū-lō-er-i-thē′mă-tŭs). Denoting lesions that are erythematous and macular, covering wide areas.

mac·u·lo·pap·ule (mak′yū-lō-pap′yūl). A lesion with a flat base surrounding a papule in the center.

mac·u·lop·a·thy (mak-yū-lop′ă-thē). Any pathological condition of the macula lutea. SYN macular retinopathy.

bull's-eye m., an ocular condition in which edema or degeneration of the sensory retina at the posterior pole of the eye causes alternating areas of light and dark, as in a target; seen in toxic, inflammatory, and hereditary conditions.

cystoid m., cystic degeneration of the central retina that may occur after cataract extraction, in senile macular degeneration, and in other retinal abnormalities.

familial pseudoinflammatory m., familial macular degeneration resembling inflammatory changes.

nicotinic acid m., m. observed in persons taking 3000 mg or more of nicotinic acid daily; normal vision returns after this medication is discontinued.

solar m., damage to the fovea centralis of the retina and the adjacent choroid due to the thermal action of infrared rays, consequent to sungazing or watching a solar eclipse without sufficient eye protection. SEE ALSO photoretinopathy. SYN eclipse blindness, solar blindness.

mad. A non-medical, pejorative term for: **1.** Rabid. **2.** Mentally ill; insane. [A.S. *gemād*]

mad·a·ro·sis (mad-ă-rō′sis). SYN milphosis. [G. a falling off of the eyelashes, fr. *madaō*, to fall off (of hair)]

mad·a·ro·sis. SYN alopecia adnata.

mad·der (mad′er). **1.** The dried and powdered root of *Rubia tinctorum* (family Rubiaceae); it contains several glycosides that upon fermentation give the red dyes, alizarin and purpurin. When m. (or alizarin) is fed to young animals, the calcium in newly deposited bone salt, hydroxyapatite, is stained red. **2.** Any dye obtained from plants of the madder family (Rubiaceae). SYN turkey red. [A.S. *maedere*]

Maddox, Ernest E., English ophthalmologist, 1860–1933. SEE M.'s *rod*.

Madelung, Otto W., German surgeon, 1846–1926. SEE M.'s *deformity, disease, neck*.

ma·des·cent (mă-des′ent). Becoming moist; slightly moist. [L. *madesco*, to become moist]

ma·di·dans (mad′i-danz). Moist; denoting certain skin lesions. [L. *madido*, pres. p. *-ans*, to moisten]

Madlener, Max, German surgeon, 1868–1951. SEE M. *operation*.

mad·ness (mad′nes). The state of being mad.

Madsen, Thorvald J.M., *1870. SEE Arrhenius-M. *theory*.

Mad·u·rel·la (mad′yū-rel′ă). A genus of fungi including a number of species, such as *M. grisea* and *M. mycetomi*, that cause mycetoma. [*Madura*, India]

ma·du·ro·my·co·sis (mad′yū-rō-mī-kō′sis). SYN mycetoma (1). [*Madura*, India, + mycosis]

mae·di (mā′dē). A chronic, progressive, contagious interstitial pneumonitis of sheep in Europe and the U.S. caused by a "slow virus" (family Lentiviridae); it is now believed that maedi and visna are two histopathological and clinical manifestations of the same viral infection. SYN ovine progressive pneumonia. [Icelandic, dyspnea]

MAF Abbreviation for macrophage-activating *factor*.

ma·fe·nide (mā′fe-nīd). α-Amino-*p*-toluenesulfonamide; a topical antibacterial agent active against anaerobic pathogens. M. acetate is the preferred salt for ointment; m. hydrochloride is the preferred salt for solution. SYN 4-homosulfanilamide.

Maffucci, Angelo, Italian physician, 1847–1903. SEE M.'s *syndrome*.

mag·al·drate (mag′al-drāt). A chemical combination of aluminum hydroxide and magnesium hydroxide, used as an antacid.

Magendie, François, French physiologist, 1783–1855. SEE M.'s *foramen;* Bell-M. *law;* M.'s *law, spaces,* under *space;* M.-Hertwig *sign, syndrome*.

ma·gen·stras·se (mag′en-stras′e). SYN gastric *canal*. [Ger. *Magen*, stomach, + *Strasse*, road]

mag·got (mag′ot). A fly larva or grub.

cheese m., SYN *Philopia casei*.

surgical m., a sterilized botfly maggot used in an obsolete therapy of wound debridement and removal of abscessed tissues.

wool m., the larva of one of several species of blowflies which deposit eggs on sheep, causing myiasis. SYN fleece worm.

mag·is·tral (maj′is-trăl). Denoting a preparation compounded according to a physician's prescription, in contrast to officinal (derived from a pharmacist's stock). [L. *magister,* master]

mag·ma (mag′mă). **1.** A soft mass left after extraction of the active principles. **2.** A salve or thick paste. [G. a soft mass or salve, fr. *massō*, to knead]

m. reticula′re, delicate noncellular strands running between the yolk sac and the outer wall of the blastocyst which is the early chorionic sac.

Magnan, Valentin J.J., Paris psychiatrist, 1835–1916. SEE M.'s trombone *movement, sign*.

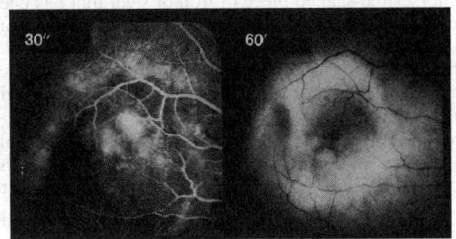

bull's-eye maculopathy
in midretina of right eye (posterior view)

mag·ne·sia (mag-nē′zhŭh). SYN *magnesium* oxide. [see magnesium]

calcined m., SYN *magnesium* oxide.

m. magma, SYN *milk* of magnesia.

mag·ne·si·um (Mg) (mag-nē′zē-ŭm). An alkaline earth element, atomic no. 12, atomic wt. 24.3050, that oxidizes to magnesia; a bioelement, many salts have clinical applications. [Mod. L. fr. G. *Magnēsia,* a region in Thessaly]

m. aluminum silicate, an antacid. SYN aluminum magnesium silicate.

m. bacteriopheophytinate, SEE bacteriochlorophyll.

m. benzoate, has been used in gout and rheumatoid arthritis.

m. carbonate, used in gastric and intestinal acidity and as a laxative.

m. chloride, $MgCl_2 \cdot 6H_2O$; has been used as a laxative.

m. citrate, $Mg_3(C_6H_5O_7)_2 \cdot 14H_2O$; a laxative; usually administered as an effervescent flavored beverage.

effervescent m. citrate, m. carbonate, citric acid, sodium bicarbonate, and sugar, moistened with alcohol, passed through a sieve, and dried to a coarse granular powder; used as a laxative.

effervescent m. sulfate, effervescent Epsom salt; m. sulfate, sodium bicarbonate, tartaric acid, and citric acid, moistened, passed through a sieve, and dried to a coarse granular powder; a purgative.

m. hydroxide, $Mg(OH)_2$; an antacid and laxative.

m. lactate, a laxative.

m. oxide, used as an antacid and laxative. SYN calcined magnesia, magnesia.

m. peroxide, decomposes in water to hydrogen peroxide; used as an ingredient in dentifrices and in antiseptic dusting powder.

m. phytinates, chlorophyll *a* and *b*. See entries under chlorophyll.

m. salicylate, a sodium-free salicylate derivative with anti-inflammatory, analgesic, and antipyretic actions; used for relief of mild to moderate pain.

m. stearate, a compound of m. with variable proportions of stearic and palmitic acids; used in the preparation of tablets, as a lubricant, and as an ingredient in some baby powders.

m. sulfate, active ingredient of most natural laxative waters; used as a promptly acting cathartic in certain poisonings, in the treatment of increased intracranial pressure and edema, as an anticonvulsant in eclampsia (when administered intravenously), and as an anti-inflammatory (when applied locally). SYN Epsom salts.

tribasic m. phosphate, $Mg_3(PO_4)_2 \cdot 5H_2O$; tertiary m. phosphate, it is used as an antacid but it does not produce systemic alkalization; 1 g is equivalent in neutralizing power to about 0.46 g of sodium bicarbonate.

m. trisilicate, $2MgO \cdot 3SiO_2 \cdot nH_2O$; a compound of m. oxide and silicon dioxide with varying proportions of water; occurs in nature as meerschaum, pararepiolite, and repiolite; a gastric antacid.

mag·net. 1. A body that has the property of attracting particles of iron, cobalt, nickel, or any of various metallic alloys and that when freely suspended tends to assume a definite direction between the magnetic poles of the earth (magnetic polarity). **2.** A

ma

bar or horseshoe-shaped piece of iron or steel that has been made magnetic by contact with another m. or, as in an electromagnet, by passage of electric current around a metallic (iron) core. **3.** An electromagnet built in a cynlindrical configuration to accommodate a patient in its core, for magnetic resonance imaging. [G. *magnēs*]

superconducting m., a m. whose coils are cooled, usually with liquid helium, to a temperature at which the metal becomes superconducting, effectively removing all electrical resistance.

mag·net·ic. 1. Relating to or characteristic of a magnet. **2.** Possessing magnetism.

mag·ne·tism (mag′nĕ-tizm). The property of mutual attraction or repulsion possessed by magnets.

animal m., a psychic force akin to the property of mutual attraction or repulsion possessed by metal magnets and once believed to be the principal factor in hypnosis, which thus was called animal m. SEE hypnosis, mesmerism.

mag·ne·to·car·di·og·ra·phy (mag′nĕ-tō-kar-dē-og′ră-fē). Measurement of the magnetic field of the heart, produced by the same ionic currents that generate the electrocardiogram, and showing characteristic P, QRS, T, and U waves.

mag·ne·to·en·ceph·a·lo·gram (MEG) (mag-nē′tō-en-sef′ă-lō-gram). A gauss-time record of the magnetic field of the brain.

mag·ne·to·en·ceph·a·log·ra·phy (mag-nē′tō-en-sef-ă-log′ră-fē). The process of recording the brain's magnetic field.

mag·ne·tom·e·ter (mag-nĕ-tom′ĕ-ter). An instrument for detecting and measuring the magnetic field.

mag·ne·ton (mag′nĕ-ton). A unit of measurement of the magnetic moment of a particle (*e.g.,* atom or subatomic particle).

Bohr m., a constant in the equation relating the difference in energies between parallel and antiparallel spin alignments of electrons in a magnetic field; the net magnetic moment of one unpaired electron; used in electron spin resonance spectrometry for detection and estimation of free radicals. SYN electron m.

electron m., SYN Bohr m.

nuclear m., a constant in the equation relating the difference in energies between parallel and antiparallel spin alignments of atomic nuclei in a magnetic field; used in nuclear magnetic resonance spectrometry.

mag·ne·to·ther·a·py (mag-nē′tō-thār′ă-pē). Attempted treatment of disease by application of magnets.

mag·ni·fi·ca·tion (mag′ni-fi-kā′shŭn). **1.** The seeming increase in size of an object viewed under the microscope; when noted, this increased size is expressed by a figure preceded by ×, indicating the number of times its diameter is enlarged. **2.** The increased amplitude of a tracing, as of a muscular contraction, caused by the use of a lever with a long writing arm, *i.e.,* one in which the fulcrum is placed nearer to the muscle than to the writing point. [L. *magnifico,* pp. *-atus,* to magnify]

mag·ni·tude (mag′ni-tūd). Size or extent.

average pulse m., the amplitude of pulse averaged throughout its duration; identical with peak amplitude for a square wave or pulse without droop.

peak m., the greatest amplitude.

mag·no·cel·lu·lar (mag′nō-sel′yū-lăr). Composed of cells of large size. [L. *magnus,* large, + cellular]

mag·num (mag′nŭm). SYN capitate (1). [L. *magnus,* large]

Magnus, Rudolph, German physiologist, 1873–1927. SEE M.'s *sign.*

mag·nus (mag′nŭs). Large; great; denoting a structure of large size. [L.]

Mahaim, I. SEE M. *fibers,* under *fiber.*

Ma·huang (mah-hwahng). Name for *Ephedra equisetina.* [Chinese]

MAI. Abbreviation for *Mycobacterium avium-intracellulare.* SEE ALSO *Mycobacterium avium-intracellulare complex.*

maid·en·head (mā′den-hed). Obsolete term for the intact hymen of a virgin.

mai·dism (mā′dizm). SYN pellagra. [*Zea mays,* maize]

Maier, Rudolf, German physician, 1824–1888. SEE M.'s *sinus.*

maim (mām). To disable or cripple by an injury.

main (man). SYN hand. [Fr.]

m. d'accoucheur, SYN accoucheur's *hand.*

m. en crochet, a permanent flexure of the fourth and fifth fingers, resembling the hand of a woman crocheting with three fingers bent to guide the thread.

m. en griffe, SYN clawhand.

m. en lorgnette, SYN opera-glass *hand.*

m. fourchée, SYN cleft *hand.*

m. succulente, SYN Marinesco's succulent *hand.*

main·frame (mān′frām). A large digital computer, such as would be used in a hospital for information management. Cf. mini.

main·stream·ing (mān′strēm-ing). Providing the least restrictive environment (socially, physically, and educationally) for chronically disabled individuals by introducing them into the natural environment rather than segregating them into homogeneous groups living in sheltered environments under constant supervision.

main·tain·er (mān-tā′ner). A device utilized to hold or keep teeth in a given position.

space m., an orthodontic appliance used to prevent the loss of space or the shifting of teeth following extraction or premature loss of teeth. SYN space retainer.

main·te·nance (mān′ten-ans). **1.** A therapeutic regimen intended to preserve benefit. Cf. compliance (2), adherence (2). **2.** The extent to which the patient continues good heath practices without supervision, incorporating them into a general life-style. Cf. compliance. [M.E., fr O.Fr., fr. Mediev. L. *manuteneo,* to hold in the hand]

maise oil (māz). SYN corn oil.

Maissiat, Jacques H., French anatomist, 1805–1878. SEE M.'s *band.*

Majocchi, Domenico, Italian dermatologist, 1849–1929. SEE M. *granulomas,* under *granuloma;* M.'s *disease.*

ma·jor (mā′jŏr). Larger or greater in size of two similar structures. [L. comparative of *magnus,* great]

Makeham, William Matthew, English actuary, †1892. SEE M.'s *hypothesis.*

mal (mahl). A disease or disorder. [Fr. fr. L. *malum,* an evil]

m. de caderas, a disease of horses in some South American countries caused by the protozoan parasite *Trypanosoma equinum* and manifested by emaciation, remittent fever, weakness (especially of the hindquarters, from which the disease gets its name), and eventually death; the trypanosome has a reservoir in the giant rodent, the capybara; cattle, sheep, and goats are only mildly affected; humans are not susceptible.

m. de Cayenne, SYN elephantiasis.

m. de la rosa, m. rosso, SYN pellagra.

m. de los pintos, SYN pinta.

m. de Meleda, endemic symmetrical keratoderma of the extremities occurring on the island of Meleda off the coast of Dalmatia.

m. de mer, SYN seasickness.

m. de San Lazaro, SYN elephantiasis.

grand m. (grahn), SYN generalized tonic-clonic *seizure.*

m. perforant, SYN perforating *ulcer* of foot.

petit m. (pĕ-tē′), type of seizure. [Fr. small]

△**mal-.** Ill, bad; opposite of eu-. Cf. dys-, caco-. [L. *malus,* bad]

ma·la (mā′lă). **1.** SYN cheek. **2.** SYN zygomatic *bone.* [L. cheek bone]

mal·ab·sorp·tion (mal-ab-sōrp′shŭn). Imperfect, inadequate, or otherwise disordered gastrointestinal absorption.

congenital selective glucose and galactose m., an inherited disorder in which D-glucose and D-galactose accumulate in the intestinal lumen and exert an osmotic effect; leads to abdominal fullness, abdominal pain, and diarrhea.

enterocyte cobalamin m., an inherited disorder of impaired transintestinal transport of cobalamin; symptoms are similar to a vitamin B_{12} deficiency.

fructose m., an inborn error in metabolism in which oral D-fructose is incompletely absorbed; results in abdominal symptoms and diarrhea.

hereditary folate m., an inherited disorder in which there is defective transport of folates in intestine and choroid plexus, results in megaloblastic anemia and neurologic abnormalities.

Malacarne, Michele V.G., Italian surgeon, 1744–1816. SEE M.'s *pyramid, space.*

mal·a·chite green (mal′ă-kīt) [C.I. 42000]. Tetramethyl-di-*p*-aminotriphenylcarbinol; a dye that has been used as a wound antiseptic, as a treatment of mycotic skin infections, and in biological staining of tissues and bacteria. [G. *malachē,* a mallow]

ma·la·cia (mă-lā′shē-ă). A softening or loss of consistency and contiguity in any of the organs or tissues. Also used as a combining form in the suffix position. SYN mollities (2). SYN malacosis. [G. *malakia,* a softness]

ma·la·cic (mă-lā′sik). SYN malacotic.

⌂malaco-. Soft, softening. [G. *malakos,* soft; *malakia,* a softness]

mal·a·co·pla·kia, mal·a·ko·pla·kia (mal′ă-kō-plā′kē-ă, mal′ă-kō-plā′kē-a). Rare lesion in the mucosa of the urinary bladder and other organs, more frequent in women, characterized by numerous mottled yellow and gray soft plaques and nodules that consist of numerous macrophages and calcospherites (Michaelis-Guttmann bodies) that may form around intracellular bacteria, usually *Escherichia coli.* [malaco- + G. *plax,* plate, plaque]

mal·a·co·sis (mal′ă-kō′sis). SYN malacia.

mal·a·cot·ic (mal′ă-kot′ik). Pertaining to or characterized by malacia. SYN malacic.

mal·a·cot·o·my (mal′ă-kot′ō-mē). Obsolete term for incision of soft parts, especially of the abdominal wall. [malaco- + G. *tomē,* incision]

ma·lac·tic (mă-lak′tik). SYN emollient. [G. *malaktikos,* softening]

ma·la·die (mal′ă-dē′). SYN malady. [Fr.]

m. de Roger, SYN Roger's *disease.* [Fr.]

m. des jambes (mal′ă-dē′ dĕ zhamb′), ill-defined disease seen among rice-growers in Louisiana.

mal·ad·just·ment (mal-ad-jŭst′ment). In the mental health professions, an inability to cope with the problems and challenges of everyday living. [mal- + *adjust,* fr. O.Fr. *adjuster,* fr. L.L. *adjuxto,* to put close to, + -ment]

social m., m. without manifest psychiatric disorder, as that occasioned by an inability to cope with social situations.

mal·a·dy (mal′ă-dē). A disease or illness. SYN maladie. [Fr. *maladie,* illness]

ma·lag·ma (mă-lag′mă). A cataplasm or emollient. [G. a poultice]

mal·aise (mă-lāz′). A feeling of general discomfort or uneasiness, an "out-of-sorts" feeling, often the first indication of an infection or other disease. [Fr. discomfort]

mal·a·lign·ment (mal-ă-līn′ment). Displacement of a tooth or teeth from a normal position in the dental arch.

ma·lar (mā′lăr). Relating to the mala, the cheek or cheek bones.

ma·lar·ia (mă-lār′ē-ă). A disease caused by the presence of the sporozoan *Plasmodium* in human or other vertebrate red blood cells, usually transmitted to humans by the bite of an infected female mosquito of the genus *Anopheles* that previously sucked the blood from a person with m. Human infection begins with the exoerythrocytic cycle in liver parenchyma cells, followed by a series of erythrocytic schizogenous cycles repeated at regular intervals; production of gametocytes in other red cells provides future gametes for another mosquito infection; characterized by episodic severe chills and high fever, prostration, occasionally fatal termination. SEE tropical *diseases,* under *disease.* SEE ALSO *Plasmodium.* SYN jungle fever, marsh fever, paludal fever, swamp fever (2). [It. *malo* (fem. *mala*), bad, + *aria,* air, referring to the old theory of the miasmatic origin of the disease]

acute m., a form of m. that may be intermittent or remittent, consisting of a chill accompanied and followed by fever with its attendant general symptoms, and terminating in a sweating stage; the paroxysms, caused by release of merozoites from infected cells, recur every 48 hours in tertian (vivax or ovale) m., every 72 hours in quartan (malariae) m., and at indefinite but frequent intervals, usually about 48 hours, in malignant tertian (falciparum) m.

algid m., a form of falciparum m. chiefly involving the gut and other abdominal viscera; gastric algid m. is characterized by persistent vomiting; dysenteric algid m. is characterized by bloody diarrheic stools in which enormous numbers of infected red blood cells are found.

autochthonous m., disease acquired by mosquito transmission in an area where m. regularly occurs.

avian m., plasmodial infections of domestic and wild birds, transmitted chiefly by culicine mosquitoes.

benign tertian m., SYN vivax m.

bilious remittent m., a form of falciparum m. characterized by bilious vomiting, bilious diarrhea, etc.

cerebral m., a form of falciparum m. characterized by cerebral involvement, with extreme hyperthermia and headache, and a case fatality rate of about 50%.

chronic m., m. that develops after frequently repeated attacks of one of the acute forms, usually falciparum m.; it is characterized by profound anemia, enlargement of the spleen, emaciation, mental depression, sallow complexion, edema of ankles, feeble digestion, and muscular weakness. SYN limnemia, malarial cachexia.

m. comato′sa, falciparum m. complicated by coma.

double tertian m., SEE quotidian m.

dysenteric algid m., SEE algid m.

falciparum m., m. caused by *Plasmodium falciparum* and characterized by malarial paroxysms of severe form that occur every 48 hours with acute cerebral, renal, or gastrointestinal manifestations in severe cases, chiefly caused by the large number of red blood cells affected and the tendency for infected red cells to become sticky and clump, thus blocking capillaries. SEE ALSO malarial *knobs,* under *knob.* SYN aestivoautumnal fever, falciparum fever, malignant tertian fever, malignant tertian m., pernicious m.

gastric algid m., SEE algid m.

induced m., m. acquired by artificial means, *e.g.,* via blood transfusion, common syringes, or malariotherapy.

intermittent m., a malarial fever, usually of the tertian or quartan type, in which there is complete apyrexia, with absence of the other symptoms, in the intervals between the paroxysms.

malariae m., a malarial fever with paroxysms that recur every 72 hours or every fourth day, reckoning the day of the paroxysm as the first; due to the schizogony and release of merozoites from infected cells, with invasion of new red blood corpuscles by *Plasmodium malariae.* SYN quartan fever, quartan m.

malignant tertian m., SYN falciparum m.

monkey m., SYN simian m.

nonan m., a malarial fever with paroxysms that occur every ninth day, *i.e.,* every eighth day following the preceding paroxysm, the day of each paroxysm being included in the computation.

ovale m., ovale tertian m., m. caused by *Plasmodium ovale.*

pernicious m., SYN falciparum m.

quartan m., SYN malariae m.

quotidian m., m. in which the paroxysms occur daily; usually a double tertian m., in which there is an infection by two distinct groups of *Plasmodium vivax* parasites sporulating alternately every 48 hours, but also may be an infection by the pernicious form of malarial parasite, *P. falciparum,* combined with *P. vivax,* or infection by two distinct *P. falciparum* generations, which mature on different days; also may develop from infection with *P. knowlesi.* SYN quotidian fever.

relapsing m., renewal of clinical activity at some interval after the primary attack.

remittent m., a malarial fever, usually of the severe falciparum type, in which the temperature falls but not to the normal level during the interval between two pronounced paroxysms.

simian m., plasmodial infection of monkeys and apes, as with human m., transmitted chiefly by anopheline mosquitoes; a number of *Plasmodium* species are responsible, with Southeast Asia and Africa being the apparent centers of evolution; among the 20 plasmodial agents described from nonhuman primates, some resemble and induce a malarial infection similar to those caused by

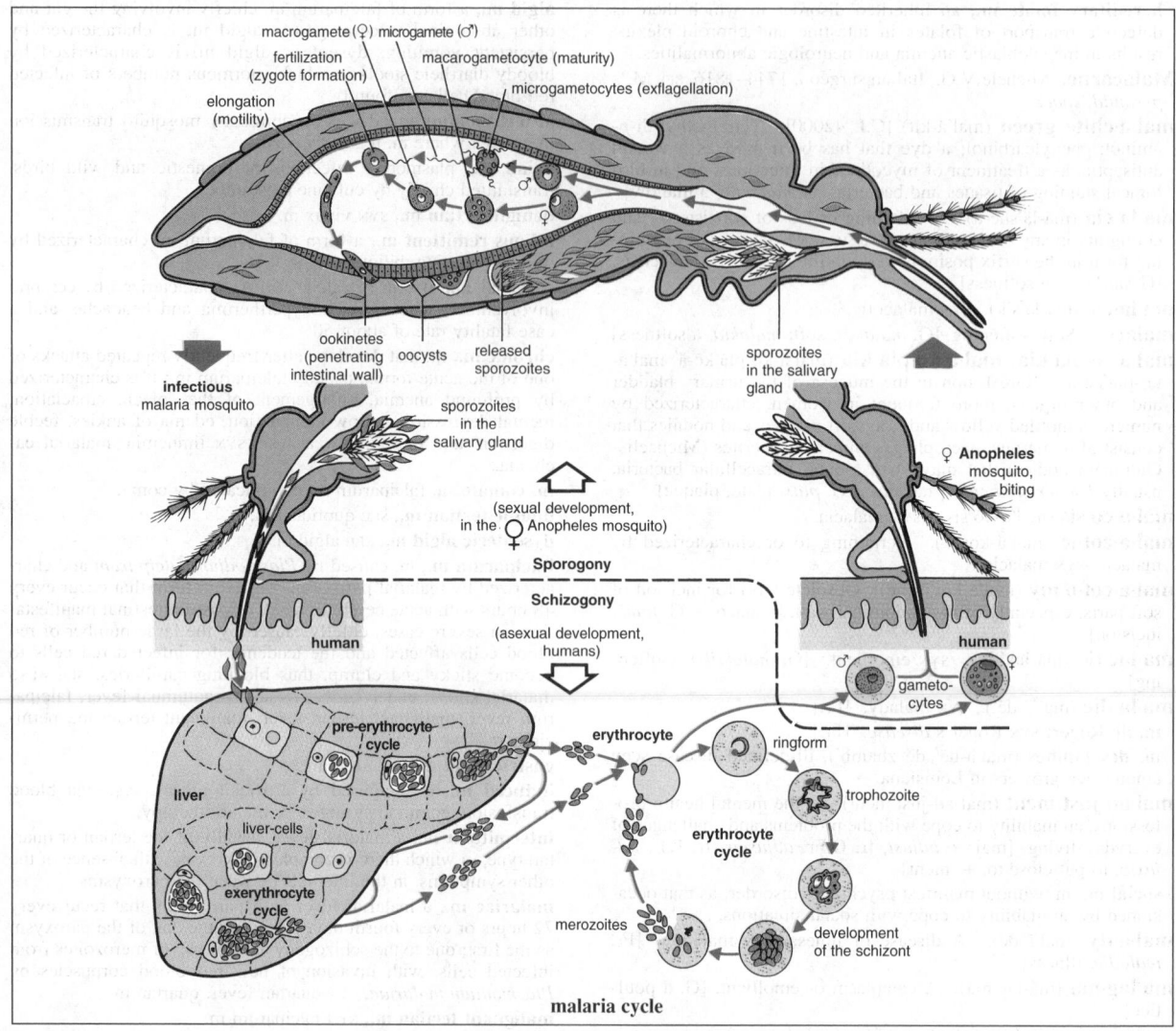

malaria cycle

the four species of *Plasmodium* from humans, from which the agents of human m. appear to be derived. SYN monkey m.

tertian m., SYN

therapeutic m., intentionally induced m., formerly used against neurosyphilis and certain other paralytic diseases; the mechanism is thought to be immunological, with *Plasmodium* antibodies cross-reacting against the spirochetes or other agents.

vivax m., a malarial fever with paroxysms that recur every 48 hours or every other day (every third day, reckoning the day of the paroxysm as the first); the fever is induced by release of merozoites and their invasion of new red blood corpuscles. SYN benign tertian m., tertian fever, tertian m., vivax fever.

ma·lar·i·al (mă-lār′ē-ăl). Pertaining to or affected with malaria.

ma·lar·i·ol·o·gy (mă-lār-ē-ol′ō-jē). A study of malaria in all aspects, with particular reference to epidemiology and control.

ma·lar·i·ous (mă-lār′ē-ŭs). Relating to or characterized by the prevalence of malaria.

Malassez, Louis C., French physiologist, 1842–1910. SEE *Malassezia;* M.'s epithelial *rests,* under *rest.*

Ma·las·sez·ia (mal-ă-sā′zē-ă). A genus of fungi (family Cryptococcaceae) of low pathogenicity that lack the ability to synthesize medium-chain and long-chain fatty acids, and require an exogenous supply of these lipids for growth as can be found in the skin. [L. C. *Malassez*]

M. fur′fur, a fungus species which causes tinea versicolor and which may cause folliculitis. SYN *Pityrosporum orbiculare.*

M. ova′lis, a species of yeast found in superficial epidermal scales and hair follicles on oily skin, of borderline pathogenicity; may cause seborrheic dermatitis associated with immune deficiency. SYN *Pityrosporum ovale.*

mal·as·sim·i·la·tion (mal′ă-sim-i-lā′shŭn). Rarely used term for incomplete or faulty assimilation; malabsorption.

ma·late (mal′āt). A salt or ester of malic acid.

m. dehydrogenase, an enzyme that catalyzes, through NAD^+ or $NADP^+$, the dehydrogenation of malate to oxaloacetate or its decarboxylation to pyruvate and CO_2. At least six are known, distinguished by their products, use of NAD^+ or $NADP^+$, and specificity of substrate (one acts on D-m.; the rest act on L-m.); one is an enzyme in the tricarboxylic acid cycle. SYN malic acid dehydrogenase, malic dehydrogenase, malic enzyme, pyruvic-malic carboxylase.

m. synthase, an enzyme catalyzing the reversible condensation of acetyl-CoA with glyoxylate and water to form L-malate and coenzyme A; an enzyme in the glyoxylate cycle. SYN glyoxylate transacetylase, malate-condensing enzyme.

mal·a·thi·on (mal-ă-thī′on, mă-lā′thī-on). *S*-(1,2-Dicarboxyethyl)-*O,O*-dimethyldithiophosphate; an organophosphorous compound used as an insecticide and veterinary ectoparasiticide; considered to be less toxic than parathion.

mal·ax·a·tion (mal′ak-sā′shŭn). **1.** Formation of ingredients into a mass for pills and plasters. **2.** A kneading process in massage. [L. *malaxo,* pp. *-atus,* to soften]

mal·di·ges·tion (mal-dī-jes′chŭn). Imperfect digestion.

Mal·do·na·do-San Jo·se stain. See under stain.

male (māl). **1.** In zoology, denoting the sex to which those belong that produce spermatozoa; an individual of that sex. **2.** SYN masculine. [L. *masculus,* fr. *mas,* male]

genetic human m., **(1)** an individual with a karyotype containing a Y chromosome; **(2)** an individual whose cell nuclei do not contain Barr sex chromatin bodies, which are normally present in females. Patients with ambiguous sexual development and those with Turner's syndrome are classed as genetic m.'s or genetic females according to the absence or presence of Barr bodies even though their sex chromosome complement may suggest otherwise.

XX m., a clear male phenotype in the presence of a 46,XX karyotype; presumably the vital parts of the Y chromosome are located elsewhere in the genome as a result of translocation at least in some of these persons.

XXY m., SEE Klinefelter's *syndrome.*

XYY m., SEE XYY *syndrome.*

Malecot, Achille-Etienne, French surgeon, *1852. SEE M. *catheter.*

ma·le·ic ac·id (mă-lē′ik). HOOC–CH=CH–COOH; (*Z*)-butenedioic acid; the *cis* isomer of fumaric acid; used for preparing maleate salts of antihistaminics and similar drugs. SYN toxilic acid.

mal·e·mis·sion (mal-ē-mish′ŭn). Failure of semen to be ejected from the penis in coitus. [mal- + L. *e-mitto,* pp. *missus,* to send out]

mal·e·rup·tion (mal-ē-rŭp′shŭn). Faulty eruption of teeth.

ma·ley·lac·e·to·ac·e·tate (mal′a-il-as′e-tō-as′ē-tāt). ‾OOC-CH=CH-ĊOCH₂COCH₂COO‾; an intermediate in L-phenylalanine and L-tyrosine catabolism; accumulates in certain inherited disorders of tyrosine metabolism.

m. *cis,trans*-isomerase, an enzyme that catalyzes the reversible conversion of m. to 4-fumarylacetoacetate; an enzyme that participates in L-tyrosine catabolism; a deficiency of this enzyme is associated with tyrosinemia type IB.

mal·for·ma·tion (mal-fōr-mā′shŭn). Failure of proper or normal development; more specifically, a primary structural defect that results from a localized error of morphogenesis; *e.g.,* cleft lip. Cf. deformation.

Arnold-Chiari m., malformed posterior fossa structures resulting from caudad traction and displacement of the rhombencephalon caused by tethering of the spinal cord; may or may not be accompanied by spina bifida and associated anomalies such as meningomyelocele; weak evidence of autosomal recessive inheritance. SYN Arnold-Chiari deformity, Arnold-Chiari syndrome, cerebellomedullary malformation syndrome.

cystic adenomatoid m., a rare developmental lung-bud abnormality which results in stillbirth, acute progressive respiratory disease of newborns, or protracted childhood pneumonias; this m. combines features of a hamartoma, dysplastic growth, and tumorous growth. Three types have been described, based chiefly on cyst diameters: Type I: up to 10 cm; Type II: less than 1.2 cm; Type III: less than 0.5 cm.

mal·func·tion (mal-fŭnk′shŭn). Disordered, inadequate, or abnormal function.

Malgaigne, Joseph F., French surgeon, 1806–1865. SEE M.'s *amputation, fossa, hernia, luxation, triangle.*

Malherbe, A. SEE M.'s calcifying *epithelioma.*

mal·ic ac·id (mal′ik, mā′lik). HOOC-CH₂-CHOH-COOH; hydroxysuccinic acid; an acid found in apples and various other tart fruits; an intermediate in the tricarboxylic acid cycle, the glyoxylate cycle, and in a shuttle system. SYN monohydroxysuccinic acid.

mal·ic ac·id de·hy·dro·gen·ase. SYN *malate* dehydrogenase.

mal·ic de·hy·dro·gen·ase. SYN *malate* dehydrogenase.

ma·lig·nan·cy (mă-lig′nan-sē). The property or condition of being malignant.

ma·lig·nant (mă-lig′nănt). **1.** Resistant to treatment; occurring in severe form, and frequently fatal; tending to become worse and leading to an ingravescent course. **2.** In reference to a neoplasm, having the property of locally invasive and destructive growth and metastasis. [L. *maligno,* pres. p. *-ans* (*ant-*), to do anything maliciously]

ma·lin·ger (mă-ling′ger). To engage in malingering.

ma·lin·ger·er (mă-ling′ger-er). One who engages in malingering.

ma·lin·ger·ing (mă-ling′ger-ing). Feigning illness or disability to escape work, excite sympathy, or gain compensation. [Fr. *malingre,* poor, weakly]

mal·in·ter·dig·i·ta·tion (mal′in-ter-dij′i-tā′shŭn). Faulty intercuspation of teeth.

Mall, Franklin Paine, U.S. anatomist and embryologist, 1862–1917. SEE M.'s *formula, ridges,* under *ridge;* periportal *space* of M.

mal·le·a·ble (mal′ē-ă-bl). Capable of being shaped by being beaten or by pressure; a property of certain metals such as gold and silver. [L. *malleus,* a hammer]

mal·le·a·tion (mal-ē-ā′shŭn). A form of tic, in which the hands twitch in a hammering motion against the thighs. [L. *malleus,* a hammer]

mal·le·brin (mal′e-brin). SYN *aluminum* chlorate nonahydrate.

mal·le·in (mal′ē-in). An allergin, analogous to tuberculin, made from the growth products of *Pseudomonas mallei,* the causative agent of glanders; used as a diagnostic agent to provoke reactions in animals affected with glanders.

mal·le·in·i·za·tion (mal′ē-in-i-zā′shŭn). Inoculation with mallein.

mal·le·o·in·cu·dal (mal′ē-ō-ing′kū-dăl). Relating to the malleus and the incus in the tympanum.

mal·le·o·lar (mă-lē′ō-lăr). Relating to one or both malleoli.

mal·le·o·lus, pl. **mal·le·o·li** (ma-lē′ō-lŭs, -lī) [NA]. A rounded bony prominence such as those on either side of the ankle joint. [L. dim. of *malleus,* hammer]

external m., SYN lateral m.

inner m., SYN medial m.

internal m., SYN medial m.

lateral m., the process at the lateral side of the lower end of the fibula, forming the projection of the lateral part of the ankle; the lateral malleolus is more inferiorly placed then the medial malleolus. SYN m. lateralis [NA], external m., extramalleolus, outer m.

m. latera′lis [NA], SYN lateral m.

medial m., the process at the medial side of the lower end of the tibia, forming the projection of the medial side of the ankle. SYN m. medialis [NA], inner m., internal m.

m. media′lis [NA], SYN medial m.

outer m., SYN lateral m.

mal·le·ot·o·my (mal′ē-ot′ō-mē). **1.** Division of the malleus. [malleus + G. *tomē,* incision] **2.** Division of the ligaments holding the malleoli in apposition in order to permit their separation in certain cases of clubfoot. [malleolus + G. *tomē,* incision]

mal·le·us, gen. and pl. **mal·lei** (mal′ē-ŭs, mal′ē-ī) [NA]. The largest of the three auditory ossicles, resembling a club rather than a hammer; it is regarded as having a head, below which is the neck, and from this diverge the handle or manubrium, and the slender, anterior process; from the base of the manubrium the short lateral process arises. The manubrium and lateral process are firmly attached to the tympanic membrane, and the head articulates with a saddle-shaped surface on the body of the incus. SYN hammer. [L. a hammer]

Mal·loph·a·ga (mă-lof′ă-gă). An order of biting lice that cause irritation by feeding on hair, feathers, and skin, and on blood and exudates when present; most species are found on birds, but some are found on common domestic animals. The genera *Menacanthus* and *Menopon* (family Menoponidae) attack domestic fowl, as do *Columbicola, Chelopistes, Lipeurus,* and other genera of the family Philopteridae, while *Bovicola, Felicola,* and *Trichodectes* (family Trichodectidae) infest domestic mammals. [G. *mallos,* wool, + *phagein,* to eat]

Ma

Mallory, Frank B., U.S. pathologist, 1862–1941. SEE M. *bodies,* under *body;* picro-M. trichrome *stain.* See entries under stain.

Mallory, G. Kenneth, U.S. pathologist, *1926. SEE M.-Weiss *lesion, syndrome, tear.*

mal·nu·tri·tion (mal-nū-trish′ŭn). Faulty nutrition resulting from malabsorption, poor diet, or overeating.

malignant m., SYN kwashiorkor.

protein m., undernutrition resulting from inadequate intake of protein; characteristic manifestations include nutritional *edema,* kwashiorkor.

mal·oc·clu·sion (mal-ō-klū′zhŭn). **1.** Any deviation from a physiologically acceptable contact of opposing dentitions. **2.** Any deviation from a normal occlusion.

mal·on·ate (măl′on-āt). The salt or ester of malonic acid.

mal·on·ate sem·i·al·de·hyde. OHC–CH$_2$–COO$^-$; the transaminated product of β-alanine; elevated in hyper-β-alaninemia.

Maloney bou·gies. See under bougie.

ma·lo·nic ac·id (mă-lō′nik, -lon′ik). HOOC–CH$_2$–COOH; a dicarboxylic acid of importance in intermediary metabolism; an inhibitor of succinate dehydrogenase. SYN propanedioic acid.

mal·o·nyl (mal′ō-nil). The divalent radical derived from malonic acid.

m. transacylase, SYN ACP-malonyltransferase.

mal·o·nyl-CoA. The condensation product of malonic acid and coenzyme A, an intermediate in fatty acid biosynthesis. SYN malonylcoenzyme A.

mal·o·nyl·co·en·zyme A (mal′ō-nil-kō-en′zīm). SYN malonyl-CoA.

mal·o·nyl·u·rea (mal′ō-nil-yū-rē′ă). SYN barbituric acid.

Malpighi, Marcello, Italian anatomist, histologist, and embryologist, 1628–1694. SEE malpighian *bodies,* under *body;* malpighian *capsule;* malpighian *cell;* malpighian *corpuscles,* under *corpuscle;* malpighian *glands,* under *gland;* malpighian *glomerulus;* malpighian *layer;* malpighian *nodules,* under *nodule;* malpighian *pyramid;* malpighian *rete;* malpighian *stigmas,* under *stigma;* malpighian *stratum;* malpighian *tubules,* under *tubule;* malpighian *tuft;* malpighian *vesicles,* under *vesicle.*

mal·pi·ghi·an (mahl-pig′ē-an). Described by or attributed to Marcello Malpighi.

mal·po·si·tion (mal-pō-zish′ŭn). SYN dystopia.

mal·prac·tice (mal-prak′tis). Mistreatment of a patient through ignorance, carelessness, neglect, or criminal intent.

mal·pre·sen·ta·tion (mal′prē-sen-tā′shŭn). Faulty presentation of the fetus; presentation of any part other than the occiput.

mal·ro·ta·tion (mal-rō-tā′shŭn). Failure during embryonic development of normal rotation of all or part of an organ or system such as gut tube or kidney.

malt (mawlt). The seed of barley or other grain, artificially germinated and dried, containing dextrin, maltose, small amounts of glucose, and amylolytic enzymes. Used in the form of an extract as a digestive and flavoring agent. [A.S. *mealt*]

malt·ase (mawl-tās). SEE α-D-glucosidase.

acid m., SYN exo-1,4-α-D-glucosidase.

mal·to·bi·ose (mawl-tō-bī′ōs). SYN maltose.

mal·tose (mawl-tōs). 4-(α-D-Glucosido)-D-glucose; a disaccharide formed in the hydrolysis of starch and consisting of two D-glucose residues bound by a 1,4-α-glycoside link. SYN malt sugar, maltobiose.

mal·to·tet·rose (mawl-tō-tet′rōs). A saccharide comprised of four D-glucose units in the α-1,4 linkage.

ma·lum (mā′lŭm). A disease. [L. an evil]

m. artic′ulorum seni′lis, arthritis in the aged.

m. cox′ae, disease of the hip joint.

m. cox′ae seni′le, deformity of the head of the femur caused by ischemic damage. SYN senile hip disease.

m. per′forans pe′dis, perforating ulcer of the foot occurring in certain neuropathies.

m. vene′reum, SYN syphilis.

m. vertebra′le suboccipita′le, SYN Rust's *disease.*

mal·un·ion (mal-yūn′yŭn). SYN vicious *union.*

ma·man·pi·an (mă-mon-pē-on′). SYN mother *yaw.* [Fr. *maman,* mother + *pian,* yaw]

mam·e·lon (mam′ĕ-lon). One of the rounded prominences, three in number, on the cutting edge of an incisor tooth when it first pierces the gum. [Fr. nipple]

mam·e·lon·at·ed (mam′ĕ-lon-āt-ed). Having rounded, teatlike elevations; nodulated. [Fr. *mamelon,* nipple]

mam·e·lo·na·tion (mam′ĕ-lŏ-nā′shŭn). The formation of rounded projections or nodules on bony and other structures.

△**mamil-, mamilli-.** The mamillae. SEE ALSO mammil-. Cf. thelo-. [L. *mamilla,* nipple]

ma·mil·la, pl. **ma·mil·lae** (mă-mil′ă, mă-mil′ē). **1.** A small rounded elevation resembling the female breast. **2.** SYN nipple. [L. nipple]

ma·mil·la·re (mam-i-lā′rē). SYN mamillary. [L.]

mam·il·lar·ia. SEE mamillary *body.*

mam·il·lary (mam′i-lār-ē). Relating to or shaped like a nipple. SYN mamillare.

mam·il·late, mam·il·lat·ed (mam′i-lāt, -lāt′ed). Studded with nipple-like projections.

mam·il·la·tion (mam-i-lā′shŭn). **1.** A nipple-like projection. **2.** The condition of being mamillated.

ma·mil·li·form (mă-mil′i-fōrm). Nipple-shaped. [L. *mamilla,* nipple, + *forma,* form]

mam·ma, gen. and pl. **mam·mae** (mam′ă, mam′ē) [NA]. SYN breast. SEE ALSO mammary *gland.* [L.]

m. accesso′ria [NA], SYN supernumerary *breast.*

m. errat′ica, a supernumerary breast aberrantly located, *i.e.,* in some part other than the milk line.

m. masculi′na [NA], SYN male *breast.*

supernumerary m., SYN supernumerary *breast.*

m. viri′lis, SYN male *breast.*

mam·mal (mam′ăl). An animal of the class Mammalia.

mam·mal·gia (mă-mal′jē-ă). SYN mastodynia. [L. *mamma,* breast, + G. *algos,* pain]

Mam·ma·lia (mă-mā′lē-ă). The highest class of living organisms; it includes all the vertebrate animals (monotremes, marsupials, and placentals) that suckle their young, possess hair, and (except for the egg-laying monotremes) bring forth living young rather than eggs. [L. *mamma,* breast]

mam·ma·plas·ty (mam′ă-plas-tē). Plastic surgery of the breast to alter its shape, size, or position, or all of these. SYN mammoplasty, mastoplasty. [L. *mamma,* breast, + G. *plastos,* formed]

Arie-Pitanguy m., SYN Arie-Pitanguy *operation.*

augmentation m., plastic surgery to enlarge the breast, often by insertion of an implant.

reconstructive m., the making of a simulated breast by plastic surgery, to replace the appearance of one that has been removed.

reduction m., plastic surgery of the breast to reduce its size and (frequently) to improve its shape and position.

mam·ma·ry (mam′ă-rē). Relating to the breasts.

mam·mec·to·my (ma-mek′tō-mē). SYN mastectomy. [L. *mamma,* breast, + *ektomē,* excision]

mam·mi·form (mam′i-fōrm). Resembling a breast; breast-shaped. SYN mammose (1). [L. *mamma,* breast, + *forma,* form]

△**mammil-, mammilli-.** The mamillae. SEE ALSO mamil-. Cf. thelo-. [L. *mammilla (mamilla),* nipple]

mam·mil·la·plas·ty (ma-mil′ă-plas-tē). Plastic surgery of the nipple and areola. SYN theleplasty. [L. *mammilla,* nipple, + G. *plastos,* formed]

mam·mil·li·tis (mam-i-lī′tis). Inflammation of the nipple. [L., *mamilla,* nipple, + G. *-itis,* inflammation]

bovine herpes m., an ulcerative disease of the skin of the bovine teat caused by bovine herpesvirus type 2. SYN bovine ulcerative m.

bovine ulcerative m., SYN bovine herpes m.

bovine vaccinia m., a poxlike disease of the skin of the bovine teat caused by vaccinia virus.

mam·mi·tis (ma-mī′tis). SYN mastitis. [L. *mamma,* breast, + G. *-itis,* inflammation]

mammo-. The breasts. Cf. masto-. [L. *mamma*, breast]

mam·mo·gram (mam′ō-gram). The record produced by mammography.

mam·mog·ra·phy (ma-mog′ră-fē). Imaging examination of the breast by means of x-rays, ultrasound, and nuclear magnetic resonance; used for screening and diagnosis of breast disease. [mammo- + G. *graphō*, to write]

> The benefit of mammography is its ability to detect cancers of the breast sometimes as early as 2 years before they become palpable and, in many cases, before they have spread to lymph nodes. For this reason, it originally appeared that x-ray mammography would provide the means for affordable mass screening, and help to minimize breast cancer deaths. Currently, guidelines established by the American College of Radiology and the American Cancer Society recommend that women be given a baseline mammogram between ages 35 and 40, and then have them every 1 to 2 years; after age 50, an annual mammogram is recommended. (High-risk women are advised to seek more frequent exams; see breast cancer.) Analysis of numerous clinical studies has revealed that mammograms may not save lives for healthy women under 50 (only 17.5% of breast cancer occurs in women under 40). The higher density of breast tissues in younger women lowers the ability to identify nonpalpable growths; mammography spots only about a third of such growths in women between ages 40 and 50. In addition, research has suggested that for a small fraction of women, exposure to radiation for mammography may actually trigger breast cancer. Mammography is never intended to replace monthly self-examination, nor, in diagnosis, to substitute for biopsy, which is still required to establish malignancy.

mam·mo·plas·ty (mam′ō-plas-tē). SYN mammaplasty. [mammo- + G. *plastos*, formed]

mam·mose (mam′mōs). 1. SYN mammiform. 2. Having large breasts.

mam·mo·so·ma·to·troph (mam′ō-sō-mat′ō-trof). A cell of the adenohypophysis that produces prolactin and somatotropin.

mam·mot·o·my (ma-mot′ō-mē). SYN mastotomy. [mammo- + G. *tomē*, incision]

mam·mo·troph (mam′ō-trof). An acidophilic cell of the adenohypophysis that produces prolactin. SYN prolactin cell.

mam·mo·tro·pic, mam·mo·tro·phic (mam-ō-trop′ik, -trof′ik). Having a stimulating effect upon the development, growth, or function of the mammary glands. [mammo- + G. *tropos*, a turning]

mam·mo·tro·pin, mam·mo·tro·phin (mam-ō-trō′pin, -trō′fin). Obsolete term for prolactin.

Man Symbol for mannose or its radicals in polysaccharides.

man·chette (man-shet′). A conical array of microtubules that invests the nucleus of a spermatid; believed to play a role in shaping the nucleus during spermatogenesis. [Fr. cuff, dim. of *manche*, sleeve, fr. L. *manicae*; fr. *manus*, hand]

man·del·ate (man′de-lāt). A salt or ester of mandelic acid.

man·del·ic ac·id (man-del′ik). $C_6H_5CHOHCOOH$; a urinary antibacterial agent (both bactericidal and bacteriostatic). SYN hydroxytoluic acid, phenylglycolic acid. [Ger. *Mandel*, almond]

Mandelin's re·a·gent. See under reagent.

man·de·lyt·ro·pine (man-de-lit′rō-pēn). SYN homatropine.

man·di·ble (man′di-bl). A U-shaped bone, forming the lower jaw, articulating by its upturned extremities with the temporal bone on either side. SYN mandibula [NA], jaw bone, lower jaw, mandibulum, submaxilla.

man·dib·u·la, pl. **man·dib·u·lae** (man-dib′yū-lă, -lē) [NA]. SYN mandible. [L. a jaw, fr. *mando*, pp. *mansus*, to chew]

man·dib·u·lar (man-dib′yū-lăr). Relating to the lower jaw. SYN inframaxillary, submaxillary (1).

man·dib·u·lec·to·my (man-dib-yū-lek′tō-mē). Resection of the lower jaw. [mandibula + G. *ektomē*, excision]

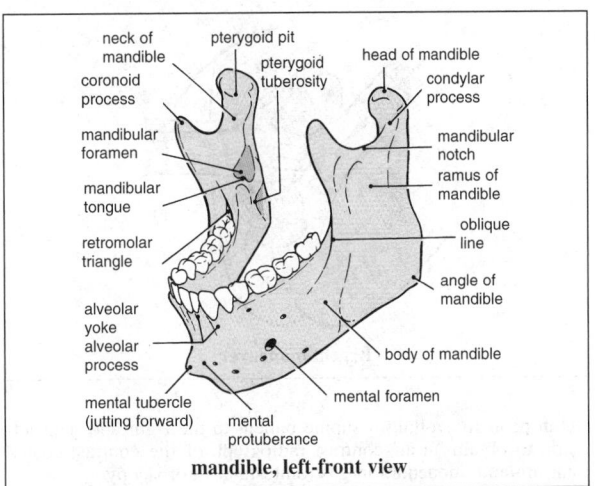

neck of mandible — pterygoid pit — head of mandible — coronoid process — pterygoid tuberosity — condylar process — mandibular foramen — mandibular notch — ramus of mandible — mandibular tongue — oblique line — retromolar triangle — angle of mandible — alveolar yoke — alveolar process — body of mandible — mental tubercle (jutting forward) — mental foramen — mental protuberance

mandible, left-front view

man·dib·u·lo·fa·cial (man-dib′yū-lō-fā′shăl). Relating to the mandible and the face.

man·dib·u·lo·oc·u·lo·fa·cial (man-dib′yū-lō-ok′yū-lō-fā′shăl). Relating to the mandible and the orbital part of the face.

man·dib·u·lo·pha·ryn·ge·al (man-dib′yū-lō-fa-rin′jē-ăl). Relating to the mandible and the pharynx; denoting the region between the pharynx and the ramus of the mandible, in which are found the internal carotid artery, the internal jugular vein, and the vagus, glossopharyngeal, accessory, and hypoglossal nerves.

man·dib·u·lum (man-dib′yū-lŭm). SYN mandible.

man·drag·o·ra (man-drag′ō-ră). The European mandrake, *Mandragora officinalis*, or *Atropa mandragora* (family Solanaceae), the mandrake of the Bible; its properties are similar to those of stramonium, hyoscyamus, and belladonna. [G. *mandragoras*]

man·drake (man′drāk). 1. SEE mandragora. 2. SEE podophyllum. [thr. L., fr. G. *mandragoras*]

wild m., SYN podophyllum *resin*.

man·drel, man·dril. 1. The shaft or spindle to which a tool is attached and by means of which it is rotated. 2. SYN mandrin. 3. In dentistry, an instrument used in a handpiece to hold a disk, stone, or cup used for grinding, smoothing, or finishing. [G. *mandra*, a stable; the bed in which a ring's stone is set]

man·drill. Common name for a species of monkey of the genus *Cynocephalus*, with a short tail and doglike head.

man·drin. A stiff wire or stylet inserted in the lumen of a soft catheter to give it shape and firmness while passing through a hollow tubular structure. SYN mandrel (2), mandril. [Fr. *mandrin*, mandrel]

ma·neu·ver (mă-nū′ver). A planned movement or procedure. [Fr. *manoeuvre*, fr. L. *manu operari*, to work by hand]

Adson m., SYN Adson's *test*.

Bill's m., forceps rotation of the fetal head at mid-pelvis before extraction of the head.

Bracht m., delivery of a fetus in breech position by extension of the legs and trunk of the fetus over the symphysis pubis and abdomen of the mother; the fetal head is born spontaneously as the legs and trunk are lifted above the maternal pelvis, and as the body of the infant is extended by the operator.

Brandt-Andrews m., the expression of the placenta by grasping the umbilical cord with one hand and placing the other hand on the abdomen, with the fingers over the anterior surface of the uterus at the junction of the lower uterine segment and the corpus uteri.

Buzzard's m., testing the patellar reflex while the sitting patient makes firm pressure on the floor with the toes.

Credé's m.'s, SYN Credé's *methods*, under *method*.

DeLee's m., SYN key-in-lock m.

Ejrup m., demonstration of collateral circulation by reduction in the prominence of activity of the greater arteries and reduced pulse volume following muscular activity.

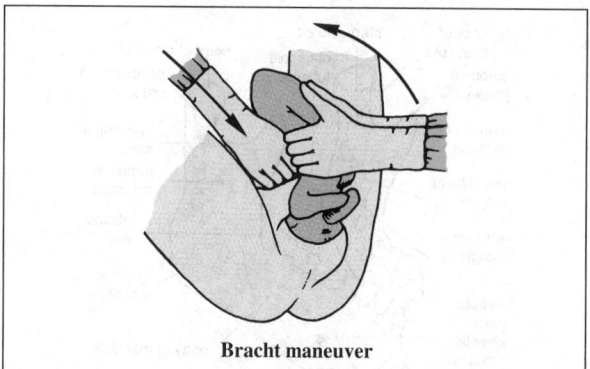
Bracht maneuver

Hampton m., rolling a supine patient to the right and then left side to obtain an air contrast radiograph of the contrast-coated antrum and duodenum in gastrointestinal fluoroscopy.

Heimlich m., a planned action designed to expel an obstructing bolus of food from the throat by placing a fist on the abdomen between the navel and the costal margin, grasping the fist with the other hand, and forcefully thrusting it inward and upward so as to force the diaphragm upward, forcing air up the trachea to dislodge the obstruction.

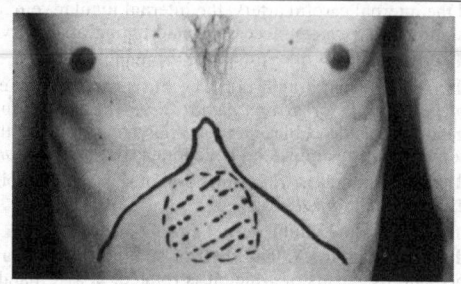
Heimlich maneuver
the pressure point is in the abdominal area, just over the stomach

Hillis-Müller m., manual pressure on the term fundus while a finger in the vagina determines the descent of the head into the pelvis.

Hueter's m., pressing the patient's tongue downward and forward with the left forefinger in passing a stomach tube.

Jendrassik's m., a method of emphasizing the patellar reflex: the subject hooks his hands together by the flexed fingers and pulls against them with all his strength.

key-in-lock m., a method by which obstetrical forceps are used to rotate the fetal head. SYN DeLee's m.

LeCompte m., a repair of double outlet right ventricle with pulmonary stenosis and other abnormalities of ventricular arterial connection and ventricular septal defect in which the LV is connected to the aorta and the RV to the pulmonary artery using a technique that does not require an extracardiac conduit. SYN LeCompte operation.

Leopold's m.'s, four m.'s employed to determine fetal position: 1) determination of what is in the fundus; 2) evaluation of the fetal back and extremities; 3) palpation of the presenting part above the symphysis; 4) determination of the direction and degree of flexion of the head.

Mauriceau-Levret m., SYN Mauriceau's m.

Mauriceau's m., a method of assisted breech delivery in which the infant's body is astraddle the right forearm, and the middle finger of the right hand is in the fetal mouth to maintain flexion

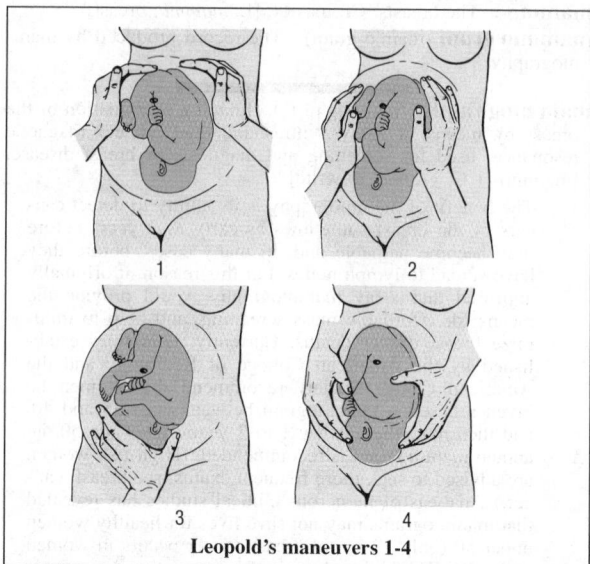
Leopold's maneuvers 1-4

while traction is made upon the shoulders by the other hand. SYN Mauriceau-Levret m.

McDonald's m., measurement of uterus from the upper border of the symphysis to a line tangential to the fundus over the abdomen with a tape to determine the height of the uterus; each centimeter approximately corresponds to the gestational age in weeks.

McRoberts m., m. to reduce a fetal shoulder dystocia by flexion of the maternal hips.

Müller's m., after a forced expiration, an attempt at inspiration is made with closed mouth and nose or closed glottis, whereby the negative pressure in the chest and lungs is made very subatmospheric; the reverse of Valsalva m.

Pajot's m., obsolete term for traction downward on the forceps lock with one hand while traction is applied with the other hand to bring the fetal head down in the axis of the birth canal.

Pinard's m., in management of a frank breech presentation, pressure on the popliteal space is made by the index finger while the other three fingers flex the leg while sliding it along the other thigh as the foot of the flexed leg is brought down and out.

Prague m., obsolete term for a technique for delivery of the fetus in breech position when the fetal occiput is posterior; one hand of the operator delivers the shoulders, while making pressure over the symphysis pubis with the other hand.

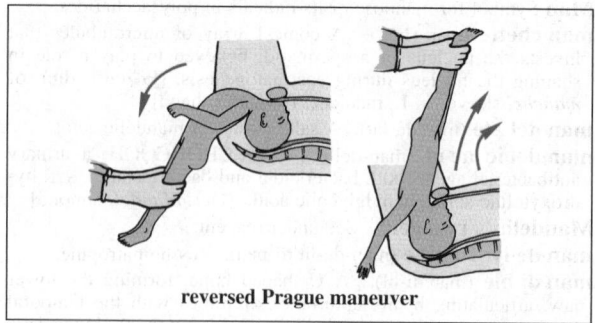
reversed Prague maneuver

Ritgen's m., delivery of a child's head by pressure on the perineum while controlling the speed of delivery by pressure with the other hand on the head.

Scanzoni's m., forceps rotation and traction in a spiral course, with reapplication of forceps for delivery.

Sellick's m., pressure applied to the cricoid cartilage, to prevent regurgitation during tracheal intubation in the anesthetized patient.

Valsalva m., any forced expiratory effort ("strain") against a closed airway, whether at the nose and mouth or at the glottis, the reverse of Müller's m.; because high intrathoracic pressure impedes venous return to the right atrium, this m. is used to study cardiovascular effects of raised peripheral venous pressure and decreased cardiac filling and cardiac output, as well as post-strain responses.

Wigand m., an assisted breech delivery with pressure above the symphysis while the fetus lies astraddle the operator's other arm.

man·ga·nese (Mn) (mang′gă-nēz). A metallic element resembling and often associated, in ores, with iron; atomic no. 25, atomic wt. 54.94; manganous salts are sometimes used in medicine. SYN manganum. [Mod. L. *manganesium, manganum,* an altered form of *magnesium*]

man·gan·ic (mang-gan′ik). Denoting the trivalent cation of manganese, Mn³⁺.

man·ga·nous (mang′gă-nŭs). Denoting the divalent cation of manganese, Mn²⁺.

man·ga·num (man′gă-nŭm). SYN manganese. [L.]

mange (mānj). A cutaneous disease of domestic and wild animals caused by any one of several genera of skin-burrowing mites; in humans, mite infestations are usually referred to as scabies. [Fr. *manger,* to eat]

chorioptic m., m. caused by mites of the genus *Chorioptes;* in many cases it involves the skin of much of the body.

demodectic m., an infestation of the hair follicles and sebaceous glands with mites of the genus *Demodex;* they occur in humans and a number of domesticated animals; although asymptomatic in most species, these mites can cause severe and extensive dermatitis ("red mange") in dogs. SYN demodectic acariasis, follicular m.

ear m., SYN otodectic m.

follicular m., SYN demodectic m.

notoedric m., m. of cats caused by the mite, *Notoedres cati.*

otodectic m., disease resulting from heavy infestation with the mite *Otodectes cynotis* in the ears of dogs, cats, foxes, and other carnivores and manifested by head shaking, continual ear scratching, and ear droop; observed in severe cases are torticollis, circling, epileptoid fits with purulent inflammation and discharge of the external ear, and possible perforation of the tympanic membrane. SEE ALSO otoacariasis. SYN ear m.

psoroptic m., hair loss or m. caused by infestation with mites of the genus *Psoroptes.*

red m., demodectic m. in dogs.

sarcoptic m., a cutaneous disease of domestic animals caused by mites of the genus *Sarcoptes* including *Sarcoptes scabiei.*

Manhold, John H., U.S. dentist, *1919 SEE Volpe-M. *Index.*

ma·nia (mā′nē-ă). An emotional disorder characterized by euphoria or irritability, increased psychomotor activity, rapid speech, flight of ideas, decreased need for sleep, distractibility, grandiosity, and poor judgment; usually occurs in bipolar disorder. SEE manic-depressive, manic *excitement.* [G. frenzy]

acute m., SYN manic *excitement.*

♻**-mania.** An abnormal love for, or morbid impulse toward, some specific object, place, or action. [G. frenzy]

ma·ni·ac (mā′nē-ak). **1.** Obsolete term for a mentally ill or disturbed person. **2.** One suffering from mania.

ma·ni·a·cal (mă-nī′ă-kăl). Relating to or characterized by mania. SEE amok. SYN manic.

man·ic (man′ik, mā′nik). SYN maniacal.

man·ic-de·pres·sive. 1. Pertaining to a manic-depressive psychosis (bipolar *disorder*). **2.** One suffering from such a disorder.

man·i·cy (man′i-sē). Behavior characteristic of the manic phase of bipolar disorder.

man·i·fes·ta·tion (man′i-fes-tā′shŭn). The display or disclosure of characteristic signs or symptoms of an illness. [L. *manifestus,* caught in the act]

behavioral m., a m. characterized by defects in personality structure and attendant behavior with minimal anxiety and little

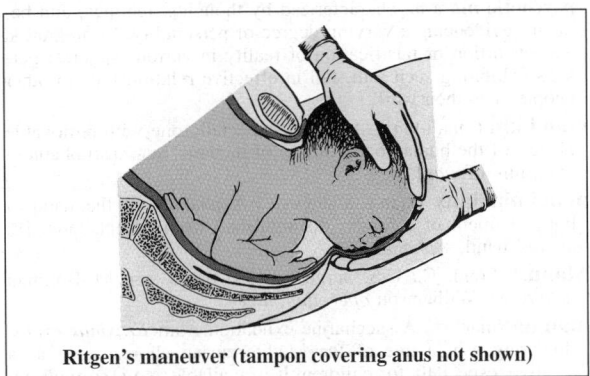

Ritgen's maneuver (tampon covering anus not shown)

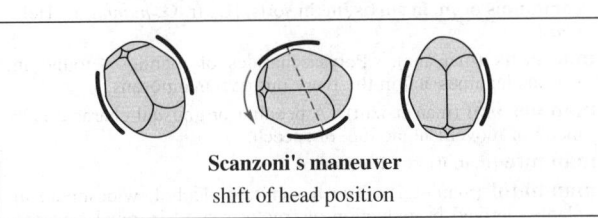

Scanzoni's maneuver
shift of head position

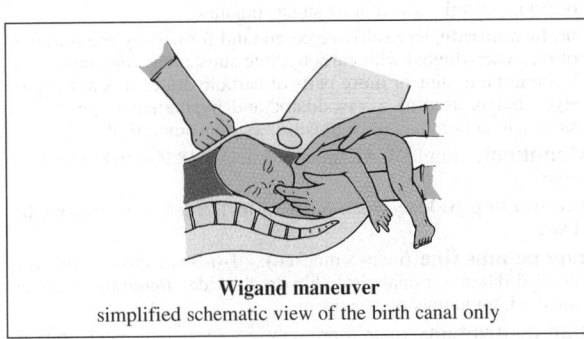

Wigand maneuver
simplified schematic view of the birth canal only

or no sense of distress, indicative of a psychiatric disorder; occasionally encephalitis or head injury will produce the clinical picture which is properly diagnosed as chronic brain disorder with behavioral m.'s.

neurotic m., a m. characterized by such defenses as conversion, dissociation, displacement, phobia formation, or repetitive thoughts and acts being utilized to handle anxiety; in contrast to psychotic m.'s, gross distortion or falsification of reality is not exhibited, and gross disintegration of the personality is not usually observed.

psychophysiologic m., a m. characterized by the visceral expression of affect, the symptoms due to a chronic and exaggerated state of the physiologic expression of emotion with the feeling repressed; such m.'s are commonly characteristic of psychosomatic disorders.

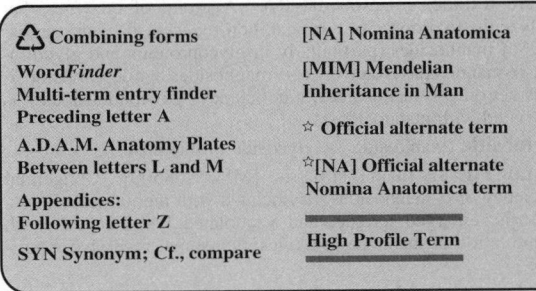

♻ Combining forms	[NA] Nomina Anatomica
Word*Finder* **Multi-term entry finder** Preceding letter A	[MIM] Mendelian **Inheritance in Man**
A.D.A.M. Anatomy Plates Between letters L and M	☆ Official alternate term
Appendices: **Following letter Z**	☆[NA] Official alternate **Nomina Anatomica term**
SYN Synonym; Cf., compare	High Profile Term

ma

psychotic m., a m. characterized by thoughts, feelings, and behavior evidencing a varying degree of personality disintegration and distortion or falsification of reality in various spheres; persons exhibiting such a m. fail in effective relationships to other people or to their work.

man·i·kin (man'i-kin). A model, especially one with removable pieces, of the human body or any of its parts. SEE ALSO phantom (2). [dim. of *man*]

man·i·pha·lanx (man'i-fā'langks). A phalanx of the hand; a bony segment of a finger; distinguished from pediphalanx. [L. *manus,* hand, + *phalanx*]

Mann, Frank C., U.S. surgeon, 1887–1962. SEE M.-Bollman *fistula;* M.-Williamson *operation, ulcer.*

man·na (man'ă). A saccharine exudation from *Fraxinus ornus,* flowering ash, a tree of the Mediterranean shores, used as a laxative, especially for children. It is available as **m. cannellata,** a flake m.; **m. in lacrimis,** m. in tears or small flakes; and **m. communis** or **m. in sortis,** m. in sorts. [L., fr. G. *manna,* fr. Heb. *mān*]

man·nans (man'anz). Polysaccharides of mannose, found in various legumes and in the ivory nut. SYN mannosans.

man·ner·ism (man'er-izm). A peculiar or unusual characteristic mode of movement, action, or speech.

man·nite (man'īt). SYN mannitol.

man·ni·tol (man'i-tol). The hexahydric alcohol, widespread in plants, derived by reduction of fructose; used in renal function testing to measure glomerular filtration, and intravenously as an osmotic diuretic. SYN manna sugar, mannite.

m. hexanitrate, an explosive compound formed by the nitration of m.; when diluted with carbohydrate substances (one part of m. hexanitrate to nine or more parts of carbohydrate) it is not explosive, and is used as a vasodilator and hypotensive agent; it is slower in action than nitroglycerin. SYN nitromannitol.

Mannkopf, Emil W., German physician, 1836–1918. SEE M.'s *sign.*

man·no·hep·tu·lose (man-ō-hep'tū-lōs). SEE D-*manno*-heptulose.

man·no·mus·tine (man-ō-mŭs'tēn). 1-6-Bis(2-chloroethylamino)-1,6-dideoxy-D-mannitol dihydrochloride; mannitol nitrogen mustard; an antineoplastic agent.

man·no·pro·teins (man'ō-prō-tēnz). Yeast cell wall components that are proteins with large numbers of mannose groups attached; highly antigenic.

man·no·sa·mine (man-ōs'a-mēn). 2-Amino-2-deoxymannose; the D-isomer is a constituent of neuraminic acids as well as mucolipids and mucoproteins.

man·no·sans (man'ō-sanz). SYN mannans.

man·nose (Man) (man'ōs). An aldohexose obtained from various plant sources (*i.e.,* from mannans).

man·nose-1-phos·phate gua·nyl·yl·trans·fer·ase (GDP). A transferase that catalyzes the transfer of GDP to the mannose of mannose-1-phosphate. SYN GDPmannose phosphorylase.

man·nose·phos·phate isom·er·ase. An enzyme that catalyzes the reversible conversion of D-mannose-6-phosphate to D-fructose-6-phosphate; a key step in the synthesis of mannose derivatives as well as the entry of mannose into the central pathways of carbohydrate metabolism.

man·no·si·dases (man-ō'si-dās'es). A group of enzymes that catalyze the hydrolysis of terminal, non-reducing D-mannose residues of mannosides (particularly in glycoproteins and glycolipids); α-mannosidases act on α-D-mannosides while β-mannosidases act on β-D-mannosides; a deficiency of α-mannosidases is associated with mannosidosis.

man·no·side (man'ō-sīd). A glycoside of mannose.

man·no·si·do·sis (man'ō-si-dō'sis) [MIM*268500]. Congenital deficiency of α-mannosidase; associated with mental retardation, kyphosis, enlarged tongue, and vacuolated lymphocytes, with accumulation of mannose in tissues; autosomal recessive inheritance.

Mann's meth·yl blue-e·o·sin stain. See under stain.

man·nu·ron·ic ac·id (man-yū-ron'ik). Uronic acid derived from the oxidation of mannose.

ma·nom·e·ter (mă-nom'ĕ-ter). An instrument for indicating the pressure of any fluid or the difference in pressure between two fluids, whether gas or liquid. [G. *manos,* thin, scanty, + *metron,* measure]

aneroid m., a m. in which the pressure is indicated by a revolving pointer moved by a diaphragm or Bourdon tube exposed to the pressure. SYN dial m.

dial m., SYN aneroid m.

differential m., any device that indicates the difference in pressure between two fluids, regardless of any changes in their absolute pressures.

mercurial m., an m. in which the varying pressures are shown by differences of elevation in a column of mercury.

man·o·met·ric (man-ō-met'rik). Relating to a manometer.

ma·nom·e·try (mă-nom'ĕ-trē). Measurement of the pressure of gases by means of a manometer. SYN manoscopy. [see manometer]

esophageal m., measurement of intra-esophageal pressures at one or more sites by intraluminal pressure-sensitive instruments.

ma·nos·co·py (mă-nos'kŏ-pē). SYN manometry.

man. pr. Abbreviation for L. *mane primo,* early morning, first thing in the morning.

Manson, Sir Patrick, English authority on tropical medicine, 1844–1922. SEE *Mansonella; Mansonia;* M.'s *disease, pyosis, schistosomiasis; Schistosoma mansoni; schistosomiasis* mansoni; M.'s eye *worm.*

Man·son·el·la (man-sō-nel'ă). A genus of filaria, widely distributed in tropical Africa and South America, that infects the peritoneal cavity, serous surfaces, or skin with unsheathed microfilariae in the skin or blood of man and other primates. The important human parasites *M. perstans* and *M. streptocerca* formerly were placed in the genera *Dipetalonema, Acanthocheilonema,* and *Tetrapetalonema.*

M. demarqua'yi, SYN *M. ozzardi.*

M. ozzar'di, a filarial parasite occurring in Yucatan, Panama, Colombia, northern Argentina, Guyana, French Guiana, and the islands of St. Vincent and Dominica, causing mansonelliasis; the microfilariae are not ensheathed, and there are no nuclei in the pointed tail; the life cycle is similar to that of *Wuchereria bancrofti;* humans are the only known definitive host, and the intermediate hosts are biting midges, *Culicoides furens* and possibly *C. paraensis.* SYN *M. demarquayi, M. tucumana.*

M. per'stans, the "persistent filaria," a species widely prevalent in tropical Africa and northern South America where it infects human peritoneal and other body cavities, but is non- or mildly pathogenic; characteristic subperiodic microfilariae occur in peripheral blood. It is transmitted in Africa by the biting midges *Culicoides austeni* and *C. grahami.*

M. streptocer'ca, a filarial species in humans that produces nonperiodic sheathless microfilariae found in the circulating blood; may cause a lichenoid condition or edema of the skin; commonly found in the corium of the skin of west African residents and transmitted by the biting midge, *Culicoides grahami.*

M. tucuma'na, SYN *M. ozzardi.*

man·so·nel·li·a·sis (man'sō-nel-ī'ă-sis). Infection with a species of *Mansonella,* transmitted to humans by biting midges of the genus *Culicoides;* adult worms live in the serous cavities, especially the peritoneal cavity, in mesenteric and perivisceral adipose tissue, and in the skin.

man·son·el·lo·sis (man-sō-nel'lō-sis). Infection with the filarial parasite *Mansonella ozzardi.*

Man·so·nia (man-sō'nē-ă). A genus of brown or black medium-sized mosquitoes (tribe Culicini), often having banded abdomen and legs; larvae and pupae have modified breathing tubes enabling them to pierce aquatic plants to obtain air. *M.* mosquitoes are distributed worldwide and, in tropical areas, are important vectors of *Brugia malayi;* in some areas they also transmit *Wuchereria bancrofti.* [P. *Manson*]

Man·so·noi·des (man-sō-noy'dēz). A subgenus of *Mansonia.*

Mantel, Nathan, U.S. biostatistician, *1927. SEE Mantel-Haenszel *test.*

man·tle (man′tl). **1.** A covering layer. **2.** SYN pallium.

brain m., SYN pallium.

myoepicardial m., the dorsal wall of the primitive pericardium which, in the early somite embryo, becomes both the epicardium and the myocardium.

Mantoux, Charles, French physician, 1877–1947. SEE M. *pit, test.*

ma·nu·bri·um, pl. **ma·nu·bria** (mă-nū′brē-ŭm, -ă) [NA]. The portion of the sternum or of the malleus that represents the handle. [L. handle]

m. mal′lei [NA], SYN m. of malleus.

m. of malleus, the handle of the malleus; the portion that extends downward, inward, and backward from the neck of the malleus; it is embedded throughout its length in the tympanic membrane. SYN m. mallei [NA].

m. ster′ni [NA], SYN m. of sternum.

m. of sternum, the upper segment of the sternum, a flattened, roughly triangular bone, occasionally fused with the body of the sternum, forming with it a slight angle, the sternal angle. SYN m. sterni [NA], episternum, presternum.

man·u·dy·na·mom·e·ter (man′yū-dī-nă-mom′ĕ-ter). In dentistry, a device for measuring the force exerted by the thrust of an instrument. [L. *manus,* hand, + G. *dynamis,* force, + *metron,* measure]

ma·nus, gen. and pl. **ma·nus** (mā′nŭs) [NA]. SYN hand. [L.]

m. ca′va, a condition of extreme concavity of the palm of the hand.

m. exten′sa, clubhand with deviation backward. SYN m. superextensa.

m. flex′a, clubhand with forward deviation.

m. pla′na, loss of normal arches of the hand. SYN flat hand.

m. superexten′sa, SYN m. extensa.

m. val′ga, clubhand with deviation to the ulnar side.

m. va′ra, clubhand with deviation to the radial side.

MAO Abbreviation for monoamine oxidase.

MAOI Abbreviation for monoamine oxidase *inhibitor.*

map. A representation of a region or structure; *e.g.,* of a stretch of DNA.

conformational m., SYN Ramachandran *plot.*

contig m., a physical m. of a chromosome or stretch of DNA constructed from sets of overlapping and order clones (contigs).

cytogenetic m., a m. in which the classical bonding pattern of a chromosome is shown.

fate m., SYN germinal *localization.*

linkage m., SYN genetic map.

physical m., a m. of a stretch of DNA with ordered landmarks a known distance from each other; the ultimate physical m. would be the base sequence of the entire chromosome.

restriction m., the order of restriction sites along a chromosome or plasmid.

sequence-tagged site (STS) m., a m. representing the order and spacing of sequence-tagged sites within a stretch of DNA.

map dis·tance. The degree of separation of two loci on a linkage map, measured in morgans or centimorgans.

map·pine (map′ēn). SYN bufotenine.

map·ping. The process of identifying the relative position of genes on chromosomes.

cardiac m., a method by which local cardiac potentials are spatially depicted in an integrated manner as a function of time (isochrone map) or potential (isopotential map).

S1 nuclease m., a method for locating the 5′ end of a transcript in a mixture of RNA.

map·ping func·tion. In linkage analysis, a formula that converts the recombination fraction (which is on the probability scale) into map distance (in morgans).

ma·pro·ti·line (ma-prō′ti-lēn). *N*-Methyl-9,10-ethanoanthracene-9(10*H*)-propylamine; a tricyclic antidepressant used in the treatment of various depressive illnesses, and for relief of anxiety associated with depression.

MAPs Abbreviation for microtubule-associated *proteins,* under *protein.*

Marañón. Gregorio, Spanish endocrinologist, 1887–1960. SEE Marañón's *sign,* syndrome.

ma·ran·tic (mă-ran′tik). SYN marasmic. [G. *marantikos,* wasting]

ma·ras·mic (mă-raz′mik). Relating to or suffering from marasmus. SYN marantic.

ma·ras·moid (mă-raz′moyd). Resembling marasmus. [G. *marasmos,* withering, + *eidos,* resemblance]

ma·ras·mus (mă-raz′mŭs). Cachexia, especially in young children, primarily due to prolonged dietary deficiency of protein and calories. SYN marantic atrophy, Parrot's disease (2), pedatrophia, pedatrophy. [G. *marasmos,* withering]

nutritional m., extreme weakness and wasting secondary to malnutrition.

marc (mark). The residue remaining after percolation of a drug. [Fr. fr. *marcher,* to trample]

Marcacci, Arturo, Italian physiologist, 1854–1915. SEE M.'s *muscle.*

Marchand, Felix, German pathologist, 1846–1928. SEE M.'s *adrenals,* under *adrenal, rest,* wandering *cell.*

Marchant, Gérard T.J., French surgeon, 1850–1903. SEE M.'s *zone.*

Marchesani, Oswald, 1900–1952. SEE Weill-M. *syndrome.*

Marchetti, Andrew A., U.S. obstetrician and gynecologist, 1901–1970. SEE Marshall-M.-Krantz *operation.*

Marchi, Vittorio, Italian physician, 1851–1908. SEE M.'s *fixative, reaction, stain, tract.*

Marchiafava, Ettore, Italian pathologist, 1847–1935. SEE M.-Bignami *disease;* M.-Micheli *anemia, syndrome.*

mar·cid (mar′sid). Emaciating; wasting away. [L. *marcidus;* fr. *marceo,* to wither]

Marcille, Maurice, 1871–1941. SEE M.'s *triangle.*

mar·cor (mar′kōr). Obsolete term for marasmus. [L. fr. *marceo,* to wither]

Marcus Gunn, Robert. SEE Gunn.

Marek, Josef, Hungarian veterinarian and pathologist, 1867–1952. SEE M.'s *disease,* disease *virus.*

Marey, Étienne Jules, French physiologist, 1830–1904. SEE M.'s *law.*

Marfan, Antoine Bernard-Jean, French pediatrician, 1858–1942. SEE M.'s *disease, law, syndrome.*

mar·fan·oid (mar′fan-oyd). An obsolete term used of those whose phenotype bears a superficial resemblence to that of Marfan's syndrome.

Marg, Elwin, U.S. physicist, *1918. SEE Mackay-M. *tonometer.*

Mar·gar·o·pus (mar-gar′ō-pŭs). A genus of ixodid ticks closely resembling *Boophilus,* but not having festoons or ornamentations; they are characterized by greatly enlarged posterior legs and a prolonged median plate. [G. *margaros,* pearl oyster, + *pous,* foot]

M. winthe′mi, the one-host South American winter horse tick; it also sometimes attacks cattle and sheep.

mar·gin (mar′jin). A boundary, edge, or border, as of a surface or structure. SEE ALSO border, edge. SYN margo [NA]. [L. *margo,* border, edge]

m. of acetabulum, the rim of bone around the acetabulum to which is attached the labrum acetabulare. SYN limbus acetabuli [NA], margo acetabularis* [NA].

anterior m., SYN anterior *border.*

articular m., SYN glenoid *labrum.*

cavity m., the periphery of a filling, the line of junction between a restoration and the external surface of a tooth.

cervical m., (1) SYN gingival m. (2) termination of a restoration in the gingival area.

cervical m. of tooth, SYN *neck* of tooth.

ciliary m. of iris, SYN ciliary *border* of iris.

ma

corneal m., SYN *limbus* of cornea.

m.'s of eyelids, the free edges of the eyelids. SEE ALSO anterior *border* of eyelids, posterior *border* of eyelids. SYN margo palpebrae.

falciform m., the sharply curved, free margin of the saphenous opening in the fascia lata; medially, it ends in a superior and an inferior horn. SYN margo falciformis [NA].

fibular m. of foot, SYN lateral *border* of foot.

m. of fossa ovalis, SYN *limbus* fossae ovalis.

free m., SYN free *border*.

free m. of eyelids, the unattached inferior edge of the upper lid and superior edge of the lower lid, where the anterior (cutaneous) surface of the eyelid meets the posterior (conjunctival) surface of the eyelid. The free m.'s of the eyelids bound the rima palpebrarum, and each free m. has an anterior and posterior border. SEE *borders* of eyelids, under *border*.

frontal m., SYN frontal *border*.

gingival m., (1) the most coronal portion of the gingiva surrounding the tooth; **(2)** the edge of the free gingiva. SYN cervical m. (1), gingival crest.

incisal m., SYN incisal *edge*.

inferior m., SYN inferior *border*.

inferolateral m., SYN *margo* inferior cerebri.

inferomedial m., SYN *margo* medialis cerebri.

infraorbital m., the inferior half of the orbital rim, or the lower border of the orbital opening, formed by the maxilla medially and the zygomatic bone laterally. SEE orbital *rim*. SYN margo infraorbitalis [NA].

interosseous m., SYN interosseous *border*.

lacrimal m. of maxilla, SYN lacrimal *border* of maxilla.

lambdoid m. of occipital bone, SYN lambdoid *border* of occipital bone.

lateral m., SYN lateral *border*.

mastoid m. of occipital bone, SYN mastoid *border* of occipital bone.

medial m., SYN medial *border*.

mesovarian m. of ovary, SYN mesovarian *border* of ovary.

nasal m. of frontal bone, SYN nasal *border* of frontal bone.

m. of orbit, SYN orbital *rim*.

occipital m., SYN occipital *border*.

orbital m. of eyelids, the outer or peripheral attached borders of the upper and lower eyelids; the "root" of the eyelids, along which it is attached to the orbital rim.

parietal m., SYN parietal *border*.

psoas m., in abdominal radiography, the appearance of the fat stripe delineating the lateral margin of the psoas muscle shadow; shows a normal retroperitoneum when visible.

pupillary m. of iris, SYN pupillary *border* of iris.

right m. of heart, SYN right *border* of heart.

m. of safety, the m. between the minimal therapeutic dose and the minimal toxic dose of a drug.

squamous m., SYN squamous *border*.

superomedial m., SYN *margo* superior cerebri.

supraorbital m., the superior half of the orbital rim, which constitutes the curved superior border of the orbital opening, formed by the frontal bone. SEE orbital *rim*. SYN margo supraorbitalis [NA], supraorbital arch, supraorbital ridge.

m. of the tongue, the lateral border that separates the dorsum from the inferior surface of the tongue on each side, the two borders meeting anteriorly at the apex. SYN margo linguae [NA].

ulnar m. of forearm, SYN medial *border* of forearm.

zygomatic m. of greater wing of sphenoid bone, SYN zygomatic *border* of greater wing of sphenoid bone.

mar·gi·nal (mar'ji-năl). Relating to a margin.

Mar·gi·nal Line Cal·cu·lus In·dex (MLC). An index which scores supragingival calculus found in cervical areas paralleling marginal gingiva.

mar·gin·a·tion (mar'ji-nā'shŭn). A phenomenon that occurs during the relatively early phases of inflammation; as a result of dilation of capillaries and slowing of the bloodstream, leukocytes tend to occupy the periphery of the cross-sectional lumen and adhere to the endothelial cells that line the vessels.

m. of placenta, SEE *placenta* marginata.

mar·gi·nes (mar'ji-nēz). Plural of margo. [L.]

mar·gi·no·plas·ty (mar'ji-nō-plas-tē). Plastic surgery of the tarsal border of an eyelid.

mar·go, gen. **mar·gi·nis,** pl. **mar·gi·nes** (mar'gō, mar'ji-nis, -nēz) [NA]. SYN margin, border. [L.]

m. acetabularis [NA], ★official alternate term for *margin* of acetabulum.

m. anterior fibulae [NA], SYN anterior *border* of fibula.

m. anterior pancreatis [NA], SYN anterior *border* of pancreas.

m. anterior pulmonis [NA], SYN anterior *border* of lung.

m. anterior radii [NA], SYN anterior *border* of radius.

m. anterior testis [NA], SYN anterior *border* of testis.

m. anterior tibiae [NA], SYN anterior *border* of tibia.

m. anterior ulnae [NA], SYN anterior *border* of ulna.

m. cilia'ris i'ridis [NA], SYN ciliary *border* of iris.

m. dex'ter cor'dis [NA], SYN right *border* of heart.

m. falcifor'mis [NA], SYN falciform *margin*.

m. fibula'ris pedis, ★official alternate term for lateral *border* of foot.

m. frontalis [NA], SYN frontal *border*.

m. frontalis ossis parietalis [NA], SYN frontal *border* of parietal bone.

m. frontalis ossis sphenoidalis [NA], SYN frontal *border* of sphenoid bone.

m. incisa'lis [NA], SYN incisal *edge*.

m. inferior, SYN inferior *border*.

m. inferior cer'ebri [NA], the irregular, discontinuous margin of the cerebral hemisphere at the junction of the inferior and superolateral surfaces. SYN m. inferolateralis★ [NA], inferolateral margin.

m. inferior hep'atis [NA], SYN inferior *border* of liver.

m. inferior pancrea'tis [NA], SYN inferior *border* of pancreas.

m. inferior pulmo'nis [NA], SYN inferior *border* of lung.

m. inferior splenis [NA], SYN inferior *border* of pancreas.

m. inferolatera'lis [NA], ★official alternate term for m. inferior cerebri.

m. inferomedia'lis [NA], ★official alternate term for m. medialis cerebri.

m. infraorbita'lis [NA], SYN infraorbital *margin*.

m. interosseus [NA], SYN interosseous *border*.

m. interos'seus fib'ulae [NA], SYN interosseous *border* of fibula.

m. interos'seus ra'dii [NA], SYN interosseous *border* of radius.

m. interos'seus tib'iae [NA], SYN interosseous *border* of tibia.

m. interos'seus ul'nae [NA], SYN interosseous *border* of ulna.

m. lacrima'lis maxillae [NA], SYN lacrimal *border* of maxilla.

m. lambdoid'eus squamae occipitalis [NA], SYN lambdoid *border* of occipital bone.

m. lateralis [NA], SYN lateral *border*.

m. latera'lis antebra'chii [NA], SYN lateral *border* of forearm.

m. latera'lis humer'ii [NA], SYN lateral *border* of humerus.

m. latera'lis pe'dis [NA], SYN lateral *border* of foot.

m. latera'lis re'nis [NA], SYN lateral *border* of kidney.

m. latera'lis scap'ulae [NA], SYN lateral *border* of scapula.

m. latera'lis un'guis [NA], SYN lateral *border* of nail.

m. liber [NA], SYN free *border*.

m. li'ber ova'rii [NA], SYN free *border* of ovary.

m. li'ber un'guis [NA], SYN free *border* of nail.

m. lin'guae [NA], SYN *margin* of the tongue.

m. mastoi'deus squamae occipitalis [NA], SYN mastoid *border* of occipital bone.

m. media'lis [NA], SYN medial *border*.

m. media'lis antebra'chii [NA], SYN medial *border* of forearm.

m. media'lis cer'ebri, the irregular border of the cerebral hemisphere at the junction of the inferior and medial surfaces. SYN m. inferomedialis★ [NA], inferomedial margin.

m. media′lis glan′dulae suprarena′lis [NA], SYN medial *border* of suprarenal gland.

m. media′lis humer′ii [NA], SYN medial *border* of humerus.

m. media′lis pe′dis [NA], SYN medial *border* of foot.

m. media′lis re′nis [NA], SYN medial *border* of kidney.

m. medialis tibiae [NA], SYN medial *border* of tibia.

m. mesova′ricus ovarii [NA], SYN mesovarian *border* of ovary.

m. nasa′lis ossis frontalis [NA], SYN nasal *border* of frontal bone.

m. occipitalis [NA], SYN occipital *border*.

m. occipita′lis os′sis parieta′lis [NA], SYN occipital *border* of parietal bone.

m. occipita′lis os′sis tempora′lis [NA], SYN occipital *border* of temporal bone.

m. occul′tus un′guis [NA], SYN proximal *border* of nail.

m. pal′pebrae, SYN *margins* of eyelids, under *margin*.

m. parieta′lis [NA], SYN parietal *border*.

m. parieta′lis os′sis fronta′lis [NA], SYN parietal *border* of frontal bone.

m. parieta′lis os′sis sphenoida′lis [NA], SYN parietal *border* of sphenoid bone.

m. parieta′lis os′sis tempora′lis [NA], SYN parietal *border* of temporal bone.

m. poste′rior fib′ulae [NA], SYN posterior *border* of fibula.

m. poste′rior par′tis petro′sae os′sis tempora′lis [NA], SYN posterior *border* of petrous part of temporal bone.

m. poste′rior ra′dii [NA], SYN posterior *border* of radius.

m. poste′rior tes′tis [NA], SYN posterior *border* of testis.

m. poste′rior ul′nae [NA], SYN posterior *border* of ulna.

m. pupilla′ris ir′idis [NA], SYN pupillary *border* of iris.

m. radia′lis antebrachii, ☆official alternate term for lateral *border* of forearm.

m. sagitta′lis ossis parietalis [NA], SYN sagittal *border* of parietal bone.

m. sphenoida′lis ossis temporalis [NA], SYN sphenoidal *border* of temporal bone.

m. squamo′sus [NA], SYN squamous *border*.

m. squamo′sus os′sis parieta′lis [NA], SYN squamous *border* of parietal bone.

m. squamo′sus os′sis sphenoida′lis [NA], SYN squamous *border* of sphenoid bone.

m. supe′rior cer′ebri, the curved margin of the cerebral hemisphere at the junction of the superolateral and medial surfaces. SYN m. superomedialis [NA], superomedial margin.

m. supe′rior glan′dulae suprarena′lis [NA], SYN superior *border* of suprarenal gland.

m. supe′rior pancrea′tis [NA], SYN superior *border* of pancreas.

m. superior par′tis petro′sae os′sis tempora′lis [NA], SYN superior *border* of petrous part of temporal bone.

m. supe′rior scap′ulae [NA], SYN superior *border* of scapula.

m. supe′rior splenis [NA], SYN superior *border* of spleen.

m. superomedia′lis [NA], SYN m. superior cerebri.

m. supraorbita′lis [NA], SYN supraorbital *margin*.

m. tibia′lis pedis [NA], ☆official alternate term for medial *border* of foot.

m. ulna′ris antebrachii [NA], ☆official alternate term for medial *border* of forearm.

m. u′teri [NA], SYN *border* of uterus.

m. zygomat′icus alae majoris [NA], SYN zygomatic *border* of greater wing of sphenoid bone.

Marie, Pierre, French neurologist, 1853–1940. SEE M.'s *ataxia;* Charcot-M.-Tooth *disease;* Bamberger-M. *disease, syndrome;* M.-Strümpell *disease;* Strümpell-M. *disease;* Brissaud-M. *syndrome;* Foix-Cavany-Marie *syndrome*.

mar·i·hua·na (mar-i-wah′nǎ). Popular name for the dried flowering leaves of *Cannabis sativa,* which are smoked as cigarettes, "joints," or "reefers." In the U.S. m. includes any part of, or any extracts from, the female plant. Alternative spellings are mariguana, marijuana. SEE ALSO cannabis. [fr. Sp. *Maria-Juana,* Mary-Jane]

Marinesco, Georges, Roumanian neurologist, 1863–1938. SEE M.'s succulent *hand;* M.-Garland *syndrome;* Marinesco-Sjögren *syndrome*.

mar·i·no·bu·fo·tox·in (mar′i-nō-bū′fō-toks-in). A poison produced by the parotid gland of *Bufo marinus* (family Bufonidae), a large toad native to Central and South America; used in tropical countries for insect control.

Marion, Georges, French urologist, 1869–1932. SEE M.'s *disease*.

Mariotte, Edmé, French physicist, 1620–1684. SEE M. *bottle;* M.'s *experiment, law,* blind *spot*.

mar·i·po·sia (mār-i-pō′zē-ǎ). Thallasoposia; rarely used term for abnormal consumption of sea water as a result of psychogenic factors. SYN thalassoposia. [L. *mare,* the sea, + G. *posis,* drinking]

Marjolin, Jean N., French physician, 1780–1850. SEE M.'s *ulcer*.

mar·jo·ram (mar′jō-ram). Sweet, leaf, or garden m. whose leaves, with and without a small portion of the flowering tops of *Majorana hortensis* (*Origanum majorana*) (family Labiatae), are used as seasoning and medicinally as a stimulant, carminative, and emmenagogue.

mark. 1. Any spot, line, or other figure on the cutaneous or mucocutaneous surface, visible through difference in color, elevation, or other peculiarity. 2. SYN infundibulum (8). [A.S. *mearc*]

alignment m., m.'s made in tracings while the kymograph or other recording apparatus is at rest in order to indicate the time relations between two tracings inscribed one above the other, *e.g.,* jugular and radial pulses.

dhobie m., SYN dhobie mark *dermatitis*.

port-wine m., SYN *nevus* flammeus.

strawberry m., SYN strawberry *nevus*.

stretch m.'s, SYN *striae* cutis distensae, under *stria*.

Unna's m., SYN nape *nevus*.

washerman's m., SYN dhobie mark *dermatitis*.

mark·er. 1. A device used to make a mark or to indicate measurement. 2. A characteristic or factor by which a cell or molecule can be recognized or identified. 3. A locus containing two or more alleles that, being harmless, are common and therefore yield high frequencies of heterozygotes which facilitate linkage *analysis*.

allotypic m., SYN allotype.

cell m., an identifying characteristic of a cell; *e.g.,* formation of rosettes with sheep erythrocytes as a m. of T lymphocytes, or the presence of surface immunoglobulin as a m. of B lymphocytes.

cell surface m., a surface protein, glycoprotein, or group of proteins that distinguish a cell or subset of cells from another defined subset of cells.

genetic m., SYN genetic *determinant*.

linkage m., a locus at which there is a high probability of heterozygotes (indispensible state for linkage analysis), but in itself perhaps of no clinical interest. SEE ALSO marker *locus*.

oncofetal m., a tumor m. produced by tumor tissue and by fetal tissue of the same type as the tumor, but not by normal adult tissue from which the tumor arises.

polymorphic genetic m.'s, inherited characteristics that occur within a given population as two or more traits.

time m., an instrument that marks the time, usually in seconds or fractions of seconds, on a kymograph record in physiologic experiments.

tumor m., a substance, released into the circulation by tumor tissue, whose detection in the serum indicates the presence and specific type of tumor.

Markov, Andrei, Russian mathematician, 1865–1922. SEE Markov *process*.

Marme's re·a·gent. See under reagent.

mar·mo·rat·ed (mar′mō-rā-ted). Denoting a condition in which the appearance of the skin is streaked like marble. SEE ALSO *cutis* marmorata. [L. *marmoratus,* marbled]

mar·mot. A woodchuck or groundhog; a hibernating rodent that

ma

marker of human T lymphocytes		
area	type of cell	marker
bone marrow	pre-T cells	TDT enzyme, T10
thymus	early thymus cells ↓	TDT, T10, T9, T11
	thymus cells ↓	T10, T11, T6, T4, T8
	mature thymocytes ↓ ↓	
	T-helper T-suppressor/ cells (T$_H$) cytotoxic cells (T$_{S/C}$)	T$_H$: T10, T11, T3, T4 T$_{S/C}$: T10, T11, T3, T8
peripheral blood, lymph nodes, spleen	T-helper T-suppressor/ cells (T$_H$) cytotoxic cells (T$_{S/C}$)	T$_H$: T11, T3, T4 T$_{S/C}$: T11, T3, T8

TDT, terminal desoxyribosyl transferase

tumor markers used in primary diagnoses	
type of tumor	marker
testicular carcinoma chorionic carcinoma	β-subunit of human choriogonadotropin (β-HCG) and α-1-fetoprotein (AFP)
multiple myeloma	immunoglobulins, Bence-Jones protein
neuroblastoma pheochromocytoma	catecholamines, vanillylmandelic acid, metanephrines
carcinoid primary liver-cell carcinoma	5-hydroxyindoleacetic acid α-1-fetoprotein
medullary thyroid gland carcinoma	calcitonin
malignant lymphoma, leukemia	surface antigens

may serve as reservoir host of plague bacillus in North America. [Fr. *marmotte*]

Maroteaux, Pierre, French medical geneticist, *1926. SEE M.-Lamy *syndrome.*

Marquis' re·a·gent. See under reagent.

mar·row (mar′ō). **1.** A highly cellular hematopoietic connective tissue filling the medullary cavities and spongy epiphyses of bones that becomes predominantly fatty with age, particularly in the long bones of the limbs. **2.** Any soft gelatinous or fatty material resembling the m. of bone. SEE ALSO medulla. [A.S. *mearh*]

bone m., the tissue filling the cavities of bones, having a stroma of reticular fibers and cells. SYN medulla ossium [NA].

red bone m., bone marrow in which the meshes contain the developmental stages of erythrocytes, leukocytes, and megakaryocytes. SYN medulla ossium rubra.

spinal m., SYN spinal *cord.*

yellow bone m., bone m. in which the meshes of the reticular network are filled with fat. SYN medulla ossium flava.

Marshall, Don, U.S. ophthalmologist, *1905. SEE M. *syndrome.*

Marshall, Eli K., U.S. pharmacologist, 1889–1966. SEE M.'s *method.*

Marshall, John, English anatomist, 1818–1891. SEE M.'s vestigial *fold,* oblique *vein.*

Marshall, Victor F., U.S. urologist, *1913. SEE M.-Marchetti-Krantz *operation.*

Mar·shal·la·gia mar·shalli (mar-sha-lā′jē-ă mar-shal′ī). One of the medium stomach worms of the nematode family Trichostrongylidae, found in the abomasum of sheep, goats, camels, and various wild ruminants.

marsh·mal·low root (marsh′mal-ō). SYN althea.

mar·su·pi·al (mar-sū′pē-ăl). **1.** A member of the order Marsupalia which includes such mammals as kangaroos, wombats, bandicoots, and opossums, the female of which has an abdominal pouch for carrying the young. **2.** Of or pertaining to marsupials. [L. *marsupium,* a pouch]

mar·su·pi·al·i·za·tion (mar-sū′pē-ăl-i-zā′shŭn). Exteriorization of a cyst or other such enclosed cavity by resecting the anterior wall and suturing the cut edges of the remaining wall to adjacent edges of the skin, thereby creating a pouch. [L. *marsupium,* pouch]

mar·su·pi·um (mar-sū′pē-ŭm). **1.** SYN scrotum. **2.** A pouch or sac; *e.g.,* in marsupials. [L. pouch]

Martegiani, J., 19th century Italian anatomist. SEE M.'s *area, funnel.*

Martin, August E., German gynecologist, 1847–1933. SEE M.'s *tube;* M.-Gruber *anastomosis.*

Martin, Henry A., U.S. surgeon, 1824–1884. SEE M.'s *bandage, disease.*

Martin, J.E. SEE Thayer-M. *medium.*

Martinotti, Giovanni, Italian physician, 1857–1928. SEE M.'s *cell.*

mar·ti·us yel·low (marsh′ē-ŭs) [C.I. 10315]. $C_{10}H_6N_2O_5$; 2,4-dinitro-α-naphthol; an acid dye used as a plasma stain in plant and animal histology, and as a light filter for photomicrography. [Karl A. *Martius,* Ger. chemist, *1920]

Martorell, Fernando Otzet, Spanish cardiologist, *1906. SEE M.'s *syndrome.*

Mar·y·land co·ma scale. SEE coma *scale.*

mas·chal·ad·e·ni·tis (mas′kăl-ad′ĕ-nī′tis). Obsolete term for inflammation of the axillary glands. [G. *maschalē,* axilla, + *adēn,* gland, + *-itis,* inflammation]

mas·cha·le (mas′kăl-ē). SYN axilla. [G.]

mas·chal·eph·i·dro·sis (mas′kăl-ef-i-drō′sis). Sweating in the axillae. [G. *maschalē,* axilla, + *ephidrōsis,* perspiration]

mas·chal·on·cus (mas-kăl-ong′kŭs). Obsolete term for a neoplasm in the axilla. [G. *maschalē,* axilla, + *onkos,* mass]

mas·chal·y·per·i·dro·sis (mas′kăl-i-per-i-drō′sis). Excessive sweating in the axillae. [G. *maschalē,* axilla, + *hyper,* over, + *hidrōs,* sweat]

mas·cu·line (mas′kyū-lin). Relating to or marked by the characteristics of the male sex or gender. SYN masculinus [NA], male (2). [L. *masculus,* male, fr. *mas,* male]

mas·cu·line pro·test. Adler's term to describe the movement of individuals from passive to active roles in a desire to escape from the feminine role.

mas·cu·lin·i·ty (mas-kyū-lin′i-tē). The qualities and characteristics of a male.

mas·cu·lin·i·za·tion (mas′kyū-lin-i-zā′shŭn). The condition marked by the attainment of male characteristics, such as facial hair, either physiologically as part of male maturation, or pathologically by individuals of either sex. [L. *masculus,* male]

mas·cu·li·nize (mas′kyū-li-nīz). To confer the qualities or characteristics peculiar to the male.

mas·cu·lin·o·vo·blas·to·ma (mas′kyū-lin-ō′vō-blas-tō′mă). Obsolete term for an ovarian neoplasm that causes varying degrees of masculinization, *e.g.,* distribution of hair, change in voice, hypertrophy of the clitoris; m. consists of cords or anastomosing columns of cells with vesicular nuclei and indistinct cytoplasm, and is usually well vascularized; m.'s are thought by some to be derived from rests of adrenal cortical tissue, and they are morphologically similar to certain types of arrhenoblastoma.

mas·cu·li·nus (mas-kyū-lī′nŭs) [NA]. SYN masculine, masculine. [L.]

Masini, Giulio, Italian physician, 1874–1937. SEE M.'s *sign.*

mask. 1. Any of a variety of disease states producing alteration or discoloration of the skin of the face. **2.** The expressionless appearance seen in certain diseases; *e.g.,* Parkinson's facies. **3.** A facial bandage. **4.** A shield designed to cover the mouth and nose for maintenance of antiseptic conditions. **5.** A device designed to cover the mouth and nose for administration of inhalation anesthetics, oxygen, or other gases.

ecchymotic m., a dusky discoloration of the head and neck occurring when the trunk has been subjected to sudden and extreme compression, as in traumatic asphyxia.

Hutchinson's m., the sensation experienced in tabetic neurosyphilis as if the face were covered with a m. or with cobwebs.

laryngeal m., a tubular oropharyngeal airway with an inflatable rim at the distal end that when inflated creates an airtight seal immediately above the larynx.

luetic m., a dirty brownish yellow pigmentation, blotchy in character, resembling that of chloasma, occurring on the forehead, temples, and sometimes the cheeks in patients with tertiary syphilis.

nonrebreathing m., a m. fitted with both an inhalation valve and an exhalation valve so that all exhaled gas is vented to the external atmosphere and inhaled gas comes only from a reservoir connected to the m.

m. of pregnancy, SYN melasma.

tropical m., SYN *chloasma* bronzinum.

masked (maskt). Concealed.

mask·ing. 1. The use of noise of any kind to interfere with the audibility of another sound. For any given intensity, low pitched tones have a greater m. effect than those of a high pitch. **2.** In audiology, the use of a noise applied to one ear while testing the hearing acuity of the other ear. **3.** The hiding of smaller rhythms in the brain wave record by larger and slower ones whose wave form they distort. **4.** In dentistry, an opaque covering used to camouflage the metal parts of a prosthesis. **5.** In radiography, superimposition of an altered positive image on the original negative to produce an enhanced copy photographically. SEE subtraction.

unsharp m., in radiography, superimposing a blurred negative of a radiograph to cancel large density differences, leaving fine detail more visible.

Maslow, Abraham H., U. S. psychologist, 1908–1970. SEE M.'s *hierarchy.*

mas·och·ism (mas′ō-kizm, maz′ō-). **1.** Passive algolagnia; a form of perversion, often sexual in nature, in which a person experiences pleasure in being abused, humiliated, or maltreated. Cf. sadism. **2.** A general orientation in life that personal suffering relieves guilt and leads to a reward. [Leopold von Sacher-*Masoch,* Austrian novelist, 1836–1895]

mas·och·ist (mas′ō-kist). The passive party in the practice of masochism.

Mason, Edward E., U.S. surgeon, *1920. SEE M. *operation.*

masque bil·i·aire (mask bil-ē-ār′). Obsolete term for periocular hyperpigmentation in middle-aged women, unrelated to any systemic disease. [Fr.]

MASS. Acronym for *m*itral valve prolapse, *a*ortic anomalies, *s*keletal changes, and *s*kin changes. SEE MASS *syndrome.*

mass (m). 1. A lump or aggregation of coherent material. **2.** In pharmacy, a soft solid preparation containing an active medicinal agent, of such consistency that it can be divided into small pieces and rolled into pills. **3.** One of the seven fundamental quantities in the SI system; its unit is the kilogram, defined as the m. of the international prototype of the kilogram, which is made of platinum-iridium and kept at the International Bureau of Weights and Measures. SYN massa [NA]. [L. *massa,* a dough-like mass]

apperceptive m., the already existing knowledge base in a similar or related area with which the new perceptual material is articulated.

filar m., SYN reticular *substance* (1).

injection m., colored solutions or suspensions injected into the vascular system to render vessels and their walls prominent; useful for gross preparations and for study under low magnification after clearing; most fluids contain warm gelatin and the coloring materials are carmine, Berlin blue, or carbon.

inner cell m., SYN embryoblast.

intermediate m., SYN interthalamic *adhesion.*

lateral m. of atlas, the thick lateral part of the atlas on each side that articulates above with the occipital condyle and below with the axis. SYN massa lateralis atlantis [NA].

lateral m. of ethmoid bone, SYN ethmoidal *labyrinth.*

molar m., SEE molecular *weight.*

molecular m., SYN molecular *weight.*

pilular m., the mixture of drug(s), excipients, diluents and binders with a suitable amount of liquid to form a plastic mass which can be rolled into a long rod and cut into the appropriate number of units for pills to be rolled from. SYN pill mass.

relative molecular m. (M_r), SYN molecular *weight.*

sclerotic cemental m., benign fibro-osseous jaw lesions of unknown etiology, occurring predominantly in middle-aged black females, which present as large painless radiopaque masses usually involving several quadrants of the jaw. SYN florid osseous dysplasia, cemental dysplasia.

tubular excretory m., the m. of functioning excretory tubules of the kidney determined from the excretion of iodopyracet, or other compounds processed in the kidney primarily by tubular secretion, when large doses are used.

mas·sa, gen. and pl. **mas·sae** (mas′ă, mas′sē) [NA]. SYN mass. [L.]

m. interme′dia, SYN interthalamic *adhesion.*

m. latera′lis atlan′tis [NA], SYN lateral *mass* of atlas.

mas·sage (mă-sahzh′). A method of manipulation of the body by rubbing, pinching, kneading, tapping, etc. SYN tripsis (2). [Fr. from G. *massō,* to knead]

cardiac m., SYN heart m.

closed chest m., rhythmic compression of the heart between sternum and spine by depressing the lower sternum backward with the heels of the hands, the patient lying supine. SYN external cardiac m.

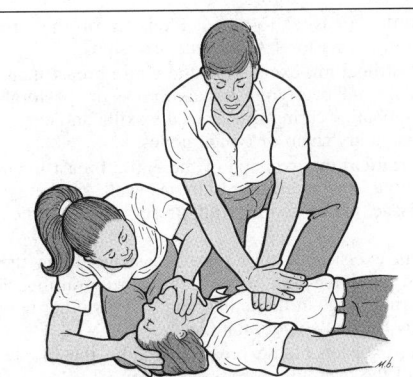

heart massage
with the heel of the right hand, push the breast bone 4 to 5 cm. toward the spine (for an adult); frequency should be 60 times per minute; after every 5 pushes a breath should be taken (by mouth-to-mouth resuscitation)

external cardiac m., SYN closed chest m.

gingival m., mechanical stimulation of the gingiva by rubbing or pressure.

heart m., rhythmic m. of the heart either in an open chest or through the chest wall to renew failed circulation during cardiac resuscitation. SYN cardiac m.

open chest m., rhythmic manual compression of the ventricles of the heart with the hand inside the thoracic cavity.

prostatic m., (1) manual expression of prostatic secretions by digital rectal technique; **(2)** the emptying of prostatic sini and ducts by repeated downward compression maneuvers, used in the treatment of various congestive and inflammatory prostatic conditions.

vibratory m., very rapid tapping of the surface effected by means of an instrument, usually with an elastic tip. SYN seismotherapy, sismotherapy, vibrotherapeutics.

Masselon, M. Julián, French physician, 1844–1917. SEE M.'s *spectacles.*

mas·se·ter. SEE masseter *muscle.*

mas·seur (mă-ser'). **1.** A man who massages. **2.** An instrument used in mechanical massage. [Fr. see *massage*]

mas·seuse (mă-sūz'). A woman who massages.

mas·si·cot (mas'i-kot). SYN *lead* monoxide.

Masson, C.L. Pierre, Canadian pathologist, 1880–1959. SEE M.'s *pseudoangiosarcoma;* M.-Fontana ammoniacal silver *stain.* See entries under stain.

mas·so·ther·a·py (mas-ō-thār'ă-pē). The therapeutic use of massage. [G. *massō,* to knead, + *therapeia,* treatment]

MAST Abbreviation for military antishock trousers.

△**mast-.** SEE masto-.

mast·ad·e·ni·tis (mast'ad-ĕ-nī'tis). SYN mastitis. [masto- + G. *adēn,* gland, + *-itis,* inflammation]

mast·ad·e·no·ma (mast'ad-ĕ-nō'mă). An adenoma of the breast. [masto- + G. *adēn,* gland, + *-ōma,* tumor]

Mast·ad·e·no·vi·rus (mast-ad'ĕ-nō-vī'rŭs). A genus of the family Adenoviridae, including adenoviruses that infect mammals, with over 40 antigenic types (species) being infective for humans. They cause respiratory infections in children, epidemic acute respiratory disease in military recruits, acute follicular conjunctivitis in adults, and epidemic keratoconjunctivitis; many infections are inapparent. [G. *mastos,* breast, hence mammal, + adenovirus]

mas·tal·gia (mas-tal'jē-ă). SYN mastodynia. [masto- + G. *algos,* pain]

mas·tat·ro·phy, mas·ta·tro·phia (mas-tat'rō-fē, mast-ă-trō'fē-ă). Atrophy or wasting of the breasts. [masto- + atrophy]

mas·tauxe (mas-tawk'sē). Hypertrophy of the breast. [masto- + G. *auxē,* increase]

mas·tec·to·my (mas-tek'tō-mē). Excision of the breast. SYN mammectomy. [masto- + G. *ektomē,* excision]

extended radical m., excision of the entire breast including the nipple, areola, and overlying skin, as well as the pectoral muscles and the lymphatic-bearing tissues of the axilla and chest wall and internal mammary chain of lymph nodes.

modified radical m., excision of the entire breast including the nipple, areola, and overlying skin, as well as the lymphatic-bearing tissue in the axilla with preservation of the pectoral muscles.

radical m., excision of the entire breast including the nipple, areola, and overlying skin, as well as the pectoral muscles, lymphatic-bearing tissue in the axilla, and various other neighboring tissues. SYN Halsted's operation (2).

simple m., excision of the breast including the nipple, areola, and most of the overlying skin. SYN total m.

subcutaneous m., excision of the breast tissues, but sparing the skin, nipple, and areola; usually followed by implantation of a prosthesis.

total m., SYN simple m.

Master, Arthur, U.S. physician, *1895. SEE M. *test;* M.'s two-step exercise *test.*

Masters, William H., U.S. gynecologist, *1915. SEE Allen-M. *syndrome.*

mas·tic (mas'tik). A resinous exudate from *Pistacia lentiscus* (family Anacardiaceae), a small tree of the Mediterranean shores; used in chewing gum, as an enteric coating, and as a

temporary filling material in dentistry. SYN mastich, mastiche. [G. *mastichē,* the resin of the mastich tree]

mas·ti·cate (mas'ti-kāt). To chew; to perform mastication.

mas·ti·ca·tion (mas-ti-kā'shŭn). The process of chewing food in preparation for deglutition and digestion; the act of grinding or comminuting with the teeth. [L. *mastico,* pp. *-atus,* to chew]

mas·ti·ca·to·ry (mas'ti-kă-tō-rē). Relating to mastication.

mas·tich, mas·ti·che (mas'tik, mas'ti-kē). SYN mastic.

Mas·ti·goph·o·ra (mas'ti-gof'ŏ-ră). The flagellates, a subphylum of Protozoa having one or more locomotory flagella, a single vesicular nucleus, and symmetric binary fission; sexual reproduction is unknown in many groups (*e.g., Volvox, Trypanosoma, Euglena*). It consists of two classes: Phytomastigophorea (to which *Euglena* belongs), which contains chlorophyll and is therefore photosynthetic and holophytic (although this has secondarily been lost in some groups), and Zoomastigophorea (including *Trypanosoma* and *Leishmania*), which lacks chromatophores and is heterotrophic. [G. *mastix* (*mastig-*), a whip, + *phoros,* bearing]

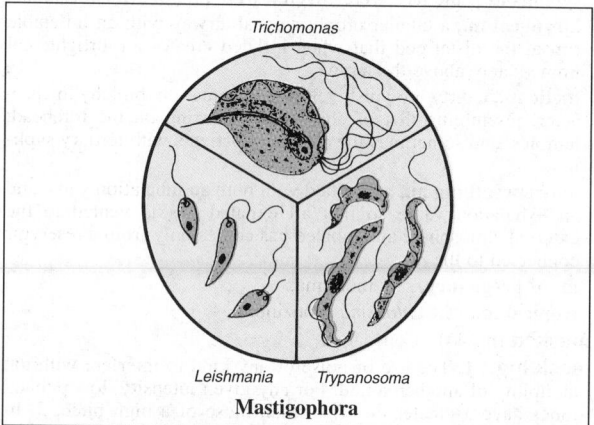

Trichomonas

Leishmania Trypanosoma

Mastigophora

mas·ti·gote (mas'ti-gōt). An individual flagellate. [G. *mastix,* a whip]

mas·ti·tis (mas-tī'tis). Inflammation of the breast. SYN mammitis, mastadenitis. [masto- + G. *-itis,* inflammation]

bovine m., a disease complex which occurs in acute, gangrenous, chronic, and subclinical forms of inflammation of the bovine udder, and is due to a variety of infectious agents; animal care, hygiene, and management are important factors in this dairy cow disease of great economic importance.

chronic cystic m., older term corresponding to fibrocystic *condition* of the breast.

gargantuan m., obsolete term for chronic inflammation of the breast with great enlargement of the gland.

glandular m., SYN parenchymatous m.

granulomatous m., a rare granulomatous inflammation of lobular breast tissue, with multinucleated giant cells; sarcoidosis is excluded by the frequent presence of neutrophils and absence of involvement of other tissues.

interstitial m., inflammation of the connective tissue of the mammary gland.

lactational m., SYN puerperal m.

m. neonator'um, m. in the secreting breast tissue of the newborn, usually staphylococcal.

ovine m., an acute inflammation of the sheep udder, usually gangrenous. SYN bluebag.

parenchymatous m., inflammation of the secreting tissue of the breast. SYN glandular m.

phlegmonous m., old term for abscess or cellulitis of the breast.

plasma cell m., a condition of the breasts characterized by tumorlike indurated masses containing numerous plasma cells, usually resulting from mammary duct ectasia; although clinically resembling malignant disease (attachment to skin and enlargement of axillary lymph nodes), it is not neoplastic.

puerperal m., m., usually suppurative, occurring in the later part of the puerperium. SYN lactational m.

retromammary m., SYN submammary m.

stagnation m., painful distention of the breast occurring during the latter days of pregnancy and the first days of lactation. SYN caked breast.

submammary m., inflammation of the tissues lying deep to the mammary gland. SYN retromammary m.

suppurative m., inflammation of the breast due to infection with pyogenic bacteria.

masto-, mast-. The breast; the mastoid. Cf. mammo-, mazo-. [G. *mastos*]

mas·toc·cip·i·tal (mast'ok-sip'-i-tǎl). SYN masto-occipital.

mas·to·cyte (mas'tō-sīt). SYN mast *cell*.

mas·to·cy·to·gen·e·sis (mas'tō-sī'tō-jen'ĕ-sis). Formation and development of mast cells. [mastocyte + G. *genesis* production]

mas·to·cy·to·ma (mas'tō-sī-tō'mǎ). A fairly well-circumscribed accumulation or nodular focus of mast cells, grossly resembling a neoplasm. [mastocyte + G. *-oma,* tumor]

mas·to·cy·to·sis (mas'tō-sī-tō'sis). Abnormal proliferation of mast cells in a variety of tissues; may be systemic, involving a variety of organs, or cutaneous (urticaria pigmentosa). [mastocyte + G. *-osis,* condition]

diffuse m., infiltration of many organ systems by mast cells with varied clinical manifestations that can include fever, weight loss, flushing, bronchospasm, rhinorrhea, palpitations, dyspnea, diarrhea, gastrointestinal bleeding, and hypotension. SYN systemic m.

diffuse cutaneous m., a benign process consisting of focal cutaneous infiltrates composed of mast cells; lesions are flat or slightly elevated, form wheals and itch when stroked; bone lesions may occur. SYN urticaria pigmentosa.

systemic m., SYN diffuse m.

mas·to·dyn·ia (mas-tō-din'ē-ǎ). Pain in the breast. SEE ALSO mammary *neuralgia.* SYN mammalgia, mastalgia, mazodynia. [masto- + G. *odynē,* pain]

mas·toid (mas'toyd). **1.** Resembling a mamma; breast-shaped. **2.** Relating to the m. process, antrum, cells, etc. SYN mastoidal. [masto- + G. *eidos,* resemblance]

mas·toi·dal (mas-toy'dǎl). SYN mastoid (2).

mas·toi·da·le (mas-toy-dā'lē). The lowest point on the contour of the mastoid process.

mas·toid·ec·to·my (mas'toy-dek'tō-mē). Hollowing out of the mastoid process by curretting, gouging, drilling, or otherwise removing the bony partitions forming the mastoid cells. [mastoid (process) + G. *ektomē,* excision]

radical m., an operation to exteriorize and join the mastoid air cells, the middle ear space, and the external meatus, often for extensive cholesteatoma. SYN tympanomeatomastoidectomy.

mas·toid·i·tis (mas-toy-dī'tis). Inflammation of any part of the mastoid process. SYN mastoid empyema.

Bezold's m., m. with perforation medially into the digastric groove and forming a deep neck abscess.

sclerosing m., a chronic m. in which the trabeculae are greatly thickened, almost or entirely obliterating the cells.

mas·ton·cus (mas-tong'kǔs). A tumor or swelling of the breasts. [masto- + G. *onkos,* mass]

mas·to·oc·cip·i·tal (mas'tō-ok-sip'i-tǎl). Relating to the mastoid portion of the temporal bone and to the occipital bone, denoting the suture uniting them. SYN mastoccipital.

mas·to·pa·ri·e·tal (mas'tō-pa-rī'ĕ-tǎl). Relating to the mastoid portion of the temporal bone and to the parietal bone, denoting the suture uniting them.

mas·top·a·thy (mas-top'ǎ-thē). Any disease of the breasts. SYN mazopathy (2), mazopathia. [masto- + G. *pathos,* suffering]

mas·to·pexy (mas'tō-pek-sē). Plastic surgery to affix sagging breasts in a more elevated and normal position, often with some improvement in shape. [masto- + G. *pēxis,* fixation]

mas·to·pla·sia (mas-tō-plā'zē-ǎ). Enlargement of the breast. [masto- + G. *plasis,* a molding]

mas·to·plas·ty (mas'tō-plas-tē). SYN mammaplasty. [masto- + G. *plastos,* formed]

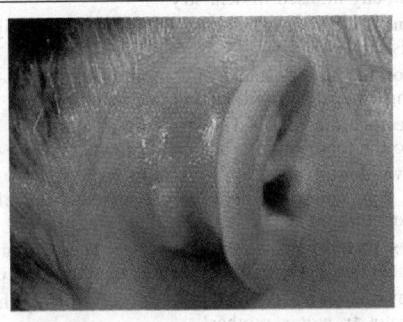

mastoiditis (ruptured retroauricular abscess)

mas·top·to·sis (mas-top-tō'sis). Ptosis or sagging of the breast. [masto- + G. *ptōsis,* a falling]

mas·tor·rha·gia (mas-tō-rā'jē-ǎ). Hemorrhage from a breast. [masto- + G. *rhēgnymi,* to burst forth]

mas·to·squa·mous (mas'tō-skwā'mǔs). Relating to the mastoid and the squamous portions of the temporal bone.

mas·to·syr·inx (mas'tō-sir'ingks). A fistula of the mammary gland. [masto- + G. *syrinx,* tube]

mas·tot·o·my (mas-tot'ō-mē). Incision of the breast. SYN mammotomy. [masto- + G. *tomē,* incision]

mas·tur·bate (mas'ter-bāt). To practice masturbation. [L. *masturbari,* pp. *masturbatus*]

mas·tur·ba·tion. Self-stimulation of the genitals for erotic pleasure, often resulting in orgasm.

false m., SYN peotillomania.

Masugi, Matazo, 20th century Japanese pathologist. SEE M.'s *nephritis.*

Matas, Rudolph, U.S. surgeon, 1860–1957. SEE M.'s *operation.*

match·ing. The process of making a study group and a comparison group in an epidemiological study comparable with respect to extraneous or confounding factors such as age, sex, weight, etc.

maté (mah-tā'). The dried leaves of *Ilex paraguayensis* and other species of *Ilex* (family Aquifoliaceae), shrubs growing in Paraguay and Brazil, which contain caffeine and tannin; used in South American countries as a beverage and medicinally as a diuretic and diaphoretic, and for the relief of headache. SYN Paraguay tea. [Sp. *maté,* a vessel in which the leaves are prepared]

mat·er (ma'ter). The "sheltering" coverings of the central nervous system. [L. mother]

ma·te·ria (mǎ-tē'rē-ǎ). Substance or matter. [L. substance]

m. al′ba, accumulation or aggregation of microorganisms, desquamated epithelial cells, blood cells and food debris loosely adherent to surfaces of plaques, teeth, gingiva or dental appliances. [L. white matter]

m. med′ica, (1) that aspect of medical science concerned with the origin and preparation of drugs, their doses, and their mode of administration; **(2)** any agent used therapeutically. SEE ALSO pharmacognosy, pharmacology. [L. medical matter]

ma·te·ri·al (mǎ-tēr'ē-ǎl). That of which something is made or composed; the constituent element of a substance. [L. *materialis,* fr. *materia,* substance]

base m., any substance from which a denture base may be made, such as shellac, acrylic resin, vulcanite, polystyrene, metal, etc.

by-product m., radioactive material produced by nuclear fission or by neutron irradiation in a nuclear reactor or similar device.

contrast m., SYN contrast *medium.*

cross-reacting m. (CRM), a substance sufficiently different from a reference substance (R) to have a perceptibly different function from R but sufficiently similar to R that it reacts with anti-R antibodies; *e.g.,* mutant factor VIII may be defective or even inert in coagulation and yet be immunologically identified as factor VIII.

ma

dental m., any m. used in dentistry.

genetic m., the carrier of hereditary information; in higher organisms it is duplex DNA.

impression m., any substance or combination of substances used for making a negative reproduction or impression.

plastic restoration m., in dentistry, any m. that may be shaped directly to the tooth cavity, such as amalgam, cement, or resin.

restorative dental m.'s, m.'s used to replace oral tissues in dentistry; *e.g.,* amalgam, gold alloys, cements, porcelain, plastics, and denture m.'s.

ma·te·ri·es mor·bi (mă-tē′rē-ēz mōr′bī). The substance acting as the immediate cause of a disease. [L. the matter of disease]

ma·ter·nal (mă-ter′năl). Relating to or derived from the mother. [L. *maternus,* fr. *mater,* mother]

ma·ter·ni·ty (mă-ter′ni-tē). Motherhood. [see maternal]

mat·ing (māt′ing). The pairing of male and female for the purpose of reproduction.

assortative m., selection of a mate with preference for (or aversion to) a particular genotype, *i.e.,* nonrandom m. SYN nonrandom m.

cross m., SEE cross.

nonrandom m., SYN assortative m.

random m., a practice of m. in a population in which at some specified locus m. patterns occur with expected frequencies predicted by the product of the frequencies of the genotypes in the population. SYN panmixis.

mat·rass (mat′răs). A long-necked glass vessel used for heating dry substances in chemical manipulations. [Fr. *matras*]

mat·ri·cal (mat′ri-kăl). Relating to any matrix. SYN matricial.

mat·ri·ca·ria (mat-ri-kā′rē-ă). The flowers of *Matricaria chamomilla* (family Compositae); used internally as a tonic and externally as a counterirritant. SEE ALSO chamomile. [L. *matrix,* womb]

ma·tri·ces (mā′tri-sēz, mat′rĭ-sēz). Plural of matrix. [L.]

ma·tri·cial (mă-trish′ăl). SYN matrical.

mat·ri·cide (mat′ri-sīd). **1.** The killing of one's mother. Cf. patricide. **2.** One who commits such an act. [L. *mater,* mother, + *caedo,* to kill]

mat·ri·lin·e·al (mat-ri-lin′ē-ăl). Denoting descent through the female line. [L. *mater,* mother, + *linea,* line]

ma·trix, pl. **ma·tri·ces** (mā′triks, mat′riks; mā′tri-sēz, mat′ri-sēz). **1** [NA]. The formative portion of a tooth or a nail. **2.** The intercellular substance of a tissue. **3.** A surrounding substance within which something is contained or embedded, *e.g.,* the fatty tissue in which blood vessels or lymph nodes lie; provides a matrix for these embedded structures. **4.** A mold in which anything is cast or swaged; a counterdie; a specially shaped instrument, plastic material, or metal strip used for holding and shaping the material used in filling a tooth cavity. **5.** A rectangular array of numbers or symbol quantities that simplify the execution of linear operations of tedious complexity, *e.g.,* the ITO method; the theory of matrices is widely used in solving simultaneous equations and in population genetics. [L. womb; female breeding animal]

amalgam m., a device used during placement of the amalgam mass within a compound cavity preparation, facilitating proper condensation and contour thereof by providing a confining wall.

bone m., the intercellular substance of bone tissue consisting of collagen fibers, ground substance, and inorganic bone salts.

cartilage m., the intercellular substance of cartilage consisting of fibers and ground substance.

cell m., SYN cytoplasmic m.

cytoplasmic m., a fluid cytoplasmic substance filling the interstices of the cytoskeleton. SYN cell m., cytomatrix.

external m., the substance occupying the space between the inner and outer membrane of any organelle (*e.g.,* mitochondria) with a double membrane.

identity m., a square m. in which the quantities on the diagonal from top left to bottom right are all equal to 1 and all the other entries are 0.

mitochondrial m., SYN m. mitochondrialis.

m. mitochondria′lis, the substance occupying the space enclosed by the inner membrane of a mitochondrion; it contains enzymes, filaments of DNA, ribosomes, granules, and inclusions of protein crystals, glycogen, and lipid. SYN mitochondrial m.

nail m., SYN nail *bed*.

nuclear m., the network of protein fibers both around the outside of the nucleus as well as inside the nucleus.

square m., a m. in which the numbers of rows and columns are equal.

territorial m., SYN cartilage *capsule*.

m. un′guis [NA], SYN nail *bed*.

mat·ter. SYN substance. SEE ALSO substance. [L. *materies,* substance]

gray m., those regions of the brain and spinal cord which are made up primarily of the cell bodies and dendrites of nerve cells rather than myelinated axons. SYN substantia grisea [NA], gray substance, substantia cinerea.

pontine gray m., SYN pontine *nuclei,* under *nucleus*.

white m., those regions of the brain and spinal cord that are largely or entirely composed of nerve fibers and contain few or no neuronal cell bodies or dendrites. SYN substantia alba [NA], alba, white substance.

mat·u·rate (mat′yū-rāt). To suppurate. [L. *maturo,* pp. *-atus,* to make ripe, fr. *maturus,* ripe]

mat·u·ra·tion (mat-yū-rā′shŭn). **1.** Achievement of full development or growth. **2.** Developmental changes that lead to maturity. **3.** Processing of a macromolecule; *e.g.,* posttranscriptional modification of RNA or posttranslational modification of proteins. [L. *maturatio,* a ripening, fr. *maturus,* ripe]

ma·ture (mă-chūr′, -tūr). **1.** Ripe; fully developed. **2.** To ripen; to become fully developed. [L. *maturus,* ripe]

ma·tu·ri·ty (mă-chūr′i-tē). A state of full development or completed growth.

Mauchart (Mauchard), Burkhard D., German anatomist, 1696–1751. SEE M.'s *ligaments,* under *ligament*.

Maurer, Georg, German physician in Sumatra, *1909. SEE M.'s *clefts,* under *cleft, dots,* under *dot*.

Mauriac, Pierre, French physician, *1882. SEE M.'s *syndrome*.

Mauriceau, François, French obstetrician, 1637–1709. SEE M.'s *maneuver;* M.-Levret *maneuver*.

Mauthner, Ludwig, Austrian ophthalmologist, 1840–1894. SEE M.'s *cell, sheath, test*.

max·il·la, gen. and pl. **max·il·lae** (mak-sil′ă, mak-sil′ē) [NA]. An irregularly shaped bone, supporting the superior teeth and taking part in the formation of the orbit, hard palate, and nasal cavity. SYN upper jaw bone, upper jaw. [L. jawbone]

max·il·lary (mak′si-lār-ē). Relating to the maxilla, or upper jaw.

max·il·lec·to·my (mak-sil-ek′tō-mē). Resection of the maxilla. [maxilla + G. *ektomē,* excision]

max·il·li·tis (mak′si-lī′tis). Inflammation of the maxilla.

max·il·lo·den·tal (mak-sil′ō-den′tăl). Relating to the upper jaw and its associated teeth.

max·il·lo·fa·cial (mak-sil′ō-fā′shăl). Pertaining to the jaws and face, particularly with reference to specialized surgery of this region.

max·il·lo·ju·gal (mak-sil′ō-jū′găl). Relating to the maxilla and the zygomatic bone.

max·il·lo·man·dib·u·lar (mak-sil′ō-man-dib′yū-lăr). Relating to the upper and lower jaws.

max·il·lo·pal·a·tine (mak-sil′ō-pal′ă-tīn). Relating to the maxilla and the palatine bone.

max·il·lot·o·my (mak-si-lot′ō-mē). Surgical sectioning of the maxilla to allow movement of all or a part of the maxilla into the desired portion. [maxilla + G. *tomē,* incision]

max·il·lo·tur·bi·nal (mak-sil′lō-ter′bi-năl). Relating to the inferior nasal concha.

Maximow, Alexander A., Russian physician in U.S., 1874–1928. SEE M.'s *stain* for bone marrow.

max·i·mum (mak′si-mŭm). The greatest amount, value, or degree attained or attainable. [L. neuter of *maximus,* greatest]

glucose transport m., the maximal rate of reabsorption of glucose from the glomerular filtrate; it amounts to approximately 320 mg/min in humans.

transport m. (Tm), the maximal rate of secretion or reabsorption of a substance by the renal tubules. SYN tubular m.

tubular m. (Tm), SYN transport m.

May, Richard, German physician. SEE M.-Hegglin *anomaly.*

May ap·ple. SYN podophyllum.

Mayer, Karl, Austrian neurologist, 1862–1932. SEE M.'s *reflex.*

Mayer, Karl, W., German gynecologist, 1795–1868. SEE M.'s *pessary.*

Mayer, Paul, German histologist, 1848–1923. SEE M.'s hemalum *stain,* mucicarmine *stain,* mucihematein *stain.*

Mayer-Rokitansky-Küster-Hauser syn·drome. See under syndrome.

May-Grünwald stain. See under stain.

may·id·ism (mā′id-izm). SYN pellagra. [*Zea mays,* maize]

Mayo, Charles H., U.S. surgeon, 1865–1939. SEE M. *bunionectomy.*

Mayo, William J., U.S. surgeon, 1861–1939. SEE M.'s *operation, vein.*

Mayo-Robson, Sir Arthur W., British surgeon, 1853–1933. SEE Mayo-Robson's *point;* Mayo-Robson's *position.*

Mayou, Marmaduke Stephen, British ophthalmologist, 1876–1934. SEE Batten-M. *disease.*

ma·za·mor·ra (maz-ă-mōr′ă). Name given in Puerto Rico to a dermatitis caused by penetration of the skin by hookworm larvae.

maze (māz). A labyrinth; frequently used to study higher functions of the nervous system in rats. [M.E. *masen,* to confuse]

ma·zin·dol (mā′zin-dol). An isoindole anorexiant that is distinctive in not having the phenethylamine chain common to sympathomimetic amines.

mazo-. The breast. SEE ALSO masto-. [G. *mazos*]

ma·zo·dyn·ia (mā-zō-din′ē-ă). SYN mastodynia. [mazo- + G. *odynē,* pain]

ma·zol·y·sis (mā-zol′i-sis). Detachment of the placenta. [G. *maza,* placenta, + *lysis,* a loosening]

ma·zop·a·thy, ma·zo·path·ia (mā-zop′ă-thē, mā-zō-path′ē-ă). 1. Any disease of the placenta. [G. *maza,* a barley cake (placenta), + *pathos,* suffering] 2. SYN mastopathy. [G. *mazos,* breast]

ma·zo·pexy (mā′zō-pek-sē). Obsolete term for mastopexy. [mazo- + G. *pēxis,* fixation]

ma·zo·pla·sia (mā-zō-plā′zē-ă). Old term for mastoplasia. [mazo- + G. *plasia,* a moulding]

Mazzoni, Vittorio, Italian physician, 1880–1940. SEE M. *corpuscle;* Golgi-M. *corpuscle.*

Mazzotti, Luigi, Mexican physician specializing in tropical medicine in mid-20th century. SEE Mazzotti *reaction,* Mazzotti *test.*

Mb, MbCO, MbO₂ Symbols for myoglobin and its combinations with CO and O₂.

MBC Abbreviation for maximum breathing *capacity.*

M.C. Abbreviation for *Magister Chirurgiae,* Master of Surgery; Medical Corps.

mc Former abbreviation for millicurie.

McArdle, Brian, 20th century British neurologist. SEE McA.'s *disease;* McA.-Schmid-Pearson *disease;* McA.'s *syndrome.*

McBurney, Charles, U.S. surgeon, 1845–1913. SEE McB.'s *incision, point, sign.*

McCarthy, Daniel J., U.S. neurologist, 1874–1958. SEE McC.'s *reflexes,* under *reflex.*

McCrea, Lowrain E., U.S. urologist, *1896. SEE McC. *sound.*

McCune, Donovan James, U.S. pediatrician, 1902–1976. SEE M.-Albright *syndrome.*

McDonald, Ellice, U.S. gynecologist, 1876–1955. SEE McD.'s *maneuver.*

McGoon, Dwight C., U.S. surgeon, *1925. SEE McG.'s *technique.*

MCH Abbreviation for mean corpuscular *hemoglobin.*

M.Ch. Abbreviation for *Magister Chirurgiae,* Master of Surgery.

MCHC Abbreviation for mean corpuscular hemoglobin *concentration.*

mCi Abbreviation for millicurie.

McKee, George Kenneth, British orthopedic surgeon, *1930. SEE McK.'s *line.*

McLean, Malcolm, U.S. obstetrician, 1848–1924. SEE Tucker-McL. *forceps.*

MCMI Abbreviation for Millon clinical multiaxial *inventory.*

McMurray, Thomas P., British surgeon, *1889. SEE McM. *test.*

m-cone. Middle wavelength sensitive c. (green c.).

MCP-1 Abbreviation for monocyte chemoattractant *protein*-1.

McPhail, M.K., Canadian physiologist, *1907. SEE McP. *test.*

MCR Abbreviation for steroid metabolic clearance *rate.*

McReynolds, John O., U.S. ophthalmologist, 1865–1942.

M-CSF Abbreviation for macrophage colony-stimulating *factor.*

MCV Abbreviation for mean corpuscular *volume.*

McVay, Chester B., U.S. surgeon, *1911. SEE McV.'s *operation.*

MD Abbreviation for methyldichloroarsine.

M.D. Abbreviation of *Medicinae Doctor,* Doctor of Medicine.

Md Symbol for mendelevium.

MDF Abbreviation for myocardial depressant *factor.*

m. dict. Abbreviation for [L] *more dicto,* as directed.

MDMA A centrally active phenethylamine derivative related to amphetamine and methamphetamine, with central nervous system excitant and hallucinogenic properties. SYN 3,4-methylenedioxymethamphetamine.

M'Dowel, Benjamin G., Irish anatomist, 1829–1885. SEE *frenulum* of M.

M.D.S. Abbreviation of Master of Dental Surgery.

Me Symbol for methyl.

Meadows, William Robert, U.S. cardiologist, *1919. SEE M.'s *syndrome.*

meal (mēl). 1. The food consumed at regular intervals or at a specified time. 2. Ground flour from a grain.

Boyden m., a m. consisting of three or four egg yolks, beaten up in milk and seasoned with sugar, port wine, etc., used to test the evacuation time of the gallbladder; two-thirds to three-quarters of the contents will be normally evacuated within 40 minutes.

test m., (1) toast and tea, or crackers and tea, or gruel or other bland food, given to stimulate gastric secretion before withdrawing gastric contents for analysis; (2) administration of food containing a substance thought to be responsible for symptoms, such as an allergic reaction.

mean (mēn). A statistical measurement of central tendency or average of a set of values, usually assumed to be the arithmetic m. unless otherwise specified. [M.E., *mene* fr. O.Fr., fr. L. *medianus,* in the middle]

arithmetic m., the m. calculated by adding a set of values and then dividing the sum by the number of values.

geometric m., the m. calculated as the antilogarithm of the arithmetic mean of the logarithms of the individual values; it can also be calculated as the *n*th root of the product of *n* values.

harmonic m., the m. calculated as the number of values being averaged, divided by the sum of their reciprocals.

regression of the m., if, for a symmetrical population with a single mode, a measurement, selected because it is extreme, is repeated, on average the second reading will be closer to the m. than the first.

standard error of the m. (SEM), a statistical index of the probability that a given sample m. is representative of the m. of the population from which the sample was drawn.

mea·sle (mē′zl). 1. The larva (*Cysticercus cellulosae*) of *Taenia* *solium,* the pork tapeworm. **2.** The larva (*Cysticercus bovis*) of *Taenia saginata,* the beef tapeworm.

mea·sles (mē'zlz). **1.** An acute exanthematous disease, caused by m. virus, a member of the family Paramyxoviridae, and marked by fever and other constitutional disturbances, a catarrhal inflammation of the respiratory mucous membranes, and a generalized maculopapular eruption of a dusky red color; the eruption occurs early on the buccal mucous membrane in the form of Koplik's *spots,* under *spot,* a manifestation utilized in early diagnosis; average incubation period is from 10 to 12 days. SYN morbilli. **2.** A disease of swine caused by the presence of *Cysticercus cellulosae,* the measle or larva of *Taenia solium,* the pork tapeworm. **3.** A disease of cattle caused by the presence of *Cysticercus bovis,* the measle or larva of *Taenia saginata,* the beef tapeworm of man. [D. *maselen*]

atypical m., sometimes severe, unusual clinical manifestation of natural m. virus infection in persons with waning vaccination immunity, particularly in those who had received formaldehyde-inactivated vaccine; an accelerated allergic reaction apparently resulting from an anamnestic antibody response, characterized by high fever, absence of Koplik's spots, a shortened prodromal period, atypical rash, and pneumonia.

black m., (1) SYN hemorrhagic m. **(2)** SYN Rocky Mountain spotted *fever.*

German m., SYN rubella.

hemorrhagic m., a severe form in which the eruption is dark in color due to effusion of blood into affected areas of the skin. SYN black m. (1).

three-day m., SYN rubella.

tropical m., a disease of uncertain character, somewhat resembling rubella, occurring in southern China.

mea·sly (mēz'lē). Pertaining to pork or beef infected with the cysticerci of the tapeworms *Taenia solium* or *Taenia saginata,* respectively.

mea·sure (mezh'er). **1.** To determine the magnitude or quantity of a substance by comparing it to some accepted standard or by calculation. **2.** A specified magnitude of a physical quantity. **3.** A graduated instrument used to measure an object or substance. [O.F. *mesure,* fr. L. *mensura,* fr. *metior,* to measure]

mea·sure·ment (mezh'ŭr-ment). Determination of a dimension or quantity.

end-point m., analytical m. at the end of a chemical reaction, as opposed to making the m. while the reaction proceeds.

kinetic m., continuous or frequent monitoring of the readings in a chemical reaction to determine its rate.

nasion-pogonion m., SYN facial *plane.*

mea·sures of cen·tral ten·den·cy. General term for several characteristics of the distribution of a set of measurements or values around a value or values at or near the middle of the set; the principal measures of central tendency are mean, median, and mode.

me·a·tal (mē-ā'tăl). Relating to a meatus.

△**meato-.** Meatus. [L. *meatus,* passage]

me·a·tom·e·ter (mē-ă-tom'ĕ-ter). An instrument for measuring the size of a meatus, especially the meatus of the urethra. [meato- + G. *metron,* measure]

me·a·to·plas·ty (mē'ă-tō-plas-tē). Plastic surgery of a meatus or canal, *e.g.,* the external auditory meatus or the urethral meatus.

me·a·tor·rha·phy (mē-ă-tōr'ă-fē). Closing by suture of the wound made by performing a meatomy. [meato- + G. *rhaphē,* suture]

me·at·o·scope (mē-at'ō-skōp). A form of speculum for examining a meatus, especially the meatus of the urethra. [meato- + G. *skopeō,* to view]

me·a·tos·co·py (mē-ă-tos'kŏ-pē). Inspection, usually instrumental, of any meatus, especially of the meatus of the urethra. [meato- + G. *skopeō,* to view]

me·at·o·tome (mē-at'ō-tōm). A knife with short cutting edge for use in meatotomy.

me·a·tot·o·my (mē-ă-tot'ō-mē). An incision made to enlarge a meatus, *e.g.,* of the urethra or ureter. [meato- + G. *tomē,* incision]

me·a·tus, pl. **me·a·tus** (mē-ā'tŭs) [NA]. A passage or channel,

especially the external opening of a canal. [L. a going, a passage, fr. *meo,* pp. *meatus,* to go, pass]

acoustic m., SYN external acoustic m.

m. acus'ticus exter'nus [NA], SYN external acoustic m.

m. acus'ticus inter'nus [NA], SYN internal acoustic m.

external acoustic m., the passage leading inward through the tympanic portion of the temporal bone, from the auricle to the tympanic membrane; it consists of a bony (inner) portion and a fibrocartilaginous (outer) portion, the cartilaginous external acoustic meatus. SYN m. acusticus externus [NA], acoustic m., antrum auris, auditory canal, external auditory m.

external auditory m., SYN external acoustic m.

fish-mouth m., a red and swollen condition of the orifice of the urethra (urinary m.) in gonorrhea.

internal acoustic m., a canal running from the opening of the internal acoustic meatus, through the petrous portion of the temporal bone, ending at the fundus where a thin plate of bone separates it from the vestibule; it gives passage to the facial and vestibulocochlear nerves together with the labyrinthine artery and veins. SYN m. acusticus internus [NA], internal auditory m.

internal auditory m., SYN internal acoustic m.

nasal m., any of three passages in the nasal cavity formed by the projection of the conchae: middle nasal m., lies below the inferior concha; middle nasal m., lies between the middle and inferior conchae; superior nasal m., lies between the superior and middle conchae. SYN m. nasi [NA].

m. na'si [NA], SYN nasal m.

m. nasopharyn'geus [NA], SYN nasopharyngeal *passage.*

ureteral m., SYN ureteric *orifice.*

m. urina'rius, SYN external urethral *orifice.*

me·ban·a·zine (mē-ban'ă-zēn). (1-Phenylethyl)methylbenzyl)-hydrazine; an antidepressant with inhibitory effect on monoamine oxidase.

me·ben·da·zole (mē-ben'dă-zōl). Methyl 5-benzoylbenzimidazole-2-carbamate; an effective broad-spectrum nematicidal agent against intestinal nematodes such as pinworm, hookworm, whipworm, and *Ascaris.*

me·bev·er·ine hy·dro·chlo·ride (mě-bev'er-ēn). 4-[Ethyl(*p*-methoxy-α-methylphenethyl)amino] butyl veratrate hydrochloride; an intestinal antispasmodic.

meb·hy·dro·line (meb-hī'drō-lēn). 5-Benzyl-2,3,4,5-tetrahydro-2-methyl-1*H*-pyrido[4,3-*b*]indole; an antihistaminic.

me·bro·phen·hy·dra·mine (mě-brō-fen-hī'dră-mēn). 2-(*p*-Bromo-α-methyl-α-phenylbenzyloxy)-*N,N*-dimethylethylamine; an antihistaminic.

me·but·a·mate (mě-byū'tă-māt). Carbamic acid 2-*sec*-butyl-2-methyltrimethylene ester; chemically, it differs only slightly from meprobamate, and possesses similar CNS-depressant properties.

mec·a·myl·a·mine hy·dro·chlo·ride (mek'ă-mil'ă-mēn). 3-Methylaminoisocamphane hydrochloride; a secondary amine that blocks transmission of impulses at autonomic ganglia (similar to but more effective than hexamethonium); used in the management of severe hypertension.

me·chan·i·cal (mě-kan'i-kăl). **1.** Performed by means of some apparatus, not manually. **2.** Explaining phenomena in terms of mechanics. **3.** Automatic. [G. *meckanikos,* relating to a machine, fr. *mēchanē,* a contrivance, machine]

me·chan·i·co·re·cep·tor (mě-kan'i-kō-rē-sep'ter, tōr). SYN mechanoreceptor.

me·chan·ics (mě-kan'iks). The science of the action of forces in promoting motion or equilibrium. [see mechanical]

body m., the study of the action of muscles in producing motion or posture of the body.

mech·a·nism (mek'ă-nizm). **1.** An arrangement or grouping of the parts of anything that has a definite action. **2.** The means by which an effect is obtained. [G. *mēchanē,* a contrivance]

association m., the cerebral m. whereby the memory of past sensations may be compared or associated with present ones.

counter-current m., a system in the renal medulla that facilitates concentration of the urine as it passes through the renal tubules. SEE countercurrent exchanger, countercurrent multiplier.

defense m., (1) a psychological means of coping with conflict or anxiety, *e.g.,* conversion, denial, dissociation, rationalization, repression, sublimation; **(2)** the psychic structure underlying a coping strategy; **(3)** immunological m. vs. non-specific defense m.

double displacement m., SYN ping-pong m.

Douglas m., m. of spontaneous evolution in transverse lie; extreme lateral flexion of the vertebral column with birth of the lateral aspect of thorax before the buttocks.

Duncan's m., passage of the placenta from the uterus with the rough side foremost.

gating m., (1) occurrence of the maximum refractory period among cardiac conducting cells approximately 2 mm proximal to the terminal Purkinje fibers in the ventricular muscle, beyond which the refractory period is shortened through a sequence of Purkinje cells, transitional cells, and muscular cells; gating m. may be a cause of ventricular aberration, bidirectional tachycardia, and concealed extrasystoles; **(2)** a m. by which painful impulses may be blocked from entering the spinal cord. Cf. gate-control *theory.*

immunological m., the groups of cells (chiefly lymphocytes and cells of the reticuloendothelial system) that function in establishing active acquired immunity (induced sensitivity, allergy).

ordered m., a scheme for substrate binding and product release for multisubstrate enzymes; for a two-substrate two-product enzyme with an ordered m., one particular substrate has to bind to the enzyme first followed by the other substrate; chemistry then occurs, products are formed and are released from the enzyme in a distinct order. More complex ordered schemes exist for enzymes having more than two substrates. Some of the dehydrogenases have such a m. SYN ordered.

ordered on-random off m., a scheme for substrate binding and product release for multisubstrate enzymes; for a two-substrate two-product enzyme with this m., the individuals have to bind to the enzyme in a distinct order; however, once the products are formed they may dissociate from the enzyme in either order. It has been suggested that pyruvate kinase has such a mechanism. The random on-ordered off m. is simply the reverse of this m.

ping-pong m., a special multisubstrate reaction in which, for a two-substrate, two-product (*i.e.,* bi-bi) system, an enzyme reacts with one substrate to form a product and a modified enzyme, the latter then reacting with a second substrate to form a second, final product, and regenerating the original enzyme. An example of such a m. is found in the aminotransferases. More complex ping-pong m.'s exist for enzymes having more than two substrates. SYN double displacement m.

pressoreceptive m., the pressoreceptor system, especially of the carotid sinuses and aortic arch.

proprioceptive m., the m. of sense of position and movement, by which muscular movements can be adjusted to a great degree of accuracy and equilibrium maintained.

random m., a scheme for substrate binding and product release for a multisubstrate enzyme; for a two-substrate two-product enzyme with this m., either substrate can bind first and, after the reaction has taken place, either product can be the first to dissociate from the enzyme. Brain hexokinase has a random m. More complex random m.'s exist for enzymes having more than two substrates.

re-entrant m., the probable basis of most arrhythmias, requiring at least three criteria in the heart: 1. a loop circuit, 2. unidirectional block, 3. slowed conduction. Impulses enter the loop circuit and divide in both directions (blocked in one direction only), negotiate the loop circuit to the area of block where the slowed conduction has allowed the impulse to arrive at a time when the tissue proximal to the unidirectional block has recovered and will permit its passage in the opposite direction.

Schultze's m., expulsion of the placenta with the fetal surface foremost.

mech·a·no·car·di·og·ra·phy (mek′ă-nō-kar-dē-og′ră-fē). Use of graphic tracings reflecting the mechanical effects of the heartbeat, such as the carotid pulse tracing or apexcardiogram; phonocardiography is also usually considered a form of m.

mech·a·no·cyte (mek′ă-nō-sīt). An *in vitro* tissue culture fibroblast.

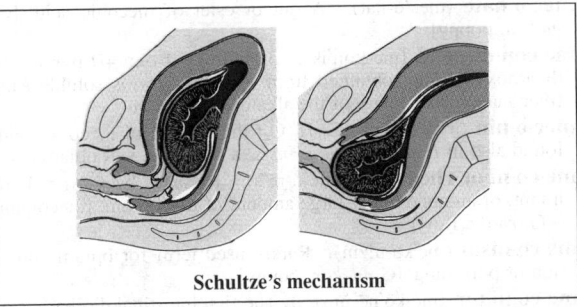

Schultze's mechanism

mech·a·no·pho·bia (mek′ă-nō-fō′bē-ă). Morbid fear of machinery. [G. *mēchanē,* machine, + *phobos,* fear]

mech·a·no·re·cep·tor (mek′ă-nō-rē-sep′tŏr). A receptor which responds to mechanical pressure or distortion; *e.g.,* receptors in the carotid sinuses, touch receptors in the skin. SYN mechanicoreceptor.

mech·a·no·re·flex (mek′ă-nō-rē′fleks). A reflex triggered by stimulation of a mechanoreceptor.

mech·a·no·ther·a·py (mek′ă-nō-thār′ă-pē). Treatment of disease by means of apparatus or mechanical appliances of any kind. [G. *mēchanē,* machine, + *therapeia,* treatment]

mèche (māsh). A strip of gauze or other material used as a tent or drain. [Fr. wick]

mech·lor·eth·a·mine hy·dro·chlo·ride (mek′lōr-eth′ă-mēn). 2,2′-Dichloro-*N*-methyldiethylamine hydrochloride; methyl-bis(β-chloroethyl)amine hydrochloride; nitrogen mustard hydrochloride; it is cytotoxic for all cells, but with a special affinity for bone marrow, lymphatic tissues, and rapidly proliferating cells of certain neoplasms. Used for the palliative treatment of Hodgkin's disease, lymphosarcoma, and certain chronic leukemias. SYN mustine hydrochloride.

me·cil·li·nam (me-sil′i-nam). SYN amdinocillin.

me·cism (mē′sizm). Abnormal elongation of the body or one or more of its parts. [G. *mēkos,* length, *-ismos,* condition]

Me·cis·to·cir·rus (mē-sis-tō-sir′ŭs). A monotypic genus of trichostrongylid nematodes (subfamily Mecistocirrinae), with the single species, *M. digitatus;* it is not grossly distinguished from *Haemonchus contortus* and has about the same effect on the host. *M.* is distributed chiefly in Asia in cattle, sheep, buffalo, bison, the stomach of pigs, and occasionally in humans. [G. *mēkistos,* very long, + L. *cirrus,* curl, the protruding male organ of a nematode]

Meckel, Johann F., the elder, German anatomist and obstetrician, 1714–1774. SEE M.'s *band, cavity, ganglion, ligament, space.*

Meckel, Johann F., the younger, German comparative anatomist and embryologist, 1781–1833. SEE M. *scan, syndrome;* M.'s *cartilage, diverticulum, plane;* M.-Gruber *syndrome.*

Mecke's re·a·gent. See under reagent.

me·clas·tine (mĕ-klas′tēn). SYN clemastine.

mec·li·zine hy·dro·chlo·ride (mek′li-zēn). 1-(*p*-Chlorobenzhydryl)-4-(*m*-methylbenzyl)piperazine dihydrochloride; an antihistaminic useful in the prevention and relief of motion sickness and symptoms caused by vestibular disorders. SYN meclozine hydrochloride.

mec·lo·fen·a·mate so·di·um (mek-lō-fen′ă-māt). Monosodium *N*-(2,6-dichloro-*m*-tolyl)anthranilate monohydrate; a nonsteroidal anti-inflammatory agent with analgesic and antipyretic actions.

mec·lo·fen·a·mic ac·id (mĕ-klō-fen-am′ik). An NSAID used for inflammatory conditions and dysmenorrhea; also antipyretic.

mec·lo·fen·ox·ate (mek′lō-fen-ok′sāt). 2-(Dimethylamino)ethyl (4-chlorophenoxy)acetate; an analeptic.

mec·lo·zine hy·dro·chlo·ride (mek′lō-zēn). SYN meclizine hydrochloride.

me·com·e·ter (mē-kom′ĕ-ter). An instrument, such as calipers with a scale attachment, for measurement of newborn infants. [G. *mēkos,* length, + *metron,* measure]

me

mec·o·nate (mek'ŏ-nāt). A salt or ester of meconic acid. [G. *mēkōn*, poppy]

me·con·ic ac·id (me-kon'ik). 3-Hydroxy-4-oxy-4*H*-pyran-2,6-dicarboxylic acid; obtained from opium; it forms soluble salts (meconates) with many of the alkaloids of opium.

mec·o·nin (mek'ŏ-nin). $C_{10}H_{10}O_4$; the lactone of meconic acid, found also in *Hydrastis canadensis*; a hypnotic. SYN opianyl.

me·co·ni·or·rhea (mē-kō'nē-ō-rē'ă). Passage, by the newborn infant, of an abnormally large amount of meconium. [meconium + G. *rhoia*, flow]

me·co·nism (mē'kō-nizm). Rarely used term for opium addiction or poisoning. [G. *mēkōn*, poppy]

me·co·ni·um (mē-kō'nē-ŭm). 1. The first intestinal discharges of the newborn infant, greenish in color and consisting of epithelial cells, mucus, and bile. 2. SYN opium. [L., fr. G. *mēkōnion*, dim. of *mēkōn*, poppy]

me·daz·e·pam hy·dro·chlo·ride (me-daz'ě-pam). 7-Chloro-2,3-dihydro-1-methyl-5-phenyl-1*H*-1,4-benzodiazepine monohydrochloride; an antianxiety agent.

med·fal·an (med'fal-an). SYN medphalan.

me·dia (mē'dē-ă). 1. SYN *tunica* media. 2. Plural of medium. [L. fem. of *medius*, middle]

me·di·ad (mē'dē-ad). Toward the middle line.

me·di·al (mē'dē-ăl). Relating to the middle or center; nearer to the median or midsagittal plane. SYN medialis [NA]. [L. *medialis*, middle]

me·di·a·lec·i·thal (mē'dē-ă-les'i-thăl). Denoting an egg with a moderate amount of yolk, as in amphibians. [L. *medialis*, medial, + G. *lekithos*, egg yolk]

me·di·a·lis (mē-dē-ā'lis) [NA]. SYN medial, medial. [L.]

me·di·an (mē'dē-an). 1. Central; middle; lying in the midline. SYN medianus [NA]. 2. The middle value in a set of measurements; like the mean, a measure of central tendency. [L. *medianus*, middle]

me·di·a·nus (mē-dē-ā'nŭs) [NA]. SYN median (1). [L.]

me·di·as·ti·nal (mē'dē-as-tī'năl). Relating to the mediastinum.

me·di·as·ti·ni·tis (mē'dē-as-ti-nī'tis). Inflammation of the cellular tissue of the mediastinum.

fibrosing m., SYN mediastinal *fibrosis.*

fibrous m., scarring of mediastinal structures of unknown origin or due to infection.

idiopathic fibrous m., SYN mediastinal *fibrosis.*

me·di·as·ti·nog·ra·phy (mē'dē-as-ti-nog'ră-fē). Radiography of the mediastinum. [mediastinum + G. *graphō*, to write]

gaseous m., radiography of the mediastinum after injection of air (artificial pneumomediastinum), an obsolete procedure.

me·di·as·tin·o·per·i·car·di·tis (me'dē-as-tin-ō-per'i-kar-dī'tis). Inflammation of the pericardium and of the surrounding mediastinal cellular tissue.

me·di·as·tin·o·scope (mē-dē-as-tin'-ō-skōp). An endoscope for inspection of mediastinum through a suprasternal incision.

me·di·as·ti·nos·co·py (mē'dē-as-ti-nos'kŏ-pē). Exploration of the mediastinum through a suprasternal incision, for biopsy of paratracheal lymph nodes. [mediastinum + G. *skopeō*, to view]

me·di·as·ti·not·o·my (mē'dē-as-ti-not'ō-mē). Incision into the mediastinum. [mediastinum + G. *tomē*, incision]

anterior m., SYN Chamberlain *procedure.*

me·di·as·ti·num (me'dē-as-tī'nŭm) [NA]. 1. A septum between two parts of an organ or a cavity. 2. The median partition of the thoracic cavity, covered by the mediastinal pleura and containing all the thoracic viscera and structures except the lungs. It is divided arbitrarily into five parts: anterior mediastinum, inferior mediastinum, middle mediastinum, posterior mediastinum, and superior mediastinum. SYN interpleural space, interpulmonary septum, mediastinal space, septum mediastinale. [Mod. L. a middle septum, fr. Mediev. L. *mediastinus*, medial, fr. L. *mediastinus*, a lower servant, fr. *medius*, middle]

anterior m., anterior m., the narrow region between the pericardium and the sternum containing the thymus or its remnants, some lymph nodes and vessels and branches of the internal thoracic artery. SYN m. anterius.

m. ante'rius, SYN anterior m.

inferior m., the region below a plane transecing the $T_{4/5}$ intervertebral disc posteriorly and the sternal angle anteriorly, demarcating the inferior limit of the superior mediastinum. It is subdivided into three regions: middle, anterior, and posterior. SYN m. inferius.

m. infe'rius, SYN inferior m.

m. me'dium, SYN middle m.

middle m., the central portion of the inferior m. which contains the pericardium and its contents and the phrenic nerves and accompanying vessels. SYN m. medium.

posterior m., lies between the pericardium and the vertebral column, below the level of the $T_{4/5}$ intervertebral disc. It contains the descending aorta, thoracic duct, esophagus, azygos veins, and vagus nerves. SYN m. posterius, postmediastinum.

m. poste'rius, SYN posterior m.

superior m., that part lying above, *i.e.*, above the pericardium; it contains the arch of the aorta and the vessels arising from it, the brachiocephalic veins, and upper portion of the superior vena cava, the trachea, the esophagus, the thoracic duct, the thymus, and the phrenic, vagus, cardiac, and left recurrent laryngeal nerves. SYN m. superius.

m. supe'rius, SYN superior m.

m. tes'tis [NA], a mass of fibrous tissue continuous with the tunica albuginea, projecting into the testis from its posterior border. SYN corpus highmori, corpus highmorianum, Highmore's body, septum of testis.

me·di·ate. 1 (mē'dē-it). Situated between; intermediate. **2** (mē'dē-āt). To effect something by means of an intermediary substance, as in complement-mediated phagocytosis. [L. *mediatus*, fr. *medio*, pp. *-atus*, to divide in the middle]

me·di·a·tion (mē-dē-ā'shŭn). The action of an intermediary substance (mediator).

me·di·a·tor (mē'dē-ā-ter, -tōr). An intermediary substance or thing.

pharmacologic m.'s of anaphylaxis, substances released from mast (and other) cells by the reaction of antigen and specific homocytotropic antibody on their surfaces; they include histamine, slow-reacting substance of anaphylaxis (SRS-A), bradykinin, and (in some species of animals) serotonin.

med·i·ca·ble (med'i-kă-bl). Treatable, with hope of a cure.

med·i·cal (med'i-kăl). 1. Relating to medicine or the practice of medicine. SYN medicinal (2). 2. SYN medicinal (1). [L. *medicalis*, fr *medicus*, physician]

med·i·cal corps. The subdivision of a military organization, such as the U.S. Army, devoted to medical care of the troops.

med·i·cal tran·scrip·tion·ist. An individual who performs machine transcription of physician-dictated medical reports concerning a patient's health care, which become part of the patient's permanent medical record; a certified m. t. (CMT) has satisfied the requirements for certification by the American Association for Medical Transcription.

me·dic·a·ment (me-dik'ă-ment, med'i-kă-ment). A medicine, medicinal application, or remedy. [L. *medicamentum*, medicine]

med·i·ca·men·to·sus (med'i-kă-men-tō'sŭs). Relating to a drug; denoting a drug eruption. [L.]

med·i·cate (med'i-kāt). 1. To treat disease by the giving of drugs. 2. To impregnate with a medicinal substance. [L. *medico*, pp. *-atus*, to heal]

med·i·cat·ed (med'i-kāt-ed). Impregnated with a medicinal substance.

med·i·ca·tion (med-i-kā'shŭn). 1. The act of medicating. 2. A medicinal substance, or medicament.

arrhenic m., treatment of disease by means of the organic preparations of arsenic, the cacodylates, and methylarsinates.

ionic m., SYN iontophoresis.

maintenance medication, m. taken to stabilize an illness or symptoms of illness.

preanesthetic m., drugs administered prior to an anesthetic to decrease anxiety and to obtain a smoother induction of, maintenance of, and emergence from anesthesia.

sublingual m., a drug dosage form intended to be used by placement under the tongue; the drug (*e.g.,* nitroglycerin) is absorbed from the mucosal tissues and bypasses the gastrointestinal tract, where it may be partially or totally degraded.

med·i·ca·tor (med'i-kā-ter, -tōr). **1.** An instrument for use in making therapeutic applications to the deeper parts of the body. **2.** One who gives medicaments for the relief of disease; sometimes applied in derision to one who prescribes drugs excessively for minor ailments.

me·di·ce·phal·ic (mē'dē-se-fal'ik). Median cephalic, denoting the communicating vessel between the median and the cephalic veins of the forearm.

me·dic·i·nal (mě-dis'i-năl). **1.** Relating to medicine having curative properties. SYN medical (2). **2.** SYN medical (1).

me·dic·i·nal scar·let red. SYN scarlet red.

med·i·cine (med'i-sin). **1.** A drug. **2.** The art of preventing or curing disease; the science concerned with disease in all its relations. **3.** The study and treatment of general diseases or those affecting the internal parts of the body, especially those not usually requiring surgical intervention. [L. *medicina,* fr. *medicus,* physician (see medicus)]

adolescent m., the branch of medicine concerned with the treatment of youth in the approximate age range of 13 to 21 years. SYN hebiatrics.

aerospace m., a branch of m. combining the areas of concern of both aviation and space m.

alternative m., a term used by practitioners of Western, clinical m. to refer to a range of approaches to health and disease, some quite ancient and widely practiced. The category is broad, and encompasses bodies of knowledge that may be founded upon anatomical observation, possession of an effective pharmacopeia, and some form of clinical practice; and which may advance self-consistent explanations for the causation and cure of disease, whether physically or supernaturally based. Alternative m. also comprises approaches with limited known effectiveness. Examples of alternative practices include acupuncture and acupressure, homeopathy, osteopathy, chiropractic, massage, meditation, imaging, relaxation techniques, biofeedback, hypnosis, exercise, life style diets, megavitamin therapy, pulse diagnosis, tongue diagnosis, iridology, rolfing, faith healing, and prayer.

aviation m., the study and practice of m. as it applies to physiologic problems peculiar to aviation. SYN aeromedicine.

behavioral m., an interdisciplinary field concerned with the development and integration of behavioral and biomedical science knowledge and techniques relevant to health and illness, and to its application to prevention, diagnosis, treatment, and rehabilitation.

clinical m., the study and practice of m. in relation to the care of patients; the art of m. as distinguished from laboratory science.

community m., the study of health and disease in a defined community; the practice of m. in such a setting.

comparative m., a field of study concentrating on similarities and differences between veterinary m. and human m.

defensive m., diagnostic or therapeutic measures conducted primarily as a safeguard against possible subsequent malpractice liability.

desmoteric m., the branch of medical practice that deals with the health problems occurring among prison inmates. [G. *desmōtērion,* prison, fr. *deo,* to bind, + -ic]

experimental m., the scientific investigation of medical problems by experimentation upon animals or by clinical research.

family m., the medical specialty concerned with providing continuous, comprehensive care to all age groups, from first patient contact to terminal care, with special emphasis on care of the family as a unit.

fetal m., study of the growth, development, care, and treatment of the fetus, and of environmental factors harmful to the fetus. SYN fetology.

folk m., treatment of ailments outside of organized medicine by remedies and simple measures based upon experience and knowledge handed on from generation to generation.

forensic m., (1) the relation and application of medical facts to legal matters; **(2)** the law in its bearing on the practice of medicine. SYN legal m., medical jurisprudence.

geriatric m., a specialty of m. that is concerned with the disease and health problems of older people, usually those over 65 years of age. Considered a subspecialty of internal medicine.

holistic m., an approach to medical care that emphasizes the study of all aspects of a person's health, especially that a person should be considered as a unit, including psychological as well as social and economic influences on health status.

hyperbaric m., the medicinal use of high barometric pressure, usually in specially constructed chambers, to increase oxygen content of blood and tissues.

internal m. (IM), the branch of m. concerned with nonsurgical diseases in adults, but not including diseases limited to the skin or to the nervous system.

legal m., SYN forensic m.

military m., the practice of m. as applied to the special circumstances associated with military life.

neonatal m., SYN neonatology.

nuclear m., the clinical discipline concerned with the diagnostic and therapeutic uses of radionuclides, excluding the therapeutic use of sealed radiation sources.

> Nuclear medicine in the 1980s pioneered treatment of cancers with radioactively conjugated monoclonal antibodies, which carry cytotoxic doses of radiation directly to target cells, which the antibodies are designed to bind to. Yoked to MoAbs or to DNA probes, radionuclides also serve as assays, to identify gene sequences or signal the presence of given types of cells. Certain imaging procedures, including PET scanning, employ radionuclides to provide real-time visuals of biochemical processes. One device, a nuclear imaging machine, employs a scintillation camera, which can rotate around the body to pick up radiation emitted by an injected substance (*e.g.,* radioactive iodine, which localizes in the thyroid, or radioactive thallium, which localizes in the heart). Through computerization, a digitized image of a particular organ is produced.

osteopathic m., SYN osteopathy (2).

patent m., a m., usually originally patented, advertised to the public.

perinatal m., SYN perinatology.

physical m., the study and treatment of disease mainly by mechanical and other physical methods. SYN physiatry.

podiatric m., SYN podiatry.

preventive m., the branch of medical science concerned with the prevention of disease and with promotion of physical and mental health, through study of the etiology and epidemiology of disease processes.

proprietary m., a medicinal compound the formula and mode of manufacture of which are the property of the maker.

psychosomatic m., the study and treatment of diseases, disorders, or abnormal states in which psychological processes resulting in physiological reactions are believed to play a prominent role.

quack m., a compound advertised falsely as curative of a certain disease or diseases.

social m., a specialized field of medical knowledge concentrating on the social, cultural and economic impact of medical phenomena.

socialized m., the organization and control of medical practice by a government agency, the practitioners being employed by the organization from which they receive standardized compensation for their services, and to which the public contributes usually in the form of taxation rather than fee-for-service.

space m., the field of m. concerned with physiologic diseases or disturbances resulting from the unique conditions of space travel.

sports m., a field of m. that uses a holistic, comprehensive, and multidisciplinary approach to health care for those engaged in a sporting or recreational activity.

me

The American College of Sports Medicine identifies ancient roots for the approach. The Indian Ayur-Veda, dating to 800 BC, prescribes exercise and massage for rheumatism, and the Greek historian Herodotus (ca. 480 BC) commented on the therapeutic benefits of physical exertion. Galen (ca. 130–201 AD) thought exercise in moderation guarded against disease. The field has burgeoned with the worldwide rise in organized sports and individual exercise, which began in the 1950s. It now embraces attempts to refine understanding of human kinesiology, to detail the physiology of exercise, and to determine the powers of exercise in preventing or reversing disease.

tropical m., the branch of m. concerned with diseases, mainly of parasitic origin, in areas having a tropical climate.

veterinary m., the field concerned with the diseases and health of all animal species other than humans.

△**medico-.** Medical. Cf. iatro-. [L. *medicus*, physician]

med·i·co·bi·o·log·ic, med·i·co·bi·o·log·i·cal (med′i-kō-bī-ō-loj′ik, -loj′i-kăl). Pertaining to the biologic aspects of medicine.

med·i·co·chi·rur·gi·cal (med′i-kō-kī-rŭr′ji-kăl). Relating to both medicine and surgery, or to both physicians and surgeons. [medico- G. *cheirourgia*, surgery]

med·i·co·le·gal (med′i-kō-lē′găl). Relating to both medicine and the law. SEE ALSO forensic *medicine*. [medico- + L. *legalis*, legal]

med·i·co·me·chan·i·cal (med′i-kō-mě-kan′i-kăl). Relating to both medicinal and mechanical measures in therapeutics.

med·i·co·phys·i·cal (med′i-kō-fiz′i-kăl). Relating to disease and the condition of the body in general; *e.g.*, a m. examination, in which a person is examined in order to determine the presence or absence of disease as well as to note the general physical condition.

med·i·co·psy·chol·o·gy (med′i-kō-sī-kol′ō-jē). Psychology in its relation to medicine. SEE medical *psychology*, health *psychology*.

△**medio-, medi-.** Middle, median. [L. *medius*]

me·di·o·car·pal (mē′dē-ō-kar′păl). SYN midcarpal. SYN midcarpal (1).

me·di·oc·cip·i·tal (mē′dē-ok-sip′i-tăl). SYN midoccipital.

me·di·o·dens (mē′dē-ō-dens). A supernumerary tooth located between the two maxillary central incisors. [medio- + L. *dens*, tooth]

me·di·o·dor·sal (mē′dē-ō-dōr′săl). Relating to the median plane and the dorsal plane.

me·di·o·lat·er·al (mē′dē-ō-lat′er-ăl). Relating to the median plane and a side.

me·di·o·ne·cro·sis (mē′dē-ō-ne-krō′sis). Necrosis of a tunica media.

m. of the aorta, SYN cystic medial *necrosis*.

m. aor′tae idiopath′ica cys′tica, SYN cystic medial *necrosis*.

me·di·o·tar·sal (mē′dē-ō-tar′săl). SYN midtarsal.

me·di·o·tru·sion (mē′dē-ō-trū′zhŭn). A thrusting of the mandibular condyle toward the midline during movement of the mandible. [medio- + L. *trudo*, pp. *trusus*, to thrust]

me·di·o·type (mē′dē-ō-tīp). SYN mesomorph.

me·di·sect (mē′di-sekt). To incise in the median line. [L. *medius*, middle, + *seco*, pp. *sectus*, to cut]

me·di·um, pl. **me·dia** (mē′dē-ŭm, -ă). **1.** A means; that through which an action is performed. **2.** A substance through which impulses or impressions are transmitted. **3.** SYN culture m. **4.** The liquid holding a substance in solution or suspension. [L. neuter of *medius*, middle]

clearing m., a m. used in histology for making specimens translucent or transparent.

complete m., a m. for an *in vitro* culture that contains the supplemental nutrients as well as the basic nutrients to support fastidious or mutant growth requirements.

contrast m., any internally administered substance that has a different opacity from soft tissue on radiography or computed tomography; includes barium, used to opacify parts of the gastrointestinal tract; water-soluble iodinated compounds, used to opacify blood vessels or the genitourinary tract; may refer to air occurring naturally or introduced into the body; also, paramagnetic substances used in magnetic resonance imaging. SYN contrast agent, contrast material.

culture m., a substance, either solid or liquid, used for the cultivation, isolation, identification, or storage of microorganisms. SYN growth m., medium (3), nutrient m.

Czapek-Dox m., SYN Czapek's solution *agar*.

dispersion m., SYN external *phase*.

Dorset's culture egg m., a m. for cultivating *Mycobacterium tuberculosis*; it consists of the whites and yolks of four fresh eggs and a solution of sodium chloride.

Eagle's basal m., a solution of various salts containing 13 naturally occurring amino acids, several vitamins, two antibiotics, and phenol red; used as a tissue culture medium.

Eagle's minimum essential m. (MEM), a tissue culture m. similar to Eagle's basal medium but with different amounts and a few exclusions (*e.g.*, antibiotics and phenol red).

Endo's m., SYN Endo *agar*.

external m., SYN external *phase*.

growth m., SYN culture m.

high osmolar contrast m. (HOCM), SYN high osmolar contrast *agent*.

Loeffler's blood culture m., a culture m. consisting of beef blood serum, sheep blood serum, and beef bouillon containing peptone, glucose, and sodium chloride; used for the isolation of *Corynebacterium diphtheriae*.

Lowenstein-Jensen m., SYN Lowenstein-Jensen culture m.

Lowenstein-Jensen culture m., primary mycobacterial recovery media composed of fresh whole eggs, defined salts, glycerol, potato flour, and malachite green (as an inhibitory agent). SYN Lowenstein-Jensen m.

motility test m., a culture m. with a concentration of agar that produces a less solid consistency than usual and allows motile organisms to grow away from the line of inoculation; used to differentiate species of bacteria.

mounting m., a substance, usually resinous, used for mounting a cover glass on histologic suspensions.

Mueller-Hinton m., an agar-based media composed of beef infusion, casamino acids, and starch useful in the isolation of gonococci and meningococci; the recommended medium for antibacterial susceptibility tests for most common aerobic and facultatively anaerobic bacteria.

nutrient m., SYN culture m.

passive m., a m. that produces no change in the specimens placed in it.

selective m., a culture m. containing ingredients that inhibit growth of contaminants or microorganisms other than that desired.

separating m., (**1**) any coating which serves to prevent one surface from adhering to another; (**2**) in dentistry, a material usually applied to a cast to facilitate separation from the resin denture base after curing; a coating on impressions to facilitate removal of the cast.

Simmons' citrate m., a diagnostic m. used in the differentiation of species of Enterobacteriaceae, based on their ability to utilize sodium citrate as the sole source of carbon.

support m., the material in which separation takes place, as in separation of components in electrophoresis.

Thayer-Martin m., SYN Thayer-Martin *agar*.

transport m., a m. for transporting clinical specimens to the laboratory for examination.

me·di·um-chain ac·yl-CoA de·hy·dro·gen·ase. SEE acyl-CoA dehydrogenase (NADPH⁺).

me·di·us (mē′dē-ŭs) [NA]. SYN middle. [L.]

MEDLARS Abbreviation for Medical Literature Analysis and Retrieval System, a computerized index system of the U.S. National Library of Medicine.

MEDLINE. [MEDLARS-on-line] A computer-based telephone linkage to MEDLARS for rapid provision of medical bibliographies.

med·pha·lan (med′fă-lan). D-Phenylalanine mustard; D-sarcolysine; D-3-[*p*-[*bis*-(2-chloroethyl)amino]phenyl]alanine; an antineoplastic agent. SYN medfalan.

med·ro·ges·tone (med-rō-jes′tōn). 6,17α-Dimethyl-4,6-pregnadiene-3,20-dione; an oral progestin.

me·drox·y·pro·ges·ter·one ac·e·tate (med-rok′sē-prō-jes′ter-ōn). 17α-Hydroxy-6α-methylprogesterone; a progestational agent that is active orally as well as parenterally, and more potent than progesterone; used, in combination with ethynyl estradiol, as an oral contraceptive.

med·ryl·a·mine (med-ril′ă-mēn). 2-(*p*-Methoxy-α-phenylbenzyloxy-*N*,*N*-dimethylethylamine; an antihistaminic.

med·ry·sone (med′ri-sōn). 11β-Hydroxy-6α-methylpregn-4-ene-3,20-dione; a glucocorticoid used topically as an anti-inflammatory agent, usually on the eye.

me·dul·la, pl. **me·dul·lae** (me-dūl′ă, me-dūl′ē) [NA]. Any soft marrow-like structure, especially in the center of a part. SEE ALSO m. oblongata. SYN substantia medullaris (1). [L. marrow, fr. *medius,* middle]

m. of adrenal gland, SYN suprarenal m.

m. glan′dulae suprarena′lis, SYN suprarenal m.

m. of hair shaft, the central axis of some hairs, containing a column of large vacuolated and keratinized cells; the medullary portion is surrounded by the cortex.

m. of kidney, SYN renal m.

m. of lymph node, the central portion of a node consisting of cordlike masses of lymphocytes, plasma cells, and macrophages in a stroma of reticular fibers separated by lymph sinuses; it reaches the surface of the node at the hilum. SYN m. nodi lymphatici.

m. no′di lymphat′ici, SYN m. of lymph node.

m. oblonga′ta [NA], the most caudal subdivision of the brainstem, immediately continuous with the spinal cord, extending from the lower border of the decussation of the pyramid to the pons; its ventral surface resembles that of the spinal cord except for the bilateral prominence of the inferior olive; the dorsal surface of its upper half forms part of the floor of the fourth ventricle. Motor nuclei of the m. oblongata include the hypoglossal nucleus, the dorsal motor nucleus, inferior salivatory nucleus, and the nucleus ambiguus; sensory nuclei include the nuclei of the posterior column (gracile and cuneate), the cochlear and vestibular nuclei, the mid and caudal portions of the spinal trigeminal nucleus, and the nucleus of the solitary tract. SEE ALSO medulla. SYN myelencephalon [NA], oblongata.

m. os′sium [NA], SYN bone *marrow.*

m. os′sium fla′va, SYN yellow bone *marrow.*

m. os′sium ru′bra, SYN red bone *marrow.*

renal m., the inner, darker portion of the kidney parenchyma consisting of the renal pyramids. SYN m. renalis [NA], m. of kidney.

m. rena′lis [NA], SYN renal m.

m. spina′lis [NA], SYN spinal *cord.*

suprarenal m., it is composed principally of anastomosing cords of cells in the core of the gland; the cells display a chromaffin reaction because of the presence of epinephrine and norepinephrine in their granules. SYN m. glandulae suprarenalis, m. of adrenal gland.

me·dul·lar (med-yūl′ăr). SYN medullary.

med·ul·lary (med′ŭ-lār-ē, mĕ-dul′er-ē, med′yū-lār-ē). Relating to the medulla or marrow. SYN medullar.

med·ul·lat·ed (med′ŭ-lā-ted, med′yū-). **1.** Having a medulla or medullary substance. **2.** SYN myelinated.

med·ul·la·tion (med′ŭ-lā′shŭn, med′yū-). **1.** Acquiring, or the act of formation of, marrow or medulla. **2.** SYN myelination.

med·ul·lec·to·my (med-ū-lek′tō-mē, med-yū-). Excision of any medullary substance. [medulla + G. *ektomē,* excision]

med·ul·li·za·tion (med′ŭ-li-zā′shŭn, med′yū-). Enlargement of the medullary spaces in rarefying osteitis.

△**medullo-.** Medulla. Cf. myel-. [L. *medulla*]

me·dul·lo·ar·thri·tis (med-ŭ-lō-ar-thrī′tis). Inflammation of the cancellous articular extremity of a long bone.

me·dul·lo·blas·to·ma (med′ŭ-lō-blas-tō′mă). A tumor consist-

ing of neoplastic cells that resemble the undifferentiated cells of the primitive medullary tube; m.'s are usually located in the vermis of the cerebellum, and may be implanted discretely or coalescently on the surfaces of the cerebellum, brainstem, and spinal cord; they comprise approximately 3% of all intracranial neoplasms, and occur most frequently in children; the neoplastic cells are compactly arranged, rounded or ovoid, with hyperchromatic nuclei and relatively scant cytoplasm, and lie in small and poorly defined groups, or, occasionally, in a pseudorosette pattern (Homer Wright rosette). A type of primitive neuroectodermal tumor.

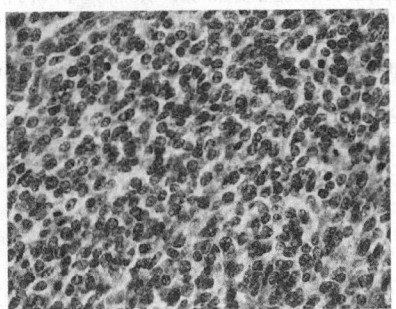

medulloblastoma
note diffuse proliferation of undifferentiated cells

desmoplastic m., subtype of m. with a biphasic pattern of compact sheets of undifferentiated cells alternating with islands of more loosely cohesive cells, generally occurs in adolescence and young adults and has a better prognosis than the usual m.

melanotic m., a rare variant of m. in which melanin-pigmented cells are present.

me·dul·lo·cell (med′ŭ-lō-sel, med′yū-). SYN myelocyte (2).

me·dul·lo·ep·i·the·li·o·ma (me′dŭ-lō-ep′ĭ-thē-lē-ō′mă). A rare, primitive, rapidly growing intracranial neoplasm thought to originate from the cells of the embryonic medullary canal and hence included with ependymoblastomas by some neuropathologists; ganglion cells and astrocyte maturation has also been reported. Tumors that occur in the ciliary body are referred to as embryonal m.'s. [medullo- + epithelium + -*oma,* tumor]

adult m., SYN malignant ciliary *epithelioma.*

embryonal m., an epitheliomatous tumor of the nonpigmented layer of the ciliary epithelium. SYN embryonal tumor of ciliary body.

me·dul·lo·my·o·blas·to·ma (med′ŭ-lō-mī′ō-blas-tō′mă). A rare histologic variant of medulloblastoma with scattered smooth and striated muscle cells incorporated into the neoplasm.

Meeh, K., 19th century German physiologist. SEE M. *formula;* M.-Dubois *formula.*

Mees, R.A., 20th century Dutch physician. SEE M.'s *lines,* under *line, stripes,* under *stripe.*

Mees' lines. See under line.

Meesman, A., German ophthalmologist, 1888–1969. SEE M. *dystrophy.*

Mees' stripes. See under stripe.

mef·e·nam·ic ac·id (me-fĕ-nam′ik). *N*-(2,3-Xylyl)anthranilic acid; an aspirin-like analgesic with anti-inflammatory properties.

me·fen·o·rex hy·dro·chlo·ride (me-fen′ō-reks). *N*-(3-Chloropropyl)-α- methylphenethylamine hydrochloride; a sympathomimetic drug with anorexic activity.

me·fex·a·mide (mĕ-fek′ă-mīd). *N*-[2-Diethylamino)ethyl]-2- (*p*-methoxyphenoxy)acet amide; an antidepressant.

mef·lo·quine (mef′lō-kwin). An antimalarial resembling quinine and chloroquine.

MEG Abbreviation for magnetoencephalogram.

△**mega-.** **1.** Combining form meaning large, oversize; opposite of micro-. SEE ALSO macro-, megalo-. **2 (M).** Prefix used in the SI and metric systems to signify one million (10^6). [G. *megas,* big]

me

meg·a·bac·te·ri·um (meg'ă-bak-tēr'ē-ŭm). A bacterium of unusually large size. SYN macrobacterium.

meg·a·ca·ly·co·sis (meg'ă-kal-ĭ-kō-sis). 1. Congenital, nonobstructive enlargement of renal calices. 2. Excessively large number of calices. [mega- + G. *kalyx*, cup of a flower, + *-osis*, condition]

meg·a·car·dia (meg-ă-kar'dē-ă). SYN cardiomegaly.

meg·a·car·y·o·blast (meg-ă-kar'ē-ō-blast). SYN megakaryoblast.

meg·a·car·y·o·cyte (meg-ă-kar'ē-ō-sīt). SYN megakaryocyte.

meg·a·ce·pha·lia (meg-ă-se-fā'lē-ă). SYN megacephaly.

meg·a·ce·phal·ic (meg'ă-se-fal'ik). Relating to or characterized by megacephaly. SYN macrocephalic, macrocephalous, megacephalous.

meg·a·ceph·a·lous (meg-ă-sef'ă-lŭs). SYN megacephalic.

meg·a·ceph·a·ly (meg-ă-sef'ă-lē). A condition, either congenital or acquired, in which the head is abnormally large; usually applied to an adult skull with a capacity of over 1450 ml. SYN leontiasis ossea, macrocephaly, macrocephalia, megacephalia, megalocephaly, megalocephalia, Virchow's disease. [mega- + G. *kephalē*, head]

meg·a·cins (meg'ă-sinz). Antibacterial proteins produced by strains of *Bacillus megaterium*.

meg·a·coc·cus, pl. **meg·a·coc·ci** (meg'ă-kok'ŭs, -kok'sī). A coccus of unusually large size. SYN macrococcus.

meg·a·co·lon (meg'ă-kō'lon). A condition of extreme dilation and hypertrophy of the colon. SYN giant colon.

acquired m., m. occurring on the basis of an acquired disease; occurs in inflammatory bowel disease (toxic m.) and Chagas' *disease* (South American *trypanosomiasis*).

congenital m., m. congen'itum, congenital dilation and hypertrophy of the colon due to absence (aganglionosis) or marked reduction (hypoganglionosis) in the number of ganglion cells of the myenteric plexus of the rectum and a varying but continuous length of gut above the rectum; also seen in dogs. SYN Hirschsprung's disease.

idiopathic m., an acquired m., found in children and adults, without distal obstruction or absence of ganglion cells; the muscle of the dilated colon is thin.

toxic m., acute nonobstructive dilation of the colon, seen in fulminating ulcerative colitis and Crohn's disease.

meg·a·cy·cle (meg'ă-sī-kl). One million cycles per second.

meg·a·cys·tis (meg'ă-sis-tis). Pathologically large bladder in children. SYN megalocystis. [mega- + *kystis*, bladder]

meg·a·dac·ty·ly, meg·a·dac·tyl·ia, meg·a·dac·tyl·ism (meg-ă-dak'ti-lē, -dak-til'ē-ă -dak'til-izm). Condition characterized by enlargement of one or more digits (fingers or toes). SYN dactylomegaly, macrodactylia, macrodactylism, macrodactyly, megalodactylia, megalodactylism, megalodactyly. [mega- + G. *daktylos*, digit]

meg·a·dol·i·cho·co·lon (meg'ă-dol'i-kō-kō'lon). Excessive length and dilation of colon. [mega- + G. *dolichos*, long, + *kōlon*, colon]

meg·a·dont (meg'ă-dont). SYN macrodont. [mega- + G. *odous* (*odont-*), tooth]

meg·a·don·tism (meg-ă-don'tizm). SYN macrodontia.

meg·a·dyne (meg'ă-dīn). One million dynes.

meg·a·e·soph·a·gus (meg'ă-ē-sof'ă-gŭs, meg'ă-e-sof'). Great enlargement of the lower portion of the esophagus, as seen in patients with achalasia and Chagas' disease.

meg·a·ga·mete (meg-ă-gam'ēt). SYN macrogamete.

meg·a·gna·thia (meg-ă-nā'thē-ă). SYN macrognathia.

meg·a·hertz (MHz) (meg'ă-hertz). One million hertz.

meg·a·kar·y·o·blast (meg-ă-kar'ē-ō-blast). The precursor of a megakaryocyte. SYN megacaryoblast.

meg·a·kar·y·o·cyte (meg-ă-kar'ē-ō-sīt). A large cell (as much as 100 μm in diameter) with a polyploid nucleus that is usually multilobed; m.'s are normally present in bone marrow, not in the circulating blood, and give rise to blood platelets. SYN megacaryocyte, megalokaryocyte, thromboblast. [mega- + G. *karyon*, nut (nucleus), + *kytos*, hollow vessel (cell)]

△**megal-.** SEE megalo-.

meg·a·lec·i·thal (meg-ă-les'i-thăl). Denoting an egg rich in yolk, as in bony fishes, reptiles, and birds. [mega- + G. *lekithos*, yolk]

meg·al·gia (meg-al'jē-ă). Very severe pain. [mega- + G. *algos*, pain]

△**megalo-, megal-.** Large; opposite of micro-. SEE ALSO macro-, mega-. [G. *megas* (*megal-*)]

meg·a·lo·blast (meg'ă-lō-blast). A large, nucleated, embryonic type of cell that is a precursor of erythrocytes in an abnormal erythropoietic process observed in pernicious anemia; a m.'s four stages of development are as follows: 1) promegaloblast, 2) basophilic m., 3) polychromatic m., 4) orthochromatic m. SEE ALSO erythroblast. [megalo- + G. *blastos*, + germ, sprout]

meg·a·lo·car·dia (meg'ă-lō-kar'dē-ă). SYN cardiomegaly. [megalo- + G. *kardia*, heart]

meg·a·lo·ceph·a·ly, meg·a·lo·ce·pha·lia (meg'ă-lō-sef'ă-lē, -sĕ-fā'lē-ă). SYN megacephaly.

meg·a·lo·chei·ria, meg·a·lo·chi·ria (meg'ă-lō-kī'rē-ă). SYN macrocheiria. [megalo- + G. *cheir*, hand]

meg·a·lo·cor·nea (meg'ă-lō-kōr'nē-ă). SYN keratoglobus.

meg·a·lo·cys·tis (meg'ă-lō-sis'tis). SYN megacystis. [megalo- + G. *kystis*, bladder]

meg·a·lo·cyte (meg'ă-lō-sīt). A large (10 to 20 μm) nonnucleated red blood cell. [megalo- + G. *kytos*, cell]

meg·a·lo·cy·the·mia (meg'ă-lō-sī-thē'mē-ă). SYN macrocythemia.

meg·a·lo·cy·to·sis (meg'ă-lō-sī-tō'sis). SYN macrocythemia.

meg·a·lo·dac·tyl·ia, meg·a·lo·dac·tyl·ism, meg·a·lo·dac·ty·ly (meg'ă-lō-dak-til'ē-ă, -dak'til-izm, -dak'ti-lē). SYN megadactyly.

meg·a·lo·dont (meg'ă-lō-dont). SYN macrodont.

meg·a·lo·don·tia (meg'ă-lō-don'shē-ă). SYN macrodontia.

meg·a·lo·en·ce·phal·ic (meg'ă-lō-en'sĕ-fal'ik). Denoting an abnormally large brain.

meg·a·lo·en·ceph·a·lon (meg'ă-lō-en-sef'ă-lon). An abnormally large brain. SYN macroencephalon. [megalo- + G. *enkephalos*, brain]

meg·a·lo·en·ceph·a·ly (meg'ă-lō-en-sef'ă-lē). Abnormal largeness of the brain. [megalo- + G. *enkephalon*, brain]

meg·a·lo·en·ter·on (meg'ă-lō-en'ter-on). Abnormal largeness of the intestine. SYN enteromegaly, enteromegalia. [megalo- + G. *enteron*, intestine]

meg·a·lo·gas·tria (meg'ă-lō-gas'trē-ă). Abnormally large size of the stomach. SYN macrogastria. [megalo- + G. *gastēr*, stomach]

meg·a·lo·glos·sia (meg'ă-lō-glos'sē-ă). SYN macroglossia. [megalo- + G. *glōssa*, tongue]

meg·a·lo·graph·ia (meg'ă-lō-graf'ē-ă). SYN macrography.

meg·a·lo·he·pat·ia (meg'ă-lo-he-pat'ē-ă). SYN hepatomegaly.

meg·a·lo·kar·y·o·cyte (meg'ă-lō-kar'ē-ō-sīt). SYN megakaryocyte.

meg·a·lo·ma·nia (meg'ă-lō-mā'nē-ă). A type of delusion in which the individual considers himself or herself possessed of greatness. He/she believes him/herself to be Christ, God, Napoleon, etc., or everyone and everything, including a lawyer, physician, clergyman, merchant, prince, ace athlete in all divisions of sport, etc. 2. Morbid verbalized overevaluation of oneself or of some aspect of oneself. [megalo- + G. *mania*, frenzy]

meg·a·lo·ma·ni·ac (meg'ă-lō-mā'nē-ak). A person exhibiting megalomania.

meg·a·lo·me·lia (meg'ă-lō-mē'lē-ă). SYN macromelia.

meg·a·lon·y·cho·sis (meg'ă-lon-i-kō'sis). SYN macronychia. [megalo- + G. *onyx*, nail, -*osis*, condition]

meg·a·loph·thal·mos (meg'ă-lof-thal'mŭs). Congenital large globe. SYN macrophthalmia, megophthalmus. [megalo- + G. *ophthalmos*, eye]

anterior m., SYN keratoglobus.

meg·a·lo·pia (meg-ă-lō'pē-ă). SYN macropsia.

meg·a·lo·po·dia (meg'ă-lō-pō'dē-ă). SYN macropodia. [megalo- + G. *pous*, foot]

meg·a·lop·sia (meg-ă-lop′sē-ă). SYN macropsia.

meg·a·lo·splanch·nic (meg′ă-lō-splangk′nik). Having abnormally large viscera. SYN macrosplanchnic. [megalo- + G. *splanchnon,* viscus]

meg·a·lo·sple·nia (meg′ă-lō-splē′nē-ă). SYN splenomegaly.

meg·a·lo·spore (meg′ă-lō-spōr). SYN macrospore.

meg·a·lo·syn·dac·ty·ly, meg·a·lo·syn·dac·tyl·ia (meg′ă-lō-sin-dak′ti-lē, -dak-til′ē-ă). Condition of webbed or fused fingers or toes of large size. [megalo- + G. *syn,* together, + *daktylos,* finger]

meg·a·lo·u·re·ter (meg′ă-lō-yū-rē′ter). An enlarged, dilated ureter. SYN megaureter.

meg·a·lo·u·re·thra (meg′ă-lō-yū-rē′thră). Congenital dilation of the urethra.

△**-megaly.** Large. [G. *megas (megal-)*]

meg·a·mer·o·zo·ite (meg′ă-mer-ō-zō′īt). SYN macromerozoite.

meg·a·nu·cle·us (meg-ă-nū′klē-ŭs). SYN macronucleus (1).

meg·a·pro·so·pia (meg′ă-prō-sō′pē-ă). SYN macroprosopia. [mega- + G. *prosōpon,* face]

meg·a·pros·o·pous (meg-ă-pros′ō-pŭs). SYN macroprosopous.

meg·a·rec·tum (meg-ă-rek′tŭm). Extreme dilation of the rectum.

meg·a·seme (meg′ă-sēm). Denoting an orbital aperture with an index above 89. [mega- + G. *sēma,* sign]

meg·a·sig·moid (meg-ă-sig′moyd). SYN macrosigmoid.

meg·a·so·mia (meg-ă-sō′mē-ă). SYN macrosomia.

meg·a·spore (meg′ă-spōr). SYN macrospore.

meg·a·throm·bo·cyte (meg-ă-throm′bō-sīt). A large blood platelet, especially a young one recently released from the bone marrow. [mega- + G. *thrombos,* clot, + *kytos,* cell]

meg·a·u·re·ter (meg-ă-yū-rē′ter). SYN megaloureter.
 primary m., independent ureteral dilation; may be nonobstructive or related to congenital distal ureteral obstruction.
 secondary m., hydroureter secondary to vesicoureteral reflux or distal obstruction.

meg·a·volt (meg′ă-vōlt). One million volts.

meg·a·volt·age (meg′ă-vol′tij). In radiation therapy, a term for voltage above one million volts.

me·ges·trol ac·e·tate (me-jes′trōl). 17α-Hydroxy-6-methyl-pregna-4,6-diene-3,20-dione acetate; a synthetic progestin with progestational effects similar to those of progesterone; used in threatened and habitual abortion, endometriosis, and menstrual disorders; claimed to be superior to 19-nor compounds as an antifertility agent because it has less effect on the endometrium and vagina; in combination with ethynyl estradiol, it acts as an oral contraceptive.

meg·lu·mine (meg′lū-mēn). USAN-approved contraction for *N*-methylglucamine.
 m. acetrizoate, a radiographic contrast medium. SEE acetrizoate sodium.
 m. diatrizoate, *N*-methylglucamine salt of 3,5-diacetamido-2,4,6-triiodobenzoic acid; a water-soluble organic iodine compound used for excretory urography, for contrast visualization of the cardiovascular system, and orally for opacification of the gastrointestinal tract. SYN methylglucamine diatrizoate.
 m. iothalamate, *N*-methylglucamine salt of iothalamic acid (60% solution); a diagnostic radiopaque medium for intravascular use in angiography and urography.

meg·ohm (meg′ōm). One million ohms.

meg·oph·thal·mus (meg-of-thal′mŭs). SYN megalophthalmos.

meg·ox·y·cyte (meg-oks′ē-sīt). SYN megoxyphil.

meg·ox·y·phil, meg·ox·y·phile (meg-oks′ē-fil, fīl). An eosinophilic leukocyte containing coarse granules. SYN megoxycyte. [mega- + G. *oxys,* acid, + *phileō,* to like]

me·grim (mē′grim). Obsolete term for migraine.

Meibom (Mei·bo·mi·us), Hendrik (Heinrich), German anatomist, 1638–1700. SEE meibomian *conjunctivitis,* meibomian *cyst,* meibomian *glands,* under *gland,* meibomian *sty.*

mei·bo·mi·an (mī-bō′mē-an). Attributed to or described by Meibom.

mei·bo·mi·tis, mei·bo·mi·a·ni·tis (mī′bō-mī′tis, mī-bō′mē-ă-nī′ tis). Inflammation of the meibomian glands.

Meier, Georg, German serologist, *1875. SEE Porges-M. *test.*

Meige, Henri, French physician, 1866–1940. SEE M.'s *disease.*

Meigs, Joe V., U.S. gynecologist, 1892–1963. SEE M.'s *syndrome.*

Meinicke, Ernst, German physician, 1878–1945. SEE M. *test.*

△**meio-.** For words beginning thus and not found here, see mio-.

mei·o·sis (mī-ō′sis). A special process of cell division comprising two nuclear divisions in rapid succession that result in four gametocytes, each containing half the number of chromosomes found in somatic cells. SYN meiotic division. [G. *meiōsis,* a lessening]

mei·ot·ic (mī-ot′ik). Pertaining to meiosis.

Meissel. SEE Wachstein-Meissel *stain* for calcium-magnesium-ATPase.

Meissner, Georg, German histologist, 1829–1905. SEE M.'s *corpuscle, plexus.*

mel. 1. SYN honey. **2.** Unit of pitch; a pitch of 1000 mels results from a simple tone of frequency 1000 Hz, 40 dB above the normal threshold of audibility.

△**mel-, melo-. 1.** Limb. [G. *melos*] **2.** A cheek. [G. *mēlon*] **3.** Honey, sugar. SEE ALSO meli-. [L. *mel, mellis,* G. *meli, melitos*] **4.** Sheep. [G. *mēlon*]

me·lag·ra (mě-lag′ră). Rheumatic or myalgic pains in the arms or legs. [G. *melos,* limb, + *agra,* seizure]

me·lal·gia (mě-lal′jē-ă). Pain in a limb; specifically, burning pain in the feet extending up the leg and even to the thigh. [G. *melos,* a limb, + *algos,* pain]

mel·a·mine form·al·de·hyde (mel′ă-mēn). SYN melamine *resin.*

△**melan-, melano-.** Black, extreme darkness of hue. [G. *melas*]

mel·an·cho·lia (mel-an-kō′lē-ă). **1.** A severe form of depression marked by anhedonia, insomnia, psychomotor changes, and guilt. **2.** A symptom occurring in other conditions, marked by depression of spirits and by a sluggish and painful process of thought. SYN melancholy. [melan- + G. *cholē,* bile. See humoral *doctrine*]
 hypochondriacal m., m. with many associated physical complaints, often with little basis in fact.
 involutional m., a depressive disorder of middle life, commonly associated with the climacteric.

mel·an·chol·ic (mel-an-kol′ik). **1.** Relating to or characteristic of melancholia. **2.** Formerly, denoting a temperament characterized by irritability and a pessimistic outlook. **3.** A person who is exhibiting melancholia.

mel·an·choly (mel′an-kol-ē). SYN melancholia.

mel·an·e·de·ma (mel′an-e-dē′mă). SYN anthracosis. [melan- + G. *oidēma,* swelling]

mel·a·ne·mia (mel-ă-nē′mē-ă). The presence of dark brown, almost black, or black granules of insoluble pigment (melanin) in the circulating blood. [melan- + G. *haima,* blood]

mel·an·i·dro·sis (mel′an-i-drō′sis). SEE chromhidrosis, pseudochromidrosis.

mel·a·nif·er·ous (mel-ă-nif′er-ŭs). Containing melanin or other black pigment. [melan- (melanin) + L. *ferro,* to carry]

mel·a·nin (mel′ă-nin). Any of the dark brown to black polymers of indole 5,6-quinone and/or 5,6-dihydroxyindole 2-carboxylic acid that normally occur in the skin, hair, pigmented coat of the retina, and inconstantly in the medulla and zona reticularis of the adrenal gland. M. may be formed *in vitro* or biologically by oxidation of L-tyrosine or L-tryptophan, the usual mechanism being the enzymatic oxidation of L-tyrosine to 3,4-dihydroxy-L-phenylalanine (dopa) and dopaquinone by monophenol monooxygenase, and the further oxidation (probably spontaneous) of this intermediate to m. Cf. eumelanin, pheomelanin. SYN melanotic pigment. [G. *melas (melan-),* black]
 artificial m., factitious m., SYN melanoid.

mel·a·nism (mel′ă-nizm). Unusually marked, diffuse, melanin pigmentation of body hair and skin (usually not affecting the iris). SEE ALSO melanosis.

☉**melano-.** SEE melan-.

mel·a·no·ac·an·tho·ma (mel'ă-nō-ak-an-thō'mă). A seborrheic keratosis with melanin pigmentation associated with proliferation of intraepidermal melanocytes. [melano- + G. *akantha*, thorn, + suffix *-ōma*, tumor]

mel·a·no·am·e·lo·blas·to·ma (mel'ă-nō-am'ĕ-lō-blas-tō'mă). SYN melanotic neuroectodermal *tumor* of infancy. [melano- + ameloblastoma]

mel·a·no·blast (mel'ă-nō-blast). A cell derived from the neural crest; it migrates to various parts of the body early in embryonic life, and then becomes a mature melanocyte capable of forming melanin. [melano- + G. *blastos*, germ, sprout]

mel·a·no·blas·to·ma (mel'ă-nō-blas-tō'mă). Obsolete term for melanoma. [melano- + G. *blastos*, germ, sprout, + *-ōma*, tumor]

mel·a·no·car·ci·no·ma (mel'ă-nō-kar-si-nō'mă). Obsolete term for melanoma.

mel·a·noc·o·mous (mel-ă-nok'ŏ-mŭs). SYN melanotrichous. [melano- + G. *komē*, hair of the head]

mel·a·no·cyte (mel'ă-nō-sīt). A pigment-producing cell located in the basal layer of the epidermis with branching processes by means of which melanosomes are transferred to epidermal cells, resulting in pigmentation of the epidermis. SYN melanodendrocyte, pigment cell of skin. [melano- + G. *kytos*, cell]

mel·a·no·cy·to·ma (mel'ă-nō-sī-tō'mă). **1.** A pigmented tumor of the uveal stroma. **2.** Usually benign melanoma of the optic disk, appearing in markedly pigmented individuals as a small deeply pigmented tumor at the edge of the disk, sometimes extending into the retina and choroid; malignant metaplasia is rare. [megalo- + cyto- + G. *-oma;* tumor]

mel·a·no·den·dro·cyte (mel'ă-nō-den'drŏ-sīt). SYN melanocyte. [melano- + G. *dendron*, tree, + *kytos*, a hollow (cell)]

mel·a·no·der·ma (mel'ă-nō-der'mă). **1.** An abnormal darkening of the skin by deposition of excess melanin. **2.** Hyperpigmentation of the skin by melanin or deposition of dark metallic substances such as silver and iron. [melano- + G. *derma*, skin]

m. cachectico'rum, m. of the cachectic, occurring in certain chronic diseases, such as malaria and tuberculosis.

m. chloas'ma, SYN melasma.

parasitic m., excoriations and m. caused by scratching the bites of the body louse, *Pediculus corporis.* SYN Greenhow's disease, vagabond's disease, vagrant's disease.

racial m., the normally dark skin of blacks and certain other races.

senile m., cutaneous pigmentation occurring in the aged. SYN melasma universale.

mel·a·no·der·ma·ti·tis (mel'ă-nō-der-mă-tī'tis). Excessive deposit of melanin in an area of dermatitis.

mel·a·no·der·mic (mel'ă-nō-der'mik). Relating to or marked by melanoderma.

me·la·no·gen (mĕ-lan'ō-jen, mel'ă-nō-jen). A colorless substance that may be converted into melanin; *e.g.,* some patients with widespread metastases of melanoma excrete m. in their urine, and melanin is formed when the urine is exposed to air (*i.e.,* oxidized) for a few hours. [melanin + G. *-gen*, producing]

mel·a·no·ge·ne·mia (mel'ă-nō-jĕ-nē'mē-ă). The presence of melanin precursors in the blood; may occur in malignant melanoma with metastasis. [melanogen + G. *haima*, blood]

mel·a·no·gen·e·sis (mel'ă-nō-jen'ĕ-sis). Formation of melanin. [melanin + G. *genesis*, production]

mel·a·no·glos·sia (mel'ă-nō-glos'ē-ă). SYN black *tongue.* [melano- + G. *glōssa*, tongue]

mel·a·noid (mel'ă-noyd). A dark pigment, resembling melanin, formed from glucosamines in chitin. SYN artificial melanin, factitious melanin.

mel·a·no·ker·a·to·sis (mel'ă-nō-ker-ă-tō'sis). Migration of conjunctival melanoblasts into the cornea. [melano- + kerato- + G. *-osis*, condition]

mel·a·no·leu·ko·der·ma (mel'ă-nō-lū-kō-der'mă). Marbled, or marmorated, skin. [melano- + G. *leukos*, white, + *derma*, skin]

m. col'li, SYN syphilitic *leukoderma.*

mel·an·o·li·ber·in (mel'ă-nō-lib'er-in). A hexapeptide similar to oxytocin; it stimulates the release of melanotropin. SYN melanotropin-releasing factor, melanotropin-releasing hormone. [melanotropin + L. *libero*, to free, + -in]

———

mel·a·no·ma (mel'ă-nō'mă). A malignant neoplasm, derived from cells that are capable of forming melanin, arising most commonly in the skin of any part of the body, or in the eye, and, rarely, in the mucous membranes of the genitalia, anus, oral cavity, or other sites; occurs mostly in adults and may originate *de novo* or from a pigmented nevus or lentigo maligna. In the early phases, the cutaneous form is characterized by proliferation of cells at the dermal-epidermal junction which soon invade adjacent tissues. The cells vary in amount and pigmentation of cytoplasm; the nuclei are relatively large and frequently bizarre in shape, with prominent acidophilic nucleoli; and mitotic figures tend to be numerous. M.'s frequently metastasize widely; regional lymph nodes, skin, liver, lungs, and brain are likely to be involved. SYN malignant m. [melano- + G. *-ōma*, tumor]

> In January 1985, the Environmental Protection Agency predicted that depletion of the Earth's ozone layer, which guards against ultraviolet radiation from space, would cause an increase in the number of skin cancer cases worldwide, including melanomas. The EPA estimated an annual increase of 2 million cases by the year 2050, when the ozone layer was expected to be diminished by 10% because of human activities, primarily the release of long-lived chlorofluorocarbons into the atmosphere (now banned in most developed countries). Public health efforts have focussed on encouraging people to use sunscreen, avoid outdoor activities during peak exposure times, perform frequent self-checks of the skin, and visit dermatologists when irregularities are noted. Exposure to higher levels of ultraviolet radiation may also promote cataracts and immune system dysfunction.

———

acral lentiginous m., a form of malignant lentigo m. that occurs in acral areas not excessively exposed to sunlight and where hair follicles are absent.

amelanotic m., an anaplastic m. consisting of cells derived from melanocytes but not forming melanin.

benign juvenile m., SYN Spitz *nevus.*

Cloudman m., a transplantable m. that arose spontaneously in a mouse of DBA strain, and which grows and metastasizes in mice of related strains.

desmoplastic malignant m. (dez-mō-plas-mik), a m. with marked fibrosis surrounding atypical spindle-shaped melanocytes in the dermis.

halo m., a rare condition in which a m. is surrounded by an irregular area of depigmentation.

Harding-Passey m., a melanin-forming tumor that arose spontaneously in a non-inbred mouse, and that is transplantable to mice of many strains but does not ordinarily metastasize.

malignant m., SYN melanoma.

malignant lentigo m., a m. arising from a malignant lentigo.

malignant m. in situ, a m. limited to the epidermis and composed of nests of atypical melanocytes and scattered single cells extending into the upper epidermis; local excision is curative although the lesion, if untreated, may soon invade the dermis. Malignant lentigo may be considered a slowly progressive type of malignant m. in situ.

minimal deviation m., a malignant m. showing less cytologic atypia than is usual in m. cells showing asymmetric expansile invasion of the dermis.

nodular m., primary cutaneous m. characterized by dermal invasion extending to the lateral margins of epidermal involvement or ulceration.

subungual m., a m. beginning in the skin at the border of or beneath the nail. SYN melanotic whitlow.

superficial spreading m., primary cutaneous m. characterized by intraepidermal growth extending laterally beyond the site of dermal invasion.

mel·a·no·ma·to·sis (mel'ă-nō-mă-tō'sis). A condition characterized by numerous, widespread lesions of melanoma. [melanoma + G. -*osis*, condition]

mel·a·no·nych·ia (mel′ă-nō-nik′ē-ă). Black pigmentation of the nails. [melano- + G. *onyx* (*onych-*), nail]

mel·a·nop·a·thy (mel′ă-nop′ă-thē). Any disease marked by abnormal pigmentation of the skin. [melano- + G. *pathos*, suffering]

mel·a·no·phage (mel′ă-nō-fāj, mĕ-lan′ō-fāj). A histiocyte that has phagocytized melanin. [melano- + G. *phagein*, to eat]

mel·a·no·phore (mel′ă-nō-fōr, mĕ-lan′ō-fōr). A dermal pigment cell that does not secrete its pigment granules but participates in rapid color changes by intracellular aggregation and dispersal of melanosomes; it is well developed in fish, amphibians, and reptiles, but absent in humans. [melano- + G. *phoros*, bearing]

mel·a·no·pla·kia (mel′ă-nō-plā′kē-ă). The occurrence of pigmented patches on the tongue and buccal mucous membrane. [melano- + G. *plax*, plate, plaque]

mel·a·no·pro·tein (mel′ă-nō-prō′tēn). A protein complex containing melanin.

mel·a·nor·rha·gia (mel′ă-nō-rā′jē-ă). SYN melena. [melano- + G. *rhēgnymi*, to burst forth]

mel·a·nor·rhea (mel′ă-nō-rē′ă). SYN melena. [melano- + G. *rhoia*, a flow]

mel·a·no·sis (mel-ă-nō′sis). Abnormal dark brown or brownblack pigmentation of various tissues or organs, as the result of melanin or, in some situations, other substances that resemble melanin to varying degrees; *e.g.,* m. of the skin may occur in widespread metastatic melanoma, sunburn, during pregnancy, and as a result of various diseases, infections, and other neoplasms. [melano- + G. -*osis*, condition]
m. circumscrip′ta precancero′sa, obsolete term for *lentigo* maligna.
m. co′li, m. of the large intestinal mucosa due to accumulation of pigment of uncertain composition within macrophages in the lamina propria.
m. cori′i degenerati′va, a congenital abnormality in which pigment is deposited in whorls and streaks; vesicles occasionally occur, and it may be associated with cardiac or neurologic disorders. Cf. *incontinentia* pigmenti, *incontinentia* pigmenti achromians.
neurocutaneous m., cutaneous giant pigmented nevi associated with m. of the leptomeninges; malignant melanomas may develop in the skin or meninges.
oculodermal m., pigmentation of the conjunctiva and skin around the eye, usually unilateral; seen especially in women of Oriental races. SYN Ota's nevus.
precancerous m. of Dubreuilh, obsolete term for *lentigo* maligna.
Riehl's m., a brown pigmentary condition of the exposed portions of the skin of the neck and face with melanin pigment in dermal macrophages, thought to result from photodermatitis due to materials, such as cosmetic ingredients, or oils encountered in various occupations.

mel·a·nos·i·ty (mel-ă-nos′i-tē). Darkness of complexion.

mel·a·no·some (mel′ă-nō-sōm). The generally oval pigment granule (0.2 by 0.6 μm) produced by melanocytes. SYN eumelanosome. [melano- + G. *sōma*, body]
giant m., a large spherical m. (1 to 6 μ in diameter) formed in the cytoplasm of melanocytes in café-au-lait spots and other melanocytic disorders. SYN macromelanosome.

mel·an·o·sta·tin. Inhibits synthesis and release of melanotropin. SYN melanotropin release-inhibiting hormone. [melanotropin + G. *states*, stationary, + -in]

mel·a·not·ic (mel′ă-not′ik). **1.** Pertaining to the presence, normal or pathologic, of melanin. **2.** Relating to or characterized by melanosis.

mel·a·no·ton·in (mel′ă-nō-tō-nin). SEE melatonin.

mel·a·not·ri·chous (mel-ă-not′ri-kŭs). Having black hair. SYN melanocomous. [melano- + G. *thrix* (*trich-*), hair]

mel·a·no·troph (mel′ă-nō-trōf). A cell of the intermediate lobe of the hypophysis that produces melanotropin. [melano- + G. *trophē*, nourishment]

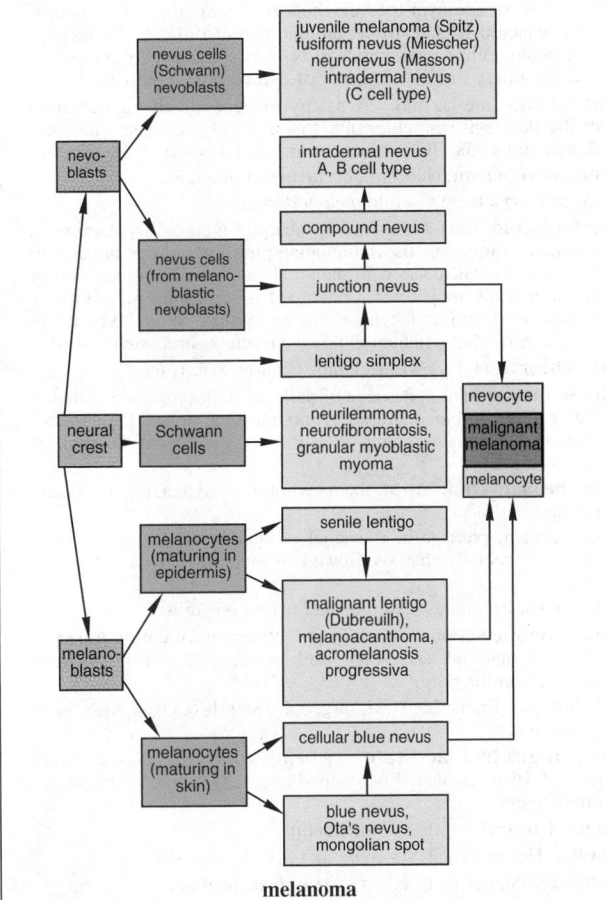

melanoma

me·la·no·tro·pin (mel′ă-nō-trōp-in). A polypeptide hormone secreted by the intermediate lobe of the hypophysis in humans (in neurohypophysis in certain other species) which causes dispersion of melanin by melanophores, resulting in darkening of the skin, presumably by promoting melanin synthesis; this effect is readily demonstated in some lower vertebrates, such as frogs and fish; α-m. is an *N*-acetylated peptide with 13 amino acids; β-m. has 22 amino acids. SYN intermedin, melanocyte-stimulating hormone, melanophore-expanding principle.

mel·a·nu·ria (mel-ă-nū′rē-ă). The excretion of urine of a dark color, resulting from the presence of melanin or other pigments or from the action of phenol, creosote, resorcin, and other coal tar derivatives. [melano- + G. *ouron*, urine]

mel·a·nu·ric (mel-ă-nū′rik). Pertaining to or characterized by melanuria.

mel·ar·so·prol (me-lar′sō-prol). 2-*p*-(4,6-Diamino-1,3,5-triazine-2-ylamino)phenyl-4-hydroxymethyl-1,3,2-dithioarsolan; used in the treatment of the meningoencephalitic stages of trypanosomiasis; may produce a fatal reactive encephalopathy.

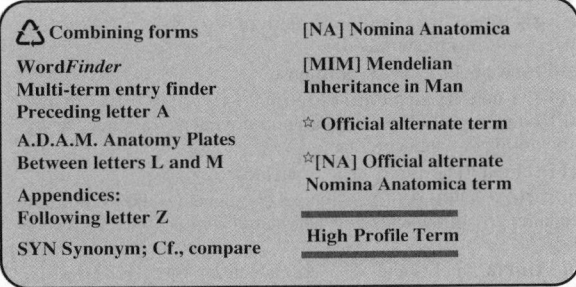

△ **Combining forms**	**[NA] Nomina Anatomica**
Word*Finder* Multi-term entry finder Preceding letter A	**[MIM] Mendelian Inheritance in Man**
A.D.A.M. Anatomy Plates Between letters L and M	☆ **Official alternate term**
Appendices: Following letter Z	☆**[NA] Official alternate Nomina Anatomica term**
SYN Synonym; Cf., compare	**High Profile Term**

me

MELAS An acronym for mitochondrial myopathy, encephalopathy, lactacidosis, and stroke; an inherited disorder of the respiratory chain, either a deficiency of NADH:ubiquinone oxidoreductase (complex I of the chain) or of cytochrome *c* oxidase.

me·las·ma (mĕ-laz′mă). A patchy or generalized pigmentation of the skin. SEE ALSO chloasma. SYN mask of pregnancy, melanoderma chloasma. [G. a black color, a black spot]

m. gravida′rum, chloasma occurring in pregnancy.

m. universa′le, SYN senile *melanoderma.*

mel·a·ton·in (mel-ă-tōn′in). *N*-Acetyl-5-methoxytryptamine; a substance formed by the mammalian pineal gland that appears to depress gonadal function in mammals and causes contraction of amphibian melanophores; a precursor is serotonin; m. is rapidly metabolized and is taken up by all tissues; it is involved in circadian rhythms. [melanophore + G. *tonos,* stretching, + -in]

Melchior. SEE Dyggve-Melchior-Clausen *syndrome.*

me·le·na (me-lē′nă). Passage of dark-colored, tarry stools, due to the presence of blood altered by the intestinal juices. Cf. hematochezia. SYN melanorrhagia, melanorrhea. [G. *melaina,* fem. of *melas,* black]

m. neonato′rum, m. of the newborn; m. occurring in young infants.

m. spu′ria, passage in the stool of blood that has been swallowed, especially that swallowed by nurslings from a fissured nipple.

m. ve′ra, true m. as distinguished from m. spuria.

mel·e·nem·e·sis (mel-ĕ-nem′ĕ-sis). Vomiting of dark-colored or blackish material. SEE ALSO black *vomit.* [G. *melas,* black, + *emesis,* vomiting]

Meleney, Frank L., U.S. surgeon, 1889–1963. SEE M.'s *gangrene, ulcer.*

mel·en·ges·trol ac·e·tate (mel-en-jes′trōl). 17α-Acetoxy-6-methyl-16-methylene-4,6-pregnadiene-3,20-dione; a progestational agent.

mel·e·tin (mel′ĕ-tin). SYN quercetin.

⚲meli-. Honey, sugar. SEE ALSO mel- (3). [G. *meli*]

mel·i·bi·ase (mel-i-bī′ās). SYN α-D-galactosidase.

mel·i·bi·ose (mel-i-bī′ōs). 6-*O*-α-D-Galactopyranosyl-D-glucose; a disaccharide formed by the hydrolysis of raffinose by β-fructofuranosidase; also present in plant juices.

mel·i·ce·ra, mel·i·ce·ris (mel-i-sē′ră, mel-i-sē′ris). A hygroma or other type of cyst that contains a relatively thick, tenacious, semifluid material. [G. *meli- kēris,* a tumor, fr. *melikēron,* honeycomb, fr. *meli,* honey, + *kēros,* wax]

mel·i·oi·do·sis (mel′ē-oy-dō′sis). An infectious disease of rodents in India and Southeast Asia that is caused by *Pseudomonas pseudomallei* and is communicable to humans. The characteristic lesion is a small caseous nodule, found generally throughout the body, which breaks down into an abscess; symptoms vary according to the tracts or organs involved. SYN pseudoglanders, Whitmore's disease. [G. *mēlis,* a distemper of asses, + *eidos,* resemblance, + -*osis,* condition]

me·lis·sa (me-lis′ă). The leaves from the tops of *Melissa officinalis* (family Labiatae), a plant of southern Europe; a diaphoretic. SYN sweet balm. [G. a bee]

me·lis·sic ac·id (me-lis′ik). Found in waxes. [G. *melissa,* bee + -ic]

me·lis·so·pho·bia (mĕ-lis′ō-fō′bē-ă). SYN apiphobia. [G. *melissa,* bee, + *phobos,* fear]

me·li·tis (mē-lī′tis). Inflammation of the cheek. [G. *mēlon,* cheek, + -*itis,* inflammation]

mel·i·tose (mel′i-tōs). SYN raffinose.

mel·i·tra·cen hy·dro·chlo·ride (mel-i-trā′sen). 9,10-Dihydro-10,10-dimethyl-9-(3-dimethylaminopropylidene) anthracene hydrochloride; an antidepressant.

mel·i·tri·ose (mel-i-trī′ōs). SYN raffinose.

mel·it·tin (mel′i-tin). The principal component in bee venom; m. contains 26 amino acids and is a hemolysin. [G. *melitta,* bee, + -in]

mel·i·tu·ria (mel-i-tū′rē-ă). Obsolete term for glycosuria. [G. *meli,* honey, + *ouron,* urine]

Melkersson, Ernst G., Swedish physician, 1898–1932. SEE M.-Rosenthal *syndrome.*

mel·li·tum, gen. **mel·li·ti,** pl. **mel·li·ta** (me-lī′tŭm, -tī, tă). A pharmaceutical preparation with honey as an excipient. [L. neut. of *mellitus,* honeyed]

Melnick, John C., U.S. radiologist, *1928. SEE M.-Needles *syndrome.*

⚲melo-. SEE mel-.

mel·o·cer·vi·co·plas·ty (mel-ō-ser′vi-kō-plas-tē). Plastic surgery of the cheek and neck. [melo- + L. *cervix,* neck, + G. *plastos,* formed]

mel·o·did·y·mus (mel′ō-did′ĭ-mus). A fetus with a supernumerary limb. [melo- + G. *didymos,* twin]

mel·o·ma·nia (mel-ō-mā′nē-ă). An abnormal fascination with or devotion to music. [L. *melos,* song + *mania,* frenzy]

mel·o·me·lia (mel-ō-mē′lē-ă). A malformation in which the fetus has one or more rudimentary limbs in addition to the normal limbs. Cf. micromelia. [G. *melos,* limb]

me·lon·o·plas·ty (mē′lon-ō-plas-tē). Obsolete spelling for meloplasty. [G. *mēlon,* cheek, + *plastos,* formed]

Me·loph·a·gus (mē-lof′ă-gŭs). A genus of louse flies (family Hippoboscidae) that includes the ectoparasite of sheep, *M. ovinus.* SEE ALSO *Hippobosca.* [G. *mēlon,* sheep, + *phagein,* to eat]

M. ovi′nus, a wingless, flattened, hairy, leathery parasitic fly found in the wool of sheep and on goats; it is widespread in sheep, in which it sucks blood and causes much skin irritation. SYN ked.

mel·o·plas·ty (mel′ō-plas-tē). Plastic surgery of the cheek. [melo- + G. *plastos,* formed]

mel·o·rhe·os·to·sis (mel′ō-rē-os-tō′sis). Rheostosis confined to the long bones. SYN osteosis eburnisans monomelica. [G. *melos,* limb, + *rheos,* stream, + *osteon,* bone, + -*ōsis*]

mel·o·sal·gia (mel-ō-sal′jē-ă). Pain in the lower limbs. [G. *melos,* limb, + *algos,* pain]

me·los·chi·sis (me-los′ki-sis). Congenital cleft in the face. [G. *mēlon,* cheek, + *schisis,* a cleaving]

me·lo·tia (me-lō′shē-ă). Congenital displacement of the auricle onto the cheek. [G. *mēlon,* cheek, + *ous,* ear]

mel·pha·lan (mel′fă-lan). L-Phenylalanine mustard; L-sarcolysine; L-3-[*p*-[*bis*(2-chloroethyl)amino]phenyl]alanine; a phenylalanine derivative of nitrogen mustard; an alkalylating antineoplastic agent.

Meltzer, Samuel J., U.S. physiologist, 1851–1920. SEE M.'s *law;* M.-Lyon *test.*

MEM Abbreviation for Eagle's minimum essential *medium.*

mem·ber. A limb. [L. *membrum*]

virile m., obsolete term for penis.

mem·bra (mem′bră) [NA]. Plural of membrum. [L.]

MEMBRANA

mem·bra·na, gen. and pl. **mem·bra·nae** (mem-brā′nă, -brā′nē) [NA]. SYN biomembrane. [L.]

m. abdom′inis, SYN peritoneum.

m. adamanti′na, SYN enamel *cuticle.*

m. adventi′tia, (1) SYN adventitia. (2) SYN *decidua* capsularis.

m. atlanto-occipita′lis ante′rior [NA], SYN anterior atlanto-occipital *membrane.*

m. atlanto-occipita′lis poste′rior [NA], SYN posterior atlanto-occipital *membrane.*

m. basa′lis duc′tus semicircula′ris [NA], SYN basal *membrane* of semicircular duct.

m. basila′ris, SYN basilar *membrane.*

m. capsula′ris, the hyaloid vascular network around the posterior pole of the lens in the embryo.

m. capsulopupilla′ris, the lateral portion of the vascular tunic of the lens of the eye in the embryo.

m. carno′sa, SYN dartos *fascia.*

m. cer′ebri, any one of the cerebral meninges.

m. choriocapilla′ris, SYN choriocapillary *layer.*

m. cor′dis, SYN pericardium.

m. cricothyroi′dea, SYN cricothyroid *membrane.*

m. decid′ua [NA], SYN deciduous *membrane.*

m. e′boris, the lining membrane of the pulp cavity of a tooth, consisting of the odontoblastic layer. SYN ivory membrane.

m. fibroelas′tica laryn′gis [NA], SYN fibroelastic *membrane* of larynx.

m. fibro′sa [NA], SYN fibrous articular *capsule.*

m. flac′cida, SYN flaccid *part* of tympanic membrane.

m. fus′ca, SYN *lamina* fusca of sclera.

m. germinati′va, SYN blastoderm.

m. granulo′sa, SYN *stratum* granulosum folliculi ovarici vesiculosi.

m. hyaloi′dea, SYN posterior limiting *layer* of cornea.

m. hyothyroi′dea, SYN thyrohyoid *membrane.*

membran′ae intercosta′lia [NA], SYN intercostal *membranes,* under *membrane.*

m. intercosta′lis exter′na [NA], SYN external intercostal *membrane.*

m. intercosta′lis inter′na [NA], SYN internal intercostal *membrane.*

m. interos′sea antebra′chii [NA], SYN interosseous *membrane* of forearm.

m. interos′sea cru′ris [NA], SYN interosseous *membrane* of leg.

m. lim′itans, (1) SYN limiting *membrane* of retina. **(2)** limiting membrane separating the neural parenchyma from the pia and blood vessels.

m. lim′itans gli′ae, SYN glial limiting *membrane.*

m. muco′sa, SYN mucosa.

m. nic′titans, SYN *plica* semilunaris conjunctivae (2).

m. obturato′ria [NA], SYN obturator *membrane.*

m. perine′i [NA], SYN inferior *fascia* of urogenital diaphragm.

m. pituito′sa, SYN nasal *mucosa.*

m. preformati′va, the thickened m. formed by fusion of Korff's fibers and the basement membrane of the ameloblasts in a developing tooth.

m. pro′pria duc′tus semicircula′ris [NA], SYN lamina *propria* of semicircular duct.

m. pupilla′ris [NA], SYN pupillary *membrane.*

m. quadrangula′ris [NA], SYN quadrangular *membrane.*

m. reticula′ris [NA], SYN reticular *membrane.*

m. sero′sa, (1) SYN serosa, chorion. **(2)** SYN serosa (2).

m. seroti′na, obsolete synonym of *decidua* basalis.

m. spira′lis [NA], ⭐official alternate term for tympanic *wall* of cochlear duct, tympanic *wall* of cochlear duct.

m. stape′dis [NA], SYN stapedial *membrane.*

m. statoconio′rum [NA], SYN statoconial *membrane.*

m. ster′ni [NA], SYN sternal *membrane.*

m. stria′ta, SYN *zona* striata.

m. succin′gens, SYN pleura. [L. *succingere,* to surround]

m. suprapleura′lis [NA], SYN suprapleural *membrane.*

m. synovia′lis [NA], SYN synovial *membrane.*

m. tecto′ria [NA], SYN tectorial *membrane.*

m. tecto′ria duc′tus cochlea′ris [NA], SYN tectorial *membrane* of cochlear duct.

m. ten′sa, SYN tense *part* of the tympanic membrane.

m. thyrohyoi′dea [NA], SYN thyrohyoid *membrane.*

m. tym′pani [NA], SYN tympanic *membrane.*

m. tym′pani secunda′ria [NA], SYN secondary tympanic *membrane.*

m. versic′olor, SYN tapetum (2).

m. vestibula′ris [NA], SYN vestibular *membrane.*

m. vi′brans, SYN tense *part* of the tympanic membrane.

m. vitelli′na, (1) the membrane enveloping the yolk; specifically,

the thickened cell membrane of large-yolked ova; SYN ovular membrane, vitelline membrane. **(2)** sometimes used to designate the zona pellucida of a mammalian ovum. SYN yolk membrane.

m. vit′rea [NA], SYN posterior limiting *layer* of cornea.

---

mem·bra·na·ceous (mem-bră-nā′shŭs). SYN membranous.

mem·bra·nate (mem′bră-nāt). Of the nature of a membrane.

MEMBRANE

---

mem·brane (mem′brān). **1.** A thin sheet or layer of pliable tissue, serving as a covering or envelope of a part, as the lining of a cavity, as a partition or septum, or to connect two structures. **2.** SYN biomembrane. [L. *membrana,* a skin or membrane that covers parts of the body, fr. *membrum,* a member]

adamantine m., SYN enamel *cuticle.*

allantoid m., SYN allantois.

alveolocapillary m., the pulmonary diffusion barrier.

alveolodental m., SYN periodontal *ligament.*

anal m., the dorsal portion of the embryonic cloacal m. after its division by the urorectal septum.

anterior atlanto-occipital m., the fibrous layer that extends from the anterior arch of the atlas to the anterior margin of the foramen magnum. SYN membrana atlanto-occipitalis anterior [NA].

arachnoid m., SYN arachnoid.

atlanto-occipital m., SEE anterior atlanto-occipital m., posterior atlanto-occipital m.

basal m. of semicircular duct, the basal m. underlying the epithelium of the semicircular duct. SYN membrana basalis ductus semicircularis [NA], basal lamina of semicircular duct.

basement m., an amorphous extracellular layer closely applied to the basal surface of epithelium and also investing muscle cells, fat cells, and Schwann cells; thought to be a selective filter and to serve both structural and morphogenetic functions. It is composed of three successive layers (lamina lucida, lamina densa, and lamina fibroreticularis), a matrix of collagen (of which type IV is unique to this membrane), and several glycoproteins. SYN basement lamina, basilemma.

basilar m., the m. extending from the bony spiral m. to the basilar crest of the cochlea; it forms the greater part of the floor of the cochlear duct separating the latter from the scala tympani and it supports the organ of Corti. SYN lamina basilaris cochleae [NA], basal lamina of cochlear, basilar lamina, membrana basilaris.

Bichat's m., the inner elastic m. of arteries.

Bogros' serous m., a m. of the episcleral space (of Tenon).

Bowman's m., SYN anterior limiting *layer* of cornea.

Bruch's m., SYN *lamina* basalis choroideae.

Brunn's m., the epithelium of the olfactory region of the nose.

bucconasal m., a thin, transient epithelial sheet separating the primitive nasal cavity from the stomodeum in the seven-week-old human embryo. SYN oronasal m.

buccopharyngeal m., a bilaminar (ectoderm and endoderm) m. derived from the prochordal plate; after the embryonic head fold has evolved it lies at the caudal limit of the stomodeum. SYN oral m., oropharyngeal m.

cell m., the protoplasmic boundary of all cells that controls permeability and may serve other functions through surface specializations; *e.g.,* active ion transport absorption by formation of pinocytotic vesicles; receptor-mediated antigen recognition, etc..; its fine structure is trilaminar and consists of the electron-dense lamina externa and lamina interna with an electron-lucent lamina intermedia. SYN cytolemma, cytomembrane, plasma m., plasmalemma, plasmolemma, Wachendorf's m. (2).

chorioallantoic m., extraembryonic m. formed by fusion of chorion and allantois.

cloacal m., a transitory m. in the caudal area of the ventral wall

me

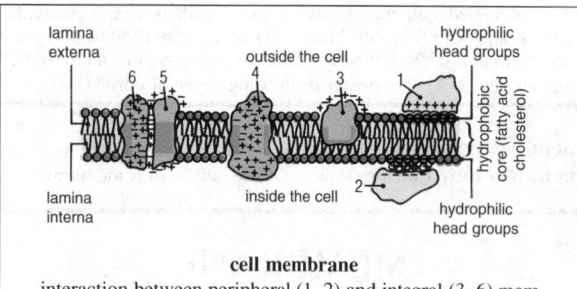

cell membrane

interaction between peripheral (1, 2) and integral (3–6) membrane proteins on the one hand, and the lipid phase on the other

of the embryo, separating the endodermal from the ectodermal cloaca; it is divided into anal and genitourinary m.'s that break down during the eighth to ninth week to establish the external opening for the alimentary and genitourinary tracts.

closing m.'s, thin sheets, composed of ectoderm externally and endoderm internally, which separate the pharyngeal pouches from the overlying branchial clefts in the early embryo. SYN pharyngeal m.'s.

Corti's m., SYN tectorial m. of cochlear duct.

cricothyroid m., one of the bilateral m.'s extending between arch and the inferior edge of the thyroid lamina one each side of the midline, occupied by the thicker cricothyroid ligament. SEE ALSO *conus* elasticus, cricothyroid *ligament.* SYN membrana cricothyroidea.

cricotracheal m., SYN cricotracheal *ligament.*

cricovocal m., SYN *conus* elasticus (1).

croupous m., SYN false m.

deciduous m., the mucous m. of the pregnant uterus that has already undergone certain changes, under the influence of the ovulation cycle, to fit it for the implantation and nutrition of the ovum; so-called because the m. is cast off after labor. SYN membrana decidua [NA], caduca, decidua, Hunter's m.

Descemet's m., SYN posterior limiting *layer* of cornea.

diphtheritic m., the false m. forming on the mucous surfaces in diphtheria.

double m., two biomembrane layers, with an intermembranal space, surrounding certain organelles (*e.g.,* mitochondria) or structures.

drum m., SYN tympanic m.

Duddell's m., SYN posterior limiting *layer* of cornea.

dysmenorrheal m., a m., resembling the decidua, cast off in cases of membranous dysmenorrhea.

egg m., the investing envelope of the ovum; a **primary egg m.** is produced from ovarian cytoplasm (*e.g.,* a vitelline m.); a **secondary egg m.** is the product of the ovarian follicle (*e.g.,* the zona pellucida); a **tertiary egg m.** is secreted by the lining of the oviduct (*e.g.,* a shell).

elastic m., a m. formed of elastic connective tissue, present as fenestrated lamellae in the coats of the arteries and elsewhere.

embryonic m., SYN fetal m.

enamel m., the internal layer of the enamel organ formed by the enamel cells.

epipapillary m., (1) a congenital m. covering the optic disk; (2) the glial remnants of Bergmeister's *papilla.*

epiretinal m., a m., usually acquired, covering a portion of the retina and composed of fibrous tissue from metaplasia of retinal pigment epithelial cells or glia.

exocelomic m., a layer of cells delaminated from the inner surface of the blastocystic cytotrophoblast and from the envelope of the primary yolk sac during the second week of embryonic life. SYN Heuser's m.

external intercostal m., the m. that replaces the external intercostal muscle anteriorly between costal cartilages. SYN membrana intercostalis externa [NA].

extraembryonic m., SYN fetal m.

false m., a thick, tough fibrinous exudate on the surface of a mucous m. or the skin, as seen in diphtheria. SYN croupous m., neomembrane, plica (2), pseudomembrane.

fenestrated m., an elastic m., as in elastic laminae of arteries.

fertilization m., a viscous m. formed on the inner surface of the vitelline m. from the cytoplasm of the egg cell after entry of the sperm, preventing the entry of additional sperm.

fetal m., a structure or tissue that develops from the fertilized ovum but does not form part of the embryo proper. SYN embryonic m., extraembryonic m.

fibroelastic m. of larynx, a layer of fibrous and elastic fibers, taking the place of the submucosa in the larynx. It is divided by the laryngeal ventricle into two parts: the quadrangular m. superiorly and the *conus* elasticus (1) inferiorly. SYN membrana fibroelastica laryngis [NA].

fibrous m., SYN fibrous articular *capsule.*

Fielding's m., SYN tapetum (2).

flaccid m., SYN flaccid *part* of tympanic membrane.

germ m., germinal m., SYN blastoderm.

glassy m., (1) the basement m. present between the stratum granulosum and the theca interna of a vesicular ovarian follicle; it becomes very prominent in large atretic follicles; (2) the basement m. and associated connective tissue of the hair follicle. SYN hyaline m. (2).

glial limiting m., a dense, resilient m. forming the true capsule of the brain and spinal cord, composed of the processes of astrocytes (macroglia cells) and covered throughout by the pia mater, which firmly adheres to it; the two m.'s are collectively called the pial-glial m. SYN membrana limitans gliae.

Henle's m., SYN *lamina* basalis choroideae.

Henle's fenestrated elastic m., SYN elastic *laminae* of arteries, under *lamina.*

Heuser's m., SYN exocelomic m.

Hunter's m., SYN deciduous m.

Huxley's m., SYN Huxley's *layer.*

hyaline m., (1) the thin, clear basement m. beneath certain epithelia; (2) SYN glassy m. (2).

hyaloid m., SYN posterior limiting *layer* of cornea.

hyoglossal m., posterior widening of the lingual septum connecting the root of the tongue to the hyoid bone; the inferior fibers of the genioglossus are attached to it and by this means to the upper anterior body of the hyoid bone near the midline.

inner m., the smaller of a double m.

intercostal m.'s, the membranous layers between ribs. SYN membranae intercostalia [NA], intercostal ligaments, ligamenta intercostalia.

internal intercostal m., the m. that replaces the internal intercostal muscle posteriorly, medial to the angles of the ribs. SYN membrana intercostalis interna [NA].

interosseous m. of forearm, the dense m. that connects the interosseous margins of the radius and ulna, forming the radioulnar syndesmosis, and with the bones separating the flexor and extensor compartments of the forearm. SYN membrana interossea antebrachii [NA].

interosseous m. of leg, the dense fibrous layer that connects the interosseous margins of the tibia and fibula, forming the upper portion of the tibiofibular syndesmosis and, with the bones and intermuscular septa, creating anterior and posterior comparments of the leg. SYN membrana interossea cruris [NA], ligamentum tibiofibulare medium.

ivory m., SYN *membrana* eboris.

Jackson's m., a thin vascular m. or veil-like adhesion, covering the anterior surface of the ascending colon from the cecum to the right flexure; it may cause obstruction by kinking of the bowel. SYN Jackson's veil.

keratogenous m., SYN nail *bed.*

limiting m. of retina, one of two layers of the retina: **internal limiting m.,** formed by the expanded inner ends of Müller's fibers; **outer limiting m.,** not a m. but a row of junctional complexes. SYN membrana limitans (1).

medullary m., SYN endosteum.

mitochondrial m., the double biomembrane surrounding the mitochondrion.

mucous m.'s, SYN mucosa.

mucous m. of tympanic cavity, SYN *mucosa* of tympanic cavity.

Nasmyth's m., SYN enamel *cuticle.*

nictitating m., SYN *plica* semilunaris conjunctivae (2).

Nitabuch's m., a layer of fibrin between the boundary zone of compact endometrium and the cytotrophoblastic shell in the placenta. SYN Nitabuch's layer, Nitabuch's stria.

nuclear m., SYN nuclear *envelope.*

obturator m., the thin m. of strong interlacing fibers filling the obturator foramen. SYN membrana obturatoria [NA].

olfactory m., that part of the nasal mucosa having olfactory receptor cells and glands of Bowman.

oral m., SYN buccopharyngeal m.

oronasal m., SYN bucconasal m.

oropharyngeal m., SYN buccopharyngeal m.

otolithic m., SYN statoconial m.

outer m., the larger of the two m.'s of a double m.

ovular m., SYN *membrana* vitellina (1).

Payr's m., a fold of peritoneum that crosses over the left flexure of the colon.

pericardiopleural m., SYN pleuropericardial *fold.*

peridental m., SYN periodontal *ligament.*

perineal m., SYN inferior *fascia* of urogenital diaphragm.

periodontal m., SYN periodontal *ligament.*

periorbital m., SYN periorbita.

pharyngeal m.'s, SYN closing m.'s.

pial-glial m., the dual outer lining of the brain and spinal cord, composed of the glial limiting m. and the pia mater.

pituitary m., SYN nasal *mucosa.*

placental m., the semipermeable layer of fetal tissue separating the maternal from the fetal blood in the placenta; composed of: 1) endothelium of the fetal vessels in the chorionic villi, 2) stromata of the villi, 3) cytotrophoblast (negligible after the fifth month of gestation), and 4) syncytial trophoblast covering the villi; the placental m. acts as a selective m. regulating passage of substances from the maternal to the fetal blood. SYN placental barrier.

plasma m., SYN cell m.

pleuropericardial m., SYN pleuropericardial *fold.*

pleuroperitoneal m., SYN pleuroperitoneal *fold.*

posterior atlanto-occipital m., the fibrous membrane that attaches between the posterior arch of the atlas and the posterior margin of the foramen magnum. SYN membrana atlanto-occipitalis posterior [NA].

postsynaptic m., that part of the plasma m. of a neuron or muscle fiber with which an axon terminal forms a synaptic junction; in many instances, at least part of such a small postsynaptic m. patch shows characteristic morphological modifications such as greater thickness and higher electron-density, believed to correspond to the transmitter-sensitive receptor site of such synapses.

presynaptic m., that part of the plasma m. of an axon terminal that faces the plasma m. of the neuron or muscle fiber with which the axon terminal establishes a synaptic junction; many synaptic junctions exhibit structural presynaptic characteristics, such as conical, electron-dense internal protrusions, that distinguish it from the remainder of the axon's plasma m. SEE ALSO synapse.

primary egg m., SEE egg m.

proligerous m., SYN *cumulus* oöphorus.

prophylactic m., SYN pyogenic m.

pupillary m., remnants of the central portion of the anterior layer of the iris stroma (the iridopupillary lamina) which occludes the pupil in fetal life, and normally atrophies about the seventh month of gestation. Persistent strands usually stretch across the pupil from one iris collarette to the other, without touching the pupillary margin. Failure to regress is a rare cause of congenital blindness. SYN membrana pupillaris [NA], Wachendorf's m. (1).

pyogenic m., a layer of pus cells lining an abscess cavity which have not yet autolyzed. SYN prophylactic m.

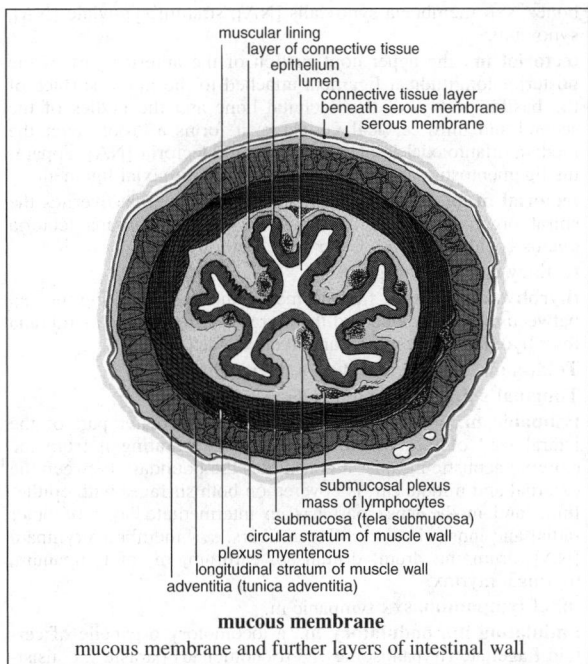

muscular lining
layer of connective tissue
epithelium
lumen
connective tissue layer
beneath serous membrane
serous membrane

submucosal plexus
mass of lymphocytes
submucosa (tela submucosa)
circular stratum of muscle wall
plexus myentencus
longitudinal stratum of muscle wall
adventitia (tunica adventitia)

mucous membrane
mucous membrane and further layers of intestinal wall

quadrangular m., the elastic fibra m. that extends from the ventricular fold of the larynx upward to the aryepiglottic fold; it attaches anteriorly to the epiglottis and posteriorly to the lateral margin of the arytenoid and corniculate cartilages. SYN membrana quadrangularis [NA], Tourtual's m.

Reissner's m., SYN vestibular m.

reticular m., the m. formed by cuticular plates of the cells of the spiral organ of Corti; it appears netlike when viewed from above. SYN membrana reticularis [NA].

Rivinus' m., SYN flaccid *part* of tympanic membrane.

Ruysch's m., SYN choriocapillary *layer.*

Scarpa's m., SYN secondary tympanic m.

schneiderian m., SYN nasal *mucosa.*

Schultze's m., SYN *region* of olfactory mucosa.

secondary egg m., SEE egg m.

secondary tympanic m., the m. closing the fenestra cochleae or rotunda. SYN membrana tympani secundaria [NA], Scarpa's m.

semipermeable m., a m. that is relatively permeable to the solvent but relatively impermeable to all or at least some of the solutes in either or both of the solutions separated by the m.

serous m., SYN serosa.

Shrapnell's m., SYN flaccid *part* of tympanic membrane.

spiral m., SYN tympanic *wall* of cochlear duct.

stapedial m., the delicate mucosal layer that bridges the space between the crura and base of the stapes. SYN membrana stapedis [NA].

statoconial m., a gelatinous m. supported by the hairs of the hair cells of the maculae of the saccule and utriculus of the inner ear; adhering to the surface are numerous crystalline particles called statoconia. SYN membrana statoconiorum [NA], otolithic m.

sternal m., interlacing fibers from the anterior costosternal ligaments covering the anterior surface of the sternum. SYN membrana sterni [NA].

striated m., SYN *zona* striata.

suprapleural m., the thickened portion of endothoracic fascia extending over the cupola of the pleura and reinforcing it; it attaches to the inner border of the first rib and to the transverse process of the seventh cervical vertebra. SYN membrana suprapleuralis [NA], Sibson's aponeurosis, Sibson's fascia.

synovial m., the connective tissue m. that lines the cavity of a synovial joint and produces the synovial fluid; it lines all internal surfaces of the cavity except for the articular cartilage of the

me

bones. SYN membrana synovialis [NA], stratum synoviale [NA], synovium.

tectorial m., the upper continuation of the anterior part of the posterior longitudinal ligament attached to the upper surface of the basilar portion of the occipital bone and the bodies of the second and third cervical vertebrae; it forms a "roof" over the median atlantoaxial joint. SYN membrana tectoria [NA], apparatus ligamentosus weitbrechti, posterior occipitoaxial ligament.

tectorial m. of cochlear duct, a gelatinous m. that overlies the spiral organ (Corti) in the inner ear. SYN membrana tectoria ductus cochlearis [NA], Corti's m., tectorium (2).

tertiary egg m., SEE egg m.

thyrohyoid m., a thin, fibrous, membranous sheet filling the gap between the hyoid bone and the thyroid cartilage. SYN membrana thyrohyoidea [NA], membrana hyothyroidea.

Toldt's m., the anterior layer of the renal fascia.

Tourtual's m., SYN quadrangular m.

tympanic m., a thin tense m. forming the greater part of the lateral wall of the tympanic cavity and separating it from the external acoustic meatus; it constitutes the boundary between the external and middle ear, is covered on both surfaces with epithelium, and in the tense part has an intermediate layer of outer radial and inner circular collagen fibers. SYN membrana tympani [NA], drum m., drum, drumhead, eardrum, m. of tympanum, myringa, myrinx.

m. of tympanum, SYN tympanic m.

undulating m., undulatory m., a locomotory organelle of certain flagellate (trypanosome and trichomonad) parasites, consisting of a finlike extension of the limiting m. with the flagellar sheath; wavelike rippling of the undulating m. produces a characteristic movement.

unit m., the trilaminar structure of the plasmalemma and other intercellular m.'s, when seen in cross-section with the electron microscope, composed of two electron-dense laminae approximately 20 Å thick separated by a less dense lamina 35 Å thick.

urogenital m., the ventral portion of the embryonic cloacal m. after its division by the urorectal septum.

urorectal m., in the embryo, urorectal septum separating the cloaca into urogenital sinus and rectum. SYN urorectal fold.

uteroepichorial m., rarely used term for *decidua* parietalis.

vaginal synovial m., SYN synovial tendon *sheath*.

vestibular m., the m. separating the cochlear duct from the vestibular canal; it consists of squamous epithelial cells with microvilli toward the ductus, a basement m., and a thin layer of connective tissue toward the scala. SYN membrana vestibularis [NA], paries vestibularis ductus cochlearis [NA], Reissner's m., vestibular wall of cochlear duct.

virginal m., obsolete term for hymen.

vitelline m., SYN *membrana* vitellina (1).

vitreous m., (1) SYN posterior limiting *layer* of cornea. **(2)** a condensation of fine collagen fibers in places in the cortex of the vitreous body; formerly thought to form a m. or capsule at its periphery; **(3)** SYN *lamina* basalis choroideae.

Wachendorf's m., (1) SYN pupillary m. **(2)** SYN cell m.

yolk m., SYN *membrana* vitellina.

Zinn's m., the anterior layer of the iris.

---

mem·bra·nec·to·my (mem-bră-nek'tō-mē). Removal of the membranes of a subdural hematoma. [membrane + G. *ektomē*, excision]

mem·bra·nelle (mem-bră-nel'). A minute membrane formed of fused cilia, found in certain ciliate protozoa.

mem·bra·ni·form (mem-brā'ni-fōrm). Of the appearance or character of a membrane. SYN membranoid.

mem·bra·no·car·ti·lag·i·nous (mem'bră-nō-kar-ti-laj'i-nŭs). **1.** Partly membranous and partly cartilaginous. **2.** Derived from both a mesenchymal membrane and cartilage; denoting certain bones.

mem·bra·noid (mem'bră-noyd). SYN membraniform.

mem·bra·nous (mem'bră-nŭs). Relating to or of the form of a membrane. SYN hymenoid (1), membranaceous.

mem·brum, pl. **mem·bra** (mem'brŭm, mem'bră) [NA]. A limb; a member. [L. member]

m. infe'rius [NA], SYN lower *limb*.

m. mulieb're, obsolete term for clitoris.

m. supe'rius [NA], SYN upper *limb*.

m. vir'ile, SYN penis.

mem·o·ry (mem'ŏ-rē). **1.** General term for the recollection of that which was once experienced or learned. **2.** The mental information processing system that receives (registers), modifies, stores, and retrieves informational stimuli; composed of three stages: encoding, storage, and retrieval. [L. *memoria*]

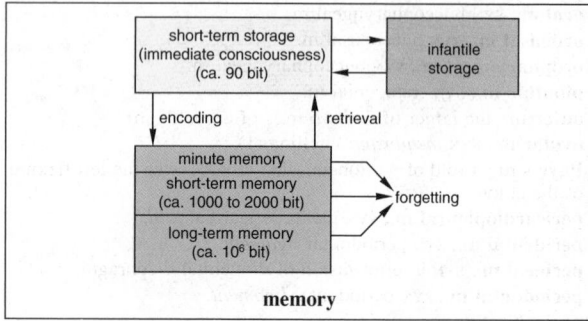

memory

affect m., the emotional element recurring whenever a significant experience is recalled.

anterograde m., m. for that which occurred after an event such as a brain injury.

long-term m. (LTM), that phase of the m. process considered the permanent storehouse of information which has been registered, encoded, passed into the short-term m., coded, rehearsed, and finally transferred and stored for future retrieval; material and information retained in LTM underlies cognitive abilities.

remote m., m. for events of long ago as opposed to recent events.

retrograde m., m. for that which occurred before an event such as a brain injury.

screen m., in psychoanalysis, a consciously tolerable m. that unwittingly serves as a cover for another associated m. which would be emotionally painful if recalled.

selective m., reception or retrieval of only some of the events in an experience.

senile m., m. that is good for remote events, often in contrast to current events; characteristically seen in aged or demented persons.

short-term m. (STM), that phase of the m. process in which stimuli that have been recognized and registered are stored briefly; decay occurs rapidly, typically within seconds, but may be held indefinitely by using rehearsal as a holding process by which to recycle material over and over through STM. SYN temporary m.

subconscious m., information not immediately available for recall.

temporary m., SYN short-term m.

mem·o·tine hy·dro·chlo·ride (mem'ō-tēn). 3,4-Dihydro-1-[(*p*-methoxyphenoxy)methyl]isoquinoline hydrochloride; an antiviral drug.

men·ac·me (me-nak'mē). The period of menstrual activity in a woman's life. [G. *mēn*, month, + *akmē*, prime]

men·a·di·ol di·ac·e·tate (men-ă-dī'ol). 2-Methyl-1,4-naphthohydroquinone diacetate; menadiol acetylated at both OH groups; a prothrombogenic vitamin. SYN acetomenaphthone, vitamin K_4.

men·a·di·ol so·di·um di·phos·phate. Tetrasodium 2-methyl-1,4-naphthalenediol-bis(dihydrogen phosphate); a dihydro derivative of menadione, with similar vitamin K activity.

men·a·di·one (men-ă-dī'ōn). 2-Methyl-1,4-naphthoquinone; the root of compounds that are 3-multiprenyl derivatives of m. and known as the menaquinones or vitamins K_2. SYN menaphthone, menaquinone, vitamin K_3.

m. reductase, SYN NADPH dehydrogenase (quinone).

m. sodium bisulfite, it possesses the same action and is used for the same purposes as m. or vitamin K; it differs, however, from m. in being water-soluble.

men·aph·thone (men-ă-naf′thōn). SYN menadione.

men·a·quin·one (MK) (men′ă-kwin′ōn, -kwī′nōn). SYN menadione.

men·a·quin·one-6 (MK-6). Hexaprenylmenaquinone; prenylmenaquinone-6; 2-methyl-3-hexaprenyl-1,4-naphthoquinone; isolated from putrified fish meal; potency is about 60% of that of phylloquinone (vitamin K_1). SYN farnoquinone, vitamin K_2, vitamin $K_2(30)$.

men·a·quin·one-7 (MK-7). Menaquinone-6 with a 3-heptaprenyl side chain. SYN vitamin $K_2(35)$.

men·ar·che (me-nar′kē). Establishment of the menstrual function; the time of the first menstrual period. [G. *mēn,* month, + *archē,* beginning]

men·ar·che·al, men·ar·chi·al (me-nar′kē-ăl). Pertaining to the menarche.

Mendel, Gregor J., Austrian geneticist, 1822–1884. SEE mendelian *character;* mendelian *inheritance;* mendelian *ratio;* M.'s first *law,* second *law.*

Mendel, Kurt, German neurologist, 1874–1946. SEE M.'s instep *reflex;* Bechterew-M. *reflex.*

Mendeléeff (Mendeleev), Dimitri (Dmitri) I., Russian chemist, 1834–1907. SEE mendelevium; M.'s *law.*

men·de·le·vi·um (Md, Mv) (men-dĕ-lē′vē-ŭm). An element, atomic no. 101, atomic wt. 258.1, prepared in 1955 by bombardment of einsteinium with alpha particles. [*D. Mendeléeff*]

men·de·li·an (men-dē′lē-ăn). Attributed to or described by Gregor Mendel; usually referring to the behavior and the mechanism of the genetic transmission of single-locus traits.

Men·de·li·an In·her·i·tance in Man. A standard, comprehensive, perpetually updated reference source for traits in humans that have been shown to be mendelian or that are thought on reasonable grounds to be so. Each entry has a six-digit catalog number. Those securely established (by molecular biology or by extensive clinical studies) are marked with an asterisk.

men·del·ism (men′del-izm). The hereditary principles of unilocal traits derived from Mendel's laws.

men·del·iz·ing (men′del-īz-ing). Denoting a pattern of inheritance of a trait that corresponds phenotypically to the segregation of known or putative genes at one genetic locus.

Mendelson, Curtis L., U.S. physician, *1913. SEE M.'s *syndrome.*

Ménétrier, Pierre E., French physician, 1859–1935. SEE M.'s *disease, syndrome.*

Menge, Karl, German gynecologist, 1864–1945. SEE M.'s *pessary.*

Ménière, Prosper, French physician, 1799–1862. SEE M.'s *disease, syndrome.*

⌂mening-. SEE meningo-.

me·nin·ge·al (mĕ-nin′jē-ăl, men′in-jē′ăl). Relating to the meninges.

me·nin·ge·o·cor·ti·cal (mĕ-nin′jē-ō-kōr′ti-kăl). SYN meningocortical.

me·nin·ge·or·rha·phy (mĕ-nin′jē-ōr′ă-fē). Suture of the cranial or spinal meninges or of any membrane. [G. *mēninx (mēning-),* membrane, + *rhaphē,* suture]

me·nin·ges (mĕ-nin′jēz). Plural of meninx.

me·nin·gi·o·an·gi·o·ma·to·sis (mĕ-nin′jē-ō-an′jē-ō-mă-tō-sis). Proliferation of vessels and meningothelial cells, associated with epilepsy and neurofibromatosis.

me·nin·gi·o·ma (mĕ-nin′jē-ō′mă). A benign, encapsulated neoplasm of arachnoidal origin, occurring most frequently in adults; most frequent form consists of elongated, fusiform cells in whorls and pseudolobules with psammoma bodies frequently present; m.'s tend to occur along the superior sagittal sinus, along the sphenoid ridge, or in the vicinity of the optic chiasm; in

addition to meningothelial m., angiomatous, chondromatous, osteomatous, lipomatous, melanotic, fibroblastic and transitional varieties are recognized. [mening- + G. *-oma,* tumor]

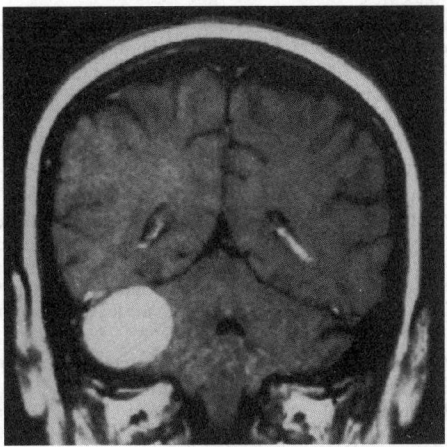

meningioma
meningioma in the cerebellopontine angle (MRI, after injection of contrast medium)

cutaneous m., a lesion in the skin and subcutis composed of meningeal cells; occurs as a developmental lesion in children or as an extension of an intracranial m. in adults.

malignant m., m. that either invades brain parenchyma or metastasizes.

psammomatous m., a firm cellular neoplasm derived from fibrous tissue of the meninges, choroid plexus, and certain other structures associated with the brain, characterized by the formation of multiple, discrete, concentrically laminated, calcareous bodies (psammoma bodies); most of these neoplasms are histologically benign, but may lead to severe symptoms as a result of compressing the brain. SYN angiolithic sarcoma, sand tumor, Virchow's psammoma.

me·nin·gi·o·ma·to·sis (mĕ-nin′jē-ō-mă-tō′sis). The presence of multiple meningiomas, sometimes seen in von Recklinghausen's disease.

me·nin·gism (men′in-jizm, mĕ-nin′jizm). A condition in which the symptoms simulate a meningitis, but in which no actual inflammation of these membranes is present. SYN pseudomeningitis.

men·in·git·ic (men′in-jit′ik). Relating to or characterized by meningitis.

men·in·gi·tis, pl. **men·in·git·i·des** (men-in-jī′tis, -jit′i-dēz; -jit′i-dēz). Inflammation of the membranes of the brain or spinal cord. SEE ALSO arachnoiditis, leptomeningitis. SYN cerebrospinal m. [mening- + G. *itis,* inflammation]

basilar m., m. at the base of the brain, due usually to tuberculosis, syphilis, or any low-grade chronic granulomatous process; may result in an internal hydrocephalus.

cerebrospinal m., SYN meningitis.

eosinophilic m., SYN angiostrongylosis.

epidemic cerebrospinal m., SYN meningococcal m.

epidural m., SYN *pachymeningitis* externa.

external m., SYN *pachymeningitis* externa.

internal m., SYN *pachymeningitis* interna.

listeria m., SYN listeriosis.

meningococcal m., an acute infectious disease affecting children and young adults, caused by *Neisseria meningitidis;* characterized by nasopharyngeal catarrh, headache, vomiting, convulsions, stiffness in the neck (nuchal rigidity), photophobia, constipation, cutaneous hyperesthesia, a purpuric or herpetic eruption, and the presence of Kernig's sign. Fulminant form may cause

me

Waterhouse-Friderichsen syndrome. SYN cerebrospinal fever, epidemic cerebrospinal m.

Mollaret's m., a recurrent aseptic m.; febrile illness accompanied by headaches, malaise, meningeal signs, and cerebrospinal fluid monocytes.

neoplastic m., infiltration of subarachnoid space by neoplastic cells, typically medulloblastoma or metastatic carcinoma. SYN neoplastic arachnoiditis.

occlusive m., leptomeningitis causing occlusion of the spinal fluid pathways.

otitic m., infection of the meninges secondary to mastoiditis or otitis media.

serous m., acute m. with secondary external hydrocephalus.

tuberculous m., inflammation of the cerebral leptomeninges marked by the presence of granulomatous inflammation; it is usually confined to the base of the brain (basilar m., internal hydrocephalus) and is accompanied in children by an accumulation of spinal fluid in the ventricles (acute hydrocephalus). SYN cerebral tuberculosis (1).

△**meningo-, mening-.** The meninges. [G. *mēninx*, membrane]

me·nin·go·cele (mĕ-ning′gō-sēl). Protrusion of the membranes of the brain or spinal cord through a defect in the skull or spinal column. [meningo- + G. *kēlē*, tumor]

spurious m., an extracranial or extraspinal accumulation of cerebrospinal fluid, due to meningeal tear. SYN traumatic m.

traumatic m., SYN spurious m.

me·nin·go·coc·ce·mia (mĕ-ning′gō-kok-sē′mē-ă). Presence of meningococci (*N. meningitidis*) in the circulating blood.

acute fulminating m., rapidly moving systemic infection with *Neisseria meningitidis*, usually without meningitis, characterized by rash, usually petechial or purpuric, high fever, and hypotension. May lead to death within hours.

me·nin·go·coc·cus, pl. **me·nin·go·coc·ci** (mĕ-ning′gō-kok′ŭs, -kok′sī). SYN *Neisseria meningitidis.* [meningo- + G. *kokkos*, berry]

me·nin·go·cor·ti·cal (mĕ-ning′gō-kōr′ti-kăl). Relating to the meninges and the cortex of the brain. SYN meningeocortical.

me·nin·go·cyte (mĕ-ning′gō-sīt). A mesenchymal epithelial cell of the subarachnoid space; it may become a macrophage. [meningo- + G. *kytos*, cell]

me·nin·go·en·ceph·a·li·tis (mĕ-ning′gō-en-sef′ăl-ī′tis). An inflammation of the brain and its membranes. SYN cerebromeningitis, encephalomeningitis. [meningo- + G. *enkephalos*, brain, + *-itis*, inflammation]

acute primary hemorrhagic m., SYN acute epidemic *leukoencephalitis.*

biundulant m., SYN tick-borne *encephalitis* (Central European subtype).

chronic progressive syphilitic m., SYN paretic *neurosyphilis.*

eosinophilic m., a disease caused by infection with the rat lungworm, *Angiostrongylus cantonensis,* whose larvae, ingested with infected slugs or land snails (or some unidentified transport host), migrate from intestine to the meninges of the brain where the disease is produced; it is usually mild, of short duration, and characterized by fever, eosinophilia, and white blood cells (rarely nematode larvae) in the spinal fluid.

herpetic m., a severe form of m. caused by herpesvirus type 1 and associated with a high mortality rate; definite diagnosis depends upon isolation of the virus or demonstration of viral antigens.

mumps m., a usually benign nervous system infection arising during the active phase of clinical mumps parotiditis.

primary amebic m., an invasive, rapidly fatal cerebral infection by soil amebae, chiefly *Naegleria fowleri,* found in man and other primates and experimentally in rodents; the disease is characterized by a high fever, neck rigidity, and symptoms associated with upper respiratory infection such as cough and nausea; although organisms have been cultured from various organs, the brain is the primary focus, especially the olfactory lobes and cerebral cortex, which are first attacked by the amebae that enter from nasal mucosa through the cribriform plate; death usually occurs two to three days after onset of symptoms.

syphilitic m., a secondary or tertiary stage manifestation of syphilis; rarely fatal.

thromboembolic m., an acute septicemic disease of cattle caused by the bacterium *Haemophilus somnus* and characterized by fever, severe depression, ataxia, blindness, coma, and rapid death.

me·nin·go·en·ceph·a·lo·cele (mĕ-ning′gō-en-sef′ă-lō-sēl). A protrusion of the meninges and brain through a congenital defect in the cranium, usually in the frontal or occipital region. SYN encephalomeningocele. [meningo- + G. *enkephalos*, brain, + *kēlē*, hernia]

me·nin·go·en·ceph·a·lo·my·e·li·tis (mĕ-ning′gō-en-sef′ă-lō-mī-ĕ-lī′tis). Inflammation of the brain and spinal cord together with their membranes. [meningo- + G. *enkephalos*, brain, + *myelos*, marrow, + *-itis*, inflammation]

granulomatous m., a sporadic disease of dogs characterized by incoordination, ataxia, cervical pain, nystagmus, circling, seizures, and depression.

me·nin·go·en·ceph·a·lop·a·thy (mĕ-ning′gō-en-sef-ă-lop′ă-thē). Disorder affecting the meninges and the brain. SYN encephalomeningopathy. [meningo- + G. *enkephalos*, brain, + *pathos*, suffering]

me·nin·go·my·e·li·tis (mĕ-ning′gō-mī′ĕ-lī′tis). Inflammation of the spinal cord and of its enveloping arachnoid and pia mater, and less commonly also of the dura mater. [meningo- + G. *myelos*, marrow, + *-itis*, inflammation]

me·nin·go·my·e·lo·cele (mĕ-ning′gō-mī′ĕ-lō-sēl). Protrusion of the spinal cord and its membranes through a defect in the vertebral column. SYN myelocystomeningocele, myelomeningocele. [meningo- + G. *myelos*, marrow, + *kēlē*, tumor]

me·nin·go·os·te·o·phle·bi·tis (mĕ-ning′gō′os-tē-ō-flĕ-bī′tis). Inflammation of the veins of the periosteum.

me·nin·go·ra·dic·u·lar (mĕ-ning′gō-ra-dik′yū-lăr). Relating to the meninges covering cranial or spinal nerve roots. [meningo- + L. *radix*, root]

me·nin·go·ra·dic·u·li·tis (mĕ-ning′gō-ra-dik-yū-lī′tis). Inflammation of the meninges and roots of the nerves.

me·nin·gor·rha·chid·i·an (mĕ-ning′gō-ra-kid′ē-an). Relating to the spinal cord and its membranes. [meningo- + G. *rhachis*, spine]

me·nin·gor·rha·gia (mĕ-ning′gō-rā′jē-ă). Hemorrhage into or beneath the cerebral or spinal meninges. [meningo- + G. *rhēgnymi*, to burst forth]

men·in·go·sis (men′ing-gō′sis). Membranous union of bones, as in the skull of the newborn. [meningo- + G. *-ōsis*, condition]

me·nin·go·vas·cu·lar (mĕ-ning′gō-vas′kyū-lăr). Concerning the blood vessels in the meninges; or the meninges and blood vessels.

men·in·gu·ria (men-ing-gū′rē-ă). The passage of membraniform shreds in the urine. [meningo- + G. *ouron*, urine]

me·ninx, gen. **me·nin·gis,** pl. **me·nin·ges** (mē′ninks, -jēz; men′ingks; mĕ-nin′jes). Any membrane; specifically, one of the membranous coverings of the brain and spinal cord. SEE ALSO arachnoidea, dura mater, pia mater. [Mod. L. fr. G. *mēninx*, membrane]

m. fibro′sa, rarely used term for dura mater.

m. primiti′va, SYN primitive m.

primitive m., the embryonic loose mesenchymatous tissue surrounding the brain and spinal cord; from it the three definite meninges (arachnoidea, dura mater, and pia mater) are derived. SYN m. primitiva.

m. sero′sa, obsolete term for arachnoidea; the arachnoid is actually not a serous membrane.

m. ten′uis, SYN leptomeninges.

vascular m., rarely used term for pia mater. SYN m. vasculosa.

m. vasculo′sa, SYN vascular m.

men·is·cec·to·my (men′i-sek′tō-mē). Excision of a meniscus, usually from the knee joint. [G. *mēniskos*, crescent (meniscus) + *ektomē*, excision]

me·nis·ci (mĕ-nis′sī). Plural of meniscus.

men·is·ci·tis (men′i-sī′tis). Inflammation of a fibrocartilaginous meniscus. [G. *mēniskos,* crescent (meniscus), + *-itis,* inflammation]

me·nis·co·cyte (mĕ-nis′kō-sīt). SYN sickle *cell.* [G. *mēniskos,* a crescent, + *kytos,* a hollow (cell)]

me·nis·co·pexy (mĕ-nis′kō-pek-sē). Surgical procedure anchoring the medial meniscus to its former attachment. SYN meniscorrhaphy. [menisco- + G. *pēxis,* fixation]

men·is·cor·rha·phy (men-is-kōr′ă-fē). SYN meniscopexy. [menisco- + G. *rhaphē,* suture]

me·nis·co·tome (mĕ-nis′kō-tōm). An instrument used in the removal of a meniscus. [G. *mēniskos,* crescent (meniscus) + *tomē,* incision]

me·nis·cus, pl. **me·nis·ci** (mĕ-nis′kŭs, mĕ-nis′sī). **1.** SYN meniscus *lens.* **2** [NA]. A crescent-shaped structure. **3.** A crescent-shaped fibrocartilaginous structure of the knee, the acromio- and sternoclavicular and the temporomandibular joints. [G. *mēniskos,* crescent]

   articular m., a crescent-shaped intra-articular fibrocartilage found in certain joints. SYN m. articularis [NA], articular crescent, intra-articular cartilage (2).

   m. articula′ris [NA], SYN articular m.

   converging m., a convexoconcave lens in which the power of the convexity exceeds that of the concavity. SYN positive m.

   diverging m., a convexoconcave lens in which the power of the concavity exceeds that of the convexity. SYN negative m.

   lateral m., attached to the lateral border of the upper articular surface of the tibia. SYN m. lateralis [NA], external semilunar fibrocartilage.

   m. latera′lis [NA], SYN lateral m.

   medial m., attached to the medial border of the upper articular surface of the tibia. SYN m. medialis [NA], falciform cartilage, internal semilunar fibrocartilage of knee joint.

   m. media′lis [NA], SYN medial m.

   negative m., SYN diverging m.

   periscopic m., SYN aplanatic *lens.*

   positive m., SYN converging m.

   tactile m., a specialized tactile sensory nerve ending in the epidermis, characterized by a terminal cuplike expansion of an intraepidermal axon in contact with the base of a single modified keratinocyte. SYN m. tactus [NA], Merkel's corpuscle, Merkel's tactile cell, Merkel's tactile disk, tactile disk.

   m. tac′tus [NA], SYN tactile m.

Menkes, John H., U.S. neurologist, *1928. SEE M.'s *syndrome.*

⌂meno-. The menses, menstruation. [G. *mēn,* month]

men·o·ce·lis (men-ō-sē′lis). A dark macular or petechial eruption sometimes occurring in cases of amenorrhea. [meno- + G. *kēlis,* spot]

men·o·me·tror·rha·gia (men′ō-mē-trō-rā′jē-ă). Irregular or excessive bleeding during menstruation and between menstrual periods. [meno- + G. *mētra,* uterus, + *rhēgnymi,* to burst forth]

men·o·pau·sal (men′ō-paw-zăl). Associated with or occasioned by the menopause.

men·o·pause (men′ō-pawz). Permanent cessation of the menses; termination of the menstrual life. [meno- + G. *pausis,* cessation]

men·o·pha·nia (men-ō-fā′nē-ă). First sign of the menses at puberty. [meno- + G. *phainō,* to show]

Men·o·pon (men′ō-pon). A genus of biting lice (family Menoponidae, order Mallophaga) found on birds; it includes important pests that infect domestic fowl, such as *M. gallinae* (*M. pallidum*), the shaft louse of poultry, a light yellow louse about 1.7 to 2.0 mm long, found on barnyard fowl, ducks, and pigeons.

men·or·rha·gia (men-ō-rā′jē-ă). SYN hypermenorrhea. [meno- + G. *rhēgnymi,* to burst forth]

men·or·rhal·gia (men-ō-ral′jē-ă). SYN dysmenorrhea. [meno- + G. *algos,* pain]

me·nos·che·sis (me-nos′ke-sis, men-ō-skē′sis). Suppression of menstruation. [meno- + G. *schesis,* retention]

me·nos·ta·sis, **men·o·sta·sis** (mĕ-nos′tă-sis, men-ō-stā′zē-ă). Obsolete term for amenorrhea. [meno- + G. *stasis,* a standing]

men·o·stax·is (men-ō-stak′sis). SYN hypermenorrhea. [meno- + G. *staxis,* a dripping]

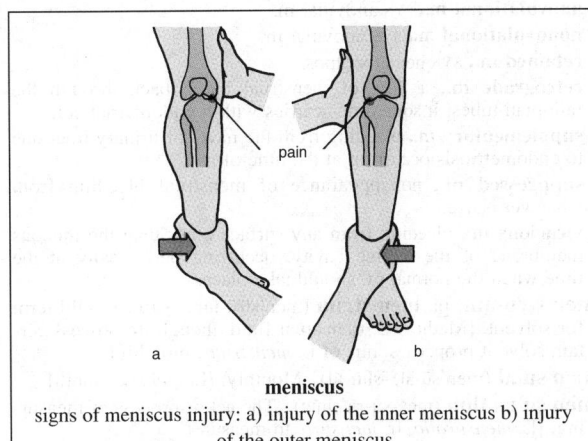

meniscus
signs of meniscus injury: a) injury of the inner meniscus b) injury of the outer meniscus

men·o·tro·pins (men-ō-trō′pinz). Extract of postmenopausal urine containing primarily the follicle-stimulating hormone. SEE ALSO human menopausal *gonadotropin,* urofollitropin.

men·o·u·ria (men-ō-yū′rē-ă). Menstruation occurring through the urinary bladder as a result of vesicouterine fistula. [meno- + G. *ouron,* urine, + *-ia,* condition]

men·o·xe·nia (men-ō-zē′nē-ă, men′ok-sē′nē-ă). Any abnormality of menstruation. [meno- + G. *xenos,* strange]

men·ses (men′sēz). A periodic physiologic hemorrhage, occurring at approximately 4-week intervals, and having its source from the uterine mucous membrane; usually the bleeding is preceded by ovulation and predecidual changes in the endometrium. SEE ALSO menstrual *cycle.* SYN catamenia, emmenia, menstrual period. [L. pl. of *mensis,* month]

men·stru·al (men′strū-ăl). Relating to the menses. SYN catamenial, emmenic. [L. *menstrualis*]

men·stru·ant (men′strū-ant). Menstruating.

men·stru·ate (men′strū-āt). To undergo menstruation. [L. *menstruo,* pp. *-atus,* to be menstruant]

men·stru·a·tion (men-strū-ā′shŭn). Cyclic endometrial shedding and discharge of a bloody fluid from the uterus during the menstrual cycle. [see menstruate]

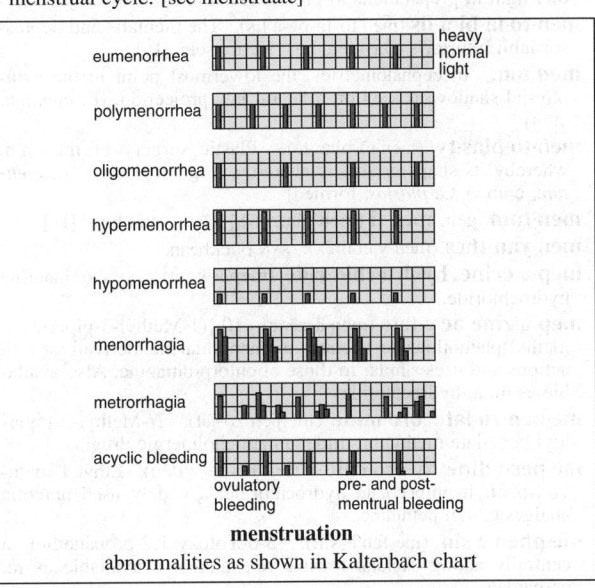

menstruation
abnormalities as shown in Kaltenbach chart

   anovular m., menstrual bleeding without recent ovulation; also occurs in subhuman primates. SYN anovulational m., nonovulational m.

me

anovulational m., SYN anovular m.

nonovulational m., SYN anovular m.

retained m., SYN hematocolpos.

retrograde m., a flow of menstrual blood back through the fallopian tubes; it sometimes carries with it endometrial cells.

supplementary m., bleeding from the navel or urinary tract due to endometriosis occurring at the time of m.

suppressed m., nonappearance of menstrual bleeding from whatever cause.

vicarious m., bleeding from any surface other than the mucous membrane of the uterine cavity, occurring periodically at the time when the normal m. should take place.

men·stru·um, pl. **men·strua** (men′strū-ŭm, -strū-ă). Old term for solvent. [Mediev. L. menstrual fluid, thought to possess certain solvent properties, ntr. of L. *menstruus,* monthly]

men·su·al (men′sū-ăl, -shū-ăl). Monthly. [L. *mensis,* month]

men·su·ra·tion (men-sū-rā′shŭn). The act or process of measuring. [L. *mensuratio,* fr. *mensuro,* to measure]

men·tag·ra (men-tag′ră). SYN sycosis. [L. tetter on the chin, fr. *mentum,* chin, + G. *agra,* a seizure]

men·tal. 1. Relating to the mind. [L. *mens* (*ment-*), mind] **2.** Relating to the chin. SYN genial, genian. [L. *mentum,* chin]

men·ta·lis (men-tā′lis). SEE mentalis *muscle.* [L.]

men·tal·i·ty (men-tal′i-tē). The functional attributes of the mind; mental activity.

men·ta·tion (men-tā′shŭn). The process of reasoning and thinking.

Menten, Maud L., Canadian pathologist in U.S., 1879–1960. SEE Michaelis-M. *constant, hypothesis.*

Men·tha (men′thă). A genus of plants of the family Labiatae. *M. piperita* is peppermint; *M. pulegium,* pennyroyal; *M. viridis,* spearmint. SYN mint. [L.]

men·thane (men′thān). 1-Isopropyl-4-methylcyclohexane; the monocyclic terpene parent of alcohols such as menthol, terpin.

men·thol. *p*-Menthan-3-ol; an alcohol obtained from peppermint oil or other mint oils, or prepared synthetically; used as an antipruritic and topical anesthetic, in nasal sprays and inhalers, and as a flavoring agent. SYN peppermint camphor.

camphorated m., a liquid obtained by triturating equal parts of camphor and m.; was used locally as a counterirritant and (diluted) as a spray in rhinitis and pharyngitis.

men·thyl sa·lic·y·late. Used as a sunscreen to filter out ultraviolet light in preparations to protect the skin from sunburn.

men·to·la·bi·a·lis (men′tō-lā-bē-ā′lis). The mentalis and depressor labii inferioris considered as one muscle. [L.]

men·ton. In cephalometrics, the lowermost point in the symphysial shadow as seen on a lateral jaw projection. [L. *mentum,* chin]

men·to·plas·ty (men′tō-plas-tē). Plastic surgery of the chin, whereby its shape or size is altered. SYN genioplasty. [L. *mentum,* chin, + G. *plastos,* formed]

men·tum, gen. **men·ti** (men′tŭm, -tī) [NA]. SYN chin. [L.]

men·yan·thes (men-yan′thēz). SYN buckbean.

mep·a·crine hy·dro·chlo·ride (mep′ă-krēn). SYN quinacrine hydrochloride.

mep·a·zine ac·e·tate (mep′ă-zēne). 10-[(1-Methyl-3-piperidyl)-methyl]phenothiazine acetate; a phenothiazine derivative with actions and uses similar to those of chlorpromazine. Also available as m. a. hydrochloride.

me·pen·zo·late bro·mide (me-pen′zō-lāt). *N*-Methyl-3-piperidyl benzilate methyl bromide; an anticholinergic drug.

me·per·i·dine hy·dro·chlo·ride (me-per′i-dēn). Ethyl 1-methyl-4-phenylisonipecotate hydrochloride; a widely used narcotic analgesic. SYN pethidine.

me·phen·e·sin (me-fen′ĕ-sin). 3-*o*-Toloxy-1,2-propanediol; a centrally acting skeletal muscle relaxant; also available as m. carbamate.

me·phen·ox·a·lone (me-fen-ok′să-lōn). 5-[(*o*-Methoxyphenoxy)methyl]-2-oxazolidinone; a mild tranquilizer and muscle relaxant.

me·phen·ter·mine (me-fen′ter-mēn). *N*-α,α-trimethylphenethylamine; a sympathomimetic amine.

m. sulfate, used topically as a nasal decongestant and systemically for its pressor effects in acute hypotensive states.

me·phen·y·to·in (mĕ-fen′i-tō-in). 5-Ethyl-3-methyl-5-phenylhydantoin; an anticonvulsant used when safer agents prove inadequate; used in drug metabolism studies.

me·phit·ic (me-fit′ik). Foul, poisonous, or noxious. [L. *mephitis,* a noxious exhalation]

meph·o·bar·bi·tal (mef-ō-bar′bi-tawl). 5-Ethyl-1-methyl-5-phenylbarbituric acid; used as a sedative and long-acting hypnotic, and as an anticonvulsant in the management of epilepsy; converted to phenobarbital in the body.

me·piv·a·caine hy·dro·chlo·ride (me-piv′ă-kān). *d*-1-*N*-Methylpipecolic acid 2,6-dimethylanilide hydrochloride; a local anesthetic agent.

me·pred·ni·sone (me-pred′ni-sōn). 17,21-Dihydroxy-16β-methylpregna-1,4-diene-3,11,20-trione; a glucocorticoid for oral use.

me·pro·ba·mate (me-prō′bă-māt). 2-Methyl-2-*n*-propyl-1,3-propanediol dicarbamate; a skeletal muscle relaxant with action similar to that produced by mephenesin but of longer duration; used in the management of certain disorders associated with abnormal motor activity, as a mild hypnotic, and as an antianxiety agent.

mep·ta·zi·nol (mep-tāz′ĭ-nol). A narcotic analgesic mixed agonist/antagonist (like pentazocine) which is about one-tenth as potent as morphine in producing analgesia. Though its abuse potential is less than that of pure agonists, the drug can precipitate an abstinence syndrome in persons dependent on opioids.

me·pyr·a·mine ma·le·ate (me-pir′ă-mēn). SYN pyrilamine maleate.

me·pyr·a·pone (me-pir′ă-pōn). SYN metyrapone.

mEq, meq Abbreviation for milliequivalent.

△-mer. 1. Chemical suffix attached to a prefix such as mono-, di-, poly-, tri-, etc., to indicate the smallest unit of a repeating structure; *e.g.,* polymer. **2.** Suffix denoting a member of a particular group; *e.g.,* isomer, enantiomer.

me·ral·gia (me-ral′jē-ă). Pain in the thigh; specifically, m. paresthetica. [G. *mēros,* thigh, + *algos,* pain]

m. paraesthet′ica, tingling, formication, itching, and other forms of paresthesia in the outer side of the lower part of the thigh in the area of distribution of the lateral femoral cutaneous nerve; there may be pain, but the skin is usually hypesthetic to the touch. SYN Bernhardt's disease, Bernhardt-Roth syndrome, Roth's disease, Roth-Bernhardt disease.

mer·al·lu·ride (mer-al′yū-rīd). *N*-[[2-Methoxy-3-[(1,2,3,6-tetrahydro-1,3-dimethyl-2,6-dioxopurin-7-yl) mercuri]propyl]-carbamoyl]succinamic acid; a mercurial diuretic.

mer·bro·min (mer-brō′min). The disodium salt of 2,7-dibromo-4-hydroxymercurifluorescein; an organic mercurial antiseptic compound that also has staining properties similar to those of eosin and phloxine, with strong affinity for cytoplasmic structures; also used histochemically to stain protein-bound sulfhydryl and disulfide groups for bright-field and fluorescence microscopy. SYN mercurochrome.

mer·cap·tal (mer-kap′tăl). A substance derived from an aldehyde by the replacement of the bivalent oxygen by two thioalkyl (−SR) groups.

mer·cap·tan (mer-kap′tan). **1.** A class of substances in which the oxygen of an alcohol has been replaced by sulfur (*e.g.,* cysteine). SYN thioalcohol. **2.** In dentistry, a class of elastic impression compounds sometimes referred to as rubber base materials.

methyl m., CH₃SH; formed in the intestines by bacterial action on sulfur-containing proteins and appears in urine after ingestion of asparagus (contributing to the characteristic odor); also used in the manufacture of various organic sulfur-containing pesticides and fungicides.

△mercapto-. Prefix indicating the presence of a thiol group, −SH.

mer·cap·to·a·ce·tic ac·id (mer-kap′tō-ă-sē′tik). SYN thioglycolic acid.

mer·cap·to·eth·a·nol (mer-kap′tō-eth′ă-nol). $SH–CH_2–CH_2–OH$; a commonly used reducing agent.

β-mercaptoethanol. SYN 2-mercaptoethanol.

2-mer·cap·to·eth·a·nol (mer-kap′tō-eth-ăn-ol). $HO–CH_2–CH_2–SH$; a reagent used to reduce disulfide bonds, particularly in proteins, and to prevent their formation. SYN β-mercaptoethanol.

mer·cap·tol (mer-kap′tol). A substance derived from a ketone by the replacement of the bivalent oxygen by two thioalkyl (–SR) groups.

3-mer·cap·to·lac·tate (mer-kap′tō-lak-tāt). A product of cysteine catabolism; formed by the action of lactate dehydrogenase on 3-mercaptopyruvate that was, in turn, formed by transamination of cysteine; present in normal human urine as a mixed disulfide with cysteine; elevated in the urine in individuals with mercaptolactate-cysteine disulfiduria.

mer·cap·to·lac·tate-cys·te·ine di·sul·fid·u·ria. Elevated levels of the mixed disulfide of 3-mercaptolactate and cysteine in the urine.

mer·cap·tom·er·in so·di·um (mer-kap-tom′ĕ-rin, mer-kap-tō-mer′in). *N*-(γ-Carboxymethylmercaptomercuri-β-methoxy)-propylcamphoramic acid disodium salt; a mercurial diuretic.

6-mer·cap·to·pu·rine (Shy) (mer-kap-tō-pūr′ēn). 6-Purinethiol; an analogue of hypoxanthine and of adenine; an antineoplastic agent.

3-mer·cap·to·py·ru·vate (mer-kap′tō-pī-rū-vāt). The transaminated product of cysteine; formed in cysteine catabolism; elevated in individuals with a deficiency of 3-m. sulfurtransferase.

3-m. sulfurtransferase, an enzyme that is a part of the cysteine catabolic pathway; it catalyzes the conversion of 3-m. to pyruvate and H_2S; a deficiency of this enzyme will result in elevated urine concentrations of 3-m. as well as of 3-mercaptolactate, both in the form of disulfides with cysteine.

mer·cap·tu·ric ac·id (mer-kap-tyūr′ik). A condensation product of L-cysteine with aromatic compounds, such as bromobenzene; formed biologically via glutathione in the liver and excreted in the urine; an *S*-substituted *N*-acetylated L-cysteine. Cf. mercapturic acid *pathway*.

Mercier, Louis A., French urologist, 1811–1882. SEE M.'s *bar, sound, valve;* median *bar* of M.

mer·co·cre·sols (mer-kō-krē′solz). A mixture consisting of equal parts by weight of *sec*-amyltricresol and *o*-hydroxyphenylmercuric chloride; it possesses fungicidal, germicidal, and bacteriostatic action.

mer·cu·ma·til·in (mer′kyū-mă-til′in, -mat′i-lin). 8-(2′-Methoxy-3′-hydroxymercuripropyl) coumarin-3-carboxylic acid (mercumallylic acid) and theophylline; a mercurial diuretic; also available as m. sodium.

mer·cu·ra·mide (mer-kū′ră-mīd). SYN mersalyl.

mer·cu·ri·al (mer-kyū′rē-ăl). **1.** Relating to mercury. **2.** Any salt of mercury used medicinally. **3.** Having the characteristic of rapid, changing moods.

mer·cu·ri·a·len·tis (mer-kyū′rē-ă-len′tis). A brown discoloration of the anterior capsule of the lens caused by mercury; early sign of mercurial poisoning.

mer·cu·ri·a·lism (mer-kyū′rē-ă-lizm). SYN mercury *poisoning.*

p-mer·cur·i·ben·zo·ate (mer-kyūr-i-ben′zō-āt). A commonly used enzyme inhibitor because of its reaction with sulfhydryl groups; usually *p*-chloromercuribenzoate or *p*-hydroxymercuribenzoate is used.

mer·cu·ric (mer-kyū′rik). Denoting a salt of mercury in which the ion of the metal is bivalent, as in corrosive sublimate, mercuric chloride, $HgCl_2$; the mercurous chloride is calomel, HgCl.

mer·cu·ric chlo·ride. $HgCl_2$; a topical antiseptic and disinfectant for inanimate objects. SYN corrosive sublimate, mercury bichloride, mercury perchloride, corrosive mercury chloride.

ammoniated m. c., SYN ammoniated *mercury.*

mer·cu·ric io·dide, red. HgI_2; has been used as an antiseptic and as a disinfectant for inanimate objects. SYN mercury biniodide, mercury deutoiodide.

mer·cu·ric ole·ate. An ointment-like preparation used in parasitic skin diseases.

mer·cu·ric ox·ide, red. The red precipitate of HgO; it has been used externally as an antiseptic in chronic skin diseases and fungus infections. SYN red precipitate.

mer·cu·ric ox·ide, yel·low. The yellow precipitate of HgO; used externally as an antiseptic in the treatment of inflammatory conditions of the eyelids and the conjunctivae. SYN yellow precipitate.

mer·cu·ric sa·lic·y·late. A powder used externally in the treatment of parasitic and fungus skin diseases. SYN mercury subsalicylate.

mer·cu·ro·chrome (mer-kur′ō-krōm). SYN merbromin.

mer·cu·ro·phen (mer-kyū′-rō-fen). Sodium hydroxymercury-*o*-nitrophenolate; a local antiseptic.

mer·cu·ro·phyl·line so·di·um (mer-kyūr-of′i-lēn). The sodium salt of β-methoxy-γ-hydroxymercuripropylamide of trimethylcyclopentanedicarboxylic acid, and theophylline; a mercurial diuretic.

mer·cu·rous (mer-kyū′rŭs, mer′kyū-rŭs). Denoting a salt of mercury in which the ion of the metal is univalent, as in calomel, mercurous chloride, HgCl; the mercuric chloride is corrosive sublimate, $HgCl_2$.

mer·cu·rous chlo·ride. SYN calomel.

mer·cu·rous io·dide. HgI; used externally as an ointment in eye diseases. SYN mercury protoiodide, yellow mercury iodide.

mer·cu·ry (Hg) (mer′kyū-rē). A dense liquid metallic element, atomic no. 80, atomic wt. 200.59; used in thermometers, barometers, manometers, and other scientific instruments; some salts and organic mercurials are used medicinally; care must be followed with its handling; ^{197}Hg (half-life of 2.672 days) and ^{203}Hg (half-life of 46.61 days) have been used in brain and renal scanning. SYN hydrargyrum, quicksilver. [L. *Mercurius,* Mercury, the god of trade, messenger of the gods; in Mediev. L., quicksilver, mercury]

ammoniated m., $HgNH_2Cl$; used in ointment for the treatment of skin diseases. SYN ammoniated mercuric chloride, white mercuric precipitate.

m. bichloride, m. perchloride, corrosive m. chloride, SYN mercuric chloride.

m. biniodide, SYN mercuric iodide, red.

m. deutoiodide, SYN mercuric iodide, red.

m. protoiodide, SYN mercurous iodide.

m. subsalicylate, SYN mercuric salicylate.

yellow m. iodide, SYN mercurous iodide.

△**mere-, mero-.** Part; also indicating one of a series of similar parts. SEE ALSO -mer. [G. *mēros,* share]

Merendino, K. Alvin, U.S. surgeon, *1914. SEE M.'s *technique.*

mer·e·prine (mer′ĕ-prēn). SYN doxylamine succinate.

mer·e·thox·yl·line pro·caine (mer-ĕ-thok′si-lēn). Dehydro-2-[*N*-(3′-hydroxymercuri-2′-methoxyethoxy)propylcarbamoyl]-phenoxyacetic acid (merethoxylline), 2-diethylaminoethyl *p*-aminobenzoate (procaine), and theophylline; a mixture of the procaine salt of merethoxylline and anhydrous theophylline; used as a mercurial diuretic.

me·rid·i·an (mĕ-rid′-ē-an). **1.** A line encircling a globular body at right angles to its equator and touching both poles, or the half of such a circle extending from pole to pole. **2.** In acupuncture, the lines connecting different anatomical sites. SYN meridianus [NA]. [L. *meridianus,* pertaining to midday, on the south side, southern]

m. of cornea, any line bisecting the cornea through its apex.

m.'s of eye, lines surrounding the surface of the eyeball passing through both anterior and posterior poles. SYN meridiani bulbi oculi [NA].

me·rid·i·ani (mĕ-rid-ē-ā′nī). Plural of meridianus.

me·rid·i·a·nus, pl. **me·rid·i·ani** (mĕ-rid′ē-ā′nŭs, -nī) [NA]. SYN meridian, meridian. [L.]

meridiani bul′bi oc′uli [NA], SYN *meridians* of eye, under *meridian.*

me·rid·i·o·nal (mĕ-rid′ē-ŏ-năl). Relating to a meridian.

me

mer·i·spore (mer′i-spōr). A secondary spore, one resulting from the segmentation of another (compound or septate) spore. [G. *meros*, a part, + *sporos*, seed]

mer·i·ste·mat·ic (mer′is-tĕ-mat′ik). Pertaining (in fungi) to an area (meristem) of the hyphae or of other specialized structures from which new growth occurs. [G. *merizein*, to divide]

me·ris·tic (mĕ-ris′tik). Symmetrical; that which can be divided evenly; denoting bilateral or longitudinal symmetry in the arrangement of parts in one organism. [G. *meristikos*, suitable for dividing]

Merkel, Friedrich S., German anatomist and physiologist, 1845–1919. SEE M. cell *tumor;* M.'s *corpuscle*, tactile *cell*, tactile *disk*.

Merkel, Karl L., German anatomist and laryngologist, 1812–1876. SEE M.'s *filtrum* ventriculi, *fossa*, *muscle*.

△**mero-.** SEE mere-.

mer·o·a·cra·nia (mer′ō-ă-krā′nē-ă). Congenital lack of a part of the cranium other than the occipital bone. [mero- + G. *a-* priv. + *kranion*, skull]

mer·o·an·en·ceph·a·ly (mer′ō-an-en-sef′ă-lē). A type of anencephaly in which the brain and cranium are present in rudimentary form. [mero- + G. *an-* priv. + *enkephalos*, brain]

mer·o·cele (mēr′ō-sēl). Obsolete term for femoral *hernia*. [G. *mēros*, thigh, + *kēlē*, hernia]

mer·o·crine (mer′ō-krin, -krīn, -krēn). SEE merocrine *gland*. [mero- + G. *krinō*, to separate]

mer·o·di·a·stol·ic (mer′ō-dī-ă-stol′ik). Partially diastolic; relating to a part of the diastole of the heart. [mero- + diastole]

mer·o·gas·tru·la (mer′ō-gas′trū-lă). The gastrula of a meroblastic ovum.

mer·o·gen·e·sis (mer-ō-jen′ĕ-sis). 1. Reproduction by segmentation. 2. Cleavage of an ovum. [mero- + G. *genesis*, origin]

mer·o·ge·net·ic, mer·o·gen·ic (mer-ō-jĕ-net′ik, -ō-jen′ik). Relating to merogenesis.

me·rog·o·ny (mĕ-rog′ō-nē). 1. The incomplete development of an ovum that has been disorganized. 2. A form of asexual schizogony, typical of sporozoan protozoa, in which the nucleus divides several times before the cytoplasm divides; the schizont divides to form merozoites in this asexual phase of the life cycle. [mero- + G. *gonē*, generation]

mer·o·me·lia (mer-ō-mē′lē-ă). Partial absence of a free limb (exclusive of girdle); *e.g.*, hemimelia, phocomelia. [mero- + G. *melos*, a limb]

mer·o·mi·cro·so·mia (mer′ō-mī′krō-sō′mē-ă). Abnormal smallness of some portion of the body; local dwarfism. [mero- + G. *mikros*, small, + *sōma*, body]

mer·o·my·o·sin (mer-ō-mī′ō-sin). A subunit of the tryptic digestion of myosin; two types are produced, H-m. and L-m.

H-m., one of the relatively heavy products (mol. wt. about 232,000) of the action of trypsin on myosin; it carries the ATPase activity of myosin. [H for "heavy"]

L-m., the relatively low-molecular-weight product (mol. wt. about 96,000) of the tryptic digestion of myosin. [L for "light"]

mer·ont (mer′ont). A stage in the life cycle of sporozoans in which multiple asexual fission (schizogony) occurs, resulting in production of merozoites. SEE ALSO schizont.

mer·o·ra·chis·chi·sis, mer·or·rha·chis·chi·sis (mer′ō-ră-kis′ki-sis). Fissure of a portion of the spinal cord. SYN mesorrhachischisis, rachischisis partialis. [mero- + G. *rhachis*, spine, + *schisis*, fissure]

me·ros·mia (me-roz′mē-ă). A condition in which the perception of certain odors is wanting; analogous to color blindness. [mero- + G. *osmē*, smell]

mer·o·spor·an·gi·um (mer′ō-spōr-ran′-jē-ŭm). A cylindrical small sporangium containing few spores and found in certain Zygomycetes. [G. *meros*, part, + sporangium]

mer·o·sys·tol·ic (mer′ō-sis-tol′ik). Partially systolic; relating to a portion of the systole of the heart. [mero- + systole]

me·rot·o·my (me-rot′ō-mē). The procedure of cutting into parts, as the cutting of a cell into separate parts to study their capacity for survival and development. [mero- + G. *tomē*, incision]

mer·o·zo·ite (mer-ō-zō′īt). The motile infective stage of sporozoan protozoa that results from schizogony or a similar type of asexual reproduction; *e.g.*, endodyogeny or endopolygeny. M.'s form at the surface of schizonts, blastophores, or invaginations into schizonts, and are responsible for the vast reproductive powers of sporozoan parasites; this is seen in human malaria, where the cyclic production of m.'s produces the typical fever and chill syndrome. SYN endodyocyte (2). [mero- + G. *zōon*, animal]

me·ro·zy·gote (mē-rō-zī′gōt). In microbial genetics, an organism that, in addition to its own original genome (endogenote), contains a fragment (exogenote) of a genome from another organism; the relatively small size of the exogenote permits a diploid condition for only a limited region of the endogenote. [mero- + *zygōtos*, yoked]

mer·pha·lan (mer′fă-lan). The racemic mixture of melphalan and medphalan; an antineoplastic agent. SYN sarcolysine.

Merrifield, R. Bruce, U.S. biochemist and Nobel laureate, *1921. SEE M. *synthesis*.

Merrifield knife. See under knife.

Merritt, Katharine K., U.S. pediatrician, *1886. SEE Kasabach-M. *syndrome*.

mer·sa·lyl (mer′să-lil). Sodium salt of (3-hydroxymercuric-2-methoxypropyl)salicylamide-*O*-acetic acid; a mercurial diuretic. SYN mercuramide.

m. acid, a mixture of *o*-carboxymethylsalicyl-(3-hydroxymercuric-2-methoxypropyl)amide and its anhydrides; same use as m.

m. theophylline, m. plus theophylline added to inhibit decomposition of m.

Méry, Jean, French anatomist, 1645–1722. SEE M.'s *gland*.

Merzbacher, Ludwig, German physician in Argentina, 1875–1942. SEE M.-Pelizaeus *disease;* Pelizaeus-M. *disease*.

△**mes-.** SEE meso-.

me·sad (mē′zad, mē′sad). Passing or extending toward the median plane of the body or of a part. SYN mesiad. [G. *mesos*, middle, + L. *ad*, to]

me·sal (mē′zăl, mē′săl). Rarely used term referring to the median plane of the body or a part. [G. *mesos*, middle]

me·sal·a·mine (me-sal′ă-mēn). A salicylate used in the treatment of active mild to moderate distal ulcerative colitis, proctosigmoiditis, and proctitis.

mes·a·me·boid (mez-ă-mē′boyd). Minot's term for a primitive, "wandering" cell derived from mesoderm, probably a hemocytoblast. [mes- + G. *amoibē*, change (ameba), + *eidos*, resemblance]

mes·an·gi·al (mes-an′jē-ăl). Referring to the mesangium.

mes·an·gi·um (mes-an′jē-ŭm). A central part of the renal glomerulus between capillaries; mesangial cells are phagocytic and for the most part separated from capillary lumina by endothelial cells. [mes- + G. *angeion*, vessel]

extraglomerular m., mesangial cells that fill the triangular space between the macula densa and the afferent and efferent arterioles of the juxtaglomerular apparatus. SYN polkissen of Zimmermann.

mes·a·or·ti·tis (mes-ā-ōr-tī′tis). Inflammation of the middle or muscular coat of the aorta. [mes- + aortitis]

mes·a·re·ic, mes·a·ra·ic (mes-ă-rā′ik). SYN mesenteric. [G. *mesaraion*, mesentery, fr. *mesos*, middle, + *araia*, flank, belly]

mes·ar·ter·i·tis (mes-ar-ter-ī′tis). Inflammation of the middle (muscular) coat of an artery. [mes- + arteritis]

me·sat·i·ce·phal·ic (mĕ-sat′i-se-fal′ik). SYN mesocephalic. [G. *mesatos*, midmost, + *kephalē*, head]

me·sat·i·pel·lic, me·sat·i·pel·vic (mĕ-sat′i-pel′ik, -pel′vik). Denoting an individual with a pelvic index between 90 and 95; the superior strait has a round appearance, with the transverse diameter longer than the anteroposterior by 1 cm or less. [G. *mesatos*, midmost, + *pellis*, a bowl (pelvis)]

mes·ax·on (mez-ak′son, mes-). The plasma membrane of the neurolemma that is folded in to surround a nerve axon. In electron micrographs this double layer resembles a mesentery in appearance.

mes·cal but·tons (mes′kal). The dried slices of the cactus *Lophophora williamsii* containing mescaline and related alkaloids.

mes·ca·line (mes′kă-lēn). 3,4,5-Trimethoxyphenethylamine; the most active alkaloid present in the buttons of a small cactus, *Lophophora williamsii*. M. produces psychotomimetic effects similar to those produced by LSD: alteration in mood, changes in perception, reveries, visual hallucinations, delusions, depersonalization, mydriasis, hippus, and increases in body temperature and blood pressure; psychic dependence, tolerance, and cross tolerance to LSD and psilocybin develop; the principal component of peyote.

me·sec·tic (me-sek′tik). Obsolete term denoting a specimen of blood that has a normal percentage saturation of oxygen at any given pressure. [mes- + G. *echō*, to have]

mes·ec·to·derm (mez-ek′tō-derm). 1. Cells in the area around the dorsal lip of the blastopore where mesoderm and ectoderm undergo a process of separation. 2. That part of the mesenchyme derived from ectoderm, especially from the neural crest in the cephalic region in very young embryos. SYN ectomesenchyme. [mes- + ectoderm]

mes·en·ce·phal·ic (mez-en′se-fal′ik). Relating to the mesencephalon.

mes·en·ceph·a·li·tis (mez′en-sef′ă-lī′tis). Inflammation of the midbrain (mesencephalon).

mes·en·ceph·a·lon (mez-en-sef′ă-lon) [NA]. That part of the brainstem developing from the middle of the three primary cerebral vesicles of the embryo (the caudal of these being the rhombencephalon or hindbrain, the rostral the prosencephalon or forebrain). In the adult, the m. is characterized by the unique conformation of its roof plate, the lamina of mesencephalic tectum, composed of the bilaterally paired superior and inferior colliculus, and by the massive paired prominence of the crus cerebri at its ventral surface. On transverse section, its patent central canal, the cerebral aqueduct, is surrounded by a prominent ring of gray matter poor in myelinated fibers; the periaqueductal gray is ventrally and laterally adjoined by the myelin-rich mesencephalic tegmentum, and covered dorsally by the lamina of mesencephalic tectum. Prominent cell groups of the m. include the motor nuclei of the trochlear and oculomotor nerves, the red nucleus, and the substantia nigra. SYN midbrain vesicle, midbrain. [mes- + G. *enkephalos*, brain]

mes·en·ceph·a·lot·o·my (mez′en-sef′ă-lot′ō-mē). 1. The sectioning of any structure in the midbrain, especially of the spinothalamic tracts for the relief of intractable pain or the cerebral peduncle for dyskinesias. 2. A mesencephalic spinothalamic tractotomy. [mesencephalon + G. *tomē*, incision]

me·sen·chy·ma (mĕ-seng′ki-mă, mĕ-zeng′). SYN mesenchyme.

me·sen·chy·mal (mĕ-seng′ki-măl, mez-eng-kī′măl). Relating to the mesenchyme.

mes·en·chyme (mez′en-kīm). 1. An aggregation of mesenchymal cells. 2. Primordial embryonic connective tissue consisting of mesenchymal cells, usually stellate in form, supported in interlaminar jelly. SYN mesenchyma. [mes- + G. *enkyma*, infusion]

    interzonal m., an area of avascular m. between adjacent skeletal elements in the embryo; it denotes the region of future joints.

    synovial m., vascular m. surrounding the interzonal m.; it develops into the synovial membrane of a joint.

mes·en·chy·mo·ma (mez′en-kī-mō′mă). A neoplasm in which there is a mixture of mesenchymal derivatives, other than fibrous tissue. A **benign m.** may contain foci of vascular, muscular, adipose, osteoid, osseous, and cartilaginous tissue; such neoplasms are sometimes classed under a compounded name, *e.g.,* angioleiomyolipoma, and the like, but the broader term may be preferred. A **malignant m.** may also occur as a similar mixture of two or more types of mesenchymal cells that are malignant (other than fibrous tissue cells).

mes·en·ter·ic (mez-en-ter′ik). Relating to the mesentery. SYN mesareic, mesaraic.

mes·en·ter·i·o·lum (mez-en-ter-ē′ō-lŭm). A small mesentery, as one of an intestinal diverticulum. SYN mesoenteriolum. [Mod. L. dim. of *mesenterium*, mesentery]

    m. proces′sus vermifor′mis, SYN mesoappendix.

mes·en·ter·i·o·pexy (mes′en-ter-ē-ō-pek′sē). Fixation or attachment of a torn or incised mesentery. SYN mesopexy. [mesentery + G. *pēxis*, fixation]

mes·en·ter·i·or·rha·phy (mez′en-ter-ē-ōr′ă-fē). Suture of the mesentery. SYN mesorrhaphy. [mesentery + G. *rhaphē*, suture]

mes·en·ter·i·pli·ca·tion (mez′en-ter-i-pli-kā′shŭn). Reducing redundancy of a mesentery by making one or more tucks in it. [mesentery + L. *plico*, pp. *-atus*, to fold]

mes·en·ter·i·tis (mez′en-ter-ī′tis). Inflammation of the mesentery.

mes·en·te·ri·um (mez′en-ter′ē-ŭm) [NA]. SYN mesentery, mesentery. [Mod. L.]

    m. dorsa′le commu′ne, SYN mesentery (2).

mes·en·ter·on (mez-en′ter-on). The midportion of the insect alimentary canal and site of digestion; the m. may possess anterior finger-like projections, the gastric ceca, and a tubular anterior midgut, followed posteriorly by the saccular ventriculus, or stomach. [mes- + G. *enteron*, intestine]

mes·en·tery (mes′en-ter-ē). 1. A double layer of peritoneum attached to the abdominal wall and enclosing in its fold a portion or all of one of the abdominal viscera, conveying to it its vessels and nerves. 2. The fan-shaped fold of peritoneum encircling the greater part of the small intestines (jejunum and ileum) and attaching it to the posterior abdominal wall at the root of the m. (radix mesenterii). SYN mesenterium dorsale commune, mesostenium. SYN mesenterium [NA]. [Mod. L. *mesenterium*, fr. G. *mesenterion*, fr. G. *mesos*, middle, + *enteron*, intestine]

    m. of appendix, SYN mesoappendix.

    m. of cecum, SYN mesocecum.

    m. of lung, SYN mesopneumonium.

    m. of sigmoid colon, SEE mesocolon.

    m. of transverse colon, SEE mesocolon.

    urogenital m., SYN diaphragmatic *ligament* of the mesonephros.

mesh·work. SEE network.

    trabecular m., SYN trabecular *reticulum*.

me·si·ad (mē′zē-ad, mes′ē-ad). SYN mesad.

me·si·al (mē′zē-ăl, mes′ē-ăl). Toward the median plane following the curvature of the dental arch, in contrast to distal (2). SYN proximal (2). [G. *mesos*, middle]

△ **mesio-.** Mesial (especially in dentistry). [G. *mesos*, middle]

me·si·o·buc·cal (mē′zē-ō-bŭk′ăl). Relating to the mesial and buccal surfaces of a tooth; denoting especially the angle formed by the junction of these two surfaces.

me·si·o·buc·co·oc·clu·sal (mē′zē-ō-bŭk′ō-ŏ-klū′săl). Relating to the angle formed by the junction of the mesial, buccal, and occlusal surfaces of a bicuspid or molar tooth.

me·si·o·buc·co·pul·pal (mē′zē-ō-bŭk′ō-pŭl′păl). Relating to the angle denoting the junction of mesial, buccal and pulpal surfaces in a tooth cavity preparation.

me·si·o·cer·vi·cal (mē′zē-ō-ser′vi-kăl). 1. Relating to the line angle of a cavity preparation at the junction of the mesial and cervical walls. 2. Pertaining to the area of a tooth at the junction of the mesial surface and the cervical region.

me·si·o·clu·sion (mē′zē-ō-klū′zhŭn). A malocclusion in which the mandibular arch articulates with the maxillary arch in a position mesial to normal; in Angle's classification, a Class III malocclusion. SYN mesial occlusion (2).

me·si·o·dens (mē′zē-ō-denz). A supernumerary tooth located in the midline of the anterior maxillae, between the maxillary central incisor teeth. [mesio- + L. *dens*, tooth]

me·si·o·dis·tal (mē′zē-ō-dis′tăl). Denoting the plane or diameter of a tooth cutting its mesial and distal surfaces.

me·si·o·dis·toc·clu·sal (MOD) (mē′zē-ō-dist′ō-klū′săl, -zăl). Denoting three-surface cavity or cavity preparation or restoration (class 2, Black classification) in the premolars (bicuspids) and molars.

me·si·o·gin·gi·val (mē′zē-ō-jin′ji-văl). Relating to the angle formed by the junction of the mesial surface with the gingival line of a tooth.

me·si·o·gnath·ic (mē′zē-ō-nath′ik). Denoting malposition of one or both jaws forward from their normal position.

me·si·o·in·ci·sal (mē′zē-ō-in-sī′săl, -zăl). Relating to the mesial and incisal surfaces of a tooth; denoting the angle formed by their junction.

me

me·si·o·la·bi·al (mē′zē-ō-lā′bē-ăl). Relating to the mesial and labial surfaces of a tooth; denoting especially the angle formed by their junction.

me·si·o·lin·gual (mē′zē-ō-ling′gwăl). Relating to the mesial and lingual surfaces of a tooth; denoting especially the angle formed by their junction.

me·si·o·lin·guo·oc·clu·sal (mē′zē-ō-ling′gwō-ŏ-klū′săl, -zăl). Denoting the angle formed by the junction of the mesial, lingual, and occlusal surfaces of a bicuspid or molar tooth.

me·si·o·lin·guo·pul·pal (mē′zē-ō-ling′gwō-pŭl′păl). Relating to the angle denoting the junction of the mesial, lingual, and pulpal surfaces in a tooth cavity preparation.

me·sio·oc·clu·sal (mē′zē-ō-ō-klū′săl, -zăl). Denoting the angle formed by the junction of the mesial and occlusal surfaces of a bicuspid or molar tooth.

me·sio·oc·clu·sion (mē′zē-ō-ō-klū′zhŭn). SYN mesial *occlusion* (1).

me·si·o·place·ment (mē′zē-ō-plās′ment). SYN mesioversion.

me·si·o·pul·pal (mē′zē-ō-pŭl′păl). Pertaining to the inner wall or floor of a cavity preparation on the mesial side of a tooth.

me·si·o·ver·sion (mē′zē-ō-ver-zhŭn). Malposition of a tooth mesial to normal, in an anterior direction following the curvature of the dental arch. SYN mesial displacement, mesioplacement.

Mesmer, F. A., Austrian physician, 1733–1815. SEE mesmerism.

mes·mer·ism (mes′mer-izm). A system of therapeutics from which were developed hypnotism and therapeutic suggestion. [F.A. *Mesmer,* Austrian physician, 1734–1815]

mes·mer·ize (mes′mer-īz). Obsolete term for hypnotize. [see mesmerism]

⚠**meso-, mes·.** 1. Middle, mean, intermediacy. 2. A mesentery, mesentery-like structure. 3. A prefix denoting a compound, containing more than one chiral center, having an internal plane of symmetry; such compounds do not exhibit optical activity (*e.g., meso*-cystine). [G. *mesos*]

mes·o·ap·pen·dix (mez′ō-ă-pen′diks) [NA]. The short mesentery of the appendix lying behind the terminal ileum, in which the appendicular artery courses. SYN mesenteriolum processus vermiformis, mesentery of appendix.

mes·o·ar·i·um (mez-ō-ār′ē-ŭm). SYN mesovarium.

mes·o·bi·lane (mez-ō-bī′lān). A reduced mesobilirubin with no double bonds between the pyrrole rings and, consequently, colorless. SEE ALSO bilirubinoids. SYN mesobilirubinogen, urobilinogen IXα.

mes·o·bi·lene, mesobilene- (mez-ō-bī′lēn). A bilirubinoid. SEE urobilin. SYN urobilin IX-α.

mes·o·bil·i·ru·bin (mez′ō-bil-i-rū′bin). A compound differing from bilirubin only in that the vinyl groups of bilirubin are reduced to ethyl groups. SEE ALSO bilirubinoids.

mes·o·bil·i·ru·bin·o·gen (mez′ō-bil-i-rū-bin′ō-jen). SYN mesobilane.

mes·o·bil·i·vi·o·lin (mez′ō-bil-i-vī-ō′lin). A bilirubinoid.

mes·o·blast (mez′ō-blast). SYN mesoderm. [meso- + G. *blastos,* germ]

mes·o·blas·te·ma (mez′ō-blas-tē′mă). All the cells collectively which constitute the early undifferentiated mesoderm. [meso- + G. *blastēma,* a sprout]

mes·o·blas·tem·ic (mez′ō-blas-tē′mik). Relating to or derived from the mesoblastema.

mes·o·blas·tic (mez′ō-blas′tik). Relating to or derived from the mesoderm.

mes·o·car·dia (mez′ō-kar′dē-ă). 1. Atypical position of the heart in a central position in the chest, as in early embryonic life. 2. Plural of mesocardium. [meso- + G. *kardia,* heart]

mes·o·car·di·um, pl. **mes·o·car·dia** (mez-ō-kar′dē-ŭm). The double layer of splanchnic mesoderm supporting the embryonic heart in the pericardial cavity. It disappears before birth. [meso- + G. *kardia,* heart]
  dorsal m., the part of the m. dorsal to the embryonic heart; it breaks down to form the transverse sinus of the pericardium.
  ventral m., the part of the m. ventral to the embryonic cardiac tube; transitory in all vertebrates; in the higher mammals, it

breaks through as soon as its component layers of epicardium make contact with each other.

mes·o·car·pal (mez′ō-kar′păl). SYN midcarpal.

mes·o·ce·cal (mez′ō-sē′kăl). Relating to the mesocecum.

mes·o·ce·cum (mez′ō-sē′kŭm). Part of the mesocolon, supporting the cecum, that occasionally persists when the ascending colon becomes retroperitoneal during fetal life. SYN mesentery of cecum. [meso- + cecum]

mes·o·ce·phal·ic (mez′ō-se-fal′ik). Having a head of medium length; denoting a skull with a cephalic index between 75 and 80 and with a capacity of 1350 to 1450 ml, or an individual with such a skull. SYN mesaticephalic, mesocephalous, normocephalic. [meso- + G. *kephalē,* head]

mes·o·ceph·a·lous (mez′ō-sef′ă-lŭs). SYN mesocephalic.

mes·o·col·ic (mez′ō-kol′ik). Relating to the mesocolon.

mes·o·co·lon (mez′ō-kō′lon) [NA]. The fold of peritoneum attaching the colon to the posterior abdominal wall; ascending m. (m. ascendens [NA]), transverse m. (m. transversum [NA]), descending m. (m. descendens [NA]), and sigmoid m. (m. sigmoideum [NA]) correspond to the respective divisions of the colon; the ascending and descending portions are usually fused to the peritoneum of the posterior abdominal wall, but can be mobilized. [meso- + *kolon,* colon]

mes·o·co·lo·pexy (mez′ō-kō′lō-pek-sē). An operation for shortening the mesocolon, for correction of undue mobility and ptosis. SYN mesocoloplication. [meso- + G. *kolon,* colon, + *pēxis,* fixation]

mes·o·co·lo·pli·ca·tion (mes′ō-kō′lō-pli-kā′shŭn). SYN mesocolopexy. [meso- + G. *kolon,* colon, + L. *plico,* pp. *-atus,* to fold]

mes·o·cord (mez′ō-kōrd). A fold of amnion that sometimes binds a segment of the umbilical cord to the placenta.

mes·o·cu·ne·i·form (mez-ō-kū′nē-i-fōrm). SYN intermediate cuneiform *bone.*

mes·o·derm (mez′ō-derm). The middle of the three primary germ layers of the embryo (the others being ectoderm and endoderm); m. is the origin of all connective tissues, all body musculature, blood, cardiovascular and lymphatic systems, most of the urogenital system, and the lining of the pericardial, pleural, and peritoneal cavities. SYN mesoblast. [meso- + G. *derma,* skin]
  branchial m., m. surrounding the primitive stomodeum and pharynx; it develops into the pharyngeal arches.
  extraembryonic m., extraembryonic ectoderm cells or tissues which, though derived from the zygote, are not part of the embryo proper and along with the m. form the fetal membranes (*e.g.,* amnion). SYN primary m.
  gastral m., m. in lower vertebrates formed by constriction from the roof of the archenteron or yolk sac.
  intermediate m., a continuous band of m. between the segmented paraxial m. medially and the lateral plate m. laterally; from it develops the nephrogenic cord.
  intraembryonic m., m. derived from the primitive streak and lying between the ectoderm and endoderm. SYN secondary m.
  lateral m., SYN lateral plate m.
  lateral plate m., the peripheral thinned-out portion of intraembryonic m. which is continuous with the extraembryonic m. beyond the margins of the embryonic disk; in it develops the intraembryonic celom. SYN lateral m.
  paraxial m., a thickened mass lying at either side of the midline embryonic notochord; on segmentation, it forms the paired somites.
  primary m., SYN extraembryonic m.
  prostomial m., m. that arises in lower vertebrates by continued proliferation at the lateral lips of the blastopore.
  secondary m., SYN intraembryonic m.
  somatic m., the m. adjacent to the ectoderm in the early embryo, after foundation of the intraembryonic celom.
  somitic m., m. derived from cells situated in or derived from somites.
  splanchnic m., the layer of lateral plate m. adjacent to the endoderm.
  visceral m., the splanchnic m. or the branchial m.

mes·o·der·mal (mez-ō-der'mal). Pertaining to the mesoderm.

mes·o·der·mic (mez-ō-der'mik). Relating to the mesoderm.

mes·o·di·a·stol·ic (mez-ō-dī-ă-stol'ik). Middiastolic.

mes·o·dont (mez'ō-dont). Having teeth of medium size; denoting a skull with a dental index between 42 and 43.9. [meso- + G. *odous*, tooth]

mes·o·du·o·de·nal (mez'ō-dū-ō-dē'năl). Relating to the mesoduodenum.

mes·o·du·o·de·num (mez'ō-dū'ō-dē'nŭm, -dū-od'ĕ-nŭm). The mesentery of the duodenum.

mes·o·en·te·ri·o·lum (mes'ō-en-ter-ē'ō-lŭm). SYN mesenteriolum.

mes·o·ep·i·did·y·mis (mez-ō-ep-i-did'i-mis). An occasional fold of the tunica vaginalis binding the epididymis to the testis. [meso- + epididymis]

mes·o·gas·ter (mez-ō-gas'ter). SYN mesogastrium.

mes·o·gas·tric (mez-ō-gas'trik). Relating to the mesogastrium.

mes·o·gas·tri·um (mez-ō-gas'trē-ŭm). In the embryo, the mesentery of the dilated portion of the enteric canal that is the future stomach; it gives rise to the greater omentum and consequently is involved in the formation of the omental bursa. The spleen and body of the pancreas develop within it, and thus the splenorenal and gastrosplenic ligaments are derivatives of the (dorsal) mesogastrium. SYN dorsal m., mesogaster. [meso- + G. *gastēr* stomach]

dorsal m., SYN mesogastrium.

ventral m., the primitive midline mesentery extending between the future stomach and proximal duodenum and the anterior abdominal wall superior to the umbilicus (umbilical vein). The liver develops within it, and consequently, the lesser omentum, coronary and falciform ligaments are derivatives of it. The umbilical vein runs in its caudal free edge, becoming the postnatal round ligament of the liver.

ventral m., the primitive midline mesentery extending between future stomach and proximal duodenum and the anterior abdominal wall superior to the umbilicus (umbilical vein). The liver develops within it, and consequently the lesser omentum, coronary and falciform ligaments are derivatives of it. The umbilical vein runs in its caudal free edge, becoming the postnatal round ligament of the liver.

mes·o·gen·ic (mez-ō-jen'ik). Denoting the virulence of a virus capable of inducing lethal infection in embryonic hosts, after a short incubation period, and an inapparent infection in immature and adult hosts; used in characterizing Newcastle disease virus, particularly strains used in parenteral vaccination of chickens. [meso- + G. *-gen*, producing]

me·sog·lia (me-sog'lē-ă). Neuroglial cells of mesodermal origin. SEE ALSO microglia. SYN mesoglial cells. [meso- + G. *glia*, glue]

mes·o·glu·te·al (mez'ō-glū'tē-ăl). Relating to the musculus gluteus medius.

mes·o·glu·te·us (mez'ō-glū-tē'ŭs). SYN gluteus medius *muscle*.

mes·o·gnath·ic (mez-ō-nath'ik, -og-nath'ik). 1. Relating to the mesognathion. 2. SYN mesognathous.

mes·o·gna·thi·on (mez'ō-nā'thē-on, -og-nā'thē-on, nath'ē-on). The lateral segment of the premaxillary or incisive bone external to the endognathion. [meso- + G. *gnathos*, jaw]

me·sog·na·thous (me-zog'nă-thŭs). Having a face with slightly projecting jaw, one with a gnathic index from 98 to 103. SYN mesognathic (2).

mes·o·il·e·um (mez-ō-il'ē-ŭm). The mesentery of the ileum.

mes·o·je·ju·num (mez'ō-je-jū'nŭm). The mesentery of the jejunum.

mes·o·lep·i·do·ma (mes'ō-lep'i-dō'mă). A neoplasm derived from the persistent embryonic mesothelium. [meso- + G. *lepis*, rind, + *-oma*, tumor]

me·sol·o·bus (me-sol'ō-bŭs). Obsolete term for *corpus callosum*. [meso- + L. *lobus*, lobe]

mes·o·lym·pho·cyte (mez-ō-lim'fō-sīt). A mononuclear leukocyte of medium size, probably a lymphocyte, with a deeply staining nucleus of large size but relatively smaller than that in most lymphocytes. [meso- + lymphocyte]

mes·o·me·lia (mez-ō-mē'lē-ă). The condition of having abnormally short forearms and lower legs. [meso- + G. *melos*, limb]

mes·o·mel·ic (mez-ō-mē'lik). Pertaining to the middle segment of a limb.

mes·o·mere (mez'ō-mēr). 1. A blastomere of a size intermediate between a macromere and a micromere. 2. The zone between an epimere and a hypomere. [meso- + G. *meros*, part]

mes·o·mer·ic (mez-ō-mer'ik). Pertaining to mesomerism.

me·som·er·ism (mě-som'er-izm). Displacement of electrons within a molecule in such a way as to create fractional charges on different parts of the molecule.

mes·o·me·tri·tis (mez'ō-mē-trī'tis). SYN myometritis. [meso- + G. *mētra*, uterus, + *-itis*, inflammation]

mes·o·me·tri·um (mez'ō-mē'trē-ŭm) [NA]. The broad ligament of the uterus, below the mesosalpinx. [meso- + G. *mētra*, uterus]

mes·o·morph (mez'ō-mōrf). A constitutional body type or build (biotype or somatotype) in which tissues that originate from the mesoderm prevail; from the morphological standpoint, there is a balance between trunk and limbs. SEE ALSO hypermorph, hypomorph, ectomorph, endomorph. SYN mediotype. [meso- + G. *morphē*, form]

mes·o·mor·phic (mez-ō-mōrf'ik). Relating to mesomorphs.

me·son (mez'on, mē'zon, mes'on). An elementary particle having a rest mass intermediate in value between the mass of an electron and that of a proton. [G. neuter of *mesos*, middle]

mes·o·neph·ric (mez-ō-nef'rik). Relating to the mesonephros.

mes·o·neph·roi (mez'ō-nef'roy). Plural of mesonephros.

mes·o·ne·phro·ma (mez'ō-ne-frō'mă). A relatively rare malignant neoplasm of the ovary and corpus uteri, thought to originate in mesonephric structures that become misplaced in ovarian tissue during embryonic development; characterized by a tubular pattern, with focal proliferation of epithelial cells with clear cytoplasm or of the hob-nail type; so-called glomeruloid structures are reported, *i.e.*, small convolutions or tufts of tiny tubate formations with capillaries extending into the spaces. SYN mesometanephric carcinoma, mesonephric adenocarcinoma, mesonephroid tumor, wolffian duct carcinoma. [mesonephros + *-oma*, tumor]

mes·o·neph·ros, pl. **mes·o·neph·roi** (mez'ō-nef'ros, -roy) [NA]. One of three excretory organs appearing in the evolution of vertebrates; in life forms with a metanephros, the m. is located between the regressing pronephros and the metanephros, cephalic to the latter. In young mammalian embryos, the m. is well developed and briefly functional until establishment of the metanephros, the definitive kidney; in older embryos, the m. undergoes regression as an excretory organ, but its duct system is retained in the male as the epididymis and ductus deferens. SYN middle kidney, wolffian body. [meso- + G. *nephros*, kidney]

mes·o·neu·ri·tis (mez'ō-nū-rī'tis). Inflammation of a nerve or of its connective tissue without involvement of its sheath.

nodular m., inflammation of the connective tissue beneath the nerve sheath, with the formation of circumscribed fibrous thickenings.

meso·on·to·morph (mez-ō-on'tō-mōrf). A broad, stocky individual. [meso- + G. *ōn*, being, + *morphē*, form]

mes·o·pexy (mez'ō-pek-sē). SYN mesenteriopexy.

mes·o·phil, mes·o·phile (mez'ō-fil, -fīl). A microorganism with an optimum temperature between 25°C and 40°C, but growing within the limits of 10°C and 45°C. [meso- + G. *philos*, fond]

mes·o·phil·ic (mez'ō-fil'ik). Pertaining to a mesophil.

mes·o·phle·bi·tis (mez'ō-flě-bī'tis). Inflammation of the middle coat of a vein. [meso- + phlebitis]

mes·o·phrag·ma (mez-ō-frag'mă). SYN M *line*. [meso- + G. *phragma*, a fence]

me·soph·ry·on (mez-of'ri-on). SYN glabella (2). [meso- + Gr. *ophrys*, eyebrow]

me·sop·ic (me-zō'pik). Pertaining to illumination between the photopic and scotopic ranges. [meso- + G. *opsis*, vision]

mes·o·pneu·mo·ni·um (mez'ō-noo-mō'nē-um). The reflection of pleura surrounding the root of the lung (including the pulmon-

me

ary ligament inferiorly) as parietal pleura becomes continuous with the visceral pleura of the lung. SYN mesentery of lung.

mes·o·por·phy·rins (mez-ō-pōr'fi-rinz). Porphyrin compounds resembling the protoporphyrins except that the vinyl side chains of the latter are reduced to ethyl side chains; *e.g.,* mesobilane.

mes·o·pro·sop·ic (mez'ō-prō-sop'ik). Having a face of moderate width, *i.e.,* with a facial index of about 90. [meso- + G. *prosōpon,* face]

mes·o·pul·mon·um (mez-ō-pŭl'mon-ŭm). The mesentery of the embryonic lung. [meso- + L. *pulmo,* lung]

me·sor·chi·al (mez-ōr'kē-ăl). Relating to the mesorchium.

me·sor·chi·um (mez-ōr'kē-ŭm). **1.** In the fetus, a fold of tunica vaginalis testis supporting the mesonephros and the developing testis. **2.** In the adult, a fold of tunica vaginalis testis between the testis and epididymis. [meso- + G. *orchis,* testis]

mes·o·rec·tum (mez'ō-rek'tŭm). The peritoneal investment of the rectum, covering the upper part only.

mes·o·rid·a·zine be·syl·ate (mez-ō-rid'ă-zēn). 10-[2-(1-Methyl-2-piperidyl)ethyl]-2-(methylsulfinyl)phenothiazone; a biotransformation product of thioridazine; an antipsychotic.

mes·or·rha·chis·chi·sis (mez'ō-ră-kis'ki-sis). SYN merorachischisis.

mes·or·rha·phy (mez-ōr'ă-fē). SYN mesenteriorrhaphy.

mes·or·rhine (mez'ō-rin). Having a nose of moderate width. Denoting a skull with a nasal index from 47 to 51 (Frankfort agreement) or 48 to 53 (Broca). [meso- + G. *rhis* (*rhin*-), nose]

mes·o·sal·pinx (mez'ō-sal'pinks) [NA]. The part of the broad ligament investing the uterine (fallopian) tube. [meso- + G. *salpinx,* trumpet]

mes·o·scope (mez'ō-skōp). An instrument for viewing objects that are larger than microscopic but cannot be seen distinctly with the naked eye. [meso- + G. *skopeō,* to view]

mes·o·seme (mez'ō-sēm). Denoting an orbital aperture with an index between 84 and 89; characteristic of the white race. [meso- + G. *sēma,* sign]

mes·o·sig·moid (mez'ō-sig'moyd). Sigmoid mesocolon. SEE mesocolon.

mes·o·sig·moid·i·tis (mes'ō-sig-moy-dī'tis). Inflammation of the mesosigmoid.

mes·o·sig·moid·o·pexy (mez-ō-sig-moy'dō-pek-sē). Surgical fixation of the mesosigmoid.

mes·o·so·ma·tous (mez'ō-so'mă-tŭs). Denoting a person of medium height.

mes·o·some (mes'ōsom). A convoluted membranous body formed by involution of the plasma membranes of certain bacteria; it functions in cellular respiration and septum formation. [meso + G. *soma,* body]

mes·o·so·mia (mez'ō-sō'mē-ă). Medium height. [meso- + G. *sōma,* body]

mes·o·ste·ni·um (mez'ō-stē'nē-ŭm). SYN mesentery (2).

mes·o·ster·num (mez'ō-ster'nŭm). SYN *body* of sternum. [meso- + G. *sternon,* chest]

mes·o·syph·i·lis (mez-ō-sif'i-lis). SYN secondary *syphilis.*

mes·o·sys·tol·ic (mez'ō-sis-tol'ik). Midsystolic.

mes·o·tar·sal (mez'ō-tar'săl). SYN midtarsal.

mes·o·ten·di·ne·um (mez'ō-ten-din'ē-ŭm) [NA]. SYN mesotendon.

mes·o·ten·don (mez'ō-ten'don). The synovial layers that pass from a tendon to the wall of a tendon sheath in certain places where tendons lie within osteofibrous canals. In most instances, the m. degenerates, leaving only the vinculae. SYN mesotendineum [NA].

mes·o·the·lia (mez-ō-thē'lē-ă). Plural of mesothelium.

mes·o·the·li·al (mez-ō-thē'lē-ăl). Relating to the mesothelium.

mes·o·the·li·o·ma (mez'ō-thē-lē-ō'mă). A rare neoplasm derived from the lining cells of the pleura and peritoneum which grows as a thick sheet covering the viscera, and is composed of spindle cells or fibrous tissue which may enclose glandlike spaces lined by cuboidal cells. [mesothelium + G. *-oma,* tumor]

benign m., SYN solitary fibrous *tumor.*

benign m. of genital tract, SYN adenomatoid *tumor.*

mes·o·the·li·um, pl. **mes·o·the·lia** (mez-ō-thē'lē-ŭm, -lē-ă). A single layer of flattened cells forming an epithelium that lines serous cavities; *e.g.,* peritoneum, pleura, pericardium. [meso- + epithelium]

mes·o·tho·ri·um (mez'ō-thōr'ē-ŭm). The first two disintegration products of thorium; mesothorium 1 is ^{228}Ra, a beta emitter with a half-life of 6.7 years, decaying into mesothorium 2, which is ^{228}Ac, a beta emitter with a half-life of 6.13 hr, which disintegrates to radiothorium (^{228}Th).

mes·o·tro·pic (mez'ō-trop'ik). Turned toward the median plane. [meso- + G. *tropē,* a turning]

mes·o·u·ran·ic (mes'ō-yū-ran'ik). Having a palatal index between 110 and 115. SYN mesuranic. [meso- + G. *ouranos,* palate]

mes·o·va·ri·um, pl. **mes·o·va·ria** (mez'ō-vā'rē-ŭm, -ă) [NA]. A short peritoneal fold connecting the anterior border of the ovary with the posterior layer of the broad ligament of the uterus. SYN mesoarium. [meso- + L. *ovarium,* ovary]

Mes·o·zoa (mez-ō-zō'ă). A small phylum of about 50 species of parasites of marine invertebrates with complex life cycles. M. are classified with the Metazoa, but they are regarded by some observers as intermediate between unicellular and multicellular animals; others consider them a degenerate group of flatworms. M. are divided into two very distinct orders, the Orthonectida and Dicyemida; the latter are nephridial parasites of squids, octopods, and cuttlefish. [meso- + G. *zōon,* animal]

mes·sen·ger (mes'en-jer). **1.** That which carries a message. **2.** Having message-carrying properties.

first m., a hormone that binds to a receptor on the surface cell and, in so doing, communicates with intracellular metabolic processes.

second m., an intermediary molecule that is generated as a consequence of hormone-receptor interaction; *e.g.,* see adenosine 3',5'-cyclic monophosphate; guanosine 3',5'-cyclic monophosphate; calcium; inositide.

mes·sen·ger RNA (mRNA). See under ribonucleic acid.

mes·tan·o·lone (mes-tan'ŏ-lōn). 17β-Hydroxy-17-methyl-5α-androstan-3-one; an androgenic steroid with anabolic properties.

mes·tene·di·ol (mes-tēn'dī-ol). SYN methandriol.

mes·tra·nol (mes'tră-nōl). 3-Methoxy-19-nor-17α-pregna-1,3,5(10)-trien-20-yn-17 -ol; the 3-methyl ether of ethynyl estradiol; an estrogen used in many oral contraceptive preparations.

me·sul·phen (mĕ-sŭl'fen). 2-7-Dimethylthianthrene; a topical scabicide with antipruritic properties.

me·su·ran·ic (mez'yū-ran'ik). SYN mesouranic.

MET Abbreviation for metabolic *equivalent.*

Met Symbol for methionine or its radicals in peptides.

△**meta-.** **1.** In medicine and biology, a prefix denoting the concept of after, subsequent to, behind, or hindmost. Cf. post-. **2.** In chemistry, an italicized prefix denoting joint, action sharing. **3** (*m*-). In chemistry, an italicized prefix denoting compound formed by two substitutions in the benzene ring separated by one carbon atom, *i.e.,* linked to the first and third, second and fourth, etc., carbon atoms of the ring. For terms beginning with *meta*-, or *m*-, see the specific name. [G. after, between, over]

met·a·anal·y·sis (met'ă-ă-nal'i-sis). The process of using statistical methods to combine the results of different studies; systematic, organized, and structured evaluation of a problem using information, commonly in the form of statistical tables, etc., from a number of different studies of the problem.

me·tab·a·sis (mĕ-tab'ă-sis). Rarely used term for a change of any kind in symptoms or course of a disease. [G. a passing over, change, fr. *metabainō,* to pass over]

met·a·bi·o·sis (met'ă-bī-ō'sis). Dependence of one organism on another for its existence. SEE ALSO commensalism, mutualism, parasitism. [meta- + G. *biōsis,* way of life]

met·a·bol·ic (met-ă-bol'ik). Relating to metabolism.

met·a·bo·lim·e·ter (met'ă-bŏ-lim'ĕ-ter). A modified calorimeter for measuring the rate of basal metabolism.

me·tab·o·lin (mĕ-tab'ŏ-lin). SYN metabolite.

me·tab·o·lism (mĕ-tab'ŏ-lizm). **1.** The sum of the chemical and physical changes occurring in tissue, consisting of anabolism, those reactions that convert small molecules into large, and catabolism, those reactions that convert large molecules into small, including both endogenous large molecules as well as biodegradation of xenobiotics. **2.** Often incorrectly used as a synonym for either anabolism or catabolism. [G. *metabolē,* change]

basal m., oxygen utilization of an individual during minimal physiologic activity while awake; an obsolete test determined by measuring oxygen consumption of a fasting subject at complete bodily and mental rest and a room temperature of 20°C. SYN basal metabolic rate.

carbohydrate m., oxidation, breakdown, and synthesis of carbohydrates in the tissues.

electrolyte m., the chemical changes that various essential minerals (*e.g.,* sodium, potassium, calcium, magnesium) undergo in the tissues.

energy m., those metabolic reactions whose role is to release or to provide energy.

fat m., oxidation, decomposition, and synthesis of fats in the tissues.

inborn error of m., a genetic biochemical disorder of a specific enzyme that forms a metabolic block, *e.g.,* phenylketonuria.

intermediary m., the sum of all metabolic reactions between uptake of foodstuffs and formation of excretory products.

oxidative m., SYN ventilation (2).

primary m., metabolic processes central to most cells; *e.g.,* biosynthesis of macromolecules, energy production, turnover, etc.

protein m., decomposition and synthesis of protein in the tissues. SYN proteometabolism.

respiratory m., the exchange of respiratory gases in the lungs, oxidation of foodstuffs in the tissues, and production of carbon dioxide and water.

secondary m., metabolic processes in which substances (such as pigments, alkaloids, terpenes, etc.) are only synthesized in certain types of tissues or cells or are only synthesized under certain conditions.

me·tab·o·lite (mě-tab′ō-līt). Any product (foodstuff, intermediate, waste product) of metabolism, especially of catabolism. SYN metabolin.

primary m., a m. synthesized in a step in primary metabolism.

secondary m., a m. synthesized in a step in secondary metabolism.

me·tab·o·lize (mě-tab′ō-līz). To undergo the chemical changes of metabolism.

met·a·car·pal (met′ă-kar′păl). **1.** Relating to the metacarpus. **2.** Any one of the metacarpal bones (I–V). SEE metacarpal *bone.*

met·a·car·pec·to·my (met′ă-kar-pek′tō-mē). Excision of one or all of the metacarpals. [metacarpus + G. *ektomē,* excision]

met·a·car·po·pha·lan·ge·al (met′ă-kar′pō-fă-lan′jē-ăl). Relating to the metacarpus and the phalanges; denoting the articulations between them.

met·a·car·pus, pl. **met·a·car·pi** (met′ă-kar′pŭs, -kar′pī) [NA]. The five bones of the hand between the carpus and the phalanges. [meta- + G. *karpos,* wrist]

met·a·cen·tric (met-ă-sen′trik). Having the centromere about equidistant from the extremities, said of a chromosome. [meta- + G. *kentron,* circle]

met·a·cer·ca·ria, pl. **met·a·cer·ca·ri·ae** (met′ă-ser-kar′ē-ă, -ē). The post-cercarial encysted stage in the life history of a fluke, prior to transfer to the definitive host. Some cercariae attach themselves to grass or other vegetation, form m., and later are ingested by herbivores, as in *Fasciola* and similar forms; others encyst in muscles of fish, as in *Clonorchis,* or in crayfish, as in *Paragonimus.* [meta- + G. *kerkos,* tail]

met·a·ces·tode (met-ă-ses′tōd). The larval stages of a tapeworm, including the metamorphosis of the oncosphere to the first evidence of sexuality in the adult worm, differentiation of the scolex, and beginning of proglottid formation; it includes the procercoid and plerocercoid stages of pseudophyllid cestodes, and the cysticercus, cysticercoid, coenurus, and hydatid stages of cyclophyllidean cestodes.

mineral metabolism				
	adults	children	adolescents	pregnant or nursing women
calcium (g)	0.8	1.0	1.2	2.0
phosphorus (g)	0.9	1.3	1.3	1.5
iron (mg)	12.0	7–12.0	15.0	15.0
sodium (g)	1.5–5.0			
potassium (g)	2.0			
magnesium (g)	0.3			
copper (mg)	2.0	0.1/kg		
zinc (mg)	10.0			
manganese (mg)	2.0–3.0			
fluoride (mg)	1.0			
iodine (mg)	0.1–0.15			

met·a·chlo·ral (met-ă-klō′răl). SYN *m*-chloral.

met·a·chro·ma·sia (met′ă-krō-mā′zē-ă). **1.** The condition in which a cell or tissue component takes on a color different from the dye solution with which it is stained. SYN metachromatism (2). **2.** A change in the characteristic color of certain basic thiazine dyes, such as toluidine blue, when the dye molecules are bound in proximate array to tissue polyanionic polymers, such as glycosaminoglycans. [meta- + G. *chrōma,* color]

met·a·chro·mat·ic (met′ă-krō-mat′ik). Denoting cells or dyes that exhibit metachromasia. SYN metachromophil, metachromophile.

met·a·chro·ma·tism (met-ă-krō′mă-tizm). **1.** Any color change, whether natural or produced by basic aniline dyes. **2.** SYN metachromasia (1). [meta- + G. *chrōma,* color]

met·a·chrom·ing (met′ă-krō′ming). The process of mixing a metal mordant with a dye before applying the dye to a tissue or fabric.

met·a·chro·mo·phil, met·a·chro·mo·phile (met-ă-krō′mō-fil, -fīl). SYN metachromatic. [meta- + G. *chrōma,* color, + *philos,* fond]

me·tach·ro·nous (mě-tak′rō-nŭs). Not synchronous; multiple separate occurrences, such as multiple primary cancers developing at intervals. [meta- + G. *chronos,* time]

met·a·chro·sis (met-ă-krō′sis). A change of color, such as occurs in certain animals, *e.g.,* the chameleon, by expansion and contraction of chromatophores. [meta- + G. *chrōsis,* a coloring]

met·a·cone (met′ă-kōn). The distobuccal cusp of an upper molar tooth. [meta- + G. *kōnos,* cone]

met·a·co·nid (met-ă-kon′id, -kō′nid). The mesolingual cusp of a lower molar tooth.

met·a·con·trast (met-ă-kon′trast). Inhibition of the brightness of illumination when an adjacent visual field is illuminated.

met·a·con·ule (met-ă-kon′yūl). The distal intermediate cusp of an upper molar tooth. [meta- + G. *kōnos,* a cone]

met·a·cre·sol (met-ă-krē′sol). SYN *m*-cresol.

met·a·cryp·to·zo·ite (met′ă-krip-tō-zō′īt). The exoerythrocytic stage that develops from merozoites formed by the first, or cryptozoite, generation; the cryptozoite and metacryptozoite generations comprise the primary exoerythrocytic stages of malaria development (prepatent period) prior to infection of red blood cells. [meta- + G. *kryptos,* hidden, + *zōon,* animal]

met·a·cy·e·sis (met-ă-sī-ē′sis). SYN ectopic *pregnancy.* [meta- + G. *kyēsis,* pregnancy]

met·a·dys·en·tery (met-ă-dis′en-tār-ē). Old term for bacillary *dysentery.*

Met·a·gon·i·mus (met-ă-gon′i-mŭs). A genus of flukes (superfamily Heterophypoidea) that encyst on fish and infect various fish-eating animals, including humans. *M. yokogawai*, an intestinal fluke widely distributed in the Far East and the Balkans and one of the smallest (1–2.5 mm) flukes infecting humans, is passed from *Semisulcospira* snails to cyprinoid fish and then to man and other fish-eating mammals and birds. [meta- + G. *gonimos*, productive]

met·a·ic·ter·ic (met-ă-ik′ter-ik). Occurring as a sequel of jaundice. [meta- + G. *ikterikos*, jaundiced]

met·a·in·fec·tive (met′ă-in-fek′tiv). Occurring subsequent to an infection; denoting specifically a febrile condition sometimes observed during convalescence from an infectious disease.

met·a·ki·ne·sis, met·a·ki·ne·sia (met′ă-ki-nē′sis, -ki-nē′sē-ă). Moving apart; the separation of the two chromatids of each chromosome and their movement to opposite poles in the anaphase of mitosis. [meta- + G. *kinēsis*, movement]

met·al (met′ăl). One of the electropositive elements, either amphoteric or basic, usually characterized by properties such as luster, malleability, ductility, the ability to conduct electricity, and the tendency to lose rather than gain electrons in chemicals. [L. *metallum*, a mine, a mineral, fr. G. *metallon*, a mine, pit]

alkali m., an alkali of the family Li, Na, K, Rb, Cs, and Fr, all of which have highly ionized hydroxides. SYN alkali (3).

alkali earth m., SEE alkaline earth *elements*, under *element*.

Babbitt m., an alloy of antimony, copper, and tin; used occasionally in dentistry.

base m., basic m., a m. that is readily oxidized; *e.g.,* iron, copper.

colloidal m., a colloidal solution of a m. obtained by passing electric sparks between terminals of the m. in distilled water. SYN electrosol.

d'Arcet's m., an alloy of lead, bismuth, and tin; used in dentistry.

fusible m., a m. with a low melting point.

heavy m., a m. with a high specific gravity, typically larger than 5; *e.g.,* Fe, Co, Cu, Mn, Mo, Zn, V.

light m., a m. with a specific gravity of less than 4.

noble m., a m. that cannot be oxidized by heat alone, nor readily dissolved by acid; *e.g.,* gold, platinum. SYN noble element (1).

rare earth m., SEE lanthanides.

respiratory m., a m. present in certain respiratory pigments; *e.g.,* iron, manganese, copper, vanadium.

met·al·de·hyde (met-al′dĕ-hīd). A polymer of acetaldehyde. [meta- + aldehyde]

me·tal·lic (mĕ-tal′ik). Relating to, composed of, or resembling metal.

⚠**metallo-.** Metal, metallic. [see metal]

me·tal·lo·cy·a·nide (mĕ-tal-ō-sī′ă-nīd). A compound of cyanogen with a metal forming an ionic radical that combines with a basic element to form a salt; *e.g.,* potassium ferricyanide, $K_3Fe(CN)_6$.

me·tal·lo·en·zyme (mĕ-tal-ō-en′zīm). An enzyme containing a metal (ion) as an integral part of its active structure; *e.g.,* cytochromes (Fe, Cu), aldehyde oxidase (Mo), catechol oxidase (Cu), carbonic anhydrase (Zn).

me·tal·lo·fla·vo·de·hy·drog·e·nase (mĕ-tal′ō-flā′vō-dē-hī′drō-jen-ās). A type of oxidizing enzyme, containing one of the flavin nucleotides as coenzyme, plus a metal ion that is also necessary to the action; the metal may be Fe (as in succinate dehydrogenase), Cu (as in urate oxidase), or Mo (as in xanthine oxidase).

me·tal·lo·fla·vo·en·zyme (mĕ-tal′ō-flā-vō-en′zīm). An enzyme that contains one of the flavin nucleotides and at least one metal ion as a required part of its active structure.

me·tal·lo·fla·vo·pro·tein (mĕ-tal′ō-flā′vō-prō-tēn). A protein containing a flavin entity and at least one metal ion.

met·al·loid (met′ă-loyd). Resembling a metal in at least one amphoteric form; *e.g.,* silicon and germanium as semiconductors. [metal + G. *eidos*, resemblance]

me·tal·lo·phil·ia (mĕ-tal′ō-fil′ē-ă). Affinity for metal salts; *e.g.,* the affinity of the cytoplasm of cells of the reticuloendothelial system for silver carbonate stain and salts of gold and iron. [metallo- + G. *philos*, fond]

me·tal·lo·pho·bia (mĕ-tal-ō-fō′bē-ă). Morbid fear of metal objects. [G. *metallon*, metal, + *phobos*, fear]

me·tal·lo·por·phy·rin (mĕ-tal-ō-pōr′fi-rin). A combination of a porphyrin with a metal, *e.g.,* Fe (hematin), Mg (as in chlorophyll), Cu (in hemocyanin), Zn.

me·tal·lo·pro·tein (mĕ-tal-ō-prō′tēn). A protein with a tightly bound metal ion or ions; *e.g.,* hemoglobin.

met·al·los·co·py (met-ă-los′kō-pē). Testing the action of various metals applied to the surface of the body. [metallo- + G. *skopeō*, to examine]

me·tal·lo·thi·o·nein (mĕ-tal-ō-thī′ō-nēn). Name proposed for a small protein, rich in cysteinyl residues, that is synthesized in the liver and kidney in response to the presence of divalent ions (zinc, mercury, cadmium, copper, etc.) and that binds these ions tightly; of importance in ion transport and detoxification; the apoprotein is thionein.

met·a·lu·et·ic (met′ă-lū-et′ik). 1. SYN metasyphilitic (1). 2. SYN metasyphilitic (2). 3. SYN parasyphilitic. [meta- + L. *lues*, pestilence]

met·a·mer (met′ă-mer). An entity that is similar to, but ultimately differentiable from, another entity. [meta- + -mer]

met·a·mere (met′ă-mēr). One of a series of homologous segments in the body. SEE ALSO somite. [meta- + G. *meros*, part]

met·a·mer·ic (met-ă-mer′ik). Relating to or showing metamerism, or occurring in a metamere.

me·tam·er·ism (me-tam′er-izm). 1. A type of anatomic structure exhibiting serially homologous metameres; in primitive forms, such as the annelids, the metameres are almost alike in structure; in vertebrates, specialization in the cephalic region masks the underlying m., which is still clearly evident in serially repeated vertebrae, ribs, intercostal muscles, and spinal nerves, and in young vertebrate embryos. 2. In chemistry, rarely used synonym for isomerism.

met·a·mor·phop·sia (met′ă-mōr-fop′sē-ă). Distortion of visual images. [meta- + G. *morphē*, shape, + *opsis*, vision]

met·a·mor·pho·sis (met-ă-mōr′fŏ-sis, -mōr-fō′sis). 1. A change in form, structure, or function. 2. Transition from one developmental stage to another. SYN allaxis, transformation (1). [G. *metamorphasos*, transformation fr. *meta*, beyond, over, + *morphē*, form]

complete m., insect development from egg, through successive larval instars, pupa, and adult; the latter is distinct from the first two forms of the insect, permitting specialization of feeding (larval) and reproductive-flying functions (adult); characteristic of the higher insect orders, such as Coleoptera (beetles), Hymenoptera (bees, wasps, ants), Diptera (two-winged flies), and Siphonaptera (fleas). SYN holometabolous m.

fatty m., the appearance of microscopically visible droplets of fat in the cytoplasm of cells. SEE ALSO fatty *degeneration*. SYN fatty change.

heterometabolous m., SYN incomplete m.

holometabolous m., SYN complete m.

incomplete m., the development of a nymph into the imago which in many respects resembles the former; characteristic of more primitive insect orders, such as Heteroptera (true bugs), Orthoptera (locusts, grasshoppers), and Blatterria (roaches). SYN heterometabolous m.

retrograde m., SYN degeneration (3). (1) SYN cataplasia.

met·a·mor·phot·ic (met′ă-mōr-fot′ik). Relating to or marked by metamorphosis.

met·a·my·el·o·cyte (met-ă-mī′el-ō-sīt). A transitional form of myelocyte with nuclear construction that is intermediate between the mature myelocyte (myelocyte C of Sabin) and the two-lobed granular leukocyte. SYN juvenile cell. [meta- + G. *myelos*, marrow, + *kytos*, cell]

met·a·neph·ric (met-ă-nef′rik). Of or pertaining to the metanephron.

met·a·neph·rine (met-ă-nef′rin). 3-O-Methylepinephrine; a catabolite of epinephrine found, together with normetanephrine, in the urine and in some tissues, resulting from the action of catechol-O-methyltransferase on epinephrine; has no sympathomimetic actions.

met·a·neph·ro·gen·ic, met·a·ne·phrog·e·nous (met′ă-nef-rō-jen′ik, -nĕ-froj′ĕ-nŭs). Applied to the more caudal part of the intermediate mesoderm which, under the inductive action of the metanephric diverticulum, has the potency to form metanephric tubules. [meta- + G. *nephros*, kidney, + *-gen*, producing]

met·a·neph·ros, pl. **met·a·neph·roi** (met-ă-nef′ros, -roy). The most caudally located of the three excretory organs appearing in the evolution of the vertebrates (the others being the pronephros and the mesonephros); in mammalian embryos, the m. develops caudal to the mesonephros during its regression, becoming the permanent kidney. SYN hind kidney. [meta- + G. *nephros*, kidney]

met·a·neu·tro·phil, met·a·neu·tro·phile (met-ă-nū′trō-fil, -fīl). Not staining true with neutral dyes. [meta- + L. *neuter*, neither, + G. *philos*, fond]

met·a·nil yel·low (mĕt′ă-nil) [C.I. 13065]. A monoazo acid dye, $C_{18}H_{14}N_3O_3SNa$, used as a cytoplasmic and connective tissue stain.

met·a·phase (met′ă-fās). The stage of mitosis or meiosis in which the chromosomes become aligned on the equatorial plate of the cell separating the centromeres. In mitosis and in the second meiotic division, the centromeres of each chromosome divide and the two daughter centromeres are directed toward opposite poles of the cell; in the first division of meiosis, the centromeres do not divide but the centromeres of each pair of homologous chromosomes become directed toward opposite poles. [meta- + G. *phasis*, an appearance]

met·a·phos·phor·ic ac·id (met′ă-fos-fōr′ik). SYN glacial *phosphoric acid*.

met·a·phy·si·al, met·a·phy·se·al (met-ă-fiz′ē-ăl). Relating to a metaphysis.

me·taph·y·sis, pl. **me·taph·y·ses** (mĕ-taf′i-sis, -sēz) [NA]. A conical section of bone between the epiphysis and diaphysis of long bones. [meta- + G. *physis*, growth]

me·taph·y·si·tis (mĕ-taf′i-sī′tis). Inflammation of the metaphysis.

met·a·pla·sia (met-ă-plā′zē-ă). Abnormal transformation of an adult, fully differentiated tissue of one kind into a differentiated tissue of another kind; an acquired condition, in contrast to heteroplasia (2). [G. *metaplasis*, transformation]
  agnogenic myeloid m., SYN primary myeloid m.
  apocrine m., alteration of acinar epithelium of breast tissue to resemble apocrine sweat glands; seen commonly in fibrocystic disease of the breasts.
  autoparenchymatous m., m. occurring in the parenchymal cells proper to the tissue.
  coelomic m., potential of coelomic epithelium to differentiate into several different histologic cell types.
  intestinal m., the transformation of mucosa, particularly in the stomach, into glandular mucosa resembling that of the intestines, although usually lacking villi.
  myeloid m., a syndrome characterized by anemia, enlargement of the spleen, nucleated red blood cells and immature granulocytes in the circulating blood, and conspicuous foci of extramedullary hemopoiesis in the spleen and liver; may develop in the course of polycythemia rubra vera; there is a high incidence of development of myeloid leukemia.
  primary myeloid m., myeloid m. occurring as the primary condition, often in association with myelofibrosis. SYN agnogenic myeloid m.
  secondary myeloid m., myeloid m. occurring in individuals with another disease. SYN symptomatic myeloid m.
  squamous m., the transformation of glandular or mucosal epithelium into stratified squamous epithelium. SYN epidermalization.
  squamous m. of amnion, SYN *amnion* nodosum.
  symptomatic myeloid m., SYN secondary myeloid m.

me·tap·la·sis (mĕ-tap′lă-sis). 1. E.H. Haeckel's term for the stage of completed growth or development of the individual. 2. SYN metaplasia. [G. a transformation]

met·a·plasm (met′ă-plazm). SYN cell *inclusions* (1), under *inclusion*. [meta- + G. *plasma*, something formed]

met·a·plas·tic (met-ă-plas′tik). Pertaining to metaplasia or metaplasis.

met·a·plex·us (met′ă-plek′sŭs). The choroid plexus in the fourth ventricle of the brain. [meta- + L. *plexus*, an interweaving]

met·a·poph·y·sis (met′ă-pof′i-sis). SYN mamillary *process*. [meta- + G. *apophysis*, a process]

met·a·pore (met′ă-pōr). Rarely used term for *apertura* mediana ventriculi quarti. [meta- + G. *poros*, pore]

met·a·pro·tein (met-ă-prō′tēn). Nondescript term for a derived protein obtained by the action of acids or alkalies, soluble in weak acids or alkalies but insoluble in neutral solutions; *e.g.,* albuminate.

met·a·pro·ter·e·nol sul·fate (met′ă-prō-ter′ĕ-nol). 3,5-Dihydroxy-α-[(isopropylamino)methyl]benzyl alcohol sulfate; a sympathomimetic bronchodilator used for the treatment of bronchial asthma and in chronic obstructive lung disease. It has relatively greater effect on β_2-adrenergic receptors than β_1, conferring some selectivity in relaxing bronchiolar smooth muscle as compared with cardiac stimulation. SYN orciprenaline sulfate.

met·a·psy·chol·o·gy (met′ă-sī-kol′ō-jē). 1. A systematic attempt to discern and describe what lies beyond the empirical facts and laws of psychology, such as the relations between body and mind, or concerning the place of the mind in the universe. 2. In psychoanalysis, or psychoanalytic m., psychology concerning the fundamental assumptions of the freudian theory of the mind, which entail five points of view: 1) dynamic, concerning psychologic forces; 2) economic, concerning psychologic energy; 3) structural, concerning psychologic configurations; 4) genetic, concerning psychologic origins; 5) adaptive, concerning psychologic relations with the environment. [G. *meta*, beyond, transcending, + psychology]

met·a·py·ret·ic (met′ă-pī-ret′ik). SYN postfebrile. [meta- + G. *pyretos*, fever]

met·a·py·ro·cat·e·chase (met′ă-pī-rō-kat′ĕ-kās). SYN catechol 2,3-dioxygenase.

met·a·ram·i·nol bi·tar·trate (met-ă-ram′i-nol). *l*-α-(1-Aminoethyl)-*m*-hydroxybenzyl alcohol hydrogen *d*-tartrate; a potent sympathomimetic amine used for the elevation and maintenance of blood pressure in acute hypotensive states and topically as a nasal decongestant.

met·a·rho·dop·sin. (met-ă-rō-dop′sin) A light-activated form of rhodopsin; m. I is formed from lumirhodopsin and is converted to m. II; m. II is the form of rhodopsin that releases all-*trans*-retinal.

met·ar·te·ri·ole (met′ar-tēr′ē-ōl). One of the small peripheral blood vessels between the arterioles and the true capillaries that contain scattered groups of smooth muscle fibers in their walls. [meta- + arteriole]

met·a·ru·bri·cyte (met-ă-rū′bri-sīt). Orthochromatic normoblast. SEE normoblast.
  pernicious anemia type m., orthochromatic megaloblast. SEE megaloblast.

met·a·sta·ble (met′ă-stā-bl). 1. Of uncertain stability; in a condition to pass into another phase when slightly disturbed; *e.g.,* water, when cooled below the freezing point may remain liquid but will at once congeal if a piece of ice is added. 2. Denoting the excited condition of the nucleus of a radionuclide isomer that reaches a lower energy state by the process of isomeric transition decay without changing its atomic number or weight; *e.g.,* $^{99m}_{43}$Tc $\rightarrow$ $^{99}_{43}$Tc + γ. [meta- + L. *stabilis*, stable]

me·tas·ta·sis, pl. **me·tas·ta·ses** (mĕ-tas′tă-sis, -sēz). 1. The shifting of a disease or its local manifestations, from one part of the body to another, as in mumps when the symptoms referable to the parotid gland subside and the testis becomes affected. 2. The spread of a disease process from one part of the body to another, as in the appearance of neoplasms in parts of the body remote from the site of the primary tumor; results from dissemination of tumor cells by the lymphatics or blood vessels or by direct extension through serous cavities or subarachnoid or other spaces. 3. Transportation of bacteria from one part of the body to another, through the bloodstream (hematogenous m.) or through lymph channels (lymphogenous m.). SYN secondaries (1). [G. a removing, fr. *meta*, in the midst of, + *stasis*, a placing]

me

biochemical m., the transportation and induction of abnormal immunochemical specificities in apparently normal organs.

calcareous m., the deposit of calcareous material in remote tissues in the event of extensive resorption of osseous tissue in caries, malignant neoplasms, and so on.

hematogenous m., SEE metastasis.

lymphogenous m., SEE metastasis.

pulsating metastases, metastases to bone, usually from hypernephromas, but occasionally from thyroid tumors; may have expansile pulsation and a continuous bruit.

satellite m., m. within the immediate vicinity of a primary malignant neoplasm; *e.g.,* skin adjacent to a melanoma.

me·tas·ta·size (mĕ-tas'tă-sīz). To pass into or invade by metastasis.

met·a·stat·ic (met-ă-stat'ik). Relating to metastasis.

met·a·ster·num (met'ă-ster'nŭm). SYN xiphoid *process.*

met·a·stron·gyle (met-ă-stron'jīl). Common name for members of the genus *Metastrongylus* or of the family Metastrongylidae.

Met·a·stron·gy·lus (met-ă-stron'jĭ-lŭs). A genus of nematode lungworms (family Metastrongylidae), the only genus in its subfamily (Metastrongylinae). The four known species are found only in pigs; transmission is by earthworm intermediate hosts. [meta- + G. *strongylos,* round]

M. a'pri, a common lungworm species that occurs in larger bronchi of wild and domestic pigs, where it is highly pathogenic, causing verminous pneumonia, consolidation of lungs, emphysema, loss of condition, and reduced growth.

M. elonga'tus, SYN *M. salmi.*

M. pudendotec'tus, a lungworm species, considerably smaller than *M. apri,* found in domestic and wild pigs.

M. sal'mi, a lungworm species that occurs in the trachea, bronchi, and bronchioles of domestic and wild pigs. SYN *M. elongatus.*

met·a·syph·i·lis (met-ă-sif'i-lis). **1.** The constitutional state due to congenital syphilis without local lesions. **2.** SYN parasyphilis.

met·a·syph·i·lit·ic (met'ă-sif-i-lit'ik). **1.** Relating to metasyphilis. SYN metaluetic (1). **2.** Following or occurring as a sequel of syphilis. SYN metaluetic (2). **3.** SYN parasyphilitic.

met·a·tar·sal (met'ă-tar'săl). Relating to the metatarsus or to one of the metatarsal bones.

met·a·tar·sal·gia (met'ă-tar-sal'jē-ă). Pain in the forefoot in the region of the heads of the metatarsals. [meta- + G. *algos,* pain]

met·a·tar·sec·to·my (met'ă-tar-sek'tō-mē). Excision of the metatarsus. [metatarsus + G. *ektomē,* excision]

met·a·tar·so·pha·lan·ge·al (met'ă-tar'sō-fă-lan'jē-ăl). Relating to the metatarsal bones and the phalanges; denoting the articulations between them.

met·a·tar·sus, pl. **me·ta·tar·si** (met'ă-tar'sŭs, -sī) [NA]. The distal portion of the foot between the instep and the toes, having as its skeleton the five long bones (metatarsal bones) articulating posteriorly with the cuboid and cuneiform bones and distally with the phalanges. [meta- + G. *tarsos,* tarsus]

m. adductova'rus, fixed deformity of the foot in which both adductus and varus vectors contribute to the resultant foot posture.

m. adduc'tus, a fixed deformity of the foot in which the forepart of the foot is angled away from the main longitudinal axis of the foot toward the midline; usually congenital in origin.

m. atav'icus, abnormal shortness of the first metatarsal bone as compared with the second.

m. la'tus, deformity caused by sinking down of the transverse arch of the foot. SYN talipes transversoplanus.

m. va'rus, fixed deformity of the foot in which the forepart of the foot is rotated on the long axis of the foot, so that the plantar surface faces the midline of the body. SYN intoe.

met·a·thal·a·mus (met'ă-thal'ă-mŭs) [NA]. The most caudal and ventral part of the thalamus, composed of the medial and lateral geniculate bodies. [meta- + G. *thalamos,* thalamus]

me·tath·e·sis (me-tath'ĕ-sis). **1.** Transfer of a pathologic product (*e.g.,* a calculus) from one place to another where it causes less inconvenience or injury, when it is not possible or expedient to remove it from the body. **2.** In chemistry, a double decomposition, wherein a compound, A-B, reacts with another compound, C-D, to yield A-C + B-D, or A-D + B-C. [meta- + G. *thesis,* a placing]

met·a·troph (met'ă-trof). An organism that requires complex organic sources of carbon and nitrogen for growth.

met·a·tro·phic (met-ă-trof'ik). Denoting the ability to undertake anabolism or to obtain nourishment from varied sources, *i.e.,* both nitrogenous and carbonaceous organic matter. [meta- + G. *trophē,* nourishment]

met·a·tro·pic (met-ă-trop'ik). Denoting a reversion to a previous state. [meta- + G. *tropē,* a turning]

met·a·typ·i·cal (met-ă-tip'i-kăl). Pertaining to tissue that is formed of elements identical to those occurring in that site under normal conditions, but the various elements are not arranged in the usual normal pattern.

me·tax·a·lone (mĕ-tak'să-lōn). 5-[(3,5-Xylyloxy)methyl]-2-oxazolidinone; 5-(3,5-dimethylphenoxymethyl)-2-oxazolidinone; a centrally acting skeletal muscle relaxant.

Met·a·zoa (met-ă-zō'ă). A subkingdom of the kingdom Animalia, including all multicellular animal organisms in which the cells are differentiated and form tissues; distinguished from the subkingdom Protozoa, or unicellular animal organisms. [meta- + G. *zōon,* animal]

met·a·zo·o·no·sis (met'ă-zō-ō-nō'sis). A zoonosis that requires both a vertebrate and an invertebrate host for completion of its life cycle; *e.g.,* the arbovirus, infections of humans and other vertebrates. [meta- + G. *zōon,* animal, + *nosos,* disease]

Metchnikoff, Elie, Russian biologist in Paris and Nobel laureate, 1845–1916. SEE M.'s theory.

met·en·ce·phal·ic (met'en-se-fal'ik). Relating to the metencephalon.

met·en·ceph·a·lon (met'en-sef'ă-lon) [NA]. The anterior of the two major subdivisions of the rhombencephalon (the posterior being the myelencephalon or medulla oblongata), composed of the pons and the cerebellum. [meta- + G. *enkephalos,* brain]

Metenier's sign. See under sign.

met·en·keph·a·lin (met-en-kef'ă-lin). SEE enkephalins.

me·te·or·ism (mē'tē-ŏ-rizm). SYN tympanites. [G. *meteōrismos,* a lifting up]

me·te·or·op·a·thy (mē'tē-ōr-op'ă-thē). Rarely used term for ill health due to climatic conditions. [G. *meteōra,* things high in the air, + *pathos,* suffering]

me·te·or·o·tro·pic (mē'tē-ōr-ō-trop'ik). Denoting diseases affected in their incidence by the weather. [G. *meteōra,* things high in the air, + G. *tropos,* a turning]

me·ter (m) (mē'ter). **1.** The fundamental unit of length in the SI and metric systems, equivalent to 39.37007874 inches. Defined to be the length of path traveled by light in a vacuum in 1/299792458 sec. **2.** A device for measuring the quantity of that which passes through it. [Fr. *metre;* G. *metron,* measure]

rate m., a device that continuously displays the magnitude of events averaged over varying time intervals.

ventilation m., a m. used to measure tidal and minute ventilatory volumes.

Venturi m., a device for measuring flow of a fluid in terms of the drop in pressure when the fluid flows into the constriction of a Venturi tube.

me·ter-can·dle (mē'ter-kan'dl). SYN lux.

met·er·ga·sia (met-er-gā'zē-ă). Change of function. [G. *meta,* denoting change, + *ergasia,* work]

me·ter·go·line (mē'ter-gō-līn). An ergot derivative with a pharmacological profile similar to methysergide; a nonselective blocker of serotonin receptors. Used as an analgesic in migraine headache. SYN methergoline.

met·es·the·si·ol·o·gist (mét'és-thē-zē-ol'ō-jíst). **1.** A proposed substitute for the term anesthesiologist to indicate the extent to which the clinical practice of a physician trained in administration of anesthetics has expanded beyond the operating room into resuscitation, critical care, management of acute and chronic pain. **2.** A physician board certified and legally qualified both to administer anesthesia and to engage in related activities outside the operating room. [G. *meta*, beyond, + anesthesiologist]

met·es·the·si·ol·o·gy (mét′és-thē-zē-ol′ō-j′e). Proposed substitute for the term anesthesiology to indicate the extent to which the specialty previously based almost completely on administration of anesthetics has come to involve equally important roles and responsibilities outside the operating room, including management of acute and chronic pain, and care of critically ill patients and women in labor. [G. *meta*, beyond, + anesthesiology]

met·es·trus, met·es·trum (met-es′trŭs, -trŭm). The period between estrus and diestrus in the estrous cycle. [meta- + estrus]

met·for·min (met-fōr′min). 1,1-Dimethylbiguanide; an oral hypoglycemic agent.

meth-, metho-. Chemical prefixes usually denoting a methyl, methoxy group.

meth·a·cho·line chlo·ride (meth′ă-kō-lēn). Acetyl-β-methylcholine chloride; a derivative of acetylcholine; a parasympathomimetic agent used as a vasodilator in peripheral vascular disease, and for inducing hyperemia in arthritis, its action being brought about locally by iontophoresis; also available as m. c. bromide.

meth·ac·ry·late res·in. See under resin.

meth·a·cryl·ic ac·id (meth′ă-kril′ik). Occurs in oil from Roman camomile; used in the manufacture of methacrylate resins and plastics. SYN methylacrylic acid.

meth·a·cy·cline hy·dro·chlo·ride (meth-ă-sī′klēn). 6-Methylene-5-hydroxytetracycline hydrochloride; an antimicrobial agent.

meth·a·done hy·dro·chlo·ride (meth′ă-dōn). 6-Dimethylamino-4,4-diphenyl-3-heptanone hydrochloride; a synthetic narcotic drug; an orally effective analgesic similar in action to morphine but with slightly greater potency and longer duration. It produces psychic and physical dependence as with morphine, but withdrawal symptoms are somewhat milder; used as a replacement (oral route) for morphine and heroin; also used during withdrawal treatment in morphine and heroin addiction.

meth·al·len·es·tril (meth′ă-len-es′tril). α,α-Dimethyl-β-ethyl-6-methoxy-2-naphthalene propionic acid; an orally effective, nonsteroid estrogenic compound.

meth·am·phet·a·mine hy·dro·chlo·ride (meth-am-fet′ă-mēn). *d*-Desoxyephedrine hydrochloride; *d*-N,α-dimethylphenethylamine hydrochloride, "speed"; a sympathomimetic agent that exerts greater stimulating effects upon the central nervous system than does amphetamine; widely used by drug abusers via the oral and intravenous ("mainlining") routes; strong psychic dependence may develop. SYN methylamphetamine hydrochloride.

meth·am·py·rone (meth-am-pī′rōn). SYN dipyrone.

meth·an·di·e·none (meth-an-dī′ĕ-nōn). SYN methandrostenolone.

meth·an·dri·ol (meth-an′drē-ol). 17-Methyl-5-androstene-3β,17β-diol; the methyl derivative of androstenediol, with similar actions and uses. SYN mestenediol.

meth·an·dro·sten·o·lone (meth-an-drō-sten′ō-lōn). 17β-Hydroxy-17α-methyl-1,4-androstadiene-3-one; a methylated dehydrotestosterone; an orally effective anabolic steroid that may promote nitrogen retention when combined with an adequate diet; in addition, it can exert typically androgenic effects. SYN methandienone.

meth·ane (meth′ān). CH_4; an odorless gas produced by the decomposition of organic matter; explosive when mixed with 7 or 8 volumes of air, constituting then the firedamp in coal mines. SYN marsh gas.

Meth·a·no·bac·te·ri·a·ce·ae (meth′ă-nō-bak-tēr-ē-ā′sē-ē). A family of bacteria containing Gram-negative and Gram-positive, motile or nonmotile, strictly anaerobic rods and cocci, which obtain energy either by the reduction of carbon dioxide to form methane or by the fermentation of compounds such as acetate and methanol with the production of methane and carbon dioxide; they are found in anaerobic habitats such as sediments of natural waters, soil, anaerobic sewage digestors, and the gastrointestinal tract of animals.

meth·an·o·gen (meth-an′ō-jen). Any methane-producing bacterium of the family Methanobacteriaceae.

meth·a·nol (meth′ă-nol). SYN *methyl* alcohol.

meth·an·the·line bro·mide (meth-an′thĕ-lēn). $C_{21}H_{26}BrNO_3$; β-diethylaminoethyl-9-xanthenecarboxylate methobromide; an anticholinergic drug.

meth·a·pyr·i·lene (meth-ă-pir′i-lēn). 2-[(2-Dimethylaminoethyl)-2-thenylamino]pyridine; an antihistamine. M. fumarate is administered topically on the skin; m. hydrochloride is the preferred salt for oral or parenteral use.

meth·a·qua·lone (meth-ă-kwā′lōn). 2-Methyl-3-o-tolyl-4(3*H*)-quinazolinone; a sedative and hypnotic, also a drug of abuse; available as the hydrochloride.

meth·ar·bi·tal (meth-ar′bi-tahl). 5,5-Diethyl-1-methylbarbituric acid; an *N*-methylated derivative of barbital with anticonvulsant properties similar to those of phenobarbital; converted to barbital in the body.

meth·ar·gen (meth′ar-jen). 2,2′-Dinaphthylmethane-3,3′-disulfonic acid disilver salt; a topical antiseptic agent.

meth·a·zo·la·mide (meth-ă-zol′ă-mīd). *N*-(4-Methyl-2-sulfamoyl-Δ²-1,3,4-thiadiazolin-5-ylidene)acetamide; a carbonic anhydrase inhibitor with uses similar to those of acetazolamide.

metHb Abbreviation for methemoglobin.

meth·dil·a·zine hy·dro·chlo·ride (meth-dil′ă-zēn). 10-(1-Methyl-3-pyrrolidylmethyl)phenothiazine hydrochloride; a phenothiazine compound with antihistaminic activity; used in the treatment of various dermatoses to relieve pruritus.

met·hem·al·bu·min (met′hēm-al-bū′min, -hem-al′bū-min). An abnormal compound formed in the blood as a result of heme combining with plasma albumin.

met·hem·al·bu·mi·ne·mia (met′hēm-al-bū-min-ē′mē-ă). The presence of methemalbumin in the circulating blood, indicative of hemoglobin breakdown; found in some patients with blackwater fever or paroxysmal nocturnal hemoglobinuria; described as a means of differentiating severe (hemorrhagic) from mild (edematous) pancreatitis, and also has been described in other acute conditions such as strangulation obstruction of intestine and mesenteric artery occlusion.

met·he·mo·glo·bin (metHb) (met-hē-mō-glō′bin). A transformation product of oxyhemoglobin because of the oxidation of the normal Fe^{2+} to Fe^{3+}, thus converting ferroprotoporphyrin to ferriprotoporphyrin; it contains water in firm union with ferric iron, thus being chemically different from oxyhemoglobin and useless for respiration; found in sanguineous effusions and in the circulating blood after poisoning with acetanilid, potassium chlorate, and other substances. SYN ferrihemoglobin.

m. reductase, a flavoenzyme catalyzing the reduction of m. to hemoglobin in the red blood cell.

met·he·mo·glo·bi·ne·mia (met-hē′mō-glō-bi-nē′mē-ă, meth′ĕ-mō-). The presence of methemoglobin in the circulating blood. [methemoglobin + G. *haima*, blood]

acquired m., m. caused by various chemical agents, such as nitrites. SYN enterogenous m., secondary m.

congenital m., (1) m. due to formation of any one of a group of abnormal α chain [MIM*141800] or β chain [MIM*141900] hemoglobins collectively known as hemoglobin M. Slate-gray cyanosis occurs in early infancy, without pulmonary or cardiac disease, and is resistant to ascorbic acid or methylene blue thera-

---

⌂ **Combining forms**	[NA] **Nomina Anatomica**
Word*Finder*	[MIM] **Mendelian**
Multi-term entry finder	**Inheritance in Man**
Preceding letter A	
	☆ **Official alternate term**
A.D.A.M. Anatomy Plates	
Between letters L and M	☆[NA] **Official alternate**
	Nomina Anatomica term
Appendices:	
Following letter Z	
	High Profile Term
SYN Synonym; Cf., compare	

me

py; autosomal dominant inheritance; **(2)** m. due to deficiency of cytochrome b_5 reductase [MIM*250790] or methemoglobin reductase [MIM*250700], the enzyme responsible for reduction of intraerythrocyte methemoglobin; cyanosis is improved by ascorbic acid or methylene blue; autosomal recessive inheritance; **(3)** one case of m. has been reported that apparently is due to a deficiency of cytochrome b_5. SYN hereditary m., hereditary methemoglobinemic cyanosis, primary m.

enterogenous m., SYN acquired m.

hereditary m., SYN congenital m.

primary m., SYN congenital m.

secondary m., SYN acquired m.

met·he·mo·glo·bi·nu·ria (met-hē′mō-glō-bi-nū′rē-ă, meth′ĕ-mō-). The presence of methemoglobin in the urine. [methemoglobin + G. *ouron*, urine]

meth·en·a·mine (me-then′ă-mēn). $C_6H_{12}N_4$; hexamethylenamine; hexamethylenetetramine; ammonioformaldehyde; a condensation product obtained by the action of ammonia upon formaldehyde; a urinary antiseptic. SYN hexamine.

m. hippurate, hexamethylenetetramine hippurate; a urinary antiseptic.

m. mandelate, $C_{14}H_{20}N_4O_3$; a urinary antiseptic.

m. salicylate, hexamethylenetetramine salicylate; a uric acid solvent and urinary antiseptic.

meth·en·a·mine-sil·ver. A hexamethylenetetramine-silver complex prepared by adding silver nitrate to methenamine; a white precipitate appears in the solution which dissolves upon shaking and is stable under refrigeration; used in various histological and histochemical staining methods. SEE ALSO Gomori's methenamine-silver *stain*, under *stain*.

meth·ene (meth′ēn). SYN methylene.

N^5,N^{10}-meth·e·nyl·tet·ra·hy·dro·fol·ic ac·id. SYN anhydroleucovorin.

N^5,N^{10}-methenyltetrahydrofolate. A one-carbon derivative of tetrahydrofolate; used in purine biosynthesis.

N^5,N^{10}-methylenetetrahydrofolate reductase, an enzyme that converts N^5,N^{10}-m ethylenetetrahydrofolate to N^5,N^{10}-methyl enyltetrahydrofolate using NADP$^+$; a deficiency of this enzyme results in an accumulation of L-homocysteine and severe neurological disturbances.

meth·er·go·line. SYN metergoline.

meth·i·cil·lin so·di·um (meth-i-sil′in). Sodium 2,6-dimethoxyphenylpenicillin monohydrate; a semisynthetic penicillin salt for parenteral administration; restriction of its use to infections caused by penicillin G-resistant staphylococci is recommended; it is less effective than penicillin G in infections caused by hemolytic streptococci, pneumococci, gonococci, and penicillin G-sensitive staphylococci. SYN sodium methicillin.

meth·im·a·zole (me-thim′ă-zōl). 1-Methylimidazole-2-thiol; an antithyroid drug similar in action to propylthiouracil.

me·thi·o·dal so·di·um (meth-ī′ō-dăl). An iodine-containing radiopaque medium, formerly used for examination of the urinary tract.

me·thi·o·nine (Met, M) (me-thī′ō-nēn). $CH_3S–CH_2CH_2CH$ $(NH_3^+)–COOCOO^-$; 2-amino-4-(methylthio)butyric acid; the L-isomer is a nutritionally essential amino acid and the most important natural source of "active methyl" groups in the body, hence usually involved in methylations *in vivo;* the DL-form is used as an adjunct in the treatment of liver diseases.

active m., SYN *S*-adenosyl-L-methionine.

m. adenosyltransferase, an enzyme catalyzing the condensation of L-methionine and ATP, forming *S*-adenosyl-L-methionine, orthophosphate, and pyrophosphate; a deficiency of the hepatic enzyme will result in hypermethionemia. SYN methionine-activating enzyme.

m. sulfoxime, a toxic derivative of m. formed when proteins containing it are treated with nitrogen chloride to give –SO(NH)-CH_3 in place of –SCH$_3$.

m. synthase, tetrahydropteroylglutamate methyltransferase; methionine-homocysteine methyltransferase; an enzyme that catalyzes the reaction of N^5-methyltetrahydrofolate with L-homocysteine to form tetrahydrofolate and L-methionine; a cobalamin-requiring enzyme; a deficiency of this enzyme results in an accumulation of L-homocysteine and neurological abnormalities. SYN tetrahydrofolate methyltransferase.

me·this·a·zone (mĕ-this′ă-zōn). *N*-Methylisatin 3-thiosemicarbazone; 1-methylindole-2,3-dione 3-thiosemicarbazone; an antiviral agent.

meth·i·tu·ral (me-thi′t-ū-ral). An intravenous thiobarbiturate resembling thiopental and used for the induction of anesthesia; exerts a brief effect due to rapid redistribution in the body after a single injection.

me·thix·ene hy·dro·chlo·ride (me-thik′sēn). 1-Methyl-3-(thioxanthen-9-ylmethyl)piperidine hydrochloride; an anticholinergic agent.

△**metho-.** SEE meth-.

meth·o·car·ba·mol (meth-ō-kar′bă-mol). 2-Hydroxy-3-*o*-methoxyphenoxypropyl carbamate; a centrally acting skeletal muscle relaxant, chemically related to mephenesin carbamate; it is slower in onset of action but of longer duration, and may be administered intravenously, intramuscularly, or orally.

METHOD

meth·od (meth′ŏd). The mode or manner or orderly sequence of events of a process or procedure. SEE ALSO fixative, operation, procedure, stain, technique. [G. *methodos;* fr. *meta*, after, + *hodos*, way]

Abbott's m., a m. of treatment of scoliosis by use of a series of plaster jackets applied after partial correction of the curvature by external force.

Abell-Kendall m., a standard m. for estimation of total serum cholesterol involving saponification of cholesterol ester by hydroxide, extraction with petroleum ether, and color development with acetic anhydride-sulfuric acid; the m. avoids interference by bilirubin, protein, and hemoglobin.

activated sludge m., a m. of sewage disposal in which the sewage is treated with 15% bacterially active, liquid sludge, which is produced by repeated vigorous aeration of fresh sewage to form floccules or sediment; when this flocculation process is complete, the resulting activated sludge contains large numbers of bacteria, together with yeasts, molds, and protozoa, which actively effect the oxidation of organic compounds; this mixture is piped to a sedimentation tank, the effluent from which is completely treated sewage.

Altmann-Gersh m., the m. of rapidly freezing a tissue and dehydrating it in a vacuum.

Anel's m., ligation of an artery immediately above (on the proximal side of) an aneurysm.

Antyllus' m., ligation of the artery above and below an aneurysm, followed by incision into and emptying of the sac.

aristotelian m., a m. of study that stresses the relation between a general category and a particular object.

Ashby m., a differential agglutination m. for estimating erythrocyte life span; compatible blood possessing a group factor that the recipient lacks is transferred to the recipient; after the transfusion, sera with potent agglutinins for the recipient's red cells are added to samples of the recipient's blood, and the unagglutinated red cells are counted; using this technique the red cell life span in normal persons is found to be 110 to 120 days.

auxanographic m., a m. for the study of bacterial enzymes in which agar is mixed with the material (*e.g.,* starch or milk) which is to serve as an indicator of the enzyme action and is inoculated and plated; if the bacteria produce enzymes digesting the admixed material, there will be a zone of clearing in the medium about each colony. SYN diffusion m.

Barraquer's m., SYN zonulolysis.

Beck's m., a permanent opening into the stomach made from its greater curvature.

Bier's m., (1) SYN intravenous regional *anesthesia*. **(2)** treatment of various surgical conditions by reactive hyperemia.

Born m. of wax plate reconstruction, the making of three-dimensional models of structures from serial sections; it depends on the building up of a series of wax plates, cut out to scaled enlargements of the individual sections involved in the region to be reconstructed.

Brasdor's m., treatment of aneurysm by ligation of the artery immediately below (on the distal side of) the tumor.

Callahan's m., SYN chloropercha m.

capture-recapture m., originally, a technique developed by biologists to track wild animal populations; now adapted for epidemiological studies of elusive human populations (*e.g.,* prostitutes, teen runaways, IV drug users).

> By comparing data from several independent overlapping sample frames, it is possible to adjust for missing cases and to generate estimates of the prevalence of a given condition, for example, AIDS infection.

Carpue's m., SYN Indian *rhinoplasty*.

Charters' m., a method of toothbrushing utilizing a restricted circular motion with the bristles inclined coronally at a 45 degree angle.

Chayes' m., a m. of replacing lost teeth utilizing a mechanical device for the fixation and stabilization of the dental prosthesis which allows "movement in function" of the abutment teeth.

chloropercha m., a m. of filling the root canals of teeth by dissolving gutta-percha cones in a chloroform-rosin medium within the root canal. SYN Callahan's m., Johnson's m.

closed circuit m., a m. for measuring oxygen consumption in which the subject rebreathes an initial quantity of oxygen through a carbon dioxide absorber and the decrease in the volume of oxygen being rebreathed is noted.

confrontation m., a m. of perimetry; the examiner compares the visual fields of the patient with his own by facing the patient who has one eye covered and the other fixed upon the corresponding (confronting) eye of the examiner. The examiner then holds his finger midway between the patient and himself and moves it slowly in different directions until the patient fails to see it. In each instance the finger is moved again toward the original position until it is just seen by the subject.

cooled-knife m., the cutting of frozen sections with a knife cooled to a few degrees below the freezing point.

copper sulfate m., a m. for the determination of specific gravity of blood or plasma in which the blood or plasma is delivered by drops into solutions of copper sulfate graded in specific gravity by increments of 0.004, each of the bottles of solution being within the expected range of the blood or plasma sample; the specific gravity of the copper sulfate solution in which the drop of blood or plasma remains suspended indefinitely indicates the specific gravity of the sample.

correlational m., a statistical m., most often used in clinical and other applied areas of psychology, to study the relationship which exists between one characteristic and another in an individual.

Credé's m.'s, (1) instillation of one drop of a 2% solution of silver nitrate into each eye of the newborn infant, to prevent ophthalmia neonatorum; **(2)** resting the hand on the fundus uteri from the moment of the expulsion of the fetus, and gently rubbing in case of hemorrhage or failing contraction; then, when the afterbirth is loosened it is expelled by firm compression or squeezing of the fundus by the hand; **(3)** use of manual pressure on a bladder, particularly a paralyzed bladder, to express urine. SYN Credé's maneuvers.

cross-sectional m., in developmental psychology, the study of the life span involving comparison of groups of individuals at different age levels. Cf. longitudinal m.

definitive m., an analytical procedure for the measurement of a specified analyte in a specified material which is known to give essentially the true value for the concentration of the analyte.

Dick m., SYN Dick *test*.

Dieffenbach's m., a plastic operation for covering a defect by sliding a flap with broad pedicle.

diffusion m., SYN auxanographic m.

direct m. for making inlays, in dentistry, an inlay technique in which the wax pattern is made directly in the prepared cavity in the tooth. SYN direct technique.

disk sensitivity m., a procedure for testing the relative effectiveness of various antibiotics; small disks of paper (or other suitable material) are impregnated with known, appropriate amounts of antibiotic, and then placed on the surface of semisolid medium that has been previously inoculated with the organism being tested; after suitable periods of incubation at 37°C, the lack of growth in zones about the various disks indicates the relative effectiveness of the antibiotic.

double antibody m., SYN double antibody *precipitation*.

Edman m., SEE phenylisothiocyanate.

Eggleston m., obsolete term for rapid digitalization by means of large doses of digitalis leaf or tincture frequently repeated.

Eicken's m., facilitation of hypopharyngoscopy by means of forward traction on the cricoid cartilage by a laryngeal probe.

encu m., a means of simplifying the calculation of risk in genetic counseling for autosomal dominant traits by converting all pertinent evidence into encu units.

ensu m., a means of simplifying the calculation of risk in genetic counseling for X-linked traits by converting all pertinent evidence into ensu units.

experimental m., in experimental psychology, control of environmental, physiological, or attitudinal factors to observe dependent changes in aspects of experience and behavior.

Fick m., in 1870 A. Fisk proposed that cardiac output can be calculated as the quotient of total body oxygen consumption divided by the difference in oxygen content of arterial blood and mixed venous blood. In the direct Fick m. all variables are measured. The indirect Fick m. employs a variety of means to avoid measuring mixed venous oxygen content. By extension, the Fick m. may be used to measure cardiac output or organ blood flow with any indicator substance for which the rate of uptake or consumption, and the arterial and mixed venous concentrations, can be measured, provided the indicator does not enter or leave the system by any route not being measured. SYN Fick principle.

flash m., sterilization of milk by raising it rapidly to a temperature of 178°F, holding it there for a short time, and reducing it rapidly to 40°F.

flotation m., any of several procedures for concentrating helminth eggs for more reliable results when eggs are difficult to find in direct examination; the flotation m.'s depend on flotation of helminth eggs on the surface of a liquid of sufficiently high specific gravity, approximately 1.180; 1 part feces mixed in about 10 parts saturated saline will float most protozoan cysts and nonpercolated helminth eggs. SEE ALSO zinc sulfate flotation centrifugation m.

Gärtner's m., a m. of measuring venous pressure, based upon Gärtner's vein phenomenon; with the patient sitting erect, a vein is selected on the back of the hand which is held dependent, well below the level of the right atrium, and then is raised slowly; when the vein is observed to collapse, the distance between its level and that of the atrium is measured with a millimeter rule; this distance gives the venous pressure in millimeters of blood; thus the vein itself is used as a manometer communicating with the right atrium; highly inaccurate, especially in elderly subjects.

Gerota's m., injection of the lymphatics with a dye that is soluble in chloroform or ether but not in water; alkannin, red sulfide of mercury, and Prussian blue are said to be suitable for this purpose.

glucose oxidase m., a highly specific m. for measurement of glucose in serum or plasma by reaction with glucose oxidase, in which gluconic acid and hydrogen peroxide are formed.

Gräupner's m., obsolete term for a test of the sufficiency of the heart muscle; if a normal subject takes a measured amount of exercise, the pulse rate rises, and after it has begun to fall the systolic blood pressure begins to rise, reaching its maximum a few minutes after the pulse rate; in the case of a weakened heart,

me

the rise in blood pressure is delayed and the amount of increase diminished; in seriously weakened hearts, a fall in blood pressure occurs.

Gruber's m., a modification of the Politzer m. in which the patient does not swallow, but says "hoc" at the instant of compression of the bag.

Hamilton-Stewart m., formula to calculate cardiac output after intravenous indicator dye injection; blood flow in liters per minute is given by dividing the amount of injectant in milligrams by the product of the average dye concentration in the initial curve of the dye concentration sampled at a given point in the circulation and multiplied by the dose of dye (in milligrams) to write the curve from appearance to disappearance (in the absence of any recirculation). SYN Hamilton-Stewart formula, Stewart-Hamilton m.

Hammerschlag's m., a hydrometric m. of determining the specific gravity of the blood by allowing a drop of blood to fall into each of a series of tubes containing mixtures of chloroform and benzene of known graded specific gravities; the specific gravity of that mixture in which the drop remains exactly suspended, neither rising nor falling, corresponds to the specific gravity of the blood sample.

hexokinase m., the most specific m. for measuring glucose in serum or plasma, wherein hexokinase plus ATP transforms glucose to glucose 6-phosphate plus ADP; glucose 6-phosphate is then reacted with NADP and glucose 6-phosphate dehydrogenase to form NADP which is measured spectrophotometrically.

Hilton's m., division of the nerves supplying a part, for the relief of pain in ulcers.

Hirschberg's m., a m. of measuring the amount of deviation of a strabismic eye, by observing the reflection of a light fixated by the straight eye on the cornea of the deviating eye.

Hung's method, SYN Wilson's m.

immunofluorescence m., any m. in which a fluorescent-labeled antibody is used to detect the presence or determine the location of the corresponding antigen.

impedance m., a m. for localizing brain structures by measuring impedance of electric current.

Indian m., SYN Indian *rhinoplasty.*

indicator dilution m., SYN Stewart-Hamilton m.

indirect m. for making inlays, a method whereby the inlay is constructed entirely on a model made from an impression of the prepared tooth or teeth in the mouth. SYN indirect technique.

indophenol m., a m. of determining quantitatively the amount of vitamin C in plant and animal tissue based on the rapid reduction of a standardized indophenol solution to a colorless compound by vitamin C in acid solution.

introspective m., in functionalism, the systematic study of mental phenomena by contemplating the processes in one's own conscious experiences.

Italian m., SYN Italian *rhinoplasty.*

ITO m., a concise matrix m. for computing the distribution of genotypes of relatives that at one locus may share no genes in common, one, or both.

Johnson's m., SYN chloropercha m.

Keating-Hart's m., fulguration in the treatment of external cancer or of the field of operation after the removal of a malignant growth.

Kety-Schmidt m., a m. for measuring organ blood flow first applied to the brain in 1944 by C. F. Schmidt and S. S. Kety. A chemically inert indicator gas is equilibrated with the tissue of the organ of interest and the rate of disappearance from the organ is measured. Blood flow is calculated on the assumption that the tissue and venous blood concentrations of the indicator gas are in diffusion equilibrium at all blood flow rates and that the rate of disappearance of the indicator from the tissue is a function of how much is in the tissue at any time, *i.e.,* it is assumed to be an exponential disappearance.

Kjeldahl m., SEE macro-Kjeldahl m., micro-Kjeldahl m.

Klapp's m., treatment of scoliosis by a series of systematic crawling movements whereby the spine is bent laterally and made more flexible.

Krause's m., SEE Krause *graft.*

Lamaze m., a technique of psychoprophylactic preparation for childbirth, designed to minimize the pain of labor.

Langendorff's m., perfusion of the isolated mammalian heart by carrying fluid under pressure into the sectioned aorta, and thus into the coronary system.

Lee-White m., a m. for determining coagulation time of venous blood in tubes of standard bore at body temperature.

Liborius' m., a m. for culturing anaerobic bacteria; a stab culture is made in the appropriate agar medium, then more of the same medium is liquefied and poured into the test tube on top of the stab culture, effectually sealing it from the air.

Ling's m., gymnastic exercises (as in Swedish movements) without the use of apparatus. SYN lingism.

Lister's m., antiseptic surgery, as first advocated by Lister in 1867; the operation was performed under a cloud of diluted carbolic acid spray, the instruments were dipped in a carbolic solution before use, and the wound was dressed with a thick layer of carbolized gauze; from this was developed the present practice of aseptic surgery. SYN listerism.

lod m., a method of linkage analysis using an examination of the common logarithm of the ratio of the likelihood for a particular value of the recombination fraction to that if the recombination fraction is 0.5 (*i.e.,* no linkage); thus, a lod score of 3 at a recombination fraction of 0.2 means that the data are 1000 times more readily explained by supposing a recombination fraction of 0.2 than by supposing the loci are unlinked and the recombination fraction is 0.5. [logarithm of the odds]

longitudinal m., in developmental psychology, the study of the life span of one individual involving comparisons of different age levels. Cf. cross-sectional m.

macro-Kjeldahl m., a procedure for analyzing the content of nitrogenous compounds in urine, serum, or other specimens, usually to determine relatively large amounts of nitrogen (*e.g.,* 20 to 100 mg); the specimen is treated with a digestion mixture (copper sulfate and sulfuric acid), heated thoroughly, and made alkaline with a solution of sodium hydroxide; ammonia is then distilled from the mixture, trapped in a boric acid-indicator solution, and titrated with standard hydrochloric or sulfuric acid.

Marshall's m., a quantitative procedure for estimating free and conjugated sulfanilamide in body fluids.

micro-Astrup m., an interpolation technique for acid-base measurement, based on pH and the use of the Siggaard-Andersen nomogram to determine the base deficit as an expression of metabolic acidosis and the arterial P_{CO_2} as an expression of respiratory acidosis or alkalosis.

micro-Kjeldahl m., a modification of the macro-Kjeldahl m. designed for the analysis of nitrogenous compounds in relatively small quantities, *e.g.,* specimens in which the total content of nitrogen is in the range of 1 to a few mg.

microsphere m., a m. for measuring organ blood flow by indicator dilution, but more importantly, a m. for measuring the distribution of cardiac output or the intraorgan distribution of blood flow. To measure distribution of flow, neutrally buoyant, chemically inert microspheres that have an indicator property (*e.g.,* radioactivity) are injected into a cardiac chamber or arterial blood. They are presumed to distribute in proportion to the distribution of arterial blood flow. Injected sphere size is selected to be large enough to embolize the vessels of interest. Injected quantity is selected to be large enough to provide statistically meaningful samples and small enough not to alter the organ blood flow under investigation. Organ samples are taken to quantify the distribution of the microspheres and hence the flow. SEE Fick m., Stewart-Hamilton m.

Moore's m., treatment of aneurysm by the introduction of silver or zinc wire into the sac to induce fibrin deposition.

Needles' split cast m., SYN split cast m.

Nikiforoff's m., the fixing of blood films by immersion for 5 to 15 minutes in absolute alcohol, a mixture of equal parts of alcohol and ether, or pure ether.

Ochsner's m., an obsolete treatment for appendicitis (by peristaltic rest), when surgery is not advisable.

Ollier's m., SEE Ollier *graft.*

open circuit m., a m. for measuring oxygen consumption and carbon dioxide production by collecting the expired gas over a known period of time and measuring its volume and composition.

Orsi-Grocco m., palpatory percussion of the heart.

Ouchterlony method, SYN Ouchterlony *test.*

Pachon's m., cardiography, carried out with the patient lying on the left side.

paracelsian m., the use of chemical agents only in the treatment of disease.

parallax m., localization of a foreign body by observing the direction of its motion on a fluoroscopic screen while moving the x-ray tube or the screen.

Pavlov m., the m. of studying conditioned reflex activity by the observation of a motor indicator, such as the salivary or electroencephalographic response.

Politzer m., inflation of the eustachian tube and tympanum by forcing air into the nasal cavity at the instant the patient swallows.

Porges m., a m. of destroying the capsule of bacteria by heating with N/4 hydrochloric acid and neutralizing with NaOH.

Purmann's m., treatment of aneurysm by extirpation of the sac.

Quick's m., SYN prothrombin *test.*

reference m., an analytical procedure sufficiently free of random or systematic error to make it useful for validating proposed new analytical procedures for the same analyte.

Rehfuss m., fractional m. of gastric activity: a fine tube with fenestrated metal tip is passed into the stomach after a test meal, and small quantities (6 or 8 ml) of the stomach contents are removed at 15-minute intervals and examined.

Reverdin's m., SEE Reverdin *graft.*

rhythm m., a natural contraceptive m. that spaces human sexual intercourse to avoid the fertile period of the menstrual cycle. SYN rhythm (2).

Rideal-Walker m., SEE Rideal-Walker *coefficient.*

Roux's m., division of the inferior maxilla in the median line, to facilitate the operation of ablation of the tongue.

Sanger m., the m. for the sequencing of DNA employing an enzyme that can polymerase DNA and labeled nucleotides.

Scarpa's m., cure of aneurysm by ligation of the artery at some distance above the sac.

Schäfer's m., an obsolete m. of resuscitation in cases of drowning or asphyxia; the patient is laid face downward and natural breathing is imitated by gentle intermittent pressure over the lower part of the thorax at the rate of about 15 times a minute.

Schede's m., filling of the defect in bone, after removal of a sequestrum or scraping away carious material, by allowing the cavity to fill with blood which may become organized (Schede's clot).

Schick m., SYN Schick *test.*

Schmidt-Thannhauser m., a m. for fractionation of nucleic acid, based upon the fact that RNA but not DNA is hydrolyzed to nucleotides by alkali; RNA can be hydrolyzed in about 2 hours in 0.75 N NaOH, but 18 hours and 0.3 N NaOH usually are used.

Schweninger's m., a method suggested to reduce obesity by restricting intake of fluid.

Shaffer-Hartmann m., an obsolete m. for the quantitative determination of glucose in biological fluids, based on the reduction of copper by the reducing group of the sugar.

Somogyi m., SEE Somogyi *unit.*

split cast m., (1) a procedure for placing indexed casts on an articulator to facilitate their removal and replacement on the instrument; **(2)** the procedure of checking the ability of an articulator to receive or be adjusted to a maxillomandibular relation record. SYN Needles' split cast m.

Stas-Otto m., a m. of extraction of alkaloids from plants and animal bodies: the substance is digested in alcohol and tartaric acid, the fatty and resinous matters are precipitated with water, the fluid is made alkaline, and the alkaloids are extracted with ether or chloroform.

Stewart-Hamilton m., SYN Hamilton-Stewart m. SYN indicator dilution m.

Stroganoff's m., obsolete term for treatment of eclampsia by morphine, chloral hydrate, shielding the patient from all external sources of irritation, and rapid delivery.

Thane's m., a m. for indicating the position of the central sulcus (Rolando's fissure) of the brain; the upper end of the sulcus corresponds to the midpoint of a line drawn from the glabella to the inion.

Theden's m., treatment of aneurysms or of large sanguineous effusions by compression of the entire limb with a roller bandage.

Thezac-Porsmeur m., heat treatment of infected wounds by focusing of sun's rays on suppurating area by means of a lens mounted in a cylinder of canvas.

Thiersch's m., SEE Thiersch *graft.*

thiochrome m., a m. for the determination of thiamin based upon the production of thiochrome when the vitamin is oxidized by alkaline ferricyanide to yield the fluorescent compound, thiochrome.

twin m., a general means of genetic analysis that capitalizes on the fact that while twins have the same age and the same intrauterine environment, identical (monozygotic) twins have the same genotype but dizygotic twins are no more alike than sibs and may be of different sex.

ultropaque m., a rapid m. for examining thick (1 to 3 mm) sections of fresh tissue with the ultramicroscope, making use of an objective built in an illuminator so that the light is reflected down upon the tissue.

u-score m., an older, simpler, but somewhat less efficient method of linkage analysis than that by maximum likelihood estimation.

Wardrop's m., treatment of aneurysm by ligation of the artery at some distance beyond the sac, leaving one or more branches of the artery between the sac and the ligature.

Westergren m., a procedure for estimating the sedimentation rate of red blood cells in fluid blood by mixing venous blood with an aqueous solution of sodium citrate and allowing it to stand in an upright standard pipet (200 mm long) filled to the zero mark; the fall of the red blood cells, in millimeters, is then observed in 1 hr; the normal rate for men is 0 to 15 mm (average, 4 mm), and for women 0 to 20 mm (average, 5 mm).

Wheeler m., a surgical procedure for correction of cicatricial ectropion.

Wilson's m., a simple saline flotation m. for concentrating helminth eggs in the feces. SEE flotation m. SYN Hung's method.

Wolfe's m., SEE Wolfe *graft.*

zinc sulfate flotation centrifugation m., a flotation m. in which the fecal specimen is suspended in tap water, strained through wet gauze, centrifuged, resuspended in tap water, washed and recentrifuged several times, and then suspended in 33% solution of zinc sulfate and centrifuged at top speed for 45 to 60 sec; a bacteriologic loop may be used to pick up the surface layer, which contains protozoan cysts and helminth eggs.

---

meth·od·ism (meth′ŏd-izm). SYN solidism.

meth·o·dol·o·gy (meth′u-dol-ō-jē). The scientific study or logical analysis of methods.

meth·o·hex·i·tal so·di·um (meth-ō-heks′i-tawl). Sodium α-*dl*-methyl-5-allyl-5-(1-methyl-2-pentynyl)barbiturate; an ultrashort-acting barbiturate used intravenously for induction and for general anesthesia of short duration.

me·tho·ni·um com·pounds. See under compound.

meth·o·phen·a·zine (me-thō-fen′ă-zēn). 3,4,5-Trimethoxybenzoic acid 2-{4-[3-(2-chlorophenothiazin-10-yl)propyl]-1-piperazinyl}ethyl ester; an antipsychotic.

meth·o·pho·line (me-thō-fō′lēn). 1-(*p*-Chlorophenethyl)-1,2,3,4-tetrahydro-6,7-dimethoxy-2-methyl isoquinoline; an analgesic.

meth·op·ter·in (meth-op′ter-in). 10-Methylfolic acid; 10-methylpteroylglutamic acid; a folic acid antagonist.

meth·or·phi·nan (meth-ōr′fi-nan). $C_{17}H_{23}NOHBr$; 3-Hydroxy-*N*-methylmorphinan; SEE dextromethorphan hydrobromide, levorphanol tartrate.

meth·o·ser·pi·dine (meth-ō-ser′pi-dēn). 10-Methoxydeserpidine; an antihypertensive agent similar in its actions to reserpine.

meth·o·trex·ate (meth-ō-trek'sāt). Methylaminopterin; 4-amino-10-methylfolic acid; a folic acid antagonist used as an antineoplastic agent. SYN amethopterin.

meth·o·tri·mep·ra·zine (meth'ō-trī-mep'ră-zēn). 10-[3-(Dimethylamino)-2-methylpropyl]-2-methoxyphenothiazine; a phenothiazine analgesic.

me·thox·a·mine hy·dro·chlo·ride (me-thok'să-mēn). α-(1-Aminoethyl)-2,5-dimethoxybenzyl alcohol hydrochloride;; β-hydroxy-β-(2,5-dimethoxyphenyl)isopropylamine hydrochloride; a sympathomimetic amine.

me·thox·sa·len (me-thok'să-len). δ-Lactone of 3-(6-hydroxy-7-methoxybenzofuranyl)acrylic acid; a methoxypsoralen derivative that increases melanin production in the skin when exposed to ultraviolet light; used orally and topically in the treatment of idiopathic vitiligo, and also as a suntan accelerator and sun protectant.

△**methoxy-.** Chemical prefix denoting substitution of a methoxyl group.

4-me·thox·y·ben·zo·ic ac·id (meth-ok'sē-ben-zō'ik). SYN anisic acid.

me·thox·y·chlor (mĕ-thok'sē-klōr). An insecticide resembling DDT; ectoparasiticide.

me·thox·y·flu·rane (me-thok-sē-flūr'ān). 2,2-Dichloro-1,1-difluoroethyl methyl ether; a potent inhalation anesthetic no longer in use because of high-output renal failure caused by increased plasma concentrations of inorganic fluoride, a metabolic breakdown product of m.

3-me·thox·y-4-hy·drox·y·man·del·ic ac·id. SEE vanillylmandelic acid.

5-me·thox·y·in·dole-3-ac·e·tate (meth-oks'ē-in-dōl). An intermediate of tryptophan and serotonin degradation; excreted as conjugates.

me·thox·yl (me-thok'sil). The group, –OCH₃.

me·thox·y·phen·a·mine hy·dro·chlo·ride (me-thok-sē-fen'ă-mēn). β-(o-Methoxyphenyl)isopropylmethylamine hydrochloride; a sympathomimetic amine.

5-me·thox·y·trypt·a·mine (meth-oks'ē-trip-ta-mēn). An intermediate in the degradation of L-tryptophan and serotonin.

meth·sco·pol·a·mine bro·mide (meth-skō-pol'ă-mēn). Epoxytropine tropate methylbromide; a parasympatholytic drug similar to atropine; the methyl nitrate has the same action and uses.

meth·sux·i·mide (meth-sŭk'si-mīd). N,2-Dimethyl-2-phenylsuccinimide; an antiepileptic effective against petit mal and psychomotor epilepsy; similar to ethosuximide.

meth·y·clo·thi·a·zide (meth'i-klō-thī'ă-zīd). 6-Chloro-3-(chloromethyl)-3,4-dihydro-2-methyl-2H-1,2,4-benzothiadiazine-7-sulfonamide 1,1-dioxide; an orally effective diuretic and antihypertensive agent of the thiazide group.

meth·yl (Me) (meth'il). The radical, –CH₃. [G. methy, wine, + hylē, wood]

active m., a m. group attached to a quaternary ammonium ion or a tertiary sulfonium ion that can take part in transmethylation reactions; e.g., m. groups in choline and in S-adenosyl-L-methionine, which are thus m. donors.

m. alcohol, CH₃OH; a flammable, toxic, mobile liquid, used as an industrial solvent, antifreeze, and in chemical manufacture; ingestion may result in severe acidosis, visual impairment, and other effects on the central nervous system. SYN carbinol, methanol, pyroligneous alcohol, pyroligneous spirit, pyroxylic spirit, wood alcohol, wood naphtha, wood spirit.

m. aldehyde, SYN formaldehyde.

angular m., a m. group attached to carbon 10 (between rings A and B) or to carbon 13 (between rings C and D) of the steroid nucleus.

m. chloride, SYN chloromethane.

m. cysteine hydrochloride, mecysteine hydrochloride; the methyl ester of cysteine hydrochloride; a mucolytic agent.

m. hydroxybenzoate, SYN methylparaben.

m. isobutyl ketone, 4-methyl-2-pentanone; in high concentra-

tions it has narcotic action; in relatively low concentrations it may be irritating to the eyes and mucous membranes.

m. methacrylate, a thermoplastic material used for denture bases.

m. nicotinate, nicotinic acid methyl ester, used as rubefacient.

m. salicylate, the methyl ester of salicylic acid, produced synthetically or distilled from Gaultheria procumbens (family Ericaceae) or from Betula lenta (family Betulaceae); used externally and internally for the treatment of various forms of rheumatism. SYN checkerberry oil, gaultheria oil, sweet birch oil, wintergreen oil.

2-meth·yl·a·ce·to·a·ce·tyl-·CoA thi·o·lase. An enzyme that is part of the L-isoleucine degradation pathway; it catalyzes the conversion of 2-methylacetoacetyl-CoA (CH₃COCH(CH₃)-COSCoA) to acetyl-CoA and propionyl-CoA. A deficiency of this enzyme leads to an accumulation of 2-methylacetoacetyl-CoA, causing episodes of severe metabolic acidosis and ketosis.

meth·yl·a·cryl·ic ac·id (meth'il-ă-kril'ik). SYN methacrylic acid.

meth·yl·am·phet·a·mine hy·dro·chlo·ride (meth'il-am-fet'ă-mēn). SYN methamphetamine hydrochloride.

meth·yl·ate (meth'i-lāt). **1.** To mix with methyl alcohol. **2.** To introduce a methyl group. **3.** A compound in which a metal ion methyl replaces the alcoholic hydrogen of alcohol.

meth·yl·a·tion (meth-i-lā'shŭn). Addition of methyl groups; in histochemistry, used to esterify carboxyl groups and remove sulfate groups by treating tissue sections with hot methanol in the presence of hydrochloric acid; the net effect being to reduce tissue basophilia and abolish metachromasia.

restriction m., the enzymatic addition of methyl groups to selected adenine and cytosine residues to protect from hydrolysis by certain restriction enzymes.

meth·yl·at·ro·pine bro·mide (meth-il-at'rō-pēn, -pin). A quaternary derivative of atropine that is less lipid soluble and hence produces fewer central nervous system actions; a cycloplegic. SYN atropine methylbromide.

meth·yl·ben·zene (meth-il-ben'zēn). SYN toluene.

meth·yl·ben·ze·tho·ni·um chlo·ride (meth'il-ben-zě-thō'nē-ŭm). Benzyldimethyl{2-[2-(p-1,1,3,3-tetramethylbutylcresoxy)-ethoxy]-ethyl}ammonium chloride; a quaternary ammonium compound having a surface action like that of other cationic detergents; generally germicidal and bacteriostatic; used to rinse infant diapers and bed linen in the prevention of ammonia dermatitis.

meth·yl blue [C.I. 42780]. A sulfonated triphenylrosaniline dye used as a stain for cytoplasm, collagen, and Negri bodies, and as an antiseptic.

meth·yl bro·mide. Used in ionization chambers; for degreasing wool; extracting oils from nuts, seeds, flowers; used as an insect fumigant for mills, warehouses, vaults, ships, freight cars; also as a soil fumigant.

N-meth·yl·car·no·sine (meth-il-kar'nō-sēn). SYN anserine (2).

meth·yl-CCNU. A nitrosourea antineoplastic agent resembling carmustine (BCNU) and lomustine (CCNU). SYN semustine.

meth·yl·cel·lu·lose (meth-il-sel'yū-lōs). A methyl ester of cellulose that forms a colorless viscous liquid when dissolved in water, alcohol, or ether; used to increase bulk of the intestinal contents, to relieve constipation, or of the gastric contents, to reduce appetite in obesity; also used dissolved in water as a spray to cover burned areas.

meth·yl·chlo·ro·form (meth-il-chlōr'ō-fōrm). SYN trichloroethane.

3-meth·yl·chol·an·threne, 20-meth·yl·chol·an·threne (meth'il-kōl-an'thrēn). A highly carcinogenic hydrocarbon that can be formed chemically from deoxycholic or cholic acids, or from cholesterol; the choice between 3- or 20- for the methyl group depends upon whether hydrocarbon (inner) or steroid (outer) numbering is chosen; in the latter case, the formal relationship to the cholic acids and cholesterol is clear.

meth·yl·cit·rate (meth-il-sit'trāt). A minor metabolite that accumulates in individuals with propionic acidemia.

meth·yl·co·bal·a·min (meth-il-kō-bal'a-mēn). SYN vitamin B₁₂.

3-meth·yl·cro·ton·yl-CoA (meth-il-krō'ton-il). (CH₃)₂C=

CHCOSCoA; an intermediate in the degradation of L-leucine; accumulates in a deficiency of 3-methylcrotonyl-CoA carboxylase.

3-methylcrotonyl-CoA carboxylase, an enzyme in the pathway of L-leucine degradation that catalyzes the reaction of 3-methylcrotonyl-CoA with CO_2, ATP, and water to form ADP, orthophosphate, and 3-methylcrotonyl-CoA; a deficiency of this enzyme causes episodes of severe metabolic acidosis.

5-meth·yl·cy·to·sine (meth'il-sī'tō-sēn). A minor base that is present in both bacterial and human DNA.

N-methyl, D-aspartic acid. SYN NMDA.

meth·yl·di·chlo·ro·ar·sine (MD) (meth'il-dī-klōr-ō-ar'sēn). CH_3ASCl_2; a vesicant; irritating to the respiratory tract and will produce lung injury and eye injury; has been used in certain military operations.

meth·yl·do·pa (meth-il-dō'pă). L-3-(3,4-Dihydroxyphenyl)-2-methylalanine; an antihypertensive agent, also used as the ethyl ester hydrochloride, with the same action and uses. SYN alpha methyl dopa.

meth·yl·ene (meth'i-lēn). The radical, $-CH_2-$. SYN methene.

meth·yl·ene az·ure. SYN *azure* I.

meth·yl·ene blue [C.I. 52015]. 3,7-Bis(dimethylamino)-phenazathionium chloride; tetramethylthionine chloride; a basic dye easily oxidized to azure, with dye mixtures; used in histology and microbiology, to stain intestinal protozoa in wet mount preparations, to track RNA and RNase in electrophoresis, and as an antidote for methemoglobinemia; its redox indicator properties are useful in milk bacteriology.

Kühne's m. b., m. b. in absolute alcohol and phenol solution.

Loeffler's m. b., a stain for diphtheria organisms that contains m. b. in dilute ethanol plus a slight amount of potassium hydroxide; dye solution gives best results when aged to a polychrome state.

new m. b. [C.I. 52030], a basic thiazin dye, $C_{18}H_{22}N_3SCl$, used for supravital staining of reticulocytes in blood smears.

polychrome m. b., an alkaline solution of m. b. which undergoes progressive oxidative demethylation with aging (ripening) to produce a mixture of m. b., azures, and methylene violet; boiling with sodium carbonate or other oxidizing agents accomplishes this result quickly, although it is not as highly regarded.

meth·yl·ene chlo·ride. Mobile liquid with a pungent odor; harmful vapor. Organic solvent used for cellulose acetate plastic; degreasing and cleaning fluids; and in food processing. Pharmaceutical aid (solvent).

3,4-methylenedioxymethamphetamine. SYN MDMA.

meth·yl·ene·suc·cin·ic ac·id (meth'il-ēn-sŭk'sin-ik). SYN itaconic acid.

meth·yl·ene white. SYN leucomethylene blue.

meth·yl·en·o·phil, meth·yl·en·o·phile (meth-i-lēn'ō-fil, -fīl). Staining readily with methylene blue; denoting certain cells and histologic structures. SYN methylenophilic, methylenophilous. [methylene + G. *philos,* fond]

meth·yl·en·o·phil·ic, meth·yl·e·noph·i·lous (meth'i-lē-nō-fil'ik, meth'il-ĕ-nof'i-lŭs). SYN methylenophil.

meth·yl·er·go·met·rine ma·le·ate (meth'il-er-gō-met'rēn). SYN methylergonovine maleate.

meth·yl·er·go·no·vine ma·le·ate (meth'il-er-gō-nō'vēn). *d*-Lysergic acid-*dl*-hydroxybutylamide-2 maleate; a partially synthesized derivative of lysergic acid with oxytocic action, used to prevent or treat postpartum uterine atony and hemorrhage. SYN methylergometrine maleate.

meth·yl·glu·ca·mine (meth-il-glū'kă-mēn). Cation commonly used in water-soluble iodinated radiographic contrast media. SYN N-methylglucamine.

m. diatrizoate, SYN *meglumine* diatrizoate.

N-meth·yl·glu·ca·mine. SYN methylglucamine.

3-meth·yl·glu·ta·con·ic ac·i·du·ria (meth-il-glū-ta-kon'ik). Elevated levels of 3-methylglutaconic acid in the urine. An inherited disorder whose mild form is a result of a deficiency of 3-methylglutaconyl-CoA hydratase, leading to delayed speech development.

3-meth·yl·glu·ta·con·yl-CoA hy·dra·tase. An enzyme that catalyzes the reaction of *trans*-3-methylglutaconyl-CoA and water to form 3-hydroxy-3-methylglutaconyl-CoA; this enzyme participates in the pathway for L-leucine degradation; a deficiency of this enzyme will result in 3-methylglutaconic aciduria.

meth·yl·gly·ox·al (meth'il-glī-ok'săl). $CH_3-CO-CHO$; Pyruvaldehyde; the aldehyde of pyruvic acid; an intermediate of carbohydrate metabolism in certain organisms. SYN pyruvic aldehyde.

m. bis(guanylhydrazone), 1,1'-[(methylethanediylidene)-dinitrilo]diguanidine; an antineoplastic agent.

meth·yl·gly·ox·a·lase (meth'il-glī-oks'ă-lās). SYN lactoylglutathione lyase.

meth·yl green [C.I. 42585]. A basic triphenylmethane dye used as a chromatin stain and, in combination with pyronin, for differential staining of RNA (red) and DNA (green); also used as a tracking dye for DNA in electrophoresis.

meth·yl·hex·ane·a·mine (meth'il-hek-sān'ă-mēn, -min). 4-Methyl-2-hexylamine; a volatile sympathetic amine base, used as an inhalant nasal decongestant.

N-meth·yl·his·tid·ine (meth'il-his'ti-dēn). A methylated derivative of histidine found in actin; in the breakdown of actin and myosin, N-methylhistidine is released into the urine; urinary output of N-methylhistidine is a reliable index of the rate of myofibrillar protein breakdown in musculature.

meth·yl·ki·nase (meth'il-kī'nās). SYN methyltransferase.

meth·yl·mal·o·nate sem·i·al·de·hyde (meth'il-mă-lon-āt). $OHC-CH(CH_3)-COO^-$; an intermediate in L-valine catabolism; elevated in certain inborn disorders.

meth·yl·ma·lon·ic ac·id (meth'il-mă-lon'ik). 2-Methylpropanedioic acid, an important intermediate in fatty acid metabolism; seen in elevated levels in cases of vitamin B_{12} deficiency. SYN isosuccinic acid.

meth·yl·ma·lon·ic ac·i·de·mia. SYN ketotic *hyperglycinemia.*

meth·yl·ma·lon·ic ac·i·du·ria. Excretion of excessive amounts of methylmalonic acid in urine owing to deficient activity of methylmalonyl-CoA mutase or deficient cobalamin reductase. Two types occur: 1) an inborn error of metabolism resulting in severe ketoacidosis shortly after birth, with long-chain urinary ketones; autosomal recessive inheritance [MIM*251000]; 2) acquired, a type due to vitamin B_{12} deficiency [MIM*251110] due to defective synthesis of adenosylcobalamin.

meth·yl·mal·o·nyl-CoA. An intermediate in the degradation of several metabolites (*e.g.,* valine, methionine, odd-chain fatty acids, threonine); elevated in cases of pernicious anemia.

m.-CoA epimerase, an enzyme that catalyzes the interconversion of D-m.-CoA and L-m.-CoA.

m.-CoA mutase, an enzyme that catalyzes a reversible interconversion of L-methylmalonyl-CoA and succinyl-CoA; a cobalamin-dependent enzyme; deficiency of this enzyme will result in methylmalonic acidemia.

meth·yl mer·cap·tan (meth'il). CH_3SH; a product of the degradation of cysteine by intestinal bacteria; it is also reduced to produce methane and H_2S.

meth·yl·mer·cu·ry. SYN dimethylmercury.

meth·yl·mor·phine. SYN codeine.

meth·yl·ol (meth'i-lol). Hydroxymethyl; the radical, $-CH_2OH$.

meth·yl or·ange [C.I. 13025]. $C_{14}H_{14}N_3O_3SNa$; a weakly acid dye used as a pH indicator (red at 3.2, yellow at 4.4). SYN helianthine.

meth·y·lose (meth'i-lōs). A sugar in which the carbon atom farthest from the carbonyl group is a methyl (CH_3).

meth·yl·par·a·ben (meth-il-par'ă-ben). Methyl*p*-hydroxybenzoate; an antifungal preservative. SYN methyl hydroxybenzoate.

meth·yl·pen·tose (meth-il-pen'tōs). A hexose (a 6-deoxyhexose) in which carbon-6 is part of a methyl group; *e.g.,* rhamnose, fucose.

meth·yl·phen·i·date hy·dro·chlo·ride (meth-il-fen'i-dāt). Methyl α-phenyl-2-piperidineacetate hydrochloride; a central nervous system stimulant used to produce mild cortical stimulation in various types of depressions; commonly used in the treat-

me

ment of hyperkinetic or hyperactive (attention deficit disorder) children.

meth·yl·pred·nis·o·lone (meth'il-pred-nis'ŏ-lōn). 6-α-Methylprednisolone; an anti-inflammatory glucocorticoid.

m. acetate, 6-methylprednisolone 21 acetate; has the same actions and uses as m.; aqueous suspensions are suitable for intrasynovial and soft tissue injection.

sodium m. succinate, sodium 6-methylprednisolone 21-succinate; it has the same metabolic and anti-inflammatory actions as the parent compound, m.; because of its solubility it can be administered in small volumes.

meth·yl red [C.I. 13020]. $C_{15}H_{15}N_3O_2$; a weakly acid dye used as a pH indicator (red at 4.8, yellow at 6.0); easily reduced with loss of color, and pH readings must be made rapidly.

5-meth·yl·res·or·cin·ol (meth'il-rē-sōr'sin-ol). SYN orcinol.

meth·yl·ros·an·i·line chlo·ride (meth'il-rō-zan'i-lēn, -lin). SYN crystal violet.

meth·yl sa·lic·y·late. Aromatic used in perfumery, for flavoring candies; Used as a component of liniments, it produces heat when rubbed into the skin (counterirritant).

methyl-*tert*-butyl ether (MTBE). Used to dissolve gallbladder stones.

meth·yl·tes·tos·ter·one (meth'il-tes-tos'ter-ōn). A methyl derivative of testosterone, with the same actions and uses, except that it is active when given orally or sublingually. Used in the treatment of hypogenitalism. SYN 17α-methyltestosterone.

17α-meth·yl·tes·tos·ter·one. SYN methyltestosterone.

N^5-meth·yl·tet·ra·hy·dro·fo·late (meth-il-tet'ra-hī-drō-fōl-āt). An active one-carbon derivative of tetrahydrofolate that participates in the S-methylation of L-homocysteine.

N^5-m.:homocysteine methyltransferase, SEE *methionine* synthase.

meth·yl·thi·o·a·den·o·sine (meth'il-thī'ō-ă-den'ō-sēn). Adenosine carrying an –SCH₃ group in place of OH at position 5'; the –SCH₃ group is transferred to α-aminobutyric acid to form L-methionine in some bacteria. M. is formed from S-adenosyl-L-methionine in the course of spermidine synthesis by loss of the alanine moiety. SYN thiomethyladenosine.

meth·yl·thi·o·u·ra·cil (meth'il-thī-ō-yū'ră-sil). 6-Methyl-2-thiouracil; an antithyroid compound with the same action as propylthiouracil, but with a smaller dose required.

meth·yl·to·col (meth-il-tō'kol). A methylated tocol; *e.g.,* tocotrienol, the tocopherols.

meth·yl·trans·fer·ase (meth-il-trans'fer-ās). Any enzyme transferring methyl groups from one compound to another. SYN demethylase, methylkinase, transmethylase.

phenylethanolamine *N*-m. (fen'il-ēth'ă-nol'ă-mēn meth'il-transfer-ās), the enzyme that catalyzes the conversion of norepinephrine to epinephrine. Phenylethanolamine-N-m. is found in the adrenal medulla and some neurons.

meth·yl vi·o·let [C.I. 42535]. Mixtures of tetra-, penta-, or pararosanilin which vary in shade of violet depending on the extent of methylation (designated R for reddish shades, B for bluish shades); the hexamethyl compound is known as crystal violet, the pentamenthyl compound as methyl violet 6B. As stains, m. v. has many bacteriological, histological, and cytological applications.

meth·yl·xan·thines (meth'il-zan'thinz). A chemical group of drugs derived from xanthine (a purine derivative); members of the group include theophylline, caffeine, and theobromine.

meth·yl yel·low. SYN butter yellow.

meth·y·pry·lon, meth·y·pry·lone (meth-i-prī'lon, -lōn). 3,3-Diethyl-2,4-dioxo-5-methylpiperidine; a sedative and hypnotic.

meth·y·ser·gide ma·le·ate (meth-i-ser'jīd). *N*-[1-(Hydroxymethyl)propyl]-1-methyl-D-lysergamide bimaleate; a serotonin antagonist, weakly adrenolytic, chemically related to methylergonovine; used in the prophylactic treatment of vascular headache (migraine); untoward effects are common.

me·thys·ti·cum (mĕ-this'ti-kŭm). The root of *Piper methysticum* (family Piperaceae), a plant of the Pacific islands, used by the natives as an intoxicant. It has been used in diarrhea and in inflammatory affection of the urogenital tract. SYN kava (1).

metMb Abbreviation for metmyoglobin.

met·my·o·glo·bin (metMb) (met'mī-ō-glō'bin). Myoglobin in which the ferrous ion of the heme prosthetic group is oxidized to ferric ion.

met·o·clo·pra·mide hy·dro·chlo·ride (met'ō-klō-pram'īd). 4-Amino-5-chloro-*N*-[2-(diethylamino)ethyl]-*o*-anisamide hydrochloride; an antiemetic agent.

met·o·cur·ine io·dide (met-ō-kyūr'ēn). (+)-*O*,*O*'-dimethylchondrocurarine diiodide; a nondepolarizing neuromuscular blocking agent used to provide relaxation during surgical operations. SYN dimethyl *d*-tubocurarine, dimethyl tubocurarine iodide.

me·tol·a·zone (me-tol'ă-zōn). 7-Chloro-1,2,3,4-tetrahydro-2-methyl-4-oxo-3-*o*-tolyl-6-quinazolinesulfonamide; a diuretic with antihypertensive activity.

me·ton·y·my (mĕ-ton'i-mē). Rarely used term for imprecise or circumscribed labeling of objects or events, said to be characteristic of the language disturbance of schizophrenics; *e.g.,* the patient speaks of having had a "menu" rather than a "meal." [meta- + G. *onyma*, name]

me·top·a·gus (mĕ-top'ă-gŭs). Conjoined twins united at the forehead. SEE conjoined *twins,* under *twin.* [G. *metōpon,* forehead, + *pagos,* something fixed]

me·top·ic (me-tō'pik, me-top'ik). Relating to the forehead or anterior portion of the cranium. [G. *metōpon,* forehead]

me·to·pi·on (mĕ-tō'pē-on). A craniometric point midway between the frontal eminences. SYN metopic point. [G. *metōpon,* forehead]

met·o·pism (met'ō-pizm). Persistence of the frontal suture in the adult. [G. *metōpon,* forehead]

met·o·po·plas·ty (met'ŏ-pō-plas-tē, me-top'ō-plas-tē). Plastic surgery of the skin or bone of the forehead. [G. *metōpon,* forehead, + *plastos,* formed]

met·o·pos·co·py (met'ŏ-pos'kŏ-pē). The study of physiognomy. [G. *metōpon,* forehead, + *skopeō,* to view]

me·to·pro·lol tar·trate (me-tō'prō-lol). 1-Isopropylamino-3-[*p*-(2-methoxyethyl)phenoxy]-2-propanol (2:1) dextrotartrate salt; a β-adrenergic blocking agent used in the treatment of hypertension; exhibits some cardioselectivity.

Met·or·chis (met-ōr'kis). A genus of opisthorchid fish-borne flukes parasitic in the gallbladder of fish-eating mammals and birds, common in north temperate regions. *M. conjunctus* is a species that occurs in dogs and cats, and occasionally in humans, in North America. [G. *meta,* behind, + *orchis,* testicle]

me·tox·e·nous (me-tok'sĕ-nŭs). SYN heterecious. [G. *meta,* beyond, + *xenos,* host]

me·tox·e·ny (me-tok'sĕ-nē). **1.** SYN heterecism. **2.** Change of host by a parasite. [G. *meta,* beyond, + *xenos,* host]

△**metr-, metra-, metro-.** The uterus. SEE ALSO hystero- (1), utero-. [G. *mētra*]

me·tra (mē'tră). SYN uterus. [G. uterus]

me·tra·to·nia (mē-tră-tō'nē-ă). Atony of the uterine walls after childbirth. [metra- + G. *a-* priv. + *tonos,* tension]

me·trat·ro·phy, me·tra·tro·phia (mē-trat'rō-fē, mē-tră-trō'fē-ă). Uterine atrophy. [metra-atrophy]

me·tria (mē'trē-ă). Pelvic cellulitis or other inflammatory affection in the puerperal period. [G. *mētra,* uterus]

met·ric (met'rik). Quantitative; relating to measurement. SEE metric *system.* [G. *metrikos,* fr. *metron,* measure]

me·tri·fo·nate (me-trī'fō-nāt). SYN trichlorfon.

met·ri·o·ce·phal·ic (met'rē-ō-se-fal'ik). Having a head well proportioned to height; denoting a skull with an index between 72 and 77. SEE ALSO orthocephalic. [G. *metrios,* moderate, fr. *metron,* measure, + *kephalē,* head]

me·tri·tis (mē-trī'tis). Inflammation of the uterus. SYN uteritis. [G. *mētra,* uterus, + *-itis,* inflammation]

contagious equine m., a highly contagious venereal disease of horses and other Equidae caused by the bacterium *Taylorella equigenitalis* that produces an endometritis, cervicitis, and vaginitis, affecting breeding and fertility.

me·triz·a·mide (me-triz'ă-mīd). SYN metrizoate sodium.

met·ri·zo·ate so·di·um (met-ri-zō'āt). Sodium 3-acetamido-5-

(*N*-methylacetamido)-2,4,6-triiodobenzoate; a diagnostic radiopaque medium. SYN metrizamide.

⌂**metro-.** SEE metr-. [G. *mētra*, uterus]

me·tro·cyte (mē'trō-sīt). SYN mother *cell*. [G. *mētēr*, mother, + *kytos*, a hollow (cell)]

me·tro·dy·na·mom·e·ter (mē-trō-dī'nă-mom'ĕ-ter). Instrument for measuring the force of uterine contractions. [metro- + G. *dynamis*, power, + *metron*, measure]

me·tro·dyn·ia (mē-trō-dī'nē-ă). SYN hysteralgia. [metro- + G. *odynē*, pain]

me·tro·fi·bro·ma (mē'trō-fī-brō'mă). A fibroma of the uterus.

me·trog·ra·phy (mē-trog'ră-fē). SYN hysterography. [metro- + G. *graphō*, to write]

me·tro·lym·phan·gi·tis (mē'trō-lim-fan-jī'tis). Inflammation of the uterine lymphatics. [metro- + lymphangitis]

me·tro·ma·la·cia (mē'trō-mă-lā'shē-ă). Obsolete term for pathologic softening of the uterine tissues. [metro- + G. *malakia*, softness]

met·ro·ma·nia (met-rō-mā'nē-ă). Rarely used term for an incessant writing of verses. [G. *metron*, measure, + *mania*, frenzy]

met·ro·ni·da·zole (met-rō-ni'dă-zōl). 2-Methyl-5-nitroimidazole-1-ethanol; an orally effective trichomonicide used in the treatment of infections caused by *Trichomonas vaginalis* and *Entamoeba histolytica*.

me·tron·o·scope (mĕ-tron'ō-skōp). A tachistoscopic apparatus that exposes for timed intervals short selections of printed matter for reading; used in testing and developing reading speed. [G. *metron*, measure, + *skopeō*, to view]

me·tro·pa·ral·y·sis (mē'trō-pă-ral'i-sis). Flaccidity or paralysis of the uterine muscle during or immediately after childbirth. [metro- + paralysis]

me·tro·path·ia (mē-trō-path'ē-ă). SYN metropathy. [L.]
  m. hemorrhag'ica, abnormal, excessive, often continuous uterine bleeding due to persistence and exaggeration of the follicular phase of the menstrual cycle; the endometrium is the seat of glandular hyperplasia with cyst formation. SEE Swiss cheese *endometrium*.

me·tro·path·ic (mē-trō-path'ik). Relating to or caused by uterine disease.

me·trop·a·thy (mē-trop'ă-thē). Any disease of the uterus, especially of the myometrium. SYN metropathia. [metro- + G. *pathos*, suffering]

me·tro·per·i·to·ni·tis (mē'trō-per-i-tō-nī'tis). Inflammation of the uterus involving the peritoneal covering. SYN perimetritis. [metro- + peritonitis]

me·tro·phle·bi·tis (mē'trō-flĕ-bī'tis). Inflammation of the uterine veins usually following childbirth. [metro- + G. *phleps*, vein, + -*itis*, inflammation]

met·ro·plas·ty (met'trō-plas-tē, mē'trō-). SYN uteroplasty.

me·tror·rha·gia (mē-trō-rā'jē-ă). Any irregular, acyclic bleeding from the uterus between periods. [metro- + G. *rhēgnymi*, to burst forth]
  m. myopath'ica, postpartum hemorrhage due to flaccidity of the uterine muscle.

me·tror·rhea (mē'trō-rē'ă). Discharge of mucus or pus from the uterus. [metro- + G. *rhoia*, a flow]

me·tror·rhex·is (mē'trō-rek'sis). SYN hysterorrhexis. [metro- + G. *rhēxis*, rupture]

me·tro·sal·pin·gi·tis (mē'trō-sal-pin-jī'tis). Inflammation of the uterus and of one or both fallopian tubes. [metro- + G. *salpinx*, trumpet (oviduct), + -*itis*, inflammation]

me·tro·sal·pin·gog·ra·phy (mē'trō-sal-pin-gog'ră-fē). SYN hysterosalpingography. [metro- + G. *salpinx*, tube, + *graphō*, to write]

me·tro·scope (mē'trō-skōp). SYN hysteroscope. [metro- + G. *skopeō*, to view]

me·tro·stax·is (mē'trō-stak'sis). Small but continuous hemorrhage of the uterine mucous membrane. [metro- + G. *staxis*, a dripping]

me·tro·ste·no·sis (mē'trō-ste-nō'sis). A narrowing of the uterine cavity. [metro- + G. *stenōsis*, a narrowing]

me·trot·o·my (mē-trot'ō-mē). SYN hysterotomy. [metro- + G. *tomē*, incision]

me·tyr·a·pone (mĕ-tir'ă-pōn). 2-Methyl-1,2-di-3-pyridyl-1-propanone; an inhibitor of adrenocortical steroid C-11 β-hydroxylation, administered orally or intravenously to determine the ability of the pituitary gland to increase its secretion of corticotropin; because 11-deoxycorticosteroids, as a consequence of m. administration, only weakly inhibit pituitary corticotropin secretion, the normal pituitary gland will appreciably increase its output of this hormone. SYN mepyrapone.

me·ty·ro·sine (mĕ-tī'rō-sin, -sēn). α-Methyl-*p*-tyrosine; an inhibitor of tyrosine hydroxylase and therefore a powerful inhibitor of catecholamine synthesis; used for controlling the manifestations of pheochromocytoma, in preoperative preparation, or in instances where surgical resection is contraindicated or incomplete.

Mev Symbol for 1 million electron-volts.

mev·a·lo·nate (mev-ă-lon'at). The salt or ester of mevalonic acid.
  m. kinase, an enzyme that catalyzes the reaction of m. and ATP to form ADP and m. 5-phosphate; this enzyme participates in the pathway for steroid synthesis; a deficiency of this enzyme will lead to mevalonic aciduria and lack of development.

mev·a·lon·ic ac·id (mev-ă-lon'ik). $HOOC-_2C(OH)(CH_3)$ CH_2CH_2OH; 3,5-dihydroxy-3-methylpentanoic acid; precursor of squalene, steroids, terpenes, and dolichol.

mev·a·lon·ic ac·i·du·ria. Elevated levels of mevalonic acid in the urine; associated with a deficiency of mevalonate kinase.

mev·a·sta·tin (mev'ă-stat-in). Fungal metabolite which is a potent inhibitor of HMG-CoA reductase, the rate-controlling enzyme in cholesterol biosynthesis. The drug, similar to lovastatin, pravastatin and simvastatin, is used in the treatment of hyperlipidemia.

me·vin·o·lin (me-vin'ō-lin). SYN lovastatin.

mex·e·none (mek'sĕ-nōn). 2-Hydroxy-4-methoxy-4'-methylbenzophenone; a sun-screening agent.

mex·il·e·tine (meks-il'ĕ-tēn). A cardiac antiarrhythmic drug used to treat ventricular arrhythmias; resembles lidocaine in its actions but is orally effective.

mex·il·e·tine hy·dro·chlo·ride (meks-il'ĕ-tēn). 1-(2,6-Dimethylphenoxy)-2-propanamine; an orally active antiarrhythmic agent used to suppress symptomatic ventricular arrhythmias; resembles lidocaine in its actions but is orally effective.

Meyenburg, H. von, Swiss pathologist, *1877. SEE M.'s *complex*, *disease*; M.-Altherr-Uehlinger *syndrome*; von M.'s *disease*.

Meyer, Adolf, U.S. psychiatrist, 1866–1950. SEE M.-Archambault *loop*.

Meyer, Edmund V., German laryngologist, 1864–1931. SEE M.'s *cartilages*, under *cartilage*.

Meyer, Georg H., Swiss anatomist, 1815–1892. SEE M.'s *line*, *sinus*.

Meyer, Hans H., German pharmacologist, 1853–1939. SEE M.-Overton *rule*, *theory* of narcosis.

Meyer, Willy, U.S. surgeon, 1854–1932. SEE M.'s *reagent*.

Meyer-Betz, Friedrich, 20th century German physician. SEE Meyer-Betz *disease*; Meyer-Betz *syndrome*.

Meyerhof, Otto F., German-U.S. biochemist and Nobel laureate, 1884–1951. SEE Embden-M. *pathway*; Embden-M.-Parnas *pathway*; M. oxidation *quotient*.

Meyer-Schwickerath, Gerhard Rudolph Edmund, German ophthalmologist, *1920.

Meynert, Theodor H., Vienna neurologist, 1833–1892. SEE M.'s retroflex *bundle*, *cells*, under *cell*, *commissures*, under *commissure*, *decussation*, *fasciculus*, *layer*.

mez·lo·cil·lin so·di·um (mez-lō-sil'in). $C_{21}H_{24}NaN_5O_8S_2$; an extended spectrum penicillin antibiotic used intravenously and intramuscularly.

Mg Symbol for magnesium.

mg Symbol for milligram.

MGP Abbreviation for matrix Gla *protein*.

MHC Abbreviation for major histocompatibility *complex*.

mho (mō). SYN siemens. [*ohm* reversed]

MHz Symbol for megahertz.

MI Abbreviation for myocardial *infarction*.

mi·an·ser·in hy·dro·chlo·ride (mē-an′ser-in). 1,2,3,4,10,14b-Hexahydro-2-methyldibenzo[*c,f*]pyrazino[1,2*a*]azepine monohydrochloride; an antihistaminic with antiserotonin activity.

Mibelli, Vittorio, Italian dermatologist, 1860–1910. SEE M.'s *angiokeratomas,* under *angiokeratoma, disease.*

MIC Abbreviation for minimal inhibitory *concentration.*

mi·ca·to·sis (mī′kă-tō-sis). Pneumoconiosis due to inhalation of mica particles.

mi·cel·lar (mī-sel′er, mi-). Having the properties of an assemblage of micelles, *i.e.,* of a gel.

mi·celle (mi-sel′, mī-sel′). **1.** Nägeli's term for elongated sub(light)microscopic particles, detected in hydrogels, of supramolecular character and crystalline structure; now defined as one of two classes of colloidal particle: those consisting of many molecules, the other class being single macromolecules light- or submicroscopic in size. A m. is thus a structural unit of the disperse phase in a gel, a unit whose repetition in three dimensions constitutes the micellar structure of the gel; it does not denote the individual particles in free suspension or solution, or the unit structure of a crystal. **2.** Any water-soluble aggregate, spontaneously and reversibly, formed from amphiphile molecules. [L. *micella,* small morsel, dim. of *mica,* morsel, grain]

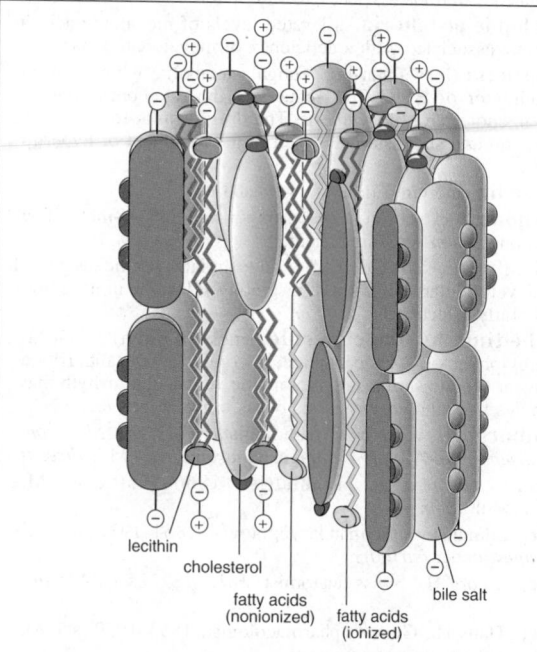

lecithin

cholesterol

fatty acids
(nonionized)

fatty acids
(ionized)

bile salt

lipid micelle

structure of mixed micelle: hydrophilic molecular groups face outward; hydrophobic molecular areas inside micelle

Michaelis, Leonor, German-U.S. chemist, 1875–1949. SEE M.-Gutmann *body;* M. *constant;* M.-Menten *constant, equation, hypothesis.*

Micheli, Ferdinando, Italian physician, 1872–1936. SEE Marchiafava-M. *anemia, syndrome.*

Michel's spur. See under spur.

mi·con·a·zole ni·trate (mī-kon′ă-zōl). 1-[2,4-Dichloro-β-[(2,4-dichlorobenzyl)oxy]phenethyl]imidazole mononitrate; an antifungal agent.

△**micr-.** SEE micro-.

mi·cra·cou·stic (mī′kră-kū′stik). **1.** Relating to faint sounds. **2.** Magnifying very faint sounds so as to make them audible. SYN microcoustic. [micro- + G. *akoustikos,* relating to hearing, fr. *akouō,* to hear]

mi·cren·ce·pha·lia (mī′kren-se-fā′lē-ă). SYN micrencephaly.

mi·cren·ceph·a·lous (mī-kren-sef′ă-lŭs). Having a small brain.

mi·cren·ceph·a·ly (mī-kren-sef′ă-lē). Abnormal smallness of the brain. SYN micrencephalia, microencephaly. [micro- + G. *enkephalos,* brain]

△**micro-, micr-.** **1.** Prefixes denoting smallness. **2.** (μ). Prefix used in the SI and metric systems to signify one-millionth (10⁻⁶) of such unit. **3.** In chemistry, prefix to terms denoting chemical examination, methods, etc. that utilize minimal quantities of the substance to be examined; *e.g.,* a drop or two in place of one or more milliliters. **4.** Combining forms meaning microscopic; opposite of macro-, megalo-. [G. *mikros,* small]

mi·cro·ab·scess (mī′krō-ab′ses). A very small circumscribed collection of leukocytes in solid tissues.

Munro's m., a microscopic collection of polymorphonuclear leukocytes found in the stratum corneum in psoriasis. SYN Munro's abscess.

Pautrier's m., a microscopic lesion in the epidermis, seen in mycosis fungoides; it is composed of the same type of atypical mononuclear cells as those that form the infiltrate in the corium. SYN Pautrier's abscess.

mi·cro·ad·e·no·ma (mī′krō-ad-ĕ-nō′mă). A pituitary adenoma less than 10 mm in diameter.

mi·cro·ae·ro·bi·on (mī′krō-ā-rō′bǐ-on). A microaerophilic microorganism.

mi·cro·aer·o·phil, mi·cro·aer·o·phile (mī-krō-ār′ō-fil, -fīl). **1.** An aerobic bacterium that requires oxygen, but less than is present in the air, and grows best under modified atmospheric conditions. **2.** Relating to such an organism. SYN microaerophilic, microaerophilous. [micro- + G. *aēr,* air, + *philos,* fond]

mi·cro·aer·o·phil·ic (mī′krō-ār-ō-fil′ik). SYN microaerophil (2).

mi·cro·aer·oph·i·lous (mī′krō-ār-ōf′i-lŭs). SYN microaerophil (2).

mi·cro·aer·o·sol (mī-krō-ār′ō-sol). A suspension in air of particles that are submicronic or, more frequently, from 1 to 10 μm in diameter.

mi·cro·a·nal·y·sis (mī′krō-ă-nal′i-sis). Analytic techniques involving unusually small samples.

mi·cro·a·nas·to·mo·sis (mī′krō-ă-nas-tō-mō′sis). Anastomosis of minute structures performed under a surgical microscope.

mi·cro·a·nat·o·mist (mī′krō-ă-nat′ŏ-mist). SYN histologist.

mi·cro·a·nat·o·my (mī′krō-ă-nat′ŏ-mē). SYN histology.

mi·cro·an·eu·rysm (mī′krō-an′yū-rizm). Focal dilation of retinal capillaries occurring in diabetes mellitus, retinal vein obstruction, and absolute glaucoma, or of arteriolocapillary junctions in many organs in thrombotic thrombocytopenic purpura.

mi·cro·an·gi·og·ra·phy (mī′krō-an-jē-og′ră-fē). Radiography of the finer vessels of an organ after the injection of a contrast medium and enlargement of the resulting radiograph. SYN microarteriography. [micro- + angiography]

mi·cro·an·gi·op·a·thy (mī′krō-an-jē-op′ă-thē). SYN capillaropathy.

thrombotic m., thrombosis within small blood vessels, as in thrombotic thrombocytopenic purpura.

mi·cro·an·gi·os·co·py (mī′krō-an-jē-os′kŏ-pē). SYN capillarioscopy.

mi·cro·ar·te·ri·og·ra·phy (mī′krō-ar-tēr-ē-og′ră-fē). SYN microangiography.

mi·cro·bal·ance (mī′krō-bal-ans). A balance designed for use in weighing unusually small samples of materials.

mi·crobe (mī′krōb). Any very minute organism. As originated, the word was intended as a collective term for the large variety of microorganisms then known in the 19th century; modern usage has retained the original collective meaning but expanded it to include both microscopic and ultramicroscopic organisms (spirochetes, bacteria, rickettsiae, and viruses). These organisms are considered to form a biologically distinctive group, in that the genetic material is not surrounded by a nuclear membrane, and mitosis does not occur during replication. [Fr., fr. G. *mikros,* small, + *bios,* life]

mi·cro·bi·al (mī-krō'bē-ăl). Relating to a microbe or to microbes. SYN microbic, microbiotic (2).

mi·cro·bi·al as·so·ci·ates (mī-krō'bē-ăl ă-sō'shē-ăts). SYN flora (2).

mi·cro·bic (mī-krō'bik). SYN microbial.

mi·cro·bi·ci·dal (mī-krō'bi-sī'dăl). Destructive to microbes. SYN microbicide (1).

mi·cro·bi·cide (mī-krō'bi-sīd). **1.** SYN microbicidal. **2.** An agent destructive to microbes; a germicide; an antiseptic. [microbe + L. *caedo,* to kill]

mi·cro·bid (mī-krō'bid). Cutaneous allergic response to superficial bacterial infection. [micro- + G. *bios,* life, + *eidēs,* resembling]

mi·cro·bi·o·log·ic (mī'krō-bī-ō-loj'ik). Relating to microbiology.

mi·cro·bi·ol·o·gist (mī'krō-bī-ol'ō-jist). One who specializes in the science of microbiology.

mi·cro·bi·ol·o·gy (mī'krō-bī-ol'ō-jē). The science concerned with microorganisms, including fungi, protozoa, bacteria, and viruses. [Fr. *microbiologie*]

mi·cro·bi·ot·ic (mī'krō-bī-ot'ik). **1.** Short-lived. **2.** SYN microbial.

mi·cro·bism (mī'krō-bizm). Infection with microbes.

latent m., the presence of pathogenic microorganisms in the body that elicit no symptoms; the condition of a pathogen carrier.

mi·cro·blast (mī'krō-blast). A small, nucleated, red blood cell. [micro- + G. *blastos,* sprout, germ]

mi·cro·ble·pha·ria, mi·cro·bleph·a·ron (mī'krō-ble-far'ē-ă, -blef'ă-ron). SYN microblepharon.

mi·cro·bleph·a·rism (-blef'ăr-izm). SYN microblepharon.

mi·cro·body (mī'krō-bod-ē). SYN peroxisome.

mi·cro·bra·chia (mī-krō-brā'kē-ă). Abnormal smallness of the arms. [micro- + G. *brachiōn,* arm]

mi·cro·bren·ner (mī-krō-bren'er). An electric cautery with needle point. [micro- + Ger. *Brenner,* burner]

mi·cro·car·dia (mī-krō-kar'dē-ă). Abnormal smallness of the heart. [micro- + G. *kardia,* heart]

mi·cro·cen·trum (mī-krō-sen'trŭm). SYN cytocentrum. [micro- + G. *kentron,* center]

mi·cro·ce·pha·lia (mī-krō-se-fā'lē-ă). SYN microcephaly.

mi·cro·ce·phal·ic (mī'krō-sĕ-fal'ik). Having a small head. SYN microcephalous, nanocephalous, nanocephalic.

mi·cro·ceph·a·lism (mī-krō-sef'ă-lizm). SYN microcephaly.

mi·cro·ceph·a·lous (mī-krō-sef'ă-lŭs). SYN microcephalic.

mi·cro·ceph·a·ly (mī-krō-sef'ă-lē). Abnormal smallness of the head; applied to a skull with a capacity below 1350 ml. Usually associated with mental retardation. SYN microcephalia, microcephalism, nanocephalia, nanocephaly. [micro- + G. *kephalē,* head]

encephaloclastic m., complex growth disturbances in the brain as a result of regressive changes in fetal life.

schizencephalic m., dysgenic process resulting in focal cerebral defects.

mi·cro·chei·lia, mi·cro·chi·lia (mī-krō-kī'lē-ă). Smallness of the lips. [micro- + G. *cheilos,* lip]

mi·cro·chei·ria, mi·cro·chi·ria (mī-krō-kī'rē-ă). Smallness of the hands. [micro- + G. *cheir,* hand]

mi·cro·chem·is·try (mī-krō-kem'is-trē). The use of chemical procedures involving minute quantities or reactions not visible to the unaided eye. Cf. macrochemistry.

mi·cro·cide (mī'krō-sīd). SYN *glucose* oxidase.

mi·cro·cin·e·ma·tog·ra·phy (mī'kro-sin-ĕ-mă-tog'ră-fē). The application of moving pictures taken through magnifying lenses to the study of an organ or system in motion; *e.g.,* the circulation in living embryos. [micro- + G. *kinēma,* movement, + *graphō,* to write]

mi·cro·cir·cu·la·tion (mī'krō-sir-kyū-lā'shŭn). Passage of blood in the smallest vessels, namely arterioles, capillaries, and venules.

Mi·cro·coc·ca·ce·ae (mī'krō-kok-ā'sē-ē). A family of bacteria (order Eubacteriales) containing Gram-positive spherical cells which occur singly or in pairs, tetrads, packets, irregular masses, or even chains. Rarely are these organisms motile. Free-living, saprophytic, parasitic, and pathogenic species occur. The type genus is *Micrococcus.*

mi·cro·coc·ci (mī'krō-kok'sī). Plural of micrococcus.

Mi·cro·coc·cus (mī'krō-kok-ŭs). A genus of bacteria (family Micrococcaceae) containing Gram-positive, spherical cells that occur in irregular masses, never in packets. Some species are motile or produce motile mutants. These organisms are saprophytic, facultatively parasitic, or parasitic but are not truly pathogenic. The type species is *M. luteus.* It is the type genus of the family Micrococcaceae. [micro- + G. *kokkos,* berry]

M. can'didus, a species found in skin secretions, milk, and dairy products.

M. conglomera'tus, a species found in infections, milk, dairy products, dairy utensils, and water.

M. cryoph'ilus, a species found in frozen meat products.

M. lu'teus, a saprophytic species found in milk and dairy products and on dust particles; it is the type species of the genus *M.*

M. morrhu'ae, former name for *Halococcus morrhuae.*

M. ure'ae, a species found in stale urine or in soil containing urine.

M. var'ians, a species found in body secretions, dairy products, dairy utensils, dust, and fresh and salt water.

mi·cro·coc·cus, pl. **mi·cro·coc·ci** (mī'krō-kok'ŭs, -kok'sī). A vernacular term used to refer to any member of the genus *Micrococcus.*

mi·cro·co·li·tis (mī'krō-kō-lī'tis). Colitis that is not seen by endoscopy, but in which microscopic examination of biopsies shows nonspecific mucosal inflammation.

mi·cro·co·lon (mī'krō-kō-lon). A small-caliber unused colon, seen in the neonate on radiographic contrast enema; usually a consequence of intestinal atresia or meconium ileus.

mi·cro·col·o·ny (mī'krō-kol-ō-nē). A colony of bacteria visible only under a low power microscope.

mi·cro·co·nid·i·um, pl. **mi·cro·co·nid·ia** (mī'krō-kō-nid'ē-ŭm, -ă). In fungi, the smaller of two distinctively different-sized types of conidia in a single species, usually single-celled and spherical, ovoid, pyriform, or clavate.

mi·cro·co·ria (mī-krō-kō'rē-ă). A congenitally small pupil with an inability to dilate. [micro- + G. *korē,* pupil]

mi·cro·cor·nea (mī'krō-kōr'nē-ă). An abnormally small cornea.

mi·cro·cou·lomb (μC) (mī-krō-kū'lom). One-millionth of a coulomb.

mi·cro·cou·stic (mī'krō-kū'stik). SYN micracoustic.

mi·cro·crys·tal·line (mī'krō-krys'tă-lin). Occurring in minute crystals.

mi·cro·cu·rie (μCi) (mī'krō-kyū'rē). One-millionth of a curie; a quantity of any radionuclide with 3.7×10^4 disintegrations per second.

mi·cro·cyst (mī'krō-sist). A tiny cyst, frequently of such dimensions that a magnifying lens or microscope is required for observation.

mi·cro·cyte (mī'krō-sīt). A small (5 μm or less) non-nucleated red blood cell. SYN microerythrocyte. [micro- + G. *kytos,* cell]

mi·cro·cy·the·mia (mī'krō-sī-thē'mē-ă). The presence of many microcytes in the circulating blood. SYN microcytosis. [microcyte + G. *haima,* blood]

mi·cro·cy·to·sis (mī'krō-sī-tō'sis). SYN microcythemia. [microcyte + G. *-osis,* condition]

mi·cro·dac·tyl·ia (mī'krō-dak-til'ē-ă). SYN microdactyly.

mi·cro·dac·ty·lous (mī-krō-dak'ti-lŭs). Relating to or characterized by microdactyly.

mi·cro·dac·ty·ly (mī-krō-dak'ti-lē). Smallness or shortness of the fingers or toes. SYN microdactylia. [micro- + G. *dactylos,* finger, toe]

mi·cro·dis·sec·tion (mī'krō-di-sek'shŭn). Dissection of tissues under a microscope or magnifying glass, usually done by teasing the tissues apart by means of needles.

mi·cro·dont (mī'krō-dont). Having small teeth; denoting a skull

mi

with a dental index below 41.9. [micro- + G. *odous* (*odont-*), tooth]

mi·cro·don·tia, mi·cro·don·tism (mī-krō-don′shē-ă, -don′ tizm). A condition in which a single tooth, or pairs of teeth, or the whole dentition, may be disproportionately small. [micro- + G. *odous,* tooth]

mi·cro·dose (mī′krō-dōs). A very small dose.

mi·cro·drep·a·no·cy·to·sis (mī′krō-drep′ă-nō-sī-tō′sis). A chronic hemolytic anemia resulting from interaction of the genes for sickle cell anemia and thalassemia. [microcytosis + drepanocytosis]

mi·cro·dys·ge·ne·sia (mī′krō-dis-ge-nē′sē-ă). Increase in partially distopic neurons in the stratum zonale, white matter, hippocampus and cerebellar cortex, producing an indistinct border between cortex and subcortical white matter and a columnar arrangement of cortical neurons; seen in patients with primary generalized epilepsy. [micro- + dys- + G. *genesis,* production]

mi·cro·e·lec·trode (mī′krō-ē-lek′trōd). An electrode of very fine caliber consisting usually of a fine wire or a glass tube of capillary diameter (10 μm to 1 mm) drawn to a fine point and filled with saline or a metal such as gallium or indium (while melted); used in physiologic experiments to stimulate or to record action currents of extracellular or intracellular origin.

microelements. SYN trace *elements,* under *element.*

mi·cro·en·ceph·a·ly (mī′krō-en-sef′ă-lē). SYN micrencephaly.

mi·cro·e·ryth·ro·cyte (mī′krō-ĕ-rith′rō-sīt). SYN microcyte.

mi·cro·ev·o·lu·tion (mī′krō-ev-ŏ-lū′shŭn). The evolution of bacteria and other microorganisms through mutations.

mi·cro·fi·bril (mi-kro-fī′bril). A very small fibril having an average diameter of 13 nm; it may be a bundle of still smaller elements, the microfilaments.

mi·cro·fil·a·ment (mī-krō-fil′ă-ment). The finest filamentous element of the cytoskeleton, having a diameter of about 5 nm and consisting primarily of actin. SEE ALSO actin *filament.*

mi·cro·fil·a·re·mia (mī′krō-fil-ă-rē′mē-ă). Infection of the blood with microfilariae. M. caused by *Wuchereria bancrofti* is characterized by sharp nocturnal periodicity, apparently tied to the nocturnal habits of the vector mosquitoes; in geographic areas where mosquitoes are not strictly night-biters (as in parts of Polynesia), the microfilarial periodicity is modified or absent. SEE ALSO periodic *filariasis.*

mi·cro·fi·lar·ia, pl. **mi·cro·fi·lar·i·ae** (mī′krō-fi-lar′ē-ă, -ē). Term for embryos of filarial nematodes in the family Onchocercidae. In the past this term has been used as a generic designation (*e.g., Microfilaria bancrofti, M. malaya*). SEE *Filaria.*

mi·cro·film (mī′krō-film). **1.** A photographic film bearing greatly reduced images of printed records. **2.** To record on microfilm.

mi·cro·flo·ra (mī′krō-flō-rā). The bacteria and fungi that inhabit an area.

mi·cro·ga·mete (mī-krō-gam′ēt). The male element in anisogamy, or conjugation of cells of unequal size; it is the smaller of the two cells and actively motile. [micro- + G. *gametēs,* husband]

mi·cro·ga·me·to·cyte (mī-krō-gam′ē-tō-sīt). The mother cell producing the microgametes, or male elements of sexual reproduction in sporozoan protozoans and fungi. SYN microgamont.

mi·cro·gam·ont (mī-krō-gam′ont). SYN microgametocyte.

mi·crog·a·my (mī-krog′ă-mē). Conjugation between two young cells, the recent product of sporulation or some other form of reproduction. [micro- + G. *gamos,* marriage]

mi·cro·gas·tria (mī-krō-gas′trē-ă). Smallness of the stomach. [micro- + G. *gastēr,* stomach]

mi·cro·gen·ia (mī-krō-jēn′ē-ă). Abnormal smallness of the chin resulting from the underdevelopment of the mental symphysis. [micro- + G. *geneion,* chin]

mi·cro·gen·i·tal·ism (mī-krō-jen′i-tal-izm). Abnormal smallness of the external genital organs.

mi·crog·lia (mī-krog′lē-ă). Small neuroglial cells, possibly of mesodermal origin, which may become phagocytic, in areas of neural damage or inflammation. SYN Hortega cells, microglia cells, microglial cells. [micro- + G. *glia,* glue]

mi·crog·li·a·cyte (mī-krōg′lē-ă-sīt). A cell, especially an embryonic cell, of the microglia. [micro- + G. *glia,* glue, + *kytos,* cell]

mi·crog·li·o·ma (mī-krog′lē-ō′mă). Obsolete term for an intracranial neoplasm of microglial cell origin that is structurally similar to lymphoma. [microglia + G. *-oma,* tumor]

mi·cro·gli·o·ma·to·sis (mī′krō-glē-ō-mă-tō′sis). Obsolete term for a condition characterized by the presence of multiple microgliomas.

mi·crog·li·o·sis (mī-krog′lē-ō′sis). Presence of microglia in nervous tissue secondary to injury. [microglia + G. *-osis,* condition]

mi·cro·glob·u·lin (mī′krō-glob′ū-lin). Any serum or urinary globulin of molecular mass below about 40 kDa, including especially Bence Jones *proteins,* under *protein.*

β-m., a polypeptide of 11,600 Da that forms the light chain of class 1 major histocompatibility antigens and can therefore be detected on all cells bearing these antigens. Free β microglobulin is found in the blood and urine of patients with certain diseases, including Wilson's *disease,* cadmium poisoning, and renal tubular *acidosis.*

$β_2$-m., the light chain of the histocompatibility class I molecule. This chain is invariant within a given species; found in elevated levels in individuals with Wilson's disease.

mi·cro·glos·sia (mī-krō-glos′ē-ă). Smallness of the tongue. [micro- + G. *glossa,* tongue]

mi·cro·gna·thia (mī-krō-nā′thē-ă, mī-krog-nath′ē-ă). Abnormal smallness of the jaws, especially of the mandible. [micro- + G. *gnathos,* jaw]

m. with peromelia, hypoplasia of the mandible with malformed and missing teeth, birdlike face, and severe deformities of the hands and forearms and sometimes of feet and legs. SYN Hanhart's syndrome.

mi·cro·gram (μg) (mī′krō-gram). One-millionth of a gram.

mi·cro·graph (mī′krō-graf). **1.** An instrument that magnifies the microscopic movements of a diaphragm by means of light interference and records them on a moving photographic film; may be used for recording various pulse curves, sound waves, and any forms of motion that may be communicated through the air to a diaphragm. **2.** SYN photomicrograph. [micro- + G. *graphō,* to write]

electron m., the image produced by the electron beam of an electron microscope, recorded on an electron-sensitive plate or film.

light m., a photograph produced by means of a light microscope.

mi·crog·ra·phy (mī-krog′ră-fē). **1.** Writing with very minute letters, sometimes observed in psychoses and in paralysis agitans. **2.** A description of objects seen with a microscope. **3.** SYN photomicrography. [micro- + G. *graphō,* to write]

mi·cro·gy·ria (mī-krō-jī′rē-ă). Abnormal narrowness of the cerebral convolutions. [micro- + G. *gyros,* convolution]

mi·cro·he·pat·ia (mī-krō-he-pat′ē-ă). Abnormal smallness of the liver. [micro- + G. *hepar* (*hepat-*), liver]

mi·cro·het·er·o·gene·i·ty (mī′krō-het′er-ō-jĕ-nē′i-tē;ne′i-tē). Slight differences in structure between essentially identical molecules; *e.g.,* in the saccharide portion of a glycoprotein.

mi·crohm (μΩ) (mī′krōm). One-millionth of an ohm. SYN micro-ohm.

mi·cro·in·cin·er·a·tion (mī′krō-in-sin′ĕ-rā′shŭn). Combustion, in a furnace, of organic constituents in a tissue section so that the remaining mineral ash can be examined microscopically. SYN spodography.

mi·cro·in·cis·ion (mī-krō-in-sizh′ŭn). An incision made with the aid of a microscope.

mi·cro·in·jec·tor (mī′krō-in-jek-tor). An instrument for infusion of very small amounts of fluids or drugs into animals or humans.

mi·cro·in·va·sion (mī′krō-in-vā′zhŭn). Invasion of tissue immediately adjacent to a carcinoma in situ, the earliest stage of malignant neoplastic invasion.

mi·cro·kat·al (mī′krō-kat′ăl). One-millionth of a katal.

mi·cro·ky·mat·o·ther·a·py (mī′krō-kī-mat′ō-thār′ă-pē). Treatment with high frequency radiations of 3,000,000,000 Hz (3000

MHz), at a wavelength of 10 cm. SYN microwave therapy. [micro- + G. *kyma,* a wave, + *therapeia,* treatment]

mi·cro·leu·ko·blast (mī-krō-lū′kō-blast). SYN micromyeloblast.

mi·cro·li·ter (μl, λ) (mī′krō-lē-ter). One-millionth of a liter.

mi·cro·lith (mī′krō-lith). A minute calculus, usually multiple and constituting a coarse sand called gravel. [micro- + G. *lithos,* stone]

mi·cro·li·thi·a·sis (mī-krō-li-thī′ă-sis). The formation, presence, or discharge of minute concretions, or gravel.

  pulmonary alveolar m., microscopic granules of calcium or bone disseminated throughout the lungs.

mi·crol·o·gy (mī-krol′ō-jē). The science concerned with microscopic objects, of which histology is a branch. [micro- + G. *logos,* study]

mi·cro·ma·nia (mī-krō-mā′nē-ă). A delusion of self-deprecation, or that one's own body is of minute size. [micro- + G. *mania,* frenzy]

mi·cro·ma·nip·u·la·tion (mī′krō-mă-nip′yū-lā′shŭn). Dissection, teasing, stimulation, etc., under the microscope, of minute structures; *e.g.,* tissue cells or unicellular organisms.

mi·cro·ma·nip·u·la·tor (mī′krō-mă-nip′yū-lā′ter, -tōr). An instrument used in micromanipulation, whereby microdissection, microinjection, and other maneuvers are performed, usually with the aid of a microscope.

mi·cro·ma·zia (mī-krō-mā′zē-ă). Condition in which the breasts are rudimentary and functionless. [micro- + G. *mazos,* breast]

mi·cro·me·lia (mī-krō-mē′lē-ă). Condition of having disproportionately short or small limbs. SEE ALSO achondroplasia. SYN nanomelia. [micro- + G. *melos,* limb]

mi·cro·mere (mī′krō-mēr). A blastomere of small size; for example, one of the blastomeres at the animal pole of an amphibian egg. [micro- + G. *meros,* a part]

mi·cro·mer·o·zo·ite (mī′krō-mer-ō-zō′īt). A small merozoite.

mi·cro·me·tas·ta·sis (mī′krō-mĕ-tas′tă-sis). A stage of metastasis when the secondary tumors are too small to be clinically detected, as in micrometastatic disease.

mi·cro·met·a·stat·ic (mī′krō-met-ă-stat′ik). Denoting or characterized by micrometastasis, as in m. disease.

mi·crom·e·ter (μm) (mī-krom′ĕ-ter). One-millionth of a meter; a device for measuring various types of objects in an accurate and precise manner; in medicine and biology, the term is usually used with reference to a glass slide or lens that is accurately marked for measuring microscopic forms. [micro- + G. *metron,* measure]

  caliper m., a gauge with a calibrated m. screw for the measurement of thin objects such as microscope cover glasses and slides.

  filar m., an ocular micrometer with a line moved by a ruled drum such that a movement of the line of 5 μm or less may be made in relation to fixed parallel lines.

  ocular m., a glass disk that fits in a microscope eyepiece and that has a ruled scale; when calibrated with a slide m., direct measurements of a microscopic object can be made.

  slide m., a scale made on a microscope slide with lines ruled in divisions, usually, of 0.01 mm; typically used to calibrate an ocular m.

mi·crom·e·try (mī-krom′ĕ-trē). Measurement of objects with some type of micrometer and a microscope.

⚠**micromicro-** (μμ). Prefix formerly used to signify one-trillionth (10^{-12}); now pico-.

mi·cro·mi·cro·gram (μμg) (mī′krō-mī′krō-gram). Former term for picogram.

mi·cro·mi·cron (μμ) (mī-krō-mī′kron). Former term for picometer.

mi·cro·min·er·als (mī-krō-min′er-ălz). SYN trace *elements,* under *element.*

mi·cro·mo·lar (μM) (mī-krō-mō′lar). Denoting a concentration of 10^{-6} mole per liter (10^{-6} M or 1 μM).

mi·cro·mole (μmol) (mī′krō-mōl). One-millionth of a mole.

mi·cro·mo·to·scope (mī′krō-mō′tō-skōp). A cinematoscope for representing the movements of amebas and other motile microscopic objects. [micro- + L. *motus,* motion, + G. *skopeō,* to view]

mi·cro·my·e·lia (mī′krō-mī-ē′lē-ă). Abnormal smallness or shortness of the spinal cord. [micro- + G. *myelos,* marrow]

mi·cro·my·el·o·blast (mī-krō-mī′el-ō-blast). A small myeloblast, often the predominating cell in myeloblastic leukemia. SYN microleukoblast.

mi·cron (μ) (mī′kron). Former term for micrometer.

mi·cro·nee·dle (mī′krō-nē′dl). A small glass needle used in micrurgical manipulation.

mi·cro·neme (mī′krō-nēm). A small, osmiophilic, cordlike twisted organelle found in the anterior region of many sporozoans; one of the characteristics that helps to define the subphylum Apicomplexa. SYN sarconeme. [micro- + G. *nēma,* thread]

mi·cron·ic (mī-kron′ik). Of the size of 1 micron (micrometer).

mi·cro·nod·u·lar (mī′krō-nod′yū-lăr). Characterized by the presence of minute nodules; denoting a somewhat coarser appearance than that of a granular tissue or substance. [G. *mikros,* small]

mi·cro·nu·cle·us (mī-krō-nū′klē-ŭs). **1.** A small nucleus in a large cell, or the smaller nuclei in cells that have two or more such structures. **2.** The smaller of the two nuclei in ciliates dividing mitotically and bearing specific inheritable material. SYN gametic nucleus, germ nucleus, gonad nucleus, karyogonad, reproductive nucleus. SEE ALSO macronucleus (2).

mi·cro·nu·tri·ents (mī-krō-nū′trē-ents). Essential food factors required in only small quantities by the body; *e.g.,* vitamins, trace minerals. SYN trace nutrient.

mi·cro·nych·ia (mī-krō-nik′ē-ă). Abnormal smallness of nails. [micro- + G. *onyx,* nail]

mi·cro·nys·tag·mus (mī′krō-nis-tag′mŭs). Nystagmus of so small an amplitude that it is not detected by the usual clinical tests. SYN minimal amplitude nystagmus. [micro- + G. *nystagmos,* a nodding].

mi·cro-ohm (mī′krō-ōm). SYN microhm.

mi·cro·or·gan·ism (mī′krō-ōr′gan-izm). A microscopic organism (plant or animal).

mi·cro·par·a·site (mī-krō-par′ă-sīt). A parasitic microorganism.

mi·cro·pa·thol·o·gy (mī′krō-pa-thol′ō-jē). The microscopic study of disease changes. [micro- + G. *pathos,* suffering, + *logos,* study]

mi·cro·pe·nis (mī-krō-pē′nis). Abnormally small penis. SYN microphallus.

mi·cro·phage (mī′krō-fāj). A polymorphonuclear leukocyte that is phagocytic. SEE ALSO phagocyte. SYN microphagocyte. [micro- + phag(ocyte)]

mi·cro·phag·o·cyte (mī-krō-fāj′ō-sīt). SYN microphage.

mi·cro·phal·lus (mī-krō-fal′ŭs). SYN micropenis.

mi·cro·pho·bia (mī-krō-fō′bē-ă). Fear of minute objects, microorganisms, germs, etc. [micro- + G. *phobos,* fear]

mi·cro·phone (mī′krō-fōn). An instrument for converting sounds to electrical impulses. [micro- + G. *phōnē,* sound]

mi·cro·pho·nia, mi·croph·o·ny (mī-krō-fō′nē-ă, mī-krof′ō-nē). SYN hypophonia. [micro- + G. *phōnē,* voice]

mi·cro·pho·no·scope (mī-krō-fō′nō-skōp). A stethoscope with a diaphragm attachment for magnifying the sound.

mi·cro·pho·to·graph (mī-krō-fō′tō-graf). A minute photograph of any object, as distinguished from a photomicrograph.

mi·croph·thal·mia (mī′krof-thal′mē-ă). SYN microphthalmos.

mi·croph·thal·mos (-thal′mos). Abnormal smallness of the eye. SYN microphthalmia, nanophthalmia, nanophthalmos. [micro + G. *ophthalmos,* eye]

mi·cro·pi·pette, mi·cro·pi·pet (mī′krō-pi-pet′, -pī-pet′). A pipette designed for the measurement of very small volumes.

mi·cro·pla·nia (mī-krō-plā′nē-ă). Decreased horizontal diameter of erythrocytes. [micro- + L. *planus,* flat]

mi·cro·pla·sia (mī-krō-plā′zē-ă). Stunted growth, as in dwarfism. [micro- + G. *plasis,* a shaping, forming]

mi·cro·pleth·ys·mog·ra·phy (mī′krō-pleth-iz-mog′ră-fē). The technique of measuring minute changes in the volume of a part as a result of blood flow into or out of it.

mi

mi·cro·po·dia (mī-krō-pō′dē-ă). Abnormal smallness of the feet. [micro- + G. *pous*, foot]

mi·cro·pore (mī′krō-pōr). An organelle formed by the pellicle of all stages of sporozoan protozoa of the subphylum Apicomplexa and also found in developmental stages that may lack the inner pellicle layer; it is composed of two concentric rings (in transverse section), the inner of which corresponds with an invagination of the outer pellicle membrane. M.'s thus far observed seem to serve as feeding organelles; their role in nonfeeding developmental forms is unknown. [micro- + G. *poros*, pore]

mi·cro·pro·my·el·o·cyte (mī′krō-prō-mī′el-ō-sīt). A cell derived from a promyelocyte.

mi·cro·pro·so·pia (mī′krō-prō-sō′pē-ă). A condition characterized by an abnormally small or imperfectly developed face. [micro- + G. *prosōpon*, face]

mi·crop·sia (mī-krop′sē-ă). Perception of objects as smaller than they are. [micro- + G. *opsis*, sight]

mi·cro·punc·ture (mī′krō-pŭnk-chūr). A puncture made with the aid of a microscope.

mi·cro·pyle (mī′krō-pīl). **1.** Minute opening believed to exist in the investing membrane of certain ova as a point of entrance for the spermatozoon. **2.** Former name for micropore. [micro- + G. *pylē*, gate]

mi·cro·ra·di·og·ra·phy (mī′krō-rā-dē-og′ră-fē). Making radiographs of histologic sections of tissue for enlargement. SEE ALSO historadiography.

mi·cro·re·frac·tom·e·ter (mī′krō-rē-frak-tom′ĕ-ter). A refractometer used in the study of blood cells.

mi·cro·res·pi·rom·e·ter (mī′krō-res-pi-rom′ĕ-ter). An apparatus for measuring the utilization of oxygen by small particles of isolated tissues or cells or particles of cells.

mi·cro·sac·cades (mī′krō-să-kādz′). Minute to and fro movements of the eyes. [micro- + Fr. *saccade*, sudden check (of a horse)]

mi·cro·scin·tig·ra·phy (mī′krō-sin-tig′ră-fē). Imaging of small anatomic structures by use of a radionuclide in conjunction with a special collimator which "magnifies" the image; for example, the use of technetium-99m in conjunction with a pinhole collimator to image the lacrimal drainage. [micro- + scintigraphy]

mi·cro·scope (mī′krō-skōp). An instrument that gives an enlarged image of an object or substance that is minute or not visible with the naked eye; usually the term denotes a compound m.; for low magnifications the term simple m., or magnifying glass, is used. [micro- + G. *skopeō*, to view]

binocular m., a m. having two eyepieces; it may be a compound m. or a stereoscopic m.

color-contrast m., a type of m. in which the condenser stop is of one color and the annulus is a complement of it so that unstained objects are observed in one color on a field of the other.

comparator m., a device constructed with one or more m.'s having micrometer eyepieces used to measure dimensional changes during setting or temperature changes.

compound m., a m. having two or more magnifying lenses.

confocal m., a m. that allows the observer to visualize objects in a single plane of focus, thereby creating a sharper image (usually the objects are fluorescent molecules); a refinement of this m. uses optical sectioning and a computer to record serial sections. This permits three-dimensional reconstruction.

dark-field m., a m. that has a special condenser and objective with a diaphragm or stop that scatters light from the object observed, with the result that the object appears bright on a dark background.

electron m., a visual and photographic m. in which electron beams with wavelengths thousands of times shorter than visible light are utilized in place of light, thereby allowing much greater resolution and magnification; in this technique, the electrons are transmitted through a very thin section of an embedded and dehydrated specimen maintained in a vacuum.

fluorescence m., SEE fluorescence *microscopy.*

flying spot m., a m. in which a moving spot of light is imaged in the object plane, the energy transmitted by the specimen being detected with a photoelectric cell; the light source may be a

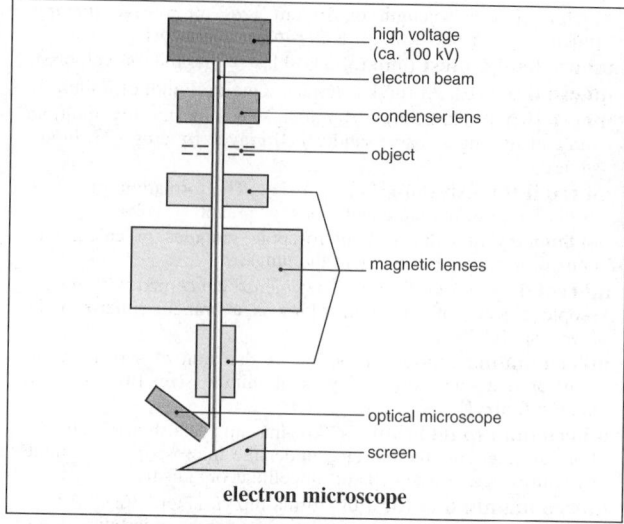

	high voltage (ca. 100 kV)
	electron beam
	condenser lens
	object
	magnetic lenses
	optical microscope
	screen

electron microscope

cathode ray tube, a scanning disk or drum, or an oscillating mirror.

infrared m., a m. that is equipped with infrared transmitting optics and that measures the infrared absorption of minute samples with the aid of photoelectric cells; images may be observed with image converters or television.

interference m., a specially constructed m. in which the entering light is split into two beams which pass through the specimen and are recombined in the image plane where the interference effects make the transparent (invisible) refractile object details become visible as intensity differences; permits measurements of light retardation, index of refraction, and thickness and mass of specimen; it is useful in the examination of living or unstained cells.

laser m., a m. in which a laser beam is focused on a microscopic field, causing it to vaporize; the emitted radiation is analyzed by means of a microspectrophotometer; at a low intensity the laser is employed as the light source in an interference m.

light m., a class of m. that forms a magnified image using visible light.

opaque m., SYN epimicroscope.

operating m., SYN surgical m.

phase m., phase-contrast m., a specially constructed m. that has a special condenser and objective containing a phase-shifting ring whereby small differences in index of refraction are made visible as intensity or contrast differences in the image; particularly useful for examining structural details in transparent specimens such as living or unstained cells and tissues.

polarizing m., a m. equipped with a polarizing filter below and above the specimen which forms an image by the influence of specimen birefringence on polarized light; the polarizing direction of the two filters is typically adjustable which, together with a graduated rotating stage, permits measurement of the angular value of different refractive indices in either biological or chemical specimens.

Rheinberg m., a modified form of dark-field m. in which the central opaque stop in the condenser is replaced by a colored filter, producing a background of contrasting color against which the specimen is illuminated.

scanning electron m., a m. in which the object in a vacuum is scanned in a raster pattern by a slender electron beam, generating reflected and secondary electrons from the specimen surface that are used to modulate the image on a synchronously scanned cathode ray tube; with this method a three-dimensional image is obtained, with both high resolution and great depth of focus.

simple m., single m., a m. that has a single magnifying lens.

stereoscopic m., a m. having double eyepieces and objectives and thus independent light paths, giving a three-dimensional image.

stroboscopic m., a m. that has a light source that flashes at a constant rate so that an analysis of the motility of an object may be made; it may be used for high speed or low speed (time-lapse) cinephotomicrography.

surgical m., a binocular m. used to obtain good visualization of fine structures in the operating field; in the standing type of m., a motorized zoom lens system operated by hand or foot controls provides an adjustable working distance; in headborne models, interchangeable oculars provide the magnification needed. SYN operating m.

television m., a m. in which the image is observed by a television camera that produces a television display; it is used for quantitative studies, display to a large audience, or examinations in ultraviolet and infrared regions of the spectrum.

ultra-m., SEE ultramicroscope.

ultrasonic m., a m. that has lenses designed to use acoustic energy so that the ultrasonic wavelengths may be utilized; by means of transducers, the information is translated to a form that may be visualized or recorded.

ultraviolet m., a m. having optics of quartz and fluorite that allow transmission of light waves shorter than those of the visible spectrum, *i.e.,* below 400 nm; the image is made visible by photography, fluorescence of special glasses, or television; in a scanning instrument the receptor is a multiplier phototube.

x-ray m., a m. in which images are obtained by using x-rays as an energy source that are recorded on a very fine-grained film, or the image is enlarged by projection; if film is used, it may be examined with the light m. at fairly high magnifications.

mi·cro·scop·ic, mi·cro·scop·i·cal (mī-krō-skop′ik, -i-kăl). **1.** Of minute size; visible only with the aid of the microscope. **2.** Relating to a microscope.

mi·cros·co·py (mī-kros′kŏ-pē). Investigation of minute objects by means of a microscope. SEE ALSO microscope.

electron m., examination of minute objects by use of an electron microscope.

fluorescence m., a procedure based on the fact that fluorescent materials emit visible light when they are irradiated with ultraviolet or violet-blue visible rays; some materials manifest this property naturally, whereas others may be treated with fluorescent solutions (somewhat analogous to staining); when the absorption of the specimen is in the relatively long ultraviolet range, a filter that transmits these radiations is used, and a yellow filter is placed on or in the ocular; the background field is then dark, and any yellow or red fluorescence becomes visible.

immersion m., SEE immersion.

immune electron m., electron m. of biological specimens to which specific antibody has been bound.

immunofluorescence m., SEE immunofluorescence.

Nomarski interference m., SEE Nomarski *optics*.

time-lapse m., m. in which the same object (*e.g.,* a cell) is photographed at regular time intervals over several hours.

mi·cro·seme (mī′krō-sēm). Denoting a skull with an orbital index below 84. [micro- + G. *sēma,* sign]

mi·cro·sides (mī′krō-sīdz). Fatty acid esters of trehalose and mannose isolated from diphtheria bacilli.

mi·cros·mat·ic (mī′kroz-mat′ik). Having a weakly developed sense of smell. [micro- + G. *osmē,* sense of smell]

mi·cro·some (mī′krō-sōm). One of the small spherical vesicles derived from the endoplasmic reticulum after disruption of cells and ultracentrifugation. [micro- + G. *sōma,* body]

mi·cro·so·mia (mī-krō-sō′mē-ă). Abnormal smallness of body, as in dwarfism or as in a fetus. SYN nanocormia. [micro- + G. *sōma,* body]

mi·cro·spec·tro·pho·tom·e·try (mī′krō-spek-trō-fō-tom′ĕ-trē). A technique for characterizing and quantitating nucleoproteins in single cells or cell organelles by their natural absorption spectra (ultraviolet) or after binding stoichiometrically in selective cytochemical staining reactions, as in the Feulgen stain for DNA. SEE ALSO cytophotometry.

mi·cro·spec·tro·scope (mī-krō-spek′trō-skōp). An instrument for observing the optical spectrum of microscopic objects.

micro·sphere (mī′krō-sfēr). Tiny globules of radiolabeled material such as macroaggregated albumin, about 15 microns in size.

mi·cro·sphe·ro·cy·to·sis (mī′krō-sfēr′ō-sī-tō′sis). A condition of the blood seen in hemolytic icterus in which small spherocytes are predominant; the red blood cells are smaller and more globular than normal.

mi·cro·sphyg·my (mī′krō-sfig′mē). Smallness of the pulse. SYN microsphyxia. [micro- + G. *sphygmos,* pulse]

mi·cro·sphyx·ia (mī-krō-sfik′sē-ă). SYN **microsphygmy.** [micro- + G. *sphyxis,* pulse]

mi·cro·splanch·nic (mī-krō-splangk′nik). Referring to smallness of the abdominal viscera. [micro- + G. *splanchna,* viscera]

mi·cro·sple·nia (mī-krō-sple′nē-ă). Abnormal smallness of the spleen.

Mi·cro·spo·ra (mī-krō-spōr′ă). A protozoan phylum that includes the genus *Nosema* and *Encephalitozoon,* and is characterized by the presence of unicellular spores with an imperforate wall and an extrusion apparatus having a polar tube and a polar cap; mitochondria are absent. They are intracellular parasites of invertebrates and lower vertebrates, with rare examples in higher vertebrates. SYN Cnidospora. [micro- + G. *sporos,* seed]

Mi·cro·spo·ra·si·da (mī-krō-spōr-as′i-dă). SYN **Microsporida.**

Mi·cro·spo·rida (mī-krō-spō′ri-dă). An order of the protozoan class Microsporea and phylum Microspora, characterized by minute spores with a single long, coiled, tubular filament enclosing the infective cell or sporoplasm. They are typically parasites of invertebrates and lower vertebrates, although fish and higher vertebrates (including man) have been infected. The order includes genera such as *Encephalitozoon* and *Nosema.* SYN Cnidosporidia, Microsporasida.

mi·cro·spor·id·ia. Common name for members of the protozoan phylum Microspora. It includes some 80 genera parasitizing all classes of vertebrates and many invertebrates, especially the insects. Several genera, such as *Encephalitozoon, Enterocytozoon, Nosema, Pleistophora,* and *Septata* have been implicated in the infection of immunocompromised humans.

mi·cro·spo·rid·i·a·sis (mī′krō-spō-ri-dī′a-sis). SEE microsporidiosis.

mi·cro·spo·rid·i·o·sis, mi·cro·spo·rid·i·a·sis (mī-krō-spō-rid-ē-ō′sis, mī′krō-spō-ri-dī′a-sis). Infection with a member of the phylum Microspora, the microsporidians.

Mi·cros·po·rum (mī-kros′pŏ-rŭm, mī-krō-spō′rŭm). A genus of pathogenic fungi causing dermatophytosis. In appropriate culture media, characteristic macroconidia are seen; microconidia are rare in most species. [micro- + G. *sporos,* seed]

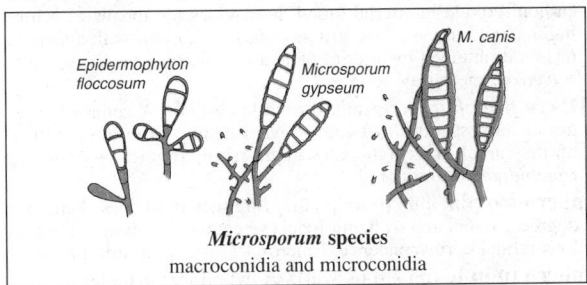

Microsporum species
macroconidia and microconidia

M. audoui′nii, an anthrophilic species that used to cause epidemic tinea capitis in children.

M. ca′nis, the principal cause of ringworm in dogs and cats and a zoophilic species causing sporadic dermatophytosis in humans, especially tinea capitis in children with cats and dogs.

M. canis, var. distor′tum, a zoophilic fungal species that causes dermatophytosis in humans and animals; seen among laboratory animal handlers.

M. ferrugin′eum, an anthropophilic species that causes dermatophytosis, primarily in Japan and the Far East.

M. ful′vum, a geophilic species that causes dermatophytosis in humans and is a member of the *M. gypseum* complex whose ascomycetous state elevates it to the rank of a specific species.

M. galli′nae, a fungal species that causes dermatophytosis in fowl and, occasionally, in man; due to its broadly clavate macro-

mi

conidia, it was until recently erroneously classified as a species of *Trichophyton*.

M. gyp′seum, a cause of ringworm in dogs and horses and occasionally other animal species; a geophilic complex of species causing sporadic dermatophytosis in humans.

M. na′num, a geophilic fungal species that is the principal cause of ringworm in pigs; rarely causes dermatophytosis in humans.

M. persic′olor, a geophilic fungal species that causes dermatophytosis in voles, field voles, and, occasionally, man; its ascomycetous state is *Nannizzia persicolor.*

M. vanbreusegh′emi, a zoophilic fungal species that causes dermatophytosis in dogs and squirrels, and occasionally in humans.

mi·cro·steth·o·phone (mī-krŏ-steth′ō-fōn). SYN microstethoscope. [micro- + G. *stēthos*, chest, + *phōnē*, sound]

mi·cro·steth·o·scope (mī-krŏ-steth′ō-skōp). A very small stethoscope that amplifies the sounds heard. SYN microstethophone.

mi·cro·sto·mia (mī-krŏ-stō′mē-ă). Smallness of the oral aperture. [micro- + G. *stoma*, mouth]

mi·cro·sur·gery (mī-krŏ-ser′jer-ē). Surgical procedures performed under the magnification of a surgical microscope.

mi·cro·su·ture (mī-krŏ-sū′chūr). Tiny caliber suture material, often 9-0 or 10-0, with an attached needle of corresponding size, for use in microsurgery.

mi·cro·sy·ringe (mī′krŏ-si-rinj′). A hypodermic syringe that has a micrometer screw attached to the piston, whereby accurately measured minute quantities of fluid may be injected.

mi·cro·the·lia (mī-krŏ-thē′lē-ă). Smallness of the nipples. [micro- + G. *thēlē*, nipple]

mi·cro·tia (mī-krŏ′shē-ă). Smallness of the auricle of the ear with a blind or absent external auditory meatus. [micro- + G. *ous*, ear]

Mi·cro·ti·nae (mī-krot′in-ē). The rodent subfamily comprising voles or lemmings.

mi·cro·tine (mī′krŏ-tēn). Relating to voles or lemmings.

mi·cro·tome (mī′krŏ-tōm). An instrument for making sections of biological tissue for examination under the microscope. SEE ALSO ultramicrotome. SYN histotome.

mi·crot·o·my (mī-krot′ō-mē). The making of thin sections of tissues for examination under the microscope. SYN histotomy. [micro- + G. *tomē*, incision]

mi·cro·to·nom·e·ter (mī′krŏ-tō-nom′ĕ-ter). A small tonometer invented by Krogh, originally intended for animals but later adapted to humans, for determining the tensions of oxygen and carbon dioxide in arterial blood; it provides the means of bringing a small bubble of air into gaseous equilibrium with a sample of blood obtained by arterial puncture. [micro- + G. *tonos*, tone, + *metron*, measure]

Mi·cro·trom·bid·i·um (mī′krŏ-trom-bid′ē-ŭm). A genus of chigger or harvest mites that cause severe itching from the presence of the larval stage (chigger) in the skin. [micro- + Mod. L. *trombidium*, a timid one]

mi·cro·tro·pia (mī-krŏ-trō′pē-ă). Strabismus of less than four degrees, associated with amblyopia, eccentric fixation, or anomalous retinal correspondence. [micro- + G. *tropē*, a turn, turning]

mi·cro·tu·bule (mī-krŏ-tū′byūl). A cylindrical cytoplasmic element, 20 to 27 nm in diameter and of variable length, that occurs widely in the cytoskeleton of plant and animal cells; m.'s increase in number during mitosis and meiosis, where they may be related to movement of the chromosomes or chromatids on the nuclear spindle during nuclear division.

subpellicular m., a m. lying beneath the unit membrane (pellicle) of many protozoans, often as a palisade of longitudinally arranged fibrils connected by fine lateral bridges that support the external cell form; in certain sporozoan stages a fixed number of m.'s are found, extending longitudinally from the polar ring. SYN subpellicular fibril.

mi·cro·ves·i·cle (mī-krŏ-ves′i-kl). A fluid-filled space formed within the epidermis that is too small to be recognized as a blister.

mi·cro·vil·lus, pl. **mi·cro·vil·li** (mī-krŏ-vil′ŭs, -vil′ī). One of the minute projections of cell membranes greatly increasing sur-

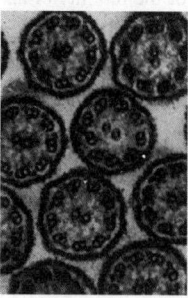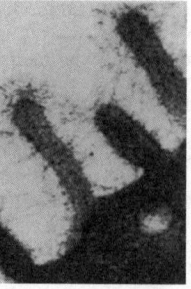

microtubules (ciliated epithelium of mouse oviduct)
left, cross-section showing characteristic arrangement; right, microvilli: length-wise section

face area; microvilli form the striated or brush borders of certain cells.

Mi·cro·vir·i·dae (mī-krŏ-vir′i-dē). Provisional name for a family of small, spherical, bacterial viruses with a genome of single-stranded DNA (MW 1.7×10^6).

mi·cro·volt (μV) (mī′krŏ-vōlt). One-millionth of a volt.

mi·cro·waves (mī′krŏ-wāvz). That portion of the radio wave spectrum of shortest wavelength, including the region with wavelengths of 1 mm to 30 cm (1000 to 300,000 megacycles per second). SYN microelectric waves.

mi·cro·weld·ing (mī-krŏ-weld′ing). A method of fastening or joining stainless steel sutures or such sutures to needles.

mi·crox·y·phil (mī-krok′si-fil). A multinuclear oxyphil leukocyte. [micro- + G. *oxys*, acid, + *philos*, fond]

mi·cro·zo·on (mī-krŏ-zō′on). A microscopic form of the animal kingdom; a protozoon. [micro- + G. *zōon*, animal]

mi·crur·gi·cal (mī-krer′ji-kăl). Relating to procedures performed on minute structures under a microscope. [micro- + G. *ergon*, work]

mic·tion (mik′shŭn). SYN urination.

mic·tu·rate (mik′chū-rāt). SYN urinate. [see micturition]

mic·tu·ri·tion (mik-chū-rish′ŭn). **1.** SYN urination. **2.** The desire to urinate. **3.** Frequency of urination. [L. *micturio*, to desire to make water]

M.I.D. Abbreviation for minimal infecting *dose.*

△ **mid-.** Middle. [A.S. *mid, midd*]

mi·daz·o·lam hy·dro·chlo·ride. 8-Chloro-6-(6-fluorophenyl)-1-methyl-4*H*-imidazo[1,5-*a*][1,4]benzodiazepine monohydrochloride; a short-acting injectable benzodiazapine central nervous system depressant used for preoperative sedation.

mid·body (mid′bod′ē). A dense stalk of residual interzonal spindle fibers (microtubules) and actin-containing filaments that is formed during anaphase of mitosis and connects daughter cells during telophase; m.'s are frequently observed between spermatids. SYN intermediate body of Flemming.

mid·brain (mid′brān). SYN mesencephalon.

mid·car·pal (mid′kar-păl). **1.** Relating to the central part of the carpus. SYN mediocarpal. **2.** Denoting the articulation between the two rows of carpal bones. SYN carpocarpal. SYN mediocarpal, mesocarpal.

mid·dle. Denoting an anatomical structure that is between two other similar structures or that is midway in position. SYN medius [NA].

mid·grac·ile (mid-gras′il). Denoting an occasional fissure dividing the gracile lobe of the cerebellum into two parts.

mid·gut (mid′gŭt). **1.** The central portion of the digestive tube; the distal duodenum, small intestine, and proximal colon. **2.** The portion of the embryonic gut tract between the foregut and the hindgut which originally is open to the yolk sac.

mid·men·stru·al (mid′men′strū-ăl). Denoting the several days midway in time between two menstrual periods.

mid·oc·cip·i·tal (mid′ok-sip′i̯-tăl). Relating to the central portion of the occiput. SYN medioccipital.

mid·pain (mid′pān). SYN intermenstrual *pain* (1).

mid·plane (mid′plān). SYN pelvic *plane* of least dimensions.

mid·riff (mid′rif). SYN diaphragm (1). [A.S. *mid*, middle, + *hrif*, belly]

mid·sec·tion (mid′sek-shŭn). A cut or section through the middle of an organ.

mid·ster·num (mid′ster′nŭm). SYN *body* of sternum.

mid·tar·sal (mid′tar′săl). Relating to the middle of the tarsus. SYN mediotarsal, mesotarsal.

mid·wife (mid′wīf). A person qualified to practice midwifery, having specialized training in obstetrics and child care. [A.S. *mid*, with, + *wif*, wife]

mid·wife·ry (mid′wīf′rē, mid′wif′ĕ-rē). Independent care of essentially normal, healthy women and infants by a midwife, antepartally, intrapartally, postpartally, and/or obstetrically in a hospital, birth center, or home setting, and including normal delivery of the infant, with medical consultation, collaborative management, and referral of cases in which abnormalities develop; strong emphasis is placed on educational preparation of parents for childbearing and childrearing, with an orientation toward childbirth as a normal physiological process requiring minimal intervention.

Miescher, Johann F., Swiss pathologist, 1811–1887. SEE M.'s *elastoma, granuloma, tubes,* under *tube.*

MIF Abbreviation for migration-inhibitory *factor.*

mife·pris·tone (mif′pris-tōn). Synthetic chemical compound with antiprogesterone properties used for early pregnancy termination; the substance binds with glucocorticoid receptors resulting in increased adrenal gland secretion. SYN RU-486.

mi·graine (mī′grān, mi-grān′). A symptom complex occurring periodically and characterized by pain in the head (usually unilateral), vertigo, nausea and vomiting, photophobia, and scintillating appearances of light. Classified as classic m., common m., cluster headache, hemiplegic m., ophthalmoplegic m., and ophthalmic m. SYN bilious headache, blind headache, hemicrania (1), sick headache, vascular headache. [through O. Fr., fr. G. *hēmikrania*, pain on one side of the head, fr. *hēmi-*, half, + *kranion*, skull]

abdominal m., m. in children accompanied by paroxysmal abdominal pain. This must be distinguished from similar symptoms requiring surgical attention.

acephalic m., a classic m. episode in which the teichopsia is not followed by a headache. SYN m. without headache.

basilar m., a m. accompanied by transient brainstem signs (vertigo, tinnitus, perioral numbness, diplopia, etc.) thought to be due to vasospastic narrowing of the basilar artery.

classic m., a form of hemicrania m. preceded by a scintillating scotoma (teichopsia).

common m., a form of m. headache without the visual prodrome, that is not limited on one side of the head but nevertheless is recognizable as m. because of the stereotyped course; the tendency to nausea, photophobia, and phonophobia; and the relief produced by sleep.

complicated m., a m. attack during which an infarction of tissue takes place.

fulgurating m., m. characterized by its abrupt commencement and the severity of the episode.

Harris' m., SYN periodic migrainous *neuralgia.*

hemiplegic m., a form associated with transient hemiplegia.

ocular m., vasospastic infarction of tissue in or about the eye during an otherwise typical m.; a form of complicated m.

ophthalmoplegic m., a form of m. associated with paralysis of the extraocular muscles.

m. without headache, SYN acephalic m.

mi·gra·tion (mī-grā′shŭn). 1. Passing from one part to another, said of certain morbid processes or symptoms. 2. SYN diapedesis. 3. Movement of a tooth or teeth out of normal position. 4. Movement of molecules during electrophoresis. [L. *migro*, pp. -*atus*, to move from place to place]

branch m., a process in which the cross connection around the position where two DNA helices are joined moves along the strands.

epithelial m., apical shift of epithelial attachment, exposing more of the tooth crown.

m. of ovum, the transperitoneal passage of an ovum from the ovarian follicle into the uterine tube.

MIH Abbreviation for melanotropin release-inhibiting *hormone.*

Mikity, Victor G., U.S. radiologist, *1919. SEE Wilson-M. *syndrome.*

Mikulicz, Johannes von-Radecki, Polish surgeon in Germany, 1850–1905. SEE M.'s *aphthae,* under *aphtha, cells,* under *cell;* M. *clamp;* M.'s *disease, drain, operation, syndrome;* M.-Vladimiroff *amputation;* Vladimiroff-M. *amputation;* Heineke-Mikulicz *pyloroplasty.*

Miles, William E., British surgeon, 1869–1947. SEE M.'s *operation;* M. *resection.*

mil·ia (mil′ē-ă). Plural of milium.

Milian, Gaston, French dermatologist, 1871–1945. SEE M.'s *disease, erythema.*

mil·i·a·ria (mil-ē-ā′rē-ă). An eruption of minute vesicles and papules due to retention of fluid at the orifices of sweat glands. SYN miliary fever (2). [L. *miliarius,* relating to millet, fr. *milium,* millet]

m. al′ba, m. with vesicles containing a milky fluid.

apocrine m., SYN Fox-Fordyce *disease.*

m. crystalli′na, a noninflammatory form of m. in which the vesicles are filled with clear fluid. SYN crystal rash, sudamina (2).

m. profun′da, pale firm papules, most commonly on the trunk; it is asymptomatic and results from severe damage to the sweat ducts after repeated episodes of m. rubra or from experimental injury.

pustular m., an eruption of pustules that occurs usually in very hot weather and mostly on the flexor aspects of the limbs, the groins, and the axillae; the lesions are situated at the orifices of sweat glands.

m. ru′bra, an eruption of papules and vesicles at the orifices of sweat glands, accompanied by redness and inflammatory reaction of the skin. SYN heat rash, lichen infantum, lichen strophulosus, prickly heat, strophulus, summer rash, tropical lichen, lichen tropicus, wildfire rash.

mil·i·a·ry (mil′ē-ā-rē, mil′yă-rē). 1. Resembling a millet seed in size (about 2 mm). 2. Marked by the presence of nodules of millet seed size on any surface. [see miliaria]

mil·ieu (mēl-yū′). 1. Surroundings; environment. 2. In psychiatry, the social setting of the mental patient, *e.g.,* the family setting or a hospital unit. [Fr. *mi,* fr. L. *medius,* middle, + *lieu,* fr. L. *locus,* place]

m. intérieur, m. inter′ne, the internal environment; the fluids bathing the tissue cells of multicellular animals.

mil·i·tar·y an·ti·shock trou·sers (MAST). A garment used to apply pressure to the lower half of body and thus increase blood volume in the upper half.

mil·i·um, pl. **mil·ia** (mil′ē-ŭm, -ē-ă). A small subepidermal keratin cyst, usually multiple and therefore commonly referred to in the plural. SYN sebaceous tubercle, tuberculum sebaceum, whitehead (1). [L. millet]

milk. 1. A white liquid, containing proteins, sugar, and lipids, secreted by the mammary glands, and designed for the nourishment of the young. SYN lac (1) [NA]. 2. Any whitish milky fluid; *e.g.,* the juice of the coconut or a suspension of various metallic oxides. 3. A pharmacopeial preparation that is a suspension of insoluble drugs in a water medium; distinguished from gels mainly in that the suspended particles of m. are larger. 4. SYN strip (1). [A.S. *meolc*]

acidophilus m., m. inoculated with a culture of *Bacillus acidophilus.*

m. of bismuth, a suspension of bismuth hydroxide and bismuth subcarbonate in water; used in gastrointestinal disorders as a protective agent.

buddeized m., SEE Budde *process.*

certified m., cow's m. that does not have more than the maximal

milk							mineral content, mg %							
	specific gravity	protein %	fat %	carbo-hydrate (lactose) %	ash %	joule/ 100 ml	Na	K	Ca	Mg	Fe	Cl	P	citric acid
human milk	1.030	1.1–1.5	2.5–4.8	6–7.1	0.20	293	14	53	30	4	0.15	30	15	120
cow's milk	1.031	3.1–4.0	3.5–4.8	4–4.8	0.75	285	45	160	126	12	0.18	126	98	250
goat's milk	1.031	3.7–4.0	4.0–4.8	4–4.8	0.80	293	79	145	128	12	0.21	128	100	150

permissible limit of 10,000 bacteria per ml at any time prior to delivery to the consumer, and that must be cooled to 10°C or less and maintained at that temperature until delivery.

certified pasteurized m., cow's m. in which the maximum permissible limit for bacteria should not be more than 10,000 bacteria per ml before pasteurization and not more than 500 bacteria per ml after pasteurization; it must be cooled to 7.2°C or less and maintained at that temperature until delivery.

condensed m., a thick liquid prepared by the partial evaporation of cow's m., with or without the addition of sugar.

crop m., SYN pigeon's m.

fortified m., m. to which some essential nutrient, usually vitamin D, has been added.

fortified vitamin D m., m. produced through direct addition of vitamin D; standardized at 400 USP units per quart.

irradiated vitamin D m., cow's m. exposed in a thin film to ultraviolet light and standardized to contain 400 USP units of vitamin D per quart.

lactobacillary m., m. inoculated with a culture of *Bacillus acidophilus, B. bulgaricus,* or other lactic acid-forming microorganism.

m. of magnesia, mixture of magnesium hydroxide; an aqueous solution of magnesium hydroxide, used as an antacid and laxative. SYN magnesia magma.

metabolized vitamin D m., m. produced by feeding irradiated yeast to cows; standardized to contain not less than 400 USP units per quart.

modified m., cow's m. altered, by increasing the fat and reducing the amount of protein, to resemble human m. in composition.

perhydrase m., m. treated by the addition of hydrogen peroxide. SEE Budde *process.*

pigeon's m., a secretion formed by glands in the mucosa of the pigeon's crop with which the young are fed; it is increased under the influence of prolactin. SYN crop m.

skim m., skimmed m., the aqueous (noncream) part of m. from which casein is isolated.

m. of sulfur, SYN precipitated *sulfur.*

uterine m., a whitish fluid secretion between the villi of the placenta, which nourishes the implanting ovum.

vitamin D m., cow's m. to which vitamin D has been added, to contain 400 USP units of vitamin D per quart.

witch's m., a secretion of colostrum-like m. sometimes occurring in the glands of newborn infants of either sex 3 to 4 days after birth and lasting a week or two; due to endocrine stimulation from the mother before birth.

Milkman, Louis A., U.S. roentgenologist, 1895–1951. SEE M.'s *syndrome.*

milk·pox (milk′poks). SYN alastrim.

Millard, Auguste L.J., French physician, 1830–1915. SEE M.-Gubler *syndrome.*

Miller, Thomas Grier, U.S. physician, *1886. SEE M.-Abbott *tube.*

Miller, Willoughby D., U.S. dentist, 1853–1907. SEE M.'s chemicoparasitic *theory.*

mil·let seed (mil′et). The seed of a grass, formerly used as a rough designation of size of about 2 mm in diameter.

△**milli- (m).** Prefix used in the SI and metric systems to signify one-thousandth (10^{-3}). [L. *mille,* one thousand]

mil·li·am·pere (ma, mA) (mil′ē-am′pēr). One thousandth of an ampere.

mil·li·bar (mil′i-bar). One-thousandth of a bar; 100 newtons/sq m; 0.75006 mm Hg; standard atmospheric pressure is 1013 millibars.

mil·li·cu·rie (mc, mCi) (mil′i-kyū′rē). A unit of radioactivity equivalent to 3.7×10^7 disintegrations per second.

mil·li·e·quiv·a·lent (mEq, meq) (mil′i-ē-kwiv′ă-lent). One-thousandth equivalent; 10^{-3} mole divided by valence.

mil·li·gram (mg) (mil′i-gram). One-thousandth of a gram.

mil·li·gram·age (mil′i-gram-āj). SYN milligram hour.

mil·li·gram hour. Obsolete term for a unit of exposure in radium therapy, *i.e.,* the application of 1 milligram of radium during 1 hour. SYN milligramage.

mil·li·lam·bert (mil-i-lam′bert). One thousandth of a lambert; a unit of brightness equal to 0.929 lumen per square foot (roughly, 1 equivalent footcandle).

mil·li·li·ter (mL, ml) (mil′i-lē-ter). One-thousandth of a liter.

mil·li·me·ter (mm) (mil′i-mē-ter). One-thousandth of a meter.

△**millimicro-.** Prefix formerly used to signify one-billionth (10^{-9}); now nano-.

mil·li·mi·cron (mμ) (mil′i-mī-kron). Former term for nanometer.

mil·li·mole (mmol) (mil′i-mōl). One-thousandth of a gram-molecule.

mil·ling-in (mil′ing-in). Refining the occlusion of teeth by the use of abrasives between their occluding surfaces while the dentures are rubbed together in the mouth or on the articulator.

mil·li·os·mole (mil′i-oz-mōl). One-thousandth of an osmole.

mil·li·pede (mil′i-pēd). A venomous nonpredaceous arthropod of the order Diplopoda, characterized by two pairs of legs per leg-bearing segment. The venom is purely defensive, oozed or squirted from pores along the body, producing irritation to the skin or severe inflammation if it reaches the eyes. [milli- + L. *pes, pedis,* foot]

mil·li·sec·ond (ms, msec) (mil′i-sek′ŏnd). One-thousandth of a second.

mil·li·volt (mV, mv) (mil′i-vōlt). One thousandth of a volt.

Millon, Auguste N.E., French chemist, 1812–1867. SEE M. *reaction;* M.'s *reagent;* M.-Nasse *test.*

mil·pho·sis (mil-fō′sis). Loss of eyelashes. SYN madarosis. [G. *milphōsis*]

mil·ri·none (mil′rĭ-nōn). A xanthine oxidase inhibitor which increases the force of contraction of the heart; used in congestive heart failure; resembles amrinone; cardiotonic.

Milroy, William F., U.S. physician, 1855–1942. SEE M.'s *disease.*

Milton, John L., English dermatologist, 1820–1898. SEE M.'s *disease.*

MIM Abbreviation for *Mendelian Inheritance in Man.*

mi·me·sis (mi-mē′sis, mī-). 1. Hysterical simulation of organic disease. 2. The symptomatic imitation of one organic disease by another. [G. *mimēsis,* imitation, fr. *mimeomai,* to mimic]

mi·met·ic (mi-met′ik, mī-). Relating to mimesis. [G. *mimētikos,* imitative]

mim·ic (mim′ik). To imitate or simulate. [G. *mimikos,* imitating, fr. *mimos,* a mimic]

mim·ma·tion (mi-mā′shŭn). A form of stammering in which the m-sound is given to various letters. [Ar. *mim,* the letter m]

min. Abbreviation for minute.

mind. **1.** The organ or seat of consciousness and higher functions of the human brain, such as cognition, reasoning, willing, and emotion. **2.** The organized totality of all mental processes and psychic activities, with emphasis on the relatedness of the phenomena. [A.S. *gemynd*]

prelogical m., SYN prelogical *thinking*.

subconscious m., SYN subliminal *self*.

mind-read·ing. SYN telepathy.

min·er·al (min′er-ăl). Any homogeneous inorganic material usually found in the earth's crust. [L. *mineralis,* pertaining to mines, fr. *mino,* to mine]

min·er·al·i·za·tion (mĭn′er-al-i-zā′shŭn). The introduction of minerals into a structure, as in the normal mineralization of bones and teeth or the pathologic mineralization of tissues, *i.e.,* dystrophic or metastatic calcification.

min·er·al·o·coid (min-er-al′ō-koyd). SYN mineralocorticoid.

min·er·al·o·cor·ti·coid (min′er-al-ō-kōr′ti-koyd). One of the steroids of the adrenal cortex that influences salt (sodium and potassium) metabolism. SYN mineraloid.

min·er·al oil. A mixture of liquid hydrocarbons obtained from petroleum, used as a vehicle in pharmaceutical preparations; occasionally used as an intestinal lubricant. SYN heavy liquid petrolatum, liquid paraffin, liquid petroleum.

min·er·al·o·tro·pic (min-er-al′ō-trō′pik). Concerning the action of or relating to mineralocorticoids.

mini (mi′nē). A moderate-sized computer that can serve many users in a department, or one dedicated to a complex computational function such as computed tomography or magnetic resonance imaging; smaller and slower than a mainframe, more complex and powerful than a personal computer. [It. *miniatura,* decoration of manuscripts, fr. L. *minium,* red lead]

min·i·lap·a·rot·o·my (min′ē-lap-ă-rot′ō-mē). Technique for sterilization by surgical ligation of the fallopian tubes, performed through a small suprapubic incision.

min·im (m). **1.** A fluid measure, $\frac{1}{60}$ of a fluidrachm; in the case of water about one drop. **2.** Smallest; least; the smallest of several similar structures. [L. *minimus,* least]

min·i·mum (min-i-mum). The smallest amount or lowest limit. [L. smallest, least]

min·i·my·o·sin (min-ē-mī′ō-sin). A protein similar to myosin in having a globular actin-binding domain and a short tail that can bind to membranes but lacking a long α-helical tail; believed to have a role in filopodium extension in the growth cone of neurons.

min·o·cy·cline (min-ō-sī′klēn). A substituted naphthacenecarboxamide; an antibacterial drug related to tetracycline.

mi·nor (mī′ner). Smaller; lesser; denoting the smaller of two similar structures. [L.]

mi·nox·i·dil (mi-nok′si-dil). 2,4-Diamino-6-piperidinopyrimidine 3-oxide; an antihypertensive agent used for treatment of premature hair loss; sometimes used topically on the scalp to increase hair growth.

mint. SYN Mentha. [G. *mintha*]

◊**mio-.** Less. [G. *meiōn*]

mi·o·did·y·mus, mi·od·y·mus (mī-ō-did′i-mŭs, mī-od′i-mŭs). Unequal conjoined twins with the head of the smaller twin fused to the occipital region of the head of the larger twin. SEE conjoined *twins,* under *twin.* [mio- + G. *didymos,* twin]

mi·o·lec·i·thal (mī-ō-les′i-thal). Denoting an egg with little yolk which is uniformly dispersed throughout the egg. [mio- + G. *lekithos,* egg yolk]

mi·o·nec·tic (mī-ō-nek′tik). An obsolete term denoting less than the normal; used especially with reference to blood that has an abnormally low percentage of saturation with oxygen at a certain pressure. [G. *meionekteō,* to have too little, fr. *meion,* less, + *echō,* to have]

mi·o·pra·gia (mī-ō-prā′jē-ă). Diminished functional activity in a part. [mio- + G. *prassō,* to do]

mi·o·pus (mī-ō′pŭs). Unequal conjoined twins with heads united in such a manner that one face is rudimentary. SEE conjoined *twins,* under *twin.* [mio- + G. *ōps,* eye]

mi·o·sis (mī-ō′sis). **1.** Contraction of the pupil. **2.** Incorrect alternative spelling for meiosis. [G. *meiōsis,* a lessening]

paralytic m., m. due to paralysis of the dilator muscle of the pupil.

spastic m., m. due to spasmodic contraction of the sphincter muscle of the pupil.

mi·o·sphyg·mia (mī′ō-sfig′mē-ă). Condition in which pulse beats are fewer than heart beats. [mio- + G. *sphygmos,* pulse]

mi·ot·ic (mī-ot′ik). **1.** Relating to or characterized by contraction of the pupil. **2.** An agent that causes the pupil to contract.

MIP Abbreviation for macrophage inflammatory *protein.*

mi·ra·cid·i·um, pl. **mi·ra·cid·ia** (mī-ră-sid′ē-ŭm, -ă). The ciliated first-stage larva of a trematode that emerges from the egg and must penetrate into the tissues of an appropriate intermediate host snail if it is to continue its life cycle; followed by development into a mother sporocyst and by production of a number of offspring of successive larval generations. SEE ALSO sporocyst (1). [G. *meirakidion,* boy]

Mirchamp's sign. See under sign.

mire (mēr). One of the test objects in the ophthalmometer; its image (also called a m.), mirrored on the corneal surface, is measured to determine the radii of curvature of the cornea. [L. *miror,* pp. *-atus,* to wonder at]

mi·rex (mī′reks). Benzene derivative used as insecticide and fire retardant for plastics, rubber, paint, paper, electrical goods; likely carcinogen.

Mirizzi, P.L., 20th century Argentinian physician. SEE M.'s *syndrome.*

mir·ror (mir′ŏr). A polished surface reflecting the rays of light from objects in front of it. [Fr. *miroir,* fr. L. *miror,* to wonder at]

concave m., a spherical reflecting surface that constitutes a segment of the interior of a sphere.

convex m., a spherical reflecting surface that constitutes a segment of the exterior of a sphere.

head m., a circular concave m. attached to a head band, used to project a beam of light into a cavity, such as the nose or larynx, for purposes of examination and permitting binocular vision.

mouth m., a small m. on a handle used to facilitate visualization in the examination of the teeth.

van Helmont's m., obsolete term for central *tendon* of diaphragm.

mir·ror-writ·ing (mir′ŏr-rīt-ing). Writing backward, from right to left, the letters appearing like ordinary writing seen in a mirror. SYN retrography.

mir·yach·it (mir-yach′it). A nervous affection observed in Siberia. SEE jumping *disease.* SYN myriachit.

MIS Abbreviation for müllerian inhibiting *substance.*

mis·an·dry (mis′an-drē). Aversion to or hatred of men. [G. *miseō,* to hate, + *anēr, andros,* male]

mis·an·thro·py (mis-an′thrō-pē). Aversion to and hatred of human beings. [G. *miseō,* to hate, + *anthrōpos,* man]

mis·car·riage (mis-kar′ij). Spontaneous expulsion of the products of pregnancy before the middle of the second trimester.

mis·car·ry (mis-kar′ē). To have a miscarriage.

mis·ce·ge·na·tion (mis′e-jĕ-nā′shŭn). Marriage or interbreeding of individuals of different races. [L. *misceo,* to mix, + *genus,* descent, race]

mis·ci·ble (mis′i-bl). Capable of being mixed and remaining so after the mixing process ceases. [L. *misceo,* to mix]

mis·di·ag·no·sis (mis′dī-ag-nō′sis). A wrong or mistaken diagnosis.

mis·e·ro·tia (mis-ĕ-rō′shi-ă). Dislike of or aversion to physical love. [G. *miseō,* to hate, + *erōs,* physical love]

mi·sog·a·my (mi-sog′ă-mē). Aversion to marriage. [G. *miseō,* to hate, + *gamos,* marriage]

mi·sog·y·ny (mi-soj′i-nē). Aversion to or hatred of women. [G. *miseō,* to hate, + *gynē,* woman]

mis·o·lo·gia (mis-ō-lō′jē-ă). Aversion to talking or to mental activity. [G. *miseō,* to hate, + *logos,* reasoning, discussion]

mis·o·ne·ism (mis-ō-nē′izm). Dislike of and disinclination to accept new ideas. [G. *miseō*, to hate, + *neos*, new]

mis·o·pe·dia, mis·op·e·dy (mis-ō-pē′dē-ă, -op′ě-dē). Aversion to or hatred of children. [G. *miseō*, to hate, + *pais* (*paid-*), child]

mi·so·pros·tol (mī-sō-prost′ol). A prostaglandin analog used in the treatment of ulcer disease; particularly useful in persons taking nonsteroidal anti-inflammatory drugs; antiulcerative.

mis·sense (mis′ens). As used in genetics, a mutation that causes a sequence such that there is a substitution of one amino acid residue for another.

m. suppression, a mutation in tRNA that allows for incorporation of an amino acid residue that allows for full function of the gene product.

mis·tle·toe (mis′l-tō). SYN viscum (1).

MIT Abbreviation for monoiodotyrosine.

Mitchell, Silas Weir, U.S. neurologist, poet, and novelist, 1829–1914. SEE M.'s *disease, treatment;* Gerhardt-Mitchell *disease;* Weir M.'s *disease;* Weir M. *treatment.*

mite (mīt). A minute arthropod of the order Acarina, a vast assemblage of parasitic and (primarily) free-living organisms. Most are still undescribed, and only a relatively small number are of medical or veterinary importance as vectors or intermediate hosts of pathogenic agents, by directly causing dermatitis or tissue damage, or by causing blood or tissue fluid loss. The six-legged larvae of trombiculid m.'s, the chigger m.'s (*Trombicula*), are parasitic of humans and many mammals and birds, and are important as vectors of scrub typhus (tsutsugamushi disease) and other rickettsial agents. Some other important m.'s are *Acarus hordei* (barley m.), *Demodex folliculorum* (follicular or mange m.), *Dermanyssus gallinae* (red hen m.), *Ornithonyssus bacoti* (tropical rat m.), *O. bursa* (tropical fowl m.), *O. sylviarum* (northern fowl m.), *Pyemotes tritici* (straw or grain itch m.), and *Sarcoptes scabiei* (itch m.). [A.S.]

mi·tel·la (mī-tel′ă). A sling for the arm. [L. dim. of *mitra*, a bandage, band]

mith·ra·my·cin (mith-ră-mī′sin). An antibiotic produced by *Streptomyces argillaceus* and *S. tanashiensis;* possesses antineoplastic activity. SYN aureolic acid, mitramycin.

mith·ri·da·tism (mith′ri-dā′tizm, mith-rid′ă-tizm). Immunity against the action of a poison produced by small and gradually increasing doses of the same. [*Mithridates*, King of Pontus (132–63 B.C.), supposedly an unsuccessful suicide (by poison) because of repeated small doses taken to become invulnerable to assassination by poison]

mi·ti·ci·dal (mī-ti-sī′dăl). Destructive to mites.

mi·ti·cide (mī′ti-sīd). An agent destructive to mites. [mite + L. *caedo,* to kill]

mit·i·gate (mit′i-gāt). SYN palliate. [L. *mitigo,* pp. *-atus,* to make mild or gentle, fr. *mitis,* mild, + *ago,* to do, make]

mi·tis (mī′tis). Mild. [L.]

mi·to·chon·dria (mī-tō-kon′drē-ă). Plural of mitochondrion.

mi·to·chon·dri·al (mī-tō-kon′drē-ăl). Relating to mitochondria.

mi·to·chon·dri·on, pl. **mi·to·chon·dria** (mī-tō-kon′drē-on, -kon′drē-ă). An organelle of the cell cytoplasm consisting of two sets of membranes, a smooth continuous outer coat and an inner membrane arranged in tubules or more often in folds that form platelike double membranes called cristae; mitochondria are the principal energy source of the cell and contain the cytochrome enzymes of terminal electron transport and the enzymes of the citric acid cycle, fatty acid oxidation, and oxidative phosphorylation. SYN Altmann's granule (2). [G. *mitos,* thread, + *chondros,* granule, grits]

m. of hemoflagellates, the "mother m.," from which smaller mitochondria appear to arise.

mi·to·gen (mī′tō-jen). A substance that stimulates mitosis and lymphocyte transformation; includes not only lectins such as phytohemagglutinins and concanavalin A, but also substances from streptococci (associated with streptolysin S) and from strains of α-toxin-producing staphylococci. SYN transforming agent. [mitosis + G. *-gen,* producing]

pokeweed m. (PWM), a m. (lectin) from *Phytolacca americana* (pokeweed) which stimulates chiefly B lymphocytes.

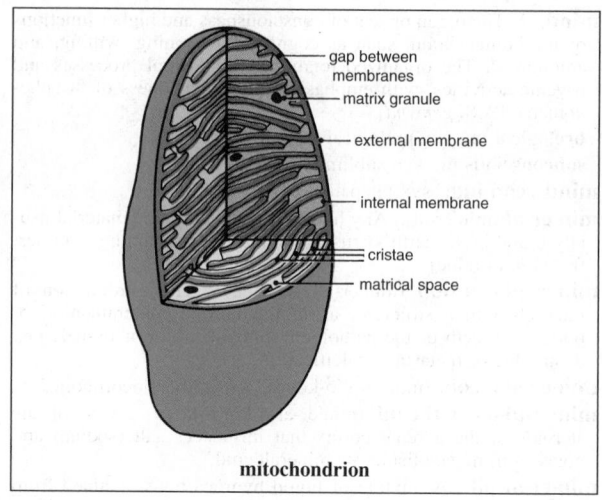

mitochondrion

mi·to·gen·e·sis (mī-tō-jen′ě-sis). The process of induction of mitosis in or transformation of a cell. [mitosis + G. *genesis,* origin]

mi·to·ge·net·ic (mī′tō-jě-net′ik). Pertaining to the factor or factors promoting cell mitosis.

mi·to·gen·ic (mī-tō-jen′ik). Causing mitosis or transformation.

mi·to·my·cin (mī-tō-mī′sin). Antibiotic produced by *Streptomyces caespitosus,* variants of which are designated m. A, m. B, etc.; m. C is an antineoplastic agent and a bacteriocide; inhibits DNA synthesis.

mi·to·plast (mī′tō-plast). A mitochondrion without its outer membrane.

mi·to·sis, pl. **mi·to·ses** (mī-tō′sis, -sēz). The usual process of somatic reproduction of cells consisting of a sequence of modifications of the nucleus (prophase, prometaphase, metaphase, anaphase, telophase) that result in the formation of two daughter cells with exactly the same chromosome and DNA content as that of the original cell. SEE ALSO cell cycle. SYN indirect nuclear division, mitotic division. [G. *mitos,* thread]

heterotype m., a variety of m. in which the halved chromosomes are united at their ends forming ring-like figures. Occurs in the first division of meiosis.

multipolar m., a pathologic form in which the spindle has three or more poles, resulting in the formation of a corresponding number of nuclei.

somatic m., the ordinary process of m. as it occurs in the somatic or body cells, characterized by the formation of the prescribed number of chromosomes, appropriate for the species (in humans the number is 46).

mi·to·tane (mī′tō-tān). 1,1-Dichloro-2-(*o*-chlorophenyl)-2-(*p*-chlorophenyl)ethane; an antineoplastic agent.

mi·tot·ic (mī-tot′ik). Relating to or marked by mitosis.

mi·to·xan·trone hy·dro·chlo·ride (mī-tō-zan′trōn). 1,4-Dihydro-5,8-bis[[2-[2-hydroxyethyl)-amino]ethyl]anthraquinone dihydrochloride; a synthetic anti-neoplastic used intravenously in the initial therapy for acute nonlymphocytic leukemia in adults.

mi·tral (mī′trăl). **1.** Relating to the mitral or bicuspid valve. **2.** Shaped like a bishop's miter; denoting a structure resembling the shape of a headband or turban. [L. *mitra,* a coif or turban]

mi·tral·i·za·tion (mī′tră-li-zā′shŭn). Straightening of the left heart border on a chest radiograph due to prominence of the left atrial appendage or the pulmonary outflow tract; an unreliable indication of mitral valve disease.

mit·ra·my·cin (mit-ră-mī′sin). SYN mithramycin.

Mitrofanoff, Paul, French pediatric surgeon, *1934. SEE Mitrofanoff *principle.*

Mitsuda, Kensuke, Japanese physician, *1876. SEE M. *antigen, reaction.*

Mitsuo, Gentaro, Japanese ophthalmologist, 1876–1913. SEE M.'s *phenomenon.*

mit·tel·schmerz (mit'el-schmärts). Abdominal pain occurring at the time of ovulation, resulting from irritation of the peritoneum by bleeding from the ovulation site. SYN intermenstrual pain (2), middle pain. [Ger. Mittelschmerz, middle + pain]

mi·vac·ur·i·um (mī'vă-kŭr'ē-ŭm). A neuromuscular blocking agent resembling *d*-tubocurarine, but having a shorter duration of action.

mix·ing (mik'sing). The mingling or blending of particles or components, especially of different kinds.

   phenotypic m., the condition in which virus particles released from a cell that is infected with two different viruses has components from both the infecting agents.

mix·o·tro·phy (miks-o'trō-fē). The property of certain microorganisms that can assimilate organic compounds as carbon sources but not as energy sources. [G. *mixis,* mixture, fr. *mignumi,* to mix, + *trophē,* nourishment]

mix·ture (miks'chŭr). 1. A mutual incorporation of two or more substances, without chemical union, the physical characteristics of each of the components being retained. A **mechanical m.** is a m. of particles or masses distinguishable as such under the microscope or in other ways; a **physical m.** is a more intimate m. of molecules, as in the case of gases and many solutions. 2. In chemistry, a mingling together of two or more substances without the occurrence of a reaction by which they would lose their individual properties, *i.e.,* without permanent gain or loss of electrons. 3. In pharmacy, a preparation, consisting of a liquid holding an insoluble medicinal substance in suspension by means of acacia, sugar, or some other viscid material. [L. *mixtura* or *mistura*]

   Bordeaux m., a plant fungicidal m., comprising copper sulfate (5 parts) and calcium oxide (5 parts) in water (400 parts) freshly mixed; the CaO is added to the CuSO$_4$ solution.

   extemporaneous m., a m. prepared at the time ordered, according to the directions of a prescription, as distinguished from a stock preparation.

   Seidlitz m., a m. of 3 parts Rochelle salt and 1 part sodium bicarbonate. Ten grams of the m. are employed with 2.17 g tartaric acid for one Seidlitz powder. The powder, which effervesces when placed in water, was widely used as a cathartic.

Miyagawa, Yoneji, Japanese bacteriologist, 1885–1959. SEE *Miyagawanella;* M. *bodies,* under *body.*

Mi·ya·ga·wa·nel·la (mē'yă-gah'wă-nel'ă). Formerly considered a genus of Chlamydiaceae, but now synonymous with *Chlamydia.* [Y. *Miyagawa*]

MK Abbreviation for menaquinone.

MK-6 Abbreviation for menaquinone-6.

MK-7 Abbreviation for menaquinone-7.

mL, ml Abbreviation for milliliter.

MLC Abbreviation for Marginal Line Calculus Index.

MLD, mld Abbreviation for minimal lethal *dose.*

mlRNA Abbreviation for messenger-like RNA.

mm Abbreviation for millimeter.

MMMT Abbreviation for malignant mixed müllerian *tumor* or malignant mixed mesodermal tumor.

M-mode. A diagnostic ultrasound presentation of the temporal changes in echoes in which the depth of echo-producing interfaces is displayed along one axis with time (T) along the second axis; motion (M) of the interfaces toward and away from the transducer is displayed. SYN TM-mode.

mmol Abbreviation for millimole.

MMPI Abbreviation for Minnesota multiphasic personality inventory *test.*

MMR Abbreviation for measles, mumps, and rubella *vaccine.*

Mn Symbol for manganese.

M'Naghten, Daniel, British criminal, tried in March, 1843. SEE M. *rule.*

MND Abbreviation for motor neuron *disease.*

mne·me (nē'mē). 1. The enduring quality in the mind that ac-

counts for the facts of memory; the engram of a specific experience. [G. *mnēmē,* memory]

mne·men·ic, mne·mic (nē-men'ik, nē'mik). Relating to memory.

mne·mism (nē'mizm). SYN mnemic *hypothesis.* [G. *mnēmē,* memory]

mne·mon·ic (nē-mon'ik). SYN anamnestic (1).

mne·mon·ics (nē-mon'iks). The art of improving the memory; a system for aiding the memory. [G. *mnēmonikos,* mnemonic, pertaining to memory]

MNSs blood group. See Blood Groups appendix.

M.O. Abbreviation for Medical Officer.

Mo Symbol for molybdenum.

^{99}Mo. Abbreviation for molybdenum-99.

MoAb Abbreviation for monoclonal *antibody.*

mo·bi·li·za·tion (mō'bi-li-zā'shŭn). 1. Making movable; restoring the power of motion in a joint. 2. The act or the result of the act of mobilizing; exciting a hitherto quiescent process into physiologic activity. [see mobilize]

   stapes m., an operation to remobilize the footplate of the stapes to relieve conductive hearing impairment caused by its immobilization through otosclerosis or middle ear disease.

mo·bi·lize (mō'bi-līz). 1. To liberate material stored in the body; more specifically, to move a substance from tissue stores into the bloodstream. 2. To excite quiescent material to physiologic activity. [Fr. *mobiliser,* to liberate, make ready, fr. L. *mobilis,* movable]

Mobitz, Woldemar, German cardiologist, *1889. SEE M. types of atrioventricular *block.*

Möbius, Paul J., German physician, 1853–1907. SEE M.'s *sign, syndrome;* Leyden-M. muscular *dystrophy.*

MOD Abbreviation for mesiodistocclusal.

mo·dal·i·ty (mō-dal'i-tē). 1. A form of application or employment of a therapeutic agent or regimen. 2. Various forms of sensation, *e.g.,* touch, vision, etc.. [Mediev. L. *modalitas,* fr. L. *modus,* a mode]

mode (mōd). In a set of measurements, that value which appears most frequently. [L. *modus,* a measure, quantity]

mod·el (mod'ĕl). 1. A representation of something, often idealized or modified to make it conceptually easier to understand. 2. Something to be imitated. 3. In dentistry, a cast. [It. *midello,* fr. L. *modus,* measure, standard]

   Adair-Koshland-Némethy-Filmer m. (AKNF), SYN Koshland-Némethy-Filmer m. SEE Koshland-Némethy-Filmer m.

   additive m., a m. in which the combined effect of several factors is the sum of the effects that would be produced by each of the factors in the absence of the others.

   animal m., study in a population of laboratory animals that uses conditions of animals analogous to conditions of humans to simulate processes comparable to those that occur in human populations.

   Bingham m., a m. representing the flow behavior of a Bingham plastic, in the idealized case.

   biomedical m., a conceptual m. of illness that excludes psychological and social factors and includes only biological factors in an attempt to understand a person's medical illness or disorder.

   biopsychosocial m., a conceptual m. that assumes that psycho-

♻ **Combining forms**

Word*Finder*
Multi-term entry finder
Preceding letter A
A.D.A.M. Anatomy Plates
Between letters L and M

Appendices:
Following letter Z

SYN Synonym; Cf., compare

[NA] Nomina Anatomica

**[MIM] Mendelian
Inheritance in Man**

☆ **Official alternate term**

☆**[NA] Official alternate
Nomina Anatomica term**

High Profile Term

mo

logical and social factors must also be included along with the biological in understanding a person's medical illness or disorder.

cloverleaf m., a m. for the structure of tRNA; so named because the structure roughly resembles a cloverleaf.

computer m., a mathematical representation of the functioning of a system, presented in the form of a computer program. SYN computer simulation.

concerted m., SYN Monod-Wyman-Changeux m.

cooperativity m., a m. used to explain the property of cooperativity observed in certain enzymes; *e.g.,* allosterism or hysteresis.

fluid mosaic m., a m. for the structure of a biomembrane, with lateral diffusibility of constituents and little, if any, flip-flop motion.

genetic m., a formalized conjecture about the behavior of a heritable structure in which the component terms are intended to have literal interpretation as standard structures of empirical genetics.

induced fit m., (1) a m. to suggest a mode of action of enzymes in which the substrate binds to the active site of the protein, causing a conformational change in the protein; **(2)** SYN Koshland-Némethy-Filmer m.

Koshland-Némethy-Filmer m. (KNF model), a m. to explain the allosteric form of cooperativity; in this m., in the absence of ligands, the protein exists in only one conformation; upon binding, the ligand induces a conformational change that may be transmitted to other subunits. SYN Adair-Koshland-Némethy-Filmer m., induced fit m. (2).

lock-and-key m., a m. used to suggest the mode of operation of an enzyme in which the substrate fits into the active site of the protein like a key into a lock.

logistic m., a statistical m.; in epidemiology, a m. of risk as a function of exposure to a risk factor.

mathematical m., representation of a system, process, or relationship in mathematical form, using equations to simulate the behavior of the system or process under study.

medical m., a set of assumptions that views behavioral abnormalities in the same framework as physical disease or abnormalities.

Monod-Wyman-Changeux m. (MWC m.), a m. used to explain the allosteric form of cooperativity; in this m., an oligomeric protein can exist in two conformational states in the absence of the ligand; these states are in equilibrium and the one that is predominant has a lower affinity for the ligand (which binds to the protein in a rapid equilibrium fashion). SYN concerted m.

multiplicative m., a m. in which the joint effect of two or more causes is the product of their effects if they were acting alone.

multistage m., a mathematical m., mainly for carcinogenesis, based on the theory that a specific carcinogen may affect one among a number of stages in the development of cancer.

MWC m., abbreviation for Monod-Wyman-Changeux m.

pathological m., an animal or animal stock that by inheritance or by artificial manipulation develops a disorder similar to some disease of interest and hence directly or by analogy furnishes evidence of its pathogenesis and may be used as a m. for the study of preventive or therapeutic measures.

statistical m., a formal representation for a class of processes that allows a means of analyzing results from experimental studies, such as the Poisson m. or the general linear m.; it need not propose a process literally interpretable in the context of the individual case.

mod·el·ing (mod′ĕl-ing). **1.** In learning theory, the acquiring and learning of a new skill by observing and imitating that behavior being performed by another individual. **2.** In behavior modification, a treatment procedure whereby the therapist or another significant person presents (models) the target behavior which the learner is to imitate and make part of his repertoire. **3.** A continuous process by which a bone is altered in size and shape during its growth by resorption and formation of bone at different sites and rates.

mod·i·fi·ca·tion (mod′i-fi-kā′shŭn). **1.** A nonhereditary change in an organism; *e.g.,* one that is acquired from its own activity or environment. **2.** A chemical or structural alteration in a molecule.

behavior m., the systematic use of principles of conditioning and learning, especially operant or instrumental conditioning, to teach certain skills or to extinguish undesirable behaviors, attitudes, or phobias.

chemical m., alteration in the structure of a molecule, typically a macromolecule such as a protein, by chemical means; often, the covalent addition by some reagent.

covalent m., alteration in the structure of a macromolecule by enzymatic means, resulting in a change in the properties of that macromolecule; frequently, this type of m. is physiologically relevant.

mo·di·o·lus, pl. **mo·di·′o·li** (mō-dī′ō-lŭs, -ō-lī). **1** [NA]. The central cone-shaped core of spongy bone about which turns the spiral canal of the cochlea. **2.** SYN m. labii. [L., the nave of a wheel]

m. la′bii, a point near the corner of the mouth where several muscles of facial expression converge. SYN columella cochleae, modiolus (2).

mod·u·la·tion (mod-yū-lā′shŭn). **1.** The functional and morphologic fluctuation of cells in response to changing environmental conditions. **2.** Systematic variation in a characteristic (*e.g.,* frequency, amplitude) of a sustained oscillation to code additional information. **3.** A change in the kinetics of an enzyme or metabolic pathway. **4.** The regulation of the rate of translation of mRNA by a modulating codon. [L. *modulor,* to measure off properly]

mo·du·lus (moj′yū-lŭs, mod′yū-). A coefficient expressing the magnitude of a physical property by a numerical value. [L. dim. of *modus,* a measure, quantity]

bulk m., SYN m. of volume elasticity.

m. of elasticity, a coefficient expressing the ratio between stress per unit area acting to deform a body and the amount of deformation that results from it.

m. of volume elasticity, a coefficient expressing the ratio between pressure acting to change the volume of a substance and the amount of change that results from it. SYN bulk m.

Young's m., a type of m. of elasticity which specifies the force applied to a body in one direction, per unit cross-sectional area of the body perpendicular to that direction, divided by the fractional change in length of the body in that direction.

Moeller, Alfred, German bacteriologist, *1868. SEE M.'s grass *bacillus.*

Moeller, Julius O.L., German surgeon, 1819–1887. SEE M.'s *glossitis.*

mo·fe·bu·ta·zone (mof-ĕ-byū′tă-zōn). 4-Butyl-1-phenyl-3,5-pyrazolidinedione; an anti-inflammatory agent used for the treatment of arthritis.

mog·i·ar·thria (moj-i-ar′thrē-ă). Speech defect due to muscular incoordination. [G. *mogis,* with difficulty, + *arthroō,* to articulate]

mog·i·graph·ia (moj-i-graf′ē-ă). SYN writer's *cramp.* [G. *mogis,* with difficulty, + *graphē,* writing]

mog·i·la·lia (moj-i-lā′lē-ă). Stuttering, stammering, or any speech defect. SYN molilalia. [G. *mogis,* with difficulty, + *lalia,* speech]

mog·i·pho·nia (moj-i-fō′nē-ă). Laryngeal spasm occurring in public speakers as a result of overuse of the voice. [G. *mogis,* with difficulty, + *phōnē,* voice]

Mohrenheim, Joseph J. Freiherr von, Austrian-Russian surgeon, 1755–1799. SEE M.'s *fossa, space.*

Mohs (mōz), Frederic E., U.S. surgeon, *1910, who as a medical student, devised a system of microscopicaly controlled removal of skin tumors. SEE M.'s fresh tissue chemosurgery *technique, chemosurgery.*

Mohs, Friedrich, German mineralogist, 1773–1839. SEE M. *scale.*

moi·e·ty (moy′i-tē). **1.** Originally, a half; now, loosely, a portion of something. **2.** Functional group. [M.E. *moite,* a half]

mol Abbreviation for mole (4).

mo·lal (mō′lăl). Denoting 1 mol of solute dissolved in 1000 g of solvent; such solutions provide a definite ratio of solute to solvent molecules. Cf. molar (4).

mo·lal·i·ty (m) (mō-lal'i-tē). Moles of solute per kilogram of solvent; the molarity is equal to mρ/(1 + mM), where m is the molality, ρ is the density of the solution, and M is the molar mass of the solute. Cf. molarity.

mo·lar (mō'lăr). **1.** Denoting a grinding, abrading, or wearing away. [L. *molaris,* relating to a mill, millstone] **2.** SYN molar *tooth.* **3.** Massive; relating to a mass; not molecular. [L. *moles,* mass] **4.** Denoting a concentration of 1 gram-molecular weight (1 mol) of solute per liter of solution, the common unit of concentration in chemistry. Cf. molal. **5.** Denoting specific quantity, *e.g.,* m. volume (volume of 1 mol).

first m., first permanent m., sixth permanent tooth or fourth deciduous tooth in the maxilla and mandible on either side of the midsagittal plane of the head following the arch form.

Moon's m.'s, small dome-shaped first m. teeth occurring in congenital syphilis.

mulberry m., a m. tooth with alternating nonanatomical depressions and rounded enamel nodules on its crown surface, usually associated with congenital syphilis.

second m., seventh permanent or fifth deciduous tooth in the maxilla and mandible on either side of the midsagittal plane of the head following the arch form.

sixth-year m., the first permanent m. tooth.

third m., eighth permanent tooth in the maxilla and mandible on each side, making it the most posterior tooth in human dentition; usually erupts between the seventeenth and twenty-third years; the roots are often fused, the separation being marked only by grooves; because it tends to erupt in an anterosuperior direction, the lower third molar often becomes impacted against the lower second molar; it is common for one or more third molar to fail to develop. SYN dens serotinus [NA], molaris tertius[*], dens sapientiae, wisdom tooth.

twelfth-year m., the second permanent m. tooth.

mo·lar·i·form (mō-lar'i-fōrm). Having the form of a molar tooth. [molar (tooth) + L. *forma,* form]

mo·la·ris ter·ti·us. [*]official alternate term for third *molar.*

mo·lar·i·ty (M) (mō-lar'i-tē). Moles per liter of solution (mol/L). Cf. molality.

mold (mōld). **1.** A filamentous fungus, generally a circular colony that may be cottony, wooly, etc., or glabrous, but with filaments not organized into large fruiting bodies, such as mushrooms. **2.** A shaped receptacle into which wax is pressed or fluid plaster is poured in making a cast. **3.** To shape a mass of plastic material according to a definite pattern. **4.** To change in shape; denoting especially the adaptation of the fetal head to the pelvic canal. **5.** The term used to specify the shape of an artificial tooth (or teeth). SYN mould.

pink bread m., SYN *Neurospora.*

mold·ing (mōld'ing). Shaping by means of a mold.

border m., the shaping of an impression material by the manipulation or action of the tissues adjacent to the borders of an impression. SYN muscle-trimming, tissue m., tissue-trimming.

compression m., (1) the act of pressing or squeezing together to form a shape in a mold; **(2)** the adaptation of a plastic material to the negative form of a split mold by pressure. SEE ALSO injection m.

injection m., the adaptation of a plastic material to the negative form of a closed mold by forcing the material into the mold through appropriate gateways. SEE ALSO compression m. (2).

tissue m., SYN border m.

mole (mōl). **1.** SYN nevus (2). **2.** SYN *nevus* pigmentosus. [A.S. *māēl* (L. *macula*), a spot] **3.** An intrauterine mass formed by the degeneration of the partly developed products of conception. [L. *moles,* mass] **4 (mol).** In the SI system, the unit of amount of substance, defined as that amount of a substance containing as many "elementary entities" as there are atoms in 0.0120 kg of carbon-12; "elementary entities" may be atoms, molecules, ions, or any describable entity or defined mixture of entities and must be specified when this term is used; in practical terms, the mole is 6.0221367×10^{23} "elementary entities." SEE ALSO Avogadro's *number.*

blood m., SYN fleshy m.

Breus m., an aborted ovum in which the fetal surface of the placenta presents numerous hematomata with an absence of blood vessels in the chorion and an ovum much smaller in size than normal in relation to the duration of the pregnancy.

carneous m., SYN fleshy m.

cystic m., SYN hydatidiform m.

false m., an intrauterine polyp.

fleshy m., a uterine mass occurring after fetal death and consisting of blood clots, fetal membranes, and placenta. SYN blood m., carneous m.

grape m., SYN hydatidiform m.

hairy m., SYN *nevus* pilosus.

hydatidiform m., hydatid m., a vesicular or polycystic mass resulting from the proliferation of the trophoblast, with hydropic degeneration and avascularity of the chorionic villi. SYN cystic m., grape m., vesicular m.

invasive m., SYN *chorioadenoma* destruens.

spider m., SYN spider *angioma.*

vesicular m., SYN hydatidiform m.

mo·lec·u·lar (mō-lek'yū-lăr). Relating to molecules.

mo·lec·u·lar·i·ty (mō-lek'yū-lār'i-tē). The number of reactants in a reaction. For example, a reaction involving one reactant is unimolecular; reactions involving two compounds are bimolecular. Molecularity and order are not synonymous. Cf. order (2).

mol·e·cule (mol'ĕ-kyūl). The smallest possible quantity of a di-, tri-, or polyatomic substance that retains the chemical properties of the substance. [Mod. L. *molecula,* dim. of L. *moles,* mass]

accessory m.'s, cell surface adhesion m.'s on T cells that are involved in binding of one cell to another cell or in signal transduction, *e.g.,* CD4.

adhesion m.'s, m.'s that are involved in T helper-accessory cell, T helper-B cell, and T cytotoxic-target cell interactions.

cell adhesion m. (CAM), proteins that hold cells together, *e.g.,* uvomorulin, and hold them to their substrates, *e.g.,* laminin.

chimeric m., a m. (usually a biopolymer) containing sequences derived from two different genes; specifically, from two different species. Cf. chimera.

endothelial-leukocyte adhesion m. (E-LAM), 115,000 M_r m. on the surface of endothelial cells that is involved in blood leukocyte attachment to vessel walls as well as emigration from the vessels into the tissues.

gram-molecule, the amount of a substance with a mass in grams equal to its molecular weight; *e.g.,* a m. of hydrogen weighs 2.016 g, that of water 18.015 g.

intercellular adhesion m.-1 (ICAM-1), a glycoprotein that is expressed on a variety of cells. It is the ligand for LFA-1 as well as the receptor for the rhinoviruses.

mol·i·la·lia (mol'i-lā'lē-ă). SYN mogilalia. [G. *molis,* with difficulty (a later form of *mogis*), + *lalia,* talking]

mo·li·men, pl. **mo·lim·i·na** (mō-lī'men, -lim'i-nă). An effort; laborious performance of a normal function. [L. an endeavor]

m. climacte'ricum vi'rile, a condition resembling neurasthenia, occurring in men of 45 to 55 years of age; may be psychosomatic or due to alteration in testicular androgen secretion.

menstrual molimina, SYN premenstrual *syndrome.*

mo·lin·done hy·dro·chlo·ride (mō-lin'dōn). 3-Ethyl-6,7-dihydro-2-methyl-5-(morpholinomethyl)indol-4(5*H*)-one monohydrochloride; an antipsychotic.

Molisch, Hans, Austrian chemist, 1856–1937. SEE M.'s *test.*

Moll, Jacob A., Dutch oculist, 1832–1914. SEE M.'s *glands,* under *gland.*

mol·li·ti·es (mō-lish'i-ēz). **1.** Characterized by a soft consistency. **2.** SYN malacia. [L. *mollis,* soft]

mol·lusc (mol'ŭsk). SYN mollusk.

Mol·lus·ca (mo-lŭs'kă). A phylum of the subkingdom Metazoa with soft, unsegmented bodies, consisting of an anterior head, a dorsal visceral mass and a ventral foot. Most forms are enclosed in a protective calcareous shell. M. includes the classes Gastropoda (snails, whelks, slugs) Pelecypoda (oysters, clams, mussels), Cephalopoda (squids, octopuses), Amphineura (chitons), Scaphopoda (tooth shells), and the class of primitive metameric

Mo

mollusks, Monoplacophora. [L. *mollusca,* a nut with a thin shell, fr. *mollis,* soft]

mol·lus·cous (mo-lŭs′kŭs). Relating to or resembling molluscum.

mol·lus·cum (mo-lŭs′kŭm). A disease marked by the occurrence of soft rounded tumors of the skin. [L. *molluscus,* soft]

m. contagio′sum, a contagious disease of the skin caused by intranuclear proliferation of a virus of the family Poxviridae and characterized by the appearance of few to numerous small, pearly, umbilicated papular expansile epidermal downgrowths that contain numerous cytoplasmic inclusion bodies (m. bodies); occurs in anthropoid apes as well as in humans. SYN m. verrucosum.

m. verruco′sum, SYN m. contagiosum.

mol·lusk (mol′ŭsk). Common name for members of the phylum Mollusca, although usually restricted to the gastropods and bivalves. SYN mollusc.

Moloney, John B., 20th century U.S. oncologist. SEE M.'s *virus.*

Moloney, Paul J., Canadian physician, 1870–1939. SEE M. *test.*

Moloy, Howard C., U.S. obstetrician, 1903–1953. SEE Caldwell-M. *classification.*

molt (mōlt). To cast off feathers, hair, or cuticle; to undergo ecdysis. SEE ALSO desquamate. SYN moult. [L. *muto,* to change]

mol wt Abbreviation for molecular *weight.*

mo·lyb·date (mō-lib′dāt). A salt of molybdic acid.

mo·lyb·den·ic, mo·lyb·de·nous (mō-lib′den-ik, -den-ŭs). Relating to molybdenum.

mo·lyb·de·num (Mo) (mō-lib′dĕ-nŭm). A silvery white metallic element, atomic no. 42, atomic wt. 95.94; a bioelement found in a number of proteins (*e.g.,* xanthine oxidase). SEE molybdenum target *tube.* [G. *molybdaina,* a piece of lead; a metal, prob. galena, fr. *molybdos,* lead]

mo·lyb·de·num-99 (⁹⁹Mo). A reactor-produced radioisotope of molybdenum with a half-life of 2.7476 days, used in radionuclide generators for the production of technetium-99m.

mo·lyb·dic (mō-lib′dik). Denoting molybdenum in the 6+ state, as in MoO_3.

mo·lyb·dic ac·id. $MoO_3 \cdot H_2O$; a yellowish crystalline acid, forming molybdates; used in the determination of phosphorus or phosphate.

mo·lyb·do·en·zymes (mō-lib′dō-en′zīmz). Enzymes that require a molybdenum ion as a component (*e.g.,* xanthine oxidase).

mo·lyb·do·fla·vo·pro·teins (mō-lib′dō-flā′vō-prō′tēnz). Proteins that require a molybdenum ion and a flavin nucleotide as a part of its naturally occurring structure (*e.g.,* aldehyde dehydrogenase).

mo·lyb·dop·ter·in (mō-lib-op′ter-in). A pterin derivative that complexes with molybdenum to form the molybdenum cofactor required by several enzymes.

mo·lyb·dous (mō-lib′dŭs). Denoting molybdenum in the 4+ state, as in MoO_2.

mo·lys·mo·pho·bia (mŏ-liz-mō-fō′bē-ă). Morbid fear of infection. [G. *molysma,* filth, infection, + *phobos,* fear]

mo·ment (mō′ment). The product of a quantity times a distance. [L. *momentum* (for *movimentum*), motion, moment, fr. *moveo,* to move]

dipole m., the product of one of the two charges of a dipole and the distance that separates them; an important measure of the degree of polarity of many biomolecules.

mom·ism (mom′izm). Rarely used term relating to excessive or overbearing mothering, especially as attributed to American cultural stereotypes.

⚠**mon-.** SEE mono-.

mo·nad (mō′nad, mon′ad). **1.** A univalent element or radical. **2.** A unicellular organism. **3.** In meiosis, the single chromosome derived from a tetrad after the first and second maturation divisions. [G. *monas,* the number one, unity]

Monakow, Constantin von, Swiss histologist, 1853–1930. SEE M.'s *bundle, nucleus, syndrome, tract.*

mon·am·ide (mon-am′id). SYN monoamide.

mon·am·ine (mon-am′in). SYN monoamine.

mon·am·i·nu·ria (mon′am-i-nū′rē-ă). SYN monoaminuria.

mon·an·gle (mon′ang-gl). Having only one angle, denoting a dental instrument that has only one angle between the handle or shaft and the working portion (blade or nib).

mon·ar·da (mon-ar′dă). The leaves of *Monarda punctata* (family Labiatae), American horsemint, a labiate plant of the U.S. east of the Mississippi; the main commercial source of natural thymol; used as a carminative in colic.

mon·ar·thric (mon-ar′thrik). SYN monarticular.

mon·ar·thri·tis (mon-ar-thrī′tis). Arthritis of a single joint.

mon·ar·tic·u·lar (mon-ar-tik′yū-lăr). Relating to a single joint. SYN monarthric, uniarticular.

mon·as·ter (mon-as′ter). The single star figure at the end of prophase in mitosis. SYN mother star. [mono- + G. *aster,* star]

mon·ath·e·to·sis (mon-ath-ĕ-tō′sis). Athetosis affecting one hand or foot.

mon·a·tom·ic (mon-ă-tom′ik). **1.** Relating to or containing a single atom. **2.** SYN monovalent (1).

mon·au·ral (mon-aw′răl). Pertaining to one ear. [mono- + L. *auris,* ear]

mon·ax·on·ic (mon-aks-on′ik). **1.** Having but one axis, being therefore elongated and slender. **2.** Having one axon. [mono- + G. *axōn,* axle]

Mönckeberg, Johann G., German pathologist, 1877–1925. SEE M.'s *arteriosclerosis, calcification, degeneration, sclerosis.*

Mondini. C., Italian physician, 1729–1803. SEE Mondini *deafness,* Mondini *dysplasia.*

Mondonesi, Filippo, Italian physician. SEE M.'s *reflex.*

Mondor, Henri, French surgeon, 1885–1962. SEE M.'s *disease.*

Mo·ne·ra (mō-ne′ră). The prokaryotes, a kingdom of primitive microbial organisms characterized by having no defined nucleus or chromosomes; DNA that is not membrane-bound; and absence of centrioles, mitotic spindle, microtubules, and mitochondria; division of the ill-defined nuclear zone (nucleoid) is by separation of two masses attached to parts of the cell membrane, then growing apart (a form of amitosis). M. includes the blue-green algae and bacteria; viruses, which lack a true cell, may have originated as "escaped nucleic acids" or "wild genes" from eukaryotic cells and are not included. [pl. of Mod. L. *moneron,* fr. G. *monērēs,* solitary]

mo·ne·ran (mō-ne′ran). A member of the prokaryote kingdom Monera.

mon·es·thet·ic (mon-es-thet′ik). Relating to a single sense or sensation. [mono- + G. *aisthēsis,* sense perception]

mon·es·trous (mon-es′trŭs). Having but one estrous cycle in a mating season.

Monge Medrano, Carlos, Peruvian professor of medicine and high altitude specialist, 1884–1970. SEE Monge's *disease.*

mon·go·li·an (mon-gō′lē-ăn). **2.** Relating to a member of the Mongolian race.

Mo·ni·e·zia ex·pan·sa (mon-i-e′zē-ă ek-span′să). The broad tapeworm (family Anoplocephalidae) of sheep and cattle, occurring in the small intestine and reaching a length of 4–5 meters; infections are usually benign. Cysticercoids develop in soil-dwelling oribatid mites commonly ingested with grass by herbivores.

mon·i·lat·ed (mon′i-lāt-ed). SYN moniliform.

mo·nil·e·thrix (mō-nil′ĕ-thriks). An autosomal dominant trichodystrophy in which brittle hairs show a series of constrictions, usually without a medulla. SYN beaded hair, moniliform hair. [L. *monile,* necklace, + G. *thrix,* hair]

Mo·nil·i·a (mo-nil′ē-ă). Generic term for a group of fungi that are commonly known as fruit molds; the sexual state is *Neurospora.* A few closely related pathogenic organisms formerly classified in this genus are now properly termed *Candida.* [L. *monile,* necklace]

Mo·nil·i·a·ce·ae (mō-nil-ē-ā′sē-ē). A family of Fungi Imperfecti (order Moniliales) which includes *Sporothrix schenckii,* the causative agent of sporotrichosis.

mo·nil·i·al (mō-nil′ē-ăl). Precisely, pertaining to the *Monilia* but, in medicine, frequently used incorrectly with reference to the genus *Candida*.

mon·i·li·a·sis (mō-ni-lī′ă-sis). SYN candidiasis.

mo·nil·i·form (mō-nil′i-fōrm). Shaped like a string of beads or beaded necklace. SYN monilated. [L. *monile*, necklace, + *forma*, appearance]

Mo·nil·i·for·mis (mō-nil-i-fōr′mis). A genus of the class (or phylum) Acanthocephala, the thorny-headed worms. *M. dubius*, the common spiny-headed worm of house rats, is transmitted by infected cockroaches, *Periplaneta americana;* a few infections in humans have been reported. *M. moniliformis* is a species normally found in rodents and is a rare parasite of humans. [L. *monile*, necklace, + *forma*, appearance]

mo·nil·i·id (mō-nil′ē-id). Minute macular or papular lesions occurring as an allergic reaction to monilial infection.

mon·ism (mō′nizm). A metaphysical system in which all of reality is conceived as a unified whole. [G. *monos*, single]

mo·nis·tic (mo-nis′tik). Pertaining to monism.

mon·i·tor (mon′i-ter, -tōr). A device that displays and/or records specified data for a given series of events, operations, or circumstances. [L., one who warns, fr. *moneo*, pp. *monitum*, to warn]

cardiac m., an electronic m. which, when connected to the patient, signals each heart beat with a flashing light, an electrocardiographic curve, an audible signal, or all three.

electronic fetal m., an instrument for continuous monitoring of the fetal heart before or during labor.

Holter m., a technique for long-term, continuous recording of electrocardiographic signals on magnetic tape for scanning and selection of significant but fleeting changes that might otherwise escape notice.

mon·i·tor·ing. 1. Performance and analysis of routine measurements aimed at detecting a change in the environment or health status of a population. **2.** Ongoing measurement of performance of a health service. **3.** Continuous oversight of implementation of an activity.

mon·key-paw (mong′kē-paw). SYN ape hand. SYN monkey hand.

mon·key·pox (mŏng′kē-poks). A disease of monkeys and, rarely, of man caused by the monkeypox virus, a member of the family Poxviridae; the human disease clinically resembles smallpox.

monks·hood (monks′hud). SEE aconite.

mono-, mon-. The participation or involvement of a single element or part. Cf. uni-. [G. *monos*, single]

mon·o·ac·yl·glyc·er·ol (mon-ō-ās-il-gli′ser-ol). Glycerol with an acyl moiety esterified to position 1 (*i.e.*, 1-m.) or position 2 (*i.e.*, 2-m.); an intermediate in the degradation and synthesis of lipids; 2 m.'s are a major end product of triacylglycerol degradation.

m. acyltransferase, an intestinal enzyme that catalyzes the reaction of 2-m. and acyl-CoA to form coenzyme A and 1,2-diacylglycerol.

m. lipase, an enzyme that catalyzes the hydrolysis of m. to produce a fatty acid anion and glycerol; a part of lipid degradation.

mon·o·a·me·lia (mon-ō-ă-mē′lē-ă). Absence of one limb.

mon·o·am·ide (mon-ō-am′īd, -id). A molecule containing one amide group. SYN monamide.

mon·o·am·ine (mon-ō-am′īn, -in). A molecule containing one amine group. SYN monamine.

mon·o·am·ine ox·i·dase (MAO). SYN *amine* oxidase (flavin-containing).

mon·o·am·i·ner·gic (mon′ō-am-i-ner′jik). Referring to nerve cells or fibers that transmit nervous impulses by the medium of a catecholamine or indolamine. [monoamine + G. *ergon*, work]

mon·o·am·i·nu·ria (mon′ō-am-i-nū′rē-ă). The excretion of any monoamine in the urine. SYN monaminuria.

mon·o·am·ni·ot·ic (mon′ō-am-nē-ot′ik). Denoting two or more progeny of a multiple pregnancy that have shared a common amniotic sac.

mon·o·as·so·ci·at·ed (mon′ō-ă-sō′shē-ā-tĕd). Denoting a germ-free organism that becomes colonized by a single microbial species.

mon·o·aux·o·troph (mon-ō-auks′ō-troph). A mutant microorganism that requires a particular nutrient that is not required by the wild type organism. Cf. auxotroph, polyauxotroph.

mon·o·bac·tam (mon-ō-bak′tam). A class of antibiotic that has a monocyclic β-lactam nucleus and is structurally different from other β-lactams; *e.g.*, aztreonam.

mon·o·ba·sic (mon-ō-bā′sik). Denoting an acid with only one replaceable hydrogen atom, or only one replaced hydrogen atom.

mon·o·ben·zone (mon-ō-ben′zōn). *p*-Benzyloxyphenol; a melanin-pigment inhibiting agent; used topically for the treatment of hyperpigmentation caused by formation of melanin.

mon·o·blast (mon′ō-blast). An immature cell that develops into a monocyte. [mono- + G. *blastos*, germ]

mon·o·bra·chi·us (mon-ō-brā′kē-ŭs). The condition of being one-armed. [mono- + G. *brachiōn*, arm]

mon·o·bro·mat·ed, mon·o·bro·mi·nat·ed (mon-ō-brō′māt-ed, -brō′min-āt-ed). Denoting a chemical compound with one atom of bromine per molecule.

mon·o·car·di·an (mon-ō-kar′dē-an). Having a heart with a single atrium and ventricle.

mon·o·ceph·a·lus (mon-ō-sef′ă-lŭs). SYN syncephalus.

mon·o·chlor·phen·am·ide (mon′ō-klōr-fen′ă-mīd). SYN clofenamide.

mon·o·cho·rea (mon′ō-kō-rē′ă). Chorea affecting the head alone or only one extremity.

mon·o·cho·ri·al (mon-ō-kō-rē′ăl). SYN monochorionic.

mon·o·cho·ri·on·ic (mon′ō-kōr-ē-on′ik). Relating to or having a single chorion; denoting monovular twins. SYN monochorial.

mon·o·chro·ic (mon-ō-krō′ik). SYN monochromatic.

mon·o·chro·ma·sia (mon′ō-krō-mā′zē-ă). SYN achromatopsia.

mon·o·chro·ma·sy (mon′ō-krō′mă-sē). SYN achromatopsia.

blue cone m., SEE incomplete *achromatopsia.*

pi cone m., SEE incomplete *achromatopsia.*

mon·o·chro·mat·ic (mon′ō-krō-mat′ik). **1.** Having but one color. **2.** Indicating a light of a single wavelength. **3.** Relating to or characterized by monochromatism. SYN monochroic, monochromic.

mon·o·chro·ma·tism (mon-ō-krō′mă-tizm). **1.** The state of having or exhibiting only one color. **2.** SYN achromatopsia. [mono- + G. *chrōma*, color]

blue cone m., SEE incomplete *achromatopsia.*

pi cone m., SEE incomplete *achromatopsia.*

rod m., SYN complete *achromatopsia.*

mon·o·chro·mat·o·phil, mon·o·chro·mat·o·phile (mon′ō-krō-mat′ō-fil, -fīl). **1.** Taking only one stain. **2.** A cell or any histologic element staining with only one kind of dye. SYN monochromophil, monochromophile. [mono- + G. *chrōma*, color, + *philos*, fond]

mon·o·chro·ma·tor (mon-ō-krō′mă-ter, -tōr). A prism or diffraction grating used in spectrophotometry to isolate a narrow spectral range.

mon·o·chro·mic (mon-ō-krō′mik). SYN monochromatic.

mon·o·chro·mo·phil, mon·o·chro·mo·phile (mon-ō-krō′mō-fil, -fīl). SYN monochromatophil.

mon·o·cis·tron·ic (mon-ō-sis-tron′ik). Referring to fully processed mRNA that codes for a single protein.

mon·o·cle (mon′ŏ-kl). A lens used for one eye, usually in the correction of presbyopia.

mon·o·clin·ic (mon-ō-klin′ik). Relating to crystals with a single oblique inclination. [mono- + G. *klinō*, to incline]

mon·o·clo·nal (mon-ō-klō′năl). In immunochemistry, pertaining to a protein from a single clone of cells, all molecules of which are the same; *e.g.*, in the case of Bence Jones protein, the chains are all κ or λ.

mon·o·clo·nal peak. A narrow band visible on electrophoresis or an abnormal arc seen on immunoelectrophoresis, thought to represent immunoglobulin of one cell clone.

mo

mon·o·cra·ni·us (mon-ō-krā'nē-ŭs). SYN syncephalus. [mono- + G. *kranion,* cranium]

mon·o·cro·ta·line (mon-ō-crō'tă-lin). An alkaloid in the seeds, leaves, and stems of *Crotalaria spectabilis* (family Leguminosae), a plant poisonous to livestock and poultry in the southern U.S. SYN crotaline.

mon·o·crot·ic (mon'ō-krot'ik). Denoting a pulse the curve of which presents no notch or subsidiary wave in its descending line. [mono- + G. *krotos,* a beat]

mon·oc·ro·tism (mon-ok'rō-tizm). The state in which the pulse is monocrotic. [mono- + G. *krotos,* a beat]

mo·noc·u·lar (mon-ok'yū-lăr). Relating to, affecting, or visible by one eye only. [mono- + L. *oculus,* eye]

mo·noc·u·lus (mon-ok'yū-lŭs). 1. SYN cyclops. 2. A bandage applied to one eye only. [L. a one-eyed man, a hybrid word fr. G. *monos,* single, + L. *oculus,* eye]

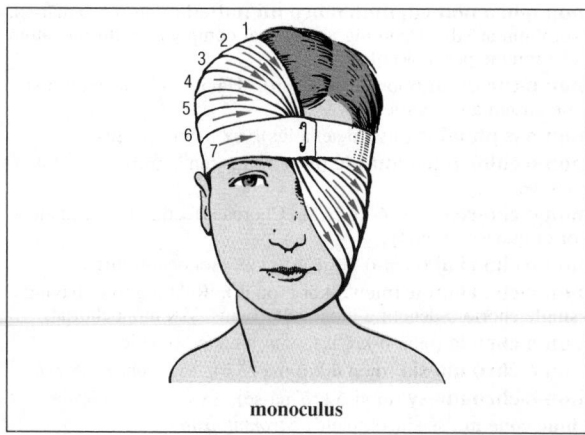

monoculus

mon·o·cyte (mon'ō-sīt). A relatively large mononuclear leukocyte (16 to 22 μm in diameter), that normally constitutes 3 to 7% of the leukocytes of the circulating blood, and is normally found in lymph nodes, spleen, bone marrow, and loose connective tissue. When treated with the usual dyes, m.'s manifest an abundant pale blue or blue-gray cytoplasm that contains numerous, fine, dustlike, red-blue granules; vacuoles are frequently present; the nucleus is usually indented, or slightly folded, and has a stringy chromatin structure that seems more condensed where the delicate strands are in contact. SEE ALSO monocytoid *cell,* endothelial *leukocyte.* [mono- + G. *kytos,* cell]

mon·o·cy·to·pe·nia (mon'ō-sī-tō-pē'nē-ă). Diminution in the number of monocytes in the circulating blood. SYN monocytic leukopenia, monopenia. [mono- + G. *kytos,* cell, + *penia,* poverty]

mon·o·cy·to·sis (mon'ō-sī-tō'sis). An abnormal increase in the number of monocytes in the circulating blood. SYN monocytic leukocytosis.

avian m., SYN bluecomb *disease* of chickens.

Mon·o·d, Jacques L., French biochemist and Nobel laureate, 1910–1976. SEE M.-Wyman-Changeux *model.*

mon·o·dac·ty·ly, mon·o·dac·tyl·ism (mon-ō-dak'ti-lē, -dak'-ti-lizm). The presence of a single finger on the hand, or a single toe on the foot. [mono- + G. *daktylos,* digit]

mon·o·der·mo·ma (mon'ō-der-mō'mă). A neoplasm composed of tissues from a single germinal layer. [mono- + G. *derma,* skin, + *-ōma,* tumor]

mon·o·dis·perse (mon'ō-dis-pers). Of relatively uniform size; said of aerosol suspensions with size variation of less than ±20%.

mon·o·eth·a·nol·a·mine (mon'ō-eth-ă-nol'ă-mēn). 2-Aminoethanol; a surfactant; the oleate is used as a sclerosing agent in the treatment of varicose veins.

mon·o·ga·met·ic (mon'ō-gă-met'ik). SYN homogametic.

mo·nog·a·my (mon-og'ă-mē). The marriage or mating system in which each partner has but one mate. [mono- + G. *gamos,* marriage]

mon·o·gen·e·sis (mon-ō-jen'ĕ-sis). 1. The production of similar organisms in each generation. 2. The production of young by one parent only, as in nonsexual generation and parthenogenesis. 3. The process of parasitizing a single host, in which the life cycle of the parasite is passed; *e.g., Boophilus annulatus,* the one-host cattle tick, or certain trematodes of the order Monogenea. [mono- + G. *genesis,* origin, production]

mon·o·ge·net·ic (mon'ō-jĕ-net'ik). Relating to monogenesis. SYN monoxenous.

mon·o·gen·ic (mon-ō-jen'ik). Relating to a hereditary disease or syndrome, or to an inherited characteristic, controlled by alleles at a single genetic locus.

mo·nog·e·nous (mŏ-noj'ĕ-nŭs). Asexually produced, as by fission, gemmation, or sporulation.

mon·o·ger·mi·nal (mon-ō-jer'mi-năl). SYN unigerminal.

mon·o·glyc·er·ide (mon-ō-gli'ser-īd). SEE monoacylglycerol.

mon·o·graph (mon'ō-graf). A treatise on a particular subject or specific aspect of a subject. [mono- + G. *graphē,* a writing]

mon·o·hy·drat·ed (mon-ō-hī'drā-ted). Containing or united with a single molecule of water per molecule of substance.

mon·o·hy·dric (mon-ō-hī'drik). Having but one hydrogen atom in the molecule.

mon·o·hy·drox·y·succinic ac·id (mon-ō-hī-droks'ē-suk-sin'ik). SYN malic acid.

mon·o·i·de·ism (mon'ō-ī-dē'izm). A marked preoccupation with one idea or subject; a slight degree of monomania. [mono- + G. *idea,* form, idea]

mon·o·in·fec·tion (mon'ō-in-fek'shŭn). Simple infection with a single variety of microorganism.

mon·o·i·o·do·ty·ro·sine (MIT) (mon'ō-ī-ō'dō-tī-rō-sēn). An intermediate in thyroid hormone synthesis.

mon·o·i·so·ni·tro·so·ac·e·tone (mon'ō-ī'sō-nī-trō'sō-as'ĕ-tōn). SYN isonitrosoacetone.

mon·o·kine (mon'ō-kīn). Polypeptides secreted by both monocytes and macrophages. These substances influence the activity of other cells. The general term cytokine is preferentially used today. SEE cytokine. [monocyte + G. *kineō,* to set in motion]

mon·o·lay·ers (mon-ō-lā'erz). 1. Films, one molecule thick, formed on water by certain substances, such as proteins and fatty acids, characterized by molecules containing some atom groupings that are soluble in water and other atom groupings that are insoluble in water. 2. A confluent sheet of cells, one cell deep, growing on a surface in a cell culture.

mon·o·loc·u·lar (mon-ō-lok'yū-lăr). Having one cavity or chamber. SYN unicameral, unicamerate. [mono- + L. *loculus,* a small place]

mon·o·ma·nia (mon-ō-mā'nē-ă). An obsession or abnormally extreme enthusiasm for a single idea or subject; a psychosis marked by the limitation of the symptoms rather strictly to a certain group, as the delusion in paranoia. [mono- + G. *mania,* frenzy]

mon·o·ma·ni·ac (mon-ō-mā'nē-ak). 1. One exhibiting monomania. 2. Characterized by or relating to monomania.

mon·o·mas·ti·gote (mon-ō-mas'ti-gōt). A mastigote having only one flagellum. [mono- + Roman *mastix, a whip*]

mon·o·mel·ic (mon-ō-mel'ik). Relating to one limb. [mono- + G. *melos,* limb]

mon·o·mer (mon'ō-mer). 1. The molecular unit that, by repetition, constitutes a large structure or polymer; *e.g.,* ethylene, $H_2C=CH_2$, is the monomer of polyethylene, $H(CH_2)_nH$. SEE ALSO subunit. 2. The protein structural unit of a virion capsid. SEE virion. 3. The protein subunit of a protein composed of several loosely associated such units, usually noncovalently bound together. [mono- + -mer]

mon·o·mer·ic (mon-ō-mer'ik). 1. Consisting of a single component. 2. In genetics, relating to a hereditary disease or characteristic controlled by genes at a single locus. 3. Consisting of monomers. [mono- + G. *meros,* part]

mon·o·me·tal·lic (mon′ō-mĕ-tal′ik). Containing one atom of a metal per molecule.

mon·o·mi·cro·bic (mon′ō-mī-krō′bik). Denoting a monoinfection.

mon·o·mo·lec·u·lar (mon′ō-mō-lek′yū-lăr). SYN unimolecular.

mon·o·mor·phic (mon′ō-mōr′fik). Of one shape; unchangeable in shape. [mono- + G. *morphē*, shape]

mon·om·pha·lus (mon-om′fă-lŭs). SYN omphalopagus. [mono- + G. *omphalos*, umbilicus]

mon·o·my·o·ple·gia (mon′ō-mī′ō-plē′jē-ă). Paralysis limited to one muscle. [mono- + G. *mys*, muscle, + *plēgē*, a stroke]

mon·o·my·o·si·tis (mon′ō-mī-ō-sī′tis). Inflammation of a single muscle.

mon·o·neme (mon′ō-nēm). An unpaired helix of nucleic acid, as occurs in a chromatid.

mon·o·neu·ral, mon·o·neu·ric (mon′ō-nū′răl, -nū′rik). **1.** Having only one neuron. **2.** Supplied by a single nerve.

mon·o·neu·ral·gia (mon′ō-nū-ral′jă). Pain along the course of one nerve.

mon·o·neu·ri·tis (mon′ō-nū-rī′tis). Inflammation of a single nerve.

mon·o·neu·rop·a·thy (mon′ō-nū-rop′ă-thē). Disorder involving a single nerve.

  m. mul′tiplex, inflammation of several nerves usually in unrelated portions of the body.

mon·o·noea (mon-ō-nē′ă). Fixation of the mind on one subject. [mono- + G. *noēsis*, idea]

mon·o·nu·cle·ar (mon-ō-nū′klē-ăr). Having only one nucleus; used especially in reference to blood cells.

mon·o·nu·cle·o·sis (mon′ō-nū-klē-ō′sis). Presence of abnormally large numbers of mononuclear leukocytes in the circulating blood, especially with reference to forms that are not normal.

  infectious m., an acute febrile illness caused by the Epstein-Barr virus, a member of the Herpesviridae family; frequently spread by saliva transfer; characterized by fever, sore throat, enlargement of lymph nodes and spleen, and leukopenia that changes to lymphocytosis during the second week; the circulating blood usually contains abnormal, large lymphocytes that have a resemblance to monocytes, and there is heterophil antibody that may be completely adsorbed on beef erythrocytes, but not on guinea pig kidney antigen. Collections of the characteristic abnormal lymphocytes may be present not only in the lymph nodes and spleen, but in various other sites, such as the meninges, brain, and myocardium. SYN benign lymphadenosis, glandular fever.

mon·o·nu·cle·o·tide (mon-ō-nū′klē-ō-tīd). SYN nucleotide.

mon·o·oc·tan·o·in (mon-ok-tan′ō-in). A semisynthetic esterified glycerol used as a solubilizing agent for radiolucent gallstones retained in the biliary tract following cholecystectomy.

mon·o·ox·y·ge·na·ses (mon-ō-ok′si-jĕ-nā-sez). Oxidoreductases that induce the incorporation of one atom of oxygen from O_2 into the substance being oxidized.

mon·o·pa·re·sis (mon′o-pa-rē′sis, -par′ĕ-sis). Paresis affecting a single extremity or part of an extremity.

mon·o·par·es·the·sia (mon′ō-par-es-thē′zē-ă). Paresthesia affecting a single region only.

mon·o·path·ic (mon-ō-path′ik). Relating to a monopathy.

mo·nop·a·thy (mon-op′ă-thē). **1.** A single uncomplicated disease. **2.** A local disease affecting only one organ or part. [mono- + G. *pathos*, suffering]

mon·o·pe·nia (mon-ō-pē′nē-ă). SYN monocytopenia.

mo·noph·a·gism (mŏ-nof′ă-jizm). Habitual eating of but one kind of food or but one meal a day when the latter is clearly an aberration. [mono- + G. *phagō*, to eat]

mon·o·pha·sia (mon-ō-fā′zē-ă). Inability to speak other than a single word or sentence. [mono- + G. *phasis*, speech]

mon·o·pha·sic (mon-ō-fā′zik). **1.** Marked by monophasia. **2.** Occurring in or characterized by only one phase or stage. **3.** Fluctuating from the baseline in one direction only.

mon·o·phe·nol mon·o·ox·y·gen·ase (mon-ō-fē′nol). **1.** A copper-containing oxidoreductase that catalyzes the oxidation of *o*-diphenols to *o*-quinones by O_2, with the incorporation of one of the two oxygen atoms in the product; it also catalyzes the oxidation of monophenols, such as L-tyrosine, to dihydroxy-L-phenylalanine (dopa), a precursor of melanin and epinephrine (catecholamines), and can act as a catechol oxidase; a deficiency of this enzyme is observed in a number of forms of albinism. SYN cresolase, monophenol oxidase, tyrosinase. **2.** SYN laccase.

mon·o·phe·nol ox·i·dase. SYN monophenol monooxygenase (1).

mon·o·pho·bia (mon-ō-fō′bē-ă). Morbid fear of solitude or of being left alone. [mono- + G. *phobos*, fear]

mon·oph·thal·mos (mon-of-thal′mos). Failure of outgrowth of a primary optic vesicle with absence of ocular tissues; the remaining eye is often maldeveloped. [mono- + G. *ophthalmos*, eye]

mon·oph·thal·mus (mon′of-thal′mŭs). SYN cyclops. [mono- + G. *ophthalmos*, eye]

mon·o·phy·let·ic (mon′ō-fī-let′ik). **1.** Having a single cell type of origin; derived from one line of descent, in contrast to polyphyletic. **2.** In hematology, relating to monophyletism. [mono- + G. *phylē*, tribe]

mon·o·phy·le·tism (mon-ō-fī′lĕ-tizm). In hematology, the theory that all the blood cells are derived from one common stem cell or histioblast. SYN monophyletic theory. [mono- + G. *phylē*, tribe]

mon·o·phy·o·dont (mon-ō-fī′ō-dont). Having one set of teeth only; without deciduous dentition. [mono- + G. *phyō*, to grow, + *odous* (*odont*-), tooth]

mon·o·plas·mat·ic (mon′ō-plas-mat′ik). Formed of but one tissue. [mono- + G. *plasma*, thing formed]

mon·o·plast (mon′ō-plast). A unicellular organism that retains the same structure or form throughout its existence. [mono- + G. *plastos*, formed]

mon·o·plas·tic (mon-ō-plas′tik). Undergoing no change in structure; relating to a monoplast.

mon·o·ple·gia (mon-ō-plē′jē-ă). Paralysis of one limb. [mono- + G. *plēgē*, a stroke]

  m. masticato′ria, unilateral paralysis of the muscles of mastication (masseter, temporal, pterygoid).

mon·o·ploid (mon′ō-ployd). SYN haploid. [mono- + G. *ploides*, in form]

mon·o·po·dia (mon-ō-pō′dē-ă). Malformation in which only one foot is externally recognizable. [mono- + G. *pous*, foot]

mon·ops (mon′ops). SYN cyclops. [mono- + G. *ōps*, eye]

mon·o·pty·chi·al (mon-ō-tī′kē-ăl). Arranged in a single but folded layer, as the cells in the epithelium of the gallbladder or certain glands. [mono- + G. *ptychē*, fold]

mon·or·chia (mon-ōr′kē-ă). SYN monorchism.

mon·or·chid·ic, mon·or·chid (mon-ōr-kid′ik, mon-ōr′kid). **1.** Having only one testis. **2.** Having apparently only one testis, the other being undescended.

mon·or·chid·ism (mon-ōr′ki-dizm). SYN monorchism.

mon·or·chism (mon′ōr-kizm). A condition in which only one testis is apparent, the other being absent or undescended. SYN monorchia, monorchidism. [mono- + G. *orchis*, testis]

mon·o·rec·i·dive (mon-o-res′i-dēv). Denoting a late or tertiary manifestation of syphilis which takes the form of an ulcerated papule located at the site of the original chancre. [mono- + L. *recidivus*, relapsing]

mon·o·rhin·ic (mon-ō-rin′ik). Single-nosed; used to characterize conjoined twins in which cephalic fusion has left only a single nose cavity evident. [mono- + G. *rhis* (*rhin*-), nose]

mon·o·sac·cha·ride (mon-ō-sak′ă-rīd). A carbohydrate that cannot form any simpler sugar by simple hydrolysis; *e.g.*, pentoses, hexoses. SYN monose.

mon·o·scel·ous (mon-ō-sel′ŭs, -skel′ŭs). Having only one leg. [mono- + G. *skelos*, leg]

mon·o·sce·nism (mon-ō-sē′nizm). Morbid concentration on some past experience. [mono- + G. *skēnē*, tent (stage drop)]

mon·ose (mon′ōs). SYN monosaccharide.

mon·o·so·di·um glu·ta·mate (MSG) (mon-ō-sō′dē-ŭm glū′tă-māt). $C_5H_8NNaO_4 \cdot H_2O$; the monosodium salt of the naturally occurring L form of glutamic acid; used as a flavor enhancer which is a cause or contributing factor to "Chinese restaurant" syndrome; also used intravenously as an adjunct in treatment of encephalopathies associated with hepatic disease.

mon·o·some (mon'ō-sōm). **1.** SYN accessory *chromosome*. **2.** Obsolete term for ribosome. [mono- + chromosome]

mon·o·so·mia (mon-ō-sō'mē-ă). In conjoined twins, a condition in which the trunks are completely merged although the heads remain separate. SEE conjoined *twins*, under *twin*. [mono- + G. *sōma*, body]

mon·o·so·mic (mon-ō-sō'mik). Relating to monosomy.

mon·o·so·mous (mon-ō-sō'mŭs). Characterized by or pertaining to monosomia.

mon·o·so·my (mon'ō-sō-mē). Absence of one chromosome of a pair of homologous chromosomes. SEE ALSO chromosomal *deletion*. [see monosome]

mon·o·spasm (mon'ō-spazm). Spasm affecting only one muscle or group of muscles, or a single extremity.

mon·o·sper·my (mon'ō-sper-mē). Fertilization by the entrance of only one spermatozoon into the egg. [mono- + G. *sperma*, seed]

Mon·o·spo·ri·um ap·i·o·sper·mum (mon-ō-spō'rē-ŭm ap'ē-ō-sper'mŭm). SYN *Scedosporium apiospermum*.

Mo·nos·to·ma (mō-nos'tō-mă, mon-ō-stō'mă). Archaic name for a genus of trematodes, based on the presence of a single sucker. [mono- + G. *stoma*, mouth]

mon·o·stome (mon'ō-stōm). Common name for digenetic trematodes that possess a single sucker, oral or ventral, rather than both. SEE ALSO *Monostoma*. [mono- + G. *stoma*, mouth]

mon·o·stot·ic (mon-os-tot'ik). Involving only one bone. [mono- + G. *osteon*, bone]

mon·o·stra·tal (mon-ō-strā'tăl). Composed of a single layer. [mono- + L. *stratum*, layer]

mon·o·sub·sti·tut·ed (mon-ō-sŭb'sti-tū-těd). In chemistry, denoting an element or radical, only one atom or unit of which is found in each molecule of a substitution compound.

mon·o·symp·to·mat·ic (mon'ō-simp-tō-mat'ik). Denoting a disease or morbid condition manifested by only one marked symptom.

mon·o·sy·nap·tic (mon'ō-si-nap'tik). Referring to direct neural connections (those not involving an intermediary neuron); *e.g.*, the direct connection between primary sensory nerve cells and motor neurons characterizing the monosynaptic reflex arc.

mon·o·syph·i·lide (mon-o-sif'i-lid). Marked by the occurrence of a single syphilitic lesion.

mon·o·ter·penes (mon-ō-ter'pēnz). Hydrocarbons or their derivatives formed by the condensation of two isoprene units, and therefore containing 10 carbon atoms; *e.g.*, camphor; often containing a cyclic structure.

mon·o·ther·mia (mon-ō-ther'mē-ă). Evenness of bodily temperature; absence of an evening rise in body temperature. [mono- + G. *thermē*, heat]

mon·o·thi·o·glyc·er·ol (mon'ō-thī-ō-glis'er-ol). α-Monothioglycerol; 3-mercapto-1,2-propanediol; used to promote wound healing. SYN thioglycerol.

mo·not·o·cous (mŏ-not'ō-kŭs). Producing a single offspring at a birth. [mono- + G. *tokos*, birth]

Mon·o·tre·ma·ta (mon-ō-trē'mă-tă). An order of egg-laying mammals that have a cloaca or common chamber which receives digestive, urinary, and reproductive products; only Australia has such forms, the duck-billed platypus (*Ornithorhynchus*) and the echidna (*Tachyglossus*). [mono- + G. *trēma*, a hole]

mon·o·treme (mon'ō-trēm). A member of the order Monotremata.

mo·not·ri·chate (mŏ-not'ri-kāt). SYN monotrichous.

mo·not·ri·chous (mŏ-not'ri-kŭs). Denoting a microorganism possessing a single flagellum or cilium. SYN monotrichate, uniflagellate.

mon·o·va·lence, mon·o·va·len·cy (mon-ō-vā'lens, -vā'len-sē).

A combining power (valence) equal to that of a hydrogen atom. SYN univalence, univalency.

mon·o·va·lent (mon-ō-vā'lent). **1.** Having the combining power (valence) of a hydrogen atom. SYN monatomic (2), univalent. **2.** Pertaining to a monovalent (specific) antiserum to a single antigen or organism.

mon·ox·e·nous (mon-oks'ĕ-nŭs). SYN monogenetic. [mono- + G. *xenos*, stranger]

mon·ox·ide (mon-ok'sīd). Any oxide having only one atom of oxygen; *e.g.*, CO.

mon·o·zo·ic (mon-ō-zō'ik). Unisegmented, as in cestodarian tapeworms. SEE polyzoic.

mon·o·zy·got·ic, mon·o·zy·gous (mon-ō-zī-got'ik, -zī'gŭs). SYN unigerminal. SEE monozygotic *twins*, under *twin*. [mono- + G. *zygōtos*, yoked]

Monro, Alexander Sr., Scottish anatomist and surgeon, 1697–1767. SEE *bursa* of M.

Monro, Alexander, Jr., Scottish anatomist, 1733–1817. SEE M.'s *doctrine, foramen, line, sulcus;* M.-Kellie *doctrine;* M.-Richter *line;* Richter-M. *line*.

mons, gen. **mon·tis,** pl. **mon·tes** (monz, mon'tis, mon'tēz) [NA]. An anatomical prominence or slight elevation above the general level of the surface. [L. a mountain]
m. pu'bis [NA], the prominence caused by a pad of fatty tissue over the symphysis pubis in the female. SYN os pubis [NA], m. veneris, pubes (3), pubic bone.
m. ure'teris, a pinkish prominence on the wall of the bladder marking each ureteral orifice.
m. ven'eris, SYN m. pubis. [L. *Venus*]

Monson, George S., U.S. dentist, 1869–1933. SEE M. *curve;* anti-M. *curve*.

mon·ster. Outmoded term for a malformed embryo, fetus, or individual. See entries beginning with terato-. SEE teras. [L. *monstrum*, an evil omen, a prodigy, a wonder]

mon·tan·ic ac·id (mon-tan'ik). SYN octacosanoic acid. [montan (wax)]

Monteggia, Giovanni B., Italian surgeon, 1762–1815. SEE M.'s *fracture*.

Montgomery, William F., Irish obstetrician, 1797–1859. SEE M.'s *follicles*, under *follicle, glands*, under *gland, tubercles*, under *tubercle*.

mon·tic·u·lus, pl. **mon·tic·u·li** (mon-tik'yū-lŭs, -lī). **1.** Any slight rounded projection above a surface. **2.** The central portion of the superior vermis forming a projection on the surface of the cerebellum; its anterior and most prominent portion is called the culmen, its posterior sloping portion, the declive. [L. dim. of *mons*, mountain]
palmar monticuli, three small elevations in the distal palm corresponding to the window-like deficiencies in the distal palmar aponeurosis between the four longitudinal bundles and proximal to the superficial transverse metacarpal ligament.

mood (mūd). The pervasive feeling, tone, and internal emotional state of an individual which, when impaired, can markedly influence virtually all aspects of a person's behavior or his or her perception of external events.

mood swing. Oscillation of a person's emotional feeling tone between periods of euphoria and depression.

Moon, Henry, English surgeon, 1845–1892. SEE M.'s *molars*, under *molar*.

Moon, Robert C., U.S. ophthalmologist, 1844–1914. SEE Laurence-M.-Biedl *syndrome*.

Moore, Charles H., English surgeon, 1821–1870. SEE M.'s *method*.

Moore, Robert Foster, British ophthalmologist, 1878–1963. SEE M.'s lightning *streaks*, under *streak*.

Mooren, Albert, German ophthalmologist, 1828–1899. SEE M.'s *ulcer*.

Mooser, Hermann, Swiss pathologist in Mexico, *1891. SEE M. *bodies*, under *body*.

MOPP Acronym for *mechlorethamine, oncovin* (vincristine), procarbazine, and *p*rednisone, a chemotherapy regimen used in the treatment of Hodgkin's disease.

Morand, Sauveur F., French surgeon, 1697–1773. SEE M.'s *foot, spur.*

Morax, Victor, French ophthalmologist, 1866–1935. SEE *Moraxella;* Morax-Axenfeld *diplobacillus.*

Mor·ax·el·la (mōr'ak-sel'ă). A genus of obligately aerobic nonmotile bacteria (family Neisseriaceae) containing Gram-negative coccoids or short rods which usually occur in pairs. They do not produce acid from carbohydrates, are oxidase-positive and penicillin-susceptible, and are parasitic on the mucous membranes of man and other mammals. The type species is *M. lacunata.* [V. *Morax*]

M. bo'vis, a bacterial species causing pinkeye in cattle.

M. catarrha'lis, a species that causes upper respiratory tract infections, particularly in immunocompromised hosts; the type species of the genus *M.* SYN *Branhamella catarrhalis.*

M. kingae, SYN *Kingella kingae.*

M. lacuna'ta, a species causing conjunctivitis in man; it is the type species of the genus *M.* SYN Morax-Axenfeld diplobacillus.

M. anatipes'tifer, a species causing a respiratory disease in ducklings.

M. nonliquefa'ciens, a species found in the respiratory tract of man, especially in the nose; usually not pathogenic, but occasionally causes sinusitis.

M. osloen'sis, a species found in the genitourinary tract, blood, spinal and chest fluids, and nose; rarely found in the respiratory tract; usually not pathogenic, although some strains have been isolated from serious pathologic conditions in humans.

M. phenylpyru'vica, a species of unknown pathogenicity found in the genitourinary tract, blood, cerebrospinal fluid, and in pus from various lesions.

mor·bid (mōr'bid). **1.** Diseased or pathologic. **2.** In psychology, abnormal or deviant. [L. *morbidus,* ill, fr. *morbus,* disease]

mor·bid·i·ty (mōr-bid'i-tē). **1.** A diseased state. **2.** The ratio of sick to well in a community. SYN morbility. SEE ALSO morbidity *rate.* **3.** The frequency of the appearance of complications following a surgical procedure or other treatment.

puerperal m., illness arising during the first 10 days of the postpartum period, *i.e.,* a temperature of 38°C (100.4°F) or more on any two days of the first 10, excluding the first 24 hours.

mor·bif·ic (mōr-bif'ik). SYN pathogenic. [L. *morbus,* disease, + *facio,* to make]

mor·big·e·nous (mor-bij'ě-nŭs). SYN pathogenic. [L. *morbus,* disease, + G. *-gen,* producing]

mor·bil·i·ty (mor-bil'i-tē). SYN morbidity (2).

mor·bil·li (mōr-bil'ī). SYN measles (1). [Mediev. L. *morbillus,* dim. of L. *morbus,* disease]

mor·bil·li·form (mōr-bil'i-fōrm). Resembling measles (1). [see morbilli]

Mor·bil·li·vi·rus (mōr-bil'i-vī'rŭs). A genus of the family Paramyxoviridae, including measles, canine distemper, and bovine rinderpest viruses.

mor·bil·lous (mōr-bil'ŭs). Relating to measles (1). [see morbilli]

mor·bus (mōr'bŭs). SYN disease (1). [L. disease]

mor·bus Ad·di·so·nii (mōr'bus ad'ĭ-son). SYN chronic adrenocortical *insufficiency.*

mor·cel (mōr-sel'). To remove piecemeal. [Fr. *morceler,* to subdivide]

mor·cel·la·tion (mōr-se-lā'shŭn). Division into and removal of small pieces, as of a tumor. SYN morcellement. [Fr. *morceler,* to subdivide]

mor·celle·ment (mōr-sel-maw'). SYN morcellation. [Fr.]

mor·dant (mōr'dant). **1.** A substance capable of combining with a dye and the material to be dyed, thereby increasing the affinity or binding of the dye; *e.g.,* a m. commonly used to promote staining with hematoxylin is alum. **2.** To treat with a m. [L. *mordeo,* to bite]

mor. dict. Abbreviation for L. *more dicto,* as directed.

Morel, Benedict A., French psychiatrist, 1809–1873. SEE M.'s *ear;* Stewart-M. *syndrome.*

Mo·re·ra·stron·gy·lus cos·tar·i·cen·sis (mōr'er-ă-stron'ji-lŭs kos'tar-i-sen'sis). SYN *Angiostrongylus costaricensis.*

mo·res (mo'rāz). A concept used in the behavioral and social sciences to refer to centrally important and accepted folkways, and cultural norms which embody the fundamental moral views of a group. [L. pl. of *mos,* custom]

Morgagni, Giovanni B., Italian anatomist and pathologist, 1682–1771. SEE morgagnian *cyst;* M.'s *appendix, cartilage, caruncle, cataract, columns,* under *column, concha, crypts,* under *crypt, disease, foramen, fossa, fovea, frenum, globules,* under *globule, humor, hydatid, lacuna, liquor, nodule, prolapse, retinaculum, sinus, spheres,* under *sphere, syndrome, tubercle, valves,* under *valve, ventricle;* M.-Adams-Stokes *syndrome; frenulum* of M.

Morgan, Harry de R., British physician, 1863–1931. SEE M.'s *bacillus.*

mor·gan (M) (mōr'găn). The standard unit of genetic distance on the genetic map: the distance between two loci such that on average one crossing over will occur per meiosis; for working purposes, the centimorgan (0.01 M) is used. [T.H. *Morgan,* U.S. geneticist, 1866–1945]

Mor·gan·el·la (mōr'gan-el'-ah). A genus of Gram-negative, facultatively anaerobic, chemoorganotrophic, straight rods that are motile by peritrichous flagella. Found in feces of human beings, other animals, and reptiles. Can cause opportunistic infections of the blood, respiratory tract, wounds, and urinary tract.

M. morganii, type (and only) species of the genus *M.* SYN *Morgan's bacillus.*

Morgan's fold. See under fold.

morgue (mōrg). **1.** A building where unidentified dead are kept pending identification before burial. **2.** A building or room in a hospital or other facility where the dead are kept pending autopsy, burial, or cremation. SYN mortuary (2). [Fr.]

mo·ria (mōr'ē-ă). **1.** Rarely used term denoting foolishness or dullness of comprehension. SYN hebetude. **2.** Rarely used term for a mental state marked by frivolity, joviality, an inveterate tendency to jest, and inability to take anything seriously. [G. *mōria,* folly, fr. *mōros,* stupid, dull]

mor·i·bund (mōr'i-bŭnd). Dying; at the point of death. [L. *moribundus,* dying, fr. *morior,* to die]

mo·rin (mōr'in) [C.I. 75660]. 2',3,4',5,7-Pentahydroxyflavone; a natural yellow dye obtained from fustic and other members of the mulberry family and often associated with the dye maclurin; used as a fluorochrome for detection of metals, particularly aluminum. Fluorescent morinates are also formed with beryllium, gallium, indium, scandium, thorium, titanium, and zirconium.

Morison, James R., British surgeon, 1853–1939. SEE M.'s *pouch.*

Mörner, Karl A.H., Swedish chemist, 1855–1917. SEE M.'s *test.*

morn·ing glo·ry (mōr'ning glō'rē). **1.** SYN *Ipomoea rubrocoerulea* var. *praecox.* **2.** SYN *Rivea corymbosa.*

morn·ing glo·ry seeds. The seeds of morning glories, *Rivea corymbosa,* have been used for mind-altering purposes; hallucinogenic; intoxicant.

Moro, Ernst, German physician, 1874–1951. SEE M. *reflex.*

mo·ron (mōr'on). An obsolete term for a subclass of mental retardation or the individual classified therein. [G. *mōros,* stupid]

mo·rox·y·dine (mŏ-rok'si-dēn). Abitilguanide; 4-morpholine-carboximidoylguanidine; an antiviral agent.

△**morph-.** SEE morpho-.

mor·pha·zin·a·mide hy·dro·chlo·ride (mōr-fă-zin'ă-mīd). Morinamide hydrochloride; *N*-(morpholinomethyl)-pyrazinecarboxamide hydrochloride; an antituberculous agent.

mor·phea (mōr-fē'ă). Cutaneous lesion(s) characterized by indurated, slightly depressed plaques of thickened dermal fibrous tissue, of a whitish or yellowish white color surrounded by a pinkish or purplish halo. SYN localized scleroderma. [G. *morphē,* form, figure]

m. acroter'ica, m. confined chiefly to the extremities.

m. al'ba, m. in which there is reduction or absence of normal skin pigmentation.

mo

m. gutta'ta, small discrete, white, waxy, indurated lesions due to localized degenerative changes in the fibrous tissue. SYN white spot disease.

m. herpetifor'mis, m. distributed along the course of distribution of a nerve, similar to the distribution of the lesions of herpes zoster.

m. linea'ris, m. in which lesions are arranged in bands.

m. pigmento'sa, localized scleroderma in which there is an increase in pigmentation.

mor·pheme (mōr'fēm). The smallest linguistic unit with a meaning. [G. *morphē,* form + *-eme,* from *phoneme,* G. *phēmē,* utterance]

mor·phine (mōr'fēn, mōr-fēn'). $C_{17}H_{19}NO_3$; the major phenanthrene alkaloid of opium; contains 9 to 14% of anhydrous m. It produces a combination of depression and excitation in the central nervous system and some peripheral tissues; predominance of either central stimulation or depression depends upon the species and dose; repeated administration leads to the development of tolerance, physical dependence, and (if abused) psychic dependence. Used as an analgesic, sedative, and anxiolytic. [L. *Morpheus,* god of dreams or of sleep]

m. hydrochloride, white acicular or cubical crystals of bitter taste, soluble in about 25 parts of water.

m. sulfate (MS), m. used for formulation of tablets as well as solutions for parenteral, epidural, or intrathecal injection to relieve pain.

△**morpho-, morph-.** Form, shape, structure. [G. *morphē*]

mor·pho·gen·e·sis (mōr-fō-jen'ĕ-sis). **1.** Differentiation of cells and tissues in the early embryo which establishes the form and structure of the various organs and parts of the body. **2.** The ability of a molecule or group of molecules (particularly macromolecules) to assume a certain shape. [morpho- + G. *genesis,* production]

mor·pho·ge·net·ic (mōr'fō-jĕ-net'ik). Relating to morphogenesis.

mor·pho·log·ic (mōr-fō-loj'ik). Relating to morphology.

mor·phol·o·gy (mōr-fol'ō-jē). The science concerned with the configuration or the structure of animals and plants. [morpho- + G. *logos,* study]

mor·pho·met·ric (mōr'fō-met'rik). Pertaining to morphometry.

mor·phom·e·try (mōr-fom'ĕ-trē). The measurement of the form of organisms or their parts. [morpho- + G. *metron,* measure]

mor·phon (mōr'fon). Any one of the individual structures entering into the formation of an organism; a morphologic element, such as a cell. [G. *morphē,* form]

mor·pho·phys·i·ol·o·gy (mōr-fō-fiz-ē-ol'ō-jē). SYN functional anatomy.

mor·pho·sis (mōr-fō'sis). Mode of development of a part. [G. formation, act of forming]

mor·pho·syn·the·sis (mōr-fō-sin'thĕ-sis). An awareness of space and of body schema represented in the parietal lobes of the cerebral cortex. [morpho- + synthesis]

mor·pho·type (mōr'fō-tīp). An infrasubspecific group of bacterial strains distinguishable from other strains of the same species on the basis of morphologic characters which may or may not be associated with a change in serologic state. [morpho- + G. *typos,* stamp, model]

Morquio, Louis, Uruguayan physician, 1867–1935. SEE M.'s *disease, syndrome;* M.-Ullrich *disease;* Brailsford-Morquio *disease.*

mor·rhu·ate so·di·um (mōr'rū-āt). The sodium salts of the fatty acids of cod liver oil; a sclerosing agent used in the treatment of varicose veins, mixed with a local anesthetic. [fr. *Gadus morrhua,* cod]

Morrison, Ashton B., Irish pathologist in the U.S., *1922. SEE Verner-M. *syndrome.*

mors, gen. **mor·tis** (mōrz, mōr'tis). SYN death. [L.]

m. thy'mica, old term for sudden death in young children, usually the result of infection; formerly erroneously attributed to an enlarged thymus. SEE ALSO sudden infant death *syndrome.*

mor·si·ca·tio (mor-sik'ă-tē-ō). Habitual nibbling of the lips (labiorum), tongue (linguae), or buccal mucosa (buccarum); often produces a shaggy white lesion. [L. biting, fr. *mordeo,* to bite]

morsicatio buccarum (mor-sik'ă-tē-ă), White elevations of buccal mucosa caused by the pressure of molar teeth. [L. chewing of the cheeks]

mor. sol. Abbreviation for L. *more solito,* as usual, as customary.

mor·su·lus (mōr'sū-lŭs). SYN troche. [Mod. L. dim. of L. *morsus,* a bite]

mor·tal (mōr'tăl). **1.** Pertaining to or causing death. **2.** Destined to die. [L. *mortalis,* fr. *mors,* death]

mor·tal·i·ty (mōr-tal'i-tē). **1.** The state of being mortal. **2.** SYN mortality *rate.* **3.** A fatal outcome. [L. *mortalitas,* fr. *mors* (*mort-*), death]

perinatal m. (per'ē-nā-tal), m. around the time of birth, conventionally limited to the period from 28 weeks gestation to one week postnatal.

mor·tar (mōr'tăr). A vessel with rounded interior in which crude drugs and other substances are crushed or bruised by means of a pestle. [L. *mortarium*]

Mor·ti·er·el·la (mōr'tē-ĕ-rel'ă). A genus of saprophytic fungi (class Zygomycetes, family Mucoraceae) commonly found in nature and occasionally causing zygomycosis in humans.

mor·ti·fi·ca·tion (mōr'ti-fi-kā'shŭn). SYN gangrene (1). [L. *mors* (*mort-*), death, + *facio,* to make]

mor·ti·fied (mōr'ti-fīd). SYN gangrenous.

mor·tise (mōr'tēs). The seating for the talus formed by the union of the fibula and the tibia at the ankle joint. [M.E., fr. O.Fr., fr. Ar. *murtazz,* fastened]

Morton, Dudley J., U.S. orthopedist, 1884–1960. SEE M.'s *syndrome.*

Morton, Samuel G., U.S. physician, 1799–1851. SEE M.'s *plane.*

Morton, Thomas G., U.S. physician, 1835–1903. SEE M.'s *neuralgia.*

mor·tu·ary (mōr'tyū-ār-ē). **1.** Relating to death or to burial. **2.** SYN morgue. [L. *mortuus,* dead, part. adj. fr. *morior,* pp. *mortuus,* to die]

mor·u·la (mōr'ū-lă, mōr'yū-). The solid mass of blastomeres resulting from the early cleavage divisions of the zygote. In ova with little yolk, the m. is a spheroidal mass of cells; in forms with considerable yolk, the configuration of the m. stage is greatly modified. [Mod. L. dim. of L. *morus,* mulberry]

mor·u·la·tion (mōr-ū-lā'shŭn, mōr-yū-). Formation of the morula.

mor·u·loid (mōr'ū-loyd, mōr'yū-). **1.** Resembling a morula. **2.** Shaped like a mulberry.

Morvan, Augustin, French physician, 1819–1897. SEE M.'s *chorea, disease.*

mo·sa·ic (mō-zā'ik). **1.** Inlaid; resembling inlaid work. **2.** The juxtaposition in an organism of genetically different tissues; it may occur normally (as in lyonization, *q.v.*), or pathologically, as an occasional phenomenon. from somatic mutation (gene mosaicism), an anomaly of chromosome division resulting in two or more types of cells containing different numbers of chromosomes (chromosome mosaicism), or chimerism (cellular mosaicism). [Mod. L. *mosaicus, musaicus,* pertaining to the Muses, artistic]

mo·sa·i·cism (mō-zā'i-sizm). Condition of being mosaic (2).

cellular m., a chimerism in which a tissue contains cells from different zygotes; *e.g.,* in humans, involving erythrocytes.

chromosome m., SEE mosaic (2).

gene m., SEE mosaic (2).

germinal m., gonadal m., a state in which cells in a sector of a gonad are of a form not present in either parent, because of mutation in an intermediate progenitor of that sector.

Moschcowitz, Eli, U.S. physician, 1879–1964. SEE M.'s *disease;* Moschcowitz *test.*

mos·chus (mos'kŭs). Musk. [G. *moschos,* musk]

Mosenthal, Herman Otto, American physician, 1878–1954. SEE Mosenthal *test.*

Mosler, Karl F., German physician, 1831–1911. SEE M.'s *diabetes, sign.*

mos·qui·to, pl. **mos·qui·toes** (mŭs-kē'tō, -tōs). A blood-sucking dipterous insect of the family Culicidae. *Aedes, Anopheles, Culex, Mansonia,* and *Stegomyia* are the genera containing most of the species involved in the transmission of protozoan and other disease-producing parasites. [Sp. dim. of *mosca,* fly, fr. L. *musca,* a fly]

Moss, Gerald, U.S. physician, *1931. SEE M. *tube.*

Moss, Melvin L., U.S. oral pathologist, *1923. SEE Gorlin-Chaudhry-M. *syndrome.*

moss. **1.** Any low growing, delicate cryptogamous plant of the class Musci. **2.** Popularly, any one of a number of lichens and seaweeds. [A.S. *meōs*]

Ceylon m., a red seaweed; a source of agar.

club m., SYN lycopodium.

Iceland m., SYN cetraria.

Irish m., SYN chondrus (2).

muskeag m., SYN sphagnum m.

pearl m., SYN chondrus (2).

peat m., SYN sphagnum m.

sphagnum m., a highly absorbent m. used as a substitute for absorbent cotton or gauze in surgical dressing and sanitary napkins. SYN muskeag m., peat m.

Mosso, Angelo, Italian physiologist, 1846–1910. SEE M.'s *ergograph, sphygmomanometer.*

Motais, Ernst, French ophthalmologist, 1845–1913. SEE M.'s *operation.*

mote (mōt). A small particle; a speck. [A.S. *mot*]

blood m.'s, SYN hemoconia.

moth·er (mŭth'er). **1.** The female parent. **2.** Any cell or other structure from which other similar bodies are formed. [A.S. *mōdor*]

surrogate m., a woman who has been contracted with to carry a pregnancy for another woman or couple.

moth·er of vin·e·gar. In vinegar, the fungus of acetous fermentation appearing as a stringy sediment. [A.S. *modder,* mud]

mo·tile (mō'til). **1.** Having the power of spontaneous movement. **2.** Denoting the type of mental imagery in which one learns and recalls most readily that which has been felt. Cf. audile, visile. **3.** A person having such mental imagery. [see motion]

mo·til·in (mō-til'in). A 22-amino acid polypeptide occurring in duodenal mucosa as a controller of normal gastrointestinal motor activity; in minute (ng) doses it induces powerful motor activity increases in the fundic gland area and antral pouches of the stomach, with an increase in pepsin output from the former. [motility + -in]

mo·til·i·ty (mō-til'i-tē). The power of spontaneous movement.

mo·tion (mō'shŭn). **1.** A change of place or position. Cf. movement (1). **2.** SYN defecation. **3.** SYN stool. [L. *motio,* movement, fr. *moveo,* pp. *motus,* to move]

brownian m., SYN brownian *movement.*

continuous passive m. (CPM), a technique in which a joint, usually the knee, is moved constantly in a mechanical splint to prevent stiffness and to increase the range of motion.

mo·ti·va·tion (mō-ti-vā'shŭn). In psychology, the aggregate of all the individual motives, needs, and drives operative in an individual at any given moment which influence will and cause behavior. [ML. *motivus,* moving]

extrinsic m., the search for satisfaction, or to avoid dissatisfaction, through non-task aspects of the environment such as seeking comfort, safety, and security from others or through the efforts of others.

intrinsic m., derivation of personal satisfaction through self-initiated achievement and behavior.

personal m., an individual's predispositions and expectations that give meaning and direction to personality functioning.

mo·tive (mō'tiv). **1.** An acquired predisposition, need, or specific state of tension within an individual which arouses, maintains, and directs behavior toward a goal. SYN learned drive. **2.** The reason attributed to or given by an individual for a behavioral act. Cf. instinct. [L. *moveo,* to move, to set in motion]

achievement m., an acquired, chronic need to succeed in the face of recognizable obstacles; its strength is usually diagnosed from recurring themes in stories told by the individual while taking a thematic apperception test or from other assessment instruments used by clinical psychologists.

mastery m., an acquired need to be assertive, to stand out in a crowd, to be dominant.

mo·to·fa·cient (mō-tō-fā'shent). Causing motion; denoting the second phase of muscular activity in which actual movement is produced. [L. *motus,* motion, + *facio,* to make]

mo·to·neu·ron (mō'tō-nū'ron). SYN motor *neuron.*

mo·tor (mō'ter). **1.** In anatomy and physiology, denoting those neural structures which by the impulses generated and transmitted by them cause muscle fibers or pigment cells to contract, or glands to secrete. SEE ALSO motor *cortex,* motor *endplate,* motor *neuron.* **2.** In psychology, denoting the organism's overt reaction to a stimulus (motor response). [L. a mover, fr. *moveo,* to move]

m. oc'uli, SYN oculomotor *nerve.*

plastic m., an artificial point of attachment on an amputation stump to which is fastened the cord or extensor by which movement is transmitted to an artificial limb; used in cinematization.

mo·tor·i·al (mō-tōr'ē-ăl). Relating to motion, to a motor nerve or the motor nucleus.

mo·tor·me·ter (mō'ter-mē'ter). A device for determining the amount, force, and rapidity of movement.

mot·tle (mot'tl). Fine inhomogeneity of an area of generally uniform opacity on a photograph or radiograph; noise. [fr. *motley,* fr. M.E. *mot,* speck]

quantum m., m. caused by the statistical fluctuation of the number of photons absorbed by the intensifying screens to form the light image on the film; faster screens produce more quantum m.

mot·tling (mot'ling). An area of skin comprised of macular lesions of varying shades or colors. [E. *motley,* variegated in color]

Motulsky dye re·duc·tion test. See under test.

mou·lage (mū-lazh'). A reproduction in wax of a skin lesion, tumor, or other pathologic state. [F. a molding]

mould (mōld). SYN mold.

moult (mōlt). SYN molt.

mound·ing (mownd'ing). SYN myoedema.

Mounier-Kuhn, P., 20th century French physician. SEE Mounier-Kuhn *syndrome.*

mount (mownt). **1.** To prepare for microscopic examination. **2.** To climb on for purposes of copulation.

mount·ing (mownt'ing). In dentistry, the laboratory procedure of attaching the maxillary and/or mandibular cast to an articulator.

split cast m., (1) a cast with key grooves on its base, mounted on an articulator for the purpose of easy removal and accurate replacement; split remounting metal plates may be used instead of grooves in casts; **(2)** a means for testing the accuracy of articulator adjustment.

mourn (mōrn). To express grief or sorrow as a result of loss. In psychoanalysis, mourning is the frequently unexpressed process of responding to loss of a cathectic object which, in contrast to melancholia, usually does not involve loss of self-esteem. [O.E. *murnan*]

mouse (mows). A small rodent belonging to the genus *Mus.*

multimammate m., an African rodent, *Praomys natalensis,* widely used in cancer research.

New Zealand mice, inbred strains of mice, either black (NZB) or white (NZW), unique among strains used in experimental immunology because of their proclivity to spontaneous immunologic abnormalities and disorders including systemic lupus erythematosus similar to that found in humans.

nude m., a hairless mutant m. with thymic hypoplasia, lacking T cells.

mouse·pox (mows'poks). SYN ectromelia (2).

mouth (mowth). **1.** SYN oral *cavity.* **2.** The opening, usually the external opening, of a cavity or canal. SEE os (2), ostium, orifice, stoma (2). [A.S. *mūth*]

mo

carp m., a m. like that of the carp, with downturning of the corners; observed in Cornelia de Lange syndrome and Silver-Russel dwarfism.

denture sore m., mucosal erythema underlying a denture base, usually representing inflammation caused by ill-fitting dentures, poor oral hygiene, or *Candida albicans*.

parrot m., a condition of the horse in which the upper jaw is relatively longer than the lower, resulting in elongation of the upper incisors.

scabby m., SYN orf.

sore m., SEE soremouth.

tapir m., protrusion of the lips due to weakness of the orbicularis oris muscles; seen with some dystrophies. SYN bouche de tapir.

trench m., SYN necrotizing ulcerative *gingivitis*.

m. of the womb, SYN external *os* of uterus.

mouth guard. A pliable plastic device, adapted to cover the maxillary teeth, which is worn to reduce potential injury to oral structures during participation in contact sports.

mouth stick. A prosthesis which is held by the teeth and utilized by handicapped persons to perform such actions as typing, painting, and lifting small objects.

mouth·wash. A medicated liquid used for cleaning the mouth and treating diseased states of its mucous membranes. SYN collutorium, collutory.

move·ment (mūv′ment). **1.** The act of motion; said of the entire body or of one or more of its members or parts. **2.** SYN stool. **3.** SYN defecation. [L. *moveo*, pp. *motus*, to move]

active m., m. effected by the organism itself, unaided by external influences.

adversive m., a rotation of the eyes, head, or trunk about the long axis of the body.

after-m., SEE aftermovement.

ameboid m., the m. characteristic of leukocytes and protozoan organisms of the superclass Rhizopoda. SEE ALSO streaming m., filopodium, lobopodium.

assistive m., in massage, a m. which the partially paralyzed muscle of the patient would be unable to perform unaided but which is effected with the graduated assistance of the operator.

associated m.'s, normal involuntary limp m.'s that accompany voluntary movement, *e.g.,* arm swing with walking.

Bennett m., the bodily lateral m. or lateral shift of the mandible during a laterotrusive m.

border m.'s, any extreme compass of mandibular m. limited by bone, ligaments, or soft tissues; usually applied to horizontal mandibular m.'s.

border tissue m.'s, the action of the muscles and other tissues adjacent to the borders of a denture.

bowel m., defecation.

brownian m., erratic, nondirectional, zigzag m. observed by ultramicroscope in certain colloidal solutions and by microscope in suspensions of light particulate matter that results from the jostling or bumping of the larger particles by the molecules in the suspending medium which are regarded as being in continuous motion. SYN brownian motion, brownian-Zsigmondy m., molecular m., pedesis.

brownian-Zsigmondy m., SYN brownian m.

cardinal ocular m.'s, eye rotations to the right and left, upward to the right and left, and downward to the right and left, to diagnose positions of gaze.

choreic m., an involuntary spasmodic twitching or jerking in groups of muscles not associated in the production of definite purposeful m.'s.

ciliary m., the rhythmic, sweeping m. of epithelial cell cilia, of ciliate protozoans, or the sculling m. of flagella, effected possibly by the alternate contraction and relaxation of contractile threads (myoids) on one side of the cilium or flagellum.

circus m., a contraction or excitation wave traveling continuously in circular fashion around a ring of muscle or through the wall of the heart. SYN circus rhythm.

cogwheel ocular m.'s, loose, jerky ocular rotations replacing smooth following rotations.

conjugate m. of eyes, rotation of the two eyes in the same direction. SEE ALSO version (4).

decomposition of m., a manifestation of cerebellar disease in which a muscular movement is not carried out smoothly but in a series of component motions.

disconjugate m. of eyes, rotation of the two eyes in opposite directions, as in convergence or divergence.

drift m.'s, SYN drifts.

fetal m., the m. characteristic of the fetus *in utero;* usually commences between the sixteenth and eighteenth weeks of pregnancy. SEE ALSO quickening.

fixational ocular m., rotation of the eyes during voluntary fixation on an object; tremors, flicks, and drifts occur.

flick m.'s, SYN flicks.

free mandibular m.'s, (1) any mandibular m.'s made without tooth interference; **(2)** any uninhibited m.'s of the mandible.

functional mandibular m.'s, all natural, proper, or characteristic m.'s of the mandible made during speech, mastication, yawning, swallowing, and other associated m.'s.

fusional m., a reflex m. that tends to move the visual axes to the object of fixation so that stereoscopic vision is possible.

hinge m., an opening or closing m. of the mandible on the hinge axis.

intermediary m.'s, in dentistry, all m.'s between the extremes of mandibular excursions.

lateral m., in dentistry, m. of the mandible to the side.

Magnan's trombone m., an involuntary forward and back m. of the tongue when it is drawn out of the mouth; may be seen in several basal ganglia disorders.

mandibular m., (1) m.'s of the lower jaw; **(2)** all changes in position of which the mandible is capable.

mass m., SYN mass *peristalsis*.

molecular m., SYN brownian m.

morphogenetic m., the streaming of cells in the early embryo to form tissues or organs.

muscular m., m. caused by the contraction of the myofibrils of the muscle cells.

neurobiotactic m., the streaming of nerve cells toward the area from which they receive the most stimuli.

non-rapid eye m. (NREM), slow oscillation of the eyes during sleep.

opening m., in dentistry, m. of the mandible executed during jaw separation.

paradoxical m. of eyelids, spontaneous, involuntary elevation or lowering of the eyelids, associated with m. of extraocular muscles or muscles of mastication (external pterygoids). SEE jaw winking.

passive m., m. imparted to an organism or any of its parts by external agency; m. of any joint effected by the hand of another person, or by mechanical means, without participation of the subject himself.

pendular m., a to-and-fro m. of the intestine, without any propelling or peristaltic action, whereby the contents are churned and thoroughly mixed with the intestinal ferments.

protoplasmic m., m. produced by the inherent power of contraction and relaxation of protoplasm; such m.'s are of three kinds: muscular, streaming, and ciliary.

rapid eye m.'s (REM), symmetrical quick scanning m.'s of the eyes occurring many times during sleep in clusters for 5 to 60 minutes; associated with dreaming.

reflex m., an involuntary m. resulting from a sensory stimulus.

resistive m., in massage, a m. made by the patient against the efforts of the operator, or one forced by the operator against the resistance of the patient.

saccadic m., (1) a quick rotation of the eyes from one fixation point to another as in reading; **(2)** the rapid correction m. of a jerky nystagmus, as in labyrinthine and optokinetic nystagmus.

streaming m., the form of m. characteristic of the protoplasm of leukocytes, amebae, and other unicellular organisms; it involves the massing of the protoplasm at a point where surface pressure is least and its extrusion in the form of a pseudopod; the protoplasm may return to the body of the cell, resulting in the retraction of the pseudopod, or the entire mass may flow into the latter and thereby result in locomotion of the cell.

Swedish m.'s, a form of kinesitherapy in which certain systematized m.'s of the body and limbs are regulated by resistance made by an attendant. SYN Swedish gymnastics.

translatory m., the motion of the body at any instant when all points within the body are moving at the same velocity and in the same direction.

vermicular m., SYN peristalsis.

Mowry's col·loi·dal iron stain. See under stain.

moxa (mok′să). A cone or cylinder of cotton wool or other combustible material, placed on the skin and ignited in order to produce counterirritation. SEE ALSO moxibustion. [Jap. *moe kusa*, burning herb]

mox·a·lac·tam. A third-generation cephalosporin with a broad spectrum of antibacterial action; causes bleeding disorders which limit its use.

mox·a·lac·tam di·so·di·um (moks-ă-lak′tam). $C_{20}H_{18}N_6$-Na_2O_9S; a broad spectrum β-lactam antibiotic related to the penicillins and cephalosporins.

mox·i·bus·tion (mok-sĭ-bŭs′chŭn). Burning of herbal agents, such as moxa, on the skin as a counterirritant in the treatment of disease; a component of traditional Chinese and Japanese medicine.

mox·i·sy·lyte (mok-sĭ′si-līt). 5-(2-Dimethylaminoethoxy)-carvacrol acetate; used as an α-adrenergic blocking agent for treatment of peripheral vascular disease. SYN thymoxamine.

m.p. 1. Abbreviation for melting *point*. **2.** Abbreviation for [L] *modo praescripto*, in the manner prescribed.

MPD Abbreviation for maximum permissible *dose*.

MPR Abbreviation for mannose-6-phosphate *receptors*, under *receptor*.

MPS Abbreviation for mononuclear phagocyte *system*.

MPTP. *N*-Methyl-4-phenyl-1,2,3,6-tetrahydropyridine; piperidine derivative which causes irreversible symptoms of parkinsonism in humans and monkeys. A by-product of illicitly manufactured meperidine that caused numerous cases of parkinsonism. Used as an experimental tool in research on parkinsonism.

MQ Former abbreviation for menaquinone; now MK.

M.R.C.P. Abbreviation for Member of the Royal College of Physicians (of England).

M.R.C.P.(E) Abbreviation for Member of the Royal College of Physicians (Edinburgh).

M.R.C.P.(I) Abbreviation for Member of the Royal College of Physicians (Ireland).

M.R.C.S. Abbreviation for Member of the Royal College of Surgeons (England).

M.R.C.S.(E) Abbreviation for Member of the Royal College of Surgeons (Edinburgh).

M.R.C.S.(I) Abbreviation for Member of the Royal College of Surgeons (Ireland).

M.R.C.V.S. Abbreviation for Member of the Royal College of Veterinary Surgeons (of the United Kingdom).

MRD, mrd Abbreviation for minimal reacting *dose*.

MRF Abbreviation for melanotropin-releasing *factor*.

MRH Abbreviation for melanotropin-releasing *hormone*.

MRI Abbreviation for magnetic resonance *imaging*.

mRNA Abbreviation for messenger RNA. See entries under ribonucleic acid.

MS Abbreviation for multiple *sclerosis*; *morphine* sulfate; mitral *stenosis*; and myasthenic *syndrome* (Lambert-Eaton syndrome).

ms Abbreviation for millisecond.

M.S.D. Abbreviation for Master of Science in Dentistry.

msec Abbreviation for millisecond.

MSG Abbreviation for monosodium glutamate.

MSH Abbreviation for melanocyte-stimulating *hormone*.

MTBE Abbreviation for methyl-*tert*-butyl ether.

MTF Abbreviation for modulation transfer *function*.

m.u. Abbreviation for mouse *unit*.

mu (myū). Twelfth letter of the Greek alphabet, μ.

mu·case (myū′kās). SYN mucinase.

Much, Hans C.R., German physician, 1880–1932. SEE M.'s *bacillus*.

Mucha, Victor, Austrian dermatologist, 1877–1919. SEE M.-Habermann *disease, syndrome*.

muci-. Mucous, mucin. SEE ALSO muco-, myxo-. [L. *mucus*]

mu·ci·car·mine (myū-si-kar′mĭn). A red stain containing aluminum chloride and carmine; used to detect epithelial mucins and mucin-secreting adenocarcinomas; also used to demonstrate the capsule of *Cryptococcus neoformans* and other fungi.

mu·cid (myū′sid). SYN muciparous.

mu·cif·er·ous (myū-sif′er-ŭs). SYN muciparous.

mu·ci·fi·ca·tion (myū′si-fi-kā′shŭn). A change produced in the vaginal mucosa of spayed experimental animals following stimulation with estrogen; characterized by the formation of tall columnar cells secreting mucus. [L. *mucus + facio,* to make]

mu·ci·form (myū′si-fōrm). Resembling mucus. SYN blennoid, mucoid (2).

mu·cig·e·nous (myū-sij′ĕ-nŭs). SYN muciparous.

mu·ci·he·ma·te·in (myū-si-hē′mă-tē-in). A violet-blue staining fluid containing aluminum chloride and hematein; used to detect connective tissue mucins.

mu·ci·lage (myū′si-lij). A pharmacopeial preparation consisting of a solution in water of the mucilaginous principles of vegetable substances; used as a soothing application to the mucous membranes and in the preparation of official and extemporaneous mixtures. [L. *mucilago*]

mu·ci·lag·i·nous (myū-sĭ-laj′i-nŭs). **1.** Resembling mucilage; *i.e.,* adhesive, viscid, sticky. **2.** SYN muciparous.

mu·cin (myū′sin). A secretion containing carbohydrate-rich glycoproteins such as that from the goblet cells of the intestine, the submaxillary glands, and other mucous glandular cells; it is also present in the ground substance of connective tissue, especially mucous connective tissue, is soluble in alkaline water, and is precipitated by acetic acid.

gastric m., a white or yellowish powder which forms a viscous opalescent fluid with water, prepared from mucosa of hog's stomach by pepsin-hydrochloric acid digestion and precipitation of the supernatant fluid with 60% alcohol; used in peptic ulcer for its protective and lubricating action.

mu·cin·ase (myū′si-nās). A term specifically applied to hyaluronate lyase, hyaluronoglucosaminidase, and hyaluronoglucuronidase (hyaluronidases), but more loosely to any enzyme that hydrolyzes mucopolysaccharide substances (mucins). SYN mucase, mucopolysaccharidase.

mu·ci·ne·mia (myū-si-nē′mē-ă). The presence of mucin in the circulating blood. SYN myxemia. [mucin + G. *haima,* blood]

mu·cin·o·gen (myū′sin-ō-jen). A glycoprotein that forms mucin through the imbibition of water. [mucin + G. *-gen,* producing]

mu·ci·noid (myū′si-noyd). **1.** SYN mucoid (1). **2.** Resembling mucin.

mu·ci·no·lyt·ic (myū′si-nō-lit′ik). Capable of bringing about the hydrolysis of mucin, as by a mucinase.

mu·ci·no·sis (myū-si-nō′sis). A condition in which mucin is present in the skin in excessive amounts, or in abnormal distribution; classified as: **metabolic m.,** diffuse or pretibial myxedema, lichen myxedematosus, gargoylism; **secondary m.,** degeneration in tumors; **localized m.,** follicular, papular, plaque-like, focal, and myxoid or synovial cyst. [mucin + G. *-osis,* condition]

cutaneous focal m., flesh-colored papules of the skin, composed of homogenous mucinous material with scattered fibroblasts.

follicular m., a relatively uncommon benign eruption of discrete erythematous lesions progressing to alopecia on the face or scalp, usually in young people, in which there are cystic mucinous changes in the epithelium of hair follicles in the involved area; may also develop in mycosis fungoides.

oral focal m., an area of myxomatous connective tissue; the mucosal counterpart of cutaneous focal m.

papular m., SYN *lichen* myxedematosus.

reticular erythematous m. (REM), SYN REM *syndrome*.

mu

mu·ci·nous (myū′si-nŭs). Relating to or containing mucin. SYN mucoid (3).

mu·ci·nu·ria (myū-si-nū′rē-ă). The presence of mucin in the urine. [mucin + G. *ouron,* urine]

mu·cip·a·rous (myū-sip′ă-rŭs). Producing or secreting mucus. SYN blennogenic, blennogenous, mucid, muciferous, mucigenous, mucilaginous (2). [mucin + L. *pario,* to bring forth, bear]

mu·ci·tis (myū-sī′tis). Inflammation of a mucous membrane.

Muckle, T.J., 20th century Canadian pediatrician. SEE M.-Wells *syndrome.*

⌂**muco-.** Mucous, mucous (mucous membrane). SEE ALSO muci-, myxo-. [L. *mucus*]

mu·co·cele (myū′kō-sēl). SYN mucous *cyst.* 3. A retention cyst of the salivary gland, lacrimal sac, paranasal sinuses, appendix, or gallbladder. [muco- + G. *kēlē,* tumor, hernia]

mu·coc·la·sis (myū-kok′lă-sis). Denudation of any mucous surface. [muco- + G. *klasis,* a breaking off]

mu·co·co·li·tis (myū-kō-kō-lī′tis). SYN mucous *colitis.*

mu·co·col·pos (myū-kō-kol′pos). Presence of mucus in the vagina. [muco- + G. *kolpos,* vagina]

mu·co·cu·ta·ne·ous (myū′kō-kyū-tā′nē-ŭs). Relating to mucous membrane and skin; denoting the line of junction of the two at the nasal, oral, vaginal, and anal orifices. SYN cutaneomucosal.

mu·co·en·ter·i·tis (myū′kō-en-ter-ī′tis). **1.** Inflammation of the intestinal mucous membrane. **2.** SYN mucomembranous *enteritis.*

mu·co·ep·i·der·moid (myū′kō-ep-i-der′moyd). Denoting a mixture of mucus-secreting and epithelial cells, as in m. carcinoma.

mu·co·glob·u·lin (myū-kō-glob′yū-lin). A glycoprotein or mucoprotein in which the protein component is a globulin.

mu·coid (myū′koyd). **1.** General term for a mucin, mucoprotein, or glycoprotein. SYN mucinoid (1). **2.** SYN muciform. **3.** SYN mucinous. [mucus + G. *eidos,* appearance]

mu·co·lip·i·do·sis, pl. **mu·co·lip·i·do·ses** (myū′kō-lip-i-dō′sis, -sēz). Any of a group of lysosomal storage diseases in which symptoms of visceral and mesenchymal mucopolysaccharide, glycoprotein, oligosaccharide, or glycolipid storage are present; clinically, they bear a superficial resemblance to the mucopolysaccharidoses; autosomal recessive inheritance. [muco- + lipid + *-osis,* condition]

m. I [MIM*256550], m. somewhat like a mild form of Hurler's *syndrome* with mild dysostosis multiplex, and moderate mental retardation due to neuraminidase deficiency; autosomal recessive inheritance. SYN lipomucopolysaccharidosis.

m. II [MIM*252500], m. of early onset and with severe symptoms like those in Hurler's *syndrome* but with normal urinary mucopolysaccharides, vacuolated lymphocytes, and inclusion bodies in cultured fibroblasts (I-cells); lysosomal enzymes are increased in serum, spinal fluid, and urine; associated with a deficiency of *N*-acetylglucosaminyl-1-phosphotransferase; autosomal recessive inheritance. SYN I-cell disease, inclusion cell disease.

m. III [MIM*252600, MIM*252600], m. with mild Hurler-like symptoms, restricted joint mobility, short stature, mild mental retardation, and dysplastic skeletal changes, especially of the hip; aortic and mitral valve disease are often present; associated with a deficiency of UDP-*N*-acetyl glucosamine; lysosomal enzyme *N*-acetylglucosaminyl-1-phosphotransferase; autosomal recessive inheritance. SYN pseudo-Hurler polydystrophy, pseudopolydystrophy.

m. IV [MIM*252650], psychomotor retardation with cloudy corneas and retinal degeneration, with inclusion cells in cultured fibroblasts; may be due to a deficiency of neuramidase, but details are uncertain; autosomal recessive inheritance.

mu·col·y·sis (myū-kol′i-sis). The solution, digestion, or liquefaction of mucus. [muco- + G. *lysis,* dissolution]

mu·co·lyt·ic (myū-kō-lit′ik). Capable of dissolving, digesting, or liquefying mucus.

mu·co·mem·bra·nous (myū′kō-mem′bră-nŭs). Relating to a mucous membrane.

mu·co·pep·tide (myū-kō-pep′tīd). A peptide found in combination with polysaccharides containing muramic or sialic acids.

m. glycohydrolase, SYN lysozyme.

mu·co·per·i·os·te·al (myū′kō-per-ē-os′tē-ăl). Relating to mucoperiosteum.

mu·co·per·i·os·te·um (myū′kō-per-ē-os′tē-ŭm). Mucous membrane and periosteum so intimately united as to form practically a single membrane, as that covering the hard palate.

mu·co·pol·y·sac·cha·ri·dase (myū′kō-pol-ē-sak′ă-ri-dās). SYN mucinase, β-*d*-glucuronidase *deficiency.*

mu·co·pol·y·sac·cha·ride (myū′kō-pol-ē-sak′ă-rīd). General term for a protein-polysaccharide complex obtained from proteoglycans and containing as much as 95% polysaccharide; m.'s include the blood group substances. A more modern term is glycosaminoglycan, as all of the known six classes contain major amounts of D-glucosamine and D-galactosamine.

mu·co·pol·y·sac·cha·ri·do·sis, mu·co·pol·y·sac·cha·ri·do·ses (myū′kō-pol-ē-sak′ă-ri-dō′sis, -sēz) [MIM*252700 to MIM* 253230]. Any of a group of lysosomal storage diseases that have in common a disorder in metabolism of mucopolysaccharides, as evidenced by excretion of various mucopolysaccharides in urine and infiltration of these substances into connective tissue, with resulting various defects of bone, cartilage, and connective tissue.

type IH m., SYN Hurler's *syndrome.*

type I H/S m., SYN Hurler-Scheie *syndrome.*

type IS m., SYN Scheie's *syndrome.*

type II m., SYN Hunter's *syndrome.*

type III m., SYN Sanfilippo's *syndrome.*

type IVA, B m., SYN Morquio's *syndrome.*

type V m., former designation for Scheie's *syndrome.*

type VI m., SYN Maroteaux-Lamy *syndrome.*

type VII m., SYN Sly *syndrome.*

type VIII m., SYN Sly *syndrome.* **(1)** SYN Di Ferrante *syndrome.*

mu·co·pol·y·sac·cha·ri·du·ria (myū′kō-pol-ē-sak′ă-ri-dū′rē-ă). The excretion of mucopolysaccharides in the urine.

mu·co·pro·tein (myū-kō-prō′tēn). General term for a protein-polysaccharide complex, usually implying that the protein component is the major part of the complex, in contradistinction to mucopolysaccharide; m.'s include the α_1- and α_2-globulins of serum (and others). Sometimes called glycoproteins, although this term usually refers to those m.'s containing less than 4% carbohydrate.

Tamm-Horsfall m., the matrix of urinary casts derived from the secretion of renal tubular cells.

mu·co·pu·ru·lent (myū-kō-pū′rū-lent). Pertaining to an exudate that is chiefly purulent (pus), but containing relatively conspicuous proportions of mucous material. SYN puromucous.

mu·co·pus (myū′kō-pŭs). A mucopurulent discharge; a mixture of mucous material and pus. SYN mycopus.

Mu·cor (myū′kōr). A genus of fungi (class Zygomycetes, family Mucoraceae), most species of which are saprobic; several are pathogenic and may cause zygomycosis in humans.

Mu·co·ra·ce·ae (myū′kōr-a′sē-ē). A family of fungi (class Zygomycetes) comprised of terrestrial, aquatic, and sometimes parasitic organisms; includes the genera *Mucor, Absidia, Rhizopus,* and *Mortierella.* Although the various species of the four genera are ordinarily saprobic, free-living forms, some of them cause zygomycosis (mucormycosis) in humans. [L. *mucor,* mold]

mu·cor·my·co·sis (myū′kōr-mī-kō′sis). SYN zygomycosis.

mu·co·sa (myū-kō′să). a mucous tissue lining various tubular structures, consisting of epithelium, lamina, propria, and, in the digestive tract, a layer of smooth muscle. SYN tunica mucosa [NA], membrana mucosa, mucosal tunics, mucous tunics, mucous membranes. [L. fem. of *mucosus,* mucous]

alveolar m., the mucous membrane apical to the attached gingiva.

m. of auditory tube, the lining coat of the auditory tube. SYN tunica mucosa tubae auditivae [NA].

m. of bronchi, the inner coat of the bronchi. SYN tunica mucosa bronchiorum [NA].

m. of ductus deferens, the inner layer of the ductus deferens. SYN tunica mucosa ductus deferentis [NA].

esophageal m., the inner coat of the esophagus. SYN tunica mucosa esophagi [NA].

m. of female urethra, the inner mucosal layer of the female urethra. SYN tunica mucosa urethrae femininae [NA].

m. of gallbladder, the inner coat of the gallbladder. SYN tunica mucosa vesicae biliaris [NA], tunica mucosa vesicae felleae☆ [NA].

gastric m., the mucous layer of the stomach. SYN tunica mucosa gastrica [ventriculi] [NA].

gingival m., that portion of the oral mucous membrane that covers and is attached to the necks of the teeth and the alveolar process of the jaws; it is demarcated from lining m. on the facial aspect by a clearly defined line which marks the mucogingival junction, and, in contrast to the lining m., is keratinized and lighter in color; on the palatal surface, the gingiva blends imperceptibly with the palatal m.

laryngeal m., the mucous coat of the larynx. SYN tunica mucosa laryngis [NA].

lingual m., mucous membrane of the tongue, the mucosa of the dorsum of the tongue appears velvety due to the presence of vast numbers of papillae; that of the inferior surface is smooth and thinner. SYN tunica mucosa linguae [NA].

nasal m., the mucous membrane of the nose; it is continuous with the skin in the vestibule of the nose and with the mucosa of the nasopharynx, the paranasal sinuses, and the nasolacrimal duct, and contains goblet cells; it is subdivided into the regio olfactoria and regio respiratoria. SYN tunica mucosa nasi [NA], membrana pituitosa, pituitary membrane, schneiderian membrane.

olfactory m., epithelium containing nerve cells whose axons form the filaments of the olfactory nerve; the lamina propria contains numerous olfactory glands (Bowman) that open to the surface.

oral m., the mucous membrane of the oral cavity, including the gingiva. SYN tunica mucosa oris [NA].

pharyngeal m., the mucous coat of the pharynx. SYN tunica mucosa pharyngis [NA].

respiratory m., pseudostratified ciliated columnar epithelium with goblet cells and a lamina propria containing, in addition to connective tissue, numerous seromucous glands and in some regions many thin-walled veins which line the airways. SEE *region* of respiratory mucosa.

m. of seminal vesicle, the mucous membrane of the seminal vesicle. SYN tunica mucosa vesiculae seminalis [NA].

m. of small intestine, the mucous coat of the small intestine. SYN tunica mucosa intestini tenuis [NA].

tracheal m., the inner mucous layer of the trachea. SYN tunica mucosa tracheae [NA].

m. of tympanic cavity, the mucous layer of the tympanic cavity and the structures in it. SYN tunica mucosa cavitatis tympani [NA], mucous membrane of tympanic cavity.

m. of ureter, the inner layer of the ureter. SYN tunica mucosa ureteris [NA].

m. of urinary bladder, the inner coat of the urinary bladder. SYN tunica mucosa vesicae urinariae [NA].

m. of uterine tube, the mucous layer of the uterine tube. SYN tunica mucosa tubae uterinae [NA].

vaginal m., the mucous membrane of the vagina. SYN tunica mucosa vaginae [NA].

mu·co·sal (myū-kō′săl). Relating to the mucosa or mucous membrane.

mu·co·san·guin·e·ous, mu·co·san·guin·o·lent (myū′kō-sang-gwin′ē-ŭs, -ŏ-lent). Pertaining to an exudate or other fluid material that has a relatively high content of blood and mucus. [muco- + L. *sanguis,* blood]

mu·co·sec·to·my (myū-kō-sek′tō-me). Excision of the mucosa, usually of the rectum prior to ileoanal anastomosis for treatment of ulcerative colitis. [mucosa + G. *ektomē,* excision]

mu·co·se·rous (myū-kō-sē′rŭs). Pertaining to an exudate or secretion that consists of both mucus and serum or a watery component.

mu·co·stat·ic (myū-kō-stat′ik). **1.** Denoting the normal relaxed condition of mucosal tissues covering the jaws. **2.** Arresting the secretion of mucus. [muco- + G. *stasis,* a standing]

mu·cous (myū′kŭs). Relating to mucus or a m. membrane. [L. *mucosus,* mucous, fr. *mucus*]

mu·co·vis·ci·do·sis (myū′kō-vis-i-dō′sis). SYN cystic *fibrosis.* [myco- + G. *toxikon,* poison, + -osis, condition]

mu·cro, pl. **mu·cron·es** (myū′krō, myū-krō′nēz). A term applied to the pointed extremity of a structure. [L. point, sword]

m. cor′dis, obsolete term for *apex* of heart.

m. ster′ni, SYN xiphoid *process.*

mu·cron (myū′kron). Attachment organelle of aseptate gregarines, similar to an epimerite; the latter is set off from the rest of the gregarine body by a septum.

mu·cro·nate (myū′krō-nāt). SYN xiphoid. [L. *mucronatus,* pointed]

mu·cus (myū′kŭs). The clear viscid secretion of the mucous membranes, consisting of mucin, epithelial cells, leukocytes, and various inorganic salts suspended in water. [L.]

glairy m., SYN pituita.

Muehrcke, Robert C. SEE M.'s *lines,* under *line.*

Mueller. U.S. manufacturer of surgical instruments. SEE Mueller electronic *tonometer.*

Muel·le·ri·us cap·il·la·ris (myū-ler′ē-ŭs kap-i-lā′ris). One of the most common species of hair lungworms (subfamily Protostrongylinae) of sheep, goats, and deer. It is smaller than *Dictyocaulus,* inhabits the smaller bronchi and lung parenchyma, and is relatively nonpathogenic to its host.

Muir, E. G. SEE M.-Torre *syndrome.*

Mules, Philip H., English ophthalmologist, 1843–1905. SEE M.'s *operation.*

mu·li·e·bria (mū′lē-ē′brē-ă). The female genital organs. [L. neut pl. of *muliebris,* relating to *mulier,* a woman]

Müller, Friedrich von, German physician, 1858–1941. SEE M.'s *sign.*

Müller, Heinrich, German anatomist, 1820–1864. SEE M.'s radial *cells,* under *cell, fibers,* under *fiber, muscle, trigone.*

Müller, Hermann F., German histologist, 1866–1898. SEE formol-M. *fixative;* M.'s *fixative.*

Müller, Johannes P., German anatomist, physiologist, and pathologist, 1801–1858. SEE M.'s *capsule, duct, law, maneuver, tubercle.*

Müller, Leopold, Czechoslovakian ophthalmologist, 1862–1936.

Müller, Peter, German obstetrician, 1836–1922. SEE Hillis-M. *maneuver.*

Müller, Walther, 20th century German physicist. SEE Geiger-M. *counter, tube.*

mül·le·ri·an (myū-ler′ē-an). Attributed to or described by Johannes Müller.

mul·ling (mŭl′ing). In dentistry, the final step of mixing dental amalgam, when the triturated mass is kneaded to complete the amalgamation.

mult·ang·u·lar (mŭl-tang′gyū-lăr). Having many angles.

△**multi-.** Many, properly joined only to words of L. derivation; SEE ALSO pluri-. Cf. poly-. [L. *multus,* much]

mul·ti·ar·tic·u·lar (mŭl′tē-ar-tik′yū-lăr). Relating to or involving many joints. SYN polyarthric, polyarticular. [multi- + L. *articulus,* joint]

mul·ti·bac·il·lary (mŭl-tē-bas′i-lār-ē). Made up of, or denoting the presence of, many bacilli.

mul·ti·cap·su·lar (mŭl-tē-kap′sū-lăr). Having numerous capsules.

mul·ti·cel·lu·lar (mŭl-tē-sel′yū-lăr). Composed of many cells.

Mul·ti·ceps (mŭl′ti-seps). A genus of taeniid tapeworms in which the larval forms in herbivores occur in the form of a coenurus (multiple scoleces invaginated within a single cyst). [multi- + L. *caput,* head]

M. mul′ticeps, a species the mature form of which occurs in the intestines of dogs; the coenurus develops in the brains of herbivorous animals, especially sheep; the cyst is often called *Coenurus cerebralis.*

mu

M. seria′lis, a species the mature form of which is found in the intestine of dogs; the coenurus is found in the subcutaneous tissues of rabbits.

mul·ti·col·lin·e·ar·i·ty (mul′tē-kol′in-ē-ar′i-tē). In multiple regression analysis, a situation in which at least some independent variables in a set are highly correlated with each other. [multi- + L. *col-lineo,* to line up together]

mul·ti-CSF Abbreviation for multi-colony-stimulating *factor.*

mul·ti·cus·pid (mŭl-tē-kŭs′pid). SYN multicuspidate (2).

mul·ti·cus·pi·date (mŭl-tē-kŭs′pi-dāt). **1.** Having more than two cusps. **2.** A molar tooth with three or more cusps or projections on the crown. SYN multicuspid.

mul·ti·en·zyme (mŭl′tī-en′zīm, mŭl′tē-). Referring to several enzymes; *e.g.,* multienzyme complex.

mul·ti·fe·ta·tion (mŭl-tē-fe-tā′shŭn). SYN superfetation.

mul·ti·fid (mŭl′tē-fid). Divided into many clefts or segments. SYN multifidus (1). [L. *multifidus,* fr. *multus,* much, + *findo,* to cleave]

mul·tif·i·dus (mŭl-tif′i-dŭs). **1.** SYN multifid. **2.** SEE multifidus *muscle.* [L.]

mul·ti·fo·cal (mŭl-tē-fō′kăl). Relating to or arising from many foci.

mul·ti·form (mŭl′ti-fōrm). SYN polymorphic.

mul·ti·glan·du·lar (mŭl-tē-glan′dyū-lăr). SYN pluriglandular.

mul·ti·grav·i·da (mŭl-tē-grav′i-dă). A pregnant woman who has been pregnant one or more times previously. [multi- + L. *gravi-da,* pregnant]

mul·ti·in·fec·tion (mŭl′tē-in-fek′shŭn). Mixed infection with two or more varieties of microorganisms developing simultaneously.

mul·ti·lo·bar, mul·ti·lo·bate, mul·ti·lobed (mŭl-tē-lō′bar, -lō′bāt, -lōbd′). Having several lobes.

mul·ti·lob·u·lar (mŭl-tē-lob′yū-lăr). Having many lobules.

mul·ti·lo·cal (mŭl-tē-lō′kăl). Denoting traits with an etiology comprising effects of multiple genetic loci operating together and simultaneously. Cf. galtonian.

mul·ti·loc·u·lar (mŭl-tē-lok′yū-lăr). Many-celled; having many compartments or loculi. SYN plurilocular.

mul·ti·mam·mae (mŭl-tē-mam′ē). SYN polymastia. [multi- + L. *mamma,* breast]

mul·ti·no·dal (mŭl-tē-nō′dăl). Having many nodes.

mul·ti·nod·u·lar, mul·ti·nod·u·late (mŭl-tē-nod′yū-lăr, -yū-lāt). Having many nodules.

mul·ti·nu·cle·ar, mul·ti·nu·cle·ate (mŭl-tē-nū′klē-ăr, -āt). Having two or more nuclei. SYN plurinuclear, polynuclear, polynucleate.

mul·ti·nu·cle·o·sis (mŭl′tē-nūk-lē-ō′sis). SYN polynucleosis.

mul·tip·a·ra (mŭl-tip′ă-ră). A woman who has given birth at least two times to an infant, liveborn or not, weighing 500 g or more, or having an estimated length of gestation of at least 20 weeks. [multi- + L. *pario,* to bring forth, to bear]

grand m., a m. who has given birth five or more times.

mul·ti·par·i·ty (mŭl-tē-păr′i-tē). Condition of being a multipara.

mul·tip·a·rous (mŭl-tip′ă-rŭs). Relating to a multipara.

mul·ti·par·tial (mŭl′tē-par′shăl). Polyvalent, with respect to an antiserum.

mul·ti·ple (mŭl′ti-pl). Manifold; repeated several times; occurring in several parts at the same time, as m. arthritis, m. neuritis. [L. *multiplex,* fr. *multus,* many, + *plico,* pp. *-atus,* to fold]

mul·ti·po·lar (mŭl-tē-pō′lăr). Having more than two poles; denoting a nerve cell in which the branches project from several points.

mul·ti·root·ed (mŭl-tē-rūt′ed). Having more than two roots.

mul·ti·ro·ta·tion (mŭl′tē-rō-tā′shŭn). SYN mutarotation.

mul·ti·sub·strate (mŭl-tī-sub′stăt, mŭl-tē′-). Referring to an enzyme, receptor, or acceptor protein, which requires two or more substrates.

mul·ti·sy·nap·tic (mŭl′tē-si-nap′tik). SYN polysynaptic.

mul·ti·va·lence, mul·ti·va·len·cy (mŭl-tē-vā′lens, -vā′len-sē). The state of being multivalent.

mul·ti·va·lent (mŭl-tē-vā′lent). **1.** In chemistry, having a combining power (valence) of more than one hydrogen atom. **2.** Efficacious in more than one direction. **3.** An antisera specific for more than one antigen or organism. SYN polyvalent (1).

mum·mi·fi·ca·tion (mŭm′i-fi-kā′shŭn). **1.** SYN dry *gangrene.* **2.** Shrivelling of a dead, retained fetus. **3.** In dentistry, treatment of inflamed dental pulp with fixative drugs (usually formaldehyde derivatives) in order to retain teeth so treated for relatively short periods; generally acceptable only for primary (deciduous) teeth. [mummy + L. *facio,* to make]

mumps (mŭmpz). SYN epidemic *parotiditis.* [dialectic Eng. *mump,* a lump or bump]

metastatic m., m. complicated by involvement of organs other than parotid glands, such as the testis, breast, or pancreas.

Münchhausen, Baron Karl F.H. von, German nobleman, soldier, and raconteur, 1720–1797. SEE Munchausen *syndrome;* Munchausen *syndrome* by proxy.

Munro, John C., U.S. surgeon, 1858–1910. SEE M.'s *point.*

Munro, William J., 19th century Australian dermatologist. SEE M.'s *abscess, microabscess.*

Munsell, Albert H., U.S. artist, 1858–1918. SEE Farnsworth-M. color *test.*

Munsell, Hazel E., U.S. chemist, *1891. SEE Sherman-M. *unit.*

Munson's sign. See under sign.

Münzer, Egmont, Austrian physician, 1865–1924. SEE *tract* of M. and Wiener.

Mur Abbreviation for muramic acid.

mu·ral (myū′răl). Relating to the wall of any cavity. [L. *muralis;* fr. *murus,* wall]

mu·ram·ic ac·id (Mur) (myū-ram′ik). 2-Amino-3-*O*-(1-carboxyethyl)-2-deoxy-D-glucose; D-Glucosamine and lactate in ether linkage between the 3 and 2 positions, respectively; a constituent of the mureins in bacterial cell walls.

mu·ram·i·dase (myū-ram′i-dās). SYN lysozyme.

mu·reins (myūr′ēnz). Peptidoglycans composing the sacculus or cell casing of bacteria, consisting of linear polysaccharides of alternating *N*-acetyl-D-glucosamine and *N*-acetylmuramic acid units, to the lactate side chains of which are linked oligopeptides; independent chains are cross-linked in three dimensions via the peptides or the 6-OH groups (the latter may be linked via phosphate to a teichoic acid). [L. *murus,* wall]

Muret, Paul-Louis, French physician, *1878. SEE Quénu-M. *sign.*

mu·rex·ide (myū-rek′sīd, -sid). The ammonium salt of purpuric acid, formerly used as a dye but superseded by the aniline colors.

mu·ri·ate (myū′rē-āt). Former term for chloride. [L. *muria,* brine]

mu·ri·at·ic (myū-rē-at′ik). Relating to brine. [L. *muriaticus,* pickled in brine, fr. *muria,* brine]

mu·ri·at·ic ac·id. SYN hydrochloric acid.

Mu·ri·dae (myū′ri-dē). The largest family of Rodentia and of mammals, embracing the Old World mice and rats. [L. *mus* (*mur-*), a mouse]

mu·ri·form (myūr′i-fōrm). Multicellular with cross and longitudinal septa; denoting an aggregation of cells fitting together like stones in a stone wall. [L. *murus,* wall, + -form]

mu·rine (myū′rīn, -rin, -rēn). Relating to animals of the family Muridae. [L. *murinus,* relating to mice, fr. *mus* (*mur-*), a mouse]

mur·mur (mer′mer). **1.** A soft sound, like that made by a somewhat forcible expiration with the mouth open, heard on auscultation of the heart, lungs, or blood vessels. SYN susurrus. **2.** An other-than-soft sound, which may be loud, harsh, frictional, etc. *e.g.,* organic cardiac m.'s may be soft or loud and harsh; pericardial m.'s usually are frictional and are more properly described as "rubs" rather than m.'s. [L.]

accidental m., an evanescent cardiac m. not due to valvular lesion.

anemic m., a nonvalvular m. heard on auscultation of the heart and large blood vessels in cases of profound anemia associated mainly with turbulent blood flow due to decreased blood viscosity.

aneurysmal m., a systolic or systolic-diastolic m. heard over some cardiac aneurysms.

aortic m., a m. produced at the aortic orifice, either obstructive or regurgitant.

arterial m., a m. heard on auscultating an artery.

atriosystolic m., SYN presystolic m.

Austin Flint m., SYN Austin Flint *phenomenon*, Flint's m.

bellows m., a blowing m.

brain m., sounds produced by intracranial aneurysms or arterial venous aneurysms in congenital dysplastic angiomatosis.

Cabot-Locke m., an early diastolic m., like that of aortic insufficiency, heard best at the left lower sternal border in severe anemia.

cardiac m., a m. produced within the heart, at one of its valvular orifices or across ventricular septal defects.

cardiopulmonary m., an innocent extracardiac m., synchronous with the heart's beat but disappearing when the breath is held, believed due to movement of air in a segment of lung compressed by the contracting heart. SYN cardiorespiratory m.

cardiorespiratory m., SYN cardiopulmonary m.

Carey Coombs m., a blubbering apical middiastolic m. occurring in the acute stage of rheumatic mitral valvulitis and disappearing as the valvulitis subsides. SYN Coombs m.

Cole-Cecil m., the diastolic m. of aortic insufficiency when well or predominantly heard in the left axilla.

continuous m., a m. that is heard without interruption throughout systole and into diastole.

cooing m., a m., usually of mitral regurgitation, of very high pitch resembling the cooing of a pigeon or a dove.

Coombs m., SYN Carey Coombs m.

crescendo m., a m. that increases in intensity and suddenly ceases; the presystolic m. of mitral stenosis is a common example.

Cruveilhier-Baumgarten m., a venous m. heard over collateral veins, connecting portal and caval venous systems, on the abdominal wall. SEE ALSO Cruveilhier-Baumgarten *sign*.

diamond-shaped m., a crescendo-decrescendo m., from the shape of the frequency intensity curve of the phonocardiogram, often audible as such.

diastolic m. (DM), a m. heard during diastole.

Duroziez' m., a two-phase m. over peripheral arteries, especially the femoral artery, due to rapid ebb and flow of blood during aortic insufficiency. SYN Duroziez' sign.

dynamic m., a heart m. due to anemia or to any cause other than a valvular lesion.

early diastolic m., a m. that begins with the second heart sound, as the m. of aortic insufficiency.

ejection m., a diamond-shaped systolic m. produced by the ejection of blood into the aorta or pulmonary artery and ending by the time of the second heart sound component produced, respectively, by closing of the aortic or pulmonic valve.

endocardial m., a m. arising, from any cause, within the heart.

extracardiac m., a bruit heard over or near the precordium originating from structures other than the heart; the term includes pericardial friction rubs and cardiopulmonary m.'s.

Flint's m., a diastolic m., similar to that of mitral stenosis, heard best at the cardiac apex in some cases of free aortic insufficiency; it is thought to be caused by the turbulent regurgitating stream from the aorta mixing into the stream simultaneously entering from the left atrium through the mitral valve, causing posterior movement of the anterior leaflet of the mitral valve with transient acceleration of blood flow through the mitral valve. SYN Austin Flint m.

Fräntzel's m., m. of mitral stenosis when louder at its beginning and end than in its midportion.

friction m., SYN friction *sound.*

functional m., a cardiac m. not associated with a significant heart lesion. SYN innocent m., inorganic m.

Gibson m., the typical continuous "machinery-like" m. of patent ductus arteriosus.

Graham Steell's m., an early diastolic m. of pulmonic insufficiency secondary to pulmonary hypertension, as in mitral stenosis and various congenital defects associated with pulmonary hypertension. SYN Steell's m.

Hamman's m., a crunching precordial sound synchronous with the heart beat; heard in mediastinal emphysema.

hemic m., a cardiac or vascular m. heard in anemic persons who have no valvular lesion, probably due to the increased blood velocity and turbulence that characterizes anemia.

Hodgkin-Key m., a musical diastolic m. associated with retroversion of an aortic cusp; often very loud.

holosystolic m., SYN pansystolic m.

hourglass m., one in which there are two areas of maximum loudness decreasing to a point midway between the two.

innocent m., SYN functional m.

inorganic m., SYN functional m.

late apical systolic m., a m. previously considered benign, or even extracardiac, with a possible relationship to pericardial disease; it often represents mitral insufficiency, often localized and of moderate severity but with propensity for developing bacterial endocarditis, and is frequently associated with systolic click and mitral prolapse (Barlow syndrome; a balloon or billowing mitral valve leaflet) often producing a click, murmur, or both, as it prolapses during systole into the left atrium.

late diastolic m., SYN presystolic m.

machinery m., the long "continuous" rumbling m. of patent ductus arteriosus.

middiastolic m., a m. beginning after the A-V valves have opened in diastole, *i.e.,* an appreciable time after the second heart sound, as the m. of mitral stenosis.

mill wheel m., churning cardiac m. produced by air embolism to the heart; also heard in pneumohydropericardium. SYN water wheel m.

mitral m., a m. produced at the mitral valve, either obstructive or regurgitant.

musical m., a cardiac or vascular m. having a high-pitched musical character.

nun's m., SYN venous *hum.*

obstructive m., a m. caused by narrowing of one of the valvular orifices.

organic m., a m. caused by an organic lesion.

pansystolic m., a m. occupying the entire systolic interval, from first to second heart sounds. SYN holosystolic m.

pericardial m., a friction sound, synchronous with the heart movements, heard in certain cases of pericarditis.

pleuropericardial m., a pleural friction sound over the pericardial region, synchronous with the heart's action, and simulating a pericardial m. (rub).

presystolic m., a m. heard at the end of ventricular diastole (during atrial systole if in sinus rhythm), usually due to obstruction at one of the atrioventricular orifices. SYN atriosystolic m., late diastolic m.

pulmonary m., pulmonic m., a m. produced at the pulmonary orifice of the heart, either obstructive or regurgitant.

regurgitant m., a m. due to leakage or backward flow at one of the valvular orifices of the heart.

respiratory m., SYN vesicular *respiration.*

Roger's m., a loud pansystolic m. maximal at the left sternal border, caused by a small ventricular septal defect. SYN bruit de Roger, Roger's bruit.

sea gull m., a m. imitating the cooing sound of a seagull nearly always due to aortic stenosis or mitral regurgitation.

seesaw m., SYN to-and-fro m.

Steell's m., SYN Graham Steell's m.

stenosal m., an arterial m. due to narrowing of the vessel from pressure or organic change.

Still's m., an innocent musical m. resembling the noise produced by a twanging string; almost exclusively in young children, of uncertain origin and ultimately disappearing.

systolic m., a m. heard during ventricular systole.

to-and-fro m., m. heard in both systole and diastole of the heart, as in aortic stenosis and insufficiency. SYN seesaw m.

tricuspid m., a m. produced at the tricuspid orifice, either obstructive or regurgitant.

vascular m., a m. originating in a blood vessel.

venous m., a m. heard over a vein.

vesicular m., SYN vesicular *respiration.*

water wheel m., SYN mill wheel m.

mu·ro·mo·nab-CD3 (myū-rō-mō′nab). A murine monoclonal antibody to the T3 (CD3) antigen of human T lymphocytes, used as an immunosuppressant in the treatment of acute allograft rejection following renal transplantation.

Murphy, John B., U.S. surgeon, 1857–1916. SEE M. *drip;* M.'s *button, percussion.*

mur·ri·na (mū-rē′nă). A disease of horses, mules, and burros in Panama caused by the protozoan parasite *Trypanosoma evansi* and characterized by emaciation, weakness, anemia, edema, ecchymotic conjunctivitis, fever, and paralysis of the hind legs. [Fr. *morine;* Sp. *morriña,* cattle plague, prob. fr. L. *morior,* to die]

Mus (mŭs). A genus of the family Muridae that includes about 16 species of mice; domesticated strains are numerous and genetically well defined, the most popular being the albino and piebald strains. [L. *mus* (mur-), a mouse]

Mus·ca (mŭs′kă). A genus of flies (family Muscidae, order Diptera) that includes the common housefly, *M. domestica,* a species universally associated with humans, particularly under unsanitary conditions; it breeds in filth and organic waste, and is involved in the mechanical transfer of numerous pathogens. [L. fly]

mus·cae vol·i·tan·tes (mŭs′sē, mŭs′kē vol-i-tan′tēs). Floaters; appearance of moving spots before the eyes, arising from remnants of the embryologic hyaloid vascular system in the vitreous humor. [L. pl. of *musca,* fly; pres. ppl. of *volito,* to fly to and fro]

mus·ca·rine (mŭs′kă-rēn, -rin). A toxin with neurologic effects, first isolated from *Amanita muscaria* (fly agaric) and also present in some species of *Hebeloma* and *Inocybe.* The quaternary trimethylammonium salt of 2-methyl-3-hydroxy-5-(aminomethyl)tetrahydrofuran, it is a cholinergic substance whose pharmacologic effects resemble those of acetylcholine and postganglionic parasympathetic stimulation (cardiac inhibition, vasodilation, salivation, lacrimation, bronchoconstriction, gastrointestinal stimulation).

mus·ca·rin·ic (mŭs-kă-rin′ik). **1.** Having a muscarine-like action, *i.e.,* producing effects that resemble postganglionic parasympathetic stimulation. **2.** An agent that stimulates the postganglionic parasympathetic receptor. SEE ALSO muscarine, nicotinic.

mus·ca·rin·ism (mŭs′kă-rin-izm). SYN mycetism.

Mus·ci (mŭs′sī). The class of plants that includes the mosses. [L. pl. of *muscus,* moss]

mus·ci·cide (mŭs′i-sīd). An agent destructive to flies. [L. *musca,* fly, + *caedo,* to kill]

Mus·ci·dae (mŭs′i-dē). The family of flies (order Diptera) that includes the houseflies (*Musca*) and stable flies (*Stomoxys*). [L. *musca,* fly]

mus·ci·mol (mŭs′sē-mol). 5-(Aminomethyl)-3(2H)-isoxazolone; pharmacologically very potent CNS depressant and agonist of γ-aminobutyric acid; isolated from *Amanita* sp. (esp. fly agaric); inhibits motor function and can lead to psychosis.

mus·ci·mol (mus-ĭ-mol). An alkaloid extracted from the poison mushroom *Amanita muscaria.* It selectively stimulates receptors for γ-aminobutyric acid (GABA); used as a molecular probe to study GABA receptors.

MUSCLE

mus·cle (mŭs′ĕl). A primary tissue, consisting predominantly of highly specialized contractile cells, which may be classified as skeletal m., cardiac m., or smooth m.; microscopically, the latter is lacking in transverse striations characteristic of the other two types; one of the contractile organs of the body by which movements of the various organs and parts are effected; typical m. is a mass of m. fibers (venter or belly), attached at each extremity, by means of a tendon, to a bone or other structure; the more proximal or more fixed attachment is called the *origin,* the more distal or more movable attachment is the *insertion;* the narrowing part of the belly that is attached to the tendon of origin is called the caput or head. For gross anatomical description, see musculus. SYN musculus [NA]. [L. *musculus*]

m.'s of abdomen, m.'s forming the wall of the abdomen including rectus abdominis, external and internal oblique m.'s, transversus abdominis, and quadratus abdominis. SYN musculi abdominis [NA].

abdominal external oblique m., SYN external oblique m.

abdominal internal oblique m., SYN internal oblique m.

abductor digiti minimi m. of foot, *origin,* lateral and medial processes of calcanean tuberosity; *insertion,* lateral side of proximal phalanx of fifth toe; *action,* abducts and flexes little toe; *nerve supply,* lateral plantar nerve. SYN musculus abductor digiti minimi pedis [NA], abductor m. of little toe, musculus abductor digiti quinti (2).

abductor digiti minimi m. of hand, *origin,* pisiform bone and pisohamate ligament; *insertion,* medial side of base of proximal phalanx of the little finger; *action,* abducts and flexes little finger; *nerve supply,* ulnar. SYN musculus abductor digiti minimi manus [NA], abductor m. of little finger, musculus abductor digiti quinti (1).

abductor m. of great toe, SYN abductor hallucis m.

abductor hallucis m., *origin,* medial process of calcaneal tuberosity, flexor retinaculum, and plantar aponeurosis; *insertion,* medial side of proximal phalanx of great toe; *action,* abducts great toe; *nerve supply,* medial plantar. SYN musculus abductor hallucis [NA], abductor m. of great toe.

abductor m. of little finger, SYN abductor digiti minimi m. of hand.

abductor m. of little toe, SYN abductor digiti minimi m. of foot.

abductor pollicis brevis m., *origin,* tubercle of trapezium and flexor retinaculum; *insertion,* lateral side of proximal phalanx of thumb; *action,* abducts thumb; *nerve supply,* median. SYN musculus abductor pollicis brevis [NA], short abductor m. of thumb.

abductor pollicis longus m., *origin,* interosseous membrane and posterior surfaces of radius and ulna; *insertion,* lateral side of base of first metacarpal bone; *action,* abducts and assists in extending thumb; *nerve supply,* radial. SYN musculus abductor pollicis longus [NA], long abductor m. of thumb, musculus extensor ossis metacarpi pollicis.

accessory flexor m. of foot, SYN quadratus plantae m.

adductor brevis m., *origin,* superior ramus of pubis; *insertion,* upper third of medial lip of linea aspera; *action,* adducts thigh; *nerve supply,* obturator. SYN musculus adductor brevis [NA], short adductor m.

adductor m. of great toe, SYN adductor hallucis m.

adductor hallucis m., *origin,* by two heads, the transverse head from the capsules of the lateral four metatarsophalangeal joints and the oblique head from the lateral cuneiform and bases of the third and fourth metatarsal bones; *insertion,* lateral side of base of proximal phalanx of great toe; *action,* adducts great toe; *nerve supply,* lateral plantar. SYN musculus adductor hallucis [NA], adductor m. of great toe.

adductor longus m., *origin,* symphysis and crest of pubis; *insertion,* middle third of medial lip of linea aspera; *action,* adducts thigh; *nerve supply,* obturator. SYN musculus adductor longus [NA], long adductor m.

adductor magnus m., *origin,* ischial tuberosity and ischiopubic ramus; *insertion,* linea aspera and adductor tubercle of femur; *action,* adducts and extends thigh; *nerve supply,* obturator and sciatic. SYN musculus adductor magnus [NA], great adductor m.

adductor minimus m., a small flat m. constituting the upper portion of the adductor magnus, *insertion,* the space above linea aspera. SYN musculus adductor minimus.

adductor pollicis m., *origin,* by two heads, the transverse head from the shaft of the third metacarpal and the oblique head from the front of the base of the second metacarpal, the trapezoid and capitate bones; *insertion,* medial side of base of proximal phalanx of thumb; *action*, adducts thumb; *nerve supply*, ulnar. SYN musculus adductor pollicis [NA], adductor m. of thumb.

adductor m. of thumb, SYN adductor pollicis m.

Aeby's m., SYN cutaneomucous m.

Albinus' m., (1) SYN risorius m. **(2)** SYN scalenus minimus m.

anconeus m., *origin*, back of lateral condyle of humerus; *insertion*, olecranon process and posterior surface of ulna; *action*, extends forearm and abducts ulna in pronation of wrist; *nerve supply*, radial. SYN musculus anconeus [NA], anconeus.

antagonistic m.'s, those having an opposite function, the contraction of one having the potential, in theory, to "neutralize" that of the other.

anterior auricular m., *origin*, galea aponeurotica; *insertion*, cartilage of auricle; *action*, draws pinna of ear upward and forward; *nerve supply*, facial. Considered by some to be the anterior part of the temporoparietal m. SYN musculus auricularis anterior [NA], musculus attrahens aurem, musculus attrahens auriculam, zygomaticoauricularis.

anterior cervical intertransversarii m.'s, *origin*, anterior tubercle of cervical transverse process; *insertion*, anterior tubercle of next superior transverse process; *action*, abducts cervical vertebrae; *nerve supply*, ventral branch of cervical nerves. SYN musculi intertransversarii anteriores cervicis [NA], anterior cervical intertransverse m.'s.

anterior cervical intertransverse m.'s, SYN anterior cervical intertransversarii m.'s.

anterior rectus m. of head, SYN rectus capitis anterior m.

anterior scalene m., SYN scalenus anterior m.

anterior serratus m., SYN serratus anterior m.

anterior tibial m., SYN tibialis anterior m.

antigravity m.'s, the m.'s that maintain the posture characteristic of a given animal species. In most mammals they are the extensor m.'s.

antitragicus m., a band of transverse muscular fibers on the outer surface of the antitragus, arising from the border of the intertragic notch and inserted into the anthelix and cauda helicis. SYN musculus antitragicus [NA], m. of antitragus.

m. of antitragus, SYN antitragicus m.

appendicular m., one of the skeletal m.'s of the limbs.

arrector pili m.'s, bundles of smooth m. fibers, attached to the deep part of the hair follicles, passing outward alongside the sebaceous glands to the papillary layer of the corium; they act to pull the hairs erect, causing "goose bumps" or "goose flesh" (cutis anserina). SYN musculi arrectores pilorum [NA], arrectores pilorum, erector m.'s of hairs.

articular m., a m. that inserts directly onto the capsule of a joint, acting to retract the capsule in certain movements. SYN musculus articularis [NA].

articular m. of elbow, SYN articularis cubiti m.

articularis cubiti m., the name applied to a small slip of the medial head of the triceps that inserts into the capsule of the elbow joint. SYN musculus articularis cubiti [NA], articular m. of elbow, subanconeus m.

articularis genu m., *origin*, lower fourth of anterior surface of shaft of femur; *insertion*, suprapatellar bursa of knee joint; *action*, retracts suprapatellar bursa, during extension of knee; *nerve supply*, femoral. SYN musculus articularis genus [NA], articular m. of knee, Dupré's m., subcrural m., subcruralis, subcrureus, subquadricipital m.

articular m. of knee, SYN articularis genu m.

aryepiglottic m., the fibers of the oblique arytenoid m. that extend from the summit of the arytenoid cartilage to the side of the epiglottis; *action*, constricts the laryngeal aperture. SYN musculus aryepiglotticus [NA].

m.'s of auditory ossicles, the m. stapedius and m. tensor tympani. SYN musculi ossiculorum auditus [NA].

axial m., one of the skeletal m.'s of the trunk or head.

axillary arch m., SYN pectorodorsalis m. SYN Langer's arch, Langer's m.

m.'s of the back, the m.'s of the back in general, including those attaching the shoulder girdle to the trunk posteriorly, the

posterior serratus m.'s, and the erector spinae. SYN musculi dorsi [NA], dorsal m.'s.

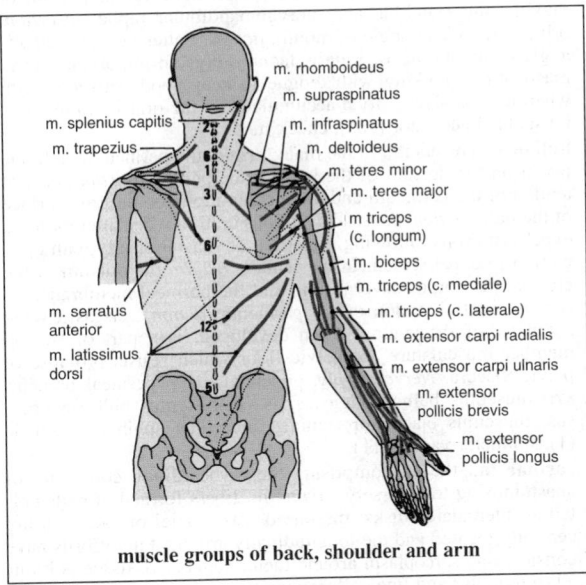

muscle groups of back, shoulder and arm

Bell's m., a band of muscular fibers, forming a slight fold in the wall of the bladder, running from the uvula to the opening of the ureter on either side, bounding the trigonum.

biceps m. of arm, SYN biceps brachii m.

biceps brachii m., *origin*, long head from supraglenoidal tuberosity of scapula, short head from coracoid process; *insertion*, tuberosity of radius; *action*, flexes and supinates forearm (it is the primary supinator of the forearm); *nerve supply*, musculocutaneous. SYN musculus biceps brachii [NA], biceps m. of arm.

biceps femoris m., *origin*, long head (caput longum) from tuberosity of ischium, short head (caput breve) from lower half of lateral lip of linea aspera; *insertion*, head of fibula; *action*, flexes knee and rotates leg laterally; *nerve supply*, long head, tibial, short head, peroneal. SYN musculus biceps femoris [NA], biceps m. of thigh, musculus biceps flexor cruris.

biceps m. of thigh, SYN biceps femoris m.

bipennate m., a muscle with a central tendon toward which the fibers converge on either side like the barbs of a feather. SYN musculus bipennatus [NA].

Bochdalek's m., SYN *musculus* triticeoglossus.

Bovero's m., SYN cutaneomucous m.

Bowman's m., SYN ciliary m.

brachial m., SYN brachialis m.

brachialis m., *origin*, lower two-thirds of anterior surface of humerus; *insertion*, coronoid process of ulna; *action*, flexes elbow; *nerve supply*, musculocutaneous, usually with a minor contribution from the radial. SYN musculus brachialis [NA], brachial m.

brachiocephalic m., SYN *musculus* brachiocephalicus.

brachioradial m., SYN brachioradialis m.

brachioradialis m., *origin*, lateral supracondylar ridge of humerus; *insertion*, front of base of styloid process of radius; *action*, flexes elbow and assists slightly in supination; *nerve supply*, (common) radial. SYN musculus brachioradialis [NA], brachioradial m.

branchiomeric m.'s, the m.'s derived from branchial arch mesoderm that provide a large portion of the musculature for the face and neck.

Braune's m., SYN puborectalis m.

broadest m. of back, SYN latissimus dorsi m.

bronchoesophageal m., muscular fascicles, arising from the wall of the left bronchus, which reinforce the musculature of the esophagus. SYN musculus bronchoesophageus [NA].

Brücke's m., the part of the ciliary m. formed by the meridional fibers. SYN Crampton's m.

buccinator m., *origin*, posterior portion of alveolar portion of maxilla and mandible and pterygomandibular raphe; *insertion*, orbicularis oris at angle of mouth; *action*, flattens cheek, retracts angle of mouth; *nerve supply*, facial. Plays an important role in mastication, working with tongue to keep food between teeth; when it is paralyzed, food accumulates in the oral vestibule. SYN musculus buccinator [NA], cheek m.

bulbocavernosus m., in the male: *origin*, the perineal membrane fascia on the dorsum of the bulb of the penis; *insertion*, central tendon of the perineum and the median raphe on the free surface of the bulb; *action*, constricts bulbous urethra when attempting to expel last drops following urination, or spasmodically with ejaculation to expel semen. In the female: *origin*, the dorsum of the clitoris, the corpus cavernosum, and the perineal membrane; *insertion*, central tendon of the perineum; *action*, acts as a weak sphincter of the vagina; when developed, is a part of "cross-member musculature" of pelvic floor which resists prolapse of pelvic viscera. *Nerve supply*, pudendal (deep perineal branch). SYN musculus bulbospongiosus [NA], musculus bulbocavernosus, musculus ejaculator seminis, musculus sphincter vaginae (1), sphincter vaginae (1).

cardiac m., the m. comprising the myocardium, consisting of anastomosing transversely striated m. fibers formed of cells united at intercalated disks; the one or two nuclei of each cell are centrally located and the longitudinally arranged myofibrils have considerable sarcoplasm around them; connective tissue is limited to reticular and fine collagenous fibers. SYN m. of heart.

Casser's perforated m., SYN coracobrachialis m.

ceratocricoid m., a fasciculus from the posterior cricoarytenoid m. inserted into the inferior horn of the thyroid cartilage. SYN musculus ceratocricoideus [NA], Merkel's m.

cervical iliocostal m., SYN iliocostalis cervicis m.

cervical interspinal m., SYN cervical interspinales m.'s.

cervical interspinales m.'s, *origin*, tubercle of spinous process of cervical vertebra; *insertion*, tubercle of spinous process of next superior vertebra; *action*, extends the neck; *nerve supply*, dorsal rami of cervical nerves. SYN musculus interspinalis cervicis [NA], cervical interspinal m.

cervical longissimus m., SYN longissimus cervicis m.

cervical rotator m.'s, SYN rotatores cervicis m.'s.

cheek m., SYN buccinator m.

chin m., SYN mentalis m.

chondroglossus m., muscular fibers from lesser horn of hyoid bone occasionally separated from the hyoglossus, but usually forming part of it. SYN musculus chondroglossus [NA], ceratoglossus, keratoglossus.

ciliary m., the smooth m. of the ciliary body; it consists of circular fibers (Müller's m.) and radiating fibers (meridional fibers, or Brücke's m.); *action*, in contracting, its diameter is reduced (like a sphincter), reducing tensile (stretching) forces on lens, allowing it to thicken for near vision (accommodation). SYN musculus ciliaris [NA], Bowman's m., ciliary ligament.

coccygeal m., SYN coccygeus m.

coccygeus m., *origin*, spine of ischium and sacrospinous ligament; *insertion*, sides of lower part of sacrum and upper part of coccyx; *action*, assists in support of pelvic floor, especially when intra-abdominal pressures increase; *nerve supply*, third and fourth sacral. SYN musculus coccygeus [NA], coccygeal m., musculus ischiococcygeus.

m.'s of coccyx, the m.'s of the coccyx considered as a group, including the musculus coccygeus and the inconstant ventral and dorsal sacrococcygeal m.'s. SYN musculi coccygei [NA].

Coiter's m., SYN corrugator supercilii m.

compressor m. of lips, SYN cutaneomucous m.

coracobrachial m., SYN coracobrachialis m.

coracobrachialis m., *origin*, coracoid process of scapula; *insertion*, middle of medial border of humerus; *action*, adducts and flexes the arm; resists downward dislocation of shoulder joint; *nerve supply*, musculocutaneous. SYN musculus coracobrachialis [NA], Casser's perforated m., coracobrachial m.

corrugator m., SYN corrugator supercilii m.

corrugator cutis m. of anus, smooth muscle fibers radiating from the anal opening superficial to the external sphincter. SYN musculus corrugator cutis ani.

corrugator supercilii m., *origin*, from orbital portion of m. orbicularis oculi and nasal prominence; *insertion*, skin of eyebrow; *action*, draws medial end of eyebrow downward and wrinkles forehead vertically; *nerve supply*, facial. SYN musculus corrugator supercilii [NA], Coiter's m., corrugator m., wrinkler m. of eyebrow.

cowl m., SYN trapezius m.

Crampton's m., SYN Brücke's m.

cremaster m., *origin*, from internal oblique m. and inguinal ligament; *insertion*, cremasteric fascia (spermatic cord); *action*, raises testicle; *nerve supply*, genital branch of genitofemoral; in the male the muscle envelops the spermatic cord and testis, in the female, the round ligament of the uterus. SYN musculus cremaster [NA], Riolan's m. (2).

cricopharyngeus m., SYN inferior constrictor m. of pharynx. SYN superior esophageal sphincter.

cricothyroid m., *origin*, anterior surface of arch of cricoid; *insertion*, the anterior or straight part passes upward to ala of thyroid; the posterior or oblique part passes more outward to inferior horn of thyroid; *action*, makes vocal folds tense increasing the pitch of voice tone; *nerve supply*, external laryngeal branch of superior laryngeal nerve (from vagus). SYN musculus cricothyroideus [NA].

cruciate m., a general type of m. in which the m.'s or bundles of m. fibers cross in an X-shaped configuration; *e.g.,* the oblique arytenoid m.'s. SYN musculus cruciatus [NA].

cutaneomucous m., the "sucking m.," a labial m. formed by sagittal fibers running from the skin to the mucous membrane. SYN Aeby's m., Bovero's m., compressor m. of lips, Klein's m., Krause's m., mucocutaneous m., musculus cutaneomucosus.

cutaneous m., a m. that lies in the subcutaneous tissue and attaches to the skin; it may or may not have a bony attachment. The m.'s of expression are the chief examples of cutaneous m.'s in the human. SYN musculus cutaneus [NA].

dartos m., SYN dartos *fascia.*

deep m.'s of back, m.'s of the back innervated by the dorsal primary rami of spinal nerves; includes erector spinae, transversospinalis, interspinal, and intertransverse m.'s; excludes the superficial back m.'s which are appendicular and are innervated by ventral rami, and the trapezius, innervated by the spinal accessory nerve. SYN true m.'s of back.

deep flexor m. of fingers, SYN flexor digitorum profundus m.

deep transverse perineal m., *origin*, ramus of ischium; *insertion*, with its fellow in a median raphe; *action*, assists sphincter urethrae with some sphincteric action on vagina in female; *nerve supply*, pudendal (dorsal nerve of penis/clitoris). SYN musculus transversus perinei profundus [NA], deep transverse m. of perineum, musculus sphincter vaginae (2), sphincter vaginae (2).

deep transverse m. of perineum, SYN deep transverse perineal m.

deltoid m., *origin*, lateral third of clavicle, lateral border of acromion process, lower border of spine of scapula; *insertion*, lateral side of shaft of humerus a little above its middle (deltoid tuberosity); *action*, abduction, flexion, extension, and rotation of arm; *nerve supply*, axillary from fifth and sixth cervical spinal cord segments through brachial plexus. SYN musculus deltoideus [NA], deltoid (2).

depressor anguli oris m., *origin*, lower border of mandible anteriorly; *insertion*, blends with other m.'s in lower lip near angle of mouth; *action*, pulls down corners of mouth; *nerve supply*, facial. SYN musculus depressor anguli oris [NA], musculus triangularis labii inferioris, musculus triangularis (2), triangular m. (2).

depressor m. of epiglottis, SYN thyroepiglottic m.

depressor m. of eyebrow, SYN depressor supercilii m.

depressor labii inferioris m., *origin*, anterior portion of lower border of mandible; *insertion*, orbicularis oris m. and skin of lower lip; *action*, depresses lower lip; *nerve supply*, facial. SYN musculus depressor labii inferioris [NA], depressor m. of lower lip, musculus quadratus labii inferioris, musculus quadratus menti.

depressor m. of lower lip, SYN depressor labii inferioris m.

depressor septi m., a vertical fasciculus from the orbicularis oris m. passing upward along the median line of the upper lip, and inserted into the cartilaginous septum of the nose; *action,* depresses septum; *nerve supply,* facial. SYN musculus depressor septi [NA], depressor m. of septum.

depressor m. of septum, SYN depressor septi m.

depressor supercilii m., fibers of the orbital part of the orbicularis oculi m. insert in the eyebrow; *action,* depresses eyebrow; *nerve supply,* facial. SYN musculus depressor supercilii [NA], depressor m. of eyebrow.

detrusor m. of urinary bladder, the muscular coat of the bladder. SYN musculus detrusor urinae.

digastric m., (1) one of the suprahyoid group of m.'s consisting of two bellies united by a central tendon which is connected to the body of the hyoid bone; *origin,* by posterior belly from the digastric groove medial to the mastoid process; *insertion,* by anterior belly into lower border of mandible near midline; *action,* elevates the hyoid when mandible is fixed; depresses the mandible when hyoid is fixed; *nerve supply,* posterior belly from facial, anterior belly by nerve to the mylohyoid from the mandibular division of trigeminal; **(2)** a m. with two fleshy bellies separated by a fibrous insertion; SYN musculus digastricus [NA], biventer mandibulae, musculus biventer mandibulae, two-bellied m.

dilator m., a m. which opens an orifice or dilates the lumen of an organ; it is the dilating or opening component of a pylorus (the other component is the sphincter m.). SYN musculus dilatator, musculus dilator.

dilator m. of ileocecal sphincter, the longitudinal muscular fibers that open the ileal orifice at the level of the cecocolic junction. SYN musculus dilator pylori ilealis.

dilator pupillae m., the radial muscular fibers extending from the sphincter pupillae to the ciliary margin; some anatomists regard them as elastic, not muscular, in humans. SYN musculus dilator pupillae [NA], dilator iridis, dilator of pupil, musculus dilator iridis.

dilator m. of pylorus, the longitudinal muscular fibers that open the gastroduodenal junction. SYN musculus dilator pylori gastroduodenalis.

dorsal m.'s, SYN m.'s of the back.

dorsal interosseous m.'s of foot, four muscles in the foot; *origin,* from sides of adjacent metatarsal bones; *insertion,* first into medial, second into lateral side of proximal phalanx of second toe, third and fourth into lateral side of proximal phalanx of third and fourth toes; *action,* abduct toes 2-4 from an axis through the second toe; *nerve supply,* lateral plantar. SYN musculi interossei dorsalis pedis [NA].

dorsal interosseous m.'s of hand, four muscles in the hand; *origin,* sides of adjacent metacarpal bones; *insertion,* proximal phalanges and extensor expansion, first on radial side of index, second on radial side of middle finger, third on ulnar side of middle finger, fourth on ulnar side of ring finger; *action,* abduct fingers 2-4 from the axis of the middle finger, *nerve supply,* ulnar. SYN musculi interossei dorsalis manus [NA].

dorsal sacrococcygeal m., SYN dorsal sacrococcygeus m.

dorsal sacrococcygeus m., an inconstant and poorly developed muscle on the dorsal surfaces of the sacrum and coccyx, the remains of a portion of the tail musculature of lower animals. SYN musculus sacrococcygeus dorsalis [NA], dorsal sacrococcygeal m., musculus extensor coccygis, musculus sacrococcygeus posterior.

Dupré's m., SYN articularis genu m.

Duverney's m., SYN lacrimal *part* of orbicularis oculi muscle. SEE orbicularis oculi m.

elevator m. of anus, SYN levator ani m.

elevator m. of prostate, SYN levator prostatae m.

elevator m. of rib, SYN levatores costarum m.'s.

elevator m. of scapula, SYN levator scapulae m.

elevator m. of soft palate, SYN levator veli palatini m.

elevator m. of thyroid gland, SYN levator m. of thyroid gland.

elevator m. of upper eyelid, SYN levator palpebrae superioris m.

elevator m. of upper lip, SYN levator labii superioris m.

elevator m. of upper lip and wing of nose, SYN levator labii superioris alaeque nasi m.

epicranial m., SYN epicranius m.

epicranius m., composed of the epicranial aponeurosis and the m.'s inserting into it, *i.e.,* the occipitofrontalis m. and temporoparietalis m. SYN musculus epicranius [NA], epicranial m., scalp m.

erector m.'s of hairs, SYN arrector pili m.'s.

erector spinae m.'s, *origin,* from sacrum, ilium, and spines of lumbar vertebrae; it divides into three columns, iliocostalis m., longissimus m., and spinalis m., which insert into ribs and vertebrae with additional muscle slips joining the columns at successively higher levels; *action,* extends vertebral column; *nerve supply,* dorsal primary rami of spinal nerves. SYN musculus erector spinae [NA], erector m. of spine, musculus sacrospinalis.

erector m. of spine, SYN erector spinae m.'s.

extensor carpi radialis brevis m., *origin,* lateral epicondyle of humerus; *insertion,* base of third metacarpal bone; *action,* extends and abducts wrist radialward; *nerve supply,* radial. SYN musculus extensor carpi radialis brevis [NA], short radial extensor m. of wrist.

extensor carpi radialis longus m., *origin,* lateral supracondylar ridge of humerus; *insertion,* back of base of second metacarpal bone; *action,* extends and deviates wrist radialward; *nerve supply,* radial. SYN musculus extensor carpi radialis longus [NA], long radial extensor m. of wrist.

extensor carpi ulnaris m., *origin,* lateral epicondyle of humerus (humeral head) and oblique line and posterior border of ulna (ulnar head); *insertion,* base of fifth metacarpal bone; *action,* extends and abducts wrist ulnarward; *nerve supply,* radial (posterior interosseous). SYN musculus extensor carpi ulnaris [NA], ulnar extensor m. of wrist.

extensor digiti minimi m., *origin,* lateral epicondyle of humerus; *insertion,* dorsum of proximal, middle, and distal phalanges of little finger; *action,* extends fingers; *nerve supply,* radial (posterior interosseous). SYN musculus extensor digiti minimi [NA], extensor m. of little finger, musculus extensor digiti quinti proprius, musculus extensor minimi digiti.

extensor digitorum m., *origin,* lateral epicondyle of humerus; *insertion,* by four tendons into the base of the proximal and middle and base of the distal phalanges; *action,* extends fingers; *nerve supply,* radial (posterior interosseous). SYN musculus extensor digitorum [NA], extensor m. of fingers, musculus extensor digitorum communis.

extensor digitorum brevis m., *origin,* dorsal surface of calcaneus; *insertion,* by four tendons fusing with those of the extensor digitorum longus, and by a slip attached independently to the base of the proximal phalanx of the great toe; *action,* extends toes; *nerve supply,* deep peroneal. SYN musculus extensor digitorum brevis [NA], musculus extensor brevis digitorum, short extensor m. of toes.

extensor digitorum brevis m. of hand, a short extensor muscle of the fingers of rare occurrence, and comparable to the short extensor of the toes. SYN musculus extensor digitorum brevis manus, Pozzi's m.

extensor digitorum longus m., *origin,* lateral condyle of tibia, upper two-thirds of anterior margin of fibula; *insertion,* by four tendons to the dorsal surfaces of the bases of the proximal, middle, and distal phalanges of the second to fifth toes; *action,*

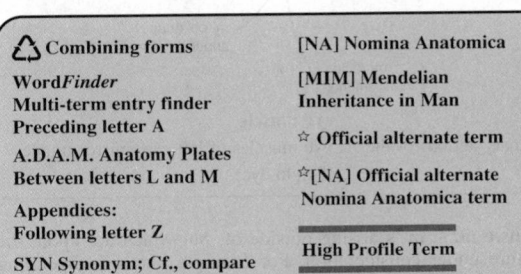

⌂ **Combining forms**	**[NA]** Nomina Anatomica
Word*Finder*	**[MIM]** Mendelian
Multi-term entry finder	**Inheritance in Man**
Preceding letter A	
A.D.A.M. Anatomy Plates	☆ Official alternate term
Between letters L and M	
Appendices:	☆**[NA]** Official alternate
Following letter Z	Nomina Anatomica term
SYN Synonym; Cf., compare	**High Profile Term**

mu

extends the four lateral toes; *nerve supply*, deep branch of peroneal. SYN musculus extensor digitorum longus [NA], long extensor m. of toes, musculus extensor longus digitorum.

extensor m. of fingers, SYN extensor digitorum m.

extensor hallucis brevis m., the medial belly of extensor digitorum brevis m., the tendon of which is inserted into the base of the proximal phalanx of the great toe. SYN musculus extensor hallucis brevis [NA], short extensor m. of great toe.

extensor hallucis longus m., *origin*, lateral surface of tibia and interosseous membrane; *insertion*, base of distal phalanx of great toe; *action*, extends the great toe; *nerve supply*, anterior tibial. SYN musculus extensor hallucis longus [NA], long extensor m. of great toe.

extensor indicis m., *origin*, dorsal surface of ulna; *insertion*, dorsal extensor aponeurosis of index finger; *action*, assists in extending the forefinger; *nerve supply*, radial. SYN musculus extensor indicis [NA], index extensor m., musculus extensor indicis proprius.

extensor m. of little finger, SYN extensor digiti minimi m.

extensor pollicis brevis m., *origin*, dorsal surface of radius; *insertion*, base of proximal phalanx of thumb; *action*, extends and abducts the thumb; *nerve supply*, radial. SYN musculus extensor pollicis brevis [NA], musculus extensor brevis pollicis, short extensor m. of thumb.

extensor pollicis longus m., *origin*, posterior surface of ulna; *insertion*, base of distal phalanx of thumb; *action*, extends distal phalanx of thumb; *nerve supply*, radial. SYN musculus extensor pollicis longus [NA], long extensor m. of thumb, musculus extensor longus pollicis.

external intercostal m.'s, each arises from lower border of one rib and pass obliquely downward and forward to be inserted into the upper border of rib below; *action*, contract during inspiration, also maintain tension in the intercostal spaces to resist mediolateral movement; *nerve supply*, intercostal. SYN musculus intercostales externi [NA].

external oblique m., *origin*, fifth to twelfth ribs; *insertion*, anterior half of lateral lip of iliac crest, inguinal ligament, and anterior layer of the rectus sheath; *action*, diminishes capacity of abdomen, draws thorax downward; *nerve supply*, thoracoabdominal nerves. SYN musculus obliquus externus abdominis [NA], abdominal external oblique m.

external obturator m., SYN obturator externus m.

external pterygoid m., SYN lateral pterygoid m.

external sphincter m. of anus, SYN external anal *sphincter.*

extraocular m.'s, the m.'s within the orbit including the four rectus muscles (superior, inferior, medial and lateral); two oblique muscles (superior and inferior), and the levator of the superior eyelid (levator palpebrae superioris). SYN musculi bulbi [NA], m.'s of eyeball, ocular m.'s.

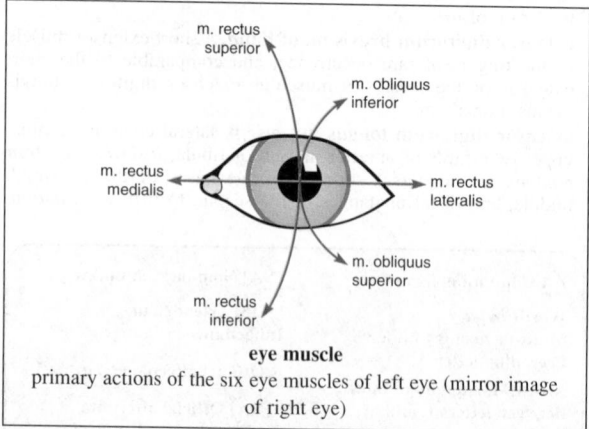

eye muscle
primary actions of the six eye muscles of left eye (mirror image of right eye)

extrinsic m.'s, m.'s arising outside of, but which act upon, the structure under consideration. For example, the m.'s operating the hand but having fleshy bellies located in the forearm.

m.'s of eyeball, SYN extraocular m.'s.

facial m.'s, SYN m.'s of facial expression.

m.'s of facial expression, the numerous m.'s supplied by the facial nerve that are attached to and move the skin of the face. Nomina Anatomica also includes the buccinator m. in this group; even though it functions primarily in mastication. SYN musculi faciales [NA], facial m.'s, mimetic m.'s.

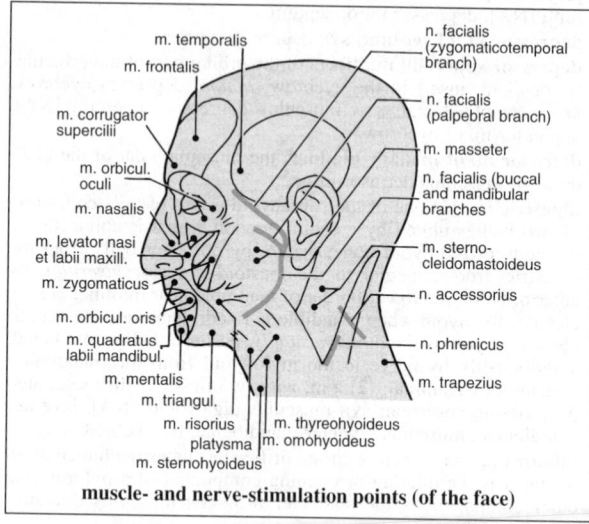

muscle- and nerve-stimulation points (of the face)

femoral m., SYN vastus intermedius m.

fixator m., a m. that acts as a stabilizer of one part of the body during movement of another part.

flexor carpi radialis m., *origin*, common flexor origin of the medial condyle of humerus; *insertion*, anterior surface of the base of the second and most often sending a slip to that of the third metacarpal bone; *action*, flexes and abducts wrist radialward; *nerve supply*, median; its tendon travels in its own canal roofed by a layer of the transverse carpal ligament. SYN musculus flexor carpi radialis [NA], radial flexor m. of wrist.

flexor carpi ulnaris m., *origin*, humeral head from medial condyle of humerus, ulnar head from olecranon and upper three-fifths of posterior border of ulna; *insertion*, pisiform bone, but is continued to the fifth metacarpal bone via the pisometacarpal ligament; *action*, flexes and abducts wrist ulnarward; *nerve supply*, ulnar. SYN musculus flexor carpi ulnaris [NA], ulnar flexor m. of wrist.

flexor digiti minimi brevis m. of foot, *origin*, base of metatarsal bone of the little toe and sheath of m. peroneus longus; *insertion*, lateral surface of base of proximal phalanx of little toe; *action*, flexes the proximal phalanx of the little toe; *nerve supply*, lateral plantar. SYN musculus flexor digiti minimi brevis pedis [NA], short flexor m. of little toe.

flexor digiti minimi brevis m. of hand, *origin*, hamulus of hamate bone; *insertion*, medial side of proximal phalanx of little finger; *action*, flexes proximal phalanx of little finger; *nerve supply*, ulnar. SYN musculus flexor digiti minimi brevis manus [NA], short flexor m. of little finger.

flexor digitorum brevis m., *origin*, medial tubercle of calcaneus and central portion of plantar fascia; *insertion*, middle phalanges of four lateral toes by tendons perforated by those of the flexor longus; *action*, flexes lateral four toes; *nerve supply*, medial plantar. SYN musculus flexor digitorum brevis [NA], musculus flexor brevis digitorum, short flexor m. of toes.

flexor digitorum longus m., *origin*, middle third of posterior surface of tibia; *insertion*, by four tendons, perforating those of the flexor brevis, into bases of distal phalanges of four lateral toes; *action*, flexes second to fifth toes; *nerve supply*, tibial nerve. SYN musculus flexor digitorum longus [NA], long flexor m. of toes, musculus flexor longus digitorum.

flexor digitorum profundus m., *origin*, anterior surface of upper third of ulna; *insertion*, by four tendons, piercing those of the superficialis, into base of distal phalanx of each finger; *action*, flexes distal interphalangeal joint of fingers; *nerve supply*, ulnar and median (anterior interosseous muscle). SYN musculus flexor digitorum profundus [NA], deep flexor m. of fingers, musculus flexor profundus.

flexor digitorum superficialis m., *origin*, humeroulnar head from the medial epicondyle of the humerus, the medial border of the coronoid process, and a tendinous arch between these points, radial head from the oblique line and middle third of the lateral border of the radius; *insertion*, by four split tendons, passing to either side of the profundus tendons, into sides of middle phalanx of each finger; *action*, flexes proximal interphalangeal joint of the fingers; *nerve supply*, median. SYN musculus flexor digitorum superficialis [NA], musculus flexor digitorum sublimis, musculus flexor sublimis, superficial flexor m. of fingers.

flexor hallucis brevis m., *origin*, medial surface of cuboid and middle and lateral cuneiform bones; *insertion*, by two tendons, embracing that of the flexor longus hallucis, into the sides of the base of the proximal phalanx of the great toe; *action*, flexes great toe; *nerve supply*, medial and lateral plantar. SYN musculus flexor hallucis brevis [NA], musculus flexor brevis hallucis, short flexor m. of great toe.

flexor hallucis longus m., *origin*, lower two-thirds of posterior surface of fibula; *insertion*, base of distal phalanx of great toe; *action*, flexes great toe; *nerve supply*, medial plantar. SYN musculus flexor hallucis longus [NA], long flexor m. of great toe, musculus flexor longus hallucis.

flexor pollicis brevis m., *origin*, superficial portion from flexor retinaculum of wrist, deep portion from ulnar side of first metacarpal bone; *insertion*, base of proximal phalanx of thumb; *action*, flexes proximal phalanx of thumb; *nerve supply*, median (superficial head) and deep branch of ulnar (deep head). Some authors consider the deep head to be the first in a series of four palmar interossei muscles of the hand. SYN musculus flexor pollicis brevis [NA], short flexor m. of thumb.

flexor pollicis longus m., *origin*, anterior surface of middle third of radius; *insertion*, distal phalanx of thumb; *action*, flexes distal phalanx of thumb; *nerve supply*, median palmar interosseous. SYN musculus flexor pollicis longus [NA], long flexor m. of thumb, musculus flexor longus pollicis.

frontalis m., SYN frontal *belly* of occipitofrontalis muscle.

fusiform m., one that has a fleshy belly, tapering at either extremity. SYN musculus fusiformis [NA], spindle-shaped m.

Gantzer's m., an accessory m. extending from the superficial flexor of the digits to the deep flexor of the digits.

gastrocnemius m., *origin*, by two heads (lateral and medial) from the lateral and medial condyles of the femur; *insertion*, with soleus by tendo calcaneus into lower half of posterior surface of calcaneus; *action*, plantar flexion of foot; *nerve supply*, tibial. SYN musculus gastrocnemius [NA], gastrocnemius.

Gavard's m., oblique fibers in the muscular coat of the stomach.

genioglossal m., SYN genioglossus m.

genioglossus m., one of the paired lingual m.'s; *origin*, mental spine of the mandible; *insertion*, lingual fascia beneath the mucous membrane and epiglottis; *action*, depresses and protrudes the tongue; *nerve supply*, hypoglossal. SYN musculus genioglossus [NA], genioglossal m., genioglossus, musculus geniohyoglossus.

geniohyoid m., *origin*, mental spine of mandible; *insertion*, body of hyoid bone; *action*, draws hyoid forward, or depresses jaw when hyoid is fixed; *nerve supply*, fibers from ventral primary rami of first and second cervical spinal nerves accompanying hypoglossal. SYN musculus geniohyoideus [NA], geniohyoid, geniohyoideus.

gluteus maximus m., *origin*, ilium behind posterior gluteal line, posterior surface of sacrum and coccyx, and sacrotuberous ligament; *insertion*, iliotibial band of fascia lata (superficial three-quarters) and gluteal ridge (deep inferior one-quarter) of femur; *action*, extends thigh, especially from the flexed position, as in climbing stairs or rising from a sitting position; *nerve supply*, inferior gluteal. SYN musculus gluteus maximus [NA].

gluteus medius m., *origin*, ilium between anterior and posterior gluteal lines; *insertion*, lateral surface of greater trochanter; *action*, abducts and rotates thigh; *nerve supply*, superior gluteal. SYN musculus gluteus medius [NA], mesogluteus.

gluteus minimus m., *origin*, ilium between anterior and inferior gluteal lines; *insertion*, greater trochanter of femur; *action*, abducts thigh; *nerve supply*, superior gluteal. SYN musculus gluteus minimus [NA].

gracilis m., *origin*, ramus of pubis near symphysis; *insertion*, shaft of tibia below medial tuberosity (see *pes* anserinus); *action*, adducts thigh, flexes knee, rotates leg medially; *nerve supply*, obturator. SYN musculus gracilis [NA], gracilis (2).

great adductor m., SYN adductor magnus m.

greater pectoral m., SYN pectoralis major m.

greater posterior rectus m. of head, SYN rectus capitis posterior major m.

greater psoas m., SYN psoas major m.

greater rhomboid m., SYN rhomboideus major m.

greater zygomatic m., SYN zygomaticus major m.

Guthrie's m., SYN *sphincter* urethrae.

hamstring m.'s, the m.'s at the back of the thigh, comprising the long head of biceps, the semitendinosus, and the semimembranosus m.

m.'s of head, the m.'s of expression, of mastication, and the suboccipital m.'s in general. SYN musculi capitis [NA].

m. of heart, SYN cardiac m.

helicis major m., a narrow band of muscular fibers on the anterior border of the helix of the auricle arising from the spine and inserted at the point where the helix becomes transverse. SYN musculus helicis major [NA], large m. of helix.

helicis minor m., a band of oblique fibers covering the crus of the helix of the auricle. SYN musculus helicis minor [NA], smaller m. of helix.

Horner's m., SYN lacrimal *part* of orbicularis oculi muscle. SEE orbicularis oculi m.

Houston's m., SYN *compressor* venae dorsalis penis.

hyoglossal m., SYN hyoglossus m.

hyoglossus m., *origin*, body and greater horn of hyoid bone; *insertion*, side of the tongue; *action*, retracts and pulls down side of tongue; *nerve supply*, motor by hypoglossal, sensory by lingual. SYN musculus hyoglossus [NA], hyoglossal m., hyoglossus.

iliac m., SYN iliacus m.

iliacus m., *origin*, iliac fossa; *insertion*, tendon of psoas, anterior surface of lesser trochanter, and capsule of hip joint; *action*, flexes thigh and rotates it medially; *nerve supply*, lumbar plexus. SYN musculus iliacus [NA], iliac m.

iliacus minor m., the fibers of the iliacus arising from the anterior or inferior iliac spine and inserted into the iliofemoral ligament, sometimes distinctly separate from the rest of the muscle. SYN musculus iliacus minor, musculus iliocapsularis.

iliococcygeal m., SYN iliococcygeus m.

iliococcygeus m., the posterior part of the levator ani arising from the tendinous arch of the levator ani muscle and inserting on the anococcygeal ligament and coccyx. SYN musculus iliococcygeus [NA], iliococcygeal m.

iliocostal m., SYN iliocostalis m.

iliocostalis m., the lateral division of the erector spinae, having three subdivisions: iliocostalis lumborum m., iliocostalis thoracis m., and iliocostalis cervicis m. SYN musculus iliocostalis [NA], iliocostal m.

iliocostalis cervicis m., *origin*, angles of upper six ribs; *insertion*, transverse processes of middle cervical vertebrae; *action*, extends, abducts, and rotates cervical vertebrae; *nerve supply*, dorsal branches of upper thoracic nerves. SYN musculus iliocostalis cervicis [NA], cervical iliocostal m., cervicalis ascendens (1), musculus cervicalis ascendens.

iliocostalis lumborum m., *origin*, with erector spinae; *insertion*, the angles of lower six ribs; *action*, extends, abducts, and rotates lumbar vertebrae; *nerve supply*, dorsal branches of thoracic and lumbar nerves. SYN musculus iliocostalis lumborum [NA], lumbar iliocostal m., musculus sacrolumbalis.

iliocostalis thoracis m., *origin*, medial side of angles of lower six ribs; *insertion*, angles of upper six ribs; *action*, extends, abducts, and rotates thoracic vertebrae; *nerve supply*, dorsal branches of thoracic nerves. SYN musculus iliocostalis thoracis [NA], musculus iliocostalis dorsi.

mu

iliopsoas m., a compound muscle, consisting of the iliacus m. and psoas major m. SYN musculus iliopsoas [NA].

index extensor m., SYN extensor indicis m.

inferior constrictor m. of pharynx, *origin,* outer surfaces of thyroid (thyropharyngeal part) and cricoid (cricopharyngeal part, musculus cricopharyngeus; superior or upper esophageal sphincter m.) cartilages; *insertion,* pharyngeal raphe in the posterior portion of wall of pharynx; *action,* narrows lower part of pharynx in swallowing, the cricopharyngeal part has a sphincteric function for the esophagus, allowing some voluntary control of eructation and reflux; *nerve supply,* pharyngeal plexus. SYN musculus constrictor pharyngis inferior [NA], cricopharyngeus m., laryngopharyngeus, musculus laryngopharyngeus.

inferior gemellus m., *origin,* tuberosity of ischium; *insertion,* tendon of m. obturator internus; *action,* rotates thigh laterally; *nerve supply,* sacral plexus. SYN musculus gemellus inferior [NA], gemellus.

inferior lingual m., SYN inferior longitudinal m. of tongue.

inferior longitudinal m. of tongue, an intrinsic m. of the tongue, cylindrical in shape, occupying the underpart on either side; *action,* shortens the lower part of the tongue; *nerve supply,* motor by hypoglossal, sensory by lingual. SYN musculus longitudinalis inferior [NA], inferior lingual m.

inferior oblique m., *origin,* orbital plate of maxilla lateral to the lacrimal groove; *insertion,* sclera between the superior and lateral recti; *action,* primary, extorsion; secondary, elevation and abduction; *nerve supply,* oculomotor (inferior branch). SYN musculus obliquus inferior [NA].

inferior oblique m. of head, SYN obliquus capitis inferior m.

inferior posterior serratus m., SYN serratus posterior inferior m.

inferior rectus m., *origin,* inferior part of the common tendinous ring; *insertion,* inferior part of sclera of the eye; *action,* primary, depression; secondary, adduction and extorsion; *nerve supply,* oculomotor (inferior branch). SYN musculus rectus inferior [NA].

inferior tarsal m., poorly developed smooth m. in the lower eyelid that acts to widen the palpebral fissure. SYN musculus tarsalis inferior [NA].

infrahyoid m.'s, the small, flat m.'s inferior to the hyoid bone including the sternohyoid, omohyoid, sternothyroid, thyrohyoid, and levator m. of the thyroid gland. SYN musculi infrahyoidei [NA], strap m.'s.

infraspinatus m., *origin,* infraspinous fossa of scapula; *insertion,* middle facet of greater tubercle of humerus; *action,* extends arm and rotates it laterally; *nerve supply,* suprascapular (from fifth to sixth cervical spinal nerves). SYN musculus infraspinatus [NA].

innermost intercostal m., a layer parallel to and essentially part of the internal intercostal m. but separated from it by the intercostal vessels and nerves. See also entries under internal intercostal muscle for attachment, action and nerve supply. SYN musculus intercostalis intimus [NA].

intermediate great m., SYN vastus intermedius m.

intermediate layer of the transversospinalis m.'s, SYN multifidus m.

intermediate vastus m., SYN vastus intermedius m.

internal intercostal m., each arises from lower border of rib and passes obliquely downward and backward to be inserted into upper border of rib below; *action,* contract during expiration, also maintain tension in the intercostal spaces to resist mediolateral movement; *nerve supply,* intercostal. SYN musculus intercostalis internus [NA].

internal oblique m., *origin,* iliac fascia deep to lateral part of inguinal ligament, anterior half of crest of ilium, and lumbar fascia; *insertion,* tenth to twelfth ribs and sheath of rectus; some of the fibers from inguinal ligament terminate in the conjoint tendon; *action,* diminishes capacity of abdomen, flexes lumbar vertebral column (bends thorax forward); *nerve supply,* lower thoracic. SYN musculus obliquus internus abdominis [NA], abdominal internal oblique m.

internal obturator m., SYN obturator internus m.

internal pterygoid m., SYN medial pterygoid m.

internal sphincter m. of anus, SYN internal anal *sphincter.*

interosseous m.'s, m.'s which arise from and run between the

long (metacarpal and metatarsal) bones of the hand and foot, extending to and producing movement of the digits. SEE ALSO dorsal interosseous m.'s of foot, dorsal interosseous m.'s of hand, palmar interosseous m., plantar interosseous m. SYN musculi interossei [NA].

interspinal m.'s, SYN interspinales m.'s.

interspinales m.'s, the paired m.'s between spinous processes of adjacent vertebrae; subdivided into cervical, thoracic, and lumbar m.'s. SYN musculi interspinales [NA], interspinal m.'s.

intertransverse m.'s, SYN intertransversarii m.'s.

intertransversarii m.'s, the paired m.'s between transverse processes of adjacent vertebrae; there are anterior and posterior m.'s in the cervical region; lateral and medial m.'s in the lumbar region; and single m.'s in the thoracic region. SYN musculi intertransversarii [NA], intertransverse m.'s.

intrinsic m.'s, m.'s fully contained (origin, belly, and insertion) within the structure under consideration. For example, the interossei and lumbrical m.'s are intrinsic m.'s of the hand.

intrinsic m.'s of foot, m.'s fully contained (origin, belly, insertion) in the foot and toes. These m.'s are arranged in four layers and all are innervated by the plantar branches of the tibial nerve. Although they may be capable of producing the actions described under their individual entries, as a group the primary function of the intrinsic m.'s of the foot is to provide dynamic support of the longitudinal arch of the foot, resisting the forces which act momentarily to spread the arch during walking and running.

involuntary m.'s, m.'s not ordinarily under control of the will; except in the case of the heart, they are smooth (nonstriated) m.'s, innervated by the autonomic nervous system.

ischiocavernous m., *origin,* ramus of ischium; *insertion,* corpus cavernosum penis (or clitoridis); *action,* compresses the crus of the penis (or clitoris) forcing blood in its sinuses into the distal part of the corpus cavernosum; *nerve supply,* perineal. SYN musculus ischiocavernosus [NA], musculus erector clitoridis, musculus erector penis.

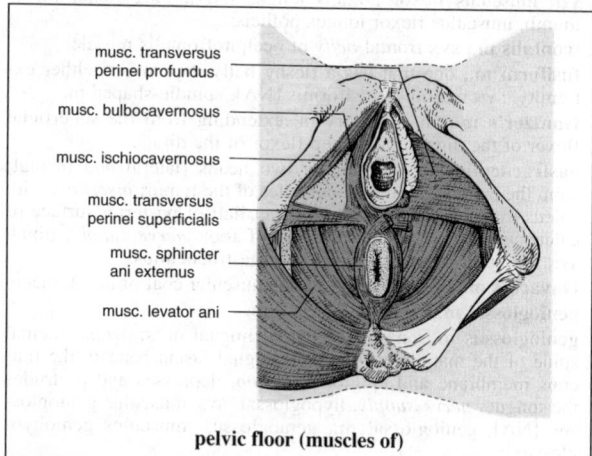

musc. transversus perinei profundus

musc. bulbocavernosus

musc. ischiocavernosus

musc. transversus perinei superficialis

musc. sphincter ani externus

musc. levator ani

pelvic floor (muscles of)

Jung's m., SYN pyramidal auricular m.

Klein's m., SYN cutaneomucous m.

Kohlrausch's m., the longitudinal m.'s of the rectal wall.

Krause's m., SYN cutaneomucous m.

Landström's m., microscopic m. fibers in the fascia behind and about the eyeball, attached anteriorly to the lids and anterior orbital fascia; its action is to draw the eyeball forward and the lids backward, resisting the pull of the four orbital m.'s.

Langer's m., SYN axillary arch m.

large m. of helix, SYN helicis major m.

m.'s of larynx, the intrinsic m.'s that regulate the length, position and tension of the vocal cords and adjust the size of the openings between the aryepiglottic folds, the ventricular folds and the vocal folds. SYN musculi laryngis [NA].

lateral cricoarytenoid m., *origin,* upper margin of arch of cricoid cartilage; *insertion*, muscular process of arytenoid; *action*, adducts vocal folds (narrows rima glottidis); *nerve supply*, recurrent laryngeal. SYN musculus cricoarytenoideus lateralis [NA].

lateral great m., SYN vastus lateralis m.

lateral lumbar intertransversarii m.'s, *origin*, transverse processes of lumbar vertebrae; *insertion*, next superior transverse process; *action*, abducts lumbar vertebrae; *nerve supply*, ventral branches of lumbar nerves. SYN musculi intertransversarii laterales lumborum [NA], lateral lumbar intertransverse m.'s.

lateral lumbar intertransverse m.'s, SYN lateral lumbar intertransversarii m.'s.

lateral pterygoid m., *origin*, inferior head from lateral lamina of pterygoid process; superior head from infratemporal crest and adjacent greater wing of the sphenoid; *insertion*, into pterygoid pit of mandible and articular disk; *action*, brings jaw forward, opens jaw; *nerve supply*, nerve to lateral pterygoid from mandibular division of trigeminal. SYN musculus pterygoideus lateralis [NA], external pterygoid m., musculus pterygoideus externus.

lateral rectus m., *origin*, lateral part of the common tendinous ring that bridges superior orbital fissure; *insertion*, lateral part of sclera of eye; *action*, abduction; *nerve supply*, abducens. SYN musculus rectus lateralis [NA], abducens oculi, musculus rectus externus.

lateral rectus m. of the head, SYN rectus capitis lateralis m.

lateral vastus m., SYN vastus lateralis m.

latissimus dorsi m., *origin*, spinous processes of lower five or six thoracic and the lumbar vertebrae, median ridge of sacrum, and outer lip of iliac crest; *insertion*, with teres major into posterior lip of bicipital groove of humerus; *action*, adducts arm, rotates it medially, and extends it; *nerve supply*, thoracodorsal. SYN musculus latissimus dorsi [NA], broadest m. of back.

lesser rhomboid m., SYN rhomboid minor m.

lesser zygomatic m., SYN zygomaticus minor m.

levator anguli oris m., *origin*, canine fossa of maxilla; *insertion*, orbicularis oris and skin at angle of mouth; *action*, raises angle of mouth; *nerve supply*, facial. SYN musculus levator anguli oris [NA], musculus caninus, musculus triangularis labii superioris.

levator ani m., formed by pubococcygeus and iliococcygeus m.'s; *origin*, posterior body of pubis, tendinous arch of the levator ani, and spine of ischium; *insertion*, anococcygeal ligament, sides of the lower part of the sacrum and of coccyx; *action*, resists prolapsing forces and draws the anus upward following defecation; supports the pelvic viscera; *nerve supply*, nerve to levator ani (fourth sacral spinal nerve). SYN musculus levator ani [NA], elevator m. of anus.

levatores costarum m.'s, SYN musculus levator costae [NA], elevator m. of rib, musculi levatores costarum. SEE long levatores costarum m.'s, short levatores costarum m.'s.

levator labii superioris m., *origin*, maxilla below infraorbital foramen; *insertion*, orbicularis oris of upper lip; *action*, elevates upper lip; *nerve supply*, facial. SYN musculus levator labii superioris [NA], caput infraorbitale quadrati labii superioris, elevator m. of upper lip.

levator labii superioris alaeque nasi m., *origin*, root of nasal process of maxilla; *insertion*, wing of nose and orbicularis oris m. of upper lip; *action*, elevates upper lip and wing of nose; *nerve supply*, facial. SYN musculus levator labii superioris alaeque nasi [NA], caput angulare quadrati labii superioris, elevator m. of upper lip and wing of nose.

levator palati m., SYN levator veli palatini m.

levator palpebrae superioris m., *origin*, orbital surface of the lesser wing of the sphenoid, above and anterior to the optic canal; *insertion*, skin of eyelid, tarsal plate, and orbital walls, by medial and lateral expansions of the aponeurosis of insertion; *action*, raises the upper eyelid; *nerve supply*, oculomotor. SYN musculus levator palpebrae superioris [NA], elevator m. of upper eyelid, musculus orbitopalpebralis, palpebralis.

levator prostatae m., in the male, the most medial fibers of the levator ani (pubococcygeus) m. that extend from the pubis into the fascia of the prostate. SYN musculus levator prostatae [NA], elevator m. of prostate.

levator scapulae m., *origin*, from posterior tubercles of transverse processes of four upper cervical vertebrae; *insertion*, into

superior angle of scapula; *action*, raises the scapula; *nerve supply*, dorsal scapular nerve. SYN musculus levator scapulae [NA], elevator m. of scapula, musculus levator anguli scapulae.

levator m. of thyroid gland, a fasciculus occasionally passing from the thyrohyoid m. to the isthmus of the thyroid gland. SYN musculus levator glandulae thyroideae [NA], elevator m. of thyroid gland, Soemmerring's m.

levator veli palatini m., *origin*, apex of petrous portion of temporal bone and lower part of cartilaginous auditory (eustachian) tube; *insertion*, aponeurosis of soft palate; *action*, raises soft palate; through the expansion of its fleshy belly during contraction, it helps to "push" open the auditory tube; *nerve supply*, pharyngeal plexus (cranial root of accessory nerve). SYN musculus levator veli palatini [NA], elevator m. of soft palate, levator palati m., musculus levator palati, musculus petrostaphylinus.

long abductor m. of thumb, SYN abductor pollicis longus m.

long adductor m., SYN adductor longus m.

long extensor m. of great toe, SYN extensor hallucis longus m.

long extensor m. of thumb, SYN extensor pollicis longus m.

long extensor m. of toes, SYN extensor digitorum longus m.

long fibular m., SYN peroneus longus m.

long flexor m. of great toe, SYN flexor hallucis longus m.

long flexor m. of thumb, SYN flexor pollicis longus m.

long flexor m. of toes, SYN flexor digitorum longus m.

long m. of head, SYN longus capitis m.

longissimus m., the intermediate division of the erector spinae m. having three subdivisions: longissimus capitis m., longissimus cervicis m., and longissimus thoracis m. SYN musculus longissimus [NA].

longissimus capitis m., *origin*, from transverse processes of upper thoracic and transverse and articular processes of lower and middle cervical vertebrae; *insertion*, into mastoid process; *action*, keeps head erect, draws it backward or to one side; *nerve supply*, dorsal primary rami of cervical spinal nerves. SYN musculus longissimus capitis [NA], musculus complexus minor, musculus trachelomastoideus, musculus transversalis capitis.

longissimus cervicis m., *origin*, transverse processes of upper thoracic vertebrae; *insertion*, transverse processes of middle and upper cervical vertebrae; *action*, extends cervical vertebrae; *nerve supply*, dorsal primary rami of lower cervical and upper thoracic spinal nerves. SYN musculus longissimus cervicis [NA], cervical longissimus m., musculus transversalis cervicis, musculus transversalis colli.

longissimus thoracis m., *origin*, with iliocostalis and from transverse processes of lower thoracic vertebrae; *insertion*, by lateral slips into most or all of the ribs between angles and tubercles and into tips of transverse processes of upper lumbar vertebrae, and by medial slips into accessory processes of upper lumbar and transverse processes of thoracic vertebrae; *action*, extends vertebral column; *nerve supply*, dorsal primary rami of thoracic and lumbar spinal nerves. SYN musculus longissimus thoracis [NA], musculus longissimus dorsi, thoracic longissimus m.

long levatores costarum m.'s, *insertion*, the second rib below their origin; *action*, raise ribs; *nerve supply*, intercostal. SYN musculi levatores costarum longi.

long m. of neck, SYN longus colli m.

long palmar m., SYN palmaris longus m.

long peroneal m., SYN peroneus longus m.

long radial extensor m. of wrist, SYN extensor carpi radialis longus m.

longus capitis m., *origin*, anterior tubercles of transverse processes of third to sixth cervical vertebrae; *insertion*, basilar process of occipital bone; *action*, twists or flexes neck anteriorly; *nerve supply*, cervical plexus. SYN musculus longus capitis [NA], long m. of head, musculus rectus capitis anticus major.

longus colli m., medial part: *origin*, the bodies of the third thoracic to the fifth cervical vertebrae; *insertion*, the bodies of the second to fourth cervical vertebrae; superolateral part: *origin*, the anterior tubercles of the transverse processes of the third to fifth cervical vertebrae; *insertion*, the anterior tubercle of the atlas; inferolateral part: *origin*, the bodies of the first to third thoracic vertebrae; *insertion*, the anterior tubercles of the transverse processes of the fifth and sixth cervical vertebrae; *action*,

mu

for all three parts, twist neck and flex neck anteriorly; *nerve supply*, for all three parts, ventral primary rami of cervical spinal nerves (cervical plexus). SYN musculus longus colli [NA], long m. of neck.

lumbar iliocostal m., SYN iliocostalis lumborum m.

lumbar interspinal m., SYN lumbar interspinales m.'s.

lumbar interspinales m.'s, *origin*, superior margin of lumbar spinous process; *insertion*, inferior margin of next superior spinous process; *action*, extends lumbar vertebrae; *nerve supply*, dorsal primary rami of lumbar spinal nerves. SYN musculus interspinalis lumborum [NA], lumbar interspinal m.

lumbar quadrate m., SYN quadratus lumborum m.

lumbar rotator m.'s, SYN rotatores lumborum m.'s.

lumbrical m. of foot, four intrinsic m.'s of the foot; *origin*, first: from tibial side of tendon to second toe of flexor digitorum longus; second, third, and fourth: from adjacent sides of all four tendons of this m.; *insertion*, tibial side of extensor tendon on dorsum of each of the four lateral toes; *action*, flex the proximal and extend the middle and distal phalanges; *nerve supply*, lateral (second to fourth lumbricals) and medial (first lumbrical) plantar. SYN musculus lumbricalis pedis [NA].

lumbrical m. of hand, four intrinsic muscles of the hand; *origin*, the two lateral: from the radial side of the tendons of the flexor digitorum profundus going to the index and middle fingers; the two medial: from the adjacent sides of the second and third, and third and fourth tendons; *insertion*, radial side of extensor tendon on dorsum of each of the four fingers; *action*, flexes metacarpophalangeal joint and extends the proximal and distal interphalangeal joint; *nerve supply*, the two radial m.'s by the median, the two ulnar m.'s by the ulnar. SYN musculus lumbricalis manus [NA].

Marcacci's m., a sheet of smooth m. fibers underlying the areola and nipple of the mammary gland.

masseter m., *origin*, superficial part: inferior border of the anterior two-thirds of the zygomatic arch; deep part: inferior border and medial surface of the zygomatic arch; *insertion*, lateral surface of ramus and coronoid process of the mandible; *action*, elevates mandible (closes jaw); *nerve supply*, masseteric branch of mandibular division of trigeminal. SYN musculus masseter [NA].

m.'s of mastication, m.'s derived from the first (mandibular) arch used in chewing; all receive innervation from the motor root of the trigeminal nerve via its mandibular division. SEE masseter m., temporalis m., lateral pterygoid m., medial pterygoid m.

medial great m., SYN vastus medialis m.

medial lumbar intertransversarii m.'s, *origin*, accessory and mamillary processes of lumbar vertebrae; *insertion*, corresponding processes of next superior vertebra; *action*, abducts lumbar vertebrae; *nerve supply*, dorsal primary rami of lumbar spinal nerves. SYN musculi intertransversarii mediales lumborum [NA], medial lumbar intertransverse m.'s.

medial lumbar intertransverse m.'s, SYN medial lumbar intertransversarii m.'s.

medial pterygoid m., *origin*, pterygoid fossa of sphenoid and tuberosity of maxilla; *insertion*, medial surface of mandible between angle and mylohyoid groove; *action*, elevates mandible closing jaw; *nerve supply*, nerve to medial pterygoid from mandibular division of trigeminal. SYN musculus pterygoideus medialis [NA], internal pterygoid m., musculus pterygoideus internus.

medial rectus m., *origin*, medial part of the anulus tendineus communis; *insertion*, medial part of sclera of the eye; *action*, adduction; *nerve supply*, oculomotor. SYN musculus rectus medialis [NA], musculus rectus internus.

medial vastus m., SYN vastus medialis m.

mentalis m., *origin*, incisor fossa of mandible; *insertion*, skin of chin; *action*, raises and wrinkles skin of chin, thus elevating the lower lip; *nerve supply*, facial. SYN musculus mentalis [NA], chin m., musculus levator labii inferioris.

Merkel's m., SYN ceratocricoid m.

middle constrictor m. of pharynx, *origin*, stylohyoid ligament, lesser cornu of the hyoid bone (chondropharyngeal part) and greater cornu of the hyoid bone (ceratopharyngeal part); *insertion*, pharyngeal raphe in the posterior wall of the pharynx;

action, narrows pharynx in the act of swallowing; *nerve supply*, pharyngeal plexus. SYN musculus constrictor pharyngis medius [NA].

middle scalene m., SYN scalenus medius m.

mimetic m.'s, SYN m.'s of facial expression.

mucocutaneous m., SYN cutaneomucous m.

Müller's m., (1) SYN orbitalis m. **(2)** SYN circular *fibers*, under *fiber*. **(3)** SYN superior tarsal m.

multifidus m., *origin*, from the sacrum, sacroiliac ligament, mamillary processes of the lumbar vertebrae, transverse processes of thoracic vertebrae, and articular processes of last four cervical vertebrae; *insertion*, into the spinous processes of all the vertebrae up to and including the axis; *action*, rotates vertebral column; *nerve supply*, dorsal primary rami of spinal nerves. SYN musculus multifidus [NA], intermediate layer of the transversospinalis m.'s, musculus multifidus spinae.

multipennate m., a m. with several central tendons toward which the m. fibers converge like the barbs of feathers. SYN musculus multipennatus [NA].

mylohyoid m., *origin*, mylohyoid line of mandible; *insertion*, upper border of hyoid bone and raphe separating m. from its fellow; *action*, elevates floor of mouth and the tongue, depresses jaw when hyoid is fixed; *nerve supply*, nerve to mylohyoid from mandibular division of trigeminal. SYN musculus mylohyoideus [NA], mylohyoideus.

nasal m., SYN nasalis m.

nasalis m., compound m. consisting of: a transverse part (pars transversa musculi nasalis [NA], musculus compressor naris) arising from the maxilla above the root of the canine tooth on each side and forming an aponeurosis across the bridge of the nose; and an alar part (pars alaris musculi nasalis [NA], musculus dilator naris) arising from the maxilla above the lateral incisor and attaching to the wing of the nose; the alar part dilates the nostril; *nerve supply*, facial. SYN musculus nasalis [NA], nasal m.

m.'s of neck, the anterolateral m.'s of the neck including the platysma, sternocleidomastoid, suprahyoid m.'s, infrahyoid m.'s, longus colli and scalene m.'s. SYN musculi colli [NA].

m. of notch of helix, an occasional m. on the cranial surface of the auricle spanning the antitragohelicine fissure. SYN musculus incisurae helicis [NA], musculus intertragicus.

oblique arytenoid m., *origin*, muscular process of arytenoid cartilage; *insertion*, summit of arytenoid cartilage of opposite side and continuing as the aryepiglottic muscle in the aryepiglottic fold to the epiglottis; *action*, narrows the interarytenoid portion of the rima glottidis; *nerve supply*, recurrent laryngeal. SYN musculus arytenoideus obliquus [NA], arytenoideus.

oblique m. of auricle, SYN oblique auricular m.

oblique auricular m., a thin band of oblique muscular fibers extending from the upper part of the eminence of the concha to the convexity of the helix, running across the groove corresponding to the inferior crus of the anthelix. SYN musculus obliquus auriculae [NA], oblique m. of auricle, Tod's m.

obliquus capitis inferior m., *origin*, spinous process of axis; *insertion*, transverse process of the atlas; *action*, rotates head; *origin*, spinous process of axis; *insertion*, transverse process of the atlas; *nerve supply*, suboccipital. SEE ALSO suboccipital m.'s. SYN musculus obliquus capitis inferior [NA], inferior oblique m. of head.

obliquus capitis superior m., *origin*, transverse process of atlas; *insertion*, lateral third of inferior nuchal line; *action*, rotates head; *nerve supply*, suboccipital. SEE ALSO suboccipital m.'s. SYN musculus obliquus capitis superior [NA], superior oblique m. of head.

obturator externus m., *origin*, lower half of margin of obturator foramen and adjacent part of external surface of obturator membrane; *insertion*, trochanteric fossa of greater trochanter; *action*, rotates thigh laterally; *nerve supply*, obturator. SYN musculus obturator externus [NA], external obturator m.

obturator internus m., *origin*, pelvic surface of obturator membrane and margin of obturator foramen; *insertion*, passes out of pelvis through lesser sciatic foramen, in so doing, making a 90° turn to insert into the medial surface of greater trochanter; *action*, rotates thigh laterally; *nerve supply*, nerve to obturator internus

movements of the eyes and muscles employed				
sideways motion (ab- and adduction)	vertical motion	oblique motion		rolling motion
dextroversion right eye: lateral rectus left eye: medial rectus	*elevation (lifting)* superior rectus inferior oblique	*dextroelevation* right eye: superior rectus left eye: inferior oblique	*levoelevation* left eye: superior rectus right eye: inferior oblique	*extorsion (outward rolling)* inferior rectus inferior oblique
levoversion right eye: medial rectus left eye: lateral rectus	*depression (lowering)* inferior rectus inferior oblique	*dextrodepression* right eye: inferior rectus left eye: superior oblique	*levodepression* left eye: inferior rectus right eye: superior oblique	*intorsion (inward rolling)* superior rectus superior oblique

(sacral plexus). SYN musculus obturator internus [NA], internal obturator m.

occipitalis m., SYN occipital *belly* of occipitofrontalis muscle.

occipitofrontal m., SYN occipitofrontalis m.

occipitofrontalis m., it is a part of m. epicranius; the occipital belly (occipitalis m.) arises from the occipital bone and inserts into the galea aponeurotica; the frontal belly (frontalis m.) arises from the galea and inserts into the skin of the eyebrow and nose; *action*, to move the scalp; *nerve supply*, facial. SYN musculus occipitofrontalis [NA], occipitofrontal m.

ocular m.'s, SYN extraocular m.'s.

Oehl's m.'s, strands of m. fibers in the chordae tendineae of the left atrioventricular valve.

omohyoid m., formed of two bellies attached to intermediate tendon; *origin*, by inferior belly from upper border of scapula between superior angle and notch; *insertion*, by superior belly into hyoid bone; *action*, depresses hyoid; *nerve supply*, upper cervical spinal nerves through ansa cervicalis. SYN musculus omohyoideus [NA], omohyoid.

opponens digiti minimi m., *origin*, hamulus of the hamate bone and transverse carpal ligament; *insertion*, shaft of fifth metacarpal; *action*, "cups" palm, drawing ulnar side of hand toward center of palm; *nerve supply*, ulnar. SYN musculus opponens digiti minimi [NA], musculus opponens digiti quinti, musculus opponens minimi digiti, opposer m. of little finger.

opponens pollicis m., *origin*, ridge of trapezium and flexor retinaculum; *insertion*, anterior surface of the full length of the shaft of the first metacarpal bone; *action*, acts at carpometacarpal joint to "cup" palm, enabling one to oppose thumb to other fingers; *nerve supply*, median. SYN musculus opponens pollicis [NA], opposer m. of thumb.

opposer m. of little finger, SYN opponens digiti minimi m.

opposer m. of thumb, SYN opponens pollicis m.

orbicular m., SYN orbicularis m.

orbicular m. of eye, SYN orbicularis oculi m.

orbicularis m., a sphincter-like sheet of m. that encircles an orifice such as the mouth or the palpebral fissures. SYN musculus orbicularis [NA], orbicular m., orbicularis (2).

orbicularis oculi m., consists of three portions: orbital part, or external portion, which arises from frontal process of maxilla and nasal process of frontal bone, encircles aperture of orbit, and is inserted near origin; palpebral part, or internal portion, which arises from medial palpebral ligament, passes through each eyelid, and is inserted into lateral palpebral raphe; lacrimal part (tensor tarsi muscle, Duverney's or Horner's muscle) arises from posterior lacrimal crest and passes across lacrimal sac to join palpebral portion; *action*, closes eye, wrinkles forehead vertically; *nerve supply*, facial. SYN musculus orbicularis oculi [NA], musculus orbicularis palpebrarum, orbicular m. of eye, sphincter oculi.

orbicularis oris m., *origin*, by nasolabial band from septum of the nose, by superior incisive bundle from incisor fossa of maxilla, by inferior incisive bundle from lower jaw each side of symphysis; *insertion*, fibers surround mouth between skin and mucous membrane of lips and cheeks, and are blended with other m.'s; *action*, closes lips; *nerve supply*, facial. SYN musculus orbicularis oris [NA], musculus sphincter oris, orbicular m. of mouth, sphincter oris.

orbicular m. of mouth, SYN orbicularis oris m.

orbital m., SYN orbitalis m.

orbitalis m., a rudimentary nonstriated m., crossing the infraorbital groove and sphenomaxillary fissure, intimately united with the periosteum of the orbit. SYN musculus orbitalis [NA], Müller's m. (1), orbital m.

palatoglossus m., forms anterior pillar of tonsillar fossa; *origin*, oral surface of soft palate; *insertion*, side of tongue; *action*, raises back of tongue and narrows fauces; *nerve supply*, pharyngeal plexus (cranial root of accessory nerve). SYN musculus palatoglossus [NA], glossopalatinus, musculus glossopalatinus, palatoglossus.

palatopharyngeal m., SYN palatopharyngeus m.

palatopharyngeus m., *origin*, soft palate; forms the posterior pillar of the fauces or tonsillar fossa; *insertion*, posterior border of thyroid cartilage and aponeurosis of pharynx; *action*, narrows fauces, depresses soft palate, elevates pharynx and larynx; *nerve supply*, pharyngeal plexus (cranial root of accessory nerve). SYN musculus palatopharyngeus [NA], musculus pharyngopalatinus, palatopharyngeal m., palatopharyngeus, pharyngopalatinus, pharyngostaphylinus.

palatouvularis m., SYN uvulae m.

palmar interosseous m., three m.'s in the hand; *origin*, first: ulnar side of second metacarpal; second and third: radial sides of fourth and fifth metacarpals; *insertion*, first: into ulnar side of index; second and third: into radial sides of ring and little fingers; *action*, adducts fingers toward axis of middle finger; *nerve supply*, ulnar. SEE ALSO flexor pollicis brevis m. SYN musculus interosseus palmaris [NA], musculus interosseus volaris.

palmaris brevis m., *origin*, ulnar side of central portion of the palmar aponeurosis; *insertion*, skin of ulnar side of hand; *action*, wrinkles skin on medial side of palm; *nerve supply*, ulnar. SYN musculus palmaris brevis [NA], short palmar m.

palmaris longus m., *origin*, medial epicondyle of humerus; *insertion*, flexor retinaculum of wrist and palmar fascia; *action*, makes palmar fascia tense and flexes the hand and forearm; is absent about 20% of the time; when tensed, its tendon stands out sharply at the wrist and overlies the median nerve; *nerve supply*, median. SYN musculus palmaris longus [NA], long palmar m.

panniculus carnosus m., (1) a sheet of m., lying beneath the skin, by which the skin can be made to shiver; it is especially well developed in the horse; (2) in man, platysma.

papillary m., one of the group of myocardial bundles which terminate in the chordae tendineae which attach to the cusps of the atrioventricular valves; each has an anterior and a posterior papillary muscle; the right ventricle sometimes has a septal papillary muscle. SYN musculus papillaris [NA].

pectinate m.'s, prominent ridges of atrial myocardium located on the inner surface of much of the right atrium and both auricles. SYN musculi pectinati [NA], pectinate fibers.

mu

pectineal m., SYN pectineus m.

pectineus m., *origin,* crest of pubis; *insertion,* pectineal line of femur; *action,* adducts thigh and assists in flexion; *nerve supply,* obturator and femoral. SYN musculus pectineus [NA], pectineal m.

pectoralis major m., *origin,* clavicular part (pars clavicularis), medial half of clavicle; sternocostal part (pars sternocostalis), anterior surface of manubrium and body of sternum and cartilages of first to sixth ribs; abdominal part (pars abdominalis), aponeurosis of external oblique; *insertion,* crest of greater tubercle of humerus; *action,* adducts and medially rotates arm; *nerve supply,* anterior thoracic. SYN musculus pectoralis major [NA], greater pectoral m.

pectoralis minor m., *origin,* third to fifth ribs at the costochondral articulations; *insertion,* tip of coracoid process of scapula; *action,* draws down scapula or raises ribs; *nerve supply,* medial pectoral nerve. SYN musculus pectoralis minor [NA], smaller pectoral m.

pectorodorsal m., SYN pectorodorsalis m.

pectorodorsalis m., an anomalous m. or tendinus slip that passes across the axilla from the pectoralis major to insert with the latissimus dorsi onto the humerus. Though to be a vestige of the panniculus carnosus muscle of lower mammals. SYN axillary arch m., axillary arch, pectorodorsal m.

pennate m., SEE bipennate m., unipennate m.

perineal m.'s, the muscles located in the perineal region; these are the external anal sphincter, the superficial transverse perineal m., ischiocavernosus m., bulbospongiosus m., deep transverse perineal m., and sphincter urethrae m. SYN musculi perinei [NA].

peroneus brevis m., *origin,* lower two-thirds of lateral surface of fibula; *insertion,* base of fifth metatarsal bone; *action,* everts foot; *nerve supply,* superficial peroneal. SYN musculus fibularis brevis [NA], musculus peroneus brevis [NA], short fibular m., short peroneal m.

peroneus longus m., *origin,* upper two-thirds of outer surface of fibula and lateral condyle of tibia; *insertion,* by tendon passing behind lateral malleolus and across sole of foot to medial cuneiform and base of first metatarsal; *action,* plantar flexes and everts foot; *nerve supply,* superficial peroneal. SYN musculus fibularis longus [NA], musculus peroneus longus [NA], long fibular m., long peroneal m.

peroneus tertius m., *origin,* in common with m. extensor digitorum longus; *insertion,* dorsum of base of fifth metatarsal bone; *nerve supply,* deep branch of peroneal; *action,* assists in dorsiflexion and eversion of foot. SYN musculus fibularis tertius [NA], musculus peroneus tertius [NA], third peroneal m.

piriform m., SYN piriformis m.

piriformis m., *origin,* margins of pelvic sacral foramina and greater sciatic notch of ilium; *insertion,* upper border of greater trochanter; *action,* rotates thigh laterally; *nerve supply,* nerve to piriformis (sciatic plexus). SYN musculus piriformis [NA], musculus pyriformis, piriform m.

plantar m., SYN plantaris m.

plantar interosseous m., three intrinsic m.'s of foot; *origin,* the medial side of the third, fourth, and fifth metatarsal bones; *insertion,* corresponding side of proximal phalanx of the same toes; *action,* adducts three lateral toes; *nerve supply,* lateral plantar. SYN musculus interosseus plantaris [NA].

plantaris m., *origin,* lateral supracondylar ridge; *insertion,* medial margin of tendo achillis and deep fascia of ankle; *action,* traditionally described as plantar flexion of foot; many investigators now believe the plantaris muscle to be primarily a proprioceptive organ; *nerve supply,* tibial nerve. SYN musculus plantaris [NA], musculus tibialis gracilis, plantar m.

plantar quadrate m., SYN quadratus plantae m.

platysma m., *origin,* subcutaneous layer and fascia covering pectoralis major and deltoid at level of first or second rib; *insertion,* lower border of mandible, risorius and platysma of opposite side; *action,* depresses lower lip, forms ridges in skin of neck and upper chest when jaws are "clenched", denoting stress, anger; *nerve supply,* cervical branch of facial. SYN platysma [NA], musculus platysma myoides, musculus platysma, musculus subcutaneus colli, musculus tetragonus.

pleuroesophageal m., muscular fasciculi, arising from the mediastinal pleura, which reinforce musculature of esophagus. SYN musculus pleuroesophageus [NA].

popliteal m., SYN popliteus m.

popliteus m., *origin,* lateral condyle of femur; *insertion,* posterior surface of tibia above oblique line; *action,* from the fully extended and "locked" position, rotates the femur medially, on the fixed (planted) tibial plateau about 5°, "unlocking" the knee to enable flexion to occur; *nerve supply,* tibial. SYN musculus popliteus [NA], popliteal m., popliteus (3).

posterior auricular m., *origin,* mastoid process; *insertion,* posterior portion of root of auricle; *action,* draws back the pinna; *nerve supply,* facial. SYN musculus auricularis posterior [NA], musculus retrahens aurem, musculus retrahens auriculam.

posterior cervical intertransversarii m.'s, *origin,* lateral part: posterior tubercle of cervical transverse process; medial part: transverse process; *insertion,* corresponding parts of next superior transverse process; *action,* abducts cervical vertebrae; *nerve supply,* lateral part: ventral primary rami of cervical spinal nerves; medial part: dorsal primary rami of cervical spinal nerves. SYN musculi intertransversarii posteriores cervicis [NA], posterior cervical intertransverse m.'s.

posterior cervical intertransverse m.'s, SYN posterior cervical intertransversarii m.'s.

posterior cricoarytenoid m., *origin,* depression on posterior surface of lamina of cricoid; *insertion,* muscular process of arytenoid; *action,* abducts vocal folds, widening rima glottidis as for taking a breath; *nerve supply,* recurrent laryngeal. SYN musculus cricoarytenoideus posterior [NA].

posterior scalene m., SYN scalenus posterior m.

posterior tibial m., SYN tibialis posterior m.

Pozzi's m., SYN extensor digitorum brevis m. of hand.

procerus m., *insertion,* into frontalis; *action,* assists frontalis; *origin,* from membrane covering bridge of nose; *nerve supply,* branch of facial. SYN musculus procerus [NA], musculus pyramidalis nasi, procerus.

pronator quadratus m., *origin,* distal fourth of anterior surface of ulna; *insertion,* distal fourth of anterior surface of radius; *action,* pronates forearm; *nerve supply,* anterior interosseous. SYN musculus pronator quadratus [NA], quadrate pronator m.

pronator teres m., *origin,* superficial (humeral) head (ulnar) from the common flexor origin on the medial epicondyle of the humerus, deep (ulnar) head from the medial side of the coronoid process of the ulna; *insertion,* middle of the lateral surface of the radius; *action,* pronates forearm; *nerve supply,* median. SYN musculus pronator teres [NA], musculus pronator radii teres, round pronator m.

psoas major m., *origin,* bodies of vertebrae and intervertebral disks from the twelfth thoracic to the fifth lumbar, and transverse processes of the lumbar vertebrae; *insertion,* forms a common insertion with iliacus m.'s into lesser trochanter of femur; *action,* flexes hip joint; *nerve supply,* lumbar plexus (ventral rami of first, second and usually third lumbar spinal nerves). SYN musculus psoas major [NA], greater psoas m.

psoas minor m., an inconstant m., absent in about 40%; *origin,* bodies of twelfth thoracic and first lumbar vertebrae and disk between them; *insertion,* iliopubic eminence via iliopectineal arch (iliac fascia); *action,* assists in flexion of lumbar spine; *nerve supply,* lumbar plexus. SYN musculus psoas minor [NA], smaller psoas m.

pubococcygeal m., SYN pubococcygeus m.

pubococcygeus m., fibers of the levator ani, arising from the pelvic surface of the body of the pubis and adjacent tendinous arch of obturator fascia, attaching to the coccyx. SYN musculus pubococcygeus [NA], pubococcygeal m.

puboprostatic m., smooth m. fibers within the puboprostatic ligament. SYN musculus puboprostaticus [NA].

puborectal m., SYN puborectalis m.

puborectalis m., the medial part of the m. levator ani (pubococcygeus muscle) that passes from the body of the pubis around the anus to form a muscular sling at the level of the anorectal junction; it contracts to increase the perineal flexure during a peristalsis to maintain fecal continence and relaxes to allow defecation. SYN musculus puborectalis [NA], Braune's m., puborectal m.

pubovaginal m., SYN pubovaginalis m.

pubovaginalis m., in the female, the most medial fibers of the levator ani (pubococcygeus) m. that extend from the pubis into the lateral walls of the vagina. SYN musculus pubovaginalis [NA], pubovaginal m.

pubovesical m., SYN pubovesicalis m.

pubovesicalis m., smooth m. fibers within the pubovesical ligament in the female. SYN musculus pubovesicalis [NA], pubovesical m.

pyramidal m., SYN pyramidalis m.

pyramidal m. of auricle, SYN pyramidal auricular m.

pyramidal auricular m., an occasional prolongation of the fibers of the tragicus to the spina helicis. SYN musculus pyramidalis auriculae [NA], Jung's m., pyramidal m. of auricle.

pyramidalis m., *origin,* crest of pubis; *insertion,* lower portion of linea alba; *action,* makes linea alba tense; *nerve supply,* subcostal. SYN musculus pyramidalis [NA], pyramidal m.

quadrate m., SYN quadratus m.

quadrate m. of loins, SYN quadratus lumborum m.

quadrate pronator m., SYN pronator quadratus m.

quadrate m. of sole, SYN quadratus plantae m.

quadrate m. of thigh, SYN quadratus femoris m.

quadrate m. of upper lip, SYN *musculus* quadratus labii superioris.

quadratus m., a m. that is more or less square in shape. SYN musculus quadratus [NA], quadrate m.

quadratus fem′oris m., *insertion,* intertrochanteric ridge; *origin,* lateral border of tuberosity of ischium; *action,* rotates thigh laterally; *nerve supply,* nerve to quadratus femoris (sacral plexus). SYN musculus quadratus femoris [NA], quadrate m. of thigh.

quadratus lumborum m., *origin,* iliac crest, iliolumbar ligament, and transverse processes of lower lumbar vertebrae; *insertion,* twelfth rib and transverse processes of upper lumbar vertebrae; *action,* abducts trunk; *nerve supply,* ventral primary rami of upper lumbar spinal nerves. SYN musculus quadratus lumborum [NA], lumbar quadrate m., quadrate m. of loins.

quadratus plantae m., *origin,* by two heads from the lateral and medial borders of the inferior surface of the calcaneus; *insertion,* tendons of flexor digitorum longus; *action,* assists long flexor; *nerve supply,* lateral plantar. SYN musculus flexor accessorius [NA], musculus quadratus plantae [NA], accessory flexor m. of foot, caro quadrata sylvii, musculus pronator pedis, plantar quadrate m., quadrate m. of sole.

quadriceps fem′oris m., *origin,* by four heads: rectus femoris, vastus lateralis, vastus intermedius, and vastus medialis; *insertion,* patella, and thence by ligamentum patellae to tuberosity of tibia; *action,* extends leg; flexes thigh by action of rectus femoris; *nerve supply,* femoral. SYN musculus quadriceps femoris [NA], musculus quadriceps extensor femoris, quadriceps m. of thigh.

quadriceps m. of thigh, SYN quadriceps femoris m.

radial flexor m. of wrist, SYN flexor carpi radialis m.

rectococcygeal m., SYN rectococcygeus m.

rectococcygeus m., a band of smooth m. fibers passing from the posterior surface of the rectum to the anterior surface of second or third coccygeal segment. SYN musculus rectococcygeus [NA], rectococcygeal m.

rectourethral m., SYN rectourethralis m.

rectourethralis m., smooth m. fibers that pass forward from the longitudinal m. layer of the rectum to the membranous urethra in the male. SYN musculus rectourethralis [NA], rectourethral m.

rectouterine m., a band of fibrous tissue and smooth muscle fibers passing between the cervix of the uterus and the rectum in the rectouterine fold, on either side. SYN musculus rectouterinus [NA].

rectovesical m., SYN rectovesicalis m.

rectovesicalis m., smooth m. fibers in the sacrogenital fold in the male; they correspond to rectouterinus m. SYN musculus rectovesicalis [NA], rectovesical m.

rectus m. of abdomen, SYN rectus abdominis m.

rectus abdominis m., m. of ventral abdominal wall, flanking the linea alba, and characterized by tendinous intersections separating its length into multiple bellies; *origin,* crest and symphysis of the pubis; *insertion,* xiphoid process and fifth to seventh costal cartilages; *action,* flexes lumbar vertebral column, draws thorax downward toward pubis; *nerve supply,* thoracoabdominal nerves. SYN musculus rectus abdominis [NA], rectus m. of abdomen.

rectus capitis anterior m., *origin,* transverse process and lateral mass of atlas; *insertion,* basilar process of occipital bone; *action,* turns and inclines head forward; *nerve supply,* ventral primary ramus of first and second cervical spinal nerve. SYN musculus rectus capitis anterior [NA], anterior rectus m. of head, musculus rectus capitis anticus minor.

rectus capitis lateralis m., *origin,* transverse process of atlas; *insertion,* jugular process of occipital bone; *action,* inclines head to one side; *nerve supply,* ventral primary ramus of first cervical spinal nerve. SYN musculus rectus capitis lateralis [NA], lateral rectus m. of the head.

rectus capitis posterior major m., *origin,* spinous process of axis; *insertion,* middle of inferior nuchal line of occipital bone; *action,* rotates and draws head backward; *nerve supply,* dorsal branch of first cervical (suboccipital). SEE ALSO suboccipital m.'s. SYN musculus rectus capitis posterior major [NA], greater posterior rectus m. of head, musculus rectus capitis posticus major.

rectus capitis posterior minor m., *origin,* from posterior tubercle of atlas; *insertion,* medial third of inferior nuchal line of occipital bone; *action,* rotates head and draws it backward; *nerve supply,* dorsal branch of first cervical (suboccipital). SEE ALSO suboccipital m.'s. SYN musculus rectus capitis posterior minor [NA], musculus rectus capitis posticus minor, smaller posterior rectus m. of head.

rectus femoris m., *origin,* anterior inferior spine of ilium and upper margin of acetabulum; *insertion,* via common tendon of quadriceps femoris into patella, and via patellar ligament to tibial tuberosity. SYN musculus rectus femoris [NA], rectus m. of thigh.

rectus m. of thigh, SYN rectus femoris m.

red m., slow-twitch m. in which small dark "red" m. fibers predominate; myoglobin is abundant and great numbers of mitochondria occur, characterized by slow, sustained (tonic) contraction. Contrast with white m.

Reisseisen's m.'s, microscopic smooth m. fibers in the smallest bronchial tubes.

rhomboideus major m., *origin,* spinous processes and corresponding supraspinous ligaments of first four thoracic vertebrae; *insertion,* medial border of scapula below spine; *action,* draws scapula toward vertebral column; *nerve supply,* dorsal of scapula nerve. SYN musculus rhomboideus major [NA], greater rhomboid m.

rhomboid minor m., *origin,* spinous processes of sixth and seventh cervical vertebrae; *insertion,* medial margin of scapula above spine; *action,* draws scapula toward vertebral column and slightly upward; *nerve supply,* dorsal nerve of scapula. SYN musculus rhomboideus minor [NA], lesser rhomboid m.

rider's m.'s, the adductor m.'s of the thigh, which come into play especially in horseback riding.

Riolan's m., (1) marginal fibers of the palpebral part of the orbicularis oculi m.; (2) SYN cremaster m.

risorius m., *origin,* from platysma and fascia of masseter; *insertion,* orbicularis oris and skin at corner of mouth; *action,* draws angle of mouth laterally, lenghtening rima oris; *nerve supply,* facial. SYN musculus risorius [NA], Albinus' m. (1), Santorini's m.

rotator m.'s, SYN rotatores m.'s.

rotatores m.'s, deepest of the three layers of transversospinalis m.'s, chiefly developed in the thoracic region; they arise from the transverse process of one vertebra and are inserted into the root of the spinous process of the next two or three vertebrae above; *action,* traditionally described as a column, it is more likely that these m.'s, provided with a very high density of m. spindles, are organs of proprioception; *nerve supply,* dorsal primary rami of the spinal nerves. SYN musculi rotatores [NA], rotator m.'s.

rotatores cervicis m.'s, the rotator m.'s attached to the cervical vertebrae. SYN musculi rotatores cervicis [NA], cervical rotator m.'s.

rotatores lumborum m.'s, the rotator m.'s of the lumbar vertebrae. SYN musculi rotatores lumborum [NA], lumbar rotator m.'s.

rotatores thoracis m.'s, the rotators of the thoracic vertebrae. SYN musculi rotatores thoracis [NA], thoracic rotator m.'s.

Rouget's m., SYN circular *fibers,* under *fiber.*

round pronator m., SYN pronator teres m.

Ruysch's m., the muscular tissue of the fundus of the uterus.

salpingopharyngeal m., SYN salpingopharyngeus m.

salpingopharyngeus m., *origin,* medial lamina of cartilaginous part of auditory tube; *insertion,* longitudinal muscular layer of pharynx in association with m. palatopharyngeus; *action,* assists in elevating pharynx and, according to some, assists in opening the auditory tube during swallowing; *nerve supply,* pharyngeal plexus. SYN musculus salpingopharyngeus [NA], salpingopharyngeal m.

Santorini's m., SYN risorius m.

sartorius m., *origin,* anterior superior spine of ilium; *insertion,* medial border of tuberosity of tibia; *action,* flexes thigh and leg, rotates leg medially and thigh laterally; *nerve supply,* femoral. SYN musculus sartorius [NA], tailor's m.

scalenus anterior m., *origin,* anterior tubercles of transverse processes of third to sixth cervical vertebrae; *insertion,* scalene tubercle of first rib; *action,* raises first rib; *nerve supply,* cervical plexus. SYN musculus scalenus anterior [NA], anterior scalene m., musculus scalenus anticus.

scalenus medius m., *origin,* costotransverse lamellae of transverse processes of second to sixth cervical vertebrae; *insertion,* first rib posterior to subclavian artery; *action,* raises first rib; *nerve supply,* cervical plexus. SYN musculus scalenus medius [NA], middle scalene m.

scalenus minimus m., an occasional independent muscular fasciculus between the scalenus anterior and medius, and having the same action and innervation. SYN musculus scalenus minimus [NA], Albinus' m. (2), Sibson's m., smallest scalene m.

scalenus posterior m., *origin,* posterior tubercles of transverse processes of fourth to sixth cervical vertebrae; *insertion,* lateral surface of second rib; *action,* elevates second rib; *nerve supply,* cervical and brachial plexuses. SYN musculus scalenus posterior [NA], musculus scalenus posticus, posterior scalene m.

scalp m., SYN epicranius m.

Sebileau's m., deep fibers of the dartos tunic which pass into the scrotal septum.

second tibial m., SYN *musculus* tibialis secundus.

semimembranosus m., *origin,* tuberosity of ischium; *insertion,* medial condyle of tibia and by membrane to tibial collateral ligament of knee joint, popliteal fascia, and via its reflected tendon of insertion (oblique popiteal ligament) lateral condyle of femur; *action,* flexes knee and rotates leg medially when knee is flexed; and contributes to the stability of extended knee by making capsule of knee joint tense; *nerve supply,* tibial. SYN musculus semimembranosus [NA].

semispinal m., SYN semispinalis m.

semispinal m. of head, SYN semispinalis capitis m.

semispinalis m., the most superficial layer of the three layers of the transversospinal m.; comprised of semispinalis capitis, semispinalis cervicis, and semispinalis thoracis m.'s. SYN musculus semispinalis [NA], semispinal m.

semispinalis capitis m., *origin,* transverse processes of five or six upper thoracic and articular processes of four lower cervical vertebrae; *insertion,* occipital bone between superior and inferior nuchal lines; *action,* rotates head and draws it backward; *nerve supply,* dorsal primary rami of cervical spinal nerves. SYN musculus semispinalis capitis [NA], musculus complexus, semispinal m. of head.

semispinalis cervicis m., continuous with m. semispinalis thoracis; *origin,* transverse processes of second to fifth thoracic vertebrae; *insertion,* spinous processes of axis and third to fifth cervical vertebrae; *action,* extends cervical spine; *nerve supply,* dorsal primary rami of cervical and thoracic spinal nerves. SYN musculus semispinalis cervicis [NA], musculus semispinalis colli, semispinal m. of neck.

semispinalis thoracis m., *origin,* transverse processes of fifth to eleventh thoracic vertebrae; *insertion,* spinous processes of first four thoracic and fifth and seventh cervical vertebrae; *action,* extends vertebral column; *nerve supply,* dorsal primary rami of cervical and thoracic spinal nerves. SYN musculus semispinalis thoracis [NA], musculus semispinalis dorsi, semispinal m. of thorax.

semispinal m. of neck, SYN semispinalis cervicis m.

semispinal m. of thorax, SYN semispinalis thoracis m.

semitendinosus m., *origin,* ischial tuberosity; *insertion,* medial surface of the upper fourth of shaft of tibia; *action,* extends thigh, flexes leg and rotates it medially; *nerve supply,* tibial. SYN musculus semitendinosus [NA].

serratus anterior m., *origin,* from center of lateral aspect of first eight to nine ribs; *insertion,* superior and inferior angles and intervening medial margin of scapula; *action,* rotates scapula and pulls it forward, elevates ribs; *nerve supply,* long thoracic from brachial plexus. SYN musculus serratus anterior [NA], anterior serratus m., costoscapularis, musculus serratus magnus.

serratus posterior inferior m., *origin,* with latissimus dorsi, from spinous processes of two lower thoracic and two upper lumbar vertebrae; *insertion,* into lower borders of last four ribs; *action,* draws lower ribs backward and downward; *nerve supply,* ninth to twelfth intercostal. SYN musculus serratus posterior inferior [NA], inferior posterior serratus m.

serratus posterior superior m., *origin,* from spinous processes of two lower cervical and two upper thoracic vertebrae; *insertion,* into lateral side of angles of second to fifth ribs; *nerve supply,* first to fourth intercostals. SYN musculus serratus posterior superior [NA], superior posterior serratus m.

shawl m., obsolete term for trapezius m.

short abductor m. of thumb, SYN abductor pollicis brevis m.

short adductor m., SYN adductor brevis m.

short extensor m. of great toe, SYN extensor hallucis brevis m.

short extensor m. of thumb, SYN extensor pollicis brevis m.

short extensor m. of toes, SYN extensor digitorum brevis m.

short fibular m., SYN peroneus brevis m.

short flexor m. of great toe, SYN flexor hallucis brevis m.

short flexor m. of little finger, SYN flexor digiti minimi brevis m. of hand.

short flexor m. of little toe, SYN flexor digiti minimi brevis m. of foot.

short flexor m. of thumb, SYN flexor pollicis brevis m.

short flexor m. of toes, SYN flexor digitorum brevis m.

short levatores costarum m.'s, *origin,* the transverse processes of last cervical and eleven thoracic vertebrae; *insertion* ribs immediately below, between angle and tubercle. SYN musculi levatores costarum breves.

short palmar m., SYN palmaris brevis m.

short peroneal m., SYN peroneus brevis m.

short radial extensor m. of wrist, SYN extensor carpi radialis brevis m.

Sibson's m., SYN scalenus minimus m.

skeletal m., grossly, a collection of striated m. fibers connected at either or both extremities with the bony framework of the body; it may be an appendicular or an axial m.; histologically, a m. consisting of elongated, multinucleated, transversely striated skeletal m. fibers together with connective tissues, blood vessels, and nerves; individual m. fibers are surrounded by fine reticular and collagen fibers (endomysium); bundles (fascicles) of m. fibers are surrounded by irregular connective tissue (perimysium); the entire m. is surrounded, except at the m. tendon junction, by a dense connective tissue (epimysium). SYN musculus skeleti.

smaller m. of helix, SYN helicis minor m.

smaller pectoral m., SYN pectoralis minor m.

smaller posterior rectus m. of head, SYN rectus capitis posterior minor m.

smaller psoas m., SYN psoas minor m.

smallest scalene m., SYN scalenus minimus m.

smooth m., one of the m. fibers of the internal organs, blood vessels, hair follicles, etc.; contractile elements are elongated, usually spindle-shaped cells with centrally located nuclei and a length from 20 to 200 µm, or even longer in the pregnant uterus; although transverse striations are lacking, both thick and thin myofibrils occur; smooth m. fibers are bound together into sheets or bundles by reticular fibers, and frequently elastic fiber nets are also abundant. SEE ALSO involuntary m.'s. SYN unstriated m., unstriped m., visceral m.

Soemmerring's m., SYN levator m. of thyroid gland.

soleus m., *origin*, posterior surface of head and upper third of shaft of fibula, oblique line and middle third of medial margin of tibia, and a tendinous arch passing between tibia and fibula over the popliteal vessels; *insertion*, with gastrocnemius by tendo calcaneus (achillis) into tuberosity of calcaneus; *action*, plantar flexion of foot; *nerve supply*, tibial. SYN musculus soleus [NA].

sphincter m., SYN sphincter.

sphincter m. of common bile duct, SYN *sphincter* of common bile duct.

sphincter m. of pancreatic duct, SYN *sphincter* of pancreatic duct.

sphincter m. of pupil, SYN *sphincter* pupillae.

sphincter m. of pylorus, SYN pyloric *sphincter*.

sphincter m. of urethra, SYN *sphincter* urethrae.

sphincter m. of urinary bladder, SYN *sphincter* vesicae.

spinal m., SYN spinalis m.

spinal m. of head, SYN spinalis capitis m.

spinalis m., the medial component of the erector spinae muscle; it is comprised of the spinalis capitis, spinalis cervicis, and spinalis thoracis muscles. SYN musculus spinalis [NA], spinal m.

spinalis capitis m., an inconstant extension of spinalis cervicis to the occipital bone, sometimes fusing with semispinalis capitis. SYN musculus spinalis capitis [NA], biventer cervicis, spinal m. of head.

spinalis cervicis m., an inconstant or rudimentary muscle; *origin*, spinous processes of sixth and seventh cervical vertebrae; *insertion*, spinous processes of axis and third cervical vertebra; *action*, extends cervical spine; *nerve supply*, dorsal primary rami of cervical. SYN musculus spinalis cervicis [NA], musculus spinalis colli, spinal m. of neck.

spinalis thoracis m., *origin*, spinous processes of upper lumbar and two lower thoracic vertebrae; *insertion*, spinous processes of middle and upper thoracic vertebrae; *action*, supports and extends vertebral column; *nerve supply*, dorsal primary rami of thoracic and upper lumbar. SYN musculus spinalis thoracis [NA], musculus spinalis dorsi, spinal m. of thorax.

spinal m. of neck, SYN spinalis cervicis m.

spinal m. of thorax, SYN spinalis thoracis m.

spindle-shaped m., SYN fusiform m.

splenius capitis m., *origin*, from ligamentum nuchae of last four cervical vertebrae and supraspinous ligament of first and second thoracic vertebrae; *insertion*, lateral half of superior nuchal line and mastoid process; *action*, rotates head and extends neck; *nerve supply*, dorsal primary rami of second to sixth cervical spinal nerves. SYN musculus splenius capitis [NA], splenius m. of head.

splenius cervicis m., *origin*, from supraspinous ligament and spinous processes of third to fifth thoracic vertebrae; *insertion*, posterior tubercles of transverse processes of first and second (sometimes third) cervical vertebrae; *action*, rotates and extends neck; *nerve supply*, dorsal primary rami of fourth to eighth cervical spinal nerves. SYN musculus splenius cervicis [NA], musculus splenius colli, splenius m. of neck.

splenius m. of head, SYN splenius capitis m.

splenius m. of neck, SYN splenius cervicis m.

stapedius m., *origin*, internal walls of pyramidal eminence in tympanic cavity; *insertion*, neck of the stapes; *action*, dampens vibration of stapes by drawing head of stapes backward as a result of a protective reflex stimulated by loud noise; *nerve supply*, facial. SYN musculus stapedius [NA], stapedius.

sternal m., SYN sternalis m.

sternalis m., an inconstant muscle, running parallel to the sternum across the costosternal origin of the pectoralis major, and usually connected with the sternocleidomastoid and rectus abdominis muscles due to their common development source. SYN musculus sternalis [NA], musculus rectus thoracis, sternal m.

sternochondroscapular m., an occasional muscle arising from the manubrium of the sternum and first costal cartilage and passing lateralward and backward to be inserted into the upper border of the scapula. SYN musculus sternochondroscapularis.

sternoclavicular m., an occasional m. a slip from the subclavius muscle, passing from the upper part of the sternum to the clavicle beneath the pectoralis major m. SYN musculus sternoclavicularis.

sternocleidomastoid m., *origin*, by two heads from anterior surface of manubrium of the sternum and sternal end of clavicle; *insertion*, mastoid process and lateral half of superior nuchal line; *action*, turns head obliquely to opposite side; when acting together, flex the neck and extend the head; *nerve supply*, motor by accessory, sensory by cervical plexus. SYN musculus sternocleidomastoideus [NA], sternomastoid m.

sternocostalis m., SYN transversus thoracis m.

sternohyoid m., *origin*, posterior surface of manubrium sterni and first costal cartilage; *insertion*, body of hyoid bone; *action*, depresses hyoid bone; *nerve supply*, upper cervical via spinal nerves(ansa cervicalis). SYN musculus sternohyoideus [NA].

sternomastoid m., SYN sternocleidomastoid m.

sternothyroid m., *origin*, posterior surface of manubrium of sternum and first or second costal cartilage; *insertion*, oblique line of thyroid cartilage; *action*, depresses larynx; *nerve supply*, upper cervical via spinal nerves (ansa cervicalis). SYN musculus sternothyroideus [NA].

strap m.'s, SYN infrahyoid m.'s.

striated m., skeletal or voluntary m. in which cross striations occur in the fibers as a result of regular overlapping of thick and thin myofilaments; contrast with smooth muscle. Although cardiac muscle (which is not voluntary muscle) is also striated in appearance, the term "striated muscle" is commonly used as a synonym for voluntary, skeletal muscle.

styloauricular m., an occasional small m. extending from the root of the styloid process to the cartilage of the meatus of the ear. SYN musculus styloauricularis.

styloglossus m., *action*, retracts tongue; *origin*, lower end of styloid process; *insertion*, side and undersurface of tongue; *nerve supply*, hypoglossal. SYN musculus styloglossus [NA].

stylohyoid m., *origin*, styloid process of temporal bone; *insertion*, hyoid bone by two slips on either side of intermediate tendon of digastric; *action*, elevates hyoid bone; *nerve supply*, facial. SYN musculus stylohyoideus [NA].

stylopharyngeal m., SYN stylopharyngeus m.

stylopharyngeus m., *origin*, root of styloid process; *insertion*, thyroid cartilage and wall of pharynx (becomes part of the longitudinal coat): *action*, elevates pharynx and larynx; *nerve supply*, glossopharyngeal. SYN musculus stylopharyngeus [NA], stylopharyngeal m.

subanconeus m., SYN articularis cubiti m.

subclavian m., SYN subclavius m.

subclavius m., *origin*, first costal cartilage; *insertion*, inferior surface of acromial end of clavicle; *action*, fixes clavicle or elevates first rib; *nerve supply*, subclavian from brachial plexus. SYN musculus subclavius [NA], subclavian m.

subcostal m., one of a number of inconstant muscles of the posterolateral thoracic wall having the same direction as the internal intercostal muscles but extending across (deep to) one or more ribs. SYN musculus subcostalis [NA], musculus infracostalis.

subcrural m., SYN articularis genu m.

suboccipital m.'s, a group of muscles located immediately below the occipital bone; they are: rectus capitis anterior muscle, rectus capitis posterior major and minor muscles, rectus capitis lateralis m., obliquus capitis superior and inferior muscles; innervated by suboccipital nerve; although actions are described, it is held by many authorities that these muscles act primarily as organs of proprioception. SYN musculi suboccipitales [NA].

subquadricipital m., SYN articularis genu m.

subscapular m., SYN subscapularis m.

subscapularis m., *origin*, subscapular fossa; *insertion*, lesser tuberosity of humerus; *action*, rotates arm medially; *nerve supply*, upper and lower subscapular from posterior cord of brachial

mu

plexus (fifth and sixth cervical spinal nerves). SYN musculus subscapularis [NA], subscapular m.

superficial back m.'s, m.'s originating from the vertebral column and having their fleshy bellies located in the back, but inserting onto the appendicular skeleton of the upper limb or the ribs. They are not innervated by dorsal primary rami of spinal nerves, as are the deep or true m.'s of the back; includes the trapezius m. (innervated by spinal accessory nerve) and latissimus dorsi, rhomboids, levator scapulae, and thoracic m.'s (innervated by ventral primary rami of spinal nerves, or derivatives thereof).

superficial flexor m. of fingers, SYN flexor digitorum superficialis m.

superficial lingual m., SYN superior longitudinal m. of tongue.

superficial transverse perineal m., an inconstant muscle; *origin*, ramus of ischium; *insertion*, central tendon of perineum; *action*, draws back and fixes the central tendon of the perineum; *nerve supply*, pudendal (perineal). SYN musculus transversus perinei superficialis [NA], superficial transverse m. of perineum, Theile's m.

superficial transverse m. of perineum, SYN superficial transverse perineal m.

superior auricular m., *origin*, galea aponeurotica; *insertion*, cartilage of auricle; *action* draws pinna of ear upward and backward; *nerve supply*, facial. Considered by some to be the posterior part of the temporoparietal muscle. SYN musculus auricularis superior [NA], attollens aurem, attollens auriculam, musculus attollens aurem, musculus attollens auriculam.

superior constrictor m. of pharynx, *origin*, medial pterygoid plate (pterygopharyngeal part), pterygomandibular raphe (buccopharyngeal part), mylohyoid line of mandible (mylopharyngeal part), and the mucous membrane of the floor of the mouth and the side of the tongue (glossopharyngeal part); *insertion*, pharyngeal raphe in the posterior wall of the pharynx; *action*, narrows pharynx; *nerve supply*, pharyngeal plexus. SYN musculus constrictor pharyngis superior [NA], musculus cephalopharyngeus.

superior gemellus m., *origin*, ischial spine and margin of lesser sciatic notch; *insertion*, tendon of m. obturator internus; *action*, rotates thigh laterally; *nerve supply*, sacral plexus. SYN musculus gemellus superior [NA], gemellus.

superior longitudinal m. of tongue, an intrinsic muscle of the tongue, running from base to tip on the dorsum just beneath the mucous membrane; *action*, shortens the upper part of the tongue; *nerve supply*, motor by hypoglossal, sensory by lingual. SYN musculus longitudinalis superior [NA], superficial lingual m.

superior oblique m., *origin*, above the medial margin of the optic canal; *insertion*, by a tendon passing through the trochlea, or pulley, and then reflected backward, downward, and laterally to the sclera between the superior and lateral recti; *action*, primary, intorsion; secondary, depression and abduction; *nerve supply*, trochlear nerve. SYN musculus obliquus superior [NA].

superior oblique m. of head, SYN obliquus capitis superior m.

superior posterior serratus m., SYN serratus posterior superior m.

superior rectus m., *origin*, superior part of common tendinous ring; *insertion*, superior part of sclera of the eye; *action*, primary, elevation; secondary, adduction and intorsion; *nerve supply*, oculomotor. SYN musculus rectus superior [NA], attollens oculi.

superior tarsal m., a well defined layer of smooth muscle that extends from the aponeurosis of the m. levator palpebrae superioris to the superior tarsus; it is innervated by sympathetic nerves and acts to hold the upper lid in an elevated position; its paralysis in Horner's syndrome result in ptosis. SYN musculus tarsalis superior [NA], Müller's m. (3).

supinator m., *origin*, lateral epicondyle of humerus radial collateral and anular ligaments, and supinator ridge of ulna; *insertion*, anterior and lateral surface of radius; *action*, supinates the forearm; *nerve supply*, radial (posterior interosseous). SYN musculus supinator [NA], musculus supinator radii brevis.

supraclavicular m., an anomalous muscular slip running from the upper edge of the manubrium of the sternum lateralward to about the middle of the upper surface of the clavicle. SYN musculus supraclavicularis.

suprahyoid m.'s, the group of muscles attached to the upper part of the hyoid bone including the digastric, stylohyoid, mylohyoid, and geniohyoid muscles. SYN musculi suprahyoidei [NA].

supraspinalis m., one of a number of muscular bands passing between the tips of the spinous processes of the cervical vertebrae. SYN musculus supraspinalis.

supraspinatus m., *origin*, supraspinous fossa of scapula; *insertion*, greater tuberosity of humerus; *action*, initiates abduction of arm; *nerve supply*, suprascapular from fifth and sixth cervical. SYN musculus supraspinatus [NA], supraspinous m.

supraspinous m., SYN supraspinatus m.

suspensory m. of duodenum, a broad flat band of smooth muscle and fibrous tissue attached to the right crus of the diaphragm and to the duodenum at its junction with the jejunum. SYN musculus suspensorius duodeni [NA], Treitz' ligament, Treitz' m.

synergistic m.'s, m.'s having a similar and mutually helpful function or action.

tailor's m., SYN sartorius m.

temporal m., SYN temporalis m.

temporalis m., *origin*, temporal fossa; *insertion*, coronoid process of mandible and anterior border of ramus; *action* elevates mandible (closes jaw); its posterior, nearly horizontally-oriented fibers are the primary retractors of the protruded mandible. *nerve supply*, deep temporal branches of mandibular division of trigeminal. SYN musculus temporalis [NA], temporal m.

temporoparietal m., SYN temporoparietalis m.

temporoparietalis m., the part of epicranius m. that arises from the lateral part of the epicranial aponeurosis and inserts in the cartilage of the auricle. SYN musculus temporoparietalis [NA], temporoparietal m.

tensor fasciae latae m., *origin*, anterior superior spine and adjacent lateral surface of the ilium; *insertion*, iliotibial band of fascia lata; *action*, tenses fascia lata; flexes, abducts and medially rotates thigh; *nerve supply*, superior gluteal. SYN musculus tensor fasciae latae [NA], musculus tensor fasciae femoris, tensor m. of fascia lata.

tensor m. of fascia lata, SYN tensor fasciae latae m.

tensor m. of soft palate, SYN tensor veli palati m.

tensor tarsi m., lacrimal part of orbicularis oculi muscle. SEE orbicularis oculi m.

tensor tympani m., *origin*, the cartilaginous part of the auditory (eustachian) tube and the walls of its hemi-canal just above the bony portion of the auditory tube; *insertion*, handle of malleus; *action*, draws the handle of the malleus medialward tensing the tympanic membrane to protect it from excessive vibration by loud sounds. *nerve supply*, branches of trigeminal through the otic ganglion. SYN musculus tensor tympani [NA], tensor m. of tympanic membrane, Toynbee's m.

tensor m. of tympanic membrane, SYN tensor tympani m.

tensor veli palati m., tensor muscle of soft palate, m. tensor palati; m. palatosalpingeus; m. sphenosalpingostaphylinus; dilator tubae; *origin*, scaphoid fossa of sphenoid, cartilaginous and membranous part of auditory (eustachian) tube and spine of sphenoid; *insertion*, posterior border of hard palate and aponeurosis of soft palate; *action*, tenses the soft palate; contributes to opening of auditory tube; *nerve supply*, branches of trigeminal nerve through the otic ganglion. SYN musculus tensor veli palatini [NA], dilator tubae, musculus palatosalpingeus, musculus sphenosalpingostaphylinus, musculus tensor palati, palatosalpingeus, tensor m. of soft palate.

teres major m., *origin*, inferior angle and lower third of border of scapula; *insertion*, medial border of intertubercular groove of humerus; *action*, adducts and extends arm and rotates it medially; *nerve supply*, lower subscapular from posterior cord of brachial plexus (fifth and sixth cervical spinal nerves). SYN musculus teres major [NA].

teres minor m., *origin*, upper two-thirds of the lateral border of scapula; *insertion*, lower facet of greater tuberosity of humerus; *action*, adducts arm and rotates it laterally; *nerve supply*, axillary (fifth and sixth cervical spinal nerves). SYN musculus teres minor [NA].

Theile's m., SYN superficial transverse perineal m.

third peroneal m., SYN peroneus tertius m.

thoracic interspinal m., SYN thoracic interspinales m.'s.

thoracic interspinales m.'s, often poorly developed or absent muscles between spinous process of thoracic vertebrae; *action*, extends thoracic vertebrae; *nerve supply*, dorsal primary rami of thoracic nerves. SYN musculus interspinalis thoracis [NA], thoracic interspinal m.

thoracic intertransversarii m.'s, *origin*, transverse processes of thoracic vertebrae; *insertion*, next superior transverse process; *action*, abducts thoracic vertebrae; *nerve supply*, dorsal primary rami of thoracic nerves. SYN musculi intertransversarii thoracis [NA], thoracic intertransverse m.'s.

thoracic intertransverse m.'s, SYN thoracic intertransversarii m.'s.

thoracic longissimus m., SYN longissimus thoracis m.

thoracic rotator m.'s, SYN rotatores thoracis m.'s.

m.'s of thorax, the muscles attaching to the rib cage including the pectoral muscles, serratus anterior, subclavius, levator muscles, intercostal muscles, transverse thoracic muscle, subcostal muscles, and diaphragm. SYN musculi thoracis [NA].

thyroarytenoid m., *origin*, inner surface of thyroid cartilage; *insertion*, muscular process and outer surface of arytenoid; *action*, decreases tension on (relaxes) vocal cords lowering the pitch of the voice tone; *nerve supply*, recurrent laryngeal. SYN musculus thyroarytenoideus [NA], musculus thyroarytenoideus externus.

thyroepiglottic m., thyroepiglottidean m., *origin*, inner surface of thyroid cartilage in common with m. thyroarytenoideus; *insertion*, aryepiglottic fold and margin of epiglottis; *action*, depresses base of epiglottis; *nerve supply*, recurrent laryngeal. SYN musculus thyroepiglotticus [NA], depressor m. of epiglottis, ventricularis (2).

thyrohyoid m., apparently a continuation of the sternothyroid; *origin*, oblique line of thyroid cartilage; *insertion*, body of hyoid bone; *action*, approximates hyoid bone to the larynx; *nerve supply*, upper cervical spinal nerves carried by hypoglossal. SYN musculus thyrohyoideus [NA].

tibialis anterior m., *origin*, upper two-thirds of lateral surface of tibia, interosseous membrane, and intermuscular septum; *insertion*, medial cuneiform and base of first metatarsal; *action*, dorsiflexion and inversion of foot; *nerve supply*, deep peroneal. SYN musculus tibialis anterior [NA], anterior tibial m., musculus tibialis anticus.

tibialis posterior m., *origin*, soleal line and posterior surface of tibia, the head and shaft of the fibula between the medial crest and interosseous border, and the posterior surface of interosseous membrane; *insertion*, navicular, three cuneiform, cuboid, and second, third, and fourth metatarsal bones; *action*, plantar flexion and inversion of foot; *nerve supply*, tibial. SYN musculus tibialis posterior [NA], musculus tibialis posticus, posterior tibial m.

Tod's m., SYN oblique auricular m.

m.'s of tongue, the extrinsic m.'s include the genioglossus, hyoglossus, chondroglossus, and styloglossus m.'s; the intrinsic muscles are the vertical, transverse, and the superior and inferior longitudinal; all are innervated by the hypoglssal nerve. SYN musculi linguae [NA].

Toynbee's m., SYN tensor tympani m.

trachealis m., the band of smooth muscular fibers in the fibrous membrane connecting posteriorly the ends of the tracheal rings. SYN musculus trachealis [NA].

tracheloclavicular m., an anomalous muscle occasionally arising from the cervical vertebrae and inserted into the lateral end of the clavicle. SYN musculus tracheloclavicularis.

tragicus m., a band of vertical muscular fibers on the outer surface of the tragus of the ear. SYN musculus tragicus [NA], m. of tragus, Valsalva's m.

m. of tragus, SYN tragicus m.

transverse m. of abdomen, SYN transversus abdominis m.

transverse arytenoid m., a band of muscular fibers passing between the two arytenoid cartilages posteriorly; *action*, narrows the intercartilaginous portion of the rima glottidis; *nerve supply*, recurrent laryngeal. SYN musculus arytenoideus transversus [NA], arytenoideus.

transverse m. of auricle, SYN transverse auricular m.

transverse auricular m., a band of sparse muscular fibers on the cranial surface of the auricle, extending from the eminence of the concha to the eminence of the scapha. SYN musculus transversus auriculae [NA], transverse m. of auricle.

transverse m. of chin, SYN transversus menti m.

transverse m. of nape, SYN transversus nuchae m.

transverse m. of thorax, SYN transversus thoracis m.

transverse m. of tongue, an intrinsic muscle of the tongue, the fibers of which arise from the septum and radiate to the dorsum and sides; *action*, decreases lateral dimension of the tongue; *nerve supply*, hypoglossal for motor, lingual for sensory. SYN musculus transversus linguae [NA].

transversospinal m., SYN transversospinalis m.

transversospinalis m., the group of muscles that originate from transverse processes of vertebrae and pass to spinous processes of higher vertebrae; they act as rotators and include the semispinalis (capitis, cervicis, thoracis), multifidus, and rotatores (cervicis, thoracis, lumborum) muscles. All are innervated by dorsal primary rami of spinal nerves. SYN musculus transversospinalis [NA], transversospinal m.

transversus abdominis m., *origin*, seventh to twelfth costal cartilages, lumbar fascia, iliac crest, and inguinal ligament; *insertion*, xiphoid cartilage and linea alba and, through the conjoint tendon, pubic tubercle and pecten; *action*, compresses abdominal contents; *nerve supply*, lower thoracic. SYN musculus transversus abdominis [NA], musculus transversalis abdominis, transverse m. of abdomen.

transversus menti m., inconstant fibers of the depressor anguli oris m. continue into the neck and cross to the opposite side inferior to the chin. SYN musculus transversus menti [NA], transverse m. of chin.

transversus nuchae m., an occasional muscle passing between the tendons of the trapezius and sternocleidomastoid, possibly a fasciculus of the posterior auricular muscle. SYN musculus transversus nuchae [NA], transverse m. of nape.

transversus thoracis m., *origin*, dorsal surface of xiphoid cartilage and lower portion of dorsal surface of body of sternum; *insertion*, second to sixth costal cartilages; *action*, contributes to depression of ribs, narrowing chest; *nerve supply*, intercostal. SYN musculus transversus thoracis [NA], musculus triangularis sterni, sternocostalis m., transverse m. of thorax.

trapezius m., *origin*, medial third of superior nuchal line, external occipital protuberance, ligamentum nuchae, spinous processes of seventh cervical and the thoracic vertebrae and corresponding supraspinous ligaments; *insertion*, lateral third of posterior surface of clavicle, anterior side of acromion, and upper and medial border of the spine of the scapula; *action*, when scapulae are fixed, portions of muscle can act independently: cervical portion elevates scapula, thoracic portion contributes to depression of scapula; upper and lowermost portions act simultaneously to rotate glenoid fossa superiorly; when the entire muscle and especially middle part contracts, the scapulae retract; draws head to one side or backward; *nerve supply*, motor by accessory, sensory by cervical plexus. SYN musculus trapezius [NA], cowl m., trapezius.

Treitz' m., SYN suspensory m. of duodenum.

triangular m., (1) a muscle that is triangular in shape; SYN musculus triangularis (1). **(2)** SYN depressor anguli oris m.

triceps m. of arm, SYN triceps brachii m.

triceps brachii m., *origin*, long or scapular head: lateral border of scapula below glenoid fossa, lateral head: lateral and posterior surface of humerus below greater tubercle, medial head: posterior surface of humerus below radial groove; *insertion*, olecranon of ulna; *action*, extends elbow; *nerve supply*, radial. SYN musculus triceps brachii [NA], triceps m. of arm.

triceps m. of calf, SYN triceps surae m.

triceps coxae m., the obturator internus and superior and inferior gemellus m.'s considered as one muscle, inserting via a single tendon into the greater trochanter of the femur. SYN musculus triceps coxae, triceps m. of hip.

triceps m. of hip, SYN triceps coxae m.

triceps surae m., the two bellies of the gastrocnemius and soleus considered as one muscle. SYN musculus triceps surae [NA], triceps m. of calf.

true m.'s of back, SYN deep m.'s of back.

two-bellied m., SYN digastric m.

ulnar extensor m. of wrist, SYN extensor carpi ulnaris m.

ulnar flexor m. of wrist, SYN flexor carpi ulnaris m.

unipennate m., a muscle with a lateral tendon to which the fibers are attached obliquely, like one half of a feather. SYN musculus unipennatus [NA].

unstriated m., unstriped m., SYN smooth m.

m. of uvula, SYN uvulae m.

uvulae m., *origin,* posterior nasal spine; *insertion,* forms chief bulk of the uvula; *action,* raises the uvula; *nerve supply,* pharyngeal plexus. SYN musculus uvulae [NA], m. of uvula, musculus azygos uvulae, palatouvularis m., uvularis.

Valsalva's m., SYN tragicus m.

vastus intermedius m., *origin,* upper three-fourths of anterior surface of shaft of femur; *insertion,* tibial tuberosity by way of common tendon of quadriceps femoris and patellar ligament; *action,* extends leg; *nerve supply,* femoral. SYN musculus vastus intermedius [NA], crureus, femoral m., intermediate great m., intermediate vastus m.

vastus lateralis m., *origin,* lateral lip of linea aspera as far as great trochanter; *insertion,* tibial tuberosity by way of common tendon of quadriceps femoris and patellar ligament; *action,* extends leg; *nerve supply,* femoral. SYN musculus vastus lateralis [NA], lateral great m., lateral vastus m., musculus vastus externus.

vastus medialis m., *origin,* medial lip of linea aspera; *insertion,* tibial tuberosity by way of common tendon of quadriceps femoris and ligamentum patellae; *action,* extends leg; *nerve supply,* femoral. SYN musculus vastus medialis [NA], medial great m., medial vastus m., musculus vastus internus.

ventral sacrococcygeal m., SYN ventral sacrococcygeus m.

ventral sacrococcygeus m., an inconstant muscle on the pelvic surfaces of the sacrum and coccyx, the remains of a portion of the tail musculature of lower animals. SYN musculus sacrococcygeus ventralis [NA], musculus sacrococcygeus anterior, ventral sacrococcygeal m.

vertical m. of tongue, an intrinsic muscle of the tongue, consisting of fibers that pass from the aponeurosis of the dorsum to the aponeurosis of the inferior surface; *action,* decreases the superior to inferior dimension of (flattens) the tongue; *nerve supply,* hypoglossal for motor, lingual for sensory. SYN musculus verticalis linguae [NA].

vestigial m., an imperfect structure in man corresponding to a functioning m. in the lower animals.

visceral m., SYN smooth m.

vocal m., SYN vocalis m.

vocalis m., *origin,* depression between the two laminae of thyroid cartilage; *insertion,* portions of vocal process of arytenoid; *action,* shortens and relaxes vocal cords; *nerve supply,* recurrent laryngeal; a number of the deeper and finer fibers of the thyroaryteroid m. attached directly to the outer side of the true vocal cord. SYN musculus vocalis [NA], musculus thyroarytenoideus internus, vocal m.

voluntary m., one whose action is under the control of the will; all the striated m.'s, except the heart, are voluntary m.'s.

white m., a rapid or fast-twitch m. in which pale large "white" fibers predominate; mitochondria and myoglobin are relatively sparse compared with red m.; involved in phasic contraction.

Wilson's m., (1) SYN *sphincter* urethrae. (2) certain fibers of the levator ani.

wrinkler m. of eyebrow, SYN corrugator supercilii m.

zygomaticus major m., *origin,* zygomatic bone anterior to temporozygomatic suture; *insertion,* muscles at angle of mouth; *action,* draws upper lip upward and laterally; *nerve supply,* facial. SYN musculus zygomaticus major [NA], greater zygomatic m., musculus zygomaticus.

zygomaticus minor m., *origin,* zygomatic bone posterior to zygomaticomaxillary suture; *insertion,* orbicularis oris of upper lip; *action,* draws upper lip upward and outward; *nerve supply,* facial. SYN musculus zygomaticus minor [NA], caput zygomaticum quadrati labii superioris, lesser zygomatic m.

---

mus·cle-bound (mŭs'ĕl-bownd). Denoting a condition in which individual muscles are overdeveloped but dyssynergic in concerted action.

mus·cle-trim·ming. SYN border *molding.*

mus·cone (mŭs'kōn). Muskone.

mus·cu·la·mine (mŭs'kyūl-ă-mēn). SYN spermine.

mus·cu·lar (mŭs'kyū-lăr). 1. Relating to a muscle or the muscles. 2. Having well developed musculature.

mus·cu·la·ris (mŭs-kyū-lā'ris). The muscular coat of a hollow organ or tubular structure. [Mod. L. muscular]
m. muco'sae, the thin layer of smooth muscle found in most parts of the digestive tube located outside the m. propria mucosae and adjacent to the tela submucosa. SYN lamina muscularis mucosae [NA], muscular layer of mucosa.

mus·cu·lar·i·ty (mŭs'kyū-lar'i-tē). The state or condition of having well developed muscles.

mus·cu·la·ture (mŭs'kyū-lă-chūr). The arrangement of the muscles in a part or in the body as a whole.

mus·cu·lo·ap·o·neu·rot·ic (mŭs'kyū-lō-ap'ō-nū-rot'ik). Relating to muscular tissue and an aponeurosis of origin or insertion.

mus·cu·lo·cu·ta·ne·ous (mŭs'kyū-lō-kyū-tā'nē-ŭs). Relating to both muscle and skin. SYN myocutaneous, myodermal.

mus·cu·lo·mem·bra·nous (mŭs'kyū-lō-mem'bră-nŭs). Relating to both muscular tissue and membrane; denoting certain muscles, such as the occipitofrontalis, that are largely membranous.

mus·cu·lo·phren·ic (mŭs'kyū-lō-fren'ik). Relating to the muscular portion of the diaphragm; denoting an artery supplying this part.

mus·cu·lo·skel·e·tal (mŭs'kyū-lō-skel'ĕ-tăl). Relating to muscles and to the skeleton, as, for example, the m. system.

mus·cu·lo·spi·ral (mŭs'kyū-lō-spī'răl). Denoting the musculospiral nerve. SEE radial *nerve.*

mus·cu·lo·ten·di·nous (mŭs'kyū-lō-ten'di-nŭs). Relating to both muscular and tendinous tissues.

mus·cu·lo·tro·pic (mŭs'kyū-lō-trop'ik). Affecting, acting upon, or attracted to muscular tissue.

MUSCULUS

mus·cu·lus, gen. and pl. **mus·cu·li** (mŭs'kyū-lŭs, -kyū-lī) [NA]. SYN muscle. For histologic description, see muscle. [L. a little mouse, a muscle, fr. *mus* (*mur*-), a mouse]

mus'culi abdom'inis [NA], SYN *muscles* of abdomen, under *muscle.*

m. abduc'tor dig'iti min'imi ma'nus [NA], SYN abductor digiti minimi *muscle* of hand.

m. abduc'tor dig'iti min'imi pe'dis [NA], SYN abductor digiti minimi *muscle* of foot.

m. abduc'tor dig'iti quin'ti, (1) SYN abductor digiti minimi *muscle* of hand. (2) SYN abductor digiti minimi *muscle* of foot.

m. abduc'tor hal'lucis [NA], SYN abductor hallucis *muscle.*

m. abduc'tor pol'licis bre'vis [NA], SYN abductor pollicis brevis *muscle.*

m. abduc'tor pol'licis lon'gus [NA], SYN abductor pollicis longus *muscle.*

m. adduc'tor bre'vis [NA], SYN adductor brevis *muscle.*

m. adduc'tor hal'lucis [NA], SYN adductor hallucis *muscle.*

m. adduc'tor lon'gus [NA], SYN adductor longus *muscle.*

m. adduc'tor mag'nus [NA], SYN adductor magnus *muscle.*

m. adduc'tor min'imus, SYN adductor minimus *muscle.*

m. adduc'tor pol'licis [NA], SYN adductor pollicis *muscle.*

m. anco'neus [NA], SYN anconeus *muscle.*

m. antitrag'icus [NA], SYN antitragicus *muscle.*

mus'culi arrecto'res pilo'rum [NA], SYN arrector pili *muscles*, under *muscle*.

m. articula'ris [NA], SYN articular *muscle*.

m. articula'ris cu'biti [NA], SYN articularis cubiti *muscle*.

m. articula'ris ge'nus [NA], SYN articularis genu *muscle*.

m. aryepiglot'ticus [NA], SYN aryepiglottic *muscle*.

m. arytenoi'deus obli'quus [NA], SYN oblique arytenoid *muscle*.

m. arytenoi'deus transver'sus [NA], SYN transverse arytenoid *muscle*.

m. aryvoca'lis, a number of the deeper fibers of the vocalis muscle attached directly to the outer side of the true vocal cord.

m. attol'lens au'rem, m. attol'lens auric'ulam, SYN superior auricular *muscle*.

m. a'ttrahens au'rem, m. a'ttrahens auric'ulam, SYN anterior auricular *muscle*.

m. auricula'ris ante'rior [NA], SYN anterior auricular *muscle*.

m. auricula'ris poste'rior [NA], SYN posterior auricular *muscle*.

m. auricula'ris supe'rior [NA], SYN superior auricular *muscle*.

m. az'ygos u'vulae, SYN uvulae *muscle*.

m. bi'ceps bra'chii [NA], SYN biceps brachii *muscle*.

m. bi'ceps fem'oris [NA], SYN biceps femoris *muscle*.

m. bi'ceps flex'or cru'ris, SYN biceps femoris *muscle*.

m. bipenna'tus [NA], SYN bipennate *muscle*.

m. biven'ter mandib'ulae, SYN digastric *muscle*.

m. brachia'lis [NA], SYN brachialis *muscle*.

m. brachiocephal'icus, in animals, a compound muscle passing from the brachium or humerus to the head and the dorsal cervical raphe; the clavicular insertion or clavicle subdivides the muscle. SYN brachiocephalic muscle.

m. brachioradia'lis [NA], SYN brachioradialis *muscle*.

m. bronchoesopha'geus [NA], SYN bronchoesophageal *muscle*.

m. buccina'tor [NA], SYN buccinator *muscle*.

m. buccopharyn'geus, SEE superior constrictor *muscle* of pharynx.

mus'culi bul'bi [NA], SYN extraocular *muscles*, under *muscle*.

m. bulbocaverno'sus, SYN bulbocavernosus *muscle*.

m. bulbospongio'sus [NA], SYN bulbocavernosus *muscle*.

m. cani'nus, SYN levator anguli oris *muscle*.

mus'culi cap'itis [NA], SYN *muscles* of head, under *muscle*.

m. cephalopharyn'geus, SYN superior constrictor *muscle* of pharynx.

m. ceratocricoi'deus [NA], SYN ceratocricoid *muscle*.

m. ceratopharyn'geus, SEE middle constrictor *muscle* of pharynx.

m. cervica'lis ascen'dens, SYN iliocostalis cervicis *muscle*.

m. chondroglos'sus [NA], SYN chondroglossus *muscle*.

m. chondropharyn'geus, SEE middle constrictor *muscle* of pharynx.

m. cilia'ris [NA], SYN ciliary *muscle*.

m. cleidoepitrochlea'ris, the anterior portion of the deltoid, arising from the clavicle.

m. cleidomastoi'deus, the portion of the sternocleidomastoid muscle passing between the clavicle and the mastoid process.

m. cleido-occipita'lis, the portion of the sternocleidomastoid muscle between the clavicle and the superior nuchal line.

mus'culi coccyg'ei [NA], SYN *muscles* of coccyx, under *muscle*.

m. coccyg'eus [NA], SYN coccygeus *muscle*.

mus'culi col'li [NA], SYN *muscles* of neck, under *muscle*.

m. complex'us, SYN semispinalis capitis *muscle*.

m. complex'us mi'nor, SYN longissimus capitis *muscle*.

m. compres'sor na'ris, SEE nasalis *muscle*.

m. compres'sor ure'thrae, SYN *sphincter* urethrae.

m. constric'tor pharyn'gis infe'rior [NA], SYN inferior constrictor *muscle* of pharynx.

m. constric'tor pharyn'gis me'dius [NA], SYN middle constrictor *muscle* of pharynx.

m. constric'tor pharyn'gis supe'rior [NA], SYN superior constrictor *muscle* of pharynx.

m. constric'tor ure'thrae, SYN *sphincter* urethrae.

m. coracobrachia'lis [NA], SYN coracobrachialis *muscle*.

m. corruga'tor cu'tis a'ni, SYN corrugator cutis *muscle* of anus.

m. corruga'tor supercil'ii [NA], SYN corrugator supercilii *muscle*.

m. cremas'ter [NA], SYN cremaster *muscle*.

m. cricoarytenoi'deus latera'lis [NA], SYN lateral cricoarytenoid *muscle*.

m. cricoarytenoi'deus poste'rior [NA], SYN posterior cricoarytenoid *muscle*.

m. cricopharyn'geus, SEE inferior constrictor *muscle* of pharynx.

m. cricothyroi'deus [NA], SYN cricothyroid *muscle*.

m. crucia'tus [NA], SYN cruciate *muscle*.

m. cutaneomuco'sus, SYN cutaneomucous *muscle*.

m. cuta'neus [NA], SYN cutaneous *muscle*.

m. deltoi'deus [NA], SYN deltoid *muscle*.

m. depres'sor an'guli o'ris [NA], SYN depressor anguli oris *muscle*.

m. depres'sor la'bii inferio'ris [NA], SYN depressor labii inferioris *muscle*.

m. depres'sor sep'ti [NA], SYN depressor septi *muscle*.

m. depres'sor supercil'ii [NA], SYN depressor supercilii *muscle*.

m. detru'sor uri'nae, SYN detrusor *muscle* of urinary bladder.

m. diaphrag'ma, SEE diaphragm.

m. digas'tricus [NA], SYN digastric *muscle*.

m. dilata'tor, SYN dilator *muscle*.

m. dila'tor, SYN dilator *muscle*.

m. dila'tor i'ridis, SYN dilator pupillae *muscle*.

m. dila'tor na'ris, SEE nasalis *muscle*.

m. dila'tor pupil'lae [NA], SYN dilator pupillae *muscle*.

m. dila'tor pylo'ri gastroduodena'lis, SYN dilator *muscle* of pylorus.

m. dila'tor pylo'ri ilea'lis, SYN dilator *muscle* of ileocecal sphincter.

m. dila'tor tu'bae, that portion of m. tensor veli palatini that attaches to the mucous membrane of the auditory tube; formerly described as a separate muscle.

mus'culi dor'si [NA], SYN *muscles* of the back, under *muscle*.

m. ejacula'tor sem'inis, SYN bulbocavernosus *muscle*.

m. epicra'nius [NA], SYN epicranius *muscle*.

m. epitrochleoanco'neus, an occasional muscle *origin*, from the back of the medial condyle of the humerus, and *insertion* into the medial side of the olecranon process.

m. erec'tor clitor'idis, SYN ischiocavernous *muscle*.

m. erec'tor pe'nis, SYN ischiocavernous *muscle*.

m. erec'tor spi'nae [NA], SYN erector spinae *muscles*, under *muscle*.

m. exten'sor bre'vis digito'rum, SYN extensor digitorum brevis *muscle*.

m. exten'sor bre'vis pol'licis, SYN extensor pollicis brevis *muscle*.

m. exten'sor car'pi radia'lis bre'vis [NA], SYN extensor carpi radialis brevis *muscle*.

m. exten'sor car'pi radia'lis lon'gus [NA], SYN extensor carpi radialis longus *muscle*.

m. exten'sor car'pi ulna'ris [NA], SYN extensor carpi ulnaris *muscle*.

m. exten'sor coccyg'is, SYN dorsal sacrococcygeus *muscle*.

m. exten'sor dig'iti min'imi [NA], SYN extensor digiti minimi *muscle*.

m. exten'sor dig'iti quin'ti pro'prius, SYN extensor digiti minimi *muscle*.

m. exten'sor digito'rum [NA], SYN extensor digitorum *muscle*.

m. exten'sor digito'rum bre'vis [NA], SYN extensor digitorum brevis *muscle*.

m. exten'sor digito'rum bre'vis ma'nus, SYN extensor digitorum brevis *muscle* of hand.

m. exten'sor digito'rum commu'nis, SYN extensor digitorum *muscle*.

m. exten'sor digito'rum lon'gus [NA], SYN extensor digitorum longus *muscle*.

m. exten′sor hal′lucis bre′vis [NA], SYN extensor hallucis brevis *muscle.*

m. exten′sor hal′lucis lon′gus [NA], SYN extensor hallucis longus *muscle.*

m. exten′sor in′dicis [NA], SYN extensor indicis *muscle.*

m. exten′sor in′dicis pro′prius, SYN extensor indicis *muscle.*

m. exten′sor lon′gus digito′rum, SYN extensor digitorum longus *muscle.*

m. exten′sor lon′gus pol′licis, SYN extensor pollicis longus *muscle.*

m. exten′sor min′imi dig′iti, SYN extensor digiti minimi *muscle.*

m. exten′sor os′sis metacar′pi pol′licis, SYN abductor pollicis longus *muscle.*

m. exten′sor pol′licis bre′vis [NA], SYN extensor pollicis brevis *muscle.*

m. exten′sor pol′licis lon′gus [NA], SYN extensor pollicis longus *muscle.*

mus′culi facia′les [NA], SYN *muscles* of facial expression, under *muscle.*

m. fibula′ris brev′is [NA], SYN peroneus brevis *muscle.*

m. fibula′ris long′us [NA], SYN peroneus longus *muscle.*

m. fibula′ris ter′tius [NA], SYN peroneus tertius *muscle.*

m. flex′or accesso′rius [NA], SYN quadratus plantae *muscle.*

m. flex′or bre′vis digito′rum, SYN flexor digitorum brevis *muscle.*

m. flex′or bre′vis hal′lucis, SYN flexor hallucis brevis *muscle.*

m. flex′or car′pi radia′lis [NA], SYN flexor carpi radialis *muscle.*

m. flex′or car′pi ulna′ris [NA], SYN flexor carpi ulnaris *muscle.*

m. flex′or dig′iti min′imi brev′is ma′nus [NA], SYN flexor digiti minimi brevis *muscle* of hand.

m. flex′or dig′iti min′imi brev′is pe′dis [NA], SYN flexor digiti minimi brevis *muscle* of foot.

m. flex′or digito′rum bre′vis [NA], SYN flexor digitorum brevis *muscle.*

m. flex′or digito′rum lon′gus [NA], SYN flexor digitorum longus *muscle.*

m. flex′or digito′rum profun′dus [NA], SYN flexor digitorum profundus *muscle.*

m. flex′or digito′rum subli′mis, SYN flexor digitorum superficialis *muscle.*

m. flex′or digito′rum superficia′lis [NA], SYN flexor digitorum superficialis *muscle.*

m. flex′or hal′lucis bre′vis [NA], SYN flexor hallucis brevis *muscle.*

m. flex′or hal′lucis lon′gus [NA], SYN flexor hallucis longus *muscle.*

m. flex′or lon′gus digito′rum, SYN flexor digitorum longus *muscle.*

m. flex′or lon′gus hal′lucis, SYN flexor hallucis longus *muscle.*

m. flex′or lon′gus pol′licis, SYN flexor pollicis longus *muscle.*

m. flex′or pol′licis bre′vis [NA], SYN flexor pollicis brevis *muscle.*

m. flex′or pol′licis lon′gus [NA], SYN flexor pollicis longus *muscle.*

m. flex′or profun′dus, SYN flexor digitorum profundus *muscle.*

m. flex′or subli′mis, SYN flexor digitorum superficialis *muscle.*

m. fronta′lis, SEE occipitofrontalis *muscle.*

m. fusifor′mis [NA], SYN fusiform *muscle.*

m. gastrocne′mius [NA], SYN gastrocnemius *muscle.*

m. gemel′lus infe′rior [NA], SYN inferior gemellus *muscle.*

m. gemel′lus supe′rior [NA], SYN superior gemellus *muscle.*

m. genioglos′sus [NA], SYN genioglossus *muscle.*

m. geniohyoglos′sus, SYN genioglossus *muscle.*

m. geniohyoi′deus [NA], SYN geniohyoid *muscle.*

m. glossopalati′nus, SYN palatoglossus *muscle.*

m. glossopharyn′geus, SEE superior constrictor *muscle* of pharynx.

m. glu′teus max′imus [NA], SYN gluteus maximus *muscle.*

m. glu′teus me′dius [NA], SYN gluteus medius *muscle.*

m. glu′teus min′imus [NA], SYN gluteus minimus *muscle.*

m. grac′ilis [NA], SYN gracilis *muscle.*

m. hel′icis ma′jor [NA], SYN helicis major *muscle.*

m. hel′icis mi′nor [NA], SYN helicis minor *muscle.*

m. hyoglos′sus [NA], SYN hyoglossus *muscle.*

m. hypopharyn′geus, SEE middle constrictor *muscle* of pharynx.

m. ili′acus [NA], SYN iliacus *muscle.*

m. ili′acus mi′nor, SYN iliacus minor *muscle.*

m. iliocapsula′ris, SYN iliacus minor *muscle.*

m. il′iococcyg′eus [NA], SYN iliococcygeus *muscle.*

m. iliocosta′lis [NA], SYN iliocostalis *muscle.*

m. iliocosta′lis cer′vicis [NA], SYN iliocostalis cervicis *muscle.*

m. iliocosta′lis dor′si, SYN iliocostalis thoracis *muscle.*

m. iliocosta′lis lumbo′rum [NA], SYN iliocostalis lumborum *muscle.*

m. iliocosta′lis thora′cis [NA], SYN iliocostalis thoracis *muscle.*

m. iliopso′as [NA], SYN iliopsoas *muscle.*

m. incisi′vus la′bii inferior′is, inferior incisive bundle of origin of orbicularis oris m.

m. incisi′vus la′bii superior′is, superior incisive bundle of origin of orbicularis oris m.

m. incisu′rae hel′icis [NA], SYN *muscle* of notch of helix.

m. infracosta′lis, pl. **musculi infracosta′les,** SYN subcostal *muscle.*

mus′culi infrahyoi′dei [NA], SYN infrahyoid *muscles,* under *muscle.*

m. infraspina′tus [NA], SYN infraspinatus *muscle.*

m. intercosta′les exter′ni, pl. **mus′culi intercosta′les exter′ni** [NA], SYN external intercostal *muscles,* under *muscle.*

m. intercosta′lis inter′nus, pl. **mus′culi intercosta′les inter′ni** [NA], SYN internal intercostal *muscle.*

m. intercosta′lis in′timus, pl. **mus′culi intercosta′les in′timi** [NA], SYN innermost intercostal *muscle.*

musculi interos′sei dorsa′lis ma′nus, pl. **mus′culi interos′sei dorsa′les ma′nus** [NA], SYN dorsal interosseous *muscles* of hand, under *muscle.*

musculi interos′sei dorsa′lis pe′dis, pl. **mus′culi interos′sei dorsa′les pe′dis** [NA], SYN dorsal interosseous *muscles* of foot, under *muscle.*

m. interos′seus palma′ris, pl. **mus′culi interos′sei palma′res** [NA], SYN palmar interosseous *muscle.*

m. interos′seus planta′ris, pl. **mus′culi interos′sei planta′res** [NA], SYN plantar interosseous *muscle.*

m. interos′seus vola′ris, SYN palmar interosseous *muscle.*

mus′culi interspina′les [NA], SYN interspinales *muscles,* under *muscle.*

m. interspina′lis cer′vicis [NA], SYN cervical interspinales *muscles,* under *muscle.*

m. interspina′lis lumbo′rum [NA], SYN lumbar interspinales *muscles,* under *muscle.*

m. interspina′lis thora′cis [NA], SYN thoracic interspinales *muscles,* under *muscle.*

m. intertra′gicus, SYN *muscle* of notch of helix.

mus′culi intertransversa′rii [NA], SYN intertransversarii *muscles,* under *muscle.*

mus′culi intertransversa′rii anterio′res cer′vicis [NA], SYN anterior cervical intertransversarii *muscles,* under *muscle.*

mus′culi intertransversa′rii latera′les lumbo′rum [NA], SYN lateral lumbar intertransversarii *muscles,* under *muscle.*

mus′culi intertransversa′rii media′les lumbo′rum [NA], SYN medial lumbar intertransversarii *muscles,* under *muscle.*

mus′culi intertransversa′rii posterio′res cer′vicis [NA], SYN posterior cervical intertransversarii *muscles,* under *muscle.*

mus′culi intertransversa′rii thora′cis [NA], SYN thoracic intertransversarii *muscles,* under *muscle.*

m. ischiocaverno′sus [NA], SYN ischiocavernous *muscle.*

m. ischiococcyg′eus, SYN coccygeus *muscle.*

m. keratopharyn′geus, SEE middle constrictor *muscle* of pharynx.

mus′culi laryn′gis [NA], SYN *muscles* of larynx, under *muscle.*

m. laryngopharyn'geus, SYN inferior constrictor *muscle* of pharynx.

m. latis'simus dor'si [NA], SYN latissimus dorsi *muscle.*

m. leva'tor a'lae na'si, portion of m. levator labii superioris alaeque nasi muscle inserting into wing of nose.

m. leva'tor an'guli o'ris [NA], SYN levator anguli oris *muscle.*

m. leva'tor an'guli scap'ulae, SYN levator scapulae *muscle.*

m. leva'tor a'ni [NA], SYN levator ani *muscle.*

m. leva'tor cos'tae, pl. mus'culi levato'res costa'rum [NA], SYN levatores costarum *muscles,* under *muscle.*

musculi levatores costarum breves, SYN short levatores costarum *muscles,* under *muscle.*

musculi levatores costarum longi, SYN long levatores costarum *muscles,* under *muscle.*

m. leva'tor glan'dulae thyroi'deae [NA], SYN levator *muscle* of thyroid gland.

m. leva'tor la'bii inferio'ris, SYN mentalis *muscle.*

m. leva'tor la'bii superio'ris [NA], SYN levator labii superioris *muscle.*

m. leva'tor la'bii superio'ris alae'que na'si [NA], SYN levator labii superioris alaeque nasi *muscle.*

m. leva'tor pala'ti, SYN levator veli palatini *muscle.*

m. leva'tor pal'pebrae superio'ris [NA], SYN levator palpebrae superioris *muscle.*

m. leva'tor pro'statae [NA], SYN levator prostatae *muscle.*

m. leva'tor scap'ulae [NA], SYN levator scapulae *muscle.*

m. leva'tor ve'li palati'ni [NA], SYN levator veli palatini *muscle.*

mus'culi lin'guae [NA], SYN *muscles* of tongue, under *muscle.*

m. longis'simus [NA], SYN longissimus *muscle.*

m. longis'simus cap'itis [NA], SYN longissimus capitis *muscle.*

m. longis'simus cer'vicis [NA], SYN longissimus cervicis *muscle.*

m. longis'simus dor'si, SYN longissimus thoracis *muscle.*

m. longis'simus thora'cis [NA], SYN longissimus thoracis *muscle.*

m. longitudina'lis infe'rior [NA], SYN inferior longitudinal *muscle* of tongue.

m. longitudina'lis supe'rior [NA], SYN superior longitudinal *muscle* of tongue.

m. lon'gus cap'itis [NA], SYN longus capitis *muscle.*

m. lon'gus col'li [NA], SYN longus colli *muscle.*

m. lumbrica'lis ma'nus, pl. mus'culi lumbrica'les ma'nus [NA], SYN lumbrical *muscle* of hand.

m. lumbrica'lis pe'dis, pl. mus'culi lumbrica'les pe'dis [NA], SYN lumbrical *muscle* of foot.

m. masse'ter [NA], SYN masseter *muscle.*

m. menta'lis [NA], SYN mentalis *muscle.*

m. multif'idus [NA], SYN multifidus *muscle.*

m. multif'idus spi'nae, SYN multifidus *muscle.*

m. multipenna'tus [NA], SYN multipennate *muscle.*

m. mylohyoi'deus [NA], SYN mylohyoid *muscle.*

m. mylopharyn'geus, SEE superior constrictor *muscle* of pharynx.

m. nasa'lis [NA], SYN nasalis *muscle.*

m. obli'quus auric'ulae [NA], SYN oblique auricular *muscle.*

m. obli'quus cap'itis infe'rior [NA], SYN obliquus capitis inferior *muscle.*

m. obli'quus cap'itis supe'rior [NA], SYN obliquus capitis superior *muscle.*

m. obli'quus exter'nus abdom'inis [NA], SYN external oblique *muscle.*

m. obli'quus infe'rior [NA], SYN inferior oblique *muscle.*

m. obli'quus inter'nus abdom'inis [NA], SYN internal oblique *muscle.*

m. obli'quus supe'rior [NA], SYN superior oblique *muscle.*

m. obtura'tor exter'nus [NA], SYN obturator externus *muscle.*

m. obtura'tor inter'nus [NA], SYN obturator internus *muscle.*

m. occipita'lis, SEE occipitofrontalis *muscle.*

m. occipitofronta'lis [NA], SYN occipitofrontalis *muscle.*

m. omohyoi'deus [NA], SYN omohyoid *muscle.*

m. oppo'nens dig'iti min'imi [NA], SYN opponens digiti minimi *muscle.*

m. oppo'nens dig'iti quin'ti, SYN opponens digiti minimi *muscle.*

m. oppo'nens min'imi dig'iti, SYN opponens digiti minimi *muscle.*

m. oppo'nens pol'licis [NA], SYN opponens pollicis *muscle.*

m. orbicula'ris [NA], SYN orbicularis *muscle.*

m. orbicula'ris oc'uli [NA], SYN orbicularis oculi *muscle.*

m. orbicula'ris o'ris [NA], SYN orbicularis oris *muscle.*

m. orbicula'ris palpebra'rum, SYN orbicularis oculi *muscle.*

m. orbita'lis [NA], SYN orbitalis *muscle.*

m. orbitopalpebra'lis, SYN levator palpebrae superioris *muscle.*

mus'culi ossiculo'rum audi'tus [NA], SYN *muscles* of auditory ossicles, under *muscle.*

m. palatoglos'sus [NA], SYN palatoglossus *muscle.*

m. palatopharyn'geus [NA], SYN palatopharyngeus *muscle.*

m. palatosalpin'geus, SYN tensor veli palati *muscle.*

m. palatostaphyli'nus, a bundle of muscular fibers from the tensor veli palatini joining the m. uvulae.

m. palma'ris bre'vis [NA], SYN palmaris brevis *muscle.*

m. palma'ris lon'gus [NA], SYN palmaris longus *muscle.*

m. papilla'ris [NA], SYN papillary *muscle.*

mus'culi pectina'ti [NA], SYN pectinate *muscles,* under *muscle.*

m. pectin'eus [NA], SYN pectineus *muscle.*

m. pectora'lis ma'jor [NA], SYN pectoralis major *muscle.*

m. pectora'lis mi'nor [NA], SYN pectoralis minor *muscle.*

mus'culi perine'i [NA], SYN perineal *muscles,* under *muscle.*

m. peroneocalca'neus, an occasional muscle arising from the shaft of the fibula and inserted into the calcaneus.

m. perone'us bre'vis [NA], SYN peroneus brevis *muscle.*

m. perone'us lon'gus [NA], SYN peroneus longus *muscle.*

m. perone'us ter'tius [NA], SYN peroneus tertius *muscle.*

m. petropharyn'geus, an occasional accessory levator muscle of the pharynx, arising from the undersurface of the petrous portion of the temporal bone and inserted into the pharynx.

m. petrostaphyli'nus, SYN levator veli palatini *muscle.*

m. pharyngopalati'nus, SYN palatopharyngeus *muscle.*

m. pirifor'mis [NA], SYN piriformis *muscle.*

m. planta'ris [NA], SYN plantaris *muscle.*

m. platys'ma, SYN platysma *muscle.*

m. platys'ma myoi'des, SYN platysma *muscle.*

m. pleuroesopha'geus [NA], SYN pleuroesophageal *muscle.*

m. poplit'eus [NA], SYN popliteus *muscle.*

m. proce'rus [NA], SYN procerus *muscle.*

m. prona'tor pe'dis, SYN quadratus plantae *muscle.*

m. prona'tor quadra'tus [NA], SYN pronator quadratus *muscle.*

m. prona'tor ra'dii te'res, SYN pronator teres *muscle.*

m. prona'tor te'res [NA], SYN pronator teres *muscle.*

m. prostat'icus, SYN muscular *substance* of prostate.

m. pso'as ma'jor [NA], SYN psoas major *muscle.*

m. pso'as mi'nor [NA], SYN psoas minor *muscle.*

m. pterygoi'deus exter'nus, SYN lateral pterygoid *muscle.*

m. pterygoi'deus inter'nus, SYN medial pterygoid *muscle.*

m. pterygoi'deus latera'lis [NA], SYN lateral pterygoid *muscle.*

m. pterygoi'deus media'lis [NA], SYN medial pterygoid *muscle.*

m. pterygopharyn'geus, SEE superior constrictor *muscle* of pharynx.

m. pterygospino'sus, a muscular slip, occasionally present, passing between the spine of the sphenoid bone and the posterior margin of the lateral pterygoid plate.

m. pubococcyg'eus [NA], SYN pubococcygeus *muscle.*

m. puboprostat'icus [NA], SYN puboprostatic *muscle.*

m. puborecta'lis [NA], SYN puborectalis *muscle.*

m. pubovagina'lis [NA], SYN pubovaginalis *muscle.*

m. pubovesica'lis [NA], SYN pubovesicalis *muscle.*

m. pyramida'lis [NA], SYN pyramidalis *muscle.*

m. pyramida'lis auric'ulae [NA], SYN pyramidal auricular *muscle.*

m. pyramida'lis na'si, SYN procerus *muscle.*

mu

m. pyrifor'mis, SYN piriformis *muscle.*

m. quadra'tus [NA], SYN quadratus *muscle.*

m. quadra'tus fem'oris [NA], SYN quadratus femoris *muscle.*

m. quadra'tus la'bii inferio'ris, SYN depressor labii inferioris *muscle.*

m. quadra'tus la'bii superio'ris, composed of three heads usually described as three separate muscles; they are the caput angulare or levator labii superioris alaeque nasi muscle; caput infraorbitale or levator labii superioris muscle; caput zygomaticum or zygomaticus minor muscle. SYN quadrate muscle of upper lip.

m. quadra'tus lumbo'rum [NA], SYN quadratus lumborum *muscle.*

m. quadra'tus men'ti, SYN depressor labii inferioris *muscle.*

m. quadra'tus plan'tae [NA], SYN quadratus plantae *muscle.*

m. quad'riceps exten'sor fem'oris, SYN quadriceps femoris *muscle.*

m. quad'riceps fem'oris [NA], SYN quadriceps femoris *muscle.*

m. rectococcyg'eus [NA], SYN rectococcygeus *muscle.*

m. rectourethra'lis [NA], SYN rectourethralis *muscle.*

m. rectouteri'nus [NA], SYN rectouterine *muscle.*

m. rectovesica'lis [NA], SYN rectovesicalis *muscle.*

m. rec'tus abdom'inis [NA], SYN rectus abdominis *muscle.*

m. rec'tus cap'itis ante'rior [NA], SYN rectus capitis anterior *muscle.*

m. rec'tus cap'itis anti'cus ma'jor, SYN longus capitis *muscle.*

m. rectus cap'itis anti'cus mi'nor, SYN rectus capitis anterior *muscle.*

m. rec'tus cap'itis latera'lis [NA], SYN rectus capitis lateralis *muscle.*

m. rec'tus cap'itis poste'rior ma'jor [NA], SYN rectus capitis posterior major *muscle.*

m. rec'tus cap'itis poste'rior mi'nor [NA], SYN rectus capitis posterior minor *muscle.*

m. rec'tus cap'itis posti'cus ma'jor, SYN rectus capitis posterior major *muscle.*

m. rec'tus cap'itis posti'cus mi'nor, SYN rectus capitis posterior minor *muscle.*

m. rec'tus exter'nus, SYN lateral rectus *muscle.*

m. rec'tus fem'oris [NA], SYN rectus femoris *muscle.*

m. rec'tus infe'rior [NA], SYN inferior rectus *muscle.*

m. rec'tus inter'nus, SYN medial rectus *muscle.*

m. rec'tus latera'lis [NA], SYN lateral rectus *muscle.*

m. rec'tus media'lis [NA], SYN medial rectus *muscle.*

m. rec'tus supe'rior [NA], SYN superior rectus *muscle.*

m. rec'tus thora'cis, SYN sternalis *muscle.*

m. ret'rahens au'rem, m. ret'rahens auric'ulam, SYN posterior auricular *muscle.*

m. rhomboatloi'deus, an occasional muscle arising with the rhomboids from the cervical and thoracic vertebrae and inserted into the atlas.

m. rhomboi'deus ma'jor [NA], SYN rhomboideus major *muscle.*

m. rhomboi'deus mi'nor [NA], SYN rhomboid minor *muscle.*

m. riso'rius [NA], SYN risorius *muscle.*

mus'culi rotato'res [NA], SYN rotatores *muscles, under muscle.*

mus'culi rotato'res cer'vicis [NA], SYN rotatores cervicis *muscles, under muscle.*

mus'culi rotato'res lumbo'rum [NA], SYN rotatores lumborum *muscles, under muscle.*

mus'culi rotato'res thora'cis [NA], SYN rotatores thoracis *muscles, under muscle.*

m. sacrococcyg'eus ante'rior, SYN ventral sacrococcygeus *muscle.*

m. sacrococcyg'eus dorsa'lis [NA], SYN dorsal sacrococcygeus *muscle.*

m. sacrococcyg'eus poste'rior, SYN dorsal sacrococcygeus *muscle.*

m. sacrococcyg'eus ventra'lis [NA], SYN ventral sacrococcygeus *muscle.*

m. sacrolumba'lis, SYN iliocostalis lumborum *muscle.*

m. sacrospina'lis, SYN erector spinae *muscles, under muscle.*

m. salpingopharyn'geus [NA], SYN salpingopharyngeus *muscle.*

m. sarto'rius [NA], SYN sartorius *muscle.*

m. scale'nus ante'rior [NA], SYN scalenus anterior *muscle.*

m. scale'nus anti'cus, SYN scalenus anterior *muscle.*

m. scale'nus me'dius [NA], SYN scalenus medius *muscle.*

m. scale'nus min'imus [NA], SYN scalenus minimus *muscle.*

m. scale'nus poste'rior [NA], SYN scalenus posterior *muscle.*

m. scale'nus posti'cus, SYN scalenus posterior *muscle.*

m. semimembrano'sus [NA], SYN semimembranosus *muscle.*

m. semispina'lis [NA], SYN semispinalis *muscle.*

m. semispina'lis cap'itis [NA], SYN semispinalis capitis *muscle.*

m. semispina'lis cer'vicis [NA], SYN semispinalis cervicis *muscle.*

m. semispina'lis col'li, SYN semispinalis cervicis *muscle.*

m. semispina'lis dor'si, SYN semispinalis thoracis *muscle.*

m. semispina'lis thora'cis [NA], SYN semispinalis thoracis *muscle.*

m. semitendino'sus [NA], SYN semitendinosus *muscle.*

m. serra'tus ante'rior [NA], SYN serratus anterior *muscle.*

m. serra'tus mag'nus, SYN serratus anterior *muscle.*

m. serra'tus poste'rior infe'rior [NA], SYN serratus posterior inferior *muscle.*

m. serra'tus poste'rior supe'rior [NA], SYN serratus posterior superior *muscle.*

m. skel'eti, SYN skeletal *muscle.*

m. sol'eus [NA], SYN soleus *muscle.*

m. sphenosalpingostaphyli'nus, SYN tensor veli palati *muscle.*

m. sphinc'ter [NA], SYN sphincter.

m. sphinc'ter ampullae hepatopancreat'icae [NA], SYN *sphincter* of hepatopancreatic ampulla.

m. sphinc'ter a'ni exter'nus [NA], SYN external anal *sphincter.*

m. sphinc'ter a'ni inter'nus [NA], SYN internal anal *sphincter.*

m. sphinc'ter duc'tus choledo'chi [NA], SYN *sphincter* of common bile duct.

m. sphinc'ter duc'tus pancreat'ici, SYN *sphincter* of pancreatic duct.

m. sphinc'ter o'ris, SYN orbicularis oris *muscle.*

m. sphinc'ter pupil'lae [NA], SYN *sphincter* pupillae.

m. sphinc'ter pylo'ri [NA], SYN pyloric *sphincter.*

m. sphinc'ter ure'thrae [NA], SYN *sphincter* urethrae.

m. sphinc'ter ure'thrae membrana'ceae, SYN *sphincter* urethrae.

m. sphinc'ter vagi'nae, (1) SYN bulbocavernosus *muscle.* (2) SYN deep transverse perineal *muscle.*

m. sphinc'ter vesi'cae, SYN *sphincter* vesicae.

m. spina'lis [NA], SYN spinalis *muscle.*

m. spina'lis cap'itis [NA], SYN spinalis capitis *muscle.*

m. spina'lis cer'vicis [NA], SYN spinalis cervicis *muscle.*

m. spina'lis col'li, SYN spinalis cervicis *muscle.*

m. spina'lis dor'si, SYN spinalis thoracis *muscle.*

m. spina'lis thora'cis [NA], SYN spinalis thoracis *muscle.*

m. sple'nius cap'itis [NA], SYN splenius capitis *muscle.*

m. sple'nius cer'vicis [NA], SYN splenius cervicis *muscle.*

m. sple'nius col'li, SYN splenius cervicis *muscle.*

m. stape'dius [NA], SYN stapedius *muscle.*

m. sterna'lis [NA], SYN sternalis *muscle.*

m. sternochondroscapula'ris, SYN sternochondroscapular *muscle.*

m. sternoclavicula'ris, SYN sternoclavicular *muscle.*

m. sternocleidomastoi'deus [NA], SYN sternocleidomastoid *muscle.*

m. sternofascia'lis, an occasional muscular slip arising from the manubrium of the sternum and inserted into the fascia of the neck.

m. sternohyoi'deus [NA], SYN sternohyoid *muscle.*

m. sternothyroi'deus [NA], SYN sternothyroid *muscle.*

m. styloauricula'ris, SYN styloauricular *muscle.*

m. styloglos'sus [NA], SYN styloglossus *muscle.*

m. stylohyoi'deus [NA], SYN stylohyoid *muscle.*

spontaneous m., a m. that arises naturally and not as a result of exposure to mutagens. SYN natural m.

suppressor m., (1) A m. that alters the anticodon in a tRNA so that it is complementary to a termination codon, thus suppressing termination of the amino acid chain. Cf. amber m., ochre m., umber m. **(2)** Genetic changes such that the effect of a m. in one place can be overcome by a second m. in another location. There are two types: intergenic suppression (occurring in a different gene) and intragenic suppression (occurring in the same gene but at a different site). SYN nonsense m.

transition m., a point m. involving substitution of one base-pair for another, *i.e.,* replacement of one purine for another and of one pyrimidine for another pyrimidine without change in the purine-pyrimidine orientation.

transversion m., a point m. involving base substitution in which the orientation of purine and pyrimidine is reversed, in contradistinction to transition m.

umber m., a m. yielding the termination codon UGA, resulting in premature termination of a polypeptide chain. Cf. suppressor m. SYN opal m.

up promoter m., a m. that increases the frequency of initiation of transcription.

mute (myūt). **1.** Unable or unwilling to speak. **2.** A person who has not the faculty of speech. [L. *mutus*]

mu·tein (myū'tēn). General, little-used term for a protein arising as a result of a mutation. [*mut*ation + prot*ein*]

mu·ti·la·tion (myū-ti-lā'shŭn). Disfigurement or injury by removal or destruction of any conspicuous or essential part of the body. [L. *mutilatio,* fr. *mutilo,* pp. *-atus,* to maim]

mut·ism (myū'tizm). **1.** The state of being silent. **2.** Organic or functional absence of the faculty of speech. [L. *mutus,* mute]

akinetic m., subacute or chronic state of altered consciousness, in which the patient appears alert intermittently, but is not responsive, although his/her descending motor pathways appear intact; due to lesions of various cerebral structures. SYN coma vigil.

elective m., m. due to psychogenic causes. SYN voluntary m.

voluntary m., SYN elective m.

mu·ton (myū'ton). In genetics, the smallest unit of a chromosome in which alteration can be effective in causing a mutation. [*mut*ation + -*on*]

mu·tu·al·ism (myū'tyū-ăl-izm). Symbiotic relationship in which both species derive benefit. Cf. commensalism, metabiosis, parasitism.

mu·tu·al·ist (myū'tyū-ăl-ist). SYN symbion. [L. *mutuus,* in return, mutual]

muz·zle (mŭz'l). The snout of an animal.

Mv Obsolete abbreviation for mendelevium.

mV, mv Abbreviation for millivolt.

MVV Abbreviation for maximum voluntary *ventilation.*

MW Abbreviation for molecular *weight.*

my·al·gia (mī-al'jē-ă). Muscular pain. SYN myodynia, myoneuralgia, myosalgia. [G. *mys,* muscle, + *algos,* pain]

epidemic m., SYN epidemic *pleurodynia.*

m. ther'mica, SYN heat *cramps,* under *cramp.*

my·as·the·nia (mī-as-thē'nē-ă). Muscular weakness. [G. *mys,* muscle, + *astheneia,* weakness]

m. angiosclerot'ica, SYN intermittent *claudication.*

m. gravis, disorder of neuromuscular transmission, marked by fluctuating weakness, especially of the oculofacial muscles and the proximal limb muscles; the weakness characteristically increases with activity; due to an immunological disorder. SYN Goldflam disease.

my·as·then·ic (mī'as-then'ik). Relating to myasthenia.

my·a·to·nia, my·at·o·ny (mī-ă-tō'nē-ă, mī-at'ō-nē). Abnormal extensibility of a muscle. [G. *mys,* muscle, + *a* priv. + *tonos,* tone]

m. congen'ita, SYN *amyotonia* congenita (1).

my·at·ro·phy (mī-at'rō-fē). SYN muscular *atrophy.*

my·ce·lia (mī-sē'lē-ă). Plural of mycelium.

my·ce·li·an (mī-sē'lē-an). Pertaining to a mycelium.

my·ce·li·oid (mī-sē'lē-oyd). Resembling a mycelium. [mycelium + G. *eidos,* resemblance]

my·ce·li·um, pl. **my·ce·lia** (mī-sē'lē-ŭm, -ă). The mass of hyphae making up a colony of fungi. [G. *mykēs,* fungus, + *hēlos,* nail, wart, excrescence on animal or plant]

aerial m., the portion of m. that grows upward or outward from the surface of the substrate, and from which propagative spores develop in or on characteristic structures that are distinctive for various generic groups.

nonseptate m., one in which there are no septa, or "cross-walls," in the hyphae; inasmuch as the latter are not divided into numerous individual cells, the multinucleated protoplasm may flow throughout the tubelike structures.

septate m., one in which septa, or "cross-walls," divide the hyphae into numerous uninucleated or multinucleated cells.

⌂**mycet-, myceto-.** Fungus. SEE ALSO myco-. [G. *mykēs,* fungus]

my·cete (mī'sēt). A fungus. [G. *mykēs,* fungus]

my·ce·tism, my·ce·tis·'mus (mī-sē-tizm, -tiz'mŭs). Poisoning by certain species of mushrooms. SYN muscarinism. [G. *mykēs,* fungus]

m. cerebra'lis, a condition characterized by transient hallucinogenic symptoms following ingestion of mushrooms such as *Psilocybe* and *Panaeolus.*

m. cholifor'mis, a severe and occasionally fatal illness due to the consumption of *Amanita phalloides* and other poisonous mushroom species.

m. gastrointestina'lis, a relatively mild type of mushroom poisoning characterized by nausea, vomiting, and diarrhea and caused by eating certain species of *Boletus, Lactarius, Entoloma,* and *Lepiota.*

m. nervo'sa, mushroom poisoning that involves the parasympathetic nervous system and causes gastrointestinal distress, after consumption of species such as *Amanita, Inocybe,* and *Clitocybe.*

m. sanguina'reus, a transient hemoglobinuria and jaundice caused by eating the mushroom *Helvella esculenta,* either raw or cooked.

my·ce·to·ge·net·ic, my·ce·to·gen·ic (mī-sē'tō-jĕ-net'ik, mī'sē-tō-; -jen'ik). Caused by fungi. SYN mycetogenous. [G. *mykēs,* fungus, + *gennētos,* begotten]

my·ce·tog·e·nous (mī-sē-toj'ĕ-nŭs). SYN mycetogenetic.

my·ce·to·ma (mī-sē-tō'mă). **1.** A chronic infection involving the feet and characterized by the formation of localized lesions with tumefactions and multiple draining sinuses. The exudate contains granules that may be yellow, white, red, brown, or black, depending upon the causative agent. M. is caused by two principal groups of microorganisms: 1) actinomycotic m. is caused by actinomycetes, including species of *Streptomyces, Actinomadurae,* and *Nocardia,* 2) eumycotic mycetoma is caused by true fungi, including species of *Madurella, Exophiala, Pseudallescheria, Curvularia, Neotestudina, Pyrenochaeta, Aspergillus, Leptosphaeria, Plemodomus, Polycytella, Fusarium, Phialophora, Corynespora, Cylindrocarpon, Pseudochaetosphaeronema, Bipolaris,* and *Acremonium.* SYN fungous foot, Madura boil, Madura foot, maduromycosis. **2.** Any tumor with draining sinuses produced by filamentous fungi.

Bouffardi's black m., an obsolete term for a chronic infection, usually involving the feet. SEE mycetoma (1).

⌂ **Combining forms**	**[NA] Nomina Anatomica**
Word*Finder*	**[MIM] Mendelian**
Multi-term entry finder	**Inheritance in Man**
Preceding letter A	
A.D.A.M. Anatomy Plates	☆ **Official alternate term**
Between letters L and M	
	☆**[NA] Official alternate**
Appendices:	**Nomina Anatomica term**
Following letter Z	
	High Profile Term
SYN Synonym; Cf., compare	

my

Bouffardi's white m., a form of mycetoma common in India and found occasionally in Somalia, caused by the organism *Streptomyces somaliensis;* in this variety, the muscles, tendons, and bones of the foot are destroyed by the disease process; numerous draining sinuses discharge yellowish grains, clustered like fish roe.

Brumpt's white m., m. caused by *Pseudallescheria boydii,* occurring in temperate and subtropical areas in India; small, white to yellow, hard to soft granules are discharged through the draining sinuses.

Carter's black m., m. caused by *Madurella mycetomatis* which is prevalent in Italy, parts of Africa, and India; the exuded granules are black.

Nicolle's white m., m. caused by a species of *Aspergillus,* and producing relatively large granules, about the size of a pea; infection occurs from barley grain.

Vincent's white m., m. caused by *Actinomadura madurae* and occurring in North Africa, India, the Argentine, and Cuba.

my·cid (mī′sid). An allergic reaction to a remote focus of mycotic infection. [G. *mykēs,* fungus, + -id]

△**myco-.** Fungus. SEE ALSO mycet-. [G. *mykēs,* fungus]

my·co·bac·te·ria (mī′kō-bak-tē′rē-ă). Organisms belonging to the genus *Mycobacterium.*

atypical m., species of mycobacteria other than *M. tuberculosis* or *M. bovis* that can cause disease in immunocompromised humans.

group I m., m. that produce a bright yellow color when grown in the presence of light. Organisms placed in this group appear to belong to the species *Mycobacterium kansasii.* SYN photochromogens.

group II m., m. that produce a yellow pigment even when grown in the dark; when grown in the light, the pigment is orange. These organisms behave as do saprophytes in humans and are nonpathogenic to laboratory animals. SYN scotochromogens.

group III m., m. that are either colorless or that slowly produce a light yellow pigment when grown in the presence of light. Organisms placed in this group belong to the species *Mycobacterium intracellulare.* SYN nonchromogens.

group IV m., m. that grow rapidly and that do not produce pigment. Organisms placed in this group belong to such species as *Mycobacterium ulcerans* and *M. marinum.*

My·co·bac·te·ri·a·ce·ae (mī′kō-bak-tēr-ē-ā′sē-ē). A family of aerobic bacteria (order Actinomycetales) containing Gram-positive, spherical to rod-shaped cells. Branching does not occur under ordinary cultural conditions. They may or may not be acid-fast. They occur in soil and dairy products and as parasites on man and other animals. The type genus is *Mycobacterium.*

my·co·bac·te·ri·o·sis (mī′kō-bak-tēr′ē-ō′sis). Infection with mycobacteria.

My·co·bac·te·ri·um (mī′kō-bak-tēr′ē-ŭm). A genus of aerobic, nonmotile bacteria (family Mycobacteriaceae) containing Gram-positive, acid-fast, slender, straight or slightly curved rods; slender filaments occasionally occur, but branched forms rarely are produced. Parasitic and saprophytic species occur. A number of species are associated with infections in immunocompromised people, especially those with AIDS. The type species is *M. tuberculosis.* It is the type genus of the family Mycobacteriaceae. [myco- + bacterium]

M. absces′sus, SYN *M. chelonae* subsp. *abscessus.*

M. a′vium, a species causing tuberculosis in fowl and other birds. Recently linked to opportunistic infections in humans. SYN tubercle bacillus (3).

M. avium-intracellulare complex, an opportunistic agent of people with AIDS. Difficult to treat because *Mycobacterium* is resistant to many antibiotics. May also cause chronic lower respiratory tract infections.

M. bo′vis, a species that is the primary cause of tuberculosis in cattle; transmissible to humans and other animals, causing tuberculosis. SYN tubercle bacillus (2).

M. chelonae, rapid-growing mycobacterium (Runyon group IV) that cause sporadic infection in any tissue or organ system in humans following cardiothoracic surgery, peritoneal- and hemo-

dialysis, augmentation mammaplasty, arthroplasty, and immunocompromised patients.

M. chelonae subsp. **abscessus,** a species originally found in a traumatic infection of the knee. SYN *M. abscessus.*

M. fortui′tum, a saprophytic species found in soil and in infections of humans, cattle, and cold-blooded animals. Causes skin abscesses.

M. intracellula′re, a species found in lung lesions and sputum of humans; may cause bone and tendon-sheath lesions in rabbits; some strains are pathogenic for mice. Recently linked to opportunistic infections in humans. SYN Battey bacillus.

M. kansas′ii, a species causing a tuberculosis-like pulmonary disease; also found to cause infections (and usually lesions) in spinal fluid, spleen, liver, pancreas, testes, hip joint, knee joint, finger, wrist, and lymph nodes.

M. lep′rae, a species that causes Hansen's disease; recently identified from wild leprous armadillos (*Dasypus novemcinctus*) in Texas. SYN Hansen's bacillus, leprosy bacillus.

M. lepraemu′rium, a bacterial species which causes rat leprosy.

M. maria′num, former name for *M. scrofulaceum.*

M. mari′num, a species causing spontaneous tuberculosis in salt water fish; it also occurs in other cold-blooded animals, in some swimming pools in which it may cause human cutaneous infection (see swimming pool *granuloma*), irrigation canals and ditches, and ocean beaches.

M. micro′ti, a species causing generalized tuberculosis in voles; transmissible to guinea pigs, rabbits, and calves, causing localized infections.

M. paratuberculo′sis, a species causing Johne's disease, a chronic enteritis in cattle. SYN Johne's bacillus.

M. phle′i, a species found in soil and dust and on plants. SYN Moeller's grass bacillus, timothy-hay bacillus.

M. scrofula′ceum, a species frequently associated with cervical adenitis in children; also found in a skin lesion of a leprosy patient.

M. smeg′matis, a saprophytic species of bacteria found in smegma from the genitalia of humans and many of the lower animals; it is also found in soil, dust, and water.

M. tuberculo′sis, a species which causes tuberculosis in man; it is the type species of the genus *M.* SYN Koch's bacillus (1), tubercle bacillus (1).

M. ul′cerans, a species causing Buruli ulcers in man; transmissible from soil, usually after an injury, and possibly by an insect vector.

M. xen′opi, a species found in a skin lesion of a cold-blooded animal, *Xenopus laevis;* a rare cause of nosocomial human pulmonary tuberculosis.

my·co·bac·tin (mī′kō-bak′tin). A complex lipid factor reported to be required for the growth of *Mycobacterium tuberculosis* in human plasma; appears to be identical with the lipid factor extracted from *M. phlei* and essential for the growth of *M. johnei.*

my·co·cide (mī′kō-sīd). SYN fungicide. [myco- + L. *caedo,* to kill]

my·co·der·ma·ti·tis (mī′kō-der-mă-tī′tis). A nonspecific term used to designate an eruption of mycotic (fungus, yeast, mold) origin.

my·co·gas·tri·tis (mī′kō-gas-trī′tis). Inflammation of the stomach due to the presence of a fungus. [myco- + G. *gastēr,* stomach, + -*itis,* inflammation]

my·col·ic ac·ids (mī-kol′ik). Long-chain cyclopropanecarboxylic acids (C_{19}–C_{21}), further substituted by long-chain (C_{24}–C_{30}) alkanes containing free hydroxyl groups, found in certain bacteria; these waxy substances appear to be responsible for the acid-fastness of the bacteria that contain them. SYN mykol.

my·col·o·gist (mī-kol′ŏ-jist). A person specializing in mycology.

my·col·o·gy (mī-kol′ō-jē). The study of fungi: their classification, edibility, cultivation, and biology. [myco- + G. *logos,* study]

medical m., the study of fungi that produce disease in humans and other animals, and of the diseases they produce, their ecology, and their epidemiology.

my·co·myr·in·gi·tis (mī′kō-mir-in-jī′tis). An obsolete term denoting an inflammation of the membrana tympani caused by the presence of *Aspergillus* or other fungus. SYN myringomycosis. [myco- + Mod. L. *myringa,* drum-membrane, + G. *-itis,* inflammation]

my·co·phage (mī′kō-fāj). A virus, the host of which is a fungus, in contradistinction to a bacteriophage, the host of which is a bacterium. SEE ALSO mycovirus. [myco- + G. *phagō,* to eat]

My·co·plas·ma (mī′kō-plaz-mă). A genus of aerobic to facultatively anaerobic bacteria (family Mycoplasmataceae) containing Gram-negative cells that do not possess a true cell wall but are bounded by a three-layered membrane; they do not revert to bacteria containing cell walls or cell wall fragments. The minimal reproductive units of these organisms are 0.2 to 0.3 μm in diameter. The cells are pleomorphic, and in liquid media appear as coccoid bodies, rings, or filaments. Colonies usually consist of a central core, growing down into the medium, surrounded by superficial peripheral growth. They require sterol for growth. They also require enrichment with serum or ascitic fluid. These organisms are found in humans and other animals and are parasitic to pathogenic. The type species is *M. mycoides.* SYN Asterococcus. [myco- + G. *plasma,* something formed (plasm)]

M. agalact′iae, a bacterial species causing contagious agalactia of sheep and goats, a common disease in the Mediterranean region.

M. bucca′le, a bacterial species which is an infrequent parasitic inhabitant of the human oropharynx; it is the predominant mycoplasma in the oropharynx of nonhuman primates.

M. conjuncti′vae subsp. *o′vis,* a bacterial subspecies associated with pinkeye of sheep.

M. fau′cium, a species which is a rare member of the normal flora of the human oropharynx; it is occasionally found in the oropharynx of nonhuman primates.

M. fermen′tans, a species found in ulcerative genital lesions associated with fusiform bacteria and spirilla and also on the apparently normal genital mucosa of humans.

M. gallisep′ticum, a bacterial species causing chronic respiratory disease of chickens and infectious sinusitis of turkeys.

M. genitalium, a species that may be a causative agent of urethritis.

M. granula′rum, former name for *Acholeplasma granularum.*

M. hominis, a species that is the causative agent of pelvic inflammatory disease and other genitourinary tract infections; can also cause chorioamnionitis and postpartum fever.

M. hyorhi′nis, a bacterial species found in the nasal cavity of swine; associated with arthritis and polyserositis in domestic pigs.

M. hyosyno′viae, a bacterial species found in the joints and respiratory tract of swine, and associated with arthritis and polyserositis in domestic pigs.

M. hyopneumo′niae, a bacterial species causing mycoplasma pneumonia of pigs.

M. laidla′wii, SYN *Acholeplasma laidlawii.*

M. meleag′ridis, a bacterial species causing air sacculitis in turkeys.

M. mycoi′des, a bacterial species containing two subspecies: *M. mycoides* subsp. *mycoides,* the type subspecies, and *M. mycoides* subsp. *capri;* the former causes contagious bovine pleuropneumonia in cattle; the latter causes contagious pleuropneumonia in sheep and goats; it is the type species of the genus *M.*

M. neuroly′ticum, a bacterial species found in normal and diseased mice; causes "rolling disease."

M. orale, a species of *M.* associated with the buccal and pharyngeal cavities of humans and animals.

M. pharyn′gis, a species occurring as a commensal in the human oropharynx.

M. pneumo′niae, a species causing primary atypical pneumonia in human beings. SYN Eaton agent.

M. saliva′rium, a species found in human saliva.

M. syno′viae, a bacterial species found in the hock joint of a fowl; causes infectious synovitis in chickens.

my·co·plas·ma, pl. **my·co·plas·ma·ta** (as′ter-ō-kok′kŭs, -plaz′

mah-tă). A vernacular term used only to refer to any member of the genus *Mycoplasma.*

My·co·plas·ma·ta·les (mī′kō-plaz′mă-tā′lēz). An order of Gram-negative bacteria containing cells which are bounded by a three-layered membrane but which do not possess a true cell wall. The minimal reproductive units are 0.2 to 0.3 μm in diameter. Pathogenic and saprophytic species occur. These organisms reproduce through the breaking up of branched filaments into coccoid, filterable elementary bodies. The order includes the so-called pleuropneumonia-like *organisms,* under *organism* (PPLO).

my·co·pus (mī′kō-pŭs). SYN mucopus.

my·cose (mī′kōs). SYN trehalose.

my·co·sis, pl. **my·co·ses** (mī-kō′sis, -sēz). Any disease caused by a fungus (filamentous or yeast). [myco- + G. *-osis,* condition]

   m. cu′tis chron′ica, a chronic dermatomycosis caused by a fungus.

   m. framboesioi′des, SYN yaws.

   m. fungoi′des, a chronic progressive lymphoma arising in the skin which initially simulates eczema or other inflammatory dermatoses; the appearance of plaques is associated with acanthosis and bandlike infiltration of the upper dermis by a pleomorphic infiltrate including atypical T lymphocytes which also collect in clear spaces in the lower epidermis (Pautrier's microabscesses); in advanced cases, ulcerated tumors and infiltrations of lymph nodes may occur.

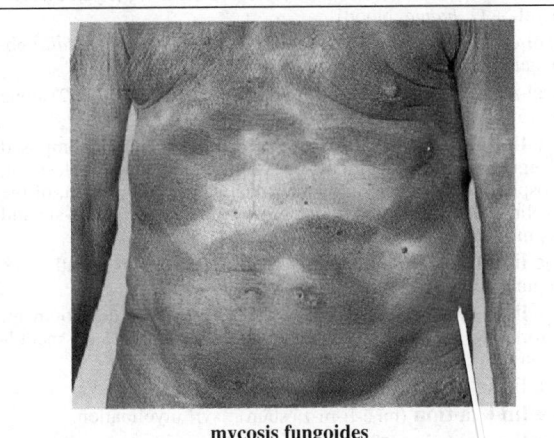

mycosis fungoides

   Gilchrist's m., obsolete term for blastomycosis.

   m. intestina′lis, gastroenteric form of anthrax, the symptoms of which are those of gastroenteritis followed by toxemia and general depression.

my·co·stat·ic (mī-kō-stat′ik). SYN fungistatic.

my·cos·ter·ols (mī-kos′ter-olz). Sterols obtained from fungi.

my·cot·ic (mī-kot′ik). Relating to or caused by a fungus.

my·co·tox·i·co·sis (mī′kō-tok-si-kō′sis). Poisoning due to the ingestion of preformed substances produced by the action of certain fungi on particular foodstuffs or ingestion of the fungi themselves; *e.g.,* ergotism. [myco- + G. *toxikon,* poison, + *-osis,* condition]

my·co·tox·ins (mī′kō-tok-sinz). Toxic compounds produced by certain fungi, some of which are used for medicinal purposes; *e.g.,* muscarine, psilocybin.

my·co·vi·rus (mī′kō-vī-rŭs). A virus that infects fungi.

my·da·le·ine (mī-dā′lē-ēn). A poisonous ptomaine formed in putrefying liver and other viscera; it acts specifically upon the heart, causing arrest of its action in diastole. [G. *mydaleos,* moldy, fr. *mydos,* dampness]

my·da·tox·in (mī-dă-tok′sin). A ptomaine from putrefying viscera and flesh. [G. *mydos,* dampness, decay, + *toxikon,* poison]

my·dri·a·sis (mi-drī′ă-sis). Dilation of the pupil. [G.]

   alternating m., m. alternately affecting each eye.

amaurotic m., a moderate widening of both pupils resulting from impaired visual input from one or both eyes.

paralytic m., pupillary dilation due to paralysis of the sphincter muscle of the pupil induced by anticholinergic drugs given topically or systemically, or resulting from lesions of the oculomotor nucleus or nerve, contusion of the eyeball, or glaucoma.

spastic m., pupillary dilation due to contraction of the dilator muscle of the pupil induced by adrenergic drugs or by stimulation of the sympathetic pathway.

myd·ri·at·ic (mi-drē-at′ik). **1.** Causing mydriasis or dilation of the pupil. **2.** An agent that dilates the pupil.

my·ec·to·my (mī-ek′tō-mē). Excision of a portion of a muscle. [G. *mys,* muscle, + *ektomē,* excision]

my·ec·to·py, my·ec·to·pia (mī-ek′tō-pē, mī-ek-tō′pē-ă). Rarely used term for dislocation of a muscle. [G. *mys,* muscle, + *ektopos,* out of place]

△**myel-, myelo-.** **1.** The bone marrow. **2.** The spinal cord and medulla oblongata. Cf. medullo-. **3.** The myelin sheath of nerve fibers. [G. *myelos,* medulla, marrow]

my·el·ap·o·plexy (mī′el-ap′ō-plek′sē). SYN hematomyelia. [myel- + G. *apoplēxia,* apoplexy]

my·el·a·te·lia (mī′el-ă-tē′lē-ă). Developmental defect of the spinal cord. [myel- + G. *ateleia,* incompleteness]

my·el·auxe (mī-el-awk′sē). Hypertrophy of the spinal cord. [myel- + G. *auxē,* increase]

my·e·le·mia (mī-ě-lē′mē-ă). Rarely used term for myelocytosis. [myel- + G. *haima,* blood]

my·el·en·ceph·a·lon (mī′el-en-sef′ă-lon) [NA]. SYN *medulla* oblongata. [myel- + G. *enkephalos,* brain]

my·el·ic (mī-el′ik). Relating to (1) the spinal cord, or (2) bone marrow.

my·e·lin (mī′ě-lin). **1.** The lipoproteinaceous material, composed of regularly alternating membranes of lipid lamellae (cholesterol, phospholipids, sphingolipids, phosphatidates) and protein, of the myelin sheath. **2.** Droplets of lipid formed during autolysis and postmortem decomposition.

my·e·li·nat·ed (mī′ě-li-nāt-ed). Having a myelin sheath. SYN medullated (2).

my·e·li·na·tion (mī′ě-li-nā′shŭn). The acquisition, development, or formation of a myelin sheath around a nerve fiber. SYN medullation (2), myelinization, myelinogenesis.

my·e·lin·ic (mī′ě-lin′ik). Relating to myelin.

my·e·lin·i·za·tion (mī′ě-li-nī-zā′shŭn). SYN myelination.

my·e·li·noc·la·sis (mī′ě-li-nok′lă-sis). Destruction of myelin. SEE ALSO demyelination, dysmyelination. [myelin + G. *klasis,* a breaking]

my·e·lin·o·gen·e·sis (mī′ě-lin-ō-jen′ě-sis). SYN myelination. [myelin + G. *genesis,* production]

my·e·li·nol·y·sis (mī′ě-li-nol′i-sis). Dissolution of the myelin sheaths of nerve fibers. [myelin + G. *lysis,* dissolution]

central pontine m., localized loss of myelin within the midbase of the pons; related to malnutrition and often to alcoholism.

my·e·lin·op·a·thy (mī′ě-lin-op′ă- thē). A disorder affecting the myelin of peripheral nerve fibers, in contrast to one affecting axons (axonopathy).

my·e·lit·ic (mī-ě-lit′ik). Relating to or affected by myelitis.

my·e·li·tis (mī-ě-lī′tis). **1.** Inflammation of the spinal cord. **2.** Inflammation of the bone marrow. [myel- + G. *-itis,* inflammation]

acute necrotizing m., a spinal cord disorder, probably a demyelinating disease, which affects persons of all ages and either sex. Presents with abrupt or more gradual onset with sensory abnormalities and upper motor neuron weakness; soon a reflexic flaccid motor paralysis and sphincter paralysis supervenes, which is permanent. In some, but not all cases, bilateral or unilateral optic neuritis is associated. In the cerebrospinal fluid, the protein is increased, and mononuclear cells are present. After autopsy, the lesion has been identified as a necrotizing hemorrhagic leukomyelitis.

acute transverse m., acute inflammation and softening of the spinal cord; involves the entire thickness of the spinal cord but of limited longitudinal extent; multiple etiologies.

ascending m., progressive inflammation involving successively higher areas of the spinal cord.

bulbar m., inflammation of the medulla oblongata.

concussion m., traumatic myelopathy.

demyelinated m., acute multiple sclerosis presenting as a myelitis.

Foix-Alajouanine m., SYN subacute necrotizing m.

funicular m., (1) inflammation involving any of the columns of the spinal cord; (2) SYN subacute combined *degeneration* of the spinal cord.

postinfectious m., spinal cord inflammation that follows a viral infection, usually one of the exanthemas.

postvaccinal m., spinal cord inflammation that follows vaccination.

radiation m., SYN radiation *myelopathy.*

subacute necrotizing m., a disorder of the lower spinal cord in adult males resulting in progressive paraplegia. SYN angiodysgenetic myelomalacia, Foix-Alajouanine m.

systemic m., inflammation confined to special tracts of the spinal cord.

transverse m., an inflammatory process involving both gray and white matter of spinal cord.

△**myelo-.** SEE myel-.

my·e·lo·ar·chi·tec·ton·ics (mī′ě-lō-ar′ki-tek-ton′iks). The pattern of myelinated nerve fibers in the brain, as distinguished from cytoarchitectonics.

my·e·lo·blast (mī′ě-lō-blast). An immature cell (10 to 18 μm in diameter) in the granulocytic series, occurring normally in bone marrow, but not in the circulating blood (except in certain diseases). When stained with the usual dyes, the cytoplasm is light blue, nongranular, and variable in amount, sometimes being only a thin rim around the nucleus; the latter is deep purple-blue with finely divided, punctate, threadlike chromatin that is somewhat condensed at the periphery. A few light blue nucleoli are usually present in the nucleus, and these generally disappear as the m. matures into a promyelocyte and then a myelocyte. M.'s ordinarily yield a negative reaction with peroxidase. [myelo- + G. *blastos,* germ]

my·e·lo·blas·te·mia (mī′ě-lō-blas-tē′mē-ă). The presence of myeloblasts in the circulating blood. [myeloblast + G. *haima,* blood]

my·e·lo·blas·to·ma (mī′ě-lō-blas-tō′mă). A nodular focus or fairly well-circumscribed accumulation of myeloblasts, as sometimes observed in acute myeloblastic leukemia and chlorosis. [myeloblast + G. *-oma,* tumor]

my·e·lo·blas·to·sis (mī′ě-lō-blas-tō′sis). The presence of unusually large numbers of myeloblasts in the circulating blood, or tissues, or both (as in acute leukemia).

avian m., fowl m., disease caused by the avian leukosis-sarcoma virus, which belongs to the family Retroviridae, characterized by progressive anemia, enormous numbers of myeloblasts in the blood, weakness, and death.

my·e·lo·cele (mī′ě-lō-sēl). **1.** Protrusion of the spinal cord in spina bifida. [myelo- + G. *kēlē,* hernia] **2.** The central canal of the spinal cord. [G. *myelos,* marrow, + *koilia,* a hollow]

my·e·lo·cyst (mī′ě-lō-sist). Any cyst (usually lined with columnar or cuboidal cells) that develops from a rudimentary medullary canal in the central nervous system. [myelo- + G. *kystis,* bladder]

my·e·lo·cyst·ic (mī′ě-lō-sist′ik). Pertaining to or characterized by the presence of a myelocyst.

my·e·lo·cys·to·cele (mī′ě-lō-sis′tō-sēl). Spina bifida containing spinal cord substance. [myelo- + G. *kystis,* bladder, + *kēlē,* tumor]

my·e·lo·cys·to·me·ning·o·cele (mī′ě-lō-sis′tō-mě-ning′gō-sēl). SYN meningomyelocele. [myelo- + G. *kystis,* bladder, + *mēninx* (*mēning-*), membrane, + *kēlē,* hernia]

Pertaining to, derived from, or manifesting the features of diseased bone marrow.

my·en·ter·ic (mī-en-ter'ik). Relating to the myenteron.

my·en·ter·on (mī-en'ter-on). The muscular coat, or muscularis, of the intestine. [G. *mys*, muscle, + *enteron*, intestine]

my·es·the·sia (mī-es-thē'zē-ă). The sensation felt in muscle when it is contracting; awareness of movement or activity in muscles or joints; sense of position or movement mediated in large part by the posterior columns and medial lemniscus. SEE ALSO bathyesthesia. SYN deep sensibility, kinesthetic sense, mesoblastic sensibility, muscular sense, myoesthesis, myoesthesia. [G. *mys*, muscle, + *aisthēsis*, sensation]

my·i·a·sis (mī-ī'ă-sis). Any infection due to invasion of tissues or cavities of the body by larvae of dipterous insects. [G. *myia*, a fly]

African furuncular m., SYN cordylobiasis.

aural m., invasion of the external, middle, or inner ear by larvae of dipterous insects.

creeping m., m. causing suppurating cutaneous sinuses which may be mistaken for the creeping eruption of cutaneous larva migrans.

cutaneous m., invasion of the skin of sheep by larvae of blowflies. SYN blowfly strike.

human botfly m., SYN dermatobiasis.

intestinal m., presence of larvae of certain dipterous insects in the gastrointestinal tract, as of *Musca domestica* (domestic housefly), the cheese mite, and *Fannia canicularis* (lesser housefly).

nasal m., fly larva invasion of the nasal passages, due most commonly in the U.S. to primary screw-worms, the larvae of *Cochliomyia hominivorax*, which develop in the nasal or aural cavity.

ocular m., invasion of the conjunctival sac or eyeball by larvae of flies, *e.g., Hypoderma bovis, H. lineata, Sarcophaga,* or *Gasterophilus intestinalis.* SYN ophthalmomyiasis.

m. oestruo'sa, m. due to a species of the family Oestridae, the gadflies or botflies.

subcutaneous m., invasion of subcutaneous tissues by the larvae of dipterous insects.

tumbu dermal m., SYN cordylobiasis.

wound m., traumatic m., the infestation of a surface wound or other open lesion by fly larvae.

my·i·tis (mī-ī'tis). SYN myositis. [G. *mys*, muscle, + *-itis*, inflammation]

my·kol (mī'kol). SYN mycolic acids.

myl·a·bris (mil'ă-bris). The dried beetle, *Mylabris phalerata;* a vesicant similar to cantharis. [G. a cockroach found in mills and bakehouses, fr. *mylē*, mill]

my·lo·hy·oid (mī'lō-hī'oyd). Relating to the molar teeth, or posterior portion of the lower jaw, and to the hyoid bone; denoting various structures. SEE nerve, muscle, region, sulcus. [G. *mylē*, a mill, in pl. *mylai*, molar teeth]

my·lo·hy·oi·de·us (mī-lō-hī-oy'dē-ŭs). SYN mylohyoid *muscle.*

myo-. Muscle. [G. *mys*, muscle]

my·o·aden·y·late de·am·i·nase (mī'ō-a-den-il-āt). Muscle AMP deaminase. SEE AMP deaminase.

my·o·al·bu·min (mī'ō-al-byū'min). Albumin in muscle tissue, possibly the same as serum albumin.

my·o·ar·chi·tec·ton·ic (mī'ō-ar'ki-tek-ton'ik). Relating to the structural arrangement of muscle or of fibers in general. [myo- + G. *architektonikos*, relating to construction]

my·o·at·ro·phy (mī-ō-at'rō-fē). SYN muscular *atrophy.*

my·o·blast (mī'ō-blast). A primitive muscle cell with the potentiality of developing into a muscle fiber. SYN sarcoblast, sarcogenic cell. [myo- + G. *blastos*, germ]

my·o·blas·tic (mī-ō-blas'tik). Relating to a myoblast or to the mode of formation of muscle cells.

my·o·blas·to·ma (mī'ō-blas-tō'mă). A tumor of immature muscle cells. [myo- + G. *blastos*, germ, + *-oma*, tumor]

granular cell m., obsolete term for granular cell *tumor.*

my·o·bra·dia (mī-ō-brā'dē-ă). Sluggish reaction of muscle following stimulation. [myo- + G. *bradys*, slow]

my·o·car·dia (mī-ō-kar'dē-ă). Plural of myocardium.

my·o·car·di·al (mī-ō-kar'dē-ăl). Relating to the myocardium.

my·o·car·di·o·graph (mī'ō-kar'dē-ō-graf). An instrument composed of a tambour with recording lever attachment, by means of which a tracing is made of the movements of the heart muscle. [myo- + G. *kardia*, heart, + *graphō*, to record]

my·o·car·di·op·a·thy (mī'ō-kar-dē-op'ă-thē). SYN cardiomyopathy. [myocardium + G. *pathos*, suffering]

alcoholic m., SYN alcoholic *cardiomyopathy.*

chagasic m. (chă'gă-sik), heart muscle disease due to Chagas' disease (caused by *Trypanosoma cruzi*) in which right bundle branch block is common.

my·o·car·di·or·rha·phy (mī'ō-kar-dē-ōr'ă-fē). Suture of the myocardium. [myocardium + G. *rhaphē*, suture]

my·o·car·di·tic (mī-ō-kar'dī-ik). Related to myocarditis (adjective).

my·o·car·di·tis (mī'ō-kar-dī'tis). Inflammation of the muscular walls of the heart.

acute isolated m., an acute interstitial m. of unknown cause, the endocardium and pericardium being unaffected. SYN Fiedler's m.

Fiedler's m., SYN acute isolated m.

fragmentation m., fragmentation of the myocardium as the result of inflammation.

giant cell m., acute isolated m. characterized by infiltration by granulomas containing giant cells.

idiopathic m., inflammation of the heart muscle of unknown origin.

indurative m., chronic m. leading to hardening of the muscular wall of the heart.

toxic m., inflammation of heart muscle caused by any noxious chemical, *e.g.,* alcohol, heavy metals.

my·o·car·di·um, pl. **my·o·car·dia** (mī-ō-kar'dē-ŭm, -kar'dē-ă) [NA]. The middle layer of the heart, consisting of cardiac muscle. [myo- + G. *kardia*, heart]

hibernating m., ventricular dysfunction following months or years of ischemia that is reversible when blood flow is restored. Must be carefully distinguished from dysfunction due to necrotic or scarred m.

stunned m., impaired myocardial contractile performance following a brief period of ischemia and ultimately reversible.

my·o·car·do·sis (mī-ō-kar-dō'sis). Obsolete term for a condition marked by symptomatic signs of cardiac trouble without any discoverable pathologic lesion and for any degenerative condition of the heart muscle except myofibrosis.

my·o·cele (mī'ō-sēl). **1.** Protrusion of muscle substance through a rent in its sheath. [myo- + G. *kēlē*, hernia] **2.** The small cavity that appears in somites. SYN somite cavity. [myo- + G. *koilia*, a cavity]

my·o·ce·li·al·gia (mī'ō-sē-lē-al'jē-ă). Obsolete term for celiomyalgia. [myo- + G. *koilia*, the belly, + *algos*, pain]

my·o·ce·li·tis (mī'ō-sē-lī'tis). Inflammation of the abdominal muscles. [myo- + G. *koilia*, belly, + *-itis*, inflammation]

my·o·cel·lu·li·tis (mī'ō-sel-yū-lī'tis). Inflammation of muscle and cellular tissue. [myo- + Mod. L. *cellularis*, cellular (tissue), + G. *-itis*, inflammation]

my·o·ce·ro·sis (mī'ō-sē-rō'sis). Waxy degeneration of the muscles. SYN myokerosis. [myo- + G. *kēros*, wax]

my·o·chrome (mī'ō-krōm). Rarely used term for cytochrome found in muscle tissue.

my·o·chron·o·scope (mī-ō-kron'ō-skōp). An instrument for timing a muscular impulse, *i.e.,* the interval between the application of the stimulus and the muscular movement in response. [myo- + G. *chronos*, time, + *skopeō*, to examine]

my·o·cin·e·sim·e·ter (mī'ō-sin-ĕ-sim'ĕ-ter). SYN myokinesimeter.

my

my·o·clo·nia (mī′ō-klō′nē-ă). Any disorder characterized by myoclonus. [myo- + G. *klonos,* a tumult]

fibrillary m., the twitching of a limited part or group of fibers of a muscle. SYN tetanilla (1).

my·o·clon·ic (mī-ō-klon′ik). Showing myoclonus.

my·oc·lo·nus (mī-ok′lō-nŭs, mī-ō-klo′nŭs). One or a series of shock-like contractions of a group of muscles, of variable regularity, synchrony, and symmetry, generally due to a central nervous system lesion. [myo- + G. *klonos,* tumult]

m. mul′tiplex, an ill-defined disorder marked by rapid and widespread muscle contractions. SYN paramyoclonus multiplex, polyclonia, polymyoclonus.

nocturnal m., frequently repeated muscular jerks occurring at the moment of dropping off to sleep.

palatal m., rhythmic contractions of the soft palate, the facial muscles, and the diaphragm, related to lesions of the olivocerebellar pathways. SEE ALSO palatal *nystagmus.*

stimulus sensitive m., m. induced by a variety of stimuli, *e.g.,* talking, calculation, loud noises, tapping, etc.

my·o·col·pi·tis (mī-ō-kol-pī′tis). Inflammation of the muscular tissue of the vagina. [myo- + G. *kolpos,* bosom (vagina), + *-itis,* inflammation]

my·o·com·ma, pl. **my·o·com·ma·ta** (mī-ō-kom′ă, -kom′ă-tă). The connective tissue septum separating adjacent myotomes. SYN myoseptum. [myo- + G. *komma,* a coin or the stamp of a coin]

my·o·cris·mus (mī-ō-kris′mŭs). A creaking sound sometimes heard on auscultation of a contracting muscle. [myo- + G. *krizō,* to squeak]

my·o·cu·ta·ne·ous (mī-ō-kyū-tā′nē-ŭs). SYN musculocutaneous. [myo- + L. *cutis,* skin]

my·o·cyte (mī′ō-sīt). A muscle cell. [myo- + G. *kytos,* cell]

Anitschkow m., SYN cardiac *histiocyte.*

my·o·cy·tol·y·sis (mī-ō-sī-tol′i-sis). Dissolution of muscle fiber. [myo- + G. *kytos,* cell, + *lysis,* a loosening]

m. of heart, local loss of myocardial syncytium as a result of a metabolic imbalance, insufficient in intensity or duration (or both) to cause stromal injury or to elicit any reactive exudation.

my·o·cy·to·ma (mī′ō-sī-tō′mă). A benign neoplasm derived from muscle.

my·o·de·gen·er·a·tion (mī′ō-dē-jen-ĕ-rā′shŭn). Muscular degeneration.

my·o·de·mia (mī-ō-dē′mē-ă). Fatty degeneration of muscle. [myo- + G. *dēmos,* tallow]

my·o·der·mal (mī-ō-der′mal). SYN musculocutaneous. [myo- + G. *derma,* skin]

my·o·di·as·ta·sis (mī′ō-dī-as′tă-sis). Separation of muscle. [myo- + G. *diastasis,* separation]

my·o·dy·na·mia (mī′ō-dī-nā′mē-ă). Muscular strength. [myo- + G. *dynamis,* power]

my·o·dy·nam·ics (mī′ō-dī-nam′iks). The dynamics of muscular action.

my·o·dy·na·mom·e·ter (mī′ō-dī-nă-mom′ĕ-ter). An instrument for determining muscular strength. [myo- + G. *dynamis,* force, + *metron,* measure]

my·o·dyn·ia (mī′ō-din′ē-ă). SYN myalgia. [myo- + G. *odynē,* pain]

my·o·dys·to·ny (mī-ō-dis′tō-nē). A condition of slow relaxation, interrupted by a succession of slight contractions, following electrical stimulation of a muscle. [myo- + G. *dys-,* difficult, + *tonos,* tone, tension]

my·o·dys·tro·phy, my·o·dys·tro·phia (mī-ō-dis′trō-fē, mī′-ō-dis-trō′fē-ă). SYN muscular *dystrophy.* [myo- + G. *dys-,* difficult, poor, + *trophē,* nourishment]

my·o·e·de·ma (mī′ō-e-dē′mă). A localized contraction of a degenerating muscle, occurring at the point of a sharp blow, independent of the nerve supply. SYN idiomuscular contraction, mounding, myoidema. [myo- + G. *oidēma,* swelling]

my·o·e·las·tic (mī′ō-e-las′tik). Pertaining to closely associated smooth muscle fibers and elastic connective tissue.

my·o·e·lec·tric (mī′ō-ē-lek′trik). Relating to the electrical properties of muscle.

my·o·en·do·car·di·tis (mī-ō-en′dō-kar-dī′tis). Inflammation of the muscular wall and lining membrane of the heart. [myo- + G. *endon,* within, + *kardia,* heart, + *-itis,* inflammation]

my·o·ep·i·the·li·al (mī′ō-ep-i-thē′lē-ăl). Relating to myoepithelium.

my·o·ep·i·the·li·o·ma (mī′ō-ep-i-thē-lē-ō′mă). A benign tumor of myoepithelial cells. [myo- + epithelium, + G. *-ōma,* tumor]

my·o·ep·i·the·li·um (mī′ō-ep-i-thē′lē-ŭm). Spindle-shaped, contractile, smooth muscle-like cells of epithelial origin that are arranged longitudinally or obliquely around sweat glands and the secretory alveoli of the mammary gland; stellate myoepithelial cells occur around lacrimal and some salivary gland secretory units. SYN muscle epithelium. [myo- + epithelium]

my·o·es·the·sis, my·o·es·the·sia (mī′ō-es-thē′sis, -thē′zē-ă). SYN myesthesia.

my·o·fas·ci·al (mī′ō-fash′ē-ăl). Of or relating to the fascia surrounding and separating muscle tissue.

my·o·fas·ci·tis (mī′ō-fă-sī′tis). SYN *myositis* fibrosa.

my·o·fi·bril (mī-ō-fī′bril). One of the fine longitudinal fibrils occurring in a skeletal or cardiac muscle fiber comprising many regularly overlapped ultramicroscopic thick and thin myofilaments. SYN muscular fibril, myofibrilla. [myo- + Mod. L. *fibrilla,* fibril]

my·o·fi·bril·la, pl. **my·o·fi·bril·lae** (mī′ō-fī-bril′ă, -bril′ē). SYN myofibril.

my·o·fib·ril·lar (mī-ō-fī-bril-ar). Pertaining or relating to myofibril.

my·o·fi·bro·blast (mī-ō-fī′brō-blast). A cell thought to be responsible for contracture of wounds; such cells have some characteristics of smooth muscle, such as contractile properties and fibrils, and are also believed to produce, temporarily, type III collagen.

my·o·fi·bro·ma (mī′ō-fī-brō′mă). A benign neoplasm that consists chiefly of fibrous connective tissue, with variable numbers of muscle cells forming portions of the neoplasm.

my·o·fi·bro·ma·to·sis (mī′-yō-fī-brō-ma- tō′sis). Solitary or multiple tumors of muscle and fibrous tissue, or tumors composed by myofibroblasts. [myo- + L. *fibra,* fiber, + G. suffix, *-ōma,* tumor, + suffix *-osis,* condition]

infantile myofibromatosis, myofibromatosis seen at birth or in infants, with multiple lytic bone lesions and involving soft tissue, or with visceral involvement.

my·o·fi·bro·sis (mī′ō-fī-brō′sis). Chronic myositis with diffuse hyperplasia of the interstitial connective tissue pressing upon and causing atrophy of the muscular tissue.

m. cor′dis, m. of the heart walls.

my·o·fi·bro·si·tis (mī′ō-fī-brō-sī′tis). Inflammation of the perimysium.

my·o·fil·a·ments (mī-ō-fil′ă-ments). The ultramicroscopic threads of filamentous proteins making up myofibrils in striated muscle. Thick ones contain myosin and thin ones actin; thick and thin m.'s also occur in smooth muscle fibers but are not regularly arranged in discrete myofibrils and thus do not impart a striated appearance to these cells.

my·o·func·tion·al (mī′ō-fŭnk′shŭn-ăl). 1. Relating to function of muscles. 2. In dentistry, relating to the role of muscle function in the etiology or correction of orthodontic problems.

my·o·gen (mī′ō-jen). Proteins extracted from muscle with cold water, largely the enzymes promoting glycolysis; from the residue, alkaline 0.6 M KCl extracts actin and myosin as actomyosin, with myosin further separable into two meromyosins by protein-ase treatment. SYN myosinogen. [myo- + G. *-gen,* producing]

my·o·gen·e·sis (mī-ō-jen′ĕ-sis). Embryonic formation of muscle cells or fibers. [myo- + G. *genesis,* origin]

my·o·ge·net·ic, my·o·gen·ic (mī-ō-jĕ-net′ik, -jen′ik). 1. Originating in or starting from muscle. 2. Relating to the origin of muscle cells or fibers. SYN myogenous.

my·og·e·nous (mī-oj′ĕ-nŭs). SYN myogenetic.

my·o·glo·bin (Mb, MbCO, MbO₂) (mī-ō-glō′bin). The oxygen-transporting and storage protein of muscle, resembling blood hemoglobin in function but containing only one subunit and one heme as part of the molecule (rather than the four of hemoglobin), and with a molecular weight approximately one-quarter that of hemoglobin. SYN muscle hemoglobin, myohemoglobin. [myo- + hemoglobin]

my·o·glo·bi·nu·ria (mī′ō-glō-bi-nū′rē-ă). Excretion of myoglobin in the urine; results from muscle degeneration, which releases myoglobin into the blood; occurs in certain types of trauma (crush syndrome), advanced or protracted ischemia of muscle, or as a paroxysmal process of unknown etiology. SYN idiopathic paroxysmal rhabdomyolysis, Meyer-Betz disease, Meyer-Betz syndrome.

paralytic m., SYN *azoturia* of horses.

my·o·glob·u·lin (mī-ō-glob′yū-lin). Globulin present in muscle tissue.

my·o·glob·u·li·nu·ria (mī′ō-glob′yū-li-nū′rē-ă). The excretion of myoglobulin in the urine.

my·og·na·thus (mī-og′nă-thŭs, mī-ō-nāth′ŭs). An unequal conjoined twin in which the rudimentary head of the parasite is attached to the lower jaw of the autosite by muscle and skin only. SEE conjoined *twins,* under *twin.* [myo- + G. *gnathos,* jaw]

my·o·gram (mī′ō-gram). The tracing made by a myograph. SYN muscle curve. [myo- + G. *gramma,* a drawing]

my·o·graph (mī′ō-graf). A recording instrument by which tracings are made of muscular contractions. [myo- + G. *graphō,* to write]

palate m., SYN palatograph.

my·o·graph·ic (mī-ō-graf′ik). Relating to a myogram, or the record of a myograph.

my·og·ra·phy (mī-og′ră-fē). **1.** The recording of muscular movements by the myograph. **2.** A description of or treatise on the muscles. SYN descriptive myology.

my·o·he·mo·glo·bin (mī′ō-hēm-ō-glō′bin). SYN myoglobin.

my·oid (mī′oyd). **1.** Resembling muscle. **2.** One of the fine, contractile, threadlike protoplasmic elements found in certain epithelial cells in lower animals. **3.** A contractile part of retinal cones in certain fish and amphibia. In mammals, the m. is the inner part of the inner segment of rods and cones; it contains microtubules, the Golgi apparatus, endoplasmic reticulum, and ribosomes, but no myofibrils. [myo- + G. *eidos,* appearance]

my·oi·de·ma (mī-oy-dē′mă). SYN myoedema. [myo- + G. *oidēma,* swelling]

my·o·i·no·si·tol (mī-ō-in-o′-si-tōl). SEE *myo*-inositol.

my·o·is·che·mia (mī′ō-is-kē′mē-ă). A condition of localized deficiency or absence of blood supply in muscular tissue.

my·o·ke·ro·sis (mī′ō-kē-rō′sis). SYN myocerosis.

my·o·ki·nase (mī-ō-kī′nās). SYN *adenylate* kinase.

my·o·kin·e·sim·e·ter (mī′ō-kin-ĕ-sim′ĕ-ter). A device for registering the exact time and extent of contraction of the larger muscles of the lower extremity in response to electric stimulation. SYN myocinesimeter. [myo- + G. *kinesis,* movement, + *metron,* measure]

my·o·ky·mia (mī-ō-kī′mē-ă). Continuous involuntary quivering or rippling of muscles at rest, caused by spontaneous, repetitive firing of groups of motor unit potentials. SYN fibrillary chorea, kymatism, Morvan's chorea. [myo- + G. *kyma,* wave]

facial m., m. that appears in the facial muscles, causing narrowing of the palpebral fissure and continuous undulation of the facial skin surface; the latter is referred to as "bag of worms" appearance and is best seen with reflected light; due to intrinsic brainstem lesion, such as a pontine glioma or multiple sclerosis.

generalized m., widespread m., present in multiple limbs and often the face; of various causes, including Isaac's syndrome, uremia, thyrotoxicosis and gold toxicity (gold-m. syndrome).

hereditary m. [MIM*160100], a syndrome consisting of m., hypoglycemia, and disturbed thyroid function.

limb m., m. present in one or more limbs; various causes, one of the more common being prior plexus radiation.

my·o·lem·ma (mī-ō-lem′ă). SYN sarcolemma.

my·o·li·po·ma (mī′ō-li-pō′mă). A benign neoplasm that consists chiefly of fat cells (adipose tissue), with variable numbers of muscle cells forming portions of the neoplasm.

my·o·lo·gia (mī′ō-lō′jē-ă) [NA]. SYN myology, myology.

my·ol·o·gist (mī-ol′ō-jist). One learned in the knowledge of muscles.

my·ol·o·gy (mī-ol′ō-jē). The branch of science concerned with the muscles and their accessory parts, tendons, aponeuroses, bursae, and fasciae. SYN myologia [NA], sarcology (1). [myo- + G. *logos,* study]

descriptive m., SYN myography (2).

my·ol·y·sis (mī-ol′i-sis). Dissolution or liquefaction of muscular tissue, frequently preceded by degenerative changes such as infiltration of fat, atrophy, and fatty degeneration. [myo- + G. *lysis,* dissolution]

cardiotoxic m., cardiomalacia occurring in fever and various systemic infections.

my·o·ma (mī-ō′mă). A benign neoplasm of muscular tissue. SEE ALSO leiomyoma, rhabdomyoma. [myo- + G. *-oma,* tumor]

my·o·ma·la·cia (mī′ō-mă-lā′shē-ă). Pathologic softening of muscular tissue. [myo- + G. *malakia,* softness]

my·o·ma·tous (mī-ō′mă-tŭs). Pertaining to or characterized by the features of a myoma.

my·o·mec·to·my (mī-ō-mek′tō-mē). Operative removal of a myoma, specifically of a uterine myoma. [myoma + G. *ektomē,* excision]

abdominal m., removal of a myoma of the uterus through an abdominal incision. SYN celiomyomectomy, laparomyomectomy.

left ventricular m., resection of myocardial tissue used in cases of idiopathic hypertrophic subaortic stenosis.

vaginal m., removal of a myoma of the uterus through the vagina. SYN colpomyomectomy.

my·o·mel·a·no·sis (mī′ō-melă-nō′sis). Abnormal dark pigmentation of muscular tissue. SEE ALSO melanosis. [myo- + G. *melanōsis,* becoming black]

my·o·mere (mī′ō-mēr). SYN myotome (4). [myo- + G. *meros,* a part]

my·om·e·ter (mī-om′ĕ-ter). An instrument for measuring the extent of a muscular contraction. [myo- + G. *metron,* measure]

my·o·me·tri·al (mī-ō-mē′trē-ăl). Relating to the myometrium.

my·o·me·tri·tis (mī′ō-mē-trī′tis). Inflammation of the muscular wall of the uterus. SYN mesometritis. [myo- + G. *mētra,* uterus, + *-itis,* inflammation]

my·o·me·tri·um (mī′ō-mē′trē-ŭm) [NA]. The muscular wall of the uterus. SYN tunica muscularis uteri [NA], muscular coat of uterus. [myo- + G. *mētra,* uterus]

my·o·mi·to·chon·dri·on, pl. **my·o·mi·to·chon·dria** (mī′ō-mī′tō-kon′drē-on, -drē-ă). A mitochondrion of a muscle fiber.

my·o·mot·o·my (mī-ō-mot′ō-mē). Incision of a myoma. [myoma + G. *tomē,* incision]

my·on (mī′on). An individual muscle unit. [G. *mys,* muscle]

my·o·ne·cro·sis (mī′ō-nĕ-krō′sis). Necrosis of muscle.

clostridial m., SYN gas *gangrene.*

my·o·neme (mī′ō-nēm). **1.** A muscle fibril. **2.** One of the contractile fibrils of certain protozoans; thought to function in an analogous fashion to metazoan muscle fibers. [myo- + G. *nēma,* thread]

my·o·neu·ral (mī-ō-nū′răl). Relating to both muscle and nerve; denoting specifically the synapse of the motor neuron with striated muscle fibers: myoneural junction or motor endplate. SEE ALSO neuromuscular. [myo- + G. *neuron,* nerve]

my·o·neu·ral·gia (mī′ō-nū-ral′jē-ă). SYN myalgia. [myo- + G. *neuron,* nerve, + *algos,* pain]

postural m., muscle pain associated with cramped position, stress of standing with improper posture, etc.

my·o·neu·ras·the·nia (mī′ō-nū-ras-thē′nē-ă). Obsolete term for muscular weakness associated with neurasthenia.

my·o·neu·ro·ma (mī′ō-nū-rō′mă). A tumefaction consisting chiefly of abnormally proliferating Schwann cells, with variable numbers of muscle cells forming portions of the mass; m.'s are probably malformations, rather than true neoplasms. [myo- + G. *neuron,* nerve, + *-oma,* tumor]

my

my·on·o·sus (mī-on'ŏ-sŭs). SYN myopathy. [myo- + G. *nosos,* disease]

my·on·y·my (mī-on'i-mē). Nomenclature of the muscles. [myo- + G. *onyma* or *onoma,* name]

my·o·pa·chyn·sis (mī'ō-pă-kin'sis). Muscular hypertrophy. [myo- + G. *pachynsis,* a thickening]

my·o·pal·mus (mī-ō-pal'mŭs). Muscle twitching. [myo- + G. *palmos,* a quivering]

my·o·pa·ral·y·sis (mī-ō-pă-ral'i-sis). Muscular paralysis.

my·o·pa·re·sis (mī'ō-pă-rē'sis, -par'ē-sis). Slight muscular paralysis.

my·o·path·ic (mī-ō-path'ik). Denoting a disorder involving muscular tissue.

my·op·a·thy (mī-op'ă-thē). Any abnormal condition or disease of the muscular tissues; commonly designates a disorder involving skeletal muscle. SYN myonosus. [myo- + G. *pathos,* suffering]

carcinomatous m., SYN Lambert-Eaton *syndrome.*

centronuclear m., slowly progressive generalized muscle weakness and atrophy beginning in childhood; on biopsy of skeletal muscle, the nuclei of most muscle fibers are seen to be located near the center of a small fiber (the normal position for a 10-week embryo) rather than at the periphery of the fiber; familial incidence. Autosomal dominant [MIM*160150] recessive [MIM*255200] and X-linked [310400] forms occur. SYN myotubular m.

distal m., m. affecting predominantly the distal portions of the limbs; onset is usually after age 40, with weakness and wasting of small muscles of the hands; The infantile form [MIM*160300] and the Swedish later-onset [MIM*160500] are autosomal dominant and there is a Japanese late-onset type [MIM*254130] that is recessive.

minicore-multicore m., an uncommon nonprogressive m. with early onset, proximal weakness, and hypotonia. Muscle fibers show focal defects of oxidative and myofibrillar adenosine triphosphatase enzymes with disorganization of myofibril ultrastructure.

mitochondrial m., weakness and hypotonia of muscles, primarily those of the neck, shoulder, and pelvic girdles, with onset in infancy or childhood; on biopsy, giant, bizarre mitochondria are seen located between muscle fibrils just beneath the sarcolemma. The dominant form is due to deletion of mitochondrial DNA [MIM*160560] and the recessive form [MIM*252010] is due to a complex deficiency.

myotubular m., SYN centronuclear m.

nemaline m., congenital, nonprogressive muscle weakness most evident in the proximal muscles; named after the characteristic nemaline (threadlike) rods seen in the muscle cells composed of Z-band material. There are two forms, dominant [MIM*161800] and recessive [MIM*256030], that are clinically indistinguishable. SYN rod m.

ocular m., SYN chronic progressive external *ophthalmoplegia.*

rod m., SYN nemaline m.

thyrotoxic m., extreme muscular weakness in severe thyrotoxicosis affecting muscles of limbs and trunk as well as those used in speech and swallowing.

my·o·per·i·car·di·tis (mī'ō-per-i-kar-dī'tis). Inflammation of the muscular wall of the heart and of the enveloping pericardium; also, perimyocarditis--choice of term determined by whether the principal involvement is pericardial or myocardial. [myo- + pericarditis]

my·o·per·i·to·ni·tis (mī'ō-per-i-tō-nī'tis). Inflammation of the parietal peritoneum with myositis of the abdominal wall.

my·o·phone (mī'ō-fōn). An instrument to enable one to hear the murmur of muscular contractions. [myo- + G. *phōnē,* sound]

my·o·phos·phor·y·lase (mī-ō-fus-fōr'i-lās). Muscle phosphorylase

my·o·pia (M) (mī-ō'pē-ă). That optical condition in which only rays from a finite distance from the eye focus on the retina. SYN near sight, nearsightedness, short sight, shortsightedness. [G. fr. *myo,* to shut, + *ōps,* eye]

axial m., m. due to elongation of the globe of the eye.

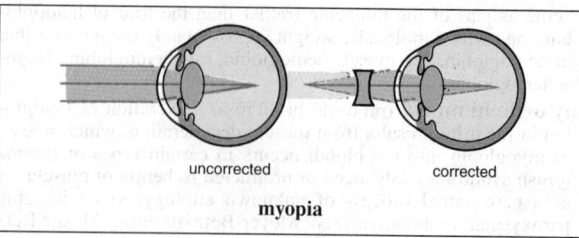

uncorrected   corrected

myopia

curvature m., m. due to refractive errors resulting from excessive corneal curvature.

degenerative m., SYN pathologic m.

index m., m. arising from increased refractivity of the lens, as in nuclear sclerosis.

malignant m., SYN pathologic m.

night m., in dark adaptation the eye becomes more sensitive to shorter wave lengths (Purkinje shift), and visual acuity depends on parafoveal blue cones. Shorter wavelengths come into focus in front of the retina, and this chromatic aberration accounts for some of the relative m. that a normal eye experiences at night; much of the remainder is due to an increase in accommodative tone in the dark.

pathologic m., progressive m. marked by fundus changes, posterior staphyloma, and subnormal corrected acuity. SYN degenerative m., malignant m.

prematurity m., m. observed in infants of low birth weight or in association with retrolental fibroplasia.

senile lenticular m., SYN second *sight.*

simple m., m. arising from failure of correlation of the refractive power of the anterior segment and the length of the eyeball.

space m., a type of m. arising when no contour is imaged on the retina.

transient m., m. observed in accommodative spasm secondary to iridocyclitis or ocular contusion.

my·o·pic (M) (mī-op'ik, -ō'pik). Relating to or suffering from myopia.

my·o·plasm (mī'ō-plazm). The contractile portion of the muscle cell, as distinguished from the sarcoplasm. [myo- + G. *plasma,* a thing formed]

my·o·plas·tic (mī-ō-plas'tik). Relating to the plastic surgery of the muscles, or to the use of muscular tissue in correcting defects.

my·o·plas·ty (mī'ō-plas-tē). Plastic surgery of muscular tissue. [myo- + G. *plastos,* formed]

my·o·po·lar (mī-ō-pō'lăr). Relating to muscular polarity, or to the portion of muscle between two electrodes.

my·o·pro·tein (mī-ō-prō'tēn). Protein occurring in muscle.

my·o·rhyth·mia (mī'ō-ridh'mē-ă). A form of hyperkinesia in which the tremor rate (2 to 4 per second) is irregular and slower than in alternating tremor, with greater frequency and higher voltage of the associated spike potentials in the electromyogram. [myo- + G. *rhythmos,* rhythm]

my·or·rha·phy (mī-ōr'ă-fē). Suture of a muscle. [myo- + G. *rhaphē,* seam]

my·or·rhex·is (mī-ō-rek'sis). Tearing of a muscle. [myo- + G. *rhēxis,* a rupture]

my·o·sal·gia (mī-ō-sal'jē-ă). SYN myalgia.

my·o·sal·pin·gi·tis (mī'ō-sal-pin-jī'tis). Inflammation of the muscular tissue of the uterine tube. [myosalpinx + G. *-itis* inflammation]

my·o·sal·pinx (mī'ō-sal'pingks). The muscular tunic of the uterine tube. [myo- + salpinx]

my·o·sar·co·ma (mī'ō-sar-kō'mă). A general term for a malignant neoplasm derived from muscular tissue. SEE ALSO leiomyosarcoma, rhabdomyosarcoma.

my·o·scle·ro·sis (mī'ō-skle-rō'sis). Chronic myositis with hyperplasia of the interstitial connective tissue.

my·o·seism (mī'ō-sīzm). Nonrhythmic spasmodic muscular contractions. [myo- + G. *seismos*, a shaking, shock, fr. *seiō*, fut. *seisō*, to shake]

my·o·sep·tum (mī-ō-sep'tŭm). SYN myocomma. [myo- + L. *saeptum*, a barrier]

my·o·sin (mī'ō-sin). A globulin present in muscle; in combination with actin, it forms actomyosin; m. forms the thick filaments in muscle.

m. light chain kinase, a calcium/calmodulin-dependent enzyme that phosphorylates the p-light chains of smooth muscle m. and initiates contraction.

my·o·sin·o·gen (mī-ō-sin'ō-jen). SYN myogen.

my·o·si·nose (mī'ō-si-nōs). A proteose formed by the partial hydrolysis of myosin.

my·o·sis (mī-ō'sis). Obsolete alternative spelling for miosis (2).

my·o·sit·ic (mī-ō-sit'ik). Relating to myositis.

my·o·si·tis (mī-ō-sī'tis). Inflammation of a muscle. SYN initis (2), myitis. [myo- + G. *-itis,* inflammation]

acute disseminated m., SYN multiple m.

cervical m., SEE posttraumatic neck *syndrome*.

epidemic m., m. epidem'ica acu'ta, SYN epidemic *pleurodynia*.

m. fibro'sa, induration of a muscle through an interstitial growth of fibrous tissue. SYN Froriep's induration, interstitial m., myofascitis.

infectious m., inflammation of the voluntary muscles, marked by swelling and pain, affecting usually the shoulders and arms, though almost the entire body may be involved.

interstitial m., SYN m. fibrosa.

multiple m., the occurrence of multiple foci of acute inflammation in the muscular tissue and overlying skin in various parts of the body, accompanied by fever and other signs of systemic infection. SEE ALSO dermatomyositis. SYN acute disseminated m., pseudotrichinosis, pseudotrichiniasis.

m. ossif'icans, ossification or deposit of bone in muscle with fibrosis, causing pain and swelling in muscles.

m. ossif'icans circumscrip'ta, local deposit of bone in a muscle, usually following prolonged trauma; *e.g.,* riders' bone.

m. ossif'icans progressi'va, a rare and frequently fatal mutation, beginning in early life, characterized by progressive ossification of the muscles; it is not strictly a m., but a noninflammatory ossification.

proliferative m., a rapidly growing benign infiltrating fibrous nodule in skeletal muscle, containing characteristic giant cells resembling ganglion cells.

m. purulen'ta trop'ica, a disease observed in Samoa and in tropical Africa, marked by pains in the extremities, fever of a remittent or intermittent type, and abscesses in the muscles in various parts of the body (may result in death from sepsis); causative organisms are *Staphylococcus aureus* and *Streptococcus pyogenes*, but usually the disease is associated with parasitic infections. SYN bungpagga, lambo lambo, tropical m., tropical pyomyositis.

tropical m., SYN m. purulenta tropica.

my·o·spasm, my·o·spas·mus (mī'ō-spazm, mī-ō-spaz'mŭs). Spasmodic muscular contraction.

cervical m., SEE posttraumatic neck *syndrome*.

my·o·spher·u·lo·sis (mī'ō-sfēr-ū-lō'sis). A chronic granulomatous reaction to undetermined spherical structures frequently contained within a microscopic cyst; first reported in cystic lesions in skeletal muscle from eastern Africa and subsequently in nasal infections in the U.S. [myo- + L. *sphaerula,* small sphere, + G. *-osis,* condition]

my·o·sthe·nom·e·ter (mī'ō-sthě-nom'ě-ter). An instrument for measuring the power of muscle groups. [myo- + G. *sthenos,* strength, + *metron,* measure]

my·o·stro·ma (mī-ō-strō'mă). The supporting connective tissue or framework of muscular tissue. [myo- + G. *strōma,* mattress]

my·o·stro·min (mī-ō-strō'min). A protein found in muscle stroma.

my·o·tac·tic (mī-ō-tak'tik). Relating to the muscular sense. [myo- + L. *tactus,* a touching]

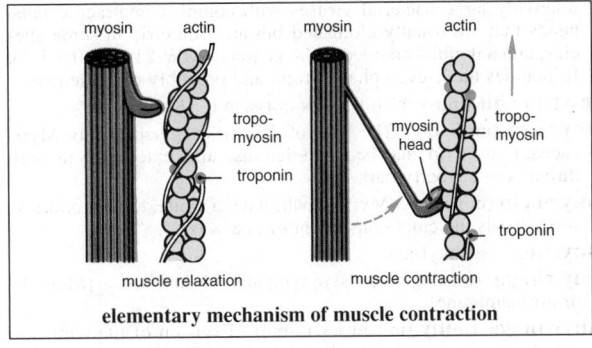

elementary mechanism of muscle contraction

my·ot·a·sis (mī-ot'ă-sis). Stretching of a muscle. [myo- + G. *tasis,* a stretching]

my·o·tat·ic (mī-ō-tat'ik). Relating to myotasis.

my·o·ten·o·si·tis (mī'ō-te-nō-sī'tis). Inflammation of a muscle with its tendon. [myo- + G. *tenōn,* tendon, + *-itis,* inflammation]

my·o·te·not·o·my (mī'ō-te-not'ō-mē). Cutting through the principal tendon of a muscle, with division of the muscle itself in whole or in part. SYN tenomyotomy, tenontomyotomy. [myo- + G. *tenōn,* tendon, + *tomē,* incision]

my·o·ther·mic (mī-ō-ther'mik). Relating to the increased temperature in muscular tissue resulting from its contraction. [myo- + G. *thermē,* heat]

my·o·tome (mī'ō-tōm). **1.** A knife for dividing muscle. **2.** In embryos, that part of the somite that develops into skeletal muscle. SYN muscle plate. **3.** All muscles derived from one somite and innervated by one segmental spinal nerve. **4.** In primitive vertebrates, the muscular part of a metamere. SYN myomere. [myo- + G. *tomos,* a cut]

my·ot·o·my (mī-ot'ō-mē). **1.** Anatomy or dissection of the muscles. **2.** Surgical division of a muscle. [myo- + G. *tomē,* excision]

cricopharyngeal m., division of the cephalad portion of the cricopharyngeus muscle, usually for treatment of Zenker's esophageal diverticulum.

Heller m., SYN esophagomyotomy.

my·o·tone (mī'ō-tōn). SYN myotony.

my·o·to·nia (mī-ō-tō'nē-ă). Delayed relaxation of a muscle after a strong contraction, or prolonged contraction after mechanical stimulation (as by percussion) or brief electrical stimulation; due to abnormality of the muscle membrane, specifically the ion channels. [myo- + G. *tonos,* tension, stretching]

m. acquisi'ta, acquired m. following exposure to certain toxins.

m. atroph'ica, SYN myotonic *dystrophy*.

m. congen'ita [MIM*160800], a hereditary disease marked by momentary tonic spasms occurring when a voluntary movement is attempted. SYN Thomsen's disease.

m. dystroph'ica, SYN myotonic *dystrophy*.

m. neonato'rum, SYN neonatal *tetany*.

my·o·ton·ic (mī-ō-ton'ik). Pertaining to or exhibiting myotonia.

my·ot·o·noid (mī-ot'ō-noyd). Denoting a muscular reaction, naturally or electrically excited, characterized by slow contraction and, especially, slow relaxation. [myo- + G. *tonos,* tone, tension, + *eidos,* resemblance]

my·ot·o·nus (mī-ot'ō-nŭs). A tonic spasm or temporary rigidity of a muscle or group of muscles. [myo- + G. *tonos,* tension, stretching]

my·ot·o·ny (mī-ot'ō-nē). Muscular tonus or tension. SYN myotone. [myo- + G. *tonos,* tension]

my·ot·ro·phy (mī-ot'rō-fē). Nutrition of muscular tissue. [myo- + G. *trophē,* nourishment]

my·o·tube (mī'ō-tūb). A skeletal muscle fiber formed by the fusion of myoblasts during a developmental stage; a few myofibrils occur at the periphery, and the central core is occupied by nuclei and sarcoplasm so that the fiber has a tubular appearance.

my·o·tu·bule (mī-ō-tū'būl). Former term for myotube.

My·o·vir·i·dae (mī-ō-vir'i-dē). Provisional name for a family of

My

relatively large bacterial viruses with complex contractile tails, heads that are usually elongated but are isometric in some species, and a double-stranded DNA genome (MW 21 to 190 × 10⁶). It includes the T-even phage group and probably other genera.

myr·ia·chit (mir-yah'chit). SYN miryachit. [Kalmuk?]

myr·i·ca (mir'i-kă). The bark of *Myrica cerifera* (family Myricaceae); used in diarrhea and icterus, and externally in sore throat. SYN bayberry bark.

myr·i·cin (mir'i-sin). Myricyl palmitate, a white, almost odorless solid that is the chief constituent of beeswax.

⟁**myring-.** SEE myringo-.

my·rin·ga (mi-ring'gă). SYN tympanic *membrane*. [Mod. L. drum membrane]

myr·in·gec·to·my (mir-in-jek'tō-mē). Excision of the tympanic membrane. [myring- + G. *ektomē*, excision]

myr·in·gi·tis (mir-in-jī'tis). Inflammation of the tympanic membrane. SYN tympanitis. [myring- + G. *-itis*, inflammation]
   m. bulbo'sa, SYN myringodermatitis.
   bullous m., painful inflammation of the tympanic membrane accompanied by bullae, probably of viral etiology.

⟁**myringo-, myring-.** The membrana tympani. [Mod. L. *myringa*]

my·rin·go·der·ma·ti·tis (mi-ring'gō-der-mă-tī'tis). Inflammation of the meatal or outer surface of the drum membrane and the adjoining skin of the external auditory canal. SYN myringitis bulbosa.

my·rin·go·my·co·sis (mi-ring'gō-mī-kō'sis). SYN mycomyringitis.

my·rin·go·plas·ty (mi-ring'gō-plas'tē). Operative repair of a damaged tympanic membrane. [myringo- + G. *plassō*, to form]

my·rin·go·sta·pe·di·o·pexy (mi-ring'gō-stā-pē'dē-ō-pek'sē). A technique of tympanoplasty in which the drum membrane or grafted drum membrane is brought into functional connection with the stapes. [myringo- + L. *stapes*, stirrup (stapes), + G. *pēxis*, fixation]

my·rin·go·tome (mi-ring'gō-tōm). A knife used for paracentesis of the tympanic membrane. [myringo- + G. *tomē*, excision]

myr·in·got·o·my (mir-ing-got'ŏ-mē). Paracentesis of the tympanic membrane. SYN tympanostomy, tympanotomy. [myringo- + G. *tomē*, excision]

my·rinx (mī'ringks, mir'ringks). SYN tympanic *membrane*. [Mod. L. *myringa*, drum membrane]

my·ris·ti·ca (mi-ris'ti-kă). SYN nutmeg. [G. *myrizō*, to anoint, fr. *myron*, an unguent]
   m. oil, SYN nutmeg oil.

my·ris·tic ac·id (mi-ris'tik). CH₃–(CH₂)₁₂–COOH; a saturated fatty acid present as an acylglycerol in milk, vegetable fats, cod liver oil, and waxes. SYN tetradecanoic acid.

my·ris·ti·cin (mī-ris'ti-sin). A constituent of nutmeg thought to be responsible, at least in part, for the bizarre central nervous system symptoms produced by the ingestion of large amounts of nutmeg.

my·ris·to·le·ic ac·id (mi-ris-tō-lē'ik). 9-Tetradecenoic acid; a 14-carbon unsaturated fatty acid with a double bond between carbons 9 and 10; the 14-carbon analog of oleic acid.

myr·me·cia (mĭr-mē'shē-ă). A form of viral wart in which the lesion has a domed surface (*i.e.*, an ant hill configuration) and is associated with pale staining intranuclear and amphophilic intracytoplasmic inclusion bodies in the epidermal cells. [G. *murmex*, ant]

my·ro·si·nase (mī-rō'si-nās). SYN thioglucosidase.

myrrh (mer). A gum resin from *Commiphora molmol* and *C. abyssinica* (family Burseraceae) and other species of *C.*, a shrub of Arabia and eastern Africa; used as an astringent, tonic, and stimulant, and locally for diseases of the oral cavity and in mouthwashes. [G. *myrrha*]

my·so·phil·ia (mī-sō-fil'ē-ă). Sexual interest in excretions. [G. *mysos*, defilement, + *philos*, fond]

my·so·pho·bia (mī-sō-fō'bē-ă). Morbid fear of dirt or defilement from touching familiar objects. [G. *mysos*, defilement, + *phobos*, fear]

my·ta·cism (mī'tă-sizm). A form of stammering in which the letter *m* is frequently substituted for other consonants. SYN mutacism. [G. *my*, the letter μ]

my·ur·ous (mī-yū'rŭs). Gradually decreasing, as a mouse's tail, in thickness; rarely used term denoting certain symptoms in process of cessation, or the heartbeat in certain cases in which it grows feebler and feebler for a while and then strengthens. [G. *mys*, mouse, + *ouros*, tail]

myx·a·de·ni'tis (mīks-ă-dē-nī'tis). SEE myxo-.
   m. labialis, SYN *cheilitis* glandularis.

myx·ad·e·no·ma (mik-sad-ĕ-nō'mă). A benign neoplasm derived from glandular epithelial tissue, *i.e.*, an adenoma, in which the loose connective tissue of the stroma resembles relatively primitive mesenchymal tissue.

myx·as·the·nia (mik-sas-thē'nē-ă). Faulty secretion of mucus. [myx- + G. *astheneia*, weakness]

myx·e·de·ma (mik-se-dē'mă). Hypothyroidism characterized by a relatively hard edema of subcutaneous tissue, with increased content of proteoglycans in the fluid; characterized by somnolence, slow mentation, dryness and loss of hair, increased fluid in body cavities such as the pericardial sac, subnormal temperature, hoarseness, muscle weakness, and slow return of a muscle to the neutral position after a tendon jerk; usually caused by removal or loss of functioning thyroid tissue. [myx- + G. *oidēma*, swelling]
   circumscribed m., nodules and plaques of mucoid edema of the skin, usually in the pretibial region, occurring in some patients with hyperthyroidism. SYN pretibial m.
   congenital m., SYN infantile *hypothyroidism*.
   infantile m., SYN infantile *hypothyroidism*.
   operative m., m. developing after thyroidectomy.
   pituitary m., m. resulting from inadequate secretion of the thyrotropic hormone; commonly occurs in association with inadequate secretion of other anterior pituitary hormones.
   pretibial m., SYN circumscribed m.

myx·e·de·ma·toid (mik-sĕ-dem'ă-toyd). Resembling myxedema.

myx·e·dem·a·tous (mik-sĕ-dem'ă-tŭs). Relating to myxedema.

myx·e·mia (mik-sĕ'mē-ă). SYN mucinemia. [myx- + G. *haima*, blood]

⟁**myxo-, myx-.** Mucus. SEE ALSO muci-, muco-. [G. *myxa*, mucus]

myx·o·chon·dro·fi·bro·sar·co·ma (mik'sō-kon'drō-fī'brō-sar-kō'mă). A malignant neoplasm derived from fibrous connective tissue, *i.e.*, a fibrosarcoma, in which there are intimately associated foci of cartilaginous and myxomatous tissue. [myxo- + G. *chondros*, cartilage, + L. *fibra*, fiber, + G. *sarx*, flesh, + *-ōma*, tumor]

myx·o·chon·dro·ma (mik'sō-kon-drō'mă). A benign neoplasm of cartilaginous tissue, *i.e.*, a chondroma, in which the stroma resembles relatively primitive mesenchymal tissue. SYN myxoma enchondromatosum. [myxo- + G. *chondros*, cartilage, + *-ōma*, tumor]

Myx·o·coc·cid·i·um steg·o·my·i·ae (mik'sō-kok-sid'ē-ŭm steg-ō-mī'ē-ē). A protozoon once found in the body of the mosquito, *Stegomyia calopus*, that had fed on the blood of a patient with yellow fever; the organism was then postulated, incorrectly, to be the causal agent of yellow fever.

myx·o·cyte (mik'sō-sīt). One of the stellate or polyhedral cells present in mucous tissue. [myxo- + G. *kytos*, cell]

myx·o·fi·bro·ma (mik'sō-fī-brō'mă). A benign neoplasm of fibrous connective tissue that resembles primitive mesenchymal tissue. SYN fibroma myxomatodes, myxoma fibrosum. [myxo- + L. *fibra*, fiber, + G. *-ōma*, tumor]

myx·o·fi·bro·sar·co·ma (mik'sō-fī'brō-sar-kō'mă). A malignant fibrous histiocytoma with a predominance of myxoid areas that resemble primitive mesenchymal tissue. [myxo- + L. *fibra*, fiber, + G. *sarx*, flesh, + *-ōma*, tumor]

myx·oid (mik'soyd). Resembling mucus. [myxo- + G. *eidos*, resemblance]

myx·o·li·po·ma (mik'sō-li-pō'mă). A benign neoplasm of adipose tissue in which portions of the tumor resemble mucoid mesenchymal tissue. SYN lipoma myxomatodes, myxoma lipomatosum. [myxo- + G. *lipos,* fat, + *-ōma,* tumor]

myx·o·ma (mik-sō'mă). A benign neoplasm derived from connective tissue, consisting chiefly of polyhedral and stellate cells that are loosely embedded in a soft mucoid matrix, thereby resembling primitive mesenchymal tissue; occurs frequently intramuscularly (where it may be mistaken for a sarcoma), also in the jaw bones, and encysted in the skin (focal mucinosis and dorsal wrist ganglion). [myxo- + G. *-ōma,* tumor]

atrial m., a primary cardiac neoplasm arising most commonly in the left atrium as a soft polypoid mass attached by a stalk to the septum; it may resemble an organized mural thrombus, and the symptoms may include cardiac murmurs, which change with alteration of body position, signs of mitral stenosis or insufficiency, with continuous danger of embolism by fragments of the tumor or its entire mass.

m. enchondromato'sum, SYN myxochondroma.

m. fibro'sum, SYN myxofibroma.

m. lipomato'sum, SYN myxolipoma.

odontogenic m., a benign, expansile, multilocular radiolucent neoplasm of the jaws consisting of myxomatous fibrous connective tissue; presumably derived from the mesenchymal components of the odontogenic apparatus.

m. sarcomato'sum, SYN myxosarcoma.

myx·o·ma·to·sis (mik'sō-mă-tō'sis). **1.** A fatal disease of European rabbits (*Oryctolagus cuniculus*) marked by purulent conjunctivitis and the development of myxomatous growths in the skin; caused by rabbit myxoma virus, a member of the family Poxviridae, and transmitted mechanically by mosquitoes; natural hosts are rabbits of the genus *Sylvilagus* in California and Brazil, in which the infection is not fatal and causes only local swelling. **2.** SYN mucoid *degeneration.* **3.** Multiple myxomas.

myx·o·ma·tous (mik-sō'mă-tŭs). **1.** Pertaining to or characterized by the features of a myxoma. **2.** Said of tissue that resembles primitive mesenchymal tissue.

myx·o·my·cete (mik'sō-mī-sēt). A member of the class Myxomycetes.

Myx·o·my·ce·tes (mik'sō-mī-sē'tēz). A class of fungi containing the slime molds, which occur on rotting vegetation but are not pathogenic for humans. [myxo- + G. *mykēs,* fungus]

myx·o·neu·ro·ma (mik'sō-nū-rō'mă). **1.** Obsolete term for a tumefaction resulting from abnormal proliferation of Schwann cells, in which focal or diffuse degenerative changes result in portions that resemble primitive mesenchymal tissue. **2.** Obsolete term for a neurilemoma, meningioma, or glioma in which the stroma is myxomatous in nature. [myxo- + G. *neuron,* nerve, + *-ōma,* tumor]

myx·o·pap·il·lo·ma (mik'sō-pap-i-lō'mă). A benign neoplasm of epithelial tissue in which the stroma resembles primitive mesenchymal tissue. [myxo- + L. *papilla,* a nipple, + G. *-ōma,* tumor]

myx·o·poi·e·sis (mik'sō-poy-ē'sis). Mucus production. [myxo- + G. *poiēsis,* a making]

myx·or·rhea (mik-sō-rē'ă). SYN blennorrhea. [myxo- + G. *rhoia,* a flow]

m. gas'trica, SYN gastromyxorrhea.

myx·o·sar·co·ma (mik'sō-sar-kō'mă). A sarcoma, usually a liposarcoma or malignant fibrous histiocytoma, with an abundant component of myxoid tissue resembling primitive mesenchyme containing connective tissue mucin. SYN myxoma sarcomatosum. [myxo- + G. *sarx,* flesh, + *-ōma,* tumor]

Myx·o·spo·ra (mik-sō-spō'ră). A subphylum of the phylum Protozoa, characterized by the presence of spores of multicellular origin, usually with two or three valves, two or more polar filaments, and an ameboid sporoplasm; parasitic in lower vertebrates, especially common in fishes. Important genera include *Ceratomyxa, Hanneguya, Leptotheca, Myxidium,* and *Myxobolus.* [myxo- + G. *sporos,* seed]

myx·o·spore (mik'sō-spōr). Obsolete term for the spore of a myxomycete. [myxo- + G. *sporos,* seed]

Myx·o·spo·rea (mik'sō-spō-rē'ă). A class of Myxozoa with spores containing one to six (usually two) polar capsules, each containing a coiled polar filament; parasitic in the celom or tissues of cold-blooded vertebrates, especially fishes. Important genera include *Ceratomyxa, Hanneguya, Leptotheca, Myxidium,* and *Myxobolus.*

myx·o·vi·rus (mik'sō-vī'rŭs). Term formerly used for viruses with an affinity for mucins, now included in the families Orthomyxoviridae and Paramyxoviridae. The m.'s included influenza virus, parainfluenza virus, respiratory syncytial virus, measles virus, and mumps virus.

Myx·o·zoa (mik-sō-zō'ă). A phylum of the subkingdom Protozoa, characterized by spores of multicellular origin (usually with two or three valves), one to six polar capsules or nematocysts (each with a coiled hollow filament), and a one- to many-nucleated ameboid sporoplasm; parasitic in annelids and other invertebrates (class Actinosporea; subclass Actinomyxa) and in lower vertebrates (class Myxosporea). [myxo- + G. *zōon,* animal]

My

ν **1.** Thirteenth letter of the Greek alphabet, nu. **2.** Symbol for kinematic *viscosity*; frequency; stoichiometric *number*. **3.** In chemistry, denotes the position of a substituent located on the thirteenth atom from the carboxyl or other functional group.

N 1. Symbol for newton; nitrogen; asparagine; nucleoside. **2.** Designation for an inherited blood factor. See MNSs blood group, Blood Groups appendix.

N/2. Symbol for seminormal.

^{13}N Symbol for nitrogen-13.

^{14}N Symbol for nitrogen-14.

^{15}N Symbol for nitrogen-15.

N_A Symbol for Avogadro's *number*.

n Symbol for nano- (2); reaction order.

N Symbol for normal *concentration*. SEE normal (3).

n. **1.** The number in a scientific study. Sample size. **2.** Symbol for refractive *index*.

n_0 Abbreviation for Loschmidt's *number*.

NA Abbreviation for Nomina Anatomica.

N.A. Abbreviation for numerical *aperture*.

Na Symbol for sodium (natrium).

^{24}Na. Symbol for sodium-24.

nab·i·lone (nab′i-lōn). (±)-3-(1,1-Dimethylheptyl-6-6aβ,7,8,10,10aα-hexahydro-1-hydroxy-6,6-dimethyl-9*H*-dibenzo[*b,d*]pyran-9-one; a synthetic cannabinoid used in the treatment of nausea and vomiting associated with cancer chemotherapy.

Naboth, Martin, German anatomist and physician, 1675–1721. SEE nabothian *cyst; follicle.*

na·cre·ous (nā′krē-ŭs). Lustrous, like mother-of-pearl; descriptive term for bacterial colonies. [Fr. *nacre,* mother-of-pearl]

NAD Abbreviation for nicotinamide adenine dinucleotide.

N.A.D. Abbreviation for no appreciable disease; nothing abnormal detected (British).

NAD⁺ Abbreviation for nicotinamide adenine dinucleotide (oxidized form).

NAD⁺ nucleosidase, an enzyme hydrolyzing NAD⁺ to nicotinamide and adenosine diphosphoribose. SYN DPNase, NADase.

NAD⁺ pyrophosphorylase, an enzyme that participates in the synthesis of NAD⁺; it reacts nicotinamide mononucleotide with ATP to produce NAD⁺ and pyrophosphate; it will also act on nicotinate mononucleotide.

NAD⁺ synthetase, an enzyme that catalyzes the reaction of ATP, L-glutamine, and nicotinate adenine dinucleotide to form NAD⁺, ADP, and L-glutamate.

NADase SYN *NAD⁺* nucleosidase.

NADH Abbreviation for nicotinamide adenine dinucleotide (reduced form).

NADH-dehydrogenase, an iron-containing flavoprotein reversibly oxidizing NADH to NAD⁺; an inherited deficiency of this complex results in overwhelming acidosis. SYN cytochrome *c* reductase.

NADH dehydrogenase (quinone), an enzyme oxidizing NADH with quinones (*e.g.,* menadione) as acceptors.

NADH-hydroxylamine reductase, an enzyme catalyzing the reaction of hydroxylamine and NADH to form ammonia, NAD⁺, and water; used in a number of clinical assays.

na·dide (nā′dīd). 3-Carbamoyl-1-β-D-ribofuranosylpyridinium hydroxide; a nicotinamide adenine dinucleotide compound used as an antagonist to alcohol and narcotics.

Nadi re·ac·tion. See under reaction.

na·do·lol (nā′dō-lol). 1-(*tert*-Butylamino)-3-[(5,6,7,8-tetrahydro-*cis*-6,7-dihydroxy-1-naphthyl)oxy]-2-propanol; a β-adrenergic blocking agent with actions similar to those of propranolol.

NADP Abbreviation for nicotinamide adenine dinucleotide phosphate.

NADP⁺ Abbreviation for nicotinamide adenine dinucleotide phosphate (oxidized form).

NADPH Abbreviation for nicotinamide adenine dinucleotide phosphate (reduced form).

NADPH-cy·to·chrome c_2 re·duc·tase. An enzyme catalyzing the reduction of 2 ferricytochrome c_2 to 2 ferrocytochrome c_2 at the expense of NADPH. SYN cytochrome c_2 reductase.

NADPH de·hy·dro·gen·ase. A flavoprotein oxidizing NADPH to NADP⁺. SYN NADPH diaphorase, old yellow enzyme, Warburg's old yellow enzyme.

NAD(P)H de·hy·dro·gen·ase (qui·none). A flavoprotein oxidizing NADH or NADPH to NAD⁺ or NADP⁺ with quinones (*e.g.,* menadione) as hydrogen acceptors.

NADPH de·hy·dro·gen·ase (qui·none). A flavoprotein similar to NADH dehydrogenase (quinone), but oxidizing NADPH. SYN DT-diaphorase, menadione reductase, phylloquinone reductase, quinone reductase.

NADPH di·aph·o·rase. SYN NADPH dehydrogenase.

NADPH-fer·ri·he·mo·pro·tein re·duc·tase (fer′ĭ-hē-mō-prō′tēn, fer′ē-). An enzyme catalyzing the reduction of 2 ferricytochrome by NADPH to 2 ferrocytochrome; the physiological acceptor is probably cytochrome P-450; hence, it has a role in steroid hydroxylations. SYN cytochrome reductase.

NAD(P)⁺ nu·cle·o·si·dase. An enzyme hydrolyzing NAD(P)⁺ to release free nicotinamide and adenosinediphosphoribose-(phosphate).

Naegeli, Oskar, Swiss physician, 1885–1959. SEE N. *syndrome.*

Naegeli, Otto, Swiss physician, 1871–1938. SEE N. type of monocytic *leukemia.*

Nae·gle·ria (nā-glē′rē-ă). A genus of free-living soil, water, and sewage ameba (order Schizopyrenida, family Vahlkampfiidae) one species of which, *N. fowleri,* has been implicated as the causative agent of the rapidly fatal primary amebic meningoencephalitis. Infection has been traced to swimming pools (including indoor chlorinated pools); entry is by the nasal mucosa, from which the amebae reach the meninges and brain through the cribriform plate and olfactory nerves. Other soil amebae that have been implicated, although of far less epidemiological significance, include the genera *Acanthamoeba* and *Hartmanella,* the latter being a suspected but unproved causative agent.

NAF Abbreviation for neutrophil activating *factor.*

naf·cil·lin (naf′sil′in). 6-(2-Ethoxy-1-naphthamido)penicillin; a semisynthetic penicillin derived from 6-aminopenicillanic acid; resistant to penicillinase, and effective against *Staphylococcus aureus.*

n. sodium, a penicillinase-resistant penicillin.

Naffziger, Howard C., U.S. surgeon, 1884–1961. SEE N. *operation, syndrome.*

naf·ro·nyl ox·a·late (naf′rō-nil). 2-(Diethylamino)ethyl tetrahydro-α-(1-naphthylmethyl)-2-furanpropionate oxalate; a vasodilator drug.

naf·ti·fine hy·dro·chlo·ride (naf′ti-fēn). (*E*)-*N*-Cinnamyl-*N*-methyl-1-naphthalenemethylamine hydrochloride; a broad spectrum antifungal agent used in the topical treatment of tinea infections.

NAG Abbreviation for *N*-acetylglutamate.

na·ga·na (nah-gah′nah). An acute or chronic disease of cattle, dogs, pigs, horses, sheep, and goats in sub-Saharan Africa; marked by fever, anemia, and cachexia, varying in severity with the parasite and the host. A collective term for diseases caused by the protozoan parasites *Trypanosoma brucei brucei, T. congolense,* and *T. vivax.*

Nagel, Willibald, A., German ophthalmologist and physiologist, 1870–1911. SEE N.'s test.

Nägele, Franz K., German obstetrician, 1777–1851. SEE N. *obliquity;* N.'s *pelvis, rule.*

Nageotte, Jean, French histologist, 1866–1948. SEE N. *cells,* under *cell.*

nail (nāl). **1.** One of the thin, horny, translucent plates covering the dorsal surface of the distal end of each terminal phalanx of fingers and toes. A nail consists of corpus or body, the visible part, and radix or root at the proximal end concealed under a fold of skin. The under part of the nail is formed from the stratum germinativum of the epidermis, the free surface from the stratum lucidum, the thin cuticular fold overlapping the lunula representing the stratum corneum. **2.** A slender rod of metal, bone, or other solid substance, used in operations to fasten together the divided extremities of a broken bone. SYN unguis [NA], nail plate, onyx. [A.S. *naegel*]

egg shell n., SYN hapalonychia.

half and half n., division of the n. by a transverse line into a proximal dull white part and a distal pink or brown part; seen in uremia.

hippocratic n.'s, the coarse curved n.'s capping clubbed digits (hippocratic fingers).

ingrown n., a toenail, one edge of which is overgrown by the nailfold, producing a pyogenic granuloma; due to faulty trimming of the toenails or pressure from a tight shoe. SYN ingrowing toenail, onychocryptosis, onyxis, unguis aduncus, unguis incarnatus.

Küntscher n., an intramedullary n. used for internal fixation of a fracture.

parrot-beak n., a markedly curved fingernail.

pincer n., transverse overcurvature of the n. that increases distally, causing the lateral borders of the n. to pinch the soft tissue with resulting tenderness; may result from a developmental anomaly or subungual exostosis.

racket n., a broad flat thumbnail resulting from a congenital shorter and wider distal phalanx of the thumb.

reedy n., a n. marked by longitudinal ridges and furrows.

shell n., bronchiectasis with excessive longitudinal curvature of the nail plate and atrophy of the nail bed and underlying bone.

Smith-Petersen n., a flanged n. for pinning a fracture of the neck of the femur.

spoon n., SYN koilonychia.

Terry's n.'s, a white, ground-glass-like opacity of the n.'s with a zone of normal pink at the distal edge of the n.'s; associated with liver disease (most commonly, cirrhosis of the liver).

yellow n., the complete or almost complete cessation of all n. growth, with thickening of the n.'s, increase in the convexity, loss of cuticles, and yellowing; the resulting onycholysis can cause loss of some of the n.'s; the condition is often associated with pulmonary disease but differs from clubbing in that the soft tissues are not hypertrophic. SYN yellow nail syndrome.

nail·ing (nāl'ing). Act of inserting or driving a nail into the ends of a fractured bone.

Najjar, Victor A., U.S. physician and biochemist, *1914. SEE Crigler-N. *syndrome.*

Nakanishi, K., Japanese physician. SEE N.'s stain.

nal·bu·phine hy·dro·chlo·ride (nal-byū'fēn). 17-(Cyclobutylmethyl)4,5α-epoxymorphinan-3,6α,14-triol hydrochloride; a synthetic opioid analgesic chemically related to oxymorphone, a narcotic, and to naloxone, a narcotic antagonist, with both agonist and antagonist narcotic properties.

na·li·dix·ic ac·id (nal-i-dik'sik). 1-Ethyl-1,4-dihydro-7-methyl-4-oxo-1,8-naphthyridine-3-carboxylic acid; an orally effective antibacterial agent used in the treatment of genitourinary tract infections.

nal·or·phine (nal-ōr'fēn). $C_{19}H_{21}NO_3$; an early antagonist of most of the depressant and stimulatory effects of morphine and related narcotic analgesics; precipitates severe withdrawal symptoms in morphine addicts, is used in the diagnosis of suspected morphine addiction, and counteracts the respiratory depression produced by morphine and related compounds; when administered in the absence of narcotics, n. has mild analgesic and respiratory depressant effects in nonaddicts; superseded by naloxone. SYN *N*-allylnormorphine.

nal·ox·one hy·dro·chlo·ride (nal-ok'sōn). 1-*N*-Allyl-7,8-

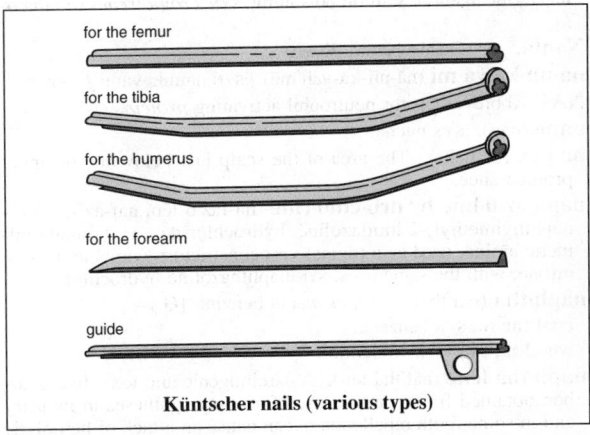

Küntscher nails (various types)

dihydro-14-hydroxymorphinone hydrochloride; a potent antagonist of endorphins and narcotics, including pentazocine; devoid of pharmacologic action when administered without narcotics.

nal·trex·one (nal-treks'ōn). 17-(Cyclopropylmethyl)-4,5-epoxy-3,14-dihydroxymorphinan-6-one; an orally active narcotic antagonist; devoid of pharmacologic action when administered in the absence of narcotics.

NAME Acronym for *n*evi, *a*trial myxoma, *m*yxoid neurofibromas, and *e*philides. SEE NAME *syndrome.*

NANDA. Acronym for North American Nursing Diagnosis Association.

nan·dro·lone (nan'drō-lōn). 17β-Hydroxy-4-estrene-3-one; a semisynthetic, parenterally administered, anabolic, androgenic steroid.

n. decanoate, an anabolic androgen.

n. phenpropionate, a moderately long-acting synthetic anabolic androgen. SYN n. phenylpropionate.

n. phenylpropionate, SYN n. phenpropionate.

nan·ism (nan'izm). Obsolete term for dwarfism. [G. *nanos;* L. *nanus,* dwarf]

mulibrey n. (mŭ'li-brā), autosomal recessive disorder with defects of liver, brain, muscle, and eyes. [taken from muscle, liver, brain, and eyes]

renal n., infantile renal osteodystrophy.

symptomatic n., dwarfism with defects in bone, dentition, and sexual development.

Nan·niz·zia (nă-niz'ē-ă). A genus of ascomycetous fungi comprised of *Microsporum* species in their perfect state.

nano-. **1.** Combining form relating to dwarfism (nanism). **2 (n).** Prefix used in the SI and metric systems to signify one-billionth (10^{-9}). [G. *nanos,* dwarf]

nan·o·ce·pha·lia (nan'ō-se-fā'lē-ă). SYN microcephaly.

nan·o·ceph·a·lous, nan·o·ce·phal·ic (nan-ō-sef'ă-lŭs, -se-fal'ik). SYN microcephalic.

nan·o·ceph·a·ly (nan-ō-sef'ă-lē). SYN microcephaly. [nano- + G. *kephalē,* head]

nan·o·cor·mia (nan-ō-kōr'mē-ă). SYN microsomia. [nano- + G. *kormos,* trunk]

nan·o·gram (ng) (nan'ō-gram). One-billionth of a gram (10^{-9} g).

nan·o·ka·tal (nkat) (nan-ō-ka-tăl'). One-billionth of a katal (10^{-9} kat).

nan·o·me·lia (nan-ō-mē'lē-ă). SYN micromelia. [nano- + G. *melos,* limb]

nan·o·me·ter (nm) (năn-om'ĕ-ter). One-billionth of a meter (10^{-9} m).

nan·oph·thal·mia, nan·oph·thal·mos (nan-of-thal'mē-ă, -mos). SYN microphthalmos. [nano- + G. *ophthalmos,* eye]

Na·no·phy·e·tus sal·min·co·la (na-nō'fī-ĕ-tŭs sal-min'kō-lă). A digenetic fish-borne fluke (family Nanophyetidae) of dogs and other fish-eating mammals; the vector of *Neorickettsia helmin-*

theca, the agent of salmon poisoning. SYN *Troglotrema salmincola*.

Nanta. SEE Gandy-Nanta *disease*.

na·nu·ka·ya·mi (nă-nū-kă-yah'mē). SYN nanukayami *fever*.

NAP Abbreviation for neutrophil activating *protein*.

nape (nāp). SYN nucha.

na·pex (nā'peks). The area of the scalp just below the occipital protuberance.

naph·az·o·line hy·dro·chlo·ride (nă-faz'ŏ-lēn, naf-az'-). 2-(1-naphthylmethyl)-2-imidazoline hydrochloride; a sympathomimetic amine, used as a topical vasoconstrictor; available as n. h. nitrate, with the same uses. SYN naphthazoline hydrochloride.

naph·tha (naf'thă). SYN *petroleum* benzin. [G.]
　coal tar n., SYN benzene.
　wood n., SYN *methyl* alcohol.

naph·tha·lene (naf'thă-lēn). A carcinogenic and toxic hydrocarbon obtained from coal tar; used for many syntheses in industry and in some moth repellents; n. can cause an attack of hemolytic anemia in individuals with a deficiency of glucose-6-phosphate dehydrogenase. SYN naphthalin, tar camphor.

naph·thal·e·nol (naf-thal'ĕ-nol). SYN naphthol.

naph·tha·lin (naf'thă-lin). SYN naphthalene.

naph·thaz·o·line hy·dro·chlo·ride (naf-thaz'ŏ-lēn). SYN naphazoline hydrochloride.

naph·thol (naf'thol). $C_{10}H_7OH$; a phenol of naphthalene, occurring in two forms: α-naphthol, a dye intermediate used in cytochemistry for L-arginine localization; β-naphthol, also known as isonaphthol, used as an anthelmintic and antiseptic. Both forms are also used in the manufacture of dyes, organic chemicals, and rubber products. SYN naphthalenol.

naph·tho·late (naf'thō-lāt). A compound of naphthol in which the hydrogen in the hydroxyl radical is substituted by a base.

naph·thol yel·low S [C.I. 10316]. 8-Hydroxy-5,7-dinitro-2-naphthalene sulfonic acid; an acid dye used as a stain for basic proteins in microspectro-photometry.

naph·tho·qui·none (naf-thō-kwin'ōn). **1.** A quinone derivative of naphthalene, reducible to naphthohydroquinone; 1,4-naphthoquinone derivatives have vitamin K activity (*e.g.*, menaquinone). **2.** A class of compounds containing the n. (1) structure.

naph·thyl (naf'thil). The radical of naphthalene, $C_{10}H_7-$.

α-naph·thyl·thi·o·u·rea (ANTU) (naf'thil-thī'ō-yū-rē'ă). 1-(1-Naphthyl)-2-thiourea; a derivative of thiourea; a highly toxic antithyroid agent, especially to small mammals, causing pulmonary edema, fatty degeneration of the liver, and low body temperature; used as a rat poison.

na·pi·er (nā'pē-er). SYN neper. [John *Napier*, Scottish mathematician, 1550–1617]

na·prap·a·thy (nă-prap'ă-thē). A system of therapeutic manipulation based on the theory that morbid symptoms are dependent upon strained or contracted ligaments in the spine, thorax, or pelvis. [Bohemian *napravit*, to correct, + G. *pathos*, suffering]

na·prox·en (nă-prok'sēn). (+)-6-Methoxy-α-methyl-2-naphthaleneacetic acid; a nonsteroidal anti-inflammatory analgesic agent used in the treatment of rheumatoid conditions.

nap·syl·ate (nap'si-lāt). USAN-approved contraction for 2-naphthalenesulfonate.

nar·ce·ine (nar'sē-ēn). An alkaloid of opium; $C_{23}H_{27}NO_8$. Ethylnarceine is a narcotic, analgesic, and antitussive.

nar·cis·sism (nar-sis'izm, nar'si-sizm). **1.** Sexual attraction toward one's own person. SYN autophilia. **2.** A state in which the individual interprets and regards everything in relation to himself and not to other persons or things. SYN autosexualism (2), narcissistic personality, self-love. [*Narkissos*, G. myth. char.]
　primary n., in psychoanalysis, the original psychic energy embodied or invested in the ego.
　secondary n., in psychoanalysis, the psychic energy once attached to external objects, but now withdrawn from those objects and reinvested in the ego.

△**narco-.** Stupor, narcosis. [G. *narkoō*, to benumb, deaden]

nar·co·a·nal·y·sis (nar'kō-ă-nal'i-sis). Psychotherapeutic treatment under light anesthesia, originally used in acute combat

cases during World War II; also has been used in the treatment of childhood trauma. SEE ALSO narcotherapy. SYN narcosynthesis.

nar·co·hyp·nia (nar-kō-hip'nē-ă). A general numbness sometimes experienced at the moment of waking. [narco- + G. *hypnos,* sleep]

nar·co·hyp·no·sis (nar'kō-hip-nō'sis). Stupor or deep sleep induced by hypnosis. [narco- + G. *hypnos,* sleep]

nar·co·lep·sy (nar'kō-lep-sē). A sleep disorder that usually appears in young adulthood, consisting of recurring episodes of sleep during the day, and often disrupted nocturnal sleep; frequently accompanied by cataplexy, sleep paralysis, and hypnagogic hallucinations; a genetically determined disease. SYN Gélineau's syndrome, paroxysmal sleep. [narco- + G. *lēpsis,* seizure]

nar·co·lep·tic (nar'kō-lep'-tik). **1.** A sleep inducing drug. **2.** A person with narcolepsy.

nar·co·sis (nar-kō'sis). General and nonspecific reversible depression of neuronal excitability, produced by a number of physical and chemical agents, usually resulting in stupor rather than in anesthesia (with which n. was once synonymous). [G. a benumbing]
　CO_2 **n.,** SYN hypoventilation *coma.*
　intravenous n., administration of opiate medication intravenously.
　nitrogen n., (1) n. produced by nitrogenous materials such as occurs in certain forms of uremia and hepatic coma; (2) the stuporous condition characterized by disorientation and by loss of judgment and skill, attributed to an increased partial pressure of nitrogen in the inspired air of deepsea divers during underwater operations. Commonly referred to as "rapture of the deep."

nar·co·syn·the·sis (nar-kō-sin'thĕ-sis). SYN narcoanalysis.

nar·co·ther·a·py (nar-kō-thār'ă-pē). Psychotherapy conducted with the patient under the influence of a sedative or narcotic.

nar·cot·ic (nar-kot'ik). **1.** Originally, any drug derived from opium or opium-like compounds with potent analgesic effects associated with both significant alteration of mood and behavior and potential for dependence and tolerance. **2.** More recently, any drug, synthetic or naturally occurring, with effects similar to those of opium and opium derivatives, including meperidine and fentanyl and its derivatives. **3.** Capable of inducing a state of stuporous analgesia. [G. *narkōtikos,* benumbing]

dl-**nar·co·tine** (nar'kō-tēn). SYN gnoscopine.

l-α-**nar·co·tine.** SYN noscapine.

nar·co·tism (nar'kō-tizm). **1.** Stuporous analgesia induced by a narcotic. **2.** Addiction to a narcotic.

na·ris, pl. **na·res** (nā'ris, -res) [NA]. SYN nostril. [L.]
　anterior n., SYN nostril.
　external n., SYN nostril.
　internal n., obsolete term for choana.
　posterior n., SYN choana.

na·sal (nā'zăl). Relating to the nose. SYN rhinal. [L. *nasus,* nose]

nas·cent (nas'ent, nā'sent). **1.** Beginning; being born or produced. **2.** Denoting the state of a chemical element at the moment it is set free from one of its compounds. [L. *nascor,* pres. p. *nascens,* to be born]

na·si·o·in·i·ac (nā'zē-ō-in'ē-ak). Relating to the nasion and inion; denoting the distance in a straight line between the frontonasal suture and the external occipital protuberance.

na·si·on (nā'zē-on) [NA]. A point on the skull corresponding to the middle of the nasofrontal suture. SYN nasal point. [L. *nasus,* nose]

Nasmyth, Alexander, London dentist, †1847. SEE N.'s *cuticle, membrane.*

△**naso-.** The nose. [L. *nasus*]

na·so·an·tral (nā'zō-an'trăl). Relating to the nose and the maxillary sinus.

na·so·cil·i·ary. Relating to nose and eyelids. SEE nasociliary *nerve.*

na·so·fron·tal (nā-zō-frŭn'tăl). Relating to the nose and forehead, or to the nasal cavity and frontal sinuses.

na·so·gas·tric (nā-zō-gas'trik). Pertaining to or involving the nasal passages and the stomach, as in n. intubation.

na·so·la·bi·al (nā-zō-lā'bē-ăl). Relating to the nose and upper lip. [naso- + L. *labium,* lip]

na·so·lac·ri·mal (nā-zō-lak'ri-măl). Relating to the nasal and the lacrimal bones, or to the nasal cavity and the lacrimal ducts.

na·so-oral (nā-zō-ō'răl). Relating to the nose and mouth.

na·so·pal·a·tine (nā'zō-pal'ă-tēn, -tin). Relating to the nose and the palate.

na·so·pha·ryn·ge·al (nā'zō-fă-rin'jē-ăl). Relating to the nose or nasal cavity and the pharynx. SYN rhinopharyngeal (1).

na·so·pha·ryn·go·la·ryn·go·scope (nā'zō-fa-ring'gō-lā-ring' gō-skōp). An instrument, often of fiberoptic type, used to visualize the upper airways and pharynx.

na·so·pha·ryn·go·scope (nā'zō-fa-ring'gō-skōp). Telescopic instrument, electrically lighted, for examination of the nasal passages and the nasopharynx.

na·so·pha·ryn·gos·co·py (nā'zō-fa-ring-gos'kŏ-pē). Examination of the nasopharynx by flexible or rigid optical instruments, or with a mirror. [nasopharynx + G. *skopeō,* to view]

na·so·pha·rynx (nā'zō-far'ingks). The part of the pharynx that lies above the soft palate; anteriorly it opens into the nasal cavity; inferiorly it communicates with the oropharynx via the pharyngeal isthmus; laterally it communicates with tympanic cavities via auditory tubes. SYN pars nasalis pharyngis [NA], epipharynx, nasal part of pharynx, nasal pharynx, pharyngonasal cavity, rhinopharynx.

na·so·ros·tral (nā'zō-ros'trăl). Relating to the nasal cavity and the rostrum of the sphenoid bone.

na·so·si·nu·si·tis (nā'zō-sī-nŭ-sī'tis). Inflammation of the nasal cavities and of the accessory sinuses.

Nasse, Christian Friedrich, German physician, 1788–1851.

Nasse's law. See under law.

na·sus (nā'sŭs) [NA]. **1.** SYN external *nose.* **2.** SYN nose. [L.]

n. exter'nus [NA], SYN external *nose.*

na·tal (nā'tăl). **1.** Relating to birth. [L. *natalis,* fr. *nascor,* pp. *natus,* to be born] **2.** Relating to the buttocks or nates. [L. *nates,* buttocks]

na·tal·i·ty (nā-tal'i-tē). The birth rate; the ratio of births to the general population. [see natal (1)]

na·ta·my·cin (nā-tă-mī'sin). SYN pimaricin.

na·tes (nā'tēz) [NA]. SYN buttocks. [L. pl. of *natis*]

na·ti·mor·tal·i·ty (nā'ti-mōr-tal'i-tē). The perinatal death rate; the proportion of fetal and neonatal deaths to the general natality. [L. *natus,* birth, + *mortalitas,* fr. *mors,* death]

Na·tion·al For·mu·lary (NF). An official compendium formerly issued by the American Pharmaceutical Association but now published by the United States Pharmacopeial Convention for the purpose of providing standards and specifications which can be used to evaluate the quality of pharmaceuticals and therapeutic agents.

na·tre·mia, na·tri·e·mia (nā-trē'mē-ă, nā'trē-ē'mē-ă). The presence of sodium in the blood. [natrium, sodium, + G. *haima,* blood]

na·trex·one hy·dro·chlo·ride (nă-treks'on). 17-(Cyclopropylmethyl)4,5α-epoxy-3,14-dihydroxymorphinan-6-one hydrochloride; an orally active narcotic antagonist used in maintenance therapy of detoxified, formerly opioid-dependent, patients.

na·trif·er·ic (nā-trif'er-ik). Tending to increase sodium transport. [natrium + L. *fero,* to carry]

na·tri·um (Na) (nā'trē-ŭm). SYN sodium. [Ar. *natrūm,* fr. G. *nitron,* carbonate of soda]

na·tri·u·re·sis (nā'trē-yū-rē'sis). Urinary excretion of sodium; commonly designates enhanced sodium excretion, which may occur in certain diseases or as a result of the administration of diuretic drugs. [natrium + G. *ouron,* urine]

na·tri·u·ret·ic (nā'trē-yū-ret'ik). **1.** Pertaining to or characterized by natriuresis. **2.** A substance that increases urinary excretion of sodium, usually as a result of decreased tubular reabsorption of sodium ions from glomerular filtrate.

na·tur·o·path (nā'chūr-ō-path). One who practices naturopathy.

na·tur·o·path·ic (nā'chūr-ō-path'ik). Relating to or by means of naturopathy.

na·tur·op·a·thy (nā-chūr-op'ă-thē). A system of therapeutics in which neither surgical nor medicinal agents are used, dependence being placed only on natural (nonmedicinal) forces.

nau·path·ia (naw-path'ē-ă). SYN seasickness. [G. *naus,* ship, + *pathos,* suffering]

nau·sea (naw'zē-ă, -zhă). Symptoms resulting from an inclination to vomit. SYN sicchasia (1). [L. fr. G. *nausia,* seasickness, fr. *naus,* ship]

epidemic n., SYN epidemic *vomiting.*

n. gravida'rum, SYN morning *sickness.*

nau·se·ant (naw'zē-ănt). **1.** Nauseating; causing nausea. **2.** An agent that causes nausea.

nau·se·ate (naw'zē-āt). To cause an inclination to vomit.

nau·se·at·ed (naw'zē-ā-ted). Affected with nausea. SYN sick (2).

nau·seous (naw'zē-ŭs, naw'shŭs). Causing nausea.

Nauta, Walle J.H., U.S. neuroscientist, *1916. SEE N.'s *stain.*

na·vel (nā'vel). SYN umbilicus. [A.S. *nafela*]

na·vic·u·la (nă-vik'yū-lă). A small boat-shaped structure. [L. dim of *navis,* ship]

na·vic·u·lar (nă-vik'yū-lăr). SYN scaphoid. [L. *navicularis,* relating to shipping]

na·vic·u·lar·thri·tis (nă-vik'yū-lar-thrī'tis). SYN navicular *disease.* [navicular + arthritis]

Nb Symbol for niobium.

NBT Abbreviation for nitroblue *tetrazolium.*

Nd Symbol for neodymium.

NDP Abbreviation for *nucleoside* diphosphate.

Ne Symbol for neon.

ne·al·bar·bi·tal (nē-al-bar'bi-tahl). 5-Allyl-5-neopentylbarbituric acid; an obsolete sedative and hypnotic.

near·sight·ed·ness (nēr'sīt-ed-nes). SYN myopia.

ne·ar·thro·sis (nē-ar-thrō'sis). A new joint; *e.g.,* a pseudarthrosis arising in an ununited fracture, or an artificial joint resulting from a total joint replacement operation. SYN neoarthrosis. [G. *neos,* new, + *arthrōsis,* a jointing]

neb·ra·my·cin (neb-ră-mī'sin). A complex of substances produced by *Streptomyces tenebrarius;* an antibacterial agent.

nebul.. Abbreviation for nebula.

neb·u·la (nebul.), pl. **neb·'u·lae** (neb'yū-lă, -lē). **1.** A translucent foglike opacity of the cornea. **2.** A class of oily preparations, intended for application by atomization. SEE spray. **3.** A spray. [L. fog, cloud, mist]

neb·u·la·rine (neb-yū-lār'in). A toxic nucleoside isolated from the mushroom *Agaricus nebularis* and from *Streptomyces* sp. SYN 9-β-ribofuranosylpurine, purine ribonucleoside, ribosylpurine.

neb·ul·in (neb'yū-lin). A very large protein, constituting about 3% of muscle protein; may aid in the organization of actin filaments as well as in actin polymerization. [L. *nebula,* mist, fog, fr. G. *nephelē,* + -in]

neb·u·li·za·tion (neb'yū-li-zā'shŭn). Spraying or vaporization. [L. *nebula,* mist]

neb·u·lize (neb'yū-līz). To break up a liquid into a fine spray or vapor; to vaporize. [L. *nebula,* mist]

neb·u·liz·er (neb'yū-līz-er). A device used to reduce liquid medication to extremely fine cloudlike particles; useful in delivering medication to deeper parts of the respiratory tract. SEE ALSO atomizer, vaporizer.

jet n., an atomizer that uses an air or gas stream to change a liquid into small particles.

spinning disk n., a n. in which water is changed into small particles as it is thrown by centrifugal force from a spinning disk.

ultrasonic n., a humidifier using high-frequency electricity to power a transducer that vibrates 1,350,000 times per second and changes water up into particles 0.5 to 3 μm in size in its nebulizing chamber; used in inhalation therapy.

Ne·ca·tor (nē-kā'tŏr). A genus of nematode hookworms (family Ancylostomatidae, subfamily Necatorinae) distinguished by two chitinous cutting plates in the buccal cavity and fused male copulatory spicules. Species include *N. americanus*, the so-called New World hookworm (although it is also prevalent in the tropics of Africa, southern Asia, and Polynesia); the adults of this species attach to villi in the small intestine and suck blood, causing abdominal discomfort, diarrhea (usually with melena) and cramps, anorexia, loss of weight, and hypochromic microcytic anemia, which may occur in advanced disease. SEE ALSO *Ancylostoma*. [L. a murderer]

ne·ca·to·ri·a·sis (nē-kā-tō-rī′ă-sis). Hookworm disease caused by *Necator*, the resulting anemia being usually less severe than that from ancylostomiasis.

neck (nek). **1.** SYN *regions* of neck, under *region*. **2.** In anatomy, any constricted portion having a fancied resemblance to the n. of an animal. **3.** The germinative portion of an adult tapeworm which develops the segments or proglottids; the region of cestode segmentation behind the scolex. [A.S. *hnecca*]

anatomical n. of humerus, a groove separating the head of the humerus from the tuberosities, giving attachment to the articular capsule. SYN collum anatomicum humeri [NA].

buffalo n., combination of moderate kyphosis with thick heavy fat pad on the n., seen especially in persons with Cushing's disease or syndrome.

bull n., a heavy thick n. caused by hypertrophied muscles or enlarged cervical lymph nodes.

dental n., SYN n. of tooth.

n. of femur, a short, constricted, strong bar projecting at an obtuse angle (about 125°) from the upper end of the shaft of the thigh bone and supporting its head. SYN collum ossis femoris [NA], collum femoris, n. of thigh bone.

n. of fibula, the slightly constricted region between the head and body of the fibula. SYN collum fibulae [NA].

n. of gallbladder, the narrow portion between the body of the gallbladder and beginning of the cystic duct. SYN collum vesicae biliaris [NA], collum vesicae felleae★.

n. of glans penis, a constriction behind the corona glandis of the penis. SYN collum glandis penis [NA].

n. of hair follicle, the narrowed part of the hair follicle between the hair bulb and the surface of the skin. SYN collum folliculi pili.

n. of humerus, SEE anatomical n. of humerus, surgical n. of humerus.

Madelung's n., multiple symmetric lipomatosis (Madelung's disease) confined to the n.

n. of malleus, the constricted portion of the malleus between the head and the manubrium. SYN collum mallei [NA].

n. of mandible, the constricted portion of the condylar process below the head of the mandible. SYN collum mandibulae [NA].

n. of radius, the narrow part of the shaft just below the head. SYN collum radii [NA].

n. of rib, the flattened portion of a rib between the head and the tuberosity. SYN collum costae [NA].

n. of scapula, a slight constriction marking the separation of that portion bearing the glenoid cavity and coracoid process from the remainder of the scapula. SYN collum scapulae [NA].

stiff n., nonspecific term for limited neck mobility, often due to muscle cramps and accompanied by pain.

surgical n. of humerus, the narrow portion below the head and tuberosities. SYN collum chirurgicum humeri [NA].

n. of talus, a constriction separating the head, or anterior portion, from the body of the talus. SYN collum tali [NA].

n. of thigh bone, SYN n. of femur.

n. of tooth, the slightly constricted part of a tooth, between the crown and the root. SYN cervix dentis [NA], cervical margin of tooth, cervical zone of tooth, collum dentis, dental n.

turkey gobbler n., large skin folds hanging under the chin.

n. of urinary bladder, the lowest part of the bladder formed by the junction of the fundus and the inferolateral surfaces. SYN cervix vesicae urinariae [NA].

n. of uterus, SYN *cervix* of uterus.

webbed n., the broad n. due to lateral folds of skin extending from the clavicle to the head but containing no muscles, bones, or other structures; occurs in Turner's syndrome and in Noonan's syndrome.

n. of womb, SYN *cervix* of uterus.

wry n., SYN torticollis.

neck·lace (nek′lăs). Term used to describe a skin rash that encircles the neck.

Casal's n., a dermatitis partly or completely encircling the lower part of the neck in pellagra.

n. of Venus, obsolete term for syphilitic *leukoderma*.

△**necr-.** SEE necro-.

nec·rec·to·my (ne-krek′tō-mē). Operative removal of any necrosed tissue. [necr- + G. *ektomē*, excision]

△**necro-, necr-.** Death, necrosis. [G. *nekros*, corpse]

nec·ro·ba·cil·lo·sis (nek′rō-bas-il-ō′sis). Any disease with which the bacterium *Fusobacterium necrophorum* is associated.

nec·ro·bi·o·sis (nek′rō-bī-ō′sis). **1.** Physiologic or normal death of cells or tissues as a result of changes associated with development, aging, or use. **2.** Necrosis of a small area of tissue. SYN bionecrosis. [necro- + G. *bios*, life]

n. lipoid′ica, n. lipoid′ica diabetico′rum, a condition, in many cases associated with diabetes, in which one or more yellow, atrophic, shiny lesions develop on the legs (typically pretibial); characterized histologically by indistinct areas of necrosis in the cutis.

nec·ro·bi·ot·ic (nek′rō-bī-ot′ik). Pertaining to or characterized by necrobiosis.

nec·ro·cy·to·sis (nek′rō-sī-tō′sis). A process that results in, or a condition that is characterized by, the abnormal or pathologic death of cells. [necro- + G. *kytos*, cell, + *-osis*, condition]

nec·ro·gen·ic (nek-rō-jen′ik). Relating to, living in, or having origin in dead matter. SYN necrogenous. [necro- + G. *genesis*, origin]

ne·crog·e·nous (ne-kroj′ĕ-nŭs). SYN necrogenic.

nec·ro·gran·u·lo·ma·tous (nek′rō-gran-yū-lō′mă-tŭs). Having the characteristics of a granuloma with central necrosis.

ne·crol·o·gist (nĕ-krol′ō-jist). A student of, or a specialist in, necrology.

ne·crol·o·gy (nĕ-krol′ō-jē). The science of the collection, classification, and interpretation of mortality statistics. [necro- + G. *logos*, study]

ne·crol·y·sis (nĕ-krol′i-sis). Necrosis and loosening of tissue. [necro- + G. *lysis*, loosening]

toxic epidermal n. (TEN), a syndrome in which a large portion of the skin becomes intensely erythematous with epidermal necrosis, and peels off in the manner of a second-degree burn, often simultaneous with the formation of flaccid bullae, resulting from drug sensitivity or of unknown cause; the level of separation is subepidermal, unlike staphylococcal scalded skin syndrome in which there is subcorneal change. SYN Lyell's syndrome.

nec·ro·ma·nia (nek-rō-mā′nē-ă). **1.** A morbid tendency to dwell with longing on death. **2.** A morbid attraction to dead bodies. [necro- + G. *mania*, frenzy]

ne·crom·e·ter (nĕ-krom′ĕ-ter). An instrument for measuring a dead body or any of its parts or organs. [necro- + G. *metron*, measure]

nec·ro·par·a·site (nek-rō-par′ă-sīt). SYN saprophyte.

ne·crop·a·thy (nĕ-krop′ă-thē). A tendency to tissue death or gangrene. [necro- + G. *pathos*, disease]

ne·croph·a·gous (nĕ-krof′ă-gŭs). **1.** Living on carrion. **2.** SYN necrophilous. [necro- + G. *phagō*, to eat]

nec·ro·phil·ia, ne·croph·i·lism (nek-rō-fil′ē-ă, nĕ-krof′i-lizm). **1.** A morbid fondness for being in the presence of dead bodies. **2.** The impulse to have sexual contact, or the act of such contact, with a dead body, usually of males with female corpses. [necro- + G. *phileō*, to love]

ne·croph·i·lous (nĕ-krof′i-lŭs). Having a preference for dead tissue; denoting certain bacteria. SYN necrophagous (2). [necro- + G. *philos*, fond]

nec·ro·pho·bia (nek-rō-fō′bē-ă). Morbid fear of corpses. [necro- + G. *phobos*, fear]

ne·crop·sy (nek′rop-sē). SYN autopsy (1). [necro- + G. *opsis*, view]

nec·ro·sa·dism (nek-rō-sād′izm). Sexual gratification derived by mutilating corpses. [necro- + sadism]

ne·cros·co·py (nĕ-kros′kŏ-pē). Rarely used term for autopsy. [necro- + G. *skopeō,* to examine]

ne·crose (nĕ-krōz′). **1.** To cause necrosis. **2.** To become the site of necrosis.

nec·ro·sec·to·my (nĕ-krō′sek-tō-mē). Resection of necrotic tissue.

ne·cro·sis (nĕ-krō′sis). Pathologic death of one or more cells, or of a portion of tissue or organ, resulting from irreversible damage; earliest irreversible changes are mitochondrial, consisting of swelling and granular calcium deposits seen by electron microscopy; most frequent visible alterations are nuclear: pyknosis, shrunken and abnormally dark basophilic staining; karyolysis, swollen and abnormally pale basophilic staining; or karyorrhexis, rupture and fragmentation of the nucleus. After such changes, the outlines of individual cells are indistinct, and affected cells may become merged, sometimes forming a focus of coarsely granular, amorphous, or hyaline material. [G. *nekrōsis,* death, fr. *nekroō,* to make dead]

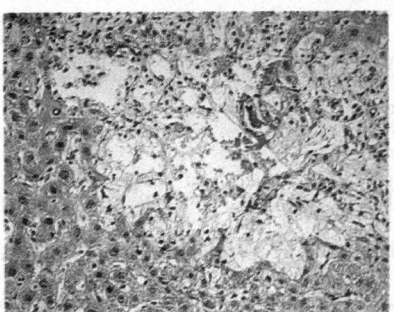

necrosis (of heart muscle tissue, after myocardial infarct)
the indistinct striation shows the homogenizing of cells without nuclei

aseptic n., n. occurring in the absence of infection.

avascular n., n. due to deficient blood supply.

bridging hepatic n., area of liver n. which bridges adjacent portal areas and central veins; subsequent post-necrotic collapse and fibrosis is likely to result in cirrhosis.

caseous n., caseation n., n. characteristic of certain inflammations (*e.g.,* tuberculosis, histoplasmosis), which represents n. with loss of separate structures of the various cellular and histologic elements; affected tissue manifests the friable, crumbly consistency and dull, opaque quality observed in cheese. SYN caseous degeneration.

central n., n. involving the deeper or inner portions of a tissue, or an organ or its units.

cerebrocortical n., SYN polioencephalomalacia.

coagulation n., a type of n. in which the affected cells or tissue are converted into a dry, dull, fairly homogeneous eosinophilic mass without nuclear staining, as a result of the coagulation of protein as occurs in an infarct; microscopically, the necrotic process involves chiefly the cells, and remnants of histologic elements (*e.g.,* elastin, collagen, muscle fibers) may be recognizable, as well as "ghosts" of cells and portions of cell membranes; may be caused by heat, ischemia, and other agents that destroy tissue, including enzymes that would continue to alter the devitalized cellular substance.

colliquative n., obsolete term for liquefactive n.

contraction band n., SYN contraction *band.*

cystic medial n., loss of elastic and muscle fibers in the aortic media, with accumulation of mucopolysaccharide, sometimes in cystlike spaces between the fibers; a disease of unknown cause, which may be inherited and which predisposes to dissecting aneurysms. SYN Erdheim disease, medionecrosis aortae idiopathica cystica, medionecrosis of the aorta, mucoid medial degeneration.

epiphysial aseptic n., aseptic n. of bony epiphyses, probably due to ischemia; it may affect the upper end of the femur (Legg-Calvé-Perthes disease), the tibial tubercle (Osgood-Schlatter disease), the tarsal navicular bone or the patella (Köhler's disease), the second metatarsal head (Freiberg's disease), vertebral bodies (Scheuermann's disease), or the capitellum of the humerus (Panner's disease).

fat n., the death of adipose tissue, characterized by the formation of small (1 to 4 mm), dull, chalky, gray or white foci; these represent small quantities of calcium soaps formed in the affected tissue when fat is hydrolyzed into glycerol and fatty acids. SYN steatonecrosis.

fibrinoid n., n. in which the necrotic tissue has some staining reactions resembling fibrin and becomes deeply eosinophilic, homogenous, and refractile.

focal n., occurrence of numerous, relatively small or tiny, fairly well-circumscribed, usually spheroidal portions of tissue that manifest coagulative, caseous, or gummatous n. and are characteristically associated with agents that are hematogenously disseminated; frequently observed only in histologic sections, but the foci may be as large as 1 to 3 mm and macroscopically visible; arbitrarily, foci larger than that are usually not termed focal n.

ischemic n., n. caused by hypoxia resulting from local deprivation of blood supply, as by infarction.

laminar cortical n., the breaking down of a definite cell layer in the cerebral cortex, encountered typically after temporary cardiac arrest or perinatal hypoxia.

liquefactive n., a type of n. characterized by a fairly well-circumscribed, microscopically or macroscopically visible lesion that consists of the dull, opaque or turbid, gray-white to yellow-gray, soft or boggy, partly or completely fluid remains of tissue that became necrotic and was digested by enzymes, especially proteolytic enzymes liberated from disintegrating leukocytes; it is classically observed in abscesses, and frequently in infarcts of the brain.

mummification n., SYN dry *gangrene.*

progressive emphysematous n., SYN gas *gangrene.*

renal papillary n., n. of renal papillae, occurring in acute pyelonephritis, especially in diabetics, or in analgesic nephropathy; renal failure may result. SYN necrotizing papillitis.

simple n., a stage of coagulation n.; the occurrence of a coarsely granular or hyaline change in the cytoplasm, and the lack of a recognizable nucleus, with the general configuration of the dead cells being relatively unchanged.

subcutaneous fat n. of newborn, indurated plaques and nodules appearing usually a few days or a few weeks after birth and usually resolving within a few months, characterized microscopically by birefringent needle-shaped crystals within necrotic fat cells; the condition remains localized, unlike sclerema neonatorum.

suppurative n., liquefactive n. with pus formation.

total n., (1) complete n. of the cytologic and histologic elements in a portion of tissue, as in caseous n.; **(2)** death of an entire organ or part.

Zenker's n., SYN Zenker's *degeneration.*

zonal n., n. predominantly affecting or limited to an anatomical zone, especially parts of the hepatic lobules defined according to proximity to either the portal tracts or central (hepatic) veins.

nec·ro·sper·mia (nek-rō-sper′mē-ă). A condition in which there are dead or immobile spermatozoa in the semen. [necro- + G. *sperma,* seed]

ne·cros·te·on, ne·cros·te·o·sis (nĕ-kros′tē-on, nĕ-kros-tē-ō′sis). Gangrene of bone. [necro- + G. *osteon,* bone]

ne·crot·ic (nĕ-krot′ik). Pertaining to or affected by necrosis.

ne·crot·o·my (ne-krot′ō-mē). **1.** SYN dissection. **2.** Operation for the removal of a necrosed portion of bone (sequestrum). [necro- + G. *tomē,* cutting]

osteoplastic n., removal of a bone sequestrum through a hinged window of bone which is then replaced.

nee·dle (nē′dl). **1.** A slender, usually sharp-pointed, instrument used for puncturing tissues, suturing, or passing a ligature around an artery. **2.** A hollow n. used for injection, aspiration, biopsy, or to guide introduction of a catheter into a vessel or other space. **3.** To separate the tissues by means of one or two n.'s, in the dissection of small parts. **4.** To perform discission of a cataract by means of a knife n. [M.E. *nedle,* fr. A.S. *nāedl*]

aneurysm n., artery n., a blunt-pointed, curved n., set in a handle, with the eye at the point, used for passing a ligature around an artery.

aspirating n., a hollow n. used for withdrawing fluid from a cavity, when combined with an aspirator tube attached to one end.

atraumatic n., an eyeless surgical n. with the suture permanently fastened into a hollow end.

biopsy n., a hollow n. used to obtain a core of tissue for histologic study.

cataract n., SYN knife n.

couching n., an obsolete instrument used in couching.

cutting n., a surgical n. with angulated surface designed to puncture tough tissue.

Deschamps n., a n. with a long shaft for passing sutures in the deep tissues.

Emmet's n., a strong n. with the eye in the point, having a wide curve, and set in a handle, used to pass a ligature around an undissected structure.

exploring n., a strong n. with a longitudinal groove, which is thrust into a tumor or cavity to determine the presence of fluid, the latter escaping externally along the groove.

Francke's n., a small lancet-shaped spring-activated n., used to evacuate a small effusion of blood.

Frazier's n., a n. for draining lateral ventricles of brain.

Gillmore n., a device for obtaining the setting time of dental cement.

Hagedorn n., a curved surgical n. flattened on the sides.

hypodermic n., a hollow n., similar to but smaller than an aspirating n., attached to a syringe; used primarily for injection.

knife n., a very narrow, needle-pointed knife used in discission of a cataract. SYN cataract n.

lumbar puncture n., a n., provided with a stylet, for entering the spinal canal or cisterna magna, with a bore of at least 1 mm and 40 mm or more in length.

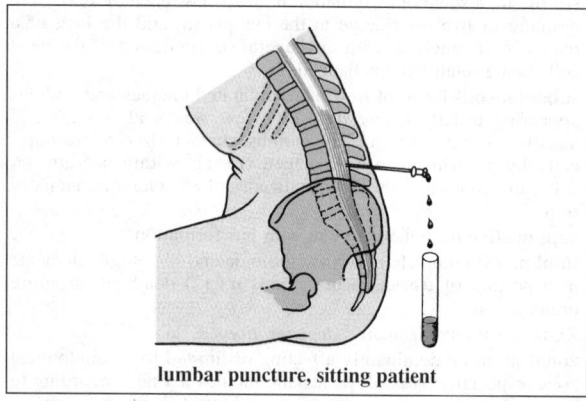

lumbar puncture, sitting patient

Millner n., a fine, non-cutting n. with eye for thread frequently used for suture of skin.

Salah's sternal puncture n., a wide-bore n. for obtaining samples of red marrow from the sternum.

spatula n., a minute n. with a flat (non-cutting) concave surface, used by eye surgeons.

stop-n., a surgical n., with the eye at the tip, the shank of which has a projecting shelf to arrest the n. when it has passed the desired distance through the tissues.

Tuohy n., a n. with a lateral opening at the distal end, designed to cause a catheter passing through the n.'s lumen to exit laterally at a 45° angle; used to place catheters into the subarachnoid or epidural space.

Veress n., a n. equipped with a spring loaded obturator that is used for insufflation of the abdomen in laparoscopic surgery.

Vicat n., a device for obtaining the setting time of plaster and other materials.

nee·dle-hold·er, nee·dle-car·ri·er, nee·dle-driv·er. An instrument for grasping a needle in suturing. SYN needle forceps.

Needles, Carl F., U.S. pediatrician, *1935. SEE Melnick-N. *syndrome.*

Needles, J.W., U.S. dentist. SEE N.'s split cast *method.*

nee·dling (nēd'ling). Discission of a soft or secondary cataract.

Neelsen, Friedrich K.A., German pathologist, 1854–1894. SEE Ziehl-N. *stain.*

ne·en·ceph·a·lon (nē-en-sef'ă-lon). Edinger's term for the higher levels of the central nervous system superimposed upon the metameric or propriospinal system (paleencephalon). SYN neonencephalon. [G. *neos,* new, + *enkephalos,* brain]

NEEP Abbreviation for negative end-expiratory *pressure.*

nef·o·pam hy·dro·chlo·ride (nef'ō-pam). 3,4,5,6-Tetrahydro-5-methyl-1-phenyl-1*H*-2,5-benzoxazocine hydrochloride; an analgesic agent.

Neftel, William B., U.S. neurologist, 1830–1906. SEE N.'s *disease.*

ne·ga·tion (nĕ-gā'shŭn). SYN denial.

neg·a·tive (neg'ă-tiv). **1.** Not affirmative; refutative; not positive; not abnormal. **2.** Denoting failure of response, absence of a reaction, or absence of an entity or condition in question. [L. *negativus,* fr. *nego,* to deny]

neg·a·tive G. Gravity in a foot-to-head direction in flying, or in standing on one's head; opposite of positive G.

neg·a·tive S. SYN flotation *constant.*

neg·a·tiv·ism (neg'ă-tiv-izm). A tendency to do the opposite of what one is requested to do, or to stubbornly resist for no apparent reason; seen in catatonic states and in toddlers.

neg·a·tron (neg'ă-tron). Term used for an electron to emphasize its negative charge in contradistinction to the positive charge carried by the otherwise similar positron.

Negri, Adelchi, Italian physician, 1876–1912. SEE N. *bodies,* under *body, corpuscles,* under *corpuscle.*

Negro, Camillo, Italian neurologist, 1861–1927. SEE N.'s *phenomenon.*

Neisser, Albert L.S., Breslau physician, 1855–1916. SEE *Neisseria;* N.'s *coccus, syringe.*

Neisser, Max, German bacteriologist, 1869–1938. SEE N.'s *stain.*

Neis·se·ria (nī-sē'rē-ă). A genus of aerobic to facultatively anaerobic bacteria (family Neisseriaceae) containing Gram-negative cocci which occur in pairs with the adjacent sides flattened. These organisms are parasites of animals. The type species is *N. gonorrhoeae.* [A. *Neisser*]

N. catarrhalis, former name for *Moraxella catarrhalis.*

N. ca'viae, a species found in the pharyngeal region of guinea pigs; may also be found in other animals.

N. fla'va, a species found in the mucous membranes of the human respiratory tract; easily confused with *N. meningitidis.* SYN *N. subflava.*

N. flaves'cens, a species found in cerebrospinal fluid in cases of meningitis; probably occurs in the mucous membranes of the human respiratory tract.

N. gonorrhoe'ae, a species that causes gonorrhea and other infections in humans; the type species of the genus *N.* SYN gonococcus, Neisser's coccus.

N. haemol'ysans, former name for *Gemella haemolysans.* SEE *Gemella.*

N. meningi'tidis, a species found in the nasopharynx of human but not in other animals; the causative agent of meningococcal meningitis; virulent organisms are strongly Gram-negative and occur singly or in pairs; in the latter case the cocci are elongated and are arranged with long axes parallel and facing sides kidney-shaped; groups characterized by serologically specific capsular polysaccharides are designated by capital letters (the main serogroups being A, B, C, and D). SYN meningococcus, Weichselbaum's coccus.

N. sic'ca, a species found in the mucous membranes of the human respiratory tract.

N. subfla'va, SYN *N. flava.*

neis·se·ria, pl. **neis·se·ri·ae** (nī-sē'rē-ă, nī-sē'rē-ē). A vernacular term used to refer to any member of the genus *Neisseria.*

Nélaton, Auguste, French surgeon, 1807–1873. SEE N.'s *catheter, dislocation, fibers,* under *fiber, line, sphincter;* Roser-N. *line.*

Nelson, Don H., U.S. internist, *1925. SEE N. *syndrome, tumor.*

nem. A nutritional unit defined as 1 gram breast milk of specific nutritional components having a caloric value equivalent to ⅔ calorie. [Ger. *Nahrungseinheit Milch,* milk nutrition unit]

⚠nema-, nemat-, nemato-. Thread, threadlike. [G. *nēma*]

nem·a·thel·minth (nem-ă-thel'minth). A member of the former phylum Nemathelminthes.

Nem·a·thel·min·thes (nem'ă-thel-min'thēz). Formerly considered a phylum to incorporate the pseudocelomate organisms, which now are divided into the distinct phyla Acanthocephala, Entoprocta, Rotifera, Gastrotricha, Kinorhyncha, Nematoda, and Nematomorpha. [nemat- + G. *helmins, helminthos,* worm]

nem·a·ti·ci·dal, nem·a·to·ci·dal (nem'ă-tī-sī'dăl -tō-sī' dăl). Destructive to nematode worms.

nem·a·ti·cide, nem·a·to·cide (ně-mat'ĭ-sīd -ō-sīd). An agent that kills nematodes. [nematode + L. *caedo,* to kill]

nem·a·ti·za·tion (nem'ă-tī-zā-shŭn). Infestation by nematodes.

nem·a·to·blast (nem'ah-to-blast). SYN spermatid. [G., *nēma,* thread + *blastos,* germ]

nem·a·to·cyst (nem'ă-tō-sist). A stinging cell of coelenterates consisting of a poison sac and a coiled barbed sting capable of being ejected and penetrating the skin of an animal on contact; of considerable consequence in large jellyfish and in the Portuguese man-of-war whose large numbers of these stinging cells can cause great pain and even death. SYN cnida, cnidocyst. [nemato- + G. *kystis,* bladder]

Nem·a·to·da (nem-ă-tō'dă). The roundworms, a large phylum that includes many of the helminths parasitic in man and a far greater number of plant-parasitic and free-living soil and aquatic nonparasitic species. For practical purposes, the parasitic nematodes may be placed in two groups, based on their adult habitat in the human body: 1) the intestinal roundworms (*e.g.,* the genera *Ascaris, Trichuris, Ancylostoma, Necator, Strongyloides, Enterobius,* and *Trichinella*); and 2) the filarial roundworms of the blood, lymphatic tissues, and viscera (*e.g.,* the genera *Wuchereria, Mansonella, Loa, Onchocerca,* and *Dracunculus*). [nemat- + G. *eidos,* form]

nem·a·tode (nem'ă-tōd). A common name for any roundworm of the phylum Nematoda.

nem·a·to·di·a·sis (nem'ă-tō-dī'ă-sis). Infection with nematode parasites.

   cerebrospinal n., invasion of the central nervous system by wandering nematode larvae; *e.g., Setaria* species in horses, *Angiostrongylus cantonensis* in rats and humans.

Nem·a·to·di·rel·la lon·gi·spi·cu·la·ta (ně'mă-tō-di-rel'ă lon'gi-spik-yū-lā'tă). One of the thread-necked trichostrongyle nematodes in the small intestine of sheep, goats, reindeer, moose, musk ox, and pronghorn.

Nem·a·to·di·rus (nem-ă-tō'di-rŭs). The genus of thread-necked or thin-necked trichostrongyles; slender, relatively elongated nematodes occurring in herbivorous animals, usually in the small intestine. Generally, they are not believed to be highly pathogenic except in poorly fed, heavily infected animals. Species include *N. abnormalis,* common in the U.S. and occurring in sheep, goats, camels, and mule deer; *N. filicollis,* occurring worldwide in sheep, goats, oxen, and various wild ruminants; *N. helvetianus,* in cattle, sheep, goats, and camels in Europe, Asia, and the Americas; *N. lanceolatus,* in sheep and pronghorns in the Americas; *N. leporis,* in domestic rabbits and wild cottontail rabbits in North America; and *N. spathiger,* the most common, widespread, and abundant species, in sheep, cattle, camels, and other ruminants.

nem·a·toid (nem'ă-toyd). Relating to nematodes.

nem·a·tol·o·gist (nem-ă-tol'ŏ-jist). A specialist in nematology.

nem·a·tol·o·gy (nem-ă-tol'ŏ-jē). The science concerned with all aspects of nematodes, their biology, and their importance to humans. [nematode + G. *logos,* study]

nem·a·to·sper·mia (nem'ă-tō-sper'mē-ă). Spermatozoa with an elongated tail, as in humans, in contrast to spherospermia. [nemat- + G. *sperma,* seed]

Némethy, George, Hungarian-U.S. biochemist, *1934. SEE Adair-Koshland-Némethy-Filmer *model;* Koshland-N.-Filmer *model.*

⚠neo-. New, recent. [G. *neos*]

ne·o·an·ti·gens (nē-ō-an'ti-jenz). SYN tumor *antigens,* under *antigen.*

ne·o·ars·phen·a·mine (nē'ō-ar-sfen'ă-mēn). Sodium arsphenamine methylenesulfoxylate; formerly used as an antisyphilitic agent.

ne·o·ar·thro·sis (nē-ō-ar-thrō'sis). SYN nearthrosis.

Ne·o·as·ca·ris vi·tu·lo·rum (nē-ō-as'kă-ris vit-yū-lō'rŭm). The large roundworm occurring in the small intestine of cattle, water buffalo, and (rarely) sheep; although uncommon in the U.S., it is a serious cattle parasite in many other areas. Experimental infection has been produced in rodents and humans.

ne·o·bi·o·gen·e·sis (nē'ō-bī-ō-jen'ě-sis). The theory that life can originate from nonliving matter. [neo- + G. *bios,* life, + *genesis,* origin]

ne·o·blas·tic (nē-ō-blas'tik). Developing in or characteristic of new tissue. [neo- + G. *blastos,* germ, offspring]

ne·o·cer·e·bel·lum (nē'ō-ser-ě-bel'ŭm) [NA]. Phylogenetic term referring to the larger lateral portion of the cerebellar hemisphere receiving its dominant input from the pontine nuclei which, in turn, are dominated by afferent nerves originating from all parts of the cerebral cortex; phylogenetically, of more recent origin than the archicerebellum and paleocerebellum, *q.v.,* the n. reaches its largest development in humans and other primates. SYN corticocerebellum.

ne·o·chy·mo·tryp·sin·o·gen (nē-ō-kī'mō-trip-sin'ō-jen). An intermediate in the conversion of chymotrypsin to α-chymotrypsin by chymotrypsin cleavage.

ne·o·cin·cho·phen (nē-ō-sin'kō-fen). The ethyl ester of 6-methyl-2-phenylquinolin-4-carboxylic acid; its action and uses are similar to those of cinchophen.

ne·o·cor·tex (nē-ō-kōr'teks). SYN isocortex.

ne·o·cys·tos·to·my (nē'ō-sis-tos'tō-mē). An operation in which the ureter is implanted into the bladder. [neo- + G. *kystis,* bladder, + *stoma,* mouth]

ne·o·dym·i·um (Nd) (nē-ō-dim'ē-ŭm). One of the rare earth elements; atomic no. 60, atomic wt. 144.24. [*neo-,* new, + G. *didymos,* twin (of lanthanum)]

ne·o·en·ceph·a·lon (nē-ō-en-sef'ă-lon). SYN neencephalon.

ne·o·fe·tal (nē-ō-fē'tăl). Relating to the neofetus or to the transition between the embryonic and fetal periods of development.

ne·o·fe·tus (nē-ō-fē'tŭs). The intrauterine organism at about 8 weeks of development.

ne·o·for·ma·tion (nē'ō-fōr-mā'shŭn). **1.** Formation of neoplasia, or a neoplasm. **2.** Sometimes used to indicate the process of regeneration, or a regenerated tissue or part.

ne·og·a·la (nē-og'ă-lă). The first milk formed in the breasts after childbirth. [neo- + G. *gala,* milk]

⚠ **Combining forms**	**[NA] Nomina Anatomica**
Word*Finder*	**[MIM] Mendelian**
Multi-term entry finder	**Inheritance in Man**
Preceding letter A	
A.D.A.M. Anatomy Plates	☆ **Official alternate term**
Between letters L and M	
	☆**[NA] Official alternate**
Appendices:	**Nomina Anatomica term**
Following letter Z	
	High Profile Term
SYN Synonym; Cf., compare	

ne·o·gen·e·sis (nē-ō-jen′ĕ-sis). SYN regeneration (1). [neo- + G. *genesis,* origin]

ne·o·ge·net·ic (nē′ō-je-net′ik). Pertaining to or characterized by neogenesis.

ne·o·ki·net·ic (nē′ō-ki-net′ik). Denoting one of the divisions of the motor system, the function of which is the transmission of isolated synergic movements of voluntary origin; it represents a more highly specialized form of movement than the paleokinetic function. [neo- + G. *kinētikos,* relating to movement]

ne·o·lal·lism (nē-ō-lal′izm). Abnormal use of neologisms in speech. [neo- + G. *laleō,* to chatter]

ne·ol·o·gism (nē-ol′ō-jizm). A new word or phrase of the patient's own making often seen in schizophrenia (*e.g.,* headshoe to mean hat), or an existing word used in a new sense; in psychiatry, such usages may have meaning only to the patient or be indicative of his condition. [neo- + G. *logos,* word]

ne·o·mem·brane (nē-ō-mem′brān). SYN false *membrane.*

ne·o·morph, ne·o·mor·phism (nē′ō-mōrf, nē′ō-mōr′fizm). A new formation; a structure found in higher organisms, only slight or no traces of which exist in lower orders. [neo- + G. *morphē,* form]

ne·o·my·cin sul·fate (nē-ō-mī′sin). The sulfate of an antibacterial antibiotic substance produced by the growth of *Streptomyces fradiae,* active against a variety of Gram-positive and Gram-negative bacteria.

ne·on (Ne) (nē′on). An inert gaseous element in the atmosphere, separated from argon by Ramsay and Travers in 1898; atomic no. 10, atomic wt. 20.1797. [G. *neos,* new]

ne·o·na·tal (nē-ō-nā′tăl). Relating to the period immediately succeeding birth and continuing through the first 28 days of life. SYN newborn. [neo- + L. *natalis,* relating to birth]

ne·o·nate (nē′ō-nāt). A neonatal infant. SYN newborn. [neo- + L. *natus,* born, fr. *nascor,* to be born]

ne·o·na·tol·o·gist (nē′ō-nā-tol′ō-jist). One who specializes in neonatology.

ne·o·na·tol·o·gy (nē′ō-nā-tol′ō-jē). The pediatric subspecialty concerned with disorders of the neonate. SYN neonatal medicine. [neo- + L. *natus,* pp. born, + G. *logos,* theory]

ne·o·pal·li·um (nē-ō-pal′ē-ŭm). SYN isocortex.

ne·op·a·thy (nē-op′ă-thē). A new lesion or pathologic process. [neo- + G. *pathos,* disease]

ne·o·pho·bia (nē-ō-fō′bē-ă). Morbid aversion to, or dread of, novelty or the unknown. [neo- + G. *phobos,* fear]

ne·o·phre·nia (nē-ō-frē′nē-ă). Rarely used term for any major mental disorder (psychosis) occurring in childhood. [neo- + G. *phrēn,* mind]

ne·o·pla·sia (nē-ō-plā′zē-ă). The pathologic process that results in the formation and growth of a neoplasm. [neo- + G. *plasis,* a molding]

cervical intraepithelial n., dysplastic changes beginning at the squamocolumnar junction in the uterine cervix which may be precursors of squamous cell carcinoma: grade 1, mild dysplasia involving the lower one-third or less of the epithelial thickness; grade 2, moderate dysplasia with one-third to two-thirds involvement; grade 3, severe dysplasia or carcinoma in situ, with two-thirds to full-thickness involvement.

lobular n., SYN noninfiltrating lobular *carcinoma.*

multiple endocrine n., type 2, SYN Sipple's *syndrome.*

prostatic intraepithelial n. (PIN), dysplastic changes involving glands and ducts of the prostate which may be a precursor of adenocarcinoma; low grade (PIN 1), mild dysplasia with cell crowding variation in nuclear size and shape, and irregular cell spacing; high grade (PIN 2 and 3), moderate to severe dysplasia with cell crowding, nucleomegaly and nucleolomegaly, and irregular cell spacing.

ne·o·plasm (nē′ō-plazm). An abnormal tissue that grows by cellular proliferation more rapidly than normal and continues to grow after the stimuli that initiated the new growth cease. N.'s show partial or complete lack of structural organization and functional coordination with the normal tissue, and usually form a distinct mass of tissue which may be either benign (benign

tumor) or malignant (cancer). SYN new growth, tumor (2). [neo- + G. *plasma,* thing formed]

histoid n., old term for a n. characterized by a cytohistologic pattern that closely resembles the tissue from which the neoplastic cells are derived.

ne·o·plas·tic (nē-ō-plas′tik). Pertaining to or characterized by neoplasia, or containing a neoplasm.

ne·op·ter·in (nē-op′trin). A pteridine present in body fluids; elevated levels result from immune system activation, malignant disease, allograft rejection, and viral infections (especially as in AIDS). [neo- + G. *pteron,* wing, + -in]

ne·o·pyr·i·thi·a·min (nē′ō-pir-i-thī′ă-min). SYN pyrithiamin.

ne·o·ret·i·nal b (nē-ō-ret′in-al). SYN 11-*cis*-retinal.

ne·o·ret·i·nene B (nē-ō-ret′i-nēn). SYN 11-*cis*-retinol.

Ne·o·rick·ett·sia hel·min·the·ca (nē′ō-ri-ket′sē-ă hel-min′thē-kă). A rickettsial organism that is the agent of salmon disease of dogs and is transmitted by the heterophyid fluke, *Nanophytes salmincola.*

Neospora canium. A protozoan parasite of dogs in the phylum Apicomplexa, an intracellular cyst-forming pathogen of neural and other tissues. Its epidemiology and life history are unknown.

ne·o·spor·o·sis (nē′ō-spōr-ō′sis). A recently recognized disease of dogs caused by the protozoan parasite *Neospora canina* and characterized by polyradiculoneuromyositis with ascending paralysis of limbs.

ne·o·stig·mine (nē-ō-stig′min). $C_{12}H_{19}BrN_2O_2$; a synthetic compound, similar in action to physostigmine (eserine); a reversible cholinesterase inhibitor, used as the bromide or methylsulfate salts in the treatment of myasthenia gravis, postoperative distention, urinary retention, and antagonist of stabilizing neuromuscular blocking drugs.

ne·os·to·my (nē-os′tō-mē). Surgical construction of a new or artificial opening. [neo- + G. *stoma,* mouth]

ne·o·stri·a·tum (nē-ō-strī-ā′tŭm). The caudate nucleus and putamen considered as one and distinguished from the globus pallidus (paleostriatum).

ne·ot·e·ny (nē-ot′ĕ-nē). Prolongation of the larval state, as in the Mexican tiger salamander or axolotl, or in certain termite castes held in the larval stage as future replacements of the queen. Cf. pedogenesis. [neo- + G. *teinō,* to stretch]

Ne·o·tes·tu·di·na ro·sa·ti (nē′ō-tes-tū-dī′nă rō-sā′tī). A species of fungus which causes white grain mycetoma in Somalia and elsewhere in Africa.

ne·o·thal·a·mus (nē-ō-thal′ă-mŭs). The portion of the thalamus projecting to the neocortex.

ne·o·ty·ro·sine (nē-ō-tī′rō-sēn). Dimethyltyrosine; a tyrosine antimetabolite.

ne·o·vas·cu·lar·i·za·tion (nē′ō-vas′kyū-lar-i-zā′shŭn). Proliferation of blood vessels in tissue not normally containing them, or proliferation of blood vessels of a different kind than usual in tissue.

ne·per (Np). A unit for comparing the magnitude of two powers, usually in electricity or acoustics; it is one half of the natural logarithm of the ratio of the two powers. SYN napier. [fr. *neperus,* latinized form of (John) *Napier*]

neph·e·lom·e·ter (nef-ĕ-lom′ĕ-ter). An instrument used in nephelometry. [G. *nephelē,* cloud, + *metron,* measure]

neph·e·lom·e·try (nef-ĕ-lom′ĕ-trē). A technique for estimation of the number and size of particles in a suspension by measurement of light scattered from a beam of light passed through the solution.

△neph·-. SEE nephro-.

neph·rad·e·no·ma (nef′rad-ĕ-nō′mă). Obsolete term for adenoma of the kidney. [nephr- + adenoma]

ne·phral·gia (ne-fral′jē-ă). Rarely used term for pain in the kidney. [nephr- + G. *algos,* pain]

ne·phral·gic (ne-fral′jik). Relating to nephralgia.

neph·ra·to·ni·a, ne·phrat·o·ny (nef-ră-tō′nē-ă, -frat′ō-nē). Obsolete term for diminished functional activity of the kidneys. [nephr- + G. *a-* priv. + *tonos,* tension]

ne·phrec·to·my (ne-frek'tō-mē). Removal of a kidney. [nephr- + G. *ektomē,* excision]

abdominal n., removal of the kidney by an incision through the anterior abdominal wall; performed by either a transperitoneal or extraperitoneal technique.

lumbar n., n. through an incision in the flank or loin, usually with the patient in the lateral position.

posterior n., retroperitoneal removal of a kidney through an incision in the posterior lumbar muscles, usually with the patient in a prone position.

neph·re·de·ma (nef-re-dē'mă). Edema caused by renal disease; rarely, edema of the kidney. [nephr- + G. *oidēma,* swelling]

neph·rel·co·sis (nef-rel-kō'sis). Ulceration of the mucous membrane of the pelvis or calices of the kidney. [nephr- + G. *helkōsis,* ulceration]

neph·ric (nef'rik). Relating to the kidney. SYN renal.

ne·phrid·i·um, pl. **ne·phrid·ia** (ne-frid'ē-ŭm, -ă). One of the paired, segmentally arranged excretory tubules of invertebrates such as the annelids. [G. *nephros,* kidney, + Mod. L. *-idium,* dim. suffix, fr. G. *-idion*]

ne·phrit·ic (ne-frit'ik). Relating to or suffering from nephritis.

ne·phri·tis, pl. **ne·phrit·i·des** (ne-frī'tis, -frit'i-dēz). Inflammation of the kidneys. [nephr- + G. *-itis,* inflammation]

acute n., SYN acute *glomerulonephritis.*

acute interstitial n., interstitial n. with variable tubular damage and infiltration by numerous neutrophils, due to bacterial infection, urinary tract obstruction, or other causes (including drugs) which may be hypersensitivity reactions; accompanied by renal failure, fever, blood or tissue eosinophilia, and rash.

analgesic n., chronic interstitial n. with renal papillary necrosis, occurring in patients with a long history of excessive consumption of analgesics, especially those containing phenacetin. SYN analgesic nephropathy.

anti-basement membrane n., glomerulonephritis produced by autologous or heterologous antibodies to the glomerular capillary basement membranes, the latter known as anti-kidney serum n.

anti-kidney serum n., experimental glomerulonephritis produced by injection of antiserum to kidney.

chronic n., SYN chronic *glomerulonephritis.*

Ellis type 1 n., SYN Ellis type 1 *glomerulonephritis.*

focal n., SYN focal *glomerulonephritis.*

glomerular n., SYN glomerulonephritis.

n. gravida'rum, n. developing in pregnancy.

hemorrhagic n., acute glomerulonephritis accompanied by hematuria.

hereditary n. [MIM*161900], familial renal disease progressing to chronic renal failure, especially in males; associated with nerve deafness. SEE ALSO Alport's *syndrome.*

immune complex n., an immune complex disease resulting from glomerular deposits, as in systemic lupus erythematosus.

interstitial n., a form of n. in which the interstitial connective tissue is chiefly affected.

lupus n., glomerulonephritis occurring in some patients with systemic lupus erythematosus, characterized by hematuria and a progressive course culminating in renal failure, often without hypertension; sometimes also applied to the nephrotic syndrome in patients with systemic lupus. Renal biopsies in patients with a progressive course show diffuse proliferative glomerulonephritis; in milder cases, there are focal proliferative glomerular lesions or mesangial nephritis.

Masugi's n., glomerulonephritis produced by injecting into rats a rabbit antiserum prepared against rat kidney tissue suspensions.

mesangial n., glomerulonephritis with an increase in glomerular mesangial cells or matrix, or mesangial deposits.

salt-losing n., a rare disorder resulting from renal tubular damage of a variety of etiologies; mimics adrenocortical insufficiency in that abnormal renal loss of sodium chloride occurs, accompanied by hyponatremia, azotemia, acidosis, dehydration, and vascular collapse. SYN salt-losing syndrome, Thorn's syndrome.

scarlatinal n., acute glomerulonephritis occurring as a complication of scarlet fever.

serum n., glomerulonephritis occurring in serum sickness or in animals injected with foreign serum protein.

subacute n., SYN subacute *glomerulonephritis.*

suppurative n., focal glomerulonephritis with abscess formation in the kidney.

syphilitic n., a rare complication of congenital and secondary syphilis, with the nephrotic syndrome, resulting from glomerular immune-complex deposits.

transfusion n., renal failure and tubular damage resulting from the transfusion of incompatible blood; the hemoglobin of the hemolyzed red cells is deposited as casts in the renal tubules.

trench n., obsolete term for glomerulonephritis occurring in soldiers subjected to cold and damp conditions in trenches.

tuberculous n., n., mainly interstitial, due to the tubercle bacillus.

tubulointerstitial n., n. affecting renal tubules and interstitial tissue, with infiltration by plasma cells and mononuclear cells; seen in lupus n., allograft rejection, and methicillin sensitization.

uranium n., an experimental n. produced by the administration of uranium nitrate.

ne·phrit·o·gen·ic (nef'ri-tō-jen'ik). Causing nephritis; said of conditions or agents. [nephritis + G. *genesis,* production]

△**nephro-, nephr-.** The kidney. SEE ALSO reno-. [G. *nephros,* kidney]

neph·ro·blas·te·ma (nef'rō-blas-tē'mă). SYN nephric *blastema.* [nephro- + G. *blastēma,* a sprout]

neph·ro·blas·to·ma (nef'rō-blas-tō'mă). SYN Wilms' *tumor.*

neph·ro·cal·ci·no·sis (nef'rō-kal-si-nō'sis). A form of renal lithiasis characterized by diffusely scattered foci of calcification in the renal parenchyma; deposits of calcium phosphate, calcium oxalate monohydrate, and similar compounds are usually demonstrable radiologically. [nephro- + calcinosis]

neph·ro·cap·sec·to·my (nef'rō-kap-sek'tō-mē). Obsolete operation for decortication, or decapsulation, of the kidney. [nephro- + L. *capsula,* a small box, + G. *ektomē,* excision]

neph·ro·car·di·ac (nef'rō-kar'dē-ak). SYN cardiorenal. [nephro- + G. *kardia,* heart]

neph·ro·cele (nef'rō-sēl). **1.** Hernial displacement of a kidney. [nephro- + G. *kēlē,* hernia] **2.** In lower vertebrates, the developmental cavity connecting the myocele with the celom. SYN nephrotomic cavity. [nephro- + G. *koilōma,* a hollow (celom)]

neph·ro·cys·to·sis (nef'rō-sis-tō'sis). Formation of renal cysts. [nephro- + G. *kystis,* cyst, + *-osis,* condition]

neph·ro·ge·net·ic, neph·ro·gen·ic (nef'rō-jĕ-net'ik, -jen'ik). Developing into kidney tissue. [nephro- + G. *genesis,* origin]

ne·phrog·e·nous (ne-froj'ĕ-nŭs). Developing from kidney tissue.

neph·ro·gram (nef'rō-gram). Radiographic examination of the kidney after the intravenous injection of a water-soluble iodinated contrast material; also, the diffuse opacification of the renal parenchyma following such injection, an indication of renal blood flow and glomerular filtration. A persistent nephrogram indicates obstruction of kidney drainage.

ne·phrog·ra·phy (ne-frog'ră-fē). Radiography of the kidney. [nephro- + G. *graphō,* to write]

neph·ro·hy·dro·sis (nef'rō-hī-drō'sis). SYN hydronephrosis.

neph·roid (nef'royd). Kidney-shaped; resembling a kidney. SYN reniform. [nephro- + G. *eidos,* resemblance]

neph·ro·lith (nef'rō-lith). SYN renal *calculus.* [nephro- + G. *lithos,* stone]

neph·ro·li·thi·a·sis (nef'rō-li-thī'ă-sis). Presence of renal calculi.

neph·ro·li·thot·o·my (nef'rō-li-thot'ō-mē). Incision into the kidney for the removal of a renal calculus. [nephro- + G. *lithos,* stone, + *tomē,* incision]

ne·phrol·o·gy (ne-frol'ō-jē). The branch of medical science concerned with medical diseases of the kidneys. [nephro- + G. *logos,* study]

ne·phrol·y·sin (ne-frol'i-sin). An antibody that causes destruction of the cells of the kidneys, formed in response to the injection of an emulsion of renal substance; it is specific for the species from which the antigen was prepared.

ne·phrol·y·sis (ne-frol'i-sis). **1.** Freeing of the kidney from inflammatory adhesions, with preservation of the capsule. **2.** Destruction of renal cells. [nephro- + G. *lysis*, dissolution]

neph·ro·lyt·ic (nef-rō-lit'ik). Pertaining to, characterized by, or causing nephrolysis. SYN nephrotoxic (2).

ne·phro·ma (ne-frō'mă). A tumor arising from renal tissue. [nephro- + G. *-oma*, tumor]

mesoblastic n., a spindle cell neoplasm of the infant and rarely adult kidney with entrapped renal tubules.

neph·ro·ma·la·cia (nef'rō-mă-lā'shē-ă). Softening of the kidneys. [nephro- + G. *malakia*, softness]

neph·ro·meg·a·ly (nef-rō-meg'ă-lē). Extreme hypertrophy of one or both kidneys. [nephro- + G. *megas*, great]

neph·ro·mere (nef'rō-mēr). That portion of the intermediate mesoderm from which segmented kidney tubules develop. SEE nephrotome. [nephro- + G. *meros*, a part]

neph·ron (nef'ron). A long convoluted tubular structure in the kidney, consisting of the renal corpuscle, the proximal convoluted tubule, the nephronic loop, and the distal convoluted tubule. SEE ALSO uriniferous *tubule*. [G. *nephros*, kidney]

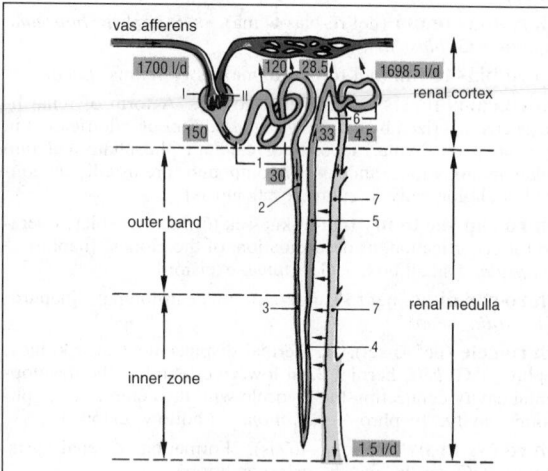

nephron structure and function

I) renal corpuscle; II) glomerulus of renal cortex (+ mesangium) (for nos. 1–7 see accompanying table; *numbers on blue bars* indicate average quantities of liquid passing through different regions daily)

neph·ro·path·ia ep·i·dem·i·ca (nef-rō-path'ē-ă ep-i-dem'i-kă). A generally benign form of epidemic hemorrhagic fever reported in Scandinavia.

neph·ro·path·ic (nef'rō-path'ik). Causing organic renal disease or impairment of renal function.

ne·phrop·a·thy (ne-frop'ă-thē). Any disease of the kidney. SYN nephrosis (1). [nephro- + G. *pathos*, suffering]

analgesic n., SYN analgesic *nephritis*.

Balkan n., interstitial chronic nephritis of unknown etiology, originally described as a disease endemic in the Balkans, characterized by insidious onset, scanty urinary findings, anemia, and acidosis. SYN Danubian endemic familial n.

Danubian endemic familial n., SYN Balkan n.

hypokalemic n., vacuolation of the epithelial cytoplasm of renal convoluted tubules in patients seriously depleted of potassium; vacuoles do not contain fat or glycogen, concentrating ability is impaired, polyuria and polydipsia are common, and pyelonephritis may develop. SYN vacuolar nephrosis.

IgA n., SYN focal *glomerulonephritis*.

IgM n., SYN mesangial proliferative *glomerulonephritis*.

reflux n., damaged renal parenchyma secondary to vesicoureteral reflux of infected urine.

neph·ro·pexy (nef'rō-pek-sē). Operative fixation of a floating or mobile kidney. [nephro- + G. *pēxis*, fixation]

neph·roph·thi·sis (nef-rof'thĭ-sis, -tĭ-sis). **1.** Suppurative nephritis with wasting of the substance of the organ. **2.** Tuberculosis of the kidney. [nephro- + G. *phthisis*, a wasting]

familial juvenile n. [MIM*256100], cystic disease of renal medulla, autosomal recessive type.

neph·rop·to·sis, neph·rop·to·sia (nef-rop-tō'sis, -tō'sē-ă). Prolapse of the kidney. [nephro- + G. *ptōsis*, a falling]

neph·ro·py·o·sis (nef'rō-pī-ō'sis). SYN pyonephrosis. [nephro- + G. *pyōsis*, suppuration]

neph·ror·rha·phy (nef-rōr'ă-fē). Nephropexy by suturing the kidney. [nephro- + G. *rhaphē*, a suture]

neph·ros (nef'ros). ⋆official alternate term for kidney.

neph·ro·scle·ro·sis (nef'rō-skle-rō'sis). Induration of the kidney from overgrowth and contraction of the interstitial connective tissue. [nephro- + G. *sklērōsis*, hardening]

arterial n., patchy atrophic scarring of the kidney due to arteriosclerotic narrowing of the lumens of large branches of the renal artery, occurring in old or hypertensive persons and occasionally causing hypertension. SYN arterionephrosclerosis, senile n.

arteriolar n., renal scarring due to arteriolar sclerosis resulting from longstanding hypertension; the kidneys are finely granular and mildly or moderately contracted, with hyaline thickening of the walls of afferent glomerular arterioles and hyaline scarring of scattered glomeruli; chronic renal failure develops infrequently. SYN arteriolonephrosclerosis, benign n.

benign n., SYN arteriolar n.

malignant n., the renal changes in malignant hypertension; subcapsular petechiae, necrosis in the walls of scattered afferent glomerular arterioles, and red blood cells and casts in the urine, with uremia as a common termination.

senile n., SYN arterial n.

neph·ro·scle·rot·ic (nef'rō-skle-rot'ik). Pertaining to or causing nephrosclerosis.

neph·ro·scope (ne-frō'skōp). An endoscope passed into the renal pelvis to view it. Route of access may be percutaneous, through a surgically exposed kidney, or retrograde via the ureter.

ne·phro·sis (ne-frō'sis). **1.** SYN nephropathy. **2.** Degeneration of renal tubular epithelium. **3.** SYN nephrotic *syndrome*. [nephro- + G. *-osis*, condition]

acute n., acute oliguric renal failure, especially that caused by certain poisons.

acute lobar n., a severe but localized bacterial infection of the renal parenchyma that may produce a mass effect simulating a renal abscess.

amyloid n., (1) SYN renal *amyloidosis*. (2) the nephrotic syndrome due to deposition of amyloid in the kidney.

cholemic n., obsolete term for the occurrence of acute renal failure in jaundiced patients; the kidneys contain tubular casts of bile and may show tubular necrosis, but there is little evidence that jaundice or bile casts directly damage the kidneys.

familial n., the nephrotic syndrome appearing in sibs in infancy, without nerve deafness.

hemoglobinuric n., acute oliguric renal failure associated with hemoglobinuria, due to massive intravascular hemolysis, *e.g.*, following an incompatible blood transfusion; the kidneys show the morphologic changes of hypoxic n.

hypoxic n., acute oliguric renal failure following hemorrhage, burns, shock, or other causes of hypovolemia and reduced renal blood flow; frequently associated with patchy tubular necrosis, tubulorrhexis, and distal tubular casts of hemoglobin.

lipoid n., idiopathic nephrotic syndrome occurring most commonly in children, in which glomeruli show minimal changes with no thickening of the basement membranes, fat vacuoles in the tubular epithelium, and fusion of glomerular foot processes. SYN minimal-change disease, nil disease.

lower nephron n., obsolete term for acute tubular necrosis.

osmotic n., swelling of renal tubular epithelium associated with glomerular filtration of sugars and dextrose; the swelling is due

renal tubule nomenclature			
1 tubulus contortus proximalis	pars proximalis tubuli nephroni (pars convoluta and recta)	principal part	
2 tubulus rectus proximalis			
tubulus attenuatus		nephronic loop (intermediate tubule)	Ansa nephroni (Henle's ansa or loop)
3 pars descendens			
4 pars ascendens			
5 tubulus rectus distalis	pars distalis tubuli nephroni (pars recta + pars convoluta [+pars conjungens = connecting part])	middle part	
6 tubulus contortus distalis			
7 tubulus renalis colligens		collecting tubule	

to formation of cytoplasmic vesicles by pinocytosis, and is reversible, probably with no dysfunction, when produced by glucose or mannitol.

toxic n., acute oliguric renal failure due to chemical poisons, septicemia, or bacterial toxemia; frequently associated with extensive necrosis of proximal convoluted tubules.

vacuolar n., SYN hypokalemic *nephropathy.*

neph·ro·spa·sia, neph·ros·pa·sis (nef-rō-spā′sē-ă, nef-ros′pă-sis). Obsolete term for floating kidney in which the organ is attached only by the blood vessels entering at the hilus. [nephro- + G. *spasis,* a pulling]

ne·phros·to·gram (ne-fros′tō-gram). A radiograph of the kidney after opacification of the renal pelvis by injecting a contrast agent through a nephrostomy tube. [nephrostomy + G. *gramma,* writing]

ne·phros·to·ma, neph·ro·stome (ne-fros′tō-mă, nef′rō-stōm). One of the ciliated funnel-shaped openings by which pronephric and some primitive mesonephric tubules communicate with the celom. [nephro- + G. *stoma,* mouth]

ne·phros·to·my (ne-fros′tō-mē). Establishment of an opening between the pelvis of the kidney through its cortex to the exterior of the body. [nephro- + G. *stoma,* mouth]

percutaneous n., drainage of the collecting system through a catheter inserted through the skin of the flank under fluoroscopic control, usually using the Seldinger technique.

neph·rot·ic (nef-rot′ik). Relating to, caused by, or similar to nephrosis.

neph·ro·tome (nef′rō-tōm). The intermediate mesoderm, sometimes so designated because it evolves into nephric primordia. [nephro- + G. *tomē,* a cutting]

neph·ro·tom·ic (nef-rō-tom′ik). Relating to the nephrotome.

neph·ro·to·mo·gram (nef-rō-tō′mō-gram). A tomographic examination of the kidneys following the intravenous administration of water-soluble iodinated contrast material for the purpose of improving demonstration of renal parenchymal abnormalities. [nephro- + G. *tomos,* a cutting + *gramma,* a writing]

neph·ro·to·mog·ra·phy (nef′rō-tō-mog′ră-fē). Tomographic examination of the kidney.

ne·phrot·o·my (ne-frot′ō-mē). Incision into the kidney. [nephro- + G. *tomē,* incision]

anatrophic n., an incision into the posterolateral renal parenchyma, gaining access to the calyceal system through an avascular plane between anterior and posterior branches of the renal artery; used for removal of calyceal and branched renal calculi, with maximum exposure yet minimal bleeding or parenchymal damage. SYN Smith-Boyce operation.

neph·ro·tox·ic (nef-rō-tok′sik). **1.** Pertaining to nephrotoxin; toxic to renal cells. **2.** SYN nephrolytic.

neph·ro·tox·ic·i·ty (nef′rō-tok-sis′i-tē). The quality or state of being toxic to kidney cells.

neph·ro·tox·in (nef-rō-tok′sin). A cytotoxin that is specific for cells of the kidney.

neph·ro·tro·phic (nef-rō-trof′ik). SYN renotrophic.

neph·ro·tro·pic (nef-rō-trop′ik). SYN renotrophic.

neph·ro·tu·ber·cu·lo·sis (nef′rō-tū-ber-kyū-lō′sis). Tuberculosis of the kidney.

neph·ro·u·re·ter·ec·to·my (nef′rō-yū-rē′ter-ek′tō-mē). Surgical removal of a kidney and its ureter. SYN ureteronephrectomy. [nephro- + ureter + G. *ektomē,* excision]

neph·ro·u·re·ter·o·cys·tec·to·my (nef′rō-yū-rē′ter-ō-sis-tek′tō-mē). Removal of kidney, ureter, and part or all of the bladder. [nephro- + ureter + G. *kystis,* bladder, + *ektomē,* excision]

nep·i·ol·o·gy (nep-ē-ol′ō-jē). Obsolete term for neonatology. [G. *nepios* (adj.), infant, + *logos,* study]

nep·tu·ni·um (Np) (nep-tū′nē-ŭm). A radioactive element; atomic no. 93; first element of the transuranian series (not found in nature); ^{237}Np has a half-life of 2.14×10^6 years. [planet, *Neptune*]

ne·ral (nē′ral). *Cis-*Citral. SEE citral.

ne·ri·ine (nē′ri-ēn). SYN conessine.

Néri's sign. See under sign.

Nernst, Walther, German physicist and Nobel laureate, 1864–1941. SEE N.'s *equation, theory.*

NERVE

nerve (nerv). A whitish cordlike structure composed of one or more bundles (fascicles) of myelinated or unmyelinated n. fibers, or more often mixtures of both, coursing outside of the central nervous system, together with connective tissue within the fascicle and around the neurolemma of individual n. fibers (endoneurium), around each fascicle (perineurium), and around the entire n. and its nourishing blood vessels (epineurium), by which stimuli are transmitted from the central nervous system to a part of the body or the reverse. Nerve branches are given in the definition of the major nerve; many are also listed and defined under branch. SYN nervus [NA]. [L. *nervus*]

abdominopelvic splanchnic n.'s, visceral branches of the sympathetic trunks conveying presynaptic sympathetic fibers to and visceral afferent fibers from the prevertebral ganglia and para-aortic/hypogastric plexuses for the innervation of viscera located below the diaphragm. The greater, lesser, lowest, lumbar, and sacral splanchnic n.'s belong to this group.

abducent n., a small motor nerve supplying the lateral rectus muscle of the eye; its origin is in the dorsal part of the tegmentum of the pons just below the surface of the rhomboid fossa, and it emerges from the brain in the fissure between the medulla oblongata and the posterior border of the pons; it enters the dura of the clivus and passes through the cavernous sinus, entering the orbit through the superior orbital fissure. SYN nervus abducens [NA], abducent (2), sixth cranial n.

nerves of the brain			
I	olfactory nerves	VII	facial n.
II	optical n.	VIII	vestibulocochlear n.
III	oculomotor n.	IX	glossopharyngeal n.
IV	trochlear n.	X	vagus n.
V	trigeminal n.	XI	accessory n.
VI	abducent n.	XII	hypoglossal n.

accelerator n.'s, certain of the cardiopulmonary splanchnic n.'s establishing the sympathetic innervation of the heart; originating from ganglion cells of the superior, middle, and inferior cervical ganglion of the sympathetic trunk, the unmyelinated efferent fibers of the accelerator n.'s stimulate an increase in the heart rate.

accessory n., arises by two sets of roots: cranial, emerging from the side of the medulla, and spinal, emerging from the ventrolateral part of the first five cervical segments of the spinal cord; these roots unite to form the accessory nerve trunk, which divides into two branches, internal and external; the internal branch, carrying fibers of the cranial root, unites with the vagus in the jugular foramen and supplies the muscles of the pharynx, larynx, and soft palate; the external branch continues independently through the jugular foramen to supply the sternocleidomastoid and trapezius muscles. SYN nervus accessorius [NA], accessorius willisii, eleventh cranial n., spinal accessory n.

accessory phrenic n.'s, accessory nerve strands that arise from the fifth cervical nerve, often as branches of the nerve to the subclavius, passing downward to join the phrenic nerve. SYN nervi phrenici accessorii [NA].

acoustic n., an archaic term sometimes used to designate the vestibulocochlear n.

afferent n., a n. conveying impulses from the periphery to the central nervous system. SYN centripetal n., esodic n.

Andersch's n., SYN tympanic n.

anococcygeal n.'s, several small nerves arising from the coccygeal plexus, supplying the skin over the coccyx. SYN nervi anococcygei [NA].

anterior ampullar n., a branch of the utriculoampullar nerve that supplies the crista ampullaris of the anterior semicircular duct. SYN nervus ampullaris anterior [NA].

anterior antebrachial n., SYN anterior interosseous n.

anterior auricular n.'s, branches of the auriculotemporal nerve that supply the tragus and upper part of the auricle. SYN nervi auriculares anteriores [NA].

anterior crural n., SYN femoral n.

anterior cutaneous n.'s of abdomen, SYN thoracoabdominal n.'s.

anterior ethmoidal n., a branch of the nasociliary nerve; passes through anterior ethmoidal foramen on superomedial wall of orbit into cranial cavity, giving rise to anterior meningeal n.'s, then passes through cribriform plates into nasal cavity, supplying anterosuperior nasal mucosa. SYN nervus ethmoidalis anterior [NA].

anterior femoral cutaneous n.'s, anterior cutaneous branches of femoral nerve; supplies distal 3/4 of skin and superficial fascia of anterior and medial thigh. SYN rami cutanei anteriores nervi femoralis [NA].

anterior interosseous n., a branch of the median arising in elbow region, running on interosseous membrane, supplying the flexor pollicis longus, part of flexor digitorum profundus and the pronator quadratus muscles, as well as radiocarpal and intercarpal joints. SYN nervus interosseus anterior [NA], ramus profundus

nervi radialis [NA], nervus antebrachii anterior☆ [NA], anterior antebrachial n., volar interosseous n.

anterior labial n.'s, branches of the ilioinguinal nerve distributed to the labia majora, mons pubis and adjacent thigh. SYN nervi labiales anteriores [NA].

anterior scrotal n.'s, the branches of the ilioinguinal nerve, distributed to the skin of the root of the penis, mons pubis, adjacent thigh and the anterior surface of the scrotum. SYN nervi scrotales anteriores [NA].

anterior supraclavicular n., SYN medial supraclavicular n.

anterior tibial n., SYN deep peroneal n.

aortic n., a branch of the vagus which ends in the aortic arch and base of the heart; composed entirely of afferent fibers; its stimulation elicits a brainstem reflex which causes slowing of the heart, dilation of the peripheral vessels, and a fall in blood pressure. SYN Cyon's n., depressor n. of Ludwig, Ludwig's n.

Arnold's n., SYN auricular *branch* of vagus nerve.

articular n., a branch of a nerve supplying a joint. SYN nervus articularis [NA].

auditory n., SYN cochlear n.

augmentor n.'s, SYN cervical splanchnic n.'s.

auriculotemporal n., a branch of the mandibular, usually arising by two roots embracing the middle meningeal artery; it passes through the parotid gland conveying post-synaptic parasympathetic secretomotor fibers from the otic ganglion, and continuing to terminate in the skin of the temple and scalp; also sends branches to the external acoustic meatus, tympanic membrane, and auricle as well as a communicating branch to the facial nerve. SYN nervus auriculotemporalis [NA].

autonomic n., a bundle of nerve fibers outside of the central nervous system belonging or relating to the autonomic nervous system.

axillary n., arises from the posterior cord of the brachial plexus in the axilla, passes laterally and posteriorly through quadrangular space with the posterior circumflex artery, winding round the surgical neck of the humerus to supply the deltoid and teres minor muscles, terminating as the superior lateral brachial cutaneous n. SYN nervus axillaris [NA], circumflex n.

baroreceptor n., SYN pressoreceptor n.

Bell's respiratory n., SYN long thoracic n.

Bock's n., SYN pharyngeal *branch* of pterygopalatine ganglion.

buccal n., a sensory branch of the mandibular division of the trigeminal nerve; it passes downward emerging from beneath the ramus of the mandible to run forward on the buccinator muscle, piercing (but not supplying) it to supply the buccal mucous membrane and skin of the cheek near the angle of the mouth. SYN nervus buccalis [NA], buccinator n., long buccal n.

buccinator n., SYN buccal n.

cardiopulmonary splanchnic n.'s, visceral branches of the sympathetic trunks conveying postsynaptic sympathetic fibers to and visceral afferent fibers from viscera located above the diaphragm, mainly via the cardiac, pulmonary, and esophageal plexuses. The cervical and upper thoracic splanchnic n.'s are part of this group.

caroticotympanic n., one of two sympathetic branches from the internal carotid plexus to the tympanic plexus. SYN nervus caroticotympanicus [NA], small deep petrosal n.

carotid sinus n., a branch of the glossopharyngeal nerve that innervates the baroreceptors in the wall of the carotid sinus and the chemoreceptors in the carotid body. SYN ramus sinus carotici [NA], carotid sinus branch, Hering's sinus n., intercarotid n., n. to carotid sinus, sinus n. of Hering.

n. to carotid sinus, SYN carotid sinus n.

cavernous n.'s of clitoris, n.'s corresponding to the cavernous n.'s of penis in the male, arising from the vesicular portion of the pelvic plexus. SYN nervi cavernosi clitoridis [NA], cavernous plexus of clitoris.

cavernous n.'s of penis, two nerves, major and minor, derived from the prostatic portion of the pelvic plexus supplying sympathetic and parasympathetic fibers to the helicine arteries and arteriorvenous anastomoses of the corpus cavernosum stimulating erection. SYN nervi cavernosi penis [NA], cavernous plexus of penis.

centrifugal n., SYN efferent n.

centripetal n., SYN afferent n.

cervical n.'s, nerves arising from the cervical segments of the spinal cord. SYN nervi cervicales [NA].

cervical splanchnic n.'s, segments of the visceral branches arising from the superior, middle, and inferior (stellate) cervical ganglia; they are part of the cardiopulmonary splanchnic n.'s. SYN augmentor n.'s.

circumflex n., SYN axillary n.

coccygeal n., a small nerve, the lowest of the spinal nerves, entering into the formation of the coccygeal plexus. SYN nervus coccygeus [NA].

cochlear n., the part of the vestibulocochlear nerve peripheral to the cochlear root it is composed of the central nerve processes of which the bipolar neurons of the spiral ganglion, which have their peripheral processes on the four rows of neuroepithelial cells (hair cells) of the spiral organ. SEE ALSO cochlear *root* of VIII nerve. SYN nervus cochlearis [NA], pars cochlearis nervi vestibulocochlearis [NA], auditory n., cochlear part of vestibulocochlear nerve, inferior part of vestibulocochlear nerve.

common fibular n., SYN common peroneal n.

common palmar digital n.'s, four nerves in the palm that send branches (proper palmar digital nerves) to adjacent sides of two digits; three are branches of the median, one is from the ulnar. SYN nervi digitales palmares communes [NA].

common peroneal n., one of the terminal divisions of the sciatic nerve, diverging from the tibial n. at the upper end of the popliteal fossa, then coursing with the biceps tendon along the lateral portion of the popliteal space to wind around the neck of the fibula where it divides into the superficial and deep peroneal nerves. The common peroneal n., or its deep branch, is the most commonly injured n., being located in a lateral subcutaneous position at the fibular neck; a lesion causes a loss of ability to dorsiflex the foot ("foot drop"). SYN nervus fibularis communis [NA], nervus peroneus communis [NA], common fibular n., lateral popliteal n.

common plantar digital n.'s, three nerves derived from the medial plantar and one from the lateral plantar that supply the skin overlying the metatarsals and terminate as proper plantar digital nerves to the side of each toe. SYN nervi digitales plantares communes [NA].

cranial n.'s, those nerves that emerge from, or enter, the cranium or skull, in contrast to the spinal nerves, which emerge from the spine or vertebral column. The twelve paired cranial nerves are the olfactory, optic, oculomotor, trochlear, trigeminal, abducent, facial, vestibulocochlear, glossopharyngeal, vagal, accessory, and hypoglossal n.'s. SYN nervi craniales [NA].

crural interosseous n., a nerve given off from one of the muscular branches of the tibial nerve which passes down over the posterior surface of the interosseous membrane supplying it and the two bones of the leg. SYN nervus interosseus cruris [NA], interosseous n. of leg.

cubital n., SYN ulnar n.

cutaneous n., a mixed nerve supplying a region of the skin, including its sensory endings, blood vessels, smooth muscle and glands. SYN nervus cutaneus [NA].

cutaneous cervical n., SYN transverse cervical n.

Cyon's n., SYN aortic n.

dead n., misnomer for nonvital dental pulp.

deep fibular n., SYN deep peroneal n.

deep peroneal n., one of the terminal branches of the common peroneal nerve, arising at the fibular neck and passing into the anterior compartment of the leg; it supplies the tibialis anterior, extensor hallucis longus, extensor digitorum longus, and peroneus tertius muscles in the leg, then crosses the ankle joint to supply the muscles on the dorsum of the foot (extensors hallucis and digitorum brevis) becoming cutaneous to innervate adjacent sides of the great and second toes. SYN nervus fibularis profundus [NA], nervus peroneus profundus [NA], anterior tibial n., deep fibular n.

deep petrosal n., the deep petrosal branch of the internal carotid plexus, which joins the greater petrosal nerve at the entrance of the pterygoid canal to provide postsynaptic fibers to nerve of the pterygoid canal. SYN nervus petrosus profundus [NA].

deep temporal n.'s, two branches, anterior and posterior, from the mandibular nerve, supplying the temporalis muscle and periosteum of the temporal fossa. SYN nervi temporales profundi [NA].

dental n., (1) layperson's term for a dental pulp; (2) branches of the inferior and superior alveolar n.'s to the teeth. SEE inferior alveolar n., superior alveolar n.'s.

depressor n. of Ludwig, SYN aortic n.

dorsal n. of clitoris, the deep terminal branch of the pudendal, supplying especially the glans clitoridis after passing through the musculature of the urogenital diaphragm, to run along the dorsum of the clitoral shaft. SYN nervus dorsalis clitoridis [NA].

dorsal digital n.'s, SYN dorsal digital n.'s of hand.

dorsal digital n.'s of foot, nerves supplying the skin of the dorsal aspect of the proximal and middle phalanges of the toes. SYN nervi digitales dorsales pedis [NA], dorsal n.'s of toes.

dorsal digital n.'s of hand, terminal branches of the radial and ulnar nerves in the hand supplying the skin of the dorsal surface of the proximal and middle phalanges of the fingers. SYN nervi digitales dorsales [NA], dorsal digital n.'s.

dorsal interosseous n., SYN posterior interosseous n.

dorsal lateral cutaneous n., SYN lateral dorsal cutaneous n.

dorsal medial cutaneous n., SYN medial dorsal cutaneous n.

dorsal n. of penis, the deep terminal branch of the pudendal which runs through the urogenital diaphragm giving branches, then runs along the dorsum of the penis, supplying the skin of the penis, the prepuce, the corpora cavernosa, and the glans. SYN nervus dorsalis penis [NA].

dorsal n. of scapula, SYN dorsal scapular n.

dorsal scapular n., arises from ventral primary rami of the fifth to seventh cervical nerves and passes downward to supply the levator scapulae and the rhomboideus major and minor muscles. SYN nervus dorsalis scapulae [NA], dorsal n. of scapula, n. to rhomboid, posterior scapular n.

dorsal n.'s of toes, SYN dorsal digital n.'s of foot.

efferent n., a n. conveying impulses from the central nervous system to the periphery. SYN centrifugal n., exodic n.

eighth n., SYN vestibulocochlear n.

eighth cranial n., SYN vestibulocochlear n.

eleventh cranial n., SYN accessory n.

esodic n., SYN afferent n.

excitor n., a n. conducting impulses that stimulate to increase function.

excitoreflex n., a visceral n. the special function of which is to cause reflex action.

exodic n., SYN efferent n.

n. of external acoustic meatus, a branch of the auriculotemporal nerve supplying the lining of the external acoustic meatus. SYN nervus meatus acustici externi [NA].

external carotid n.'s, a number of sympathetic nerve fibers conveyed via the cephalic arterial ramus of the sympathetic trunk which extends from the superior cervical ganglion to the external carotid artery, forming the external carotid plexus. SYN nervi carotici externi [NA].

external respiratory n. of Bell, SYN long thoracic n.

external saphenous n., SYN sural n.

external spermatic n., SYN genital *branch* of genitofemoral nerve.

facial n., its origin is in the tegmentum of the lower portion of the pons, and it emerges from the brain at the posterior border of the pons; it leaves the cranial cavity through the internal acoustic meatus where it is joined by the intermediate n., traverses the facial canal in the petrous portion of the temporal bone, and makes its exit through the stylomastoid foramen; it passes through the parotid gland forming the intraparotid plexus, the various branches of which pass to the muscles of facial expression. SYN nervus facialis [NA], motor n. of face, seventh cranial n.

femoral n., arises from the second, third, and fourth lumbar nerves in the substance of the psoas muscle and enters the thigh

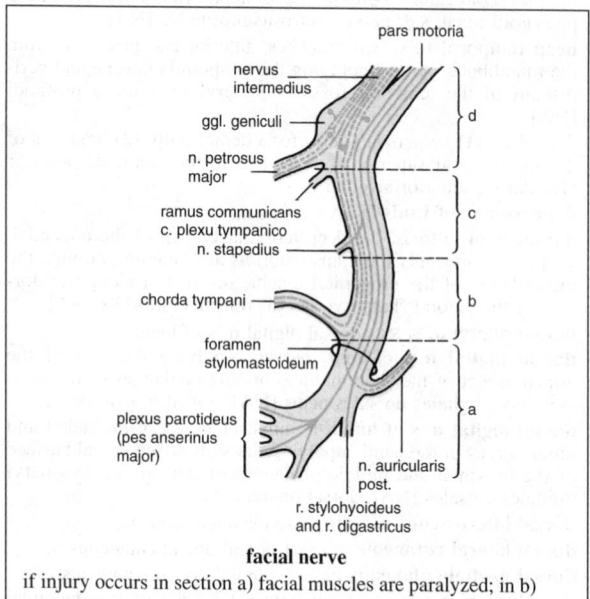

facial nerve

if injury occurs in section a) facial muscles are paralyzed; in b) additional loss of sense of taste and saliva secretion; in c) hearing loss, and d) loss of tear secretion

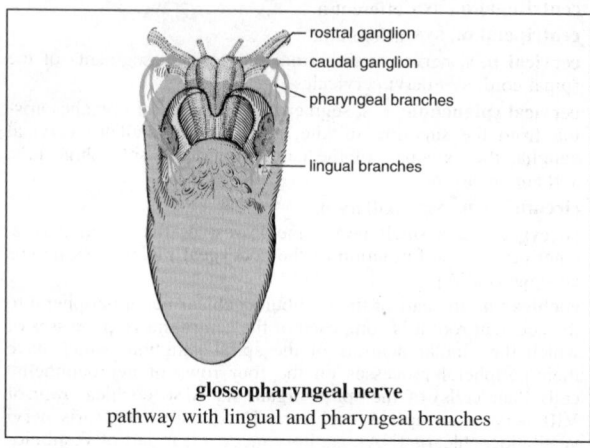

glossopharyngeal nerve
pathway with lingual and pharyngeal branches

via the muscular lacuna beneath the inguinal ligament, lateral to the femoral vessels; it arborizes within the femoral triangle into muscle branches to the sartorius, pectineus and quadriceps muscles and anterior femoral cutaneous n.'s to the skin of the anterior and medial region of the thigh; its terminal branch is the saphenous n. by which it supplies the skin of the medial leg and foot anterior region of the thigh. SYN nervus femoralis [NA], anterior crural n.

fifth cranial n., SYN trigeminal n.

first cranial n., SYN olfactory n.'s.

fourth cranial n., SYN trochlear n.

fourth lumbar n., the ventral branch of the n. is forked to enter into the formation of both lumbar and sacral plexuses. SYN furcal n., nervus furcalis.

frontal n., a branch of the ophthalmic nerve which divides within the orbit into the supratrochlear and the supraorbital nerves. SYN nervus frontalis [NA].

furcal n., SYN fourth lumbar n.

Galen's n., SYN communicating *branch* of superior laryngeal nerve with recurrent laryngeal nerve.

gangliated n., a sympathetic n.

genitocrural n., SYN genitofemoral n.

genitofemoral n., arises from the first and second lumbar nerves, passes distad along the anterior surface of psoas major muscle and divides into genital and femoral branches. SYN nervus genitofemoralis [NA], genitocrural n.

glossopharyngeal n., it emerges from the rostral end of the medulla and passes through the jugular foramen to supply sensation to the pharynx and posterior third of the tongue; it also carries somatic motor fibers to the stylopharyngeus muscle and presynaptic parasympathetic fibers to the otic ganglion. SYN nervus glossopharyngeus [NA], ninth cranial n.

great auricular n., arises from the ventral primary rami of the second and third cervical, spinal nerves, supplies the skin of part of the auricle, adjacent portion of the scalp, and that overlying the angle of the jaw; it also innervates the parotid sheath, conveying from it the pain fibers stimulated by stretching of the sheath during parotitis (mumps). SYN nervus auricularis magnus [NA].

greater occipital n., medial branch of the dorsal primary ramus of the second cervical nerve; sends branches to the semispinalis capitis and multifidus cervicis, but is mainly cutaneous, supplying the back part of the scalp. SYN nervus occipitalis major [NA].

greater palatine n., a branch of the pterygopalatine ganglion that passes downward through the greater palatine canal to supply the mucosa and glands of the hard palate, and the anterior part of the soft palate. SYN nervus palatinus major [NA].

greater petrosal n., SYN greater superficial petrosal n.

greater splanchnic n., uppermost of the abdominopelvic splanchnic which arises from the fifth or sixth to the ninth or tenth thoracic sympathetic ganglia in the thorax and passes downward along the bodies of the thoracic vertebrae, penetrating the diaphragm to join the celiac plexus; conveys presynaptic sympathetic fibers to the celiac ganglia, and visceral afferent fibers from the celiac plexus. SYN nervus splanchnicus major [NA].

greater superficial petrosal n., the parasympathetic root of the pterygopalatine ganglion; a branch from the genu of the facial nerve exiting via the hiatus of the facial canal and running in a groove on the anterior surface of the petrous part of the temporal bone beside the foramen lacerum to join the deep petrosal n., thus forming the n. of the pterygoid canal, which passes through the pterygoid canal to reach the pterygopalatine ganglion. SYN nervus petrosus major [NA], greater petrosal n.

great sciatic n., SYN sciatic n.

hemorrhoidal n.'s, SEE superior rectal *plexus*, middle rectal *plexuses*, under *plexus*, inferior rectal n.'s.

Hering's sinus n., SYN carotid sinus n.

hypogastric n., one of the two nerve trunks (right and left) which lead from the superior hypogastric plexus into the pelvis to join the inferior hypogastric plexuses. SYN nervus hypogastricus [NA].

hypoglossal n., arises from an oblong nucleus in the medulla and emerges by several root filaments between the pyramid and the olive; it passes through the hypoglossal canal, then courses downward and forward to supply the intrinsic and four of five extrinsic muscles of the tongue. SYN nervus hypoglossus [NA], twelfth cranial n.

iliohypogastric n., arises from the first lumbar nerve; it supplies the abdominal muscles and the skin of the lower part of the anterior abdominal wall. SYN nervus iliohypogastricus [NA].

ilioinguinal n., arises from the first lumbar nerve, passes through the inguinal canal and superficial inguinal ring to supply the skin of the upper medial thigh, mons pubis, and scrotum or labia majora. SYN nervus ilioinguinalis [NA].

inferior alveolar n., one of the terminal branches of the mandibular, it enters the mandibular canal to be distributed to the lower teeth, periosteum, and gingiva of the mandible; a branch, the mental nerve, passes through the mental foramen to supply the skin and mucosa of the lower lip and chin. SYN nervus alveolaris inferior [NA], inferior dental n.

inferior cervical cardiac n., a nerve passing from the stellate ganglion to the cardiac plexus. SYN nervus cardiacus cervicalis inferior [NA].

inferior cluneal n.'s, branches of the posterior femoral cutaneous nerve emerging from beneath the inferior border of the gluteus maximus to supply the skin of the lower half of the gluteal region. SYN nervi clunium inferiores [NA].

inferior dental n., SYN inferior alveolar n.

inferior gluteal n., arises from the fifth lumbar and first and second sacral nerves, and supplies the gluteus maximus muscle. It is subject to injury by compression and ischemia in sedentary individuals, resulting in difficulty in rising from a sitting position and difficulty climbing stairs. SYN nervus gluteus inferior [NA].

inferior hemorrhoidal n.'s, SYN inferior rectal n.'s.

inferior laryngeal n., the terminal branch of the recurrent laryngeal nerve; it supplies the laryngeal mucosa inferior to the vocal folds and all laryngeal muscles except the cricothyroid. SYN nervus laryngeus inferior [NA].

inferior lateral brachial cutaneous n., a branch of the radial nerve supplying the skin of the lower lateral aspect of the arm; it frequently is a branch of the posterior antebrachial nerve. SYN nervus cutaneus brachii lateralis inferior [NA], lower lateral cutaneous n. of arm.

inferior maxillary n., SYN mandibular n.

inferior rectal n.'s, several branches of the pudendal nerve that pass to the external and sphincter anoderm and skin of the anal region. SYN nervi rectales inferiores [NA], inferior hemorrhoidal n.'s.

inferior vesical n.'s, several small n.'s once considered to pass from the pudendal plexus to the bladder. (obsolete)

infraorbital n., the continuation of the maxillary nerve after it has entered the orbit, via the infraorbital fissure, traversing the infraorbital canal to reach the face; it supplies the mucosa of the maxillary sinus, the upper incisors, canine and premolars, the upper gums, the inferior eyelid and conjunctiva, part of the nose and the superior lip. SYN nervus infraorbitalis [NA].

infratrochlear n., a terminal branch of the nasociliary nerve running beneath the pulley of the superior oblique muscle to the front of the orbit, and supplying the skin of the eyelids and root of the nose. SYN nervus infratrochlearis [NA].

inhibitory n., a n. conveying impulses that diminish functional activity in a part.

intercarotid n., SYN carotid sinus n.

intercostal n.'s, ventral primary rami of the thoracic nerves. SYN nervi intercostales [NA].

intercostobrachial n.'s, lateral cutaneous branches of the second and third intercostal nerves which pass to the skin of the medial side of the arm. SYN nervi intercostobrachiales [NA], intercostohumeral n.'s.

intercostohumeral n.'s, SYN intercostobrachial n.'s.

intermediary n., SYN *nervus* intermedius.

intermediate n., SYN *nervus* intermedius.

intermediate dorsal cutaneous n., the lateral terminal branch of the superficial peroneal nerve, supplying the dorsum of the foot and dorsal nerves to the toes (except for adjacent parts of great and second toes). SYN nervus cutaneus dorsalis intermedius [NA].

intermediate supraclavicular n., one of several nerves arising from the C-3–C-4 part of the cervical plexus which run across the top of the shoulder and pass down across the clavicle to supply the skin of the top of the shoulder and in the infraclavicular region. SYN nervus supraclavicularis intermedius [NA], middle supraclavicular n.

internal carotid n., the cephalic arterial ramus conveying postsynaptic sympathetic fibers from the superior cervical ganglion to the internal carotid artery to form the internal carotid plexus. SYN nervus caroticus internus [NA].

internal saphenous n., SYN saphenous n.

interosseous n. of leg, SYN crural interosseous n.

Jacobson's n., SYN tympanic n.

jugular n., a communicating branch between the superior cervical ganglion of the sympathetic nerve, the superior ganglion of the vagus nerve, and the inferior ganglion of the glossopharyngeal nerve. SYN nervus jugularis [NA].

lacrimal n., a branch of the ophthalmic nerve supplying sensory fibers to the lateral part of the upper eyelid, conjunctiva, and lacrimal gland. The secretomotor fibers of the latter were conveyed to the lacrimal n. by the communicating branch of the zygomatic n. (a branch of the maxillary n.). SYN nervus lacrimalis [NA].

Latarget's n., (1) SYN superior hypogastric *plexus*. **(2)** terminal branch of anterior vagal trunk which runs along lesser curvature of the stomach to within a few centimeters of the gastroduodenal junction, but apparently never reaching the pyloric sphincter.

lateral ampullar n., a branch of the utriculoampullar nerve that supplies the crista ampullaris of the lateral semicircular duct. SYN nervus ampullaris lateralis [NA].

lateral antebrachial cutaneous n., the terminal cutaneous branch of the musculocutaneous nerve that emerges between biceps brachii and brachialis muscles to supply the skin of the radial side of the forearm. SYN nervus cutaneus antebrachii lateralis [NA], lateral cutaneous n. of forearm.

lateral anterior thoracic n., SYN lateral pectoral n.

lateral cutaneous n. of calf, SYN lateral sural cutaneous n.

lateral cutaneous n. of forearm, SYN lateral antebrachial cutaneous n.

lateral cutaneous n. of thigh, SYN lateral femoral cutaneous n.

lateral dorsal cutaneous n., the continuation of the sural nerve in the foot, supplying the lateral margin and dorsum. SYN nervus cutaneus dorsalis lateralis [NA], dorsal lateral cutaneous n.

lateral femoral cutaneous n., arises from the second and third lumbar nerves, supplies the skin of the anterolateral and lateral surfaces of the thigh. SYN nervus cutaneus femoris lateralis [NA], lateral cutaneous n. of thigh.

lateral pectoral n., a nerve that arises from the lateral cord of the brachial plexus usually passing medial to pectoralis minor to supply the sternoclavicular head of pectoralis major. SYN nervus pectoralis lateralis [NA], lateral anterior thoracic n.

lateral plantar n., one of the two terminal branches of the tibial nerve; it courses along the lateral side of the sole, dividing into superficial and deep branches; it supplies the skin of the lateral aspect of the sole and the lateral one and one-half toes; it innervates the intrinsic muscles of the plantar part of the foot with the exception of the abductor hallucis and the flexor digitorum brevis; its distribution in the foot is very similar to that of the ulnar n. in the hand. SYN nervus plantaris lateralis [NA].

lateral popliteal n., SYN common peroneal n.

lateral supraclavicular n., one of several branches of the C-3–C-4 portion of the cervical plexus which descend to the skin over the acromion and deltoid region. SYN nervus supraclavicularis lateralis [NA], posterior supraclavicular n.

lateral sural cutaneous n., it arises from the common peroneal in the popliteal space and is distributed to the skin of the inferolateral surface of the calf. SYN nervus cutaneus surae lateralis [NA], lateral cutaneous n. of calf.

lesser internal cutaneous n., SYN medial brachial cutaneous n.

lesser occipital n., arises from the ventral primary rami of the second and third cervical nerves; supplies the skin of the posterior surface of the auricle and the adjacent portion of the scalp. posterior to the auricle. SYN nervus occipitalis minor [NA].

lesser palatine n.'s, usually two, these nerves emerge through the lesser palatine foramina and supply the mucosa and glands of the soft palate and uvula; they are branches of the pterygopalatine ganglion and contain postsynaptic parasympathetic and sensory fibers of the maxillary n. SYN nervi palatini minores [NA].

lesser petrosal n., SYN lesser superficial petrosal n.

lesser splanchnic n., one of the abdominopelvic splanchnic n.'s arising in the thorax from the last two thoracic sympathetic ganglia and passing through the diaphragm to the aorticorenal ganglion; conveys presynaptic sympathetic fibers and visceral afferent fibers. SYN nervus splanchnicus minor [NA].

lesser superficial petrosal n., the parasympathetic root of the otic ganglion, derived from the tympanic plexus; it leaves the tympanic cavity through the canal for the lesser petrosal nerve and passes within the cranium to the sphenopetrosal fissure, or to the foramen ovale, or to the petrosal foramen through which it descends to reach the otic ganglion; conveys presynaptic parasympathetic fibers from the glossopharyngeal nerve concerned with secretomotor innervation of the perotid gland. SYN nervus petrosus minor [NA], lesser petrosal n.

lingual n., one of the branches of the mandibular nerve, passing medial to the lateral pterygoid muscle, between the medial pterygoid and the mandible, and beneath the mucous membrane of the floor of the mouth to the side of the tongue over the anterior two-thirds of which it is distributed: it supplies also the mucous membrane of the floor of the mouth. It passes close to the lingual side of the roots of the second and third lower molar teeth and is endangered during tooth extractions. SYN nervus lingualis [NA].

long buccal n., SYN buccal n.

long ciliary n., one of two or three branches of the nasociliary nerve, which by-pass the ciliary ganglion, supplying post-synaptic sympathetic fibers for the dilator pupillae muscle and sensory fibers for the ciliary muscles, iris, and cornea. SYN nervus ciliaris longus [NA].

long saphenous n., SYN saphenous n.

long subscapular n., SYN thoracodorsal n.

long thoracic n., arises from the fifth, sixth, and seventh cervical nerves (roots of brachial plexus), descends the neck behind the brachial plexus, and is distributed to the serratus anterior muscle; it is somewhat unusual in that it courses on the superficial aspect of the muscle is supplies; its paralysis results in "winged scapula". SYN nervus thoracicus longus [NA], Bell's respiratory n., external respiratory n. of Bell, posterior thoracic n.

lower lateral cutaneous n. of arm, SYN inferior lateral brachial cutaneous n.

lowest splanchnic n., one of the abdominopelvic splanchnic n.'s arising in the thorax and penetrating the diaphragm to supply presynaptic sympathetic fibers for the renal plexus; often combined with the lesser splanchnic nerve, but occasionally existing as an independent nerve. SYN nervus splanchnicus imus [NA], smallest splanchnic n.

Ludwig's n., SYN aortic n.

lumbar n.'s, five bilaterally-paired nerves emerging from the lumbar portion of the spinal cord; the first four nerves enter into the formation of the lumbar plexus, the fourth and fifth into that of the sacral plexus. SYN nervi lumbales [NA].

lumbar splanchnic n.'s, branches from the lumbar sympathetic trunks that pass anteriorly to convey presynaptic sympathetic fibers to, and visceral afferents from, the celiac, intermesenteric, aortic, and superior hypogastric plexuses. SYN nervi splanchnici lumbales [NA].

lumboinguinal n., femoral branch of genitofemoral n. SEE genitofemoral n.

mandibular n., the third division of the trigeminal nerve formed by the union of sensory fibers from the trigeminal ganglion and the motor root in the foramen ovale, through which the nerve emerges; its branches are: meningeal, masseteric, deep temporal, lateral and medial pterygoid, buccal, auriculotemporal, lingual, and inferior alveolar; its sensory fibers are distributed to the auricle, external acoustic meatus, tympanic membrane, temporal region, cheek, skin overlying the mandible (except its angle); anterior 2/3 of tongue, floor of mouth, lower teeth and gingiva; its motor fibers innervate all the muscles of mastication plus the mylohyoid, anterior belly of the digestive and the tensores veli palati and tympani. SYN nervus mandibularis [NA], inferior maxillary n.

masseteric n., a muscular branch of the mandibular nerve passing through the mandibular notch to the medial surface of the masseter muscle which it supplies and the temporomandibular joint. SYN nervus massetericus [NA].

masticator n., SYN motor *root* of trigeminal nerve.

maxillary n., the second division of the trigeminal nerve, passing from the trigeminal ganglion through the foramen rotundum into the pterygopalatine fossa, where it gives off ganglionic branches to the pterygopalatine ganglion and continues forward to give off the zygomatic nerve and enter the orbit, where it is named the infraorbital nerve. Its sensory fibers are distributed to the skin and conjunctiva of the lower eyelid, the skin and mucosa of the upper lip and cheek, the palate, upper teeth and gingiva, the maxillary sinus, wings of the nose and posterior/interior nasal cavity. SYN nervus maxillaris [NA], superior maxillary n.

medial antebrachial cutaneous n., arises from the medial cord of the brachial plexus, passes downward in company with the brachial artery and then the basilic vein, and supplies the skin of

the anterior and ulnar surfaces of the forearm. SYN nervus cutaneus antebrachii medialis [NA], medial cutaneous n. of forearm.

medial anterior thoracic n., SYN medial pectoral n.

medial brachial cutaneous n., arises from the medial cord of the brachial plexus, unites in the axilla with the lateral cutaneous branch of the second intercostal nerve, and supplies the skin of the medial side of the arm. SYN nervus cutaneus brachii medialis [NA], lesser internal cutaneous n., medial cutaneous n. of arm, Wrisberg's n. (1).

medial cutaneous n. of arm, SYN medial brachial cutaneous n.

medial cutaneous n. of forearm, SYN medial antebrachial cutaneous n.

medial cutaneous n. of leg, SYN medial sural cutaneous n.

medial dorsal cutaneous n., the medial terminal branch of the superficial peroneal nerve, supplying the dorsum of the foot and dorsal nerves to the toes (except adjacent sides of great and second toes). SYN nervus cutaneus dorsalis medialis [NA], dorsal medial cutaneous n.

medial pectoral n., a nerve that arises from the medial cord of the brachial plexus to supply the pectoral muscles; usually pierces pectoralis minor, then continues to supply mainly the sternocostal portion of pectoralis major. SYN nervus pectoralis medialis [NA], medial anterior thoracic n.

medial plantar n., one of the two terminal branches of the tibial nerve; it courses along the medial aspect of the sole to supply the abductor hallucis and flexor digitorum brevis and, by way of common and proper digital branches, to innervate the skin of the medial part of the foot and medial three and one-half toes. SYN nervus plantaris medialis [NA].

medial popliteal n., SYN tibial n.

medial supraclavicular n., one of several nerves arising from the cervical plexus which supply the skin over the upper medial part of the thorax. SYN nervus supraclavicularis medialis [NA], anterior supraclavicular n.

medial sural cutaneous n., arises from the tibial in the popliteal space, passes down the calf between the two heads of the gastrocnemius and unites in the middle of the leg with the communicating branch of the common peroneal to form the sural nerve, distributed to the skin of the distal and lateral surfaces of the leg and ankle. SYN nervus cutaneus surae medialis [NA], medial cutaneous n. of leg, popliteal communicating n., tibial communicating n.

median n., formed by the union of medial and lateral roots from the medial and lateral cords of the brachial plexus, respectively; it supplies all the muscles in the anterior compartment of the forearm with the exception of the flexor carpi ulnaris and ulnar half of the flexor digitorum profundus; it passes through the carpal tunnel to supply the thenar muscles (except adductor pollicis and the deep head of flexor pollicis brevis) via its recurrent thenar branch; its sensory fibers are distributed to the skin of the palmar and distal dorsal aspects of the radial 3 1/2 digits and adjacent palm. The median n. is most commonly injured through compression in carpal tunnel syndrome, resulting in a loss of ability to oppose the thumb ("ape hand") and loss of sensation over the radial portion of the hand. SYN nervus medianus [NA].

mental n., a branch of the inferior alveolar nerve, arising in the mandibular canal and passing through the mental foramen to the chin and lower lip. SYN nervus mentalis [NA].

middle cervical cardiac n., one of the cardiopulmonary splanchnic nerves conveying postsynaptic sympathetic fibers running downward, from the middle cervical ganglion along the subclavian artery (on the left) or the brachiocephalic (on the right side) to join the cardiac plexus. SYN nervus cardiacus cervicalis medius [NA].

middle cluneal n.'s, terminal branches of the dorsal primary rami of the sacral nerves, supplying the skin of the mid-gluteal region. SYN nervi clunium medii [NA].

middle meningeal n., SYN middle meningeal *branch* of maxillary nerve.

middle supraclavicular n., SYN intermediate supraclavicular n.

mixed n., a n. containing both afferent and efferent fibers.

motor n., an efferent n. conveying an impulse that excites mus cular contraction; motor n.'s in the autonomic nervous system also elicit secretions from glandular epithelia.

motor n. of face, SYN facial n.

musculocutaneous n., arises from lateral cord of the brachial plexus, passes through the coracobrachialis muscle, and then downward between the brachialis and biceps, supplying these three muscles and being prolonged as the lateral cutaneous nerve of the forearm. SYN nervus musculocutaneus [NA].

musculocutaneous n. of leg, SYN superficial peroneal n.

musculospiral n., SYN radial n.

myelinated n., a peripheral nerve whose axons are surrounded by layers of Schwann cell membranes that form the myelin sheath; also called medullated n.'s.

mylohyoid n., a small branch of the inferior alveolar nerve given off posteriorly just before the nerve enters the mandibular foramen, distributed to the anterior belly of the digastric muscle and to the mylohyoid muscle. SYN nervus mylohyoideus [NA], n. to mylohyoid.

n. to mylohyoid, SYN mylohyoid n.

nasal n., SYN nasociliary n.

nasociliary n., a branch of the ophthalmic nerve in the superior orbital fissure, passing through the orbit, giving rise to the communicating branch to the ciliary ganglion, the long ciliary nerves, the posterior and anterior ethmoidal nerves, and terminating as the infratrochlear and nasal branches, which supply the mucous membrane of the nose, the skin of the tip of the nose, and the conjunctiva. SYN nervus nasociliaris [NA], nasal n.

nasopalatine n., a branch from the pterygopalatine ganglion, passing through the sphenopalatine foramen, crossing to and then down the nasal septum, and through the incisive foramen to supply the mucous membrane of the hard palate. SYN nervus nasopalatinus [NA].

ninth cranial n., SYN glossopharyngeal n.

obturator n., arises from the second, third, and fourth lumbar nerves in the psoas muscle, crosses the brim of the pelvis, and enters the thigh through the obturator canal; it supplies muscles of the medial compartment of the thigh (adductors of thigh at the hip joint) and terminates as the cutaneous branch of the obturator n., supplying a small area of medial thigh above knee. SYN nervus obturatorius [NA].

oculomotor n., it supplies all the extrinsic muscles of the eye, except the lateral rectus and superior oblique; it also supplies the levator palpebrae superioris, and conveys presynaptic parasympathetic fibers to the ciliary ganglion for innervation of the ciliary muscle and sphincter pupillae; its origin is in the midbrain below the cerebral aqueduct; it emerges from the brain in the interpeduncular fossa, pierces the dura mater to the side of the posterior clinoid process, passes in the lateral wall of the cavernous sinus and enters the orbit through the superior orbital fissure. SYN nervus oculomotorius [NA], motor oculi, oculomotorius, third cranial n.

olfactory n.'s, collective term denoting the numerous olfactory filaments: slender fascicles each composed of the thin, unmyelinated axons of 8 to 12 of the bipolar olfactory receptor cells in the olfactory portion of the nasal mucosa; the olfactory filaments pass through the cribriform plate of the ethmoid bone and enter the olfactory bulb, where they terminate in synaptic contact with mitral cells, tufted cells, and granule cells. SEE ALSO olfactory *tract.* SYN nervi olfactorii [NA], fila olfactoria, first cranial n., n. of smell, olfactory fila.

ophthalmic n., a branch of the trigeminal nerve that passes forward from the trigeminal ganglion in the lateral wall of the cavernous sinus, entering the orbit through the superior orbital fissure; through its branches, frontal, lacrimal, and nasociliary, it supplies sensation to the orbit and its contents, the anterior part of the nasal cavity, and the skin of the nose and forehead. SYN nervus ophthalmicus [NA].

optic n., originating from the ganglion cells of the retina, it passes out of the orbit through the optic canal to the chiasm, where part of the fibers cross to the opposite side and pass through the optic tract to the geniculate bodies, superior colliculus, and the pretectum. SYN nervus opticus [NA], second cranial n.

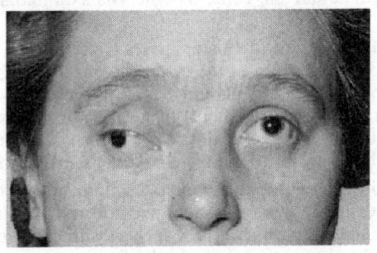

oculomotor paralysis
partial paralysis of oculomotor nerve (right side, after skull/brain injury)

orbital n., SYN zygomatic n.

parasympathetic n., one of the n.'s of the parasympathetic nervous system.

pathetic n., SYN trochlear n.

pelvic splanchnic n.'s, visceral branches from the ventral primary rami of the second, third, and fourth sacral spinal nerves that join the inferior hypogastric plexus, to form the pelvic plexuses to and from which they convey presynaptic parasympathetic and sensory fibers, respectively. SYN nervi pelvici splanchnici [NA], nervi erigentes* [NA].

perineal n.'s, the superficial terminal branches of the pudendal nerve, supplying most of the muscles of the perineum (deep branch) as well as the skin of that region (superficial branch). SYN nervi perineales [NA].

peroneal communicating n., SYN peroneal communicating *branch.*

phrenic n., arises from the cervical plexus, chiefly from the fourth cervical nerve, passes downward in front of the anterior scalene muscle and enters the thorax between the subclavian artery and vein behind the sternoclavicular articulation; it then passes in front of the root of the lung to the diaphragm; it is mainly the motor nerve of the diaphragm but sends sensory fibers to the mediastinal parietal pleura, the pericardium, the diaphragmatic pleura and peritoneum, and branches (phrenicoabdominales branches) that communicate with branches from the celiac plexus. SYN nervus phrenicus [NA].

pneumogastric n., SYN vagus n.

popliteal communicating n., SYN medial sural cutaneous n.

posterior ampullar n., a branch of the vestibular part of the eighth nerve that supplies the crista ampullaris of the posterior semicircular duct. SYN nervus ampullaris posterior [NA].

posterior antebrachial n., SYN posterior interosseous n.

posterior antebrachial cutaneous n., a branch of the radial nerve supplying the skin of the dorsal surface of the forearm. SYN nervus cutaneus antebrachii posterior [NA], posterior cutaneous n. of forearm.

posterior auricular n., the first extracranial branch of the facial nerve, it passes behind the ear, supplying the posterior auricular muscle and intrinsic muscles of the auricle and, through its occipital branch, innervating the occipital belly of the occipitofrontalis muscle. SYN nervus auricularis posterior [NA].

posterior brachial cutaneous n., a branch of the radial nerve supplying the skin of the posterior surface of the arm. SYN nervus cutaneus brachii posterior [NA], posterior cutaneous n. of arm.

posterior cutaneous n. of arm, SYN posterior brachial cutaneous n.

posterior cutaneous n. of forearm, SYN posterior antebrachial cutaneous n.

posterior cutaneous n. of thigh, SYN posterior femoral cutaneous n.

posterior ethmoidal n., a branch of the nasociliary nerve providing sensory innervation to the sphenoidal sinus and the posterior ethmoidal air cells. SYN nervus ethmoidalis posterior [NA].

posterior femoral cutaneous n., arises from the first three sacral nerves, supplies the skin of the posterior surface of the thigh and of the popliteal region (S1 and S2 component); it gives off a perineal branch (S3 component) that passes to the lateral aspect of the scrotum or labia majora. SYN nervus cutaneus femoris posterior [NA], posterior cutaneous n. of thigh, small sciatic n.

posterior interosseous n., the deep terminal branch of the radial nerve, arises in the cubital region, penetrating and supplying the supinator and continuing with the posterior interosseous artery to supply all the extensor muscles in the forearm. SYN nervus interosseus posterior [NA], nervus antebrachii posterior★ [NA], deep branch of the radial nerve, dorsal interosseous n., nervus interosseus dorsalis, posterior antebrachial n.

posterior labial n.'s, terminal branches of the superficial perineal nerve, supplying the skin of the posterior portion of the labia and the vestibule of the vagina, corresponding to the posterior scrotal nerves in the male. SYN nervi labiales posteriores [NA].

posterior scapular n., SYN dorsal scapular n.

posterior scrotal n.'s, several terminal branches of the superficial perineal nerve supplying the skin of the posterior portion of the scrotum, corresponding to the posterior labial nerves in the female. SYN nervi scrotales posteriores [NA].

posterior supraclavicular n., SYN lateral supraclavicular n.

posterior thoracic n., SYN long thoracic n.

presacral n., SYN superior hypogastric *plexus.*

pressor n., an afferent n., stimulation of which excites a reflex vasoconstriction, thereby raising the blood pressure.

pressoreceptor n., a n. composed of afferent fibers the endings of which are sensitive to increases in mechanical pressure; the term specifically refers to sensory n.'s innervating the walls of hollow organs. SYN baroreceptor n.

proper palmar digital n.'s, the palmar nerves of the digits of the hand derived from common palmar digital nerves; each nerve supplies a palmar quadrant of a digit and a part of the dorsal surface of the distal phalanx. SYN nervi digitales palmares proprii [NA].

proper plantar digital n.'s, the ten nerves derived from the common plantar digital nerves; each nerve supplies a plantar quadrant of a toe and part of the dorsal surface of the distal phalanx. SYN nervi digitales plantares proprii [NA].

pterygoid n., one of two motor branches, lateral and medial, of the mandibular nerve, supplying the lateral and medial pterygoid muscles with fibers of the motor root of the trigeninal nerve. SYN nervus pterygoideus [NA].

n. of pterygoid canal, the nerve constituting the parasympathetic and sympathetic root of the pterygopalatine ganglion; it is formed in the region of the foramen lacerum by the union of the greater superficial petrosal and the deep petrosal nerves, and runs through the pterygoid canal to the pterygopalatine fossa. SYN nervus canalis pterygoidei [NA], radix facialis [NA], facial root, vidian n.

pterygopalatine n.'s, SYN ganglionic *branches* of maxillary nerve, under *branch.*

pudendal n., formed by fibers from the ventral primary rami of the second, third, and fourth sacral spinal nerves; it exits the pelvis via the greater sciatic foramen, passes posterior to the sacrospinous ligament, and accompanies the internal pudendal artery, into the perineum via the lesser sciatic foramen; it gives off inferior rectal nerves, then courses through the pudendal canal in the lateral wall of the ischiorectal fossa, terminating as the dorsal nerve of the penis or of the clitoris. SYN nervus pudendus [NA], plexus pudendus nervosus, pudic n.

pudic n., SYN pudendal n.

radial n., arises from the posterior cord of the brachial plexus; it curves round the posterior surface of the humerus and passes down to the cubital fossa where it divides into its two terminal branches, the superficial branch and the deep branch; it supplies muscular and cutaneous branches to the posterior compartments of the arm and forearm. The radial n. is most commonly injured by fractures of the middle 1/3 of the humerus, resulting in a loss

of extension at the wrist ("wrist drop"). SYN nervus radialis [NA], musculospiral n.

recurrent n., SYN recurrent laryngeal n.

recurrent laryngeal n., a branch of the vagus nerve curving upward, on the right side round the root of the subclavian artery, on the left side round the arch of the aorta, then passing up behind the common carotid artery and between the trachea and the esophagus to the larynx; it supplies cardiac, tracheal, and esophageal branches terminating as the inferior laryngeal nerve. SYN nervus laryngeus recurrens [NA], recurrent n.

recurrent meningeal n., meningeal branches of 1) mandibular, 2) maxillary, 3) ophthalmic, and 4) spinal nerves.

n. to rhomboid, SYN dorsal scapular n.

saccular n., a branch of the vestibular nerve going to the macula of the sacculus. SYN nervus saccularis [NA].

sacral n.'s, five nerves issuing from the sacral foramina on either side; the ventral branches of the first three enter into the formation of the sacral plexus, and the last two into the coccygeal plexus. SYN nervi sacrales [NA].

sacral splanchnic n.'s, branches from the sacral sympathetic trunk that pass to the inferior hypogastric plexus; part of the abdominopelvic (sympathetic) splanchnic nerves, but their specific function is unclear. They tend to be confused with the pelvic splanchnic nerves, which are much more significant structures. SYN nervi splanchnici sacrales [NA].

saphenous n., a branch of the femoral, extending from the femoral triangle to the foot, becoming subcutaneous on the medial side of the knee; it supplies cutaneous branches to the skin of the leg and foot, by way of infrapatellar and medial crural branches. SYN nervus saphenus [NA], internal saphenous n., long saphenous n.

sciatic n., arises from the sacral plexus, passes through the greater sciatic foramen and down the thigh, deep to the long head of biceps femoris n.; at the apex of the popliteal fossa it divides into the common peroneal and tibial nerves, although the two may separate at higher levels. SYN nervus ischiadicus [NA], nervus sciaticus★, great sciatic n.

second cranial n., SYN optic n.

secretomotor n., SYN secretory n.

secretory n., a n. conveying impulses that excite functional activity in a gland. SYN secretomotor n.

sensory n., an afferent n. conveying impulses that are processed by the central nervous system so as to become part of the organism's perception of self and its environment.

seventh cranial n., SYN facial n.

short ciliary n., one of a number of branches of the ciliary ganglion, supplying the ciliary muscles, iris, and tunics of the eyeball. SYN nervus ciliaris brevis [NA].

short saphenous n., SYN sural n.

sinus n. of Hering, SYN carotid sinus n.

sinuvertebral n.'s, SYN meningeal *branch* of spinal nerves.

sixth cranial n., SYN abducent n.

small deep petrosal n., SYN caroticotympanic n.

smallest splanchnic n., SYN lowest splanchnic n.

small sciatic n., SYN posterior femoral cutaneous n.

n. of smell, SYN olfactory n.'s.

somatic n., one of the n.'s of parietal sensation or voluntary motion, as distinguished from the visceral sensory, involuntary motor and secretory n.'s.

space n., one of the branches of the vestibulocochlear n. distributed to the semicircular canals.

spinal n.'s, the nerves emerging from the spinal cord; there are 31 pairs, each attached to the cord by two roots, anterior and posterior, or ventral and dorsal; the latter is provided with a circumscribed enlargement, the dorsal root (spinal) ganglion; the two roots unite in the intervertebral foramen, and the mixed spinal nerve almost immediately divides again into ventral and dorsal primary rami, the former supplying the anterolateral trunk and the limbs, the latter the true muscles and overlying skin of the back. SYN nervi spinales [NA].

spinal accessory n., SYN accessory n.

splanchnic n., one of the n.'s supplying the viscera. There are three groups of splanchnic nerves: cardiopulmonary splanchnic n.'s, abdominopelvic n.'s, and pelvic splanchnic n.'s. See also entries under the individual listings for the splanchnic nerves mentioned.

n. to stapedius muscle, a branch of the facial arising in the facial canal and innervating the stapedius muscle. SYN nervus stapedius [NA].

statoacoustic n., SYN vestibulocochlear n.

subclavian n., a branch from the superior trunk of the brachial plexus supplying the subclavius muscle. SYN nervus subclavius [NA].

subcostal n., the ventral ramus of the twelfth thoracic nerve; it courses below the last rib, supplies parts of the abdominal muscles and gives off cutaneous branches to the skin of the lowermost ventrolateral abdominal wall and to the superolateral gluteal region. SYN nervus subcostalis [NA].

sublingual n., a branch of the lingual to the sublingual gland and mucous membrane of the floor of the mouth. SYN nervus sublingualis [NA].

suboccipital n., dorsal ramus of the first cervical nerve, passing through the suboccipital triangle and sending branches to the rectus capitis posterior major and minor, obliquus capitis superior and inferior, rectus capitis lateralis, and semispinalis capitis; the first cervical spinal n. is generally considered to have only motor fibers, but the suboccipital n. receives sensory fibers for proprioception via a communicating branch from the second cervical spinal nerve. SYN nervus suboccipitalis [NA].

subscapular n.'s, two branches of the posterior cord of the brachial plexus, an upper and lower, supplying the subscapularis muscle; the lower subscapular nerve also supplies the teres major muscle. SYN nervi subscapulares [NA].

sudomotor n.'s, n.'s containing autonomic (general visceral efferent - postganglionic) fibers that innervate sweat glands.

superficial cervical n., SYN transverse cervical n.

superficial fibular n., SYN superficial peroneal n.

superficial peroneal n., a branch of the common peroneal nerve which passes downward in the lateral compartment of the leg to supply the peroneus longus and brevis muscles and terminate as the intermediate and medial dorsal cutaneous n.'s supplying the skin of the dorsum of the foot and toes (except for adjacent sides of great and second toes). SYN nervus fibularis superficialis [NA], nervus peroneus superficialis [NA], musculocutaneous n. of leg, superficial fibular n.

superior alveolar n.'s, three branches (posterior, middle, and anterior) of the maxillary nerve (or its continuation as the infraorbital n.) that enter the maxilla to supply the mucosa of the maxillary sinus, upper teeth and gingiva. SYN nervi alveolares superiores [NA], superior dental n.'s.

superior cervical cardiac n., the uppermost of the cardiopulmonary splanchnic n.'s which arises from the lower part of the superior cervical ganglion and passes down to form, with branches of the vagus, the cardiac plexus. SYN nervus cardiacus cervicalis superior [NA].

superior cluneal n.'s, terminal branches of the dorsal primary rami of the lumbar nerves, supplying the skin of the upper half of the gluteal region. SYN nervi clunium superiores [NA].

superior dental n.'s, SYN superior alveolar n.'s.

superior gluteal n., arises from the fourth and fifth lumbar and first sacral nerves, and supplies the gluteus medius and minimus and tensor fasciae latae muscles (abductors and medial rotators of the hip joint). A lesion of this n. causes the pelvis to drop on the unsupported side when the foot is lifted off the ground (Trendelenburg sign). SYN nervus gluteus superior [NA].

superior laryngeal n., a branch of the vagus nerve at the inferior ganglion; at the thyroid cartilage it divides into two branches; the internal laryngeal nerve, a sensory branch which supplies the mucous membrane of the larynx superior to the vocal folds, and the external laryngeal nerve, a motor branch which supplies the inferior pharyngeal constrictor and the cricothyroid muscle. SYN nervus laryngeus superior [NA].

superior lateral brachial cutaneous n., the terminal branch of the axillary n. supplying the skin over the lower portion of the deltoid and for a distance below its insertion. SYN nervus cutane-

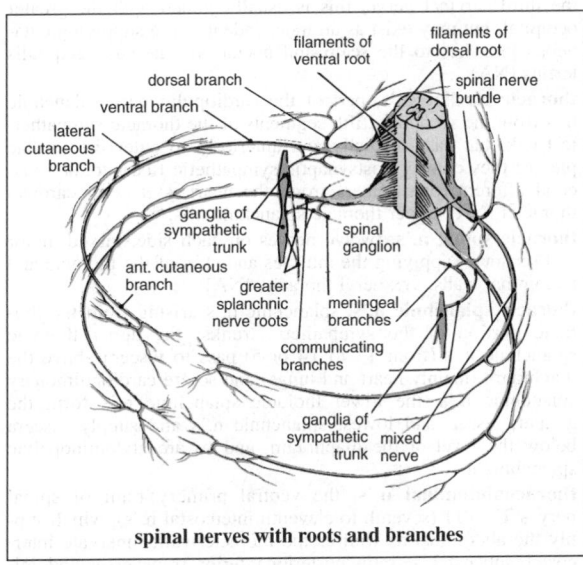

spinal nerves with roots and branches

us brachii lateralis superior [NA], upper lateral cutaneous n. of arm.

superior maxillary n., SYN maxillary n.

supraorbital n., a branch of the frontal n. leaving the orbit through the supraorbital foramen or notch and dividing into branches distributed to the forehead and scalp, upper eyelid, and frontal sinus. SYN nervus supraorbitalis [NA].

suprascapular n., arises from the upper trunk of the brachial plexus (fifth and sixth cervical spinal n.'s), passes downward parallel to the cords of the brachial plexus, then through the scapular notch, supplying the supraspinatus and infraspinatus muscles, and also sending branches to the shoulder joint. It is vulnerable to injury in fractures of the middle 1/3 of the clavicle; a lesion of the suprascapular n. results in a loss of lateral rotation at the shoulder so that when relaxed the limb rotates medially (waiter's tip position); ability to initiate abduction is also affected. SYN nervus suprascapularis [NA].

supratrochlear n., a branch of the frontal n. supplying the medial part of the upper eyelid, the central part of the skin of the forehead, and the root of the nose. SYN nervus supratrochlearis [NA].

sural n., formed by the union of the medial sural cutaneous from the tibial and the peroneal communicating branch of the common peroneal nerve, usually about the middle of the calf, although this is highly variable; thence it accompanies the small saphenous vein around the lateral malleolus to the dorsum of the foot as the lateral dorsal cutaneous n. SYN nervus suralis [NA], external saphenous n., short saphenous n.

sympathetic n., one of the n.'s of the sympathetic nervous system.

temporomandibular n., SYN zygomatic n.

n. of tensor tympani muscle, a branch of the mandibular n. conveying fibers from the motor root of the trigeminal n. which pass through the otic ganglion without synapse to supply the tensor tympani muscle. SYN nervus tensoris tympani [NA].

n. of tensor veli palatini muscle, a branch of the mandibular n.conveying fibers from the motor root of the trigeminal n. which pass through the otic ganglion without synapse to supply the tensor veli palatini muscle. SYN nervus tensoris veli palatini [NA].

tenth cranial n., SYN vagus n.

tentorial n., the tentorial branch, a branch arising in a recurrent fashion from the intracranial portion of the ophthalmic nerve supplying the tentorium and supratentorial falx cerebri. SYN ramus tentorii [NA], nervus tentorii.

terminal n.'s, SYN *nervi* terminales, under *nervus*.

third cranial n., SYN oculomotor n.

third occipital n., medial branch of the dorsal primary ramus of the third cervical nerve; this is usually joined with the greater occipital, but may exist as an independent nerve supplying cutaneous branches to the scalp and nucha. SYN nervus occipitalis tertius [NA].

thoracic cardiac n.'s, part of the cardiopulmonary splanchnic n.'s from the second to fifth segments of the thoracic sympathetic trunk that pass medially and anteriorly to enter the cardiac plexus; they convey postsynaptic sympathetic fibers to, and visceral afferent (pain) fibers from, the heart. SYN nervi cardiaci thoracici [NA], upper thoracic splanchnic n.'s.

thoracic spinal n.'s, twelve nerves on each side, mixed motor and sensory, supplying the muscles and skin of the thoracic and abdominal walls. SYN nervi thoracici [NA].

thoracic splanchnic n.'s, splanchnic n.'s arising from the thoracic portion of the sympathetic trunks; the upper thoracic splanchnic n.'s (from T1 to T4 or 5) pass to viscera above the diaphragm (mainly heart and lungs) and so are cardiopulmonary splanchnic n.'s; the lower thoracic splanchnic n.'s form the greater, lesser, and lowest splanchnic n.'s and supply viscera below the level of the diaphragm, and so are abdominopelvic splanchnic n.'s.

thoracoabdominal n.'s, the ventral primary rami of spinal nerves T7–T11 (seventh to eleventh intercostal n.'s), which supply the abdominal as well as the thoracic wall; innervate intercostal, subcostal, serratus posterior inferior, transversus abdominis, external and internal oblique, and rectus abdominis muscles, and provide sensory branches to the periphery of the diaphragm, and parietal pleura and peritoneum. SYN rami cutanei anteriores pectoralis et abdominalis nervorum intercostalium [NA], ramus cutaneus anterior (pectoralis et abdominalis) nervorum thoracicorum [NA], anterior cutaneous n.'s of abdomen, pectoral and abdominal anterior cutaneous branch of intercostal nerves.

thoracodorsal n., arises from the posterior cord of the brachial plexus; it contains fibers from the sixth, seventh, and eighth cervical nerves and supplies the latissimus dorsi muscle. SYN nervus thoracodorsalis [NA], long subscapular n.

n. to thyrohyoid muscle, the thyrohyoid branch, contains fibers of the first and second cervical nerves that have accompanied the hypoglossal nerve to the suprahyoid region, then branch from it to reach the thyrohyoid muscle. SYN ramus thyrohyoideus ansae cervicalis [NA].

tibial n., one of the two major divisions of the sciatic nerve, it courses down the back of the leg to terminate as the medial and lateral plantar nerves in the foot; it supplies the hamstring muscles, the muscles of the back of the leg (the dorsiflexors and invertors of the foot) and the plantar aspect of the foot, as well as the skin on the back of the leg and sole of the foot. SYN nervus tibialis [NA], medial popliteal n.

tibial communicating n., SYN medial sural cutaneous n.

Tiedemann's n., a sympathetic n. accompanying the central artery of the retina in the optic n.

transverse cervical n., a branch of the cervical plexus that supplies the skin over the anterior triangle of the neck. SYN nervus transversus colli [NA], cutaneous cervical n., nervus cervicalis superficialis, superficial cervical n., transverse n. of neck.

transverse n. of neck, SYN transverse cervical n.

trifacial n., SYN trigeminal n.

trigeminal n., the chief sensory nerve of the face and the motor nerve of the muscles of mastication; its nuclei are in the mesencephalon and in the pons extending down into the cervical portion of the spinal cord; it emerges by two roots, sensory and motor, from the lateral portion of the surface of the pons, and enters a cavity of the dura mater, the trigeminal cave, at the apex of the petrous portion of the temporal bone, where the sensory root expands to form the trigeminal ganglion; from there the three divisions (ophthalmic, maxillary, and mandibular n.'s) arise. SYN nervus trigeminus [NA], fifth cranial n., trifacial n.

trochlear n., supplies the superior oblique muscle of the eye; its origin is in the midbrain below the cerebral aqueduct, its fibers decussate in the superior medullary velum, and emerge from the brain at the side of the frenulum, the only cranial n. to arise from the dorsal aspect of the brain stem; it therefore has the longest intracranial course, entering the dura in the free edge of the tentorium, close to the posterior clinoid process, and passing in

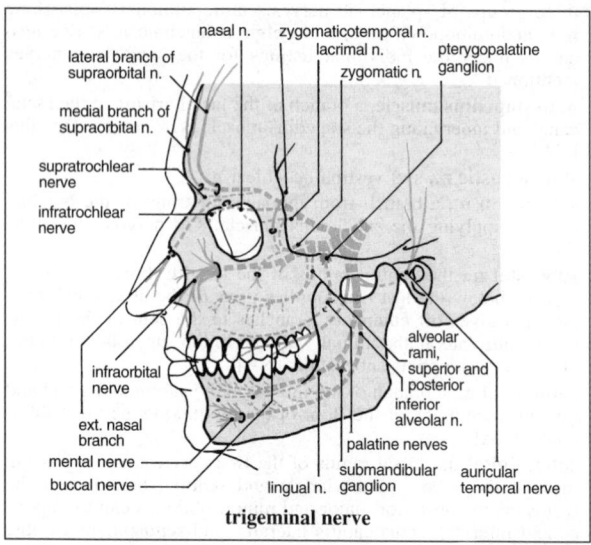

trigeminal nerve

the lateral wall of the cavernous sinus to enter the orbit through the superior orbital fissure. SYN nervus trochlearis [NA], fourth cranial n., pathetic n.

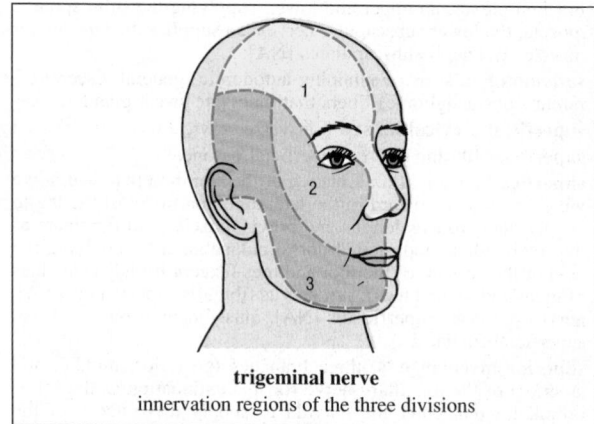

trigeminal nerve
innervation regions of the three divisions

twelfth cranial n., SYN hypoglossal n.

tympanic n., a nerve from the inferior ganglion of the glossopharyngeal nerve, passing through the tympanic canaliculus to the tympanic cavity, forming there the tympanic plexus which supplies the mucous membrane of the tympanic cavity, mastoid cells, and auditory tube; presynaptic parasympathetic fibers also pass through the tympanic nerve via the lesser superficial petrosal nerve to the otic ganglion, where they synapse with postsynaptic fibers that continue to supply the parotid gland. SYN nervus tympanicus [NA], Andersch's n., Jacobson's n.

n. of tympanic membrane, SYN *branch* of auriculotemporal nerve to tympanic membrane.

ulnar n., arises from the medial cord of the brachial plexus and passes down the arm, behind the medial epicondyle of the humerus, and down the ulnar side of the anterior compartment of the forearm to the hand; it gives off muscular branches in the forearm to the flexor carpi ulnaris muscle and the ulnar portion of flexor digitorum profundus and supplies hypothenar, interosseous, medial lumbricals, adductor pollicis and deep head of flexor hallucis brevis; intrinsic muscles of the hand and the skin of the small finger and medial side of the ring finger and adjacent portions of the palm of the hand. The ulnar n. is most vulnerable to injury where it passes subcutaneously behind the medial epicondyle of the humerus. Mild injury here produces "crazy bone" sensation. An ulnar n. lesion here results in loss of flexion of metacarpophalangeal joints and of extension at the interphalangeal joints ("claw hand"). SYN nervus ulnaris [NA], cubital n.

unmyelinated n., a n. made up largely, or exclusively, of unmyelinated fibers; a n. composed of axons having no myelin covering, but lying in troughs in Schwann cells; a slow conducting n.

upper lateral cutaneous n. of arm, SYN superior lateral brachial cutaneous n.

upper subscapular n., SEE subscapular n.'s.

upper thoracic splanchnic n.'s, SYN thoracic cardiac n.'s.

utricular n., a branch of the utriculoampullar nerve, supplying the macula of the utricle. SYN nervus utricularis [NA].

utriculoampullar n., a division of the vestibular part of the eighth cranial nerve; it gives off branches to the macula of the utricle (utricular n.) and to the cristae of the ampullae of the anterior and lateral semicircular ducts (anterior and lateral ampullary n.'s). SYN nervus utriculoampullaris [NA].

vaginal n.'s, several nerves passing from the uterovaginal plexus to the vagina. SYN nervi vaginales [NA].

vagus n., a mixed nerve that arises by numerous small roots from the side of the medulla oblongata, between the glossopharyngeal above and the accessory below; it leaves the cranial cavity by the jugular foramen and passes down to supply the pharynx; larynx, trachea, lungs, heart, and the gastrointestinal tract as far as the left colic (splenic) flexure. SYN nervus vagus [NA], pneumogastric n., tenth cranial n., vagus.

Valentin's n., a n. that connects the pterygopalatine ganglion with the abducens n.

vascular n., a small nerve filament that supplies the wall of a blood vessel. SYN nervus vascularis [NA].

vasomotor n., a motor n. effecting or inhibiting contraction of the blood vessels.

vertebral n., a branch from the stellate ganglion that ascends along the vertebral artery to the level of the axis or atlas, giving branches to the cervical nerves and meninges. SYN nervus vertebralis [NA].

vestibular n., the part of the vestibulocochlear n. peripheral to the vestibular root; it is composed of the central processes of bipolar neurons which have their terminals of their peripheral processes on the hair cells in the ampullae of the semicircular ducts and the maculae of the saccule and utricle, and cell bodies of the vestibular ganglion. SEE ALSO vestibular *root*. SYN nervus vestibularis [NA], pars vestibularis nervi vestibulocochlearis [NA], superior part of vestibulocochlear nerve, vestibular part of vestibulocochlear nerve.

vestibulocochlear n., a composite sensory nerve innervating the receptor cells of the membranous labyrinth; it consists of two major, anatomically and functionally distinct components each of which have different central connections: the vestibular nerve and cochlear nerve. SYN nervus vestibulocochlearis [NA], eighth cranial n., eighth n., nervus acusticus, nervus octavus, nervus statoacusticus, octavus, statoacoustic n.

vidian n., SYN n. of pterygoid canal.

visceral n., a term describing n.'s conveying autonomic (general visceral efferent) fibers.

volar interosseous n., SYN anterior interosseous n.

Wrisberg's n., (1) SYN medial brachial cutaneous n. **(2)** SYN nervus intermedius.

zygomatic n., a branch of the maxillary n. in the inferior orbital fissure through which it passes; it gives rise to two sensory branches, the zygomaticotemporal and zygomaticofacial, which supply the skin of the temporal and zygomatic regions and is continued as the communicating branch of the lacrimal n. with the zygomatic n. SYN nervus zygomaticus [NA], orbital n., temporomandibular n.

nerve root sleeve. in myelography, the funnel-shaped extension of the opacified subarachnoid space that surrounds each nerve root as it enters its neural foramen.

ner·vi (ner'vī) [NA]. Plural of nervus. [L.]

ner·vi·mo·til·i·ty (ner-vi-mō-til'i-tē). Capability of movement in response to a nervous stimulus. SYN neuromotility.

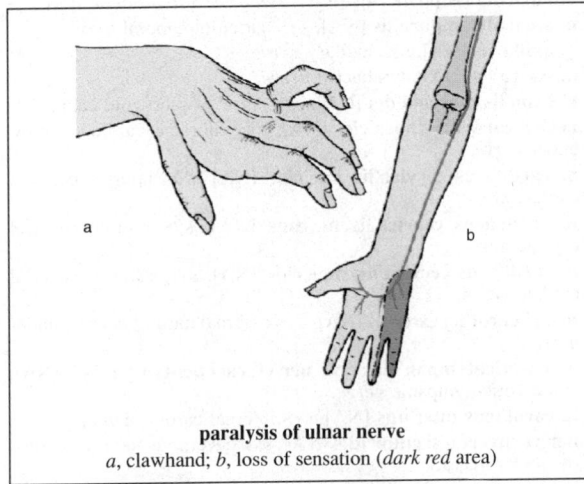

paralysis of ulnar nerve
a, clawhand; *b*, loss of sensation (*dark red* area)

ner·vi·mo·tion (ner-vi-mō'shŭn). Movement in response to a nervous stimulus.

ner·vi·mo·tor (ner-vi-mō'ter). Relating to a motor nerve. SYN neurimotor.

ner·vine (ner'vīn). Acting therapeutically, especially as a sedative, upon the nervous system.

ner·vone (ner'vōn). A cerebroside containing a nervonyl moiety.

ner·von·ic ac·id (ner-von'-ik). *cis*-15-Tetracosanoic acid; a 24-carbon straight-chain fatty acid unsaturated between C-15 and C-16; occurs in cerebrosides such as nervone.

ner·vo·sism (ner'vō-sizm). **1.** Rarely used term for neurasthenia. **2.** Hypothetical dependence of psychiatric conditions upon alterations of nerve force. [L. *nervosus,* nervous]

ner·vous (ner'vŭs). **1.** Relating to a nerve or the nerves. **2.** Easily excited or agitated; suffering from mental or emotional instability; tense or anxious. **3.** Formerly, denoting a temperament characterized by excessive mental and physical alertness, rapid pulse, excitability, often volubility, but not always fixity of purpose. [L. *nervosus*]

ner·vous break·down. Nonmedical term for an emotional or mental illness; often a euphemism for a psychiatric disorder.

ner·vous·ness (ner'vŭs-nes). A condition of being nervous (2).

NERVUS

ner·vus, gen. and pl. **ner·vi** (ner'vŭs, -vī) [NA]. SYN nerve. [L.]

n. abdu'cens [NA], SYN abducent *nerve.*

n. accesso'rius [NA], SYN accessory *nerve.*

n. acu'sticus, SYN vestibulocochlear *nerve.*

ner'vi alveola'res superio'res [NA], SYN superior alveolar *nerves,* under *nerve.*

n. alveola'ris infe'rior [NA], SYN inferior alveolar *nerve.*

n. ampulla'ris ante'rior [NA], SYN anterior ampullar *nerve.*

n. ampulla'ris latera'lis [NA], SYN lateral ampullar *nerve.*

n. ampulla'ris poste'rior [NA], SYN posterior ampullar *nerve.*

ner'vi anococcyg'ei [NA], SYN anococcygeal *nerves,* under *nerve.*

n. antebra'chii anter'ior [NA], ✩official alternate term for anterior interosseous *nerve.*

n. antebra'chii poste'rior [NA], ✩official alternate term for posterior interosseous *nerve.*

n. articula'ris [NA], SYN articular *nerve.*

ner'vi auricula'res anterio'res [NA], SYN anterior auricular *nerves,* under *nerve.*

n. auricula'ris mag'nus [NA], SYN great auricular *nerve.*

n. auricula′ris poste′rior [NA], SYN posterior auricular *nerve*.

n. auriculotempora′lis [NA], SYN auriculotemporal *nerve*.

n. axilla′ris [NA], SYN axillary *nerve*.

n. bucca′lis [NA], SYN buccal *nerve*.

n. cana′lis pterygoi′dei [NA], SYN *nerve* of pterygoid canal.

ner′vi cardi′aci thora′cici [NA], SYN thoracic cardiac *nerves*, under *nerve*.

n. cardi′acus cervica′lis infe′rior [NA], SYN inferior cervical cardiac *nerve*.

n. cardi′acus cervica′lis me′dius [NA], SYN middle cervical cardiac *nerve*.

n. cardi′acus cervica′lis supe′rior [NA], SYN superior cervical cardiac *nerve*.

ner′vi carot′ici exter′ni [NA], SYN external carotid *nerves*, under *nerve*.

n. caroticotympan′icus, pl. **ner′vi caroticotympan′ici** [NA], SYN caroticotympanic *nerve*.

n. carot′icus inter′nus [NA], SYN internal carotid *nerve*.

ner′vi caverno′si clitor′idis [NA], SYN cavernous *nerves* of clitoris, under *nerve*.

ner′vi caverno′si pe′nis [NA], SYN cavernous *nerves* of penis, under *nerve*.

ner′vi cervica′les [NA], SYN cervical *nerves*, under *nerve*.

n. cervica′lis superficia′lis, SYN transverse cervical *nerve*.

n. cilia′ris bre′vis, pl. **ner′vi cilia′res bre′ves** [NA], SYN short ciliary *nerve*.

n. cilia′ris lon′gus, pl. **ner′vi cilia′res lon′gi** [NA], SYN long ciliary *nerve*.

ner′vi clu′nium inferio′res [NA], SYN inferior cluneal *nerves*, under *nerve*.

ner′vi clu′nium me′dii [NA], SYN middle cluneal *nerves*, under *nerve*.

ner′vi clu′nium superio′res [NA], SYN superior cluneal *nerves*, under *nerve*.

n. coccyg′eus [NA], SYN coccygeal *nerve*.

n. cochlea′ris [NA], SYN cochlear *nerve*. SEE ALSO cochlear *root* of vestibulocochlear nerve.

n. commu′nicans fibula′ris, SYN peroneal communicating *branch*.

n. commu′nicans perone′us, SYN peroneal communicating *branch*.

ner′vi crania′les [NA], SYN cranial *nerves*, under *nerve*.

n. cuta′neus [NA], SYN cutaneous *nerve*.

n. cuta′neus antebra′chii latera′lis [NA], SYN lateral antebrachial cutaneous *nerve*.

n. cuta′neus antebra′chii media′lis [NA], SYN medial antebrachial cutaneous *nerve*.

n. cuta′neus antebra′chii poste′rior [NA], SYN posterior antebrachial cutaneous *nerve*.

n. cuta′neus bra′chii latera′lis infe′rior [NA], SYN inferior lateral brachial cutaneous *nerve*.

n. cuta′neus bra′chii latera′lis supe′rior [NA], SYN superior lateral brachial cutaneous *nerve*.

n. cuta′neus bra′chii media′lis [NA], SYN medial brachial cutaneous *nerve*.

n. cuta′neus bra′chii poste′rior [NA], SYN posterior brachial cutaneous *nerve*.

n. cuta′neus dorsa′lis interme′dius [NA], SYN intermediate dorsal cutaneous *nerve*.

n. cuta′neus dorsa′lis latera′lis [NA], SYN lateral dorsal cutaneous *nerve*.

n. cuta′neus dorsa′lis media′lis [NA], SYN medial dorsal cutaneous *nerve*.

n. cuta′neus fem′oris latera′lis [NA], SYN lateral femoral cutaneous *nerve*.

n. cuta′neus fem′oris poste′rior [NA], SYN posterior femoral cutaneous *nerve*.

n. cuta′neus su′rae latera′lis [NA], SYN lateral sural cutaneous *nerve*.

n. cuta′neus su′rae media′lis [NA], SYN medial sural cutaneous *nerve*.

ner′vi digita′les dorsa′les [NA], SYN dorsal digital *nerves* of hand, under *nerve*.

ner′vi digita′les dorsa′les pe′dis [NA], SYN dorsal digital *nerves* of foot, under *nerve*.

ner′vi digita′les palma′res commu′nes [NA], SYN common palmar digital *nerves*, under *nerve*.

ner′vi digita′les palma′res pro′prii [NA], SYN proper palmar digital *nerves*, under *nerve*.

ner′vi digita′les planta′res commu′nes [NA], SYN common plantar digital *nerves*, under *nerve*.

ner′vi digita′les planta′res pro′prii [NA], SYN proper plantar digital *nerves*, under *nerve*.

n. dorsa′lis clitor′idis [NA], SYN dorsal *nerve* of clitoris.

n. dorsa′lis pe′nis [NA], SYN dorsal *nerve* of penis.

n. dorsa′lis scap′ulae [NA], SYN dorsal scapular *nerve*.

ner′vi erigen′tes [NA], ✻official alternate term for pelvic splanchnic *nerves*, under *nerve*.

n. ethmoida′lis ante′rior [NA], SYN anterior ethmoidal *nerve*.

n. ethmoida′lis poste′rior [NA], SYN posterior ethmoidal *nerve*.

n. facia′lis [NA], SYN facial *nerve*.

n. femora′lis [NA], SYN femoral *nerve*.

n. fibula′ris commu′nis [NA], SYN common peroneal *nerve*.

n. fibula′ris profun′dus [NA], SYN deep peroneal *nerve*.

n. fibula′ris superficia′lis [NA], SYN superficial peroneal *nerve*.

n. fronta′lis [NA], SYN frontal *nerve*.

n. furca′lis, SYN fourth lumbar *nerve*.

n. genitofemora′lis [NA], SYN genitofemoral *nerve*.

n. glossopharyn′geus [NA], SYN glossopharyngeal *nerve*.

n. glu′teus infe′rior [NA], SYN inferior gluteal *nerve*.

n. glu′teus supe′rior [NA], SYN superior gluteal *nerve*.

n. hemorrhoida′lis, SEE superior rectal *plexus*, inferior rectal *nerves*, under *nerve*.

n. hypogas′tricus [NA], SYN hypogastric *nerve*.

n. hypoglos′sus [NA], SYN hypoglossal *nerve*.

n. iliohypogas′tricus [NA], SYN iliohypogastric *nerve*.

n. ilioinguina′lis [NA], SYN ilioinguinal *nerve*.

n. im′par, SYN terminal *filum*.

n. infraorbita′lis [NA], SYN infraorbital *nerve*.

n. infratrochlea′ris [NA], SYN infratrochlear *nerve*.

ner′vi intercosta′les [NA], SYN intercostal *nerves*, under *nerve*.

ner′vi intercostobrachia′les [NA], SYN intercostobrachial *nerves*, under *nerve*.

n. interme′dius [NA], a root of the facial nerve containing sensory fibers for taste from the anterior 2/3 of tongue whose cell bodies are located in the geniculate ganglion and presynaptic parasympathetic autonomic fibers whose cell bodies are located in the superior salivatory nucleus, i.e., the fibers eventually conveyed via the chorda tympani branch of the facial n. to the lingual nerve. SYN intermediary nerve, intermediate nerve, portio intermedia, Wrisberg's nerve (2).

n. interos′seus ante′rior [NA], SYN anterior interosseous *nerve*.

n. interos′seus cru′ris [NA], SYN crural interosseous *nerve*.

n. interos′seus dorsa′lis, SYN posterior interosseous *nerve*.

n. interos′seus poste′rior [NA], SYN posterior interosseous *nerve*.

n. ischia′dicus [NA], SYN sciatic *nerve*.

n. jugula′ris [NA], SYN jugular *nerve*.

ner′vi labia′les anterio′res [NA], SYN anterior labial *nerves*, under *nerve*.

ner′vi labia′les posterio′res [NA], SYN posterior labial *nerves*, under *nerve*.

n. lacrima′lis [NA], SYN lacrimal *nerve*.

n. laryn′geus infe′rior [NA], SYN inferior laryngeal *nerve*.

n. laryn′geus recur′rens [NA], SYN recurrent laryngeal *nerve*.

n. laryn′geus supe′rior [NA], SYN superior laryngeal *nerve*.

n. lingua′lis [NA], SYN lingual *nerve*.

ner′vi lumba′les [NA], SYN lumbar *nerves*, under *nerve*.

n. mandibula′ris [NA], SYN mandibular *nerve*.

n. masseter′icus [NA], SYN masseteric *nerve*.

n. maxilla'ris [NA], SYN maxillary *nerve*.

n. mea'tus acus'tici exter'ni [NA], SYN *nerve* of external acoustic meatus.

n. media'nus [NA], SYN median *nerve*.

n. menta'lis [NA], SYN mental *nerve*.

n. musculocuta'neus [NA], SYN musculocutaneous *nerve*.

n. mylohyoi'deus [NA], SYN mylohyoid *nerve*.

n. nasocilia'ris [NA], SYN nasociliary *nerve*.

n. nasopalati'nus [NA], SYN nasopalatine *nerve*.

ner'vi nervo'rum, nerves distributed to the sheaths of nerve trunks.

n. obturato'rius [NA], SYN obturator *nerve*.

n. occipita'lis ma'jor [NA], SYN greater occipital *nerve*.

n. occipita'lis mi'nor [NA], SYN lesser occipital *nerve*.

n. occipita'lis ter'tius [NA], SYN third occipital *nerve*.

n. octa'vus, SYN vestibulocochlear *nerve*.

n. oculomoto'rius [NA], SYN oculomotor *nerve*.

ner'vi olfacto'rii [NA], SYN olfactory *nerves*, under *nerve*. SEE ALSO olfactory *tract*.

n. ophthal'micus [NA], SYN ophthalmic *nerve*.

n. op'ticus [NA], SYN optic *nerve*.

ner'vi palati'ni mino'res [NA], SYN lesser palatine *nerves*, under *nerve*.

n. palati'nus ma'jor [NA], SYN greater palatine *nerve*.

n. pectora'lis latera'lis [NA], SYN lateral pectoral *nerve*.

n. pectora'lis media'lis [NA], SYN medial pectoral *nerve*.

ner'vi pelvici splanch'nici [NA], SYN pelvic splanchnic *nerves*, under *nerve*.

ner'vi perinea'les [NA], SYN perineal *nerves*, under *nerve*.

n. perone'us commu'nis [NA], SYN common peroneal *nerve*.

n. perone'us profun'dus [NA], SYN deep peroneal *nerve*.

n. perone'us superficia'lis [NA], SYN superficial peroneal *nerve*.

n. petro'sus ma'jor [NA], SYN greater superficial petrosal *nerve*.

n. petro'sus mi'nor [NA], SYN lesser superficial petrosal *nerve*.

n. petro'sus profun'dus [NA], SYN deep petrosal *nerve*.

ner'vi phren'ici accesso'rii [NA], SYN accessory phrenic *nerves*, under *nerve*.

n. phren'icus [NA], SYN phrenic *nerve*.

n. planta'ris latera'lis [NA], SYN lateral plantar *nerve*.

n. planta'ris media'lis [NA], SYN medial plantar *nerve*.

n. presacra'lis [NA], ☆official alternate term for superior hypogastric *plexus*.

n. pterygoi'deus [NA], SYN pterygoid *nerve*.

ner'vi pterygopalati'ni, SYN ganglionic *branches* of maxillary nerve, under *branch*.

n. puden'dus [NA], SYN pudendal *nerve*.

n. radia'lis [NA], SYN radial *nerve*.

ner'vi recta'les inferio'res [NA], SYN inferior rectal *nerves*, under *nerve*.

n. saccula'ris [NA], SYN saccular *nerve*.

ner'vi sacra'les [NA], SYN sacral *nerves*, under *nerve*.

n. saphe'nus [NA], SYN saphenous *nerve*.

n. sciaticus, ☆official alternate term for sciatic *nerve*.

ner'vi scrota'les anterio'res [NA], SYN anterior scrotal *nerves*, under *nerve*.

ner'vi scrota'les posterio'res [NA], SYN posterior scrotal *nerves*, under *nerve*.

n. spermat'icus exter'nus, SYN genital *branch* of genitofemoral nerve.

ner'vi sphenopalati'ni, SYN ganglionic *branches* of maxillary nerve, under *branch*.

ner'vi spina'les [NA], SYN spinal *nerves*, under *nerve*.

n. spinosus, SYN meningeal *branch* of mandibular nerve.

ner'vi splanch'nici lumba'les [NA], SYN lumbar splanchnic *nerves*, under *nerve*.

ner'vi splanch'nici sacra'les [NA], SYN sacral splanchnic *nerves*, under *nerve*.

n. splanch'nicus i'mus [NA], SYN lowest splanchnic *nerve*.

n. splanch'nicus ma'jor [NA], SYN greater splanchnic *nerve*.

n. splanch'nicus mi'nor [NA], SYN lesser splanchnic *nerve*.

n. stape'dius [NA], SYN *nerve* to stapedius muscle.

n. statoacus'ticus, SYN vestibulocochlear *nerve*.

n. subcla'vius [NA], SYN subclavian *nerve*.

n. subcosta'lis [NA], SYN subcostal *nerve*.

n. sublingua'lis [NA], SYN sublingual *nerve*.

n. suboccipita'lis [NA], SYN suboccipital *nerve*.

nervi subscapula'res [NA], SYN subscapular *nerves*, under *nerve*.

n. supraclavicula'ris interme'dius [NA], SYN intermediate supraclavicular *nerve*.

n. supraclavicula'ris latera'lis [NA], SYN lateral supraclavicular *nerve*.

n. supraclavicula'ris media'lis [NA], SYN medial supraclavicular *nerve*.

n. supraorbita'lis [NA], SYN supraorbital *nerve*.

n. suprascapula'ris [NA], SYN suprascapular *nerve*.

n. supratrochlea'ris [NA], SYN supratrochlear *nerve*.

n. sura'lis [NA], SYN sural *nerve*.

ner'vi tempora'les profun'di [NA], SYN deep temporal *nerves*, under *nerve*.

n. tenso'ris tym'pani [NA], SYN *nerve* of tensor tympani muscle.

n. tenso'ris ve'li palati'ni [NA], SYN *nerve* of tensor veli palatini muscle.

n. tento'rii, SYN tentorial *nerve*.

ner'vi termina'les [NA], delicate plexiform nerve strands passing parallel and medial to the olfactory tracts, distributing peripherally with the olfactory nerves and passing centrally into the anterior perforated substance; they are considered to have an autonomic function but the exact nature of this is unknown. SYN terminal nerves.

ner'vi thora'cici [NA], SYN thoracic spinal *nerves*, under *nerve*.

n. thora'cicus lon'gus [NA], SYN long thoracic *nerve*.

n. thoracodorsa'lis [NA], SYN thoracodorsal *nerve*.

n. tibia'lis [NA], SYN tibial *nerve*.

n. transver'sus col'li [NA], SYN transverse cervical *nerve*.

n. trigem'inus [NA], SYN trigeminal *nerve*.

n. trochlea'ris [NA], SYN trochlear *nerve*.

n. tympan'icus [NA], SYN tympanic *nerve*.

n. ulna'ris [NA], SYN ulnar *nerve*.

n. utricula'ris [NA], SYN utricular *nerve*.

n. utriculoampulla'ris [NA], SYN utriculoampullar *nerve*.

ner'vi vagina'les [NA], SYN vaginal *nerves*, under *nerve*.

n. va'gus [NA], SYN vagus *nerve*.

n. vascula'ris [NA], SYN vascular *nerve*.

n. vertebra'lis [NA], SYN vertebral *nerve*.

n. vestibula'ris [NA], SYN vestibular *nerve*. SEE ALSO vestibular *root* of vestibulocochlear nerve.

n. vestibulocochlea'ris [NA], SYN vestibulocochlear *nerve*. See entries under radix.

n. zygomat'icus [NA], SYN zygomatic *nerve*.

ne·sid·i·ec·to·my (ne-sid'ē-ek'tō-mē). Excision of islet tissue of the pancreas. [G. *nēsidion,* islet, dim. of *nēsos,* island, + *ektomē,* excision]

ne·sid·i·o·blast (ne-sid'ē-ō-blast). A pancreatic islet-forming cell. [G. *nēsidion,* dim. of *nēsos,* island, + *blastos,* germ]

ne·sid·i·o·blas·to·ma (ne-sid'ē-ō-blas-tō'mă). SYN islet cell *adenoma*. [nesidioblast + G. *-oma,* tumor]

ne·sid·i·o·blas·to·sis (ne-sid'ē-ō-blas-tō'sis). Hyperplasia of the cells of the islets of Langerhans. [nesidioblast + G. *-osis,* tumor]

Nessler, A., German chemist, 1827–1905. SEE N.'s *reagent*.

ness·ler·ize (nes'ler-īz). To treat with Nessler's reagent; used in the determination of urea nitrogen in the blood and in the urine.

nest. A group or collection of similar objects. SEE ALSO nidus. [A.S.]

Brunn's n.'s, glandlike invaginations of surface transitional epithelium in the mucosa of the lower urinary tract.

cell n.'s, a small focus or accumulation of one type of cell that is different from the other cells in the tissue.

epithelial n., SYN keratin *pearl.*

isogenous n., a clone of cartilage cells all from one progenitor cell and occurring as a cluster.

net. SYN network (1).

Chiari's n., abnormal fibrous or lacelike strands in the right atrium, extending from the margins of the coronary or caval valves and attaching to the atrial wall along the line of the crista terminalis; results when resorption of the septum spurium is markedly less than normal.

chromidial n., a reticulum of basophilic-staining material in the cytoplasm of certain cells.

Netherton, Earl W., 20th century U.S. dermatologist. SEE N.'s *syndrome.*

net·il·mi·cin sul·fate (net-il-mī′sin). $(C_{21}H_{41}N_5O_7)_2\cdot5H_2SO_4$; a parenteral aminoglycoside antibiotic used for short-term treatment of serious or life-threatening bacterial infections.

net·tle (net′l). SYN urtica. [A.S. *netele*]

net·work (net′werk). **1.** A structure bearing a resemblance to a woven fabric. A network of nerve fibers or small vessels. SYN rete (1) [NA], net. SEE ALSO reticulum. **2.** The persons in a patient's environment, especially as significant for the course of the illness.

acromial arterial n., a vascular n. between the acromion and the skin of the shoulder, formed by anastomoses of the acromial branch of the suprascapular artery with the acromial branch of the thoracoacromial artery. SYN rete acromiale [NA], acromial plexus.

arteriolar n., a vascular network formed by anastomoses between minute arteries just before they become capillaries. SYN rete arteriosum [NA].

articular n., SYN articular vascular n. SEE plane *joint.*

articular vascular n., a vascular n. in the neighborhood of a joint, where such arrangements are common, enabling a collateral circulation by which blood will be supplied distal to the joint regardless of compromises resulting from joint position. SYN circulus articularis vasculosus [NA], rete vasculosum articulare [NA], articular n.

articular vascular n. of elbow, vascular networks in the region of the elbow, composed of anastomoses between branches of the radial and middle collateral, superior and inferior ulnar collateral, radial recurrent, interosseous recurrent, and recurrent ulnar arteries. SYN rete articulare cubiti [NA].

articular vascular n. of knee, an arterial network over the front and sides of the knee, formed by branches of the descending genicular artery, of the five genicular arteries from the popliteal, of the anterior tibial recurrent, and of the fibular circumflex branch of the posterior tibial. SYN rete articulare genus [NA].

calcaneal arterial n., a superficial network over the calcaneus, formed by branches of the peroneal and posterior tibial arteries and twigs from the malleolar retia. SYN rete calcaneum [NA].

chromatin n., the appearance of basophilic material in the nuclei of many cells after fixation. SEE ALSO chromatin.

dorsal carpal n., a vascular network over the dorsal surface of the carpal joints, formed by anastomoses of branches of the anterior and posterior interosseous, and dorsal carpal branches of the radial and ulnar arteries. SYN rete carpi dorsale [NA], rete carpi posterius.

dorsal venous n. of foot, a superficial network of fine veins on the dorsum of the foot. SYN rete venosum dorsale pedis [NA].

dorsal venous n. of hand, a superficial network of veins on the dorsum of the hand emptying into the cephalic and the basilic veins. SYN rete venosum dorsale manus [NA].

lateral malleolar n., a network over the lateral malleolus formed by branches of the posterior lateral malleolar, anterior lateral malleolar, peroneal, and lateral tarsal arteries. SYN rete malleolare laterale [NA].

linin n., SEE linin (3).

medial malleolar n., a network over the medial malleolus formed by branches from the anterior and posterior medial mal-

leolar and medial tarsal arteries. SYN rete malleolare mediale [NA].

neurofibrillar n., the intertwined patterns formed by neurofibrils in the neuron.

patellar n., the superficial portion of the articular vascular network of the knee. SYN rete patellae [NA].

peritarsal n., the lymphatic vessels along the margin of the eyelid.

plantar venous n., a fine superficial venous network in the sole of the foot. SYN rete venosum plantare [NA].

Purkinje's n., the n. formed by Purkinje's fibers beneath the endocardium.

subpapillary n., the capillary blood vessels in the deeper layers of the skin.

trabecular n., SYN trabecular *reticulum.*

NeuAc. Abbreviation for *N*-acetylneuraminic acid.

Neubauer, Johann E., German anatomist, 1742–1777. SEE N.'s *artery.*

Neufeld, Fred, German bacteriologist, 1869–1945. SEE N. *reaction,* capsular *swelling.*

Neumann, Ernst F.C., German histologist, anatomist, and pathologist, 1834–1918. SEE N.'s *cells,* under *cell, sheath;* Rouget-N. *sheath.*

Neumann, Franz E., German physicist, 1798–1895. SEE N.'s *law.*

Neumann, Isidor Edler von Heilwart, Austrian dermatologist, 1832–1906. SEE N.'s *disease.*

neur-, neuri-, neuro-. Nerve, nerve tissue, the nervous system. [G. *neuron*]

neu·rag·mia (nū-rag′mē-ă). Rupture or tearing asunder of a nerve. [neur- + G. *agmos,* fracture]

neu·ral (nūr′ăl). **1.** Relating to any structure composed of nerve cells or their processes, or that on further development will evolve into nerve cells. **2.** Referring to the dorsal side of the vertebral bodies or their precursors, where the spinal cord is located, as opposed to hemal (2). [G. *neuron,* nerve]

neu·ral·gia (nū-ral′jē-ă). Pain of a severe, throbbing, or stabbing character in the course or distribution of a nerve. SYN neurodynia. [neur- + G. *algos,* pain]

atypical facial n., SYN atypical trigeminal n.

atypical trigeminal n., periodic pain in any region of the face, teeth, tongue, and occasionally in the occipital or shoulder area, which lasts several minutes to several days but has no trigger point and lacks the paroxysmal character of tic douloureux. SYN atypical facial n.

epileptiform n., SYN trigeminal n.

facial n., SYN trigeminal n.

n. facia′lis ve′ra, SYN geniculate n.

Fothergill's n., SYN trigeminal n.

geniculate n., a severe paroxysmal lancinating pain deep in the ear, on the anterior wall of the external meatus, and on a small area just in front of the pinna. SYN geniculate otalgia, Hunt's n., n. facialis vera.

glossopharyngeal n., paroxysmal lancinating pain in the throat or palate. SYN glossopharyngeal tic.

hallucinatory n., an impression of local pain persisting after an attack of n. has ceased.

Hunt's n., SYN geniculate n.

idiopathic n., nerve pain not due to any apparent cause.

intercostal n., pain in the chest wall due to n. of one or more of the intercostal nerves.

mammary n., n. of the intercostal nerve or nerves supplying the breast.

Morton's n., n. of an interdigital nerve, usually the anastomotic branch between the medial and lateral plantar nerves, resulting from compression of the nerve by the metatarsophalangeal joint.

occipital n., SEE posttraumatic neck *syndrome.*

periodic migrainous n., recurrent facial pain and headache, more common in men than in women. SYN Harris' migraine.

red n., SYN erythromelalgia.

sciatic n., SYN sciatica.

Sluder's n., SYN sphenopalatine n.

sphenopalatine n., n. of the lower half of the face, with pain referred to the root of the nose, upper teeth, eyes, ears, mastoid, and occiput, in association with nasal congestion and rhinorrhea occurring in infection of the nasal sinuses, and produced by lesions of the sphenopalatine ganglion; ocular hyperemia and excessive lacrimation may occur. SYN Sluder's n.

stump n., pain experienced as coming from an absent part, caused by irritation of neuromas in the scarred tissue of an amputation stump.

suboccipital n., SEE posttraumatic neck *syndrome.*

supraorbital n., n. of the supraorbital nerve.

symptomatic n., n. occurring as a symptom of some local or systemic disease not involving primarily nerve structures.

trifacial n., SYN trigeminal n.

trigeminal n., severe, paroxysmal bursts of pain in one or more branches of the trigeminal nerve; often induced by touching trigger points in or about the mouth. SYN epileptiform n., facial n., Fothergill's disease (1), Fothergill's n., prosopalgia, prosopo-neuralgia, tic douloureux, trifacial n., trismus dolorificus.

neu·ral·gic (nū-ral′jik). Relating to, resembling, or of the character of, neuralgia.

neu·ral·gi·form (nū-ral′ji-fōrm). Resembling or of the character of neuralgia.

neur·am·e·bim·e·ter (nūr′am-ĕ-bim′ĕ-ter). An instrument for measuring the rapidity of response of a nerve to any stimulus. [neur- + G. *amoibē,* exchange, return, answer, + *metron,* measure]

neur·a·min·ic ac·id (nūr′ă-min′ik). 5-amino-3,5-dideoxy-D-*glycero*-D-*galacto*-2-nonulopyranosonic acid; an aldol product of D-mannosamine and pyruvic acid, linking the C-1 of the former to the C-3 of the latter. The *N*- and *O*-acyl derivatives of n. a. are known as sialic acids and are constituents of gangliosides and of the polysaccharide components of muco- and glycoproteins from many tissues, secretions, and species. SYN prehemataminic acid.

neur·a·min·i·dase (nūr-ă-min′i-dās). SYN sialidase.

α₂-neur·a·mi·no·gly·co·pro·tein (nūr-ă-min′ō-glī-kō-prō′tēn). A glycoprotein that contains neuraminic acid and which during electrophoresis migrates with the α₂ portion of serum proteins. SEE ALSO C1 esterase *inhibitor.*

neur·an·a·gen·e·sis (nūr′an-ă-jen′ĕ-sis). Regeneration of a nerve. [neur- + G. *ana,* up, again, + *genesis,* origin]

neur·a·poph·y·sis (nūr-ă-pof′i-sis). SYN *lamina* of vertebral arch. [neur- + G. *apophysis,* offshoot]

neur·a·prax·ia (nūr-ă-prak′sē-ă). The mildest type of focal nerve lesion that produces clinical deficits; localized loss of conduction along a nerve without axon degeneration; caused by a focal lesion, usually demyelinating, and followed by a complete recovery. Term often misspelled (neuropraxia), and often used, incorrectly, as a synonym for nerve lesion. SEE ALSO axonotmesis. [neur- + G. a- priv. + *praxis,* action]

neur·ar·chy (nūr′ar-kē). The dominant action of the nervous system over the physical processes of the body. [neur- + G. *archē,* dominion]

neur·as·the·nia (nūr-as-thē′nē-ă). An ill-defined condition, commonly accompanying or following depression, characterized by vague fatigue believed to be brought on by psychological factors. [neur- + G. *astheneia,* weakness]

angiopathic n., angioparalytic n., a form of mild n. in which the chief complaint is of a universal throbbing or sense of pulsation throughout the body. SYN pulsating n.

gastric n., a condition marked by vague epigastric atony and distention, and mild neurasthenic symptoms.

n. gra′vis, a condition of extreme and lasting n.

n. prae′cox, a form of nervous exhaustion appearing in the adolescent period. SYN primary n.

primary n., SYN n. praecox.

pulsating n., SYN angiopathic n.

sexual n., a form in which sexual erethism, weakness, or perversion is a marked symptom.

traumatic n., SYN posttraumatic *syndrome.*

neur·as·then·ic (nūr-as-then′ik). Relating to, or suffering from, neurasthenia.

neur·as·then·ic hel·met. A feeling of pressure over the entire cranium in certain cases of neurasthenia.

neur·ax·is (nū-rak′sis). The axial, unpaired part of the central nervous system: spinal cord, rhombencephalon, mesencephalon, and diencephalon, in contrast to the paired cerebral hemisphere, or telencephalon.

neur·ax·on, neur·ax·one (nū-rak′son, -sōn). Obsolete term for axon. [neur- + G. *axōn,* axis]

neur·ec·ta·sis, neur·ec·ta·sia, neur·ec·ta·sy (nū-rek′tă-sis, nūr-ek-tā′zē-ă, -ek′tă-sē). The operation of stretching a nerve or nerve trunk. SYN neurotension. [neur- + G. *ektasis,* extension]

neu·rec·to·my (nū-rek′tō-mē). Excision of a segment of a nerve. SYN neuroectomy. [neur- + G. *ektomē,* excision]

occipital n., excision of greater occipital nerve for the treatment of occipital neuralgia.

presacral n., cutting of the presacral nerve to relieve severe dysmenorrhea. SYN Cotte's operation, presacral sympathectomy.

retrogasserian n., SYN trigeminal *rhizotomy.*

neur·ec·to·pia, neur·ec·to·py (nūr-ek-tō′pē-ă, -ek′tō-pē). **1.** Dislocation of a nerve trunk. **2.** A condition in which a nerve follows an anomalous course. [neur- + G. *ektopos,* fr. *ek,* out of, + *topos,* place]

neur·ep·i·the·li·um (nūr′ep-i-thē′lē-ŭm). SYN neuroepithelium.

neu·rer·gic (nū-rer′jik). Relating to the activity of a nerve. [neur- + G. *ergon,* work]

neur·ex·er·e·sis (nūr-ek-ser′ĕ-sis). Tearing out or evulsion of a nerve. [neur- + G. *exairesis,* a taking out, fr. *haireō,* to grasp, take]

△**neuri-.** SEE neur-.

neu·ri·dine (nūr′i-dēn). SYN spermine.

neu·ri·lem·ma (nūr-i-lem′ă). A cell that enfolds one or more axons of the peripheral nervous system; in myelinated fibers its plasma membrane forms the lamellae of myelin. SYN neurolemma, sheath of Schwann. [neuri + G. *lemma,* husk]

neu·ri·le·mo·ma (nūr′i-lē-mō′mă). SYN schwannoma. [neurilemma + G. *-oma,* tumor]

acoustic n., schwannoma arising from cranial nerve eight.

Antoni type A n., relatively solid or compact arrangement of neoplastic tissue that consists of Schwann cells arranged in twisting bundles and associated with delicate reticulin fibers; the nuclei of the Schwann cells are frequently grouped in parallel rows (so-called palisades), and the nuclei and fibers sometimes form exaggerated tactile corpuscles, called Verocay bodies.

Antoni type B n., relatively soft or loose arrangement of neoplastic tissue that consists of Schwann cells in a haphazard or nondescript type of arrangement among reticulin fibers and tiny cystlike foci; fat-laden macrophages may be observed in some of the larger neoplasms.

neu·ril·i·ty (nū-ril′i-tē). The property, inherent in nerves, of conducting stimuli.

neu·ri·mo·til·i·ty (nūr′i-mō-til′i-tē). SYN nervimotility.

neu·ri·mo·tor (nūr-i-mō′ter). SYN nervimotor.

neu·rine (nūr′ēn). $CH_2{=}CH{-}N^+(CH_3)_3OH$; a toxic amine that is a product of decomposing animal matter (dehydration of choline) and a poisonous constituent of mushrooms.

neu·ri·no·ma (nūr-i-nō′mă). Obsolete term for schwannoma.

acoustic n., obsolete term for acoustic *schwannoma.*

neu·rit, neu·rite (nūr′it, nūr′īt). Obsolete term for axon. [G. *neuritēs,* of a nerve]

neu·rit·ic (nū-rit′ik). Relating to neuritis.

neu·ri·tis, pl. **neu·ri·ti·des** (nū-rī′tis, nū-rit′i-dēz). **1.** Inflammation of a nerve. **2.** SYN neuropathy. [neuri- + G. *-itis,* inflammation]

adventitial n., inflammation of the sheath of a nerve. SEE ALSO perineuritis.

ascending n., inflammation progressing upward along a nerve trunk in a direction away from the periphery.

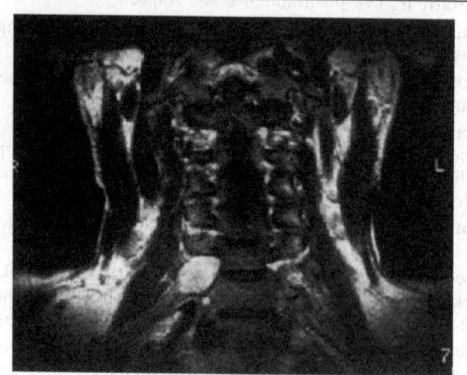

neurinoma of the nerve root of C₇
(MRI, after injection of contrast medium)

axial n., SYN parenchymatous n.

brachial n., SYN brachial plexus *neuropathy*.

central n., SYN parenchymatous n.

descending n., inflammation progressing downward along a nerve trunk in a direction toward the periphery.

Eichhorst's n., SYN interstitial n.

endemic n., SYN beriberi.

fallopian n., SYN facial *paralysis*.

interstitial n., inflammation of the connective tissue framework of a nerve. SYN Eichhorst's n.

intraocular n., inflammation of the retinal portion of the optic nerve.

Leyden's n., fatty degeneration of the fibers of the affected nerve.

multiple n., SYN polyneuropathy.

occipital n., SEE posttraumatic neck *syndrome*.

optic n., inflammation of the optic nerve. SEE ALSO *neuromyelitis* optica, retrobulbar n., papillitis.

parenchymatous n., inflammation of the nervous substance proper, the axons, and myelin. SYN axial n., central n.

retrobulbar n., optic n. without swelling of the optic disk.

sciatic n., SYN sciatica.

segmental n., (1) inflammation occurring at several points along the course of a nerve; (2) segmental demyelinating neuropathy

suboccipital n., SEE posttraumatic neck *syndrome*.

toxic n., n. caused by an endogenous or exogenous toxin.

traumatic n., nerve lesion following an injury.

⌂**neuro-.** SEE neur-.

neu·ro·al·ler·gy (nūr-ō-al′er-jē). An allergic reaction in nervous tissue.

neu·ro·an·as·to·mo·sis (nūr′ō-an-as-tō-mō′sis). Surgical formation of a junction between nerves.

neu·ro·a·nat·o·my (nūr′ō-ă-nat′ō-mē). The anatomy of the nervous system, usually specific to the central nervous system.

neu·ro·ar·throp·a·thy (nūr′ō-ar-throp′ă-thē). A joint disorder caused by loss of joint sensation. SEE Charcot's *joint*. [neuro- + G. *arthron,* joint, + *pathos,* suffering, disease]

neu·ro·aug·men·ta·tion (nūr′ō-awg-men-tā′shŭn). Use of electrical stimulation to supplement activity of the nervous system.

neu·ro·aug·men·tive (nūr′ō-awg-men′tiv). Related to neuro-augmentation.

neur·o·bi·ol·o·gy. The biology of the nervous system.

neu·ro·bi·o·tax·is. The theory that nerve cell bodies may move toward, or their axons may grow toward, the area from which they receive the most stimuli. [G. *neuron,* nerve + *bios,* life + *taxis,* arrangement]

neu·ro·blast (nūr′ō-blast). An embryonic nerve cell. [neuro- + G. *blastos,* germ]

neu·ro·blas·to·ma (nūr′ō-blas-tō′mă). A malignant neoplasm characterized by immature, only slightly differentiated nerve cells of embryonic type, *i.e.,* neuroblasts; typical cells are relatively small (10 to 15 μm in diameter) with disproportionately large, darkly staining, vesicular nuclei and scant, palely acidophilic cytoplasm; they may be arranged in sheets, irregular clumps, or cordlike groups, as well as occurring individually and in pseudorosettes (with nuclei arranged peripherally about the centrally directed cytoplasmic processes); ordinarily, the stroma is sparse, and foci of necrosis and hemorrhage are not unusual. N.'s occur frequently in infants and children in the mediastinal and retroperitoneal regions (approximately 30% associated with the adrenal glands); widespread metastases to the liver, lungs, lymph nodes, cranial cavity, and skeleton are very common.

olfactory n., a rare, often slowly growing malignant tumor of primitive nerve cells, usually arising in the olfactory area of the nasal cavity. SYN olfactory esthesioneuroblastoma.

neu·ro·bor·re·li·o·sis (noor′ō-bōr-rel′ē-ō′sis). Inflammation or disease caused by infection of the central nervous system by a member of the genus *Borrelia.* It is frequently a late stage in the disease process, particularly in immunosuppressed individuals, such as those suffering from AIDS.

neu·ro·car·di·ac (nūr-ō-kar′dē-ak). **1.** Relating to the nerve supply of the heart. **2.** Relating to a cardiac neurosis. [neuro- + G. *kardia,* heart]

neu·ro·cele (nūr′ō-sēl). Rarely used collective term for the central cavity of the cerebrospinal axis; the combined ventricles of the brain and central canal of the spinal cord. [neuro- + G. *koilos,* hollow]

neu·ro·chem·is·try (nūr-ō-kem′is-trē). The science concerned with the chemical aspects of nervous system structure and function.

neu·ro·chi·tin (nūr-ō-kī′tin). SYN neurokeratin. [neuro- + G. *chitōn,* tunic]

neu·ro·cho·ri·o·ret·i·ni·tis (nūr-ō-kōr′ē-ō-ret-in-ī′tis). Inflammation of the choroid, the retina, and the optic nerve.

neu·ro·cho·roi·di·tis (nūr′ō-kō-roy-dī′tis). Inflammation of the choroid and the optic nerve.

neu·roc·la·dism (nū-rok′lă-dizm). The outgrowth of axons from the central stump to bridge the gap in a cut nerve. SYN odogenesis. [neuro- + G. *klados,* a young branch]

neu·ro·cra·ni·um (nūr-ō-krā′nē-ŭm). Those bones of the skull enclosing the brain, as distinguished from the bones of the face. SYN braincase, cranial vault, cranium cerebrale, cerebral cranium. [neuro- + G. *kranion,* skull]

cartilaginous n., in the embryo, that part of the base of the skull first laid down in cartilage and then ossified.

membranous n., the vault of the embryonic skull which is ossified in membrane.

neu·ro·cris·top·a·thy (nūr′ō-kris-top′ă-thē). Developmental anomaly of the neural crest manifested by abnormal development and tumors of the neural axis. [neuro- + L. *crista,* crest, + G. *pathos,* suffering]

neu·ro·cyte (nūr′ō-sīt). SYN neuron (1). [neuro- + G. *kytos,* cell]

neu·ro·cy·tol·y·sis (nūr′ō-sī-tol′i-sis). Destruction of neurons. [neuro- + G. *kytos,* cell, + *lysis,* dissolution]

neu·ro·cy·to·ma (nūr′ō-sī-tō′mă). A tumor of neuronal differentiation usually intraventricular in location, consisting of sheets of cells with uniform nuclei and occasional perivascular-pseudorosette formation. [neuro- + G. *kytos,* cell, + *-oma,* tumor]

neu·ro·den·drite (nūr-ō-den′drīt). SYN dendrite (1).

neu·ro·den·dron (nūr-ō-den′dron). SYN dendrite (1).

neu·ro·der·ma·ti·tis (nūr′ō-der-mă-tī′tis). A chronic lichenified skin lesion, localized or disseminated; if generalized, a term loosely applied to atopic dermatitis. SYN neurodermatosis. [neuro- + G. *derma,* skin, + *-itis,* inflammation]

neu·ro·der·ma·to·sis (nūr′ō-der-mă-tō′sis). SYN neurodermatitis.

neu·ro·dy·nam·ic (nūr′ō-dī-nam′ik). Pertaining to nervous energy. [neuro- + G. *dynamis,* force]

neu·ro·dyn·ia (nūr-ō-din′ē-ă). SYN neuralgia. [neuro- + G. *odynē,* pain]

neu·ro·ec·to·derm (nūr-ō-ek′tō-derm). That central region of the early embryonic ectoderm which on further development forms the brain and spinal cord, and also evolves into the nerve cells and neurilemma or Schwann cells of the peripheral nervous system.

neu·ro·ec·to·der·mal (nūr′ō-ek-tō-der′măl). Relating to the neuroectoderm.

neu·ro·ec·to·my (nūr-ō-ek′tō-mē). SYN neurectomy.

neu·ro·en·ceph·a·lo·my·e·lop·a·thy (nūr′ō-en-sef′ă-lō-mī-ĕ-lo-p′ă-thē). Disease of the brain, spinal cord, and nerves.

neu·ro·en·do·crine (nūr-ō-en′dō-krin). **1.** Pertaining to the anatomical and functional relationships between the nervous system and the endocrine apparatus. **2.** Descriptive of cells that release a hormone into the circulating blood in response to a neural stimulus. Such cells may comprise a peripheral endocrine gland (*e.g.,* the insulin-secreting beta cells of the islets of Langerhans in the pancreas and the adrenaline-secreting chromaffin cells of the adrenal medulla); others are neurons in the brain (*e.g.,* the neurons of the supraoptic nucleus that release antidiuretic hormone from their axon terminals in the posterior lobe of the hypophysis).

neu·ro·en·do·crin·ol·o·gy (nūr-ō-en′dō-krin-ol′ō-jē). The specialty concerned with the anatomical and functional relationships between the nervous system and the endocrine apparatus.

neu·ro·ep·i·the·li·al (nūr′ō-ep-i-thē′lē-ăl). Relating to the neuroepithelium.

neu·ro·ep·i·the·li·um (nūr′ō-ep-i-thē′lē-ŭm) [NA]. Epithelial cells specialized for the reception of external stimuli. Most neuroepithelial cells, notably the hair cells of the inner ear and the receptor cells of the taste buds, are not true neurons but transducer cells that stand in synaptic contact with the peripheral endings of sensory ganglion cells. The neuroepithelial receptor cells of the olfactory epithelium, by contrast, are true peripheral neurons whose extremely thin, unmyelinated axons compose the olfactory filaments that enter the olfactory bulb of the cerebral hemisphere. The NA also applies the term to the rods and cones of the retina. SYN neurepithelium, neuroepithelial cells.

n. of ampullary crest, the specialized sensory hair cells in the ampullary crest of the ampulla of each semicircular duct. SYN n. cristae ampullaris [NA].

n. cris′tae ampulla′ris [NA], SYN n. of ampullary crest.

n. of macula, the specialized sensory hair cells of the epithelium of the macula sacculi and macula utriculi. SYN n. maculae [NA].

n. mac′ulae [NA], SYN n. of macula.

neu·ro·fi·bril (nūr-ō-fī′bril). A filamentous structure seen with the light microscope in the nerve cell's body, dendrites, axon, and sometimes synaptic endings, as aggregations of much finer ultramicroscopic elements, the neurofilaments and microtubules; their functional significance remains to be established.

neu·ro·fi·bril·lar (nūr-ō-fī′bri-lĕr). Relating to neurofibrils.

neu·ro·fi·bro·ma (nūr′ō-fī-brō′mă). A moderately firm, benign, encapsulated tumor resulting from proliferation of Schwann cells in a disorderly pattern that includes portions of nerve fibers; in neurofibromatosis, n.'s are multiple. SYN fibroneuroma.

plexiform n., a type of n., representing an anomaly rather than a true neoplasm, in which the proliferation of Schwann cells occurs from the inner aspect of the nerve sheath, thereby resulting in an irregularly thickened, distorted, tortuous structure; in some instances, the process extends along the course of the nerve and may eventually involve the spinal roots and the spinal cord; seen most frequently in neurofibromatosis. SYN fibrillary neuroma, plexiform neuroma.

storiform n., SYN pigmented *dermatofibrosarcoma protuberans.*

neu·ro·fi·bro·ma·to·sis (nūr′ō-fī-brō-mă-tō′sis) [MIM*162200]. Under this heading, it is now appreciated, are grouped two distinct major (and some minor) hereditary disorders, formerly labeled peripheral and central n., but now entitled n. type 1 and type 2. Type 1 (peripheral) n., by far the most common of the two types, is characterized clinically by the combination of patches of hyperpigmentation in both cutaneous and subcutaneous tumors. The hyperpigmented skin areas, present from birth and found anywhere on the body surface, can vary markedly in size and color; those that are dark brown are called café-au-lait spots. The multiple cutaneous and subcutaneous tumors, nerve

sheath neoplasms, called neurofibromas, can develop anywhere along the peripheral nerve fibers, from the roots, distally. Neurofibromas can become quite large, causing a major disfigurement, eroding bone, and compressing various peripheral nerve structures; a small hamartoma (Lisch nodule) can be found in the iris of almost all patients.

Type 1 n., also called von Recklinghausen's disease, has dominant inheritance, with a gene locus on the proximal long arm of chromosome 17. Type 2 (central) n. has few cutaneous manifestations, and consists primarily of bilateral (less often, unilateral) acoustic neuromas, causing deafness, often accompanied by other intracranial/paraspinal neoplasms, such as meningiomas and gliomas. Type 2 n. also has autosomal dominant inheritance, but the gene locus is on the distal long arm of chromosome 22.

abortive n., SYN incomplete n.

central type n., type I neurofibromatosis.

incomplete n., multiple neurofibromas with minimal manifestations, perhaps limited to café-au-lait spots; individuals with minimal lesions may have offspring with severe involvement. SYN abortive n.

neu·ro·fil·a·ment (nūr-ō-fil′ă-ment). A class of intermediate filaments found in neurons.

neu·ro·gang·li·on (nūr-ō-gang′lē-on). SYN ganglion (1).

neu·ro·gas·tric (nūr-ō-gas′trik). Relating to the innervation of the stomach.

neu·ro·gen·e·sis (nūr-ō-jen′ĕ-sis). Formation of the nervous system. [neuro- + G. *genesis,* production]

neu·ro·gen·ic, neu·ro·ge·net·ic (nūr-ō-jen′ik, -jĕ-net′ik). **1.** Originating in, starting from, or caused by, the nervous system or nerve impulses. SYN neurogenous. **2.** Relating to neurogenesis.

neu·rog·e·nous (nū-roj′ĕ-nŭs). SYN neurogenic (1).

neu·rog·li·a (nū-rog′lē-ă). Non-neuronal cellular elements of the central and peripheral nervous system; formerly believed to be merely supporting cells but now thought to have important metabolic functions, since they are invariably interposed between neurons and the blood vessels supplying the nervous system. In central nervous tissue they include oligodendroglia cells, astrocytes, ependymal cells, and microglia cells. The satellite cells of ganglia and the neurolemmal or Schwann cells around peripheral nerve fibers can be interpreted as the oligodendroglia cells of the peripheral nervous system. SYN glia, Kölliker's reticulum, reticulum (2). [neuro- + G. *glia,* glue]

neu·rog·li·a·cyte (nū-rog′lē-ă-sīt). A neuroglia cell. SEE neuroglia. [neuro- + G. *glia,* glue, + *kytos,* cell]

neu·rog·li·al, neu·rog·li·ar (nū-rog′lē-ăl, -lē-ăr). Relating to neuroglia.

neu·rog·li·o·ma·to·sis (nū-rog′lē-ō-mă-tō′sis). SYN gliomatosis.

neu·ro·gram (nūr′ō-gram). The imprint on the brain substance theoretically remaining after every mental experience, *i.e.,* the engram or physical register of the mental experience, stimulation of which retrieves and reproduces the original experience, thereby producing memory. [neuro- + G. *gramma,* something written]

neu·rog·ra·phy (nū-rog′ră-fē). A method of depicting the state of a peripheral nerve, such as electrical recording or radiographic visualization by contrast media. [neuro- + G. *graphō,* to write]

neu·ro·he·mal (nūr-ō-hē′măl). Descriptive of structures containing neurosecretory neurons, whose axons form no synapses with other neurons and whose axonal endings are modified to permit storage and release into the circulation of neurosecretory material. [neuro- + G. *haima*, blood + suffix -in, material]

neu·ro·his·tol·o·gy (nūr′ō-his-tol′ō-jē). The microscopic anatomy of the nervous system. SYN histoneurology.

neu·ro·hor·mone (nūr-ō-hōr′mōn). A hormone formed by neurosecretory cells and liberated by nerve impulses (*e.g.*, norepinephrine).

neu·ro·hu·mor (nūr-ō-hyū′mer). Obsolete term for the active chemical substance liberated at nerve endings with exciting effect on adjacent structures.

neu·ro·hy·po·phys·i·al (nūr′ō-hī-pō-fiz′ē-ăl). Relating to the neurohypophysis.

neu·ro·hy·poph·y·sis (nūr′ō-hī-pof′i-sis) [NA]. It is composed of the infundibulum and the nervous lobe of hypophysis. SEE ALSO hypophysis. SYN lobus posterior hypophyseos✲ [NA], neural part of hypophysis, pars nervosa hypophyseos, posterior lobe of hypophysis. [neuro- + hypophysis]

neu·roid (nūr′oyd). Resembling a nerve; nervelike. [neuro- + G. *eidos*, resemblance]

neu·ro·ker·a·tin (nūr-ō-kār′ă-tin). **1.** The proteinaceous network that remains of the myelin sheath of axons following fixation and the removal of the fatty material; the reticular appearance is probably a fixation artifact. **2.** The insoluble protein matter of brain remaining after extraction with solvents following proteolytic digestion; it is unrelated to the keratins. SYN neurochitin. [neuro- + G. *keras*, horn]

neu·ro·lem·ma (nūr-ō-lem′ă). SYN neurilemma. [neuro- + G. *lemma*, husk]

neu·ro·lept·an·al·ge·sia (nūr′ō-lept-an-ăl-jē′zē-ă). An intense analgesic and amnesic state produced by administration of narcotic analgesics and neuroleptic drugs; unconsciousness may or may not occur, and cardiorespiratory function may be altered.

neu·ro·lept·an·es·the·sia (nūr′ō-lept-an-es-thē′zē-ah). A technique of general anesthesia based upon intravenous administration of neuroleptic drugs, together with inhalation of a weak anesthetic with or without neuromuscular relaxants.

neu·ro·lep·tic (nūr-ō-lep′tik). **1.** SYN neuroleptic *agent*. **2.** Denoting a condition similar to that produced by such an agent. **3.** Any of a class of psychotropic drugs used to treat psychosis, particularly schizophrenia; includes the phenothiazine, thioxanthene, and butyrophenone derivatives and the dihydroindolones. SEE ALSO antipsychotic *agent*. [neuro- + G. *lēpsis*, taking hold]

neu·ro·lin·guis·tics (nur′ō-ling-gwis′tiks). The branch of medical science concerned with the neuroanatomical basis of speech and its disorders.

neu·rol·o·gist (nū-rol′ō-jist). A specialist in the diagnosis and treatment of disorders of the neuromuscular system: the central, peripheral, and autonomic nervous systems, the neuromuscular junction, and muscle.

neu·rol·o·gy (nū-rol′ō-jē). The branch of medical science concerned with the various nervous systems (central, peripheral, and autonomic, plus the neuromuscular junction and muscle) and its disorders. [neuro- + G. *logos*, study]

neu·ro·lymph (nūr′ō-limf). Obsolete term for cerebrospinal *fluid*. [neuro- + L. *lympha*, clear water]

neu·ro·lym·pho·ma·to·sis (nūr′ō-lim-fō-mă-tō′sis). Lymphoblastic invasion of a nerve.

n. gallina′rum, SEE avian *lymphomatosis*.

neu·rol·y·sin (nŭ-rol′i-sin). An antibody causing destruction of ganglion and cortical cells, obtained by the injection of brain substance. SYN neurotoxin (1).

neu·rol·y·sis (nū-rol′i-sis). **1.** Destruction of nerve tissue. **2.** Freeing of a nerve from inflammatory adhesions. [neuro- + G. *lysis*, dissolution]

neu·ro·lyt·ic (nūr-ō-lit′ik). Relating to neurolysis.

neu·ro·ma (nū-ro′mă). General term for any neoplasm derived from cells of the nervous system; on the basis of newer knowledge pertaining to cytologic and histologic characteristics, a variety of neoplasms, formerly placed in the general category of n., may now be classified in more specific categories, *e.g.*, ganglio-

neuroma, neurilemoma, pseudoneuroma, and others. [neuro- + G. *-oma*, tumor]

acoustic n., SYN acoustic *schwannoma*.

amputation n., SYN traumatic n.

n. cu′tis, neurofibroma of the skin.

false n., SYN traumatic n.

fibrillary n., SYN plexiform *neurofibroma*.

plexiform n., SYN plexiform *neurofibroma*.

n. telangiecto′des, a neurofibroma with a conspicuous number of blood vessels, some of which have unusually large lumens (in proportion to the thickness of the walls).

traumatic n., the non-neoplastic proliferative mass of Schwann cells and neurites that may develop at the proximal end of a severed or injured nerve. SYN amputation n., false n., pseudoneuroma.

Verneuil's n., a nodular enlargement of the cutaneous nerves.

neu·ro·ma·la·cia (nūr′ō-mă-lā′shē-ă). Pathologic softening of nervous tissue. [neuro- + G. *malakia*, softness]

neu·ro·mast (nūr′ō-mast). SEE lateral line sense *organ*.

neu·ro·ma·to·sis (nūr′ō-mă-tō′sis). The presence of multiple neuromas, as in neurofibromatosis.

neu·ro·mel·a·nin (nūr-ō-mel′ă-nin). A modified form of melanin pigment normally found in certain neurons of the nervous system, especially in the substantia nigra and locus ceruleus.

neu·ro·men·in·ge·al (nūr-ō-mě-nin′jē- ăl). Related to involvement of nervous tissue and the meninges.

neu·ro·mere (nūr′ō-mēr). Elevations in the wall of the developing neural tube, especially the rhombencephalon/rhombomeres; that segment of the developing spinal cord to which dorsal and ventral roots are attached. SYN neural segment, neurotome (2). [neuro- + G. *meros*, part]

neu·ro·mi·me·sis (nūr′ō-mi-mē′sis). Obsolete term for hysterical or neurotic simulation of disease. [neuro- + G. *mimēsis*, imitation]

neu·ro·mi·met·ic (nūr′ō-mi-met′ik). Relating to the action of a drug that mimics the response of an effector organ to nerve impulses.

neu·ro·mus·cu·lar (nūr-ō-mŭs′kyū-lăr). Referring to the relationship between nerve and muscle, in particular to the motor innervation of skeletal muscles and its pathology (*e.g.*, neuromuscular disorders). SEE ALSO myoneural.

neu·ro·my·as·the·nia (nūr′ō-mī-as-thē′nē-ă). Obsolete term for muscular weakness, usually of emotional origin. [neuro- + G. *mys*, muscle, + *a-* priv. + *sthenos*, strength]

epidemic n., an epidemic disease characterized by stiffness of the neck and back, headache, diarrhea, fever, and localized muscular weakness; restricted almost exclusively to adults, affecting women more than men; probably viral in origin. SYN Akureyri disease, benign myalgic encephalomyelitis, epidemic myalgic encephalomyelitis, Iceland disease.

neu·ro·my·e·li·tis (nūr′ō-mī-el-ī′tis). Neuritis combined with spinal cord inflammation. SYN myeloneuritis. [neuro- + G. *myelos*, marrow, + *-itis*, inflammation]

n. op′tica, a demyelinating disorder consisting of a transverse myelopathy and optic neuritis. SYN Devic's disease.

neu·ro·my·op·a·thy (nūr′ō-mī-op′ă-thē). **1.** A disorder of muscle due to disorder of its nerve supply. **2.** Simultaneous disorders of nerve and muscles. [neuro- + G. *mys*, muscle, + *pathos*, disease]

carcinomatous n., n. associated with carcinoma, especially of the lung.

neu·ro·my·o·si·tis (nūr′ō-mī-ō-sī′tis). Obsolete term for polymyositis. [neuro- + G. *mys*, muscle, + *-itis*, inflammation]

neu·ron (nūr′on). **1.** The morphological and functional unit of the nervous system, consisting of the nerve cell body, the dendrites, and the axon. SYN nerve cell, neurocyte, neurone. **2.** Obsolete term for axon. [G. *neuron*, a nerve]

autonomic motor n., SEE motor n.

bipolar n., a n. that has two processes arising from opposite poles of the cell body.

gamma motor n.'s, SYN gamma *loop*.

ganglionic motor n., SEE motor n.

Golgi type I n., nerve cells whose long axons leave the gray matter of which they form a part.

Golgi type II n., nerve cells with short axons which ramify in the gray matter.

intercalary n., SYN internuncial n.

internuncial n., a n. interposed between and connecting two other n.'s. SYN intercalary n.

lower motor n., clinical term used to indicate the final motor n.'s that innervate the skeletal muscles; distinguished from upper motor n.'s of the motor cortex that contribute to the pyramidal or corticospinal tract. SEE ALSO motor n.

motor n., a nerve cell in the spinal cord, rhombencephalon, or mesencephalon characterized by having an axon that leaves the central nervous system to establish a functional connection with an effector (muscle or glandular) tissue; **somatic motor n.'s** directly synapse with striated muscle fibers by motor endplates; **visceral motor n.'s** or **autonomic motor n.'s** (preganglionic m. n.'s), by contrast, innervate smooth muscle fibers or glands only by the intermediary of a second, peripheral, n. (postganglionic or ganglionic m. n.) located in an autonomic ganglion. SEE ALSO motor *endplate*, autonomic nervous *system*. SYN anterior horn cell, motoneuron.

multipolar n., a n. with several processes, usually an axon and three or more dendrites.

NANC n., abbreviation for non-adrenergic, non-cholinergic n.

non-adrenergic, non-cholinergic n. (NANC n.), autonomic efferent neuron whose transmission is not blocked by blocking adrenergic and cholinergic transmission. Nitric oxide may be the transmitter in some cases.

polymorphic n., occurring in many shapes. SEE ALSO multipolar *cell*.

postganglionic motor n., SEE motor n.

preganglionic motor n., SEE motor n.

pseudounipolar n., SYN unipolar n.

sensory n., a n. conveying information originating from sensory receptors or nerve endings; afferent neuron, may be general or special sensory.

somatic motor n., SEE motor n.

unipolar n., a n. whose cell body emits a single axonal process resulting from the fusion of two polar processes during development; at a variable distance from the cell body, the process divides into a peripheral axon branch extending outward as a peripheral afferent (sensory) nerve fiber, and a central axon branch that enters into synaptic contact with n.'s in the spinal cord or brainstem. With the single known exception of the n.'s composing the mesencephalic nucleus of the trigeminus, unipolar n.'s are the exclusive neural elements of the sensory ganglia. The lack of dendritic processes of these primary sensory n.'s is only apparent: the dendritic pole of the unipolar n. is represented by the unmyelinated terminal ramifications of the peripheral axon branch. SYN pseudounipolar cell, pseudounipolar n., unipolar cell.

upper motor n., clinical term indicating those n.'s of the motor cortex that contribute to the formation of the pyramidal or corticospinal and corticobulbar tracts, as distinguished from the lower motor n.'s innervating the skeletal muscles. Although not motor n.'s in the strict sense, these cortical n.'s became colloquially classified as motor n.'s because their stimulation produces movement and their destruction causes severe disorders of movement. SEE ALSO motor n., motor *cortex*.

visceral motor n., SEE motor n.

neu·ro·nal (nūr′ō-năl, nū-rō′năl). Pertaining to a neuron.

neu·rone (nūr′ōn). SYN neuron (1).

neu·ro·neph·ric (nūr-ō-nef′rik). Relating to the nerve supply of the kidney. [neuro- + G. *nephros*, kidney]

neu·ro·ne·vus (nūr-ō-nē′vŭs). A variety of intradermal nevus in adults in which nests of atrophic nevus cells in the lower dermis are hyalinized and resemble nerve bundles.

neu·ron·i·tis (nūr-ŏ-nī′tis). Inflammatory disorder of the neuron.

vestibular n., a paroxysmal attack of severe vertigo, not accompanied by deafness or tinnitus, which affects young to middle-aged adults, often following a nonspecific upper respiratory in-

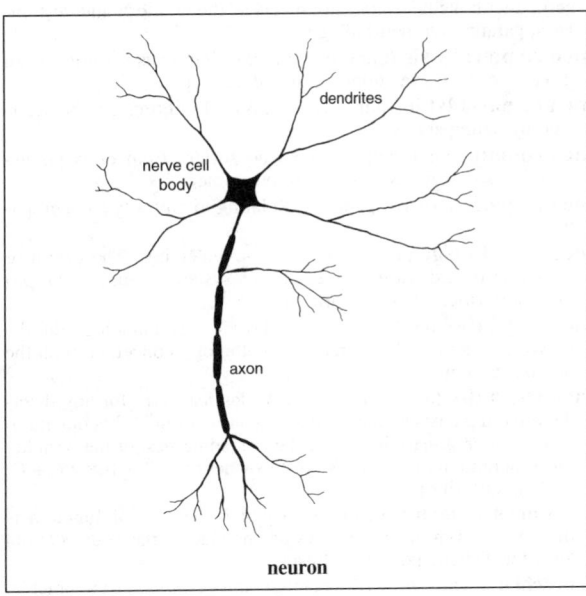

neuron

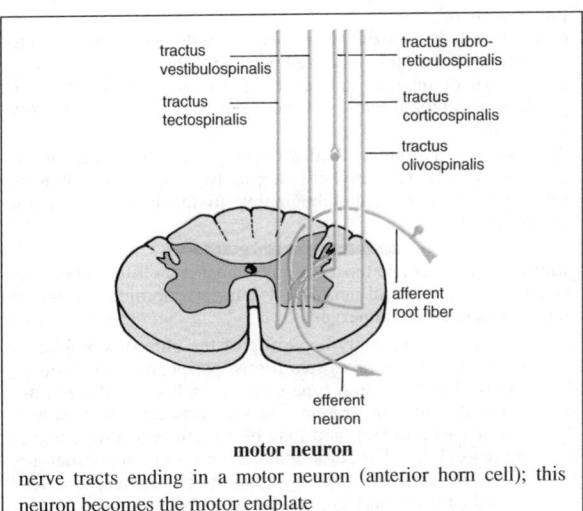

motor neuron

nerve tracts ending in a motor neuron (anterior horn cell); this neuron becomes the motor endplate

fection; due to unilateral vestibular dysfunction. SYN endemic paralytic vertigo, epidemic vertigo, Gerlier's disease, kubisagari, kubisagaru, paralyzing vertigo.

neu·ro·nop·a·thy (nūr-ō-nop′ă-thē). Disorder, often toxic, of the neuron (1).

sensory n., n. confined to dorsal root and gasserian ganglia.

neu·ron·o·phage (nū-ron′ō-fāj). A phagocyte that ingests neuronal elements. SEE microglia. [neuron + G. *phago*, to eat]

neu·ron·o·pha·gia, neu·ro·noph·a·gy (nūr′on′ō-fā′jē-ă, nūr-ō-nof′ă-jē). Phagocytosis of nerve cells. [neuron + G. *phago*, to eat]

neu·ro·nyx·is (nūr-ō-nik′sis). Acupuncture of a nerve. [neuro- + G. *nyxis*, pricking]

neu·ro·on·col·o·gy (nūr′ō-on-kol′ō-jē). The branch of medicine concerned with the direct and indirect effects of neoplasms on the nervous system, neuromuscular junction, and muscle. [neuro- + onco- + G. *logos*, study]

neu·ro·oph·thal·mol·o·gy (nūr′ō-of-thal-mol′ō-jē). That branch of medicine concerned with the neurological aspects of the visual apparatus.

neu·ro·otol·o·gy (nūr′ō-ō-tol′ō-jē). The branch of medicine concerned with the neurological aspects of the auditory and vestibular apparatus. SYN neurotology.

neu·ro·pa·ral·y·sis (nūr'ō-pă-ral'i-sis). Paralysis resulting from disease of the nerve supplying the affected part.

neu·ro·par·a·lyt·ic (nūr'ō-pa-ră-lit'ik). Denoting or characterized by neuroparalysis.

neu·ro·path (nūr'ō-path). One who suffers from or is predisposed to some disease of the nervous system.

neu·ro·path·ic (nūr-ō-path'ik). Relating in any way to neuropathy.

neu·ro·path·o·gen·e·sis (nūr'ō-path-ō-jen'ě-sis). The origin or causation of a disease of the nervous system. [neuro- + G. *pathos,* suffering, + *genesis,* origin]

neu·ro·pa·thol·o·gy (nūr'ō-pa-thol'ō-jē). **1.** Pathology of the nervous system. **2.** That branch of pathology concerned with the nervous system.

neu·rop·a·thy (nū-rop'ă-thē). **1.** A classical term for any disorder affecting any segment of the nervous system. **2.** In contemporary usage, a disease involving the cranial nerves, or the peripheral or autonomic nervous sytems. SYN neuritis (2). [neuro- + G. *pathos,* suffering]

asymmetric motor n., (1) n. in which the loss of function is more marked in the extremities of one side of the body; **(2)** old term for diabetic polyradiculopathy.

brachial plexus n., SYN neuralgic *amyotrophy.* SYN brachial neuritis.

chronic interstitial hypertrophic n., SYN progressive hypertrophic *polyneuropathy.*

compression n., a focal nerve lesion produced when sustained pressure is applied to a localized portion of the nerve, either from an external or internal source; the main source of injury is the pressure differential that exists between one portion of the nerve and another.

dapsone n., a peripheral n. that develops in patients taking dapsone (4,4-diaminodiphenylsulfone); unusual features include being a pure motor n., and beginning in the hands, sometimes asymmetrically.

———

diabetic n., a generic term for any diabetes mellitus-related disorder of the peripheral nervous system, autonomic nervous system, and some cranial nerves.

> This most commonly occurring of the chronic complications of diabetes takes two forms, peripheral and autonomous. The peripheral type causes a dulling of the sensations of pain, temperature, and pressure, especially in the lower legs and feet, and may be treated with drugs (e.g., amitriptyline). The autonomous type results in alternating bouts of diarrhea and constipation, impotence, and reduced cardiac function, and is more refractory.

———

diphtheritic n., a rapidly developing peripheral n. caused by a toxin elaborated by *Corynebacterium diphtheriae.*

entrapment n., a focal nerve lesion produced by constriction or mechanical distortion of the nerve, within a fibrous or fibro-osseous tunnel, or by a fibrous band; with these lesions, stretching and angulation of the nerve may be as important a source of injury as compression; entrapment n.'s tend to occur at particular sites in the body.

familial amyloid n. [MIM*176300, various kinds], a disorder in which various peripheral nerves are infiltrated with amyloid and their functions disturbed, an abnormal prealbumin is also formed and is present in the blood; characteristically, it begins during mid-life and is found largely in persons of Portuguese descent; autosomal dominant inheritance. Other rare clinical types occur. SYN familial amyloidosis, hereditary amyloidosis.

giant axonal n., a rare disorder beginning at or after the third year of life, and presenting clinically with kinky hair, progressive painless clumsiness, muscle weakness and atrophy, sensory loss, and areflexia. Pathologically, both myelinated and unmyelinated nerve fibers contain axonal spheroids packed with neurofilaments; sporadic in nature.

Graves' optic n., visual dysfunction due to optic nerve compression in Graves' orbitopathy.

heavy metal n., peripheral nervous system disorders attributed to intoxication of one of the heavy metals: arsenic, gold, lead, mercury, platinum and thallium.

hereditary hypertrophic n. [MIM*165000], SYN progressive hypertrophic *polyneuropathy.*

hereditary sensory radicular n. [MIM*162400], n. characterized by the occurrence of severe, relapsing foot ulcerations of neuropathic origin, destruction of terminal digits of feet and hands, and a loss of sensation; autosomal dominant inheritance is associated with onset in the second decade or later.

hypertrophic interstitial n., sensorimotor neuropathy characterized pathologically by collections of Schwann cell processes arranged concentrically around one or more nerve fibers. No genetic factors are known in its etiology. For hereditary types, see hereditary hypertrophic n..

ischemic n., n. resulting from acute or chronic ischemia of the involved nerves.

ischemic optic n., optic nerve n. secondary to hypoperfusion of the low pressure posterior ciliary arteries supplying the optic nerve head (nonarteritic) or to temporal arteritis (arteritic).

isoniazid n., an axonal form of n. seen in some patients treated with isoniazid.

lead n., a peripheral n. reportedly seen in chronic lead intoxication; reputedly characterized by wrist-drop, but no convincing modern reports of this are available.

leprous n., a slowly developing granulomatous n., commonly seen in leprosy, caused by *Mycobacterium leprae.*

motor dapsone n., a peripheral n. due to ingestion of 4,4-deaminodiphenylsulphone.

onion bulb n., designation for any of several demyelinating polyneuropathies in which the nerves are enlarged, due to onion bulb formation—whorls of overlapping Schwann cell processes encircling bare medullated axons, *e.g.,* progressive hypertrophic polyneuropathy. SEE hypertrophic interstitial n.

symmetric distal n., SYN polyneuropathy.

vitamin B$_{12}$ n., SYN subacute combined *degeneration* of the spinal cord.

neu·ro·pep·tide (nūr-ō-pep'tīd). Any of a variety of peptides found in neural tissue; *e.g.,* endorphins, enkephalins.

n. Y, a 36 amino acid peptide neurotransmitter found in the brain and autonomic nervous system. It augments the vasoconstrictor effects of noradrenergic neurons.

neu·ro·phar·ma·col·o·gy (nūr'ō-far'mă-kol'ō-jē). The study of drugs that affect neuronal tissue.

neu·ro·phil·ic (nūr-ō-fil'ik). SYN neurotropic. [neuro- + G. *philos,* fond]

neu·ro·pho·nia (nūr-ō-fō'nē-ă). A spasm or tic of the muscles of phonation causing involuntary sounds or cries. [neuro- + G. *phōnē,* voice]

neu·ro·phy·sins (nūr-ō-fiz'inz). A family of proteins synthesized in the hypothalamus as part of the large precursor protein that includes vasopressin and oxytocin in the neurosecretory granules; n. function as carriers in the transport and storage of neurohypophysial hormones.

neu·ro·phys·i·ol·o·gy (nūr'ō-fiz-ē-ol'ō-jē). Physiology of the nervous system.

neu·ro·pil, neu·ro·pile (nūr'ō-pil, -pīl). The complex, feltlike net of axonal, dendritic, and glial arborizations that forms the bulk of the central nervous system's gray matter, and in which the nerve cell bodies lie embedded. [neuro- + G. *pilos,* felt]

neu·ro·plasm (nūr'ō-plazm). The protoplasm of a nerve cell.

neu·ro·plas·ty (nūr'ō-plas-tē). Plastic surgery of the nerves. [neuro- + G. *plastos,* formed]

neu·ro·ple·gic (nūr-ō-plē'jik). Pertaining to paralysis due to nervous system disease. [neuro- + G. *plēgē,* a stroke]

neu·ro·plex·us (nū'rō-plek'sus). A plexus or network of nerve cells or fibers.

neu·ro·po·dia (nūr-ō-pō'dē-ă). SYN axon *terminals,* under *terminal.* [pl. of *neuropodium* or *neuropodion,* fr. neuro- + G. *podion,* little foot]

neu·ro·pore (nūr'ō-pōr). An opening in the embryo leading from the central canal of the neural tube to the exterior of the tube. [neuro- + G. *poros,* pore]

anterior n., SYN rostral n.

caudal n., the temporary opening at the extreme caudal end of the neural tube in early embryos; closes at the 25th somite stage. SYN posterior n.

cranial n., SYN rostral n.

posterior n., SYN caudal n.

rostral n., the temporary opening at the extreme rostral (cephalic) end of the early embryonic forebrain; closes at the 20th somite stage. SYN anterior n., cranial n.

neu·ro·prax·ia. Commonly used misspelling of neurapraxia.

neu·ro·psy·chi·a·try (nūr′ō-sī-kī′ă-trē). The specialty dealing with both organic and psychic disorders of the nervous system; earlier term for psychiatry.

neu·ro·psy·cho·log·ic, neu·ro·psy·cho·log·i·cal (nūr′ō-sī-kō-loj′ik, -loj′i-kăl). Pertaining to neuropsychology.

neu·ro·psy·chol·o·gy (nūr′ō-sī-kol′ō-jē). A specialty of psychology concerned with the study of the relationships between the brain and behavior, including the use of psychological tests and assessment techniques to diagnose specific cognitive and behavioral deficits and to prescribe rehabilitation strategies for their remediation.

neu·ro·psy·cho·path·ic (nūr′ō-sī-kō-path′ik). Relating to neuropsychopathy.

neu·ro·psy·chop·a·thy (nūr′ō-sī-kop′ă-thē). An emotional illness of neurologic and/or functional origin.

neu·ro·psy·cho·phar·ma·col·o·gy (nūr′ō-sī′kō-far-mă-kol′ō-jē). SYN psychopharmacology.

neu·ro·ra·di·ol·o·gy (nūr′rō-rā-dē-ol′ō-jē). The clinical subspecialty concerned with the diagnostic radiology of diseases of the central nervous system, head, and neck.

neu·ro·re·lapse (nūr′ō-rē-laps′). Obsolete term for the recurrence of neurological symptoms upon initiation of therapy, especially with antisyphilitic drugs.

neu·ro·ret·i·ni·tis (nūr′ō-ret-i-nī′tis). An inflammation affecting the optic nerve head and the posterior pole of the retina, with cells in the nearby vitreous, usually producing a macular star. SYN papilloretinitis.

Leber's idiopathic stellate n., SYN stellate n.

stellate n., a unilateral n. with perifoveal exudates in Henle's nerve fiber layer producing a macular star and spontaneous regression in a few months. SYN Leber's idiopathic stellate n.

neu·ror·rha·phy (nūr-ōr′ă-fē). Joining together, usually by suture, of the two parts of a divided nerve. SYN nerve suture, neurosuture. [neuro- + G. *rhaphē,* suture]

neu·ro·sar·co·clei·sis (nūr′ō-sar-kō-klī′sis). An operation for the relief of neuralgia, consisting of resection of one of the walls of an osseous canal traversed by the nerve and transposition of the nerve into the soft tissues. [neuro- + G. *sarx,* flesh, + *kleisis,* closure]

neu·ro·sar·coid·o·sis (nūr′ō-sar-koy-dō′sis). A granulomatous disease of unknown etiology involving the central nervous system, usually with concomitant systemic involvement.

neu·ro·sar·co·ma (nū′rō-sar-kō′mā). A sarcoma with neuromatous elements; includes neurofibrosarcoma, neurogenic sarcoma, and malignant schwannoma.

neu·ro·schwan·no·ma (nūr′ō-shwah-nō′mă). SYN schwannoma.

neu·ro·sci·enc·es (nūr-ō-sī′en-sez). The scientific disciplines concerned with the development, structure, function, chemistry, pharmacology, clinical assessments, and pathology of the nervous system.

neu·ro·se·cre·tion (nūr′ō-sē-krē′shŭn). The release of a secretory substance from the axon terminals of certain nerve cells in the brain into the circulating blood. The secretory product may be a true hormone, *e.g.,* the antidiuretic hormone released from the axon terminals of the neurons composing the supraoptic nucleus of the hypothalamus; in the case of the so-called releasing-factor neurons of the hypothalamus the cell product is not a systemic hormone in its own right but elicits the release of trophic hormones by the anterior lobe of the hypophysis, substances that in turn stimulate peripheral endocrine glands to release their systemically active hormones.

neu·ro·se·cre·to·ry (nūr′ō-sē′krĕ-tōr-ē, -sē-krē′tōr-ē). Relating to neurosecretion.

neu·ro·sis, pl. **neu·ro·ses** (nū-rō′sis, -sēz). **1.** A psychological or behavioral disorder in which anxiety is the primary characteristic; defense mechanisms or any of the phobias are the adjustive techniques which an individual learns in order to cope with this underlying anxiety. In contrast to the psychoses, persons with a n. do not exhibit gross distortion of reality or disorganization of personality. **2.** A functional nervous disease, or one for which there is no evident lesion. **3.** A peculiar state of tension or irritability of the nervous system; any form of nervousness. [neuro- + G. *-osis,* condition]

accident n., SYN traumatic n.

anxiety n., chronic abnormal distress and worry to the point of panic followed by a tendency to avoid or run from the feared situation, associated with overaction of the sympathetic nervous system.

association n., a n. in which association of ideas causes mental repetition of an experience.

battle n., SYN war n.

cardiac n., anxiety concerning the state of the heart, as a result of palpitation, chest pain, or other symptoms not due to heart disease; a form of hypochondriasis. SEE ALSO neurocirculatory *asthenia.* SYN cardioneurosis.

character n., a subclass of personality disorders.

combat n., SEE war n., battle *fatigue,* posttraumatic stress *disorder.*

compensation n., the development of symptoms of n. believed to be motivated by the desire for, and hope of, monetary or interpersonal gain.

compulsive n., SYN obsessive-compulsive n.

conversion n., SYN conversion *hysteria.*

conversion hysteria n., SYN conversion *hysteria.*

depressive n., SEE depression, dysthymia.

expectation n., a condition in which anticipation of an event produces neurotic symptoms.

experimental n., a behavior disorder produced experimentally, as when an organism is required to make a discrimination of extreme difficulty and "breaks down" in the process.

hypochondriacal n., SYN hypochondriasis.

hysterical n., a bona fide disorder characterized by an alteration or loss of physical functioning, such as blurred vision, numbness or paralysis of limbs, coordination difficulties, etc., that suggests a physical disorder, but that instead is apparently an expression of a psychological conflict or need. Also called conversion disorder. SEE ALSO hysteria.

military n., SYN war n.

noogenic n., in existential psychiatry, the neurotic symptomatology resulting from existential frustration.

obsessional n., SYN obsessive-compulsive personality *disorder.*

obsessive-compulsive n., a disorder characterized by the persistent and repetitive intrusion of unwanted thoughts, urges, or actions that the individual is unable to prevent; the compulsive thoughts may consist of single words, ideas, or ruminations often perceived by the sufferer as nonsensical; the repetitive urges or actions vary from simple movements to complex rituals; anxiety or distress is the underlying emotion or drive state, and the ritualistic behavior is a learned method of reducing the anxiety. SYN compulsive n.

obsessive-compulsive n., SYN obsessive-compulsive *disorder.*

occupational n., professional n., a disorder of a group of muscles used chiefly in one's occupation, marked by the occurrence of spasm, paresis, or incoordination on attempt to repeat the habitual movements; *e.g.,* writer's cramp; probably a focal dystonia. SYN craft palsy, functional spasm.

oedipal n., continuation of the Oedipus complex into adulthood.

pension n., a type of compensation n., motivated by the desire for premature retirement on pension.

postconcussion n., a type of traumatic n. following a cerebral concussion.

posttraumatic n., SYN traumatic n.

n. tar′da, neurotic patterns developing in older people, related to organic cerebral lesions.

torsion n., SYN *dysbasia* lordotica progressiva.

transference n., in psychoanalysis, the phenomenon of the patient's developing a strong emotional relationship with the analyst, symbolizing an emotional relationship with a family figure; analysis of this n. comprises an important part of psychoanalytic treatment.

traumatic n., any functional nervous disorder following an accident or injury. SEE posttraumatic stress *disorder.* SYN accident n., posttraumatic n.

vasomotor n., a group of trophic disorders in which pathological changes occur in blood vessels, often due to autonomic nervous system dysfunction; includes Raynaud's disease, acrocyanosis, erythromelalgia, Buerger's disease, causalgia, and trench foot; archaic concept. SYN angioneurosis, vasoneurosis.

war n., a stress condition or mental disorder induced by conditions existing in warfare. SEE ALSO battle *fatigue.* SYN battle n., military n.

neu·ro·splanch·nic (nūr-ō-splangk′nik). SYN neurovisceral. [neuro- + G. *splanchnon,* a viscus]

neu·ro·spon·gi·um (nūr-ō-spon′jē-ŭm, nūr-ō-spŭn′jē-ŭm). **1.** Obsolete term for the plexus of neurofibrils within nerve cells. **2.** Obsolete designation for the reticular layer of the retina. [neuro- + G. *spongion,* small sponge]

Neu·ros·po·ra (nū-ros′pōr-ă). A genus of fungi (class Ascomycetes) grown in cultures and used in research in genetics and cellular biochemistry. SYN pink bread mold. [neuro- + G. *spora,* seed]

neu·ro·stim·u·la·tor (nūr-ō-stim′yū-lā-ter). A device for electrical excitation of the central or peripheral nervous system.

neu·ro·sur·geon (nūr-ō-ser′jŭn). A surgeon specializing in operations on the nervous system.

neu·ro·sur·gery (nūr-ō-ser′jer-ē). Surgery of the nervous system.

functional n., destruction or chronic excitation of a part of the brain to treat disordered behavior or function.

neu·ro·su·ture (nūr-ō-sū′chūr). SYN neurorrhaphy.

neu·ro·syph·i·lis (nūr-ō-sif′i-lis). Infection of the central nervous system by *Treponema pallidum,* or syphilis; there are several subdivisions, including asymptomatic n., meningeal n., meningovascular n., paretic n., and tabetic n.

asymptomatic n., clinically inapparent (except for possible abnormal pupils) syphilitic meningeal infection, diagnosed by examination of the cerebrospinal fluid; if untreated, often develops into some form of symptomatic n.

meningeal n., syphilitic meningeal infection producing an afebrile clinical meningitis, with headache, stiff neck, obtusion, etc., and abnormal CSF findings. Most often develops within 2 years of initial infection.

meningovascular n., syphilitic meningeal infection accompanied by changes (inflammation, fibrous thickening) in the walls of the subarachnoid arteries, manifested as a stroke, with sudden onset of symptoms such as hemiplegia, aphasia, visual disturbances, etc., and abnormal CSF findings.

paretic n., syphilitic infection manifested as dementia (often with delusional features), dysarthria, seizures, myoclonic jerks, action tremor, impaired walking and standing, pupillary abnormalities, and abnormal CSF findings. SYN chronic progressive syphilitic meningoencephalitis.

tabetic n., type of n. in which the posterior roots of the spinal cord, especially in the lumbosacral area, are the principal sites of infection, resulting in ataxia, hypotonia, impotence, constipation, hypotonic bladder, areflexia, and Romberg's sign; other findings include lancinating pains (most often in the legs), visceral crises, Argyll-Robinson pupils, optic atrophy, and Charcot joints; in most patients, the CSF is abnormal. SYN myelosyphilis, posterior sclerosis, posterior spinal sclerosis, tabes dorsalis, tabes spinalis.

neu·ro·tax·is (nūr′ō-tak′sis). Neuronal elongation in the direction of a target. [neuro- + *taxis,* arrangement]

neu·ro·ten·di·nous (nūr-ō-ten′di-nŭs). Relating to both nerves and tendons.

neu·ro·ten·sin (nū-rō-ten′sin). A 13-amino acid peptide neurotransmitter found in synapsomes in the hypothalamus, amygdala, basal ganglia, and dorsal gray matter of the spinal cord; it plays a role in pain perception, but its analgesic effects are not blocked by opioid antagonists; it also affects pituitary hormone release and gastrointestinal function.

neu·ro·ten·sion (nūr-ō-ten′shŭn). SYN neurectasis.

neu·ro·the·ke·o·ma (nūr-ō-thē′kē-ō-mă). A benign myxoma of cutaneous nerve sheath origin. [neuro- + G. *thēkē,* box, sheath, + *-oma,* tumor]

neu·ro·the·le (nūr′ō-thēl). SYN nerve *papilla.* [neuro- + G. *thēlē,* nipple]

neu·ro·ther·a·peu·tics, neu·ro·ther·a·py (nūr′ō-thār′ă-pyū′ tiks, -thār′ă-pē). The treatment of psychological, psychiatric, and nervous disorders.

neu·ro·thlip·sis, neu·ro·thlip·sia (nūr-ō-thlip′sis, -sē-ă). Pressure on one or more nerves. [neuro- + G. *thlipsis,* pressure]

neu·rot·ic (nū-rot′ik). Relating to or suffering from a neurosis. SEE neurosis.

neu·rot·i·cism (nū-rot′i-sizm). The condition or psychological trait of being neurotic.

neu·rot·i·za·tion (nūr′ō-ti-zā′shŭn). The acquisition of nervous substance; the regeneration of a nerve.

neu·ro·tize (nūr′ō-tīz). To provide with nerve substance.

neu·rot·me·sis. A type of axon loss lesion resulting from focal peripheral nerve injury in which, at the lesion site, the nerve stroma is damaged to varying degrees, as well as the axon and myelin, which degenerate from that point distally; with the most severe n. lesions, the gross continuity of the nerve is disrupted. SEE axonotmesis, neurapraxia.

neu·ro·tol·o·gy (nūr-ō-tol′ō-jē). SYN neuro-otology. [neuro- + G. *ous (ot-),* ear, + *logos,* study]

neu·ro·tome (nūr′ō-tōm). **1.** A very slender knife or needle, used for teasing apart nerve fibers in microdissection. **2.** SYN neuromere. [neuro- + G. *tomē,* a cutting]

neu·rot·o·my (nū-rot′ō-mē). Operative division of a nerve. [neuro- + G. *tomē,* a cutting]

retrogasserian n., SYN trigeminal *rhizotomy.*

neu·ro·ton·ic (nūr-ō-ton′ik). **1.** Relating to neurotony. **2.** Strengthening or stimulating impaired nervous action. **3.** An agent that improves the tone or force of the nervous system.

neu·ro·tox·ic (nūr-ō-tok′sik). Poisonous to nervous substance.

neu·ro·tox·in (nūr-ō-tok′sin). **1.** SYN neurolysin. **2.** Any toxin that acts specifically on nervous tissue.

neu·ro·trans·mis·sion (nūr′ō-trans-mish′ŭn). SYN neurohumoral *transmission.*

neu·ro·trans·mit·ter (nūr′ō-trans-mit′er). Any specific chemical agent (including acetylcholine, 5 amines, 4 amino acids, 2 purines, and more than 28 peptides) released by a presynaptic cell, upon excitation, that crosses the synapse to stimulate or inhibit the postsynaptic cell. More than one may be released at any given synapse. The n.'s released by presynaptic cells may modulate transmitter release from presynaptic cells. NO may be a retrograde n., released from postsynaptic cells, to act on presynaptic cells. [neuro- + L. *transmitto,* to send across]

adrenergic n., a n. formed in sympathetic postganglionic synapses (*e.g.,* norepinephrine).

cholinergic n., a n. formed in pre- and postganglionic synapses of the parasympathetic nervous system (*e.g.,* acetylcholine).

neu·ro·trau·ma (nūr-ō-traw′mă). **1.** Trauma of the nervous system. **2.** Trauma or wounding of a nerve. SYN neurotrosis. [neuro- + G. *trauma,* injury]

neu·ro·trip·sy (nūr-ō-trip′sē). Operative crushing of a nerve. [neuro- + G. *tripsis,* a rubbing]

neu·ro·tro·phic (nūr-ō-trof′ik). Relating to neurotrophy.

neu·rot·ro·phy (nū-rot′rō-fē). Nutrition and metabolism of tissues under nervous influence. [neuro- + G. *trophē,* nourishment]

neu·ro·tro·pic (nūr-ō-trop′ik). Having an affinity for the nervous system. SYN neurophilic.

neu·rot·ro·py, neu·rot·ro·pism (nū-rot′rō-pē, -pizm). **1.** Affinity of basic dyes for nervous tissue. **2.** The attraction of certain pathogenic microorganisms, poisons, and nutritive substances toward the nerve centers. [neuro- + G. *trope,* a turning]

neu·ro·tro·sis (nūr-ō-trō′sis). SYN neurotrauma (2). [neuro- + G. *trōsis,* a wounding]

neu·ro·tu·bule (nūr′ō-tū-byūl). One of the microtubules, 10 to 20 nm in diameter, occurring in the cell body, dendrites, axon, and in some synaptic endings of neurons.

neu·ro·vac·cine (nūr-ō-vak′sēn). A fixed or standardized vaccine virus of definite strength, obtained by continued passage through the brain of rabbits.

neu·ro·var·i·co·sis, neu·ro·var·i·cos·i·ty (nūr′ō-var-i-kō′sis, -var-i-kos′i-tē). A condition marked by multiple swellings along the course of a nerve. [neuro- + L. *varix,* varicosis]

neu·ro·vas·cu·lar (nūr-ō-vas′kyū-lăr). Relating to both nervous and vascular systems; relating to the nerves supplying the walls of the blood vessels, the vasomotor nerves.

neu·ro·veg·e·ta·tive (nūr-ō-vej′ĕ-tā-tiv). SYN neurovisceral.

neu·ro·vi·rus (nūr-ō-vī′rŭs). Vaccine virus modified by means of passage into and growth in nervous tissue.

neu·ro·vis·cer·al (nūr-ō-vis′er-ăl). Referring to the innervation of the internal organs by the autonomic nervous system. SYN neurosplanchnic, neurovegetative. [neuro- + L. *viscera,* the internal organs]

neu·ru·la, pl. **neu·ru·lae** (nūr′ū-lă, -lē). Stage in embryonic development after the gastrula state, in which the prominent processes are the formation of the neural plate and the plate's closure to form the neural tube. [neur- + L. *-ulus,* small one]

neu·ru·la·tion (nūr-ū-lā′shŭn). Processes involved in the formation of the neurula stage. [see neurula]

Neusser, Edmund von, Austrian physician, 1852–1912. SEE N.'s *granules,* under *granule.*

neu·tral (nū′trăl). **1.** Exhibiting no positive properties; indifferent. **2.** In chemistry, neither acid nor alkaline, *i.e.,* $[OH^-] = [H^+]$. [L. *neutralis,* fr. *neuter,* neither]

neu·tral·i·za·tion (nū′trăl-i-zā′shŭn). **1.** The change in reaction of a solution from acid or alkaline to neutral by the addition of just a sufficient amount of an alkaline or of an acid substance, respectively. **2.** The rendering ineffective of any action, process, or potential.

viral n., the elimination of viral infectivity as with specific antibodies.

neu·tra·lize (nū′tră-līz). To effect neutralization.

neu·tral red [C.I. 50040]. $N^8,N^8,3$-trimethyl-2,8-phenazinediamine monohydrochloride; used as an indicator (red at pH 6.8, yellow at 8.0), as a vital dye to stain granules and vacuoles in living cells, in testing the secretion of acid by the stomach (given with a test meal), and in general histologic staining. SYN toluylene red.

△ **neutro-, neutr-.** Neutral. [L. *neutralis,* fr. *neuter,* neither]

neu·tro·clu·sion (nū-trō-klū′zhŭn). A malocclusion in which there is a normal anteroposterior relationship between the maxilla and mandible; in Angle's classification, a Class I malocclusion. SYN neutral occlusion (2). [neutro- + occlusion]

neu·tron (nū′tron). An electrically neutral particle in the nuclei of all atoms (except hydrogen-1) with a mass slightly larger than that of a proton; in isolation, it breaks down to a proton and an electron with a half-life of about 10.3 minutes. [L. *neuter,* neither]

epithermal n., a n. having an energy in the range immediately above the thermal range, *i.e.,* having an energy between a few hundredths and approximately 100 ev.

neu·tro·pe·nia (nū-trō-pē′nē-ă). The presence of abnormally small numbers of neutrophils in the circulating blood. SYN neutrophilic leukopenia, neutrophilopenia. [neutrophil + G. *penia,* poverty]

cyclic n., SYN periodic n.

periodic n., n. recurring at regular intervals (14 to 45 days), in association with various types of infectious diseases, *e.g.,* stomatitis, cutaneous ulcers, furuncles, arthritis, and others. SYN cyclic n.

neu·tro·phil, neu·tro·phile (nū′trō-fil, -fīl). **1.** A mature white blood cell in the granulocytic series, formed by myelopoietic tissue of the bone marrow (sometimes also in extramedullary sites), and released into the circulating blood, where they normally represent from 54% to 65% of the total number of leukocytes. When stained with the usual Romanovsky type of dyes, n.'s are characterized by: 1) a nucleus that is dark purple-blue, lobated (three to five distinct lobes joined by thin strands of chromatin), and with a rather coarse network of fairly dense chromatin; 2) a cytoplasm that is faintly pink (sharply contrasted with the nucleus) and contains numerous fine pink or violet-pink granules, *i.e.,* not acidophilic or basophilic (as in eosinophils or basophils). The precursors of n.'s, in order of increasing maturity, are: myeloblasts, promyelocytes, myelocytes, metamyelocytes, and band forms. Although the terms neutrophilic leukocytes and neutrophilic granulocytes include younger cells in which neutrophilic granules are recognized, the two expressions are frequently used as synonyms for n.'s, which are mature forms unless otherwise indicated by a modifying term, such as immature n. SEE ALSO leukocyte, leukocytosis. **2.** Any cell or tissue that manifests no special affinity for acid or basic dyes, *i.e.,* the cytoplasm stains approximately equally with either type of dye. [neutro- + G. *philos,* fond]

band n., SYN band *cell.*

hypersegmented n., an aged and degenerated n. in which there may be 6 to 10 lobes in the nucleus.

immature n., a young n.; the term is usually used with reference to stab n.'s (or other "juvenile" n.'s), neutrophilic granulocytes in which the nucleus is indented but not distinctly segmented.

juvenile n., any cell of the granulocytic series in which the neutrophilic granules are recognizable and the nucleus is indented (the first phase of segmentation).

mature n., SYN segmented n.

segmented n., a fully matured n. that has at least 2 (and as many as 5) distinct lobes in the nucleus and manifests active ameboid motion. SYN mature n.

stab n., SYN band *cell.*

neu·tro·phil·ia (nū-trō-fil′ē-ă). An increase of neutrophilic leukocytes in blood or tissues; also frequently used synonymously with leukocytosis, inasmuch as the latter is generally the result of an increased number of neutrophilic granulocytes in the circulating blood (or in the tissues, or both). N. is usually absolute, *i.e.,* there is an increase in the total number of leukocytes as well as an increased percentage of neutrophils; in some instances, n. may be relative, *i.e.,* there is an increased percentage of neutrophils, but the total number of all types of leukocytes may be within the normal range. SYN neutrophilic leukocytosis.

neu·tro·phil·ic (nū-trō-fil′ik). **1.** Pertaining to or characterized by neutrophils, such as an exudate in which the predominant cells are n. granulocytes. **2.** Characterized by a lack of affinity for acid or basic dyes, *i.e.,* staining approximately equally with either type. SYN neutrophilous.

neu·tro·phil·o·pe·nia (nū′trō-fil-ō-pē′nē-ă). SYN neutropenia. [neutrophil + G. *penia,* poverty]

neu·troph·i·lous (nū-trof′i-lŭs). SYN neutrophilic (2).

neu·tro·tax·is (nū-trō-tak′sis). A phenomenon in which neutrophilic leukocytes are stimulated by a substance in such a manner that they are either attracted, and move toward it (**positive neutrotaxis**), or they are repelled, and move away from it (**negative neutrotaxis**); in some instances, there is no effect (sometimes called **indifferent neutrotaxis**). [neutrophil + G. *taxis,* arrangement]

ne·vi (nē′vī). Plural of nevus. [L.]

ne·vo·cyte (nē′vō-sīt). SYN nevus *cell.*

ne·void (nē′voyd). Resembling a nevus. SYN nevose (2), nevous. [L. *naevus,* mole (nevus), + G. *eidos,* resemblance]

ne·vo·li·po·ma (nē′vō-li-pō′mă). Unsatisfactory terms for a lesion that is basically a melanocytic nevus, mixed adipose cells in the dermis. SYN nevus lipomatodes, nevus lipomatosus. [nevus + lipoma]

ne·vose, ne·vous (nē′vōs, -vŭs). **1.** Marked with nevi. **2.** SYN nevoid.

ne·vo·xan·tho·en·do·the·li·o·ma (nē′vō-zan′thō-en′dō-thē-lē-ō′mă). SYN juvenile *xanthogranuloma.* [nevus + G. *xanthos,* yellow, + endothelioma]

ne·vus, pl. **ne·vi** (nē′vŭs, -vī). **1.** A circumscribed malformation of the skin, especially if colored by hyperpigmentation or increased vascularity; a n. may be predominantly epidermal, adnexal, melanocytic, vascular, or mesodermal, or a compound overgrowth of these tissues. **2.** A benign localized overgrowth of melanin-forming cells of the skin present at birth or appearing early in life. SYN mole (1). SYN spiloma. [L. *naevus,* mole, birthmark]

acquired n., a melanocytic n. that is not visible at birth, but appears in childhood or adult life.

n. ane′micus, a functional developmental defect in vascular filling characterized by pale, round or oval, flat lesions, indistinguishable from surrounding normal skin on diascopy.

n. angiectodes, SYN capillary *hemangioma.*

n. arachnoi′deus, SYN spider *angioma.*

n. ara′neus, SYN spider *angioma.*

balloon cell n., a n. in which many of the cells are large, with clear cytoplasm.

basal cell n. [MIM*109400], a hereditary disease noted in infancy or adolescence, characterized by lesions of the eyelids, nose, cheeks, neck, and axillae, appearing as uneroded flesh-colored papules, some becoming pedunculated, and histologically indistinguishable from basal cell epithelioma; also noted are punctate keratotic lesions of the palms and soles; the lesions usually remain benign, but in some cases ulceration and invasion occur and are evidence of malignant change; autosomal dominant inheritance.

bathing trunk n., a large hairy congenital pigmented n. with a predilection for the entire lower trunk; malignant melanoma may develop in childhood. SYN giant pigmented n., Tierfellnaevus.

Becker's n., a n. first seen as an irregular pigmentation of the shoulders, upper chest, or scapular area, gradually enlarging irregularly and becoming thickened and hairy. SYN pigmented hair epidermal n.

blue n., a dark blue or blue-black n. covered by smooth skin and formed by heavily pigmented spindle-shaped or dendritic melanocytes in the reticular dermis. SYN Jadassohn-Tièche n.

blue rubber-bleb nevi, a syndrome characterized by erectile, easily compressible, thin-walled hemangiomatous nodules, widely distributed in the skin and in the alimentary canal, and sometimes in other tissues; lesions in the gut may perforate or cause hemorrhage, and the patient may be anemic from continual bleeding.

capillary n., capillary hemangioma of the skin.

n. caverno′sus, SYN cavernous *angioma.*

cellular blue n., a large, acquired blue n. in which melanocytes are often clear and large, alternating with pigmented spindle cells and which may expand deeply into the subcutis; malignant change is very rare.

n. comedon′icus, comedo n., congenital or childhood linear keratotic cystic invaginations of the epidermis, with failure of development of normal pilosebaceous follicles. SYN n. follicularis keratosis.

compound n., a n. in which there are nests of melanocytes in the epidermal-dermal junction and in the dermis.

congenital n., a melanocytic n. that is visible at birth, is often larger than an acquired n., and more frequently involves deeper structures.

dysplastic n., SEE dysplastic nevus *syndrome.*

n. elas′ticus of Lewandowski, obsolete term for plaques of smooth or nodular papules, skin- or ivory-colored, occurring symmetrically on the trunk or extremities; now known to be a collagenous n.

epidermic-dermic n., SYN junction n.

epithelioid cell n., SYN Spitz n.

faun tail n., a circumscribed growth of hair of the lumbosacral area, associated with diastematomyelia.

n. flam′meus, flame n., a large congenital vascular n. having a purplish color; it is usually found on the head and neck and persists throughout life. SEE ALSO Sturge-Weber *syndrome.* SYN port-wine mark, port-wine stain.

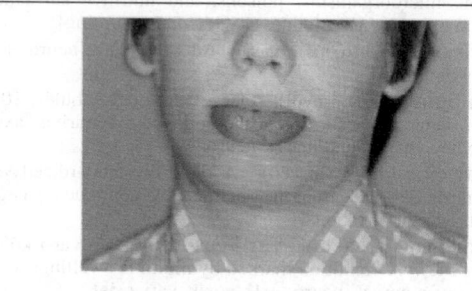
nevus flammeus

n. follicula′ris kerato′sis, SYN n. comedonicus.

giant pigmented n., SYN bathing trunk n.

halo n., a benign, sometimes multiple, melanocytic n. in which involution occurs with a central brown mole surrounded by a uniformly depigmented zone or halo. SYN leukoderma acquisitum centrifugum, Sutton's disease (1), Sutton's n.

intradermal n., a n. in which nests of melanocytes are found in the dermis, but not at the epidermal-dermal junction; benign pigmented nevi in adults are most commonly intradermal.

Ito's n., pigmentation of skin innervated by lateral branches of the supraclavicular nerve and the lateral cutaneous nerve of the arm, due to scattered, heavily pigmented, dendritic melanocytes in the dermis.

Jadassohn's n., SYN n. sebaceus.

Jadassohn-Tièche n., SYN blue n.

junction n., consisting of nests of melanocytes in the basal cell zone, at the junction of the epidermis and dermis, appearing as a slightly raised, small, flat, nonhairy pigmented (brown or black) tumor. SYN epidermic-dermic n.

linear epidermal n., SYN n. unius lateris.

n. lipomato′des, n. lipomato′sus, SYN nevolipoma.

n. lymphat′icus, a cutaneous lymphangioma.

nape n., a pale vascular birthmark found on the nape of the neck in 25 to 50% of normal persons. SYN Unna's mark.

oral epithelial n., SYN white sponge n.

organoid n., SYN n. sebaceus.

Ota's n., SYN oculodermal *melanosis.*

n. papillomato′sus, a prominent wartlike mole.

pigmented hair epidermal n., SYN Becker's n.

n. pigmento′sus, a benign pigmented melanocytic proliferation; raised or level with the skin, present at birth or arising early in life. SYN mole (2).

n. pilo′sus, a mole covered with an abundant growth of hair. SYN hairy mole.

n. sanguineus, SYN capillary *hemangioma.*

n. seba′ceus, congenital papillary acanthosis of the epidermis, with hyperplasia of sebaceous glands developing at puberty and presence of apocrine glands in non-apocrine areas of the skin (commonly the scalp). A variety of epithelial tumors may arise from a n. sebaceus in adult life, most commonly basal cell carcinoma. SYN Jadassohn's n., organoid n.

spider n., SYN spider *angioma.*

n. spi′lus, a form of (flat) nevus pigmentosus. SYN spilus.

spindle cell n., SYN Spitz n.

Spitz n., a benign, slightly pigmented or red superficial small skin tumor composed of spindle-shaped, epithelioid, and multinucleated cells that may appear atypical; most common in children, but also appearing in adults. SYN benign juvenile melanoma, epithelioid cell n., spindle cell n.

strawberry n., a small n. vascularis (capillary hemangioma) resembling a strawberry in size, shape, and color; it usually disappears spontaneously in early childhood. SEE capillary *hemangioma.* SYN strawberry birthmark, strawberry mark.

Sutton's n., SYN halo n.

systematized n., a developmental dysplasia of the skin; extensive, patterned, and usually unilateral.

n. u'nius lat'eris, a congenital systematized linear n. limited to one side of the body or to portions of the extremities on one side; lesions are often extensive, forming wave-like bands on the trunk and spiraling streaks on the extremities. SYN linear epidermal n.

n. vascula'ris, n. vasculo'sus, SYN capillary *hemangioma.*

n. veno'sus, a n. formed of a patch of dilated venules.

verrucous n., a skin-colored or darker wartlike, often linear, lesion appearing at birth or early in childhood, and occurring in various sizes and locations, single or multiple.

white sponge n. [MIM*193900], an autosomal dominant condition of the oral cavity characterized by soft, white or opalescent, thickened and corrugated folds of mucous membrane; other mucosal sites are occasionally involved simultaneously. SYN familial white folded dysplasia, oral epithelial n.

woolly-hair n. [MIM*194300], a circumscribed patch of fine, curly hair in an otherwise normal scalp appearing during childhood and enlarging for a period of 2 to 3 years; autosomal dominant inheritance. There is another, mostly sporadic form that may be autosomal recessive [MIM*278150]. SYN allotrichia circumscripta.

new·bery·ite (nū′ber-ē-īt). $MgHPO_4 \cdot 3H_2O$; the trihydrate of magnesium hydrogen phosphate; found in some renal calculi. Cf. bobierrite, struvite. [J. Cosmo *Newberry*, Australian mineralogist, + -ite 4.]

new·born (nū′bōrn). SYN neonatal, neonate.

New·cas·tle dis·ease. See under disease.

Newcomer's fix·a·tive. See under fixative.

New Hamp·shire rule. See under rule.

Newton, Sir Isaac, English physicist, 1642–1727. SEE newton; newtonian *aberration;* Newtonian *constant* of gravitation; newtonian *flow;* newtonian *viscosity;* N.'s *disk, law.*

new·ton (N) (nū′tŏn). Derived unit of force in the SI system, expressed as meters-kilograms per second squared ($m \cdot kg \cdot s^{-2}$); equivalent to 10^5 dynes in the CGS system. [I. *Newton*]

new·ton-me·ter. A unit of the MKS system, expressed as energy expended, or work done, by a force of 1 newton acting through a distance of 1 meter; equal to 1 joule = 10^7 ergs.

nex·us, pl. **nex·us** (nek′sŭs). SYN gap *junction.* [L. interconnection]

Nezelof, C., French pathologist, *1922. SEE N. *syndrome,* type of thymic *alymphoplasia.*

NF Abbreviation for National Formulary.

ng Abbreviation for nanogram.

NGF Abbreviation for nerve growth *factor.*

N.H.S. Abbreviation for National Health Service (England).

NH₂-ter·mi·nal. SYN amino-terminal.

Ni Symbol for nickel.

ni·a·cin (nī′ă-sin). SYN nicotinic acid.

ni·a·cin·a·mide (nī′ă-sin-am′īd). SYN nicotinamide.

ni·al·a·mide (nī-al′ă-mīd). *N*-Benzyl-β-(isonicotinoylhydrazine) propionamide; a monoamine oxidase inhibitor used in the treatment of depressive disorders.

nib. In dentistry, the portion of a condensing instrument that comes into contact with the restorative material being condensed; its end, the face, is smooth or serrated.

ni·car·di·pine (nī-kar′dē-pēn). A calcium channel blocker of the

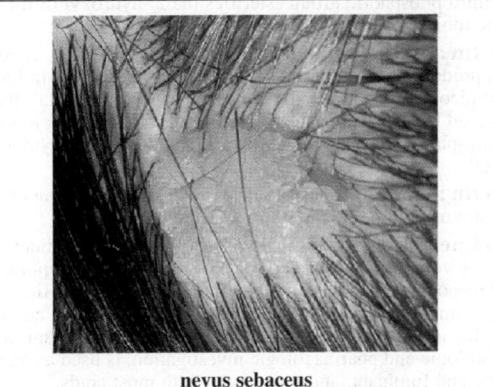
nevus sebaceus

dihydropyridine series; used as an antihypertensive and antianginal agent.

niche (nitch, nēsh). **1.** In contrast radiography, an eroded or ulcerated area, especially gastrointestinal or vascular, which can be detected when it fills with contrast medium. **2.** An ecological term for the position occupied by a species in a biotic community, particularly its relationships to various other competitor, predator, prey, and parasite species. [Fr.]

enamel n., SYN enamel *crypt.*

Haudek's n., an archaic term for the radiographic appearance in profile of contrast material filling a gastric ulcer in the wall of the stomach.

nick (nik). In molecular biology, a hydrolytic cleavage of a phosphodiester bond in one strand of a double-stranded polynucleic acid. Cf. cut.

nick·el (Ni) (nik′l). A metallic bioelement, atomic no. 28, atomic wt. 58.6934, closely resembling cobalt and often associated with it. Protects ribosome structure against heat denaturation. A deficiency of n. causes changes in the ultrastructure of the liver. [abbrev. fr. Ger. *kupfer-nickel,* name of copper-colored ore from which nickel was first obtained; *nickel,* the Ger. word for a dwarfish imp]

nick·el·o·plas·min (nik′l-ō-plas-mēn). A nickel-containing protein found in human sera.

Nickerson-Kveim test. See under test.

nick·ing (nik′ing). Localized constrictions in retinal blood vessels.

arteriovenous n., constriction of a retinal vein at an artery-vein crossing.

ni·clo·sa·mide (ni-klō′să-mīd). *N*-(2′-Chloro-4′-nitrophenyl)-5-chlorosalicylamide; a teniacide effective against intestinal cestodes.

ni·co·fu·ra·nose (ni-kō-fyū′ră-nōs). Fructose 1,3,4,6-tetranicotinate; a peripheral vasodilator.

Nicol, William, Scottish physicist, 1768–1851. SEE N. *prism.*

Nicolas, Joseph, French physician, *1868. SEE N.-Favre *disease.*

Nicolle, J.H., French microbiologist and Nobel laureate, 1866–1936. SEE N.'s white *mycetoma, stain* for capsules.

nic·o·tin·a·mide (nik-ō-tin′ă-mīd). pyridine-3-carboxamide; the biologically active amide of nicotinic acid, used in the prevention and treatment of pellagra. SYN niacinamide, nicotinic acid amide.

nic·o·tin·a·mide ad·e·nine di·nu·cle·o·tide (NAD). Ribosylnicotinamide 5′-phosphate (NMN) and adenosine 5′-phosphate (AMP) linked by phosphoanhydride linkage between the two phosphoric groups; binds as a coenzyme to proteins, serves in respiratory metabolism (hydrogen acceptor and donor) through alternate oxidation and reduction (NAD⁺-NADH). See also entries under NAD and NADP.. SYN diphosphopyridine nucleotide.

nic·o·tin·a·mide ad·e·nine di·nu·cle·o·tide phos·phate (NADP). A coenzyme of many oxidases (dehydrogenases), in which the reaction $NADP^+ + 2H \leftrightarrow NADPH + H^+$ takes place;

the third phosphoric group esterifies the 2'-hydroxyl of the adenosine moiety of NAD.

nic·o·tin·a·mide mon·o·nu·cle·o·tide (NMN). A condensation product of nicotinamide and ribose 5-phosphate, linking the N of nicotinamide to the (β) C-1 of the ribose; in NAD⁺, the ring is linked by the 5'-phosphoryl residue of the ribose moiety to the 5'-phosphoryl residue of AMP; a precursor in the synthesis of NAD⁺.

nic·o·tin·ate (nik'ō-ti-nāt). Salt or ester of nicotinic acid; some n.'s are used in ointments as rubefacients.

nic·o·tine (nik'ō-tēn). 1-Methyl-2-(3-pyridyl)pyrrolidine; a poisonous volatile alkaloid derived from tobacco (*Nicotiana* spp.) and responsible for many of the effects of tobacco; it first stimulates (small doses) then depresses (large doses) at autonomic ganglia and myoneural junctions. N. is an important tool in physiologic and pharmacologic investigation, is used as an insecticide and fumigant, and forms salts with most acids.

nic·o·tine·hy·drox·am·ic ac·id me·thi·o·dide (nik'ō-tēn-hī'drok-sam'ik as'id mĕ-thī'ō-dīd). An effective cholinesterase reactivator, with actions that are most marked at the skeletal neuromuscular junction; antidotal effects are less striking at autonomic effector sites, and insignificant in the central nervous system.

nic·o·tin·ic (nik-ō-tin'ik). Relating to the stimulating action of acetylcholine and other nicotine-like agents on autonomic ganglia, adrenal medulla, and the motor end-plate of striated muscle.

nic·o·tin·ic ac·id. pyridine-3-carboxylic acid; a part of the vitamin B complex; used in the prevention and treatment of pellagra, as a vasodilator, and as an HDL-raising agent. SYN anti-black-tongue factor, antipellagra factor, niacin, pellagra-preventing factor, vitamin PP.

nic·o·tin·ic ac·id am·ide. SYN nicotinamide.

nic·o·tin·ic al·co·hol. SYN nicotinyl alcohol.

nic·o·tin·o·mi·met·ic (nik-ō-tin'ō-mi-met'ik). Mimicking the action of nicotine.

nic·o·ti·nyl al·co·hol (nik-ō-tin'il). 3-pyridinemethanol; same action and use as nicotinyl tartrate. SYN nicotinic alcohol.

nic·o·ti·nyl tar·trate. 3-Pyridinemethanol tartrate; a relatively weak peripheral vasodilator related to nicotinic acid; used in peripheral vascular disorders such as Raynaud's disease, acrocyanosis, and chilblains.

ni·cou·ma·lone (ni-kū'mă-lōn). SYN acenocoumarol.

nic·ta·tion (nik-tā'shŭn). SYN nictitation.

nic·ti·tate (nik'ti-tāt). To wink. [see nictitation]

nic·ti·ta·tion (nik-ti-tā'shŭn). Winking. SYN nictation. [L. *nicto*, pp. *-atus*, to wink, fr. *nico*, to beckon]

ni·dal (nī'dăl). Relating to a nidus, or nest.

ni·da·tion (nī-dā'shŭn). Embedding of the early embryo in the uterine endometrium. [L. *nidus*, nest]

NIDDM Abbreviation for non-insulin-dependent *diabetes* mellitus.

ni·do·gen (nī'dō-jen). SYN entactin. [L. *nidus*, nest, + -gen 1.]

ni·dus, pl. **ni·di** (nī'dŭs, nī'dī). **1.** A nest. **2.** The nucleus or central point of origin of a nerve. **3.** A focus of infection. **4.** The nucleus of a crystal; the coalescence of molecules or small particles that is the beginning of a crystal or similar solid deposit. **5.** The focus of reduced density at the center of an osteoid osteoma, on bone radiographs. [L. nest]

n. a'vis, a deep depression on each side of the inferior surface of the cerebellum, between the uvula and the biventral lobe, in which the tonsil rests. SYN n. hirundinis. [L. bird's nest]

n. hirun'dinis, SYN n. avis. [L. swallow's nest]

Nieden's syn·drome. See under syndrome.

Niemann, Albert, German physician, 1880–1921. SEE N.-Pick *cell, disease;* N. *disease;* N.'s *splenomegaly.*

Niewenglowski, Gaston H., 19th century French scientist. SEE N. *rays,* under *ray.*

ni·fed·i·pine (ni-fed'i-pēn). 1,4-Dihydro-2,6-dimethyl-4-(2-nitrophenyl)-3,5-pyridinedicarboxylic acid dimethyl ester; a calcium channel-blocking agent of the dihydropyridine type; coronary vasodilator.

ni·fen·a·zone (ni-fen'ă-zōn). *N*-Antipyrinylnicotinamide; an analgesic and antipyretic.

ni·fur·al·de·zone (nī-fyūr-al'dĕ-zōn). 5-Nitro-2-furaldehyde semioxamazone; an antibacterial agent.

ni·fu·ra·tel (nī-fyū'ră-tel). Methylmercadone 5-[(methylthio)methyl]-3-[(5-nitrofurfurylidene)amino]-2-oxazolidinone; trichomonacide.

ni·fu·rox·ime (nī-fyū-rok'sēm, -sim). *Anti*-5-nitro-2-furaldoxime; a furan derivative, principally effective against *Candida albicans.*

ni·ge·rose (nī'jĕ-rōs). 3-*O*-α-D-Glucopyranosyl-D-glucose; a disaccharide obtained by the hydrolysis of amylopectins, consisting of two D-glucose residues bound in an α1–3 linkage. [fr. *nigeran,* a polysaccharide synthesized by *Aspergillus niger*]

night·guard (nīt'gard). A device used to stabilize the teeth and reduce the traumatic effects of bruxism.

Nightingale, Florence, 1820-1910. Founder of modern nursing. Originated environmental model for nursing.

night·mare (nīt'mār). A terrifying dream, as in which one is unable to cry for help or to escape from a seemingly impending evil. SYN incubus (2), oneirodynia gravis. [*A.S. nyht,* night, + *mara,* a demon]

night·shade (nīt'shād). Any of a number of plants of the genus *Solanum* (family Solanaceae) and of some other genera of the family Solanaceae.

deadly n., SYN belladonna.

night-ter·rors (nīt'tār-erz). A disorder allied to nightmare, occurring in children, in which the child awakes screaming with fright, the distress persisting for a time during a state of semiconsciousness. SYN pavor nocturnus, sleep terror.

nig·ra (nī'gră). In neuroanatomy, the *substantia* nigra. [L. fr. *niger,* black]

ni·gri·cans (nī'gri-kanz). Blackish. [L. fr. *niger,* black]

ni·gri·ti·es (nī-grish'i-ēz). A black pigmentation. [L. blackness, fr. *niger,* black]

n. lin'guae, SYN black *tongue.*

ni·gro·sin, ni·gro·sine (nī'grō-sin, -sēn) [C.I. 50420]. A variable mixture of blue-black aniline dyes; used as a histologic stain for nervous tissue and as a negative stain for studying bacteria and spirochetes; also used to discriminate between live and dead cells in dye-exclusion staining.

Ni·gros·po·ra (nī-gros'pōr-ă). A genus of rapidly growing fungi that produces shiny, black conidia in cultures; it is a common contaminant in laboratory cultures and is nonpathogenic for humans.

ni·gro·stri·a·tal (nī'grō-strī-ā'tăl). Referring to the efferent connection of the substantia nigra with the striatum. SEE *substantia* nigra.

NIH Abbreviation for National Institutes of Health (U.S. Public Health Service).

ni·hil·ism (nī'i-lizm, nī'hi-lizm). **1.** In psychiatry, the delusion of the nonexistence of everything, especially of the self or part of the self. **2.** Engagement in acts which are totally destructive to one's own purposes and those of one's group. [L. *nihil,* nothing]

therapeutic n., a disbelief in the efficacy or value of therapy, as of drugs, psychotherapy, etc.

ni·keth·a·mide (nī-keth'ă-mīd). *N,N*-Diethylpyridine-3-carboxamide; *N,N*-diethylnicotinamide; it acts mainly on the central nervous system, as a respiratory and cardiovascular stimulant.

Nikiforoff, Mikhail, Russian dermatologist, 1858–1915. SEE N.'s *method.*

Nikolsky, Pyotr V., Russian dermatologist, 1858–1940. SEE N.'s *sign.*

Nile blue A [C.I. 51180]. A basic oxazin dye, $C_{20}H_{20}N_3OCl$, used as a fat and vital stain, and in Kittrich's stain; as an indicator, it changes from blue to purplish red at pH 10 to 11.

ni·mo·di·pine (nī-mō'dī-pēn). A calcium channel blocking drug of the dihydropyridine series used as a vasodilator.

ni·mus·tine (nī'mŭs-tīn). A nitrosourea antineoplastic similar to carmustine (BCNU)

nin·hy·drin (nin-hī'drin). 2,2-Dihydroxy-1,3-indanedione; reacts with free amino acids to yield CO_2, NH_3, and an aldehyde, the NH_3 produced yielding a colored product (diketohydrindylidene-diketohydrinamine, a bi-indanedione derivative). SEE ALSO ninhydrin *reaction.*

ni·o·bi·um (Nb) (nī-ō'bē-ŭm). A rare metallic element, atomic no. 41, atomic wt. 92.90638, usually found with tantalum. [*Niobe,* daughter of Tantalus]

nip·ple (nip'l). A wartlike projection at the apex of the breast on the surface of which the lactiferous ducts open; it is surrounded by a circular pigmented area, the areola. SYN papilla mammae [NA], mamilla (2), papilla of breast, teat (1), thele, thelium (3). [dim. of A.S. *neb,* beak, nose (?)]

aortic n., colloq. term for the radiographic appearance of the left superior intercostal or accessory hemiazygos vein as a bump on the aortic knob.

ni·ri·da·zole (nī-rid'ă-zōl). 1-(5-Nitro-2-thiazolyl)-2-imidazolidinone; used for the treatment of schistosomiasis, amebiasis, and dracontiasis.

nisol·di·pine (nī-sol'dī-pēn). A calcium channel blocker of the dihydropyridine series; used as an antihypertensive and antianginal agent.

Nissen, Rudolf, Swiss surgeon, *1896. SEE N.'s *operation.*

Nissl, Franz, German neurologist, 1860–1919. SEE N. *bodies,* under *body, degeneration, granules,* under *granule, substance;* N.'s *stain.*

nit. **1.** The ovum of a body, head, or crab louse; it is attached to human hair or clothing by a layer of chitin. **2.** A unit of luminance; a luminous intensity of 1 candela per square meter of orthogonally projected surface. [A.S. *knitu*]

Nitabuch, Raissa, 19th century German physician. SEE N.'s *layer, membrane, stria.*

ni·ter (nī'ter). SYN *potassium* nitrate. [G. *nitron,* soda, formerly not distinguished from potash]

cubic n., SYN *sodium* nitrate.

ni·ton (nī'ton). Archaic term for radon.

ni·trate (nī'trāt). A salt of nitric acid.

ni·tra·ze·pam (nī-trā'zě-pam). 1,3-Dihydro-7-nitro-5-phenyl-2*H*-1,4-benzodiazepin-2-one; a hypnotic and sedative of the benzodiazepine class.

ni·tren·di·pine (nī-tren-dī-pēn). A calcium channel blocker of the dihydropyridine series; used as an antihypertensive.

ni·tric ac·id (nī'trik). HNO_3; a strong acid oxidant and corrosive.

fuming n. a., contains about 91% n. a.; used as a caustic.

ni·tric ox·ide (NO). A colorless, free-radical gas; it reacts rapidly with O_2 to form other nitrogen oxides (*e.g.,* $NO_2\cdot$, N_2O_3, and N_2O_4) and ultimately is converted to nitrite (NO_2^-) and nitrate (NO_3^-); physiologically, it is a naturally occurring vasodilator (endothelium-derived relaxing factor) derived from L-arginine in endothelial cells, macrophages, neutrophils, platelets, etc. A gaseous mediator of cell-to-cell communication formed in bone, brain, endothelium, granulocytes, pancreatic β-cells and peripheral nerves by a constitutive nitric oxide synthase. In hepatocytes, Kupffer cells, macrophages, and smooth muscle it is formed by an inducible nitric oxide synthase (*e.g.,* induced by endotoxin). NO activates soluble guanylate cyclase. In endothelial cells it is an endothelium-derived relaxing factor (EDRF); it mediates penile erection, and may be the first known retrograde neurotransmitter. neurotransmitter.

Physiologically, the short-lived NO molecule is manufactured by tissues, and plays a role in various processes, primarily by interacting between endothelium and smooth muscle cells. It is involved in dilation of blood vessels and penile erection, and possibly affects immune reactions and memory. Shortage or inactivation of NO may contribute to high blood pressure and formation of atherosclerotic plaque. An excess of NO, which is a free radical, is toxic to brain cells, and NO is also responsible for the precipitate, often fatal, drop in blood pressure accompanying septic shock. The question of NO's medical importance represents a growing area of interest.

nitric oxide reductase, an enzyme oxidizing N_2 with some acceptor to $2NO\cdot$, a first step in the fixing of atmospheric nitrogen by bacteria.

nitric oxide synthase (NO synthase), an enzyme that catalyzes the reaction of L-arginine with $2O_2$ and $1.5NADPH$ to form $NO\cdot$, L-citrulline, $1.5NADP^+$, and $2H_2O$; there is both an inducible and a constitutive form of this enzyme, the latter requiring calmodulin. Both forms of the enzyme play significant roles in vasodilation, renal function, vascular tone, etc. The constitutive form of the enzyme in bone, brain, endothelium, granulocytes, pancreatic β-cells, and peripheral nerves is calcium-calmodulin dependent. In brain the enzyme is cytosolic; in endothelium it is membrane-bound. The inducible form of the enzyme (*e.g.,* by endotoxin) in hepatocytes, Kupffer cells, macrophages, and smooth muscle is not calcium-calmodulin dependent.

ni·tric ox·ide syn·thase (NO syn·thase). See under nitric oxide.

ni·trid·a·tion (nī-tri-dā'shŭn). Formation of nitrides; formation of nitrogen compounds through the action of ammonia (analogous to oxidation).

ni·tride (nī'trīd). A compound of nitrogen and one other element; *e.g.,* magnesium nitride, Mg_3N_2.

ni·tri·fi·ca·tion (nī'tri-fi-kā'shŭn). **1.** Bacterial conversion of nitrogenous matter into nitrates. **2.** Treatment of a material with nitric acid.

ni·trile (nī'tril). An alkyl cyanide. Individual n.'s are named for the acid formed on hydrolysis; *e.g.,* CH_3CN is acetonitrile rather than methyl cyanide.

△**nitrilo-.** Prefix indicating a tervalent nitrogen atom attached to three identical groups; *e.g.,* nitrilotriacetic acid, $N(CH_2COOH)_3$.

ni·tri·mu·ri·at·ic ac·id (nī'tri-myū-rē-at'ik). SYN nitrohydrochloric acid.

ni·trite (nī'trīt). A salt of nitrous acid.

ni·tri·tu·ria (nī-tri-tū'rē-ă). The presence of nitrites in the urine, as a result of the action of *Escherichia coli, Proteus vulgaris,* and other microorganisms that may reduce nitrates.

△**nitro-.** Prefix denoting the group $-NO_2$. [G. *nitron,* sodium carbonate.]

ni·tro·cel·lu·lose (nī-trō-sel'yū-lōs). SYN pyroxylin.

ni·tro·chlo·ro·form (nī-trō-klōr'ō-fōrm). SYN chloropicrin.

ni·tro·fu·rans (nī-trō-fyū'ranz). Antimicrobials (*e.g.,* nitrofurazone) effective against Gram-positive and Gram-negative organisms.

ni·tro·fu·ran·to·in (nī'trō-fyū-ran'tō-in). *N*-(5-Nitro-2-furfurylidene)-1-aminohydantoin; a urinary antibacterial agent with a wide range of activity against both Gram-positive and Gram-negative organisms; also available as n. sodium for injection.

ni·tro·fu·ran·to·in (nī'trō-fū-ran'tō-in). A nitrofuran compound (*O*-[5-nitrofurfurylideneamino]hydantoin) with antimicrobial activity against a wide spectrum of Gram-positive and -negative bacteria.

ni·tro·fu·ra·zone (nī-trō-fyū'ră-zōn). 5-Nitro-2-furaldehyde semicarbazone; a topical bacteriostatic and bactericidal agent.

ni·tro·gen (N) (nī'trō-jen). **1.** A gaseous element, atomic no. 7, atomic wt. 14.00674; forms about 78.084% by volume of the dry atmosphere. **2.** The molecular form of n., N_2. **3.** Pharmaceutical grade N_2, containing not less than 99.0% by volume of N_2; used as a diluent for medicinal gases, and for air replacement in pharmaceutical preparations. [L. *nitrum,* niter, + *-gen,* to produce]

blood urea n. (BUN), n., in the form of urea, in the blood; the most prevalent of nonprotein nitrogenous compounds in blood; blood normally contains 10 to 15 mg of urea/100 ml. SEE ALSO urea n.

filtrate n., nonprotein n. in various compounds that normally pass through the glomerular filtration, or through a filter in the laboratory (after proteins are precipitated).

heavy n., SYN nitrogen-15.

n. monoxide, SYN nitrous oxide.

nonprotein n. (NPN), the n. content of other than protein bod-

main components of nonprotein nitrogen
normal values given in mEq/100mL

	whole blood	plasma/serum
total nonprotein nitrogen	20–40	18–29 (40)
nonprotein, nonurea nitrogen	16–26	6–18
unidentified nitrogen compounds	5–18	—
free amino acids (nonprotein amino acids)	4.6–6.8	3.4–5.9
ammonia	0.07–0.1	0.1–0.2
creatine	1.0–1.6	—
creatinine	—	0.5–1.3
ergothioneine	0.03	—
glutathione	4.6	—
uric acid	0.3–1.3	0.7–1.3
urea (BUN, blood urea nitrogen)	8.5–15	9.6–17.6
nucleotides	4.4–7.4	—

ies; *e.g.,* about one-half the nonprotein n. in the blood is contained in urea. SYN rest n.

rest n., SYN nonprotein n.

undetermined n., the n. of blood, urine, etc., other than urea, uric acid, amino acids, etc., that can be directly estimated; in blood it amounts to about 25 mg per 100 ml.

urea n., the portion of n. in a biological sample, such as blood or urine, that derives from its content of urea. SEE ALSO blood urea n.

urinary n., n. excreted as urea, amino acids, uric acid, etc., in the urine; 1 g of urinary n. indicates the breakdown in the body of 6.25 g of protein. SEE ALSO nitrogen *equivalent.*

ni·tro·gen-13 (^{13}**N**). A cyclotron-produced, positron-emitting radioisotope of nitrogen with a half-life of 9.97 minutes; used in protein metabolism studies and in positron-emission tomography.

ni·tro·gen-14 (^{14}**N**). The common nitrogen isotope, making up 99.63% of natural nitrogen.

ni·tro·gen-15 (^{15}**N**). The less common stable nitrogen isotope, making up 0.37% of natural nitrogen. SYN heavy nitrogen.

ni·tro·ge·nase (nī′trō-jĕ-nās). Formerly a general term used to describe enzyme systems that catalyze the reduction of molecular nitrogen to ammonia in nitrogen-fixing bacteria; now specifically applied to enzymes that carry out this reaction with reduced ferredoxin and ATP; typically n. consists of two components, the first of which reduces N_2 while the second transfers electrons.

ni·tro·gen dis·tri·bu·tion. SYN nitrogen partition.

ni·tro·gen group. Five trivalent or quinquivalent elements whose hydrogen compounds are basic and whose oxyacids vary from monobasic to tetrabasic: nitrogen, phosphorus, arsenic, antimony, and bismuth.

ni·tro·gen lag. The length of time after the ingestion of a given protein before the amount of nitrogen equal to that in the protein has been excreted in the urine.

ni·tro·gen mus·tards. See under mustard.

ni·trog·e·nous (nī-troj′ĕ-nŭs). Relating to or containing nitrogen.

ni·tro·gen par·ti·tion. Determination of the distribution of nitrogen in the urine among the various constituents. SYN nitrogen distribution.

ni·tro·glyc·er·in (nī-trō-glis′er-in). $O_2NOCH_2CH(ONO_2)CH_2ONO_2$; an explosive yellowish oily fluid formed by the action of sulfuric and nitric acids on glycerin; used as a vasodilator, especially in angina pectoris. SYN glonoin, glyceryl trinitrate, trinitroglycerin.

ni·tro·hy·dro·chlo·ric ac·id (nī′trō-hī-drō-klōr′ik). An extremely caustic mixture that contains 18 parts nitric acid and 82 parts hydrochloric acid. SYN aqua regia, aqua regalis, nitrimuriatic acid.

ni·tro·man·ni·tol (nī-trō-man′i-tol). SYN *mannitol* hexanitrate.

ni·tro·mer·sol (nī-trō-mer′sol). The anhydride of 4-nitro-3-hydroxymercuriorthocresol; a synthetic organic mercurial compound, used as an antiseptic for skin and mucous membranes.

ni·trom·e·ter (nī-trom′ĕ-ter). A device for collecting and measuring the nitrogen set free in a chemical reaction. [nitrogen + G. *metron,* measure]

ni·tron (nī′tron). 1,4-Diphenyl-3-phenylamino-1,2,4-triazolium hydroxide (inner salt); a reagent for the determination of nitric acid, perchlorate, and rhenium, as it is one of the few substances to form an insoluble nitrate.

ni·tro·phen·yl·sul·fen·yl (Nps) (nī′trō-fen′il-sŭl-fēn′il). $O_2N-C_6H_4-S-$; Nitrophenylthio; a radical easily attached to amino groups; used in peptide synthesis and protein chemistry.

ni·tro·prus·side (nī-trō-prŭs′īd). The anion $[Fe(CN)_5NO]^=$; as in sodium n.; used as a vasodilator by the intravenous route.

ni·tros·a·mines (nī-trōs′am-ēnz). Amines substituted by a nitroso (NO) group, usually on a nitrogen atom, to yield *N*-nitrosamines (R–NH–NO or R_2N–NO); can be formed by direct combination of an amine and nitrous acid (can be formed from nitrites in the acidic gastric juice); some are mutagenic and/or carcinogenic.

⚫**nitroso-.** Prefix denoting a compound containing nitrosyl. [L. *nitrosus*]

ni·tro·sou·rea (nī-trō′sō-ūr′ē-ă). Alkylating agent used in the treatment of many neoplasms; an example is BCNU [*N,N′-Bis(2-chloroethyl)-N-nitrosourea;* carmustine].

ni·tro·syl (nī′trō-sil). A univalent radical or atom group, –N=O, forming the nitroso compounds.

ni·trous (nī′trŭs). Denoting a nitrogen compound containing one less atom of oxygen than the nitric compounds; one in which the nitrogen is present in its trivalent state.

ni·trous ac·id. HNO_2; a standard biologic and clinical laboratory reagent.

ni·trous ox·ide. N_2O; a nonflammable, nonexplosive gas that will support combustion; widely used as a rapidly acting, rapidly reversible, nondepressant, and nontoxic inhalation analgesic to supplement other anesthetics and analgesics; its anesthetic potency alone is inadequate to provide surgical anesthesia. SYN dinitrogen monoxide, nitrogen monoxide.

ni·tro·xan·thic ac·id (nī-trō-zan′thik). SYN picric acid.

ni·trox·o·line (nī-trok′sō-lēn). 5-Nitro-8-quinolinol; an antibacterial agent.

ni·trox·y (nī-trok′sē). The –O–NO_2 radical. [contraction of nitryloxy]

ni·trox·yl (nī-trok′sil). The nitrosyl hydride, HNO.

ni·tryl (nī′tril). The radical –NO_2 of the nitro compounds.

ni·zat·i·dine (ni-zat′i-den). *N*-[2-[[[2-[(Dimethylamino)methyl]-4-thiazdyl]methyl]thio]ethyl]-*N′*-methyl-2-nitro-1,1-ethenediamine; a histamine H_2 antagonist used to treat active duodenal ulcers.

njo·ve·ra (nyŏ-ver′ă). A nonvenereal disease of children in Zimbabwe, indistinguishable from syphilis, due to an organism apparently identical with *Treponema pallidum;* probably the same as bejel. [Native]

N.K. Abbreviation for Nomenklatur Kommission.

nkat Abbreviation for nanokatal.

NKSF. Abbreviation for natural killer cell stimulating *factor.*

Nle Abbreviation for norleucine.

NLN. Abbreviation for National League for Nursing.

nM Abbreviation for nanomolar (10^{-9} M).

nm Symbol for nanometer.

NMDA Abbreviation for *N*-methyl D-aspartate. SYN *N*-methyl, D-aspartic acid.

NMDA. Excitotoxic amino acid used to identify a specific subset of glutamate (an excitatory amino acid) receptors.

NMN Abbreviation for nicotinamide mononucleotide.

NMP Abbreviation for nucleoside 5′-monophosphate.

NMR Abbreviation for nuclear magnetic *resonance.*

NO· Symbol for nitric oxide.

No Symbol for nobelium.

Noack, M., 20th century German physician. SEE N.'s *syndrome.*

no·bel·i·um (No) (nō-bel′ē-ŭm). An unstable transuranium element, atomic no. 102, prepared by bombardment of curium with carbon-12 nuclei and similar heavy ions on other elements of the transuranium series. [*Nobel* Institute for Physics and A.B. Nobel, Swedish inventor, 1833–1896]

Noble, Charles P., U.S. gynecologist, 1863–1935. SEE N.'s *position.*

Noble, Robert L., Canadian physiologist, *1910. SEE N.-Collip *procedure.*

Noble's stain. See under stain.

Nocard, Edmund I.E., French veterinarian, 1850–1903. SEE *Nocardia; Nocardiaceae; Preisz-N. bacillus.*

No·car·dia (nō-kar′dē-ă). A genus of aerobic nonmotile actinomycetes (family Nocardiaceae, order Actinomycetales), transitional between bacteria and fungi, containing variably acid-fast, slender rods or filaments, frequently swollen and occasionally branched, forming a mycelium. Coccus or bacillary forms are produced by these organisms, which are mainly saprophytic but may produce disease in human beings and other animals. The type species is *N. farcinica.* [E. *Nocard*]

N. asteroi′des, a species of aerobic, Gram-positive, partially acid-fast, branching organisms causing nocardiosis and possibly mycetoma in humans. SYN *N. leishmanii.*

N. brasilien′sis, a species that closely resembles *N. asteroides* and is a cause of mycetoma in humans.

N. ca′viae, a species that causes mycetoma in humans; it closely resembles *N. asteroides* but differs by its ability to decompose xanthine and by formation of acid from inositol and mannitol.

N. farci′nica, a species causing bovine farcy; it is the type species of the genus *N.*

N. gibso′nii, SYN *Streptomyces gibsonii.*

N. leishma′nii, SYN *N. asteroides.*

N. lurida, Former name for *Amycolatopsis orientalis* subsp. *lurida.*

N. lu′tea, a species found in a case of actinomycosis of the lacrimal gland.

N. madurae, former name for *Actinomadura madurae.*

N. mediterra′nei, a species that produces rifamycin.

N. orienta′lis, a species that produces vancomycin.

no·car·dia, pl. **no·car·di·ae** (nō-kar′dē-ă, nō-kar′dē-ē). A vernacular term used to refer to any member of the genus *Nocardia.*

No·car·di·a·ce·ae (nō-kar-dē-ā′sē-ē). A family of acid-fast, Gram-positive, aerobic bacteria (order Actinomycetales) that includes the genus *Nocardia.* [E. *Nocard*]

no·car·di·a·sis (nō-kar-dī′ă-sis). SYN nocardiosis.

no·car·di·o·form (nō-kar′dē-ō-fōrm). Denoting an organism that morphologically and culturally resembles members of the genus *Nocardia.*

no·car·di·o·sis (nō-kar-dē-ō′sis). A generalized disease in humans and other animals caused by *Nocardia asteroides* and *Nocardia brasiliensis* (or occasionally by *Nocardia farcinica*) and characterized by primary pulmonary lesions which may be subclinical or chronic with hematogenous spread, and usually with involvement of the central nervous system. SYN nocardiasis.

granulomatous n., a form of n. characterized by emaciation, abdominal distention, and replacement of lymphoid tissue in lymph nodes and spleen by granulomatous tissue.

⚠**noci-.** Hurt, pain, injury. [L. *noceo*]

no·ci·cep·tive (nō-si-sep′tiv). Capable of appreciation or transmission of pain. [see nociceptor]

no·ci·cep·tor (nō-si-sep′ter, -tōr). A peripheral nerve organ or mechanism for the reception and transmission of painful or injurious stimuli. [noci- + L. *capio,* to take]

no·ci·fen·sor (nō-si-fen′ser). Denoting processes or mechanisms

that act to protect the body from injury; specifically, a system of nerves in the skin and mucous membranes that react to adjacent injury by causing vasodilation. [noci- + L. *fendo* (only in compounds), to strike, ward off]

no·ci·in·flu·ence (nō′si-in′flū-ens). Injurious or harmful influence.

no·ci·per·cep·tion (nō′si-per-sep′shŭn). The appreciation of injurious influences, referring to nerve centers. [noci- + perception]

⚠**noct-.** Nocturnal. SEE ALSO nycto-. [L. *nox,* night]

noc·tal·bu·min·ur·ia (nok′tal-bū′mi-nu′rē-ă). A pathological increase of albumin in urine excreted during the evening, a rarely observed event. [L. *nox,* night, + albuminuria]

noc·tam·bu·la·tion (nok′tam-byū-lā′shŭn). SYN somnambulism (1).

noc·tam·bu·lism (nok-tam′byū-lizm). SYN somnambulism (1).

noc·ti·pho·bia (nok′tē-fō′bē-ă). Morbid dread of night and its darkness and silence. [noct- + phobia]

noct. maneq. Abbreviation for L. *nocte maneque,* at night and in the morning.

noc·to·graph (nok′tō-graf). SYN scotograph. [noct- + G. *graphō,* to write]

noc·tu·ria (nok-tū′rē-ă). Urinating at night, often because of increased nocturnal secretion of urine resulting from failure of suppression of urine production during recumbency from obstructive lesions in the lower urinary tract or from detrusor instability. SYN nycturia. [noct- + G. *ouron,* urine]

noc·tur·nal (nok-ter′năl). Pertaining to the hours of darkness; opposite of diurnal (1). [L. *nocturnus,* of the night]

no·dal (nō′dăl). Relating to any node.

NODE

node (nōd). **1.** A knob or nodosity; a circumscribed swelling; in anatomy, a circumscribed mass of tissue. **2.** A circumscribed mass of differentiated tissue. **3.** A knuckle, or finger joint. SYN nodus [NA]. [L. *nodus,* a knot]

anterior tibial n., SYN anterior tibial *lymph node.*

n. of Aschoff and Tawara, SYN atrioventricular n.

atrioventricular n. (A-V n.), a small node of modified cardiac muscle fibers located near the ostium of the coronary sinus; it gives rise to the atrioventricular bundle of the conduction system of the heart. SYN nodus atrioventricularis [NA], n. of Aschoff and Tawara, Tawara's n.

Babès' n.'s, collections of lymphocytes in the central nervous system found in rabies.

buccinator n., buccal n., SYN buccal *lymph node.*

n. of Cloquet, one of the deep inguinal lymph n.'s located in or adjacent to the femoral canal; sometimes mistaken for a femoral hernia when enlarged. SYN Rosenmüller's gland, Rosenmüller's n.

coronary n., the uppermost part of the atrioventricular n.

cystic n., SYN cystic *lymph node.*

delphian n., a midline prelaryngeal lymph node, adjacent to the thyroid gland, enlargement of which is indicative of thyroid disease or early metastasis from the subglottic larynx.

diaphragmatic n.'s, SYN superior phrenic *lymph nodes,* under *lymph node.*

ductus n.'s, the highest nodes in a left pneumonectomy specimen that lie on the upper aspect of the left main branches and are accessed by dividing the ligamentum arteriosum.

Dürck's n.'s, perivascular chronic inflammatory infiltrates in the brain, occurring in human trypanosomiasis.

epitrochlear n.'s, SYN cubital *lymph nodes,* under *lymph node.*

fibular n., SYN fibular *lymph node.*

Flack's n., SYN sinuatrial n.

foraminal n., SYN foraminal *lymph node.*

Haygarth's n.'s, exostoses from the margins of the articular surfaces and from the periosteum and bone in the neighborhood of the joints of the fingers, leading to ankylosis and associated with lateral deflection of the fingers toward the ulnar side, which occur in rheumatoid arthritis. SYN Haygarth's nodosities.

Heberden's n.'s, exostoses about the size of a pea or smaller, found on the terminal phalanges of the fingers in osteoarthritis, which are enlargements of the tubercles at the articular extremities of the distal phalanges. SYN Heberden's nodosities, Rosenbach's disease (1), tuberculum arthriticum (1).

hemal n., a lymphoid structure in which the blood sinuses are present in place of lymph sinuses; hemal n.'s occur in ruminants and some other mammals, but their presence in humans is questioned. SYN hemal gland, hemolymph gland, hemolymph n., vascular gland.

hemolymph n., SYN hemal n.

Hensen's n., SYN primitive n.

intermediate lacunar n., SYN intermediate lacunar *lymph node.*

jugulodigastric n., SYN jugulo-digastric *lymph node.*

jugulo-omohyoid n., SYN jugulo-omohyoid *lymph node.*

Keith and Flack n., SYN sinuatrial n.

Keith's n., SYN sinuatrial n.

Koch's n., SYN sinuatrial n.

lateral lacunar n., SYN lateral lacunar *lymph node.*

left gastro-omental n.'s, SYN left gastroepiploic *lymph nodes,* under *lymph node.*

n. of ligamentum arteriosum, a lymph n. of the anterior mediastinal group located adjacent to the ligamentum arteriosum. SYN nodus ligamenti arteriosi [NA], lymph node of ligamentum arteriosum.

lymph n., SEE lymph node.

malar n., SYN malar *lymph node.*

mandibular n.'s, SYN mandibular *lymph node.*

medial lacunar n., SYN medial lacunar *lymph node.*

middle rectal n., SYN middle rectal *lymph node.*

milkers' n.'s, SYN milkers' *nodules,* under *nodule.*

nasolabial n., SYN nasolabial *lymph node.*

Osler n., a tender cutaneous lesion, probably of immunopathic origin, characteristic of subacute bacterial endocarditis; small, raised, and discolored, these n.'s usually appear in the pads of fingers or toes.

parietal n.'s, SYN parietal *lymph nodes,* under *lymph node.*

peroneal n., SYN fibular *lymph node.*

posterior tibial n., SYN posterior tibial *lymph node.*

primitive n., a local thickening of the blastoderm at the cephalic end of the primitive streak of the embryo. SYN Hensen's knot, Hensen's n., Hubrecht's protochordal knot, primitive knot, protochordal knot.

Ranvier's n., a short interval in the myelin sheath of a nerve fiber, occurring between each two successive segments of the myelin sheath; at the n., the axon is invested only by short, finger-like cytoplasmic processes of the two neighboring Schwann cells or, in the central nervous system, oligodendroglia cells. SEE ALSO myelin *sheath.*

retropyloric n.'s, SYN retropyloric *lymph nodes,* under *lymph node.*

Rosenmüller's n., SYN n. of Cloquet.

n. of Rouviere, one of the lateral group of retropharyngeal lymph nodes. SEE retropharyngeal *lymph nodes,* under *lymph node.*

S-A n., abbreviation for sinoatrial n.

signal n., a firm supraclavicular lymph n., especially on the left side, sufficiently enlarged that it is palpable from the cutaneous surface; such a lymph n. is so termed because it may be the first recognized *presumptive* evidence of a malignant neoplasm in one of the viscera. A signal n. that is *known* to contain a metastasis from a malignant neoplasm is sometimes designated by an old eponym, Troisier's ganglion. SYN jugular gland, Virchow's n.

singer's n.'s, SYN vocal cord *nodules,* under *nodule.*

sinoatrial n. (S-A n.), SYN sinuatrial n.

sinuatrial n., the mass of specialized cardiac muscle fibers that normally acts as the "pacemaker" of the cardiac conduction sys-

tem; it lies under the epicardium at the upper end of the sulcus terminalis. SYN nodus sinuatrialis [NA], atrionector, Flack's n., Keith and Flack n., Keith's n., Koch's n., sinoatrial n., sinus n.

sinus n., SYN sinuatrial n.

subdigastric n., SYN jugulo-digastric *lymph node.*

subpyloric n., SYN subpyloric *lymph nodes,* under *lymph node.*

suprapyloric n., SYN suprapyloric *lymph node.*

Tawara's n., SYN atrioventricular n.

teachers' n.'s, SYN vocal cord *nodules,* under *nodule.*

Troisier's n., SYN Troisier's *ganglion.*

Virchow's n., SYN signal n.

visceral n.'s, SYN visceral *lymph nodes,* under *lymph node.*

vital n., SYN noeud vital.

no·di (nō′dī). Plural of nodus. [L.]

no·dose (nō′dōs). Having nodes or knotlike swellings. SYN nodous, nodular, nodulate, nodulated, nodulous. [L. *nodosus*]

no·do·si·tas (nō-dos′i-tas). SYN nodosity. [L. fr. *nodus,* a knot]

n. crin′ium, SYN *trichorrhexis* nodosa.

no·dos·i·ty (nō-dos′i-tē). **1.** A node; a knoblike or knotty swelling. **2.** The condition of being nodose. SYN nodositas. [L. *nodositas*]

Haygarth's n.'s, SYN Haygarth's *nodes,* under *node.*

Heberden's n.'s, SYN Heberden's *nodes,* under *node.*

no·dous, nod·u·lar, nod·u·late, nod·u·lat·ed (nō′dŭs, nod′yū-lăr, nod′yū-lāt, -lā′ted). SYN nodose.

nod·u·la·tion (nod-yū-lā′shŭn). The formation or the presence of nodules.

nod·ule (nod′yūl). A small node. a small node. SEE ALSO nodule. SYN nodulus (1) [NA]. [L. *nodulus,* dim. of *nodus,* knot]

aggregated lymphatic n.'s, SYN Peyer's *patches,* under *patch.*

Albini's n.'s, minute fibrous n.'s on the margins of the mitral and tricuspid valves of the heart, sometimes present in the neonate and representing fetal tissue rests; described previously by Cruveilhier. Cf. n. of semilunar valve.

apple jelly n.'s, descriptive term for the papular lesions of lupus vulgaris, as they appear on diascopy.

Arantius' n., SYN n. of semilunar valve.

Aschoff n.'s, SYN Aschoff *bodies,* under *body.*

Bianchi's n., SYN n. of semilunar valve.

Bohn's n.'s, tiny multiple cysts in newborns. They are found at the junction of the hard and soft palates and along buccal and lingual parts of the dental ridges and are derived from epithelial remnants of mucous gland tissue.

Caplan's n.'s, SYN Caplan's *syndrome.*

cold n., a thyroid n. with a much lower uptake of radioactive iodine than the surrounding parenchyma; about one in four prove to be malignant.

Dalen-Fuchs n.'s, collections of epithelial cells lying between Bruch's membrane and the retinal pigment epithelium in sympathetic ophthalmia and rarely in other granulomatous intraocular inflammations.

enamel n., SYN enameloma.

Gamna-Gandy n.'s, SYN Gamna-Gandy *bodies,* under *body.*

Hoboken's n.'s, gross dilations on the outer surface of the umbilical arteries. SEE ALSO Hoboken's *valves,* under *valve.* SYN Hoboken's gemmules.

hot n., a thyroid n. with a much higher uptake of radioactive iodine than the surrounding parenchyma; usually benign but sometimes causing hyperthyroidism.

Jeanselme's n.'s, a form of tertiary yaws that is characterized by the occurrence of n.'s on the arms and legs, situated usually near the joints. SYN juxta-articular n.'s.

juxta-articular n.'s, SYN Jeanselme's n.'s.

Lisch n., iris hamartomas typically seen in type 1 neurofibromatosis. SYN Sakurai-Lisch n.

lymph n., SYN lymph *follicle.* SYN lymphatic n.

lymphatic n., SYN lymph n.

malpighian n.'s, SYN splenic lymph *follicles,* under *follicle.*

milkers' n.'s, an infection of cows' udders by pseudocowpox virus, a member of the Poxviridae, that is transmitted to the fingers and hands of milkers, producing nodules and lymphangitis, and occasionally widespread papular or papulovesicular eruptions; human infection is transferable to uninfected cows. SYN milkers' nodes, paravaccinia, pseudocowpox.

Morgagni's n., SYN n. of semilunar valve.

picker's n.'s, lichenified skin n.'s seen in prurigo nodularis.

primary n., a lymphatic n. having small lymphocytes and lacking a germinal center.

pulp n., SYN endolith.

rheumatoid n.'s, subcutaneous n.'s, occurring most commonly over bony prominences, in some patients with rheumatoid arthritis; microscopically, the n.'s are foci of fibrinoid necrosis, surrounded by a palisade of fibroblasts.

Sakurai-Lisch n., SYN Lisch n.

Schmorl's n., prolapse of the nucleus pulposus through the vertebral body endplate into the spongiosa of the vertebra.

secondary n., a lymphatic n. having a germinal center.

n. of semilunar valve, a nodule at the center of the free border of each semilunar valve at the beginning of the pulmonary artery and aorta. SYN nodulus valvulae semilunaris [NA], Arantius' n., Bianchi's n., corpus arantii, Morgagni's n.

siderotic n.'s, SYN Gamna-Gandy *bodies,* under *body.*

singer's n.'s, SYN vocal cord n.'s.

Sister Joseph's n., a malignant intra-abdominal neoplasm metastatic to the umbilicus.

solitary n.'s of intestine, SYN solitary lymphatic *follicles,* under *follicle.*

splenic lymph n.'s, SYN splenic lymph *follicles,* under *follicle.*

vocal cord n.'s, small, circumscribed, bilateral, beadlike enlargements on the vocal cords caused by overuse or abuse of the voice; often reversible by voice therapy. SYN singer's nodes, singer's n.'s, teachers' nodes.

nod·u·lous (nod′yū-lŭs). SYN nodose.

no·du·lus, pl. **no·du·li** (nod′yū-lŭs, nod′yū-lī) [NA]. **1.** SYN nodule. **2.** The posterior extremity of the inferior vermis of the cerebellum, forming with the posterior medullary velum the central portion of the flocculonodular lobe. [L. dim. of *nodus*]

n. carot′icus, SYN carotid *body.*

n. lymphat′icus, SYN lymph *follicle.*

n. val′vulae semiluna′ris, pl. **nod′uli valvula′rum semiluna′rium** [NA], SYN *nodule* of semilunar valve.

no·dus, pl. **no·di** (nō′dŭs, -dī) [NA]. SYN node. [L. a knot]

n. atrioventricula′ris [NA], SYN atrioventricular *node.*

n. buccinato′rius [NA], SYN buccal *lymph node.*

n. cys′ticus [NA], SYN cystic *lymph node.*

n. fibula′ris [NA], SYN fibular *lymph node.*

n. foraminalis [NA], SYN foraminal *lymph node.*

n. jugulodigas′tricus [NA], SYN jugulo-digastric *lymph node.*

n. jugulo-omohyoi′deus [NA], SYN jugulo-omohyoid *lymph node.*

n. lacuna′ris interme′dius [NA], SYN intermediate lacunar *lymph node.*

n. lacuna′ris latera′lis [NA], SYN lateral lacunar *lymph node.*

n. lacuna′ris media′lis [NA], SYN medial lacunar *lymph node.*

n. ligamen′ti arterio′si [NA], SYN *node* of ligamentum arteriosum.

n. mala′ris [NA], SYN malar *lymph node.*

n. mandibula′ris [NA], SYN mandibular *lymph node.*

n. nasolabia′lis [NA], SYN nasolabial *lymph node.*

n. recta′lis me′dius, SYN middle rectal *lymph node.*

no′di retropylo′rici [NA], SYN retropyloric *lymph nodes,* under *lymph node.*

n. sinuatria′lis [NA], SYN sinuatrial *node.*

no′di subpylo′rici [NA], SYN subpyloric *lymph nodes,* under *lymph node.*

n. suprapylo′ricus [NA], SYN suprapyloric *lymph node.*

n. tibia′lis ante′rior [NA], SYN anterior tibial *lymph node.*

n. tibia′lis poste′rior [NA], SYN posterior tibial *lymph node.*

no′di viscera′les [NA], SYN visceral *lymph nodes,* under *lymph node.*

NODUS LYMPHATICUS

no·dus lym·pha·ti·cus, pl. **no·di lym·pha·ti·ci** (nō′dŭs lim′fat′ē-kus, -nō′dī) [NA]. SYN lymph node. [lympho- + L. *nodus,* node]

nodi lymphatici abdom′inis viscera′les [NA], SYN *lymph nodes* of abdominal organs, under *lymph node.*

nodi lymphatici anorecta′les [NA], ☆official alternate term for pararectal *lymph nodes,* under *lymph node.*

nodi lymphatici appendicula′res [NA], SYN appendicular *lymph nodes,* under *lymph node.*

l. ar′cus ve′nae az′ygos [NA], SYN *lymph node* of azygos arch.

nodi lymphatici axilla′res [NA], SYN axillary *lymph nodes,* under *lymph node.*

nodi lymphatici axillares apicales [NA], SYN apical group of axillary *lymph nodes,* under *lymph node.*

nodi lymphatici axillares subscapulares [NA], SYN subscapular group of axillary *lymph nodes,* under *lymph node.*

nodi lymphatici axillaris pectorales [NA], SYN pectoral group of axillary *lymph nodes,* under *lymph node.*

nodi lymphatici brachia′les [NA], SYN lateral group of axillary *lymph nodes,* under *lymph node.*

nodi lymphatici bronchopulmona′les, SYN bronchopulmonary *lymph nodes,* under *lymph node.*

nodi lymphat′ici centra′les, SYN superior mesenteric *lymph nodes,* under *lymph node.*

nodi lymphatici cervicales anterio′res [NA], SYN anterior cervical *lymph nodes,* under *lymph node.*

nodi lymphatici cervicales anterio′res profun′di, SYN anterior deep cervical *lymph nodes,* under *lymph node.*

nodi lymphatici cervicales anterio′res superficia′les, SYN anterior superficial cervical *lymph nodes,* under *lymph node.*

nodi lymphatici cervicales laterales profundi [NA], SYN lateral deep cervical *lymph nodes,* under *lymph node.*

nodi lymphatici cervicales laterales superficiales [NA], SYN lateral superficial cervical *lymph nodes,* under *lymph node.*

nodi lymphatici coeliaci [NA], SYN celiac *lymph nodes,* under *lymph node.*

nodi lymphatici col′ici, SYN colic *lymph nodes,* under *lymph node.*

nodi lymphatici col′ici dex′tri [NA], SYN right colic *lymph nodes,* under *lymph node.*

nodi lymphatici col′ici me′dii [NA], SYN middle colic *lymph nodes,* under *lymph node.*

nodi lymphatici col′ici sinis′tri [NA], SYN left colic *lymph nodes,* under *lymph node.*

nodi lymphatici comitan′tes ner′vi accesso′rii, SYN accessory nerve *lymph nodes,* under *lymph node.*

nodi lymphatici cubitales [NA], SYN cubital *lymph nodes,* under *lymph node.*

nodi lymphatici epigastrici inferiores [NA], SYN inferior epigastric *lymph nodes,* under *lymph node.*

nodi lymphatici faciales [NA], SYN facial *lymph nodes,* under *lymph node.*

nodi lymphatici gastrici dextri [NA], SYN right gastric *lymph nodes,* under *lymph node.*

nodi lymphatici gastrici sinistri [NA], SYN left gastric *lymph nodes,* under *lymph node.*

nodi lymphatici gastro-omentales dextri [NA], SYN right gastroepiploic *lymph nodes,* under *lymph node.*

nodi lymphatici gastro-omentales sinistri [NA], SYN left gastroepiploic *lymph nodes,* under *lymph node.*

nodi lymphatici gluteales [NA], SYN gluteal *lymph nodes,* under *lymph node.*

no

nodi lymphatici hepatici [NA], SYN hepatic *lymph nodes*, under *lymph node*.

nodi lymphatici ileocolici [NA], SYN ileocolic *lymph nodes*, under *lymph node*.

nodi lymphatici iliaci communes [NA], SYN common iliac *lymph nodes*, under *lymph node*.

nodi lymphatici iliaci externi [NA], SYN external iliac *lymph nodes*, under *lymph node*.

nodi lymphatici iliaci externi media′les, SEE external iliac *lymph nodes*, under *lymph node*.

nodi lymphatici iliaci interni [NA], SYN internal iliac *lymph nodes*, under *lymph node*.

nodi lymphatici inguinales profundi [NA], SYN deep inguinal *lymph nodes*, under *lymph node*.

nodi lymphatici inguinales superficiales [NA], SYN superficial inguinal *lymph nodes*, under *lymph node*.

nodi lymphatici intercostales [NA], SYN intercostal *lymph nodes*, under *lymph node*.

nodi lymphatici interiliaci [NA], SYN interiliac *lymph nodes*, under *lymph node*.

nodi lymphatici interpectorales [NA], SYN interpectoral *lymph nodes*, under *lymph node*.

nodi lymphatici jugulares anteriores [NA], SYN anterior jugular *lymph nodes*, under *lymph node*.

nodi lymphatici jugulares laterales [NA], SYN lateral jugular *lymph nodes*, under *lymph node*.

nodi lymphatici juxta-esophageales pulmonales [NA], SYN juxta-esophageal pulmonary *lymph nodes*, under *lymph node*.

nodi lymphatici juxta-intestinales [NA], SYN juxta-intestinal *lymph nodes*, under *lymph node*.

nodi lymphatici lienales [NA], ✫official alternate term for splenic *lymph nodes*, under *lymph node*.

nodi lymphatici linguales [NA], SYN lingual *lymph nodes*, under *lymph node*.

nodi lymphatici lumbales dextri [NA], SYN right lumbar *lymph nodes*, under *lymph node*.

nodi lymphatici lumbales intermedii [NA], SYN intermediate lumbar *lymph nodes*, under *lymph node*.

nodi lymphatici lumbales sinistri [NA], SYN left lumbar *lymph nodes*, under *lymph node*.

nodi lymphatici mastoidei [NA], SYN retroauricular *lymph nodes*, under *lymph node*.

nodi lymphatici mediastinales anteriores [NA], SYN anterior mediastinal *lymph nodes*, under *lymph node*.

nodi lymphatici mediastinales posteriores [NA], SYN posterior mediastinal *lymph nodes*, under *lymph node*.

nodi lymphatici mesenterici [NA], SYN mesenteric *lymph nodes*, under *lymph node*.

no′di lymphat′ici mesenter′ici inferio′res [NA], SYN inferior mesenteric *lymph nodes* >, under *lymph node*.

no′di lymphat′ici mesenter′ici superio′res [NA], SYN superior mesenteric *lymph nodes*, under *lymph node*.

nodi lymphatici mesocolici [NA], SYN mesocolic *lymph nodes*, under *lymph node*.

nodi lymphatici obturatorii [NA], SYN obturator *lymph nodes*, under *lymph node*.

nodi lymphatici occipitales [NA], SYN occipital *lymph nodes*, under *lymph node*.

nodi lymphatici pancreatici [NA], SYN pancreatic *lymph nodes*, under *lymph node*.

nodi lymphatici pancreatici inferio′res, inferior pancreatic lymph nodes. SEE pancreatic *lymph nodes*, under *lymph node*.

nodi lymphatici pancreatici superio′res, superior pancreatic lymph nodes. SEE pancreatic *lymph nodes*, under *lymph node*.

nodi lymphatici pancreaticoduodenales [NA], SYN pancreatico-duodenal *lymph nodes*, under *lymph node*.

nodi lymphatici pancreticolienales, SYN pancreaticosplenic *lymph nodes*, under *lymph node*.

nodi lymphatici paracolici, SYN mesocolic *lymph nodes*, under *lymph node*.

nodi lymphatici paramammarii [NA], SYN paramammary *lymph nodes*, under *lymph node*.

nodi lymphatici pararectales [NA], SYN pararectal *lymph nodes*, under *lymph node*.

nodi lymphatici parasternales [NA], SYN parasternal *lymph nodes*, under *lymph node*.

nodi lymphatici paratracheales [NA], SYN paratracheal *lymph node*.

nodi lymphatici parauterini [NA], SYN parauterine *lymph nodes*, under *lymph node*.

nodi lymphatici paravaginales [NA], SYN paravaginal *lymph nodes*, under *lymph node*.

nodi lymphatici paravesiculares [NA], SEE paravesical *lymph nodes*, under *lymph node*.

no′di lymphatici parieta′les [NA], SYN parietal *lymph nodes*, under *lymph node*.

nodi lymphatici parotid′ei intraglandulares [NA], SYN intra-glandular deep parotid *lymph nodes*, under *lymph node*.

nodi lymphatici parotid′ei profundi [NA], SYN deep parotid *lymph nodes*, under *lymph node*.

nodi lymphatici parotid′ei profundi infra-auricula′res [NA], SYN infra-auricular deep parotid *lymph nodes*, under *lymph node*.

nodi lymphatici parotidei profundi preauriculares [NA], small lymph nodes located deep to the parotid fascia and in front of the ear. SYN preauricular deep parotid lymph nodes.

nodi lymphatici parotid′ei superficiales [NA], SYN superficial parotid *lymph nodes*, under *lymph node*.

nodi lymphatici pericardiales laterales [NA], SYN lateral peri-cardiac *lymph nodes*, under *lymph node*.

nodi lymphatici phrenici inferiores [NA], SYN inferior phrenic *lymph nodes*, under *lymph node*.

nodi lymphatici phrenici superiores [NA], SYN superior phrenic *lymph nodes*, under *lymph node*.

nodi lymphatici popliteales [NA], SYN popliteal *lymph nodes*, under *lymph node*.

nodi lymphatici postcavales, SEE right lumbar *lymph nodes*, under *lymph node*.

nodi lymphatici postvesiculares, SEE paravesical *lymph nodes*, under *lymph node*.

nodi lymphatici prececales [NA], SYN prececal *lymph nodes*, under *lymph node*.

nodi lymphatici prelaryngeales [NA], SYN prelaryngeal *lymph nodes*, under *lymph node*.

nodi lymphatici prepericardiales [NA], SYN prepericardiac *lymph nodes*, under *lymph node*.

nodi lymphatici pretracheales [NA], SYN pretracheal *lymph nodes*, under *lymph node*.

nodi lymphatici prevertebrales [NA], SYN prevertebral *lymph nodes*, under *lymph node*.

nodi lymphatici prevesiculares, SEE paravesical *lymph nodes*, under *lymph node*.

nodi lymphatici promontorii [NA], SYN promontory common iliac *lymph nodes*, under *lymph node*.

nodi lymphatici pulmonales, SYN pulmonary *lymph nodes*, under *lymph node*.

nodi lymphatici pylorici [NA], SYN pyloric *lymph nodes*, under *lymph node*.

nodi lymphatici rectales superiores [NA], SYN superior rectal *lymph nodes*, under *lymph node*.

nodi lymphatici retrocecales [NA], SYN retrocecal *lymph nodes*, under *lymph node*.

nodi lymphatici retropharyngeales [NA], SYN retropharyngeal *lymph nodes*, under *lymph node*.

nodi lymphatici sacrales [NA], SYN sacral *lymph nodes*, under *lymph node*.

nodi lymphatici sigmoidei [NA], SYN sigmoid *lymph nodes*, under *lymph node*.

nodi lymphatici splenici [NA], SYN splenic *lymph nodes*, under *lymph node*.

nodi lymphatici subaortici [NA], SYN subaortic *lymph nodes*, under *lymph node*.

nodi lymphatici submandibulares [NA], SYN submandibular *lymph nodes*, under *lymph node*.

nodi lymphatici submentales [NA], SYN submental *lymph nodes*, under *lymph node*.

nodi lymphatici superiores centrales [NA], SYN middle group of mesenteric *lymph nodes*, under *lymph node*.

nodi lymphatici supraclaviculares [NA], SYN supraclavicular *lymph nodes*, under *lymph node*.

nodi lymphatici thyroidei [NA], SYN thyroid *lymph nodes*, under *lymph node*.

nodi lymphatici tracheobronchiales inferiores [NA], SYN inferior tracheobronchial *lymph nodes*, under *lymph node*.

nodi lymphatici tracheobronchiales superiores [NA], SYN superior tracheobronchial *lymph nodes*, under *lymph node*.

nodi lymphatici vesicales laterales, SEE paravesical *lymph nodes*, under *lymph node*.

NOE Abbreviation for nuclear Overhauser *effect*.

no·e·mat·ic (nō-ē-mat′ik). Rarely used term relating to the mental processes. SYN noetic. [G. *noēma*, perception, a thought]

no·e·sis (nō-ē′sis). Cognition, especially through direct and self-evident knowledge. [G. *noēsis*, thought, intelligence]

no·et·ic (nō-et′ik). SYN noematic.

no·eud vi·tal (nū vē-tal′). A circumscript region in the lower part of the medulla oblongata, near the apex of the calamus scriptorius, interpreted by M. Flourens (1858) as a nerve center controlling respiration. SYN vital knot, vital node. [Fr.]

No·gu·chia (nō-gū′chē-ă). A genus of aerobic to facultatively anaerobic, motile, peritrichous bacteria (family Brucellaceae) containing small, slender, Gram-negative, encapsulated rods. These organisms are present in the conjunctiva of man and other animals affected by a follicular type of disease. The type species is *N. granulosis*. [Hideyo *Noguchi*, Japanese bacteriologist, 1876–1928]

N. cunic′uli, a species which causes conjunctival folliculosis in rabbits.

N. granulo′sis, a species regarded by some as a cause of trachoma in man; it produces a granular conjunctivitis in monkeys and apes; it is the type species of the genus *N.*

N. sim′iae, a species which causes conjunctival folliculosis in monkeys (*Macacus rhesus*).

noise (noyz). **1.** Unwanted additions to a signal not arising at its source; *e.g.,* the 60-cycle frequency wave in an electrocardiogram; includes visual n. on imaging studies; largely eliminated from modern (post-1980) machines. SEE signal-to-noise *ratio*. **2.** Extraneous uncontrolled variables influencing the distibution of measurements in a set of data. [M.E., fr. O.Fr., fr. L.L. *nausea*, seasickness]

structured n., in radiology, the signals from anatomic structures which interfere with the detection of significant pathology.

no·ma (nō′mă). A gangrenous stomatitis, usually beginning in the mucous membrane of the corner of the mouth or cheek, and then progressing fairly rapidly to involve the entire thickness of the lips or cheek (or both), with conspicuous necrosis and complete sloughing of tissue; usually observed in poorly nourished children and debilitated adults, especially in lower socioeconomic groups, and frequently preceded by another disease, *e.g.,* kala azar, dysentery, or scarlet fever. A similar process (n. pudendi, n. vulvae) also may involve the labia majora. Several organisms are usually found in the necrotic material, but fusiform bacilli, *Borrelia* organisms, staphylococci, and anaerobic streptococci are most frequently observed. SYN cancrum oris, corrosive ulcer, stomatonecrosis, stomatonoma, water canker. [G. *nomē*, a spreading (sore)]

Nomarski, Georges, 20th century French optical inventor. SEE N. *optics*.

no·ma·to·pho·bia (nō′ma-tō-fō′bē-ă). SYN onomatophobia.

no·men·cla·ture (nō′men-klā-chūr, nō-men′klă-chūr). A set system of names used in any science, as of anatomic structures, organisms, etc. [L. *nomenclatura*, a listing of names, fr. *nomen*, name, + *calo*, to proclaim]

binary n., binomial n., SYN linnaean *system* of nomenclature.

Cleland n., a n. for representing the binding mechanisms of enzyme-catalyzed reactions; in this n., substrates are represented by the letters A, B, C, etc., while products are represented by P, Q, R, etc., enzyme by E, and modified forms of the enzyme by F, G, etc.; in addition, the number of substrates or products is represented by uni, bi, ter, etc.; thus, an aminotransferase reaction (*e.g.,* alanine transaminase) has a ping-pong bi bi mechanism; glutamine synthetase has been reported to have a random ter ter mechanism. See also entries under subentries under mechanism.

No·men·kla·tur Kom·mis·sion (N.K.). Committee on Nomenclature of the German Anatomical Society, appointed to revise or supplement the BNA (1895).

no·mi·fen·sine ma·le·ate (nō-mi-fen′sēn). 8-Amino-1,2,3,4-tetrahydro-2-methyl-4-phenylisoquinoline maleate; an antidepressant.

Nom·i·na An·a·tom·i·ca (NA) (nom′i-nă an-ă-tom′i-kă, nō′mi-nă an′ă-tō′mi-kă). The modification of the Basle Nomina Anatomica or BNA system of anatomical terminology adopted in 1955 by the International Congress of Anatomists in Paris, France. The International Anatomical Nomenclature Committee is responsible for continued revisions of the NA which are reviewed and adopted by the International Congress of Anatomists meeting at five-year intervals since 1950.

nom·o·gram (nom′ō-gram). A form of line chart showing scales for the variables involved in a particular formula in such a way that corresponding values for each variable lie in a straight line intersecting all the scales. SYN nomograph (2). [G. *nomos*, law, + *gramma*, something written]

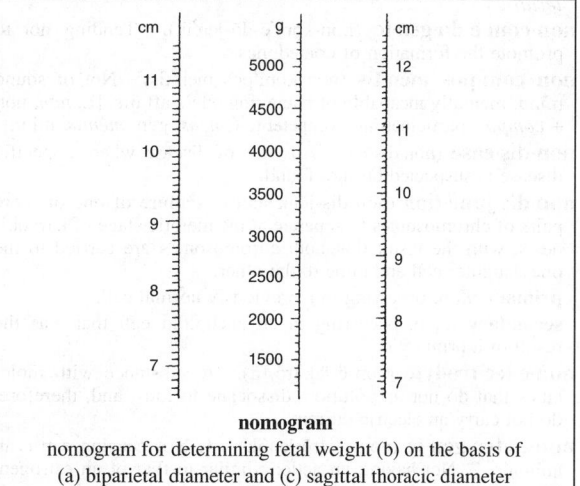

nomogram
nomogram for determining fetal weight (b) on the basis of
(a) biparietal diameter and (c) sagittal thoracic diameter

blood volume n., a n. used to predict blood volume on the basis of the individual's weight and height.

cartesian n., a n. based on rectangular coordinates, representing two variables, on which a family of isopleths is superimposed for each of the additional variables involved. [from R. Descartes, French philosopher and mathematician, 1596–1650]

d'Ocagne n., an alignment chart consisting of an arrangement of three or more graduated lines (straight or curved), each constituting a scale of values of a variable, constructed so that any straight line crossing these scales connects the simultaneously compatible values; from values for any two variables, the values of all other variables can be determined.

Radford n., a n. used to predict necessary tidal volume for artificial respiration on the basis of respiratory rate, body weight, and sex; correction factors are supplied for activity, fever, altitude, metabolic acidosis, and alterations in dead space.

Siggaard-Andersen n., a n. used to predict acid-base composition of blood by the slope and position of a buffer line constructed when P_{CO_2} on a logarithmic scale is plotted against pH.

nom·o·graph (nom′ō-graf). **1.** A graph consisting of three co-planar curves, usually parallel, each graduated for a different variable so that a straight line cutting all three curves intersects the related values of each variable. **2.** SYN nomogram. [G. *nomos,* law, + *graphō,* to write]

nom·o·thet·ic (nom-ō-thet′ik). Denoting the generalizations pertaining to the behavior of groups of individuals as groups, as opposed to idiographic. [G. *nomos,* law, + *thesis,* a placing]

no·mo·top·ic (nō-mō-top′ik). Relating to, or occurring at, the usual or normal place. [G. *nomos,* law, custom, + *topos,* place]

non·al·lele (non-ă-lēl′). Used of genes that are not competitors at the same locus; how independently they will behave depends on whether their loci are linked. At least when first formed (for instance, as a result of unequal crossing-over) two nonalleles may be identical.

no·nan (nō′nan). Occurring on the ninth day. [L. *nonus,* ninth]

n-**non·a·no·ic ac·id** (non-ă-nō′ik). SYN pelargonic acid.

non·a·pep·tide (non-a-pep′tīd). An oligopeptide containing nine amino acid residues (*e.g.,* oxytocin).

non·bur·sate (non-ber′sāt). Denoting a nontaxonomic division of Nematoda embracing those in which the male copulatory bursa is only a skin fold containing no fleshy ribs, as seen in the hookworms, and other bursate nematodes. [L. *non,* not, + Mediev. L. *bursa,* purse]

non·car·i·o·gen·ic (non-kă′rē-ō-jen′ik). Not caries-producing.

non·cel·lu·lar (non-sel′yū-lăr). **1.** Lacking cellular organization, as applied to viruses, which can only replicate within a cell, whether prokaryotic or eukaryotic. SYN subcellular. **2.** SYN acellular (1).

non·chro·mo·gens (non-krō′mō-jenz). SYN group III *mycobacteria.*

non·com·e·do·gen·ic (non-kom′ē-dō-jen′ik). Tending not to promote the formation of comedones.

non com·pos men·tis (non kom′pos men′tis). Not of sound mind; mentally incapable of managing one's affairs. [L. *non,* not, + *compos,* participating, competent, + *mens,* gen. *mentis,* mind]

non·dis·ease (non′dis-ēz). Absence of disease when a specific disease is suspected but not found.

non·dis·junc·tion (non-dis-jŭnk′shŭn). Failure of one or more pairs of chromosomes to separate at the meiotic stage of karyokinesis, with the result that both chromosomes are carried to the one daughter cell and none to the other.

primary n., n. occurring in a previously normal cell.

secondary n., n. occurring in an aneuploid cell that was the result of a primary n.

non·e·lec·tro·lyte (non-ē-lek′trō-līt). A substance with molecules that do not, in solution, dissociate to ions, and, therefore, do not carry an electric current.

non·es·tro·gen·ic (non-es-trō-jen′ik). **1.** Not causing estrus in animals. **2.** Not having an action similar to that of an estrogen. Cf. nonuterotropic. SYN nonoestrogenic.

non·im·mune (non-i-myūn′). Pertaining to an individual that is not immune or to a serum from such an individual.

non·im·mun·i·ty (non-i-myūn′i-tē). SYN aphylaxis.

non·in·fec·tious (non′in-fek′shŭs). Not infectious; not able to spread disease.

non·in·va·sive (non-in-vā′siv). Denoting a procedure that does not require insertion of an instrument or device through the skin or a body orifice for diagnosis or treatment.

non·ion·ic (non-ī-on′ik). A class of radiographic contrast media which do not ionize in solution, thereby decreasing effective osmolarity and toxicity.

non·ma·lef·i·cence (non-mal′ef-ĭ-sens). The ethical principle of doing no harm, based on the Hippocratic maxim, *primum non nocere,* first do no harm. [non- + L. *maleficencia,* evildoing, fr. *male,* badly, wrongly, + *facio,* to do, act]

non·med·ul·lat·ed (non-med′yū-lāt-ed). SYN unmyelinated.

non·my·e·li·nat·ed (non-mī′ĕ-li-nāt′ed). SYN unmyelinated.

non·ne·o·plas·tic (non′nē-ō-plas′tik). Not neoplastic.

non·nu·cle·at·ed (non-nū′klē-ā-ted). Having no nucleus.

non·oc·clu·sion (non-ŏ-klū′shŭn). Failure of a tooth to contact an opposing tooth.

non·oes·tro·gen·ic. SYN nonestrogenic.

non·ose (non′ōs). A sugar with nine carbon atoms. [L. *nonus,* ninth]

non·ox·y·nol 9 (non′noks-ĭ-nol). A group of compounds which are surface acting agents, used in spermicidal preparations such as contraceptive foam and diaphragm jelly.

non·par·ous (non-par′ŭs). SYN nulliparous.

non·pen·e·trance (non-pen′ĕ-trans). The state in which a genetic trait, although present in the appropriate genotype (*i.e.,* homozygous, hemizygous, or heterozygous according to the state of dominance and mode of inheritance), fails to manifest itself in the phenotype because of nongenetic mechanisms. Cf. hypostasis.

non·pro·pri·e·tary name (non-prō-prī′ĕ-tār-ē). A short name (often called a generic name) of a chemical, drug, or other substance that is not subject to trademark (proprietary) rights but is, in contrast to a trivial name, recognized or recommended by government agencies (*e.g.,* Federal Food and Drug Administration) and by quasi-official organizations (*e.g.,* U.S. Adopted Names Council) for general public use. Like a proprietary name, it is almost always a coined designation derived without using set criteria. Cf. trivial name, proprietary name, semisystematic name, systematic name.

non·pro·te·o·gen·ic (non-prō′tē-ō-jen′ik). Not leading to the production of proteins.

non·re·set no·dus si·nu·a·tri·a·lis (non-rē′set nō′dŭs sī′nū-ā-trē-ā′lis). Nonreset of the sinoatrial node produced by a premature atrial depolarizaton when the sum of the duration of the premature cycle and the return cycle is fully compensatory, *i.e.,* twice the duration of the spontaneous cycle length. Cf. reset nodus sinuatrialis.

non·ro·ta·tion (non-rō-tā′shŭn). Failure of normal rotation.

n. of intestine, a developmental anomaly resulting in the small intestine being on the right of the abdomen and the colon on the left.

n. of kidney, a developmental anomaly in which the hilum of the kidney retains its original position, facing ventrally.

non·sa·pon·i·fi·a·ble ((non-să-pon-i-fī′a-bl). Not subject to saponification; *e.g.,* triacylglycerols are saponifiable but cholesterol is n.

non·se·cre·tor (non-sē-krē′tŏr, -tōr). An individual whose saliva does not contain antigens of the ABO blood group. SEE ALSO secretor.

non·sense. As used in genetics, relating to a mutation that causes a sequence such that the growing peptide chain terminates, often after several incorrect amino acid residues are incorporated.

nonsense suppression, mutant tRNAs that read a chain termination codon as the signal for incorporation of a specific amino acid residue.

non·un·ion (non′yūn-yŭn). Failure of normal healing of a fractured bone.

non·uter·o·tro·pic (non-yū-ter-ō-trō′pik). Not causing an effect on the uterus. Cf. nonestrogenic.

non·va·lent (non-vā′lent). Having no valency; not capable of entering into chemical composition.

non·vas·cu·lar (non-vas′kyū-lăr). SYN avascular.

non·ver·bal (non-ver′bl). Denoting communication without sounds or words; *e.g.,* by signs, symbols, facial expressions, gestures, posture.

non·vi·a·ble (non-vī′ă-bl). **1.** Incapable of independent existence; often denoting a prematurely born fetus. **2.** Denoting a microorganism or parasite incapable of metabolic or reproductive activity.

Noonan, Jacqueline A., U.S. pediatric cardiologist, *1921. SEE N.'s *syndrome.*

△**nor-.** **1.** Chemical prefix denoting 1) elimination of one methylene group from a chain, the highest permissible locant being used; 2) contraction of a (steroid) ring by one CH_2 unit, the locant being the capital letter identifying the ring. Elimination of two methylene groups is denoted by the prefix dinor-; three groups, by trinor-, etc. **2.** Chemical prefix denoting "normal," *i.e.,* unbranched chain of carbon atoms in aliphatic compounds, as opposed to branched with the same number of carbon atoms; *e.g.,* norleucine, leucine.

nor·a·dren·a·line (nor-ă-dren′ă-lin). SYN norepinephrine.

n. acid tartrate, SYN *norepinephrine* bitartrate.

n. bitartrate, SYN *norepinephrine* bitartrate.

nor·da·ze·pam (nor′daz-pam). An active sedative/hypnotic of the benzodiazepine class. An active metabolite of diazepam, chlorazepate, and several other benzodiazepines. Has a long biological half-life (40–80 hours).

nor·def·rin hy·dro·chlo·ride (nor-def′rin). *dl*-α(1-Aminoethyl)-3,4-dihydrobenzyl alcohol hydrochloride; a sympathomimetic and vasoconstrictor.

nor·ep·i·neph·rine (nor′ep-i-nef′rin). *l*-(–)-α-(aminomethyl)-3,4-dihydroxybenzyl alcohol; a catecholamine hormone of which the natural form is D, although the L form has some activity; the base is considered to be the postganglionic adrenergic mediator, acting on alpha and beta receptors; it is stored in chromaffin granules in the adrenal medulla, in much smaller amounts than epinephrine, and secreted in response to hypotension and physical stress; in contrast to epinephrine it has little effect on bronchial smooth muscle, metabolic processes, and cardiac output, but has strong vasoconstrictive effects and is used pharmacologically as a vasopressor, primarily as the bitartrate salt. SYN levarterenol, noradrenaline.

n. bitartrate, (-)-α-(aminomethyl)-3,4-dihydroxybenzyl alcohol tartrate. For actions and uses, see n. SYN levarterenol bitartrate, noradrenaline acid tartrate, noradrenaline bitartrate.

nor·eth·an·dro·lone (nor-eth-an′drō-lōn). 17α-Ethyl-19-nortestosterone; 17α-ethyl-17-hydroxy-19-nor-androst-4-en-3-one; an androgenic steroid similar chemically and pharmacologically to testosterone.

nor·eth·in·drone (nor-eth′in-drōn). 19-norethisterone; 19-nor-17α-ethinyltestosterone; 17α-ethynl-17β-hydroxy-4-estren-3-one; a potent orally effective progestational agent with some estrogenic and androgenic activity; used as a substitute for progesterone and, in combination with an estrogen, as an oral contraceptive. SYN norethisterone.

n. acetate, 17-hydroxy-19-nor-17α-pregn-4-en-20-yn-3-one acetate; an orally active progestin with some estrogenic and androgenic activity, used to treat endometriosis and, with an estrogen, as an oral contraceptive.

nor·eth·is·ter·one (nor-eth-is′ter-ōn). SYN norethindrone.

nor·e·thyn·o·drel (nor-ĕ-thī′nō-drel). An orally active progestin with some estrogenic activity; used as a progestational agent and, in combination with mestranol, as an oral contraceptive.

nor·flox·a·cin (nor-floks′ă-sin). 1-Ethyl-6-fluoro-1,4-dihydro-4-oxo-7-(1-piperazinyl)-3-quinolinecarboxylic acid; an oral broad spectrum quinoline antibacterial agent used in the treatment of urinary tract infections.

nor·ges·trel (nor-jes′trel). (±)-13-Ethyl-17-hydroxy-18,19-di-nor-17α-pregn-4-en-20-yn-3-one; a progestin used in oral contraceptive products.

nor·leu·cine (Nle) (nor-lū′sin). α-amino-*n*-caproic acid; 2-aminohexanoic acid; an α-amino acid, isomer of leucine and isoleucine, but not found in proteins; a deamination product of L-lysine, to which it is linked in collagens. SYN glycoleucine.

norm. 1. The usual value. **2.** The desirable value or behavior.

nor·ma, pl. **nor·mae** (nor′mă, nor′mē) [NA]. SYN profile (1). [L. a carpenter's square]

n. ante′rior, SYN n. facialis.

n. facia′lis [NA], the outline of the skull viewed from in front. SYN n. anterior, n. frontalis.

n. fronta′lis, SYN n. facialis.

n. infe′rior, SYN external *base* of skull.

n. latera′lis [NA], the profile of the skull; the outline of the skull viewed from either side. SYN n. temporalis.

n. occipita′lis [NA], the outline of the skull viewed from behind. SYN n. posterior.

n. poste′rior, SYN n. occipitalis.

n. sagitta′lis, the outline of a sagittal section through the skull.

n. supe′rior, SYN n. verticalis.

n. tempora′lis, SYN n. lateralis.

n. ventra′lis, SYN external *base* of skull.

n. verti′calis [NA], the outline of the surface of the skull viewed from above. SYN n. superior.

nor·mal (nor′măl). **1.** Typical; usual; according to the rule or standard. **2.** In bacteriology, nonimmune; untreated; denoting an animal, or the serum or substance contained therein, that has not been experimentally immunized against any microorganism or its products. **3.** Denoting a solution containing 1 equivalent of replaceable hydrogen or hydroxyl per liter; *e.g.,* 1 M HCl is 1 N, but 1 M H_2SO_4 is 2 N. **4.** In psychiatry and psychology, denoting a level of effective functioning which is satisfactory to both the individual and his social milieu. [L. *normalis,* according to pattern]

nor·mal·i·za·tion (nor′mal-i-zā′shŭn). **1.** Making normal or according to the standard. **2.** Reducing or strengthening of a solution to make it normal. **3.** Adjusting one curve to another by multiplication of the points of the one by some arbitrary factor.

nor·mal·ize (nor′măl-īz). To effect normalization.

nor·ma·tive. Pertaining to the normal or usual.

nor·me·per·i·dine (nor-mep′er-ĭ-dīn). A metabolite of meperidine in which the *N*-methyl group has been removed. The compound possesses convulsant properties.

nor·met·a·neph·rine (nor-met′ă-nef′rin). 3-*O*-Methylnorepinephrine; a catabolite of norepinephrine found, together with metanephrine, in the urine and some tissues, resulting from the action of catechol-*O*-methyltransferase on norepinephrine; has no sympathomimetic actions.

nor·meth·a·done (nor-meth′ă-dōn). Desmethylmethadone; phenyldimazone; 6-dimethylamino-4,4-diphenyl-3-hexanone; an antitussive with narcotic properties.

△**normo-.** Normal, usual. [L. *normalis,* according to pattern]

nor·mo·bar·ic (nor-mō-bar′ik). Denoting a barometric pressure equivalent to sea level pressure. [normo- + G. *baros,* weight]

nor·mo·blast (nor′mō-blast). A nucleated red blood cell, the immediate precursor of a normal erythrocyte in humans. Its four stages of development are: 1) pronormoblast, 2) basophilic n., 3) polychromatic n., and 4) orthochromatic n. SEE erythroblast. [normo- + G. *blastos,* sprout, germ]

nor·mo·blas·to·sis. Excessive production of normoblasts by the bone marrow.

nor·mo·cap·nia (nor-mō-kap′nē-ă). A state in which the arterial carbon dioxide pressure is normal, about 40 mm Hg. SEE ALSO eucapnia. [normo- + G. *kapnos,* vapor]

nor·mo·ce·phal·ic (nor′mō-se-fal′ik). SYN mesocephalic. [normo- + G. *kephalē,* head]

nor·mo·chro·mia (nor-mō-krō′mē-ă). Normal color; referring to blood in which the amount of hemoglobin in the red blood cells is normal. [normo- + G. *chrōma,* color]

nor·mo·chro·mic (nor-mō-krō′mik). Being normal in color; referring especially to red blood cells that possess the normal quantity of hemoglobin.

nor·mo·cyte (nor′mō-sīt). A non-nucleated erythrocyte of normal size (average 7.5 μm); a normal, healthy red blood cell. SYN normoerythrocyte. [normo- + G. *kytos,* cell]

nor·mo·cy·to·sis (nor′mō-sī-tō′sis). A normal state of the blood with regard to its component formed elements.

nor·mo·e·ryth·ro·cyte (nor′mō-ĕ-rith′rō-sīt). SYN normocyte.

nor·mo·gly·ce·mia (nor′mō-glī-sē′mē-ă). SYN euglycemia.

nor·mo·gly·ce·mic (nor′mō-glī-sē′mik). SYN euglycemic.

nor·mo·ka·le·mia, nor·mo·ka·li·e·mia (nor′mō-kă-lē′mē-ă, -ka-lē-ē′mē-ă). A normal level of potassium in the blood.

nor·mo·pla·sia (nor-mō-plā′zē-ă). A specific differentiation characteristic of a cell within normal limits. [normo- + G. *plasis,* a forming]

nor·mo·sthe·nu·ria (nor′mō-sthē-nū′rē-ă). Condition in which specific gravity of urine is normal. [normo- + G. *sthenos,* strength, + *ouron,* urine]

nor·mo·ten·sive (nōr-mō-ten'siv). Indicating a normal arterial blood pressure. SYN normotonic (2).

nor·mo·ther·mia (nōr-mō-ther'mē-ă). Environmental temperature that does not cause increased or depressed activity of body cells. [normo- + G. *thermē*, heat]

nor·mo·ton·ic (nōr-mō-ton'ik). 1. Relating to or characterized by normal muscular tone. SYN eutonic. 2. SYN normotensive.

nor·mo·to·pia (nōr-mō-tō'pē-ă). The state of being in the normal place; used in reference to normal placement of an organ. [normo- + G. *topos*, place]

nor·mo·top·ic (nōr-mō-top'ik). Relating to normotopia; in the right place.

nor·mo·vol·e·mia (nōr'mō-vol-ē'mē-ă). A normal blood volume. [normo- + volume, + G. *haima*, blood]

nor·mox·ia (nōr-mok'sē-ă). A state in which the partial pressure of oxygen in the inspired gas is equal to that of air at sea level, about 150 mm Hg. [normo- + oxygen]

nor·oph·thal·mic ac·id (nōr'of-thal-mik). *N*-[*N*-(γ-Glutamyl)-alanyl]glycin e; a tripeptide analogue of glutathione (L-cysteine replaced by L-alanine), found in the lens of the eye.

nor·pi·pa·none (nōr-pip'ă-nōn). 4,4-Diphenyl-6-(1-piperidyl)-3-hexanone; an analgesic agent.

Norrie, Gordon, Danish ophthalmologist, 1855–1941. SEE N.'s *disease*.

Norris, Richard, English physiologist, 1831–1916. SEE N.'s *corpuscles*, under *corpuscle*.

nor·ster·oids (nōr-stēr'oydz). Steroids in which an angular methyl group is missing; most commonly, the group between the A and B rings (C-19).

nor·sym·pa·tol (nōr-sim'pă-tōl). SYN octopamine.

nor·sy·neph·rine (nōr-si-nef'rin). SYN octopamine.

Norton, U.F., U.S. obstetrician. SEE N.'s *operation*.

nor·trip·ty·line hy·dro·chlo·ride (nōr-trip'ti-lēn). 10,11-Dihydro-*N*-methyl-5*H*-dibenzol[a,d]cycloheptene-Δ⁵,γ-propylamine hydrochloride; an antidepressant.

nor·val·ine (Nva) (nōr-val'ēn, -vā'lēn). CH₃(CH₂)₂CH(NH₃)⁺COO⁻; α-Aminovaleric acid; the straight chain analogue of valine; not found in proteins.

nos·ca·pine (nos'kă-pēn). 2-methyl-8-methoxy-6,7-methylenedioxy-1-(6,7-dimethoxy-3-phthalidyl)-1,2,3,4-tetrahydroisoquinoline; an isoquinoline alkaloid, occurring in opium, with papaverine-like action on smooth muscle; suppresses the cough reflex and is used as an antitussive; it appears to be without addiction liability. SYN *l*-α-narcotine, opianine.

nose (ENT) (nōz). That portion of the respiratory pathway above the hard palate; includes both the external nose and the nasal cavity. SYN nasus (2) [NA]. [A.S. *nosu*]

brandy n., SYN rhinophyma.

cleft n., a n. with a furrow where the bridge is normally present; due to failure of complete convergence of the paired primordia.

copper n., SYN rhinophyma.

dog n., SYN goundou.

external n., the visible portion of the nose which forms a prominent feature of the face; it consists of a root, dorsum and apex from above downward and is perforated inferiorly by two nostrils separated by a septum. SYN nasus externus [NA], nasus (1) [NA].

hammer n., SYN rhinophyma.

potato n., SYN rhinophyma.

rum n., SYN rhinophyma.

saddle n., a n. with markedly depressed bridge, seen in congenital syphilis or after injury from trauma or operation.

toper's n., SYN rhinophyma.

nose·bleed (nōs'blēd). SYN epistaxis.

No·se·ma (nō-sē'mă). A protozoan genus (family Nosematidae, order Microsporida, phylum Microspora) with species (*N. apis*, *N. bombycis*, and others) pathogenic for invertebrates of economic importance (bees, silkworms); others are being studied as possible agents of biological control of pest insects or other target invertebrates. *N. connori* infects human fat tissue, diaphragm, myocardium, liver and other tissues of the immunosuppressed individuals. [G. *nosēma*, plague, fr. *noseō*, to be sick, fr. *nosos*, disease]

N. corneum, a cause of keratoconjunctivitis and diffuse punctate keratopathy in AIDS patients.

No·se·mat·i·dae (nō-sē-mat'i-dē). A family of the class Microsporida that includes the genera *Encephalitozoon* and *Nosema*, containing several pathogenic and economically important species.

no·sem·a·to·sis (nō-sē'ma-tō'sis). An infection of rabbits with the protozoan parasite *Encephalitozoon cuniculi* that can cause a focal interstitial nephritis; one case of n. has been reported in humans.

nose·piece (nōs'pēs). A microscope attachment, consisting of several objectives surrounding a central pivot.

nos·e·ti·ol·o·gy (nōs'ē-tē-ol'ō-jē). Rarely used term for the study of the causes of disease. [G. *nosos*, disease, + *aitia*, cause, + *logos*, study]

⌂**noso-.** Disease. SEE ALSO path-. [G. *nosos*]

nos·och·tho·nog·ra·phy (nos'ok-thō-nog'ră-fē). SYN geomedicine. [noso- + G. *chthōn*, the earth, + *graphē*, a description]

nos·o·co·mi·al (nos-ō-kō'mē-ăl). 1. Relating to a hospital. 2. Denoting a new disorder (not the patient's original condition) associated with being treated in a hospital, such as a hospital-acquired infection. [G. *nosokomeion*, hospital, fr. *nosos*, disease, + *komeō*, to take care of]

nos·o·gen·e·sis, no·sog·e·ny (nos-ō-jen'ē-sis, no-soj'ĕ-nē). Rarely used terms for pathogenesis. [noso- + G. *genesis*, production]

nos·o·gen·ic (nos-ō-jen'ik). SYN pathogenic.

nos·o·ge·og·ra·phy (nos'ō-jē-og'ră-fē). SYN geomedicine.

nos·o·graph·ic (nos-ō-graf'ik). Relating to nosography, or the description of diseases.

no·sog·ra·phy (nō-sog'ră-fē). 1. Assignment of names to each disease entity in a group that has been classified according to a systematic nosology. 2. A treatise on pathology or the practice of medicine. [noso- + G. *graphē*, description]

nos·o·log·ic (nos-ō-loj'ik). Relating to nosology.

no·sol·o·gy (nō-sol'ō-jē). The science of classification of diseases. SYN nosonomy, nosotaxy. [noso- + G. *logos*, study]

psychiatric n., SYN psychonosology.

no·sol·o·gy (nō-sol'ō-jē). 1. The science of classification of diseases. 2. Classification of ill persons into groups, whatever the criteria for the classification, and agreement as to the boundaries of the group.

nos·o·ma·nia (nos-ō-mā'nē-ă). An unfounded morbid belief that one is suffering from some special disease. [noso- + G. *mania*, insanity]

no·som·e·try (nō-som'ĕ-trē). Measurement of morbidity or of the sickness rate in occupations and social conditions. [noso- + G. *metron*, measure]

nos·o·my·co·sis (nos'ō-mī-kō'sis). Any disease caused by a fungus. [noso- + G. *mykēs*, fungus]

no·son·o·my (nō-son'ō-mē). SYN nosology. [noso- + G. *nomos*, law]

nos·o·phil·ia (nos-ō-fil'ē-ă). A morbid desire to be sick. [noso- + G. *phileō*, to love]

nos·o·pho·bia (nos-ō-fō'bē-ă). An inordinate dread and fear of disease. SYN pathophobia. [noso- + G. *phobos*, fear]

nos·o·phyte (nos'ō-fīt). A pathogenic microorganism of the plant kingdom. [noso- + G. *phyton*, plant]

nos·o·poi·et·ic (nos'ō-poy-et'ik). SYN pathogenic. [noso- + G. *poiēsis*, a making]

Nos·o·psyl·lus (nos-ō-sil'ŭs). A flea genus commonly found on rodents. *N. fasciatus*, the northern rat flea, is a species that infrequently transmits the plague bacillus to humans. [noso- + G. *psylla*, flea]

nos·o·taxy (nos'ō-tak-sē). SYN nosology. [noso- + G. *taxis*, arrangement]

nos·o·tox·ic (nos-ō-tok'sik). Relating to a nosotoxin or to nosotoxicosis.

nos·o·tox·i·co·sis (nos′ō-tok-si-kō′sis). A morbid state caused by a toxin. SEE ALSO toxicosis. [noso- + G. *toxikon,* poison]

nos·o·tox·in (nos-ō-tok′sin). Rarely used term for any toxin associated with a disease.

no·sot·ro·phy (nos-ot′rō-fē). Rarely used term for care of the sick. [noso- + G. *trophē,* nourishment]

nos·o·tro·pic (nos-ō-trop′ik). Directed against the pathologic changes or symptoms of a disease. [noso- + G. *tropē,* a turning]

nos·tal·gia (nos-tal′jē-ă). The longing to return home, to a former time in one's life, or to familiar people and surroundings. Cf. apodemialgia. [G. *nostos,* a return (home), + *algos,* pain]

nos·to·ma·nia (nos-tō-mā′nē-ă). An obsessive or abnormal interest in nostalgia, especially as an extreme manifestation of homesickness. [G. *nostos,* return, homecoming, + *mania,* frenzy]

nos·to·pho·bia (nos-tō-fō′bē-ă). Morbid fear of returning home. [G. *nostos,* return, homecoming, + *phobos,* fear]

nos·tril. Anterior opening to either side of the nasal cavity. SYN naris [NA], anterior naris, external naris, prenaris.

    internal n., SYN secondary *choana.*

nos·trum (nos′trŭm). General term for a therapeutic agent, sometimes patented but usually of secret composition, offered to the general public as a specific remedy for any disease or class of diseases. [L. neuter of *noster,* our, "our own remedy"]

NO syn·thase Abbreviation for nitric oxide synthase.

no·tal (nō′tăl). Relating to the back. [G. *nōtos,* the back]

no·tal·gia (nō-tal′jē-ă). Obsolete term for dorsalgia. [G. *nōtos,* the back, + *algos,* pain]

    n. paresthet′ica, localized pruritus in the oval-shaped area in the inferomedial border of the scapula, with no demonstrable changes in the skin except for what results from repeated and prolonged scratching.

no·tan·ce·pha·lia (nō′tan-se-fā′lē-ă). Fetal malformation characterized by a bony deficiency, *i.e.,* absence of the occipital bone of the cranium. [G. *nōtos,* back, + *an-* priv. + *kephalē,* head]

no·tan·en·ce·pha·lia (nō′tan-en-se-fā′lē-ă). Absence of the cerebellum. [G. *nōtos,* back, + *an-* priv. + *enkephalos,* brain]

no·ta·tin (nō-tā′tin). A protein (glucose oxidase) that has specifically been isolated from *Penicillium notatum.* [from *Penicillium notatum*]

NOTCH

notch. An indentation at the edge of any structure. SYN incisura [NA], emargination, incisure.

    acetabular n., a gap in the inferior the margin of the acetabulum. SYN incisura acetabuli [NA], cotyloid n.

    angular n., a sharp angular depression in the lesser curvature of the stomach at the junction of the body with the pyloric canal. SYN incisura angularis [NA], sulcus angularis.

    antegonial n., the highest point of the n. or concavity of the lower border of the ramus where it joins the body of the mandible.

    anterior cerebellar n., a wide, shallow notch on the anterior surface of the cerebellum occupied laterally by the superior cerebellar peduncles and the inferior quadrigeminal bodies medially. SYN anterior n. of cerebellum, incisura cerebelli anterior, semilunar n. (1).

    anterior n. of cerebellum, SYN anterior cerebellar n.

    anterior n. of ear, a notch between the supratragic tubercle and the crus of the helix. SYN incisura anterior auris [NA], anterior auricular groove, auricular n. (1), sulcus auriculae anterior.

    aortic n., the n. in a sphygmographic tracing caused by rebound following closure of the aortic valves.

    n. of apex of heart, a slight notch near the apex of the heart where the anterior interventricular sulcus reaches the diaphragmatic surface of the heart. SYN incisura apicis cordis [NA].

    auricular n., (1) SYN anterior n. of ear. **(2)** SYN terminal n. of auricle.

    cardiac n., a deep notch between the esophagus and fundus of the stomach. SYN incisura cardiaca [NA].

    cardiac n. of left lung, the notch in the anterior border of the superior lobe of the left lung which accommodates the pericardium. SYN incisura cardiaca pulmonis sinistri [NA].

    n.'s in cartilage of external acoustic meatus, (usually) two vertical fissures in the anterior portion of the cartilage of the external auditory meatus, filled by fibrous tissue. SYN incisurae cartilaginis meatus acustici externi [NA], Duverney's fissures, incisurae santorini, Santorini's fissures, Santorini's incisures.

    clavicular n. of sternum, a hollow on either side of the upper surface of the manubrium sterni which articulates with the clavicle. SYN incisura clavicularis [NA], clavicular facet.

    costal n., one of the notches or facets on the lateral edge of the sternum for articulation with a costal cartilage. SYN incisura costalis [NA].

    cotyloid n., SYN acetabular n.

    craniofacial n., a defect in the osseous partition between the orbital and nasal cavities.

    dicrotic n. (dī-krot-ik), the acute drop in arterial pressure pulse curves following the systolic peak, corresponding to the incisura of the displacement pulse curve.

    digastric n., SYN mastoid *groove.*

    ethmoidal n., an oblong gap between the orbital parts of the frontal bone in which the ethmoid bone is lodged. SYN incisura ethmoidalis [NA].

    fibular n., a hollow on the lateral surface of the lower end of the tibia in which the fibula is lodged. SYN incisura fibularis [NA].

    frontal n., a small notch, sometimes a foramen, on the orbital margin of the frontal bone medial to the supraorbital notch. SYN incisura frontalis [NA].

    greater sciatic n., the deep indentation in the posterior border of the hip bone at the point of union of the ilium and ischium. SYN incisura ischiadica major [NA], iliosciatic n., sacrosciatic n.

    hamular n., SYN pterygomaxillary n.

    Hutchinson's crescentic n., the semilunar n. on the incisal edge of Hutchinson's teeth, encountered in congenital syphilis.

    iliosciatic n., SYN greater sciatic n.

    inferior thyroid n., a shallow notch in the middle of the lower border of the thyroid cartilage. SYN incisura thyroidea inferior [NA].

    interarytenoid n., the indentation of posterior portion of the aditus laryngis between the two arytenoid cartilages. SYN incisura interarytenoidea [NA].

    interclavicular n., SYN suprasternal n.

    intercondyloid n., SYN intercondylar *fossa.*

    intertragic n., the deep notch in the lower part of the auricle between the tragus and antitragus. SYN incisura intertragica [NA], incisura tragica.

    intervertebral n., SYN vertebral n.

    ischiatic n., SEE greater sciatic n., lesser sciatic n.

    jugular n. of occipital bone, the notch in the occipital bone which forms one boundary of the jugular foramen. SYN incisura jugularis ossis occipitalis [NA].

    jugular n. of temporal bone, the notch in the temporal bone

---

♻ **Combining forms**	**[NA] Nomina Anatomica**
Word*Finder* **Multi-term entry finder** Preceding letter A	**[MIM] Mendelian** **Inheritance in Man**
A.D.A.M. Anatomy Plates **Between letters L and M**	☆ **Official alternate term**
Appendices: **Following letter Z**	☆**[NA] Official alternate** **Nomina Anatomica term**
SYN Synonym; Cf., compare	**High Profile Term**

which forms one boundary of the jugular foramen. SYN incisura jugularis ossis temporalis [NA].

Kernohan's n., a n. in the cerebral peduncle due to displacement of the brainstem against the incisura of the tentorium by a transtentorial herniation.

lacrimal n., the notch on the frontal process of the maxilla into which the lacrimal bone fits. SYN incisura lacrimalis [NA].

lesser sciatic n., the notch in the posterior border of the ischium below the ischial spine. SYN incisura ischiadica minor [NA].

mandibular n., the deep notch between the condylar and coronoid processes of the mandible. SYN incisura mandibulae [NA], sigmoid n.

marsupial n., SYN posterior cerebellar n.

mastoid n., SYN mastoid *groove*.

nasal n., the notch in the medial border of the maxilla anteriorly which, with its fellow, forms most of the piriform opening of the nasal cavity. SYN incisura nasalis [NA].

pancreatic n., a notch separating the uncinate process of the head of the pancreas from the neck. SYN incisura pancreatis [NA].

parietal n., the angle posteriorly between the squamous and petrous parts of the temporal bone. SYN incisura parietalis [NA].

parotid n., the space between the ramus of the mandible and the mastoid process of the temporal bone.

popliteal n., SYN intercondylar *fossa*.

posterior cerebellar n., a narrow notch between the cerebellar hemispheres posteriorly, occupied by the falx cerebelli. SYN incisura cerebelli posterior, marsupial n., posterior n. of cerebellum.

posterior n. of cerebellum, SYN posterior cerebellar n.

preoccipital n., an indentation in the ventrolateral border of the temporal lobe of the cerebral hemisphere. SYN incisura preoccipitalis [NA].

presternal n., SYN suprasternal n.

pterygoid n., SYN pterygoid *fissure*.

pterygomaxillary n., the n. or fissure between the tuberosity of the maxilla and the hamulus of the pterygoid process of the sphenoid bone. SYN hamular n.

radial n., the concavity on the lateral aspect of the coronoid process of the ulna which articulates with the head of the radius. SYN incisura radialis [NA].

Rivinus' n., SYN tympanic n.

n. for round ligament of liver, the notch in the inferior border of the liver that accommodates the round ligament. SYN incisura ligamenti teretis hepatis [NA], incisura umbilicalis, umbilical n.

sacrosciatic n., SYN greater sciatic n.

scapular n., a n. on the superior border of the scapula through which the suprascapular nerve passes. SYN incisura scapulae [NA], suprascapular n.

semilunar n., (1) SYN anterior cerebellar n. (2) SYN trochlear n.

sigmoid n., SYN mandibular n.

sphenopalatine n., the deep notch between the orbital and sphenoidal processes of the palatine bone which is converted into the foramen of the same name by the undersurface of the sphenoid bone. SYN incisura sphenopalatina [NA].

sternal n., SYN suprasternal n.

superior thyroid n., a deep notch in the middle of the upper border of the thyroid cartilage. SYN incisura thyroidea superior [NA].

supraorbital n., a groove in the orbital margin of the frontal bone, about the junction of the medial and intermediate thirds, through which pass the supraorbital nerve and artery. SEE ALSO supraorbital *foramen*. SYN incisura supraorbitalis [NA].

suprascapular n., SYN scapular n.

suprasternal n., the large notch in the superior margin of the sternum. SYN incisura jugularis sternalis [NA], interclavicular n., presternal n., sternal n.

tentorial n., the triangular opening in the tentorium cerebelli through which the brainstem extends from the posterior into the middle cranial fossa. SYN incisura tentorii [NA], n. of tentorium.

n. of tentorium, SYN tentorial n.

terminal n. of auricle, a deep notch separating the lamina tragi and cartilage of the external auditory meatus from the main

auricular cartilage, the two being connected below by the isthmus. SYN incisura terminalis auris [NA], auricular n. (2).

trochlear n., the large semicircular notch at the proximal extremity of the ulna between the olecranon and coronoid processes that articulates with the trochlea of the humerus. SYN incisura trochlearis [NA], incisura semilunaris ulnae, semilunar n. (2).

tympanic n., the notch in the superior part of the tympanic ring bridged by the flaccid part of the tympanic membrane. SYN incisura tympanica [NA], incisura rivini, Rivinus' incisure, Rivinus' n., tympanic incisure.

ulnar n., the concave surface on the medial side of the distal end of the radius which articulates with the head of the ulna. SYN incisura ulnaris [NA].

umbilical n., SYN n. for round ligament of liver.

vertebral n., one of the two concavities above (superior) and below (inferior) the pedicle of a vertebra; the notches of two adjacent vertebrae (plus the intervertebral disc) form an intervertebral foramen. SYN incisura vertebralis [NA], intervertebral n.

---

notched. SYN emarginate.

no·ten·ceph·a·lo·cele (nō-ten-sef′ă-lō-sēl). Malformation in the occipital portion of the cranium with protrusion of brain substance. [G. *nōtos,* back, + *enkephalos,* brain, + *kēlē,* hernia]

Nothnagel, C.W. Hermann, Austrian physician, 1841–1905. SEE N.'s *syndrome.*

no·to·chord (nō′tō-kōrd). **1.** In primitive vertebrates, the primary axial supporting structure of the body, derived from the notochordal or head process of the early embryo; an important organizer for determining the final form of the nervous system and related structures. **2.** In embryos, the axial fibrocellular cord about which the vertebral primordia develop; vestiges of it persist in the adult as the nuclei pulposi of the intervertebral discs. SYN chorda dorsalis. [G. *nōtos,* back, + *chordē,* cord, string]

no·to·chor·dal (nō-tō-kōr′dăl). Relating to the notochord.

No·to·ed·res ca·ti (nō-tō-ed′rēz kā′tī). Sarcoptic mange mite of cats.

nou·men·al (nū′men-ăl). Intellectually, not sensuously, intuitional; relating to the object of pure thought divorced from all concepts of time or space. [G. *nooumenos,* perceived, fr. *noeō,* to perceive, think]

nour·ish·ment (ner′ish-ment). A substance used to feed or to sustain life and growth of an organism. SYN aliment (1).

nous (nūs, nows). A word originally used by Anaxagoras to mean an all-knowing, all-pervading spirit or force; in later Greek philosophy it came to mean simply mind, reason, or intellect. [G. mind, reason]

no·vo·bi·o·cin (nō-vō-bī′ō-sin). An antibiotic antibacterial substance produced by fermentation from cultures of *Streptomyces niveus* or *S. spheroides,* effective against penicillin-resistant *Staphylococcus* and *Proteus;* also available as n. calcium and n. sodium. SYN streptonivicin.

Novy, Frederick G., U.S. bacteriologist, 1864–1957. SEE N. and MacNeal's blood *agar.*

noxa (nok′să). Anything that exerts a harmful influence, such as trauma, poison, etc. [L. injury, fr. *noceo,* to injure]

nox·ious (nok′shŭs). Injurious; harmful. [L. *noxius,* injurious, fr. *noceo,* to injure]

nox·y·thi·o·lin (nok-sē-thī′ō-lin). 1-(Hydroxymethyl)-3-methyl-2-thiourea; an antibacterial and antifungal agent.

Np 1. Symbol for neptunium. **2.** Abbreviation for neper.

NPN Abbreviation for nonprotein *nitrogen.*

NPO, n.p.o.. Abbreviation for L. *non per os* or *nil per os,* nothing by mouth.

Nps Abbreviation for nitrophenylsulfenyl.

NREM Abbreviation for non-rapid eye *movement.*

nRNA Abbreviation for nuclear RNA.

NSAID Abbreviation for nonsteroidal anti-inflammatory *drugs,* under *drug; e.g.,* aspirin, ibuprofen.

NSF Abbreviation for National Science Foundation.

NSILA Abbreviation for nonsuppressible insulin-like *activity.*

NTMI Abbreviation for nontransmural myocardial *infarction*.

NTNG Abbreviation for nontoxic nodular goiter.

NTP Abbreviation for nucleoside 5′-triphosphate.

NTS Abbreviation for *nucleus* tractus solitarii.

nu (nū). Thirteenth letter of the Greek alphabet, ν (q.v.).

nu·bec·u·la (nū-bek′yū-lă). A faint cloud or cloudiness. [L. dim. of *nubes,* cloud]

Nuc Abbreviation for nucleoside.

nu·cha (nū′kă) [NA]. The back of the neck. SYN nape. [Fr. *nuque*]

nu·chal (nū′kăl). Relating to the nucha.

Nuck, Anton, Dutch anatomist, 1650–1692. SEE N.'s *diverticulum, hydrocele; canal* of N.

⚠ **nucl-.** SEE nucleo-.

nu·cle·ar (nū′klē-er). Relating to a nucleus, either cellular or atomic; in the latter sense, usually referring to radiation emanating from atomic nuclei (α, β, or γ) or to atomic fission.

nu·cle·ase (nū′klē-ās). General term for enzymes that catalyze the hydrolysis of nucleic acid into nucleotides or oligonucleotides by cleaving phosphodiester linkages. For n.'s not listed below, see the specific term. Cf. exonuclease, endonuclease.

azotobacter n., endonuclease (*Serratia marcescens*).

micrococcal n., SYN micrococcal *endonuclease.*

mung bean n., endonuclease S₁ (*Aspergillus*).

nu·cle·ate (nū′klē-āt). A salt of a nucleic acid.

nu·cle·at·ed (nū′klē-ā-ted). Provided with a nucleus, a characteristic of all true cells.

nu·cle·a·tion (nū-klē-ā′shŭn). Process of forming a nidus (4).

heterogeneous n., n. about a nidus composed of material other than that precipitating.

homogeneous n., n. about a nidus composed of material identical with that precipitating.

nu·clei (nū′klē-ī). Plural of nucleus.

nu·cle·ic ac·id (nū-klē′ik, -klā′ik). A family of macromolecules, of molecular masses ranging upward from 25,000, found in the chromosomes, nucleoli, mitochondria, and cytoplasm of all cells, and in viruses; in complexes with proteins, they are called nucleoproteins. On hydrolysis they yield purines, pyrimidines, phosphoric acid, and a pentose, either D-ribose or D-deoxyribose; from the last, the n. a.'s derive their more specific names, ribonucleic acid and deoxyribonucleic acid. N. a.'s are linear (*i.e.,* unbranched) chains of nucleotides in which the 5′-phosphoric group of each one is esterified with the 3′-hydroxyl of the adjoining nucleotide.

infectious n. a., viral n. a. that can infect cells and bring about the production of viruses.

nu·cle·i·form (nū′klē-i-fōrm). Shaped like or having the appearance of a nucleus. SYN nucleoid (1).

nu·cle·in·ase (nū′klē-in-ās). Obsolete term for nuclease.

⚠ **nucleo-, nucl-.** Nucleus, nuclear. SEE ALSO karyo-, caryo-. [L. *nucleus*]

nu·cle·o·cap·sid (nū′klē-ō-kap′sid). SEE virion.

nu·cle·o·chy·le·ma (nū-klē-ō-kī-lē′mă). SYN karyolymph. [nucleo- + G. *chylos,* juice]

nu·cle·o·chyme (nū′klē-ō-kīm). SYN karyolymph.

nu·cle·o·fil·a·ments (nū′klē-ō-fil-a-ments). A filamentous form of chromosome formed in low ionic strength solutions; fibers are about 100 Å wide and have a string-of-beads appearance.

nu·cle·of·u·gal (nū-klē-of′yū-găl). **1.** Moving within the cell body in a direction away from the nucleus. **2.** Moving in a direction away from a nerve nucleus; said of nerve transmission. [nucleo- + L. *fugio,* to flee]

nu·cle·o·his·tone (nū′klē-ō-his′tōn). A complex of histone and deoxyribonucleic acid, the form in which the latter is usually found in the nuclei of cells; n. may be viewed as a salt between the basic protein and the acidic nucleic acid.

nu·cle·oid (nū′klē-oyd). **1.** SYN nucleiform. **2.** A nuclear inclusion body. **3.** SYN nucleus (2). [nucleo- + G. *eidos,* resemblance]

Lavdovsky's n., SYN astrosphere.

nu·cle·o·lar (nū-klē′ō-lăr). Relating to a nucleolus.

nu·cle·o·li (nū-klē′ō-lī). Plural of nucleolus.

nu·cle·o·li·form (nū-klē′ō-lē-fōrm). Resembling a nucleolus. SYN nucleoloid.

nu·cle·o·loid (nū-klē′ō-loyd). SYN nucleoliform. [nucleolus + G. *eidos,* resemblance]

nu·cle·o·lo·ne·ma (nū-klē′ō-lō-nē′mă). The irregular network or rows of fine ribonucleoprotein granules or microfilaments forming most of the nucleolus. [nucleolus + G. *nēma,* thread]

nu·cle·o·lus, pl. **nu·cle·o·li** (nū-klē′ō-lŭs, -lī). **1.** A small rounded mass within the cell nucleus where ribonucleoprotein is produced; it is usually single, but there may be several accessory nucleoli besides the principal one. The n. is composed of a meshwork (nucleolonema) of microfilaments and granules and the pars amorpha, now shown to have microfilaments also. **2.** A more or less central body in the vesicular nucleus of certain protozoa in which an endosome is lacking but one or more Feulgen-positive (DNA+) nucleoli are present; characteristic of certain sporozoans, flagellates, opalinids, dinoflagellates, and radiolarians among the Protozoa. The chromatin material is distributed throughout the nucleus rather than peripherally, as in the endosome type of nucleus of *Entamoeba.* [L. dim of *nucleus,* a nut, kernel]

chromatin n., SYN karyosome.

false n., SYN karyosome.

nu·cle·o·mi·cro·some (nū′klē-ō-mī′krō-sōm). SYN karyomicrosome.

nu·cle·on (nū′klē-on). **1.** One of the subatomic particles of the atomic nucleus; *i.e.,* either a proton or a neutron. **2.** Slang term for specialist in nuclear medicine. [nucleus + -on]

nu·cle·op·e·tal (nū-klē-op′ě-tăl). **1.** Moving in the cell body in a direction toward the nucleus. **2.** Moving in a direction toward a nerve nucleus; said of a nervous impulse. [nucleo- + L. *peto,* to seek]

Nu·cle·oph·a·ga (nū-klē-of′ă-gă). A microsporan parasite of amebae which destroys the nucleus of its host. [nucleo- + G. *phagō,* to eat]

nu·cle·o·phil, nu·cle·o·phile (nū′klē-ō-fil, -fīl). **1.** The electron pair donor atom in a chemical reaction in which a pair of electrons is picked up by an electrophil. **2.** Relating to a nucleophil. SYN nucleophilic (1). [nucleo- + G. *philos,* fond]

nu·cle·o·phil·ic (nū′klē-ō-fil′ik). **1.** SYN nucleophil (2). **2.** A reaction involving a nucleophile.

nu·cle·o·phos·pha·tas·es (nū′klē-ō-fos′fă-tās-ez). SYN nucleotidases.

nu·cle·o·plasm (nū′klē-ō-plazm). The protoplasm of the nucleus of a cell.

nu·cle·o·plas·min (nū′klē-ō-plas′min). Contents of resting (interphase) nucleus. [nucleo- + plasma + -in]

nu·cle·o·pro·tein (nū′klē-ō-prō′tēn). A complex of protein and nucleic acid, the form in which essentially all nucleic acids exist in nature; chromosomes and viruses are largely n.

nu·cle·o·re·tic·u·lum (nū′klē-ō-rē-tik′yū-lŭm). The intranuclear network of chromatin or linin. [nucleo- + L. *reticulum,* dim. of *rete,* net]

nu·cle·or·rhex·is (nū′klē-ō-rek′sis). Fragmentation of a cell nucleus. [nucleo- + G. *rhēxis,* rupture]

nu·cle·o·si·das·es (nū′klē-ō-sī′dās-ez). Enzymes (particularly EC subgroup 3.2.2) that catalyze the hydrolysis or phosphorolysis of nucleosides, releasing the purine or pyrimidine base.

nu·cle·o·side (Nuc, N) (nū′klē-ō-sīd). A compound of a sugar (usually ribose or deoxyribose) with a purine or pyrimidine base by way of an *N*-glycosyl link.

n. bisphosphate, a n. that carries two independent (*i.e.,* not linked to each other) phosphoric residues. Cf. n. diphosphate.

n. diphosphate (NDP), the pyrophosphoric ester of a n., *i.e.,* a n. in which the H of one of the ribose hydroxyls (usually the 5′) is replaced by a pyrophosphoric (diphosphoric) radical; *e.g.,* adenosine 5′-diphosphate. Cf. n. bisphosphate.

n. monophosphate, a nucleotide, *e.g.,* AMP.

n. triphosphate, a n. in which the H of one of the ribose hydroxyls (usually the 5′) is replaced by a triphosphoric group,

–PO(OH)–O–PO(OH)–O–PO(OH)$_2$; *e.g.,* adenosine triphosphate.

nu·cle·o·side di·phos·phate ki·nase. A phosphotransferase reversibly catalyzing the transfer of one phosphoryl group from ATP to a nucleoside diphosphate to yield a nucleoside triphosphate and ADP.

nu·cle·o·side di·phos·phate sug·ars. Nucleoside diphosphates linked through the 5′-diphosphoric group with simple or complex carbohydrates; *e.g.,* GDP-mannose, UDP-glucose (UDPG), dTDP-glucosamine.

nu·cle·o·some (nū′klē-ō-sōm). A localized aggregation of histone and DNA that is evident when chromatin is in the uncondensed stage. SYN nu body. [nucleo- + G. *sōma,* body]

nu·cle·o·spin·dle (nū′klē-ō-spin′dl). The fusiform body in mitosis.

nu·cle·o·ti·da·ses (nū′klē-ō-tī-dās-ez). Enzymes (EC class 3.1.3) that catalyze the hydrolysis of nucleotides into phosphoric acid and nucleosides; specificities are indicated by prefixes 3′- and 5′ -. SYN nucleophosphatases.

nu·cle·o·tide (nū′klē-ō-tīd). Originally a combination of a (nucleic acid) purine or pyrimidine, one sugar (usually ribose or deoxyribose), and a phosphoric group; by extension, any compound containing a heterocyclic compound bound to a phosphorylated sugar by an *N*-glycosyl link (*e.g.,* adenosine monophosphate, NAD⁺). For individual n.'s see specific names. SYN mononucleotide.

   cyclic n., a nucleoside monophosphate in which the phosphoryl group is linked twice to the sugar moiety; *e.g.,* adenosine 3′,5′-cyclic monophosphate (cAMP).

   flavin n., SEE flavin.

nu·cle·o·tid·yl·trans·fer·as·es (nū′klē-ō-tī′dil-trans′fer-ās-ez). Enzymes (EC class 2.7.7) transferring nucleotide residues (nucleotidyls) from nucleoside di- or triphosphates into dimer or polymer forms. Some n.'s bear specific names (*e.g.,* adenylyl-transferases), or trivial names indicating the linkage hydrolyzed in the synthesis (pyrophosphorylases, phosphorylases), or names of the material synthesized (RNA or DNA polymerase).

nu·cle·o·tox·in (nū′klē-ō-tok′sin). A toxin acting upon the cell nuclei.

NUCLEUS

nu·cle·us, pl. **nu·clei** (nū′klē-ŭs, nū′klē-ī). **1.** In cytology, typically a rounded or oval mass of protoplasm within the cytoplasm of a plant or animal cell; it is surrounded by a nuclear envelope, which encloses euchromatin, heterochromatin, and one or more nucleoli, and undergoes mitosis during cell division. SYN karyon. **2.** By extension, because of similar function, the genome of microorganisms (microbes) that is relatively simple in structure, lacks a nuclear membrane, and does not undergo mitosis during replication. SYN nucleoid (3). SEE ALSO virion. 3 [NA]. In neuroanatomy, a group of nerve cells in the brain or spinal cord that can be demarcated from neighboring groups on the basis of either differences in cell type or the presence of a surrounding zone of nerve fibers or cell-poor neuropil. **4.** Any substance (*e.g.,* foreign body, mucus, crystal) around which a urinary or other calculus is formed. **5.** The central portion of an atom (composed of protons and neutrons) where most of the mass and all of the positive charge are concentrated. [L. a little nut, the kernel, stone of fruits, the inside of a thing, dim. of *nux,* nut]

   abducens n., n. of abducent nerve, n. abducen′tis, a group of motor neurons in the lower part of the pons, innervating the lateral rectus muscle of the eye; unique among motor cranial nerve nuclei in that it consists of two distinct populations of neurons: neurons that give rise to fibers forming the abducens nerve root and those internuclear neurons whose processes cross the midline, ascend in the opposite medial longitudinal fasciculus, and terminate upon specific oculomotor neurons; considered a primary center for mechanisms controlling conjugate horizontal gaze. SYN n. nervi abducentis [NA].

   accessory cuneate n., a cell group lateral to the cuneate n. which receives posterior-root fibers corresponding to the proprioceptive innervation of the arm and hand; it projects to the cerebellum by way of the cuneocerebellar tract, and can be considered the upper-extremity equivalent of the thoracic n. SYN n. cuneatus accessorius [NA], external cuneate n., lateral cuneate n., Monakow's n.

   accessory olivary nuclei, SEE dorsal accessory olivary n., medial accessory olivary n.

   n. accum′bens sep′ti, the region of fusion between the head of the caudate n. and the putamen, covered on the ventral side by the olfactory tubercle. The name ("a nucleus leaning against the septum") refers to a medial, hook-shaped expansion of this anteroventral region of the striatum which curves under the floor of the frontal horn of the lateral ventricle and ascends for some distance into the ventral half of the septal region.

   n. acu′sticus, obsolete term for the combined vestibular and cochlear nuclei.

   n. a′lae cine′reae, SYN dorsal n. of vagus nerve.

   almond n., SYN amygdaloid *body.*

   ambiguous n., SYN n. ambiguus.

   n. ambig′uus [NA], a very slender, longitudinal column of motor neurons in the ventrolateral medulla oblongata; its efferent fibers leave with the vagus and glossopharyngeal nerve and innervate the striated muscle fibers of the pharynx (including the musculus levator veli palatini) and the vocal cord muscles of the larynx. SYN ambiguous n.

   n. amyg′dalae, SYN amygdaloid *body.*

   amygdaloid n., SYN amygdaloid *body.*

   nu′clei anterio′res thal′ami [NA], SYN anterior nuclei of thalamus.

   anterior nuclei of thalamus, collective term for three groups of nerve cells which together form the anterior thalamic tubercle: the anteroventral nuclei, a relatively large n.; the anteromedial nuclei; and the anterodorsal nuclei, a small (but large-celled) n. The nuclei receive the mamillothalamic tract from the mamillary body, and additional afferents by way of the fornix; they project collectively to the cortex of the cingulate and parahippocampal gyrus. SYN nuclei anteriores thalami [NA].

   n. anterodorsa′lis [NA], SYN anterodorsal thalamic n.

   anterodorsal thalamic n., SYN n. anterodorsalis [NA]. SEE anterior nuclei of thalamus.

   n. anteromedia′lis [NA], SYN anteromedial thalamic n.

   anteromedial thalamic n., SYN n. anteromedialis [NA]. SEE anterior nuclei of thalamus.

   n. anteroventra′lis [NA], SYN anteroventral thalamic n.

   anteroventral thalamic n., SYN n. anteroventralis [NA]. SEE anterior nuclei of thalamus.

   arcuate n., (1) SYN posterior periventricular n. SYN arcuate n. of thalamus. **(2)** a cell group in the hypothalamus, located in the lowest part of the infundibulum adjacent to the median eminence.

   arcuate nuclei, a variable assembly of small cell groups, probably outlying components of the pontine nuclei, on the ventral and medial aspects of the pyramid in the medulla oblongata. SYN nuclei arcuati [NA].

   arcuate n. of thalamus, the small ventral region of the ventral posteromedial n. of thalamus in which the fibers of the gustatory lemniscus and secondary trigeminal tracts terminate; it projects to the lower part of the postcentral gyrus of the cerebral cortex. SYN arcuate n. (1), n. arcuatus thalami, n. arcuatus, semilunar n. of Flechsig, thalamic gustatory n.

   nu′clei arcua′ti [NA], SYN arcuate nuclei.

   n. arcua′tus, SYN arcuate n. of thalamus.

   n. arcua′tus thal′ami, SYN arcuate n. of thalamus.

   auditory n., SEE nuclei nervi vestibulocochlearis.

   autonomic nuclei, nuclei located in the spinal cord (T1–L2, S2–S4) and in the brainstem (Edinger-Westphal n., superior and inferior salivatory nuclei, dorsal vagal n. and parts of the ambiguus n.) from which general visceral efferent preganglionic fibers arise; may be sympathetic (T1-L2) or parasympathetic (craniosacral); hypothalamic nuclei/areas function in concert with autonomic nuclei.

basal nuclei, n. of the cerebral hemisphere that originally included the caudate and lenticular nuclei, the claustrum and the amygdaloid body (complex); functionally the term basal nuclei now specifies the caudate and lenticular nuclei and adjacent cell groups having important connections therewith (subthalamic n.; substantia nigra, partes compacta and reticulata); amygdaloid complex now known to be part of the limbic system; SYN nuclei basales.

nuclei basales, SYN basal nuclei.

basal n. of Ganser, a large group of large cells in the innominate substance, ventral to the lentiform n. SYN n. basalis of Ganser.

n. basa′lis of Ganser, SYN basal n. of Ganser.

Bechterew's n., (1) SEE vestibular n. **(2)** SYN n. centralis tegmenti superior.

benzene n., the six conjugated carbon atoms of the benzene ring.

Blumenau's n., the lateral cuneate n. of the medulla oblongata.

branchiomotor nuclei, collective term for those motoneuronal nuclei of the brainstem (n. ambiguus, facial motor n., motor n. of the trigeminus) that develop from the branchiomotor column of the embryo and innervate striated muscle fibers (muscles of mastication, facial musculature, pharynx and vocal cord muscles) developed from the mesenchyme of the branchial arches. SYN special visceral efferent nuclei, special visceral motor nuclei.

Burdach's n., SYN cuneate n.

caudate n., an elongated curved mass of gray matter, consisting of an anterior thick portion, the caput or head, which protrudes into the anterior horn of the lateral ventricle, a portion extending along the floor of the body of the lateral ventricle, known as the corpus or body, and an elongated curved thin portion, the cauda or tail, which curves downward, backward, and forward in the temporal lobe in the wall of the lateral ventricle. SYN n. caudatus [NA], caudate (2), caudatum.

n. cauda′tus [NA], SYN caudate n.

n. centra′lis latera′lis thal′ami, SYN central lateral n. of thalamus.

n. centra′lis tegmen′ti supe′rior, one of the nuclei raphes. SYN Bechterew's n. (2).

central lateral n. of thalamus, the most lateral of the intralaminar nuclei of the thalamus. SYN n. centralis lateralis thalami.

centromedian n., a large, lentil-shaped cell group, the largest and most caudal of the intralaminar nuclei, located within the lamina medullaris interna of the thalamus between the mediodorsal n. and ventrobasal n.; so called by Luys because of its prominent appearance on frontal sections midway between the anterior and posterior pole of the human thalamus. The n. receives numerous fibers from the internal segment of the globus pallidus by way of the thalamic fasciculus, ansa lenticularis, and lenticular fasciculus as well as projections from area 4 of the motor cortex; its major efferent connection is with the putamen although collaterals reach broad areas of the cerebral cortex. SYN n. centromedianus [NA], centre médian de Luys, centrum medianum.

n. centromedia′nus [NA], SYN centromedian n.

cerebellar nuclei, collective term for the dentate, globosus, and emboliform nuclei, and the tectal and fastigial nuclei of the cerebellum.

ceruleus n., a widely used term designating the locus ceruleus; SEE *locus* ceruleus.

Clarke's n., SYN thoracic n.

cochlear nuclei, SYN nuclei cochleares.

nu′clei cochlea′res [NA], the n. cochlearis dorsalis and n. cochlearis ventralis, located on the dorsal and lateral surface of the inferior cerebellar peduncle, in the floor of the lateral recess of the rhomboid fossa. They receive the incoming fibers of the cochlear part of the vestibulocochlear nerve and are the major source of origin of the lateral lemniscus or central auditory pathway. SYN cochlear nuclei, nuclei nervi cochlearis.

n. collic′uli inferio′ris [NA], SYN n. of inferior colliculus.

convergence n. of Perlia, SYN Perlia's n.

n. cor′poris genicula′ti media′lis [NA], SYN n. of medial geniculate body.

nu′clei cor′poris mamilla′ris [NA], SYN nuclei of mamillary body.

nuclei of cranial nerves, groups of nerve cells associated with the cranial nerves either as motor nuclei (nuclei originis) or sensory nuclei (nuclei terminationis). SYN nuclei nervorum cranialium [NA].

cuneate n., the larger Burdach's n.; one of the three nuclei of the posterior column of the spinal cord; located near the dorsal surface of the medulla oblongata at and below the level of the obex, the n. receives posterior root fibers corresponding to the sensory innervation of the arm and hand of the same side; together with its medial companion, the gracile n., it is the major source of origin of the medial lemniscus. SYN n. cuneatus [NA], Burdach's n., n. funiculi cuneati, n. of cuneate fasciculus.

n. of cuneate fasciculus, SYN cuneate n.

n. cunea′tus [NA], SYN cuneate n.

n. cunea′tus accesso′rius [NA], SYN accessory cuneate n.

n. of Darkschewitsch, an ovoid cell group in the ventral central gray substance rostral to the oculomotor nucleus, receiving fibers from the vestibular nuclei by way of the medial longitudinal fasciculus; projections are not known, although some cross in the posterior commissure.

Deiters' n., SEE vestibular n.

dentate n. of cerebellum, the most lateral and largest of the cerebellar nuclei; it receives the axons of the Purkinje cells of the neocerebellum (lateral areas of cerebellar cortex); together with the more medially located globosus and emboliform nuclei it is the major source of fibers composing the massive superior cerebellar peduncle or brachium conjunctivum. SYN n. dentatus cerebelli [NA], corpus dentatum, dentatum.

n. denta′tus cerebel′li [NA], SYN dentate n. of cerebellum.

descending n. of the trigeminus, SYN spinal trigeminal n.

diploid n., a n. containing the diploid or normal double complement of chromosomes for one somatic cell.

dorsal n., SYN thoracic n.

dorsal accessory olivary n., a detached part of the olivary n. dorsal to the latter's main body. SYN n. olivaris accessorius dorsalis [NA].

n. dorsa′lis, SYN thoracic n.

n. dorsa′lis cor′poris trapezoi′dei [NA], SYN dorsal n. of trapezoid body.

n. dorsa′lis ner′vi va′gi [NA], SYN dorsal n. of vagus nerve.

dorsal motor n. of vagus, SYN dorsal n. of vagus nerve.

dorsal n. of trapezoid body, a circumscript, bipartite cell group located ventrolaterally in the lower pontine tegmentum, immediately dorsal to the trapezoid body; the n. receives fibers from both the ipsilateral and contralateral cochlear nuclei, and contributes fibers to the lateral (auditory) lemniscus of both sides. It is believed to be prominently involved in the function of spatial localization of sound. SYN n. dorsalis corporis trapezoidei [NA], oliva superior, superior olivary n., superior olive.

dorsal vagal n., SYN dorsal n. of vagus nerve.

dorsal n. of vagus, SYN dorsal n. of vagus nerve.

dorsal n. of vagus nerve, the visceral motor n. located in the vagal trigone (ala cinerea) of the floor of the fourth ventricle. It gives rise to the parasympathetic fibers of the vagus nerve innervating the heart muscle and the smooth musculature and glands of the respiratory and intestinal tracts. SYN n. dorsalis nervi vagi [NA], dorsal motor n. of vagus, dorsal n. of vagus, dorsal vagal n., n. alae cinereae.

dorsomedial n., SYN medial n. of thalamus.

dorsomedial hypothalamic n., SYN dorsomedial n. of hypothalamus.

dorsomedial n. of hypothalamus, an oval cluster of cells located dorsal to the ventromedial hypothalamic n. SYN n. dorsomedialis hypothalami [NA], dorsomedial hypothalamic n.

n. dorsomedia′lis hypothal′ami [NA], SYN dorsomedial n. of hypothalamus.

droplet nuclei, particles 1–10 m in diameter, implicated in spread of airborne infection; the dried residue formed by evaporation of droplets coughed or sneezed into the atmosphere or by aerosolization of infective material.

Edinger-Westphal n., a small group of preganglionic parasympathetic motor neurons in the midline near the rostral pole of the oculomotor n. of the midbrain; the axons of these motor neurons leave the brain with the oculomotor nerve and synapse on the cells of the ciliary ganglion which in turn innervate the sphincter muscle of the pupil and ciliary muscle. Destruction of this n. or its efferent fibers causes maximal paralytic dilation of the pupil; also demonstrated to project fibers to lower levels of the brainstem and all spinal levels.

emboliform n., a small wedge-shaped n. in the central white substance of the cerebellum just internal to the hilus of the dentate n.; receives axons of Purkinje cells of the intermediate area of the cerebellar cortex; axons of these cells exit the cerebellum via the superior cerebellar peduncle. SYN n. emboliformis [NA], embolus (2).

n. embolifor′mis [NA], SYN emboliform n.

external cuneate n., SYN accessory cuneate n.

facial n., a group of motor neurons located in the ventrolateral region of the lower pontine tegmentum and innervating the facial muscles, the stapedius muscle in the middle ear, the posterior limb of the musculus digastricus, and the stylohyoid muscle. SYN n. nervi facialis [NA], facial motor n., motor n. of facial nerve, n. facialis.

n. facia′lis, SYN facial n.

facial motor n., SYN facial n.

n. fascic′uli gra′cilis, SYN gracile n.

fastigial n., the most medial of the cerebellar nuclei, lying medial to the interpositus n., near the midline, in the white matter underneath the vermis of the cerebellar cortex. It receives the axons of Purkinje cells from all parts of the vermis. Its major projection is to the vestibular nuclei and medullary reticular formation. SYN n. fastigii [NA], fastigatum, n. tecti, roof n., tectal n.

n. fasti′gii [NA], SYN fastigial n.

n. fibro′sus lin′guae, SYN *septum* of tongue.

filiform n., SYN paraventricular n.

n. filifor′mis, SYN paraventricular n.

n. funic′uli cunea′ti, SYN cuneate n.

n. funic′uli gra′cilis, SYN gracile n.

gametic n., SYN micronucleus (2).

n. gelatino′sus, SYN n. pulposus.

gelatinous n., SYN n. pulposus.

geniculatus lateralis n., SEE lateral geniculate *body*.

germ n., SYN micronucleus (2).

n. gigantocellula′ris medul′lae oblonga′tae, SYN gigantocellular n. of medulla oblongata.

gigantocellular n. of medulla oblongata, one of the three major nuclei of the reticular formation of the brainstem. SYN n. gigantocellularis medullae oblongatae.

n. globo′sus [NA], SYN globosus n.

globosus n., a group of two or three small masses of gray substance in the white central core of the cerebellum, medial to the emboliform n.; receives axons of Purkinje cells of the intermediate area of the cerebellar cortex; axons of these cells exit the cerebellum via the superior cerebellar peduncle. SYN n. globosus [NA], spherical n.

n. of Goll, SYN gracile n.

gonad n., SYN micronucleus (2).

gracile n., the medial one of the three nuclei of the dorsal column, the remaining two being the cuneate n. and the accessory cuneate n., which corresponds to the clava; it receives dorsal-root fibers conveying sensory innervation of the leg, and lower trunk, and projects, by way of the medial lemniscus, to the ventral n. posterior n. of the thalamus. SYN n. gracilis [NA], n. fasciculi gracilis, n. funiculi gracilis, n. of Goll.

n. gra′cilis, [NA], SYN gracile n.

Gudden's tegmental nuclei, SYN tegmental nuclei.

gustatory n., SEE rhombencephalic gustatory n., thalamic gustatory n.

n. haben′ulae [NA], SYN habenular n.

habenular n., the gray matter of the habenula, composed of a small-celled medial and a larger-celled lateral habenular n.; both nuclei receive fibers from basal forebrain regions (septum, basal n., lateral preoptic n.); the lateral habenular n. receives an additional projection from the medial segment of the globus pallidus. Both nuclei project by way of the retroflex fasciculus to the interpeduncular n. and a medial zone of the midbrain tegmentum. SYN n. habenulae [NA], ganglion habenulae.

hypoglossal n., the motor n. innervating the intrinsic and four of the five extrinsic muscles of the tongue; it is located in the medulla oblongata near the midline, immediately beneath the floor of the inferior recess of the rhomboid fossa. SYN n. nervi hypoglossi [NA], n. of hypoglossal nerve.

n. of hypoglossal nerve, SYN hypoglossal n.

n. of inferior colliculus, the nerve cell groups composing the colliculus inferior. SYN n. colliculi inferioris [NA].

inferior olivary n., a large aggregate of small densely packed nerve cells arranged in folded laminae shaped like a purse with the opening (hilum) directed medially. It corresponds in position to the oliva, projects to all parts of the contralateral half of the cerebellar cortex by way of the olivocerebellar tract, and is the only source of cerebellar climbing fibers. Its afferent connections include fibers from the spinal cord, the dentate nucleus and motor cortex, but its major input appears to be the central tegmental tract originating from multiple nuclei at midbrain levels. SYN n. olivaris [NA].

inferior salivary n., SYN inferior salivatory n.

inferior salivatory n., a group of preganglionic parasympathetic motor neurons located in the reticular formation of the medulla oblongata dorsal to the n. ambiguus; its axons leave the brain with the glossopharyngeal nerve and govern secretion from the parotid gland by the intermediary of the ganglion oticum; cells of the inferior and superior n. are scattered and overlapping in lateral regions of the reticular formation. SYN n. salivatorius inferior [NA], inferior salivary n.

inferior vestibular n., n. vestibularis inferior. SEE ALSO vestibular n.

intercalated n., a small collection of nerve cells in the medulla oblongata lying lateral to the hypoglossal n. SYN n. intercalatus [NA], Staderini's n.

n. intercala′tus [NA], SYN intercalated n.

intermediolateral n., the cell column that forms the lateral horn of the spinal cord's gray matter. Extending from the first thoracic through the second lumbar segment, the column contains the autonomic motor neurons that give rise to the preganglionic fibers of the sympathetic system. SYN intermediolateral cell column of spinal cord, n. intermediolateralis.

n. intermediolatera′lis, SYN intermediolateral n.

intermediomedial n., a small group of scattered visceral motor neurons immediately ventral to the thoracic n. in the thoracic and upper two lumbar segments of the spinal cord; considered to receive visceral afferent fibers at all spinal levels. SYN n. intermediomedialis.

n. intermediomedia′lis, SYN intermediomedial n.

interpeduncular n., a median, unpaired, ovoid cell group at the base of the midbrain tegmentum between the cerebral peduncles; it receives the retroflex fasciculus from the habenula, and projects to the raphe region (raphe nuclei) and periaqueductal gray substance of the midbrain. SYN n. interpeduncularis [NA], ganglion isthmi, Gudden's ganglion, intercrural ganglion, interpeduncular ganglion.

n. interpeduncula′ris [NA], SYN interpeduncular n.

n. interpos′itus, SYN interpositus n.

interpositus n., collective term denoting the combined globosus nuclei and emboliform nuclei of the cerebellum; more correctly used as interposed nuclei as it identifies two cell groups. SYN n. interpositus.

interstitial n., a group of widely spaced, medium-sized neurons in the dorsomedial region of the upper mesencephalic tegmentum, immediately lateral to the n. of Darkschewitsch; together with the latter, the interstitial n. is closely associated with the medial longitudinal fasciculus, via which it receives fibers from the vestibular nuclei and projects crossed fibers via the posterior commissure to the oculomotor n.; also projects fibers to all spinal levels. It is believed to be involved in the integration of head and eye movements, particularly eye movements of a vertical or oblique nature. SYN n. interstitialis [NA], interstitial n. of Cajal.

interstitial n. of Cajal, SYN interstitial n.

n. interstitia′lis [NA], SYN interstitial n.

nu′clei intralamina′res thal′ami [NA], SYN intralaminar nuclei of thalamus.

intralaminar nuclei of thalamus, collective term denoting several cell groups embedded in the internal medullary lamina of the thalamus: central lateral n., paracentral n., and farthest caudally, the large centromedian n. The first two of these receive afferents from the cerebral cortex, brainstem, reticular formation, cerebellum, and spinal cord, and project more or less diffusely to large regions of the frontal and parietal cortex. SEE ALSO centromedian n. SYN nuclei intralaminares thalami [NA].

Klein-Gumprecht shadow nuclei, shadow nuclei in degenerating lymphoidocytes and macrolymphocytes in leukemia.

lateral cervical nuclei, diffusely arranged n. located in the dorsal portions of the lateral funiculus in about cervical levels C1-C3; synaptic station for the spinocervicothalamic tract.

lateral cuneate n., SYN accessory cuneate n.

n. of lateral geniculate body, n. of the thalamus characterized by six layers of cells, two parvicellular, four magnocellular, alternating with thin layers of fibers; receives bilateral visual input, projects to calcarine cortex.

n. latera′lis medul′lae oblonga′tae [NA], SYN lateral n. of medulla oblongata.

n. latera′lis thal′ami [NA], SYN lateral n. of thalamus.

n. of lateral lemniscus, a substantial cell mass embedded in the lateral lemniscus, immediately below the latter's entry into the inferior colliculus; the n. represents a synaptic way-station for part of the fibers of the lateral lemniscus. SYN n. lemnisci lateralis [NA].

lateral n. of medulla oblongata, a group of cells in the medulla oblongata, located between the inferior olive and the descending trigeminal n., receiving fibers from the spinal cord and motor cortex and projecting to the cerebellum. SYN n. lateralis medullae oblongatae [NA], lateral reticular n.

lateral preoptic n., a vaguely defined group of nerve cells in the lateral zone of the preoptic region. SYN n. preopticus lateralis [NA].

lateral reticular n., SYN lateral n. of medulla oblongata.

lateral n. of thalamus, the largest of the major subdivisions of the thalamus; the composite lateral n. includes, from before backward, the n. lateralis anterior or dorsalis, n. lateralis intermedius, n. lateralis posterior, and pulvinar; together, these cell groups form most of the free dorsal surface of the posterior half of the thalamus and project to a very large region of parietal, occipitoparietal, and temporal cortex; its afferent connections are largely obscure, but the n. lateralis posterior and the pulvinar receive a projection from the superior colliculus. SYN n. lateralis thalami [NA].

lateral tuberal nuclei, SYN tuberal nuclei.

lateral vestibular n., n. vestibularis lateralis. SEE vestibular n.

n. lemnis′ci latera′lis [NA], SYN n. of lateral lemniscus.

n. of lens, SYN n. lentis.

lenticular n., lentiform n., the large cone-shaped mass of gray matter forming the central core of the cerebral hemisphere. The convex base of the cone, oriented laterally and rostrally, is formed by the putamen which together with the caudate nucleus composes the striatum; the apical part, oriented medially and caudally, consists of the two segments of the globus pallidus. The n. is ventral and lateral to the thalamus and caudate n., from which it is separated by the internal capsule, and together with the caudate n. composes the striate body. SYN n. lentiformis [NA], lenticula (1).

n. lentifor′mis [NA], SYN lenticular n.

n. len′tis [NA], the core or inner dense portion of the lens of the eye. SYN n. of lens.

n. of Luys, SYN subthalamic n.

n. of the mamillary body, SYN nuclei of mamillary body.

nuclei of mamillary body, a single large-celled lateral n. and a larger bipartite medial n. together comprising the mamillary body; present in the caudal hypothalamus. SYN nuclei corporis mamillaris [NA], n. of the mamillary body.

n. masticato′rius, SYN motor n. of trigeminal nerve.

masticatory n., SYN motor n. of trigeminal nerve.

medial accessory olivary n., a detached part of the olivary n. medial to the latter's main body, against the lateral side of the medial lemniscus and pyramidal tract. SYN n. olivaris accessorius medialis [NA].

medial central n. of thalamus, a small cell group in the interthalamic adhesion of the thalamus, occupying the midline region of the internal medullary lamina, between the left and the right paracentral n. SYN n. medialis centralis thalami [NA].

n. of medial geniculate body, the nerve cell groups composing the medial geniculate body (corpus geniculatum mediale). SYN n. corporis geniculati medialis [NA].

n. media′lis centra′lis thal′ami [NA], SYN medial central n. of thalamus.

n. media′lis thal′ami [NA], SYN medial n. of thalamus.

medial preoptic n., a group of nerve cells forming the medial zone of the preoptic region. SYN n. preopticus medialis [NA].

medial n. of thalamus, a large, composite cell group in the dorsomedial region of the thalamus having reciprocal connections with the entire extent of the frontal cortex anterior to the motor cortex (area 4) and premotor cortex (area 6). The afferent connections of the medial n. also include projections from the olfactory cortex and amygdala. SYN n. medialis thalami [NA], dorsomedial n., mediodorsal n.

medial vestibular n., n. vestibularis medialis. SEE vestibular n.

mediodorsal n., SYN medial n. of thalamus.

mesencephalic n. of trigeminal nerve, a long, narrow plate of unipolar neurons extending throughout the length of the midbrain, in and along the lateral angle of the central gray substance. The n. is the single known instance of primary sensory neurons enclosed in the central nervous system instead of in a peripheral sensory ganglion. Its peripheral axonal processes pass with the trigeminal nerve, give collaterals to the trigeminal motor n., and terminate in the muscles of mastication. SYN n. tractus mesencephali nervi trigemini [NA].

Monakow's n., SYN accessory cuneate n.

motor nuclei, SYN nuclei of origin.

motor n. of facial nerve, SYN facial n.

n. moto′rius ner′vi trigem′ini [NA], SYN motor n. of trigeminal nerve.

motor n. of trigeminal nerve, a group of motor neurons innervating the muscles of mastication (masseter, temporalis, internal and external pterygoid muscles) and the musculi tensor tympani and tensor veli palatini. The n. lies in the upper pontine tegmentum medial to the main sensory n. of the trigeminus. SYN n. motorius nervi trigemini [NA], masticatory n., motor n. of trigeminus, n. masticatorius.

motor n. of trigeminus, SYN motor n. of trigeminal nerve.

n. ner′vi abducen′tis [NA], SYN abducens n.

nu′clei ner′vi cochlea′ris [NA], SYN nuclei cochleares.

n. ner′vi facia′lis [NA], SYN facial n.

n. ner′vi hypoglos′si [NA], SYN hypoglossal n.

n. ner′vi oculomoto′rii [NA], SYN oculomotor n.

n. ner′vi trochlea′ris [NA], SYN trochlear n.

nu′clei ner′vi vestibulocochlea′ris [NA], SYN vestibulocochlear nuclei.

nu′clei nervo′rum crania′lium [NA], SYN nuclei of cranial nerves.

n. ni′ger, SYN *substantia* nigra.

oculomotor n., the composite group of motor neurons innervating all of the external eye muscles except the musculus rectus lateralis and musculus obliquus superior, and including the musculus levator palpebrae superioris; the most rostral component of the n. is the Edinger-Westphal n. which innervates the musculi sphincter pupillae and ciliaris via the ciliary ganglion. The oculomotor n. lies in the rostral half of the midbrain, near the midline in the most ventral part of the central gray substance; fibers of the medial longitudinal fasciculus form its lateral borders. SYN n. nervi oculomotorii [NA], n. of oculomotor nerve.

n. of oculomotor nerve, SYN oculomotor n.

n. oliva′ris [NA], SYN inferior olivary n.

n. oliva′ris accesso′rius dorsa′lis [NA], SYN dorsal accessory olivary n.

n. oliva′ris accesso′rius media′lis [NA], SYN medial accessory olivary n.

Onuf's n., small somatic motor neurons in the ventral horn of the spinal cord at sacral 2 level which innervate the vesicorectal sphincters, that is, the external anal and the urethral sphincter; O.'s n. has been identified in the cat, dog, and humans.

nuclei of origin, collections of motor neurons (forming a continuous column in the spinal cord, discontinuous in the medulla and pons) giving origin to the spinal and cranial motor nerves. SYN nuclei originis [NA], motor nuclei.

nu′clei ori′ginis [NA], SYN nuclei of origin.

parabrachial nuclei, the cell groups flanking the brachium conjunctivum at levels immediately caudal to the inferior colliculus; they serve as way-stations in the pathways ascending from the n. of solitary tract to the thalamus and hypothalamus, and receive afferent fibers from the hypothalamus and amygdaloid body. SYN nuclei parabrachiales.

nuclei parabrachia′les, SYN parabrachial nuclei.

n. paracentra′lis thal′ami, SYN paracentral n. of thalamus.

paracentral n. of thalamus, one of the intralaminar nuclei of the thalamus, medial to the central lateral n. SYN n. paracentralis thalami.

paraventricular n., a triangular group of large magnocellular neurons in the periventricular zone of the anterior half of the hypothalamus. The cells of the n. are similar to those of the supraoptic n.; the axons of about 20% of their number join in the formation of the supraopticohypophysial tract and are functionally associated with the posterior lobe of the hypophysis; they project fibers to the brainstem nuclei (dorsal motor n. and solitary n.) and to the intermediolateral cell column of the spinal cord at thoracic, lumbar, and spinal levels; similar descending autonomic fibers arise from the lateral and posterior hypothalamic nuclei. SYN n. paraventricularis [NA], filiform n., n. filiformis.

n. paraventricula′ris [NA], SYN paraventricular n.

perihypoglossal nuclei, nuclei found in the floor of the 4th ventricle in relation to the hypoglossal nucleus, includes the prepositus and intercalated nuclei and the n. of Roller.

Perlia's n., a small cell group located between the somatic cell columns of the oculomotor nuclei. Since it is placed between the groups of motor neurons innervating, respectively, the left and right medial rectus muscles, the n. is considered to possibly represent an integrating mechanism for ocular convergence. SYN convergence n. of Perlia, Spitzka's n.

phenanthrene n., misnomer for tetracyclic steroid n.

phrenic n., a n. comprised of motor neurons located in medial areas of the ventral horn of the spinal cord from about C3 to C6; axons of neurons in this n. innervate the diaphragm.

pontine nuclei, the massive gray matter filling the basilar pons. The nuclei are of fairly homogeneous architecture and project to the cortex of the contralateral cerebellar hemisphere by way of the middle cerebellar peduncle. Their main afferents come from the entire extent of the cerebral neocortex by way of the longitudinal pontine bundles (corticopontine fibers); thus, the pontine nuclei form a major way-station in the impulse conduction from the cerebral cortex of one hemisphere to the posterior lobe of the opposite cerebellum. SYN nuclei pontis [NA], pontine gray matter.

nu′clei pon′tis [NA], SYN pontine nuclei.

pontis nervi trigeminalis n., SEE principal sensory n. of trigeminal nerve.

n. poste′rior hypothal′ami [NA], SYN posterior hypothalamic n.

posterior hypothalamic n., a large, periventricular hypothalamic n. located dorsal to the mamillary body, continuous with the central gray substance of the mesencephalon. SYN n. posterior hypothalami [NA].

posterior periventricular n., SYN arcuate n. (1).

n. preop′ticus latera′lis [NA], SYN lateral preoptic n.

n. preop′ticus media′lis [NA], SYN medial preoptic n.

prerubral n., the gray matter of field H₂; SEE *fields* of Forel, under *field*.

pretectal n., group of cells, constituting several subnuclei, located rostral to the superior colliculus in the "pretectal" area; receive input from retinal ganglion cells (via the optic tract) and project bilaterally to the Edinger-Westphal n.; relay center for pupillary light reflex pathway.

principal sensory n. of trigeminal nerve, the term commonly used to designate the nucleus pontis nervi trigeminalis [NA]; located in pons lateral to the motor trigeminal n.; receives primary sensory (touch and pressure) input via the trigeminal nerve, projects to ventral posteromedial n. of thalamus. SYN n. sensorius principalis nervi trigemini [NA], n. sensorius superior nervi trigemini, principal sensory n. of the trigeminus.

principal sensory n. of the trigeminus, SYN principal sensory n. of trigeminal nerve.

n. pulpo′sus [NA], the soft fibrocartilage central portion of the intervertebral disk; regarded as a derivative of the notochord. SYN gelatinous n., n. gelatinosus, vertebral pulp.

pulvinar n., the large caudal portion of the lateral thalamic nuclear group; may be divided into oral, inferior, medial and lateral parts based on cytoarchitecture and connections; functionally related to the visual system.

n. pyramida′lis, obsolete term for n. olivaris accessorius medialis.

pyrrole n., of porphyrins, a cyclic tetrapyrrole; four pyrrole groups joined into a ring structure by way of −CH= (methylidyne) bridges between the α (2) position of one pyrrole and the α′ (5) position of another pyrrole, the fourth pyrrole being joined to the first. SEE ALSO porphin, porphyrin.

raphe nuclei, collective term denoting a variety of unpaired nerve cell groups in and along the median plane of the mesencephalic and rhombencephalic tegmentum: the n. centralis tegmenti superior, and the n. raphes dorsalis, n. raphes pontis, n. raphes magnus, n. raphes pallidus, and n. raphes obscurus. These nuclei include neurons characterized by their containing the indolamine transmitter agent serotonin; their serotonin-carrying axons extend rostrally to the hypothalamus, septum, hippocampus, and cingulate gyrus and include projections to brainstem, cerebellum, and spinal cord. SYN nuclei raphes, superior central tegmental n.

nu′clei raph′es, SYN raphe nuclei.

red n., a large, well defined, somewhat elongated cell mass, of reddish-gray hue in the fresh brain, located in the rostral mesencephalic tegmentum. The n. receives a massive projection from the contralateral half of the cerebellum by way of the superior cerebellar peduncle, and an additional projection from the ipsilateral motor cortex. Projections from the anterior interposed n. and motor cortex to the red nucleus are somatopically organized. Its efferent connections are with the contralateral rhombencephalic reticular formation and spinal cord by way of the rubrobulbar and rubrospinal tracts. Rubrospinal fibers have somatotopic origin. SYN n. ruber [NA].

reduction n., a n. that degenerates in the cell during the changes incident to fertilization.

reproductive n., SYN micronucleus (2).

reticular nuclei of the brainstem, the vaguely delineated cell groups composing the gray matter of the reticular formation of the rhombencephalon and mesencephalon. In general, large-celled territories occupy the medial two-thirds of the reticular formation: gigantocellular n. of medulla oblongata, nuclei tegmenti pontis caudalis and oralis. Smaller groups of reticular nuclei are found laterally and in paramedian locations; lateral nuclei receive sensory collaterals and project medially; paramedian reticular nuclei largely project to the cerebellum. SEE ALSO reticular *formation*.

n. reticula′ris thal′ami [NA], SYN reticular n. of thalamus.

reticular n. of thalamus, a sheet of fairly large neurons covering the lateral, ventral, and rostral surfaces of the thalamus; its reticular appearance is caused by the numerous fascicles of the thalamic peduncles which traverse the n. The n. receives numerous fibers from the cerebral cortex but it has no cortical projection. SYN n. reticularis thalami [NA].

rhombencephalic gustatory n., the rostral one-third of the n. of solitary tract, receiving afferents from the facial, glossopharyngeal, and vagus nerves conveying impulses originating from the receptor cells of the taste buds.

Roller's n., (1) lateral n. of the accessory nerve; **(2)** a small bulbar n. lying immediately anterior to the hypoglossal n., considered one of the perihypoglossal nuclei.

roof n., SYN fastigial n.

n. ru'ber [NA], SYN red n.

n. salivato'rius infe'rior [NA], SYN inferior salivatory n.

n. salivato'rius supe'rior [NA], SYN superior salivatory n.

Schwalbe's n., SEE vestibular n.

secondary sensory nuclei, SYN terminal nuclei.

segmentation n., (1) the compound n. in the impregnated ovum, formed by conjugation of the nuclei of the ovum and spermatozoon (female and male pronuclei); **(2)** the zygote nucleus after it commences the first cleavage division.

semilunar n. of Flechsig, SYN arcuate n. of thalamus.

n. senso'rius principa'lis ner'vi trigem'ini [NA], SYN principal sensory n. of trigeminal nerve.

n. senso'rius supe'rior ner'vi trigem'ini, SYN principal sensory n. of trigeminal nerve.

sensory nuclei, a group of cell bodies that receive afferent (sensory) input from the periphery.

shadow n., a n. that has lost its pigment and staining properties.

sole nuclei, an accumulation of skeletal muscle fiber nuclei at the myoneural junction.

n. of solitary tract, a slender cell column extending sagittally through the dorsal part of the medulla oblongata, beneath the floor of the rhomboid fossa, immediately lateral to the limiting sulcus. It is the visceral sensory (visceral afferent) n. of the brainstem, receiving the afferent fibers of the vagus, glossopharyngeal, and facial nerves by way of the solitary tract. The caudal two-thirds of the n. processes impulses originating in the pharynx, larynx, intestinal and respiratory tracts, and heart and large blood vessels; its rostral one-third receives impulses from the taste buds and is known as the rhombencephalic gustatory n. SYN n. tractus solitarii [NA].

somatic n., SYN macronucleus (2).

somatic motor nuclei, collective term indicating the motor nuclei innervating the tongue musculature (hypoglossal n.) and the extraocular eye muscles (abducens n., trochlear n., and oculomotor n.).

special visceral efferent nuclei, SYN branchiomotor nuclei.

special visceral motor nuclei, SYN branchiomotor nuclei.

sperm n., the head of the spermatozoon, which becomes spheroidal, after entering the ovum. SEE ALSO male *pronucleus*.

spherical n., SYN globosus n.

spinal n. of accessory nerve, a slender column of motor neurons extending longitudinally through the central part of the ventral horn of the upper five segments of the spinal cord, giving origin to the spinal part of the accessory nerve. SYN n. spinalis nervi accessorii [NA].

n. spina'lis ner'vi accesso'rii [NA], SYN spinal n. of accessory nerve.

spinal trigeminal n., the long sensory n. extending from the caudal border of the pontine sensory n. of the trigeminus down through the lateral region of the rhombencephalon into the upper three segments of the spinal cord's dorsal horn; it receives the fibers of the sensory root of the trigeminal nerve which descend along its lateral border as the spinal tract of trigeminal nerve. SYN n. tractus spinalis nervi trigemini [NA], descending n. of the trigeminus, spinal n. of the trigeminus.

spinal n. of the trigeminus, SYN spinal trigeminal n.

Spitzka's n., SYN Perlia's n.

Staderini's n., SYN intercalated n.

steroid n., SYN tetracyclic steroid n.

Stilling's n., SYN thoracic n.

subceruleus n., diffusely organized n. of noradrenergic cells located ventral to the n. (locus) ceruleus.

subthalamic n., a circumscript n., shaped like a biconvex lens, located in the ventral part of the subthalamus on the dorsal surface of the peduncular part of the internal capsule immediately rostral to the substantia nigra. The n. receives a massive topographic projection from the lateral segment of the globus pallidus, and a somatopically organized projection from the ipsilateral motor cortex; a smaller bundle of afferents from the centromedian n. of the thalamus terminate in the rostral part of the n. The subthalamic n. projects to both pallidal segments, to the pars reticulata of the substantia nigra, and in a small way to the ipsilateral pedunculopontine nucleus. SYN n. subthalamicus [NA], corpus luysi, Luys' body, n. of Luys.

n. subthalam'icus [NA], SYN subthalamic n.

superior central tegmental n., SYN raphe nuclei.

superior olivary n., SYN dorsal n. of trapezoid body.

superior salivary n., SYN superior salivatory n.

superior salivatory n., a group of preganglionic parasympathetic motor neurons situated rostral and lateral to the inferior salivatory n.; it governs secretion of the lacrimal, sublingual, and submaxillary glands by way of the facial nerve and the sphenopalatine and submandibular ganglia. SYN n. salivatorius superior [NA], superior salivary n.

superior vestibular n., n. vestibularis superior. SEE vestibular n.

n. suprachiasmatica, small n. located dorsal to the optic chiasm; receives input from retina, influences hypothalamic neuroendocrine function; closely associated with regulation of circadian rhythmicity.

supraoptic n., SYN supraoptic n. of hypothalamus.

supraoptic n. of hypothalamus, a large-celled neurosecretory n. in the hypothalamus, located over the lateral border of the optic tract, from which the supraopticohypophysial tract arises; its neurons produce and transport vasopressin released into the general circulation from the axon terminals in the supraopticohypophysial tract. SYN n. supraopticus hypothalami [NA], supraoptic n.

n. supraop'ticus hypothal'ami [NA], SYN supraoptic n. of hypothalamus.

tectal n., SYN fastigial n.

n. tec'ti, SYN fastigial n.

tegmental nuclei, collective term for two small round cell groups in the caudal part of the midbrain (caudal pontine tegmental nucleus, n. tegmenti pontis caudalis and oral pontine tegmental nucleus, n. tegmenti pontis oralis), associated with the mamillary body by way of the mamillary peduncle and mamillotegmental tract. SYN nuclei tegmenti [NA], Gudden's tegmental nuclei.

nu'clei tegmen'ti [NA], SYN tegmental nuclei.

terminal nuclei, nuclei termina'les, collective term indicating those nerve cell groups in the rhombencephalon and spinal cord in which the afferent fibers of the spinal and cranial nerves terminate. SYN nuclei terminationis [NA], secondary sensory nuclei.

nu'clei terminatio'nis [NA], SYN terminal nuclei.

tetracyclic steroid n., the group of four fused rings forming the framework or parent substance of the steroids. SYN perhydrocyclopenta[*a*]phenanthrene, steroid n.

thalamic gustatory n., SYN arcuate n. of thalamus.

thoracic n., a column of large neurons located in the base of the posterior gray column of the spinal cord, extending from the first thoracic through the second lumbar segment; it gives rise to the dorsal spinocerebellar tract of the same side. SYN n. thoracicus [NA], Clarke's column, Clarke's n., dorsal n., n. dorsalis, Stilling's column, Stilling's n.

n. thorac'icus [NA], SYN thoracic n.

n. trac'tus mesenceph'ali ner'vi trigem'ini [NA], SYN mesencephalic n. of trigeminal nerve.

n. trac'tus solita'rii (NTS) [NA], SYN n. of solitary tract.

n. trac'tus spina'lis ner'vi trigem'ini [NA], SYN spinal trigeminal n.

triangular n., alternative term for the medial vestibular n.

trochlear n., a group of motor neurons innervating the superior oblique muscle of the contralateral eye. The n. lies in the caudal half of the midbrain, behind the oculomotor n., in the most ventral part of the central gray substance, near the midline. SYN n. nervi trochlearis [NA], n. of trochlear nerve.

n. of trochlear nerve, SYN trochlear n.

trophic n., SYN macronucleus (2).

tuberal nuclei, two or three small, encapsulated, round or ovoid clusters of cells in the lateral hypothalamic area along the surface of the tuber cinereum; their connections and functional significance are unknown. SYN nuclei tuberales [NA], lateral tuberal nuclei.

nu'clei tubera'les [NA], SYN tuberal nuclei.

ventral anterior n. of thalamus, the most rostral of the subdivisions of the ventral n., receiving projections from the globus pallidus and projecting to the premotor and frontal cortex. SYN n. ventralis anterior thalami.

ventral intermediate n. of thalamus, the composite middle third of the ventral n. receiving in its various parts distinctive projections from the contralateral half of the cerebellum (by way of the superior cerebellar peduncle) and the ipsilateral globus pallidus; nearly all parts of the n. projects to the motor cortex. SYN n. ventralis intermedius thalami [NA], n. ventralis lateralis, ventral lateral n. of thalamus.

n. ventra'lis ante'rior thal'ami, SYN ventral anterior n. of thalamus.

n. ventra'lis cor'poris trapezoi'dei [NA], SYN ventral n. of trapezoid body.

n. ventra'lis interme'dius thal'ami [NA], SYN ventral intermediate n. of thalamus.

n. ventra'lis latera'lis, SYN ventral intermediate n. of thalamus.

n. ventra'lis poste'rior interme'dius thal'ami, intermediate part of the ventrobasal nuclear complex. SEE ventral posterior n. of thalamus. SYN ventral posterior intermediate n. of thalamus.

n. ventra'lis poste'rior thal'ami, SYN ventral posterior n. of thalamus.

n. ventra'lis posterolatera'lis thal'ami [NA], SYN ventral posterolateral n. of thalamus.

n. ventra'lis posteromedia'lis thal'ami [NA], SYN ventral posteromedial n. of thalamus.

n. ventra'lis thal'ami [NA], SYN ventral n. of thalamus.

ventral lateral n. of thalamus, SYN ventral intermediate n. of thalamus.

ventral posterior intermediate n. of thalamus, SYN n. ventralis posterior intermedius thalami. SEE ventral posterior n. of thalamus.

ventral posterior n. of thalamus, the large posterior part of the ventral n. of the thalamus receiving the somatic sensory lemnisci (medial lemniscus, spinothalamic tract, trigeminal lemniscus) and the ascending gustatory (taste) lemniscus, and projecting in turn by way of the internal capsule to the cortex of the postcentral gyrus. The n. is somatotopically organized and subdivided into a ventral posterolateral n. of thalamus representing the leg, a ventral posterior intermediate n. of thalamus representing the arm, a ventral posteromedial n. of thalamus representing the face, and an arcuate n. of thalamus receiving the gustatory lemniscus. SYN n. ventralis posterior thalami, ventrobasal n.

ventral posterolateral n. of thalamus, ventral posterior lateral n. of thalamus, lateral part of the ventrobasal nuclear complex. SEE ventral posterior n. of thalamus. SYN n. ventralis posterolateralis thalami [NA].

ventral posteromedial n. of thalamus, posterior medial n. of thalamus, medial part of the ventrobasal nuclear complex. SEE ventral posterior n. of thalamus. SYN n. ventralis posteromedialis thalami [NA].

ventral n. of thalamus, a large, complex cell mass the external border of which forms the ventral and much of the lateral boundary, as well as the rostral border, of the thalamus; it can be subdivided into an anterior, intermediate, and posterior part. SYN n. ventralis thalami [NA].

ventral tier thalamic nuclei, collective term for nuclei in the ventral part of the lateral nuclear group, *e.g.,* ventral anterior, lateral, posterolateral, and posteromedial nuclei and the medial and lateral geniculate bodies. The basoventral nuclear complex constitutes the caudal part of the ventral tier thalamic nuclei.

ventral n. of trapezoid body, a cell group embedded among the fibers of the trapezoid body, the major decussation of the central auditory pathway, in the lower pons. The n. receives fibers from the contralateral cochlear nuclei and contributes fibers to the ascending auditory system or lateral lemniscus. SYN n. ventralis corporis trapezoidei [NA].

ventrobasal n., SYN ventral posterior n. of thalamus.

ventromedial n. of hypothalamus, a circumscript ovoid group of small neurons in the medial zone of the tuberal region of the hypothalamus. Bilateral destruction of this n. in the rat leads to severe obesity. It receives numerous fibers from the amygdala via the terminal stria; its efferent connections are obscure. SYN n. ventromedialis hypothalami [NA].

n. ventromedia'lis hypothal'ami [NA], SYN ventromedial n. of hypothalamus.

vestibular n., one of a group of four main nuclei that includes: the lateral vestibular n. (Deiters' n.), medial vestibular n. (Schwalbe's n.), superior vestibular n. (Bechterew's n.), and inferior vestibular n., located in the lateral region of the hindbrain beneath the floor of the rhomboid fossa. They receive primary fibers of the vestibular nerve, are reciprocally connected with the flocculonodular lobe of the cerebellum, and project by way of the medial longitudinal fasciculus to the abducens, trochlear, and oculomotor nuclei and to the ventral horn of the spinal cord. The lateral vestibular n. projects to the ipsilateral ventral horn of the spinal cord by the vestibulospinal tract. SYN n. vestibularis [NA].

n. vestibula'ris [NA], SYN vestibular n.

vestibulocochlear nuclei, the combined cochlear and vestibular nuclei in the brainstem that receive the incoming fibers of the eighth cranial nerve. SEE vestibular n. SYN nuclei nervi vestibulocochlearis [NA].

---

nu·clide (nū'klīd). A particular (atomic) nuclear species with defined atomic mass and number. SEE ALSO isotope.

Nuel, Jean P., Belgian ophthalmologist and otologist, 1847–1920. SEE N.'s *space.*

NUG Abbreviation for necrotizing ulcerative *gingivitis.*

Nuhn, Anton, German anatomist, 1814–1889. SEE N.'s *gland.*

nul·li·grav·i·da (nŭl-i-grav'i-dă). A woman who has never conceived a child. [L. *nullus,* none, + *gravida,* pregnant]

nul·lip·a·ra (nŭ-lip'ă-ră). A woman who has never borne children. [L. *nullus,* none, + *pario,* to bear]

nul·li·par·i·ty (nŭl-i-par'i-tē). Condition of having borne no children.

nul·lip·a·rous (nŭl-ip'ă-rŭs). Never having borne children. SYN nonparous.

num·ber (nŭm'ber). **1.** A symbol expressive of a certain value or of a specific quantity determined by count. **2.** The place of any unit in a series.

atomic n. (Z), the number of protons in the nucleus of an atom; it indicates the position of the element in the periodic system.

Avogadro's n. (Λ, N_A), the n. of molecules in one gram-molecular weight (1 mol) of any compound; defined as the number of atoms in 0.0120 kg of pure carbon-12; equivalent to 6.0221367×10^{23}. SYN Avogadro's constant.

Brinell hardness n. (BHN), a n. related to the size of the permanent impression made by a ball indenter of specified size (usually 10 mm in diameter) pressed into the surface of the material under a specified load:

$$\text{BHN} = \frac{P}{\frac{\pi D}{2}(D - \sqrt{D^2 - d^2})}$$

where P = applied load in kg, D = diameter of the ball in mm, and d = diameter of the impression in mm.

CT n., a normalized value of the calculated x-ray absorption coefficient of a pixel (picture element) in a computed tomogram, expressed in Hounsfield units, where the CT n. of air is −1000 and that of water is zero. SYN Hounsfield n.

electronic n., the n. of electrons in the outermost orbit (valence shell) of an element.

gold n., SYN gold *equivalent.*

Hehner n., the weight or percentage of the nonvolatile fatty acids yielded by 5 g of a saponified fat or oil. SYN Hehner value.

Hogben n., unique personal identifying number constructed by using a sequence of digits for birth date, sex, birthplace, and other identifiers; invented by and named for Lancelot Hogben, British mathematician; Hogben n.'s are the basis for identification n.'s in many primary care facilities and are used in many record linkage systems.

Hounsfield n., SYN CT n.

hydrogen n., the quantity of hydrogen that 1 g of fat will absorb; it is a measurement of the amount of unsaturated fatty acids in the fat. SEE ALSO iodine n.

iodine n., an indication of the quantity of unsaturated fatty acids present in a fat; it represents the number of grams of iodine absorbed by each 100 g of fat. SEE ALSO hydrogen n. SYN iodine value.

Kestenbaum's n., the difference between the two pupil diameters when each eye is measured in bright light with the other eye tightly covered; an indicator of the relative afferent pupillary defect in patients with two normally innervated irises.

Knoop hardness n. (KHN), a n. obtained by dividing the load in kg applied to a pyramid-shaped diamond of specific size divided by the projected area of the impression: $KHN = L/A$, where $A=$ the projected area of the impression in mm^2 and $L=$ the load in kg; used for measurements of hardness of any materials, especially very hard and brittle substances such as tooth dentin and enamel.

Koettstorfer n., SYN saponification n.

linking n. (L), a property of a long biopolymer (such as duplex DNA) equal to the number of twists (related to the frequency of turns around the central axis of the helix) plus the writhing n.

Loschmidt's n. (n_0), the n. of molecules in 1 cm^3 of ideal gas at 0°C and 1 atmosphere of pressure; Avogadro's n. divided by 22,414 (*i.e.,* 2.6868×10^{19} cm^{-3}).

Mach n., a n. representing the ratio between the speed of an object moving through a fluid medium, such as air, and the speed of sound in the same medium.

mass n., the mass of the atom of a particular isotope relative to hydrogen-1 (or to $\frac{1}{12}$ the mass of carbon-12), generally very close to the whole number represented by the sum of the protons and neutrons in the atomic nucleus of the isotope (indicated in the name or symbol of the isotope; *e.g.,* oxygen-16, ^{16}O); not to be confused with the atomic weight of an element, which may include a number of isotopes in natural proportion.

MIM n., the catalog assignment for a mendelian trait in the MIM system. If the initial digit is 1, the trait is deemed autosomal dominant; if 2, autosomal recessive; if 3, then X-linked. Wherever a trait defined in this dictionary has a MIM n. the n. from the tenth edition of MIM is given in square brackets with or without an asterisk as appropriate *e.g.,* Pelizaeus-Merzbacher disease [MIM*169500] is a well-established, autosomal, dominant, mendelian disorder.

Polenské n., the n. of milliliters of 0.1 N KOH required to neutralize the nonvolatile fatty acids obtained from 5 g of a saponified fat or oil.

Reichert-Meissl n., an index of the volatile acid content of a fat; the n. of milliliters of 0.1 N KOH required to neutralize the soluble volatile fatty acids in 5 g of fat that has been saponified, acidified to liberate the fatty acids, and then steam-distilled. SYN volatile fatty acid n.

Reynolds n., a dimensionless n. that describes the tendency for a flowing fluid, such as blood, to change from laminar flow to turbulent flow or vice versa.

saponification n., the n. of milligrams of KOH required to saponify 1 g of fat; an approximate measure of the average molecular weight of a fat, with which it varies inversely. SYN Koettstorfer n.

stoichiometric n. (v), the n. associated with a reactant or product participating in a defined chemical reaction; usually an integer.

thiocyanogen n., the n. of grams of thiocyanogen taken up by 100 g of fat; analogous to the iodine n., except that thiocyanogen will not add to all the double bonds in polyunsaturated fatty acids as will iodine. SYN thiocyanogen value.

transport n., the fraction of the total current carried through a solution by a particular type of ion present in that solution.

turnover n. (k_{cat}), the number of substrate molecules converted into product in an enzyme-catalyzed reaction under saturating conditions per unit time per unit quantity of enzyme; *e.g.,* $k_{cat} = V_{max}/[E_{total}]$.

volatile fatty acid n., SYN Reichert-Meissl n.

wave n., the n. of waves (of any wave form such as light or sound) per unit length.

writhing n., the n. of times a DNA duplex axis crosses over itself in space.

numb·ness (nŭm'nes). Indefinite term for abnormal sensation, including absent or reduced sensory perception as well as paresthesias.

num·mi·form (nŭm'i-fōrm). SYN nummular.

num·mu·lar (nŭm'yū-ler). **1.** Discoid or coin-shaped; denoting the thick mucous or mucopurulent sputum in certain respiratory diseases, so called because of the disc shape assumed when it is flattened on the bottom of a sputum mug containing water or transparent disinfectant. **2.** Arranged like stacks of coins, denoting the lining up of the red blood cells into rouleaux formation. SYN nummiform. [L. *nummulus,* small coin, dim. of *nummus,* coin]

num·mu·la·tion (nŭm-yū-lā'shŭn). Formation of nummular masses.

nun·na·tion (nŭ-nā'shŭn). A form of stammering in which the *n* sound is given to other consonants. [Ar. *nūn,* the letter n.]

nurse (ners). **1.** To breast feed. **2.** To provide care of the sick. **3.** One who is educated in the scientific basis of nursing under defined standards of education and is concerned with the diagnosis and treatment of human responses to actual or potential health problems. [O. Fr. *nourice,* fr. L. *nutrix,* wet-nurse, nurse, fr. *nutrio,* to sucke, to tend]

certified registered n. anesthetist (C.R.N.A.), a registered professional nurse with additional education in the administration of anesthetics. Certification achieved through a program of study recognized by the American Association of Nurse Anesthetists.

charge n., a n. administratively responsible for a designated hospital unit on an 8 hour basis. SYN head n. (2).

clinical n. specialist, a registered n. with at least a master's degree who has advanced education in a particular area of clinical practice such as oncology, psychiatry. Usually employed in a hands-on clinical setting such as a hospital.

community n., SYN public health n.

community health n., SYN public health n.

dry n., a woman who cares for newborn infants without breast feeding them, as opposed to a wet n.

n. epidemiologist, a registered n. with additional education in the monitoring and prevention of nosocomial infections in the client population in an agency. SYN infection control n.

flight n., a n. who cares for clients during transport in any type of aircraft.

general duty n., n. who accepts assignment to any unit of a hospital other than an intensive care unit.

graduate n., a n. who has received a degree, most often a bachelor's degree, from a school or college of nursing.

head n., (1) a n. administratively responsible for a designated hospital unit on a 24 hour basis; **(2)** SYN charge n.

home health n., a n. who is responsible for a group of clients in the home setting. Visits clients on a routine basis to assist client and family with care as needed and to teach family the care needed so that the client may remain in his/her home. SYN visiting n.

hospital n., a registered n. working in a hospital.

infection control n., SYN n. epidemiologist.

licensed practical n. (L.P.N.), a n. who has graduated from an accredited school of practical (vocational) nursing, passed the state examination for licensure and been licensed to practice by a state authority. Program is generally one year in length. SYN licensed vocational n.

licensed vocational n. (L.V.N.), SYN licensed practical n.

practical n., a graduate of a specific educational program that prepares the individual for a career in nursing with less responsibility than a graduate or registered n.

private n., SYN private duty n.

private duty n., (1) a n. who is not a member of a hospital staff, but is hired by the client or his/her family on a fee-for-service basis to care for the client; **(2)** a n. who specializes in the care of patients with diseases of a particular class, *e.g.,* surgical cases, tuberculosis, children's diseases. SYN private n.

public health n., a n. who provides care to individuals or groups in a community outside of institutions. Usually works through the auspices of a state or city health department. SYN community health n., community n.

registered n. (R.N.), a n. who has graduated from an accredited nursing program, has passed the state exam for licensure, and been registered and licensed to practice by a state authority.

school n., a n., usually an RN, working in a school or similar institution.

scrub n., a n. who has scrubbed arms and hands, donned sterile gloves and, usually, a sterile gown, and assists an operating surgeon, primarily by passing instruments.

special n., a n., who might be a registered nurse or a practical nurse, assigned to limited, specialized functions; usually synonymous with private duty nurse.

student n., a student in a program leading to certification in a form of nursing; usually applied to students in an RN or practical n. program.

visiting n., SYN home health n.

wet n., a woman who breast-feeds a child not her own.

nurse prac·ti·tion·er (ners prak-tish′ŭ-ner). A registered nurse with at least a master's degree in nursing and advanced education in the primary care of particular groups of clients. Capable of independent practice in a variety of settings.

> Nurse practitioners have been recognized in the U.S. since 1955, and currently are seen as a possible means of reducing health care costs. They are able to carry out 60–90% of the tasks required of a primary health care provider, including taking medical histories, performing physical exams and laboratory tests, and treating common illnesses and injuries. In this way they free physicians to address more acute illnesses, or, especially in rural regions without a local primary care physician, allow patients to receive treatment for most medical problems without having to travel long distances. Generally, nurse practitioners emphasize preventive health care and close management of chronic disorders.

nurs·ing (ner′sing). **1.** Feeding an infant at the breast; tending and caring for a child. **2.** The scientific application of principles of care related to prevention of illness and care during illness.

n. assignment, the method(s) by which the patient care load is distributed among the n. personnel available to provide care.

n. audit, a defined procedure used to evaluate the quality of n. care provided within an agency to its clients.

n. model, a set of abstract and general statements about the concepts that serve to provide a framework for organizing ideas about clients, their environment, health and nursing.

n. plan of care, the written framework that provides direction for the delivery of n. care.

n. process, a five-part systematic decision-making method focusing on identifying and treating responses of individuals or groups to actual or potential alterations in health. Includes assessment, n. diagnosis, planning, implementation, and evaluation. The first phase of the n. process is assessment, which consists of data collection by such means as interviewing, physical examination, and observation. It requires collection of both objective and subjective data. The second phase is n. diagnosis, a clinical judgment about individual, family or community n. responses to actual or potential health problems/life processes. Provides the basis for selection of n. intervention to achieve outcomes for which the nurse is accountable (NANDA, 1990). The third phase is planning, which requires establishment of outcome criteria for the client's care. The fourth phase is imple-

mentation (intervention). This phase involves demonstrating those activities that will be provided to and with the client to allow achievement of the expected outcomes of care. Evaluation is the fifth and final phase of the n. process. It requires comparison of client's current state to the stated expected outcomes and results in revision of the plan of care to enhance progress toward the stated outcomes.

nurs·ing home. A convalescent home or private facility for the care of individuals who do not require hospitalization and who cannot be cared for at home.

Nussbaum, Johann von, German surgeon, 1829–1890. SEE N.'s *bracelet.*

Nussbaum, Moritz, German histologist, 1850–1915. SEE N.'s *experiment.*

nu·ta·tion (nū-tā′shŭn). The act of nodding, especially involuntary nodding. [L. *annuo,* to nod]

nut·gall (nŭt′gahl). An excrescence on the oak, *Quercus infectoria* (family Fagaceae) and other species of *Quercus,* caused by the deposit of the ova of a fly, *Cynips gallae tinctorae;* an astringent and styptic, by virtue of the tannin it contains. SYN gall (3), galla, oak apple.

nut·meg (nŭt′meg). The dried ripe seed of *Myristica fragrans* (family Myristicaceae), deprived of its seed coat and arillode; an aromatic stimulant, carminative, condiment, and source of volatile and expressed nutmeg oils; it is consumed for its bizarre central nervous system effects. SEE ALSO myristicin. SYN myristica.

nut·meg oil. The volatile oil distilled from the dried kernels of the ripe seeds of *Myristica fragrans;* used as a flavoring agent and a carminative; in large quantities, it may produce narcosis and delirium; the fixed oil expressed from *M. fragrans* is used as a rubefacient. SYN myristica oil.

nu·tri·ent (nū′trē-ent). A constituent of food necessary for normal physiologic function. [L. *nutriens,* fr. *nutrio,* to nourish]

essential n.'s, nutritional substances required for optimal health. They must be in the diet since they are not formed metabolically within the body.

trace n., SYN micronutrients.

nu·tri·lites (nū′tri-līts). Essential nutritional factors. [L. *nutrio,* to suckle, nourish]

nu·tri·tion (nū-trish′ŭn). **1.** A function of living plants and animals, consisting in the taking in and metabolism of food material whereby tissue is built up and energy liberated. SYN trophism (2). **2.** The study of the food and liquid requirements of human beings or animals for normal physiologic function, including energy, need, maintenance, growth, activity, reproduction, and lactation. [L. *nutritio,* fr. *nutrio,* to nourish]

total parenteral n. (TPN), n. maintained entirely by intravenous injection or other nongastrointestinal route.

nu·tri·tive (nū′tri-tiv). **1.** Pertaining to nutrition. **2.** Capable of nourishing. SYN alible.

nu·tri·ture (nū′tri-chūr). State or condition of the nutrition of the body; state of the body with regard to nourishment. [L. *nutritura,* a nursing, fr. *nutrio,* to nourish]

Nuttall, G. H. F., U.S. biologist, 1862–1937. SEE *Nuttallia.*

Nut·tal·lia (nŭ-tal′ē-ă). Former name for *Babesia.*

nux vom·i·ca (nŭks vom′i-kă). Poison nut or Quaker button, the seed of *Strychnos nux-vomica* (family Logeniaceae), a tree of tropical Asia; it contains two alkaloids, strychnine and brucine; it has been used as a bitter tonic and central nervous system stimulant. [Mod. L. emetic nut, fr. L. *nux,* nut, + *vomo,* to vomit]

Nva Abbreviation for norvaline.

nyct-. SEE nycto-.

nyc·tal·gia (nik-tal′jē-ă). Denoting especially the osteocopic pains of syphilis occurring at night. SYN night pain. [nyct- + G. *algos,* pain]

nyc·ta·lo·pia (nik-tă-lō′pē-ă). Decreased ability to see in reduced illumination. Seen in patients with impaired rod function; often associated with a deficiency of vitamin A. SYN day sight, night blindness, nocturnal amblyopia, nyctanopia. [nyct- + G. *alaos,* obscure, + *ōps,* eye]

n. with congenital myopia [MIM*310500], an abnormality of

X-linked inheritance characterized by low visual acuity, strabismus, or nystagmus.

nyc·ta·no·pia (nik-tă-nō′pē-ă). SYN nyctalopia. [nyct- + G. *an*-priv. + *opsis*, sight]

nyc·ter·ine (nik′ter-īn, -in). **1.** By night. **2.** Dark or obscure. [G. *nykterinos*]

nyc·ter·o·hem·er·al (nik′ter-ō-hē′mer-ăl). SYN nyctohemeral. [G. *nykteros*, by night, nightly, + *hēmera*, day]

⚠nycto-, nyct-. Night, nocturnal. SEE ALSO noct-. [G. *nyx*]

nyc·to·hem·er·al (nik-tō-hē′mer-ăl). Both daily and nightly. SYN nycterohemeral. [nycto- + G. *hēmera*, day]

nyc·to·phil·ia (nik-tō-fil′ē-ă). Preference for the night or darkness. SYN scotophilia. [nycto- + G. *philos*, fond]

nyc·to·pho·bia (nik-tō-fō′bē-ă). Morbid fear of night or of the dark. SYN scotophobia. [nycto- + G. *phobos*, fear]

Nyc·to·the·rus (nik-tō-thē′rŭs). A genus of Ciliophora, one species of which, *N. faba*, has been reported, though rarely, from the human intestine; it is generally found in amphibia. [G. *nyktothēras*, one who hunts by night, fr. *thērao*, to hunt, fr. *thēr*, wild beast]

nyc·tu·ria (nik-tū′rē-ă). SYN nocturia.

Nyhan, William L. U.S. pediatrician, *1926. SEE Lesch-N. *syndrome*.

ny·li·drin hy·dro·chlo·ride (nī′li-drin, nil′). 1-(*p*-Hydroxyphenyl)-2-(1-methyl-3-phenylpropylamino) propanol hydrochloride; a sympathomimetic agent, similar to isoproterenol, that produces vasodilation of arterioles of skeletal muscles and increases muscle blood flow; used in the treatment of peripheral vascular diseases.

nymph (nimf). **1.** The earliest series of stages in metamorphosis following hatching in the development of hemimetabolous insects (*e.g.*, locusts); the n. resembles the adult in many respects, but lacks full wing or genitalia development; it grows through successive instars without any intermediate or pupal stage into the imago or adult form. SEE ALSO incomplete *metamorphosis*, complete *metamorphosis*. **2.** The third stage in the life cycle of a tick, between the larva and the adult. [G. *nymphē*, maiden]

nym·pha, pl. **nym·phae** (nim′fă, nim′fē). One of the labia minora. [Mod. L., fr. G. *nymphē*, a bride]

nym·phal (nim′făl). **1.** Pertaining to a nymph. **2.** Pertaining to the labia minora (nymphae).

nym·phec·to·my (nim-fek′tō-mē). Surgical removal of hypertrophied labia minora. [nympha + G. *ektomē*, excision]

nym·phi·tis (nim-fī′tis). Inflammation of the labia minora. [nympha + G. *-itis*, inflammation]

⚠nympho-, nymph-. The nymphae (labia minora). [L. *nympha*]

nym·pho·la·bi·al (nim′fō-lā′bē-ăl). Relating to the labia minora (nymphae) and the labia majora; denoting a furrow between the two labia on each side.

nym·pho·lep·sy (nim-fō-lep′sē). Demoniac frenzy, especially of an erotic nature. [nympho- + G. *lēpsis*, a seizure]

nym·pho·ma·nia (nim-fō-mā′nē-ă). An insatiable impulse to engage in sexual intercourse in a female; the counterpart of satyriasis in a male. [nympho- + G. *mania*, frenzy]

nym·pho·ma·ni·ac (nim-fō-mā′nē-ak). A female exhibiting nymphomania.

nym·pho·ma·ni·a·cal (nim′fō-mă-nī′ă-kăl). Pertaining to, or exhibiting, nymphomania.

nym·phon·cus (nim-fong′kŭs). Swelling or hypertrophy of one or both labia minora. [nympho- + G. *onkos*, tumor]

nym·phot·o·my (nim-fot′ō-mē). Incision into the labia minora or the clitoris. [nympho- + G. *tomē*, incision]

nys·tag·mic (nis-tag′mik). Relating to or suffering from nystagmus.

nys·tag·mi·form (nis-tag′mi-fōrm). SYN nystagmoid.

nys·tag·mo·gram (nis-tag′mō-gram). The tracing produced by a nystagmograph.

nys·tag·mo·graph (nis-tag′mō-graf). An apparatus for measuring the amplitude, periodicity, and velocity of ocular movements in nystagmus, by measuring the change in the resting potential of the eye as the eye moves. [nystagmus + G. *graphō*, to write]

nys·tag·mog·ra·phy (nis-tag-mog′ră-fē). The technique of recording nystagmus.

nys·tag·moid (nis-tag′moyd). Resembling nystagmus. SYN nystagmiform. [nystagmus + G. *eidos*, resemblance]

nys·tag·mus (nis-tag′mŭs). Rhythmical oscillation of the eyeballs, either pendular or jerky. [G. *nystagmos*, a nodding, fr. *nystazō*, to be sleepy, nod]

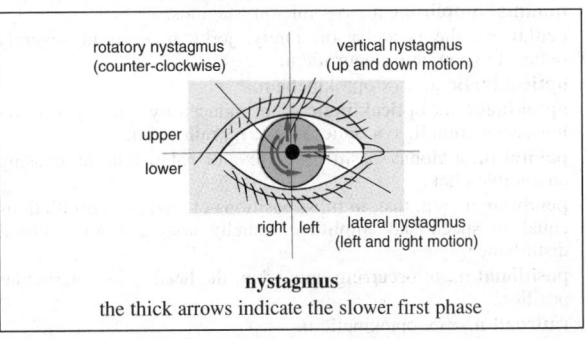

nystagmus
the thick arrows indicate the slower first phase

after-n., n. occurring after the abrupt cessation of rotation in the opposite direction of the rotatory n.

amaurotic n., SYN ocular n.

Bruns' n., a fine, jerking (vestibular) n. on horizontal gaze in one direction, together with a slower, larger amplitude (gaze, paretic) n. on looking in the opposite direction; due to lateral brainstem compression, usually by a cerebellar-pontine angle mass such as an acoustic neuroma.

caloric n., jerky n. induced by labyrinthine stimulation with hot or cold water in the ear. SEE ALSO Bárány's *sign*.

cervical n., n. arising from a lesion of the proprioceptive mechanism of the neck.

compressive n., a jerky n. resulting from unilateral changes of pressure in semicircular canals.

congenital n., (1) n. present at birth or caused by lesions sustained *in utero* or at the time of birth; **(2)** inherited n., usually X-linked, without associated neurologic lesions and nonprogressive; all three patterns of mendelian inheritance may occur: autosomal dominant [MIM*164100, *164150, *124170], autosomal recessive [MIM*257400], [MIM*310800, *310700]; **(3)** the n. associated with albinism, achromatopsia, and hypoplasia of the macula.

conjugate n., a n. in which the two eyes move simultaneously in the same direction.

convergence-retraction n., irregular, jerky n. combining convergence and retraction of the eye into the orbit, especially on attempting an upward gaze. SYN Koerber-Salus-Elschnig syndrome.

deviational n., SYN end-point n.

dissociated n., a n. in which the movements of the two eyes are dissimilar in direction, amplitude, and periodicity. SYN dysjunctive n., incongruent n., irregular n.

downbeat n., a vertical n. with a rapid component downward, occurring in lesions of the lower part of the brainstem or cerebellum.

dysjunctive n., SYN dissociated n.

end-point n., a jerky, physiologic n. occurring in a normal individual when attempts are made to fixate a point at the limits of the field of fixation. SYN deviational n.

fixation n., n. aggravated or induced by ocular fixation, arising as optokinetic n., or resulting from midbrain lesions.

galvanic n., n. involving galvanic stimulation of the labyrinth.

gaze paretic n., n. occurring in partial gaze paralysis when an attempt is made to look in the direction of the gaze paresis.

incongruent n., SYN dissociated n.

irregular n., SYN dissociated n.

jerky n., n. in which there is a slow drift of the eyes in one direction, followed by a rapid recovery movement, always described in the direction of the recovery movement; it usually arises from labyrinthine or neurologic lesions or stimuli.

labyrinthine n., SYN vestibular n.

latent n., jerky n. that is brought out by covering one eye. The fast phase is always away from the covered eye.

miner's n., n. occurring in 19th century coal miners and thought at the time to be related to lack of illumination as well as other factors. SYN miner's disease (1).

minimal amplitude n., SYN micronystagmus.

ocular n., the pendular or, rarely, jerky n. seen in severely reduced vision. SYN amaurotic n.

opticokinetic n., SYN optokinetic n.

optokinetic n., opticokinetic n., n. induced by looking at moving visual stimuli. SYN opticokinetic n., railroad n.

palatal n., a clonic spasm of the levator palati muscle, causing an audible click.

pendular n., a n. that, in most positions of gaze, has oscillations equal in speed and amplitude, usually arising from a visual disturbance.

positional n., n. occurring only when the head is in a particular position.

railroad n., SYN optokinetic n.

rotational n., jerky n. arising from stimulation of the labyrinth by rotation of the head around any axis and induced by change of motion.

rotatory n., a movement of the eyes around the visual axis.

seesaw n., a n. in which one eye moves upward as the other moves downward, often combined with a torsional rotation (down and out, up and in—as in a see-saw).

upbeat n., a vertical jerky n. with a rapid component upward, occurring with brainstem lesions.

vertical n., an up-and-down oscillation of the eyes.

vestibular n., n. resulting from physiological stimuli to the labyrinth that may be rotatory, caloric, compressive, or galvanic, or due to labyrinthal lesions. SEE ALSO Bárány's *sign*. SYN labyrinthine n.

voluntary n., pendular n. in which the individual causes an extremely fine and rapid horizontal oscillation of the eyes. The n. consists of back-to-back saccades and is seldom done for more than a few seconds at a time.

nys·tat·in (nī-stat′in, nis′tă-tin). An antibiotic substance isolated from cultures of *Streptomyces noursei*, effective in the treatment of all forms of candidiasis, particularly candidal infections of the intestine, skin, and mucous membranes. SYN fungicidin. [*New York State* + -in]

Nysten, Pierre H., French physician, 1771–1818. SEE N.'s *law*.

nyx·is (nik′sis). A pricking; paracentesis. [G.]

O

Ω **1.** Twenty-fourth and last letter of the Greek alphabet, omega. **2.** Symbol for Ohm.

O 1. Symbol for oxygen; orotidine. **2.** Abbreviation for opening (in formulas for electrical reactions). **3.** Symbol for a blood group in the ABO system. See ABO blood group, Blood Groups appendix. **4.** An abbreviation derived from *ohne Hauch* (without a film), used as a designation for: 1) antigens that occur in the bacterial cell, in contrast to those in the flagella; 2) specific antibodies for such somatic antigens; 3) the agglutinative reaction between somatic antigen and its antibody.

^{15}**O.** Symbol for oxygen-15.

^{16}**O.** Symbol for oxygen-16.

^{17}**O.** Symbol for oxygen-17.

^{18}**O.** Symbol for oxygen-18.

o- In chemistry, the abbreviation for ortho- (2).

oak ap·ple. SYN nutgall.

oari-, oario-. Obsolete term for an ovary. SEE oo-, oophor-, ovario-. [G. *ōarion*, a small egg, dim. of *ōon*, egg]

oath (ōth). A solemn affirmation or attestation. SEE Hippocratic Oath, Veterinarian's Oath.

OB Abbreviation for obstetrics.

ob·dor·mi·tion (ob-dōr-mish'ŭn). Numbness of an extremity, due to pressure on the sensory nerve. [L. *ob-dormio*, pp. *-itus,* to sleep]

O'Beirne, James, Irish surgeon, 1786–1862. SEE O'B.'s *sphincter.*

obe·li·ac (ō-bē'lē-ak). Relating to the obelion.

obe·li·ad (ō-bē'lē-ad). Toward the obelion.

obe·li·on (ō-bē'lē-on). A craniometric point on the sagittal suture between the parietal foramina near the lambdoid suture. [G. *obelos,* a spit]

Obermayer, Friedrich, Austrian physician, 1861–1925. SEE O.'s *test.*

Obermeier, Otto H.F., German physician, 1843–1873. SEE O.'s *spirillum.*

Obersteiner, H., Austrian neurologist, 1847–1922. SEE O.-Redlich *line, zone.*

obese (ō-bēs'). Excessively fat. SYN corpulent. [L. *obesus,* fat, partic. adj., fr. *ob-edo,* pp. *-esus,* to eat away, devour]

obe·si·ty (ō-bē'si-tē). An abnormal increase of fat in the subcutaneous connective tissues. SYN adiposity (1), corpulence, corpulency.

hypothalamic o., o. caused by disease of the hypothalamus.

hypothalamic o. with hypogonadism, SYN *dystrophia* adiposogenitalis.

morbid o., o. sufficient to prevent normal activity or physiologic function, or to cause the onset of a pathologic condition.

simple o., o. resulting when caloric intake exceeds energy expenditure.

obex (ō'beks) [NA]. The point on the midline of the dorsal surface of the medulla oblongata that marks the caudal angle of the rhomboid fossa or fourth ventricle. It corresponds to a small, transverse medullary fold overhanging the calamus scriptorius. [L. barrier]

ob·fus·ca·tion (ob-fus-kā'shŭn). **1.** A rendering dark or obscure. **2.** A deliberate attempt to confuse or to prevent understanding. [L. *ob-fusco,* pp. *-atus,* to darken, fr. *fuscus,* dark, tawny]

OB/GYN Abbreviation for obstetrics and gynecology.

ob·i·dox·ime chlo·ride (ob'ē-dok-sēm). A cholinesterase reactivator much like 2-PAM.

ob·ject (ob'jekt). **1.** Anything to which thought or action is directed. **2.** In psychoanalysis, that through which an instinct can achieve its aim. **3.** In psychoanalysis, often used synonymously with person.

good o., in psychoanalysis, the good or supporting aspects of an important person in the patient's life, especially of a parent or parent-surrogate.

sex o., a person toward whom another is sexually attracted; a term usually used by a female to indicate that a male narrowly views her as a vehicle for sex while completely disregarding the rest of her persona.

test o., (1) an o. having very fine surface markings, mounted on a slide, used to determine the defining power of the objective lens of a microscope; (2) the target in measurement of the visual field.

ob·ject choice. In psychoanalysis, the object (usually a person) upon which psychic energy is centered.

ob·jec·tive (ob-jek'tiv). **1.** The lens or lenses in the lower end of the body tube of a microscope, by means of which the rays coming from the object examined are brought to a focus. SYN object glass. **2.** Viewing events or phenomena as they exist in the external world, impersonally, or in an unprejudiced way; open to observation by oneself and by others. Cf. subjective. [L. *ob- jicio,* pp. *-jectus,* to throw before]

achromatic o., an o. that is corrected for two colors chromatically, and one color spherically.

apochromatic o., an o. in which chromatic aberration is corrected for three colors and spherical aberration is corrected for two.

immersion o., a high power o. used with a drop of oil between the lens and the specimen on the slide, allowing a greater numerical aperture; similar lenses are available for use with water as the immersing liquid.

ob·jec·tive as·sess·ment da·ta. Those facts presented by the client that show his/her perception, understanding and interpretation of what is happening.

ob·li·gate (ob'li-gāt). Without an alternative system or pathway. [L. *ob-ligo,* pp. *-atus,* to bind to]

ob·lique (ob-lēk'). Slanting; deviating from the perpendicular, horizontal, sagittal, or coronal plane of the body. In radiography, a projection that is neither frontal nor lateral. [L. *obliquus*]

ob·liq·ui·ty (ob-lik'wi-tē). SYN asynclitism.

Litzmann o., inclination of the fetal head so that the biparietal diameter is oblique in relation to the plane of the pelvic brim, the posterior parietal bone presenting to the parturient canal. SYN posterior asynclitism.

Nägele o., inclination of the fetal head in cases of flat pelvis, so that the biparietal diameter is oblique in relation to the plane of the pelvic brim, the anterior parietal bone presenting to the parturient canal. SYN anterior asynclitism.

ob·li·qu·us (ob-lī'kwŭs). Denoting a structure having an oblique course or direction; a name given, with further qualification, to several muscles. SEE muscle. [L. slanting, oblique]

ob·lit·er·a·tion (ob-lit-er-ā'shŭn). Blotting out, especially by filling of a natural space or lumen by fibrosis or inflammation. In radiology, disappearance of the contour of an organ when the adjacent tissue has the same x-ray absorption. [L. *oblittero,* to blot out]

ob·lon·ga·ta (ob-long-gah'tă). SYN *medulla* oblongata. [L. fem. of *oblongatus,* from *oblongus,* rather long]

ob·nu·bi·la·tion (ab-nū'bil-ā'shun). A clouded mental state. [L. *ob-nubilo,* to becloud, obscure, fr. *nubes,* cloud]

OBS. SYN organic brain *syndrome.*

ob·ser·ver (ob-zer'ver). One who perceives, notices, or watches; in behavioral research with humans, the investigator or his/her surrogate. [L. *observo,* to watch]

nonparticipant o., an investigator who studies a group of subjects engaged in certain activities but does not directly participate in these activities, presumably being able to study them more objectively.

participant o., an investigator who while studying the activities of a group of subjects also participates in their activities, presumably being able to gain more detailed, relevant information but with less objectivity.

ob·ses·sion (ob-sesh'ŭn). A recurrent and persistent idea,

1235

thought, or impulse to carry out an act that is ego-dystonic, that is experienced as senseless or repugnant, and that the individual cannot voluntarily suppress. [L. *obsideo*, pp. -*sessus*, to besiege, fr. *sedeo*, to sit]

impulsive o., an o. accompanied by action, sometimes becoming a mania.

inhibitory o., an o. involving an impediment to action, usually representing a phobia.

ob·ses·sive-com·pul·sive. Having a tendency to perform certain repetitive acts or ritualistic behavior to relieve anxiety, as in obsessive-compulsive neurosis (*e.g.*, a compulsive, ritualistic need to wash one's hands many dozens of times per day).

ob·so·les·cence (ob-sō-les'ens). Falling into disuse; denoting the abolition of a function. [L. *obsolesco*, to grow out of use]

ob·stet·ric, ob·stet·ri·cal (ob-stet'rik, -ri-kăl). Relating to obstetrics.

ob·ste·tri·cian (ob-stĕ-trish'ŭn). A physician specializing in the medical care of women during pregnancy and childbirth. [see obstetrics]

ob·stet·rics (OB) (ob-stet'riks). The specialty of medicine concerned with the care of women during pregnancy, parturition, and the puerperium. SYN tocology. [L. *obstetrix*, a midwife, fr. *ob-sto*, to stand before, denoting the position formerly taken by the midwife]

ob·sti·nate (ob'sti-năt). **1.** Firmly adhering to one's own purpose, opinion, etc. even when wrong; not yielding to argument, persuasion, or entreaty. SYN intractable (2), refractory (2). **2.** SYN refractory (1). [L. *obstinatus*, determined]

ob·sti·pa·tion (ob-sti-pā'shŭn). Intestinal obstruction; severe constipation. [L. *ob*, against, + *stipo*, pp. -*atus*, to crowd]

ob·struc·tion (ob-strŭk'shŭn). Blockage or clogging, *e.g.*, by occlusion or stenosis. [L. *obstructio*]

closed-loop o., o. of a segment of intestine by rotation on a fixed point (volvulus); frequently impairs venous circulation of the affected bowel segment, resulting in strangulation and gangrene; the segment of intestine contained in a hernia can also become a closed-loop o. when sufficient compression occurs at the neck of the sac.

ureteropelvic junction o., an impediment to drainage of urine from kidney usually to partial or intermittent blockage of renal collecting system of the junction of renal pelvis and ureter.

ureteropelvic o., a blocking or stenosis, usually congenital, at the junction of the renal pelvis and ureter, usually resulting in stasis, pelvocaliectasis, hydronephrosis, or calyceal clubbing.

ureterovesical o., o. of the lower ureter at its entrance into the bladder.

ob·struc·tive pul·mo·nary over·in·fla·tion. Emphysema caused by obstruction of airways that has greater effect on expiration than inspiration; occurs reversibly with bronchospasm of asthma; localized process can be due to aspiration of a foreign body.

ob·stru·ent (ob'strū-ent). **1.** Rarely used term for obstructing or clogging. **2.** Rarely used term for an agent that obstructs or prevents a normal discharge, especially a discharge from the bowels. [L. *ob-struo*, to build against, obstruct]

ob·tund (ob-tŭnd'). To dull or blunt, especially to blunt sensation or deaden pain. [L. *ob-tundo*, pp. -*tusus*, to beat against, blunt]

ob·tu·ra·tion (ob-tū-rā'shŭn). Obstruction or occlusion. [see obturator]

intermittent self-o., passage of a blunt object in a lumen or meatus to occlude it or to dilate it.

ob·tu·ra·tor (ob'tū-rā-tŏr). **1.** Any structure that occludes an opening. **2.** Denoting the obturator foramen, the obturator membrane, or any of several parts in relation to this foramen. **3.** A prosthesis used to close an opening of the hard palate, usually a cleft palate. **4.** The stylus or removable plug used during the insertion of many tubular instruments. [L. *obturo*, pp. -*atus*, to occlude or stop up]

ob·tuse (ob-tūs'). **1.** Dull in intellect; of slow understanding. **2.** Blunt; not acute. [see obtund]

ob·tu·sion (ob-tū'zhŭn). **1.** Dullness of sensibility. **2.** A dulling or deadening of sensibility.

Occam's ra·zor. the principle of scientific parsimony. William of Occam (14th Century) stated it thus: "The assumptions introduced to explain a thing must not be multiplied beyond necessity."

oc·cip·i·tal (ok-sip'i-tăl). Relating to the occiput. referring to the occipital bone or to the back of the head. SYN occipitalis [NA].

oc·ci·pi·ta·lis (ok'sip-i-tā'lis) [NA]. SYN occipital. [L.]

oc·cip·i·tal·i·za·tion (ok'sip'i-tăl-i-zā'shŭn). Bony ankylosis between the atlas and occipital bone.

△**occipito-.** The occiput, occipital structures. [L. *occiput*]

oc·cip·i·to·at·loid (ok-sip'i-tō-at'loyd). Relating to the occipital bone and the atlas; denoting the articulation between the two bones.

oc·cip·i·to·ax·i·al, oc·cip·i·to·ax·oid (ok-sip'i-tō-ak'sē-ăl, -ak' soyd). Relating to the occipital bone and the axis, or epistropheus.

oc·cip·i·to·breg·mat·ic (ok-sip'i-tō-breg-mat'ik). Relating to the occiput and the bregma; denoting a measurement in craniometry.

oc·cip·i·to·fa·cial (ok-sip'i-tō-fā'shăl). Relating to the occiput and the face.

oc·cip·i·to·fron·tal (ok-sip'i-tō-frŭn'tăl). **1.** Relating to the occiput and the forehead. **2.** Relating to the occipital and frontal lobe of the cerebral cortex and association pathways that interconnect these regions.

oc·cip·i·to·fron·ta·lis (ok-sip'i-tō-frŭn-tā'lis). SEE occipitofrontalis *muscle*. [L.]

oc·cip·i·to·mas·toid (ok-sip'i-tō-mas'toyd). Relating to the occipital bone and the mastoid process.

oc·cip·i·to·men·tal (ok-sip'i-tō-men'tăl). Relating to the occiput and the chin.

oc·cip·i·to·pa·ri·e·tal (ok-sip'i-tō-pă-rī'ĕ-tăl). Relating to the occipital and the parietal bones.

oc·cip·i·to·tem·po·ral (ok-sip'i-tō-tem'pŏ-răl). Relating to the occiput and the temple, or the occipital and the temporal bones.

oc·cip·i·to·tha·lam·ic (ok-sip'i-tō-tha-lam'ik). Relating to the nerve fibers leading from the occipital lobe of the cerebral cortex to the thalamus.

oc·ci·put, gen. **oc·cip·i·tis** (ok'si-put, ok-sip'i-tis) [NA]. The back of the head. [L.]

oc·clude (ŏ-klūd'). **1.** To close or bring together. **2.** To enclose, as in an occluded *virus*. [see occlusion]

oc·clud·er (ŏ-klūd'er). In dentistry, a name given to some articulators.

oc·clu·sal (ŏ-klū'zăl). **1.** Pertaining to occlusion or closure. **2.** In dentistry, pertaining to the contacting surfaces of opposing occlusal units (teeth or occlusion rims), or the masticating surfaces of the posterior teeth.

oc·clu·sion (ŏ-klū'zhŭn). **1.** The act of closing or the state of being closed. **2.** In chemistry, the absorption of a gas by a metal or the inclusion of one substance within another (as in a gelatinous precipitate). **3.** Any contact between the incising or masticating surfaces of the upper and lower teeth. **4.** The relationship between the occlusal surfaces of the maxillary and mandibular teeth when they are in contact. [L. *oc-cludo*, pp. -*clusus*, to shut up, fr. *ob*, against, + *claudo*, to close]

abnormal o., an arrangement of the teeth which is not considered to be within the normal range of variation.

afunctional o., a malocclusion which does not permit normal function of the dentition.

anterior o., (1) the o. of anterior teeth; (2) SYN mesial o. (1).

balanced o., the simultaneous contacting of the upper and lower teeth on the right and left and in the anterior and posterior occlusal areas in centric and eccentric positions within the functional range; used primarily in reference to the mouth, but also arranged and observed on articulators, developed to prevent a tipping or rotating of the denture bases in relation to the supporting structures. SYN balanced articulation, balanced bite.

bimaxillary protrusive o., an o. in which both the maxilla and mandible protrude, causing the long axes of the maxillary anterior teeth to be at an extremely acute angle to the mandibular teeth; may be secondary to a skeletal or dental deformity, or both; seen commonly in blacks.

buccal o., (1) malposition of a tooth toward the cheek; **(2)** the o. as seen from the buccal side of the teeth.

centric o., (1) the relation of opposing occlusal surfaces which provides the maximum planned contact and/or intercuspation; **(2)** the o. of the teeth when the mandible is in centric relation to the maxillae. SYN centric contact.

coronary o., blockage of a coronary vessel, usually by thrombosis or atheroma, often leading to myocardial infarction.

distal o., (1) a tooth occluding in a position distal to normal; SYN disto-occlusion, postnormal o., retrusive o. (2). **(2)** SYN distocclusion.

eccentric o., any o. other than centric.

edge-to-edge o., an o. in which the anterior teeth of both jaws meet along their incisal edges when the teeth are in centric o. SYN edge-to-edge bite, end-to-end bite, end-to-end o.

end-to-end o., SYN edge-to-edge o.

functional o., (1) any tooth contacts made within the functional range of the opposing teeth surfaces; **(2)** o. which occurs during function.

gliding o., SYN dental *articulation.*

hyperfunctional o., occlusal stress of tooth or teeth exceeding normal physiologic demands.

labial o., (1) malposition of a tooth in a labial direction; **(2)** the o. as seen from the labial side of the arches.

lateral o., malposition of a tooth or an entire dental arch in a direction away from the midline.

lingual o., (1) SYN linguoclusion. **(2)** interdigitation of the teeth as seen from the internal or lingual aspect.

mechanically balanced o., a balanced o. without reference to physiologic considerations, as on an articulator.

mesenteric artery o., obstruction of arterial flow in the mesenteric circulation by an embolus or thrombus; usually refers to o. of the superior mesenteric artery, although atherosclerotic narrowing may involve all three major splanchnic branches (celiac, superior, and inferior mesenteric).

mesial o., (1) o. in which the mandibular teeth articulate with the maxillary teeth in a position anterior to normal; SYN anterior o. (2), mesio-occlusion. **(2)** SYN mesioclusion.

neutral o., (1) an arrangement of teeth such that the maxillary and mandibular first permanent molars are in normal anteroposterior relation; SYN normal o. (2). **(2)** SYN neutroclusion.

normal o., (1) that arrangement of teeth and their supporting structure which is usually found in health and which approaches an ideal or standard arrangement; SYN normal bite. **(2)** SYN neutral o. (1).

pathogenic o., an occlusal relationship capable of producing pathologic changes in the supporting tissues.

physiologic o., o. in harmony with functions of the masticatory system.

physiologically balanced o., a balanced o. that is in harmony with the temporomandibular joints and the neuromuscular system.

posterior o., the most effective contact of the molar and bicuspid teeth of both jaws which allows for all the natural movements of the jaws essential to normal mastication and closure. SYN posteroclusion.

postnormal o., SYN distal o. (1).

protrusive o., o. which results when the mandible is protruded forward from centric position.

o. of pupil, the presence of an opaque membrane closing the pupillary area.

retrusive o., (1) a biting relationship in which the mandible is forcefully or habitually placed more distally than the patient's centric o.; **(2)** SYN distal o. (1).

spherical form of o., an arrangement of teeth which places their occlusal surfaces on the surface of an imaginary sphere (usually 8 inches in diameter) with its center above the level of the teeth. SEE ALSO Monson *curve.*

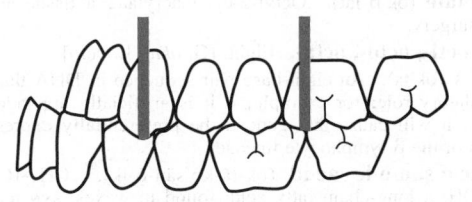

mesial occlusion
articulation of the side teeth in sagittal direction

torsive o., SYN torsiversion.

traumatic o., SYN traumatogenic o.

traumatogenic o., a malocclusion capable of producing injury to the teeth and/or associated structures. SYN traumatic o.

working o., SYN working *contacts,* under *contact.*

oc·clu·sive (ŏ-klū′siv). Serving to close; denoting a bandage or dressing that closes a wound and excludes it from the air.

oc·clu·som·e·ter (ok-lū-som′ĕ-ter). SYN gnathodynamometer.

oc·cult (ŏ-kŭlt′, ok′ŭlt). **1.** Hidden; concealed; not manifest. **2.** Denoting a concealed hemorrhage, the blood being inapparent or localized to a site where it is not visible. SEE occult *blood.* **3.** In oncology, a clinically unidentified primary tumor with recognized metastases. [L. *oc-culo,* pp. *-cultus,* to cover, hide]

Oce·an·o·spi·ril·lum (ō′shen-ō-spī-ril′ŭm). A genus of motile, nonsporeforming, aerobic bacteria (family Spirillaceae) containing Gram-negative, rigid, helical cells which are 0.3 to 1.2 μm in diameter. Motile cells contain bipolar fascicles of flagella. There is no growth anaerobically with nitrate. These organisms are chemoorganotrophic and possess a strictly respiratory metabolism; they neither oxidize nor ferment carbohydrates; found in marine environments. There are at present five species in this genus, of which the type species is *O. linum.* [L. *oceanus,* ocean, + *spirillum,* coil]

ocel·lus, pl. **ocel·li** (ō-sel′ŭs, -lī). **1.** The simple eye found in many invertebrates. SYN eyespot (2). **2.** Facet of the compound eye of an insect. [L. dim. of *oculus,* eye]

och·lo·pho·bia (ok-lō-fō′bē-ă). Morbid fear of crowds. [G. *ochlos,* a crowd, + *phobos,* fear]

Ochoa, Severo, Spanish-U.S. biochemist and Nobel laureate, *1905. SEE O.'s *law.*

Ochoa's law. See under law.

ochra·tox·ins (ō-kra-toks′ins). Mycotoxins produced by *Aspergillus ochraceus* during food spoilage.

ochro·der·mia (ō-krō-der′mē-ă). Yellow discoloration of the skin. [G. *ōchros,* pale yellow, + *derma,* skin]

ochrom·e·ter (ō-krom′ĕ-ter). An instrument for determining the capillary blood pressure; one of two adjacent fingers is compressed by a rubber balloon until blanching of the skin occurs, after which the force necessary to accomplish this color change is read in millimeters of mercury. [G. *ōchros,* pale yellow, + *metron,* measure]

ochro·no·sis (o-kron-ō′sis). A pathologic condition observed in certain persons with alkaptonuria, characterized by pigmentation of the cartilages and sometimes tissues such as muscle, epithelial cells, and dense connective tissue; may affect also the sclera, mucous membrane of the lips, and skin of the ears, face, and hands, and cause standing urine to be dark-colored and contain pigmented casts; pigmentation is thought to result from oxidized homogentisic acid, and cartilage degeneration results in osteoarthritis, particularly of the spine. [G. *ōchros,* pale yellow, + *nosos,* disease]

exogenous o., pigmentation of the skin of the face and elsewhere from prolonged topical exposure to hydroquinone-containing bleaching creams.

ochro·not·ic (ō-kron-ot′ik). Relating to or characterized by ochronosis.

Ochsner, Albert J., U.S. surgeon, 1858–1925. SEE O. *clamp;* O.'s *method.*

oc·ry·late (ok'ri-lāt). Octyl-2-cyanoacrylate; a tissue adhesive for surgery.

oct-, octi-, octo-, octa-. Eight. [G. *oktō*, L. *octo*]

OCTA (ok'ta). An eight-base pair sequence in DNA that has a regulatory role; for example, if it is artificially appended to a gene, it will cause that gene to be preferentially expressed in cells of the β-lymphocyte lineage.

oc·tac·o·san·o·ic ac·id (ok-tă-kō'săn-ō-ik). $CH_3–(CH_2)_{26}–$COOH; a long-chain fatty acid; found in waxes. SYN montanic acid.

oc·tad (ok'tad). **1.** SYN octavalent. **2.** An octavalent element or radical. [L. *octo*, eight]

oc·ta·meth·yl py·ro·phos·phor·a·mide (OMPA) (ok-tă-meth'il pī'rō-fos-fōr'ă-mīd). SYN schradan.

oc·ta·myl·a·mine (ok-tă-mil'ă-mēn). *N*-Isopentyl-1,5-dimethylhexylamine; an anticholinergic agent.

oc·tan (ok'tan). Applied to fever, the paroxysms of which recur every eighth day, the day of a paroxysm being counted as the first in the computation. [L. *octo*, eight]

oc·tan·di·o·ic ac·id. SYN suberic acid.

oc·ta·no·ate (ok'tă-nō-āt). SYN caprylate.

oc·ta·no·ic ac·id (ok'tă-nō-ik). SYN caprylic acid.

oc·ta·no·yl-CoA syn·the·tase (ok'tăn-ō-il sin-thē'tās). SYN butyrate-CoA ligase.

oc·ta·pep·tide (ok-tă-pep'tīd). A peptide made up of eight amino acid residues.

oc·ta·ploi·dy (ok'tă-ploy'dē). SEE polyploidy.

oc·ta·pres·sin (ok-tă-pres'in). SYN felypressin.

oc·ta·va·lent (ok'tă-vā'lent, ok-tav'ă-lent). Denoting a chemical element or radical having a combining power (valency) of eight. SYN octad (1).

oc·ta·vus (ok-tā'vŭs). SYN vestibulocochlear *nerve*. [L.]

octi-. SEE oct-.

octo-. SEE oct-.

Oc·to·mit·i·dae (ok-tō-mit'i-dē). A family in the protozoan class Zoomastigophorea; flagellates with six to eight flagella arranged in pairs and a body that is bilaterally symmetric; it includes the common human intestinal parasite *G. lamblia*. [octo- + G. *mitos*, thread]

Oc·tom·i·tus hom·i·nis (ok-tom'i-tŭs hom'i-nis). *Pentatrichomonas hominis*.

oc·to·pa·mine (ok-tō'pă-mēn). α-(aminomethyl)-*p*-hydroxybenzyl alcohol; a sympathomimetic amine; a false neurotransmitter produced by noradrenergic neurons in the presence of monoamine oxidase inhibitors. SYN norsympatol, norsynephrine.

oc·tose (ok'tōs). A sugar containing eight carbon atoms.

oc·tox·y·nol (ok-tok'si-nol). Polyethylene glycol mono[*p*-(1,1,3,3,-tetramethylbutyl)phenyl]ether; a surfactant.

oc·tu·lose (ok'tū-lōs). An eight-carbon monoketose.

oc·tu·lo·son·ic ac·id (ok'tū-lō-son'ik). The -onic acid formally formed by oxidation of carbon atom 1 of octulose to a carboxylic acid group; a condensation product of D-arabinose and phosphoenolpyruvate analogous to neuraminic acid. It forms part of the repeating unit of the polysaccharides of the complex lipopolysaccharides of the Enterobacteriaceae constituting the characteristic somatic octose antigens.

oc·tyl gal·late (ok'til gal'āt). Octyl 3,4,5-trihydroxybenzoate; an antioxidant.

oc·tyl·phe·noxy pol·y·eth·ox·y·eth·a·nol (ok'til-fe-nok'sē pol'ē-eth-ok'sē-eth'ă-nol). Mono-*p*-isooctyl phenyl ether of polyethylene glycol; a surface-active (wetting) agent.

oc·u·lar (ok'yū-lăr). **1.** SYN ophthalmic. **2.** The eyepiece of a microscope, the lens or lenses at the observer end of a microscope, by means of which the image focused by the objective is viewed. [L. *oculus*, eye]

compensating o., an o. that compensates and corrects for the effects of chromatic aberration in the objective.

Huygens' o., the compound o. of a microscope, composed of two planoconvex lenses so arranged that the plane side of each is directed toward the observer.

o. motor, relating to or causing movements of the eyeball.

Ramsden's o., an eyepiece of a microscope, consisting of two planoconvex lenses with convexities turned to each other.

wide field o., an o. that gives a larger than usual field of view and a high eyepoint.

oc·u·lar·ist (ok'yū-lăr-ist). One skilled in the design, fabrication, and fitting of artificial eyes and the making of prostheses associated with the appearance or function of the eyes. [L. *oculus*, eye]

o·cu·len·tum, pl. **o·cu·len·ta** (ok-yū-len'tŭm, -tă). SYN ophthalmic *ointment*. [Mod. L., fr. L. *oculus*, eye]

oc·u·li (ok'yū-lī). Plural of oculus. [L.]

oc·u·list (ok'yū-list). SYN ophthalmologist. [L. *oculus*, eye]

oculo-. The eye, ocular. SEE ALSO ophthalmo-. [L. *oculus*]

oc·u·lo·au·ric·u·lo·ver·te·bral (ok'yū-lō-aw-rik'yū-lō-ver'tĕ-brăl). Relating to the eyes, ears, and vertebrae.

oc·u·lo·car·di·ac (ok'yū-lō-kar'dē-ak). Relating to the eyes and heart.

oc·u·lo·cer·e·bro·re·nal (ok'yū-lō-ser'ē-brō-rē'năl). Relating to the eyes, brain, and kidneys.

oc·u·lo·cu·ta·ne·ous (ok'yū-lō-kyū-tā'nē-ŭs). Relating to the eyes and the skin.

oc·u·lo·den·to·dig·i·tal (ok'yū-lō-den'tō-dij'i-tăl). Relating to the eyes, teeth, and fingers.

oc·u·lo·der·mal (ok'yū-lō-der'măl). Relating to the eyes and skin.

oc·u·lo·dyn·ia. Pain in the eyeball. SYN ophthalmalgia. [ophthalmo- + G. *algos*, pain]

oc·u·lo·fa·cial (ok-yū-lō-fā'shăl). Relating to the eyes and the face.

oc·u·lo·g·ra·phy (ok-yū-log'ră-fē). A method of recording eye position and movements. [oculo- + G. *graphē*, a writing]

photosensor o., o. in which photocells are directed to the surface of the eye to record rotations.

oc·u·lo·gy·ria (ok'yū-lō-jī'rē-ă). The limits of rotation of the eyeballs. [oculo- + G. *gyros*, circle]

oc·u·lo·gy·ric (ok'yū-lō-jī'rik). Referring to rotation of the eyeballs; characterized by oculogyria.

oc·u·lo·man·dib·u·lo·dys·ceph·a·ly (ok'yū-lō-man-dib'yū-lō-dis-sef'ă-lē). SYN *dyscephalia* mandibulo-oculofacialis.

oc·u·lo·mo·tor (ok'yū-lō-mō'tŏr). Pertaining to the o. cranial nerve. [L. *oculomotorius*, fr. oculo- + L. *motorius*, moving]

o·cu·lo·mo·to·ri·us (ok'yū-lō-mō-tō'rē-ŭs). SYN oculomotor *nerve*. [L.]

oc·u·lo·na·sal (ok'yū-lō-nā'săl). Relating to the eyes and the nose. [oculo- + L. *nasus*, nose]

oc·u·lop·a·thy (ok-yū-lop'ă-thē). SYN ophthalmopathy.

oc·u·lo·pleth·ys·mog·ra·phy (ok'yū-lō-pleth-iz-mog'ră-fē). Indirect measurement of the hemodynamic significance of internal carotid artery stenosis or occlusion by demonstration of an ipsilateral delay in the arrival of ocular pressure transmitted from branches of the ophthalmic artery. [oculo- + G. *plēthymos*, increase, + *graphē*, to write]

oc·u·lo·pneu·mo·pleth·ys·mog·ra·phy (ok'yū-lō-nū'mō-pleth-iz-mog'ră-fē). A method of bilateral measurement of ophthalmic artery pressure that reflects pressure and flow in the internal carotid artery. SEE oculoplethysmography.

oc·u·lo·pu·pil·lary (ok'yū-lō-pū'pi-lăr-ē). Pertaining to the pupil of the eye.

oc·u·lo·sym·pa·thet·ic (ok'ū-lō-sim-pa-the'tik). Pertaining to the sympathetic pathway to the eye, damage to which produces Horner's *syndrome*.

oc·u·lo·ver·te·bral (ok'yū-lō-ver'tĕ-brăl). Relating to the eyes and vertebrae.

oc·u·lo·zy·go·mat·ic (ok'yū-lō-zī-gō-mat'ik). Relating to the orbit or its margin and the zygomatic bone.

oc·u·lus, gen. and pl. **oc·u·li** (ok'yū-lŭs, -lī) [NA]. SYN eye (1). [L.]

ocy-. SEE oxy-.

ocy·toc·in (ō-si-tō'sin). SYN oxytocin. [G. *okytokos*, fast birth, prompt delivery]

OD Abbreviation for overdose; optical *density* (see absorbance).

O.D. Abbreviation for L. *oculus dexter*, right eye. **2.** Abbreviation for Doctor of Optometry. SEE optometrist.

o.d. Abbreviation for L. *omni die*, every day.

od. A force assumed to be exerted upon the nervous system by magnets. [G. *hodos*, way]

odax·es·mus (ō′dak-sez′mŭs). A biting sensation; a form of paresthesia. [G. *odaxēsmos*, an irritation, fr. *odax* (adv.), by biting.]

odax·et·ic (ō′dak-set′ik). **1.** Causing formication or itching. **2.** A substance or agent that causes formication or itching. [G. *odaxēsmos*, an irritation]

Oddi, Ruggero, Italian physician; 1864–1913. SEE O.'s *sphincter*.

od·di·tis (od-ī′tis). Inflammation of the junction of the duodenum and common bile duct at the sphincter of Oddi.

odds. The ratio of probability of occurrence to non-occurrence of an event. [pl. of *odd*, fr. M.E. *odde*, fr. O.Norse *oddi*, odd number]

△-odes. Having the form of, resembling. [G. *eidos*, form, resemblance]

Odland body. See under body.

odo·gen·e·sis (ō-dō-jen′ĕ-sis). SYN neurocladism. [G. *hodos*, path, + *genesis*, source]

△odont-, odonto-. A tooth, teeth (properly used in words formed from G. roots). [G. *odous* (*odont-*)]

odon·tag·ra (ō-don-tag′ră). Obsolescent term for toothache thought to be of gouty origin. [odonto- + G. *agra*, seizure]

odon·tal·gia (ō-don-tal′jē-ă). SYN toothache. [odont- + G. *algos*, pain]

o. denta′lis, reflex pain in the ear due to dental disease, usually propagated along the auriculotemporal nerve.

odon·tal·gic (ō-don-tal′jik). Relating to or marked by toothache.

odon·tec·to·my (ō-don-tek′tō-mē). Removal of teeth by the reflection of a mucoperiosteal flap and excision of bone from around the root or roots before the application of force to effect the tooth removal. [odont- + G. *ektomē*, excision]

odon·ter·ism (ō-don′ter-izm). Chattering of the teeth. [odont- + G. *erismos*, quarrel]

odon·ti·a·sis (ō-don-tī′ă-sis). SYN teething.

odon·ti·noid (ō-don′ti-noyd). **1.** Resembling dentin. **2.** A small excrescence from a tooth, most common on the root or neck. **3.** Toothlike.

odon·ti·tis (ō-don-tī′tis). SYN pulpitis.

△odonto-. SEE odont-.

odon·to·am·e·lo·blas·to·ma (ō-don′tō-am′ĕ-lō-blas-tō′mă). SYN ameloblastic *odontoma*.

odon·to·blast (ō-don′tō-blast). One of the dentin-forming cells, derived from mesenchyme of neural crest origin, lining the pulp cavity of a tooth; o.'s are arranged in a peripheral layer in the dental pulp, forming the dentinal matrix, with odontoblastic processes extending from each cell into a dentinal tubule; the cells generally are columnar in the coronal pulp but are more cuboidal in the radicular area and adjacent to tertiary dentin. [odonto- + G. *blastos*, sprout, germ]

odon·to·blas·to·ma (ō-don′tō-blas-tō′mă). **1.** A tumor composed of neoplastic epithelial and mesenchymal cells that may differentiate into cells able to produce calcified tooth substances. **2.** An odontoma in its early formative stage. [odontoblast + G. *-oma*, tumor]

odon·to·clast (ō-don′tō-klast). One of the cells believed to produce resorption of the roots of the deciduous teeth. [odonto- + G. *klastos*, broken]

odon·to·dyn·ia (ō-don-tō-din′ē-ă). SYN toothache. [odonto- + G. *odynē*, pain]

odon·to·dys·pla·sia (ō-don′tō-dis-plā′zē-ă). A developmental disturbance of one or of several adjacent teeth, of unknown etiology, characterized by deficient formation of enamel and dentin which results in an abnormally large pulp chamber and imparts a ghostlike radiographic image to the teeth; such teeth exhibit delayed eruption into the oral cavity. SYN odontogenesis imperfecta, odontogenic dysplasia.

odon·to·gen·e·sis (ō-don-tō-jen′ĕ-sis). The process of development of the teeth. SYN odontogeny, odontosis. [odonto- + G. *genesis*, production]

o. imperfec′ta, SYN odontodysplasia.

odon·tog·e·ny (ō-don-toj′ĕ-nē). SYN odontogenesis.

odon·toid (ō-don′toyd). **1.** Shaped like a tooth. SYN dentoid. **2.** Relating to the toothlike o. process of the second cervical vertebra. [odont- + G. *eidos*, resemblance]

odon·tol·o·gy (ō-don-tol′ŏ-jē). SYN dentistry. [odonto- + G. *logos*, study]

forensic o., SYN forensic *dentistry*.

odon·to·lox·ia, odon·to·loxy (ō-don-tō-lok′sē-ă, ō-don-tol′ok-sē). SYN odontoparallaxis. [odonto- + G. *loxos*, slanting]

odon·tol·y·sis (ō-don-tol′i-sis). SYN erosion (3). [odonto- + G. *lysis*, dissolution]

odon·to·ma (ō-don-tō′mă). **1.** A tumor of odontogenic origin. **2.** A hamartomatous odontogenic tumor comprised of enamel, dentin, cementum, and pulp tissue that may or may not be arranged in the form of a tooth. [odonto- + G. *-oma*, tumor]

ameloblastic o., a benign mixed odontogenic tumor comprised of an undifferentiated component histologically identical to an ameloblastoma and a well differentiated component identical to an odontoma; appears as a mixed radiolucent-radiopaque lesion and presents clinically as an ameloblastoma. SYN odontoameloblastoma.

complex o., an o. in which the various odontogenic tissues are organized in a haphazard arrangement with no resemblance to teeth.

compound o., an o. in which the odontogenic tissues are organized and resemble anomalous teeth.

odon·to·neu·ral·gia (ō-don′tō-nū-ral′jē-ă). Facial neuralgia caused by a carious tooth.

odon·ton·o·my (ō-don-ton′ō-mē). Dental nomenclature. [odonto- + G. *onoma*, name]

odon·to·no·sol·o·gy (ō-don′tō-nō-sol′ŏ-jē). SYN dentistry. [odonto- + G. *nosos*, disease, + *logos*, study]

odon·to·par·al·lax·is (ō-don′tō-par-ă-lak′sis). Irregularity of the teeth. SYN odontoloxia, odontoloxy. [odonto- + G. *parallax*, alternately]

odon·top·a·thy (ō-don-top′ă-thē). Any disease of the teeth or of their sockets. [odonto- + G. *pathos*, suffering]

odon·to·pho·bia (ō-don-tō-fō′bē-ă). Morbid fear of teeth. [odonto- + G. *phobos*, fear]

odon·to·plas·ty (ō-don′tō-plas-tē). Surgical contouring of tooth surface to enhance plaque control and gingival morphology. [odonto- + G. *plassō*, to mold]

odon·top·ri·sis (ō-don-top′ri-sis). Grinding together of the teeth. SEE ALSO bruxism. [odonto- + G. *prisis*, a sawing, a grinding]

odon·top·to·sis (ō-don-top-tō′sis, -tō-tō′sis). Downward movement of an upper tooth due to the loss of its lower antagonist(s). SEE ALSO supereruption. [odonto- + G. *ptōsis*, a falling]

odon·tor·rha·gia (ō-don-tō-rā′jē-ă). Profuse bleeding from the socket after the extraction of a tooth. [odonto- + G. *rhēgnymi*, to burst forth]

odon·to·schism (ō-don′tō-skizm, -sizm). Fissure of a tooth. [odonto- + G. *schisma*, a cleft]

odon·to·scope (ō-don′tō-skōp). An optical device, similar to a closed circuit television system, that projects a view of the oral cavity onto a screen for multiple viewing.

odon·tos·co·py (ō-don-tos′kŏ-pē). **1.** Examination of the oral cavity by means of the odontoscope. **2.** Examination of the markings in prints of the cutting edges of the teeth; used, like fingerprints, as a method of personal identification. [odonto- + G. *skopeō*, to view]

odon·to·sis (ō-don-tō′sis). SYN odontogenesis.

odon·to·ther·a·py (ō-don-tō-thar′ă-pē). Treatment of diseases of the teeth.

odon·tot·o·my (ō-don-tot′ō-mē). Cutting into the crown of a tooth. [odonto- + G. *tomē*, incision]

od

prophylactic o., a preventive operation in which imperfectly formed developmental grooves, pits, and fissures are opened up by means of a bur and filled in order to obviate future decay.

odor (ō'dŏr). Emanation from any substance that stimulates the olfactory cells in the organ of smell. SYN scent, smell (3). [L.]

odor·ant (ō'dŏr-ant). A substance with an odor.

odor·a·tism (ō-dŏr'ă-tizm). SEE lathyrism, osteolathyrism. [fr. *Lathyrus odoratus,* sweet pea]

odor·if·er·ous (ō-dŏ-rif'er-ŭs). Having a scent, perfume, or odor. SYN odorous. [odor + L. *fero,* to bear]

odor·im·e·ter (ō'dŏ-rim'ĕ-ter). Instrument for performing odorimetry.

odo·rim·e·try (ō'dŏ-rim'ĕ-trē). The determination of the comparative power of different substances in exciting olfactory sensations. [odor + G. *metron,* measure]

odor·i·vec·tion (ō'dŏr-i-vek'shŭn). Conveying or bearing an odor, as on the air. [odor + L. *vector,* a carrier]

odor·og·ra·phy (ō'dŏ-rog'ră-fē). Description of odors. [odor + G. *graphē,* a description]

odor·ous (ō'dŏr-ŭs). SYN odoriferous.

O'Dwyer, Joseph P., U.S. physician, 1841–1898. SEE O'D.'s *tube.*

△ **odyn-, odyno-.** Pain. [G. *odynē*]

odyn·a·cu·sis (ō-din'ă-kū'sis). Hypersensitiveness of the organ of hearing, so that noises cause actual pain. [odyn- + G. *akouō,* to hear]

ody·nom·e·ter (ō-di-nom'ĕ-ter). SYN algesiometer. [odyno- + G. *metron,* measure]

odyn·o·pha·gia (ō-din-ō-fā'jē-ă). Pain on swallowing. [odyno- + G. *phagō* to eat]

odyn·o·pho·nia (ō-din-ō-fō'nē-ă). Pain on using the voice. [odyno- + G. *phonē,* sound, voice]

Oe Symbol for oersted.

△ **oe-.** For words so beginning and not found here, see e-.

oe·di·pism (ed'i-pizm). **1.** Self-infliction of injury to the eyes, usually an attempt at evulsion. **2.** Manifestation of the Oedipus complex. [*Oedipus,* G. myth. char.]

Oehl, Eusebio, Italian anatomist, 1827–1903. SEE O.'s *muscles,* under *muscle.*

Oehler, Johannes, German physician, *1879. SEE O.'s *symptom.*

oe·nan·thal (ē-nan'thăl). SYN heptanal.

oer·sted (Oe) (er'sted). A unit of magnetic field intensity; the magnetic field intensity that exerts a force of 1 dyne on unit magnetic pole; equal to $(1000/4\pi)$ A·m^{-1}. [Hans-Christian *Oersted* Danish physicist, 1777–1851]

oe·soph·a·go·sto·mi·a·sis (ē-sof'ă-gō-stō-mī'ă-sis). Infection with nematode parasites of the genus *Oesophagostomum.* SYN esophagostomiasis. [G. *oi-sophagos,* gullet (esophagus), + *stoma,* mouth, + *-iasis,* condition]

Oe·soph·a·gos·to·mum (ē-sof-ă-gos'tō-mŭm). A genus of strongyle nematodes (subfamily Oesophagostominae) that encyst in the intestinal wall of herbivores and primates, causing nodular disease. Larvae appear to stimulate a host reaction in the intestinal wall, forming nodules in which the worms complete their development (unless the host is immune); they then leave the nodule and feed as adults in the lumen of the large intestine. [G. *oisophagos,* gullet (esophagus), + *stoma,* mouth]

O. apios'tomum, a primate species that has been reported in northern Nigeria and central Africa to encyst under the submucosa of the human intestine and occasionally cause dysentery; a common parasite of monkeys and apes, both in captivity and in the wild.

O. brevicau'dum, a species that occurs in the cecum and colon of pigs in North America and India.

O. brump'ti, a species described from African monkeys and reported occasionally in humans.

O. columbia'num, a species that occurs in sheep, goats, and wild African antelopes; except when present in large numbers, it does not appear to seriously affect the health of the host.

O. denta'tum, a species that affects the colon of swine; the lesions are similar to those in sheep.

O. georgia'num, a species that occurs in the cecum and colon of pigs in the U.S.

O. quadrispinula'tum, a species that occurs in the cecum and colon of pigs in the Americas, Europe, and Southeast Asia.

O. radia'tum, a species that occurs worldwide in cattle and water buffalo; the lesions are similar to those of sheep.

O. stephanos'tomum, a species occurring in chimpanzees, monkeys, and gorillas in Africa, but also reported from humans and monkeys in Brazil.

O. venulo'sum, a species that occurs worldwide in the cecum and colon of cattle, sheep, goats, deer, and many other ruminants.

oest·ra·di·ol (es-tră-dī'ol). SYN estradiol.

oest·rids (est'ridz). Common name for botflies of the family Oestridae, such as *Oestrus.* [G. *oistros,* gadfly]

oes·tri·ol (es'trē-ol). SYN estriol.

oest·ro·gen (es'trō-jen). SYN estrogen.

oest·rone (es'trōn). SYN estrone.

oes·tro·sis (es-trō'sis). Infection of small ruminants and rarely humans with larvae of the fly *Oestrus ovis.*

Oes·trus (es'tŭs). A genus of tissue-invading flies that cause myiasis in sheep; the head botflies in the family Oestridae. *O. ovis* (a nose fly) is a grayish brown, robust, hairy, beelike botfly, imported from Europe, and now a serious pest in parts of the U.S.; larvae are deposited by the adult fly in the nostrils of sheep, and inch-long larvae develop in the paranasal sinuses, causing considerable mucous discharge and distress in old or weak sheep. [G. *oistros,* gadfly]

of·fi·cial (ŏ-fish'ăl). Authoritative; denoting a drug or a chemical or pharmaceutical preparation recognized as standard in the pharmacopeia. Cf. officinal. [L. *officialis,* fr. *officium,* a favor, service, fr. *opus,* work, + *facio,* to do]

of·fic·i·nal (ŏ-fis'i-năl). Denoting a chemical or pharmaceutical preparation kept in stock, in contrast to magistral (prepared extemporaneously according to a physician's prescription); an o. preparation is often, though not necessarily, official. [L. *officina,* shop]

Ogino, Kyusaka, 20th century Japanese physician. SEE O.-Knaus *rule.*

Ogston, Sir Alexander, Scottish surgeon, 1844–1929. SEE O.'s *line;* O.-Luc *operation.*

Oguchi, Chita, Japanese ophthalmologist, 1875–1945. SEE O.'s *disease.*

Ogura, Joseph H., U.S. otolaryngologist, *1915. SEE O. *operation.*

O'Hara, Michael, Jr., U.S. surgeon, 1869–1926. SEE O'H. *forceps.*

OHI Abbreviation for Oral Hygiene Index.

OHI-S Abbreviation for Simplified Oral Hygiene Index.

Ohm (Ω), Georg S., German physicist, 1787–1854. SEE ohm; O.'s *law.*

ohm (ōm). The practical unit of electrical resistance; the resistance of any conductor allowing 1 ampere of current to pass under the electromotive force of 1 volt. [G.S. *Ohm*]

ohm·am·me·ter (ōm-am'ĕ-ter). A combined ohmmeter and ammeter.

ohm·me·ter (ōm'ĕ-ter). An instrument for determining the resistance, in ohms, of a conductor.

oh·ne Hauch (ō'nă howch). Term used to designate the nonspreading growth of nonflagellated bacteria on agar media; also applied to somatic agglutination. SEE ALSO O *antigen.* [Ger. without breath]

Ohngren's line. See under line.

△ **oi-.** For words so beginning and not found here, see e-.

△ **-oid.** Resemblance to, joined properly to words formed from G. roots; equivalent to Eng. -form. [G. *eidos,* form, resemblance]

oid·ia (ō-id'ēă). Plural of oidium.

oid·i·o·my·cin (ō-id'ē-ō-mī'sin). An antigen used to demonstrate cutaneous hypersensitivity in patients infected with one of the Candida species; one of a series of antigens used to demonstrate an immunocompromised patient's capacity to react to any cutaneous antigen. [oidium + G. *mykēs,* fungus, + -in]

oid·i·um, pl. **oid·ia** (ō-id′ē-ŭm, ō-id′ē-ă). Formerly used term for arthroconidium. [Mod. L. dim. of G. *ōon,* egg]

oil (oyl). An inflammable liquid, of fatty consistence and unctuous feel, that is insoluble in water, soluble or insoluble in alcohol, and freely soluble in ether. O.'s are variously classified as animal, vegetable, and mineral o.'s according to their source (the mineral o.'s probably being of remote animal and vegetable origin); into fatty (fixed) and volatile o.'s; and into drying and nondrying (fatty) o.'s, the former becoming gradually thicker when exposed to the air and finally drying to a varnish, the latter not drying but liable to become rancid on exposure. Many of the o.'s, both fixed and volatile, are used in medicine. For individual o.'s, see the specific names. [L. *oleum;* G. *elaion,* originally olive oil]

absolute o.'s, essential o.'s that are obtained by the removal of insoluble compounds from concrete oils.

o. of anise, volatile o. derived from the dried ripe fruit of *Pimpinella anisum* (family Umbelliferae) or of *Illicium verum,* (family Magnoliaceae) (Chinese star anise); has a characteristic anise aroma, resembling fennel. Used in manufacture of liqueurs, and as flavoring for candies, cookies, dentifrices. Pharmaceutical aid (flavor). Carminative.

o. of bay, volatile o. derived by steam distillation of the dried leaves of *Pimenta (Myrcia) acris* (family Myrtaceae); o. of myrcia; used as an aromatic in the manufacture of bay rum and as a pharmaceutical aid.

o. of bergamot, volatile o. derived by steam distillation from the rind of the fresh fruit of *Citrus aurantium* or *C. bergamia;* contains *l*-linalyl acetate, *l*-linalool; *d*-limonene, dipentene, bergaptene; used as a deodorant in preparations containing malodorous ingredients and as an aromatic in perfumes, hairdressings, and pomades.

betula oil (bet′yū-lă), oil of sweet birch, a volatile oil obtained by distillation from the bark of *Betula lenta* (sweet birch); used as a flavoring agent and as a counterirritant liniment. SEE ALSO *methyl* salicylate.

o. of bitter almond, volatile o. from the dried ripe kernels of bitter almonds or from other kernels containing amygdalin, such as apricots, peaches, plums and cherries; obtained by steam distillation subsequent to maceration of the source with water. Formerly used as an antipruritic; poisonous—releases hydrocyanic acid (hydrogen cyanide). Only the oil free of hydrogen cyanide may be used to flavor liquors and foods.

o. of bitter orange, volatile o. obtained by steam distillation from the fresh peel of *Citrus aurantium* (family Rutaceae). Aromatic material used as a flavoring agent in pharmaceuticals and foods and liquors; also used in perfumes.

o. of cardamom, volatile o. obtained by steam distillation from the seeds of *Elettaria cardamomum* (family Zingiberacea.) A flavoring agent in pharmaceuticals (syrups), liquors, sauces, confections and baked goods; formerly used as a carminative.

o. of chenopodium, volatile o. from the fresh above ground part of the flower, American wormseed, *Chenopodium ambrosioides,* or *C. anthelminticum.* Used as an anthelmintic. SYN oil of American o.

o. of cherry laurel, volatile o. derived by steam distillation from *Prunus laurocerasus* (family Rosaceae); similar to o. of bitter almond; highly toxic due to hydrogen cyanide content.

o. of cinnamon, volatile o. obtained by steam distillation from the leaves and twigs of *Cinnamomum cassia* (family Lauracea). A flavor in foods and perfumes.

o. of citronella, volatile o. obtained by steam distillation of fresh lemon grass. Contains citranellol; used as an insect repellent either on the skin or in the form of incense; also used as a perfume.

o. of clove, volatile o. obtained by steam distillation of the dried flower buds of *Eugenia caryophyllata* (family Myrtacea). Contains about 85% eugenol along with other constituents. Used in dentistry as a local anesthetic and component of temporary fillings of the teeth. Also used to flavor foods; strong, pungent odor. SYN clove oil.

concrete o.'s, essential o.'s obtained by extraction with organic solvents; contain waxes and paraffins.

o. of coriander, volatile o. from the dried ripe fruit of *Coriandrum sativum* (family Umbelliferae). Flavoring in foods and alcoholic beverages.

o. of cubeb, volatile o. of the unripe fruit of *Piper cubeba* (family Piperaceae). Formerly used as a urinary antiseptic.

o. of dwarf pine needles, volatile o. from the fresh leaves of *Pinus montana* (family Pinaceae). Pleasant pine odor; used as a pharmaceutical aid (flavor and perfume). Has been used as an expectorant.

essential o.'s, plant products, usually somewhat volatile, giving the odors and tastes characteristic of the particular plant, thus possessing the essence, *e.g.,* citral, pinene, camphor, menthane, terpenes; usually, the steam distillates of plants or oils of plants obtained by pressing out the rinds of a particular plant. SEE ALSO volatile o.

ethereal o., SYN volatile o.

o. of eucalyptus, volatile o. from the fresh leaves of *Eucalyptus globulus* (family Myrtaceae) and some other species of *Eucalyptus;* native to Australia; pungent o. with a spicy, cooling taste. Has been used as an aromatic in inhalants, as an expectorant, anthelmintic, and local antiseptic.

fatty o., an o. derived from both animals and plants; chemically, a glyceride of a fatty acid which, by substitution of the glycerine by an alkaline base, is converted into a soap; a fatty o., in contrast to a volatile o., is permanent, leaving a stain on an absorbent surface, and thus is not capable of distillation; it is obtained by expression or extraction; the consistency varies with the temperature, some being liquid (o.'s proper), others semisolid (fats), and others solid (tallows) at ordinary temperatures; both liquid and semisolid o.'s are congealed by cold and the solids are liquified by heat. SYN fixed o.

o. of fennel, volatile o. from the dried fruit of *Foeniculum vulgare* (family Umbelliferae). An aromatic o. with the odor and taste of fennel, similar to anise; used as a flavoring agent in pharmaceuticals. Has been used as a carminative.

fixed o., SYN fatty o.

fusel o., a mixture of side products of alcoholic fermentation; consists primarily of alcohols (*e.g.,* amyl, propyl, isoamyl, and isobutyl alcohols).

joint o., SYN synovial *fluid.*

jojoba o., a liquid wax ester mixture extracted from ground or crushed seeds from *Simmondsia chinensis* and *S. californica* (family Buxaceae), desert shrubs native to Arizona, California, and northern Mexico. Used extensively in cosmetics for alleged skin softening and lubricating properties; other uses include as lubricant, fuel, chemical feedstock, substitute for sperm whale oil. SYN oil of jojoba.

o. of juniper, volatile o. from the dried ripe fruit (berries) of *Juniperus communis* (family Cupressaceae). Formerly used as a diuretic. Used in perfumery. SYN juniper berry oil.

o. of lavender, volatile o. from fresh flowering tops of *Lavandula officinalis* (family Labiatae). Aromatic o. used in perfume and as a flavoring agent. Has been used as a carminative.

o. of lemon, volatile o. expressed from fresh peel of *Citrus limonum* (family Rutaceae). Aromatic o. used for flavoring pharmaceuticals, liqueurs, pastry, foods, beverages, and in perfumes.

△ Combining forms	[NA] Nomina Anatomica
Word*Finder*	**[MIM] Mendelian**
Multi-term entry finder	**Inheritance in Man**
Preceding letter A	
A.D.A.M. Anatomy Plates	☆ **Official alternate term**
Between letters L and M	
Appendices:	☆[NA] **Official alternate**
Following letter Z	**Nomina Anatomica term**
SYN Synonym; Cf., compare	**High Profile Term**

o. of lemon grass, volatile o. from *Cymbopogon citratus* and of *C. flexuosus* (family Gramineae). Used in perfumery and as a source of citral for the synthesis of vitamin A.

oil of American o., SYN o. of chenopodium.

oil of crispmint, SYN o. of spearmint.

oil of curled mint, SYN o. of spearmint.

oil of jojoba, SYN jojoba o.

palm o., an o. obtained from the seeds of *Elaeis guineensis* (family Palmae); used in the manufacture of soap, liniments, and ointments; also in foods.

o. of pennyroyal, either American or European. The former is a volatile o. derived from the flowering tops and leaves of *Hedeoma pulegioides* (family Labiatae). Contains pulegone and ketones. European is o. of pulegium; a volatile o. from *Mentha pulegium* (family Labiatae); about 85% pulegone. Has been used as an aromatic carminative, abortifacient and insect repellent.

o. of peppermint, a volatile o. containing menthol (not less than 50% of total) obtained by steam distillation from the fresh flowering plant *Mentha piperita* (family Labiatae). Used as a pharmaceutical aid (flavor) and in flavoring liqueurs; a carminative.

o. of rose, a volatile o. from the fresh flowers of *Rosa gallica* and *R. damascena* and other members of the Rosaceae family. Used largely in perfumery; ointments, and toilet preparations. SYN attar of rose, essence of rose, otto of rose.

o. of spearmint, volatile o. from the flowering tops of *Mentha spicata* (family Labiatae, pharmaceutical aid (flavor) and a carminative. SYN oil of crispmint, oil of curled mint.

sweet birch o., SYN *methyl* salicylate.

o. of turpentine, volatile o. distilled from the oleoresin and obtained from *Pinus palastris* (family Pinaceae) and other species of *Pinus* yielding terpene oils. Solvent for o.'s, resins, varnishes; vehicle, thinner and remover of o.-based paints. Rubefacient; has been used as a counterirritant in liniments.

volatile o., a substance of oily consistency and feel, derived from a plant and containing the principles to which the odor and taste of the plant are due (essential o.); in contrast to a fatty o., a volatile o. evaporates when exposed to the air and thus is capable of distillation; it may also be obtained by expression or extraction; many volatile o.'s, identical to or closely resembling the natural o.'s, can be made synthetically. Volatile o.'s are used in medicine as stimulants, stomachics, correctives, carminatives, and for purposes of flavoring (*e.g.*, peppermint oil). SYN ethereal o.

o. of wormwood, volatile o. from leaves and tops of *Artemisia absinthium* (family Compositae). Thujol alcohol and acetate; thujone (a powerful convulsant), phellandrene, cadinene; also a blue o. Used in flavoring of vermouth; formerly in absinthe.

oil red O [C.I. 26125]. 1-8-[4-(Dimethylphenylazo)-dimethylphenylazo]-2-naphthalenol; a weakly acid diazo oil-soluble dye, used in histologic demonstration of neutral fats.

oil of vit·ri·ol. SYN sulfuric acid.

oint·ment (oynt′ment). A semisolid preparation usually containing medicinal substances and intended for external application. O. bases used as vehicles fall into four general classes: 1) Hydrocarbon bases (oleaginous o. bases) keep medicaments in prolonged contact with the skin, act as occlusive dressings, and are used chiefly for emollient effects. 2) Absorption bases either permit the incorporation of aqueous solutions with the formation of a water-in-oil emulsion or are water-in-oil emulsions that permit the incorporation of additional quantities of aqueous solutions; such bases permit better absorption of some medicaments and are useful as emollients. 3) Water-removable bases (creams) are oil-in-water emulsions containing petrolatum, anhydrous lanolin, or waxes; they may be washed from the skin with water, and are thus more acceptable for cosmetic reasons; they favor absorption of serous discharges in dermatological conditions. 4) Water-soluble bases (greaseless ointment bases) contain only water-soluble substances. SEE ALSO cerate. SYN salve, uncture, unguent. [O. Fr. *oignement*; L. *unguo*, pp. *unctus*, to smear]

blue o., a grease-based o. containing 20% finely divided metallic mercury, formerly widely used for local application to the skin for the destruction of body lice. Risk is associated with trans-

dermal absorption of mercury and a local dermatitis. SYN mild mercurial ointment.

eye o., SYN ophthalmic o.

hydrophilic o., an o. base consisting of 25% each of white petrolatum and stearyl alcohol, 12% propyl glycol emulsified in 37% water by 1% of lauryl sulfate; preserved with paraben. Suitable for the incorporation of numerous drugs intended for local application; a washable o. base.

mild mercurial ointment, SYN blue o.

ophthalmic o., a special o. for application to the eye that must be free from particles and must be nonirritating to the eye. SYN eye o., oculentum.

Okazaki, Reiji and Tuneko, 20th century Japanese biochemists. SEE O. *fragment.*

⚠️**-ol.** Suffix denoting that a substance is an alcohol or a phenol.

ol·a·mine (ōl′ă-mēn). USAN-approved contraction for ethanolamine.

o·le·ag·i·nous (ō-lē-aj′i-nŭs). Oily or greasy. [L. *oleagineus,* pertaining to *olea,* the olive tree]

ole·an·der (ō-lē-an′der). The bark and leaves of *Nerium oleander* (family Apocynaceae), a shrub of the eastern Mediterranean; formerly used as a diuretic and heart tonic.

ole·an·do·my·cin phos·phate (ō-lē-an-dō-mī′sin). An antibiotic substance produced by species of *Streptomyces antibioticus;* effective against staphylococci, streptococci, pneumococci, and some Gram-negative bacteria.

ole·ate (ō′lē-āt). 1. A salt of oleic acid. 2. A pharmacopeial preparation consisting of a combination or solution of an alkaloid or metallic base in oleic acid, used as an inunction.

olec·ra·non (ō-lek′ră-non, ō′lē-krā′non) [NA]. The prominent curved proximal extremity of the ulna, the upper and posterior surface of which gives attachment to the tendon of the triceps muscle, the anterior surface entering into the formation of the trochlear notch. SYN elbow bone, olecranon process, point of elbow, tip of elbow. [G. the head or point of the elbow, fr. *ōlenē,* ulna, + *kranion,* skull, head]

ole·fin (ō′lĕ-fin). SYN alkene.

ole·ic ac·id (ō-lē′ik). *cis*-9-Octadecenoic acid; an unsaturated fatty acid that is the most widely distributed and abundant fatty acid in nature; used commercially in the preparation of oleates and lotions, and as a pharmaceutical solvent. Cf. elaidic acid. [L. *oleum,* oil]

ole·in (ō′lē-in). trioleoyl glycerol; glyceryl trioleate; a triacylglycerol, solely containing oleoyl moieties, found in fats and oils. SYN triolein.

⚠️**oleo-.** Oil. SEE ALSO eleo-. [L. *oleum*]

ole·o·go·men·ol (ō′lē-ō-gō′men-ol). SYN gomenol.

ole·o·gran·u·lo·ma (ō′lē-ō-gran-yū-lō′mă). SYN lipogranuloma.

ole·o·ma (ō-lē-ō′mă). SYN lipogranuloma.

ole·om·e·ter (ō-lē-om′ĕ-ter). An instrument, similar to a hydrometer, for determining the specific gravity of oils. SYN eleometer. [oleo- + G. *metron,* measure]

ole·o·pal·mi·tate (ō′lē-ō-pal′mi-tāt). A double salt of oleic and palmitic acids.

ole·o·res·in (ō′lē-ō-rez′in). 1. A compound of an essential oil and resin, present in certain plants. 2. A pharmaceutical preparation. SEE aspidium, capsicum, ginger. 3. SYN balsam.

ole·o·sac·cha·rum, pl. **ole·o·sac·cha·ra** (ō′lē-ō-sak′ă-rŭm). A class of preparations made by the trituration of a volatile oil (anise, fennel, lemon, etc.) with sugar; used as a diluent or corrigent of powerful or bad tasting drugs in powder form. SYN oil sugar. [oleo- + G. *saccharon,* sugar]

ole·o·ste·a·rate (ō′lē-ō-stē′ă-rāt). A double salt of oleic and stearic acids.

ole·o·sus (ō-lē-ō′sŭs). Greasy; relating to abnormality of the sebaceous apparatus. [L., fr. *oleum,* oil]

ole·o·ther·a·py (ō′lē-ō-thār′ă-pē). Treatment of disease by an oil given internally or applied externally. SYN eleotherapy. [oleo- + G. *therapeia,* therapy]

ole·o·vi·ta·min (ō′lē-ō-vī′tă-min). A solution of a vitamin in an edible oil.

o. A and D, a solution of vitamins A and D in fish liver oil or in an edible vegetable oil.

ole·um ter·e·bin·thin·ae (ō′lē-um ter-ē-ben′thin-ī). SYN turpentine oil.

ole·yl al·co·hol (ō-lē′il). A mixture of aliphatic alcohols consisting chiefly of $CH_3(CH_2)_7CH=CH(CH_2)_7CH_2OH$; used as an emulsifying aid and in the preparation of cold cream; found in fish oils.

ole·yl-CoA (ō-lē-il). A product of the Δ^9-desaturase enzyme system in the biosynthesis of monounsaturated fatty acids. SYN oleyl-coenzyme A.

ole·yl-co·en·zyme A. SYN oleyl-CoA.

ol·fac·tie, ol·fac·ty (ol-fak′tē). The unit of smell; the threshold of olfactory stimulation, or the point where the smell is just received in the olfactometer. SYN olfacty. [see olfaction]

ol·fac·tion (ol-fak′shŭn). **1.** The sense of smell. SYN smell (2). **2.** The act of smelling. SYN osmesis, osphresis. [L. *ol- facio,* pp. *-factus,* to smell]

ol·fac·tol·o·gy (ol′fak-tol′-ō-jē). Study of the sense of smell. [olfaction + G. *logos,* study]

ol·fac·tom·e·ter (ol′fak-tom′ĕ-ter). A device for estimating the keenness of the sense of smell. [L. *olfactus,* smell, + G. *metron,* measure]

ol·fac·tom·e·try (ol′fak-tom′ĕ-trē). Determination of the degree of sensibility of the olfactory organ.

ol·fac·to·pho·bia (ol-fak-tō-fō′bē-ă). Morbid fear of odors. SYN osmophobia, osphresiophobia. [L. *olfactus,* smell, + G. *phobos,* fear]

ol·fac·to·ry (ol-fak′tŏ-rē). Relating to the sense of smell. SYN osmatic, osphretic. [see olfaction]

ol·fac·ty (ol-fak′tē). SYN olfactie.

olib·a·num (ō-lib′ă-nŭm). A gum resin from several trees of the genus *Boswellia* (family Burseraceae); has been used as a stimulant expectorant in bronchitis, for fumigations, and as incense. SYN frankincense, thus. [Ar. *al,* the, + *lubān,* frankincense]

olig-. SEE oligo-.

ol·i·gam·ni·os (ol-i-gam′nē-os). SYN oligohydramnios.

ol·i·ge·mia (ol-i-gē′mē-ă). A deficiency in the amount of blood in the body or any organ or tissue. [oligo- + G. *haima,* blood]

ol·i·ge·mic (ol-i-gē′mik). Pertaining to or characterized by oligemia.

ol·ig·he·mia (ol-ig-hē′mē-ă). Obsolete term for oligemia.

ol·ig·hid·ria, ol·ig·id·ria (ol-ig-hid′rē-ă, -id′rē-ă). Scanty perspiration. [oligo- + G. *hidrōs,* sweat]

oligo-, olig-. **1.** A few, a little; too little, too few. **2.** In chemistry, used in contrast to "poly-" in describing polymers; *e.g.,* oligosaccharide. [G. *oligos,* few]

ol·i·go·am·ni·os (ol′i-gō-am′nē-os). SYN oligohydramnios. [oligo- + amnion]

ol·i·go·cho·lia (ol′i-gō-kō′lē-ă). A deficient secretion of bile. [oligo- + G. *cholē,* bile]

ol·i·go·chy·li·a (ol′i-gō-kī′lē-ă). A deficiency of gastric juice. [oligo- + G. *chylos,* juice]

ol·i·go·chy·mia (ol′i-gō-kī′mē-ă). A deficiency of chyme. [oligo- + G. *chymos,* juice]

ol·i·go·cys·tic (ol′i-gō-sis′tik). Consisting of only a few cysts, as occasionally observed in certain examples of hydatidiform mole and other lesions that ordinarily have numerous cysts. [oligo- + G. *kystis,* bladder, cyst]

ol·i·go·dac·ty·ly, ol·i·go·dac·tyl·ia (ol′i-gō-dak′ti-lē, -dak′til′ē-ă). Presence of fewer than five digits on one or more limbs. [oligo- + G. *daktylos,* finger or toe]

ol·i·go·den·dria (ol′i-gō-den′drē-ă). SYN oligodendroglia.

ol·i·go·den·dro·blast (ol′i-gō-den′drō-blast). A primitive glial cell that is the normal precursor cell of the oligodendrocyte.

ol·i·go·den·dro·blas·to·ma (ol′i-gō-den′drō-blas-tō′mă). Obsolete term for oligodendroglioma. [oligo- + G. *dendron,* tree, + *blastos,* germ, + -oma]

ol·i·go·den·dro·cyte (ol′i-gō-den′drō-sīt). A cell of the oligodendroglia.

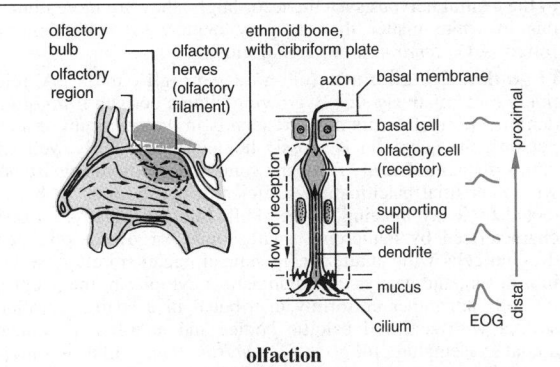

olfaction

left, nose-throat area, sagittal view, with olfactory region and air flow; *right,* olfactory cell in mucous membrane of nose (curves taken by electroolfactography, EOG)

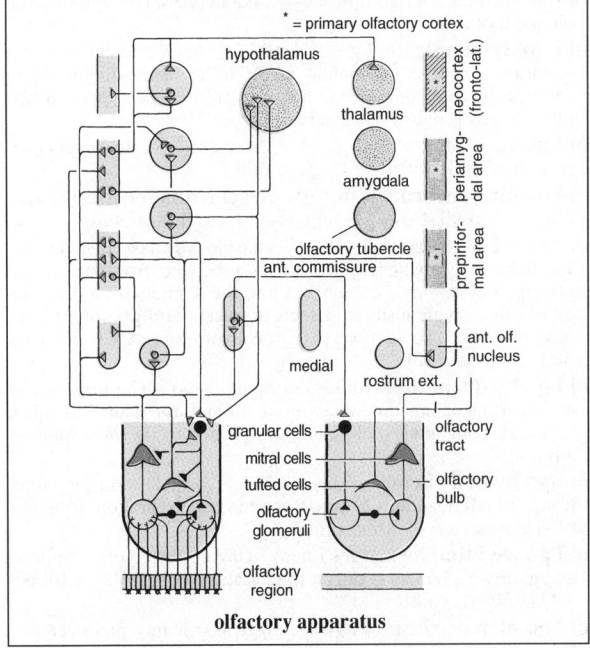

olfactory apparatus

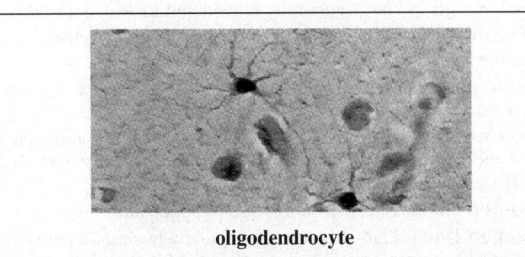

oligodendrocyte

ol·i·go·den·drog·lia (ol′ĭ-gō-den-drog′lē-ă). One of the three types of glia cells (the other two being macroglia or astrocytes, and microglia) that, together with nerve cells, compose the tissue of the central nervous system. O. cells are characterized by variable numbers of veillike or sheetlike processes that are wrapped each around individual axons to form the myelin sheath of nerve fibers in the central nervous system (compared with Schwann cells in the peripheral nervous system); forms myelin in the central nervous system; accordingly, they are more numerous in white matter than in gray matter. SYN oligodendria. [oligo- + G. *dendron,* tree, + *glia,* glue]

ol·i·go·den·dro·gli·o·ma (ol'i-gō-den'drō-glī-ō'mǎ). A relatively rare, relatively slowly growing glioma derived from oligodendrocytes that occurs most frequently in the cerebrum of adult persons; the neoplasm is grossly homogeneous, fairly well circumscribed, moderately firm, and somewhat gritty in consistency with interstitial calcification sufficiently dense so as to be detected by x-ray imaging of the skull. Microscopically, an o. is characterized by numerous, small, round, or ovoid, oligodendroglial cells with small, deeply stained nuclei (rarely observed in mitosis), and palely stained, indistinct cytoplasm; the neoplastic cells are rather uniformly distributed in a sparse, fibrillary stroma with scattered calcific bodies and an often prominent arcuate vasculature. [oligo- + G. *dendron,* tree, + glia, + -oma]

anaplastic o., an aggressive o. characterized by prominent nuclear pleomorphism, mitoses, and increased cellularity. SYN pleomorphic o.

pleomorphic o., SYN anaplastic o.

ol·i·go·dip·sia (ol'i-gō-dip'sē-ǎ). Abnormal lack of thirst. SEE ALSO hypodipsia. [oligo- + G. *dipsa,* thirst]

ol·i·go·don·tia (ol'i-gō-don'shē-ǎ). SYN hypodontia. [oligo- + G. *odous,* tooth]

ol·i·go·dy·nam·ic (ol'i-gō-dī-nam'ik). Active in very small quantity; *e.g.,* the germicidal effect of an exceedingly dilute solution (such as one to one hundred million) of copper in distilled water. [oligo- + G. *dynamis,* power]

ol·i·go·ga·lac·tia (ol'i-gō-gǎ-lak'tē-ǎ, -shē-ǎ). Slight or scant secretion of milk. [oligo- + G. *gala,* milk]

ol·i·go·glu·can-branch·ing gly·co·syl·trans·fer·ase (ol'i-gō-glū'kan). SYN 1,4-α-D-glucan 6-α-D-glucosyltransferase.

ol·i·go-α1,6-glu·co·si·dase. A glucanohydrolase cleaving α-1,6 links in isomaltose and dextrins produced from starch and glycogen by α-amylase; secreted into the duodenum; a deficiency of this enzyme leads to defects in intestinal digestion of limit dextrins. SEE ALSO sucrose α-D-glucohydrolase. SYN isomaltase, limit dextrinase (2).

ol·i·go·hy·dram·ni·os (ol'i-gō-hī-dram'nē-os). The presence of an insufficient amount of amniotic fluid (less than 300 ml at term). SYN oligamnios, oligoamnios. [oligo- + G. *hydōr,* water, + amnion]

ol·i·go·hy·dru·ria (ol'i-gō-hī-drū'rē-ǎ). Obsolete term for excretion of small quantities of urine, as seen in dehydration. [oligo- + G. *hydōr,* water, + *ouron,* urine]

ol·i·go·lec·i·thal (ol'i-gō-les'i-thal). Having little yolk; denoting an egg in which there is only a little scattered deutoplasm. [oligo- + G. *lekithos,* yolk]

ol·i·go·men·or·rhea (ol'i-gō-men-ō-rē'ǎ). Scanty menstruation. [oligo- + menorrhea]

ol·i·go·mer (ol'i-gō-mer). A polymer containing only a few repeating units, a "few" generally considered as less than 20.

ol·i·go·mor·phic (ol'-i-gō-mōr'fik). Presenting few changes of form; not polymorphic. [oligo- + G. *morphē,* form]

ol·i·go·neph·ron·ic (ol'i-gō-nef-ron'ik). Characterized by a reduced number of nephrons.

ol·i·go·nu·cle·o·tide (ol'i-gō-nū'klē-ō-tīd). A compound made up of the condensation of a small number (typically less than twenty) of nucleotides. Cf. polynucleotide.

ol·i·go·pep·sia (ol'i-gō-pep'sē-ǎ). SYN hypopepsia.

ol·i·go·pep·tide (ol'igō-pep-tīd). A peptide whose molecule contains a few amino acid residues up to about 20.

ol·i·go·pep·tide 20. A compound made up of the condensation of a small number (typically less than 20) of amino acids. Cf. polypeptide.

ol·i·go·phre·nia (ol'i-gō-frē'nē-ǎ). SYN mental *retardation.*

phenylpyruvate oligophrenia, SYN phenylketonuria.

ol·i·go·plas·tic (ol'i-gō-plas'tik). Deficient in reparative power. [oligo- + G. *plassō,* to form]

ol·i·gop·nea (ol'i-gop-nē'ǎ, -gop'nē-ǎ). SYN hypopnea. [oligo- + G. *pnoē,* breath]

ol·i·go·pty·a·lism (ol'i-gō-tī'ǎ-lizm, ol'i-gop-tī'). A scanty secretion of saliva. SYN oligosialia. [oligo- + G. *ptyalon,* saliva]

ol·i·gor·ia (ol-i-gōr'ē-ǎ). An abnormal indifference toward or dislike of persons or things. [G. *oligōria,* negligence, slight esteem, fr. *oligos,* little, + *ōra,* care, regard]

ol·i·go·sac·cha·ride (ol'i-gō-sak'ǎ-rīd). A compound made up of the condensation of a small number of monosaccharide units. Cf. polysaccharide.

ol·i·go·si·a·lia (ol'i-gō-sī-ā'lē-ǎ). SYN oligoptyalism. [oligo- + G. *sialon,* saliva]

ol·i·go·sper·mia, ol·i·go·sper·ma·tism (ol-i-gō-sper'mē-ǎ, -mǎ-tizm). A subnormal concentration of spermatozoa in the penile ejaculate. SYN oligozoospermatism, oligozoospermia. [oligo- + G. *sperma,* seed]

ol·i·go·symp·to·mat·ic (ol'i-gō-simp-tō-mat'ik). Having few or minor symptoms.

ol·i·go·sy·nap·tic (ol'i-gō-si-nap'tik). Referring to neural conduction pathways that are interrupted by only a few synaptic junctions, *i.e.,* made up of a sequence of only few nerve cells, in contrast to polysynaptic pathways. SYN paucisynaptic.

ol·i·go·thy·mia (ol'i-gō-thī'mē-ǎ). Rarely used term for a poverty or loss of affect. [oligo- + -thymia]

ol·i·go·trich·ia (ol'i-gō-trik'ē-ǎ). SYN hypotrichosis.

ol·i·go·tri·cho·sis (ol'i-gō-tri-kō'sis). SYN hypotrichosis.

ol·i·go·tro·phia, ol·i·got·ro·phy (ol'i-gō-trō'fē-ǎ, -got'rō-fē). Deficient nutrition. [oligo- + G. *trophē,* nourishment]

ol·i·go·zo·o·sper·ma·tism, ol·i·go·zo·o·sper·mia (ol'i-gō-zō'ō-sper'mǎ-tizm, -sper'mē-ǎ). SYN oligospermia. [oligo- + G. *zōon,* animal, + *sperma,* seed]

ol·i·gu·re·sia, ol·i·gu·re·sis (ol-i-gū-rē'sē-ǎ, -rē'sis). SYN oliguria. [oligo- + G. *ourēsis,* urination]

ol·i·gu·ria (ol-i-gū'rē-ǎ). Scanty urine production. SYN oliguresia, oliguresis. [oligo- + G. *ouron,* urine]

oli·va, pl. **oli'vae** (ō-lī'vǎ) [NA]. A smooth oval prominence of the ventrolateral surface of the medulla oblongata lateral to the pyramidal tract, corresponding to the inferior olivary nucleus. SYN corpus olivare, inferior olive, olivary body, olivary eminence, olive (1). [L.]

o. infe'rior, the oliva.

o. supe'rior, SYN dorsal *nucleus* of trapezoid body.

ol·i·vary (ol'i-vār-ē). 1. Relating to the oliva. 2. Relating to or shaped like an olive.

ol·ive (ol'iv). 1. SYN oliva. 2. Common name for a tree of the genus *Olea* (family Oleaceae) or its fruit. [L. *oliva*]

inferior o., SYN oliva.

superior o., SYN dorsal *nucleus* of trapezoid body.

ol·ive oil. The expressed oil of the fruit of *Olea europaea;* used as a cholagogue, laxative, and emollient, in the preparation of liniments, and in the preparation of foods.

ol·i·vif·u·gal (ol'i-vif'yū-gǎl). In a direction away from the olive. [oliva + L. *fugio,* to flee]

ol·i·vip·e·tal (ol'i-vip'ě-tǎl). In a direction toward the olive. [oliva + L. *peto,* to seek]

ol·i·vo·co·chle·ar (ol'i-vō-kok'lē-ǎr). SEE olivocochlear *bundle.*

ol·i·vo·pon·to·cer·e·bel·lar (ol'i-vō-pon'tō-sār-ě-bel'ar). Relating to the olivary nucleus, basis pontis, and cerebellum.

Ollendorf, Helene, German dermatologist, fl. 1928. SEE Buschke-O. *syndrome.*

Ollier, Louis X.E.L., French surgeon, 1830–1900. SEE O. *graft;* O.'s *disease, method, theory;* O.-Thiersch *graft.*

△**-ology.** SEE -logia.

olo·liu·qui (ō-lō-lyū'kē). A hallucinogen used in ceremonies by the Aztec Indians in Mexico; contains ergot alkaloids and derivatives of lysergic acid. SEE ALSO *Rivea corymbosa, Ipomoea rubrocoerulea* var. *praecox.*

olo·pho·nia (ol'ō-fō'nē-ǎ). Impaired speech due to an anatomical defect in the vocal organs. [G. *oloos,* destroyed, lost, + *phōnē,* voice]

Olszewski, Jerzy, Polish-Canadian neuropathologist, †1966. SEE Steele-Richardson-O. *disease, syndrome.*

△**-oma.** A tumor or neoplasm (added to words from G. roots). [G. -*ōma*]

oma·si·tis (ō-mă-sī′tis). Inflammation of the omasum.

oma·sum (ō-mā′sŭm). The third stomach division of a ruminant. SYN psalterium (2). [L. bullock's tripe]

△**-omata.** Plural of -oma.

Ombrédanne, Louis, French surgeon, 1871–1956. SEE O. *operation.*

om·bro·pho·bia (om-brō-fō′bē-ă). Morbid fear of rain. [G. *ombros,* rainstorm, + *phobos,* fear]

Omenn, Gilbert S., U.S. internist, *1941. SEE O.'s *syndrome.*

omen·tal (ō-men′tăl). Relating to the omentum. SYN epiploic.

omen·tec·to·my (ō-men-tek′tō-mē). Resection or excision of the omentum. SYN omentumectomy. [omentum + G. *ektomē,* excision]

omen·ti·tis (ō-men-tī′tis). Peritonitis involving the omentum. [L. *omentum* + G. -*itis,* inflammation]

△**omento-, oment-.** The omentum. SEE ALSO epiplo-. [L. *omentum*]

omen·to·fix·a·tion (ō-men′tō-fik-sā′shŭn). SYN omentopexy.

omen·to·pexy (ō-men′tō-pek-sē). **1.** Suture of the great omentum to the abdominal wall to induce collateral portal circulation. **2.** Suture of the omentum to another organ to increase arterial circulation. SEE ALSO omentoplasty. SYN omentofixation. [omento- + G. *pēxis,* fixation]

omen·to·plas·ty (ō-men′tō-plas-tē). Use, of the greater omentum to cover or fill a defect, augment arterial or portal venous circulation, absorb effusions, or increase lymphatic drainage. SEE ALSO omentopexy. [omento- + G. *plastos,* formed]

omen·tor·rha·phy (ō-men-tōr′ă-fē). Suture of an opening in the omentum. [omento- + G. *rhaphē,* suture]

omen·to·vol·vu·lus (ō-men-tō-vol′vyū-lŭs). Twisting of the omentum.

omen·tu·lum (ō-men′tyū-lŭm). SYN lesser *omentum.* [Mod. L. dim. of *omentum*]

omen·tum, pl. **omen·ta** (ō-men′tŭm, -tă) [NA]. A fold of peritoneum passing from the stomach to another abdominal organ. [L. the membrane that encloses the bowels]

gastrocolic o., SYN greater o.

gastrohepatic o., SYN lesser o.

gastrosplenic o., SYN gastrosplenic *ligament.*

greater o., a peritoneal fold passing from the greater curvature of the stomach to the transverse colon, hanging like an apron in front of the intestines. SYN o. majus [NA], caul (2), cowl, epiploon, gastrocolic o., pileus, velum (3).

lesser o., a peritoneal fold passing from the margins of the porta hepatis and the bottom of the fissure of the ductus venosus to the lesser curvature of the stomach and to the the upper border of the duodenum for a distance of about 2 cm beyond the gastroduodenal pylorus. SYN o. minus [NA], gastrohepatic o., omentulum.

o. ma′jus [NA], SYN greater o.

o. mi′nus [NA], SYN lesser o.

omen·tum·ec·to·my (ō-men-tŭ-mek′tō-mē). SYN omentectomy.

ome·pra·zole (ō-mē′prā-zol). A drug which blocks the transport of hydrogen ions into the stomach and is used as an antiulcerative, and in treatment of Zollinger-Ellison syndrome.

Ommaya, Ayub, 20th century U.S. neurosurgeon. SEE O. *reservoir.*

omn. hor. Abbreviation for L. *omni hora,* every hour.

om·nip·o·tence of thought (om-nip′ō-tens). A childish or magical thought process whereby instantaneous gratification of fantasies and wishes is believed to be imminent.

om·niv·o·rous (om-niv′ō-rŭs). Living on food of all kinds, upon both animal and vegetable food. [L. *omnis,* all, + *voro,* to eat]

△**omo-.** The shoulder (sometimes including the upper arm). [G. *ōmos,* shoulder]

omo·cla·vic·u·lar (ō′mō-kla-vik′yū-lăr). Relating to the shoulder and the clavicle; denoting an anomalous muscle attached to the coracoid process or upper edge of the scapula and to the clavicle.

omo·hy·oid (ō-mō-hī′oyd). SYN omohyoid *muscle.*

omo·pha·gia (ō-mō-fā′jē-ă). The eating of raw food, especially of raw flesh. [G. *ōmos,* raw, + *phagō,* to eat]

omo·thy·roid (ō-mō-thī′royd). Denoting a band of muscular fibers passing between the superior cornu of the thyroid cartilage and the omohyoid muscle.

OMP Abbreviation for oligo-*N*-methylmorpholinium propylene oxide; orotidylic acid; orotidylate; *orotidine* 5′-monophosphate.

OMPA Abbreviation for octamethyl pyrophosphoramide.

OMP de·car·box·yl·ase. SYN *orotidylic acid* decarboxylase.

△**omphal-, omphalo-.** The umbilicus, the navel. [G. *omphalos,* navel (umbilicus)]

om·pha·lec·to·my (om-fă-lek′tō-mē). Excision of the umbilicus or of a neoplasm connected with it. [omphal- + G. *ektomē,* excision]

om·phal·el·co·sis (om′fal-el-kō′sis). Ulceration at the umbilicus. [omphal- + G. *helkōsis,* ulceration]

om·phal·ic (om-fal′ik). SYN umbilical. [G. *omphalos,* umbilicus]

om·pha·li·tis (om-fă-lī′tis). Inflammation of the umbilicus and surrounding parts.

△**omphalo-.** SEE omphal-.

om·pha·lo·an·gi·op·a·gus (om′fă-lō-an-jē-op′ă-gŭs). Unequal conjoined twins in which the parasite derives its blood supply from the placenta of the autosite. SEE conjoined *twins,* under *twin.* SYN allantoidoangiopagus. [omphalo- + G. *angeion,* vessel, + *pagos,* something fixed]

om·phal·o·cele (om′fal-ō-sēl, om′fă-lō-). Congenital herniation of viscera into the base of the umbilical cord, with a covering membranous sac of peritoneum-amnion. The umbilical cord is inserted into the sac here, in contradistinction to its attachment in gastroschisis. SEE ALSO umbilical *hernia.* SYN amniocele, exomphalos (3), exumbilication (3). [omphalo- + G. *kēlē,* hernia]

om·pha·lo·en·ter·ic (om′fă-lō-en-tār-ik). Relating to the umbilicus and the intestine.

om·pha·lo·mes·en·ter·ic (om′fă-lō-mez-en-tār′ik). **1.** Term denoting relationship of the midgut to the yolk sac. As the head and tail folds of the embryo continue to form, this relationship is diminished and is represented by a narrow yolk stalk or vitelline duct. **2.** Relating to the vitelline duct.

om·pha·lop·a·gus (om′fă-lop′ă-gŭs). Conjoined twins united at their umbilical regions. SEE conjoined *twins,* under *twin.* SYN monomphalus. [omphalo- + G. *pagos,* something fixed]

om·pha·lo·phle·bi·tis (om′fă-lō-fle-bī′tis). Inflammation of the umbilical veins. [omphalo- + G. *phleps,* vein, + -*itis,* inflammation]

om·pha·lor·rha·gia (om′fă-lō-rā′jē-ă). Bleeding from the umbilicus. [omphalo- + G. *rhēgnymi,* to burst forth]

om·pha·lor·rhea (om′fă-lō-rē′ă). A serous discharge from the umbilicus. [omphalo- + G. *rhoia,* flow]

om·pha·lor·rhex·is (om′fă-lō-rek′sis). Rupture of the umbilical cord during childbirth. [omphalo- + G. *rhēxis,* rupture]

om·pha·los (om′fă-los). Rarely used term for umbilicus. [G. navel]

om·pha·lo·site (om′fă-lō-sīt). Underdeveloped twin of allantoidoangiopagus twin; joined by umbilical vessels. SYN placental parasitic twin. [omphalo- + G. *sitos,* food]

om·pha·lo·spi·nous (om′fă-lō-spī′nŭs). Denoting a line connecting the umbilicus and the anterior superior spine of the ilium, on which lies McBurney's point.

om·pha·lot·o·my (om-fă-lot′ō-mē). Cutting of the umbilical cord at birth. [omphalo- + G. *tomē,* incision]

om·pha·lo·trip·sy (om′fă-lō-trip′sē). Crushing, instead of cutting, the umbilical cord after childbirth. [omphalo- + G. *tripsis,* a rubbing]

om·pha·lo·ves·i·cal (om′fă-lō-ves′i-kăl). SYN vesicoumbilical.

om·pha·lus (om′fă-lŭs). Rarely used term for umbilicus. [G. *omphalos,* navel]

OMP py·ro·phos·pho·ryl·ase. SYN *orotate* phosphoribosyltransferase.

OMS Abbreviation for organic mental *syndrome.*

onan·ism (ō'nan-izm). **1.** The act of a male to spill his seed on the ground; withdrawal of the penis before ejaculation, in order to prevent insemination and fecundation of the ovum. **2.** Incorrectly used as a synonym of masturbation. [*Onan,* son of Judah, who practiced it. Genesis 38:9]

⌂ **oncho-.** SEE onco-.

On·cho·cer·ca (ong-kō-ser'kă). A genus of elongated filariform nematodes (family Onchocercidae) that inhabit the connective tissue of their hosts, usually within firm nodules in which these parasites are coiled and entangled. SYN *Oncocerca.* [G. *onkos,* a barb, + *kerkos,* tail]

O. cervica'lis, a species common in the ligamentum nuchae of horses, mules, and asses, where it has been suspected of playing a role in fistulous withers and poll evil.

O. gibso'ni, a species that infects the subcutaneous tissues of cattle, buffalo, and sheep.

O. liena'lis, a species that inhabits the connective tissue around the ligamentum nuchae, tibiofemoral ligament, spleen capsule, and other sites in cattle and buffalo; although widely distributed, it is not common in the U.S.

O. vol'vulus, the blinding nodular worm, a species that causes onchocerciasis.

on·cho·cer·ci·a·sis (ong'kō-ser-kī'ă-sis). Infection with *Onchocerca* (especially *O. volvulus,* a filarial nematode transmitted from person to person by black flies of the genus *Simulium*), marked by nodular swellings forming a fibrous cyst enveloping the coiled parasites; microfilariae move freely out of the nodule and escape into the intercellular lymph in the dermis. Dermatological changes often develop, especially in Africa, resulting in intense pruritus, scaly or lichenoid skin, depigmentation, and destruction of elastic fibers. Most important are the ocular complications that may develop after a long chronic course, with blindness frequently occurring in advanced cases, due to the presence of living or dead microfilariae seen by slit lamp biomicroscopy. SYN blinding disease, onchocercosis, volvulosis.

ocular o., ocular complications, such as keratitis, iridocyclitis, or retrobulbar neuritis, caused by the microfilariae of *Onchocerca volvulus.* SYN river blindness.

on·cho·cer·cid (ong-kō-ser'kid). Common name for members of the family Onchocercidae.

On·cho·cer·ci·dae (ong-kō-ser'ki-dē). A family of nematode parasites (superfamily Filarioidea) characterized by production of microfilariae; it includes the genera *Onchocerca, Wuchereria, Brugia, Loa,* and *Mansonella.*

on·cho·cer·co·sis (ong'kō-ser-kō'sis). SYN onchocerciasis.

⌂ **onco-, oncho-.** A tumor. [G. *onkos,* bulk, mass]

On·co·cer·ca (ong-kō-ser'kă). SYN *Onchocerca.*

on·co·cyte (ong'kō-sīt). A large, granular, acidophilic tumor cell containing numerous mitochondria; a neoplastic oxyphil cell. [onco- + G. *kytos,* cell]

on·co·cy·to·ma (ong'kō-sī-tō'mă). A glandular tumor composed of large cells with cytoplasm that is granular and eosinophilic due to the presence of abundant mitochondria; occurs uncommonly in the kidney, salivary glands, and endocrine glands. SYN oxyphil adenoma. [onco- + G. *kytos,* cell, + *-oma,* tumor]

on·co·fe·tal (ong-kō-fē'tăl). Relating to tumor-associated substances present in fetal tissue, as o. antigens.

on·co·gene (ong'kō-jēn). **1.** Any of a family of genes which under normal circumstances code for proteins involved in cell growth or regulation (*e.g.,* protein kinases, GTPases, nuclear proteins, growth factors) but may foster malignant processes if mutated or activated by contact with retroviruses. Identified oncogenes include the ras, originally associated with bladder tumors, and the p53, a mutated version of a gene on chromosome 17 which normally corrects for mutations caused by ultraviolet radiation. p53 now has been shown to be involved in cancers of the breast, cervix, ovary, and lung, among others. Oncogenes often work in concert to produce cancer, and their action may be exacerbated by retroviruses, jumping genes, or inherited genetic mutations. SEE antioncogene. **2.** Found in certain DNA tumor viruses. It is required for viral replication. SYN transforming gene. [onco- + gene]

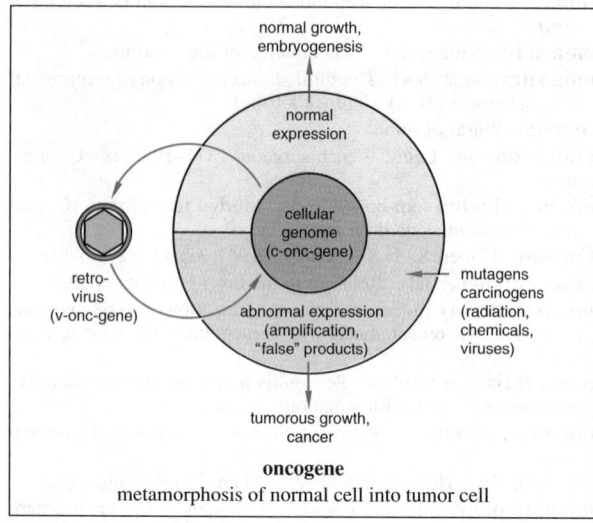

oncogene
metamorphosis of normal cell into tumor cell

on·co·gen·e·sis (ong-kō-jen'ě-sis). Origin and growth of a neoplasm. [onco- + G. *genesis,* production]

on·co·gen·ic (ong-kō-jen'ik). SYN oncogenous.

on·cog·en·ous (ong-koj'ě-nŭs). Causing, inducing, or being suitable for the formation and development of a neoplasm. SYN oncogenic.

on·co·graph (ong'kō-graf). A recording oncometer, or the recording portion of an oncometer. [onco- + G. *graphē,* a record]

on·cog·ra·phy (ong'kog'ră-fē). Graphic representation, by means of a special apparatus, of the size and configuration of an organ.

on·coi·des (ong-koy'dēz). Intumescence or turgescence. [onco- + G. *eidos,* resemblance]

on·col·o·gist (ong-kol'ō-jist). A specialist in oncology.

radiation o., SYN radiotherapist.

on·col·o·gy (ong-kol'ō-jē). The study or science dealing with the physical, chemical, and biologic properties and features of neoplasms, including causation, pathogenesis, and treatment. [onco- + G. *logos,* study]

radiation o., the medical specialty of radiation therapy; the study of radiation treatment of neoplasms.

on·col·y·sis (ong-kol'i-sis). Destruction of a neoplasm; sometimes used with reference to the reduction of any swelling or mass. [onco- + G. *lysis,* dissolution]

on·co·lyt·ic (ong-kō-lit'ik). Pertaining to, characterized by, or causing oncolysis.

On·co·me·la·nia (ong'kō-mě-lā'nī-ă). A medically important genus of amphibious freshwater operculate snails of the family Hydrobiidae (subfamily Hydrobiinae; subclass Prosobranchiata). In the Orient, several subspecies of *O. hupensis* serve as intermediate hosts of the oriental blood fluke, *Schistosoma japonicum.* [onco- + G. *melas (melan-),* black]

on·com·e·ter (ong-kom'ě-ter). **1.** An instrument for measuring the size and configuration of the kidneys and other organs. **2.** The measuring, as distinguished from the recording part of the oncograph. [onco- + G. *metron,* measure]

on·co·met·ric (ong-kō-met'rik). Relating to oncometry.

on·com·e·try (ong-kom'ě-trē). Measurement of the size of an organ.

on·cor·na·vi·rus·es (ong-kōr'nă-vī'rŭs-ez). SYN Oncovirinae.

on·co·sis (ong-kō'sis). A condition characterized by the formation of one or more neoplasms or tumors. [G. *onkōsis,* swelling, fr. *onkos,* bulk, mass]

on·co·sphere (ong'-kō-sfēr). SYN hexacanth. [onco- + G. *sphaira,* sphere]

on·co·ther·a·py (ong-kō-thār'ă-pē). Treatment of tumors.

on·cot·ic (ong-kot′ik). Relating to or caused by edema or any swelling (oncosis).

on·cot·o·my (ong-kot′ō-mē). Rarely used term for incision of an abscess, cyst, or other tumor. [onco- + G. *tomē*, incision]

on·co·tro·pic (ong′kō-trop′ik). Manifesting a special affinity for neoplasms or neoplastic cells. SYN tumoraffin. [onco- + G. *tropē*, a turning]

On·co·vir·i·nae (ong-kō-vir′i-nē). A subfamily of viruses (family Retroviridae) composed of the RNA tumor viruses that contain two identical plus stranded RNA molecules. Subgroups are based on antigenicity, host range, and kind of malignancy induced (avian, feline, hamster, or murine leukemia-sarcoma complex; murine mammary tumor virus; primate oncoviruses). Like other retroviruses, the oncoviruses contain RNA-dependent DNA polymerases (reverse transcriptases). Virions, on the basis of morphology and antigenicity, are of four types: 1) type A, found only within infected cells and seemingly immature in that there is no electron-dense nucleoid; 2) type B, having an eccentric electron-dense nucleoid and associated with the Bittner mammary tumor; 3) type C, having a centrally located, electron-dense nucleoid and associated with leukemia-sarcoma complexes of various species; 4) type D, having a central electron-dense nucleoid but differing in other respects from type C. An important aspect of these viruses seems to be utilization of viral reverse transcriptase to make DNA which can be integrated into the DNA of the host cell and will replicate along with cellular DNA. SYN oncornaviruses.

on·co·vi·rus (ong′kō-vī′rŭs). Any virus of the subfamily Oncovirinae. SEE ALSO oncogenic *virus*.

on·dan·se·tron (ŏn-dan′sĕ-tron). A serotonin 5-HT$_3$ receptor antagonist used as an antiemetic, particularly in patients undergoing chemotherapy or radiation treatment for cancer.

Ondine, German mythological character.

-one. Suffix indicating a ketone (–CO–) group.

onei·ric (ō-nī′rik). 1. Pertaining to dreams. 2. Pertaining to the clinical state of oneirophrenia. SYN oniric. [G. *oneiros*, dream]

onei·rism (ō-nī′rizm). A waking dream state. [G. *oneiros*, dream]

onei·ro·crit·i·cal (ō-nī-rō-krit′i-kăl). Rarely used term pertaining to the logic of dreams. [G. *oneiros*, dream, + *kritikos*, skilled in judgment]

onei·ro·dyn·ia (ō-nī-rō-din′ē-ă). Rarely used term for an unpleasant or painful dream. [G. *oneiros*, dream, + *odynē*, pain]

o. acti′va, SYN somnambulism (1).

o. gra′vis, SYN nightmare.

onei·rog·mus (ō′nī-rog′mŭs). Nocturnal emission of semen, often related to erotic dreams. SEE ALSO wet *dream*. [G. *oneirōgmos*, an effusion of semen during sleep]

onei·rol·o·gy (ō-nī-rol′ō-jē). The study of dreams and their content. [G. *oneiros*, dream, + *logos*, study]

onei·ro·phre·nia (ō-nī-rō-frē′nē-ă). A state in which hallucinations occur, caused by such conditions as prolonged deprivation of sleep, sensory isolation, and a variety of drugs. [G. *oneiros*, dream, + *phrēn*, mind]

onei·ros·co·py (ō-nī-ros′kŏ-pē). Rarely used term for the diagnosis of a person's mental state by an analysis of his dreams. [G. *oneiros*, dream, + *skopeō*, to examine]

oni·o·ma·nia (ō′nē-ō-mā′nē-ă). Rarely used term for the morbidly exaggerated need or urge to buy beyond the realistic needs of the individual. [G. *ōnios*, for sale, + *mania*, insanity]

oni·ric (ō-nī′rik). SYN oneiric.

-onium. Suffix indicating a positively charged radical; *e.g.*, ammonium, NH_4^+.

onko-. SEE onco-.

on·lay (on′lā). 1. A metal (usually gold) cast restoration of the occlusal surface of a posterior tooth or the lingual surface of an anterior tooth, the entire surface of which is in dentin without side walls; retention in the anterior tooth is by pins and in the posterior by pins and/or boxes in retentive grooves in the buccal and lingual walls. 2. A graft applied on the exterior of a bone.

Onodi, A., 20th century Hungarian laryngologist. SEE Onodi *cell*.

on·o·mat·o·ma·nia (on′ō-mat-ō-mā′nē-ă). An abnormal impulse to dwell upon certain words and their supposed significance, or to frantically try to recall a particular word. [G. *onoma*, name, + *mania*, frenzy]

on·o·mat·o·pho·bia (on′ō-mat-ō-fō′bē-ă). Abnormal dread of certain words or names because of their supposed significance. SYN nomatophobia. [G. *onoma*, name, + *phobos*, fear]

on·o·mat·o·poi·e·sis (on′ō-mat′ō-poy-ē′sis). The making of a name or word, especially to express or imitate a natural sound (*e.g.*, hiss, crash, boom); in psychiatry, the tendency to make new words of this type is said to characterize some persons with schizophrenia. SEE ALSO neologism. [G. *onoma*, name, + *poiēsis*, making]

on·to·gen·e·sis (on-tō-jen′ĕ-sis). SYN ontogeny.

on·to·ge·net·ic, on·to·gen·ic (on′tō-jĕ-net′ik, -jen′ik). Relating to ontogeny.

on·tog·e·ny (on-toj′ĕ-nē). Development of the individual, as distinguished from phylogeny, which is evolutionary development of the species. SYN ontogenesis. [G. *ōn*, being, + *genesis*, origin]

on·tol·o·gy (on-tol′ō-jē). A traditional branch of metaphysics that deals with problems of being, existence, inner nature, meaning, etc. It is fundamental to problems involving normality and disease, individuality, responsibility, and the analysis of values. In recent years, it has been slowly assuming a place as a branch of medicine proper.

Onufrowicz (on-ū-frō′-wikz), Wladislaus, Swiss anatomist, 1836–1900. SEE Onuf's *nucleus*.

on·y·al·ai (on-i-al′ā). An acute disease affecting natives of Central Africa, characterized by bloody vesicles of the mouth and other mucous surfaces, hematuria, and melena; defective nutrition may be the cause. SYN akembe, kafindo.

onych-. SEE onycho-.

on·y·chal·gia (on-i-kal′jē-ă). Pain in the nails. [onycho- + G. *algos*, pain]

on·y·cha·tro·phia, on·ych·at·ro·phy (on′i-kă-trō′fē-ă, on-ik-at′rō-fē). Atrophy of the nails. [onycho- + G. *atrophia*, atrophy]

on·y·chaux·is (on-i-kawk′sis). Marked overgrowth of the fingernails or toenails. [onycho- + G. *auxē*, increase]

on·y·chec·to·my (on-i-kek′tō-mē). Ablation of a toenail or fingernail. [onycho- + G. *ektomē*, excision]

onych·ia (ō-nik′ē-ă). Inflammation of the matrix of the nail. SYN onychitis, onyxitis. [onycho- + G. -*ia*, condition]

o. latera′lis, SYN paronychia.

o. malig′na, acute o. occurring spontaneously in debilitated patients, or in response to slight trauma. SYN Wardrop's disease.

o. periungua′lis, SYN paronychia.

o. sic′ca, a condition characterized by brittle nails.

on·y·chi·tis (on-i-kī′tis). SYN onychia.

onycho-, onych-. A finger nail, a toenail. [G. *onyx*, nail]

on·y·choc·la·sis (on-i-kok′lă-sis). Breaking of the nails. [onycho- + G. *klasis*, breaking]

on·y·cho·cryp·to·sis (on′i-kō-krip-tō′sis). SYN ingrown *nail*. [onycho- + G. *kryptō*, to conceal]

on·y·cho·dys·tro·phy (on′i-kō-dis′trō-fē). Dystrophic changes in the nails occurring as a congenital defect or due to any illness or injury that may cause a malformed nail. [onycho- + G. *dys-*, bad, + *trophē*, nourishment]

on·y·cho·graph (on′i-kō-graf). An instrument for recording the capillary blood pressure as shown by the circulation under the nail. [onycho- + G. *graphō*, to write]

on·y·cho·gry·pho·sis (on′i-kō-gri-fō′sis). SYN onychogryposis.

on·y·cho·gry·po·sis (on′i-kō-gri-pō′sis). Enlargement with increased thickening and curvature of the fingernails or toenails. SYN grypisis unguium, onychogryphosis. [onycho- + G. *grypō-sis*, a curvature]

on·y·cho·het·er·o·to·pia (on′i-kō-het-er-ō-tō′pē-ă). Abnormal placement of nails.

on·y·choid (on′i-koyd). Resembling a fingernail in structure or form. [onycho- + G. *eidos*, resemblance]

on·y·chol·o·gy (on-i-kol′ō-jē). Study of the nails. [onycho- + G. *logos,* treatise]

on·y·chol·y·sis (on-i-kol′i-sis). Loosening of the nails, beginning at the free border, and usually incomplete. [onycho- + G. *lysis,* loosening]

on·y·cho·ma (on-i-kō′mă). A tumor arising from the nail bed. [onycho- + G. *-ōma,* tumor]

on·y·cho·ma·de·sis (on′i-kō-mă-dē′sis). Complete shedding of the nails, usually associated with systemic disease. [onycho- + G. *madēsis,* a growing bald, fr. *madaō,* to be moist, (of hair) fall off]

on·y·cho·ma·la·cia (on′i-kō-mă-lā′shē-ă). Abnormal softness of the nails. [onycho- + G. *malakia,* softness]

on·y·cho·my·co·sis (on′i-kō-mī-kō′sis). Very common fungus infections of the nails, causing thickening, roughness, and splitting, often caused by *Trichophyton rubrum* or *T. mentagrophytes, Candida* in the immunodeficient, and molds in the elderly. SYN ringworm of nails. [onycho- + G. *mykēs,* fungus, + *-ōsis,* condition]

on·y·chon·o·sus (on-i-kon′ō-sŭs). SYN onychopathy. [onycho- + G. *nosos,* disease]

on·y·cho-os·te·o·dys·pla·sia (on′i-kō-os′tē-ō-dis-plā′zē-ă). Obsolete term for the nail-patella *syndrome.*

on·y·cho·path·ic (on′i-kō-path′ik). Relating to or suffering from any disease of the nails.

on·y·cho·pa·thol·o·gy (on′i-kō-pă-thol′ō-jē). Study of diseases of the nails.

on·y·chop·a·thy (on-i-kop′ă-thē). Any disease of the nails. SYN onychonosus, onychosis. [onycho- + G. *pathos,* suffering]

on·y·choph·a·gy, on·y·cho·pha·gia (on-i-kof′ă-jē, on′i-kō-fā′jē-ă). Habitual nailbiting. [onycho- + G. *phago,* to eat]

on·y·cho·pho·sis (on′i-kō-fō′sis). A growth of horny epithelium in the nail bed. [onycho- + G. *phōs,* light, + *-osis,* condition]

on·y·cho·phy·ma (on′i-kō-fī′mă). Swelling or hypertrophy of the nails. [onycho- + G. *phyma,* growth]

on·y·cho·plas·ty (on′i-kō-plas-tē). A corrective or plastic operation on the nail matrix. [onycho- + G. *plastos,* formed, shaped]

on·y·chop·to·sis (on′i-kop-tō′sis). Falling off of the nails. [onycho- + G. *ptōsis,* a falling]

on·y·chor·rhex·is (on′i-kō-rek′sis). Abnormal brittleness of the nails with splitting of the free edge. [onycho- + G. *rhēxis,* a breaking]

on·y·cho·schiz·ia (on′i-kō-skiz′ē-ă). Splitting of the nails in layers. [onycho- + G. *schizō,* to divide, + *-ia,* condition]

on·y·cho·sis (on-i-kō′sis). SYN onychopathy.

on·y·cho·stro·ma (on′i-kō-strō′mă). SYN nail *bed.* [onycho- + G. *strōma,* bedding]

on·y·chot·il·lo·ma·nia (on′i-kot′i-lo-mā′nē-ă). A tendency to pick at the nails. [onycho- + G. *tillō,* to pluck, + *mania,* insanity]

on·y·chot·o·my (on-i-kot′ō-mē). Incision into a toenail or fingernail. [onycho- + G. *tomē,* cutting]

on·y·chot·ro·phy (on-i-kot′rō-fē). Nutrition of the nails. [onycho- + G. *trophē,* nourishment]

on·yx (on′iks). SYN nail. [G. nail]

on·yx·is (on-iks′is). SYN ingrown *nail.*

on·yx·i·tis (on-iks-ī′tis). SYN onychia.

△**oo-.** Egg, ovary. SEE ALSO oophor-, ovario-, ovi-, ovo-. [G. *ōon,* egg. OO-]

oo·cy·e·sis (ō-ō-sī-ē′sis). SYN ovarian *pregnancy.* [G. *ōon,* egg, + *kyēsis,* pregnancy]

oo·cyst (ō′ō-sist). The encysted form of the fertilized macrogamete, or zygote, in coccidian Sporozoea in which sporogonic multiplication occurs; results in the formation of sporozoites, infectious agents for the next stage of the sporozoan life cycle. [G. *ōon,* egg, + *kystis,* bladder]

oo·cyte (ō′ō-sīt). The immature ovum. SYN ovocyte. [G. *ōon,* egg, + *kytos,* a hollow (cell)]

primary o., an o. during its growth phase and before it completes the first maturation division.

secondary o., an o. in which the first meiotic division is com-

pleted; the second meiotic division usually stops short of completion unless fertilization occurs.

oo·gen·e·sis (ō-ō-jen′ĕ-sis). Process of formation and development of the ovum. SYN ovigenesis, ovogenesis. [G. *ōon,* egg, + *genesis,* origin]

oo·ge·net·ic (ō-ō-jĕ-net′ik). Producing ova. SYN oogenic, oogenous, ovigenetic, ovigenic, ovigenous.

oo·gen·ic, oog·e·nous (ō-ō-jen′ik, ō-oj′ĕ-nŭs). SYN oogenetic.

oo·go·ni·um, pl. **oo·go·nia** (ō-ō-gō′nē-ŭm, -ă). **1.** Primitive germ cells; proliferate by mitotic division. All oogonia develop into primary oocytes prior to birth; no oogonia are present after birth. **2.** In fungi, the female gametangium bearing one or more oospores. [G. *ōon,* egg, + *gonē,* generation]

oo·ki·ne·sis, oo·ki·ne·sia (ō-ō′ki-nē′sis, -zē-ă). Chromosomal movements of the egg during maturation and fertilization. [G. *ōon,* egg, + *kinēsis,* movement]

oo·ki·nete (ō′ō-ki-ne′t, -kī′ne′t). The motile zygote of the malarial organism that penetrates the mosquito stomach to form an oocyst under the outer gut lining; the contents of the oocyst subsequently divide to produce numerous sporozoites. SYN vermicule (2). [G. *ōon,* egg, + *kinētos,* motile]

oo·lem·ma (ō-ō-lem′ă). Plasma membrane of the oocyte. [G. *ōon,* egg, + *lemma,* sheath]

oo·my·co·sis (ō′ō-mī-kō′sis). A mycosis caused by fungi belonging to the class Oomycetes; *e.g.,* rhinosporidiosis, pythiosis.

oo·pha·gia, ooph·a·gy (ō-ō-fā′jē-ă, ō-of′ă-jē). The habitual eating of eggs; subsisting largely on eggs. [G. *ōon,* egg, + *phagō,* to eat]

△**oophor-, oophoro-.** The ovary. SEE ALSO oo-, ovario-. [Mod. L. *oophoron,* ovary, fr. G. *ōophoros,* egg-bearing]

ooph·or·al·gia (ō-of-ōr-al′jē-ă). SYN ovarialgia. [oophor- + G. *algos,* pain]

ooph·o·rec·to·my (ō-of-ōr-ek′tō-mē). SYN ovariectomy. [G. *ōon,* egg, + *phoros,* bearing, + *ektomē,* excision]

ooph·or·i·tis (ō-of-ōr-ī′tis). Inflammation of an ovary. SYN ovaritis. [G. *ōon,* egg, + *phoros,* a bearing, + *-itis,* inflammation]

△**oophoro-.** SEE oophor-.

ooph·or·o·cys·tec·to·my (ō-of′ōr-ō-sis-tek′tō-mē). Excision of an ovarian cyst.

ooph·or·o·cys·to·sis (ō-of′ōr-ō-sis-tō′sis). Ovarian cyst formation.

ooph·or·o·hys·ter·ec·to·my (ō-of′ōr-ō-his-ter-ek′tō-mē). SYN ovariohysterectomy.

ooph·or·o·ma (ō-of-ōr-ō′mă). An ovarian tumor. SYN ovariocus.

ooph·or·on (ō-of′ōr-on). Rarely used term for ovary. [G. *ōon,* egg, + *phoros,* bearing]

ooph·or·op·a·thy (ō-of-ōr-op′ă-thē). SYN ovariopathy.

ooph·or·o·pel·i·o·pexy (ō-of′ōr-ō-pel′i-ō-pek-sē). SYN oophororrhaphy. [oophoro- + G. *pellis,* pelvis, + *pēxis,* fixation]

ooph·or·o·pexy (ō-of′ōr-ō-pek-sē). Surgical fixation or suspension of an ovary. [oophoro- + G. *pēxis,* fixation]

ooph·or·o·plas·ty (ō-of′ōr-ō-plas-tē). Plastic operation upon an ovary. [oophoro- + G. *plastos,* formed, shaped]

ooph·o·ror·rha·phy (ō-of-ō-rōr′ă-fē). Suspension of the ovary by attachment to pelvic the wall. SYN oophoropeliopexy. [oophoro- + G. *rhaphē,* suture]

ooph·or·o·sal·pin·gec·to·my (ō-of′ōr-ō-sal-pin-jek′tō-mē). SYN ovariosalpingectomy.

ooph·or·o·sal·pin·gi·tis (ō-of′ōr-ō-sal-pin-jī′tis). SYN ovariosalpingitis. [oophoro- + salpingitis]

ooph·or·os·to·my (ō-of-ōr-os′tō-mē). SYN ovariostomy. [oophoro- + G. *stoma,* mouth]

ooph·or·ot·o·my (ō-of-ōr-ot′ō-mē). SYN ovariotomy. [oophoro- + G. *tomē,* incision]

ooph·or·rha·gia (ō-of-ōr-rā′jē-ă). Ovarian hemorrhage. [oophor- + G. *rhēgnymi,* to burst forth]

oo·plasm (ō′ō-plazm). Protoplasmic portion of the ovum. [G. *ōon,* egg, + *plasma,* a thing formed]

oo·some (ō'ō-sōm). A cytoplasmic body in the ovum that passes into the germ cell. [G. *ōon,* egg + *sōma,* body]

oo·spo·ran·gi·um (ō'ō-spō-ran'jē-ŭm). Obsolete term for oogonium (2). [oospore + G. *angeion,* vessel]

oo·spore (ō'ō-spōr). A thick-walled fungus spore which develops from a female gamete either through fertilization or parthenogenesis in an oogonium. [see *Oospora*]

oo·the·ca (ō-oth-ē'kǎ). **1.** An egg case found in some lower animals. **2.** Rarely used term for ovary. [G. *ōon,* egg, + *thēkē,* box, case]

oo·tid (ō'ō-tid). The nearly mature ovum after the first meiotic division has been completed and the second initiated; in most higher mammals, the second meiotic division is not completed unless fertilization occurs. [G. *ōotidion,* a diminutive egg. See -id (2)]

oo·type (ō'ō-tīp). The central portion of the ovarian complex of trematodes and cestodes in which fertilization takes place and the vitellarian or eggshell materials are coated over the egg; this occurs in a rapid, stamping-mill sequence, after which eggs pass into the uterus for tanning of the shell, storage, and passage toward the genital pore. [G. *ōon,* egg, + *typos,* stamp, print]

opac·i·fi·ca·tion (ō-pas'i-fi-kā'shŭn). **1.** The process of making opaque. **2.** The formation of opacities. [L. *opacus,* shady]

opac·i·ty (ō-pas'i-tē). **1.** A lack of transparency; an opaque or nontransparent area. **2.** On a radiograph, a more transparent area is interpreted as an o. to x-rays in the body. **3.** Mental dullness. [L. *opacitas,* shadiness]

  nodular o., a solitary, round, circumscribed shadow found in the lung on chest radiograph; causes include granuloma, primary or metastatic carcinoma, benign tumor, vascular malformation. SYN coin lesion of lungs.

  snowball o., a spherical, white body seen in the vitreous in asteroid hyalosis.

opal·es·cent (ō-pǎ-les'ent). Resembling an opal in the display of various colors; denoting certain bacterial cultures. [Fr. fr. L. *opalus,* opal]

Opalski, Adam, Polish physician, 1897–1963. SEE O. *cell.*

opaque (ō-pāk'). Impervious to light; not translucent or only slightly so. Cf. radiopaque. [Fr. fr. L. *opacus,* shady]

o·pei·do·scope (op-ī'dō-skōp). An apparatus for study of voice vibrations by which the vibrations of a diaphragm, started by the voice, move a mirror by which a ray of light is reflected on a screen. [G. *ops* (*op-*), a voice, + *eidos,* appearance, + *skopeō,* to view]

open (ō'pen). **1.** Not closed; exposed, said of a wound. **2.** To enter or expose, as a wound or cavity. [A.S.]

open·ing (ō'pen-ing). SYN aperture. SEE ALSO aperture, fossa, ostium, orifice.

  access o., SYN access.

  aortic o., SYN aortic *hiatus.*

  cardiac o., SYN cardiac *orifice.*

  o. to cerebral aqueduct, SYN *anus* cerebri.

  esophageal o., SYN esophageal *hiatus.*

  o. of external acoustic meatus, the orifice of the external acoustic meatus in the tympanic portion of the temporal bone. SYN porus acusticus externus [NA], external acoustic foramen, external acoustic pore, external auditory pore, external auditory foramen, orifice of external acoustic meatus.

  external o. of urethra, SYN external urethral *orifice.*

  femoral o., SYN adductor *hiatus.*

  ileocecal o., SYN ileocecal *orifice.*

  o. of inferior vena cava, the orifice through which the inferior vena cava opens into the right atrium. SYN ostium venae cavae inferioris [NA], orifice of inferior vena cava.

  o. of internal acoustic meatus, the inner opening of the internal acoustic meatus on the posterior surface of the petrous part of the temporal bone. SYN porus acusticus internus [NA], internal acoustic foramen, internal acoustic pore, auditory pore, internal auditory foramen, orifice of internal acoustic meatus.

  internal urethral o., SYN internal urethral *orifice.*

  lacrimal o., SYN lacrimal *punctum.*

  orbital o., the somewhat quadrangular anterior entrance to the orbit which forms the base of the pyramid-shaped orbital cavity. It is bounded by the sharp supra-, infra-, and lateral orbital margins and a less obvious medial margin on each side of the upper nose. SYN aditus orbitae [NA], aperture of orbit.

  pharyngeal o. of auditory tube, an opening in the upper part of the nasopharynx about 1.2 cm behind the posterior extremity of the inferior concha on each side. SYN ostium pharyngeum tubae auditivae [NA], pharyngeal o. of eustachian tube.

  pharyngeal o. of eustachian tube, SYN pharyngeal o. of auditory tube.

  piriform o., SYN anterior nasal *aperture.*

  o. of pulmonary trunk, the o. of the pulmonary trunk from the right ventricle, guarded by the pulmonary valve. SYN ostium trunci pulmonalis [NA], pulmonary orifice.

  o.'s of pulmonary veins, the orifices of the pulmonary veins, usually two on each side, in the wall of the left atrium. SYN ostia venarum pulmonalium [NA].

  saphenous o., the opening in the fascia lata inferior to the medial part of the inguinal ligament through which the saphenous vein passes to enter the femoral vein. SYN hiatus saphenus [NA], fossa ovalis (2), saphenous hiatus.

  o. of the sphenoidal sinus, one of the pair of openings in the body of the sphenoid bone through which the sphenoid sinuses communicate with the sphenoethmoidal recess of the nasal cavity. SYN apertura sinus sphenoidalis [NA], sphenoidal sinus aperture.

  o. of superior vena cava, the point of entry of the superior vena cava into the right atrium. SYN ostium venae cavae superioris [NA], orifice of superior vena cava.

  tendinous o., SYN adductor *hiatus.*

  tympanic o. of auditory tube, an opening in the anterior part of the tympanic cavity below the canal for the tensor tympani muscle. SYN ostium tympanicum tubae auditivae [NA], tympanic o. of eustachian tube.

  tympanic o. of canaliculi for chorda tympani, the small canal opening found lateral to the pyramidal eminence in the posterior wall of the middle ear cavity from which the chorda tympani nerve emerges to pass anteriorly between the ossicles accompanied by a branch of the stylomastoid artery. SYN apertura tympanica canaliculi chordae tympani [NA].

  tympanic o. of eustachian tube, SYN tympanic o. of auditory tube.

  ureteral o., SYN ureteric *orifice.*

  urethral o.'s, SEE external urethral *orifice,* internal urethral *orifice.*

  uterine o. of uterine tubes, SYN uterine *ostium* of uterine tubes.

  o. of uterus, SYN external *os* of uterus.

  vaginal o., SYN vaginal *orifice.*

  vertical o., SYN vertical *dimension.*

op·er·a·ble (op'er-ǎ-bl). Denoting a patient or condition on which a surgical procedure can be performed with a reasonable expectation of cure or relief.

op·er·ant (op'er-ănt). In conditioning, any behavior or specific response chosen by the experimenter; its frequency is intended to increase or decrease by the judicious pairing with it of a reinforcer when it occurs. SYN target behavior (1), target response.

op·er·ate (op'er-āt). **1.** To work upon the body by the hands or by means of cutting or other instruments to correct a surgical problem. **2.** To cause a movement of the bowels; said of a laxative or cathartic remedy. [L. *operor,* pp. *-atus,* to work, fr. *opus,* work]

OPERATION

op·er·a·tion (op-er-ā'shŭn). **1.** Any surgical procedure. **2.** The act, manner, or process of functioning. SEE ALSO method, procedure, technique.

Abbe o., use of an Abbe flap in plastic surgery of the lips.

Arie-Pitanguy o., a procedure to reduce a large breast by a lozenge-shaped resection of tissue from its inferior pole. SYN Arie-Pitanguy mammaplasty.

Arlt's o., transplantation of the eyelashes back from the edge of the lid in trichiasis.

arterial switch o., o. for complete transposition of the great arteries; the most common way to repair this defect consists of switching the aorta and pulmonary arteries and implanting the coronary arteries into the neoaorta (the original pulmonary artery).

Baldy's o., an obsolete o. for retrodisplacement of the uterus, consisting of bringing the round ligaments through the perforated broad ligaments and attaching them to each other and to the back of the uterus. SYN Webster's o.

Ball's o., division of the sensory nerve trunks supplying the anus, for relief of pruritus ani.

Barkan's o., goniotomy for congenital glaucoma under direct observation of the anterior chamber angle.

Bassini's o., an o. for an inguinal hernia repair; after reduction of the hernia, the sac is twisted, ligated, and cut off, then a new inguinal canal is made by uniting the edge of the internal oblique muscle to the inguinal ligament, placing on this the cord, and covering the latter by the external oblique muscle.

Baudelocque's o., an incision through the posterior cul-de-sac of the vagina for the removal of the ovum, in extrauterine pregnancy.

Belsey Mark IV o., a transthoracic anti-reflux procedure; it restores a 3 to 4 cm length of intraabdominal esophagus, maintains a narrow diameter of the distal esophagus by a gastric fundoplication.

Billroth's o. I, excision of the pylorus with end-to-end anastomosis of stomach and duodenum. SYN Billroth I anastomosis.

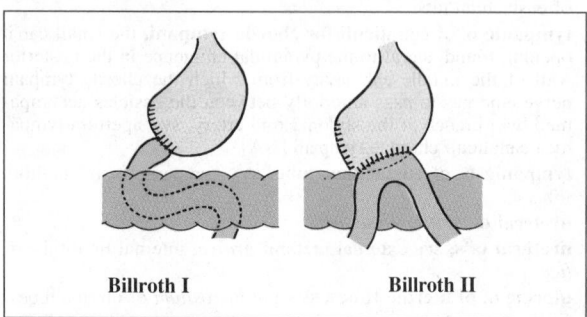

Billroth I   Billroth II

Billroth's o. II, resection of the pylorus with the greater part of the lesser curvature of the stomach, closure of the cut ends of the duodenum and stomach, followed by a gastrojejunostomy. SYN Billroth II anastomosis.

Blalock-Hanlon o., the creation of a large atrial septal defect as a palliative procedure for complete transposition of the great arteries.

Blalock-Taussig o., an o. for congenital malformations of the heart, in which an abnormally small volume of blood passes through the pulmonary circuit; blood from the systemic circulation is directed to the lungs by anastomosing the right or left subclavian artery to the right or left pulmonary artery.

bloodless o., an o. performed with negligible loss of blood.

Bozeman's o., an o. for uterovaginal fistula, the cervix uteri being attached to the bladder and opening into its cavity.

Bricker o., an o. utilizing an isolated segment of ileum to collect urine from the ureters and conduct it to the skin surface.

Brock o., transventricular valvotomy for relief of pulmonic valvar stenosis. Obsolete procedure.

Brunschwig's o., SYN total pelvic *exenteration*.

Burow's o., an o. in which triangles of skin adjacent to a sliding flap are excised to facilitate movement of the flap.

Caldwell-Luc o., an intraoral procedure for opening into the maxillary antrum through the supradental (canine) fossa above the maxillary premolar teeth. SYN intraoral antrostomy, Luc's o.

capital o., obsolete term for an o. of such magnitude or involving vital organs to such an extent that it is *per se* dangerous to life.

Carmody-Batson o., reduction of fractures of the zygoma and zygomatic arch through an intraoral incision above the maxillary molar teeth.

Caslick's o., an o. for the correction of faulty conformation of the vulva of the mare, a frequent cause of low-grade vaginitis and infertility; consists of surgical closure of the dorsal portion of the vulva.

cesarean o., SEE cesarean *section*, cesarean *hysterectomy*.

commando o., SYN commando *procedure*.

concrete o.'s, in the psychology of Piaget, a stage of development in thinking, occurring approximately between 7 and 11 years of age, during which a child becomes capable of reasoning about concrete situations.

Cotte's o., SYN presacral *neurectomy*.

Dana's o., SYN posterior *rhizotomy*.

Dandy o., SEE third *ventriculostomy*, trigeminal *rhizotomy*.

Daviel's o., extracapsular cataract extraction.

debulking o., excision of a major part of a malignant tumor which cannot be completely removed, so as to enhance the effectiveness of subsequent radio- or chemotherapy.

decompression o.'s, SEE decompression.

Doyle's o., paracervical uterine denervation.

Dupuy-Dutemps o., a modified dacryocystorhinostomy for stenosis of the lacrimal duct.

Elliot's o., trephining of the eyeball at the corneoscleral margin to relieve tension in glaucoma.

Emmet's o., SYN trachelorrhaphy.

Esser o., SEE inlay *graft*.

Estes o., an o. for sterility in which a portion of an ovary is implanted on one uterine cornu.

Estlander o., use of an Estlander flap in plastic surgery of the lips.

fenestration o., a rarely used surgical procedure producing an opening from the external auditory canal to the membranous labyrinth to improve hearing in hearing impairment of the conduction type.

Filatov's o., obsolete eponym for penetrating *keratoplasty*.

filtering o., a surgical procedure for creation of a fistula between the anterior chamber of the eye and the subconjunctival space in treatment of glaucoma.

Finney's o., gastroduodenostomy which creates, by the technique of closure, a large opening to insure free emptying from the stomach.

flap o., (1) SYN flap *amputation*. (2) in dental surgery, an o. in which a portion of the mucoperiosteal tissues is surgically detached from the underlying bone or impacted tooth for better access and visibility in exploring the area covered by the tissue. SEE ALSO flap.

Foley o., SYN Foley Y-plasty *pyeloplasty*.

Fontan o., SYN Fontan *procedure*.

formal o.'s, in the psychology of Piaget, a stage of development in thinking, occurring approximately between 11 and 15 years of age, during which a child becomes capable of reasoning about abstract situations; reasoning at this stage is comparable to that of normal adults but less sophisticated.

Fothergill's o., SYN Manchester o.

Frazier-Spiller o., SEE trigeminal *rhizotomy*.

Fredet-Ramstedt o., SYN pyloromyotomy.

Freund's o., (1) total abdominal hysterectomy for uterine cancer; (2) chondrotomy to relieve Freund's anomaly.

Gigli's o., SYN pubiotomy.

Gilliam's o., an o. for retroversion of the uterus by suturing round ligaments to abdominal wall fascia.

Gillies' o., a technique for reducing fractures of the zygoma and the zygomatic arch through an incision in the temporal region above the hairline.

Gil-Vernet o., SYN extended *pyelotomy*.

op

Glenn's o., anastomosis between the superior vena cava and the right main pulmonary artery to increase pulmonary blood flow as a palliative correction for tricuspid atresia.

Graefe's o., (1) removal of cataract by a limbal incision with capsulotomy and iridectomy. Both operations were landmarks in the field of ophthalmic surgery; (2) iridectomy for glaucoma.

Gritti's o., SYN Gritti-Stokes *amputation.*

Halsted's o., (1) an o. for the radical correction of inguinal hernia; (2) SYN radical *mastectomy.*

Hartmann's o., resection of the rectosigmoid colon beginning at or just above the peritoneal reflexion and extending proximally, with closure of the rectal stump and end-colostomy.

Heaney's o., technique for vaginal hysterectomy.

Heller o., esophagomyotomy at the gastro-esophageal region.

Hill o., repair of hiatus hernia; narrowing the esophagogastric junction and attaching it to the right medial arcuate ligament.

Hoffa's o., in congenital dislocation of the hip, hollowing out the acetabulum and reduction of the head of the femur after severing the muscles inserted into the upper portion of the bone.

Hofmeister's o., partial gastrectomy with closure of a portion of the lesser curvature and retrocolic anastomosis of the remainder to jejunum.

Huggins' o., orchidectomy performed for palliation or cure of cancer of the prostate. SYN castration (1).

Hummelsheim's o., transplantation of a normal ocular rectus muscle, to substitute for a paralyzed muscle.

Hunter's o., ligation of the artery proximal and distal to an aneurysm.

Indian o., SYN Indian *rhinoplasty.*

interval o., an o. performed during a period of quiescence or of intermission in the condition necessitating surgery.

Italian o., SYN Italian *rhinoplasty.*

Jacobaeus o., obsolete term for pleurolysis.

Jansen's o., an o. for frontal sinus disease, the lower wall and lower portion of the anterior wall being removed and the mucous membrane curetted away.

Kasai o., SYN portoenterostomy.

Kazanjian's o., surgical extension of the vestibular sulcus of edentulous ridges to increase their height and to improve denture retention. SEE ALSO ridge *extension.*

Keen's o., removal of sections of the posterior branches of the spinal nerves to the affected muscles, and of the spinal accessory nerve, as a cure for torticollis.

Keller-Madlener o., an o. for treatment of gastric ulcer located in the proximal cardia that involves 75% gastrectomy and gastro-jejunostomy.

Kelly's o., (1) correction of retroversion of the uterus by plication of uterosacral ligaments; (2) correction of urinary stress incontinence by vaginally placing sutures beneath the bladder neck.

Killian's o., an o. for frontal sinus disease in which the entire anterior wall is removed and the mucous membrane is curetted away; the ethmoid cells are scraped out through an opening in the nasal process of the maxillary bone, and the upper wall of the orbit is removed as well.

Koerte-Ballance o., operative anastomosis of the facial and hypoglossal nerves for the treatment of facial paralysis.

Kondoleon o., excision of strips of subcutaneous connective tissue for the relief of elephantiasis.

Kraske's o., removal of the coccyx and excision of the left wing of the sacrum in order to afford approach for resection of the rectum for cancer or stenosis.

Krönlein o., orbital decompression through the anterior lateral wall of the orbit.

Ladd's o., division of Ladd's band to relieve duodenal obstruction in malrotation of the intestine.

Lambrinudi o., a form of triple arthrodesis done in such a manner as to prevent foot drop, usually as occurs in poliomyelitis.

Laroyenne's o., puncture of Douglas pouch to evacuate the pus and to secure drainage in cases of pelvic suppuration.

Lash's o., removal of a wedge of the internal cervical os with suturing of the internal os into a tighter canal structure.

LeCompte o., SYN LeCompte *maneuver.*

Leriche's o., SYN periarterial *sympathectomy.*

Lisfranc's o., SYN Lisfranc's *amputation.*

Longmire's o., intrahepatic cholangiojejunostomy with partial hepatectomy for biliary obstruction.

Luc's o., SYN Caldwell-Luc o.

Madlener o., tubal sterilization by clamp and tie.

major o., an extensive, relatively difficult surgical procedure involving vital organs and/or in itself hazardous to life.

Manchester o., a vaginal o. for prolapse of the uterus, consisting of cervical amputation and parametrial fixation (cardinal ligaments) anterior to the uterus. SYN Fothergill's o. [*Manchester, England*]

Mann-Williamson o., an o. performed on experimental animals (dogs) in research on peptic ulcer, the duodenum with its alkaline secretions being transplanted into the ileum and the cut end of the jejunum anastomosed to the pylorus; the animals develop ulcers in the jejunum which directly receives the gastric juice.

Marshall-Marchetti-Krantz o., an o. for urinary stress incontinence, performed retropubically.

Mason o., SYN gastric *bypass.*

Matas' o., obsolete term for aneurysmoplasty.

Mayo's o., an o. for the radical cure of umbilical hernia; the neck of the sac is exposed by two elliptical incisions, the gut is returned to the abdomen, the sac and adherent omentum are cut away, and the fascial edges of the opening are overlapped with mattress sutures.

McIndoe o., o. for the development of a neovagina using a split thickness skin graft over a vaginal mold.

McVay's o., repair of inguinal and femoral hernias by suture of the transversus abdominis muscle and its associated fasciae (transversus layer) to the pectineal ligament.

mika o., the establishment of a permanent fistula in the bulbous portions of the urethra in order to render the man incapable of procreating; said to be a practice among certain Australian aborigines. [Australian native term]

Mikulicz' o., excision of bowel in two stages: 1) exteriorizing the diseased area, suturing efferent and afferent limbs together, and closing the abdomen around them, after which the diseased part is excised; 2) at a later time, cutting the spur with an enterotome and closing the stoma extraperitoneally.

Miles' o., combined abdominoperineal resection for carcinoma of the rectum. SYN Miles resection.

minor o., a surgical procedure of relatively slight extent and not in itself hazardous to life.

morcellation o., vaginal hysterectomy in which the uterus is removed in multiple pieces after being split or partitioned.

Motais' o., transplantation of the middle third of the tendon of the superior rectus muscle of the eyeball into the upper lid, between the tarsus and skin, to supplement the action of the levator muscle in ptosis.

Mules' o., evisceration of the eyeball followed by the insertion within the sclera of a spherical prosthesis to support an artificial eye.

Mustard o., correction, at the atrial level, of hemodynamic abnormality due to transposition of the great arteries by an intraatrial baffle to direct pulmonary venous blood through the tricuspid orifice into the right ventricle and the systemic venous blood through the mitral valve into the left ventricle. SYN Mustard procedure.

Naffziger o., orbital decompression for severe malignant exophthalmos by removal of the lateral and superior orbital walls.

Nissen's o., SYN fundoplication.

Norton's o., extraperitoneal cesarean section by a paravesical approach.

Norwood's o., in infants with subaortic stenosis and tricuspid atresia; the pulmonary artery is divided and both ends are attached to the aorta, the distal end via a prosthetic graft.

Ogston-Luc o., an o. for frontal sinus disease; a skin incision is made from the inner third of the edge of the orbit toward the root of the nose or outward; the periosteum is pushed upward and outward, and the sinus is opened on the outer side of the median line; then a wide opening is made by curetting the nasofrontal duct, interior of the sinus, and anterior ethmoid cells.

Ogura o., orbital decompression by removal of the floor of the orbit through an opening made in the supradental (canine) fossa.

Ombrédanne o., a technique whereby the mobilized testis is brought down into the scrotum and through the scrotal septum, to be affixed to the tissues in the contralateral scrotal pouch. SYN transseptal orchiopexy.

Payne o., a jejunoileal bypass for morbid obesity utilizing end-to-side anastomosis of the upper jejunum to the terminal ileum, with closure of the proximal end of the bypassed intestine.

plastic o., SEE plastic *surgery*.

Pólya's o., SYN Pólya *gastrectomy*.

Pomeroy's o., excision of a ligated portion of the fallopian tubes.

Porro o., SYN cesarean *hysterectomy*.

Potts' o., direct side-to-side anastomosis between aorta and pulmonary artery as a palliative procedure in congenital malformation of the heart. SYN Potts' *anastomosis*.

pubovaginal o., operative procedure for urinary incontinence. A strip of tissue, usually autologous rectus abdominis fascia, is used to suspend or elevate bladder neck and posterior urethra toward pubic symphysis.

Putti-Platt o., a procedure for recurrent dislocation of shoulder joint. SYN Putti-Platt procedure.

radical o. for hernia, an o. by which the hernia is not only reduced, but the hernial defect is also repaired.

Ramstedt o., SYN pyloromyotomy.

Rastelli's o., an o. for transposition of the great arteries plus ventricular septal defect and LV outflow obstruction; employs an intraventricular tunnel repair and a rerouting valved extracardiac conduit.

Rastelli's o., for "anatomic" repair of transposition of the great arteries (ventriculoarterial discordance) with ventricular septal defect and left ventricular outflow tract obstruction; conduits are used to create left ventricular to aortic continuity and right ventricular to pulmonary artery continuity. All septal defects are obliterated as are any previously constructed palliative shunts.

Récamier's o., curettage of the uterus.

Ridell's o., removal of the entire anterior and inferior walls of the frontal sinus, for chronic inflammation of that cavity.

Roux-en-Y o., anastomosis of the distal end of the divided upper jejunum to the stomach, esophagus, biliary tract, or other structure and anastomosis of the proximal end to the side of the jejunum a little further distal.

Saenger's o., cesarean section followed by careful closure of the uterine wound by three tiers of sutures.

Schauta vaginal o., an extensive extirpation of the uterus and the adnexa, using the vaginal approach facilitated by Schuchardt's o.

Schönbein's o., the use of a flap of mucous membrane from the posterior wall of the pharynx to the soft palate closing off the flow of air from the nose to the mouth.

Schroeder's o., excision of diseased endocervical mucosa.

Schuchardt's o., a paravaginal rectal displacement incision, a surgical technique of making the upper vagina accessible for fistula closure or radical surgery via the vagina.

scleral buckling o., an o. performed in retinal detachment to indent the sclerochoroidal wall.

Scott o., a jejunoileal bypass for morbid obesity utilizing end-to-end anastomosis of the upper jejunum to the terminal ileum, with the bypassed intestine closed proximally and anastomosed distally to the colon.

second-look o., exploratory celiotomy within a year after apparently curative resection of intra-abdominal cancer, in patients with no sign or symptom of recurrence, to resect an occult tumor if present.

Senning o., an atrial switch o. for patients with transposition of the great arteries that employs a septal flap instead of excising the atrial septum as in the Mustard o., thus minimizing foreign material and allowing for growth.

seton o., an o. for advanced glaucoma; passage of a tube or seton into the anterior chamber to act as a wick.

Shirodkar o., a cerclage procedure done by purse-string suturing of an incompetent cervical os with a nonabsorbent suture material.

Sistrunk o., excision of the thyroglossal cyst and duct including the midportion of the hyoid bone through, or near, which the duct traverses.

Smith-Boyce o., SYN anatrophic *nephrotomy*.

Smith-Indian o., a surgical technique for removal of cataract within the capsule. SYN Smith's o.

Smith-Robinson o., interbody spinal fusion through an anterior cervical approach.

Smith's o., SYN Smith-Indian o.

Soave o., endorectal pull-through for treatment of congenital megacolon.

Spinelli o., an o. splitting the anterior wall of the prolapsed uterus and reversing the organ preliminary to reduction.

stapes mobilization o., now infrequently used o. involving fracture of tissue immobilizing the stapes to restore hearing; especially used in patients with otosclerosis.

Stoffel's o., division of certain motor nerves for the relief of spastic paralysis.

Stookey-Scarff o., SEE third *ventriculostomy*.

Sturmdorf's o., conical removal of the endocervix.

subcutaneous o., an o., as for the division of a tendon, performed without incising the skin other than by a minute opening made by the entering knife.

Syme's o., SYN Syme's *amputation*.

tagliacotian o., SYN Italian *rhinoplasty*.

talc o., an obsolete o. in which magnesium silicate (talc) powder is applied to the epicardium to create a sterile granulomatous pericarditis and thus promote pericardial anastomoses with the coronary circulation. SYN poudrage (2).

TeLinde o., SYN modified radical *hysterectomy*.

Thiersch's o., the application of a partial thickness skin graft. SYN Thiersch's graft o.

Thiersch's graft o., SYN Thiersch's o.

Torek o., a two-stage o. for bringing down an undescended testicle.

Trendelenburg's o., a pulmonary embolectomy.

Urban's o., extended radical mastectomy, including *en bloc* resection of internal mammary lymph nodes, part of the sternum, and costal cartilages.

Waters' o., an extraperitoneal cesarean section with a supravesical approach.

Waterston o., a surgically created anastomosis between the pulmonary artery and the ascending aorta to palliate adult tetralogy of Fallot.

Webster's o., SYN Baldy's o.

Weir's o., obsolete eponym for appendicostomy.

Wertheim's o., a radical o. for carcinoma of the uterus in which as much as possible of the vagina is excised and there is wide lymph node excision.

Wheelhouse's o., obsolete term for external *urethrotomy*.

Whipple's o., SYN pancreatoduodenectomy.

Whitehead's o., excision of hemorrhoids by two circular incisions above and below involved veins, allowing normal mucosa to be pulled down and sutured to anal skin.

op·er·a·tive (op'er-ă-tiv). **1.** Relating to, or effected by means of an operation. **2.** Active or effective.

op·er·a·tor (op'er-ā-tor). **1.** One who performs an operation or operates equipment. **2.** In genetics, a sequence of DNA that interacts with a repressor of operon to control the expression of adjacent structural genes. SEE operator *gene*. **3.** A symbol representing a mathematical operation. [L. worker, fr *operor*, to work]

oper·cu·lar (ō-per'kyū-lăr). Relating to an operculum.

oper·cu·lat·ed (ō-per'kyū-lā-ted). Provided with a lid (operculum); denoting members of the mollusk class Gastropoda (the snails), subclass Prosobranchiata (operculate snails), and the eggs of certain parasitic worms such as the digenetic trematodes (except the schistosomes) and the broad fish tapeworm, *Diphyllobotrium latum*.

oper·cu·li·tis (ō-perk-yū-lī'tis). Originating under an operculum. [operculum + G. -*itis*, inflammation]

oper·cu·lum, gen. **oper·cu·li**, pl. **oper·cu·la** (ō-per'kyū-lŭm, -lī, -lă). **1.** Anything resembling a lid or cover. **2** [NA]. In anatomy, the portions of the frontal, parietal, and temporal lobes bordering the lateral sulcus and covering the insula. **3.** Mucus sealing the endocervical canal of the uterus after conception has taken place. **4.** In parasitology, the lid or caplike cover of the shell opening of operculated freshwater snails in the subclass Prosobranchiata, and of the eggs of certain trematode and cestode parasites. **5.** The attached flap in the tear of retinal detachment. **6.** The mucosal flap partially or completely covering an unerupted tooth. [L. cover or lid, fr. *operio*, pp. *opertus*, to cover]
o. il'ei, SYN ileal *sphincter.*

occipital o., a portion of the occipital lobe of the brain demarcated by the simian fissure (*sulcus* lunatus cerebri) when present in humans.

trophoblastic o., the mushroom-shaped plug of fibrin that fills the aperture in the endometrium made by the implanting ovum.

op·er·on (op'er-on). A genetic functional unit that controls production of a messenger RNA; it consists of an operator gene and two or more structural genes located in sequence in the *cis* position on one chromosome. [L. *operor*, to work, act, + -on]

Lac o., a collection of adjacent bacterial genes responsible for the entry and metabolism of lactose; contains the genes coding for three enzymes and is flanked by a repressor and a promoter region to control expression.

ophi·a·sis (ō-fī'ă-sis). A form of alopecia areata in which the loss of hair occurs in bands along the scalp margin partially or completely encircling the head. [G., fr. *ophis*, snake]

Ophid·ia (ō-fid'ē-ă). The snakes, a suborder of the class Reptilia, including the families Colubridae, Crotalidae, Elapidae, Hydrophyidae, and Viperidae. [G. *ophidion*, dim. of *ophis*, a serpent]

ophi·di·a·sis (ō'fi-dī'ă-sis). Poisoning by a snake. SYN ophidism. [G. *ophidion*, dim. of *ophis*, a serpent]

ophid·i·o·pho·bia (ō-fid'ē-ō-fō'bē-ă). Morbid fear of snakes. [G. *ophidion*, a small snake, + *phobos*, fear]

ophid·ism (ō'fid-izm). SYN ophidiasis.

oph·ri·tis (of-rī'tis). Dermatitis in the region of the eyebrows. SYN ophryitis. [G. *ophrys*, eyebrow, + -*itis*, inflammation]

oph·ry·i·tis (of-rē-ī'tis). SYN ophritis.

oph·ry·og·e·nes (of'rē-yō-jen-'enz). Related to the eyebrows. [Mod. L., fr. G. *ophrys*, eyebrow, + suffix -*genēs*, arising from]

oph·ry·on (of'rē-on). The point on the midline of the forehead just above the glabella (1). SYN supranasal point, supraorbital point. [G. *ophrys*, eyebrow]

Oph·ry·o·sco·lec·i·dae (of'rē-ō-skō-les'i-dē). A family of ciliate protozoa occurring in the rumen and reticulum of ruminant animals, characterized by having cilia arranged in spiral membranelles around the mouth (adoral) and in some genera also in a dorsal (metoral) position. The most important genera are *Entodinium*, *Diplodinium*, *Epidinium*, and *Ophryoscolex*, which are thought to contribute to ruminant nutrition by converting cellulose in plant material ingested by the ruminant into readily digestible animal protein of their own bodies. [G. *ophrys*, eyebrow, + *skōlēx*, a worm]

oph·ry·o·sis (of-rē-ō'sis). Spasmodic twitching of the upper portion of the orbicularis palpebrarum muscle causing a wrinkling of the eyebrow. [G. *ophrys*, eyebrow, + -*osis*, condition]

ophthalm-. SEE ophthalmo-.

ophthalmalgia (of'thal-mal'jē-ă). SYN oculodynia. [ophthalmo- + G. *algos*, pain]

oph·thal·mia (of-thal'mē-ă). **1.** Severe, often purulent, conjunctivitis. **2.** Inflammation of the deeper structures of the eye. [G.]

catarrhal o., a mild form of conjunctivitis with mucopurulent secretion.

caterpillar-hair o., SYN o. nodosa.

o. eczemato'sa, obsolete term for phlyctenular *conjunctivitis.*

Egyptian o., SYN trachoma.

gonorrheal o., acute purulent conjunctivitis excited by *Neisseria gonorrhoeae*. SYN blennophthalmia (2), blennorrhea conjunctivalis, gonorrheal conjunctivitis.

granular o., SYN trachoma.

infectious o., SYN infectious bovine *keratoconjunctivitis.*

metastatic o., **(1)** sympathetic o; **(2)** choroiditis in septicemia.

o. neonato'rum, a conjunctival inflammation occurring within the first 10 days of life; causes include *Neisseria gonorrhoeae*, *Staphylococcus*, *Streptococcus pneumoniae*, and *Chlamydia trachomatis*. SYN blennorrhea neonatorum, infantile purulent conjunctivitis, neonatal conjunctivitis.

o. niva'lis, SYN ultraviolet *keratoconjunctivitis.*

o. nodo'sa, the presence of nodular swellings on the conjunctiva, due to penetration of ocular tissues by the hairs of caterpillars. SYN caterpillar-hair o.

periodic o., an acute iridocyclitis of horses, involving one or both eyes; it subsides only to recur at intervals of varying length and usually ends in blindness; the cause is uncertain but some have associated it with leptospires; does not appear to be contagious. SYN moon blindness.

phlyctenular o., SYN phlyctenular *conjunctivitis.*

purulent o., purulent conjunctivitis, usually of gonorrheal origin.

spring o., SYN vernal *conjunctivitis.*

sympathetic o., a serous or plastic uveitis caused by a perforating wound of the uvea followed by a similar severe reaction in the other eye that may lead to bilateral blindness. SYN transferred o.

transferred o., SYN sympathetic o.

oph·thal·mic (of-thal'mik). Relating to the eye. SYN ocular (1). [G. *ophthalmikos*]

oph·thal·mic ac·id. A tripeptide occurring in lens, similar to glutathione but differing in the replacement of cysteine by α-amino-*n*-butyric acid (*i.e.*, in the replacement of –SH by –CH₃); a potent inhibitor of glyoxalase. Cf. norophthalmic acid.

ophthalmo-, ophthalm-. Relationship to the eye. SEE ALSO oculo-. [G. *ophthalmos*]

oph·thal·mo·dy·na·mom·e·ter (of-thal'mō-dī-nă-mom'ĕ-ter). An instrument to measure the blood pressure in the retinal vessels. [ophthalmo- + G. *dynamis*, power, + *metron*, measure]

Bailliart's o., an instrument used to measure the blood pressure of the central retinal artery; of value in diagnosing occlusion of the proximal carotid artery.

suction o., an o. with a suction disk which increases ocular pressure during ophthalmoscopic observation of the retinal artery.

oph·thal·mo·dy·na·mom·e·try (of-thal'mō-dī-nă-mom'ĕ-trē). The measurement of blood pressure in the retinal vessels by means of an ophthalmodynamometer. [ophthalmo- + G. *dynamis*, power, + *metron*, measure]

oph·thal·mo·lith (of-thal'mō-lith). SYN dacryolith. [ophthalmo- + G. *lithos*, stone]

oph·thal·mol·o·gist (of-thal-mol'ō-jist). A specialist in ophthalmology. SYN oculist.

oph·thal·mol·o·gy (of-thal-mol'ō-jē). The medical specialty concerned with the eye, its diseases, and refractive errors. [ophthalmo- + G. *logos*, study]

oph·thal·mo·ma·la·cia (of-thal'mō-mă-lā'shē-ă). Abnormal softening of the eyeball. [ophthalmo- + G. *malakia*, softness]

oph·thal·mo·mel·a·no·sis (of-thal'mō-mel-ă-nō'sis). Melanotic discoloration of the conjunctiva and adjoining tissues.

oph·thal·mom·e·ter (of-thal-mom'ĕ-ter). SYN keratometer. [ophthalmo- + G. *metron*, measure]

oph·thal·mo·my·co·sis (of-thal'mō-mī-kō'sis). Any disease of the eye or its appendages caused by a fungus. [ophthalmo- + G. *mykēs*, fungus, + -*osis*, condition]

op

oph·thal·mo·my·i·a·sis (of-thal′mō-mī-ī′ă-sis). SYN ocular *myiasis*.

oph·thal·mop·a·thy (of-thal-mop′ă-thē). Any disease of the eyes. SYN oculopathy. [ophthalmo- + G. *pathos,* suffering]

endocrine o., SYN Graves' o.

external o., any disease of the conjunctiva, cornea, or adnexa of the eye.

Graves' o., exophthalmos caused by increased water content of retro-ocular orbital tissues; associated with thyroid disease, usually hyperthyroidism. SYN endocrine o., Graves' orbitopathy.

internal o., any disease of the internal structures of the eyeball.

oph·thal·mo·ple·gia (of-thal-mō-plē′jē-ă). Paralysis of one or more of the ocular muscles. [ophthalmo- + G. *plēgē,* stroke]

chronic progressive external o., a specific type of slowly worsening weakness of the ocular muscles, usually associated with a pigmentary retinopathy. SEE Kearns-Sayre *syndrome,* oculopharyngeal *dystrophy.* SYN ocular myopathy.

exophthalmic o., o. with protrusion of the eyeballs due to increased water content of orbital tissues incidental to thyroid disorders, usually hyperthyroidism.

o. exter′na, paralysis affecting one or more of the extrinsic eye muscles. SYN external o.

external o., SYN o. externa.

fascicular o., o. due to a lesion within the brainstem.

fibrotic o. [MIM*135700], o. that may be congenital in association with blepharoptosis in and autosomal dominant disorder.

o. inter′na, paralysis affecting only the sphincter muscle of the pupil and the ciliary muscle. SYN internal o.

internal o., SYN o. interna.

o. internuclea′ris, o. in lesions of the medial longitudinal fasciculus, with failure of adduction in horizontal gaze but with retention of convergence.

nuclear o., o. due to a lesion of the nuclei of origin of the motor nerves of the eye.

orbital o., o. due to a lesion within the orbit.

Parinaud's o., SYN Parinaud's *syndrome.*

o. partia′lis, incomplete o. involving only one or two of the extrinsic or intrinsic ocular muscles.

o. progressi′va, progressive upper bulbar palsy, due to degeneration of the nuclei of the motor nerves of the eye.

o. tota′lis, paralysis of both the extrinsic and intrinsic ocular muscles.

oph·thal·mo·ple·gic (of-thal-mō-plē′jik). Relating to or marked by ophthalmoplegia.

oph·thal·mo·scope (of-thal′mō-skōp). A device for studying the interior of the eyeball through the pupil. SYN funduscope. [ophthalmo- + G. *skopeō,* to examine]

binocular o., an o. that provides a stereoscopic view of the fundus.

demonstration o., an o. by which the fundus may be seen simultaneously by more than one observer.

direct o., an instrument designed to visualize the interior of the eye, with the instrument relatively close to the subject's eye and the observer viewing an upright magnified image.

indirect o., an instrument designed to visualize the interior of the eye, with the instrument at arm's length from the subject's eye and the observer viewing an inverted image through a convex lens located between the instrument and the subject's eye.

oph·thal·mo·scop·ic (of′thal-mō-skop′ik). Relating to examination of the interior of the eye.

oph·thal·mos·co·py (of-thal-mos′kŏ-pē). Examination of the fundus of the eye by means of the ophthalmoscope. SYN funduscopy.

direct o., o. performed with a direct ophthalmoscope.

indirect o., o. performed with an indirect ophthalmoscope.

o. with reflected light, examination of that part of the fundus adjacent to an area illuminated by a sharply focused light.

oph·thal·mo·trope (of-thal′mō-trōp). A model of the two eyes, to each of which are attached weighted cords pulling in the direction of the six extrinsic eye muscles; used to demonstrate

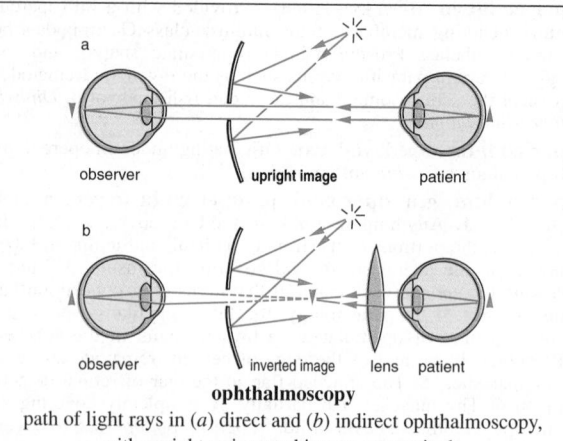

ophthalmoscopy
path of light rays in (*a*) direct and (*b*) indirect ophthalmoscopy, with upright or inverted image, respectively

the action of the ocular muscles singly or in various combinations. [ophthalmo- + G. *tropos,* a turning]

oph·thal·mo·vas·cu·lar (of-thal′mō-vas′kyū-lăr). Relating to the blood vessels of the eye.

-opia. Vision. [G. *ōps,* eye]

opi·a·nine (ō-pī′ă-nēn). SYN noscapine.

opi·a·nyl (ō′pī-ă-nil). SYN meconin.

opi·ate (ō′pē-āt). Any preparation or derivative of opium.

opine (ō′pēn). A derivative of basic amino acids, produced by crown-gall tumors in plants.

opi·oid (ō′pē-oyd). Originally, a term denoting synthetic narcotics resembling opiates but increasingly used to refer to both opiates and synthetic narcotics.

opi·o·mel·a·no·cor·tin (ō′pē-ō-mel′ă-nō-kōr′tin). A linear polypeptide of the pituitary gland that contains in its sequence the sequences of endorphins, MSH, ACTH, and the like, which are split off enzymically; the nucleotide sequences coding has been determined for several species.

opip·ra·mol hy·dro·chlo·ride (ō-pip′ră-mōl). 4-[3-(5*H*-Dibenz[*b.f*]azepin-5-yl)propyl]-1-piperazineethanol dihydrochloride; an antidepressant agent.

opis·the·nar (ō-pis′thē-nar). Dorsum of the hand. [G. back of the hand, from *opisthen,* behind, + *thenar,* palm of the hand]

opis·thi·o·ba·si·al (ō-pis′thē-ō-bā′sē-ăl). Relating to both opisthion and basion; denoting a line connecting the two, or the distance between them.

opis·thi·on (ō-pis′thē-on) [NA]. The middle point on the posterior margin of the foramen magnum, opposite the basion. [G. *opisthios,* posterior]

opis·thi·o·na·si·al (ō-pis′thē-ō-nā′zē-ăl). Relating to the opisthion and the nasion; denoting the distance between the two points.

opistho-. Backward, behind, dorsal. [G. *opisthen,* at the rear, behind]

op·is·tho·chei·lia, op·is·tho·chi·lia (op′is-thō-kī′lē-ă). Recession of the lips. [opistho- + G. *cheilos,* lip]

opis·tho·mas·ti·gote (ō-pis-thō-mas′ti-gōt). Term now used instead of herpetomonad for the stage of development of certain insect and plant parasitizing flagellates to avoid confusion between the stage and the genus *Herpetomonas.* In this stage the flagellum arises from the kinetoplast located behind the nucleus and emerges from the anterior end of the organism; an undulating membrane is absent. [opistho- + G. *mastix,* whip]

opis·tho·po·reia (ō-pis′thō-pō-rī′ă, -rē′ă). Involuntary backward gait; frequently connected with parkinsonism. [opistho- + G. *poreia,* a walking, fr. *poreuō,* to go, walk]

op·is·thor·chi·a·sis (op′is-thōr-kī′ă-sis). Infection with the Asiatic liver fluke, *Opisthorchis viverrini,* or other opisthorchids.

op·is·thor·chid (op-is-thōr′kid). Common name for members of the family Opisthorchiidae.

Opis·thor·chi·i·dae (op′is-thōr-kē′i-dē). A family of trematodes that includes the genera *Opisthorchis* and *Clonorchis*.

Opis·thor·chis (op-is-thōr′kis). Genus of digenetic trematodes (family Opisthorchiidae) found in the bile ducts or gallbladder of fish-eating mammals, birds, and fish. [opistho- + G. *orchis*, testis]

O. felin′eus, the cat liver fluke, a species frequently found as a parasite of man in Eastern Europe, Siberia, India, Japan, and Southeast Asia; adults are lancet-shaped, thin, relatively transparent, and hermaphroditic, with sizes ranging from 7 to 12 by 2 to 3 mm; ingested eggs hatch in *Bithynia* snails, and cercariae encyst on various species of freshwater fish; man acquires the infection by ingesting raw or inadequately cooked fish; the parasites sometimes cause no evidence of disease, but cholangitis, biliary cirrhosis, and chronic pancreatitis may occur.

O. sinen′sis, SYN *Clonorchis sinensis.*

O. viverri′ni, a species closely related to *O. felineus,* very common in man in Thailand; causes opisthorchiasis.

op·is·thotic (op-is-thō′tik). Behind the ear. [opistho- + G. *ous* (ōt-), ear]

op·is·thot·on·ic (op-is-thot′ō-nik, ō-pis′thō-ton′ik). Relating to or characterized by opisthotonos.

op·is·thot·o·noid (op-is-thot′ō-noyd). Resembling opisthotonos.

op·is·thot·o·nos, op·is·thot·o·nus (op-is-thot′ō-nŭs). A tetanic spasm in which the spine and extremities are bent with convexity forward, the body resting on the head and the heels. SYN tetanus dorsalis, tetanus posticus. [opistho- + G. *tonos,* tension, stretching]

Opitz, John M., U.S. pediatrician, *1935. SEE Smith-Lemli-O. *syndrome.*

opi·um (ō′pē-ŭm). The air-dried milky exudation obtained by incising the unripe capsules of *Papaver somniferum* (family Papveraceae) or its variety, *P. album.* Contains some 20 alkaloids, including morphine, 9 to 16%; noscapine, 4 to 8%; codeine, 0.8 to 2.5%; papaverine, 0.5 to 2.5%; and thebaine, 0.5 to 2%. Used as an analgesic, hypnotic, and diaphoretic, and in diarrhea and spasmodic conditions. SYN gum opium, meconium (2). [L. fr. G. *opion,* poppy-juice]

Boston o., o. so diluted after importation as barely to meet the official requirements. SYN pudding o.

deodorized o., denarcotized o., powdered o. treated with purified petroleum benzine which removes certain nauseating and odorous constituents.

granulated o., o. dried and reduced to a coarse powder; it contains 10 to 10.5% anhydrous morphine.

powdered o., dried and finely powdered o. containing 10% morphine.

pudding o., SYN Boston o.

⚠**opo-.** The face; an eye. SEE ALSO fascio-. 2. Juice, balm. [G. *ōps*]

op·o·bal·sa·mum (op-ō-bal′sa-mŭm). SYN *balm* of Gilead. [G. *opobalsamon,* the juice of the balsam tree, fr. *opos,* juice, + *balsamon*]

op·o·did·y·mus (op-ō-did′i-mŭs). Conjoined twins with a single body having two heads fused at the back with partially separated facial regions. SEE conjoined *twins,* under *twin.* [G. *ōps,* eye, face, + *didymos,* twin]

Oppenheim, Hermann, Berlin neurologist, 1858–1919. SEE O.'s *disease, reflex, syndrome;* Ziehen-O. *disease.*

op·pi·la·tion (op-i-lā′shŭn). Obstruction or closing of the pores. [L. *oppilatio,* fr. *op-pilo* (obp-), pp. *-atus,* to stop up, fr. *pilo,* to ram down]

op·pi·la·tive (op-i-lā′tiv). Obstructive to any secretion.

op·po·nens (ŏ-pō′nens). A name given to several muscles of the fingers or toes, by the action of which these digits are opposed to the others. The opponens muscles of the hands act at the carpometacarpal joints, cupping the palm; this enables flexion at the metacarpophalangeal joints to oppose the thumb to the small finger or vice versa. Although comparable muscles in the foot are called "opponens" no opposition occurs in the foot. [L. *op-pono* (obp-), pres. p. *-ens,* to place against, oppose]

op·por·tun·is·tic (op′ŏr-tū-nis′tik). **1.** Denoting an organism capable of causing disease only in a host whose resistance is

lowered, *e.g.,* by other diseases or by drugs. **2.** Denoting a disease caused by such an organism.

op·po·sure (op′pō-shŭr). Bringing together of tissue during suturing.

op·sin. The protein portion of the rhodopsin molecule; at least three separate o.'s are located in cone cells.

op·sin·o·gen (op-sin′ō-jen). A substance that stimulates the formation of opsonin, such as the antigen contained in a suspension of bacteria used for immunization. SYN opsogen. [opsonin + -gen]

op·si·u·ria (op-sē-ū′rē-ă). A more rapid excretion of urine during fasting than after a full meal. [G. *opsi,* late, + *ouron,* urine]

op·so·clo·nus (op′sō-klō′nŭs). Rapid, irregular, nonrhythmic movements of the eye in horizontal and vertical directions. [G. *ōps, ōpos,* eye, + *klonos,* confused motion]

op·so·gen (op′sō-jen). SYN opsinogen.

op·so·ma·nia (op′sō-mā′nē-ă). A longing for a particular article of diet, or for highly seasoned food. [G. *opson,* seasoning, + *mania,* frenzy]

op·son·ic (op-son′ik). Relating to opsonins or to their utilization.

op·so·nin (op′sŏ-nin). A substance that binds to antigens, enhancing phagocytosis (*e.g.,* C3b of the complement system). [G. *opson,* boiled meat, provisions, fr. *hepsō,* to boil, + -in]

common o., SYN normal o.

immune o., SYN specific o.

normal o., that normally present in the blood, *i.e.,* without stimulation by a known, specific antigen such as certain complement components; it is relatively thermolabile and reacts with various organisms. SYN common o., thermolabile o.

specific o., antibodies formed in response to stimulation by a specific antigen, either as a result of an attack of a disease, or injections with a suitably prepared suspension of the specific microorganism. SYN immune o., thermostable o.

thermolabile o., SYN normal o.

thermostable o., SYN specific o.

op·son·i·za·tion (op′sŏ-nī-zā′shŭn). The process by which bacteria are altered in such a manner that they are more readily and more efficiently engulfed by phagocytes.

op·so·no·cy·to·pha·gic (op′sŏ-nō-sī′tō-fā′jik). Pertaining to the increased efficiency of phagocytic activity of the leukocytes in blood that contains specific opsonin. [opsonin + G. *kytos,* a hollow (cell), + *phagō,* to eat]

op·so·nom·e·try (op-sŏ-nom′ĕ-trē). Determination of the opsonic index or the opsonocytophagic activity.

op·so·no·phil·ia (op-sŏ-nō-fil′ē-ă). The condition in which bacteria readily unite with opsonins, thereby sensitizing them for more effective phagocytosis. [opsonin + G. *phileō,* to love]

op·so·no·phil·ic (op-sŏ-nō-fil′ik). Pertaining to, characterized by, or resulting in opsonophilia.

op·tic, op·ti·cal (op′tik, op′ti-kăl). Relating to the eye, vision, or optics. [G. *optikos*]

op·ti·cian (op-tish′an). One who practices opticianry.

op·ti·cian·ry (op-tish′an-rē). The professional practice of filling prescriptions for ophthalmic lenses, dispensing spectacles, and making and fitting contact lenses.

⚠**optico-.** SEE opto-.

op·ti·co·cil·i·a·ry (op′ti-kō-sil′ē-ār-ē). Relating to the optic and ciliary nerves.

op·ti·co·pu·pil·lary (op′ti-kō-pyū′pi-lār-ē). Relating to the optic nerve and the pupil.

op·tics (op′tiks). The science concerned with the properties of light, its refraction and absorption, and the refracting media of the eye in that relation. [G. *optikos,* fr. *ōps,* eye]

Nomarski o., an optical system for differential interference contrast microscopy.

schlieren o., an optical system, often used in diffusion and centrifugation studies, which observes the refractive index gradient in solutions containing macromolecules.

op·ti·mism (op′ti-mizm). The tendency to look on the bright side of everything, to believe that there is good in everything. [L. *optimus,* best] therapeutic o., a belief in the efficacy of drugs and other therapeutic agents in the treatment of diseases.

op·ti·mum (op′ti-mŭm). The best or most suitable; *e.g.,* denoting the dose of a remedy likely to give most benefit with fewest side effects, the temperature or pH at which an enzyme has maximal activity. [L. ntr. sing. of *optimus,* best]

△**opto-, optico-.** Optical; optic; ocular. [G. *optikos,* optical, from *ōps,* eye]

op·to·ki·net·ic (op′tō-ki-net′ik). SEE optokinetic *nystagmus.* [opto- + G. *kinēsis,* movement]

op·to·me·ninx (op′tō-mē′ninks). SYN retina. [opto- + G. *mēninx,* membrane]

op·tom·e·ter (op-tom′ĕ-ter). An instrument for determining the refraction of the eye. [opto- + G. *metron,* measure]
objective o., SYN refractometer.

op·tom·e·trist (op-tom′ĕ-trist). One who practices optometry.

op·tom·e·try (op-tom′ĕ-trē). **1.** The profession concerned with the examination of the eyes and related structures to determine the presence of vision problems and eye disorders, and with the prescription and adaptation of lenses and other optical aids or the use of visual training for maximum visual efficiency. **2.** The use of an optometer.

op·to·my·om·e·ter (op′tō-mī-om′ĕ-ter). An instrument for determining the relative power of the extrinsic muscles of the eye. [opto- + G. *mys,* muscle, + *metron,* measure]

op·to·types (op′tō-tīps). Test letters. SEE test types. [opto- + G. *typos,* type]

OPV Abbreviation for oral poliovirus *vaccine.* SEE poliovirus *vaccines,* under *vaccine.*

ora (ō′ră). Plural of L. *os,* the mouth. [L.]

ora, pl. orae (ō′ră, ō′rē) [NA]. An edge or a margin. [L.]
o. serra′ta [NA], the serrated extremity of the optic part of the retina, located a little behind the ciliary body and marking the limits of the percipient portion of the membrane.

or·ad (ad-ō′răl). **1.** In a direction toward the mouth. **2.** Situated nearer the mouth in relation to a specific reference point; opposite of aborad. [L. *os,* mouth, + *ad,* to]

oral (ōr′ăl). Relating to the mouth. [L. *os* (*or-*), mouth]

ora·le (ō-rā′lē). A point at the lingual side of the alveolar termination of the premaxillary suture. [Mod. L. punctum *orale,* oral point, fr. L. *os* (*or-*), mouth]

Oral Hy·giene In·dex (OHI). An index used in epidemiological studies of dental disease, to evaluate dental plaque and dental calculus separately.

oral·i·ty (ōr-al′i-tē). In freudian psychology, a term used to denote the psychic organization derived from, and characteristic of, the oral period of psychosexual development.

Oram, S., 20th century English cardiologist. SEE Holt-O. *syndrome.*

or·ange (ōr′enj). **1.** The fruit of the orange tree, *Citrus aurantium* (family Rutaceae). **2.** A color between yellow and red in the spectrum. For individual orange dyes, see specific name. [O.F. *orenge,* fr. Ar. *nāranj,* the initial *n* being absorbed in Fr. article *une*]
bitter o. peel, the dried rind of the unripe but fully grown fruit; a flavoring agent.
bitter o. peel, dried, the dried outer part of the pericarp of the ripe, or nearly ripe, fruit; it contains not less than 2.5% v/w of volatile oil.
bitter o. peel, fresh, the outer part of the pericarp of the ripe, or nearly ripe, fruit; used to prepare the tincture and the syrup.
bitter o. peel oil, a volatile oil obtained by expression from the fresh peel of the bitter o.

or·ange G [C.I. 16230]. An azo dye, $C_{16}H_{10}N_2O_7S_2Na_2$, used as a cytoplasmic stain in histologic techniques.

or·ange wood. A soft wood used in dentistry for placement of bridges, crowns, etc. by biting pressure, also used as a burnishing point in the polishing of root surfaces.

Orbeli, Leon A., Russian physiologist, 1882–1958. SEE O. *effect.*

or·bic·u·lar (or-bik′yū-lăr). Similar in form to an orb; circular in form. [L. *orbiculus,* a small disk, dim. of *orbis,* circle]

or·bic·u·la·re (ōr-bik-yū-lā′rē). SYN lenticular *process* of incus. [L., fr. *orbiculus,* a small disk]

or·bic·u·la·ris (ōr-bik′yū-lā′ris). **1.** Circular; denoting a circular or disk-shaped structure. **2.** SYN orbicularis *muscle.* [L. fr. *orbiculus,* a small disk]

or·bi·cu·lus cil·i·ar·is (ōr-bik′yū-lŭs sil-ē-ār′is) [NA]. The darkly pigmented posterior zone of the ciliary body continuous with the retina at the ora serrata. SYN ciliary disk, ciliary ring, pars plana. [Mod. L.]

or·bit (ōr′bit). The bony cavity containing the eyeball and its adnexa; it is formed of parts of seven bones: the frontal, maxillary, sphenoid, lacrimal, zygomatic, ethmoid, and palatine bones. SYN orbita [NA], eye socket, orbital cavity.

or·bi·ta, gen. or·bi·tae (ōr′bi-tă, -tē) [NA]. SYN orbit. [L. a wheel-track, fr. *orbis,* circle]

or·bi·tal (ōr′bi-tăl). Relating to the orbits.

or·bi·ta·le (ōr-bi-tā′lē). In cephalometrics, the lowermost point in the lower margin of the bony orbit that may be felt under the skin. [L. of an orbit]

or·bi·tog·ra·phy (ōr′bi-tog′ră-fē). Radiographic evaluation of the orbit. [L. *orbita,* orbit, + G. *graphō,* to write]
positive contrast o., o. with injection of a water soluble iodinated compound into the muscle cone or along the orbital floor.

or·bi·to·na·sal (ōr′bi-tō-nā′săl). Relating to the orbit and the nose or nasal cavity.

or·bi·to·nom·e·ter (ōr′bi-tō-nom′ĕ-ter). An instrument that measures the resistance offered to pressing the eyeball backwards into its socket. [L. *orbita,* orbit, + G. *metron,* measure]

or·bi·to·nom·e·try (ōr′bi-tō-nom′ĕ-trē). Measurement by means of the orbitonometer.

or·bi·top·a·gus (ōr-bi-top′ă-gŭs). Unequal conjoined twins in which the parasite, usually very imperfectly developed, is attached at an orbit of the autosite. SEE conjoined *twins,* under *twin.* SYN teratoma orbitae. [L. *orbita,* orbit, + G. *pagos,* something fixed]

or·bi·top·a·thy. disease of the orbit and its contents.
Graves' orbitopathy, SYN Graves' *ophthalmopathy.*

or·bi·to·sphe·noid (ōr′bi-tō-sfe′noyd). Relating to the orbit and the sphenoid bone.

or·bi·tot·o·my (ōr-bi-tot′ō-mē). Surgical incision into the orbit. [L. *orbita,* orbit, + *tomē,* a cutting]

Or·bi·vi·rus (ōr′bi-vī-rŭs). A genus of viruses of vertebrates (family Reoviridae) that multiply in insects, including certain viruses formerly included with the arboviruses. They are antigenically distinct from other groups of viruses and are characterized by an indistinct but rather large outer layer of capsomeres which give the appearance of rings (hence the name). The genus includes, among others, Colorado tick fever virus of man, bluetongue virus of sheep, and African horse sickness virus. [L. *orbis,* ring, + virus]

or·ce·in (ōr′sē-in) [old C.I. 1242]. A natural dye derived from orcinol by treatment with air and ammonia, which as a purple dye complex is used in various histologic staining methods.

or·chec·to·my (ōr-kek′tō-mē). SYN orchiectomy.

or·chel·la (ōr-kel′ă) [old C.I. 1242]. SYN archil.

△**orcheo-.** SEE orchio-.

△**orchi-, orchido-, orchio-.** The testes. [G. *orchis,* testis]

or·chi·al·gia (ōr-kē-al′jē-ă). Pain in the testis. SYN orchiodynia, orchioneuralgia, testalgia. [orchi- + G. *algos,* pain]

or·chi·cho·rea (ōr′kē-kō-rē′ă). Involuntary rising and falling movements of the testis. [orchi- + G. *choreia,* a dance]

or·chi·dec·to·my (ōr-ki-dek′tō-mē). SYN orchiectomy.

or·chid·ic (ōr-kid′ik). Relating to the testis.

or·chi·di·tis (ōr-ki-dī′tis). SYN orchitis.

△**orchido-.** SEE orchi-.

or·chi·dom·e·ter (ōr-ki-dom′ĕ-ter). **1.** A caliper device used to measure the size of testes. **2.** A set of sized models of testes for comparison of testicular development. [orchido- + G. *metron,* measure]

or·chi·dop·to·sis (ōr'ki-dop-tō'sis). Ptosis of the male gonads. [orchido- + G. *ptōsis,* a falling]

or·chi·dor·ra·phy (ōr-ki-dōr'ă-fē). SYN orchiopexy.

or·chi·ec·to·my (ōr-kē-ek'tō-mē). Removal of one or both testes. SYN orchectomy, orchidectomy, testectomy. [orchi- + G. *ektomē,* excision]

or·chi·ep·i·did·y·mi·tis (ōr'kē-ep'i-did'i-mī'tis). Inflammation of the testis and epididymis. [orchi- + epididymis, + G. *-itis,* inflammation]

or·chil (ōr'kil) [old C.I. 1242]. SYN archil.

◇**orchio-.** SEE orchi-.

or·chi·o·cele (ōr'kē-ō-sēl). A testis retained in the inguinal canal. [orchio- + G. *kēlē,* hernia, tumor]

or·chi·o·coc·cus (ōr'kē-ō-kok'ŭs). An old term for any Gram-negative diplococcus that resembles the gonococcus but is more easily cultivated on ordinary media; it is sometimes found in vaginal secretions. Such bacteria are now classified as species of *Neisseria,* along with *N. gonorrhoeae.* [orchio- + G. *kokkos,* berry (coccus)]

or·chi·o·dyn·ia (ōr'kē-ō-din'ē-ă). SYN orchialgia. [orchi- + G. *odynē,* pain]

or·chi·on·cus (ōr-kē-ong'kŭs). A neoplasm of the testis. [orchio- + G. *onkos,* bulk, mass]

or·chi·o·neu·ral·gia (ōr'kē-ō-nū-ral'jē-ă). SYN orchialgia. [orchio- + G. *neuron,* nerve, + *algos,* pain]

or·chi·op·a·thy (ōr-kē-op'ă-thē). Disease of a testis. [orchio- + G. *pathos,* suffering]

or·chi·o·pexy (ōr'kē-ō-pek'sē). Surgical treatment of an undescended testicle by freeing it and implanting it into the scrotum. SYN cryptorchidopexy, orchidorraphy, orchiorrhaphy. [orchio- + G. *pēxis,* fixation]

    transseptal o., SYN Ombrédanne *operation.*

or·chi·o·plas·ty (ōr'kē-ō-plas-tē). Surgical reconstruction of the testis. [orchio- + G. *plastos,* formed]

or·chi·or·rha·phy (ōr-kē-ōr'ă-fē). SYN orchiopexy. [orchio- + G. *rhaphē,* a suture]

or·chi·o·ther·a·py (ōr'kē-ō-thār'ă-pē). Treatment with testicular extracts.

or·chi·ot·o·my (ōr-kē-ot'ō-mē). Incision into a testis. SYN orchotomy. [orchio- + G. *tomē,* incision]

or·chis, pl. **or·chis·es** (ōr'kis, ōr'ki-sēz). SYN testis. [G. *testis,* an orchid]

or·chit·ic (ōr-kit'ik). Denoting orchitis.

or·chi·tis (ōr-kī'tis). Inflammation of the testis. SYN orchiditis, testitis. [orchi- + G. *-itis,* inflammation]

    o. parotid'ea, o. associated with mumps.

    traumatic o., simple inflammation of the testis caused by mechanical injury.

    o. variolo'sa, o. complicating smallpox.

or·chot·o·my (ōr-kot'ō-mē). SYN orchiotomy.

or·cin (ōr'sin). SYN orcinol.

or·cin·ol (ōr'sin-ol). 3,5-dihydroxytoluene; the parent substance of the natural dye orcein, obtained from certain colorless lichens (*Lecanora tinctoria, Rocella tinctoria*) by treatment with boiling water; used as an external antiseptic in various skin diseases and in chemistry as a reagent for pentoses. SYN 5-methylresorcinol, orcin.

or·ci·pren·a·line sul·fate (ōr-si-pren'ă-lēn). SYN metaproterenol sulfate.

ORD Abbreviation for optical rotatory *dispersion.*

Ord Symbol for orotidine.

or·deal bean (ōr'dē-ăl). SYN physostigma.

or·der (ōr'der). **1.** In biological classification, the division just below the class (or subclass) and above the family. **2.** In a reaction, o. is the sum of the exponents of all the concentration terms in that reaction's rate expression. For example, for the natural decomposition of nitrogen pentoxide, the rate expression is $v = -d[N_2O_5]/dt = k_1[N_2O_5]$. Thus, this is a first-order reaction. A reaction involving two different compounds is often a second-order reaction (but not necessarily so). Pseudo-first-order reac-

tions are multi-order reactions in which one of the reactants is in substoichiometric amounts. Cf. molecularity. [L. *ordo,* regular arrangement]

    pecking o., in some species of birds and primates the establishment of a graded dominance in members of a group by the use of aggression.

or·dered (ord'erd). SYN ordered *mechanism.*

or·der·ly (ōr'der-lē). An attendant in a hospital unit who assists in the care of patients.

or·di·nate (ōr'di-nāt). In a plane cartesian coordinate system, the vertical axis (*y*). Cf. abscissa.

orec·tic (ō-rek'tik). Pertaining to or characterized by orexia.

orex·ia (ō-rek'sē-ă). **1.** The affective and conative aspects of an act, in contrast to the cognitive aspect. **2.** SYN appetite. [G. *orexis,* appetite]

orex·i·gen·ic (ō-rek-si-jen'ik). Appetite-stimulating.

orf. A specific disease of sheep and goats, caused by the orf virus. This virus is transmissible to man and characterized by vesiculation and ulceration of the infected site. SYN contagious ecthyma, contagious pustular dermatitis, scabby mouth, soremouth. [O.E. *orfcwealm,* murrain, fr. *orf,* cattle, + *cwealm,* destruction]

or·gan (ōr'găn). Any part of the body exercising a specific function, as of respiration, secretion, digestion. SYN organum [NA], organon. [L. *organum,* fr. G. *organon,* a tool, instrument]

    accessory o.'s, (1) SYN supernumerary o.'s. **(2)** SYN accessory o.'s of the eye.

    accessory o.'s of the eye, the eyelids, with lashes and eyebrows, lacrimal apparatus, conjunctival sac, and extrinsic muscles of the eyeball. SYN organa oculi accessoria [NA], accessory o.'s (2), accessory visual apparatus, adnexa oculi, appendages of eye.

    annulospiral o., SYN annulospiral *ending.*

    auditory o., archaic term for gustatory o.

    Chievitz' o., a normal epithelial structure, possibly a neurotransmitter, found at the angle of the mandible with branches of the buccal nerve.

    circumventricular o.'s, four small areas in or near the base of the brain that have fenestrated capillaries and are outside the blood-brain barrier. They are neurohypophysis, area postrema, organum vasculosum of the lamina terminalis and subfornical organ (SFO). The neurohypophysis is a neurohemal organ. The other three are chemoreceptors: area postrema triggers vomiting in response to chemical changes in plasma, organum vasculosum of the lamina terminalis senses osmolality and alters vasopressin secretion and SFO initiates drinking in response to angiotensin II.

    Corti's o., SYN spiral o.

    critical o., the o. or physiologic system that for a given source of radiation would first reach its legally defined maximum permissible radiation exposure as the dose of radiopharmaceutical is increased; *e.g.,* the kidney is the critical o. when [197]Hg-chlormerodrin is given.

    enamel o., a circumscribed mass of ectodermal cells budded off from the dental lamina; it becomes cup-shaped and develops on its internal face the ameloblast layer of cells that produce the enamel cap of a developing tooth.

    end o., the special structure containing the terminal of a nerve fiber in peripheral tissue such as muscle, tissue, skin, mucous membrane, or glands. SEE ALSO ending.

    external female genital o.'s, the external feminine genital o.'s, the vulva and clitoris. SYN organa genitalia feminina externa.

    external male genital o.'s, the external masculine genital o.'s, the penis and scrotum. SYN organa genitalia masculina externa.

    floating o., SYN wandering o.

    flower-spray o. of Ruffini, SYN flower-spray *ending.*

    genital o.'s, the organs of reproduction or generation, external and internal. SYN organa genitalia [NA], genitalia, genitals.

    Golgi tendon o., a proprioceptive sensory nerve ending embedded among the fibers of a tendon, often near the musculotendinous junction; it is compressed and activated by any increase of the tendon's tension, caused either by active contraction or passive stretch of the corresponding muscle. SYN neurotendinous o., neurotendinous spindle.

gustatory o., located in the papillae of the mucous membrane of the tongue, chiefly in the vallate papillae. SYN organum gustus [NA], o. of taste.

o. of hearing, SYN cochlear *labyrinth*.

internal female genital o.'s, the internal feminine genital organs, the ovaries, uterine tubes, uterus, and vagina. SYN organa genitalia feminina interna.

internal male genital o.'s, the internal masculine genital organs, the testes, epididymides, deferent ducts, seminal vesicles, prostate, and bulbourethral glands. SYN organa genitalia masculina interna.

intromittent o., SYN penis.

Jacobson's o., SYN vomeronasal o.

lateral line sense o., a structure in fish consisting of a long groove or canal extending along each side of the trunk and tail and branching in the head region; the groove or tube is lined with neuroepithelial cells, some of which are in groups known as neuromasts; its function appears to be the detection of vibrations of low frequency. SYN neuromast o.

neurohemal o.'s, brain areas from which substances enter blood *e.g.,* the neurohypophysis from which oxytocin and vasopressin enter blood.

neuromast o., SYN lateral line sense o.

neurotendinous o., SYN Golgi tendon o.

olfactory o., the olfactory region in the superior portion of the nasal cavity. SYN organum olfactus [NA], o. of smell.

ptotic o., SYN wandering o.

o. of Rosenmüller, SYN epoöphoron.

sense o.'s, the organs of special sense, including the eye, ear, olfactory organ, taste organs, and the accessory structures associated with these organs. SYN organa sensuum [NA].

o. of smell, SYN olfactory o.

spiral o., a prominent ridge of highly specialized epithelium in the floor of the cochlear duct overlying the basilar membrane of cochlea, containing one inner row and three outer rows of hair cells, or cells of Corti (the auditory receptor cells innervated by the cochlear nerve) supported by various columnar cells: the pillars of Corti, cells of Hensen, and cells of Claudius; the spiral o. is partly overhung by an awning-like shelf, the tectorial membrane, the free marginal zone of which is covered by a gelatinous substance in which the stereocilia of the outer hair cells are embedded. SYN organum spirale [NA], acoustic papilla, Corti's o.

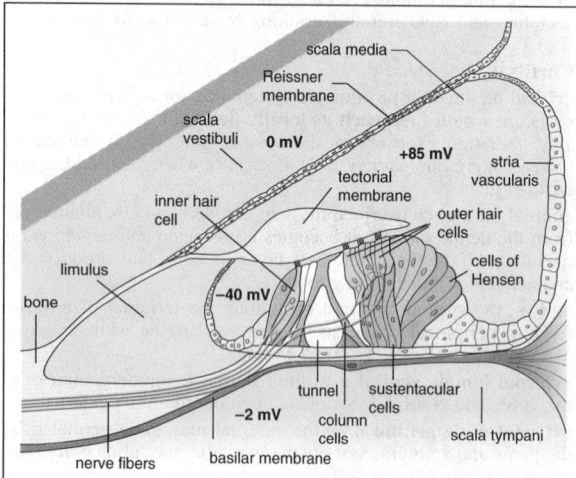

spiral organ
schematic representation of a histological cross-section of the spiral organ. The electrical potentials indicated in the scala vestibuli, etc. are relative to neutral points in the body.

subcommissural o., a microscopic organ, made up of columnar

ciliated ependymal cells, located in the cerebral aqueduct beneath the posterior commissure of the brain; it is believed to have a neurosecretory function.

subfornical o. (SFO), the intercolumnar tubercle. One of the circumventricular o.'s. SFO has fenestrated capillaries and is outside the blood-brain barrier. It is thought to be a chemoreceptor zone involving in cardiovascular regulation.

supernumerary o.'s, o.'s exceeding the normal number, which may develop from multiple foci of organization in an organformative field larger (originally) than that of the definitive main o.; such o.'s are aberrant but frequently not a cause of disease; illness may persist if they are left in the body after therapeutic removal of the main o., *e.g.,* accessory spleen. SYN accessory o.'s (1).

tactile o., SYN o. of touch.

target o., a tissue or o. upon which a hormone exerts its action; generally, a tissue or organ with appropriate receptors for a hormone. SYN target (3).

o. of taste, SYN gustatory o.

o. of touch, any one of the sensory end o.'s. SYN organum tactus, tactile o.

urinary o.'s, organs involved with the formation, storage, and excretion of urine. SYN organa urinaria [NA].

vestibular o., collective term for the utricle, saccule, and semicircular ducts of the membranous labyrinth, each having a single patch of ciliated receptor epithelium innervated by the vestibular nerve: macula of sacculus, macula of utriculus, and cristae of the semicircular ducts.

vestibulocochlear o., the external, middle, and internal ear. SYN organum vestibulocochleare [NA].

vestigial o., a rudimentary structure in humans corresponding to a functional structure or o. in the lower animals.

o. of vision, SYN visual o.

visual o., the eye and its adnexa. SYN organum visus [NA], o. of vision.

vomeronasal o., a fine vestigal horizontal canal, ending in a blind pouch, in the mucous membrane of the nasal septum, beginning just behind and above the incisive duct; a structure which usually regresses after the 6th month of gestation. In many lower animals if functions as an accessory olfactory organ. SYN organum vomeronasale [NA], Jacobson's o.

wandering o., an o. with loose attachments, permitting its displacement. SYN floating o., ptotic o.

Weber's o., SYN prostatic *utricle*.

o.'s of Zuckerkandl, SYN para-aortic *bodies,* under *body.*

or·ga·na (ōr'gă-nă). Plural of organum.

or·gan·elle (or'gă-nel). One of the specialized parts of a protozoan or tissue cell; these subcellular units include mitochondria, the Golgi apparatus, nucleus and centrioles, granular and agranular endoplasmic reticulum, vacuoles, microsomes, lysosomes, plasma membrane, and certain fibrils, as well as plastids of plant cells. SYN cell o., organoid (3). [G. *organon,* organ, + Fr. *-elle,* dim. suffix, fr. L. *-ella*]

cell o., SYN organelle.

paired o.'s, SYN rhoptry.

or·gan·ic (ōr-gan'ik). **1.** Relating to an organ. **2.** Relating to or formed by an organism. **3.** Organized; structural. **4.** SEE organic *compound.* [G. *organikos*]

or·gan·i·cism (ōr-gan'i-sizm). A theory that attributes all diseases, in particular, all mental disorders, as organic in origin.

or·gan·i·cist (ōr-gan'i-sist). One who believes in, or subscribes to the views of, organicism.

or·gan·i·din. SYN iodinated *glycerol.*

or·ga·nism (ōr'gă-nizm). Any living individual, whether plant or animal, considered as a whole.

calculated mean o. (CMO), a hypothetical o. whose characters are the means of both the positive and negative characters of the o.'s which belong to the same taxon as the CMO, as opposed to the hypothetical mean o.

defective o., SYN auxotrophic *mutant.*

fastidious o., a bacterial organism having complex nutritional requirements.

hypothetical mean o. (HMO), a hypothetical o. whose characters are the means of the positive characters of the organisms which belong to the same taxon as the HMO, as opposed to the calculated mean o.

pleuropneumonia-like o.'s (PPLO), the original name given to a group of bacteria which did not possess cell walls; these o.'s, isolated from man and other animals, soil, and sewage, are now assigned to the order Mycoplasmatales.

or·ga·ni·za·tion (ōr′gan-i-zā′shŭn). **1.** An arrangement of distinct but mutually dependent parts. **2.** The conversion of coagulated blood, exudate, or dead tissue into fibrous tissue.

health maintenance o., a prepaid health plan that provides its members a full range of health services from a limited group of doctors and hospitals.

preferred provider o. (PPO), a health care delivery model which uses a panel of eligible physicians.

pregenital o., in psychoanalysis, the o. or arrangement of the libido in the stages prior to that of genital primacy.

or·ga·nize (ōr′gan-īz). To provide with, or to assume, a structure.

or·ga·niz·er (ōr′gan-ī-zer). **1.** Originally applied to a group of cells on the dorsal lip of the blastopore, which induce differentiation of cells in the embryo and control growth and development of adjacent parts. **2.** Any group of cells having such a controlling influence, the effects being brought about through the action of an evocator.

nucleolar o., the region of the satellites on the acrocentric chromosomes that is active in nucleolus formation. SYN nucleolar zone, nucleolus o.

nucleolus o., SYN nucleolar o.

primary o., the o. situated on the dorsal lip of the blastopore.

procentriole o., SYN deuterosome.

organo-. Organ; organic. [G. *organon*]

or·ga·no·ax·i·al (ōr-gă′no-aks′ē-ăl). Rotation around the long axis of the organ; a type of gastric volvulus.

or·gan·o·fer·ric (ōr′gă-nō-fār′ik). Relating to an organic compound containing iron.

or·gan·o·gel (ōr-gan′ō-jel). A hydrogel with an organic liquid instead of water as the dispersion means.

or·ga·no·gen·e·sis (ōr′gă-nō-jen′ĕ-sis). Formation of organs during development. SYN organogeny. [organo- + G. *genesis,* origin]

or·ga·no·ge·net·ic, or·ga·no·gen·ic (ōr′gă-nō-jĕ-net′ik, -jen′ik). Relating to organogenesis.

or·ga·nog·e·ny (ōr-gan-oj′ĕ-nē). SYN organogenesis.

or·ga·nog·ra·phy (ōr′gă-nog′ră-fē). A treatise on, or description of, the organs of the body. [organo- + G. *graphē,* a writing]

or·gan·oid (ōr′gă-noyd). **1.** Resembling in superficial appearance or in structure any of the organs or glands of the body. **2.** Composed of glandular or organic elements, and not of a single tissue; pertaining to certain neoplasms (*e.g.,* an adenoma) that contain cytologic and histologic elements arranged in a pattern that closely resembles or is virtually identical to a normal organ. SEE ALSO histoid. **3.** SYN organelle. [organo- + G. *eidos,* resemblance]

or·ga·no·lep·tic (ōr′gă-nō-lep′tik). **1.** Stimulating any of the organs of sensation. **2.** Susceptible to a sensory stimulus. [organo- + G. *lēptikos,* disposed to accept]

or·ga·nol·o·gy (ōr-gă-nol′ō-jē). Branch of science concerned with the anatomy, physiology, development, and functions of the various organs. [organo- + G. *logos,* study]

or·ga·no·ma (ōr-gă-nō′mă). Obsolete term for a neoplasm that contains cytologic and histologic elements in such an arrangement that specific types of tissue, *e.g.,* thyroid glands, intestinal mucosa, ovarian stroma and follicles, may be identified in various parts. SEE ALSO teratoma. [organo- + G. *-oma,* tumor]

or·ga·no·meg·a·ly (ōr′gă-nō-meg′ă-lē). SYN visceromegaly.

or·gan·o·mer·cur·i·al (ōr-gan′ō-mer-kyū′rē-ăl). Any organic mercurial compound; *e.g.,* merbromin, thimerosal.

or·ga·no·me·tal·lic (ōr′gă-nō-me-tal′ik). Denoting an organic compound containing one or more metallic atoms in its structure.

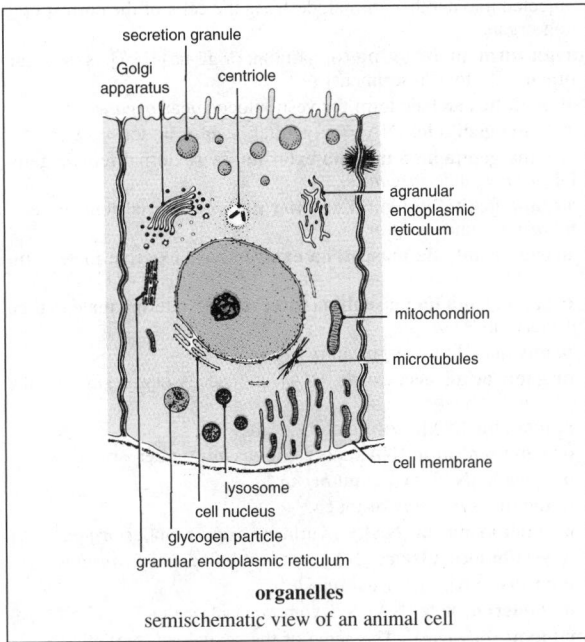

secretion granule
Golgi apparatus
centriole
agranular endoplasmic reticulum
mitochondrion
microtubules
cell membrane
lysosome
cell nucleus
glycogen particle
granular endoplasmic reticulum

organelles
semischematic view of an animal cell

or·ga·non, pl. **or·ga·na** (ōr′gă-non, ōr′gă-nă). SYN organ. [G. organ]

or·ga·non·o·my (ōr-gă-non′ō-mē). The body of laws regulating the life processes of organized beings. [organo- + G. *nomos,* law]

or·ga·non·y·my (ōr′gă-non′i-mē). The nomenclature of the organs of the body, as distinguished from toponymy. [organo- + G. *onyma,* name]

or·ga·nop·a·thy (ōr-gă-nop′ă-thē). Any disease especially affecting one of the organs of the body. [organo- + G. *pathos,* suffering]

or·ga·no·pexy, or·ga·no·pex·ia (ōr′gă-nō-pek-sē, -pek′sē-ă). Fixation by suture or otherwise of a floating or ptotic organ. [organo- + G. *pēxis,* fixation]

or·ga·no·phil·ic (ōr′gă-nō-fil′ik). Pertaining to organophilicity.

or·ga·no·phi·lic·i·ty (ōr′gă-nō-fi-li′si-tē). Attraction of nonpolar substances (organic molecules) to each other.

or·ga·no·phos·phates (ōr-gă-nō-fos′fāts). A series of phosphorus-containing organic compounds usually also containing a halide ion which reacts with cholinesterase. Organophosphates phosphorylate cholinesterase and thus irreversibly inhibit it. Used as insecticides; have also been used as war gases.

or·gan·o·sol (ōr-gan′ō-sol). A hydrosol with an organic liquid instead of water as the dispersion means.

or·ga·no·tax·is (ōr′gă-nō-tak′sis). The tendency to migrate to a certain organ selectively. [organo- + G. *taxis,* orderly arrangement]

or·ga·no·ther·a·py (ōr′gă-nō-thār′ă-pē). Treatment of disease by preparations made from animal organs; now frequently by synthetic preparations instead of extracts of a gland.

or·ga·no·tro·phic (ōr′gă-nō-trof′ik). **1.** Pertaining to the nourishment of an organ. **2.** Pertaining to a microorganism that uses organic sources as a reducing power. [organo- + G. *trophē,* nourishment]

or·ga·no·tro·pic (ōr′gă-nō-trop′ik). Pertaining to or characterized by organotropism.

or·ga·not·ro·pism (ōr-gă-not′rō-pizm). The special affinity of particular drugs, pathogens, or metastatic tumors for particular organs or their component parts. Cf. parasitotropism. SYN organotropy. [organo- + G. *tropē,* a turning]

or·ga·not·ro·py (ōr-gă-not′rō-pē). SYN organotropism.

or·gan-spe·cif·ic. Denoting or pertaining to a serum produced by the injection of the cells of a certain organ or tissue that, when injected into another animal, destroys the cells of the corresponding organ.

or·ga·num, pl. **or·ga·na** (ōr′gă-nŭm, ōr′gă-nă) [NA]. SYN organ, organ. [L. tool, instrument]

o. audi′tus, archaic term for vestibulocochlear *organ*.

or′gana genita′lia [NA], SYN genital *organs*, under *organ*.

organa genita′lia femini′na exter′na, SYN external female genital *organs*, under *organ*.

organa genita′lia femini′na inter′na, SYN internal female genital *organs*, under *organ*.

organa genita′lia masculi′na exter′na, SYN external male genital *organs*, under *organ*.

organa genita′lia masculi′na inter′na, SYN internal male genital *organs*, under *organ*.

o. gus′tus [NA], SYN gustatory *organ*.

or′gana oc′uli accesso′ria [NA], SYN accessory *organs* of the eye, under *organ*.

o. olfac′tus [NA], SYN olfactory *organ*.

or′gana sen′suum [NA], SYN sense *organs*, under *organ*.

o. spira′le [NA], SYN spiral *organ*.

o. tac′tus, SYN *organ* of touch.

or′gana urina′ria [NA], SYN urinary *organs*, under *organ*.

o. vestibulocochlea′re [NA], SYN vestibulocochlear *organ*.

o. vi′sus [NA], SYN visual *organ*.

o. vomeronasa′le [NA], SYN vomeronasal *organ*.

or·gasm (ōr′gazm). The acme of the sexual act. SYN climax (2). [G. *orgaō*, to swell, be excited]

or·gas·mic, or **gas·tic** (ōr-gaz′mik, -gas′tik). Relating to, characteristic of, or tending to produce an orgasm.

or·i·en·ta·tion (ōr-ē-en-tā′shŭn). **1.** The recognition of one's temporal, spatial, and personal relationships and environment. **2.** The relative position of an atom with respect to one to which it is connected, *i.e.,* the direction of the bond connecting them. [Fr. *orienter,* to set toward the East, therefore in a definite position]

or·i·en·to·my·cin (or′ē-en-tō-mī′sin). SYN cycloserine.

or·i·fice (or′i-fis). Any aperture or opening. SYN orificium [NA]. [L. *orificium*]

anal o., SYN anus.

aortic o., the opening from the left ventricle into the ascending aorta; it is guarded by the aortic valve. SYN ostium aortae [NA], aortic ostium.

cardiac o., the trumpet-shaped opening of the esophagus into the stomach. SYN ostium cardiacum [NA], cardiac opening, esophagogastric o.

esophagogastric o., SYN cardiac o.

o. of external acoustic meatus, SYN *opening* of external acoustic meatus.

external urethral o., (1) the slitlike opening of the urethra in the glans penis; **(2)** the external orifice of the urethra (in the female) in the vestibule, usually upon a slight elevation, the papilla urethrae. SYN ostium urethrae externum [NA], external opening of urethra, meatus urinarius, orificium urethrae externum.

gastroduodenal o., SYN pyloric o.

golf-hole ureteral o., a retracted funnel-shaped condition of the ureteral o. in the wall of the bladder, due often to tuberculosis or a secondary sclerosis of the ureter.

ileocecal o., the opening of the terminal ileum into the large intestine at the transition between the cecum and the ascending colon. SYN ostium ileocecale [NA], ileocecal opening.

o. of inferior vena cava, SYN *opening* of inferior vena cava.

o. of internal acoustic meatus, SYN *opening* of internal acoustic meatus.

internal urethral o., the internal opening or orifice of the urethra, at the anterior and inferior angle of the trigone. SYN ostium urethrae internum [NA], internal urethral opening.

mitral o., an atrioventricular opening which leads from the left atrium into the left ventricle of the heart. SYN ostium atrioventriculare sinistrum [NA], ostium arteriosum.

pulmonary o., SYN *opening* of pulmonary trunk.

pyloric o., the opening between the stomach and the superior

part of the duodenum. SYN ostium pyloricum [NA], gastroduodenal o.

root canal o., an opening in the pulp chamber leading to the root canal.

o. of superior vena cava, SYN *opening* of superior vena cava.

tricuspid o., an atrioventricular opening which leads from the right atrium into the right ventricle of the heart. SYN ostium atrioventriculare dextrum [NA], ostium venosum cordis.

ureteric o., the opening of the ureter in the bladder, situated one at each lateral angle of the trigone; wide gaping of the o. usually indicates vesicoureteral reflux. SYN ostium ureteris [NA], orificium ureteris, ureteral meatus, ureteral opening.

vaginal o., the narrowest portion of the canal, in the floor of the vestibule posterior to the urethral orifice. SYN ostium vaginae [NA], orificium vaginae, vaginal opening.

or·i·fi·cial (ōr-i-fish′ăl). Relating to an orifice of any kind.

or·i·fi·ci·um, pl. **or·i·fi·cia** (ōr-i-fish′ē-ŭm, -ă) [NA]. SYN orifice, orifice. [L.]

o. exter′num u′teri, SYN external *os* of uterus.

o. inter′num u′teri, SYN *isthmus* of uterus.

o. ure′teris, SYN ureteric *orifice*.

o. ure′thrae exter′num, SYN external urethral *orifice*.

o. vagi′nae, SYN vaginal *orifice*.

orig·a·num oil (ŏ-rig′ă-nŭm). The volatile oil (which contains carvacrol) obtained from various species of *Origanum* (family Labiatae); used as a rubefacient, as a constituent in veterinary liniments, and in microscopic techniques.

or·i·gin (or′i-jin). **1.** The less movable of the two points of attachment of a muscle, that which is attached to the more fixed part of the skeleton. **2.** The starting point of a cranial or spinal nerve. The former have two o.'s: the **ental o., deep o.,** or **real o.,** the cell group in the brain or medulla, whence the fibers of the nerve begin, and the **ectal o., superficial o.,** or **apparent o.,** the point where the nerve emerges from the brain. [L. *origo,* source, beginning, fr. *orior,* to rise]

o. of replication, a sequence of the bacterial genome required for the initiating of a replicating fork by leading strand synthesis.

ori·za·ba jal·ap root (ŏ-riz′ă-bă ja′lap). SYN ipomea.

Ormond, John K., U.S. urologist, *1886. SEE O.'s *disease*.

Orn Symbol for ornithine or its radical.

or·nate (ōr′nāt). A term that refers to the patterning of the scutum (gray or white markings on a dark background) in ixodid ticks. [L. *ornatus,* decorated]

Ornish, Dean, U.S. physician, *1953. SEE O. reversal *diet*.

or·ni·thine (Orn) (ōr′ni-thēn, -thin). $NH_2(CH_2)_3CH(NH_2)$ COOH; 2,5-Diaminovaleric acid; the L-isomer is the amino acid formed when L-arginine is hydrolyzed by arginase; not a constituent of proteins, but an important intermediate in the urea cycle; elevated levels seen in certain defects of the urea cycle.

o. acetyltransferase, SYN *glutamate* acetyltransferase.

o. δ-aminotransferase, an enzyme that will reversibly catalyze the reaction of α-ketoglutarate and L-o. to form L-glutamate and L-glutamate γ-semialdehyde; a deficiency of this enzyme will result in gyrate atrophy of the choroid and retina. SYN o. transaminase.

o. carbamoyltransferase, an enzyme catalyzing formation of L-citrulline and orthophosphate from L-o. and carbamoyl phosphate; a part of the urea cycle; a deficiency of this enzyme will result in ammonia intoxication and impaired urea formation. SYN o. transcarbamoylase.

o. decarboxylase, an enzyme catalyzing the decarboxylation of L-o. to putrescine and CO_2; first step in polyamine biosynthesis.

o. transaminase, SYN o. δ-aminotransferase.

o. transcarbamoylase, SYN o. carbamoyltransferase.

or·ni·thi·ne·mia (ōr′ni-thi-nē″mē-ă). A toxic condition occasionally producing localized cerebral swelling, caused by abnormal amounts of ammonia in the blood. [ornithine + G. *haima,* blood]

or·ni·thi·nu·ria (ōr′ni-thi-nū″rē-ă). Excretion of excessive amounts of ornithine in the urine.

Or·ni·thod·o·ros (ōr-ni-thod′ŏ-rŭs). A genus of soft ticks (family

Argasidae) several species of which are vectors of pathogens of various relapsing fevers. They are characterized by a capitulum hidden below the hood and by disks and mamillae of the integument that are continuous from dorsal to ventral surfaces in a variety of patterns. [G. *ornis* (*ornith-*), bird, + *doros,* a leather bag]

O. coria′ceus, a species common in the mountainous coastal areas of California; adults readily attack deer, cattle, and humans, and have an irritating, painful, sometimes toxic bite. Transmits epizootic bovine abortion to cattle. SYN pajaroello.

O. errat′icus, a species the small variety of which is the vector of *Borrelia crocidurae* in Africa, the Near East, and central Asia; the large variety is the vector of *B. hispanica* in the Spanish peninsula and adjacent north Africa.

O. herm′si, a species that is a rodent parasite and vector of relapsing fever spirochetes, such as *Borrelia hermsii,* in the western U.S. and Canada.

O. lahoren′sis, a species that possibly transmits *Borrelia persica,* the agent of Persian relapsing fever.

O. mouba′ta complex, a group of four species in Africa; the taxonomy and ecology of this complex is of great significance because its members are vectors of relapsing fever spirochetes; members of the complex include *O. moubata* (various hosts), *O. compactus* (tortoises), *O. apertus* (porcupines), and *O. porcinus* (warthogs); a domestic subspecies of *O. porcinus,* in turn, forms three strains that feed chiefly on humans, fowl, and swine.

O. pappil′ipes, the "Persian bug," a species found in the former USSR and the Near East that transmits *Borrelia persica,* the pathogen in Iran of Persian relapsing fever.

O. par′keri, a species found in the western U.S. and a vector of *Borrelia parkeri.*

O. ru′dis, a species that is an important vector of relapsing fever spirochetes in Central and South America; possibly another complex similar to the *O. moubata* complex.

O. savi′gni, a species transmitting *Borrelia,* an agent of relapsing fever of eastern Africa, southern Egypt, Ethiopia, and southwestern Asia.

O. talajé, a species found in Mexico and in Central and South America, where it feeds on wild rodents, domestic animals, and humans; it delivers a painful, irritating bite and is a vector of *Borrelia mazzottii,* a cause of relapsing fever.

O. tholoza′ni, a species transmitting *Borrelia persica,* an agent of relapsing fever in the Middle East and central Asia.

O. turica′ta, a species that readily attacks man and other animals in the southern portion of the U.S. and Mexico; it is a vector of *Borrelia turicatae,* an agent of relapsing fever; the bite is painful and irritating.

O. venezuelen′sis, a species that is the vector of *Borrelia venezuelensis,* agent of relapsing fever in Colombia, Venezuela, and mountainous parts of South America.

O. verruco′sus, vector of *Borrelia caucasica.*

Or·ni·tho·nys·sus (ōr-i-thon′i-sŭs). A genus of bird and rodent mites; species include *O. bacoti,* the tropical rat mite, a possible vector of murine typhus and a cause of human dermatitis; *O. bursa,* the tropical fowl mite; and *O. sylviarum,* the northern fowl mite. [G. *ornis* (*ornith-*), bird, + *nyssus,* to prick]

or·ni·tho·sis (ōr-ni-thō′sis). Originally, a disease in nonpsittacine birds (domestic fowls, ducks, pigeons, turkeys, and many wild birds) caused by *Chlamydia psittaci;* now, generally referred to as psittacosis. [G. *ornis* (*ornith-*), bird, + *-osis,* condition]

Oro Symbol for orotic acid or orotate.

⟁**oro-.** **1.** The mouth. [L. *os, oris,* mouth] **2.** Obsolete alternative spelling is orrho-. SEE sero-. [G. *orrhos,* whey, serum]

or·o·dig·i·to·fa·cial (ōr′ō-dij′i-tō-fā′shăl). Relating to the mouth, fingers, and face.

or·o·fa·cial (ōr-ō-fā′shăl). Relating to the mouth and face.

or·o·lin·gual (ōr-ō-ling′gwăl). Relating to the mouth and tongue.

or·o·na·sal (ōr-ō-nā′săl). Relating to the mouth and nose.

or·o·pha·ryn·ge·al (ōr-ō-fă-rin′jē-ăl). Relating to the oropharynx.

or·o·phar·ynx (ōr′ō-far′ingks). The portion of the pharynx that lies posterior to the mouth; it is continuous above with the nasopharynx via the pharyngeal isthmus and below with the laryngopharynx. SYN pars oralis pharyngis [NA], oral part of pharynx, oral pharynx. [L. *os* (*or-*), mouth]

or·o·so·mu·coid (ōr′ō-sō-myū′koyd). α_1-acid glycoprotein; a subgroup of the α_1-globulin fraction of blood; increased plasma levels are associated with inflammation. SYN α_1-acid glycoprotein, acid seromucoid.

or·o·tate (Oro) (ōr′ō-tāt). A salt or ester of orotic acid.

o. phosphoribosyltransferase, a phosphoribosyltransferase synthesizing orotidylate and pyrophosphate from orotate and 5-phospho-α-D-ribosyl-1-pyrophosphate; this enzyme is a part of pyrimidine biosynthesis; a deficiency of this enzyme is associated with orotic aciduria type I. Cf. *uridylic acid* synthase. SYN OMP pyrophosphorylase, orotidylic acid phosphorylase, orotidylic acid pyrophosphorylase.

orot·ic ac·id (Oro) (ōr-ot′ik). 6-Carboxyuracil; uracil-6-carboxylic acid; an important intermediate in the formation of the pyrimidine nucleotides; elevated in certain inherited defects of pyrimidine biosynthesis. SYN uracil-6-carboxylic acid.

orot·ic ac·i·du·ria [MIM*258900]. A rare disorder of pyrimidine metabolism characterized by hypochromic anemia with megaloblastic changes in bone marrow, leukopenia, retarded growth, and urinary excretion of orotic acid; autosomal recessive inheritance. [orotic acid + G. *ouron,* urine]

orot·i·dine (O, Ord) (ō-rot′i-dēn). orotic acid-3-β-D-ribonucleoside; uridine-6-carboxylic acid; elevated in cases of orotidinuria. SYN 1-ribosylorotate.

o. 5′-monophosphate (OMP), SYN orotidylic acid.

orot·i·di·nu·ria (ō-rot′i-dēn-yū′rē-ă). Elevated levels of orotidine in the urine; has been observed in defects in and inhibition of orotidylic acid decarboxylase.

orot·i·dyl·ate (OMP) (ō-rot-i-dil′āt). A salt or ester of orotidylic acid.

orot·i·dyl·ic ac·id (OMP) (ō-rot-i-dil′ik). Orotidine 5′-monophosphate; an intermediate in the biosynthesis of the pyrimidine nucleosides (cytidine and uridine) that are found in nucleic acids. SYN orotidine 5′-monophosphate.

o. a. decarboxylase, an enzyme that catalyzes the conversion of OMP to UMP and CO_2; a defect or inhibition of this enzyme will result in orotic aciduria and orotidinuria; this enzyme is a part of pyrimidine biosynthesis. Cf. *uridylic acid* synthase. SYN OMP decarboxylase.

o. a. phosphorylase, SYN *orotate* phosphoribosyltransferase.

o. a. pyrophosphorylase, SYN *orotate* phosphoribosyltransferase.

or·phan (ōr′făn). SEE orphan *products,* under *product.* [G. *orphanos*]

or·phen·a·drine cit·rate (ōr-fen′ă-drēn). An antihistaminic that also has the same action and use as orphenadrine hydrochloride.

or·phen·a·drine hy·dro·chlo·ride. *N,N*-Dimethyl-2(*o*-methyl-α-phenylbenzoyloxy)ethylamine hydrochloride; the *o*-methyl analogue of diphenhydramine hydrochloride; it reduces spasm of voluntary muscles, probably by action on the cerebral motor areas; used in the symptomatic treatment of paralysis agitans and drug-induced parkinsonism.

⟁**orrho-.** OBSOLETE serum. SEE sero-. [G. *orrhos, oros,* whey, serum]

♲ **Combining forms**	**[NA] Nomina Anatomica**
Word*Finder*	**[MIM] Mendelian**
Multi-term entry finder	**Inheritance in Man**
Preceding letter A	
A.D.A.M. Anatomy Plates	☆ **Official alternate term**
Between letters L and M	
	☆**[NA] Official alternate**
Appendices:	**Nomina Anatomica term**
Following letter Z	
SYN Synonym; Cf., compare	**High Profile Term**

or·ris (ōr'is). SYN iris.

or·seil·lin BB (ōr-sīl-in) [C.I. 26670]. A red diazo acid dye, $C_{24}H_{18}N_4O_7S_2Na_2$, used as a fungal and bacterial stain.

Orsi, Francesco, Italian physician, 1828–1890. SEE O.-Grocco *method.*

Orth, Johannes J., German pathologist, 1847–1923. SEE O.'s *fixative, stain.*

orth-. SEE ortho-.

orth·er·ga·sia (ōrth-er-ga'zē-ă). Rarely used term for normal intellectual and emotional adjustment. [G. *orthos,* straight, correct, + *ergasia,* work]

or·the·sis (ōr-thē'sis). Rarely used term for an orthopedic brace, splint, or appliance. [ortho- + *-esis,* process]

or·thet·ics (ōr-thet'iks). SYN orthotics.

ortho-, orth-. **1.** Prefix denoting straight, normal, in proper order. **2** (*o-*). In chemistry, italicized prefix denoting that a compound has two substitutions on adjacent carbon atoms in a benzene ring. For terms beginning *ortho-* or *o-,* see the specific name. [Gr. *orthos* correct]

or·tho·ac·id (ōr'thō-as'id). An acid in which the number of hydroxyl groups equals the valence of the acid-forming element; *e.g.,* $C(OH)_4$, orthocarbonic acid. When there is no such acid, the one that most nearly approaches this condition is sometimes called an o.; *e.g.,* $OP(OH)_3$, orthophosphoric acid.

or·tho·ar·te·ri·ot·o·ny (ōr'thō-ar-tēr-ē-ot'ō-nē). Normal blood pressure. [ortho- + G. *artēria,* artery, + *tonos,* tension]

or·tho·bi·o·sis (ōr'thō-bī-ō'sis). Rarely used term for correct living, both hygienically and morally. [ortho- + G. *biōsis,* life]

or·tho·caine (ōr'thō-kān). The methyl ester of 3-amino-4-hydroxybenzoic acid; a surface anesthetic agent usually used in dusting powder form.

or·tho·ce·phal·ic (ōr'thō-sě-fal'ik). Having a head well proportioned to height; denoting a skull with a vertical index between 70 and 75. SEE ALSO metriocephalic. SYN orthocephalous. [ortho- + G. *kephalē,* head]

or·tho·ceph·a·lous (ōr-thō-sef'ă-lŭs). SYN orthocephalic.

or·tho·cho·rea (ōr'thō-kōr-ē'ă). A form of chorea in which the spasms occur only or chiefly when the patient is in the erect posture.

or·tho·chro·mat·ic (ōr'thō-krō-mat'ic). Denoting any tissue or cell that stains the color of the dye used, *i.e.,* the same color as the dye solution with which it is stained. SYN euchromatic (1), orthochromophil, orthochromophile. [ortho- + G. *chrōma,* color]

or·tho·chro·mo·phil, or·tho·chro·mo·phile (ōr-thō-krō'mō-fil, -fīl). SYN orthochromatic. [ortho- + G. *chrōma,* color, + *philos,* fond]

or·tho·cra·sia (ōr-thō-krā'sē-ă). Obsolete term for condition in which there is a normal reaction to drugs, articles of diet, etc. [ortho- + G. *krasis,* a mixing, temperament]

or·tho·cy·to·sis (ōr'thō-sī-tō'sis). A condition in which all of the cellular elements in the circulating blood are mature forms, irrespective of the proportions of various types and total numbers. [ortho- + G. *kytos,* cell, + *-osis,* condition]

or·tho·den·tin (ōr-thō-den'tin). Straight tubed dentin as seen in the teeth of mammals.

or·tho·de·ox·ia. Fall in arterial blood oxygen upon assuming the upright posture. Usually due to right-to-left cardiac or vascular shunting with a posturally induced fall in left sided pressure permitting a corresponding gradient across the shunt.

or·tho·di·gi·ta (or-tho-dij'ĭ-tah). Correction of malformations of fingers or toes. [ortho- + L. *digitus,* finger or toe]

or·tho·don·tia (ōr-thō-don'shē-ă). SYN orthodontics.

or·tho·don·tics (ōr-thō-don'tiks). That branch of dentistry concerned with the correction and prevention of irregularities and malocclusion of the teeth. SYN dental orthopedics, orthodontia. [ortho- + G. *odous,* tooth]

surgical o., the correction of occlusal abnormalities by the surgical repositioning of segments of the mandible or maxillae containing one to several teeth; or the bodily repositioning of entire jaws to improve function and esthetics. SYN orthognathic surgery.

or·tho·dont·ist. A dental specialist who practices orthodontics.

or·tho·dro·mic (ōr-thō-drō'mik). Denoting the propagation of an impulse along an axon in the normal direction. Cf. antidromic. SYN dromic. [ortho- + G. *dromos,* course]

or·tho·gen·e·sis (ōr-thō-jen'ě-sis). The doctrine that evolution is governed by intrinsic factors and occurs in predictable directions. [ortho- + G. *genesis,* origin]

or·tho·gen·ic (ōr-thō-jen'ik). Relating to orthogenesis.

or·tho·gen·ics (ōr-thō-jen'iks). SYN eugenics.

or·thog·nath·ia (ōr-thō-nath'ē-ă). The study of the causes and treatment of conditions related to malposition of the bones of the jaws. [ortho- + G. *gnathos,* jaw]

or·thog·nath·ic, or·thog·na·thous (ōr-thō-nath'ik, ōr-thog'năthŭs). **1.** Relating to orthognathia. **2.** Having a face without projecting jaw, one with a gnathic index below 98. [ortho- + G. *gnathos,* jaw]

or·tho·grade (ōr'thō-grād). Walking or standing erect; denoting the posture of man; opposed to pronograde. [ortho- + L. *gradior,* pp. *gressus,* to walk]

or·tho·ker·a·tol·o·gy (ōr'thō-ker-ă-tol'ō-jē). A method of molding the cornea with contact lenses to improve unaided vision. [ortho- + G. *keras,* horn (cornea), + *logos,* science]

or·tho·ker·a·to·sis (ōr'thō-ker-ă-tō'sis). Formation of an anuclear keratin layer, as in the normal epidermis. [ortho- + G. *keras,* horn, + *-osis,* condition]

or·tho·ki·net·ics (ōr-thō-ki-net'iks). A method advocated for the treatment of hypertrophic osteoarthritis in which an attempt is made to change muscular action from one group of muscles to another set of muscles to protect the diseased joint. [ortho- + G. *kinētikos,* movable, fr. *kineō,* to move]

or·tho·me·chan·i·cal (ōr-thō-mě-kan'i-kăl). Pertaining to braces, prostheses, orthotic devices, and appliances. [ortho- + mechanical]

or·tho·me·chan·o·ther·a·py (ōr'thō-mě-kan-ō-thār'ă-pē). Treatment with braces, prostheses, orthotic devices, or appliances. [ortho- + G. *mēchanē,* machine, + *therapeia,* medical treatment]

or·tho·me·lic (ōr-thō-mē'lik). Correcting malformations of arms or legs. [ortho- + G. *melos,* limb]

or·thom·e·ter (ōr-thom'ě-ter). SYN exophthalmometer. [ortho- + G. *metron,* measure]

or·tho·mo·lec·u·lar (ōr'thō-mō-lek'yū-lăr). L.C. Pauling's term denoting a therapeutic approach designed to provide an optimum molecular environment for body functions, with particular reference to the optimum concentrations of substances normally present in the human body, whether formed endogenously or ingested.

Or·tho·myx·o·vir·i·dae (ōr'thō-mik-sō-vir'i-dē). The family of viruses that comprises the three groups of influenza viruses, types A, B, and C. Virions are roughly spherical or filamentous, the former (the more common form) are 80 to 120 nm in diameter and ether-sensitive; envelopes are studded with surface projections; nucleocapsids are of helical symmetry, 6 to 9 nm in diameter, and contain single-stranded, segmented RNA. The nucleoprotein antigen of each type of virus is common to all strains of the type but distinct from those of the other two types; the mosaic of surface antigens varies from strain to strain. Nucleocapsids seem to be formed in the nuclei of infected cells, hemagglutinin and neuraminidase in the cytoplasm; virus maturation occurs during budding of the cell membrane. The only recognized genus is *Influenzavirus,* which comprises the strains of virus types A and B, both of which are subject to mutation resulting in epidemics. Influenza virus type C differs from types A and B somewhat (*e.g.,* the "receptor-destroying enzyme" seems not to be a neuraminidase) and probably belongs to a separate genus. SEE ALSO *Influenzavirus.*

or·tho·pae·dic, or·tho·pe·dic (ōr-thō-pē'dik). Relating to orthopaedics.

or·tho·pae·dics, or·tho·pe·dics (ōr-thō-pē'diks). The medical specialty concerned with the preservation, restoration, and development of form and function of the musculoskeletal system, extremities, spine, and associated structures by medical, surgical, and physical methods. SYN orthopedics. [ortho- + G. *pais* (*paid-*), child]

or·tho·pae·dist, or·tho·pe·dist (ōr-thō-pē′dist). One who practices orthopaedics.

or·tho·pe·dics (ōr-thō-pē′diks). SYN orthopaedics.

dental o., SYN orthodontics.

functional jaw o., utilization of muscle forces to effect changes in jaw position and tooth alignment by removable appliances. SYN functional orthodontic therapy.

or·tho·per·cus·sion (ōr′thō-per-kŭsh′ŭn). Very light percussion of the chest, made in a sagittal direction (*i.e.,* anteroposteriorly, and not perpendicularly to the wall of the chest); used to determine the size of the heart, the faint percussion sound disappearing when the heart is reached even though that may be overlapped by a layer of the lung.

or·tho·pho·ria (ōr-thō-fōr′ē-ă). Absence of heterophoria; the condition of binocular fixation in which the lines of sight meet at a distant or near point of reference in the absence of a fusion stimulus. [ortho- + G. *phora,* motion]

or·tho·phor·ic (ōr-thō-fōr′ik). Pertaining to orthophoria.

or·tho·phos·phate (ōr-thō-fos′fāt). A salt or ester of orthophosphoric acid.

inorganic o. (P$_i$, P$_1$), any ion or salt form of phosphoric acid. SYN inorganic phosphate.

or·tho·phos·phor·ic ac·id (ōr′thō-fos-fōr′ik). Phosphoric acid, O=P(OH)$_3$, distinguished by ortho- from meta- and pyrophosphoric acids, (HPO$_3$)$_n$ and OP(OH$_2$)OP(OH)$_2$O, respectively, which are anhydrides of H$_3$PO$_4$; the ultimate anhydride is phosphorus pentoxide, P$_2$O$_5$.

or·tho·phre·nia (ōr-thō-frē′nē-ă). 1. Rarely used term for soundness of mind. 2. Rarely used term for a condition of normal interpersonal relationships. [ortho- + G. *phrēn,* mind]

or·thop·nea (ōr-thop-nē′ă, ōr-thop′nē-ă). Discomfort in breathing which is brought on or aggravated by lying flat. Cf. platypnea. [ortho- + G. *pnoē,* a breathing]

or·thop·ne·ic (or′thop-ne′ik). Relating to or characterized by orthopnea.

Or·tho·pox·vi·rus (ōr-thō-poks′vī-rŭs). The genus of the family Poxviridae which comprises the viruses of alastrim, vaccinia, variola, cowpox, ectromelia, monkeypox, and rabbitpox.

or·tho·pros·the·sis (ōr′thō-pros′thĕ-sis, -pros-thē′sis). An appliance used in the management of prosthetic problems related to alignment of teeth.

or·tho·psy·chi·a·try (ōr′thō-sī-kī′ă-trē). A cross-disciplinary science combining child psychiatry, developmental psychology, pediatrics, and family care devoted to the discovery, prevention, and treatment of mental and psychological disorders in children and adolescents.

Or·thop·tera (ōr-thop′ter-ă). A large order of hemimetabolous insects that includes the locusts, grasshoppers, mantids, walking sticks, and related forms. [ortho- + G. *pteron,* a wing]

or·thop·tic (ōr-thop′tik). Relating to orthoptics.

or·thop·tics (ōr-thop′tiks). The study and treatment of defective binocular vision, of defects in the action of the ocular muscles, or of faulty visual habits. [*ortho-* straightened + G. *optikos,* sight]

or·thop·tist (ōr-thop′tist). One skilled in orthoptics.

or·tho·scope (ōr′thō-skōp). 1. An instrument by means of which one is able to draw the outlines of the various normas of the skull. [ortho- + G. *skopeō,* to view]

or·tho·sis, pl. **or·tho·ses** (ōr-thō′sis, -sēz). An external orthopaedic appliance, as a brace or splint, that prevents or assists movement of the spine or the limbs. [G. *orthōsis,* a making straight]

or·tho·stat·ic (ōr-thō-stat′ik). Relating to an erect posture or position.

or·tho·ster·e·o·scope (ōr-thō-ster′ē-ō-skōp). A rarely used instrument for viewing stereoscopic radiographs.

or·tho·sym·pa·thet·ic (ōr′thō-sim-pa-thet′ik). Referring to the sympathetic component of the autonomic nervous system, as distinguished from parasympathetic. SEE autonomic nervous *system.*

or·tho·tha·na·sia (ōr′thō-thă-na′zē-ă). 1. A normal or natural manner of death and dying. 2. Sometimes used to denote the deliberate stopping of artificial or heroic means of maintaining life. [ortho- + G. *thanatos,* death]

or·thot·ics (ōr-thot′iks). The science concerned with the making and fitting of orthopaedic appliances. SYN orthetics.

or·tho·tist (ōr′thō′tist). A maker and fitter of orthopaedic appliances.

or·tho·tol·i·dine (ōr-thō-tō′li-dēn). *o*-Tolidine; 3,3′-dimethylbenzidine; in the presence of peroxidase, o. (like benzidine) is oxidized to a blue color; since hemoglobin behaves like a peroxidase, o. has been used as an *in vitro* aid for the detection of occult blood in feces.

or·thot·o·nos, or·thot·o·nus (ōr-thot′ŏ-nos, -ŏ-nŭs). A form of tetanic spasm in which the neck, limbs, and body are held fixed in a straight line. [ortho- + G. *tonos,* tension]

or·tho·top·ic (ōr-thō-top′ik). In the normal or usual position. [ortho- + G. *topos,* place]

or·tho·tro·pic (ōr-thō-trop′ik). Extending or growing in a straight, especially a vertical, direction. [ortho- + G. *tropē,* a turn]

or·tho·vol·tage (ōr-thō-vōl′tij). In radiation therapy, a vague term for voltage between 400 and 600 kv.

Orton, S.T., U.S. neurologist, 1879–1975. SEE Wolf-O. *bodies,* under *body.*

or·y·ce·nin (ōr-ē-sen′in). A glutelin in rice. [G. *oryza,* rice, + -in]

O.S. Abbreviation for L. *oculus sinister,* left eye.

Os Symbol for osmium.

os, gen. **o′ris,** pl. **ora.** 1 [NA]. The mouth. 2. Term applied sometimes to an opening into a hollow organ or canal, especially one with thick or fleshy edges. [L. mouth]

external o. of uterus, the vaginal opening of the uterus. SYN ostium uteri [NA], mouth of the womb, opening of uterus, orificium externum uteri, o. uteri externum, ostium uteri externum.

incompetent cervical o., a defect in the strength of the internal o. allowing premature dilation of the cervix.

Scanzoni's second o., SYN pathologic retraction *ring.*

o. u′teri exter′num, SYN external o. of uterus.

o. u′teri inter′num, SYN *isthmus* of uterus.

OS

os, gen. **os·sis,** pl. **os·sa** (os, os′is, os′ă) [NA]. SYN bone. For histological description, see bone. [L. bone]

o. acromia′le, an acromion that is joined to the scapular spine by fibrous rather than by bony union.

o. basila′re, SYN basilar *bone.*

o. bre′ve [NA], SYN short *bone.*

o. cal′cis, SYN calcaneus (1).

o. capita′tum [NA], SYN capitate (1).

os′sa car′pi [NA], SYN carpal *bones,* under *bone.*

o. centra′le [NA], a small bone occasionally found at the dorsal aspect of the wrist between the scaphoid, capitate, and trapezoid; it is developed as an independent cartilage in early fetal life but usually becomes fused with the scaphoid; it occurs normally in most monkeys. SYN central bone.

o. centra′le tar′si, SYN navicular *bone.*

o. clitor′idis, a small bone located in the clitoris of many carnivorous mammals. It is homologous with the o. penis of many male mammals.

o. coc′cygis [NA], SYN coccyx.

o. costa′le [NA], SYN Rib.

o. cox′ae [NA], SYN hip *bone.*

ossa cra′nii [NA], SYN *bones* of skull, under *bone.*

o. cuboi′deum [NA], SYN cuboid *bone.*

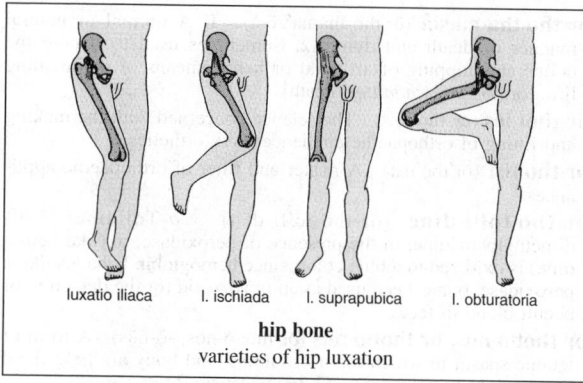

luxatio iliaca   l. ischiada   l. suprapubica   l. obturatoria

hip bone
varieties of hip luxation

o. cuneifor′me interme′dium [NA], SYN intermediate cuneiform *bone.*

o. cuneifor′me latera′le [NA], SYN lateral cuneiform *bone.*

o. cuneifor′me media′le [NA], SYN medial cuneiform *bone.*

os′sa digito′rum [NA], SYN *bones* of digits, under *bone.* SEE ALSO phalanx (1).

o. ethmoida′le [NA], SYN ethmoid *bone.*

os′sa facie′i [NA], SYN facial *bones*, under *bone.*

o. fem′oris [NA], SYN femur.

o. fronta′le [NA], SYN frontal *bone.*

o. hama′tum [NA], SYN hamate *bone.*

o. hyoi′deum [NA], SYN hyoid *bone.* SEE ALSO hyoid *apparatus.*

o. iliacum, ✩official alternate term for ilium.

o. il′ium [NA], SYN ilium.

o. in′cae, SYN o. interparietale.

o. incisi′vum [NA], the anterior and inner portion of the maxilla, which in the fetus and sometimes in the adult is a separate bone; the incisive suture runs from the incisive canal between the lateral incisor and the canine tooth; according to K. Albrecht, the o. incisivum is further divided by a suture between the two incisor teeth on each side into two bones, the endognathion and the mesognathion. SYN incisive bone, intermaxilla, intermaxillary bone, o. intermaxillare, o. premaxillare, premaxilla (1), premaxillary bone.

o. innomina′tum, SYN hip *bone.*

o. intermaxilla′re, SYN o. incisivum.

o. interme′dium, SYN lunate *bone.*

o. intermetatar′seum, a supernumerary bone at the base of the first metatarsal, or between the first and second metatarsal bones, usually fused with one or the other or with the medial cuneiform bone. SYN intermetatarseum.

o. interparieta′le [NA], the upper part of the squama of the occipital bone, developed in membrane instead of in cartilage as is the rest of the occipital, and occasionally (especially in ancient Peruvian skulls) existing as a separate bone, separated from the remainder of the occipital by the sutura mendosa. SYN incarial bone, interparietal bone, o. incae.

o. irregula′re [NA], SYN irregular *bone.*

o. is′chii [NA], SYN ischium.

o. japon′icum, a bipartite or tripartite zygomatic bone, found with greater frequency in the Japanese than in other races.

o. lacrima′le [NA], SYN lacrimal *bone.*

o. lon′gum [NA], SYN long *bone.*

o. luna′tum [NA], SYN lunate *bone.*

o. mag′num, SYN capitate (1).

o. mala′re, SYN zygomatic *bone.*

os′sa mem′bri inferio′ris [NA], SYN *bones* of lower limb, under *bone.*

os′sa mem′bri superio′ris [NA], SYN *bones* of upper limb, under *bone.*

o. metacarpa′le, pl. **os′sa metacarpa′lia** [NA], SYN metacarpal *bone.*

o. metatarsa′le, pl. **os′sa metatarsa′lia** [NA], SYN metatarsal *bone.*

o. multan′gulum ma′jus, SYN trapezium.

o. multan′gulum mi′nus, SYN trapezoid *bone.*

o. nasa′le [NA], SYN nasal *bone.*

o. navicula′re [NA], SYN navicular *bone.*

o. navicula′re ma′nus, SYN scaphoid *bone.*

o. occipita′le [NA], SYN occipital *bone.*

o. odontoi′deum, the dens of the axis when anomalously not fused with the body of the axis.

o. orbicula′re, SYN lenticular *process* of incus.

o. palati′num [NA], SYN palatine *bone.*

o. parieta′le [NA], SYN parietal *bone.*

o. pe′nis, a bone of variable size and shape, located in the glans penis or glans clitoridis of all animals, except man, ungulates, elephants, whales, and a few others; it is particularly well developed in carnivora, and in the dog may reach a length of more than 10 cm; its size and shape are often a characteristic of a species. SYN baculum, penis bone.

o. pisifor′me [NA], SYN pisiform *bone.*

o. pla′num [NA], SYN flat *bone.*

o. pneumat′icum [NA], SYN pneumatic *bone.*

o. premaxilla′re, SYN o. incisivum.

o. pterygoi′deum, SYN pterygoid *process.*

o. pu′bis [NA], SYN *mons* pubis.

o. pyramida′le, SYN triquetral *bone.*

o. sa′crum [NA], SYN sacrum.

o. scaphoi′deum, SYN scaphoid *bone.*

o. sesamoi′deum, pl. **os′sa sesamoi′dea** [NA], SYN sesamoid *bone.*

o. sphenoida′le [NA], SYN sphenoid *bone.*

o. subtibia′le, an inconstant bone found very rarely in the distal articular end of the tibia.

o. suprasterna′le, pl. **os′sa suprasterna′lia** [NA], one of the small ossicles occasionally found in the ligaments of the sternoclavicular articulation. SYN Breschet's bones, episternal bone, suprasternal bone.

os′sa sutura′rum [NA], SYN sutural *bones*, under *bone.*

o. syl′vii, SYN lenticular *process* of incus.

os′sa tar′si [NA], SYN tarsal *bones*, under *bone.*

o. tempora′le [NA], SYN temporal *bone.*

o. tibia′le poste′rius, o. tibia′le posti′cum, a sesamoid bone in the tendon of the tibialis posterior muscle, occasionally fused with the tuberosity of the navicular. SYN tibiale posticum.

o. trape′zium [NA], SYN trapezium.

o. trapezoi′deum [NA], SYN trapezoid *bone.*

o. triangula′re, (1) SYN o. trigonum. **(2)** SYN triquetral *bone.*

o. tribasila′re, the single bone resulting from the fusion in infancy of the occipital and temporal bones at the base of the cranial cavity.

o. trigo′num [NA], an independent ossicle sometimes present in the tarsus; usually it forms part of the talus, constituting the lateral tubercle of the posterior process. SYN o. triangulare (1), triangular bone.

o. trique′trum [NA], SYN triquetral *bone.*

o. un′guis, SYN lacrimal *bone.*

o. vesalia′num, the tuberosity of the fifth metatarsal bone sometimes existing as a separate bone. SYN vesalianum, Vesalius' bone.

o. zygomat′icum [NA], SYN zygomatic *bone.*

---

osa·zone (ō′să-zōn). The compound formed by certain sugars (*e.g.,* glucose, galactose, fructose) with excess hydrazines, possessing two hydrazones on carbons 1 and 2 instead of only one at C-1, as in the ordinary hydrazone; o.'s formed with phenylhydrazine (phenylosazones) are used to characterize and identify certain sugars. SYN dihydrazone.

△**osche-, oscheo-.** The scrotum. [G. *oschē*]

os·che·al (os′kē-ăl). SYN scrotal.

os·che·i·tis (os-kē-ī′tis). Inflammation of the scrotum. [osche- + G. -itis, inflammation]

osch·el·e·phan·ti·a·sis (osk′el-ĕ-fan-tī′ă-sis). An enlargement or elephantiasis of the scrotum. [osche- + elephantiasis]

os·che·o·hy·dro·cele (os-kē-ō-hī′drō-sēl). Scrotal hydrocele. [oscheo- + G. hydōr, water, + kēlē, tumor]

os·che·o·plas·ty (os′kē-ō-plas-tē). SYN scrotoplasty. [oscheo- + plastos, formed]

os·cil·la·tion (os-i-lā′shŭn). **1.** A to-and-fro movement. **2.** A stage in the vascular changes in inflammation in which the accumulation of leukocytes in the small vessels arrests the passage of blood and there is simply a to-and-fro movement at each cardiac contraction. [L. oscillatio, fr. oscillo, to swing]

os·cil·la·tor (os′si-lā-ter). **1.** An apparatus somewhat like a vibrator, used to give a form of mechanical massage. **2.** An electric circuit designed to generate alternating current at a particular frequency. **3.** Any device that produces oscillation.

os·cil·lo·graph (ŏ-sil′ō-graf). An instrument that records oscillations, usually electrical.

os·cil·log·ra·phy (os-i-log′ră-fē). The study of the records made by an oscillograph.

os·cil·lom·e·ter (os-i-lom′ĕ-ter). An apparatus for measuring oscillations of any kind, especially those of the bloodstream in sphygmometry. SEE ALSO sphygmo-oscillometer. [L. oscillo, to swing, + G. metron, measure]

os·cil·lo·met·ric (os′i-lō-met′rik). Relating to the oscillometer or the records made by its use.

os·cil·lom·e·try (os-i-lom′ĕ-trē). The measurement of oscillations of any kind with an oscillometer.

os·cil·lop·sia (os-i-lop′sē-ă). The subjective sensation of oscillation of objects viewed. SYN oscillating vision. [L. oscillo, to swing, + G. opsis, vision]

os·cil·lo·scope (ŏ-sil′ō-skōp). An oscillograph in which the record of oscillations is continuously visible.

    cathode ray o. (CRO), the common form of o., in which a varying electrical signal (y) vertically deflects an electron beam impinging on a fluorescent screen, while some other function (x or time) deflects the beam horizontally; the result is a visual graph of y plotted against x or time with negligible distortion by inertia.

    storage o., a cathode ray o. in which the visual record of oscillations persists on the fluorescent screen until erased electrically.

os·ci·tate (os′i-tāt). To yawn; to gape. [L. oscito, fr. os, mouth, + cieo, to put in motion]

os·ci·ta·tion (os′i-tā′shŭn). SYN yawning. [L. oscitatio]

os·cu·lum, pl. **os·cu·la** (os′kyū-lŭm, -lă). A pore or minute opening. [L. dim. of os, mouth]

△**-ose. 1.** In chemistry, a terminator usually indicating a carbohydrate. **2.** Suffix appended to some Latin roots, with significance of the more common -ous (2). [L. -osus, full of, abounding] **3.** Full of, having much of.

△**-oses.** Plural of -osis.

Osgood, Robert B., U.S. orthopedic surgeon, 1873–1956. SEE O.-Schlatter disease; Schlatter-O. disease.

OSHA Abbreviation for Occupational Safety and Health Administration of the U.S. Department of Labor, responsible for establishing and enforcing safety and health standards in the workplace.

△**-osis**, pl. **-oses.** Suffix, properly added only to words formed from G. roots, meaning a process, condition, or state, usually abnormal or diseased. It denotes primarily any production or increase, physiologic or pathologic, and secondarily an invasion, and increase within the organism, of parasites; in the latter sense, it is similar to and often interchangeable with G. -iasis, as seen in trichinosis, trichiniasis. [G.]

Osler, Sir William, Canadian physician in U.S. and England, 1849–1919. SEE O.'s disease; O. node; O.'s sign; Rendu-O.-Weber syndrome.

os·mate (os′māt). A salt of osmic acid.

os·mat·ic (oz-mat′ik). SYN olfactory. [G. osmē, smell]

os·me·sis (oz-mē′sis). SYN olfaction. [G. osmēsis, smelling]

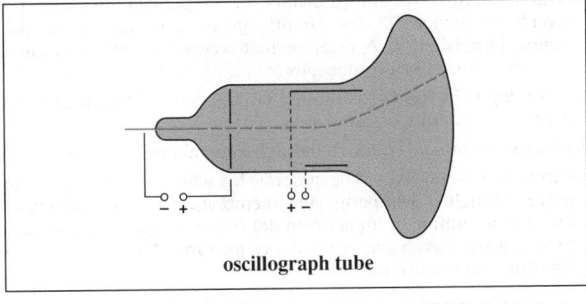
oscillograph tube

os·mic ac·id (oz′mik). OsO₄; a volatile caustic and strong oxidizing agent; colorless crystals, poorly soluble in water, but soluble in organic solvents; the aqueous solution is a fat and myelin stain and a general fixative for electron microscopy. SYN osmium tetroxide.

os·mi·cate (oz′mi-kāt). To stain or fix with osmic acid.

os·mi·ca·tion, os·mi·fi·ca·tion (os′mi-kā′shŭn, os′mi-fi-kā′ shŭn). The fixation of tissue with an osmic acid solution; also serves as a stain for both light and electron microscopy.

os·mics (oz′miks). The science of olfaction. [G. osmē, smell]

os·mi·dro·sis (oz-mi-drō′sis). SYN bromidrosis. [G. osmē, smell, + hidrōs, sweat]

os·mi·o·phil·ic (oz′mi-ō-fil′ik). Readily stained with osmic acid. [osmium + G. phileō, to love]

os·mi·o·pho·bic (oz′mi-ō-fō′bik). Not readily stained with osmic acid. [osmium + G. phobos, fear]

os·mi·um (Os) (oz′mē-ŭm). A metallic element of the platinum group, atomic no. 76, atomic wt. 190.2. [G. osmē, smell, because of the strong odor of the tetroxide]

    o. tetroxide, SYN osmic acid.

△**osmo-. 1.** Osmosis. [G. ōsmos, impulsion] **2.** Smell, odor. [G. osmē]

os·mo·cep·tor (os-mō-sep′ter, tōr). SYN osmoreceptor.

os·mo·dys·pho·ria (oz′mō-dis-fōr′ē-ă). An abnormal dislike of certain odors. [G. osmē, smell, + dys-, bad, + phora, a carrying]

os·mo·gram (oz′mō-gram). SYN electro-olfactogram. [G. osmē, smell, + gramma, a drawing]

os·mo·lal·i·ty (os-mō-lal′i-tē). The concentration of a solution expressed in osmoles of solute particles per kilogram of soluent.

    calculated serum osmolality, the calculation of serum osmolality from serum sodium, glucose, and urea nitrogen values by a variety of formulae, the most common of which is: $1.86 × [Na^{30}] + glucose(mg/dl)/18 + BUN(mg/dl)/2.8$

os·mo·lar (os-mō′lăr). SYN osmotic.

os·mo·lar·i·ty (os-mō-lār′i-tē). The osmotic concentration of a solution expressed as osmoles of solute per liter of solution.

os·mole (os′mōl). The molecular weight of a solute, in grams, divided by the number of ions or particles into which it dissociates in solution.

os·mol·o·gy (os-mol′ō-jē). **1.** The study of odors, their production, and their effects. SYN osphresiology. **2.** The study of osmosis.

os·mom·e·ter (os-mom′ĕ-ter). An instrument for measuring osmolality by freezing point depression or vapor pressure elevation techniques.

os·mom·e·try (os-mom′ĕ-trē). Measurement of osmolality by use of an osmometer.

os·mo·phil, os·mo·phil·ic (os′mō-fil, -fil′ik). Flourishing in a medium of high osmotic pressure. [osmo(sis) + G. phileō, to love]

os·mo·pho·bia (oz-mō-fō′bē-ă). SYN olfactophobia. [G. osmē, smell, + phobia]

os·mo·phore (oz′mō-fōr). The group of atoms in the molecule of a compound that is responsible for the compound's characteristic odor. [G. osmē, smell, + phonos, bearing]

os·mo·re·cep·tor (os′mō-rē-sep′ter, -tōr). **1.** A receptor in the central nervous system (probably the hypothalamus) that responds to changes in the osmotic pressure of the blood. [G. *osmos,* impulsion] **2.** A receptor that receives olfactory stimuli. [G. *osmē,* smell] SYN osmoceptor.

os·mo·reg·u·la·to·ry (os-mō-reg′yū-lă-tōr-ē). Influencing the degree and rapidity of osmosis.

os·mose (os′mōs). To move through a membrane by osmosis.

os·mo·sis (os-mō′sis). The process by which solvent tends to move through a semipermeable membrane from a solution of lower to a solution of higher osmolal concentration of the solutes to which the membrane is relatively impermeable. [G. *ōsmos,* a thrusting, an impulsion]

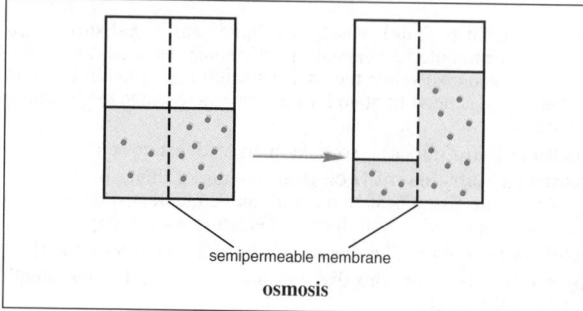

semipermeable membrane

osmosis

reverse o., movement of solvent in the opposite direction from o., *i.e.,* pressure filtration of solvent through a semipermeable membrane that will hold back the solutes; commonly replaced by filtration or ultrafiltration when speaking of capillary membranes, as in the renal glomerulus.

os·mos·i·ty (os-mos′i-tē). An indirect measure of the osmotic characteristics of a solution, in terms of a comparable sodium chloride solution, now rendered obsolete by the more precisely defined term osmolality.

os·mo·ther·a·py (os′mō-thār′ă-pē). Dehydration by means of intravenous injections of hypertonic solutions of sodium chloride, dextrose, urea, mannitol, or other osmotically active substances, or by oral administration of glycerine, isosorbide, glycine, etc.; used in the treatment of cerebral edema and increased intracranial pressure. [osmosis + therapy]

os·mot·ic (os-mot′ik). Relating to osmosis. SYN osmolar.

△**osphresio-.** Odor; sense of smell. [G. *osphrēsis,* smell]

os·phre·si·o·lag·nia (os-frē′zē-ō-lag′nē-ă). Sexual excitement produced by odors. [osphresio- + G. *lagneia,* lust]

os·phre·si·o·log·ic (os-frē-zē-ō-loj′ik). Relating to osphresiology.

os·phre·si·ol·o·gy (os-frē′zē-ol′ŏ-jē). SYN osmology (1). [osphresio- + G. *logos,* study]

os·phre·si·o·phil·ia (os-frē′zē-ō-fil′ē-ă). An unusual interest in odors. [osphresio- + G. *phileō,* to love]

os·phre·si·o·pho·bia (os-frē′zē-ō-fō′bē-ă). SYN olfactophobia. [osphresio- + G. *phobos,* fear]

os·phre·sis (os-frē′sis). SYN olfaction. [G. *osphrēsis,* smell]

os·phret·ic (os-fret′ik). SYN olfactory.

os·sa (os′ă). Plural of L. *os,* bone. [L.]

os·se·in, os·se·ine (os′ē-in). SYN collagen. [L. *os,* bone]

os·se·let (os′ĕ-let). A periostitis of the anterior margin of the third metacarpal bone or first phalanx near the fetlock, characterized first by a painful, soft swelling and later by exostosis; a cause of lameness in horses, particularly young race horses in training. [L. dim. of *os,* bone]

△**osseo-.** Bony. SEE ALSO ossi-, osteo-. [L. *osseus*]

os·se·o·car·ti·lag·i·nous (os′ē-ō-kar-ti-laj′i-nŭs). Relating to, or composed of, both bone and cartilage. SYN osteocartilaginous, osteochondrous.

os·se·o·mu·cin (os′ē-ō-myū′sin). The ground substance of bony tissue.

os·se·o·mu·coid (os′ē-ō-myū′koyd). A mucoid derived from ossein.

os·se·ous (os′ē-ŭs). Bony, of bone-like consistency or structure. SYN osteal. [L. *osseus*]

△**ossi-.** Bone. SEE ALSO osseo-, osteo-. [L. *os*]

os·si·cle (os′i-kl). A small bone; specifically, one of the bones of the tympanic cavity or middle ear. SYN ossiculum [NA], bonelet. [L. *ossiculum,* dim. of *os,* bone]

Andernach's o.'s, SYN sutural *bones,* under *bone.*

auditory o.'s, the small bones of the middle ear; they are articulated to form a chain for the transmission of sound from the tympanic membrane to the oval window. SYN ossicula auditus [NA], ear bones, ossicular chain.

Bertin's o.'s, SYN sphenoidal *conchae,* under *concha.*

epactal o.'s, SYN sutural *bones,* under *bone.*

Kerckring's o., SYN Kerckring's *center.*

os·sic·u·la (ŏ-sik′yū-lă). Plural of ossiculum. [L.]

os·sic·u·lar (ŏ-sik′yū-lăr). Pertaining to an ossicle.

os·sic·u·lec·to·my (os′i-kyū-lek′tō-mē). Removal of one or more of the ossicles of the middle ear. [L. *ossiculum,* ossicle, + G. *ektomē,* excision]

os·si·cu·lot·o·my (os′i-kyū-lot′ō-mē). Division of one of the processes of the ossicles of the middle ear, or of a fibrous band causing ankylosis between any two ossicles. [L. *ossiculum,* ossicle, + G. *tomē,* incision]

os·sic·u·lum, pl. **os·sic·u·la** (ŏ-sik′yū-lŭm, -lă) [NA]. SYN ossicle. [L. dim. of *os,* bone]

ossicula audi′tus [NA], SYN auditory *ossicles,* under *ossicle.*

ossic′ula menta′lia, small nodules of bone that appear at the symphysis menti shortly before birth and fuse with the mandible after birth.

os·sif·er·ous (ŏ-sif′er-ŭs). Containing or producing bone. [ossi- + L. *fero,* to bear]

os·sif·ic (o-sif′ik). Relating to a change into, or formation of, bone.

os·si·fi·ca·tion (os′i-fi-kā′shŭn). **1.** The formation of bone. **2.** A change into bone. [L. *ossificatio,* fr. *os,* bone, + *facio,* to make]

endochondral o., formation of osseous tissue by the replacement of calcified cartilage; long bones grow in length by endochondral o. at the epiphysial cartilage plate where osteoblasts form bone trabeculae on a framework of calcified cartilage.

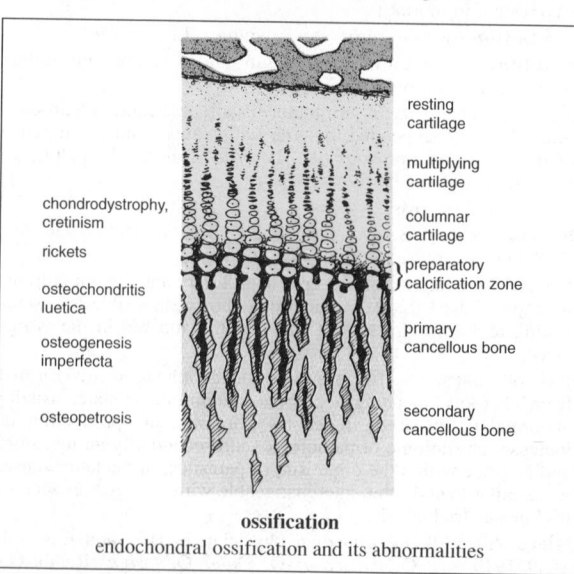

resting cartilage

multiplying cartilage

columnar cartilage

preparatory calcification zone

primary cancellous bone

secondary cancellous bone

chondrodystrophy, cretinism

rickets

osteochondritis luetica

osteogenesis imperfecta

osteopetrosis

ossification
endochondral ossification and its abnormalities

intramembranous o., SYN membranous o.

membranous o., intramembranous o., development of osseous tissue within mesenchymal tissue without prior cartilage formation, such as occurs in the frontal and parietal bones. SYN intramembranous o.

metaplastic o., the formation of irregular foci of bone (sometimes including bone marrow) in various soft structures, such as the muscles, lungs, brain, and other sites where osseous tissue is abnormal.

os·si·form (os′i-fōrm). SYN osteoid (1). [ossi- + L. *forma,* form]

os·si·fy (os′i-fī). To form bone or convert into bone. [ossi- + L. *facio,* to make]

⚕**ost-.** SEE osteo-.

os·te·al (os′tē-ăl). SYN osseous. [G. *osteon,* bone]

os·te·al·gia (os-tē-al′jē-ă). Pain in a bone. SYN osteodynia. [osteo- + G. *algos,* pain]

os·te·al·gic (os-tē-al′jik). Relating to or marked by bone pain.

os·te·an·a·gen·e·sis (os′tē-an-ă-jen′ĕ-sis). SYN osteoanagenesis.

os·te·a·naph·y·sis (os′tē-ă-naf′i-sis). SYN osteoanagenesis. [osteo- + G. *anaphysis,* a growing again]

os·tec·to·my (os-tek′tō-mē). **1.** Surgical removal of bone. **2.** In dentistry, resection of supporting osseous structure to eliminate periodontal pockets. SYN osteoectomy. [osteo- + G. *ektomē,* excision]

os·te·in, os·te·ine (os′tē-in). SYN collagen. [G. *osteon,* bone]

os·te·it·ic (os-tē-it′ik). Relating to or affected by osteitis. SYN ostitic.

os·te·i·tis (os-tē-ī′tis). Inflammation of bone. SYN ostitis. [osteo- + G. *-itis,* inflammation]

alveolar o., SYN alveoalgia.

caseous o., tuberculous caries in bone.

central o., (1) SYN osteomyelitis. (2) SYN endosteitis.

o. condensans ilii (con-den′sanz il′ē-ī), symmetric benign osteosclerosis of the portion of the iliac bones adjacent to the sacroiliac joints.

condensing o., SYN sclerosing o.

cortical o., periostitis with involvement of the superficial layer of bone.

o. defor′mans, SYN Paget's *disease* (1).

o. fibro′sa cir′cumscrip′ta, SYN monostotic fibrous *dysplasia.*

o. fibro′sa cys′tica, increased osteoclastic resorption of calcified bone with replacement by fibrous tissue, due to primary hyperparathyroidism or other causes of the rapid mobilization of mineral salts. SYN parathyroid osteosis, Recklinghausen's disease of bone.

o. fibro′sa disseminat′a, SYN polyostotic fibrous *dysplasia.*

focal condensing o., SYN chronic focal sclerosing *osteomyelitis.*

hematogenous o., any o. caused by infection carried in the bloodstream.

localized o. fibro′sa, SYN monostotic fibrous *dysplasia.*

multifocal o. fibro′sa, SYN polyostotic fibrous *dysplasia.*

o. pubis, osteosclerosis of the pubic bone next to the symphysis, caused by trauma to that region, from pregnancy or instrumentation.

renal o. fibro′sa, SYN renal *rickets.*

sclerosing o., fusiform thickening or increased density of bones, of unknown cause; it has been considered a form of chronic nonsuppurative osteomyelitis. SYN condensing o., Garré's disease.

o. tuberculo′sa mul′tiplex cys′tica, an o. of tuberculous origin, marked by numerous small cavities in the osseous substance. SYN Jüngling's disease.

os·tem·bry·on (os-tem′brē-on). Archaic term for lithopedion. [osteo- + G. *embryon,* embryo]

os·te·mia (os-tē′mē-ă). Congestion or hyperemia of a bone. [osteo- + G. *haima,* blood]

os·tem·py·e·sis (os′tem-pī-ē′sis). Suppuration in bone. [osteo- + G. *empyēsis,* suppuration]

⚕**osteo-, ost-, oste-.** Bone. SEE ALSO osseo-, ossi-. [G. *osteon*]

os·te·o·an·a·gen·e·sis (os′tē-ō-an-ă-jen′ĕ-sis). Regeneration of bone. SYN osteanagenesis, osteanaphysis. [osteo- + G. *ana,* again, + *genesis,* generation]

os·te·o·ar·thri·tis (os′tē-ō-ar-thrī′tis). Arthritis characterized by

erosion of articular cartilage, either primary or secondary to trauma or other conditions, which becomes soft, frayed, and thinned with eburnation of subchondral bone and outgrowths of marginal osteophytes; pain and loss of function result; mainly affects weight-bearing joints, is more common in older persons. SYN degenerative arthritis, degenerative joint disease, hypertrophic arthritis, osteoarthrosis.

hyperplastic o., SYN hypertrophic pulmonary *osteoarthropathy.*

os·te·o·ar·throp·a·thy (os′tē-ō-ar-throp′ă-thē). A disorder affecting bones and joints. [osteo- + G. *arthron,* joint, + *pathos,* suffering]

hypertrophic pulmonary o., expansion of the distal ends, or the entire shafts, of the long bones, sometimes with erosions of the articular cartilages and thickening and villous proliferation of the synovial membranes, and frequently clubbing of fingers; the disorder occurs in chronic pulmonary disease, in heart disease, and occasionally in other acute and chronic disorders; also occurs in dogs as a result of *Spirocerca lupi* infection of the esophagus. SYN Bamberger-Marie disease, Bamberger-Marie syndrome, hyperplastic osteoarthritis, pneumogenic o., pulmonary o.

idiopathic hypertrophic o., o. not secondary to pulmonary or other progressive lesions, which may occur alone (acropathy) or as part of the syndrome of pachydermoperiostosis.

pneumogenic o., SYN hypertrophic pulmonary o.

pulmonary o., SYN hypertrophic pulmonary o.

os·te·o·ar·thro·sis (os′tē-ō-ar-thrō′sis). SYN osteoarthritis. [osteo- + G. *arthron,* joint, + *-osis,* condition]

os·te·o·blast (os′tē-ō-blast). A bone-forming cell that is derived from mesenchyme (fibroblast) and forms an osseous matrix in which it becomes enclosed as an osteocyte. SYN osteoplast. [osteo- + G. *blastos,* germ]

os·te·o·blas·tic (os′tē-ō-blas′tik). Relating to the osteoblasts; describes any region of increased radiographic bone density, in particular, metastases that stimulate o. activity.

os·te·o·blas·to·ma (os′tē-ō-blas-tō′mă). An uncommon benign tumor of osteoblasts with areas of osteoid and calcified tissue, occurring most frequently in the spine of a young person. SYN giant osteoid osteoma.

os·te·o·cal·cin. A protein found in bone and dentin; contains γ-carboxyglutamyl residues; has a role in mineralization and calcium ion homeostasis. SYN bone Gla protein.

os·te·o·car·ci·no·ma (os′tē-ō-kar′si-nō′mă). Undesirable and obsolete nonspecific term for a metastasis of carcinoma in a bone, or a carcinoma that contains foci of osseous tissue (as a result of metaplasia).

os·te·o·car·ti·lag·i·nous (os′tē-ō-kar-ti-laj′i-nŭs). SYN osseocartilaginous.

os·te·o·chon·dri·tis (os′tē-ō-kon-drī′tis). Inflammation of a bone and its cartilage. [osteo- + G. *chondros,* cartilage, + *-itis,* inflammation]

o. defor′mans juveni′lis, SYN Legg-Calvé-Perthes *disease.*

o. defor′mans juveni′lis dor′si, SYN Scheuermann's *disease.*

o. dis′secans, complete or incomplete separation of a portion of joint cartilage and underlying bone, usually involving the knee, associated with epiphyseal aseptic necrosis.

syphilitic o., inflammation of the epiphysial line associated with congenital syphilis. SYN Wegner's disease.

os·te·o·chondro·dys·pla·sia. SYN camptomelic *syndrome.*

os·te·o·chon·dro·dys·tro·phia de·for·mans (os′tē-ō-kon′drō-dis-trō′fē-ă dē-fōr′manz). SYN chondro-osteodystrophy.

os·te·o·chon·dro·dys·tro·phy (os′tē-ō-kon′drō-dis′trō-fē). SYN chondro-osteodystrophy.

os·te·o·chon·dro·ma (os′tē-ō-kon-drō′mă). A benign cartilaginous neoplasm that consists of a pedicle of normal bone (protruding from the cortex) covered with a rim of proliferating cartilage cells; may originate from any bone that is preformed in cartilage, but is most frequent near the ends of long bones, usually in patients who are 10 to 25 years of age; the lesion is frequently not noticed, unless it is traumatized or of large size; multiple o.'s are inherited and referred to as hereditary multiple exostoses. SYN solitary osteocartilaginous exostosis. [osteo- + G. *chondros,* cartilage, + *-oma,* tumor]

os·te·o·chon·dro·ma·to·sis (os'tē-ō-kon-drō-mă-tō'-sis). SYN hereditary multiple *exostoses,* under *exostosis.*

synovial o., SYN synovial *chondromatosis.*

os·te·o·chon·dro·sar·co·ma (os'tē-ō-kon'drō-sar-kō'-mă). Chondrosarcoma arising in bone. Sarcomas in bone containing foci of neoplastic cartilage as well as bone are classified as osteogenic sarcomas. [osteo- + G. *chondros,* cartilage, + *sarx,* flesh, + *-oma,* tumor]

os·te·o·chon·dro·sis (os'tē-ō-kon-drō'sis). Any of a group of disorders of one or more ossification centers in children, characterized by degeneration or aseptic necrosis followed by reossification; includes the various forms of epiphysial aseptic necrosis. [osteo- + G. *chondros,* cartilage, + *-osis,* condition]

os·te·o·chon·drous (os'tē-ō-kon'drŭs). SYN osseocartilaginous. [osteo- + G. *chondros,* cartilage]

os·te·oc·la·sis, os·te·o·cla·sia (os'tē-ok'lă-sis, os'tē-ō-klā'zē-ă). Intentional fracture of a bone in order to correct deformity. SYN diaclasis, diaclasia. [osteo- + G. *klasis,* fracture]

os·te·o·clast (os'tē-ō-klast). **1.** A large multinucleated cell, possibly of monocytic origin, with abundant acidophilic cytoplasm, functioning in the absorption and removal of osseous tissue. SYN osteophage. **2.** An instrument used to fracture a bone to correct a deformity. [osteo- + G. *klastos,* broken]

os·te·o·clas·tic (os'tē-ō-klas'tik). Pertaining to osteoclasts, especially with reference to their activity in the absorption and removal of osseous tissue.

os·te·o·clas·to·ma (os'tē-ō-klas-tō'mă). SYN giant cell *tumor* of bone.

os·te·o·cra·ni·um (os'tē-ō-krā'nē-ŭm). The cranium of the fetus after ossification of the membranous cranium has made it firm. [osteo- + G. *kranion,* skull]

os·te·o·cys·to·ma (os'tē-ō-sis-tō'mă). SYN solitary bone *cyst.*

os·te·o·cyte (os'tē-ō-sīt). A cell of osseous tissue that occupies a lacuna and has cytoplasmic processes that extend into canaliculi and make contact by means of gap junctions with the processes of other osteocytes. SYN bone cell, bone corpuscle, osseous cell. [osteo- + G. *kytos,* cell]

os·te·o·den·tin (os'tē-ō-den'tin). Rapidly formed tertiary dentin that contains entrapped odontoblasts and few dentinal tubules, thereby superficially resembling bone. [osteo- + L. *dens,* tooth]

os·te·o·der·ma·to·poi·ki·lo·sis (os'tē-ō-der'mă-tō-poy-ki-lō'sis) [MIM*166700]. Osteopoikilosis with skin lesions, most commonly small elastic fibrous nodules on the posterior aspects of the thighs and buttocks; irregular autosomal dominant inheritance. SYN Buschke-Ollendorf syndrome. [osteo- + G. *derma,* skin, + *poikilos,* dappled, + *-osis,* condition]

os·te·o·der·ma·tous (os'tē-ō-der'mă-tŭs). Pertaining to or characterized by osteodermia.

os·te·o·der·mia (os'tē-ō-der'mē-ă). SYN *osteoma* cutis. [osteo- + G. *derma,* skin]

os·te·o·des·mo·sis (os'tē-ō-dez-mō'sis). Transformation of tendon into bony tissue. [osteo- + G. *desmos,* a band (tendon), + *-osis,* condition]

os·te·o·di·as·ta·sis (os'tē-ō-dī-as'tă-sis). Separation of two adjacent bones, as of the cranium. [osteo- + G. *diastasis,* a separation]

os·te·o·dyn·ia (os-tē-ō-din'ē-ă). SYN ostealgia. [osteo- + G. *odynē,* pain]

os·te·o·dys·plas·ty (os'tē-ō-dis'plas-tē). A generalized skeletal dysplasia with prominent forehead and small mandible; radiographically, there are irregular ribbon-like constrictions of the ribs and tubular bones; probably autosomal dominant inheritance. There are arguably two forms, autosomal recessive [MIM*249420] and X-linked [MIM*309350]. SYN Melnick-Needles syndrome. [osteo- + G. *dys-,* bad, + *plastos,* formed]

os·te·o·dys·tro·phia (os'tē-ō-dis-trō'fē-ă). SYN osteodystrophy.

os·te·o·dys·tro·phy (os'tē-ō-dis'trō-fē). Defective formation of bone; common in dogs with chronic nephritis. SYN osteodystrophia. [osteo- + G. *dys,* difficult, imperfect, + *trophē,* nourishment]

Albright's hereditary o., an inherited form of hyperparathyroidism associated with ectopic calcification and ossification and skeletal defects, notably the small fourth metacarpals, but intelligence is normal. There are dominant [MIM*103580 and *139320.001], recessive [MIM*203330] and X-linked [MIM*300800] forms. SEE ALSO pseudohypoparathyroidism. SYN Albright's syndrome (2).

renal o., generalized bone changes resembling osteomalacia and rickets or osteitis fibrosa, occurring in children or adults with chronic renal failure.

os·te·o·ec·ta·sia (os'tē-ō-ek-tā'zē-ă). Bowing of bones, particularly of the legs. [osteo- + G. *ektasis,* a stretching]

os·te·o·ec·to·my (os-tē-ō-ek'tō-mē). SYN ostectomy.

os·te·o·e·piph·y·sis (os'tē-ō-e-pif'i-sis). An epiphysis of a bone.

os·te·o·fi·bro·ma (os'tē-ō-fī-brō'mă). A benign lesion of bone, probably not a true neoplasm, consisting chiefly of fairly dense, moderately cellular, fibrous connective tissue in which there are small foci of osteogenesis. Most examples of this condition, especially in the maxilla and mandible, probably represent foci of fibrous dysplasia; a few examples of fibrous lesions with foci of osteogenesis, especially in vertebral bodies, may be neoplasms.

os·te·o·fi·bro·sis (os'tē-ō-fī-brō'sis). Fibrosis of bone, mainly involving red bone marrow.

periapical o., SYN periapical cemental *dysplasia.*

os·te·o·gen (os'tē-ō-jen). A bone matrix-producing tissue or layer. [osteo- + G. *-gen,* producing]

os·te·o·gen·e·sis (os'tē-ō-jen'ĕ-sis). The formation of bone. SYN osteogeny, osteosis (2), ostosis (2). [osteo- + G. *genesis,* production]

o. imperfec'ta, a large and miscellaneous group of conditions of abnormal fragility and plasticity of bone, with recurring fractures on trivial trauma; variable associated features include deformity of long bones, blueness of sclerae [MIM 166200], laxity of ligaments, and otosclerosis; inheritance is autosomal dominant in most families [MIM*120150, *120160, 166200, 166210–166230], but rare autosomal recessive types also exist [MIM 259400–259450]; there is an alteration in procollagen and collagen. In **o. imperfecta congenita,** a more severe form [MIM 166230], the fractures occur before or at birth; in **o. imperfecta tarda,** a less severe form, the fractures occur later in childhood. More recently classified as o. imperfecta types I, II, III, and IV based on the mode of inheritance as well as on clinical and biochemical criteria. SYN brittle bones.

os·te·o·gen·ic, os·te·o·ge·net·ic (os'tē-ō-jen'ik, -jĕ-net'ik). Relating to osteogenesis. SYN osteogenous, osteoplastic (1).

os·te·og·e·nous (os-tē-oj'ĕ-nŭs). SYN osteogenic.

os·te·og·e·ny (os-tē-oj'ĕ-nē). SYN osteogenesis.

os·te·og·ra·phy (os'tē-og'ră-fē). A treatise on or description of the bones. [osteo- + G. *graphē,* a writing]

os·te·o·ha·li·ste·re·sis (os'tē-ō-hal'is-ter-ē'sis). Softening of the bones through absorption or insufficient supply of the mineral portion. [osteo- + G. *hals,* salt, + *sterēsis,* privation]

os·te·o·hy·per·tro·phy (os'tē-ō-hī-per'trō-fē). Condition characterized by overgrowth of bones. [osteo- + G. *hyper-* over, + *trophē,* nourishment]

os·te·oid (os'tē-oyd). **1.** Relating to or resembling bone. SYN ossiform. **2.** Newly formed organic bone matrix prior to calcification. [osteo- + G. *eidos,* resemblance]

os·te·o·lath·y·rism (os'tē-ō-lath'i-rizm). An experimental disease in rats, swine, turkeys, and other animals fed the seeds of certain species of *Lathyrus* (*e.g.,* L. *odoratus,* sweet pea), or such nitriles as aminoacetonitrile or β-aminopropionitrile; the chief pathologic changes occur in connective tissue structures, as follows: 1) fibroblastic, chondroblastic, and osteoblastic proliferative changes in the periosteum; 2) degeneration, necrosis, and atypical proliferation of epiphysial cartilages; 3) an increase in adipose tissue of the bone marrow; 4) sometimes proliferation of synovial membranes; 5) relatively large foci of extensive destruction of elastic fibers in the aorta, especially in the thoracic aorta. [osteo- + lathyrism]

os·te·o·lip·o·chon·dro·ma (os'tē-ō-lip'ō-kon-drō'mă). A benign neoplasm of cartilaginous tissue, in which metaplasia occurs and foci of adipose cells and osseous tissue are formed. [osteo- + G. *lipos,* fat, + *chondros,* cartilage, + *-oma,* tumor]

os·te·o·lo·gia (os-tē-ō-lō′jē-ă) [NA]. SYN osteology, osteology. [L.]

os·te·ol·o·gist (os′tē-ol′ŏ-jist). A specialist in osteology.

os·te·ol·o·gy (os′tē-ol′ŏ-jē). The anatomy of the bones; the science concerned with the bones and their structure. SYN osteologia [NA]. [osteo- + G. *logos,* study]

os·te·ol·y·sis (os-tē-ol′i-sis). Softening, absorption, and destruction of bony tissue, a function of the osteoclasts. [osteo- + G. *lysis,* dissolution]

os·te·o·lyt·ic (os-tē-ō-lit′ik). Pertaining to, characterized by, or causing osteolysis.

os·te·o·ma (os-tē-ō′mă). A benign slow-growing mass of mature, predominantly lamellar bone, usually arising from the skull or mandible. [osteo- + G. *-oma,* tumor]

o. cu′tis, cutaneous ossification usually secondary to calcification in foci of degeneration in tumors or inflammatory lesions or rarely primary new bone formation with normal skin. SYN dermostosis, osteodermia, osteosis cutis.

dental o., an exostosis arising from the root of a tooth.

giant osteoid o., SYN osteoblastoma.

o. medulla′re, an o. containing spaces that are filled (or partly filled) with various elements of bone marrow.

osteoid o., a painful benign neoplasm that usually originates in one of the bones of the lower extremities, especially the femur or tibia of adolescent and young adult persons; characterized by a nidus (usually no larger than 1 cm in diameter) that consists of osteoid material, vascularized osteogenic stroma, and poorly formed bone; around the nidus there is a relatively large zone of reactive thickening of the cortex.

o. spongio′sum, an o. that consists chiefly of cancellous bone tissue.

os·te·o·ma·la·cia (os′tē-ō-mă-lā′shē-ă). A disease characterized by a gradual softening and bending of the bones with varying severity of pain; softening occurs because the bones contain osteoid tissue which has failed to calcify due to lack of vitamin D or renal tubular dysfunction; more common in women than in men, o. often begins during pregnancy. SYN adult rickets, late rickets, rachitis tarda. [osteo- + G. *malakia,* softness]

infantile o., juvenile o., SYN rickets.

senile o., osteoporosis in the aged.

os·te·o·ma·lac·ic (os′tē-ō-mă-lā′sik). Relating to, or suffering from, osteomalacia.

os·te·o·ma·toid (os-tē-ō′mă-toyd). An abnormal nodule or small mass of overgrowth of bone, usually occurring bilaterally and symmetrically, in juxtaepiphysial regions, especially in long bones of the lower extremities; lesions are not actually neoplasms, but represent anomalous developments in which there are outpouchings of the cortex (in contrast to a growth superimposed on the cortex), and are more properly termed exostoses. [osteoma + G. *eidos,* appearance, form]

os·te·o·mere (os′tē-ō-mēr). One of the series of bone segments, such as the vertebrae. [osteo- + G. *meros,* a part]

os·te·om·e·try (os-tē-om′ĕ-trē). The branch of anthropometry concerned with the relative size of the different parts of the skeleton. [osteo- + G. *metron,* measurement]

os·te·o·my·e·li·tis (os′tē-ō-mī-ĕ-lī′tis). Inflammation of the bone marrow and adjacent bone. SYN central osteitis (1). [osteo- + G. *myelos,* marrow, + *-itis,* inflammation]

chronic diffuse sclerosing o., a proliferative reaction of bone to a low-grade infection of the jaws; most often seen in middle-aged or older black women as extensive, often bilateral radio-opacities of the mandible and maxilla.

chronic focal sclerosing o., a reaction of bone to a mild bacterial infection, often the result of a carious tooth, in persons with a high degree of tissue resistance; results in a localized radio-opacity. SYN focal condensing osteitis.

Garré's o., chronic o. with proliferative periostitis. A focal gross thickening of the periosteum with peripheral reactive bone formation resulting from mild infection.

---

etiology of osteomalacia

vitamin D deficiency

malnutrition (in developing nations, slums, vegetarians, older persons)

reduced absorption due to impaired digestion (gastrectomy, reduced bile secretion, pancreatic insufficiency, malabsorption (sprue, intestinal resections)

reduced formation of vitamin D_3 due to lack of UV light (rickets in children)

disrupted metabolism of vitamin D

disruption of calcidiol formation in liver (antiepileptic therapy, hepatic cirrhosis)

disruption of 1-hydroxylation in the kidneys (kidney failure, pseudovitamin D deficiency, rickets)

disrupted phosphate metabolism

phosphaturia (phosphate diabetes, congenital and acquired)

cystinosis (congenital and acquired)

renal tubular acidosis

tumor-induced forms (with bone tumors and mesenchymal tumors)

phosphate deficiency

hypophosphatasia (congenital: autosomal recessive)

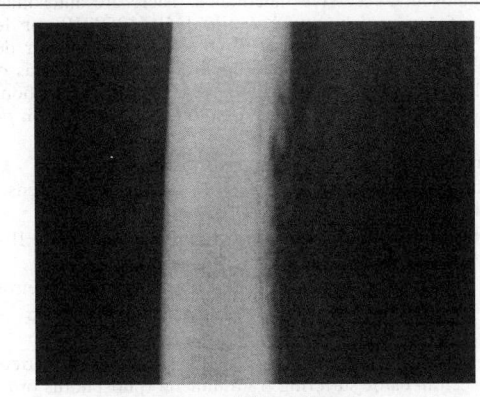

osteomyelitis on femur

os·te·o·my·e·lo·dys·pla·sia (os′tē-ō-mī′ĕ-lō-dis-plā′-zē-ă). A disease characterized by enlargement of the marrow cavities of the bones, thinning of the osseous tissue, large, thin-walled vascular spaces, leukopenia, and irregular fever. [osteo- + G. *myelos,* marrow, + dysplasia]

os·te·on, os·te·one (os′tē-on, -ōn). A central canal containing blood capillaries and the concentric osseous lamellae around it occurring in compact bone. SYN haversian system. [G. *osteon,* bone]

os·te·on·cus (os-tē-ong′kŭs). An osteoma, sometimes used with reference to any neoplasm of a bone. [osteo- + G. *onkos,* bulk (swelling)]

os·te·o·ne·cro·sis (os′tē-ō-ne-krō′sis). The death of bone in mass, as distinguished from caries ("molecular death") or relatively small foci of necrosis in bone. [osteo- + G. *nekrōsis,* death]

os·te·o·nec·tin. A protein (MW 39,000-40,000) found in bone and nonmineralized tissues and believed to play a role in mineralization.

os·te·o·path (os′tē-ō-path). SYN osteopathic *physician.*

os·te·o·path·ia (os′tē-ō-path′ē-ă). SYN osteopathy (1).

   o. conden′sans, SYN osteopoikilosis.

   o. hemorrha′gica infan′tum, SYN infantile *scurvy.*

   o. stria′ta, linear striations seen radiographically in the metaphyses of long bones and also flat bones; it may be a variant of osteopoikilosis. SYN Voorhoeve's disease.

os·te·o·path·ic (os-tē-ō-path′ik). Relating to osteopathy.

os·te·o·pa·thol·o·gy (os′tē-ō-pa-thol′ŏ-jē). Study of diseases of bone.

os·te·op·a·thy (os-tē-op′ă-thē). **1.** Any disease of bone. SYN osteopathia. **2.** A school of medicine based upon a concept of the normal body as a vital machine capable, when in correct adjustment, of making its own remedies against infections and other toxic conditions; practitioners use the diagnostic and therapeutic measures of conventional medicine in addition to manipulative measures. SYN osteopathic medicine. [osteo- + G. *pathos,* suffering]

   alimentary o., bone disease due to dietary deficiency.

os·te·o·pe·di·on (os′tē-ō-pē′dē-on). Archaic term for lithopedion. [osteo- + G. *paidion,* dim. of *pais,* a child]

os·te·o·pe·nia (os′tē-ō-pē′nē-ă). **1.** Decreased calcification or density of bone; a descriptive term applicable to all skeletal systems in which such a condition is noted; carries no implication about causality. **2.** Reduced bone mass due to inadequate osteoid synthesis. [osteo- + G. *penia,* poverty]

os·te·o·per·i·os·ti·tis (os′tē-ō-per′ē-os-tī′tis). Inflammation of the periosteum and of the underlying bone.

os·te·o·pe·tro·sis (os′tē-ō-pe-trō′sis) [MIM*166600]. Excessive formation of dense trabecular bone and calcified cartilage, especially in long bones, leading to obliteration of marrow spaces and to anemia, with myeloid metaplasia and hepatosplenomegaly, beginning in infancy and with progressive deafness and blindness; autosomal recessive inheritance. There are autosomal recessive forms which may be mild [MIM*259310] or lethal [MIM*259720] and sometimes involves a renal tubular defect [MIM*259730]. A milder, autosomal domimant form has onset in childhood and no neurologic sequelae. SYN Albers-Schönberg disease, marble bone disease, marble bones. [osteo- + G. *petra,* stone, + *-osis,* condition]

   o. ac′ro-osteoly′tica, SYN pyknodysostosis.

   o. gallina′rum, a virus-induced bone tumor of chickens. SEE ALSO avian *leukosis.*

   o. with renal tubular acidosis, SYN carbonic anhydrase II deficiency *syndrome.*

os·te·o·pe·trot·ic (os′tē-ō-pe-trot′ik). Relating to osteopetrosis.

os·te·o·phage (os′tē-ō-fāj). SYN osteoclast (1). [osteo- + G. *phagō,* to eat]

os·te·o·pha·gia (os′tē-ō-fā′jē-ă). Eating of bones; perverted appetite seen in cattle suffering from mineral (phosphorus or calcium) deficiency. [osteo- + G. *phagō,* to eat]

os·te·o·phle·bi·tis (os′tē-ō-fle-bī′tis). Inflammation of the veins of a bone. [osteo- + G. *phleps,* vein, + *-itis,* inflammation]

os·te·oph·o·ny (os′tē-of′ō-nē). SYN bone *conduction.*

os·te·o·phy·ma (os-tē-ō-fī′mă). SYN osteophyte. [osteo- + G. *phyma,* tumor]

os·te·o·phyte (os′tē-ō-fīt). A bony outgrowth or protuberance. SYN osteophyma. [osteo- + G. *phyton,* plant]

os·te·o·plaque (os′tē-ō-plak). Any osseous layer. [osteo- + Fr. *plaque,* plate]

os·te·o·plast (os′tē-ō-plast). SYN osteoblast. [osteo- + G. *plastos,* formed]

os·te·o·plas·tic (os-tē-ō-plas′tik). **1.** SYN osteogenic. **2.** Relating to osteoplasty.

os·te·o·plas·ty (os′tē-ō-plas-tē). **1.** Bone grafting; reparative or plastic surgery of the bones. **2.** In dentistry, resection of osseous structure to achieve acceptable gingival contour. [osteo- + G. *plastos,* formed]

os·te·o·poi·ki·lo·sis (os′tē-ō-poy-ki-lō′sis). Mottled or spotted bones caused by widespread small foci of compact bone in the substantia spongiosa; autosomal dominant inheritance [MIM*166700]. SEE ALSO *osteopathia* striata, dermatofibrosis lenticularis disseminata. SYN osteopathia condensans. [osteo- + G. *poikilos,* dappled, + *-osis,* condition]

os·te·o·po·nin. A protein produced by osteoblasts of unknown function.

os·te·o·pon·tin. A secreted phosphoprotein, produced by many epithelial cell types, that is highly negatively charged and frequently associated with mineralization processes. It is found in plasma, urine, milk, and bile. Transformed cells express o. in elevated levels.

os·te·o·po·ro·sis (os′tē-ō-pō-rō′sis). Reduction in the quantity of bone or atrophy of skeletal tissue; occurs in postmenopausal women and elderly men, resulting in bone trabeculae that are scanty, thin, and without osteoclastic resorption. [osteo- + G. *poros,* pore, + *-osis,* condition]

   o. circumscrip′ta cra′nii, localized cranial o. often seen in Paget's disease.

   juvenile o., idiopathic o. with onset before puberty, leading to pain or fractures, with spontaneous remission within a few years.

   posttraumatic o., SYN Sudeck's *atrophy.*

os·te·o·po·rot·ic (os′tē-ō-pŏ-rot′ik). Pertaining to, characterized by, or causing a porous condition of the bones.

os·te·o·ra·di·ol·o·gist (os′tē-ō-rā-dē-ol′ō-jist). A physician who specializes in radiology of the bones and joints. [osteo- + radiologist]

os·te·o·ra·di·ol·o·gy. The clinical subspecialty of diagnostic bone radiology.

os·te·o·ra·di·o·ne·cro·sis (os′tē-ō-rā′dē-ō-ne-krō′sis). Necrosis of bone produced by ionizing radiation; may be planned or unplanned. [osteo- + radionecrosis]

os·te·or·rha·phy (os-tē-ōr′ă-fē). Wiring together the fragments of a broken bone. SYN osteosuture. [osteo- + G. *rhaphē,* suture]

os·te·o·sar·co·ma (os′tē-ō-sar-kō′mă). SYN osteogenic *sarcoma.*

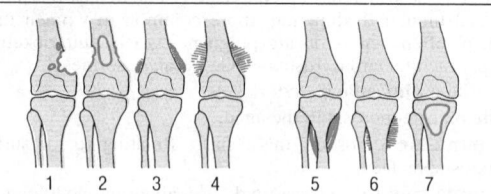

osteosarcoma

characteristic x-ray views (*1–4*) osteolytic, osteoclastic, osteophytic, and combined tumor growth; (*5–7*) Ewing's tumor: lamellae (layers), spiculae (spikes), and osteolysis

   parosteal o., low grade o. arising on the surface of bone without involvement of the underlying marrow, usually occurring as a heavily ossified mass of the distal femur in women in the third and fourth decades of life.

   periosteal o., chondroblastic o. occurring on the surface of bones without involvement of the marrow; usually presents in adolescents and young adults as a lucent defect with bone spicules extending into soft tissues. Histologically, the tumor is intermediate to high grade, and the cartilage is lobulated.

os·te·o·scle·ro·sis (os′tē-ō-skle-rō′sis). Abnormal hardening or eburnation of bone. [osteo- + G. *sklērōsis,* hardness]

os·te·o·scle·rot·ic (os′tē-ō-skle-rot′ik). Relating to, due to, or marked by hardening of bone substance.

os·te·o·sis (os-tē-ō′sis). **1.** A morbid process in bone. SYN ostosis (1). **2.** SYN osteogenesis. [osteo- + G. *-osis,* condition]

   o. cu′tis, SYN osteoma cutis.

   o. eburni′sans monomel′ica, SYN melorheostosis.

   parathyroid o., SYN *osteitis* fibrosa cystica.

   renal fibrocystic o., SYN renal *rickets.*

os·te·o·spon·gi·o·ma (os′tē-ō-spon′jē-ō′mă). General nonspecific term for a neoplasm in bone that results in thinning and fragmentation (thus, in softening) of the cortex. [osteo- + G. *spongos,* sponge, + *-oma,* tumor]

os·te·o·ste·a·to·ma (os′tē-ō-stē′ă-tō′mă). A benign mass, usually a lipoma or sebaceous cyst, in which small foci of bony elements are present. [osteo- + G. *stear,* suet, fat, + *-oma,* tumor]

os·te·o·su·ture (os-tē-ō-sū′chŭr). SYN osteorrhaphy.

os·te·o·syn·the·sis (os-tē-ō-sin′thē-sis). Internal fixation of a fracture by means of a mechanical device, such as a pin, screw, or plate.

os·te·o·throm·bo·sis (os′tē-ō-throm-bō′sis). Thrombosis in one or more of the veins of a bone.

os·te·o·tome (os′tē-ō-tōm). An instrument for use in cutting bone. [osteo- + G. *tomē,* incision]

os·te·ot·o·my (os-tē-ot′ō-mē). Cutting a bone, usually by means of a saw or chisel. [osteo- + G. *tomē,* incision]

"C" sliding o., an extraoral o. in the shape of a "C" performed bilaterally in the mandibular rami for the correction of retrognathia and/or apertognathia.

horizontal o., an o. performed intraorally for genioplasty; the inferior aspect of the anterior mandible is advanced or retruded by movement of the free segment.

Le Fort o., an o. often done to correct a maxillary skeletal deformity. Classified as Le Fort o. I, II, or III, depending upon the location.

sagittal split mandibular o., an intraoral surgical procedure for correction of retrognathism, apertognathia, and prognathism; the mandibular rami and posterior body are sectioned in the sagittal plane.

segmental alveolar o., an intraoral surgical procedure in which segments of alveolar bone containing teeth are sectioned between, and apically to, the teeth for the repositioning of the alveolus and teeth; it may be maxillary or mandibular, and may be combined with ostectomy.

sliding oblique o., an oral surgical procedure in which the mandibular ramus is cut vertically from the sigmoid notch to the angle to facilitate posterior repositioning of the mandible in correction of mandibular prognathism; it may be performed extraorally or intraorally, and is similar to vertical o.

vertical o., an oral surgical procedure similar to sliding oblique o.

os·te·o·tribe (os′tē-ō-trīb). An instrument for crushing off bits of necrosed or carious bone. [osteo- + G. *tribō,* to bruise, to grind down]

os·te·o·trite (os′tē-ō-trīt). An instrument with conical or olive-shaped tip having a cutting surface, resembling a dental burr, used for the removal of carious bone. [osteo- + L. *tritus,* a grinding, a wearing off]

os·te·ot·ro·phy (os-tē-ot′rō-fē). Nutrition of osseous tissue. [osteo- + G. *trophē,* nourishment]

os·te·o·tym·pan·ic (os′tē-ō-tim-pan′ik). SYN otocranial. [osteo- + G. *tympanon,* drum]

Os·ter·ta·gia (os-ter-tā′jē-ă). The medium or brown stomach worm; a genus of small, slender, bloodsucking trichostrongyle nematodes found in the abomasum (rarely in the small intestine) of sheep, goats, cattle, and other ruminants. Species include *O. bisonis* in bison, cattle, and deer; *O. circumcincta,* the most economically important species found in sheep, which occurs worldwide in sheep, goats, camels, and wild ruminants; *O. lyrata* in cattle and wild ruminants; *O. occidentalis* in sheep, goats, pronghorn, mule deer, and other ruminants; *O. orloffi* in sheep, cattle, mule deer, and Barbary sheep in North America and the area formerly known as the USSR; *O. ostertagi,* in cattle, sheep, and many wild ruminants; and *O. trifurcata* in sheep and goats, also reported from many wild ruminants. [R. von *Ostertag*]

os·tia (os′tē-ă). Plural of ostium. [L.]

os·ti·al (os′tē-ăl). Relating to any orifice, or ostium.

os·ti·tic (os-tī′tik). SYN osteitic.

os·ti·tis (os-tī′tis). SYN osteitis.

os·ti·um, pl. **os·tia** (os′tē-ŭm, -ă) [NA]. A small opening, espe-

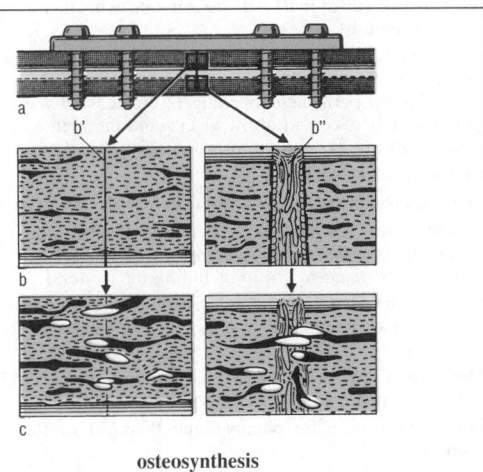

osteosynthesis
primary angiogenic healing of fracture in stable osteosynthesis
b' + c = contact healing; b" + c = gap healing

cially one of entrance into a hollow organ or canal. [L. door, entrance, mouth]

o. abdomina′le tu′bae uteri′nae [NA], SYN abdominal o. of uterine tube.

abdominal o. of uterine tube, the fimbriated or ovarian extremity of an oviduct. SYN o. abdominale tubae uterinae [NA].

o. aor′tae [NA], SYN aortic *orifice.*

aortic o., SYN aortic *orifice.*

o. appen′dicis vermifor′mis [NA], SYN o. of vermiform appendix.

o. arterio′sum, SYN mitral *orifice.*

o. atrioventricula′re dex′trum [NA], SYN tricuspid *orifice.*

o. atrioventricula′re sinis′trum [NA], SYN mitral *orifice.*

o. cardi′acum [NA], SYN cardiac *orifice.*

o. ileoceca′le [NA], SYN ileocecal *orifice.*

o. inter′num, SYN uterine o. of uterine tubes.

o. pharyn′geum tu′bae auditi′vae [NA], SYN pharyngeal *opening* of auditory tube.

o. pri′mum, SYN interatrial *foramen* primum.

o. pylor′icum [NA], SYN pyloric *orifice.*

o. secun′dum, SYN interatrial *foramen* secundum.

o. trun′ci pulmona′lis [NA], SYN *opening* of pulmonary trunk.

o. tympan′icum tu′bae auditi′vae [NA], SYN tympanic *opening* of auditory tube.

o. ure′teris [NA], SYN ureteric *orifice.*

o. ure′thrae exter′num [NA], SYN external urethral *orifice.*

o. ure′thrae inter′num [NA], SYN internal urethral *orifice.*

o. u′teri [NA], SYN external *os* of uterus.

o. u′teri exter′num, SYN external *os* of uterus.

o. u′teri inter′num, SYN *isthmus* of uterus.

uterine o. of uterine tubes, the uterine opening of the oviduct. SYN o. uterinum tubae [NA], o. internum, uterine opening of uterine tubes.

o. uteri′num tu′bae [NA], SYN uterine o. of uterine tubes.

o. vagi′nae [NA], SYN vaginal *orifice.*

o. ve′nae ca′vae inferio′ris [NA], SYN *opening* of inferior vena cava.

o. ve′nae ca′vae superio′ris [NA], SYN *opening* of superior vena cava.

os′tia vena′rum pulmona′lium [NA], SYN *openings* of pulmonary veins, under *opening.*

o. veno′sum cordis, SYN tricuspid *orifice.*

o. of vermiform appendix, the opening of the vermiform appendix into the lumen of the cecum. SYN o. appendicis vermiformis [NA].

os·to·mate (os'tō-māt). Term for one who has an ostomy. [L. *ostium,* mouth]

os·to·my (os'tō-mē). **1.** An artificial stoma or opening into the urinary or gastrointestinal canal, or the trachea. **2.** Any operation by which a permanent opening is created between two hollow organs or between a hollow viscus and the skin externally, as in tracheostomy. [L. *ostium,* mouth]

⌂-ostomy. SEE -stomy.

os·to·sis (os-tō'sis). **1.** SYN osteosis (1). **2.** SYN osteogenesis.

os·tra·ceous (os-trā'shŭs). Denoting the heaping up of scales seen in psoriasis, which resembles the stratification of oyster shells. [*Ostraeacea,* group including the oysters]

os·tre·o·tox·ism (os'trē-ō-tok'sizm). Poisoning from eating infected or contaminated oysters. [G. *ostreon,* oyster, + *toxikon,* poison]

Ostwald, Friedrich Wilhelm, German physical chemist and Nobel laureate, 1853–1932. SEE O.'s solubility *coefficient.*

OT Abbreviation for occupational therapist or therapy; Koch's old *tuberculin.*

⌂ot-. The ear. SEE ALSO auri-. [G. *ous*]

Ota, Masao T., Japanese dermatopathologist, 1885–1945. SEE Ota's *nevus.*

otal·gia (ō-tal'jē-ă). SYN earache. [ot- + G. *algos,* pain]

geniculate o., SYN geniculate *neuralgia.*

reflex o., pain referred to the ear from disease in another part, most commonly laryngeal, tonsillar, or nasopharyngeal.

otal·gic (ō-tal'jik). **1.** Relating to otalgia, or earache. **2.** A remedy for earache.

OTC Abbreviation for *over the counter,* pertaining to a drug available without a prescription.

oth·er-di·rect·ed (odh'er-di-rek'ted). Pertaining to a person readily influenced by the attitudes of others.

otic (ō'tik). Relating to the ear. [G. *otikos,* fr. *ous,* ear]

Otis, Arthur Brooks, U.S. respiratory physiologist, *1913. SEE Rahn-O. *sample.*

otit·ic (ō-tit'ik). Relating to otitis.

oti·tis (ō-tī'tis). Inflammation of the ear. [ot- + G. *-itis,* inflammation]

adhesive o., inflammation of the middle ear caused by prolonged eustachian tube dysfunction resulting in permanent retraction of the eardrum and obliteration of the middle ear space.

aviation o., SYN aerotitis media.

o. desquamati′va, o. externa with a copious brawny desquamation.

o. exter′na, inflammation of the external auditory canal. SYN swimmer's ear.

o. inter′na, SYN labyrinthitis.

o. me′dia, inflammation of the middle ear, or tympanum.

parasitic o., SYN otoacariasis.

reflux o. me′dia, o. media caused by passage of nasopharyngeal secretions through the eustachian tube.

secretory o. me′dia, SYN serous o.

serous o., inflammation of middle ear mucosa, often accompanied by accumulation of fluid, secondary to eustachian tube obstruction. SYN secretory o. media.

⌂oto-. The ear. SEE ALSO auri-. [G. *ous*]

oto·ac·a·ri·a·sis (ō'tō-ak-ă-rī'ă-sis). An infestation of the auditory canal of cats, dogs, foxes, and other animals by auricular mites, chiefly *Otodectes cynotis,* which infest the ears and cause considerable discomfort and tenderness; in extreme cases, they cause symptoms such as loss of appetite, wasting, and fits. SEE ALSO otodectic *mange.* SYN parasitic otitis.

oto·acous·tic (ō'tō-a-ku-stik). Referring to the very faint sounds produced by the ear; thought to represent mechanical vibrations in the cochlea.

oto·bi·o·sis (ō'tō-bī-ō'sis). Presence of larvae and the characteristic spiny nymphs of *Otobius megnini* in the external auditory canal of cattle, horses, cats, dogs, deer, coyotes, and other domestic and wild animals; they may remain in the ear for several months before dropping out to pupate and mature. Several records of human infection are known.

Oto·bi·us (ō-tō′bē-ŭs). A genus of argasid ticks similar to *Ornithodoros* but characterized by a granulated integument, a hypostome that is vestigial in the adult but well developed in the spiny nymphs, and the absence of eyes and hood. Two species are recognized: *O. lagophilus* (the face tick of rabbits), and *O. megnini,* the spinose ear tick that causes otobiosis in horses, cattle, sheep, dogs, and some wild animals; it occurs in southwestern parts of the U.S., where it is an important pest, and is also distributed worldwide.

oto·ceph·a·ly (ō-tō-sef′ă-lē). Malformation characterized by markedly defective development of the lower jaw (micrognathia or agnathia) and the union or close approach of the ears (synotia) on the front of the neck. [oto- + G. *kephalē,* head]

oto·cer·e·bri·tis (ō-tō-ser-ĕ-brī′tis). SYN otoencephalitis.

oto·co·nia, sing. **oto·co·ni·um** (ō-to-kō′nē-ă, -ŭm). SYN statoliths.

oto·cra·ni·al (ō-tō-krā′nē-ăl). Relating to the otocranium. SYN osteotympanic.

oto·cra·ni·um (ō′tō-krā′nē-um). The bony case of the internal and middle ear, consisting of the petrous portion of the temporal bone. [oto- + G. *kranion,* cranium]

oto·cyst (ō′tō-sist). **1.** Embryonic auditory vesicle. **2.** A balancing organ, analogous to the utricle of mammals, possessed by certain invertebrates and containing grains of calcareous material or of sand. [oto- + G. *kystis,* a bladder]

Oto·dec·tes (ō-tō-dek′tēz). A genus of ear mites (family Psoroptidae) consisting of a single species, *O. cynotis,* the cause of otodectic mange in dogs, cats, and other carnivores; the entire lifespan of this mite is spent in the ears (rarely on the body) of the host, where it feeds on epidermal debris; it can be found in the encrusted material scraped from infected ears. [oto- + *dektēs,* beggar, receiver]

oto·dec·tic (ō-tō-dek′tik). Of, relating to, or caused by mites of the genus *Otodectes.*

oto·dyn·ia (ō-tō-din′ē-ă). SYN earache. [oto- + G. *odynē,* pain]

oto·en·ceph·a·li·tis (ō′tō-en-sef-ă-lī′tis). Inflammation of the brain by extension of the process from the middle ear and mastoid cells. SYN otocerebritis. [oto- + G. *enkephalos,* brain, + *-itis,* inflammation]

oto·gang·li·on (ō′tō-gang′glē-on). SYN otic *ganglion.*

oto·gen·ic, otog·e·nous (ō′tō-jen′ik, ō-toj′ĕ-nŭs). Of otic origin; originating within the ear, especially from inflammation of the ear. [oto- + G. *-gen,* producing]

oto·lar·yn·gol·o·gist (ō′tō-lar-ing-gol′ŏ-jist). A physician who specializes in otolaryngology.

oto·lar·yn·gol·o·gy (ō′tō-lar-ing-gol′ŏ-jē). The combined specialties of diseases of the ear and larynx, often including upper respiratory tract and many diseases of the head and neck, tracheobronchial tree, and esophagus. [oto- + G. *larynx,* + *logos,* study]

oto·liths, oto·lites (ō′tō-lith, ō′tō-līt). SYN statoliths. [oto- + G. *lithos,* stone]

oto·log·ic (ō′tō-loj′ik). Relating to otology.

otol·o·gist (ō-tol′ŏ-jist). A specialist in otology.

otol·o·gy (ō-tol′ŏ-jē). The branch of medical science concerned with the study, diagnosis, and treatment of diseases of the ear and related structures. [oto- + G. *logos,* study]

oto·mu·cor·my·co·sis (ō-tō-myŭ′kŏr-mī-kō′sis). Mucormycosis of the ear.

⌂-otomy. SEE -tomy.

oto·my·co·sis (ō′tō-mī-kō′sis). An infection due to a fungus in the external auditory canal, usually unilateral, with scaling, itching, and pain as the primary symptoms.

oto·neu·ral·gia (ō′tō-nū-ral′jē-ă). Earache of neuralgic origin, not caused by inflammation. [oto- + G. *neuron,* nerve, + *algos,* pain]

oto·pal·a·to·dig·i·tal (ō′tō-pal′ă-tō-dij′i-tăl). Relating to the ears, palate, and fingers.

otop·a·thy (ō-top′ă-thē). Any disease of the ear. [oto- + G. *pathos,* suffering]

oto·pha·ryn·ge·al (ō'tō-fa-rin'jē-ăl). Relating to the middle ear and the pharynx.

oto·plas·ty (ō'tō-plas-tē). Reparative or plastic surgery of the auricle of the ear. [oto- + G. *plastos,* formed]

oto·rhi·no·lar·yn·gol·o·gy (ō'tō-rī'nō-lar-ing -gol'ŏ-jē). The combined specialties of diseases of the ear, nose, and larynx; including diseases of related structures of the head and neck. SEE ALSO otolaryngology. [oto- + G. *rhis,* nose, + *larynx,* larynx, + *logos,* study]

otor·rhea (ō-tō-rē'ă). A discharge from the ear. [oto- + G. *rhoia,* flow]

  cerebrospinal fluid o., discharge of cerebrospinal fluid through the external auditory meatus or through the eustachian tube into the nasopharynx.

oto·sal·pinx (ō-tō-sal'pingks). SYN auditory *tube.* [oto- + G. *salpinx,* trumpet]

oto·scle·ro·sis (ō'tō-sklē-rō'sis). A new formation of spongy bone about the stapes and fenestra vestibuli (ovalis), resulting in progressively increasing deafness, without signs of disease in the eustachian tube or tympanic membrane. SEE ALSO Bezold's *triad.* [oto- + G. *sklērosis,* hardening]

oto·scope (ō'tō-skōp). An instrument for examining the drum membrane or auscultating the ear. [oto- + G. *skopeō,* to view]

  Siegle's o., an ear speculum with a bulb attachment by which the air pressure can be varied, thus imparting movement to the membrana tympani, if intact, while under inspection.

otos·co·py (ō-tos'kŏ-pē). Inspection of the ear, especially of the drum membrane. [oto- + G. *skopeō,* to view]

  pneumatic o., inspection of the ear with a device capable of varying air pressure against the eardrum. Imparting movement to the tympanic membrane suggests normal middle ear compliance; the lack of movement indicates either increased impedance or eardrum perforation.

otos·te·al (ō-tos'tē-ăl). Relating to the ossicles of the ear. [oto- + G. *osteon,* bone]

oto·tox·ic (ō'tō-tok'sik). Having a toxic action upon the ear. [oto- + G. *toxikon,* poison]

oto·tox·ic·i·ty (ō-tō-tok-sis'i-te). The property of being ototoxic.

Otto, Adolph W., German surgeon, 1786–1845. SEE O. *pelvis;* O.'s *disease.*

ot·to of rose. SYN *oil* of rose.

Ottoson, David, 20th century Swedish physiologist. SEE O. *potential.*

O.U. Abbreviation for Latin *oculus uterque,* each eye or both eyes.

oua·ba·gen·in (wă'bă-jen-in). The aglycon obtained from the hydrolysis of the cardiac glycoside, ouabain; exerts cardiotonic activity.

oua·ba·in (wah'bān, wah'bah-in). $C_{29}H_{44}O_{12}8H_2O$; G-strophanthin; acocantherin; a glycoside and African arrow poison from ouabaio, obtained from the wood of *Acocanthera ouabaio* or from the seeds of *Strophanthus gratus;* its action is qualitatively identical to that of strophanthus and the digitalis glycosides; used for rapid digitalization; often used in pharmacological studies due to water solubility.

Ouchterlony, Orjan, Swedish bacteriologist, *1914. SEE O. method, *technique, test, technique.*

△ **oul-.** For words beginning thus, see ulo-.

ounce (oz.) (owns). A weight containing 480 gr., or $\frac{1}{12}$ pound troy and apothecaries' weight, or $437\frac{1}{2}$ gr., $\frac{1}{16}$ pound avoirdupois. The apothecary oz. (used in the USP) contains 8 dr. and is equivalent to 31.10349 g; the avoirdupois oz. is equivalent to 28.35 g. [L. *uncia,* the twelfth part (of a pound or foot) hence also inch]

△ **-ous. 1.** Chemical suffix attached to the name of an element in one of its lower valencies. Cf. -ic (1). **2.** Having much of. [L. *-osus,* full of, abounding]

out·let (owt'let). An exit or opening of a passageway.

  pelvic o., SYN inferior pelvic *aperture.*

out·li·er (owt'lē-er). An observation that differs so widely from all others in a set as to justify the conclusion that a gross error has occurred or that it comes from a different population.

out·pa·tient (owt'pā'shent). A patient treated in a hospital dispensary or clinic instead of in a room or ward.

out of phase. Not in phase, moving in opposite directions at the same time; 180° out of phase; a possible characteristic of two simultaneous oscillations of similar frequency.

out·put (owt'put). The quantity produced, ejected, or excreted of a specific entity in a specified period of time or per unit time, *e.g.,* urinary sodium o.; the opposite of intake or input.

  cardiac o., the amount of blood ejected by the heart in a unit of time (*i.e.,* the minute volume), usually expressed in liters per minute. SYN minute o.

  minute o., SYN cardiac o.

  pacemaker o., electrical energy delivered into a standard load (500 ohms resistance).

  stroke o., SYN stroke *volume.*

ova (ō'vă). Plural of ovum. [L.]

oval (ō'văl). **1.** Relating to an ovum. **2.** Egg-shaped, resembling in outline the longitudinal section of an egg.

ov·al·bu·min (ō-văl-byū'min). The chief protein occurring in the white of egg and resembling serum albumin; also found in phosphorylated form. SYN albumen, egg albumin.

oval·o·cyte (ō'văl-ō-sīt). SYN elliptocyte. [L. *ovalis,* oval, + G. *kytos,* cell]

oval·o·cy·to·sis (ō'vă-lō-sī-tō'sis). SYN elliptocytosis.

ovar·i·al·gia (ō-var-ē-al'jē-ă). Pain in an ovary. SYN oophoralgia. [ovario- + G. *algos,* pain]

ovar·i·an (ō-var'ē-an). Relating to the ovary.

ovar·i·ec·to·my (ō-var-ē-ek'tō-mē). Excision of one or both ovaries. SYN oophorectomy, ovariosteresis. [ovario- + G. *ektomē,* excision]

△ **ovario-, ovari-.** Ovary. SEE ALSO oo-, oophor-. [L. *ovarium*]

ovar·i·o·cele (ō-var'ē-ō-sēl). Hernia of an ovary. [ovario- + G. *kēlē,* hernia]

ovar·i·o·cen·te·sis (ō-var'ē-ō-sen-tē'sis). Puncture of an ovary or an ovarian cyst. [ovario- + G. *kentēsis,* puncture]

ovar·i·o·cy·e·sis (ō-var'ē-ō-sī-ē'sis). SYN ovarian *pregnancy.* [ovario- + G. *kyēsis,* pregnancy]

ovar·i·o·dys·neu·ria (ō-var'ē-ō-dis-nū'rē-ă). Ovarian pain or neuralgia. [ovario- + G. *dys-,* bad, + *neuron,* nerve]

ovar·i·o·gen·ic (ō-var'ē-ō-jen'ik). Originating in the ovary. [ovario- + G. *-gen,* producing]

ovar·i·o·hys·ter·ec·to·my (ō-var'ē-ō-his-ter-ek'tō-mē). Removal of ovaries and uterus. SYN oophorohysterectomy. [ovario- + G. *hystera,* uterus, + *ektomē,* excision]

ovar·i·o·lyt·ic (ō-var'ē-ō-lit'ik). Destructive to the ovary. [ovario- + G. *lysis,* dissolution]

ovar·i·on·cus (ō-var-ē-ong'kŭs). SYN oophoroma. [ovario- + G. *onkos,* tumor]

ovar·i·op·a·thy (ō-var-ē-op'ă-thē). Any disease of the ovary. SYN oophoropathy. [ovario- + G. *pathos,* suffering]

ovar·i·or·rhex·is (ō-var'ē-ō-rek'sis). Rupture of an ovary. [ovario- + G. *rhēxis,* rupture]

ovar·i·o·sal·pin·gec·to·my (ō-var'ē-ō-sal-pin-jek'tō-mē). Operative removal of an ovary and the corresponding oviduct. SYN oophorosalpingectomy. [ovario- + salpingectomy]

ovar·i·o·sal·pin·gi·tis (ō-var'ē-ō-sal-pin-jī'tis). Inflammation of ovary and oviduct. SYN oophorosalpingitis. [ovario- + salpingitis]

ovar·i·o·ste·re·sis (ō-var'ē-ō-stĕ-rē'sis). SYN ovariectomy. [ovario- + G. *sterēsis,* deprivation, loss]

ovar·i·os·to·my (ō-var-ē-os'tō-mē). Establishment of a temporary fistula for drainage of a cyst of the ovary. SYN oophorostomy. [ovario- + G. *stoma,* mouth]

ovar·i·ot·o·my (ō-var-ē-ot'ō-mē). An incision into an ovary, *e.g.,* a biopsy or a wedge excision. SYN oophorotomy. [ovario- + G. *tomē,* incision]

  normal o., historically, removal of an apparently healthy ovary.

ova·ri·tis (ō-vă-rī'tis). SYN oophoritis.

ovar·i·um, pl. **ova·ria** (ō-vār'ē-ŭm, -ă) [NA]. SYN ovary. [Mod. L. fr. *ovum,* egg]

o. biparti'tum, an ovary separated into two distinct parts.

o. disjunc'tum, an ovary partially or completely divided into two sections.

o. gyra'tum, an ovary showing curved or irregular grooves or furrows.

o. loba'tum, an ovary demarcated by deep furrows into two or more lobes.

o. masculi'num, SYN testicular *appendage.*

ova·ry (ō'vă-rē). One of the paired female reproductive glands containing the ova or germ cells; the o.'s stroma is a vascular connective tissue containing numbers of ovarian follicles enclosing the ova; surrounding this stroma is a more condensed layer of stroma called the tunica albuginea. SYN ovarium [NA], female gonad, genital gland (2). [Mod. L. *ovarium,* fr. *ovum,* egg]

mulberry o., the type of o. produced by the administration of anterior pituitary extracts to immature rats; such an o. contains many more follicles than normal, with the follicles in various stages of development and with prominent corpora lutea on their surfaces, thus the perceived resemblance to a mulberry.

polycystic o., enlarged cystic o.'s, pearl white in color, with thickened tunica albuginea, characteristic of the Stein-Leventhal syndrome; clinical features are abnormal menses, obesity, and evidence of masculinization, such as hirsutism.

third o., an accessory o.

over·bite (ō'ver-bīt). SYN vertical *overlap.*

over·clo·sure (ō'ver-klō-zher). A decrease in occlusal vertical dimension.

over·com·pen·sa·tion (ō'ver-kom-pen-sā'shŭn). **1.** An exaggeration of personal capacity by which one overcomes a real or imagined inferiority. **2.** The process in which a psychologic deficiency inspires exaggerated correction. SEE compensation.

over·cor·rec·tion (ō'ver-kŏ-rek'shŭn). In behavior modification treatment programs, especially those involving mentally retarded individuals, overlearning the desired target behavior beyond the set criterion to assure that the behavior will continue to meet the established criterion when the post-learning decrements and forgetting occur.

over·den·ture (ō-ver-den'chŭr). SYN overlay *denture.*

over·de·ter·mi·na·tion (ō'ver-dē-ter'min-ā'shŭn). In psychoanalysis, ascribing the cause of a single behavioral or emotional reaction, mental symptom, or dream to the operation of two or more forces, that is, it is overdetermined (*e.g.,* ascribing the nature of an emotional outburst not only to the immediate precipitant but also to a lingering inferiority complex).

over·dom·i·nance (ō-ver-dom'i-năns). That state in which the heterozygote has greater phenotype value and perhaps is more fit than the homozygous state for either of the alleles that it comprises. Cf. balanced *polymorphism.*

over·dom·i·nant (ō-ver-dom'i-nănt). Denoting heterozygous states that exhibit overdominance.

over·drive (ō-ver-drīv). An electrophysiologic pacing technique to exceed the rate of an abnormal pacemaker and so capture the territory controlled by that pacemaker (usually atrial).

over·e·rup·tion (ō'ver-ē-rŭp'shŭn). Occlusal projection of a tooth beyond the line of occlusion.

over·ex·ten·sion (ō-ver-eks-ten'shŭn). SYN hyperextension.

over·graft·ing (ō'ver-graft'ing). Placing a second or additional grafts over a previously healed graft from which the epithelium has been removed, as with dermabrasion, to strengthen a split-thickness *graft.*

over·hang (ō'ver-hang). An excess of dental filling material beyond the cavity margin or normal tooth contour.

over·head pro·jec·tor. SYN epidiascope.

over·hy·dra·tion (ō'ver-hī-drā'shŭn). SYN hyperhydration.

over·jet, over·jut (ō'ver-jet, ō'ver-jŭt). SYN horizontal *overlap.*

over·lap (ō'ver-lap). **1.** Suturing of one layer of tissue above or under another to gain strength. **2.** An extension or projection of one tissue over another.

horizontal o., the projection of the upper anterior and/or posterior teeth beyond their antagonists in a horizontal direction. SYN overjet, overjut.

vertical o., (1) the extension of the upper teeth over the lower teeth in a vertical direction when the opposing posterior teeth are in contact in centric occlusion; **(2)** the distance that teeth lap over their antagonists vertically, especially for the distance that the upper incisal edges drop below the lower ones, but may also describe the vertical relations of opposing cusps; **(3)** the relationship of the maxillary incisors to the mandibular incisors when the incisal edges pass each other in centric occlusion. SYN overbite.

over·lay (ō'ver-lā). An addition to an already existing condition.

emotional o., the emotional or psychological concomitant of an organic disability.

over·learn·ing (ō'ver-lern'ing). In the psychology of memory, continuation of practice beyond the point where one is able to perform according to the specified criterion; typically, retention is longer after o. as compared with retention after practice only to the point of performance meeting the specified criterion.

over·re·sponse (ō'ver-rē-spons'). An abnormally strong reaction to a stimulus.

over·rid·ing (ō'ver-rī'ding). **1.** Slippage of the lower fragment of a broken long bone upward and alongside the proximal portion. **2.** Obsolete term denoting a fetal head which is palpable above the symphysis because of cephalopelvic disproportion.

over·sens·ing (ō'ver-sen'sing). Sensing of electrical or magnetic signals, which normally should not be sensed by a pacemaker, but result in inappropriate inhibition of the pacemaker's output.

over·shoot (ō'ver-shŭt). **1.** Generally, any initial change, in response to a sudden step change in some factor, that is greater than the steady-state response to the new level of that factor; common in systems in which inertia or a time lag in negative feedback outweighs any damping that may be present. Changes in a negative direction are sometimes distinguished by the term undershoot, and the two may alternate in an oscillatory fashion, as in the transient oscillations of a pendulum when released from an initial displacement. **2.** Momentary reversal of the membrane potential of a cell (inside becoming positive rather than negative relative to the outside) during an action potential; considered a form of overshoot (1) because, before discovery of overshoot (2), excitation was thought merely to depolarize the membrane to zero transmembrane potential.

Overton, Charles E., German biologist in Sweden, 1865–1933. SEE Meyer-O. *rule, theory* of narcosis.

over·tone (ō'ver-tōn). Any of the tones, other than the lowest or fundamental tone, of which a sound is composed.

psychic o., the mental associations related to any stimulus.

over·ven·ti·la·tion (ō'ver-ven-ti-lā'shŭn). SYN hyperventilation.

over·win·ter·ing (ō'ver-win'ter-ing). Persistence of an infectious agent in its vector for extended periods, such as the cooler winter months, during which the vector has no opportunity to be reinfected or to infect another host.

ovi-. Egg. SEE ALSO oo-, ovo-. [L. *ovum*]

ovi·ci·dal (ō-vi-sī'dăl). Causing death of the ovum. [ovi- + L. *caedo,* to kill]

ovi·du·cal (ō-vi-dū'kăl). SYN oviductal.

ovi·duct (ō'vi-dŭkt). SYN uterine *tube.* [ovi- + L. *ductus,* a leading, fr. *duco,* pp. *ductus,* to lead]

ovi·duc·tal (ō-vi-dŭk'tăl). Relating to a uterine tube. SYN oviducal.

ovif·er·ous (ō-vif'er-ŭs). Carrying, containing, or producing ova. SYN ovigerous. [ovi- + L. *fero,* to carry]

ovi·form (ō'vi-fōrm). SYN ovoid (2).

ovi·gen·e·sis (ō-vi-jen'ě-sis). SYN oogenesis.

ovi·ge·net·ic, ovi·gen·ic (ō-vi-jě-net'ik, -jen'ik). SYN oogenetic.

ovig·e·nous (ō-vij'ě-nŭs). SYN oogenetic.

ovig·er·ous (ō-vij'er-ŭs). SYN oviferous.

ovi·ge·rus. SYN *cumulus* oöphorus.

ovine (ō'vīn). Relating to sheep; sheeplike. [L. *ovinus,* relating to a sheep]

ovin·ia (ō-vin'ē-ă). SYN sheep-pox. [L. *ovinus,* relating to a sheep]

o·vi·par·i·ty (ō-vi-par′i-tē). The quality of being oviparous. [ovi- + L. *pario,* to bear]

o·vip·a·rous (ō-vip′ă-rŭs). Egg-laying; denoting those birds, fish, amphibians, reptiles, monotreme mammals, and invertebrates whose young develop in eggs outside of the maternal body. [L. *oviparus,* fr. *ovum,* egg, + *pario,* to bear]

o·vi·pos·it (ō′vi-poz′it). To lay eggs; applied especially to insects. [ovi- + L. *pono,* pp. *positus,* to place]

o·vi·po·si·tion (ō′vi-pō-zish′ŭn). Act of laying or depositing eggs by insects.

o·vi·pos·i·tor (ō-vi-poz′i-tŏr, -tōr). A specialized female organ especially well developed in insects for laying or depositing eggs.

o·vist (ō′vist). A preformationist who believed that the female sex cell contained a miniature body susceptible to growth when stimulated by semen.

ovo-. Egg. SEE ALSO oo-, ovi-. [L. *ovum*]

o·vo·cyte (ō′vō-sīt). SYN oocyte. [ovo- + G. *kytos,* a hollow (cell)]

o·vo·fla·vin (ō-vō-flā′vin). Riboflavin found in eggs.

o·vo·gen·e·sis (ō-vō-jen′ĕ-sis). SYN oogenesis.

o·vo·glob·u·lin (ō-vō-glob′yū-lin). Globulin in the white of egg.

o·vo·go·ni·um (ō-vō-gō′nē-ŭm). Obsolete term for oogonium. [ovo- + G. *gonē,* generation]

o·void (ō′voyd). 1. An oval or egg-shaped form. 2. Resembling an egg. SYN oviform. [ovo- + G. *eidos,* resemblance]

fetal o., the form of the fetus *in utero;* its length is about one-half of the length of the extended fetus.

Manchester o., an egg-shaped radium applicator for placement in the lateral vaginal fornices. [University of *Manchester,* England]

o·vo·lar·vip·a·rous (ō′vō-lar-vip′ă-rŭs). Denoting certain nematodes and other invertebrates in which the eggs are hatched within the female, and the larvae developed or protected within the uterus until the correct time for their emergence. [ovo- + L. *larva,* a mask, + *pario,* to bear]

o·vo·mu·cin (ō-vō-myū′sin). A glycoprotein in the white of egg.

o·vo·mu·coid (ō-vō-myū′koyd). A mucoprotein obtained from the white of egg.

o·vo·plasm (ō′vō-plazm). Protoplasm of an unfertilized egg.

o·vo·pro·to·gen (ō-vō-prō′tō-jen). SYN lipoic acid.

o·vo·sis·ton (ō-vō-sis′ton). An oral contraceptive that consists of a mixture of a progestin and an estrogen.

o·vo·tes·tis (ō′vō-tes′tis). Gonad in which both testicular and ovarian components are present; a form of hermaphroditism.

o·vo·trans·fer·rin (ō′vō-trans-fār′in). SYN conalbumin.

o·vo·vi·tel·lin (ō′vō-vī-tel′in). SYN vitellin. [ovo- + L. *vitellus,* yolk]

o·vo·vi·vip·ar·ous (ō′vō-vī-vip′ă-rŭs). Denoting those fish, amphibians, and reptiles that produce eggs which hatch within the body of the parent. [ovo- + L. *viviparus,* bringing forth alive, fr. *vivus,* alive, + *pario,* to bear]

o·vu·lar (ov′yū-lăr, ō′vyū-). Relating to an ovule.

o·vu·la·tion (ov′yū-lā′shŭn, ō′vyū-). Release of an ovum from the ovarian follicle.

anestrous o., discharge of ova occurring in animals without estrus.

paracyclic o., o. occurring in the menstrual cycle at any time other than the normally anticipated time; believed to be usually a psychogenic phenomenon.

o·vu·la·to·ry (ov′yū-lă-tō-rē, ō′vyū-). Relating to ovulation.

o·vule (ov′yūl, ō′vyū-). 1. The ovum of a mammal, especially while still in the ovarian follicle. 2. A small beadlike structure bearing a fancied resemblance to an o. SYN ovulum. [Mod. L. *ovulum,* dim. of L. *ovum,* egg]

o·vu·lo·cy·clic (ov′yū-lō-sī′klik, ō′vyū-). Denoting any recurrent phenomenon associated with and occurring at a certain time within the ovulatory cycle, as, for example, ovulocyclic porphyria.

o·vu·lum, pl. **ovu·la** (ov′yū-lŭm, ō′vyū-; -lă). SYN ovule.

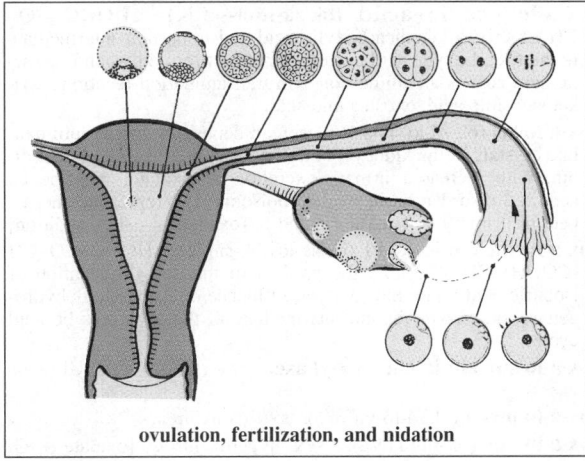

ovulation, fertilization, and nidation

o·vum, gen. **ovi,** pl. **ova** (ō′vŭm, -vī, -vă). The female sex cell. When fertilized by a spermatozoon, an o. is capable of developing into a new individual of the same species; during maturation, the o., like the spermatozoon, undergoes a halving of its chromosomal complement so that, at its union with the male gamete, the species number of chromosomes (46 in humans) is maintained; yolk contained in the ova of different species varies greatly in amount and distribution, which influences the pattern of the cleavage divisions. [L. egg]

alecithal o., an o. in which the yolk is nearly absent, consisting of only a few particles.

blighted o., a fertilized o. whose development has ceased at an early stage.

centrolecithal o., one in which the yolk is mostly located near the center of the egg, as in arthropods.

fertilized o., an o. impregnated by a spermatozoon.

isolecithal o., an o. in which the yolk is evenly distributed throughout the cytoplasm.

Peters' o., an o. with a presumptive fertilization age of about 13 days; for many years, it was one of very few young human embryos recovered in good condition and its study furnished many facts regarding early embryonic changes.

telolecithal o., an o. in which there is a large amount of yolk massed at the vegetative pole, as in the eggs of birds and reptiles.

Owen, Sir Richard, English anatomist, 1804–1892. SEE O.'s *lines,* under *line;* contour *lines* of O., under *line;* interglobular *space* of O.

Owren, Paul A., Norwegian hematologist, *1905. SEE O.'s *disease.*

oxa-. Combining form inserted in names of organic compounds to signify the presence or addition of oxygen atom(s) in a chain or ring (as in ethers), not appended to either (as in ketones and aldehydes). SEE ALSO hydroxy-, oxo-, oxy-. [English. *oxygen*]

ox·a·cil·lin so·di·um (ok-să-sil′in). 5-Methyl-3-phenyl-4-isoxazolylpenicillin sodium; a semisynthetic penicillin used in the oral therapy of penicillin-resistant staphylococcal infections.

ox·al·al·de·hyde (ok-să-lal′dĕ-hīd). SYN glyoxal.

ox·a·late (ok′să-lāt). A salt of oxalic acid.

ox·a·le·mia (ok-să-lē′mē-ă). The presence of an abnormally large amount of oxalates in the blood. [oxalate + G. *haima,* blood]

ox·al·ic ac·id (ok-sal′ik). An acid, HOOC–COOH, found in many plants and vegetables, particularly in buckwheat (family Polygoniaceae) and *Oxalis* (family Oxalidaceae); used as a hemostatic in veterinary medicine, but toxic when ingested by man; also used in the removal of ink and other stains, and as a general reducing agent; salts of o. are found in renal calculi; accumulates in cases of primary hyperoxaluria.

ox·a·lo (ok′să-lō). The monoacyl radical, HOOC–C(O)–.

ox·a·lo·ac·e·tate trans·ac·e·tase (ok′să-lō-as′ĕ-tāt trans-as′ĕ-tās). SYN *citrate* synthase.

ox·a·lo·a·ce·tic ac·id (oks′ă-lō-ă-sē′tik). HOOC–CO–CH₂COOH; a ketodicarboxylic acid and important intermediate in the tricarboxylic acid cycle; the product formed when L-aspartic acid acts as an amine donor in transamination reactions. SYN ketosuccinic acid, oxosuccinic acid.

ox·a·lo·sis (ok-să-lō′sis). Widespread deposition of calcium oxalate crystals in the kidneys, bones, arterial media, and myocardium, with increased urinary excretion of oxalate; may be an acquired disorder, as in oxalate poisoning, or represent one aspect of primary hyperoxaluria and o. [oxalate + -osis, condition]

ox·a·lo·suc·cin·ic ac·id (ok′să-lō-sŭk-sin′ik). HOOC–CO–CH (COOH)–CH₂–CO OH; the product of the dehydrogenation of isocitric acid under the catalytic influence of isocitrate dehydrogenase; an enzyme-bound intermediate of the tricarboxylic acid cycle.

ox·a·lo·suc·cin·ic car·box·yl·ase. SYN *isocitrate* dehydrogenase.

ox·a·lo·u·rea (ok′să-lō-yū-rē′ă). SYN oxalylurea.

ox·a·lu·ria (ok-să-lū′rē-ă). SYN hyperoxaluria. [oxalate + G. *ouron*, urine]

ox·a·lur·ic ac·id (ok-să-lūr′ik). NH₂CONHCOCOOH; the ureide of oxalic acid, derived from uric acid or oxalylurea.

ox·a·lyl (ok′să-lil). The diacyl radical, –CO–CO– .

ox·a·lyl·u·rea (ok-să-lil-yū-rē′ă). The cyclic (end-to-end) amide anhydride of oxaluric acid; an oxidation product of uric acid. SYN oxalourea, parabanic acid.

ox·am·ni·quine (oks-am′ni-quin). C₁₄H₂₁N₃O₃; a tetrahydroquinoline derivative, similar to hycanthone and lucanthone, effective against *Schistosoma mansoni;* now largely superseded by the broad spectrum anthelmintic drug praziquantel.

ox·an·a·mide (ok-san′ă-mīd). 2-Ethyl-3-propylglycidamide; a sedative.

ox·an·dro·lone (ok-san′drō-lōn). 17β-Hydroxy-17α-methyl-2-oxa-5α-androstan-3-one (C-2 replaced by O in the androstane nucleus); an androgenic anabolic steroid.

ox·a·phen·a·mide (ok-să-fen′ă-mīd). 4′-Hydroxysalicylanilide; a choleretic.

ox·a·ze·pam (ok-să′ze-pam). 7-Chloro-1,3-dihydro-3-hydroxy-5-phenyl-2*H*-1,4-benzodiazepin-2-one; a benzodiazepine chemically and pharmacologically related to chlordiazepoxide and diazepam; an antianxiety agent.

ox·a·zin (ok′să-zin). C₁₂H₁₀ON₂; Oxyiminodiphenylimine; parent substance of a series of biological dyes, *e.g.,* gallocyanin, brilliant cresyl blue, cresyl violet acetate.

ox·a·zole (ok′să-zōl). The fundamental ring system.

ox·a·zo·li·dine·di·ones (ok-să-zō-lid′īn-dē-onz). An obsolescent chemical class of antiepileptic drugs useful in the treatment of absence (petit mal) seizures; examples include trimethadione and paramethadione.

ox·el·a·din (ok-sel′ă-din). 2-Ethyl-2-phenylbutyric acid 2-(2-diethylaminoethoxy)ethyl ester; an antitussive agent.

ox·i·con·a·zole (ok′se-kō′nă-zōl). Broad spectrum antifungal agent resembling ketoconazole.

ox·i·dant (ok′si-dant). The substance that is reduced and that, therefore, oxidizes the other component of an oxidation-reduction system.

ox·i·dase (ok′si-dās). Classically, one of a group of enzymes, now termed oxidoreductases (EC class 1), that bring about oxidation by the addition of oxygen to a metabolite or by the removal of hydrogen or of one or more electrons. O. is now used for those cases in which O₂ acts as an acceptor (of H or of electrons); those removing hydrogen are now termed dehydrogenases. For individual o.'s, see the specific names.
  direct o., originally, an o. catalyzing the transfer of O₂ directly to other bodies; now termed oxygenase.
  indirect o., originally, an o. that acts by reducing a peroxide; now termed peroxidase.
  terminal o., the last protein in the electron transport, respiratory chain. In mammals this is cytochrome *c* oxidase.

ox·i·da·sis (ok-si-dā′sis). Oxidation by an oxidase.

ox·i·da·tion (ok-si-dā′shŭn). **1.** Combination with oxygen; increasing the valence of an atom or ion by the loss from it of hydrogen or of one or more electrons thus rendering it more electropositive, as when iron is changed from the ferrous (2+) to the ferric (3+) state. **2.** In bacteriology, the aerobic dissimilation of substrates with the production of energy and water; in contrast to fermentation, the transfer of electrons in the o. process is accomplished via the respiratory chain, which utilizes oxygen as the final electron acceptor.
  alpha-o., α-oxidation, a form of o. of fatty acids in which carbons are removed one at a time in the form of CO₂; the α-carbon is first hydroxylated and then converted into a carbonyl; a deficiency of this pathway is associated with Refsum's disease.
  beta-o., β-oxidation, (1) o. of the β-carbon (carbon 3) of a fatty acid, forming the β-keto (β-oxo) acid analog; of importance in fatty acid catabolism; **(2)** the entire pathway for the catabolism of saturated fatty acids containing an even number of carbon atoms; beta-o. (1) is a part of this pathway; acetyl-CoA is a major product of this pathway.
  end o., the last o. step in a catabolic pathway. SYN terminal o.
  omega-o., ω-oxidation, o. at the carbon atom farthest removed (ω-carbon) from the carboxyl group (carbon 1); thus, in this pathway, a dicarboxylic acid is formed; an important pathway in the degradation of prostaglandins.
  terminal o., SYN end o.

ox·i·da·tion-re·duc·tion. Any chemical oxidation or reduction reaction, which must, *in toto,* comprise both oxidation and reduction; the basis for calling all oxidative enzymes (formerly oxidases) oxidoreductases. Often shortened to "redox."

ox·i·da·tive (ok-si-dā′tiv). Having the power to oxidize; denoting a process involving oxidation.

ox·ide (ok′sīd). A compound of oxygen with another element or a radical; *e.g.,* mercuric o., HgO.
  acid o., an acid anhydride; an o. of an electronegative element or radical; it can combine with water to form an acid.
  basic o., a base anhydride; an o. of an electropositive element or radical; it can combine with water to form a base.
  indifferent o., SYN neutral o.
  neutral o., an o. that is neither an acid nor a base; *e.g.,* water (hydrogen oxide, H₂O). SYN indifferent o.

ox·i·dize (ok′si-dīz). To combine or cause an element or radical to combine with oxygen or to lose electrons.

ox·i·do·re·duc·tase (ok′si-dō-rē-dŭk′tās). An enzyme (EC class 1) catalyzing an oxidation-reduction reaction. Trivial names for o.'s include dehydrogenase, reductase, oxidase (where O₂ is the H acceptor), oxygenase (where O₂ is incorporated into the substrate), peroxidase (H₂O₂ is the acceptor; catalase is an exception), hydroxylase (coupled oxidation of two donors). SEE ALSO oxidase.

ox·ime (ok′sēm). A compound resulting from the action of hydroxylamine, NH₂OH, on a ketone or an aldehyde to yield the group =N–OH attached to the former carbonyl carbon atom.
  amide o.'s, SYN amidoximes.

ox·im·e·ter (ok-sim′ĕ-ter). An instrument for determining photoelectrically the oxygen saturation of a sample of blood.
  cuvette o., an o. that reads the percentage of oxygen saturation of the blood as it passes through a cuvette outside the body.

ox·im·e·try (ok-sim′ĕ-trē). Measurement with an oximeter of the oxygen saturation of hemoglobin in a sample of blood.

oxi·rane (oks′ē-rān). SYN *ethylene* oxide.

oxo-. Prefix denoting addition of oxygen; used in place of keto- in systematic nomenclature. SEE ALSO hydroxy-, oxa-, oxy-.

oxo·ace·tic ac·id (ok′sō-a-sē′tik). SYN glyoxylic acid.

oxo ac·id (ok′sō). SYN keto acid.

3-ox·o·ac·id-CoA trans·fer·ase. An enzyme catalyzing the reversible conversion of acetoacetyl-CoA and succinate into succinyl-CoA and acetoacetate; malonyl-CoA can substitute for succinyl-CoA and a few other 3-oxo acids for the acetoacetate; an important step in order for the ketone bodies to serve as a fuel for extrahepatic tissues. SYN 3-ketoacid-CoA transferase, acetoacetyl-succinic thiophorase.

3-ox·o·ac·yl-ACP re·duc·tase (ok′sō-as′il). A part of the fatty acid synthase complex; an enzyme reversibly reacting 3-oxoacyl-

ACP with NADPH to form D-3-hydroxyacyl-ACP and NADP⁺. SYN β-ketoacyl-ACP reductase.

3-ox·o·ac·yl-ACP syn·thase. An enzyme condensing malonyl-ACP and acyl-cys-protein to 3-oxoacyl-ACP + cys-protein + CO_2, and similar reactions, as steps in fatty acid synthesis; cys-protein is also a part of the fatty acid synthase complex. SYN acyl-malonyl-ACP synthase, β-ketoacyl-ACP synthase.

2-ox·o·glu·tar·ate de·hy·dro·gen·ase (ok'sō-glū-tar'āt). SYN α-*ketoglutarate* dehydrogenase.

2-ox·o·glu·tar·ic ac·id (oks'-ō-glū-tar-ik). SYN α-ketoglutaramic acid.

2-oxo-5-guanidovaleric ac·id (gwan-ē'dō-va-ler'ik). The deaminated derivative of arginine.

ox·ol·a·mine (ok-sol'ă-mēn). 5-(2-Diethylaminoethyl)-3-phenyl-1,2,4-oxadiazole; used for treatment of bronchopulmonary infections.

ox·o·lin·ic ac·id (ok-sō-lin'ik). 5-Ethyl-5,8-dihydro-8-oxo-1,3-dioxolo[4,5-*g*]quinoline-7-carboxylic acid; a quinolone antibacterial agent used in the treatment of urinary tract infections.

ox·o·phen·ar·sine hy·dro·chlo·ride (ok'sō-fen-ar'sēn). 3-Amino-4-hydroxyphenylarsineoxide hydrochloride; an antisyphilitic and antitrypanosomal agent.

5-ox·o·pro·lin·ase. An enzyme that catalyzes the ATP-dependent hydrolysis of L-5-oxoproline (ATP + L-5-oxoproline → ADP + P_i + L-glutamate) a deficiency of this enzyme will result in 5-oxoprolinuria.

5-ox·o·pro·line (Glp) (oks'ō-prō'lēn). A keto derivative of proline that is formed nonenzymatically from glutamate, glutamine, and γ-glutamylated peptides; it is also produced by the action of γ-glutamylcyclotransferase; elevated levels of 5-o. are often associated with problems of glutamine or glutathione metabolism. SYN 5-pyrrolidone-2-carboxylic acid, pyroglutamic acid, pyrrolidone-5-carboxylate.

4-ox·o·pro·line re·duc·tase. SYN *4-hydroxyproline* oxidase.

5-ox·o·pro·lin·ur·ia (oks'ō-prō'lēn-yūr-ē-ă). Elevated levels of 5-oxoproline in the urine.

17-ox·o·ste·roids (ok-sō-stēr'oydz). SYN 17-ketosteroids.

ox·o·suc·cin·ic ac·id (ok'sō-sŭk-sin'ik). SYN oxaloacetic acid.

ox·o·tre·mo·rine (ok'sō-trem'er-ēn). An active metabolite of tremorine. Used as a pharmacological tool for producing a parkinson-like tremor.

ox·pren·o·lol hy·dro·chlo·ride (oks-pren'ō-lol). 1-[*o*-(Allyloxy)phenoxy]-3-(isopropylamino)-2-propanol hydrochloride; a β-receptor blocking agent with coronary vasodilator activity.

OXT Abbreviation for oxytocin.

ox·tri·phyl·line (oks-trī'fi-lin, oks'trī-fil'in). A true salt of theophylline; it has mild diuretic, myocardial stimulating vasodilator, and bronchodilator actions, with the same uses as theophylline, but is better absorbed and less irritating. SYN choline theophyllinate.

△oxy-. **1.** Combining form denoting shrill; sharp, pointed; quick (incorrectly used for ocy-, from G. *ōkys*, swift). **2.** In chemistry, combining form denoting the presence of oxygen, either added or substituted, in a substance. SEE ALSO hydroxy-, oxa-, oxo-. [G. *oxys*, keen]

ox·y·a·coia, ox·y·a·koia (ok'sē-ă-koy'ă). Increased sensitiveness to noises, occurring in facial paralysis, especially when the stapedius muscle is paralyzed. [G. *oxys*, acute, + *akoē*, hearing]

ox·y·a·phia (ok-sē-ā'fē-ă). SYN hyperaphia. [G. *oxys*, acute, + *haphē*, touch]

ox·y·bar·bi·tu·rates (ok'sē-bar-bit'yūr-āts). Hypnotics of the barbiturate group in which the atom attached at the carbon-2 position is oxygen; virtually all hypnotic barbituates are o.'s.

ox·y·ben·zone (ok-sē-ben'zōn). 2-Hydroxy-4-methoxybenzophenone; an ultraviolet screen for use in skin ointments and lotions.

ox·y·bi·o·tin (ok-sē-bī'ō-tin). An analogue and antimetabolite of biotin, in which the sulfur atom is replaced by oxygen.

ox·y·bu·ty·nin chlo·ride (ok-sē-byū'ti-nin). α-Phenylcyclohex-

aneglycolic acid 4-(diethylamino)-2-butynyl ester hydrochloride; an intestinal antispasmodic.

ox·y·cal·o·rim·e·ter (ok'sē-kal-ō-rim'ĕ-ter). A calorimeter measuring energy content of substances in terms of oxygen consumed.

ox·y·cel·lu·lose (ok-sē-sel'yū-lōs). Cellulose that has been oxidized by NO_2 or other oxidizing agents to the point where all or most of the glucose residues have been converted to glucuronic acid residues; used as an adsorbent in chromatography or other adsorption processes. SEE ALSO oxidized *cellulose*.

ox·y·ce·pha·lia (ok'sē-se-fā'lē-ă). SYN oxycephaly.

ox·y·ce·phal·ic, ox·y·ceph·a·lous (ok-sē-se-fal'ik, -sef'ă-lŭs). Relating to or characterized by oxycephaly. SYN acrocephalic, acrocephalous.

ox·y·ceph·a·ly (ok-sē-sef'ă-lē). A type of craniosynostosis in which there is premature closure of the lambdoid and coronal sutures, resulting in an abnormally high, peaked, or conically shaped skull. SYN acrocephalia, acrocephaly, hypsicephaly, hypsocephaly, oxycephalia, steeple skull, tower skull, turricephaly. [G. *oxys*, pointed, + *kephalē*, head]

ox·y·chlo·ride (ok-sē-klōr'īd). A compound of oxygen with a metallic chloride; *e.g.,* a chlorate or perchlorate.

ox·y·chro·mat·ic (ok'sē-krō-mat'ik). SYN acidophilic. [G. *oxys*, sour, acid, + *chrōma*, color]

ox·y·chro·ma·tin (ok-sē-krō'mă-tin). Chromatin that stains with acid dyes, as in interphase nuclei. SYN oxyphil chromatin.

ox·y·co·done (ok-sē-kō'dōn). 14-Hydroxydihydrocodeinone; a narcotic analgesic.

11-ox·y·cor·ti·coids (ok-sē-kōr'ti-koydz). Corticosteroids bearing an alcohol or ketonic group on carbon-11; *e.g.,* cortisone, cortisol.

ox·y·es·the·sia (ok'sē-es-thē'zē-ă). SYN hyperesthesia. [G. *oxys*, acute, + *aisthēsis*, sensation]

ox·y·gen (O) (ok'sē-jen). **1.** A gaseous element, atomic no. 8, atomic wt. 15.9994 on basis of $^{12}C = 12.0000$; an abundant and widely distributed chemical element, which combines with most of the other elements to form oxides and is essential to animal and plant life. **2.** The molecular form of o., O_2. **3.** A medicinal gas that contains not less than 99.0%, by volume, of O_2. [G. *oxys*, sharp, acid and *genes*, forming]

heavy o., SYN oxygen-18.

hyperbaric o., high pressure o., o. at a pressure greater than 1 atmosphere. SEE ALSO hyperbaric *oxygenation.*

singlet o., an excited or higher energy form of o. characterized by the spin of a pair of electrons in opposite directions, whereas electron spin is unidirectional in normal molecular o. Because of its great reactivity, singlet o. is a probable intermediate in most photo-oxidation reactions. Although it exists for no more than 0.1 sec, it may react with atmospheric pollutants to foster smog formation and may have harmful biological effects.

triplet o., the normal unexcited state of O_2 in the atmosphere, in which the unpaired pair of electrons are so displaced that their magnetic fields are oriented in the same direction, resulting in paramagnetism; each of the heat-generated spectral lines of such o. can be split by a magnetic field into a triplet. Cf. singlet o.

ox·y·gen-15 (^{15}O). A cyclotron-produced, positron-emitting radioisotope of oxygen with a half-life of 122.2 seconds; used in studies of respiratory function and in positron emission tomography.

ox·y·gen-16 (^{16}O). The common oxygen isotope, making up 99.76% of natural oxygen.

ox·y·gen-17 (^{17}O). The rarest of the stable oxygen isotopes, making up 0.04% of natural oxygen.

ox·y·gen-18 (^{18}O). A stable oxygen isotope making up 0.20% of natural oxygen; used in mass spectrometry and in NMR studies of tissue. SYN heavy oxygen.

ox·y·gen·ase (ok'sē-jĕ-nās). One of a group of enzymes (EC subclass 1.13) catalyzing direct incorporation of O_2 into substrates; *e.g.,* tryptophan 2,3-dioxygenase (tryptophan pyrolase) catalyzing reaction between O_2 and L-tryptophan to form *N*-L-formylkynurenine. Cf. dioxygenase, monooxygenases.

mixed function o., any monooxygenase that catalyzes AH + O_2 + $DH_2 \rightarrow AOH + H_2O + D$.

ox·y·gen·ate (ok′sē-jĕ-nāt). To accomplish oxygenation.

ox·y·gen·a·tion (ok′sē-jĕ-nā′shŭn). Addition of oxygen to any chemical or physical system.

apneic o., SYN diffusion *respiration*.

hyperbaric o., an increased amount of oxygen in organs and tissues resulting from the administration of oxygen in a compression chamber at an ambient pressure greater than 1 atmosphere.

ox·y·gen·ic (ok-sē-jen′ik). Pertaining to or containing oxygen.

ox·y·gen·ize (ok′sē-jen-īz). To oxidize with oxygen.

ox·y·geu·sia (ok-sē-gū′sē-ă). SYN hypergeusia. [G. *oxys,* acute, + *geusis,* taste]

ox·y·heme (ok′sē-hēm). SYN hematin.

ox·y·he·mo·chro·mo·gen (ok′sē-hēm′ō-krō′mō-jen). SYN hematin.

ox·y·he·mo·glo·bin (HbO₂) (ok′sē-hē-mō-glō′bin). Hemoglobin in combination with oxygen, the form of hemoglobin present in arterial blood, scarlet or bright red when dissolved in water. SYN oxygenated hemoglobin.

ox·y·i·o·dide (ok-sē-ī′ō-dīd). A compound of oxygen with a metallic iodide, *e.g.,* an iodate or periodate.

ox·y·krin·in (ok-sē-krin′in). SYN secretin.

ox·y·luc·i·fer·in (oks′ē-lū-si′fer-in). The activated derivative of luciferin formed in bioluminescence.

ox·y·mes·ter·one (ok-sē-mes′te-rōn). 4,17β-Dihydroxy-17-methylandrost-4-en-3-one; an anabolic steroid.

ox·y·met·az·o·line hy·dro·chlo·ride (ok′sē-mĕ-taz′ŏ-lēn). 6-Tert-butyl-3-(2-imidazolin-2-ylmethyl)-2,4-dimentylphenol hydrochloride; a vasoconstrictor used topically to reduce swelling and congestion of the nasal mucosa.

ox·y·meth·o·lone (ok-sē-meth′ŏ-lōn). 17β-Hydroxy-2-(hydroxymethylene)-17-methyl-5α-androstan-3-one; an androgenic anabolic steroid.

ox·y·mor·phone hy·dro·chlo·ride (ok-sē-mōr′fōn). 14-Hydroxydihydromorphinone hydrochloride; a semisynthetic narcotic analgesic closely related chemically to hydromorphone hydrochloride; its actions are similar to those of morphine, but more potent.

ox·y·my·o·glo·bin (MbO₂) (ok′sē-mī-ō-glō′bin). Myoglobin in its oxygenated form, analogous in structure to oxyhemoglobin.

ox·y·ner·vone (ok′sē-ner′vōn). SYN hydroxynervone.

ox·y·neu·rine (ok-sē-nūr′ēn). SYN betaine.

ox·yn·tic (ok-sin′tik). Acid-forming, *e.g.,* the parietal cells of the gastric glands. [G. *oxynō,* to sharpen, make sour, acid]

ox·y·os·mia (ok-sē-oz′mē-ă). SYN hyperosmia. [G. *oxys,* acute + *osmē,* sense of smell]

ox·y·os·phre·sia (ok′sē-os-frē′zē-ă). SYN hyperosmia. [G. *oxys,* acute, + *osphrēsis,* smell]

ox·y·per·tine (ok-sē-per′tēn). 5,6-Dimethoxy-2-methyl-3-[2-(4-phenyl-1-piperazinyl)ethyl]indole; an antianxiety agent; also available as the hydrochloride.

ox·y·phen·bu·ta·zone (ok′sē-fen-bū′tă-zōn). 1-(p-Hydroxyphenyl)-2-phenyl-4-butyl-3,5-pyrazolidine-dione monohydrate; an orally effective analgesic and anti-inflammatory agent used (usually in short courses) for rheumatoid arthritis and gout.

ox·y·phen·cy·cli·mine hy·dro·chlo·ride (ok′sē-fen-sī′klī-mēn). The hydrochloride of 1,4,5,6-tetrahydro-1-methylpyrimidin-2-ylmethyl-α-cyclohexyl-α-hydroxy-α-phenylacetate; an anticholinergic agent.

ox·y·phe·ni·sa·tin ac·e·tate (ok′sē-fe-nī′să-tin). endophenolphthalein; diacetyldiphenolisatin; 3,3-bis(p-acetoxyphenyl)-oxindole; a cathartic with pharmacologic properties resembling those of phenolphthalein, except that it is not absorbed from the gastrointestinal tract.

ox·y·phe·no·ni·um bro·mide (ok′sē-fe-nō′nē-ŭm). Diethyl(2-hydroxyethyl)methylammonium bromide α-phenyl-α-cyclohexylglycolate; a quaternary ammonium compound with anticholinergic action.

ox·y·phil, ox·y·phile (ok′sē-fil, -fīl). **1.** Oxyphil *cell.* **2.** SYN

eosinophilic *leukocyte.* **3.** SYN oxyphilic. [G. *oxys,* sour, acid, + *philos,* fond]

ox·y·phil·ic (ok-sē-fil′ik). Having an affinity for acid dyes; denoting certain cell or tissue elements. SYN oxyphil (3), oxyphile.

ox·y·pho·nia (ok-sē-fō′nē-ă). Shrillness or high pitch of the voice. [G. *oxys,* sharp, + *phōnē,* voice]

ox·y·pol·y·gel·a·tin (ok′sē-pol-ē-jel′ă-tin). A modified gelatin used as a plasma extender in transfusions.

ox·y·pu·rine (ok-sē-pyūr′ēn). A purine containing oxygen; *e.g.,* hypoxanthine, xanthine, uric acid.

ox·y·pu·ri·nol (ok-sē-pūr′ĭ-nol). Alloxanthine and inhibitor of xanthine oxidase; an active metabolite of allopurinol. The drug inhibits the formation of uric acid and is used in the treatment of gout.

ox·y·rhine (ok′sē-rīn). Having a sharp-pointed nose. [G. *oxys,* sharp, + *rhis* (rhin-), nose]

ox·y·ryg·mia (ok-sē-rig′mē-ă). Obsolete term for eructation of acid fluid. [G. *oxys,* acid, + *erygmos,* eructation]

Ox·y·spi·ru·ra man·so·ni (ok′-sē-spī-rū′ră man-sō′nī). A widely distributed spiruroid nematode parasite found under the nictitating membrane in the eye of turkeys, chickens, peafowl, quail, and grouse; larvae develop to the infective stage in cockroaches. SYN Manson's eye worm.

ox·y·ta·lan (ok-sit′ă-lan). A type of connective tissue fiber histochemically distinct from collagen or elastic fibers described in the periodontal ligament and gingivae. [G. *oxys,* acid, + *talas,* suffering, resisting; coined term probably intended to mean "resistant to acid hydrolysis"]

ox·y·tet·ra·cy·cline (ok′sē-tet-ră-sī′klēn). An antibiotic produced by the actinomycete, *Streptomyces rimosus,* present in the soil; its actions and uses are similar to those of tetracycline; available as the dihydrate, hydrochloride, and calcium.

ox·y·thi·a·min (ok-sē-thī′ă-min). A molecule similar to that of thiamin but with a hydroxyl group replacing the amino group on the pyrimidine ring; a thiamin antagonist capable of inducing symptoms of thiamin deficiency on administration; increases thiamin excretion.

ox·y·to·cia (ok-sē-tō′sē-ă). Rapid parturition. [G. *okytokos,* swift birth]

ox·y·to·cic (ok-sē-tō′sik). **1.** Hastening childbirth. **2.** SYN parturifacient (2).

ox·y·to·cin (OXT) (ok-sē-tō′sin). A nonapeptide neurohypophysial hormone, differing from human vasopressin in having leucine at position 8 and isoleucine at position 3, that causes myometrial contractions at term and promotes milk release during lactation; used for the induction or stimulation of labor, in the management of postpartum hemorrhage and atony, and to relieve painful breast engorgement. SYN ocytocin. [G. *okytokos,* swift birth]

arginine o., o. with arginine at position 8 (identical with arginine vasotocin). SEE ALSO arginine *vasopressin.*

ox·y·u·ri·a·sis (ok-sē-yū-rī′ă-sis). Infection with nematode parasites of the genus *Oxyuris.*

ox·y·u·ri·cide (ok′sē-yū′ri-sīd). An agent that destroys pinworms. [oxyurid + L. *caedo,* to kill]

ox·y·u·rid (ok-sē-yū′rid). Common name for members of the family Oxyuridae. [see *Oxyuris*]

Ox·y·u·ri·dae (ok-sē-yū′ri-dē). A family of parasitic nematodes (superfamily Oxyuroidea) found in the large intestine or cecum of vertebrates and the intestine of invertebrates, especially insects and millipedes; it includes the genera *Aspiculurus, Enterobius, Oxyuris, Passalurus, Syphacia,* and *Thelandros.*

Ox·y·u·ris (ok′sē-yū′ris). A genus of nematodes commonly called seatworms or pinworms (although the pinworm of humans is the closely related form, *Enterobius vermicularis*). *O. equi,* the horse pinworm, is a common parasite of horses in all parts of the world, inhabiting the large intestine. [G. *oxys,* sharp, + *oura,* tail]

△**-oyl.** Suffix denoting an acyl radical; -yl replaces -ic in acid names.

oz. Abbreviation for ounce.

oze·na (ō-zē′nă). A disease characterized by intranasal crusting, atrophy, and fetid odor. [G. *ozaina,* a fetid polypus, fr. *ozō,* to smell]

oze·nous (ō′zē-nŭs). Relating to ozena.

ozo·ce·rite (ō-zō-sē′rīt). SYN ozokerite.

ozo·chro·tia (ō-zō-krō′shē-ă). SYN bromidrosis. [G. *ozō,* to smell, + *chroa,* skin]

ozo·ker·ite (ō-zō-kēr′ĭt). A mixture of paraffinic and cycloparaffinic hydrocarbons occurring in nature; it has a higher melting point than synthetic paraffin, and is used as a substitute for beeswax. SYN ozocerite.

purified o., SYN ceresin.

ozon·a·tor (ō′zō-nā-ter, -tōr). An apparatus for generating ozone and diffusing it in the atmosphere of a room.

ozone (ō′zōn). O_3; a powerful oxidizing agent; air containing a perceptible amount of O_3 formed by an electric discharge or by the slow combustion of phosphorus, and has an odor suggestive of Cl_2 or SO_2; also formed by the action of solar UV radiation on atmospheric O_2. [G. *ozō,* to smell]

ozo·nide (ō′zō-nīd). The unstable intermediate formed by the reaction of ozone with an unsaturated organic compound, especially with unsaturated fatty acids.

ozon·ol·y·sis (ō-zō-nol′ĭ-sis). The splitting of a double bond in a hydrocarbon chain upon treatment with ozone, with the formation of two aldehydes (an ozonide is the unstable intermediate); has been used to determine the structure of unsaturated fatty acids. [ozone + G. *lysis,* dissolution]

ozon·om·e·ter (ō-zō-nom′ĕ-ter). A modified form of ozonoscope, in which by a series of test papers the amount of ozone in the atmosphere may be estimated.

ozo·no·scope (ō-zō′nō-skōp). Filter paper saturated with starch and potassium iodide or with litmus and potassium iodide; turns blue in the presence of ozone.

ozo·sto·mia (ō-zō-stō′mē-ă). SYN halitosis. [G. *ozō,* to smell, + *stoma,* mouth]

OZ

π. 1. pi, The sixteenth letter of the Greek alphabet. **2.** Symbol for circumference of circle divided by diameter, 3.14159.

Π Symbol for osmotic *pressure*.

Φ The 21st letter of the Greek alphabet. Symbol for phenyl.

φ. Symbol for quantum *yield*.

Ψ, Ψrd. 1. psi, The 23rd letter of the Greek alphabet. **2.** Symbol for pseudouridine; psi (pounds per square inch); psychology.

P$_i$ Symbol for inorganic *orthophosphate* (should not be used when covalently linked to another moiety).

P$_{CO_2}$, pCO$_2$ Symbol for partial pressure (tension) of carbon dioxide. SEE partial *pressure*.

^{32}P. Symbol for phosphorus-32.

^{33}P Symbol for phosphorus-33.

P$_{700}$. The pigment in chloroplasts bleached by light of wavelengths about 700 nm.

P$_1$ Abbreviation for parental *generation*; symbol for inorganic *orthophosphate* (should *not* be used when covalently linked to another moiety).

P$_B$ Symbol for barometric *pressure*.

P 1. Symbol for peta-; phosphorus; pressure or partial *pressure*; proline; product; power; frequently with subscripts indicating location and/or chemical species. **2.** Followed by a subscript, 1) refers to the plasma concentration of the substance indicated by the subscript; 2) permeability *constant*. **3.** A blood group designation. See P blood group, Blood Groups appendix. **4.** Symbol for probability; when followed by the sign for "less than" (<) this indicates that a test statistic, *e.g.*, a chi-square test gives a result unlikely to occur by chance.

P$_{O_2}$, pO$_2$ Symbol for the partial pressure (tension) of oxygen. SEE partial *pressure*.

P In nucleic acid terminology, symbol for phosphoric residue.

p 1. Abbreviation for pupil; optic *papilla*. **2.** In polynucleotide symbolism, phosphoric ester or phosphate. **3.** Symbol for pico-(2); momentum (in italics). **4.** In cytogenetics, symbol for the short arm of a chromosome. [fr. Fr. *petit,* small]

p$_{870}$. The pigment in bacterial chromatophores bleached by light of wavelengths about 870 nm.

p- Abbreviation for para- (4).

P.A. Abbreviation for physician assistant.

Pa Symbol for pascal; protactinium.

Paas, H.R., German physician, *1900. SEE P.'s *disease*.

PABA Abbreviation for *p*-aminobenzoic acid.

pab·lum (pab'lŭm). A precooked infant food, a mixture of wheat, oat, and corn meals, wheat embryo, alfalfa leaves, brewers' yeast, iron, and sodium chloride. [L. *pabulum,* nourishment, fr. *pasco,* to nourish]

pab·u·lar (pab'yū-lăr). Relating to, or of the nature of, pabulum.

pab·u·lum (pab'yū-lŭm). Food or nutriment. [L.]

Pacchioni, Antonio, Italian anatomist, 1665–1726. SEE pacchionian *bodies,* under *body,* pacchionian *corpuscles,* under *corpuscle,* pacchionian *depressions,* under *depression,* pacchionian *glands,* under *gland,* pacchionian *granulations,* under *granulation.*

pac·chi·o·ni·an (pak-ē-ō'nē-an). Attributed to or described by Pacchioni.

pace·fol·low·er (pās'fawl-ō-er). Any cell in excitable tissue that responds to stimuli from a pacemaker.

pace·mak·er (pās'mā-ker). **1.** Biologically, any rhythmic center that establishes a pace of activity; **2.** An artificial regulator of rate activity. **3.** In chemistry, the substance whose rate of reaction sets the pace for a series of chain reactions; the rate-limiting reaction itself; *e.g.*, in a metabolic pathway, the enzyme catalyzing the slowest or rate-limiting reaction in that pathway. [L. *passus,* step, pace]

artificial p., any device that substitutes for the normal p. and controls the rhythm of the organ; especially an electronic cardiac

p., which may be implanted in the chest, with electrodes attached to the external cardiac surface, or passed through the venous circulation into the right side of the heart (pervenous p.).

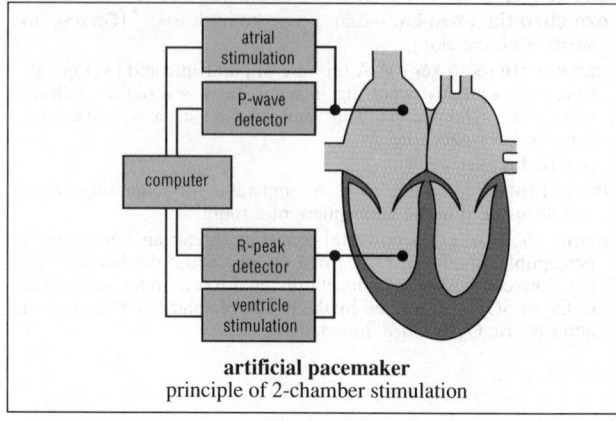

artificial pacemaker
principle of 2-chamber stimulation

demand p., a form of artificial p. usually implanted into cardiac tissue because its output of electrical stimuli can be inhibited by endogenous cardiac electrical activity.

diaphragmatic p., a device that paces the diaphragm, used in patients with chronic ventilatory insufficiency resulting from malfunction of the respiratory control center on certain types of phrenic nerve malfunction.

ectopic p., any p. other than the sinus node.

electric cardiac p., an electric device that can substitute for the normal cardiac p., controlling the heart's rhythm by artificial electric discharges. SYN electronic p.

electronic p., SYN electric cardiac p.

external p., an artificial cardiac p. whose electrodes for delivering rhythmical electrical stimuli to the heart are placed on the chest wall.

fixed-rate p., an artificial p. that emits electrical stimuli at a constant frequency.

nuclear p., a nuclear-powered unit used to generate the electrical current for artificially pacing the heart; replaced by units using long-life nickel-cadmium and other power sources.

pervenous p., an artificial p. passed through the venous circulation into the right side of the heart.

runaway p., rapid heart rates over 140/min caused by electronic circuit instability in an implanted pulse generator.

shifting p., SYN wandering p.

subsidiary atrial p., secondary source for rhythmic control of the heart, available for controlling cardiac activity if the sinoatrial pacemaker fails; located within the crista terminalis and atrial free wall near the inferior vena cava.

transthoracic p., artificial p. delivering stimuli through the chest wall usually applied as a temporizing measure in patients with atrioventricular block.

wandering p., a disturbance of the normal cardiac rhythm in which the site of the controlling p. shifts from beat to beat, usually between the sinus and A-V nodes, often with gradual sequential changes in P waves between upright and inverted in a given ECG lead. SYN shifting p.

pa·chom·e·ter (pa-kom'ĕ-ter). SYN pachymeter.

Pachon, Michel V., French physiologist, 1867–1938. SEE P.'s *method, test.*

pachy-. Thick. [G. *pachys,* thick]

pach·y·bleph·a·ron (pak'ē-blef'ă-ron). Thickening of the tarsal border of the eyelid. SYN tylosis ciliaris. [pachy- + G. *blepharon,* eyelid]

pach·y·ce·pha·lia (pak'ē-se-fā'lē-ă). SYN pachycephaly.

pach·y·ce·phal·ic, pach·y·ceph·a·lous (pak'ē-se-fal'ik, -sef'ă-lŭs). Relating to or marked by pachycephaly.

pach·y·ceph·a·ly (pak-i-sef'ă-lē). Abnormal thickness of the skull. SYN pachycephalia. [pachy- + G. *kephalē,* head]

pach·y·chei·lia, pach·y·chi·lia (pak-i-kī'lē-ă). Swelling or abnormal thickness of the lips. [pachy- + G. *cheilos,* lip]

pach·y·cho·lia (pak-i-kō'lē-ă). Inspissation of the bile. [pachy- + G. *cholē,* bile]

pach·y·chro·mat·ic (pak'ē-krō-mat'ik). Having a coarse chromatin reticulum.

pach·y·chy·mia (pak-i-kī'mē-ă). Inspissation of the chyme. [pachy- + G. *chymos,* juice]

pach·y·dac·tyl·ia (pak'ē-dak-til'ē-ă). SYN pachydactyly.

pach·y·dac·ty·lous (pak-i-dak'ti-lŭs). Relating to or characterized by pachydactyly.

pach·y·dac·ty·ly (pak-i-dak'ti-lē). Enlargement of the fingers or toes, especially extremities; often seen in neurofibromatosis. SYN pachydactylia. [pachy- + G. *daktylos,* finger or toe]

pach·y·der·ma (pak-i-der'mă). Abnormally thick skin. SEE ALSO elephantiasis. SYN pachydermatosis, pachydermia. [pachy- + G. *derma,* skin]

p. laryn′gis, a circumscribed connective tissue hyperplasia at the posterior commissure of the larynx.

p. lymphangiectat′ica, elephantiasis due to lymph stasis.

p. verruco′sa, chronic wart-like elephantiasis due to lymph stasis.

p. vesi′cae, elephantiasis with nodules comprised of lymph vesicles on the skin surface.

pach·y·der·mat·o·cele (pak'ē-der-mat'ō-sēl). **1.** SYN *cutis* laxa. **2.** Obsolete term for a huge neurofibroma. [pachy- + G. *derma,* skin, + *kēlē,* tumor]

pach·y·der·ma·to·sis (pak-i-der'mă-tō'sis). SYN pachyderma.

pach·y·der·ma·tous (pak-i-der'mă-tŭs). Relating to pachyderma. SYN pachydermic.

pach·y·der·mia (pak-i-der'mē-ă). SYN pachyderma.

pach·y·der·mic (pak-i-der'mik). SYN pachydermatous.

pach·y·der·mo·per·i·os·to·sis (pak-i-der'mō-per'ē-os-tō'sis) [MIM*167100]. A syndrome of clubbing of the digits, periosteal new bone formation, especially over the distal ends of the long bones (idiopathic hypertrophic osteoarthropathy), and coarsening of the facial features with thickening, furrowing, and oiliness of the skin of the face and forehead (cutis verticis gyrata); there is seborrheic hyperplasia with open sebaceous pores filled with plugs of sebum; often of autosomal dominant inheritance, usually more severe in males. SYN acropachyderma, Brugsch's syndrome. [pachy- + G. *derma,* skin, + periostosis]

pach·y·glos·sia (pak-i-glos'ē-ă). An enlarged thick tongue. [pachy- + G. *glōssa,* tongue]

pa·chyg·na·thous (pă-kig'nath-ŭs). Characterized by a large or thick jaw. [pachy- + G. *gnathos,* jaw]

pach·y·gy·ria (pak-i-jī'rē-ă). Condition in which the convolutions of the cerebral cortex are abnormally large; there are fewer sulci than normal and in some cases the amount of brain substance is somewhat increased. SYN macrogyria. [pachy- + G. *gyros,* circle]

pach·y·hy·me·nia (pak'ē-hī-me'nē-ă). SYN pachymenia. [pachy- + G. *hymēn,* membrane]

pach·y·hy·men·ic (pak'ē-hī-men'ik). SYN pachymenic.

pach·y·lep·to·men·in·gi·tis (pak'i-lep'tō-men-in-jī'tis). Inflammation of all the membranes of the brain or spinal cord. [G. *pachys,* thick, + *leptos,* thin, + *mēninx* (*mēning-*), membrane, + *-itis,* inflammation]

pach·y·lo·sis (pak-i-lō'sis). A condition of roughness, dryness and thickening of the skin, usually on the lower extremities. [G. *pachylos,* rather coarse]

pach·y·me·nia (pak-i-mē'nē-ă). Thickening of the skin or contiguous membranes. SYN pachyhymenia. [pachy- + G. *hymēn,* a membrane]

pach·y·men·ic (pak-i-men'ik). Marked by or relating to pachymenia. SYN pachyhymenic.

pach·y·men·in·gi·tis (pak'i-men'in-jī'tis). Inflammation of the dura mater. SYN perimeningitis. [pachy- + G. *mēninx,* membrane, + *-itis,* inflammation]

p. exter′na, inflammation of the outer surface of the dura mater. SYN epidural meningitis, external meningitis.

hemorrhagic p., subdural *hemorrhage* associated with pachymeningitis. SEE ALSO subdural *hemorrhage.*

hypertrophic cervical p., a fibrotic and inflammatory thickening of spinal pachymeninges, particularly in the cervical region, resulting in spinal nerve radiculopathy; believed to be of syphilitic etiology.

p. inter′na, inflammation of the inner surface of the dura mater. SYN internal meningitis.

pyogenic p., suppurative inflammation of the dura, often spreading from a neighboring osteomyelitis.

pach·y·me·nin·gop·a·thy (pak'ē-mĕ-ning-gop'ă-thē). Disease of the dura mater. [pachy- + G. *mēninx* (*mēning-*), membrane, + *pathos,* disease]

pach·y·me·ninx (pak'i-mē'ningks). The dura mater. [pachy- + G. *mēninx,* membrane]

pa·chym·e·ter (pă-kim'ē-ter). An instrument for measuring the thickness of any object, especially of thin objects such as a plate of bone or a membrane. SYN pachometer. [pachy- + G. *metron,* measure]

optical p., a lens and/or mirror used to measure corneal thickness.

pach·y·ne·ma (pak-ē-nē'mă). SYN pachytene. [pachy- + G. *nēma,* thread]

pa·chyn·sis (pă-kin'sis). Any pathologic thickening. [G. a thickening]

pa·chyn·tic (pă-kin'tic). Relating to pachynsis.

pach·y·o·nych·ia (pak'ē-ō-nik'ē-ă). Abnormal thickness of the fingernails or toenails. [pachy- + G. *onyx,* nail]

p. congen′ita [MIM*167200], a syndrome of ectodermal dysplasia of abnormal thickness and elevation of nail plates with palmar and plantar hyperkeratosis; the tongue is whitish and glazed owing to papillary atrophy; autosomal dominant inheritance. SYN Jadassohn-Lewandowski syndrome.

pach·y·o·tia (pak-i-ō'shē-ă). Thickness and coarseness of the auricles of the ears. [pachy- + G. *ous,* ear]

pach·y·per·i·os·ti·tis (pak'i-per'ē-ōs-tī'tis). Proliferative thickening of the periosteum caused by inflammation. [pachy- + periostitis]

pach·y·per·i·to·ni·tis (pak'i-per'i-tō-nī'tis). Inflammation of the peritoneum with thickening of the membrane. SYN productive peritonitis. [pachy- + peritonitis]

pach·y·pleu·ri·tis (pak'ē-plū-rī'tis). Inflammation of the pleura with thickening of the membrane. SYN productive pleurisy. [pachy- + pleura + G. *-itis,* inflammation]

pa·chyp·o·dous (pă-kip'ō-dŭs). Having large thick feet. [pachy- + G. *pous,* foot]

pach·y·sal·pin·gi·tis (pak'ē-sal-pin-jī'tis). SYN chronic interstitial *salpingitis.*

pach·y·sal·pin·go-o·va·ri·tis (pak-i-sal'pin-gō-ō-va-rī'tis). Chronic parenchymatous inflammation of the ovary and fallopian tube. [pachy- + salpinx + Mod. L. *ovarium,* ovary, + G. *-itis,* inflammation]

pach·y·so·mia (pak-i-sō'mē-ă). Pathologic thickening of the soft parts of the body, notably in acromegaly. [pachy- + G. *sōma,* body]

pach·y·tene (pak'i-tēn). The stage of prophase in meiosis in which pairing of homologous chromosomes is complete and the paired homologues may twine about each other as they continue to shorten; longitudinal cleavage occurs in each chromosome to form two sister chromatids so that each homologous chromosome pair becomes a set of four intertwined chromatids. SYN pachynema. [pachy- + G. *tainia,* band, tape]

pach·y·vag·i·nal·i·tis (pak'i-vaj'i-năl-ī'tis). Chronic inflammation with thickening of the tunica vaginalis testis. [pachy- + Mod. L. (tunica) *vaginalis,* + G. *-itis,* inflammation]

pach·y·vag·i·ni·tis (pak'i-vaj'i-nī'tis). Chronic vaginitis with thickening and induration of the vaginal walls. [pachy- + vagina + G. -*itis,* inflammation]

p. cys′tica, SYN *vaginitis* emphysematosa.

Pacini, Filippo, Italian anatomist, 1812–1883. SEE pacinian *corpuscles,* under *corpuscle;* Vater-P. *corpuscles,* under *corpuscle.*

pa·ci·ni·an (pa-sin′ē-an, pa-chin′). Attributed to or described by Pacini.

pa·cin·i·tis (pa-sin-ī′tis, pa-chin-). Inflammation of the pacinian corpuscles.

pack (pak). **1.** To fill, stuff, or tampon. **2.** To enwrap or envelop the body in a sheet, blanket, or other covering. **3.** To apply a dressing or covering to a surgical site. **4.** The items used above. [M.E. *pak,* fr. Germanic]

cold p., a p. of cloth or other material soaked in cold water or encasing ice.

dry p., a p. enveloping one in dry, warmed blankets in order to induce profuse perspiration.

hot p., a p. of cloth or other material soaked in hot water, or producing moist heat by another means.

wet p., the usual form of p. using hot or cold moisture.

pack·er (pak′er). **1.** An instrument for tamponing. **2.** SYN plugger.

pack·ing (pak′ing). **1.** Filling a natural cavity, a wound, or a mold with some material. **2.** The material so used. **3.** The application of a pack.

denture p., filling and compressing a denture base material into a mold in a flask.

pac·li·tax·el (pac-lē-taks′el). Antitumor agent that promotes microtubule assembly by preventing depolymerization; currently used in salvage therapy for metastatic carcinoma of ovary.

PACS Acronym for *picture archive and communication system,* a computer network for digitized radiologic images and reports.

pad. 1. Soft material forming a cushion, used in applying or relieving pressure on a part, or in filling a depression so that dressings can fit snugly. **2.** A more or less encapsulated body of fat or some other tissue serving to fill a space or act as a cushion in the body.

abdominal p., SYN laparotomy p.

dinner p., a p. of moderate thickness placed over the pit of the stomach before the application of a plaster jacket; after the plaster has set the p. is removed, leaving space for varying degrees of abdominal distention.

fat p., SEE fat-pad.

knuckle p.'s, (1) an autosomal dominant trait, in which thick p.'s of skin appear over the proximal phalangeal joints; occasionally associated with leukonychia and deafness or Dupuytren's contracture; **(2)** a callus reaction in persons predisposed to producing callus and as the result of occupational or self-inflicted trauma.

laparotomy p., a p. made from several layers of gauze folded into a rectangular shape; used as a sponge, for packing off the viscera in abdominal operations, and in other ways. SYN abdominal p.

Passavant's p., SYN Passavant's *cushion.*

periarterial p., SYN juxtaglomerular *body.*

pharyngoesophageal p.'s, SYN pharyngoesophageal *cushions,* under *cushion.*

retromolar p., a cushioned mass of tissue, frequently pear-shaped, located on the alveolar process of the mandible behind the area of the last natural molar tooth. SYN pear-shaped area.

sucking p., suctorial p., SYN buccal *fat-pad.*

Padykula-Herman stain for my·o·sin ATPase. See under stain.

Pae·ci·lo·my·ces (pē-sil-ō-mī′sēz). A genus of saprophytic imperfect fungi whose conidia-bearing hyphae superficially resemble the penicillus of *Penicillium;* isolated as contaminants, extremely rare pathogen.

pae·ci·loy·co·sis (pē-sil′ō-ē-cō′sis). A systemic (mainly pulmonary) mycosis of humans and various lower animals caused by fungi of the genus *Paecilomyces.*

△**paed-.** SEE ped-.

PAF Abbreviation for platelet-aggregating *factor.*

PAGE Abbreviation for polyacrylamide gel *electrophoresis.*

Pagenstecher, Alexander, German ophthalmologist, 1828–1879. SEE P.'s *circle.*

Paget, Sir James, English surgeon, 1814–1899. SEE P.'s *cells,* under *cell, disease;* extramammary P. *disease;* Paget-von Schrötter *syndrome.*

Paget-Eccleston stain. See under stain.

pa·get·ic (pa-jet′ik). Relating to or suffering from Paget's disease.

pag·et·oid (paj′ě-toyd). Resembling or characteristic of Paget's disease.

pa·go·pha·gia (pā-gō-fā′jē-ă). Compulsive and repeated ingestion of ice; sometimes associated with iron deficiency anemia. [G. *pagos,* frost, + *phagō,* to eat]

△**-pagus.** Conjoined twins, the first element of the word denoting the parts fused. SEE ALSO -didymus, -dymus. [G. *pagos,* something fixed, fr. *pēgnymi,* to fasten together]

PAH Abbreviation for *p*-aminohippuric acid.

pai·dol·o·gy (pā-dol′ō-jē). SYN pedology.

pain (pān). **1.** An unpleasant sensation associated with actual or potential tissue damage, and mediated by specific nerve fibers to the brain where its conscious appreciation may be modified by various factors. **2.** Term used to denote a painful uterine contraction occurring in childbirth. [L. *poena,* a fine, a penalty]

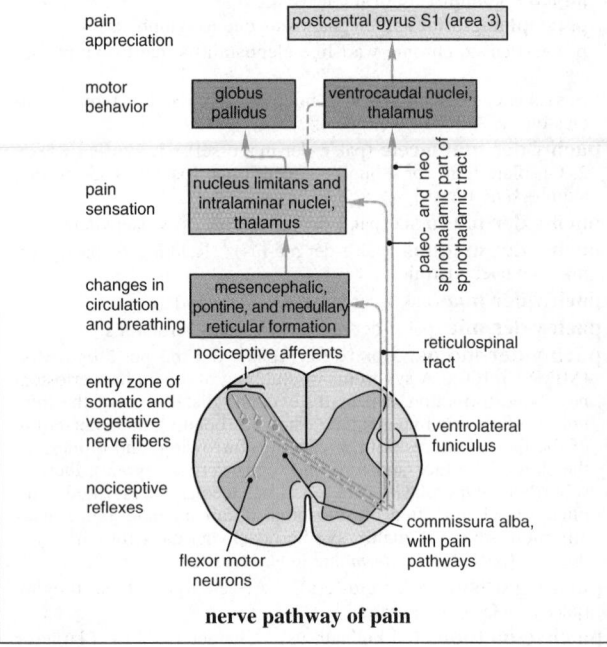

nerve pathway of pain

after-p.'s, SEE afterpains.

bearing-down p., a uterine contraction accompanied by straining and tenesmus; usually appearing in the second stage of labor.

dream p., SYN hypnalgia.

expulsive p.'s, effective labor p.'s, associated with contraction of the uterine muscle.

false p.'s, ineffective uterine contractions, preceding and sometimes resembling true labor, but distinguishable from it by the lack of progressive effacement and dilation of the cervix.

girdle p., a painful sensation encircling the body like a belt, occurring in tabes dorsalis or other spinal cord disease.

growing p.'s, aching p.'s, frequently felt at night, in the limbs of growing children; attributed variously to growth, rheumatic state, faulty posture, fatigue, or ill-defined psychic causes.

hunger p., cramp in the epigastrium associated with hunger.

intermenstrual p., (1) pelvic discomfort occurring approximately at the time of ovulation, usually at the midpoint of the menstrual cycle; SYN midpain. **(2)** SYN mittelschmerz.

intractable p., p. resistant or refractory to ordinary analgesic agents.

labor p.'s, rhythmical uterine contractions which under normal conditions increase in intensity, frequency, and duration, culminating in vaginal delivery of the infant. SYN parodynia.

middle p., SYN mittelschmerz.

mind p., SYN psychalgia (1).

nerve p., obsolete term for neuralgia.

night p., SYN nyctalgia.

organic p., pain caused by an organic lesion.

phantom limb p., SEE phantom *limb.*

postprandial p., p. occurring after eating, typical of malignancy in esophagus or stomach.

psychogenic p., somatoform p.; p. which is associated or correlated with a psychological, emotional, or behavioral stimulus. SYN psychalgia (2), somatoform p.

referred p., p. from deep structures perceived as arising from a surface area remote from its actual origin; the area where the pain is appreciated is innervated by the same spinal segment(s) as the deep structure. SYN synalgia, telalgia.

rest p., p. occurring usually in the extremities during rest in the sitting or lying position.

somatoform p., SYN psychogenic p.

soul p., SYN psychalgia (1).

paint (pānt). A solution or suspension of one or more medicaments applied to the skin with a brush or large applicator; usually used in the treatment of widespread eruptions.

carbol-fuchsin p., a p. containing boric acid, phenol, resorcinol, fuchsin, acetone, and alcohol in water; used in the treatment of superficial mycotic infections. SYN Castellani's p.

Castellani's p., SYN carbol-fuchsin p.

pair (pār). Two objects considered together because of similarity, for a common purpose, or because of some attracting force between them.

---

base p., the complex of two heterocyclic nucleic acid bases, one a pyrimidine and the other a purine, brought about by hydrogen bonding between the purine and the pyrimidine; base pairing is the essential element in the structure of DNA proposed by Watson and Crick in 1953; usually guanine is paired with cytosine (G·C), and adenine with thymine (A·T) or uracil (A·U). SYN nucleoside p., nucleotide p.

> The particular sequence of the complementary bases in either strand of a two-stranded DNA molecule codes for amino acids used in the manufacture of proteins. Trios of bases (codons) specify each of 20 amino acids. During protein synthesis (translation), messenger RNA and ribosomes read the order of amino acids from strings of DNA to create protein chains, which are then released into the cell.

---

buffer p., an acid and its conjugate base (anion).

chromosome p., two chromosomes of the full diploid karyotype that are similar in form and function but that usually differ in content, one normally being inherited from each parent and one being transmitted to each progeny; in the heteromorphic sex (in humans, the male), one pair, the sex chromosomes, differ markedly in appearance, content, and function.

conjugate acid-base p., in prototonic solvents (*e.g.*, H_2O, NH_3, acetic acid), two molecular species differing only in the presence or absence of a hydrogen ion (*e.g.*, carbonic acid/bicarbonate ion or ammonium ion/ammonia); the basis of buffer action.

line p.'s, a unit of resolution of radiographic screens and films or photographic films.

nucleoside p., nucleotide p., SYN base p.

p. production, creation of a positron and electron, each of mass 0.511 MeV, when an incident photon of energy greater than 1.02 MeV is absorbed by matter; occurs in high energy radiotherapy.

pa·ja·roe·llo (pah-har-wā′ō). SYN *Ornithodoros coriaceus.* [Am. Sp. *pajahuello,* fr. Sp. *paja,* straw, + *huello,* undersurface of hoof]

Pajot, Charles, French obstetrician, 1816–1896. SEE P.'s *maneuver.*

Palade, George E., Roumanian-U.S. cell biologist and Nobel laureate, *1912. SEE P. *granule;* Weibel-P. *bodies,* under *body.*

pal·a·tal (pal′ă-tăl). Relating to the palate or the palate bone. SYN palatine.

pal·ate (pal′ăt). The bony and muscular partition between the oral and nasal cavities. SYN palatum [NA], roof of mouth, uraniscus. [L. *palatum,* palate]

bony p., a concave elliptical bony plate, constituting the roof of the oral cavity, formed of the palatine process of the maxilla and the horizontal plate of the palatine bone on either side. SYN palatum osseum [NA].

Byzantine arch p., incomplete fusion of the palatal process with the nasal spine.

cleft p., a congenital fissure in the median line of the p., often associated with cleft lip. Often occurs as a feature of a syndrome or generalized condition, *e.g.,* diastrophic dwarfism or spondyloepiphyseal dysplasia congenita; its general genetic behavior resembles that of cleft *lip.* SYN palatoschisis, palatum fissum.

falling p., SYN uvuloptosis.

Gothic p., an abnormally highly arched p.

hard p., (1) the anterior part of the palate, consisting of the bony p. covered above by the mucous membrane of the floor of the nasal cavity and below by the mucoperiosteum of the roof of the mouth which contains the palatine vessels, nerves, and mucous glands; (2) in cephalometrics, a line connecting the anterior and posterior nasal spines to represent the position of the bony p. SYN palatum durum [NA].

pendulous p., SYN palatine *uvula.*

primary p., in the early embryo, the mesoderm-filled shelf, formed from the medial nasal process, that anteriorly separates the oral cavity below from the primitive nasal cavities above. SYN primitive p.

primitive p., SYN primary p.

secondary p., the posterior portion of the embryonic p., which forms from the palatal processes of the embryonic maxilla and develops into the hard p.

soft p., the posterior muscular portion of the palate, forming an incomplete septum between the mouth and the oropharynx, and between the oropharynx and the nasopharynx. SYN palatum molle [NA], velum palatinum★ [NA], velum pendulum palati.

pa·lat·i·form (pă-lat′i-fōrm). Palate-shaped; resembling the palate.

pa·lat·i·nase (pă-lat′i-nās). A maltase in the intestinal mucosa that hydrolyzes palatinose; probably oligo-1,6-glucosidase.

pal·a·tine (pal′ă-tīn). SYN palatal.

pa·lat·i·nose (pă-lat′i-nōs). A disaccharide consisting of D-glucose and D-fructose in α-1,6 linkage (sucrose is α-1,2).

pal·a·ti·tis (pal-ă-tī′tis). Inflammation of the palate. SYN uranisconitis.

△**palato-.** Palate. [L. *palatum,* palate]

pal·a·to·glos·sal (pal′ă-tō-glos′ăl). Relating to the palate and the tongue, or to the palatoglossus muscle.

pal·a·to·glos·sus (pal-ă-tō-glos′ŭs). SYN palatoglossus *muscle.*

pal·a·tog·na·thous (pal′ă-tog′nă-thŭs). Having a cleft palate. [palato- + G. *gnathos,* jaw]

pal·a·to·gram (pal′ă-tō-gram). A registration of tongue action against the palate made by placing soft wax or powder on a baseplate.

pal·a·to·graph (pal′ă-tō-graf). An instrument used in recording the movements of the soft palate in speaking and during respiration. SYN palate myograph, palatomyograph. [palato- + G. *graphō,* to record]

pal·a·to·max·il·lary (pal′ă-tō-mak′si-lār-ē). Relating to the palate and the maxilla.

pal·a·to·my·o·graph (pal′ă-tō-mī′ō-graf). SYN palatograph. [G. palato- + *mys,* muscle, + *graphō,* to record]

pal·a·to·na·sal (pal-ă-tō-nā′sal). Relating to the palate and the nasal cavity.

pal·a·to·pha·ryn·ge·al (pal′ă-tō-fa-rin′jē-ăl). Relating to palate and pharynx.

pal·a·to·pha·ryn·ge·us (pal′ă-tō-far-in-jē′ŭs). SYN palatopharyngeus *muscle.* [L.]

pa

pal·a·to·pha·ryn·go·plas·ty (pal'ă-tō-fa-rin'gō-plas-tē). Surgical resection of unnecessary palatal and oropharyngeal tissue in selected cases of snoring, with or without sleep apnea. SYN uvulopalatopharyngoplasty, uvulopalatoplasty. [palato- + pharynx, + plastos, formed]

> This technique has proven effective in approximately 50% of cases, when undertaken to cure sleep apnea. Pharmacological treatment of apnea generally fails to correct the problem, thus surgery has offered the best recourse in extreme cases. New mechanical devices which prevent the pharynx from collapsing also appear promising.

pal·a·to·pha·ryn·gor·rha·phy (pal'ă-tō-far'in-gōr'ă-fē). SYN staphylopharyngorrhaphy. [palato- + pharynx + G. rhaphē, suture]

pal·a·to·plas·ty (pal'ă-tō-plas-tē). Surgery of the palate to restore form and function. SYN staphyloplasty, uraniscoplasty, uranoplasty. [palato- + G. plassō, to form]

pal·a·to·ple·gia (pal'ă-tō-plē'jē-ă). Paralysis of the muscles of the soft palate. SYN staphyloplegia. [palato- + G. plēgē, stroke]

pal·a·tor·rha·phy (pal-ă-tōr'ă-fē). Suture of a cleft palate. SYN staphylorrhaphy, uraniscorrhaphy, uranorrhaphy, velosynthesis. [palato- + G. rhaphē, suture]

pa·la·to·sal·pin·ge·us (pal'ă-tō-sal-pin-jē'ŭs). SYN tensor veli palati muscle. [L.]

pal·a·tos·chi·sis (pal-ă-tos'ki-sis). SYN cleft palate. [palato- + G. schisis, fissure]

pa·la·tum, pl. **pa·la·ti** (pă-lā'tŭm) [NA]. SYN palate. [L.]

p. du'rum [NA], SYN hard palate.

p. fis'sum, SYN cleft palate.

p. mol'le [NA], SYN soft palate.

p. os'seum [NA], SYN bony palate.

pa·le·en·ceph·a·lon (pā'lē-en-sef'ă-lon). L. Edinger's term for the metameric nervous system. Excludes cerebral cortex. [paleo- + G. enkephalos, brain]

△**paleo-, pale-.** Old, primitive, primary, early. [G. palaios, old, ancient]

pa·le·o·cer·e·bel·lum (pā'lē-ō-ser'ĕ-bel'ŭm) [NA]. Phylogenetic term referring to the portion of the cerebellum including most of the vermis and the adjacent zones of the cerebellar hemispheres rostral to the primary fissure; p. is equated with the anterior lobe and corresponds to the zone of distribution of the spinocerebellar tracts and is sometimes called spinocerebellum; in phylogenetic age, it is thought to be intermediate between the archicerebellum and the neocerebellum. SYN spinocerebellum. [paleo- + L. cerebellum]

pa·le·o·cor·tex (pā'lē-ō-kōr'teks). The phylogenetically oldest part of the cortical mantle of the cerebral hemisphere, represented by the olfactory cortex.

pa·le·o·ki·net·ic (pā'lē-ō-ki-net'ik). Denoting the primitive motor mechanisms underlying muscular reflexes and automatic, stereotyped movements. [paleo- + G. kinētikos, relating to movement]

pa·le·o·pa·thol·o·gy (pā'lē-ō-pa-thol'ō-jē). The science of disease in prehistoric times as revealed in bones, mummies, and archaeologic artifacts. [paleo- + pathology]

pa·le·o·stri·a·tal (pā'lē-ō-strī-ā'tăl). Relating to the paleostriatum.

pa·le·o·stri·a·tum (pā'lē-ō-strī-ā'tŭm). Term denoting the globus pallidus and expressing the hypothesis that this component of the striate body developed earlier in evolution than the "neostriatum" or striatum (caudate nucleus and putamen) and that it is a diencephalic derivative. [paleo- + L. striatum]

pa·le·o·thal·a·mus (pā'lē-ō-thal'ă-mŭs). The intralaminar nuclei, believed to have been the earliest components of the thalamus to evolve; they lack reciprocal connections with the isocortex.

Palfyn (Palfin), Jean, Belgian surgeon and anatomist, 1650–1730. SEE P.'s sinus.

pal·i·ki·ne·sia, pal·i·ci·ne·sia (pal-i-ki-nē'zē-ă, -si-nē'zē-ă). Involuntary repetition of movements. [G. palin, again, + kinēsis, movement]

pal·i·la·lia (pal-i-lā'lē-ă). SYN paliphrasia. [G. palin, again, + lalia, a form of speech]

pal·i·nal (pal'i-năl). Moving backward. [G. palin, backward]

pal·in·drome (pal'in-drōm). In molecular biology, a self-complementary nucleic acid sequence; a sequence identical to its complementary strand, if both are "read" in the same 5'- to 3' direction, or inverted repeating sequences running in opposite directions (but same 5'- to 3'- direction) on either side of an axis of symmetry; p.'s occur at sites of important reactions (e.g., binding sites, sites cleaved by restriction enzymes); imperfect p.'s exist as do interrupted p.'s which allow the formation of loops. [G. palindromos, a running back]

pal·in·dro·mia (pal-in-drō'mē-ă). A relapse or recurrence of a disease. [G. palindromos, a running back, + -ia, condition]

pal·in·drom·ic (pal-in-drom'ik). Recurring.

pal·i·nop·sia (pal-i-nop'sē-ă). Abnormal recurring visual hallucinations. [G. palin, again, + opsis, vision]

pal·i·phra·sia (pal-i-frā'zē-ă). In speech, involuntary repetition of words or sentences. SEE ALSO echolalia. SYN palilalia. [G. palin, again, + phrasis, speech]

pal·i·sade (pal'i-sād). In pathology, a row of elongated nuclei parallel to each other. [Fr. palissade, fr. L. palus, a pale, stake]

pal·la·di·um (Pd) (pă-lā'dē-ŭm). A metallic element resembling platinum, atomic no. 46, atomic wt. 106.42. [fr. the asteroid, Pallas; G. Pallas, goddess of wisdom]

pall·an·es·the·sia (pal'an-es-thē'zē-ă). Absence of pallesthesia. SYN apallesthesia. [G. pallō, to quiver, + anaisthēsia, insensibility]

pal·les·cense (pal-es'ens). SYN pallor. [L. pallesco, to become pale, fr. palleo, to be pale]

pall·es·the·sia (pal'es-thē'zē-ă). The appreciation of vibration, a form of pressure sense; most acute when a vibrating tuning fork is applied over a bony prominence. SYN bone sensibility, pallesthetic sensibility, vibratory sensibility. [G. pallō, to quiver, + aisthēsis, sensation]

pall·es·thet·ic (pal-es-thet'ik). Pertaining to pallesthesia.

pal·li·al (pal'ē-ăl). Relating to the pallium.

pal·li·ate (pal'ē-āt). To reduce the severity of; to relieve slightly. SYN mitigate. [L. palliatus (adj.), dressed in a pallium, cloaked]

pal·li·a·tive (pal-ē-ă-tiv). Reducing the severity of; denoting the alleviation of symptoms without curing the underlying disease.

pal·li·dal (pal'i-dăl). Relating to the pallidum.

pal·li·dec·to·my (pal'i-dek'tō-mē). Excision or destruction of the globus pallidus, usually by stereotaxy; a prefix may indicate the method used, e.g., chemopallidectomy (destruction by a chemical agent), cryopallidectomy (destruction by cold). [pallidum + G. ektomē, excision]

pal·li·do·a·myg·da·lot·o·my (pal'i-dō-ă-mig'dă-lot'ō-mē). Production of lesions in the globus pallidus and amygdaloid nuclei. [pallidum + amygdala (1) + G. tomē, a cutting]

pal·li·do·an·sot·o·my (pal'i-dō-an-sot'ō-mē). Production of lesions in the globus pallidus and ansa lenticularis.

pal·li·dot·o·my (pal-i-dot'ō-mē). A destructive operation on the globus pallidus, done to relieve involuntary movements or muscular rigidity. [pallidum + G. tomē, incision]

pal·li·dum (pal'i-dŭm). SYN globus pallidus. [L. pallidus, pale]

pal·li·um (pal'ē-ŭm) [NA]. The cerebral cortex with the subjacent white substance. SYN brain mantle, mantle (2). [L. cloak]

pal·lor (pal'ŏr). Paleness, as of the skin. SYN pallescense. [L.]

cachectic p., SYN achromasia (1).

palm (pahm, pawlm). The flat of the hand; the flexor or anterior surface of the hand, exclusive of the thumb and fingers; the opposite of the dorsum. SYN palma [NA]. [L. palma]

liver p., exaggerated erythema of the thenar and hypothenar eminences.

pal·ma, pl. **pal·mae** (pawl'mă, pawl'mē) [NA]. SYN palm, palm. [L.]

p. ma'nus [NA], palm of the hand. SEE palm.

pal·mar (pawl'măr). Referring to the palm of the hand; volar. SYN palmaris [NA]. [L. *palmaris,* fr. *palma*]

pal·mar·is (pawl-măr'is) [NA]. SYN palmar, palmar. [L.]

pal·mel·lin (pal'mel-in). A red coloring matter formed by an alga, *Palmella cruenta.*

Palmer, Walter L., U.S. physician, *1896. SEE P. acid *test* for peptic ulcer.

palm·ic (pal'mik). Beating; throbbing; relating to a palmus.

pal·mi·tal·de·hyde (pal-mi-tal'dĕ-hīd). $CH_3(CH_2)_{14}CHO$; Hexadecanal(dehyde); the 16-carbon aldehyde analog of palmitic acid; a constituent of plasmalogens.

pal·mi·tate (pal'mi-tāt). A salt of palmitic acid.

pal·mit·ic ac·id (pal-mit'ik). $CH_3-(CH_2)_{14}-$ COOH; a common saturated fatty acid occurring in palm oil and olive oil as well as many other fats and waxes. SYN hexadecanoic acid.

pal·mi·tin (pal'mi-tin). The triglyceride of palmitic acid occurring in palm oil. SYN tripalmitin.

pal·mit·o·le·ic ac·id (pal'mi-tō-lē'ik). 9-Hexadecenoic acid; a monounsaturated 16-carbon acid; one of the common constituents of the triacylglycerols of human adipose tissue. SYN zoomaric acid.

pal·mi·tyl al·co·hol (pal'mi-til). SYN *cetyl* alcohol.

pal·mod·ic (pal-mod'ik). Relating to palmus (1).

pal·mos·co·py (pal-mos'kŏ-pē). Examination of the cardiac pulsation. [G. *palmos,* pulsation, + *skopeō,* to examine]

pal·mus, pl. **pal·mi** (pal'mŭs, -mī). **1.** SYN facial *tic.* **2.** Rhythmical fibrillary contractions in a muscle. SEE ALSO jumping *disease.* **3.** The heart beat. [G. *palmos,* pulsation, quivering]

pal·pa·ble (pal'pă-bl). **1.** Perceptible to touch; capable of being palpated. **2.** Evident; plain. [see palpation]

pal·pate (pal'pāt). To examine by feeling and pressing with the palms of the hands and the fingers.

pal·pa·tion (pal-pā'shŭn). **1.** Examination with the hands, feeling for organs, masses, or infiltration of a part of the body, feeling the heart or pulse beat, vibrations in the chest, etc. **2.** Touching, feeling, or perceiving by the sense of touch. [L. *palpatio,* fr. *palpo,* pp. -*atus,* to touch, stroke]

    bimanual p., use of both hands to feel organs or masses, especially in the abdomen or pelvis.

    light-touch p., a method of determining the outlines of organs or masses by lightly palpating the surface with the tip of a finger.

pal·pa·to·per·cus·sion (pal'pă-tō-per-kŭsh'ŭn). Examination by means of combined palpation and percussion.

pal·pe·bra, pl. **pal·pe·brae** (pal-pē'bră, pē'brē) [NA]. SYN eyelid. [L.]

    p. III, SYN *plica* semilunaris conjunctivae (2).

    p. infe'rior [NA], SYN lower *eyelid.*

    p. supe'rior [NA], SYN upper *eyelid.*

    p. ter'tia, SYN *plica* semilunaris conjunctivae (2).

pal·pe·bral (pal'pē-brăl). Relating to an eyelid or the eyelids.

pal·pe·bra·lis (pal'pē-brā'lis). SYN levator palpebrae superioris *muscle.* [L.]

pal·pe·brate (pal'pē-brāt). **1.** Having eyelids. **2.** To wink. [L. *palpebra,* eyelid]

pal·pe·bra·tion (pal-pē-brā'shŭn). Winking. [L. *palpebratio*]

pal·pi·ta·tio cor·dis (pal-pi-tā'shē-ō kōr'dis). Palpitation of the heart.

pal·pi·ta·tion (pal-pi-tā'shŭn). Forcible or irregular pulsation of the heart, perceptible to the patient, usually with an increase in frequency or force, with or without irregularity in rhythm. SYN trepidatio cordis. [L. *palpito,* to throb]

pal·sy (pawl'zē). Paralysis or paresis. [a corruption of O. Fr. fr. L. and G. *paralysis*]

    Bell's p., paresis or paralysis, usually unilateral, of the facial muscles, caused by dysfunction of the 7th cranial nerve; probably due to a viral infection; usually demyelinating in type. SYN peripheral facial paralysis.

    birth p., indefinite term for any motor abnormality in the infant caused by or attributed to the birthing process; includes obstetrical paralysis, infantile hemiplegia, etc. SYN infantile hemiplegia.

    brachial birth p., paralysis of the infant's arm due to injury received at birth usually resulting from a shoulder dystocia; three types are recognized: 1) whole arm; 2) upper arm (Erb's p.); 3) forearm (Klumpke's paralysis).

    bulbar p., SYN progressive bulbar *paralysis.*

    cerebral p., defect of motor power and coordination related to damage of the brain.

    craft p., SYN occupational *neurosis.*

    creeping p., SYN amyotrophic lateral *sclerosis.*

    crutch p., SYN crutch *paralysis.*

    Dejerine-Klumpke p., SYN Klumpke p.

    diver's p., SYN decompression *sickness.*

    Erb p., a type of brachial birth p. in which there is paralysis of the muscles of the upper arm and shoulder girdle (deltoid, biceps, brachialis, and brachioradialis muscles) due to a lesion of the upper trunk of the brachial plexus or of the roots of the fifth and sixth cervical roots. SYN Duchenne-Erb paralysis, Erb paralysis.

    extrapyramidal cerebral p., SYN athetosis.

    facial p., SYN facial *paralysis.*

    Klumpke p., a type of brachial birth p. in which there is paralysis of the muscles of the distal forearm and hand (all ulnar innervated muscles, plus more distal radial and median-innervated muscles), due to a lesion of the lower trunk of the brachial plexus, or of the C8 and T1 cervical roots. SYN Dejerine-Klumpke p., Dejerine-Klumpke syndrome, Klumpke's paralysis.

    lead p., paralysis of the extensor muscles of the wrist causing wrist-drop; occurs in lead poisoning. SYN lead paralysis.

    obstetrical p., a brachial plexus lesion sustained by the infant during the birthing process; three types are recognized: 1) upper plexus type, affects the shoulder and upper arm (Erb p.); 2) total plexus type, involves the whole arm; 3) lower plexus type, involves the forearm and hand (Klumpke p.). SYN obstetrical paralysis.

    posticus p., paralysis of the cricoarytenoideus posticus muscle, resulting in the vocal cord being held in or near the midline.

    pressure p., SYN pressure *paralysis.*

    progressive bulbar p., one of the subgroups of motor neuron disease; a progressive degenerative disorder of the motor neurons of primarily the brainstem, manifested as weakness (and wasting) of the various bulbar muscles, resulting in dysarthria and dysphagia—fluid regurgitation is an outstanding symptom and can cause aspiration; tongue weakness and wasting is usually evident, and often the fasciculation potentials are present in the tongue and facial muscles. SYN glossopalatolabial paralysis, glossopharyngeolabial paralysis.

    progressive supranuclear p., a progressive neurologic disorder in the sixth decade characterized by a supranuclear paralysis of vertical gaze, retraction of eyelids, exophoria under cover, dysarthria, and dementia. SYN Steele-Richardson-Olszewski disease, Steele-Richardson-Olszewski syndrome.

    scrivener's p., SYN writer's *cramp.*

    shaking p., trembling p., SYN parkinsonism (1).

    wasting p., SYN amyotrophic lateral *sclerosis.*

pal·u·dal (pal'ū-dăl). Obsolete term for malarial. [L. *palus,* marsh]

2-PAM Abbreviation for 2-pralidoxime.

pam·a·brom (pam'ă-brom). 8-Bromotheophylline compound with 2-amino-2-methyl-1-propanol; an obsolete diuretic.

pam·a·quine (pam'ă-kwēn). An antimalarial agent, active against avian malaria and against the gametocytes of all malarial forms in humans; it is more toxic than chloroquine or primaquine and has been replaced by primaquine.

pam·o·ate (pam'ō-āt). USAN-approved contraction for 4,4'-methylenebis(3-hydroxy-2-naphthoate).

pam·pin·i·form (pam-pin'i-fōrm). Having the shape of a tendril; denoting a vinelike structure. [L. *pampinus,* a tendril, + *forma,* form]

pam·pin·o·cele (pam-pin'ō-sēl). SYN varicocele. [L. *pampinus,* tendril, + G. *kēlē,* tumor]

Pan. Genus of anthropoid apes including the gorilla and chimpanzee. *P. panisus* and *P. troglodytes* are chimpanzee species used in biologic experiments. [G. myth. god of forest]

Pa

⌂**pan-.** All, entire (properly affixed to words derived from G. roots). SEE ALSO pant-. [G. *pas,* all]

pan·a·cea (pan-ă-sē'ă). A cure-all; a remedy claimed to be curative of all diseases. [G. *panakeia,* universal remedy, fr. Panacea, Aesculapius' daughter]

pan·ag·glu·ti·na·ble (pan-ă-glū'ti-nă-bl). Agglutinable with all types of human serum; denoting erythrocytes having this property.

pan·ag·glu·ti·nins (pan-ă-glū'ti-ninz). Agglutinins that react with all human erythrocytes. [pan + L. *agglutino,* to glue]

pan·an·gi·i·tis (pan'an-jē-ī'tis). Inflammation involving all the coats of a blood vessel. [pan- + angiitis]

pan·ar·ter·i·tis (pan'ar-ter-ī'tis). An inflammatory disorder of the arteries characterized by involvement of all structural layers of the vessels. SYN endoperiarteritis. [pan- + L. *arteria,* artery, + G. *-itis,* inflammation]

pan·ar·thri·tis (pan-ar-thrī'tis). **1.** Inflammation involving all the tissues of a joint. **2.** Inflammation of all the joints of the body.

pan·at·ro·phy (pan-at'rō-fē). **1.** Atrophy of all the parts of a structure. **2.** General atrophy of the body. SYN pantatrophia, pantatrophy.

pan·blas·tic (pan-blas'tik). Relating to all the primary germ layers. [pan- + G. *blastos,* germ]

pan·bron·chi·ol·i·tis (pan'bron-kē-ō-lī'tis). Idiopathic inflammation and obstruction of bronchioles, eventually accompanied by bronchiectasis; cases reported almost entirely from Japan. SYN diffuse panbronchiolitis.

diffuse panbronchiolitis, SYN panbronchiolitis.

pan·car·di·tis (pan-kar-dī'tis). Inflammation of all the structures of the heart.

Pancoast, Henry K., U.S. roentgenologist, 1875–1939. SEE P. *syndrome, tumor.*

Pancoast, Joseph, U.S. surgeon, 1805–1882. SEE P.'s *suture.*

pan·co·lec·to·my (pan'kō-lek'tō-mē). Extirpation of the entire colon.

pan·cre·as, pl. **pan·cre·a·ta** (pan'krē-as, pan-krē-ā'tă) [NA]. An elongated lobulated retroperitoneal gland, devoid of capsule, extending from the concavity of the duodenum to the spleen; it consists of a flattened head (caput) within the duodenal concavity, an elongated three-sided body extending transversely across the abdomen, and a tail in contact with the spleen. The gland secretes from its exocrine part pancreatic juice that is discharged into the intestine and from the its endocrine part the internal secretions, insulin and glucagon. [G. *pankreas,* the sweetbread, fr. *pas (pan),* all, + *kreas,* flesh]

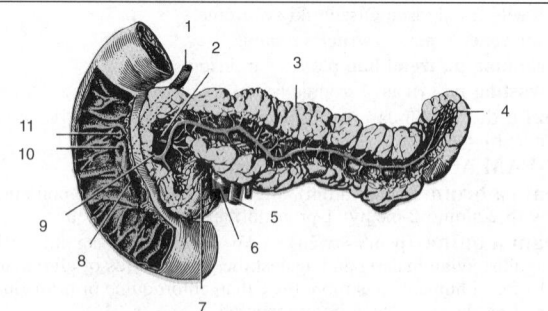

pancreas (and part of duodenum)

1) ductus choledochus 2) ductus pancreaticus accessorius; 3) and 4) body and tail of pancreas; 5) and 6) arteria and vena mesenterica superiores; 7) uncinate process; 8) fold of duodenum; 9) ductus pancreaticus; 10) and 11) papillae duodeni major and minor

p. accesso'rium [NA], SYN accessory p.

accessory p., a detached portion of pancreatic tissue, usually the uncinate process, and hence most often found in the vicinity of the head of the pancreas, but may occur within the gut wall (stomach or duodenum). SYN p. accessorium [NA].

annular p., a ring of p. encircling the duodenum, caused by a failure of the embryologic ventral pancreas to migrate to the right of the duodenum.

Aselli's p., SYN Aselli's *gland.*

p. divi'sum, a bifid, or divided, p. resulting from a congenital failure of the embryonic primordia to unite completely; each of the portions has its own duct.

dorsal p., that portion of the pancreatic primordium of the embryo that arises as a dorsal bud from the foregut endoderm above the hepatic diverticulum.

lesser p., SYN uncinate *process* of pancreas.

p. mi'nus, SYN uncinate *process* of pancreas.

small p., SYN uncinate *process* of pancreas.

uncinate p., unciform p., SYN uncinate *process* of pancreas.

ventral p., that portion of the primordium of the pancreas that develops, together with the hepatic diverticulum, as a ventral bud from the foregut endoderm.

Willis' p., SYN uncinate *process* of pancreas.

Winslow's p., SYN uncinate *process* of pancreas.

⌂**pancreat-, pancreatico-, pancreato-, pancreo-.** The pancreas. [G. *pankreas,* pancreas]

pan·cre·a·tal·gia (pan'krē-ă-tal'jē-ă). Pain arising from the pancreas or felt in or near the region of the pancreas. [pancreat- + G. *algos,* pain]

pan·cre·a·tec·to·my (pan'krē-ă-tek'tō-mē). Excision of the pancreas. SYN pancreectomy. [pancreat- + G. *ektomē,* excision]

pan·cre·at·em·phrax·is (pan'krē-at-em-frak'sis). Obstruction in the pancreatic duct, causing swelling of the gland. [pancreat- + G. *emphraxis,* a stoppage]

pan·cre·at·ic (pan-krē-at'ik). Relating to the pancreas.

⌂**pancreatico-.** SEE pancreat-.

pan·cre·at·i·co·du·o·de·nal (pan-krē-at'i-kō-dū'ō-dē'năl, -dū-od'ĕ-năl). Relating to the pancreas and the duodenum.

pan·cre·a·tin (pan'krē-ă-tin). A mixture of the enzymes from the pancreas of the ox or hog, used internally as a digestive, and also as a peptonizing agent in preparing predigested foods; it contains the proteolytic trypsin, the amylolytic amylopsin, and the lipolytic steapsin.

pan·cre·a·ti·tis (pan'krē-ă-tī'tis). Inflammation of the pancreas.

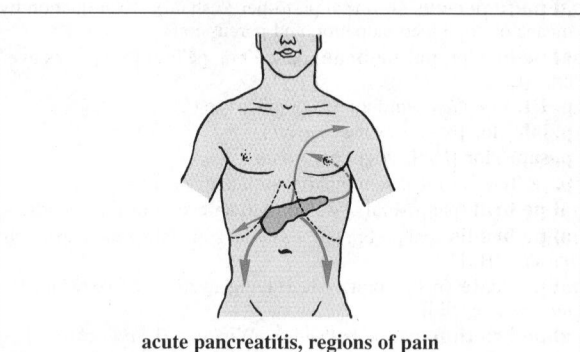

acute pancreatitis, regions of pain

acute hemorrhagic p., an acute inflammation of the pancreas accompanied by the formation of necrotic areas and hemorrhages into the substance of the gland; clinically marked by sudden severe abdominal pain, nausea, fever, and leukocytosis; areas of fat necrosis are present on the surface of the pancreas and in the omentum due to the action of the escaped pancreatic enzyme (trypsin and lipase).

calcareous p., chronic p. with appearance of areas of calcification, seen by x-ray. SYN calcific p.

calcific p. (kal'sif-ik), SYN calcareous p.

chronic p., inflammatory disease of the pancreas characterized by fibrosis and irreversible loss of exocrine function.

chronic fibrosing p., inflammation of the pancreas consisting of fibrosis, acinar atrophy, and calcification. Clinically, it follows a protracted course with relapses and remissions, and is usually due to alcohol abuse or malnutrition.

chronic relapsing p., repeated exacerbations of p. in patient with chronic inflammation of that organ. Relapses are usually due to persistence of etiologic factor or repeated exposure to it, such as occurs with partial ductal obstruction or chronic alcoholism.

△pancreato-. SEE pancreat-.

pan·cre·at·o·cho·le·cys·tos·to·my (pan-krē-at′ō-kō-lē-sis-tos′ tō-mē, pan′krē-ă-tō-). A rarely performed surgical anastomosis between a pancreatic cyst or fistula and the gallbladder.

pan·cre·at·o·du·o·de·nec·to·my (pan-krē-at′ō-dū-ō-dē-nek′tō-mē, pan′krē-ă-tō-). Excision of all or part of the pancreas together with the duodenum. SYN Whipple's operation.

pan·cre·at·o·du·o·de·nos·to·my (pan-krē-at′ō-dū-ō-dē-nos′tō-mē, pan′krē-ă-tō-). Surgical anastomosis of a pancreatic duct, cyst, or fistula to the duodenum.

pan·cre·at·o·gas·tros·to·my (pan-krē-at′ō-gas-tros′tō-mē, pan′ krē-ă-tō-). Surgical anastomosis of a pancreatic cyst or fistula to the stomach.

pan·cre·a·to·gen·ic, pan·cre·a·tog·en·ous (pan′krē-ă-tō-jen′ ik, -toj′ĕ-nŭs). Of pancreatic origin; formed in the pancreas. [pancreato- + G. *genesis,* origin]

pan·cre·a·tog·ra·phy (pan′krē-ă-tog′ră-fē). Radiographic demonstration of the pancreatic ducts, after retrograde injection of radiopaque material into the distal duct. [pancreato- + G. *graphō,* to write]

pan·cre·a·to·je·ju·nos·to·my (pan-krē-at′ō-je-jū-nos′tō-mē, pa-n′krē-ă-tō-). Surgical anastomosis of a pancreatic duct, cyst, or fistula to the jejunum.

pan·cre·at·o·lith (pan-krē-at′ō-lith). SYN pancreatic *calculus.* [pancreato- + G. *lithos,* stone]

pan·cre·at·o·li·thec·to·my (pan-krē-at′ō-li-thek′tō-mē, pan′krē-ă-tō-). SYN pancreatolithotomy. [pancreato- + G. *lithos,* stone, + *ektomē,* excision]

pan·cre·at·o·li·thi·a·sis (pan-krē-at′ō-li-thī′ă-sis, pan′krē-ă-tō-). Stones in the pancreas, usually found in the pancreatic duct system.

pan·cre·at·o·li·thot·o·my (pan-krē-at′ō-li-thot′ō-mē, pan′krē-ă-tō-). Removal of a pancreatic concretion. SYN pancreatolithectomy. [pancreato- + G. *lithos,* stone, + *tomē,* incision]

pan·cre·a·tol·y·sis (pan′krē-ă-tol′i-sis). Destruction of the pancreas. [pancreato- + G. *lysis,* dissolution]

pan·cre·a·to·lyt·ic (pan′krē-ă-tō-lit′ik). Denoting pancreatolysis.

pan·cre·a·to·meg·a·ly (pan′krē-ă-tō-meg′ă-lē). Abnormal enlargement of the pancreas. [pancreato- + G. *megas,* great]

pan·cre·at·o·my (pan′krē-at′ō-mē). SYN pancreatotomy.

pan·cre·a·top·a·thy (pan′krē-ă-top′ă-thē). Any disease of the pancreas. SYN pancreopathy. [pancreato- + G. *pathos,* suffering]

pan·cre·a·to·pep·ti·dase E (pan′krē-ă-tō-pep′ti-dās). SEE elastase.

pan·cre·a·tot·o·my (pan′krē-ă-tot′ō-mē). Incision of the pancreas. SYN pancreatomy. [pancreato- + G. *tomē,* incision]

pan·cre·a·tro·pic (pan′krē-ă-trop′ik). Exerting an action on the pancreas. [pancreat- + G. *tropikos,* relating to a turning]

pan·cre·ec·to·my (pan-krē-ek′tō-mē). SYN pancreatectomy.

pan·cre·li·pase (pan-krē-lip′ās, -lī′pās). A concentrate of pancreatic enzymes standardized for lipase content; a lipolytic used for substitution therapy. SYN lipancreatin.

△pancreo-. SEE pancreat-.

pan·cre·o·lith (pan′krē-ō-lith). SYN pancreatic *calculus.* [pancreo- + G. *lithos,* stone]

pan·cre·op·a·thy (pan-krē-op′ă-thē). SYN pancreatopathy.

pan·cre·o·priv·ic (pan′krē-ō-priv′ik). Without a pancreas (obsolete term). [pancreo- + L. *privus,* deprived of]

pan·cre·o·zy·min (pan′krē-ō-zī′min). SYN cholecystokinin.

pan·cu·ro·ni·um bro·mide (pan-kyūr-ō′nē-ŭm). 2β,16β-Dipiperidino-5α-androstane-3α,17β-diol diacetate dimethobromide; a nondepolarizing steroidal neuromuscular blocking agent

acute pancreatitis: frequency of etiological factors

I. principal causes

1. cholecystolithiasis, choledocholithiasis
2. alcoholism
3. abdominal surgery — postoperative pancreatitis
4. endoscopy of biliary and pancreatic ducts
5. blunt abdominal injury

II. less-frequent causes

1. endocrine diseases (polyadenomatosis, hyperparathyroidism, Cushing's syndrome)
2. pregnancy, hyperlipoproteinemia, pancreatitis due to ingestion of birth-control pills
3. drug effects (corticosteroids, diuretics)
4. immunological-allergic causes
5. neurogenic pancreatitis
6. hereditary pancreatitis
7. viral pancreatitis
8. parasitic pancreatitis

III. pancreatitis due to shock and acidosis

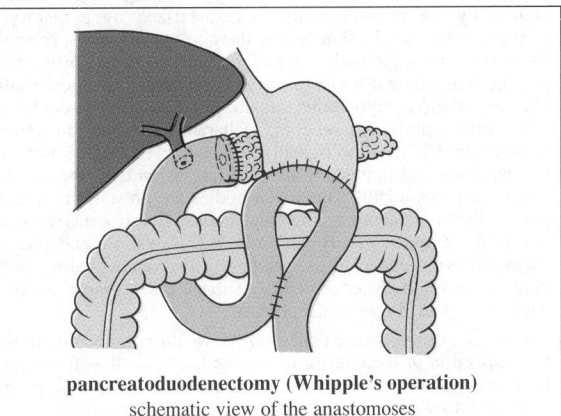

pancreatoduodenectomy (Whipple's operation)
schematic view of the anastomoses

resembling curare but without its potential for ganglionic blockade, histamine release, or hypotension.

pan·cy·to·pe·nia (pan′sī-tō-pē′nē-ă). Pronounced reduction in the number of erythrocytes, all types of white blood cells, and the blood platelets in the circulating blood. [pan- + G. *kytos,* cell, + *penia,* poverty]

congenital p., SYN Fanconi's *anemia.* SYN Fanconi's p.

Fanconi's p., SYN congenital p.

tropical canine p., SYN canine *ehrlichiosis.*

pan·dem·ic (pan-dem′ik). Denoting a disease affecting or attacking the population of an extensive region, country, continent; extensively epidemic. [pan- + G. *dēmos,* the people]

pan·de·mic·i·ty (pan-dĕ-mis′i-tē). The state or condition of being pandemic.

pan·dic·u·la·tion (pan-dik-yū-lā′shŭn). The act of stretching, as when awaking. [L. *pandiculor,* to stretch oneself, fr. *pando,* to spread out]

Pandy, Kalman, Hungarian neurologist, *1868. SEE P.'s *test, reaction.*

Pa

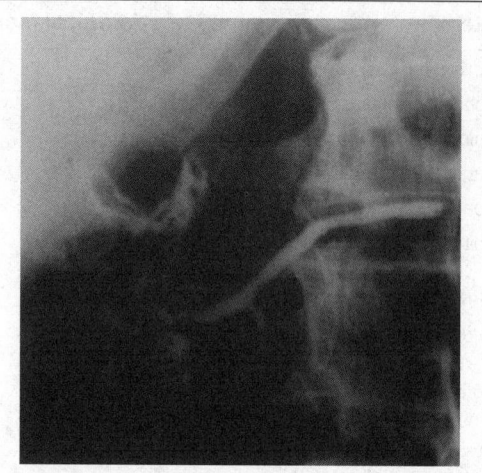

endoscopic retrograde cholangio-pancreatography (ERCP)
a neoplasm on body of the pancreas with secondary
pseudocyst ruptured duct also visible

pan·en·ceph·a·li·tis (pan'en-sef-ă-lī'tis). A diffuse inflammation of the brain.

nodular p., probably a form of subacute sclerosing p. SYN Pette-Döring disease.

subacute sclerosing p. (SSPE), a rare chronic, progressive encephalitis that affects primarily children and young adults, caused by the measles virus. Characterized by a history of primary measles infection before the age of two years, followed by several asymptomatic years, and then gradual, progressive psychoneurological deterioration, consisting of personality change, seizures, myoclonus, ataxia, photosensitivity, ocular abnormalities, spasticity, and coma. Characteristic periodic activity is seen on EEG; pathologically, the white matter of both the hemispheres and brainstem are affected, as well as the cerebral cortex, and eosinophilic inclusion bodies are present in the cytoplasm nuclei of neurons and glial cells. Death usually occurs within three years. SYN Bosin's disease, Dawson's encephalitis, inclusion body encephalitis, sclerosing leukoencephalitis, subacute inclusion body encephalitis, subacute sclerosing leukoencephalitis, Van Bogaert encephalitis.

pan·en·do·scope (pan-en'dō-skōp). An illuminated instrument for inspection of the interior of the urethra as well as the bladder by means of a foroblique lens system. [pan- + G. *endon,* within, + *skopeō,* to view]

pan·es·the·sia (pan-es-thē'zē-ă). The sum of all the sensations experienced by a person at one time. SEE ALSO cenesthesia. [pan- + G. *aisthēsis,* sensation]

Paneth, Josef, Austrian physician, 1857–1890. SEE P.'s granular *cells,* under *cell.*

pang. A sudden sharp, brief pain.

breast p., SYN *angina* pectoris.

pan·glos·sia (pan-glos'ē-ă). Abnormal or pathologic garrulousness. SEE logorrhea. [pan- + G. *glōssa,* tongue]

pan·hi·dro·sis (pan-hi-drō'sis). SYN panidrosis.

pan·hy·drom·e·ter (pan-hī-drom'ĕ-ter). A hydrometer for determining the specific gravity of any liquid. [pan- + G. *hydōr,* water, + *metron,* measure]

pan·hy·per·e·mia (pan'hī-per-ē'mē-ă). Universal congestion or hyperemia. [pan- + G. *hyper,* over, + *haima,* blood]

pan·hy·po·pi·tu·i·tar·ism (pan-hī'pō-pi-tū'i-tă-rizm). A state in which the secretion of all anterior pituitary hormones is inadequate or absent; caused by a variety of disorders that result in destruction or loss of function of all or most of the anterior pituitary gland. Rare forms of PHP are inherited as autosomal recessive [MIM*262600] or as an X-linked recessive

[MIM*312000]. SYN ateliotic dwarfism, hypophyseal cachexia, hypophysial cachexia.

pan·ic (pan'ik). Extreme and unreasoning anxiety and fear, often accompanied by disturbed breathing, increased heart activity, vasomotor changes, sweating, and a feeling of dread. SEE anxiety. [fr. G. myth. char., *Pan*]

homosexual p., an acute, severe attack of anxiety based on unconscious conflicts regarding homosexuality.

pan·i·dro·sis (pan-i-drō'sis). Sweating of the entire surface of the body. SYN panhidrosis. [pan- + G. *hidros,* sweat]

pan·im·mu·ni·ty (pan-i-myū'ni-tē). A general immunity to all infectious diseases.

pan·leu·ko·pe·nia (pan'lū-kō-pē'nē-ă). A highly contagious and fatal disease of cats, particularly young cats, caused by feline panleukopenia virus, a member of the family Parvoviridae, and manifested by severe leukopenia, prostration, fever, vomiting and diarrhea. SYN distemper (2), feline agranulocytosis, feline distemper, feline infectious enteritis.

pan·mix·is (pan-mik'sis). SYN random *mating.* [pan- + G. *mixis,* intercourse]

pan·my·e·loph·thi·sis (pan'mī-ĕ-lof'thi-sis). SYN myelophthisis (2).

pan·my·e·lo·sis (pan'mī-ĕ-lō'sis). Myeloid metaplasia with abnormal immature blood cells in the spleen and liver, associated with myelofibrosis. [pan- + G. *myelos,* marrow, + *-osis,* condition]

Panner, H.J., Danish radiologist, 1871–1930. SEE P.'s *disease.*

pan·neu·ri·tis (pan-nū-rī'tis). Rarely used term meaning extreme polyneuritis.

p. endem'ica, SYN beriberi.

pan·ni (pan'ī). Plural of pannus.

pan·nic·u·lec·to·my (pa-nik-yū-lek'tō-mē). Surgical excision of redundant paniculus adiposus, usually of the abdomen. [panniculus + G. *ektomē,* a cutting out]

pan·nic·u·li·tis (pă-nik'yū-lī'tis). Inflammation of subcutaneous adipose tissue. [panniculus + G. *-itis,* inflammation]

α-1 antitrypsin deficiency p., multiple painful subcutaneous nodules occurring in patients with severe antitrypsin deficiency; biopsies show lobular p. with neutrophils and foamy histiocytes. Some patients formerly diagnosed with Weber-Christian disease show this deficiency.

cytophagic histiocytic p., chronic lobular p. with infiltration by histiocytes that have phagocytized red blood cells, leukocytes, and platelets; a hemorrhagic diathesis or T cell lymphoma may result.

lupus erythematosus p., p. characterized by erythematous or flesh-colored nodules associated with lupus erythematosus, especially of the discoid variety, on the face, upper extremities, and trunk, and with nodular infiltration of lymphocytes and plasma cells in the fat lobules.

nodular nonsuppurative p., SYN relapsing febrile nodular nonsuppurative p.

poststeroid p., subcutaneous nodules developing in children within a month after withdrawal of corticosteroids given to treat the nephrotic syndrome or rheumatic fever; microscopically identical to subcutaneous fat necrosis of the newborn, the condition resolves spontaneously or with steroid readministration.

relapsing febrile nodular nonsuppurative p., nodular fat necrosis of a variety of possible causes. SYN Christian's disease (2), nodular nonsuppurative p., Weber-Christian disease.

subacute migratory p., non-scarring plaques of changing configuration on the lateral aspect of one or both legs, of many months duration. SYN erythema nodosum migrans.

pan·nic·u·lus, pl. **pan·nic·u·li** (pă-nik'yū-lŭs, -lī) [NA]. A sheet or layer of tissue. [L. dim. of *pannus,* cloth]

p. adipo'sus [NA], the superficial fascia which contains an abundance of fat deposit in its areolar substance.

p. carno'sus, the skeletal muscle layer in the superficial fascia represented in humans by the platysma muscle; it is much more extensive in lower mammals.

pan·nus, pl. **pan·ni** (pan'ŭs, pan'ī). A membrane of granulation tissue covering a normal surface: **1.** The articular cartilages in rheumatoid arthritis and in chronic granulomatous diseases such as tuberculosis; **2.** The cornea in trachoma. SEE ALSO corneal p. [L. cloth]

corneal p., fibrovascular connective tissue that proliferates in the anterior layers of the peripheral cornea in inflammatory corneal disease, particularly trachoma in which the p. involves the superior cornea. Three forms occur: **p. crassus** (thick), in which there are many blood vessels and the opacity is very dense; **p. siccus** (dry), p. with dry, glossy surface; **p. tenuis** (thin), in which there are few blood vessels and the opacity is slight.

phlyctenular p., p. occurring in phlyctenular conjunctivitis.

trachomatous p., p. of the superior cornea associated with trachoma.

pan·od·ic (pan-od′ik). Denoting a wide and extreme diffusion of a nerve impulse. SYN panthodic, pollodic. [pan- + G. *hodos*, way]

pan·oph·thal·mitis (pan′of-thal′mē-ă). Purulent inflammation of all layers of the eye. [pan- + G. *ophthalmos*, eye]

pan·op·tic (pan-op′tik). All-revealing, denoting the effect of multiple or differential staining. [pan- + G. *optikos*, relating to vision]

pan·o·ste·i·tis. Inflammation of an entire bone.

canine p., a disease of dogs characterized by intermittent shifting lameness and spontaneous remission.

pan·o·ti·tis (pan′ō-tī′tis). General inflammation of all parts of the ear; specifically, a disease which begins as an otitis interna, the inflammation subsequently extending to the middle ear and neighboring structures. [pan- + G. *ous*, ear, + *-itis*, inflammation]

pan·pho·bia (pan-fō′bē-ă). Fear of everything. [pan- + G. *phobos*, fear]

pan·ple·gia (pan-plē′jē-ă). Paralysis of the four extremities. [pan- + G. *plēgē*, stroke]

Pansch, Adolf, German anatomist, 1841–1887. SEE P.'s *fissure*.

pan·scle·ro·sis (pan-skle-rō′sis). Universal sclerosis of an organ or part.

pan·sin·u·i·tis (pan-sin-yū-ī′tis). SYN pansinusitis.

pan·si·nu·si·tis (pan-sī-nŭ-sī′tis). Inflammation of all the accessory sinuses of the nose on one or both sides. SYN pansinuitis.

pan·sper·mia, pan·sper·ma·tism (pan-sper′mē-ă, -sper′mă-tizm). The hypothetical doctrine of the omnipresence of minute forms and spores of animal and vegetable life, thus accounting for apparent spontaneous generation. [pan- + G. *sperma*, seed]

pan·spor·o·blast (pan-spō′rō-blast). The reproductive sporoblast that gives rise to more than one spore in the order Myxosporida (class Myxosporea, phylum Myxozoa). [pan- + G. *sporos*, seed, + *blastos*, germ]

pan·spo·ro·blas·tic (pan′spō-rō-blas′tik). Referring to a pansporoblast.

pan·sys·tol·ic (pan′sis-tol′ik). Lasting throughout systole, extending from first to second heart sound. SYN holosystolic.

pant. To breathe rapidly and shallowly. [Fr. *panteler*, to gasp]

△ **pant-, panto-.** Entire (properly affixed to words derived from G. roots). SEE ALSO pan-. [G. *pas*, all]

pan·ta·chro·mat·ic (pan′tă-krō-mat′ik). Obsolete term meaning completely achromatic.

pan·tal·gia (pan-tal′jē-ă). Pain involving the entire body. [pant- + G. *algos*, pain]

pan·ta·mor·phia (pan-tă-mōr′fē-ă). Shapelessness; general or over-all malformation. [pant- + G. *a-* priv. + *morphē*, shape]

pan·ta·mor·phic (pan-tă-mōr′fik). Relating to or characterized by pantamorphia.

pan·tan·en·ceph·a·ly, pan·tan·en·ce·pha·lia (pan′tan-en-sef′ă-lē, -se-fā′lē-ă). Congenital absence of the brain. [pant- + G. *an-* priv. + *enkephalos*, brain]

pan·tan·ky·lo·bleph·a·ron (pan′tan-kī-lō-blef′ă-ron). Obsolete term for blepharosynechia.

pan·ta·pho·bia (pan-tă-fō′bē-ă). Absolute fearlessness. [pant- + G. *a-* priv. + *phobos*, fear]

pan·ta·tro·phia, pan·tat·ro·phy (pan-tă-trō′fē-ă, pan-tat′rō-fē). SYN panatrophy. [pant- + atrophy]

pan·te·the·ine (pan-tĕ-thē′in). The condensation product of pantothenic acid and aminoethanethiol, *N*-pantothenyl-2-aminoethanethiol, $HOCH_2C(CH_3)_2CHOH$–CO–NH–CH$_2CH_2CO$–NH–CH_2CH_2SH; an intermediate in biosynthesis of coenzyme A via 4′-phosphopantetheine (phosphate on the terminal –CH$_2$O group) and ATP. SYN *Lactobacillus bulgaricus* factor.

p. kinase, an enzyme that catalyzes the phosphorylation of pantetheine by ATP to pantetheine 4′-phosphate; a step in coenzyme A biosynthesis.

p. 4′-phosphate, SYN 4′-phosphopantetheine.

pan·te·thine (pan′tĕ-thin). The disulfide formed from two pantetheines.

pan·the·nol (pan′thĕ-nol). SYN dexpanthenol.

pan·thod·ic (pan-thod′ik). SYN panodic.

△ **panto-.** SEE pant-.

pan·to·ate (pan′tō-āt). A salt or ester of pantoic acid.

pan·to·graph (pan′tō-graf). **1.** An instrument for reproducing drawings by a system of levers whereby a recording pencil is made to follow the movements of a stylet passing along the lines of the original. **2.** In dentistry, an instrument used to record mandibular border movements that may be transferred to make equivalent settings on an articulator. [panto- + G. *graphō*, to record]

pan·to·ic ac·id (pan-tō′ik). 2,4-Dihydroxy-3,3-dimethylbutyric acid; $hOCH_2C(CH_3)_2CHOH$–COOH, the β-alanine amide of which is pantothenic acid; a coenzyme A precursor.

pan·to·mo·gram (pan′tō-mō-gram). A panoramic radiographic record of the maxillary and mandibular dental arches and their associated structures, obtained by a pantomograph. [pan- + tomogram]

pan·to·mo·graph (pan′tō-mō-graf). A panoramic radiographic instrument that permits visualization of the entire dentition, alveolar bone, and contiguous structures on a single extraoral film.

pan·to·mog·ra·phy (pan-tō-mog′ră-fē). A method of radiography by which a radiograph (pantomogram) of the maxillary and mandibular dental arches and their contiguous structures may be obtained on a single film.

pan·to·mor·phia (pan-to-mōr′fē-ă). **1.** The condition of an organism, such as an ameba, that is capable of assuming all shapes. **2.** Perfect shapeliness or symmetry. [panto- + G. *morphē*, shape]

pan·to·mor·phic (pan-tō-mōr′fik). Capable of assuming all shapes.

pan·to·nine (pan′tō-nēn). An amino acid identified in *Escherichia coli* that may be an intermediate in the biosynthesis of pantothenic acid by that organism, containing NH_2 in place of the α-OH group of pantothenic acid.

pan·to·scop·ic (pan-tō-skop′ik). Designed for observing objects at all distances; denoting bifocal lenses. [panto- + G. *skopeō*, to view]

pan·to·the·nate (pan-tō-then′āt). A salt or ester of pantothenic acid.

p. synthetase, an enzyme that converts pantoate and β-alanine to p. with cleavage of ATP to AMP and PP$_i$; a key step in coenzyme A biosynthesis. SYN pantoate-activating enzyme.

pan·to·then·ic ac·id (pan-tō-then′ik). $HOCH_2C(CH_3)_2 CHOH$–CO–NH– CH_2CH_2COOH; *N*-(2,4-dihydroxy-3,3-dimethylbutyryl)-3-aminopropionic acid; the β-alanine amide of pantoic acid. A growth substance widely distributed in plant and animal tissues, and essential for growth of a number of organisms; deficiency in diet causes a dermatitis in chicks and rats and achromotrichia in the latter; a precursor to coenzyme A. SYN antidermatitis factor.

pan·to·then·yl (pan-tō-then′il). The acyl radical of pantothenic acid.

p. alcohol, SYN dexpanthenol.

pan·to·yl (pan′tō-il). The acyl radical of pantoic acid.

pan·to·yl·tau·rine (pan′tō-il-taw′rin, -rēn). Pantothenic acid in which the carboxyl group is replaced by a sulfonic acid group; analogous to pantothenic acid in structure, except that taurine replaces β-alanine in the molecule. SYN thiopanic acid.

Panum, Peter L., Danish physiologist, 1820–1885. SEE P.'s *area*.

Pa

pan·zer·herz (pahn'zer-härtz). SYN armored *heart*. [Ger. *Panzerherz*]

PAP Acronym for *p*eroxidase *a*nti*p*eroxidase complex. Abbreviation for 3'-phosphoadenosine 5'-phosphate. SEE PAP *technique*.

pap. A food of soft consistency, like that of breadcrumbs soaked in milk or water.

pa·pa·in, pa·pa·in·ase (pa-pā'in, -ās). A proteolytic enzyme, or a crude extract containing it, obtained from papaya latex. It has esterase, thiolase, transamidase, and transesterase activities, and is used as a protein digestant, meat tenderizer, and to prevent adhesions. SYN papayotin.

Papanicolaou, George N., Greek-U.S. physician, anatomist, and cytologist, 1883–1962. SEE Pap *smear*; Pap *test*; P. *examination*, *smear*, *smear test*, *stain*.

Pa·pav·er (pă-pā'ver, pă-pav'er). A genus of plants, one species of which, *P. somniferum* (family Papaveraceae), furnishes opium. SYN poppy. [L. poppy]

pa·pav·er·e·tum (pă-pav-er-ē'tŭm). A preparation of water soluble opium alkaloids, including 50% anhydrous morphine. [L. *papaver*, poppy]

pa·pav·er·ine (pa-pav'er-ēn). A benzylisoquinoline alkaloid of opium that is not a narcotic but has mild analgesic action and is a powerful spasmolytic; does not evoke tolerance and has no addiction liability. Also available as p. hydrochloride. [L. *papaver*, poppy]

pa·paw (pă-paw'). SEE papaya.

pa·pa·ya (pă-pī'yah, pă-pā'yah). The fruit of the papaw (pawpaw), *Carica papaya* (family Caricaceae), a tree of tropical America; it possesses a proteolytic action and is the source of papain. SYN carica. [Sp.]

pap·a·yo·tin (pap-ā'yō-tin). SYN papain.

pa·per (pā'per). **1.** A square of p. folded over so as to form an envelope containing a dose of any medicinal powder. **2.** A piece of blotting p. or filter p. impregnated with a medicinal solution, dried, and burned; formerly, the fumes were inhaled in the treatment of asthma and other respiratory affections. [L. *papyrus*; G. *papyros*, a kind of rush, from which writing paper was made]

articulating p., SYN occluding p.

chromatography p., used in p. chromatography. SYN high quality filter p.

Congo red p., p. impregnated with Congo red; used as a pH indicator, changing from blue-violet at 3.0 to red at 5.0.

filter p., an unsized p. used in pharmacy and chemistry for filtering solutions; many varieties are used for p. chromatography.

high quality filter p., SYN chromatography p.

niter p., p. impregnated with potassium nitrate that is ignited to produce fumes inhaled as treatment for asthma. SYN potassium nitrate p., saltpeter p.

occluding p., an inked p. or ribbon interposed between natural or artificial teeth to determine tooth contacts. SYN articulating p.

potassium nitrate p., SYN niter p.

saltpeter p., SYN niter p.

Papez, J.W., U.S. anatomist, 1883–1958. SEE P. *circuit*.

PAPILLA

pa·pil·la, pl. **pa·pil·lae** (pă-pil'ă, -pil'ē) [NA]. Any small nipple-like process. SYN teat (3). [L. a nipple, dim. of *papula*, a pimple]

acoustic p., SYN spiral *organ*.

Bergmeister's p., a small mass of glial tissue that forms during fetal life a temporary conical investment of the hyaloid artery at its emergence into the vitreous chamber; vestiges of it may persist as a prepapillary membrane.

bile p., SYN major duodenal p.

p. of breast, SYN nipple.

circumvallate p., SYN vallate p.

clavate papillae, SYN fungiform papillae.

conic papillae, SYN conical papillae.

papil'lae con'icae [NA], SYN conical papillae.

conical papillae, numerous projections on the dorsum of the tongue, scattered among the filiform papillae and similar to them, but shorter. SYN papillae conicae [NA], conic papillae.

papil'lae co'rii [NA], ⁕official alternate term for dermal papillae.

papillae of corium, SYN dermal papillae.

dental p., a projection of the mesenchymal tissue of the developing jaw into the cup of the enamel organ; its outer layer becomes a layer of specialized columnar cells, the odontoblasts, that form the dentin of the tooth. SYN p. dentis [NA], dentinal p.

dentinal p., SYN dental p.

p. den'tis [NA], SYN dental p.

dermal papillae, the superficial projections of the dermis (corium) that interdigitate with recesses in the overlying epidermis; they contain vascular loops and specialized nerve endings, and are arranged in ridgelike lines best developed in the hand and foot. SYN papillae dermis [NA], papillae corii ⁕ [NA], papillae of corium.

papil'lae der'mis [NA], SYN dermal papillae.

p. duode'ni ma'jor [NA], SYN major duodenal p.

p. duode'ni mi'nor [NA], SYN minor duodenal p.

filiform papillae, numerous elongated conical keratinized projections on the dorsum of the tongue. SYN papillae filiformes [NA].

papil'lae filifor'mes [NA], SYN filiform papillae.

papil'lae folia'tae [NA], SYN foliate papillae.

foliate papillae, numerous projections arranged in several transverse folds upon the lateral margins of the tongue just in front of the palatoglossus muscle. SYN papillae foliatae [NA], folia linguae.

fungiform papillae, numerous minute elevations on the dorsum of the tongue, of a fancied mushroom shape, the tip being broader than the base; the epithelium of many of these papillae has taste buds. SYN papillae fungiformes [NA], clavate papillae.

papil'lae fungifor'mes [NA], SYN fungiform papillae.

hair p., SYN p. pili.

p. incisi'va [NA], SYN incisive p.

incisive p., a slight elevation of the mucosa at the anterior extremity of the raphe of the palate. SYN p. incisiva [NA], palatine p.

interdental p., the gingiva that fills the interproximal space between two adjacent teeth. SYN gingival septum, interproximal p.

interproximal p., SYN interdental p.

lacrimal p., a slight projection from the margin of each eyelid near the medial commisure, in the center of which is the lacrimal punctum (opening of the lacrimal duct). SYN p. lacrimalis [NA].

p. lacrima'lis [NA], SYN lacrimal p.

lenticular papillae, SYN *folliculi* linguales, under *folliculus*.

lingual p., (1) one of numerous variously shaped projections of the mucous membrane of the dorsum of the tongue; SYN p. lingualis [NA]. (2) the lingual portion of the gingiva filling the interproximal space between adjacent teeth; in molar and premolar areas, there may be separate lingual and buccal interdental papillae. SEE ALSO interdental p.

p. lingua'lis, pl. **papil'lae lingua'les** [NA], SYN lingual p. (1).

major duodenal p., point of opening of the common bile duct and pancreatic duct into the duodenum; it is located posteriorly in the descending part of the duodenum. SYN p. duodeni major [NA], bile p., p. of Vater, Santorini's major caruncle.

p. mam'mae [NA], SYN nipple.

minor duodenal p., the site of the opening of the accessory pancreatic duct into the duodenum, located anterior to and slightly superior to the major p. SYN p. duodeni minor [NA], Santorini's minor caruncle.

nerve p., one of the papillae in the dermis containing a tactile corpuscle or other form of end organ. SYN neurothele.

p. ner'vi op'tici, SYN optic *disk*.

optic p. (p), SYN optic *disk*.

palatine p., SYN incisive p.

parotid p., the projection at the opening of the parotid duct into the vestibule of the mouth opposite the neck of the upper second molar tooth. SYN p. parotidea [NA].

p. parotid'ea [NA], SYN parotid p.

p. pi'li, a knoblike indentation of the bottom of the hair follicle, upon which the hair bulb fits like a cap; it is derived from the corium and contains vascular loops for the nourishment of the hair root. SYN hair p.

renal p., the apex of a renal pyramid that projects into a minor calyx; some 10 to 25 openings of papillary ducts occur on its tip, forming the area cribrosa. SYN p. renalis [NA].

p. rena'lis, pl. **papil'lae rena'les** [NA], SYN renal p.

retrocuspid p., a small tissue tag located on the mandibular gingiva lingual to the cuspid teeth; usually occurs bilaterally, is more commonly identified in children, and is considered a normal anatomic structure.

tactile p., one of the papillae of the dermis containing a tactile cell or corpuscle.

urethral p., p. urethra'lis, the slight projection often present in the vestibule of the vagina marking the urethral orifice.

p. valla'ta, pl. **papil'lae valla'tae** [NA], SYN vallate p.

vallate p., one of eight or ten projections from the dorsum of the tongue forming a row anterior to and parallel with the sulcus terminalis; each p. is surrounded by a circular trench (fossa) having a slightly raised outer wall (vallum); on the sides of the vallate p. and the opposed margin of the vallum are numerous taste buds. SYN p. vallata [NA], circumvallate p.

vascular papillae, dermal papillae containing vascular loops.

p. of Vater, SYN major duodenal p.

---

pap·il·lary, pap·il·late (pap′i-lār-ē, -i-lāt). Relating to, resembling, or provided with papillae.

pap·il·lec·to·my (pap-i-lek′tō-mē). Surgical removal of any papilla. [papilla + G. *ektomē*, excision]

pa·pil·le·de·ma (pă-pil-e-dē′mă). Edema of the optic disk, often due to increased intracranial pressure. SYN choked disk. [papilla + edema]

pap·il·lif·er·ous (pap-i-lif′er-ŭs). Provided with papillae. [papilla + L. *fero*, to bear]

pa·pil·li·form (pă-pil′i-fōrm). Resembling or shaped like a papilla.

pap·il·li·tis (pap-i-lī′tis). 1. Optic neuritis with swelling of the optic disk. 2. Inflammation of the renal papilla. [papilla + G. *-itis*, inflammation]

foliate p., inflamed vestigial foliate papillae on the posterior lateral tongue.

necrotizing p., SYN renal papillary *necrosis*.

△ **papillo-.** A papilla, papillary. [L. *papilla*]

pap·il·lo·ad·e·no·cys·to·ma (pap′i-lō-ad′ĕ-nō-sis-tō′mă). A benign epithelial neoplasm characterized by glands or glandlike structures, formation of cysts, and finger-like projections of neoplastic cells covering a core of fibrous connective tissue.

pap·il·lo·car·ci·no·ma (pap′i-lō-kar-si-nō′mă). 1. A papilloma that has become malignant. 2. A carcinoma that is characterized by papillary, finger-like projections of neoplastic cells in association with cores of fibrous stroma as a supporting structure. [papilla + G. *karkinōma*, cancer]

pap·il·lo·ma (pap-i-lō′mă). A circumscribed benign epithelial tumor projecting from the surrounding surface; more precisely, a benign epithelial neoplasm consisting of villous or arborescent outgrowths of fibrovascular stroma covered by neoplastic cells. SYN papillary tumor, villoma. [papilla + G. *-oma*, tumor]

p. acumina'tum, obsolete term for *condyloma* acuminatum.

basal cell p., SYN seborrheic *keratosis*.

p. canalic'ulum, a papillomatous benign tumor arising within the duct of a gland.

canine oral p., warts affecting mucous membranes of young dogs; caused by a papillomavirus.

p. diffu'sum, widespread occurrence of p.'s.

duct p., SYN intraductal p.

p. du'rum, a wart, corn, or cutaneous horn. SYN hard p.

hard p., SYN p. durum.

Hopmann's p., a papillomatous overgrowth of the nasal mucous membrane. SYN Hopmann's polyp.

infectious p. of cattle, single or multiple rough nodules on the skin and mucous membranes caused by a papillomavirus; in young cattle, which are most susceptible, they are most numerous on the head, neck, and shoulders; in cows they usually affect the udder and teats. SYN cattle warts.

p. inguina'le trop'icum, a cutaneous eruption, occurring in Colombia, characterized by numerous slender pink vegetations in the inguinal region.

intracystic p., a p. growing within a cystic adenoma, filling the cavity with a mass of branching epithelial processes.

intraductal p., a small, often nonpalpable, benign p. arising in a lactiferous duct and frequently causing bleeding from the nipple. SYN duct p.

inverted p., a mucosal tumor of the urinary bladder or nasal cavity in which proliferating epithelium is invaginated beneath the surface and is more smoothly rounded than in other p.'s.

p. mol'le, SYN soft p.

Shope p., a papillomatous growth found in wild cottontail rabbits that is caused by a virus in the family Papovaviridae and can be transferred to domestic rabbits where it will cause similar growths. A high percentage of these growths may become malignant.

soft p., a p. with only a thin layer of horny epithelium. SYN p. molle.

transitional cell p., a benign papillary tumor of transitional epithelium; in the urinary tract, frequently called transitional cell carcinoma, grade 1, because of the likelihood of its recurrence.

p. vene'reum, obsolete term for *condyloma* acuminatum.

villous p., a p. composed of slender, finger-like excrescences occurring in the bladder or large intestine, or from the choroid plexus of the cerebral ventricles; villous p.'s of the colon are usually sessile and frequently become malignant. SYN villous tumor.

zymotic p., SYN yaws.

pap·il·lo·ma·to·sis (pap′i-lō-mă-tō′sis). 1. The development of numerous papillomas. 2. Papillary projections of the epidermis forming a microscopically undulating surface.

confluent and reticulate p., discrete and confluent gray-brown papules of the anterior and posterior mid-chest, spreading gradually; *Malassezia furfur* has been found in the keratin layer. SYN Gougerot-Carteaud syndrome.

florid oral p., diffuse involvement of the lips and oral mucosa with benign squamous papillomas; microscopically, it resembles verrucous carcinoma, but is not invasive or localized to a specific area of the oral mucosa.

juvenile p., a form of fibrocystic disease of the breast in young women, with florid and sclerosing adenosis that microscopically may suggest carcinoma.

laryngeal p., multiple squamous papillomas of the larynx, seen most commonly in young children, usually due to infection by the human papilloma virus which may be transmitted at birth from the maternal condylomata; recurrences are common, with remission after several years.

palatal p., SYN inflammatory papillary *hyperplasia*.

subareolar duct p., a benign tumor which may clinically resemble Paget's disease, but which is a papillary or solid growth of columnar and myoepithelial cells producing a florid pseudoinfiltrative pattern. SYN adenoma of nipple, erosive adenomatosis of nipple.

pap·il·lo·ma·tous (pap-i-lō′mă-tŭs). Relating to a papilloma.

Pa·pil·lo·ma·vi·rus (pap-i-lō′mă-vī-rŭs). A genus of viruses (family Papovaviridae) containing DNA (MW 5×10^6), having virions about 55 nm in diameter, and including the papilloma and warts viruses of man and other animals, some of which are associated with inductions of carcinoma. Over 70 types are known to infect man and are differentiated by DNA homology. SYN papilloma virus.

Papillon, M.M., 20th century French dermatologist. SEE P.-Lefèvre *syndrome*.

Papillon-Léage, E., 20th century French dentist. SEE Papillon-Léage and Psaume *syndrome*.

pap·il·lo·ret·i·ni·tis (pap'i-lō-ret-i-nī'tis). SYN neuroretinitis.

pap·il·lot·o·my (pă-pi-lot'ō-mē). An incision into the major duodenal papilla. [papilla + G. *tomē*, incision]

pa·pil·lu·la, pl. **pa·pil·lu·lae** (pă-pil'yū-lă, -lē). A small papilla. [Mod. L. dim. of L. *papilla*]

Pa·po·va·vir·i·dae (pă-po'vă-vir'i-dē). A family of small, antigenically distinct viruses that replicate in nuclei of infected cells; most have oncogenic properties. Virions are 45 to 55 nm in diameter, nonenveloped, and ether-resistant; capsids are icosahedral with 72 capsomeres, and they contain double-stranded DNA (MW 3 to 5 × 10⁶). The family includes the genera *Papillomavirus* and *Polyomavirus*. [*papilloma* + *polyoma* + *va*cuolating]

pa·po·va·vi·rus (pă-pō'vă-vī'rŭs). Any virus of the family Papovaviridae.

PAPP Abbreviation for *p*-aminopropiophenone.

Pappenheim, Artur, German physician, 1870–1916. SEE P.'s *stain;* Unna-P. *stain*.

Pap·pen·hei·mer. A.M., U.S. pathologist, 1878–1955. His work in experimental pathology was extensive and included studies of the thymus, identification of the role of lice transmission in trench *fever*, development of an experimental model for rickets, and evaluation of viral infections in animals. SEE Pappenheimer *bodies*, under *body*.

Pappenheimer bod·ies. See under body.

pap·pose, pap·pous (pap'pōs, pap'pŭs). Downy. [G. *pappos*, down]

pap·pus (pap'ŭs). The first downy growth of beard. [G. *pappos*, down]

PAPS Abbreviation for adenosine 3'-phosphate 5'-phosphosulfate; 3'-phosphoadenosine 5'-phosphosulfate.

pap·u·la, pl. **pap·u·lae** (pap'yū-lă, -lē). SYN papule. [L.]

pap·u·lar (pap'yū-lăr). Relating to papules.

pap·u·la·tion (pap-yū-lā'shŭn). The formation of papules.

pap·ule (pap'yūl). A small, circumscribed, solid elevation on the skin. SYN papula. [L. *papula*, pimple]

    Celsus' p.'s, SYN *lichen* agrius.

    follicular p., a papular lesion arising about a hair follicle; not specific for any condition.

    moist p., mucous p., SYN *condyloma* latum.

    piezogenic pedal p., pressure-induced papules of the heel, occurring probably as a result of herniation of fat tissue.

    pruritic urticarial p.'s and plaques of pregnancy (PUPPP), intensely pruritic papulovesicles that begin on the abdomen in the third trimester and spread peripherally, resolves rapidly after delivery and does not affect the fetus.

    split p.'s, p.'s at commissures of the mouth seen in some cases of secondary syphilis.

pap·u·lif·er·ous (pap-yū-lif'er-ŭs). Having papules. [papule + L. *fero*, to bear]

papulo-. Papule. [L. *papula*, papule]

pap·u·lo·er·y·them·a·tous (pap'yū-lō-er-i-them'ă-tŭs, -thē'mă-tŭs). Denoting an eruption of papules on an erythematous surface.

pap·u·lo·pus·tu·lar (pap'yū-lō-pŭs'tū-lăr). Denoting an eruption composed of papules and pustules.

pap·u·lo·pus·tule (pap'yū-lō-pŭs'tyūl). A small semisolid skin elevation which rapidly evolves into a pustule.

pa·pu·lo·sis (pap-yū-lō'sis). The occurrence of numerous widespread papules.

    bowenoid p., a clinically benign form of intraepithelial neoplasia that microscopically resembles Bowen's disease or carcinoma in situ, occurring in young individuals of both sexes on the genital or perianal skin usually as multiple well-demarcated pigmented warty papules.

lymphomatoid p., a chronic papular and ulcerative variant of pityriasis lichenoides et varioliformis acuta characterized by dermal perivascular infiltration by atypical T lymphocytes suggestive of a lymphoma; it is usually benign, but transformation to lymphoma has been reported.

malignant atrophic p., a cutaneovisceral syndrome characterized by pathognomonic umbilicated porcelain-white papules with elevated telangiectatic annular borders, followed by the development of intestinal ulcers which perforate, causing peritonitis; arterioles in the lesions are occluded by thrombosis without inflammatory cells, leading to infarction, progressive neurological disability, and death. SYN Degos' disease, Degos' syndrome.

pap·u·lo·squa·mous (pap'yū-lō-skwă'mŭs). Denoting an eruption composed of both papules and scales. [papulo- + L. *squamosus,* scaly (squamous)]

pap·u·lo·ves·i·cle (pap'yū-lō-ves'i-kl). A small semisolid skin elevation which evolves into a blister.

pap·u·lo·ve·sic·u·lar (pap'yū-lō-ve-sik'yū-lăr). Denoting an eruption composed of papules and vesicles.

pap·y·ra·ceous (pap-i-rā'shŭs). Like parchment or paper. [L. *papyraceus,* made of *papyrus*]

par. A pair; specifically a pair of cranial nerves, *e.g.,* p. nonum, ninth pair, glossopharyngeal; p. vagum, the vagus or tenth pair. [L. equal]

para (par'ă). A woman who has given birth to one or more infants. Para followed by a roman numeral or preceded by a Latin prefix (primi-, secundi-, terti-, quadri-, etc.) designates the number of times a pregnancy has culminated in a single or multiple birth; *e.g.,* **para I,** primipara; a woman who has given birth for the first time; **para II,** secundipara; a woman who has given birth for the second time to one or more infants. Cf. gravida. [L. *pario,* to bring forth]

para-. 1. Prefix denoting a departure from the normal. 2. Prefix denoting involvement of two like parts or a pair. 3. Prefix denoting adjacent, alongside, near, etc. 4 (*p*-). In chemistry, and italicized prefix two substitutions in the benzene ring arranged symmetrically, *i.e.,* linked to opposite carbon atoms in the ring. For words beginning with *para*- or *p*-, see the specific name. [G. alongside of, near]

para·ac·ti·no·my·co·sis (par-ă-ak'ti-nō-mī- kō'sis). Chronic infection, usually pulmonary, resembling actinomycosis; ordinarily caused by nocardiosis. SYN pseudoactinomycosis.

par·a·ami·no·ben·zo·ic ac·id (par'ă-mē'nō). SYN *p*-aminobenzoic acid.

para·ap·pen·di·ci·tis (par'ă-ă-pen-di-sī'tis). SYN periappendicitis.

par·a·bal·lism (par-ă-bal'izm). Severe jerking movements of both legs. [para- + G. *ballismos,* jumping about]

par·a·ban·ic ac·id (par'ă-ban-ik). SYN oxalylurea.

par·a·bi·o·sis (par-ă-bī-ō'sis). 1. Fusion of whole eggs or embryos, as occurs in conjoined twins. 2. Surgical joining of the vascular systems of two organisms. [para- + G. *biōsis,* life]

par·a·bi·ot·ic (par-ă-bī-ot'ik). Relating to, or characterized by, parabiosis.

par·a·bu·lia (par-ă-bū'lē-ă). Perversion of volition or will in which one impulse is checked and replaced by another. [para- + G. *boulē,* will]

par·ac·an·tho·ma (par'ak-an-thō'mă). A neoplasm arising from abnormal hyperplasia of the prickle cell layer of the skin. [para- + G. *akantha,* a thorn, + *-oma,* tumor]

par·ac·an·tho·sis (par'ak-an-thō'sis). 1. The development of paracanthomas. 2. A division of tumors that includes the cutaneous epitheliomas.

par·a·car·mine. SEE paracarmine *stain*.

par·a·ca·se·in (par-ă-kā'sē-in). The compound produced by the action of rennin upon κ-casein (which liberates a glycoprotein), and that precipitates with calcium ion as the insoluble curd.

Paracelsus, Aureolus Theophrastus Bombastus von Hohenheim, Swiss physician, 1493–1541. SEE paracelsian *method*.

par·a·ce·nes·the·sia (par'ă-sē-nes-thē'zē-ă). Deterioration in one's sense of bodily well-being, *i.e.,* of the normal functioning of one's organs. [para- + G. *koinos,* common, + *aisthēsis,* feeling]

par·a·cen·te·sis (par'ă-sen-tē'sis). The passage into a cavity of a trocar and cannula, needle, or other hollow instrument for the purpose of removing fluid; variously designated according to the cavity punctured. SYN tapping (2). [G. *parakentēsis,* a tapping for dropsy, fr. *para,* beside, + *kentēsis,* puncture]

par·a·cen·tet·ic (par-ă-sen-tet'ik). Relating to paracentesis.

par·a·cen·tral (par-ă-sen'trăl). Close to or alongside the center or some structure designated "central."

par·a·cer·vi·cal (par-ă-ser'vi-kăl). Connective tissue adjacent to the uterine cervix.

par·a·cer·vix (par-ă-ser'viks) [NA]. The connective tissue of the pelvic floor extending from the fibrous subserous coat of the cervix of the uterus laterally between the layers of the broad ligament.

par·ac·e·tal·de·hyde (par-as-ĕ-tal'dĕ-hīd). SYN paraldehyde.

par·a·cet·a·mol (par-ă-set'ă-mol). SYN acetaminophen.

par·a·chlo·ro·phe·nol (par'ă-klōr-ō-fē'nol). A disinfectant effective against most Gram-negative organisms; also available as camphorated p. SYN *p*-chlorophenol.

par·a·chol·er·a (par-ă-kol'er-ă). A disease clinically resembling Asiatic cholera but due to a vibrio specifically different from *Vibrio cholerae.*

par·a·chor·dal (par-ă-kōr'dăl). Alongside the anterior portion of the notochord in the embryo; designating the bilateral cartilaginous bars that enter into the formation of the base of the skull. [para- + G. *chordē,* cord]

par·a·chro·ma (par-ă-krō'mă). Abnormal coloration of the skin. SYN parachromatosis. [para- + G. *chrōma,* color]

par·a·chro·ma·to·sis (par-ă-krō-mă-tō'sis). SYN parachroma.

par·a·chy·mo·sin (par-ă-kī'mō-sin). An enzyme resembling chymosin.

par·a·ci·ne·sia, par·a·ci·ne·sis (par'ă-si-nē'zē-ă, -nē'sis). SYN parakinesia.

par·ac·ma·sis (par-ak'mă-sis). SYN paracme.

par·ac·mas·tic (par-ak-mas'tik). Relating to the paracme.

par·ac·me (par-ak'mē). 1. The stage of subsidence of a fever. 2. The period of life beyond the prime; the decline or stage of involution of an organism. SYN paracmasis. [G. the point at which the prime is past; fr. *para,* beyond, + *akmē,* highest point, prime]

Par·a·coc·cid·i·oi·des bra·sil·i·en·sis (par'ă-kok-sid-ē-oy'dēz bră-sil-ē-en'sis). A dimorphic fungus that causes paracoccidioidomycosis. In tissues and on enriched culture medium at 37°C, it grows as large spherical or oval cells which bear single or several buds, and usually is identified by this characteristic; at lower temperatures, it grows slowly as a white mold with minimal sporulation and is noncharacteristic.

par·a·coc·cid·i·oi·din (par'ă-kok-sid-ē-oy'din). A filtrate antigen prepared from the filamentous form of the pathogenic fungus, *Paracoccidioides brasiliensis;* used for demonstrating delayed type dermal hypersensitivity in populations and useful in demonstrating endemic areas in different geographic regions.

par·a·coc·cid·i·oi·do·my·co·sis (par'ă-kok-sid-ē-oy'dō-mī-kō'sis). A chronic mycosis characterized by primary pulmonary lesions with dissemination to many visceral organs, conspicuous ulcerative granulomas of the buccal and nasal mucosa with extensions to the skin, and generalized lymphangitis; caused by *Paracoccidioides brasiliensis.* SYN Almeida's disease, Lutz-Splendore-Almeida disease, paracoccidioidal granuloma, South American blastomycosis.

par·a·co·li·tis (par'ă-kō-lī'tis). Inflammation of the peritoneal coat of the colon.

par·a·col·pi·tis (par'ă-kol-pī'tis). SYN paravaginitis. [para- + G. *kolpos,* vagina, + *-itis,* inflammation]

par·a·col·pi·um (par-ă-kol'pē-ŭm). The tissues alongside the vagina. [para- + G. *kolpos,* vagina]

par·a·cone (par'ă-kōn). The mesiobuccal cusp of an upper molar tooth. [para- + G. *kōnos,* cone]

par·a·co·nid (par-ă-kon'id). The mesiobuccal cusp of a lower molar tooth.

par·a·cor·tex (par-ă-kōr'teks). The area of a lymph node between the subcapsular cortex and the medullary cords; it contains mostly the long-lived lymphocytes derived from the thymus. SYN deep cortex, tertiary cortex, thymus-dependent zone.

par·a·cou·sis (par-ă-kū'sis). SYN paracusis.

par·a·crine (par'ă-krin). Relating to a kind of hormone function in which the effects of the hormone are restricted to the local environment. Cf. endocrine. [para- + G. *krinō,* to separate]

par·a·cu·sis, par·a·cu·sia (par'ă-kū'sis, -kū'sē-ă). 1. Impaired hearing. 2. Auditory illusions or hallucinations. SYN paracousis. [para- + G. *akousis,* hearing]

false p., the apparent increase in auditory acuity of a deaf person to conversation in noisy surroundings due to his companion unconsciously raising his voice. SYN Willis' p.

p. loci, loss or diminution of the power of determining the direction of sound.

Willis' p., SYN false p.

par·a·cy·e·sis (par-ă-sī-ē'sis). SYN ectopic *pregnancy.* [para- + G. *kyēsis,* pregnancy]

par·a·cys·tic (par-ă-sis'tik). Alongside or near a bladder, specifically the urinary bladder. SYN paravesical. [para- + G. *kystis,* bladder]

par·a·cys·ti·tis (par'ă-sis-tī'tis). Inflammation of the connective tissue and other structures about the urinary bladder. [para- + G. *kystis,* bladder, + *-itis,* inflammation]

par·a·cys·ti·um (par-ă-sis'tē-ŭm). The tissues adjacent to the urinary bladder. [para- + G. *kystis,* bladder]

par·a·cy·tic (par-ă-sī'tik). 1. Relating to cells other than those normal to the part where they are found. 2. Between or among, but independent of, cells. [para- + G. *kytos,* cell]

par·ad·e·ni·tis (par'ad'ĕ-nī'tis). Inflammation of the tissues adjacent to a gland. [para- + G. *adēn,* gland, + *-itis,* inflammation]

par·a·den·tal (par-ă-den'tăl). SYN periodontal.

par·a·den·ti·um (par-ă-den'tē-ŭm). SYN periodontal *ligament.*

par·a·did·y·mal (par-ă-did'i-măl). 1. Relating to the paradidymis. 2. Alongside the testis.

par·a·did·y·mis, pl. **par·a·did·y·mi·des** (par'ă-did'i-mis, -didim'i-dēz) [NA]. A small body sometimes attached to the front of the lower part of the spermatic cord above the head of the epididymis; the remnants of tubules of the mesonephros. Its equivalent in the female is the paroöphoron. SYN parepididymis. [para- + G. *didymos,* twin, in pl. *didymoi,* testes]

par·a·dip·sia (par-ă-dip'sē-ă). A perverted appetite for fluids, ingested without relation to bodily need. [para- + G. *dipsa,* thirst]

par·a·dox (par'ă-doks). That which is apparently, though not actually, inconsistent with or opposed to the known facts in any case. [G. *paradoxos,* incredible, beyond belief, fr. *doxa,* belief]

Weber's p., if a muscle is loaded beyond its power to contract it may elongate.

par·a·es·the·sia (par-es-thē'zē-ă). SYN paresthesia.

par·af·fin (par'ă-fin). 1. One of the methane series of acyclic hydrocarbons. 2. SYN hard p. [L. *parum,* little, + *affinis,* neighboring, akin, so called because of its slight tendency to chemical reaction]

chlorinated p., a solvent for dichloramine-T.

hard p., a purified mixture of solid hydrocarbons derived from petroleum. SYN paraffin (2).

liquid p., SYN mineral oil.

white soft p., SYN white *petrolatum.*

yellow soft p., SYN petrolatum.

par·af·fi·no·ma (par'ă-fi-nō'mă). A tumefaction, usually a granuloma, caused by the prosthetic or therapeutic injection of paraffin into the tissues; sometimes used with reference to similar lesions resulting from the injection of any oil, wax, or the like. SEE ALSO lipogranuloma. SYN paraffin tumor.

Par·a·fi·lar·ia mul·ti·pa·pil·lo·sa (par'ă-fi-lā'rē-ă mul'ti-pap-ilō'să). A common filarial parasite that causes dermatorrhagia parasitica.

par·a·fla·gel·la (par'ă-fla-jel'ă). Plural of paraflagellum.

par·a·flag·el·late (par-ă-flaj'ĕ-lāt). **1.** Having one or more paraflagella. **2.** SYN paramastigote.

par·a·fla·gel·lum, pl. **par·a·fla·gel·la** (par'ă-fla-jel'ŭm, -ă). A minute accessory flagellum sometimes present in addition to the ordinary flagellum of certain protozoans.

par·a·fol·lic·u·lar (par-ă-fo-lik'yū-lăr). Associated spatially with a follicle.

par·a·for·mal·de·hyde (par-ă-fōr-mal'dĕ-hīd). A polymer of formaldehyde, used as a disinfectant. SYN trioxymethylene.

par·a·fuch·sin (par-ă-fuk'sin). SYN pararosanilin.

par·a·gam·ma·cism (par'ă-gam'ă-sizm). Substitution of another letter sound for the g sound. SEE ALSO gammacism. [para- + G. *gamma*, the letter g]

par·a·gan·glia (par-ă-gang'glē-ă). Plural of paraganglion.

par·a·gan·gli·o·ma (par'ă-gang-glē-ō'mă). A neoplasm usually derived from the chromoreceptor tissue of a paraganglion, such as the carotid body, or the medulla of the adrenal gland; the latter is usually termed a chromaffinoma or pheochromocytoma.

nonchromaffin p., SYN chemodectoma.

par·a·gan·gli·on, pl. **par·a·gan·glia** (par-ă-gang'glē-on, -ă). A small, roundish body containing chromaffin cells; a number of such bodies may be found retroperitoneally near the aorta and in organs such as the kidney, liver, heart, and gonads. SYN chromaffin body.

par·a·gene (par'ă-jēn). SYN plasmid.

par·a·gen·i·tal (par-ă-jen'i-tal). Alongside the gonads.

par·a·geu·sia (par-ă-gyū'sē-ă, -jū'sē-ă). Disordered or perverted sense of taste. [para- + G. *geusis*, taste]

par·a·geu·sic (par-ă-gyū'sik). Relating to parageusia.

pa·rag·na·thus (pa-rag'na-thŭs). **1.** A developmental defect resulting in an individual with an accessory lower jaw. **2.** A parasitic fetus attached to the jaw of the autosite. [para- + G. *gnathos*, jaw]

par·ag·no·men (par-ag-nō'men). An unexpected reaction. [para- + G. *gnōmēn, gnōmē*, judgment]

par·a·gon·i·mi·a·sis (par'ă-gon-i-mī'ă-sis). Infection with a worm of the genus *Paragonimus*, especially *P. westermani*. SYN pulmonary distomiasis.

Par·a·gon·i·mus (par-ă-gon'i-mŭs). A genus of lung flukes, parasitic in man and a wide variety of mammals, that feed upon crustacea carrying the metacercariae. [para- + G. *gonimos*, with generative power]

P. kellicot'ti, a species prevalent in certain wild animals, such as raccoons, and occurring in dogs, in the Great Lakes region of the U.S.; it is morphologically similar to *P. westermani*.

P. rin'geri, SYN *P. westermani*.

P. westerman'i, the bronchial or lung fluke; a species that causes paragonimiasis, found chiefly in Japan, Korea, Taiwan, China, the Philippines, and Thailand; eggs are coughed up in sputum or swallowed and passed in the feces; miracidia invade *Melania* snails, and produce large numbers of stumpy-tailed cercariae that leave the snail and crawl into muscles and viscera of crayfish or crabs and encyst; in humans the excysted worms invade the wall of the gut and migrate through the diaphragm into the lungs; the developing parasites cause an intense inflammatory reaction and eventually induce fibrous-walled nodules that usually contain a pair of adult worms, along with exudate, eggs, and remains of red blood cells; the fibroparasitic nodules may become contiguous and form multiloculated cystlike structures; in some instances, the flukes involve the brain, liver, peritoneum, intestine, or skin. SYN *P. ringeri*.

par·a·gon·or·rhe·al (par'ă-gon-ō-rē'ăl). Indirectly related to or consequent to gonorrhea.

par·a·gram·ma·tism (par-ă-gram'ă-tizm). SYN paraphasia.

par·a·graph·ia (par-ă-graf'ē-ă). **1.** Loss of the power of writing from dictation, although the words are heard and comprehended. **2.** Writing one word when another is intended. [para- + G. *graphō*, to write]

par·a·he·mo·phil·ia (par'ă-hē-mō-fil'ē-ă). An obsolete term for Owren's *disease*

par·a·he·pat·ic (par-ă-he-pat'ik). Adjacent to the liver.

par·a·hi·dro·sis (par'ă-hi-drō'sis). SYN paridrosis.

par·a·hor·mone (par-ă-hōr'mōn). A substance, product of ordinary metabolism, not produced for a specific purpose, that acts like a hormone in modifying the activity of some distant organ; *e.g.,* the action of carbon dioxide on the control of breathing.

par·a·hyp·no·sis (par'ă-hip-nō'sis). Disordered sleep, such as caused by nightmare or somnambulism.

par·a·hy·poph·y·sis (par'ă-hī-pof'i-sis). A small mass of pituitary tissue, or tissue resembling in structure the anterior lobe of the hypophysis, occasionally found in the dura mater lining of the sella turcica.

par·a·kap·pa·cism (par'ă-kap'ă-sizm). Substitution of another letter sound for that of k. SEE ALSO kappacism. [para- + G. *kappa*, the letter k]

par·a·ker·a·to·sis (par'ă-ker-ă-tō'sis). Retention of nuclei in the cells of the stratum corneum of the epidermis, observed in many scaling dermatoses such as psoriasis and subacute or chronic dermatitis.

p. ostra'cea, SYN p. scutularis.

porcine p., a skin disease of young pigs characterized by a hard, scaly proliferation of the surface layers of the skin. The extremities are commonly affected first, but it may involve the entire body.

p. psoriasifor'mis, an eruption marked by the presence of thick scales resembling those of psoriasis.

p. pustulo'sa, idiopathic subungual keratosis with nail deformity or pitting and with pustular or well-demarcated scaling eczematous changes of the fingertips; usually seen in young girls.

p. scutula'ris, a disease of the scalp marked by the formation of crusts that envelop the hairs. SYN p. ostracea.

p. variega'ta, SYN *poikiloderma* atrophicans vasculare.

par·a·ki·ne·sia, par·a·ki·ne·sis (par'ă-ki-nē'zē-ă, -ki-nē'sis). Any motor abnormality. SYN paracinesia, paracinesis. [para- + G. *kinēsis*, movement]

par·a·la·lia (par-ă-lā'lē-ă). Any speech defect; especially one in which one letter is habitually substituted for another. [para- + G. *lalia*, talking]

p. litera'lis, SYN stammering.

par·a·lamb·da·cism (par-ă-lam'dă-sizm). Mispronunciation of the letter l, or the substitution of some other letter for it. SEE ALSO lambdacism. [para- + G. *lambda*, letter l]

par·al·de·hyde (par-al'dĕ-hīd). $(CH_3CHO)_3$; a cyclic polymer of acetaldehyde; a potent hypnotic sedative, and anticonvulsant suitable for oral, rectal, intravenous, and intramuscular administration; its offensive odor limits its use; effective in suppressing abstinence from alcohol dependence. SYN paracetaldehyde.

par·a·lep·ro·sis (par-ă-lĕ-prō'sis). Presence of certain trophic or nerve changes suggesting an attenuated form of leprosy in regions where the disease has long prevailed.

par·a·lep·sy (par'ă-lep-sē). **1.** A temporary attack of mental inertia and hopelessness. **2.** A sudden alteration in mood or emotional tension. [G. para- + *lēpsis*, seizure]

par·a·lex·ia (par-ă-lek'sē-ă). Misapprehension of written or printed words, other meaningless words being substituted for them in reading. [para- + G. *lexis*, speech]

par·al·ge·sia (par-al-jē'zē-ă). Painful paresthesia; any disorder or abnormality of the sense of pain. [para- + G. *algēsis*, the sense of pain]

par·al·gia (par-al'jē-ă). Abnormal or unusual pain. [para- + G. *algos*, pain]

par·a·lip·o·pho·bia (par'ă-lip-ō-fō'bē-ă). Morbid fear of neglect or omission of some duty. [G. *paraleipō*, to omit, pass over, + *phobos*, fear]

par·al·lac·tic (par-ă-lak'tik). Relating to a parallax.

par·al·lax (par'ă-laks). **1.** The apparent displacement of an object that follows a change in the position from which it is viewed. **2.** SEE phi *phenomenon*. [G. alternately, fr. *par-allassō*, to make alternate, fr. *allos*, other]

binocular p., the difference in the angles formed by the lines of sight to two objects situated at different distances from the eyes; a factor in the visual perception of depth. SYN stereoscopic p.

heteronymous p., the apparent movement of an object toward the closed eye; noted in exophoria.

homonymous p., the apparent movement of an object toward the open eye when one is closed; noted in esophoria.

stereoscopic p., SYN binocular p.

vertical p., the relative vertical displacement of the image when each eye is closed in turn; seen in vertical diplopia, or heterophoria.

par·al·lel·ism (par′ă-lel-izm). **1.** The state of being structurally parallel. **2.** In psychology, the mind-body doctrine that for every conscious process there is a corresponding or parallel organic process, without asserting a causal interrelation between the two. [para- + G. *allēlōn,* of one another, fr. *allos,* other]

par·al·lel·om·e·ter (par′ă-lel-om′ĕ-ter). An apparatus used for paralleling the attachments and abutments for fixed or removable partial dentures.

par·al·ler·gic (par-ă-ler′jik). Denoting an allergic state in which the body becomes predisposed to nonspecific stimuli following original sensitization with a specific allergen.

par·a·lo·gia, pa·ral·o·gism, pa·ral·o·gy (par-ă-lō′jē-ă, pă-ral′ō-jizm, -ral′ō-jē). False reasoning, involving self-deception. [G. *paralogia,* a fallacy, fr. *para,* beside, + *logos,* reason]

thematic p., false reasoning in relation chiefly to one theme or subject, upon which the mind dwells insistently.

pa·ral·y·sis, pl. **pa·ral·y·ses** (pă-ral′i-sis, -sēz). **1.** Loss of power of voluntary movement in a muscle through injury to or disease of its nerve supply. **2.** Loss of any function, as sensation, secretion, or mental ability. [G. fr. para- + *lysis,* a loosening]

acute ascending p., a p. of rapid course beginning in the legs and involving progressively the trunk, arms, and neck, ending sometimes in death in from one to three weeks. SYN ascending p.

acute atrophic p., SYN acute anterior *poliomyelitis.*

p. ag′itans, obsolete term for parkinsonism (1).

ascending p., SYN acute ascending p.

Brown-Séquard's p., SYN Brown-Séquard's *syndrome.*

bulbar p., SYN progressive bulbar p.

central p., p. due to a lesion in the brain or spinal cord.

Chastek p., a disease of foxes and mink caused by feeding on raw fish of certain types which contain an enzyme destructive of thiamin; the thiamin deficiency causes loss of appetite, emaciation, and finally paralysis and death.

compression p., p. due to external presure on a nerve.

coonhound p., a polyradiculoneuritis of dogs (especially raccoon-hunting breeds) following a raccoon bite and characterized by weakness, hindlimb hyporeflexia, and a flaccid symmetrical tetraplegia.

crossed p., SYN alternating *hemiplegia.*

crutch p., a form of pressure p. affecting the arm, and caused by compression of the brachial plexus or radial nerve by the crosspiece of a crutch. SYN crutch palsy.

diphtheritic p., SYN postdiphtheritic p.

diver's p., lay term for decompression *sickness.*

Duchenne-Erb p., SYN Erb *palsy.*

Erb p., SYN Erb *palsy.*

Erb spinal p., chronic myelitis of syphilitic origin.

facial p., paresis or p. of the facial muscles, usually unilateral, due to either 1) a lesion involving either the nucleus or the facial nerve peripheral to the nucleus (peripheral facial paralysis), or 2) a supranuclear lesion in the cerebrum or upper brainstem (central facial paralysis); with the latter, facial weakness is usually partial and the upper portion of the face is relatively spared, due to bilateral cortical connections. SYN facial palsy, facioplegia, fallopian neuritis, prosopoplegia.

familial periodic p., one of the inherited muscle disorders manifested as recurrent episodes of marked generalized weakness. SEE hyperkalemic periodic p., hypokalemic periodic p., normokalemic periodic p.

faucial p., SYN isthmoparalysis.

flaccid p., p. with a loss of muscle tone. Cf. spastic *diplegia.*

fowl p., SEE avian *lymphomatosis.*

generalized p., SYN global p.

ginger p., SYN jake p.

global p., p. of both whole sides of the body; survival is usually of short duration. SYN generalized p.

glossolabiolaryngeal p., glossolabiopharyngeal p., SYN progressive bulbar p.

glossopalatolabial p., SYN progressive bulbar *palsy.*

glossopharyngeolabial p., SYN progressive bulbar *palsy.*

Gubler's p., SYN Gubler's *syndrome.*

hyperkalemic periodic p., a form of periodic p. in which the serum potassium level is elevated during attacks; onset occurs in infancy, attacks are frequent but relatively mild, and myotonia is often present; autosomal dominant inheritance.

hypokalemic periodic p. [type I MIM 17066, *170600, *311700], a form of periodic p. in which the serum potassium level is low during attacks; onset usually occurs between the ages of 7 and 21 years; attacks may be precipitated by exposure to cold, high carbohydrate meal, or alcohol, may last hours to days, and may cause respiratory p.; autosomal dominant or X-linked inheritance.

hysterical p., a psychosomatic numbness of a limb sometimes to the point of p. SEE hysteria.

immune p., the induction of tolerance in mice due to injection of large amounts of polysaccharide. The polysaccharide is poorly metabolized and the p. remains only during the persistence of the above.

immunological p., lack of specific antibody production after exposure to large doses of the antigen; immunological p. disappears when the antigen is eliminated. SEE ALSO immunologic *tolerance.*

infectious bulbar p., SYN pseudorabies.

jake p., neuropathy produced by drinking synthetic Jamaican ginger (or "jake" in the vernacular) containing triorthocresylphosphate. SYN ginger p.

Klumpke's p., SYN Klumpke *palsy.*

lambing p., SYN pregnancy *disease* of sheep.

Landry's p., SYN acute idiopathic *polyneuritis.*

lead p., SYN lead *palsy.*

mimetic p., p. of the facial muscles.

mixed p., combined motor and sensory p.

motor p., loss of the power of muscular contraction.

musculospiral p., p. of the muscles of the forearm due to injury of the radial (musculospiral) nerve.

myogenic p., SYN acute anterior *poliomyelitis.*

normokalemic periodic p. [type III MIM 170600], a form of periodic p. in which the serum potassium level is within normal limits during attacks; onset usually occurs between the ages of 2 and 5 years; there is often severe quadriplegia, usually improved by the administration of sodium salts; autosomal dominant inheritance. SYN sodium-responsive periodic p.

obstetrical p., SYN obstetrical *palsy.*

ocular p., p. of extraocular and intraocular muscles.

parturient p., SYN milk *fever* (2).

periodic p., term for a group of diseases characterized by recurring episodes of muscular weakness or flaccid p. without loss of consciousness, speech, or sensation; attacks begin when the patient is at rest, and there is apparent good health between attacks. SEE hyperkalemic periodic p., hypokalemic periodic p., normokalemic periodic p.

peripheral facial p., SYN Bell's *palsy.*

postdiphtheritic p., p. affecting the uvula most frequently, but also any other muscle, due to toxic neuritis; usually appears in the second or third week following the beginning of the attack of diphtheria. SYN diphtheritic p.

posti′cus p., p. of the posterior cricothyroid muscles.

Pott's p., SYN Pott's *paraplegia.*

pressure p., p. due to compression of a nerve, nerve trunk, or spinal cord. SYN pressure palsy.

progressive bulbar p., progressive weakness and atrophy of the muscles of the tongue, lips, palate, pharynx, and larynx, usually occurring in later life; most often caused by motor neuron disease. SYN bulbar palsy, bulbar p., Duchenne's disease (2), Erb disease, glossolabiolaryngeal p., glossolabiopharyngeal p.

pa

pseudobulbar p., p. of the lips and tongue, simulating progressive bulbar p., but due to supranuclear lesions with bilateral involvement of the upper motor neurons; characterized by speech and swallowing difficulties, emotional instability, and spasmodic, mirthless laughter.

sensory p., loss of sensation; anesthesia.

sleep p., brief episodic loss of voluntary movement that occurs when falling asleep (hypnagogic sleep p.) or when awakening (hypnopompic sleep p.). One of the narcoleptic tetrad. SYN sleep dissociation.

sodium-responsive periodic p., SYN normokalemic periodic p.

spastic spinal p., SYN spastic *diplegia.*

spinal p., loss of motor power due to a lesion of the spinal cord. SYN myeloparalysis, myeloplegia, rachioplegia.

supranuclear p., p. due to lesions above the primary motor neurons.

tick p., an ascending p. caused by the continuing presence of *Dermacentor* and *Ixodes* ticks attached in the occipital region or on the upper neck of humans, often hidden under long hair; reported from the western U.S., British Columbia, and other regions; occurs mainly in children, but also in animals.

Todd's p., p. of temporary duration (normally not more than a few days) that occurs in the limb or limbs involved in jacksonian epilepsy after the seizure. SYN Todd's postepileptic p.

Todd's postepileptic p., SYN Todd's p.

vasomotor p., SYN vasoparesis.

wasting p., SYN amyotrophic lateral *sclerosis.*

Zenker's p., paresthesia and p. in the area of the external popliteal nerve.

pa·ra·lys·sa (par′ă-lis′ă). A paralytic form of rabies caused by the bite of the vampire bat (*Desmodus*). [paralysis + G. *lyssa,* madness (rabies)]

par·a·lyt·ic (par-ă-lit′ik). Relating to paralysis or to suffering from paralysis.

par·a·ly·zant (pă-ral′i-zant). 1. Causing paralysis. 2. Any agent, such as curare, that causes paralysis.

par·a·lyze (par′ă-līz). To render incapable of movement.

par·a·mag·net·ic (par′ă-mag-net′ik). Having the property of paramagnetism; in magnetic resonance imaging, contrast media are chosen for their p. property, which shortens relaxation time.

par·a·mag·ne·tism (par-ă-mag′nĕ-tizm). The property of having a strong magnetic moment from one or more unpaired electrons, causing orientation in a magnetic field; most significant in imaging are ions of certain transition metals such as gadolinium, iron, and manganese, or organic compounds which are stable free radicals; molecular oxygen also exhibits p.

par·a·mas·ti·gote (par-ă-mas′ti-gōt). A mastigote having two flagella, one long and one short. SYN paraflagellate (2). [para- + G. *mastix,* whip]

par·a·mas·toid (par-ă-mas′toyd). Near the mastoid process.

Par·a·me·ci·um (par-ă-mē′shē-ŭm, -sē-ŭm). An abundant genus of freshwater holotrichous ciliates, characteristically slipper-shaped and often large enough to be visible to the naked eye; commonly used for genetic and other studies. [G. *paramēkēs,* rather long, fr. *mēkos,* length]

par·a·me·di·an (par-ă-mē′dē-an). Near the middle line. SYN paramesial.

par·a·med·ic (par-ă-med′ik). A person trained and certified to provide emergency medical care.

par·a·med·i·cal (par-ă-med′i-kăl). 1. Related to the medical profession in an adjunctive capacity, *e.g.,* denoting allied health fields such as physical therapy, speech pathology, etc. 2. Relating to a paramedic.

par·a·me·nia (par-ă-mē′nē-ă). Any disorder or irregularity of menstruation. [para- + G. *mēn,* month]

par·a·me·si·al (par-ă-mē′sē-ăl). SYN paramedian.

par·a·mes·o·neph·ric (par-ă-mes-ō-nef′rik). Close to or alongside the embryonic mesonephros. SEE paramesonephric *duct.*

pa·ram·e·ter (pă-ram′ĕ-ter). 1. One of many dimensions or ways of measuring or describing an object or evaluating a subject: **1.** In a mathematical expression, an arbitrary constant that can possess different values, each value defining other expressions, and can determine the specific form but not the general nature of the

expression; *e.g.,* in the equation $y = a + bx$, a and b are p.'s. **2.** In statistics, a term used to define a characteristic of a population, in contrast to a sample from that population; *e.g.,* the mean and standard deviation of a total population. **3.** In psychoanalysis, any tactic, other than interpretation, used by the analyst to further the patient's progress. [para- + G. *metron,* measure]

enzyme p.'s, those factors and constants that govern the rate of an enzyme-catalyzed reaction, *e.g.,* V_{max} and K_m.

par·a·meth·a·di·one (par′ă-meth-ă-dī′ōn). 3,5-Dimethyl-5-ethyloxazolidine-2,4-dione; an anticonvulsant used in petit mal epilepsy.

par·a·meth·a·sone (par-ă-meth′ă-sōn). 6α-Fluoro-11β,17,21-trihydroxy-16α-methyl-1,4-pregnadiene-3,20-dione; a glucocorticoid with anti-inflammatory effects and toxicity similar to those of prednisone.

p. acetate, acetic ester of p. at C-21; a glucocorticoid useful in the treatment of rheumatoid arthritis and other collagen diseases, allergic conditions, and certain hematologic disorders.

par·a·me·tri·al (par-ă-mē′trē-ăl). Pertaining to the parametrium.

par·a·met·ric (par-ă-met′rik). Relating to the parametrium, or structures immediately adjacent to the uterus.

par·a·me·tris·mus (par′ă-mĕ-triz′mŭs). Painful spasm of the muscular fibers in the broad ligaments. [parametrium + G. *trismos,* a creaking]

par·a·me·trit·ic (par′ă-me-trit′ik). Relating to parametritis.

par·a·me·tri·tis (par′ă-me-trī′tis). Inflammation of the tissue adjacent to the uterus, particularly in the broad ligament. SYN pelvic cellulitis. [parametrium + G. -*itis,* inflammation]

par·a·me·tri·um, pl. **par·a·me·tria** (par-ă-mē′trē-ŭm, -ă) [NA]. The connective tissue of the pelvic floor extending from the fibrous subserous coat of the supracervical portion of the uterus laterally between the layers of the broad ligament. [para- + G. *mētra,* uterus]

par·a·mim·ia (par-ă-mim′ē-ă). The use of gestures unsuited to the words which they accompany. [para- + G. *mimia,* imitation]

par·am·ne·sia (par-am-nē′zē-ă). False recollection, as of events that have never occurred. [para- + G. *amnēsia,* forgetfulness]

Par·a·moe·ba (par-ă-mē′bă). Former name for *Entamoeba.*

par·a·mo·lar (par-ă-mō-lăr). A supernumerary tooth lying among, lingual, or buccal to the maxillary or mandibular molars.

par·a·mor·phine (par-ă-mōr′fēn). SYN thebaine.

Par·am·phis·to·mat·i·dae (par′am-fis-tō-mat′i-dē). A family of parasitic trematodes characterized by large fleshy bodies with a large posterior sucker; included are the genera *Paramphistomum, Gastrodiscoides,* and *Watsonius.*

par·am·phis·to·mi·a·sis (par′am-fis-tō-mī′ă-sis). Infection of animals and humans with trematodes of the family Paramphistomatidae; human disease is caused by *Gastrodiscoides hominis* in Asia and *Watsonius watsoni* in Africa.

Par·am·phis·to·mum (par-am-fis′tō-mŭm). The rumen fluke, a genus of digenetic trematodes (family Paramphistomatidae) parasitic in the rumen or paunch of cattle; species include *P. microbothrioides, P. cervi,* and *P. liorchis.* [para- + G. *amphistomos,* having a double mouth, fr. *amphi,* two-sided, + *stoma,* mouth]

par·a·mu·sia (par-ă-mū′zē-ă). Loss of the ability to read or to render music correctly. [para- + G. *mousa,* music, + -*ia*]

par·am·y·loi·do·sis (par-am′ĭ-loy-dō′sis). 1. Deposition in tissues of an amyloid-like protein resembling light chains of immunoglobulins in primary amyloidosis or (particularly) in atypical amyloidosis of multiple myeloma. 2. Various hereditary amyloidoses (Portuguese amyloidosis, Indiana amyloidosis) characterized by progressive hypertrophic polyneuritis with sensory changes, ataxia, paresis, and muscle atrophy due to amyloid deposits in peripheral and visceral nerves.

par·a·my·oc·lo·nus mul·ti·plex (par′ă-mī-ok′lō-nŭs). SYN *myoclonus* multiplex. [para- + G. *mys,* muscle, + *klonos,* a tumult]

par·a·my·o·to·nia (par′ă-mī-ō-tō′nē-ă). An atypical form of myotonia. SYN paramyotonus.

ataxic p., a disorder characterized by a tonic muscular spasm on attempted movement, associated with slight paresis and ataxia.

congenital p., p. congen′ita [MIM*168300], a nonprogressive myotonia induced by exposure of muscles to cold; there are episodes of intermittent flaccid paralysis, but no atrophy or hypertrophy of muscles; autosomal dominant inheritance. There is a variant autosomal dominant form [MIM*168350] in which cold is not a provoking factor. SYN Eulenburg's disease.

par·a·my·ot·o·nus (par-ă-mī-ot′ō-nŭs). SYN paramyotonia.

Par·a·myx·o·vir·i·dae (par-ă-mik′sō-vir′i-dē). A family of RNA-containing viruses about twice the size of the influenza viruses (Orthomyxoviridae) but similar to them in morphology. Virions are 150 to 300 nm in diameter, enveloped, ether-sensitive, and contain RNA-dependent RNA polymerase. Nucleocapsids are helical, considerably larger than those of the influenza viruses, and contain single-stranded unsegmented RNA. Three genera are recognized: *Paramyxovirus, Morbillivirus,* and *Pneumovirus,* all of which cause cell fusion and produce cytoplasmic eosinophilic inclusions.

Par·a·myx·o·vi·rus (par-ă-mik′sō-vī′rŭs). A genus of viruses (family Paramyxoviridae) that includes Newcastle disease, mumps, and parainfluenza viruses (types 1 to 4). They all have hemagglutinating and hemadsorbing activities, but only Newcastle disease and mumps viruses grow well in embryonated eggs.

par·an·al·ge·sia (par-an-ăl-jē′zē-ă). Analgesia of the lower half of the body. [para- + analgesia]

par·a·na·sal (par-ă-nā′săl). Alongside the nose.

par·a·ne·o·pla·sia (par′ă-nē-ō-plā′zē-ă). Hormonal, neurological, hematological, and other clinical and biochemical disturbances associated with malignant neoplasms but not directly related to invasion by the primary tumor or its metastases.

par·a·ne·o·plas·tic (par′ă-nē-ō-plas′tik). Relating to or characteristic of paraneoplasia.

par·a·neph·ric (par-ă-nef′rik). **1.** Relating to the paranephros. **2.** SYN pararenal.

par·a·neph·ros, pl. **par·a·neph·roi** (par-ă-nef′ros, -nef′roy). SYN suprarenal *gland.* [para- + G. *nephros,* kidney]

par·an·es·the·sia (par-an-es-thē′zē-ă). Anesthesia of the lower half of the body. [para- + anesthesia]

par·a·neu·ral (par-ă-nūr′ăl). Near or alongside a nerve. [para- + G. *neuron,* nerve]

par·a·neu·rone (par-ă-nūr′ōn). A gland or aggregate of cells containing neurosecretory granules. SYN neuroendocrine cell (2).

pa·ran·gi (pă-rang′gē, -ran′jē). A disease similar to yaws, occurring in Sri Lanka.

par·a·noia (par-ă-noy′ă). A severe but relatively rare mental disorder characterized by the presence of systematized delusions, often of a persecutory character involving being followed, poisoned, or harmed by other means, in an otherwise intact personality. SEE ALSO paranoid *personality.* [G. derangement, madness, fr. para- + *noeō,* to think]

  acute hallucinatory p., a form in which periods of hallucination occur in addition to the delusions.

  litigious p., SYN p. querulans.

  p. origina′ria, a form occurring in children.

  p. quer′ulans, a morbid state characterized by discontent and the disposition to complain of imaginary slights. SYN litigious p.

par·a·noi·ac (par-ă-noy′ak). **1.** Relating to or affected with paranoia. **2.** One who is suffering from paranoia.

par·a·noid (par′ă-noyd). **1.** Relating to or characterized by paranoia. **2.** Having delusions of persecution.

par·a·no·mia (par-ă-nō′mē-ă). A form of aphasia in which objects are called by the wrong names. [para- + G. *onoma,* name]

par·a·nu·cle·ar (par-ă-nū′klē-ăr). **1.** SYN paranucleate. **2.** Outside, but near the nucleus.

par·a·nu·cle·ate (par′ă-nū′klē-āt). Relating to or having a paranucleus. SYN paranuclear (1).

par·a·nu·cle·o·lus (par′ă-nū-klē′ō-lŭs). SEE sex *chromatin.*

par·a·nu·cle·us (par-ă-nū′klē-ŭs). An accessory nucleus or small mass of chromatin lying outside, though near, the nucleus.

par·a·om·phal·ic (par′ă-om-fal′ik). SYN paraumbilical. [para- + G. *omphalos,* umbilicus]

par·a·op·er·a·tive (par-ă-op′er-ă-tiv). SYN perioperative.

par·a·o·ral (par-ă-ō′răl). Near or adjacent to the mouth. [para- + L. *os (or-),* mouth]

par·a·o·var·i·an (par′ă-ō-var′ē-an). SYN parovarian (2).

par·a·ox·on (par-ă-ok′son). Diethyl-4-nitrophenyl phosphate; an organophosphorous cholinesterase inhibitor used in insecticides; parathion is converted in the liver to p.

par·a·pan·cre·at·ic (par′ă-pan-krē-at′ik). Near or alongside of the pancreas.

par·a·pa·re·sis (par-ă-pă-rē′sis). Weakness affecting the lower extremities. [para- + paresis]

par·a·pa·ret·ic (par′ă-pă-ret′ik). **1.** Relating to paraparesis. **2.** A person with paraparesis.

par·a·pe·de·sis (par′ă-pĕ-dē′sis). Excretion or secretion through an abnormal channel. [para- + G. *pēdēsis,* a bending, deflection]

par·a·per·i·to·ne·al (par′ă-per′i-tō-nē′ăl). Outside of or alongside the peritoneum.

par·a·pes·tis (par-ă-pes′tis). SYN ambulant *plague.* [para- + L. *pestis,* plague]

par·a·pha·sia (par-ă-fā′zē-ă). A form of aphasia in which a person has lost the ability to speak correctly, substituting one word for another, and jumbling words and sentences unintelligibly. SYN jargon (2), paragrammatism, paraphrasia, pseudoagrammatism. [para- + G. *phasis,* speech]

  thematic p., incoherent speech that wanders from the theme or subject under discussion.

par·a·pha·sic (par-ă-fā′sik). Relating to paraphasia.

pa·ra·phia (pa-rā′fē-ă). Any disorder of the sense of touch. SYN parapsia, pseudaphia, pseudesthesia (1), pseudoesthesia (1). [para- + G. *haphē,* touch]

par·a·phil·ia (par-ă-fil′ē-ă). A mental disorder characterized by sexual deviation. [para- + G. *philos,* fond]

par·a·phi·mo·sis (par′ă-fī-mō′sis). **1.** Painful constriction of the glans penis by a phimotic foreskin, which has been retracted behind the corona. **2.** SEE p. palpebrae. [para- + G. phimosis]

  p. palpe′brae, total spastic eversion of the upper and lower eyelids.

par·a·pho·nia (par-ă-fō′nē-ă). Any disorder of the voice, especially a change in its tone. [para- + G. *phōnē,* voice]

pa·raph·o·ra (pă-raf′ō-ră). A slight emotional disturbance. [G. a going aside, derangement]

par·a·phra·sia (par-ă-frā′zē-ă). SYN paraphasia. [para- + G. *phrasis,* speech]

par·a·phys·i·al, par·a·phys·e·al (par-ă-fiz′ē-ăl). Pertaining to the paraphysis.

pa·raph·y·sis, pl. **pa·raph·y·ses** (pă-raf′i-sis, -sēz). A median organ developing from the roofplate of the diencephalon in certain lower vertebrates. Present in the human embryo and fetus for a short time. SYN paraphysial body. [G. an offshoot]

par·a·pin·e·al (par-ă-pin′ē-ăl). Beside the pineal; denoting the visual or photoreceptive portion of the pineal body present, if not functioning, in certain lizards.

par·a·plasm (par′ă-plazm). **1.** Obsolete term for hyaloplasm. **2.** Malformed or abnormal tissue. [para- + G. *plasma,* a thing formed]

par·a·plas·tic (par-ă-plas′tik). Relating to paraplasm.

par·a·plec·tic (par-ă-plek′tik). SYN paraplegic. [G. *paraplēktikos,* paralyzed]

par·a·ple·gia (par-ă-plē′jē-ă). Paralysis of both lower extremities and, generally, the lower trunk. [para- + *plēgē,* a stroke]

  ataxic p., progressive ataxia and paresis of the leg muscles due to sclerosis of the lateral and posterior funiculi of the spinal cord.

  congenital spastic p., a spastic paralysis of the lower extremities occurring in the infant. SYN infantile spastic p.

  p. doloro′sa, paralysis of the lower extremities in which the affected parts, in spite of loss of motion and sensation, are the seat of excruciating pain; occurs in certain cases of cancer of the spinal cord. SYN painful p.

  p. in extension, paralysis of the legs, maintained in an extended position by hypertonic extensor muscles.

  p. in flexion, the fixation of the paralyzed legs in a flexed posture; usually in transection of the spinal cord.

  infantile spastic p., SYN congenital spastic p.

  painful p., SYN p. dolorosa.

  Pott's p., paralysis of the lower part of the body and the extremities, due to pressure on the spinal cord as the result of tuberculous spondylitis. SYN Pott's paralysis.

spastic p., paresis of the lower extremities with increased muscle tone and spasmodic contraction of the muscles. SYN Erb-Charcot disease (2).

superior p., paralysis of both arms.

par·a·ple·gic (par-ă-plē′jik). Relating to or suffering from paraplegia. SYN paraplectic.

Par·a·pox·vi·rus (par-ă-poks′vī-rŭs). The genus of viruses (family Poxviridae) that includes the contagious ecthyma of sheep, bovine papular stomatitis, and paravaccinia viruses. They possess the nucleoprotein antigen common to all viruses included in the family but differ from other poxviruses in morphology (e.g., virions are smaller and have thicker external coats) and by not multiplying in embryonated eggs.

par·a·prax·ia (par-ă-prak′sē-ă). A condition analogous to paraphasia and paragraphia in which there is a defective performance of purposive acts; e.g., slips of the tongue, or mislaying of objects. [para- + G. praxis, a doing]

par·a·proc·ti·tis (par′ă-prok-tī′tis). Inflammation of the cellular tissue surrounding the rectum. [para- + G. prōktos, anus, + -itis, inflammation]

par·a·proc·ti·um, pl. **par·a·proc·tia** (par′ă-prok′shē-um, -tē-ŭm; -ă). The cellular tissue surrounding the rectum. [para- + G. prōktos, anus]

par·a·pros·ta·ti·tis (par′ă-pros-tă-tī′tis). Inflammation of the tissue around the prostate gland. [para- + L. prostata, prostate, + -itis, inflammation]

par·a·pro·tein ((par-a-prō′tēn). **1.** A monoclonal immunoglobulin of blood plasma, observed electrophoretically as an intense band in γ, β, or α regions, due to an isolated increase in a single immunoglobulin type as a result of a clone of plasma cells arising from the abnormal rapid multiplication of a single cell. The finding of a paraprotein in a patient's serum indicates the presence of a proliferating clone of immunoglobulin-producing cells and may be seen in a variety of malignant, benign, or nonneoplastic diseases. **2.** SYN monoclonal immunoglobulin. [para + protein, fr. G. protos, first]

par·a·pro·tein·e·mia (par′ă-prō-tēn-ē′mē-ă). The presence of abnormal proteins in the blood.

pa·rap·sia (pă-rap′sē-ă). SYN paraphia. [para- + G. hapsis, touch]

par·a·pso·ri·a·sis (par′ă-sō-rī′ă-sis). A heterogenous group of skin disorders including pityriasis lichenoides and small and large plaque variants.

p. en plaque, a form of large plaque parapsoriasis in middle age which frequently develops into mycosis fungoides. Affecting the trunk and proximal extremities, the lesions exceed 5 cm in diameter and are often symmetrical. Small plaques p. en plaque is a benign variant, also called digitate dermatosis.

p. gutta′ta, SYN pityriasis lichenoides.

p. lichenoi′des, SYN poikiloderma atrophicans vasculare.

p. lichenoi′des et variolifor′mis acu′ta, SYN pityriasis lichenoides et varioliformis acuta.

small plaque p., SYN digitate dermatosis.

p. variolifor′mis, SYN pityriasis lichenoides et varioliformis acuta.

par·a·psy·chol·o·gy (par′ă-sī-kol′ō-jē). The study of extrasensory perception, such as thought transference (telepathy) and clairvoyance.

par·a·quat (par′ă-kwaht). 1,1′-Dimethyl-4,4′-dipyridilium; a weedkiller that produces delayed toxic effects on the liver, kidneys, and lungs when ingested; progressive interstitial pneumonia with proliferation of alveolar lining cells may develop.

par·a·ra·ma (par-ă-rā′mă). Painful or crippling disease of the fingers, first described in Brazilian rubber workers, produced by accidental contact with setae of the larva of the moth, Premolis semirufa; immediate pruritus, hyperemia, and local edema may be followed by chronic swelling and immobility that may lead to loss of one or more fingers, presenting a clinical picture corresponding to ankylosis.

par·a·rec·tal (par-ă-rek′tăl). Near the rectum or rectus muscle.

par·a·re·flex·ia (par′ă-rē-flek′sē-ă). A condition characterized by abnormal reflexes.

par·a·re·nal (par-ă-rē′năl). Near or adjacent to the kidneys. SYN paranephric (2).

par·a·rho·ta·cism (par′ă-rō′tă-sizm). Substitution of another sound for that of r. SEE ALSO rhotacism. [para- + G. rho, letter r]

par·a·ro·san·i·lin (par′ă-rō-san′i-lin) [C.I. 42500]. A tri-(aminophenyl)methane hydrochloride; an important red biologic stain used in Schiff's reagent to detect cellular DNA (Feulgen stain), mucopolysaccharides (PAS stain), and proteins (ninhydrin-Schiff stain). SYN parafuchsin.

par·ar·rhyth·mia (par-ă-ridh′mē-ă). A cardiac dysrhythmia in which two independent rhythms coexist, but not as a result of A-V block; p. thus includes parasystole and A-V dissociation (2), but not complete A-V block. [para- + G. rhythmos, rhythm]

par·a·sac·ral (par-ă-sā′krăl). Alongside the sacrum.

par·a·sal·pin·gi·tis (par′ă-sal-pin-jī′tis). Inflammation of the tissues surrounding the fallopian or the eustachian tube. [para- + salpinx + G. -itis, inflammation]

Par·as·ca·ris equo·rum (pa-ras′ka-ris ē-kwō′rŭm). A large heavy-bodied ascarid nematode extremely common in the small intestine of horses and other equids. Larvae may develop in man or mice, but do not reach the adult stage. SYN Ascaris equorum.

par·a·scar·la·ti·na (par′ă-skar-lă-tē′nă). SYN Filatov Dukes' disease.

par·a·se·cre·tion (par′ă-sē-krē′shŭn). Obsolete term for abnormal secretion.

par·a·sex·u·al·i·ty (par′ă-sek-shŭ-al′i-tē). Abnormal or perverted sexuality.

par·a·sig·ma·tism (par-ă-sig′mă-tizm). SYN lisping. [para- + G. sigma, the letter s]

par·a·si·noi·dal (par′ă-sī-noy′dăl). Near a sinus, particularly a cerebral sinus.

par·a·site (par′ă-sīt). **1.** An organism that lives on or in another and draws its nourishment therefrom. **2.** In the case of a fetal inclusion or conjoined twins, the usually incomplete twin that derives its support from the more nearly normal autosite. [G. parasitos, a guest, fr. para, beside, + sitos, food]

autistic p., a p. descended from the tissues of the host. SYN autochthonous p.

autochthonous p., SYN autistic p.

commensal p., SEE commensal (2).

euroxenous p., a p. with a broad or nonspecific host range.

facultative p., an organism that may either lead an independent existence or live as a p., in contrast to obligate p.

heterogenetic p., a p. whose life cycle involves an alternation of generations.

heteroxenous p., a p. that has more than one obligatory host in its life cycle.

incidental p., a p. that normally lives on a host other than its present host.

inquiline p., SEE inquiline.

malignant tertian malarial p., SYN Plasmodium falciparum.

obligate p., a p. that cannot lead an independent nonparasitic existence, in contrast to facultative p.

quartan p., SYN Plasmodium malariae.

specific p., a p. that habitually lives in its present host and is particularly adapted for the host species.

stenoxous p., a p. with a narrow or specific host range.

temporary p., an organism accidentally ingested that survives briefly in the intestine.

tertian p., SYN Plasmodium vivax.

par·a·si·te·mia (păr′ă-sī-tē′mē-ă). The presence of parasites in the circulating blood; used especially with reference to malarial and other protozoan forms, and microfilariae.

par·a·sit·ic (par-ă-sit′ik). **1.** Relating to or of the nature of a parasite. **2.** Denoting organisms that normally grow only in or on the living body of a host.

par·a·sit·i·ci·dal (par′ă-sit-i-sī′dăl). Destructive to parasites.

par·a·sit·i·cide (par-ă-sit′i-sīd). An agent that destroys parasites. [parasite + L. *caedo*, to kill]

par·a·sit·ism (par′ă-si-tizm). A symbiotic relationship in which one species (the parasite) benefits at the expense of the other (the host). Cf. mutualism, commensalism, symbiosis, metabiosis.

multiple p., a condition in which parasites of different species parasitize a single host, in contrast to superparasitism (2) or hyperparasitism.

par·a·si·tize (par′ă-si-tīz). To invade as a parasite.

par·a·si·to·ce·nose (par-ă-sī′tō-sē-nōz). Complex of all parasite species and individuals associated with a specific host. SYN parasite-host ecosystem. [parasite + G. *koinos*, common, together]

par·a·si·to·gen·e·sis (par′ă-sī-tō-jen′ĕ-sis). The evolution of relationships between parasite and host.

par·a·si·to·gen·ic (par′-ă-sī-tō-jen′ik). 1. Caused by certain parasites. 2. Favoring parasitism. [parasite + G. *-gen*, producing]

par·a·si·toid (par-ă-sī′toyd). Denoting a feeding relationship intermediate between predation and parasitism, in which the p. eventually destroys its host; refers especially to parasitic wasps (order Hymenoptera) whose larvae feed on and finally destroy a grub or other arthropod host stung by the mother wasp prior to laying its egg(s) on the host. [parasite + G. *eidos*, appearance]

par·a·si·tol·o·gist (par′ă-si-tol′ŏ-jist). One who specializes in the science of parasitology.

par·a·si·tol·o·gy (par′ă-si-tol′ō-jē). The branch of biology and of medicine concerned with all aspects of parasitism. [parasite + G. *logos*, study]

par·a·si·tome (par′ă-sī-tōm). The total mass or number of individuals of all developmental stages of a single parasite species in one host. [parasite + *-ome* (fr. G. *-ōma*), group, mass]

par·a·si·to·pho·bia (par′ă-sī-tō-fō′bē-ă). Morbid fear of parasites. [parasite + G. *phobos*, fear]

par·a·sit·o·sis (par′ă-sī-tō′sis). Infestation or infection with parasites.

par·a·si·to·tro·pic (par′ă-sī-tō-trop′ik). Pertaining to or characterized by parasitotropism.

par·a·si·tot·ro·pism (par′ă-sī-tot′rō-pizm). The special affinity of particular drugs or other agents for parasites rather than for their hosts, including microparasites that infect a larger parasite. Cf. organotropism. SYN parasitotropy. [parasite + G. *tropē*, a turning]

par·a·si·tot·ro·py (par′ă-sī-tot′rō-pē). SYN parasitotropism.

par·a·som·nia (par-ă-som′nē-ă). Any dysfunction associated with sleep, *e.g.*, somnambulism, pavor nocturnus, enureseis, or nocturnal seizures.

par·a·sta·sis (par-ă-stā′sis). A reciprocal relationship among causal mechanisms that can compensate for, or mask defects in, each other; in genetics, a relationship between non-alleles (classified by some as a form of epistasis). [G. standing shoulder to shoulder]

par·a·ster·nal (par-ă-ster′năl). Alongside the sternum.

Par·a·stron·gy·lus (par′a-stron′ji-lus). SYN *Angiostrongylus.*

par·a·stru·ma (par-ă-strū′mă). Obsolete term for a goitrous tumefaction resulting from enlargement of a parathyroid gland. [para- + L. *struma*, a scrofulous tumor]

par·a·sym·pa·thet·ic (par-ă-sim-pa-thet′ik). Pertaining to a division of the autonomic nervous system. SEE autonomic nervous *system.*

par·a·sym·pa·tho·lyt·ic (par-ă-sim′pă-thō-lit′ik). Relating to an agent that annuls or antagonizes the effects of the parasympathetic nervous system; *e.g.*, atropine.

par·a·sym·pa·tho·mi·met·ic (par-ă-sim′pă-thō-mi-met′ik). Relating to drugs or chemicals having an action resembling that caused by stimulation of the parasympathetic nervous system. SEE ALSO cholinomimetic. [para- + G. *sympatheia*, sympathy, + *mimētikos*, imitative]

par·a·sym·pa·tho·to·nia (par-ă-sim′pă-thō-tō′nē-ă). SYN vagotonia.

par·a·sy·nap·sis (par′ă-si-nap′sis). Union of chromosomes side to side in the process of reduction. [para- + G. *synapsis*, a connection, junction]

par·a·sy·no·vi·tis (par′ă-si-nō-vī′tis). Inflammation of the tissues immediately adjacent to a joint. [para- + synovitis]

par·a·syph·i·lis (par-ă-sif′i-lis). Any condition indirectly due to syphilis. SYN metasyphilis (2), parasyphilosis, quaternary syphilis.

par·a·syph·i·lit·ic (par′ă-sif-i-lit′ik). Denoting certain diseases supposed to be indirectly due to syphilis but presenting none of the recognized lesions of that infection. SYN metaluetic (3). SYN metasyphilitic (3).

par·a·syph·i·lo·sis (par′ă-sif-i-lō′sis). SYN parasyphilis.

par·a·sys·to·le (par-ă-sis′tō-lē). A second automatic rhythm existing simultaneously with normal sinus or other dominant rhythm, the parasystolic center being protected from the dominant rhythm's impulses so that its basic rhythm is undisturbed, although it may be manifest in the ECG only at various multiples of its basic periodicity. SYN parasystolic beat. [para- + G. *systolē*, a contracting]

par·a·tax·ia (par-ă-tak′sē-ă). SYN parataxis.

par·a·tax·ic (par-ă-tak′sik). Pertaining to parataxis.

par·a·tax·is (par-ă-tak′sis). The psychological state or repository of attitudes, ideas, and experiences accumulated during personality development that are not effectively assimilated or integrated into the growing mass and residue of the other attitudes, ideas, and experiences of an individual's personality. SYN parataxia. [para- + G. *taxis*, orderly arrangement]

par·a·te·ne·sis (par-ă-te-nē′sis). Passage of an infective agent by one or a series of paratenic hosts in which the agent is transported between hosts but does not undergo further development. [parasite + L. *teneo*, to hold, maintain]

par·a·ten·on (par-ă-ten′on). The tissue, fatty or synovial, between a tendon and its sheath. [para- + G. *tenōn*, tendon]

par·a·ter·mi·nal (par-ă-ter′mi-năl). Near or alongside any terminus.

par·a·thi·on (par-ă-thī′on). Phosporothioic acid *O,O*-diethyl*O*-(4-nitrophenyl) ester; an organic phosphate insecticide, highly toxic to animals and humans, that is an irreversible inhibitor of cholinesterases.

par·a·thor·mone (par-ă-thōr′mōn). SYN parathyroid *hormone.*

par·a·thy·mia (par-ă-thī′mē-ă). Misdirection of the emotional faculties; disordered mood. [para- + G. *thymos*, soul, mind]

par·a·thy·rin (par-ă-thī′rin). SYN parathyroid *hormone.*

par·a·thy·roid (par-ă-thī′royd). 1. Adjacent to the thyroid gland. 2. SYN parathyroid *gland.*

par·a·thy·roid·ec·to·my (pa′ră-thī-roy-dek′to-mē). Excision of the parathyroid glands. [parathyroid + G. *ektomē*, excision]

par·a·thy·ro·tro·pic, par·a·thy·ro·tro·phic (par′ă-thī-rō-trop′ik, -trof′ik). Influencing the growth or activity of the parathyroid glands. [parathyroid + G. *tropē*, a turning; *trophē*, nourishment]

par·a·tope (par′a-tōp). That part of an antibody molecule composed of the variable regions of both the light and heavy chains that combine with the antigen. SYN antibody combining site, antigen-binding site, combining site. [para- + *-tope*]

par·a·tri·cho·sis (par′ă-tri-kō′sis). Any disorder in the growth of the hair, with particular reference to quantity. [para- + G. *trichōsis*, making or being hairy, fr. *thrix* (trich-), hair]

par·a·trip·sis (par′ă-trip′sis). Chafing. [G. friction, fr. *para*, beside, + *tripsis*, rubbing]

par·a·trip·tic (par-ă-trip′tik). Causing or caused by chafing.

par·a·tro·phic (par-ă-trof′ik). Deriving sustenance from living organic material. SEE ALSO metatrophic, prototrophic. [para- + G. *trophē*, nourishment]

par·a·tu·ber·cu·lo·sis (pa-ra-too-ber-kyū-lō′sis). SYN Johne's *disease.*

par·a·typh·li·tis (par′ă-tif-lī′tis). Inflammation of the connective tissue adjacent to the cecum. [para- + G. *typhlon*, cecum, + *-itis*, inflammation]

par·a·ty·phoid (par-ă-tī′foyd). SYN paratyphoid *fever.*

par·a·um·bil·i·cal (par′ă-ŭm-bil′i-kal). Near the umbilicus. SYN paraomphalic, parumbilical.

par·a·u·re·thral (par′ă-yū-rē′thrăl). Alongside the urethra.

par·a·vac·cin·ia (par'ă-vak-sin'ē-ă). SYN milkers' *nodules*, under *nodule*.

par·a·vag·i·nal (par-ă-vaj'i-năl). Alongside the vagina.

par·a·vag·i·ni·tis (par'ă-vaj-i-nī'tis). Inflammation of the connective tissue alongside the vagina. SYN paracolpitis.

par·a·val·vu·lar (par-ă-val'vyū-lăr). Alongside or in the vicinity of a valve.

par·a·ve·nous (par'ă-vē'nŭs). Beside a vein.

par·a·ver·te·bral (par-ă-ver'tĕ-brăl). Alongside a vertebra or the vertebral column.

par·a·ves·i·cal (par-ă-ves'i-kăl). SYN paracystic.

par·ax·i·al (par-ak'sē-ăl). By the side of the axis of any body or part.

par·ax·on (par-ak'son). A collateral branch of an axon. [para- + G. *axōn*, axis]

Par·a·zoa (par-ă-zō'ă). A subkingdom that includes the sponges (phylum Porifera), considered by many zoologists to be intermediate between the subkingdoms Protozoa and Metazoa.

par·a·zo·on (par-ă-zō'on). **1.** An animal parasite. **2.** A member of the subkingdom Parazoa. [para- + G. *zōon*, animal]

parch·ment crack·ling (parch'ment krak'ling). The sensation as of the crackling of stiff paper or parchment, noted on palpation of the skull in cases of craniotabes.

Paré, Ambroise, French surgeon, 1510–1590. SEE P.'s *suture*.

par·ec·ta·sis, par·ec·ta·sia (par-ek'tă-sis, -ek-tă'zē-ă). Obsolete term for extreme distention of a cavity or other part. [G. *parektasis*, extrusion, fr. *para*, beside, + *ektasis*, extension]

par·ec·tro·pia (par-ek-trō'pē-ă). SYN apraxia. [G. *par-ektropē*, a turning aside]

par·e·gor·ic (par-ĕ-gōr'ik). Camphorated opium tincture, an antiperistaltic agent containing powdered opium, anise oil, benzoic acid, camphor, glycerin, and diluted alcohol. [G. *parēgorikos*, soothing]

pa·rei·ra (pă-rā'ē-ră). Pareira brava, the root of *Chondodendron tomentosum* and other species of *Chondodendron* (family Menispermaceae), a vine of tropical America; one of the chief sources of *d*-tubocurarine; it has diuretic and urinary antiseptic properties. [Pg. *parreira*, vine trained against a wall]

par·e·lec·tro·nom·ic (par'ĕ-lek-trō-nom'ik). Not subject to the laws of electricity, *i.e.,* not excited by an electric stimulus. [para- + G. *ēlektron*, amber (electricity), + *nomos*, law]

par·en·ce·pha·lia (par'en-se-fā'lē-ă). Congenital defect of brain. [para- + G. *enkephalos*, brain]

par·en·ceph·a·li·tis (par'en-sef-ă-lī'tis). Inflammation of the cerebellum. [parencephalon + G. *-itis*, inflammation]

par·en·ceph·a·lo·cele (par-en-sef'ă-lō-sēl). Protrusion of the cerebellum through a defect in the cranium. [parencephalon + G. *kēlē*, hernia]

par·en·ceph·a·lous (par-en-sef'ă-lŭs). Relating to parencephalia.

pa·ren·chy·ma (pă-reng'ki-mă). **1.** The distinguishing or specific cells of a gland or organ, contained in and supported by the connective tissue framework, or stroma. **2.** The endoplasm of a protozoan cell. [G. anything poured in beside, fr. *parencheō*, to pour in beside]
   p. tes'tis [NA], the parenchyma of the testis, consisting of the seminiferous tubules located within the lobules.

pa·ren·chy·mal (pă-reng'ki-măl). SYN parenchymatous.

pa·ren·chy·ma·ti·tis (pă-reng'ki-mă-tī'tis). Inflammation of the parenchyma or differentiated substance of a gland or organ.

par·en·chym·a·tous (par'eng-kim'ă-tŭs). Relating to the parenchyma. SYN parenchymal.

par·ent (par'ent). **1.** An individual who has produced at least one offspring through sexual reproduction. **2.** Any source or basis, as for the elaboration of a substance. [L. *parens*, fr. *pario*, to bring forth]

par·en·ter·al (pă-ren'ter-ăl). By some other means than through the gastrointestinal tract; referring particularly to the introduction of substances into an organism by intravenous, subcutaneous,

intramuscular, or intramedullary injection. [para- + G. *enteron*, intestine]

par·ep·i·cele (par-ep'i-sēl). The lateral recess of the fourth ventricle of the brain. [para- + G. *epi*, upon, + *koilia*, a hollow]

par·ep·i·did·y·mis (par'ep'i-did'i-mis). SYN paradidymis.

par·ep·i·thy·mia (par'ep-i-thī'mē-ă). A morbid longing; an abnormal desire or craving. [para- + G. *epithymia*, desire]

par·e·re·thi·sis (par-ĕ-rēth'i-sis). Abnormal or morbid excitement. [para- + G. *erethizō*, to excite]

par·er·ga·sia (par-er-gā'zē-ă). Obsolete term for schizophrenia. [para- + G. *ergasia*, work]

pa·re·sis (pă-rē'sis, par'ĕ-sis). **1.** Partial or incomplete paralysis. **2.** A disease of the brain, syphilitic in origin, marked by progressive dementia, tremor, speech disturbances, and increasing muscular weakness; in a large proportion of cases there is a preliminary stage of irritability often followed by exaltation and delusions of grandeur. SYN Bayle's disease, general p. [G. a letting go, slackening, paralysis, fr. *paritēmi*, to let go]
   general p., SYN paresis (2).
   parturient p., SYN milk *fever* (2).

par·es·the·sia (par-es-thē'zē-ă). An abnormal sensation, such as of burning, pricking, tickling, or tingling. SYN paraesthesia. [para- + G. *aisthēsis*, sensation]

par·es·thet·ic (par-es-thet'ik). Relating to or marked by paresthesia; denoting numbness and tingling in an extremity which usually occurs on the resumption of the blood flow to a nerve following temporary pressure or mild injury.

pa·ret·ic (pa-ret'ik). Relating to or suffering from paresis.

pa·reu·nia (par-yū'nē-ă). SYN coitus. [G. *pareunos*, lying beside, fr. *para*, beside, + *eunē*, a bed]

par·gy·line hy·dro·chlo·ride (par'ji-lēn). *N*-Methyl-*N*-(2-propynyl)-benzylamine hydrochloride; a nonhydrazine monoamine oxidase inhibitor, used as an antihypertensive agent.

par·i·dro·sis (par-i-drō'sis). Any derangement of perspiration. SYN parahidrosis. [para- + G. *hidrōsis*, sweating]

par·i·es, gen. **pa·ri·e·tis,** pl. **pa·ri·e·tes** (par'i-ēz, pā'rī-ēz; pă-rī'ĕ-tēz) [NA]. SYN wall. [L. wall]
   p. ante'rior gas'tris [NA], SYN anterior *wall* of stomach.
   p. ante'rior vagi'nae [NA], SYN anterior *wall* of vagina.
   p. carot'icus ca'vi tym'pani [NA], SYN anterior *wall* of tympanic cavity.
   p. exter'nus duc'tus cochlea'ris [NA], SYN external *wall* of cochlear duct.
   p. infe'rior or'bitae [NA], SYN *floor* of orbit.
   p. jugula'ris ca'vi tym'pani [NA], SYN *floor* of tympanic cavity.
   p. labyrin'thicus ca'vi tym'pani [NA], SYN medial *wall* of tympanic cavity.
   p. latera'lis or'bitae [NA], SYN lateral *wall* of orbit.
   p. mastoi'deus ca'vi tym'pani [NA], SYN posterior *wall* of tympanic cavity.
   p. media'lis or'bitae [NA], SYN medial *wall* of orbit.
   p. membrana'ceus ca'vi tym'pani [NA], SYN lateral *wall* of tympanic cavity.
   p. membrana'ceus tra'cheae [NA], SYN membranous *wall* of trachea.
   p. poste'rior gas'tris [NA], SYN posterior *wall* of stomach.
   p. poste'rior va'ginae [NA], SYN posterior *wall* of vagina.
   p. supe'rior or'bitae [NA], SYN roof of orbit.
   p. tegmenta'lis ca'vi tym'pani [NA], SYN roof of tympanic cavity.
   p. tympan'icus duc'tus cochlea'ris [NA], SYN tympanic *wall* of cochlear duct.
   p. vestibula'ris duc'tus cochlea'ris [NA], SYN vestibular *membrane*.

pa·ri·e·tal (pă-rī'ĕ-tăl). **1.** Relating to the wall of any cavity. **2.** SYN somatic (1). **3.** SYN somatic (2). **4.** Relating to the parietal bone.

pa·ri·e·tes (pă-rī'ĕ-tēz). Plural of paries. [L.]

△**parieto-.** A wall (of the body, *e.g.,* the abdominal wall); a parietal bone. [L. *paries*, wall]

pa·ri·e·to·fron·tal (pa-rī′ĕ-tō-fron′tăl). Relating to the parietal and the frontal bones or the parts of the cerebral cortex corresponding thereto.

pa·ri·e·tog·ra·phy (pa-rī′ĕ-tog′ră-fē). Rarely used term for a radiographic examination of the wall of the stomach using a combination of pneumoperitoneum and intraluminal air and barium. [parieto- + G. *graphē*, a writing]

pa·ri·e·to·mas·toid (pă-rī′ĕ-to-mas′toyd). Relating to the parietal bone and the mastoid portion of the temporal bone.

pa·ri·e·to·oc·cip·i·tal (pă-rī′ĕ-tō-ok-sip′i-tăl). Relating to the parietal and occipital bones or to the parts of the cerebral cortex corresponding thereto.

pa·ri·e·to·sphe·noid (pă-rī′ĕ-tō-sfē′noyd). Relating to the parietal and the sphenoid bones.

pa·ri·e·to·splanch·nic (pă-rī′ĕ-tō-splangk′nik). SYN parietovisceral.

pa·ri·e·to·squa·mo·sal (pă-rī′ĕ-tō-skwā-mō′săl). Relating to the parietal bone and the squamous portion of the temporal bone.

pa·ri·e·to·tem·po·ral (pă-rī′ĕ-tō-tem′pŏ-răl). Relating to the parietal and the temporal bones.

pa·ri·e·to·vis·cer·al (pă-rī′ĕ-tō-vis′er-ăl). Relating to the wall of a cavity and to the contained viscera. SYN parietosplanchnic.

Parinaud, Henri, French ophthalmologist, 1844–1905. SEE P.'s *conjunctivitis*, *ophthalmoplegia*, *syndrome*, oculoglandular *syndrome*.

Par·is green. Cupric acetoarsenite, used as an insecticide and as a pigment.

Par·is yel·low [C.I. 77600]. SYN chrome yellow.

par·i·ty (par′ĭ-tē). The condition of having given birth to an infant or infants, alive or dead; a multiple birth is considered as a single parous experience. [L. *pario*, to bear]

Park, Henry, British surgeon, 1744–1831. SEE P.'s *aneurysm*.

Park, William H., U.S. bacteriologist, 1863–1939. SEE P.-Williams *bacillus*, *fixative*.

Parker, Edward Mason, U.S. surgeon, 1860–1941. SEE P.-Kerr *suture*.

Parkinson, James, British physician, 1755–1824. SEE parkinsonism (1); P.'s *disease*, *facies*.

Parkinson, Sir John, British cardiologist, *1885. SEE Wolff-P.-White *syndrome*.

par·kin·so·ni·an (par-kin-sō′nē-an). Relating to or the suffering from parkinsonism (1).

par·kin·son·ism (par′kin-son-izm). **1.** A neurological syndrome usually resulting from deficiency of the neurotransmitter dopamine as the consequence of degenerative, vascular, or inflammatory changes in the basal ganglia; characterized by rhythmical muscular tremors, rigidity of movement, festination, droopy posture, and masklike facies. SYN Parkinson's disease, shaking palsy, trembling palsy. **2.** A syndrome similar to p. appearing as a side effect of certain antipsychotic drugs. [J. *Parkinson*]

Parnas, Jakob Karol, Polish physiologic chemist, 1884–1955. SEE Embden-Meyerhof-P. *pathway*.

par·oc·cip·i·tal (par′ok-sip′i-tăl). Near or beside the occipital bone or the occiput. [para- + occipital]

par·o·don·ti·tis (par′ō-don-tī′tis). Obsolete term for periodontitis.

pa·ro·don·ti·um (par-ō-don′shē-ŭm). SYN periodontal *ligament*. [para- + G. *odous*, tooth]

par·o·dyn·ia (par-ō-din′ē-ă). SYN labor *pains*, under *pain*. [L. *pario*, to bear, + G. *odynē*, pain]

pa·role (pă-rōl′). In psychiatry, term for conditional release of a formally committed patient from a mental hospital prior to formal discharge, so that the patient may be returned to the hospital if necessary without fresh legal action. [Fr., fr. L. *parabola*, discourse, fr G. *parabolē*]

par·ol·fac·to·ry (par-ol-fak′tōr-ē). Associated with or related to the olfactory system.

par·ol·i·vary (par-ol′i-văr-ē). By the side of or near the oliva. [para- + L. *oliva*, olive]

par·o·mo·my·cin sul·fate (par′ō-mō-mī′sin). A broad spectrum

antibiotic produced by *Streptomyces rimosus* forma *paromomycinus;* used in the treatment of bacterial enteritis and amebiasis, and for preoperative suppression of intestinal bacteria.

par·om·pha·lo·cele (par-om′fă-lō-sēl). **1.** A tumor near the umbilicus. **2.** A hernia through a defect in the abdominal wall near the umbilicus. [para- + G. *omphalos*, umbilicus, + *kēlē*, tumor, hernia]

Parona, Francesco, 19th century Italian surgeon. SEE P.'s *space*.

par·o·nei·ria, par·o·ni·ria (par-ō-nī′rē-ă). Rarely used term for disagreeable or terrifying dreams. [para- + G. *oneiros*, dream]
   p. sa′lax, rarely used term denoting restlessness in sleep, with lascivious dreams and nocturnal emissions.

par·o·nych·ia (par-ō-nik′ē-ă). Suppurative inflammation of the nail fold surrounding the nail plate; may be due to bacteria or fungi, most commonly staphylococci and streptococci. SYN onychia lateralis, onychia periungualis. [para- + G. *onyx*, nail]

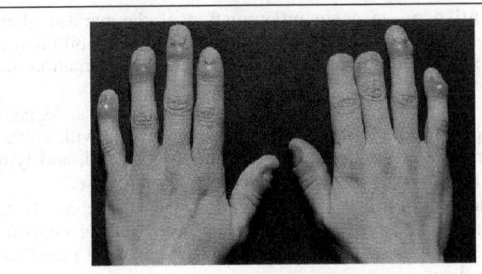

paronychia (chronic form)

par·o·nych·i·al (par-ō-nik′ē-ăl). Relating to paronychia.

par·o·oph·o·ri·tis (par′ō-of′ō-rī′tis). Inflammation of tissues adjacent to the ovaries. [paroophoron + G. *-itis*, inflammation]

par·o·öph·o·ron (par-ō-of′ōr-on) [NA]. Remnants of the tubules and glomeruli of the lower part of the mesonephros appearing as a few scattered tubules in the broad ligament between the epoöphoron and the uterus. Its equivalent in the male is the paradidymis. SYN parovarium. [para- + oophoron, ovary]

par·or·chid·i·um (par-ōr-kid′ē-ŭm). SYN testis *ectopia*. [para- + G. *orchis*, testis]

par·or·chis (par-ōr′kis). SYN epididymis. [para- + G. *orchis*, testis]

par·o·rex·ia (par-ō-rek′sē-ă). An abnormal or disordered appetite. [para- + G. *orexis*, appetite]

par·os·mia (par-oz′mē-ă). Any disorder of the sense of smell, especially subjective perception of nonexistent odors. SYN parosphresia. [para + G. *osmē*, sense of smell]

par·os·phre·sia (par-os-frē′zē-ă). SYN parosmia. [para- + G. *osphrēsis*, smell]

par·os·te·al (par-os′tē-ăl). Relating to the tissues immediately adjacent to the periosteum of a bone.

par·os·te·i·tis (păr-os-tē-ī′tis). Inflammation of the tissues immediately adjacent to a bone. SYN parostitis. [para- + G. *osteon*, bone, + *-itis*, inflammation]

par·os·te·o·sis, par·os·to·sis (par′os-tē-ō′sis, -os-tō′sis). **1.** Development of bone in an unusual location, as in the skin. **2.**

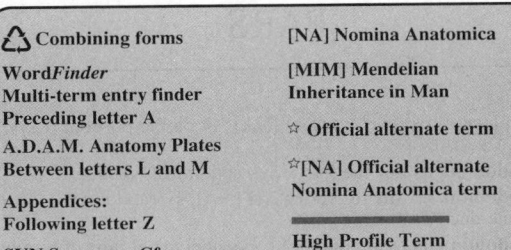

♲ Combining forms	[NA] Nomina Anatomica
WordFinder	[MIM] Mendelian
Multi-term entry finder	Inheritance in Man
Preceding letter A	
A.D.A.M. Anatomy Plates	☆ Official alternate term
Between letters L and M	
	☆[NA] Official alternate
Appendices:	Nomina Anatomica term
Following letter Z	
	High Profile Term
SYN Synonym; Cf., compare	

Abnormal or defective ossification. [para- + G. *osteon*, bone, + *-osis*, condition]

par·os·ti·tis (par-os-tī'tis). SYN parosteitis.

pa·rot·ic (pă-rot'ik). Near or beside the ear. [para- + G. *ous*, ear]

pa·rot·id (pă-rot'id). Situated near the ear; denoting several structures in this neighborhood. Usually refers to the p. salivary gland. [G. *parōtis* (*parōtid-*), the gland beside the ear, fr. *para*, beside, + *ous* (*ōt-*), ear]

pa·rot·i·dec·to·my (pă-rot'i-dek'tō-mē). Surgical removal of the parotid gland. [parotid + G. *ektomē*, excision]

pa·rot·i·di·tis (pă-rot-i-dī'tis). Inflammation of the parotid gland. SYN parotitis.

epidemic p., an acute infectious and contagious disease caused by a Paramyxovirus and characterized by fever, inflammation and swelling of the parotid gland, sometimes of other salivary glands, and occasionally by inflammation of the testis, ovary, pancreas, or meninges. SYN mumps.

postoperative p., an acute inflammation of the parotid gland occurring in the postoperative period, especially in debilitated or dehydrated patients; frequently results in abscess formation and rapidly spreading cellulitis that may become fatal.

punctate p., recurrent or chronic p. with terminal sialectasis, giving a punctate pattern on sialography; associated with epithelial hyperplasia of intralobular ducts, atrophy of acini, and lymphocytic infiltration, characteristic in Sjögren's *disease*.

pa·ro·ti·do·au·ri·cu·la·ris (pă-rot'i-dō-aw-rik-yū-lā'ris). **1.** An occasional band of muscle fibers passing from the surface of the parotid gland to the auricle. **2.** Relating to the parotid gland and the external ear.

par·o·tin (par'ō-tin). A globulin obtained from parotid glands, that causes hypocalcemia, has effects on mesenchymal tissues, produces first leukopenia and then leukocytosis, and promotes calcification of dentin. SYN salivary gland hormone.

par·o·ti·tis (par-o-tī'tis). SYN parotiditis.

par·ous (par'ŭs). Pertaining to parity. [L. *pario*, to bear]

par·o·var·i·an (par-ō-var'ē-an). **1.** Relating to the paroöphoron. **2.** Beside or in the neighborhood of the ovary. SYN paraovarian.

par·o·var·i·ot·o·my (par'ō-var-ē-ot'ō-mē). Incision into or removal of a tumor of the parovarium. [parovarium + G. *tomē*, incision]

par·o·va·ri·tis (par'ō-var-ī'tis). Inflammation of the parovarium.

par·o·var·i·um (par-ō-var'ē-ŭm). SYN paroöphoron. [para- + L. *ovarium*, ovary]

par·ox·y·pro·pi·one (par-ok-si-prō'pē-ōn). *p*-Hydroxypropiophenone; an inhibitor of pituitary gonadotropic hormone.

par·ox·ysm (par'ok-sizm). **1.** A sharp spasm or convulsion. **2.** A sudden onset of a symptom or disease, especially one with recurrent manifestations such as the chills and rigor of malaria. [G. *paroxysmos*, fr. *paroxynō*, to sharpen, irritate, fr. *oxys*, sharp]

par·ox·ys·mal (par-ok-siz'măl). Relating to or occurring in paroxysms.

par·ri·cide (par'i-sīd). **1.** The killing of one's parent (patricide or matricide). **2.** One who commits such an act. [L. *parricidium*, killing of close kin]

Parrot, Jules, French physician, 1829–1883. SEE P.'s *disease*.

Parry, Caleb H., English physician, 1755–1822. SEE P.'s *disease*.

PARS

pars, pl. **par·tes** (pars, par'tēz) [NA]. A part; a portion. [L. *pars* (*part-*) a part]

p. abdomina′lis aor′tae [NA], SYN abdominal *aorta*.

p. abdomina′lis duc′tus thora′cici [NA], SYN abdominal *part* of thoracic duct.

p. abdomina′lis esoph′agi [NA], SYN abdominal *part* of esophagus.

p. abdomina′lis ure′teris [NA], SYN abdominal *part* of ureter.

p. ala′ris mus′culi nasa′lis [NA], SYN alar *part* of nasalis muscle. SEE nasalis *muscle*.

p. alveola′ris mandib′ulae [NA], SYN alveolar *part* of mandible.

p. amor′pha, the part of the nucleolus that occupies irregular spaces in the nucleolonema and contains finely filamentous substance. SEE ALSO p. granulosa.

p. annula′ris vagi′nae fibro′sae [NA], SYN annular *part* of fibrous digital sheath.

p. ante′rior [NA], SYN anterior *part*.

p. ante′rior commissu′rae anterio′ris cere′bri, SYN anterior *part* of anterior commissure of brain.

p. ante′rior commissu′rae rostra′lis [NA], ☆official alternate term for anterior *part* of anterior commissure of brain.

p. ante′rior facie′i diaphrag′matis hepa′tis [NA], SYN anterior *part* of diaphragmatic surface of liver.

p. ante′rior for′nicis vagi′nae [NA], SYN anterior *part* of fornix of vagina.

p. ascen′dens aor′tae, SYN ascending *aorta*.

p. ascen′dens duode′ni, SYN ascending *part* of duodenum.

p. atlan′tica [NA], SEE vertebral *artery*.

p. autonom′ica [NA], SYN autonomic nervous *system*.

p. basa′lis arte′riae pulmona′lis [NA], SEE right pulmonary *artery*, left pulmonary *artery*.

p. basila′ris os′sis occipita′lis [NA], SYN basilar *part* of the occipital bone.

p. basila′ris pon′tis, SYN ventral *part* of pons.

p. buccopharyn′gea mu′sculi constricto′ris phary′ngei superio′ris [NA], SYN buccopharyngeal *part* of superior pharyngeal constrictor. SEE superior constrictor *muscle* of pharynx.

p. cardi′aca gas′tris [NA], SYN cardiac *part* of stomach.

p. cardi′aca ventric′uli [NA], ☆official alternate term for cardiac *part* of stomach.

p. cartilagin′ea sep′ti na′si, SYN nasal septal *cartilage*.

p. cartilagin′ea tu′bae auditi′vae [NA], SYN cartilaginous *part* of auditory tube.

p. cartilagino′sa system′atis skeleta′lis [NA], SYN cartilaginous *part* of skeletal system.

p. caverno′sa, SYN spongy *urethra*.

p. caverno′sa arte′riae caro′tidis inter′nae [NA], SYN cavernous *part* of internal carotid artery.

p. ce′ca ret′inae, the embryological anterior part of the retina that evolves into the p. ciliaris retinae and p. iridica retinae.

p. centra′lis [NA], SYN central nervous *system*.

p. centra′lis ventric′uli latera′lis [NA], the body of the lateral ventricle of the brain, extending from the interventricular foramen (of Monro) to the collateral trigone (*i.e.*, junction of posterior and inferior horns). SYN cella media.

p. ceratopharyn′gea mu′sculi constricto′ris phary′ngis me′dii [NA], SYN ceratopharyngeal *part* of middle pharyngeal constrictor. SEE middle constrictor *muscle* of pharynx.

p. cerebra′lis arte′riae caro′tidis inter′nae [NA], SYN cerebral *part* of internal carotid artery.

p. cervica′lis arte′riae caro′tidis inter′nae, SYN cervical *part* of internal carotid artery.

p. cervica′lis duc′tus thora′cici, SYN cervical *part* of thoracic duct.

p. cervica′lis esoph′agi, SYN cervical *part* of esophagus.

p. cervica′lis medul′lae spina′lis, SYN cervical *part* of spinal cord.

p. chondropharyn′gea muscu′li constricto′ris pharynge′a me′di′i [NA], SYN chondropharyngeal *part* of middle pharyngeal constrictor. SEE middle constrictor *muscle* of pharynx.

p. cilia′ris ret′inae [NA], SYN ciliary *part* of retina. SEE retina.

p. clavicula′ris mus′culi pectora′lis major′is [NA], SYN clavicular *part* of pectoralis major muscle. SEE pectoralis major *muscle*.

p. coccyg′ea medul′lae spina′lis [NA], SYN coccygeal *part* of spinal cord.

p. cochlea′ris ner′vi vestibulocochlea′ris [NA], SYN cochlear *nerve*.

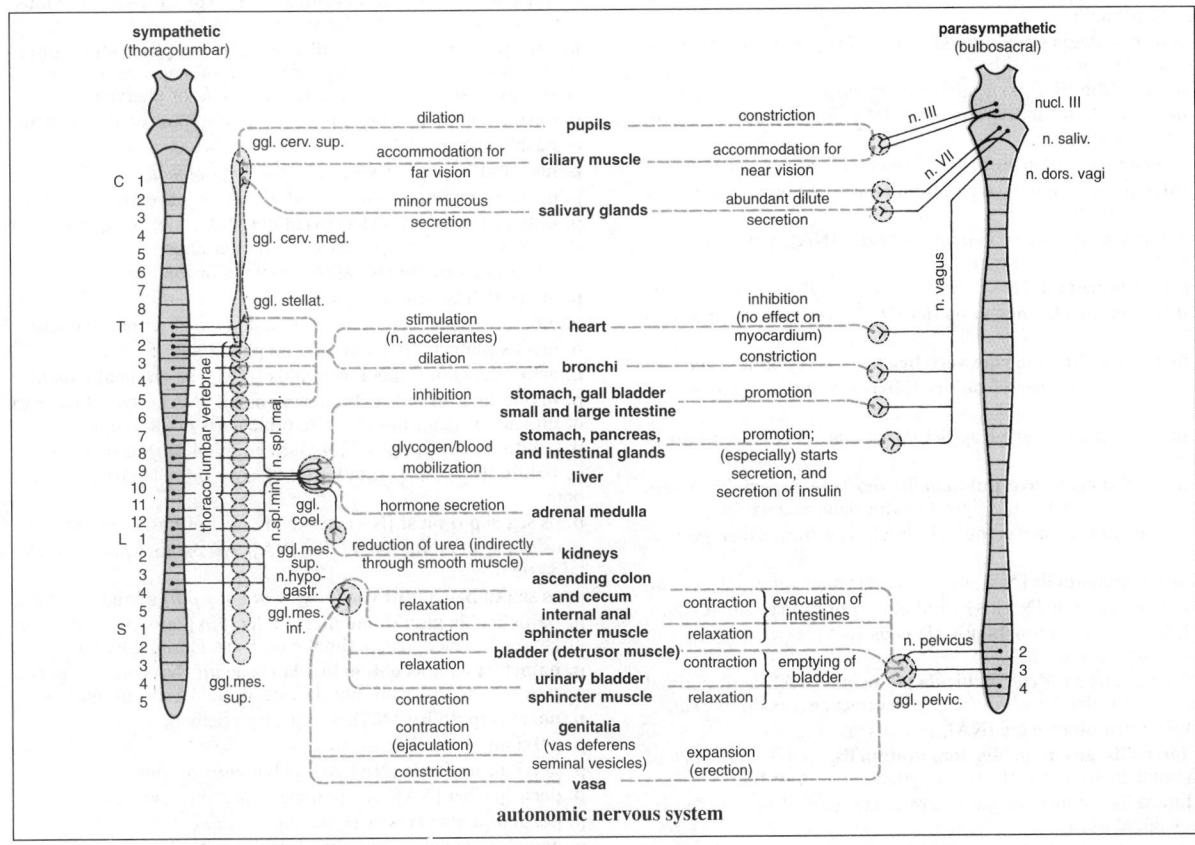

autonomic nervous system

p. convolu′ta lo′buli cortica′lis re′nis [NA], SYN convoluted *part* of kidney lobule.

p. corneoscle′ra′lis reti′culi trabecula′ris [NA], SYN corneoscleral *part* of trabecular reticulum.

par′tes cor′poris huma′ni [NA], SYN *parts* of human body, under *part*.

p. cortica′lis [NA], SYN cortical *part*. SEE middle cerebral *artery*, posterior cerebral *artery*.

p. cortica′lis arteri′ae cerebra′lis medi′ae [NA], ⋆official alternate term for cortical *part* of middle cerebral artery. SEE middle cerebral *artery*.

p. costa′lis diaphrag′matis [NA], SYN costal *part* of diaphragm.

p. cricopharyn′gea mus′culi constricto′ris pharyn′gis inferio′ris [NA], SYN cricopharyngeal *part* of inferior pharyngeal constrictor. SEE inferior constrictor *muscle* of pharynx.

p. crucifor′mis vagi′nae fibro′sae [NA], SYN cruciform *part* of fibrous digital sheath.

p. cupula′ris reces′sus epitympan′ici [NA], SYN cupular *part* of epitympanic recess.

p. cys′tica, the smaller caudal division of the primitive embryonic hepatic bud, developing into the gallbladder and cystic duct.

p. descen′dens aor′tae [NA], SYN descending *aorta*.

p. descen′dens duode′ni, SYN descending *part* of duodenum. SEE duodenum.

p. dex′tra facie′i diaphragma′ticae hepa′tis [NA], SYN right *part* of diaphragmatic surface of liver.

p. dista′lis [NA], SYN distal *part* of anterior lobe of hypophysis.

p. dorsa′lis pon′tis [NA], SYN dorsal *part* of pons.

p. endocri′na pancrea′tis, SEE pancreas.

p. exocri′na pancrea′tis, SYN exocrine *part* of pancreas. SEE pancreas.

p. feta′lis placen′tae [NA], SYN fetal *placenta*.

p. flac′cida membra′nae tym′pani [NA], SYN flaccid *part* of tympanic membrane.

p. fronta′lis cor′poris callo′si, SYN minor *forceps*.

par′tes genita′les femini′nae exter′nae, outmoded term for external female genital *organs*, under *organ*.

par′tes genita′les masculi′nae exter′nae, outmoded term for external male genital *organs*, under *organ*.

p. glossopharyn′gea mus′culi constricto′ris pharyn′gis superi′or′is [NA], SYN glossopharyngeal *part* of superior pharyngeal constrictor. SEE superior constrictor *muscle* of pharynx.

p. granulo′sa, the granular and filamentous part of the nucleolonema of the nucleolus.

p. hepat′ica, the larger cranial division of the primitive embryonic hepatic bud, developing into the liver proper.

p. horizonta′lis duode′ni [NA], SYN horizontal *part* of duodenum. SEE duodenum.

p. infe′rior [NA], SYN inferior *part*.

p. infe′rior duode′ni, SYN horizontal *part* of duodenum.

p. infe′rior gang′lii vestibula′ris [NA], SYN inferior *part* of vestibular ganglion.

p. infe′rior ra′mi lingula′ris, ⋆official alternate term for inferior *part* of lingular branch of left pulmonary vein.

p. infraclavicula′ris plex′us brachia′lis [NA], SYN infraclavicular *part* of brachial plexus.

p. infraloba′ris ra′mi posterio′ris ve′nae pulmona′lis dex′trae [NA], SYN infralobar *part* of posterior branch of right pulmonary vein.

p. infrasegmenta′lis, SYN intersegmental *veins*, under *vein*.

p. infundibula′ris, SYN p. tuberalis.

p. insula′ris [NA], SYN insular *part*.

p. insularis arte′riae cerebra′lis me′diae, SYN insular *part* of middle cerebral artery. SEE middle cerebral *artery*.

p. interarticula′ris (in-ter-ar-tik′u-lar-is), the segment of bone between the superior and inferior articular facets, especially in the lumbar spine.

p. intercartilagin′ea ri′mae glot′tidis [NA], SYN intercartilaginous *part* of rima glottidis.

p. interme′dia [NA], SYN intermediate *part*.

p. interme′dia adenohypophys′eos [NA], SYN intermediate *part* of adenohypophysis.

p. interme′dia bulbo′rum, SYN *commissure* of vestibular bulb.

p. interme′dia commissu′ra bulbo′rum [NA], SYN *commissure* of vestibular bulb.

p. intermembrana′cea ri′mae glot′tidis [NA], SYN intermembranous *part* of rima glottidis.

p. intersegmenta′lis [NA], SYN infrasegmental *veins*, under *vein*.

p. intracanalic′ulus ner′vi op′tici [NA], SYN intracanicular *part* of optic nerve.

p. intracrania′lis arte′riae vertebra′lis, SEE vertebral *artery*.

p. intracrania′lis ner′vi op′tici [NA], SYN intracranial *part* of optic nerve.

p. intralamina′ris ner′vi op′tici [NA], SYN intralaminar *part* of optic nerve.

p. intraloba′ris ve′nae pulmona′lis dex′trae superio′ris [NA], SYN intralobar *part* of the right superior pulmonary vein.

p. intraocula′ris ner′vi op′tici [NA], SYN intraocular *part* of optic nerve.

p. intrasegmenta′lis [NA], SYN intrasegmental *veins*, under *vein*.

p. irid′ica ret′inae [NA], SYN iridial *part* of retina. SEE retina.

p. labia′lis mus′culi orbicula′ris o′ris [NA], SYN labial *part* of orbicularis oris muscle.

p. lacrima′lis mus′culi orbicula′ris oc′uli [NA], SYN lacrimal *part* of orbicularis oculi muscle. SEE orbicularis oculi *muscle*.

p. laryn′gea pharyn′gis [NA], SYN laryngopharynx.

p. latera′lis ar′cus pe′dis longitudina′lis, SYN lateral *part* of longitudinal arch of foot. SEE longitudinal *arch* of foot.

p. latera′lis for′nicis va′ginae, SYN lateral *part* of vaginal fornix. SEE vaginal *fornix*.

p. latera′lis mus′culorum intertransversa′riorum posterio′rum cer′vicis, SYN lateral *part* of posterior cervical intertransversarii muscles. SEE posterior cervical intertransversarii *muscles*, under *muscle*.

p. latera′lis os′sis occipita′lis [NA], SYN lateral *part* of occipital bone.

p. latera′lis os′sis sa′cri [NA], SYN lateral *part* of sacrum.

p. latera′lis ra′mi lo′bi medi′i ve′nae pulmona′lis dex′ter superi′or [NA], SYN lateral *part* of middle lobar branch of right superior pulmonary vein.

p. lumba′lis diaphrag′matis [NA], SYN lumbar *part* of diaphragm.

p. lumba′lis medul′lae spina′lis [NA], SYN lumbar *part*.

p. margina′lis mus′culi orbicula′ris o′ris [NA], SYN marginal *part* of orbicularis oris muscle.

p. mastoi′dea os′sis tempora′lis [NA], SYN mastoid *part* of the temporal bone.

p. media′lis ar′cus pe′dis longitudina′lis, SYN medial *part* of longitudinal arch of foot. SEE longitudinal *arch* of foot.

p. media′lis mus′culorum intertransversa′riorum posterior′um cer′vicis, SYN medial *part* of posterior cervical intertransversarii muscles. SEE posterior cervical intertransversarii *muscles*, under *muscle*.

p. media′lis ra′mi lobi′i me′dii ve′nae pulmo′nis dex′trae superio′ris [NA], SYN medial *part* of middle lobar branch of right superior pulmonary vein.

p. mediastina′lis pulmo′nis [NA], SYN mediastinal *surface* of lung.

p. membrana′cea sep′ti atrio′rum, SYN atrioventricular *septum*.

p. membrana′cea sep′ti interventricula′ris [NA], SYN membranous *part* of interventricular septum.

p. membrana′cea sep′ti na′si [NA], SYN membranous *part* of nasal septum.

p. membrana′cea ure′thrae masculi′nae [NA], SYN membranous *part* of male urethra.

p. mo′bilis sep′ti na′si [NA], SYN mobile *part* of nasal septum.

p. muscula′ris sep′ti interventricula′ris cor′dis [NA], SYN muscular *part* of interventricular septum of heart.

p. mylopharyn′geus mus′culi constricto′ris pharyn′gis superio′ris [NA], SYN mylopharyngeal *part* of superior pharyngeal constrictor. SEE superior constrictor *muscle* of pharynx.

p. nasa′lis os′sis fronta′lis [NA], SYN nasal *part* of frontal bone.

p. nasa′lis pharyn′gis [NA], SYN nasopharynx.

p. nervo′sa hypophys′eos, SYN neurohypophysis.

p. nervo′sa ret′inae [NA], SYN nervous *part* of retina. SEE retina.

p. obli′qua mus′culi cricothyroi′dei [NA], SYN oblique *part* of cricothyroid muscle. SEE cricothyroid *muscle*.

p. occipita′lis cor′poris callo′si, SYN major *forceps*.

p. opercula′ris, SYN opercular *part*.

p. op′tica ret′inae [NA], SYN cerebral *layer* of retina. SEE retina.

p. ora′lis pharyn′gis [NA], SYN oropharynx.

p. orbita′lis glan′dulae lacrima′lis [NA], SEE lacrimal *gland*.

p. orbita′lis mus′culi orbicula′ris oc′uli [NA], SYN orbital part of orbicularis oculi muscle. SEE orbicularis oculi *muscle*.

p. orbita′lis ner′vi op′tici [NA], SYN orbital *part* of optic nerve.

p. orbita′lis os′sis fronta′lis [NA], SYN orbital *part* of frontal bone.

p. os′sea sep′ti na′si [NA], SYN bony *part* of nasal septum.

p. os′sea system′atis skeleta′lis [NA], SYN osseous *part* of skeletal system.

p. os′sea tu′bae audeti′vae [NA], SYN bony *part* of auditory tube.

p. palpebra′lis glan′dulae lacrima′lis [NA], SYN palpebral *part* of lacrimal gland. SEE lacrimal *gland*. SEE lacrimal *gland*.

p. palpebra′lis mus′culi orbicula′ris oc′uli [NA], SYN palpebral *part* of orbicularis oculi muscle. SEE orbicularis oculi *muscle*.

p. parasympath′ica [NA], SYN parasympathetic *part*.

p. pelvi′na, SYN pelvic *part*.

p. pelvi′na ure′teris [NA], SYN pelvic *part* of ureter.

p. peripher′ica [NA], SYN peripheral nervous *system*.

p. perpendicula′ris, SYN perpendicular *plate*.

p. petro′sa arte′riae caro′tidis inter′nae [NA], SYN petrous *part* of internal carotid artery. SEE internal carotid *artery*.

p. petro′sa os′sis tempora′lis [NA], SYN petrous *part* of temporal bone. SEE temporal *bone*.

p. phal′lica, the lower portion of the urogenital sinus, related to the base of the genital tubercle.

p. pharyn′gea hypophys′eos, SYN pharyngeal *hypophysis*.

p. pigmento′sa [NA], SYN pigmented *part* of retina. SEE retina. SYN pigment epithelium of optic retina.

p. pla′na, SYN orbiculus ciliaris.

p. postcommunica′lis arte′ria cere′bri anteri′or [NA], SYN pericallosal *artery*.

p. poste′rior commissu′rae anterio′ris, the posterior portion of the anterior commissure of the brain.

p. poste′rior facie′i diaphrag′matis hep′atis [NA], SYN posterior *part* of the diaphragmatic surface of the liver.

p. poste′rior for′nicis vagi′nae, SEE vaginal *fornix*.

p. postlamina′ris ner′vi op′tici [NA], SYN postlaminar *part* of optic nerve.

p. postsulca′lis [NA], SEE *dorsum* of tongue.

p. precommunica′lis arteri′ae cere′bri anteri′or [NA], SYN precommunical *part* of anterior cerebral artery. SEE anterior cerebral *artery*.

p. prelamina′ris ner′vi op′tici [NA], SYN prelaminar *part* of optic nerve.

p. presulca′lis [NA], SEE *dorsum* of tongue.

p. profun′da glan′dulae parotid′eae [NA], SEE parotid *gland*.

p. profun′da mus′culi masse′teri [NA], SYN deep *part* of masseter muscle.

p. profun′da mus′culi sphinc′teri a′ni exter′ni [NA], SYN deep *part* of external anal sphincter. SEE external anal *sphincter*.

p. prostat′ica ure′thrae [NA], SYN prostatic *urethra*.

p. pterygopharyn′gea mus′culi constricto′ris pharyn′gis superio′ris [NA], SYN pterygopharyngeal *part* of superior constrictor muscle of pharynx. SEE superior constrictor *muscle* of pharynx.

p. pylo'rica gas'tris [NA], SYN pyloric *part* of stomach.

p. pylo'rica ventric'uli [NA], ✫official alternate term for pyloric *part* of stomach.

p. quadra'ta hepa'tis [NA], SYN quadrate *part* of liver.

p. radia'ta lo'buli cortica'lis re'nis [NA], SYN medullary *ray*.

p. rec'ta mus'culi cricothyroi'dei [NA], SEE cricothyroid *muscle*.

p. retrolentifor'mis cap'sulae inter'nae [NA], SYN retrolenticular *part* of internal capsule.

p. sacra'lis medul'lae spina'lis [NA], SYN sacral *part* of spinal cord.

p. sella'ris, SYN *sella* turcica.

p. sphenoida'lis arteri'ae cerebra'lis me'diae [NA], SYN sphenoidal *part* of middle cerebral artery. SEE middle cerebral *artery*.

p. spina'lis ner'vi accesso'rii, ✫official alternate term for spinal *root* of accessory nerve.

p. spongio'sa ure'thrae masculi'nae [NA], SYN spongy *urethra*.

p. squamo'sa os'sis tempora'lis [NA], SYN squamous *part* of temporal bone.

p. sterna'lis diaphrag'matis [NA], SYN sternal *part* of diaphragm.

p. sternocosta'lis mus'culi pectora'lis majo'ris [NA], SYN sternocostal *part* of pectoralis major muscle. SEE pectoralis major *muscle*.

p. subcuta'nea mus'culi sphinc'teri a'ni exter'ni [NA], SYN subcutaneous *part* of external anal sphincter. SEE external anal *sphincter*.

p. sublentifor'mis cap'sulae inter'nae [NA], SYN sublenticular *part* of internal capsule.

p. superficia'lis glan'dulae parotid'eae, SYN superficial *part* of parotid gland. SEE parotid *gland*.

p. superficia'lis mus'culi masse'teri, SYN superficial *part* of masseter muscle. SEE masseter *muscle*.

p. superficia'lis mus'culi sphinc'teri a'ni exter'ni, SYN superficial *part* of external anal sphincter. SEE external anal *sphincter*.

p. supe'rior duode'ni [NA], SYN superior *part* of duodenum. SEE duodenum.

p. supe'rior facie'i diaphrag'maticae hep'atis, SYN superior *part* of diaphragmatic surface of liver.

p. supe'rior gan'glii vestibula'ris [NA], SYN superior *part* of vestibular ganglion.

p. supe'rior ra'mi lingula'ris ve'nae pulmo'nis sin'istri [NA], SYN superior *part* of lingular branch of left pulmonary vein.

p. supraclavicula'ris plex'us brachia'lis [NA], SYN supraclavicular *part* of brachial plexus.

p. sympath'ica [NA], SYN sympathetic nervous *system*.

p. tec'ta, obsolete term; **p. tecta duodeni,** the part of duodenum covered by the root of the transverse mesocolon, the coalescence of the ascending mesocolon, and the root of the mesentery; **p. tecta pancreatis,** hidden portion of the pancreas; part of the pancreas covered by the root of the transverse mesocolon, the coalescence of the ascending mesocolon, and the root of the mesentery; **p. tecta renalis,** hidden portion of the kidney; part of the kidney covered by the root of the transverse mesocolon; **p. tecta ureteralis,** hidden portion of the ureter; part of the right ureter covered (crossed) by the root of the mesentery, and of the left ureter covered (crossed) by the root of the sigmoid mesocolon. SYN hidden part.

p. ten'sa membra'nae tym'pani [NA], SYN tense *part* of the tympanic membrane.

p. termina'lis [NA], SEE middle cerebral *artery*, posterior cerebral *artery*. SYN terminal part.

p. thorac'ica aor'tae [NA], SYN thoracic *aorta*.

p. thorac'ica duc'tus thorac'ici [NA], SYN thoracic *part* of thoracic duct. SEE thoracic *duct*.

p. thorac'ica esoph'agi [NA], SYN thoracic *part* of esophagus.

p. thorac'ica medul'lae spina'lis [NA], SYN thoracic *part* of spinal cord.

p. thyropharyn'gea mus'culi constricto'ris pharyn'gis inferio'ris [NA], SYN thyropharyngeal *part* of inferior pharyngeal constrictor muscle. SEE inferior constrictor *muscle* of pharynx.

p. tibiocalca'nea ligamen'ti media'lis [NA], SYN tibiocalcaneal *ligament*.

p. tibionavicula'ris ligamen'ti media'lis [NA], SYN tibionavicular *ligament*.

p. tibiotala'ris ante'rior ligamen'ti media'lis [NA], SYN anterior tibiotalar *ligament*.

p. tibiotala'ris poste'rior ligamen'ti media'lis [NA], SYN posterior tibiotalar *ligament*.

p. transver'sa mus'culi nasa'lis [NA], SYN transverse *part* of nasalis muscle. SEE nasalis *muscle*.

p. transver'sa ra'mi si'nistri ve'nae por'tae hepa'tis [NA], SYN transverse *part* of left branch of portal vein.

p. transversa'ria arte'riae vertebra'lis [NA], SEE vertebral *artery*.

p. triangula'ris, SYN triangular *part*.

p. tubera'lis [NA], the upward extension of the anterior lobe that wraps around the infundibular stalk; its cells, mostly gonadotropic, are arranged in cords and clusters; it is supplied by the superior hypophyseal arteries and contains the first capillary bed and the venules of a portal system that carries neurosecretory factors from the hypothalamus to a second capillary bed in the adenohypophysis where they regulate the release of hormones. SEE ALSO hypophysis. SYN infundibular part, p. infundibularis.

p. tympan'ica os'sis tempora'lis [NA], SYN tympanic *plate* of temporal bone.

p. umbilica'lis ra'mi si'nistri ve'nae por'tae hepa'tis [NA], SYN umbilical *part* of left branch of portal vein.

p. uteri'na placen'tae [NA], the part of the placenta derived from the uterine tissue. SEE ALSO placenta. SYN maternal placenta, placenta uterina.

p. uteri'na tu'bae uteri'nae [NA], SYN uterine *part* of uterine tube.

p. uvea'lis reti'culi trabecula'ris [NA], SYN uveal *part* of trabecular reticulum.

p. vaga'lis ner'vi accesso'rii [NA], SYN cranial *root* of accessory nerve.

p. ventra'lis pon'tis [NA], SYN ventral *part* of pons.

p. vertebra'lis fa'ciei costa'lis pulmo'nis [NA], SYN vertebral *part* of the costal surface of the lungs.

p. vestibula'ris ner'vi vestibulocochlea'ris [NA], SYN vestibular *nerve*.

pars-pla·ni·tis (parz'plā-nī'tis). A clinical syndrome consisting of inflammation of the peripheral retina and/or pars plana, exudation into the overlying vitreous base, and edema of the optic disk and adjacent retina.

part. A portion.

abdominal p. of aorta, SYN abdominal *aorta*.

abdominal p. of esophagus, the part of the esophagus inferior to the diaphragm. SEE esophagus. SYN pars abdominalis esophagi [NA].

abdominal p. of thoracic duct, the part of the thoracic duct between the cisterna chyli and the aortic hiatus of the diaphragm. SYN pars abdominalis ductus thoracici [NA].

abdominal p. of ureter, the part of the ureter between the renal pelvis and the brim of the pelvis. SYN pars abdominalis ureteris [NA].

alar p. of nasalis muscle, SEE nasalis *muscle*. SYN pars alaris musculi nasalis [NA].

alveolar p. of mandible, the portion of the body of the mandible that surrounds and supports the lower teeth. SYN pars alveolaris mandibulae [NA].

annular p. of fibrous digital sheath, one of the two circular fibrous bands of the fibrous sheaths of the fingers and toes attached to the shaft of the proximal and middle phalanges. SYN pars annularis vaginae fibrosae [NA], annular pulley, annulus of fibrous sheath, ligamentum annulare digitorum.

anterior p., the portion of a structure that tlies most forward, or closest to the front surface relative to other parts; in human anatomy, the ventral portion of a structure. SEE anterior p. of anterior commissure of brain, anterior p. of diaphragmatic surface of liver, anterior p. of fornix of vagina. SYN pars anterior [NA].

anterior p. of anterior commissure of brain, the anterior part of the anterior or rostral commissure of the brain; SYN pars anterior commissurae rostralis✶ [NA], pars anterior commissurae anterioris cerebri.

anterior p. of diaphragmatic surface of liver, the part of the diaphragmatic surface of the liver deep to the costal arches and the xiphoid process. SYN pars anterior faciei diaphragmatis hepatis [NA].

anterior p. of fornix of vagina, the portion of the fornix of the vagina anterior to the uterine cervix. SYN pars anterior fornicis vaginae [NA].

anterior p. of pons, SYN ventral p. of pons.

anterior tibiotalar p. of deltoid ligament, SYN anterior tibiotalar *ligament.*

ascending p. of aorta, SYN ascending *aorta.*

ascending p. of duodenum, the terminal or fourth p. of the duodenum, ascending from the horizontal p. to the jejunum. SYN pars ascendens duodeni.

atlantic p. of vertebral artery, suboccipital part of vertebral artery. SEE vertebral *artery.*

autonomic p., SYN autonomic nervous *system.*

basal p. of occipital bone, SYN basilar p. of the occipital bone.

basal p. of pulmonary artery, SEE right pulmonary *artery,* left pulmonary *artery.*

basilar p. of the occipital bone, the part of the occipital bone that lies anterior to the foramen magnum and joins with the body of the sphenoid bone. SYN pars basilaris ossis occipitalis [NA], basal p. of occipital bone, basilar apophysis, basilar process of occipital bone, basilar process, basiocciput.

basilar p. of pons, SYN ventral p. of pons.

bony p. of auditory tube, the portion of the auditory tube that passes from the tympanic cavity anteromedially through the semicanal for auditory tube. SYN pars ossea tubae auditivae [NA].

bony p. of external acoustic meatus, the medial two-thirds of the external acoustic meatus which is formed as the tympanic plate of the temporal bone develops; it extends approximately 16 mm. from its junction with the cartilaginous part to the tympanic membrane.

bony p. of nasal septum, the major portion of the nasal septum supported by the vomer and the perpendicular plate of the ethmoid. SYN pars ossea septi nasi [NA].

buccopharyngeal p. of superior pharyngeal constrictor, SEE superior constrictor *muscle* of pharynx. SYN pars buccopharyngea musculi constrictoris pharyngei superioris [NA].

cardiac p. of stomach, the area of the stomach close to the esophageal opening (cardiac orifice or cardia) which contains the cardiac glands. SYN pars cardiaca gastris [NA], pars cardiaca ventriculi✶ [NA], cardia, gastric cardia.

cartilaginous p. of auditory tube, that portion of the auditory tube that is supported by cartilage; it continues anteromedially from the osseous part to open into the nasopharynx. SYN pars cartilaginea tubae auditivae [NA].

cartilaginous p. of external acoustic meatus, the lateral third of the external acoustic meatus which is continuous with the auricular cartilage and attached to the circumference of the bony part.

cartilaginous p. of skeletal system, the part of the skeleton composed of cartilage. SYN pars cartilaginosa systematis skeletalis [NA].

cavernous p. of internal carotid artery, the tortuous portion of the internal carotid artery located within the cavernous sinus; it has numerous small branches. SYN pars cavernosa arteriae carotidis internae [NA].

ceratopharyngeal p. of middle pharyngeal constrictor, SEE middle constrictor *muscle* of pharynx. SYN pars ceratopharyngea musculi constrictoris pharyngis medii [NA].

cerebral p. of arachnoid, SYN *arachnoid* of brain.

cerebral p. of dura mater, SYN *dura mater* of brain.

cerebral p. of internal carotid artery, the portion of the internal carotid artery that supplies the brain; its branches are: superior hypophyseal, clival, ophthalmic, anterior choroidal, anterior cerebral, and middle cerebral. SYN pars cerebralis arteriae carotidis internae [NA].

cervical p. of esophagus, the p. of the esophagus located in the neck. SEE esophagus. SYN pars cervicalis esophagi.

cervical p. of internal carotid artery, the unbranched portion located in the neck. SYN pars cervicalis arteriae carotidis internae.

cervical p. of spinal cord, the p. of the spinal cord that consists of the eight cervical segments and gives rise to the first eight pairs of spinal nerves. SYN pars cervicalis medullae spinalis.

cervical p. of thoracic duct, the portion of the thoracic duct above the first rib. SYN pars cervicalis ductus thoracici.

chondropharyngeal p. of middle pharyngeal constrictor, SEE middle constrictor *muscle* of pharynx. SYN pars chondropharyngea musculi constrictoris pharyngea medii [NA].

ciliary p. of retina, SYN pars ciliaris retinae [NA]. SEE retina.

clavicular p. of pectoralis major muscle, SYN pars clavicularis musculi pectoralis majoris [NA], clavicular head of pectoralis major muscle. SEE pectoralis major *muscle.*

coccygeal p. of spinal cord, the terminal part of the spinal cord consisting of the three coccygeal segments of the spinal cord from which the three pairs of coccygeal nerves originate. SYN pars coccygea medullae spinalis [NA], segmenta medullae spinalis coccygea.

cochlear p. of vestibulocochlear nerve, SYN cochlear *nerve.*

convoluted p. of kidney lobule, proximal and distal convoluted tubules and the associated renal corpuscles supplied by branches of the interlobular arteries. SYN labyrinthus [NA], pars convoluta lobuli corticalis renis [NA], labyrinth (3), Ludwig's labyrinth, renal labyrinth.

corneoscleral p. of trabecular reticulum, the anterior part of the trabecular reticulum, located between the sinus venosus sclerae, the scleral spur, and the posterior limiting membrane of the cornea. SYN pars corneoscleralis reticuli trabecularis [NA].

cortical p., SYN pars corticalis [NA]. SEE middle cerebral *artery,* posterior cerebral *artery.*

cortical p. of middle cerebral artery, SEE middle cerebral *artery.* SYN pars corticalis arteriae cerebralis mediae✶ [NA].

costal p. of diaphragm, the part of the diaphragm that arises from the inner aspect of the lower six costal cartilages and the lower four ribs and inserts on the anterolateral part of the central tendon. SYN pars costalis diaphragmatis [NA].

cricopharyngeal p. of inferior pharyngeal constrictor, SEE inferior constrictor *muscle* of pharynx. SYN pars cricopharyngea musculi constrictoris pharyngis inferioris [NA].

cruciform p. of fibrous digital sheath, the fibers of the fibrous sheath of the fingers and toes which form X-shaped patterns over the region of the interphalangeal joints. SYN pars cruciformis vaginae fibrosae [NA], crucial ligament (4), cruciform p. of fibrous sheath, cruciform pulley, ligamenta cruciata digitorum.

cruciform p. of fibrous sheath, SYN cruciform p. of fibrous digital sheath.

cupular p. of epitympanic recess, the dome-shaped, highest portion of the epitympanic recess. SYN pars cupularis recessus epitympanici [NA].

deep p. of external anal sphincter, SYN pars profunda musculi sphincteri ani externi [NA]. SEE external anal *sphincter.*

deep p. of flexor retinaculum, SYN transverse carpal *ligament.*

deep p. of masseter muscle, SYN pars profunda musculi masseteri [NA]. SEE masseter *muscle.*

deep p. of parotid gland, SEE parotid *gland.*

descending p. of aorta, SYN descending *aorta.*

descending p. of duodenum, SYN pars descendens duodeni. SEE duodenum.

descending p. of facial canal, second portion of the facial canal, after the horizontal parts, beginning at the posterior end of the lateral crus where the canal begins to descend. It runs vertically downward, ending at the stylomastoid foramen. Anteriorly, the descending part of the facial canal communicates with the tympanic cavity via the canaliculus for the nerve to the stapedius muscle and the posterior canaliculus of the chorda tympani. SEE ALSO facial *canal.*

distal p. of anterior lobe of hypophysis, the larger part of the adenohypophysis composed of cords of epithelial cells individually specialized to secrete various tropic hormones that exert their effect on several target organs in the body. The secretory activity of these cells is under the control of either releasing or inhibiting factors elaborated by hypothalamic neurons and transported to the adenohypophysis by the hypothalamo-hypophysial portal system. SYN pars distalis [NA].

dorsal p. of pons, the part of the pons bounded laterally by the middle cerebellar peduncles and anteriorly by the ventral part of pons; it is continuous with the tegmentum of the mesencephalon and contains long tracts such as the medial and lateral lemnisci, cranial nerve nuclei, and reticular formation. SYN pars dorsalis pontis [NA], tegmentum of pons.

endocrine p. of pancreas, SEE pancreas.

exocrine p. of pancreas, SYN pars exocrina pancreatis. SEE pancreas.

flaccid p. of tympanic membrane, triangular loose p. of tympanic membrane between the malleolar folds. SYN pars flaccida membranae tympani [NA], flaccid membrane, membrana flaccida, Rivinus' membrane, Shrapnell's membrane.

frontal p. of corpus callosum, SYN minor *forceps.*

glossopharyngeal p. of superior pharyngeal constrictor, SEE superior constrictor *muscle* of pharynx. SYN pars glossopharyngea musculi constrictoris pharyngis superioris [NA].

hidden p., SYN *pars* tecta.

horizontal p. of duodenum, SYN pars horizontalis duodeni [NA], inferior p. of duodenum, pars inferior duodeni. SEE duodenum.

horizontal p. of facial canal, first portion of facial canal, between beginning of canal (at the introitus of the facial canal at the end of the internal auditory meatus) and the point at which it turns to descend, beginning the *descending part.* There are two components (crura) of the horizontal part: the medially-located, anteriorly-directed medial crus and the laterally-placed, posteriorly-directed lateral crus, the two being continuous at a sharp bend, the genu of the facial canal. This lateral part is where the genicular ganglion is located and which communicates with the middle cranial fossa via the hiatus of the facial canal, through which the greater superficial petrosal nerve passes.

p.'s of human body, the head, neck, trunk, and limbs. SYN partes corporis humani [NA].

inferior p., the lowermost portion of a structure relative to the other parts; portion closest to the soles of the feet. SEE inferior p. of duodenum, inferior p. of lingular branch of left pulmonary vein, inferior p. of vestibular ganglion. SYN pars inferior [NA].

inferior p. of duodenum, SYN horizontal p. of duodenum.

inferior p. of lingular branch of left pulmonary vein, the vein draining the inferior lingular bronchopulmonary segment of the left lung. SYN pars inferior rami lingularis[*].

inferior p. of vestibular ganglion, the lower part of the vestibular ganglion that receives fibers from the macula of the saccule and the ampulla of the posterior semicircular duct. SYN pars inferior ganglii vestibularis [NA].

inferior p. of vestibulocochlear nerve, SYN cochlear *nerve.*

infraclavicular p. of brachial plexus, the part of the brachial plexus that extends from the level of the clavicle downward into the axilla; it includes the cords of the plexus and their branches. SYN pars infraclavicularis plexus brachialis [NA].

infralobar p. of posterior branch of right pulmonary vein, the vein draining the posterior segment of the right lung that emerges inferior to the superior lobe; tributary to the posterior branch of the right superior pulmonary vein. SYN pars infralobaris rami posterioris venae pulmonalis dextrae [NA].

infrasegmental p., SYN intersegmental *veins,* under *vein.*

infundibular p., SYN *pars* tuberalis.

insular p., SYN pars insularis [NA]. SEE middle cerebral *artery.*

insular p. of middle cerebral artery, SYN pars insularis arteriae cerebralis mediae. SEE middle cerebral *artery.*

intercartilaginous p. of glottic opening, SYN intercartilaginous p. of rima glottidis.

intercartilaginous p. of rima glottidis, the opening between the vocal processes of the arytenoid cartilages. SYN pars intercartila-

ginea rimae glottidis [NA], glottis respiratoria, intercartilaginous p. of glottic opening.

intermediate p., central portion; the portion located between extreme portions of a structure; an interposed or intervening part. SEE intermediate p. of adenohypophysis, intermediate p. of vestibular bulb. SYN pars intermedia [NA].

intermediate p. of adenohypophysis, the part of the adenohypophysis located between the pars distalis and the nervous lobe; poorly developed in humans. SYN pars intermedia adenohypophyseos [NA].

intermediate p. of vestibular bulb, SYN *commissure* of vestibular bulb.

intermembranous p. of glottic opening, SYN intermembranous p. of rima glottidis.

intermembranous p. of rima glottidis, the portion of the opening anterior to the vocal processes of the arytenoid cartilages bounded by the vocal ligaments. SYN pars intermembranacea rimae glottidis [NA], glottis vocalis, intermembranous p. of glottic opening.

intersegmental p. of pulmonary vein, SYN intersegmental *veins,* under *vein.*

intracanicular p. of optic nerve, the part of the optic nerve lying within the optic canal. SYN pars intracanaliculus nervi optici [NA].

intracranial p. of optic nerve, the portion of the optic nerve between the optic canal and the optic chiasm. SYN pars intracranialis nervi optici [NA].

intracranial p. of vertebral artery, SEE vertebral *artery.*

intralaminar p. of optic nerve, the portion of the optic nerve as it passes through the lamina cribrosa of the sclera. SYN pars intralaminaris nervi optici [NA].

intralobar p. of the right superior pulmonary vein, the vein draining the apical and posterior segments of the right lung; tributary to the posterior branch of the right superior pulmonary vein. SYN pars intralobaris venae pulmonalis dextrae superioris [NA].

intraocular p. of optic nerve, the part of the optic nerve within the eye; it is divided into intralaminar, postlaminar, and prelaminar parts. SYN pars intraocularis nervi optici [NA].

intrasegmental p., SYN intrasegmental *veins,* under *vein.*

iridial p. of retina, SYN pars iridica retinae [NA]. SEE retina.

labial p. of orbicularis oris muscle, the major p. of the orbicularis oris muscle within the body of the lips. SYN pars labialis musculi orbicularis oris [NA].

lacrimal p. of orbicularis oculi muscle, SEE orbicularis oculi *muscle.* SYN pars lacrimalis musculi orbicularis oculi [NA], Duverney's muscle, Horner's muscle, musculus tensor tarsi.

laryngeal p. of pharynx, SYN laryngopharynx.

lateral p. of longitudinal arch of foot, SYN longitudinal *arch* of foot. SYN pars lateralis arcus pedis longitudinalis.

lateral p. of middle lobar branch of right superior pulmonary vein, the vein draining the lateral bronchopulmonary segment of the middle lobe of the right lung. SYN pars lateralis rami lobi medii venae pulmonalis dexter superior [NA].

lateral p. of occipital bone, the part of the occipital bone that lies on either side of the foramen magnum. SYN pars lateralis ossis occipitalis [NA], exoccipital bone.

lateral p. of posterior cervical intertransversarii muscles, SYN pars lateralis musculorum intertransversariorum posteriorum cervicis. SEE posterior cervical intertransversarii *muscles,* under *muscle.*

lateral p. of sacrum, the lateral mass of the sacrum formed by the fused costal elements. SYN pars lateralis ossis sacri [NA].

lateral p. of vaginal fornix, SYN pars lateralis fornicis vaginae. SEE vaginal *fornix.*

lumbar p., that p. of the cord that consists of the five lumbar segments and gives rise to the five pairs of lumbar nerves. SYN pars lumbalis medullae spinalis [NA].

lumbar p. of diaphragm, the portion of the diaphragm that arises from the upper lumbar vertebrae and from the medial and lateral arcuate ligaments. SEE right *crus* of diaphragm, left *crus* of diaphragm, lateral arcuate *ligament,* medial arcuate *ligament.* SYN pars lumbalis diaphragmatis [NA], vertebral p. of diaphragm.

lumbar p. of spinal cord, portion of spinal cord which consists of the five lumbar segments (L_1–L_5) and from which five pairs of lumbar spinal nerves originate; in the adult it is located in the T_{10}–L_1 portion of the vertebral canal, and is enlarged relative to other parts of the cord due to its involvement in innervation of the lower limb.

marginal p. of orbicularis oris muscle, the p. of the orbicularis oris muscle located in the margin of the lips, *i.e.,* the red area. SYN pars marginalis musculi orbicularis oris [NA].

mastoid p. of the temporal bone, the portion of the petrous part of the temporal bone bearing the mastoid process. SYN pars mastoidea ossis temporalis [NA].

medial p. of longitudinal arch of foot, SYN pars medialis arcus pedis longitudinalis. SEE longitudinal *arch* of foot.

medial p. of middle lobar branch of right superior pulmonary vein, the vein draining the medial bronchopulmonary segment of the middle lobe of the right lung. SYN pars medialis rami lobii medii venae pulmonis dextrae superioris [NA].

medial p. of posterior cervical intertransversarii muscles, SYN pars medialis musculorum intertransversariorum posteriorum cervicis [NA]. SEE posterior cervical intertransversarii *muscles,* under *muscle.*

mediastinal p. of lung, SYN mediastinal *surface* of lung.

membranous p. of interventricular septum, p. of the fibrous skeleton of the heart which is seen as a small, thin, round or oval nonmuscular area at the superior end of the interventricular septum; it lies just below and is continuous with the portion of the fibrous ring of the aortic valve supporting the anterior and posterior cusps, and with the right fibrous trigone; the atrioventricular bundle of conducting tissue courses along its dorsal margin and bifurcates at its inferior margin into the right and left crura. SYN pars membranacea septi interventricularis [NA], membranous septum (2), septum membranaceum ventriculorum.

membranous p. of male urethra [NA], the portion of the male urethra, about 1 cm in length, extending from the prostate to the beginning of the urethra in the corpus spongiosum just beyond the bulb. SYN pars membranacea urethrae masculinae [NA], membranous urethra.

membranous p. of nasal septum, the small portion of the nasal septum anterior to the portion supported by the cartilage of the nasal septum. SYN pars membranacea septi nasi [NA], membranous septum (1).

mobile p. of nasal septum, the anterior movable part of the nasal septum formed by the medial crus of the greater alar cartilage on each side. SYN pars mobilis septi nasi [NA], septum mobile nasi.

muscular p. of interventricular septum of heart, the thick muscular portion which comprises most of the interventricular septum of the heart. SYN pars muscularis septi interventricularis cordis [NA], septum musculare ventriculorum.

mylopharyngeal p. of superior pharyngeal constrictor, SEE superior constrictor *muscle* of pharynx. SYN pars mylopharyngeus musculi constrictoris pharyngis superioris [NA].

nasal p. of frontal bone, nasal portion of the frontal bone which lies between the two orbital parts anteriorly and forms part of the roof of the nasal cavity. SYN pars nasalis ossis frontalis [NA].

nasal p. of pharynx, SYN nasopharynx.

nervous p. of retina, SYN pars nervosa retinae [NA]. SEE retina.

neural p. of hypophysis, SYN neurohypophysis.

oblique p. of cricothyroid muscle, SEE cricothyroid *muscle.* SYN pars obliqua musculi cricothyroidei [NA].

occipital p. of corpus callosum, SYN major *forceps.*

opercular p., one of the three small cortical convolutions together forming a cover for the insular region. Opercular convolutions are frontal, temporal, and parietal. SYN pars opercularis.

optic p. of retina, SYN cerebral *layer* of retina.

oral p. of pharynx, SYN oropharynx.

orbital p. of frontal bone, the portion of the frontal bone that contributes to the formation of the orbits; the most rostral of three cortical convolutions that togetther form the inferior frontal gyrus. SYN pars orbitalis ossis frontalis [NA].

orbital p. of lacrimal gland, SEE lacrimal *gland.*

orbital p. of optic nerve, the part of the optic nerve between the eye and the optic canal. SYN pars orbitalis nervi optici [NA].

orbital p. of orbicularis oculi muscle, SYN *pars* orbitalis musculi orbicularis oculi. SEE orbicularis oculi *muscle.*

osseous p. of skeletal system, the part of the skeleton composed of bone. SYN pars ossea systematis skeletalis [NA].

palpebral p. of lacrimal gland, SYN pars palpebralis glandulae lacrimalis [NA]. SEE lacrimal *gland.*

palpebral p. of orbicularis oculi muscle, SYN pars palpebralis musculi orbicularis oculi [NA]. SEE orbicularis oculi *muscle.*

parasympathetic p., the parasympathetic p. of the autonomic nervous system. SEE autonomic nervous *system.* SYN pars parasympathica [NA], bulbosacral system, craniosacral system.

pelvic p., the portion of a structure which is located within or is related to the pelvis. SEE pelvic p. of ureter. SYN pars pelvina.

pelvic p. of ureter, the p. of the ureter between the brim of the pelvis and the urinary bladder; the upper pelvic portion of the embryologic urogenital sinus. SYN pars pelvina ureteris [NA].

peripheral p., SYN peripheral nervous *system.*

petrous p. of internal carotid artery, the part of the internal carotid artery in the carotid canal; its branches are carotidotympanic arteries and the artery of the pterygoid canal. SYN pars petrosa arteriae carotidis internae [NA], petrous bone.

petrous p. of temporal bone, the part of the temporal bone that contains the structures of the inner ear and the second part of the internal carotid artery; in antenatal life it appears as a separate ossification center. SYN pars petrosa ossis temporalis [NA], periotic bone, petrosal bone, petrous pyramid.

pigmented p. of retina, SYN pars pigmentosa [NA]. SEE retina.

postcommunical p. of anterior cerebral artery, SYN pericallosal *artery.*

posterior p., the posterior portion of the anterior commissure of the brain.

posterior p. of the diaphragmatic surface of the liver, that portion of the diaphragmatic surface of the liver that includes the bare area and the caudate lobe. SYN pars posterior faciei diaphragmatis hepatis [NA].

posterior tibiotalar p. of deltoid ligament, SYN posterior tibiotalar *ligament.*

postlaminar p. of optic nerve, the portion of the optic nerve posterior to the lamina cribrosa of the sclera. SYN pars postlaminaris nervi optici [NA].

postsulcal p. of tongue, SEE *dorsum* of tongue.

precommunical p. of anterior cerebral artery, SYN pars precommunicalis arteriae cerebri anterior [NA]. SEE anterior cerebral *artery.*

prelaminar p. of optic nerve, the portion of the optic nerve anterior to the lamina cribrosa of the sclera. SYN pars prelaminaris nervi optici [NA].

presulcal p. of tongue, SEE *dorsum* of tongue.

prevertebral p. of vertebral artery, SEE vertebral *artery.*

pterygopharyngeal p. of superior constrictor muscle of pharynx, SYN pars pterygopharyngea musculi constrictoris pharyngis superioris [NA]. SEE superior constrictor *muscle* of pharynx.

pyloric p. of stomach, that portion of the stomach between the angular notch and the pylorus; its mucosa contains pyloric glands. SYN pars pylorica gastris [NA], pars pylorica ventriculi ☆ [NA].

quadrate p. of liver, the part of the medial segment of the liver which includes the quadrate lobe. SYN pars quadrata hepatis [NA].

retrolenticular p. of internal capsule, that portion of the capsule caudal to the lentiform nucleus which contains large parts of the optic or geniculocalcarine radiation and other fiber systems. SYN pars retrolentiformis capsulae internae [NA], retrolenticular limb of internal capsule.

right p. of diaphragmatic surface of liver, the part of the diaphragmatic surface of the liver deep to the bodies of the lower ribs on the right side. SYN pars dextra faciei diaphragmaticae hepatis [NA].

sacral p. of spinal cord, the part of the cord from which consists of the five sacral segments of the spinal cord (S_1–S_5) and from which five pairs of sacral nerves originate. SYN pars sacralis medullae spinalis [NA], segmenta medullae spinalis sacralia.

soft p.'s, the nonbony and noncartilaginous tissues of the body.

sphenoidal p. of middle cerebral artery, SYN pars sphenoidalis arteriae cerebralis mediae [NA]. SEE middle cerebral *artery*.

spinal p. of accessory nerve, SYN spinal *root* of accessory nerve.

spinal p. of arachnoid, SYN *arachnoid* of spinal cord.

spongy p. of the male urethra, SYN spongy *urethra*.

squamous p. of frontal bone, the broad curved portion of the frontal bone forming the forehead. SYN squama frontalis [NA].

squamous p. of occipital bone, the tabular or squamous portion of occipital bone. SYN squama occipitalis, occipital squama [NA], frontal squama.

squamous p. of temporal bone, the broad, flat, thin (scale-like) anterior and superior portion of the temporal bone forming part of the lateral wall of the cranial vault. SYN pars squamosa ossis temporalis [NA], squama temporalis, temporal squama.

sternal p. of diaphragm, the small slip on each side that arises from the inner surface of the xiphoid process and inserts on the central tendon. SYN pars sternalis diaphragmatis [NA].

sternocostal p. of pectoralis major muscle, SYN pars sternocostalis musculi pectoralis majoris [NA], sternocostal head of pectoralis major muscle. SEE pectoralis major *muscle*.

straight p. of cricothyroid muscle, SEE cricothyroid *muscle*.

subcutaneous p. of external anal sphincter, SYN pars subcutanea musculi sphincteri ani externi [NA], subcutaneous portion of external anal sphincter. SEE external anal *sphincter*.

sublenticular p. of internal capsule, the part of the internal capsule below the caudal third of the lentiform nucleus that contains the auditory radiation as well as that part of the optic radiation representing the upper part of the contralateral half of the binocular visual field. SYN pars sublentiformis capsulae internae [NA], sublenticular limb of internal capsule.

suboccipital p. of vertebral artery, SEE vertebral *artery*.

superficial p. of duodenum, SEE duodenum.

superficial p. of external anal sphincter, SYN pars superficialis musculi sphincteri ani externi. SEE external anal *sphincter*.

superficial p. of masseter muscle, SYN pars superficialis musculi masseteri. SEE masseter *muscle*.

superficial p. of parotid gland, SYN pars superficialis glandulae parotideae. SEE parotid *gland*.

superior p. of diaphragmatic surface of liver, the convex superior portion of the diaphragmatic surface of the liver. SYN pars superior faciei diaphragmaticae hepatis.

superior p. of duodenum, SYN pars superior duodeni [NA]. SEE duodenum.

superior p. of lingular branch of left pulmonary vein, the vein that drains the superior lingular bronchopulmonary segment of the left lung. SYN pars superior rami lingularis venae pulmonis sinistri [NA].

superior p. of vestibular ganglion, rostral part, the superior part of the vestibular ganglion that receives fibers from the maculae of the utricle and the saccule and the ampullae of the anterior and lateral semicircular ducts. SYN pars superior ganglii vestibularis [NA].

superior p. of vestibulocochlear nerve, SYN vestibular *nerve*.

supraclavicular p. of brachial plexus, the part of the brachial plexus, including the roots, trunks, and divisions, that gives rise to the dorsal scapular, long thoracic, suprascapular and subclavian nerves. SYN pars supraclavicularis plexus brachialis [NA].

sympathetic p., SYN sympathetic nervous *system*.

tense p. of the tympanic membrane, the greater portion of the tympanic membrane which is tense and firm, contrasting with the small triangular flaccid part of tympanic membrane. SYN pars tensa membranae tympani [NA], membrana tensa, membrana vibrans.

terminal p., SYN *pars* terminalis. SEE middle cerebral *artery*, posterior cerebral *artery*.

thoracic p. of aorta, SYN thoracic *aorta*.

thoracic p. of esophagus, the p. of the esophagus between the superior thoracic aperture and the diaphragm. SYN pars thoracica esophagi [NA].

thoracic p. of spinal cord, the p. of the spinal cord which consists of the twelve thoracic segments of the spinal cord from which the twelve pairs of thoracic nerves originate. SYN pars thoracica medullae spinalis [NA], segmenta medullae spinalis thoracica.

thoracic p. of thoracic duct, SYN pars thoracica ductus thoracici [NA]. SEE thoracic *duct*.

thyropharyngeal p. of inferior pharyngeal constrictor muscle, SYN pars thyropharyngea musculi constrictoris pharyngis inferioris [NA]. SEE inferior constrictor *muscle* of pharynx.

tibiocalcaneal p. of deltoid ligament, SYN tibiocalcaneal *ligament*.

tibionavicular p. of deltoid ligament, SYN tibionavicular *ligament*.

transversarial p. of vertebral artery, SEE vertebral *artery*.

transverse p. of left branch of portal vein, the long unbranched portion of the left branch of the portal vein. SYN pars transversa rami sinistri venae portae hepatis [NA].

transverse p. of nasalis muscle, SEE nasalis *muscle*. SYN pars transversa musculi nasalis [NA].

triangular p., the middle one of three small convolutions which together compose the inferior frontal gyrus of the cerebral cortex; the other two being the orbital part and opercular part. SYN pars triangularis.

tympanic p. of temporal bone, SYN tympanic *plate* of temporal bone.

umbilical p. of left branch of portal vein, the highly branched part of the left branch of the portal vein; the round and venous ligaments attach to this part. SYN pars umbilicalis rami sinistri venae portae hepatis [NA].

uterine p. of uterine tube, the part of the uterine tube located within the wall of the uterus. SYN pars uterina tubae uterinae [NA].

uveal p. of trabecular reticulum, the posterior part of the trabecular reticulum, located between the scleral spur, the ciliary body, and the anterior surface of the iris. SYN pars uvealis reticuli trabecularis [NA].

vagal p., SYN cranial *root* of accessory nerve.

vagal p. of accessory nerve, SYN cranial *root* of accessory nerve.

ventral p. of pons, the large ventral p. of the pons occupied by the nuclei pontis, traversed longitudinally by corticopontine, corticobulbar, and corticospinal fibers, and transversely by pontocerebellar fibers. Pontocerebellar fibers converging laterally form the middle cerebellar peduncle or brachium pontis. SYN pars ventralis pontis [NA], anterior p. of pons, basilar p. of pons, pars basilaris pontis.

vertebral p. of the costal surface of the lungs, the p. of the medial surface of the lung in contact with the vertebral bodies. SYN pars vertebralis faciei costalis pulmonis [NA].

vertebral p. of diaphragm, SYN lumbar p. of diaphragm.

vestibular p. of vestibulocochlear nerve, SYN vestibular *nerve*.

part. aeq. Abbreviation for L. *partes aequales*, in equal parts (amounts).

par·tes (par′tēz). Plural of pars.

par·the·no·gen·e·sis (par′the-nō-jen′ĕ-sis). A form of nonsexual reproduction, or agamogenesis, in which the female reproduces its kind without fecundation by the male. SYN apogamia, apogamy, apomixia, virgin generation. [G. *parthenos*, virgin, + *genesis*, product]

par·the·no·pho·bia (par′the-nō-fō′bē-ă). Morbid fear of girls. [G. *parthenos*, virgin, + *phobos*, fear]

par·ti·cle (par′ti-kl). A very small piece or portion of anything. [L. *particula*, dim. of *pars*, part]

alpha p. (α), a p. consisting of two neutrons and two protons, with a positive charge (2e⁺); emitted energetically from the nuclei of unstable isotopes of high atomic number (elements of mass number from 82 up); identical to the helium nucleus. SYN alpha ray.

beta p., an electron, either positively (positron, β^+) or negatively (negatron, β^-) charged, emitted during beta decay of a radionuclide. SEE ALSO cathode *rays*, under *ray*. SYN beta ray.

chromatin p.'s, fine bluish dots thought to represent remnants of the nucleus, occasionally seen in stained erythrocytes.

core p., p. released by partial enzymatic digestion of chromatin.

Dane p.'s, the larger spherical forms of hepatitis-associated antigens; they comprise the virion of hepatitis B virus, containing a 27-nm "core" in which DNA-dependent DNA polymerase and circular, double-stranded DNA have been found.

defective interfering p., an incomplete virus that is unable to replicate and interferes with replication of an infectious virus.

D.I. p., abbreviation for defective interfering p.

electron transport p.'s (ETP), fragments of mitochondria still capable of transporting electrons. SYN submitochondrial p.'s.

elementary p., (1) SYN platelet. **(2)** one of the units occurring on the matrical surface of mitochondrial cristae; the head of the p., which measures about 9 nm, attaches to the membrane of the crista by a stalk 5 nm in length; the p.'s may be concerned with the electron transport system.

kappa p.'s, inheritable cytoplasmic symbionts, once thought to be p.'s mainly or exclusively of DNA, occurring in some strains of *Paramecium;* capable of producing a product lethal to other strains.

signal recognition p. (SRP), a small RNA-protein complex that interacts with the signal sequence of nascent secretory proteins. Binding of the signal recognition p. results in arrest of translation until interaction with docking protein, an integral part of the endoplasmic reticulum membrane.

submitochondrial p.'s, SYN electron transport p.'s.

Zimmermann's elementary p., SYN platelet.

par·tic·u·late (par-tik'yū-lāt). Relating to or occurring in the form of fine particles.

par·tic·u·lates (par-tik'yū-lats). Formed elements, discrete bodies, as contrasted with the surrounding liquid or semiliquid material; *e.g.,* granules or mitochondria in cells.

par·tu·ri·ent (par-tū'rē-ent). Relating to or in the process of childbirth. [L. *parturio,* to be in labor]

par·tu·ri·fa·cient (par-tūr-ē-fā'shent). **1.** Inducing or accelerating labor. **2.** An agent that induces or accelerates labor. SYN oxytocic (2). [L. *parturio,* to be in labor, + *facio,* to make]

par·tu·ri·om·e·ter (par-tūr-ē-om'ĕ-ter). Device for determining the force of the uterine contractions in childbirth. [L. *parturitio,* parturition, + G. *metron,* measure]

par·tu·ri·tion (par-tūr-ish'ŭn). SYN childbirth. [L. *parturitio,* fr. *parturio,* to be in labor]

part. vic. Abbreviation for L. *partes vicibus,* in divided doses.

pa·ru·lis, pl. **pa·ru·li·des** (pă-rū'lis, -li-dēz). SYN gingival *abscess.* [G. *paroulis,* gumboil, fr. *para,* beside, + *oulon,* gum]

par·um·bil·i·cal (par'ŭm-bil'i-kăl). SYN paraumbilical.

par·u·re·sis (par-yū-rē'sis). Inhibited urination, especially in the presence of strangers. [para- + G. *ourēsis,* urination]

par·val·bu·min (par-val-byū'min). A small water-soluble calcium-binding protein distinct from calmodulin and other calcium-binding proteins; found in the brain, skeletal muscle, and retina, but not in the heart, liver, or spleen, of various species. [L. *parvus,* small, + albumin]

Par·vo·bac·te·ri·a·ce·ae (par'vō-bak-tēr-ē-ā'sē-ē). A family name regarded as a former name for the bacterial family Brucellaceae. No type genus has ever been proposed for the family P.

par·vo·cel·lu·lar (par-vi-sel'yū-lăr). Relating to or composed of cells of small size. [L. *parvus,* small, + Mod. L. *cellularis,* cellular]

par·vo·line (par'vō-lēn). A ptomaine, $C_9H_{13}N$, from decaying fish.

Par·vo·vir·i·dae (par-vō-vir'i-dē). A family of small viruses containing single-stranded DNA. Virions are 18 to 26 nm in diameter, are not enveloped, and are ether-resistant. Capsids are of cubic symmetry, with 32 capsomeres. Replication and assembly occur in the nucleus of infected cells. Three genera are recognized: *Parvovirus, Densovirus,* and *Dependovirus,* which includes the adeno-associated satellite virus.

Par·vo·vi·rus (par'vō-vī-rŭs). A genus of viruses (family Parvoviridae) that replicate autonomously in suitable cells. Strain B19

infects humans, causing erythema infectiosum and aplastic crisis in hemolytic anemia. [L. *parvus,* small, + virus]

canine P. 2, a virus causing canine parvovirus disease in dogs, an acute enteritis with panleukopenia and myocarditis. SEE canine parvovirus *disease.*

goose P., a virus causing goose viral hepatitis in geese and Muscovy ducks.

porcine P., a virus causing stillbirths, abortions, fetal deaths, mummifications, and infertility in swine.

Par·vo·vi·rus B 19. A small 20 mm single stranded DNA virus belonging to the family Parvoviridae that is associated with erythema infectiosum (fifth disese) and aplastic crisis in patients with hemolytic anemia.

par·vule (par'vūl). A very small pill. [L. *parvulus,* very small, fr. *parvus,* small]

par·vus (par'vŭs). Small. [L.]

PAS Abbreviation for *p*-aminosalicylic acid; periodic acid-Schiff *stain.*

PASA Abbreviation for *p*-aminosalicylic acid.

Pascal, Blaise, French scientist, 1623–1662. SEE pascal; P.'s *law.*

pas·cal (Pa) (pas'kăl). A derived unit of pressure or stress in the SI system, expressed in newtons per square meter; equal to 10^{-5} bar or 7.50062×10^{-3} torr. [B. *Pascal*]

Pascheff (Pashev), Constantin (Konstantin), Bulgarian ophthalmologist, 1873–1961. SEE P.'s *conjunctivitis.*

Paschen, Enrique, German pathologist, 1860–1936. SEE P. *bodies,* under *body.*

Pashev. SEE Pascheff.

Pasini, Augustine, 20th century Argentinian dermatologist. SEE *atrophoderma* of P. and Pierini.

pas·i·ni·a·zide (pas-i-nī'ă-zīd). Isoniazid 4-aminosalicylate; an antituberculostatic agent.

pas·pal·ism (pas'păl-izm). Poisoning by seeds of a species of grass, *Paspalum scrobiculatum.* [G. *paspalos,* a kind of millet, fr. *pas,* all, + *palē,* meal]

pas·sage (pas'ij). **1.** The act of passing. **2.** A discharge, as from the bowels or of urine. **3.** Inoculation of a series of animals with the same strain of a pathogenic microorganism whereby the virulence is increased, but is sometimes diminished. **4.** A channel, duct, pore, or opening. [Mediev. L. *passo,* to pass]

blind p., successive transfer of an agent through cultures or animals without incidence of either replication or disease.

nasopharyngeal p., the posterior part of the nasal cavity from the posterior limits of the conchae to the choanae. SYN meatus nasopharyngeus [NA].

oropharyngeal p., SYN fauces.

serial p., successive transfer of an infectious agent through a series of cultures or experimental animals, usually to attenuate pathogenicity.

Pas·sal·u·rus am·big·u·us (pa-sal'yū-rŭs am-big'yū-ŭs). The rabbit pinworm, an oxyurid nematode found abundantly in the cecum and large intestine of rabbits.

Passavant, Philippas G., German physician, 1815–1893. SEE P.'s *bar, cushion, pad, ridge.*

Passey, R.D., 20th century British pathologist. SEE Harding-P. *melanoma.*

pas·si·flo·ra (pas-i-flō'ră). The passion-flower, *Passiflora incarnata* (family Passifloraceae), a climbing herb of the southern U.S.; the dried flowering and fruiting top has been used in neuralgia, dysmenorrhea, and insomnia, and as an application to hemorrhoids and for burns. [L. *passio,* passion, + *flos (flor-),* flower]

pas·sion (pash'ŭn). **1.** Intense emotion. **2.** Obsolete term for suffering or pain. [L. *passio,* fr. *patior,* pp. *passus,* to suffer]

pas·sive (pas'iv). Not active; submissive. [L. *passivus,* fr. *patior,* to endure]

pas·siv·ism (pas'iv-izm). **1.** An attitude of submission. **2.** A form of sexual perversion in which the subject, usually male, is submissive to the will of the partner, male or female, in sexual practices which usually require the consent of both participants (*e.g.,* anal intercourse). SEE ALSO pathic. [see passive]

pas·siv·i·ty (pas-iv′i-tē). **1.** The condition of a metal having formed a protective oxide coating; *e.g.,* rustless metals and aluminum become passive in air. **2.** In dentistry, the quality or condition of inactivity or rest assumed by the teeth, tissues, and denture when a removable partial denture is in place but not under masticatory pressure.

pas·ta, gen. and pl. **pas·tae** (pas′tă, -tē). SYN paste. [L.]

paste (pāst). A soft semisolid of firmer consistency than pap, but soft enough to flow slowly and not to retain its shape. SYN pasta. [L. *pasta*]

dermatologic p., a class of preparations consisting of starch, dextrin, sulfur, calcium carbonate, or zinc oxide made into a p. with glycerin, soft soap, petrolatum, or some fat, with which is incorporated some medicinal substance.

desensitizing p., an ointment, usually caustic, coagulating or cytotoxic, formulated to be applied to the cervix of a tooth for the purpose of obtunding pain from sensitive, exposed cementum or dentin.

past·er (pā′ster). The segment forming the part for near vision in two-piece bifocal lenses.

pas·tern. The part of the leg of a horse and similar animals that lies between the fetlock joint and the hoof. [O. Fr. *pasturon,* pasture; because the shackle of a horse out at pasture is attached to this part of the leg]

Pasteur, Louis, French chemist and bacteriologist, 1822–1895. SEE P. *vaccine;* P.'s *effect;* P. *pipette.*

Pas·teu·rel·la (pas-ter-el′ă). A genus of aerobic to facultatively anaerobic, nonmotile bacteria (family Brucellaceae) containing small, Gram-negative, ellipsoidal to elongated rods which, with special methods, show bipolar staining. These organisms are parasites of humans and other animals, including birds. The type species is *P. multocida.* [L. *Pasteur*]

P. anatipes′tifer, former name for *Moraxella anatipestifer.*

P. haemolyt′ica, a species associated with pneumonia in sheep, goats, and cattle, and causing mastitis in ewes.

P. multoci′da, a species that causes fowl cholera and hemorrhagic septicemia in warm-blooded animals and may infect dog or cat bites or scratches and cause cellulitis and septicemia in humans with chronic disease. Most common pathogen associated with cat and dog bites. Cause of pasteurellosis. It is the type species of the genus *P.*

P. novici′da, a species pathogenic for white mice, guinea pigs, and hamsters; it produces lesions in experimental animals similar to those found in cases of tularemia; it is not known to infect humans.

P. pes′tis, SYN *Yersinia pestis.*

P. pfaf′fii, a species found in an epidemic of septicemia in canaries where it caused a necrotic enteritis; pathogenic for canaries, sparrows, pigeons, white mice, guinea pigs, and rabbits; not pathogenic for chickens.

P. pseudotuberculo′sis, SYN *Yersinia pseudotuberculosis.*

P. septicae′miae, a species which causes fatal septicemia in young geese.

P. tularen′sis, SYN *Francisella tularensis.*

pas·teu·rel·la, pl. **pas·teu·rel·lae** (pas-ter-el′ă, pas-ter-el′ē). A vernacular term used to refer to any member of the genus *Pasteurella.*

pas·teu·rel·lo·sis (pas′ter-ĕ-lō′sis). Infection with bacteria of the genus *Pasteurella.*

pas·teur·i·za·tion (pas′ter-i-zā′shŭn). The heating of milk, wines, fruit juices, etc., for about 30 minutes at 68°C (154.4°F) whereby living bacteria are destroyed, but the flavor or bouquet is preserved; the spores are unaffected, but are kept from developing by immediately cooling the liquid to 10°C (50°F) or lower. SEE ALSO sterilization. [L. *Pasteur*]

pas·teur·ize (pas′ter-īz). To treat by pasteurization.

pas·teur·iz·er (pas′ter-ī-zer). An apparatus used in pasteurization.

Pastia, C., 20th century Roumanian physician. SEE P.'s *sign.*

pas·til, pas·tille (pas′til, pas-tēl′). **1.** A small mass of benzoin and other aromatic substances to be burned for fumigation. **2.**

SYN troche. [Fr. *pastille;* L. *pastillus,* a roll (of bread), dim. of *panis,* bread]

Sabouraud's p.'s, disks containing barium platinocyanide which undergo a color change when exposed to x-rays; previously used to indicate the administered dose.

past-point·ing (past′poynt′ing). A test of the integrity of the vestibular apparatus of the ear and of cerebellar function: the patient, seated in a revolving chair, is rotated to the right ten times with eyes closed; then with the arm held horizontal, the right index finger is brought in touch with the tip of the examiner's finger; the arm is then raised vertically and the patient is instructed to touch the examiner's finger on bringing the arm once more to the horizontal; if the vestibular apparatus is normal, the finger will be brought down several inches to the right of the examiner's finger because the patient is still responding to the sensation of rotation to the left; the reverse is true on rotation to the left. In cerebellar disease, a patient attempting to reach a point with the finger will overshoot it. The test is also used in connection with caloric stimulation.

pa·ta·gi·um, pl. **pa·ta·gia** (pă-tā′jē-ŭm, -ă). A winglike membrane. [L. a gold edging on a woman's gown]

cervical p., obsolete term for *pterygium* colli.

Patau, Klaus, 20th century U.S. cytogeneticist. SEE P.'s *syndrome.*

patch. A small circumscribed area differing in color or structure from the surrounding surface.

butterfly p., SYN butterfly (2).

p. clamping, a technique used in the study of ion channels in which the movement of ions across a small p. of isolated membrane is measured when the membrane is electrically polarized or hyperpolarized and maintained at that potential. SYN patch clamp.

cotton-wool p.'s, white, fuzzy areas on the surface of the retina (accumulations of cellular organelles) caused by damage (usually infarction) of the retinal fiber layer. SYN cotton-wool spots.

herald p., the initial rapidly enlarging oval-shaped red papulosquamous lesion, usually on the trunk, heralding the widespread eruption of pityriasis rosea, and preceding the latter by 7–14 days.

Hutchinson's p., SYN salmon p.

moth p., SYN chloasma.

mucous p., an oval to round, yellow-gray to white, membrane-covered lesion or lesions occurring on the mucous membranes; usually seen in secondary syphilis.

opaline p., a mucous p. of silver-gray appearance.

Peyer's p.'s, collections of many lymphoid follicles closely packed together, forming oblong elevations on the mucous membrane of the small intestine. SYN folliculi lymphatici aggregati [NA], aggregate glands, aggregated lymphatic follicles, aggregated lymphatic nodules, agmen peyerianum, agminate glands, agminated glands, Peyer's glands.

salmon p., interstitial or parenchymatous keratitis giving rise to neovascularization of the cornea. SYN Hutchinson's p.

shagreen p., SYN shagreen skin.

smoker's p.'s, obsolete term for leukoplakia.

soldier's p.'s, SYN milk *spots* (1), under *spot.*

pat·e·fac·tion (pat-ĕ-fak′shŭn). Obsolete term for a laying open. [L. *pate-facio,* pp. *-factus,* to make lie open, fr. *pateo,* to lie open]

Patein, G., French physician, 1857–1928. SEE P.'s *albumin.*

pa·tel·la, gen. and pl. **pa·tel·lae** (pa-tel′ă, -ē) [NA]. The large sesamoid bone, in the combined tendon of the extensors of the leg, covering the anterior surface of the knee. SYN kneecap. [L. a small plate, the kneecap, dim. of *patina,* a shallow disk, fr. *pateo,* to lie open]

floating p., a p. riding high on effusion of the knee.

slipping p., spontaneous or easily provoked dislocation of the p.

pa·tel·lal·gia (pa-tĕ-lal′jē-ă). A painful condition involving the patella. [patella + G. *algos,* pain]

pa·tel·lar (pa-tel′ăr). Relating to the patella.

pat·el·lec·to·my (pat′ĕ-lek′tō-mē). Excision of the patella. [patella + G. *ektomē,* excision]

pa

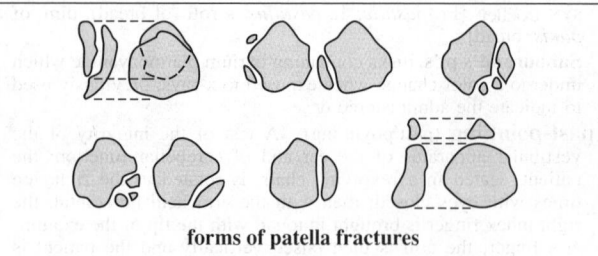

forms of patella fractures

pa·tel·li·form (pa-tel'i-fōrm). Of the shape of the patella.

pat·el·lom·e·ter (pat'ĕ-lom'ĕ-ter). Instrument for measuring the patellar reflex. [patella + G. *metron*, measure]

pa·ten·cy (pā'ten-sē). The state of being freely open or exposed.
   probe p., (of foramen ovale), a term introduced by B.M. Patten to cover incomplete fibrous adhesion of an adequate valvula foraminis ovalis in the postnatal closure of the foramen ovale.

pa·tent (pa'tent, pā'tent). Open or exposed. SYN patulous. [L. *patens*, pres. p. of *pateo*, to lie open]

pa·tent blue V. SYN leuco patent blue.

Paterson, Donald R., English otolaryngologist, 1863–1939. SEE P.-Kelly *syndrome;* Paterson-Brown-Kelly *syndrome.*

path. A road or way; the course taken by an electric current or by nervous impulses. SEE ALSO pathway. [A.S. *paeth*]
   condyle p., the p. traveled by the mandibular condyle in the temporomandibular joint during the various mandibular movements.
   generated occlusal p., a registration of the p.'s of movement of the occlusal surfaces of mandibular teeth on a plastic or abrasive surface attached to the maxillary arch. SEE ALSO functional chew-in *record.*
   incisal p., SYN incisal *guidance.*
   p. of insertion, the direction in which a dental prosthesis is placed upon or removed from the supporting tissues or abutment teeth.
   milled-in p.'s, (1) contours carved by various mandibular movements into the occluding surface of an occlusion rim, by teeth or studs placed in the opposing occlusion rim; the curves or contours may be carved into wax, modeling plastic, or plaster of Paris; **(2)** occlusal curves developed by masticatory or gliding movements of occlusion rims which are composed of materials including abrasives. SEE ALSO functional chew-in *record.* SYN milled-in curves.
   occlusal p., (1) a gliding occlusal contact; **(2)** the p. of movement of an occlusal surface.

☊ path-, -pathy, patho-, path·ic. Disease. [G. *pathos*, feeling, suffering, disease]

pa·the·ma (pă-thē'mă). Obsolete term for a disease or morbid condition. [G. *pathēma*, suffering]

path·er·ga·sia (path-er-gā'zē-ă). Obsolete term for a physiologic or anatomical defect that limits normal emotional adjustment. [G. *pathos*, disease, + *ergasia*, work]

path·er·gy (path'er-jē). Those reactions resulting from a state of altered activity, both allergic (immune) and nonallergic. [G. *pathos*, disease, + *ergon*, work]

pa·thet·ic (pă-thet'ik). **1.** Denoting the fourth cranial nerve (pathetic nerve), the trochlear nerve. **2.** Denoting that which arouses sorrow or pity. [G. *pathētikos*, relating to the feelings]

path·find·er (path'fīn-der). A filiform bougie for introduction through a narrow stricture end to serve as a guide for the passage of a larger sound or catheter.

path·ic (path'ik). A person who assumes the passive role in less frequently engaged sexual acts. SEE ALSO passivism (2). [G. *pathikos*, remaining passive]

☊ patho-. SEE path-.

path·o·am·ine (path-ō-am'ēn). A ptomaine; a toxic amine causing disease or resulting from a disease process.

path·o·bi·ol·o·gy (path'ō-bī-ol'ō-jē). Pathology with emphasis more on the biological than on the medical aspects.

path·o·ci·din (path-ō-sī'din). 8-Azaguanine

path·o·clis·is (path-ō-klis'is). A specific tendency to sensitivity to special toxins; a tendency for toxins to attack certain organs. [patho- + G. *klisis,* bending, proneness]

path·o·crin·ia (path-ō-krin'ē-ă). Obsolete term for any disorder of the endocrine glands. [patho- + G. *krinō,* to separate]

path·o·dix·ia (path-ō-dik'sē-ă). Rarely used term for a morbid desire to exhibit one's injured or diseased part. [patho- + G. *deiknumi,* to show]

path·o·don·tia (path-ō-don'shē-ă). The science concerned with diseases of the teeth. [patho- + G. *odous,* tooth]

path·o·for·mic (path-ō-fōr'mik). Relating to the beginning of disease; denoting especially certain symptoms occurring in the transition period between a normal and a diseased state. [patho- + L. *formo,* to form]

path·o·gen (path'ō-jen). Any virus, microorganism, or other substance causing disease. [patho- + G. *-gen,* to produce]
   behavioral p., the personal habits and lifestyle behaviors of an individual which are associated with an increased risk of physical illness and dysfunction. SEE ALSO risk *factor.* Cf. behavioral *immunogen.*
   opportunistic p., an organism that is capable of causing disease only when the host's resistance is lowered, *e.g.,* by other diseases or drugs.

path·o·gen·e·sis (path-ō-jen'ĕ-sis). The pathologic, physiologic, or biochemical mechanism resulting in the development of a disease or morbid process. Cf. etiology. [patho- + G. *genesis,* production]
   drug p., the production of morbid symptoms by drugs.

path·o·gen·ic, path·o·ge·net·ic (path-ō-jen'ik, -jĕ-net'ik). Causing disease or abnormality. SYN morbific, morbigenous, nosogenic, nosopoietic.

path·o·ge·nic·i·ty (path'ō-jĕ-nis'i-tē). The condition or quality of being pathogenic, or the ability to cause disease.

pa·thog·e·ny (pă-thoj'ĕ-nē). Rarely used synonym for pathogenesis.

path·og·no·mon·ic (path'og-nō-mon'ik). Characteristic or indicative of a disease; denoting especially one or more typical symptoms, findings, or pattern of abnormalities specific for a given disease and not found in any other condition. [see pathognomy]

path·og·no·my (pă-thog'nō-mē). Rarely used term for diagnosis by means of a study of the typical symptoms of a disease, or of the subjective sensations of the patient. [patho- + G. *gnōmē,* a mark, a sign]

path·og·nos·tic (path-og-nos'tik). Rarely used synonym for pathognomonic. [patho- + G. *gnōstikos,* pertaining to knowledge]

pa·thog·ra·phy (pă-thog'ră-fē). Rarely used term for a treatise on or description of disease; a treatise on pathology. [patho- + G. *graphē,* a description]

path·o·le·sia (path-ō-lē'sē-ă). Rarely used term for any impairment or abnormality of the will. [path- + G. *lēsis,* choice, will]

path·o·log·ic, path·o·log·i·cal (path-ō-loj'ik, -i-kăl). **1.** Pertaining to pathology. **2.** Morbid or diseased; resulting from disease.

pa·thol·o·gist (pa-thol'ō-jist). A specialist in pathology; a physician who practices, evaluates, or supervises diagnostic tests, using materials removed from living or dead patients, and functions as a laboratory consultant to clinicians, or who conducts experiments or other investigations to determine the causes or nature of disease changes.

pa·thol·o·gy (pa-thol'ō-jē). The medical science, and specialty practice, concerned with all aspects of disease, but with special reference to the essential nature, causes, and development of abnormal conditions, as well as the structural and functional changes that result from the disease processes. [patho- + G. *logos,* study, treatise]
   anatomical p., the subspecialty of p. that pertains to the gross and microscopic study of organs and tissues removed for biopsy or during postmortem examination, and also the interpretation of the results of such study. SYN pathological anatomy.
   cellular p., (1) the interpretation of diseases in terms of cellular

alterations, *i.e.,* the ways in which cells fail to maintain homeostasis; (**2**) sometimes used as a synonym for cytopathology (1).

clinical p., (**1**) any part of the medical practice of p. as it pertains to the care of patients; (**2**) the subspecialty in p. concerned with the theoretical and technical aspects (*i.e.,* the methods or procedures) of chemistry, immunohematology, microbiology, parasitology, immunology, hematology, and other fields as they pertain to the diagnosis of disease and the care of patients, as well as to the prevention of disease.

comparative p., the p. of diseases of animals, especially in relation to human p.

dental p., SYN oral p.

functional p., p. pertaining to abnormalities in function of a tissue, organ, or part, with or without associated changes in structure.

humoral p., the thesis that disorders in the fluids of the body, especially the blood, are the basic factors in disease.

medical p., p. pertaining to various diseases not suitable for treatment by surgery.

molecular p., the study of biochemical and biophysical cellular mechanisms as the basic factors in disease.

oral p., the branch of dentistry concerned with the etiology, pathogenesis, and clinical, gross, and microscopic aspects of oral and paraoral disease, including oral soft tissues, the teeth, jaws, and salivary glands. SYN dental p.

speech p., the science concerned with functional and organic speech defects and disorders.

surgical p., a field in anatomical p. concerned with examination of tissues removed from living patients for the purpose of diagnosis of disease and guidance in the care of patients.

path·o·met·ric (path-ō-met′rik). Relating to pathometry.

pa·thom·e·try (pă-thom′ĕ-trē). Determination of the proportionate number of individuals affected with a certain disease at a given time, and of the conditions leading to an increase or decrease in this number. [patho- + G. *metron,* measure]

path·o·mi·me·sis (path′ō-mi-mē′sis). Mimicry of a disease or dysfunction, whether intentional or unconscious. SYN pathomimicry. [patho- + G. *mimēsis,* imitation]

path·o·mim·ic·ry (path-ō-mim′i-krē). SYN pathomimesis.

path·o·mi·o·sis (path-ō-mī-ō′sis). The attitude that leads a patient to minimize his/her disease. [patho- + G. *meiōsis,* a lessening]

path·o·mor·phism (path-ō-mōr′fizm). Abnormal morphology.

path·o·no·mi·a, pa·thon·o·my (path-ō-nō′mē-ă, pă-thon′ō-mē). The science of the laws of morbid changes. [patho- + G. *nomos,* law]

path·o·pho·bia (path-ō-fō′bē-ă). SYN nosophobia. [patho- + G. *phobos,* fear]

path·o·phys·i·ol·o·gy (path′ō-fiz-ē-ol′ō-jē). Derangement of function seen in disease; alteration in function as distinguished from structural defects.

path·o·poi·e·sis (path′ō-poy-ē′sis). Rarely used term for the mode of production of disease. [patho- + G. *poiēsis,* making]

pa·tho·sis (pă-thō′sis). Rarely used term for a state of disease, diseased condition, or disease entity. [patho- + G. *-osis,* condition]

pa·thot·ro·pism (pa-thot′rō-pizm). Attraction of drugs toward diseased structures. [patho- + G. *tropos,* a turning]

path·way (path′wā). **1.** A collection of axons establishing a conduction route for nerve impulses from one group of nerve cells to another group or to an effector organ composed of muscle or gland cells. **2.** Any sequence of chemical reactions leading from one compound to another; if taking place in living tissue, usually referred to as a **biochemical p.**.

4-aminobutyrate p., the p. that ultimately converts 4-aminobutyrate to succinate; succinate is then converted to α-ketoglutarate, via the tricarboxylic acid cycle, which is then acted upon by glutamate dehydrogenase; glutamate is then decarboxylated to reform 4-aminobutyrate; an important p. for those cells which make this neuroactive molecule. SYN GABA p.

auditory p., neural paths and connections within the central nervous system, beginning at the organ of Corti's hair cells,

continuing along the eighth nerve, and terminating at the auditory cortex.

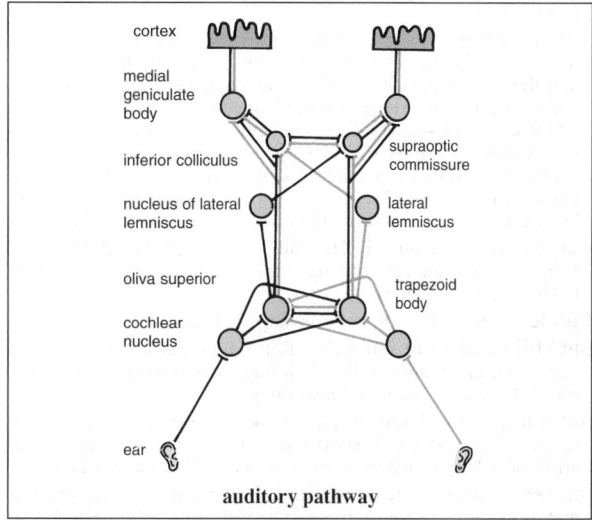

auditory pathway

Embden-Meyerhof p., the anaerobic glycolytic p. by which D-glucose (most notably in muscle) is converted to lactic acid. Cf. glycolysis. SYN Embden-Meyerhof-Parnas p.

Embden-Meyerhof-Parnas p., SYN Embden-Meyerhof p.

Entner-Douderoff p., a degradative p. for carbohydrates in certain microorganisms (*e.g., Pseudomonas* sp.) that lack hexokinase, phosphofructokinase, and glyceraldehyde-3-phosphate dehydrogenase.

GABA p., SYN 4-aminobutyrate p.

hexose monophosphate p., SYN pentose phosphate p.

mercapturic acid p., a glutathione-dependent p. for the detoxification of a number of compounds, including arene oxides; an *S*-substituted glutathione is formed and ultimately converted to a mercapturic acid (an *S*-substituted *N*-acetylated L-cysteine), which is excreted; the leukotrienes are believed to be degraded through this p.

pentose phosphate p., a secondary p. for the oxidation of D-glucose (not occurring in skeletal muscle), generating reducing power (NADPH) in the cytoplasm outside the mitochondria and synthesizing pentoses and a few other sugars. It also provides a means of converting pentoses and certain other sugars into intermediates of the glycolytic p. It proceeds from D-glucose 6-phosphate to D-ribulose and D-ribose phosphates, thence (with D-xylulose 5-phosphate) to D-sedoheptulose 7-phosphate and D-glyceraldehyde 3-phosphate; carbon dioxide is released in the gluconate-ribulose step. In plants, it participates in the formation of D-glucose from carbon dioxide in the dark reactions of photosynthesis. This p. is defective in certain inherited diseases, *e.g.,* glucose-6-phosphate dehydrogenase deficiency. SYN Dickens shunt, hexose monophosphate p., hexose monophosphate shunt, pentose monophosphate shunt, pentose phosphate cycle, phosphogluconate p., Warburg-Dickens-Horecker shunt, Warburg-Lipmann-Dickens-Horecker shunt.

phosphogluconate p., SYN pentose phosphate p.

polyol p., SYN sorbitol p.

salvage p., the utilization of preformed purine and pyrimidine bases to synthesize nucleotides.

sorbitol p., a p. responsible for D-fructose formation from sorbitol; increases in activity as the glucose concentration rises in diabetes. SYN polyol p.

visual p., neural paths and connections within the central nervous system, beginning with the retina and terminating in the occipital cortex.

△**-pathy.** SEE path-.

pa·tient (pā′shent). One who is suffering from any disease or behavioral disorder and is under treatment for it. Cf. case (1). [L. *patiens,* pres. p. of *patior,* to suffer]

target p., in group therapy, the p. being analyzed in turn by another member p.

Patient Zero. The individual identified in 1982 by the Centers for Disease Control as responsible for introducing the HIV virus into the U.S. population. A Canadian citizen, Patient Zero was a homosexual airline steward who claimed to have had as many as 2,500 sexual encounters. CDC epidemiologists located 19 men in Los Angeles, 22 in New York City, and 8 in other cities who had contracted AIDS from contact with Patient Zero, the earliest known cases of the disease in the U.S. Revealed to be Gaetan Dugas, Patient Zero died in 1984 due to AIDS-related illness.

pat·ri·cide (pat′ri-sīd). **1.** The killing of one's father. **2.** One who commits such an act. SEE parricide. Cf. matricide. [L. *pater,* father, + *caedō,* to kill]

Patrick, Hugh T., U.S. neurologist, 1860–1938. SEE P.'s *test.*

pat·ri·lin·e·al (pat-ri-lin′ē-ăl). Related to descent through the male line; inheritance of the Y chromosome is exclusively patrilineal. [L. *pater,* father, + *linea,* line]

pat·ten (pat′en). A support placed under one shoe to equalize leg length when one leg is shorter than the other, or when one is artificially lengthened by a brace or splint. [Fr. *patin,* a clog]

pat·tern (pat′ern). **1.** A design. **2.** In dentistry, a form used in making a mold, as for an inlay or partial denture framework.

airspace-filling p., SYN alveolar p.

airway p., chest radiographic appearance of thickened bronchial walls, bronchiectasis, bronchiolitis, or acinar consolidation.

alveolar p., cloudy to dense opacities, obscuring vascular markings, on chest radiographs. SYN airspace-filling p.

ballerina-foot p., a vigorous posteromedial contraction of the left ventricle coupled with convexity anteriorly sometimes resulting from poor contraction of the opposing anterior wall; it is the most frequent dyssynergy observed in the prolapsed mitral valve leaflet syndrome (even with a normal anterior wall) and produces a configuration of angiographic dye in the right anterior oblique projection resembling a ballerina's foot; sometimes called dancer's foot malformation.

butterfly p., bilateral, symmetric, pulmonary alveolar opacities sparing the periphery, on chest radiographs; usually caused by pulmonary edema.

ground-glass p., radiographic or CT appearance of hazy opacity which fails to obscure pulmonary vascular markings.

honeycomb p., dense, slightly irregular circular shadows, most common next to the pleura at the lung base, on chest radiographs or CT; caused by chronic interstitial fibrosis of diverse causes.

hourglass p., a vigorous ringlike contraction observed angiographically in the left ventricular angiogram in the right anterior oblique projection, resembling an hourglass; it is seen in the prolapsed mitral valve leaflet syndrome.

interstitial p., one of several chest radiographic patterns associated with interstitial infiltration or thickening, including honeycomb p., miliary p., reticulonodular p., or septal lines.

juvenile p., a precordial T-wave inversion, sometimes with J-ST elevations in an electrocardiogram, resembling that seen in normal children, which occurs as a normal variant in some adults, especially blacks, and especially in leads V_1, V_2, and V_3.

miliary p., a chest radiographic pattern of fine, rounded opacities, typical of hematogenous dissemination of tuberculosis; size has some relationship to that of a millet seed.

mosaic p., on high-resolution CT scans of the lungs, a p. of brighter and darker regions corresponding to differences in perfusion or aeration; found in some cases of chronic thromboembolism or of bronchiolitis obliterans. Cf. oligemia.

occlusal p., SYN occlusal *form.*

reticulonodular p. (re-tik′yū-lō-nod′yū-lăr), a somewhat net-like chest radiographic p., with nodular thickening at the intersections of the lines; a nonspecific interstitial p.

wax p., a p. of wax that, when invested and burned out or otherwise eliminated, will produce a mold in which a casting may be made. SYN wax form.

pat·u·lin (pat′yū-lin). 4-Hydroxy-4*H*- furo[3,2-*c*]pyran-2(6*H*)-

one; an antibiotic derived from metabolites of fungi, such as species of *Aspergillus, Penicillium,* and *Gymnoascus;* has carcinogenic activity.

pat·u·lous (pat′yū-lŭs). SYN patent. [L. *patulus,* fr. *pateo,* to lie open]

pau·ci·bac·il·lary (paw-sē-bas′i-lār-ē). Made up of, or denoting the presence of, few bacilli.

pau·ci·sy·nap·tic (paw′sē-si-nap′tik). SYN oligosynaptic. [L. *paucus,* few, + synapse]

Paul, Gustav, Austrian physician, 1859–1935. SEE P.'s *reaction, test;* P.-Bunnell *test.*

Pauli, Wolfgang, Austrian-U.S. physicist and Nobel laureate, 1900–1958. SEE P.'s exclusion *principle.*

Pauling, Linus C., U.S. chemist and Nobel laureate, 1901–1994. SEE P.'s *theory;* P.-Corey *helix.*

paunch (pawnch). SYN rumen.

pause (pawz). Temporary stop. [G. *pausis,* cessation]

apneic p., cessation of air flow for more than 10 seconds. SEE sleep *apnea.*

compensatory p., the p. following an extrasystole, when the p. is long enough to compensate for the prematurity of the extrasystole; the short cycle ending with the extrasystole plus the p. following the extrasystole together equal two of the regular cycles.

postextrasystolic p., the somewhat prolonged cycle immediately following an extrasystole.

preautomatic p., a temporary p. in cardiac activity before an automatic pacemaker escapes. SEE ALSO escape.

respiratory p., cessation of air flow for less than 10 seconds. SEE sleep *apnea.*

sinus p., a spontaneous interruption in the regular sinus rhythm, the p. lasting for a period that is not an exact multiple of the sinus cycle. SEE ALSO sinus *arrest,* sinus *standstill.*

Pautrier, Lucien M.A., French dermatologist, 1876–1959. SEE P.'s *abscess, microabscess.*

Pauzat, Jean E., 19th century French physician. SEE P.'s *disease.*

pa·vex (pā′veks). An apparatus for producing passive vascular exercise in peripheral circulatory disorders by means of alternate positive and negative pressure. [*passive vascular exercise*]

Pavlov, Ivan, Russian physiologist and Nobel laureate, 1849–1936. SEE pavlovian *conditioning;* P. *method, pouch, stomach;* P.'s *reflex.*

pav·or noc·tur·nus (pā′vōr nok-ter′nŭs). SYN night-terrors. [L.]

Pavy, Frederick W., English physician, 1829–1911. SEE P.'s *disease.*

paw·paw. SEE papaya.

Paxton, Francis V., English physician, 1840–1924. SEE P.'s *disease.*

Payne, J. Howard, U.S. surgeon, *1916. SEE P. *operation.*

Payr, Erwin, German surgeon, 1871–1946. SEE P.'s *clamp, membrane, sign.*

Pb Symbol for lead (plumbum).

PBG. Abbreviation for porphobilinogen.

PBI Abbreviation for protein-bound *iodine.*

p. c. Abbreviation for L. *post cibum,* after a meal.

PCA Abbreviation for passive cutaneous *anaphylaxis;* patient controlled *analgesia.*

pCa. A way of reporting calcium ion levels; equal to $-\log[Ca^{2+}]$.

PCB. Abbreviation for polychlorinated *biphenyl.*

PCIS Acronym for *patient care information system,* the interactive computer system used to store medical records in a hospital.

PCMB, *p*CMB Abbreviation for *p*-chloromercuribenzoate.

P-con·gen·i·ta·le (kon-jen-i-tā′lē). The P-wave pattern in the electrocardiogram seen in some cases of congenital heart disease, consisting of tall peaked P waves in leads I, II, aVF, and aVL (usually largest in lead II) with predominant positivity of diphasic waves in V1-2. SEE ALSO spannungs-P.

PCP Abbreviation for phencyclidine; *Pneumocystis carinii* pneumonia.

PCR Abbreviation for polymerase chain *reaction.*

PCT 1. Abbreviation for *porphyria* cutanea tarda. **2.** Abbreviation for patient care technician.

PCWP Abbreviation for pulmonary capillary wedge *pressure*.

PD Abbreviation for phenyldichloroarsine.

Pd Symbol for palladium.

p.d. Abbreviation of prism *diopter*.

P-dex·tro·car·di·a·le (deks-trō-kar-dē-ā′lē). An electrocardiographic syndrome characteristic of overloading of the right atrium, often erroneously called P-pulmonale because the syndrome can result from any overloading of the right atrium (*e.g.,* tricuspid stenosis) and independently of cor pulmonale.

PDGF Abbreviation for platelet-derived growth *factor*.

PDI Abbreviation for Periodontal Disease Index.

PDL. Abbreviation for pulsed dye *laser*.

PDLL Abbreviation for poorly differentiated lymphocytic *lymphoma*.

peach ker·nel oil (pēch ker′nĕl). SEE persic oil.

peak (pēk). The top or upper limit of a graphic tracing or of any variable. [M.E. *peke, pike,* fr. Sp. *pico,* beak, fr. L. *picus,* magpie]

juxtaphrenic p. (jŭks-tă-fren′ik pēk), on chest radiograph, a triangular density on top of the right diaphragmatic shadow, probably caused by tension of the phrenic nerve on the pleura over the diaphragm.

pea·nut oil (pē′nŭt). Oil extracted from the kernels of one or more cultivated varieties of *Arachis hypogaea* (family Leguminosae); used as a solvent for intramuscular injections and in the preparation of foods. SYN arachis oil.

pearl (perl). **1.** A concretion formed around a grain of sand or other foreign body within the shell of certain mollusks. **2.** One of a number of small tough masses, such as mucus occurring in the sputum in asthma.

Elschnig p.'s, the proliferated anterior capsule of the lens of the eye after surgical capsulotomy or injury.

enamel p., SYN enameloma.

epithelial p., SYN keratin p.

Epstein's p.'s, multiple small white epithelial inclusion cysts found in the midline of the palate in newborn infants.

gouty p., a concretion of sodium urate on the cartilage of the ear, occurring in the gouty.

keratin p., a focus of central keratinization within concentric layers of abnormal squamous cells; seen in squamous cell carcinoma. SYN epithelial nest, epithelial p., squamous p.

Laënnec's p.'s, obsolete term for small, round, translucent, tenacious bodies in the sputum of some persons with asthma; when floated in water, they become unfurled and are then recognizable as Curschmann's spirals.

squamous p., SYN keratin p.

pearl-ash. SYN potash.

Pearson, Karl, English mathematician, 1857–1936. SEE Poisson-P. *formula;* McArdle-Schmid-P. *disease.*

peau d'orange (pō-dŏ-rahnj′). A swollen pitted skin surface overlying carcinoma of the breast in which there is both stromal infiltration and lymphatic obstruction with edema. [Fr. orange peel]

pec·cant (pek′ant). Unhealthy; producing disease. [L. *peccans* (-*ant*-), pres. p. of *pecco,* to sin]

pec·ca·ti·pho·bia (pek′kă-ti-fō′bē-ă). Morbid fear of sinning. [L. *peccatum,*, sin, + G. *phobos,* fear]

⚐**pecilo-.** SEE poikilo-.

pe·cil·o·cin (pĕ-sil′ō-sin). 1-(8-Hydroxy-6-methyl-1-oxo-2,4,6-dodecatrienyl)-2-pyrrolidinone; an antifungal agent.

Pecquet, Jean, French anatomist, 1622–1674. SEE P.'s *cistern, duct; receptaculum* pecqueti; P.'s *reservoir.*

pec·tase (pek′tās). An enzyme that converts pectin to D-galacturonic acid (pectic acid); used in the treatment of certain foodstuffs. SYN pectinesterase.

pec·ten (pek′ten). **1** [NA]. A structure with comblike processes or projections. **2.** SYN anal p. [L. comb]

anal p., the middle third of the anal canal. SYN p. analis [NA], pecten (2).

p. ana′lis [NA], SYN anal p.

p. os′sis pu′bis [NA], SYN p. pubis.

p. pu′bis, the continuation on the superior ramus pubis of the linea terminalis, forming a sharp ridge. SYN p. ossis pubis [NA], pectineal line of pubis.

pec·ten·i·tis (pek-ten-ī′tis). Inflammation of the sphincter ani. [L. *pecten,* a comb, + G. -*itis,* inflammation]

pec·ten·o·sis (pek-ten-ō′sis). Exaggerated enlargement of the pecten band.

pec·tic (pek′tik). Relating to any of the substances or materials now referred to as pectin. [G. *pēktos,* stiff, curdled]

pec·tic ac·id. SYN D-galacturonic acid.

pec·tin (pek′tin). Broad generic term for what are now called pectic substances or materials; specifically, a gelatinous substance, consisting largely of long chains of mostly D-galacturonic acid units (typically α-1,4 linkages and sometimes present as methyl esters), that is extracted from fruits where it is presumed to exist as protopectin (pectose). Commercial p.'s are sometimes called pectinic acid and are used in the preparation of jams, jellies, and similar food products; therapeutically, they are used to control diarrhea (usually in conjunction with other agents), as a plasma expander, and as a protectant; p.'s bind calcium ions and are highly hydrated.

p. lyase, an enzyme that catalyzes the elimination of 6-methyl-Δ-4,5-D-galacturonate residues from pectin; thus, it brings about depolymerization; it does not act on de-esterified p.; used in the treatment of certain foodstuffs.

pec·tin·ase (pek′tin-ās). SYN polygalacturonase.

pec·ti·nate (pek′ti-nāt). **1.** Combed; comb-shaped. SYN pectiniform. **2.** In fungi, used to describe a particular type of branching hyphae in cultures of dermatophytes.

pec·tin·e·al (pek-tin′ē-ăl). Ridged; relating to the os pubis or to any comblike structure. SYN pectineus (1).

pec·tin·es·ter·ase (pek-tin-es′ter-ās). SYN pectase.

pec·ti·ne·us (pek′ti-nē′ŭs). **1.** SYN pectineal. **2.** SEE pectineus *muscle.* [L.]

pec·tin·ic ac·ids (pek-tin′ik). Term sometimes used for commercial pectins.

pec·tin·i·form (pek-tin′i-fōrm). SYN pectinate (1).

pec·ti·za·tion (pek-ti-zā′shŭn). In colloidal chemistry, coagulation. [G. *pēktikos,* curdling]

pec·to·ral (pek′tŏ-răl). Relating to the chest. [L. *pectoralis;* fr. *pectus,* breast bone]

pec·to·ral·gia (pek-tō-ral′jē-ă). Pain in the chest. [L. *pectus* (*pector-*), chest, + G. *algos,* pain]

pec·to·ril·o·quy (pek-tō-ril′ō-kwē). Increased transmission of the voice sound through the pulmonary structures, so that it is clearly audible on auscultation of the chest; usually indicates consolidation of the underlying lung parenchyma. SYN pectorophony. [L. *pectus,* chest, + *loquor,* to speak]

aphonic p., SYN Baccelli's *sign.*

whispered p., whispering p., p. of whispered sounds in the same fashion as that of voice sounds. SYN whispered bronchophony.

pec·to·roph·o·ny (pek-tō-rof′ō-nē). SYN pectoriloquy. [L. *pectus,* chest, + G. *phōnē,* voice]

pec·tose (pek′tōs). SEE pectin, protopectin.

pec·tous (pek′tŭs). **1.** Relating to or consisting of pectin or pectose. **2.** Denoting a firm coagulated condition sometimes assumed by a gel, which is permanent in that the substance cannot be made to reassume the gel form.

pec·tus, gen. **pec·to·ris,** pl. **pec·to·ra** (pek′tŭs, pek′tō-ris, pek′tō-ră) [NA]. SYN chest. [L.]

p. carina′tum, flattening of the chest on either side with forward projection of the sternum resembling the keel of a boat. SYN chicken breast, keeled chest, pigeon breast, pigeon chest.

p. excava′tum, a hollow at the lower part of the chest caused by a backward displacement of the xiphoid cartilage. SYN chonechondrosternon, foveated chest, funnel chest, funnel breast, koilosternia, p. recurvatum, trichterbrust.

p. recurva′tum, SYN p. excavatum.

△**ped-, pedi-, pedo-. 1.** Child. [G. *pais,* child] **2.** Foot, feet. [L. *pes,* foot]

ped·al (ped′ăl). Relating to the feet, or to any structure called pes. [L. *pedalis,* fr. *pes (ped-),* a foot]

pe·da·tro·phia, pe·dat·ro·phy (ped-ă-trō′fē-ă, -at′rō-fē). SYN marasmus. [G. *pais (paid-),* child, + atrophy]

ped·er·ast (ped′er-ast). One who practices pederasty.

ped·er·as·ty (ped′er-as-tē). Homosexual anal intercourse, especially when practiced on boys. [G. *paiderastia;* fr. *pais (paid-),* boy, + *eraō,* to long for]

Pedersen's spec·u·lum. See under speculum.

pe·de·sis (pē-dē′sis). SYN brownian *movement.* [G. *pēdēsis,* a leaping]

△**pedi-.** SEE ped-.

pe·di·at·ric (pē-dē-at′rik). Relating to pediatrics. [G. *pais (paid-),* child, + *iatrikos,* relating to medicine]

pe·di·a·tric·ian (pē′dē-ă-trish′ăn). A specialist in pediatrics. SYN pediatrist.

pe·di·at·rics (pē-dē-at′riks). The medical specialty concerned with the study and treatment of children in health and disease during development from birth through adolescence. [G. *pais (paid-),* child, + *iatreia,* medical treatment]

pe·di·at·rist (pē-dē-at′rist). SYN pediatrician.

ped·i·at·ry (pē′dē-at-rē, pē-dī′ă-trē). A rarely used term for pediatrics

ped·i·cel (ped′i-sel). The secondary process of a podocyte, which helps form the visceral capsule of a renal corpuscle. SYN foot process, footplate (2), foot-plate. [Mod. L. *pedicellus,* dim. of L. *pes,* foot]

ped·i·cel·late (ped′i-sel-lāt). SYN pediculate.

ped·i·cel·la·tion (ped′i-sĕ-lā′shŭn). Formation of a pedicle or peduncle.

ped·i·cle (ped′ĭ-kl). **1.** A constricted portion or stalk. SYN pediculus (1) [NA]. **2.** A stalk by which a nonsessile tumor is attached to normal tissue. SYN pedunculus [NA], peduncle (2). **3.** A stalk through which a flap receives nourishment until its transfer to another site results in the nourishment coming from that site. [L. *pediculus,* dim. of *pes,* foot]

p. of arch of vertebra, the constricted portion of the arch on either side extending from the body to the lamina; bound intervertebral foramina superiorly and inferiorly. SYN pediculus arcus vertebrae [NA], radix arcus vertebrae.

Filatov-Gillies tubed p., SYN tubed *flap.*

vascular p., the tissues containing arteries and veins of an organ, specifically in chest radiology, the (width of the) mediastinum at the level of the aortic arch and superior vena cava.

pe·dic·u·lar (pĕ-dik′yū-lăr). Relating to pediculi, or lice. [L. *pedicularis*]

pe·dic·u·late (pĕ-dik′yū-lāt). Not sessile, having a pedicle or peduncle. SYN pedicellate, pedunculate. [L. *pediculatus*]

pe·dic·u·la·tion (pĕ-dik′yū-lā′shŭn). Infestation with lice. [L. *pediculus,* louse]

pe·dic·u·li (pĕ-dik′yū-lī). Plural of pediculus. [L.]

pe·dic·u·li·cide (pĕ-dik′yū-li-sīd). An agent used to destroy lice. [L. *pediculus,* louse, + *caedo,* to kill]

Pe·dic·u·loi·des ven·tri·co·sus (pĕ-dik-yū-loy′dēz ven-tri-kō′sŭs). SYN *Pyemotes tritici.* [Mod. L., fr. L. *pediculus,* louse, + *venter,* belly]

pe·dic·u·lo·pho·bia (pē-dik′yū-lō-fō′bē-ă). Morbid fear of infestation with lice. SYN phthiriophobia. [L. *pediculus,* louse, + G. *phobos,* fear]

pe·dic·u·lo·sis (pē-dik′yū-lō′sis). The state of being infested with lice. SYN lousiness. [L. *pediculus,* louse, + G. *-osis,* condition]

p. cap′itis, the presence of lice on the scalp, seen especially in children, with nits attached to hairs. SYN pthiriasis capitis.

p. cor′poris, the presence of body lice which live in the seams of clothing. Biting causes pruritus and excoriations. SEE ALSO parasitic *melanoderma.* SYN p. vestimenti, p. vestimentorum, pthiriasis corporis.

p. palpebra′rum, the presence of lice in the eyelashes.

p. pu′bis, infestation with the pubic or crab louse, *Pthirus pubis,* especially in pubic hair, causing pruritus and maculae ceruleae. SYN pthiriasis.

p. vestimen′ti, p. vestimento′rum, SYN p. corporis.

pe·dic·u·lous (pě-dik′yū-lŭs). Infested with lice. SYN lousy.

Pe·dic·u·lus (pĕ-dik′yū-lŭs). A genus of parasitic lice (family Pediculidae) that live in the hair and feeds periodically on blood. Important species include *P. humanus,* the species of louse infecting man; *P. humanus* var. *capitis,* the head louse of man; *P. humanus* var. *corporis* (also called *P. vestimenti* or *P. corporis*), the body louse or clothes louse, which lives and lays eggs (nits) in clothing and feeds on the human body; and *P. pubis.* [L.]

pe·dic·u·lus, pl. **pe·dic·u·li** (pě-dik′yū-lŭs, -lī) [NA]. **1.** SYN pedicle (1). [L. pedicle] **2.** A louse. SEE *Pediculus.* [L.]

p. ar′cus ver′tebrae [NA], SYN *pedicle* of arch of vertebra.

ped·i·cure (ped′i-kyūr). Care and treatment of the feet. [L. *pes (ped-),* foot, + *cura,* treatment]

ped·i·gree (ped′i-grē). Ancestral line of descent, especially as diagrammed on a chart to show ancestral history; used in genetics to analyze inheritance. [M.E. *pedegra* fr. O.Fr. *pie de grue,* foot of crane]

ped·i·lu·vi·um (ped′i-lū′vē-ŭm). A foot bath. [L. *pes (ped-),* foot, + *luo,* to wash]

ped·i·o·nal·gia (ped′ē-ō-nal′jē-ă). Rarely used term for podalgia. SYN pedioneuralgia. [G. *pedion,* a plain, sole of the foot, metatarsus, + *algos,* pain]

ped·i·o·neu·ral·gia (ped′ē-ō-nū-ral′jē-ă). SYN pedionalgia.

pe·di·o·pho·bia (pē′dē-ō-fō′bē-ă). Morbid fear aroused by the sight of a child or of a doll. [G. *paidion,* a little child, + *phobos,* fear]

ped·i·pha·lanx (ped′i-fā′langks). A phalanx of the foot, distinguished from maniphalanx. [L. *pes (ped-),* foot, + phalanx]

△**pedo-.** SEE ped-.

pe·do·don·tia (pē-dō-don′shē-ă). SYN pedodontics.

pe·do·don·tics (pē-dō-don′tiks). The branch of dentistry concerned with the dental care and treatment of children. SYN pediatric dentistry, pedodontia. [G. *pais,* child, + *odous,* tooth]

pe·do·don·tist (pē-dō-don′tist). A dentist who practices pedodontics.

ped·o·dy·na·mom·e·ter (ped′ō-dī-nă-mom′ě-ter). An instrument for measuring the strength of the leg muscles. [L. *pes (ped-),* foot, + G. *dynamis,* force, + G. *metron,* measure]

pe·do·gen·e·sis (pē-dō-jen′ě-sis). Permanent larval stage with sexual development, as in certain gall midges (genus *Miastor*). Cf. neoteny. [G. *pais (paid-),* child, + *genesis,* origin]

ped·o·gram (ped′ō-gram). A record made by the pedograph.

ped·o·graph (ped′ō-graf). An instrument for recording and studying the gait. [L. *pes (ped-),* foot, + G. *graphō,* to write]

pe·dog·ra·phy (pě-dog′ră-fē). Production of a record as made by a pedograph.

pe·dol·o·gist (pē-dol′ō-jist). A specialist in pedology.

pe·dol·o·gy (pē-dol′ō-jē). A rarely used term for the branch of biology and of sociology concerned with the child in his physical, mental, and social development. SYN paidology. [G. *pais (paid-),* child, + *logos,* study]

pe·dom·e·ter (pě-dom′ě-ter). An instrument for measuring the distance covered in walking. SYN podometer. [L. *pes (ped-),* foot]

pe·do·mor·phism (pē-dō-mōr′fizm). Description of adult behavior in terms appropriate to child behavior. [G. *pais (paid),* child, + *morphē,* form]

pe·do·phil·ia (pē-dō-fil′ē-ă). In psychiatry, an abnormal attraction to children by an adult for sexual purposes. [G. *pais,* child, + *philos,* fond]

pe·do·phil·ic (pē-dō-fil′ik). Relating to or exhibiting pedophilia.

pe·dun·cle (pe-dŭng′kl, pē′dŭng-kl). **1.** In neuroanatomy, term loosely applied to a variety of stalklike connecting structures in the brain, composed either exclusively of white matter (*e.g.,* cerebellar p.) or of white and gray matter (*e.g.,* cerebral p. **2.** SYN pedicle (2). [Mod. L. *pedunculus,* dim. of *pes,* foot]

cerebral p., originally denoting either of the two halves of the midbrain (a relatively narrow "neck" connecting the forebrain to the hindbrain); this term has been variably used to designate only those large bundles of corticofugal fibers forming the *crus* cerebri, or to designate the crus cerebri plus the midbrain tegmentum; this latter more inclusive usage (crus cerebri and midbrain tegmentum) is preferred; the substantia nigra, while a part of the base of the p. (basis pedunculi), is considered a structure separating the midbrain tegmentum from the crus cerebri. SEE ALSO *crus* cerebri. SYN pedunculus cerebri [NA].

p. of corpus callosum, SYN subcallosal *gyrus.*

p. of flocculus, the bundle of afferent and efferent nerve fibers connecting the flocculus and the nodule of the cerebellum; part of its course is in the inferior medullary velum. SYN pedunculus flocculi [NA].

inferior cerebellar p., large paired bundles of nerve fibers which develop on the dorsolateral surfaces of the upper medulla, extend under the lateral recesses of the rhomboid fossa and curve dorsally into the cerebellum medial to the middle cerebellar peduncle; composed of a larger (lateral) bundle, the restiform body, and a small (medial) bundle, the juxtarestiform body. Fibers forming this composite bundle originate from spinal neurons and medullary relay nuclei. The largest constituent (restiform body) is crossed fibers from the inferior olive; it also contains the dorsal spinocerebellar tract and cerebellar projections from the lateral reticular nucleus, the accessory cuneate nucleus, the paramedian reticular nuclei and the perihypoglossal nuclei. Vestibulocerebellar fibers are placed medially in the inferior cerebellar p. and are usually separately identified as the juxtarestiform body. SYN pedunculus cerebellaris inferior [NA].

inferior thalamic p., a large fiber bundle emerging from the anterior part of the thalamus in the ventral direction, in part joining the medial fibers of the internal capsule, in other part curving laterally around the medial margin of the capsule into the innominate substance. Many of its fibers establish a reciprocal connection of the mediodorsal nucleus of the thalamus with the orbital gyri of the frontal lobe, but numerous other fibers constitute a conduction system from the amygdala and olfactory cortex to the mediodorsal nucleus. SEE ALSO *ansa* peduncularis. SYN pedunculus thalami inferior [NA].

lateral thalamic p., the massive group of fibers that emerges from the laterodorsal side of the thalamus to join the corona radiata; it reciprocally connects the lateral nucleus and the geniculate bodies of the thalamus with the corresponding regions of the cerebral cortex. SYN pedunculus thalami lateralis.

p. of mamillary body, a fascicle of nerve fibers passing to the mamillary body along the ventral surface of the midbrain; it consists of fibers that originate from the dorsal and ventral tegmental nuclei. SYN pedunculus corporis mamillaris [NA], fasciculus pedunculomamillaris, pedunculomamillary fasciculus.

middle cerebellar p., the largest of three paired cerebellar p.'s, composed mainly of fibers that originate in the pontine nuclei, cross the midline in the ventral part of pons, and emerge on the opposite side as a massive bundle arching dorsally along the lateral side of the pontine tegmentum into the cerebellum; its fibers are distributed chiefly to the cortex of the cerebellar hemisphere. SYN pedunculus cerebellaris medius [NA], brachium pontis.

olfactory p., SYN olfactory *tract.*

superior cerebellar p., a large bundle of nerve fibers that originate from the dentate and interpositus nuclei and emerges from the cerebellum in the rostral direction, along the lateral wall of the fourth ventricle. The bundle submerges from the dorsal surface of the brainstem into the mesencephalic tegmentum, where all of its fibers cross in the massive decussation of the superior cerebellar p.'s. Part of the bundle terminates in the contralateral red nucleus; the bulk of the fibers continue rostrally to parts of the ventral intermediate nucleus of thalamus, ventral posterolateral nucleus of thalamus, and central lateral nucleus of thalamus.

SYN pedunculus cerebellaris superior [NA], brachium conjunctivum cerebelli.

ventral thalamic p., the massive system of fiber bundles emerging through the ventral, lateral, and anterior borders of the thalamus to join the internal capsule and parts of the corona radiata; it contains the fibers reciprocally connecting the ventral thalamic nuclei with the precentral and postcentral gyri of the cerebral cortex. SYN pedunculus thalami ventralis.

pe·dun·cu·lar (pĕ-dŭng′kyū-lăr). Relating to a pedicle or peduncle.

pe·dun·cu·late (pĕ-dŭng′kyū-lāt). SYN pediculate.

pe·dun·cu·lot·o·my (pĕ-dŭng′kyū-lot′ō-mē). **1.** A total or partial section of a cerebral peduncle. **2.** A mesencephalic pyramidal tractotomy. [peduncle + G. *tomē,* incision]

pe·dun·cu·lus, pl. **pe·dun·cu·li** (pe-dŭng′kyū-lŭs, -kyū-lī) [NA]. SYN pedicle (2). [Mod. L. dim. of *pes,* foot]

  p. cerebella′ris infe′rior [NA], SYN inferior cerebellar *peduncle.*

  p. cerebella′ris me′dius [NA], SYN middle cerebellar *peduncle.*

  p. cerebella′ris supe′rior [NA], SYN superior cerebellar *peduncle.*

  p. cer′ebri [NA], SYN cerebral *peduncle.*

  p. cor′poris callo′si [NA], SYN subcallosal *gyrus.*

  p. cor′poris mamilla′ris [NA], SYN *peduncle* of mamillary body.

  p. floc′culi [NA], SYN *peduncle* of flocculus.

  p. of pineal body, SEE habenula (2).

  p. thal′ami infe′rior [NA], SYN inferior thalamic *peduncle.*

  p. thal′ami latera′lis, SYN lateral thalamic *peduncle.*

  p. thal′ami ventra′lis, SYN ventral thalamic *peduncle.*

  p. vitelli′nus, obsolete term for yolk *stalk.*

peel. To remove hair from; to remove the outer layer of.

  face p., removal of skin blemishes such as wrinkles, freckles, or acne scars by chemical agents producing injury (trichloracetic, phenol, or other organic acids) or solid carbon dioxide.

peel·ing (pēl′ing). A stripping off or loss of epidermis, as in sunburn or toxic epidermal necrolysis. [M.E. *pelen*]

  chemical p., SYN chemexfoliation.

pee·nash (pē′nash). Rhinitis caused by insect larvae in the nasal passages. [East Indian]

PEEP Abbreviation for positive end-expiratory *pressure.*

peer re·view. process of p. r. of research proposals, manuscripts submitted for publication, abstracts submitted for presentation at a scientific meeting, whereby these are judged for technical and scientific merit by other scientists in the same field.

peg. A cylindrical projection.

  rete p.'s, SYN rete *ridges,* under *ridge.*

PEGs Abbreviation for polyethylene glycols.

Peiffer, J., German physician, *1922. SEE Hirsch-P. *stain.*

pe·jor·ism (pē′jōr-izm). A pessimistic attitude. [L. *pejor,* worse]

PEL. Abbreviation for permissible exposure *limit.*

Pel, Pieter K., Dutch physician, 1852–1919. SEE P.-Ebstein *disease, fever.*

pe·lade (pĕ-lad′, -lahd′). SYN alopecia. [Fr. *peler,* to remove the hair from a hide]

pel·age (pel′ij). The hairy covering of the body of animals; *e.g.,* the fur or coat. [Fr.]

pel·ar·gon·ic ac·id (pel-ar-gon′ik). $CH_3(CH_2)_7COOH$; used in the manufacture of lacquers and plastics; produced in the oxidative cleavage of oleic acid. SYN *n*-nonanoic acid.

Pelger, Karel, Dutch physician, 1885–1931. SEE P.-Huët nuclear *anomaly.*

pe·lid·no·ma (pē-lid-nō′mă). A circumscribed, elevated, livid patch on the skin. SYN pelioma. [G. *pelidnos,* livid, + *-oma,* tumor]

pe·li·o·ma (pē-lē-ō′mă). SYN pelidnoma.

pe·li·o·sis (pē-lē-ō′sis, pel-). SYN purpura. [G. *peliōsis,* a livid spot, livor]

  bacterial p., bacterial infection of hemorrhagic cysts of the liver, spleen, or lymph nodes, seen in immunocompromised persons, caused by *Rochalimaea henselae.*

p. hep′atis, the presence throughout the liver of blood-filled cavities which may become lined by endothelium or become organized.

Pelizaeus, Friedrich, German neurologist, 1850–1917. SEE Merzbacher-P. *disease;* P.-Merzbacher *disease.*

pel·lag·ra (pĕ-lag′ră, pĕ-lā′gră). An affection characterized by gastrointestinal disturbances, erythema (particularly of exposed areas) followed by desquamation, and nervous and mental disorders; may occur because of a poor diet, alcoholism, or some other disease causing impairment of nutrition; commonly seen when corn (maize) is a main nutrient in the diet, resulting in a deficiency of niacin. SYN Alpine scurvy, maidism, mal de la rosa, mal rosso, mayidism, psychoneurosis maidica, Saint Ignatius' itch. [It. *pelle,* skin, + *agra,* rough]

infantile p., SYN kwashiorkor.

secondary p., p. resulting from any morbid condition that impairs nutrition by increasing the requirement or reducing the available supply of vitamins.

p. si′ne p., p. without the characteristic skin lesions.

pel·lag·roid (pĕ-lag′royd). Resembling pellagra.

pel·lag·rous (pĕ-lag′rŭs). Relating to or suffering from pellagra.

Pellegrini, Augusto, Italian surgeon, *1877. SEE P.'s *disease;* P.-Stieda *disease.*

pel·let (pel′et). **1.** A pilule, or very small pill. **2.** A small rod-shaped or ovoid dosage form that is sterile and is composed essentially of pure steroid hormones in compressed form, intended for subcutaneous implantation in body tissues; serves as a depot providing for the slow release of the hormone over an extended period of time. [Fr. *pelote;* L. *pila,* a ball]

pel·li·cle (pel′i-kl). **1.** Literally and nonspecifically, a thin skin. **2.** A film or scum on the surface of a liquid. **3.** Cell boundary of sporozoites and merozoites among members of the protozoan subphylum Apicomplexa (Sporozoa), consisting of an outer unit membrane and an inner layer of two unit membranes. [L. *pellicula,* dim of *pellis,* skin]

acquired p., a thin film (about 1 μm), derived mainly from salivary glycoproteins, which forms over the surface of a cleansed tooth crown when it is exposed to the saliva. SYN acquired cuticle, acquired enamel cuticle, brown p., posteruption cuticle.

brown p., SYN acquired p.

pel·lic·u·lar, pel·lic·u·lous (pe-lik′yū-lăr, -lŭs). Relating to a pellicle.

Pellizzari, Pietro, Italian dermatologist, 1823–1892. SEE Jadassohn-P. *anetoderma.*

Pellizzi, G.B., 19th-20th century Italian physician. SEE P.'s *syndrome.*

pe·llo·te (pā-yō′tā). SYN peyote. [Aztec, *peyotl*]

pel·lu·cid (pe-lū′sid). Allowing the passage of light. [L. *pellucidus*]

pel·ma (pel′mă). SYN sole. [G.]

pel·mat·ic (pel-mat′ik). Relating to the sole of the foot. [G. *pelma,* sole]

pel·mat·o·gram (pel-mat′ō-gram). An imprint of the sole of the foot, made by resting the inked foot on a sheet of paper, or by pressing the greased foot on a plaster of Paris paste. [G. *pelma* (*pelmat-*), sole of the foot, + *gramma,* a picture]

pe·lop·a·thy (pē-lop′ă-thē). SYN pelotherapy. [G. *pēlos,* mud, + *pathos,* suffering]

pe·lo·ther·a·py (pē′lō-thār-ă-pē). Application of peloids, such as mud, peat, or clay, to all or part of the body. SYN pelopathy. [G. *pēlos,* mud, + *therapeia,* treatment]

pelt. The hide of animals on which the hair, fur, or wool is left.

pel·ta (pel′tă). A crescentic, silver-staining, membranous organelle located anteriorly near the base of the flagella in certain flagellate protozoa, as in *Trichomonas.* [L. a shield]

pel·ta·tion (pel-tā′shŭn). Protection provided by inoculation with an antiserum or with a vaccine. [L. *pelta,* a light shield, fr. G. *peltē*]

△**pelvi-, pelvio-, pelvo-.** The pelvis. Cf. pyelo-, pelyco-. [L. *pelvis,* basin (pelvis)]

pel·vic (pel′vik). Relating to a pelvis.

pel·vic di·rec·tion (pel′vik dī-rek′shŭn). The direction of the axis of the pelvis.

pel·vi·ceph·a·log·ra·phy (pel′vi-sef-ă-log′ră-fē). SYN cephalopelvimetry. [pelvi- + G. *kephalē,* head, + *graphō,* to write]

pel·vi·ceph·a·lom·e·try (pel′vi-sef-ă-lom′ĕ-trē). Measurement of the female pelvic diameters in relation to those of the fetal head. [pelvi- + G. *kephalē,* head, + *metron,* measure]

pel·vi·fix·a·tion (pel-vi-fik-sā′shŭn). Surgical attachment of a floating pelvic organ to the wall of the pelvic cavity.

pel·vi·graph (pel′vi-graf). Obsolete term for an instrument for drawing the contour and dimensions of the pelvis; may be drawn to scale. [pelvi- + G. *graphō,* to write]

pel·vi·li·thot·o·my (pel′vi-li-thot′ō-mē). SYN pyelolithotomy. [pelvi- + G. *lithos,* stone, + *tomē,* incision]

pel·vim·e·ter (pel-vim′ĕ-ter). Obsolete term for instrument shaped like calipers for measuring the diameters of the pelvis.

pel·vim·e·try (pel-vim′ĕ-trē). Measurement of the diameters of the pelvis. SYN radiocephalpelvimetry. [pelvi- + G. *metron,* measure]

manual p., measurement of the essential diameters of the bony pelvis using the hands.

radiographic p., obsolete procedure for measurement of the bony pelvis and fetal head using anteroposterior and lateral radiographs, with a device for the correction of magnification.

△**pelvio-.** SEE pelvi-.

pel·vi·o·li·thot·o·my (pel-vē-ō-li-thot′ō-mē). SYN pyelolithotomy.

pel·vi·o·per·i·to·ni·tis (pel′vē-ō-per-i-tō-nī′tis). SYN pelvic *peritonitis.*

pel·vi·o·plas·ty (pel′vē-ō-plas-tē). **1.** Symphysiotomy or pubiotomy for enlargement of the female pelvic outlet. **2.** SYN pyeloplasty. [pelvio- + G. *plastos,* formed]

pel·vi·os·co·py (pel-vē-os′kŏ-pē). Examination of the pelvis for any purpose, usually by endoscopy. SYN pelvoscopy. [pelvio- + G. *skopeō,* to view]

pel·vi·ot·o·my, pel·vit·o·my (pel′vē-ot′ō-mē). **1.** SYN symphysiotomy. **2.** SYN pubiotomy. **3.** SYN pyelotomy. [pelvio- + G. *tomē,* incision]

pel·vi·per·i·to·ni·tis (pel-vē-per-i-tō-nī′tis). SYN pelvic *peritonitis.*

PELVIS

pel·vis, pl. **pel·ves** (pel′vis, pel′vēz). **1** [NA]. The massive cup-shaped ring of bone, with its ligaments, at the lower end of the trunk, formed of the hip bone (the pubic bone, ilium, and ischium) on either side and in front, and the sacrum, and coccyx posteriorly. **2.** Any basin-like or cup-shaped cavity, as the p. of the kidney. [L. basin]

android p., a masculine or funnel-shaped p.

anthropoid p., an apelike p., with a long anteroposterior diameter and a narrow transverse diameter.

assimilation p., a deformity in which the transverse processes of the last lumbar vertebra are fused with the sacrum, or the last sacral with the first coccygeal body.

beaked p., SYN osteomalacic p.

brachypellic p., a p. in which the transverse diameter is more than 1 cm longer but less than 3 cm longer than the anteroposterior diameter. SYN transverse oval p.

caoutchouc p., in osteomalacia, a p. in which the bones are still soft. SYN rubber p.

contracted p., a p. with less than normal measurements in any diameter.

cordate p., cordiform p., a p. with sacrum projecting forward between the ilia, giving to the brim a heart shape. SYN heart-shaped p.

Deventer's p., a p. with shortened anteroposterior diameter.

dolichopellic p., a p. in which the anteroposterior diameter is longer than the transverse. SYN longitudinal oval p.

dwarf p., a very small p., in which the several bones are united by cartilage as in the infant. SYN p. nana.

false p., SYN greater p.

flat p., a p. in which the anteroposterior diameter is uniformly contracted, the sacrum being dislocated forward between the iliac bones. SYN p. plana.

frozen p., a condition in which the true p. is indurated throughout, especially by carcinoma. SYN hardened p.

funnel-shaped p., a p. in which the pelvic inlet dimensions are normal, but the outlet is contracted in the transverse or in both transverse and anteroposterior diameters.

p. of gallbladder, SYN Hartmann's *pouch.*

greater p., the expanded portion of the p. above the brim. SYN p. major [NA], false p., large p., p. spuria.

gynecoid p., the normal female p.

hardened p., SYN frozen p.

heart-shaped p., SYN cordate p.

inverted p., split p. with separation at pubis.

p. jus'to ma'jor, a symmetrical p. with greater than normal measurements in all diameters.

p. jus'to mi'nor, a p. of the female type, but with all its diameters smaller than normal.

juvenile p., a p. justo minor in which the bones are slender.

kyphoscoliotic p., a p. with marked anteroposterior curvature of the spine combined with lateral spinal curvature, usually due to severe rickets.

kyphotic p., backward curvature of the lumbar spine causing contraction of pelvic measurements.

large p., SYN greater p.

lesser p., the cavity of the p. below the brim or superior aperture. SYN p. minor [NA], p. vera, small p., true p.

longitudinal oval p., SYN dolichopellic p.

lordotic p., a deformed p. associated with lordosis.

p. ma'jor [NA], SYN greater p.

masculine p., (1) a p. justo minor in which the bones are large and heavy; (2) a slight degree of funnel-shaped p. in the woman, in which the shape approximates that of the male p.

mesatipellic p., obsolete term for one in which the anteroposterior and transverse diameters are equal or the transverse diameter is not more than 1 cm longer than the anteroposterior diameter. SYN round p.

p. mi'nor [NA], SYN lesser p.

Nägele's p., an obliquely contracted or unilateral synostotic p., marked by arrest of development of one lateral half of the sacrum, usually ankylosis of the sacroiliac joint on that side, rotation of the sacrum toward the same side, and deviation of the symphysis pubis to the opposite side.

p. na'na, SYN dwarf p.

p. obtec'ta, a form of kyphotic p. in which the angular curvature of the spine is low and extreme so that the spinal column projects horizontally across the inlet of the p.

osteomalacic p., a pelvic deformity in osteomalacia; the pressure of the trunk on the sacrum and lateral pressure of the femoral heads produce a pelvic aperture that is three-cornered or has the shape of a heart or cloverleaf, while the pubic bone becomes beak-shaped. SYN beaked p., rostrate p.

Otto p., SYN Otto's *disease.*

p. pla'na, SYN flat p.

platypellic p., flat oval p., in which the transverse diameter is more than 3 cm longer than the anteroposterior diameter.

platypelloid p., simple flat p.

Prague p., SYN spondylolisthetic p.

pseudo-osteomalacic p., an extreme degree of rachitic p., resembling the puerperal osteomalacic p., in which the pelvic canal is obstructed by a forward projection of the sacrum, and an approximation of the acetabula.

rachitic p., a contracted and deformed p., most commonly a flat p., occurring from rachitic softening of the bones in early life.

renal p., a flattened funnel-shaped expansion of the upper end of the ureter receiving the calices, the apex being continuous with the ureter. SYN p. renalis [NA], ureteric p.

p. rena'lis [NA], SYN renal p.

reniform p., a modified cordate p., with a long transverse diameter, giving the brim a kidney shape.

Robert's p., obsolete term for a p. which is narrowed transversely in consequence of the almost entire absence of the alae of the sacrum.

Rokitansky's p., SYN spondylolisthetic p.

rostrate p., SYN osteomalacic p.

round p., SYN mesatipellic p.

rubber p., SYN caoutchouc p.

scoliotic p., a deformed p. associated with lateral curvature of the spine.

small p., SYN lesser p.

spider p., narrow calices of renal p.

split p., a p. in which the symphysis pubis is absent, the pelvic bones being separated by quite an interval; usually associated with exstrophy of the bladder.

spondylolisthetic p., a p. whose brim is more or less occluded by a forward dislocation of the body of the lower lumbar vertebra. SYN Prague p., Rokitansky's p.

p. spu'ria, SYN greater p.

transverse oval p., SYN brachypellic p.

true p., SYN lesser p.

ureteric p., SYN renal p.

p. ve'ra, SYN lesser p.

---

pel·vi·sa·cral (pel-vi-sā'krăl). Relating to both the pelvis, or hip bones, and the sacrum.

pel·vi·scope (pel'vi-skōp). Endoscopic instrument for examining the interior of the pelvis. [pelvi- + G. *skopeō,* to view]

pel·vi·therm (pel'vi-therm). Instrument for applying heat to the pelvic organs. [pelvi- + G. *thermē,* heat]

pel·vi·u·re·ter·og·ra·phy (pel-vi-yū-rē-ter-og'ră-fē). SYN pyelography.

△**pelvo-.** SEE pelvi-.

pel·vo·ceph·a·log·ra·phy (pel'vō-sef-ă-log'ră-fē). SYN cephalopelvimetry.

pel·vos·co·py (pel-vos'cŏ-pē). SYN pelvioscopy.

pel·vo·spon·dy·li·tis os·sif·i·cans (pel'vō-spon-di-lī'tis os-if'i-kanz). Deposit of bony substance between the vertebrae of the sacrum. [L. *pelvis,* basin, + G. *spondylos,* vertebra, + *-itis;* L. *os,* bone, + *facio,* to make]

△**pelyco-.** RARE the pelvis. SEE pelvi-. [G. *pelyx,* bowl (pelvis)]

pem·o·line (pem'ō-lēn). 2-Imino-5-phenyl-4-oxazolidinone; a psychostimulant used in the treatment of attention deficit disorder (hyperactivity) in children.

pem·phi·goid (pem'fi-goyd). 1. Resembling pemphigus. 2. A disease resembling pemphigus but significantly distinguishable histologically (nonacantholytic) and clinically (generally benign course). [G. *pemphix,* blister, + *eidos,* resemblance]

benign mucosal p., SYN cicatricial p.

bullous p., a chronic, generally benign disease, most commonly of old age, characterized by tense nonacantholytic bullae in which serum antibodies are localized to the epidermal basement membrane, causing detachment of the entire thickness of the epidermis.

cicatricial p., a chronic disease that produces adhesions and progressive cicatrization and shrinkage of the conjunctival, oral, and vaginal mucous membranes. SYN benign mucosal p.

localized p. of Brunsting-Perry, a variant of p., primarily on the scalp and face, with some scar formation.

ocular p., a conjunctivitis with transient small vesicles, a viscid ropy discharge, symblepharon, xerosis, and trichiasis, eventually becoming bilateral.

pem·phi·gus (pem'fi-gŭs). 1. Auto-immune bullous diseases with acantholysis: p. vulgaris, p. foliaceus, p. erythematosus, or

p. vegetans. **2.** A nonspecific term for blistering skin diseases. [G. *pemphix*, a blister]

p. acu′tus, obsolete term for a pyogenic infection due to local trauma, that responds to antibiotic therapy; if untreated, the condition may become extensive and the patient seriously ill. SYN bullous fever.

benign familial chronic p. [MIM*169600], recurrent eruption of vesicles and bullae that become scaling and crusted lesions with vesicular borders, predominantly of the neck, groin, and axillary regions; autosomal dominant inheritance, presenting in late adolescence or early adult life. SYN Hailey-Hailey disease.

Brazilian p., SYN fogo selvagem.

p. contagio′sus, obsolete term for a superficial pyogenic infection. SYN Manson's pyosis.

p. erythemato′sus, an eruption involving sun-exposed skin, especially the face; the lesions are scaling erythematous macules and blebs, combining the clinical features of both lupus erythematosus and p. vulgaris; bullae are subcorneal; probably a variant of p. foliaceus. SYN Senear-Usher disease, Senear-Usher syndrome.

p. folia′ceus, a generally chronic form of p. in which extensive exfoliative dermatitis, with no perceptible blistering, may be present in addition to the bullae; serum autoantibodies induce bullae and crusted acantholytic superficial epidermal lesions.

p. gangreno′sus, (1) SYN *dermatitis* gangrenosa infantum. **(2)** SYN bullous *impetigo* of newborn.

p. lepro′sus, an eruption of bullae, occurring sometimes in the course of anesthetic leprosy.

p. veg′etans, (1) a form of p. vulgaris in which vegetations develop on the eroded surfaces left by ruptured bullae; new bullae continue to form; SYN Neumann's disease. **(2)** a chronic benign vegetating form of p., with lesions commonly in the axillae and perineum; spontaneous remissions and occasionally permanent healing occur. SYN Hallopeau's disease (2).

p. vulga′ris, a serious form of p., occurring in middle age, in which cutaneous flaccid acantholytic suprabasal bullae and oral mucosal erosions may be localized a few months before becoming generalized; blisters break easily and are slow to heal; results from the action of autoimmune antibodies that localize to intercellular sites of stratified squamous epithelium.

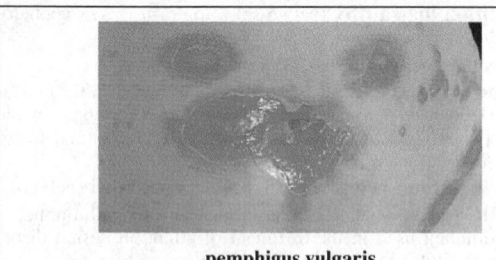

pemphigus vulgaris

pem·pi·dine (pem′pi-dēn). Secondary amine of the mecamylamine group, effective as a ganglionic blocking agent; also available as p. tartrate, with the same uses.

pen·del·luft (pen-del-lŭft′). Transient movement of gas out of some alveoli and into others when flow has just stopped at the end of inspiration, or such movement in the opposite direction just at the end of expiration; occurs when regions of the lung differ in compliance, airway resistance, or inertance so that the time constants of their filling (or emptying) in response to a change of transpulmonary pressure are not the same. [Ger. *Pendel*, pendulum, + *Luft*, air]

Pendred, Vaughan, English surgeon, 1869–1946. SEE P.'s *syndrome*.

pe·nec·to·my (pē-nek′tō-mē). SYN phallectomy. [L. *penis* + G. *ektomē*, excision]

pe·nes. Plural of penis, as in diphallus.

pen·e·trance (pen′ĕ-trans). The frequency, expressed as a fraction or percentage, of individuals who are phenotypically affect-

ed, among persons of an appropriate genotype (*i.e.,* homozygous or hemizygous for recessives, heterozygotes or homozygotes for dominants); factors affecting expression may be environmental, or due to purely random variation; contrasted with hypostasis where the condition has a genetic origin and therefore tends to cause correlation in relatives. [see penetration]

genetic p. (pen′ĕ-trans), the extent to which a genetically determined condition is expressed in an individual.

pen·e·trate (pen′ĕ-trāt). To pierce; to pass into the deeper tissues or into a cavity.

pen·e·tra·tion (pen-ĕ-trā′shŭn). **1.** A piercing or entering. **2.** Mental acumen. **3.** SYN focal *depth*. [L. *penetratio*, fr. *penetro*, pp. *-atus*, to enter]

pen·e·trom·e·ter (pen-ĕ-trom′ĕ-ter). An obsolete instrument for measuring the penetrating power of x-rays from any given source. [penetration + G. *metron*, measure]

△-penia. Deficiency. [G. *penia*, poverty]

pe·ni·al (pē′nē-ăl). SYN penile.

pe·ni·a·pho·bia (pē′nē-ă-fō′bē-ă). Morbid fear of poverty. [G. *penia*, poverty, + *phobos*, fear]

pen·i·cil·la·mine (pen-i-sil′ă-mēn). β-thiovaline; a degradation product of penicillin; a chelating agent used in the treatment of lead poisoning, hepatolenticular degeneration, and cystinuria, and in the removal of excess copper in Wilson's disease; also available as p. hydrochloride. SYN β, β-dimethylcysteine.

pen·i·cil·la·nate (pen-i-sil′ă-nāt). A salt of penicillanic acid.

pen·i·cil·lan·ic ac·id (pen-i-si-lan′ik). A penicillin without the characterizing R group (with H– replacing ROONH–) of penicillin.

pen·i·cil·lar·y (pen-i-sil′ă-rē). Denoting a penicillus (1).

pen·i·cil·late (pen-i-sil′āt). **1.** Pertaining to a penicillus. **2.** Having a tuftlike structure.

pen·i·cil·lic ac·id (pen-i-sil′ik). An antibiotic produced by *Penicillium puberulum*, a mold found on maize, and from *P. cyclopium;* active against Gram-positive and Gram-negative bacteria but toxic to animal tissues.

pen·i·cil·lin (pen-i-sil′in). **1.** Originally, an antibiotic substance obtained from cultures of the molds *Penicillium notatum* or *P. chrysogenum.* **2.** One of a family of natural or synthetic variants of penicillic acid. They are mainly bactericidal in action, are especially active against Gram-positive organisms, and, with the exception of hypersensitivity reactions, show a particularly low toxic action on animal tissue. [see penicillus]

aluminum p., the trivalent aluminum salt of an antibiotic substance or substances produced by the growth of the molds *Penicillium notatum* or *P. chrysogenum;* used for oral or sublingual administration.

p. amidase, an enzyme that catalyzes the hydrolysis of the amide bond in the p.'s, producing a carboxylic acid anion and penicin; penicin is the precursor of many synthetic p.'s.

p. B, SYN phenethicillin potassium.

benzyl p., SYN p. G.

buffered crystalline p. G, crystalline potassium p. G or crystalline sodium p. G buffered with not less than 4% and not more than 5% of sodium citrate.

chloroprocaine p. O, a crystalline salt of 2-chloroprocaine and p. O, insoluble in water; the level of the antibiotic in the blood persists for 24 hours; its antibacterial activity is similar to that of p. O and G.

p. G, R=$C_6H_5CH_2$–; a commonly used p. compound; it comprises 85% of the p. salts: sodium, potassium, aluminum, and procaine, with the latter exerting prolonged action on intramuscular injection, due to limited solubility. An antibiotic obtained from the mold *Penicillium chrysogenum* used orally and parenterally; primarily active against Gram-positive staphylococci and streptococci; destroyed by bacterial beta lactamase. SYN benzyl p., benzylpenicillin.

p. G benzathine, a benzylpenicillin compound with *N,N*-dibenzylethylenediamine (2:1); a relatively insoluble preparation that may remain in the body for 1 to 2 weeks.

p. G hydrabamine, a dipenicillin compound, a mixture of p. G salts consisting chiefly of the salt of the diacidic base *N,N '*-bis-(dehydroabietyl) ethylenediamine.

p. G potassium, potassium benzylpenicillin; the potassium salt of p. G, containing 85 to 90% p. G.

p. G procaine, procaine p; procaine benzylpenicillin; the procaine salt of p. G; it has a more prolonged action than p. G.

p. G sodium, sodium benzylpenicillin; the sodium salt of p. G, containing not less than 85% p. G.

p. N, SYN *cephalosporin* N.

p. O, R–=CH_2=$CHCH_2SCH_2$–; produced by growing the mold in a medium containing allylmercaptomethylacetic acid; also available as the potassium and sodium salts. SYN allylmercaptomethylpenicillin.

p. phenoxymethyl, SYN p. V.

p. V, R=$C_6H_5OCH_2$–; obtained from *Penicillium chrysogenum* Q 176; a crystalline nonhydroscopic acid, very stable even in high humidity; it resists destruction by gastric juice; the potassium salt is used orally; precursor for the synthesis of analogs of cephalosporin C. SYN p. phenoxymethyl, phenoxymethylpenicillin.

p. V benzathine, benzathine phenoxymethylpenicillin; p. for oral use.

p. V hydrabamine, hydrabamine phenoxymethylpenicillin; a compound with preparation and uses analogous to those of p. G hydrabamine.

pen·i·cil·li·nase (pen-i-sil′i-nās). **1.** SYN β-lactamase. **2.** A purified enzyme preparation obtained from cultures of a strain of *Bacillus cereus;* formerly used in the treatment of slowly developing or delayed penicillin reactions.

pen·i·cil·li·nate (pen-i-sil′i-nāt). A salt of a penicillic acid (*i.e.,* of a penicillin).

pen·i·cil·li·o·sis (pen-ē-sil-ē-ō′sis). Infection with fungi of the genus *Penicillium* and characterized in dogs by chronic sneezing and a nasal discharge.

Pen·i·cil·li·um (pen-i-sil′ē-ŭm). A genus of fungi (class Ascomycetes, order Aspergillales), species of which yield various antibiotic substances and biologicals; *e.g., citrinum* yields citrinin; *P. claviforme, P. expansum,* and *P. patulum* yield patulin; *P. chrysogenum* yields penicillin; *P. griseofulvum* yields griseofulvin; *P. notatum* yields penicillin and notatin; *P. cyclopium* and *P. puberulum* yield penicillic acid; *P. purpurogenum* and *P. rubrum* yield rubratoxin. *P. marneffei* is a true pathogen in Southeast Asia and in the bamboo rats. [see penicillus]

pen·i·cil·lo·ic ac·id (pen′i-si-lō′ik). Alkali and bacterial degradation product of a penicillin, resulting from hydrolysis of the 1,7 bond.

pen·i·cil·lo·yl pol·y·ly·sine (pen-i-sil′ō-il). A preparation of polylysine and a penicillic acid, used intradermally in the diagnosis of penicillin sensitivity; sensitive persons may react with systemic manifestations, including generalized cutaneous eruptions.

pen·i·cil·lus, pl. **pe·ni·cil·li** (pen-i-sil′ŭs, -sil′ī). **1** [NA]. One of the tufts formed by the repeated subdivision of the minute arterial twigs in the spleen. **2.** In fungi, one of the branched conidiophores bearing chains of conidia in *Penicillium* species. [L. paint brush]

pen·i·cin (pen′i-sin). SYN 6-aminopenicillanic acid.

pe·nile (pē′nīl). Relating to the penis. SYN penial.

pe·nil·lic ac·ids (pe-nil′ik). Acid degradation products of penicillins, produced by cleavage of the 1,7 bond, forming penicilloic acid, and formation of a bond between the exocyclic carbonyl carbon and N-1 with elimination of H_2O from those two and the exocyclic NH.

pen·in (pen′in). 6-Aminopenicillanic acid (NH_2 replacing RCONH– in penicillin); an intermediate in the synthesis of penicillins.

pe·nis, pl. **pe·nes** (pē′nis) [NA]. The organ of copulation in the male; it is formed of three columns of erectile tissue, two arranged laterally on the dorsum (corpora cavernosa p.) and one median below (corpus spongiosum); the urethra traverses the latter; the extremity (glans p.) is formed by an expansion of the corpus spongiosum, and is more or less completely covered by a

free fold of skin (preputium). SYN intromittent organ, membrum virile, phallus, priapus, virga. [L. tail]

bifid p., SYN diphallus.

buried p., normal p. obscured by suprapubic fat.

clubbed p., a deformity of the erect p. marked by a curve to one side or toward the scrotum.

concealed p., usually a complication of circumcision wherein the anastomotic line between shaft skin and preputial collar closes like an iris or cicatrix over glans (some equate this to buried penis).

p. femin′eus, obsolete term for clitoris.

gryposis p., SYN chordee (1).

p. luna′tus, SYN chordee (1).

p. mulie′bris, obsolete term for clitoris.

p. palma′tus, SYN webbed p.

webbed p., deficient ventral penile shaft skin which is buried in scrotum or tethered to scrotal midline by a fold or web of skin. The urethra and erectile bodies are usually normal. SYN p. palmatus, penoscrotal transposition.

pe·nis·chi·sis (pē-nis′ki-sis). A fissure of the penis resulting in an abnormal opening into the urethra, either above (epispadias), below (hypospadias), or to one side (paraspadias). [L. *penis* + G. *schisis,* fissure]

pe·ni·tis (pē-nī′tis). Obsolete term for inflammation of the penis. SYN phallitis.

pen·nate (pen′āt). Feathered; resembling a feather. SYN penniform. [L. *pennatus,* fr. *penna,* feather]

pen·ni·form (pen′i-fŏrm). SYN pennate. [L. *penna,* feather, + *forma,* form]

pen·ny·roy·al (pen′ē-roy-ăl). A name in folk medicine given to *Mentha pulegium* (an aromatic p.), or to *Hedeoma pulegeoides* (American p.) (family Labiatae); an aromatic stimulant formerly used as an emmenagogue.

pe·no·scro·tal (pē′nō-skrō′tăl). Relating to both penis and scrotum.

pe·not·o·my (pē-not′o-mē). SYN phallotomy. [L. *penis* + G. *tomē,* a cutting]

Penrose, Charles B., U.S. gynecologist, 1862–1925. SEE P. drain.

penta-. Combining form denoting five. [G. *pente,* five]

pen·ta·ba·sic (pen-tă-bā′sik). Denoting an acid having five replaceable hydrogen atoms. [penta- + G. *basis,* base]

pen·ta·chlo·ro·phe·nol (pen-tă-klōr-ō-fen′ol). Insecticide for termite control; pre-harvest defoliant; general herbicide. Has been recommended for use in the preservation of wood, wood products, starches, dextrins, glues. No longer available for consumer use; a powerful irritant.

pen·tad. 1. A collection of five things in some way related. **2.** In chemistry, a pentavalent element. [G. *pentas,* the number five]

Reynolds p., abdominal pain, fever, jaundice, shock, and depression of central nervous system function; usually indicative of acute suppurative cholangitis.

pen·ta·dac·tyl, pen·ta·dac·tyle (pen-tă-dak′til). Having five fingers or toes on each hand or foot. SYN quinquedigitate. [penta- + G. *daktylos,* finger]

pen·ta·e·ryth·ri·tol (pen-tă-ĕ-rith′ri-tol). C($CH_2OH)_4$; Tetrakis-(hydroxymethyl)methane; the tetranitrate is a coronary vasodilator with action similar to that of other slow acting organic nitrates.

pen·ta·e·ryth·ri·tol tet·ra·ni·trate. An organic nitrate used as a vasodilator in the treatment of angina pectoris. Exerts a longer duration of action than nitroglycerin.

pen·ta·gas·trin (pen-tă-gas′trin). The substituted pentapeptide, BOC-β-Ala-Trp-Met-Asp-Phe(NH₂); a gastric acid stimulator.

pen·tal·o·gy (pen-tal′ŏ-jē). A rarely used term for a combination of five elements, such as five concurrent symptoms. [penta- + G. *logos,* treatise, word]

p. of Cantrell, a type of sternal anomaly associated with midline abdominal defects, a pericardial defect, a cardiac anomaly, and ectopia cordis.

p. of Fallot, Fallot's tetralogy with, in addition, a patent foramen ovale or atrial septal defect.

pen·ta·mer (pen′tă-mer). SEE virion. [penta- + G. *meros,* part]

pen·ta·me·tho·ni·um bro·mide (pen′tă-me-thō′nē-ŭm). Pentamethylene-*bis*[trimethylammonium bromide]; a ganglionic blocking agent with the same antihypertensive use as hexamethonium chloride.

pen·tam·i·dine is·e·thi·o·nate (pen-tam′i-dēn). *p,p′*-(Pentamethylenedioxy)dibenzamidinebis(β-hydroxyethanesulfonate); a toxic but effective drug used in the prophylaxis and treatment of early stages of both types of African sleeping sickness (Gambian and Rhodesian trypanosomiasis). It does not cross the blood-brain barrier and is not effective in the treatment of the advanced (neurological) stage of the disease. Also used to treat leishmaniasis that does not respond to therapy with pentavalent antimonials and in the treatment of pneumonia caused by *Pneumocystis carinii.*

pen·ta·no·ic ac·id (pen-tă-nō′ik). SYN valeric acid.

pen·ta·pep·tide (pen′tă-pep′tīd). A compound containing five amino acid residues linked via peptide bonds.

pen·ta·pip·er·ide fu·ma·rate (pen-tă-pip′er-īd). 3-Methyl-2-phenylvaleric acid 1-methyl-4-piperidyl ester fumarate; an intestinal antispasmodic.

pen·ta·pi·per·i·um meth·yl·sul·fate (pen′tă-pī-per′ē-ŭm). 4-Hydroxy-1,1-dimethylpiperidinium methyl sulfate 3-methyl-2-phenylvalerate; an anticholinergic agent.

pen·ta·quine (pen′tă-kwīn). 8-(5-Iso-propylamino)-6-methoxy-quinoline)-an antimalarial agent closely related chemically to pamaquine but less toxic and more effective; it is administered with quinine, the two drugs acting synergically; active against *Plasmodium vivax* infections.

Pen·tas·to·ma (pen-tas′tō-mă). Older name for a genus of Pentastomida, now called *Linguatula.* The species described as *P. denticulatum* proved to be the larva of *Linguatula rhinaria,* sometimes parasitic in the nose of humans and other mammals; adults are found in the lungs of reptiles. [penta- + G. *stoma,* mouth]

pen·ta·sto·mi·a·sis (pen′tă-stō-mī′ă-sis). Infection of herbivorous animals, swine, and man with larval tongue worms; lesions occur principally in the lymph nodes of the digestive tract, where they often resemble those of tuberculosis.

Pen·ta·stom·i·da (pen-tă-stom′i-dă). The tongue worms, a group of parasitic wormlike animals considered to form a distinct phylum thought to be descended from primitive arthropods, though modified by parasitism to form elongate, pseudosegmented, wormlike organisms with two to three pairs of budlike degenerate limbs in the larva and anterior, hollow, fanglike hooks in the adult. Adults are usually parasitic in the lungs or respiratory tract of vertebrates, usually in snakes and other reptiles, though one group parasitizes the air sacs of birds and one family (Linguatulidae) has become adapted to the lungs of mammal carnivores (families Felidae and Canidae). Larvae are found in the viscera of many hosts that serve as prey of the final hosts (insects, fish, amphibians, chiefly frogs, and mammals, chiefly rodents). Dogs may develop adult *Linguatula serrata* in their nasal passages from infective larvae (nymphs) in the viscera of sheep, cattle, or rabbits, which became infected from water or vegetation contaminated with eggs passed by infected dogs; humans also can develop a larval infection from this source. Human infection of liver, spleen, and lungs has been reported in

Africa from *Armillifer armillatus* and in China by *A. moniliformis* from contaminated water or vegetation or from handling infected snakes. [see *Pentastoma*]

pent·a·tom·ic (pent′ă-tom-ik). Denoting five atoms per molecule. [penta- + atomic]

Pen·ta·trich·o·mon·as (pen′tă-trik-ŏ-mō′nas, pen′tă-trī-kom′ŏ-nas). A genus of parasitic protozoan flagellates, formerly part of the genus *Trichomonas* but now separated as a distinct genus by the presence of five anterior flagella and a granular parabasal body. The species *Pentatrichomonas hominis* lives as a commensal in the colon of man and other primates, dogs, cats, oxen, and various rodents. [penta- + *Trichomonas*]

pen·ta·va·lent (pen-tă-vā′lent, pen-tav′ă-lent). Having a combining power (valence) of five. SYN quinquevalent.

pen·taz·o·cine (pen-taz′ō-sēn). 1,2,3,4,5,6-Hexahydro-6,11-dimethyl-3-(3-methyl-2-butenyl)   -2,6-methano-3-benzazocin-8-ol; a potent opioid agonist/antagonist analgesic with some addiction liability but only rare withdrawal syndrome and tolerance; available as the hydrochloride and lactate salts.

pen·te·tate tri·so·di·um cal·ci·um (pen′tĕ-tāt). The calcium trisodium salt of pentetic acid. SYN calcium trisodium pentetate.

pen·tet·ic ac·id (pen-tet′ik). A pentaacetic acid triamine with affinity for heavy metals; used as the calcium sodium chelate in the treatment of iron-storage disease and poisoning from heavy metals and radioactive metals. SEE ALSO ethylenediaminetetraacetic acid.

pen·thi·e·nate bro·mide (pen-thī′ĕ-nāt). 2-Diethylaminoethyl-α-cyclopentyl-2-thiopheneglycolate methylbromide; an anticholinergic agent.

pen·tif·yl·line (pen-tif′i-lēn). 1-Hexyltheobromine; a vasodilator; has more lipid solubility than theobromine.

pen·ti·tol (pen′ti-tol). A reduced pentose; *e.g.,* ribitol, lyxitol, xylitol.

pen·to·bar·bi·tal (pen-tō-bar′bi-tahl). 5-(Ethyl-5-methylbutyl)-barbituric acid; an oral and intravenous sedative and short-acting hypnotic barbiturate; largely replaced by benzodiazepines.

pen·to·lin·i·um tar·trate (pen-tō-lin′ē-ŭm). Pentamethylene-1,1′-bis-(1-methylpyrrolidinium bitartrate; a quaternary ammonium compound with potent ganglionic blocking action; used in the management of severe and malignant hypertension and peripheral vasospastic diseases.

pen·ton (pen′tŏn). The pentagonal capsomere (p. base) along with the protruding fiber at each of the 12 vertices of the adenovirus capsid; antigenically, the p. base differs from the fiber, and both differ from the other (hexagonal) capsomeres.

pen·to·san (pen′tō-san). A poly- or oligosaccharide of a pentose; *e.g.,* arabans, xylans.

pen·tose (pen′tōs). A monosaccharide containing five carbon atoms in the molecule; *e.g.,* arabinose, lyxose, ribose, xylose, xylulose.

p. nucleotide, a nucleotide having a p. as the sugar component.

pen·to·sta·tin (pen′tō-stat′in). An antineoplastic; a potent inhibitor of adenosine deaminase; interferes with the synthesis of nicotinamide adenine dinucleotide. SYN 2-deoxycoformycin.

pen·to·su·ria (pen-tō-sū′rē-ă). The excretion of one or more pentoses in the urine.

alimentary p., the urinary excretion of L-arabinose and L-xylose, as the result of the excessive ingestion of fruits containing these pentoses.

essential p. [MIM*260800], a benign heritable disorder in which the urinary output of L-xylulose is 1 to 4 g per 24 hr; it occurs principally in Ashkenazi Jewish; autosomal recessive inheritance. SYN L-xylulosuria, primary p.

primary p., SYN essential p.

pen·tox·ide (pen-tok′sīd). An oxide containing five oxygen atoms; *e.g.,* phosphorus p., P₂O₅.

pen·tox·if·yl·line (pen-toks-if′i-lēn). 1-(5-Oxohexyl)-theobromine; a dimethylxanthine derivative that decreases blood viscosity and improves blood flow; used in the treatment of intermittent claudication.

pen·tu·lose (pen′tyū-lōs). A ketopentose; *e.g.,* ribulose, xylulose.

pen·tyl (pen'til). **1.** SYN amyl. **2.** The $CH_3(CH_2)_3CH_2-$ moiety.

pen·ty·lene·tet·ra·zol (pen'ti-lēn-tet'ră-zol). $C_6H_{10}N_4$; a powerful stimulant to the central nervous system; has been used to cause generalized convulsion in the shock treatment of emotional states and as a respiratory stimulant; mainly used in experimental studies of seizure mechanisms.

pe·num·bra (pe-nŭm'bră). The region of partial illumination or radiation caused by light or x-rays not originating from a point source; also called geometric unsharpness. [Mod. L., fr. L. *paene*, almost, + *umbra*, shadow]

pe·o·til·lo·ma·nia (pē'ō-til-ō-mā'nē-ă). Rarely used term for a nervous tic consisting of a constant pulling of the penis. SYN false masturbation, pseudomasturbation. [G. *peos*, penis, + *tillō*, to pull out (of hair), + *mania*, frenzy]

pep·lo·mer (pep'lō-mer). A part or subunit of the peplos of a virion, the assemblage of which produces the complete peplos, produced from the peplos by detergent treatment. [see peplos]

pep·los (pep'lōs). The coat or envelope of lipoprotein material that surrounds certain virions. [G. an outer garment worn by women]

Pepper, William, Jr., U.S. physician, 1874–1947. SEE P. *syndrome*.

pep·per·mint (pep'er-mint). The dried leaves and flowering tops of *Mentha piperita* (family Labiatae); a carminative and antiemetic.

p. camphor, SYN menthol.

p. oil, the volatile oil distilled with steam from the fresh, overground parts of the flowering plant of *Mentha piperita*, rectified by distillation and neither partially nor wholly dementholized; a flavor.

pep·sic (pep'sik). SYN peptic.

pep·sin (pep'sin). P. A is the principal digestive enzyme (protease) of gastric juice, formed from pepsinogen; it hydrolyzes peptide bonds at low pH values (is alkali-labile), preferably adjacent to phenylalanyl and leucyl residues, thus reducing proteins to smaller molecules (proteoses and peptones); p. B (gelatinase) is similar to p. A, but formed from porcine pepsinogen B and has a more restricted specificity; p. C (gastricsin is human p. C) is also similar to p. A, and structurally related to it, having a more restricted specificity. [G. *pepsis*, digestion]

pep·si·nate (pep'si-nāt). To mix pepsin with.

pep·si·nif·er·ous (pep-si-nif'er-ŭs). SYN pepsinogenous.

pep·sin·o·gen (pep-sin'ō-jen). A proenzyme formed and secreted by the chief cells of the gastric mucosa; the acidity of the gastric juice and pepsin itself remove 42 amino acid residues from p. to form active pepsin. SYN propepsin. [pepsin + G. *-gen*, producing]

pep·sin·og·e·nous (pep-sin-oj'ĕ-nŭs). Producing pepsin. SYN pepsiniferous.

pep·si·nu·ria (pep-si-nū'rē-ă). Excretion of pepsin in the urine. [pepsin + G. *ouron*, urine]

pep·sta·tin (pep-sta'tin). An inhibitor peptide from actinomycetes that inhibits pepsin and cathepsin D.

pep·tic (pep'tik). Relating to the stomach, to gastric digestion, or to pepsin A. SYN pepsic. [G. *peptikos*, fr. *peptō*, to digest]

pep·ti·dase (pep'ti-dās). Any enzyme capable of hydrolyzing one of the peptide links of a peptide; *e.g.*, carboxypeptidases, aminopeptidases. SYN peptide hydrolase.

p. D, SYN *proline* dipeptidase.

p. P, SYN peptidyl dipeptidase A.

pep·tide (pep'tīd). A compound of two or more amino acids in which a carboxyl group of one is united with an amino group of another, with the elimination of a molecule of water, thus forming a peptide bond, –CO–NH–; *i.e.*, a substituted amide. Cf. eupeptide *bond*, isopeptide *bond*.

adrenocorticotropic p., a p. with ACTH activity, isolated from pituitary extracts.

anionic neutrophil activating p. (ANAP), SYN interleukin-8.

atrial natriuretic p. (ANP) (na'trē-ū-ret'ik), a 28 amino acid p. (α-ANP), derived from cardiac atria, several smaller fragments of α-ANP, and a dimer of α-ANP with 56 amino acids (β-ANP)

that are present in plasma in heart failure. ANP actions include increasing capillary filtration, and renal salt and water excretion, and decreasing arterial pressure and the secretion of renin, angiotensin, aldosterone, and antidiuretic hormone. SYN atriopeptin, cardionatrin.

bitter p.'s, p.'s that have a bitter taste and may spoil certain foods; often contain high proportions of leucyl, valyl, and aromatic amino acid residues.

bradykinin-potentiating p., SYN teprotide.

calcitonin gene related p. (CGRP) (kal'sĭ-tō'nin), a second product transcribed from the calcitonin gene. Calcitonin gene related p. is found in a number of tissues including nervous tissue. It is a vasodilator that may participate in the cutaneous triple response.

corticotropin-like intermediate-lobe p. (CLIP), product of propiomelanocortin with unknown function.

cyclic p., a p. that forms a ring structure; *e.g.*, tyrocidin A, an antibiotic, is a cyclic decapeptide; valinomycin is a cyclic depsipeptide.

gastric inhibitory p. (GIP), SYN gastric inhibitory *polypeptide*.

heterodetic p., a p. that contains p. bonds as well as covalent linkages between certain amino acid residues that are not p. bonds; *e.g.*, valinomycin, oxytocin. [hetero- + G. *detos*, bound, fr. *deō*, to bind, + -ic]

heteromeric p., a p. which, on hydrolysis, yields substances other than amino acids in addition to amino acids; *e.g.*, pteroylglutamic acid.

homodetic p., a p. in which all of the covalent linkages between the constituent amino acids are p. bonds; *e.g.*, bradykinin. [homo- + G. *detos*, bound, fr. *deō*, to bind, + -ic]

homomeric p., **(1)** a p. which, on hydrolysis, yields only amino acids; *e.g.*, glutathione; **(2)** a p. which consists of only one particular amino acid; *e.g.*, alanylalanylalanine.

p. hydrolase [EC subclass 3.4], SYN peptidase.

phenylthiocarbamoyl p., PTC p., the p. formed by combination of phenylisothiocyanate and an α-amino group of a peptide. SEE ALSO phenylthiohydantoin.

S p., SEE S *protein*.

sigma p., a p. with one end bonded to a point within the chain, usually by means of the disulfide group of a cystine residue, so that only one end of the p. is free; so called since the p. chain has then the rough shape of the Greek letter sigma; *e.g.*, oxytocin.

p. synthetase [EC sub-subclass 6.3.2], any enzyme that catalyzes the synthesis of peptide bonds, with the hydrolysis of a nucleoside triphosphate.

vasoactive intestinal p., SYN vasoactive intestinal *polypeptide*.

pep·ti·der·gic (pep-ti-der'jik). Referring to nerve cells or fibers that are believed to employ small peptide molecules as their neurotransmitter. [peptide + G. *ergon*, work]

pep·ti·do·gly·can (pep'ti-dō-glī'kan). A compound containing amino acids (or peptides) linked to sugars, with the latter preponderant. Cf. glycopeptide.

pep·ti·doid (pep'ti-doyd). A condensation product of two amino acids involving at least one condensing group other than the α-carboxyl or α-amino group; *e.g.*, glutathione.

pep·ti·do·lyt·ic (pep'ti-dō-lit'ik). Causing the cleavage or digestion of peptides. [peptide + G. *lytikos*, solvent]

pep·ti·dyl di·pep·ti·dase A (pep'ti-dil). A hydrolase cleaving C-terminal dipeptides from a variety of substrates, including angiotensin I, which is converted to angiotensin II and histidylleucine. An important step in the metabolism of certain vasopressor agents. SYN carboxycathepsin, dipeptidyl carboxypeptidase, kinase II, peptidase P.

pep·tid·yl·trans·fer·ase (pep-tī'dil-trans'fer-ās). The enzyme responsible for the formation of the peptide bond on the ribosome during protein biosynthesis, peptidyl-$tRNA^1$ + aminoacyl-$tRNA^2$ → $tRNA^1$ + peptidylaminoacyl-$tRNA^2$.

pep·ti·za·tion (pep-ti-zā'shŭn). In colloid chemistry, an increase in the degree of dispersion, tending toward a uniform distribution of the dispersed phase.

Pep·to·coc·ca·ce·ae (pep'tō-kok-ā'sē-ē). A family of nonmotile, nonsporeforming, anaerobic bacteria (order Eubacteriales) containing Gram-positive (staining may be equivocal) cocci, 0.5 to

1.6 μm in diameter, which occur singly, in pairs, tetrads, and irregular masses but not in three-dimensional, cubic packets. These organisms are chemoorganotrophic and have complex nutritional requirements. Carbohydrates may or may not be fermented by these organisms, which produce gas, principally CO_2 and usually H_2, from amino acids, or carbohydrates, or both. They are found in the mouth and intestinal and respiratory tracts of man and other animals; they are frequently found in normal and pathologic human female urogenital tracts. The type genus is *Peptococcus.*

Pep·to·coc·cus (pep′tō-kok′ŭs). A genus of nonmotile, anaerobic, chemoorganotrophic bacteria (family Peptococcaceae) containing Gram-positive, spherical cells that occur singly, in pairs, tetrads, or irregular masses, rarely in short chains. They are frequently found in association with pathologic conditions. The type species is *P. niger.* [G. *peptō,* to digest, + *kokkos,* berry]

P. aero′genes, former name for *Peptostreptococcus asaccharolyticus.*

P. asaccharolyt′icus, former name for *Peptostreptococcus asaccharolyticus.*

P. constellatus, a species found in tonsils, purulent pleurisy, appendix, the nose, throat, and gums, and infrequently on the skin and in the vagina.

P. ni′ger, a species found once, in the urine of an aged woman; type species of the genus *P.*

pep·to·crin·ine (pep-tō-krin′ēn). An extract of the intestinal mucosa resembling secretin.

pep·to·gen·ic, pep·tog·e·nous (pep-tō-jen′ik, pep-toj′ĕ-nŭs). **1.** Producing peptones. **2.** Promoting digestion.

pep·toid (pep′tŏyd). A peptide with one or more non-amino acyl groups (*e.g.,* sugar, lipid, etc.) covalently linked to the peptide.

pep·to·lide (pep′tō-līd). **1.** A cyclic depsipeptide; *e.g.,* valinomycin. **2.** A heteromeric depsipeptide.

pep·tol·y·sis (pep-tol′i-sis). The hydrolysis of peptones.

pep·to·lyt·ic (pep-tō-lit′ik). **1.** Pertaining to peptolysis. **2.** Denoting an enzyme or other agent that hydrolyses peptones.

pep·tone (pep′tōn). Descriptive term applied to intermediate polypeptide products, formed in partial hydrolysis of proteins, that are soluble in water, diffusible, and not coagulable by heat; used in bacterial culture media.

pep·ton·ic (pep-ton′ik). Relating to or containing peptone.

pep·to·ni·za·tion (pep′ton-i-zā′shŭn). Conversion by enzymic action of native protein into soluble peptone.

Pep·to·strep·to·coc·cus (pep′tō-strep-tō-kok′ŭs). A genus of nonmotile, anaerobic, chemoorganotrophic bacteria (family Peptococcaceae) containing spherical to ovoid, Gram-positive cells which occur in pairs and short or long chains. These organisms are found in normal and pathologic female genital tracts and blood in puerperal fever, in respiratory and intestinal tracts of normal humans and other animals, in the oral cavity, and in pyogenic infections, putrefactive war wounds, and appendicitis; they may be pathogenic. The type species is *P. anaerobius.* [G. *peptō,* to digest, + *streptos,* curved, + *kokkos,* berry]

P. anaero′bius, a species found in the mouth, intestinal and respiratory tracts, and cavities, especially the vagina, of humans and other animals; it may be pathogenic; it is the type species of the genus *P.*

P. asaccharoly′ticus, a species found in the human large intestine, buccal cavity, pleura, uterus, and vagina. Also found in cases of puerperal fever.

P. evolu′tus, a species found in the human respiratory tract, mouth, and vagina.

P. foe′tidus, a species found in abscesses, blood, the intestinal tract, vagina, and mouth of humans and other animals; it is sometimes fatal.

P. interme′dius, a species found in the human respiratory and digestive tracts, oral cavity, and vagina; it has been isolated from various pathologic conditions.

P. mag′nus, a species found in putrefying butcher's meat and in a case of appendicitis.

P. mi′cros, a species found in natural cavities of humans and other animals; it has been isolated from various pathologic conditions.

P. morbillo′rum, a species found in the nose, throat, eyes, ears, mucous secretions, and blood in cases of measles, being irrelevant, however, to the etiology of measles; probably present normally, developing as a secondary invader.

P. paleopneumo′niae, a species found in the buccal pharyngeal cavity and the upper respiratory tract of humans.

P. par′vulus, a species isolated from the mouth and the respiratory tract.

P. plagarumbel′li, a species commonly found in septic war wounds.

P. produc′tus, a species found in natural cavities of humans, especially respiratory cavities.

P. pu′tridus, a species found in the human mouth and intestinal tract but especially in the human vagina.

△**per-.** **1.** Through, conveying intensity. **2.** In chemistry, a prefix denoting either 1) more or most, with respect to the amount of a given element (usually oxygen, as in perchloric acid) or radical contained in a compound, or 2) the degree of substitution for hydrogen, as in peroxides, peroxy acids (*e.g.,* hydrogen peroxide, peroxyformic acid). SEE ALSO peroxy-. [L. through, throughout, extremely]

per·a·ceph·a·lus (per-ă-sef′ă-lŭs). An omphalosite lacking head and arms, and with a defective thorax; typically, the body consists of little more than pelvis and legs. [per- + G. *a-* priv. + *kephalē,* head]

per·ac·id (per-as′id). An acid containing a peroxide group (–O–OH); *e.g.,* peracetic acid. SYN peroxy acid.

per·a·cute (per-ă-kyut′). Very acute; said of a disease. [L. *peracutus,* very sharply]

per an·um (per ā′nŭm). By or through the anus. [L.]

per·ar·tic·u·la·tion (per′ar-tik′yū-lā′shŭn). SYN synovial *joint.* [per- + L. *articulatio,* joint]

per·a·to·dyn·ia (per′ă-tō-din′ē-ă). Obsolete term for pyrosis. [G. *peratos,* on the opposite side, + *odynē,* pain]

per·ax·il·lary (per-ak′si-lār-ē). Through the axilla.

per·a·zine (per′ă-zēn). 10-[3-(4-Methyl-1-piperazinyl)propyl]-phenothiazine; an antipsychotic.

per·cen·tile (per-sen′tīl). The rank position of an individual in a serial array of data, stated in terms of what percentage of the group he/she equals or exceeds.

per·cept (per′sept). **1.** That which is perceived; the complete mental image, formed by the process of perception, of an object or idea. **2.** In clinical psychology, a single unit of perceptual report, such as one of the responses to an inkblot in the Rorschach test. [L. *perceptum,* a thing perceived]

per·cep·tion (per-sep′shun). The mental process of becoming aware of or recognizing an object or idea; primarily cognitive rather than affective or conative, although all three aspects are manifested. SYN esthesia (1).

depth p., the visual ability to judge depth or distance.

extrasensory p. (ESP), p. by means other than through the ordinary senses; *e.g.,* telepathy, clairvoyance, precognition.

simultaneous p., a combination of two slightly dissimilar images into a single image.

per·cep·tive (per-sep′tiv). Relating to or having a higher than normal power of perception.

per·cep·tiv·i·ty (per-sep-tiv′i-tē). The power of perception.

per·cep·to·ri·um (per-sep-tōr′ē-ŭm). SYN sensorium (2).

per·co·la·tion (per-kō-lā′shŭn). **1.** SYN filtration. **2.** Extraction of the soluble portion of a solid mixture by passing a solvent liquid through it. **3.** Passage of saliva or other fluids into the interface between tooth structure and restoration; sometimes induced by thermal changes. [L. *percolatio,* fr. per- + *colare,* to strain]

per·co·la·tor (per′kō-lā-ter). A funnel-shaped vessel used for the process of percolation in pharmacy.

per·co·morph oil (per-kō-mōrf). A liver oil from fish of the order Percomorphi, with a standardized amount of vitamins A and D.

per·con·tig·u·um (per kon-tig′yū-ŭm). In contiguity; denoting the mode by which an inflammation or other morbid process spreads into an adjacent contiguous structure. [per- + L. *contiguus*, touching, fr. *tango*, to touch]

per·con·tin·u·um (per kon-tin′yū-ŭm). In continuity; continuous; denoting the mode by which an inflammation or other morbid process spreads from one part to another through continuous tissue. [per- + L. *continuus*, holding together, continuous, fr. *teneo*, to hold]

per·cuss (per-kŭs′). To perform percussion.

per·cus·sion (per-kŭsh′ŭn). **1.** A diagnostic procedure designed to determine the density of a part by the sound produced by tapping the surface with the finger or a plessor; performed primarily over the chest to determine presence of normal air content in the lungs and over the abdomen to evaluate air in the loops of intestine. **2.** A form of massage, consisting of repeated blows or taps of varying force. [L. *percussio*, fr. *per-cutio*, pp. *-cussus*, to beat, fr. *quatio*, to shake, beat]

auscultatory p., auscultation of the chest or other part at the same time that p. is made, to aid in hearing the sound made by p.

bimanual p., immediate p. in which the finger of one hand taps the other hand; a form of mediate p.

clavicular p., p., usually direct, along the entire clavicle to demonstrate dullness, particularly in apical pulmonary tuberculosis.

deep p., heavy p. to obtain information about deeply situated organs or structures.

direct p., SYN immediate p.

finger p., p. in which a finger of one hand is used as a plessimeter and one of the other hand as a plessor.

immediate p., the striking of the part under examination directly with the finger or a plessor, without the intervention of another finger or plessimeter. SYN direct p.

mediate p., p. effected by the intervention of a finger or a plessimeter between the striking finger or plessor and the part percussed.

Murphy's p., examination for dullness by striking the chest wall directly with the fingertips of one hand successively, beginning with the fifth finger. SYN piano p.

palpatory p., finger p. in which attention is focused upon the resistance and reverberation of the tissues under the finger as well as upon the sound elicited. SYN plessesthesia.

piano p., SYN Murphy's p.

threshold p., p. effected by means of a glass rod as a plessimeter, the rod being inclined to the wall of the chest or abdomen and touching it only by one extremity.

per·cus·sor (per-kŭs′er). SYN plessor.

per·cu·ta·ne·ous (per-kyū-tā′nē-ŭs). Denoting the passage of substances through unbroken skin, as in absorption by inunction; also passage through the skin by needle puncture, including introduction of wires and catheters by Seldinger *technique*. SYN diadermic, transcutaneous, transdermic.

p. transhepatic cholangiography (PTHC), contrast radiographic examination of biliary system performed by injection through a percutaneously placed needle inserted into an intrahepatic bile duct.

per·en·ceph·a·ly (per-en-sef′ă-lē). A condition marked by one or more cerebral cysts. [G. *pēra*, a purse, a wallet, + *enkephalos*, brain]

Perez, Bernard, French physician, 1836–1903. SEE P. *reflex*.

Perez, George V., Spanish physician, †1920. SEE P.'s *sign*.

per·fec·tion·ism (per-fek′shŭn-izm). A tendency to set rigid high standards of performance for oneself.

per·fla·tion (per-flā′shŭn). Blowing air into or through a cavity or canal in order to force apart its walls or to expel any contained material. [L. *per-flo*, pp, *-flatus*, to blow through]

per·flu·bron (per-flū′bron). Generic name for perflurooctyl bromide.

per·flu·o·ro·octyl bro·mide (PFOB) (per-flū′ro-ok-til brō′mīd). A bromine-substituted fluorocarbon, prepared as a particulate emulsion, used as a CT, MR, and ultrasound contrast medium.

per·fo·rans (per′fō-rans). A term applied to several muscles and nerves which, in their course, perforate other structures. [L. perforating]

per·fo·rat·ed (per′fō-rāt-ed). Pierced with one or more holes. [L. *perforatus*, fr. *per-foro*, pp. *-atus*, to bore through]

per·fo·ra·tion (per-fō-rā′shŭn). Abnormal opening in a hollow organ or viscus. SYN tresis. [see perforated]

per·fo·ra·tor (per′fōr-ā-ter). An instrument for perforation of cranium.

per·fo·ra·to·ri·um (per-fōr-ă-tōr′ē-ŭm). A rod or fibrous cone located between the acrosome and the anterior pole of the nucleus in the spermatozoa of toads and birds; no corresponding structure evident in the subacrosomal space of mammalian spermatozoa. [L. *per-foro*, pp. *-foratum*, to bore, + *-orium*, instrumental suffix]

per·fo·rin (per′fōr-in). A protein found in the cytoplasmic granules of both T cytotoxic lymphocytes and natural killer cells. This protein is implicated in target cell lysis by the above cells. [L. *per-foro*, to bore, pierce, + *-in*]

per·for·mic ac·id (per-fōr′mik). H–CO–O–OH; an organic peracid used in cleaving disulfide links in peptides by oxidizing cysteine and cystine to cysteic acid. SYN peroxyformic acid.

per·frig·er·a·tion (per-frij-er-ā′shŭn). A minor degree of frostbite. [L. *per-frigero*, pp. *-atus*, to make cold, fr. *frigus*, cold]

per·fus·ate (per′fyū-sāt). The fluid used for perfusion; sometimes more broadly applied to fluid that has been forced through any more or less porous membrane or material. [see perfuse]

per·fuse (per-fyŭs′). To force blood or other fluid to flow from the artery through the vascular bed of a tissue or to flow through the lumen of a hollow structure (*e.g.*, an isolated renal tubule). Cf. perifuse, superfuse. [L. *perfusio*, fr. per- + *fusio*, a pouring]

per·fu·sion (per-fyū′zhŭn). **1.** The act of perfusing. **2.** The flow of blood or other perfusate per unit volume of tissue, as in ventilation/perfusion ratio.

regional p., p. of part of the body, especially a limb, and particularly with chemotherapeutic agents, for treatment of a malignant tumor, primary, recurrent, or metastatic.

per·go·lide mes·y·late (per′go-līd). 8β-[(Methylthio)methyl]-6-propylergoline monomethanesulfonate; an ergot derivative with dopaminergic properties.

per·hex·il·ine ma·le·ate (per-hek′si-lēn). 2-(2,2-Dicyclohexylethyl)piperidine maleate; a coronary vasodilator and diuretic.

per·hy·dro·cy·clo·pen·ta[a]phen·an·threne. SYN tetracyclic steroid *nucleus*.

△**peri-.** Around, about, near. Cf. circum-. [G. around]

per·i·ac·i·nal, per·i·ac·i·nous (per-ē-as′i-năl, -i-nŭs). Surrounding an acinus.

per·i·ad·e·ni·tis (per′ē-ad-ĕ-nī′tis). Inflammation of the tissues surrounding a gland. [peri- + G. *adēn*, gland, + *-itis*, inflammation]

p. muco′sa necrot′ica recur′rens, SYN *aphthae* major, under *aphtha*.

per·i·a·nal (per-ē-ā′năl). SYN circumanal.

per·i·an·gi·o·cho·li·tis (per′ē-an′jē-ō-kō-lī′tis). SYN pericholangitis. [peri- + G. *angeion*, vessel, + *cholē*, bile, + *-itis*, inflammation]

per·i·an·gi·tis (per′ē-an-jī′tis). Inflammation of the adventitia of a blood vessel or of the tissues surrounding it or a lymphatic vessel. SEE ALSO periarteritis, periphlebitis, perilymphangitis. SYN perivasculitis. [peri- + G. *angeion*, a vessel, + *-itis*, inflammation]

per·i·a·or·tic (per′ē-ā-ōr′tik). Surrounding or adjacent to the aorta.

per·i·a·or·ti·tis (per′ē-ā-ōr-tī′tis). Inflammation of the adventitia of the aorta and of the tissues surrounding it.

per·i·a·pex (per′ē-ā′peks). The periapical structures, particularly periodontal membrane and adjacent bone. [peri- L. *apex*, tip]

per·i·ap·i·cal (per-ē-ap′i-kăl). **1.** At or around the apex of a root of a tooth. **2.** Denoting the periapex.

per·i·ap·pen·di·ci·tis (per′ē-ă-pen-di-sī′tis). Inflammation of the tissue surrounding the vermiform appendix. SYN para-appendicitis.

p. decidua′lis, the presence of decidual cells in the peritoneum of the vermiform appendix in cases of right tubal pregnancy with adhesions between the fallopian tube and the appendix.

per·i·ap·pen·dic·u·lar (per′ē-ap-en-dik′yū-lăr). Surrounding an appendix, especially the vermiform appendix.

per·i·ar·te·ri·al (per′ē-ar-tē′rē-ăl). Surrounding an artery.

per·i·ar·te·ri·tis (per′ē-ar-ter-ī′tis). Inflammation of the adventitia of an artery. SYN exarteritis.

p. nodo′sa, SYN *polyarteritis* nodosa.

per·i·ar·thric (per′ē-ar′thrik). SYN circumarticular.

per·i·ar·thri·tis (per′ē-ar-thrī′tis). Inflammation of the parts surrounding a joint. [peri- + arthritis]

per·i·ar·tic·u·lar (per′ē-ar-tik′yū-lăr). SYN circumarticular.

per·i·a·tri·al (per′ē-ā′trē-ăl). Surrounding the atrium of the heart. SYN periauricular (1).

per·i·au·ric·u·lar (per′ē-aw-rik′yū-lăr). **1.** SYN periatrial. **2.** SYN periconchal. **3.** Around the external ear.

per·i·ax·i·al (per′ē-ak′sē-ăl). Surrounding an axis.

per·i·ax·il·lary (per′ē-ak′sē-lār-ē). SYN circumaxillary.

per·i·ax·o·nal (per′ē-ak′sō-năl). Surrounding the axon of a nerve. [peri- + G. *axōn,* axis]

per·i·blast (per′i-blast). A specialized region of yolk surface immediately peripheral to the blastoderm in telolecithal eggs. [peri- + G. *blastos,* germ]

per·i·bron·chi·al (per-i-brong′kē-ăl). Surrounding a bronchus or the bronchi.

per·i·bron·chi·o·lar (per-i-brong′kē-ō′lăr). Surrounding the bronchioles.

per·i·bron·chi·o·li·tis (per′i-brong′kē-ō-lī′tis). Inflammation of the tissues surrounding the bronchioles.

per·i·bron·chi·tis (per′i-brong-kī′tis). Inflammation of the tissues surrounding the bronchi or bronchial tubes.

per·i·buc·cal (per′i-bŭk′ăl). Surrounding the cheek.

per·i·bul·bar (per-i-bŭl′băr). Surrounding any bulb, especially the eyeball or the bulb of the urethra. SYN circumbulbar.

per·i·bur·sal (per-i-ber′săl). Surrounding a bursa.

per·i·can·a·lic·u·lar (per′i-kan-ă-lik′yū-lăr). Surrounding a canaliculus.

per·i·car·dec·to·my (per′i-kar-dek′tō-mē). SYN pericardiectomy.

per·i·car·dia (per-i-kar′dē-ă). Plural of pericardium.

per·i·car·di·ac, per·i·car·di·al (per-i-kar′dē-ak, -dē-ăl). **1.** Surrounding the heart. **2.** Relating to the pericardium.

per·i·car·di·cen·te·sis (per-i-kar′dē-sen-tē′sis). Needle drainage of the pericardium, usually accompanied by placement of an indwelling catheter for continuing drainage. SYN pericardial tap, pericardiocentesis.

per·i·car·di·ec·to·my (per′i-kar-dē-ek′tō-mē). Excision of a portion of the pericardium. SYN pericardectomy. [pericardium + G. *ektomē,* excision]

radical p., excision of almost the entire pericardium.

pe·ri·car·dii (per-i-kar′dē-ī). Plural of pericardium.

per·i·car·di·o·cen·te·sis (per-i-kar′dē-ō-sen-tē′sis). SYN pericardicentesis. [peri- + G. *kardia,* heart, + *kentēsis,* puncture]

per·i·car·di·o·per·i·to·ne·al (per-i-kar′dē-ō-per-i-tō-nē′ăl). Relating to the pericardial and peritoneal cavities.

per·i·car·di·o·phren·ic (per-i-kar′dē-ō-fren′ik). Relating to the pericardium and the diaphragm. [pericardium + G. *phrēn,* diaphragm]

per·i·car·di·o·pleur·al (per-i-kar′dē-ō-plūr′ăl). Relating to the pericardial and pleural cavities.

per·i·car·di·or·rha·phy (per′i-kar-dē-ōr′ă-fē). Suture of the pericardium. [pericardium + G. *rhaphē,* suture]

per·i·car·di·os·to·my (per·i-kar-dē-os′tō-mē). Establishment of an opening into the pericardium. [pericardium + G. *stoma,* mouth]

per·i·car·di·ot·o·my (per′i-kar-dē-ot′ō-mē). Incision into the

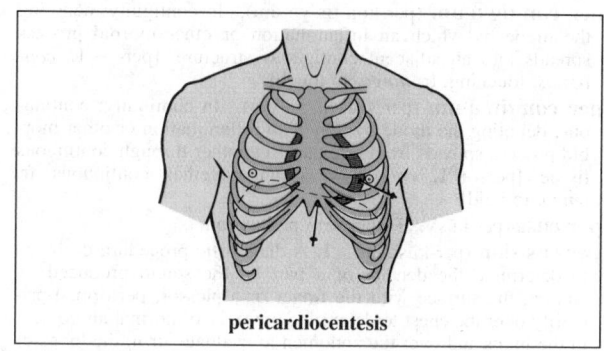

pericardiocentesis

pericardium. SYN coleotomy (1), pericardotomy. [pericardium + G. *tomē,* incision]

per·i·car·dit·ic (per′i-kar-dit′ik). Relating to pericarditis.

per·i·car·di·tis (per′i-kar-dī′tis). Inflammation of the pericardium. SYN Dressler's syndrome, postmyocardial infarction p.

acute fibrinous p., the usual lesion of acute p. in which inflammation produces large quantities of fibrin.

adhesive p., p. with adhesions between the two pericardial layers, between the pericardium and heart, or between the pericardium and neighboring structures. SYN adherent pericardium.

bacterial p., p. produced by bacterial infection.

p. calculosa, pericardial calcification owing to antecedent p.

carcinomatous p., p. due to infiltration of carcinomatous cells, usually from surrounding structures.

chronic constrictive p., tuberculous or other infection of the pericardium, with thickening of the membrane and constriction of the cardiac chambers.

constrictive p., postinflammatory thickening and scarring of the membrane producing constriction of the cardiac chambers; may be acute, subacute, or chronic. Formerly called chronic constrictive p.

dry p., pericardial inflammation in the absence of demonstrable pericardial effusion.

p. with effusion, pericardial inflammation producing excess pericardial fluid.

p. epistenocardica, p. accompanying transmural myocardial infarction and limited to the area over the infarct.

fibrinous p., acute p. with fibrinous exudate. SEE ALSO bread-and-butter *pericardium.* SYN hairy heart, p. villosa, shaggy pericardium.

fibrous p., scarring, usually with adhesions, of all or most of the pericardium.

hemorrhagic p., p. with bloodstained effusion.

internal adhesive p., SYN concretio cordis.

p. oblit′erans, inflammation of the pericardium leading to adhesion of the two layers, obliterating the sac. SEE ALSO adhesive p.

obliterating p., complete obliteration by postinflammatory adhesions of the pericardial cavity.

postmyocardial infarction p., SYN pericarditis.

postpericardiotomy p., a syndrome characterized by fever, substernal chest pain, and pericardial rub following cardiac surgery.

posttraumatic p., pericardial inflammation developing following injury to the chest.

purulent p., p., usually bacterial, with pus in the sac.

rheumatic p., fibrinous p. occurring in acute rheumatic fever.

p. sic′ca, fibrinous p. without significant pericardial effusion.

tuberculous p., p. caused by tuberculosis infection.

uremic p., fibrinous p. seen in chronic renal failure.

p. villo′sa, SYN fibrinous p.

viral p., p. due to a viral infection.

per·i·car·di·um, pl. **per·i·car·dia** (per-i-kar′dē-ŭm, -ă) [NA]. The fibroserous membrane, consisting of mesothelium and submesothelial connective tissue, covering the heart and beginning of the great vessels. It is a closed sac having two layers: the visceral layer (epicardium), immediately surrounding the heart, and the outer parietal layer, forming the sac, composed of strong fibrous tissue, the fibrous p. fibrosum, lined with serous membrane, serous pericardium. The phrenic nerve divides the p. into antephrenic and retrophrenic portions; the pulmonary hilum divides both of these portions into suprahilar, hilar, and infrahilar portions. SYN capsula cordis, heart sac, membrana cordis, theca cordis. [L. fr. G. *pericardion,* the membrane around the heart]

adherent p., SYN adhesive *pericarditis.*

bread-and-butter p., fibrinous pericarditis in which the visceral and parietal surfaces of the p. resemble those of two pieces of buttered bread that have been pressed together and then pulled apart, when they are separated at surgery or necropsy.

p. fibro´sum [NA], SYN fibrous p.

fibrous p., SEE pericardium. SYN p. fibrosum [NA].

hydrops pericardii (hī´drops per-i-kar´dē-ī), an obsolete term for pericardial *effusion.*

periaccretio pericardii (per´i-ă-krē´shē-ō per-i-kar´dē-ī), adhesion of the p. or part of it to the cardiac surface due to antecedent inflammation.

p. sero´sum [NA], serous p.

serous p., SEE pericardium.

shaggy p., SYN fibrinous *pericarditis.*

visceral p., the layer of the pericardial sac on the epicardial surface of the heart. It is composed mainly of a single layer of mesothelium.

per·i·car·dot·o·my (per-i-kar-dot´ō-mē). SYN pericardiotomy.

per·i·ce·cal (per´i-sē´kăl). Surrounding the cecum. SYN perityphlic.

per·i·cel·lu·lar (per-i-sel´yū-lăr). Surrounding a cell. SYN pericytial.

per·i·ce·men·tal (per´i-sē-men´tăl). SYN periodontal.

per·i·ce·men·ti·tis (per´i-sē-men-tī´tis). Obsolete term for periodontitis.

per·i·cen·tral (per-i-sen´trăl). Surrounding the center.

per·i·cha·reia (per´i-kă-rī´ă). Rarely used term for delirious rejoicing. [G. excessive joy, fr. *chairō,* to rejoice]

per·i·cho·lan·gi·tis (per´i-kō-lan-jī´tis). Inflammation of the tissues around the bile ducts. SYN periangiocholitis. [peri- + G. *cholē,* bile, + *angeion,* vessel, + *-itis,* inflammation]

per·i·chon·dral, per·i·chon·dri·al (per-i-kon´drăl, -kon´drē-ăl). Relating to the perichondrium.

per·i·chon·dri·tis (per´i-kon-drī´tis). Inflammation of the perichondrium.

peristernal p., SYN Tietze's *syndrome.*

relapsing p., SYN relapsing *polychondritis.*

per·i·chon·dri·um (per-i-kon´drē-ŭm) [NA]. The dense irregular connective tissue membrane around cartilage. [peri- + G. *chondros,* cartilage]

per·i·chord (per´i-kōrd). Sheath of the notochord.

per·i·chor·dal (per´i-kōr´dăl). Relating to the perichord.

per·i·cho·roi·dal (per-i-kŏ-roy´dăl). Surrounding the choroid coat of the eye.

per·i·chrome (per´i-krōm). Denoting a nerve cell in which the chromophil substance, or stainable material, is scattered throughout the cytoplasm. [peri- + G. *chrōma,* a color]

per·i·col·ic (per´i-kol´ik). Surrounding or encircling the colon.

per·i·co·li·tis (per´i-kō-lī´tis). Inflammation of the connective tissue or peritoneum surrounding the colon. SYN pericolonitis, serocolitis.

p. dex´tra, p. involving the ascending colon.

p. sinis´tra, SYN perisigmoiditis.

per·i·co·lon·i·tis (per´i-kō-lon-ī´tis). SYN pericolitis.

per·i·col·pi·tis (per´i-kol-pī´tis). SYN perivaginitis. [peri- + G. *kolpos,* bosom (vagina), + *-itis,* inflammation]

per·i·con·chal (per´i-kong´kăl). Surrounding the concha of the auricle. SYN periauricular (2).

per·i·cor·ne·al (per-i-kōr´nē-ăl). Surrounding the cornea. SYN circumcorneal, perikeratic.

per·i·cor·o·nal (per-i-kōr´ŏ-năl). Around the crown of a tooth.

per·i·cor·o·ni·tis (per´i-kōr-ŏ-nī´tis). Inflammation around the

crown of a tooth, usually one that is incompletely erupted into the oral cavity. [peri- + L. *corona,* crown, + G. *-itis,* inflammation]

per·i·cra·ni·al (per-i-krā´nē-ăl). Relating to the pericranium; surrounding the skull.

per·i·cra·ni·tis (per´i-krā-nī´tis). Inflammation of the pericranium.

per·i·cra·ni·um (per´i-krā´nē-ŭm) [NA]. The periosteum of the skull. SYN periosteum cranii. [peri- + G. *kranion,* skull]

per·i·cy·a·zine (per-i-sī´ă-zēn). 10-[3-(4-Hydroxypiperidinyl)-propyl]phenothiazine-2-carbonitrile; an antipsychotic.

per·i·cys·tic (per´i-sis´tik). **1.** Surrounding the urinary bladder. **2.** Surrounding the gallbladder. **3.** Surrounding a cyst. SYN perivesical. [peri- + G. *kystis,* bladder]

per·i·cys·ti·tis (per´i-sis-tī´tis). Inflammation of the tissues surrounding a bladder, especially the urinary bladder.

per·i·cys·ti·um (per-i-sis´tē-ŭm). **1.** The tissues surrounding the urinary bladder or gallbladder. **2.** A vascular investment of a cystic tumor. [peri- + G. *kystis,* bladder, cyst]

per·i·cyte (per´i-sīt). One of the slender mesenchymal-like cells found in close association with the outside wall of postcapillary venules; it is relatively undifferentiated and may become a fibroblast, macrophage, or smooth muscle cell. SYN adventitial cell, pericapillary cell, perithelial cell. [peri- + G. *kytos,* cell]

capillary p., SYN Rouget *cell.*

per·i·cy·ti·al (per´i-sish´ē-ăl, -sit´ē-ăl). SYN pericellular.

per·i·dens (per´i-denz). A supernumerary tooth appearing elsewhere than the midline of the dental arch. [peri- + L. *dens,* tooth]

per·i·den·tal (per´i-den´tăl). SYN periodontal.

per·i·den·ti·tis (per´i-den-tī´tis). Obsolete term for periodontitis.

per·i·den·ti·um (per´i-den´tē-ŭm). SYN periodontal *ligament.*

per·i·derm, per·i·der·ma (per´i-derm, -i-der´mă). The outermost layer of the epidermis of the embryo and fetus to the sixth month of intrauterine life; desquamated epitrichial cells are a considerable component of the vernix caseosa. SYN epitrichium. [peri- + G. *derma,* skin]

per·i·der·mal, per·i·der·mic (per-i-der´măl, -mik). Relating to the periderm.

per·i·des·mic (per-i-dez´mik). **1.** Surrounding a ligament. **2.** Relating to the peridesmium. SYN periligamentous.

per·i·des·mi·tis (per´i-dez-mī´tis). Inflammation of the connective tissue surrounding a ligament. [peri- + G. *desmos,* band, + *-itis,* inflammation]

per·i·des·mi·um (per-i-dez´mē-ŭm). The connective tissue membrane surrounding a ligament. [peri- + G. *desmion (desmos),* band]

per·i·did·y·mis (per-i-did´i-mis). SYN *tunica* albuginea of testis. [G. *didymos,* twin, pl. *didymoi,* testes]

per·i·did·y·mi·tis (per´i-did-i-mī´tis). Inflammation of the perididymis.

pe·rid·i·um (pe-rid´ē-ŭm). In fungi, the hyphal structure which surrounds the asci. [G. *pēridion,* dim. of *pēra,* leather pouch]

per·i·di·ver·tic·u·li·tis (per´i-dī´ver-tik´yū-lī´tis). Inflammation of the tissues around an intestinal diverticulum.

per·i·du·o·de·ni·tis (per´i-dū´ō-dē-nī´tis). Inflammation around the duodenum.

per·i·du·ral (per-i-dū´răl). SYN epidural.

per·i·en·ceph·a·li·tis (per´ē-en-sef-ă-lī´tis). Inflammation of the cerebral membranes, particularly leptomeningitis or inflammation of the pia mater with involvement of the underlying cortex. [peri- + G. *enkephalos,* brain]

per·i·en·ter·ic (per-ē-en-ter´ik). Surrounding the intestine. SYN circumintestinal.

per·i·en·ter·i·tis (per´ē-en-ter-ī´tis). Inflammation of the peritoneal coat of the intestine. SYN seroenteritis.

per·i·e·pen·dy·mal (per´ē-e-pen´di-măl). Surrounding the ependyma.

per·i·e·soph·a·ge·al (per´ē-e-sof´ă-jē´ăl). Surrounding the esophagus.

pe

per·i·e·soph·a·gi·tis (per′ē-e-sof′ă-jī′tis). Inflammation of the tissues surrounding the esophagus.

per·i·fo·cal (per-i-fō′kăl). Surrounding a focus; denoting tissues, or the blood that they contain, in the vicinity of an infective focus.

per·i·fol·lic·u·lar (per′i-fŏ-lik′yū-lăr). Surrounding a hair follicle; usually used to describe the histopathologic appearance of the infiltrate surrounding a hair follicle.

per·i·fol·lic·u·li·tis (per′i-fŏ-lik′yū-lī′tis). The presence of an inflammatory infiltrate surrounding hair follicles; frequently occurs in conjunction with folliculitis.

p. absce′dens et suffo′diens, a chronic dissecting folliculitis of the scalp. SYN dissecting cellulitis.

superficial pustular p., SYN follicular *impetigo.*

per·i·fuse (per′i-fyūs). To flush a fresh supply of bathing fluid around all of the outside surfaces of a small piece of tissue immersed in it. Cf. perfuse, superfuse. [peri- + L. *fusio,* a pouring]

per·i·fu·sion (per-i-fyū′shŭn). The act of perifusing.

per·i·gan·gli·on·ic (per′i-gang-glē-on′ik). Surrounding a ganglion, especially a nerve ganglion.

per·i·gas·tric (per-i-gas′trik). Surrounding the stomach. [peri- + G. *gastēr,* belly, stomach]

per·i·gas·tri·tis (per′i-gas-trī′tis). Inflammation of the peritoneal coat of the stomach.

per·i·gem·mal (per′i-jem′ăl). SYN circumgemmal. [peri- + L. *gemma,* bud]

per·i·glan·du·li·tis (per′i-glan-dū-lī′tis). Inflammation of the tissues surrounding a gland.

per·i·glot·tic (per-i-glot′ik). Around the tongue, especially around the base of the tongue and the epiglottis, or around the glottis (laryngis), the rima glottidis. [peri- + G. *glōssa* or *glōtta,* tongue]

per·i·glot·tis (per-i-glot′is). The mucous membrane of the tongue. [G. *periglōttis,* covering of the tongue]

per·i·he·pat·ic (per-i-he-pat′ik). Surrounding the liver. [peri- + G. *hēpar,* liver]

per·i·hep·a·ti·tis (pĕr′i-hep-ă-tī′tis). Inflammation of the serous, or peritoneal, covering of the liver. SYN hepatic capsulitis, hepatitis externa, hepatoperitonitis. [peri- + G. *hēpar,* liver, + *-itis,* inflammation]

per·i·her·ni·al (per-i-her′nē-ăl). Surrounding a hernia.

peri-im·plan·to·cla·sia (per′ē-im-plan′tō-klā′zē-ă). In dentistry, a general term implying disease of the supporting bone involving an implant; the disease may be exfoliative, resorptive, traumatic, or ulcerative in nature. [peri- + L. *im,* in, + *planto,* to plant, + G. *klasis,* breaking up]

per·i·je·ju·ni·tis (per′i-jĕ-jū-nī′tis). Inflammation around the jejunum.

per·i·kar·y·on, pl. **per·i·kar·ya** (per-i-kar′ē-on, -ă). **1.** The cytoplasm around the nucleus, such as that of the cell body of nerve cells. **2.** The body of the odontoblast, excluding the dentinal fiber. **3.** The cell body of the nerve cell, as distinguished from its axon and dendrites. [peri- + G. *karyon,* kernel]

per·i·ke·rat·ic (per-i-ke-rat′ik). SYN pericorneal. [peri- + G. *keras,* horn]

per·i·ky·ma·ta, sing. **per·i·ky·ma** (per-i-kī′mă-tă, -kī′mă). The transverse ridges and grooves on the surface of tooth enamel. [peri- + G. *kyma,* wave]

per·i·lab·y·rin·thi·tis (per′i-lab′ī-rin-thī′tis). Inflammation of the parts about the labyrinth.

per·i·la·ryn·ge·al (per′i-lă-rin′jē-ăl). Surrounding the larynx.

per·i·len·tic·u·lar (per-i-len-tik′yū-lăr). Surrounding the lens of the eye. SYN circumlental.

per·i·lig·a·men·tous (per′i-lig-ă-men′tŭs). SYN peridesmic.

per·i·lymph (per′i-limf). The fluid contained within the osseus labyrinth, surrounding and protecting the membranous labyrinth; perilymph resembles extracellular fluid in composition (sodium salts are the predominate positive electrolyte) and, via the perilymphatic duct, is in continuity with cerebrospinal fluid. SYN perilympha [NA], Cotunnius' liquid, liquor cotunnii.

per·i·lym·pha (per′i-lim′fă) [NA]. SYN perilymph. [peri- + L. *lympha,* a clear fluid (lymph)]

per·i·lym·phan·gi·al (per′i-lim-fan′jē-ăl). Surrounding a lymphatic vessel.

per·i·lym·phan·gi·tis (per′i-lim-fan-jī′tis). Inflammation of the tissues surrounding a lymphatic vessel.

per·i·lym·phat·ic (per′i-lim-fat′ik). **1.** Surrounding a lymphatic structure (node or vessel). **2.** The spaces and tissues surrounding the membranous labyrinth of the inner ear.

per·i·men·in·gi·tis (per′i-men-in-jī′tis). SYN pachymeningitis.

per·i·men·o·pause (per′i-men′ō-paws). The three to five year period prior to menopause during which estrogen levels begin to drop.

Studies have revealed that estrogen replacement therapy may be more effective if started during perimenopause, particularly in preventing bone loss, which immediately accelerates as soon as overall estrogen is reduced. For the bone-saving benefits of estrogen replacement therapy to be seen during the period between age 70 and 80, when the risk of breakage is high, it apparently must be begun during perimenopause and continued for many years.

pe·rim·e·ter (pe-rim′ĕ-ter). **1.** A circumference, edge, or border. **2.** An instrument, usually half a circle or sphere, used to measure the field of vision. [G. *perimetros,* circumference, fr. *peri,* around, + *metron,* measure]

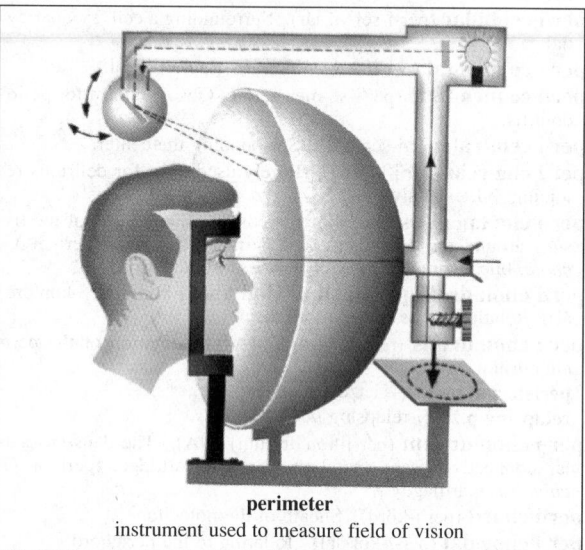

perimeter
instrument used to measure field of vision

arc p., a p. consisting of a semicircular frame at the center of which the patient looks while a white object is moving along the arc, the exact point where it becomes visible or invisible being noted and recorded on a chart.

Goldmann p., a projection p. that adds further precision by controlling the surrounding illumination.

projection p., a p. that uses as target a spot of light that can be adjusted rapidly as to size, brightness, and color, and moves silently at any desired speed.

Tübinger p., a bowl p. in which a static stimulus was increased in intensity until detected. [*Tübingen,* German city]

per·i·met·ric (per-i-met′rik). **1.** Surrounding the uterus; relating to the perimetrium. SYN periuterine. [G. *peri,* around, + *mētra,* uterus] **2.** Relating to the circumference of any part or area. [G. *perimetros,* circumference] **3.** Relating to perimetry.

per·i·me·trit·ic (per-i-me-trit′ik). Relating to or marked by perimetritis.

per·i·me·tri·tis (per′i-me-trī′tis). SYN metroperitonitis. [perimetrium + G. *-itis,* inflammation]

per·i·me·tri·um, pl. **per·i·me·tria** (per-i-mē′trē-ŭm, -ă) [NA]. The serous (peritoneal) coat of the uterus. SYN tunica serosa uteri [NA]. [peri- + G. *mētra*, uterus]

pe·rim·e·try (pe-rim′ĕ-trē). 1. The determination of the limits of the visual field. 2. The mapping of the sensitivity contours of the visual field. [G. *perimetros*, circumference]

computed p., determination of the visual field by means of a programmed routine of static stimuli.

flicker p., a technique of p. using the criterion of critical fusion frequency. SYN flicker fusion frequency technique.

kinetic p., mapping of the visual field by using a moving rather than a static test object.

mesopic p., exploration of the visual field in dim illumination.

objective p., determination of the visual field by pupillary constriction, electroencephalography, or eye movements.

quantitative p., a plotting of the visual field in isopters of equal retinal sensitivity.

scotopic p., p. of a dark-adapted eye.

static p., determination of the visual field by using test objects at fixed positions and gradually increasing luminance to the threshold of visibility.

per·i·mol·y·sis (per-ē-mol′i-sis). Decalcification of the teeth from exposure to gastric acid in individuals with chronic vomiting. [=perimylolysis, fr. peri- + G. *mylos*, molar + *lysis*, loosening, dissolving, fr. *luō*, to loosen]

per·i·my·e·lis (per-i-mī′ĕ-lis). SYN endosteum. [peri- + G. *myelos*, marrow]

per·i·my·e·li·tis (per′i-mī-ĕ-lī′tis). SYN endosteitis.

per·i·my·o·car·di·tis (per-i-mī′ō-kar-dī′tis). Simultaneous pericarditis and myocarditis usually due to the same etiologic agent.

per·i·my·o·si·tis (per′i-mī-ō-sī′tis). Inflammation of the loose cellular tissue surrounding a muscle. SYN perimysiitis (2), perimysitis.

per·i·my·si·al (per-i-mis′ē-ăl, -miz′ē-ăl). Relating to the perimysium; surrounding a muscle.

per·i·my·si·i·tis, per·i·my·si·tis (per′i-mis-ē-ī′tis, -mī-sī′tis). 1. Inflammation of the perimysium. 2. SYN perimyositis.

per·i·my·si·um, pl. **per·i·my·sia** (per-i-mis′ē-ŭm, -miz′ē-ŭm; -ē-ă) [NA]. The fibrous sheath enveloping each of the primary bundles of skeletal muscle fibers. [peri- + G. *mys*, muscle]

p. exter′num, SYN epimysium.

p. inter′num, in the older literature, a term referring to the connective tissue around secondary and tertiary fascicles and individual fibers and also to the supporting framework of the myocardium.

per·i·na·tal (per-i-nā′tăl). Occurring during, or pertaining to, the periods before, during, or after the time of birth; *i.e.*, before delivery from the 28th week of gestation through the first 7 days after delivery. [peri- + L. *natus*, pp. of *nascor*, to be born]

per·i·nate (per′i-nāt). An infant in the perinatal period.

per·i·na·tol·o·gist (per-i-nā-tol′ō-jist). An obstetrician who subspecializes in perinatology.

per·i·na·tol·o·gy (per-i-nā-tol′ō-jē). A subspeciality of obstetrics concerned with care of the mother and fetus during pregnancy, labor, and delivery, particularly when the mother and/or fetus are at a high risk for complications. SYN perinatal medicine.

per·i·ne·al (per′i-nē′ăl). Relating to the perineum.

△**perineo-**. The perineum. [L. fr. G. *perineos, perinaion*]

per·i·ne·o·cele (per-i-nē′ō-sēl). A hernia in the perineal region, either between the rectum and the vagina or the rectum and the bladder, or alongside the rectum. [perineo- + G. *kēlē*, hernia]

per·i·ne·om·e·ter (per′i-nē-om′ĕ-ter). Instrument used to measure the strength of voluntary muscle contractions of the perineum. [perineo- + G. *metron*, measure]

per·i·ne·o·plas·ty (per-i-nē′ō-plas-tē). Plastic surgery of the perineum. [perineum + G. *plastos*, formed]

per·i·ne·or·rha·phy (per-i-nē-ōr′ă-fē). Suture of the perineum, performed in perineoplasty. [perineum + G. *rhaphē*, a sewing]

per·i·ne·o·scro·tal (per-i-nē′ō-skrō′tăl). Relating to the perineum and the scrotum.

per·i·ne·os·to·my (per-i-nē-os′tō-mē). Urethrostomy through the perineum. [perineo- + G. *stoma*, mouth]

per·i·ne·o·syn·the·sis (per′i-nē-ō-sin′thĕ-sis). Rarely used term for perineoplasty in a case of extensive laceration of the perineum.

per·i·ne·ot·o·my (per-i-nē-ot′ō-mē). Incision into the perineum to facilitate childbirth. SEE ALSO episiotomy.

per·i·ne·o·vag·i·nal (per-i-nē′ō-vaj′i-năl). Relating to the perineum and the vagina.

per·i·neph·ri·al (per′i-nef′rē-ăl). Relating to the perinephrium.

per·i·neph·ric (per′i-nef′rik). Surrounding the kidney in whole or part. SYN circumrenal, perirenal.

per·i·neph·ri·tis (per′i-ne-frī′tis). Inflammation of perinephric tissue.

per·i·neph·ri·um, pl. **per·i·neph·ria** (per′i-nef′rē-ŭm, -nef′rē-ă). The connective tissue and fat surrounding the kidney. [peri- + G. *nephros*, kidney]

per·i·ne·um, pl. **per·i·nea** (per′i-nē′ŭm, -nē′ă). 1 [NA]. The area between the thighs extending from the coccyx to the pubis and lying below the pelvic diaphragm. 2. The external surface of the central tendon of the perineum, lying between the vulva and the anus in the female and the scrotum and the anus in the male. [L. fr. G. *perineon, perinaion*]

watering-can p., a p. riddled with fistulas resulting from urethral stricture.

per·i·neu·ral (per′i-nū′răl). Surrounding a nerve. [peri- + G. *neuron*, nerve]

per·i·neu·ri·al (per′i-nū′rē-ăl). Relating to the perineurium.

per·i·neu·ri·tis (per′i-nū-rī′tis). Inflammation of the perineurium. SEE ALSO adventitial *neuritis*.

per·i·neu·ri·um, pl. **per·i·neu·ria** (per′i-nū′rē-ŭm, -rē-ă). One of the supporting structures of peripheral nerve trunks, consisting of layers of flattened cells and collagenous connective tissue, which surround the nerve fasciculi and form the major diffusion barrier within the nerve; with the endoneurium and epineurium, composes the peripheral nerve stroma. [L. fr. peri- + G. *neuron*, nerve]

per·i·nu·cle·ar (per-i-nū′klē-ăr). Surrounding a nucleus. SYN circumnuclear.

per·i·oc·u·lar (per-i-ok′yū-lăr). SYN circumocular.

pe·ri·od (pēr′ē-ŏd). 1. A certain duration or division of time. 2. One of the stages of a disease, *e.g.*, p. of incubation, p. of convalescence. SEE ALSO stage, phase. 3. Colloquialism for menses. [G. *periodos*, a way round, a cycle, fr. *peri*, around, + *hodos*, way]

absolute refractory p., the p. following excitation when no response is possible regardless of the intensity of the stimulus.

critical p., (1) in the first hours after birth, the p. of maximum imprintability; the period before and after which imprinting is difficult or impossible; (2) in animals, a p. following birth when the processes underlying the capacity for socialization are activated or stamped in.

eclipse p., the time between infection by (or induction of) a bacteriophage, or other virus, and the appearance of mature virus within the cell; an interval of time during which viral infectivity cannot be recovered. SYN eclipse phase.

effective refractory p., the p. during which impulses may appear but are too weak to be conducted; the longest interval between adequate stimuli, falling just short of the time necessary to allow a propagated response to be evoked in a tissue by the second stimulus; it differs from the functional refractory p. in that it is a measure of stimulus interval rather than response interval of time.

ejection p., SYN sphygmic *interval*.

extrinsic incubation p. (eks-trin′sik), time required for the development of a disease agent in a vector, from the time of uptake of the agent to the time when the vector is infective.

fertile p., the p. in a regularly menstruating woman's cycle, during which conception is most likely.

functional refractory p., the minimum interval possible between successive responses to stimulation of a tissue.

Gap₁ p., the p. of the cell cycle after cell division when there is synthesis of RNA and protein; it may last for a few hours in rapidly growing tissue or a lifetime in non-renewing cells such as nerve cells. SYN Gap₁ phase, postmitotic phase.

Gap₂ p., the p. in the cell cycle when synthesis of DNA is completed but before mitosis begins. SYN Gap₂ phase, premitotic phase.

incubation p., (1) time interval between invasion of the body by an infecting organism and the appearance of the first sign or symptom it causes; SYN incubative stage, latent p. (2). **(2)** in a disease vector, the p. between entry of the disease organism and the time at which the vector is capable of transmitting the disease to another human host.

induction p., the p. required for a specific agent to produce a disease; the interval from the causal action of a factor to initiation of disease, *e.g.,* the interval between exposure to radiation and the onset of leukemia; the interval between an initial injection of antigen and the appearance of demonstrable antibodies in the blood.

intrapartum p., in obstetrics, the p. from the onset of labor to the end of the third stage of labor.

isoelectric p., the p. occurring in the electrocardiogram between the end of the S wave and the beginning of the T wave during which electrical forces are acting in directions such as to neutralize each other so that there is no difference in potential under the two electrodes.

isometric p. of cardiac cycle, that p. in which the muscle fibers do not shorten although the cardiac muscle is excited and the pressure in the ventricles rises, extending from the closure of the atrioventricular valves to the opening of the semilunar valves (isovolumic constriction) or the reverse (isovolumic relaxation).

isometric contraction p., the time between closure of the atrioventricular valves and opening of the semilunar valves.

isometric relaxation p., early ventricular diastole beginning with closure of the aortic and pulmonic valves and preceding opening of the atrioventricular valves.

latency p., SYN latency *phase*.

latent p., (1) the p. elapsing between the application of a stimulus and the response, *e.g.,* contraction of a muscle; **(2)** SYN incubation p. (1).

masticatory silent p., a pause in electromyographic patterns associated with tooth contacts during chewing and biting; a part of the complex feedback mechanism of mandibular control involving receptors in the periodontal ligament and muscles.

menstrual p., SYN menses.

missed p., the failure of menstruation to occur in any month at the expected time.

mitotic p., the p. of the cell cycle in which all phases of mitosis occur. SYN M phase.

oedipal p., SYN oedipal *phase*.

preejection p., the interval between onset of QRS complex and cardiac ejection; electromechanical systole minus ejection time.

prepatent p., in parasitology, the p. equivalent to the incubation period of microbial infections; it is biologically different, however, because the parasite is undergoing developmental stages in the host.

prodromal p., the time during which a disease process has begun but is not yet clinically manifest.

puerperal p., the p. elapsing between the termination of labor and the return of the generative tract to its normal condition; the 6 weeks following the completion of labor.

pulse p., the reciprocal of the repetition rate; *e.g.,* the interval between leading edges of successive pulses.

quarantine p., the time during which an infected individual or an area is kept isolated, avoiding contact with uninfected individuals; can be any specified p. of time, varying with the disease in question. The term is derived from the Italian word for forty, since the period of isolation of individuals suspected of plague in the Middle Ages was forty days.

refractory p., (1) the p. following effective stimulation, during which excitable tissue such as heart muscle and nerve fails to respond to a stimulus of threshold intensity (*i.e.,* excitability is depressed); **(2)** a period of temporary psychophysiologic resis-

tance to further sexual stimulation which occurs immediately following orgasm.

refractory p. of electronic pacemaker, the time required to restore full sensitivity after detecting cardiac activity or delivering a pacing impulse.

relative refractory p., the p. between the effective refractory p. and the end of the refractory p.; fibers then respond only to high intensity stimuli and the impulses conduct more slowly than normally.

silent p., (1) the time during which there is no electrical activity in a muscle following its rapid unloading; **(2)** any pause in an otherwise continuous series of electrophysiologic events.

synthesis p., the p. of the cell cycle when there is synthesis of DNA and histone; it occurs between Gap₁ and Gap₂. SYN S phase.

total refractory p., the absolute refractory p. plus the relative refractory p.

vulnerable p., vulnerable p. of heart, a brief time during the cardiac cycle when stimuli are particularly likely to induce repetitive activity like tachycardia, flutter, or fibrillation which persists after the stimulus has ceased; for the ventricle, it occurs during the latter part of systole, during the relative refractory period coincident with the inscription of the latter half of the T wave of the electrocardiogram.

Wenckebach p., a sequence of cardiac cycles in the electrocardiogram ending in a dropped beat due to A-V block, the preceding cycles showing progressively lengthening P-R intervals; the P-R interval following the dropped beat is again shortened.

per·i·o·date (per-ī′ō-dāt). A salt of periodic acid.

pe·ri·od·ic (pēr-ē-od′ik). **1.** Recurring at regular intervals. **2.** Denoting a disease with regularly recurring exacerbations or paroxysms.

pe·ri·od·ic ac·id (per-ī′ō-dik). HIO₄, but existing in solution usually in hydrated form; used in carbohydrate detection and analysis.

per·i·o·dic·i·ty (pēr′ē-ō-dis′i-tē). Tendency to recurrence at regular intervals.

diurnal p., a circadian rhythm with primary expression of the p. during daylight hours, as in the release of microfilariae of *Loa loa* into the peripheral blood during the day, with far fewer released at night; associated with the day-biting habits of the vector, *Chrysops* species.

filarial p., the circadian rhythm observed in the appearance of filarial microfilariae in the peripheral blood. SEE ALSO diurnal p., nocturnal p.

lunar p., any rhythmic phenomenon that follows a lunar or monthly cycle.

malarial p., a clinical rhythmicity reflected in periodic fevers and chills recurring at approximately 48-hour intervals in tertian malaria (*Plasmodium vivax* or *P. ovale*) or at 72-hour intervals in quartan malaria (*P. malariae*); the rhythm of tertian or 48-hour cycles is frequently modified in malignant tertian or falciparum malaria (*P. falciparum*); associated with release of merozoites from red cells during erythrocytic schizogony, although the controlling mechanism for the synchronous release is unknown.

nocturnal p., a circadian rhythm with the p. expressed during nighttime hours, as in the night release of microfilariae of the human filaria *Wuchereria bancrofti* into the peripheral blood; this type of p. is found in regions where the vector mosquito is a night-biting species.

subperiodic p., a modified circadian rhythm in which the p. is not clearcut, as in certain zoonotic strains of Malayan filariasis caused by *Brugia malayi;* as in examples of strict filarial p., this response is correlated with the biting habits of the vector insect (mosquito), although the precise mechanism inducing this microfilarial response is not clearly established.

per·i·o·don·tal (per′ē-ō-don′tăl). Around a tooth. SYN paradental, pericemental, peridental. [peri- + G. *odous,* tooth]

Per·i·o·don·tal Dis·ease In·dex (PDI). An index used for estimating the degree of periodontal disease based on the measurement of six representative teeth for gingival inflammation, pocket depth, calculus and plaque, attrition, mobility, and lack of contact.

Per·i·o·don·tal In·dex (PI). An index for the epidemiological classification of periodontal disease.

per·i·o·don·tia (per'ē-ō-don'shē-ă). **1.** Plural of periodontium. **2.** SYN periodontics.

per·i·o·don·tics (per'ē-ō-don'tiks). The branch of dentistry concerned with the study of the normal tissues and the treatment of abnormal conditions of the tissues immediately about the teeth. SYN periodontia (2). [peri- + G. *odous,* tooth]

per·i·o·don·tist (per'ē-ō-don'tist). A dentist who specializes in periodontics.

per·i·o·don·ti·tis (per'ē-ō-don-tī'tis). **1.** Inflammation of the periodontium. **2.** A chronic inflammatory disease of the periodontium occurring in response to bacterial plaque on the adjacent teeth; characterized by gingivitis, destruction of the alveolar bone and periodontal ligament, apical migration of the epithelial attachment resulting in the formation of periodontal pockets, and ultimately loosening and exfoliation of the teeth. [periodontium + G. *-itis,* inflammation]

apical p., inflammation of the periodontal ligament surrounding the root apex of a tooth; usually a consequence of pulpal inflammation or necrosis.

p. com′plex, vertical resorption of the alveolar process with pockets of uneven depth on adjacent teeth, and with traumatic occlusion as a factor.

juvenile p., a degenerative periodontal disease of adolescents in which the periodontal destruction is out of proportion to the local irritating factors present on the adjacent teeth; inflammatory changes become superimposed, and bone loss, migration, and extrusion are observed. Two forms are recognized: 1) localized, in which the destruction is limited to the incisors and first molars; 2) generalized, involving all of the teeth. SYN periodontosis.

p. sim′plex, horizontal resorption of the alveolar process with pockets of even depth on adjacent teeth; traumatic occlusion is not a factor.

suppurative p., p. accompanied by purulent exudate.

per·i·o·don·ti·um, pl. **per·i·o·don·tia** (per'ē-ō-don'shē-ŭm, -shē-ă) [NA]. SYN periodontal *ligament.* [L. fr. peri- + G. *odous,* tooth]

per·i·o·don·to·cla·sia (per'ē-ō-don-tō-klā'zē-ă). Destruction of periodontal tissues, gingiva, pericementum, alveolar bone, and cementum. SYN periodontolysis. [periodontium + *klasis,* breaking]

per·i·o·don·tol·y·sis (per'ē-ō-don-tol'i-sis). SYN periodontoclasia. [periodontium + G. *lysis,* dissolution]

per·i·o·don·to·sis (per'ē-ō-don-tō'sis). SYN juvenile *periodontitis.* [periodontium + G. *-osis,* condition]

per·i·om·phal·ic (per'ē-om-fal'ik). SYN periumbilical. [peri- + G. *omphalos,* umbilicus]

per·i·o·nych·ia (per-ē-ō-nik'ē-ă). **1.** Inflammation of the perionychium. SYN perionyxis. **2.** Plural of perionychium.

per·i·o·nych·i·um, pl. **per·i·o·nych·ia** (per-ē-ō-nik'ē-ŭm, -nik'ē-ă). SYN eponychium (2). [peri- + G. *onyx,* nail]

per·i·on·yx (per-ē-on'iks) [NA]. Remnant of the eponychium remaining in the narrow fold overlapping the proximal part of the lunula found beginning in the 8th month of pregancy and remaining throughout life. [peri- + G. *onyx,* nail]

per·i·o·nyx·is (per'ē-ō-nik'sis). SYN perionychia (1).

per·i·o·o·pho·ri·tis (per'ē-ō-of'ō-rī'tis). Inflammation of the peritoneal covering of the ovary. SYN periovaritis. [peri- + Mod. L. *oophoron,* ovary, + *-itis,* inflammation]

per·i·o·pho·ro·sal·pin·gi·tis (per'ē-ō-of'ō-rō-sal-pin-jī'tis). Inflammation of the peritoneum and other tissues around the ovary and oviduct. SYN perisalpingo-ovaritis. [peri- + Mod. L. *oophoron,* ovary, + *salpinx,* trumpet, + *-itis,* inflammation]

per·i·op·er·a·tive (per-ē-op'er-ă-tiv). Around the time of operation. SYN paraoperative.

per·i·oph·thal·mic (per'ē-of-thal'mik). SYN circumocular. [peri- + G. *ophthalmos,* eye]

per·i·oph·thal·mi·tis (per'ē-of-thal-mī'tis). Inflammation of the tissues surrounding the eye.

per·i·o·ple (per'ē-ō-pl). A region of the pododerm; the thin, hard,

relatively impervious, outer layer of the horn wall of the hoof of an animal. SYN corium limbi. [G. *peri,* around, + *hoplon,* implement, shield]

per·i·op·lic (per-ē-op'lik). Pertaining to the periople.

per·i·o·ral (per-ē-ō'răl). Around the mouth. SYN circumoral, peristomal, peristomatous.

per·i·or·bit (per-ē-ōr'bit). SYN periorbita.

pe·ri·or·bi·ta (per'ē-ōr'bi-tă) [NA]. The periosteum of the orbit. SYN periorbit, periorbital membrane. [peri- + L. *orbita,* orbit]

per·i·or·bi·tal (per-ē-ōr'bi-tăl). **1.** Relating to the periorbita. **2.** SYN circumorbital.

per·i·or·chi·tis (per'ē-ōr-kī'tis). Inflammation of the tunica vaginalis testis. [peri- + G. *orchis,* testis, + *-itis,* inflammation]

p. hemorrha′gica, chronic hematocele of the tunica vaginalis testis.

per·i·ost (per'ē-ost). SYN periosteum.

pe·ri·os·tea (per-ē-os'tē-ă). Plural of periosteum.

per·i·os·te·al (per-ē-os'tē-ăl). Relating to the periosteum. SYN periosteous.

per·i·os·te·i·tis (per'ē-os-tē-ī'tis). SYN periostitis.

△**periosteo-.** The periosteum. [Mod. L. *periosteum*]

per·i·os·te·o·ma (per'ē-os'tē-ō'mă). A neoplasm derived from the periosteum. SYN periosteophyte, periostoma.

per·i·os·te·o·med·ul·li·tis (per-ē-os'tē-ō-med-yū-lī'tis). SYN periosteomyelitis. [periosteo- + L. *medulla,* marrow, + G. *-itis,* inflammation]

per·i·os·te·o·my·e·li·tis (per-ē-os'tē-ō-mī-ĕ-lī'tis). Inflammation of the entire bone, with the periosteum and marrow. SYN periosteomedullitis. [periosteo- + G. *myelos,* marrow, + *-itis,* inflammation]

per·i·os·te·op·a·thy (par'ē-os-tē-op'ă-thē). Any disease of the periosteum.

per·i·os·te·o·phyte (per-ē-os'te-ō-fīt). SYN periosteoma. [periosteo- + G. *phyton,* growth]

per·i·os·te·o·sis (per'ē-os-tē-ō'sis). The formation of a periosteoma. SYN periostosis.

per·i·os·te·o·tome (per'ē-os'tē-ō-tōm). A strong scapel-shaped knife, for cutting the periosteum. SYN periostotome.

per·i·os·te·ot·o·my (per'ē-os-tē-ot'ō-mē). The operation of cutting through the periosteum to the bone. SYN periostotomy. [periosteo- + G. *tomē,* incision]

per·i·os·te·ous (per-ē-os'tē-ŭs). SYN periosteal.

per·i·os·te·um, pl. **pe·ri·os·tea** (per-ē-os'tē-ŭm, -ă) [NA]. The thick fibrous membrane covering the entire surface of a bone except its articular cartilage. In young bones, it consists of two layers: an inner cellular layer that is osteogenic, forming new bone tissue, and an outer fibrous connective tissue layer conveying the blood vessels and nerves supplying the bone; in older bones, the osteogenic layer is reduced. SEE ALSO perichondral *bone.* SYN periost. [Mod. L. fr. G. *periosteon,* ntr. of adj. *periosteos,* around the bones, fr. *peri,* around, + *osteon,* bone]

alveolar p., p. alveola′re, SYN periodontal *ligament.*

p. cra′nii, SYN pericranium.

per·i·os·ti·tis (per'ē-os-tī'tis). Inflammation of the periosteum. SYN periosteitis.

per·i·os·to·ma (per'ē-os-tō'mă). SYN periosteoma.

per·i·os·to·sis, pl. **per·i·os·to·ses** (per'ē-os-tō'sis, -sēz). SYN periosteosis.

per·i·os·tos·te·i·tis (per'ē-os'tos-tē-ī'tis). Inflammation of a bone with involvement of the periosteum. [periosteum + G. *osteon,* bone, + *-itis,* inflammation]

per·i·os·to·tome (per-ē-os'tō-tōm). SYN periosteotome.

per·i·os·tot·o·my (per-ē-os-tot'ō-mē). SYN periosteotomy.

per·i·o·tic (per'ē-ō'tik, -ot'ik). Surrounding the internal ear; referring to the petrous portion of the temporal bone, or the spaces and tissues in the bony labyrinth that surround the membranous labyrinth. [peri- + G. *ous,* ear]

per·i·o·va·ri·tis (per'ē-ō-vă-rī'tis). SYN perioophoritis.

per·i·o·vu·lar (per'ē-ō'vyū-lăr). Surrounding the ovum.

per·i·pach·y·men·in·gi·tis (per'i-pak'ē-men-in-jī'tis). Inflammation of the area between the dura and bony covering of the central nervous system. [peri- + pachymeninx (dura mater) + G. -itis, inflammation]

per·i·pan·cre·a·ti·tis (per'i-pan'krē-ă-tī'tis). Inflammation of the peritoneal coat of the pancreas.

per·i·pap·il·lary (per-i-pap'i-lār-ē). Surrounding a papilla.

per·i·pa·tet·ic (per'i-pă-tet'ik). Walking around; formerly used to describe a patient with "walking" typhoid fever. [G. peripatēsis, a walking about]

per·i·pe·ni·al (per-i-pē'nē-ăl). Surrounding the penis.

per·i·pha·ryn·ge·al (per'i-fă-rin'jē-ăl). Surrounding the pharynx.

pe·riph·er·ad (pĕ-rif'ĕ-rad). In a direction toward the periphery. [G. periphereia, periphery, + L. ad, to]

pe·riph·e·ral (pĕ-rif'ĕ-răl). 1. Relating to or situated at the periphery. 2. Situated nearer the periphery of an organ or part of the body in relation to a specific reference point; opposite of central (centralis). SYN peripheralis [NA], eccentric (3).

pe·ri·phe·ra·lis (pĕ-rif-ĕ-rā'lis) [NA]. SYN peripheral, peripheral.

per·i·phe·rin (peröi-fer-in). A protein that apparently is needed to maintain the shape of the outer segment disk membranes of rods and cones; it is thought by many investigators that a defect in p. is associated with certain types of blindness.

pe·riph·e·ro·cen·tral (pĕ-rif'ĕ-rō-sen'trăl). Relating to both the periphery and the center of the body or any part.

pe·riph·e·ry (pĕ-rif'ĕ-rē). 1. The part of a body away from the center; the outer part or surface. 2. SYN denture border. [G. periphereia, fr. peri, around, + pherō, to carry]

per·i·phle·bit·ic (per'i-fle-bit'ik). Relating to periphlebitis.

per·i·phle·bi·tis (per'i-fle-bī'tis). Inflammation of the outer coat of a vein or of the tissues surrounding it. [peri- + G. phleps, vein, + -itis, inflammation]

Per·i·pla·ne·ta (per-i-pla-nē'tă). A genus of large cockroaches including several cosmopolitan household pests found wherever food is available, especially in moist protected areas. P. americana (American cockroach), a very large brownish-chestnut species, 30 to 40 mm long, is probably native to Africa but now universally distributed; P. fuliginosa (the smoky-brown cockroach) is a common household pest in the eastern and southeastern U.S. [peri- + G. planētēs, a roamer]

per·i·plasm (per'i-plazm). The space between the outer and inner membranes, shared with the cell wall, in Gram-negative bacteria; contains proteins secreted by the cell.

pe·rip·lo·cin (pe-rip'lō-sin). Glucoperiplocymarin; a cardiotonic glycoside obtained from the bark and stems of Periploca graeca (family Asclepiadaceae), a plant of southern Europe. [G. periplokē, a winding around, fr. plekō, to twine, plait]

per·i·po·lar (per-i-pō'lăr). Surrounding the pole or poles of any body, or any electric or magnetic poles.

per·i·po·le·sis (per'i-pō-lē'sis). Penetration of migrating cells between fixed tissue cells that are normally in close contact. [peri- + G. poleomai, to wander]

per·i·po·ri·tis (per'i-pŏ-rī'tis). Miliary papules and papulovesicles with staphylococcic infection; most frequently on the face and in infants. [peri- + G. poros, pore, + -itis, inflammation]

per·i·por·tal (per-i-pōr'tăl). Surrounding the portal vein. SYN peripylic.

per·i·proc·tic (per'ē-prok'tik). SYN circumanal. [peri- + G. prōktos, anus]

per·i·proc·ti·tis (per'i-prok-tī'tis). Inflammation of the areolar tissue about the rectum. SYN perirectitis.

per·i·pros·tat·ic (per'i-pros-tat'ik). Surrounding the prostate.

per·i·pros·ta·ti·tis (per'i-pros-tă-tī'tis). Inflammation of the tissues surrounding the prostate.

per·i·py·le·phle·bi·tis (per-i-pī'lĕ-fle-bī'tis). Inflammation of the tissues around the portal vein. [peri- + G. pylē, gate, + phleps, vein, + -itis, inflammation]

per·i·py·lic (per-i-pī'lik). SYN periportal. [peri- + G. pylē, portal, gate]

per·i·py·lor·ic (per'i-pī-lōr'ik, -pĕ-lōr'ik). Surrounding the pylorus.

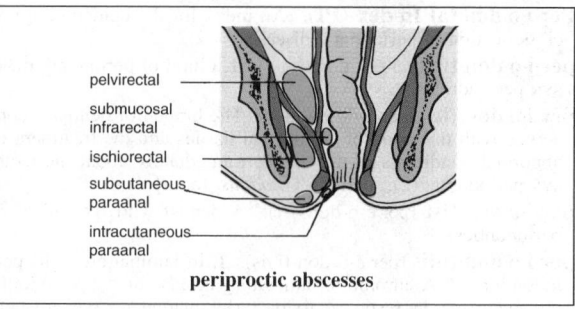
periproctic abscesses

per·i·rec·tal (per'i-rek'tăl). Surrounding the rectum.

per·i·rec·ti·tis (per'i-rek-tī'tis). SYN periproctitis.

per·i·re·nal (per'i-rē'năl). SYN perinephric. [peri- + L. ren, kidney]

per·i·rhi·nal (per'i-rī'năl). Around the nose or nasal cavity. [peri- + G. rhis, nose]

per·i·rhi·zo·cla·sia (per'ē-rī-zō-klā'zē-ă). Inflammatory destruction of tissues immediately around the root of a tooth, i.e., pericementum, cementum, and approximating layers of alveolar bone. [peri- + G. rhiza, root, + klasis, destruction]

per·i·sal·pin·gi·tis (per-i-sal-pin-jī'tis). Inflammation of the peritoneum covering the fallopian tube. [peri- + G. salpinx, trumpet, + -itis, inflammation]

per·i·sal·pin·go-ova·ri·tis (per'i-sal-ping'gō-ō-vă-rī'tis). SYN perioophorosalpingitis. [peri- + G. salpinx, trumpet, + ovary + G. -itis, inflammation]

per·i·sal·pinx (per'i-sal'pingks). The peritoneal covering of the uterine tube. [peri- + G. salpinx (salping-), trumpet]

per·i·scop·ic (per'i-skop'ik). Denoting that which gives the ability to see objects to one side as well as in the direct axis of vision. [peri- + G. skopeō, to view]

per·i·sig·moi·di·tis (per'i-sig-moy-dī'tis). Inflammation of the connective tissues surrounding the sigmoid flexure, giving rise to symptoms, referable to the left iliac fossa, similar to those of perityphlitis in the right iliac fossa. SYN pericolitis sinistra.

per·i·sin·u·ous (per'i-sin'yū-ŭs). Surrounding a sinus, especially a sinus of the dura mater.

per·i·sper·ma·ti·tis (per'i-sper-mă-tī'tis). Inflammation of the tissues around the spermatic cord.

p. sero'sa, hydrocele of the spermatic cord.

per·i·splanch·nic (per'i-splangk'nik). Surrounding any viscus or viscera. SYN perivisceral. [peri- + G. splanchna, viscera]

per·i·splanch·ni·tis (per'i-splangk-nī'tis). Inflammation surrounding any viscus or viscera. [peri- + G. splanchna, viscera, + -itis, inflammation]

per·i·splen·ic (per-i-splen'ik). Around the spleen.

per·i·sple·ni·tis (per'i-sple-nī'tis). Inflammation of the peritoneum covering the spleen.

per·i·spon·dyl·ic (per-i-spon-dil'ik). SYN perivertebral. [peri- + G. spondylos, vertebra]

per·i·spon·dy·li·tis (per-i-spon-di-lī'tis). Inflammation of the tissues about a vertebra. [peri- + G. spondylos, vertebra, + -itis, inflammation]

pe·ris·so·dac·tyl, pe·ris·so·dac·ty·lous (pĕ-ris'ō-dak-til, -til-ŭs). 1. Having an odd number of toes or digits on each foot or hand. SYN imparidigitate. 2. Any mammal of the order Perissodactyla, comprising the odd-toed hoofed quadrupeds and including the tapirs, rhinoceroses, and horses. [G. perissos, odd, + daktylos, finger or toe]

per·i·stal·sis (per-i-stal'sis). The movement of the intestine or other tubular structure, characterized by waves of alternate circular contraction and relaxation of the tube by which the contents are propelled onward. SYN vermicular movement. [peri- + G. stalsis, constriction]

mass p., forcible peristaltic movements of short duration, occurring only three or four times a day, which move the contents of the large intestine from one division to the next, as from the ascending to the transverse colon. SYN mass movement.

reversed p., a wave of intestinal contraction in a direction the reverse of normal, by which the contents of the intestine are forced backward. SYN antiperistalsis.

per·i·stal·tic (per-i-stal'tik). Relating to peristalsis.

pe·ris·ta·sis (pĕ-ris'tă-sis). Phases of inactivity of vasoconstriction in inflammation. SYN peristatic hyperemia. [peri- + G. *stasis,* a standing still]

pe·ris·to·le (pĕ-ris'tō-lē). The tonic activity of the walls of the stomach whereby the organ contracts about its contents; contrasting with the peristaltic waves passing from the cardia toward the pylorus (peristalsis). [peri- + G. *stellō,* to contract]

per·i·stol·ic (per-i-stol'ik). Relating to peristole.

pe·ris·to·ma (pe-ris'tō-mă, per-i-stō'mă). SYN peristome.

per·i·sto·mal, per·i·sto·ma·tous (per'i-stō'măl, -stō'mă-tŭs). SYN perioral.

per·i·stome (per'i-stōm). A groove leading from the cytostome in ciliates and certain other forms of protozoa. SYN peristoma. [peri- + G. *stoma,* mouth]

per·i·stru·mous (per'i-strū'mŭs). Situated about or near a goiter. [peri- + L. *struma,* goiter]

per·i·syn·o·vi·al (per'i-si-nō'vē-ăl). Around a synovial membrane.

per·i·sys·tol·ic (per-i-sis-tol'ik). Descriptive of events occurring before and after ventricular systole.

per·i·tec·to·my (per'i-tek'tō-mē). **1.** The removal of a paracorneal strip of the conjunctiva for the relief of corneal disease. **2.** SYN circumcision (2). [peri- + G. *ektomē,* excision]

pe·ri·ten·di·ne·um, pl. **pe·ri·ten·di·nea** (per-i-ten-din'ē-ŭm, -ē-ŭ) [NA]. One of the fibrous sheaths surrounding the primary bundles of fibers in a tendon. [L. fr. peri- + G. *tenōn,* tendon]

per·i·ten·di·ni·tis (per'i-ten-di-nī'tis). Inflammation of the sheath of a tendon. SYN peritenonitis.

    p. calca'rea, a calcium (chalky) deposit around a tendon.

    p. sero'sa, SYN ganglion (2).

per·i·ten·on (per'i-ten-on). SYN tendon *sheath* of extensor carpi ulnaris muscle. [peri- + G. *tenōn,* tendon]

per·i·ten·on·ti·tis (per'i-ten-on-tī'tis). SYN peritendinitis.

per·i·the·ci·um, pl. **per·i·the·cia** (per-i-thē'sē-ŭm, -sē-ă). In fungi, a flask-shaped ascocarp, one of the many shapes of structures which bear asci and ascospores; useful as an aid in identifying a fungus. [peri- + G. *thēkē,* flask]

per·i·the·li·o·ma (per'i-thē-lē-ō'mă). Obsolete term for hemangiopericytoma.

per·i·the·li·um, pl. **per·i·the·lia** (per-i-thē'lē-ŭm, -ă). The connective tissue that surrounds smaller vessels and capillaries. [peri- + G. *thēlē,* nipple]

    Eberth's p., an incomplete layer of connective tissue cells encasing the blood capillaries.

per·i·tho·rac·ic (per-i-thō-ras'ik). Surrounding or encircling the thorax.

per·i·thy·roi·di·tis (per'i-thī-roy-dī'tis). Inflammation of the capsule or tissues surrounding the thyroid gland.

pe·rit·o·mist (pe-rit'ō-mist). One who performs circumcision.

pe·rit·o·my (pe-rit'ō-mē). **1.** A circum-corneal incision through the conjunctiva. **2.** SYN circumcision (1). [G. *peritomē,* fr. *peri,* around, + *tomē,* incision]

per·i·to·ne·al (per'i-tō-nē'ăl). Relating to the peritoneum.

per·i·to·ne·al·gia (per'i-tō-nē-al'jē-ă). A rarely used term for pain in the peritoneum. [peritoneum + G. *algos,* pain]

⌂**peritoneo-.** The peritoneum. [L. *peritoneum*]

per·i·to·ne·o·cen·te·sis (per'i-tō-nē'ō-sen-tē'sis). Paracentesis of the abdomen. [peritoneum + G. *kentēsis,* puncture]

per·i·to·ne·oc·ly·sis (per'i-tō-nē-ok'li-sis). Irrigation of the abdominal cavity. [peritoneum, + G. *klysis,* a washing out]

per·i·to·ne·op·a·thy (per'i-tō-nē-op'ă-thē). A rarely used term for inflammation or other disease of the peritoneum. [peritoneum, + *pathos,* suffering]

per·i·to·ne·o·per·i·car·di·al (per'i-tō-nē'ō-per'i-kar'dē-ăl). Relating to the peritoneum and the pericardium.

per·i·to·ne·o·pexy (per'i-tō-nē'ō-pek-sē). A suspension or fixation of the peritoneum. [peritoneum + G. *pēxis,* fixation]

per·i·to·ne·o·plas·ty (per'i-tō-nē'ō-plas-tē). Loosening adhesions and covering the raw surfaces with peritoneum to prevent reformation. [peritoneum + G. *plastos,* formed]

per·i·to·ne·o·scope (per'i-tō-nē'ō-skōp). SYN laparoscope. [peritoneum + G. *skopeō,* to view]

per·i·to·ne·os·co·py (per'i-tō-nē-os'kŏ-pē). Examination of the contents of the peritoneum with a peritoneoscope passed through the abdominal wall. SEE laparoscopy. SYN abdominoscopy, celioscopy, ventroscopy.

per·i·to·ne·ot·o·my (per'i-tō-nē-ot'ō-mē). Incision of the peritoneum. [peritoneum + G. *tomē,* incision]

per·i·to·ne·um, pl. **per·i·to·nea** (per'i-tō-nē'ŭm, -ă) [NA]. The serous sac, consisting of mesothelium and a thin layer of irregular connective tissue, that lines the abdominal cavity and covers most of the viscera contained therein; it forms two sacs: the peritoneal (or greater) sac and the omental bursa (lesser sac) connected by the epiploic foramen. SYN membrana abdominis. [Mod. L. fr. G. *peritonaion,* fr. *periteinō,* to stretch over]

    parietal p., the layer of p. lining the abdominal walls. SYN p. parietale [NA].

    p. parieta'le [NA], SYN parietal p.

    visceral p., the layer of p. investing the abdominal organs. SYN p. viscerale [NA].

    p. viscera'le [NA], SYN visceral p.

per·i·to·nism (per'i-tō-nizm). A rarely used term for: **1.** A symptom complex marked by vomiting, pain, and shock associated with inflammation of any of the abdominal viscera in which the peritoneum is involved. **2.** A neurosis in which the symptoms simulate those of peritonitis. SYN pseudoperitonitis.

per·i·to·ni·tis (per'i-tō-nī'tis). Inflammation of the peritoneum.

    adhesive p., a form of p. in which a fibrinous exudate occurs, matting together the intestines and various other organs.

    benign paroxysmal p., SYN familial paroxysmal *polyserositis.*

    bile p., inflammation of the peritoneum caused by the escape of bile to the free peritoneal cavity. SYN choleperitonitis.

    chemical p., p. due to the escape of bile, contents of the gastrointestinal tract, or pancreatic juice into the peritoneal cavity; the contents of the fluid causes chemical injury, shock, and peritoneal exudation prior to occurrence of any associated infection.

    chyle p., p. due to free chyle in the peritoneal cavity.

    circumscribed p., SYN localized p.

    p. defor'mans, a chronic p. in which thickening of the membrane and contracting adhesions cause shortening of the mesentery and kinking and retraction of the intestines.

    diaphragmatic p., p. affecting mainly the peritoneal surface of the diaphragm.

    diffuse p., SYN general p.

    p. encap'sulans, a localized fibrous or adhesive p. remaining after a generalized p. has nearly disappeared; it is marked by pain, constipation, and a palpable tumor.

    feline infectious p., a chronic progressive disease of domestic cats and other Felidae caused by a coronavirus and manifested by a variety of clinical syndromes with or without an effusive p.

    fibrocaseous p., p. characterized by caseation and fibrosis, usually caused by the tubercle bacillus.

    gas p., inflammation of the peritoneum accompanied by an intraperitoneal accumulation of gas.

    general p., p. throughout the peritoneal cavity. SYN diffuse p.

    localized p., p. confined to a demarcated region of the peritoneal cavity. SYN circumscribed p.

    meconium p., p. caused by intestinal perforation in the fetus or newborn; associated with congenital obstruction or fibrocystic disease of the pancreas.

    pelvic p., generalized inflammation of the peritoneum surrounding the uterus and fallopian tubes. SYN pelvioperitonitis, pelviperitonitis.

    periodic p., SYN familial paroxysmal *polyserositis.*

productive p., SYN pachyperitonitis.

tuberculous p., p. caused by the tubercle bacillus.

per·i·ton·sil·lar (per′i-ton′si-lăr). Around a tonsil or the tonsils.

per·i·ton·sil·li·tis (per′i-ton′si-lī′tis). Inflammation of the connective tissue above and behind the tonsil.

per·i·tra·che·al (per-i-trā′kē-ăl). About the trachea.

pe·rit·ri·chal, pe·rit·ri·chate, per·i·trich·ic (pe-rit′ri-kăl, -rit′ri-kāt, per-i-trik′ik). SYN peritrichous (2).

Per·i·trich·i·da (per-i-trik′i-dă). An order of ciliates (subclass Peritrichia, phylum Ciliophora) characterized by a cylindrical shape with the cilia usually limited to the zone surrounding the mouth opening; includes the suborder Mobilina, whose members are all ecto- or endoparasites of aquatic invertebrates and vertebrates, of which the genus *Trichodina* includes economically important gill parasites of fish. [peri- + G. *thrix,* hair]

pe·rit·ri·chous (pe-rit′ri-kŭs). **1.** Relating to cilia or other appendicular organs projecting from the periphery of a cell. **2.** Having flagella uniformly distributed over a cell; used especially with reference to bacteria. SYN peritrichal, peritrichate, peritrichic. [peri- + G. *thrix,* hair]

per·i·tro·chan·ter·ic (per′i-trō′kan-ter′ik). Around a trochanter.

per·i·typh·lic (per′i-tif′lik). SYN pericecal. [peri- + G. *typhlon,* cecum]

per·i·typh·li·tis (per′ĭ-tif-lī′tis). Inflammation of the peritoneum surrounding the cecum.

perityphlitis p. (per′ĭ-tif-lī-tis ak′ti-nō-mī-kot-ĭ-kă), abdominal infection, predominantly around the cecum, with Actinomycetes, usually *Actinomyces israelii.*

per·i·um·bil·i·cal (per′i-ŭm-bil′i-kăl). Around or near the umbilicus. SYN periomphalic.

per·i·un·gual (per′i-ŭng′gwăl). Surrounding a nail; involving the nail folds. [peri- + L. *unguis,* nail]

per·i·u·re·ter·al, per·i·u·re·ter·ic (per′i-yū-rē′ter-ăl, -yū′rē-ter′ik). Surrounding one or both ureters.

per·i·u·re·ter·i·tis (per′i-yū-rē′ter-ī′tis). Inflammation of the tissues about a ureter. [peri- + ureter + G. *-itis,* inflammation]

p. plas′tica, SYN retroperitoneal *fibrosis.*

per·i·u·re·thral (per′i-yū-rē′thrăl). Surrounding the urethra.

per·i·u·re·thri·tis (per′i-yū-rē-thrī′tis). Inflammation of the tissues about the urethra. [peri- + urethra + G. *-itis,* inflammation]

per·i·u·ter·ine (per′i-yū′ter-in). SYN perimetric (1).

per·i·u·vu·lar (per′i-yū′vyū-lăr). Around the uvula.

per·i·vag·i·ni·tis (per′i-vaj-i-nī′tis). Inflammation of the connective tissue around the vagina. SYN pericolpitis.

per·i·vas·cu·lar (per′i-vas′kyū-lăr). Surrounding a blood or lymph vessel. SYN circumvascular. [peri- + L. *vasculum,* vessel]

per·i·vas·cu·li·tis (per′i-vas-kū-lī′tis). SYN periangitis.

per·i·ve·nous (per-i-vē′nŭs). Surrounding a vein.

per·i·ver·te·bral (per-i-ver′te-brăl). Around a vertebra or vertebrae. SYN perispondylic.

per·i·ves·i·cal (per-i-ves′i-kăl). SYN pericystic. [peri- + L. *vesica,* bladder]

per·i·vis·cer·al (per-ivis′er-ăl). SYN perisplanchnic.

per·i·vis·cer·i·tis (per′i-vis-er-ī′tis). Inflammation surrounding any viscus or viscera. [peri- + L. *viscera,* internal organs, + G. *-itis,* inflammation]

per·i·vi·tel·line (per′i-vi-tel′in, -īn). Surrounding the vitellus or yolk. [peri- + L. *vitellus,* yolk]

per·i·win·kle (per′i-wing-kl). SYN Vinca rosea.

per·kin·ism (per′kin-izm). A form of quackery purporting to treat disease by applying metals with magnetic and magic properties.

Perkins, Elisha, U.S. physician, 1741–1799. SEE perkinism.

per·lèche (per-lesh′). SYN angular *cheilitis.* [Fr. *per,* intensive, + *lécher,* to lick]

Perlia, Richard, 19th century German ophthalmologist. SEE P.'s *nucleus;* convergence *nucleus* of P.

per·lin·gual (per-ling′gwăl). Through or by way of the tongue,

denoting a method of medication. [L. *per,* through, + *lingua,* tongue]

Perls, Max, German pathologist, 1843–1881. SEE P.'s Prussian blue *stain, test.*

per·man·ga·nate (per-mang′gă-nāt). A salt of permanganic acid.

per·man·gan·ic ac·id (per-mang-gan′ik). An acid, HMnO₄, derived from manganese, forming permanganates with bases. SEE ALSO *potassium* permanganate.

per·me·a·bil·i·ty (per′mē-ă-bil′i-tē). The property of being permeable.

per·me·a·ble (per′mē-ă-bl). Permitting the passage of substances (*e.g.,* liquids, gases, heat), as through a membrane or other structure. SYN pervious. [L. *permeabilis* (see permeate)]

per·me·ant (per′mē-ănt). Able to pass through a particular semipermeable membrane. [L. *permeabilis* (see permeate)]

per·me·ase (per′mē-ās). Any of a group of membrane-bound carriers (enzymes) that effect the transport of solute through a semipermeable membrane; this term is not used with eukaryotes.

per·me·ate (per′mē-āt). **1.** To pass through a membrane or other structure. **2.** That which can so pass. [L. *permeo,* to pass through]

per·me·a·tion (per-mē-ā′shŭn). The process of spreading through or penetrating, as the extension of a malignant neoplasm by proliferation of the cells continuously along the blood vessels or lymphatics. [L. *per-meo,* pp. *-meatus,* to pass through]

per·nic·i·o·si·form (per-nish′ē-o′si-fōrm). Rarely used term meaning apparently pernicious, denoting a condition or disease that appears to be pernicious or malignant.

per·ni·cious (per-nish′ŭs). Destructive; harmful; denoting a disease of severe character and usually fatal without appropriate treatment. [L. *perniciosus,* destructive, fr. *pernicies,* destruction]

per·ni·o·sis (per-nē-ō′sis). SYN chilblain. [L. *pernio,* chilblain, + G. *-osis,* condition]

⌂pero-. Maimed, malformed. [G. *pēros*]

pe·ro·bra·chi·us (pē-rō-brā′kē-ŭs). An individual with a congenital malformation of one or both hands and forearms. [pero- + G. *brachiōn,* arm]

pe·ro·ceph·a·lus (pē-rō-sef′ă-lŭs). An individual with congenitally defective face and head. [pero- + G. *kephalē,* head]

pe·ro·chi·rus (pē-rō-kī′rŭs). An individual with a congenital malformation of one or both hands. [pero- + G. *cheir,* hand]

pe·ro·dac·ty·ly, pe·ro·dac·tyl·ia (pē-rō-dak′ti-lē, -dak-til′ē-ă). An individual with congenitally malformed fingers or toes. [pero- + G. *daktylos,* finger or toe]

per·o·gen (per′ō-jen). A preparation of sodium perborate that, when mixed with the accompanying catalyzer, liberates 10% of the oxygen in the salt.

pe·ro·me·lia, pe·rom·e·ly (pē-rō-mē′lē-ă, pĕ-rom′ĕ-lē). Severe congenital malformations of extremities, including absence of hand or foot. [pero- + G. *melos,* limb]

per·o·ne (per-ō′nē). SYN fibula. [G. *peronē,* brooch, the small bone of the arm or leg, the fibula, fr. *peirō,* to pierce]

per·o·ne·al (per-ō-nē′ăl). Relating to the fibula, to the lateral side of the leg, or to the muscles there present. [L. *peroneus,* fr. G. *peronē,* fibula]

per·o·ne·o·tib·i·al (per′ō-nē′ō-tib′ē-ăl). SYN tibiofibular.

pe·ro·pus (pē′rō-pŭs). A person with a congenital malformation of one or both feet. [pero- + G. *pous,* foot]

per·o·ral (per-ō′răl). Through the mouth, denoting a method of medication or an approach. [L. *per,* through, + *os* (*or-*), mouth]

per os. By or through the mouth, denoting a method of medication. [L.]

pe·ro·sis (pē-rō′sis). A nutritional disease of young birds (*e.g.,* chicks and turkeys) characterized by shortening and thickening of the limb bones and a deformity known as "slipped tendon," overcrowding, confinement, and wire floors without roosts are predisposing factors. [pero- + G. *-osis,* condition]

pe·ro·splanch·nia (pē-rō-splank′nē-ă). Congenital malformation of the viscera. [pero- + G. *splanchnon,* viscus]

per·os·se·ous (per-os′ē-ŭs). Through bone. [L. *per,* through, + *os,* bone]

peroxi-. SEE peroxy-.

per·ox·i·das·es (per-ok'si-dās-ez) [EC subclass 1.11]. Hydrogen peroxide reducing oxidoreductases; enzymes in animal and plant tissues that catalyze the dehydrogenation (oxidation) of various substances in the presence of hydrogen peroxide, which acts as hydrogen acceptor, being converted to water in the process; if the oxidized substance is iodide, yielding iodine, the enzyme is termed iodide peroxidase (*i.e.,* iodide + $2H_2O \rightarrow$ iodine + $2H_2$) and be involved in the iodination of tyrosine (as tyrosine iodinase or thyroid peroxidase).

horseradish p., an enzyme used in immunohistochemistry to label the antigen-antibody complex.

per·ox·ide (per-ok'sīd). That oxide of any series that contains the greatest number of oxygen atoms; applied most correctly to compounds containing an –O–O– link, as in hydrogen peroxide (H–O–O–H); a hydroperoxide is R–O–O–H.

per·ox·i·some (per-ok'si-sōm). A membrane-bound organelle occurring in nearly all eukaryotic cells that often has an electron-dense crystalline inclusion containing catalase, urate oxidase, and other oxidative enzymes relating to the formation and degradation of H_2O_2; thought to be important in detoxifying various molecules and in catalyzing the breakdown of fatty acids to acetyl-CoA; an absence of p.'s is found in individuals with Zellweger's syndrome. SYN microbody. [peroxide + G. *sōma,* body]

peroxy-. Prefix denoting the presence of an extra O atom, as in peroxides, peroxy acids (*e.g.,* hydrogen peroxide, peroxyformic acid). Often shortened to per-.

per·ox·y·a·ce·tyl ni·trate (per-ok-sē-ă-sē'til). The major pollutant responsible for eye and nose irritation in smog.

per·oxy ac·id (per-ok'sē). SYN peracid.

per·ox·y·for·mic ac·id (per-ok'sē-fōr'mik). SYN performic acid.

per·ox·yl (per-ok'sil). H–O–O; one of the free radicals presumed formed as a result of the bombardment of tissue by high energy radiation.

per·phe·na·zine (per-fen'ă-zēn). 2-Chloro-10-{3-[4-(2-hydroxyethyl)piperazinyl]propyl}phenothiazine; an antipsychotic.

per pri·mam (per prī'mam in-ten-shē-ō'nem). By first intention. SEE *healing* by first intention. [L.]

per rec·tum (per rek'tŭm). By or through the rectum, denoting a method of medication. [L.]

per·salt (per'sawlt). In chemistry, any salt that contains the greatest possible amount of the acid radical.

per sal·tum (per sal'tŭm). At a leap; at one bound; not gradually or through different stages. [L.]

per·sev·er·a·tion (per-sev-er-ā'shŭn). **1.** The constant repetition of a meaningless word or phrase. **2.** The duration of a mental impression, measured by the rapidity with which one impression follows another as determined by the revolving of a two-colored disk. **3.** In clinical psychology, the uncontrollable repetition of a previously appropriate or correct response, even though the repeated response has since become inappropriate or incorrect. [L. *persevero,* to persist]

per·sic oil (per'sik). The fixed oil expressed from the kernels of varieties of *Prunus armeniaca* (apricot kernel oil) or *Prunus persica* (peach kernel oil); used as a vehicle.

per·sis·tence (per-sis'tens). Obstinate continuation of characteristic behavior, or of existence in spite of opposition or adverse environmental conditions. [L. *persisto,* to abide, stand firm]

lactase p., an inherited trait (autosomal dominant) in which the levels of lactase do not decline after weaning. Cf. lactase *restriction.*

microbial p., the phenomenon of survival, in high concentration of an antimicrobial substance, of microbes that seem not to be resistant variants (mutants) since their progeny are fully susceptible.

per·sist·er (per-sis'ter). That which, or one who, is capable of persistence; especially a bacteria that exhibits microbial persistence.

per·so·na (per-sō'nă). A term that embodies the totality of the individual, the total constellation of the physical, psychological, and behavioral attributes of each unique individual; in jungian psychology, the outer aspect of character, as opposed to anima (2); the assumed personality used to mask the true one. [L. *per,* through, + *sonare,* to sound: from the small megaphone in ancient dramatic masks, to aid in projecting the actor's voice]

per·son·al·i·ty (per-sŏn-al'i-tē). **1.** The unique self; the organized system of attitudes and behavioral predispositions by which one feels, thinks, acts, and impresses and establishes relationships with others. **2.** An individual with a particular p. pattern.

allotropic p., SEE allotropic.

anancastic p., obsolete term for obsessive-compulsive personality *disorder.*

antisocial p., a p. disorder characterized by a continuous and persistent pattern of aggressive behavior in which the rights of others are violated. SEE psychopath, sociopath. SYN psychopathic p.

asthenic p., a p. type characterized by low energy level, easy fatigability, incapacity for enjoyment, lack of enthusiasm, and oversensitivity to physical and emotional stress. When appearing in marked form it becomes a psychological disorder (asthenic personality *disorder*), also called dependent p. SYN asthenic personality disorder, dependent personality disorder.

authoritarian p., a cluster of p. traits reflecting a desire for security and order, *e.g.,* rigidity, highly conventional outlook, unquestioning obedience, scapegoating, desire for structured lines of authority.

avoidant p., a p. characterized by a hypersensitivity to potential rejection, humiliation, or shame, an unwillingness to enter into relationships without unusually strong guarantees of uncritical acceptance, social withdrawal in spite of a desire for affection and acceptance, and low self-esteem.

basic p., SEE basic personality *type.*

borderline p., SEE borderline personality *disorder.*

compulsive p., a p. characterized by rigidity, extreme inhibition, perfectionism, and excessive concern with conformity and adherence to standards of conscience either for the individual or for others.

cyclothymic p., a p. disorder in which a person experiences regularly alternating periods of elation and depression, usually not related to external circumstances. SYN cyclothymic personality disorder.

dependent p., a p. in which a person passively allows others to assume responsibility for making decisions affecting him/her, characterized by a lack of self-confidence and an inability to function independently.

dual p., a mental disturbance in which a person assumes alternately two different identities without either p. being consciously aware of the other. SEE ALSO multiple p.

histrionic p., hysterical p., a p. in which a person, typically immature, dependent, self-centered, and often vain, exhibits unstable, overreactive, and excitable behavior intended to gain attention even though he or she may not be aware of this intent.

inadequate p., a p. disorder, characterized by personal and social ineptness plus emotional and physical instability, which renders the individual unable to cope with the normal vicissitudes of life.

masochistic p., a p. disorder in which the individual accepts exploitation and sacrifices self-interest while at the same time feeling morally superior or feigning moral superiority, attempting to elicit sympathy, and inducing guilt in others.

multiple p., a dissociative disorder in which two or more distinct conscious p.'s alternately prevail in the same person, without any p. being aware of the other. SEE ALSO dual p.

narcissistic p., SYN narcissism.

neurasthenic p., an obsolete term for a condition characterized by some of the following features: poor appetite or overeating, insomnia or hypersomnia, low energy or fatigue, low self esteem, poor concentration or difficulty making decisions, and feelings of hopelessness. In its most severe form it may become a chronic disturbance of mood called dysthymia (depressive neurosis) in which a depressive mood accompanies the features listed above.

obsessive p., SYN obsessive-compulsive p.

pe

obsessive-compulsive p., the p. of an individual whose overriding personal needs are manifested by a rigid, pervasive pattern of perfectionism and inflexibility, as he or she continually strives for clearly unattainable goals, to the point that such behavior frequently interferes with the actual completion of tasks and projects. SYN obsessive p.

paranoid p., a p. disorder characterized by hypersensitivity, rigidity, unwarranted suspicion, jealousy, and a tendency to blame others and ascribe evil motives to them; though neither a neurosis or psychosis, it interferes with the individual's ability to maintain interpersonal relationships.

passive-aggressive p., a p. disorder in which aggressive feelings are manifested in passive ways, especially through mild obstructionism and stubbornness.

psychopathic p., SYN antisocial p.

schizoid p., a disorder characterized by social withdrawal, emotional coldness or aloofness, and indifference to praise or criticism from others.

schizotypical p., a personality disorder characterized by eccentricities in thinking, appearance, and behavior; although not psychotic, individuals with such a disorder have unusual ideas and have difficulty relating to others.

shut-in p., a person who responds inadequately to contacts with other people.

syntonic p., a stable p., one characterized by even temperament.

type A p., type B p., SEE type A *behavior*, type B *behavior*.

per·son-years. The sum of the number of years that each member of a population has been afflicted by a certain condition; *e.g.,* years of treatment with a certain drug.

pers·pi·ra·tion (pers-pi-rā'shŭn). **1.** The excretion of fluid by the sweat glands of the skin. SYN diaphoresis, sudation, sweating. SEE ALSO Sweat. **2.** All fluid loss through normal skin, whether by sweat gland secretion or by diffusion through other skin structures. **3.** The fluid excreted by the sweat glands; it consists of water containing sodium chloride and phosphate, urea, ammonia, ethereal sulfates, creatinine, fats, and other waste products; the average daily quantity is estimated at about 1500 g. SYN sudor. SEE ALSO sweat (1). [L. *per-spiro,* pp. *-atus,* to breathe everywhere]

insensible p., p. that evaporates before it is perceived as moisture on the skin; the term sometimes includes evaporation from the lungs.

sensible p., the p. excreted in large quantity, or when there is much humidity in the atmosphere, so that it appears as moisture on the skin.

per·stil·la·tion (per-sti-lā'shŭn). SEE pervaporation. [L. *per,* through, + *stillo,* to trickle, distil]

per·sua·sion (per-swā'zhŭn). The act of influencing the mind of another, by authority, argument, reason, or personal insight; an important element in most types of psychotherapy. [L. *persuasio,* fr. *persuadeo,* to persuade]

per·sul·fate (per-sŭl'fāt). A salt of persulfuric acid.

per·sul·fide (per-sŭl'fīd). **1.** That one of a series of sulfides that contains more atoms of sulfur than any other. **2.** The sulfur analog of a peroxide.

per·sul·fu·ric ac·id (per-sŭl-fyūr'ik). H_2SO_5; Peroxymonosulfuric acid; an oxidizing agent.

per·tech·ne·tate (per-tek-ne-tāt). Anionic form of technetium used widely in nuclear scanning; $^{99m}TcO4$.

sodium p., Na 99mTcO₄; a radiopharmaceutical used for brain, thyroid, and salivary gland scanning.

Perthes, Georg C., German surgeon, 1869–1927. SEE P. *disease;* P.'s *test;* Calvé-P. *disease;* Legg-Calvé-P. *disease.*

△**perthio-.** Prefix denoting substitution of sulfur for every oxygen in a compound; *e.g.,* perthiocarbonic acid, H_2CS_3.

Pertik, Otto, Hungarian pathologist, 1852–1913. SEE P.'s *diverticulum.*

per tu·bam (per tū'băm). Through a tube. [L.]

per·tus·sis (per-tŭs'is). An acute infectious inflammation of the larynx, trachea, and bronchi caused by *Bordetella pertussis;* characterized by recurrent bouts of spasmodic coughing that continues until the breath is exhausted, then ending in a noisy inspi-

ratory stridor (the "whoop") caused by laryngeal spasm. SYN pertussis syndrome, whooping cough. [L. *per,* very (intensive), + *tussis,* cough]

Pe·ru·vi·an bark. SYN cinchona.

per·vap·o·ra·tion (per'vap-ōr-ā'shŭn). The heating of a liquid within a dialyzing bag suspended over a hot plate, evaporation taking place rapidly through the membrane; any colloids in solution remain within the bag while crystalloids diffuse out and crystallize on the outer surface of the bag (perstillation). [L. *per,* through, + *vapor,* steam]

per·ver·sion (per-ver'zhŭn). A deviation from the norm, especially concerning sexual interests or behavior. [L. *perversio,* fr. *per-verto,* pp. *-versus,* to turn about]

polymorphous p., (1) in psychoanalytic theory, a child's variegated sexual activity and interests; (2) in general, the manifold p.'s shown by an adult.

sexual p., SYN sexual *deviation.*

per·vert. One who practices perversions. SEE ALSO deviant (2).

per·vert·ed. Abnormal, deviant, or disordered.

per vi·as na·tu·ra·les (per vī'as nach'er-ā'lēz). Through the natural passages; *e.g.,* denoting a normal delivery, as opposed to cesarean section, or the passage in stool of a foreign body instead of its surgical removal. [L.]

per·vi·gi·li·um (per-vi-jil'ē-ŭm). Wakefulness; sleeplessness. [L. a watching all night]

per·vi·ous (per'vē-ŭs). SYN permeable. [L. *pervius,* fr. *per,* through, + *via,* a way]

pes, gen. **pe·dis,** pl. **pe·des** (pes, pē'dis, -dēz). **1** [NA]. SYN foot (1). **2.** Any footlike or basal structure or part. **3.** Talipes. In this sense, p. is always qualified by a word expressing the specific type. [L.]

p. abduc'tus, SYN *talipes* valgus.

p. adduc'tus, SYN *talipes* varus.

p. anseri'nus, (1) SYN intraparotid *plexus* of facial nerve. **(2)** the combined tendinous expansions of the sartorius, gracilis, and semitendinosus muscles at the medial border of the tuberosity of the tibia.

p. ca'vus, SYN *talipes* cavus.

p. equi'noval'gus, SYN *talipes* equinovalgus.

p. equi'nova'rus, SYN *talipes* equinovarus.

p. febric'itans, obsolete term for elephantiasis.

p. gi'gas, SYN macropodia.

p. hippocam'pi [NA], SYN *foot* of hippocampus.

p. pla'nus, a condition in which the longitudinal arch is broken down, the entire sole touching the ground. SYN flatfoot, talipes planus.

p. prona'tus, SYN *talipes* valgus.

p. val'gus, SYN *talipes* valgus.

p. va'rus, SYN *talipes* varus.

pes·sa·ry (pes'ă-rē). **1.** An appliance of varied form, introduced into the vagina to support the uterus or to correct any displacement. **2.** A medicated vaginal suppository. [L. *pessarium,* fr. G. *pessos,* an oval stone used in certain games]

cube p., plastic or rubber p. in a cube shape particularly suitable for elderly women with uterine prolapse.

diaphragm p., a ring with a covered opening, used as a platform to support uterus, bladder, or rectum, or to prevent conception.

Dumontpallier's p., an elastic ring p. SYN Mayer's p.

Gariel's p., a hollow inflatable rubber p. made in the form of a ring or a pear.

Hodge's p., a double-curve oblong p. employed for the correction of retrodeviations of the uterus.

Mayer's p., SYN Dumontpallier's p.

Menge's p., a ring p. with a central horizontal bar into which a detachable handle is inserted.

ring p., a ring of rubber, plastic, or metal in which the cervix rests; designed to support the uterus and to correct prolapse of that organ.

pes·si·mism (pes'i-mizm). A tendency to see or anticipate the worst. [L. *pessimus,* worst, irreg. superl. of *malus,* bad]

therapeutic p., a disbelief in the curative virtues of remedies in general and especially of drugs.

pest. SYN plague (2). [L. *pestis*]

fowl p., SYN fowl *plague.*

swine p., SYN hog *cholera.*

peste des pe·tits ru·mi·nants (pest′ dā pe-tē room-ē-nan′). A highly contagious systemic disease of sheep and goats in West Africa, caused by the p. d. p. r. virus and characterized by fever, anorexia, a necrotic stomatitis with gingivitis, and diarrhea.

pes·ti·ce·mia (pes-ti-sē′mē-ă). Bacteremia due to *Yersinia pestis.* [L. *pestis*, plague, + G. *haima*, blood]

pes·ti·cide (pes′ti-sīd). General term for an agent that destroys fungi, insects, rodents, or any other pest.

pes·tif·er·ous (pes-tif′ĕ-rŭs). SYN pestilential.

pes·ti·lence (pes′ti-lens). **1.** SYN plague (2). **2.** A virulent outbreak of any disease. [L. *pestilentia*]

pes·ti·len·tial (pes-ti-len′shăl). Relating to or tending to produce a pestilence. SYN pestiferous.

pes·tis. SYN plague (2). [L.]

p. am′bulans, SYN ambulant *plague.*

p. bubonica (pes′tis bū′bōn′ik-ă), SYN bubonic *plague.*

p. ful′minans, SYN bubonic *plague.*

p. ma′jor, SYN bubonic *plague.*

p. mi′nor, SYN ambulant *plague.*

p. sid′erans, SYN septicemic *plague.*

Pes·ti·vi·rus (pes′ti-vī′rŭs). A genus of viruses (family Togaviridae) composed of the hog cholera virus and related viruses. [L. *pestis*, plague, + virus]

pes·tle (pes′l). An instrument in the shape of a rod with one rounded and weighted extremity, used for bruising, breaking, grinding, and mixing substances in a mortar. [L. *pistillum*, fr. *pinso*, or *piso*, to pound]

PET Abbreviation for positron emission *tomography.*

⟳**peta- (P).** Prefix used in the SI and metric systems to signify one quadrillion (10^{15}).

⟳**-petal.** Seeking; movement toward the part indicated by the main portion of the word. [L. *peto*, to seek, strive for]

pe·te·chi·ae, sing. **pe·te·chia** (pe-tē′kē-ē, -tek′-; pe-tē′kē-ă). Minute hemorrhagic spots, of pinpoint to pinhead size, in the skin, which are not blanched by diascopy. [Mod. L. form of It. *petecchie*]

calcaneal p., traumatic hemorrhage into the stratum corneum of the heel which may persist for several weeks as centrally confluent black dots. SYN black heel.

Tardieu's petechiae, SYN Tardieu's *ecchymoses,* under *ecchymosis.*

pe·te·chi·al (pē-tē′kē-ăl, pē-tek′-). Relating to, accompanied by, or characterized by petechiae.

pe·te·chi·a·sis (pe-te-kī′ă-sis). Formation of petechiae or purpura.

Peters, Albert, German physician, 1862–1938. SEE P.'s *anomaly.*

Peters, Hubert, Austrian obstetrician, 1859–1934. SEE P.'s *ovum.*

Petersen, C.F., German surgeon, 1845–1908. SEE P.'s *bag.*

peth·i·dine (peth′ĭ-dēn). SYN meperidine hydrochloride.

pet·i·o·late, pet·i·o·lat·ed (pet′ē-ō-lāt, -lāt-ed). Having a stem or pedicle. SYN petioled. [L. *petiolus*]

pet·i·ole (pet′ē-ōl). SYN petiolus.

pet·i·oled (pet′ē-ōld). SYN petiolate.

pe·ti·o·lus (pe-tī′ō-lŭs). A stem or pedicle. SYN petiole. [L. dim. of *pes* (foot), the stalk of a fruit]

p. epiglot′tidis [NA], SYN *stalk* of epiglottis.

Petit, Alexis T., French physicist, 1791–1820. SEE Dulong-P. *law.*

Petit, Antoine, French surgeon and anatomist, 1718–1794. SEE P.'s *ligament.*

Petit, Francois du, French surgeon and anatomist, 1664–1741. SEE P.'s *canals, canal, sinus.*

Petit, Jean L., Paris surgeon, 1674–1750. SEE P.'s *hernia, herniotomy,* lumbar *triangle.*

Petit, Paul, French anatomist, *1889. SEE P.'s *aponeurosis.*

Petri, Julius, German bacteriologist, 1852–1921. SEE P. *dish.*

pet·ri·fac·tion (pet-ri-fak′shŭn). Fossilization, as in conversion into stone. [L. *petra*, rock + *facio*, to make]

pé·tris·sage (pā-trē-sazh′). A manipulation in massage, consisting in a kneading of the muscles. [Fr. kneading]

⟳**petro-.** Stone; stone-like hardness. [L. *petra*, rock; G. *petros*, stone]

pet·roc·cip·i·tal (pet′rok-sip′i-tăl). SYN petro-occipital.

pe·tro·la·tum (pet-rō-lā′tŭm). A yellowish mixture of the softer members of the paraffin or methane series of hydrocarbons, obtained from petroleum as an intermediate product in its distillation; used as a soothing application to burns and abrasions of the skin, and as a base for ointments. SYN petroleum jelly, yellow soft paraffin.

heavy liquid p., SYN mineral oil.

hydrophilic p., p. composed of cholesterol 30 g, stearyl alcohol 30 g, white wax 80 g, and white p. 860 g, to make 1000 g.

light liquid p., light mineral oil.

white p., of the same composition as p. except that it is decolorized by treatment with activated charcoal; used for the same purposes as p. SYN white soft paraffin.

pe·tro·le·um (pě-trō′lē-ŭm). A mixture of liquid hydrocarbons found in the earth in various parts of the world and believed to be derived from fossilized animal and plant remains; the source of petrolatum, in addition to its use for lighting and heating purposes. SYN coal oil, rock oil. [L. *petra*, rock, + *oleum*, oil]

p. benzin, purified, low boiling fractions distilled from p. consisting of hydrocarbons, chiefly of the methane series; it is highly flammable, and its vapors, when mixed with air and ignited, may explode; used as a solvent. SYN benzin, benzine, naphtha, p. ether.

p. ether, SYN p. benzin.

liquid p., SYN mineral oil.

pe·tro·le·um jel·ly. SYN petrolatum.

pet·ro·mas·toid (pet′rō-mas′toyd). Relating to the petrous and the squamous portions of the temporal bone, which are usually united at birth by the petrosquamosal suture. SYN petrosomastoid.

pet·ro·oc·cip·i·tal (pet′rō-ok-sip′i-tăl). Denoting the cranial suture between the occipital bone and the petrous portion of the temporal. SYN petroccipital.

pet·ro·pha·ryn·ge·us. SEE *musculus* petropharyngeus.

pe·tro·sa, pl. **pe·tro·sae** (pe-trō′să, -sē). The petrous portion of the temporal bone. [L. fr. *petra*, rock]

pe·tro·sal (pe-trō′săl). Relating to the petrosa. SYN petrous (2).

pe·tro·sal·pin·go·sta·phy·li·nus (pet′rō-sal′pin-gō-staf-i-lī′nŭs). Obsolete term for the levator veli palatini muscle. [petrosa + G. *salpinx*, trumpet, + *staphylē*, uvula]

pet·ro·si·tis (pet-rō-sī′tis). An inflammation involving the petrous portion of the temporal bone and its air cells. SYN petrousitis.

pet·ro·so·mas·toid (pet-rō′sō-mas′toyd). SYN petromastoid.

pet·ro·sphe·noid (pet′rō-sfē′noyd). Relating to the petrous portion of the temporal bone and to the sphenoid bone.

pet·ro·squa·mo·sal, pet·ro·squa·mous (pet′rō-skwā-mō′săl, -skwā′mŭs). Relating to the petrous and the squamous portions of the temporal bone. SYN squamopetrosal.

pe·tro·sta·phy·li·nus (pet′rō-staf-i-lī′nŭs). Obsolete term for the levator veli palatini *muscle.* [G. *petra*, stone, + *staphylē*, uvula]

pet·rous (pet′rŭs, pē′trŭs). **1.** Of stony hardness. **2.** SYN petrosal. [L. *petrosus*, fr. *petra*, a rock]

pet·rou·si·tis (pet-rū-sī′tis). SYN petrositis.

Pette, H.H. German neuropathologist, 1887–1964. SEE P.-Döring *disease.*

Pettit, Auguste, French physician, 1869–1939. SEE Bachman-P. *test.*

Peutz, J.L.A., Dutch physician. SEE P.-Jeghers *syndrome;* Jeghers-P. *syndrome.*

pex·in (pek′sin). SYN chymosin.

pex·in·o·gen (pek-sin′ō-jen). SYN prochymosin.

pex·is (pek′sis). Fixation of substances in the tissues. [G. *pēxis,* fixation]

⌂-pexy. Fixation, usually surgical. [G. *pēxis,* fixation]

Peyer, Johann K., Swiss anatomist, 1653–1712. SEE P.'s *glands,* under *gland, patches,* under *patch.*

pe·yo·te, pe·yo·tl (pā-yō′tē, pā-yō′tl). Aztec name for *Lophophora williamsii;* principal active component of p. is mescaline. SYN pellote. [Sp.]

Peyronie, Francois de la, French surgeon, 1678–1747. SEE P.'s *disease.*

Peyrot, Jean J., French surgeon, 1843–1918. SEE P.'s *thorax.*

Pezzer, O. de. SEE de Pezzer.

Pfannenstiel, Hermann Johann, German gynecologist, 1862–1909. SEE P.'s *incision.*

Pfaundler, Meinhard von, German physician, 1872–1947. SEE P.-Hurler *syndrome.*

Pfeiffer, Richard F.J., German physician, 1858–1945. SEE *Pfeifferella;* P.'s blood *agar, bacillus, phenomenon, syndrome.*

Pfeif·fer·el·la (fī-fer-el′lă). An obsolete genus of bacteria, the type species of which, *P. mallei,* formerly was placed in the genus *Actinobacillus* and presently is placed in the genus *Pseudomonas.* [R. F. J. *Pfeiffer*]

PFFD Abbreviation for proximal femoral focal *deficiency.*

Pflüger, Eduard F.W., German anatomist and physiologist, 1829–1910. SEE P.'s *law.*

PFOB Abbreviation for perfluorooctyl bromide.

Pfuhl, Eduard, German physician, 1852–1905. SEE P.'s *sign.*

PG Abbreviation for prostaglandin

pg Symbol for picogram.

PGA, PGB, PGC, PGD. Abbreviations, with numerical subscripts according to structure, often used for prostaglandins. Letters A, B, etc. indicate the nature of the cyclopentane ring (substituents, double bonds, orientation); numerical subscripts indicate the number of double bonds in the alkyl chains.

PGR Abbreviation for psychogalvanic *response.*

P₂Gri Symbol for diphosphoglycerate.

1,3-P₂Gri Symbol for 1,3-diphosphoglycerate.

2,3-P₂Gri Symbol for 2,3-diphosphoglycerate.

Ph Symbol for phenyl.

Ph1. Abbreviation for Philadelphia *chromosome.*

pH Symbol for the negative logarithm of the H^+ ion concentration (measured in moles per liter); a solution with pH 7.00 (1×10^{-7} gram molecular weight of hydrogen per liter) is neutral at 22°C (*i.e.,* $[H^+] = [OH^-]$), one with a pH of more than 7.0 is alkaline, one with a pH lower than 7.00 is acid. At a temperature of 37°C, neutrality is at a pH value of 6.8. Cf. dissociation *constant* of water. [p (power or potency) of H^+]

blood pH, pH of arterial blood; normal is 7.4 (normal range 7.36–7.44).

critical pH, the pH range, about 5.5, at which saliva ceases to be saturated with respect to calcium and phosphate, and below which tooth mineral will dissolve.

optimum pH, the pH at which an enzymatic or any other reaction or process is most effective.

PHA Abbreviation for phytohemagglutinin.

⌂phaco-. **1.** Lens-shaped, relating to a lens; **2.** Birthmark; as in phacomatosis. [G. *phakos,* lentil (lens), anything shaped like a lentil]

phac·o·an·a·phy·lax·is (fak′ō-an-ă-fī-lak′sis). Hypersensitivity to protein of the lens of the eye.

phac·o·cele (fak′ō-sēl). Hernia of the lens of the eye through the sclera. [phaco- + G. *kēlē,* hernia]

phac·o·cyst (fak′ō-sist). SYN lens *capsule.* [phaco- + G. *kystis,* bladder]

phac·o·cys·tec·to·my (fak′ō-sis-tek′tō-mē). Rarely used term for surgical removal of a portion of the capsule of the lens of the eye. [phaco- + G. *kystis,* bladder, + *ektomē,* excision]

phac·o·don·e·sis (fak′ō-don-ē′sis). Tremulousness of the lens of the eye. [phaco- + G. *doneō,* to shake to and fro]

phac·o·e·mul·si·fi·ca·tion (fak′ō-ē-mŭl-si-fi-kā′shŭn). A method of emulsifying and aspirating a cataract with a low frequency ultrasonic needle.

phac·o·er·y·sis (fak-ō-er′i-sis). Extraction of the lens of the eye by means of a suction cup called the erysophake. [phaco- + G. *erysis,* pulling, drawing off]

phac·o·frag·men·ta·tion (fak′ō-frag′men-tā′shŭn). Rupture and aspiration of the lens.

pha·coid (fak′oyd). Of lentil shape. [phaco- + G. *eidos,* resemblance]

pha·col·y·sis (fă-kol′i-sis). Operative breaking down and removal of the lens. [phaco- + G. *lysis,* dissolution]

pha·co·lyt·ic (fak-ō-lit′ik). Characterized by or referring to phacolysis.

pha·co·ma (fa-kō′mă). A hamartoma found in phacomatosis; often refers to a retinal hamartoma in tuberous sclerosis. SYN phakoma. [phaco- + G. *-oma,* tumor]

pha·co·ma·la·cia (fak′ō-mă-lā′shē-ă). Softening of the lens, as may occur in hypermature cataract. [phaco- + G. *malakia,* softness]

phac·o·ma·to·sis (fak′ō-mă-tō′sis). A generic term for a group of hereditary diseases characterized by hamartomas involving multiple tissues; *e.g.,* von Hippel-Lindau's disease, neurofibromatosis, Sturge-Weber syndrome, tuberous sclerosis. SYN phakomatosis. [Van der Hoeve's coinage fr. G. *phakos,* mother-spot]

phac·o·scope (fak′ō-skōp). An instrument in the form of a dark chamber for observing the changes in the lens during accommodation. [phaco- + G. *skopeō,* to view]

Phae·ni·cia ser·i·ca·ta (fen-ī′sē-ă ser-i-kā′tă). A common species of yellowish or metallic green blowfly (family Calliphoridae, order Diptera); an abundant scavenger feeding on carrion or excrement, and implicated in sheep strike and other forms of myiasis. SYN *Lucilia sericata.*

⌂phaeo-. SEE pheo-.

phae·o·hy·pho·my·co·sis (fē′ō-hī′fō-mī-kō′sis). A group of superficial and deep infections caused by fungi that form pigmented hyphae and yeastlike cells in tissue, *i.e.,* dematiaceous fungal infections other than chromoblastomycosis and mycetomas. In humans, cats, and horses, p. is caused by *Drechslera spicifera;* in chickens and turkeys by *Dactylaria gallopava.* [G. *phaios,* dusky, + *hyphē,* web, + mycosis]

phage (fāj). SYN bacteriophage.

β **p.,** SYN β *corynebacteriophage.*

defective p., SYN defective *bacteriophage.*

Lambda p., a bacteriophage used extensively in experimental systems.

⌂-phage, -phagia, -phagy. Eating, devouring. [G. *phagō,* to eat]

phag·e·de·na (faj-ĕ-dē′nă). An ulcer that rapidly spreads peripherally, destroying the tissues as it increases in size. [G. *phagedaina,* a canker]

p. gangreno′sa, severe gangrene with sloughing.

p. nosocomia′lis, gangrene arising in a hospital from cross infection.

sloughing p., SYN decubitus *ulcer.*

p. trop′ica, the tropical ulcer of Old World cutaneous leishmaniasis.

phag·e·den·ic (faj-ĕ-den′ik). Relating to or having the characteristics of phagedena.

⌂phago-. Eating, devouring. [G. *phagō,* to eat]

phag·o·cyte (fag′ō-sīt). A cell possessing the property of ingesting bacteria, foreign particles, and other cells. P.'s are divided into two general classes: 1) microphages, polymorphonuclear leukocytes that ingest chiefly bacteria; 2) macrophages, mononucleated cells (histiocytes and monocytes) that are largely scavengers, ingesting dead tissue and degenerated cells. SYN carrier cell, scavenger cell. [phago- + G. *kytos,* cell]

phag·o·cyt·ic (fag-ō-sit′ik). Relating to phagocytes or phagocytosis.

phag·o·cy·tin (fag-ō-sī′tin). A very labile bactericidal substance that may be isolated from polymorphonuclear leukocytes.

phag·o·cy·tize (fag′ō-si-tīz). SYN phagocytose.

phag·o·cy·to·blast (fag-ō-sī′tō-blast). A primitive cell developing into a phagocyte. [phagocyte + G. *blastos,* germ]

phag·o·cy·tol·y·sis (fag′ō-sī-tol′i-sis). **1.** Destruction of phagocytes, or leukocytes, occurring in the process of blood coagulation or as the result of the introduction of certain antagonistic foreign substances into the body. SYN phagolysis. **2.** A spontaneous breaking down of the phagocytes, preliminary (according to Metchnikoff) to the liberation of cytase, or complement. [phagocyte + G. *lysis,* dissolution]

phag·o·cy·to·lyt·ic (fag′ō-sī-tō-lit′ik). Relating to phagocytolysis. SYN phagolytic.

phag·o·cy·tose (fag′ō-si-tōz). To perform phagocytosis, denoting the action of phagocytic cells. SYN phagocytize.

phag·o·cy·to·sis (fag′ō-sī-tō′sis). The process of ingestion and digestion by cells of solid substances, *e.g.,* other cells, bacteria, bits of necrosed tissue, foreign particles. SEE ALSO endocytosis. [phagocyte + G. *-osis,* condition]

induced p., p. occurring when bacteria subjected to the action of blood serum are brought in contact with leukocytes.

spontaneous p., p. occurring when a culture of bacteria is brought in contact with washed leukocytes in an indifferent medium, such as a physiologic salt solution.

phag·o·dy·na·mom·e·ter (fag′ō-dī-nă-mom′ĕ-ter). A device for measuring the force required to chew various foods. [phago- + G. *dynamis,* force, + *metron,* measure]

pha·gol·y·sis (fa-gol′i-sis). SYN phagocytolysis (1).

phag·o·ly·so·some (fag-ō-lī′sō-sōm). A body formed by union of a phagosome or ingested particle with a lysosome having hydrolytic enzymes.

phag·o·lyt·ic (fag-ō-lit′ik). SYN phagocytolytic.

phag·o·ma·nia (fag-ō-mā′nē-ă). Rarely used term for a morbid desire to eat. SEE ALSO bulimia. [phago- + G. *mania,* frenzy]

phag·o·pho·bia (fag-ō-fō′bē-ă). Morbid fear of eating. [phago- + G. *phobos,* fear]

phag·o·some (fag′ō-sōm). A vesicle that forms around a particle (bacterial or other) within the phagocyte that engulfed it, separates from the cell membrane, and then fuses with and receives the contents of cytoplasmic granules (lysosomes), thus forming a phagolysosome in which digestion of the engulfed particle occurs. [phago- + G. *sōma,* body]

phag·o·type (fag′ō-tīp). In microbiology, a subdivision of a species distinguished from other strains therein by sensitivity to a certain bacteriophage or set of bacteriophages. [phago- + G. *typos,* type]

△ **-phagy.** SEE -phage.

△ **phako-.** For words so beginning and not listed here, see phaco-.

pha·ko·ma (fa-kō′mă). SYN phacoma.

phak·o·ma·to·sis (fak′ō-mă-tō′sis). SYN phacomatosis.

pha·lan·ge·al (fă-lan′jē-ăl). Relating to a phalanx.

phal·an·gec·to·my (fal-an-jek′tō-mē). Excision of one or more of the phalanges of hand or foot. [phalang- + G. *ektomē,* excision]

pha·lan·ges (fă-lan′jēz) [NA]. Plural of phalanx. [L.]

pha·lanx, gen. **pha·lan·gis,** pl. **pha·lan·ges** (fā′langks, fă-langks′; fă-lan′jis; -jēz). **1** [NA]. One of the long bones of the digits, 14 in number for each hand or foot, two for the thumb or great toe, and three each for the other four digits; designated as proximal, middle, and distal, beginning from the metacarpus. **2.** One of a number of cuticular plates, arranged in several rows, on the surface of the spiral organ (of Corti), which are the heads of the outer row of pillar cells and of phalangeal cells; between them are the free ends of the hair cells. [L. fr. G. *phalanx* (*-ang-*), line of soldiers, bone between two joints of the fingers and toes]

tufted p., one of the terminal phalanges of the fingers in acromegaly; it has an expanded extremity resembling a sheaf of wheat.

ungual p., the distal p. of each of the digits; so called because of the flattened tuberosity at its termination which supports the nail.

△ **phall-, phalli-, phallo-.** The penis. [G. *phallos*]

phal·lal·gia (fal-al′jē-ă). SYN phallodynia. [phall- + G. *algos,* pain]

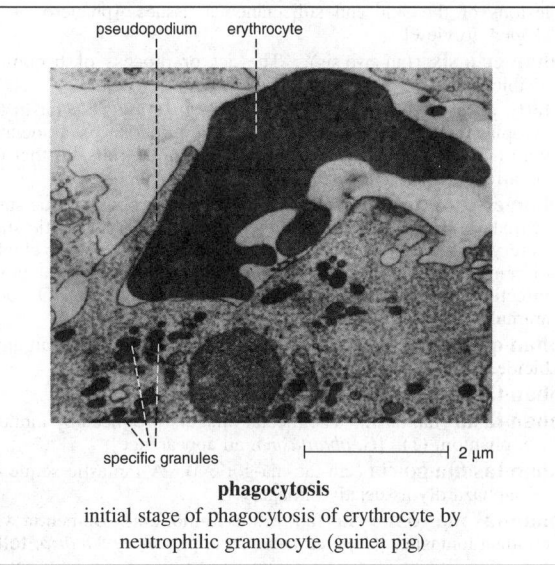

phagocytosis
initial stage of phagocytosis of erythrocyte by
neutrophilic granulocyte (guinea pig)

phal·lec·to·my (fal-ek′tō-mē). Surgical removal of the penis. SYN penectomy. [phall- + G. *ektomē,* excision]

phal·lic (fal′ik). **1.** Relating to the penis. **2.** In psychoanalysis, relating to the penis, especially during the phases of infantile psychosexuality. SEE ALSO phallic *phase.* [G. *phallos,* penis]

phal·li·cism (fal′i-sizm). Worship of the male genitalia. SYN phallism.

phal·li·form (fal′i-fōrm). SYN phalloid.

phal·lism (fal′i-sizm). SYN phallicism.

phal·li·tis (fal-ī′tis). SYN penitis.

△ **phallo-.** SEE phall-.

phal·lo·camp·sis (fal-ō-kamp′sis). Curvature of the erect penis. SEE ALSO chordee. [phallo- + G. *kampsis,* a bending]

phal·lo·cryp·sis (fal-ō-krip′sis). Dislocation and retraction of the penis. [phallo- + G. *krypsis,* concealment]

phal·lo·dyn·ia (fal-ō-din′ē-ă). Pain in the penis. SYN phallalgia. [phallo- + G. *odynē,* pain]

phal·loid (fal′oyd). Resembling in shape a penis. SYN phalliform. [phallo- + G. *eidos,* resemblance]

phal·loi·din (fă-loy′din). Best known of the toxic cyclic peptides produced by the poisonous mushroom, *Amanita phalloides;* closely related to amanitin.

phal·lol·y·sin (fă-lol′i-sin). A glycoprotein that is the heat-sensitive (destroyed in cooking) toxin of the mushroom *Amanita phalloides.*

phal·lon·cus (fal-ong′kŭs). A tumor or swelling of the penis. [phallo- + G. *onkos,* mass]

phal·lo·plas·ty (fal′ō-plas-tē). Surgical reconstruction of the penis. [phallo- + G. *plastos,* formed]

phal·lot·o·my (fal-ot′ō-mē). Surgical incision into the penis. SYN penotomy. [phallo- + G. *tomē,* a cutting]

phal·lo·tox·ins (fal′ō-toks′in). A class of heterodetic cyclic heptapeptides present in *Amanita phalloides;* together with the amatoxins, the main toxin components of this fungus.

phal·lus, pl. **phalli** (fal′ŭs, fal′ī). SYN penis. [L.; G. *phallos*]

△ **phanero-.** Visible, obvious. [G. *phaneros*]

phan·er·o·gen·ic (fan′er-ō-jen′ik). Denoting a disease, the etiology of which is manifest. Cf. cryptogenic. [phanero- + G. *genesis,* origin]

phan·er·o·ma·nia (fan′er-ō-mā′nē-ă). Rarely used term for constant preoccupation with some external part, as plucking the beard, pulling the lobe of the ear, picking at a pimple, etc. [phanero- + G. *mania,* frenzy]

phan·er·o·scope (fan′er-ō-skōp). A lens used to concentrate the light from a lamp upon the skin, to facilitate examination of

ph

lesions of the skin and subcutaneous tissues. [phanero- + G. *skopeō*, to view]

phan·er·o·sis (fan-er-ō′sis). The act or process of becoming visible. [phanero- + G. *osis*, condition]

fatty p., presumed unmasking of previously invisible fat in the cytoplasm of cells; marked fatty metamorphosis is associated with an absolute increase in the fat content of cells, so that the occurrence of p. is doubted.

phan·er·o·zo·ite (fan′er-ō-zō′īt). An exoerythrocytic tissue stage of malaria infection other than the primary exoerythrocytic stages (cryptozoite and metacryptozoite generations); consists chiefly of reinfection of the liver by merozoites produced by a blood infection (not found in falciparum malaria). [phanero- + G. *zōon*, animal]

phan·quone (fan′kwōn). 4,7-Phenanthroline-5,6-dione; an amebicide.

phan·ta·sia (fan-tā′zē-ă). SYN fantasy. [G. appearance]

phan·tasm (fan′tazm). The mental imagery produced by fantasy. SYN phantom (1). [G. *phantasma*, an appearance]

phan·tas·ma·go·ria (fan-taz-mă-gōr′ē-ă). A fantastic sequence of haphazardly associative imagery.

phan·tas·ma·to·mo·ria (fan-taz′mă-tō-mōr′ē-ă). Dementia with childish fantasies. [G. *phantasma*, an appearance, + *mōria*, folly]

phan·tas·mol·o·gy (fan-tas-mol′ō-jē). The study of spiritualistic manifestations and of apparitions. [G. *phantasma*, an appearance, + *logos*, study]

phan·tas·mo·sco·pia, phan·tas·mos·co·py (fan-taz-mō-skō′pē-ă, -mos′kō-pē). The delusion of seeing phantoms. [G. *phantasma*, an appearance, + *skopeō*, to view]

phan·tom (fan′tŏm). 1. SYN phantasm. 2. A model, especially a transparent one, of the human body or any of its parts. SEE ALSO manikin. 3. In radiology, a mechanical or computer-originated model for predicting irradiation dosage deep in the body. [G. *phantasma*, an appearance]

Schultze's p., a model of a female pelvis used in demonstrating the mechanism of childbirth and the application of forceps.

phan·tom·ize (fan′tŏm-īz). In psychiatry, to create mental imagery by fantasy.

phar·ma·cal (far′mă-kăl). SYN pharmaceutic.

phar·ma·ceu·tic, phar·ma·ceu·ti·cal (far-mă-sū′tik, sū′ti-kăl). Relating to pharmacy or to pharmaceutics. SYN pharmacal. [G. *pharmakeutikos*, relating to drugs]

phar·ma·ceu·tics (far-mă-sū′tiks). 1. SYN pharmacy (1). 2. The science of pharmaceutical systems, *i.e.*, preparations, dosage forms, etc.

phar·ma·ceu·tist (far-mă-sū′tist). SYN pharmacist.

phar·ma·cist (far′mă-sist). One who is licensed to prepare and dispense drugs and compounds and is knowledgeable concerning their properties. SYN pharmaceutist. [G. *pharmakon*, a drug]

△**pharmaco-.** Drugs. [G. *pharmakon*, medicine]

phar·ma·co·chem·is·try (far′mă-kō-kem′is-trē). SYN pharmaceutical *chemistry*.

phar·ma·co·di·ag·no·sis (far′mă-kō-dī-ag-nō′sis). Use of drugs in diagnosis.

phar·ma·co·dy·nam·ic (far′mă-kō-dī-nam′ik). Relating to drug action.

phar·ma·co·dy·nam·ics (far′mă-kō-dī-nam′iks). The study of uptake, movement, binding, and interactions of pharmacologically active molecules at their tissue site(s) of action. [pharmaco- + G. *dynamis*, force]

phar·ma·co·en·do·cri·nol·o·gy (far′mă-kō-en′dō-krin-ol′ō-jē). The pharmacology of endocrine function.

phar·ma·co·ep·i·dem·i·ol·o·gy (far′mă-kō-ep-i-dē-mē- ol′ō-jē). The study of the distribution and determinants of drug-related events in populations, and the application of this study to efficacious drug treatment.

phar·ma·co·ge·net·ics (far′mă-kō-jĕ-net′iks). The study of genetically determined variations in responses to drugs in humans or in laboratory organisms.

phar·ma·cog·no·sist (far-ma-kog′nō-sist). One skilled in pharmacognosy.

phar·ma·cog·no·sy (far-mă-kog′nō-sē). A branch of pharmacology concerned with the physical characteristics and botanical and animal sources of crude drugs. SYN pharmaceutical biology. [pharmaco- + G. *gnōsis*, knowledge]

phar·ma·cog·ra·phy (far-mă-kog′ră-fē). A treatise on or description of drugs. [pharmaco- + G. *graphē*, description]

phar·ma·co·ki·net·ic (far′mă-kō-ki-net′ik). Relating to the disposition of drugs in the body (*i.e.*, their absorption, distribution, metabolism, and elimination).

phar·ma·co·ki·net·ics (far′mă-kō-ki-net′iks). Movements of drugs within biological systems, as affected by uptake, distribution, binding, elimination, and biotransformation; particularly the rates of such movements. [pharmaco- + G. *kinēsis*, movement]

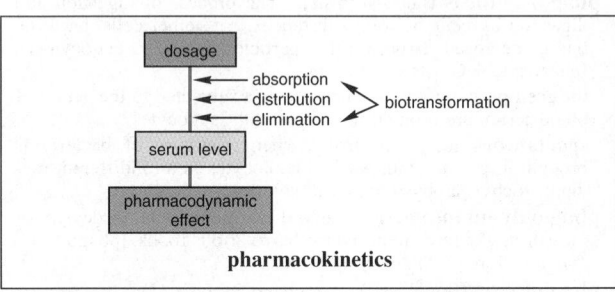

pharmacokinetics

phar·ma·co·log·ic, phar·ma·co·log·i·cal (far′mă-kō-loj′ik, -loj′i-kăl). 1. Relating to pharmacology or to the composition, properties, and actions of drugs. 2. Sometimes used in physiology to denote a dose (of a chemical agent that either is or mimics a hormone, neurotransmitter, or other naturally-occurring agent) that is so much larger or more potent than would occur naturally that it might have qualitatively different effects. Cf. homeopathic (2), physiologic (4), supraphysiologic.

phar·ma·col·o·gist (far-mă-kol′ō-jist). A specialist in pharmacology.

clinical p., a p. who has undergone training in basic pharmacology, clinical pharmacology, and one of several specialities of medical practice.

phar·ma·col·o·gy (far-mă-kol′ō-jē). The science concerned with drugs, their sources, appearance, chemistry, actions, and uses. [pharmaco- + G. *logos*, study]

biochemical p., a branch of p. concerned with the biochemical mechanisms responsible for the actions of drugs.

clinical p., the branch of p. concerned with the p. of therapeutic agents in the prevention, treatment, and control of disease in humans.

marine p., a branch of p. concerned with pharmacologically active substances present in aquatic plants and animals; its objective is to find and develop new therapeutic agents.

phar·ma·co·ma·nia (far′mă-kō-mā′nē-ă). Morbid impulse to take drugs. [pharmaco- + G. *mania*, frenzy]

phar·ma·co·pe·dics, phar·ma·co·pe·dia (far′mă-kō-pē′diks, -pē′dē-ă). The teaching of pharmacy and pharmacodynamics. [pharmaco- + G. *paideia*, instruction, fr. *pais* (*paid-*), a child]

Phar·ma·co·pe·ia, Phar·ma·co·poe·ia (far′mă-kō-pē′ă). A work containing monographs of therapeutic agents, standards for their strength and purity, and their formulations. The various national pharmacopeias are referred to by abbreviations, of which the following are the most frequently encountered: *USP*, the Pharmacopeia of the United States of America (United States Pharmacopeia); *BP*, British Pharmacopoeia; *Codex medicamentarius*, the French Pharmacopeia; *I.C. Add.* (or *BA*), the Indian and Colonial Addendum to the BP; *IP*, International Pharmacopeia; *Pharmacopeia Austr.*, the Austrian Pharmacopeia; *Ph.G.*, the German Pharmacopeia (D.A.B.); *Pharmacopeia Helv.*, the Swiss Pharmacopeia. The first edition of the USP was compiled in 1820 and was made a legal standard by the terms of the National Food and Drugs Act in January, 1907. [G. *pharmakopoiia*, fr. *pharmakon*, a medicine, + *poieo*, to make]

phar·ma·co·pe·ial (far′mă-kō-pē′ăl). Relating to the Pharmacopeia; denoting a drug in the list of the Pharmacopeia. SEE ALSO official.

phar·ma·co·phi·lia (far′mă-kō-fil′ē-ă). Morbid fondness for taking drugs. [pharmaco- + G. *phileō,* to love]

phar·ma·co·pho·bia (far′mă-kō-fō′bē-ă). Morbid fear of taking drugs. [pharmaco- + G. *phobos,* fear]

phar·ma·co·psy·cho·sis (far′mă-kō-sī-kō′sis). Rarely used term for a psychosis causally related to taking a drug. [pharmaco- + psychosis]

phar·ma·co·ther·a·py (far′mă-kō-thār′ă-pē). Treatment of disease by means of drugs. SEE ALSO chemotherapy. [pharmaco- + G. *therapeia,* therapy]

phar·ma·cy (far′mă-sē). **1.** The practice of preparing and dispensing drugs. SYN pharmaceutics (1). **2.** A drugstore. [G. *pharmakon,* drug]

   clinical p., a branch of p. practice that emphasizes the therapeutic use of drugs rather than the preparation and dispensing of drugs.

Pharm. D. Abbreviation for Doctor of Pharmacy.

♺**pharyng-.** SEE pharyngo-.

pha·ryn·ge·al (fă-rin′jē-ăl). Relating to the pharynx. SYN pharyngeus. [Mod. L. *pharyngeus*]

phar·yn·gec·to·my (far′in-jek′tō-mē). Resection of the pharynx. [pharyng- + G. *ektomē,* excision]

phar·yn·gei (far-in′jē-ī) [NA]. SYN pharyngeal *branches,* under *branch.*

pha·ryn·ges (fă-rin′jēz). Plural of pharynx.

pha·ryn·ge·us (far′in-jē′ŭs). SYN pharyngeal. [Mod. L.]

phar·yn·gis·mus (far-in-jiz′mŭs). Spasm of the muscles of the pharynx. SYN pharyngospasm.

phar·yn·git·ic (far-in-jit′ik). Relating to pharyngitis.

phar·yn·gi·tis (far-in-jī′tis). Inflammation of the mucous membrane and underlying parts of the pharynx. [pharyng- + G. *-itis,* inflammation]

   atrophic p., chronic p. accompanied by a varying degree of atrophy of the mucous glands and absence of their secretion. SYN p. sicca.

   gangrenous p., gangrenous inflammation of the pharyngeal mucous membrane.

   membranous p., inflammation accompanied by a fibrinous exudate, forming a nondiphtheritic false membrane.

   p. sic′ca, SYN atrophic p.

   ulcerative p., inflammation of the pharynx marked by ulceration of the mucosa; may have a viral etiology.

   ulceromembranous p., inflammation of the pharyngeal mucosa with membranous debris overlying the ulcerative lesions.

♺**pharyngo-, pharyng-.** The pharynx. [Mod. L. fr. G. *pharynx*]

pha·ryn·go·cele (fă-ring′gō-sēl). A diverticulum from the pharynx. [pharyngo- + G. *kēlē,* hernia]

pha·ryn·go·ep·i·glot·tic, pha·ryn·go·ep·i·glot·tid·e·an (fă-ring′gō-ep′i-glot′ik, -glo-tid′ē-an). Relating to the pharynx and the epiglottis.

pha·ryn·go·e·soph·a·ge·al (fă-ring′gō-ē-sof′ă-jē′ăl). Relating to the pharynx and the esophagus.

pha·ryn·go·e·soph·a·go·plas·ty (fă-ring′gō-ē-sof′ă-gō-plas-tē). Plastic surgery of the pharynx and esophagus. [pharyngo- + esophago- + G. *plastos,* formed]

pha·ryn·go·glos·sal (fă-ring′gō-glos′ăl). Relating to the pharynx and the tongue.

pha·ryn·go·glos·sus (fă-ring-gō-glos′ŭs). SEE superior constrictor *muscle* of pharynx.

pha·ryn·go·la·ryn·ge·al (fă-ring′gō-lă-rin′jē-ăl). Relating to both the pharynx and the larynx.

pha·ryn·go·lar·yn·gi·tis (fă-ring′gō-lar-in-jī′tis). Inflammation of both the pharynx and the larynx.

pha·ryn·go·lith (fă-ring′gō-lith). A concretion in the pharynx. SYN pharyngeal calculus. [pharyngo- + G. *lithos,* stone]

pha·ryn·go·max·il·lary (fă-ring′gō-mak′si-lār-ē). Relating to the pharynx and the maxilla.

pha·ryn·go·my·co·sis (fă-ring′gō-mī-kō′sis). Invasion of the

mucous membrane of the pharynx by fungi. [pharyngo- + G. *mykēs,* a fungus]

pha·ryn·go·na·sal (fă-ring′gō-nā′săl). Relating to the pharynx and the nasal cavity.

pha·ryn·go·oral (fă-ring′gō-ō′răl). Relating to the pharynx and the mouth; oropharyngeal. [pharyngo- + L. *os* (*or-*), mouth]

pha·ryn·go·pal·a·tine (fă-ring′gō-pal′ă-tīn). Relating to the pharynx and the palate.

pha·ryn·go·pa·la·ti·nus (fă-ring′gō-pal-ă-tī′nŭs). SYN palatopharyngeus *muscle.* [L.]

pha·ryn·go·plas·ty (fă-ring′gō-plas-tē). Plastic surgery of the pharynx. [pharyngo- + G. *plastos,* formed]

   Hynes p., an operation to narrow the pharynx in order to improve speech by cross-rotating two superiorly based flaps to produce a horizontal shelf above Passavant's *ridge.*

pha·ryn·go·ple·gia (fă-ring′gō-plē′jē-ă). Paralysis of the muscles of the pharynx. [pharyngo- + G. *plēgē,* stroke]

pha·ryn·go·rhi·nos·co·py (fă-ring′gō-rī-nos′kŏ-pē). Inspection of the rhinopharynx and posterior nares by means of the rhinoscopic mirror. [pharyngo- + G. *rhis,* nose, + *skopeō,* to view]

pha·ryn·go·scope (fă-ring′gō-skōp). An instrument like a laryngoscope, used for inspection of the mucous membrane of the pharynx. [pharyngo- + G. *skopeō,* to view]

phar·yn·gos·co·py (far′ing-gos′kŏ-pē). Inspection and examination of the pharynx. [pharyngo- + G. *skopeō,* to view]

pha·ryn·go·spasm (fă-ring′gō-spazm). SYN pharyngismus.

pha·ryn·go·sta·phy·li·nus (fă-ring′gō-staf-i-lī′nŭs). SYN palatopharyngeus *muscle.* [L. fr. pharyngo- + G. *staphylē,* uvula]

pha·ryn·go·ste·no·sis (fă-ring′gō-ste-nō′sis). Stricture of the pharynx. [pharyngo- + G. *stenōsis,* a narrowing]

phar·yn·got·o·my (far′ing-got′ō-mē). Any cutting operation upon the pharynx either from without or from within. [pharyngo- + G. *tomē,* incision]

pha·ryn·go·ton·sil·li·tis (fă-ring′gō-ton-si-lī′tis). Inflammation of the pharynx and tonsils. [pharyngo- + tonsillitis]

phar·ynx, gen. **pha·ryn·gis,** pl. **pha·ryn·ges** (far′ingks, fă-rin′jis, fă-rin′jēz) [NA]. The upper expanded portion of the digestive tube, between the esophagus below and the mouth and nasal cavities above and in front. [Mod. L. fr. G. *pharynx* (*pharyng-*), the throat, the joint opening of the gullet and windpipe]

   laryngeal p., SYN laryngopharynx.

   nasal p., SYN nasopharynx.

   oral p., SYN oropharynx.

phase (fāz). **1.** A stage in the course of change or development. **2.** A homogeneous, physically distinct, and separable portion of a heterogeneous system; *e.g.,* oil, gum, and water are three p.'s of an emulsion. **3.** The time relationship between two or more events. **4.** A particular part of a recurring time pattern or wave form. SEE ALSO stage, period. [G. *phasis,* an appearance]

   anal p., in psychoanalytic personality theory, the stage of psychosexual development, occurring when a child is between 1 and 3 years, during which activities, interests, and concerns are centered around the anal zone.

   aqueous p., the water portion of a system consisting of two liquid p.'s, one mainly water, the other a liquid immiscible with water (*e.g.,* benzene, ether).

   cis p., SEE coupling p.

♺ **Combining forms**	**[NA] Nomina Anatomica**
Word*Finder* **Multi-term entry finder** Preceding letter A **A.D.A.M. Anatomy Plates** Between letters L and M **Appendices:** Following letter Z **SYN** Synonym; Cf., compare	**[MIM] Mendelian** **Inheritance in Man** ☆ **Official alternate term** ☆**[NA] Official alternate** **Nomina Anatomica term** ▬▬▬▬▬▬▬▬▬ **High Profile Term**

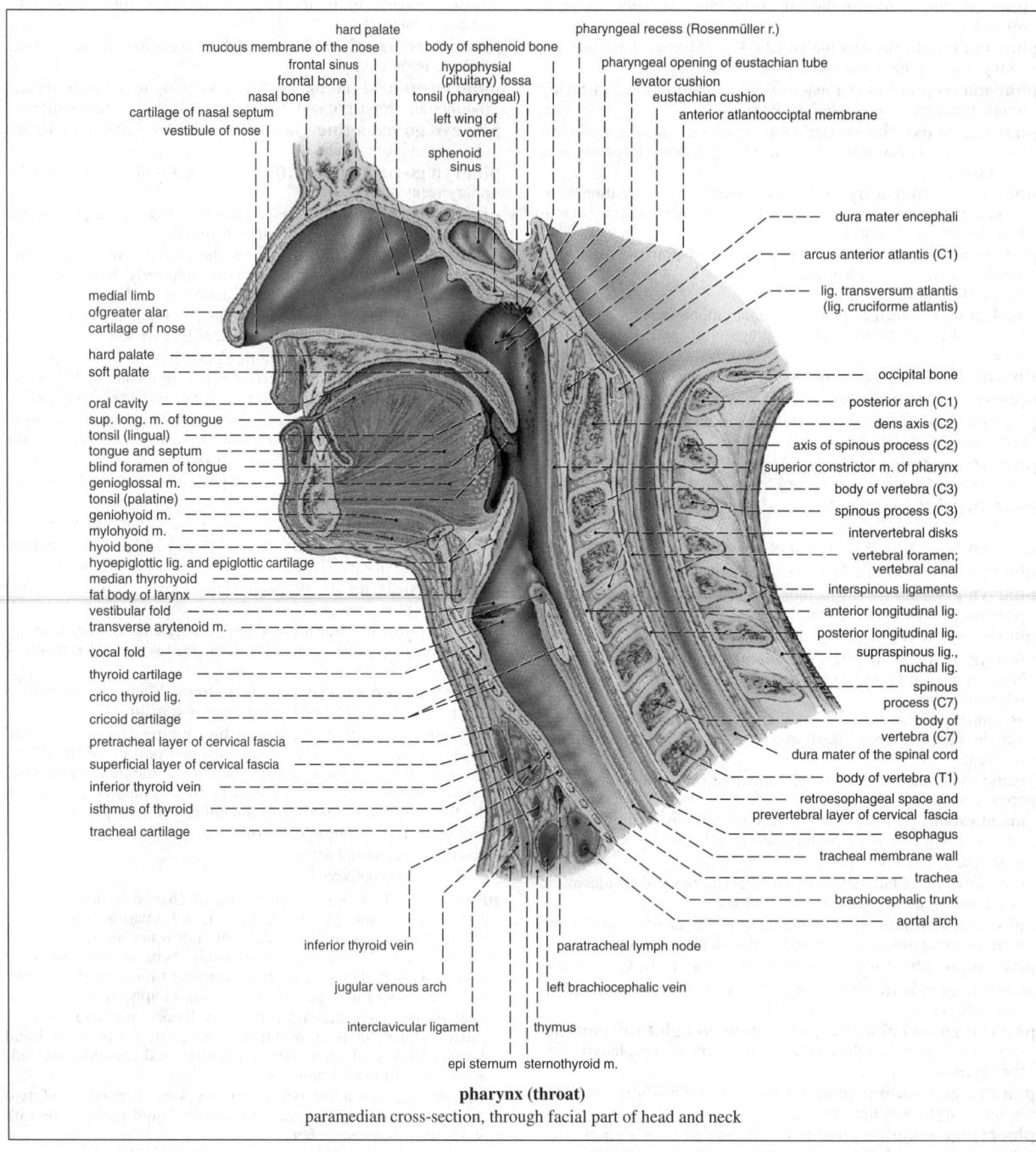

hard palate
mucous membrane of the nose
frontal sinus
frontal bone
nasal bone
cartilage of nasal septum
vestibule of nose

body of sphenoid bone
hypophysial (pituitary) fossa
tonsil (pharyngeal)
left wing of vomer
sphenoid sinus

pharyngeal recess (Rosenmüller r.)
pharyngeal opening of eustachian tube
levator cushion
eustachian cushion
anterior atlantoocciptal membrane

medial limb ofgreater alar cartilage of nose
hard palate
soft palate
oral cavity
sup. long. m. of tongue
tonsil (lingual)
tongue and septum
blind foramen of tongue
genioglossal m.
tonsil (palatine)
geniohyoid m.
mylohyoid m.
hyoid bone
hyoepiglottic lig. and epiglottic cartilage
median thyrohyoid
fat body of larynx
vestibular fold
transverse arytenoid m.
vocal fold
thyroid cartilage
crico thyroid lig.
cricoid cartilage
pretracheal layer of cervical fascia
superficial layer of cervical fascia
inferior thyroid vein
isthmus of thyroid
tracheal cartilage

dura mater encephali
arcus anterior atlantis (C1)
lig. transversum atlantis (lig. cruciforme atlantis)
occipital bone
posterior arch (C1)
dens axis (C2)
axis of spinous process (C2)
superior constrictor m. of pharynx
body of vertebra (C3)
spinous process (C3)
intervertebral disks
vertebral foramen; vertebral canal
interspinous ligaments
anterior longitudinal lig.
posterior longitudinal lig.
supraspinous lig., nuchal lig.
spinous process (C7)
body of vertebra (C7)
dura mater of the spinal cord
body of vertebra (T1)
retroesophageal space and prevertebral layer of cervical fascia
esophagus
tracheal membrane wall
trachea
brachiocephalic trunk
aortal arch

inferior thyroid vein
jugular venous arch
interclavicular ligament
paratracheal lymph node
left brachiocephalic vein
thymus
epi sternum sternothyroid m.

pharynx (throat)
paramedian cross-section, through facial part of head and neck

continuous p., SYN external p.

coupling p., the physical relationship of two syntenic genes. If they are on the same chromosome, they are said to be "in coupling" or "in the cis p."; if on opposite members of a chromosome pair, "in repulsion" or "in the trans p."

discontinuous p., SYN internal p.

dispersed p., SYN internal p.

dispersion p., SYN external p.

eclipse p., SYN eclipse *period.*

p. encoding, in magnetic resonance imaging, the technique of inducing a gradient in the magnetic field in the *Y*-axis to induce phase differences with location. SYN gradient encoding.

eruptive p., that period in the tooth formation which includes the development of the roots, periodontal ligament, and dentogingival junction of the tooth.

external p., the medium or fluid in which a disperse is suspended. SYN continuous p., dispersion medium, dispersion p., external medium.

Gap$_1$ p., SYN Gap$_1$ *period.*

Gap$_2$ p., SYN Gap$_2$ *period.*

genital p., in psychoanalytic personality theory, the final stage of psychosexual development, occurring during puberty, in which the individual's psychosexual development is so organized that sexual gratification can be achieved from genital-to-genital contact and the capacity exists for a mature affectionate relationship with an individual of the opposite sex. SEE phallic p.

growth p., a stage in the enlargement of a neoplasm.

ph

horizontal growth p., an early stage of development of cutaneous melanoma by intraepidermal spread of atypical melanocytes.

internal p., the particles contained in a colloid solution. SYN discontinuous p., dispersed p.

lag p., a brief period in the course of the growth of a bacterial culture, especially at the beginning, during which the growth is very slow or scarcely appreciable.

latency p., in psychoanalytic personality theory, the period of psychosexual development in children, extending from about age 5 to the beginning of adolescence at age 12, during which the apparent cessation of sexual preoccupation during this period stems from a strong, aggressive blockade of libidinal and sexual impulses in an effort to avoid oedipal relationships; during this p., boys and girls are inclined to choose friends and join groups of their own sex. SYN latency period.

logarithmic p., exponential, a period in the course of growth of a bacterial culture in which maximal multiplication is occurring by geometrical progression; thus, if the logarithms of their numbers are plotted against time, they will form a straight upward line.

luteal p., that portion of the menstrual cycle extending from the time of formation of the corpus luteum to the onset of menses, usually 14 days in length; **short luteal p.,** a period of 10 days or less between ovulation and the onset of menses, frequently associated with infertility.

M p., SYN mitotic *period*.

meiotic p., the stage of nuclear changes in the sexual cells during which reduction of the chromosomes takes place; it embraces the cell generations of the spermatocytes and oocytes. SYN reduction p.

negative p., the period during which the opsonic index is lowered following the injection of a vaccine.

oedipal p., in psychoanalysis, a stage in the psychosexual development of the child, characterized by erotic attachment to the parent of the opposite sex, repressed because of fear of the parent of the same sex; usually occurring between the ages of 3 and 6 years. SYN oedipal period.

oral p., in psychoanalytic personality theory, the earliest stage in psychosexual development, lasting through the first 18 months of life, during which the oral zone is the center of the infant's needs, expression, gratification, and pleasurable erotic experiences; has a strong influence on the organization and development of the child's psyche.

phallic p., in psychoanalytic personality theory, the stage in psychosexual development, occurring when a child is between 2 and 6 years of age, during which interest, curiosity, and pleasurable experiences are centered around the penis in boys and the clitoris in girls. SEE genital p.

positive p., the period following the negative p., during which the opsonic index rises.

postmeiotic p., the stage following that of reduction of the chromosomes in the sexual cells, representing the mature forms of these cells, ending with the conjugation of the nuclei in the impregnated ovum. SYN postreduction p.

postmitotic p., SYN Gap$_1$ *period*.

postreduction p., SYN postmeiotic p.

poststationary p., the period in the growth of a bacterial culture in which growth is declining.

pregenital p., in psychoanalysis, the collective psychosexual development p.'s preceding the genital p.

premeiotic p., the stage of nuclear changes in the sexual cells before the reduction of the chromosomes, embracing the cell generations up to that of the spermatogonia and oogonia. SYN prereduction p.

premitotic p., SYN Gap$_2$ *period*.

pre-oedipal p., in psychoanalysis, the collective p.'s of psychosexual development preceding the oedipal p.

prereduction p., SYN premeiotic p.

radial growth p., the early pattern of growth of cutaneous malignant melanoma, in which tumor cells spread laterally in the epidermis.

reduction p., SYN meiotic p.

S p., SYN synthesis *period*.

stationary p., (1) the period in the course of growth of a bacterial culture during which the multiplication of the organisms becomes gradually less and the bacteria undergoing division are in equilibrium with those dying; (2) referring to the usually solid, nonmobile component in partition chromatography.

supernormal recovery p., a brief period during the recovery of cardiac muscle following excitation when diseased muscle is more (*i.e.,* less abnormally) excitable; corresponds to the end of the T wave in the ECG.

synaptic p., SYN synapsis.

trans p., SEE coupling p.

vertical growth p., spread of melanoma cells from the epidermis into the dermis and later the subcutis, from which site metastasis may take place.

vulnerable p., a period in the cardiac cycle during which an ectopic impulse may lead to repetitive activity such as flutter or fibrillation of the affected chamber.

phas·mid (faz′mid). **1.** One of a pair of caudal chemoreceptors seen in nematodes of the class Secernentasida (Phasmidia). **2.** Common name for a member of the class Phasmidia, now Secernentasida.

Phas·mid·ia (faz-mid′ē-ă). SYN Secernentasida. [G. *phasma,* appearance]

phas·mo·pho·bia (fas-mō-fō′bē-ă). Morbid fear of ghosts. [G. *phasma,* apparition, + *phobos,* fear]

phat·nor·rha·gia (fat-nō-rā′jē-ă). Hemorrhage from a dental alveolus. [G. *phatnōma,* manger (alveolus), + G. *rhēgnymi,* to burst forth]

Ph.D. Abbreviation for Doctor of Philosophy.

Phe Symbol for phenylalanine or its radical.

Phemister, Dallas B., American surgeon, 1882–1951. SEE P. *graft.*

△**phen-, pheno-.** **1.** Combining form denoting appearance. **2.** In chemistry, combining form denoting derivation from benzene (phenyl-). [fr. G. *phainō,* to appear, show forth]

phen·a·caine hy·dro·chlo·ride (fen′ă-kān). Bis-(*p*-ethoxyphenyl)acetamidine hydrochloride; a potent local surface anesthetic used in ophthalmology.

phen·ac·e·mide (fe-nas′ĕ-mīd). An anticonvulsant used in the treatment of epilepsy. SYN phenylacetylurea.

phen·ac·e·tin (APC) (fĕ-nas′ĕ-tin). $C_2H_5O–C_6H_4 –NHCOCH_3$; *p*-acetaminophenetide; *p*-acetphenetidine; an analgesic and antipyretic; the "P" in APC, an analgesic combination also containing aspirin and caffeine. SYN acetophenetidin.

phen·ac·e·to·lin (fen′ă-set′ō-lin). A red powder, $(C16H12)2$; used as an indicator. It has a pH range of 5 to 6; being yellow at 5 and red at 6.

phen·ac·e·tur·ic ac·id (fĕ-nas-ĕ-tūr′ik). $C_6H_5CH_2CO–NH–CH_2COOH$; an end product of the metabolism of phenylated fatty acids with even numbers of carbon atoms. SYN phenylaceturic acid.

phen·ac·ri·dane chlo·ride (fe-nas′ri-dān). 9-[*p*-(Hexyloxy)-phenyl]-10-methylacridinium chloride; topical antiseptic.

phen·a·cy·cla·mine (fen-ă-sī′klă-mēn). SYN phenetamine.

phen·a·gly·co·dol (fen-ă-glī′kō-dol). 2-*p*-Chlorophenyl-3-methyl-2,3-butanediol; a central nervous system depressant used in the treatment of anxiety and simple neuroses.

phen·an·threne (fĕ-nan′thrēn). $C_{14}H_{10}$; a compound isomeric with anthracene, derived from coal tar; a major component of steroids, as cyclopenta[α]phenanthrene. Used as a basis for the synthesis of various dyes and drugs.

phen·ar·sen·a·mine (fen-ar-sen-am′ēn). SYN arsphenamine.

phen·ar·sone sulf·ox·y·late (fen-ar′sŏn sŭl-fok′si-lāt). Sodium 3-amino-4-hydroxyphenylarsonate-*N*-methanolsulfoxylate; a pentavalent arsenical used in trichomonal vaginitis.

phe·nate (fē′nāt). A salt or ester of phenol (carbolic acid). SYN carbolate (1).

phen·az·a·cil·lin (fen-az-ă-sil′in). SYN hetacillin.

phe·naz·o·cine (fen-ā′zō-sēn). 2′-Hydroxy-5,9-dimethyl-2-phenethyl-6,7-benzomorphan; a potent analgesic when given intramuscularly or intravenously, less effective orally.

phen·az·o·line hy·dro·chlo·ride (fen-az′ŏ-lēn). SYN antazoline hydrochloride.

phen·az·o·pyr·i·dine hy·dro·chlo·ride (fen-ā-zō-pēr′i-dēn). 2,6-Diamino-3-(phenylazo)pyridine hydrochloride; an orally administered urinary tract analgesic.

phen·cy·cli·dine (PCP) (fen-sī′kli-dēn). 1-(1-Phenylcyclohexyl)piperidine; a substance of abuse, used for its hallucinogenic properties, which can produce profound psychological and behavioral disturbances; the hydrochloride has analgesic and anesthetic properties.

phen·di·me·tra·zine tar·trate (fen-di-met′ră-zēn). (d-3,4-Dimethyl-2-phenylmorpholine)-bitartrate; an anorexic agent.

phen·el·zine sul·fate (fen′el-zēn). (2-Phenethyl) hydrazine sulfate; a monoamine oxidase inhibitor used as an antidepressant.

phe·net·a·mine (fĕ-net′ă-mēn). 2-(Cyclohexylbenzyl)$N,N,N′,N′$-tetraethyl-1,3-propanediamine; an intestinal antispasmodic. SYN phenacyclamine.

phen·e·thar·bi·tal (fen-ĕ-thar′bi-tahl). N-Phenylbarbital; 5,5-diethyl-1-phenylbarbituric acid; an obscure anticonvulsant agent.

phe·neth·i·cil·lin po·tas·si·um (fĕ-neth-i-sil′in). A penicillin preparation that is stable in gastric acid and is rapidly but only partially absorbed from the gastrointestinal tract. SYN α-phenoxyethylpenicillin potassium, penicillin B.

phen·eth·yl al·co·hol (fĕ-neth′il). SYN phenylethyl alcohol.

phe·net·sal (fĕ-net′sal). SYN acetaminosalol.

phe·net·u·ride (fĕ-net′yū-rīd). Phenylethylacetylurea; (2-phenylbutyryl)urea; an antiepileptic similar in action to phenacemide.

phen·for·min hy·dro·chlo·ride (fen-fōr′min). 1-Phenylbiguanide monohydrochloride; an oral hypoglycemic agent no longer used in the U.S. because of the high incidence of fatal lactic acidosis associated with its use.

phen·glu·tar·i·mide hy·dro·chlo·ride (fen-glū-tar′i-mīd). The hydrochloride of α-2-diethylaminoethyl-α-phenylglutarimide; an antihistaminic used to decrease or prevent motion sickness, and to control Ménière's disease and vomiting.

phen·go·pho·bia (fen-gō-fō′bē-ă). Morbid fear of daylight. [G. *phengos*, daylight, + *phobos*, fear]

phen·i·car·ba·zide (fen-i-kar′bă-zīd). 1-Phenylsemicarbazide; an antipyretic.

phe·nin·da·mine tar·trate (fĕ-nin′dă-mēn). 2-Methyl-9-phenyltetrahydro-1-pyridindene tartrate; an antihistaminic.

phen·in·di·one (fĕ-nin-dī′ōn). 2-Phenyl-1,3-indanedione: a synthetic anticoagulant with action and uses similar to those of bishydroxycoumarin. SYN phenylindanedione.

phen·ir·a·mine ma·le·ate (fĕ-nir′ă-mēn, -min). 1-phenyl-1-(2-pyridyl)-3-dimethylaminopropane maleate; an antihistaminic. SYN prophenpyridamine maleate.

phen·meth·y·lol (fen-meth′il-ol). SYN *benzyl* alcohol.

phen·met·ra·zine hy·dro·chlo·ride (fen-met′ră-zēn). 2-Phenyl-3-methyltetrahydro-1,4-oxazine hydrochloride; an anorexic agent with sympathomimetic properties.

⌂**pheno-.** SEE phen-.

phe·no·bar·bi·tal (fĕ-nō-bar′bi-tahl). $CO(NHCO)_2C(C_2H_5)(C_6H_5)$; a long-acting oral or parenteral sedative anticonvulsant and hypnotic; available as a soluble sodium salt; also used in therapeutic management of epilepsy and induction of hepatic microsomal enzymes. SYN phenylethylbarbituric acid, phenylethylmalonylurea.

phe·no·bu·ti·o·dil (fen′ō-byū-tī′ō-dil). 2-(2,4,6-Triiodophenoxy)butyric acid; a radiographic contrast medium for cholecystography.

phe·no·copy (fē′nō-kop′ē). 1. A set of clinical and laboratory characteristics that would ordinarily warrant the diagnosis of a specific genetic abnormality, but are of environmental rather than genetic etiology. 2. A condition of environmental etiology that mimics one usually of genetic etiology. [G. *phainō*, to display, + copy]

phe·no·din (fē′nō-din). SYN hematin.

phe·nol (fē′nol). C_6H_5OH; an antiseptic and disinfectant; locally escharotic in concentrated form and neurolytic in 3 to 4% solu-

tions; internally, a powerful escharotic poison. SYN carbolic acid, phenyl alcohol.

camphorated p., camphorated carbolic acid, consisting of p., camphor, and liquid petrolatum; used as a local anesthetic and for the relief of toothache.

liquefied p., liquefied carbolic acid, p. liquefied by the addition of 10% of water.

p. oxidase, SYN laccase.

phe·no·lase (fē′nō-lās). SYN laccase.

phe·no·lat·ed (fē′nō-lāt-ed). Impregnated or mixed with phenol. SYN carbolated.

phe·nol·e·mia (fē-nol-ē′mē-ă). The presence of phenols in the blood. [phenol + G. *haima*, blood]

phe·nol·o·gy (fe-nol′ō-jē). The study of the biological rhythms of plants and animals, particularly those rhythms showing seasonal variation. [G. *phainō*, to appear, + *logos*, study]

phe·nol·phthal·e·in (fē-nol-thal′ē-in, -thal′ēn). Obtained by the action of phenol on phthalic anhydride; used as a hydrogen ion indicator and as a laxative.

phe·nol red. SYN phenolsulfonphthalein.

phe·nol·sul·fon·phthal·e·in (PSP) (fē′nol-sŭl-fōn-thal′ē-in, -thal′ēn). Occurs as a bright to dark red crystalline powder; used as an indicator in tissue culture media (yellow at pH 6.8, red at pH 8.4); in the past given by parenteral injection as a test for renal function. SYN phenol red.

phe·nol·u·ria (fē-nol-yū′rē-ă). The excretion of phenols in the urine.

phe·nom·e·nol·o·gy (fē-nom-ĕ-nol′ō-jē). 1. The systematic description and classification of phenomena without attempt at explanation or interpretation. 2. The study of human experiences, irrespective of objective-subjective distinctions. SEE ALSO existential *psychology*. [phenomenon, + G. *logos*, study]

PHENOMENON

phe·nom·e·non, pl. **phe·nom·e·na** (fē-nom′ĕ-non, -nă). 1. A symptom; an occurrence of any sort, whether ordinary or extraordinary, in relation to a disease. 2. Any unusual fact or occurrence. [G. *phainomenon*, fr. *phainō*, to cause to appear]

adhesion p., a p. manifested by the adherence of antigen-antibody-complement complex to "indicator cells" (microorganisms, platelets, leukocytes, or erythrocytes), the reaction being sensitive and specific for the antigen and antibody in the complex. SYN erythrocyte adherence p., immune adherence p., red cell adherence p.

AFORMED p., as induced pulsus alternans progresses, a state in which alternating heart depolarizations fail to eject any blood, thus allowing longer diastolic filling; the subsequent beat is then able to produce a significant ejection; at high rates the cardiac minute volume and blood pressure may appear normal. [Alternating, *f*ailure *o*f *r*esponse, *m*echanical, to *e*lectrical *d*epolarization]

Anrep p., homeometric autoregulation of the heart whereby cardiac performance improves as the afterload (aortic pressure) is increased.

aqueous influx p., the filling of the aqueous vein, which normally carries blood and aqueous, with aqueous, when the junction of the aqueous vein and the recipient vein is partially occluded. SYN Ascher's aqueous influx p.

Arias-Stella p., focal, unusual, decidual changes in endometrial epithelium, consisting of intraluminal budding, and nuclear enlargement and hyperchromatism with cytoplasmic swelling and vacuolation; may be associated with ectopic or uterine pregnancy. SYN Arias-Stella effect, Arias-Stella reaction.

arm p., SYN Pool's p. (2).

Arthus p., a form of immediate hypersensitivity resulting in erythema, edema, hemorrhage, and necrosis observed in rabbits after injection of antigen to which the animal has already been sensitized and has specific IgG antibodies. The reaction is caused by the inflammation that results from the deposition of antigen-antibody complexes in tissue spaces and in blood vessel walls that activate complement, most of the damage seemingly being due to the polymorphonuclear leukocytes that phagocytize the deposits and release lysosomal enzymes. The p., described by Arthus, was in rabbits, but similar reactions (Arthus-type reactions) are observed in guinea pigs, rats, and dogs, as well as in humans. SEE ALSO Arthus *reaction* (2). SYN Arthus reaction (1).

Ascher's aqueous influx p., SYN aqueous influx p.

Aschner's p., SYN oculocardiac *reflex*.

Ashman's p., aberrant ventricular conduction of a beat ending a short cycle that is preceded by a longer cycle most commonly during atrial fibrillation.

Aubert's p., a p. in which a bright perpendicular line appears to incline to one side when the observer turns the head to the opposite side in a dark room.

Austin Flint p., the murmur of relative mitral stenosis during significant aortic regurgitation owing to narrowing of the mitral orifice by pressure of the aortic regurgitant flow on the anterior mitral leaflet. SYN Austin Flint murmur.

autoscopic p., the encountering of an image of oneself, the image being an illusion, a hallucination, or a vivid fantasy.

Babinski's p., SYN Babinski's *sign* (1).

Bell's p., a patient with peripheral facial paralysis cannot close the eyelids of the affected side without at the same time moving the eyeball upward and outward.

Bombay p., a rare recessive trait at a locus that ordinarily manufactures H substance, the precursor from which the A and B phenotypes are elaborated; the mutant causes failure to produce H substance and no matter what the genotype at the ABO locus, the phenotype is O. The Bombay p. is epistatic to the ABO locus. [*Bombay,* India, where first reported]

Bordet-Gengou p., the p. of complement fixation; when alexin (complement)-containing serum is added to a mixture of bacteria and specific antibody, the alexin is removed (fixed) and is not available to lyse subsequently added erythrocytes sensitized with specific antibody. SEE ALSO Gengou p.

breakoff p., breakaway p., the occurrence, during high-altitude flight, of a sensation of being totally detached from the earth and from other people.

Brücke-Bartley p., the sensation of glare in response to successive stimuli at frequencies just below the fusion point.

Capgras' p., SYN Capgras' *syndrome*.

cervicolumbar p., a sense of weakness in the lower extremities on movement of the neck when a lesion is present in the upper portion of the spinal cord; or sensations referred to the neck when a lesion exists in the lower portion of the cord.

cogwheel p., a sudden brief halt in usually smooth respiration or other motor activity. SYN Negro's p.

constancy p., in perception, the tendency for brightness, color, size, or shape to remain relatively perceptually constant despite real changes in color, size, shape or other conditions of observation.

crossed phrenic p., hemisection of the cord above the exit of the phrenic nerve paralyzes the ipsilateral half of the diaphragm; if the contralateral phrenic nerve is then sectioned or blocked, contractions on the ipsilateral side are resumed.

Cushing p., a rise in systemic blood pressure when the intracranial pressure acutely increases, usually in excess of 50% of the systolic arterial pressure. SYN Cushing effect, Cushing response.

Danysz p., reduction of the neutralizing effect of an antitoxin when toxin is mixed with it in divided portions, rather than adding the same total quantity of toxin in one step.

dawn p., abrupt increases in fasting levels of plasma glucose concentrations between 5 and 9 a.m., in the absence of antecedent hypoglycemia; occurs in diabetic patients receiving insulin therapy.

Debré p., in measles, the failure of the rash to develop at the site of immune serum injection.

declamping p., shock or hypotension following abrupt release of clamps from a large portion of the vascular bed, as from the aorta; apparently caused by transient pooling of blood in a previously ischemic area. SYN declamping shock.

déjà vu p., the mental impression that a new experience (*e.g.,* a scene, sight, sound, or action) has happened before; a common p. in normal persons that may occur more frequently or continuously in certain emotional or organic disorders. Also variously referred to as déjà entendu, déjà éprouvé, déjà fait, déjà pensé, déjà raconté, déjà vécu, or déjà voulu, depending on the experience or sense that is evoked.

Dejerine-Lichtheim p., SYN Lichtheim's *sign*.

Dejerine's hand p., clonic contractions of the flexors of the hand (wrist) on tapping the dorsum of the hand or the volar side of the forearm near the wrist; occurs in normal persons but is exaggerated in pyramidal tract lesions. SYN Dejerine's reflex.

Denys-Leclef p., enhanced phagocytosis by leukocytes of microorganisms in the presence of immune serum.

d'Herelle p., SYN Twort-d'Herelle p.

dip p., complete disappearance of ventricular excitability followed by progressive recovery within a few microseconds at the end of excitation; the muscle as a whole repolarizes somewhat inhomogeneously, so that this period is one of special sensitivity to exogenous or endogenous stimuli and reentry.

Donath-Landsteiner p., the hemolysis which results in a sample of blood of a subject of paroxysmal hemoglobinuria when the sample is cooled to around 5°C and then warmed again.

Doppler p., SYN Doppler *effect*.

Duckworth's p., respiratory arrest before cardiac arrest as a result of intracranial disease.

Ehret's p., a sudden throb felt by the finger on the brachial artery, as the pressure in the cuff falls during a blood pressure estimation; said to indicate fairly accurately the diastolic pressure.

Ehrlich's p., the difference between the amount of diphtheria toxin that will exactly neutralize one unit of antitoxin and that which, added to one unit of antitoxin, will leave one lethal dose free is greater than one lethal dose of toxin; *i.e.,* it is necessary to add more than one lethal dose of toxin to a neutral mixture of toxin and antitoxin to make the mixture lethal (the basis of the L_+ dose).

erythrocyte adherence p., SYN adhesion p.

escape p., failure of the pupil in an eye with optic neuritis to maintain constriction as both eyes are alternately stimulated with light.

facialis p., facial spasm produced by light rubbing of the skin or a tap on the zygoma; sometimes percussion above the zygoma causes contraction of the lip only; observed in tetany and sometimes in exophthalmic goiter.

finger p., a sign of organic hemiplegia; with the patient's elbow resting on a table, the patient's wrist is grasped by the examiner's hand, the thumb of which is used to exert pressure on the radial side of the patient's pisiform bone; if the hemiplegia is organic, some or all of the patient's fingers become extended and spread out in a fanlike form. SYN Gordon's sign.

Flynn p., SYN paradoxical pupillary *reflex*.

Friedreich's p., the tympanitic percussion sound over a pulmonary cavity is slightly raised in pitch on deep inspiration.

Galassi's pupillary p., SYN eye-closure pupil *reaction*.

Gallavardin's p., dissociation between the noisy and musical elements of the murmur of aortic stenosis, the musical element being better heard at the left sternal border and at the cardiac apex while the noisy element is better heard at the aortic area.

gap p., a short period in the cycle of the atrioventricular or intraventricular conduction allowing passage of an impulse which at other times would be blocked in transit. SYN excitable gap.

Gärtner's vein p., fullness of the veins of the arm and hand held below heart level and collapse at a certain variable distance above that level.

generalized Shwartzman p., when both the primary injection of endotoxin-containing filtrate and the secondary injection are given intravenously 24 hours apart, the animal usually dies within 24 hours after the second inoculation; the characteristic lesions in the rabbit include widespread hemorrhages in the lung, liver, and other organs and bilateral cortical necrosis of the kidney. This reaction has no immunological basis. SYN Sanarelli p., Sanarelli-Shwartzman p.

Gengou p., an extension of the Bordet-Gengou p.; noncellular antigens, when mixed with specific antibody, also fix alexin (complement).

gestalt p., SEE gestalt.

Glover p., nonrandom (*i.e.,* haphazard) variation among communities in rates of performing common elective procedures, such as tonsillectomy, hysterectomy, attributable to local variations in medical and surgical practices.

Goldblatt p., SYN Goldblatt *hypertension.*

Grasset-Gaussel p., SYN Grasset's p.

Grasset's p., in organic paralysis of the lower extremity, the patient, lying on his back, can raise either limb separately, but not both together. SYN Grasset-Gaussel p.

Gunn p., SYN jaw-winking *syndrome.*

Hamburger's p., SYN chloride *shift.*

Hill's p., SYN Hill's *sign.*

hip p., SYN Joffroy's *reflex.*

hip-flexion p., when a hemiplegic attempts to rise from a lying posture, the hip on the paralyzed side is flexed first; the same movement takes place on lying down.

Hoffmann's p., excessive irritability of the sensory nerves to electrical or mechanical stimuli in tetany.

Houssay p., SEE Houssay *animal.*

hunting p., SYN hunting *reaction.*

Hunt's paradoxical p., in dystonia musculorum deformans, if an attempt is made at plantar flexion of the foot when the foot is in dorsal spasm the only response is an increase of the extensor, or dorsal, spasm; if, however, the patient is told to extend the foot which is already in a state of strong dorsal flexion, there will be a sudden movement of plantar flexion; the same p., *mutatis mutandis,* is observed when there is a condition of strong plantar flexion.

immune adherence p., SYN adhesion p.

jaw-winking p., SYN jaw-winking *syndrome.*

Jod-Basedow p., induction of thyrotoxicosis in a previously euthyroid individual as a result of exposure to large quantities of iodine; occurs most often in areas of endemic iodine-deficient goiter and in patients with multinodular goiter; also can develop following use of iodine-containing agents for diagnostic studies. SYN iodine-induced hyperthyroidism.

knee p., SYN patellar *reflex.*

Köbner's p., an isomorphic reaction seen in response to trauma in previously uninvolved sites of patients with skin diseases including psoriasis and lichen planus, typically with lesions in a linear pattern at sites of scratching or a scar. SYN isomorphic response.

Koch's p., (1) the p. of infection immunity; living tubercle bacilli (*Mycobacterium tuberculosis*) do not cause reinfection when inoculated into tuberculous guinea pigs (*i.e.,* the animals are "immune" to reinfection) even though the original infections continue to develop and eventually cause death of the animals; (2) rise of temperature and increase of the local lesion, in a tuberculous subject, following an injection of tuberculin.

Kohnstamm's p., SYN aftermovement.

Kühne's p., when a constant current is passed through a muscle, an undulation is seen to pass from the positive to the negative pole.

LE p., the formation of LE cells in bone marrow or blood on adding serum from patients with disseminated lupus erythematosus.

Leede-Rumpel p., Rumpel-Leede p.

leg p., SYN Pool's p. (1).

Leichtenstern's p., SYN Leichtenstern's *sign.*

Lucio's leprosy p., SYN Lucio's *leprosy.*

Marcus Gunn p., SYN jaw-winking *syndrome.*

misdirection p., SYN aberrant *regeneration.*

Mitsuo's p., restoration of the normal color of the fundus with dark adaptation in Oguchi's disease.

Negro's p., SYN cogwheel p.

no reflow p., absence of blood flow in a portion of the brain which has been damaged, usually by ischemia.

on-off p., a state in the treatment of Parkinson's disease by *l*-dopa, in which there is a rapid fluctuation of akinetic (off) and choreoathetotic (on) movements.

orbicularis p., SYN eye-closure pupil *reaction.*

paradoxical diaphragm p., in pyopneumothorax, hydropneumothrax, and some cases of injury, the diaphragm on the affected side rises during inspiration and falls during expiration.

paradoxical pupillary p., SYN paradoxical pupillary *reflex.*

peroneal p., tapping the peroneal nerve below the head of the fibula causes dorsiflexion and abduction of the foot.

Pfeiffer's p., the alteration and complete disintegration of cholera vibrios when introduced into the peritoneal cavity of an immunized guinea pig, or into that of a normal one if immune serum is injected at the same time; extended to include bacteriolysis in general.

phi p., an illusion of movement, which occurs by means of successive visual impressions at intervals of $\frac{1}{15}$ to $\frac{1}{20}$ sec; when an occluder is passed from one eye to the other while a small distant light is observed, the light seems to move with the occluder in exophoria, but in an opposite direction in esophoria.

Pool's p., (1) in tetany, spasm both of the extensor muscles of the knee and of the calf muscles when the extended leg is flexed at the hip; SYN leg p., Pool-Schlesinger sign, Schlesinger's sign. (2) in tetany, contraction of the arm muscles following the stretching of the brachial plexus by elevation of the arm above the head with the forearm extended, resembles the contraction resulting from stimulation of the ulnar nerve. SYN arm p.

pseudo-Graefe's p., retraction of the upper eyelid on downward movement of the eyes.

psi p., a p. that includes both psychokinesis and extrasensory perception; the extrasensory mental processes involved in the alleged ability to send or receive telepathic messages.

Purkinje's p., in the light-adapted eye, the region of maximal brightness is in the yellow; in the dark-adapted eye, the region of maximal brightness is in the green. SYN Purkinje effect, Purkinje shift.

quellung p., SYN Neufeld capsular *swelling.*

radial p., dorsal flexion of the hand occurring involuntarily with palmar flexion of the fingers.

Raynaud's p., spasm of the digital arteries, with blanching and numbness or pain of the fingers, often precipitated by cold.

rebound p., (1) SYN Stewart-Holmes *sign.* (2) generally, any p. in which a variable that has been displaced from its normal state by a disturbing influence temporarily deviates from normal in the opposite direction when the disturbing influence is suddenly removed, before finally stabilizing at its normal state, *i.e.,* a p. involving undershoot; *e.g.,* the subsequent hypoglycemia that may follow injection of glucose, because the initial hyperglycemia caused excessive secretion of insulin.

reclotting p., SYN thixotropy.

red cell adherence p., SYN adhesion p.

reentry p., SEE reentry.

release p., the increased tonus and hyperirritability of muscle-stretch reflexes which occur following damage of the upper portions of the extrapyramidal system.

Ritter-Rollet p., on equal electrical stimulation of motor nerve trunks, the flexor and abductor muscle groups react more readily than the extensors and adductors.

R-on-T p., a premature ventricular (QRS) complex in the electrocardiogram interrupting the T wave of the preceding beat; often predisposes to serious ventricular arrhythmias.

Rumpel-Leede p., appearance of petechiae in an area following application of vascular constriction, such as by a tourniquet, usually after 10 minutes but can appear after shorter period, such as following application of tourniquet to draw blood specimen or use of blood pressure cuff. Due to capillary fragility or abnormal platelet numbers (e.g. thrombocytopenia) or function.

Rust's p., in cancer or caries of the upper cervical vertebrae, the patient will always support the head by the hands when changing from the recumbent to the sitting posture or the reverse.

Sanarelli p., SYN generalized Shwartzman p.

Sanarelli-Shwartzman p., SYN generalized Shwartzman p.

Schellong-Strisower p., a reduction of the systolic blood pressure, accompanied sometimes by vertigo, on rising from the horizontal to the erect posture.

Schiff-Sherrington p., when the spinal cord is transected in the midthoracic region or a little lower, the stretch and other postural reflexes of the upper extremity become exaggerated; if the transection is made in the sacral cord, a similar effect is observed in the lower limbs. The effect is regarded as a release p., *i.e.,* release from an inhibitory influence normally exerted by the spinal segments below the transection.

Schüller's p., in cases of functional hemiplegia the patient usually turns to the sound side in walking, but to the affected side in case of an organic lesion.

Schultz-Charlton p., SYN Schultz-Charlton *reaction.*

Sherrington p., after the muscles of the leg have been deprived of their motor innervation by sectioning the ventral roots containing fibers for the sciatic nerve, and allowing time for the degeneration of the fibers to occur, stimulation of the sciatic nerve causes slow contraction of the muscles.

shot-silk p., SYN shot-silk *retina.*

Shwartzman p., a rabbit is injected intradermally with a small quantity of lipopolysaccharide (endotoxin) followed by a second intravenous injection 24 hours later and will develop a hemorrhagic and necrotic lesion at the site of the first injection. SEE ALSO generalized Shwartzman p. SYN Shwartzman reaction.

Somogyi p., a rebound p. of reactive hyperglycemia following a period of relative hypoglycemia, which may be subclinical and difficult to detect; the hyperglycemia induces use of more insulin, thus aggravating the problem. SYN posthypoglycemic hyperglycemia.

Soret's p., in a solution kept in a long, upright tube at room temperature, the upper part, being the warmer, is also the more concentrated.

sparing p., SYN sparing *action.*

Splendore-Hoeppli p., radiating or annular eosinophilic deposits of host-derived materials, and possibly of parasite antigens, which form around fungi, helminths, or bacterial colonies in tissue.

staircase p., SYN treppe.

Staub-Traugott p., the increased rate of removal of loads of glucose given shortly after administration of an initial glucose load.

steal p., SEE steal.

Strassman's p., in the third stage of labor, failure of placental detachment indicated by transmission of pressure from the fundus uteri to the umbilical vein which becomes engorged; obsolete term.

Strümpell's p., dorsal flexion of the great toe, sometimes of the entire foot, in a paralyzed limb when the extremity is drawn up against the body, flexing both knee and hip. SYN tibial p.

symbiotic fermentation p., "two organisms, neither of which alone produces gas fermentation in certain carbohydrates, may do so when living in symbiosis or when artificially mixed" (Castellani).

Theobald Smith's p., a p. observed in guinea pigs that had survived use for diphtheria antitoxin standardization, the animals having been rendered highly susceptible to subsequent inoculation of horse serum.

tibial p., SYN Strümpell's p.

toe p., SYN Babinski's *sign* (1).

tongue p., SYN Schultze's *sign.*

Tournay's p., dilation of the pupil in the abducting eye on extreme lateral gaze. This is present in only a small percentage of the normal popupation and has no known association with disease. SYN Tournay sign.

Tullio's p., momentary vertigo caused by any loud noise, notably occurring in cases of active labyrinthine fistula.

Twort p., SYN Twort-d'Herelle p.

Twort-d'Herelle p., the lysis of bacteria by bacteriophage. SYN bacteriophagia, d'Herelle p., Twort p.

Tyndall p., the visibility of floating particles in gases or liquids when illuminated by a ray of sunlight and viewed at right angles to the illuminating ray. SYN Tyndall effect.

vacuum disk p., the appearance of a radiolucent stripe in an intervertebral disk, a manifestation of disk degeneration; a misnomer since there is gas present.

Wenckebach p., progressive lengthening of conduction time in any cardiac tissue (most often the A-V node or junction) with ultimate dropping of a beat (A-V Wenckebach) or reversion to the initial conduction time (as in QRS Wenckebach).

Westphal-Piltz p., SYN eye-closure pupil *reaction.*

Westphal's p., SYN Erb-Westphal *sign.*

Wever-Bray p., the action potentials in the acoustic nerve that correspond to auditory stimuli reaching the cochlea.

ph

phe·no·per·i·dine (fen-ō-per'i-dēn). 1-(3-Hydroxy-3-phenylpropyl)-4-phenylisonipecotic acid ethyl ester; an analgesic.

phe·no·thi·a·zine (fē-nō-thī'ă-zēn). A compound formerly used extensively for the treatment of intestinal nematodes in animals; without central nervous system depressant activity itself, it serves as the parent compound for synthesis of a large number of antipsychotic compounds, including chlorpromazine, thioridazine, perphenazine, and fluphenazine. SYN dibenzothiazine, thiodiphenylamine.

phe·no·type (fē'nō-tīp). Manifestation of a genotype or the combined manifestation of several different genotypes. The discriminating power of the p. in identifying the genotype depends on its level of subtlety; thus special methods of detecting carrier distinguish them from normal subjects from whom they are inseparable on simple physical examination. P. is the immediate cause of genetic disease and object of genetic selection. [G. *phainō,* to display, + *typos,* model]

phe·no·typ·ic (fē'nō-tip'ik, fen-ō-). Relating to phenotype.

phen·ox·a·zine (fe-nok'să-zēn). Phenothiazine in which S is replaced by O; as the 3-oxo derivative (phenoxazone), p. is the chromophore of actinomycins.

phen·ox·a·zone (fe-nok'să-zōn). SEE phenoxazine.

phe·nox·y·ben·za·mine hy·dro·chlo·ride (fĕ-nok'si-ben'ză-mēn). (2-Chloroethyl)-*N*-(1-methyl-2-phenoxyethyl benzylamine hydrochloride; a potent adrenergic (α-receptor) blocking agent of the β-haloalkylamines; selectively blocks the excitatory response of smooth muscle and exocrine glands to epinephrine; used in the treatment of peripheral vascular diseases.

2-phe·nox·y·eth·a·nol (fĕ-nok-si-eth'ă-nol). 1-Hydroxy-2-phenoxyethane; an antibacterial agent used in the topical treatment of wound infections; it is active against Gram-negative bacteria that are resistant to most other antiseptics.

α-phe·nox·y·eth·yl·pen·i·cil·lin po·tas·si·um (fē-nok'sē-eth'il-pen-i-sil'in). SYN phenethicillin potassium.

phe·nox·y·meth·yl·pen·i·cil·lin (fĕ-nok'si-meth'il-pen-i-sil'in). SYN *penicillin* V.

α-phe·nox·y·pro·pyl·pen·i·cil·lin po·tas·si·um (fē'nok-sē-prō'pil-pen-i-sil'in). SYN propicillin.

phe·no·zy·gous (fē'nō-zī'gŭs, fe-noz'i-gŭs). Having a narrow cranium as compared with the width of the face, so that when the skull is viewed from above, the zygomatic arches are visible. [G. *phainō,* to show, + *zygon,* yoke]

phen·pen·ter·mine tar·trate (fen-pen'ter-mēn). α,α,β-Trimethylphenethylamine; an anorexigenic agent.

phen·pro·ba·mate (fen-prō'bă-māt). 3-phenylpropyl carbamate; a skeletal muscle relaxant with antianxiety action. SYN proformiphen.

phen·pro·cou·mon (fen-prō-kū'mon). 3-(1'-Phenylpropyl)-4-hydroxycoumarin; a long-acting orally effective anticoagulant.

phen·pro·pi·o·nate (fen-prō'pē-ō-nāt). USAN-approved contraction for 3-phenylpropionate.

phen·sux·i·mide (fen-sŭk'si-mīd). *N*-Methyl-2-phenylsuccinimide; an anticonvulsant drug used in the treatment of petit mal epilepsy.

phen·ter·mine (fen'ter-mēn). α,α-Dimethylphenethylamine; an anorexic agent; also available as the hydrochloride.

phen·tol·a·mine hy·dro·chlo·ride (fen-tol′ă-mēn). 2-(N ′-p-Tolyl-N ′-m-hydroxyphenylaminomethyl)-imidazoline hydrochloride; an adrenergic (α-receptor) blocking agent.

phen·tol·a·mine mes·y·late. Phentolamine methanesulfonate; the same actions as phentolamine hydrochloride, for intravenous use only.

phen·yl (Ph, Φ) (fen′il). The univalent radical, C_6H_5-, of benzene.

p. alcohol, SYN phenol.

p. aminosalicylate, p-aminosalicylic acid phenyl ester; an antituberculous drug.

p. salicylate, the salicylic ester of phenol; the phenylic ester of salicylic acid; an intestinal analgesic and antipyretic; it has been used in the treatment of rheumatism, diarrhea, and pharyngitis, as an enteric coating for tablets, and in ointments for sunburn prevention. SYN salol.

phen·yl·a·ce·tic ac·id (fen′il-ă-sē′tik). $C_6H_5CH_2COOH$; an abnormal product of phenylalanine catabolism, appearing in the urine in individuals with phenylketonuria.

phen·yl·a·ce·tur·ic ac·id (fen′il-as-ě-tūr′ik). SYN phenaceturic acid.

phen·yl·a·ce·tyl·u·rea (fen-il-as′ě-til-yū-rē′ă). SYN phenacemide.

phen·yl·a·cryl·ic ac·id (fen′il-ă-kril′ik). SYN cinnamic acid.

phen·yl·al·a·nin·ase (fen-il-al′ă-nin-ās). Phenylalanine 4- monooxygenase.

phen·yl·al·a·nine (Phe, F) (fen-il-al′ă-nēn). $C_6H_5CH_2CH(NH_3)^+COO^-$; 2-Amino-3-phenylpropionic acid; the L-isomer is one of the common amino acids in proteins; a nutritionally essential amino acid.

p. ammonia-lyase, a nonmammalian enzyme that catalyzes the conversion of L-p. to trans-cinnamate and ammonia; it has been used in the treatment of phenylketonuria.

p. 4-hydroxylase, SYN p. 4-monooxygenase.

p. 4-monooxygenase, an enzyme that catalyzes the oxidation of L-phenylalanine to L-tyrosine with O_2 and tetrahydrobiopterin (the latter forming the dihydro derivative) which is reduced by NADPH and a reductase to the active form; a deficiency of either of these enzymes will result in phenylketonuria. SYN p. 4-hydroxylase.

phen·yl·a·mine (fe-nil′ă-mēn). SYN aniline.

phen·yl·ben·zene (fen-il-ben′zēn). SYN diphenyl.

phen·yl·bu·ta·zone (fen-il-byū′tă-zōn). 1,2-Diphenyl-4-butyl-3,5-pyrazolidinedione; a pyrazolone derivative; an analgesic, antipyretic, anti-inflammatory, and uricosuric agent.

phen·yl·car·bi·nol (fen-il-kar′bi-nol). SYN benzyl alcohol.

phen·yl·di·chlo·ro·ar·sine (PD) (fen′il-dī-klōr-ō-ar′sēn;). $C_6H_5A_5Cl_2$; A toxic liquid that has been used as a blister and vomiting agent by certain military and police organizations; it was first used in a limited manner in World War I.

phen·yl·eph·rine hy·dro·chlo·ride (fen-il-ef′rin). (-)-m-Hydroxy-α-[(methylamino)methyl]benzyl alcohol hydrochloride; a sympathomimetic amine; a powerful vasoconstrictor, used as a nasal decongestant and mydriatic.

phen·yl·eth·a·no·la·mine N-meth·yl·trans·fer·ase (fē-nil-eth-an-ol-a-mēn). A key enzyme in catecholamine biosynthesis that catalyzes the conversion of norepinephrine to epinephrine, using S-adenosyl-L-methionine; this enzyme's biosynthesis is induced by cortisol.

phen·yl·eth·yl al·co·hol (fen-il-eth′il). $C_6H_5CH_2CH_2OH$; 2-phenylethanol; a natural constituent of some volatile oils (rose, geranium, neroli); used as an antibacterial agent in ophthalmic solutions. SYN benzyl carbinol, phenethyl alcohol.

phen·yl·eth·yl·bar·bi·tur·ic ac·id (fen′il-eth′il-bar-bi-tyūr′ik). SYN phenobarbital.

phen·yl·eth·yl·ma·lo·na·mide (fen-il-eth′il-mal-on-ă-mīd). A metabolite of primidone, an antiepileptic agent. P. has anticonvulsant activity in animals but has not been evaluated as an antiepileptic agent in humans.

phen·yl·eth·yl·mal·o·nyl·u·rea (fen′il-eth′il-mal′ō-nil-yū-rē′ă). SYN phenobarbital.

phen·yl·gly·col·ic ac·id (fen′il-glī-kol′ik). SYN mandelic acid.

phen·yl·in·dane·di·one (fen′il-in-dān′dī-ōn). SYN phenindione.

phen·yl·i·so·thi·o·cy·a·nate (PITC, PhNCS) (fen′il-ī′sō-thī-ō-sī′ă-nāt). $C_6H_5-N=C=S$, a reagent that condenses with the free N-terminal amino group of a peptide chain to form a phenylthiohydantoin in the Edman method of identifying N-terminal amino acids. SYN Edman's reagent.

phen·yl·ke·to·nu·ria (PKU) (fen′il-kē′tō-nū′rē-ă). Congenital deficiency of phenylalanine 4-monooxygenase [MIM*261600] or occasionally of dihydropherine reductase [MIM*261630] or of dihydrobiopterin synthetase [MIM*261640]; it causes inadequate formation of L-tyrosine, elevation of serum L-phenylalanine, urinary excretion of phenylpyruvic acid and other derivatives, and accumulation of phenylalanine and its metabolites, which can produce brain damage resulting in severe mental retardation, often with seizures, other neurologic abnormalities such as retarded myelination, and deficient melanin formation leading to hypopigmentation of the skin and eczema. There are several kinds, all with autosomal recessive inheritance. Another more remote form is deficiency of guanidine triphosphate cyclohydrolase 1 [MIM*233910]. Cf. hyperphenylalaninemia. SYN Folling's disease, phenylpyruvate oligophrenia. [phenyl + ketone + G. ouron, urine]

nonclassical p., SYN malignant hyperphenylalaninemia.

phen·yl·lac·tic ac·id (fen-il-lak′tik). $C_6H_5CH_2CHOH=COOH$; a product of phenylalanine catabolism, appearing prominently in the urine in individuals with phenylketonuria.

phen·yl·mer·cu·ric ac·e·tate (fen′il-mer-kyū′rik). Acetoxyphenylmercury; a bacteriostatic preservative, fungicide, and herbicide (especially for crabgrass).

phen·yl·mer·cu·ric ni·trate. Basic phenylmercuric nitrate; a mixture of phenylmercuric nitrate and phenylmercuric hydroxide; an antiseptic used for the prophylactic disinfection of the intact skin or of minor wounds.

phen·yl·pro·pa·nol·a·mine (fen′il-prō-pă-nol′ă-mēn). α-(1-Aminoethyl)-benzyl alcohol; a sympathomimetic amine, used as a nasal decongestant and bronchodilator.

phe·nyl·py·ru·vic ac·id (fen′il-pī-rū′vik). $C_6H_5-CH_2COCOOH$; the transaminated product of the action of phenylalanine aminotransferase; elevated in the urine in individuals with phenylketonuria.

phen·yl·thi·o·car·ba·mide (fen′il-thī-ō-kar′bă-mīd). SYN phenylthiourea.

phen·yl·thi·o·car·bam·o·yl (PTC). SEE phenylthiocarbamoyl peptide.

phen·yl·thi·o·hy·dan·to·in (PTH) (fen′il-thī′ō-hī-dan′tō-in). The compound formed from an amino acid in the Edman method of protein degradation, in which phenylisothiocyanate reacts with the amino moiety of the N-terminal amino acid to form a phenylthiocarbamoyl peptide or protein, on which weak acids act to release the p. containing the N-terminal amino acid.

phen·yl·thi·o·u·rea (fen′il-thī′ō-yū-rē′ă) [MIM*171200]. A substance that tastes bitter to some persons but is tasteless to others. The ability to taste it is unilocal and dominant. P. contains the N–C=S group upon which the taste peculiarity apparently depends, for goitrogenic or antithyroid substances (e.g., thiourea and thiouracil), which also contain this group, possess the same property with respect to taste. SYN phenylthiocarbamide.

phen·yl·to·lox·a·mine (fen′il-tol-ok′să-mēn). N,N-dimethyl-2-(α-phenyl-o-tolyloxy)-ethylamine; an antihistaminic.

phen·yl·tri·meth·yl·am·mo·ni·um (PTMA) (fen′il-trī-meth′il-ă-mō′nē-ŭm). A highly selective stimulant of the motor end-plates of skeletal muscle.

phen·y·ram·i·dol hy·dro·chlo·ride (fen-i-ram′i-dol). α-(2-Pyridylaminomethyl)benzyl alcohol hydrochloride; an analgesic and a muscle relaxant.

phen·yt·o·in (fen′i-tō-in). An anticonvulsant used in the treatment of generalized tonic clonic and complex partial epilepsy. Also available as p. sodium, with the same uses as p. SYN 5,5-diphenylhydantoin.

△**pheo-. 1.** Prefix denoting the same substituents on a phorbin or phorbide (porphyrin) residue as are present in chlorophyll, excluding any ester residues and Mg. **2.** Combining form meaning gray, dark-colored. [G. *phaios*, dusky]

phe·o·chrome (fē'ō-krōm). **1.** SYN chromaffin. **2.** Staining darkly with chromic salts. [G. *phaios*, dusky, + *chrōma*, color]

phe·o·chro·mo·blast (fē-ō-krō'mō-blast). A primitive chromaffin cell which, with sympathetoblasts, enters into the formation of the adrenal gland. [G. *phaios*, dusky, + *chrōma*, color, + *blastos*, germ]

phe·o·chro·mo·blas·to·ma (fē'ō-krō'mō-blas-tō'mă). Obsolete term for pheochromocytoma.

phe·o·chro·mo·cyte (fē-ō-krō'mō-sīt). A chromaffin cell of a sympathetic paraganglion, medulla of an adrenal gland, or of a pheochromocytoma. SYN pheochrome cell (2). [pheochrome + G. *kytos*, cell]

phe·o·chro·mo·cy·to·ma (fē'ō-krō'mō-sī-tō'mă). A functional chromaffinoma, usually benign, derived from adrenal medullary tissue cells and characterized by the secretion of catecholamines, resulting in hypertension, which may be paroxysmal and associated with attacks of palpitation, headache, nausea, dyspnea, anxiety, pallor, and profuse sweating. P. is often hereditary, not only in phacomas such as Hippel-Lindau disease, neurofibromatosis, and familial endocrine neoplasia, but also as an isolated defect in its own right [MIM*171300] as an autosomal dominant trait. SEE ALSO paraganglioma.

phe·o·mel·a·nin (fē-ō-mel'ă-nin). A type of melanin found in red hair; it contains sulfur and is alkali-soluble; elevated levels are found in the rufous type of oculocutaneous albinism. Cf. eumelanin. [G. *phaios*, dusky, + *melos* (*melan-*), black]

phe·o·mel·a·no·gen·e·sis (fē'ō-mel'ă-nō-jen'ĕ-sis). The formation of pheomelanin by living cells.

phe·o·mel·a·no·some (fē-ō-mel'ă-nō-sōm). A spherical melanosome of pheomelanin in red hair.

phe·re·sis (fe-rē'sis). A procedure in which blood is removed from a donor, separated, and a portion retained, with the remainder returned to the donor. SEE ALSO leukapheresis, plateletpheresis, plasmapheresis. [G. *aphairesis*, a withdrawal]

pher·o·mones (fer'ō-mōnz). A type of ectohormone secreted by an individual and perceived by a second individual of the same species, thereby producing a change in the sexual or social behavior of that individual. Cf. allelochemicals, allomones, kairomones. [G. *pherō*, to carry, + *hormaō*, to excite, stimulate]

Ph.G. 1. Abbreviation for *Pharmacopoeia Germanica;* German Pharmacopoeia. **2.** Abbreviation for Graduate in Pharmacy, a degree no longer offered in the U.S.

phi (φ, Φ) (fī). **1.** The 21st letter of the Greek alphabet. **2.** (Φ) Symbol for phenyl; potential energy; magnetic flux. **3.** (φ) Symbol for plane angle; volume fraction; quantum yield; the dihedral angle of rotation about the N–C$_\alpha$ bond associated with a peptide bond.

phi·al (fī'ăl). SYN vial. [G. *phialē*, a broad flat vessel]

phi·a·lide (fī'ă-līd). In fungi, a conidiogenous cell in which the meristematic end remains unchanged as successive conidia are extruded out to form chains. [G. *phialē*, a broad, flat vessel]

phi·a·lo·co·nid·i·um, pl. **phi·a·lo·co·nid·ia** (fī'ă-lō-ko-nid'ē-ŭm, fī'ă-lō-kō-nid'ē-ă). A conidium produced by a phialide.

Phi·a·loph·o·ra (fī-ă-lof'ō-ră). A genus of fungi of which at least two species, *P. verrucosa* and *P. dermatitidis*, cause chromoblastomycosis. [G. *phialē*, a broad, flat vessel, + *phoreō*, to carry]

△**-phil, -phile, -philic, -philia.** Affinity for, craving for. SEE ALSO philo-. [G. *philos*, fond, loving; *phileō*, to love]

phil·i·a·ter (fil'ē-ā'ter, fi-lī'ă-ter). Rarely used term for one interested in the study of medicine. [G. *philos*, fond, + *iatreia*, practice of medicine]

Philip, Sir Robert W., Scottish physician, 1857–1939. SEE P.'s *glands*, under *gland*.

Philippe, Claudien, French pathologist, 1866–1903. SEE P.'s *triangle*.

Phillips, Charles, French urologist, 1809–1871. SEE P.'s *catheter*.

Phillipson's re·flex. See under reflex.

△**philo-.** SEE -phil. [G. *philos*, fond, loving; *phileō*, to love]

phi·lo·mi·me·sia (fil'ō-mĭ-mē'sē-ă). Rarely used term for a morbid impulse to imitate or mimic. [philo- + G. *mimēsis*, imitation]

Phil·o·pia ca·sei (fil-ō'pē-ă kā'sē-ī). A species that may cause temporary intestinal myiasis. SYN cheese maggot.

phil·o·pro·gen·i·tive (fil'ō-prō-jen'i-tiv). **1.** Procreative, producing offspring. **2.** In psychiatry, manifesting an erotic or abnormal love for children. [philo- + L. *progenies*, offspring, progeny]

phil·trum, pl. **phil·tra** (fil'trŭm, -tră). **1.** A philter or love potion. **2** [NA]. The infranasal depression; the groove in the midline of the upper lip. [L., fr. G. *philtron*, a love-charm, depression on upper lip, fr. *phileō*, to love]

phi·mo·sis, pl. **phi·mo·ses** (fī-mō'sis, -sēz). Narrowness of the opening of the prepuce, preventing its being drawn back over the glans. [G. a muzzling, fr. *phimos*, a muzzle]

  p. clitor'idis, agglutination of the clitoral folds.

  p. vagina'lis, narrowness of the vagina.

phi·mot·ic (fī-mot'ik). Pertaining to phimosis.

△**phleb-.** SEE phlebo-.

phle·bal·gia (flĕ-bal'jē-ă). Pain originating in a vein. [phlebo- + G. *algos*, pain]

phleb·ec·ta·sia (fleb-ek-tā'zē-ă). Vasodilation of the veins. SYN venectasia. [phlebo- + G. *ektasis*, a stretching]

phle·bec·to·my (fle-bek'tō-mē). Excision of a segment of a vein, performed sometimes for the cure of varicose veins. SEE ALSO strip (2). SYN venectomy. [phlebo- + G. *ektomē*, excision]

phleb·eu·rysm (fleb'yū-rizm). Pathologic dilation (varix) of a vein. [phlebo- + G. *eurys*, wide]

phle·bit·ic (fle-bit'ik). Relating to phlebitis.

phle·bi·tis (fle-bī'tis). Inflammation of a vein. [phlebo- + G. -*itis*, inflammation]

  adhesive p., a form of p. in which the walls adhere, leading to obliteration of the vessel.

  p. nodula'ris necroti'sans, obsolete term for p. in which tuberculous nodules are formed in the skin; the lesions spread peripherally and undergo central necrosis.

  puerperal p., SYN *phlegmasia* alba dolens.

  septic p., inflammation of a vein due to bacterial infection.

  sinus p., inflammation of a cerebral sinus.

△**phlebo-, phleb-.** Vein [G. *phleps*]

phleb·o·cly·sis (flĕ-bok'li-sis). Intravenous injection of an isotonic solution of dextrose or other substances in quantity. SYN venoclysis. [phlebo- + G. *klysis*, a washing out]

  drip p., intravenous injection of a liquid drop by drop, by the drip method.

phleb·o·dy·nam·ics (fleb'ō-dī-nam'iks). Laws and principles governing blood pressures and flow within the venous circulation. [phlebo- + G. *dynamis*, force]

phleb·o·gram (fleb'ō-gram). A tracing of the jugular or other venous pulse. SYN venogram (2). [phlebo- + G. *gramma*, something written]

phleb·o·graph (fleb'ō-graf). A venous sphygmograph; an instrument for making a tracing of the venous pulse. [phlebo- + G. *graphō*, to write]

△ **ph**

phle·bog·ra·phy (fle-bog′ră-fē). **1.** The recording of the venous pulse. **2.** SYN venography. [phlebo- + G. *graphē*, a writing]

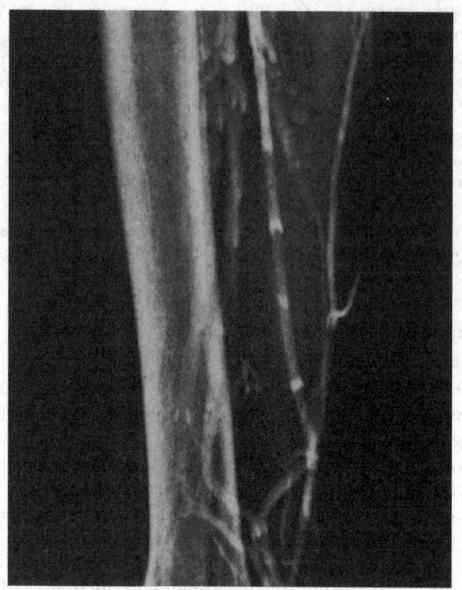

phlebography
side view (partial) of left tibia; venous valves are clearly visible

phleb·oid (fleb′oyd). **1.** Resembling a vein. **2.** SYN venous. **3.** Containing many veins. [phlebo- + G. *eidos*, resemblance]

phleb·o·lite (fleb′ō-līt). SYN phlebolith.

phleb·o·lith (fleb′ō-lith). A calcific deposit in a venous wall or thrombus; commonly seen on abdominal radiographs in the lower pelvic region. SYN phlebolite, vein stone. [phlebo- + G. *lithos*, stone]

phleb·o·li·thi·a·sis (fleb′ō-li-thī′ă-sis). The formation of phleboliths.

phle·bol·o·gy (flĕ-bol′ō-jē). The branch of medical science concerned with the anatomy and diseases of the veins. [phlebo- + G. *logos*, study]

phle·bo·ma·nom·e·ter (fleb′ō-mă-nom′ĕ-ter). A manometer for measuring venous blood pressure.

phleb·o·me·tri·tis (fleb′ō-mē-trī′tis). Inflammation of the uterine veins. [phlebo- + G. *mētra*, uterus, + *-itis*, inflammation]

phleb·o·my·o·ma·to·sis (fleb′ō-mī-ō-mă-tō′sis). Thickening of the walls of a vein by an overgrowth of muscular fibers arranged irregularly, intersecting each other without any definite relation to the axis of the vessel. [phlebo- + myoma + G. *-osis*, condition]

phleb·o·phle·bos·to·my (fleb′ō-fle-bos′tō-mē). SYN venovenostomy.

phleb·o·plas·ty (fleb′ō-plas-tē). Repair of a vein. [phlebo- + G. *plastos*, formed]

phleb·or·rha·gia (fleb-ō-rā′jē-ă). Obsolete term for venous hemorrhage. [phlebo- + G. *rhēgnymi*, to burst forth]

phle·bor·rha·phy (fle-bōr′ă-fē). Suture of a vein. [phlebo- + G. *rhaphē*, seam]

phleb·or·rhex·is (fleb-ō-rek′sis). Obsolete term for rupture of a vein. [phlebo- + G. *rhēxis*, rupture]

phleb·o·scle·ro·sis (fleb′ō-skle-rō′sis). Fibrous hardening of the walls of the veins. SYN venofibrosis, venosclerosis. [phlebo- + G. *sklērōsis*, hardening]

phle·bos·ta·sis (fle-bos′tă-sis). **1.** Abnormally slow motion of blood in veins, usually with venous distention. **2.** Treatment of congestive heart failure by compressing proximal veins of the extremities with tourniquets. SYN bloodless phlebotomy. SYN venostasis. [phlebo- + G. *stasis*, a standing still]

phleb·o·ste·no·sis (fleb′ō-stĕ-nō′sis). Narrowing of the lumen of a vein from any cause. [phlebo- + G. *stenōsis*, a narrowing]

phleb·o·strep·sis (fle-ō-strep′sis). Obsolete term for twisting the cut or torn end of a vein to arrest hemorrhage. [phlebo- + G. *strepsis*, a twisting]

phleb·o·throm·bo·sis (fleb′ō-throm-bō′sis). Thrombosis, or clotting, in a vein without primary inflammation. [phlebo- + thrombosis]

phle·bot·o·mine (flĕ-bot′ō-mēn). Relating to sand flies of the genus *Phlebotomus*.

phle·bot·o·mist (fle-bot′ō-mist). An individual trained and skilled in phlebotomy.

Phle·bot·o·mus (fle-bot′ō-mŭs). A genus of very small blood-sucking sandflies of the subfamily Phlebotominae, family Psychodidae. [phlebo- + G. *tomos*, cutting]

P. argen′tipes, the vector of kala azar in India.

P. chinen′sis, the vector of kala azar in China.

P. flaviscutel′latus, SYN *Lutzomyia flaviscutellata*.

P. longipal′pis, a vector of kala azar in South America. SYN *Lutzomyia longipalpis*.

P. ma′jor, a vector of kala azar in the Mediterranean region.

P. nogu′chi, the transmitter of *Bartonella* organisms, the causal agent of Oroya fever.

P. orienta′lis, a vector of kala azar in the Sudan.

P. papata′sii, transmitter of the virus of phlebotomus fever; also a vector of *Leishmania tropica* in the Mediterranean area.

P. pernicio′sus, a vector of kala azar in the Mediterranean region.

P. sergen′ti, a vector of *Leishmania tropica*, the cause of anthroponotic cutaneous leishmaniasis.

P. verruca′rum, a form found in Peru that transmits *Bartonella* organisms, the causal agent of Oroya fever.

phle·bot·o·my (fle-bot′ō-mē). Incision into a vein for the purpose of drawing blood. SYN venesection, venotomy. [phlebo- + G. *tomē*, incision]

bloodless p., SYN phlebostasis (2).

Phleb·o·vi·rus (fleb′ō-vī-rŭs). A genus of virus (family Bunyaviridae) that contains over 30 viruses which constitute a single serological group; transmitted by arthropods primarily of the genus *Phlebotomus*.

phlegm (flem). **1.** Abnormal amounts of mucus, especially as expectorated from the mouth. **2.** One of the four humors of the body, according to the ancient Greek humoral *doctrine*. [G. *phlegma*, inflammation]

phleg·ma·sia (fleg-mā′zē-ă). Obsolete term for inflammation, especially when acute and severe. [G. fr. *phlegma*, inflammation]

p. al′ba do′lens, an extreme edematous swelling of the leg following childbirth, due to thrombosis of the iliofemoral veins. SYN leukophlegmasia dolens, milk leg, puerperal phlebitis, thrombotic p., white leg.

cellulitic p., inflammatory swelling of the leg, following childbirth, due to septic inflammation of the connective tissue. SYN p. dolens.

p. ceru′lea do′lens, thrombosis of the veins of a limb, with sudden severe pain with swelling, cyanosis, and edema of the part, followed by circulatory collapse and shock.

p. do′lens, SYN cellulitic p.

p. malabar′ica, SYN elephantiasis.

thrombotic p., SYN p. alba dolens.

phleg·mat·ic (fleg-mat′ik). Relating to the heavy one of the four ancient Greek humors (see phlegm), and therefore calm, apathetic, unexcitable. [G. *phlegmatikos*, relating to phlegm]

phleg·mon (fleg′mon). Obsolete term for an acute suppurative inflammation of the subcutaneous connective tissue. [G. *phlegmonē*, inflammation]

diffuse p., a diffuse inflammation of the subcutaneous tissues accompanied by constitutional symptoms of sepsis.

emphysematous p., SYN gas *gangrene*.

gas p., SYN gas *gangrene*.

phleg·mon·ous (fleg′mon-ŭs). Denoting phlegmon.

phlo·gis·ton (flō-jis′ton). A hypothetical substance of negative mass that, according to the theory of Stahl was given off by a substance when it underwent combustion, thus accounting for the decrease in mass of the ash over the original substance; abandoned after the discoveries of Priestley and Lavoisier concerning oxygen. [G. *phlogistos,* inflammable]

phlo·go·cyte (flō′gō-sīt). Obsolete term for one of a number of cells present in the tissues during the course of an inflammation. [G. *phlogōsis,* inflammation, + *kytos,* a hollow (cell)]

phlo·go·cy·to·sis (flō′gō-sī-tō′sis). Obsolete term for a blood state in which there are many phlogocytes in the peripheral circulation.

phlo·go·gen·ic, phlo·gog·e·nous (flō-gō-jen′ik, flō-goj′ĕ-nŭs). Obsolete term for exciting inflammation. [G. *phlox* (*phlog*-), flame, + *-gen,* producing]

phlo·go·sin (flō′gō-sin). A substance, isolated from cultures of pus-producing cocci, injections of sterilized solutions of which will excite suppuration. [G. *phlogōsis,* inflammation]

phlo·go·ther·a·py (flō′gō-thār′ă-pē). SYN nonspecific *therapy.* [G. *phlogōsis,* inflammation, + therapy]

phlo·rid·zin. A dihydrochalcone occurring in many parts of the apple tree; used experimentally to produce glycosuria in animals. SYN phlorizin.

phlo·ri·zin. SYN phloridzin.

phlor·o·glu·cin, phlor·o·glu·cin·ol, phlor·o·glu·col (flōr-ō-glū′sin, -glū′sin-ol, -glū′kol). 1,3,5-Trihydroxybenzene; an isomer of pyrogallol, obtained from resorcinol by fusion with caustic soda; used as a reagent with vanillin, as a decalcifier of bone specimens, and as an antispasmodic. [phloridzin + G. *glykys,* sweet, + -in]

phlox·ine (flok-sēn, -sin) [C.I. 45405]. Dichloro- or tetrachlorotetrabromofluorescein; a red acid dye used as a cytoplasmic stain in histology.

phlyc·te·na, pl. **phlyc·te·nae** (flik-tē′nă, -nē). A small vesicle, especially one of a number of small blisters following a first degree burn. [G. *phlyktaina,* a blister made by a burn]

phlyc·te·nar (flik′tĕ-năr). Relating to or marked by the presence of phlyctenae. SYN phlyctenous.

phlyc·te·noid (flik′tĕ-noyd). Resembling a phlyctena. [G. *phlyktaina,* blister, + *eidos,* resemblance]

phlyc·te·no·sis (flik-tĕ-nō′sis). The occurrence of phlyctenae; a disease marked by a phlyctenar eruption.

phlyc·te·nous (flik′tĕ-nŭs). SYN phlyctenar.

phlyc·ten·u·la, pl. **phlyc·ten·u·lae** (flik-ten′yū-lă). A small red nodule of lymphoid cells, with ulcerated apex, occurring in the conjunctiva. SYN phlyctenule. [Mod. L. dim. of G. *phlyktaina,* blister]

phlyc·ten·u·lar (flik-ten′yū-lăr). Relating to a phlyctenula.

phlyc·ten·ule (flik′ten-yūl). SYN phlyctenula.

phlyc·ten·u·lo·sis (flik-ten′yū-lō′sis). A nodular hypersensitive affection of corneal and conjunctival epithelium due to endogenous toxin.

PhNCS Symbol for phenylisothiocyanate.

pho·ban·thro·py (fō-ban′thrō-pē). SYN anthropophobia. [G. *phobos,* fear, + *anthrōpos,* man]

PHOBIA

pho·bia (fō′bē-ă). Any objectively unfounded morbid dread or fear that arouses a state of panic. The word is used as a combining form in many terms expressing the object that inspires the fear. [G. *phobos,* fear]
   alcoholism, alcoholophobia.
   animals, zoophobia.
   bees, apiphobia, melissophobia.
   being beaten, rhabdophobia.
   being buried alive, taphophobia.
   being dirty, automysophobia.

being locked in, clithrophobia.
being stared at, scopophobia.
birth of malformed fetus, teratophobia.
blood, hemophobia.
blushing, ereuthophobia.
cancer, cancerophobia, carcinophobia.
cats, ailurophobia.
childbirth, tocophobia.
children, pediophobia.
choking, pnigophobia.
climbing, climacophobia.
cold, psychrophobia.
colors, chromatophobia, chromophobia.
confinement, claustrophobia.
corpses, necrophobia.
crossing a bridge, gephyrophobia.
crowds, ochlophobia.
dampness, hygrophobia.
darkness, nyctophobia, scotophobia.
dawn, eosophobia.
daylight, phengophobia.
death, thanatophobia.
deep places, bathophobia.
deserted places, eremophobia.
dirt, mysophobia, rhypophobia.
disease, nosophobia, pathophobia.
disorder, ataxiophobia.
dogs, cynophobia.
dolls, pediophobia.
drafts, aerophobia, anemophobia.
drugs, pharmacophobia.
eating, phagophobia.
electricity, electrophobia.
enclosed space, claustrophobia.
error, hamartophobia.
everything, panphobia.
excrement, coprophobia.
fatigue, ponophobia, kopophobia.
fever, pyrexiophobia.
filth, rhypophobia.
fire, pyrophobia.
fish, ichthyophobia.
food, cibophobia.
forests, hylephobia.
fur, doraphobia.
germs, microphobia.
ghosts, phasmophobia.
girls, parthenophobia.
glare of light, photaugiaphobia.
glass, crystallophobia, hyalophobia.
God, theophobia.
hair, trichophobia, trichopathophobia.
heart disease, cardiophobia.

heat, thermophobia.
heights, acrophobia.
home, returning to, nostophobia.
human companionship, anthropophobia, phobanthropy.
ideas, ideophobia.
infection, molysmophobia.
insects, entomophobia.
itching, acarophobia.
jealousy, zelophobia.
lice, pediculophobia, phthiriophobia.
light, photophobia.
lightning, astrapophobia, keraunophobia.
machinery, mechanophobia.
malignancy, cancerophobia, carcinophobia.
many things, polyphobia.
marriage, gamophobia.
men, (males), androphobia.
metal objects, metallophobia.
microorganisms, microphobia.
minute objects, microphobia.
mirrors, spectrophobia.
missiles, ballistophobia.
moisture, hygrophobia.
movements, kinesophobia.
nakedness, gymnophobia.
names, nomatophobia, onomatophobia.
neglect of duty, omission of duty, paralipophobia.
night, nyctophobia.
novelty, neophobia.
odors, olfactophobia, osmophobia, osphresiophobia, bromidosiphobia.
open spaces, agoraphobia.
pain, algophobia.
parasites, parasitophobia.
phobias, phobophobia.
places, topophobia.
pleasure, hedonophobia.
pointed objects, aichmophobia.
poisoning, toxicophobia, iophobia.
poverty, peniaphobia.
precipices, cremnophobia.
pregnancy, maieusiophobia.
radiation, radiophobia.
rain, ombrophobia.
rectal disease, proctophobia, rectophobia.
religious objects, sacred objects, hierophobia.
responsibility, hypengyophobia.
rivers, potamophobia.
robbers, harpaxophobia.
school p., a young child's sudden aversion to or fear of attending school, usually considered a manifestation of separation anxiety.
sea, thalassophobia.
self, autophobia.
semen, loss of, spermatophobia.
sexual intercourse, coitophobia, cypridophobia.
sexual love, erotophobia.
sharp objects, belonephobia.
sin, hamartophobia.
sinning, pecattiphobia.
skin of animals, doraphobia.
skin diseases, dermatophobia.
sleep, hypnophobia.
snakes, ophidiophobia.
solitude, eremophobia, autophobia, monophobia.
sounds, acousticophobia, phonophobia.
speaking, laliophobia.

spiders, arachnephobia.
stairs, climacophobia
stealing, kleptophobia.
strangers, xenophobia.
stuttering, laliophobia.
sun, heliophobia.
teeth, odontophobia.
thirteen, triskaidekaphobia.
thunder, keraunophobia, tonitrophobia, brontophobia.
time, chronophobia.
touching, being touched, aphephobia, haphephobia.
traveling, hodophobia.
trembling, tremophobia.
uncleanliness, automysophobia.
vaccination, vaccinophobia.
vehicles, amaxophobia, hamaxophobia.
venereal disease, cypridophobia, venereophobia.
voices, phonophobia.
walking, basiphobia.
water, aquaphobia.
wind, anemophobia.
women, (females), gynephobia.
work, ergasiophobia.
worms, helminthophobia.
writing, graphophobia.

pho·bic (fō′bik). Pertaining to or characterized by phobia.

pho·bo·pho·bia (fō-bō-fō′bē-ă). Morbid dread of developing some phobia. [G. *phobos,* fear]

pho·co·me·lia, pho·com·e·ly (fō-kō-mē′lē-ă, fō-kom′ĕ-lē). Defective development of arms or legs, or both, so that the hands and feet are attached close to the body, resembling the flippers of a seal. [G. *phōkē,* a seal, + *melos,* extremity]

phol·co·dine (fol′kō-dēn). 3-(2-Morpholinoethyl)morphine; a narcotic with little or no analgesic or euphorigenic activity, used mainly as an antitussive.

phol·e·drine (fōl′ĕ-drēn). *p*-[2-(Methylamino)propyl]phenol; a sympathomimetic agent for the treatment of shock; also an adrenergic and vasopressor.

Pho·ma (fō′mă). A genus of rapidly growing fungi that are common laboratory contaminants and common plant pathogens.

△**phon-.** SEE phono-.

pho·nac·o·scope (fō-nak′ō-skōp). An instrument for increasing the intensity of the percussion note or of the voice sounds, the examiner's ear or the stethoscope being placed on the opposite side of the chest. [phon- + G. *akouō,* to listen, + *skopeō,* to view]

pho·na·cos·co·py (fō-nă-kos′kŏ-pē). Examination of the chest by means of the phonacoscope.

pho·nal (fō′năl). Relating to sound or to the voice. [G. *phōnē,* voice]

pho·nar·te·ri·o·gram (fōn-ar-tēr′ē-ō-gram). An obsolete technique for recording sound created in arteries.

pho·nar·ter·i·og·ra·phy (fōn-ar-tēr′ē-og′ră-fē). The procedure of obtaining a phonarteriogram.

phon·as·the·nia (fō-nas-thē′nē-ă). Difficult or abnormal voice production, the enunciation being too high, too loud, or too hard. SYN functional vocal fatigue. [phon- + G. *astheneia,* weakness]

pho·na·tion (fō-nā′shŭn). The utterance of sounds by means of vocal folds. [G. *phōnē,* voice]

pho·na·tory (fō′nă-tōr-ē). Relating to phonation.

pho·neme (fō′nēm). The smallest sound unit which, in terms of the phonetic sequences of sound, controls meaning. [G. *phōnēma,* a voice]

pho·ne·mic (fō-nē′mik). Pertaining to or having the characteristics of a phoneme.

pho·nen·do·scope (fō-nen′dō-skōp). A stethoscope that intensifies the auscultatory sounds by means of two parallel resonating plates, one resting on the patient's chest or attached to a stethoscope tube, the other vibrating in unison with it. [phon- + G. *endon,* within, + *skopeō,* to view]

pho·net·ic (fō-net′ik). Relating to speech or to the voice. SEE ALSO phonic. [G. *phōnētikos*]

pho·net·ics (fō-net′iks). The science of speech and of pronunciation. SYN phonology.

pho·ni·at·rics (fō-nē-at′riks). The study of speech habits; the science of speech. [phon- + G. *iatrikos,* of the healing art]

phon·ic (fon′ik, fō′nik). Relating to sound or to the voice. SEE ALSO phonetic.

♻**phono-, phon-.** Sound, speech, or voice sounds. [G. *phōnē*]

pho·no·an·gi·og·ra·phy (fō′nō-an-jē-og′ră-fē). Recording and analysis of the audible frequency-intensity components of the bruit of turbulent arterial blood flow through a stenotic lesion. [phono- + G. *angeion,* vessel, + *graphō,* to write]

pho·no·car·di·o·gram (fō-nō-kar′dē-ō-gram). A record of the heart sounds made by means of a phonocardiograph.

pho·no·car·di·o·graph (fō-nō-kar′dē-ō-graf). An instrument, utilizing microphones, amplifiers, and filters, for graphically recording the heart sounds, which are displayed on an oscilloscope or analog tracing.

linear p., a p. that records all chest wall vibrations resulting from cardiac activity, with emphasis on low frequency vibrations due to its filter characteristics.

logarithmic p., a p. that records only theoretically audible vibrations with emphasis on the higher frequencies due to filter characteristics designed to imitate the logarithmic frequency-intensity response of the human auditory apparatus.

spectral p., an instrument for recording the heart sounds in which the electrical changes created by the latter pass from a microphone through a series of filters, each of which is tuned to a particular frequency band; output from each filter activates a separate light source of brightness proportional to the intensity of the sound transmitted through that filter; the lights are arranged vertically in descending order of frequencies. A record is obtained by photographing the vertical row of lights.

stethoscopic p., a p. that records all sound vibrations, audible and inaudible, conveyed by the stethoscope; however, very low frequency vibrations (in the range of body movements) are filtered out.

pho·no·car·di·og·ra·phy (fō′nō-kar-dē-og′ră-fē). **1.** Recording of the heart sounds with a phonocardiograph. **2.** The science of interpreting phonocardiograms. [phono- + G. *kardia,* heart, + *graphō,* to record]

pho·no·cath·e·ter (fō-nō-kath′ĕ-ter). A cardiac catheter with diminutive microphone housed in its tip, for recording sounds and murmurs from within the heart and great vessels.

pho·no·gram (fō′nō-gram). A graphic curve depicting the duration and intensity of a sound. [phono- + G. *gramma,* diagram]

pho·nol·o·gy (fō-nol′ō-jē). SYN phonetics. [phono- + G. *logos,* study]

pho·no·ma·nia (fō-nō-mā′nē-ă). Rarely used term for a homicidal mania. [G. *phonos,* murder, + *mania,* frenzy]

pho·nom·e·ter (fō-nom′ĕ-ter). An instrument for measuring the pitch and intensity of sounds. [phono- + G. *metron,* measure]

pho·no·my·oc·lo·nus (fō′nō-mī-ok′lō-nŭs). Clonic spasms of muscles in response to aural stimuli. [phono- + G. *mys,* muscle, + *klonos,* tumult]

pho·no·my·og·ra·phy (fō′nō-mī-og′ră-fē). The recording of the varying sounds made by contracting muscular tissue. [phono- + G. *mys,* muscle, + *graphē,* drawing]

pho·nop·a·thy (fō-nop′ă-thē). Any disease of the vocal organs affecting speech. [phono- + G. *pathos,* suffering]

pho·no·pho·bia (fō-nō-fō′bē-ă). Morbid fear of one's own voice, or of any sound. [phono- + G. *phobos,* fear]

pho·no·phore (fō′nō-fōr). A form of binaural stethoscope with a bell-shaped chest piece into which project the recurved extremities of the sound tubes. [phono- + G. *phoros,* carrying]

pho·no·pho·tog·ra·phy (fō′nō-fō-tog′ră-fē). The recording on a

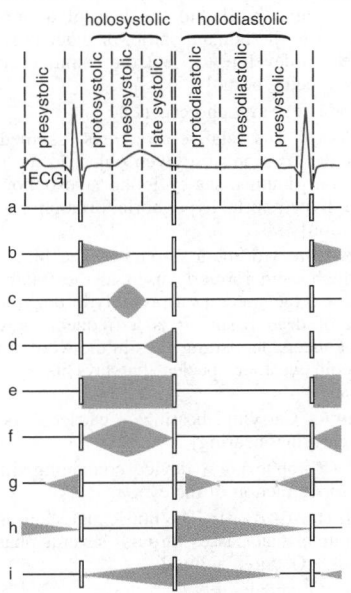

phonocardiography

typical heart sound pictures: a) temporal sequence of first and second heart sounds; b) protosystolic decrescendo m. (e.g., in mitral and tricuspid insufficiency); c) mesosystolic spindle m. (e.g., in aortic stenosis); d) late systolic crescendo m. (e.g., vestigial pericardial friction; in mitral valve insufficiency); e) holosystolic band-shaped m. (e.g., in ventricular septal defect, mitral valve insufficiency); f) holosystolic diamond-shaped m. (e.g., in pulmonary stenosis); g) presystolic crescendo and early diastolic decrescendo m.'s – latter is distinct from the second heart sound by a free interval (Flint's m., in mitral stenosis); h) holodiastolic decrescendo m., beginning immediately after second heart sound (as in aortal insufficiency); and i) continous m. (e.g., with patent ductus arteriosus or atrioventricular aneurysm)

moving photographic plate of the movements imparted to a diaphragm by sound waves. [phono- + photography]

pho·nop·sia (fō-nop′sē-ă). A condition in which the hearing of certain sounds gives rise to a subjective sensation of color. [phono- + G. *opsis,* vision]

pho·no·re·cep·tor (fō′nō-rē-sep′ter). A receptor for sound stimuli.

pho·no·scope (fō′nō-skōp). Obsolete term for an instrument for recording auscultatory percussion; originally used for photographic recording of heart sounds. [phono- + G. *skopeō,* to view]

pho·nos·co·py (fō-nos′kǒ-pē). The recording made by a phonoscope.

pho·no·sur·gery (fō′nō-ser′jer-ē). A group of operations designed to improve or alter a patient's voice.

♻**phor-.** SEE phoro-.

phor·bin (fōr′bin). The parent hydrocarbon of chlorophyll; differs from porphin (porphyrin) in the presence of an isocyclic ring formed by the addition of a two-carbon group bridging the 13 and 15 positions of porphin (porphyrin) and by saturation of the 17-18 double bond (with realignment of conjugated double bonds). Addition of hydrocarbon side-chains in specific locations yields p.'s characterized by prefixes; *e.g.,* phenophorbin.

phor·bol (fōr′bol). The parent alcohol of the cocarcinogens, which are 12,13(9,9a) diesters of p. found in croton oil; the hydrocarbon skeleton is a cyclopropa-benzazulene; p. esters mimic 1,2-diacylglycerol as activators of protein kinase C.

pho·re·sis (fōr′ē-sis, fō-rē′sis). **1.** SYN electrophoresis. **2.** A biological association in which one organism is transported by another, as in the attachment of the eggs of *Dermatobia hominis,* a human and cattle botfly, to the legs of a mosquito, which transports them to the human, cattle, or other host in which the botfly larvae can develop. SYN epizoic commensalism, phoresy. [G. *phorēsis,* a being borne]

phor·e·sy (for′ĕ-sē). SYN phoresis (2).

phor·ia (fōr′ē-ă). The relative directions assumed by the eyes during binocular fixation of a given object in the absence of an adequate fusion stimulus. SEE cyclophoria, esophoria, exophoria, heterophoria, hyperphoria, hypophoria, orthophoria. [G. *phora,* a carrying, motion]

Phor·mia re·gi·na (fōr′mē-ă re-jī′nă). The black blowfly, the larvae of which were formerly used in the treatment of septic wounds because they secrete a proteolytic enzyme that aids in the removal of dead tissue; it is a frequent cause of maggot infestation of sheep, depositing eggs in the wool, and is a widely distributed cold weather species that lays its eggs on dead or decaying tissues.

phoro-, phor-. Carrying, bearing; a carrier, a bearer; phobia. [G. *phoros,* carrying, bearing]

Pho·rop·tor (fŏ-rop′ter). A device containing different lenses that is used for refraction of the eye.

phor·o·zo·on (fōr-ō-zō′on). The nonsexual stage in the life history of an animal that passes through several phases in its life cycle. [phoro- + G. *zōon,* animal]

phos-. Light. [G. *phōs*]

phos·gene (CG) (fos′jēn). O=CCl₂; Carbonyl chloride; a colorless liquid below 8.2°C, but an extremely poisonous gas at ordinary temperatures; it is an insidious gas, since it is not immediately irritating, even when fatal concentrations are inhaled; more than 80% of World War I chemical agent fatalities were caused by p.

p. oxime (CX), Cl₂CNOH; a blister agent stored by the military of some governments; a powerful irritant that produces immediate pain. SYN dichloroformoxime.

phosph-, phospho-, phosphor-, phosphoro-. Prefixes indicating the presence of phosphorus in a compound. See phospho- for specific usage of that prefix. [G. *phōs,* light; *phoros,* carrying]

phos·pha·gen (fos′fă-jen). Energy-rich guanidinium or amidine phosphate, serving as an energy store in muscle and brain; *e.g.,* phosphocreatine in mammals, phosphoarginine in invertebrates.

phos·pha·gen·ic (fos-fă-jen′ik). Phosphate-producing.

phos·pham·ic ac·id (fos-fam′ik). R–NH–PO₃H₂, one of the three types of high energy phosphates (the others being phosphophosphoric acids and phosphosulfuric acids).

phos·pham·i·dase (fos-fam′i-dās). SYN phosphoamidase.

phos·pha·stat (fos′fă-stat). A conceptual mechanism whereby the parathyroid hormone is increased when the levels of phosphorus rise to an above-normal level; there is as yet no satisfactory evidence for its existence. [phosphate + L. *status,* a standing]

phos·pha·tase (fos′fă-tās). Any of a group of enzymes (EC subsubclass 3.1.3) that liberate inorganic phosphate from phosphoric esters. SEE ALSO phosphohydrolases.

acid p., a p. with an optimum pH of less than 7.0 (for several isozymes, it is 5.4), notably present in the prostate gland; demonstrable in lysosomes with Gomori's nonspecific acid p. stain; it hydrolyzes many orthophosphoric monoesters.

alkaline p., a p. with an optimum pH of above 7.0 (*e.g.,* 8.6), present ubiquitously; localized cytochemically in membranes by modifications of Gomori's nonspecific alkaline p. stain; it hydrolyzes many orthophosphoric monoesters; low levels of this enzyme are seen in cases of hypophosphatasia.

phos·phate (fos′fāt). A salt or ester of phosphoric acid. For individual p.'s not listed here, see under the name of the base.

bone p., SYN tribasic *calcium* phosphate.

codeine p., a water-soluble salt of codeine often used in the pharmaceutical preparation of codeine-containing liquid medications.

cyclic p., SYN adenosine 3′,5′-cyclic monophosphate.

dihydrogen p., one-third-neutralized phosphoric acid; *e.g.,* NaH₂PO₄, KH₂PO₄.

disodium p., na₂HPO₄.

energy-rich p.'s, SYN high energy p.'s.

high energy p.'s, those p.'s that, on hydrolysis, yield an unusually large amount of energy; *e.g.,* nucleotide polyphosphates such as ATP, enol p.'s such as phospho*enol*pyruvate. SEE ALSO high energy *compounds,* under *compound.* SYN energy-rich p.'s.

inorganic p., SYN inorganic *orthophosphate.*

monopotassium p., KH₂PO₄; a dihydrogen p. used as a reagent; commonly used in buffers.

monosodium p., NaH₂PO₄; a dihydrogen p. used as a reagent; commonly used in buffers.

normal p., a salt of phosphoric acid in which all the hydrogen atoms are displaced; *e.g.,* Na₃PO₄, Na₄P₂O₇.

organic p., an ester of phosphoric acid; *e.g.,* glycerol p., adenosine p., hexose p.

triple p., (1) magnesium ammonium p., MgNH₄PO₄; **(2)** a crude phosphate fertilizer product from phosphate rock and phosphoric acid.

trisodium p., Na₃PO₄; used to emulsify fats, oil, and grease; an irritant.

phos·phate ace·tyl·trans·fer·ase. An enzyme catalyzing transfer of an acetyl moiety from acetyl-CoA to orthophosphate, forming acetyl phosphate and coenzyme A. SYN phosphoacylase, phosphotransacetylase.

phos·phat·ed (fos′fāt-ed). Containing phosphates.

phos·pha·te·mia (fos-fă-tē′mē-ă). An abnormally high concentration of inorganic phosphates in the blood. [phosphate + G. *haima,* blood]

phos·phat·ic (fos-fat′ik). Relating to or containing phosphates.

phos·pha·ti·dal (fos-fă-tī′dăl). Older trivial name for alk-1-enylglycerophospholipid.

phos·pha·ti·dase (fos-fă-tī′dās). SYN *phospholipase A₂.*

phos·pha·ti·date (fos-fă-tī′dāt). A salt or ester of a phosphatidic acid.

p. phosphatase, an enzyme that catalyzes the hydrolysis of p. producing inorganic phosphate and 1,2-diacylglycerol; this enzyme participates in phospholipid and triacylglycerol metabolism.

phos·pha·tide (fos′fă-tīd). Former name for 1) phosphatidic acid and 2) phosphatidate.

phos·pha·tid·ic ac·id (fos′fă-tid′ik). 1,2-diacylglycerol phosphate; a derivative of glycerophosphoric acid in which the two remaining hydroxyl groups of the glycerol are esterified with fatty acids; *e.g.,* phosphatidic acids attached to choline are phosphatidylcholines (lecithins).

phos·pha·ti·do·lip·ase (fos′fă-tī-dō-lip′ās). SYN *phospholipase A₂.*

phos·pha·ti·dyl (Ptd) (fos-fă-tī′dĭl). The radical of a phosphatidic acid; *e.g.,* phosphatidylcholine.

phos·pha·ti·dyl·cho·line (PtdCho) (fos-fă-tī′dĭl-kō′lēn). SEE lecithin.

phos·pha·ti·dyl·eth·a·nol·a·mine (PtdEth) (fos-fă-tī′dĭl-eth-ă-nol′ă-mēn). The condensation product of a phosphatidic acid and ethanolamine; found in biomembranes. SEE ALSO cephalin.

p. cytidylyltransferase, a key enzyme in the biosynthesis of cephaline; it catalyzes the reaction of phosphoethanolamine and CTP to form CDP-ethanolamine and pyrophosphate.

phos·phat·i·dyl·glyc·er·ol (fos-fă-tī′dĭl-glis′er-ol). A phosphatidic acid in which a second glycerol molecule replaces the usual choline, or ethanolamine or serine; a constituent in human amniotic fluid that denotes fetal lung maturity when present in the last trimester.

phos·pha·ti·dyl·in·o·si·tol (PtdIns) (fos-fă-tī′dĭl-in-ō′si-tol). A phosphatidic acid combined with inositol found in biomembranes and a precursor to certain cellular signals. Sometimes referred to as inositide. SYN phosphoinositide.

p. 4,5-bisphosphate (PIP₂, PtdIns(4,5)P₂), p. with two additional sites of phosphorylation; an important constituent of cell membrane phospholipids as well as a precursor of the second messengers, diacylglycerol and inositol 1,4,5-trisphosphate.

p. 4-phosphate, the intermediate in the biosynthesis of p. 4,5-bisphosphate from p.

p. synthase, an enzyme that catalyzes the reaction of CDP-diacylglycerol with inositol to form CMP and p.; found in the endoplasmic reticulum.

phos·pha·ti·dyl·ser·ine (PtdSer) (fos-fă-tī′dĭl-ser′ēn). The condensation product of phosphatidic acid and serine; found in biomembranes. SEE ALSO cephalin.

phos·pha·tu·ria (fos-fă-tū′rē-ă). Excessive excretion of phosphates in the urine. SYN phosphoruria, phosphuria. [phosphate + G. *ouron,* urine]

phos·phene (fos′fēn). Sensation of light produced by mechanical or electrical stimulation of the peripheral or central optic pathway of the nervous system. [G. *phōs,* light, + *phainō,* to show]

accommodation p., a p. occurring during accommodation, caused by sudden relaxation of the ciliary muscle.

phos·phide (fos′fīd). A compound of phosphorus with valence −3; *e.g.,* sodium phosphide, Na_3P.

phos·phine (fos′fēn, -fin). PH_3; a colorless poisonous war gas with a characteristic garlic-like odor; also the active agent in some rodenticides; formed in small quantities in the putrefaction of organic matter containing phosphorus. SYN hydrogen phosphide, phosphureted hydrogen.

phosphinico-. In chemistry, symmetrically doubly substituted phosphinic acid, $R_2P(O)OH$.

phos·phite (fos′fīt). A salt of phosphorous acid.

phospho-. Prefix for *O*-phosphono-, which may replace the suffix phosphate; *e.g.,* glucose phosphate is *O*-phosphonoglucose or phosphoglucose. SEE ALSO phosph-, phosphoryl-.

phos·pho·ac·y·lase (fos-fō-as′i-lās). SYN phosphate acetyltransferase.

3′-phos·pho·aden·o·sine 5′-phos·phate (PAP) (fos′fō-a-den′ō-sēn). A product in sulfuryl transfer reactions.

3′-phos·pho·aden·o·sine 5′-phos·pho·sul·fate (PAPS) (fos′fō-a-dēn′ō-sēn). SEE adenosine 3′-phosphate 5′-phosphosulfate.

phos·pho·am·i·dase (fos-fō-am′i-dās). An enzyme catalyzing the hydrolysis of phosphorus-nitrogen bonds, notably the hydrolysis of *N*-phosphocreatine to creatine and orthophosphate. SYN phosphamidase.

phos·pho·am·ides (fos-fō-am′īdz). Amides of phosphoric acid (phosphoramidic acids) and their salts or esters (phosphoramidates), of the general formula $(HO)_2P(O)–NH_2$; *e.g.,* creatine phosphate.

phos·pho·ar·gi·nine (fos-fō-ar′gi-nēn). A compound (in particular, a phosphagen) of L-arginine with phosphoric acid containing the phosphoamide bond; a source of energy in the contraction of muscle in invertebrates, corresponding to phosphocreatine in the muscles of vertebrates. Cf. phosphocreatine. SYN arginine phosphate.

phos·pho·cho·line (fos-fō-kō′lēn). $(CH_3)_3N^+– CH_2\ CH_2–OPO_3 H^-$; choline *O*-phosphate; important in choline metabolism, *e.g.,* as in cytidinediphosphocholine and in the biosynthesis of lecithins. SYN *O*-phosphocholine, phosphorylcholine.

p. cytidylyltransferase, an enzyme that catalyzes the reaction of p. with CTP to form pyrophosphate and CDP-choline; the rate-limiting step of lecithin biosynthesis; the cytosolic form of the enzyme is inactive (a phosphorylated form of the enzyme).

p. diacylglycerol transferase, an enzyme in lecithin biosynthesis that catalyzes the reaction of 1,2-diacylglycerol with CDP-choline to form CMP and phosphatidylcholine.

***O*-phos·pho·cho·line.** SYN phosphocholine.

phos·pho·cre·a·tine (fos-fō-krē′ă-tēn). $^{2-}O_2P–NHC(NH)N (CH_3)CH_2COO^-$; a phosphagen; a compound of creatine (through its NH_2 group) with phosphoric acid; a source of energy in the contraction of vertebrate muscle, its breakdown furnishing phosphate for the resynthesis of ATP from ADP by creatine kinase. Cf. phosphoarginine. SYN creatine phosphate.

phos·pho·di·es·ter (fos′fō-dī-es′ter). A diesterified orthophosphoric acid, $RO–(PO_2H)–OR'$, as in the nucleic acids.

p. hydrolases, SYN phosphodiesterases.

phos·pho·di·es·ter·as·es (fos′fō-dī-es′ter-ās-ez). Enzymes (EC sub-subclass 3.1.4) cleaving phosphodiester bonds, such as those in cAMP or between nucleotides in nucleic acids, liberating smaller poly- or oligonucleotide units or mononucleotides but not inorganic phosphate. SYN phosphodiester hydrolases.

spleen p., SYN micrococcal *endonuclease*.

phos·pho·dis·mu·tase (fos-fō-dis′myū-tās). SYN phosphomutase.

phos·pho·enol·py·ru·vate car·box·y·kin·ase. SYN *phosphoenolpyruvic acid* carboxykinase.

phos·pho·e·nol·pyr·u·vic ac·id (fos′fō-ē′nol-pī-rū′vik). $CH_2= C(OPO_3H_2)–COOH$; the phosphoric ester of pyruvic acid in the latter's enol form; an intermediate in the conversion of GLUCOSE to pyruvic acid and an example of a high energy phosphate ester.

p. a. carboxykinase, an enzyme that catalyzes the reaction of oxaloacetate and GTP to form p. a., CO_2, and GDP; a key enzyme in gluconeogenesis; the biosynthesis of this enzyme is decreased by insulin. SYN phosphoenolpyruvate carboxykinase.

phos·pho·eth·a·no·la·mine (fos′fō-eth-an-ol′-a-mēn). $^{2-}O_3POCH_2CH_2NH_3^+$; a key intermediate in the formation of cephalins; formed in liver and brain by phosphorylation of ethanolamine.

p. cytidylyltransferase, a key enzyme in the biosynthesis of cephalins; it catalyzes the reaction of p. and CTP to form CDP-ethanolamine and pyrophosphate.

1-phos·pho·fruc·tal·do·lase (fos′-fō-frŭk-tal′dō-lās). SYN fructose-bisphosphate aldolase.

1-phos·pho·fruc·to·ki·nase (fos′fō-frŭk-tō-kī′nās). Fructose-1-phosphate kinase; an enzyme catalyzing phosphorylation of D-fructose 1-phosphate by ATP (or other NTP) to D-fructose 1,6-bisphosphate and ADP (or other NDP); a key step in the metabolism of D-fructose; a deficiency of the muscle enzyme can result in glycogen storage disease type VII.

6-phos·pho·fruc·to·ki·nase. phosphofructokinase I; an enzyme that catalyzes the phosphorylation of D-fructose 6-phosphate by ATP (or other NTP) to fructose 1,6-bisphosphate and ADP (or other NDP); this enzyme catalyzes a step in glycolysis; it is inhibited by elevated levels of either ATP or citrate; a deficiency of this enzyme can lead to hemolytic anemia. SYN phosphohexokinase.

phos·pho·ga·lac·to·i·som·er·ase (fos′fō-gă-lak′tō-ī-som′er-ās). SYN UDPglucose–hexose-1-phosphate uridylyltransferase.

phos·pho·glu·co·ki·nase (fos′fō-glū-kō-kī′nās). An enzyme that, in the presence of ATP, catalyzes the phosphorylation of D-glucose 1-phosphate to form D-glucose 1,6-bisphosphate and ADP; found in yeast and muscle; D-glucose 1,6-bisphosphate is a required cofactor of one of the enzymes in glycogenolysis. SYN glucose-1-phosphate kinase.

phos·pho·glu·co·mu·tase (fos′fō-glū-kō-myū′tās). An enzyme that catalyzes the reaction, α-D-glucose 1-phosphate → α-D-glucose 6-phosphate, with glucose 1,6-bisphosphate a necessary cofactor; one of the steps in glycogenolysis. SYN glucose phosphomutase.

phos·pho·glu·co·nate de·hy·dro·gen·ase (fos-fō-glū′kŏ-nāt). 6-phosphogluconic dehydrogenase; an enzyme catalyzing the reaction of 6-phospho-D-gluconate and $NAD(P)^+$ to form 6-phospho-2-keto-D-gluconate and NAD(P)H; a deficiency of this enzyme has been reported, but no cell disruption has been observed.

phos·pho·glu·co·nate de·hy·dro·gen·ase (de·car·box·y·lat·ing). An enzyme, which is part of the pentose phosphate shunt, that catalyzes the reaction of 6-phospho-D-gluconate and $NADP^+$ to produce CO_2, NADPH, and D-ribulose 5-phosphate.

6-phos·pho·glu·co·no·lac·to·nase (fos′fō-glū′kŏ-nō-lak′tō-nās). A hydrolase that catalyzes the hydrolysis of 6-phospho-D-glucono δ-lactone to 6-phospho-D-gluconate; this enzyme is a part of the pentose phosphate shunt.

6-phos·pho·D-glu·co·no δ-lac·tone. An intermediate in the pentose phosphate pathway that is synthesized from D-glucose 6-phosphate.

phos·pho·glyc·er·ac·e·tals (fos′fō-glis-er-as′ĕ-tălz). SYN plasmalogens.

phos·pho·glyc·er·ate ki·nase (fos-fō-glis′er-āt). An enzyme catalyzing the formation of 3-phospho-D-glyceroyl phosphate and ADP from 3-phospho-D-glycerate and ATP; this enzyme is a part of the glycolytic pathway; a deficiency of p. k. (an X-linked disorder) results in impaired glycolysis in most cells.

phos·pho·gly·cer·ic ac·id (fos′fō-gli-ser′ik, -glis′er-ik). **1.** $HOCH_2$–CH(OH)CO– OPO_3H_2; glyceroyl phosphoric acid; glyceroyl phosphate; an acid anhydride between glyceric acid and phosphoric acid. **2.** $HOCH_2$–CH(OPO_3H_2) COOH; 2-phosphoglyceric acid; the deprotonated form, 2-phosphoglycerate, is an intermediate in glycolysis. **3.** $H_2O_3POCH_2$–CH (OH)COOH; 3-phosphoglyceric acid; the deprotonated form, 3-phosphoglycerate, is an intermediate in glycolysis.

phos·pho·glyc·er·ides (fos-fō-glis′er-īdz). Acylglycerol and diacylglycerol phosphates; constituents of nerve tissue, and involved in fat transport and storage.

phos·pho·glyc·er·o·mu·tase (fos′fō-glis′er-ō-myū′tās). An isomerizing enzyme catalyzing the reversible interconversion of 2-phosphoglycerate and 3-phosphoglycerate with 2,3-bisphosphoglycerate present as a cofactor; a deficiency of this enzyme, which plays a role in glycolysis, is an inherited disorder that results in an intolerance for strenuous exercise.

phos·pho·hex·o·ki·nase (fos′fō-hek-sō-kī′nās). SYN 6-phosphofructokinase.

phos·pho·hex·o·mu·tase (fos′fō-hek-sō-myū′tās). SYN glucose-phosphate isomerase.

phos·pho·hex·ose isom·er·ase (fos-fō-hek′sōs). SYN glucose-phosphate isomerase.

phos·pho·hy·dro·las·es (fos-fō-hī′drō-lās-ez). Phosphoric monoester hydrolases; enzymes (EC sub-subclass 3.1.3) cleaving phosphoric acid (as orthophosphate) from its esters; trivial names usually end in phosphate.

phos·pho·in·o·si·tide (fos′fō-in-ō′si-tīd). SYN phosphatidylinositol.

phos·pho·ki·nase (fos-fō-kī′nās). A phosphotransferase or a kinase.

phos·pho·li·pase (fos-fō-lip′ās). An enzyme that catalyzes the hydrolysis of a phospholipid. SYN lecithinase.

p. A_1, an enzyme that hydrolyzes a lecithin (1,2-diacylglycerophosphocholine) to a 2-acylglycerophosphocholine and a fatty acid anion.

p. A_2, an enzyme that catalyzes the hydrolysis of a lecithin to a lysolecithin by removing the 2-acyl group; also acts on other phospholipids by removing a fatty acid from the 2-position; this enzyme has an important role in prostaglandin and leukotriene biosynthesis. SYN lecithinase A, phosphatidase, phosphatidolipase.

p. B, (1) SYN lysophospholipase. **(2)** there are reports that p. B is a mixture of p. A_1 and p. A_2.

p. C, *Clostridium welchii* α-toxin; *Clostridium oedematiens* β- and γ-toxins; an enzyme that catalyzes the hydrolysis of phosphatidylcholine (and perhaps other phospholipids) to produce choline phosphate and 1,2-diacylglycerol; also acts on sphingomyelin; a key enzyme in the formation of inositol 1,4,5-trisphosphate. SYN lecithinase C, lipophosphodiesterase I.

p. D, an enzyme that hydrolyzes phosphatidylcholine to produce choline and a phosphatidate; also acts on other phosphatidyl esters. SYN choline phosphatase, lecithinase D, lipophosphodiesterase II.

phos·pho·lip·id (fos-fō-lip′id). A lipid containing phosphorus, thus including the lecithins and other phosphatidyl derivatives, sphingomyelin, and plasmalogens; the basic constituents of biomembranes.

phos·pho·mu·tase (fos-fō-myū′tās). One of a number of enzymes (mutases) (EC sub-subclass 5.4.2) that apparently catalyze intramolecular transfer because the donor is regenerated (*e.g.,* phosphoglyceromutase, phosphoglucomutase). SYN phosphodismutase.

phos·pho·ne·cro·sis (fos-fō-ne-krō′sis). Necrosis of the osseous tissue of the jaw, as a result of poisoning by inhalation of phosphorus fumes, occurring especially in persons who work with the element. [phosphorus + G. *nekrōsis,* death (necrosis)]

phos·pho·ni·um (fos-fō′nē-ŭm). The radical, $(PR_4)^+$.

△**O-phosphono-.** Prefix indicating a phosphonic acid radical ($–PO_3H_2$) attached through an oxygen atom, hence a phosphoric ester. SEE ALSO phospho-.

4′-phos·pho·pan·te·the·ine (fos′fō-pan-tĕ-thē′in). The prosthetic group of the acyl carrier protein in the fatty acid synthase complex. SYN pantetheine 4′-phosphate.

phos·pho·pen·ia (fos′fō-pē′nē-aă). Low serum phosphate levels. SYN phosphorpenia. [phospho- + G. *penia,* poverty]

phos·pho·pen·tose ep·i·mer·ase (fos-fō-pen′tōs ē-pim-er-ās). An enzyme that catalyzes the reversible epimerization of a number of phosphorylated, five-carbon sugars; most notably ribulose 5-phosphate to xylulose 5-phosphate in the pentose phosphate pathway.

phos·pho·pen·tose isom·er·ase (fos-fō-pen′tōs). SYN *ribose-5-phosphate* isomerase.

phos·pho·pho·rin (fos-fō-fōr′in). A protein (MW 155,000) found in dentin that is believed to have a role in mineralization.

phos·pho·pro·tein (fos-fō-prō′tēn). A protein containing phosphoryl groups attached directly to the side chains of some of its constituent amino acids, usually to the hydroxyl group of an L-seryl residue or an L-threonyl residue; *e.g.,* casein, vitellin, ovalbumin.

phos·pho·py·ru·vate hy·dra·tase (fos-fō-pī′rū-vāt). SYN enolase.

phos·phor (fos′fōr). A chemical substance that transforms incident electromagnetic or radioactive energy into light, as in scintillation radioactivity determinations or radiographic intensifying screens or image amplifiers. [G. *phōs,* light, + *phoros,* bearing]

photostimulable p., the chemical coating the p. plate in a computed radiography system; the latent image is recovered by laser scanning.

△**phosphor-, phosphoro-.** SEE phosph-.

phos·phor·at·ed (fos′fōr-āt-ed). Forming a compound with phosphorus.

phos·pho·res·cence (fos-fŏ-res′ens). The quality or property of emitting light without active combustion or the production of heat, generally as the result of prior exposure to radiation, which persists after the inciting cause is removed. [G. *phōs,* light, + *phoros,* bearing]

phos·pho·res·cent (fos′fŏ-res′ent). Having the property of phosphorescence.

phos·phor·hi·dro·sis (fos′fōr-hī-drō′sis). The excretion of luminous sweat. SYN phosphoridrosis. [G. *phōs,* light, + *phoros,* bearing, + *hidrōsis,* sweating]

phos·pho·ri·bo·i·som·er·ase (fos′fō-rī′bō-ī-som′er-ās). SYN *ribose-5-phosphate* isomerase.

5-phos·pho·ri·bose 1-di·phos·phate. SYN 5-phospho-α-D-ribosyl 1-pyrophosphate.

5-phos·pho·ri·bo·syl·am·ine (fos′fō-rī-bō-sil-a-mēn). An intermediate in purine biosynthesis.

phos·pho·ri·bo·syl·gly·cine·a·mide syn·the·tase (fos′fō-rī′bō-sil-gli-sin′ă-mīd). Glycinamide ribonucleotide synthetase; an enzyme that reacts glycine with ribosylamine 5-phosphate and ATP to form ADP, orthophosphate, and phosphoribosylglycineamide in the course of purine biosynthesis.

5-phos·pho-α-D-ri·bo·syl 1-py·ro·phos·phate (PPRibp, PPRP, PRPP). 5-Phosphoribosyl 1-diphosphate; D-Ribose carrying a phosphate group on ribose carbon-5 and a pyrophosphate group on ribose carbon-1; an intermediate in the formation of the pyrimidine and purine nucleotides as well as NAD^+. SYN 5-phosphoribose 1-diphosphate.

phos·pho·ri·bo·syl·trans·fer·ase (fos′fō-rī′bō-sil-trans′fer-ās). One of a group of enzymes (EC sub-subclass 2.4.2, pentosyltransferases) that transfers D-ribose 5-phosphate from 5-phospho-α-D-ribosyl pyrophosphate to a purine, pyrimidine, or pyridine acceptor, forming a 5′-nucleotide and inorganic pyrophosphate, or D-ribose from D-ribosyl phosphate to a base, forming a nucleoside, or similar pentose transfers; important in nucleotide biosynthesis. Specific p.'s are preceded by the name of the acceptor base, *e.g.,* uracil phosphoribosyltransferase (*i.e.,* uracil + PRPP ↔ UMP + pyrophosphate).

phos·pho·ri·bu·lo·ki·nase (fos'fō-rī'byū-lō-kī'nās). An enzyme that, in the presence of ATP, catalyzes the phosphorylation of D-ribulose 5-phosphate to D-ribulose 1,5-bisphosphate and ADP, a reaction of importance in the carbon dioxide fixation cycle of photosynthesis.

phos·pho·ri·bu·lose ep·i·mer·ase (fos-fō-rī'byū-lōs). SYN ribulose-phosphate 3-epimerase.

phos·phor·ic ac·id (fos-fōr'ik). O=P(OH)₃; Orthophosphoric acid; a strong acid of industrial importance; m.p. 42.35°C; dilute solutions have been used as urinary acidifiers and as dressings to remove necrotic debris. In dentistry, it comprises about 60% of the liquid used in zinc phosphate and silicate cements; solutions are used for conditioning enamel surfaces prior to applications of various types of resins.

cyclic p. a., (1) in general, a linear polymer of phosphoric acid residues in pyrophosphate linkage in which the α and ω residues are similarly linked to make one endless loop or cyclic compound; (2) specifically, a generic term applied to compounds in which one phosphoric acid residue is esterified to two hydroxyl groups of a single carbon chain, as in adenosine 3′,5′-phosphoric acid, adenosine 2′,3′-phosphoric acid, etc.

dilute p. a., a solvent containing 10% H_3PO_4.

glacial p. a., $(HPO_3)_n$; an anhydride of phosphoric acid used as a reagent, and in the manufacture of zinc oxyphosphate cement for dentistry. SYN metaphosphoric acid.

phos·phor·i·dro·sis (fos'fōr-i-drō'sis). SYN phosphorhidrosis.

phos·phor·ism (fos'fōr-izm). Chronic poisoning with phosphorus.

phos·phor·ized (fos'fōr-īzd). Containing phosphorus.

phos·pho·rol·y·sis (fos'fō-rol'i-sis). A reaction analogous to hydrolysis except that the elements of phosphoric acid, rather than of water, are added in the course of splitting a bond; *e.g.,* the formation of glucose 1-phosphate from glycogen. SYN phosphoroclastic cleavage.

phos·pho·rous (fos'fōr-ŭs, fos-fōr'ŭs). 1. Relating to, containing, or resembling phosphorus. 2. Referring to phosphorus in its lower (+3) valence state.

phosphorous ac·id. H_3PO_3; its salts are phosphites.

phos·phor·pen·ia (fos'fōr-pē'nē-aă). SYN phosphopenia.

phos·phor·u·ria (fos-fō-rū'rē-ă). SYN phosphaturia.

phos·pho·rus (P) (fos'fōr-ŭs). A nonmetallic chemical element, atomic no. 15, atomic wt. 30.973762, occurring extensively in nature always in combination as phosphates, phosphites, etc., and as the phosphate in every living cell; the elemental form is extremely poisonous, causing intense inflammation and fatty degeneration; repeated inhalation of p. fumes may cause necrosis of the jaw (phosphonecrosis); the approximate fatal dose is 50 to 100 mg. [G. *phosphoros,* fr. *phōs,* light, + *phoros,* bearing]

amorphous p., red p., an allotropic form of p. formed by heating ordinary p., in the absence of oxygen, to 260°C; it occurs as an amorphous dark red mass or powder, nonpoisonous, and much less flammable than ordinary p.; it may be reconverted to the latter by heating to 454.4°C in nitrogen gas.

p. pentoxide, P_2O_5; the ultimate anhydride of orthophosphoric acid; a drying and dehydrating agent; corrosive.

phos·pho·rus-32 (^{32}P). Radioactive phosphorus isotope; beta emitter with half-life of 14.28 days; used as tracer in metabolic studies and in the treatment of certain diseases of the osseous and hematopoietic systems.

phos·pho·rus-33 (^{33}P). A radioactive isotope of phosphorus with a half-life of 25.3 days; used as a tracer in metabolic studies.

phos·pho·ryl (fos'fŏ-ril). The radical, O=P–, as in phosphoryl chloride, $POCl_3$.

△**phosphoryl-.** Prefix incorrectly used to signify a phosphate (*e.g.,* phosphorylcholine) in place of the correct *O*-phosphono- or phospho-.

phos·pho·ryl·ase (fos-fōr'i-lās). A phosphorylated enzyme cleaving poly(1,4-α-D-glucosyl)ₙ with inorganic phosphate to form poly(1,4-α- D-glucosyl)ₙ₋₁ and α-D-glucose 1-phosphate. SYN α-glucan phosphorylase, glycogen phosphorylase, P enzyme, p. *a,* polyphosphorylase.

p. *a*, SYN phosphorylase.

p. *b*, dephosphorylated p. *a.* Under most conditions, the inactive form of p.; active in the presence of AMP. SEE p. phosphatase.

p. kinase, an enzyme that uses ATP to phosphorylate p. *b* and thus reform p. *a,* the active form of p.; the active form of p. kinase is itself a phosphorylated protein; upon dephosphorylation of p. kinase, the enzyme is inactivated; it can be rephosphorylated with a cAMP-dependent protein kinase; p. kinase is deficient in certain types of glycogen storage disease.

p. phosphatase, an enzyme catalyzing the conversion of one p. *a* into two p. *b,* with the release of four phosphates. SYN phosphorylase-rupturing enzyme.

phos·pho·ryl·as·es (fos-fōr'i-lās-ez). 1. General term for enzymes transferring an inorganic phosphate group to some organic acceptor, hence belonging to the transferases. 2. Specifically, enzymes that release a single glucosyl residue from a polyglucose as D-glucose 1-phosphate, the phosphate coming from inorganic orthophosphate; *e.g.,* phosphophorylase, sucrose p., cellobiose p.

nucleoside p., enzymes that catalyze the phosphorolysis of a nucleoside, forming the free purine or pyrimidine plus ribose (or deoxyribose 1-phosphate); *e.g.,* purine-nucleoside phosphorylases.

phos·pho·ryl·a·tion (fos'fōr-i-lā'shŭn). Addition of phosphate to an organic compound, such as glucose to produce glucose monophosphate, through the action of a phosphotransferase (phosphorylase) or kinase.

oxidative p., formation of high energy phosphoric bonds (*e.g.,* in pyrophosphates) from the energy released by the flow of electrons to O_2 and the dehydrogenation (*i.e.,* oxidation) of various substrates, most notably isocitric acid, α-ketoglutaric acid, succinic acid, and malic acid in the tricarboxylic acid cycle.

substrate-level p., the synthesis of ATP (or other NTP) not involving electron transport coupled with oxidative p. or with photophosphorylation.

phos·pho·ryl·cho·line (fos'fōr-il-kō'lēn). SYN phosphocholine.

phos·pho·ryl·eth·a·nol·a·mine glyc·er·ide·trans·fer·ase (fos'fōr-il-eth-ă-nol'ă-mēn). SYN ethanolaminephosphotransferase.

***O*-phos·pho·ser·ine** (fos-fō-ser'ēn). $^{2-}O_3$ P– OCH_2CH $(NH_3)^+COO^-$; the phosphoric ester of serine; found as a constituent in many proteins (*e.g.,* phosphorylase *a* and phosvitin).

phos·pho·sphin·go·sides (fos-fō-sfing'gō-sīdz). SYN sphingomyelins.

phos·pho·sug·ar (fos-fō-shug'er). A phosphorylated saccharide; any sugar containing an alcoholic group esterified with phosphoric acid.

phos·pho·trans·a·cet·y·lase (fos'fō-trans-ă-set'i-lās). SYN phosphate acetyltransferase.

phos·pho·trans·fer·as·es (fos-fō-trans'fer-ās-ez). Transphosphatase; a subclass of transferases (EC subclass 2.7) transferring phosphorus-containing groups. P.'s include the "kinases" (2.7.1) transferring phosphate to alcohols, to carboxyl groups (2.7.2), to nitrogenous groups (2.7.3), or to another phosphate group (2.7.4). Phosphomutases (5.4.2) catalyze apparent intramolecular transfers; pyrophosphokinases (2.7.6) catalyze transfer of the pyrophosphate group; nucleotidyltransferases (2.7.7) catalyze transfer of the nucleotide (nucleotidyl) groups (including polyribonucleotide nucleotidyltransferase) and other similar groups (2.7.8). SYN transphosphatases.

phos·pho·tri·ose isom·er·ase (fos-fō-trī'ōs). SYN triosephosphate isomerase.

phos·pho·tung·stic ac·id (PTA) (fos-fō-tŭng'stik). A mixture of phosphoric and tungstic acids, approximately 24 WO_3, 2 H_3PO_4, 48 H_2O; a protein precipitant and reagent for arginine, lysine, histidine, and cystine; used with hematoxylin for nuclear and muscle staining; also used in electron microscopy as a stain for collagen and as a negative stain.

phos·pho·vi·tin. SYN phosvitin.

phos·phu·re·sis (fos'fū-rē'sis). Excretion of excessive amounts of phosphate in the urine. [phospho- + G. *ourēsis,* urination]

phos·phu·ria (fos-fū'rē-ă). SYN phosphaturia.

phos·vi·tin (fos-vī'tin). A phosphated protein constituting about 7% of the protein of egg yolk; it is about 60% serine, largely as *O*-phosphoserine, and has anticoagulant properties; an anticoagulant. SYN phosphovitin.

phot (fōt). A unit of illumination; 1 p. equals 1 lumen/cm^2 of surface. [G. *phōs* (*phōt*-), light]

Ophot-. SEE photo-.

pho·tal·gia (fō-tal'jē-ă). Light-induced pain, especially of the eyes. For example, in uveitis, the light-induced movement of the iris may be painful. SYN photodynia. [phot- + G. *algos,* pain]

pho·tau·gi·a·pho·bia (fō-taw'jē-ă-fō'bē-ă). Morbid fear of, or overreaction to, a glare of light. [G. *phōtaugeia,* glare of light, + *phobos,* fear]

pho·tes·the·sia (fō-tes-thē'zē-ă). Perception of light. [photo- + G. *aisthēsis,* sensation]

pho·tic (fō'tik). Relating to light.

pho·tism (fō'tizm). Production of a sensation of light or color by a stimulus to another sense organ, such as of hearing, taste, or touch. SYN pseudophotesthesia.

Ophoto-, phot-. Light. [G. *phōs* (*phōt*-)]

pho·to·ab·la·tion (fō'tō-ab-lā'shun). The process of photoablative decomposition of tissue by laser light, *e.g.,* in photorefractive keratectomy.

pho·to·ac·tin·ic (fō'tō-ak-tin'ik). Denoting radiation that produces both luminous and chemical effects. [photo- + G. *aktis,* ray]

pho·to·al·ler·gy (fō'tō-al'er-jē). SEE photosensitization.

pho·to·au·to·troph (fō'tō-aw'tō-trōf). An organism that depends solely on light for its energy and principally on carbon dioxide for its carbon. Cf. photoheterotroph, photolithotroph, phototroph. [photo- + G. *autos,* self, + *trophē,* nourishment]

pho·to·au·to·tro·phic (fō-tō-aw'tō-trof'ik). Pertaining to a photoautotroph.

pho·to·bac·te·ria (fō'tō-bak-tēr'ē-ă). Plural of photobacterium.

Pho·to·bac·te·ri·um (fō'tō-bak-tēr'ē-ŭm). A genus of motile and nonmotile, aerobic to facultatively anaerobic bacteria (family Pseudomonadaceae) containing Gram-negative coccobacilli and occasional rods; under adverse conditions pleomorphic forms frequently occur. Motile cells have polar flagella. The metabolism of these organisms is fermentative. They are usually luminescent and occur symbiotically in tissues of luminous organs of cephalopods and deep-sea fishes and on the skin and in the intestines of some marine fish. The type species is *P. phosphoreum.*

P. harve'yi, SYN *Lucibacterium harveyi.*

P. phospho'reum, a luminescent species found on dead fish and in sea water; it is the type species of the genus *P.*

pho·to·bac·te·ri·um, pl. **pho·to·bac·te·ria** (fō'tō-bak-tēr'ē-ŭm, -bak-tēr'ē-ă). A vernacular term used to refer to any member of the genus *Photobacterium.*

pho·to·bi·ol·o·gy (fō'tō-bī-ol'ō-jē). The study of the effects of light upon plants and animals.

pho·to·bi·ot·ic (fō'tō-bī-ot'ik). Living or flourishing only in the light. [photo- + G. *bios,* life]

pho·to·bleach (fō'tō-blēch). To lose color or make white by the action of light; *e.g.,* the use of a laser to bleach a fluorescent dye covalently linked to a macromolecule.

pho·to·cat·a·lyst (fō-tō-kat'ă-list). A substance that helps bring about a light-catalyzed reaction; *e.g.,* chlorophyll. [photo- + G. *katalysis,* dissolution (catalysis)]

pho·to·cep·tor (fō'tō-sep'ter, -tōr). SYN photoreceptor.

pho·to·chem·i·cal (fō-tō-kem'i-kăl). Denoting chemical changes caused by or involving light.

pho·to·chem·is·try (fō-tō-kem'is-trē). The branch of chemistry concerned with the chemical changes caused by or involving light.

pho·to·che·mo·ther·a·py (fō'tō-kem-ō-thār'ă-pē, -kē-mō-). SYN photoradiation.

pho·to·chro·mo·gens (fō'tō-krō'mō-jenz). SYN group I mycobacteria. [photo- + G. *chrōma,* color, + *-gen,* producing]

pho·to·co·ag·u·la·tion (fō'tō-kō-ag'yū-lā'shŭn). A method by which a beam of electromagnetic energy is directed to a desired tissue under visual control; localized coagulation results from absorption of light energy and its conversion to heat or conversion of tissue to plasma (atoms stripped of electrons). [photo- + L. *coagulo,* pp. *-atus,* to curdle]

pho·to·co·ag·u·la·tor (fō'tō-kō-ag'yū-lā'ter, tōr). The apparatus used in photocoagulation.

laser p., a high-energy source of electromagnetic radiation. SEE laser.

xenon-arc p., a p. in which a xenon-arc bulb delivers radiation from the visible and near-infrared spectrum.

pho·to·der·ma·ti·tis (fō'tō-der-mă-tī'tis). Dermatitis caused or elicited by exposure to sunlight; may be phototoxic or photoallergic, and can result from topical application, ingestion, inhalation, or injection of mediating phototoxic or photoallergic material. SEE ALSO photosensitization. SYN actinic dermatitis, actinodermatitis (1). [photo- + G. *derma,* skin, + *-itis,* inflammation]

pho·to·dis·tri·bu·tion (fō'tō-dis-tri-byū'shŭn). Areas on the skin that receive the greatest amount of exposure to sunlight, and which are involved in eruptions due to photosensitivity.

pho·tod·ro·my (fō-tod'rō-mē). In the induced or spontaneous clarification of certain suspensions, the settlement of particles on the side nearest the light (**positive p.**) or on the dark side (**negative p.**). [photo- + G. *dromos,* a running]

pho·to·dy·nam·ic (fō'tō-dī-nam'ik). Relating to the energy or force exerted by light. [photo- + G. *dynamis,* force]

pho·to·dyn·ia (fō-tō-din'ē-ă). SYN photalgia. [photo- + G. *odynē,* pain]

pho·to·dys·pho·ria (fō'tō-dis-fōr'ē-ă). Extreme photophobia. [photo- + G. *dysphoria,* extreme discomfort]

pho·to·e·lec·tric (fō'tō-ē-lek'trik). Denoting electronic or electric effects produced by the action of light. SEE photoelectric *effect,* photoelectric *absorption.*

pho·to·e·lec·trom·e·ter (fō'tō-ē-lek-trom'ě-ter). A device employing a photoelectric cell for measuring the concentration of substances in solution.

pho·to·e·lec·tron (fō'tō-ē-lek'tron). An electron freed by the action of light.

pho·to·er·y·the·ma (fō'tō-er-i-thē'mă). Erythema caused by exposure to light. [photo- + G. *erythēma,* flush]

pho·to·es·thet·ic (fō'tō-es-thet'ik). Sensitive to light. [photo- + G. *aisthēsis,* sensation]

pho·to·flu·o·rog·ra·phy (fō'tō-flūr-og'ră-fē). Miniature radiographs made by contact photography of a fluoroscopic screen, formerly used in mass radiographic examination of the lungs. SYN fluorography, fluororoentgenography. [photo- + L. *fluor,* a flow, + G. *graphē,* a writing]

pho·to·gas·tro·scope (fō'tō-gas'trō-skōp). An instrument for taking photographs of the interior of the stomach. [photo- + G. *gastēr,* stomach, + *skopeō,* to view]

pho·to·gen (fō'tō-jen). A microorganism that produces luminescence. [photo- + G. *gen-,* producing]

pho·to·gen·e·sis (fō-tō-jen'ě-sis). Production of light, as by bacteria, insects, or phosphorescence. [photo- + G. *genesis,* production]

pho·to·gen·ic, pho·tog·e·nous (fō-tō-jen'ik, fō-toj'ě-nŭs). Denoting or capable of photogenesis.

pho·to·he·mo·ta·chom·e·ter (fō'tō-hē'mō-tă-kom'ě-ter). An appliance for recording photographically the rapidity of the blood current. [photo- + G. *haima,* blood, + *tachos,* speed, + *metron,* measure]

pho·to·het·er·o·troph (fō'tō-het'er-ō-trof, -trōf). An organism that depends on light for most of its energy and principally on organic compounds for its carbon. Cf. photoautotroph, photolithotroph, phototroph. [photo- + G. *heteros,* other, + *trophē,* nourishment]

pho·to·het·er·o·tro·phic (fō'tō-het'er-ō-trof'ik). Pertaining to a photoheterotroph.

pho·to·in·ac·ti·va·tion (fō'tō-in-ak-ti-vā'shŭn). Inactivation by light; *e.g.,* as in the treatment of herpes simplex by local application of a photoactive dye followed by exposure to a fluorescent lamp.

pho·to·ker·a·to·scope (fō'tō-ker'ah-tō-skōp). A keratoscope fitted with a still film camera.

pho·to·ki·ne·sis (fō'tō-ki-nē'sis). Alteration of random movements of motile organisms in response to light. [photo- + G. *kinēsis*, movement]

pho·to·ki·net·ic (fō'tō-ki-net'ik). **1.** Pertaining to photokinesis. **2.** Pertaining to photokinetics.

pho·to·ki·net·ics (fō'tō-ki-net'iks). The changes in rate of a chemical reaction in response to light. [photo- + G. *kinētikos*, relating to movement]

pho·to·ky·mo·graph (fō-tō-kī'mō-graf). A device for moving film at a constant speed so that a continuous record of a physiologic event may be obtained, as by a beam of light shining on the film. [photo- + G. *kyma*, wave, + *graphō*, to record]

pho·to·lith·o·troph (fō'tō-lith'ō-trof). An organism that requires inorganic compounds and that uses light for most of its energy need. Cf. photoautotroph, photoheterotroph, phototroph. [photo- + G. *lithos*, stone, mineral, + *trophē*, nourishment]

pho·tol·o·gy (fō-tol'ō-jē). The science of light production and energy, especially in its therapeutic application. [photo- + G. *logos*, study]

pho·to·lu·mi·nes·cent (fō'tō-lū-mi-nes'ent). Having the ability to become luminescent upon exposure to visible light. [photo- + L. *lumen*, light]

pho·to·ly·ase (fō-tō-lī'ās). SEE deoxyribodipyrimidine photolyase. [photo- + G. *lyo*, to loosen, + -ase]

pho·tol·y·sis (fō-tol'i-sis). Decomposition of a chemical compound by the action of light. [photo- + G. *lysis*, dissolution]

pho·to·lyte (fō'tō-līt). Any product of decomposition by light.

pho·to·lyt·ic (fō-tō-lit'ik). Pertaining to photolysis.

pho·to·mac·rog·ra·phy (fō'tō-mă-krog'ră-fē). A technique for investigating and recording conditions and procedures involving small objects that ordinarily would be inspected through a loupe rather than a microscope. [photo- + G. *makros*, large, + *graphō*, to write]

pho·to·ma·nia (fō-tō-mā'nē-ă). Morbid or exaggerated desire for light. [photo- + G. *mania*, frenzy]

pho·tom·e·ter (fō-tom'ĕ-ter). An instrument designed to measure the intensity of light or to determine the light threshold. [photo- + G. *metron*, measure]

flame p., an instrument that uses flame emission spectrophotometry to measure the intensity and other properties of light.

flicker p., an instrument that compares two variable visual stimuli through control of the frequency of a flickering light.

pho·tom·e·try (fō-tom'ĕ-trē). The measurement of the intensity of light.

pho·to·mi·cro·graph (fō'tō-mī'krō-graf). An enlarged photograph of an object viewed with a microscope, as distinguished from microphotograph. SYN micrograph (2). [photo- + G. *mikros*, small, + *graphē*, a record]

pho·to·mi·crog·ra·phy (fō'tō-mī-krog'ră-fē). The production of a photomicrograph. SYN micrography (3).

pho·to·my·oc·lo·nus (fō'tō-mī-ok'lō-nŭs). Clonic spasms of muscles in response to visual stimuli. [photo- + G. *mys*, muscle, + *klonos*, confused motion]

hereditary p. [MIM*172500], p. associated with diabetes mellitus, deafness, nephropathy, and cerebral dyfunction.

pho·ton (hν, γ) (fō'ton). In physics, a corpuscle of energy or particle of light; a quantum of light or other electromagnetic radiation.

pho·ton·cia (fō-ton'sē-ă). Any swelling resulting from the intense action of light. [photo- + G. *onkos*, a mass (tumor)]

pho·ton·o·sus (fō-ton'ō-sŭs). Any disease caused by excessive exposure to or unusual intensity of light, or resulting from phototoxicity or photoallergy. SYN photopathy. [photo- + G. *nosos*, disease]

pho·top·a·thy (fō-top'ă-thē). SYN photonosus. [photo- + G. *pathos*, suffering]

pho·to·peak (fō'tō-pēk). The characteristic energies of photons emitted by a radionuclide, used to set scanning parameters.

pho·to·per·cep·tive (fō'tō-per-sep'tiv). Capable of both receiving and perceiving light.

pho·to·pe·ri·od·ism (fō'tō-pēr'ē-ō-dizm). The periodic (seasonal or diurnal) activities, behavior, or changes in plants or animals brought about by the action of light.

pho·to·pho·bia (fō-tō-fō'bē-ă). Morbid dread and avoidance of light. Although often an expression of undue anxiety about the eyes, photosensitivity and photalgia, past or present, should be considered. [photo- + G. *phobos*, fear]

pho·to·pho·bic (fō-tō-fō'bik). Relating to or suffering from photophobia.

pho·to·phore (fō'tō-fōr). **1.** A lamp with reflector used in laryngoscopy and in the examination of other internal parts of the body. **2.** In bacteriology, the organ producing intracellular bioluminescence in certain organisms. [photo- + G. *phoros*, bearing]

pho·to·pho·re·sis. SEE extracorporeal p.

extracorporeal p., destruction of cells separated from blood in an extracorporeal flow system by ultraviolet activation of chemotherapeutic agents such as psoralens.

pho·to·phos·pho·ry·la·tion (fō-tō-fos'fōr-i-lā'shŭn). Formation of ATP as a result of absorption of light.

pho·toph·thal·mia (fō'tof-thal'mē-ă). Keratoconjunctivitis caused by ultraviolet energy, as in snow blindness, exposure to an ultraviolet lamp, arc welding, or the short circuit of a high-tension electric current. SEE ALSO photoretinopathy. [photo- + G. *ophthalmos*, eye]

pho·to·pia (fō-tō'pē-ă). SYN photopic *vision*. [photo- + G. *opsis*, vision]

pho·top·ic (fō-top'ik). Pertaining to photopic vision.

pho·top·sia (fō-top'sē-ă). A subjective sensation of lights, sparks, or colors due to electrical or mechanical stimulation of the ocular system. SEE ALSO Moore's lightning *streaks*, under *streak*. SYN photopsy. [photo- + G. *opsis*, vision]

pho·top·sin (fō-top'sin). The protein moiety (opsin) of the pigment (iodopsin) in the cones of the retina.

pho·top·sy (fō-top'sē). SYN photopsia.

pho·to·ptar·mo·sis (fō'tō-tar-mō'sis). Reflex sneezing that occurs when bright light stimulates the retina. [photo- + G. *ptarmos*, a sneezing, + -osis, condition]

pho·to·ra·di·a·tion (fō'tō-rā-dē-ā'shŭn). Treatment of cancer by intravenous injection of a photosensitizing agent, such as hematoporphyrin, followed by exposure to visible light of superficial tumors or of deep tumors by a fiberoptic probe. SYN photochemotherapy, photoradiation therapy.

pho·to·re·ac·tion (fō'tō-rē-ak'shŭn). A reaction caused or affected by light; *e.g.,* a photochemical reaction, photolysis, photosynthesis, phototropism, thymine dimer formation.

pho·to·re·ac·ti·va·tion (fō'tō-rē-ak-ti-vā'shŭn). Activation by light of something or of some process previously inactive or inactivated; *e.g.,* pyrimidine dimers, formed in polynucleic acids by the action of UV light, can be monomerized by UV light of a different wavelength.

pho·to·re·cep·tive (fō'tō-rē-sep'tiv). Functioning as a photoreceptor.

pho·to·re·cep·tor (fō'tō-rē-sep'ter, tōr). A receptor that is sensitive to light, *e.g.,* a retinal rod or cone. SYN photoceptor. [photo- + L. *re-cipio*, pp. *-ceptus*, to receive, fr. *capio*, to take]

pho·to·res·pir·a·tion (fō'tō-res-pir-ā'shŭn). Light enhanced respiration in photosynthetic organisms; *i.e.,* light increases O_2 utilization.

pho·to·ret·i·ni·tis (fō'tō-ret'i-nī'tis). SEE photoretinopathy.

pho·to·ret·i·nop·a·thy (fō'tō-ret'i-nop'ă-thē). A macular burn from excessive exposure to sunlight or other intense light (*e.g.,* the flash of a short circuit); characterized subjectively by reduced visual acuity. SEE ALSO solar *maculopathy*. SYN electric retinopathy, solar retinopathy. [photo- + retina, + G. *pathos*, suffering]

pho·to·scan (fō'tō-skan). SYN scintiscan.

pho·to·sen·si·tive (fō-tō-sensi-tiv). **1.** An abnormally heightened reactivity of the skin to sunlight. **2.** Responding to light,

ph

e.g., ,as by a photocell. [photo + L. *sensus,* a feeling, fr. *sentio,* to feel]

pho·to·sen·si·tiv·i·ty (fō'tō-sen-si-tiv'i-tē). Abnormal sensitivity to light, especially of the eyes. For example, light may irritate the eyelids, conjunctiva, cornea or, in excess, the retina; when scattered by a cataractous lens light may produce glare; it can produce a migraine headache or a temporary exotropia. SEE photophobia, photalgia, photesthesia.

pho·to·sen·si·ti·za·tion (fō'tō-sen-si-ti-zā'shŭn). **1.** Sensitization of the skin to light, usually due to the action of certain drugs, plants, or other substances; may occur shortly after administration of the drug (phototoxic sensitivity), or may occur only after a latent period of from days to months (photoallergic sensitivity, or photoallergy). **2.** SYN photodynamic *sensitization.*

pho·to·sen·sor (fō'tō-sen'ser, sōr). A device designed to respond to light and to transmit resulting impulses for interpretation, movement, or operating control. SEE sensor.

pho·to·sta·ble (fō'tō-stā-bl). Not subject to change upon exposure to light.

pho·to·steth·o·scope (fō-tō-steth'ō-skōp). Device that converts sound into flashes of light; used for continuous observation of the fetal heart.

pho·to·stress (fō'tō-stres). Exposure to intense illumination. SEE ALSO photostress *test.*

pho·to·syn·the·sis (fō-tō-sin'thĕ-sis). **1.** The compounding or building up of chemical substances under the influence of light. **2.** The process by which green plants, using chlorophyll and the energy of sunlight, produce carbohydrates from water and carbon dioxide, liberating molecular oxygen in the process. [photo- + G. *synthesis,* a putting together]

bacterial p., a primitive form of p. observed in some bacteria using only one photosystem and some reducing agent other than water.

pho·to·tax·is (fō-tō-tak'sis). Reaction of living protoplasm to the stimulus of light, involving bodily motion of the whole organism toward (**positive p.**) or away from (**negative p.**) the stimulus. Cf. phototropism. [photo- + G. *taxis,* orderly arrangement]

pho·to·ther·a·py (fō-tō-thār'ă-pē). Treatment of disease by means of light rays. SYN light treatment, lucotherapy.

pho·to·ther·mal (fō-tō-ther'măl). Relating to radiant heat. [photo- + G. *thermē,* heat]

pho·to·tim·er (fō-tō-tīm'ĕr). An electronic device in radiography that measures the radiation that has passed through the patient and terminates the x-ray exposure when it is sufficient to form an image.

pho·to·tox·ic (fō-tō-tok'sik). Relating to, characterized by, or causing phototoxis.

pho·to·tox·is (fō-tō-tok'sis). The condition resulting from an overexposure to ultraviolet light, or from the combination of exposure to certain wavelengths of light and a phototoxic substance. SEE ALSO photosensitization. [photo- + G. *toxikon,* poison]

pho·to·troph (fō'tō-trōf). An organism that uses light for its energy needs. Cf. photoautotroph, photoheterotroph, photolithotroph.

pho·tot·ro·pism (fō-to'trō-pizm). Movement of a part of an organism toward (**positive p.**) or away from (**negative p.**) the stimulus of light. Cf. phototaxis. [photo- + G. *tropē,* a turning]

pho·tu·ria (fō-tū'rē-ă). The passage of phosphorescent urine. [photo- + G. *ouron,* urine]

phrag·mo·plast (frag'mō-plast). Barrel-shaped enlargement of the spindle associated with formation of the new cell membrane during telophase in plant cells. [G. *phragma,* hedge, enclosure, + *plassō,* to form]

phren (fren). **1.** SYN diaphragm (1). **2.** The mind. [G. *phrēn,* the diaphragm, mind, heart (as seat of emotions)]

△**phren-.** SEE phreno-.

phre·nal·gia (fre-nal'jē-ă). **1.** SYN psychalgia (1). **2.** Pain in the diaphragm. [phren- + G. *algos,* pain]

phre·nec·to·my (fre-nek'tō-mē). SYN phrenicectomy.

phren·em·phrax·is (fren'em-frak'sis). SYN phreniclasia. [phren- + G. *emphraxis,* a stoppage]

phre·net·ic (frĕ-net'ik). **1.** Frenzied; maniacal. **2.** An individual exhibiting such behavior. [G. *phrenitikos,* frenzied]

△**phreni-.** SEE phreno-.

△**-phrenia.** The diaphragm. 2. The mind. SEE phreno-. [G. *phrēn,* the diaphragm, mind, heart (as seat of emotions)]

phren·ic (fren'ik). **1.** SYN diaphragmatic. **2.** Relating to the mind.

phren·i·cec·to·my (fren-i-sek'tō-mē). Exsection of a portion of the phrenic nerve, to prevent reunion such as may follow phrenicotomy. SYN phrenectomy, phrenicoexeresis, phreniconeurectomy. [phreni- + G. *ektomē,* excision]

phren·i·cla·sia (fren-i-klā'zē-ă). Crushing of a section of the phrenic nerve to produce a temporary paralysis of the diaphragm. SYN phrenemphraxis, phrenicotripsy. [phreni- + G. *klasis,* a breaking away]

phren·i·co·col·ic (fren'i-kō-kol'ik). Relating to the diaphragm and the colon. SYN phrenocolic.

phren·i·co·ex·er·e·sis (fren'i-kō-ek-ser'ĕ-sis). SYN phrenicectomy. [phrenico- + G. *exairesis,* a taking out, fr. *haireō,* to take, grasp]

phren·i·co·gas·tric (fren'i-kō-gas'trik). Relating to the diaphragm and the stomach. SYN phrenogastric.

phren·i·co·glot·tic (fren'i-kō-glo'tik). Relating to the diaphragm and the glottis; denoting a spasm involving the diaphragm and the vocal cords.

phren·i·co·he·pa·tic (fren'i-kō-he-pa'tik). Relating to the diaphragm and the liver. SYN phrenohepatic.

phren·i·co·neu·rec·to·my (fren'i-kō-nū-rek'tō-mē). SYN phrenicectomy.

phren·i·co·splen·ic (fren'i-kō-splen'ik). Relating to the diaphragm and the spleen.

phren·i·cot·o·my (fren-i-kot'ō-mē). Section of the phrenic nerve in order to induce unilateral paralysis of the diaphragm, which is then pushed up by the abdominal viscera and exerts compression upon a diseased lung. [phrenico- + G. *tomē,* incision]

phren·i·co·trip·sy (fren'i-kō-trip'sē). SYN phreniclasia. [phrenico- + G. *tripsis,* a rubbing]

△**phreno-, phren-, phreni-, phrenico-.** The diaphragm; the mind; the phrenic nerve. [G. *phrēn,* diaphragm, mind, heart (as seat of emotions)]

phren·o·car·dia (fren-ō-kar'dē-ă). Precordial pain and dyspnea of psychogenic origin, often a symptom of anxiety neurosis. SEE cardiac *neurosis.* SYN cardiophrenia. [phreno- + G. *kardia,* heart]

phren·o·col·ic (fren'ō-kol'ik). SYN phrenicocolic. [phreno- + G. *kolon,* colon]

phren·o·col·o·pexy (fren-ō-kol'ō-pek-sē, -kō'lō-). An obsolete procedure involving suture of a displaced or prolapsed transverse colon to the diaphragm. [phreno- + G. *kolon,* colon, + *pēxis,* fixation]

phren·o·gas·tric (fren-ō-gas'trik). SYN phrenicogastric. [phreno- + G. *gastēr,* stomach]

phren·o·graph (fren'ō-graf). An instrument for recording graphically the movements of the diaphragm. [phreno- + G. *graphō,* to record]

phren·o·he·pat·ic (fren'ō-hĕ-pat'ik). SYN phrenicohepatic. [phreno- + G. *hepar,* liver]

phre·nol·o·gist (frĕ-nol'ō-jist). One who claims to be able to diagnose mental and behavioral characteristics by a study of the external configuration of the skull. [see phrenology]

phre·nol·o·gy (frĕ-nol'ō-jē). An obsolete doctrine that each of the mental faculties is located in a definite part of the cerebral cortex, the size of which part varies in a direct ratio with the development and strength of the corresponding faculty, this size being indicated by the external configuration of the skull. SYN craniognomy, Gall's craniology. [phreno- + G. *logos,* study]

phren·o·ple·gia (fren-ō-plē'jē-ă). Paralysis of the diaphragm. [phreno- + G. *plēgē,* stroke]

phren·op·to·sia (fren-op-tō'sē-ă). An abnormal sinking down of the diaphragm. [phreno- + G. *ptōsis,* a falling]

phren·o·sin (fren'ō-sin). A cerebroside abundant in white matter of the brain, composed of cerebronic acid, D-galactose, and sphingosine. SYN cerebron.

phren·o·sin·ic ac·id (fren-ō-sin′ik). SYN cerebronic acid.

phren·o·spasm (fren′ō-spazm). SYN esophageal *achalasia*. [phreno- + G. *spasmos*, spasm]

phren·o·tro·pic (fren-ō-trop′ik). Affecting or working through the mind or brain. [phreno- + G. *tropē*, a turning]

phric·to·path·ic (frik′tō-path′ik). Relating to a peculiar sensation, accompanied by shuddering, provoked by stimulation of a hysterical anesthetic area during the process of recovery. [G. *phriktos*, causing a shudder, fr. *phrissō*, to bristle, shudder, + *pathos*, suffering]

phryn·o·der·ma (frin-ō-der′mă). A follicular hyperkeratotic eruption thought to be due to deficiency of vitamin A. SYN toad skin. [G. *phrynos*, toad, + *derma*, skin]

phry·nol·y·sin (frĭ-nol′ĭ-sin). The poison of the fire-toad (*Bombinator igneus*). [G. *phrynos*, toad, + *lysis*, solution]

PHS Abbreviation for Public Health Service.

pH-stat. A device for continuously sensing the pH of a solution and automatically adding acid or alkali as necessary to keep the pH constant; used to follow the time course of reactions that liberate an acid or alkali.

o-phtha·lal·de·hyde (thal-al′de-hīd). $C_6H_4(CHO)_2$; a reagent used in the identification and the detection of amino acid. SYN *o*-benzenedialdehyde.

phthal·ein (thal′ē-in). One of a group of highly colored compounds based on a triphenylmethyl base; *e.g.*, phenolphthalein.

phthal·ic ac·id (thal′ik). *o*-Benzenedicarboxylic acid; $C_6H_4(COOH)_2$.

phthal·o·yl (thal′ō-il). $-OC-C_6H_4-CO-$; the diacyl radical of phthalic acid.

phthal·yl (thal′il). $-OC-C_6H_4-COOH$; the monoacyl radical of phthalic acid.

phthal·yl·sul·fa·cet·a·mide (thal′il-sŭl-fă-set′ă-mīd). N^1-acetyl-N^4-phthalylsulfanilamide; a sulfonamide used in the treatment of enteric infections.

phthal·yl·sul·fa·thi·a·zole (thal′il-sŭl-fă-thī′ă-zōl). 2-(N^4-Phthalylsulfanilamido)thiazole; a sulfonamide used in the treatment of enteric infections.

phthin·oid (thin′oyd). **1.** Obsolete term for wasting; consumptive; relating to or resembling phthisis. **2.** SYN chest. [G. *phthinōdēs*, consumptive]

phthi·ri·o·pho·bia (thī′rē-ō-fō′bē-ă). SYN pediculophobia. [G. *phtheir*, louse, + *phobos*, fear]

Phthi·rus (thī′rŭs). SEE *Pthirus*. [L. *phthir*; G. *phtheir*, a louse]

phthis·ic, phthis·i·cal (tiz′ik, -i-kăl). Obsolete terms relating to phthisis. [G. *phthisikos*, consumptive]

△**phthisio-.** Obsolete phthisis (tuberculosis). [G. *phthisis*, a wasting]

phthis·i·ol·o·gist (tī-ē-ō-ol′ō-jist). Obsolete term for specialist in tuberculosis.

phthi·sis (thī′sis, tī′sis). **1.** Obsolete term for a wasting or atrophy, local or general. **2.** Obsolete term for consumption or, specifically, tuberculosis of the lungs. [G. a wasting]

    aneurysmal p., the clinical picture of chest pain, cough with or without sputum, and hemoptysis sometimes produced by aortic aneurysm; reminiscent of an advanced tuberculous syndrome.

    p. bul′bi, shrinkage of the eyeball after uveitis or other inflammatory disease.

    essential p. bul′bi, a softening of the eyeball (ophthalmomalacia) and reduction in size, not due to inflammation.

    marble cutters' p., obsolete term for calcicosis.

△**phyco-.** Seaweed. [G. *phykos*]

Phy·co·my·ce·tes (fī′kō-mī-sē′tēz). SYN Zygomycetes. [phyco- + G. *mykēs*, fungus]

phy·co·my·ce·to·sis (fī′kō-mī-sē-tō′sis). SYN zygomycosis.

phy·co·my·co·sis (fī′kō-mī′kō-sis). SYN zygomycosis.

    subcutaneous p., SYN entomophthoramycosis.

phy·go·ga·lac·tic (fī-gō-gă-lak′tik). SYN lactifuge. [G. *phygē*, flight, + *gala* (*galakt*-), milk]

phy·lac·a·gog·ic (fī-lak-ă-goj′ik). Stimulating the production of protective antibodies. [G. *phylaxis*, a guarding, protection, + *agogos*, leading]

phy·lax·is (fī-lak′sis). Protection against infection. [G. a guarding, protection]

phy·let·ic (fī-let′ik). Denoting the evolution of sequential changes in a line of descent by which one species is transformed into a new species. [G. *phyletikos*, tribal, fr. *phylē*, a tribe]

△**phyllo-.** A leaf; leaf-like; chlorophyll. [G. *phyllon*, foliage]

phyl·lode (fil′ōd). A flattened leaflike petiole; applied to any structure resembling a leaf, especially to a cross section of a neoplasm with a foliated structure, such as cystosarcoma phyllodes. [G. *phyllōdēs*, like leaves, fr. *phyllon*, leaf, + *eidos*, resemblance]

phyl·lo·qui·none (K), phyl·lo·qui·none K (fil-ō-kwin′ōn, -kwī′nōn). Vitamin K_1 or $K_1(20)$; 2-methyl-3-phytyl-1,4-naphthoquinone; 3-phytylmenaquinone; isolated from alfalfa; also prepared synthetically; major form of vitamin K found in plants. SYN phytomenadione, phytonadione, vitamin K_1, vitamin $K_1(20)$.

    p. reductase, SYN NADPH dehydrogenase (quinone).

△**phylo-.** Tribe, race; a taxonomic phylum. [G. *phylon*, tribe]

phy·lo·a·nal·y·sis (fī′lō-ă-nal′i-sis). **1.** The study of bioracial origins. **2.** A rarely used term for a method of investigating individual and collective behavioral disorders putatively arising from impaired tensional processes. [phylo- + analysis]

phy·lo·gen·e·sis (fī-lō-jen′ĕ-sis). SYN phylogeny. [phylo- + G. *genesis*, origin]

phy·lo·ge·net·ic, phy·lo·gen·ic (fī′lō-jĕ-net′ik, -jen′ik). Relating to phylogenesis.

phy·log·e·ny (fī-loj′ĕ-nē). The evolutionary development of species, as distinguished from ontogeny, development of the individual. SYN phylogenesis.

phy·lum, pl. **phy·la** (fī′lŭm, fī′lă). A taxonomic division below the kingdom and above the class. [Mod. L. fr. G. *phylon*, tribe]

phy·ma (fī′mă). A nodule or small rounded tumor of the skin. [G. a tumor]

phy·ma·toid (fī′mă-toyd). Resembling a neoplasm. [G. *phyma*, a tumor, + *eidos*, resemblance]

phy·ma·tor·rhy·sin (fi′mă-tōr′i-sin). A variety of melanin obtained from certain melanotic neoplasms, and from hair and other heavily pigmented parts. [G. *phyma* (*phymat*-), tumor, + *rhysis*, a flowing]

phy·ma·to·sis (fī-mă-tō′sis). The growth or the presence of phymas or small nodules in the skin.

Phy·sa (fī′să). Type genus of the freshwater pulmonate snails (family Physidae), which includes several common American species such as *P. parkeri, P. gyrina,* and *P. integra;* they are intermediate hosts of a number of bird and animal trematodes, including several that cause schistosome dermatitis in humans. [G. a pair of bellows; an air bubble; bladder]

phys·a·lif·er·ous (fis-ă-lif′er-ŭs). SYN physaliphorous.

phy·sal·i·form (fi-sal′i-fōrm). Like a bubble or small bleb. [G. *physallis*, bladder, bubble, + L. *forma*, form]

phy·sal·i·phore (fi-sal′i-fōr). A mother cell, or giant cell containing a large vacuole, in a malignant growth. [G. *physallis*, bladder, bubble, + *phoros*, bearing]

phys·a·liph·or·ous (fis-ă-lif′ŏr-ŭs). Having bubbles or vacuoles.

△ Combining forms	[NA] Nomina Anatomica
Word*Finder*	[MIM] Mendelian
Multi-term entry finder	**Inheritance in Man**
Preceding letter A	
A.D.A.M. Anatomy Plates	☆ **Official alternate term**
Between letters L and M	
Appendices:	☆[NA] **Official alternate**
Following letter Z	**Nomina Anatomica term**
SYN Synonym; Cf., compare	**High Profile Term**

SYN **physaliferous.** [G. *physallis,* bladder, bubble, + *phoros,* bearing]

phys·a·lis (fis'ă-lis). A vacuole in a giant cell found in certain malignant neoplasms, such as chordoma. [G. *physallis,* a bladder]

Phy·sa·lop·tera (fī'să-lop'ter-ă, fis-). A large genus of spiruroid roundworms parasitic in the stomach and duodenum of vertebrates, especially birds and mammals; they are transmitted via insect and annelid intermediate hosts and are frequently pathogenic, causing erosions and catarrhal gastritis. *P. caucasica* is a species reported in man in the southern part of the area formerly known as the USSR; *P. mordens* is a species from tropical Africa found only rarely in the esophagus, stomach, and intestine of man (probably cases of temporary infection from ingestion of infected insects). [G. *physallis,* bladder, + *pteron,* wing]

phy·sa·lop·ter·i·a·sis (fī'să-lop-ter-ī'ă-sis). Infection of animals and man with nematodes of the genus *Physaloptera.*

phys·e·al (fiz'ē-ăl). Pertaining to the physis, or growth cartilage area, separating the metaphysis and the epiphysis.

⌂**physi-.** SEE physio-.

phys·i·at·ric·i·an (fix'ē-ă-trish'ŭn). A physician who specializes in physiatry (rehabilitation medicine).

phys·i·at·rics (fiz-ē-at'riks). **1.** Old term for physical *therapy.* **2.** Rehabilitation management. [G. *physis,* nature, + *iatrikos,* healing]

phys·i·a·trist (fiz-ī'ă-trist). A physician who specializes in physical medicine.

phys·i·a·try (fi-zī'ă-trē). SYN physical *medicine.*

phys·ic (fiz'ik). **1.** The art of medicine. **2.** A medicine; often a lay term for a cathartic. [G. *physikos,* natural, physical]

phys·i·cal (fiz'i-kăl). Relating to the body, as distinguished from the mind. [Mod. L. *physicalis,* fr. G. *physikos*]

phy·si·cian (fi-zish'ŭn). **1.** A doctor; a person who has been educated, trained, and licensed to practice the art and science of medicine. **2.** A practitioner of medicine, as contrasted with a surgeon. [Fr. *physicien,* a natural philosopher]

attending p., (1) p. responsible for the care of a patient; (2) p. supervising the care of patients by interns, residents, and/or medical students. (3) a doctor who has completed internship and residency.

family p., a p. who specializes in family practice.

osteopathic p., a practitioner of osteopathy. SYN osteopath.

resident p., SYN resident.

phy·si·cian as·sis·tant (P.A.). A person who is trained, certified, and licensed to perform history taking, physical examination, diagnosis, and treatment of commonly encountered medical problems, and certain technical skills, under the supervision of a licensed physician, and who thereby extends the physician's capacity to provide medical care. Many subspecialties exist, such as orthopedist's assistant, sports injury assistant, pediatrician's assistant, etc.

Physick, Philip Syng, U.S. surgeon, 1768–1837. SEE P.'s *pouches,* under *pouch.*

phys·i·co·chem·i·cal (fiz'i-kō-kem'i-kăl). Relating to the field of physical chemistry.

phys·ics (fiz'iks). The branch of science concerned with the phenomena of matter and energy and their interactions. SEE physic.

radiation p., the scientific discipline of the application of p. to the use of ionizing radiation in therapy and in diagnostic radiology; including, by extension, nuclear medicine applications, ultrasound, and magnetic resonance imaging.

⌂**physio-, physi-.** Physical, physiological; 2. Natural, relating to physics. [G. *physis,* nature]

phys·i·o·gen·ic (fiz'ē-ō-jen'ik). Related to or caused by physiologic activity. [physio- + G. *genesis,* origin]

phys·i·og·no·my (fiz-ē-og'nō-mē). **1.** The physical appearance of one's face, countenance, or habitus, especially regarded as an indication of character. **2.** Estimation of one's character and mental qualities by a study of the face and other external bodily features. [physio- + G. *gnōmōn,* a judge]

phys·i·og·no·sis (fiz-ē-og-nō'sis). Diagnosis of disease based upon a study of the facial appearance or bodily habitus. [physio- + G. *gnōsis,* knowledge]

phys·i·o·log·ic, phys·i·o·log·i·cal (fiz-ē-ō-loj'ik, -loj'i-kăl). **1.** Relating to physiology. **2.** Normal, as opposed to pathologic; denoting the various vital processes. **3.** Denoting something that is apparent from its functional effects rather than from its anatomical structure; *e.g.,* a p. sphincter. **4.** Denoting a dose or the effects of such a dose (of a chemical agent that either is or mimics a hormone, neurotransmitter, or other naturally occurring agent) that is within the range of concentrations or potencies that would occur naturally. Cf. homeopathic (2), pharmacologic (2), supraphysiologic.

phys·i·o·log·i·co·an·a·tom·i·cal (fiz'ē-ō-loj'i-kō-an-ă-tom'i-kăl). Relating to both physiology and anatomy.

phys·i·ol·o·gist (fiz-ē-ol'ō-jist). A specialist in physiology.

phys·i·ol·o·gy (fiz-ē-ol'ō-jē). The science concerned with the normal vital processes of animal and vegetable organisms, especially as to how things normally function in the living organism rather than to their anatomical structure, their biochemical composition, or how they are affected by drugs or disease. [L. or G. *physiologia,* fr. G. *physis,* nature, + *logos,* study]

comparative p., the science concerned with the differences in the vital processes in different species of organisms, particularly with a view to the adaptation of the processes to the specific needs of the species, to illuminating the evolutionary relationships among different species, or to establishing other interspecific generalizations and relationships.

general p., the science of the functions or vital processes common to almost all living things, whether animal or plant, as opposed to aspects of p. peculiar to particular types of animals or plants, or to the application of p. to applied sciences such as medicine and agriculture.

hominal p., p. as applied to the elucidation of the normal functions of the human being.

pathologic p., that part of the science of disease concerned with disordered function, as distinguished from anatomical lesions. SYN physiopathology.

phys·i·o·med·i·cal (fiz-ē-ō-med'i-kăl). Denoting the use of physical rather than medicinal measures in the treatment of disease.

phys·i·o·path·o·log·ic (fiz'ē-ō-path-ō-loj'ik). Relating to pathologic physiology.

phys·i·o·pa·thol·o·gy (fiz'ē-ō-pă-thol'ō-jē). SYN pathologic *physiology.*

phys·i·o·psy·chic (fiz'ē-ō-sī'kik). Pertaining to both mind and body.

phys·i·o·py·rex·i·a (fiz'ē-ō-pī-rek'sē-ă). Fever produced by a physical agent. [physio- + G. *pyrexis,* feverishness]

phys·i·o·ther·a·peu·tic (fiz'ē-ō-thār-ă-pyū'tik). Pertaining to physical *therapy.*

phys·i·o·ther·a·pist (fiz'ē-ō-thār'ă-pist). A physical therapist. SEE physical *therapy* (2).

phys·i·o·ther·a·py (fiz'ē-ō-thār'ă-pē). SYN physical *therapy* (1). [physio- + G. *therapeia,* treatment]

oral p., the use of a toothbrush, interdental stimulator, floss, irrigating device, or other adjunctive aid to maintain oral health.

phy·sique (fi-zēk'). constitutional type; the physical or bodily structure; the "build." [Fr.]

phy·sis (fī'sis). A term sometimes used in referring to the epiphysial cartilage. [G. growth]

⌂**physo-.** **1.** Tendency to swell or inflate. **2.** Relation to air or gas. [G. *physaō,* to inflate, distend]

phy·so·cele (fī'sō-sēl). **1.** A circumscribed swelling due to the presence of gas. **2.** A hernial sac distended with gas. [physo- + G. *kēlē,* tumor, hernia]

Phy·so·ceph·a·lus sex·a·la·tus (fī'sō-sef'ă-lŭs sek'să-lā'tŭs). A small species of spiruroid nematodes (family Spiruridae) found in the stomach of pigs, horses, camels, rabbits, and hares; worldwide in distribution, and especially prevalent in hogs. [G. *physa,* bellows, + *kephalē,* head]

phy·so·ceph·a·ly (fī-sō-sef'ă-lē). Swelling of the head resulting from introduction of air into the subcutaneous tissues. [physo- + G. *kephalē,* head]

phy·so·me·tra (fī-sō-mē'tră). Distention of the uterine cavity with air or gas. SYN uterine tympanites. [physo- + G. *mētra,* uterus]

Phy·sop·sis (fī-sop'sis). A subgenus of the genus *Bulinus,* most species of which transmit the human blood fluke, *Schistosoma haematobium,* and some animal schistosomes in Africa south of the Sahara. [G. *physis,* growth, + *opsis,* aspect, appearance]

phy·so·py·o·sal·pinx (fī'sō-pī-ō-sal'pingks). Pyosalpinx accompanied by a formation of gas in a fallopian tube. [physo- + G. *pyon,* pus, + *salpinx,* trumpet]

phy·so·stig·ma (fī-sō-stig'mă). The dried seed of *Physostigma venenosum* (family Leguminosae), a vine of western Africa; it contains the alkaloids physostigmine (eserine), eseramine, eseridine (geneserine) and physovenine; in toxic doses it causes vomiting, colic, salivation, diarrhea, convulsions, sweating, dyspnea, vertigo, slow pulse, and extreme prostration. SYN Calabar bean, ordeal bean. [G. *physa,* bellows, + *stigma,* a mark, spot; so called because of the shape of the stigma]

phy·so·stig·mine (fī-sō-stig'mēn, -min). An alkaloid of physostigma; it is a reversible inhibitor of the cholinesterases, and prevents destruction of acetylcholine; used as a cholinergic agent, and experimentally to enhance the action of acetylcholine at any of its sites of liberation. SYN eserine.

p. salicylate, used by conjunctival instillation to reduce tension in glaucoma, in the treatment of postoperative intestinal atony and urinary retention, in the management of myasthenia gravis, and to counteract excessive doses of tubocurarine; also available as p. sulfate, with the same uses. SYN eserine salicylate.

phyt-. SEE phyto-.

phy·tan·ate (fī'tan-āt). The anion of phytanic acid.

p. α-oxidase, An enzyme that oxidizes phytanic acid, removing the carboxyl group.

phy·tan·ic ac·id (fī-tan'ik). 3,7,11,15-Tetramethylhexadecanoic acid; an acid that accumulates in the serum and tissues in Refsum's disease and attributed to the hereditary absence of phytanate α-oxidase; arises from phytol and acts as an inhibitor of the α-oxidation of palmitic (hexadecanoic) acid; it also accumulates in a number of other disorders, notably peroxisomal disorders.

6-phy·tase (fī'tās). Phytate 6-phosphate; an enzyme hydrolyzing phytic acid, removing the 6-phosphoric group, thus producing orthophosphate and 1L-*myo*-1,2,3,4,5-pentakisphosphate.

phy·tate (fī'tāt). A salt or ester of phytic acid.

phy·tic ac·id (fī'tik). The hexakisphosphoric ester of *myo*-inositol; the mixed salt with magnesium and calcium is phytin.

phy·tin (fī'tin). The calcium magnesium salt of phytic acid; a dietary supplement used to provide calcium, organic phosphorus, and *myo*-inositol.

phyto-, phyt-. Plants. [G. *phyton,* a plant]

phy·to·ag·glu·ti·nin (fī'tō-ă-glū'ti-nin). A lectin that causes agglutination of erythrocytes or of leukocytes.

phy·to·be·zoar (fī-tō-bē'zōr). A gastric concretion formed of vegetable fibers, with the seeds and skins of fruits, and sometimes starch granules and fat globules. SYN food ball. [phyto- + bezoar]

phy·to·chem·is·try (fī-tō-kem'is-trē). The biochemical study of plants; concerned with the identification, biosynthesis, and metabolism of chemical constituents of plants; especially in regard to natural products.

phy·to·der·ma·ti·tis (fī'tō-der-mă-tī'tis). Dermatitis caused by various mechanisms including mechanical and chemical injury, allergy, or photosensitization (phytophotodermatitis) at skin sites previously exposed to plants.

Phy·to·fla·gel·la·ta (fī'tō-flaj-ĕ-lā'tă). A subclass of Phytomastigophorea, the members of which have yellow or green chromatophores. [phyto- + L. *flagellum,* a whip]

phy·to·hem·ag·glu·ti·nin (PHA) (fī'tō-hēm-ă-glū'ti-nin). A phytomitogen from plants that agglutinates red blood cells. The term is commonly used specifically for the lectin obtained from the red kidney bean (*Phaseolus vulgaris*) which is also a mitogen

that stimulates T lymphocytes more vigorously than B lymphocytes. SYN phytolectin.

phy·toid (fī'toyd). Resembling a plant; denoting an animal having many of the biologic characteristics of a vegetable. [G. *phytōdēs,* fr. *phyton,* plant, + *eidos,* resemblance]

phy·tol (fī'tol). 3,7,11,15-tetramethyl-2-hexadecen-1-ol; an unsaturated primary alcohol derived from the hydrolysis of chlorophyll; a constituent of vitamins E and K_1. SYN phytyl alcohol.

phy·to·lec·tin (fī-tō-lek'tin). SYN phytohemagglutinin.

Phy·to·mas·ti·gi·na (fī'tō-mas-ti-jī'nă). Former term for plant-like flagellates, originally classified as a suborder or order, raised to the class Phytomastigophorea (Phytomastigophorasida) in recent classifications. [phyto- + G. *mastix,* whip]

Phy·to·mas·ti·go·pho·ras·i·da (fī'tō-mas'ti-gō-fō-ras'i-dă). SYN Phytomastigophorea.

Phy·to·mas·ti·goph·o·rea (fī'tō-mas'ti-gof-ō-rē'ă). A class of the subphylum Mastigophora (flagellates) within the phylum Sarcomastigophora (flagellate and ameboid protozoans), consisting mostly of free-living plantlike flagellates with or without chloroplasts, and usually with one or two flagella. Cf. Zoomastigophorea. SYN Phytomastigophorasida. [phyto- + G. *mastix,* whip, + *phoros,* bearing]

phy·to·men·a·di·one (fī'tō-men-ă-dī'ōn). SYN phylloquinone.

phy·to·mi·to·gen (fī-tō-mī'tō-jen). A mitogenic lectin causing lymphocyte transformation accompanied by mitotic proliferation of the resulting blast cells identical to that produced by antigenic stimulation; *e.g.,* phytohemagglutinin, concanavalin A.

phy·to·na·di·one (fī'tō-nā-dī'ōn). SYN phylloquinone.

phy·toph·a·gous (fī-tof'ă-gŭs). Plant-eating; vegetarian. [phyto- + G. *phagō,* to eat]

phy·to·phlyc·to·der·ma·ti·tis (fī'tō-flik'tō-der-mă-tī'tis). SYN meadow *dermatitis.* [phyto- + G. *phlyktaina,* blister, + dermatitis]

phy·to·pho·to·der·ma·ti·tis (fī'tō-fō'tō-der-mă-tī'tis). Phytodermatitis resulting from photosensitization.

phy·to·pneu·mo·co·ni·o·sis (fī'tō-nū'mō-kō-nē-ō'sis). A chronic fibrous reaction in the lungs due to the inhalation of dust particles of vegetable origin. [phyto- + pneumoconiosis]

phy·to·por·phy·rin (fī-tō-pōr'fī-rin). A porphyrin similar to the pheophorbide of the chlorophylls but with the vinyl group replaced by an ethyl group, with no methoxycarbonyl group, and minus two hydrogen atoms, producing one more double bond in ring D.

phy·to·sis (fī-tō-sis). A disease process caused by infection with a vegetable organism, such as a fungus.

phy·to·sphin·go·sine (fī-tō-sfing'gō-sēn, -sin). 4D-hydroxysphinganine; 4-hydroxydihydrosphingosine; a sphingosine derivative isolated from various plants.

phy·to·ste·rol (fi-tō-stēr'ol). Generic term for the sterols of plants.

phy·to·ste·ro·lem·ia (fī-tō-stēr'ol-ē-mē-ă). An inherited disorder in which there is a hyperabsorption of phytosterols and shell-fish sterols resulting in tendon and tuberous xanthomata.

phy·to·tox·ic (fī-tō-tok'sik). **1.** Poisonous to plant life. **2.** Pertaining to a phytotoxin.

phy·to·tox·in (fī-tō-tok'sin). A substance similar in its properties to an extracellular bacterial toxin. SYN plant toxin. [phyto- + G. *toxikon,* poison]

phy·to·trich·o·be·zoar (fī'tō-trik'ō-bē'zōr). SYN trichophytobezoar.

phy·tyl (fī'til). The radical, –CH₂–CH=C(CH₃)–CH₂-[-CH₂–CH₂–CH(CH₃)–CH₂-]₃H, found in phylloquinone (vitamin K_1); a tetraprenyl radical, reduced in 3 of the 4 prenyl groups.

phy·tyl al·co·hol. SYN phytol.

PI Abbreviation for Periodontal Index.

Pi. Abbreviation for inorganic *phosphate.*

pI The pH value for the isoelectric *point* of a given substance.

pi (π) (pī). **1.** 16th Letter of the Greek alphabet. **2.** (Π). Symbol for osmotic pressure; in mathematics, symbol for the product of a series. **3.** (π). Symbol for the ratio of the circumference of a circle to its diameter (approximately 3.14159265). **4.** Symbol for pros.

pia (pī′ă, pē′ă). SYN pia mater. [L. fem. of *pius,* tender]

pia-a·rach·ni·tis (pī′ă-ă-rak-nī′tis). SYN leptomeningitis.

pia-a·rach·noid (pī′ă-ă-rak′noyd, pē′ă-). SYN leptomeninges.

pi·al (pī′al, pē′al). Relating to the pia mater.

pia mat·er (pī′ă mā′ter, pē′ă mah′ter). A delicate vasculated fibrous membrane firmly adherent to the glial capsule of the brain (**p. m. cranialis [encephali]** [NA]) and spinal cord (**p. m. spinalis** [NA] or membrana limitans gliae); following exactly the outer markings of the cerebrum and also the ependymal lining circumference of the choroid membranes and plexus, it invests the cerebellum but not so intimately as it does the cerebrum, not dipping down into all the smaller sulci. The p. m. and the arachnoid are collectively called leptomeninges, as distinguished from dura mater or pachymeninx. SYN pia. [L. tender, affectionate mother]

pi·an (pē-an′, pī′an). SYN yaws.

p. bois, a form of New World cutaneous leishmaniasis caused by *Leishmania braziliensis guyanensis* in the Amazon delta; a small proportion of cases are said to metastasize to the nasal mucosa with espundia-like involvement. SYN bosch yaws, bush yaws, forest yaws.

hemorrhagic p., SYN *verruca* peruana.

pi·a·rach·noid (pī′ă-rak′noyd). SYN leptomeninges.

pi·blok·to, pi·blok·tog (pib-lok′tō). A hysterical dissociative state, usually occurring in Eskimo women, in which the individual screams, tears off clothes, and runs out into the snow; afterward, there is no memory of the episode. [Native]

pi·ca (pī′kă, pē′kă). A perverted appetite for substances not fit as food or of no nutritional value; *e.g.,* clay, dried paint, starch, ice. [L. *pica,* magpie]

Picchini. Luigi, late 19th century Italian physician. SYN Picchini′s *syndrome.*

Pick, Arnold, Czechoslovakian psychiatrist, 1851–1924. SEE P.'s *atrophy, bundle, disease.*

Pick, Friedel, German physician, 1867–1926. SEE P.'s *bodies,* under *body, disease, syndrome.*

Pick, Ludwig, German physician, 1868–1935. SEE P. *cell;* P.'s tubular *adenoma;* Niemann-P. *cell, disease.*

pick·ling (pik′ling). In dentistry, the process of cleansing metallic surfaces of the products of oxidation and other impurities by immersion in acid.

Pickworth, F.A. SEE Lepehne-P. *stain.*

△**pico-.** **1.** Combining form meaning small. **2 (p).** Prefix used in the SI and metric systems to signify one-trillionth (10^{-12}). SYN bicro-. [It. *piccolo*]

pi·co·gram (pg) (pī′kō-gram, pē′kō-gram). One-trillionth of a gram.

pi·co·ka·tal (pkat) (pī′kō-kat′ăl; pē′ko-kat′ăl). One trillionth of a katal (10^{-12} katal).

pi·co·lin·ic ac·id (pik-ō-lin′ik). Pyridine-4-carboxylic acid; an isomer of nicotinic acid.

pi·co·li·nur·ic ac·id (pik-ō-li-nūr′ik). *N*-Picolinoylglycine; the amide, with glycine, of picolinic acid; a hippuric acid analog in which picolinic acid, rather than benzoic acid, is conjugated with glycine and excreted.

pi·com·e·ter (pm) (pī′kō-mē-ter). One-trillionth of a meter. SYN bicron.

pi·co·mole (pmol) (pē′kō-mōl; pī′kō-mol). One-trillionth of a mole (10^{-12} mole).

Pi·cor·na·vir·i·dae (pi-kōr-nă-vir′i-dē). A family of very small (20 to 30 nm) ether-resistant, nonenveloped viruses having a core of single-stranded RNA enclosed in a capsid of icosahedral symmetry with 32 capsomeres. Numerous species (including the polioviruses, coxsackieviruses, and echoviruses) are included in the family. There are four accepted genera: *Enterovirus, Rhinovirus, Cardiovirus,* and *Aphtovirus.* [It. *piccolo,* very small, + RNA + -viridae]

pi·cor·na·vi·rus (pi-kōr-nă-vī′rŭs). A virus of the family Picornaviridae.

pic·ram·ic ac·id (pī-kram′ik). 2-Amino-4,6-dinitrophenol; red crystals sometimes found in the blood of persons poisoned with picric acid; formed as a result of partial reduction of the latter.

Pic·ras·ma (pi-kraz′mă). SEE quassia. [L., fr. G. *pikrasmos,* bitterness]

pic·rate (pik′rāt). A salt of picric acid.

pic·ric ac·id (pik′rik). $C_6H_2(NO_2)_3OH$; 2,4,6-Trinitrophenol; has been used as an application in burns, eczema, erysipelas, and pruritus. SYN carbazotic acid, nitroxanthic acid. [G. *pikros,* bitter]

pic·ro·car·mine (pik-rō-kar′min, -mēn). SEE picrocarmine *stain.*

pic·ro·for·mol (pik′rō-fōr′mol). SEE picroformol *fixative.*

pic·ro·ni·gro·sin (pik′rō-nī′grō-sin). SEE picronigrosin *stain.*

pic·ro·tox·in (pik′rō-tok′sin). A very bitter neutral principle derived from the fruit of *Anamirta cocculus* (family Menispermaceae); a central nervous system stimulant, used as an antidote for poisoning by barbiturates and certain other CNS-depressant drugs; a convulsant and GABA antagonist used extensively in experimental procedures studying seizure mechanisms. SYN cocculin. [G. *pikros,* bitter, + *toxicon,* poison]

pic·ro·tox·in·in (pik-rō-tok′si-nin). $C_{15}H_{16}O_6$; a lactone breakdown product of picrotoxin; pharmacological properties resemble those of picrotoxin.

pic·ryl (pik′ril). 2,4,6-Trinitrophenyl; the organic radical derived from picric acid by removal of the hydroxyl group.

pic·to·graph (pik′tō-graf). A vision test chart for illiterates.

PID Abbreviation for pelvic inflammatory *disease.*

pie·bald·ism (pī′bawld-izm). SYN piebaldness.

pie·bald·ness (pī′bawld-ness) [MIM*172800]. Patchy absence of the pigment of scalp hair, giving a streaked appearance; patches of vitiligo may be present in other areas sue to absence of melanocytes; often transmitted as an autosomal dominant trait and may be associated with neurological defects [MIM*172850] or eye changes [MIM 172870]. Cf. Waardenburg *syndrome.* SYN piebald skin, piebaldism.

piece (pēs). A part or portion.

end p., a part of the spermatozoon consisting of an axoneme surrounded only by the flagellar membrane.

Fab p., SYN Fab *fragment.*

Fc p., SYN Fc *fragment.*

middle p., a part of the spermatozoon characterized by an axoneme and by a sheath of mitochondria arranged in a tight helix.

principal p., the principal part of the spermatozoon, which is about 45 μm long and has a characteristic fibrous sheath surrounding the axoneme.

pie·dra (pē-ā′dră). A fungus disease of the hair characterized by the formation of numerous waxy, small, firm, nodular masses on the hair shaft. SEE ALSO trichosporosis. [Sp. a stone]

black p., p. involving the hairs of the scalp, caused by *Piedraia hortae* and characterized by firmly adherent black, hard, gritty nodules composed of an organized, firmly cemented mass of fungus cells; the fungal growth is always located above the level of the hair follicles; the disease occurs in humid tropical countries of the Americas, Africa, Southeast Asia, and Indonesia, and attacks chimpanzees and other primates as well as humans.

p. nos′tras, a condition similar to p., but affecting the hair of the beard.

white p., p. of the beard, moustache, and genital areas, as well as the scalp, caused by *Trichosporon beigelii* and found in South America, Europe, and Japan; characterized by soft, mucilaginous, white to light brown nodules, within as well as on the hairs. SYN trichosporosis.

Pi·e·dra·ia (pī′ĕ-drī′ă). A genus of fungi, based on *P. hortae,* which is probably the only species and which causes black piedra. [see piedra]

pieds ter·mi·naux (pē-e′ter-mē-nō′). SYN axon *terminals,* under *terminal.* [Fr., end feet]

Pierini, Luigi, 20th century Argentinian dermatologist. SEE *atrophoderma* of Pasini and P.

Pierre Robin. SEE Robin.

pi·e·ses·the·sia (pī-ē-ses-thē′zē-ă). SYN pressure *sense*. [G. *piesis*, pressure, + *aisthēsis*, sensation]

pi·e·sim·e·ter, pi·e·som·e·ter (pī-ē-sim′ĕ-ter, pī-ē-som′ĕ-ter). An instrument for measuring the pressure of a gas or a fluid. SYN piezometer. [G. *piesis*, pressure]

Hales' p., a glass tube inserted into an artery at right angles to its axis, the pressure being shown by the height to which the blood ascends in the tube.

pi·e·sis (pī′ĕ-sis). SYN blood *pressure*. [G. pressure]

pi·e·zo·chem·is·try (pī-ĕ-zō-kem′is-trē). The study of the effect of very high pressures on chemical reactions.

pi·e·zo·e·lec·tric (pī′ĕ-zō-ē-lek′trik). Pertaining to piezoelectricity.

pi·e·zo·e·lec·tric·i·ty (pī′ĕ-zō-ē-lek-tris′i-tē). Electric currents generated by pressure upon certain crystals, *e.g.,* quartz, mica, calcite. [G. *piezo,* to press, squeeze, + electricity]

pi·e·zo·gen·ic (pī′ĕ-zō-jen′ik). Resulting from pressure. [G. *piezo,* to press, squeeze, + *genesis,* origin]

pi·e·zom·e·ter (pī-ĕ-zom′ĕ-ter). SYN piesimeter.

PIF Abbreviation for prolactin-inhibiting *factor.*

PIG. A container, usually made of lead, used for shielding vials or syringes containing radioactive materials. [jargon]

pig·bel. A type of necrotizing enteritis endemic in the Papua New Guinea highlands caused by the B toxin of *Clostridium perfringens* type C; occurs predominantly in children because of poor immunity to B toxin and a low level of intestinal proteases resulting from a diet low in protein and high in sweet potatoes.

pig·ment. 1. Any coloring matter, as that of the red blood cells, hair, iris, etc., or the stains used in histologic or bacteriologic work, or that in paints. **2.** A medicinal preparation for external use, applied to the skin like paint. [L. *pigmentum,* paint]

bile p.'s, coloring matter in the bile derived from porphyrins by rupture of a methane bridge; *e.g.,* bilirubin, biliverdin.

chymotropic p., a p. dissolved in the vacuole of a plant cell. [G. *chymos,* juice, + *tropē,* turning, inclination, + -ic]

formalin p., a p. formed when acid aqueous solutions of formaldehyde act on blood-rich tissues; characterized by rotation of the plane of polarized light, withstanding extraction in aqueous and lipid solvents, being bleached in acids and hydrogen peroxide; not formed when tissue is fixed with formaldehyde buffered to pH levels above 6.

hematogenous p., a p. derived from the hemoglobin of the red blood cells.

hepatogenous p., bile p. derived from the destruction of hemoglobin in the liver.

malarial p., a dark brown, granular p. which rotates the plane of polarized light and has other properties similar to formalin p.; occurs in parasites, such as *Plasmodium malariae,* around brain capillaries, and in fixed macrophages of spleen, liver, bone marrow, and lymph nodes. SEE malarial pigment *stain.*

melanotic p., SYN melanin.

natural p., a naturally occurring colored compound; absorbs light in the visible range of the electromagnetic spectrum. Cf. structural *color.* SYN biochrome.

respiratory p.'s, the oxygen-carrying (colored) substances in blood and tissues (hemoglobin, myoglobin, hemocyanin, etc.).

visual p.'s, the photopigments in the retinal cones and rods that absorb light and initiate the visual process.

wear-and-tear p., lipofuscin that accumulates in aging or atrophic cells as a residue of lysosomal digestion.

pig·men·tary (pig′men-tār-ē). Relating to a pigment.

pig·men·ta·tion (pig-men-tā′shŭn). Coloration, either normal or pathologic, of the skin or tissues resulting from a deposit of pigment.

arsenic p., generalized but spotty increased melanin p. of the skin in chronic arsenic poisoning.

exogenous p., discoloration of the skin or tissues by a pigment introduced from without.

pig·ment·ed (pig′men-ted). Colored as the result of a deposit of pigment.

pig·men·to·ly·sin (pig-men-tol′i-sin). An antibody causing destruction of pigment. [L. *pigmentum,* pigment, + G. *lysis,* a loosening]

pig·men·tum ni·grum (pig-men′tŭm nī′grŭm). Melanin of the choroid coat of the eye.

pig·my (pig′mē). SYN pygmy.

Pignet, Maurice-C.J., French surgeon, *1871. SEE P.'s *formula.*

PIH Abbreviation for prolactin-inhibiting *hormone.*

pi·lar, pi·la·ry (pī′lăr, pil′ă-rē). SYN hairy. [L. *pilus,* hair]

pile (pīl). **1.** A series of plates of two different metals imposed alternately one on the other, separated by a sheet of material moistened with a dilute acid solution, used to produce a current of electricity. [L. *pila,* pillar] **2.** An individual hemorrhoidal tumor. SEE hemorrhoids. [L. *pila,* ball]

sentinel p., a circumscribed thickening of the mucous membrane at the lower end of a fissure of the anus.

thermoelectric p., SYN thermopile.

pi·le·ous (pī′lē-ŭs). SYN hairy. [L. *pilus,* hair]

piles (pīlz). SYN hemorrhoids. [L. *pila,* a ball]

pi·le·us (pī′lē-ŭs). SYN greater *omentum.* [L. *pileum* or *pileus,* a felt cap]

pi·li (pī′lī) [NA]. Plural of pilus. [L.]

pi·li·mic·tion (pī-li-mik′shŭn). Passage of hairs in the urine, as in cases of dermoid tumors, or of threads of mucus in the urine. [L. *pilus,* hair, + *mictio,* urination]

pil·in (pī′lin). The protein component of bacterial adhesive appendages that help the bacterium to stick to tissue or container surfaces, often the glycoproteins on the surface of eucaryotic cells. [pilus 2. + -in]

pill. A small globular mass of some coherent but soluble substance, containing a medicinal substance to be swallowed. SEE ALSO tablet. [L. *pilula;* dim. of *pila,* ball]

bread p., a placebo made of bread crumbs or other inactive substances.

pep p.'s, colloquialism for tablets containing a central nervous system stimulant, especially amphetamine.

pil·lar (pil′ăr). A structure or part having a resemblance to a column or pillar. [L. *pila*]

anterior p. of fauces, SYN palatoglossal *arch.*

anterior p. of fornix, SYN column of fornix.

Corti's p.'s, SYN pillar *cells,* under *cell.*

p.'s of fauces, SEE palatoglossal *arch,* palatopharyngeal *arch.*

p.'s of fornix, the columna fornicis and crus fornicis.

p. of iris, SYN trabecular *reticulum.*

posterior p. of fauces, SYN palatopharyngeal *arch.*

posterior p. of fornix, SYN *crus* fornicis.

pil·let (pil′et). A small pill.

pill mass. SYN pilular *mass.*

pill-roll·ing (pil′rōl′ing). A circular movement of the opposed tips of the thumb and the index finger appearing as a form of tremor in paralysis agitans.

⌂pilo-. Hair. [L. *pilus*]

pi·lo·be·zoar (pī-lō-bē′zōr). SYN trichobezoar. [pilo- + bezoar]

pi·lo·car·pine (pī-lō-kar′pēn). An alkaloid obtained from the leaves of *Pilocarpus; Microphyllus* or *P. jaborandi* (family Rutaceae), shrubs of the West Indies and tropical America; a parasympathomimetic agent used as a diaphoretic, sialogogue, and stimulant of intestinal motility, and externally as a miotic and in the treatment of glaucoma; used as the hydrochloride and the nitrate salts. [G. *pilos,* a felt hat, + *karpos,* fruit]

pi·lo·car·pus (pil′ō-kar-pŭs). A genus of trees and shrubs found in Central and South America and in the West Indies. Constitutes the botanical source for pilocarpine, an alkaloid which activates cholinergic muscarinic receptors. Pilocarpine is used in the treatment of glaucoma where it is instilled in the eye. Sudorific; miotic. SYN Jaborandi.

pi·lo·cys·tic (pi′lō-sis′tik). Denoting a dermoid cyst containing hair. [pilo- + G. *kystis,* bladder]

pi·lo·e·rec·tion (pī′lō-ē-rek′shŭn). Erection of hair due to action of arrectores pilorum muscles.

pigmentation anomalies

hyperpigmentation melanoderma

congenital	acquired	
circumscribed	circumscribed	diffuse
nevi pigmentosi	(ephelides)	melanoses:
nevi spili	nevi tardi	arsenic
ephelides	chloasma gravidarum	idiopathic hemochromatosis
lentigines	linea fusca	bronze diabetes
combined nevi	chloasma virginum peribuccale	cirrhosis of liver
bathing-trunks nevi	Riehl's melanosis	vagabond skin
systematized nevi	melanodermatitis toxica	Addison's disease
neurofibromatosis	poikilodermia reticulata	Graves' disease
Peutz-Jeghers syndrome	angiodermatitis pigmentosa et purpurica	melanoma
Albright's disease	postlesionary hyerpigmentation	pellagra
xeroderma pigmentosum	phytophotodermatoses	sprue
nevus ceruleus	Berloque-dermatitis	tuberculosis
mongolian spots	Cologne pigmentation	pernicious anemia
diffuse	lichen ruber, impetigo etc., after psoriasis	catatonic schizophrenia, etc.
racial and constitutional hyperpigmentation	incontinentia pigmenti	

hypopigmentation, leukodermas

congenital	acquired	
circumscribed	circumscribed	diffuse
nevus achromicus	vitiligo	canities praecox
poliosis	halo nevus	Simmonds-Sheehan syndrome
albinoidism	postlesionary hypopigmentation	sudden graying and skin depigmentation
diffuse	leukoderma psoriaticum	Werner's syndrome
albinism	leukoderma syphiliticum	
albinoidism	vitiligo gravior, in leprosy	
	pinta	
	kwashiorkor	
	toxic depigmentation by hydroquinone monobenzyl ether, etc.	
	dyschromia parasitica	
	pityriasis versicolor alba	
	streptodermia alba simplex	
	Vogt-Koyanagi syndrome	

pi·loid (pī'loyd). Hairlike; resembling hair. [pilo- + G. *eidos,* resemblance]

pi·lo·jec·tion (pī-lō-jek'shŭn). Process of shooting shafts of stiff mammalian hair into a saccular aneurysm in the brain in order to produce thrombosis. [pilo- + injection]

pi·lo·ma·trix·o·ma (pī'lō-mā-trik-sō'mă). A benign solitary hair follicle tumor, often starting in childhood, containing cells resembling basal cell carcinoma and areas of epithelial necrosis forming eosinophilic ghost cells with variable calcification and foreign body giant cell reaction in the fibrous stroma. SYN Malherbe's calcifying epithelioma. [pilo- + matrix + G. *-oma,* tumor]

pi·lo·mo·tor (pī'lō-mō'ter). Moving the hair; denoting the arrectores pilorum muscles of the skin and the postganglionic sympathetic nerve fibers innervating these small smooth muscles. [pilo- + L. *motor,* mover]

pi·lo·ni·dal (pī-lō-nī'dăl). Denoting the presence of hair in a dermoid cyst or in a sinus opening on the skin. [pilo- + L. *nidus,* nest]

pi·lose (pī'lōs). SYN hairy. [L. *pilosus*]

pi·lo·se·ba·ceous (pī'lō-sē-bā'shŭs). Relating to the hair follicles and sebaceous glands. [pilo- + L. *sebum,* suet]

pi·lo·sis (pī-lō'sis). SYN hirsutism. [pilo- + G. *-osis,* condition]

Piltz, Jan, Polish neurologist, 1870–1931. SEE P. *sign;* Westphal-P. *phenomenon.*

pil·u·la, gen. and pl. **pil·u·lae** (pil'yū-lă, -lē). A pill or pilule. [L. dim. of *pila,* a ball]

pil·u·lar (pil'yū-lăr). Relating to a pill.

pil·ule (pil'yūl). A small pill. [L. *pilula*]

pi·lus, pl. **pi·li** (pī'lŭs, pī'lī). **1** [NA]. One of the fine, keratinized filamentous epidermal growths arising from the skin of the body of mammals except the palms, soles, and flexor surfaces of the joints; the full length and texture of the hair varies markedly in different body sites. SYN crinis, hair (1). **2.** A fine filamentous appendage, somewhat analogous to the flagelium, that occurs on some bacteria. Pili consist only of protein and are shorter, straighter, much more numerous, and may be chemically similar to flagella; specialized pili (F pili, I pili, and other conjugative pili) seem to mediate bacterial conjugation. SYN fimbria (2). SEE ALSO conjugative *plasmid.* [L.]

pi'li annula'ti, SYN ringed *hair.*

F pili, SEE pilus (2).

F p., a structure responsible for attachment of individual male (F⁺) to female (F⁻) bacteria, forming conjugal pairs.

I pili, SEE pilus (2).

pi'li multigem'ini, the presence of several hairs in a single follicle.

R pili, specialized pili found on bacterial cells, similar to F pili and associated with R plasmids.

pi'li tor'ti, a condition in which many hair shafts are twisted on the long axis, congenital or acquired as a result of distortion of the follicles from a scarring inflammatory process, mechanical stress, or cicatrizing alopecia; the hair shafts resemble spangles in reflected light, are brittle, and break at varying lengths with many areas appearing bald with a dark stubble; as a developmental defect it can be manifested in such syndromes as Bjornstad's, Crandall's, and Menkes'. SYN twisted hairs.

pi·mar·i·cin (pi-mar'i-sin). $C_{34}H_{49}NO_{14}$; an antifungal antibiotic for topical use, produced by *Streptomyces natalensis;* effective against *Aspergillus, Candida,* and *Mucor* species. SYN natamycin.

pi·mel·ic ac·id (pǐ-mel'ik). HOOC–$(CH_2)_5$–COOH; Heptanedioic acid; an intermediate in the oxidation of oleic acid in some microorganisms; a precursor of biotin.

⚠**pimelo-.** Fat, fatty. [G. *pimelē,* soft fat, lard, fr. *piar,* fat]

pim·e·lor·rhea (pim'ě-lō-rē'ă). SYN fatty *diarrhea.* [pimelo- + G. *rhoia,* a flux]

pim·e·lor·thop·nea (pim'ě-lōr-thop'nē-ă, -nē'ă). Orthopnea; difficulty breathing in any but the erect posture, due to obesity. SYN piorthopnea. [pimelo- + G. *orthos,* straight, + *pnoē,* breath]

pi·men·ta, pi·men·to (pi-men'tă, -tō). The dried fruit of *Pimenta officinalis* (family Myrtaceae), a tree native in Jamaica and other parts of tropical America, used as a carminative and aromatic spice; p. oil comprises 3 to 4% of the dried fruit. [Sp. fr. L. *pigmentum,* paint (Mediev. L. spice)]

p. oil, comprises 3 to 4.5% of the dried fruit. SYN allspice oil.

pim·o·zide (pim'ō-zīd). 1-[1-[4,4-bis(*p*-Fluorophenyl)butyl]-4-piperidyl]-2-benzimidazolinone; a tranquilizing drug.

pim·ple (pim'pl). A papule or small pustule; usually meant to denote an inflammatory lesion of acne.

PIN Abbreviation for prostatic intraepithelial *neoplasia.*

pin. A metal rod used in surgical treatment of bone fractures. SEE ALSO nail. [O.E. *pinn,* fr. L. *pinna,* feather]

Steinmann p., a p. that is used to transfix bone for traction or fixation.

pin·a·cy·a·nol (pin-ă-sī'ă-nol) [old C.I. 808]. A basic dye, $C_{25}H_{25}N_2I$, used as a color sensitizer (violet red in water, blue in alcohol) in photography and for vital staining of leukocytes.

Pinard, Adolphe, French obstetrician, 1844–1934. SEE P.'s *maneuver.*

pince·ment (pans-mon'). A pinching manipulation in massage. [Fr. pinching]

Pindborg, Jens J., Danish oral pathologist, *1921. SEE P. *tumor.*

pin·do·lol (pin'dō-lol). 1-(Indol-4-yloxy)-3-(isopropylamino)-2-propanol; a β-adrenergic blocking agent used in the treatment of hypertension; also possesses intrinsic sympathomimetic activity.

pine (pīn). An evergreen coniferous tree of the genus *Pinus* (family Pinaceae), various species of which yield tar, turpentine, resin, and volatile oils. [L. *pinus,* a pine tree]

p.-needle oil, a volatile oil distilled with steam from the fresh leaf of *Pinus mugo;* has been used by inhalation and spray in catarrhal affections of the air passages, and locally in rheumatism; also used as a flavoring and in perfumery.

p. oil, the volatile oil from the wood of *Pinus palustris* and other species of *Pinus;* used as a deodorant and disinfectant.

p. tar, obtained by the destructive distillation of the wood of *Pinus palustris* and other species of *Pinus;* used internally as an expectorant, and externally in the treatment of skin diseases. SYN liquid pitch.

white p., the dried inner bark of *Pinus strobus,* used as an ingredient in cough syrups.

pin·e·al (pin'ē-ăl). **1.** Shaped like a pine cone. SYN piniform. **2.** Pertaining to the pineal body. [L. *pineus,* relating to the pine, *pinus*]

pin·e·al·ec·to·my (pin'ē-ă-lek'tō-mē). Removal of the pineal body. [pineal + G. *ektomē,* excision]

pin·e·a·lo·cyte (pin-ē'al-ō-sīt). A cell of the pineal body with long processes ending in bulbous expansions. P.'s receive a direct innervation from sympathetic neurons that form recognizable synapses. The club-shaped endings of pinealocyte processes terminate in perivascular spaces surrounding capillaries. SYN chief cell of corpus pineale, parenchymatous cell of corpus pineale. [pineal + G. *kytos,* cell]

pin·e·a·lo·ma (pin'ē-ă-lō'mă). A term that has been variably used to designate germ cell tumors, pineocytomas and pineoblastomas of the pineal gland. [pineal + G. *-oma,* tumor]

ectopic p., an obsolete term for an undifferentiated neoplasm resembling a p., usually found near the pituitary gland; believed by some to be an undifferentiated teratoma.

extrapineal p., obsolete term for ectopic p.

pin·e·a·lop·a·thy (pin'ē-ă-lop'ă-thē). Disease of the pineal gland. [pineal + G. *pathos,* disease]

pine·ap·ple (pīn'ap-ĕl). The fruit of *Ananas sativa* or *Bromelia ananas* (family Bromeliaceae); it contains a proteolytic and milk-clotting enzyme, bromelain.

Pinel, Philippe, French psychiatrist, 1745–1826. SEE P.'s *system.*

pin·e·o·blas·to·ma (pin'ē-ō-blas-tō'mă). A poorly differentiated tumor of the pineal gland most frequently occurring in the first three decades of life consisting of small cells with a scant amount of cytoplams and often forming pseudorosettes. Histologically resembles a medulloblastoma. A type of primitive neuroectodermal tumor. [pineal + G. *blastos,* germ, + *-oma,* tumor]

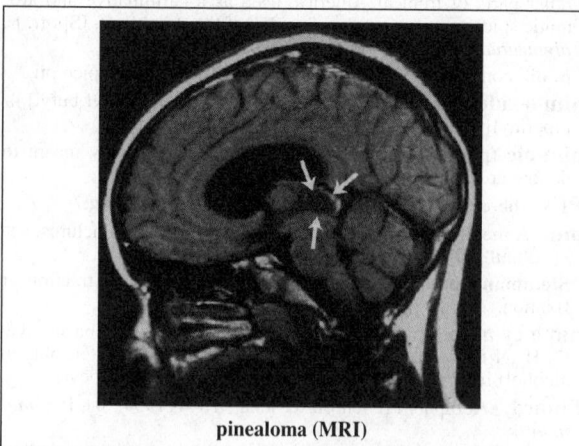

pinealoma (MRI)

pin·e·o·cy·to·ma (pin'ē-ō-cī'tō- mă). A tumor arising in the pineal gland that resembles normal pineal parenchyma.

ping-pong (ping'pong). SEE ping-pong *mechanism*. [Ping-Pong, trademark for table tennis]

pin·guec·u·la, pin·guic·u·la (ping-gwek'yū-lă). A yellowish accumulation of connective tissue that thickens the conjunctiva; occurs in the aged. [L. *pinguiculus,* fattish, fr. *pinguis,* fat]

pin·i·form (pin'i-fōrm, pī'ni-). SYN pineal (1). [L. *pinus,* pine, + *forma,* form]

pink·eye (pink'ī). **1.** SYN acute contagious *conjunctivitis.* **2.** SYN infectious bovine *keratoconjunctivitis.* **3.** In horses, a form of equine viral *arteritis.*

pin·ledge (pin'ledj). A cast metal dental restoration or technique that employs parallel pins as part of the casting to increase retention of the restoration.

pin·na, pl. **pin·nae** (pin'ă, pin'ē). **1.** SYN auricle (1). **2.** A feather, wing, or fin. [L. *pinna* or *penna,* a feather, in pl. a wing]
p. na'si, SYN *wing* of nose.

pin·nal (pin'ăl). Relating to the pinna.

pin·ni·ped (pin'i-ped). A member of the suborder Pinnipedia, aquatic carnivorous mammals with all four limbs modified into flippers (*e.g.,* seal, walrus). [L. *pinna,* feather (wing), + *pes* (*ped-*), foot]

pin·o·cyte (pin'ō-sīt, pī'nō-). A cell that exhibits pinocytosis. [G. *pineō,* to drink, + *kytos,* cell]

pin·o·cy·to·sis (pin'ō-sī-tō'sis, pī'nō-). The cellular process of actively engulfing liquid, a phenomenon in which minute incuppings or invaginations are formed in the surface of the cell membrane and close to form fluid-filled vesicles; it resembles phagocytosis. [pinocyte + G. *-osis,* condition]

pin·o·some (pin'ō-sōm, pī'nō-). A fluid-filled vacuole formed by pinocytosis. [G. *pineō,* to drink, + *sōma,* body]

Pins, Emil, Austrian physician, 1845–1913. SEE P.'s *sign, syndrome.*

pint (pīnt). A measure of quantity (U.S. liquid), containing 16 fluid ounces, 28.875 cubic inches; 473.1765 cc. An imperial p. contains 20 British fluid ounces, 34.67743 cubic inches; 568.2615 cc.

pin·ta (pin'tă, pēn'tă). A disease caused by a spirochete, *Treponema carateum,* endemic in Mexico and Central America, and characterized by a small primary papule followed by an enlarging plaque and disseminated secondary macules of varying color called pintids that finally become white. SEE ALSO nonvenereal *syphilis.* SYN azul, carate, mal de los pintos, spotted sickness. [Sp. painted]

pin·tids. Eruptions of plaque-like lesions in the secondary phase of pinta; the lesions, which vary in color (hypochromic, hyperchromic, and erythematosquamous), result in depigmentation. [pinta + -id(1)]

pin·toid (pin'toyd). Resembling pinta.

pi·nus (pī'nŭs). SYN pineal *body.* [L. a pine tree]

pin·worm (pin'werm). A member of the genus *Enterobius* or related genera of nematodes in the family Oxyuridae, abundant in a large variety of vertebrates, including such species as *Oxyuris equi* (the horse p.), *Enterobius vermicularis* (the human p.), *Syphacia* and *Aspiculuris* species (the mouse p.), *Passalurus ambiguus* (the rabbit p.), and *Syphacia muris* (the rat p.). SYN seatworm.

Pi·oph·i·la ca·sei (pī-of'i-lă kā'sē-ī). The cheese fly, a species of muscoid flies whose eggs are deposited on exposed cheese, cured meats, and other foods and are thus ingested, sometimes giving rise to temporary intestinal myiasis, with diarrhea, colicky pains, and vomiting. [L., fr. G. *piōn,* fat, + *philos,* fond; L. *caseus,* cheese]

pi·or·thop·nea (pī-ōr-thop'nē-ă, -nē'ă). SYN pimelorthopnea. [G. *piōn,* fat, + *orthos,* straight, + *pnoē,* breath]

PIP₂ Abbreviation for *phosphatidylinositol* 4,5-bisphosphate.

pi·pam·a·zine (pi-pam'ă-zēn). 1-[3-(2-Chlorophenothiazin-10-yl)propyl]isonipectoamide; a phenothiazine analogue with antiemetic and tranquilizing properties.

pi·pam·per·one (pi-pam'per-ōn). 1'-[3-(*p*-Fluorobenzoyl)-propyl]-[1,4'-bipiperidine]-4'-carboxamide; an antipsychotic tranquilizer.

pi·paz·e·thate (pi-paz'ĕ-thāt). 2-(2-Piperidinoethoxy)ethyl 10*H*-pyridol[3,2-*b*][1,4]benzothiazine-10-carboxylate; an antitussive agent.

pip·e·co·lic ac·id (pip'ĕ-kō'lik, -kol'ik). dihydrobaikiaine; 2-piperidinecarboxylic acid; saturated picolinic acid; the L-isomers of the Δ^1- and Δ^6-dehydropipecolic acids are intermediates in the catabolism of L-lysine; p. a. accumulates in disorders of the peroxisomes. SYN homoproline, pipecolinic acid.

pip·e·co·lin·ic ac·id (pip-ĕ-kō-lin'ik, -kol'i-nik). SYN pipecolic acid.

pip·e·cur·o·ni·um (pip'ĕ-kyūr-ō'nē-ŭm). A nondepolarizing steroid muscle relaxant structurally related to pancuronium and characterized by long duration of action.

pip·e·cu·ron·i·um bro·mide (pī-pĕ-kur-ō'nē-ŭm brō'mīd). A neuromuscular blocking agent with nondepolarizing properties, thus resembling d-tubocurarine but having a shorter duration of paralytic action.

pi·pen·zo·late meth·yl·bro·mide (pi-pen'zō-lāt). 1-Ethyl-3-piperidyl benzilate methylbromide; an anticholinergic drug.

Piper, E.B., U.S. obstetrician-gynecologist, 1881–1935. SEE P.'s *forceps.*

pip·er (pī'per). Black pepper, the dried unripe fruit of *Piper nigrum* (family Piperaceae), a climbing plant of the East Indies; used as a condiment, diaphoretic, stimulant, and carminative, and locally as a counterirritant. [L. pepper]

pi·per·a·cet·a·zine (pi-per-ă-set'ă-zēn). 10-{3-[4-(2-Hydroxyethyl)piperidino]-propyl}phenothiazin-2-yl methyl ketone; a tranquilizer.

pi·per·a·cil·lin so·di·um (pi-per'ă-sil'in). $C_{23}H_{26}N_5NaO_7S$; a semisynthetic extended spectrum penicillin active against a wide variety of Gram-positive and Gram-negative bacteria.

pi·per·a·zine (pī-per'ă-zēn, -zin). pyrazine hexahydride; its former use in gout was based upon its property of dissolving uric acid *in vitro,* but it is ineffective in increasing uric acid excretion; its compounds are now used as anthelmintics in oxyuriasis and ascariasis. SYN diethylenediamine.
p. adipate, a veterinary anthelmintic and filaricide.
p. calcium edetate, (ethylenedinitrilo)tetraacetic acid piperazine calcium salt; an anthelmintic.
p. citrate, a vermifuge for pinworms and roundworms.
p. estrone sulfate, a purified preparation of natural estrone sulfate; the p. acts as a buffer to increase the stability of estrone sulfate.

pi·per·a·zine di·eth·ane·sul·fon·ic ac·id (PIPES). One of several aminosulfonic acids (like HEPES) used in biological buffers; active range 6.0–8.5.

pi·per·a·zine tar·trate. An anthelmintic useful in the treatment of nematode infestation.

pi·per·i·dine (pǐ′per-i-dēn). **1.** $C_5H_{11}N$; Hexahydropyridine; a compound from which are derived phenothiazine antipsychotics such as thioridazine hydrochloride and mesoridazine besylate. **2.** One of a class of alkaloids containing a p. (1) moiety.

pi·per·i·do·late hy·dro·chlo·ride (pi-per′i-dō-lāt). 1-Ethyl-3-piperidyl diphenylacetate hydrochloride; an anticholinergic agent.

pi·per·o·caine hy·dro·chlo·ride (pip′er-ō-kān, pī′per-). 3-(2-Methyl-1-piperidino)propyl benzoate hydrochloride; a rapidly acting local anesthetic for infiltration and nerve blocks.

pi·per·ox·an hy·dro·chlo·ride (pip-er-ok′san). 2-(1-piperidylmethyl)-1,4-benzodioxane hydrochloride; an adrenergic (α-receptor blocking agent of the Fourneau series of benzodioxanes); used as a diagnostic test for pheochromocytoma. SYN Fourneau 933.

PIPES Abbreviation for piperazine diethanesulfonic acid.

pi·pette, pi·pet (pǐ-pet′, pī-pet′). A graduated tube (marked in ml) used to transport a definite volume of a gas or liquid in laboratory work. [Fr. dim. of *pipe*, pipe]

blowout p., a p. calibrated to deliver its nominal volume by permitting it first to drain and then blowing out the last drop held in the tip.

graduated p., a p. with a plain, narrow tube drawn out to a tip and graduated uniformly along its length. Calibration marks may be confined to the stem (Mohr p.) or extend to the tip (serologic p.). SYN Mohr p., serologic p.

Mohr p., SYN graduated p.

Pasteur p., a cotton-plugged, glass tube drawn out to a fine tip, used for the sterile transfer of small volumes of fluid.

serologic p., SYN graduated p.

pip·o·bro·man (pip-ō-brō′man). 1,4-Bis(3-bromopropionyl)-piperazine; an alkylating agent used in polycythemia vera and chronic granulocytic leukemia.

pi·po·sul·fan (pi-pō-sŭl′fan). 1,4-Dihydracryloylpiperazine dimethanesulfonate; an antineoplastic agent.

pi·pra·drol hy·dro·chlo·ride (pip′ră-drol). α-[2-Piperidyl]-benzhydrol hydrochloride; a central nervous system stimulant.

pi·prin·hy·dri·nate (pip-rin-hī′dri-nāt). *N*-Methylpiperidyl 4-benzhydryl ether (diphenylpyralimine) 8-chlorotheophyllinate; an antihistaminic and antiemetic.

pip·syl (Ips) (pip′sil). *p*-Iodophenylsulfonyl, the radical of p. chloride that combines with the amino groups of amino acids and proteins.

pir·bu·ter·ol (pir-byū′ter-ol). α⁶[(*tert*-Butylamino)methyl]-3-hydroxy-2,6-pyridine-dimethanol; a selective $β_2$-adrenergic bronchodilator used in the treatment of asthma.

Pi·re·nel·la (pir-ě-nel′ă). A genus of marine and brackish water operculate (prosobranch) snails. *P. conica* is the initial intermediate host of *Heterophyes heterophyes*, the fish-borne fluke of humans and fish-eating birds and mammals along the Mediterranean and Red Sea coasts.

pi·ren·zep·ine (pǐ-ren′zě-pēn). An anticholinergic agent exhibiting relative specificity for suppression of gastric hydrochloric acid secretion; relatively free of anticholinergic side effects; used in the treatment of ulcer disease.

pi·ret·a·nide (pǐ-ret′ă-nīd). High ceiling loop diuretic similar to bumetanide and furosemide; used as a diuretic in hypertension and congestive heart failure.

pi·rib·ed·il (pǐ-rib′ě-dil). An agent that stimulates dopamine receptors in the brain and also exerts a peripheral vasodilator effect.

Pirie, George A., Scottish radiologist, 1864–1929. SEE P.'s *bone.*

pir·i·form (pir′i-fōrm, pī′rē-). Pear-shaped. SYN pyriform. [L. *pirum*, pear, + *forma*, form]

Pirogoff, Nikolai I., Russian surgeon, 1810–1881. SEE P.'s *amputation, angle, triangle.*

pir·o·men (pir′ō-men, pī′rō-). A sterile, nonprotein, nonanaphylactogenic extract of *Pseudomonas aeruginosa* and *Proteus vulgaris.* The active components are bacterial polysaccharides of low toxicity; used in the treatment of certain allergic, dermatologic, and ophthalmic disorders. SYN pyromen.

Pi·ro·plas·ma (pir′ō-plaz′mă, pī′rō-). Former name for *Babesia.* [L. *pirum*, pear, + G. *plasma*, a thing formed]

Pi·ro·plas·mi·da (pi′rō-plaz-mī′dă). An order of sporozoan protozoa (subclass Piroplasmia, class Sporozoea) consisting of the families Habesiidae, Theileriidae, and Dactylosomatidae; includes heteroxenous tick-borne blood parasites of vertebrates with reduced apical complex, lacking spores, and with asexual reproduction by binary fission or schizogony.

pir·o·plas·mo·sis (pir′ō-plas-mō′sis). SYN babesiosis.

pir·ox·i·cam ol·a·mine (pir-oks′i-kam). 4-Hydroxy-2-methyl-*N*-2-pyridyl-2*H*-1,2-benzothiazine-3-carboxamide-1,1-dioxide; a nonsteroidal anti-inflammatory agent with analgesic and antipyretic actions.

pir·pro·fen (pir-prō′fen). 3-Chloro-4-(3-pyrrolin-1-yl)-hydratropic acid; an anti-inflammatory agent used in the treatment of rheumatoid arthritis.

Pirquet von Cesenatico, Clemens P., Austrian physician, 1874–1929. SEE Pirquet's *reaction;* Pirquet's *test.*

Pis·ces (pis′ēz, pī′sēz). A superclass of vertebrates, generally known as fish; the term is sometimes confined to the bony fishes. [L. pl. of *piscis*, a fish]

pis·i·form (pis′i-fōrm). Pea-shaped or pea-sized. [L. *pisum*, pea, + *forma*, appearance]

pit. 1. Any natural depression on the surface of the body, such as the axilla. Cf. dimple. **2.** One of the pinhead-sized depressed scars following the pustule of acne, chickenpox, or smallpox (pockmark). **3.** A sharp-pointed depression in the enamel surface of a tooth, due to faulty or incomplete calcification or formed at the confluent point of two or more lobes of enamel. **4.** To indent, as by pressure of the finger on the edematous skin; to become indented, said of the edematous tissues when pressure is made with the fingertip. [L. *puteus*]

anal p., SYN proctodeum (1).

articular p. of head of radius, SYN *fovea* of the radial head.

p. of atlas for dens, SYN *facet* of atlas for dens.

auditory p.'s, paired depressions, one on either side of the head of the embryo, marking the location of the future auditory vesicles. SYN otic p.'s.

buccal p., a structural depression found on the buccal enamel of molars.

central p., SYN central retinal *fovea.*

coated p., specialized depressions on the cell surface involved in receptor-mediated endocytosis; the visible proteinaceous layer on the cytosolic side of the depression provides the coated appearance.

commisural p.'s, similar to lip p.'s but found at the labial commisures.

costal p. of transverse process, SYN transverse costal *facet.*

gastric p., one of the numerous small pits in the mucous membrane of the stomach that are the mouths of the gastric glands. SYN foveola gastrica [NA].

granular p.'s, pits on the inner surface of the skull, along the course of the superior sagittal sinus, in which are lodged the arachnoidal granulations. SYN foveolae granulares [NA], pacchionian depressions.

p. of head of femur, SYN *fovea* of the femoral head.

inferior articular p. of atlas, SYN inferior articular *facet* of atlas.

inferior costal p., SYN inferior costal *facet.*

iris p.'s, colobomas affecting the stroma of the iris with pigment epithelium intact.

lens p.'s, the paired depressions formed in the superficial ectoderm of the embryonic head as the lens placodes sink in toward the optic cup; the external openings of the p.'s are closed as the lens vesicles are formed.

lip p.'s, malformations of the lip seen in unilateral or bilateral depressions or fistulae. May be hereditary or associated with cleft lip and/or palate.

Mantoux p., shallow 2–3 mm depressions of the palms and soles in basal cell nevus syndrome.

nail p.'s, small punctate depressions on the surface of the nail plate due to defective nail formation; seen in psoriasis and other disorders. SEE ALSO geographic *stippling* of nails.

pi

nasal p.'s, the paired depressions formed when the nasal placodes come to lie below the general external contour of the developing face as a result of the rapid growth of the adjacent nasal elevations; the p.'s are the primordia of the rostral portions of the nasal chambers. SYN olfactory p.'s.

oblong p. of arytenoid cartilage, SYN oblong *fovea* of arytenoid cartilage.

olfactory p.'s, SYN nasal p.'s.

optic p., a congenital structural defect of the optic nerve head.

otic p.'s, SYN auditory p.'s.

postnatal p. of the newborn, SYN *fovea* coccygis.

primitive p., the depression in the primitive node that serves to connect the notochordal canal with the surface ectoderm and the yolk sac. These connections are referred to as the neurenteric canal.

pterygoid p., SYN pterygoid *fovea.*

p. of stomach, SYN epigastric *fossa.*

sublingual p., SYN sublingual *fossa.*

superior articular p. of atlas, SYN superior articular *facet* of atlas.

superior costal p., SYN superior costal *facet.*

suprameatal p., a small depression on the mastoid part of the temporal bone, posterior to the suprameatal spine. SYN foveola suprameatica [NA], mastoid fossa, fossa mastoidea, supramastoid fossa.

triangular p. of arytenoid cartilage, SYN triangular *fovea* of arytenoid cartilage.

trochlear p., SYN trochlear *fovea.*

PITC Abbreviation for phenylisothiocyanate.

pitch (pich). A resinous substance obtained from tar after the volatile substances have been expelled by boiling. SYN pix. [L. *pix*]

Burgundy p., a resinous exudation from the spruce fir or Norway spruce, *Picea excelsa;* has been used as a counterirritant in the form of a plaster. SYN white p.

liquid p., SYN *pine* tar.

white p., SYN Burgundy p.

pitch·blende (pich'blend). A mineral of pitchlike appearance, chiefly uranium dioxide, the main source of uranium and elements, such as radium, produced as a result of the radioactive breakdown of that element. SYN uraninite.

pith. 1. The center of a hair. 2. The spinal cord and medulla oblongata. 3. To pierce the medulla of an animal with a sharp instrument introduced at the base of the skull. [A.S. *pitha*]

pith·e·coid (pith'ē-koyd). Resembling an ape. [G. *pithēkos,* ape, + *eidos,* resemblance]

pith·ode (pith'ōd). The nuclear spindle in karyokinesis. [G. *pithōdēs,* like a jar, fr. *pithos,* earthenware wine-jar, + *eidos,* resemblance]

Pitot, Henri, French engineer, 1695–1771. SEE P. *tube.*

Pitres, Jean A., French physician, 1848–1927. SEE P.'s *area, sign.*

Pi·tressin (pi-tres'in). SYN vasopressin.

pit·ting. In dentistry, the formation of well defined, relatively deep depressions in a surface, usually used in describing defects in surfaces (often golds, solder joints, or amalgam). It may arise from a variety of causes, although the clinical occurrence is often associated with corrosion. SEE ALSO pitting *edema,* nail *pits,* under *pit.*

pi·tu·i·cyte (pi-tū'i-sīt). The primary cell of the posterior lobe of the pituitary gland, a fusiform cell closely related to neuroglia. [pituitary + G. *kytos,* cell]

pi·tu·i·cy·to·ma (pi-tū'i-sī-tō'mă). A rare gliogenous neoplasm derived from pituicytes, occurring in the posterior lobe of the pituitary gland and characterized by cells with relatively small, round or oval nuclei and long branching processes that form a complex network of cytoplasmic material, in which numerous small droplets of fat may be demonstrated. [pituicyte + G. *-oma,* tumor]

pi·tu·i·ta (pi-tū'i-tă) [NA]. A thick nasal secretion. SYN glairy mucus. [L. phlegm or thick mucous secretion]

pi·tu·i·tar·ism (pi-tū'i-tār-izm). Pituitary dysfunction. SEE hyperpituitarism, hypopituitarism.

pi·tu·i·ta·ri·um (pi-tū-i-tā'rē-ŭm). SYN pituitary. [Mod. L.]

pi·tu·i·tary (pi-tū'i-tār-ē). Relating to the pituitary gland (hypophysis). SYN pituitarium. [L. *pituita*]

anterior p., the dried, partially defatted, and powdered anterior lobe of the p. gland of cattle, sheep, or swine; now rarely used therapeutically.

desiccated p., SYN posterior p.

pharyngeal p., the embryonic remnant of the oral end of Rathke's pouch that is cut off from the adenohypophysis by the developing sphenoid bone; composed chiefly of chromophobes and, under normal conditions, considered physiologically inactive. SEE hypophysis.

posterior p., the cleaned, dried, and powdered posterior lobe obtained from the p. body of domestic animals used for food by humans; an oxytocic, vasoconstrictor, antidiuretic, and a stimulant of intestinal motility. SYN desiccated p., hypophysis sicca.

pi·tu·i·tous (pi-tū'i-tŭs). Relating to pituita.

pit·y·ri·a·sic (pit-i-rī'ă-sik). Relating to or suffering from pityriasis.

pit·y·ri·a·sis (pit-i-rī'ă-sis). A dermatosis marked by branny desquamation. [G. fr. *pityron,* bran, dandruff]

p. al'ba, patchy hypopigmentation of the skin resulting from mild dermatitis.

p. al'ba atroph'icans, a scaling condition of the skin followed by atrophy.

p. amianta'cea, SYN *tinea* amiantacea.

p. cap'itis, SYN dandruff.

p. circina'ta, SYN p. rosea.

p. lichenoi'des, a self-limited skin disorder of children and adults, usually divided into p. lichenoides et varioliformis acuta and p. lichenoides chronica. SYN parapsoriasis guttata.

p. lichenoi'des et variolifor'mis acu'ta (PLEVA), an acute dermatitis affecting children and young adults that runs a relatively mild course and is self-limited, although persistence of lesions and recurrence of attacks are not uncommon; vesicles, papules, and crusted lesions eventually produce smallpox-like scars. SYN Mucha-Habermann disease, Mucha-Habermann syndrome, parapsoriasis lichenoides et varioliformis acuta, parapsoriasis varioliformis.

p. lin'guae, SYN geographic *tongue.*

p. macula'ta, SYN p. rosea.

p. ni'gra, SYN *tinea* nigra.

p. ro'sea, a self-limited eruption of macules or papules involving the trunk and less frequently extremities, scalp, and face; the lesions are usually oval and follow the crease lines of the skin; the onset is frequently preceded by a single larger scaling lesion known as the herald patch. SYN p. circinata, p. maculata.

p. ru'bra, SYN exfoliative *dermatitis.*

p. ru'bra pila'ris, an uncommon chronic pruritic eruption of the hair follicles, which become firm, red, surmounted with a horny plug, and often confluent to form scaly plaques; it is most conspicuously noted on the dorsa of the fingers and on the elbows and knees, and is associated with erythema, thickening of the palms and soles, and opaque thickening of the nails.

p. sic'ca, SYN dandruff.

p. versic'olor, SYN *tinea* versicolor.

pit·y·ri·a·sis li·che·noi·des chron·i·ca (līk'en-noyd'dēz kron'ik- ă). An eruption lasting up to a few years, of reddish-brown papules with central scaling, that clears without scarring. [lichenoides Mod. L., fr. G. *leichēn,* lichen, a lichen-like eruption, + *eidos,* resemblance chronica Mod. L. chronic, fr. G. *chronikos,* pertaining to time; fr. *chronos,* time]

pit·y·roid (pit'i-royd). SYN furfuraceous. [G. *pityrōdēs,* branlike, fr. *pityron,* bran, + *eidos,* resemblance]

Pit·y·ro·spo·rum (pit-i-ros'pō-rŭm, pit'i-rō-spō'rŭm). A genus of nonpathogenic fungi found in dandruff and seborrheic dermatitis. [G. *pityron,* bran, + *sporos,* seed]

P. orbicula're, SYN *Malassezia furfur.*

P. ova'le, SYN *Malassezia ovalis.*

piv·a·late (pĭv′ă-lāt). USAN-approved contraction for trimethylacetate, $(CH_3)_3C–CO_2$.

piv·ot (pĭv′ŏt). A post upon which something hinges or turns.

    adjustable occlusal p., an occlusal p. which may be adjusted vertically by means of a screw or by other means.

    occlusal p., an elevation contrived on the occlusal surface, usually in the molar region, designed to act as a fulcrum and to induce sagittal mandibular rotation.

pix, gen. **pi·cis** (piks, pī′sis). SYN pitch. [L]

pix·el (pĭk′sel). A contraction for picture element, a two-dimensional representation of a volume element (voxel) in the display of the CT or MR image, usually 512 by 512 or 256 by 256 pixels respectively.

PK Abbreviation for *pyruvate* kinase.

pK$_2$. The negative logarithm of the ionization constant (K_a) of an acid; the pH at which equal concentrations of the acid and conjugate base forms of a substance (often a buffer) are present.

pkat Abbreviation for picokatal.

PKU Abbreviation for phenylketonuria.

pkV, pkv Abbreviation for peak kilovoltage, the nominal voltage setting of an x-ray machine.

pkv. SEE pkV.

PL Abbreviation for placental lactogen.

pla·ce·bo (plă-sē′bō). **1.** An inert substance given as a medicine for its suggestive effect. **2.** An inert compound identical in appearance to material being tested in experimental research, which may or may not be known to the physician and/or patient, administered to distinguish between drug action and suggestive effect of the material under study. SYN active p. [L. I will please, future of *placeo*]

    active p., SYN placebo.

PLACENTA

---

pla·cen·ta (plă-sen′tă) [NA]. Organ of metabolic interchange between fetus and mother. It has a portion of embryonic origin, derived from a highly developed area of the outermost embryonic membrane (chorion frondosum), and a maternal portion formed by a modification of the part of the uterine mucosa (decidua basalis) in which the chorionic vesicle is implanted. Within the p., the chorionic villi, with their contained capillaries carrying blood of the embryonic circulation, are exposed to maternal blood in the intervillous spaces in which the villi lie; no direct mixing of fetal and maternal blood occurs, but the intervening tissue (the placental membrane) is sufficiently thin to permit the absorption of nutritive materials, oxygen, and some harmful substances, like viruses, into the fetal blood and the release of carbon dioxide and nitrogenous waste from it. At term, the human p. is disk-shaped, about 4 cm in thickness and 18 cm in diameter, and averages about ⅙ to ⅐ the weight of the fetus; its fetal surface is smooth, being formed by the adherent amnion, with the umbilical cord normally attached near its center; the maternal surface of a detached p. is rough because of the torn decidual tissue adhering to the chorion and shows lobular elevations called cotyledons or lobes. [L. a cake]

    accessory p., a mass of placental tissue distinct from the main p. SYN succenturiate p., supernumerary p.

    p. accre′ta, the abnormal adherence of the chorionic villi to the myometrium, associated with partial or complete absence of the decidua basalis and, in particular, the stratum spongiosum. SEE ALSO p. percreta.

    p. accre′ta ve′ra, the term applied when villi are juxtaposed to the myometrium.

    adherent p., a p. that fails to separate cleanly from the uterus after delivery.

    annular p., a p. in the form of a band encircling the interior of the uterus. SYN zonary p.

    battledore p., a p. in which the umbilical cord is attached at the

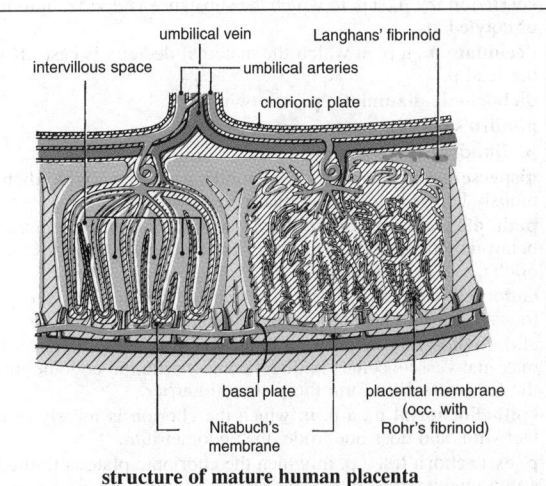

umbilical vein — Langhans' fibrinoid
intervillous space — umbilical arteries
chorionic plate
basal plate — placental membrane (occ. with Rohr's fibrinoid)
Nitabuch's membrane

structure of mature human placenta
arteries in *red*, veins in *blue*; on *left*, chorionic stems only; on *right*, whole chorionic complex with intervillous capillary system

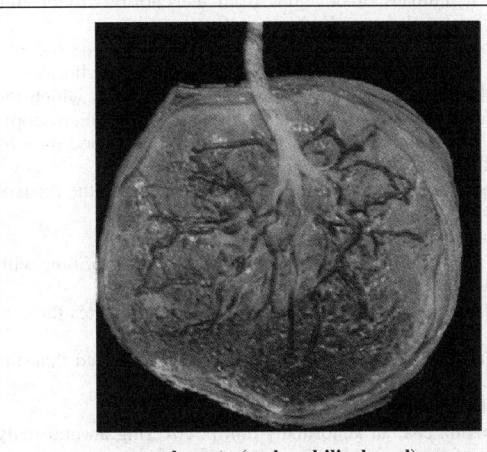

placenta (and umbilical cord)

border; so-called because of the fancied resemblance to the racquet (racket) used in battledore, a precursor to badminton.

    bidiscoidal p., a p. with two separate disc-shaped portions attached to opposite walls of the uterus, normal for certain monkeys and shrews, and occasionally found in humans.

    p. bilo′ba, a p. duplex in which the two parts are separated by a constriction. SYN p. bipartita.

    p. biparti′ta, SYN p. biloba.

    central p. previa, SYN p. previa centralis.

    chorioallantoic p., a p. (such as that of primates) in which the chorion is formed by the fusion of the allantoic mesoderm and vessels to the inner face of the serosa.

    chorioamnionic p., a form of placentation in which the amnion is fused to the inside of the chorion, thus permitting interchange of water and electrolytes between mother and fetus.

    choriovitelline p., a p. (seen in some lower animals) in which the chorion is formed by the fusion of yolk-sac mesoderm and vessels to the inner face of the serosa.

    p. circumvalla′ta, a cup-shaped p. with raised edges, having a thick, round, white, opaque ring around its periphery; a portion of the decidua separates the margin of the p. from its chorionic plate; the remainder of the chorionic surface is normal in appearance, but the fetal vessels are limited in their course across the p. by the ring. SEE ALSO p. marginata, p. reflexa.

cotyledonary p., a p. in which the substance is divided into lobes or cotyledons.

deciduate p., a p. in which the maternal decidua is cast off with the fetal p.

dichorionic diamniotic p., SEE twin p.

p. diffu′sa, SYN p. membranacea.

p. dimidia′ta, SYN p. duplex.

disperse p., a p. in which the umbilical arteries divide dichotomously before entering the placental substance.

p. du′plex, a p. consisting of two parts, almost entirely detached, being united only at the point of attachment of the cord. SEE p. biloba. SYN p. dimidiata.

endotheliochorial p., a p. in which the chorionic tissue penetrates to the endothelium of the maternal blood vessels.

endothelio-endothelial p., a p. in which the endothelium of the maternal vessels comes in direct contact with the endothelium of the fetal vessels to form the placental barrier.

epitheliochorial p., a p. in which the chorion is merely in contact with, and does not erode, the endometrium.

p. extrachora′les, a p. in which the chorionic plate is limited by a thin membranous fold at the edge.

p. fenestra′ta, a p. in which there are areas of thinning, sometimes extending to entire absence of placental tissue.

fetal p., p. feta′lis, the chorionic portion of the placenta, containing the fetal blood vessels, from which the funis develops; specifically, in humans, it develops from the chorion frondosum. SYN pars fetalis placentae [NA].

hemochorial p., the type of p., as in humans and some rodents, in which maternal blood is in direct contact with the chorion.

hemoendothelial p., the type of p., as in rabbits, in which the trophoblast becomes so attenuated that, by light microscopy, maternal blood appears to be separated from fetal blood only by the endothelium of the chorionic capillaries.

horseshoe p., an exaggerated p. reniformis curved in the form of a horseshoe; present in some twin pregnancies.

incarcerated p., SYN retained p.

p. incre′ta, a form of p. accreta in which the chorionic villi invade the myometrium.

labyrinthine p., a p. in which maternal blood circulates through channels within the fetal syncytiotrophoblast.

p. margina′ta, a p. with raised edges, less pronounced than the p. circumvallata. SEE ALSO p. reflexa.

maternal p., SYN *pars* uterina placentae.

p. membrana′cea, an abnormally thin p. covering an unusually large area of the uterine lining. SYN p. diffusa.

monochorionic diamniotic p., SEE twin p.

monochorionic monoamniotic p., SEE twin p.

p. multilo′ba, a p. having more than three lobes separated from each other by simple constrictions, the fetus being single. SYN placental multipartita.

nondeciduous p., a p. in which the fetal p. is cast off, leaving the uterine mucosa intact (*e.g.,* an epitheliochorial p.).

p. pandurafor′mis, a form of p. dimidiata with the two halves placed side by side in a shape suggestive of a lutelike musical instrument (pandura).

p. percre′ta, the term applied when the villi have invaded the full thickness of myometrium to or through the serosa of the uterus, causing incomplete or complete uterine rupture, respectively. SEE ALSO p. accreta.

p. pre′via, the condition in which the p. is implanted in the lower segment of the uterus, extending to the margin of the internal os of the cervix or partially or completely obstructing the os. SYN placental presentation.

p. pre′via centra′lis, p. previa in which the p. entirely covers the internal os of the cervix. SYN central p. previa, total p. previa.

p. pre′via margina′lis, p. previa in which the p. comes to the margin of, but does not occlude, the internal os of the cervix.

p. pre′via partia′lis, p. previa in which the internal os of the cervix is partially covered by placental tissue.

p. reflex′a, an anomaly of the p. in which the margin is thickened so as to appear turned back upon itself. SEE ALSO p. circumvallata, p. marginata.

p. renifor′mis, a kidney-shaped p.

retained p., incomplete separation of the p. and its failure to be expelled at the usual time after delivery of the child. SYN incarcerated p.

Schultze's p., a p. that appears at the vulva with the glistening fetal surface (amnion) presenting.

p. spu′ria, a mass of placental tissue which has no vascular connection with the main p.

succenturiate p., SYN accessory p.

supernumerary p., SYN accessory p.

syndesmochorial p., in ruminant animals, a type of p. in which the chorion is attached to maternal connective tissue.

total p. pre′via, SYN p. previa centralis.

p. tri′loba, SYN p. tripartita.

p. triparti′ta, a p. consisting of three parts almost entirely separate, being joined together only by the blood vessels of the umbilical cord; the fetus is single. SYN p. triloba, p. triplex.

p. tri′plex, SYN p. tripartita.

twin p., the placenta(s) of a twin pregnancy; if dizygotic, the p.'s may be separate or fused, the latter retaining two amniotic and two chorionic sacs (dichorionic diamniotic p.); if monozygotic, the p. may be a **monochorionic monoamniotic p.** or monochorionic diamniotic p., depending on the stage at which twinning took place; if twinning occurs early, there may be a fused p. with two chorionic and two amniotic membranes.

p. uteri′na, SYN *pars* uterina placentae.

p. velamento′sa, a p. in which the umbilical cord is attached to the adjoining membranes, with the umbilical vessels spread out and entering the p. independently.

villous p., a p. in which the chorion forms villi.

zonary p., SYN annular p.

---

pla·cen·ta·go·nad·o·trop·in. SYN chorionic *gonadotropin.*

pla·cen·tal (pla-sen′tăl). Relating to the placenta.

p. multipartita, SYN *placenta* multiloba.

pla·cen·tal dys·ma·ture. Immature development of the placenta so that normal function does not occur.

Pla·cen·ta·lia (plas-en-tā′lē-ă). SEE Eutheria. [L. *placenta*]

pla·cen·ta·scan (pla-sen′tă-skan). Obsolete method of determining the location of the placenta by means of injected radioactive material and its localization and display by a scintillation detector.

plac·en·ta·tion (plas-en-tā′shŭn). The structural organization and mode of attachment of fetal to maternal tissues in the formation of the placenta. Types of p. are defined under placenta.

plac·en·ti·tis (plas-en-tī′tis). Inflammation of the placenta.

plac·en·tog·ra·phy (plas-en-tog′ră-fē). Obsolete term for radiography of the placenta following intrauterine injection of a radiopaque contrast medium. [placenta + G. *graphō,* to write]

indirect p., obsolete term for radiographic determination of the presence of placenta previa by estimating the distance between the presenting fetal part and the bladder filled with contrast medium.

plac·en·to·ma (plas-en-tō′mă). SYN deciduoma.

pla·cen·to·ther·a·py (plă-sen′tō-thār′ă-pē). Therapeutic use of an extract of placental tissue.

Placido da Costa, Antonio, Portuguese ophthalmologist, 1848–1916. SEE P. da C.'s *disk.*

plac·ode (plak′ōd). Local thickening in the embryonic ectoderm layer; the cells of the p. ordinarily constitute a primordial group from which a sense organ or ganglion develops. [G. *plakōdēs,* fr. *plax,* anything flat or broad, + *eidos,* like]

auditory p.'s, paired ectodermal p.'s that sink below the general level of the superficial ectoderm to form the auditory vesicles. SYN otic p.'s.

epibranchial p.'s, ectodermal thickenings associated with the more dorsal parts of the embryonic branchial grooves; their cells are believed to contribute to formation of the cranial ganglia, especially those of nerves IX and X.

lens p.'s, paired ectodermal p.'s that become invaginated to form the embryonic lens vesicles. SYN optic p.'s.

nasal p.'s, SYN olfactory p.'s.

olfactory p.'s, paired ectodermal p.'s which come to lie in the bottom of the olfactory pits as the pits are deepened by the growth of the surrounding medial and lateral nasal processes. SYN nasal p.'s.

optic p.'s, SYN lens p.'s.

otic p.'s, SYN auditory p.'s.

plad·a·ro·ma, plad·a·ro·sis (plad-ă-rō′mă, -rō′sis). A soft wartlike growth on the eyelid. [G. *pladaros,* wet, damp, flaccid, + *-oma,* tumor]

pla·fond (plă-fon′). A ceiling, especially the ceiling of the ankle joint, *i.e.,* the articular surface of the distal end of the tibia. [Fr. ceiling]

⚠**plagio-.** Oblique, slanting. [G. *plagios*]

pla·gi·o·ce·phal·ic (plă′jē-ō-se-fal′ik). Relating to or marked by plagiocephaly. SYN plagiocephalous.

pla·gi·o·ceph·a·lism (plă′jē-ō-sef′ă-lizm). SYN plagiocephaly.

pla·gi·o·ceph·a·lous (plă′jē-ō-sef′ă-lŭs). SYN plagiocephalic.

pla·gi·o·ceph·a·ly (plă′jē-ō-sef′ă-lē). An asymmetric craniostenosis due to premature closure of the lambdoid and coronal sutures on one side; characterized by an oblique deformity of the skull. SYN plagiocephalism. [G. *plagios,* oblique, + *kephalē,* head]

plague (plăg). **1.** Any disease of wide prevalence or of excessive mortality. **2.** An acute infectious disease caused by the bacterium *Yersinia pestis* and marked clinically by high fever, toxemia, prostration, a petechial eruption, lymph node enlargement, and pneumonia, or hemorrhage from the mucous membranes; primarily a disease of rodents, transmitted to man by fleas that have bitten infected animals. In man the disease takes one of four clinical forms: bubonic *p.,* septicemic *p.,* pneumonic *p.,* or ambulant *p.*. SYN pest, pestilence (1), pestis. [L. *plaga,* a stroke, injury]

ambulant p., ambulatory p., a mild form of bubonic p. characterized by symptoms such as mild fever and lymphadenitis. SYN larval p., parapestis, pestis ambulans, pestis minor.

black p., SEE black *death.*

bubonic p., the usual form of p. marked by inflammatory enlargement of the lymphatic glands in the groins, axillae, or other parts. SYN glandular p., pestis bubonica, pestis fulminans, pestis major, polyadenitis maligna.

cattle p., SYN rinderpest.

duck p., a viral enteritis of ducks and other waterfowl in Europe, Asia, and the U.S. caused by an anatid herpes virus 1; manifested by weakness, lethargy, and diarrhea accompanied by catarrhal hemorrhagic enteritis and echymotic hemorrhages in organs and muscles. SYN duck viral enteritis.

fowl p., a highly fatal and highly transmissible disease of gallinaceous and passerine birds, pigeons, ducks, and geese, caused by avian influenza virus type A; symptoms include dyspnea, edema of head and neck, cyanosis, diarrhea, and sometimes disturbances of the central nervous system. SYN avian influenza, fowl pest.

glandular p., SYN bubonic p.

hemorrhagic p., the hemorrhagic form of bubonic p.

larval p., SYN ambulant p.

Pahvant Valley p., SYN tularemia.

pneumonic p., a rapidly progressive and frequently fatal form of p. in which there are areas of pulmonary consolidation, with chill, pain in the side, bloody expectoration, and high fever. SYN plague pneumonia, pulmonic p.

pulmonic p., SYN pneumonic p.

rabbit p., SYN rabbitpox.

septicemic p., a generally fatal form of p. in which there is an intense bacteremia with symptoms of profound toxemia. SYN pestis siderans.

sylvatic p., bubonic p. in rats and other wild animals.

plak·al·bu·min (plak-al-byū′min). The product of the action of subtilisin upon egg albumin, removing a hexapeptide.

pla·kins (plă′kinz). Bactericidal substances similar to leucins

extracted from blood platelets. [G. *plax, plakos,* anything flat, + -in]

⚠**plan-.** SEE plano-.

pla·na (plă′nă). Plural of planum. [L.]

plan·chet (plan′shet). A small, flat plate or dish used to support a sample for radioactivity determination; the sample is usually evaporated on (in) the p. [Fr. *planchette,* dim. of *planche,* plank]

Planck, Max, German physicist and Nobel laureate, 1858–1947. SEE P.'s *constant, theory.*

PLANE

pl

plane (plān). **1.** A flat surface. SEE planum. **2.** An imaginary surface formed by extension through any axis or two definite points in reference especially to craniometry and to pelvimetry. [L. *planus,* flat]

Addison's clinical p.'s, a series of p.'s used as landmarks in thoracoabdominal topography; the trunk is divided vertically by a *median p.* from the upper border of the manubrium of the sternum to the pubic symphysis, by a *lateral p.* drawn vertically on either side through a point half way between the anterior superior iliac spine and the median p. at the interspinal p., and by an *interspinal p.* passing vertically through the anterior superior iliac spine on either side; transversely the trunk is divided by a *transthoracic p.* passing across the thorax 3.2 cm above the lower border of the body of the sternum, by a *transpyloric p.* midway between the jugular notch of the sternum and the pubic symphysis, corresponding to the disc between the first and second lumbar vertebrae, and by an *intertubercular p.* passing through the iliac tubercles and cutting usually the fifth lumbar vertebra; the p.'s formed on these lines, and also on transverse p.'s cutting the upper edge of the manubrium and the upper edge of the pubic symphysis, constitute the clinical p.'s of Addison.

Aeby's p., in craniometry, a p. perpendicular to the median p. of the cranium, cutting the nasion and the basion.

auriculo-infraorbital p., SYN orbitomeatal p.

axial p., transverse plane, as in CT scanning. SYN transaxial p.

axiolabiolingual p., a p. parallel to the long axis of a tooth and extending in a labiolingual direction.

axiomesiodistal p., a p. parallel to the long axes of the teeth and extending in a mesiodistal direction.

bite p., SYN occlusal p.

Bolton p., a roentgenographic cephalometric p. extending from the Bolton point to nasion. SYN Bolton-Broadbent p., Bolton-nasion line, Bolton-nasion p.

Bolton-Broadbent p., SYN Bolton p.

Bolton-nasion p., SYN Bolton p.

Broca's visual p., a p. drawn through the visual axes of each eye.

Camper's p., a p. running from the tip of the anterior nasal spine (acanthion) to the center of the bony external auditory meatus on the right and left sides.

canthomeatal p., p. passing through the two lateral angles of the eye and the center of the external acoustic meatus; this p. lies approximately midway between the Frankfort and the supraorbitomeatal p.'s.

coronal p., a vertical p. at right angles to a sagittal p., dividing the body into anterior and posterior portions. SYN frontal p.

cove p., a classic description of terminal inversion of the electrocardiographic T wave with the initial portion arched above the baseline and the terminal portion below it, the former being rounded and the latter pointed.

datum p., an arbitrary p. used as a base from which to make craniometric measurements.

Daubenton's p., the p. of the foramen magnum. SEE ALSO Daubenton's *angle,* Daubenton's *line.*

equatorial p., in metaphase of mitosis, the p. that touches all of the centromeres and their spindle attachments.

eye-ear p., SYN orbitomeatal p.

facial p., a measurement of the bony profile of the face. SYN nasion-pogonion measurement.

first parallel pelvic p., SYN superior pelvic *aperture*.

fourth parallel pelvic p., SYN inferior pelvic *aperture*.

Frankfort p., SYN orbitomeatal p.

Frankfort horizontal p., SYN orbitomeatal p.

frontal p., SYN coronal p.

guide p., a fixed or removable device used to displace a single tooth, an arch segment, or an entire arch toward an improved relationship.

horizontal p., SYN transverse p.

p. of incidence, the p. perpendicular to a lens surface that contains the incident light ray.

infraorbitomeatal p., SYN orbitomeatal p.

p. of inlet, SYN superior pelvic *aperture*.

interspinal p., a horizontal plane passing through the anterior superior iliac spines; it marks the boundary between the lateral and umbilical regions superiorly and the inguinal and pubic regions inferiorly. SYN planum interspinale [NA], Lanz's line.

intertubercular p., a horizontal plane passing through the iliac tubercles. SYN planum intertuberculare [NA].

labiolingual p., a p. parallel to the labial and lingual surfaces of the teeth.

p. of least pelvic dimensions, SYN pelvic p. of least dimensions.

mean foundation p., the mean of the various irregularities in form and inclination of the basal seat; the ideal condition for denture stability exists when the mean foundation p. is most nearly at right angles to the direction of force.

Meckel's p., a craniometric p. cutting the alveolar and the auricular points.

median p., a vertical p. through the midline of the body that divides the body into right and left halves. SEE ALSO Addison's clinical p.'s. SYN midsagittal p.

p. of midpelvis, SYN pelvic p. of least dimensions.

midsagittal p., SYN median p.

Morton's p., a p. passing through the summits of the parietal and occipital protuberances.

nasion-postcondylar p., a p. passing through the nasion anteriorly and to a point immediately behind each condylar process of the mandible, posteriorly.

nodal p., the p. corresponding to the optical center of a simple lens. SEE nodal *point*.

nuchal p., the external surface of the squamous part of the occipital bone below the superior nuchal line, giving attachment to the muscles of the back of the neck.

occipital p., the external surface of the occipital bone above the superior nuchal line. SYN planum occipitale.

occlusal p., p. of occlusion, an imaginary surface which is related anatomically to the cranium and which theoretically touches the incisal edges of the incisors and the tips of the occluding surfaces of the posterior teeth; it is not a p. in the true sense of the word but represents the mean of the curvature of the surface. SEE ALSO *curve* of occlusion. SYN bite p.

orbital p., the orbital surface of the maxilla, lying perpendicular to the orbitomeatal p. at the orbitale. SYN planum orbitale.

orbitomeatal p., a standard craniometric reference p. passing through the right and left porion and the left orbitale; drawn on the profile radiograph or photograph from the superior margin of the acoustic meatus to the orbitale. SYN auriculo-infraorbital p., eye-ear p., Frankfort horizontal p., Frankfort p., infraorbitomeatal p.

p. of outlet, SYN inferior pelvic *aperture*.

parasagittal p., any p. parallel to the mid-sagittal p. or anteroposterior median p. SEE sagittal p.

p. of pelvic canal, SYN pelvic *axis*.

pelvic p. of greatest dimensions, the p. extending from the middle of the posterior surface of the pubic symphysis to the junction of the second and third sacral vertebrae, and laterally passing through the ischial bones over the middle of the acetabulum. SYN second parallel pelvic p., wide p.

pelvic p. of inlet, SYN superior pelvic *aperture*.

pelvic p. of least dimensions, the p. that extends from the end of the sacrum to the inferior border of the pubic symphysis; it is bounded posteriorly by the end of the sacrum, laterally by the ischial spines, and anteriorly by the inferior border of the pubic symphysis. SYN midplane, p. of least pelvic dimensions, p. of midpelvis, third parallel pelvic p.

pelvic p. of outlet, SYN inferior pelvic *aperture*.

popliteal p. of femur, SYN popliteal *surface* of femur.

principal p., the theoretic p. of a compound lens system. SEE principal *point*.

p.'s of reference, p.'s which act as a guide to the location of other p.'s.

p. of regard, an imaginary p. through which the point of regard moves as the eyes are turned from side to side.

sagittal p., originally (and strictly speaking) the sagittal plane is the median plane, and any other plane parallel to it is a parasagittal plane; in contemporary usage and in a broad sense, s. p. is used for any p. parallel to the median, *i.e.,* as a synonym for parasagittal.

second parallel pelvic p., SYN pelvic p. of greatest dimensions.

spectacle p., the p. at which spectacles are worn.

sternal p., a p. indicated by the front surface of the sternum. SYN planum sternale.

subcostal p., a horizontal plane passing through the inferior limits of the costal margin, *i.e.,* the tenth costal cartilages; it marks the boundary between the hypochondriac and epigastric regions superiorly and the lateral and umbilical regions inferiorly. SYN planum subcostale [NA], infracostal line.

supracrestal p., SYN supracristal p.

supracristal p., a horizontal plane passing through the summits of the iliac crests; it usually passes through the fourth lumbar spinous process. SYN planum supracristale [NA], supracrestal p.

supraorbitomeatal p., a p. passing the superior orbital margins and the superior margin of the external acoustic meatuses; it makes an angle of approximately 25 to 30 degrees with the Frankfort p. and is the p. in which routine CT (computed tomography) scans of the brain are made.

suprasternal p., a horizontal p. passing through the body at the level of the superior margin of the manubrium of the sternum.

temporal p., a slightly depressed area on the side of the cranium, below the inferior temporal line, formed by the temporal and parietal bones, the greater wing of the sphenoid, and a part of the frontal bone. SYN planum temporale.

third parallel pelvic p., SYN pelvic p. of least dimensions.

tooth p., any one of the imaginary p.'s of section of a tooth, such as the axial, horizontal, or vertical.

transaxial p., SYN axial p.

transpyloric p., a horizontal plane midway between the superior margins of the manubrium sterni and the symphysis pubis; the pylorus is not usually located on this plane in life. SYN planum transpyloricum [NA].

transverse p., a p. across the body at right angles to the coronal and sagittal p.'s. SYN horizontal p.

wide p., SYN pelvic p. of greatest dimensions.

---

plani-. SEE plano-.

pla·nig·ra·phy (pla-nig′ră-fē). SYN tomography. [L. *planum*, plane, + G. *graphē*, a writing]

pla·nim·e·ter (plă-nim′ĕ-ter). An instrument formed of jointed levers with a recording index, used for measuring the area of any surface, by tracing its boundaries. [L. *planum*, plane, + G. *metron*, measure]

pla·nim·et·ry (plă-nim′e-trē). The measurement of surface areas and perimeters by tracing the boundaries. Planimetry on photomicrographs or projected images may be used to evaluate the size of cells.

plan·ing (plăn′ing). SYN dermabrasion.

plan·i·tho·rax (plan′i-thō′raks). A diagram of the chest showing the front and back in plane projection, after the manner of Mercator's projection of the earth's surface.

plank·ter (plangk'ter). Any type of plankton.

plank·ton (plangk'ton). A general term for many floating marine forms, mostly of microscopic or minute size, which are moved passively by winds, waves, tides, or currents; it includes diatoms, algae, copepods, and many protozoans, crustacea, mollusks, and worms. [G. *planktos,* wandering]

plank·ton·ic (plangk-ton'ik). Relating to plankton; plankton-like.

plano-, plan-, plani-. **1.** A plane; flat, level. [L. *planum,* plane; *planus,* flat] **2.** Wandering. [G. *planos,* roaming]

pla·no·cel·lu·lar (plā-nō-sel'yū-lăr). Relating to or composed of flat cells. [L. *planus,* flat, + cellular]

pla·no·con·cave (plā'nō-kon'kāv). Flat on one side and concave on the other; denoting a lens of that shape.

pla·no·con·vex (plā'nō-kon'veks). Flat on one side and convex on the other; denoting a lens of that shape.

pla·nog·ra·phy (pla-nog'ră-fē). SYN tomography.

plan·o·ma·nia (plan-ō-mā'nē-ă). The morbid impulse to leave home and discard social restraints. [G. *planos,* wandering, + *mania,* frenzy]

Pla·nor·bis (plan-ōr'bis). A European and North African genus of freshwater snails (family Planorbidae), including *P. planorbis,* intermediate host of the sheep and cattle fluke, *Paramphistoma cervi.* [G. *planos,* wandering, + L. *orbis,* circle, ring]

plan·o·top·o·ki·ne·sia (plan'ō-top'ō-ki-nē'zē-ă). Loss of orientation in space. [G. *planos,* wandering, + *topos,* place, + *kinēsis,* motion]

pla·no·val·gus (plā-nō-val'gŭs). A condition in which the longitudinal arch of the foot is flattened and everted. [plano- + L. *valgus,* turned outward]

plan·ta, gen. and pl. **plan·tae** (plan'tă, plan'tē) [NA]. SYN sole. [L.]

p. pe'dis [NA], SYN *sole* of foot.

plan·ta·go (plan-tā'gō). The root and leaves of the common or large-leaved plantain, *Plantago major* (family Plantaginaceae). [L. plantain]

p. ovata coating, the separated outer mucilaginous layers of *Plantago ovata* seeds; used in simple constipation associated with lack of sufficient bulk.

p. seed, SYN psyllium seed.

plan·tain seed. SYN psyllium seed.

plan·tal·gia (plan-tal'jē-ă). Pain on the plantar surface of the foot over the plantar fascia. [L. *planta,* sole of foot, + G. *algos,* pain]

plan·tar (plan'tăr). Relating to the sole of the foot. SYN plantaris [NA]. [L. *plantaris*]

plan·tar·is (plan-tār'is) [NA]. SYN plantar, plantar. [L.]

plan·ti·grade (plan'ti-grād). Walking with the entire sole and heel of the foot on the ground, as do man and bears. Cf. digitigrade. [L. *planta,* sole, + *gradior,* to walk]

plan·u·la, pl. **plan·u·lae** (plan'yū-lă, -lē). Name given by Lankester to a coelenterate embryo when it consists of the two primary germ layers only, the ectoderm and endoderm. [L. dim. of *planum,* flat surface]

invaginate p., SYN gastrula.

pla·num, pl. **pla·na** (plā'nŭm, plā'nă). A plane or flat surface. SEE ALSO plane. [L. plane]

p. interspina'le [NA], SYN interspinal *plane.* SEE ALSO Addison's clinical *planes,* under *plane.*

p. intertubercula're [NA], SYN intertubercular *plane.* SEE ALSO Addison's clinical *planes,* under *plane.*

p. occipita'le, SYN occipital *plane.*

p. orbita'le, SYN orbital *plane.*

p. poplit'eum, SYN popliteal *surface* of femur.

p. semiluna'tum, the area of epithelium bounding the sensory area of the crista ampullaris.

p. sphenoida'le, SYN *jugum* sphenoidale.

p. sterna'le, SYN sternal *plane.*

p. subcosta'le [NA], SYN subcostal *plane.*

p. supracrista'le [NA], SYN supracristal *plane.*

p. tempora'le, SYN temporal *plane.*

p. transpylo'ricum [NA], SYN transpyloric *plane.* SEE Addison's clinical *planes,* under *plane.*

pla·nu·ria (plă-nū'rē-ă). **1.** Extravasation of urine. **2.** The voiding of urine from an abnormal opening. [G. *planos,* wandering, + *ouron,* urine]

plaque (plak). **1.** A patch or small differentiated area on a body surface (*e.g.,* skin, mucosa, or arterial endothelium) or on the cut surface of an organ such as the brain. **2.** An area of clearing in a flat confluent growth of bacteria or tissue cells, such as is caused by the lytic action of bacteriophage in an agar plate culture of bacteria, by the cytopathic effect of certain animal viruses in a sheet of cultured tissue cells, or by antibody (hemolysin) produced by lymphocytes cultured in the presence of erythrocytes and to which complement has been added. **3.** A sharply defined zone of demyelination characteristic of multiple sclerosis. **4.** SEE dental p. [Fr. a plate]

atheromatous p., a well-demarcated yellow area or swelling on the intimal surface of an artery; produced by intimal lipid deposit.

bacterial p., in dentistry, a mass of filamentous microorganisms and large variety of smaller forms attached to the surface of a tooth which, depending on bacterial activity and environmental factors, may give rise to caries, calculus, or inflammatory changes in adjacent tissue. SYN dental p. (2), mucous p., mucinous p.

bacteriophage p., a clear circular zone in an otherwise confluent growth of bacteria on an agar surface resulting from bacterial lysis by bacterial viruses.

dental p., **(1)** the noncalcified accumulation mainly of oral microorganisms and their products, that adheres tenaciously to the teeth and is not readily dislodged; **(2)** SYN bacterial p.

Hollenhorst p.'s, glittering, orange-yellow, atheromatous emboli in the retinal arterioles that contain cholesterin crystals and originate in the carotid artery or great vessels.

mucous p., mucinous p., SYN bacterial p.

neuritic p., SYN senile p.

pleural p., fibrous thickening of the parietal pleura, characteristically caused by inhalation exposure to asbestos.

Randall's p.'s, mineral concentrations of renal papillae.

senile p., a spherical mass comprised primarily of amyloid fibrils and interwoven neuronal processes, frequently, although not exclusively, observed in Alzheimer's disease. SYN neuritic p.

Plaque In·dex. An index for estimating the status of oral hygiene by measuring dental plaque which occurs in the areas adjacent to the gingival margin.

-plasia. Formation (especially of cells). SEE plasma-. [G. *plassō,* to form]

plasm (plazm). SYN plasma.

plas·ma (plaz'mă). **1.** The fluid (noncellular) portion of the circulating blood, as distinguished from the serum obtained after coagulation. SYN blood p. **2.** The fluid portion of the lymph. **3.** A "fourth state of matter" in which, owing to elevated temperature (*ca.* 10^6 degrees), atoms have broken down to form free electrons and more or less stripped nuclei; produced in the laboratory in connection with hydrogen fusion (thermonuclear) research. SYN plasm. [G. something formed]

antihemophilic p., human p. in which the labile antihemophilic globulin component, present in fresh p., has been preserved; it is used to temporarily relieve dysfunction of the hemostatic mechanism in hemophilia.

blood p., SYN plasma (1).

fresh frozen p. (FFP), separated p., frozen within 6 hours of collection, used in hypovolemia and coagulation factor deficiency.

p. hydrolysate, an artificial digest of protein derived from bovine blood p. prepared by a method of hydrolysis sufficient to provide more than half of the total nitrogen present in the form of α-amino nitrogen; used when high protein intake is indicated and cannot be accomplished through ordinary foods. SEE ALSO protein hydrolysate.

p. mari'num, sea water diluted to make it isotonic with p.

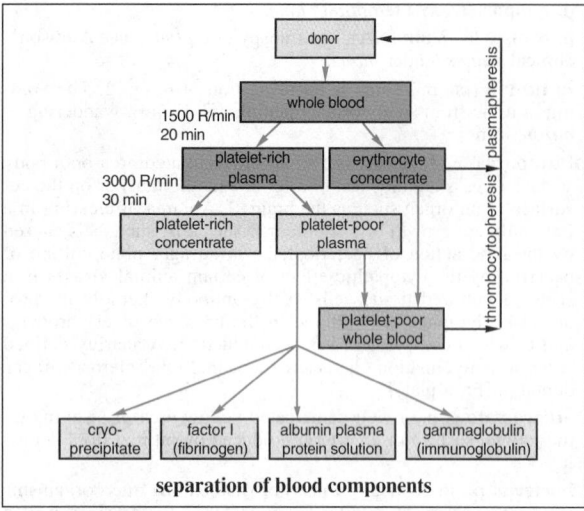

separation of blood components

blood plasma		
selected components of plasma or serum: normal parameters		
ammonia-*N* (whole blood)	53-143	µmol/l
bicarbonate	21-25	mmol/l
bilirubin (total)	5.1-18.8	µmol/l
bilirubin (direct)	up to 6.8	µmol/l
lead (whole blood)	up to 2.0	µmol/l
blood sugar: see glucose		
calcium	2.2-2.7	mmol/l
chloride	94-111	mmol/l
cholesterin	3.36-6.72*	mmol/l
creatine	♂ 23-61	µmol/l
	♀ 23-92	
creatinine	♂ 62-106	µmol/l
	♀ 44-88	
iron	♂ 16.1-25.1	µmol/l
	♀ 14.3-21.5	
iron binding capacity		
–total	♂ 53.7-71.6	µmol/l
	♀ 44.8-62.7	
–free	♂ 35.8-53.7	µmol/l
	♀ 26.9-44.8	
protein, total	67-87	g/l
fat, total	3.6-8.2*	g/l
fatty acids, free	200-900	µmol/l
fructose	up to 0.55	mmol/l
galactose	up to 0.24	mmol/l
glucose	3.33-5.55*	mmol/l
glycerine, total	0.27-2.88	mmol/l
glycerine, free	up to 0.25	mmol/l
uric acid	♂ 155-404	µmol/l
(enzymatic)	♀ 119-375	
urea	3.33-6.66	mmol/l
potassium	4.1-5.6	mmol/l
copper	♂ 11.0-22.0	µmol/l
	♀ 13.4-24.4	g/l
β-lipoproteide	3.6-6.4*	µmol/l
lithium	0.4-6.3	mmol/l
magnesium	0.66-0.90	mmol/l
lactate	1.00-1.78	mmol/l
sodium	137-148	mmol/l
phosphatide	1.74-3.94	mmol/l
inorganic phosphorus	0.81-1.55	nmol/l
thyroxine	66-187	mmol/l
triglyceride	0.97-2.70*	
*age-dependent		

muscle p., an alkaline fluid in muscle that is spontaneously coagulable, separating into myosin and muscle serum.

normal human p., sterile p. obtained by pooling approximately equal amounts of the liquid portion of citrated whole blood from eight or more adult humans who have been certified as free from any disease which is tranmissible by transfusion, and treating it with ultraviolet irradiation to destroy possible bacterial and viral contaminants.

salted p., the fluid portion of blood drawn from the vessels, which is prevented from coagulating by being drawn into a solution of sodium or magnesium sulfate. SYN salted serum.

plasma-, plasmat-, plasmato-, plasmo-. Formative, organized; plasma. [G. *plasma,* something formed]

plas·ma·blast (plaz'mă-blast). Precursor of the plasma cell. SYN plasmacytoblast. [plasma + G. *blastos,* germ]

plas·ma cell dys·cra·sia. A diverse group of diseases characterized by the proliferation of a single clone of cells producing a monoclonal immunoglobulin or immunoglobulin fragment (a serum M component). The cells usually have plasma cell morphology, but may have lymphocytic or lymphoplasmacytic morphology. This group includes multiple myeloma, Waldenström's macroglobulinemia, the heavy chain disease, benign monoclonal gammopathy, and immunocytic amyloidosis.

plas·ma·crit (plaz'mă-krit). A measure of the percentage of the volume of blood occupied by plasma, in contrast to a hematocrit. [plasma + G. *krinō,* to separate]

plas·ma·cyte (plaz'mă-sīt). SYN plasma *cell.*

plas·ma·cy·to·blast (plas-mă-sī'tō-blast). SYN plasmablast.

plas·ma·cy·to·ma (plaz'mă-sī-tō'mă). A discrete, presumably solitary mass of neoplastic plasma cells in bone or in one of various extramedullary sites; in man, such lesions are probably the initial phase of developing plasma cell myeloma. [plasmacyte + G. *-oma,* tumor]

plas·ma·cy·to·sis (plaz'mă-sī-tō'sis). **1.** Presence of plasma cells in the circulating blood. **2.** Presence of unusually large proportions of plasma cells in the tissues or exudates. [plasmacyte + G. *-osis,* condition]

plas·ma ex·pand·er (plaz'mă eks-pan'der). SYN plasma *substitute.*

plas·ma·gene (plaz'mă-jēn). A determinant of an inherited character located in the cytoplasm. SYN cytogene. [plasma + gene]

plas·ma·ki·nins (plaz'mă-kīn'inz). A group of highly active oligopeptides found in sera that act upon smooth muscle of blood vessels, uterus, bronchi, etc.; *e.g.,* bradykinin, kallidin.

plas·ma·lem·ma (plaz-mă-lem'ă). SYN cell *membrane.* [plasma + G. *lemma,* husk]

plas·mal·o·gens (plaz-mal'ō-jenz). Generic term for glycerophospholipids in which the glycerol moiety bears a 1-alkenyl ether group (on rarer occasions, a 1-alkyl ether group); *e.g.,* alk-

1-enylglycerophospholipid; p. synthesis is reduced in disorders of the peroxisome. SYN phosphoglyceracetals.

plas·mals (plaz'mălz). Long-chain aldehydes occurring in plasmalogens; *e.g.,* stearaldehyde, palmitaldehyde.

plas·ma·phe·re·sis (plaz'mă-fĕ-rē'sis). Removal of whole blood from the body, separation of its cellular elements by centrifugation, and reinfusion of them suspended in saline or some other plasma substitute, thus depleting the body's own plasma without depleting its cells. [plasma + G. *aphairesis,* a withdrawal]

plas·ma·phe·ret·ic (plaz'mă-fĕ-ret'ik). Relating to plasmapheresis.

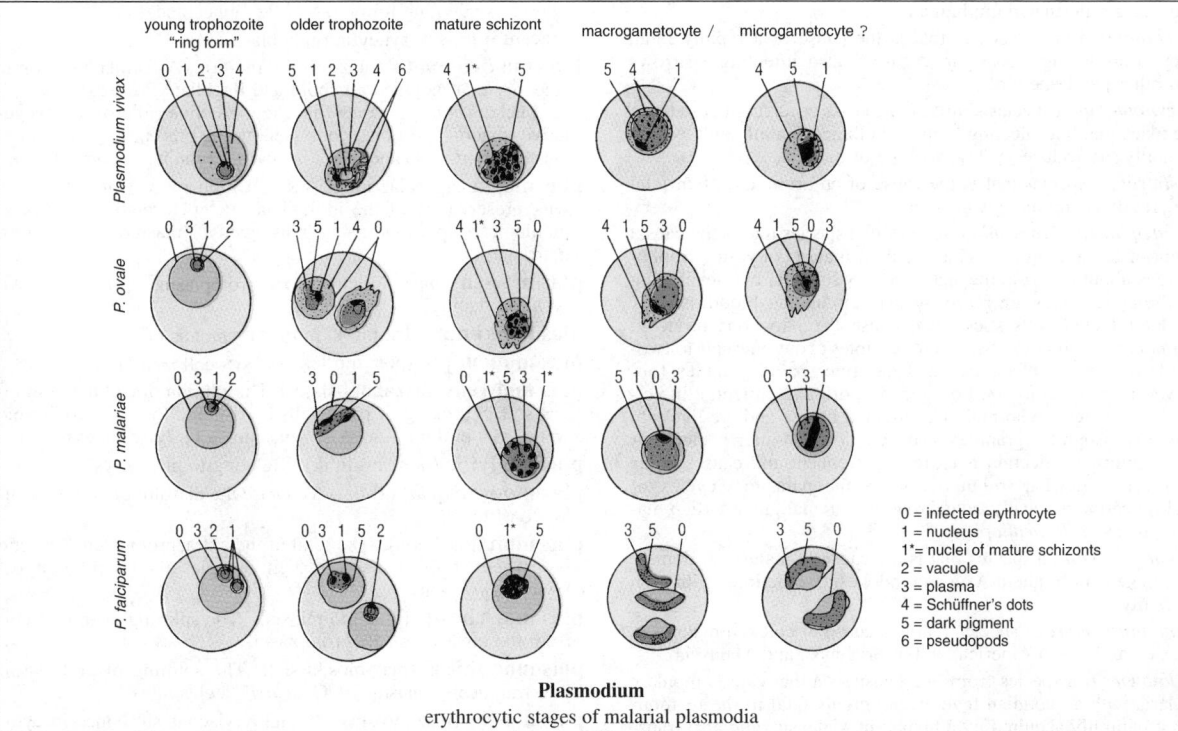

Plasmodium
erythrocytic stages of malarial plasmodia

0 = infected erythrocyte
1 = nucleus
1* = nuclei of mature schizonts
2 = vacuole
3 = plasma
4 = Schüffner's dots
5 = dark pigment
6 = pseudopods

plasmat-. SEE plasma-.

plas·mat·ic (plaz-mat'ik). Relating to plasma. SYN plasmic.

plas·ma·tog·a·my (plaz-mă-tog'ă-mē). SYN plasmogamy.

plas·men·ic ac·id (plaz'men-ik). Proposed name for phosphatidates such as alk-1-enylglycerol (lipid).

plas·mic (plaz'mik). SYN plasmatic.

plas·mid (plaz'mid). A genetic particle physically separate from the chromosome of the host cell (chiefly bacterial) that can stably function and replicate; not essential to the cell's basic functioning. SYN extrachromosomal element, extrachromosomal genetic element, paragene. [cyto*plasm* + -id]

bacteriocinogenic p.'s, bacterial p.'s responsible for the elaboration of bacteriocins. SYN bacteriocin factors, bacteriocinogens.

conjugative p., a p. that can effect its own intercellular transfer by means of conjugation; this transfer is accomplished by a bacterium being rendered a donor, usually with specialized pili. SYN infectious p., transmissible p.

F p., the prototype conjugative p. associated with conjugation in the K-12 strain of *Escherichia coli.* SYN F agent, F factor, F genote, F-genote, fertility agent, fertility factor, sex factor.

infectious p., SYN conjugative p.

nonconjugative p., a p. that cannot effect conjugation and self-transfer to another bacterium (bacterial strain); transfer depends upon mediation of another (and conjugative) p.

R p.'s, SYN resistance p.'s.

resistance p.'s, p.'s carrying genes responsible for antibiotic (or antibacterial drug) resistance among bacteria (notably Enterobacteriaceae); they may be conjugative or nonconjugative p.'s, the former possessing transfer genes (resistance transfer factor) lacking in the latter. SYN R factors, R p.'s, resistance factors, resistance-transferring episomes.

transmissible p., SYN conjugative p.

plas·min (plaz'min). An enzyme hydrolyzing peptides and esters of L-arginine and L-lysine, and converting fibrin to soluble products; occurs in plasma as the precursor of plasminogen (profibrinolysin) and is activated to plasmin by organic solvents, which remove an inhibitor, and by streptokinase, trypsin, and

plasminogen activator, all cleaving a single arginyl-valyl bond; p. is responsible for the dissolution of blood clots. SYN fibrinase (2), fibrinolysin.

plas·min·o·gen (plaz-min'ō-jen). **1.** A precursor of plasmin. There is an autosomal dominant deficiency of p. [MIM*173350] that may promote thrombosis. SEE plasmin.

plas·min·o·ki·nase (plaz'min-ō-ki'nās). SYN streptokinase.

plas·min·o·plas·tin (plaz'min-ō-plas'tin). Term proposed for activator agents that produce plasmin by direct action on plasminogen; *e.g.,* staphylokinase, plasminogen activator.

plasmo-. SEE plasma-.

plas·mo·dia (plaz-mō'dē-ă). Plural of plasmodium. [L.]

plas·mo·di·al (plaz-mō'dē-ăl). **1.** Relating to a plasmodium. **2.** Relating to any species of the genus *Plasmodium.*

plas·mo·di·o·tro·pho·blast (plaz-mō'dē-ō-trō'fō-blast). SYN syncytiotrophoblast. [plasmodium + G. *trophē,* nourishment, + *blastos,* germ]

Plas·mo·di·um (plaz-mō'dē-ŭm). A genus of the protozoan family Plasmodiidae (suborder Haemosporina, subclass Coccidia), blood parasites of vertebrates, characterized by separate microgametes and macrogametes, a motile ookinete, sporogony in the invertebrate host, and merogony (schizogony) in the vertebrate host; includes the causal agents of malaria in man and other animals, with an asexual cycle occurring in liver and red blood cells of vertebrates and a sexual cycle in mosquitoes, the latter cycle resulting in the production of large numbers of infective sporozoites in the salivary glands of the vector, which are transmitted when the mosquito bites and draws blood. Primate malaria is transmitted by various species of *Anopheles* mosquitoes, bird malaria by species of *Aedes, Culex, Anopheles,* and *Culiseta.* [Mod. L. from G. *plasma,* something formed, + *eidos,* appearance]

P. aethio'picum, SYN *P. falciparum.*

P. ber'ghei, a species that is the etiologic agent of rodent malaria from central Africa; an important source of experimental nonprimate mammal malaria.

P. brazilian'um, a species found in New World monkeys of the family Cebidae in northern South America and Panama which can cause mild malaria in humans.

P. catheme'rium, a species that is the cause of a rapidly fatal, anemia-producing disease in canaries, also infecting sparrows and other passerine birds.

P. cynomol'gi, a species similar to *P. vivax* occurring naturally in the macaque, but infecting humans both accidentally and experimentally; it produces a *P.-vivax* type of malaria.

P. du'rae, a species that is the cause of an acute and often fatal malaria of young turkeys in Africa.

P. falcip'arum, Laverania falciparum, a species that is the causal agent of falciparum (malignant tertian) malaria; a young trophozoite is about one-fifth the size of an erythrocyte, but developing erythrocytic stages are rarely seen in circulating blood, as they render infected cells sticky and cause them to concentrate in pulmonary capillaries; a schizont occupies about one-half to two-thirds of the red blood cell and has fine sparse granules (observed in peripheral blood only from moribund patients); infected erythrocytes are normal or contracted in size and are likely to contain basophilic granules and red dots (Maurer's clefts or dots); multiple infection is extremely frequent and causes bouts of fever somewhat irregularly since the parasites' cycles of multiplication is usually asynchronous. SYN malignant tertian malarial parasite, *P. aethiopicum.*

P. gallina'ceum, a species that is the cause of malaria in domestic chickens in southern Asia and Indonesia, sometimes with high mortality.

P. juxtanuclea're, a species that is a cause of chicken malaria in Mexico and South America, and in Sri Lanka and Malaysia.

P. knowles'i, a species from Southeast Asia that causes monkey malaria with a quotidian fever cycle; highly fatal in rhesus monkeys; naturally acquired by a human in Malaysia, and also transmitted to humans experimentally.

P. ko'chi, a *P.* species now recognized as *Hepatocystis kochi.*

P. mala'riae, a species that is the causal agent of quartan malaria; a ring-stage trophozoite is triangular, ovoid, or slightly bean-shaped, with fine or coarse black granules, approximately one-third the size of an eythrocyte; the schizont is oval or rounded and nearly fills the red blood cell; infected erythrocytes are normal or slightly contracted in size, usually with no stippling (the two most important characteristics that distinguish it from *P. vivax,* although extremely fine Ziemann's dots may be observed; multiple infection is extremely rare, thus bouts of fever occur fairly regularly at 72-hour intervals; prolonged asymptomatic parasitemia is characteristic of the species and recrudescence of fever may occur 10 years or more after the initial episode. SYN quartan parasite.

P. ova'le, a species that is the agent of the least common form of human malaria; resembles *P. vivax* in its earlier stages, but often modifies the cell membrane, causing it to form a fimbriated outline, and often assume an oval shape; Schüffner's dots are abundant and appear early, host cells are normal or only slightly enlarged, and only about 8 to 10 grapelike merozoites are produced; fever is tertian (every 48 hours), and relapses are infrequent.

P. relic'tum, a species of worldwide distribution found in pigeons, doves, ducks, swans, and a great variety of other birds; it is highly pathogenic in pigeons, game birds, and others to which this strain is poorly adapted, causing anemia, weakness, and often death.

P. vi'vax, a species that is the most common malarial parasite of man (except in west Africa, where lack of the Duffy antigen protects most of the resident populations, which has permitted *P. ovale* to replace *P. vivax*); the early trophozoite is irregular and ameboid in shape, one-fourth to one-third the size of a red blood cell, and contains several fine granules; the schizont is irregular in shape, fills the enlarged erythrocyte, and contains numerous yellow-brown pigment granules; affected red blood cells are pale, enlarged, and contain Schüffner's dots in the later stages of growth; causes bouts of fever fairly regularly at 48-hour intervals; but multiple infection is common. SYN tertian parasite.

plas·mo·di·um, pl. **plas·mo·dia** (plaz-mō'dē-ŭm, -dē-ă). A protoplasmic mass containing several nuclei, resulting from

multiplication of the nucleus with cell division. [Mod. L. fr. G. *plasma,* something formed, + *eidos,* appearance]

placental p., SYN syncytiotrophoblast.

Plas·mo·dro·ma·ta (plaz-mō-drō'mă-tă). A former taxonomic category that included ameboid and flagellate Protozoa in which the nucleus is not separated into reproductive (micro-) and vegetative (macro-) portions; equivalent to the present phylum Sarcomastigophora. [plasmo- + G. *dromos,* a running, a course]

plas·mog·a·my (plaz-mog'ă-mē). Union of two or more cells with preservation of the individual nuclei; formation of a plasmodium. SYN plasmatogamy, plastogamy. [plasmo- + G. *gamos,* marriage]

plas·mo·gen (plaz'mō-jen). SYN protoplasm. [plasmo- + G. *-gen,* producing]

plas·mo·ki·nin (plaz-mō-kī'nin). SYN *factor* VIII.

plas·mo·lem·ma (plaz-mō-lem'ă). SYN cell *membrane.*

plas·mol·y·sis (plaz-mol'i-sis). **1.** Dissolution of cellular components. **2.** Shrinking of plant cells by osmotic loss of cytoplasmic water. SYN protoplasmolysis. [plasmo- + G. *lysis,* dissolution]

plas·mo·lyt·ic (plaz-mō-lit'ik). Relating to plasmolysis.

plas·mo·lyze (plaz'mō-līz). To cause the dissolution of the cellular constituents.

plas·mon (plaz'mon). The total of the extrachromosomal genetic properties of the eukaryotic cell cytoplasm. SYN plasmotype. [cyto*plasm* + -on]

plas·mor·rhex·is (plaz-mō-rek'sis). The splitting open of a cell from the pressure of the protoplasm.

plas·mos·chi·sis (plaz-mos'ki-sis). The splitting of protoplasm into fragments. [plasmo- + G. *schisis,* a cleaving]

plas·mo·sin (plaz'mō-sin). A highly viscous substance in cytoplasm containing discrete fibers of considerable length; a nucleoprotein regarded as the structural foundation of the cell.

plas·mot·o·my (plaz-mot'ō-mē). A form of mitosis in multinuclear protozoan cells in which the cytoplasm divides into two or more masses, later reproducing, in some cases by sporulation. [plasmo- + G. *tomē,* incision]

plas·mo·tro·pic (plaz-mō-trop'ik). Pertaining to or manifesting plasmotropism.

plas·mot·ro·pism (plaz-mot'rō-pizm). A condition in which the bone marrow, spleen, and liver are sites for the destruction of the erythrocytes, as opposed to destruction in the circulating blood. [plasmo- + G. *tropē,* a turning]

plas·mo·type (plaz'mō-tīp). SYN plasmon.

plas·mo·zyme (plaz'mō-zīm). SYN prothrombin. [plasmo- + G. *zymē,* leaven]

plas·tein (plas'tē-in). Insoluble polypeptide formed through the random condensation of amino acids or peptides under the catalytic influence of a proteinase-like chymotrypsin; molecular weights as high as 500,000 are reported.

plas·ter. 1. A solid preparation which can be spread when heated, and which becomes adhesive at the temperature of the body; used to keep the edges of a wound in apposition, to protect raw surfaces, and, when medicated, to redden or blister the skin or to apply drugs to the surface to obtain their systemic effects. **2.** In dentistry, colloquialism for p. of Paris. [L. *emplastrum;* G. *emplastron,* plaster or mold]

p. of Paris, exsiccated calcium sulfate from which the water of crystallization has been expelled by heat, but which, when mixed with water, will form a paste which subsequently sets.

plas·tic (plas'tik). **1.** Capable of being formed or molded. **2.** A material that can be shaped by pressure or heat to the form of a cavity or mold. [G. *plastikos,* relating to molding]

Bingham p., a material that, in the idealized case, does not flow until a critical stress (yield stress) is exceeded, and then flows at a rate proportional to the excess of stress over the yield stress; real materials probably only approach this ideal model.

modeling p., a thermoplastic material usually composed of gum damar and prepared chalk, used especially for making dental impressions. SYN impression compound, modeling composition, modeling compound.

plas·tic·i·ty (plas-tis′i-tē). The capability of being formed or molded; the quality of being plastic.

plas·tid (plas′tid). **1.** One of the differentiated structures in cytoplasm of plant cells where photosynthesis or other cellular processes are carried on; p.'s contain DNA and are self-replicating. SYN trophoplast. **2.** One of the granules of foreign or differentiated matter, food particles, fat, waste material, chromatophores, trichocysts, etc., in cells. **3.** A self-duplicating virus-like particle that multiplies within a host cell, such as kappa particles in certain paramecia. [G. *plastos,* formed, + -id]

blood p., any basic, morphologic unit in the biologic composition of blood, *e.g.,* an erythrocyte.

plas·to·chro·man·ol-3, plas·to·chro·ma·nol E₃ (plas-tō-krō′man-ol). A γ-tocotrienol. SEE tocotrienol.

plas·to·chro·men·ol-8 (plas-tō-krō′men-ol). The chromenol (isomeric) form of plastoquinone-9. SYN solanochromene.

plas·tog·a·my (plas-tog′ă-mē). SYN plasmogamy.

plas·to·quin·one (PQ) (plas-tō-kwin′ōn, -kwī′nōn). 2,3-Dimethyl-1,4-benzoquinone with a multiprenyl side chain; a trivial name sometimes used for plastoquinone-9.

plas·to·quin·one-9 (PQ-9), plas·to·quin·one E₉. 2,3-Dimethyl-6-nonaprenyl-1,4-benzoquinone; one of a group of vitamins E and K and coenzymes Q; the isomeric form is plastochromenol-8; a participant in photosynthetic electron transport.

plas·tron. The sternum with costal cartilages attached. [Fr. a breastplate]

plas·ty (plas′tē). Surgical procedure for repair of a defect or restoration of form and/or function of a part. [G. *plastos,* formed]

△-plasty. Molding, shaping or the result thereof, as of a surgical procedure. [G. *plastos,* formed, shaped]

plate (plāt). **1.** In anatomy, a thin, flat, structure, such as a lamina or lamella. **2.** A metal bar applied to a fractured bone in order to maintain the ends in apposition. **3.** The agar layer within a Petri dish or similar vessel. **4.** To form a very thin layer of a bacterial culture by streaking it on the surface of an agar p. (usually within a Petri dish) in order to isolate individual organisms from which a colonial clone will develop. [O.Fr. *plat,* a flat object, fr. G. *platys,* flat, broad]

alar p. of neural tube, SYN alar *lamina* of neural tube.

anal p., the anal portion of the cloacal p.

axial p., the primitive streak of an embryo.

basal p. of neural tube, SYN basal *lamina* of neural tube.

base p., SEE baseplate.

blood p., SYN platelet.

bone p., a metal bar with perforations for the insertion of screws; used to immobilize fractured segments.

buttress p., a metal p. used to support the internal fixation of a fracture.

cardiogenic p., the thickened layer of splanchnic mesoderm from which the cardiopericardial primordia of very young embryos are derived.

cell p., a non-cellulose structure that is the precursor to the cell wall; it forms between daughter nuclei during mitosis.

chorionic p., that portion of the chorionic wall in the region of its uterine attachment; it consists of the mesoderm that lines the chorionic vesicle and, on the maternal side, of the trophoblast that lines the intervillous spaces; in the last half of gestation, the mesodermal connective tissue is largely replaced by fibrinoid material, and the amniotic membrane is adherent to the fetal side of the plate.

cloacal p., a p., composed of a layer of cloacal endoderm in contact with a layer of proctodeal ectoderm, which subsequently ruptures, forming the anal and urogenital openings of the embryo.

cribriform p. of ethmoid bone, a horizontal p. from which are suspended the labyrinth, on either side, and the p. perpendicularis in the center; it fits into the ethmoidal notch of the frontal bone and supports the olfactory lobes of the cerebrum, being pierced with numerous openings for the passage of the olfactory nerves. SYN lamina cribrosa ossis ethmoidalis [NA], cribrum, sieve bone, sieve p.

cutis p., SYN dermatome (2).

dorsal p. of neural tube, SYN roof p.

dorsolateral p. of neural tube, SYN alar *lamina* of neural tube.

end p., SEE endplate.

epiphysial p., the disc of cartilage between the metaphysis and the epiphysis of an immature long bone permitting growth in length. SYN cartilago epiphysialis [NA], epiphysial cartilage.

equatorial p., the assembly of chromosomes in mitosis.

ethmovomerine p., the central portion of the ethmoid bone, forming a distinct element at birth.

flat p., jargon for plain *film.*

floor p., ventral midline thinning of the developing neural tube, a continuity between the basal laminae of either side; opposite of roof plate. SYN ventral p.

foot p., SEE footplate.

frontal p., in the fetus, a cartilage p. between the lateral parts of ethmoid cartilage and the developing sphenoid bone.

horizontal p. of palatine bone, the part of the palatine bone that forms the posterior part (approximately one third) of the bony palate. SYN lamina horizontalis ossis palatini [NA].

Kühne's p., the endplate of a motor nerve fiber in a muscle spindle.

Lane's p.'s, flattened, narrow, metal p.'s of various shapes and sizes, perforated for screws; used to hold the fragments of a fractured bone in apposition.

lateral p., a nonsegmented mass of mesoderm on the lateral periphery of the embryonic disk.

lateral pterygoid p., the larger and more lateral of the two bony plates extending downward from the point of union of the body and greater wing of the sphenoid bone on either side; forms medial wall of intfratemporal fossa and gives origin to pterygoid muscles. SYN lamina lateralis processus pterygoidei [NA], lateral p. of pterygoid process.

lateral p. of pterygoid process, SYN lateral pterygoid p.

lingual p., SYN linguoplate.

medial pterygoid p., the smaller and more medial of the two bony plates extending downward from the point of union of the body and greater wing of the sphenoid bone on either side. ending inferiorly in the pterygoid hamulus. SYN lamina medialis processus pterygoidei [NA], medial p. of pterygoid process.

medial p. of pterygoid process, SYN medial pterygoid p.

medullary p., SYN neural p.

p. of modiolus, a bony plate, the continuation of the modiolus and of the septum between the convolutions of the spiral canal of the cochlea extending upward toward the cupola, forming with the hamulus the helicotrema. SYN lamina modioli [NA].

motor p., a motor endplate.

muscle p., SYN myotome (2).

nail p., SYN nail.

neural p., the unpaired neuroectodermal region of the early embryo's dorsal surface which in later development is transformed into the neural tube and neural crest. SYN medullary p.

neutralization p., a metal p. used for the internal fixation of a long bone fracture to neutralize the forces producing displacement.

notochordal p., the sheet of notochordal cells that are intercalated in the endodermal roof of the primitive yolk sac. SEE ALSO head *process.*

oral p., a circumscribed area of fusion of foregut endoderm and stomodeal ectoderm in the embryo which breaks through early in development to establish the oral opening. SEE ALSO buccopharyngeal *membrane.*

orbital p., SYN orbital p. of ethmoid bone.

orbital p. of ethmoid bone, a thin plate of ethmoid bone forming part of the medial wall of the orbit and the lateral wall for the ethmoidal labyrinth. SYN lamina orbitalis ossis ethmoidalis [NA], lamina papyracea, orbital lamina of ethmoid bone, orbital layer of ethmoid bone, orbital p., paper p., papyraceous p.

palatal p., a partial denture major connector that has an anteroposterior width in excess of two maxillary premolars.

paper p., papyraceous p., SYN orbital p. of ethmoid bone.

plate 1380 **platymorphia**

parachordal p., the cartilage primordia of the base of the skull situated on either side of the cephalic part of the notochord.

parietal p., (1) the outer of the two layers of the lateral plate mesoderm, which becomes associated with the ectoderm; the ectoderm and parietal plate mesoderm together constitute the somatopleure; **(2)** the lamina of the ethmoid bone that forms the nasal septum.

perpendicular p., flat portion of a bone which lies within or closely approximates a vertical plane. SEE perpendicular p. of ethmoid bone, perpendicular p. of palatine bone. SYN lamina perpendicularis [NA], pars perpendicularis, vertical p.

perpendicular p. of ethmoid bone, a thin plate of bone projecting downward from the crista galli of the ethmoid; it forms part of the nasal septum. SYN lamina perpendicularis ossis ethmoidalis [NA].

perpendicular p. of palatine bone, the part of the palatine bone that extends vertically upward from the horizontal lamina; it forms part of the lateral wall of the nasal cavity. SYN lamina perpendicularis ossis palatini [NA].

phosphor p., the coated p. used in place of a radiographic film cassette in a computed radiography system.

polar p.'s, condensed platelike bodies at the ends of the spindle during mitosis of certain types of cells.

prechordal p., SYN prochordal p.

prochordal p., a small area immediately rostral to the cephalic tip of the notochord where ectoderm and endoderm are in contact; when turned under the growing head, it forms the pharyngeal membrane. SEE ALSO oral p. SYN prechordal p.

pterygoid p.'s, SEE lateral pterygoid p., medial pterygoid p.

quadrigeminal p., SYN *lamina* of mesencephalic tectum.

roof p., the thin layer of the embryonic neural tube connecting the alar p.'s dorsally. SYN dorsal p. of neural tube.

secondary spiral p., SYN secondary spiral *lamina*.

segmental p., SYN segmental *zone*.

sieve p., SYN cribriform p. of ethmoid bone.

spiral p., SYN osseous spiral *lamina*.

suction p., in dentistry, a p. held in place by atmospheric pressure.

tarsal p.'s, SEE superior *tarsus*, inferior *tarsus*.

terminal p., SYN *lamina* terminalis of cerebrum.

tympanic p. of temporal bone, the bony p. forming the greater part of the anterior wall of the bony part of the external acoustic meatus and the tympanic cavity and the posterior wall of the mandibular fossa. SYN pars tympanica ossis temporalis [NA], tympanic part of temporal bone.

urethral p., an endodermal p. located ventromedially in the developing genital tubercle of a young embryo; it later opens to form the lining of the penile urethra.

ventral p., SYN floor p.

ventral p. of neural tube, SYN basal *lamina* of neural tube.

vertical p., SYN perpendicular p.

visceral p., the inner of the two layers of the lateral mesoderm; the splanchnic mesoderm that becomes associated with the endoderm and together with it constitutes the splanchnopleure.

wing p., SYN alar *lamina* of neural tube.

Plateau, Joseph Antoine Ferdinand, Belgian physicist, 1801–1883. SEE P.-Talbot *law*.

pla·teau (plă-tō). A flat elevated segment of a graphic record. [Fr.]

ventricular p., a level diastolic portion of the intraventricular blood pressure curve, representing graphically an equilibrium or final state of filling.

plate·let (plāt′let). An irregularly shaped disklike cytoplasmic fragment of a megakaryocyte that is shed in the marrow sinus and subsequently found in the peripheral blood where it functions in clotting. A p. contains granules in the central part (granulomere) and, peripherally, clear protoplasm (hyalomere), but no definite nucleus; is about one-third to one-half the size of an erythrocyte; and contains no hemoglobin. SYN Bizzozero's corpuscle, blood disk, blood plate, Deetjen's bodies, elementary bodies (2), elementary particle (1), Hayem's hematoblast, hemolamella, third corpuscle, thrombocyte, thromboplastid (1), Zim-

mermann's corpuscle, Zimmermann's elementary particle, Zimmermann's granule. [see plate]

plate·let·phe·re·sis (plāt′let-fĕ-rē′sis). Removal of blood from a donor with replacement of all blood components except platelets. [platelet + G. *aphairesis*, a withdrawal]

plat·ing (plāt′ing). **1.** Sowing of bacteria on a solid medium in a Petri dish or similar container; the making of a plate culture. **2.** Application of a metal strip to keep the ends of a fractured bone in apposition. **3.** Electrolytic deposition of a metal.

compression p., a technique for internal fixation of fractures in which plates and screws are applied so as to produce compression of the line of fracture.

replica p., a procedure for producing an accurate copy of bacterial colonies from one agar plate to another.

pla·tin·ic (pla-tin′ik). Relating to platinum; denoting a compound containing platinum in its higher valency.

plat·i·nous (plat′i-nŭs). Relating to platinum; denoting a compound containing platinum in its lower valency.

plat·i·num (Pt) (plat′i-nŭm). A metallic element, atomic no. 78, atomic wt. 195.08, used for making small parts for chemical apparatus because of its resistance to acids; in powdered form (**p. black**) it is an important catalyst in hydrogenation. Some of its salts have been used in the treatment of syphilis. A derivative, cisplatin, is used as an antineoplastic agent. [Mod. L., originally *platina*, fr. Sp. *plata*, silver]

plat·i·num foil. Pure platinum rolled into extremely thin sheets; its high fusing point makes it suitable as a matrix for various soldering procedures in dentistry, and also suitable for providing internal form to porcelain restorations during their fabrication.

plat·i·num group. A group of six amphoteric elements: iridium, osmium, palladium, platinum, rhodium, and ruthenium.

Platt, Sir Harry, British surgeon, *1886. SEE Putti-P. *operation, procedure*.

△**platy-.** Width; flatness. [G. *platys*, flat, broad]

plat·y·ba·sia (plat-i-bā′sē-ă). A developmental anomaly of the skull or an acquired softening of the skull bones so that the floor of the posterior cranial fossa bulges upward in the region about the foramen magnum. SYN basilar invagination. [platy- + G. *basis*, ground]

plat·y·ceph·a·ly (plat′i-sef′ă-lē). Flatness of the skull, a condition in which the vertical cranial index is below 70. SYN platycrania. [platy- + G. *kephalē*, head]

plat·yc·ne·mia (plat′ik-nē′mē-ă). A condition in which the tibia is abnormally broad and flat. SYN platycnemism. [platy- + G. *knēmē*, leg]

plat·yc·ne·mic (plat′ik-nē′mik). Relating to or marked by platycnemia.

plat·yc·ne·mism (plat′ik-nē′mizm). SYN platycnemia.

plat·y·cra·nia (plat′i-krā′nē-ă). SYN platycephaly. [platy- + G. *kranion*, skull]

plat·y·cyte (plat′i-sīt). A relatively small giant cell sometimes formed in tubercles. [platy- + G. *kytos*, cell]

plat·y·glos·sal (plat′i-glos′ăl). Having a broad, flattened tongue. [platy- + G. *glōssa*, tongue]

plat·y·hel·minth (plat-i-hel′minth). Common name for any flatworm of the phylum Platyhelminthes; any cestode (tapeworm) or trematode (fluke). [platy- + G. *helmins*, worm]

Plat·y·hel·min·thes (plat′i-hel-min′thēz). A phylum of flatworms that are bilaterally symmetric, flattened, and acelomate. There is no digestive tract in some platyhelminths (Cestoda), or the gut may be incomplete (without an anus), as in the Trematoda; most of the forms are hermaphroditic. There are three major classes, but the parasitic species of medical and veterinary importance are in the subclass Cestoda (the true tapeworms) of the class Cestoidea, and in the subclass Digenea (the digenetic flukes) of the class Trematoda.

plat·y·hi·er·ic (plat-i-hī-er′ik). Having a broad sacrum. [platy- + G. *heiron*, sacrum]

plat·y·me·ric (plat-i-mē′rik, -mer′ik). Having a broad femur. [platy- + G. *mēros*, thigh]

plat·y·mor·phia (plat′i-mōr′fē-ă). Having a flat shape; term denoting an eye with a short anteroposterior axis. [platy- + G. *morphē,* shape]

plat·y·o·pia (plat′i-ō′pē-ă). Broadness of the face; denoting a condition in which the orbitonasal index is less than 107.5. [platy- + G. *ōps,* eye, face]

plat·y·op·ic (plat′i-op′ik, -ō′pik). Relating to or characterized by platyopia.

plat·y·pel·lic (plat-i-pel′ik). Having a broad pelvis, with an index below 90°. SEE platypellic *pelvis.* SYN platypelloid. [platy- + G. *pellis,* bowl (pelvis)]

plat·y·pel·loid (plat-ē-pel′oyd). SYN platypellic.

pla·typ·nea (plă-tip′nē-ă). Difficulty in breathing when erect, relieved by recumbency. Cf. orthopnea. [platy- + G. *pnoē,* a breathing]

plat·yr·rhine (plat′i-rīn). **1.** Characterized by a nose of large width in proportion to its length. **2.** Denoting a skull with a nasal index between 53 and 58. [platy- + G. *rhis,* nose]

plat·yr·rhi·ny (plat′i-rī-nē). A condition in which the nose is wide in proportion to its length.

pla·tys·ma, pl. **pla·tys·mas, pla·tys·ma·ta** (plă-tiz′mă, -tiz′mă-tă) [NA]. SYN platysma *muscle.* [G. *platysma,* a flatplate]

plat·y·spon·dyl·ia, plat·y·spon·dyl·i·sis (plat-i-spon-dil′ē-ă, plat′i-spon-dil′i-sis). Flatness of the bodies of the vertebrae. [platy- + G. *spondylos,* vertebra]

pla·tys·ten·ceph·a·ly (plă-tis′ten-sef′ă-lē). Extreme width of the skull in the occipital region, with narrowing anteriorly and prognathism. [G. *platystos,* widest, superl. of *platys,* wide, + *enkephalē,* brain]

Plaut, Hugo K., German physician, 1858–1928. SEE P.'s *bacillus.*

Pleasure, Max A., U.S. dentist. SEE P. *curve.*

plec·trid·i·um (plek-trid′ē-ŭm). A bacterial rod-shaped cell that contains a spore at one end, imparting a drumstick shape to the cell, such as the spore-containing cells in the organism causing tetanus, *Clostridium tetani.* [Mod. L. dim. of G. *plēktron,* an instrument to strike with]

pled·get (plej′et). A tuft of wool, cotton, or lint.

⌂**-plegia.** Paralysis. [G. *plēgē,* stroke]

⌂**pleio-.** Rarely used alternative spelling for pleo-.

plei·o·tro·pic (plī-ō-trop′ik). Denoting, or characterized by, pleiotropy. SYN polyphenic.

plei·ot·ro·py, plei·o·tro·pia (plī-ot′rō-pē, plī′ō-trō′pē-ă). Production by a single mutant gene of apparently unrelated multiple effects at the clinical or phenotypic level. [pleio- + G. *tropos,* turning]

functional p., the p. due to the participation of the same allelic change in multiple otherwise distinct processes; *e.g.,* heparin is active in many body reactions including coagulation and the metabolism of fat.

structural p., a p. that occurs when two or more regions of a polypeptide may have quite distinct and unrelated biological functions which share nothing in common except that they are transcribed and translated at the same time.

Pleis·to·pho·ra (plīs-tof′er-ah). A genus of microsporidians in the protozoan phylum Microspora, commonly found in fish and insects, with mononucleate, thick-walled spores in clusters of more than eight. An undescribed but distinct species of P. was implicated as the cause of a disseminated microsporidial myositis in an immunocompromised male patient.

⌂**pleo-.** more. [G. *pleiōn*]

ple·o·chro·ic (plē-ō-krō′ik). SYN pleochromatic. [pleo- + G. *chroa,* color]

ple·och·ro·ism (plē-ok′rō-izm). SYN pleochromatism.

ple·o·chro·mat·ic (plē-ō-krō-mat′ik). Relating to pleochromatism. SYN pleochroic.

ple·o·chro·ma·tism (plē-ō-krō′mă-tizm). Property of showing changes of color when illuminated along different axes, as certain crystals or liquids. SYN pleochroism. [pleo- + G. *chrōma,* color]

ple·o·cy·to·sis (plē′ō-sī-tō′sis). Presence of more cells than normal, often denoting leukocytosis and especially lymphocytosis or round cell infiltration; orginally applied to the lymphocytosis of the cerebrospinal fluid present in syphilis of the central nervous system. [pleo- + G. *kytos,* cell, + *-ōsis,* condition]

ple·o·mas·tia, ple·o·ma·zia (plē-ō-mas′tē-ă, -mā′zē-ă). SYN polymastia. [pleo- + G. *mastos,* breast]

ple·o·mor·phic (plē-ō-mōr′fik). **1.** SYN polymorphic. **2.** Among fungi, having two or more spore forms; also used to describe a sterile mutant dermatophyte resulting from degenerative changes in culture.

ple·o·mor·phism (plē-ō-mōr′fizm). SYN polymorphism. [pleo- + G. *morphē,* form]

ple·o·mor·phous (plē-ō-mōr′fŭs). SYN polymorphic.

ple·o·nasm (plē′ō-nazm). Excess in number or size of parts. [G. *pleonasmos,* exaggeration, excessive, fr. *pleiōn,* more]

ple·o·nec·tic (plē-ō-nek′tik). Obsolete term denoting specifically a blood that has a percentage saturation of oxygen above normal at any given pressure. SEE ALSO mesectic, mionectic.

ple·o·nex·ia (plē-ō-nek′sē-ă). Rarely used term for excessive greediness. [pleo- + G. *echō,* fut. *hexō,* to have]

ple·on·os·te·o·sis (plē′on-os-tē-ō′sis). Superabundance of bone formation. [pleo- + G. *osteon,* bone, + *-osis,* condition]

Leri′'s p., SYN dyschondrosteosis.

ple·op·tics (plē-op′tiks). A term introduced by Bangerter to include all forms of treatment for amblyopia, particularly that associated with eccentric fixation. [pleo- + optics]

ple·op·to·phor (plē-op′tō-fōr). An instrument for the treatment of amblyopia. [pleo- + G. *optos,* visible, + *phoros,* bearing]

ple·ro·cer·coid (plē-rō-ser′koyd). A stage in the development of a tapeworm following the procercoid stage, which develops in an animal serving as the second or subsequent intermediate host; a wormlike nonsegmented larva with an invaginated scolex at one end, usually unencysted in the flesh of various fishes, reptiles, or amphibians, the ingestion of which transmits the parasite to the final host. SEE ALSO *Diphyllobothrium latum.* [G. *plērēs,* full, complete, + *kerkos,* tail]

⌂**plesio-.** Nearness, similarity. [G. *plēsios,* close, near]

Ples·i·o·mo·nas. A genus of Gram-negative, facultatively anaerobic, chemoorganotrophic, rod-shaped, motile bacteria. It possesses the enterobacterial common antigen. This genus is found in fish and other aquatic animals and in some other animals. Associated with diarrhea and occasional opportunistic infection in humans.

P. shigelloides, species that is an enteric pathogen and an etiologic agent of various extraintestinal infections transmitted to humans in contaminated food, water, or as a colonizer of various animals. This is the only species in the genus and has also been referred to as *Pseudomonas s., Aeromonas s.,* C57, and *Vibrio s.*

ple·si·o·mor·phic (plē′sē-ō-mōr′fik). Similar in form. SYN plesiomorphous.

ple·si·o·mor·phism (plē′sē-ō-mōr′fizm). Similarity in form. [plesio- + G. *morphē,* form]

ple·si·o·mor·phous (plē′sē-ō-mōr′fŭs). SYN plesiomorphic.

⌂**pless-, plessi-.** A striking, especially percussion. [G. *plēssō,* to strike]

ples·ses·the·sia (ples-es-thē′zē-ă). SYN palpatory *percussion.* [G. *plēssō,* to strike, + *aisthēsis,* sensation]

ples·sim·e·ter (ple-sim′ě-ter). An oblong flexible plate used in

---

⌂ **Combining forms**	**[NA] Nomina Anatomica**
Word*Finder*	**[MIM] Mendelian**
Multi-term entry finder	**Inheritance in Man**
Preceding letter A	
A.D.A.M. Anatomy Plates	☆ **Official alternate term**
Between letters L and M	
Appendices:	☆**[NA] Official alternate**
Following letter Z	**Nomina Anatomica term**
SYN Synonym; Cf., compare	**High Profile Term**

pl

mediate percussion by being placed against the surface and struck with the plessor. SYN pleximeter, plexometer. [G. *plēssō,* to strike, + *metron,* measure]

ples·si·met·ric (ples-i-met′rik). Relating to a plessimeter.

ples·sor (ples′er). A small hammer, usually with soft rubber head, used to tap the part directly, or with a plessimeter, in percussion of the chest or other part. SYN percussor, plexor. [G. *plēssō,* to strike]

pleth·o·ra (pleth′ŏ-ră). **1.** SYN hypervolemia. **2.** An excess of any of the body fluids. SYN repletion (2). [G. *plēthōrē,* fullness, fr. *plēthō,* to become full]

pleth·o·ric (ple-thŏr′ik, pleth′ŏ-rik). Relating to plethora. SYN sanguine (1), sanguineous (2).

ple·thys·mo·graph (plĕ-thiz′mō-graf). A device for measuring and recording changes in volume of a part, organ, or whole body. [G. *plēthysmos,* increase, + *graphō,* to write]

body p., a chamber apparatus surrounding the entire body, commonly used in studies of respiratory function.

digital p., p. applied to a digit of a hand or foot in order to measure skin blood flow.

pressure p., (1) a p. applied to part of the body, *e.g.,* a limb segment, and arranged so that volume is measured during temporary application of sufficient pressure to the part to empty its blood vessels; **(2)** a body p. in which changes of body volume are measured in terms of the consequent changes in air pressure in the body p.

volume-displacement p., a p., usually a body p., in which changes in volume displace a corresponding volume into or out of a very compliant measuring device, such as a Krogh spirometer or integrating flowmeter.

pleth·ys·mog·ra·phy (pleth-iz-mog′ră-fē). Measuring and recording changes in volume of an organ or other part of the body by a plethysmograph. [G. *plēthysmos,* increase, + *graphē,* a writing]

impedance p., recording changes in electrical impedance between electrodes placed on opposite sides of a part of the body, as a measure of volume changes in the path of the current. SYN dielectrography.

venous occlusion p., measurement of the rate of arterial inflow into an organ or limb segment by measuring its initial rate of increase in volume when its venous outflow is suddenly occluded.

pleth·ys·mom·e·try (pleth-iz-mom′ĕ-trē). Measuring the fullness of a hollow organ or vessel, as of the pulse. [G. *plēthysmos,* increase, + *metron,* measure]

△**pleur-, pleura-, pleuro-.** Rib, side, pleura. [G. *pleura;* a rib, the side]

pleu·ra, gen. and pl. **pleu·rae** (plūr′ă, plūr′ē) [NA]. The serous membrane enveloping the lungs and lining the walls of the pleural cavity. SYN membrana succingens. [G. *pleura,* a rib, pl. the side]

cervical p., SYN pleural *cupula.*

costal p., the layer of parietal p. lining the chest walls. SYN p. costalis [NA].

p. costa′lis [NA], SYN costal p.

diaphragmatic p., the layer of parietal p. covering the upper surface of the diaphragm, except along its costal attachments and where it is covered with the pericardium. SYN p. diaphragmatica [NA], phrenic p., p. phrenica.

p. diaphragmat′ica [NA], SYN diaphragmatic p.

mediastinal p., the continuation of the costal p. passing from the sternum to the vertebral column which covers the side of the mediastinum. SYN p. mediastinalis [NA].

p. mediastina′lis [NA], SYN mediastinal p.

parietal p., that which lines the different parts of the wall of the pleural cavity; called costal, diaphragmatic, and mediastinal, according to the parts invested. SYN p. parietalis [NA].

p. parieta′lis [NA], SYN parietal p.

p. pericardi′aca, pericardial p., that portion of the mediastinal p. which is fused with the pericardium.

phrenic p., SYN diaphragmatic p.

p. phren′ica, SYN diaphragmatic p.

p. pulmona′lis [NA], ☆official alternate term for visceral p.

pulmonary p., SYN visceral p.

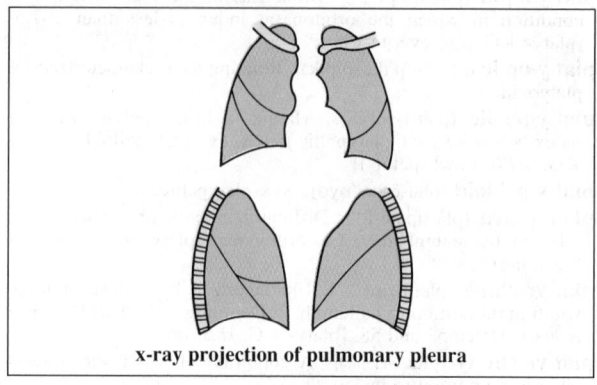

x-ray projection of pulmonary pleura

visceral p., the layer investing the lungs and dipping into the fissures between the several lobes. SYN p. pulmonalis ☆ [NA], p. visceralis, pulmonary p.

p. viscera′lis, SYN visceral p.

pleu·ra·cen·te·sis (plūr′ă-sen-tē′sis). SYN thoracentesis.

pleu·ral (plūr′ăl). Relating to the pleura.

pleu·ral crac·kles (krăk′lz). Sounds heard on auscultation of the chest as a result of inflammation of the pleura with fibrinous exudate.

pleu·ral·gia (plū-ral′jē-ă). Rarely used synonym for pleurodynia (2). [pleur- + G. *algos,* pain]

pleur·a·poph·y·sis (plūr′ă-pof′i-sis). A rib, or the process on a cervical or lumbar vertebra corresponding thereto. Cf. diapophysis. [pleur- + G. *apophysis,* process, offshoot]

pleu·rec·to·my (plū-rek′tō-mē). Excision of pleura, usually parietal. [pleur- + G. *ektomē,* excision]

pleu·ri·sy (plūr′i-sē). Inflammation of the pleura. SYN pleuritis. [L. *pleurisis,* fr. G. *pleuritis*]

adhesive p., SYN dry p.

benign dry p., SYN epidemic *pleurodynia.*

bilateral p., inflammation of the pleura on both sides of the thorax. SYN double p.

chronic p., vague or indefinite term for long-standing inflammation of the pleura of any etiology (*e.g.,* tuberculosis).

costal p., inflammation of the pleura lining the thoracic walls.

diaphragmatic p., SYN epidemic *pleurodynia.*

double p., SYN bilateral p.

dry p., p. with a fibrinous exudation, without an effusion of serum, resulting in adhesion between the opposing surfaces of the pleura. SYN adhesive p., fibrinous p., plastic p.

encysted p., a form of serofibrinous p., in which adhesions occur at various points, circumscribing the serous effusion.

epidemic benign dry p., SYN epidemic *pleurodynia.*

epidemic diaphragmatic p., SYN epidemic *pleurodynia.*

fibrinous p., SYN dry p.

hemorrhagic p., p. with an effusion of blood-stained serum.

interlobular p., inflammation limited to the pleura in the sulci between the pulmonary lobes.

mediastinal p., inflammation of the portion of the pleura lining the mediastinal surface of the lung.

plastic p., SYN dry p.

productive p., SYN pachypleuritis.

proliferating p., p. with a tendency for the proliferation of inflammatory exudate.

pulmonary p., inflammation of the pleura covering the lungs. SYN visceral p.

purulent p., p. with empyema. SYN suppurative p.

sacculated p., p. with the inflammatory exudate divided into separate regions by adhesions or inflammatory changes.

serofibrinous p., the more common form of p., characterized by a fibrinous exudate on the surface of the pleura and an extensive effusion of serous fluid into the pleural cavity.

serous p., SYN p. with effusion.

suppurative p., SYN purulent p.

typhoid p., obsolete term for acute or subacute p. with typhoid symptoms.

visceral p., SYN pulmonary p.

wet p., SYN p. with effusion.

p. with effusion, p. accompanied by serous exudation. SYN serous p., wet p.

pleu·rit·ic (plū-rit′ik). Pertaining to pleurisy.

pleu·ri·tis (plū-rī′tis). SYN pleurisy. [G. fr. *pleura*, side, + *-itis*, inflammation]

pleur·i·tog·e·nous (plūr-i-toj′ĕ-nŭs). Tending to produce pleurisy. [G. *pleuritis*, pleurisy, + *genesis*, origin]

pleuro-. SEE pleur-.

pleu·ro·cele (plūr′ō-sēl). SYN pneumonocele. [pleuro- + G. *kēlē*, hernia]

pleu·ro·cen·te·sis (plūr′ō-sen-tē′sis). SYN thoracentesis. [pleuro- + G. *kentēsis*, puncture]

pleu·ro·cen·trum (plūr′ō-sen′trŭm). One of the lateral halves of the body of a vertebra. [pleuro- + G. *kentron*, center]

pleu·roc·ly·sis (plūr-ok′li-sis). Washing out of the pleural cavity. [pleuro- + G. *klysis*, a washing out]

pleu·rod·e·sis (plūr-od′e-sis). The creation of a fibrous adhesion between the visceral and parietal layers of the pleura, thus obliterating the pleural cavity; it is performed surgically by abrading the pleura or by inserting a sterile irritant into the pleural canal, and applied as treatment in cases of recurrent spontaneous pneumothorax, malignant pleural effusion, and chylothorax. [pleuro- + G. *desis*, a binding together]

pleu·ro·dyn·ia (plūr-ō-din′ē-ă). **1.** Pleuritic pain in the chest. **2.** A painful affection of the tendinous attachments of the thoracic muscles, usually of one side only. SYN costalgia. [pleuro- + G. *odynē*, pain]

epidemic p., an acute infectious disease usually occurring in epidemic form, characterized by paroxysms of pain, usually in the chest, and associated with strains of *Enterovirus* coxsackievirus type B. SYN benign dry pleurisy, Bornholm disease, Daae's disease, devil's grip, diaphragmatic pleurisy, epidemic benign dry pleurisy, epidemic diaphragmatic pleurisy, epidemic myalgia, epidemic myositis, myositis epidemica acuta, epidemic transient diaphragmatic spasm, Sylvest's disease.

pleu·ro·gen·ic (plūr-ō-jen′ik). Of pleural origin; beginning in the pleura. SYN pleurogenous (1). [pleuro- + G. *-gen*, producing]

pleu·rog·e·nous (plūr-oj′ĕ-nŭs). **1.** SYN pleurogenic. **2.** In fungi, denoting spores or conidia developed on the sides of a conidiophore or hypha.

pleu·rog·ra·phy (plūr-og′ră-fē). Radiography of the pleural cavity after injecting contrast medium. [pleuro- + G. *graphō*, to write]

pleu·ro·hep·a·ti·tis (plūr′ō-hep-ă-tī′tis). Hepatitis with extension of the inflammation to the neighboring portion of the pleura. [pleuro- + G. *hēpar*, liver, + *-itis*, inflammation]

pleu·ro·lith (plūr′ō-lith). A concretion in the pleural cavity. SYN pleural calculus. [pleuro- + G. *lithos*, stone]

pleu·rol·y·sis (plūr-ol′i-sis). Locating pleural adhesions by the aid of an endoscope and then dividing them with the electric cautery. [pleuro- + G. *lysis*, dissolution]

pleu·ro·per·i·car·di·al (plūr′ō-per-i-kar′dē-ăl). Relating to both pleura and pericardium.

pleu·ro·per·i·car·di·tis (plūr′ō-per-i-kar-dī′tis). Combined inflammation of the pericardium and of the pleura. [pleuro- + pericardium + G. *-itis*, inflammation]

pleu·ro·per·i·to·ne·al (plūr′ō-per-i-tō-nē′ăl). Relating to both pleura and peritoneum.

pleu·ro·pneu·mo·nia (plūr′ō-nū-mō′nē-ă). Specific infectious diseases in domestic ruminants, characterized by inflammation of the lungs and pleura; caused by the bacterium *Mycoplasma mycoides* sp. *mycoides*.

contagious bovine p. (CBPP), a highly infectious disease of cattle caused by *Mycoplasma mycoides* sp. *mycoides* and occurring in acute, subacute, and chronic septicemic forms.

contagious caprine p., an acute disease of goats caused by *Mycoplasma mycoides* sp. *capri.*

pleu·ro·pul·mo·nary (plūr-ō-pul′mō-ner-ē). Relating to the pleura and the lungs.

pleu·ros·co·py (plūr-ōs′kō-pē). SYN thoracoscopy. [pleuro- + G. *skopeō*, to inspect]

pleu·ro·thot·o·nos, pleu·ro·thot·o·nus (plūr-ō-thot′ō-nŭs). Tetanus lateralis; lateral bending of the body; formerly seen as a common symptom of conversion hysteria. [G. *pleurothen*, from the side, + *tonos*, tension]

pleu·rot·o·my (plū-rot′ō-mē). SYN thoracotomy. [pleuro- + G. *tomē*, incision]

pleu·ro·ty·phoid (plur-ō-tī′foyd). Typhoid fever in which the early stage is masked by the physical signs of pleurisy.

pleu·ro·vis·cer·al (plūr′ō-vis′er-ăl). SYN visceropleural.

PLEVA. Acronym for *pityriasis* lichenoides et varioliformis acuta.

plex·al (plek′săl). Relating to a plexus.

plex·ect·o·my (plek-sek′tō-mē). Surgical excision of a plexus. [plexus + G. *ektomē*, excision]

plex·i·form (plek′si-fōrm). Weblike, or resembling or forming a plexus. [plexus + L. *forma*, form]

plex·im·e·ter (plek-sim′i-ter). SYN plessimeter. [G. *plēxis*, stroke]

plex·i·tis (plek-sī′tis). Inflammation of a plexus.

brachial p., SYN neuralgic *amyotrophy.*

plex·o·gen·ic (plek′sō-jen-ik). Giving rise to weblike or plexiform structures. [plexus + G. *-gen*, producing]

plex·om·e·ter (plek-som′ĕ-ter). SYN plessimeter.

plex·or (plek′ser). SYN plessor. [G. *plēxis*, a stroke]

PLEXUS

plex·us, pl. **plex·us, plex·us·es** (plek′sŭs, -sŭs-ez) [NA]. A network or interjoining of nerves and blood vessels or of lymphatic vessels. [L. a braid]

abdominal aortic p., an autonomic p. surrounding the abdominal aorta, directly continuous with the thoracic aortic p. above and continued inferior to the bifurcaion of the aorta as the superior or hypogastric plexus. SYN p. aorticus abdominalis [NA].

acromial p., SYN acromial arterial *network.*

annular p., a nerve p. near the corneoscleral junction from which myelinated and unmyelinated nerves pass to the cornea. SYN p. annularis.

p. annula′ris, SYN annular p.

p. of anterior cerebral artery, an autonomic p. accompanying the anterior cerebral artery, derived from the internal carotid p. SYN p. arteriae cerebri anterioris.

anterior coronary p., the part of the cardiac p. that accompanies the coronary arteries on the anterior aspect of the heart.

aortic lymphatic p., a p. of lymph nodes and connecting vessels lying along the lower portion of the abdominal aorta. SYN p. aorticus.

p. aor′ticus, SYN aortic lymphatic p.

p. aor′ticus abdomina′lis [NA], SYN abdominal aortic p.

p. aor′ticus thora′cicus [NA], SYN thoracic aortic p.

areolar venous p., a venous p. in the areola surrounding the nipple, formed by the mammary veins, and sending its blood to the lateral thoracic vein. SYN p. venosus areolaris [NA], circulus venosus halleri, Haller's circle (2), vascular circle (2), venous circle of mammary gland.

p. arte′riae cer′ebri anterio′ris, SYN p. of anterior cerebral artery.

p. arte′riae cer′ebri me′diae, SYN p. of middle cerebral artery.

p. arte′riae choroi′deae, SYN p. of choroid artery.

ascending pharyngeal p., an autonomic p. on the artery of the same name, formed of fibers from the superior cervical ganglion. SYN p. pharyngeus ascendens.

Auerbach's p., SYN myenteric p.

p. auricula'ris poste'rior, SYN posterior auricular p.

autonomic plexuses, p.'s of nerves in relation to blood vessels and viscera, the component fibers of which are sympathetic, parasympathetic, and sensory. SYN p. autonomici [NA].

p. autono'mici [NA], SYN autonomic plexuses.

p. axilla'ris, SYN axillary p.

axillary p., a lymphatic p. formed of the lymph nodes, with their afferent and efferent vessels, in the axilla. SYN p. axillaris.

basilar p., a venous p. on the clivus, connected with the cavernous and petrosal sinuses and the internal vertebral (epidural) venous p. SYN p. basilaris [NA], basilar sinus.

p. basila'ris [NA], SYN basilar p.

Batson's p., SYN vertebral venous *system*.

brachial p., major nerve p. formed of the ventral primary rami of the fifth cervical to first thoracic spinal nerves for innervation of the upper limb. The ventral primary rami entering into formation of the p. constitute the roots of the p.; the roots are located in the posterior triangle of the neck, converging to emerge from the scalenus anterior and medius muscles. As they emerge from the scalene hiatus, the C_5 and C_6 roots combine to form the superior trunk, C_7 remains alone as the middle trunk and the C_8 and T_1 roots combine to form the inferior trunk of the p. The trunks pass beneath the clavicle, passing from the neck into the axilla through the cervicoaxillary canal. As they cross the first rib, all three trunks divide into anterior and posterior divisions of the p. Nerve fibers contained within anterior divisions are destined for the anterior aspect of the limb; those contained within the posterior divisions are destined for the posterior aspect of the limb. Within the axilla, the anterior divisions of the superior and middle trunks merge to form the lateral cord of the p.; the anterior division of the inferior trunk becomes the medial cord of the p., and the posterior divisions of all three trunks become the posterior cord, the cords being named for their position in relation to the axillary artery, which they run parallel to and surround. The cords of the brachial p. give rise to most of the named peripheral nerves which are the products of the p. formation. The major nerves of the lateral cord are the musculocutaneous nerve and the lateral root of the median nerve. The medial cord gives rise to the ulnar and medial root of the median nerve. The lateral and medial roots of the median nerve merge to form the medial nerve. The posterior cord of the p. gives rise to the radial and axillary nerves. SYN p. brachialis [NA].

p. brachia'lis [NA], SYN brachial p.

cardiac p., a wide-meshed network of anastomosing cardiopulmonary and splanchnic nerves arising from the afferent and autonomic nerve fibers (sympathetic) and vagus (parasympathetic) nerves, surrounding the arch of the aorta, the pulmonary artery, and continuing to the atria, ventricles, and coronary vessels. SYN p. cardiacus [NA].

p. cardi'acus [NA], SYN cardiac p.

p. cardi'acus profun'dus, SYN deep cardiac p.

p. cardi'acus superficia'lis, SYN superficial cardiac p.

p. carot'icus commu'nis [NA], SYN common carotid p.

p. carot'icus exter'nus [NA], SYN external carotid p.

p. carot'icus inter'nus, SYN internal carotid venous p.

p. caverno'si concha'rum [NA], SYN cavernous p. of conchae.

p. caverno'sus, SYN intracavernous p.

cavernous p. of clitoris, SYN cavernous *nerves* of clitoris, under *nerve*.

cavernous p. of conchae, erectile tissue in the mucous membrane covering the conchae of the nasal cavity. SYN p. cavernosi concharum [NA], corpus cavernosum conchae.

cavernous p. of penis, SYN cavernous *nerves* of penis, under *nerve*.

celiac p., a network related to the celiac trunk. SEE celiac (nervous) p., celiac (lymphatic) p.

celiac (lymphatic) p., a network formed of the efferent and afferent lymphatic vessels of the celiac lymph nodes and related

to the celiac trunk; the afferent lymphatic vessels bring lymph primarily from structures served by the celiac artery (stomach, duodenum, pancreas, and visceral aspect of the liver); the efferent vessels drain into the cisterna chyli/thoracic duct via the intestinal lymph trunks.

celiac (nervous) p., the most substantial, superior portion of the abdominal aortic plexus lying anterior to the aorta at the level of origin of the celiac trunk (vertebral level T-12); the celiac ganglia lie within the plexus; it is formed by contributions from the greater splanchnic and vagus (especially the posterior or right vagus) nerves and communicating branches to and from the superior mesenteric and renal plexuses and ganglia; most sympathetic, parasympathetic and visceral afferent fibers serving the abdominal viscera pass through this plexus. SYN p. celiacus [NA], solar p.

p. celi'acus [NA], SYN celiac (nervous) p.

cervical p., formed by loops joining the adjacent ventral primary rami of the first four cervical nerves and receiving gray communicating rami from the superior cervical ganglion; it lies deep to the sternocleidomastoid muscle, and sends out numerous cutaneous, muscular, and communicating rami. SYN p. cervicalis [NA].

p. cervica'lis [NA], SYN cervical p.

choroid p., a vascular proliferation or fringe of the tela choroidea in the third, fourth and lateral cerebral ventricles; it secretes cerebrospinal fluid thereby regulating to some degree the intraventricular pressure. SYN p. choroideus [NA], tela vasculosa.

p. of choroid artery, an autonomic p. accompanying the artery of the same name, derived from the internal carotid p. SYN p. arteriae choroideae.

p. choroi'deus [NA], SYN choroid p.

p. choroi'deus ventric'uli latera'lis [NA], SYN choroid p. of lateral ventricle.

p. choroi'deus ventric'uli quar'ti [NA], SYN choroid p. of fourth ventricle.

p. choroi'deus ventric'uli ter'tii [NA], SYN choroid p. of third ventricle.

choroid p. of fourth ventricle, one of two vascular fringes of pia mater projecting on either side from the lower part of the roof of the fourth cerebral ventricle. SYN p. choroideus ventriculi quarti [NA].

choroid p. of lateral ventricle, the vascular fringe that projects from the choroidal fissure into each lateral ventricle. SYN p. choroideus ventriculi lateralis [NA].

choroid p. of third ventricle, the double row of vascular projections from the undersurface of the tela choroidea where it roofs over the third ventricle. SYN p. choroideus ventriculi tertii [NA].

ciliary ganglionic p., an autonomic p. lying on the ciliary muscle, derived from the oculomotor, trigeminal, and sympathetic. SYN p. gangliosus ciliaris.

coccygeal p., a small p. formed by the fifth sacral and the coccygeal nerves; it gives origin to the anococcygeal nerves. SYN p. coccygeus [NA].

p. coccyg'eus [NA], SYN coccygeal p.

common carotid p., an autonomic p. accompanying the artery of the same name formed by fibers from the middle cervical ganglion. SYN p. caroticus communis [NA].

p. corona'rius cor'dis, SYN coronary p.

coronary p., the continuation of the cardiac p. onto the coronary arteries. SYN p. coronarius cordis.

Cruveilhier's p., a nerve p. formed by communications between the dorsal primary rami of the first three cervical nerves; it lies deep to the semispinalis capitis muscle.

deep cardiac p., the deeper part of the cardiac p. SYN p. cardiacus profundus.

deferential p., an autonomic p. on the seminal vesicle and ampulla of the ductus deferens on each side, derived from the inferior hypogastric p. SYN p. deferentialis [NA].

p. deferentia'lis [NA], SYN deferential p.

p. denta'lis infe'rior [NA], SYN inferior dental p.

p. denta'lis supe'rior [NA], SYN superior dental p.

enteric p., the autonomic p. in the wall of the intestine; it consists of three parts, submucosal, myenteric, and subserosal;

ganglionic cells are scattered through the myenteric and submucosal plexus. SYN p. entericus [NA].

p. enter′icus [NA], SYN enteric p.

esophageal p., one of two nervous p.'s, posterior and anterior on the walls of the esophagus; the first is formed by branches from the right vagus and left recurrent, the second by the anastomosing trunks of the vagus after leaving the pulmonary p.'s; branches supply the mucous and muscular coats of the esophagus. SYN p. esophageus [NA], p. gulae.

p. esopha′geus [NA], SYN esophageal p.

Exner's p., a p. formed by tangential nerve fibers in the superficial plexiform or molecular layer of the cerebral cortex.

external carotid p., an autonomic p. formed by the external carotid nerves surrounding the artery of the same name, and giving origin to a number of secondary p.'s along the branches of this artery and to branches to the carotid body. SYN p. caroticus externus [NA].

external iliac p., a lymphatic p. formed by the lymph nodes along the external iliac artery on either side, and their afferent and efferent vessels. SYN p. iliacus externus.

external maxillary p., SYN facial p.

facial p., an autonomic p. on the facial artery derived from the external carotid p.; it sends a branch to the submandibular ganglion. SYN external maxillary p., p. maxillaris externus.

femoral p., an autonomic p. surrounding the femoral artery, derived from the iliac p. SYN p. femoralis [NA].

p. femora′lis [NA], SYN femoral p.

p. ganglio′sus cilia′ris, SYN ciliary ganglionic p.

gastric plexuses of autonomic system, the p.'s along the greater and lesser curvatures of the stomach derived from the celiac p.; also known as inferior and superior p. SYN p. gastrici systematis autonomici [NA].

p. gas′trici syste′matis autono′mici [NA], SYN gastric plexuses of autonomic system.

p. gu′lae, SYN esophageal p.

Haller's p., a nervous p. of sympathetic filaments and branches of the external laryngeal nerve on the surface of the inferior constrictor muscle of the pharynx.

Heller's p., p. of small arteries in the wall of the intestine.

hemorrhoidal p., SYN rectal venous p. SEE ALSO inferior rectal plexuses, middle rectal plexuses, superior rectal p.

hepatic p., an unpaired autonomic p. lying on the hepatc artery and its branches in the liver. SYN p. hepaticus [NA].

p. hepat′icus [NA], SYN hepatic p.

p. hypogas′tricus infe′rior [NA], SYN inferior hypogastric p.

p. hypogas′tricus supe′rior [NA], SYN superior hypogastric p.

iliac p., the autonomic p. lying on the iliac arteries, derived from the aortic p. SYN p. iliaci [NA].

p. ili′aci [NA], SYN iliac p.

p. ili′acus exter′nus, SYN external iliac p.

inferior dental p., formed by branches of the inferior alveolar nerve interlacing before they supply the teeth; it gives off interior dental branches to the teeth and inferior gingival branches to the gums. SYN p. dentalis inferior [NA].

inferior hemorrhoidal plexuses, SYN inferior rectal plexuses.

inferior hypogastric p., one of the bilateral autonomic p. in the pelvis distributed to the pelvic viscera; it receives the hypogastric nerves and the pelvic splanchnic nerves. SYN p. hypogastricus inferior [NA], p. pelvinus✶ [NA], pelvic p.

inferior mesenteric p., an autonomic p., derived from the abdominal aortic p., surrounding the inferior mesenteric artery and sending branches to the descending colon, sigmoid, and rectum. SYN p. mesentericus inferior [NA].

inferior rectal plexuses, the autonomic p.'s along the anus derived from the inferior hypogastric p. SYN p. rectales inferiores [NA], inferior hemorrhoidal plexuses.

inferior thyroid p., an autonomic p. on the artery of this name, derived from the subclavian p. SYN p. thyroideus inferior.

inferior vesical p., a venous p. in the female corresponding to the prostatic venous p. in the male. SYN p. vesicalis inferior.

inguinal p., a lymphatic p. formed of 10 to 15 lymph nodes with their connecting vessels lying superficially near the termination of the great saphenous vein and more deeply along the femoral artery and vein. SEE superficial inguinal *lymph nodes*, under *lymph node*. SYN p. inguinalis.

p. inguina′lis, SYN inguinal p.

intermesenteric p., the part of the aortic p. lying between the superior and inferior mesenteric p.'s. SYN p. intermesentericus [NA].

p. intermesenter′icus [NA], SYN intermesenteric p.

internal carotid (nervous) p., (1) an autonomic p. surrounding the internal carotid artery in the carotid canal and cavernous sinus, and sending branches to the tympanic p., sphenopalatine ganglion, abducens and oculomotor nerves, the cerebral vessels, and the ciliary ganglion; **(2)** SYN internal carotid venous p.

internal carotid venous p., a venous network around the internal carotid artery in the carotid canal of the temporal bone, connecting with the cavernous sinus and internal jugular vein. SYN p. venosus caroticus internus [NA], internal carotid (nervous) p. (2), p. caroticus internus.

internal mammary p., SYN internal thoracic p.

internal maxillary p., SYN periarterial p. of maxillary artery.

internal thoracic p., an autonomic p. on the internal thoracic artery derived from the subclavian p. SYN internal mammary p., p. mammarius internus.

internal thoracic lymphatic p., a lymphatic p., including the parasternal; (internal thoracic) lymph nodes, with their vessels, situated along the course of the internal thoracic veins. SYN mammary p., p. mammarius.

intracavernous p., the portion of the internal carotid p. in the cavernous sinus. SYN p. cavernosus, Walther's p.

p. intraparoti′deus [NA], SYN intraparotid p. of facial nerve.

intraparotid p. of facial nerve, the diverging branches of the facial nerve passing through the substance of the parotid gland, connected by numerous looped anastomoses. SYN p. intraparotideus [NA], pes anserinus (1).

ischiadic p., SYN sacral p.

Jacobson's p., SYN tympanic p.

Jacques' p., a nerve p. within the muscular coat of the uterine (fallopian) tube.

jugular p., a lymphatic p. which includes the deep cervical group of lymph nodes, with their afferent and efferent vessels, extending along the internal jugular vein. (carotid sheath). SYN p. jugularis.

p. jugula′ris, SYN jugular p.

Leber's p., a small venous p. in the eye between the venous sinuses of the sclera (of Schlemm) and the spaces of the iridocorneal angle (of Fontana).

p. liena′lis [NA], ✶official alternate term for splenic p.

lingual p., an autonomic p. on the artery of this name, derived from the external carotid p. SYN p. lingualis.

p. lingua′lis, SYN lingual p.

p. lumba′lis, SYN lumbar p.

lumbar p., (1) a nervous p., formed by the ventral rami of the first four lumbar nerves; it lies in the substance of the psoas muscle; **(2)** a lymphatic p. formed of about twenty lymph nodes and connecting vessels situated along the lower portion of the aorta and the common iliac vessels. SYN p. lumbalis.

lumbosacral p., formed by the union of the anterior rami of the lumbar and sacral nerves; it is divided into lumbar and sacral p.'s. SYN p. lumbosacralis [NA].

p. lumbosacra′lis [NA], SYN lumbosacral p.

lymphatic p., a p. of lymphatic capillaries, usually without valves, that opens into one or more larger lymphatic vessels. SYN p. lymphaticus [NA].

p. lymphat′icus [NA], SYN lymphatic p.

p. mamma′rius, SYN internal thoracic lymphatic p.

p. mamma′rius inter′nus, SYN internal thoracic p.

mammary p., SYN internal thoracic lymphatic p.

p. maxilla′ris exter′nus, SYN facial p.

p. maxilla′ris inter′nus, SYN periarterial p. of maxillary artery.

maxillary p., SYN periarterial p. of maxillary artery.

Meissner's p., SYN submucosal p.

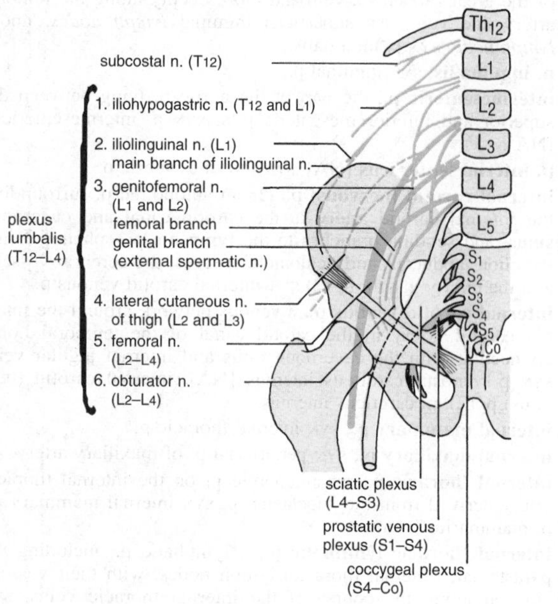
Th12
L1
L2
L3
L4
L5
S1
S2
S3
S4
S5
Co
subcostal n. (T12)
1. iliohypogastric n. (T12 and L1)
2. ilioliguinal n. (L1)
main branch of iliolinguinal n.
3. genitofemoral n.
(L1 and L2)
femoral branch
genital branch
(external spermatic n.)
plexus
lumbalis
(T12–L4)
4. lateral cutaneous n.
of thigh (L2 and L3)
5. femoral n.
(L2–L4)
6. obturator n.
(L2–L4)
sciatic plexus
(L4–S3)
prostatic venous
plexus (S1–S4)
coccygeal plexus
(S4–Co)

lumbosacral plexus

meningeal p., a nerve p. on the cerebral meninges, derived from the external carotid p. SYN p. meningeus.

p. menin′geus, SYN meningeal p.

p. mesenter′icus infe′rior [NA], SYN inferior mesenteric p.

p. mesenter′icus supe′rior [NA], SYN superior mesenteric p.

p. of middle cerebral artery, an autonomic p. accompanying the middle cerebral artery, derived from the internal carotid p. SYN p. arteriae cerebri mediae.

middle hemorrhoidal plexuses, SYN middle rectal plexuses.

middle rectal plexuses, the autonomic p.'s along the rectum derived from the inferior hypogastric p. SYN p. rectales medii [NA], middle hemorrhoidal plexuses.

middle sacral p., a lymphatic p. formed of lymph nodes and connecting vessels situated chiefly in the mesorectum anterior and inferior to the sacral promontory. SYN p. sacralis medius.

myenteric p., a p. of unmyelinated fibers and postganglionic autonomic cell bodies lying in the muscular coat of the esophagus, stomach, and intestines; it communicates with the subserous and submucous p.'s, all subdivisions of the enteric p. SYN p. myentericus [NA], Auerbach's p.

p. myenter′icus [NA], SYN myenteric p.

nerve p., a p. formed by the interlacing of nerves by means of numerous communicating branches. SYN p. nervosus.

p. nervo′rum spina′lium [NA], SYN p. of spinal nerves.

p. nervo′sus, SYN nerve p.

occipital p., an autonomic p. on the occipital artery derived from the external carotid p. SYN p. occipitalis.

p. occipita′lis, SYN occipital p.

ophthalmic p., an autonomic p., entering the orbit in company with the ophthalmic artery, derived from the internal carotid p. SYN p. ophthalmicus.

p. ophthal′micus, SYN ophthalmic p.

ovarian p., an autonomic p. derived from the aortic p. and accompanying the ovarian artery to the ovary, broad ligament, and uterine tube. SYN p. ovaricus [NA].

p. ova′ricus [NA], SYN ovarian p.

pampiniform p., a p. formed, in the male, by veins from the testicle and epididymis, consisting of eight or ten veins lying in front of the ductus deferens and forming part of the spermatic cord; in the female the ovarian veins form this p. between the layers of the broad ligament; in the male it is part of the thermoregulatory system of the testis, helping to keep the testis at a constant temperature slightly lower than the other body temperature. SYN p. pampiniformis [NA].

p. pampinifor′mis [NA], SYN pampiniform p.

pancreatic p., the autonomic p. that accompanies the pancreatic arteries. SYN p. pancreaticus [NA].

p. pancreat′icus [NA], SYN pancreatic p.

pelvic p., SYN inferior hypogastric p.

p. pelvi′nus [NA], ☆official alternate term for inferior hypogastric p.

periarterial p., an autonomic p. that accompanies an artery, surrounding it in a network of autonomic nerve fibers. SYN p. periarterialis [NA].

p. periarteria′lis [NA], SYN periarterial p.

periarterial p. of maxillary artery, an autonomic p. on the maxillary artery derived from the external carotid p. SYN internal maxillary p., maxillary p., p. maxillaris internus.

periarterial p. of vertebral artery, a p. of autonomic nerves on the vertebral artery derives from the subclavian p. SYN p. vertebralis [NA], vertebral p.

pharyngeal p., (1) the p. of nerves including branches of the glossopharyngeal, vagus, and accessory nerves (cranial root), that lies along the posterior wall of the pharynx; **(2)** a venous p. on the posteriolateral walls of the pharynx, emptying through the pharyngeal veins into the internal jugular. SYN p. pharyngeus [NA].

p. pharyn′geus [NA], SYN pharyngeal p.

p. pharyn′geus ascen′dens, SYN ascending pharyngeal p.

phrenic p., p. phren′icus, an autonomic p. surrounding the inferior phrenic artery.

popliteal p., p. poplit′eus, a nerve p. surrounding the popliteal artery, derived from the femoral p.

posterior auricular p., an autonomic p. on the artery of this name, derived from the external carotid p. SYN p. auricularis posterior.

posterior coronary p., the portion of the cardiac p. that accompanies branches of the coronary arteries on the posteroinferior surface of the heart.

prostatic p., an autonomic p. of nerves intimately associated with the capsule of the prostate, derived from the inferior hypogastric p., and giving rise to the cavernous nerves to the erectile tissue of the penis; surgical injury of this plexus ofter results in impotency. SYN p. prostaticus [NA].

prostaticovesical p., a venous p. which includes the prostatic venous plexus around the prostate gland and that of the neck of the bladder; it communicates with the vesical and pudendal p.'s, receives the deep dorsal vein of the penis, and empties. by one or more efferent vessels into the internal iliac (hypogastric) vein; it corresponds to the inferior vesical p. in the female. SYN p. prostaticovesicalis.

p. prostaticovesica′lis, SYN prostaticovesical p.

p. prostat′icus [NA], SYN prostatic p.

prostatic venous p., a venous p., arising chiefly from the dorsal vein of the penis, situated below the base of the bladder at the sides of the prostate. SEE ALSO prostaticovesical p. SYN p. venosus prostaticus [NA], p. pudendalis, Santorini's labyrinth.

pterygoid p., a venous p. occupying the infratemporal fossa receiving veins accompanying the branches of the maxillary artery, and terminating posteriorly in the maxillary vein; anteriorly the pterygoid plexus drains via the deep facial vein into the facial vein. SYN p. pterygoideus [NA].

p. pterygoi′deus [NA], SYN pterygoid p.

p. pudenda′lis, SYN prostatic venous p.

p. puden′dus nervo′sus, SYN pudendal ***nerve***.

p. pulmona′lis [NA], SYN pulmonary p.

pulmonary p., one of two autonomic p.'s, anterior and posterior, at the hilus of each lung, formed by cardiopulmonary splanchnic nerves of the sympathetic trunk and bronchial branches of the vagus nerve; from them various branches accompany the bronchi and arteries into the lung. SYN p. pulmonalis [NA].

Quénu's hemorrhoidal p., lymphatic p.'s in the skin about the anus.

Ranvier's p., a subbasal stroma p. of the cornea. SEE stroma p.

rectal plexuses, SEE inferior rectal plexuses, middle rectal plexuses, superior rectal p.

p. recta′les inferio′res [NA], SYN inferior rectal plexuses.

p. recta′les me′dii [NA], SYN middle rectal plexuses.

p. recta′lis supe′rior [NA], SYN superior rectal p.

rectal venous p., a venous p. resting upon the posterior and lateral walls of the rectum; it drains into the superior rectal vein to the portal, the middle rectal to the internal iliac and the inferior rectal to the internal pudendal. SYN p. venosus rectalis [NA], hemorrhoidal p.

Remak's p., SYN submucosal p.

renal p., the autonomic p. surrounding the renal artery and extending with it into the substance of the kidney. SYN p. renalis [NA].

p. rena′lis [NA], SYN renal p.

sacral p., formed by the fourth and fifth lumbar (lumbosacral trunk) and first, second, and third sacral nerves; it lies on the inner surface of the posterior wall of the pelvis usually embedded in the piriformis muscle; its nerves supply the lower limbs, its major product being the sciatic nerve. SYN p. sacralis [NA], ischiadic p., sciatic p.

p. sacra′lis [NA], SYN sacral p.

p. sacra′lis me′dius, SYN middle sacral p.

sacral venous p., a venous p. on the pelvic surface of the sacrum, formed by tributaries to the lateral sacral veins. SYN p. venosus sacralis [NA].

Santorini's p., venous p. on ventral and lateral prostatic surfaces.

Sappey's p., a network of lymphatics in the areola of the nipple.

sciatic p., SYN sacral p.

solar p., SYN celiac (nervous) p.

spermatic p., SYN testicular p.

p. of spinal nerves, an intermingling of fiber fascicles from adjacent spinal nerves to form a network; the major p.'s are the cervical, brachial, and lumbosacral. SYN p. nervorum spinalium [NA].

splenic p., the p. of autonomic nerves along the splenic artery. SYN p. lienalis✩ [NA], p. splenicus.

p. sple′nicus, SYN splenic p.

Stensen's p., the venous network surrounding the parotid (Stensen's) duct.

stroma p., a p. of nerves in the parenchyma of the cornea consisting of the primary or deep p., in the substance of the cornea, and the subbasal or superficial p. just beneath the anterior limiting membrane.

subclavian p., SYN subclavian periarterial p.

subclavian periarterial p., the autonomic p. accompanying the artery of this name, formed by fibers from the stellate ganglion, and giving off secondary p.'s along the branches of the subclavian. SYN p. subclavius [NA], subclavian p.

p. subcla′vius [NA], SYN subclavian periarterial p.

submucosal p., a ganglated p. of unmyelinated nerve fibers, derived chiefly from the superior mesenteric p., ramifying in the intestinal submucosa. SYN p. submucosus [NA], Meissner's p., Remak's p.

p. submuco′sus [NA], SYN submucosal p.

suboccipital venous p., the extensive p. of veins in the suboccipital region. SYN p. venosus suboccipitalis [NA].

p. subsero′sus [NA], SYN subserous p.

subserous p., the subserous part of the enteric plexus of autonomic nerves. SYN p. subserosus [NA].

superficial cardiac p., the superficial and smaller subdivision of the cardiac p., formed by the left superior cardiac nerves from the left vagus and cervical sympathetic trunk; it is found beneath the aortic arch, between the arch and the bifurcation of the pulmonary trunk. SYN p. cardiacus superficialis.

superficial temporal p., an autonomic p. of nerves on the artery of this name, derived from the external carotid p. SYN p. temporalis superficialis.

superior dental p., formed by branches of the infraorbital nerve, it gives off superior dental branches to the upper and superior gingival branches to the gums. SYN p. dentalis superior [NA].

superior hemorrhoidal p., SYN superior rectal p.

superior hypogastric p., the continuation of the aortic p. inferior to the aortic bifurcation across the fifth lumbar vertebra into the pelvis where it divides into two hypogastric nerves at the sides of the rectum; these join the pelvic splanchnic nerves to form the inferior hypogastric p.'s supplying pelvic viscera. SYN p. hypogastricus superior [NA], nervus presacralis✩ [NA], Latarget's nerve (1), presacral nerve.

superior mesenteric p., an autonomic p., a continuation of the abdominal aortic p., sending nerves to the intestines and forming with the vagus the subserous, myenteric, and submucous p.'s; this periarterial plexus is so dense that it results in the appearance of a characteristic perivascular "collar" distinguishing the superior mesenteric artery from the superior mesenteric vein in several imaging modalities such as with ultra sound. SYN p. mesentericus superior [NA].

superior rectal p., the autonomic p. derived as a continuation of the inferior mesenteric p. that accompanies the superior rectal artery. SYN p. rectalis superior [NA], superior hemorrhoidal p.

superior thyroid p., an autonomic p. on the artery of the same name, derived from the external carotid p. SYN p. thyroideus superior.

suprarenal p., an autonomic p. formed mainly by branches from the celiac ganglion, lying at the hilus of the suprarenal gland. SYN p. suprarenalis [NA].

p. suprarena′lis [NA], SYN suprarenal p.

sympathetic plexuses, autonomic plexuses, in which postsynaptic sympathetic nerve fibers are predominant.

p. tempora′lis superficia′lis, SYN superficial temporal p.

testicular p., the autonomic p. derived from the aortic p. and accompanying the testicular artery. SYN p. testicularis [NA], spermatic p.

p. testicula′ris [NA], SYN testicular p.

thoracic aortic p., an autonomic p. surrounding the thoracic aorta and passing with it through the aortic opening in the diaphragm, to become continuous with the abdominal aortic p. SYN p. aorticus thoracicus [NA].

p. thyroi′deus im′par [NA], a venous p. in front of the lower portion of the trachea formed by anastomoses between the inferior laryngeal veins and veins emerging from the caudal border of the thyroid; it terminates in the unpaired inferior thyroid vein.

p. thyroi′deus infe′rior, SYN inferior thyroid p.

p. thyroi′deus supe′rior, SYN superior thyroid p.

tympanic p., a p. on the promontory of the labyrinthine wall of the tympanic cavity, formed by the tympanic nerve, an anastomotic branch of the facial, and sympathetic branches from the internal carotid p.; it supplies the mucosa of the middle ear, mastoid cells, and auditory (eustachian) tube, and gives off the lesser superficial petrosal nerve to the otic ganglion. SYN p. tympanicus [NA], Jacobson's p.

p. tympan′icus [NA], SYN tympanic p.

ureteric p., the autonomic p. derived from the celiac p. that accompanies the ureter. SYN p. uretericus [NA].

p. ureter′icus [NA], SYN ureteric p.

uterine venous p., the plexiform veins that lie along the sides of the uterus in the broad ligament. SYN p. venosus uterinus [NA].

uterovaginal p., a ganglated autonomic p. on each side of the cervix of the uterus, derived from the inferior hypogastric p. SYN p. uterovaginalis [NA], Frankenhäuser's ganglion, Lee's ganglion.

p. uterovagina′lis [NA], SYN uterovaginal p.

vaginal venous p., the p. of veins that surrounds the vagina. SYN p. venosus vaginalis [NA].

vascular p., a vascular network formed by frequent anastomoses between the blood vessels (arteries or veins) of a part. SYN p. vasculosus [NA].

p. vasculo′sus [NA], SYN vascular p.

p. veno′sus [NA], SYN venous p.

p. veno′sus areola′ris [NA], SYN areolar venous p.

p. veno′sus cana′lis hypoglos′si [NA], SYN venous p. of hypoglossal canal.

pl

p. veno′sus carot′icus inter′nus [NA], SYN internal carotid venous p.

p. veno′sus foram′inis ova′lis [NA], SYN venous p. of foramen ovale.

p. veno′sus prostat′icus [NA], SYN prostatic venous p.

p. veno′sus recta′lis [NA], SYN rectal venous p.

p. veno′sus sacra′lis [NA], SYN sacral venous p.

p. veno′sus suboccipita′lis [NA], SYN suboccipital venous p.

p. veno′sus uteri′nus [NA], SYN uterine venous p.

p. veno′sus vagina′lis [NA], SYN vaginal venous p.

p. veno′sus vertebra′lis [NA], SYN vertebral venous *system*.

p. veno′sus vesica′lis [NA], SYN vesicular venous p.

venous p., a vascular network formed by numerous anastomoses between veins. SYN p. venosus [NA].

venous p. of bladder, SYN vesicular venous p.

venous p. of foramen ovale, a venous network around the mandibular nerve connecting the cavernous sinus and the pterygoid p. SYN p. venosus foraminis ovalis [NA], rete foraminis ovalis.

venous p. of hypoglossal canal, a small venous network around the hypoglossal nerve, connecting with the occipital sinus, inferior petrosal sinus, and internal jugular vein. SYN p. venosus canalis hypoglossi [NA], circellus venosus hypoglossi, rete canalis hypoglossi.

vertebral p., SYN periarterial p. of vertebral artery.

p. vertebra′lis [NA], SYN periarterial p. of vertebral artery.

vertebral venous p., SYN vertebral venous *system*.

vesical p., an autonomic p. on the bladder, derived from the inferior hypogastric p. SYN p. vesicalis [NA].

p. vesica′lis [NA], SYN vesical p.

p. vesica′lis infe′rior, SYN inferior vesical p.

vesicular venous p., a p. of veins around the fundus and sides of the bladder. SYN p. venosus vesicalis [NA], venous p. of bladder.

Walther′s p., SYN intracavernous p.

PLICA

pli·ca, gen. and pl. **pli·cae** (plī′kă, plī′sē). **1** [NA]. One of several anatomical structures in which there is a folding over of the parts. **2.** SYN false *membrane*. SEE ALSO fold. [Mod. L. a plait or fold]

pli′cae adipo′sae, lobules of fat enveloped in the pleura, chiefly in the neighborhood of the costomediastinal sinus. SYN adipose folds of the pleura.

pli′cae ala′res [NA], SYN alar *folds*, under *fold*.

pli′cae ampulla′res tu′bae uteri′nae, SYN ampullary *folds* of uterine tube, under *fold*.

p. aryepiglot′tica [NA], SYN aryepiglottic *fold*.

p. axilla′ris, SYN axillary *fold*.

pli′cae ceca′les [NA], SYN cecal *folds*, under *fold*.

p. ceca′lis vascula′ris [NA], SYN vascular *fold* of the cecum.

p. chor′dae tym′pani [NA], SYN *fold* of chorda tympani.

p. choroi′dea, in the embryo, an infolding of the chorion from which the choroid plexus develops.

pli′cae cilia′res [NA], SYN ciliary *folds*, under *fold*.

pli′cae circula′res [NA], the numerous folds of the mucous membrane of the small intestine, running transversely for about two-thirds of the circumference of the gut. SYN circular folds, Kerckring′s folds, Kerckring′s valves, valvulae conniventes.

p. duodena′lis infe′rior [NA], SYN inferior duodenal *fold*.

p. duodena′lis supe′rior [NA], SYN superior duodenal *fold*.

p. duodenojejuna′lis [NA], ☆official alternate term for superior duodenal *fold*.

p. duodenomesocol′ica [NA], ☆official alternate term for inferior duodenal *fold*.

p. epigas′trica, SYN lateral umbilical *fold*.

pli′cae epiglot′tica, SYN epiglottic *folds*, under *fold*.

p. fimbria′ta [NA], one of several folds running outward from the frenulum on the undersurface of the tongue. SYN fimbriated fold.

pli′cae gas′tricae [NA], SYN *rugae* of stomach, under *ruga*.

pli′cae gastropancreat′icae [NA], SYN gastropancreatic *folds*, under *fold*.

p. glossoepiglot′tica latera′lis [NA], SYN lateral glossoepiglottic *fold*.

p. glossoepiglot′tica media′na [NA], SYN median glossoepiglottic *fold*.

p. guberna′trix, SYN genitoinguinal *ligament*.

p. hypogas′trica, SYN medial umbilical *fold*.

p. ileoceca′lis [NA], SYN ileocecal *fold*.

p. incu′dis [NA], SYN incudal *fold*.

p. inguina′lis, an embryonic mesodermal thickening that joins the caudal end of the urogenital ridge to the anterior abdominal wall; the gubernaculum of the testis develops in it. SYN inguinal fold.

p. interdigita′lis, SYN *web* of fingers/toes.

p. interureter′ica [NA], SYN interureteric *fold*.

pli′cae ir′idis [NA], SYN *folds* of iris, under *fold*.

p. lacrima′lis [NA], SYN lacrimal *fold*.

p. longitudina′lis duode′ni [NA], SYN longitudinal *fold* of duodenum.

p. luna′ta, SYN p. semilunaris conjunctivae.

p. mallea′ris [NA], SYN mallear *fold*.

p. membra′nae tym′pani, SYN mallear *fold*.

p. ner′vi laryn′gei [NA], SYN *fold* of superior laryngeal nerve.

p. palati′na transver′sa [NA], SYN transverse palatine *fold*.

pli′cae palma′tae [NA], SYN palmate *folds*, under *fold*.

p. palpebronasa′lis [NA], SYN epicanthal *fold*.

p. paraduodena′lis [NA], SYN paraduodenal *fold*.

pli′cae rec′ti, SYN transverse rectal *folds*, under *fold*.

p. rectouteri′na [NA], SYN sacrouterine *fold*.

p. rectovagina′lis, SYN sacrovaginal *fold*.

p. salpingopalatin′a [NA], SYN salpingopalatine *fold*.

p. salpingopharyn′gea [NA], SYN salpingopharyngeal *fold*.

p. semiluna′ris [NA], SYN semilunar *fold*.

p. semiluna′ris of colon [NA], one of the folds of the wall of the colon between sacculations. SYN p. sigmoidea, semilunar fold of colon.

p. semiluna′ris conjuncti′vae, **(1)** [NA], the semilunar fold formed by the palpebral conjunctiva at the medial angle of the eye; **(2)** a fold of the conjunctival mucous membrane found in many animals; normally partially hidden in the medial canthus of the eye when at rest, it may be extended to cover part or all of the cornea in a winking-like action to clean the cornea, as in birds. SYN membrana nictitans, nictitating membrane, palpebra III, palpebra tertia, third eyelid. SYN p. lunata, p. semilunaris of eye, semilunar conjunctival fold.

p. semilunaris of eye, SYN p. semilunaris conjunctivae.

p. sigmoi′dea, SYN p. semilunaris of colon.

p. spira′lis duc′tus cys′tici [NA], SYN spiral *fold* of cystic duct.

p. stape′dis [NA], SYN stapedial *fold*.

p. sublingua′lis [NA], SYN sublingual *fold*.

p. synovia′lis [NA], SYN synovial *fold*.

p. synovia′lis infrapatella′ris [NA], SYN infrapatellar synovial *fold*.

p. synovia′lis patella′ris, SYN infrapatellar synovial *fold*.

pli′cae transversa′les rec′ti [NA], SYN transverse rectal *folds*, under *fold*.

p. triangula′ris [NA], SYN triangular *fold*.

pli′cae tuba′riae tu′bae uteri′nae [NA], SYN tubal *folds* of uterine tubes, under *fold*.

p. tubopalati′na, SYN salpingopalatine *fold*.

pli′cae tu′nicae muco′sae vesi′cae fel′leae [NA], SYN mucosal *folds* of gallbladder, under *fold*.

p. umbilica′lis latera′lis [NA], SYN lateral umbilical *fold*.

p. umbilica′lis me′dia, SYN median umbilical *fold.*

p. umbilica′lis media′lis [NA], SYN medial umbilical *fold.*

p. umbilica′lis media′na [NA], SYN median umbilical *fold.*

p. ura′chi, SYN median umbilical *fold.*

p. ureter′ica, SYN interureteric *fold.*

p. uterovesica′lis, SYN uterovesical *ligament.*

p. ve′nae ca′vae sinis′trae [NA], SYN *fold* of left vena cava.

p. ventricula′ris, SYN vestibular *fold.*

p. vesica′lis transver′sa [NA], SYN transverse vesical *fold.*

p. vesicouteri′na, SYN uterovesical *ligament.*

p. vestibula′ris [NA], SYN vestibular *fold.*

p. vestib′uli, a fold of mucous membrane forming a ridge on the septum of the nose.

p. villo′sa [NA], one of the ridges of the mucous membrane of the stomach in the region of the pylorus.

p. voca′lis [NA], SYN vocal *fold.*

pli·cate (plī′kāt). Folded; pleated; tucked.

pli·ca·tion (plī-kā′shŭn, pli-). A folding or putting together in pleats; specifically, an operation for reducing the size of a hollow viscus by taking folds or tucks in its walls. [L. *plico,* pp. *-atus,* to fold]

pli·cot·o·my (plī-kot′ō-mē). Division of the plica mallearis. [plica + G. *tomē,* incision]

Plimmer, Henry G., English protozoologist, 1857–1918. SEE P.'s *bodies,* under *body.*

-ploid. Multiple in form; its combinations are used both adjectivally: and substantively of a (specified) multiple of chromosomes. [G. *-plo-, -fold,* + *-ides,* in form; L. *-ploïdeus*]

ploi·dy (ploy′dē). The number of haploid sets in a cell. Gametes normally contain one; autosomal cells two. SEE ALSO polyploidy. [-ploid + *-y,* condition]

plom·bage (plom-bahzh′). Formerly, the use of an inert material in collapse of the lung in the surgical treatment of pulmonary tuberculosis. [Fr. lit. lead-work]

plo·sive (plō′siv). Speech sound made by impounding the air stream for a moment and then suddenly releasing it.

plot (plot). A graphical representation.

double-reciprocal p., a graphical representation of enzyme kinetic data in which 1/v (on the vertical axis) is plotted as a function of the reciprocal of the substrate concentration (1/[S]). SYN Lineweaver-Burk p., Woolf-Lineweaver-Burk p.

Eadie-Hofstee p., a graphical representation of enzyme kinetic data in which velocities are plotted on the vertical axis as a function of the v/[S] ratio on the horizontal axis. Sometimes referred to as the Eadie-Augustinsson p. or Woolf-Eadie-Augustinsson-Hofstee p.

Hanes p., a graphical representation of enzyme kinetic data in which the substrate concentration divided by the velocity (*i.e.,* the [S]/v ratio) is plotted on the vertical axis as a function of [S]. Sometimes referred to as the Hanes-Wilkinson p.

Hill p., a graphical representation of enzyme kinetic data or of binding phenomena to assess the degree of cooperativity of a system; the vertical axis in a Hill plot is log [Y/(1-Y)] in which Y is the degree of saturation (for enzymes the vertical axis is log[v/(V$_{max}$ − v)] and the horizontal axis is the logarithm of the ligand concentration.

Lineweaver-Burk p., SYN double-reciprocal p.

Ramachandran p., a graphical representation in which the dihedral angle of rotation about the α-carbon to carbonyl-carbon bond in polypeptides is plotted against the dihedral angle of rotation about the α-carbon to nitrogen bond. SYN conformational map.

Scatchard p., (1) a graphical representation used in the analysis of binding phenomena in which the concentration of bound ligand divided by the concentration of free ligand is plotted against

the concentration of bound ligand; (2) similar to (1), except the concentration of the bound ligand is on the vertical axis.

Woolf-Lineweaver-Burk p., SYN double-reciprocal p.

Plotz, Harry, U.S. physician, 1890–1947. SEE P. *bacillus.*

PLP Abbreviation for *pyridoxal* 5′-phosphate; parathyroid hormonelike *protein.*

plug (plŭg). Any mass filling a hole or closing an orifice.

Dittrich's p.'s, minute, dirty-grayish, ill-smelling masses of bacteria and fatty acid crystals in the sputum in pulmonary gangrene and fetid bronchitis. SYN Traube's p.'s.

epithelial p., a mass of epithelial cells temporarily occluding an embryonic opening; the term is most commonly used with reference to the external nares.

laminated epithelial p., SYN *keratosis* obturans.

mucous p., a mass of mucus and cells filling the cervical canal between periods or during pregnancy; a mass of mucous occluding a main or lobar bronchus.

Traube's p.'s, SYN Dittrich's p.'s.

vaginal p., a p. formed by the coagulation of semen; found in the vagina after copulation in certain animals, such as the baboon, rat, and squirrel.

plug·ger. A dental instrument used for condensing gold (foil), amalgam, or any plastic material in a cavity, and which is operated by hand or by mechanical means. SYN packer (2), plugging instrument.

automatic p., a mechanically or electrically activated device used to provide condensing pressure in the placement of amalgam or gold foil in a cavity preparation. SYN automatic condenser.

back-action p., an instrument for condensing gold foil or amalgam in areas that cannot be reached directly.

foot p., a p. the shape of which resembles a foot, used for condensing gold foil; the working surface may be flat or curved in the heel-toe direction.

root canal p., fine-tapered root canal instrument, blunt at the tip, used for pressing or forcing a gutta percha cone into a root canal.

plum·ba·go (plŭm-bā′gō). SYN graphite. [L. *plumbago,* black lead]

plum·bic (plŭm′bik). **1.** Relating to or containing lead. **2.** Denoting the higher valence of the lead ion, Pb^{4+}. [L. *plumbum,* lead]

plum·bism (plŭm′bizm). SYN lead *poisoning.* [L. *plumbum,* lead]

plum·bum (plŭm′bŭm). SYN lead. [L.]

Plummer, Henry S., U.S. physician, 1874–1937. SEE P.'s *dilator, disease;* P.-Vinson *syndrome.*

plu·mose (plū′mōs). Feathery. [L. *pluma,* feather]

pluri-. Several, more. SEE ALSO multi-, poly-. [L. *plus, pluris*]

plu·ri·cau·sal (plūr-i-kaw′zăl). Having two or more causes; used in reference to the etiology of a disease; often indicates that a given disease develops only when two or more causative factors are operative simultaneously.

---

plu·ri·glan·du·lar (plū-ri-glan′dū-lăr). Denoting several glands or their secretions. SYN multiglandular, polyglandular.

plu·ri·loc·u·lar (plū-ri-lok′yū-lăr). SYN multilocular.

plu·ri·nu·cle·ar (plū-ri-nū′klē-ăr). SYN multinuclear.

plu·rip·o·tent, plu·ri·po·ten·tial (plū-rip′ō-tent, plū′rē-pō-ten′shăl). **1.** Having the capacity to affect more than one organ or tissue. **2.** Not fixed as to potential development. SEE ALSO pluripotent *cells,* under *cell.*

plu·ri·re·sis·tant (plū′ri-rē-sis′tănt). Having multiple aspects of resistance.

plu·to·ma·nia (plū-tō-mā′nē-ă). A delusion that one has great wealth. [G. *ploutos,* wealth, + *mania,* frenzy]

plu·to·nism (plū′ton-izm). Effects produced, as demonstrated in experimental animals, by means of exposure to the radioactive element plutonium present in atomic piles; they consist of hepatic damage, bone changes, and graying of the hair.

plu·to·ni·um (Pu) (plū-tō′nē-ŭm). A transuranium artificial radioactive element, atomic no. 94, atomic wt. 244.064. The best-known α-emitting isotope is ^{239}Pu (half-life 24,110 years) which, like ^{235}U, is fissionable and can be used in atomic bombs and nuclear power plants; ^{238}Pu (half-life 87.74 years) is used as an energy source in pacemakers. Pu ions are bone-seekers; ingestion is a radiation hazard as with radium and radiostrontium. [planet, *Pluto*]

Pm Symbol for promethium.

pM Abbreviation for picomolar (10^{-12} M).

pm Symbol for picometer.

P-mit·ra·le (mī-tra′lē). Broad, notched P waves in several or many leads of the electrocardiogram with a prominent late negative component to the P wave in lead V_1, presumed to be characteristic of mitral valvular disease. (Although this term is extensively used in electrocardiographic literature, it is actually a misnomer and would be more appropriately called P-sinistrocardiale, as it results from overload of the left atrium regardless of the cause and may occur independently of disease of the mitral valve.)

PML Abbreviation for progressive multifocal *leukoencephalopathy.*

pmol Abbreviation for picomole.

PMR Abbreviation for proportional mortality ratio.

PMS Abbreviation for premenstrual *syndrome.*

PMSG Abbreviation for pregnant mare's serum *gonadotropin.*

-pnea. Breath, respiration. [G. *pneō,* to breathe]

pneo-. Combining form denoting breath or respiration. SEE ALSO pneum-, pneumo-. [G. *pneō,* to breathe]

pne·o·dy·nam·ics (nē′ō-dī-nam′iks). SYN pneumodynamics.

pne·om·e·ter (nē-om′ĕter). Obsolete term for spirometer. [pneo- + G. *metron,* measure]

pne·om·e·try (nē-om′ĕ-trē). Obsolete term for spirometry.

pne·o·scope (nē′ō-skōp). SYN pneumatoscope (1).

pneum-, pneuma-, pneumat-, pneumato-. Presence of air or gas, the lungs, or breathing. SEE ALSO pneo-, pneumo-. [G. *pneuma, pneumatos,* air, breath]

pneu·ma (nū′mă). In ancient Greek philosophy and medicine: **1.** Air or an all-pervading fiery essence in the air (which today would be identified with oxygen) which was the creative and animating spirit of the universe; drawn into the body through the lungs it generated and sustained the innate heat in the left ventricle of the heart and was distributed by the arteries to the brain and all parts of the body. **2.** Soul or psyche. [G. *pneuma,* air, breath]

pneu·marth·ro·gram (nū-marth′rō-gram). Film records of pneumarthrography.

pneu·marth·rog·ra·phy (nū-marth-rog′ră-fē). Radiographic examination of a joint following the introduction of air, with or without another contrast medium.

pneu·mar·thro·sis (nū-mar-thrō′sis). Presence of air in a joint. [G. *pneuma,* air, + *arthron,* joint, + *-osis,* condition]

pneu·mat·ic (nū-mat′ik). **1.** Relating to air or gas, or to a structure filled with air. **2.** Relating to respiration. [G. *pneumatikos*]

pneu·mat·ic an·ti·shock gar·ment. an inflatable suit used to apply pressure to the peripheral circulation, thus reducing blood flow and fluid exudation into tissues, to maintain central blood flow in the presence of shock.

pneu·mat·ics (nū-mat′iks). The science concerned with the physical properties of air or gases. [G. *pneuma,* air or gas]

pneu·ma·ti·nu·ria (nū-mă-ti-nū′rē-ă). SYN pneumaturia.

pneu·ma·tism (nū′mă-tizm). The doctrine of the pneumatists.

pneu·ma·tists (nū′mă-tists). The followers of the school whose physiology centered around the pneuma and who conceived the causes of disease as disturbances of this vital principle.

pneu·ma·ti·za·tion (nū′mă-ti-zā′shŭn). The development of air cells such as those of the mastoid and ethmoidal bones. [G. *pneuma,* air]

pneu·ma·tized (nū′mă-tīzd). Containing air.

pneumato-. SEE pneum-.

pneu·ma·to·car·dia (nū′mă-tō-kar′dē-ă). Presence of air bubbles or gas in the blood of the heart; produced by air embolism.

pneu·ma·to·cele (nū′mă-tō-sēl). **1.** An emphysematous or gaseous swelling. **2.** SYN pneumonocele. **3.** A thin-walled cavity within the lung, one of the characteristic sequelae of staphylococcus pneumonia. [G. *pneuma,* air, + *kēlē,* tumor, hernia]
    extracranial p., collection of gas beneath the galea aponeurotica, usually due to fracture into the paranasal sinuses. SYN extracranial pneumocele.
    intracranial p., a collection of gas within the skull, in the brain, or in the meninges. SYN intracranial pneumocele.

pneu·ma·to·en·ter·ic. SYN celomic *bay.*

pneu·ma·to·he·mia (nū′mă-tō-hē′mē-ă). SYN pneumohemia.

pneu·ma·tom·e·ter (nū-mă-tom′ĕ-ter). Obsolete term for spirometer.

pneu·ma·tor·rha·chis (nū-mă-tōr′ă-kis). SYN pneumorrhachis. [G. *pneuma,* air, + *rhachis,* spine]

pneu·ma·to·scope (nū′mă-tō-skōp, nū-mat′ō-skōp). **1.** Obsolete term for an instrument for measuring the extent of the respiratory excursions of the chest. SYN pneoscope. **2.** Obsolete term for an instrument for use in auscultatory percussion, the percussion sounds of the chest being heard at the mouth. SYN pneumoscope. [G. *pneuma,* air, + *skopeō,* to examine]

pneu·ma·to·sis (nū-mă-tō′sis). Abnormal accumulation of gas in any tissue or part of the body. [G. a blowing out]
    p. coli, a usually benign condition in which gas is seen radiographically in the wall of the colon; sometimes associated with obstructive lung disease.
    p. cystoi′des intestina′lis, a condition of unknown cause characterized by the occurrence of gas cysts in the intestinal mucous membrane; may produce intestinal obstruction. SYN intestinal emphysema.

pneu·ma·tu·ria (nū-mă-tū′rē-ă). The passage of gas or air from the urethra during or after urination, resulting from decomposition of bladder urine or, more commonly, from an intestinal fistula. SYN pneumatinuria. [G. *pneuma,* air, + *ouron,* urine]

pneu·ma·type (nū′mă-tīp). A device for determining the permeability of the nasal fossae by exhaling through the nose against a plate of cooled glass. [G. *pneuma,* breath, + *typos,* type]

pneumo-, pneumon-, pneumono-. The lungs, air or gas, respiration, or pneumonia. SEE ALSO aer-, pneo-, pneum-. [G. *pneumōn, pneumonos,* lung]

pneu·mo·an·gi·og·ra·phy (nū′mō-an-jē-og′ră-fē). Obsolete term for a radiographic contrast study of the pulmonary blood vessels. [pneumo- + G. *angeion,* vessel, + *graphō,* to write]

pneu·mo·ar·throg·ra·phy (nū′mō-ar-throg′ră-fē). Radiography of a joint after injection of air and usually a water-soluble contrast medium. [G. *pneuma,* air, + *arthron,* joint, + *graphō,* to write]

pneu·mo·ba·cil·lus (nū′mō-bă-sil′ŭs). SYN *Klebsiella pneumoniae.*

pneu·mo·bul·bar (nū-mō-bŭl′bar). Relating to the lungs and their connection with the medulla oblongata by way of the vagus nerve. [G. *pneumōn*, lung, + L. *bulbus*, bulb]

pneu·mo·car·di·al (nū′mō-kar′dē-ăl). SYN cardiopulmonary.

pneu·mo·cele (nū′mō-sēl). SYN pneumonocele.

extracranial p., SYN extracranial *pneumatocele.*

intracranial p., SYN intracranial *pneumatocele.*

pneu·mo·cen·te·sis (nū′mō-sen-tē′sis). SYN pneumonocentesis.

pneu·mo·ceph·a·lus (nū-mō-sef′ă-lŭs). Presence of air or gas within the cranial cavity. [G. *pneuma*, air, + *kephalē*, head]

pneu·mo·cho·le·cys·ti·tis (nū′mō-kō′lē-sis-tī′tis). Cholecystitis with gas-forming organisms giving rise to gas in the gallbladder.

pneu·mo·coc·cal (nū-mō-kok′ăl). Pertaining to or containing the pneumococcus.

pneu·mo·coc·ce·mia (nū′mō-kok-sē′mē-ă). The presence of pneumococci in the blood. [pneumococcus + G. *haima*, blood]

pneu·mo·coc·ci·dal (nū′mō-kok-sī′dăl). Destructive to pneumococci. [pneumococcus + L. *caedo*, to kill]

pneu·mo·coc·col·y·sis (nū′mō-kok-ol′i-sis). Lysis or destruction of pneumococci. [pneumococcus + G. *lysis*, dissolution]

pneu·mo·coc·co·sis (nū′mō-kok-ō′sis). Rarely used term for infection with pneumococci.

pneu·mo·coc·co·su·ria (nū′mō-kok-o-sū′rē-ă). The presence of pneumococci or their specific capsular substance in the urine. [pneumococcus + G. *ouron*, urine]

pneu·mo·coc·cus, pl. **pneu·mo·coc·ci** (nū-mō-kok′ŭs, -kok′sī). SYN *Streptococcus pneumoniae.* [G. *pneumōn*, lung, + *kokkos*, berry (coccus)]

Fraenkel's p., SYN *Streptococcus pneumoniae.*

Fraenkel-Weichselbaum p., SYN *Streptococcus pneumoniae.*

pneu·mo·co·lon (nū-mō-kō′lŏn). Gas in the colon or interstitial gas in the wall of the colon. [G. *pneuma*, air, + *kolon*, colon]

pneu·mo·co·ni·o·sis, pneu·mo·ko·ni·o·sis, pl. **pneu·mo·co·ni·o·ses** (nū′mō-kō-nē-ō′sis, -sēz). Inflammation commonly leading to fibrosis of the lungs caused by the inhalation of dust incident to various occupations; characterized by pain in the chest, cough with little or no expectoration, dyspnea, reduced thoracic excursion, sometimes cyanosis, and fatigue after slight exertion; degree of disability depends on the types of particles inhaled, as well as the level of exposure to them. SYN anthracotic tuberculosis, pneumonoconiosis, pneumonokoniosis. [G. *pneumōn*, lung, + *konis*, dust, + *-osis*, condition]

bauxite p., a condition due to the occupational inhalation of bauxite fumes emitted during the manufacture of alumina abrasives; characterized by cough, shortness of breath, a combined obstructive and restrictive breathing pattern, and impairment of diffusing capacity. SYN Shaver's disease.

p. of coal workers, p. seen in coal miners, for example anthracosis, black lung disease (pneumomelanosis).

collagenous p., a disease of the lungs, characterized by interstitial fibrosis, caused by inhalation of dusts or toxins in the workplace.

p. siderotica (sid-er-ot′ĭ-kă), p. caused by inhalation of iron dust. SYN pulmonary siderosis.

pneu·mo·cra·ni·um (nū-mō-krā′nē-ŭm). Air present between the cranium and the dura mater; the term is commonly used to indicate extradural or subdural air. [G. *pneuma*, air, + *kranion*, skull]

Pneu·mo·cys·tis ca·ri·nii (nū-mō-sis′tis kă-rī′nē-ī). The microorganism that causes pneumocystis pneumonia in debilitated patients. Microbiologists differ as to the taxnomic position of this agent. Recent studies indicate that the RNA of the 16s-like ribosomal RNA of *P. carinii* shares substantial sequence homology with some species of the ascomycetes by the 5s-ribosomal RNA from *P. carinii* showed that the phylogenetic position is closer to Rhizopoda (amoeba) and the slime net or the flagellated aquatic fungi and zygomycetes. [G. *pneuma*, air, breathing, + *kystis*, bladder, pouch]

pneu·mo·cys·tog·ra·phy (nū′mō-sis-tog′ră-fē). Radiography of the bladder following injection of air. [G. *pneuma*, air, + *kystis*, bladder, + *graphō*, to write]

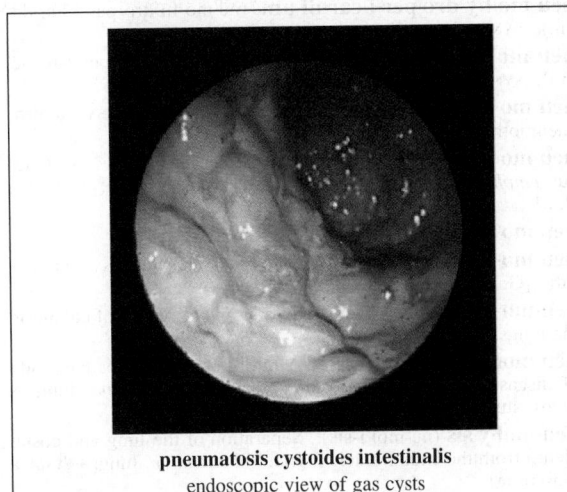

pneumatosis cystoides intestinalis
endoscopic view of gas cysts

pneu·mo·cys·to·sis (nū′mō-sis-tō′sis). SYN *Pneumocystis carinii* pneumonia.

pneu·mo·cyte (nū′mō-sīt). SYN alveolar *cell.* [pneumo- + G. *kytos,* cell]

pneu·mo·der·ma (nū-mō-der′mă). SYN subcutaneous *emphysema.* [G. *pneuma*, air, + *derma*, skin]

pneu·mo·dy·nam·ics (nū′mō-dī-nam′iks). The mechanics of respiration. SYN pneodynamics. [G. *pneuma*, breath, + *dynamis*, force]

pneu·mo·em·py·e·ma (nū′mō-em′pī-ē′mă). A rarely used term for pyopneumothorax.

pneu·mo·en·ceph·a·lo·gram (nū′mō-en-sef′ă-lō-gram). Radiographs obtained by pneumoencephalography.

pneu·mo·en·ceph·a·log·ra·phy (nū′mō-en-sef′ă-log′ră-fē). Radiographic visualization of cerebral ventricles and subarachnoid spaces by use of gas such as air; no longer used because of CT and MRI. [G. *pneuma*, air, + *enkephalos*, brain, + *graphō*, to write]

pneu·mo·gas·tric (nū-mō-gas′trik). 1. Relating to the lungs and the stomach. 2. Obsolete term denoting the nervus vagus. SYN gastropneumonic, gastropulmonary. [G. *pneumōn*, lung, + *gastēr*, stomach]

pneu·mo·gas·trog·ra·phy (nū′mō-gas-trog′ră-fē). Rarely used radiographic study of stomach after injection of air. [G. *pneuma*, air, + *gastēr*, stomach, + *graphō*, to write]

pneu·mo·gram (nū′mō-gram). 1. The record or tracing made by a pneumograph. 2. Radiographic record of pneumography. [G. *pneumōn*, lung, + *gramma*, a drawing]

pneu·mo·graph (nū′mō-graf). Generic term for any device that records respiratory excursions from movements on the body surface; *e.g.,* an impedance p., which applies the principles of impedance plethysmography to the chest. [G. *pneumōn*, lung, + *graphō*, to write]

pneu·mog·ra·phy (nū-mog′ră-fē). 1. Examination with a pneumograph. 2. A general term indicating radiography after injection of air. SYN pneumoradiography, pneumoroentgenography. [G. *pneumōn*, lung, + *graphō*, to write]

pneu·mo·he·mia (nū-mō-hē′mē-ă). Presence of air in blood vessels. SEE ALSO air *embolism.* SYN pneumatohemia. [G. *pneuma*, air, + *haima*, blood]

pneu·mo·he·mo·per·i·car·di·um (nū′mō-hē-mō-per-i-kar′dē-ŭm). SYN hemopneumopericardium.

pneu·mo·he·mo·thor·ax (nū′mō-hē-mō-thōr′aks). SYN hemopneumothorax.

pneu·mo·hy·dro·me·tra (nū′mō-hī-drō-mē′tră). The presence of gas and serum in the uterine cavity. [G. *pneuma*, air, + *hydōr* (hydr-), water, + *mētra*, uterus]

pneu·mo·hy·dro·per·i·car·di·um (nū'mō-hī'drō-pār-i-kar'dē-ŭm). SYN hydropneumopericardium.

pneu·mo·hy·dro·per·i·to·ne·um (nū'mō-hī-drō-per-i-tō-nē'ŭm). SYN hydropneumoperitoneum.

pneu·mo·hy·dro·thor·ax (nū-mō-hī-drō-thōr'aks). SYN hydropneumothorax.

pneu·mo·hy·po·der·ma (nū'mō-hī-pō-der'mă). SYN subcutaneous *emphysema*. [G. *pneuma*, air, + *hypo*, beneath, + *derma*, skin]

pneu·mo·ko·ni·o·sis. SEE pneumoconiosis.

pneu·mo·lith (nū'mō-lith). A calculus in the lung. SYN pulmolith. [G. *pneumōn*, lung, + *lithos*, stone]

pneu·mo·li·thi·a·sis (nū-mō-li-thī'ă-sis). Formation of calculi in the lungs.

pneu·mol·o·gy (nū-mol'ō-jē). A rarely used term for the study of diseases of the lung and air passages. [G. *pneuma*, lung, + *logos*, study]

pneu·mol·y·sis (nū-mol'i-sis). Separation of the lung and costal pleura from the endothoracic fascia. [G. *pneumōn*, lung, + *lysis*, a loosening]

pneu·mo·ma·la·cia (nū-mō-mă-lā'shē-ă). Softening of the lung tissue. [G. *pneumōn*, lung, + *malakia*, softness]

pneu·mo·mas·sage (nū'mō-mă-sahzh'). Compression and rarefaction of the air in the external auditory meatus, causing movement of an intact tympanic membrane. [G. *pneuma*, air, + massage]

pneu·mo·me·di·as·ti·num (nū'mō-mē'dē-ă-stī'nŭm). Escape of air into mediastinal tissues, usually from interstitial emphysema or from a ruptured pulmonary bleb. [G. *pneuma*, air, + mediastinum]

pneu·mo·mel·a·no·sis (nū'mō-mel-ă-nō'sis). Blackening of the lung tissue from the inhalation of coal dust or other black particles. SYN pneumonomelanosis. [G. *pneumōn*, lung, + *melanosis*, a becoming black]

pneu·mom·e·ter (nū-mom'ĕ-ter). Obsolete term for spirometer.

pneu·mom·e·try (nū-mom'ĕ-trē). Obsolete term for spirometry.

pneu·mo·my·co·sis (nū'mō-mī-kō'sis). Obsolete term denoting any disease of the lungs caused by the presence of fungi. SYN pneumonomycosis. [G. *pneumōn*, lung, + *mykēs*, fungus]

pneu·mo·my·e·log·ra·phy (nū'mō-mī'ĕ-log'ră-fē). Rarely used radiographic examination of spinal canal after injection of air or gas into the subarachnoid space. [G. *pneuma*, air, + *myelos*, marrow, + *graphō*, to write]

△**pneumon-.** SEE pneumo-.

pneu·mo·nec·to·my (nū'mō-nek'tō-mē). Removal of all pulmonary lobes from a lung in one operation. SYN pulmonectomy. [G. *pneumōn*, lung, + *ektomē*, excision]

pneu·mo·nia (nū-mō'nē-ă). Inflammation of the lung parenchyma characterized by consolidation of the affected part, the alveolar air spaces being filled with exudate, inflammatory cells, and fibrin. Most cases are due to infection by bacteria or viruses, a few to inhalation of chemicals or trauma to the chest wall, and a small minority to rickettsias, fungi, and yeasts. Distribution may be lobar, segmental, or lobular; when lobular, in association with bronchitis, it is termed bronchopneumonia. SEE ALSO pneumonitis. [G. fr. *pneumōn*, lung, + *-ia*, condition]

acute interstitial p., a severe and usually fatal form of p. occurring primarily in infants usually considered a form of hypersensitivity *pneumonitis.*

alcoholic p., p. occurring in patient with alcoholism, usually after a period of intoxication with stupor, resulting in aspiration.

anthrax p., SYN pulmonary *anthrax.*

apex p., apical p., p. of the apex or apices.

aspiration p., bronchopneumonia resulting from the inhalation of foreign material, usually food particles or vomit, into the bronchi; p. developing secondary to the presence in the airways of fluid, blood, saliva, or gastric contents. SYN deglutition p.

atypical p., SYN primary atypical p.

bacterial p., infection of the lung with any of a large variety of bacteria, especially *Streptococcus pneumoniae*(pneumococcus).

bilious p., p. following aspiration of gastric contents containing bile.

bronchial p., SYN bronchopneumonia.

caseous p., a form of severe pulmonary tuberculosis in which tubercles are not prominent, but with a diffuse extensive cellular infiltration that undergoes caseation affecting large areas of lung.

central p., a form of p. in which exudation is confined for a time to the central portion of a lobe or the hilar region. SYN core p.

chemical p., p. caused by inhalation of toxic gas, such as the war gases phosgene or chlorine; exudation into alveoli causes the lungs to be edematous and hemorrhagic; large amounts of fluid that fill the air passages block gaseous exchange; recovery occurs, permanent damage of the lungs remains, and recurrent pulmonary infections are common.

chronic p., vague or indefinite term for long-standing inflammation of pulmonary tissue of any etiology.

chronic eosinophilic p., a disease characterized by night sweats, exertional dyspnea, occasional wheezing, and peripheral eosinophilia. X-rays show peripheral, non-segmental pulmonary infiltrates that can be nodular with cavitation. Responds to treatment with corticosteroids. SYN Carrington's disease.

congenital p., p. in the newborn, infection being contracted prenatally.

contusion p., inflammation of the lungs following a severe blow on or compression of the chest, or following a wound of the lung itself. SYN traumatic p.

core p., SYN central p.

deglutition p., SYN aspiration p.

desquamative p., relatively rare form of p. with homogeneous filling of alveolar air spaces with macrophages and a few type II epithelial lining cells, some alveolar septal infiltration with inflammatory and connective tissue cells. Usually idiopathic but some cases have been reported in association with drugs or underlying systemic connective tissue disease. Rarely progresses to end-stage lung disease.

desquamative interstitial p. (D.I.P.), diffuse proliferation of alveolar epithelial cells, which desquamate into the air sacs and become filled with macrophages, accompanied by interstitial cellular infiltration and fibrosis; gradual onset of dyspnea and nonproductive cough occurs.

p. dis'secans, SYN p. interlobularis purulenta.

double p., lobar p. involving both lungs.

Eaton agent p., SYN primary atypical p.

embolic p., infarction following embolization of a pulmonary artery or arteries.

enzootic p., a p. of sheep caused by the bacterium *Pasteurella haemolytica.*

eosinophilic p., an immunologic disorder characterized by radiologic evidence of infiltrates accompanied by either peripheral blood eosinophilia or histopathologic evidence of eosinophilic infiltrates in lung tissue. SYN eosinophilic pneumonopathy.

fibrous p., a process affecting pulmonary tissue and leading to deposition of collagen, either interstitially or in alveolar sacs.

Friedländer's p., a form of p. caused by infection with *Klebsiella pneumoniae* (Friedländer's bacillus), characteristically severe and lobar in distribution.

Friedländer's bacillus p., p. caused by *Klebsiella pneumoniae*, the Friedländer bacillus.

gangrenous p., gangrene of the lungs.

giant cell p., a rare complication of measles, with the postmortem finding of multinucleated giant cells lining alveoli. SYN Hecht's p., interstitial giant cell p.

Hecht's p., SYN giant cell p.

hypostatic p., p. resulting from infection developing in the dependent portions of the lungs due to decreased ventilation of those areas, with resulting failure to drain bronchial secretions; occurs primarily in the aged or those debilitated by disease who lie in the same position for long periods.

influenzal p., (1) p. complicating influenza; (2) p. due to *Haemophilus influenzae.*

influenzal virus p., serious, often fatal form of p. caused by a virus of the influenzal type. Occurs in epidemics and pandemics.

p. interlobula′ris purulen′ta, p. in which the lobules of the lung are separated by collections of purulent exudate. SYN p. dissecans.

interstitial giant cell p., SYN giant cell p.

interstitial plasma cell p., SYN *Pneumocystis carinii* p.

intrauterine p., fetal p. contracted *in utero* and manifesting itself in the early neonatal period.

lipid p., lipoid p., pulmonary condition marked by inflammatory and fibrotic changes in the lungs due to the inhalation of various oily or fatty substances, particularly liquid petrolatum, or resulting from accumulation in the lungs of endogenous lipid material, either cholesterol from obstructive pneumonitis or following fracture of a bone; phagocytes containing lipid are usually present. SYN oil p.

lobar p., p. affecting one or more lobes, or part of a lobe, of the lung in which the consolidation is virtually homogeneous; commonly due to infection by *Streptococcus pneumoniae;* sputum is scanty and usually of a rusty tint from altered blood.

lymphocytic interstitial p. (LIP), SYN lymphocytic interstitial *pneumonitis.*

lymphoid interstitial p. (LIP), SYN lymphocytic interstitial *pneumonitis.*

p. malleosa (ma-lē′ō-să), p. associated with glanders.

purulent p., p. caused by an organism that produces pus, implying that there can be destruction of lung tissue with permanent changes; usually sputum contains pus. *Staphylococci,* hemolytic *streptococci,* under *streptococcus,* and Friedländer's *bacillus* are typical causes, as opposed to *Streptococcus pneumoniae,* which is rarely a cause of purulent p.

metastatic p., a purulent inflammation in the lungs due to infected emboli.

migratory p., a form of p. in which successive areas of the lung are affected; may occur in bronchopulmonary aspergillosis. SYN wandering p.

moniliasis p., p. due to species of *Candida,* usually *C. albicans.*

mycoplasmal p., SYN primary atypical p.

mycoplasma p. of pigs, a worldwide chronic p. usually involving only the anterior lobes; it seldom causes death but is responsible for much unthriftiness; it is caused by the bacterium *Mycoplasma hyopneumoniae.* SYN virus p. of pigs.

obstructive p., infection of lung resulting from obstruction of airway, by narrowing resulting from previous disease process, persistent bronchospasm, thick secretions or by aspiration of a foreign body.

oil p., SYN lipid p.

organized p., unresolved p. in which fibrous tissue forms in the alveoli.

ovine progressive pneumonia, SYN maedi.

Pittsburgh p., a variant of Legionnaires' disease caused by *Legionella midadei.*

plague p., SYN pneumonic *plague.*

pleuritic p., p. associated with inflammation of the overlying pleura. SYN pneumonopleuritis.

pneumococcal p., p. due to infection by *Streptococcus pneumoniae;* often of lobar distribution.

***Pneumocystis carinii* p. (PCP),** pneumonia resulting from infection with *Pneumocystis carinii,* frequently seen in the immunologically compromised, such as persons with AIDS, or steroid-treated individuals, the elderly, or premature or debilitated babies during their first three months. In AIDS patients the tissue damage is usually restricted to the pulmonary parenchyma, while in the infantile form of the disease the alveoli are filled with a honeycomb-like or foamy network of acidophilic material, apparently not fibrin and not stainable with silver, within which the organisms, individually or in aggregates, are enmeshed; throughout the alveolar walls and pulmonary sputa there is a diffuse infiltration of mononuclear inflammatory cells, chiefly plasma cells and macrophages, as well as a few lymphocytes. Patients may be only slightly febrile (or even afebrile), but are likely to be extremely weak, dyspneic, and cyanotic. This is a major cause of morbidity among patients with AIDS. SYN interstitial plasma cell p., pneumocystosis.

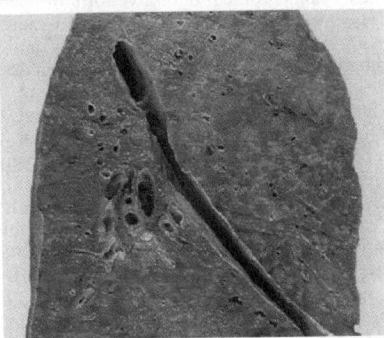

lobar pneumonia
note the numerous yellow-gray foci, unevenly distributed and varying in shape from acinous to lobular

postoperative p., p. following surgery due to viral or bacterial infection or pulmonary atelectasis.

primary atypical p., an acute systemic disease with involvement of the lungs, caused by *Mycoplasma pneumoniae* and marked by high fever, cough, relatively few physical signs, and scattered densities on x-rays; usually associated with development of cold agglutinins and antibodies to the bacteria. SYN atypical p., Eaton agent p., mycoplasmal p.

progressive p., a chronic progressive, viral disease of sheep and goats manifested as maedi or visna in different parts of the world. SEE maedi, visna.

rheumatic p., p. rarely occurring in severe acute rheumatic fever, even when the disease was common; consolidation occurs, the lungs being of a rubbery consistency, with fibrin exudate and small hemorrhages, as well as edema from left ventrical failure.

septic p., SYN suppurative p.

staphylococcal p., p., usually caused by *Staphylococcus aureus,* usually commencing as a bronchopneumonia, and frequently leading to suppuration and destruction of lung tissue.

streptococcal p., p. due to *Streptococcus pyogenes.*

suppurative p., any p. associated with the formation of pus and destruction of pulmonary tissue; abscess formation may occur. SYN septic p.

terminal p., p. occurring in the course of some other disease near its fatal termination.

traumatic p., SYN contusion p.

tularemic p., tularemia with pulmonary lesions.

typhoid p., p. complicating typhoid fever.

unresolved p., p. in which the alveolar exudate persists and eventually undergoes fibrosis.

uremic p., (1) SYN uremic *lung.* **(2)** terminal infective p. occurring in a patient with uremia.

usual interstitial p. of Liebow (UIP), a progressive inflammatory condition starting with diffuse alveolar damage and resulting in fibrosis and honeycombing over a variable time period; also a common feature of collagen-vascular diseases. SYN fibrosing alveolitis, Hamman-Rich syndrome, idiopathic interstitial fibrosis.

virus p. of pigs, SYN mycoplasma p. of pigs.

wandering p., SYN migratory p.

wool-sorter's p., SYN pulmonary *anthrax.*

pneu·mon·ic (nū-mon′ik). **1.** SYN pulmonary. **2.** Relating to pneumonia.

pneu·mo·ni·tis (nū-mō-nī′tis). Inflammation of the lungs. SEE ALSO pneumonia. SYN pulmonitis. [G. *pneumōn,* lung, + *-itis,* inflammation]

acute interstitial p., usually considered a form of hypersensitivity p.

feline p., an infectious respiratory illness of domesticated cats caused by the bacterium *Chlamydia psittaci.*

hypersensitivity p., chronic progressive form of pneumonia with wheezing, dyspnea, diffuse infiltrates seen on radiographs; occurs following exposure to any of a variety of antigens, sometimes occupational and many names are given to cases with known types of exposure (such as farmer's lung, maple bark stripper's lung, chicken plucker's lung, bagassosis, byssinosis, humidifier lung, etc.); biopsy findings usually showing patchy infiltration of alveolar walls with lymphocytes, plasma cells, and other inflammatory cells; can progress to irreversible interstitial fibrotic disease with restrictive pattern on pulmonary function, but in early disease most manifestations are reversible if offending antigen is identified and removed from environment.

lymphocytic interstitial p., a rare disease characterized by interstitial accumulation of lymphocytes in the lungs and late fibrosis; usually a result of a lymphoma, occasionally seen in AIDS, esp. in children. Sometimes seen as an autoimmune disorder. SYN lymphocytic interstitial pneumonia, lymphoid interstitial pneumonia , lymphoid interstitial pneumonia.

radiation p., the interstitial pneumonia and fibrosis that follow pulmonary irradiation at radiotherapeutic doses.

uremic p., SYN uremic *lung.*

♻ **pneumono-.** SEE pneumo-.

pneu·mo·no·cele (nū-mōn'ō-sēl). Protrusion of a portion of the lung through a defect in the chest wall. SYN pleurocele, pneumatocele (2), pneumocele.

pneu·mo·no·cen·te·sis (nū'mō-nō-sen-tē'sis). Rarely used term for paracentesis of the lung. SYN pneumocentesis. [G. *pneumōn,* lung, + *kentēsis,* puncture]

pneu·mo·no·coc·cal (nū'mō-nō-kok'ăl). Relating to or associated with *Streptococcus pneumoniae.*

pneu·mo·no·coc·cus (nū'mō-nō-kok'ŭs). SYN *Streptococcus pneumoniae.*

pneu·mo·no·co·ni·o·sis, pneu·mo·no·ko·ni·o·sis (nū'mō-nō-kō-nē-ō'sis). SYN pneumoconiosis.

pneu·mo·no·cyte (nū'mō-nō-sīt). Nonspecific term referring to cells lining alveoli in the respiratory part of the lung. [G. *pneumōn,* lung, + *kytos,* cell]

granular p.'s, SYN great alveolar *cells,* under *cell.*

phagocytic p., an alveolar phagocyte containing hemosiderin, carbon, or other foreign particles.

pneu·mo·no·ko·ni·o·sis. SEE pneumonoconiosis.

pneu·mo·no·mel·a·no·sis (nū'mō-nō-mel-ă-nō'sis). SYN pneumomelanosis.

pneu·mo·no·mon·i·li·a·sis (nū'mō-nō-mon-i-lī'ă-sis). Rarely used term for candidiasis of the lung.

pneu·mo·no·my·co·sis (nū'mō-nō-mī-kō'sis). SYN pneumomycosis.

pneu·mo·nop·a·thy (nū'mō-nop'ă-thē). Disease of the lung.

eosinophilic p., SYN eosinophilic *pneumonia.*

pneu·mo·no·pexy (nū'mō-nō-pek-sē). Fixation of the lung by suturing the costal and pulmonary pleurae or otherwise causing adhesion of the two layers. SYN pneumopexy. [G. *pneumōn,* lung, + *pēxis,* fixation]

pneu·mo·no·pleur·i·tis (nūmō'nō-plū- rī'tis). SYN pleuritic *pneumonia.*

pneu·mo·nor·rha·phy (nū-mō-nōr'ă-fē). Suture of the lung. [G. *pneumōn,* lung, + *rhaphē,* suture]

pneu·mo·not·o·my (nū-mō-not'ō-mē). Incision of the lung. SYN pneumotomy. [G. *pneumōn,* lung, + *tomē,* incision]

Pneu·mo·nys·sus si·mi·co·la (nū-mō-nis'ŭs si-mik'ō-lă). A small mite (family Halarachnidae) that causes pulmonary acariasis in monkeys. [pneumon- + G. *hyssos,* javelin; L. *simia,* ape, + *-cola,* inhabitant]

pneu·mo·or·bi·tog·ra·phy (nū'mō-ōr'bi-tog'ră-fē). Radiographic visualization of the orbital contents following injection of a gas, usually air.

pneu·mo·per·i·car·di·um (nū'mō-per-i-kar'dē-ŭm). Presence of gas in the pericardial sac. [G. *pneuma,* air, + pericardium]

pneu·mo·per·i·to·ne·um (nū'mō-per-i-tō-nē'ŭm). Presence of air or gas in the peritoneal cavity as a result of disease, or produced artificially in the abdomen to achieve exposure during laparoscopy and laparoscopic surgery for treatment of pulmonary or intestinal tuberculosis, bronchiectasis, tuberculous empyema, and certain other conditions. [G. *pneuma,* air, + peritoneum]

pneu·mo·per·i·to·ni·tis (nū'mō-per-i-tō-nī'tis). Inflammation of the peritoneum with an accumulation of gas in the peritoneal cavity. [G. *pneuma,* air, + peritonitis]

pneu·mo·pexy (nū'mō-pek-sē). SYN pneumonopexy.

pneu·mo·pha·gia (nū-mō-fā'jē-ă). SYN aerophagia.

pneu·mo·pleu·ri·tis (nū'mō-plū-ī'tis). Pleurisy with air or gas in the pleural cavity. [G. *pneuma,* air, + pleur- + *-itis,* inflammation]

pneu·mo·py·e·log·ra·phy (nū'mō-pī-ĕ-log'ră-fē). Radiography of the kidney after air or gas has been injected into the renal pelvis. [G. *pneuma,* air, + *pyelos,* pelvis, + *graphō,* to write]

pneu·mo·py·o·thor·ax (nū'mō-pī-ō-thōr'aks). SYN pyopneumothorax.

pneu·mo·ra·di·og·ra·phy (nu'mo-ra-dī-og'ră-fī). SYN pneumography (2).

pneu·mo·re·sec·tion (nū'mō-rē-sek'shŭn). Excision of part of a lung. [G. *pneumōn,* lung, + resection]

pneu·mo·ret·ro·per·i·to·ne·um (nū'mō-ret'rō-per-i-tō-nē'ŭm). Escape of air into the retroperitoneal tissues.

pneu·mo·roent·gen·og·ra·phy (nū'mō-rent'gĕ-nog'ră-fē). SYN pneumography (2).

pneu·mor·rha·chis (nū-mō-rā'kis, nū-mōr'ă-kis). The presence of gas in the spinal canal. SYN pneumatorrhachis. [G. *pneuma,* air, + *rhachis,* spinal column]

pneu·mo·scope (nū'mō-skōp). SYN pneumatoscope.

pneu·mo·ser·o·thor·ax (nū'mō-sēr-ō-thōr'aks). SYN hydropneumothorax.

pneu·mo·sil·i·co·sis (nū'mō-sil'i-kō'sis). SYN silicosis.

pneu·mo·tach·o·gram (nū-mō-tak'ō-gram). A recording of respired gas flow as a function of time, produced by a pneumotachograph. [G. *pneuma,* air, + *tachys,* swift, + *gramma,* something written]

pneu·mo·tach·o·graph (nū-mō-tak'ō-graf). An instrument for measuring the instantaneous flow of respiratory gases. SYN pneumotachometer.

Fleisch p., a p. that measures flow in terms of the proportional pressure drop across a resistance consisting of numerous capillary tubes in parallel.

Silverman-Lilly p., a p. that measures flow in terms of the proportional pressure drop across a resistance consisting of a very fine mesh screen.

pneu·mo·ta·chom·e·ter (nū'mō-tă-kom'ĕ-ter). SYN pneumotachograph. [G. *pneuma,* air, + *tachys,* swift, + *metron,* measure]

pneu·mo·ther·mo·mas·sage (nū-mō-ther'mō-mă-sahzh'). Application to the body of hot air under varying degrees of pressure. [G. *pneuma,* air, + *thermē,* heat, + Fr. *massage*]

pneu·mo·thor·ax (nū-mō-thōr'aks). The presence of air or gas in the pleural cavity. [G. *pneuma,* air, + thorax]

artificial p., p. produced by the injection of air, or a more slowly absorbed gas such as nitrogen, into the pleural space to collapse the lung.

extrapleural p., the presence of a gas between the endothoracic fascia-pleural layer and the adjacent chest wall.

open p., a free communication between the atmosphere and the pleural space either via the lung or through the chest wall. SYN sucking wound.

pressure p., SYN tension p.

p. sim'plex, p., without known cause, in an otherwise healthy person.

spontaneous p., p. occurring secondary to parenchymal lung disease, usually from an emphysematous bulla which ruptures or occasionally from a lung abscess.

tension p., a variety of spontaneous p. in which air enters the pleural cavity and is trapped during expiration; intrathoracic pressure builds to values higher than atmospheric pressure, compresses the lung, and may displace the mediastinum and its structures toward the opposite side, with consequent disadvantageous effects on blood flow. SYN pressure p., valvular p.

therapeutic p., p. designed to create some pulmonary parenchymal collapse, diaphragmatic immobilization, or both.

valvular p., SYN tension p.

pneu·mot·o·my (nū-mot′ō-mē). SYN pneumonotomy.

pneu·mo·ven·tri·cle (nū-mō-ven′tri-kl). Air in the ventricular system of the brain; occurs as a complication of a fracture of the skull which passes through the accessory nasal sinuses.

Pneu·mo·vi·rus (nū′mō-vī′rŭs). A genus of viruses (family Paramyxoviridae) including respiratory syncytial virus, which causes severe lower respiratory tract disease in infants. Nucleocapsids are 12 to 15 nm in diameter and thus intermediate in size between other Paramyxoviridae and the Orthomyxoviridae; cytoplasmic inclusions are considerably more dense than those of other viruses in the family.

pneu·sis (nū′sis). SYN breathing. [G. *pneō,* to breathe]

pni·go·pho·bia (nī-gō-fō′bē-ă). Morbid fear of choking. [G. *pnigos,* choking, + *phobos,* fear]

PNMT Abbreviation for phenylethanolamine *N-methyltransferase.*

PNP Abbreviation for psychogenic nocturnal *polydipsia.*

PNPB Abbreviation for positive-negative pressure *breathing.*

Po Symbol for polonium.

pock (pok). The specific pustular cutaneous lesion of smallpox. [A.S. *poc,* a pustule]

pock·et (pok′et). **1.** A cul-de-sac or pouchlike cavity. **2.** A diseased gingival attachment; a space between the inflamed gum and the surface of a tooth, limited apically by an epithelial attachment. **3.** To enclose within a confined space, as the stump of the pedicle of an ovarian or other abdominal tumor between the lips of the external wound. **4.** A collection of pus in a nearly closed sac. **5.** To approach the surface at a localized spot, as with the thinned out wall of an abscess which is about to rupture. [Fr. *pochette*]

gingival p., a diseased gingival attachment in which the increased depth of the sulcus is due to an increase in the bulk of its gingival wall.

infrabony p., intrabony p., SYN subcrestal p.

periodontal p., a pathologic deepening of the gingival sulcus resulting from detachment of the gingiva from the tooth.

Rathke's p., SYN pituitary *diverticulum.*

Seessel's p., the part of the embryonic foregut extending cephalad to the level of the oral plate and caudal to the pituitary diverticulum (Rathke's pouch). SYN preoral gut.

subcrestal p., a p. extending apically below the level of the adjacent alveolar crest. SYN infrabony p., intrabony p.

Tröltsch's p.'s, SYN anterior *recess* of tympanic membrane, posterior *recess* of tympanic membrane.

pock·mark (pok′mark). The small depressed scar left after the healing of the smallpox pustule.

po·cu·lum (pok′yū-lŭm). SYN cup (1). [L.]

p. diog′enis, SYN *cup* of palm.

△**pod-, podo-.** Foot, foot-shaped. Cf. ped-. [G. *pous, podos*]

po·dag·ra (pō-dag′ră). Severe pain in the foot, especially that of typical gout in the great toe. [G. fr. *pous,* foot, + *agra,* a seizure]

po·dag·ral, po·dag·ric, po·dag·rous (pod′ă-grăl, pō-dag′rik, pod′ă-grŭs). Relating to or characterized by podagra.

po·dal·gia (pō-dal′jē-ă). Pain in the foot. SYN pododynia, tarsalgia. [pod- + G. *algos,* pain]

po·dal·ic (pō-dal′ik). Relating to the foot. [G. *pous* (*pod*-), foot]

pod·ar·thri·tis (pod-ar-thrī′tis). Inflammation of any of the tarsal or metatarsal joints. [pod- + arthritis]

pod·e·de·ma (pod-e-dē′mă). Edema of the feet and ankles.

po·di·a·tric (pō-dī′ă-trik). Relating to podiatry.

po·di·a·trist (pō-dī′ă-trist). A practitioner of podiatry. SYN chiropodist, podologist. [pod- + G. *iatros,* physician]

po·di·a·try (pō-dī′ă-trē). The specialty concerned with the diagnosis and/or medical, surgical, mechanical, physical, and adjunctive treatment of the diseases, injuries, and defects of the human foot. SYN chiropody, podiatric medicine, podology. [pod- + G. *iatreia,* medical treatment]

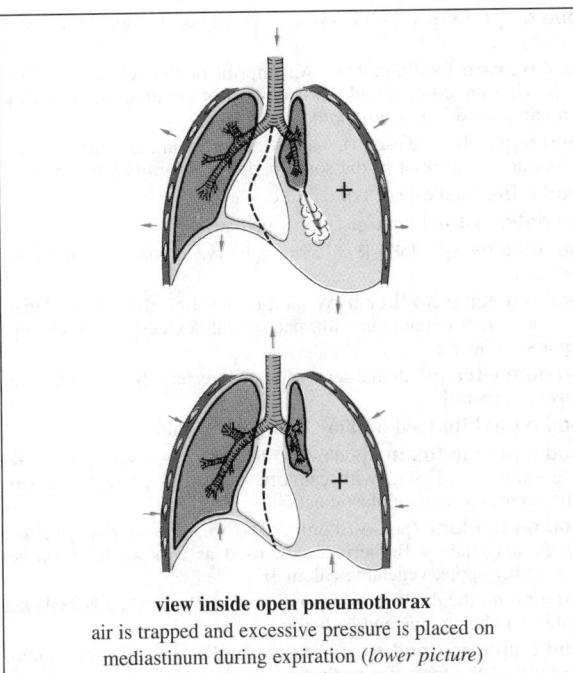

view inside open pneumothorax
air is trapped and excessive pressure is placed on mediastinum during expiration (*lower picture*)

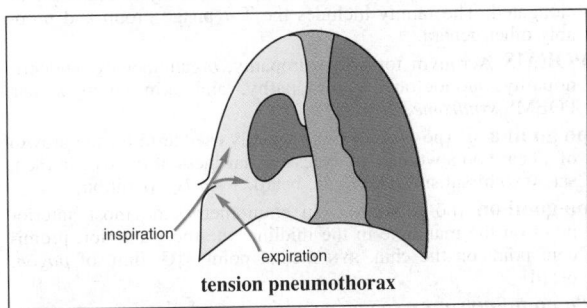

tension pneumothorax

po·dis·mus (pō-diz′mŭs). SYN podospasm.

po·di·tis (pō-dī′tis). An inflammatory disorder of the foot. [pod- + G. *-itis,* inflammation]

tourniquet p., postischemic acute inflammatory edema in the foot (or paw), as the result of complete obstruction of the circulation to that member by use of a tourniquet; produced experimentally in animals as a means of evaluating the anti-inflammatory efficacy of drugs.

△**podo-.** SEE pod-.

pod·o·bro·mi·dro·sis (pod′ō-brō-mi-drō′sis). Foul-smelling perspiration of the feet. [podo- + G. *brōmos,* a foul smell, + *hidrōs,* sweat]

pod·o·cyte (pod′ō-sīt). An epithelial cell of the visceral layer of Bowman's capsule in the renal corpuscle, attached to the outer surface of the glomerular capillary basement membrane by cytoplasmic foot processes (pedicels); believed to play a role in the ultrafiltration of blood. [podo- + G. *kytos,* a hollow (cell)]

pod·o·derm (pod′ō-derm). The corium of the foot; that portion of the skin which lies under the hoof and secretes the horny structure. The regions of the p. are the periople (corium limbi), coronary band (corium coronae), wall (corium parietis), and sole (corium solae). SYN corium ungulae. [podo- + G. *derma,* skin]

pod·o·der·ma·ti·tis (pod′ō-der-mă-tī′tis). Inflammation of the pododerm. SEE ALSO laminitis (2).

pod·o·dy·na·mom·e·ter (pod′ō-dī′nă-mom′ĕ-ter). An instrument for measuring the strength of the muscles of the foot or leg. [podo- + G. *dynamis,* force, + *metron,* measure]

po

pod·o·dyn·ia (pod-ō-din′ē-ă). SYN podalgia. [podo- + G. *odynē*, pain]

pod·o·gram (pod′ō-gram). An imprint of the sole of the foot, showing the contour and the condition of the arch, or an outline tracing. [podo- + G. *gramma*, written]

pod·o·graph (pod′ō-graf). A device for taking an outline at the foot and an imprint of the sole. [podo- + G. *graphō*, to write]

pod·o·lite (pod′ō-līt). SYN dahllite.

po·dol·o·gist (pō-dol′ō-jist). SYN podiatrist.

po·dol·o·gy (pō-dol′ō-jē). SYN podiatry. [podo- + G. *logos*, study]

pod·o·mech·a·no·ther·a·py (pod-ō-mek′ă-nō-thār′ă-pē). Treatment of foot conditions with mechanical devices; *e.g.*, arch supports, orthoses.

po·dom·e·ter (pō-dom′ĕ-ter). SYN pedometer. [podo- + G. *metron*, measure]

pod·o·phyl·lin (pod-ō-fil′in). SYN podophyllum *resin*.

pod·o·phyl·lo·tox·in (pod′ō-fil-ō-tok′sin). A toxic polycyclic substance, $C_{22}H_{22}O_8$, with cathartic properties present in podophyllum; has antineoplastic action.

pod·o·phyl·lum (pod-ō-fil′ŭm). The rhizome of *Podophyllum peltatum* (family Berberidaceae), used as a powerful laxative. SYN May apple, vegetable calomel.

Indian p., the dried rhizome and roots of *P. emodi*, a Himalayan plant; a cholagogue and cathartic.

pod·o·spasm, pod·o·spas·mus (pod′ō-spazm, -spaz-mŭs). Spasm of the foot. SYN podismus. [podo- + G. *spasmos*, spasm]

Po·do·vir·i·dae (po-dō-vir′i-dē). Provisional name for a family of bacterial viruses with short tails and genomes of double-stranded DNA (MW 12 to 73 × 10⁶); heads may be isometric or elongated. The family includes the T-7 phage group and probably other genera.

POEMS Acronym for *p*olyneuropathy, *o*rganomegaly, *e*ndocrinopathy, *m*onoclonal gammopathy, and *s*kin changes. SEE POEMS *syndrome*.

po·go·ni·a·sis (pō-gō-nī′ă-sis). A rarely used term for the growth of a beard on a woman, or excessive hairiness of the face in men. SEE ALSO hirsutism. [G. *pōgōn*, beard, + *-iasis*, condition]

po·go·ni·on (pō-gō′ni-on). In craniometry, the most anterior point on the mandible in the midline; the most anterior, prominent point on the chin. SYN mental point. [G. dim. of *pōgōn*, beard]

Po·go·no·myr·mex (pō-gō′nō-mir′meks, -mer′meks). A genus of ants that attack humans and small animals. SYN harvester ant. [G. *pōgōn*, beard, + *myrmex*, ant]

pOH. The negative logarithm of the OH⁻ concentration (in moles per liter).

△-poiesis. Production; producing. [G. *poiēsis*, a making]

poi·e·tin. Suffix used with words to indicate a stimulatory effect on growth or multiplication of cells, such as erythropoietin, etc. [G. *poietēs*, maker, + *-in*]

△poikilo-. Irregular, varied. [G. *poikilos*, many colored, varied]

poi·ki·lo·blast (poy′ki-lō-blast). A nucleated red blood cell of irregular shape. [poikilo- + G. *blastos*, germ]

poi·ki·lo·cyte (poy′ki-lō-sīt). A red blood cell of irregular shape. [poikilo- + G. *kytos*, cell]

poi·ki·lo·cy·the·mia (poy′ki-lō-sī-thē′mē-ă). SYN poikilocytosis. [poikilocyte + G. *haima*, blood]

poi·ki·lo·cy·to·sis (poy′ki-lō-sī-tō′sis). The presence of poikilocytes in the peripheral blood. SYN poikilocythemia. [poikilocyte + G. *-osis*, condition]

poi·ki·lo·den·to·sis (poy′ki-lō-den-tō′sis). Hypoplastic defects or mottling of enamel due to excessive fluoride in the water supply. [poikilo- + L. *dens*, tooth, + G. *-osis*, condition]

poi·ki·lo·der·ma (poy′ki-lō-der′mă). A variegated hyperpigmentation and telangiectasia of the skin, followed by atrophy. [poikilo- + G. *derma*, skin]

p. atroph′icans and cataract, SYN Rothmund's *syndrome*.

p. atroph′icans vascula′re, a rare condition that simulates chronic radiodermatitis in appearance; may eventuate as mycosis fungoides. SYN parakeratosis variegata, parapsoriasis lichenoides.

p. of Civatte, reticulated pigmentation and telangiectasia of the sides of the cheeks and neck; common in middle-aged women. SYN Civatte's disease.

p. congenita′le, SYN Rothmund's *syndrome*.

poi·ki·lo·therm (poy′ki-lō-therm). A poikilothermic animal. SYN allotherm, cold-blooded animal.

poi·ki·lo·ther·mic, poi·ki·lo·ther·mal, poi·ki·lo·ther·mous (poy′ki-lō-ther′mic, -măl, -mŭs). **1.** Varying in temperature according to the temperature of the surrounding medium; denoting the so-called cold-blooded animals, such as the reptiles and amphibians, and the plants. **2.** Capable of existence and growth in mediums of varying temperatures. Cf. heterothermic, homeothermic. SYN cold-blooded, hematocryal. [poikilo- + G. *thermē*, heat]

poi·ki·lo·ther·my, poi·ki·lo·ther·mism (poy′ki-lō-ther′mē, -therm′izm). The condition of plants and cold-blooded animals, the temperature of which varies with the changes in the temperature of the surrounding medium. [poikilo- + G. *thermē*, heat]

poi·ki·lo·throm·bo·cyte (poy′ki-lō-throm′bō-sīt). A blood platelet of abnormal shape. [poikilo- + G. *thrombos*, clot, + *kytos*, cell]

poi·ki·lo·thy·mia (poy′ki-lō-thī′mē-ă). A mental state marked by abnormal variations in mood. [poikilo- + G. *thymos*, mind]

POINT

point (poynt). **1.** SYN punctum. **2.** A sharp end or apex. **3.** A slight projection. **4.** A stage or condition reached, as the boiling p. **5.** To become ready to open, said of an abscess or boil the wall of which is becoming thin and is about to break. [Fr.; L. *punctum*, fr. *pungo*, pp. *punctus*, to pierce]

p. A, SYN subspinale.

absorbent p.'s, cones of paper or paper products used for drying or maintaining medicaments during root canal therapy.

alveolar p., SYN prosthion.

anterior focal p., the p. where parallel rays from the retina are focused.

apophysary p., apophysial p., (1) SYN subnasal p. **(2)** SYN Trousseau's p.

auricular p., SYN auriculare.

axial p., SYN nodal p.

p. B, SYN supramentale.

boiling p. (b.p.), the temperature at which the vapor pressure of a liquid equals the ambient atmospheric pressure.

Cannon's p., the location in the mid-transverse colon at which innervation by superior and inferior mesenteric plexuses overlap at the junction of the primitive midgut and hindgut, frequently resulting in narrowing evident on barium enema. SEE Cannon's *ring*. SYN Cannon's ring.

Capuron's p.'s, the iliopubic eminences and the sacroiliac joints, constituting four fixed p.'s in the pelvic inlet.

cardinal p.'s, (1) the four p.'s in the pelvic inlet toward one of which the occiput of the baby is usually directed in case of head presentation: two sacroiliac articulations and the two iliopectineal eminences corresponding to the acetabula; **(2)** six p.'s of a compound optical system: the anterior focal p., the posterior focal p., the two principal p.'s, and the two nodal p.'s.

central-bearing p., the contact p. of a central-bearing device.

Clado's p., a p. at the junction of the interspinous and right semilunar lines, at the lateral border of the rectus abdominis muscle, where marked tenderness on pressure is felt in some cases of appendicitis.

cold-rigor p., the degree of lowered temperature at which the activity of a cell ceases and the cell passes into the narcotic or hibernating state.

congruent p.'s, the p. in each retina referred to the same external stimulus.

conjugate p., a p. so related to another that an object at one is imaged at the other.

contact p., SYN contact *area.*

p.'s of convergence, SEE convergence.

craniometric p.'s, fixed p.'s on the skull used as landmarks in craniometry.

critical p., a p. at which two phases become identical; thus, at a given critical temperature and critical pressure, the liquid and gaseous state of a particular substance can no longer be differentiated.

dew p., the temperature at and below which moisture will condense for a specific humidity.

p. of elbow, SYN olecranon.

end p., the completion of a reaction; usually evident by the first perceptible alteration of the color of an added indicator.

equivalence p., SYN equivalence *zone.*

far p., that p. in conjugate focus with the retina when the eye is not accommodating. SYN punctum remotum.

p. of fixation, the p. on the retina at which the rays coming from an object regarded directly are focused. SYN p. of regard.

flash p., the lowest temperature at which vapors of a liquid may be ignited by a flame.

focal p., SEE anterior focal p., posterior focal p.

freezing p., the temperature at which a liquid solidifies.

fusing p., SEE fusion *temperature* (wire method).

Guéneau de Mussy's p., a p., painful on pressure, at the junction of a line prolonging the left border of the sternum and a horizontal line at the level of the end of the bony portion of the tenth rib; it is present in cases of diaphragmatic pleurisy.

gutta-percha p.'s, cones of a gutta percha compound used for filling root canals in conjunction with a cement, paste, or plastic.

Hallé's p., a p. at the intersection of a horizontal line touching the anterior superior spine of the ilium and a perpendicular line drawn from the spine of the pubis; here the ureter can be most readily palpated.

heat-rigor p., the degree of elevated temperature at which coagulation of protoplasm occurs with death of the cell.

incident p., the p. at which a light ray enters an optical system.

incisal p., the p. located between the incisal edges of the lower central incisors; the graphic projection of the excursions of the incisal p. in certain planes is generally used to illustrate the envelope of motion of mandibular movement.

isoelectric p. (I.P., i.p., pI), the pH at which an amphoteric substance, such as protein or an amino acid, is electrically neutral.

isoionic p., the pH at which a zwitterion has an equal number of positive and negative charges; in water and in the absence of other solutes, this is the isoelectric p.

isosbestic p., in applied spectroscopy, a wavelength at which absorbance of two substances, one of which can be converted into the other, is the same.

J p., the p. marking the end of the QRS complex and the beginning of the S or T wave in the electrocardiogram. SYN ST junction.

jugal p., SYN jugale.

lower alveolar p., SYN infradentale.

malar p., apex of the tuberosity of the zygomatic (malar) bone.

p. of maximal impulse, the p. on the chest wall at which the maximal cardiac impulse is seen and/or felt.

maximum occipital p., the p. on the squama of the occipital bone farthest from the glabella.

Mayo-Robson's p., a p. just above and to the right of the umbilicus, where tenderness on pressure exists in disease of the pancreas.

McBurney's p., a p. between 1½ and 2 inches superomedial to the anterior superior spine of the ilium, on a straight line joining that process and the umbilicus, where pressure elicits tenderness in acute appendicitis.

median mandibular p., a p. on the anteroposterior center of the mandibular ridge in the median sagittal plane.

melting p. (m.p., IEP, T_m), (1) the temperature at which a solid becomes a liquid; **(2)** the temperature at which 50% of a macromolecule becomes denatured.

mental p., SYN pogonion.

metopic p., SYN metopion.

motor p., a p. on the skin where the application of an electrical stimulus, via an electrode, will cause the contraction of an underlying muscle.

Munro's p., a p. at the right edge of the rectus abdominis muscle, between the umbilicus and the anterior superior spine of the ilium, where pressure elicits tenderness in appendicitis.

nasal p., SYN nasion.

near p., that p. in conjugate focus with the retina when the eye exerts maximal accommodation. SYN punctum proximum.

neutral p., the p. at which a solution is neither acid nor alkaline (pH 7 at 22°C for aqueous solutions).

nodal p., one of two p.'s in a compound optical system so related that a ray directed toward the first p. will appear to have passed through the second p. parallel to its original direction. SYN axial p.

occipital p., the most prominent posterior p. on the occipital bone above the inion.

p. of ossification, SYN *center* of ossification.

painful p., SEE Valleix's p.'s.

posterior focal p., the p. of a compound optical system where parallel rays entering the system are focused.

power p., in dentistry, the vertical dimension at which the greatest masticatory force may be registered.

preauricular p., a p. of the posterior root of the zygomatic arch lying immediately in front of the upper end of the tragus.

pressure p., a cutaneous locus having pressure-sensitive elements which when compressed, pressure is appreciated.

primary p. of ossification, SYN primary *center* of ossification.

principal p., one of two p.'s on an optic axis so related that an object at one is exactly imaged at the other without magnification, minification, or inversion.

p. of proximal contact, SYN contact *area.*

p. of regard, SYN p. of fixation.

retention p., a provision made within a cavity preparation of a tooth to hold in place the first pieces of gold when placing a direct gold restoration.

secondary p. of ossification, SYN secondary *center* of ossification.

silver p., a solid core cone of silver used in filling root canals in conjunction with a cement or paste.

spinal p., SYN subnasal p.

subnasal p., the center of the root of the anterior nasal spine. SYN apophysary p. (1), apophysial p., spinal p.

Sudeck's critical p., region in the colon between the supply of the sigmoid arteries and that of the superior rectal artery.

supra-auricular p., a craniometric p. on the posterior root of the zygomatic process of the temporal bone directly above the auricular p.

supranasal p., SYN ophryon.

supraorbital p., SYN ophryon.

sylvian p., the nearest p. on the skull to the lateral (sylvian) fissure, about 30 mm behind the zygomatic process of the frontal bone.

tender p.'s, SYN Valleix's p.'s.

trigger p., a specific p. or area where, if stimulated by touch, pain, or pressure, a painful response will be induced. SYN dolorogenic zone, trigger area, trigger zone.

triple p., the temperature at which all three phases (*i.e.,* solid, liquid, and gas) are in equilibrium; the triple p. of water (273.16 K) is a fundamental fixed point in temperature scales.

Trousseau's p., a painful p., in neuralgia, at the spinous process of the vertebra below which arises the offending nerve. SYN apophysary p. (2), apophysial p.

Valleix's p.'s, various p.'s in the course of a nerve, pressure upon which is painful in cases of neuralgia; these p.'s are: 1) where the nerve emerges from the bony canal; 2) where it pierces a muscle or aponeurosis to reach the skin; 3) where a superficial nerve rests upon a resisting surface where compression is easily made; 4) where the nerve gives off one or more branches; and 5) where the nerve terminates in the skin. SYN tender p.'s.

Weber's p., a p. situated 1 cm below the promontory of the sacrum; believed by Weber to represent the center of gravity of the body.

zygomaxillary p., SYN zygomaxillare.

---

poin·til·lage (pwan-tē-yazh′). A massage manipulation with the tips of the fingers. [Fr. dotting, stippling]

point·ing (poynt′ing). Preparing to open spontaneously, said of an abscess or a boil.

point source. In photometry, a very small source of light which is regarded as a geometrical point from which light emanates in straight lines in all directions.

Poirier, Paul J., French surgeon, 1853–1907. SEE P.'s *gland, line.*

poise (poyz, pwahz). In the CGS system, the unit of viscosity equal to 1 dyne-second per square centimeter and to 0.1 pascal-second. [J. *Poiseuille*]

Poiseuille, Jean Léonard Marie, French physiologist and physicist, 1797–1869. SEE poise; P.'s viscosity *coefficient, law, space.*

poi·son (poy′zŭn). Any substance, either taken internally or applied externally, that is injurious to health or dangerous to life. [Fr., fr. L. *potio,* potion, draught]

acrid p., a p. that causes a destructive local irritation as well as systemic effects.

arrow p., (1) SYN curare. **(2)** any natural toxin used for coating arrows, spears, and darts (*e.g.,* extracts containing aconitin, ouabain, cardiac glycosides, batrachotoxin, curare, etc.).

fish p., (1) SYN ichthyotoxicon. **(2)** SYN fugu p.

fugu p. (fū′gū), a p. in the roe and other parts of various species of *Diodon, Triodon,* and *Tetradon,* fishes of eastern Asiatic waters. SYN fish p. (2). [Jap. *fugu,* a poisonous fish]

respiratory p., SYN respiratory *inhibitor.*

poi·son·ing (poy′zŏn-ing). **1.** The administering of poison. **2.** The state of being poisoned. SYN intoxication (1).

ackee p., an acute and frequently fatal vomiting disease associated with central nervous system symptoms and marked hypoglycemia, caused by eating unripe ackee fruit of *Blighia spaida,* a tree common in Jamaica. SYN Jamaican vomiting sickness.

bacterial food p., a term commonly used to refer to conditions limited to enteritis or gastroenteritis (excluding the enteric fevers and the dysenteries) caused by bacterial multiplication per se or by a soluble bacterial exotoxin.

blister beetle p., p., most often of horses, by ingestion of blister beetles (*Epicauta* spp.) in hay; the causative toxin is cantharidin, which produces salivation, shock, pollakiuria, and colic.

blood p., SEE septicemia, pyemia.

bracken p., SYN enzootic *hematuria.*

carbon disulfide p., acute or chronic intoxication by CS_2, an industrial condition encountered among rubber workers and makers of artificial silk (rayon) by the viscose process; characterized by insomnia, listlessness, and irritability, followed by paralyses, impaired vision, peptic ulcer, and psychoses.

carbon monoxide p., a potentially fatal acute or chronic intoxication caused by inhalation of carbon monoxide gas which competes favorably with oxygen for binding with hemoglobin (carboxyhemoglobinemia) and thus interferes with the transportation of oxygen and carbon dioxide by the blood.

chocolate p., p., most commonly of dogs, by ingestion of excessive quantities of chocolate (especially unsweetened baker's chocolate); the causative toxin is theobromine which produces thirst, vomiting, diarrhea, urinary incontinence, chronic muscle spasms, seizures, and coma.

clay pigeon p., SYN pitch p.

crotalaria p., p. of humans and animals with alkaloids of the plants *Senecio* (ragwort), *Crotalaria* (rattlebox), and *Helio-*

tropum; produces a veno-occlusive disease of the liver similar to Chiari's disease. SYN crotalism.

cyanide p., a fairly common disease of herbivorous animals, caused by eating cyanogenic plants containing glucosides which are hydrolyzed, yielding hydrocyanic acid; some farm chemicals, such as fungicides or insecticides, may be causes of cyanide p.; hydrogen cyanide and its salts are extremely poisonous to humans, either by inhalation or by ingestion.

Datura p., p. resulting from ingestion of plants of the genus *Datura;* symptoms are parasympatholytic in nature and in severe p. include central nervous system depression, circulatory failure, and respiratory depression.

djenkol p., p. believed to result from eating excessive amounts of a bean, *Pitecolobium lobatum;* symptoms are pain in the renal region, dysuria, and later anuria; the djenkol bean has a high vitamin B content and is used for food despite its toxic qualities.

ergot p., a syndrome brought on by the consumption of bread (notably rye) contaminated by the ergot fungus, *Claviceps purpurea* (rye smut), the source of numerous ergot alkaloids. The effects observed include peripheral vascular constriction leading to gangrene, partial paralysis with numbing, tingling and burning in the limbs, feeble pulse, restlessness, stupor or delirium. Can prove fatal.

fescue p., SYN fescue *foot.*

food p., poisoning in which the active agent is contained in ingested food.

lead p., acute or chronic intoxication by lead or any of its salts; symptoms of **acute lead p.** usually are those of acute gastroenteritis in adults or encephalopathy in children; **chronic lead p.** is manifested chiefly by anemia, constipation, colicky abdominal pain, neuropathy with paralysis with wrist-drop involving the extensor muscles of the forearm, bluish lead line of the gums, and interstitial nephritis; saturnine gout, convulsions, and coma may occur. SYN plumbism, saturnism.

lecheguilla p., a plant toxemia of sheep and goats in western Texas, southeastern New Mexico, and northern Mexico caused by eating *Agave lecheguilla;* there is liver damage resulting in icterus, sometimes hemoglobinuria, and often death, and photosensitivity with edema, swelling, and crusting of the face and ears. SYN swellhead (1).

mercury p., a disease usually caused by the ingestion of mercury or mercury compounds, which are toxic in relation to their ability to produce mercuric ions; usually **acute mercury p.** is associated with ulcerations of the stomach and intestine and toxic changes in the renal tubules; anuria and anemia may occur; usually **chronic mercury p.** is a result of industrial p. and causes gastrointestinal or central nervous system manifestations including stomatitis, diarrhea, ataxia, tremor, hyperreflexia, sensorineural impairment, and emotional instability (Mad Hatter syndrome). SYN hydrargyria, hydrargyrism, mercurialism.

mushroom p., SEE mycetism.

oxygen p., SYN oxygen *toxicity.*

pitch p., a highly fatal disease of swine, usually caused by the ingestion of fragments of the clay pigeons used as targets by shooting clubs; some cases have been caused by consumption of other bituminous substances, such as road tar and tar paper. SYN clay pigeon p.

radiation p., SYN radiation *sickness.*

salmon p., a disease of dogs and other canids in the northwest coastal region of the U.S., resulting from eating infected salmon and trout from streams flowing into the Pacific Ocean; these fish carry the encysted form or metacercaria of *Nanophyetus salmincola,* which infects the intestine and carries with it *Neorickettsia helmintheca,* the actual agent of the disease. SYN salmon disease.

Salmonella food p., gastroenteritis caused by various strains of *Salmonella* that multiply freely in the gastrointestinal tract but do not produce septicemia; symptoms usually begin within 8 to 24 hours and include fever, headache, nausea, vomiting, diarrhea, and abdominal pain.

salt p., an often fatal disease of animals, especially pigs fed on garbage, resulting from the ingestion of excessive quantities of ordinary table salt, sodium chloride; this usually does not occur if the animals have access to sufficient quantities of fresh drinking water.

scombroid p., p. from ingestion of heat-stable toxins produced by bacterial action on inadequately preserved dark-meat fish of the order Scombroidea (tuna, bonito, mackerel, albacore, skipjack); characterized by epigastric pain, nausea and vomiting, headache, thirst, difficulty in swallowing, and urticaria.

selenium p., chronic p. of horses, cattle, and swine, caused by ingestion of grains and forage raised on soils high in selenium; it occurs only in arid regions, from eating certain plants which are selenium accumulators.

silver p., SYN argyria.

Staphylococcus food p., outbreaks commonly caused by staphylococcal enterotoxin and characterized by an abrupt onset of gastroenteritis within several hours after ingestion of the food contaminated with the preformed exotoxin; vomiting is usually more severe and diarrhea less severe than in infectious forms of bacterial food p.

sweet clover p., a hemorrhagic disease of herbivores, especially cattle, occurring as a result of consuming damaged hay or silage containing sweet clover, but never as a result of eating freshly cut plants or pasturing on sweet clover. The causative agent is the anticoagulant, dicumarol, which is formed in the spoilage process from the harmless coumarin.

systemic p., SYN toxicosis.

tetraethyl p., SEE tetraethyllead.

thallium p., a condition characterized by vomiting, diarrhea, leg pains, and severe sensorimotor polyneuropathy; about three weeks after p., temporary extensive loss of hair typically occurs; usually occurs after accidental ingestion of a rodenticide.

turpentine p., p. from oil of turpentine; symptoms include hematuria, albuminuria, and coma; the urine may have an odor of violets. SYN terebinthinism.

wheat pasture p., SYN grass *tetany*.

poi·son ivy, poi·son oak, poi·son su·mac. 1. SEE *Toxicodendron*. **2.** Common name for the cutaneous eruption (rhus dermatitis) caused by contact with these species of *Toxicodendron*.

poi·son·ous (poy′zŭn-ŭs). Characterized by, having the characteristics of, or containing a poison. SYN toxic (1), toxicant (1), toxiferous, venenous.

Poisson, Siméon Denis, French mathematician, 1781–1840. SEE P. *distribution;* P.-Pearson *formula.*

po·lar (pō′lăr). **1.** Relating to a pole. **2.** Having poles, said of certain nerve cells having one or more processes. [Mod. L. *polaris,* fr. *polus,* pole]

po·lar·im·e·ter (pō′lăr-im′ě-ter). An instrument for measuring the angle of rotation in polarization or the amount of polarized light. [Mod. L. *polaris,* polar, + G. *metron,* measure]

po·lar·im·e·try (pō′lăr-im′ě-trē). Measurement by polarimeter.

po·lar·i·scope (pō-lar′i-skōp). An instrument for studying the phenomena of the polarization of light. [Mod. L. *polaris,* polar, + G. *skopeō,* to examine]

po·lar·i·scop·ic (pō-lar-i-skop′ik). Relating to the polariscope or to polariscopy.

po·lar·is·co·py (pō′lă-ris′kŏ-pē). Use of the polariscope in studying properties of polarized light.

po·lar·i·ty (pō-lar′i-tē). **1.** The property of having two opposite poles, as that possessed by a magnet. **2.** The possession of opposite properties or characteristics. **3.** The direction or orientation of positivity relative to negativity. **4.** The direction along a polynucleotide chain, or any biopolymer, or macro-structure (*e.g.,* microtubules). [Mod. L. *polaris,* polar]

po·lar·i·za·tion (pō′lăr-i-zā′shŭn). **1.** In electricity, coating of an electrode with a thick layer of hydrogen bubbles, with the result that the flow of current is weakened or arrested. **2.** A change effected in a ray of light passing through certain media, whereby the transverse vibrations occur in one plane only, instead of in all planes as in an ordinary light ray. **3.** Development of differences in potential between two points in living tissues, as between the inside and outside of a cell wall.

po·lar·ize (pō′lăr-īz). To put into a state of polarization.

po·lar·iz·er (pō′lă-rīz′er). The first element of a polariscope that polarizes the light, as distinguished from the analyzer, the second polarizing element.

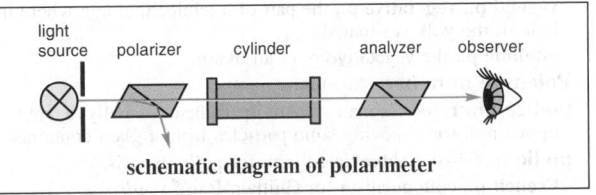

schematic diagram of polarimeter

po·lar·og·ra·phy (pō′lă-rog′ră-fē). That branch of electrochemistry concerned with the variation in current flowing through a solution as the voltage is varied; this will vary with the ionic concentration of reducible substances so that p. can be used in chemical analysis. P. is commonly employed in the form of a reduction at a dropping mercury electrode. [Mod. L. *polaris,* polar, + G. *graphō,* to write]

pol·dine meth·yl·sul·fate (pōl′dēn). 2-Benziloyloxymethyl-1,1-dimethylpyrrolidinium methylsulfate; an anticholinergic agent.

pole (pōl). **1.** One of the two points at the extremities of the axis of any organ or body. **2.** Either of the two points on a sphere at the greatest distance from the equator. **3.** One of the two points in a magnet or an electric battery or cell having extremes of opposite properties; the negative p. is a cathode, the positive p. an anode. SYN polus [NA]. [L. *polus,* the end of an axis, pole, fr. G. *polos*]

abapical p., in an ovum, the p. opposite the animal p. (*i.e.,* vegetal p.).

animal p., the point in a telolecithal egg opposite the yolk, where most of the protoplasm is concentrated and where the nucleus is located; from this region, the polar bodies are extruded during maturation. SYN germinal p.

anterior p. of eyeball, the center of the corneal curvature of the eye. SYN polus anterior bulbi oculi [NA].

anterior p. of lens, the central point on the anterior surface of the lens of the eye. SYN polus anterior lentis [NA].

cephalic p., the head end of the fetus.

frontal p., SYN frontal p. of cerebrum.

frontal p. of cerebrum, the most anterior promontory of each cerebral hemisphere. SYN polus frontalis cerebri [NA], frontal p.

germinal p., SYN animal p.

inferior p., for a structure having a vertically-oriented long axis, the point at the lower end of the axis, nearest the soles of the feet; the lowest point of a structure's surface. SEE inferior p. of kidney, inferior p. of testis. SYN extremitas inferior [NA], inferior extremity (1).

inferior p. of kidney, the inferior end of the kidney. SYN extremitas inferior renis [NA].

inferior p. of testis, the inferior end of the testis. SYN extremitas inferior testis [NA].

lateral p., SYN tubal *extremity* of ovary.

medial p. of ovary, SYN uterine *extremity* of ovary.

occipital p., SYN occipital p. of cerebrum.

occipital p. of cerebrum, the most posterior promontory of each cerebral hemisphere; the apex of the occipital lobe. SYN polus occipitalis cerebri [NA], occipital p.

pelvic p., the breech end of the fetus.

posterior p. of eyeball, the center of the posterior curvature of the eye. SYN polus posterior bulbi oculi [NA].

posterior p. of lens, the central point on the posterior surface of the lens. SYN polus posterior lentis [NA].

superior p. of kidney, the superior end of the kidney. SYN extremitas superior renis [NA].

superior p. of testis, the superior end of the testis. SYN extremitas superior testis [NA].

temporal p., SYN temporal p. of cerebrum.

temporal p. of cerebrum, the most prominent part of the anterior or extremity of the temporal lobe of each cerebral hemisphere, a short distance below the fissure of Sylvius. SYN polus temporalis cerebri [NA], temporal p.

po

vegetal p., vegetative p., the part of a telolecithal egg where the bulk of the yolk is situated.

vitelline p., the vegetative p. of an ovum.

Polenské num·ber. See under number.

po·lice·man (pō-lēs′man). An instrument, usually a rubber-tipped rod, for removing solid particles from a glass container.

po·lio (pō′lē-ō). Abbreviated term for poliomyelitis.

French p., colloquialism for Guillain-Barré *syndrome*.

⌂**polio-.** Gray; gray matter (substantia grisea). [G. *polios*]

po·li·o·clas·tic (pō′lē-ō-klas′tik). Destructive to gray matter of the nervous system. [polio- + G. *klastos*, broken]

po·li·o·dys·tro·phia (pō′lē-ō-dis-trō′fē-ă). SYN poliodystrophy.

p. cer′ebri progressi′va infanti′lis [MIM*203700], familial progressive spastic paresis of extremities with progressive mental deterioration, with development of seizures, blindness and deafness, beginning during the first year of life, and with destruction and disorganization of nerve cells of the cerebral cortex. SYN Alpers disease, Christensen-Krabbe disease, progressive cerebral poliodystrophy.

po·li·o·dys·tro·phy (pō′lē-ō-dis′trō-fē). Wasting of the gray matter of the nervous system. SYN poliodystrophia. [polio- + G. *dys-*, bad, + *trophē*, nourishment]

progressive cerebral p., SYN *poliodystrophia* cerebri progressiva infantilis.

po·li·o·en·ceph·a·li·tis (pō′lē-ō-en-sef′ă-lī′tis). Inflammation of the gray matter of the brain, either of the cortex or of the central nuclei; as contrasted to inflammation of the white matter. [polio- + G. *enkephalos*, brain, + *-tis*, inflammation]

p. infecti′va, SYN von Economo's *disease*.

inferior p., p. with predominantly bulbar paralysis.

superior p., p. with ophthalmoplegia.

superior hemorrhagic p., SYN Wernicke's *syndrome*.

po·li·o·en·ceph·a·lo·ma·la·cia (pō′lē-ō-en-sef′a-lō-ma-lā′shē-a). A noninfectious disease of ruminants characterized by a tissue-thiamine deficiency and by amaurosis and strabismus, followed by recumbency, opisthotonos, and convulsions. SYN cerebrocortical necrosis.

po·li·o·en·ceph·a·lo·me·nin·go·my·e·li·tis (pō′lē-ō-en-sef′ă-lō-mĕ-ning′gō-mī-ĕ-lī′tis). Inflammation of the gray matter of the brain and spinal cord and of the meningeal covering of the parts. [polio- + G. *enkephalos*, brain, + *mēninx*, membrane, + *myelon*, marrow, + *-itis*, inflammation]

po·li·o·en·ceph·a·lo·my·e·li·tis (pō′lē-ō-en-sef′ă-lō-mī′ĕ-lī′tis). SYN poliomyeloencephalitis.

feline p., a chronic disease of cats characterized by paraparesis and ataxia.

porcine p., SYN Teschen *disease*.

po·li·o·en·ceph·a·lop·a·thy (pō′lē-ō-en-sef′ă-lop′ă-thē). Any disease of the gray matter of the brain. [polio- + G. *enkephalos*, brain, + *pathos*, suffering]

po·li·o·my·el·en·ceph·a·li·tis (pō′lē-ō-mī′el-en-sef′ă-lī′tis). SYN poliomyeloencephalitis.

po·li·o·my·e·li·tis (pō′lē-ō-mī′ĕ-lī′tis). An inflammatory process involving the gray matter of the cord. [polio- + G. *myelos*, marrow, + *-itis*, inflammation]

acute anterior p., inflammation of the anterior cornua of the spinal cord; an acute infectious disease caused by the poliomyelitis virus and marked by fever, pains, and gastroenteric disturbances, followed by a flaccid paralysis of one or more muscular groups, and later by atrophy. SYN acute atrophic paralysis, myogenic paralysis.

acute bulbar p., poliomyelitis virus infection affecting nerve cells in the medulla oblongata and producing paralysis of the lower motor cranial nerves.

chronic anterior p., muscular atrophy of the upper extremities and neck, in which there are long intermissions of quiescence or improvement; not to be confused with poliomyelitis virus infections.

mouse p., SYN mouse *encephalomyelitis*.

po·li·o·my·e·lo·en·ceph·a·li·tis (pō′lē-ō-mī′ĕ-lō-en-sef′ă-lī′tis). Acute anterior poliomyelitis with pronounced cerebral signs. SYN

polioencephalomyelitis, poliomyelencephalitis. [polio- + G. *myelon*, marrow, + *enkephalos*, brain, + *-itis*, inflammation]

po·li·o·my·e·lop·a·thy (pō′lē-ō-mī′ĕ-lop′ă-thē). Any disease of the gray matter of the spinal cord. [polio- + G. *myelon*, marrow, + *pathos*, suffering]

po·li·o·sis (po-le-ō′sis). A patchy absence or lessening of melanin in hair of the scalp, brows, or lashes, due to lack of pigment in the epidermis; it occurs in several hereditary syndromes but may be caused by inflammation, irradiation, or infection such as herpes zoster. SYN trichopoliosis. [G., fr. *polios*, gray]

ciliary p., SYN piebald *eyelash*.

po·li·o·sis (pō-lē-ō′sis). SYN piebald *eyelash*.

po·li·o·vi·rus. SYN poliomyelitis *virus*.

po·li·o·vi·rus hom·i·nis (pō′lē-ō-vī′rŭs hom′i-nis). SYN poliomyelitis *virus*.

pol·ish·ing. In dentistry, the act or process of making a restoration smooth and glossy.

Politzer, Adam, Austrian otologist, 1835–1920. SEE P. *bag, method;* P.'s luminous *cone.*

pol·itz·er·i·za·tion (pol′it-zer-i-zā′shŭn). Inflation of the eustachian tube and middle ear by the Politzer method.

negative p., withdrawal of secretions from a cavity by suction, effected by attaching a compressed Politzer bag or rubber bulb to a tube inserted in the cavity.

pol·kis·sen of Zimmermann (pōl′kis-en). SYN extraglomerular *mesangium*. [Ger. *Polkissen*, pole + cushion]

poll (pōl). The occipital region of an animal, especially the horse; high point of the head between the ears.

pol·la·ki·dip·sia (pol′ă-ki-dip′sē-ă). Rarely used term for unduly frequent thirst. [G. *pollakis*, often, + *dipsa*, thirst]

pol·la·ki·u·ria (pol′ă-kē-yū′rē-ă). Rarely used term for extraordinary urinary frequency. [G. *pollakis*, often, + *ouron*, urine]

pol·len (pol′en). Microspores of seed plants carried by wind or insects prior to fertilization; important in the etiology of hay fever and other allergies. [L. fine dust, fine flour]

pol·le·no·sis (pol-ĕ-nō′sis). SYN pollinosis.

pol·lex, gen. **pol·li·cis,** pl. **pol·li·ces** (pol′eks, pol′i-sis, -sēz) [NA]. SYN thumb. [L.]

p. pe′dis, SYN hallux.

pol·li·ci·za·tion (pol′i-si-zā′shŭn). Construction of a substitute thumb. [L. *pollex*, thumb, + *-ize*, to make like, + *-ation*, state]

pol·li·no·sis (pol-i-nō′sis). Hay fever excited by the pollen of various plants. SYN pollenosis. [L. *pollen*, pollen, + G. *-osis*, condition]

pol·lo·dic (pŏ-lō′dik). SYN panodic. [G. *polloi*, many, + *hodos*, way]

pol·lu·tant (pŏ-lū′tănt). An undesired contaminant that results in pollution.

pol·lu·tion (pŏ-lū′shŭn). Rendering unclean or unsuitable by contact or mixture with an undesired contaminant. [L. *pollutio*, fr. *pol-luo*, pp. *-lutus*, to defile]

air p., contamination of air by smoke and harmful gases, mainly oxides of carbon, sulfur, and nitrogen, as from automobile exhausts, industrial emissions, burning rubbish, etc. SEE ALSO smog.

noise p., annoying or physiologically damaging environmental noise levels, as from automobile engines, industrial machinery, amplified music, etc.

po·lo·cyte (pō′lō-sīt). SYN polar *body*. [G. *polos*, pole, + *kytos*, cell]

po·lo·ni·um (Po) (pō-lō′nē-ŭm). A radioactive element, atomic no. 84, isolated from pitchblende; the longest-lived isotope is ^{209}Po (half-life 102 years); ^{210}Po is radium F (half-life 138.38 days), the only readily accessible isotope. [L. fr. *Polonia*, Poland, native country of Mme. Curie who with her husband discovered the substance]

pol·ox·a·lene (pŏl-ok′să-lēn). An oxyalkylene polymer, nonionic surface-active agent similar in actions and uses to dioctyl sodium sulfosuccinate; used in constipation due to hard dry stools. SYN poloxalkol.

pol·ox·al·kol (pŏl-ok′sal-kol). SYN poloxalene.

pol·ster (pōl'ster). A bulge of smooth muscle cells, as in the penile arteries and veins, formerly thought to regulate blood flow. [G. cushion, bolster]

po·lus, pl. **po·li** (pō'lŭs, -lī) [NA]. SYN pole. [L. pole]

p. ante'rior bul'bi oc'uli [NA], SYN anterior *pole* of eyeball.

p. ante'rior len'tis [NA], SYN anterior *pole* of lens.

p. fronta'lis cer'ebri [NA], SYN frontal *pole* of cerebrum.

po'li liena'lis infe'rior et supe'rior, SEE anterior *extremity,* posterior *extremity.*

p. occipita'lis cer'ebri [NA], SYN occipital *pole* of cerebrum.

p. poste'rior bul'bi oc'uli [NA], SYN posterior *pole* of eyeball.

p. poste'rior len'tis [NA], SYN posterior *pole* of lens.

poli rena'lis infe'rior et supe'rior, SEE superior *pole* of kidney, inferior *pole* of kidney.

p. tempora'lis cer'ebri [NA], SYN temporal *pole* of cerebrum.

poly (pol'ē). Abbreviated form and colloquialism for polymorphonuclear *leukocyte.*

⌂ **poly-. 1.** Prefix denoting many; multiplicity. Cf. multi-, pluri-. **2.** In chemistry, prefix meaning "polymer of," as in polypeptide, polysaccharide, polynucleotide; often used with symbols, as in poly(A) for poly(adenylic acid), poly(Lys) for poly(L-lysine). [G. *polys,* much, many]

Pólya, Jenö (Eugene), Hungarian surgeon, 1876–1944. SEE Pólya *gastrectomy;* P.'s *operation;* Reichel-P. stomach *resection.*

pol·y·(A) 1. Abbreviation for poly(adenylic acid). **2.** Iridoid indole alkaloid isolated from *Vinca* sp.; may have pharmacological applications; falling in this class are vinblastine and vincristine. **3.** Excretion of D-glyceric acid in the urine; found in renal calculi. **4.** An inborn error in metabolism resulting in D-glyceric aciduria (1). **5.** A class of basic antibiotic peptides, found in neutrophils, that apparently kill bacteria by causing membrane damage.

poly(A) polymerase, an enzyme that catalyzes the formation of a poly(adenylic acid) sequence.

pol·y·ac·id (pol-ē-as'id). An acid capable of liberating more than one hydrogen ion per molecule; *e.g.,* H_2SO_4, citric acid. [G. *polys,* much, many + acid]

pol·y·ac·ry·la·mide (pol-ē-a-kril'a-mīd). A branched polymer of acrylamide ($H_2C=CHCONH_2$) that is used in gel electrophoresis; *e.g.,* R–CH_2–CH($CONH_2$)–CH(CONHRCH(CONHR')–R".

pol·y·ad·e·ni·tis (pol'ē-ad-ĕ-nī'tis). Inflammation of many lymph nodes, especially with reference to the cervical group.

p. malig'na, SYN bubonic *plague.*

pol·y·ad·e·nop·a·thy (pol'ē-ad-ĕ-nop'ă-thē). Adenopathy affecting many lymph nodes. SYN polyadenosis.

pol·y·ad·e·no·sis (pol'ē-ad-ĕ-nō'sis). SYN polyadenopathy.

pol·y·ad·e·nous (pol-ē-ad'ĕ-nŭs). Pertaining to or involving many glands.

pol·y·ad·e·nyl·a·tion. 1. The process of formation of poly(adenylic acid). **2.** The covalent modification of a macromolecule (*e.g.,* mRNA) by the formation of a polyadenylyl moiety covalent linked to the macromolecule.

pol·y·(ad·en·yl·ic ac·id) (pol·y·(A)) (pol-ē-ă-dē-nil'ik). A homopolymer of adenylic acid; often seen at the 3' end of many eukaryotic mRNAs.

pol·y·al·co·hol (pol-ē-al'kō-hol). An aliphatic or alicyclic molecule characterized by the presence of two or more hydroxyl groups; *e.g.,* glycerol, inositol. [G. *polys,* much, many + alcohol]

pol·y(al·co·hol) (pol-ē-al'kō-hol). A polymer of an alcohol. SEE poly- (2).

pol·y·al·lel·ism (pol'ē-ă-lēl'izm). The existence of multiple alleles at a genetic locus.

pol·y·a·mine (pol-ē-am'ēn). Class name for substances of the general formula $H_2N(CH_2)_nNH_2$, $H_2N(CH_2)_nNH(CH_2)_nNH_2$, $H_2N(CH_2)_nNH(CH_2)_nNH(CH_2)_nNH_2$, where n = 3, 4, or 5. Many p.'s arise by bacterial action on protein; many are normally occurring body constituents of wide distribution, or are essential growth factors for microorganisms. [G. *polys,* much, many + amine]

pol·y(amine) (pol-ē-ă-mēn, am'ēn). A polymer of an amine. SEE poly- (2).

p. oxidase, an enzyme of liver peroxisomes that uses molecular oxygen to oxidize spermidine to psemidine and spermidine to putrescine, in both cases also producing H_2O_2 and β-aminopropionaldehyde. A part of the catabolic pathway of p.'s.

pol·y(ami·no ac·ids). Polypeptides that are polymers of aminoacyl groups, *i.e.,* of –NH–CHR–CO–; typically, a term used with homopolymers. SEE poly- (2).

pol·y·an·gi·i·tis (pol'ē-an-jē-ī'tis). Inflammation of multiple blood vessels involving more than one type of vessel, *e.g.,* arteries and veins, or arterioles and capillaries.

pol·y·an·i·on (pol-ē-an'ī-on). Anionic sites on proteoglycans in the renal glomeruli that restrict filtration of anionic molecules and facilitate filtration of cationic proteins; loss of p. may cause albuminuria in lipoid nephrosis.

pol·y·ar·ter·i·tis (pol'ē-ar-ter-ī'tis). Simultaneous inflammation of a number of arteries.

p. nodo'sa, segmental inflammation, with infiltration by eosinophils, and necrosis of medium-sized or small arteries, most common in males, with varied symptoms related to involvement of arteries in the kidneys, muscles, gastrointestinal tract, and heart. SYN arteritis nodosa, Kussmaul's disease, periarteritis nodosa.

pol·y·ar·thric (pol-ē-ar'thrik). SYN multiarticular.

pol·y·ar·thri·tis (pol'ē-ar-thrī'tis). Simultaneous inflammation of several joints. [poly- + G. *arthron,* joint, + -*itis,* inflammation]

p. chron'ica, obsolete term for rheumatoid *arthritis.*

p. chron'ica villo'sa, a chronic inflammation confined to the synovial membrane, involving a number of joints; it occurs in women at the menopause and in children.

epidemic p., a mild febrile illness of humans in Australia characterized by polyarthralgia and rash, caused by the Ross River virus, a member of the family Togaviridae, and transmitted by mosquitoes. SYN epidemic exanthema, Murray Valley rash, Ross River fever.

p. rheumat'ica acu'ta, obsolete term for p. associated with rheumatic fever.

vertebral p., inflammation of a number of the intervertebral disks without involvement of the vertebral bodies.

pol·y·ar·tic·u·lar (pol-ē-ar-tik'yū-lăr). SYN multiarticular. [poly- + L. *articulus,* joint]

pol·y·aux·o·troph (pol-ē-awks'ō-trōf). A mutant organism that requires several nutrients that are not required by the wild type organism. Cf. auxotroph, monoauxotroph.

pol·y·a·vi·ta·min·o·sis (pol'ē-ā'vī-tă-mi-nō'sis). Avitaminosis with multiple deficiencies.

pol·y·ba·sic (pol-ē-bās'ik). Having more than one replaceable hydrogen atom, denoting an acid with a basicity greater than 1.

pol·y·blast (pol'ē-blast). One of a group of ameboid, mononucleated, wandering phagocytic cells found in inflammatory exudates. [poly- + G. *blastos,* germ]

pol·y·blen·nia (pol-ē-blen'ē-ă). Excessive production of mucus. [poly- + G. *blennos,* mucus]

pol·y·car·bo·phil (pol-ē-kar'bō-fil). A polyacrylic acid crosslinked with divinyl glycol; used as a gastrointestinal absorbent.

pol·y·car·dia (pol-ē-kar'dē-ă). SYN tachycardia.

pol·y·cen·tric (pol-ē-sen'trik). Having several centers.

pol·y·chei·ria, pol·y·chi·ria (pol-ē-kī'rē-ă). Presence of supernumerary hands. [poly- + G. *cheir,* hand]

⌂ **Combining forms**

Word*Finder*
Multi-term entry finder
Preceding letter A
A.D.A.M. Anatomy Plates
Between letters L and M

Appendices:
Following letter Z

SYN Synonym; **Cf.,** compare

[NA] **Nomina Anatomica**

[MIM] **Mendelian Inheritance in Man**

☆ **Official alternate term**

☆[NA] **Official alternate Nomina Anatomica term**

High Profile Term

po

pol·y·chon·dri·tis (pol′ē-kon-drī′tis). A widespread disease of cartilage. [poly- + G. *chondros,* cartilage, + *-itis,* inflammation]

chronic atrophic p., SYN relapsing p.

relapsing p., a degenerative disease of cartilage producing a bizarre form of arthritis, with collapse of the ears, the cartilaginous portion of the nose, and the tracheobronchial tree; death may occur from chronic infection or suffocation because of loss of stability in the tracheobronchial tree of autosomal origin. SYN chronic atrophic p., generalized chondromalacia, Meyenburg's disease, Meyenburg-Altherr-Uehlinger syndrome, relapsing perichondritis, systemic chondromalacia, von Meyenburg's disease.

pol·y·chro·ma·sia (pol′ē-krō-mā′zē-ă). SYN polychromatophilia.

pol·y·chro·mat·ic (pol-ē-krō-mat′ik). Multicolored.

pol·y·chro·mat·o·cyte (pol′ē-krō-mat′ō-sīt). SYN polychromatophil (2).

pol·y·chro·ma·to·phil, pol·y·chro·ma·to·phile (pol-ē-krō′mă-tō-fil, -fīl). **1.** Staining readily with acid, neutral, and basic dyes; denoting certain cells, especially certain red blood cells. SYN polychromatophilic. **2.** A young or degenerating erythrocyte that manifests acid and basic staining affinities. SYN polychromatocyte. SYN polychromophil. [poly- + G. *chrōma,* color, + *phileō,* to love]

pol·y·chro·ma·to·phil·ia (pol-ē-krō′mă-tō-fil′ē-ă). **1.** A tendency of certain cells, such as the red blood cells in pernicious anemia, to stain with basic and also acid dyes. **2.** Condition characterized by the presence of many red blood cells that have an affinity for acid, basic, or neutral stains. SYN polychromasia, polychromatosis, polychromophilia.

pol·y·chro·ma·to·phil·ic (pol-ē-krō′mă-tō-fil′ik). SYN polychromatophil (1).

pol·y·chro·ma·to·sis (pol′ē-krō-mă-tō′sis). SYN polychromatophilia.

pol·y·chro·me·mia (pol-ē-krō-mē′mē-ă). An increase in the total amount of hemoglobin in the blood.

pol·y·chro·mia (pol-ē-krō′mē-ă). Increased pigmentation in any part.

pol·y·chro·mo·phil (pol-ē-krō′mō-fil). SYN polychromatophil.

pol·y·chro·mo·phil·ia (pol-ē-krō-mō-fil′ē-ă). SYN polychromatophilia.

pol·y·chy·lia (pol-ē-kī′lē-ă). An increased production of chyle. [poly- + G. *chylos,* chyle, + *-ia,* condition]

pol·y·cin·e·ma·to·som·nog·ra·phy (pol′ē-sin′ē-mă-tō-som-nog′ră-fē). SYN somnocinematography.

pol·y·cis·tron·ic (pol-ē-sis-tron′ik). Pertaining to mRNA carrying information for the synthesis of more than one protein.

pol·y·clin·ic (pol-ē-klin′ik). A dispensary for the treatment and study of diseases of all kinds. [poly- + G. *klinē,* bed]

pol·y·clo·nal (pol-ē-klō′năl). In immunochemistry, pertaining to proteins from more than a single clone of cells, in contradistinction to monoclonal.

pol·y·clo·nia (pol′ē-klō′nē-ă). SYN *myoclonus* multiplex. [poly- + G. *klonos,* tumult]

pol·y·co·ria (pol-ē-kō′rē-ă). The presence of two or more pupils in one iris. [poly- + G. *korē,* pupil]

pol·y·crot·ic (pol-ē-krot′ik). Relating to or marked by polycrotism.

po·lyc·ro·tism (pol-ik′rō-tizm). A condition in which the sphygmographic tracing shows several upward breaks in the descending wave. [poly- + G. *krotos,* a beat]

pol·y·cy·e·sis (pol′ē-sī-ē′sis). SYN multiple *pregnancy.* [poly- + G. *kyēsis,* pregnancy]

pol·y·cys·tic (pol-ē-sis′tik). Composed of many cysts.

pol·y·cy·the·mia (pol′ē-sī-thē′mē-ă). An increase above the normal in the number of red cells in the blood. SYN erythrocythemia. [poly- + G. *kytos,* cell, + *haima,* blood]

compensatory p., a secondary p. resulting from anoxia, *e.g.,* in congenital heart disease, pulmonary emphysema, or prolonged residence at a high altitude.

p. hyperton′ica, p. associated with hypertension, but without splenomegaly. SYN Gaisböck's syndrome.

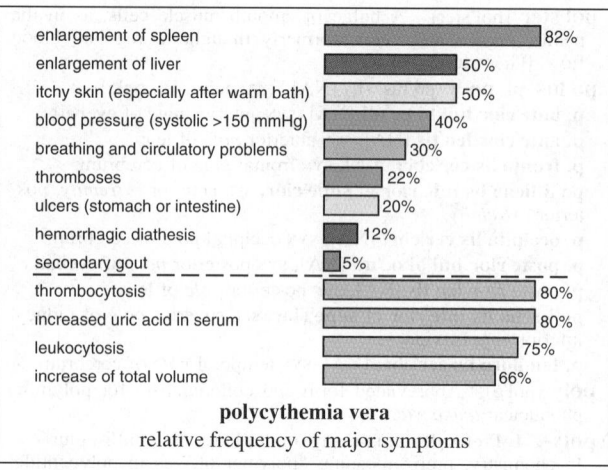

enlargement of spleen	82%
enlargement of liver	50%
itchy skin (especially after warm bath)	50%
blood pressure (systolic >150 mmHg)	40%
breathing and circulatory problems	30%
thromboses	22%
ulcers (stomach or intestine)	20%
hemorrhagic diathesis	12%
secondary gout	5%
thrombocytosis	80%
increased uric acid in serum	80%
leukocytosis	75%
increase of total volume	66%

polycythemia vera
relative frequency of major symptoms

relative p., a relative increase in the number of red blood cells as a result of loss of the fluid portion of the blood.

p. ru′bra, SYN p. vera.

p. ru′bra ve′ra, SYN p. vera.

p. ve′ra, A chronic form of polycythemia of unknown cause; characterized by bone marrow hyperplasia, an increase in blood volume as well as in the number of red cells, redness or cyanosis of the skin, and splenomegaly. SYN erythremia, Osler's disease (1), Osler-Vaquez disease, p. rubra vera, p. rubra, Vaquez' disease.

pol·y·dac·tyl·ism (pol-ē-dak′ti-lizm). SYN polydactyly.

pol·y·dac·tyl·ous (pol-ē-dak′til-ŭs). Relating to polydactyly.

pol·y·dac·ty·ly (pol-ē-dak′ti-lē). Presence of more than five digits on hand or foot. SYN polydactylism. [poly- + G. *daktylos,* finger]

pol·y·den·tia (pol-ē-den′shē-ă). SYN polyodontia. [poly- + L. *dens,* tooth]

pol·y·dip·sia (pol-ē-dip′sē-ă). Excessive thirst that is relatively prolonged. [poly- + G. *dipsa,* thirst]

hysterical p., SYN psychogenic p.

psychogenic p., excessive fluid consumption resulting from a disorder of the personality, without demonstrable organic lesion. SYN hysterical p.

psychogenic nocturnal p. (PNP), SEE psychogenic nocturnal polydipsia *syndrome.*

pol·y·dis·per·soid (pol′ē-dis-per′soyd). A colloid system in which the dispersed phase is composed of particles having different degrees of dispersion.

pol·y·dys·pla·sia (pol′ē-dis-plā′zē-ă). Tissue development abnormal in several respects. [poly- + G. *dys-,* bad, + *plasis,* a molding]

pol·y·dys·tro·phic (pol′ē-dis-trof′ik). Relating to polydystrophy.

pol·y·dys·tro·phy (pol·ē-dis′trō-fē). A condition characterized by the presence of many congenital anomalies of the connective tissues. [poly- + dystrophy]

pseudo-Hurler p., SYN *mucolipidosis* III.

pol·y·em·bry·o·ny (pol-ē-em-brē′ō-nē). Condition of a zygote's giving rise to two or more embryos. [poly- + G. *embryon,* embryo]

pol·y·en·do·crin·op·athy (pol′ē-en′dō-krĭ- nop′ă-thē). A disease usually caused by insufficiency of multiple endocrine glands. SEE multiple endocrine deficiency *syndrome.*

pol·y·ene (pol-ē-ēn′). A chemical compound having a series of conjugated (alternating) double bonds; *e.g.,* the carotenoids.

pol·y·e·nic ac·ids (pol-ē-ē′nik). SYN polyenoic acids.

pol·y·e·no·ic ac·ids (pol-ē-en′ik). Fatty acids with more than one double bonds in the carbon chain; *e.g.,* linoleic, linolenic, and arachidonic acids. SYN polyenic acids.

pol·y·er·gic (pol-ē-er'jik). Capable of acting in several different ways. [poly- + G. *ergon*, work]

pol·y·es·the·sia (pol-ē-es-thē'zē-ă). A disorder of sensation in which a single touch or other stimulus is felt as several. [poly- + G. *aisthēsis*, sensation]

pol·y·es·tra·di·ol phos·phate (pol'ē-es-tră-dī'ol). An estradiol phosphate polymer, used as a long-acting estrogen for treatment of prostatic carcinoma.

pol·y·es·trous (pol-ē-es'trŭs). Having two or more estrous cycles in a mating season.

pol·y·eth·y·lene gly·cols (PEGs) (pol-ē-eth'i-lēn). Poly-(oxyethylene) glycols; condensation polymers of ethylene oxide and water, of the general formula $HO(CH_2CH_2O)_nH$, where n equals the average number of oxyethylene groups (300–6,000); they vary in consistency based on molecular size; PEG 300 is a viscous liquid; PEG 600 is a waxlike solid; PEGs are soluble in water, and are used as pharmaceutic aids.

pol·y·fruc·tose (pol-ē-frŭk'tōs). SYN fructosan.

pol·y·ga·lac·tia (pol'ē-gă-lak'tē-ă, -shē-ă). Excessive secretion of breast milk, especially at the weaning period. [poly- + G. *gala*, milk]

pol·y·ga·lac·tu·ro·nase (pol'ē-gă-lak'tū-ron-ās). Pectin depolymerase; an enzyme catalyzing the random hydrolysis of 1,4-α-D-galactosiduronic linkages in pectate and other galacturonans. SYN pectinase.

pol·y·gan·gli·on·ic (pol'ē-gang-glē-on'ik). Containing or involving many ganglia.

pol·y·gene (pol'ē-jēn). One of many genes that contribute to the phenotypic value of a measurable phenotype.

pol·y·gen·ic (pol-ē-jen'ik). Relating to a hereditary disease or normal characteristic controlled by the added effects of genes at multiple loci.

pol·y·glan·du·lar (pol-ē-glan'dū-lăr). SYN pluriglandular.

poly-β-glu·co·sa·min·i·dase. SYN chitinase.

pol·y·glu·ta·mate (pol-ē-glū'tă-māt). SYN poly(glutamic acid).

pol·y(glu·tam·ic ac·id) (pol'ē-glū-tam'ik). A polymer of glutamic acid residues in the usual peptide linkage (α-carboxyl to α-amino). SEE poly- (2). SEE ALSO poly(γ-glutamic acid). SYN polyglutamate.

pol·y(γ-glu·tam·ic ac·id). A polypeptide formed of glutamic acid residues, the γ-carboxyl group of one glutamic acid being condensed to the amino group of its neighbor; occurs naturally in the anthrax bacillus capsule.

poly(gly·col·ic ac·id) (pol'ē-glī-kol'ik). A polymer of glycolic acid, used in absorbable surgical sutures. [see poly- (2)]

pol·y·gna·thus (pol-ē-nath'ŭs, pŏ-lig'na-thŭs). Unequal conjoined twins in which the parasite is attached to the jaw of the autosite. SEE conjoined *twins*, under *twin*. [poly- + G. *gnathos*, jaw]

pol·y·graph (pol'ē-graf). **1.** An instrument to obtain simultaneous tracings from several different sources; *e.g.*, radial and jugular pulse, apex beat of the heart, phonocardiogram, electrocardiogram. The ECG is nearly always included for timing. **2.** An instrument for recording changes in respiration, blood pressure, galvanic skin response, and other physiological changes while the person is questioned about some matter or asked to give associations to relevant and irrelevant words; the physiological changes are presumed to be indicators of emotional reactions, and thus whether the person is telling the truth. SYN lie detector. [poly- + G. *graphō*, to write]

Mackenzie's p., an instrument consisting of a system of tambours and a time-marker for recording simultaneously the jugular and arterial pulses and the apex beat; formerly used in the clinical investigation of cardiac arrhythmias.

pol·y·gy·ria (pol-ē-jī'rē-ă). Condition in which the brain has an excessive number of convolutions. [poly- + G. *gyros*, circle, gyre]

pol·y·he·dral (pol-ē-hē'drăl). Having many sides or facets. [G. *polyedros*, many-sided, fr. poly- + G. *hedra*, seat, facet]

pol·y·hex·os·es (pol-ē-heks'ōs-ez). SYN hexosans.

pol·y·hi·dro·sis (pol'ē-hī-drō'sis). SYN hyperhidrosis.

pol·y·hy·brid (pol-ē-hī'brid). The offspring of parents differing from each other in more than three characters.

pol·y·hy·dram·ni·os (pol'ē-hī-dram'nē-os). Excess amount of amniotic fluid. [poly- + G. *hydōr*, water, + amnion]

pol·y·hy·dric (pol-ē-hī'drik). Containing more than one hydroxyl group, as in polyhydric alcohols (glycerol, $C_3H_5(OH)_3$) or polyhydric acids (*o*-phosphoric acid, $OP(OH)_3$).

pol·y·hy·per·men·or·rhea (pol-ē-hī'per-men-ō-rē'ă). Frequent and excessive menstruation. [poly- + G. *hyper*, above, + *mēn*, month, + *rhoia*, flow]

pol·y·hy·po·men·or·rhea (pol-ē-hī'pō-men-ō-rē'ă). Frequent but scanty menstruation. [poly- + G. *hypo*, below, + *mēn*, month, + *rhoia*, a flow]

pol·y·i·dro·sis (pol'ē-i-drō'sis). SYN hyperhidrosis.

pol·y·iso·pre·nes (pol-ē-ī'sō-prēnz). SYN polyterpenes.

pol·y·iso·pre·noids (pol-ē-i-sō-prē-nōydz). SYN polyterpenes.

pol·y·kar·y·o·cyte (pol-ē-kar'ē-ō-sīt). A cell containing many nuclei, such as the osteoclast. [poly- + G. *karyon*, kernel, + *kytos*, cell]

pol·y·lac·to·sa·mines (pol-ē-lak-tōs'a-mēnz). A class of glycoproteins containing repeating lactosamine units in their oligosaccharide components; the I/i blood group substances belong to this class.

pol·y·lep·tic (pol-ē-lep'tik). Denoting a disease occurring in many paroxysms, *e.g.*, malaria, epilepsy. [poly- + G. *lēpsis*, a seizing]

pol·y·link·er (pol-ē-link'er). An inserted sequence of DNA in recombinant DNA vectors consisting of a cluster of numerous restriction endonuclease sites unique in the plasmid; also called restriction site bank and polycloning site.

pol·y·lo·gia (pol-ē-lō'jē-ă). Continuous and often incoherent speech. [poly- + G. *logos*, word]

pol·y·mas·tia (pol-ē-mas'tē-ă). In humans, a condition in which more than two breasts are present. SYN hypermastia (1), multi-mammae, pleomastia, pleomazia, polymazia. [poly- + G. *mastos*, breast]

pol·y·mas·ti·gote (pol-ē-mas'ti-gōt). A mastigote having several grouped flagella. [poly- + G. *mastix*, a whip]

pol·y·ma·zia (pol-ē-mā'zē-ă). SYN polymastia. [poly- + G. *mazos*, breast]

pol·y·meg·eth·ism (pol'ē-meg'-ĕ-thism). A greater than normal variation in the size of the cells of the human corneal endothelium.

pol·y·me·lia (pol-ē-mē'lē-ă). A developmental defect in which there are supernumerary limbs or parts of limbs. [poly- + G. *melos*, limb]

pol·y·men·or·rhea (pol-ē-men-ō-rē'ă). Occurrence of menstrual cycles of greater than usual frequency. [poly- + G. *mēn*, month, + *rhoia*, flow]

pol·y·mer (pol'i-mer). A substance of high molecular weight, made up of a chain of repeated units sometimes called "mers." SEE ALSO biopolymer. [see -mer (1)]

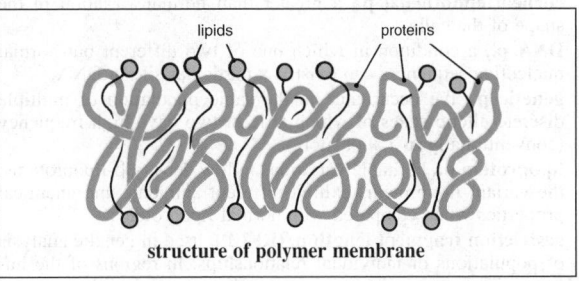

structure of polymer membrane

cross-linked p., a p. in which long-chain molecules are attached to each other, forming a two- or three-dimensional network. SYN cross-linked resin.

pol·y·mer·ase (po-lim'er-ās). General term for any enzyme catalyzing a polymerization, as of nucleotides to polynucleotides, thus belonging to EC class 2, the transferases.

p. alpha, a class of mammalian DNA p.'s in the nucleus that function in chromosome replication. SYN polymerase α.

p. beta, a class of mammalian DNA p.'s in the nucleus that do not have a role in replication but may function in DNA repair. SYN polymerase β.

p. gamma, a class of mammalian DNA p.'s in the mitochondria responsible for replication of the mitochondrial genome. SYN polymerase γ.

Taq p., a temperature-resistant DNA polymerase isolated from *Thermus aquaticus* that can extend primers at high temperatures; used in the p. chain reaction.

pol·y·mer·ase γ. SYN *polymerase* gamma.

pol·y·mer·ase α. SYN *polymerase* alpha.

pol·y·mer·ase β. SYN *polymerase* beta.

pol·y·me·ria (pol-ē-mēr′ē-ă). Condition characterized by an excessive number of parts, limbs, or organs of the body. [poly- + G. *meros,* part]

pol·y·mer·ic (pol-i-mer′ik). **1.** Having the properties of a polymer. **2.** Relating to or characterized by polymeria. **3.** Rarely used synonym for polygenic.

po·lym·er·id (po-lim′er-id). An obsolete synonym for polymer.

po·lym·er·i·za·tion (po-lim′er-i-za′shŭn). A reaction in which a high-molecular-weight product is produced by successive additions to or condensations of a simpler compound; *e.g.,* polystyrene may be produced from styrene, or rubber from isoprene, or a polynucleotide from mononucleotides, or microtubules from tubulin.

po·lym·er·ize (pol′i-mer-īz, po-lim′er-īz). To bring about polymerization.

pol·y·met·a·car·pa·lia, pol·y·met·a·car·pa·lism (pol′ē-met-ă-kar-pā′lē-ă, -kar′pă-lizm). Congenital anomaly characterized by the presence of supernumerary metacarpal bones.

pol·y·met·a·tar·sa·lia, pol·y·met·a·tar·sa·lism (pol′ē-met-ă-tar-sā′lē-ă, -tar′să-lizm). Congenital anomaly characterized by the presence of supernumerary metatarsal bones.

pol·y·mi·cro·lip·o·ma·to·sis (pol-ē-mī′krō-lip′ō-mă-tō′sis). The occurrence of multiple, small, nodular, fairly discrete masses of lipid in the subcutaneous connective tissue. [poly- + G. *mikros,* small, + lipoma + G. -*osis,* condition]

po·lym·i·tus (pŏ-lim′i-tŭs). SYN exflagellation. [poly- + G. *mitos,* thread]

pol·y·morph (pol′ē-mōrf). Colloquial term for polymorphonuclear *leukocyte.*

pol·y·mor·phic (pol-ē-mōr′fik). Occurring in more than one morphologic form. SYN multiform, pleomorphic (1), pleomorphous, polymorphous. [G. *polymorphos,* multiform]

pol·y·mor·phism (pol-ē-mōr′fizm). Occurrence in more than one form; existence in the same species or other natural group of more than one morphologic type. SYN pleomorphism.

balanced p., a unilocal trait in which two alleles are maintained at stable frequencies because the heterozygote is more fit than either of the homozygotes. SEE ALSO overdominance.

corneal endothelial p., a greater than normal variation in the shape of the cells.

DNA p., a condition in which one of two different but normal nucleotide sequences can exist at a particular site in DNA.

genetic p., the occurrence in the same population of multiple discrete allelic states of which at least two have high frequency (conventionally of 1% or more).

lipoprotein p., heritable variations in low density β-lipoproteins; the variant lipoproteins exhibit different antigenic and chemical properties when compared with normal lipoproteins.

restriction fragment length p. (RFLP), used in genetic analysis of populations or individual relationships. In regions of the human genome not coding for proteins there is often wide sequence variety between individuals that can be measured.

restriction length p., fragment length p., the existence of allelic forms recognizable by the length of fragments that result when the nucleotide chain is treated by a specific restriction enzyme that cleaves wherever a particular sequence of nucleo-

tides occurs. A mutation in this sequence changes cleaving and hence the number of fragments.

restriction-site p., dNA p. in which the sequence of one form of the p. contains a recognition site for a particular endonuclease, but the sequence of the other form lacks such a site.

pol·y·mor·pho·cel·lu·lar (pol-ē-mōr′fō-sel′yū-lăr). Relating to or formed of cells of several different kinds. [G. *polymorphos,* multiform, + L. *cellula,* cell]

pol·y·mor·pho·nu·cle·ar (pol′ē-mōr-fō-nū′klē-ăr). Having nuclei of varied forms; denoting a variety of leukocyte. [G. *polymorphos,* multiform, + L. *nucleus,* kernel]

pol·y·mor·phous (pol-ē-mōr′fŭs). SYN polymorphic.

pol·y·my·al·gia (pol′ē-mī-al′jē-ă). Pain in several muscle groups. [poly- + G. *mys,* muscle, + *algos,* pain]

p. arterit′ica, p. rheumatica resulting from arteritis, especially disseminated giant cell arteritis.

p. rheumat′ica, a syndrome within the group of collagen diseases different from spondylarthritis or from humeral scapular periarthritis by the presence of an elevated sedimentation rate; much commoner in women than in men.

pol·y·my·oc·lo·nus (pol′ē-mī-ok′lō-nŭs). SYN *myoclonus* multiplex.

pol·y·my·o·si·tis (pol′ē-mī-ō-sī′tis). Inflammation of a number of voluntary muscles simultaneously. [poly- + G. *mys,* muscle, + -*itis,* inflammation]

pol·y·myx·in (pol-ē-mik′sin). A mixture of antibiotic substances obtained from cultures of *Bacillus polymyxa* (*B. serosporus*), an organism found in water and soils, and obtainable as a crystalline hydrochloride; polypeptides containing various amino acids and a branched chain fatty acid, (+)-6-methyloctanoic acid. There are several p.'s, *e.g.,* designated A, B_1, C, D, E, M, T, etc., which are about equally effective against Gram-negative bacteria, but which differ in toxicity, p. E (colistin) and p. B being the least toxic. SEE ALSO *colistin* sulfate, colistimethate sodium.

p. B sulfate, an antibacterial effective in tularemia, brucellosis, *Pseudomonas* infections, and urinary tract infections, but used systemically only for severe infections not responsive to less toxic agents; it is also used locally. P. B is a mixture of p. B_1 and p. B_2.

pol·y·ne·sic (pol-i-nē′sik). Occurring in many separate foci; denoting certain forms of inflammation or infection. [poly- + G. *nēsos,* island]

pol·y·neu·ral (pol-ē-nū′răl). Relating to, supplied by, or affecting several nerves. [poly- + G. *neuron,* nerve]

pol·y·neu·ral·gia (pol′ē-nū-ral′jē-ă). Neuralgia of several nerves simultaneously.

pol·y·neu·ri·tis (pol′ē-nū-rī′tis). SYN polyneuropathy (2).

acute idiopathic p., a neurological syndrome, probably an immune-mediated disorder, often a sequela of certain virus infections, marked by paresthesia of the limbs and muscular weakness or a flaccid paralysis; the characteristic laboratory finding is increased protein in the cerebrospinal fluid without increase in cell count. SYN acute inflammatory polyneuropathy, Guillain-Barré syndrome, infectious p., Landry syndrome, Landry's paralysis, Landry-Guillain-Barré syndrome, myeloradiculopolyneuronitis, postinfectious p.

chronic familial p., inflammation of nerves related to infiltration by amyloid.

infectious p., SYN acute idiopathic p.

postinfectious p., SYN acute idiopathic p.

pol·y·neu·ro·ni·tis (pol′ē-nū-rō-nī′tis). Inflammation of several groups of nerve cells.

pol·y·neu·rop·a·thy (pol′ē-nū-rop′ă-thē). **1.** A disease process involving a number of peripheral nerves (literal sense). **2.** A nontraumatic generalized disorder of peripheral nerves, affecting the distal fibers most severely with proximal shading (*i.e.,* feet, before, or more severe, than hands), and typically symmetrical; most often affects motor and sensory fibers almost equally, but can involve either one solely or very disproportionately; classified as axon degenerating (axonal), or demyelinating; many causes, particularly metabolic and toxic; familial or sporadic in nature. SYN polyneuritis. SYN multiple neuritis, symmetric distal neuropathy. [poly- + G. *neuron,* nerve, + *pathos,* disease]

acute inflammatory p., SYN acute idiopathic *polyneuritis.*

alcoholic p., a nutritional axon loss p. associated with chronic alcoholism.

arsenical p., an axon loss p. that results from subacute or chronic arsenic poisoning; almost always preceded by gastrointestinal symptoms; one of the heavy metal neuropathies.

axonal p., SYN axon loss p.

axon loss p., a type of p. in which axon degeneration is the sole/predominant feature; many etiologies, particularly toxic and metabolic; on nerve conduction studies, affects amplitudes of the responses, but does not cause conduction slowing or block. SYN axonal p.

buckthorn p., ascending p. resulting from ingestion of the fruit of *Karwinskia humboldtiana.*

chronic inflammatory demyelinating p. (CIDP), an uncommon, acquired, demyelinating sensorimotor p. clinically characterized by insidious onset, and slow evolution, (either steady progression or stepwise), and chronic course; symmetrical weakness is a predominant symptom, often involving proximal leg muscles, accompanied by paresthesias, but not pain; CSF examination shows elevated protein, while electrodiagnostic studies reveal evidence of a demyelinating process, primarily conduction slowing rather than block; sometimes responds to prednisone.

critical illness p., a diffuse axon loss sensorimotor p. seen in severely ill patients, usually in the intensive care unit; most patients have been on multiple drugs, and cannot be weaned from ventilatory support; electrodiagnostic studies show evidence of an axon loss p., predominantly motor; of unknown etiology.

demyelinating p., a type of p. in which almost solely the peripheral nerve myelin is affected; can be both familial (*e.g.,* Charcot-Marie Tooth disease, type 1), or acquired (*e.g.,* Guillain-Barré syndrome); on motor nerve conduction studies, manifested as conduction slowing or block. SYN segmental demyelinating p.

diabetic p., a distal, symmetrical, generally sensorimotor p. that is a frequent complication of diabetes mellitus.

isoniazid p., an axonal loss p. seen in some patients treated with isoniazid.

nitrofurantoin p., an axon loss p., often severe, seen in some patients treated with nitrofurantoin, particularly patients with chronic renal failure.

nutritional p., a disorder of multiple peripheral nerves, noted in beriberi, chronic alcoholism, and other clinical states, resulting from thiamin deficiency.

progressive hypertrophic p., SYN Dejerine-Sottas *disease.* SYN chronic interstitial hypertrophic neuropathy, hereditary hypertrophic neuropathy.

segmental demyelinating p., SYN demyelinating p.

uremic p., a distal sensory and motor p. without conspicuous inflammation and ascribed to the metabolic effects of chronic renal failure.

pol·y·nox·y·lin (pol-ē-nok′si-lin). Poly{methylenebis[*N,N′*-di-(hydroxymethyl)urea]}; a polymer of urea with formaldehyde, used as a topical antiseptic.

pol·y·nu·cle·ar, pol·y·nu·cle·ate (pol-ē-nū′klē-ăr, -klē-āt). SYN multinuclear.

pol·y·nu·cle·o·sis (pol′ē-nū-klē-ō′sis). The presence of numbers of polynuclear, or multinuclear, cells in the peripheral blood. SYN multinucleosis.

pol·y·nu·cle·o·ti·das·es (pol′ē-nū′klē-ō-ti′dās-ez). **1.** Enzymes catalyzing the hydrolysis of polynucleotides to oligonucleotides or to mononucleotides; *e.g.,* phosphodiesterases, nucleases. **2.** Terms once applied to the two polynucleotide phosphatases, 2′(3′)- and 5′-, which do not cleave internucleotide links.

pol·y·nu·cle·o·tide (pol-ē-nū′klē-ō-tīd). A linear polymer containing an indefinite (usually large) number of nucleotides, linked from one ribose (or deoxyribose) to another via phosphoric residues. Cf. oligonucleotide.

p. methyltransferases, enzymes that catalyze the methylation of purine and/or pyrimidine bases of p.'s, or of the sugars of p.'s. SYN polynucleotide methylases.

p. phosphorylase, SYN polyribonucleotide nucleotidyltransferase.

p. thioltransferases, enzymes that catalyze specific thiolation reaction of purine and/or pyrimidine bases in p.'s.

pol·y·nu·cle·o·tide meth·yl·ases. SYN *polynucleotide* methyltransferases.

pol·y·o·don·tia (pol-ē-ō-don′shē-ă). Presence of supernumerary teeth. SYN polydentia. [poly- + G. *odous,* tooth]

pol·y·ol (pol′ē-ol). Polyhydroxy alcohol; a sugar that contains many –OH (-ol) groups, such as the sugar alcohols and inositols.

p. dehydrogenases, oxidizing enzymes that catalyze the dehydrogenation of sugar alcohols to monosaccharides (in EC class 1.1), specifically L-iditol dehydrogenase and aldose reductase.

Pol·y·o·ma·vi·rus (pol-ē-ō′mă-vī′rŭs). A genus of viruses (family Papovaviridae) containing DNA (MW 3×10^6), having virions about 45 nm in diameter, and including viruses oncogenic for animals; includes the polyoma virus of rodents, vacuolating viruses (SV40) of primates, and the BK and JC viruses of humans. [poly- + G. *-ōma,* tumor]

pol·y·on·co·sis, pol·y·on·cho·sis (pol′ē-ong-kō′sis). Formation of multiple tumors. [poly- + G. *onkos,* tumor, + *-osis,* condition]

pol·y·o·nych·ia (pol-ē-ō-nik′ē-ă). Presence of supernumerary nails on fingers or toes. SYN polyunguia. [poly- + G. *onyx,* nail]

pol·y·o·pia, pol·y·op·sia (pol′ē-ō′pē-ă, -op′sē-ă). The perception of several images of the same object. SYN multiple vision. [poly- + G. *ōps,* eye]

pol·y·or·chism, pol·y·or·chid·ism (pol-ē-ōr′kizm, -ōr′kid-izm). Presence of one or more supernumerary testes. [poly- + G. *orchis,* testis]

pol·y·os·tot·ic (pol′ē-os-tot′ik). Involving more than one bone. [poly- + G. *osteon,* bone]

pol·y·o·tia (pol-ē-ō′shē-ă). Presence of a supernumerary auricle on one or both sides of the head. [poly- + G. *ous,* ear]

pol·y·ov·u·lar (pol-ē-ō′vyū-lăr). Containing more than one ovum.

pol·y·ov·u·la·tory (pol-ē-ō′vyū-lă-tōr-ē). Discharging several ova in one ovulatory cycle. SYN polyzygotic.

pol·y·ox·yl 40 ste·a·rate (pol-ē-ok′sil). A mixture of the monostearate and distearate esters of a condensation polymer, $H(OCH_2CH_2)_n·OCOC_{16}H_{32}CH_3$ (*n* is approximately 40); it is a nonionic surface-active agent used as an emulsifying agent in hydrophilic ointment and other emulsions.

pol·yp (pol′ip). A general descriptive term used with reference to any mass of tissue that bulges or projects outward or upward from the normal surface level, thereby being macroscopically visible as a hemispheroidal, spheroidal, or irregular moundlike structure growing from a relatively broad base or a slender stalk; p.'s may be neoplasms, foci of inflammation, degenerative lesions, or malformations. SYN polypus. [L. *polypus;* G. *polypous,* contr. fr. G. *polys,* many, + *pous,* foot]

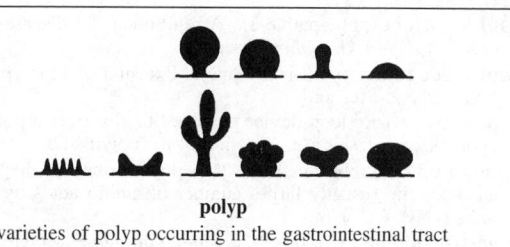

polyp
varieties of polyp occurring in the gastrointestinal tract

adenomatous p., a p. that consists of benign neoplastic tissue derived from glandular epithelium. SYN cellular p., polypoid adenoma.

bleeding p., SYN vascular p.

bronchial p., a p. growing from the bronchial mucosa.

cardiac p., usually a rounded thrombus attached to the endocardium.

cellular p., SYN adenomatous p.

choanal p., an antral-choanal p. that extends into the nasopharynx; generally originates in the antrum.

cystic p., a pedunculated cyst. SYN hydatid p.

dental p., SYN hyperplastic *pulpitis*.

fibrinous p., a misnomer for a mass of fibrin retained within the uterine cavity after childbirth.

fibroepithelial p. (fī′brō-ep-the′lē- ăl), SYN skin *tag*.

fibrous p., a p. consisting chiefly of cellular fibrous tissue, frequently with foci of fairly dense collagen or hyaline material (or both).

fleshy p., SYN myomatous p.

gelatinous p., (1) a p. that consists of delicate, loose, edematous connective tissue; (2) a polypoid myxoma.

Hopmann's p., SYN Hopmann's *papilloma*.

hydatid p., SYN cystic p.

hyperplastic p., a benign small sessile p. of the large bowel showing lengthening and cystic dilation of mucosal glands; also applied to non-neoplastic gastric mucosal p.'s. SYN metaplastic p.

inflammatory p., SYN pseudopolyp.

juvenile p., a smoothly rounded mucosal hamartoma of the large bowel, which may be multiple and cause rectal bleeding, especially in the first decade of life; it is not precancerous. SYN retention p.

laryngeal p., a p. projecting from the surface of one of the vocal cords.

lipomatous p., (1) a p. consisting chiefly of adipose tissue; (2) lipoma that bulges from the surface or is attached by means of a stalk.

lymphoid p., benign p. consisting of aggregates of lymphocytes in the rectum.

metaplastic p., SYN hyperplastic p.

mucous p., (1) an adenomatous p. in which conspicuous amounts of mucin are formed; (2) a polypoid cyst that contains mucus.

myomatous p., a p. that consists of benign neoplastic tissue derived from nonstriated (smooth) muscle. SYN fleshy p.

nasal p., an inflammatory or allergic p., arising from one of the paranasal sinuses, which projects into the nasal cavity.

osseous p., a p. consisting in part of bony tissue.

pedunculated p., any form of p. that is attached to the base tissue by means of a slender stalk.

placental p., a p. developed from a piece of retained placenta.

pulp p., SYN hyperplastic *pulpitis*.

regenerative p., a hyperplastic p. of the gastric mucosa.

retention p., SYN juvenile p.

sessile p., any form of p. that has a relatively broad base.

tooth p., SYN hyperplastic *pulpitis*.

vascular p., a bulging or protruding angioma of the nasal mucous membrane. SYN bleeding p.

pol·y·pap·il·lo·ma (pol′ē-pap-i-lō′mă). **1.** Multiple papillomas. **2.** SYN yaws.

pol·y·path·ia (pol-ē-path′ē-ă). A multiplicity of diseases or disorders. [poly- + G. *pathos*, disease]

pol·y·pec·to·my (pol-i-pek′tō-mē). Excision of a polyp. [polyp + G. *ektomē*, excision]

p. snare, a wire loop device designed to slip over a polyp and, upon closure, result in transection of the polyp stalk.

pol·y·pep·tide (pol-ē-pep′tīd). A peptide formed by the union of an indefinite (usually large) number of amino acids by peptide links (–NH–CO–).

gastric inhibitory p. (GIP), a peptide hormone, secreted by the stomach, that stimulates insulin release as part of the digestive process; GIP inhibits the secretion of acids and of pepsin. SYN gastric inhibitory peptide.

pancreatic p., (1) a 36-amino acid peptide secreted by islet cells of the pancreas in response to a meal and of uncertain physiologic function; (2) a family of gastrointestinal peptides, which includes pancreatic polypeptide, neuropeptide Y, and peptide YY.

trefoil p., a group of p.'s that share the trefoil moiety of a highly stable three-loop structure held together by disulfide bonds based on cysteine residues; they are widely expressed in gastrointestinal tissues and secreted by mucous cells; their functions are as yet unknown.

vasoactive intestinal p. (VIP), a p. hormone secreted most commonly by non-beta islet cell tumors of the pancreas, producing copious watery diarrhea and fecal electrolyte loss, particularly hypokalemia; VIP increases the rates of glycogenolysis; stimulates pancreatic bicarbonate secretion. SYN vasoactive intestinal peptide.

pol·y·pha·gia (pol-ē-fā′jē-ă). Excessive eating; gluttony. [poly- + G. *phagō*, to eat]

pol·y·pha·lan·gism (pol′ē-fă-lan′jizm). SYN hyperphalangism.

pol·y·phal·lic (pol-ē-fal′ik). Pertaining to the fantasy of possessing multiple penises.

pol·y·phar·ma·cy (pol-ē-far′mă-sē). The administration of many drugs at the same time. SEE ALSO shotgun *prescription*.

pol·y·phen·ic (pol-ē-phēn′ik). SYN pleiotropic. [poly- + G. *phainō*, to display]

pol·y·phe·nol ox·i·dase (pol-ē-fē′nol). SYN laccase.

pol·y·pho·bia (pol-ē-fō′bē-ă). Morbid fear of many things; a condition marked by the presence of many phobias. [poly- + G. *phobos*, fear]

pol·y·phos·phor·y·lase (pol′ē-fos-fōr′i-lās). SYN phosphorylase.

pol·y·phra·sia (pol-ē-frā′zē-ă). Extreme talkativeness. SEE logorrhea. [poly- + G. *phrasis*, speech]

pol·y·phy·let·ic (pol′ē-fī-let′ik). **1.** Derived from more than one source, or having several lines of descent, in contrast to monophyletic. **2.** In hematology, relating to polyphyletism.

pol·y·phy·le·tism (pol-ē-fī′lĕ-tizm). In hematology, the theory that blood cells are derived from several different stem cells, depending on the particular cell type. SYN polyphyletic theory. [poly- + G. *phylē*, tribe]

pol·y·phy·o·dont (pol-ē-fī′ō-dont). Having several sets of teeth formed in succession throughout life. [poly- + G. *phyō*, to produce, + *odous* (*odont-*), tooth]

po·ly·pi (pol′i-pī). Plural of polypus.

pol·yp·i·form (po-lip′i-fōrm). SYN polypoid.

pol·y·plas·mia (pol-ē-plaz′mē-ă). SYN hydremia.

pol·y·plas·tic (pol-ē-plas′tik). **1.** Formed of several different structures. **2.** Capable of assuming several forms. [poly- + G. *plastikos*, plastic]

Pol·y·plax (pol′ē-plaks). A sucking louse (order Anoplura) of rats and mice. The species *P. serratus* (the mouse louse) has been shown experimentally to be capable of transmitting tularemia and may also be a vector for murine typhus and *Trypanosoma lewisi*. [poly- + G. *plax*, plate, plaque]

pol·yp·loid (pol′ē-ployd). Characterized by or pertaining to polyploidy.

pol·y·ploi·dy (pol′ē-ploy′dē). The state of a cell nucleus containing three or more haploid sets. Cells containing three, four, five, or six multiples are referred to, respectively, as triploid, tetraploid, pentaploid, hexaploid, etc. [poly- + G. *ploides*, in form]

pol·yp·nea (pol-ip-nē′ă). SYN tachypnea. [poly- + G. *pnoia*, breath]

pol·y·po·dia (pol-i-pō′dē-ă). Presence of supernumerary feet.

pol·yp·oid (pol′i-poyd). Resembling a polyp in gross features. SYN polypiform. [polyp + G. *eidos*, resemblance]

po·lyp·or·ous (pol-ip′ōr-ŭs). SYN cribriform. [poly- + G. *poros*, pore]

Pol·y·po·rus (po-lip′ō-rŭs). A genus of mushrooms. SEE agaric. [poly- + G. *poros*, pore]

pol·y·po·sia (pol-ē-pō′zē-ă). Rarely used term for sustained, excessive consumption of liquids. [poly- + G. *posis*, drinking]

pol·yp·o·sis (pol′i-pō′sis). Presence of several polyps. [polyp + G. *-osis*, condition]

p. co′li, SYN multiple intestinal p. (1).

familial intestinal p., SYN multiple intestinal p.

multiple intestinal p., (1) begins usually in late childhood; polyps increase in numbers, causing symptoms of chronic colitis, and carcinoma of the colon almost invariably develops in untreated cases; autosomal dominant inheritance. In the Gardner syndrome there are extracolonic changes (desmoid tumors, etc.); SYN p. coli. (2) hamartomatous p. of the small or large intestine, Peutz-Jeghers syndrome [MIM*175200] with melanin spots on the lips, less common; (3) [MIM 175400–175510], miscellaneous, rare, and doubtful occurrences. SYN familial intestinal p.

po·lyp·o·tome (po-lip′ō-tōm). An instrument used for cutting away a polyp. [polyp + G. *tomos,* cutting]

pol·yp·o·trite (pol-ip′ō-trīt). An instrument for crushing polyps. [polyp + L. *tero,* pp. *tritus,* to rub]

pol·y·pous (pol′i-pŭs). Pertaining to, manifesting the gross features of, or characterized by the presence of a polyp or polyps.

pol·y·prag·ma·sy (pol-ē-prag′mă-sē). Administration of many different remedies at the same time. [poly- + G. *pragma,* a thing]

pol·y·pre·nols (pol-ē-prēn-olz). Acyclic polyisoprene alcohols.

pol·yp·tych·i·al (pol-ē-tik′ē-ăl). Folded or arranged so as to form more than one layer. [G. *polyptychos,* having many folds or layers, fr. poly- + *ptychē,* fold or layer]

pol·y·pus, pl. **po·ly·pi** (pol′i-pŭs, -pī). SYN polyp. [L.]

pol·y·ra·dic·u·li·tis (pol′ē-ra-dik′yū-lī′tis). SYN polyradiculopathy.

pol·y·ra·dic·u·lo·my·op·a·thy (pol′ē-ra-dik′yū-lō-mī-op′ă-thē). Coexisting polyradiculopathy and myopathy.

pol·y·ra·dic·u·lo·neu·rop·a·thy (pol-ē-ra-dik′yū-lō-nū-rop′ă-thē). Coexisting polyradiculopathy and polyneuropathy.

pol·y·ra·dic·u·lop·a·thy (pol-ē-ra-dik′yū-lop′ă-thē). Diffuse root involvement; seen with, among other disorders, diabetic neuropathy (diabetic polyradiculopathy). SYN polyradiculitis.

diabetic p., an inclusive term for several types of diabetic neuropathy other than a polyneuropathy; includes diabetic amyotrophy and diabetic thoracic radiculopathy; attributed to diabetes-induced injury of one or more roots, often sequential in the lumbar, thoracic, or occasionally, cervical region; affects primarily older males.

pol·y·ri·bo·nu·cle·o·tide nu·cle·o·tid·yl·trans·fer·ase (pol′ē-rī-bō-nū′klē-ō-tīd). An enzyme catalyzing phosphorolysis of polyribonucleotides or of RNA, yielding nucleoside diphosphates (or the reverse, the first artificial polynucleotide formation discovered). SYN polynucleotide phosphorylase.

pol·y·ri·bo·somes (pol-ē-rī′bō-sōmz). Conceptually, two or more ribosomes connected by a molecule of messenger RNA; structures satisfying this concept can be seen in electron micrographs and can be sedimented at rates consistent with aggregates of ribosomes (whence it is often, sometimes incorrectly, assumed that aggregates containing ribosomes are true p.); p. are active in protein synthesis. SYN polysomes.

pol·yr·rhea (pol-i-rē′ă). Profuse discharge of serous or other fluid. [poly- + G. *rhoia,* a flow]

pol·y·sac·char·ide (pol-ē-sak′ă-rīd). A carbohydrate containing a large number of saccharide groups; *e.g.,* starch. Cf. oligosaccharide. SYN glycan.

pneumococcal p., SYN specific capsular *substance.*

specific soluble p., SYN specific capsular *substance.*

pol·y·sce·lia (pol-ē-sē′lē-ă). A form of polymelia involving the presence of more than two legs. [poly- + G. *skelos,* leg]

pol·y·scope (pol′ē-skōp). SYN diaphanoscope.

pol·y·ser·o·si·tis (pol′ē-sēr-ō-sī′tis). Chronic inflammation with effusions in several serous cavities resulting in fibrous thickening of the serosa and constrictive pericarditis. SYN Bamberger's disease (2), Concato's disease, multiple serositis. [poly- + L. *serum,* serum, + G. *-itis,* inflammation]

familial paroxysmal p. [MIM*249100], transient recurring attacks of abdominal pain, fever, pleurisy, arthritis, and rash; the condition is asymptomatic between attacks; autosomal recessive inheritance. There is an autosomal dominant recessive [MIM*134610] in which amyloidosis in common. SYN benign paroxysmal peritonitis, familial Mediterranean fever, familial recurrent p., Mediterranean fever (2), periodic peritonitis, periodic p.

familial recurrent p., SYN familial paroxysmal p.

periodic p., SYN familial paroxysmal p.

recurrent p., familial Mediterranean *fever.*

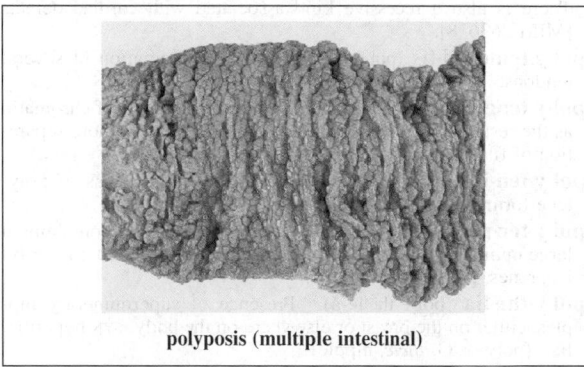
polyposis (multiple intestinal)

pol·y·si·nu·si·tis (pol′ē-sī-nŭ-sī′tis). Simultaneous inflammation of two or more sinuses.

pol·y·somes (pol′ē-sōmz). SYN polyribosomes.

pol·y·so·mia (pol-ē-sō′mē-ă). Fetal malformation involving two or more imperfect and partially fused bodies. [poly- + G. *sōma,* body]

pol·y·so·mic (pol-ē-sō′mik). Pertaining to or characterized by polysomy.

pol·y·som·no·gram (pol-ē-som′nō-gram). The recorded physiologic function(s) obtained in polysomnography. [poly- + L. *somnus,* sleep, + G. *gramma,* diagram]

pol·y·som·nog·ra·phy (pol′ē-som-nog′ră-fē). Simultaneous and continuous monitoring of relevant normal and abnormal physiological activity during sleep. [poly- + L. *somnus,* sleep, + G. *graphō,* to write]

pol·y·so·my (pol-ē-sō′mē). State of a cell nucleus in which a specific chromosome is represented more than twice. Cells containing three, four, or five homologous chromosomes are referred to, respectively, as trisomic, tetrasomic, or pentasomic. Cf. polyploidy. [poly- + G. *sōma,* body (chromosome)]

pol·y·sor·bate 80 (pol-ē-sōr′bāt). Polyoxethylene (20) sorbitan monooleate; a mixture of polyoxethylene ethers of mixed partial oleic esters of sorbitol anhydrides; used as an emulsifier, as in the preparation of pharmacologic products.

pol·y·sper·mia, pol·y·sper·mism (pol-ē-sper′mē-ă, -sper′mizm). **1.** SYN polyspermy. **2.** An abnormally profuse spermatic secretion.

pol·y·sper·my (pol′ē-sper-mē). The entrance of more than one spermatozoon into the ovum. SYN polyspermia (1), polyspermism.

pol·y·sple·nia (pol-ē-sple′nē-ă) [MIM*208530]. A condition in which splenic tissue is divided into nearly equal masses or totally absent; congenital heart disease and lung symmetry are common. The condition may be related to situs inversus. Most cases are sporadic. SEE ALSO bilateral *left-sidedness.* [poly- + G. *splēn,* spleen]

pol·y·ster·ax·ic (pol′ē-ster-ak′sik). Denoting behavior characterized by its socially provocative quality.

pol·y·stich·ia (pol-ē-stik′ē-ă). Arrangement of the eyelashes in two or more rows. [poly- + G. *stichos,* row]

pol·y·sul·fide rub·ber (pol-ē-sŭl′fīd). Synthetic rubber used as a dental impression material.

pol·y·sus·pen·soid (pol-ē-sŭs-pen′soyd). A colloid system of solid phases having different degrees of dispersion.

pol·y·sym·brach·y·dac·ty·ly (pol′ē-sim-brak-ē-dak′ti-lē). Malformation of the hand or foot in which the shortened digits are syndactylous and polydactylous. [poly- + symbrachydactyly]

pol·y·syn·ap·tic (pol′ē-si-nap′tik). Referring to neural pathways formed by a chain of a large number of synaptically connected nerve cells, as distinguished from oligosynaptic conduction systems. SYN multisynaptic.

pol·y·syn·dac·ty·ly (pol′ē-sin-dak′ti-lē). Syndactyly of several fingers or toes. There are several forms: a simple one [MIM*174700] and one with skull defects [MIM*175700].

There is also a recessive kind associated with cardiac defects [MIM 263638].

pol·y·ten·di·ni·tis (pol'ē-ten-di-nī'tis). Inflammation of several tendons.

pol·y·tene (pol'i-tēn). Consisting of many filaments of chromatin as the result of repeated division of chromonema without separation of filaments.

pol·y·ten·i·za·tion (pol'ē-ten-i-zā'shŭn). The process of polytene formation without separation.

pol·y·ter·penes (pol-ē-ter'pēnz). Acyclic polymers containing a large number of isoprene subunits, usually unsaturated. SYN polyisoprenes, polyisoprenoids.

pol·y·the·lia (pol-ē-thē'lē-ă). Presence of supernumerary nipples, either on the breast or elsewhere on the body. SYN hyperthelia. [poly- + G. *thēlē*, nipple]

pol·y·thi·a·zide (pol-ē-thī'ă-zīd). 6-Chloro-3,4-dihydro-2-methyl-3-[(2,2,2-trifluoroethylthio)methyl]-2*H*-1,2,4,-benzothiazine-7-sulfonamide 1,1-dioxide; a diuretic and antihypertensive of the benzothiadiazine group.

po·lyt·o·cous (pŏ-lit'ŏ-kŭs). Producing multiple young at a birth. [poly- + G. *tokos*, birth]

pol·y·to·mog·ra·phy (pol-i-tō-mog'ră-fē). Body section radiography using a machine designed to effect complex motion; images a thinner tissue plane compared to simple linear or circular tomography.

pol·y·trich·ia (pol-ē-trik'ē-ă). Excessive hairiness. SYN polytrichosis. [poly- + G. *thrix* (*trich*-), hair]

pol·y·tri·cho·sis (pol'ē-tri-kō'sis). SYN polytrichia.

pol·y·tro·phic (pol'ē-trō-fik). Exhibiting an attraction, trophism, for multiple organs; usually used for a virus which affects multiple organ systems.

pol·y·(u) Abbreviation for poly(uridylic acid).

pol·y·un·guia (pol-ē-ŭng'gwē-ă). SYN polyonychia. [poly- + L. *unguis*, nail]

pol·y·u·ria (pol-ē-yū'rē-ă). Excessive excretion of urine resulting in profuse micturition. [poly- + G. *ouron*, urine]

pol·y·(uri·dyl·ic ac·id) (pol·y·(u)). A homopolymer of uridylic acids.

pol·y·uro·nides (pol-ē-yūr'ō-nīdz). Polymers of uronic acids (*e.g.,* glucuronic acid, galacturonic acid); the pectins are p.

pol·y·va·lent (pol-ē-vā'lent). **1.** SYN multivalent. **2.** Pertaining to a polyvalent antiserum.

pol·y·vi·done (pol-ē-vī'dōn). SYN povidone.

pol·y·vi·nyl (pol-ē-vī'năl). Referring to a compound containing a number of vinyl groups in polymerized form.

pol·y·vi·nyl al·co·hol. A compound, $CH_2(CHOH)_n$, that is soluble in water; an adhesive and emulsifier.

pol·y·vi·nyl chlo·ride (PVC). A substance used as a rubber substitute in many industrial applications, and suspected of being carcinogenic in humans. SYN chlorethene homopolymer.

pol·y·vi·nyl·pyr·rol·i·done (PVP) (pol-ē-vī'nil-pi-rol'i-dōn). SYN povidone.

pol·y·vi·nyl·pyr·rol·i·done-io·dine com·plex. SYN povidone iodine.

pol·y·zo·ic (pol-ē-zō'ik). Segmented body form, as in the higher tapeworms, subclass Cestoda. SEE ALSO strobila, monozoic.

pol·y·zy·got·ic (pol-ē-zī-got'ik). SYN polyovulatory. [poly- + G. *zygōtos*, yoked]

po·made (pō-mād', pō-mahd'). An ointment or cream containing medicaments; usually used on the hair. SYN pomatum. [Fr. *pomade*, fr. L. *pomum*, apple]

po·ma·tum (pō-mā'tŭm). SYN pomade. [Mod. L.]

POMC Abbreviation for pro-opiomelanocortin.

pome·gran·ate (pom'gran-at). Fruit of *Punica granatum* (family Punicaceae), a reddish yellow fruit the size of an orange, containing many seeds enclosed in a reddish acidic pulp; used in diarrhea for its astringent properties; the bark of the tree and of the root contains pelletierine and other alkaloids, and has been used as a teniacide. SYN granatum. [L. *pomum*, apple, + *granatus,* many seeded, fr. *granum*, grain or seed]

Pomeroy, Ralph H., U.S. obstetrician-gynecologist, 1867–1925. SEE P.'s *operation.*

POMP Abbreviation for Purinethol (6-mercaptopurine), Oncovin (vincristine sulfate), methotrexate, and prednisone, a cancer chemotherapy regimen.

Pompe, J.C., 20th century Dutch physician. SEE P.'s *disease.*

pom·pho·lyx (pom'fō-liks). SYN dyshidrosis. [G. a bubble, fr. *pomphos,* a blister]

pom·phus (pom'fŭs). A wheal or blister. [G. *pomphos,* blister]

pon·ceau D xy·li·dine (pon-sō' dĕ zī'li-dēn) [C.I.-16151]. A monoazo acid dye originally employed as a red histological counterstain in Masson's trichrome stain.

Ponfick, Emil, German pathologist, 1844–1913. SEE P.'s *shadow.*

☐pono-. Bodily exertion, fatigue, overwork, pain. [G. *ponos,* toil, fatigue, pain]

po·no·graph (pō'nō-graf). An instrument for recording graphically the progressive fatigue of a contracting muscle. [pono- + G. *graphō,* to write]

po·no·pal·mo·sis (pō'nō-pal-mō'sis). Rarely used term for a condition of irritable heart in which palpitation is excited by slight exertion. [pono- + G. *palmos,* palpitation]

po·no·pho·bia (pō-nō-fō'bē-ă). Morbid fear of overwork or of becoming fatigued. [pono- + G. *phobos,* fear]

po·nos (pō'nos). A disease occurring in young children in certain of the islands of Greece, characterized by enlargement of the spleen, hemorrhages, fever, and cachexia; possibly the infantile form of visceral leishmaniasis. [G. toil, fatigue, pain]

pons, pl. **pon·tes** (ponz, pon'tēz). **1** [NA]. In neuroanatomy, the pons varolii or pons cerebelli; that part of the brainstem between the medulla oblongata caudally and the mesencephalon rostrally, composed of the ventral part of pons and the tegmentum pontis. On the ventral surface of the brain the ventral part of pons, the white pontine protuberance, is demarcated from both the medulla oblongata and the mesencephalon by distinct transverse grooves. SYN p. cerebelli, p. varolii. **2.** Any bridgelike formation connecting two more or less disjoined parts of the same structure or organ. [L. bridge]

p. cerebel'li, SYN pons (1).

p. hep'atis, a bridge of liver tissue that sometimes overlaps the fossa of the inferior vena cava, converting it into a canal. SYN ponticulus hepatis.

p. varo'lii, SYN pons (1).

pon·tes (pon'tēz). Plural of pons. [L.]

pon·tic (pon'tik). An artificial tooth on a fixed partial denture; it replaces the lost natural tooth, restores its functions, and usually occupies the space previously occupied by the natural crown. SYN dummy.

pon·ti·cu·lus (pon-tik'yū-lŭs). A vertical ridge on the eminentia conchae giving insertion to the auricularis posterior muscle. [L. dim. of *pons,* bridge]

p. hep'atis, SYN *pons* hepatis.

p. na'si, bridge of the nose.

p. promonto'rii, SYN *subiculum* promontorii.

pon·tile, pon·tine (pon'tīl, -tīn; -tēn). Relating to a pons.

Pool, Eugene H., U.S. surgeon, 1874–1949. SEE P.'s *phenomenon;* P.-Schlesinger *sign.*

pool (pūl). **1.** A collection of blood or other fluid in any region of the body; p. of blood results from dilation and retardation of the circulation in the capillaries and veins of the part. **2.** A combination of resources. [A.S. *pōl*]

abdominal p., the volume of blood within the abdomen.

gene p., the set of the genes that are available for inheritance in a particular mating population.

metabolic p., the quantity of a given chemical compound or group of related compounds participating in metabolic reactions; may constitute only a portion of the total bodily content of such compounds.

vaginal p., the secretions and material that accumulate in the posterior fornix of the vagina; used for sampling, principally for evaluation after premature rupture of the membranes.

pop·les (pop′lēz) [NA]. SYN popliteal *fossa*. SEE ALSO popliteal *fossa*. [L. the ham of the knee]

pop·lit·e·al (pop-lit′ē-ăl, pop-li-tē′ăl). Relating to the popliteal fossa. SYN popliteus (1).

pop·li·te·us (pop-li-tē′ŭs). **1.** SYN popliteal. **2.** SYN popliteal *fossa*. **3.** SYN popliteus *muscle*. [L.]

POPOP Abbreviation for 1,4-bis(5-phenyloxazol-2-yl)benzene, a liquid scintillator.

pop·py (pop′ē). SYN Papaver.

    p. oil, a fixed (drying) oil expressed from the seed of *Papaver somniferum;* sometimes used in the preparation of liniments and as a solvent of iodine in iodized oil.

pop·u·la·tion (pop-yū-lā′shŭn). Statistical term denoting all the objects, events, or subjects in a particular class. Cf. sample. [L. *populus,* a people, nation]

POR Abbreviation for problem-oriented *record*.

⌂**por-.** SEE poro-.

por·ce·lain (pōr′sĕ-lin). A powder composed of a clay, silica, and a flux which, when mixed with water, forms a paste that is molded to form artificial teeth, inlays, jacket crowns, and dentures. When heated, the materials fuse to form a ceramic.

por·cine (pōr′sīn, -sin). Relating to pigs. [L. *porcinus,* fr. *porcus,* a hog]

pore (pōr). **1.** An opening, hole, perforation, or foramen. A pore, meatus, or foramen. **2.** SYN sweat p. [G. *poros,* passageway]

    dilated p., an enlarged follicular opening of the skin, with a keratinous plug and occasional lanugo or mature hair. SYN acquired trichoepithelioma.

    external acoustic p., external auditory p., SYN *opening* of external acoustic meatus.

    gustatory p., the minute opening of a taste bud on the surface of the oral mucosa through which the gustatory hairs of the specialized neuroepithelial gustatory cells project. SYN porus gustatorius [NA], taste p.

    interalveolar p.'s, openings in the interalveolar septa of the lung. SYN Kohn's p.'s.

    internal acoustic p., auditory p., SYN *opening* of internal acoustic meatus.

    Kohn's p.'s, SYN interalveolar p.'s.

    nuclear p., an octagonal opening, about 70 nm across, where the inner and outer membranes of the nuclear envelope are continuous.

    skin p., SYN sweat p.

    slit p.'s, the intercellular clefts between the interdigitating pedicels of podocytes; they are part of the filtration barrier of renal corpuscles. SYN filtration slits.

    sweat p., the surface opening of the duct of a sweat gland. SYN porus sudoriferus [NA], porus [NA], pore (2), skin p.

    taste p., SYN gustatory p.

por·en·ce·pha·lia (pōr′en-se-fā′lē-ă). SYN porencephaly.

por·en·ce·phal·ic (pōr′en-se-fal′ik). Relating to or characterized by porencephaly. SYN porencephalous.

por·en·ceph·a·li·tis (pōr′en-sef-ă-lī′tis). Chronic inflammation of the brain with the formation of cavities in the organ's substance. [G. *poros,* pore, + *enkephalos,* brain, + *-itis,* inflammation]

por·en·ceph·a·lous (pōr-en-sef′ă-lŭs). SYN porencephalic.

por·en·ceph·a·ly (pōr-en-sef′ă-lē). The occurrence of cavities in the brain substance, communicating usually with the lateral ventricles. SYN porencephalia, splencephaly. [G. *poros,* pore, + *enkephalos,* brain]

Porges, Otto, Austrian bacteriologist, *1879. SEE P. *method;* P.-Meier *test.*

po·ri (pō′rī). Plural of porus.

po·ria (pōr′ē-ă). Plural of porion.

Po·rif·era (pō-rif′er-ă). The sponges; a phylum of the Metazoa, comprising a group of sessile, aquatic animals possessing an endoskeleton and many branching canals, lined by flagellated collar cells; communication of the canals with the surface is made through many pores or through larger openings and oscula. SEE ALSO Parazoa. [L. *porus,* pore, + *fero,* to bear]

po·rins (pōr′inz). Proteins found in the outer membrane of a double membrane that allow permeability in most small molecules. [G. *poros,* passageway, + -in]

por·i·o·ma·nia (pōr′ē-ō-mā′nē-ă). A morbid impulse to wander or journey away from home. [G. *poreia,* a journey, + *mania,* frenzy]

por·i·on, pl. **po·ria** (pōr′ē-on, -ē-ă). The central point on the upper margin of the external auditory meatus; as a cephalometric landmark, it is located in the middle of the metal rods of the cephalometer. [G. *poros,* a passage]

por·no·lag·nia (pōr-nō-lag′nē-ă). Sexual attraction toward prostitutes. [G. *pornē,* prostitute, + *lagneia,* lust]

⌂**poro-, por-. 1.** A pore, a duct, an opening. [G. *poros* (L. *porus*), passageway] **2.** A doing through, a passing through. [G. *poreia,* a journey, passage] **3.** A callus; an induration. [G. *poros,* a kind of marble, a stone]

po·ro·cele (pōr′ō-sēl). Obsolete term for a hernia with indurated coverings. [G. *pōros,* callus, + *kēlē,* hernia]

po·ro·ceph·a·li·a·sis (pō′rō-sef-ă-lī′ă-sis). Infection with a species of the tongue worms *Porocephalus.* SYN porocephalosis.

Po·ro·ce·phal·i·dae (pō′rō-se-fal′i-dē). A family of parasitic tongue worms (order Porocephalida, phylum Pentastomida) characterized by four hooks arranged in a curved line on either side of the mouth. Adults are found in the lungs of reptiles, and larvae or nymphs are found in the tissues of a great variety of vertebrates, including humans. SEE ALSO Linguatulidae, *Armillifer, Linguatula.* [G. *poros,* pore, + *kephalē,* head]

po·ro·ceph·a·lo·sis (pō′rō-sef-ă-lō′sis). SYN porocephaliasis.

Po·ro·ceph·a·lus (pō-rō-sef′ă-lŭs). A genus of tongue worms of the family Porocephalidae, of which the adult worms or larvae cause porocephaliasis in a number of animal species including humans. [G. *poros,* pore, + *kephalē,* head]

    P. armilla′tus, SYN *Armillifer armillatus.*

po·ro·co·nid·i·um (pōr′ō-kŏ-nid′ē-ŭm). In fungi, a conidium produced through the microscopic pore of the condidiophore. SYN porospore.

po·ro·ker·a·to·sis (pō′rō-ker-ă-tō′sis). A rare dermatosis in which there is a thickening of the stratum corneum with an annular keratotic rim or cornoid lamella surrounding progressive centrifugal atrophy; cutaneous carcinoma has been reported to arise in the lesions. SYN hyperkeratosis eccentrica, hyperkeratosis figurata centrifuga atrophica, keratoatrophoderma, keratoderma eccentrica, Mibelli's disease. [G. *poros,* pore, + keratosis]

    actinic p., a lesion which occurs on exposed areas of extremities primarily; bears a resemblance to actinic keratosis but the histologic features are those of p.

po·ro·ma (pō-rō′mă). **1.** SYN callosity. **2.** SYN exostosis. **3.** Induration following a phlegmon. **4.** A tumor of cells lining the skin openings of sweat glands. [G. *pōrōma,* callus, fr. *pōros,* stone]

    eccrine p., a p. or acrospiroma of the eccrine sweat glands, usually occurring on the sole of the foot.

po·ro·sis, pl. **po·ro·ses** (pō-rō′sis, -sēz). A porous condition. SYN porosity (1). [L. *porosus,* porous]

    cerebral p., a porous condition of the brain caused by postmortem growth of *Clostridium perfringens* or other gas-forming organisms in the tissue.

po·ros·i·ty (pō-ros′i-tē). **1.** SYN porosis. **2.** A perforation. [G. *poros,* pore]

po·ro·spore (pōr′ō-spōr). SYN poroconidium.

po·rot·ic (pō-rot′ik). Porous, as in osteoporotic.

po·rous (pō′rŭs). Having openings that pass directly or indirectly through the substance.

por·phin, por·phine (pōr′fin). The unsubstituted cyclic tetrapyrrole nucleus that is the basis of the porphyrins. SEE ALSO porphyrins. Cf. chlorin, phorbin, corrin. SYN porphyrin.

por·pho·bi·lin (pōr′fō-bī′lin). General term denoting intermediates between the monopyrrole, porphobilinogen, and the cyclic tetrapyrrole of heme (a porphin derivative). SEE ALSO bilin.

por·pho·bi·lin·o·gen (PBG) (pōr′fō-bī-lin′ō-jen). 5-Aminomethyl-4-carboxymethylpyrrole-3-propionic acid; a porphyrin

po

precursor of porphyrinogens, porphyrins, and heme; found in the urine in large quantities in cases of acute or congenital porphyria.

p. synthase, a liver enzyme catalyzing the formation of porphobilinogen and water from 2 molecules of δ-aminolevulinate, an important reaction in porphyrin biosynthesis; inhibited by lead in cases of lead poisoning; a deficiency of this enzyme results in elevated levels of δ-aminolevulinate and results in neurological disturbances. SYN δ-aminolevulinate dehydratase.

por·phyr·ia (pōr-fir′ē-ă). A group of disorders involving heme biosynthesis, characterized by excessive excretion of porphyrins or their precursors; may be inherited or may be acquired, as from the effects of certain chemical agents (*e.g.,* hexachlorobenzene).

acute intermittent p., acute p., SYN intermittent acute p.

δ-aminolevulinate dehydratase p., an inherited disorder in which there is a deficiency of porphobilinogen synthase; δ-aminolevulinate levels are elevated, leading to neurological disturbances. SYN porphobilinogen synthase p.

bovine p., p. as a mendelian recessive trait in certain breeds of cattle.

congenital erythropoietic p. [MIM*263700], enhanced porphyrin formation by erythroid cells in bone marrow, leading to severe porphyrinuria, often with hemolytic anemia and persistent cutaneous photosensitivity; caused by a deficiency of uroporphyrinogen III cosynthetase; autosomal recessive inheritance; there is an overproduction of type I porphyrin isomers.

p. cuta′nea tar′da (PCT) [MIM*176090, MIM*176100], familial or sporadic p. characterized by liver dysfunction and photosensitive cutaneous lesions, with hyperpigmentation and scleroderma-like changes in the skin, and increased excretion of uroporphyrin; caused by a deficiency of uroporphyrinogen decarboxylase induced in sporadic cases by chronic alcoholism; autosomal dominant inheritance in familial cases. SYN symptomatic p.

p. cuta′nea tar′da heredita′ria, SEE p. cutanea tarda.

p. cuta′nea tar′da symptoma′tica, SEE p. cutanea tarda.

erythropoietic p., a classification of p. that includes congenital erythropoietic p. and erythropoietic protoporphyria.

hepatic p. [MIM*176100.0002], a category of p. that includes p. cutanea tarda, variegate p., and coproporphyria. SYN p. hepatica.

p. hepatica (he-pat′ĭ-kă), SYN hepatic p.

hepatoerythropoietic p., an autosomal recessive disorder in which there is a deficiency or absence of uroporphyrinogen decarboxylase; results in photosensitivity and excessive hepatic production of 8- and 7-carboxylate porphyrins.

intermittent acute p. (IAP) [MIM*176000], p. caused by hepatic overproduction of δ-aminolevulinic acid, with greatly increased urinary excretion of it and of porphobilinogen, and some increase of uroporphyrin, due to a deficiency of porphobilinogen deaminase; characterized by intermittent acute attacks of hypertension, abdominal colic, psychosis, and polyneuropathy, but with no photosensitivity; autosomal dominant inheritance; exacerbation caused by ingestion of certain drugs (*e.g.,* barbiturates). SYN acute intermittent p., acute p.

ovulocyclic p., acute episodic exacerbations of p. occurring in the premenstrual period.

porphobilinogen synthase p., SYN δ-aminolevulinate dehydratase p.

South African type p., SYN variegate p.

squirrel p., p. as an apparently normal metabolic state seen in the Florida fox squirrel (*Sciurus niger*).

swine p., p. as a dominant trait seen in swine.

symptomatic p., SYN p. cutanea tarda.

variegate p. (VP) [MIM*176200], p. characterized by abdominal pain and neuropsychiatric abnormalities, by dermal sensitivity to light and mechanical trauma, by increased fecal excretion of proto- and coproporphyrin, and by increased urinary excretion of δ-aminolevulinic acid, porphobilinogen, and porphyrins; due to a deficiency of protoporphyrinogen oxidase; autosomal dominant inheritance. SYN protocoproporphyria hereditaria, South African type p.

por·phy·rin (pōr′fi-rin). SYN porphin.

por·phy·rin·o·gens (pōr-fi-rin′ō-jenz). Intermediates in the biosynthesis of heme, as follows: four porphobilinogens condense to form uroporphyrinogens I and III (giving rise to side products

uroporphyrins I and III) which are decarboxylated to form coproporphyrinogens I and III (giving rise to side products coproporphyrins I and III); coproporphyrinogen III is oxidized to protoporphyrinogen III (IX) which is then oxidized to form protoporphyrin III (IX) (this last intermediate adds ferrous iron to yield heme); certain p. are elevated in certain porphyrias.

por·phy·ri·nop·a·thy (pōr′fir-in-op′ă-thē). A syndrome which results from abnormal porphyrin metabolism such as acute porphyria. SYN porphyrism. [porphyrin + G. *pathos,* disease]

por·phy·rins (pōr′fi-rinz). Pigments widely distributed throughout nature (*e.g.,* heme, bile pigments, cytochromes) consisting of four pyrroles joined in a ring (porphin) structure. They are substitution products of porphin (porphyrin) and comprise several varieties, differing for the most part in the sidechains (methyl, ethyl, vinyl, formyl, carboxyethyl, carboxymethyl, etc.) present at the eight available positions on the pyrrole rings. Depending on the nature of the side chains, the prefixes dentero-, etio-, meso-, proto-, etc., are attached to p.; distribution within each class is given by type I, II, III, and IV. P. combine with various metals (iron, copper, magnesium, etc.) to form metalloporphyrins, and with nitrogenous substances.

por·phy·ri·nu·ria (pōr′fir-i-nū′rē-ă). Excretion of porphyrins and related compounds in the urine. SYN porphyruria, purpurinuria.

por·phy·rism. SYN porphyrinopathy.

por·phy·ri·za·tion (pōr′fi-ri-zā′shŭn). Grinding in a mortar (formerly on a slab of porphyry).

por·phy·ru·ria (pōr-fi-rū′rē-ă). SYN porphyrinuria.

por·ri·go (pō-rī′gō). Obsolete term for any disease of the scalp; *e.g.,* ringworm, favus, eczema. [L. scurf, dandruff]

p. decal′vans, obsolete term for *alopecia* areata.

p. favo′sa, SYN favus.

p. fur′furans, SYN *tinea* tonsurans.

p. larva′lis, eczema of the scalp.

p. lupino′sa, SYN favus.

p. scutula′ta, SYN favus.

Porro, Edoardo, Italian obstetrician, 1842–1902. SEE P. *hysterectomy, operation.*

por·ta, pl. **por·tae** (pōr′tă, -tē). **1.** SYN hilum (1). **2.** SYN interventricular *foramen.* [L. gate]

p. hep′atis [NA], a transverse fissure on the visceral surface of the liver between the caudate and quadrate lobes, lodging the portal vein, hepatic artery, hepatic nerve plexus, hepatic ducts, and lymphatic vessels. SYN caudal transverse fissure, portal fissure.

p. lie′nis, SYN *hilum* of spleen.

p. pulmo′nis, SYN *hilum* of lung.

p. re′nis, SYN *hilum* of kidney.

por·ta·ca·val (pōr′tă-kā′văl). Concerning the portal vein and the inferior vena cava.

por·tal (pōr′tăl). **1.** Relating to any porta or hilus, specifically to the porta hepatis and the p. vein. **2.** The point of entry into the body of a pathogenic microorganism. [L. *portalis,* pertaining to a porta (gate)]

anterior intestinal p., SYN *fovea* cardiaca.

posterior intestinal p., in young embryos, the communications from the midgut to the hindgut.

Porter, Curt C., U.S. biochemist, *1914. SEE P.-Silber *chromogens,* under *chromogen, reaction,* chromogens *test.*

Porter, Thomas C., British scientist, 1860–1933. SEE Ferry-P. *law.*

Porter, William H., Irish surgeon, 1790–1861. SEE P.'s *fascia.*

por·tio, pl. **por·ti·o·nes** (pōr′shē-ō, -ō′nēz) [NA]. A part. [L. portion]

p. interme′dia, SYN *nervus* intermedius.

p. ma′jor ner′vi trigem′ini, SYN sensory *root* of trigeminal nerve.

p. mi′nor ner′vi trigem′ini, SYN motor *root* of trigeminal nerve.

p. supravagina′lis [NA], SYN supravaginal *portion* of cervix.

p. vagina′lis [NA], SYN vaginal *portion* of cervix.

por·tion (pōr′shun). Part or division.

accessory p. of spinal accessory nerve, SYN cranial *root* of accessory nerve.

mesenteric p. of small intestine, SYN *intestinum* tenue mesenteriale.

subcutaneous p. of external anal sphincter, SYN subcutaneous *part* of external anal sphincter. SEE external anal *sphincter.*

supravaginal p. of cervix, the part of the cervix of the uterus lying above the attachment of the vagina. SYN portio supravaginalis [NA].

vaginal p. of cervix, the part of the cervix uteri contained within the vagina. SYN portio vaginalis [NA].

por·ti·plex·us (pōr-ti-plek′sŭs). The union of the choroid plexus of the lateral ventricle with that of the third ventricle at the interventricular foramen (of Monro).

⌂**porto-.** Portal. [L. *porta,* gate]

por·to·bil·i·o·ar·te·ri·al (pōr′tō-bil′ē-ō-ar-tēr′ē-ăl). Relating to the portal vein, biliary ducts, and hepatic artery, which have similar distributions. SEE ALSO portal *triad.*

por·to·en·ter·os·to·my (pōr′tō-en-ter-os′tō-mē). An operation for biliary atresia in which a Roux-en-Y loop of jejunum is anastomosed to the hepatic end of the divided extravascular portal structures, including rudimentary bile ducts. SYN Kasai operation.

por·to·gram (pōr′tō-gram). Radiographic record of portography. [porto- + G. *gramma,* a writing]

por·tog·ra·phy (pōr-tog′ră-fē). Delineation of the portal circulation by roentgenograms, using radiopaque material, usually introduced into the spleen or into the portal vein at operation. SYN portovenography. [porto- + G. *graphō,* to write]

por·to·sys·tem·ic (pōr′tō-sis-tem′ik). Relating to connections between the portal and systemic venous systems.

por·to·ve·nog·ra·phy (pōr′tō-vē-nog′ră-fē). SYN portography.

po·rus, pl. **po·ri** (pō′rŭs, -rī) [NA]. SYN sweat *pore.* SEE ALSO opening. [L. fr. G. *poros,* passageway]

p. acus′ticus exter′nus [NA], SYN *opening* of external acoustic meatus.

p. acus′ticus inter′nus [NA], SYN *opening* of internal acoustic meatus.

p. crotaphy′tico-buccinato′rius, an occasional foramen in the sphenoid bone through which passes the motor portion of the trigeminal nerve; it is formed by ossification of a ligament below and lateral to the foramen ovale. SYN Hyrtl's foramen.

p. gustato′rius [NA], SYN gustatory *pore.*

p. op′ticus, SYN optic *disk.*

p. sudorif′erus [NA], SYN sweat *pore.*

Posadas, Alejandro, Argentinian parasitologist, 1870–1902. SEE P. *disease.*

POSITION

---

po·si·tion (pŏ-zish′ŭn). **1.** An attitude, posture, or place occupied. **2.** Posture or attitude assumed by a patient for comfort and to facilitate the performance of diagnostic, surgical, or therapeutic procedures. **3.** In obstetrics, the relation of an arbitrarily chosen portion of the fetus to the right or left side of the mother; with each presentation there may be a right or left p.; the fetal occiput, chin, and sacrum are the determining points of p. in vertex, face, and breech presentations, respectively. Cf. presentation. [L. *positio,* a placing, position, fr. *pono,* to place]

anatomical p., the erect p. of the body with the face directed forward (skull aligned in orbitomeatal or Frankfort plane); the arms at the side and the palms of the hands directed forward; the terms posterior, anterior, lateral, medial, etc., are applied to the parts as they stand related to each other and to the axis of the body when in this p.

Bozeman's p., knee-elbow p., the patient being strapped to supports.

Casselberry p., a prone p. assumed when drinking, after intubation, in order to prevent the entrance of fluid into the tube.

centric p., the p. of the mandible in its most retruded unstrained relation to the maxillae. SEE ALSO centric jaw *relation.*

condylar hinge p., (1) the p. of the condyles in the temporomandibular joints from which a hinge movement is possible; **(2)** the maxillomandibular relation from which a consciously stimulated true hinge movement can be executed.

dorsal p., SYN supine p.

dorsosacral p., SYN lithotomy p.

eccentric p., SYN eccentric *relation.*

electrical heart p., a description of the heart's assumed electrical habitus based upon the form of the QRS complexes in leads aVL, aVF, V_1, and V_6. Sometimes loosely (and inaccurately) used to describe the frontal plane electric axis. SYN heart p.

Elliot's p., a supine p. upon a double inclined plane or on a single inclined plane, with a cushion under the back at the level of the liver; used to facilitate abdominal section.

English p., SYN Sims' p.

flank p., a lateral recumbent p., but with the lower leg flexed, the upper leg extended, and convex extension of the upper side of the body; used for nephrectomy.

Fowler's p., an inclined p. obtained by raising the head of the bed about 60 to 90 cm to promote better dependent drainage after an abdominal operation.

frontoanterior p., a cephalic presentation of the fetus with its forehead directed toward the right (**right frontoanterior,** RFA) or to the left (**left frontoanterior,** LFA) of the acetabulum of the mother.

frontoposterior p., a cephalic presentation of the fetus with its forehead directed toward the right (**right frontoposterior,** RFP) or to the left (**left frontoposterior,** LFP) sacroiliac articulation of the mother.

frontotransverse p., a cephalic presentation of the fetus with its forehead directed toward the right (**right frontotransverse,** RFT) or to the left (**left frontotransverse,** LFT) iliac fossa of the mother.

genucubital p., SYN knee-elbow p.

genupectoral p., SYN knee-chest p.

heart p., SYN electrical heart p.

hinge p., in dentistry, the orientation of parts in a manner permitting hinge movement between them.

intercuspal p., the p. of the mandible when the cusps and sulci of the maxillary and mandibular teeth are in their greatest contact and the mandible is in its most closed position.

knee-chest p., a prone posture resting on the knees and upper part of the chest, assumed for gynecologic or rectal examination. SYN genupectoral p.

knee-elbow p., a prone p. resting on the knees and elbows, assumed for gynecologic or rectal examination or operation. SYN genucubital p.

lateral recumbent p., SYN Sims' p.

leapfrog p., a stooping p., such as that taken by children in playing leapfrog, assumed for rectal examination.

lithotomy p., a supine p. with buttocks at the end of the operating table, the hips and knees being fully flexed with feet strapped in p. SYN dorsosacral p.

mandibular hinge p., any p. of the mandible which exists when the condyles are so situated in the temporomandibular joints that opening or closing movements can be made on the hinge axis.

Mayo-Robson's p., a supine p. with a thick pad under the loins, causing a marked lordosis in this region; used in operations on the gallbladder.

mentoanterior p., a cephalic presentation of the fetus with its chin pointing to the right (**right mentoanterior,** RMA) or to the left (**left mentoanterior,** LMA) acetabulum of the mother.

mentoposterior p., a cephalic presentation of the fetus with its chin pointing to the right (**right mentoposterior,** RMP) or to the left (**left mentoposterior,** LMP) sacroiliac articulation of the mother.

mentotransverse p., a cephalic presentation of the fetus with its chin pointing to the right (**right mentotransverse**, RMT) or to the left (**left mentotransverse**, LMT) iliac fossa of the mother.

Noble's p., patient standing and bent slightly forward; useful for inspection of a swelling of the loin that may occur with pyelonephritis.

obstetric p., the p. assumed by the parturient woman, either dorsal recumbent or lateral recumbent.

occipitoanterior p., a cephalic presentation of the fetus with its occiput turned toward the right (**right occipitoanterior**, ROA) or to the left (**left occipitoanterior**, LOA) acetabulum of the mother.

occipitoposterior p., a cephalic presentation of the fetus with its occiput turned toward the right (**right occipitoposterior**, ROP) or to the left (**left occipitoposterior**, LOP) sacroiliac joint of the mother.

occipitotransverse p., a cephalic presentation of the fetus with its occiput turned toward the right (**right occipitotransverse**, ROT) or to the left (**left occipitotransverse**, LOT) iliac fossa of the mother.

occlusal p., the relationship of the mandible and maxillae when the jaws are closed and the teeth are in contact; it may or may not coincide with centric occlusion.

orthopnea p., SYN orthopneic p.

orthopneic p., the p. assumed by patients with orthopnea, namely sitting propped up in bed by several pillows. SYN orthopnea p.

physiologic rest p., the usual p. of the mandible when the patient is resting comfortably in the upright p. and the condyles are in a neutral unstrained p. in the glenoid fossae. SEE ALSO rest *relation*. SYN postural p., postural resting p., rest p.

postural p., postural resting p., SYN physiologic rest p.

prone p., lying face down.

protrusive p., a forward p. of the mandible produced by muscular effort.

rest p., SYN physiologic rest p.

reverse Trendelenburg p., supine position without flexing or extending, in which the head is higher than the feet.

Rose's p., the patient lies on his back with the head falling down over the end of the table; used in operations within the mouth or pharynx.

sacroanterior p., a breech presentation of the fetus with the sacrum pointing to the right (**right sacroanterior**, RSA) or to the left (**left sacroanterior**, LSA) acetabulum of the mother.

sacroposterior p., a breech presentation of the fetus with the sacrum pointing to the right (**right sacroposterior**, RSP) or to the left (**left sacroposterior**, LSP) sacroiliac articulation of the mother.

sacrotransverse p., a breech presentation of the fetus with its sacrum pointing to the right (**right sacrotransverse**, RST) or to the left (**left sacrotransverse**, LST) sacroiliac articulation of the mother.

Scultetus' p., a supine p. on an inclined plane with head low, recommended by Scultetus for herniotomy and castration.

semiprone p., SYN Sims' p.

Simon's p., a p. for vaginal examination; a supine p. with hips elevated, thighs and legs flexed, and thighs widely separated.

Sims' p., a p. to facilitate a vaginal examination, the patient lying on the side with the under arm behind the back, the thighs flexed, the upper one more than the lower. SYN English p., lateral recumbent p., semiprone p.

supine p., lying upon the back. SYN dorsal p.

terminal hinge p., the mandibular hinge p. from which further opening of the mandible would produce translatory rather than hinge movement.

Trendelenburg's p., a supine p. on the operating table, which is inclined at varying angles so that the pelvis is higher than the head with the knees flexed and legs hanging over the end of the table; used during and after operations in the pelvis or for shock.

Valentine's p., a supine p. on a table with double inclined plane so as to cause flexion at the hips; used to facilitate urethral irrigation.

Walcher p., obsolete term for a supine p. of the parturient woman with the lower extremities falling over the edge of the table.

po·si·tion·er (pŏ-zish'ŭn-er). A resilient elastoplastic or rubber removable appliance fitting over the occlusal surface of the teeth, to obtain limited tooth movement and/or stabilization, usually used at the end of orthodontic treatment.

pos·i·tive (poz'i-tiv). **1.** Affirmative; definite; not negative. **2.** Denoting a response, the occurrence of a reaction, or the existence of the entity or condition in question. **3.** Having a value greater than zero. [L. *positivus*, settled by arbitrary agreement, fr. *pono*, pp. *positus*, to set, place]

pos·i·tive G. Gravity or acceleration in the usual head-to-foot direction in flying or in standing upright; the reverse of negative G.

pos·i·tron (β⁺) (poz'i-tron). A subatomic particle of mass and charge equal to the electron but of opposite (*i.e.*, positive) charge. SYN positive electron.

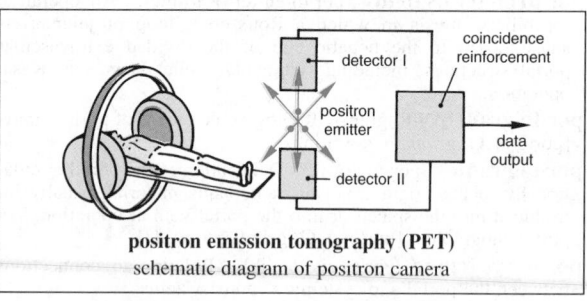

positron emission tomography (PET)
schematic diagram of positron camera

po·so·log·ic (pō-sō-loj'ik). Relating to posology.

po·sol·o·gy (pō-sol'ō-jē). The branch of pharmacology and therapeutics concerned with a determination of the doses of remedies; the science of dosage. [G. *posos*, how much, + *logos*, study]

post (pōst). In dentistry, a dowel or pin inserted into the root canal of a natural tooth as an attachment for an artificial crown.

⚠ **post-.** After, behind, posterior; opposite of anti-. Cf. meta-. [L. *post*]

post·ac·e·tab·u·lar (pōst'as-ĕ-tab'yū-lăr). Posterior to the acetabular cavity.

post·ad·o·les·cence (pōst-ad-ō-les'ens). The period after adolescence or puberty.

post·a·nal (pōst-ā'năl). Posterior to the anus.

post·an·es·thet·ic (pōst'an-es-thet'ik). Occurring after anesthesia.

post·ap·o·plec·tic (pōst'ap-ō-plek'tik). Occurring after an attack of apoplexy.

post·ax·i·al (pōst-ak'sē-ăl). **1.** Posterior to the axis of the body or any limb, the latter being in the anatomical position. **2.** Denoting the portion of a limb bud that lies caudal to the axis of the limb: the ulnar aspect of the upper limb and the fibular aspect of the lower limb.

post·bra·chi·al (pōst'brā'kē-ăl). On or in the posterior part of the upper arm.

post·car·di·nal (pōst'kar'di·năl). Relating to the posterior cardinal veins.

post·ca·va (pōst'kā'vă). SYN inferior *vena* cava.

post·ca·val (pōst'kā'văl). Relating to the inferior vena cava.

post·cen·tral (pōst-sen'trăl). Referring to the cerebral convolution forming the posterior bank of the central sulcus: the postcentral gyrus.

post·chrom·ing (pōst'krōm'ing). SYN afterchroming.

post·ci·bal (pōst-sī'bă). After a meal or the taking of food. [L. *cibum*, food]

post·cla·vic·u·lar (pōst'kla-vik'yū-lăr). Posterior to the clavicle.

post·co·i·tal (pōst-kō'i-tăl). After coitus.

post·co·i·tus (pōst-kō'i-tŭs). The time immediately after coitus.

post·cor·dial (pōst′kōr′jăl). Posterior to the heart. [L. *cor* (*cord-*), heart]

post·cos·tal (pōst-kos′tăl). Behind the ribs.

post·crown. A crown, replacing the natural crown, which is retained on the stump of the root of a tooth from which the pulp has been removed, by a post or pin integral with the crown and sealed in the treated root canal with a cement.

post·cu·bi·tal (pōst′kyū′bi-tăl). On or in the posterior or dorsal part of the forearm.

post·dam. SYN posterior palatal *seal*.

post·di·a·stol·ic (pōst′dī-ă-stol′ik). Following diastole.

post·di·crot·ic (pōst-dī-krot′ik). Following the dicrotic wave in a sphygmogram; denoting an additional variation in the descending line of the pulse tracing.

post·diph·the·rit·ic (pōst′dif-the-rit′ik). Following or occurring as a sequel of diphtheria.

post·dor·mi·tal (pōst-dōr′mi-tăl). Relating to the postdormitum.

post·dor·mi·tum (pōst-dōr′mi-tŭm). The period of increasing consciousness between sound sleep and waking. [L. *dormio,* to sleep]

post·duc·tal (pōst-dŭk′tăl). Relating to that part of the aorta distal to the aortic opening of the ductus arteriosus.

post·en·ceph·a·lit·ic (pōst-en-sef′ă-lit′ik). Following encephalitis.

post·ep·i·lep·tic (pōst′ep-i-lep′tik). Following an epileptic seizure.

pos·te·ri·or (pos-tēr′ē-ŏr). **1.** After, in relation to time or space. **2** [NA]. In human anatomy, denoting the back surface of the body. Often used to indicate the position of one structure relative to another, *i.e.,* nearer the back of the body. SYN dorsalis [NA], dorsal (2), posticus. **3.** Near the tail or caudal end of certain embryos. **4.** An undesirable and confusing substitute for caudal in quadrupeds; in veterinary anatomy, p. is used only to denote some structures of the head. [L. comparative of *posterus,* following]

pos·te·ri·us (pos-tēr′ē-ŭs). Neuter of posterior. [L.]

⚠**postero-.** Posterior; at the back of. [L. *posterior*]

pos·ter·o·an·te·ri·or (pos′ter-ō-an-tēr′ē-ŏr). A term denoting the direction of view or progression, from posterior to anterior, through a part.

pos·ter·o·clu·sion (pos′ter-ō-klū′shŭn). SYN posterior *occlusion.*

pos·ter·o·ex·ter·nal (pos′ter-ō-ek-ster′năl). SYN posterolateral.

pos·ter·o·in·ter·nal (pos′ter-ō-in-ter′năl). SYN posteromedial.

pos·ter·o·lat·er·al (pos′ter-ō-lat′ĕ-răl). Behind and to one side, specifically to the outer side. SYN posteroexternal.

pos·ter·o·me·di·al (pos′ter-ō-mē′dē-ăl). Behind and to the inner side. SYN posterointernal.

pos·ter·o·me·di·an (pos′ter-ō-mē′dē-an). Occupying a central position posteriorly.

pos·ter·o·pa·ri·e·tal (pos′ter-ō-pa-rī′ĕ-tăl). Relating to the posterior portion of the parietal lobe of the cerebrum.

pos·ter·o·su·pe·ri·or (pos′ter-ō-sū-pē′rē-ŏr). Situated behind and at the upper part.

pos·ter·o·tem·po·ral (pos′ter-ō-tem′po-răl). Relating to or lying in the posterior portion of the temporal lobe of the cerebrum.

post·e·soph·a·ge·al (pōst′ē-sof′ă-jē′ăl, ē-sŏ-faj′ē-ăl). Behind the esophagus.

post·es·trus, post·es·trum (pōst-es′trŭs, -trŭm). The period in the estrus cycle following estrus; characterized by the growth of the corpus luteum and physiologic changes related to the production of progesterone.

post·feb·rile (pōst-fē′brĭl). Occurring after a fever. SYN metapyretic.

post·gan·gli·on·ic (pōst′gang-glē-on′ik). Distal to or beyond a ganglion; referring to the unmyelinated nerve fibers originating from cells in an autonomic ganglion.

post·hem·i·ple·gic (pōst′hem-i-plē′jik). Following hemiplegia.

post·hem·or·rha·gic (pōst-hem-ŏ-raj′ik). Following a hemorrhage.

post·he·pat·ic (pōst-he-pat′ik). Behind the liver.

pos·thet·o·my (pos-thet′ō-mē). Dorsal slit of foreskin. [G. *posthē,* prepuce, + *tomē,* incision]

pos·thi·o·plas·ty (pos′thē-ō-plas-tē). Surgical reconstruction of the prepuce. [G. *posthion,* dim. form of *posthē,* prepuce, + *plastos,* formed]

pos·thi·tis (pos-thī′tis). Inflammation of the prepuce. [G. *posthē,* prepuce, + *-itis,* inflammation]

ulcerative p., a contagious disease of sheep and goats caused by the bacterium *Corynebacterium renale* in the presence of high levels of urinary urea and characterized by ulceration, with scab formation, of the prepuce. SYN enzootic balanoposthitis, pizzle rot, sheath rot.

pos·tho·lith (pos′thō-lith). SYN preputial *calculus.* [G. *posthē,* prepuce, + *lithos,* stone]

post·hy·oid (pōst-hī′oyd). Behind the hyoid bone.

post·hyp·not·ic (pōst-hip-not′ik). Following hypnotism; denoting an act suggested during hypnosis that is to be carried out at some time after the hypnotized subject is awakened.

post·ic·tal (pōst-ik′tăl). Following a seizure, *e.g.,* epileptic.

pos·ti·cus (pos-tī′kŭs). SYN posterior (2). [L. fr. *post,* after]

post·in·flu·en·zal (pōst′in-flū-en′zăl). Occurring as a sequel to influenza.

post·is·chi·al (pōst-is′kē-ăl). Posterior to the ischium.

post·ma·lar·i·al (pōst-mă-lār′ē-ăl). Occurring as a sequel to malaria.

post·mas·toid (pōst-mas′toyd). Posterior to the mastoid process.

post·ma·ture (pōst-mă-tūr′, mă-tyūr′). The fetus that remains in the uterus longer than the normal gestational period; *i.e.,* longer than 42 weeks (288 days) in humans.

post·me·di·an (pōst′mē′dē-an). Posterior to the median plane.

post·me·di·as·ti·nal (pōst′mē′dē-as′ti-năl, -mē′dē-ă-stī′năl). **1.** Posterior to the mediastinum. **2.** Relating to the posterior mediastinum.

post·me·di·as·ti·num (pōst′mē′dē-ă-stī′nŭm). SYN posterior *mediastinum.*

post·men·o·pau·sal (pōst-men-ō-paw′săl). Relating to the period following the menopause.

post·min·i·mus (pōst-min′i-mŭs). A small accessory appendage attached to the side of the fifth finger or toe; it may resemble a normal digit or be merely a fleshy mass. [post- + L. *minimus,* smallest (finger)]

post·mor·tem (pōst-mōr′tem). **1.** Pertaining to or occurring during the period after death. **2.** Colloquialism for autopsy (1). [post- + L. acc. case of *mors* (*mort-*), death]

post·na·ri·al (pōst′nā′rē-ăl). Relating to the posterior nares or choanae.

post·na·ris (pōst′nā′ris). SYN choana.

post·na·sal (pōst′nā′săl). **1.** Posterior to the nasal cavity. **2.** Relating to the posterior portion of the nasal cavity.

post·na·tal (pōst-nā′tăl). Occurring after birth. [L. *natus,* birth]

post·ne·crot·ic (post-ne-krot′ik). Subsequent to the death of a tissue or part of the body.

post·neu·rit·ic (pōst-nū-rit′ik). Following neuritis.

post·oc·u·lar (pōst′ok′yū-lăr). Posterior to the eyeball. [L. *oculus,* eye]

post·op·er·a·tive (pōst-op′er-ă-tiv). Following an operation.

post·o·ral (pos-tō′răl). In the posterior part of, or posterior to, the mouth. [L. *os* (*or-*), mouth]

post·or·bi·tal (pōst′ōr′bi-tăl). Posterior to the orbit.

post·pal·a·tine (pōst′pal′ă-tīn). Posterior to the palatine bones. Usually used to refer to the soft palate.

post·par·a·lyt·ic (pōst′par-ă-lit′ik). Following or consequent upon paralysis.

post·par·tum (pōst-par′tŭm). After childbirth. Cf. antepartum, intrapartum. [L. *partus,* birth (noun), fr. *pario,* pp. *partus,* to bring forth]

post·pha·ryn·ge·al (pōst′fă-rin′jē-ăl). Posterior to the pharynx.

post·pneu·mon·ic (pōst-nū-mon′ik). Following or occurring as a sequel to pneumonia.

po

post·pran·di·al (pōst-pran'dē-ăl). Following a meal. [L. *prandium,* breakfast]

post·pu·ber·al, post·pu·ber·tal (pōst-pū'ber-ăl, -ber-tăl). SYN postpubescent.

post·pu·ber·ty (pōst-pū'ber-tē). The period after puberty.

post·pu·bes·cent (pōst-pū-bes'ent). Subsequent to the period of puberty. SYN postpuberal, postpubertal.

post·pyk·not·ic (pōst-pik-not'ik). Following the stage of pyknosis in a red cell, denoting the disappearance of the nucleus (chromatolysis).

post·ro·lan·dic (pos'trō-lan'dik). Behind the fissure of Rolando, or central sulcus. SEE postcentral.

post·sa·cral (pōst'sā'krăl). Referring to the coccyx.

post·scap·u·lar (pōst-skap'yū-lăr). Posterior to the scapula.

post·scar·la·ti·nal (pōst'skar-lă-tē'năl). Occurring as a sequel to scarlatina.

post·sphyg·mic (pōst-sfig'mik). Occurring after the pulse wave. [G. *sphygmos,* pulse]

post·splen·ic (pōst'splen'ik). Posterior to the spleen.

post·syn·ap·tic (pōst-si-nap'tik). Pertaining to the area on the distal side of a synaptic cleft.

post·tar·sal (pōst'tar'săl). Relating to the posterior portion of the tarsus.

post·tec·ta (pōst'tek'tă). Aboral to the hidden part of the duodenum.

post·tib·i·al (pōst'tib'ē-ăl). Posterior to the tibia; situated in the posterior portion of the leg.

post·trans·crip·tion·al (pōst-tran-skrip'shŭn-al). Referring to events that occur after transcription.

post·trans·la·tion·al (pōst-trans-lă'shŭn-al). Referring to events that occur after translation.

post·trans·verse (pōst-tranz'vers). Behind a transverse process.

post·trau·mat·ic (pōst-traw-mat'ik). Temporally and implied causally, related to a trauma.

post·tre·mat·ic (pōst-trē-mat'ik). Relating to the caudal surface of a branchial cleft. [post- + G. *trēma,* perforation]

post·tus·sis (pōst-tŭs'is). After coughing; referring usually to certain auscultatory sounds. [L. *tussis,* cough]

post·ty·phoid (pōst-tī'foyd). Occurring as a sequel of typhoid fever.

pos·tu·late (pos'tyū-lăt). A proposition that is taken as self-evident or assumed without proof as a basis for further analysis. SEE ALSO hypothesis, theory. [L. *postulo,* pp. *-atus,* to demand]

Ampère's p., SYN Avogadro's *law.*

Avogadro's p., SYN Avogadro's *law.*

Ehrlich's p., SYN side-chain *theory.*

Koch's p.'s, to establish the specificity of a pathogenic microorganism, it must be present in all cases of the disease, inoculations of its pure cultures must produce disease in animals, and from these it must be again obtained and be propagated in pure cultures. SYN Koch's law.

pos·tur·al (pos'tyū-răl, pos'cher-ăl). Relating to or affected by posture.

pos·ture (pos'chūr, pos'cher). The position of the limbs or the carriage of the body as a whole. [L. *positura,* fr. *pono,* pp. *positus,* to place]

Stern's p., a supine position with the head extended and lowered over the end of the table, by which the murmur is developed or made more distinct in cases of tricuspid insufficiency.

pos·tur·og·ra·phy (pos-tyur-og'ra-fē). A force platform that evaluates somatosensory and visual influences on posture and equilibrium. SYN dynamic platform p. [posture + G. *graphō,* to write]

dynamic platform p., SYN posturography.

post·u·ter·ine (pōst-yū'ter-in). Posterior to the uterus.

post·vac·ci·nal (pōst-vak'si-năl). After vaccination.

post·val·var, post·val·vu·lar (pōst-val'văr, -val'vyū-lăr). Relating to a position distal to the pulmonary or aortic valves.

po·ta·ble (pō'tă-bl). Drinkable; fit to drink. [L. *potabilis,* fr. *poto,* to drink]

Potain, Pierre C.E., French physician, 1825–1901. SEE P.'s *sign.*

pot·a·mo·pho·bia (pot'ă-mō-fō'bē-ă). Morbid fears aroused by the sight, and sometimes thought, of a river or any flow of water. [G. *potamos,* river, + *phobos,* fear]

pot·ash. Impure potassium carbonate. SYN pearl-ash. [E. pot-ashes]

caustic p., SYN *potassium* hydroxide.

sulfurated p., a mixture composed chiefly of potassium polysulfides and potassium thiosulfate; used externally in scabies, acne, and psoriasis; used in the manufacture of "white lotion". SYN liver of sulfur.

po·tas·sic (pŏ-tas'ik). Relating to or containing potassium.

po·tas·si·um (K) (pō-tas'ē-ŭm). An alkaline metallic element, atomic no. 19, atomic wt. 39.0983, occurring abundantly in nature but always in combination; its salts are used medicinally. For organic p. salts not listed below, see the name of the anion. SYN kalium. [Mod. L., fr. Eng. potash (fr. pot + ashes) + *-ium*]

p. acetate, $KC_2H_3O_2$; a diuretic, diaphoretic, and systemic and urinary alkalizer. SYN sal diureticum.

p. acid tartrate, SYN p. bitartrate.

p. alum, SYN *aluminum* potassium sulfate.

p. aminosalicylate, SEE *p*-aminosalicylic acid.

p. antimonyltartrate, SYN *antimony* potassium tartrate.

p. atractylate, the p. salt of atractylic acid, the natural source of the latter.

p. bicarbonate, $KHCO_3$; used as a diuretic to decrease the acidity of the urine, and as an electrolyte replenisher.

p. bitartrate, $KHC_4H_4O_6$; a diuretic and laxative. SYN cream of tartar, p. acid tartrate.

p. bromide, KBr; an obsolescent sedative and hypnotic (sodium bromide is usually preferred).

p. chlorate, chlorate of potash, $KClO_3$, used as a mouthwash and gargle in stomatitis and follicular pharyngitis; it is incompatible in the dry state with all easily oxidizable substances.

p. chloride, used to correct p. deficiency.

p. citrate, $K_3C_6H_5O_7$; a deliquescent powder, soluble in water; used as a diuretic, diaphoretic, expectorant, and systemic and urinary alkalizer. SYN Rivière's salt.

p. cyanide, KCN; a commercial fumigant.

dibasic p. phosphate, SYN p. phosphate.

p. dichromate, p. bichromate, $K_2Cr_2O_7$; used externally as an astringent, antiseptic, and caustic.

effervescent p. citrate, a mixture of p. citrate, citric acid, sodium bicarbonate, and tartaric acid; used as a gastric antacid and urinary alkalizer.

p. ferrocyanide, $K_4Fe(CN)_6 3H_2O$; yellow prussiate of potash, used in the preparation of various cyanides and in medicine as an antidote to copper sulfate.

p. gluconate, gluconic acid p. salt, used in hypokalemia as a replenisher.

p. guaiacolsulfonate, $C_6H_3OHOCH_3SO_3K$; used as an expectorant.

p. hydroxide, KOH; a strong, penetrating caustic. SYN caustic potash.

p. hypophosphite, KH_2PO_2; formerly believed to have a tonic effect upon the nervous system; may be explosive if triturated or heated with oxidizing agents.

p. iodate, KIO_3; an oxidizing agent and disinfectant.

p. iodide, KI; used as an alterative and expectorant, and in certain mycoses.

p. metaphosphate, $(KPO_3)_n$; a pharmaceutical aid (buffer).

monobasic p. phosphate, KH_2PO_4; used as a urinary acidifier and buffer.

p. nitrate, KNO_3; sometimes used as a diuretic and diaphoretic; formerly it was included in asthmatic powders containing stramonium leaves. SYN niter, saltpeter.

penicillin G p., SEE *penicillin* G potassium.

p. perchlorate, $KClO_4$; occasionally used, as an alternative to a thiouracil derivative, in the control of hyperthyroidism.

p. permanganate, $KMnO_4$; a strong oxidizing agent, used in solution as an antiseptic and deodorizing application for foul lesions, and as a gastric lavage in poisoning from morphine, strychnine, aconite, and picrotoxin; in electron microscopy, it stains cytomembranes well and gives results similar to lead hydroxide staining; also used as a fixative (Luft's).

p. phosphate, K_2HPO_4; a mild saline cathartic and diuretic. SYN dibasic p. phosphate, dipotassium phosphate.

p. rhodanate, SYN p. thiocyanate.

p. sodium tartrate, $KNaC_4H_4O_6$; a mild saline cathartic, used as an ingredient in compound effervescent powders. SYN Rochelle salt, Seignette's salt, sodium potassium tartrate.

p. sorbate, 2,4-hexadienoic acid potassium salt; a mold and yeast inhibitor, used as a preservative.

p. succinate, a deliquescent powder used as a hemostatic.

p. sulfate, K_2SO_4; an obsolete laxative.

p. sulfocyanate, SYN p. thiocyanate.

p. tartrate, $K_2C_4H_4O_6 \cdot \frac{1}{2} H_2O$; a mild purgative and diuretic. SYN soluble tartar.

p. thiocyanate, formerly used in the treatment of essential hypertension and as a reagent in the detection of copper, iron, and silver. SYN p. rhodanate, p. sulfocyanate.

po·tas·si·um-40 (^{40}K). A naturally occurring (0.0117%) radioactive potassium isotope; beta emitter with half-life of 1.26 billion years; chief source of natural radioactivity of living tissue.

po·tas·si·um-42 (^{42}K). An artificial potassium isotope; beta emitter with half-life of 12.36 hr, used as a tracer in studies of potassium distribution in body fluid compartments and in localization of brain tumors.

po·tas·si·um-43 (^{43}K). An artificial potassium isotope; a beta emitter with a half-life of 22.3 hr, used as a tracer in myocardial perfusion studies.

po·ten·cy (pō′ten-sē). **1.** Power, force, or strength; the condition or quality of being potent. **2.** Specifically, sexual p. **3.** In therapeutics, the relative pharmacological activity of a compound. [L. *potentia*, power]

sexual p., the ability to carry out and consummate sexual intercourse, usually referring to the male.

po·tent (pō′tent). **1.** Possessing force, power, strength. **2.** Indicating the ability of a primitive cell to differentiate. SEE ALSO totipotent, pluripotent, unipotent. **3.** In psychiatry, possessing sexual potency.

po·ten·tial (pō-ten′shăl). **1.** Capable of doing or being, although not yet doing or being; possible, but not actual. **2.** A state of tension in an electric source enabling it to do work under suitable conditions; in relation to electricity, p. is analogous to the temperature in relation to heat. [L. *potentia*, power, potency]

action p., the change in membrane p. occurring in nerve, muscle, or other excitable tissue when excitation occurs.

after-p., SEE afterpotential.

bioelectric p., electrical p.'s occurring in living organisms.

biotic p., a theoretical measurement of the capacity of a species to survive or to compete successfully.

brain p., the electrical charge of the brain as compared to a point on the body; the p. may be steady (DC p.) or may fluctuate at specific frequencies when recorded against time, giving rise to the electroencephalogram.

chemical p. (μ), a measure of how the Gibbs free energy of a phase depends on any change in the composition of that phase.

demarcation p., the difference in p. recorded when one electrode is placed on intact nerve fibers or muscle fibers and the other electrode is placed on the injured ends of the same fibers; the intact portion is positive with reference to the injured portion. SYN injury p.

early receptor p. (ERP), a voltage arising across the eye from a charge displacement within photoreceptor pigment, in response to an intense flash of light.

evoked p., an event-related potential, elicited by, and time-locked to a stimulus. SEE ALSO evoked *response*.

excitatory junction p. (EJP), discrete partial depolarization of smooth muscle produced by stimulation of excitatory nerves;

similar to small end-plate p.'s. They summate with repeated stimuli.

excitatory postsynaptic p. (EPSP), the change in p. which is produced in the membrane of the next neuron when an impulse which has an excitatory influence arrives at the synapse; it is a local change in the direction of depolarization; summation of these p.'s can lead to discharge of an impulse by the neuron.

generator p., local depolarization of the membrane p. at the end of a sensory neurone in graded response to the strength of a stimulus applied to the associated receptor organ, *e.g.*, a pacinian corpuscle; if the generator p. becomes large enough (because the stimulus is at least of threshold strength), it causes excitation at the nearest node of Ranvier and a propagated action p.

inhibitory junction p. (IJP), hyperpolarization of smooth muscle produced by stimulation of inhibitory nerves.

inhibitory postsynaptic p. (IPSP), the change in p. produced in the membrane of the next neuron when an impulse which has an inhibitory influence arrives at the synapse; it is a local change in the direction of hyperpolarization; the frequency of discharge of a given neuron is determined by the extent to which impulses that lead to excitatory postsynaptic p.'s predominate over those that cause inhibitory postsynaptic p.'s.

injury p., SYN demarcation p.

membrane p., the p. inside a cell membrane, measured relative to the fluid just outside; it is negative under resting conditions and becomes positive during an action p. SYN transmembrane p.

myogenic p., action p. of muscle.

oscillatory p., the variable voltage in the positive deflection of the electroretinogram (B-wave) of the dark-adapted eye arising from amacrine cells.

Ottoson p., SYN electro-olfactogram.

oxidation-reduction p. (E_h), the p. in volts of an inert metallic electrode measured in a system of an arbitrarily chosen ratio of [oxidant] to [reductant] and referred to the normal hydrogen electrode at absolute temperature; it is calculated from the following equation:

$$E_h = E_0 + \frac{RT}{nF} \ln \frac{[\text{oxidant}]}{[\text{reductant}]},$$

where R is the gas constant expressed in electrical units, T the absolute temperature (Kelvin), n the number of electrons transferred, F the faraday and E_0 the normal symbol for the p. of the system at pH 0; for biological systems E_0' is often used (in which pH = 7). Cf. Nernst's *equation*. SYN redox p.

pacemaker p., the voltage inscribed by impulses from an artificial electronic pacemaker.

redox p., SYN oxidation-reduction p.

S p., prolonged, slow, depolarizing or hyperpolarizing responses to illumination; initiated between the photoreceptor and ganglion cell layers of the retina.

somatosensory evoked p., the computer-averaged cortical and subcortical responses to repetitive stimulation of peripheral nerve sensory fibers.

spike p., the main wave in the action p. of a nerve; it is followed by negative and positive afterpotentials.

thermodynamic p., SEE free *energy*.

transmembrane p., SYN membrane p.

visual evoked p., voltage fluctuations that may be recorded from the occipital area of the scalp as the result of retinal stimulation by a light flashing at $\frac{1}{4}$-second intervals; commonly summated and averaged by computer.

zeta p., the degree of negative charge on the surface of a red blood cell; *i.e.*, the p. difference between the negative charges on the red cell and the cation in the fluid portion of the blood.

zoonotic p., the p. for infections of subhuman animals to be transmissible to humans.

po·ten·ti·a·tion (pō-ten′shē-ā′shŭn). Interaction between two or more drugs or agents resulting in a pharmacologic response greater than the sum of individual responses to each drug or agent.

po·ten·ti·a·tor (pō-ten′shē-ā-ter, -tōr). In chemotherapy, a drug used in combination with other drugs to produce deliberate potentiation.

po·ten·ti·om·e·ter (pō-ten-shē-om′ĕ-ter). **1.** An instrument used for measuring small differences in electrical potential. **2.** An electrical resistor of fixed total resistance between two terminals, but with a third terminal attached to a slider that can make contact at any desired point along the resistance. [L. *potentia,* power, + G. *metron,* measure]

po·tion (pō'shŭn). A draft or large dose of liquid medicine. [L. *potio, potus,* fr. *poto,* to drink]

Pott, Sir Percivall, English surgeon, 1713–1788. SEE P.'s *abscess, aneurysm, curvature, disease, fracture, gangrene, paralysis, paraplegia,* puffy *tumor.*

Potter, Edith L., U.S. perinatal pathologist, *1901. SEE P.'s *disease, facies, syndrome.*

Potter, Irving White, U.S. obstetrician, 1868–1956. SEE P.'s *version.*

Potts, Willis J., U.S. pediatric surgeon, 1895–1968. SEE P.'s *anastomosis, clamp, operation.*

pouch (powch). A pocket or cul-de-sac.

antral p., a p. made in the antrum of the stomach of experimental animals.

branchial p.'s, SYN pharyngeal p.'s.

Broca's p., SYN pudendal *sac.*

celomic p.'s, lateral mesoderm-lined diverticula lying at either side of the notochord in the developing *Amphioxus.*

deep perineal p., SYN deep perineal *space.*

Denis Browne's p., a pocket formed between Scarpa's and external oblique fascia adjacent to external inguinal ring; a common lodging site for undescended testes (as in cryptorchism). SYN superficial inguinal p.

p. of Douglas, SYN rectouterine p.

Douglas' p., SYN rectouterine p.

endodermal p.'s, SYN pharyngeal p.'s.

guttural p., a structure in the horse which is a diverticulum of the auditory (eustachian) tube; subject to chronic infections and inflammation and frequently necessitating surgery for relief.

Hartmann's p., a spheroid or conical p. at the junction of the neck of the gallbladder and the cystic duct. SYN ampulla of gallbladder, fossa provesicalis, pelvis of gallbladder.

Heidenhain p., a small sac or p. of the stomach, vagally denervated and closed off from the main cavity but with an opening through the abdominal wall, fashioned for the purpose of obtaining gastric juice and for studying gastric secretion in physiologic experiments.

hepatorenal p., SYN hepatorenal *recess.*

hypophyseal p., SYN pituitary *diverticulum.*

ileoanal p. (il'ē-ō-ā'nal), a p. constructed from the ileum and anastomosed to the proximal anus for restoration of normal continence after proctocolectomy.

Kock p., a continent ileostomy with a reservoir and valved opening fashioned from doubled loops of ileum. SYN Kock ileostomy.

laryngeal p., SYN *saccule* of larynx.

Morison's p., SYN hepatorenal *recess.*

paracystic p., SYN paravesical *fossa.*

pararectal p., SYN pararectal *fossa.*

paravesical p., SYN paravesical *fossa.*

Pavlov p., a section of the stomach of a dog, retaining its vagal innervation but shut off from all communication with the main part of the organ and connected with the outside by a fistula; used in studies of gastric secretions. SYN miniature stomach, Pavlov stomach.

pharyngeal p.'s, paired evaginations of embryonic pharyngeal endoderm, between the branchial arches, extending toward the corresponding ectodermally lined branchial grooves; during development they evolve into epithelial tissues and organs, such as thymus and thyroid glands. SYN branchial p.'s, endodermal p.'s.

Physick's p.'s, proctitis with mucous discharge and burning pain, involving especially the sacculations between the rectal valves.

Prussak's p., SYN superior *recess* of tympanic membrane.

Rathke's p., SYN pituitary *diverticulum.*

rectouterine p., a pocket formed by the deflection of the perito-

neum from the rectum to the uterus. SYN excavatio rectouterina [NA], cavum douglasi, cul-de-sac (2), Douglas' cul-de-sac, Douglas' p., p. of Douglas, rectovaginouterine p.

rectovaginouterine p., SYN rectouterine p.

rectovesical p., a pocket formed by the deflection of the peritoneum from the rectum to the bladder in the male. SYN excavatio rectovesicalis [NA], Proust's space.

Seessel's p., SEE Seessel's *pocket.*

superficial inguinal p., SYN Denis Browne's p.

superficial perineal p., SYN superficial perineal *space.*

ultimobranchial p., a transient fifth pharyngeal p.; it is now considered to be incorporated into the caudal pharyngeal complex, the cells of which become the parafollicular cells (C cells) of the thyroid.

uterovesical p., a pocket formed by the deflection of the peritoneum from the bladder to the uterus in the female. SYN excavatio vesicouterina [NA], cavum vesicouterinum, vesicouterine p.

vesicouterine p., SYN uterovesical p.

Willis' p., obsolete term for lesser *omentum*

pouch·i·tis (pow-chī'tis). Acute inflammation of the mucosa of an ileal reservoir or pouch that has been surgically created, usually following total colectomy for inflammatory bowel disease or multiple polyposis. [pouch + -*itis,* inflammation]

pou·drage (pū-drahzh'). **1.** Powdering. **2.** SYN talc *operation.* [F.]

pleural p., covering the opposing pleural surfaces with a slightly irritating powder in order to secure adhesion.

poul·tice (pōl'tis). A soft magma or mush prepared by wetting various powders or other absorbent substances with oily or watery fluids, sometimes medicated, and usually applied hot to the surface; it exerts an emollient, relaxing, or stimulant, counterirritant effect upon the skin and underlying tissues. SYN cataplasm. [L. *puls* (*pult-*), a thick pap; G. *poltos*]

pound (pownd). A unit of weight, containing 12 ounces, apothecaries' weight, or 16 ounces, avoirdupois. [A.S. *pund;* L. *pondus,* weight]

pound·al (pownd'ăl). The force required to give a mass of 1 lb. an acceleration of 1 ft/sec^2; equal to 0.138255 newtons.

Poupart, François, French anatomist, 1616–1708. SEE P.'s *ligament, line.*

po·vi·done (pō'vi-dōn). poly[1-(2-oxo-1-pyrrolidinyl)ethylene]; a synthetic polymer consisting mainly of linear 1-vinyl-2-pyrrolidone groups, with mean molecular weights ranging from 10,000 to 70,000; used as a dispersing and suspending agent; p. with molecular weight between 20,000 and 40,000 has been used as a plasma extender. It is not metabolized, but is excreted unchanged by the kidney. SYN polyvidone, polyvinylpyrrolidone.

po·vi·done-io·dine. SYN povidone *iodine.*

pow·der. 1. A dry mass of minute separate particles of any substance. **2.** In pharmaceutics, a homogenous dispersion of finely divided, relatively dry, particulate matter consisting of one or more substances; the degree of fineness of a p. is related to passage of the material through standard sieves. **3.** A single dose of a powdered drug, enclosed in an envelope of folded paper. **4.** To reduce a solid substance to a state of very fine division. [Fr. *poudre;* L. *pulvis*]

bleaching p., SYN chlorinated lime.

pow·er. 1. In optics, the refractive vergence of a lens. **2.** In physics and engineering, the rate at which work is done.

back vertex p., the effective p. of a lens as measured from a surface toward the eye; a standard for measurement of ophthalmic lenses.

carbon dioxide combining p., a measurement of the total CO_2 that can be bound as HCO_2 at a PCO_2 of 40 mmHg at 25 C by serum, plasma, or whole blood.

equivalent p., the p. equal to an infinitely thin lens as measured on an optical bench.

resolving p., (1) definition of a lens; in a microscope objective lens it is calculated by dividing the wavelength of the light used by twice the numerical aperture of the objective. SEE ALSO definition. **(2)** analogies to other modalities, *e.g.,* two-point discrimination in neurological examination. Commonly misinterpreted as random error, although it has none of its properties. (**3**) SYN resolution (2).

statistical p., in Neyman-Pearson hypothesis testing, the probability of rejecting the null hypothesis when it is false; the complement of an *error* of the second kind.

pox (poks). **1.** An eruptive disease, usually qualified by a descriptive prefix; *e.g.,* smallpox, cowpox, chickenpox. See the specific term. **2.** An eruption, first papular then pustular, occurring in chronic antimony poisoning. **3.** Archaic or colloquial term for syphilis. [var. of pl. *pocks*]

Kaffir p., SYN alastrim.

Pox·vir·i·dae (poks-vir′i-dē). A family of large complex viruses, with a marked affinity for skin tissue, that are pathogenic for man and other animals. Virions are large, up to 250 by 400 nm and enveloped (double membranes). Replication occurs entirely in the cytoplasm of infected cells. Capsids are of complex symmetry and contain double-stranded DNA (MW 160×10^6), the nucleoprotein antigen being common to all members of the family. A number of genera are recognized including: *Orthopoxvirus, Avipoxvirus, Capripoxvirus, Leporipoxvirus,* and *Parapoxvirus.*

pox·vi·rus (poks′vī-rŭs). Any virus of the family Poxviridae.

p. officina′lis, SYN vaccinia *virus.*

Pozzi, Samuel J., French gynecologist and anatomist, 1846–1918. SEE P.'s *muscle.*

PP Abbreviation for pyrophosphate.

PP$_i$ Abbreviation for inorganic pyrophosphate.

P.p. Abbreviation for *punctum* proximum.

ppb Abbreviation for parts per billion.

PPCA Abbreviation for proserum prothrombin conversion *accelerator.*

PPCF Abbreviation for plasmin prothrombins conversion *factor.*

PPD Abbreviation for purified protein derivative of *tuberculin.*

PPLO Abbreviation for pleuropneumonia-like *organisms,* under *organism.*

ppm Abbreviation for parts per million.

PPO Abbreviation for 2,5-diphenyloxazole, a liquid scintillator; preferred provider *organization.*

PPPPPP A mnemonic of 6 P's designating the symptom complex of acute arterial occlusion. [*pain, pallor, paraesthesia, pulselessness, paralysis, prostration*]

PPRibp, PPRP Abbreviation for 5-phospho-α-D-ribosyl 1-pyrophosphate

P-pul·mo·na·le (pul-mō-nā′lē). Tall, narrow, peaked P waves in electrocardiographic leads II, III, and aVF, and often a prominent initial positive P wave component in V_1, presumed to be characteristic of cor pulmonale. (Although this term is extensively used in the electrocardiographic literature, it is actually a misnomer and would be more appropriately called P-dextrocardiale, since it results from overload of the right atrium regardless of the cause, as in tricuspid stenosis, and may occur independently of cor pulmonale.) In lung disease, P-pulmonale is usually transient, occurring during exacerbations.

PQ Abbreviation for plastoquinone.

PQ-9 Abbreviation for plastoquinone-9.

P.r. Abbreviation for *punctum* remotum.

Pr 1. Abbreviation for presbyopia. **2.** Symbol for praseodymium; propyl.

PRA Abbreviation for plasma renin *activity*; phosphoribosylamine.

prac·tice (prak′tis). The exercise of the profession of medicine or one of the allied health professions. [Mediev. L. *practica,* business, G. *praktikos,* pertaining to action]

extramural p., delivery of health care services by university faculties or full-time hospital staff to persons beyond the physical confines of their respective medical centers.

family p., a specialty of medicine in which the physician takes responsibility for the health and medical care of all members of a family group, regardless of age or gender, but usually does limited amounts of obstetrics and surgery.

general p., a relatively obsolete term for physicians who care for all types of medical problems, including internal medical, pediat-

ric, obstetrical, and surgical diseases. Post-graduate training for general practitioners was limited and there was no specialty certification; the field has been replaced by more extensively trained family practitioners.

group p., the cooperative p. of medicine by a group of physicians, each of whom as a rule specializes in some particular field; such a group often shares a common suite of consulting rooms, laboratories, staff, equipment, etc.

intramural p., delivery of health care services by university faculties or full-time hospital staff conducted within the physical confines of their respective medical centers.

prac·ti·tion·er (prak-tish′ŭn-er). A person who practices medicine or one of the allied health care professions.

prac·to·lol (prak′tō-lol). 4′-[2-Hydroxy-3-(isopropylamino)-propoxy]acetanilide; a β-receptor blocking drug for treatment of cardiac arrhythmias.

Prader, Andrea, Swiss pediatrician, *1919. SEE P.-Willi *syndrome.*

△**prae-.** SEE pre-.

prag·mat·ag·no·sia (prag′mat-ag-nō′sē-ă). Rarely used term for loss of the power of recognizing objects. [G. *pragma (pragmat-),* thing done, a deed, fr. *prassō,* to do, + *agnōsia,* ignorance]

prag·mat·am·ne·sia (prag′mat-am-nē′zē-ă). Rarely used term for loss of the memory of the appearance of objects. [G. *pragma,* a thing done, + *amnēsia,* forgetfulness]

prag·mat·ics (prag-mat′iks). A branch of semiotics; the theory that deals with the relation between signs and their users, both senders and receivers. [G. *pragmatikos,* fr. *pragma,* thing done]

prag·ma·tism (prag′mă-tizm). A philosophy emphasizing practical applications and consequences of beliefs and theories, that the meaning of ideas or things is determined by the testability of the idea in real life. [G. *pragma (pragmat-),* thing done]

2-pra·li·dox·ime (2-PAM). One of several oximes which are effective in reversing cholinesterase inhibition by organophosphates. The 2-PAM facilitates the hydrolysis of the phosphorylated enzyme so as to regenerate active cholinesterase.

pral·i·dox·ime chlo·ride (pral-i-dok′sēm, prā-li-). 2-Formyl-1-methylpyridinium chloride oxime; used to restore the inactivated cholinesterase activity resulting from organophosphate poisoning; has some limited value as an antagonist of the carbamate type of cholinesterase inhibitors that are used in the treatment of myasthenia gravis. Dizziness, blurred vision, drowsiness, nausea, tachycardia, and muscular weakness may occur.

pra·mox·ine hy·dro·chlo·ride (pră-mok′sēn, -sin). 4-[3-(*p*-Butoxyphenoxy)propyl]morpholine hydrochloride; a nonester, nonamide local anesthetic for dermal and rectal use.

pran·di·al (pran′dē-ăl). Relating to a meal. [L. *prandium,* breakfast]

pra·se·o·dym·i·um (Pr) (prā-sē-ō-dim′ē-ŭm). An element of the lanthanide or "rare earth" group; atomic no. 59, atomic wt. 140.90765. [G. *prasios,* leekgreen, fr. *prason,* a leek, + *didymos,* twin]

Pratt, Joseph H., U.S. physician, 1872–1956. SEE P.'s *symptom.*

Prausnitz, Otto Carl, German hygienist, 1876–1963. SEE P.-Küstner *antibody, reaction;* reversed P. reaction.

prav·a·sta·tin. An inhibitor of the enzyme 3-hydroxy-3-methyglutaryl coenzyme A (HMG-CoA), the rate-limiting enzyme in the biosynthesis of cholesterol. Used in the treatment of hypercholesteremia. Similar to lovastatin and simvastatin.

prax·i·ol·o·gy (prak-sē-ol′ō-jē). The science or study of behavior; it excludes the study of consciousness and similiar non-objective metaphysical concepts. [G. *praxis,* action, + *logos,* study]

prax·is (prak′sis). The performance of an action. [G. *praxis,* action]

pra·ze·pam (prā′zē-pam). 7-Chloro-1-(cyclopropylmethyl)-1,3-dihydro-5-phenyl-2 *H*-1,4-benzodiazepin-2-one; an antianxiety agent of the benzodiazepine class; a prodrug for nordiazepam.

pra·zi·quan·tel (prā-zi-kwahn′tel). $C_{19}H_{24}N_2O_2$; a pyrazinoisoquinoline derivative; a synthetic heterocyclic broad spectrum anthelmintic agent effective against all schistosome species of man as well as most other trematodes and adult cestodes.

pr

pra·zo·sin hy·dro·chlo·ride (prā′zō-sin). 1-(4-Amino-6,7-dimethoxy-2-quinazolinyl)-4-(2-furoyl)piperazine monohydrochloride; an antihypertensive agent.

⌂**pre-.** Anterior; before (in time or space). SEE ALSO ante-, pro- (1). [L. *prae*]

pre·ag·o·nal (prē-ag′ō-năl). Immediately preceding death. [pre- + G. *agōn*, struggle (agony)]

pre·al·bu·min (prē-al-byū′min). A protein component of plasma having a molecular weight of about 55,000 and containing 1.3% carbohydrate; estimated plasma concentration is 0.3 g/100 ml; abnormal levels of p. are found in cases of familial amyloidosis. SYN transthyretin.

thyroxine-binding p. (TBPA), a protein located in the "prealbumin" zone upon electrophoretic analysis of plasma proteins; its affinity for binding thyroxine is less than that of thyroxine-binding globulin but greater than that of albumin. SYN thyroxine-binding protein (2).

pre·a·nal (prē-ā′năl). Anterior to the anus.

pre·an·es·thet·ic (prē-an-es-thet′ik). Before anesthesia.

pre·an·ti·sep·tic (prē′an-ti-sep′tik). Denoting the period, especially in relation to surgery, before the adoption of the principles of antisepsis.

pre·a·or·tic (prē′ā-ōr′tik). Anterior to the aorta; denoting certain lymph nodes so situated.

pre·a·sep·tic (prē-ă-sep′tik). Denoting the period, especially the early antiseptic period in relation to surgery, before the principles of asepsis were known or adopted.

pre·a·tax·ic (prē-ă-tak′sik). Denoting the early stages of tabetic neurosyphilis prior to the appearance of ataxia.

pre·au·ric·u·lar (prē-aw-rik′yū-lăr). Anterior to the auricle of the ear; denoting lymphatic nodes so situated.

pre·ax·i·al (prē-ak′sē-ăl). **1.** Anterior to the axis of the body or a limb, the latter being in the anatomical position. **2.** Denoting the portion of a limb bud which lies cranial to the axis of the limb: the radial aspect of the upper limb and the tibial aspect of the lower limb.

pre·cal·cif·er·ol (prē-kal-si′fer-ol). The immediate precursor of ergocalciferol and lumisterol.

pre·can·cer (prē-kan′ser). A lesion from which a malignant neoplasm is believed to develop in a significant number of instances, and which may or may not be recognizable clinically or by microscopic changes in the affected tissue.

pre·can·cer·ous (prē-kan′ser-ŭs). Pertaining to any lesion that is interpreted as precancer. SYN premalignant.

pre·cap·il·lary (prē-kap′i-lār-ē). Preceding a capillary; an arteriole or venule.

pre·car·di·ac (prē-kar′dē-ak). Anterior to the heart.

pre·car·di·nal (prē-kar′di-năl). Relating to the anterior cardinal veins.

pre·car·ti·lage (prē-kar′ti-lij). A closely packed aggregation of mesenchymal cells just prior to their differentiation into embryonic cartilage.

pre·ca·va (prē-kā′vă). SYN superior *vena* cava.

pre·cen·tral (prē-sen′trăl). Referring to the cerebral convolution immediately anterior to the central sulcus: precentral gyrus.

pre·chor·dal (prē-kōr′dăl). SYN prochordal.

pre·chrom·ing (prē-krōm′ing). Treatment of a tissue or fabric first with a metal mordant, followed by a dye.

pre·cip·i·ta·ble (prē-sip′i-tă-bl). Capable of being precipitated.

pre·cip·i·tant (prē-sip′i-tant). Anything causing a precipitation from a solution.

pre·cip·i·tate (prē-sip′i-tāt). **1.** To cause a substance in solution to separate as a solid. **2.** A solid separated out from a solution or suspension; a floc or clump, such as that resulting from the mixture of a specific antigen and its antibody. **3.** Accumulation of inflammatory cells on the corneal endothelium in uveitis (keratic precipitates). [L. *praecipito*, pp. *-atus*, to cast headlong]

keratic p.'s, inflammatory cells on the corneal endothelium. SYN punctate keratitis, keratitis punctata.

mutton-fat keratic p.'s, coalescent p.'s forming small plaques that gradually become more translucent.

precancers		
organ or tissue system	preneoplasm	later malignancy
A) chronic irritation		
skin	photodermatitis	"light cancer"
	x-ray dermatitis	x-ray cancer
	tar dermatitis	pitch-worker's cancer
	arsenic dermatitis	arsenic cancer
	lupus dermatitis	lupus cancer
	senile keratosis	
	Paget's disease	skin cancer
	condylomata	
scars	burn scar	
	syphilitic scar	
	fistula scar	scar cancer
	ulcus cruris scar	
ulcers	chronic ulcer	ulcer cancer
	varicose ulcer	
	bone fistula	
	rectal fistula	fistula cancer
stomach	gastric ulcer	carcinoma ex ulcere
	gastritis	
liver, gall bladder	cholelithiasis	adeno carcinoma, scirrhous carcinoma, gall bladder carcinoma
vagina	kraurosis vulvae	vulvar carcinoma
B) systemic diseases, tissue deformities, benign neoplasms		
skin	nevus pigmentosus	malignant melanoma
	Bowen dermatosis	
	xeroderma	skin carcinomas and sarcomas
	pigmentosum	
	erythroplasia	
mucous membrane	leukoplakia	tongue cancer cheek cancer palate cancer penis cancer
bones	Paget's disease of bone	osteosarcoma
	exostoses	chondrosarcoma
	ecchondroma	
	ostitis fibrosa	osteosarcoma
	leontiasis ossea	osteosarcoma
nervous system	neurofibromatosis	fibrosarcoma
stomach/ intestine	polyposis	adenocarcinoma
uterus	hydatidiform mole	chorionic epithelioma
	adenomatous hyperplasia	cancers of uterus and cervix
	carcinoma *in situ*	
thyroid gland	struma nodosa	thyroid cancer

pigmented keratic p.'s, p.'s that occur in eyes with brown irides or after prolonged inflammation.

red p., SYN mercuric oxide, red.

sweet p., SYN calomel.

white mercuric p., SYN ammoniated *mercury*.

yellow p., SYN mercuric oxide, yellow.

pre·cip·i·ta·tion (prē-sip-i-tā′shŭn). **1.** The process of formation of a solid previously held in solution or suspension in a liquid. **2.** The phenomenon of clumping of proteins in serum produced by the addition of a specific precipitin. [see precipitate]

double antibody p., a method of separating antibody-bound antigen (*e.g.,* insulin) from free antigen by precipitating the former with antibody specific for immunoglobulin. SYN double antibody immunoassay, double antibody method.

immune p., SYN immunoprecipitation.

pre·cip·i·tin (prē-sip′i-tin). An antibody that under suitable conditions combines with and causes its specific and soluble antigen to precipitate from solution. SYN precipitating antibody.

pre·cip·i·tin·o·gen (prē-sip-i-tin′ō-jen). **1.** An antigen that stimulates the formation of specific precipitin when injected into an animal body. **2.** A precipitable soluble antigen. SYN precipitogen. [precipitin + G. *-gen,* producing]

pre·cip·i·tin·o·ge·noid (prē-sip-i-tin′ō-jĕ-noyd). A precipitinogen that is altered by means of heating, thereby resulting in a substance that combines with the specific precipitin, but does not lead to the formation of a precipitate.

pre·cip·i·to·gen (prē-sip′i-tō-jen). SYN precipitinogen.

pre·cip·i·toid (prē-sip′i-toyd). A heat-treated precipitin that when mixed with specific precipitinogen does not cause a precipitate and also interferes with the precipitating effect of additional nonheated precipitin. [precipitin + G. *eidos,* resemblance]

pre·cip·i·to·phore (prē-sip′i-tō-fōr). In Ehrlich's side chain theory, the portion of a precipitin molecule that is required in the formation of a precipitate, as distinguished from the haptophore group. [precipitin + G. *phoros,* bearing]

pre·ci·sion. 1. The quality of being sharply defined or stated; one measure of precision is the number of distinguishable alternatives to a measurement. **2.** In statistics, the inverse of the variance of a measurement or estimate. **3.** Reproducibility of a quantifiable result; an indication of the random error.

pre·clin·i·cal (prē-klin′i-kăl). **1.** Before the onset of disease. **2.** A period in medical education before the student becomes involved with patients and clinical work.

pre·co·cious (prē-kō′shŭs). Developing unusually early or rapidly. [L. *praecox,* premature]

pre·coc·i·ty (prē-kos′i-tē). Unusually early or rapid development of mental or physical traits. [see precocious]

pre·cog·ni·tion (prē-kog-nish′ŭn). Advance knowledge, by means other than the normal senses, of a future event; a form of extrasensory perception. [L. *praecogito,* to ponder before]

pre·con·scious (prē-kon′shŭs). In psychoanalysis, one of the three divisions of the psyche according to Freud's topographical psychology, the other two being the conscious and unconscious; includes all ideas, thoughts, past experiences, and other memory impressions that with effort can be consciously recalled. Cf. foreconscious.

pre·con·vul·sive (prē-kon-vŭl′siv). Denoting the stage in an epileptic paroxysm preceding convulsions (*e.g.,* aura).

pre·cor·dia (prē-kōr′dē-ă). The epigastrium and anterior surface of the lower part of the thorax. SYN antecardium. [L. *praecordia* (ntr. pl. only), the diaphragm, the entrails, fr. *prae,* before, + *cor* (*cord-*), heart]

pre·cor·di·al (prē-kōr′dē-ăl). Relating to the precordia.

pre·cor·di·al·gia (prē-kōr-dē-al′jē-ă). Pain in the precordial region. [precordia + G. *algos,* pain]

pre·cor·di·um (prē-kōr′dē-ŭm). Singular of precordia.

pre·cos·tal (prē-kos′tăl). Anterior to the ribs. [pre- + L. *costa,* rib]

pre·crit·i·cal (prē-krit′i-kăl). Relating to the phase before a crisis.

pre·cu·ne·al (prē-kū′nē-ăl). Anterior to the cuneus.

pre·cu·ne·ate (prē-kū′nē-āt). Relating to the precuneus.

pre·cu·ne·us (prē-kū′nē-ŭs) [NA]. A division of the medial surface of each cerebral hemisphere between the cuneus and the paracentral lobule; it lies above the subparietal sulcus and is bounded anteriorly by the marginal part of the cingulate sulcus and posteriorly by the parietooccipital sulcus. SYN lobulus quad-

ratus (2), quadrate lobe (3), quadrate lobule (2). [pre- + L. *cuneus,* a wedge]

pre·cur·sor (prē-ker′ser). That which precedes another or from which another is derived, applied especially to a physiologically inactive substance that is converted to an active enzyme, vitamin, hormone, etc., or to a chemical substance that is built into a larger structure in the course of synthesizing the latter. [L. *praecursor,* fr. *prae-,* pre- + *curro,* to run]

pre·de·cid·u·al (prē-dē-sid′yū-ăl). Relating to the premenstrual or secretory phase of the menstrual cycle.

pre·den·tin (prē-den′tin). The organic fibrillar matrix of the dentin before its calcification.

pre·di·a·be·tes (prē′dī-ă-bē′tēz). A state of potential diabetes mellitus, with normal glucose tolerance but with an increased risk of developing diabetes; (*e.g.,* family history).

pre·di·as·to·le (prē-dī-as′tō-lē). The interval in the cardiac rhythm immediately preceding diastole. SYN late systole.

pre·di·a·stol·ic (prē-dī-ă-stol′ik). Late systolic, relating to the interval preceding cardiac diastole.

pre·di·crot·ic (prē-dī-krot′ik). Preceding the dicrotic notch.

pre·di·ges·tion (prē-dī-jes′chŭn). The artificial initiation of digestion of proteins (proteolysis) and starches (amylolysis) before they are eaten.

pre·dis·pose (prē′dis-pōz). To render susceptible.

pre·dis·po·si·tion (prē′dis-pō-zish′ŭn). A condition of special susceptibility to a disease.

pred·nis·o·lone (pred-nis′ō-lōn). Metacortandrolone; Δ^1-dehydrocortisol; Δ^1-hydrocortisone; hydroretrocortine; 11β,17,21-trihydroxy-1,4-pregnadiene-3,20-dione; a dehydrogenated analogue of cortisol with the same actions and uses as cortisol; a potent glucocorticoid.

p. acetate, prednisolone 21-acetate; same uses as p.; suitable for intramuscular administration.

p. butylacetate, SYN p. tebutate.

p. sodium phosphate, prednisolone 21-(disodium phosphate); more soluble than p. and the other p. esters and useful when a rapid onset or a short duration of action is desired; suitable for intrasynovial, parenteral, and topical administration.

p. succinate, p. compound suitable for intramuscular, intravenous, or rectal administration.

p. tebutate, same actions and uses as p. but with longer duration of action and suitable for intrasynovial and soft tissue injection. SYN p. butylacetate.

pred·ni·sone (pred′ni-sōn). Metacortandracin; deltacortisone; Δ^1-cortisone; retrocortine; 17α,21-dihydroxy-1,4-pregnadiene-3,11,20-trione; a dehydrogenated analogue of cortisone with the same actions and uses; must be converted to prednisolone before active; inhibits proliferation of lymphocytes.

pred·nyl·i·dene (prēd-nil′i-dēn). 16-Methyleneprednisolone; 11β,17,21-trihydroxy-16-methylenepregna-1,4-diene-3,20-dione; a glucocorticoid.

pre·dor·mi·tal (prē-dōr′mi-tăl). Pertaining to the predormitum.

pre·dor·mi·tum (prē-dōr′mi-tŭm). The stage of semi-unconsciousness preceding actual sleep. [pre- + L. *dormio,* to sleep]

pre·duc·tal (prē-dŭk′tăl). Relating to that part of the aorta proximal to the aortic opening of the ductus arteriosus.

pre·e·clamp·sia (prē-ē-klamp′sē-ă). Development of hypertension with proteinuria or edema, or both, due to pregnancy or the influence of a recent pregnancy; it usually occurs after the 20th week of gestation, but may develop before this time in the presence of trophoblastic disease. [pre- + G. *eklampsis,* a shining forth (eclampsia)]

superimposed p., the development of p. or eclampsia in a patient with chronic hypertensive vascular or renal disease; when the hypertension antedates the pregnancy as established by previous blood pressure recordings, a rise in the systolic pressure of 30 mm Hg or a rise in the diastolic pressure of 15 mm Hg and the development of proteinuria or edema, or both, are required during pregnancy to establish the diagnosis. SYN superimposed eclampsia.

pre·ep·i·glot·tic (prē′ep-i-glot′ik). Anterior to the epiglottis.

pr

pre·e·rup·tive (prē-e-rŭp′tiv). Denoting the stage of an exanthematous disease preceding the eruption.

pre·ex·ci·ta·tion (prē′ek-sī-tā′shŭn). Premature activation of part of the ventricular myocardium by an impulse that travels by an anomalous path and so avoids physiological delay in the atrioventricular junction; an intrinsic part of the Wolff-Parkinson-White syndrome.

pre·for·ma·tion. SEE preformation *theory*.

pre·fron·tal (prē-fron′tăl). **1.** Denoting the anterior portion of the frontal lobe of the cerebrum. **2.** Denoting the granular frontal cortex rostral to the premotor area.

pre·gan·gli·on·ic (prē′gang-glē-on′ik). Situated proximal to or preceding a ganglion; referring specifically to the preganglionic motor neurons of the autonomic nervous system (located in the spinal cord and brainstem) and the preganglionic, myelinated nerve fibers by which they are connected to the autonomic ganglia.

preg·nan·cy (preg′nan-sē). The condition of a female after conception until the birth of the baby. SYN fetation, gestation, gravidism, graviditas. [L. *praegnans* (*praegnant-*), pregnant, fr. *prae*, before, + *gnascor*, pp. *natus*, to be born]

abdominal p., the implantation and development of the ovum in the peritoneal cavity, usually secondary to an early rupture of a tubal p.; very rarely, primary implantation may occur in the peritoneal cavity. SYN abdominocyesis (1), intraperitoneal p.

aborted ectopic p., SYN tubal *abortion*.

ampullar p., tubal p. situated near the midportion of the oviduct.

bigeminal p., SYN twin p.

cervical p., the implantation and development of the impregnated ovum in the cervical canal.

combined p., coexisting uterine and ectopic p.

compound p., development of a uterine p. in addition to a previously existing ectopic pregnancy (usually a lithopedion).

cornual p., the implantation and development of the impregnated ovum in one of the cornua of the uterus.

ectopic p., the development of an impregnated ovum outside the cavity of the uterus. SYN eccyesis, extrauterine p., metacyesis, paracyesis.

extraamniotic p., a p. in which the chorion is intact, but the amnion has ruptured and shrunk. SYN graviditas examnialis.

extrachorial p., p. in which the membranes rupture and shrink, causing the fetus to develop outside the chorionic sac but within the uterus. SYN graviditas exochorialis.

extramembranous p., a p. in which during the course of gestation the fetus has broken through its envelopes, coming directly in contact with the uterine walls.

extrauterine p., SYN ectopic p.

fallopian p., SYN tubal p.

false p., a condition in which some signs and symptoms suggest pregnancy, although the woman is not pregnant. SYN hysterical p., pseudocyesis, pseudopregnancy (1), spurious p.

heterotopic p., a p. not in the uterine cavity.

hydatid p., the presence of a hydiform mole in the pregnant uterus.

hysterical p., SYN false p.

interstitial p., SYN intramural p.

intraligamentary p., p. within the broad ligament.

intramural p., development of the fertilized ovum in the uterine portion of the fallopian tube. SYN interstitial p., tubouterine p.

intraperitoneal p., SYN abdominal p.

mesometric p., ectopic p. beginning as a tubal p., the amniotic sac being eventually formed by the mesometrium.

molar p., p. marked by a neoplasm within the uterus, whereby part or all of the chorionic villi are converted into a mass of clear vesicles.

multiple p., condition of bearing two or more fetuses simultaneously. SYN plural p., polycyesis.

mural p., p. in uterine muscular wall.

ovarian p., development of an impregnated ovum in an ovarian follicle. SEE ALSO Spiegelberg's *criteria*, under *criterion*. SYN oocyesis, ovariocyesis.

ovarioabdominal p., ovarian p. which, as the result of the embryo's growth, becomes abdominal.

persistent ectopic p., an ectopic p. which has persistent viable tissue, secreting hCG after conservative surgery.

phantom p., obsolete term for false p.

plural p., SYN multiple p.

secondary abdominal p., a condition in which the embryo or fetus continues to grow in the abdominal cavity after its expulsion from the fallopian tube or other seat of its primary development. SYN abdominocyesis (2).

spurious p., SYN false p.

tubal p., development of an impregnated ovum in the fallopian tube. SYN fallopian p., salpingocyesis.

tuboabdominal p., development of an ectopic p. partly in the fallopian tube and partly in the abdominal cavity.

tubo-ovarian p., development of the ovum at the fimbriated extremity of the fallopian and involving the ovary.

tubouterine p., SYN intramural p.

twin p., a p. that may result from the fertilization of two separate ova or of a single ovum. SEE ALSO twin. SYN bigeminal p.

uterine p., development of fetus within the uterus.

uteroabdominal p., development of the ovum primarily in the uterus and later, in consequence of the rupture of the uterus, in the abdominal cavity.

preg·nane (preg′nān). Parent hydrocarbon of two series of steroids stemming from 5α-pregnane (originally allopregnane) and 5β-pregnane (17β-ethylietiocholane). 5β-Pregnane is the parent of the progesterones, pregnane alcohols, ketones, and several adrenocortical hormones and is found largely in urine as a metabolic product of 5β-pregnane compounds. For structure, see steroids.

preg·nane·di·ol (preg-nān-dī′ol). 5β-Pregnane-3α,20α-diol; the chief steroid metabolite of progesterone that is biologically inactive and occurs as p. glucuronate in the urine.

preg·nane·di·one (preg-nān-dī′ōn). 5β-Pregnane-3,20-dione; a metabolite of progesterone, formed in relatively small quantities, that occurs in 5α and 5β isomeric forms.

preg·nane·tri·ol (preg-nān-trī′ol). 5β-Pregnane-3α,17α,20α-triol; a urinary metabolite of 17-hydroxyprogesterone and a precursor in the biosynthesis of cortisol; its excretion is enhanced in certain diseases of the adrenal cortex and following administration of corticotropin.

preg·nant. Denoting a gestating female. SYN gravid. [see pregnancy]

preg·nene (preg′nēn). An unsaturated steroid of primarily terminological importance; utilized in systematic nomenclature of appropriate 21-carbon steroids.

preg·nen·in·o·lone (preg-nēn-in′ō-lōn, preg-nēn′in-). SYN ethisterone.

preg·nen·o·lone (preg-nēn′ō-lōn). 3β-Hydroxy-5-pregnen-20-one; a steroid that serves as an intermediate in the biosynthesis of numerous hormones, including progesterone.

p. succinate, a corticosteroid used for the treatment of rheumatoid arthritis.

pre·hal·lux (prē-hal′ŭks). A supernumerary digit, usually only partial, attached to the medial border of the great toe. [pre- + Mod. L. *hallux*, great toe]

pre·hel·i·cine (prē-hel′i-sēn). In front of the helix of the pinna.

pre·he·ma·ta·min·ic ac·id (prē′hēm-ă-tin′ik). SYN neuraminic acid.

pre·hem·i·ple·gic (prē′hem-i-plē′jik). Preceding the occurrence of hemiplegia.

pre·hen·sile (prē-hen′sil). Adapted for taking hold of or grasping. [L. *prehendo*, pp. *-hensus*, to lay hold of, seize]

pre·hen·sion (prē-hen′shŭn). The act of grasping, or taking hold of.

pre·hor·mone (prē-hōr′mōn). A glandular secretory product, having little or no inherent biological potency, that is converted peripherally to an active hormone. Cf. prohormone (1).

pre·hy·oid (prē-hī′oyd). Anterior or superior to the hyoid bone;

denoting certain accessory thyroid glands lying superior to the mylohyoid muscle.

pre·ic·tal (prē-ik′tăl). Occurring before a seizure or stroke. [pre- + L. *ictus,* a stroke]

pre·in·duc·tion (prē-in-dŭk′shŭn). A modification in the third generation resulting from the action of environment on the germ cells of one or both individuals of the grandparental generation. An effect from the action of environment on the germ cells of progenitors upon their grandchildren. [L. *prae,* before, + *inductio,* a bringing in, fr. *induco,* to lead in]

Preisz, Hugo von, Hungarian bacteriologist, 1860–1940. SEE P.-Nocard *bacillus.*

pre·kal·li·kre·in (prē-kal-ĭ-krē′in). A plasma glycoprotein which in complex with kininogen serves as a cofactor in the activation of factor XII. P. also serves as the proenzyme for plasma kallikrein. SYN Fletcher factor.

pre·lac·ri·mal (prē-lak′ri-măl). Anterior to the lacrimal sac.

pre·la·ryn·ge·al (prē-lă-rin′jē-ăl). Anterior to the larynx; denoting especially one or two small lymphatic nodes.

pre·lep·to·tene (prē-lep′tō-tēn). The earliest stage of prophase in meiosis, characterized by physiochemical changes in cytoplasm and karyoplasm and beginning contraction of chromosomes. [pre- + leptotene, fr. G. *leptos,* slender, + *tainia,* band]

pre·leu·ke·mia (prē-lū-kē′mē-ă). A syndrome that in time may develop into overt leukemia. It is characterized by bone marrow dysfunction manifested by anemia, neutropenia, and thrombocytopenia.

pre·lim·bic (prē-lim′bik). Anterior to the limbus of the fossa ovalis.

pre·load (prē′lōd). **1.** The load to which a muscle is subjected before shortening. **2.** SYN ventricular p.
ventricular p., formerly, the end-diastolic pressure stretching the ventricular walls, which determines the end-diastolic fiber length at the onset of ventricular contraction, or some other measure of this load on the muscle fibers before contraction; now, more rigorously expressed in terms of the wall stress at this moment, related to the tension per unit cross-sectional area in the ventricular muscle fibers (calculated by Laplace's law from internal radius and pressure modified by wall thickness) that balances this transmural pressure at the moment before contraction begins. SYN preload (2).

pre·ma·lig·nant (prē-mă-lig′nănt). SYN precancerous.

pre·ma·ni·a·cal (prē-mă-nī′ă-kăl). Preceding a manic attack.

pre·ma·ture (prē-mă-tūr′, -chūr). **1.** Occurring before the usual or expected time. **2.** Denoting an infant born at a gestational age of less than 37 weeks; birth weight is no longer considered a critical criterion for use of this designation. [L. *praematurus,* too early, fr. *prae-,* pre- + *maturus,* ripe (mature)]

pre·ma·tu·ri·ty (prē-mă-tūr′i-tē, -chūr′i-tē). **1.** The state of being premature. **2.** In dentistry, deflective occlusal *contact.*

pre·max·il·la (prē-mak-sil′ă). **1.** SYN os incisivum. **2.** The central isolated bony part in a complete bilateral cleft of the lip. [pre- + L. *maxilla,* jawbone]

pre·max·il·lary (prē-mak′si-lār-ē). **1.** Anterior to the maxilla. **2.** Denoting the premaxilla.

pre·med·i·ca·tion (prē′med-i-kā′shŭn). **1.** Administration of drugs prior to anesthesia to allay apprehension, produce sedation, and facilitate the administration of anesthesia. **2.** Drugs used for such purposes.

pre·mel·a·no·some (prē-mel′ă-nō-sōm). A nonpigmented membrane-bound vesicle in a melanocyte that contains tyrosine and matures into the melanin-filled melanosome; prominent in melanocytes of albinos.

pre·men·stru·al (prē-men′strū-ăl). Relating to the period of time preceding menstruation.

pre·men·stru·um (prē-men′strū-ŭm). The few days preceding menstruation. [pre- + L. *menstruum,* ntr. of *menstruus,* monthly, pertaining to menstruation]

pre·mi·to·chon·dria (prē-mī-tō-kon′drē-ă). SYN promitochondria.

pre·mo·lar (prē-mō′lăr). **1.** Anterior to a molar tooth. **2.** A bicuspid tooth.

pre·mon·o·cyte (prē-mon′ō-sīt). An immature monocyte not normally seen in the circulating blood. SYN promonocyte.

pre·mor·bid (prē-mōr′bid). Preceding the occurrence of disease. [pre- + L. *morbidus,* ill, fr. *morbus,* disease]

pre·mu·ni·tion (pre-mū-nish′ŭn). A state of existing resistance of a host to infection or reinfection with a parasite; used especially in malaria epidemiology. [L. *praemunitio,* fortification in advance, fr. *prae-,* + *munio,* to fortify]

pre·mu·ni·tive (prē-mū′ni-tiv). Relating to premunition.

pre·my·e·lo·blast (prē-mī′ĕ-lō-blast). The earliest recognizable precursor of the myeloblast.

pre·my·e·lo·cyte (prē-mī′ĕ-lō-sīt). SYN promyelocyte.

pre·na·ris, pl. **pre·na·res** (prē-nā′ris, nā′rēz). SYN nostril.

pre·na·tal (prē-nā′tăl). Preceding birth. SYN antenatal. [pre- + L. *natus,* born]

pre·ne·o·plas·tic (prē′nē-ō-plas′tik). Preceding the formation of any neoplasm, benign or malignant; a p. condition is not always precancerous, although the term is frequently used erroneously in that sense. [pre- + G. *neos,* new, + *plastikos,* formative]

Prentice, Charles F., U.S. optician, 1854–1946. SEE P.'s *rule.*

pren·yl (pren′il). $(CH_3)_2C=CH–CH_2–$; 3-Methyl-2-buten-1-yl; poly- or multiprenyl residues or derivatives thereof, apparently formed by end-to-end polymerization of isoprene molecules; found in the isoprenoids in nature.

pre·nyl·a·mine (pre-nil′ă-mēn). N-(3,3-Diphenylpropyl)-α-methylphenethylamine; an antianginal agent.

pre·nyl·a·tion (pren′il-ā′shŭn). The covalent addition of prenyl and multiprenyl residues to a macromolecule. SYN isoprenylation.

pre·op·er·a·tive (prē-op′er-ă-tiv). Preceding an operation.

pre·op·tic (prē-op′tik). Referring to the preoptic *region.*

pre·o·ral (prē-ō′răl). In front of the mouth. [pre- + L. *os (or-),* mouth]

pre·os·te·o·blast (prē-os′tē-ō-blast). SYN osteoprogenitor *cell.*

pre·ox·y·gen·a·tion (prē′ok-sĕ-jĕ-nā′shŭn). Denitrogenation with 100% oxygen prior to induction of general anesthesia.

pre·pal·a·tal (prē-pal′ă-tăl). Relating to the anterior part of the palate, or anterior to the palate bone.

pre·par·a·lyt·ic (prē-par-ă-lit′ik). Before the appearance of paralysis.

prep·a·ra·tion (prep-ă-rā′shŭn). **1.** A getting ready. **2.** Something made ready, as a medicinal or other mixture, or a histologic specimen. [L. *praeparatio,* fr. *prae,* before, + *paro,* pp. *-atus,* to get ready]
cavity p., **(1)** removal of dental caries and surgical p. of the remaining tooth structure to receive a dental restoration; **(2)** the final form of an excavation in a tooth resulting from such p.
corrosion p., a p. in which the hollow parts such as ducts, vessels, or alveoli of the lung are filled with a substance that hardens and persists after dissolving the tissues by digestion.
cytologic filter p., a cytologic specimen made by depositing a watery sample (obtained by a variety of methods from many body sites) upon a filter having pores of uniform size smaller than the cellular material to be concentrated; this is followed by

---

△ **Combining forms**

Word*Finder*
Multi-term entry finder
Preceding letter A

A.D.A.M. Anatomy Plates
Between letters L and M

Appendices:
Following letter Z

SYN Synonym; Cf., compare

[NA] Nomina Anatomica

[MIM] Mendelian
Inheritance in Man

☆ **Official alternate term**

☆**[NA] Official alternate**
Nomina Anatomica term

High Profile Term

pr

fixation and staining, usually with 95% ethyl alcohol and Papanicolaou stain.

heart-lung p., an animal p. in which blood (rendered incoagulable) circulates through the heart and lungs and through an artificial system of vessels representing the systemic circulation; the latter is connected with the divided aorta on the one hand and with the superior vena cava on the other; used in physiologic studies of the heart and circulation.

pre·par·tu·ri·ent (prē-par-tū′rē-ent). Relating to the period before birth.

pre·pa·tel·lar (prē-pă-tel′ăr). Anterior to the patella.

pre·per·i·to·ne·al (prē′per-i-tō-nē′ăl). Denoting a fatty layer between the peritoneum and the transversalis fascia in the lower anterior abdominal wall.

pre·phe·nic ac·id (prē-fē′nik, -fen′ik). 1-Carboxy-4-hydroxy-2,5-cyclohexadiene-1-pyruvic acid; an intermediate in the microbial conversion of shikimic acid to L-phenylalanine and L-tyrosine.

pre·pla·cen·tal (prē-pla-sen′tăl). Before formation of a placenta.

pre·po·ten·tial (prē-pō-ten′shăl). A gradual rise in potential between action potentials as a phasic swing in electric activity of the cell membrane, which establishes its rate of automatic activity, as in the ureter or cardiac pacemaker.

pre·pro·col·la·gen (prē-prō-kol-ō-jen). The precursor of collagen that is synthesized on ribosomes; procollagen with a leader or signal sequence that directs the polypeptide chain into the vesicular space of the endoplasmic reticulum.

pre·pro·in·su·lin (prē-prō-in′sū-lin). The precursor protein to proinsulin. SEE preprotein.

pre·pro·pro·tein (prē-prō-prō′tēn). A precursor to an inactive secretory proprotein.

pre·pro·tein (prē-prō′tēn). A secretory protein with a signal peptide region attached.

pre·psy·chot·ic (prē-sī-kot′ik). 1. Relating to the period antedating the onset of psychosis. 2. Denoting a potential for a psychotic episode, one that appears imminent under continued stress.

pre·pu·ber·al, pre·pu·ber·tal (prē-pyū′ber-ăl, -ber-tăl). Before puberty.

pre·pu·bes·cent (prē-pyū-bes′ent). Immediately prior to the commencement of puberty.

pre·puce (prē′pūs). The free fold of skin that covers more or less completely the glans penis. SYN preputium [NA], foreskin. [L. praeputium, foreskin]

p. of clitoris, the external fold of the labia minora, forming a cap over the clitoris. SYN preputium clitoridis [NA].

hooded p., incomplete circumferential formation of foreskin with a dorsal component (the dorsal hood) but an absent or incomplete ventral portion. Typically seen in boys with hypospadias or isolated chordee. In the rare condition of epispadias, the hooded portional p. may be ventral.

pre·pu·ti·al (prē-pyū′shē-ăl). Relating to the prepuce.

pre·pu·ti·ot·o·my (prē-pyū′shē-ot′ō-mē). Incision of prepuce. [preputium + G. tomē, incision]

pre·pu·ti·um, pl. **pre·pu·tia** (prē-pyū′shē-ŭm, shē-ă) [NA]. SYN prepuce. [L. praeputium]

p. clitor′idis [NA], SYN prepuce of clitoris.

pre·py·lor·ic (prē-pī-lōr′ik). Anterior to or preceding the pylorus; denoting a temporary constriction of the wall of the stomach separating the fundus from the antrum during digestion.

pre·rec·tal (prē-rek′tăl). Anterior to or preceding the rectum.

pre·re·duced (prē-rē-dūsd′). Pertaining to bacteriologic media that are boiled, tubed under oxygen-free gas with chemical reducing agents and colorimetric redox indicator in stoppered tubes or bottles, and then sterilized.

pre·re·nal (prē-rē′năl). Anterior to a kidney. [L. ren, kidney]

pre·ret·i·nal (prē-ret′i-nal). Anterior to the retina.

pre·sa·cral (prē-sā′krăl). Anterior to or preceding the sacrum.

△**presby-, presbyo-.** Old age. SEE ALSO gero-. [G. presbys, old man]

pres·by·a·cou·sia (prez-bē-ă-kū′sē-ă). SYN presbyacusis.

pres·by·a·cu·sis, pres·by·a·cu·sia (prez′bē-ă-kū′sis). Loss of ability to perceive or discriminate sounds as a part of the aging process; the pattern and age of onset may vary. SYN presbyacousia, presbycusis. [presby- + G. akousis, hearing]

pres·by·at·rics (prez-bē-at′riks). Rarely used terms for geriatrics. [presby- + G. iatreia, medical treatment]

pres·by·cu·sis (prez-bē-kū′sis). SYN presbyacusis.

pres·by·o·pia (Pr) (prez-bē-ō′pē-ă). The physiologic loss of accommodation in the eyes in advancing age, said to begin when the near point has receded beyond 22 cm (9 inches). [presby- + G. ōps, eye]

pres·by·op·ic (prez′bē-op′ik, -ō′pik). Relating to or suffering from presbyopia.

pre·scribe (prē-skrīb). To give directions, either orally or in writing, for the preparation and administration of a remedy to be used in the treatment of any disease. [L. prae-scribo, pp. -scriptus, to write before]

pre·scrip·tion (prē-skrip′shŭn). 1. A written formula for the preparation and administration of any remedy. 2. A medicinal preparation compounded according to formulated directions, said to consist of four parts: 1) superscription, consisting of the word recipe, take, or its sign, ℞; 2) inscription, the main part of the p., containing the names and amounts of the drugs ordered; 3) subscription, directions for mixing the ingredients and designation of the form (pill, powder, solution, etc.) in which the drug is to be made, usually beginning with the word, misce, mix, or its abbreviation, M.; 4) signature, directions to the patient regarding the dose and times of taking the remedy, preceded by the word signa, designate, or its abbreviation, S. or Sig. [L. praescriptio; see prescribe]

shotgun p., a p. containing many ingredients, some of which may be useless, in an attempt to cover all possible types of therapy that may be needed; a pejorative term.

pre·se·nile (prē-sē′nīl). Prior to the usual onset of senility, as in the milder, presenile dementia.

pre·se·nil·i·ty (prē-sĕ-nil′i-tē). Premature old age; the condition of an individual, not old in years, who displays the physical and mental characteristics of old age but not to the extent of senility. [pre- + L. senilis, old]

pre·se·ni·um (prē-sē′nē-ŭm). The period preceding old age.

pre·sent (prē-zent′). 1. To precede or appear first at the os uteri, said of the part of the fetus first felt during examination. 2. To appear for examination, treatment, etc., said of a patient. [L. praesens (-sent-), pres. p. of prae-sum, to be before, be at hand]

pre·sen·ta·tion (prē′zen-tā′shŭn, prez′). That part of the fetus presenting at the superior strait of the maternal pelvis; occiput, chin, and sacrum are, respectively, the determining points in vertex, face, and breech p. SEE ALSO position (3). See also entries under position. [see present]

acromion p., SYN shoulder p.

breech p., p. of any part of the pelvic extremity of the fetus, the nates, knees, or feet; more properly only of the nates; frank breech p. occurs when the fetus presents by the pelvic extremity; the thighs may be flexed and the legs extended over the anterior surfaces of the body; in **full breech p.,** the thighs may be flexed on the abdomen and the legs upon the thighs, in **footling p.,** foot p. the feet may be the lowest part; in **incomplete foot p., incomplete knee p.,** one leg may retain the position which is typical of one of the above-mentioned presentations, while the other foot or knee may present. SYN pelvic p.

brow p., SEE cephalic p.

cephalic p., p. of any part of the fetal head, usually the upper and back part as a result of flexion such that the chin is in contact with the thorax in vertex p.; there may be degrees of flexion so that the presenting part is the large fontanel in sincipital p., the brow in brow p., or the face in face p. SYN head p.

face p., SEE cephalic p.

footling p., foot p., SEE breech p.

frank breech p., SEE breech p.

head p., SYN cephalic p.

incomplete foot p., SEE breech p.

knee p., SEE breech p.

pelvic p., SYN breech p.

placental p., SYN *placenta* previa.

polar p., the p. of either pole of the fetal oval; may be either a cephalic or breech p., or a longitudinal lie.

shoulder p., transverse p. with the shoulder as the presenting part. SYN acromion p.

sincipital p., SEE cephalic p.

transverse p., an abnormal p., neither head nor breech, in which the fetus lies transversely in the uterus across the axis of the parturient canal.

vertex p., SEE cephalic p.

pre·ser·va·tive (prē-zer′vă-tiv). A substance added to food products or to an organic solution to prevent chemical change or bacterial action.

pre·so·mite (prē-sō′mīt). Relating to the embryonic stage before the appearance of somites (before day 19 in the human).

pre·sphe·noid (prē-sfē′noyd). In front of the sphenoid bone or cartilage.

pre·sphyg·mic (prē-sfig′mik). Preceding the pulse beat; denoting a brief interval following the filling of the ventricles with blood before their contraction forces open the semilunar valves, corresponding to the isovolumic contraction period. [pre- + G. *sphygmos,* pulse]

pre·spi·nal (prē-spī′năl). Anterior to the spine.

pre·spon·dy·lo·lis·the·sis (prē-spon-di-lō-lis′thē-sis). A condition predisposing to spondylolisthesis, consisting of a defect in the laminae of a lumbar vertebra but before development of any displacement of the vertebral body. SEE spondylolysis.

pres·sor (pres′er, -ōr). Exciting to vasomotor activity; producing increased blood pressure; denoting afferent nerve fibers which, when stimulated, excite vasoconstrictors which increase peripheral resistance. SYN hypertensor. [L. *premo,* pp. *pressus,* to press]

pres·so·re·cep·tive (pres′ō-rē-sep′tiv). Capable of receiving as stimuli changes in pressure, especially changes of blood pressure. SYN pressosensitive.

pres·so·re·cep·tor (pres′ō-rē-sep′ter, -tōr). SYN baroreceptor.

pres·so·sen·si·tive (pres-ō-sen′si-tiv). SYN pressoreceptive.

pres·so·sen·si·tiv·i·ty (pres′ō-sen-si-tiv′i-tē). The state of being able to perceive changes in pressure. SEE ALSO pressoreceptive.

reflexogenic p., p. also capable of initiating the regulation of heart rate, vascular tone, and blood pressure.

pres·sure (P) (presh′ŭr). **1.** A stress or force acting in any direction against resistance. **2** (P, frequently followed by a subscript indicating location). In physics and physiology, the force per unit area exerted by a gas or liquid against the walls of its container or that would be exerted on a wall immersed at that spot in the middle of a body of fluid.

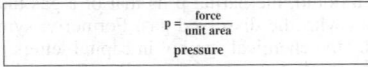

$$P = \frac{force}{unit\ area}$$
pressure

The p. can be considered either relative to some reference p., such as that of the ambient atmosphere (imagined to be on the other side of the wall), or in absolute terms (relative to a perfect vacuum). [L. *pressura,* fr. *premo,* pp. *pressus,* to press]

abdominal p., p. surrounding the bladder; estimated from rectal, gastric, or intraperitoneal p.

absolute p., p. measured with respect to zero p. Cf. gauge p.

acoustic p., in ultrasound, the instantaneous value of the total pressure minus the ambient pressure; unit is pascal (Pa).

atmospheric p., SYN barometric p.

back p., p. exerted upstream in the circulation as a result of obstruction to forward flow, as when congestion in the pulmonary circulation results from stenosis of the mitral valve or failure of the left ventricle.

barometric p. (P_B), the absolute p. of the ambient atmosphere, varying with weather, altitude, etc.; expressed in millibars (meteorology) or mm Hg or torr (respiratory physiology); at sea level, one atmosphere (atm, 760 mm Hg or torr) is equivalent to:

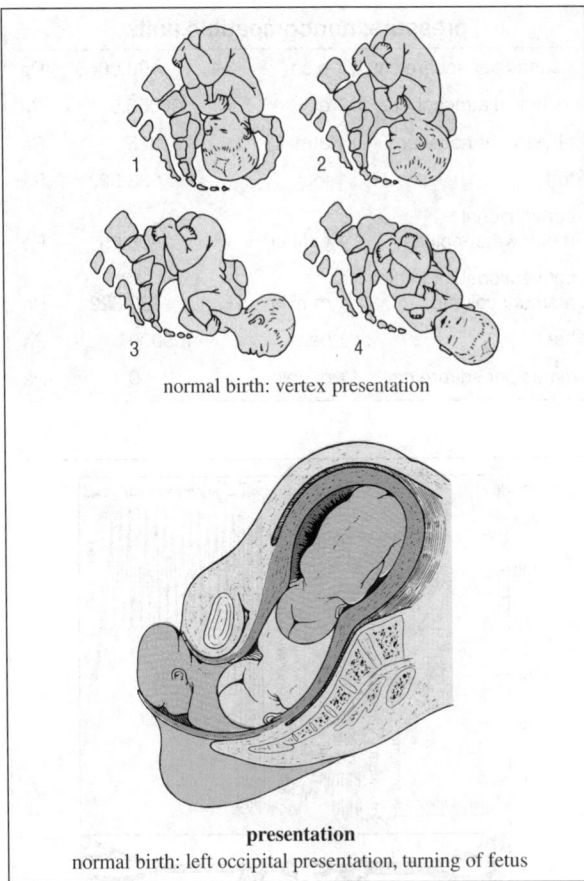

normal birth: vertex presentation

presentation
normal birth: left occipital presentation, turning of fetus

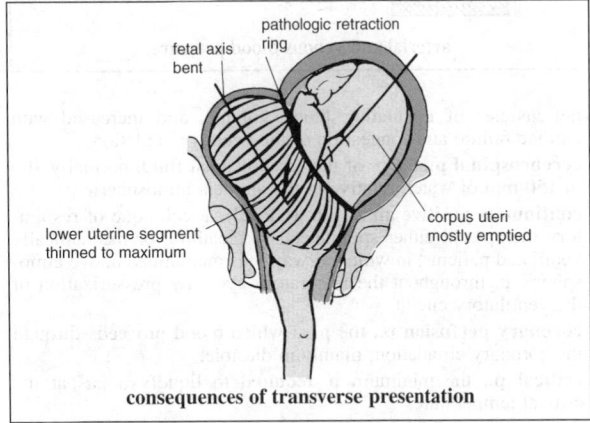

consequences of transverse presentation

14.69595 lb/sq in, 1013.25 millibars, 1013.25×10^6 dynes/cm^2, and, in SI units, 101,325 pascals (Pa). SYN atmospheric p.

biting p., SYN occlusal p.

blood p. (BP), the p. or tension of the blood within the systemic arteries, maintained by the contraction of the left ventricle, the resistance of the arterioles and capillaries, the elasticity of the arterial walls, as well as the viscosity and volume of the blood; expressed as relative to the ambient atmospheric p. SYN arteriotony, piesis.

central venous p. (CVP), the p. of the blood within the venous system in the superior and inferior vena cava, normally between 4 and 10 cm of water; it is depressed in circulatory shock and

pressure: noncompatible units

pounds per square cm	: 1 p/cm²	=	98.0665	Pa
technical atmosphere	: 1 at	=	98066.5	Pa
physical atmosphere	: 1 atm	=	101325	Pa
torr	: 1 torr	=	133.322	Pa
conventional meter water-column	: 1 m H₂O	=	9806.65	Pa
conventional millimeter mercury column	: 1 mmHg	=	133.322	Pa
bar	: 1 bar	=	100000	Pa
dynes per square cm	: 1 dyne/cm²	=	0.1	Pa

intracardial pressure (mmHg)

	A wave	X trough	V wave	Y trough	average
right atrium	up to 5	0	up to 5	0	up to 4
left atrium	ca. 8	0	ca. 10	0	ca. 6–8
	systolic		early diastolic		late diastolic
right ventricle	20–30		0		up to 5
left ventricle	ca. 120		0		ca. 7–10

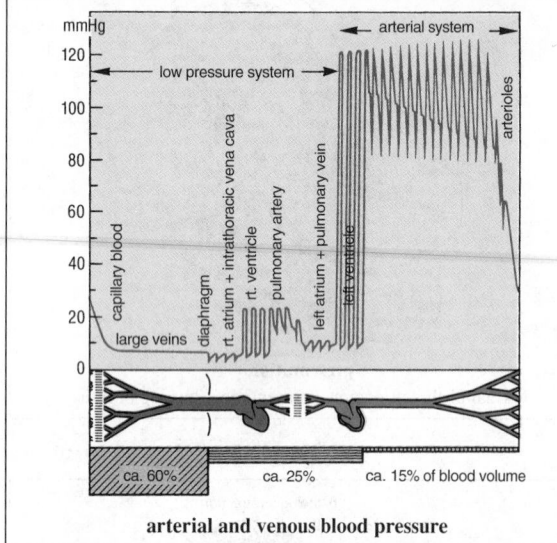

arterial and venous blood pressure

ry, usually a semipermeable membrane; it is commonly represented by the product of the total osmotic p. of the solution and the ratio (corrected for activities) of the number of dissolved particles that do not permeate the bounding membrane to the total number of particles in the solution; equivalent in meaning to tonicity; commonly expressed in equivalent units of osmolality rather than p. per se.

gauge p., p. measured relative to ambient atmospheric p.; at sea level, it is 1 atm less than the p. in the atmosphere. Cf. absolute p.

hydrostatic p., the p. exerted by a liquid as a result of its potential energy, ignoring its kinetic energy; frequently used to distinguish a true p. from an osmotic p. or to emphasize the variation in p. in a column of fluid due to the effect of gravity.

intracranial p. (ICP), p. within the cranial cavity.

intraocular p., the p. (usually measured in millimeters of mercury) of the intraocular fluid within the eye, measured by means of a manometer.

leak point p., storage p. in bladder at which leakage occurs passively, usually in patients with neuropathic bladder.

negative p., p. less than that of the ambient atmosphere.

negative end-expiratory p. (NEEP), a subatmospheric p. at the airway at the end of expiration.

occlusal p., any force exerted upon the occlusal surfaces of teeth. SYN biting p.

oncotic p., osmotic p. exerted by colloids in solution.

osmotic p. (Π), the p. that must be applied to a solution to prevent the passage into it of solvent when solution and pure solvent are separated by a membrane permeable only to the solvent. (Sometimes less correctly viewed as the force with which the solution attracts solvent through the semipermeable membrane.)

partial p. (P), the p. exerted by a single component of a mixture of gases, commonly expressed in mm Hg or torr; for a gas dissolved in a liquid, the partial p. is that of a gas that would be in equilibrium with the dissolved gas. Formerly, symbolized by p, followed by the chemical symbol in capital letters (*e.g.,* pCO_2, pO_2); now, in respiratory physiology, P, followed by subscripts denoting location and/or chemical species (*e.g.,* P_{CO_2}, P_{O_2}, PA_{CO_2}).

pleural p., the p. in the pleural space between the visceral and parietal pleurae.

positive end-expiratory p. (PEEP), a technique used in respiratory therapy in which airway p. greater than atmospheric p. is achieved at the end of exhalation by introduction of a mechanical impedance to exhalation.

pulmonary p., the blood p. in the pulmonary artery.

pulmonary capillary wedge p. (PCWP), the p. obtained when a catheter is passed from the right side of the heart into the pulmonary artery as far as it will go and "wedged" into an end artery. PCWP is measured by letting pulmonary blood flow guide a balloon-flotation catheter into a small pulmonary end artery. The p. distal to the wedged catheter is an approximation of cardiac left atrial p. The p. recorded with the balloon deflated is pulmonary artery p.

pulp p., the p. in the dental pulp cavity associated with extracellular fluid p., but showing pulsatile variations during the cardiac cycle because of the encasement of the pulp within the tooth.

pulse p., the variation in blood p. occurring in an artery during

deficiencies of circulating blood volume, and increased with cardiac failure and congestion of the venous circulation.

cerebrospinal p., the p. of the cerebrospinal fluid, normally 100 to 150 mm of water, relative to the ambient atmospheric p.

continuous positive airway p. (CPAP), a technique of respiratory therapy, in either spontaneously breathing or mechanically ventilated patients, in which airway p. is maintained above atmospheric p. throughout the respiratory cycle by pressurization of the ventilatory circuit.

coronary perfusion p., the p. at which blood proceeds through the coronary circulation, mainly in diastole.

critical p., the minimum p. required to liquefy a gas at the critical temperature.

detrusor p., that component of intravesical pressure created by the tension (active and passive) exerted by the bladder wall; the transmural p. across the bladder wall estimated by subtracting abdominal p. from intravesical p.

diastolic p., the intracardiac p. during or resulting from diastolic relaxation of a cardiac chamber; the lowest arterial blood p. reached during any given ventricular cycle.

differential blood p., the arterial blood p. at corresponding points on the two sides of the body.

Donders' p., an increase of about 6 mm Hg shown by a manometer connected with the trachea when the thorax of the dead body is opened; it is caused by the collapse of the lungs when air is admitted to the thorax.

effective osmotic p., that part of the total osmotic p. of a solution that governs the tendency of its solvent to pass across a bounda-

the cardiac cycle; it is the difference between the systolic or maximum and diastolic or minimum p.'s.

selection p., impact of effective reproduction due to environmental impact on the phenotype.

solution p., the force driving atoms or molecules to leave a solid particle and enter into solution (*i.e.,* to dissolve).

standard p., the absolute p. to which gases are referred under standard conditions (STPD), *i.e.,* 760 mm Hg, 760 torr, or 101,325 newtons/m² (*i.e.,* 101,325 Pa).

systolic p., the intracardiac p. during or resulting from systolic contraction of a cardiac chamber; the highest arterial blood pressure reached during any given ventricular cycle.

transmural p., p. across the wall of a cardiac chamber or of a blood vessel. In the heart, transmural p. is the resultant of the intracavitary p. minus the extracavitary (*i.e.,* pericardial) p. and is the distending, *i.e.,* true filling, p. of the cardiac chamber of measurement when this is done during diastole. Since the pericardial p. normally approximates zero, the filling p. (usually equal to ventricular diastolic mean p.), obviating the complexities of measuring pericardial p.

transpulmonary p., the difference between the p. of the respired gas at the mouth and the pleural p. around the lungs, measured when the airway is open; thus, it includes not only the transmural p. of the lung but also any drop in p. along the tracheobronchial tree during flow.

transthoracic p., the p. in the pleural space measured relative to the p. of the ambient atmosphere outside the chest; the transmural p. across the chest wall.

vapor p., the partial p. exerted by the vapor phase of a liquid.

ventricular filling p., the p. in the ventricle as it fills with blood, ordinarily equivalent to the mean atrial p. when there is no A-V valvular gradient. Atrial p. can be used in place of transmural p. because pericardial pressure usually varies between −2 and +2 mm Hg and hence is negligible. During cardiac tamponade, pericardial and atrial p.'s equilibrate so that transmural p. is zero and the high atrial p.'s cannot be "filling" p.'s.

wedge p., the intravascular pressure reading obtained when a fine catheter is advanced until it completely occludes a small blood vessel or is sealed in place by inflation of a small cuff; commonly measured in the lung to estimate left atrial pressure.

zero end-expiratory p. (ZEEP), airway p. which, at the end of expiration, equals atmospheric p.

pre·ster·num (prē'ster'nŭm). SYN *manubrium* of sternum.

pre·sup·pu·ra·tive (prē-sŭp'yū-rā-tiv). Denoting an early stage in an inflammation prior to the formation of pus.

pre·syn·ap·tic (prē'si-nap'tik). Pertaining to the area on the proximal side of a synaptic cleft.

pre·sys·to·le (prē-sis'tō-lē). That part of diastole immediately preceding systole. SYN late diastole.

pre·sys·tol·ic (prē-sis-tol'ik). Late diastolic, relating to the interval immediately preceding systole.

pre·tar·sal (prē-tar'săl). Denoting the anterior, or inferior, portion of the tarsus.

pre·tec·ta (prē-tek'tă). Orad to the hidden part of the duodenum.

pre·tec·tum (prē-tek'tŭm). SYN pretectal *area.*

pre·thy·roid, pre·thy·roi·de·al, pre·thy·roi·de·an (prē-thī'royd, -thī-roy'dē-ăl, -thī-roy'dē-an). Anterior to or preceding the thyroid gland or cartilage.

pre·tib·i·al (prē-tib'ē-ăl). Relating to the anterior portion of the leg; denoting especially certain muscles.

pre·tra·che·al (prē-trā'kē-al). Anterior to the trachea; denoting especially the middle layer of deep cervical fascia.

pre·tre·mat·ic (prē-trē-mat'ik). Relating to the cranial surface of a branchial cleft. [pre- + G. *trēma,* perforation]

pre·tym·pan·ic (prē-tim-pan'ik). Anterior to the drum of the ear.

prev·a·lence (prev'ă-lens). The number of cases of a disease existing in a given population at a specific period of time (*period p.*) or at a particular moment in time (*point p.*).

pre·ven·tive (prē-ven'tiv). SYN prophylactic (1). [L. *prae-venio,* pp. *-ventus,* to come before, prevent]

pre·ver·te·bral (prē-ver'tĕ-brăl). Anterior to the body of a vertebra or of the vertebral column; denoting especially the deepest layer of deep cervical fascia and the muscles on the anterior aspect of the vertebral column.

pre·ves·i·cal (prē-ves'i-kăl). Anterior to the bladder; denoting especially the retropubic space. [pre- + L. *vesica,* bladder]

pre·vi·us (prē'vē-ŭs). Obstructing; denoting anything blocking the passages in childbirth. [L. *prae,* before, + *via,* way]

Pre·vo·tel·la (prev'ō-tel'ah). Newly created genus of Gram-negative, nonmotile, nonsporeforming, obligately anaerobic, chemoorganotrophic, and pleomorphic rods.

P. di'siens, SYN *Bacteroides disiens.*

P. melani'noge'nica, a species found in the mouth, feces, infections of the mouth, soft tissue, respiratory tract, urogenital tract, and the intestinal tract. Implicated in periodontal disease; seen in aspiration. The type species of *Pretovella.* SYN *Bacteroides melaninogenicus.*

P. ora'lis, SYN *Bacteroides oralis.*

P. o'ris, SYN *Bacteroides oris.*

pre·zone (prē'zōn). SYN prozone.

PRF Abbreviation for prolactin-releasing *factor.*

PRH Abbreviation for prolactin-releasing *hormone.*

pri·a·pism (prī'ă-pizm). Persistent erection of the penis, accompanied by pain and tenderness, resulting from a pathologic condition rather than sexual desire; a term loosely used as a synonym for satyriasis. [see priapus]

pri·a·pus (prī'ă-pŭs). SYN penis. [L. fr. *Priapus* (G. *Priapos*), god of procreation]

Prib·now (prib'now). David, 20th-century U.S. molecular biologist. SEE Pribnow *box.*

Price, Ernest Arthur, English biochemist, *1882. SEE Carr-P. *reaction.*

Price-Jones, Cecil, English hematologist, 1863–1943. SEE Price-Jones *curve.*

Priestley, John Gillies, British physiologist, 1880–1941. SEE Haldane-P. *sample.*

pril·o·caine hy·dro·chlo·ride (pril'ō-kān). 2-(propylamino)-*o*-propionotoluidide hydrochloride; a local anesthetic of the amide type, related chemically and pharmacologically to lidocaine hydrochloride; used for peridural, caudal, and nerve blocks, and for regional and infiltration anesthesia. SYN propitocaine hydrochloride.

pri·ma·cy (prī'mă-sē). The state of being primary, or foremost in rank or importance. [see primary]

genital p., in psychoanalysis, the primary characteristic of the genital phase of psychosexual development, *i.e.,* the libido becomes preponderantly concentrated in the penis.

oral p., in psychoanalysis, the primary characteristic of the oral phase of psychosexual development, *i.e.,* the libido is concentrated mainly in the oral zone.

pri·mal (prī'măl). **1.** First or primary. **2.** SYN primordial (2).

pri·mal scene. In psychoanalysis, the actual or fantasied observation by a child of sexual intercourse, particularly between the parents.

pri·ma·quine phos·phate (prī'mă-kwin). 8-[(4-Amino-1-methylbutyl)amino]-6-methoxyquinoline phosphate (1:2); an antimalarial agent especially effective against *Plasmodium vivax,* terminating relapsing vivax malaria; usually administered with chloroquine.

p. p. sensitivity, a sensitivity to p. p. observed in individuals with glucose-6-phosphate dehydrogenase deficiency.

pri·mary (prī'mār-ē). **1.** The first or foremost, as a disease or symptoms to which others may be secondary or occur as complications. **2.** Relating to the first stage of growth or development. SEE primordial. [L. *primarius,* fr. *primus,* first]

pri·mary re·nin·ism (ren'in-izm). Overproduction of renin by juxtaglomerular cells in the absence of a stimulus (such as decreased renal perfusion); leads to hyperaldosteronism, hypertension, hypokalemia, and edema.

pri·mase (prī'mās). SYN dnaG. [*prim*er + -ase]

pri·mate (prī'māt). An individual of the order Primates. [L. *primus,* first]

Pri·ma·tes (prī-ma'tēz). The highest order of mammals, including man, monkeys, and lemurs. [L. *primus,* first]

prim·er (prī'mer). **1.** A molecule (which may be a small polymer) that initiates the synthesis of a larger structure. SYN starter. **2.** A pheromone that causes a long-term physiological change.

pri·mer·ite (prī'mě-rīt). SYN protomerite. [L. *primus,* first, + G. *meros,* part]

pri·mi·done (prī'mi-dōn). 5-ethyldihydro-5-phenyl-4,6-(1*H*,5*H*)- pyrimidenedione; an anticonvulsant drug used in the management of generalized tonic clonic and complex partial epilepsy.

pri·mi·grav·i·da (prī-mi-grav'i-dă). SEE gravida. [L. fr. *primus,* first, + *gravida,* a pregnant woman]

pri·mip·a·ra (prī-mip'ă-ră). SEE para. [L. fr. *primus,* first, + *pario,* to bring forth]

pri·mi·par·i·ty (prī-mi-par'i-tē). Condition of being a primipara.

pri·mip·a·rous (prī-mip'ă-rŭs). Denoting a primipara.

pri·mite (prī'mīt). The anterior member of a pair of gregarine gamonts in syzygy.

prim·i·tive (prim'i-tiv). SYN primordial (2). [L. *primitivus,* fr. *primus,* first]

pri·mor·dia (prī-mōr'dē-ă). Plural of primordium.

pri·mor·di·al (prī-mōr'dē-ăl). **1.** Relating to a primordium. **2.** Relating to a structure in its first or earliest stage of development. SYN primal (2), primitive.

pri·mor·di·um (prī-mōr'-dē-ŭm). An aggregation of cells in the embryo indicating the first trace of an organ or structure. SYN anlage (1). [L. origin, fr. *primus,* first, + *ordior,* to begin]

frontonasal p., SYN frontonasal *prominence.*

lateral nasal p., SYN lateral nasal *prominence.*

medial nasal p., SYN medial nasal *prominence.*

prim·o·some (prī-mō-sōm). A complex of proteins that bind with primase at specific sequences of DNA that serve as the sites for the formation of RNA primers; a part of the replisome. [*prim*er + -some]

prim·u·la (prim'yū-lă). The rhizome and roots of a number of species of *Primula* (family Primulaceae), primrose or cowslip; has been used as expectorant, diuretic, and anthelmintic. In some sensitive persons contact with the plant causes a rash. [Mediev. L. primrose, fem. of L. *primulus,* first]

pri·mu·lin (prī'myū-lin) [C.I. 49000]. An acid yellow thiazole dye, $C_{21}H_{14}N_3O_3Na$, used as a fluorescent vital stain.

pri·mus (prī'mŭs). First; denoting the first of a series of similar structures. [L.]

prin·ceps, pl. **prin·ci·pes** (prin'seps, -si-pēz). Principal; in anatomy, term used to distinguish several arteries. [L. chief, fr. *primus,* first, + *capio,* to take, choose]

p. cervi'cis, SYN descending *branch* of occipital artery.

p. pol'licis, SYN princeps pollicis *artery.*

Princeteau, L.R., French physician, *1884. SEE P.'s *tubercle.*

prin·ci·ple (prin'si-pl). **1.** A general or fundamental doctrine or tenet. SEE ALSO law, rule, theorem. **2.** The essential ingredient in a substance, especially one that gives it its distinctive quality or effect. [L. *principium,* a beginning, fr. *princeps,* chief]

active p., a constituent of a drug, usually an alkaloid or glycoside, upon the presence of which the characteristic therapeutic action of the substance largely depends.

antianemic p., the material in liver (and certain other tissues) that stimulates hemopoiesis in pernicious anemia; for practical purposes, the antianemic effect of extracts from such tissues is approximately equivalent to the content of vitamin B_{12}.

azygos vein p., a p. based on the observation that animals can survive prolonged vena caval occlusion without sequelae: if blood from the azygos vein alone is permitted to enter the heart, patients are perfused during cardiac and pulmonary bypass at

flows much less than the normal resting cardiac output. SYN low flow p.

Bernoulli's p., SYN Bernoulli's *law.*

bitter p.'s, a class of plant substances with a bitter taste that produce a reflexive increase in saliva secretion as well as secretion of digestive juices.

closure p., in psychology, the p. that when one views fragmentary stimuli forming a nearly complete figure (*e.g.,* an incomplete rectangle) one tends to ignore the missing parts and perceive the figure as whole. SEE gestalt.

consistency p., in psychology, the desire of the human being to be consistent, especially in his attitudes and beliefs; theories of attitude formation and change based on the consistency p. include balance theory, which suggests that the individual seeks to avoid incongruity in his various attitudes. SEE ALSO cognitive dissonance *theory.*

Fick p., SYN Fick *method.*

follicle-stimulating p., SYN follitropin.

founder p., the conditional probabilities of the frequencies of a set of genes at any future date depend on the initial composition of the founders of the population and have in general no tendency to revert to the composition of the population from which the founders were themselves derived.

hematinic p., the p. previously thought to be produced by the action of Castle's intrinsic factor upon an extrinsic factor in food, now recognized as vitamin B_{12}.

Huygens' p., used in ultrasound technology; the p. that any wave phenomenon can be analyzed as the sum of many simple sources properly chosen with regard to phase and amplitude.

p. of inertia, SYN repetition-compulsion p.

Le Chatelier's p., SYN Le Chatelier's *law.*

low flow p., SYN azygos vein p.

luteinizing p., SYN lutropin.

melanophore-expanding p., SYN melanotropin.

Mitrofanoff p., SYN appendicovesicostomy.

nirvana p., in psychoanalysis, the p. that expresses the tendency toward the death instinct.

organic p., SYN proximate p.

pain-pleasure p., a psychoanalytic concept that, in a human's psychic functioning, he/she tends to seek pleasure and avoid pain; a term borrowed by experimental psychology to denote the same tendency of an animal in a learning situation. SYN pleasure p.

Pauli's exclusion p., the theory limiting the number of electrons in the orbit or shell of an atom; that it is not possible for any two electrons to have all four quantum numbers identical.

pleasure p., SYN pain-pleasure p.

proximate p., in chemistry, an organic compound that may exist already formed as a part of some other more complex substance (*e.g.,* various sugars, starches, and albumins). SYN organic p.

reality p., the concept that the pleasure p. in personality development is modified by the demands of external reality; the p. or force that compels the growing child to adapt to the demands of external reality.

repetition-compulsion p., in psychoanalysis, the impulse to redramatize or reenact earlier emotional experiences or situations. SYN p. of inertia.

Stewart-Hamilton p., used to determine blood flow from the concentration of dye or temperature dilution.

ultimate p., one of the chemical elements.

Pringle, John J., English dermatologist, 1855–1922. SEE P.'s *disease;* Bourneville-Pringle *disease.*

Prinzmetal, Myron, U.S. cardiologist, *1908. SEE P.'s *angina.*

---

pri·on (prī'on). SYN prion *protein.* [proteinaceous infectious particle]

The word, for proteinaceous infectious agent, was coined in 1982 by neurologist Stanley Prusiner as part of a hypothesis regarding ailments bearing etiologic resemblance to those caused by slow viruses (for instance, kuru). The hypothesis has been borne out by investigation. Prions are now believed responsible for several transmissible neurodegenerative diseases.

prism (prizm). A transparent solid, with sides that converge at an angle, that deflects a ray of light toward the thickest portion (the base) and splits white light into its component colors; in spectacles, a p. corrects ocular muscle imbalance. [G. *prisma*]

enamel p.'s, SYN *prismata* adamantina, under *prisma.*

Fresnel p., a p. composed of concentric annular rings.

Nicol p., a p. that transmits only polarized light.

Risley's rotary p., a p. with a circular base that is rotated in a metal frame marked with a scale; used in examination of ocular muscle imbalance.

pris·ma, pl. **pris·ma·ta** (priz′mă, priz′mah-tă). A structure resembling a prism. [G. something sawed, a prism]

pris′mata adamanti′na, the calcified, microscopic rods radiating from the surface of the dentin, forming the substance of the enamel of a tooth. SYN enamel fibers, enamel prisms, enamel rods.

pris·mat·ic (priz-mat′ik). Relating to or resembling a prism.

prism bar. A graduated series of p. b.'s mounted on a frame and used in ocular diagnosis.

pri·va·cy (prī′vă-sē). **1.** Being apart from others; seclusion; secrecy. **2.** Especially in psychiatry and clinical psychology, respect for the confidential nature of the therapist-patient relationship.

PRL Abbreviation for prolactin.

p.r.n. Abbreviation for L. pro re nata, as the occasion arises; when necessary.

Pro Symbol for proline or its radicals.

⚠**pro-.** **1.** Prefix denoting before, forward. SEE ALSO ante-, pre-. **2.** In chemistry, prefix indicating precursor of. SEE ALSO -gen. [L. and G. *pro*]

pro·ac·cel·er·in (prō-ak-sel′er-in). SYN *factor* V.

pro·ac·ro·sin (prō-ak′rō-sin). A precursor protein of acrosin.

pro·ac·ro·so·mal (prō-ak-rō-sō′măl). Relating to an early stage in the development of the acrosome.

pro·ac·tin·i·um (prō-ak-tin′ē-ŭm). SYN protactinium.

pro·ac·ti·va·tor (prō-ak′ti-vā-ter). A substance that, when chemically split, yields a fragment (activator) capable of rendering another substance enzymatically active.

C3 p., SYN properdin *factor* B.

C3 p. convertase, SYN properdin *factor* D.

pro·al (prō′ăl). Relating to a forward movement.

pro·am·ni·on (prō-am′nē-on). An area of the extraembryonic membranes beneath, and in front of, the developing head of a young embryo which remains without mesoderm for some time.

pro·at·las (prō-at′las). A vertebral element intercalated between the atlas and occipital bone in crocodiles and alligators, traces of which are sometimes seen as an anomaly on the undersurface of the occipital bone in humans.

prob·a·bil·i·ty (P) (pro-bă-bil′ĭ-tē). **1.** A measure, ranging from zero to 1, of the degree of belief in a hypothesis or statement. **2.** The limit of the relative frequency of an event in a sequence of N random trials as N approaches infinity.

conditional p., a p. quoted when the range of choices admitted is restricted, *i.e.,* conditional; thus, the p. of the child of a color-blind man inheriting the gene is 1/2 if the child is female and almost zero if the child is male.

joint p., the p. that two or more outcomes are realized jointly; the p. that the child is both male and affected is 1/4.

objective p., a p. of an outcome based either on unassailable theory or extensive empirical experience of exactly the same combination of circumstances; the notion also implies that the realization concerned has not been effected and therefore even in principle not known with certainty.

personal p., an idiosyncratic judgment about the outcome of an event; it may include evidence too subtle to be disposed of in a subjective p.

posterior p., the best rational assessment of the p. of an outcome

on the basis of established knowledge modified and brought up to date. Cf. Bayes *theorem.*

prior p., the best rational assessment of the p. of an outcome on the basis of established knowledge before the present information is included. For instance, the prior p. of the daughter of a carrier of hemophilia being herself hemophiliac is 1/2. But if she already has one child, an affected son, the posterior p. that she is a carrier is unity, whereas if she has one child, a normal one, the posterior p. that she is a carrier is 1/3. SEE Bayes *theorem.*

subjective p., a fair statement of the odds that a rational, well-informed person would give or take for the outcome of an experiment. The experiment may be unique and not rationally understood (precluding both theoretically sound predication and empirical experience). The formulation is applicable to experiments that have been carried out but the outcome unknown. (For instance, a certain statement about the sex of the fetus early in pregnancy is established but perhaps not accessible until amniocentesis can be done.) Unlike personal p., the subjective p. should be the same from all competent counselors in possession of the same evidence.

pro·bac·te·ri·o·phage (prō-bak-tēr′ē-ō-fāj). The stage of a temperate bacteriophage in which the genome is incorporated in the genetic apparatus of the bacterial host. SYN prophage.

defective p., SEE defective *bacteriophage.*

pro·band (prō′band). In human genetics, the patient or member of the family that brings a family under study. SYN index case. [L. *probo,* to test, prove]

probe (prōb). **1.** A slender rod of flexible material, with blunt bulbous tip, used for exploring sinuses, fistulas, other cavities, or wounds. **2.** A device or agent used to detect or explore a substance; *e.g.,* a molecule used to detect the presence of a specific fragment of DNA or RNA or of a specific bacterial colony. **3.** To enter and explore, as with a p. [L. *probo,* to test]

> Probes are essential tools for DNA analysis. Every DNA molecule possesses some unique nucleotide sequences that differentiate it from all others, and these can be used as identifying markers or "fingerprints." Probes are used to test for the presence of cloned genes in bacterial or yeast colonies, for specific nucleotide sequences in samples of DNA, or for select genes upon the chromosomes. See allele, DNA fingerprinting, DNA markers.

Bowman's p., a double-ended p. for the lacrimal duct.

nucleic acid p., a nucleic acid fragment, labeled by a radioisotope, biotin, etc., that is complementary to a sequence in another nucleic acid (fragment) and that will, by hydrogen binding to the latter, locate or identify it and be detected; a diagnostic technique based on the fact that every species of microbe possesses some unique nucleic acid sequences which differentiate it from all others, and thus can be used as identifying markers or "fingerprints."

periodontal p., a calibrated instrument used to measure the depth and topography of periodontal pockets.

radioactive p., SEE nucleic acid p.

vertebrated p., a p. made up of a series of short sections hinged together for flexibility in penetrating convoluted tracts.

viral p., SEE nucleic acid p.

pro·ben·e·cid (prō-ben′ĕ-sid). *p*-Carboxy-*N,N*-diisopropyl-sulfonamide; a competitive inhibitor of the secretion of penicillin or *p*-aminohippurate by kidney tubules; a uricosuric agent used in chronic gouty arthritis.

pro·bil·i·fus·cins (prō-bil′i-fŭs′in). SEE bilirubinoids.

pro·bi·o·sis (prō-bī-ō′sis). An association of two organisms that enhances the life processes of both. Cf. antibiosis (1), symbiosis, mutualism. [pro- + G. *biōsis,* life]

pro·bi·ot·ic (prō-bī-ot′ik). Relating to probiosis.

prob·lem. In the mental health professions, a term often used to denote life problems (the difficulties or challenges of life); sometimes used in preference to the terms mental illness or mental disorder. [G. *problēma,* proposition, topic, fr. *proballo,* to put forward]

pr

pro·bos·cis, pl. **pro·bos·ci·des**, **pro·bos·ci·ses** (prō-bos'is, prō-bos'i-dēz, -sēz). **1.** A long flexible snout, such as that of a tapir or an elephant. **2.** In teratology, a cylindrical protuberance of the face which, in cyclopia or ethmocephaly, represents the nose. [G. *proboskis,* a means of providing food, fr. pro- + *boskein,* to feed]

Probst·y·may·ria vi·vip·a·ra (prob-sti-mā'rē-ă vi-vip'ă-ră). A nematode (family Atractidae) closely related to the true pinworms (family Oxyuridae) and still commonly considered the horse pinworm; it is distributed worldwide and is found often in tremendous numbers, because of internal autoreinfection, in the colon of horses and other equids.

pro·bu·col (prō'byū-kōl). Acetone bis(3,5-di-*tert*-butyl-4-hydroxyphenyl)mercaptole; an antihyperlipoproteinemic agent.

pro·cain·a·mide hy·dro·chlo·ride (pro-kān'ă-mīd, pro'kān-am'īd, -id). *p*-Amino-*N*-[2-(diethylamino)ethyl]benzamide hydrochloride; differs chemically from procaine by containing the amide group (CONH) instead of the ester group (COO). It depresses the irritability of the cardiac muscle, having a quinidine-like action upon the heart, and is used in ventricular arrhythmias.

pro·caine hy·dro·chlo·ride (prō'kān). 2-Diethylaminoethyl *p*-aminobenzoate monohydrochloride; a local anesthetic for infiltration and spinal anesthesia; previously widely used but now infrequently employed.

pro·cap·sid (prō-kap'sid). A protein shell lacking a virus genome.

pro·car·ba·zine hy·dro·chlo·ride (prō-kar'bă-zēn). Ibenzmethyzin hydrochloride; *N*-isopropyl-α-(2-methylhydrazino)-*p*-toluamide monohydrochloride; an antineoplastic agent.

pro·car·box·y·pep·ti·dase (prō'kar-bok-sē-pep'ti-dās). Inactive precursor of a carboxypeptidase.

pro·car·cin·o·gens (prō-kar-sin'-ō-jens). Inactive xenobiotics that are converted to carcinogens in the organism.

Pro·car·y·o·tae (pro-kar-ē-ō'tē). syn Prokaryotae. [pro- + G. *karyon,* kernel, nut]

pro·car·y·ote (pro-kar'ē-ōt). syn prokaryote. [pro- + G. *karyon,* kernel, nut]

pro·car·y·ot·ic (prō'kar-ē-ot'ik). syn prokaryotic.

pro·cat·arc·tic (prō-kă-tark'tik). Rarely used term for denoting the exciting cause of a disease. [G. *prokatarktikos,* beginning beforehand]

pro·cat·arx·is (prō-kă-tark'sis). **1.** syn exciting *cause.* **2.** The beginning of a disease under the influence of the exciting cause, a predisposing cause already existing. [G. a beginning beforehand, fr. *prokatararchomi,* to begin first, fr. *pro,* before, + *kata,* upon, + *archō,* to begin]

pro·ce·dure (prō-sē'jŭr). Act or conduct of diagnosis, treatment, or operation. see also method, operation, technique.

Belsey Mark IV p., a transthoracic hiatal hernia repair that restores the lower esophageal sphincter zone to the high pressure region below the diaphragm.

Belsey Mark V p., a modified Belsey Mark IV p. often employing pledgetted sutures performed for patients with hiatal hernia plus disordered esophageal motility in whom an esophageal myotomy is also needed.

Chamberlain p., a limited left anterior thoracostomy for biopsy of the mediastinal nodes out of reach by cervical mediastinoscopy. syn anterior mediastinotomy.

Clagett p. for empyema, a two-stage surgical p. for expediting treatment of chronic empyema.

Collis-Belsey p., a surgical method of treating esophageal structure by creation of a neoesophagus and a fundoplication antireflux p.

commando p., an operation for malignant tumors of the floor of the oral cavity, involving resection of portions of the mandible in continuity with the oral lesion and radical neck dissection. syn commando operation.

Damus-Kaye-Stancel p., a p. for subaortic stenosis, entails the creation of an end-to-side pulmonary trunk/aortic anastomosis, performed along with a Fontan p., particularly for patients with a double inlet left ventricle. syn Damus-Stancel-Kaye anastomosis.

dideoxy p. (di'dē-ōks-ē), an enzymatic procedure for sequencing

of DNA employing dideoxy nucleotides as chain terminators. see Sanger *method.*

Dor p., syn Jatene p.

Eloesser p., transposition of a tonguelike pedicled skin flap from the chest wall into the depths of an incision that communicates with an empyema or peripheral lung abscess; used to prevent scar closure of the tract to insure long-term mandatory dependent drainage.

endorectal pull-through p., removal of diseased rectal mucosa along with resection of the lower bowel, followed by anastomosis of the proximal stump to the anus, in order to spare rectal muscle function.

Ewart's p., elevation of the larynx between the thumb and forefinger to elicit tracheal tugging.

Fontan p., placement of a conduit (usually valved) from the right atrium to the main pulmonary artery as a bypass to a hypoplastic right ventricle, as in tricuspid atresia. syn Fontan operation.

Girdlestone p., complete resection or excision of the head and neck of the femur.

Jatene p., a method of repairing congenital tunnel-type subaortic stenosis and narrowing of the left ventricular-aortic junction by aortoventriculoplasty and prosthetic valve replacement. syn Dor p.

Konno p., a method of repairing congenital tunnel-type subaortic stenosis and narrowing of the left ventricular-aortic junction by aortoventriculoplasty and prosthetic valve replacement.

Konno-Rastan p., an aortoventriculoplasty used to enlarge the aortic annular size, especially when subaortic fibromuscular stenosis is present.

loop electrocautery excision p. (LEEP), electrocautery excisional biopsy of abnormal cervical tissue.

Mustard p., syn Mustard *operation.*

Nick's p., enlarges the aortic annulus by incising the noncoronary sinus and the roof of the left atrium.

Noble-Collip p., obsolete p. in which shock in rats is induced by rotating them in a drum.

Norwood p., a complex p. designed to treat aortic atresia with hypoplastic left heart syndrome; sometimes performed in two stages.

Puestow p., longitudinal pancreaticojejunostomy for treatment of chronic pancreatitis.

push-back p., a surgical maneuver designed to reposition the soft palate posteriorly and reestablish velopharyngeal competence.

Putti-Platt p., syn Putti-Platt *operation.*

Rittenhouse-Manogian p., enlarges the aortic annulus by incising the left coronary-noncoronary commissure down unto the anterior leaflet of the mitral valve.

shelf p., insertion of a graft from the ilium into the roof of the acetabulum for congenital dislocation of the hip.

Snow p., syn autoaugmentation.

Stanley Way p., a radical vulvectomy.

Sugiura p., esophageal transection with paraesophageal devascularization, for esophageal varices.

Thal p., correction of a benign stricturing of the lower esophagus in which the narrowed area is opened to full-thickness longitudinally and the adjacent external gastric wall is patch sutured over this defect to restore luminal circumference and continuity.

Vineberg p., implantation of the internal mammary artery into the myocardium to improve blood flow to the heart.

V-Y p., syn V-Y-plasty.

W p., syn W-plasty.

Z p., syn Z-plasty.

pro·ce·lia (prō-sē'lē-ă). A lateral ventricle of the brain; the hollow of the prosencephalon. [pro- + G. *koilia,* a hollow]

pro·ce·lous (prō-sē'lŭs). Concave anteriorly. [pro- + G. *koilos,* hollow]

pro·cen·tri·ole (prō-sen'trē-ōl). The early phase in development *de novo* of centrioles or basal bodies from the centrosphere; p.'s form in relation to deuterosomes (p. organizers).

pro·ce·phal·ic (prō-se-fal'ik). Relating to the anterior part of the head. [pro- + G. *kephalē*, head]

pro·cer·coid (prō-ser'koyd). The first stage in the aquatic life cycle of certain tapeworms, such as the pseudophyllideans (family Diphyllobothriidae), following ingestion of the newly hatched larva (coracidium) by a copepod (water flea). The p. develops into a tailed larva in the body cavity of the crustacean first intermediate host; when the p. and its host are ingested by a fish, the p. enters the new host's tissues and becomes a plerocercoid. SEE ALSO *Diphyllobothrium latum*, Pseudophyllidea. [pro- + G. *kerkos*, tail, + *eidos*, resemblance]

pro·ce·rus (prō-sē'rŭs). SYN procerus *muscle*. [L. long, stretched out]

PROCESS

pro·cess (pros'es, prō'ses). **1.** A method or mode of action used in the attainment of a certain result. A process; in anatomy, a projection or outgrowth. In anatomy, a projection or outgrowth. SYN processus [NA]. **2.** A method or mode of action used in the attainment of a certain result. **3.** An advance, progress, or method as of a desease. SEE processus. **4.** A pathologic condition or disease. **5.** In dentistry, a series of operations that convert a wax pattern, such as that of a denture base, into a solid denture base of another material. SEE dental *curing*. [L. *processus,* an advance, progress, process, fr. *pro-cedo,* pp. *-cessus,* to go forward]

A.B.C. p., purification of water or deodorization of sewage by a mixture of *alum*, *blood*, and *charcoal*.

accessory p., a small apophysis at the posterior part of the base of the transverse process of each of the lumbar vertebrae. SYN processus accessorius [NA], accessory tubercle.

acromial p., SYN acromion.

agene p., bleaching of flour with nitrogen trichloride (prohibited in the United States).

alar p., SYN *wing* of crista galli.

alveolar p., the projecting ridge on the inferior surface of the body of the maxilla containing the tooth sockets; the term is also applied to the superior aspect of the body of the mandible, containing the tooth sockets of the lower jaw. SYN processus alveolaris [NA], alveolar body, alveolar bone (1), alveolar border (2), alveolar ridge, basal ridge (1), dental p.

anterior p. of malleus, a slender spur running anteriorward from the neck of the malleus toward the petrotympanic fissure. SYN processus anterior mallei [NA], Folli's p., follian p., long p. of malleus, processus gracilis, processus ravii, Rau's p., Ravius' p., slender p. of malleus.

apical p., the dendritic p. extending from the apex of a pyramidal cell of the cerebral cortex toward the surface. SYN apical dendrite.

articular p., one of the small flat projections on the surfaces of the arches of the vertebrae on either side, at the point where the pedicles and laminae join, forming the zygapophysial joint surfaces; superior articular process, diapophysis; one of the articular processes on the superior surface of the vertebral arch; inferior articular p., one of the articular p.'s on the inferior surface of the vertebral arch. SYN processus articularis [NA], zygapophysis* [NA].

ascending p., SYN *processus* ascendens.

auditory p., the roughened edge of the tympanic plate giving attachment to the cartilaginous portion of the external acoustic meatus.

axonal p., obsolete term for axon.

basilar p., SYN basilar *part* of the occipital bone.

basilar p. of occipital bone, SYN basilar *part* of the occipital bone.

binary p., a random event with two exhaustive and mutually exclusive outcomes; a Bernoulli p.

Budde p., a method of milk sterilization; to the fresh milk, hydrogen peroxide is added in the proportion of 15 ml of a 3% solution to 1 liter of milk, and the mixture is heated to 51°or 52°C (124°F) for 3 hours, by which time the peroxide is decomposed and the nascent oxygen acts as an efficient germicide; the milk is then rapidly cooled and put into sealed bottles.

Burns' falciform p., SYN superior *horn* of falciform margin of saphenous opening.

calcaneal p. of cuboid bone, the process projecting posteriorly from the plantar surface of the cuboid; it supports the anterior end of the calcaneus. SYN processus calcaneus ossis cuboidei [NA].

caudate p., a narrow band of hepatic tissue connecting the caudate and right lobes of the liver posterior to the porta hepatis. SYN processus caudatus [NA].

ciliary p., one of the radiating pigmented ridges, usually seventy in number, on the inner surface of the ciliary body, increasing in thickness as they advance from the orbiculus ciliaris to the external border of the iris; these, together with the folds (plicae) in the furrows between them, constitute the corona ciliaris. SYN processus ciliaris [NA].

Civinini's p., SYN pterygospinous p.

clinoid p., one of three pairs of bony projections from the sphenoid bone: anterior clinoid p., the recurved posterior angle of the lesser wing; middle clinoid p., a little spur of bone on the body of the sphenoid, posterolateral to the tuberculum sellae; posterior clinoid p., a spur of bone at each superior angle of the dorsum sellae. SYN processus clinoideus [NA], clinoid (2).

cochleariform p., SYN *processus* cochleariformis.

complex learning p.'s, those p.'s that require the use of symbolic manipulations, as in reasoning.

condylar p., the articular process of the ramus of the mandible; it includes the head of the mandible, the neck of the mandible and pterygoid fovea. SYN processus condylaris [NA], condyloid p., mandibular condyle.

condyloid p., SYN condylar p.

conoid p., SYN conoid *tubercle*.

coracoid p., a long curved projection from the neck of the scapula overhanging the glenoid cavity; it gives attachment to the short head of the biceps, the coracobrachialis, and the pectoralis minor muscles, and the conoid and coracoacromial ligaments. SYN processus coracoideus [NA].

coronoid p., a sharp triangular projection from a bone; coronoid p. of the mandible, the triangular anterior process of the mandibular ramus, giving attachment to the temporal muscle; coronoid p. of the ulna, a bracket-like projection from the anterior portion of the proximal extremity of the ulna; its anterior surface gives attachment to the brachialis, its proximal surface enters into the formation of the trochlear notch. SYN processus coronoideus [NA].

costal p., an apophysis extending laterally from the transverse process of a lumbar vertebra; it is the homologue of the rib. SYN processus costalis [NA].

dendritic p., SYN dendrite (1).

dental p., SYN alveolar p.

ensiform p., SYN xiphoid p.

ethmoidal p., a projection of the inferior concha, situated behind the lacrimal process and articulating with the uncinate process of the ethmoid. SYN processus ethmoidalis [NA].

falciform p., a continuation of the inner border of the sacrotuberous ligament upward and forward on the inner aspect of the ramus of the ischium. SYN processus falciformis [NA], falciform ligament, ligamentum falciforme.

follian p., SYN anterior p. of malleus.

Folli's p., SYN anterior p. of malleus.

foot p., SYN pedicel.

frontal p. of maxilla, the upward extension from the body of the maxilla, which articulates with the frontal bone. SYN nasal p., processus frontalis maxillae.

frontal p. of zygomatic bone, the p. of the zygomatic bone which extends upward to form the lateral margin of the orbit and articulates with the frontal bone and greater wing of the sphenoid bone. SYN frontosphenoidal p., processus frontalis ossis zygomatici.

frontonasal p., SYN frontonasal *prominence*.

frontosphenoidal p., SYN frontal p. of zygomatic bone.

funicular p., the tunica vaginalis surrounding the spermatic cord.

globular p., obsolete term for intermaxillary *segment*.

hamular p. of lacrimal bone, SYN lacrimal *hamulus*.

hamular p. of sphenoid bone, SYN pterygoid *hamulus*.

head p., the primordium for the notochord. SEE ALSO notochordal p.

intrajugular p., a small pointed process of bone extending from the middle of the jugular notch in both the occipital and the temporal bones, the two being joined by a ligament and dividing the jugular foramen into two portions. SYN processus intrajugularis [NA].

jugular p., a short process jutting out from the posterior part of the condyle of the occipital bone, its anterior border forming the posterior boundary of the jugular foramen. SYN processus jugularis [NA].

lacrimal p., a projection from the anterior edge of the inferior concha which articulates with the lower border of the lacrimal bone. SYN processus lacrimalis [NA].

lateral p. of calcaneal tuberosity, the lateral projection from the posterior part of the calcaneus. SYN processus lateralis tuberis calcanei [NA].

lateral p. of malleus, a short projection from the base of the manubrium of the malleus, attached firmly to the drum membrane. SYN processus lateralis mallei [NA], processus brevis, short p. of malleus, tuberculum mallei.

lateral nasal p., SYN lateral nasal *prominence*.

lateral p. of talus, a projection on the lateral side of the talus below the malleolar articular surface. SYN processus lateralis tali [NA].

Lenhossék's p.'s, short p.'s ("aborted axons") possessed by some ganglion cells.

lenticular p. of incus, a knob at the tip of the long limb of the incus which articulates with the stapes. SYN processus lenticularis incudis [NA], lenticular apophysis, lenticular bone, orbicular bone, orbicular p., orbiculare, os orbiculare, os sylvii.

long p. of malleus, SYN anterior p. of malleus.

malar p., SYN zygomatic p. of maxilla.

mamillary p., a small apophysis or tubercle on the dorsal margin of the superior articular process of each of the lumbar vertebrae and usually of the twelfth thoracic vertebra. SYN processus mamillaris [NA], mamillary tubercle, metapophysis.

mandibular p., SYN mandibular *arch*.

Markov p., a stochastic p. such that the conditional probability distribution for the state at any future instant, given the present state, is unaffected by any additional knowledge of the past history of the system.

mastoid p., the nipple-like projection of the petrous part of the temporal bone. SYN processus mastoideus [NA], mastoid bone, temporal apophysis.

maxillary p., a thin plate of irregular form projecting from the middle of the upper border of the inferior concha, articulating with the maxilla bone and partly closing the orifice of the maxillary sinus. SYN processus maxillaris [NA].

medial p. of calcaneal tuberosity, the medial projection from the posterior part of the calcaneus. SYN processus medialis tuberis calcanei [NA].

medial nasal p., SYN medial nasal *prominence*.

mental p., SYN mental *protuberance*.

muscular p. of arytenoid cartilage, the blunt lateral projection of the arytenoid cartilage giving attachment to the lateral and posterior cricoarytenoid muscles of the larynx. SYN processus muscularis cartilaginis arytenoidei [NA].

nasal p., SYN frontal p. of maxilla.

notochordal p., in the embryo, a midline column of cells that migrate forward from the primitive node to form the notochord. SEE ALSO head p.

odontoblastic p., the extension of the odontoblast which lies within the dentinal tubule; application of stimuli to dentin may cause aspiration of odontoblast contents into the p.

odontoid p., SYN dens (2).

odontoid p. of epistropheus, SYN dens (2).

olecranon p., SYN olecranon.

orbicular p., SYN lenticular p. of incus.

orbital p., the anterior and larger of the two processes at the upper extremity of the vertical plate of the palatine bone, articulating with the maxilla, ethmoid, and sphenoid bones. SYN processus orbitalis [NA].

packing p., the method of placing denture base material in a flask for processing.

palatine p., in the embryo, medially directed shelves from the oral surface of the maxillae; they develop into the secondary palate after midline fusion. SYN processus palatinus [NA].

papillary p., the left lower angle of the caudate lobe of the liver, opposite the caudate process. SYN processus papillaris [NA].

paramastoid p., an occasional process of bone extending downward from the jugular process of the occipital bone in humans. SYN processus paramastoideus [NA], paroccipital p.

paroccipital p., SYN paramastoid p.

posterior p. of septal cartilage, the tapering extension of the septal cartilage that lies between the perpendicular plate of the ethmoid and the vomer. SYN processus posterior cartilaginis septi nasi [NA], processus sphenoidalis cartilaginis septi nasi, sphenoid p. of septal cartilage.

posterior p. of talus, a projection of the talus bearing medial and lateral tubercles; it is posterior and inferior to the trochlea. SYN processus posterior tali [NA], Stieda's p.

primary p., in psychoanalysis, the mental p. directly related to the functions of the primitive life forces associated with the id and characteristic of unconscious mental activity; marked by unorganized, illogical thinking and by the tendency to seek immediate discharge and gratification of instinctual demands. Cf. secondary p.

progressive p.'s, p.'s that continue after they no longer serve the needs of the organism, and after cessation of the stimulus that evoked the p.

pterygoid p., a long process extending downward from the junction of the body and great wing of the sphenoid bone on either side; it is formed of two plates (lateral and medial), united anteriorly but separated below to form the pterygoid notch; the pterygoid fossa is formed by the divergence of these two plates posteriorly. SYN processus pterygoideus [NA], os pterygoideum.

pterygospinous p., a sharp projection from the posterior edge of the lateral pterygoid plate of the sphenoid bone. SYN processus pterygospinosus [NA], Civinini's p.

pyramidal p., the portion of the palatine bone passing lateral and posterior from the angle formed by the vertical and horizontal plates. SYN processus pyramidalis [NA].

Rau's p., SYN anterior p. of malleus.

Ravius' p., SYN anterior p. of malleus.

retromandibular p. of parotid gland, that portion of the parotid salivary gland that is located behind the mandible and occupies the space between the ramus of the mandible and the mastoid process extending as far medially as the pharyngeal wall. SYN processus retromandibularis glandulae parotidis, processus retromandibularis.

secondary p., in psychoanalysis, the mental p. directly related to the learned and acquired functions of the ego and characteristic of conscious and preconscious mental activities; marked by logical thinking and by the tendency to delay gratification by regulation of the discharge of instinctual demands. Cf. primary p.

sheath p. of sphenoid bone, SYN vaginal p. of sphenoid bone.

short p. of malleus, SYN lateral p. of malleus.

slender p. of malleus, SYN anterior p. of malleus.

sphenoid p., SYN sphenoid p. of palatine bone.

sphenoid p. of palatine bone, the posterior and smaller of the two processes at the extremity of the vertical plate of the palatine bone; *processus* sphenoidalis cartilaginis septi nasi, p. posterior cartilaginis septi nasi. SYN processus sphenoidalis [NA], sphenoid p.

sphenoid p. of septal cartilage, SYN posterior p. of septal cartilage.

spinous p., (1) the dorsal projection from the center of a vertebral arch; **(2)** SYN sphenoidal *spine*.

spinous p. of tibia, SYN intercondylar *eminence*.

Stieda's p., SYN posterior p. of talus.

stochastic p., a p. that incorporates some element of randomness. [G. *stochastikos*, pertaining to guessing, fr. *stochazomai*, to guess]

styloid p. of fibula, SYN *apex* of head of fibula.

styloid p. of radius, a thick, pointed, palpable projection on the lateral side of the distal extremity of the radius. SYN processus styloideus radii [NA].

styloid p. of temporal bone, a slender pointed projection running downward and slightly forward from the base of the inferior surface of the petrous portion of the temporal bone where it joins the tympanic portion; it gives attachment to the styloglossus, stylohyoid, and stylopharyngeus muscles and the stylohyoid and stylomandibular ligaments. SYN processus styloideus ossis temporalis [NA].

styloid p. of third metacarpal bone, a pointed projection from the dorsolateral angle of the base of the third metacarpal bone; it sometimes exists as a separate ossicle. SYN processus styloideus ossis metacarpalis III [NA].

styloid p. of ulna, a cylindrical, pointed palpable projection from the medial and posterior aspect of the head of the ulna, to the tip of which is attached the ulnar collateral ligament of the wrist. SYN processus styloideus ulnae [NA].

superior articular p. of sacrum, the large process on each side of the sacrum posteriorly that articulates with the corresponding inferior articular process of the fifth lumbar vertebra. SYN processus articularis superior ossis sacri [NA].

supracondylar p., an occasional spine projecting from the anteromedial surface of the humerus about 5 cm above the medial epicondyle to which it is joined by a fibrous band. The supracondylar foramen thus formed transmits the brachial artery and median nerve. SYN processus supraepicondylaris humeri [NA], supraepicondylar p.

supraepicondylar p., SYN supracondylar p.

temporal p., the posterior projection of the zygomatic bone articulating with the zygomatic process of the temporal bone to form the zygomatic arch. SYN processus temporalis [NA].

Tomes' p.'s, p.'s of the enamel cells.

transverse p., a bony protrusion on either side of the arch of a vertebra, from the junction of the lamina and pedicle, which functions as a lever for attached muscles. SYN processus transversus [NA].

trochlear p., SYN peroneal *trochlea* of calcaneus.

uncinate p. of ethmoid bone, a sickle-shaped process of bone on the medial wall of the ethmoidal labyrinth below the middle concha; it articulates with the ethmoidal process of the inferior concha and partly closes the orifice of the maxillary sinus. SYN processus uncinatus ossis ethmoidalis [NA].

uncinate p. of pancreas, a portion of the head of the pancreas that hooks around posterior to the superior mesenteric vessels, sometimes into the "nutcracker" formed by the superior mesenteric artery and abdominal aorta. SYN processus uncinatus pancreatis [NA], lesser pancreas, pancreas minus, small pancreas, uncinate pancreas, unciform pancreas, Willis' pancreas, Winslow's pancreas.

vaginal p., SYN *sheath* of styloid process.

vaginal p. of peritoneum, SYN *processus* vaginalis of peritoneum.

vaginal p. of sphenoid bone, a thin lamina of bone that extends medially under the body of the sphenoid bone from the medial lamina of the pterygoid process; it articulates with the vomer and the palatine bone. SYN processus vaginalis ossis sphenoidalis [NA], sheath p. of sphenoid bone.

vaginal p. of testis, SYN *processus* vaginalis of peritoneum.

vermiform p., SYN vermiform *appendix*.

vocal p., SYN vocal p. of arytenoid cartilage.

vocal p. of arytenoid cartilage, the lower end of the anterior margin of the arytenoid cartilage to which the vocal cord is attached. SYN processus vocalis cartilaginis arytenoidei [NA], vocal p.

xiphoid p., the cartilage at the lower end of the sternum. SYN processus xiphoideus [NA], ensiform p., ensisternum, metasternum, mucro sterni, xiphisternum, xiphoid cartilage.

zygomatic p. of frontal bone, the massive projection of the frontal bone that joins the zygomatic bone to form the lateral margin of the orbit. SYN processus zygomaticus ossis frontalis.

zygomatic p. of maxilla, the rough projection from the maxilla that articulates with the zygomatic bone. SYN malar p., processus zygomaticus maxillae.

zygomatic p. of temporal bone, the anterior process of the temporal bone that articulates with the temporal process of the zygomatic bone to form the zygomatic arch. SYN processus zygomaticus ossis temporalis.

pro·cess·ing (pros'es-ing). **1.** Posttranslational modification of proteins, particularly secretory proteins and proteins targeted for membranes or specific cellular locations. SYN trafficking. **2.** Posttranscriptional modification of polynucleic acids.

PROCESSUS

pro·ces·sus, pl. **pro·ces·sus** (prō-ses'ŭs) [NA]. SYN process (1). [L. see process]

p. accesso′rius [NA], SYN accessory *process*.

p. alveola′ris [NA], SYN alveolar *process*. SEE ALSO alveolar *bone* (2).

p. ante′rior mal′lei [NA], SYN anterior *process* of malleus.

p. articula′ris [NA], SYN articular *process*.

p. articula′ris supe′rior os′sis sa′cri [NA], SYN superior articular *process* of sacrum.

p. ascen′dens, an upward extension of the embryonic pterygoquadrate cartilage; it develops into the greater wing of the sphenoid bone. SYN ascending process.

p. bre′vis, SYN lateral *process* of malleus.

p. calca′neus os′sis cuboi′dei [NA], SYN calcaneal *process* of cuboid bone.

p. cauda′tus [NA], SYN caudate *process*.

p. cilia′ris [NA], SYN ciliary *process*.

p. clinoi′deus [NA], SYN clinoid *process*.

p. cochlearifor′mis [NA], a bony angular process (the termination of the septum of the auditory tube) above the anterior end of the vestibular window, forming a pulley over which the tendon of the tensor tympani muscle plays. SYN cochleariform process, p. trochleariformis.

p. condyla′ris [NA], SYN condylar *process*.

p. coracoi′deus [NA], SYN coracoid *process*.

p. coronoi′deus [NA], SYN coronoid *process*.

p. costa′lis [NA], SYN costal *process*.

p. ethmoida′lis [NA], SYN ethmoidal *process*.

p. falcifor′mis [NA], SYN falciform *process*.

p. ferrei′ni, SYN medullary *ray*.

p. fronta′lis maxil′lae, SYN frontal *process* of maxilla.

p. fronta′lis os′sis zygomat′ici, SYN frontal *process* of zygomatic bone.

p. grac′ilis, SYN anterior *process* of malleus.

p. intrajugula′ris [NA], SYN intrajugular *process*.

p. jugula′ris [NA], SYN jugular *process*.

p. lacrima′lis [NA], SYN lacrimal *process*.

p. latera′lis mal′lei [NA], SYN lateral *process* of malleus.

p. latera′lis ta′li [NA], SYN lateral *process* of talus.

p. latera′lis tu′beris calca′nei [NA], SYN lateral *process* of calcaneal tuberosity.

p. lenticula′ris incu′dis [NA], SYN lenticular *process* of incus.

p. mamilla′ris [NA], SYN mamillary *process*.

p. mastoi′deus [NA], SYN mastoid *process*.

p. maxilla′ris [NA], SYN maxillary *process*.

pr

p. media′lis tu′beris calca′nei [NA], SYN medial *process* of calcaneal tuberosity.

p. muscula′ris cartila′ginis arytenoi′dei [NA], SYN muscular *process* of arytenoid cartilage.

p. orbita′lis [NA], SYN orbital *process.*

p. palati′nus [NA], SYN palatine *process.*

p. papilla′ris [NA], SYN papillary *process.*

p. paramastoi′deus [NA], SYN paramastoid *process.*

p. poste′rior cartila′ginis sep′ti na′si [NA], SYN posterior *process* of septal cartilage.

p. poste′rior ta′li [NA], SYN posterior *process* of talus.

p. pterygoi′deus [NA], SYN pterygoid *process.*

p. pterygospino′sus [NA], SYN pterygospinous *process.*

p. pyramida′lis [NA], SYN pyramidal *process.*

p. ra′vii, SYN anterior *process* of malleus.

p. retromandibula′ris, SYN retromandibular *process* of parotid gland.

p. retromandibula′ris glan′dulae paroti′dis, SYN retromandibular *process* of parotid gland.

p. sphenoida′lis [NA], SYN sphenoid *process* of palatine bone.

p. sphenoida′lis cartila′ginis sep′ti na′si, SYN posterior *process* of septal cartilage.

p. spino′sus [NA], SYN sphenoidal *spine.*

p. styloi′deus os′sis metacarpa′lis III [NA], SYN styloid *process* of third metacarpal bone.

p. styloi′deus os′sis tempora′lis [NA], SYN styloid *process* of temporal bone.

p. styloi′deus ra′dii [NA], SYN styloid *process* of radius.

p. styloi′deus ul′nae [NA], SYN styloid *process* of ulna.

p. supraepicondyla′ris hu′meri [NA], SYN supracondylar *process.*

p. tempora′lis [NA], SYN temporal *process.*

p. transver′sus [NA], SYN transverse *process.*

p. trochleariform′is, SYN p. cochleariformis.

p. trochlea′ris, SYN peroneal *trochlea* of calcaneus.

p. uncina′tus os′sis ethmoida′lis [NA], SYN uncinate *process* of ethmoid bone.

p. uncina′tus pancrea′tis [NA], SYN uncinate *process* of pancreas.

p. vagina′lis os′sis sphenoida′lis [NA], SYN vaginal *process* of sphenoid bone.

p. vagina′lis peritone′i, SYN p. vaginalis of peritoneum.

p. vaginalis of peritoneum, a peritoneal diverticulum in the embryonic lower anterior abdominal wall that traverses the inguinal canal; in the male it forms the tunica vaginalis testis and normally loses its connection with the peritoneal cavity; a persistent p. vaginalis in the female is known as the canal of Nuck. SYN Nuck's diverticulum, p. vaginalis peritonei, vaginal process of peritoneum, vaginal process of testis.

p. vermifor′mis, SYN vermiform *appendix.*

p. voca′lis cartila′ginis arytenoi′dei [NA], SYN vocal *process* of arytenoid cartilage.

p. xiphoi′deus [NA], SYN xiphoid *process.*

p. zygomat′icus maxil′lae, SYN zygomatic *process* of maxilla.

p. zygomat′icus os′sis fronta′lis, SYN zygomatic *process* of frontal bone.

p. zygomat′icus os′sis tempora′lis, SYN zygomatic *process* of temporal bone.

---

pro·chei·lia, pro·chi·lia (prō-kī′lē-ă). Protruding lips. [pro- + G. *cheilos,* lip]

pro·chei·lon, pro·chi·lon (prō-kī′lon). SYN labial *tubercle.*

pro·chi·ral (prō-kī′ral). Refers to an atom in a molecule (usually a carbon atom) that would become chiral if one of two identical substituents is replaced by a new ligand; *i.e.,* an atom that has two enantiotopic groups linked to it. For example, carbon-1 of ethanol is a prochiral carbon.

pro·chi·ral·i·ty (prō-ki-ral′i-tē). The property of being prochiral.

pro·chlor·per·a·zine (prō-klōr-per′ă-zēn). 2-Chloro-10-[3-(1-methyl-4-piperazinyl)propyl]phenothiazine; a phenothiazine compound similar in structure, actions, and uses to chlorpromazine; used as a tranquilizer and antiemetic; available as the edisylate for oral and intramuscular administration and as the maleate for oral administration.

pro·chon·dral (prō-kon′drăl). Denoting a developmental stage prior to the formation of cartilage. [pro- + G. *chondros,* cartilage]

pro·chor·dal (prō-kōr′dăl). Located cephalic to the notochord. SYN prechordal.

pro·chy·mo·sin (prō-kī′mō-sin). The precursor of chymosin. SYN chymosinogen, pexinogen, prorennin, renninogen, rennogen.

pro·ci·den·tia (pros-i-den′shē-ă, prō′si-). A sinking down or prolapse of any organ or part. [L. a falling forward, fr. *procido,* to fall forward]

p. u′teri, SEE *prolapse* of the uterus.

pro·col·la·gen (prō-kol′ă-jen). Soluble precursor of collagen formed by fibroblasts and other cells in the process of collagen synthesis; unstable type III p. is associated with Ehlers-Danlos syndrome type IV.

p. aminoproteinase, an extracellular enzyme that participates in the processing of collagen, removing the extension peptide at the amino-terminal end of p.

p. carboxyproteinase, an extracellular enzyme that participates in the processing of collagen, removing the extension peptide at the carboxy-terminal end of p.

pro·con·ver·tin (prō-kon-ver′tin). SYN *factor* VII.

pro·cre·ate (prō′krē-āt). To beget; to produce by the sexual act; said usually of the male parent. [L. *pro-creo,* pp. *-creatus,* to beget]

pro·cre·a·tion (prō-krē-ā′shŭn). SYN reproduction (2).

pro·cre·a·tive (prō′krē-ā-tiv). Having the power to beget or procreate.

△**proct-.** SEE procto-.

proc·tag·ra (prok-tag′ră). Obsolete term for proctalgia. [proct- + G. *agra,* a seizure]

proc·tal·gia (prok-tal′jē-ă). Pain at the anus, or in the rectum. SYN proctodynia, rectalgia. [proct- + G. *algos,* pain]

p. fu′gax, painful spasm of the muscle about the anus without known cause; probably a neurosis. SYN anorectal spasm.

proc·ta·tre·sia (prok-tă-trē′zē-ă). SYN anal *atresia.* [proct- + G. *a-* priv. + *trēsis,* a boring]

proc·tec·ta·sia (prok′tek-tā′zē-ă). Rarely used term for dilation of the anus or rectum. [proct- + G. *ektasis,* extension]

proc·tec·to·my (prok-tek′tō-mē). Surgical resection of the rectum. SYN rectectomy. [proct- + G. *ektomē,* excision]

proc·ten·clei·sis, proc·ten·cli·sis (prok-ten-klī′sis). Obsolete term for proctostenosis. [proct- + G. *enkleisis,* enclosure]

proc·teu·ryn·ter (prok-tū-rin′ter). Obsolete term for an inflatable bag for dilating the rectum. [proct- + G. *eurynō,* to dilate, fr. *eurys,* wide]

proc·ti·tis (prok-tī′tis). Inflammation of the mucous membrane of the rectum. SYN rectitis. [proct- + G. *-itis,* inflammation]

chronic ulcerative p., SYN idiopathic p.

epidemic gangrenous p., a generally fatal disease affecting chiefly children in the tropics, characterized by gangrenous ulceration of the rectum and anus, accompanied by frequent watery stools and tenesmus. SYN bicho, caribi, Indian sickness.

idiopathic p., probably a variant of ulcerative colitis involving the rectum; some cases progress to involve the remainder of the colon as well. SYN chronic ulcerative p.

△**procto-, proct-.** Anus; (more frequently) rectum; Cf. recto-. [G. *prōktos*]

proc·to·cele (prok′tō-sēl). Prolapse or herniation of the rectum. SYN rectocele. [procto- + G. *kēlē,* tumor]

proc·to·cly·sis (prok-tok′li-sis). Slow continuous administration of saline solution by instillation into the rectum and sigmoid colon. SYN Murphy drip, rectoclysis. [procto- + G. *klysis,* a washing out]

proc·to·coc·cy·pexy (prok-tō-kok′si-pek-sē). Suture of a prolapsing rectum to the tissues anterior to the coccyx. SYN rectococcypexy. [procto- + G. *kokkyx,* coccyx, + *pēxis,* fixation]

proc·to·co·lec·to·my (prok′tō-kō-lek′tō-mē). Surgical removal of the rectum together with part or all of the colon. [procto- + G. *kolon*, colon, + *ektomē*, excision]

proc·to·co·li·tis (prok'tō-kō-lī'tis). SYN coloproctitis.

proc·to·co·lo·nos·co·py (prok'tō-kō'lō-nos'kŏ-pē). Inspection of interior of rectum and colon. [procto- + G. *kolon*, colon, + *skopeō*, to view]

proc·to·col·po·plas·ty (prok'tō-kol'pō-plas-tē). Surgical closure of a rectovaginal fistula. [procto- + G. *kolpos*, bosom (vagina), + *plastos*, formed]

proc·to·cys·to·cele (prok'tō-sis'tō-sēl). Herniation of the bladder into the rectum. [procto- + G. *kystis*, bladder, + *kēlē*, hernia]

proc·to·cys·to·plas·ty (prok'tō-sis'tō-plas-tē). Surgical closure of a rectovesical fistula. [procto- + G. *kystis*, bladder, + *plastos*, formed]

proc·to·cys·tot·o·my (prok'tō-sis-tot'ō-mē). Incision into the bladder from the rectum. [procto- + G. *kystis*, bladder, + *tomē*, incision]

proc·to·de·al (prok'tō-dē-ăl). Relating to the proctodeum.

proc·to·de·um, pl. **proc·to·dea** (prok-tō-dē'ŭm, -dē'ă). **1.** An ectodermally lined depression under the root of the tail, adjacent to the terminal part of the embryonic hindgut; at its bottom, proctodeal ectoderm and cloacal endoderm form the cloacal plate. When this epithelial plate ruptures, the anal and urogenital external orifices are established. SYN anal pit. **2.** Terminal portion of the insect alimentary canal, extending from the pylorus (area of malpighian tubule attachment) to the anal opening; in certain diptera (flies) and other insects, the p. is divided into a tubular anterior intestine and an enlarged posterior intestine, or rectum, ending at the anus. [L. fr. G. *prōktos*, anus + *hodaios*, on the way, fr. *hodos*, a way]

proc·to·dyn·ia (prok'tō-din'ē-ă). SYN proctalgia. [procto- + G. *odynē*, pain]

proc·to·el·y·tro·plas·ty (prok-tō-el'i-trō-plas-tē). Obsolete term for proctocolpoplasty. [procto- + G. *elytron*, sheath (vagina), + *plastos*, formed]

proc·to·log·ic (prok-tō-loj'ik). Relating to proctology.

proc·tol·o·gist (prok-tol'ō-jist). A specialist in proctology.

proc·tol·o·gy (prok-tol'ō-jē). Surgical specialty concerned with the anus and rectum and their diseases. [procto- + G. *logos*, study]

proc·to·pa·ral·y·sis (prok'tō-pa-ral'i-sis). Paralysis of the anus, leading to incontinence of feces.

proc·to·per·i·ne·o·plas·ty (prok'tō-per-i-nē'ō-plas-tē). Plastic surgery of the anus and perineum. SYN proctoperineorrhaphy, rectoperineorrhaphy. [procto- + perineum, + G. *plastos*, formed]

proc·to·per·i·ne·or·rha·phy (prok'tō-per-i-nē-ōr'a-fē). SYN proctoperineoplasty. [procto- + perineum, + G. *rhaphē*, suture]

proc·to·pexy (prok'tō-pek-sē). Surgical fixation of a prolapsing rectum. SYN rectopexy. [procto- + G. *pēxis*, fixation]

proc·to·pho·bia (prok-tō-fō'bē-ă). A morbid fear of rectal disease. SYN rectophobia. [procto- + G. *phobos*, fear]

proc·to·plas·ty (prok'tō-plas-tē). Plastic surgery of the anus or rectum. SYN rectoplasty. [procto- + G. *plastos*, formed]

proc·to·ple·gia (prok'tō-plē'jē-ă). Paralysis of the anus and rectum occurring with paraplegia. [procto- + G. *plēge*, stroke]

proc·to·pol·y·pus (prok-tō-pol'i-pŭs). Polypus of the rectum.

proc·top·to·sia, proc·top·to·sis (prok-top-tō'sē-ă, -tō'sis). Prolapse of the rectum and anus. [procto- + G. *ptōsis*, a falling]

proc·tor·rha·gia (proc-tō-rā'jē-ă). State characterized by having a bloody discharge from the anus. [procto- + G. *rhēgnymi*, to burst forth]

proc·tor·rha·phy (prok-tōr'ă-fē). Repair by suture of a lacerated rectum or anus. SYN rectorrhaphy. [procto- + G. *rhaphē*, suture]

proc·tor·rhea (prok-tō-rē'ă). A mucoserous discharge from the rectum. [procto- + G. *rhoia*, a flow]

proc·to·scope (prok'tō-skōp). A rectal speculum. SYN rectoscope. [procto- + G. *skopeō*, to view]

Tuttle's p., a tubular rectal speculum illuminated at its distal extremity; after introduction, the obturator is withdrawn and a glass window is inserted in the proximal end; then, by means of a rubber bulb and tube connected with the p., the rectal ampulla may be inflated.

proc·tos·co·py (prok-tos'kŏ-pē). Visual examination of the rectum and anus, as with a proctoscope. SYN rectoscopy.

proc·to·sig·moid (prok'tō-sig'moyd). The area of the anal canal and sigmoid colon, usually used to describe the region visualized by sigmoidoscopy.

proc·to·sig·moi·dec·to·my (prok'tō-sig-moy-dek'tō-mē). Excision of the rectum and sigmoid colon. [procto- + sigmoid, + G. *ektomē*, excision]

proc·to·sig·moi·di·tis (prok'tō-sig-moy-dī'tis). Inflammation of the sigmoid colon and rectum. [procto- + sigmoid + G. *-itis*, inflammation]

proc·to·sig·moi·do·scope (prok'-tō-sig-moid'ō-skōp). Instrument used for examination of the sigmoid colon and rectum.

proc·to·sig·moi·dos·co·py (prok'tō-sig-moy-dos'kŏ-pē). Direct inspection through a sigmoidoscope of the rectum and sigmoid colon. [procto- + sigmoid + G. *skopeō*, to view]

proc·to·spasm (prok'tō-spazm). **1.** Spasmodic stricture of the anus. **2.** Spasmodic contraction of the rectum. [procto- + G. *spasmos*, spasm]

proc·to·sta·sis (prok-tos'tă-sis). Constipation with stasis in the rectum. [procto- + G. *stasis*, a standing]

proc·to·stat (prok'tō-stat). A tube containing radium for insertion through the anus in the treatment of rectal cancer; obsolete. [procto- + G. *statos*, standing]

proc·to·ste·no·sis (prok'tō-stě-nō'sis). Stricture of the rectum or anus. SYN rectostenosis. [procto- + G. *stenōsis*, a narrowing]

proc·tos·to·my (prok-tos'tō-mē). The formation of an artificial opening into the rectum. SYN rectostomy. [procto- + G. *stoma*, mouth]

proc·to·tome (prok'tō-tōm). An instrument for use in proctotomy. SYN rectotome.

proc·tot·o·my (prok-tot'ō-mē). An incision into the rectum. SYN rectotomy. [procto- + G. *tomē*, incision]

proc·to·tre·sia (prok-tō-trē'zē-ă). Operation for correction of an imperforate anus. [procto- + G. *trēsis*, a boring]

proc·to·val·vot·o·my (prok'tō-val-vot'ō-mē). Incision of rectal valves.

pro·cum·bent (prō-kŭm'bent). Rarely used term denoting in a prone position; lying face down. [L. *procumbens*, falling or leaning forward]

pro·cur·va·tion (prō-ker-vā'shŭn). Rarely used term for a bending forward. [L. *pro-curvo*, to bend forward]

pro·cy·cli·dine hy·dro·chlo·ride (prō-sī'kli-dēn). 1-Cyclohexyl-1-phenyl-3-pyrrolidino-1-propanol hydrochloride; an anticholinergic agent used in the treatment of paralysis agitans and drug-induced parkinsonism.

pro·cy·cli·dine meth·o·chlo·ride. 1-(3-cyclohexyl-3-hydroxy-3-phenylpropyl)-1-methylpyrrolidinium chloride; an anticholinergic drug used in the treatment of functional gastrointestinal spasm. SYN tricyclamol chloride.

pro·dig·i·os·in (prō-dij'ē-ō-sin). A red pigment synthesized by the bacterium *Serratia marcescens*. An antifungal agent.

α-pro·dine hy·dro·chlo·ride. SEE alphaprodine.

pro·dro·mal (prō-drō'măl, prod'rō'măl). Relating to a prodrome. SYN prodromic, prodromous, proemial.

pro·drome (prō'drōm). An early or premonitory symptom of a disease. SYN prodromus. [G. *prodromos*, a running before, fr. pro- + *dromos*, a running, a course]

pro·dro·mic, pro·dro·mous (prō-drō'-mik, prod'rō-; -mŭs). SYN prodromal.

prod·ro·mus, pl. **prod·ro·mi** (prod'rō-mŭs, -mī). SYN prodrome.

pro·drug (prō'drŭg). A class of drugs, the pharmacologic action of which results from conversion by metabolic processes within the body (biotransformation).

pro·duct (prod'ŭkt). **1.** Anything produced or made, either naturally or artificially. **2.** In mathematics, the result of multiplication. [L. *productus*, fr. *pro-duco*, pp. *-ductus*, to lead forth]

cleavage p., a substance resulting from the splitting of a molecule into two or more simpler molecules.

double p., the p. of systolic blood pressure multiplied by the heart frequency; a measure of heart work load. SEE Robinson *index*.

end p., the final p. in a metabolic pathway.

fibrin/fibrinogen degradation p.'s (FDP), several poorly characterized small peptides, designated X, Y, D, and E, that result following the action of plasmin on fibrinogen and fibrin in the fibrinolytic process.

fission p., an atomic species produced in the course of the fission of a larger atom such as ^{235}U.

natural p.'s, naturally occurring compounds that are end p.'s of secondary metabolism; often, they are unique compounds for particular organisms or classes of organisms.

orphan p.'s, drugs, biologicals, and medical devices (including diagnostic *in vitro* tests) that may be useful in common or rare diseases but which are not considered commercially viable. SYN orphan drugs.

spallation p., an atomic species produced in the course of the spallation of any atom.

substitution p., a p. obtained by replacing one atom or group in a molecule with another atom or group.

pro·duc·tive (prō-dŭk′tiv). Producing or capable of producing; denoting especially an inflammation leading to the production of new tissue with or without an exudate. [see product]

pro·elas·tase (prō-ĕ-las′tās). The precursor protein of elastase; formed in the pancreas (in vertebrates) and converted to elastase by the action of trypsin.

pro·e·mi·al (prō-ē′mē-ăl). SYN prodromal. [L. *prooemium*, fr. G. *prooimion*, prelude]

pro·en·ceph·a·lon (prō-en-sef′ă-lon). SYN prosencephalon.

pro·en·keph·a·lin (prō-en-kef′ă-lin). A precursor protein that contains several enkephalin sequences. Cf. propiocortin.

pro·en·zyme (prō-en′zīm). The precursor of an enzyme, requiring some change (usually the hydrolysis of an inhibiting fragment that masks an active grouping) to render it active; *e.g.,* pepsinogen, trypsinogen, profibrolysin. SYN zymogen.

pro·e·ryth·ro·blast (prō-ĕ-rith′rō-blast). SYN pronormoblast.

pro·e·ryth·ro·cyte (prō-ĕ-rith′rō-sīt). The precursor of an erythrocyte; an immature red blood cell with a nucleus.

pro·es·tro·gen (prō-es′trō-jen). A substance that acts as an estrogen only after it has been metabolized in the body to an active compound.

pro·es·trum (prō-es′trŭm). SYN proestrus.

pro·es·trus (prō-es′trŭs). The period in the estrus cycle preceding estrus, characterized by the growth of the graafian follicles and physiologic changes related to estrogen production. SYN proestrum.

pro·fen·a·mine hy·dro·chlo·ride (pro-fen′ă-mēn). SYN ethopropazine hydrochloride.

Profeta, Giuseppe, Italian dermatologist, 1840–1910. SEE P.'s *law*.

pro·fi·bri·nol·y·sin (prō′fī-bri-nol′i-sin). SEE plasmin.

pro·fi·lac·tin (prō-fil-ak′tin). A complex of actin and profilin. Cf. profilin.

pro·file (prō′fīl). **1.** An outline or contour, especially one representing a side view of the human head. SYN norma [NA]. **2.** A summary, brief account, or record. [It. *profilo*, fr. L. *pro*, forward, + *filum*, thread, line (contour)]

biochemical p., a combination of biochemical tests usually performed with automated instrumentation upon admission of a patient to a hospital or clinic.

biophysical p., technique for evaluating fetal status using fetal heart rate monitoring and ultrasound assessment of amniotic fluid volume, fetal movement, and fetal breathing motion.

facial p., (1) the outline form of the face from a lateral view; **(2)** the sagittal outline form of the face.

personality p., (1) a method by which the results of psychological testing are presented in graphic form; **(2)** a vignette or brief personality description.

test p., a combination of laboratory tests usually performed by automated methods and designed to evaluate organ systems of patients upon admission to a hospital or clinic.

urethral pressure p., the continual recording of pressure through a hole in the side of a small catheter as it is pulled (at a constant rate while either water or a gas is infused through the hole) from a point within the bladder, through the vesical neck, and down the entire urethra; a form of resistance measurement which gives a tracing indicative of the functional length of the urethra and the points of maximal urethral resistance.

pro·fi·lin (prō-fil′in). A small protein that binds to monomeric actin (thus becoming profilactin), preventing premature polymerization of actin.

pro·fi·lom·e·ter (prō′fi-lom′ĕ-ter). An instrument for measuring the roughness of a surface, *e.g.,* of teeth.

pro·fla·vine (hem·i)sul·fate (prō-flā′vin, -vēn). The neutral sulfate of 3,6-diaminoacridine; a compound closely allied to acriflavine, having similar antiseptic properties.

pro·for·mi·phen (prō-fōr′mi-fen). SYN phenprobamate.

pro·fun·da (prō-fŭn′dă). The deep one; a term applied to structures (muscles, nerves, veins, and arteries, etc.) which lie deep in the tissues, especially when contrasted with a similar, more superficial (sublimis) structure. [L. fem. of *profundus,* deep]

pro·fun·dus (prō-fŭn′dŭs) [NA]. Situated at a deeper level in relation to a specific reference point. Cf. superficialis. SYN deep. [L.]

pro·fu·sion (prō-fyū′zhŭn). A score reflecting the number of visible lesions in a region on chest radiographs of individuals with pneumoconiosis. SEE International Labour Organization *Classification*. [L. *profusio,* a pouring forth, fr. *profundo,* to pour forth]

pro·ga·bide (prō′gă-bīd). (4-{[(4-chlorophenyl, 5-fluoro-2-hydroxyphenyl) methylene]amino}-butabeamide; an anticonvulsant which is a lipid-soluble derivative of the amidated form of γ-aminobutyric acid (GABAmide) that, unlike γ-aminobutyric acid (GABA) itself, is able to cross the blood-brain barrier. Once inside the brain the drug is converted to several metabolites, some of which are active forms of GABA or related compounds which act on GABA receptors to increase inhibition in the brain.

pro·gas·trin (prō-gas′trin). Precursor of gastric secretion in the mucous membrane of the stomach.

pro·ge·nia (prō-jē′nē-ă). SYN prognathism. [pro- + L. *gena,* cheek]

pro·ge·ni·ta·lis (prō-jen-i-tā′lis). On any of the exposed surfaces of the genitalia. [L. prefix *pro-,* before, in front of, + *genitalis,* pertaining to the reproductive organs, fr. *gigno,* to bear]

pro·gen·i·tor (prō-jen′i-ter, -tōr). A precursor, ancestor; one who begets. [L.]

prog·e·ny (proj′ĕ-nē). Offspring; descendants. [L. *progenies,* fr. *progigno,* to beget]

pro·ge·ria (prō-jēr′ē-ă) [MIM*176670]. A condition in which normal development in the first year is followed by gross retardation of growth, with a senile appearance characterized by dry wrinkled skin, total alopecia, and bird-like facies; genetics unclear. SYN Hutchinson-Gilford disease, Hutchinson-Gilford syndrome, premature senility syndrome. [pro- + G. *gēras,* old age]

p. with cataract, p. with microphthalmia, SYN *dyscephalia mandibulo-oculofacialis.*

pro·ges·ta·tion·al (prō′jes-tā′shŭn-ăl). **1.** Favoring pregnancy; conducive to gestation; capable of stimulating the uterine changes essential for implantation and growth of a fertilized ovum. **2.** Referring to progesterone, or to a drug with progesterone-like properties.

pro·ges·ter·one (prō-jes′ter-ōn). 4-pregnene-3,20-dione; an antiestrogenic steroid, believed to be the active principle of the corpus luteum, isolated from the corpus luteum and placenta or synthetically prepared; used to correct abnormalities of the menstrual cycle and as a contraceptive and to control habitual abortion. SYN corpus luteum hormone, luteohormone, pregnancy hormone, progestational hormone.

pro·ges·tin (prō-jes′tin). **1.** A hormone of the corpus luteum. **2.** Generic term for any substance, natural or synthetic, that effects some or all of the biological changes produced by progesterone. **3.** SYN gestagen. [pro- + gestation + -in]

pro·ges·to·gen (prō-jes'tō-jen). **1.** Any agent capable of producing biological effects similar to those of progesterone; most p.'s are steroids like the natural hormones. **2.** A synthetic derivative from testosterone or progesterone that has some of the physiologic activity and pharmacologic effects of progesterone; progesterone is antiestrogenic, whereas some p.'s have estrogenic or androgenic properties in addition to progestational activity. [pro- + gestation + G. -gen, producing]

pro·glos·sis (prō-glos'is). The anterior portion, or tip, of the tongue. [pro- + G. glōssa, tongue]

pro·glot·tid (prō-glot'id). One of the segments of a tapeworm, containing the reproductive organs. SYN proglottis. [pro- + G. glōssa, tongue]

pro·glot·tis, pl. **pro·glot·ti·des** (prō-glot'is, -i-dēz). SYN proglottid.

prog·nath·ic (prog-nath'ik, -nā'thik). **1.** Having a projecting jaw; having a gnathic index above 103. **2.** Denoting a forward projection of either or both of the jaws relative to the craniofacial skeleton. SYN prognathous. [pro- + G. gnathos, jaw]

prog·na·thism (prog'nă-thizm). The condition of being prognathic; abnormal forward projection of one or of both jaws beyond the established normal relationship with the cranial base; the mandibular condyles are in their normal rest relationship to the temporomandibular joints. SYN progenia.

basilar p., the concave facial profile, or forward position of the chin, resembling mandibular p., created by the prominence of the bone of the chin or menton.

prog·na·thous (prog'nă-thŭs). SYN prognathic.

prog·nose (prog-nōs', -nōz'). SYN prognosticate.

prog·no·sis (prog-nō'sis). A forecast of the probable course and/or outcome of a disease. [G. prognōsis, fr. pro, before, + gignōskō, to know]

denture p., an opinion or judgment, given in advance of treatment, of the prospects for success in the construction and usefulness of a denture or restoration.

prog·nos·tic (prog-nos'tik). **1.** Relating to prognosis. **2.** A symptom upon which a prognosis is based, or one indicative of the likely outcome. [G. prognōstikos]

prog·nos·ti·cate (prog-nos'ti-kāt). To give a prognosis. SYN prognose.

prog·nos·ti·cian (prog-nos-tish'ŭn). One skilled in prognosis.

pro·gon·o·ma (prō-gon-ō'mă). A nodule or mass resulting from displacement of tissue when atavism occurs in embryonic development; represents a reversion to structures not normally occurring in the individuals of a species, but observed in ancestral forms of that species. [pro- + G. gonos, offspring, + -oma, tumor]

p. of jaw, SYN melanotic neuroectodermal tumor of infancy.

melanotic p., a pigmented hairy nevus.

pro·grade. In the normal direction of flow.

pro·gram. **1.** A formal set of procedures for conducting an activity. **2.** An ordered list of instructions directing a computer to carry out a desired sequence of operations required to solve a problem.

pro·gran·u·lo·cyte (prō-gran'yŭ-lō-sīt). SYN promyelocyte.

pro·gress. **1** (prog'res). An advance; the course of a disease. **2** (prō-gres'). To advance; to go forward; said of a disease, especially, when unqualified, of one taking an unfavorable course. [L. pro-gredior, pp. -gressus, to go forth, fr. gradior, to step, go, fr. gradus, a step]

pro·gress·ive (prō-gres'iv). Going forward; advancing; denoting the course of a disease, especially, when unqualified, an unfavorable course.

pro·gua·nil hy·dro·chlo·ride (prō-gwah'nil). SYN chloroguanide hydrochloride.

pro·hor·mone (prō-hōr'mōn). **1.** An intraglandular precursor of a hormone; e.g., proinsulin. Cf. prehormone. **2.** Obsolete term formerly used to designate a substance developed in serum that antagonizes a specific antihormone, and thus enhances the action of the corresponding hormone.

pro·in·su·lin (prō-in'sŭ-lin). A single-chain precursor of insulin.

pro·i·o·sys·tol·ia (prō-ē-ō-sis-tōl'ē-ă). Condition in which proiosystoles occur.

pro·jec·tion (prō-jek'shŭn). **1.** A pushing out; an outgrowth or protuberance. **2.** The referring of a sensation to the object producing it. **3.** A defense mechanism by which a repressed complex in the individual is denied and conceived as belonging to another person, as when faults which the person tends to commit are perceived in or attributed to others. **4.** The conception by the consciousness of a mental occurrence belonging to the self as of external origin. **5.** Localization of visual impressions in space. **6.** In neuroanatomy, the system or systems of nerve fibers by which a group of nerve cells discharges its nerve impulses ("projects") to one or more other cell groups. **7.** The image of a three dimensional object on a plane; as in a radiograph. **8.** In radiography, standardized views of parts of the body, described by body part position, the direction of the x-ray beam through the body part, or by eponym. SYN salient (1), view. [L. projectio; fr. pro- jicio, pp. -jectus, to throw before]

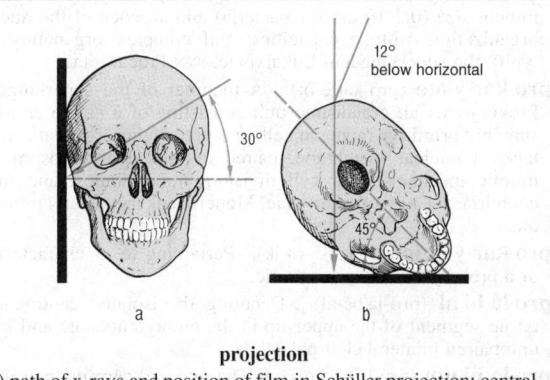

projection
a) path of x-rays and position of film in Schüller projection; central ray enters at 30° above horizontal, causing blurred picture of other ear; b) in Stenvers projection, ray enters at 12° below horizontal

anteroposterior p., SYN AP p.

AP p., the alternative frontal radiographic p., used mainly in bedside or portable radiography. SYN anteroposterior p.

apical lordotic p., SYN backprojection.

axial p., a radiographic p. devised to obtain direct visualization of the base of the skull. SYN axial view, base p., base view, submental vertex p., submentovertical p., verticosubmental view.

base p., SYN axial p.

Caldwell p., inclined PA radiographic p. devised to permit visualization of orbital structures unobstructed by the petrous ridges. SYN Caldwell view.

cross-table lateral p., lateral p. radiography of a supine subject using a horizontal x-ray beam.

enamel p., extension of enamel into furcation.

erroneous p., SYN false p.

false p., the faulty visual sensation arising secondarily to underaction of an ocular muscle. SYN erroneous p.

Fischer p., SEE sugars.

frog-leg lateral p., a lateral p. of the femoral neck made with the thigh maximally abducted.

Granger p., g. view, reversed half-axial view; uncommonly used PA view of the skull.

half-axial p., SYN Towne p.

Haworth p., SEE sugars.

lateral p., radiographic p. with the x-ray beam in a coronal plane.

oblique p., any radiographic p. between frontal and lateral.

occipitomental p., SYN Waters' p.

PA p., the standard frontal chest film p.; radiographic skull p. with the petrous ridge superimposed on the orbits. SYN posteroanterior p.

posteroanterior p., SYN PA p.

Rhese p., oblique radiographic view of the skull to show the optic foramen.

Stenvers p., oblique radiographic p. of the skull devised to provide an unobstructed view of the petrous bone, bony labyrinth, internal auditory canal, and meatus. SYN Stenvers view.

submental vertex p., SYN axial p.

submentovertical p., SYN axial p.

Towne p., reverse tilted AP radiographic p. devised to permit demonstration of the entire occipital bone, foramen magnum, and dorsum sellae, as well as the petrous ridges. SYN half axial view, half-axial p., Towne view.

visual p., a perceptual synthesis involving visual mechanisms.

Waters' p., a PA radiographic view of the skull made with the orbitomeatal line at an angle of 37° from the plane of the film, to show the orbits and maxillary sinuses. SYN occipitomental p., Waters' view.

Pro·kar·y·o·tae (pro-kar-ē-ō'tē). A superkingdom of cellular organisms that includes the kingdom Monera (bacteria and blue-green algae) and is characterized by the prokaryotic condition, minute size (0.2-10 μm for bacteria) and absence of the nuclear organization, mitotic capacities, and complex organelles that typify the superkingdom Eukaryotae. SYN Procaryotae.

pro·kar·y·ote (prō-kar'ē-ōt). A member of the superkingdom Prokaryotae; an organismic unit consisting of a single and presumably primitive moneran cell, or a precellular organism, which lacks a nuclear membrane, paired organized chromosomes, a mitotic mechanism for cell division, microtubules, and mitochondria. SEE ALSO Prokaryotae, Monera, eukaryote. SYN procaryote.

pro·kar·y·ot·ic (prō'kar-ē-ot'ik). Pertaining to or characteristic of a prokaryote. SYN procaryotic.

pro·la·bi·al (prō-lā'bē-ăl). Denoting the isolated central soft-tissue segment of the upper lip in the embryonic state and in an unrepaired bilateral cleft palate.

pro·la·bi·um (prō-lā'bē-ŭm). 1. The exposed carmine margin of the lip. 2. The isolated central soft-tissue segment of the upper lip in the embryonic state and in an unrepaired bilateral cleft palate. [pro- + L. labium, lip]

pro·lac·tin (PRL) (prō-lak'tin). A protein hormone of the anterior lobe of the hypophysis that stimulates the secretion of milk and possibly, during pregnancy, breast growth. SYN galactopoietic factor, galactopoietic hormone, lactation hormone, lactogenic factor, lactogenic hormone, lactotropin, mammotropic factor, mammotropic hormone. [pro- + L. laclact-, milk, + -in]

pro·lac·ti·no·ma (prō-lak-ti-nō'mă). SYN prolactin-producing adenoma.

pro·lac·to·lib·er·in (prō-lak-tō-lib'er-in). A substance of hypothalamic origin that stimulates the release of prolactin. SYN prolactin-releasing factor, prolactin-releasing hormone. [prolactin + L. libero, to free, + -in]

pro·lac·to·stat·in (prō-lak-tō-stat'in). A substance of hypothalamic origin capable of inhibiting the synthesis and release of prolactin. SYN prolactin-inhibiting factor, prolactin-inhibiting hormone. [prolactin + G. stasis, standing still, + -in]

pro·lam·ines (prō-lam'ēnz, prō'lă-mēnz, -minz). Proteins insoluble in water or neutral salt solutions, soluble in dilute acids or alkalies, and in 50 to 90% alcohol; e.g., gliadin, zein, hordein; all have relatively high proline contents.

pro·lapse (prō-laps'). 1. To sink down, said of an organ or other part. 2. A sinking of an organ or other part, especially its appearance at a natural or artificial orifice. SEE ALSO procidentia, ptosis. [L. prolapsus, a falling]

p. of the corpus luteum, ectropion of the corpus luteum, due to eversion of the granulosa membrane through the opening in the ruptured follicle; this occurs normally in certain animals.

mitral valve p., excessive retrograde movement of one or both mitral valve leaflets into the left atrium during left ventricular systole, often allowing mitral regurgitation; responsible for the click-murmur of Barlow syndrome, and rarely may be due to rheumatic carditis, a connective tissue disorder such as Marfan's syndrome or ruptured chorda tendinea ("flail mitral leaflet").

Morgagni's p., chronic inflammation of Morgagni's ventricle.

p. of umbilical cord, presentation of part of the umbilical cord ahead of the fetus; it may cause fetal death due to compression of the cord between the presenting part of the fetus and the maternal pelvis.

p. of the uterus, downward movement of the uterus due to laxity and atony of the muscular and fascial structures of the pelvic floor, usually resulting from injuries of childbirth or advanced age; p. occurs in three forms; **first degree p.,** the cervix of the prolapsed uterus is well within the vaginal orifice; **second degree p.,** the cervix is at or near the introitus; **third degree p.** (procidentia uteri), the cervix protrudes well beyond the vaginal orifice. SYN descensus uteri, falling of the womb.

valvular p., SYN click syndrome.

pro·lec·tive (prō'lek-tiv). Pertaining to data collected by planning in advance proportional mortality ratio. Number of deaths from a given cause in a specified period, per 100 or per 1000 total deaths. [pro- + L. lego, pp. lectum, to gather]

pro·lep·sis (prō-lep'sis). Recurrence of the paroxysm of a periodical disease at regularly shortening intervals. [G. prolēpsis, anticipation]

pro·lep·tic (prō-lep'tik). Relating to prolepsis. SYN subintrant.

pro·leu·ko·cyte (prō-lū'kō-sīt). SYN leukoblast.

pro·li·dase (prō'li-dās). SYN proline dipeptidase.

pro·lif·er·ate (prō-lif'ĕ-rāt). To grow and increase in number by means of reproduction of similar forms. [L. proles, offspring, + fero, to bear]

pro·lif·er·a·tion (prō-lif-ĕ-rā'shŭn). Growth and reproduction of similar cells.

diffuse mesangial p., SYN mesangial proliferative glomerulonephritis.

gingival p., SYN gingival hyperplasia.

pro·lif·er·a·tive, pro·lif·er·ous (prō-lif'er-ă-tiv, -er-ŭs). Increasing the numbers of similar forms.

pro·lif·ic (prō-lif'ik). Fruitful; bearing many children. [L. proles, offspring, + facio, to make]

pro·lig·er·ous (prō-lij'er-ŭs). Germinating; producing offspring. [L. proles, offspring, + gero, to bear]

pro·li·nase (prō'li-nās). SYN prolyl dipeptidase.

pro·line (Pro) (prō'lēn). Pyrrolidine-2-carboxylic acid; the L-isomer is an amino acid that is found in proteins, especially the collagens. SYN pyrrolidine-2-carboxylate.

p. aminopeptidase, SYN p. iminopeptidase.

p. dehydrogenase, SYN pyrroline-2-carboxylate reductase, pyrroline-5-carboxylate reductase.

p. dipeptidase, an enzyme cleaving aminoacyl-L-proline bonds in dipeptides containing a C-terminal prolyl residue; a deficiency of this enzyme results in hyperimidodipeptiduria. SYN imidodipeptidase, peptidase D, prolidase.

p. iminopeptidase [EC 3.4.11.5], a hydrolase cleaving L-proline residues from the N-terminal position in peptides. SYN p. aminopeptidase.

p. oxidase, SYN pyrroline-2-carboxylate reductase, pyrroline-5-carboxylate reductase.

p. racemase, an enzyme that reversibly converts D-proline to L-proline.

D-p. reductase, an oxidoreductase reversibly reacting D-proline with NADH to produce 5-aminovalerate and NAD⁺.

pro·lyl (prō'lil). The acyl radical of proline.

p. dipeptidase, an enzyme cleaving L-prolyl-amino acid bonds in dipeptides containing N-terminal prolyl residues. SYN iminodipeptidase, prolinase, prolylglycine dipeptidase.

p. hydroxylase, an enzyme that catalyzes the hydroxylation of certain p. residues in collagen precursors using molecular oxygen, ferrous ion, ascorbic acid, and α-keotglutarate; a vitamin C deficiency directly affects the activity of this enzyme; one form of this enzyme (p. 4-hydroxylase) synthesizes 4-hydroxyprolyl residues while another produces 3-hydroxyprolyl residues.

pro·lyl·gly·cine di·pep·ti·dase (prō'lil-glī'sēn). SYN prolyl dipeptidase.

pro·mas·ti·gote (prō-mas'ti-gōt). Term now generally used instead of "leptomonad" or "leptomonad stage," to avoid confusion with the flagellate genus *Leptomonas.* It denotes the flagellate stage of a trypanosomatid protozoan in which the flagellum arises from a kinetoplast in front of the nucleus and emerges from the anterior end of the organism; usually an extracellular phase, as in the insect intermediate host (or in culture) of *Leishmania* parasites. [pro- + G. *mastix,* whip]

pro·ma·zine hy·dro·chlo·ride (prō′mă-zēn). 10-(3-Dimethylaminopropyl)phenothiazine hydrochloride; a phenothiazine tranquilizing agent with actions and uses similar to those of chlorpromazine.

pro·meg·a·lo·blast (prō-meg′ă-lō-blast). The earliest of four maturation stages of the megaloblast. SEE erythroblast. SYN pernicious anemia type rubriblast.

pro·met·a·phase (prō-met′ă-fāz). The stage of mitosis or meiosis in which the nuclear membrane disintegrates and the centrioles reach the poles of the cell, while the chromosomes continue to contract.

pro·meth·a·zine hy·dro·chlo·ride (prō-meth′ă-zēn). 10-(2-Dimethylaminopropyl)phenothiazine hydrochloride; an antihistaminic with antiemetic properties.

pro·meth·a·zine the·o·clate (prō-meth′ă-zēn). Promethiazine salt of 8-chlorotheophylline; an antihistaminic drug used for motion sickness.

pro·meth·es·trol di·pro·pi·o·nate (prō-meth′es-trol dī-prō′pē-ō-nāt). Dimethylhexestrol dipropionate; 4,4′-(1,2-diethylethylene)di-*o*-cresol dipropionate; a synthetic estrogen derived from stilbene.

pro·me·thi·um (Pm) (prō-mē′thē-ŭm). A radioactive element of the rare earth series, atomic no. 61; first chemically identified in 1945; ^{145}Pm has the longest known half-life (17.7 years). [*Prometheus,* a Titan of G. myth who stole fire to give to mortals]

prom·i·nence (prom′i-nens). In anatomy, tissues or parts that project beyond a surface. SYN prominentia [NA]. [L. *prominentia*]

Ammon's p., an external p. in the posterior pole of the eyeball during early embryogenesis.

canine p., SYN canine *eminence.*

cardiac p., the conspicuous external bulge appearing on the ventral aspect of the human embryo as early as at the fourth week, indicative of the precocious development of the heart.

p. of facial canal, the prominence on the medial wall of the tympanic cavity above the vestibular (oval) window produced by the presence of the facial canal. SYN prominentia canalis facialis [NA].

forebrain p., SYN frontonasal p.

frontonasal p., the unpaired embryonic prominence between the medial nasal elevations, which eventually merges with them to contribute to the bridge of the nose and the underlying nasal septum. SYN forebrain eminence, forebrain p., frontonasal primordium, frontonasal process.

hepatic p., the conspicuous external bulge appearing dorsocaudal to the cardiac p. on the body of the human embryo at about the fourth week, indicating the precocious development of the liver.

hypothenar p., SYN hypothenar *eminence.*

laryngeal p., the projection on the anterior portion of the neck formed by the thyroid cartilage of the larynx; serves as an external indication of the level of the fifth cervical vertebra. SYN prominentia laryngea [NA], Adam's apple, protuberantia laryngea, thyroid eminence.

lateral nasal p., an ectodermally covered mesenchymal swelling separating the embryonic olfactory pit from the developing eye. SYN lateral nasal fold, lateral nasal primordium, lateral nasal process.

p. of lateral semicircular canal, the slight bulge in the medial wall of the epitympanic recess caused by the proximity of the lateral semicircular canal. SYN prominentia canalis semicircularis lateralis [NA].

mallear p., a small prominence at the upper end of the stria mallearis produced by the lateral process of the malleus. SYN prominentia mallearis [NA].

medial nasal p., an ectodermally covered mesenchymal swelling lying medial to the olfactory placode or pit in the embryo. SYN medial nasal fold, medial nasal primordium, medial nasal process.

spiral p., a projecting portion of the spiral ligament of the cochlea, bounding the lower edge of the stria vascularis and containing within it a blood vessel, the vas prominens. SYN prominentia spiralis [NA].

styloid p., a rounded eminence on the posterior (mastoid) wall of the tympanic cavity corresponding to the base of the styloid process. SYN prominentia styloidea [NA].

thenar p., SYN thenar *eminence.*

tubal p., SYN *torus* tubarius.

p. of venous valvular sinus, a slight eminence on the external wall of a vein correlating with the valvular sinus immediately proximal to the leaflets of the venous valve. SYN agger valvae venae.

pro·mi·nens (prom′i-nens). Prominent; in anatomy, denoting a prominence. [L.]

prom·i·nen·tia, pl. **prom·i·nen·ti·ae** (prom-i-nen′shē-ă, -shē-ē) [NA]. SYN prominence. [L. fr. *promineo,* to jut out, be prominent]

p. cana′lis facia′lis [NA], SYN *prominence* of facial canal.

p. cana′lis semicircula′ris latera′lis [NA], SYN *prominence* of lateral semicircular canal.

p. laryn′gea [NA], SYN laryngeal *prominence.*

p. mallea′ris [NA], SYN mallear *prominence.*

p. spira′lis [NA], SYN spiral *prominence.*

p. styloi′dea [NA], SYN styloid *prominence.*

pro·mi·to·chon·dria (prō-mī-tō-kon′drē-ă). Mitochondrial precursors with little internal structure (*e.g.,* no cristae) and no proteins of electron transport. SYN premitochondria.

pro·mon·o·cyte (prō-mon′ō-sīt). SYN premonocyte.

prom·on·to·ri·um, pl. **prom·on·to·ria** (prom′on-tō′rē-ŭm, -rē-ă) [NA]. SYN promontory. [L. a mountain ridge, a headland, fr. *promineo,* to jut out]

p. ca′vi tym′pani, SYN *promontory* of tympanic cavity.

p. os′sis sa′cri, SYN sacral *promontory.*

prom·on·to·ry (prom′on-tō-rē). An eminence or projection. A projection of a part. SEE promontory. SYN promontorium [NA]. [L. *promontorium*]

pelvic p., SYN sacral p.

sacral p., the most prominent anterior projection of the base of the sacrum. SYN pelvic p., promontorium ossis sacri, p. of the sacrum.

p. of the sacrum, SYN sacral p.

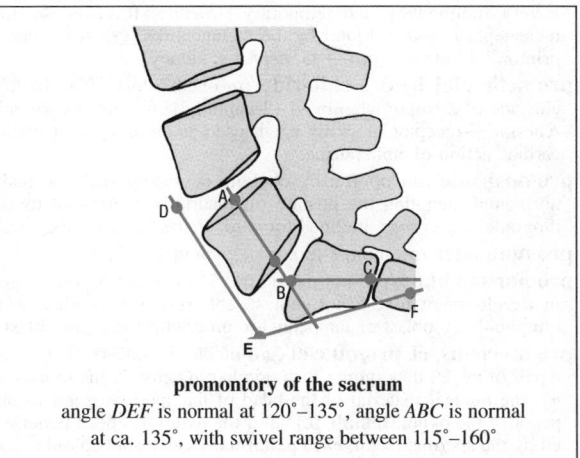

promontory of the sacrum
angle *DEF* is normal at 120°–135°, angle *ABC* is normal at ca. 135°, with swivel range between 115°–160°

tympanic p., SYN p. of tympanic cavity.

p. of tympanic cavity, a rounded eminence on the labyrinthine wall of the middle ear, caused by the first coil of the cochlea. SYN promontorium cavi tympani, tuber cochleae, tympanic p.

pro·mot·er (prō-mō'ter). **1.** In chemistry, a substance that increases the activity of a catalyst. **2.** In molecular biology, a DNA sequence at which RNA polymerase binds and initiates transcription.

pro·mo·tion (prō-mō'shŭn). Stimulation of tumor induction, following initiation, by a promoting agent which may of itself be noncarcinogenic.

health p., according to the World Health Organization, the process of enabling people to increase control over and improve their health; it involves the population as a whole in the context of their everyday lives, rather than focusing on people at risk for specific diseases, and is directed towards action on the determinants or causes of health.

pro·my·e·lo·cyte (prō-mī'ě-lō-sīt). **1.** The developmental stage of a granular leukocyte between the myeloblast and myelocyte, when a few specific granules appear in addition to azurophilic ones. **2.** A large uninuclear cell occurring in the circulating blood of persons with myelocytic leukemia. SYN premyelocyte, progranulocyte. [pro- + G. *myelos,* marrow, + *kytos,* cell]

pro·na·si·on (prō-nā'zē-on). The point of the angle between the septum of the nose and the surface of the upper lip, found at the point where a tangent applied to the nasal septum meets the upper lip. [pro- + L. *nasus,* nose]

pro·nate (prō'nāt). **1.** To assume, or to be placed in, a prone position. **2.** To perform pronation of the forearm or foot. [L. *pronatus,* fr. *prono,* pp. *-atus,* to bend forward, fr. *pronus,* bent forward]

pro·na·tion (prō-nā'shŭn). The condition of being prone; the act of assuming or of being placed in a prone position.

p. of foot, eversion and abduction of the foot, raising the lateral edge.

p. of forearm, rotation of the forearm in such a way that the palm of the hand faces backward when the arm is in the anatomical position, or downward when the arm is extended at a right angle to the body.

pro·na·tor (prō-nā'ter, tōr). A muscle which turns a part into the prone position. SEE muscle. [L.]

pro·na·tus (prō-nā'tis). A baby born prematurely. [L. *pro,* before, + *nascor,* pp. *natus,* to be born]

prone (prōn). Denoting: **1.** The body when lying face downward. **2.** Pronation of the forearm or of the foot. [L. *pronus,* bending down or forward]

pro·neph·ros, pl. **pro·neph·roi** (prō-nef'ros, -roy). **1.** The definitive excretory organ of primitive fishes. SYN head kidney. **2.** In the embryos of higher vertebrates, a vestigial structure consisting of a series of tortuous tubules emptying into the cloaca by way of the primary nephric duct; in the human embryo, the p. is a very rudimentary and temporary structure, followed by the mesonephros and still later by the metanephros. SYN forekidney, primordial kidney. [pro- + G. *nephros,* kidney]

pro·neth·a·lol hy·dro·chlo·ride (prō-neth'ă-lol). The hydrochloride of 2-isopropylamino-1-(2-naphthyl)ethanol; an early adrenergic β-receptor blocking agent used as an antagonist of the cardiac action of epinephrine.

pro·no·grade (prō'nō-grād). Walking or resting with the body horizontal, denoting the posture of quadrupeds; opposed to orthograde. [L. *pronus,* inclined forward, + *gradior,* to walk]

pro·nom·e·ter (prō-nom'ě-ter). SYN goniometer (3).

pro·nor·mo·blast (prō-nōr'mō-blast). The earliest of four stages in development of the normoblast. SEE ALSO erythroblast. SYN lymphoid hemoblast of Pappenheim, proerythroblast, rubriblast.

pro·nu·cle·us, pl. **pro·nu·clei** (prō-nū'klē-ŭs, -klē-ī). **1.** One of a pair of nuclei undergoing fusion in karyogamy. **2.** In embryology, the nuclear material of the head of the spermatozoon (**male p.**) or of the ovum (**female p.**), after the ovum has been penetrated by the spermatozoon; each p. normally carries a haploid set of chromosomes, so that the merging of the pronuclei in fertilization reestablishes the diploidy.

proof·read·ing (pruf'rēd-ing). The property of certain polymerases *e.g.,* DNA polymerase, to use their exonuclease activity to remove erroneously introduced bases and to replace them with the correct bases.

pro·-opi·o·mel·a·no·cor·tin (POMC) (prō-ō'pē-ō-mel'ă-nō-kōr'tin). A large molecule found in the anterior and intermediate lobes of the pituitary gland, the hypothalamus, and other parts of the brain as well as in the lungs, gastrointestinal tract, and placenta; the precursor of ACTH, CLIP, β-LPH, γ-MSH, β-endorphin, and met-enkephalin.

pro·o·tic (prō-ō'tik). In front of the ear. [pro- + G. *ous,* ear]

pro·ox·i·dants (prō-oks'i-dănts). Compounds or agents capable of generating toxic oxygen species. Cf. antioxidant.

pro·pa·fen·one (prō-paf'ě-nōn). Antiarrhythmic agent classified as a class I$_C$ type, thus resembling flecainide and encainide. Blocks fast sodium channels and has been used in the treatment of ventricular cardiac arrhythmias.

prop·a·gate (prop'ă-gāt). **1.** To reproduce; to generate. **2.** To move along a fiber, *e.g.,* propagation of the nerve impulse. [L. *propago,* pp. *-atus,* to generate, reproduce]

prop·a·ga·tion (prop-ă-gā'shŭn). The act of propagating.

prop·a·ga·tive (prop-ă-gā'tiv). Relating to or concerned in propagation; denoting the sexual part of an animal or plant as distinguished from the soma.

pro·pal·i·nal (prō-pal'i-năl). Back and forth; denoting a forward and backward movement. [pro- + G. *palin,* backward]

pro·pam·i·dine (prō-pam'i-dēn). 4,4'-Diamidino-1,3-diphenoxypropane; active against *Trypanosoma gambiense* infections; also markedly bacteriostatic; used as a local anti-infective agent in 0.1% aqueous solution, and against systemic fungal infections such as blastomycosis.

pro·pane (prō'pān). $CH_3CH_2CH_3$; one of the alkane series of hydrocarbons.

pro·pane·di·o·ic ac·id (prō-pān-dī'ō-ik). SYN malonic acid.

1,2,3-pro·pane·tri·ol (prō-pān-trī'ol). SYN glycerol.

pro·pan·i·did (prō-pan'i-did). Propyl{4-[(diethylcarbamoyl)-methoxy]-3-methoxyphenyl}acetate; a short-acting eugenol used intravenously for induction of general anesthesia.

pro·pa·no·ic ac·id (prō-pă-nō'ik). SYN propionic acid.

pro·pa·nol (prō'pă-nol). SYN *propyl* alcohol.

pro·pa·no·yl (prō'pă-nō-ĭl). SYN propionyl.

pro·pan·the·line bro·mide (pro-pan'thě-lēn). β-Diisopropylmethylaminoethyl-9-xanthine carboxylate bromide; the isopropyl analogue of methantheline bromide; an anticholinergic agent.

pro·par·a·caine hy·dro·chlo·ride (prō-par'ă-kān). 2-diethylaminoethyl-3-amino-4-propoxybenzoate hydrochloride; a surface anesthetic agent used in ophthalmology. SYN proxymetacaine hydrochloride.

pro·pa·tyl ni·trate (prō'pă-til). 2-Ethyl-2-(hydroxymethyl)-1,3-propanediol trinitrate; a coronary vasodilator.

pro·pene (prō'pēn). SYN propylene.

pro·pent·dy·o·pents (prō-pent-dī'ō-pentz). SEE bilirubinoids.

pro·pe·nyl (prō'pē-nil). The radical, –CH=CH–CH$_3$.

pro·pep·sin (prō-pep'sin). SYN pepsinogen.

pro·pep·tone (prō-pep'tōn). A nondescript mixture of intermediate products in the conversion of native protein into peptone.

pro·per·din (prō-per'din). A group of proteins involved in resistance to infection that participate, in conjunction with other factors, in an alternate pathway to the activation of the terminal components of complement; a deficiency of p. results in the lack of stabilization of the alternative C3-cleaving enzyme (an X-linked recessive disorder). SEE ALSO properdin *system, component* of complement. [pro- + L. *perdo,* to destroy]

pro·per·i·to·ne·al (prō'per-i-tō-nē'ăl). In front of the peritoneum.

pro·phage (prō'fāj). SYN probacteriophage.

defective p., SEE defective *bacteriophage.*

pro·phase (prō'fāz). The first stage of mitosis or meiosis, consisting of linear contraction and increase in thickness of the chromosomes (each composed of two chromatids) accompanied by migration of the two daughter centrioles and their asters toward the poles of the cell. In meiosis, p. is complex and can be subdivided into stages: preleptotene, leptotene, zygotene, pachytene, diplotene, and diakinesis. [G. *prophasis,* from *prophainō,* to foreshadow]

pro·phen·py·rid·a·mine ma·le·ate (prō'fen-pi-rid'ă-mēn). SYN pheniramine maleate.

pro·phlo·gis·tic (prō-flō-jis'tik). Causing or producing tissue inflammation. [pro- + G. *phlogōsis,* inflammation]

pro·phy·lac·tic (prō-fi-lak'tik). **1.** Preventing disease; relating to prophylaxis. SYN preventive. **2.** An agent that acts to prevent a disease. [G. *prophylaktikos;* see prophylaxis]

pro·phy·lax·is, pl. **pro·phy·lax·es** (prō-fi-lak'sis, -sēz). Prevention of disease or of a process that can lead to disease. [Mod. L. fr. G. *pro-phylassō,* to guard before, take precaution]

   active p., use of an antigenic (immunogenic) agent to actively stimulate the immunological mechanism.

   chemical p., the administration of chemicals or drugs to members of a community to reduce the number of carriers of a disease and to prevent others contracting the disease.

   dental p., a series of procedures whereby calculus, stain, and other accretions are removed from the clinical crowns of the teeth, and the enamel surfaces are polished.

   passive p., use of an antiserum from another person or animal to provide temporary (a week to 10 days) protection against a specific infectious or toxic agent.

pro·pi·cil·lin (prō-pi-sil'in). A semisynthetic acid-stable penicillin that may be more effective than penicillin G. SYN α-phenoxypropylpenicillin potassium.

pro·pi·o·cor·tin (prō-pē-ō-kōr'ten). An endogenous polypeptide that might be a precursor to the enkephalins. Cf. proenkephalin.

pro·pi·o·lac·tone (prō'pē-ō-lak'tōn). β-Propiolactone; hydracrylic acid β-lactone; used to sterilize plasma, vaccines, and tissue grafts.

pro·pi·o·nate (prō'pē-ō-nāt). A salt or ester of propionic acid.

Pro·pi·on·i·bac·te·ri·um (prō-pē-on-i-bak-tēr'ē-ŭm). A genus of nonmotile, nonsporeforming, anaerobic to aerotolerant bacteria (family Propionibacteriaceae) containing Gram-positive rods which are usually pleomorphic, diphtheroid, or club-shaped with one end rounded, the other tapered or pointed. Some cells may be coccoid, elongate, bifid, or even branched. The cells usually occur singly, in pairs, in V and Y configurations, short chains, or clumps in "Chinese character" arrangement. The metabolism of these organisms is fermentative, and the products of fermentation include combinations of propionic and acetic acids. These organisms occur in dairy products, on the skin of man, and in the intestinal tract of man and other animals. They may be pathogenic. The type species is *P. freudenreichii.*

   P. ac'nes, a species of bacteria commonly found in acne pustules, although it occurs in other types of lesions in humans and even as a saprophyte in the intestine, skin, hair follicles, and in sewage. SYN acne bacillus.

   P. freudenrei'chii, a species found in raw milk, Swiss cheese, and other dairy products; it is the type species of the genus *P.*

   P. jensen'ii, a species found in dairy products, silage, and occasionally in infections.

   P. propion'icus, SYN *Arachnia propionica.*

pro·pi·on·ic ac·id (prō-pē-on'ik). CH_3CH_2COOH; methylacetic acid; ethylformic acid; found in sweat. SYN propanoic acid.

pro·pi·on·ic ac·i·de·mia (prō-pē-on'ik-as-i-dē'mē-ă). SYN ketotic *hyperglycinemia.*

pro·pi·o·nyl (prō'pē-ō-nil). CH_3CH_2CO-; the acyl radical of propionic acid. SYN propanoyl.

pro·pi·o·nyl-CoA (prō'pē-ō-nil-kō-ā). The coenzyme A thioester derivative of propionic acid; an intermediate in the degradation of L-valine, L-isoleucine, L-threonine, L-methionine, and odd-chain fatty acids; a precursor for the synthesis of odd-chain fatty acids; it accumulates in individuals with a deficiency of p.-CoA carboxylase.

   p.-CoA carboxylase, an enzyme that catalyzes the reaction of p.-CoA with CO_2 and ATP to produce ADP, inorganic phosphate, and D-methylmalonyl-CoA; a biotin-dependent enzyme; an in-

herited deficiency of this enzyme will lead to propionic acidemia and developmental retardation.

pro·pi·o·nyl·gly·cine (prō'pē-ō-nil-glī'sēn). CH_3CH_2 $CONHCH_2COOH$; a minor metabolite that accumulates in individuals with propionic acidemia.

pro·pit·o·caine hy·dro·chlo·ride (prō-pit'ō-kān). SYN prilocaine hydrochloride.

pro·pla·sia (prō-plā'zē-ă). That state of cell or tissue in which activity is increased above that of euplasia, *i.e.,* characterized by stimulation, repair, or regeneration. [pro- + G. *plassō,* to form]

pro·plas·ma·cyte (prō-plaz'mă-sīt). A cell in the process of differentiating from a plasmablast to a mature plasma cell.

pro·plex·us (prō-plek'sŭs). The choroid plexus in the lateral ventricle of the brain.

pro·po·fol (prō'pō-fōl). An oil-in-water emulsion of 1,6-diisopropylphenol, a hypnotic with rapid onset and short duration of action; used intravenously for induction and maintenance of general anesthesia. SYN 2,6-diisopropyl phenol.

pro·pos·i·tus, pl. **pro·po·si·ti** (prō'poz'i-tŭs, -tī). **1.** Proband distinguished by sex. Cf. consultand. **2.** A premise; an argument. [L. fr. *propono,* pp. *-positus,* to lay out, propound]

pro·pox·y·phene hy·dro·chlo·ride (prō-pok'si-fēn). (+)-α-4-(dimethylamino)-3-methyl-1,2-diphenyl-2-butanol propionate hydrochloride; a nonantipyretic, orally effective weak narcotic analgesic structurally related to methadone and used for the relief of mild to moderate pain; it is less effective than codeine. SYN dextropropoxyphene hydrochloride.

pro·pox·y·phene nap·syl·ate (prō-pok'si-fēn). mono-2-naphthalenesulfonate monohydrate salt of propoxyphene; a weak narcotic analgesic. SYN dextropropoxyphene napsylate.

pro·pran·o·lol hy·dro·chlo·ride (prō-pran'ō-lōl). 1-(isopropylamino)-3-(1-naphthyloxy)-2-propanol hydrochloride; an adrenergic β-receptor blocking agent.

pro·pri·e·tary name (prō-prī'ě-tār-ē). The protected brand name or trademark, registered with the U.S. Patent Office, under which a manufacturer markets his product. It is written with a capital initial letter and is often further distinguished by a superscript R in a circle (®). Cf. generic name, nonproprietary name. [L. *proprietarius*]

pro·pri·o·cep·tion (prō-prē-ō-sep'shun). A sense or perception, usually at a subconscious level, of the movements and position of the body and especially its limbs, independent of vision; this sense is gained primarily from input from sensory nerve terminals in muscles and tendons (muscle spindles) and the fibrous capsule of joints combined with input from the vestibular apparatus.

pro·pri·o·cep·tive (prō'prē-ō-sep'tiv). Capable of receiving stimuli originating in muscles, tendons, and other internal tissues. [L. *proprius,* one's own, + *capio,* to take]

pro·pri·o·cep·tor (prō'prē-ō-sep'ter). One of a variety of sensory end organs (such as the muscle spindle and Golgi's tendon organ) in muscles, tendons, and joint capsules.

pro·pri·o·spi·nal (prō'prē-ō-spī'năl). Relating especially or wholly to the spinal cord; specifically, denoting those nerve cells and their fibers that connect the different segments of the spinal cord with each other (*e.g.,* spino-spinalis).

pro·pro·teins (prō'prō-tenz). Inactive protein precursors; *e.g.,* proinsulin.

prop·tom·e·ter (prop-tom'ě-ter). SYN exophthalmometer. [pro- + G. *ptōsis,* a falling, + *metron,* measure]

prop·to·sis (prop-tō'sis). SYN exophthalmos. [G. *proptōsis,* a falling forward]

prop·tot·ic (prop-tot'ik). Referring to proptosis.

pro·pul·sion (prō-pŭl'shun). The tendency to fall forward; responsible for the festination in paralysis agitans. [G. *pro-pello,* pp. *-pulsus,* to drive forth]

pro·pyl (Pr) (prō'pil). The alkyl radical of propane, $CH_3CH_2CH_2-$.

   p. alcohol, $CH_3CH_2CH_2OH$; ethylcarbinol; a solvent for resins and cellulose esters. SYN propanol.

   p. gallate, propyl 3,4,5-trihydroxybenzoate; an antioxidant for emulsions.

pr

p. hydroxybenzoate, SYN propylparaben.

pro·pyl·car·bi·nol (prō-pil-kar′bi-nol). Primary butyl alcohol. SEE *butyl* alcohol.

pro·py·lene (prō′pi-lēn). $CH_2=CHCH_3$; methylethylene; a gaseous olefinic hydrocarbon. SYN propene.

p. glycol, $CH_3CHOHCH_2OH$; 1,2-propanediol; 1,2-dihydroxypropane; a solvent for several water-insoluble drugs intended for parenteral administration; an ingredient of hydrophilic ointment; a viscous organic solvent frequently used in pharmaceutical preparations to dissolve drug substances with limited aqueous solubility; used in part for preparing injectable solutions of diazepam, phenytoin, pentobarbital and other drugs.

pro·pyl·hex·e·drine (prō-pil-hek′se-drēn). *N*,α-Dimethylcyclohexaneethylamine; 1-cyclohexyl-2-methylaminopropane; a sympathomimetic and local vasoconstrictor.

pro·pyl·i·o·done (prō-pil-ī′ō-dōn). Propyl-3,5-diiodo-4-oxo-1(4*H*)pyridineacetate; a radiopaque medium formerly used for bronchography.

pro·pyl·par·a·ben (prō-pil-par′ă-ben). *p*-hydroxybenzoic acid propyl ester; an antifungal agent and pharmaceutical preservative. SYN propyl hydroxybenzoate.

pro·pyl·thi·o·ur·a·cil (PTU) (prō′pil-thī-ō-yū′ră-sil). 6-Propyl-2-thiouracil; an antithyroid agent that inhibits the synthesis of thyroid hormones; used in the treatment of hyperthyroidism; a goitrogen.

pro·py·ro·ma·zine (prō-pi-rō′mă-zēn). 1-Methyl-1-[1-(phenothiazin-10-ylcarbonyl)ethyl]pyrrolidinium bromide; an intestinal antispasmodic with anticholinergic properties.

pro rat. aet. Abbreviation for L. *pro ratione aetatis,* according to (patient's) age.

pro re na·ta (p.r.n.) (prō rē nā′tă). As the occasion arises; as necessary. [L.]

pro·ren·nin (prō-ren′in). SYN prochymosin.

pror·sad (prōr′sad). In a forward direction. [L. *prorsum,* forward, + *ad,* to]

pro·ru·bri·cyte (prō-rū′bri-sīt). Basophilic normoblast. SEE erythroblast. [pro- + rubricyte]

pernicious anemia type p., basophilic megaloblast. SEE erythroblast, megaloblast.

pros (pros). **1.** (π) Referring to the nitrogen atom in the imidazole ring in histidine that is closest to the β-carbon. Cf. tele. **2.** *pros-*; Prefix for near or in front. [G. near]

pro·scil·lar·i·din (prō-si-lar′i-din). Desglucotransvaaline; scillarenin 3β-rhamnoside 14-hydroxy-3β-(rhamnosyloxy)bufa-4,20,22-trienolide; prepared from squill, the sea onion *Urginea maritima;* a cardiotonic agent, used for the treatment of congestive heart failure.

pro·sco·lex (prō-skō′leks). Seldom used term for the embryonic form of a tapeworm. [pro- + G. *skōlex,* a worm]

pro·se·cre·tin (prō-sē-krē′tin). Unactivated secretin.

pro·sect (prō-sekt′). To dissect a cadaver or any part, that it may serve for a demonstration of anatomy before a class. [L. *proseco,* pp. *-sectus,* to cut]

pro·sec·tor (prō′sek′ter). One who prosects, or prepares the material for a demonstration of anatomy before a class.

pro·sec·to·ri·um (prō′sek-tō′rē-ŭm). A dissecting room; a place in which anatomical preparations are made for demonstration or for preservation in a museum. [L.]

pros·en·ceph·a·lon (pros-en-sef′ă-lon) [NA]. The anterior primitive cerebral vesicle and the most rostral of the three primary brain vesicles of the embryonic neural tube; it subdivides to form the diencephalon and telencephalon. SYN forebrain vesicle, forebrain, proencephalon. [G. *prosō,* forward, + *enkephalos,* brain]

Proskauer, Bernhard, German bacteriologist, 1851–1915. SEE Voges-P. *reaction.*

pros·o·dem·ic (pros-ō-dem′ik). Denoting a disease that is transmitted directly from person to person. [G. *prosō,* forward, + *dēmos,* people]

△**prosop-.** SEE prosopo-.

pros·o·pag·no·sia (pros′ō-pag-nō′sē-ă). Difficulty in recognizing familiar faces. [prosop- + G. *a-* priv. + *gnōsis,* recognition]

pro·sop·a·gus (pro-sop′ă-gŭs). SYN prosopopagus.

pros·o·pal·gia (pros-ō-pal′jē-ă). SYN trigeminal *neuralgia.* [prosop- + G. *algos,* pain]

pros·o·pal·gic (pros-ō-pal′jik). Relating to or suffering from trigeminal neuralgia.

pros·o·pec·ta·sia (pros′ō-pek-tā′zē-ă). Enlargement of the face, as in acromegaly. [prosop- + G. *ektasis,* extension]

pros·o·pla·sia (pros-ō-plā′zē-ă). Progressive transformation, such as the change of cells of the salivary ducts into secreting cells. SEE cytomorphosis. [G. *prosō,* forward, + *plasis,* a molding]

△**prosopo-, prosop-.** The face. SEE ALSO facio-. [G. *prosōpon*]

pros·o·po·a·nos·chi·sis (pros′ō-pō-ă-nos′ki-sis). SYN facial *cleft.* [prosopo- + G. *anō,* upward, + *schisis,* fissure]

pros·o·po·di·ple·gia (pros′ō-pō-dī-plē′jē-ă). Paralysis affecting both sides of the face. [prosopo- + diplegia]

pros·o·po·neu·ral·gia (pros′ō-pō-nū-ral′jē-ă). SYN trigeminal *neuralgia.*

pros·o·pop·a·gus (pros-ō-pop′ă-gŭs). Unequal conjoined twins in which the parasite, in the form of a tumor-like mass, is attached to the orbit or cheek of the autosite. SEE conjoined *twins,* under *twin.* SYN prosopagus. [prosopo- + G. *pagos,* something fastened]

pros·o·po·ple·gia (pros′ō-pō-plē′jē-ă). SYN facial *paralysis.* [prosopo- + G. *plēgē,* stroke]

pros·o·po·ple·gic (pros′ō-pō-plē′jik). Relating to, or suffering from, facial paralysis.

pros·o·pos·chi·sis (pros-ō-pos′ki-sis). Congenital facial cleft from mouth to the inner canthus of the eye. SYN oblique facial cleft. [prosopo- + G. *schisis,* fissure]

pros·o·po·spasm (pros′ō-pō-spazm). SYN facial *tic.* [prosopo- + G. *spasmos,* spasm]

pros·o·po·thor·a·cop·a·gus (pros′ō-pō-thōr-ă-kop′ă-gŭs). Conjoined twins attached by the face and chest; a variety of cephalothoracopagus. SEE conjoined *twins,* under *twin.* [prosopo- + G. *thōrax,* chest, + *pagos,* something fastened]

pro·sper·mia (prō-sper′mē-ă). Rarely used term for premature *ejaculation.* [pro- + G. *sperma,* seed]

pros·ta·cy·clin (pros-tă-sī′klin). Prostaglandin I_2; a potent natural inhibitor of platelet aggregation and a powerful vasodilator. SYN epoprostenol, epoprostenol sodium.

pros·ta·glan·din (PG) (pros-tă-glan′din). Any of a class of physiologically active substances present in many tissues, with effects such as vasodilation, vasoconstriction, stimulation of intestinal or bronchial smooth muscle, uterine stimulation, and antagonism to hormones influencing lipid metabolism. P.'s are prostanoic acids with side chains of varying degrees of unsaturation and varying degrees of oxidation. Often abbreviated PGA, PGB, PGC, PGD, etc. with numerical subscripts, according to structure. [fr. genital fluids and accessory glands where discovered]

p. E_1, SYN alprostadil.

p. E_2, SYN dinoprostone.

p. endoperoxide synthase, a protein complex that catalyzes two steps in p. biosynthesis; the cyclooxygenase activity (which is inhibited by aspirin and indomethacin) converts arachidonate and $2O_2$ to p. G_2; the hydroperoxidase activity uses glutathione to convert p. G_2 to p. H_2. SYN cyclooxygenase.

p. $F_{2\alpha}$, SYN dinoprost.

p. $F_{2\alpha}$ tromethamine, SYN *dinoprost* tromethamine.

pros·ta·no·ic ac·id (pros′tă-nō-ik). 7-[2-(1-Octanyl)-cyclopentyl]heptanoic acid; the 20-carbon acid that is the skeleton of the prostaglandins, with various hydroxyl and keto substitutions at positions 9, 11, and 15, and double bonds in the long aliphatic chains.

pros·ta·noids (pros′tă-nōids). Derivatives of prostanoic acid; *e.g.,* prostaglandins, thromboxanes, etc.

△**prostat-.** SEE prostato-.

pros·ta·ta (pros'tah-tă) [NA]. SYN prostate. [Mod. L. from G. *prostatēs*, one standing before]

pros·ta·tal·gia (pros-tă-tal'jē-ă). A rarely used term for pain in the area of the prostate gland. [prostat- + G. *algos*, pain]

pros·tate (pros'tāt). A chestnut-shaped body, surrounding the beginning of the urethra in the male, that consists of two lateral lobes connected anteriorly by an isthmus and posteriorly by a middle lobe lying above and between the ejaculatory ducts. In structure, the prostate consists of 30 to 50 compound tubuloalveolar glands between which is abundant stroma consisting of collagen and elastic fibers and many smooth muscle bundles. The secretion of the glands is a milky fluid that is discharged by excretory ducts into the prostatic urethra at the time of the emission of semen. SYN prostata [NA], glandula prostatica, prostate gland.

female p., term sometimes applied to the periurethral glands in the upper part of the urethra in the female.

pros·ta·tec·to·my (pros-tă-tek'tō-mē). Removal of a part or all of the prostate. [prostat- + G. *ektomē*, excision]

pros·tat·ic (pros-tat'ik). Relating to the prostate.

pros·tat·i·co·ves·i·cal (pros-tat'i-kō-ves'i-kăl). Relating to the prostate and the bladder.

pros·ta·tism (pros'tă-tizm). A clinical syndrome, occurring mostly in older men, usually caused by enlargement of the prostate gland and manifested by irritative (nocturia, frequency, decreased voided volume, sensory urgency, and urgency incontinence) and obstructive (hesitancy, decreased stream, terminal dribbling, double voiding, and urinary retention) symptoms.

pros·ta·ti·tis (pros-tă-tī'tis). Inflammation of the prostate. [prostat- + G. *-itis*, inflammation]

prostato-, prostat-. The prostate gland. [Med. L. *prostata* fr. G. *prostatēs*, one who stands before, protects]

pros·ta·to·cys·ti·tis (pros'tă-tō-sis-tī'tis). Inflammation of the prostate and the bladder; cystitis by extension of inflammation from the prostatic urethra. [prostato- + G. *kystis*, bladder, + *-itis*, inflammation]

pros·ta·to·dyn·ia (pros'tă-tō-din'ē-ă). A rarely used term for prostatalgia. [prostato- + G. *odynē*, pain]

pros·tat·o·lith (pros-tat'ō-lith). SYN prostatic *calculus*. [prostato- + G. *lithos*, stone]

pros·ta·to·li·thot·o·my (pros'tă-tō-li-thot'ō-mē, pros-tat'ō-). Incision of the prostate for removal of a calculus. [prostato- + G. *lithos*, stone, + *tomē*, incision]

pros·ta·to·meg·a·ly (pros'tă-tō-meg'ă-lē). Enlargement of the prostate gland. [prostato- + G. *megas*, large]

pros·tat·o·my (pros-tat'ō-mē). SYN prostatotomy.

pros·ta·tor·rhea (pros'tă-tō-rē'ă). An abnormal discharge of prostatic fluid. [prostato- + G. *rhoia*, a flow]

pros·ta·to·sem·i·nal·ve·sic·u·lec·to·my (pros'tă-tō-sem'i-năl-ve-sik-yū-lek'tō-mē). SYN prostatovesiculectomy.

pros·ta·tot·o·my (pros'tă-tot'ō-mē). An incision into the prostate. SYN prostatomy. [prostato- + G. *tomē*, incision]

pros·ta·to·ve·sic·u·lec·to·my (pros'tă-tō-ve-sik'yū-lek'tō-mē). Surgical removal of the prostate gland and seminal vesicles. SYN prostatoseminalvesiculectomy.

pros·ta·to·ve·sic·u·li·tis (pros'tă-tō-ve-sik'yū-lī'tis). Inflammation of the prostate gland and seminal vesicles.

pros·ter·na·tion (pros-ter-nā'shŭn). SYN camptocormia.

pros·the·on (pros'thē-on). SYN prosthion.

pros·the·sis, pl. **pros·the·ses** (pros'thē-sis, -sēz; pros-thē'sis). Fabricated substitute for a diseased or missing part of the body. [G. an addition]

cardiac valve p., SEE valve (2).

cochlear p., SYN cochlear *implant*.

definitive p., a dental p. to be used over a prescribed period of time.

dental p., an artificial replacement of one or more teeth and/or associated structures. SEE ALSO denture.

heart valve p., replacement of a cardiac valve removed for disease by either a mechanical or a biologically derived artificial valve.

hybrid p., SYN overlay *denture*.

mandibular guide p., a p. with an extension designed to direct a resected mandible into a functional relation with the maxilla.

ocular p., an artificial eye or implant.

provisional p., an interim dental p. worn for varying periods of time.

surgical p., an appliance prepared as an aid or as a part of a surgical proceeding, such as a heart valve or cranial plate.

testicular p., SYN testicular *implant*.

tilting disc valve p., a low profile artificial heart valve with excellent flow characteristics.

pros·thet·ic (pros-thet'ik). **1.** Relating to a prosthesis or to an artificial part. **2.** SEE prosthetic *group*.

pros·thet·ics (pros-thet'iks). The art and science of making and adjusting artificial parts of the human body.

dental p., SYN prosthodontics.

maxillofacial p., that branch of dentistry which provides prostheses or devices to treat or restore tissues of the stomatognathic system and associated facial structures that have been affected by disease, injury, surgery, or congenital defect, to provide all possible function and esthetics.

pros·the·tist (pros'the-tist). One skilled in constructing and fitting prostheses.

pros·the·to·phac·os (pros'thĕ-tō-fak'ōs). SYN lenticulus. [G. *prosthesis*, an addition, + *phakos*, lens]

pros·thi·on (pros'thē-on). The most anterior point on the maxillary alveolar process in the midline. SYN alveolar point, prostheon. [G. ntr. of *prosthios*, foremost]

pros·tho·don·tia (pros-thō-don'shē-ă). SYN prosthodontics. [L.]

pros·tho·don·tics (pros-thō-don'tiks). The science of and art of providing suitable substitutes for the coronal portions of teeth, or for one or more lost or missing teeth and their associated parts, in order that impaired function, appearance, comfort, and health of the patient may be restored. SYN dental prosthetics, prosthetic dentistry, prosthodontia. [L. *prosthodontia*, fr. G. *prosthesis* + *odous* (*odont-*), tooth]

pros·tho·don·tist (pros-thō-don'tist). A dentist engaged in the practice of prosthodontics.

Pros·tho·gon·i·mus ma·cror·chis (pros'thō-gon'i-mŭs mak-rōr'kis). A digenetic trematode (family Prosthogonimidae) located in the oviduct and bursa fabricii of poultry in North America, particularly common in states bordering the Great Lakes. [G. *prosthe*, in front of, + *gonos*, seed, offspring; macro- + *orchis*, testicle]

pros·tho·ker·a·to·plas·ty (pros'thō-ker'ă-tō-plas-tē). The surgical technique involved in utilizing a keratoprosthesis.

pros·tra·tion (pros-trā'shŭn). A marked loss of strength, as in exhaustion. [L. *pro-sterno*, pp. *-stratus*, to strew before, overthrow]

heat p., SEE heat *exhaustion*.

prot-. SEE proteo-, proto-.

prot·ac·tin·i·um (Pa) (prō-tak-tin'ē-ŭm). A radioactive element, atomic no. 91, atomic wt. 231.03588, formed in the decay of uranium and thorium; its most long-lived isotope, ^{231}Pa, has a half-life of 32,500 years. SYN proactinium, protoactinium. [G. *protos*, first]

pro·tal·bu·mose (prō-tal'byū-mōs). Intermediate products of

Combining forms	[NA] Nomina Anatomica
Word*Finder* Multi-term entry finder Preceding letter A	[MIM] Mendelian Inheritance in Man
A.D.A.M. Anatomy Plates Between letters L and M	☆ Official alternate term
Appendices: Following letter Z	☆[NA] Official alternate Nomina Anatomica term
SYN Synonym; Cf., compare	High Profile Term

protein digestion, derived from hemialbumose; soluble in water and not coagulable by heat, but precipitated by ammonium sulfate, cupric sulfate, and sodium chloride. SYN protoalbumose.

pro·tam·i·nase (prō-tam'i-nās). SYN carboxypeptidase B.

prot·a·mine (prō'tă-mēn, -min). Any of a class of proteins, highly basic because rich in L-arginine and simpler in constitution than the albumins and globulins, etc., found in fish spermatozoa in combination with nucleic acid; neutralizes anticoagulant action of heparin.

p. sulfate, a purified mixture of simple protein principles from the sperm or testes of suitable species of fish; it is a heparin antagonist used in certain hemorrhagic states associated with increased amounts of heparin-like substances in the circulation and for the treatment of heparin overdosage.

pro·ta·nom·a·ly (prō'tă-nom'ă-lē). A deficiency of color perception in which the red-sensitive pigment in cones is decreased. [G. *prōtos*, first, + *anōmalia*, anomaly]

pro·ta·no·pia (prō'tă-nō'pē-ă). A form of dichromatism characterized by absence of the red-sensitive pigment in cones, decreased luminosity for long wavelengths of light, and confusion in recognition of red and green. [G. *prōtos*, first, + *a*- priv. + *ōps* (*ōp*-) eye]

pro·te·an (prō'tē-an). Changeable in form; having the power to change body form, like the ameba. [G. *Prōteus*, a god having the power to change his form]

pro·te·ase (prō'tē-ās). Descriptive term for proteolytic enzymes, both endopeptidases and exopeptidases.

Lon p. (prō'tē-ās), an enzyme that degrades a bacterial protein and stops cell division until chromosomal repair is completed.

pro·tec·tion (prō-tek'shŭn). SYN protective *block*. [see protective]

Pro·tee·ae (prō'tē-ē). A tribe within the bacterial family Enterobacteriaceae that includes the three genera: *Proteus, Morganella,* and *Providencia.*

pro·te·id (prō'tē-id). Obsolete name for conjugated *protein.*

pro·tein (prō'tēn, prō'tē-in). Macromolecules consisting of long sequences of α-amino acids [H₂N–CHR–COOH] in peptide (amide) linkage (elimination of H_2O between the α-NH_2 and α-COOH of successive residues). P. is three-fourths of the dry weight of most cell matter and is involved in structures, hormones, enzymes, muscle contraction, immunological response, and essential life functions. The amino acids involved are generally the 20 α-amino acids (glycine, L-alanine, etc.) recognized by the genetic code. Cross-links yielding globular forms of p. are often effected through the –SH groups of two sulfur-containing L-cysteinyl residues, as well as by noncovalent forces (hydrogen bonds, lipophilic attractions, etc.). [G. *protos*, first, + -in]

p. 4.1, a peripheral p. that binds tightly to spectrin in the red cell membrane; it also binds to certain glycophorins and helps determine the shape and flexibility of the red blood cell.

acyl carrier p. (ACP), one of the p.'s of the complex in cytoplasm that contains all of the enzymes required to convert acetyl-CoA (and, in certain cases, butyryl-CoA or propionyl-CoA) and malonyl-CoA to palmitic acid. This complex is tightly bound together in mammalian tissues and in yeast, but that from *Escherichia coli* is readily dissociated. The ACP thus isolated is a heat-stable p. with a molecular weight of about 10,000. It contains a free –SH that binds the acyl intermediates in the synthesis of fatty acids as thioesters. This –SH group is part of a 4'-phosphopantetheine, added to the apoprotein by ACP phosphodiesterase, which thus plays the same role that it does in coenzyme A. ACP is involved in every step of the fatty acid synthetic process.

amyloid p., SEE amyloid.

androgen binding p. (ABP), a p. secreted by testicular Sertoli cells along with inhibin and müllerian inhibiting substance. Androgen binding p. probably maintains a high concentration of androgen in the seminiferous tubules.

antitermination p., a p. that permits RNA polymerase to transcribe through certain termination sites.

antitumor p., a p. that inhibits tumor growth.

antiviral p. (AVP), a human or animal factor, induced by interferon in virus-infected cells, which mediates interferon inhibition of virus replication.

autologous p., any p. found normally in the fluids or tissues of the body.

basic p.'s, p.'s that are rich in basic amino acids; *e.g.,* histones.

Bence Jones p.'s, p.'s with unusual thermosolubility found in the urine of patients with multiple myeloma, consisting of monoclonal immunoglobulin light chains. SEE Bence Jones *reaction.* SEE ALSO immunoglobulin.

bone Gla p. (BGP), SYN osteocalcin.

p. C, a vitamin K-dependent plasma p. that inhibits coagulation by enzymatic cleavage of the activated forms of factors V and VIII, and thus interferes with the regulation of intravascular clot formation; a deficiency of p. C leads to impaired regulation of blood coagulation. There is an autosomal dominant deficiency [MIM*176860] that, like antithrombin III deficiency and plasminogen deficiency, is associated with an increased risk of severe or premature thrombosis.

cAMP receptor p. (CRP), SYN catabolite (gene) activator p.

capping p.'s, p.'s that bind to one end of actin filaments, preventing both addition and loss of actin monomers.

catabolite (gene) activator p. (CAP), a p. that can be activated by cAMP, whereupon it affects the action of RNA polymerase by binding it with it or near it on the DNA to be transcribed. SYN cAMP receptor p., catabolite gene activator.

cholesterol ester transport p.'s, a p. that transports cholesterol esters from HDL to VLDL and LDL; a deficiency of this protein is associated with elevated HDL cholesterol.

***cis*-acting p.,** a p. that acts on the molecule of DNA from which it was expressed.

compound p., SYN conjugated p.

conjugated p., p. attached to some other molecule or molecules (not amino acid in nature) otherwise than as a salt; *e.g.,* flavoproteins; chromoproteins, hemoglobins. SEE ALSO prosthetic *group.* Cf. simple p. SYN compound p.

copper p., a p. containing one or more copper ions; *e.g.,* cytochrome *c* oxidase, phenol oxidase.

corticosteroid-binding p., SYN transcortin.

C-reactive p. (CRP), a β-globulin found in the serum of various persons with certain inflammatory, degenerative, and neoplastic diseases; although the p. is not a specific antibody, it precipitates *in vitro* the C polysaccharide present in all types of pneumococci.

denatured p., a p. whose characteristics or properties have been altered in some way, as by heat, enzyme action, or chemicals, and, in so doing, has lost its biological activity.

derived p., a derivative of p. effected by chemical change, *e.g.,* hydrolysis.

docking p., in the process of translating p.'s that are to be secreted from the cell, translation is arrested until the growing polypeptide chain that is complexed by a specific particle (signal recognition particle) comes in contact with this integral p. of the endoplasmic reticulum.

encephalithogenic p., an important protein in the central nervous system. SYN myelin p. A1.

extrinsic p.'s, SYN peripheral p.'s.

fatty acid binding p., SYN Z-p.

fibrous p., any insoluble p., including the collagens, elastins, and keratins, involved in structural or fibrous tissues.

foreign p., a p. that differs from any p. normally found in the organism in question. SYN heterologous p.

G p.'s, intracellular membrane-associated p.'s activated by several (*e.g.,* beta adrenergic) receptors; they serve as second messengers or transducers of the receptor-initiated response to intracellular elements such as enzymes to initiate an effect. These p.'s have a high affinity for guanine nucleotides and hence are named "G" p.'s. SYN G-p., GTP binding p.'s.

G-p., SYN G p.'s.

globular p., any p. soluble in water, usually with added acid, alkali, salt, or ethanol, and roughly so classified (albumins, globulins, histones, protamines), in contrast to fibrous p.

GTP binding p.'s, SYN G p.'s.

heat shock p.'s (hsp), specific p.'s whose synthesis is increased immediately after sudden elevation of temperature; their function is to help diminish the harmful effects of high temperature.

heterologous p., SYN foreign p.

homologous p.'s, p.'s having a very similar primary, secondary, and tertiary structure.

immune p., SYN antibody.

integral p.'s, p.'s that cannot be easily separated from a biomembrane. SYN intrinsic p.'s.

intrinsic p.'s, SYN integral p.'s.

iron-sulfur p.'s, p.'s containing one or more iron atoms that are linked to sulfur bridges and/or sulfur of cysteinyl residues; *e.g.,* certain p.'s in the electron transport pathway.

p. kinases, a class of enzymes that phosphorylates other p.'s; many of these kinases are responsive to other effectors (*e.g.,* cAMP, cGMP, insulin, epidermal growth factor, calcium and calmodulin, calcium and phospholipids, etc.).

M p., (1) SYN Streptococcus M *antigen.* SEE ALSO β-hemolytic *streptococci,* under *streptococcus, Streptococcus pneumoniae.* **(2)** SYN monoclonal *immunoglobulin.*

macrophage inflammatory p. (mak'rō-fāj in'flam-mă-to-rē), a member of the chemokine family that is chemotactic for certain lymphocyte subsets such as T cytotoxic cells.

matrix Gla p. (MGP), a calcium binding p.

microtubule-associated p.'s (MAPs), p.'s that have a specific association with α- and/or β-tubulin; *e.g.,* tau, MAP1, MAP2; several have been found in the plaques observed in Alzheimer's disease.

mild p. protein, a complex prepared by the reaction of p. oxide with either gelatin or serum albumin. Black shiny crystals liberate p. and it was formerly widely used as a topical anti-infective on mucous membranes. Contains from 19 to 25% p., only a small fraction of which is ionizable. Can produce black or brown pigmentation due to deposition of reduced p. in the tissues. SYN argyrol, silvol.

monoclonal p., SYN monoclonal *immunoglobulin.*

monocyte chemoattractant p.-1 (MCP-1) (mon'ō-sīt kē'mō- ă-trak'tănt), secreted by endothelial cells of a blood vessel wall; it induces extravasation of monocytes.

muscle p.'s, p.'s present in muscle.

myelin p. A1, SYN encephalithogenic p.

myeloblastic p., SEE human leukemia-associated *antigens,* under *antigen.*

native p., the concept of a p. in its natural state, in the cell, unaltered by heat, chemicals, enzyme action, or the exigencies of extraction.

neutrophil activating p. (NAP), SYN interleukin-8.

non-heme iron p., any p. containing iron but not any heme iron; *e.g.,* NADH dehydrogenase.

nonspecific p., a p. substance that elicits a response not mediated by specific antigen-antibody reaction.

odorant binding p., p.'s in nasal mucus that bind lipophilic odor-producing molecules and transfer them to the olfactory receptors. Similar p.'s may mediate taste.

parathyroid hormonelike p. (PLP), a 140 amino acid p. secreted by some cancer cells; it causes hypercalcemia.

pathological p.'s, SEE paraprotein.

peripheral p.'s, p.'s that can be easily removed from a biomembrane (*e.g.,* by altering the pH or the ionic strength). SYN extrinsic p.'s.

phenylthiocarbamoyl p., formed by the reaction of phenylisothiocyanate with a terminal α-amino group of a peptide or p. SEE ALSO phenylisothiocyanate, phenylthiohydantoin. SYN PhNCS p., PTC p.

PhNCS p., SYN phenylthiocarbamoyl p.

p. phosphatases, a class of enzymes that catalyze the dephosphorylation of specific phosphorylated p.'s.

placenta p., SYN human placental *lactogen.*

plasma p.'s, dissolved p.'s (more than 100) of blood plasma, mainly albumins and globulins (normally 6 to 8 g/100 ml); they hold fluid in blood vessels by osmosis and include antibodies and blood-clotting p.'s. SYN serum p.'s.

prion p., small, infectious proteinaceous particle, of non-nucleic

acid composition because of its resistance to nucleases; the causative agent, either on a sporadic, genetic, or infectious basis, of six neurodegenerative diseases in animals, and four in humans; the latter include the spongiform encephalopathies of kuru, Creutzfeldt-Jakob disease, Gerstmann-Straussler-Scheinker syndrome and fatal familial insomnia. The gene encoding for the PrP is found on chromosome 20. SYN prion.

protective p., SYN antibody.

PTC p., SYN phenylthiocarbamoyl p.

purified placental p., SYN human placental *lactogen.*

receptor p., an intracellular p. (or p. fraction) that has a high specific affinity for binding a known stimulus to cellular activity, such as a steroid hormone or adenosine 3′,5′-cyclic phosphate.

retinol-binding p., a plasma p. that binds and transports retinol.

S p., the major fragment produced from pancreatic ribonuclease by the limited action of subtilisin, which cleaves the ribonuclease between residues 20 and 21; the smaller fragment (residues 1-20) is S peptide.

p. S, a vitamin K-dependent antithrombotic p. that functions as a cofactor with activated p. C.

serum p.'s, SYN plasma p.'s.

simple p., p. that yields only α-amino acids or their derivatives by hydrolysis; *e.g.,* albumins, globulins, glutelins, prolamines, albuminoids, histones, protamines. Cf. conjugated p.

stimulatory p. 1 (SP1), an RNA polymerase II transcription factor in vertebrates; binds to DNA in regions rich in G and C residues; a general promoter-binding factor necessary for the activation of many genes.

strong silver p., SEE strong *silver* protein.

structure p.'s, p.'s whose role is for structure and support in tissue and within the cell; *e.g.,* the collagens.

Tamm-Horsfall p., SEE Tamm-Horsfall *mucoprotein.*

thyroxine-binding p. (TBP), (1) SYN thyroxine-binding *globulin.* **(2)** SYN thyroxine-binding *prealbumin.*

unwinding p.'s, enzymes that uncoil the DNA allowing recombination events to occur.

vitamin D-binding p. (DBP), a plasma p. that binds vitamin D.

whey p., the soluble p. contained in the whey of milk clotted by rennin; *e.g.,* lactoglobulin, α-lactalbumin, lactoferrin.

Z-p., a fatty acid-binding protein that participates in the intracellular movement of fatty acids. SYN fatty acid binding p.

pro·tein·a·ceous (prō'tē-nā'shŭs, prō'tē-i-nā'shŭs). Resembling a protein; possessing, to some degree, the physicochemical properties characteristic of proteins.

pro·tein·ase. SYN endopeptidase.

pro·tein hy·drol·y·sate. A sterile solution of amino acids and soft chain peptides prepared from a suitable protein by acid or enzymatic hydrolysis; used intravenously for the maintenance of positive nitrogen balance in severe illness, and after surgery involving the alimentary tract; or used orally in the diets of infants allergic to milk or as a supplement when high protein intake from ordinary foods cannot be accomplished.

pro·tein·o·gen·ic (prō'ten-ō-jen'ik). SYN proteogenic.

pro·tein·oids (prō'tēn-oydz; prō'tē-in-oyds). Artificially synthesized heteropoly(amino acids).

pro·tein·o·sis (pro-tē-nō'sis, prō'tē-i-nō'sis). A state characterized by disordered protein formation and distribution, particularly as manifested by the deposition of abnormal proteins in tissues. [protein + G. *-osis,* condition]

lipoid p. [MIM*247100], a disturbance of lipid metabolism in which there are deposits of a protein-lipid complex on the oral tongue and sublingual and faucial areas, and translucent keratotic papillomatous eyelid lesions; autosomal recessive inheritance, frequently with intracranial calcifications. SYN hyalinasis cutis et mucosae, lipoidosis cutis et mucosae, Urbach-Wiethe disease.

pulmonary alveolar p., a chronic progressive lung disease of adults, characterized by alveolar accumulation of granular proteinaceous material that is PAS-positive and lipid rich, with little inflammatory cellular exudate; the cause is unknown.

pro·tein·u·ria (prō-tē-nū'rē-ă, prō'tē-i-nū'rē-ă). **1.** Presence of urinary protein in concentrations greater than 0.3 g in a 24-hour urine collection or in concentrations greater than 1 g/l (1+ to 2+

plasma proteins				
	physiological function	concentration in plasma or serum (mg/L)	electrophoretic activity	molecular weight (daltons)
transport proteins				
albumin	oncotic pressure, transport of many substances	35,000–55,000	5.92	66,300
prealbumin	thyroxine binding	100–400	7.6	55,000
transcortin	cortisone binding	70	α_1	55,700
haptoglobin (types 1-1, 2-1, 2-2)	hemoglobin binding, acute phase protein	410–2,460	α_2 4.5	100,000–400,000
hemopexin	binds heme	500–1,150	β_1 3.1	57,000
retinol-binding protein	binds vitamin A	30–60	α_2	21,000
transcobalamins I-III	vitamin B_{12} transport		α_1–β_1	
α_2-macroglobulin	hormone transport, enzyme inhibition, acute phase protein	1,500–4,200	α_2 4.2	725,000
transferrin	iron transport	2,000–4,000	β_1 3.1	76,500
acidic α_1-glycoprotein	acute phase protein	550–1,400	α_1 5.7	41,000
(C-reactive protein)	acute phase protein, stimulation of phagocytosis	<1		135,000–140,000
immunoglobulins (Ig)				
IgM	early antibodies	600–2,800	β/γ 2.1	950,000
IgG	late antibodies	8,000–18,000	γ 1.2	150,000
IgA	secretory antibodies	900–4,500	β/γ 2.1	160,000 and multiples
IgD	regulatory antibodies	<150	β/γ <2.1	175,000
IgE	reagins, allergic antibodies	0.3	β/γ 2.3	190,000
complement system				
C1q		190	γ_2	400,000
C1r		100	β	190,000
C1s		120	α_2	85,000
C2		30	β_2	117,000
C3		1,300	β_1	180,000
C4	(see under "complement")	430	β_1	206,000
C5		75	β_1	180,000
C6		60	β_2	128,000
C7		10	β_2	121,000
C8		10	γ_1	153,000
C9		10	α_2	79,000
activators of alternate pathways				
properdin	complement activation	10–20	β–γ_2	224,000
C3-proactivator (C3-PA)	through surface-bonded polysaccharides	225	β_2	93,000
C3-PA convertase		trace		22,000
				continued

plasma proteins (continued)				
	physiological function	concentration in plasma or serum (mg/L)	electrophoretic activity	molecular weight (daltons)
enzyme				348,000
cholinesterase	hydrolysis of cholinesters	5–15	α_2 3.1	132,000
ceruloplasmin	oxidase, Cu-binding	150–600	α_2 4.6	91,000
plasminogen	fibrinolysis (proenzyme)	100–300	β_1 3.7	~15,000
lysozyme	protease	5–15	α_1	?
lipoprotein lipase	fat transport	varies	?	?
adenosine desaminase	nucleotide metabolism	trace	α/β	
enzyme inhibitors				
C1-esterase inhibitor	inactivation	150–350	α_2	104,000
α_1-antitrypsin	trypsin inhibition	2,000–4,000	α_1 5.42	45,000–54,000
inter-α-trypsin inhibitor	trypsin inhibition	200–700	α_1/α_2	~160,000
antichymotrypsin	chymotrypsin inhibition	300–600	α_1	68,000
antithrombin III	thrombin inhibition	170–300	α_2	65,000
coagulation factors				
factor I, fibrinogen	formation of coagulants, endphase	2,000–4,500	$\beta/\gamma = \phi\ 2.1$	340,000
factor II, prothrombin	proenzyme	50–100	α	69,000
factors III–XIII	see under coagulation (diagram); see also factor...			
lipoproteins				
α_1-lipoprotein, HDL$_2$	lipid transport	400–1,200	α_1	
α_1-lipoprotein, HDL$_3$	lipid transport	220–2,700	α_1	
α_2-lipoprotein, pre-β, very low density lipoprotein, VLDL	lipid transport	150–2,300	α_2	
β-lipoprotein, low density lipoprotein, LDL	lipid transport	250–8,000	β	

by standard turbidometric methods) in a random urine collection on two or more occasions at least 6 hours apart; specimens must be clean, voided midstream, or obtained by catheterization. **2.** SYN albuminuria. [protein + G. *ouron,* urine]

Bence Jones p., presence of Bence Jones proteins in the urine, usually indicative of a neoplastic process such as multiple myeloma, amyloidosis, or Waldenström's macroglobulinemia.

gestational p., the presence of p. during or under the influence of pregnancy in the absence of hypertension, edema, renal infection, or known intrinsic renovascular disease.

isolated p., p. in a patient who is asymptomatic, has normal renal function and urinary sediment, and has no manifestation of systemic disease upon initial examination.

nonisolated p., p. associated with other abnormalities.

orthostatic p., postural p., SYN orthostatic *albuminuria.*

pro·ten·si·ty (prō-ten′si-tē). The time attribute of a mental process; the attribute of a mental process characterized by its temporality or movement forward in time. [L. *protendo* (-*tensum*), to extend]

⚫**proteo-, prot-.** Protein.

pro·te·o·clas·tic (prō′tē-ō-klas′tik). SYN proteolytic. [proteo- + G. *klastos,* broken]

pro·te·o·gen·ic (prō′tē-ō-jen-ik). Capable of producing proteins. SYN proteinogenic.

pro·te·o·gly·can I. SYN biglycan.

pro·te·o·gly·cans (prō′tē-ō-glī′kanz). Glycoaminoglycans (mucopolysaccharides) bound to protein chains in covalent complexes; occur in the extracellular matrix of connective tissue.

pro·te·o·hor·mone (prō′tē-ō-hōr′mŏn). Obsolete term for a hormone possessing a protein structure.

pro·te·o·lip·ids (prō′tē-ō-lip′idz). A class of lipid-soluble proteins found in brain tissue, insoluble in water but soluble in chloroform-methanol-water mixtures.

pro·te·ol·y·sis (prō-tē-ol′i-sis). The decomposition of protein; primarily via the hydrolysis of peptide bonds, both enzymatically and nonenzymatically. [proteo- + G. *lysis,* dissolution]

pro·te·o·lyt·ic (prō′tē-ō-lit′ik). Relating to or effecting proteolysis. SYN proteoclastic.

pro·te·o·met·a·bol·ic (prō′tē-ō-met′ă-bol′ik). Relating to the metabolism of proteins.

pro·te·o·me·tab·o·lism (prō′tē-ō-mě-tab′ō-lizm). SYN protein *metabolism.*

Pro·te·o·myx·id·ia (prō′tē-ō-mik-sid′ē-ă). Former name for Eumycetozoea. [*Proteus* + G. *myxa,* mucus]

pro·te·o·pec·tic, pro·te·o·pex·ic (prō′tē-ō-pek′tik, -pek′sik). Relating to proteopexis.

pro·te·o·pep·sis (prō'tē-ō-pep'sis). The digestion of protein. [proteo- + G. *pepsis,* digestion]

pro·te·o·pex·is (prō'tē-ō-pek'sis). The fixation of protein in the tissues. [proteo- + G. *pēxis,* fixation]

pro·te·ose (prō'tē-ōs). A nondescript mixture of intermediate products of proteolysis between protein and peptone.

primary p., the first result of hydrolysis of metaprotein; two stages, protoproteose and heteroproteose, have been distinguished.

secondary p., p. derived from primary p. by further hydrolysis.

Pro·teus (prō'tē-ŭs). **1.** A former genus of the Sarcodina, now termed *Amoeba.* **2.** A genus of motile, peritrichous, non-sporeforming, aerobic to facultatively anaerobic bacteria (family Enterobacteriaceae) containing Gram-negative rods; coccoid forms, large irregular involution forms, filaments, and spheroplasts occur under certain conditions. The metabolism is fermentative, producing acid or acid and visible gas from glucose; lactose is not fermented, and they rapidly decompose urea and deaminate phenylalanine. *P.* occurs primarily in fecal matter and in putrefying materials. The type species is *P. vulgaris.* [G. *Proteus,* a sea god, who had the power to change his form]

P. incon'stans, a species found in urinary tract infections and in sporadic cases of diarrhea in man; some strains cause gastroenteritis.

P. mirab'ilis, a species found in putrid meat, infusions, and abscesses; also reported to be a cause of gastroenteritis and urinary tract infections.

P. morgan'ii, a species found in the intestinal canal and in normal and diarrheal stools.

P. rettge'ri, SYN *Providencia rettgeri.*

P. vulgar'is, the type species of the genus *P.,* found in putrefying materials and in abscesses; it is pathogenic for fish, dogs, guinea pigs, and mice; certain strains, the X strains of Weil and Felix, are agglutinated by typhus serum and are therefore of great importance in the diagnosis of typhus; strain X-19 is strongly agglutinated. SEE ALSO Weil-Felix *reaction.*

pro·thi·pen·dyl (prō-thī'pen-dil). 10-(3-Dimethylaminopropyl)-10*H*-pyrido-[3,2-*b*][1,4]benzothiazine; an antipsychotic.

pro·throm·base (prō-throm'bās). SEE *factor* X.

pro·throm·bin (prō-throm'bin). A glycoprotein, molecular weight approximately 69,000, formed and stored in the parenchymal cells of the liver and present in blood in a concentration of approximately 20 mg/100 ml. In the presence of thromboplastin and calcium ion, p. is converted to thrombin, which in turn converts fibrinogen to fibrin, this process resulting in coagulation of blood; a deficiency of p. leads to impaired blood coagulation. SYN plasmozyme, serozyme, thrombinogen, thrombogen.

pro·throm·bin·ase (prō-throm'bi-nās). SYN *factor* X.

pro·throm·bi·no·gen (prō-throm'bi-nō-jen). SYN *factor* VII.

pro·throm·bi·no·pe·nia (prō-throm'bi-nō-pē'nē-ă). SYN hypoprothrombinemia.

pro·throm·bo·ki·nase (prō'throm-bō-kī'nās). SYN *factor* V, *factor* VIII.

pro·thy·mia (prō-thī'mē-ă). Rarely used term for mental alertness. [G. eagerness, fr. *pro,* before, + *thymos,* mind]

pro·tide (prō'tīd). Obsolete term for protein.

pro·ti·re·lin (prō-tī'rĕ-lin). 5-Oxo-L-prolyl-L-histidyl-L-prolinamide; a synthetic form of thyroliberin.

pro·tist (prō'tist). A member of the kingdom Protista.

Pro·tis·ta (prō-tis'tă). A kingdom of both plantlike and animal-like eucaryotic unicellular organisms, either in the form of solitary, *e.g.,* protozoa, or colonies of cells lacking true tissues. [G. ntr. pl. of *prōtistos,* the first of all]

pro·tis·tol·o·gist (prō-tis-tol'ō-jist). Obsolete term for microbiologist.

pro·tis·tol·o·gy (prō-tis-tol'ō-jē). Obsolete term for microbiology. [G. *prōtistos,* first, + *logos,* study]

pro·ti·um (prō'tē-ŭm). SYN hydrogen-1.

⌂**proto-, prot-.** The first in a series; the highest in rank (properly prefixed to words derived from G. roots). [G. *prōtos,* first]

pro·to·ac·tin·i·um (prō'tō-ak-tin'ē-um). SYN protactinium.

pro·to·al·bu·mose (prō-tō-al'byū-mōs). SYN protalbumose.

pro·to·al·ka·loid (prō-tō-al'kă-loyd). A biogenic amine serving as a precursor of an alkaloid.

pro·tobe (prō'tōb). F. d'Herelle's term for bacteriophage. [proto- + G. *bios,* life]

pro·to·bi·ol·o·gy (prō'tō-bī-ol'ō-jē). SYN bacteriophagology.

pro·to·cat·e·chu·ic ac·id (prō'tō-kat'ĕ-chū'ik, -kū'ik). 3,4-Dihydroxybenzoic acid; 4-carboxycatechol; oxidation product of epinephrine.

pro·to·col (prō'tō-kol). A precise and detailed plan for the study of a biomedical problem or for a regimen of therapy.

pro·to·cone (prō'tō-kōn). The mesiolingual cusp of an upper molar tooth in a mammal. [proto- + G. *kōnos,* cone]

pro·to·co·nid (prō-tō-kon'id). The mesiolingual cusp of a lower molar tooth in a mammal.

pro·to·cop·ro·por·phyr·ia (prō'tō-kop'rō-pōr-fir'ē-ă). Enhanced fecal excretion of proto- and coproporphyrins.

p. heredita'ria, SYN variegate *porphyria.*

Pro·toc·tis·ta (prō-tok-tis'tă). A kingdom of eukaryotes incorporating the algae and the protozoans that comprise the presumed ancestral stocks of the fungi, plant, and animal kingdoms; they lack the developmental pattern stemming from a blastula, typical of animals, the pattern of embryo development typical of plants, and development from spores as in the fungi. Included in P. are the nucleated algae and seaweeds, the flagellated water molds, slime molds and slime nets, and the protozoa; unicellular, colonial, and multicellular organisms are included, but the complex development of tissues and organs of plants and animals is absent. The term P. replaces the term Protista, which connotes single-celled or acellular organisms, whereas the basal pre-plant (Protophyta) and pre-animal (Protozoa) assemblages incorporated in P. include many multicellular forms, since multicellularity appears to have evolved independently a number of times within these primitive groups. [G. *prōtos,* the first, + *ktizō,* to establish]

pro·to·derm (prō'tō-derm). The undifferentiated cells of very young embryos, from which the primary germ layers will evolve. [proto- + G. *derma,* skin]

pro·to·di·a·stol·ic (prō'tō-dī-ă-stol'ik). Early diastolic, relating to the beginning of cardiac diastole.

pro·to·du·o·de·num (prō'tō-dū-ō-dē'nŭm, -dū-od'ĕ-nŭm). The first part of the duodenum which extends from the gastroduodenal pylorus as far as the major duodenal papilla and develops from the caudal foregut of the embryo; it has no plicae circulares and is the seat of the duodenal glands.

pro·to·e·ryth·ro·cyte (prō'tō-ĕ-rith'rō-sīt). A primitive erythroblast.

pro·to·fil·a·ment (prō-tō-fil'ă-ment). Basic element of a contractile flagellar microtubule, approximately 5 nm thick. [proto- + L. *filum,* a thread]

pro·to·gen, pro·to·gen A (prō'tō-jen). SYN lipoic acid.

pro·to·gon·o·plasm (prō-tō-gon'ō-plazm). A differentiated mass of cytoplasm in a protozoan, which forms the substance of later developing reproductive bodies. [proto- + G. *gonos,* seed, + *plasma,* a thing formed]

pro·to·ky·lol hy·dro·chlo·ride (prō-tō-kī'lōl). α-[(α-Methyl-3,4-methylenedioxyphenethylamino)methyl]protocatechuyl alcohol hydrochloride; a derivative of isoproterenol with the selective β-receptor-stimulating activity of the parent compound; it is effective orally and is more stable in the body than isoproterenol; used as a bronchodilator in the treatment of bronchial asthma and status asthmaticus.

pro·to·leu·ko·cyte (prō-tō-lū'kō-sīt). A primitive leukocyte; a leukocyte of the bone marrow.

pro·tol·y·sate (prō-tol'i-sāt). Rarely used term for a protein hydrolysate.

pro·tom·er (prō'tō-mer). A structural subunit of a larger structure. P.'s may themselves consist of subunits. For example, tubulin, an αβ dimer, is the protomer for microtubules. [G. *prōtos,* first, + -mer 1]

pro·tom·e·rite (prō-tom'ĕ-rīt, prō'tō-mēr'īt). The second segment (lacking a nucleus) of a septate gregarine, between the epimerite and the deutomerite; it becomes the anterior end of the gamont after it has broken free of its host cell, leaving the epimerite embedded (usually in the gut wall of an infected invertebrate). SYN primerite. [proto- + G. *meros,* part]

pro·to·me·tro·cyte (prō-tō-mē′trō-sīt). The ancestor cell of the protoleukocyte and protoerythrocyte, or of the cells of the leukocytic and erythrocytic series. [proto- + G. *mētēr,* mother, + *kytos,* cell]

pro·ton (prō′ton). The positively charged unit of the nuclear mass; p.'s form part (or in hydrogen-1 the whole) of the nucleus of the atom around which the negative electrons revolve. [G. ntr. of *prōtos,* first]

pro·to·neu·ron (prō-tō-nūr′on). Hypothetical primitive neuron lacking polarization. [proto- + G. *neuron,* nerve]

pro·to·on·co·gene (prō-tō-on′kō-jēn). A gene conserved long on the evolutionary scale present in the normal human genome, that appears to have a role in normal cellular physiology and is often involved in regulation of normal cell growth or proliferation; as a result of somatic mutations these genes may become oncogenic; products of p.-o.'s may have important roles in normal cellular differentiation.

pro·to·path·ic (prō-tō-path′ik). Denoting a supposedly primitive set or system of peripheral sensory nerve fibers conducting a low order of pain and temperature sensibility which is poorly localized. Cf. epicritic. [proto- + G. *pathos,* suffering]

pro·to·pec·tin (prō-tō-pek′tin). SEE pectin.

pro·to·pi·an·o·ma (prō′tō-pē-an-ō′mă). SYN mother *yaw.*

pro·to·plasm (prō′tō-plazm). 1. Living matter, the substance of which animal and vegetable cells are formed. SEE ALSO cytoplasm, nucleoplasm. 2. The total cell material, including cell organelles. Cf. cytoplasm, cytosol, hyaloplasm. SYN plasmogen. [proto- + G. *plasma,* thing formed]

totipotential p., living matter with the least recognizable differentiation of structure but with the greatest potential, all cell organs being formable by it.

pro·to·plas·mat·ic, pro·to·plas·mic (prō′tō-plaz-mat′ik, -plaz′ mik). Relating to protoplasm.

pro·to·plas·mol·y·sis (prō′tō-plaz-mol′i-sis). SYN plasmolysis.

pro·to·plast (prō′tō-plast). 1. Archaic term meaning the first individual of a type or race. 2. A bacterial cell from which the rigid cell wall has been completely removed; the bacterium loses its characteristic form. [proto- + G. *plastos,* formed]

pro·to·por·phyr·ia (prō′tō-pōr-fir′ē-ă). Enhanced fecal excretion of protoporphyrin.

erythropoietic p. [MIM*177000], a benign disorder of porphyrin metabolism due to a deficiency of ferrochelatase and characterized by enhanced fecal excretion of protoporphyrin and increased protoporphyrin IX in red blood cells, plasma, and feces; acute solar urticaria or more chronic solar eczema develops quickly on exposure to sunlight; autosomal dominant inheritance.

pro·to·por·phy·rin·o·gen type III (prō-tō-pōr′fi-rin′ō-jen). The immediate precursor of protoporphyrin III in heme biosynthesis; elevated in cases of variegate porphyria.

p. t. III oxidase, a mitochondrial enzyme that uses O_2 to convert p. t. III to protoporphyrin type III in heme biosynthesis; a deficiency of this enzyme is associated with variegate porphyria.

pro·to·por·phy·rin type III (prō-tō-pōr′fi-rin). 2,7,12,18-Tetramethyl-3,8-divinylporphin-13,17dipropionic acid; the principal protoporphyrin found in nature (one of 15 possible isomers), characterized by the presence of 4 methyl groups, 2 vinyl groups, and 2 propionic acid side chains; a porphyrin derivative that, with iron, forms the heme of hemoglobin and the prosthetic groups of myoglobin, catalase, cytochromes, etc.

pro·to·pro·te·ose (prō-tō-prō′tē-ōs). SEE primary *proteose.*

pro·to·salt (prō′tō-sawlt). SYN acid *salt.*

pro·to·spore (prō′tō-spōr). The initial product of progressive cleavage, in which a multinucleate spore is produced. [proto- + G. *sporos,* seed]

pro·to·sto·ma. SYN blastopore.

pro·tos·tome. SYN blastopore. [proto- + G. *stoma,* mouth]

Pro·to·stron·gy·lus ru·fes·cens (prō-tō-stron′ji-lŭs rū-fes′ens).

The small lungworm of sheep, goats, and deer that occurs in the smaller bronchioles, where it causes plugging of the air passages by its presence and the formation of multiple areas of bronchopneumonia; symptoms produced generally are milder than those induced by the large lungworm, *Dictyocaulus filaria.* [proto- + G. *strongylos,* round]

pro·to·sul·fate (prō-tō-sŭl′fāt). A compound of sulfuric acid with a protoxide of the metal.

pro·to·tax·ic (prō-tō-tak′sik). In interpersonal psychiatry, a term referring to the earliest form of experience characteristic of the infant which is undifferentiated, global, and unorganized. [proto- + G. *taxis,* order, arrangement]

Pro·to·the·ca (prō-tō-thē′kă). A genus of microbes transitional between the fungi and achlorophyllous mutants of the green alga, *Chlorella.* Two species, *P. zopfii* and *P. wickerhamii,* cause protothecosis.

pro·to·the·co·sis (prō′tō-thē-kō′sis). A rare verrucous cutaneous or disseminated disease caused by *Prototheca zopfii* and *Prototheca wickerhamii.*

pro·to·troph (prō′tō-trof, -trōf). A bacterial strain that has the same nutritional requirements as the wild-type strain from which it was derived. SEE ALSO wild-type *strain.* [proto- + G. *trophē,* nourishment]

pro·to·tro·phic (prō-tō-trof′ik). 1. Pertaining to a prototroph. 2. Denoting the ability to undertake anabolism or to obtain nourishment from a single source, as with iron, sulfur, or nitrifying bacteria or photosynthesizing plants.

pro·to·tro·phism (prō-tō-trōf′izm). The property of being phototrophic.

pro·to·type (prō′tō-tīp). The primitive form; the first form to which subsequent individuals of the class or species conform. [proto- + G. *typos,* type]

pro·to·ver·a·trine A and B (prō-tō-ver′ă-trēn). A mixture of two alkaloids isolated from *Veratrum album;* they exert their main effect upon the cardiovascular system through the carotid sinus receptors and vagal sensory endings in the heart; they cause vasodilation and are thought to bring about a redistribution to all vascular beds and thus to induce a fall in blood pressure; used in certain forms of hypertension; the maleates have the same actions.

pro·to·ver·te·bra (prō-tō-ver′tě-bră). 1. In the older literature, a mesodermic somite. 2. More recently applied to the caudal half of each sclerotomal concentration, which is the primordium of the centrum of a vertebra. SYN provertebra.

pro·to·ver·te·bral (prō-tō-ver′tě-brăl). Relating to a protovertebra.

prot·ox·ide (prō-tok′sīd). SYN suboxide.

Pro·to·zoa (prō-tō-zō′ă). Formerly considered a phylum, now regarded as a subkingdom of the animal kingdom, including all of the so-called acellular or unicellular forms. They consist of a single functional cell unit or aggregation of nondifferentiated cells, loosely held together and not forming tissues, as distinguishes the Animalia or Metazoa, which include all other animals. P. were formerly divided into four classes: Sarcodina, Mastigophora, Sporozoa, and Ciliata; new classifications employ higher taxa (phyla, subphyla, and superclasses) and a number of major subdivisions. [proto- + G. *zōon,* animal]

pro·to·zo·al (prō-tō-zō′ăl). SYN protozoan (2).

pro·to·zo·an (prō-tō-zō′an). 1. A member of the phylum Protozoa. SYN protozoon. 2. Relating to protozoa. SYN protozoal.

pro·to·zo·i·a·sis (prō′tō-zō-ī′ă-sis). Infection with protozoans.

pro·to·zo·i·cide (prō-tō-zō′i-sīd). An agent used to kill protozoa. [protozoa + L. *caedo,* to kill]

pro·to·zo·ol·o·gist (prō′tō-zō-ol′ō-jist). A biologist who specializes in protozoology.

pro·to·zo·ol·o·gy (prō′tō-zō-ol′ō-jē). The science concerned with all aspects of the biology and human interest in protozoa. [protozoa + G. *logos,* study]

pro·to·zo·on, pl. **pro·to·zoa** (prō-tō-zō′on, -zō′ă). SYN protozoan (1).

pro·to·zo·o·phage (prō-tō-zō′ō-fāj). A phagocyte that ingests protozoa. [protozoa + G. *phagō,* to eat]

pro·trac·tion (prō-trak′shŭn). In dentistry, the extension of teeth or other maxillary or mandibular structures into a position anterior or to normal. [see protractor]

mandibular p., a type of facial anomaly in which the gnathion lies anterior to the orbital plane.

maxillary p., a type of facial anomaly in which the subnasion lies anterior to the orbital plane.

pro·trac·tor (prō-trak′ter, -tōr). A muscle drawing a part forward, as antagonistic to a retractor; *e.g.,* the serratus anterior muscle is a protractor of the scapula; the lateral pterygoid muscle is a protractor of the mandible. [L. *pro-traho,* pp. *-tractus,* to draw forth]

pro·trip·ty·line hy·dro·chlo·ride (prō-trip′ti-lēn). *N*-Methyl-5*H*-dibenzo[*a,d*]cycloheptene-5-propylamine hydrochloride; an antidepressant.

pro·trude (prō-trūd′). To thrust forward or project.

pro·tru·sio ac·e·tab·u·li (prō-trū′sē-ō as-ĕ-tab′yū-lī). SYN Otto's *disease.*

pro·tru·sion (prō-trū′zhŭn). 1. The state of being thrust forward or projected. 2. In dentistry, a position of the mandible forward from centric relation. [L. *protrusio*]

bimaxillary p., the excessive forward projection of both the maxilla and the mandible in relation to the cranial base. SYN double p.

bimaxillary dentoalveolar p., the positioning of the entire dentition forward with respect to the facial profile.

double p., SYN bimaxillary p.

pro·tryp·sin (prō-trip′sin). SYN trypsinogen.

pro·tu·ber·ance (prō-tū′ber-ans). A swelling or knoblike outgrowth. A bulging, swelling, or protruding part. SEE ALSO protuberance. SYN protuberantia [NA]. [Mod. L. *protuberantia*]

Bichat's p., SYN buccal *fat-pad.*

external occipital p., a prominence about the center of the outer surface of the squamous portion of the occipital bone, giving attachment to the ligamentum nuchae. SYN protuberantia occipitalis externa [NA].

internal occipital p., a projection from about the center of the cruciform eminence on the inner surface of the occipital bone. SYN protuberantia occipitalis interna [NA].

mental p., the prominence of the chin at the anterior part of the mandible. SYN protuberantia mentalis [NA], mental process.

pro·tu·be·ran·tia (prō-tū-ber-an′shē-ă) [NA]. SYN protuberance. SEE ALSO protuberance, prominence, eminence. [Mod. L. fr. *protubero,* to swell out, fr. *tuber,* a swelling]

p. laryn′gea, SYN laryngeal *prominence.*

p. menta′lis [NA], SYN mental *protuberance.*

p. occipita′lis exter′na [NA], SYN external occipital *protuberance.*

p. occipita′lis inter′na [NA], SYN internal occipital *protuberance.*

pro·ur·o·kin·ase (prō-yūr-ō-kī′nās). The precursor of an activator of plasminogen, urokinase.

Proust, Louis J., French chemist, 1755–1826. SEE P.'s *law.*

Proust, T., 19th century French physician. SEE P.'s *space.*

pro·ven·tri·cu·lus (prō-ven-trik′yū-lŭs). 1. In birds, the thin-walled glandular stomach preceding the muscular gizzard. 2. In insects, the portion of the stomodeum that lies in front of the ventriculus or stomach; it is modified into a small proventricular valve in many diptera (flies). [L. *pro,* before, + *ventriculus,* dim. of *venter* (*ventr-*) belly]

pro·ver·te·bra (prō-ver′tĕ-bră). SYN protovertebra.

Pro·vi·den·cia (prov′i-den′sē-ă). A genus of motile, peritrichous, nonsporeforming, aerobic or facultatively anaerobic bacteria (family Enterobacteriaceae) containing Gram-negative rods. These organisms do not hydrolyze urea or produce hydrogen sulfide; they produce indole and grow on Simmons' citrate medium. They do not decarboxylate lysine, arginine, or ornithine. These organisms occur in specimens from extraintestinal sources, particularly urinary tract infections; they have also been isolated from small outbreaks and sporadic cases of diarrheal disease. The type species is *P. alcalifaciens.*

P. alcalifa′ciens, a species found in extraintestinal sources, particularly in urinary tract infections; it has also been isolated from small outbreaks and sporadic cases of diarrheal disease; it is the type species of the genus *P.*

P. rettger′i, species that is found in chicken cholera and human gastroenteritis. SYN *Proteus rettgeri.*

P. stuar′tii, a species isolated from urinary tract infections and from small outbreaks and sporadic cases of diarrheal disease.

pro·vi·rus (prō-vī′rŭs). The precursor of an animal virus; theoretically analogous to the prophage in bacteria, the p. being integrated in the nucleus of infected cells.

pro·vi·ta·min (prō-vī′tă-min). A substance that can be converted into a vitamin.

p. A, trivial name for carotenoids exhibiting qualitatively the biological activity of β-carotene, *i.e.,* vitamin A precursors (α-, β-, and γ-carotene and cryptoxanthin); contained in fish liver oils, spinach, carrots, egg yolk, milk products, and other green leaf or yellow vegetables and fruits.

p. D_2, any substance that can give rise to ergocalciferol (vitamin D_2); *e.g.,* ergosterol.

p. D_3, SYN 7-dehydrocholesterol.

Prowazek, Stanislas J.M. von, German protozoologist, 1876–1915. SEE *Prowazekia; P.* bodies, under *body;* P.-Greeff *bodies,* under *body;* Halberstaedter-P. *bodies,* under *body.*

Pro·wa·ze·kia (prō-vă-zē′kē-ă). A genus of coprozoic flagellate protozoans, formerly part of the genus *Bodo;* the organisms may be parasitic but are not, so far as is known, pathogenic. [S. Prowazek]

Prower. Surname of the patient in whom the Stuart-Prower *factor* was first discovered.

△**prox-.** SEE proximo-.

prox·em·ics (prok-sem′iks). The scientific discipline concerned with the various aspects of urban overcrowding. [L. *proximus,* nearest, next]

△**proxi-.** SEE proximo-.

prox·i·mad (prok′si-mad). In a direction toward a proximal part, or toward the center; not distad. [L. *proximus,* nearest, next, + *ad,* to]

prox·i·mal (prok′si-măl). 1. Nearest the trunk or the point of origin, said of part of a limb, of an artery or a nerve, etc., so situated. 2. SYN mesial. 3. In dental anatomy, denoting the surface of a tooth in relation with its neighbor, whether mesial or distal, *i.e.,* nearer to or farther from the anteroposterior median plane. SYN proximalis [NA]. [Mod. L. *proximalis,* fr. L. *proximus,* nearest, next]

prox·i·ma·lis (prok-si-mā′lis) [NA]. SYN proximal. [Mod. L.]

prox·i·mate (prok′si-māt). Immediate; next; proximal.

△**proximo-, prox-, proxi-.** Proximal. [L. *proximus,* nearest, next (to)]

prox·i·mo·a·tax·ia (prok′si-mō-ă-tak′sē-ă). Ataxia or lack of muscular coordination in the proximal portions of the extremities, *i.e.,* arms and forearms, thighs and legs. Cf. acroataxia. [proximo- + ataxia]

prox·i·mo·buc·cal (prok′si-mō-bŭk′ăl). Relating to the proximal and buccal surfaces of a tooth; denoting the angle formed by their junction.

prox·i·mo·la·bi·al (prok′si-mō-lā′bē-ăl). Relating to the proximal and labial surfaces of a tooth; denoting the angle formed by their junction.

prox·i·mo·lin·gual (prok′si-mō-ling′gwăl). Relating to the proximal and lingual surfaces of a tooth; denoting the angle formed by their junction.

prox·y·met·a·caine hy·dro·chlo·ride (prok-si-met′ă-kān). SYN proparacaine hydrochloride.

pro·za·pine (prō′ză-pēn). 1-(3,3-diphenylpropyl)hexamethyleneimine; an intestinal antispasmodic with choleretic properties. SYN hexadiphane.

pro·zone (prō′zōn). In the case of agglutination and of precipitation, the phenomenon in which visible reaction does not occur in mixtures of specific antigen and antibody because of antibody excess. SYN prezone.

pro·zy·go·sis (prō-zī-gō′sis). SYN syncephaly. [G. *pro,* before, + *zygōsis,* a yoking]

PrP Abbreviation for prion *protein.*

PRPP Abbreviation for 5-phospho-α-D-ribosyl 1-pyrophosphate.

PRPP syn·the·tase. An enzyme that catalyzes the reaction of α-D-ribose-5-phosphate and ATP to produce PRPP and AMP; a regulatory enzyme in purine and pyrimidine biosynthesis; enhanced activity of this enzyme results in an increase in purine biosynthesis leading to gout.

prune (prūn). The dried ripe fruit of *Prunus domestica* (family Rosaceae), a tree cultivated in warm temperate regions; a food with laxative properties.

Pru·nus (prū′nŭs). A genus of trees (family Rosaceae) including the cherry, plum, peach, and apricot trees. [L. a plum-tree]

P. seroti′na, the wild black cherry; a botanical source of wild cherry. SEE *P. virginiana.*

P. virginia′na, **(1)** wild black cherry bark, the bark of *P. serotina,* used as a tonic and in cough mixtures as a bronchial sedative; **(2)** the choke cherry; the chief substitute and adulterant of *P. serotina.*

pru·rig·i·nous (prū-rij′i-nŭs). Relating to or suffering from prurigo. [L. *pruriginosus,* having the itch]

pru·ri·go (prū-rī′gō). A chronic disease of the skin marked by a persistent eruption of papules that itch intensely. [L. itch, fr. *prurio,* to itch]

actinic p., SYN p. aestivalis.

p. aestiva′lis, a form recurring each summer, becoming very severe as long as the hot weather continues. SYN actinic p., summer p.

p. a′gria, SYN Hebra's p.

Besnier's p., an atopic form which may be associated with asthma, hay fever, or other allergic conditions.

p. fe′rox, SYN Hebra's p. [L. wild, cruel]

p. gestatio′nis, a pruritic papular skin disease occurring in pregnant women, without adversely affecting pregnancy or the fetus.

Hebra's p., a severe form of chronic dermatitis with secondary infection in which there are constantly recurring, intensely itchy papules and nodules, often associated with atopy. SYN p. agria, p. ferox.

p. infanti′lis, SYN papular *urticaria.*

p. mi′tis, a mild form of a chronic dermatitis characterized by recurring, intensely itching papules and nodules, probably atopic.

p. nodula′ris, an eruption of hard nodules (Picker's nodules) in the skin caused by rubbing and accompanied by intense itching. SYN Hyde's disease.

p. sim′plex, a mild form of p. having a pronounced tendency to relapse.

summer p., SYN p. aestivalis.

pru·rit·ic (prū-rit′ik). Relating to pruritus.

pru·ri·tus (prū-rī′tŭs). **1.** SYN itching. **2.** SYN itch (3). SYN itch (3). [L. an itching, fr. *prurio,* to itch]

p. aestiva′lis, p. occurring during hot weather; may be associated with prickly heat. SYN summer itch.

p. a′ni, itching of varying intensity at the anus; may be paroxysmal or constant, associated with seborrheic dermatitis or moniliasis, with irritated and enlarged hemorrhoidal veins, or may occur independently of any cutaneous lesions in association with systemic disease.

aquagenic p., intense itching produced by brief contact with water at any temperature without visible changes in the skin.

p. bal′nea, SYN bath p.

bath p., itching produced by inadequate rinsing off of soap or by overdrying of skin from excessive bathing. SYN bath itch, p. balnea.

essential p., itching that occurs independently of skin lesions.

p. hiema′lis, SYN *dermatitis* hiemalis.

p. seni′lis, senile p., itching associated with dryness of the skin in the aged.

symptomatic p., itching occurring as a symptom of some systemic disease.

p. vul′vae, itching of the external female genitalia, caused by a variety of factors, *e.g.,* seborrheic dermatitis, allergy to local contactants, senile atrophy of the vulva, and occasionally systemic disease.

Prussak, Alexander, Russian otologist, 1839–1897. SEE P.'s *fibers,* under *fiber, pouch, space.*

Prus·sian blue [C.I. 77510]. SYN Berlin blue.

prus·si·ate (prŭsh′ē-āt, prŭs′ē-āt). **1.** A cyanide; a salt of hydrocyanic acid. **2.** A ferricyanide or ferrocyanide.

prus·sic ac·id (prŭs′ik). SYN hydrocyanic acid.

PSA Abbreviation for prostate-specific *antigen.*

psal·ter·i·al (sawl-ter′ē-ăl). Relating to the psalterium.

psal·ter·i·um, pl. **psal·ter·ia** (sawl-ter′ē-ŭm, sawl-ter′ē-ă). **1.** SYN *commissura* fornicis. **2.** SYN omasum. [G. *psaltērion,* harp]

△psammo-. Sand. [G. *psammos*]

psam·mo·car·ci·no·ma (sam′ō-kar-si-nō′mă). Obsolete term for a carcinoma that contains calcified foci resembling psammoma bodies.

psam·mo·ma (sa-mō′mă). Obsolete term for psammomatous *meningioma* or meningioma. [psammo- + G. *-oma,* tumor]

Virchow's p., SYN psammomatous *meningioma.*

psam·mo·ma·tous (sa-mō′mă-tŭs). Possessing or characterized by the presence of psammoma bodies; refers usually to certain types of meningioma or to meningeal hyperplasia with psammoma bodies.

psam·mous (sam′ŭs). Sandy. [G. *psammos,* sand]

Psaume, J., 20th century French physician. SEE Papillon-Léage and P. *syndrome.*

pse·laph·e·sis, pse·la·phe·sia (se-laf′e·sis, sel-ă-fē′zē-ă; sel-ă-fē′sis). The higher tactile sense, including the muscle sense. [G. *psēlaphēsis,* a touching]

psel·lism (sel′izm). SYN stammering. [G. *psellismos,* a stammering]

△pseud-. SEE pseudo-.

pseud·ac·ro·meg·a·ly (sū-dak-rō-meg′ă-lē). Enlargement of the extremities and face, not caused by acromegaly.

pseud·a·graph·ia (sū-dă-graf′ē-ă). Partial agraphia in which one can do no original writing, but can copy correctly. SYN pseudoagraphia. [pseud- + G. *a-* priv. + *graphō,* to write]

pseud·al·bu·min·u·ria (sū′dal-byū-mi-nū′rē-ă). Albuminuria which is not associated with renal disease. SYN pseudoalbuminuria.

Pseud·al·les·che·ria boy·dii (sūd′al-es-kē′rē-ă boy′dē-ī). A species of fungus that causes eumycotic mycetoma and pseuallescheriasis; its conidial (asexual) state is *Scedosporium apiospermum.* SYN *Allescheria boydii.*

pseud·al·les·che·ri·a·sis (sūd′al-es-kē′ri-ă-sis). A variety of clinical diseases resulting from infection with *Pseudallescheria boydii; e.g.,* pulmonary colonization, fungoma, and invasive pneumonitis, as well as mycotic keratitis, endophthalmitis, endocarditis, meningitis, sinusitis, brain abscesses, cutaneous and subcutaneous infections, and disseminated systemic infections.

Pseu·dam·phis·to·mum (sū-dam-fis′tō-mŭm). A genus of digenetic flukes of the family Opisthorchiidae; *P. truncatum* is a species that infects the bile ducts of the dog and cat (rarely of humans) in Europe and India. [pseud- + G. *amphi,* two-sided, + *stoma,* mouth]

pseud·an·gi·na (sū′dan-jī′nă, sū-dan′ji-nă). SYN *angina* pectoris vasomotoria.

pseud·an·ky·lo·sis (sū-dang′ki-lō′sis). SYN fibrous *ankylosis.*

pseud·aph·ia (sū-daf′e-ă). SYN paraphia. [G. *haphē,* a touch]

pseud·ar·thro·sis (sū-dar-thrō′sis). A new, false joint arising at the site of an ununited fracture. SYN false joint, pseudoarthrosis. [pseud- + G. *arthrōsis,* a joint]

pseu·del·minth (sū-del′minth). Anything having the appearance of an intestinal worm. [pseud- + G. *helmins,* worm]

pseud·es·the·sia (sū-des-thē′zē-ă). **1.** SYN paraphia. **2.** A subjective sensation not arising from an external stimulus. SYN pseudoesthesia (2). **3.** SYN phantom *limb.* [pseud- + G. *aisthēsis,* sensation]

pseu·di·no·ma (sū-di-nō′mă). Obsolete term for an indurated swelling that grossly resembles a fibroma. [pseud- + G. *is* (*in*), fiber, + *-oma,* tumor]

⚱**pseudo- (psi), pseud-.** False (often used about a deceptive resemblance). [G. *pseudēs*]

pseu·do·ac·an·tho·sis ni·gri·cans (sū′dō-ak-an-thō′sis nī′gri-kanz). Acanthosis nigricans secondary to maceration of the skin from excessive sweating, or occurring in obese and dark-complexioned adults, or in association with endocrine disorders; not associated with visceral cancer.

pseu·do·a·ceph·a·lus (sū′dō-ă-sef′ă-lŭs). An apparently headless placental parasitic twin which, however, has rudimentary cephalic structures that can be demonstrated by dissection. [pseudo- + G. *a-* priv. + *kephalē,* head]

pseu·do·a·chon·dro·pla·sia (sū′dō-ă-kon-drō-plā′sē-ă). Dwarfism with short limbs and a relatively long trunk as in achondroplasia, but not evident at birth; autosomal dominant [MIM*177150 *177170] and recessive [MIM*264150 and *264160] forms occur.

pseu·do·ac·tin·o·my·co·sis (sū′dō-ak′ti-nō-mī- kō′sis). SYN para-actinomycosis.

pseu·do·ag·glu·ti·na·tion (sū′dō-ă-glū-ti-nā′shŭn). **1.** Agglomeration of particles in solution which does not involve antigen-antibody combination. SYN false agglutination (1). **2.** SYN rouleaux *formation.*

pseu·do·a·gram·ma·tism (sū′dō-ă-gram′ă-tizm). SYN paraphasia. [pseudo- + G. *a-* priv. + *gramma,* writing, + *-ismos,* condition]

pseu·do·a·graph·ia (sū′dō-ă-graf′ē-ă). SYN pseudagraphia.

pseu·do·ai·nhum (sū′dō-in′yŭm). Nonspontaneous amputation of a digit, caused by a variety of disorders such as neural leprosy, syringomyelia, and palmoplantar keratoderma.

pseu·do·al·bu·mi·nu·ria (sū′dō-al-byū′mi-nū′rē-ă). SYN pseudalbuminuria.

pseu·do·al·ka·loids (sū′dō-al-kă-loydz). A group of compounds that are structurally similar to alkaloids.

pseu·do·al·lel·ic (sū′dō-ă-le′lik). Relating to pseudoallelism.

pseu·do·al·lel·ism (sū-dō-ă-lē′lizm). Relationship of two or more loci that are difficult to distinguish from a single locus by classical genetic analysis. For instance, the states of the D, D, and E components of the Rh blood locus [MIM*111700] is so far unresolved.

pseu·do·al·o·pe·cia ar·e·a·ta (sū′dō-al-ō-pē′shē-ă ar-ē-ā′tă). Alopecia in which mild inflammatory changes develop at the orifices of the affected hair follicles.

pseu·do·an·a·phy·lac·tic (sū′dō-an-ă-fī-lak′tik). SYN anaphylactoid.

pseu·do·an·a·phy·lax·is (sū′dō-an-ă-fī-lak′sis). A condition resembling anaphylaxis, but not due to specific antigen-antibody reaction. SYN anaphylactoid crisis (2).

pseu·do·a·ne·mia (sū′dō-ă-nē′mē-ă). Pallor of the skin and mucous membranes without the blood changes of anemia. SYN false anemia.

pseu·do·an·eu·rysm (sū-dō-an′yū-rizm). **1.** A cavity due to ruptured myocardial infarction that has been contained by an intact parietal pericardium and communicates with the left ventricle by a narrow neck; **2.** A dilation of an artery with actual disruption of one or more layers of its walls, as at the site of puncture as a complication of precutaneous arterial catheterization, rather than with expansion of all layers of the wall. SYN communicating hematoma, pulsatile hematoma.

pseu·do·an·gi·na (sū′dō-an′ji-nă, -an-jī′nă). SYN *angina* pectoris vasomotoria.

pseu·do·an·gi·o·sar·co·ma (sū′dō-an′jē-ō-sar-kō′mă). A benign vascular lesion that microscopically may be mistaken for an angiosarcoma.

    Masson's p., SYN intravascular papillary endothelial *hyperplasia.*

pseu·do·an·o·don·tia (sū′dō-an-o-don′shē-ă). Clinical absence of teeth due to a failure in eruption. [pseudo- + G. *an-* priv. + *odous,* tooth]

pseu·do·ap·o·plexy (sū-dō-ap′ŏ-plek-sē). A condition simulating apoplexy, not due to a cerebral vascular event. SYN pseudoplegia.

pseu·do·ap·pen·di·ci·tis (sū′dō-ă-pen-di-sī′tis). A symptom-complex simulating appendicitis without inflammation of the appendix.

pseu·do·a·prax·ia (sū′dō-ă-prak′sē-ă). A condition of exaggerated awkwardness in which the person makes wrong use of objects.

pseu·do·ar·thro·sis (sū′dō-ar-thrō′sis). SYN pseudarthrosis.

pseu·do·a·tax·ia (sū′dō-ă-tak′sē-ă). SYN pseudotabes.

pseu·do·au·then·tic·i·ty (sū′dō-aw-then-ti′si-tē). False or copied expression of thoughts and feelings. [pseudo- + G. *authentikos,* original]

pseu·do·ba·cil·lus (sū′dō-bă-sil′ŭs). Any microscopic object, such as a poikilocyte, resembling a bacillus.

pseu·do·bac·te·ri·um (sū′dō-bak-tēr′ē-ŭm). Any microscopic object resembling a small bacillary organism or other bacterial form.

pseu·do·bul·bar (sū-dō-bŭl′bar). Denoting a supranuclear paralysis of the bulbar nerves.

pseu·do·car·ti·lage (sū-dō-kar′ti-lij). SYN chondroid *tissue* (1).

pseu·do·car·ti·lag·i·nous (sū′dō-kar-ti-laj′i-nŭs). Composed of a substance resembling cartilage in texture.

pseu·do·cast (sū′dō-kast). SYN false *cast.*

pseu·do·cele (sū′dō-sēl). SYN *cavity* of septum pellucidum. [pseudo- + G. *koilia,* cavity]

pseu·do·ce·lom (sū-dō-sē′lom). A partial or false celom, typical of Nematoda (roundworms) and related phyla, in which the body cavity is lined by mesoderm along only one surface (hypodermis, under the cuticular body wall). Cf. celom, acelom. [pseudo- + G. *koilōma,* hollow]

pseu·do·ceph·a·lo·cele (sū-dō-sef′ă-lō-sēl). Acquired herniation of intracranial tissues caused by injury or disease. [pseudo- + G. *kephalē,* head, + *kēlē,* tumor]

pseu·do·chan·cre (sū-dō-shang′ker). A nonspecific indurated sore, usually located on the penis, resembling a chancre.

pseu·do·cho·lin·es·ter·ase (sū′dō-kol-in-es′ter-ās). SYN cholinesterase.

    atypical p. [MIM*177400, MIM*177500, MIM*177600], a genetic variant of cholinesterase that fails to catalyze the hydrolysis of succinylcholine. SEE ALSO dibucaine number, fluoride number.

    typical p., a cholinesterase formed in the liver and present in plasma; it catalyzes the hydrolysis of succinylcholine, first into succinylmonocholine and choline, and then into choline and succinic acid.

pseu·do·cho·rea (sū-dō-kōr-ē′ă). A spasmodic affection or extensive tic resembling chorea.

pseu·do·chro·mes·the·sia (sū′dō-krō-mes-thē′zē-ă). **1.** An anomaly in which each vowel in the printed word is seen as colored. SEE ALSO photism. **2.** SYN color *hearing.* [pseudo- + G. *chrōma,* color, + *aisthēsis,* sensation]

pseu·do·chro·mi·dro·sis, pseu·do·chrom·hi·dro·sis (sū′dō-krō-mi-drō′sis, -hi-drō′sis). The presence of pigment on the skin in association with sweating, but due to the local action of pigment-forming bacteria and not to the excretion of colored sweat. [pseudo- + G. *chrōma,* color, + *hidrōs,* sweat]

pseu·do·chy·lous (sū-dō-kī′lŭs). Resembling chyle.

pseu·do·cir·rho·sis (sū′dō-si-rō′sis). SYN cardiac *cirrhosis.*

pseu·do·clo·nus (sū-dō-klō′nŭs). Unsustained clonic response despite continued force to elicit it.

pseu·do·co·arc·ta·tion (sū′dō-kō-ark-tā′shŭn). Distortion, often with slight narrowing, of the aortic arch at the level of insertion of the ligamentum arteriosum. SYN buckled aorta, kinked aorta.

pseu·do·col·loid (sū-dō-kol′oyd). A colloid-like or mucoid substance found in ovarian cysts, in the lips, and elsewhere.

    p. of lips, SYN Fordyce's *spots,* under spot.

pseu·do·col·lu·sion (sū′dō-co-lū′zhŭn). In psychoanalysis, a merely apparent sense of closeness emanating from a transference. [pseudo- + Fr. *collusion,* fr. L. *colludo,* to play together]

pseu·do·co·ma (sū-dō-kō′mă). SYN locked-in *syndrome.*

pseu·do·cow·pox (sū-dō-kow′poks). SYN milkers' *nodules*, under *nodule*.

pseu·do·cox·al·gia (sū′dō-kok-sal′jē-ă). SYN Legg-Calvé-Perthes *disease*. [pseudo- + L. *coxa*, hip, + G. *algos*, pain]

pseu·do·cri·sis (sū-dō-krī′sis). A temporary fall of the temperature in a disease usually ending by crisis; not a true crisis.

pseu·do·croup (sū-dō-krūp′). SYN *laryngismus* stridulus.

pseu·do·cryp·tor·chism (sū-dō-krip′tŏr-kizm). A condition in which the testes descend to the scrotum but continue to move up and down, rising high in the inguinal canal at one time and descending to the scrotum at another. [pseudo- + G. *kryptos*, hidden, + *orchis*, testis]

pseu·do·cu·mene (sū-dō-kū′mēn). trimethyl benzene; a colorless liquid obtained from coal tar; used in the sterilization of catgut. SYN pseudocumol.

pseu·do·cu·mol (sū-dō-kū′mol). SYN pseudocumene.

pseu·do·cy·e·sis (sū′dō-sī-ē′sis). SYN false *pregnancy*. [pseudo- + G. *kyēsis*, pregnancy]

pseu·do·cyl·in·droid (sū-dō-sil′in-droyd). A shred of mucus or other substance in the urine resembling a renal cast.

pseu·do·cyst (sū′dō-sist). **1.** An accumulation of fluid in a cystlike loculus, but without an epithelial or other membranous lining. SYN adventitious cyst, false cyst. **2.** A cyst whose wall is formed by a host cell and not by a parasite. **3.** A mass of 50 or more *Toxoplasma* bradyzoites, found within a host cell, frequently in the brain; formerly called a p., but now considered a true cyst enclosed in its own membrane within the host cell that may rupture to release particles that form new cysts, and apparently is infective to another vertebrate host. SEE ALSO bradyzoite. [pseudo- + G. *kystis*, bladder]

pseu·do·de·cid·u·o·sis (sū′dō-de-sid-yū-ō′sis). A decidual response of endometrium in the absence of pregnancy. [pseudo- + L. *deciduus*, falling off]

pseu·do·de·men·tia (sū′dō-dē-men′shē-ă). A condition resembling dementia but usually due to a depressive disorder rather than brain dysfunction.

pseu·do·dex·tro·car·dia (sū′dō-deks′trō-kar′dē-ă). Displacement of the heart to the right, either congenital or due to trauma, with all the chambers and vessels in their correct positions.

pseu·do·di·a·be·tes (sū′dō-dī-ă-bē′tēz). A condition in which a false positive test for sugar in the urine occurs.

pseu·do·di·a·stol·ic (sū′dō-dī-as-tol′ik). Seemingly associated with cardiac diastole.

pseu·do·dig·i·tox·in (sū′dō-dij-i-tok′sin). SYN gitoxin.

pseu·do·diph·the·ria (sū′dō-dif-thēr′ē-ă). SYN diphtheroid (1).

pseu·do·dip·sia (sū-dō-dip′sē-ă). SYN false *thirst*. [pseudo- + G. *dipsa*, thirst]

pseu·do·di·ver·tic·u·lum (sū′dō-dī-ver-tik′yū-lŭm). An outpouching from the lumen into an area of central necrosis within a large smooth muscle tumor, along any part of the intestinal wall.

pseu·do·dys·en·tery (sū-dō-dis′en-tār-ē). Occurrence of symptoms indistinguishable from those of bacillary dysentery, due to causes other than the presence of the specific microorganisms of bacillary dysentery.

pseu·do·e·de·ma (sū′dō-e-dē′mă). A puffiness of the skin not due to a fluid accumulation. [pseudo- + G. *oidēma*, a swelling (edema)]

pseu·do·e·phed·rine hy·dro·chlo·ride (sū′dō-e-fed′rin). *d*-Pseudoephedrine hydrochloride; the naturally occurring isomer of ephedrine; a sympathomimetic amine with actions and uses similar to those of ephedrine.

pseu·do·er·y·sip·e·las (sū′dō-er-i-sip′e-lăs). SYN erysipeloid.

pseu·do·es·the·sia (sū-dō-es-thē′zē-ă). **1.** SYN paraphia. **2.** SYN pseudesthesia (2). **3.** SYN phantom *limb*.

pseu·do·ex·fo·li·a·tion (sū′dō-eks-fō-lē-ā′shŭn). A condition simulating exfoliation in some respects, but in which the surface layer is not actually detached.

p. of lens capsule, deposition in all parts of the eye, including the lens capsule, of a material derived from basement membranes. If this material clogs the trabecular meshwork, impeding the outflow of aqueous humor from the eye, glaucoma may result. SEE exfoliation *syndrome*, capsular *glaucoma*.

pseu·do·fluc·tu·a·tion (sū′dō-flŭk-chū-ā′shŭn). A wavelike sensation, resembling fluctuation, obtained by tapping muscular tissue.

pseu·do·fol·lic·u·li·tis (sū′dō-fo-lik-yū-lī′tis). Erythematous follicular papules or, less commonly, pustules resulting from close shaving of very curly hair; growing tips of hairs consequently reenter the skin adjacent to the follicle producing ingrown hairs; p. of the beard area is very common in blacks.

pseu·do·frac·ture (sū-dō-frak′chūr). A condition in which a radiograph shows formation of new bone with thickening of periosteum at site of an injury to bone.

pseu·do·fruc·tose (sū-dō-fruk′tōs). SYN psicose.

pseu·do·gan·gli·on (sū-dō-gang′glē-on). A localized thickening of a nerve trunk having the appearance of a ganglion.

pseu·do·gene (sū′dō-jēn). **1.** A sequence of nucleotides that is not transcribed and therefore has no phenotypic effect. **2.** An inactive DNA segment that arose by a mutation of a parental active gene.

pseu·do·geu·ses·the·sia (sū′dō-gyū-ses-thē′zē-ă). SYN color *taste*. [pseudo- + G. *geusis*, taste, + *aisthēsis*, sensation]

pseu·do·geu·sia (sū-dō-gyū′sē-ă). A subjective taste sensation not produced by an external stimulus. [pseudo- + G. *geusis*, taste]

pseu·do·glan·ders (sū-dō-glan′derz). SYN melioidosis.

pseu·do·gli·o·ma (sū′dō-glī-ō′mă). Any intraocular opacity liable to be mistaken for retinoblastoma.

pseu·do·glob·u·lin (sū′dō-glob′ū-lin). The fraction of the serum globulin that is more soluble in an ammonium sulfate solution than is the euglobulin fraction.

pseu·do·glo·mer·u·lus (sū′dō-glō-mer′yū-lŭs). A structure within a neoplasm microscopically resembling a renal glomerulus but not representing renal glomerular differentiation.

pseu·do·glu·co·sa·zone (sū′dō-glū-kō′să-zōn). A substance sometimes present in normal urine which gives a reaction in the phenylhydrazine test.

pseu·do·gout (sū′dō-gowt) [MIM*118600]. Acute episodes of synovitis caused by deposits of calcium pyrophosphate crystals rather than urate crytals as in true gout; associated with articular chondrocalcinosis. SYN calcium gout.

pseu·do·gy·ne·co·mas·tia (sū′dō-gī-ně-kō-mas′tē-ă, -jin-ě-kō-). Enlargement of the male breast by an excess of adipose tissue without any increase in breast tissue. [pseudo- + G. *gynē*, woman, + *mastos*, breast]

pseu·do·he·ma·tu·ria (sū′dō-hem-ă-tū′rē-ă, -he-mă-). A red pigmentation of urine caused by certain foods or drugs, and thus not actually hematuria. SYN false hematuria.

pseu·do·he·mop·ty·sis (sū′dō-hē-mop′ti-sis). Spitting of blood that does not come from the lungs or bronchial tubes. [pseudo- + G. haima, blood, + *ptysis*, a spitting]

pseu·do·her·maph·ro·dite (sū′dō-her-maf′rō-dīt). An individual exhibiting pseudohermaphroditism.

pseu·do·her·maph·ro·dit·ism (sū′dō-her-maf′rō-dī-tizm). A state in which the individual is of an unambiguous gonadal sex (*i.e.*, possesses either testes or ovaries) but has ambiguous external genitalia. Cf. *steroid* 5α-reductase. SYN false hermaphroditism.

female p. [MIM*264270], p. with skeletal and genital anomalies but with female gonads and an XX karyotype. SYN androgynism, androgyny (1).

male p. [MIM*261550, MIM*264300, MIM*312100], p. in which the gonads are male and the karyotype is XY but with genital anomalies.

pseu·do·her·nia (sū-dō-her′nē-ă). Inflammation of the scrotal tissues or of an inguinal gland, simulating a strangulated hernia.

pseu·do·het·er·o·to·pia (su′dō-het-er-ō-tō′pē-ă). A seeming displacement of certain tissues observed postmortem; actually an artifact, rather than a true heterotopia.

pseu·do·hy·dro·ceph·a·ly (sū′dō-hī-drō-sef′ă-lē). Condition characterized by an enlargement of the head without concomitant enlargement of the ventricular system.

pseu·do·hy·dro·ne·phro·sis (sū'dō-hī-drō-ne-frō'sis). Presence of a cyst near the kidney, simulating hydronephrosis.

pseu·do·hy·per·kal·e·mia (sū'dō-hī'per-kal-ē'ē-ă). A spurious elevation of the serum concentration of potassium occurring when potassium is released in vitro from cells in a blood sample collected for a potassium measurement. This may be a consequence of disease (*i.e.*, myeloproliferative disorders with marked leukocytosis or thrombocytosis) or as a result of improper collection technique with in vitro hemolysis. [pseudo + G. *hyper*, above + L. *kalium*, potassium, G. *haima*, blood]

pseu·do·hy·per·par·a·thy·roid·ism (sū'dō-hī'per-par-ă-thī'roy-dizm). Hypercalcemia in a patient with a malignant neoplasm in the absence of skeletal metastases or primary hyperparathyroidism; believed to be due to formation of parathyroid-like hormone by nonparathyroid tumor tissue.

pseu·do·hy·per·tel·or·ism (sū'dō-hī-per-tel'ōr-izm). An appearance of excessive distance between the eyes (ocular telorism) due to lateral displacement of the inner canthi. SEE Waardenburg *syndrome*.

pseu·do·hy·per·tro·phic (sū'dō-hī-per-trof'ik). Relating to or marked by pseudohypertrophy.

pseu·do·hy·per·tro·phy (sū'dō-hī-per'trō-fē). Increase in size of an organ or a part, due not to increase in size or number of the specific functional elements but to that of some other tissue, fatty or fibrous. SYN false hypertrophy.

pseu·do·hy·pha (sū-dō-hī'fă). A chain of easily disrupted fungal cells that is intermediate between a chain of budding cells and a true hypha, marked by constrictions rather than septa at the junctions. [pseudo- + G. *hyphē*, a web (hypha)]

pseu·do·hy·po·na·tre·mia (sū'dō-hī-pō-nă-trē'mē-ă). A low serum sodium concentration due to volume displacement by massive hyperlipidemia or hyperproteinemia; also used to describe the low serum sodium concentration which may occur with high blood glucose.

pseu·do·hy·po·par·a·thy·roid·ism (sū'dō-hī'pō-par-ă-thī'roydizm) [MIM*103500]. A disorder resembling hypoparathyroidism, with high serum phosphate and low calcium levels, but with normal or elevated serum parathyroid hormone levels; due to lack of end-organ responsiveness to parathyroid hormone; type I shows lack of renal tubular response to exogenous parathyroid hormone, with increase in urinary cAMP; in type II the defect is at a locus after cAMP production; type Ia has associated skeletal defects characteristic of Albright's hereditary *osteodystrophy* (shortened metacarpals and metatarsals, short stature, round face, calcification of basal ganglia, ectopic bone formation, mental deficiency, sex-linked dominant inheritance, a demonstrable defect in red cell membrane G protein subunit, and resistance to therapeutic amounts of exogenous parathyroid hormone). Cf. thyrotropin *resistance*.
p. type Ia, p. believed to be due to a defect in the G-protein associated with adenylate cyclase (probably autosomal dominant).
p. type Ib, p. due to a defect in the adenylate cyclase complex.

pseu·do·ic·ter·us (sū-dō-ik'ter-ŭs). Yellowish discoloration of the skin not due to bile pigments, as in Addison's disease. SYN pseudojaundice.

pseu·do·il·e·us (sū-dō-il'ē-ŭs). Absolute obstipation, stimulating ileus, due to paralysis of the intestinal wall.

pseu·do·in·farc·tion (sū-dō-in-fark'shŭn). Any condition mimicking myocardial infarction, for example, acute pericarditis, dissecting aneurysm of the aorta, etc.

pseu·do·in·flu·en·za (sū'dō-in-flū-en'ză). An epidemic catarrh simulating influenza, but less severe.

pseu·do·in·tra·lig·a·men·tous (sū-dō-in'tră-lig-ă-men'tŭs). Falsely giving the impression of lying within the broad ligament; *e.g.*, a p. tumor.

pseu·do·i·so·chro·mat·ic (sū'dō-ī-sō-krō-mat'ik). Apparently of the same color; denoting certain charts containing colored spots mixed with figures printed in confusion colors; used in testing for color vision deficiency.

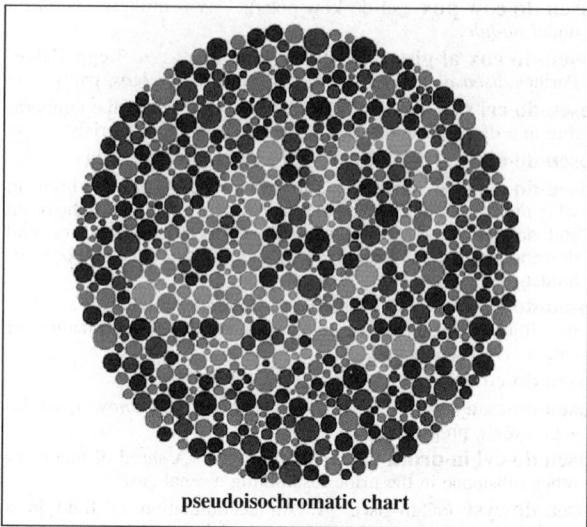
pseudoisochromatic chart

pseu·do·iso·en·zymes (sū'dō-ī-sō-en'zīmz). Multiple forms of enzymes that catalyze the same reaction and have the same amino acid sequence; differences are due to effects of some posttranslational modification.

pseu·do·jaun·dice (sū-dō-jawn'dis). SYN pseudoicterus.

pseu·do·ker·a·tin (sū-dō-kār'ă-tin). A protein extracted from epidermis and nervous tissue (glial fibrils), probably involved in keratinization.

pseu·do·li·po·ma (sū'dō-li-pō'mă). Any circumscribed, soft, smooth, usually movable swelling or tumefaction that grossly resembles a lipoma.

pseu·do·li·thi·a·sis (sū'dō-li-thī'ă-sis). A disorder resembling one of the syndromes associated with a stone in a hollow viscus or elsewhere. [pseudo- + G. *lithos,* stone]

pseu·do·lo·gia (sū-dō-lō'jē-ă). Pathological lying in speech or writing. [pseudo- + G. *logos,* word]
p. phantas'tica, an elaborate and often fantastic account of a patient's exploits, which are completely false but which the patient appears to believe.

pseu·do·lym·pho·cyte (sū-dō-lim'fō-sīt). A small neutrophilic leukocyte with a single round nucleus, characteristic of the rare homozygous Pelger-Huët anomaly.

pseu·do·lym·pho·ma (sū'dō-lim-fō'mă). A benign infiltration of lymphoid cells or histiocytes which microscopically resembles a malignant lymphoma.
Spiegler-Fendt p., SYN benign *lymphocytoma* cutis.

pseu·do·ly·so·gen·ic (sū'dō-lī-sō-jen'ik). Pertaining to pseudolysogeny.

pseu·do·ly·sog·e·ny (sū'dō-lī-soj'ĕ-nē). The condition in which a bacteriophage is maintained (carried) in a culture of a bacterial strain by infecting susceptible variants of the strain, in contradistinction to true lysogeny in which the bacteriophage genome multiplies as an integral part of the bacterial genome.

pseu·do·ma·lig·nan·cy (sū'dō-mă-lig'nan-sē). A benign tumor that appears, clinically or histologically, to be a malignant neoplasm. SEE ALSO pseudotumor.

pseu·do·mam·ma (sū-dō-mam'ă). A glandular structure resembling the mammary gland, occurring in dermoid cysts.

pseu·do·ma·nia (sū-dō-mā'nē-ă). 1. A factitious mental disorder. 2. A mental disorder in which the patient alleges to have committed a crime, but of which he or she is innocent. 3. Generally, the morbid impulse to falsify or lie, as in pseudologia.

pseu·do·mas·tur·ba·tion (sū'dō-mas-ter-bā'shŭn). SYN peotillomania.

pseu·do·meg·a·col·on. Enlargement of the distal colon with sluggish muscular function without the neurologic abnormalities of congenital megacolon (Hirschsprung's *disease*).

pseu·do·mel·a·no·sis (sū′dō-mel-ă-nō′sis). A dark greenish or blackish postmortem discoloration of the surface of the abdominal viscera, resulting from the action of sulfureted hydrogen upon the iron of disintegrated hemoglobin. [pseudo- + G. *melas,* black]

pseu·do·mem·brane (sū-dō-mem′brān). SYN false *membrane.*

pseu·do·mem·bra·nous (sū-dō-mem′bră-nŭs). Relating to or marked by the presence of a false membrane.

pseu·do·men·in·gi·tis (sū′dō-men-in-jī′tis). SYN meningism.

pseu·do·men·stru·a·tion (sū′dō-men-strū-ā′shŭn). Uterine bleeding without the typical premenstrual endometrial changes.

pseu·do·met·a·pla·sia (sū′dō-met-ă-plā′zē-ă). SYN histologic *accommodation.*

pseu·dom·ne·sia (sū-dom-nē′zē-ă). A subjective impression of memory of events that have not occurred. [pseudo- + G. *mnēsis,* memory]

pseu·do·mo·nad (sū-dō-mō′nad). A vernacular term used to refer to any member of the genus *Pseudomonas.*

Pseu·do·mo·nas (sū-dō-mō′nas). A genus of motile, polar flagellate, nonsporeforming, strictly aerobic bacteria (family Pseudomonadaceae) containing straight or curved, but not helical, Gram-negative rods which occur singly. The metabolism is respiratory, never fermentative. They occur commonly in soil and in fresh water and marine environments. Some species are plant pathogens. Others are involved in human infections. The type species is *P. aeruginosa.* [pseudo- + G. *monas,* unit, monad]

P. acido′vorans, a species found in soil and occasionally in clinical specimens.

P. aerugino′sa, a species found in soil, water, and commonly in clinical specimens (wound infections, infected burn lesions, urinary tract infections); the causative agent of blue pus; occasionally pathogenic for plants; usually causes infections in humans only where there is a defect in host defense mechanisms. It is the type species of the genus *P.* SYN blue pus bacillus.

P. cepa′cia, a species found in rotted onions and in clinical specimens.

P. diminu′ta, a species found primarily in clinical specimens, rarely in water.

P. fluores′cens, a species found in soil and water; it is frequently found in clinical specimens and is commonly associated with food spoilage (eggs, cured meats, fish, and milk).

P. mal′lei, a species infectious to horses and donkeys, causing glanders and farcy. SYN glanders bacillus.

P. maltophil′ia, SYN *Xanthomonas maltophilia.*

P. piscici′da, a species pathogenic for fish.

P. pseudoalcalig′enes, a species found in a sinus discharge.

P. pseudomal′lei, a species found in cases of melioidosis in humans and other animals and in soil and water in tropical regions. SYN Whitmore's bacillus.

P. putrefa′ciens, former for term for *Alteromonas putrefaciens.*

P. stut′zeri, a species found in soil and water, frequently in clinical specimens.

P. vesicula′ris, a species found in the medicinal leech (*Hirudo medicinalis*) and in water from a stream.

pseu·do·mon·o·mo·lec·u·lar. SYN pseudounimolecular.

pseu·do·morph (sū′dō-mōrf). A mineral found crystallized in a form that is not proper to it but to some other mineral. [pseudo- + G. *morphē,* form]

pseu·do·my·ce·li·um (sū′dō-mī-se′lē-ŭm). A mycelium-like mass of pseudohyphae.

pseu·do·my·o·pia (sū′dō-mī-ō′pē-ă). A condition simulating myopia and due to spasm of the ciliary muscle.

pseu·do·myx·o·ma (sū′dō-mik-sō′mă). A gelatinous mass resembling a myxoma but composed of epithelial mucus.

p. peritone′i, the accumulation of large quantities of mucoid or mucinous material in the peritoneal cavity, either as a result of rupture of a mucocele of the appendix, or rupture of benign or malignant cystic neoplasms of the ovary; it will frequently persist because of the growth of mucus-secreting cells scattered on serosal surfaces, leading to intestinal adhesions and obstruction. SYN gelatinous ascites.

pseu·do·nar·cot·ic (sū′dō-nar-kot′ik). Inducing sleep by reason of a sedative effect, but not directly narcotic.

pseu·do·ne·o·plasm (sū-dō-nē′ō-plazm). SYN pseudotumor.

pseu·do·neu·ro·ma (sū-dō-nū-rō′mă). SYN traumatic *neuroma.*

pseu·do·nit (sū′dō-nit). SYN hair *cast.*

pseu·do-os·te·o·ma·la·cia (sū-dō-os′tē-ō-mă-lā′shē-ă). Rachitic softening of bone.

pseu·do-os·te·o·ma·la·cic (sū-dō-os′tē-ō-mă-lā′sik). Marked by pseudo-osteomalacia.

pseu·do·pap·il·le·de·ma (sū′dō-pap-il-e-dē′mă). Anomalous elevation of the optic disk; seen in severe hyperopia and optic nerve drusen.

pseu·do·pa·ral·y·sis (sū′dō-pă-ral′i-sis). Apparent paralysis due to voluntary inhibition of motion because of pain, to incoordination, or other cause, but without actual paralysis. SYN pseudoparesis (1).

arthritic general p., a disease, occurring in arthritic subjects, having symptoms resembling those of general paresis, the lesions of which consist of diffuse changes of a degenerative and noninflammatory character due to intracranial atheroma.

congenital atonic p., SYN *amyotonia* congenita (1).

pseu·do·par·a·ple·gia (sū′dō-par-ă-plē′jē-ă). Apparent paralysis in the lower extremities, in which the tendon and skin reflexes and the electrical reactions are normal; the condition is sometimes observed in rickets.

Basedow's p., weakness of the thigh muscles in thyrotoxicosis; may occur suddenly and cause the patient to fall.

pseu·do·par·a·site (sū-dō-par′ă-sīt). A false parasite; may be either a commensal or a temporary parasite (the latter being an organism accidentally ingested and surviving briefly in the intestine).

pseu·do·pa·ren·chy·ma (sū′dō-pă-reng′ki-mă). In fungi, a tissue-like mass of modified hyphae.

pseu·do·pa·re·sis (sū′dō-pa-rē′sis, -par′ĕ-sis). **1.** SYN pseudoparalysis. **2.** A condition marked by the pupillary changes, tremors, and speech disturbances suggestive of early paresis, in which, however, the serologic tests are negative.

pseu·do·pe·lade (sū′dō-pĕ-lahd′). A scarring type of alopecia; usually occurs in scattered irregular patches; of uncertain cause. SYN p. of Brocq. [pseudo- + Fr. *pelade,* disease that causes sporadic falling of hair]

p. of Brocq, SYN pseudopelade.

pseu·do·per·i·car·di·tis (sū′dō-per-i-kar-dī′tis). An artifact of auscultation resembling a friction rub, but due to movement of the tissue in the intercostal space when the diaphragm of the stethoscope is placed over the apex beat.

pseu·do·per·i·to·ni·tis (sū′dō-per′i-tō-nī′tis). SYN peritonism (2).

pseu·do·per·ox·i·dase (sū′dō-per-oks-i-dās). Referring to the nonenzymatic, heat-stable peroxidase activity associated with hemeproteins.

pseu·do·phac·os (sū′dō-fak′ōs). SYN lenticulus. [pseudo- + G. *phakos,* lens]

pseu·do·pha·kia (sū-dō-fak′ē-ă). An eye in which the natural lens is replaced with an intraocular lens. [pseudo- + *phakos,* lentil (lens)]

pseu·do·pha·ko·do·ne·sis (sū-dō-fā′kō-dō-nē′sis). Excessive mobility of an intraocular lens implant.

pseu·do·phleg·mon (sū-dō-fleg′mon). A noninflammatory circumscribed redness of the skin. [pseudo- + G. *phlegmonē,* inflammation]

Hamilton's p., a trophic affection of the subcutaneous connective tissue, marked by a circumscribed swelling which may become indurated and red, but never suppurates.

pseu·do·pho·tes·the·sia (sū′dō-fō-tes-thē′zē-ă). SYN photism. [pseudo- + G. *phōs,* light, + *aisthēsis,* sensation]

pseu·do·phyl·lid (sū-dō-fī′lid). Common name for members of the order Pseudophyllidea.

Pseu·do·phyl·lid·ea (sū′dō-fi-lid′ē-ă). An order of tapeworms with an aquatic life cycle, passing through coracidium, procercoid, and plerocercoid stages before developing into adults in fish, marine mammals, or fish-eating mammals; includes the broad fish tapeworm of humans, *Diphyllobothrium latum.* [pseudo- + G. *phyllon,* leaf]

pseu·do·plate·let (sū-dō-plāt′let). Any of the fragments of neutrophils which may be mistaken for platelets, especially in peripheral blood smears of leukemic patients.

pseu·do·ple·gia (sū-dō-plē′jē-ă). SYN pseudoapoplexy. [pseudo- + G. *plēgē,* a stroke]

pseu·do·pock·et (sū′dō-pok′et). A pocket, adjacent to a tooth, resulting from gingival hyperplasia and edema but without apical migration of the epithelial attachment.

pseu·do·pod (sū′dō-pod). SYN pseudopodium.

pseu·do·po·di·um, pl. **pseu·do·po·dia** (sū-dō-pō′dē-ŭm, -pō′dē-ă). A temporary protoplasmic process, put forth by an ameboid stage or amebic protozoan for locomotion or for prehension of food. SYN pseudopod. [pseudo- + G. *pous,* foot]

pseu·do·pol·y·dys·tro·phy (sū′dō-pol-ē-dis′trō-fē). SYN *mucolipidosis* III.

pseu·do·pol·yp (sū-dō-pol′ip). A projecting mass of granulation tissue, large numbers of which may develop in ulcerative colitis; may become covered by regenerating epithelium. SYN inflammatory polyp.

pseu·do·por·phyr·ia (sū′dō-pōr-fir′ē-ă). A condition clinically and ultrastructurally identical to porphyria but with no abnormality in porphyrin excretion, consequent to drug ingestion or hemodialysis.

pseu·do·preg·nan·cy (sū-dō-preg′nan-sē). **1.** SYN false *pregnancy.* **2.** A condition in which symptoms resembling those of pregnancy are present, but which is not pregnancy; occurs after sterile copulation in mammalian species in which copulation induces ovulation, and also in dogs, in which the estrus cycle includes a marked luteal phase.

pseu·do·prog·na·thism (sū-dō-prog′nă-thizm). An acquired projection of the mandible due to occlusal disharmonies which force the mandible forward; the mandibular condyles are forward of their expected functional position.

pseu·do·pte·ryg·i·um (sū′dō-tě-rij′ē-ŭm). Adhesion of the conjunctiva to the cornea, occurring after injury.

pseu·dop·to·sis (sū-dō-tō′sis, sū-dop′tō-sis). A condition resembling an inability to elevate the eyelid, due to blepharophimosis, blepharochalasis, or some other affection. SYN false blepharoptosis. [pseudo- + G. *ptōsis,* a falling]

pseu·do·pu·ber·ty (sū-dō-pyū′ber-tē). Condition characterized by the development of a varying number of the somatic and functional changes typical of puberty; commonly caused by the hormonal secretions of a tumor and typically arises before the chronological age of puberty.

precocious p., the development of p. in very young children; commonly characterized by secretion of gonadal hormones, without stimulation of gametogenesis.

pseu·do·ra·bies (sū-dō-rā′bēz). A highly contagious disease affecting cattle, horses, dogs, swine, and other mammalian species, caused by porcine herpes virus 1, which has its reservoir in swine. In species other than swine, it is highly fatal. SYN Aujeszky's disease, infectious bulbar paralysis, mad itch. [pseudo- + rabies]

pseu·do·re·ac·tion (sū′dō-rē-ak′shŭn). A false reaction; one not due to specific causes in a given test.

pseu·do·rep·li·ca (sū-dō-rep′li-kă). A specimen for electron microscopic examination obtained by depositing particles from a virus-containing suspension on an agarose surface, covering the surface with a plastic-containing solution, and, after evaporation of the solvent, removing the film along with enmeshed particles by floating it onto the surface of a uranyl acetate solution.

pseu·do·ret·i·ni·tis pig·men·to·sa (sū′dō-ret-i-nī′tis pig-men-tō′să). A widespread pigmentary mottling of the retina that may follow severe eye trauma, especially from a penetrating injury.

pseu·do·rheu·ma·tism (sū-dō-rū′mă-tizm). Joint or muscle symptoms without objective findings and with no apparent underlying causes.

pseu·do·rick·ets (sū-dō-rik′ets). SYN renal *rickets.*

pseu·do·ro·sette (sū′dō-rō-zet′). Perivascular radial arrange-

ment of neoplastic cells around a small blood vessel. SEE rosette (2).

pseu·do·ru·bel·la (sū′dō-rū-bel′ă). SYN *exanthema* subitum.

pseu·do·sar·co·ma (sū-dō-sar-kō′mă). A bulky polyploid malignant tumor of the esophagus, composed of spindle cells with a focus of squamous cell carcinoma; spindle cells may be epithelial or metaplastic malignant fibroblasts.

pseu·do·scar·la·ti·na (sū′dō-skar-lă-tē′nă). Erythema with fever, due to causes other than *Streptococcus pyogenes.*

pseu·do·scle·ro·sis (sū′dō-sklēr-ō′sis). **1.** Inflammatory induration or fatty or other infiltration simulating fibrous thickening. **2.** SYN Wilson's *disease* (1). [pseudo- + G. *sklērōsis,* hardening]

Westphal's p., SYN Wilson's *disease* (1).

Westphal-Strümpell p., SYN Wilson's *disease* (1).

pseu·do·sei·zure (sū′dō-sē′zher). A psychogenic seizure.

pseu·do·small·pox (sū-dō-smawl′poks). SYN alastrim.

pseu·dos·mia (sū-doz′mē-ă). Subjective sensation of an odor that is not present. [pseudo- + G. *osmē,* smell]

Pseu·do·ster·ta·gia bul·lo·sa (sū′dō-ster-tā′jē-ă bŭl-ō′să). One of the medium stomach worms located in the abomasum of sheep, goats, and pronghorn; it is found chiefly in the western U.S.

pseu·dos·to·ma (sū-dos′tō-mă). An apparent opening in a cell, membrane, or other tissue, due to a defect in staining or other cause. [pseudo- + G. *stoma,* mouth]

pseu·do·stra·bis·mus (sū-dō-stra-biz′mŭs). The appearance of strabismus caused by epicanthus, abnormality in interorbital distance, or corneal light reflex not corresponding to the center of the pupil. [pseudo- + G. *strabismos,* a squinting]

pseu·do·ta·bes (sū-dō-tā′bēz). A syndrome having the characteristics of tabetic neurosyphilis but not due to syphilis. SYN Leyden's ataxia, peripheral tabes, pseudoataxia.

pupillotonic p., SYN Adie *syndrome.*

pseu·do·trich·i·no·sis, pseu·do·trich·i·ni·a·sis (sū′dō-trik-i-nō′sis, -trik-i-nī′ă-sis). SYN multiple *myositis.*

pseu·do·trun·cus ar·te·ri·o·sus (sū-dō-trŭng′kŭs ar-tēr-ē-ō′sŭs). Congenital cardiovascular deformity with atresia of the pulmonic valve and absence of the main pulmonary artery; the lungs are supplied with blood either through a patent ductus or via bronchial arteries arising from the aorta. A characteristic of the most severe form of tetralogy of Fallot.

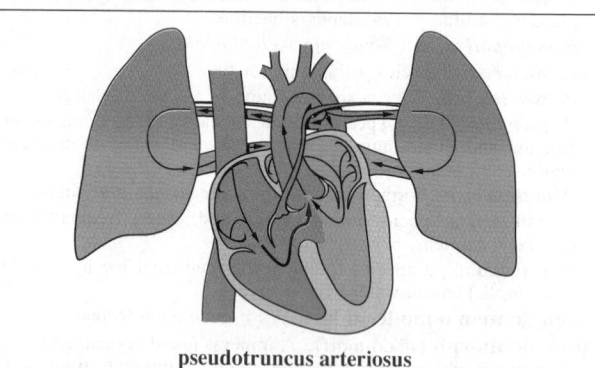

pseudotruncus arteriosus

pseu·do·tu·ber·cle (sū-dō-tū′ber-kl). A nodule histologically similar to a tuberculous granuloma, but due to infection by some microorganism other than *Mycobacterium tuberculosis.*

pseu·do·tu·ber·cu·lo·sis (sū′dō-tū-ber′kyū-lō′sis). A disease of a wide variety of animal species caused by the bacterium *Yersinia pseudotuberculosis.* Epizootics of p. are commonly seen in birds and rodents, often with high case fatality rates. In man, seven clinical entities are recognized: primary focalized infections (pseudoappendicitis, acute mesenteric lymphadenitis, or acute terminal ileitis), primary generalized infections (septicemia or scarlatiniform fever), and secondary immunological phenomena (erythema nodosum or arthralgia). SYN pseudotubercular yersiniosis.

pseu·do·tu·mor (sū′dō-tū-mer). **1.** An enlargement of nonneoplastic character which clinically resembles a true neoplasm so closely as to often be mistaken for such. **2.** A condition, commonly associated with obesity in young females, of cerebral edema with narrowed small ventricles but with increased intracranial pressure and frequently papilledema. SYN pseudoneoplasm.

p. cer′ebri, a condition of the brain simulating the presence of an intracranial tumor. SEE pseudotumor (2).

inflammatory p., a tumor-like mass in the lungs or other sites, composed of fibrous or granulation tissue infiltrated by inflammatory cells.

pseu·do·uni·mo·lec·u·lar (sū′dō-ū-nē-mō-lek-ū-lar). Referring to a reaction whose rate appears to be dependent on the concentration of only one substrate; usually due to a constant, saturating level of the other compounds. SYN pseudomonomolecular.

pseu·do·u·ri·dine (Ψ, Q) (sū-dō-yū′ri-dēn, -din). 5-β-D-Ribosyluracil; a naturally occurring isomer of uridine found in transfer ribonucleic acids; unique in that the ribosyl is attached to carbon (C-5) rather than to nitrogen; excreted in urine.

pseu·do·vac·u·ole (sū-dō-vak′yū-ōl). An apparent vacuole in a cell, either an artifact or an intracellular parasite.

pseu·do·va·ri·o·la (sū′dō-vă-rī′ō-lă). SYN alastrim. [pseudo- + L. *variola,* smallpox]

pseu·do·ven·tri·cle (sū-dō-ven′tri-kl). SYN *cavity* of septum pellucidum.

pseu·do·vi·ta·min (sū-dō-vī′tă-min). A substance having a chemical structure very similar to that of a given vitamin, but lacking the usual physiologic action.

p. B₁₂, cobamide cyanide phosphate, 3′-ester with 7-α-D-ribofuranosyladenine, inner salt; vitamin B₁₂ with adenine replacing dimethylbenzimidazole; one of several substances produced during anaerobic fermentation by certain organisms in bovine rumen contents; it is chemically closely similar to vitamin B₁₂ (cyanocobalamin) but without, in humans, the physiologic action of the vitamin.

pseu·do·vom·it·ing (sū-dō-vom′i-ting). Regurgitation of matter from the esophagus or stomach without expulsive effort.

pseu·do·xan·tho·ma elas·ti·cum (sū′dō-zan-thō′mă e-las′ti-kŭm) [MIM*177850, MIM*264800, MIM*264810]. An inherited disorder of connective tissue characterized by slightly elevated yellowish plaques on the neck, axillae, abdomen, and thighs, developing in the second or third decade, associated with angioid streaks of the retina and similar elastic tissue degeneration and calcification in arteries; autosomal dominant and autosomal recessive types have been described.

psi (sī) **1.** 23rd Letter of the Greek alphabet (ψ). **2.** (ψ) Symbol for pseudouridine; pseudo-; wave function; the dihedral angle of rotation about the C₁–Cα bond associated with a peptide bond.

psi·cose (sī′kōs). ribo-2-hexulose; a ketohexose; D-p. is epimeric with D-fructose. SYN pseudofructose, ribo-2-hexulose.

psi·lo·cin (sī′lō-sin). 3-[2-(Dimethylamino)ethyl]indol-4-ol; a hallucinogenic agent related to psilocybin.

Psil·o·cy·be (sī-lō-sī′bē). A genus of mushrooms (family Agaricaceae) containing many species with psychotropic or hallucinogenic properties, including *P. mexicana,* of which the fruiting bodies are a source of the hallucinogen, psilocybin.

psi·lo·cy·bin (sī-lō-sī′bin, -sib′in). 3-(2-dimethylamino)-ethylindol-4-ol dihydrogen phosphate; the *N′,N′* -dimethyl derivative of 4-hydroxytryptamine; obtained from the fruiting bodies of the fungus *Psilocybe mexicana* and other species of *Psilocybe* and *Stropharia.* P. is a congener of 5-hydroxytryptamine, with striking central nervous system effects, and is readily hydrolyzed to 4-hydroxybufotenine; used as a hallucinogenic agent (and by Mexican aborigines to induce trances). SYN indocybin.

psi·lo·sis (sī-lō′sis). Falling out of the hair. [G. *psilōsis,* a stripping, fr. *psilos,* bare]

psi·lo·thin (sil′ō-thin). A depilatory plaster applied when warm to a hairy surface, and ripped off when cool, causing removal of the hairs. [see psilosis]

psi·lot·ic (sī-lot′ik). **1.** Relating to psilosis. **2.** SYN epilatory (1).

P-sin·is·tro·car·di·a·le (sin-is-trō-kar-dē-ā′lē). An electrocardiographic P-wave characteristic of overloading of the left atrium; often erroneously called P-mitrale, as the syndrome can result from any overloading of the left atrium from any cause.

psit·ta·cine (sit′ă-sēn). Referring to birds of the parrot family (parrots, parakeets, and budgerigars).

psit·ta·co·sis (sit-ă-kō′sis). An infectious disease in psittacine birds and man caused by the bacterium *Chlamydia psittaci.* Avian infections are mainly inapparent or latent, although acute disease does occur; human infections may result in mild disease with a flu-like syndrome or in severe disease, especially in older persons, with symptoms of bronchopneumonia. SYN parrot disease, parrot fever. [G. *psittakos,* a parrot, + *-osis,* condition]

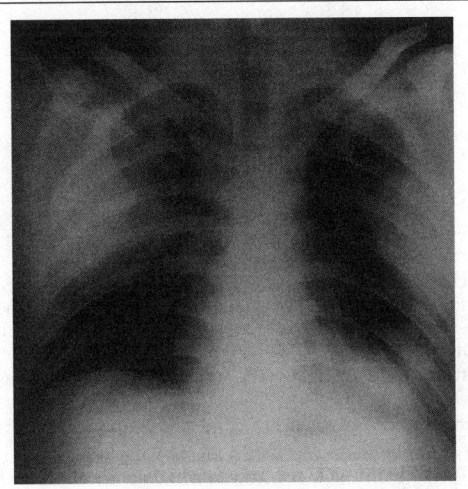

psittacosis
alveolar and interstitial infiltrates in both lobes of lungs

pso·as (sō′as). SEE psoas major *muscle,* psoas minor *muscle.* [G. *psoa,* the muscles of the loins]

pso·mo·pha·gia, pso·moph·a·gy (sō-mō-fā′jē-ă, sō-mof′ă-jē). The practice of swallowing the food without thorough mastication. [G. *psōmos,* morsel, bit, + *phagō,* to eat]

pso·ra (sō′ră). SYN psoriasis. [G. *psōra,* itch]

psor·a·len (sōr′ă-len). Furo[3,2-*g*]coumarin; a phototoxic drug used by topical or oral administration for the treatment of vitiligo and psoriasis. Also present in oil of bergamot perfume, and in fruits and vegetables such as limes, which may cause photosensitization. SEE ALSO PUVA.

pso·rel·co·sis (sō-rel-kō′sis). Ulceration resulting from scabies of the skin. [G. *psōra,* itch, + *helkōsis,* ulceration]

psor·en·ter·i·tis (sōr′en-ter-ī′tis). Inflammatory swelling of the solitary lymphatic follicles of the intestine. [G. *psōra,* itch (scabies), + *enteron,* intestine, + *-itis,* inflammation]

Psor·er·ga·tes (psŏ-rer′gă-tēz). A genus of itch mites (family Cheyletidae) parasitic on cattle, sheep, and goats. *P. bos* is the itch mite of cattle, described in New Mexico; *P. ovis* is the small itch mite of sheep in the U.S., Australia, New Zealand, and South Africa. [G. *psōra,* itch]

pso·ri·a·sic (sō-rī′ă-sik). SYN psoriatic.

pso·ri·a·si·form (sō-rī′ă-si-fōrm). Resembling psoriasis.

pso·ri·a·sis (sō-rī′ă-sis). A common multifactorial inherited condition characterized by the eruption of circumscribed, discrete and confluent, reddish, silvery-scaled maculopapules; the lesions occur predominantly on the elbows, knees, scalp, and trunk, and microscopically show characteristic parakeratosis and elongation of rete ridges with shortening of epidermal keratinocyte transit time due to decreased cyclic guanosine monophosphate. SYN psora. [G. *psōriasis,* fr. *psōra,* the itch]

p. annula′ris, p. annula′ta, SYN p. circinata.

p. arthrop′ica, p. associated with severe arthritis resembling rheumatoid arthritis, although serum rheumatoid factor is absent.

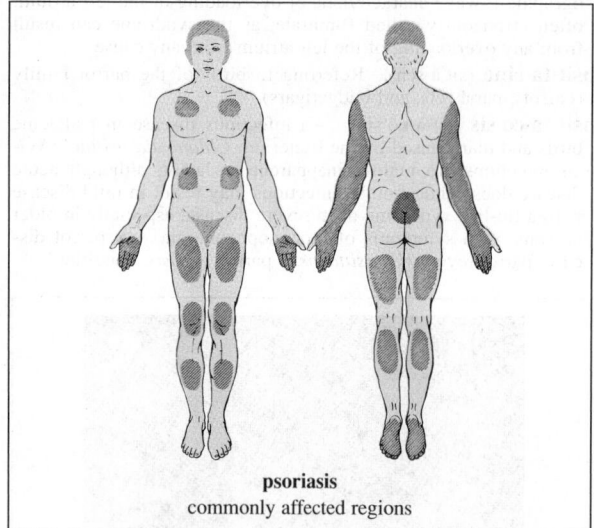

psoriasis
commonly affected regions

p. circina′ta, p. in which healing is taking place at the center of the lesion while the process continues at the periphery, producing a ring-shaped or annular lesion. SYN p. annularis, p. annulata, p. orbicularis.

p. diffu′sa, diffused p., a form of p. with extensive coalescence of the lesions.

p. discoi′dea, p. in which the lesions are discrete and disklike. SYN p. nummularis.

generalized pustular p. of Zambusch, SYN pustular p. (1).

p. geograph′ica, p. gyrata in which the lesions suggest the coast outline on a map.

p. gutta′ta, p. occurring abruptly in round patches of small size; seen in young persons following streptococcal infections.

p. gyra′ta, p. circinata in which there is a coalescence of the rings giving rise to figures of various outlines.

p. invetera′ta, p. in which the lesions are confluent, the affected skin being thickened, indurated, and scaly.

p. nummula′ris, SYN p. discoidea.

p. orbicula′ris, SYN p. circinata.

p. ostrea′cea, p. with concentric tiers of scales which give the appearance of the layering of an oyster shell. SYN p. rupioides.

p. puncta′ta, p. in which the individual lesions are papules, each red in color, and tipped with a single white scale.

pustular p., (1) an extensive exacerbation of p., with pustule formation in the normal and psoriatic skin, fever, and granulocytosis; sometimes precipitated by oral steroids; SYN generalized pustular p. of Zambusch. **(2)** a local pustular eruption of the palms and soles, occurring most commonly in a patient with p.; difficult to distinguish from acrodermatitis continua.

p. rupioi′des, SYN p. ostreacea.

p. spondylit′ica, p. associated with an ankylosing spondylitis.

p. universa′lis, a generalized p.

pso·ri·at·ic (sō-rē-at′ik). Relating to psoriasis. SYN psoriasic.

pso·ric (sō′rik). Relating to scabies. SYN psorous.

pso·roid (sō′royd). Resembling scabies. [G. *psōra,* itch (scabies), + *eidos,* resemblance]

Pso·rop·tes (sō-rop′tēz). A genus of itch or mange mites (family Cheyletidae), including the species *P. cuniculi* (the scab mite of rabbits), *P. equi* (the mange or body mite of horses), and *P. ovis* (the common scab mite of sheep and cattle). [G. *psōra,* itch]

pso·rous (sō′rŭs). SYN psoric.

PSP Abbreviation for phenolsulfonphthalein.

△**psych-.** SEE psycho-.

psy·cha·go·gy (sī′kă-go-jē). Rarely used term for psychotherapeutic reeducation stressing social adjustment of the individual. [psych- + G. *agōgia,* a tutor's office]

psy·chal·ga·lia (sī-kal-gā′lē-ă). SYN psychalgia (1).

psy·chal·gia (sī-kal′jē-ă). **1.** Distress attending a mental effort, noted especially in melancholia. SYN algopsychalia, mind pain, phrenalgia (1), psychalgalia, soul pain. **2.** SYN psychogenic *pain.* [psych- + G. *algos,* pain]

psy·cha·lia (sī-kā′lē-ă). An emotional condition characterized by auditory and visual hallucinations.

psy·cha·nop·sia (sī′kă-nop′sē-ă). SYN mind *blindness.* [psych- + G. *an-* priv, + *opsis,* vision]

psy·cha·tax·ia (sī-kă-tak′sē-ă). Mental confusion; inability to fix one's attention or to make any continued mental effort. [psych- + G. *ataxia,* confusion]

psy·che (sī′kē). Term for the subjective aspects of the mind, self, soul; the psychological or spiritual as distinct from the bodily nature of persons. [G. mind, soul]

△**psyche-.** SEE psycho-.

psy·che·del·ic (sī-kĕ-del′ik). **1.** Pertaining to a rather imprecise category of drugs with mainly central nervous system action, and with effects said to be the expansion or heightening of consciousness, *e.g.,* LSD, hashish, mescaline. **2.** A hallucinogenic substance, visual display, music, or other sensory stimulus having such action. [psyche- + G. *dēloō,* to manifest]

psy·chen·to·nia (sī-ken-tō′nē-ă). Rarely used term for mental tension. [psych- + G. *en,* in, + *tonos,* tension]

psy·chi·at·ric (sī-kē-at′rik). Relating to psychiatry.

psy·chi·at·rics (sī-kē-at′riks). SYN psychiatry.

psy·chi·at·ric trend. Benign or morbid emotional interests, urges, and tendencies as revealed by postures, gestures, actions, or speech.

psy·chi·a·trist (sī-kī′ă-trist). A physician who specializes in psychiatry.

psy·chi·a·try (sī-kī′ă-trē). **1.** The medical specialty concerned with the diagnosis and treatment of mental disorders. **2.** The diagnosis and treatment of mental disorders. For some types of p. not listed below, see also subentries under therapy, psychotherapy, psychoanalysis. SYN psychiatrics. [psych- + G. *iatreia,* medical treatment]

analytic p., SYN psychoanalytic p.

biological p., a branch of p. that emphasizes molecular, genetic, and pharmacologic approaches in the diagnosis and treatment of mental disorders.

community p., p. focusing on the detection, prevention, early treatment, and rehabilitation of individuals with emotional disorders and social deviance as they develop in the community rather than as encountered one-on-one, in private practice, or at larger centralized psychiatric facilities; particular emphasis is placed on the social-interpersonal-environmental factors that contribute to mental illness.

contractual p., psychiatric intervention voluntarily assumed by the patient, who is prompted by his personal difficulties or suffering and who retains control over his participation with the psychiatrist.

cross-cultural p., a field of p. with interest in the study of psychological and psychiatric phenomena as differentially expressed in the cultures of different countries.

descriptive p., that aspect of the practice of psychiatry that deals with the diagnosis of mental disorders.

dynamic p., SYN psychoanalytic p.

existential p., SYN existential *psychotherapy.*

forensic p., legal p., the application of p. in courts of law, *e.g.,* in determinations for commitment, competency, fitness to stand trial, responsibility for crime.

industrial p., the application of the principles of p. to problems in business and industry.

orthomolecular p., an approach to p. that focuses on the use of megavitamins and nutrition in the treatment of such mental illnesses as the schizophrenic disorders.

psychoanalytic p., psychiatric theory and practice emphasizing the principles of psychoanalysis. SYN analytic p., dynamic p.

social p., an approach to psychiatric theory and practice emphasizing the cultural and sociological aspects of mental disorder and treatment; the application of p. to social problems. SEE ALSO community p.

psy·chic (sī'kik). **1.** Relating to the phenomena of consciousness, mind, or soul. SYN psychical. **2.** A person supposedly endowed with the power of communicating with spirits; a spiritualistic medium. [G. *psychikos*]

psy·chi·cal (sī'ki-kăl). SYN psychic (1).

psy·chism (sī'kizm). The theory that a principle of life pervades all nature. [G. *psychē*, soul]

△**psycho-, psych-, psyche-.** The mind; mental; psychological. [G. *psychē*, soul, mind]

psy·cho·a·cous·tics (sī'kō-ă-kūs'tiks). **1.** A discipline combining experimental psychology and physics that deals with the physical features of sound as related to audition, as well as with the physiology and psychology of sound recepter processes. **2.** The science pertaining to the psychologic factors that influence one's awareness of sound. [psycho- + G. *akoustikos*, relating to hearing]

psy·cho·ac·tive (sī-kō-ak'tiv). Possessing the ability to alter mood, anxiety, behavior, cognitive processes, or mental tension; usually applied to pharmacologic agents.

psy·cho·al·ler·gy (sī-kō-al'er-jē). A sensitization to emotionally charged symbols.

psy·cho·a·nal·y·sis (sī'kō-ă-nal'i-sis). **1.** A method of psychotherapy, originated by Freud, designed to bring preconscious and unconscious material to consciousness primarily through the analysis of transference and resistance. SYN psychoanalytic therapy. SEE ALSO freudian p. **2.** A method of investigating the human mind and psychological functioning, interpretations of resistances, and the patient's emotional reactions to the analyst plus use of free association and dream analysis in the psychoanalytic situation. **3.** An integrated body of observations and theories on personality development, motivation, and behavior. **4.** An institutionalized school of psychotherapy, as in jungian or freudian p. [psycho- + analysis]

active p., p. in which the analyst intervenes directly and actively in the patient's life, *e.g.,* by making prohibitions, assigning tasks.

adlerian p., SYN individual *psychology.*

freudian p., the theory and practice of p. and psychotherapy as developed by Freud, based on: 1) his theory of personality, which postulates that psychic life is made up of instinctual and socially acquired forces, or the id, the ego, and a superego, each of which must constantly accommodate to the other; 2) his discovery that the free association technique of verbalizing for the analyst all thoughts without censoring any of them is the therapeutic tactic which reveals the areas of conflict within a patient's personality; 3) that the vehicle for gaining this insight and next, on this basis, readjusting one's personality is the learning a patient does as he first develops a stormy emotional bond with the analyst (transference relationship) and next successfully learns to break his bond.

jungian p., the theory of psychopathology and the practice of psychotherapy, according to the principles of Jung, which utilizes a system of psychology and psychotherapy emphasizing man's symbolic nature, and differs from freudian p. especially in placing less significance upon instinctual (sexual) urges. SYN analytical psychology.

psy·cho·an·a·lyst (sī-kō-an'ă-list). A psychotherapist, usually a psychiatrist or clinical psychologist, trained in psychoanalysis and employing its methods in the treatment of emotional disorders.

psy·cho·an·a·lyt·ic (sī'kō-an-ă-lit'ik). Pertaining to psychoanalysis.

psy·cho·au·di·to·ry (sī-kō-aw'di-tōr-ē). Relating to the mental perception and interpretation of sounds. SEE psychoacoustics. [psycho- + L. *auditorius*, relating to hearing]

psy·cho·bi·ol·o·gy (sī'kō-bī-ol'ō-jē). **1.** The study of the interrelationships of the biology and psychology in cognitive functioning, including intellectual, memory, and related neurocognitive processes. **2.** Adolf Meyer's term for psychiatry.

psy·cho·ca·thar·sis (sī'kō-kă-thar'sis). SYN catharsis (2).

psy·cho·chrome (sī'kō-krōm). A certain color mentally conceived in response to a sense impression. SEE ALSO psychochromesthesia. [psycho- + G. *chrōma*, color]

psy·cho·chro·mes·the·sia (sī'kō-krō-mes-thē'zē-ă). A form of synesthesia in which a certain stimulus to one of the special organs of sense produces the mental image of a color. SEE ALSO photism, color *taste*, pseudogeusesthesia. [psycho- + G. *chrōma*, color, + *aisthēsis*, sensation]

psy·cho·del·ic (sī'-kō-del-ik). A property of a drug or chemical which produces hallucinations or other bizarre aberrations in mental functioning. SYN hallucinogenic.

psy·cho·di·ag·no·sis (sī'kō-dī-ag-nō'sis). **1.** Any method used to discover the factors which underlie behavior, especially malajusted or abnormal behavior. **2.** A subspecialty within clinical psychology that emphasizes the use of psychological tests and techniques for assessing psychopathology.

Psy·chod·i·dae (sī-kod'i-dē). A family of small flies or gnats characterized by hairy mothlike body and the presence of 7 to 11 long parallel wing veins lacking cross-veins; includes the sandflies, *Phlebotomus* and *Lutzomyia*, vectors of all known forms of leishmaniasis. [G. *Psychē*, a Greek nymph, sometimes represented as a butterfly]

psy·cho·dom·e·try (sī-kō-dom'ĕ-trē). The measurement of the rapidity of mental action. [psycho- + G. *hodos*, way, + *metron*, measure]

psy·cho·dra·ma (sī'kō-drah-mā). A method of psychotherapy in which patients act out their personal problems by spontaneously enacting without rehearsal diagnostically specific roles in dramatic performances put on before their patient peers.

psy·cho·dy·nam·ics (sī'kō-dī-nam'iks). The systematized study and theory of the psychological forces that underlie human behavior, emphasizing the interplay between unconscious and conscious motivation and the functional significance of emotion. SEE role-playing. [psycho- + G. *dynamis*, force]

psy·cho·en·do·cri·nol·o·gy (sī'kō-en'dō-krĭ-nol'ō-jē). Study of the interrelationships between endocrine function and mental states.

psy·cho·ex·plor·a·tion (sī'kō-eks-plōr-ā'shŭn). Study of the attitudes and emotional life of a person.

psy·cho·gal·van·ic (sī'kō-gal-van'ik). Relating to changes in electric properties of the skin; *e.g.,* a change in skin resistance induced by psychologic stimulus.

psy·cho·gal·va·nom·e·ter (sī'kō-gal-vă-nom'ĕ-ter). A galvanometer that records changes in skin resistance related to emotional stress.

psy·cho·gen·der (sī-kō-jen'der). The attitudes adopted by an individual related to his or her personal identification as either a male or a female. SEE ALSO gender *role.*

psy·cho·gen·e·sis (sī-kō-jen'ĕ-sis). The origin and development of the psychic processes including mental, behavioral, emotional, personality, and related psychological processes. SYN psychogeny. [psycho- + G. *genesis*, origin]

psy·cho·gen·ic, psy·cho·ge·net·ic (sī'kō-jen'ik, -jĕ-net'ik). **1.** Of mental origin or causation. **2.** Relating to emotional and related psychological development or to psychogenesis.

psy·chog·e·ny (sī-koj'ĕ-nē). SYN psychogenesis.

psy·cho·geu·sic (sī-kō-gū'sik). Pertaining to the mental perception and interpretation of taste. [psycho- + G. *geusis*, taste]

psy·cho·gog·ic (sī-kō-goj'ik). Acting as a stimulant to the emotions. [psycho- + G. *agōgos*, a leading away]

psy·cho·graph·ic (sī-kō-graf'ik). Relating to psychography.

psy·chog·ra·phy (sī-kog'ră-fē). The literary characterization of an individual, real or fictional, that uses psychoanalytical and psychological categories and theories; a psychological biography or character description. [psycho- + G. *graphē*, a writing]

psy·cho·his·to·ry (sī-kō-his'tōr-ē). The combined use of psychology (especially psychoanalysis) and history in the writing, especially of biography, as in the work of Erik Erikson. SEE ALSO psychography.

psy·cho·ki·ne·sis, psy·cho·ki·ne·sia (sī'kō-ki-nē'sis, -nē'zē-ă). **1.** The influence of mind upon matter, as the use of mental "power" to move or distort an object. **2.** Impulsive behavior. [psycho- + G. *kinēsis*, movement]

psy·cho·kym (sī'kō-kīm). Rarely used term for the physiologic substrate of psychic processes. [psycho- + G. *kyma*, wave]

synopsis of three great psychological theories			
	psychoanalysis (depth psychology)	behaviorism	cognitive psychology
central area of research	unconscious drives and content of the unconscious	external behavior (reactions, reflexes)	consciousness
determining factors of behavior	(unconscious) complexes, fixations	environmental conditions (stimulus, reinforcement)	structrues of consciousness
image of the human being	human being is a prisoner of drives	freedom and reason are pre-scientific concepts; human behavior is completely determined by the environment and its stimuli	humans possess insight and foresight and thereby have responsibility and freedom of choice
preferred method of research	search for symbolic contents of the unconscious in speech and nonlinguistic expression	assessment of stimuli and reactions	open questioning
preferred method of treatment	enlightenment about traumas, complexes, and suppressions	behavior modification through planning of stimuli and reinforcement	counsel, assistance toward self-reflexion and self-control

psy·cho·lag·ny (sī-kō-lag'nē). Rarely used term for sexual excitement and satisfaction from mental imagery. [psycho- + G. *lagneia,* lust]

psy·cho·lep·sy (sī'kō-lep-sē). Rarely used term for sudden mood changes accompanied by feelings of hopelessness and inertia. [psycho- + G. *lēpsis,* seizure]

psy·cho·lin·guis·tics (sī'kō-ling-gwi'stiks). Study of a host of psychological factors associated with speech, including voice, attitudes, emotions, and grammatical rules, that affect communication and understanding of language. [psycho- + L. *lingua,* tongue]

psy·cho·log·ic, psy·cho·log·i·cal (sī-kō-loj'ik, -loj'i-kăl). **1.** Relating to psychology. **2.** Relating to the mind and its processes. SEE psychology.

psy·chol·o·gist (sī-kol'ō-jist). A specialist in psychology licensed to practice professional psychology (*e.g.,* clinical p.), or qualified to teach psychology as a scholarly discipline (academic p.), or whose scientific specialty is a subfield of psychology (research p.).

psy·chol·o·gy (Ψ) (sī-kol'ō-jē). The profession (*e.g.,* clinical p.), scholarly discipline (academic p.), and science (research p.) concerned with the behavior of humans and animals, and related mental and physiological processes. [psycho- + G. *logos,* study]

adlerian p., SYN individual p.

analytical p., SYN jungian *psychoanalysis.*

animal p., a branch of p. concerned with the study of the behavior and physiological responses of animal organisms as a means of understanding human behavior; some synonyms include comparative psychology, experimental psychology, and physiological psychology.

atomistic p., any psychologic system based on the doctrine that mental processes are built up through the combination of simple elements; *e.g.,* psychoanalysis, behaviorism.

behavioral p., SYN behaviorism.

behavioristic p., a branch of psychology that uses behavioral approaches such as desensitization and flooding in contrast to counseling and other psychodynamic approaches to the treatment of psychological disorders. SEE ALSO behavior *therapy.*

child p., a branch of p. the theories and applications of which focus on the cognitive and intellectual development of the child in contrast to the adult; subspecialties include developmental psychology, child clinical psychology, pediatric psychology, and pediatric neuropsychology.

clinical p., a branch of p. that specializes in both discovering new knowledge and in applying the art and science of p. to persons with emotional or behavioral disorders; subspecialties include clinical child p. and pediatric p.

cognitive p., a branch of p. that attempts to integrate into a whole the disparate knowledge from the subfields of perception, learning, memory, intelligence, and thinking.

community p., the application of p. to community programs, *e.g.,* in the schools, correctional and welfare systems, and community mental health centers.

comparative p., a branch of p. concerned with the study and comparison of the behavior of organisms at different levels of phylogenic development to discover developmental trends.

constitutional p., the p. of the individual as related to body habitus.

counseling p., p. with emphasis on facilitating the normal development and growth of the individual in coping with important problems of everyday living, as initally contrasted with clinical p.

criminal p., the study of the mind and its workings in relation to crime. SEE forensic p.

depth p., the p. of the unconscious, especially in contrast with older (19th century) academic p. dealing only with conscious mentation; sometimes used synonymously with psychoanalysis.

developmental p., the study of the psychological, physiological, and behavioral changes in an organism that occur from birth to old age.

dynamic p., a psychologic approach that concerns itself with the causes of behavior.

educational p., the application of p. to education, especially to problems of teaching and learning.

environmental p., the study and application by behavioral scientists and architects of how changes in physical space and related physical stimuli impact upon the behavior of individuals. SEE ALSO personal *space.*

existential p., a theory of p., based on the philosophies of phenomenology and existentialism, which holds that the proper study of p. is an individual's experience of the sequence, spatiality, and organization of his or her existence in the world.

experimental p., (1) a subdiscipline within the science of p. that is concerned with the study of conditioning, learning, perception, motivation, emotion, language, and thinking; **(2)** also used in relation to subject-matter areas in which experimental, in contrast to correlational or socio-experiential, methods are emphasized.

forensic p., the application of p. to legal matters in a court of law.

genetic p., a science dealing with the evolution of behavior and the relation to each other of the different types of mental activity.

gestalt p., SEE gestaltism.

health p., the aggregate of the specific educational, scientific, and professional contributions of the discipline of p. to the promotion and maintenance of health, the prevention and treatment of illness, the identification of etiologic and diagnostic correlates of health, illness, and related dysfunction, and the analysis and improvement of the health care system.

holistic p., any psychologic system which postulates that the human mind or any mental process must be studied as a unit; *e.g.,* gestaltism, existential p.

humanistic p., an existential approach to psychology which emphasizes humans' uniqueness, subjectivity, and capacity for psychological growth.

individual p., a theory of human behavior emphasizing humans' social nature, strivings for mastery, and drive to overcome, by compensation, feelings of inferiority. SYN adlerian psychoanalysis, adlerian p.

industrial p., the application of the principles of p. to problems in business and industry.

medical p., the branch of p. concerned with the application of psychologic principles to the practice of medicine; the application of clinical p. or clinical health p., usually in a hospital setting.

objective p., p. as studied by observation of the behavior and mental functions in others.

subjective p., the study of one's own mind and its various modes of action as a basis for psychologic deductions.

psy·cho·met·rics (sī-kō-met′riks). SYN psychometry.

psy·chom·e·try (sī-kom′ĕ-trē). The discipline pertaining to psychological and mental testing, and to any quantitative analysis of an individual's psychological traits or attitudes or mental processes. SYN psychometrics. [psycho- + G. *metron,* measure]

psy·cho·mo·tor (sī-kō-mō′ter). **1.** Relating to the psychological processes associated with muscular movement, and to the production of voluntary movements. **2.** Relating to the combination of psychic and motor events, including disturbances. [psycho- + L. *motor,* mover]

psy·cho·neu·ro·im·mun·o·logy (sī′kō-nū-rō-im′yū- nol′ō-jē). An area of study that focuses on emotional and other psychological states that affect the immune system, rendering the individual more susceptible to disease or the course of a disease. [psycho- + neuro- + immunology]

psy·cho·neu·ro·sis (sī′kō-nū-rō′sis). **1.** A mental or behavioral disorder of mild or moderate severity. **2.** Formerly a classification of neurosis that included hysteria, psychasthenia, neurasthenia, and the anxiety and phobic disorders. [psycho- + G. *neuron,* nerve, + *-osis,* condition]

p. mai′dica, SYN pellagra.

psy·cho·neu·rot·ic (sī′kō-nū-rot′ik). Pertaining to or suffering from psychoneurosis.

psy·cho·nom·ic (sī-kō-nom′ik). Relating to psychonomy.

psy·chon·o·my (sī-kon′ō-mē). A rarely used term referring to the branch of psychology concerned with the laws of behavior. [psycho- + G. *nomos,* law]

psy·cho·no·sol·o·gy (sī′kō-nō-sol′ō-jē). The classification of mental illnesses and behavioral disorders. SYN psychiatric nosology. [psycho- + G. *nosos,* disease, + *logos,* study]

psy·cho·nox·ious (sī-kō-nok′shŭs). Rarely used term for: **1.** Having an unfavorable effect on the emotional life and reactions mediated by higher levels of the central nervous system; may be endogenous or exogenous. **2.** Denoting persons or situations that elicit fear, pain, anxiety, or anger in an individual. [psycho- + L. *noxius,* harmful]

psy·cho·-on·col·o·gy (sī-kō-ong-kol′ō-jē). The psychological aspects of the treatment and management of the patient with cancer; it combines elements of psychiatry, psychology, and medicine with special concern for the psychosocial needs of the patient and his/her family.

psy·cho·path (sī′kō-path). Former designation for an individual with an antisocial type of personality disorder. SEE ALSO antisocial *personality,* sociopath. [psycho- + G. *pathos,* disease]

psy·cho·path·ic (sī-kō-path′ik). Relating to or characteristic of psychopathy.

psy·chop·a·thist (sī-kop′ă-thist). Obsolete term for psychiatrist.

psy·cho·pa·thol·o·gist (sī′kō-pă-thol′ō-jist). One who specializes in psychopathology.

psy·cho·pa·thol·o·gy (sī′kō-pă-thol′ō-jē). **1.** The science concerned with the pathology of the mind and behavior. **2.** The science of mental and behavioral disorders, including psychiatry and abnormal psychology. [psycho- + G. *pathos,* disease, + *logos,* study]

psy·chop·a·thy (sī-kop′ă-thē). Obsolete and inexact term referring to a pattern of antisocial or manipulative behavior engaged in by a psychopath. SEE ALSO personality *disorder.* [psycho- + G. *pathos,* disease]

psy·cho·phar·ma·ceu·ti·cals (sī′kō-far-mă-sū′ti-kălz). Drugs used in the treatment of emotional disorders.

psy·cho·phar·ma·col·o·gy (sī′kō-far′mă-kol′ō-jē). **1.** The use of drugs to treat mental and psychological disorders. **2.** The science of drug-behavior relationships. SYN neuropsychopharmacology. [psycho- + G. *pharmakon,* drug, + *logos,* study]

With the explosive advance of brain science since 1970 has come understanding of the role neurotransmitters play in emotion, mood, and psychological states and of how errors in the production or uptake of these chemicals may cause or contribute to neurological disease and mental illness. Using radionuclide-tagged molecules as probes, neurochemists have identified the major neural pathways and functions of many neurotransmitters, more than 60 of which are currently known. Building on this knowledge, neuropsychopharmacologists have succeeded in designing potent new psychoactive drugs. Most successful to date have been those for treating psychoses, obsessive-compulsive disorders, anxiety states, and clinical depression. The new drugs have underscored the biological bases of mental disorders, at once bolstering modern materialistic theories that hold that all mental states are a function of brain activity, and undercutting Cartesian dualism, which argues that the mind originates from nonmaterialistic sources.

psy·cho·phys·i·cal (sī-kō-fiz′i-kăl). **1.** Relating to the mental perception of physical stimuli. SEE psychophysics. **2.** SYN psychosomatic.

psy·cho·phys·ics (sī-kō-fiz′iks). The science of the relation between the physical attributes of a stimulus and the measured, quantitative attributes of the mental perception of that stimulus (*e.g.,* the relationship between changes in decibel level and the corresponding changes in the human's perception of the sound).

psy·cho·phys·i·o·log·ic (sī′kō-fiz-ē-ō-loj′ik). **1.** Pertaining to psychophysiology. **2.** Denoting a so-called psychosomatic illness. **3.** Denoting a somatic disorder with significant emotional or psychological etiology.

psy·cho·phys·i·ol·o·gy (sī′kō-fiz-ē-ol′ō-jē). The science of the relation between psychological and physiological processes; *e.g.,* conscious elements of autonomic nervous system activity activated by emotion.

psy·cho·pro·phy·lax·is (sī′kō-prō-fi-lak′sis). Psychotherapy directed toward the prevention of emotional disorders and the maintenance of mental health. [psycho- + prophylaxis]

psy·cho·re·lax·a·tion (sī′kō-rē-lak-sā′shŭn). A method of treating anxiety and tension by practicing general bodily relaxation, as in systematic desensitization.

psy·chor·mic (sī-kōr′mik). SYN psychostimulant. [psycho- + G. *hormaō,* to set in motion]

psy·chor·rhea (sī-kō-rē′ă). Rarely used term for a psychiatric syndrome characterized by incoherent and strange philosophical theories; a manifestation of schizophrenia. [psycho- + G. *rhoia,* flow]

psy·chor·rhyth·mia, psy·cho·rhyth·mia (sī-kō-rith′mē-ă). Rarely used term for an involuntary repetition of formerly voluntary acts. [psycho- + G. *rhythmos,* rhythm]

psy·cho·sen·so·ry, psy·cho·sen·so·ri·al (sī′kō-sen′sōr-ē, -sen-sōr′ē-ăl). **1.** Denoting the mental perception and interpretation of sensory stimuli. **2.** Denoting a hallucination which by effort the mind is able to distinguish from reality.

psy·cho·sex·u·al (sī-kō-sek′shū-ăl). Pertaining to the relation-

psychopharmacology	
I. psychotropic agents in the broad sense	
1. hypnotics	
2. sedatives	
3. anticonvulsants	
4. psychostimulants	
II. psychotropic agents in the narrow sense	
1. neuroleptics	nonsedating tranquilizers, non-hypnotic calming agents with antipsychotic/antischizophrenic effect
2. tranquilizers	nonsedating tranquilizers without antipsychotic/antischizophrenic effect
3. antidepressants	psychotropic agents with antidepressant effect
thymoleptics	antidepressants, predominantly mood elevating
thymoeretics	antidepressants, predominantly inhibition reducing
III. psychotropic agents with psychotomimetic effect	
psycholytics	drugs that elicit experimental psychoses, which can also be used as an aid in therapy

ships among the emotional, mental physiologic, and behavioral components of sex or sexual development.

psy·cho·sine (sī'kō-sēn). Galactosylsphingosine, a constituent of cerebrosides, formed from UDPgalactose and sphingosine by UDPgalactose-sphingosine β-D-galactosyltransferase.

psy·cho·sis, pl. **psy·cho·ses** (sī-kō'sis, -sēz). **1.** A mental and behavioral disorder causing gross distortion or disorganization of a person's mental capacity, affective response, and capacity to recognize reality, communicate, and relate to others to the degree of interfering with the person's capacity to cope with the ordinary demands of everyday life. The psychoses are divided into two major classifications according to their origins: 1) those associated with organic brain syndromes (*e.g.,* Korsakoff's syndrome); 2) those less strictly organic and having some functional component(s) (*e.g.,* the schizophrenias, bipolar disorder). **2.** Generic term for any of the so-called insanities, the most common forms being the schizophrenias. **3.** A severe emotional and behavioral disorder. [G. an animating]

affective p., p. with predominant affective features. SYN manic p.

alcoholic psychoses, mental disorders that result from alcoholism and that involve organic brain damage, as in delirium tremens and Korsakoff's syndrome.

amnestic p., SYN Korsakoff's *syndrome.*

arteriosclerotic p., psychotic disturbance in elderly persons suffering from cerebral arteriosclerosis.

bipolar p., a mental disorder characterized by one or more episodes of mania (manic depression) which is usually accompanied by one or more episodes of depression (major depressive episode). SEE endogenous *depression,* manic-depressive.

Cheyne-Stokes p., a mental state characterized by anxiety and restlessness, accompanying Cheyne-Stokes respiration.

climacteric p., obsolete term for involutional p. associated with the climacteric.

depressive p., a major disorder of mood in which biologic factors are believed to play a prominent role. SEE depression.

drug p., p. following or precipitated by ingestion of a drug, *e.g.,* LSD.

dysmnesic p., SYN Korsakoff's *syndrome.*

exhaustion p., rarely used term for a confusional emotional state following an exhausting event.

febrile p., SYN infection-exhaustion p.

functional p., an obsolete term once used to denote schizophrenia and other severe mental disorders before modern science discovered a biological component to some aspects of each of the disorders.

gestational p., obsolete term for psychotic reaction with morbid depressive features associated with pregnancy. SEE postpartum p., puerperal p.

hysterical p., **(1)** a psychotic disturbance with predominantly hysterical symptoms; **(2)** a mental disorder resembling conversion hysteria but of psychotic severity; **(3)** a brief reactive p., often culture bound.

ICU p., psychotic episode(s), classically occurring in coronary care patients, occurring within 24 hours after entering the ICU in individuals with no previous history of p.; related to sleep deprivation, overstimulation in the ICU, and time spent on life support systems, and should be distinguished from exacerbation of a pre-existing p. or an organic p. such as delirium.

infection-exhaustion p., a p. following an acute infection, shock, or chronic intoxication; begins as delirium followed by pronounced mental confusion with hallucinations and unsystematized delusions, and sometimes stupor. SYN febrile p.

involutional p., obsolete term for mental disturbance occurring during the menopause or later life.

Korsakoff's p., SYN Korsakoff's *syndrome.*

manic-depressive p., SYN bipolar *disorder.*

manic p., SYN affective p. SEE bipolar *disorder.*

polyneuritic p., SYN Korsakoff's *syndrome.*

posthypnotic p., p. following or precipitated by hypnosis.

postinfectious p., psychotic disturbance following acute febrile disease such as pneumonia or typhoid fever.

postpartum p., an acute mental disorder with depression in the mother following childbirth. SYN puerperal p.

posttraumatic p., p. following trauma, especially to the head. Cf. traumatic p.

pseudo p., a condition resembling p.; may be a factitious or malingering disorder.

puerperal p., SYN postpartum p.

schizo-affective p., psychotic disturbance in which there is a mixture of schizophrenic and manic-depressive symptoms.

senile p., mental disturbance occurring in old age and related to degenerative cerebral processes.

situational p., a transitory but severe emotional disorder caused in a predisposed person by a seemingly unbearable situation.

toxic p., a p. caused by some toxic substance, whether endogenous or exogenous.

traumatic p., a p. resulting from physical injury or emotional shock. Cf. posttraumatic p.

Windigo p., Wittigo p., severe anxiety neurosis with special reference to food, manifested in melancholia, violence, and obsessive cannibalism, occurring among Canadian Indians.

psy·cho·so·cial (sī-kō-sō'shăl). Involving both psychological and social aspects; *e.g.,* age, education, marital and related aspects of a person's history.

psy·cho·so·mat·ic (sī'kō-sō-mat'ik). Pertaining to the influence of the mind or higher functions of the brain (emotions, fears, desires, etc.) upon the functions of the body, especially in relation to bodily disorders or disease. SEE psychophysiologic. SYN psychophysical (2). [psycho- + G. *sōma,* body]

psy·cho·so·mi·met·ic (sī-kō'sō-mi-met'ik). SYN psychotomimetic.

psy·cho·stim·u·lant (sī-kō-stim'yū-lant). An agent with antidepressant or mood-elevating properties. SYN psychormic.

psy·cho·sur·ger·y (sī-kō-ser'jer-ē). The treatment of mental disorders by operation upon the brain, *e.g.,* lobotomy.

psy·cho·syn·the·sis (sī-kō-sin'thĕ-sis). A lay movement, the opposite of psychoanalysis, stressing therapy aimed at restoring useful inhibitions and restoring the id to its rightful place in relation to the ego. [psycho- + synthesis]

psy·cho·tech·nics (sī-kō-tek′niks). Practical application of psychologic methods in the study of economics, sociology, and other subjects. [psycho- + G. *technē,* art, skill]

psy·cho·ther·a·peu·tic (sī′kō-thār-ă-pyū′tik). Relating to psychotherapy.

psy·cho·ther·a·peu·tics (sī′kō-thār-ă-pyū′tiks). SYN psychotherapy.

psy·cho·ther·a·pist (sī-kō-thār′ă-pist). A person, usually a psychiatrist or clinical psychologist, professionally trained and engaged in psychotherapy. Currently, the term is also applied to social workers, nurses, and others whose state licensing practice acts include psychotherapy.

psy·cho·ther·a·py (sī-kō-thār′ă-pē). Treatment of emotional, behavioral, personality, and psychiatric disorders based primarily upon verbal or nonverbal communication and interventions with the patient, in contrast to treatments utilizing chemical and physical measures. See entries under psychoanalysis; psychiatry; psychology; therapy. SYN psychotherapeutics. [psycho- + G. *therapeia,* treatment]

anaclitic p., a psychotherapeutic method characterized by encouragement and utilization of the patient's tendency to depend and lean upon the therapist as an authority figure; often contrasted with psychoanalytic therapy, which seeks to dissolve, rather than exploit, this phenomenon.

autonomous p., a type of psychoanalytic p. placing special emphasis on the value of the patient's self-determination in both the therapeutic situation and in real life.

brief p., any form of psychotherapy or counseling designed to produce emotional or behavioral therapeutic change within a minimal amount of time (generally not more than 20 sessions). Brief therapy is usually active and directive; it is more clearly indicated when there are clearly defined symptoms or problems, and where the goals are limited and specific.

contractual p., p. based on a firm agreement, or "contract," between therapist and patient as to the role of each in the therapeutic situation.

directive p., p. utilizing the authority of the therapist to direct the course of the patient's therapy, as contrasted with nondirective p.

dyadic p., a psychotherapeutic session involving only two persons, the therapist and the patient. Cf. group p. SYN individual therapy.

dynamic p., SYN psychoanalytic p.

existential p., a type of therapy, based on existential philosophy, emphasizing confrontation, primarily spontaneous interaction, and feeling experiences rather than rational thinking, with less attention given to patient resistances; the therapist is involved on the same level and to the same degree as the patient. SYN existential psychiatry.

group p., a type of psychological treatment involving several patients participating together in the presence of one or more psychotherapists who facilitate both emotional and rational cognitive interaction to effect uniquely targeted changes in the maladaptive behavior of the individual patient in his or her everyday interpersonal exchanges. See also entries under group.

heteronomous p., term embracing all forms of p. that foster the patient's dependence on others, especially dependence on the psychotherapist, in contrast to autonomous p.

hypnotic p., p. based on hypnosis.

intensive p., p. involving thorough exploration of the patient's life history, conflicts, and related psychodynamics; often contrasted with supportive p.

marathon group p., a type of group p. characterized by uninterrupted sessions for periods of hours or days, with minimal interruptions for food and rest.

nondirective p., p. in which the therapist follows the lead of the patient during the interview rather than introducing her or his own theories and directing the course of the interview. SEE ALSO client-centered *therapy.*

psychoanalytic p., p. utilizing freudian principles. SEE ALSO psychoanalysis. SYN dynamic p.

reconstructive p., a form of therapy, such as psychoanalysis,

that seeks not only to alleviate symptoms but also to produce alterations in maladaptive character structure and to expedite new adaptive potentials; this aim is achieved by bringing into consciousness an awareness of and insight into conflicts, fears, inhibitions, and their manifestations.

suggestive p., p. utilizing the influence and authority of the therapist. SEE ALSO directive p.

supportive p., p. aiming at bolstering the patient's psychological defenses and providing him or her reassurance, as in crisis intervention, rather than probing provocatively into his or her conflicts.

transactional p., p. with central emphasis on the actual day-to-day interactions (transactions) between the patient and other people in his life.

psy·chot·ic (sī-kot′ik). Relating to or affected by psychosis.

psy·chot·o·gen (sī-kot′ŏ-jen). A drug that produces psychotic manifestations. [psychotic + G. *-gen,* producing]

psy·chot·o·gen·ic (sī-kot-ō-jen′ik). Capable of inducing psychosis; particularly referring to drugs of the LSD series and similar substances.

psy·chot·o·mi·met·ic (sī-kot′ŏ-mi-met′ik). **1.** A drug or substance that produces psychological and behavioral changes resembling those of psychosis; *e.g.,* LSD. **2.** Denoting such a drug or substance. SYN psychosomimetic. [psychosis + G. *mimetikos,* imitative]

psy·cho·tro·pic (sī-kō-trop′ik). Capable of affecting the mind, emotions, and behavior; denoting drugs used in the treatment of mental illnesses. [psycho- + G. *tropē,* a turning]

⌂**psychro-.** Cold. SEE ALSO cryo-, crymo-. [G. *psychros*]

psy·chro·al·gia (sī-krō-al′jē-ă). A painful sensation of cold. [psychro- + G. *algos,* pain]

psy·chro·es·the·sia (sī′krō-es-thē′zē-ă). **1.** The form of sensation that perceives cold. **2.** A sensation of cold although the body is warm; a chill. [psychro- + G. *aisthēsis,* sensation]

psy·chrom·e·ter (sī-krom′ĕ-ter). A device for measuring the humidity of the atmosphere by the difference in temperature between two thermometers, the bulb of one kept moist, the other dry. Evaporation from the moist bulb lowers the reading of that thermometer; the greater the difference in readings, the drier the air; no difference indicates 100% relative humidity. SYN wet and dry bulb thermometer. [psychro- + G. *metron,* measure]

sling p., wet and dry bulb thermometers mounted on a hand sling, for use when a small portable psychrometer is required.

psy·chrom·e·try (sī-krom′ĕ-trē). The calculation of relative humidity and water vapor pressures from wet and dry bulb temperatures and barometric pressure; whereas relative humidity is the value ordinarily employed, the vapor pressure is the measurement of physiological significance. SYN hygrometry. [psychro- + G. *metron,* measure]

psy·chro·phile, psy·chro·phil (sī′krō-fīl). An organism which grows best at a low temperature (0 to 32°C; 32 to 86°F), with optimum growth occurring at 15 to 20°C (59 to 68°F). [psychro- + G. *phileō,* to love]

psy·chro·phil·ic (sī-krō-fil′ik). Pertaining to a psychrophile. [psychro- + G. *phileō,* to love]

psy·chro·pho·bia (sī-krō-fō′bē-ă). **1.** Extreme sensitivity to cold. **2.** A morbid dread of cold. [psychro- + G. *phobos,* fear]

⌂ **Combining forms**	[NA] Nomina Anatomica
Word*Finder*	[MIM] Mendelian
Multi-term entry finder	**Inheritance in Man**
Preceding letter A	
A.D.A.M. Anatomy Plates	☆ **Official alternate term**
Between letters L and M	
Appendices:	☆[NA] **Official alternate**
Following letter Z	**Nomina Anatomica term**
SYN Synonym; Cf., compare	**High Profile Term**

psy·chro·phore (sī'krō-fōr). A double catheter through which cold water is circulated to apply cold to the urethra or another canal or cavity. [psychro- + G. *phoros,* bearing]

psyl·li·um hy·dro·phil·ic mu·cil·loid (sil'ē-ŭm). SEE *plantago* seed.

psyl·li·um seed (sil'ē-ŭm). The cleaned, dried ripe seed of *Plantago indica* or of *P. ovata.* A mild cathartic that acts by absorbing water and providing indigestible mucilaginous bulk for the intestines. Must not be used in intestinal obstruction. SYN plantago seed, plantain seed.

PT Abbreviation for physical *therapy* or physical therapist; prothrombin *time.*

Pt Symbol for platinum.

PTA Abbreviation for plasma thromboplastin *antecedent*; phosphotungstic acid; percutaneous transluminal *angioplasty.*

PTAH Abbreviation for phosphotungstic acid *hematoxylin.*

ptar·mic (tar'mik). SYN sternutatory. [G. *ptarmikos,* causing to sneeze, fr. *ptarmos,* a sneezing]

ptar·mus (tar'mŭs). Sneezing. [G. *ptarmos,* a sneezing]

PTC Abbreviation for plasma thromboplastin *component*; phenylthiocarbamoyl.

PTCA Abbreviation for percutaneous transluminal coronary *angioplasty.*

Ptd Abbreviation for phosphatidyl.

PtdCho Abbreviation for phosphatidylcholine.

PtdEth Abbreviation for phosphatidylethanolamine.

PtdIns Abbreviation for phosphatidylinositol.

PtdIns(4,5)P₂. Symbol for *phosphatidylinositol* 4,5-bisphosphate.

PtdSer Abbreviation for phosphatidylserine.

PTE Abbreviation for pulmonary thromboembolism or pulmonary thromboendarterectomy.

PTEA Abbreviation for pulmonary thromboendarterectomy.

△**pter-, ptero-.** Combining form meaning wing; feather. [G. *pteron,* wing, feather]

pter·i·dine (ter'i-dēn, -din). Azinepurine; benzotetrazine; pyrazino[2,3-*d*]pyrimidine; a two-ring heterocyclic compound found as a component of pteroic acid and the pteroylglutamic acids (folic acids, pteropterin, etc.); simple p. derivatives (*e.g.,* xanthopterin, leucopterin) occur as pigments in butterfly wings, whence the name.

pter·in (ter'in). Term loosely used for any of the compounds containing pteridine; specifically, 2-amino-4-hydroxypteridine. Some pteridines (*e.g.,* xanthopterin, leucopterin) still retain the pterin root.

p. deaminase, an aminohydrolase catalyzing hydrolytic deamination of 2-amino-4-hydroxypteridine to form 2,4-dihydroxypteridine and ammonia.

pter·i·on (tē'rē-on). A craniometric point in the region of the sphenoid fontanelle, at the junction of the greater wing of the sphenoid, the squamous temporal, the frontal, and the parietal bones; it intersects the course of the anterior division of the middle meningeal artery. [G. *pteron,* wing]

pte·ro·ic ac·id (tě-rō'ik). A constituent of folic acid, containing *p*-aminobenzoic acid and pteridine linked by a –CH₂– group between the amino group of the former and C-6 of the latter.

pter·op·ter·in (ter-op'ter-in). pteroyl-γ-glutamyl-γ-glutamyl-glutamic acid; a folic acid conjugate, a principle chemically similar to folic acid except that it contains three molecules of glutamic acid instead of one, in γ linkage. SYN fermentation *Lactobacillus casei* factor, pteroyltriglutamic acid.

pter·o·yl·mon·o·glu·tam·ic ac·id (ter'ō-il-mon-ō'glū-tam'ik). SYN folic acid (2).

pter·o·yl·tri·glu·tam·ic ac·id (ter'ō-il-trī'glū-tam'ik). SYN pteropterin.

pte·ryg·i·um (tě-rij'ē-ŭm). **1.** A triangular patch of hypertrophied bulbar subconjunctival tissue, extending from the medial canthus to the border of the cornea or beyond, with apex pointing toward the pupil. SYN web eye. **2.** Forward growth of the cuticle over the nail plate, seen most commonly in lichen planus. SYN p.

unguis. **3.** An abnormal skin web. [G. *pterygion,* anything like a wing, a disease of the eye, dim. of *pteryx,* wing]

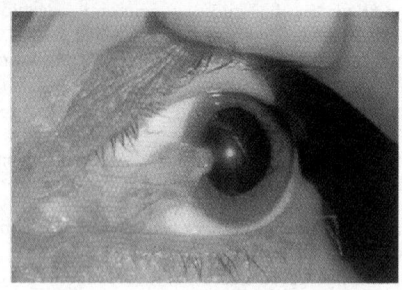

pterygium
vessels and tissue have grown from the conjunctiva over the edge of the cornea

p. col'li, a congenital, usually bilateral, web or tight band of skin of the neck extending from the acromion to the mastoid seen in Turner's syndrome and Noonan's syndrome.

p. un'guis, SYN pterygium (2).

△**pterygo-.** Wing-shaped, usually the pterygoid process. [G. *pteryx, pterygos,* wing]

pter·y·goid (ter'i-goyd). Wing-shaped; resembling a wing; a term applied to various anatomical parts relating to the sphenoid bone. [G. *pteryx* (*pteryg-*), wing, + *eidos,* resemblance]

pter·y·go·man·dib·u·lar (ter'i-gō-man-dib'yū-lăr). Relating to the pterygoid process and the mandible.

pte·ry·go·max·il·la·re (ter'i-gō-mak-si-lār'ē). The point where the pterygoid process of the sphenoid bone and the pterygoid process of the maxilla begin to form the pterygomaxillary fissure; the lowest point of the opening is used in cephalometrics.

pter·y·go·max·il·lary (ter'i-gō-mak'si-lār-ē). Relating to the pterygoid process and the maxilla.

pter·y·go·pal·a·tine (ter'i-gō-pal'ă-tīn). Relating to the pterygoid process and the palatine bone.

pter·y·go·qua·drate (ter'i-gō-kwah'drāt). Relating to the pterygoid and quadrate bones in the upper jaw of lower vertebrates.

PTF Abbreviation for plasma thromboplastin *factor.*

PTH Abbreviation for parathyroid *hormone*; phenylthiohydantoin.

PTHC Abbreviation for *percutaneous* transhepatic cholangiography.

pthi·ri·a·sis (thī-rī'a-sis). SYN *pediculosis* pubis. [G. *phtheiriasis,* fr. *phtheir,* a louse]

p. cap'itis, SYN *pediculosis* capitis.

p. cor'poris, SYN *pediculosis* corporis.

p. pu'bis, presence of crab lice in the pubis and other hairy areas of the trunk, and in the eyelashes of infants and young children.

Pthir·us (thī'rŭs). A genus of lice (family Pediculidae) formerly grouped in the genus *Pediculus.* The main species is *P. pubis* (*Pediculus pubis*), the crab or pubic louse, a parasite that infests the pubis and neighboring hairy parts of the body. Often incorrectly spelled *Phthirus* or *Phthirius.* [irreg. fr. G. *phtheir,* louse]

PTMA Abbreviation for phenyltrimethylammonium.

pto·maine (tō'mān). An indefinite term applied to poisonous substances, *e.g.,* toxic amines, formed in the decomposition of protein by the decarboxylation of amino acids by bacterial action. SYN ptomatine. [G. *ptōma,* a corpse]

pto·mai·ne·mia (tō-mā-nē'mē-ă). A condition resulting from the presence of a ptomaine in the circulating blood. [ptomaine + G. *haima,* blood]

pto·ma·tine (tō'mă-tēn). SYN ptomaine.

pto·mat·ro·pine (tō-mat'rō-pēn). A ptomaine characterized by poisonous properties similar to those of atropine; formed by the action of bacteria in the decarboxylation of amino acids.

ptosed (tōzd). SYN ptotic.

pto·sis, pl. **pto·ses** (tō′sis, tō′sēz). **1.** A sinking down or prolapse of an organ. **2.** SYN blepharoptosis. [G. *ptōsis*, a falling]

p. adipo′sa, SYN blepharochalasis.

p. sympathet′ica, SYN Horner's *syndrome*.

-ptosis. A sinking down or prolapse of an organ. 2. Blepharoptosis. [G. *ptōsis*, a falling]

pto·tic (tot′ik). Relating to or marked by ptosis. SYN ptosed.

6-PTS Abbreviation for 6-pyruvoyltetrahydropterin synthase.

PTT Abbreviation for partial thromboplastin *time*.

PTU Abbreviation for propylthiouracil.

ptyal-, ptyalo-. The salivary glands, saliva. SEE ALSO sialo-. [G. *ptyalon*]

pty·al·a·gogue (tī-al′ă-gog). SYN sialagogue.

pty·a·lec·ta·sis (tī′ă-lek′tă-sis). SYN sialectasis. [ptyal- + G. *ektasis*, a stretching out]

pty·a·lin (tī′ă-lin). SYN α-amylase.

pty·a·lism (tī′al-izm). SYN sialism. [G. *ptyalismos*, spitting]

pty·a·lo·cele (tī′ă-lō-sēl). SYN ranula (2).

pty·a·log·ra·phy (tī-ă-log′ră-fē). SYN sialography.

pty·a·lo·lith (tī′ă-lō-lith). SYN sialolith.

pty·a·lo·li·thi·a·sis (tī′ă-lō-li-thī′ă-sis). SYN sialolithiasis.

pty·a·lo·li·thot·o·my (tī′ă-lō-li-thot′ō-mē). SYN sialolithotomy.

pty·cho·tis oil (tī-kō′tis). SYN ajowan oil.

pty·oc·ri·nous (tī-ok′ri-nŭs). Secreting by discharge of the contents of the cell, as in mucous cells. [G. *ptyō*, to spit out, + *krinō*, to separate]

Pu Symbol for plutonium.

pu·bar·che (pyū-bar′kē). Onset of puberty, particularly as manifested by the appearance of pubic hair. [puberty + G. *archē*, beginning]

pu·ber·al, pu·ber·tal (pyū′ber-ăl, -ber-tăl). Relating to puberty.

pu·ber·tas prae·cox (pyū′ber-tahs prē′koks). SYN precocious *puberty*. [L.]

pu·ber·ty (pyū′ber-tē). Sequence of events by which a child becomes a young adult, characterized by the beginning of gametogenesis, secretion of gonadal hormones, development of secondary sexual characters and reproductive functions; sexual dimorphism is accentuated. In girls, the first signs of p. may be evident at age 8 with the process largely completed by age 16; in boys, p. commonly begins at ages 10 to 12 and is largely completed by age 18. Ethnic and geographical factors may influence the time at which various events typical of p. occur. In law, the ages of presumptive puberty are 12 years in girls and 14 years in boys. [L. *pubertas*, fr. *puber*, grown up]

precocious p., condition in which pubertal changes begin at an unexpectedly early age; often the result of a pathological process involving a gland capable of secreting estrogens or androgens, *e.g.*, the ovary or the adrenal cortex. SYN pubertas praecox.

pu·bes (pyū′bis). **1.** The anteroinferior portion of the hip bone, distinct at birth but later becoming fused with the ilium and ischium; it is composed of a body which articulates with its fellow at the symphysis pubis, and two rami; the superior ramus enters into the formation of the acetabulum, the inferior ramus fuses with the ramus of the ischium to form the ischiopubic ramus. **2** [NA]. One of the pubic hairs; the hair of the pubic region just above the external genitals. **3.** SYN *mons* pubis. [L. *pubes*, the hair on the genitals; the genitals]

pu·bes·cence (pyū-bes′ens). **1.** The approach of the age of puberty or sexual maturity. [L. *pubesco*, to attain puberty] **2.** Presence of downy or fine, short hair. [L. *pubes*, pubic hair]

pu·bes·cent (pyū-bes′ent). Pertaining to pubescence.

pu·bic (pyū′bik). Relating to the os pubis.

pu·bi·ot·o·my (pyū-bē-ot′ō-mē). Severance of the pubic bone a few centimeters lateral to the symphysis, in order to increase the capacity of a contracted pelvis sufficiently to permit the passage of a living child. SYN Gigli's operation, pelviotomy (2), pelvitomy. [L. *pubis*, pubic bone, + G. *tomē*, incision]

Pub·lic Health Ser·vice (PHS). SEE United States Public Health Service.

pubo-. Pubic, pubis. [L. *pubes*]

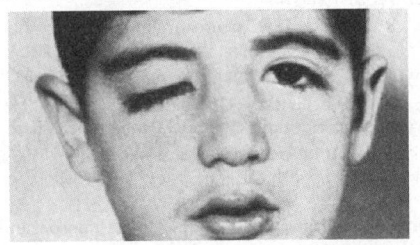
congenital ptosis (blepharoptosis)

temporal sequence of events in puberty		
age in years	girls	boys
9–10	widening of pelvis, rounding of hips, adrenarche	
11	thelarche, pubarche	adrenarche
12	gonadarche, peak of growth spurt	
13	menarche, axillary hair	gonadarche, enlargement of testes
14		peak of growth spurt, gynecomastia of puberty
15	regular menstruation, with ovulation	voice change, axillary hair, beard growth
16–17	cessation of long-bone growth	male pubic hair, more bodily hair
18–19		cessation of long-bone growth

pu·bo·cap·su·lar (pyū′bō-kap′sū-lăr). Relating to the pubis and the capsule of the hip joint.

pu·bo·coc·cy·ge·al (pyū-bō-kok-sij′ē-ăl). Relating to the pubis and the coccyx.

pu·bo·fem·o·ral (pyū′bō-fem′ŏ-răl). Relating to the os pubis and the femur.

pu·bo·ma·de·sis (pyū′bō-mă-dē′sis). SYN pubic *baldness*. [L. *pubes*, pubic hair, + G. *madesis*, baldness]

pu·bo·pros·tat·ic (pyū′bō-pros-tat′ik). Relating to the pubic bone and the prostate.

pu·bo·rec·tal (pyū′bō-rek′tăl). Relating to the pubis and the rectum.

pu·bo·ves·i·cal (pyū′bō-ves′i-kăl). Relating to the pubic bone and the bladder.

Puchtler-Sweat stains. SEE Puchtler-Sweat *stain* for basement membranes, Puchtler-Sweat *stain* for hemoglobin and hemosiderin.

pu·den·da (pyū-den′dă). Plural of pudendum. [L.]

pu·den·dal (pyū-den′dăl). Relating to the external genitals. SYN pudic.

pu·den·dum, pl. **pu·den·da** (pyū-den′dŭm, -dă). The external genitals, especially the female genitals (vulva). Used also in the plural. [L. ntr. of *pudendus*, particip. adj. of *pudeo*, to feel ashamed]

p. femini′num [NA], SYN vulva.

p. mulieb′re, SYN vulva.

Pudenz, Robert H., U.S. neurosurgeon, *1911. SEE Heyer-P. *valve.*

pu·dic (pyū′dik). SYN pudendal. [L. *pudicus,* modest]

Pud·lak, P., 20th century Czech physician. SEE Hermansky-Pudlak *syndrome;* Hermansky-P. *syndrome* type VI.

pu·er·pera, pl. **pu·er·per·ae** (pyū-er′per-ă, -per-ē). A woman who has just given birth. [L., fr. *puer,* child, + *pario,* to bring forth]

pu·er·per·al (pyū-er′per-ăl). Relating to the puerperium, or period after childbirth. SYN puerperant (1).

pu·er·per·ant (pyū-er′per-ant). **1.** SYN puerperal. **2.** A puerpera.

pu·er·pe·ri·um, pl. **pu·er·pe·ria** (pyū-er-pēr′ē-ŭm, -ē-ă). Period from the termination of labor to complete involution of the uterus, usually defined as 42 days. [L. childbirth, fr. *puer,* child, + *pario,* to bring forth]

Puestow, Charles B., U.S. surgeon, 1902–1973. SEE P. *procedure.*

puff (pŭf). A short blowing sound heard on auscultation, usually a systolic murmur heard over the heart. SEE ALSO *chromosome* puffs.

veiled p., a faint pulmonary murmur, simulating the muffled flapping of a cloth in the wind.

puff·ball (pŭf′bawl). SYN *Lycoperdon.*

Pu·lex (pyū′leks). A genus of fleas (family Pulicidae, order Siphonaptera). [L. flea]

P. che′opis, former name for *Xenopsylla cheopis.*

P. fascia′tus, former name for *Nosopsyllus fasciatus.*

P. ir′ritans, the human flea, a common flea that infests humans, many domestic animals (especially swine), and wild mammals and birds; a poor vector of plague.

P. pen′etrans, incorrect name for *Tunga penetrans.*

P. serra′ticeps, former name for *Ctenocephalides canis.*

pu·lic·i·cide, pu·li·cide (pyū-lis′i-sīd, pyū′li-sīd). A chemical agent destructive to fleas. [L. *pulex (pulic-),* flea, + *caedo,* to kill]

pul·ley (pŭl′ē). SEE trochlea.

annular p., SYN annular *part* of fibrous digital sheath.

cruciform p., SYN cruciform *part* of fibrous digital sheath.

p. of humerus, SYN *trochlea* of humerus.

muscular p., a fibrous loop through which the tendon of a muscle passes; the intermediate tendon of the digastric and omohyoid muscles pass through such a p. SYN trochlea muscularis [NA].

peroneal p., SYN peroneal *trochlea* of calcaneus.

p. of talus, SYN *trochlea* of the talus.

pul·lu·la·nase (pul′yŭ-lă-nās). SYN α-dextrin endo-1,6-α-glucosidase.

pul·lu·late (pŭl′yū-lāt). To undergo pullulation.

pul·lu·la·tion (pŭl-yū-lā′shŭn). The act of sprouting, or of budding as seen in yeast. [L. *pullulo,* pp. *-atus,* to sprout forth]

pul·mo, gen. **pul·mo·nis,** pl. **pul·mo·nes** (pŭl′mō, pŭl-mō′nis, -mō′nēz) [NA]. SYN lung. [L.]

p. dex′ter [NA], right lung.

p. sinis′ter [NA], left lung.

⌂**pulmo-, pulmon-, pulmono-.** The lungs. SEE ALSO pneum-, pneumo-. [L. *pulmo,* lung]

pul·mo·a·or·tic (pŭl′mō-ā-ōr′tik). Relating to the pulmonary artery and the aorta.

pul·mo·lith (pŭl′mō-lith). SYN pneumolith. [L. *pulmo,* long, + G. *lithos,* stone]

pul·mom·e·ter (pŭl-mom′ĕ-ter). Obsolete term for spirometer. [L. *pulmo,* lung, + G. *metron,* measure]

pul·mom·e·try (pŭl-mom′ĕ-trē). Obsolete term for spirometry.

pul·mo·nary (pŭl′mō-nār-ē). Relating to the lungs, to the pulmonary artery, or to the aperture leading from the right ventricle into the pulmonary artery. SYN pneumonic (1), pulmonic (1). [L. *pulmonarius,* fr. *pulmo,* lung]

pul·mo·nec·to·my (pŭl-mō-nek′tō-mē). SYN pneumonectomy. [L. *pulmo (pulmon-),* lung, + G. *ektomē,* excision]

pul·mon·ic (pŭl-mon′ik). **1.** SYN pulmonary. **2.** Obsolete term for a remedy for diseases of the lungs.

pul·mo·ni·tis (pŭl-mō-nī′tis). SYN pneumonitis.

pul·mo·tor (pŭl′mō-ter). A medically obsolete term still used occasionally by lay personnel to refer to volume-limited or, more rarely, pressure-limited devices for the rhythmical inflation of lungs during resuscitation outside of hospitals. [L. *pulmo,* lung, + motor]

pulp (pŭlp). **1.** A soft, moist, coherent solid. SYN pulpa [NA]. **2.** SYN dental p. **3.** SYN chyme. [L. *pulpa,* flesh]

coronal p., that portion of the dental p. contained within the pulp chamber or crown cavity of the tooth. SYN pulpa coronalis [NA].

dead p., SYN necrotic p.

dental p., dentinal p., the soft tissue within the pulp cavity, consisting of connective tissue containing blood vessels, nerves and lymphatics, and at the periphery a layer of odontoblasts capable of internal repair of the dentin. SYN pulpa dentis [NA], pulp (2), tooth p.

digital p., SYN p. of finger.

enamel p., a layer of stellate cells in the enamel organ.

exposed p., p. that has been exposed or laid bare by a pathologic process, trauma, or a dental instrument.

p. of finger, the fleshy mass at the extremity of the finger. SYN digital p.

mummified p., a misnomer for a p. treated with a formaldehyde derivative.

necrotic p., necrosis of the dental p. which clinically does not respond to thermal stimulation; the tooth may be asymptomatic or sensitive to percussion and palpation. SYN dead p., nonvital p.

nonvital p., SYN necrotic p.

putrescent p., a decomposed p., often infected.

radicular p., that part of the dental p. contained within the apical or root portion of the tooth. SYN pulpa radicularis [NA].

red p., splenic p. seen grossly as a reddish brown substance, due to its abundance of red blood cells, consisting of splenic sinuses and the tissue intervening between them (splenic cords).

splenic p., the soft cellular substance of the spleen. SYN pulpa splenica [NA], pulpa lienis.

tooth p., SYN dental p.

vertebral p., SYN *nucleus* pulposus.

vital p., a p. composed of viable tissue, either normal or diseased, that responds to electric stimuli and to heat and cold.

white p., that part of the spleen that consists of nodules and other lymphatic concentrations.

pul·pa (pŭl′pă) [NA]. SYN pulp (1). [L. pulp]

p. corona′lis [NA], SYN coronal *pulp.*

p. den′tis [NA], SYN dental *pulp.*

p. lie′nis, SYN splenic *pulp.*

p. radicula′ris [NA], SYN radicular *pulp.*

p. splen′ica [NA], SYN splenic *pulp.* SEE ALSO red *pulp,* white *pulp.*

pul·pal (pŭl′păl). Relating to the pulp.

pul·pal·gia (pŭl-pal′jē-ă). Pain arising from the dental pulp. [L. *pulpa,* pulp, + G. *algos,* pain]

pul·pa·tion (pŭl-pā′shŭn). Obsolete term for pulpifaction.

pulp·ec·to·my (pŭl-pek′tō-mē). Removal of the entire pulp structure of a tooth, including the pulp tissue in the roots. [L. *pulpa,* pulp, + G. *ektomē,* excision]

pul·pi·fac·tion (pŭl-pi-fak′shŭn). Reduction to a pulpy condition. [L. *pulpa,* pulp, + *facio,* pp. *factus,* to make]

pulp·i·form (pŭl′pi-fōrm). Resembling pulp; pulpy.

pulp·i·fy (pŭl′pi-fī). To reduce to a pulpy state.

pulp·i·tis (pŭl-pī′tis). Inflammation of the pulp of a tooth. SYN odontitis. [L. *pulpa,* pulp, + G. *-itis,* inflammation]

hyperplastic p., hyperplastic granulation tissue growing out of the exposed pulp chamber of a grossly decayed tooth. SYN dental polyp, pulp polyp, tooth polyp.

hypertrophic p., a misnomer for hyperplastic p.

irreversible p., inflammation of the dental pulp from which the pulp is unable to recover; clinically, may be asymptomatic or characterized by pain which persists after thermal stimulation; microscopically, characterized by marked acute or chronic inflammation, sometimes with partial pulpal necrosis.

reversible p., minor inflammation from which the pulp is able to recover; characterized clinically by pain which disappears rapidly upon removal of thermal stimulation; characterized microscopically by vasodilation, hyperemia, and edema with minimal diapedesis of leukocytes.

suppurative p., obsolete term for a purulent irreversible p.

pulp·less. 1. Without a pulp. **2.** Denoting a tooth in which the pulp has died or from which the pulp has been removed. **3.** Denoting a tooth that gives no response to an electric pulp test or thermal test.

pulp·o·don·tia (pŭl-pō-don'shē-ă). The science of root canal therapy. SEE ALSO endodontics. [L. *pulpa,* pulp, + G. *odous,* tooth]

pul·po·sus (pŭl-pō'sŭs). SYN pulpy. [L.]

pulp·ot·o·my (pŭl-pot'ō-mē). Removal of a portion of the pulp structure of a tooth, usually the coronal portion. SYN pulp amputation. [L. *pulpa,* pulp, + G. *tomē,* incision]

pulpy (pŭl'pē). In the condition of a soft, moist solid. SYN pulposus.

pul·sate (pŭl'sāt). To throb or beat rhythmically; said of the heart or an artery. [L. *pulso,* pp. *-atus,* to beat]

pul·sa·tile (pŭl'să-til). Throbbing or beating.

pul·sa·tion (pŭl-sā'shŭn). A throbbing or rhythmical beating, as of the pulse or the heart. [L. *pulsatio,* a beating]

balloon counter p., a form of circulatory assistance in which a balloon inflates in the aorta during diastole to improve diastolic pressure and deflates during systole to reduce left ventricular after load.

suprasternal p., any p. in the suprasternal notch at the anterior route of the neck.

pul·sa·tor (pŭl-sā'ter, -tōr). A machine or device that operates in a throbbing, vibrating, or rhythmic manner.

pulse (pŭls). Rhythmical dilation of an artery, produced by the increased volume of blood thrown into the vessel by the contraction of the heart. A p. may also at times occur in a vein or a vascular organ, such as the liver. SYN pulsus. [L. *pulsus*]

abdominal p., the soft, compressible aortic p. occurring in certain abdominal disorders. SYN pulsus abdominalis.

alternating p., mechanical alternation, a pulse regular in time but with alternate beats stronger and weaker, often detectable only with the sphygmomanometer and usually indicating serious myocardial disease. SYN pulsus alternans.

anacrotic p., anadicrotic p., a p. wave showing one or more notches or indentations on its rising limb that are sometimes detectable by palpation. SYN pulsus anadicrotus.

bigeminal p., a p. in which the beats occur in pairs. SYN bigemina, coupled p., pulsus bigeminus.

bisferious p. (bis-fer'ē-ŭs), an arterial p. with peaks that may be palpable. SYN pulsus bisferiens.

bulbar p., a jugular p. supposed to indicate tricuspid insufficiency.

cannonball p., SYN water-hammer p.

capillary p., the alternate rhythmical blanching and reddening of a capillary area, as seen under the nails or in the lip, upon gentle compression; a sign of arteriolar dilation, well seen in aortic insufficiency.

carotid p., the p. of the carotid arteries in the neck.

catacrotic p., a p. in which there is an upward notch interrupting the descending limb of the sphygmogram. SYN pulsus catacrotus.

catadicrotic p., a catacrotic p. in which there are two interrupting upward notches. SYN pulsus catadicrotus.

collapsing p., SYN water-hammer p.

cordy p., SYN tense p.

Corrigan's p., SYN Corrigan's sign.

coupled p., SYN bigeminal p.

dicrotic p., a p. which is marked by a double beat, the second, due to a palpable dicrotic wave, being weaker than the first. SYN pulsus duplex.

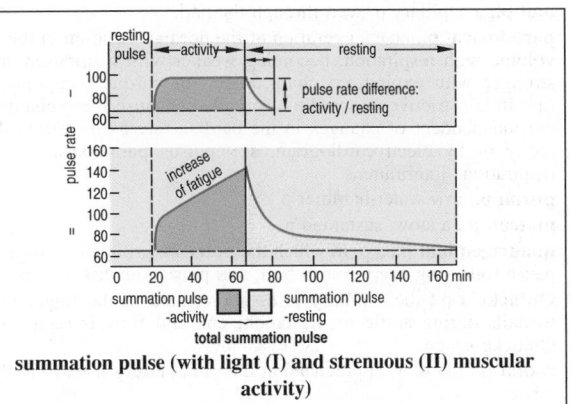

summation pulse (with light (I) and strenuous (II) muscular activity)

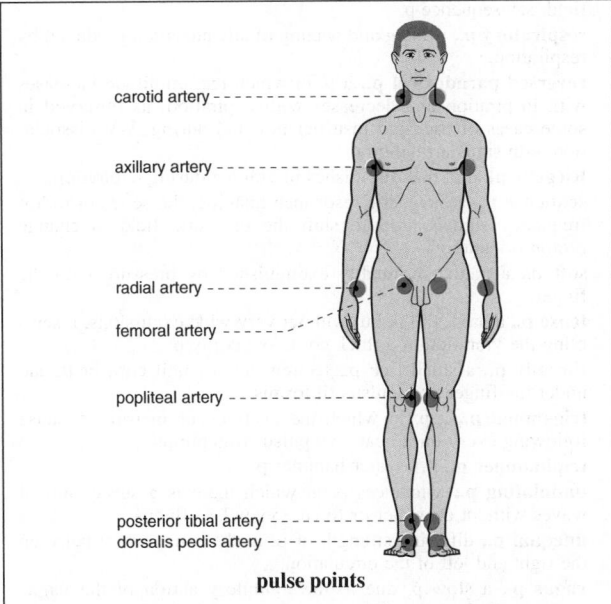

pulse points

entoptic p., an intermittent phose synchronous with the p.

filiform p., a thready p.

gaseous p., a soft, full, but feeble p.

guttural p., a pulsation felt in the throat.

hard p., a p. that strikes forcibly against the tip of the finger and is with difficulty compressed, suggesting hypertension. SYN pulsus durus.

intermittent p., irregularity of the heart due to extrasystoles which are too weak to open the semilunar valves; often owing to the long pause following the premature beat, extra long pauses equal to two regular cycles occur from time to time between p. beats. SYN pulsus intercidens.

irregular p., variation in rate of impulses in an artery due to cardiac arrhythmia.

jugular p., the venous p. as observed in the jugular veins of the neck, usually the deep jugular veins.

Kussmaul's p., reduction or disappearance of the p. during inspiration.

Kussmaul's paradoxical p., SEE paradoxical p.

labile p., frequent changes in p. rate.

long p., a p. in which the impact is felt longer than usual.

monocrotic p., a p. without any perceptible dicrotism. SYN pulsus monocrotus.

mousetail p., SYN *pulsus* myurus.

movable p., the lateral movement of a strongly pulsating tortuous artery.

nail p., a capillary p. seen through the nail.

paradoxical p., an exaggeration of the normal variation in the p. volume with respiration, becoming weaker with inspiration and stronger with expiration; characteristic of cardiac tamponade, rare in constrictive pericarditis; so called because these changes are independent of changes in the cardiac rate as measured directly or by electrocardiogram. SYN pulsus paradoxus, pulsus respiratione intermittens.

piston p., SYN water-hammer p.

plateau p., a slow, sustained p.

quadrigeminal p., a p. in which the beats are grouped in fours, a pause following every fourth beat. SYN pulsus quadrigeminus.

Quincke's p., the capillary p. as appreciated in the finger and toenails during aortic regurgitation; ebb and flow is seen. SYN Quincke's sign.

radial p., the p. as appreciated at the radial artery usually in the wrist.

radiofrequency p., in nuclear magnetic resonance, a short electromagnetic signal used to change the direction of the magnetic field. SEE sequence p.

respiratory p., waxing and waning of any pulsation produced by respiration.

reversed paradoxical p., a p. in which the amplitude increases with inspiration and decreases with expiration, as observed in some cases of tricuspid insufficiency and during A-V dissociation with sinus arrhythmia.

Riegel's p., a p. that diminishes in volume during expiration.

sequence p., in magnetic resonance imaging, the series of radiofrequency signals used to shift the magnetic field to change proton orientation.

soft p., a p. that is readily extinguished by pressure with the finger.

tense p., a hard, full p. but without very wide excursions, resembling the vibration of a thick cord. SYN cordy p.

thready p., a small fine p., feeling like a small cord or thread under the finger. SYN pulsus filiformis.

trigeminal p., a p. in which the beats occur in trios, a pause following every third beat. SYN pulsus trigeminus.

triphammer p., SYN water-hammer p.

undulating p., a toneless p. in which there is a succession of waves without character or force. SYN pulsus fluens.

unequal p., differing strength of p. in the same artery between the right and left of the circulation.

vagus p., a slow p. due to the inhibitory action of the vagus nerve on the heart.

venous p., a pulsation occurring in the veins, especially the internal jugular vein. SYN pulsus venosus.

vermicular p., a small rapid p., giving a wormlike sensation to the finger.

water-hammer p., a p. with forcible impulse but immediate collapse, characteristic of aortic incompetency. SEE ALSO Corrigan's *sign.* SYN cannonball p., collapsing p., piston p., pulsus celerrimus, triphammer p.

wiry p., a small, fine, incompressible p.

pul·sel·lum (pŭl-sel'ŭm). A posterior flagellum constituting the organ of locomotion in certain protozoa. [Mod. L. dim. of L. *pulsus,* a stroking]

pul·sim·e·ter, pul·som·e·ter (pŭl-sim'ĕ-ter, -som'ĕ-ter). An instrument for measuring the force and rapidity of the pulse. [L. *pulsus,* pulse, + *metron,* measure]

pul·sion (pŭl'shŭn). A pushing outward or swelling. [L. *pulsio*]

pul·sus (pŭl'sŭs). SYN pulse. [L. a stroke, pulse]

p. abdomina′lis, SYN abdominal *pulse.*

p. alter′nans, SYN alternating *pulse.*

p. anadic′rotus, SYN anacrotic *pulse.*

p. bigem′inus, SYN bigeminal *pulse.*

p. bisfer′iens, SYN bisferious *pulse.*

p. cap′risans, a bounding leaping pulse, irregular in both force and rhythm.

p. catac′rotus, SYN catacrotic *pulse.*

p. catadic′rotus, SYN catadicrotic *pulse.*

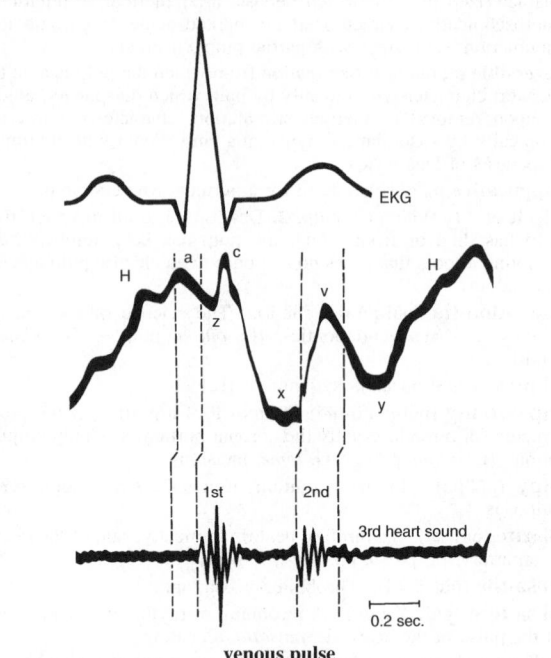

venous pulse

H = small waves, in long-lasting diastole; a = "atrial wave" (by atrial contraction); 2 = small plateau immediately preceding contraction of the right ventricle; c = wave by atrial dilation; x = suction, by change of ventricular level, during atrial expulsion ("systolic collapse"); v = wave at the opening of the mitral valve; y = tricuspid valve opening ("diastolic collapse")

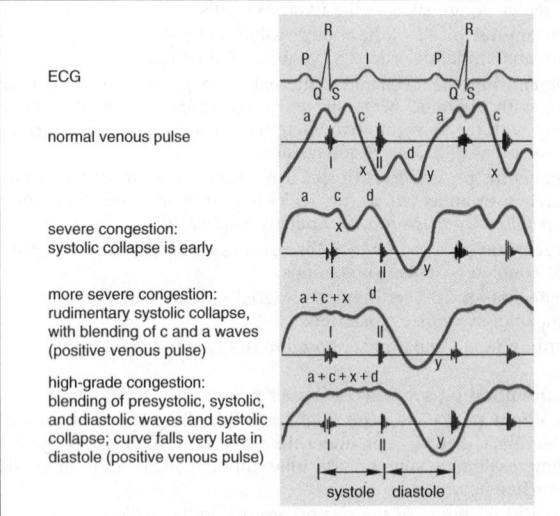

development of positive venous pulse

p. cel′er, a pulse beat swift to rise and fall.

p. celer′rimus, SYN water-hammer *pulse.*

p. cor′dis, the apex beat of the heart.

p. deb′ilis, a weak pulse.

p. dif′ferens, a condition in which the pulses in the two radial or other corresponding arteries differ in strength. SYN p. incongruens.

p. du′plex, SYN dicrotic *pulse.*

p. du′rus, SYN hard *pulse.*

p. filifor′mis, SYN thready *pulse.*

p. flu′ens, SYN undulating *pulse.*

p. for′micans, a very small, nearly imperceptible pulse, the impression it gives to the finger being compared to formication.

p. for′tis, a full strong pulse.

p. fre′quens, a rapid pulse.

p. heterochron′icus, an arrhythmic pulse.

p. inaequa′lis, a pulse irregular in rhythm and force.

p. incon′gruens, SYN p. differens.

p. infre′quens, a slow pulse.

p. inter′cidens, SYN intermittent *pulse.*

p. intercur′rens, an occasional strong dicrotic pulse wave giving the impression of an intercurrent ventricular contraction.

p. irregula′ris perpet′uus, permanently irregular pulse often caused by, or characteristic of, atrial fibrillation; it may also be produced by a wide variety of other chaotic rhythms.

p. mag′nus, a large full pulse.

p. mol′lis, a soft, easily compressible pulse.

p. monoc′rotus, SYN monocrotic *pulse.*

p. myu′rus, a pulse marked by a wave, the apex of which is reached suddenly and which then subsides very gradually. SYN mousetail pulse.

p. paradoxus (pŭl′sŭs par′ă-doks-ŭs), SYN paradoxical *pulse.*

p. par′vus, a pulse of small amplitude, as in aortic stenosis.

p. parvus et tardus (pŭl′sŭs par′vŭs ā tar′dŭs), small, late pulse considered typical of severe aortic stenosis.

p. quadrigem′inus, SYN quadrigeminal *pulse.*

p. ra′rus, SYN p. tardus.

p. respiratio′ne intermit′tens, SYN paradoxical *pulse.*

p. tar′dus, a pulse with pathologically gradual upstroke typical of severe aortic stenosis. SEE ALSO plateau *pulse.* SYN p. rarus.

p. trem′ulus, a feeble fluttering pulse.

p. trigem′inus, SYN trigeminal *pulse.*

p. vac′uus, a very weak pulse hardly distending the arterial wall.

p. veno′sus, SYN venous *pulse.*

pul·ta·ceous (pŭl-tā′shŭs). Macerated; pulpy. [G. *poltos,* porridge]

pul·ver·i·za·tion (pŭl′ver-i-zā′shŭn). Reduction to powder.

pul·ver·ize (pŭl′ver-īz). To reduce to a powder. [L. *pulverizo,* fr. *pulvis, pulveris,* dust]

pul·ver·u·lent (pŭl-ver′yū-lent). In a state of powder; powdery.

pul·vi·nar (pŭl-vī′năr) [NA]. The expanded posterior extremity of the thalamus which forms a cushion-like prominence overlying the geniculate bodies. [L. a couch made from cushions, fr. *pulvinus,* cushion]

pul·vi·nate (pŭl′vi-nāt). Raised or convex, denoting a form of surface elevation of a bacterial culture. [L. *pulvinus,* cushion]

pum·ice (pŭm′is). Volcanic cinders ground to particles of varying sizes; used in dentistry for polishing restorations or teeth; an abrasive. [L. *pumex* (*pumic*-), a pumice stone]

pump (pŭmp). **1.** An apparatus for forcing a gas or liquid from or to any part. **2.** Any mechanism for using metabolic energy to accomplish active transport of a substance.

breast p., a suction instrument for withdrawing milk from the breast.

calcium p., a membranal protein that can transport calcium ions across the membrane using energy from ATP.

calf p., muscular activity of calf that promotes venous flow towards the heart.

Carrel-Lindbergh p., a perfusion device designed for use in culture of whole organs.

constant infusion p., an electrically driven device for delivery from a reservoir of a constant, often very small, volume of solution over a prolonged period of time.

dental p., SYN saliva *ejector.*

hydrogen p., molecular mechanism for acid secretion from gastric parietal cells based on the activity of a H^+-K^+-ATPase.

intra-aortic balloon p., a pump connected to a balloon device which is inserted into the descending aorta as a counterpulsation

device to provide temporary cardiac assistance in the management of left ventricular failure.

ion p., a membranal complex of proteins that is capable of transporting ions against a concentration gradient using the energy from ATP.

jet ejector p., a suction p. in which fluid under high pressure is forced through a nozzle into an abruptly larger tube where a high velocity jet, at a low pressure in accordance with Bernoulli's law, entrains gas or liquid from a side tube opening just beyond the end of the nozzle to create suction; *e.g.,* the p. by which steam is used to evacuate an autoclave, a water aspirator.

proton p., molecular mechanism for the net transport of protons across a membrane; usually involves the activity of an ATPase.

saliva p., SYN saliva *ejector.*

sodium p., a biologic mechanism that uses metabolic energy from ATP to achieve active transport of sodium across a membrane; sodium p.'s expel sodium from most cells of the body, sometimes coupled with the transport of other substances, and also serve to move sodium across multicellular membranes such as renal tubule walls.

sodium-potassium p., a membrane-bound transporter that maintains the high potassium and low sodium intracellular concentrations relative to the extracellular medium. This exchange is accomplished at the expense of cellular energy in the form of ATP.

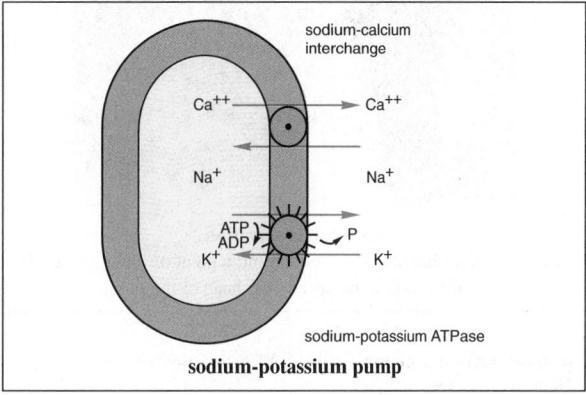

sodium-potassium pump

stomach p., an apparatus for removing the contents of the stomach by means of suction.

pump-ox·y·gen·a·tor (pŭmp-ok′si-je-nā′ter). A mechanical device that can substitute for both the heart (pump) and the lungs (oxygenator) during open heart surgery.

pu·na (pū′nă). SYN altitude *sickness* (1). [Sp., fr. Quechua *puna,* a high, dry Andean plateau]

punch (pŭnch). An instrument for making a hole or indentation in some solid material or for driving out a foreign body in such material. [L. *pungo,* pp. *punctus,* to stick, to punch]

punch·drunk (pŭnch′drŭnk). SEE punchdrunk *syndrome.*

punc·ta (pŭngk′tă). Plural of punctum. [L.]

punc·tate (pŭngk′tāt). Marked with points or dots differentiated from the surrounding surface by color, elevation, or texture. [L. *punctum,* a point]

punc·ti·form (pŭngk′ti-fōrm). Very small but not microscopic, having a diameter of less than 1 mm. [L. *punctum,* a point, + *forma,* shape]

punc·tum, gen. **punc·ti,** pl. **punc·ta** (pŭngk′tŭm, -tī, -tă) [NA]. **1.** The tip of a sharp process. **2.** A minute round spot differing in color or otherwise in appearance from the surrounding tissues. **3.** A point on the optic axis of an optical system. SEE ALSO point. SYN point (1). [L. a prick, point, pp. ntr. of *pungo,* to prick, used as noun]

p. ce′cum, the blind spot in the visual field corresponding to the location of the optic disk.

p. coxa′le, the highest point of the crest of the ilium.

p. doloro′sum, SEE Valleix's *points,* under *point.*

lacrimal p., the minute circular opening of the lacrimal canaliculus, on the margin of each eyelid near the medial commissure. SYN p. lacrimale [NA], lacrimal opening.

p. lacrima′le [NA], SYN lacrimal p.

p. lu′teum, SYN *macula* retinae.

p. ossificatio′nis [NA], SYN *center* of ossification.

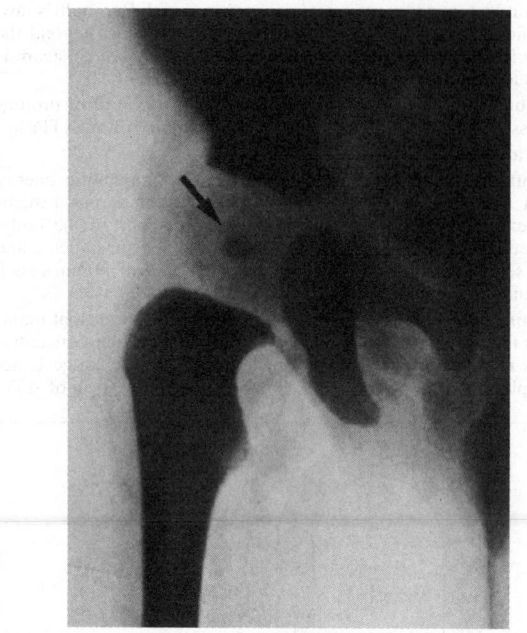

center of ossification
x-ray image of hip of a 4 mo. old infant; a point of (endochondral) ossification can be seen in the head of the femur

p. ossificatio′nis prima′rium [NA], SYN primary *center* of ossification.

p. ossificatio′nis secunda′rium [NA], SYN secondary *center* of ossification.

p. prox′imum (P.p.), SYN near *point.*

p. remo′tum (P.r.), SYN far *point.*

p. vasculo′sum, one of the minute dots seen on section of the brain, due to small drops of blood at the cut extremities of the arteries.

punc·ture (pŭnk′chūr). **1.** To make a hole with a small pointed object, such as a needle. **2.** A prick or small hole made with a pointed instrument. [L. *punctura,* fr. *pungo,* pp. *punctus,* to prick]

Bernard's p., SYN diabetic p.

cisternal p., passage of a hollow needle through the posterior atlantooccipital membrane into the cisterna cerebellomedullaris.

diabetic p., a p. at a point in the floor of the fourth ventricle of the brain which causes glycosuria. SYN Bernard's p.

lumbar p., a p. into the subarachnoid space of the lumbar region to obtain spinal fluid for diagnostic or therapeutic purposes. SYN Quincke's p., rachicentesis, rachiocentesis, spinal p., spinal tap.

Quincke's p., SYN lumbar p.

spinal p., SYN lumbar p.

sternal p., removal of bone marrow from the manubrium by needle.

pun·gent (pŭn′jent). Sharp; said of the taste or odor of a substance. [L. *pungo,* pres. p. *-ens* (*-ent-*), to pierce]

PUO Abbreviation for pyrexia of unknown (or uncertain) origin, a term applied to febrile illness before diagnosis has been established; also referred to as FUO (fever of unknown origin).

pu·pa, pl. **pu·pae** (pyū′pă, -pē). The stage of insect metamor-

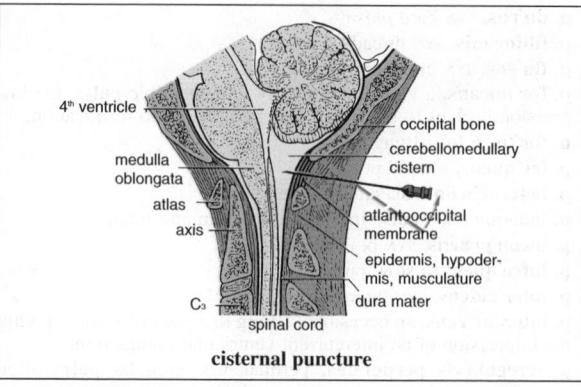

cisternal puncture

phosis following the larva and preceding the imago. SEE ALSO complete *metamorphosis.* [L. *pupa,* doll]

pu·pil (p) (pyū′pĭl). The circular orifice in the center of the iris, through which the light rays enter the eye. SYN pupilla [NA]. [L. *pupilla*]

Adie's p., SYN Adie *syndrome.*

amaurotic p., p. in an eye that is blind because of ocular or optic nerve disease; this p. will not contract to light except when the normal fellow eye is stimulated with light.

Argyll Robertson p., a form of reflex iridoplegia characterized by miosis, irregular shape, and a loss of the direct and consensual pupillary reflex to light, with normal pupillary constriction to a near vision effort (light-near dissociation); often present in tabetic neurosyphilis. SYN Robertson p.

artificial p., an opening made by excision of a portion of the iris in order to improve the vision in cases of central opacity of the cornea or lens.

Bumke's p., dilation of the p. in response to anxiety or other psychic stimuli.

catatonic p., transient pupillary dilation with absence of pupillary reaction to light and convergence.

cat's-eye p., a distorted, elongated p.; usually due to anterior segment anomaly.

fixed p., a stationary pupil unresponsive to all stimuli.

Gunn p., SYN Marcus Gunn p.

Holmes-Adie p., SYN Adie *syndrome.*

Horner's p., constricted p. due to impairment of sympathetic nerve innervation of the dilator muscle of the pupil. SEE ALSO Horner's *syndrome.*

Hutchinson's p., dilation of the p. on the side of the lesion as part of a third nerve palsy; often due to herniation of the uncus of the temporal lobe through the tentorial notch.

keyhole p., a p. with a coloboma.

Marcus Gunn p., relative afferent *pupillary* defect. SYN Gunn p.

paradoxical p., SEE paradoxical pupillary *reflex.*

pinhole p., an extremely constricted p.

Robertson p., SYN Argyll Robertson p.

seclusion of p. (se-klū′zhŭn), the condition resulting from posterior annular synechia, in which the iris is bound down throughout the entire pupillary margin, but the pupil is not occluded. SYN exclusion of pupil.

tadpole-shaped p., an intermittent, brief distortion and dilation of a pupil that draws one part of the iris into a peak so that the p. resembles a tadpole; a temporary, benign condition associated with migraine that may leave the patient with a Horner's syndrome.

tonic p., a general term for a p. with delayed, slow, long-lasting contractions to light and to a near vision effort, often with light-near dissociation; due to denervation and aberrant reinnervation of the iris sphincter; seen in various autonomic neuropathies and in Adie *syndrome.*

pu·pil·la, pl. **pu·pil·lae** (pyū-pil′ă, pyū-pil′ē) [NA]. SYN pupil. [L. dim. of *pupa,* a girl or doll]

pu·pil·lary (pyū′pi-lār-ē). Relating to the pupil.

p. light-near dissociation, a stronger near pupil response than light response; due to weak pupillomotor input, Argyll Robertson *pupil,* dorsal midbrain syndrome, or to misdirection of ciliary muscle fibers into the iris sphincter. SYN light-near dissociation.

relative afferent p. defect, an asymmetry of the pupillomotor input between the two eyes; tested by alternating the light from one eye to the other and comparing the direct light reactions.

pu·pil·lary ruff. The dark-brown, wrinkled rim of the normal pupil. This is the posterior pigment epithelium of the iris showing itself at the pupillary margin.

pupillo-. The pupils. [L. *pupilla,* pupil]

pu·pil·log·ra·phy (pyū'pi-log'ră-fē). The recording of pupillary reactions. [pupillo- + G. *graphō,* to write]

pu·pil·lom·e·ter (pyū'pi-lom'ĕ-ter). An instrument for measuring and recording the diameter of the pupil. [pupillo- + G. *metron,* measure]

pu·pil·lom·e·try (pyū'pi-lom'ĕ-trē). Measurement of the pupil.

pu·pil·lo·mo·tor (pyū'pĭ-lō-mō'ter). Relating to the autonomic nerve fibers that supply the smooth muscle of the iris. SYN iridomotor. [pupillo- + L. *motor,* mover]

pu·pil·lo·sta·tom·e·ter (pyū'pi-lō-stă-tom'ĕ-ter). An instrument for measuring the distance between the centers of the pupils. [pupillo- + G. *statos,* placed, + *metron,* measure]

pu·pip·a·rous (pyū-pip'ă-rŭs). Pupae-bearing; denoting those insects that give birth to late-stage larvae that have already passed their larval development within the body of the female, as in flies of the family Hippoboscidae and in the Glossinidae (tsetse flies). [pupa + L. *pario,* to give birth]

PUPPP Acronym for *p*ruritic *u*rticarial *p*apules and *p*laques of *p*regnancy, an intensely pruritic, occasionally vesicular, eruption of the trunk and arms appearing in the third trimester of pregnancy; spontaneous involution occurs within 10 days of term.

Pur Abbreviation for purine.

pure (pyūr). Unadulterated; free from admixture or contamination with any extraneous matter. [L. *purus*]

pure·bred (pyūr'bred). An animal whose ancestors on both sides have been members of a recognized breed, and usually officially registered as such.

pur·ga·tion (per-gā'shŭn). Evacuation of the bowels with the aid of a purgative or cathartic. SYN catharsis (1). [L. *purgatio*]

pur·ga·tive (per'gă-tiv). An agent used for purging the bowels. SEE ALSO cathartic (2). [L. *purgativus,* purging]

saline p., epsom salt, Rochelle salt, or any salt having p. properties.

purge (perj). **1.** To cause a copious evacuation of the bowels. **2.** A cathartic remedy. [L. *purgo,* to cleanse, fr. *purus,* pure, + *ago,* to do]

purg·ing cas·sia (perj'ing kash'yă). SYN cassia fistula.

pu·ri·form (pyū'ri-fōrm). Resembling pus. [L. *pus (pur-),* pus, + *forma,* form]

pu·rine (Pur) (pyūr'ēn, -rin). The parent substance of adenine, guanine, and other naturally occurring p. "bases"; not known to exist as such in mammals.

p.-nucleoside phosphorylase, a ribosyltransferase that reversibly catalyzes the phosphorolysis of a p. nucleoside with inorganic phosphate to produce a p. and α-D-ribose 1-phosphate; an inherited deficiency of this enzyme leads to cellular immunodeficiency.

p. ribonucleoside, SYN nebularine.

pu·ri·ne·mia (pyū-ri-nē'mē-ă). The presence of purine or xanthine bases in the circulating blood. [purine + G. *haima,* blood]

pu·ri·ty (pyūr'i-tē). The state of being pure, free from contaminants or pollutants. [L. *puritas,* fr. *purus,* clean, undefiled]

radiochemical p., the proportion of the total activity of a specific radionuclide in a specific chemical or biological form.

radioisotopic p., a loose term commonly used to denote radionuclidic p.

radionuclidic p., the proportion of the total radioactivity that is present as a specific radionuclide.

radiopharmaceutical p., the sterility and apyrogenicity of a radioactive tracer for human use.

Purkinje, Johannes E. von (Jan E. Purkyne), Bohemian anatomist and physiologist, 1787–1869. SEE P. *conduction, images,* under *image, shift, system;* P.'s *cells,* under *cell, corpuscles,* under *corpuscle, fibers,* under *fiber, figures,* under *figure, layer, network, phenomenon;* P.-Sanson *images,* under *image.*

Purmann, Matthaeus G., German surgeon, 1648–1721. SEE P.'s *method.*

pu·ro·mu·cous (pyū-rō-myū'kŭs). SYN mucopurulent. [L. *pus (pur-),* pus, + *mucus,* mucus]

pu·ro·my·cin (pyū-rō-mī'sin). 6-Dimethylamino-9-(3'-*p*-methoxy-L-phenylalanylamino-β-D-ribofuranosyl) purine; an antibiotic produced by the growth of *Streptomyces alboniger;* formerly used in the treatment of amebiasis and trypanosomiasis.

pur·ple (per'pl). A color formed by a mixture of blue and red. For individual purple dyes see specific name. [L. *purpura*]

Ruhemann's p., a blue-violet dye formed in the reaction of ninhydrin with amino acids.

visual p., SYN rhodopsin.

pur·pu·ra (pŭr'pū-ră). A condition characterized by hemorrhage into the skin. Appearance of the lesions varies with the type of p., the duration of the lesions, and the acuteness of the onset. The color is first red, gradually darkens to purple, fades to a brownish yellow, and usually disappears in 2 or 3 weeks; color of residual permanent pigmentation depends largely on the type of unabsorbed pigment of the extravasated blood; extravasations may occur also into the mucous membranes and internal organs. SYN peliosis. [L. fr. G. *porphyra,* purple]

acute vascular p., SYN Henoch-Schönlein p.

allergic p., nonthrombocytopenic p. due to sensitization to foods, drugs, and insect bites. SYN anaphylactoid p. (1).

anaphylactoid p., **(1)** SYN allergic p. **(2)** SYN Henoch-Schönlein p.

p. angioneurot'ica, an eruption marked by angioneurotic edema, petechiae, and hyperesthesia of the skin and gastric mucous membrane.

p. annula'ris telangiecto'des, asymptomatic annular lesions, principally of the lower extremities of adolescent males, in which the peripheral portion is composed of purpura or petechiae with brawny staining of hemosiderin deposits and minute telangiectasia. SYN Majocchi's disease.

equine nonthrombocytopenic p., an immune-mediated vasculitis of horses due to immune complex deposition, characteristically as a sequela of strangles.

factitious p., self-induced, often painful, ecchymoses.

fibrinolytic p., p. in which the bleeding is associated with rapid fibrinolysis of the clot.

p. ful'minans, a severe and rapidly fatal form of p. hemorrhagica, occurring especially in children, with hypotension, fever, and disseminated intravascular coagulation, usually following an infectious illness.

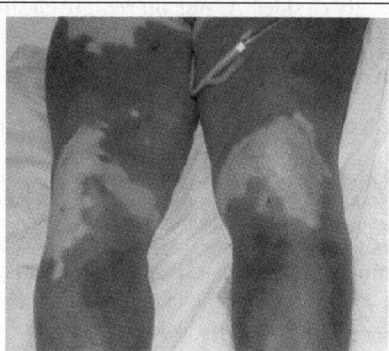

purpura fulminans (in 78 year old patient)

p. hemorrhag'ica, **(1)** SYN idiopathic thrombocytopenic p. **(2)** a noncontagious malady of horses, which occurs following suppurative infections, characterized by multiple hemorrhages and edema of the subcutaneous and submucous tissues. SYN petechial fever.

Henoch's p., SYN Henoch-Schönlein p.

Henoch-Schönlein p., an eruption of nonthrombocytopenic purpuric lesions due to dermal leukocytoclastic vasculitis with IgA in vessel walls associated with joint pain and swelling, colic, and passage of bloody stools, and occurring characteristically in young children; glomerulonephritis may occur during an initial episode or develop later. SYN acute vascular p., anaphylactoid p. (2), hemorrhagic exudative erythema, Henoch's p., Henoch-Schönlein syndrome, p. nervosa, p. rheumatica, Schönlein's disease, Schönlein's p., Schönlein-Henoch syndrome.

hyperglobulinemic p., SYN Waldenström's *macroglobulinemia.*

idiopathic thrombocytopenic p. (ITP), a systemic illness characterized by extensive ecchymoses and hemorrhages from mucous membranes and very low platelet counts; resulting from platelet destruction by macrophages due to an antiplatelet factor; childhood cases are usually brief and rarely present with intracranial hemorrhages, but adult cases are often recurrent and have a higher incidence of grave bleeding, especially intracranial. SYN immune thrombocytopenic p., p. hemorrhagica (1), thrombopenic p.

immune thrombocytopenic p., SYN idiopathic thrombocytopenic p.

p. iod′ica, iodic p., an eruption of discrete miliary petechiae, usually confined to the lower extremities, appearing in rare instances on administration of any of the iodides.

p. nervo′sa, SYN Henoch-Schönlein p.

nonthrombocytopenic p., SYN p. simplex.

psychogenic p., SYN autoerythrocyte sensitization *syndrome.*

p. pu′licans, p. pulico′sa, petechiae caused by the bites of insects and animal parasites.

p. rheumat′ica, SYN Henoch-Schönlein p.

Schönlein's p., SYN Henoch-Schönlein p.

p. seni′lis, the occurrence of petechiae and ecchymoses on the atrophic skin of the legs in aged and debilitated subjects.

p. sim′plex, the eruption of petechiae or larger ecchymoses, usually unaccompanied by constitutional symptoms and not associated with systemic illness. SYN nonthrombocytopenic p.

p. symptomat′ica, a petechial eruption in scarlet fever and other exanthemas.

thrombocytopenic p., SEE idiopathic thrombocytopenic p.

thrombopenic p., SYN idiopathic thrombocytopenic p.

thrombotic thrombocytopenic p., a rapidly fatal or occasionally protracted disease with varied symptoms in addition to p., including signs of central nervous system involvement, due to formation of fibrin or platelet thrombi in arterioles and capillaries in many organs. SYN Moschcowitz' disease.

p. urti′cans, p. simplex accompanied by an urticarial eruption.

Waldenström's p., SYN Waldenström's *macroglobulinemia.*

pur·pu·rea gly·co·sides A, pur·pu·rea gly·co·sides B (per′pŭ-rē′ă glī′kō-sīdz). The cardioactive precursor glycosides of *Digitalis purpurea;* they are structurally identical with desacetyllanatosides A and B, respectively. SEE ALSO lanatosides A, B, and C.

pur·pu·ric (pŭr-pū′rik). Relating to or affected with purpura.

pur·pu·rin (per′pyū-rin). 1. SYN uroerythrin. 2 [C.I. 58205]. A violet stain related to alizarin by addition of a 4-OH group to alizarin; found in madder root and other members of the *Rubiaceae;* used to detect calcium salts, boron, and as a histological stain. SYN alizarin purpurin.

pur·pu·ri·nu·ria (per′pyū-ri-nū′rē-ă). SYN porphyrinuria.

purr (per). A low vibratory murmur. SYN frémissement cattaire.

Purtscher, Otmar, German ophthalmologist, 1852–1927. SEE P.'s *disease.*

pu·ru·lence, pu·ru·len·cy (pyūr′ŭ-lens, -len-sē; pyūr′yū-lens). The condition of containing or forming pus. [L. *purulentia,* a festering, fr. *pus (pur-),* pus]

pu·ru·lent (pyūr′ŭ-lent, pyūr′yū-). Containing, consisting of, or forming pus.

pu·ru·loid (pyū′rŭ-loyd). Resembling pus.

pus (pŭs). A fluid product of inflammation, consisting of a liquid containing leukocytes and the debris of dead cells and tissue elements liquefied by the proteolytic and histolytic enzymes (*e.g.,* leukoprotease) that are elaborated by polymorphonuclear leukocytes. [L.]

blue p., p. tinged with pyocyanin, a product of *Pseudomonas aeruginosa.*

cheesy p., a very thick almost solid p. resulting from the absorption of the liquor puris.

curdy p., p. containing flakes of caseous matter.

green p., blue p. when, as sometimes happens, it has more of a green hue.

ichorous p., thin p. containing shreds of sloughing tissue, and sometimes of a fetid odor.

laudable p., an obsolete term used when suppuration was considered unlikely to lead to pyemia (blood poisoning) but more likely to remain localized.

sanious p., ichorous p. stained with blood.

pus·tu·lant (pŭs′chū-lant). 1. Causing a pustular eruption. 2. An agent producing pustules.

pus·tu·lar (pŭs′chū-lăr). Relating to or marked by pustules.

pus·tu·la·tion (pŭs′chū-lā′shŭn). The formation or the presence of pustules.

pus·tule (pŭs′chūl). A small circumscribed elevation of the skin, containing purulent material. [L. *pustula*]

malignant p., SYN cutaneous *anthrax.*

postmortem p., obsolete term for an ulcer, usually on the knuckle, resulting from infection during a dissection or the performance of an autopsy.

spongiform p. of Kogoj, an epidermal p. formed by infiltration of neutrophils into necrotic epidermis in which the cell walls persist as a spongelike network; seen in pustular psoriasis.

pus·tu·li·form (pŭs′chū-li-fōrm). Having the appearance of a pustule.

pus·tu·lo·crus·ta·ceous (pŭs′chū-lō-krŭs-tā′shŭs). Marked by pustules crusted with dry pus.

pus·tu·lo·sis (pŭs-chū-lō′sis). 1. An eruption of pustules. 2. Term occasionally used to designate acropustulosis. [L. *pustula,* pustule, + G. *-osis,* condition]

p. palmar′is et plantar′is, a sterile pustular eruption of the fingers and toes, variously attributed to dyshidrosis, pustular psoriasis, and unidentified bacterial infection. SYN acrodermatitis continua, acrodermatitis perstans, dermatitis repens, Hallopeau's disease (1).

p. vaccinifor′mis acu′ta, SYN *eczema* herpeticum.

pu·ta·men (pyū-tā′men) [NA]. The outer, larger, and darker gray of the three portions into which the lenticular nucleus is divided by laminae of white fibers; it is connected with the caudate nucleus by bridging bands of gray substance that penetrate the internal capsule. Its histological structure is similar to that of the caudate nucleus together with which it composes the striatum. SEE ALSO striate *body,* lenticular *nucleus.* [L. that which falls off in pruning, fr. *puto,* to prune]

Putnam, James J., U.S. neurologist, 1846–1918. SEE P.-Dana *syndrome.*

pu·tre·fac·tion (pyū-tri-fak′shŭn). Decomposition or rotting, the breakdown of organic matter usually by bacterial action, resulting in the formation of other substances of less complex constitution with the evolution of ammonia or its derivatives and hydrogen sulfide; characterized usually by the presence of toxic or malodorous products. SYN decay (2), decomposition. [L. *putrefacio,* pp. *-factus,* to make rotten]

pu·tre·fac·tive (pyū-tri-fak′tiv). Relating to or causing putrefaction.

pu·tre·fy (pyū′tri-fī). To cause to become, or to become, putrid.

pu·tres·cence (pyū-tres′ens). The state of putrefaction.

pu·tres·cent (pyū-tres′ent). Denoting, or in the process of, putrefaction. [L. *putresco,* to grow rotten, fr. *puter,* rotten]

pu·tres·cine (pyū-tres′ēn). $NH_2(CH_2)_4NH_2$; 1,4-Diaminobutane; a poisonous polyamine formed from the amino acid, arginine, during putrefaction; found in urine and feces; in certain cells, p. is a precursor to γ-aminobutyrate.

pu·trid (pyū′trid). **1.** In a state of putrefaction. **2.** Denoting putrefaction. [L. *putridus*]

Putti, Vittorio, Italian surgeon, 1880–1940. SEE P.-Platt *operation, procedure.*

PUVA Acronym for oral administration of *p*soralen and subsequent exposure to long wavelength *u*ltraviolet light (*uv-a*); used to treat psoriasis.

PVC Abbreviation for polyvinyl chloride.

PVP Abbreviation for polyvinylpyrrolidone.

P with a sub·script for the ion. Abbreviation for permeability *constant.*

PWM Abbreviation for pokeweed *mitogen.*

py·ar·thro·sis (pī-ar-thrō′sis). SYN suppurative *arthritis.* [G. *pyon,* pus, + *arthrōsis,* a jointing]

△**pycno-.** SEE pykno-.

△**pyel-.** SEE pyelo-.

py·e·lec·ta·sis, py·e·lec·ta·sia (pī-ĕ-lek′tă-sis, pī-ĕ-lek-tā′zē-ă). Dilation of the pelvis of the kidney. [pyel- + G. *ektasis,* extension]

py·e·lit·ic (pī-ĕ-lit′ik). Relating to pyelitis.

py·e·li·tis (pī-ĕ-lī′tis). **1.** Inflammation of the renal pelvis. **2.** Obsolescent term for pyelonephritis. [pyel- + G. *-itis,* inflammation]

△**pyelo-, pyel-.** Pelvis, usually the renal pelvis. [G. *pyelos,* trough, tub, vat]

py·e·lo·cal·i·ce·al (pī′ĕ-lō-kal′i-sē′ăl). Relating to the renal pelvis and calices. SYN pyelocalyceal.

py·e·lo·cal·i·ec·ta·sis (pī′ĕ-lō-kal′ē-ek′tă-sis). SYN caliectasis.

py·e·lo·cal·y·ce·al (pī′ĕ-lō-kal′i-sē′ăl). SYN pyelocaliceal.

py·e·lo·cys·ti·tis (pī-ĕ-lō-sis-tī′tis). Inflammation of the renal pelvis and the bladder. [pyelo- + G. *kystis,* bladder, + *-itis,* inflammation]

py·e·lo·flu·o·ros·co·py (pī′ĕ-lō-flūr-os′kŏ-pē). Fluoroscopic examination of the renal pelves and ureters, following administration of contrast medium. [pyelo- + L. *fluo,* to flow, + G. *skopeō,* to view]

py·el·o·gram (pī′el-ō-gram). A radiograph or series of radiographs of the renal pelvis and ureter, following injection of contrast medium.

py·e·log·ra·phy (pī′ĕ-log′ră-fē). Radiologic study of the kidney, ureters, and usually the bladder, performed with the aid of a contrast agent either injected intravenously, or directly through a ureteral or nephrostomy catheter or percutaneously. SYN pelviureterography, pyeloureterography, ureteropyelography. [pyelo- + G. *graphō,* to write]

   antegrade p., antegrade urography in which the contrast medium is injected into the renal calices or pelvis.

   intravenous p. (IVP), former name for intravenous *urography.*

   retrograde p., p. in which contrast material is injected into the ureters from an endoscope in the bladder.

py·e·lo·li·thot·o·my (pī′ĕ-lō-li-thot′ō-mē). Operative removal of a calculus from the kidney through an incision in the renal pelvis. SYN pelvilithotomy, pelviolithotomy. [pyelo- + G. *lithos,* stone, + *tomē,* incision]

py·e·lo·lym·phat·ic (pī′ĕ-lō-lim-fat′ik). Pertaining to the lymphatics of the renal pelvis.

py·e·lo·ne·phri·tis (pī′ĕ-lō-ne-frī′tis). Inflammation of the renal parenchyma, calyces, and pelvis, particularly due to local bacterial infection. [pyelo- + G. *nephros,* kidney, + *-itis,* inflammation]

   acute p., acute inflammation of the renal parenchyma and pelvis characterized by small cortical abscesses and yellowish streaks in the medulla due to pus in the collecting tubules and interstitial tissue.

   ascending p., p. due to bacterial infection from the lower urinary tract, particularly by reflux of infected urine.

   chronic p., chronic inflammation of the renal parenchyma and pelvis resulting from bacterial infection, characterized by calyce-

al deformities and overlying large flat renal scars with patchy distribution.

   contagious bovine p., a specific necrotizing inflammation of the renal pelvis and ureters of cattle, caused by infection with *Corynebacterium renale.*

   xanthogranulomatous p., a chronic inflammatory condition diffusely involving the entire kidney and usually resulting in a grossly enlarged and functionless kidney which can grossly resemble a neoplasm or tuberculosis; histologically, it is characterized by an inflammatory reaction with numerous lipid-laden, foamy histiocytes mixed with lymphocytes and plasma cells to form multiple granulomas.

py·e·lo·ne·phro·sis (pī′ĕ-lō-ne-frō′sis). Obsolete term for any disease of the pelvis of the kidney. [pyelo- + G. *nephros,* kidney, + *-osis,* condition]

py·e·lo·plas·ty (pī′e-lō-plas-tē). Surgical reconstruction of the kidney pelvis to correct an obstruction. SYN pelvioplasty (2). [pyelo- + G. *plastos,* formed]

   Anderson-Hynes p., disjoined or dismembered p.

   capsular flap p., a reconstructive procedure for correction of uteropelvic obstruction, whereby a flap of renal capsule is swung down from the renal hilus to enlarge an obstructed intrarenal pelvis and upper ureter; used to correct situations involving loss of renal pelvic tissue which preclude the use of renal pelvis for the reconstruction.

   Culp p., a reconstructive technique for correction of uteropelvic obstruction, whereby a spiral flap of renal pelvis is brought down and interposed into a vertical incision in the ureter. SEE ALSO Scardino vertical flap p.

   disjoined p., dismembered p., a reconstructive procedure for correction of ureteropelvic obstruction, whereby the obstructed segment is resected and the upper ureter reanastomosed into the lower renal pelvis, usually utilizing a modified elliptical anastomotic technique.

   Foley Y-plasty p., a reconstructive procedure for correction of ureteropelvic obstruction, whereby a Y-shaped flap of renal pelvis is advanced downward into a vertical incision in the upper ureter, thereby widening the ureteropelvic junction. SYN Foley operation.

   Scardino vertical flap p., a reconstructive technique for correction of uteropelvic obstruction, whereby a vertical flap of renal pelvis is brought down and interposed into a vertical incision in the ureter. Cf. Culp p.

py·e·lo·pli·ca·tion (pī′ĕ-lō-pli-kā′shŭn). An obsolete procedure of taking tucks in the wall of the renal pelvis when unduly dilated by a hydronephrosis. [pyelo- + L. *plico,* to fold]

py·e·los·co·py (pī-ĕ-los′kŏ-pē). Fluoroscopic observation of the pelvis and calices of the kidney, and the ureter, after the injection through the ureter of an opaque solution. [pyelo- + G. *skopeō,* to view]

py·e·los·to·my (pī-ĕ-los′tō-mē). Formation of an opening into the kidney pelvis to establish urinary drainage. [pyelo- + G. *stoma,* mouth]

py·e·lot·o·my (pī-ĕ-lot′ō-mē). Incision into the pelvis of the kidney. SYN pelviotomy (3), pelvitomy. [pyelo- + G. *tomē,* incision]

   extended p., extension of a standard p. into the lower pole infundibulum through the avascular plane between the posterior and basilar segmental renal arteries. SYN Gil-Vernet operation.

py·e·lo·u·re·ter·ec·ta·sis (pī′ĕ-lō-yū-rē′ter-ek′tă-sis). Dilation of kidney pelvis and ureter, seen in hydronephrosis due to obstruction in the lower urinary tract. [pyelo- + ureter + G. *ektasis,* a stretching]

py·e·lo·u·re·ter·og·ra·phy (pī′ĕ-lō-yū-rē′ter-og′ră-fē). SYN pyelography.

py·e·lo·ve·nous (pī′ĕ-lō-vē′nŭs). Denoting the phenomenon of drainage from the renal pelvis into the renal veins from increased intrapelvic pressure. [pyelo- + venous]

py·em·e·sis (pī-em′ĕ-sis). The vomiting of pus. [G. *pyon,* pus, + *emesis,* vomiting]

py·e·mia (pī-ē′mē-ă). Septicemia due to pyogenic organisms causing multiple abscesses. SYN pyogenic fever. [G. *pyon*, pus, + *haima*, blood]

cryptogenic p., p. whose source is not evident.

portal p., suppurative pylephlebitis.

tick p., a disease of lambs caused by the bacterium *Staphylococcus aureus* in association with infestations of the tick *Ixodes ricinus* and characterized by pyemic abscesses in joints.

py·e·mic (pī-ē′mik). Relating to or suffering from pyemia.

Py·e·mo·tes tri·ti·ci (pī-ĕ-mō′tēz tri-tī′kī). The straw or grain itch mite, a common parasite of insects in stored grain and a frequent cause of straw or grain itch from their bites; not to be confused with *P. t. ventricosus*, often called the straw itch mite, which is associated with the furniture beetle *Anobium punctatum* and is harmless to humans. SYN *Pediculoides ventricosus*.

py·en·ceph·a·lus (pī-en-sef′ă-lŭs). SYN pyocephalus. [G. *pyon*, pus, + *enkephalos*, brain]

py·e·sis (pī-ē′sis). SYN suppuration. [G. *pyon*, pus, + *-esis*, condition or process]

△**pyg-.** SEE pygo-.

py·gal (pī′găl). Relating to the buttocks. [G. *pygē*, buttocks]

py·gal·gia (pī-gal′jē-ă). Rarely used term meaning pain in the buttocks. [pyg- + G. *algos*, pain]

pyg·ma·li·on·ism (pig-māl′yon-izm). Rarely used term for the state of being in love with an object of one's own creation. [Pygmalion, G. myth. char.]

pyg·my (pig′mē) [MIM*177850, MIM*177860, MIM*265850]. A physiologic dwarf; especially one of a race of similar people, such as the p.'s of central Africa. SYN pigmy. [G. *pygmaios*, dwarfish, fr. *pygmē*, fist, also a measure of length from elbow to knuckles]

△**pygo-, pyg-.** The buttocks. [G. *pygē*]

py·go·a·mor·phus (pī′gō-ă-mōr′fŭs). Conjoined twins in which the parasite, attached to the buttocks of the autosite, is reduced to a formless mass or embryoma. SEE conjoined *twins*, under *twin*. [pygo- + G. *a-* priv. + *morphē*, form]

py·go·did·y·mus (pī-gō-did′i-mŭs). Conjoined twins fused in the cephalothoracic region but with the buttocks and parts below doubled. SEE conjoined *twins*, under *twin*. SEE ALSO *duplicitas* posterior. [pygo- + G. *didymos*, twin]

py·gom·e·lus (pī-gom′ĕ-lŭs). Unequal conjoined twins in which the parasite is represented by a fleshy mass, or by a more fully developed limb, attached to the sacral or coccygeal region of the autosite. SEE conjoined *twins*, under *twin*. [pygo- + G. *melos*, part]

py·gop·a·gus (pī-gop′ă-gŭs). Conjoined twins in which the two individuals are joined at the buttocks, most often back to back. SEE conjoined *twins*, under *twin*. [pygo- + G. *pagos*, something fixed]

△**pyk-.** SEE pykno-.

pyk·nic (pik′nik). Denoting a constitutional body type characterized by well rounded external contours and ample body cavities; virtually synonymous with endomorphic. [G. *pyknos*, thick]

△**pykno-, pyk-.** Thick, dense, compact. [G. *pyknos*]

pyk·no·dys·os·to·sis (pik′nō-dis-os-tō′sis). A condition characterized by short stature, delayed closure of the fontanels, and hypoplasia of the terminal phalanges. Autosomal recessive inheritance. SYN osteopetrosis acro-osteolytica. [pykno- + G. *dys-*, difficult, + *osteon*, bone, + *-osis*, condition]

pyk·no·ep·i·lep·sy, pyk·no·lep·sy (pik′nō-ep-i-lep-sē, pik′nō-lep-sē). Obsolete terms for absence. [pykno- + G. *lepsis*, seizure]

pyk·no·lep·sy. SYN childhood absence *epilepsy*.

pyk·no·mor·phous (pik′nō-mōr′fŭs). Denoting a cell or tissue that stains deeply because the stainable material is closely packed. [pykno- + G. *morphē*, form, shape]

pyk·no·phra·sia (pik′nō-frā′zē-ă). Thickness of utterance. [pykno- + G. *phrasis*, speech]

pyk·no·sis (pik-nō′sis). A thickening or condensation; specifically, a condensation and reduction in size of the cell or its nucleus, usually associated with hyperchromatosis; nuclear p. is a stage of necrosis. [pykno- + G. *-osis*, condition]

pyk·not·ic (pik-not′ik). Relating to or characterized by pyknosis.

py·la (pī′lă). The orifice of communication between the third ventricle and cerebral aqueduct (of Sylvius). [G. *pylē*, gate]

py·lar (pī′lăr). Relating to the pyla.

py·lem·phrax·is (pī-lem-frak′sis). Obsolete term for obstruction of the portal vein. [G. *pylē*, gate, + *emphraxis*, a stoppage]

py·le·phle·bec·ta·sis, py·le·phle·bec·ta·sia (pī′lē-fle-bek′tă-sis, -bek-tā′sē-ă). Obsolete term for dilation of the portal vein. [G. *pylē*, gate, + *phleps* (*phleb-*), vein, + *ektasis*, extension]

py·le·phle·bi·tis (pī′lē-fle-bī′tis). Inflammation of the portal vein or any of its branches. [G. *pylē*, a gate, + *phleps*, vein, + *-itis*, inflammation]

py·le·throm·bo·phle·bi·tis (pī-lē-throm′bō-phle-bī′tis). Inflammation of the portal vein with the formation of a thrombus. [G. *pylē*, gate, + *thrombos*, a clot, + *phleps*, vein, + *-itis*, inflammation]

py·le·throm·bo·sis (pī′lē-throm-bō′sis). Thrombosis of the portal vein or its branches. [G. *pylē*, gate, + *thrombos*, a clot, + *-osis*, condition]

py·lic (pī′lik). Relating to the portal vein.

py·lon (pī′lon). A simple prosthesis, usually without joints, for a lower limb amputation. [G. gateway]

△**pylor-.** SEE pyloro-.

py·lo·ral·gia (pī-lō-ral′jē-ă). Rarely used term for pain in the pyloric region of the stomach. [pylor- + G. *algos*, pain]

py·lo·rec·to·my (pī′lōr-ek′tō-mē). Excision of the pylorus. SYN gastropylorectomy, pylorogastrectomy. [pylor- + G. *ektomē*, excision]

py·lo·ri (pī-lōr′ī). Plural of pylorus. [L.]

py·lor·ic (pī-lōr′ik). Relating to the pylorus.

py·lo·ri·ste·no·sis (pī-lōr′i-ste-nō′sis). Stricture or narrowing of the orifice of the pylorus. SYN pylorostenosis. [pylor- + G. *stenōsis*, a narrowing]

py·lo·ri·tis (pī-lō-rī′tis). Inflammation of the pyloric end of the stomach. [pylor- + G. *-itis*, inflammation]

△**pyloro-, pylor-.** The pylorus. [G. *pyloros*, gatekeeper]

py·lo·ro·di·o·sis (pī-lōr′ō-dī-ō′sis). Obsolete term for operative dilation of the pylorus. [pyloro- + G. *diōsis*, pushing apart]

py·lo·ro·du·o·de·ni·tis (pī-lōr′ō-dū′od-ĕ-nī′tis). Inflammation involving the pyloric outlet of the stomach and the duodenum. [pyloro- + duodenitis]

py·lo·ro·gas·trec·to·my (pī-lōr′ō-gas-trek′tō-mē). SYN pylorectomy.

py·lo·ro·my·ot·o·my (pī-lōr′ō-mī-ot′ō-mē). Longitudinal incision through the anterior wall of the pyloric canal to the level of the submucosa, to treat hypertrophic pyloric stenosis. SYN Fredet-Ramstedt operation, Ramstedt operation. [pyloro- + G. *mys*, muscle, + *tomē*, incision]

py·lo·ro·plas·ty (pī-lōr′ō-plas-tē). Widening of the pyloric canal and any adjacent duodenal stricture by means of a longitudinal incision closed transversely. [pyloro- + G. *plastos*, formed]

Finney p., extension of a long full-thickness incision into the duodenum and proximally into the gastric antrum, with a C-shaped closure to provide a wider opening between stomach and duodenum.

Heineke-Mikulicz p., p. in which a short longitudinal incision is made over the pylorus and closed transversely.

Jaboulay p., a side-to-side gastroduodenostomy, useful when the pylorus and proximal duodenum are extensively scarred or indurated by peptic ulcer disease.

py·lor·op·to·sis, py·lor·op·to·sia (pī-lōr-ō-tō′sis, -tō′sē-ă). Downward displacement of the pyloric end of the stomach. [pyloro- + G. *ptōsis*, a falling]

py·lo·ro·spasm (pī-lōr′ō-spazm). Spasmodic contraction of the pylorus.

py·lo·ro·ste·no·sis (pī-lōr′ō-stĕ-nō′sis). SYN pyloristenosis.

py·lo·ros·to·my (pī-lō-ros′tō-mē). Establishment of a fistula from the abdominal surface into the stomach near the pylorus. [pyloro- + G. *stoma*, mouth]

py·lo·rot·o·my (pī-lō-rot′ō-mē). Incision of the pylorus. [pyloro- + G. *tomē*, incision]

py·lo·rus, pl. **py·lo·ri** (pī-lōr'ŭs, pī-lōr'ī) [NA]. **1.** A muscular or myovascular device to open (musculus dilator) and to close (musculus sphincter) an orifice or the lumen of an organ. **2.** The muscular tissue surrounding and controlling the aboral outlet of the stomach. [L. fr. G. *pylōros,* a gatekeeper, the pylorus, fr. *pylē,* gate, + *ouros,* a warder]

Pym, Sir William, English physician, 1772–1861. SEE P.'s *fever.*

△**pyo-.** Suppuration, accumulation of pus. [G. *pyon,* pus]

py·o·cele (pī'ō-sēl). An accumulation of pus in the scrotum. [pyo- + G. *kēlē,* tumor, hernia]

py·o·ce·lia (pī'ō-sē'lē-ă). SYN pyoperitoneum. [pyo- + G. *koilia,* a cavity]

py·o·ceph·a·lus (pī'ō-sef'ă-lŭs). A purulent effusion within the cranium. SYN pyencephalus. [pyo- + G. *kephalē,* head]

  circumscribed p., abscess of the brain.

  external p., meningeal suppuration.

  internal p., intraventricular suppuration.

py·o·che·zia (pī-ō-kē'zē-ă). A discharge of pus from the bowel. [pyo- + G. *chezō,* to defecate]

py·o·cin (pī'ō-sin). Bacteriocin produced by strains of *Pseudomonas pyocyaneus.*

py·o·coc·cus (pī'ō-kok'ŭs). One of the cocci causing suppuration, especially *Streptococcus pyogenes.* [pyo- + G. *kokkos,* berry (coccus)]

py·o·col·po·cele (pī-ō-kol'pō-sēl). A vaginal tumor or cyst containing pus. [pyo- + G. *kolpos,* bosom (vagina), + *kēlē,* tumor, hernia]

py·o·col·pos (pī-ō-kol'pos). Accumulation of pus in the vagina. [pyo- + G. *kolpos,* bosom (vagina)]

py·o·cy·an·ic (pī'ō-sī-an'ik). Relating to blue pus or the organism that causes blue pus, *Pseudomonas aeruginosa.* [pyo- + G. *kyanos,* blue]

py·o·cy·a·no·gen·ic (pī'ō-sī'ă-nō-jen'ik). Causing blue pus. [pyo- + G. *kyanos,* blue, + *-gen,* producing]

py·o·cy·a·nol·y·sin (pī'ō-sī-ă-nol'i-sin). A hemolysin formed by *Pseudomonas aeruginosa.*

py·o·cyst (pī'ō-sist). A cyst with purulent contents. [pyo- + G. *kystis,* bladder]

py·o·cys·tis (pī-ō-sis'tis). Chronic development and retention of excessive amounts of purulent matter in a urinary bladder that has been defunctionalized by prior supravesical diversion. [pyo- + G. *kystis,* bladder]

py·o·cyte (pī'ō-sīt). SYN pus *corpuscle.* [pyo- + G. *kytos,* cell]

py·o·der·ma (pī-ō-der'mă). Any pyogenic infection of the skin; may be primary, as impetigo, or secondary to a previously existing condition. SYN pyodermatitis, pyodermatosis. [pyo- + G. *derma,* skin]

  chancriform p., a persistent, necrotizing, ulcerated, single pyogenic lesion, usually on the face or genitalia.

  p. gangreno'sum, a chronic non-infective eruption of spreading, undermined ulcers showing central healing, with diffuse dermal neutrophil infiltration; often associated with ulcerative colitis.

  primary p., a p., such as impetigo, in which pus formation is an essential part of the disease.

  secondary p., a p. in which an existing skin lesion (eczema, herpes, seborrheic dermatitis, etc.) becomes secondarily infected.

  p. veg'etans, SYN *dermatitis* vegetans.

py·o·der·ma·ti·tis (pī'ō-der-mă-tī'tis). SYN pyoderma. [pyo- + G. *derma,* skin, + *-itis,* inflammation]

py·o·der·ma·to·sis (pī'ō-der-mă-tō'sis). SYN pyoderma. [pyo- + G. *derma,* skin, + *-osis,* condition]

py·o·gen (pī'ō-jen). An agent that causes pus formation. [pyo- + G. *-gen,* producing]

py·o·gen·e·sis (pī'ō-jen'ě-sis). SYN suppuration. [pyo- + G. *genesis,* production]

py·o·gen·ic, py·o·ge·net·ic (pī-ō-jen'ik, -jě-net'ik). Pus-forming; relating to pus formation. SYN pyogenous.

py·og·e·nous (pī-oj'ě-nŭs). SYN pyogenic.

py·o·he·mia (pī-ō-hě'mē-ă). A rarely used term for pyemia.

py·o·he·mo·tho·rax (pī'ō-hē-mō-thōr'aks). Presence of pus and blood in the pleural cavity. [pyo- + G. *haima,* blood, + thorax]

py·oid (pī'oyd). Resembling pus. [G. *pyōdēs,* fr. *pyon,* pus, + *eidos,* resemblance]

py·o·me·tra (pī-ō-mē'tră). Accumulation of pus in the uterine cavity. [pyo- + G. *mētra,* uterus]

py·o·me·tri·tis (pī'ō-mē-trī'tis). Inflammation of uterine musculature associated with pus in the uterine cavity. [pyo- + G. *mētra,* womb, + *-itis,* inflammation]

py·o·my·o·si·tis (pī'ō-mī-ō-sī'tis). Abscesses, carbuncles, or infected sinuses lying deep in muscles. [pyo- + G. *mys,* muscle, + *-itis,* inflammation]

  tropical p., SYN *myositis* purulenta tropica.

py·o·ne·phri·tis (pī-ō-ne-frī'tis). Suppurative inflammation of the kidney. [pyo- + G. *nephros,* kidney, + *-itis,* inflammation]

py·o·neph·ro·li·thi·a·sis (pī'ō-nef'rō-li-thī'ă-sis). Presence in the kidney of pus and calculi. [pyo- + G. *nephros,* kidney, + *lithos,* stone, + *-iasis,* condition]

py·o·ne·phro·sis (pī'ō-ne-frō'sis). Distention of the pelvis and calices of the kidney with pus, usually associated with obstruction. SYN nephropyosis. [pyo- + G. *nephros,* kidney, + *-osis,* condition]

pyo-ova·ri·um (pī'ō-ō-var'ē-ŭm). Presence of pus in the ovary; an ovarian abscess.

py·o·per·i·car·di·tis (pī'ō-per-i-kar-dī'tis). Suppurative inflammation of the pericardium.

py·o·per·i·car·di·um (pī'ō-per-i-kar'dē-ŭm). An accumulation of pus in the pericardial sac. SYN empyema of the pericardium.

py·o·per·i·to·ne·um (pī'ō-per-i-tō-nē'ŭm). An accumulation of pus in the peritoneal cavity. SYN pyocelia. [G. *pyon,* pus]

py·o·per·i·to·ni·tis (pī'ō-per-i-tō-nī'tis). Suppurative inflammation of the peritoneum. [pyo- + peritonitis]

py·o·phy·so·me·tra (pī'ō-fī-sō-mē'tră). Presence of pus and gas in the uterine cavity. [pyo- + G. *physa,* air, + *mētra,* uterus]

py·o·pneu·mo·cho·le·cys·ti·tis (pī'ō-nū'mō-kō'lē-sis-tī'tis). Combination of pus and gas in an inflamed gallbladder caused by gas-producing organisms or by the entry of air from the duodenum through the biliary tree. [pyo- + G. *pneuma,* air, + cholecystitis]

py·o·pneu·mo·hep·a·ti·tis (pī'ō-nū'mō-hep-ă-tī'tis). Combination of pus and air in the liver, usually in association with an abscess. [pyo- + G. *pneuma,* air, + hepatitis]

py·o·pneu·mo·per·i·car·di·um (pī'ō-nū'mō-per-i-kar'dē-ŭm). Presence of pus and gas in the pericardial sac. [pyo- + G. *pneuma,* air, + pericardium]

py·o·pneu·mo·per·i·to·ne·um (pī'ō-nū'mō-per-i-tō-nē'ŭm). Presence of pus and gas in the peritoneal cavity. [pyo- + G. *pneuma,* air, + peritoneum]

py·o·pneu·mo·per·i·to·ni·tis (pī'ō-nū'mō-per-i-tō-nī'tis). Peritonitis with gas-forming organisms or with gas introduced from a ruptured bowel. [pyo- + G. *pneuma,* air, + peritonitis]

py·o·pneu·mo·tho·rax (pī'ō-nū-mō-thōr'aks). The presence of gas together with a purulent effusion in the pleural cavity. SYN pneumopyothorax. [pyo- + G. *pneuma,* air, + thorax]

  subdiaphragmatic p., subphrenic p., subphrenic abscess associated with perforation of one of the hollow viscera, with gas in the chest and abdomen.

py·o·poi·e·sis (pī'ō-poy-ē'sis). SYN suppuration. [pyo- + G. *poiēsis,* a making]

py·o·poi·et·ic (pī'ō-poy-et'ik). Pus-producing.

py·op·ty·sis (pī-op'ti-sis). A rarely used term for a purulent expectoration. [pyo- + G. *ptysis,* a spitting]

py·o·py·e·lec·ta·sis (pī'ō-pī-ě-lek'tă-sis). Dilation of the renal pelvis with pus-producing inflammation. [pyo- + G. *pyelos,* pelvis, + *ektasis,* a stretching]

py·or·rhea (pī-ō-rē'ă). A purulent discharge. [pyo- + G. *rhoia,* a flow]

py·o·sal·pin·gi·tis (pī'o-sal-pin-ji'tis). Suppurative inflammation of the fallopian tube. [pyo- + salpingitis]

py·o·sal·pin·go-ooph·o·ri·tis (pī-ō-sal'ping-gō-ō-of'ō-rī'tis).

Suppurative inflammation of the fallopian tube and the ovary. SYN pyosalpingo-oothecitis. [pyo- + G. *salpinx,* trumpet (tube), + oophoritis]

py·o·sal·pin·go-oo·the·ci·tis (pī-ō-sal'ping-gō-ō'ō-thē-sī'tis). SYN pyosalpingo-oophoritis. [pyo- + G. *salpinx,* trumpet (tube), + Mod. L. *ootheca,* ovary, + G. *-itis,* inflammation]

py·o·sal·pinx (pī-ō-sal'pingks). Distention of a fallopian tube with pus. SYN pus tube. [pyo- + G. *salpinx,* trumpet (tube)]

py·o·se·mia (pī-ō-sē'mē-ă). Presence of pus in seminal fluid, often associated with chronic prostatitis or other inflammatory conditions of the male genital tract. SYN pyospermia. [pyo- + L. *semen,* seed (of man)]

py·o·sep·ti·ce·mia (pī'ō-sep-ti-sē'mē-ă). Infection of the blood with several forms of bacteria, so-called pyogenic and also nonpyogenic organisms. [pyo- + G. *sēptikos,* putrefying, + *haima,* blood]

py·o·sis (pī-ō'sis). SYN suppuration. [G.]

Manson's p., SYN *pemphigus* contagiosus.

p. palma'ris, an affection observed in children in the East Indies, characterized by the presence of numerous discrete pustules on the palms.

p. trop'ica, an affection seen in Sri Lanka, marked by the presence of dirty yellowish or blackish lesions, covered with a crust, the removal of which leaves a shallow granulating ulcer. SYN Kurunegala ulcers.

py·o·sper·mia (pī-ō-sper'mē-ă). SYN pyosemia. [pyo- + G. *sperma,* seed, + *ia,* condition]

py·o·stat·ic (pī-ō-stat'ik). **1.** Arresting the formation of pus. **2.** An agent that arrests the formation of pus. [pyo- + G. *statikos,* causing to stand]

py·o·sto·ma·ti·tis (pī'ō-stō-mă-tī'tis). A suppurating inflammatory eruption of the mouth. [pyo- + G. *stoma,* mouth, + *-itis,* inflammation]

p. veg'etans, confluent pustular lesions of the mouth, with proliferative and verrucose eruptions of the buccal mucous membrane; associated with ulcerative colitis and other wasting diseases.

py·o·tho·rax (pī-ō-thōr'aks). Empyema in a pleural cavity.

py·o·u·ra·chus (pī-ō-yū'ră-kŭs). A purulent accumulation in the urachus.

py·o·u·re·ter (pī-ō-yū-rē'ter). Distention of a ureter with pus.

py·o·xan·thin (pī'ō-zan'thin). A reddish yellow pigment obtained from blue pus by oxidation.

py·o·xan·those (pī'ō-zan'thōs). A yellowish pigment obtained from blue pus by oxidation.

Pyr Abbreviation for pyrimidine; pyroglutamic acid.

⌂**pyr-.** Fire, heat. SEE ALSO pyreto-, pyro- (1). [G. *pyr*]

pyr·a·cin (pir'ă-sin). Pyridoxolactone, the lactone of 4-pyridoxic acid.

pyr·a·mid (pir'ă-mid). **1.** A term applied to a number of anatomical structures having a more or less pyramidal shape. SYN pyramis [NA]. **2.** An obsolete term denoting the petrous portion of the temporal bone. [G. *pyramis (pyramid-),* a pyramid]

anterior p., SYN p. of medulla oblongata.

cerebellar p., SYN p. of vermis.

Ferrein's p., SYN medullary *ray.*

Lallouette's p., SYN pyramidal *lobe* of thyroid gland.

p. of light, a triangular area at the anterior inferior part of the tympanic membrane, running from the umbo to the periphery, where there is seen a bright reflection of light. SYN cone of light, light reflex (3), Politzer's luminous cone, red reflex, Wilde's triangle.

Malacarne's p., a lobule on the undersurface of the cerebellum, the posterior portion of the vermis.

malpighian p., SYN renal p.

p. of medulla oblongata, an elongated, white prominence on the ventral surface of the medulla oblongata on either side along the anterior median fissure, corresponding to the pyramidal tract. SYN pyramis medullae oblongatae [NA], anterior column of medulla oblongata, anterior p.

medullary p., SYN renal p.

olfactory p., a small area of gray matter situated between the roots of the olfactory tracts; it is continuous caudally with the anterior perforated substance.

petrous p., SYN petrous *part* of temporal bone.

population p., graphical representation of the age and sex composition of a population, constructed by computing the percentage distribution of the population in each age and sex class.

posterior p. of the medulla, SYN *fasciculus* gracilis.

renal p., one of a number of pyramidal masses seen on longitudinal section of the kidney; collectively, they constitute the renal medulla, and contain part of the secreting tubules and the collecting tubules. SYN pyramis renalis [NA], malpighian p., medullary p.

p. of thyroid, SYN pyramidal *lobe* of thyroid gland.

p. of tympanum, SYN *eminentia* pyramidalis.

p. of vermis, a subdivision of the inferior vermis of the cerebellum between the tuber and the uvula. SYN pyramis vermis [NA], cerebellar p.

p. of vestibule, the upper triangular extremity of the crista vestibuli. SYN pyramis vestibuli [NA].

py·ram·i·dal (pi-ram'i-dal). **1.** Of the shape of a pyramid. **2.** Relating to any anatomical structure called pyramid.

py·ra·mi·da·le (pi-ram'i-dā'lē). SYN triquetral *bone.* [Mod. L.]

py·ra·mi·da·lis. SEE pyramidalis *muscle.*

py·ram·i·dot·o·my (pi-ram'i-dot'ō-mē). Section of pyramidal tracts, in the spinal cord, for the relief of involuntary movements. [G. *pyramis,* pyramid, + *tomē,* incision]

medullary p., a medullary pyramidal tractotomy.

spinal p., a spinal pyramidal tractotomy.

pyr·a·min, pyr·a·mine (pir'ă-min). SYN toxopyrimidine.

pyr·a·mis, pl. **py·ra·mi·des** (pir'ă-mis, pi-ram'i-dēz) [NA]. SYN pyramid (1). [Mod. L. fr. G. pyramid]

p. medul'lae oblonga'tae [NA], SYN *pyramid* of medulla oblongata.

p. rena'lis, pl. **pyram'ides rena'les** [NA], SYN renal *pyramid.*

p. tym'pani, SYN *eminentia* pyramidalis.

p. ver'mis [NA], SYN *pyramid* of vermis.

p. vestib'uli [NA], SYN *pyramid* of vestibule.

py·ran (pī'ran). A cyclic compound that may be considered the formal parent of sugars with an oxygen bridge from carbon atoms 1 to 5 (the pyranoses).

pyr·a·none (pir'ă-nōn, pī'-). SYN pyrone.

pyr·a·nose (pir'ă-nōs, pī'-). A cyclic form of a sugar in which the oxygen bridge forms a pyran.

py·ran·tel pam·o·ate (pi-ran'tel). (*E*)-1,4,5,6-Tetrahydro-1-methyl-2-[2-(2-thienyl)vinyl]pyrimidine pamoate; an anthelmintic, especially useful drug for single or mixed intestinal nematode infections such as *Ascaris,* hookworm, pinworm, and *Trichostrongylus* species.

pyr·a·thi·a·zine hy·dro·chlo·ride (pir-ă-thī'ă-zēn). 10-[2-(1-Pyrrolidyl)ethyl]phenolthiazine hydrochloride; an antihistaminic.

pyr·a·zin·a·mide (pir-ă-zin'ă-mīd). Pyrazinoic acid amide; pyrazinecarboxamide; an antituberculous agent; the rapid development of resistance is delayed when given in combination with isoniazid; p. may produce hepatic damage.

pyr·az·o·lone (pir-ă-zō'lōn). A class of nonsteroidal anti-inflammatory agents used in the treatment of arthritic conditions; *e.g.,* phenylbutazone.

py·rec·tic (pī-rek'tik). SYN febrile.

py·re·ne·mia (pī-rĕ-nē'mē-ă). A condition characterized by the presence of nucleated red blood cells. [G. *pyrēn,* the pit of a fruit, + *haima,* blood]

Py·re·no·chae·ta ro·me·roi (pī'rĕ-nō-kē'tă rō'mĕ-roy). One of the numerous species of true fungi capable of causing mycetoma in humans.

py·re·noid (pī'rē-noyd). One of the minute luminous bodies sometimes visualized in the chromatophores of some protozoa, such as *Euglena viridis.* [G. *pyrēn,* pit of a fruit, + *eidos,* resemblance]

py·re·thrins (pī-reth'rinz). Insecticidal constituents of pyrethrum flowers.

py·re·throids. Synthetic pyrethrin derivatives that are used as insecticides; as a class these agents are less toxic to mammals than are other effective insecticides.

py·re·thro·lone (pī-reth′rō-lōn). 2-Methyl-4-oxo-3-(2,4-pentanedienyl)-2-cyclopentenol, a constituent of the pyrethrins.

py·re·thrum (pī-rē′thrŭm). The root of *Anacyclus pyrethrum* (family Compositae), a shrub native to Morocco; has been used as a sialogogue; its flowers are a source of pyrethrins. [G. *pyrethron,* feverfew, fr. *pyr,* fire, from the hot-tasting root]

py·ret·ic (pī-ret′ik). SYN febrile. [G. *pyretikos*]

pyreto-. Fever. SEE ALSO pyr-, pyro- (1). [G. *pyretos,* fever, fr. *pyr,* fire]

py·ret·o·gen (pī-ret′ō-jen). Rarely used term for pyrogen. [pyreto- + G. *-gen,* producing]

py·re·to·gen·e·sis (pī′rĕ-tō-jen′ĕ-sis, pir′ĕ-tō-). Rarely used term for the origin and mode of production of fever. [pyreto- + G. *genesis,* origin]

py·re·to·ge·net·ic, py·re·to·gen·ic (pī′rĕ-tō-jĕ-net′ik, -jen′ik). SYN pyrogenic.

py·re·tog·e·nous (pī-rĕ-toj′ĕ-nŭs). **1.** Causing fever. **2.** SYN pyrogenic.

py·re·to·ther·a·py (pī′rĕ-tō-thār′ă-pē). **1.** Obsolete synonym for pyrotherapy. **2.** Treatment of fever. SYN artificial fever, induced fever. [pyreto- + G. *therapeia,* treatment]

py·rex·ia (pī-rek′sē-ă). SYN fever. [G. *pyrexis,* feverishness]

py·rex·i·al (pī-rek′sē-ăl). Relating to fever.

py·rex·i·o·pho·bia (pī-rek′sē-ō-fō′bē-ă). Morbid fear of fever. [G. *pyrexis,* feverishness, + *phobos,* fear]

pyr·i·ben·zyl meth·yl sul·fate (pir-i-ben′zil). SYN bevonium methyl sulfate.

pyr·i·dine (pir′i-dēn, -din). C₅H₅N; a colorless volatile liquid of empyreumatic odor and burning taste, resulting from the dry distillation of organic matter containing nitrogen; used as an industrial solvent, in analytical chemistry, and for denaturing alcohol.

pyr·i·dof·yl·line (pir-i-dof′i-lin). 7-(2-Hydroxyethyl)-theophylline hydrogen sulfate compound with pyridoxol; a coronary vasodilator.

pyr·i·do·stig·mine bro·mide (pir′i-dō-stig′mēn). 3-Hydroxy-1-methylpyridinium bromide dimethylcarbamate; a cholinesterase inhibitor useful in the treatment of myasthenia gravis.

pyr·i·dox·al (pir′i-dok′săl). 4-Formyl-3-hydroxy-5-hydroxymethyl-2-methylpyridine; the 4-aldehyde of pyridoxine, having a similar physiologic action. SEE ALSO pyridoxine.

p. kinase, an enzyme that catalyzes the phosphorylation by ATP of p. to p. 5′-phosphate and ADP, thus converting the nutrient to the active coenzyme.

p. 5′-phosphate (PLP), a coenzyme essential to many reactions in tissue, notably transaminations and amino acid decarboxylations. SYN codecarboxylase.

pyr·i·dox·a·mine (pir-i-dok′să-mēn). The amine of pyridoxine (–CH₂NH₂ replacing –CH₂OH at position 4), having a similar physiologic action. SEE pyridoxine.

p. 5′-phosphate, the amine of pyridoxal 5′-phosphate (–CH₂NH₂ replacing -CHO at position 4) it is the intermediate formed in many enzyme-catalyzed reactions that utilize pyridoxal 5′-phosphate.

pyr·i·dox·a·mine-phos·phate ox·i·dase. An oxidoreductase catalyzing oxidative deamination of pyridoxamine 5′-phosphate (with O₂ and H₂O) to form pyridoxal 5′-phosphate, H₂O₂, and NH₃.

4-pyr·i·dox·ic ac·id (pir-i-dok′sik). The principal product of the metabolism of pyridoxal (–COOH replaces –CHO at position 4), appearing in the urine.

pyr·i·dox·ine (pir-i-dok′sēn, -sin). 3-Hydroxy-4,5-bis-(hydroxymethyl)-2-methylpyridine (with CH₂OH replacing CHO in pyridoxal); the original vitamin B₆, which term now includes pyridoxal and pyridoxamine, associated with the utilization of unsaturated fatty acids. In rats, deficiency produces a nutritional dermatitis and acrodynia; in humans, deficiency may result in increased irritability, convulsions, and peripheral neuritis. The

hydrochloride is used in pharmaceutical preparations; the chief form in vegetables.

pyr·i·dox·ine 4-de·hy·dro·gen·ase. An oxidoreductase catalyzing oxidation of pyridoxine with NADP⁺ to pyridoxal and NADPH.

pyr·i·form (pir′i-fōrm). SYN piriform. [L. *pyrum* (prop. *pirum*), pear, + *forma,* form]

py·ril·a·mine ma·le·ate (pī-ril′ă-mēn, pir′i-lă-). 2-[(2-dimethylaminoethyl) (*p*-methoxybenzyl)amino]pyridine maleate; an antihistaminic. SYN mepyramine maleate.

py·ri·meth·a·mine (pir-i-meth′ă-mēn). 2,4-Diamino-5-*p*-chlorophenyl-6-ethylpyrimidine; a potent folic acid antagonist used as an antimalarial agent effective against *Plasmodium falciparum;* a valuable suppressant, active against the asexual erythrocytic and tissue forms; also used in the treatment of toxoplasmosis.

py·rim·i·dine (Pyr) (pī-rim′i-dēn). 1,3-diazine; a heterocyclic substance, the formal parent of several "bases" present in nucleic acids (uracil, thymine, cytosine) as well as of the barbiturates.

p. 5′-nucleotidase, an enzyme that catalyzes the hydrolysis of a pyrimidine-nucleoside 5′-monophosphate to produce inorganic phosphate and the pyrimidine nucleoside; a deficiency of this enzyme results in accumulation of pyrimidine nucleotides leading to hemolytic anemia.

p. transferase, SYN *thiamin* pyridinylase.

pyr·i·thi·a·min (pir′i-thī′ă-min). A thiamin antimetabolite, differing from thiamin in that the thiazole ring of the thiamin molecule is replaced by a pyridine ring. SYN neopyrithiamin.

pyro-. **1.** Combining form denoting fire, heat, or fever. SEE ALSO pyr-, pyreto-. **2.** In chemistry, combining form denoting derivatives formed by removal of water (usually by heat) to form anhydrides. SEE ALSO anhydro-. [G. *pyr,* fire]

py·ro·bor·ic ac·id (pī-rō-bōr′ik). SYN tetraboric acid.

py·ro·cal·cif·er·ol (pī′rō-kal-sif′er-ol). 10α-Ergosta-5,7,22-trien-3β-ol; 9-α-lumisterol; a thermal decomposition product of calciferol.

py·ro·cat·e·chase (pī-rō-kat′ĕ-kās). SYN catechol 1,2-dioxygenase.

py·ro·cat·e·chin (pī-rō-kat′ĕ-kin). SYN pyrocatechol.

py·ro·cat·e·chol (pī-rō-kat′ĕ-kol). 1,2-benzenediol; a constituent of the catecholamines, epinephrine and norepinephrine, and dopa; used externally as an antiseptic. SYN catechol (1), pyrocatechin.

py·ro·gal·lic ac·id (pī-rō-gal′ik). SYN pyrogallol.

py·ro·gal·lol (pī-rō-gal′ol). C₆H₃(OH)₃; 1,2,3-trihydroxybenzene; used externally in the treatment of psoriasis, ringworm, and other skin affections. SYN pyrogallic acid.

py·ro·gal·lol·phthal·e·in (pī′rō-gal-ō-thal′ē-in, -thāl′ē-in). SYN gallein.

py·ro·gen (pī′rō-jen). A fever inducing agent that causes a rise in temperature; p.'s are produced by bacteria, molds, viruses, and yeasts, and commonly occur in distilled water. [pyro- + G. *-gen,* producing]

endogenous p. (EP), proteins that induce fever. Several (about 11) have been identified, including cytokines formed by components of the immune system, especially macrophages (*e.g.,* interleukins 1 and 6, interferons and tumor necrosis factors). SYN leukocytic p.'s.

exogenous p., drugs or substances that are formed by microorganisms and induce fever. Among the latter are lipopolysaccharides and lipoteichoic acid.

leukocytic p.'s, SYN endogenous p.

py·ro·gen·ic (pī-rō-jen′ik). Causing fever. SEE ALSO febrifacient. SYN pyretogenetic, pyretogenic, pyretogenous (2).

py·ro·glob·u·lins (pī-rō-glob′yū-linz). Serum proteins (immunoglobulins), usually associated with multiple myeloma or macroglobulinemia, which precipitate irreversibly when heated to 56°C.

py·ro·glu·tam·ic ac·id (Pyr) (pī′rō-glū-ta′mik). SYN 5-oxoproline.

py·ro·lag·nia (pī-rō-lag′nē-ă). Sexual gratification from setting fires. [pyro- + G. *lagneia*, lust]

py·ro·lig·ne·ous (pī-rō-lig′nē-ŭs). Relating to or produced by the dry distillation of wood. [pyro- + L. *lignum*, wood]

py·rol·y·sis (pī-rol′i-sis). Decomposition of a substance by heat. [pyro- + G. *lysis*, dissolution]

py·ro·ma·nia (pī-rō-mā′nē-ă). A morbid impulse to set fires. SYN incendiarism. [pyro- + G. *mania*, frenzy]

py·ro·ma·ni·ac (pī-rō-mā′nē-ak). One affected with pyromania; arsonist.

py·ro·men (pī′rō-men). SYN piromen.

py·rom·e·ter (pī-rom′ĕ-ter). An instrument for measuring very high degrees of heat, beyond the capacity of a mercury or gas thermometer. [pyro- + G. *metron*, measure]

resistance p., SYN resistance *thermometer*.

py·rone (pī′rōn). A keto derivative of pyran. SYN pyranone.

py·ro·nin (pī′rō-nin). A fluorescent red basic xanthene dye, the chloride of tetramethyldiaminoxanthene, **p. Y** or **p. G** (C.I. 45005), or of tetraethyldiaminoxanthene, **p. B** (C.I. 45010). These dyes, especially p. Y, are used in combination with methyl green for differential staining of RNA (red) and DNA (green); difference in staining result is probably due to the higher degree of polymerization of DNA; p. Y is also used as a tracking dye for RNA in electrophoresis.

py·ro·ni·no·phil·ia (pī′rō-nin-ō-fil′ē-ă). An affinity for the basic pyronin dyes; a useful indicator of intense protein synthesis accompanying RNA synthesis, as in the cytoplasm of an active plasma cell. [pyronin + G. *philos*, fond]

py·ro·pho·bia (pī-rō-fō′bē-ă). Morbid dread of fire. [pyro- + G. *phobos*, fear]

py·ro·phos·pha·tase (pī-rō-fos′fă-tās). Any enzyme cleaving a pyrophosphate bond between two phosphoric groups, leaving one on each of the two fragments; *e.g.*, inorganic p., NAD⁺ p. (cleaves NAD, etc., to mononucleotides), ATP p. (cleaves inorganic pyrophosphate from ATP, leaving AMP). SEE ALSO *flavin* adenine dinucleotide.

inorganic p., a phosphohydrolase catalyzing hydrolysis of inorganic pyrophosphate to two orthophosphates.

py·ro·phos·phate (PP) (pī-rō-fos′fāt). A salt of pyrophosphoric acid; accumulates in cases of hypophosphatasia; sometimes referred to as inorganic p. (PP$_i$). SYN diphosphate.

⁹⁹ᵐTc p., a radionuclide tracer used for imaging ischemic myocardium in nuclear medicine. SEE technetium-99m.

py·ro·phos·pho·ki·nas·es (pī′rō-fos-fō-kī′nās-ez). Enzymes (sub-subclass EC 2.7.6) transferring a pyrophosphoric group (*e.g.*, phospho-α-D-ribosyl pyrophosphate synthetase). SYN pyrophosphotransferases.

py·ro·phos·phor·ic ac·id (pī′rō-fos-fōr′ik). $H_4P_2O_7$; an anhydride of phosphoric acid obtained by heating phosphoric acid to 213°C; it forms pyrophosphates with bases, and its esters are important in energy metabolism and in biosynthesis.

py·ro·phos·pho·ryl·as·es (pī′rō-fos-fōr′il-ās-ez). Trivial name applied to the nucleotidyltransferases that catalyze the transfer of the AMP of ATP to another residue with the release of inorganic pyrophosphate, or the attachment of a nucleoside pyrophosphate to a polynucleotide with release of inorganic orthophosphate.

py·ro·phos·pho·trans·fer·as·es (pī′rō-fos-fō-trans′fer-ās-ez). SYN pyrophosphokinases.

py·ro·poi·ki·lo·cy·to·sis (pī′rō-pōy-kil-ō-si-tō-sis). A rare recessive disorder manifested by severe hemolysis, marked poikilocytosis, and a characteristic sensitivity of the red cells to heat-induced fragmentation *in vitro;* apparently due to a defect in spectrin self-association. SYN hereditary pyropoikilocytosis.

hereditary pyropoikilocytosis, SYN pyropoikilocytosis.

py·rop·to·thy·mia (pī-rop-tō-thī′mē-ă). Rarely used term for a delusion in which one imagines being surrounded by flames. [pyro- + G. *ptoeō*, to frighten, + *thymos*, mind]

py·ro·scope (pī′rō-skōp). An instrument for measuring temperature by comparing the light of a heated object with a light standard. [pyro- + G. *skopeō*, to view]

py·ro·sis (pī-rō′sis). Substernal pain or burning sensation, usually associated with regurgitation of acid-peptic gastric juice into the esophagus. SYN heartburn. [G. a burning]

py·ro·ther·a·py (pī′rō-thār′ă-pē). Treatment of disease by inducing an artificial fever in the patient. SYN therapeutic fever.

py·rot·ic (pī-rot′ik). **1.** Relating to pyrosis. **2.** SYN caustic.

py·ro·tox·in (pī′rō-tok′sin). A supposed toxic substance produced in the tissues during the progress of a fever.

pyr·o·val·er·one hy·dro·chlo·ride (pir-ō-val′er-ōn). 4′-Methyl-2-(1-pyrrolidinyl)valerophenone hydrochloride; an analeptic.

pyr·ox·y·lin (pī-rok′si-lin). Consists chiefly of cellulose tetranitrate, obtained by the action of nitric and sulfuric acids on cotton; used in the preparation of collodion. SYN colloxylin, dinitrocellulose, nitrocellulose, soluble gun cotton, xyloidin. [pyro- + G. *xylon*, wood]

pyr·ro·bu·ta·mine phos·phate (pir-ō-byū′tă-mēn). 1-[4-(*p*-Chlorophenyl)-3-phenyl-2-butenyl]-pyrrolidine diphosphate; an antihistamine.

pyr·ro·lase (pir′ō-lās). SYN *tryptophan* 2,3-dioxygenase.

pyr·rol blue (pir′ol) [C.I. 42700]. $C_4OH_3ON_3O_6Na$; an acid triarylmethane dye employed as a vital dye and as an elastin stain. SYN Isamine blue.

pyr·role (pir′ōl). divinylenimine; a heterocyclic compound found in many biologically important substances. SYN azole, imidole.

pyr·rol·i·dine (pi-rol′i-dēn). **1.** Tetrahydropyrrole; pyrrole to which four H atoms have been added; the structural basis of proline and hydroxyproline. **2.** A class of alkaloids containing a p. (1) moiety or a p. derivative.

pyr·rol·i·dine·-2-car·box·yl·ate. SYN proline.

pyr·rol·i·done (pi-rol′i-dōn). 2-Pyrrolidinone; 2-ketopyrrolidine; 2-oxopyrrolidine; an industrial solvent, plasticizer, and coalescing agent.

pyr·rol·i·done·-5-car·box·yl·ate (pi-rol′i-dōn). SYN 5-oxoproline.

5-pyr·ro·li·done-2-car·box·yl·ic ac·id. SYN 5-oxoproline.

pyr·ro·line (pir′ō-lēn). A group of isomers of pyrrole to which two H atoms have been added; 1-p. has a double bond between the nitrogen and an adjacent carbon.

1-pyr·ro·line·-5-car·box·y·late de·hy·dro·gen·ase. An enzyme that catalyzes the reversible reaction of 1-pyrroline-5-carboxylate and NAD⁺ to form L-glutamate and NADH; this enzyme plays a role in proline and ornithine metabolism; 1-pyrroline-5-carboxylate is in equilibrium with glutamate γ-semialdehyde; a deficiency of this enzyme is associated with type II hyperprolinemia.

pyr·ro·line-2-car·box·yl·ate re·duc·tase. An oxidoreductase reducing 1-pyrroline-2-carboxylate to L-proline with NAD(P)H. SYN proline dehydrogenase, proline oxidase.

pyr·ro·line-5-car·box·y·late re·duc·tase. An oxidoreductase reversibly reducing 1-pyrroline-5-carboxylate to L-proline with NAD(P)H; a deficiency of this enzyme is associated with type I hyperprolinemia. SYN proline dehydrogenase, proline oxidase.

pyr·rol·ni·trin (pir-ol-nī′trin). 3-Chloro-4-(3-chloro-2-nitrophenyl)pyrrole; an antifungal agent.

py·ru·val·dox·ine (pī′rū-văl-dok′sēn). SYN isonitrosoacetone.

py·ru·vate (pī′rū-vāt). A salt or ester of pyruvic acid.

active p., an intermediate formed in the oxidative decarboxylation of pyruvate. Cf. p. dehydrogenase (lipoamide). SYN α-lactylthiamin pyrophosphate.

p. carboxylase, ligase catalyzing reaction of ATP, p., and HCO_3^{2-}, to form ADP, inorganic phosphate, and oxaloacetate; biotin and acetyl-CoA are involved; an absence of this enzyme results in neuronal loss in the cerebral cortex, leading to mental retardation.

p. decarboxylase, α-carboxylase; α-ketoacid carboxylase; a carboxylase of yeast catalyzing decarboxylation of a 2-oxoacid (*e.g.*, p.) to an aldehyde (*e.g.*, acetaldehyde) without oxidoreduction and without lipoamide, in contrast to p. dehydrogenase (lipoamide); thiamin pyrophosphate dependent.

p. dehydrogenase, a structurally distinct collection of enzymes containing p. dehydrogenase (lipoamide), dihydrolipoyl transacetylase, and dihydrolipoyl dehydrogenase.

p. dehydrogenase (cytochrome), an oxidoreductase catalyzing reaction between ferricytochrome b_1 and p. to yield acetate and CO_2, and ferrocytochrome b_1.

p. dehydrogenase (lipoamide), an oxidoreductase catalyzing conversion of p. and (oxidized) lipoamide to CO_2 and S^6-acetyldihydrolipoamide in two successive reactions: the first between p. and thiamin pyrophosphate to yield CO_2 and α-hydroxyethylthiamin pyrophosphate (active p.); the second between the last named and lipoamide to regain the thiamin pyrophosphate and yield S^6-acetylhydrolipoamide. Cf. α-ketodecarboxylase.

p. kinase (PK), phospho*enol*pyruvate kinase; a phosphotransferase catalyzing transfer of phosphate from phospho*enol*pyruvate to ADP, forming ATP and p.; other nucleoside phosphates can participate in the reaction; a key step in glycolysis; a deficiency in p. kinase will lead to hemolytic anemia.

p. oxidase [EC 1.2.3.3], an oxidoreductase catalyzing the reaction of p., phosphate, and O_2 to yield acetyl phosphate, CO_2, and H_2O_2.

py·ru·vic ac·id (pī-rū′vik). CH_3–CO–COOH; 2-Oxopropanoic acid; α-ketopropionic acid; acetylformic acid; pyroacemic acid; the simplest α-keto acid; an intermediate compound in the metabolism of carbohydrate; in thiamin deficiency, its oxidation is retarded and it accumulates in the tissues, especially in nervous structures. The enol form, *enol* pyruvic acid, CH_2=C(OH)–COOH, when phosphorylated, plays an important metabolic role. SEE phosphoenolpyruvic acid.

py·ru·vic al·de·hyde. SYN methylglyoxal.

py·ru·vic-mal·ic car·box·yl·ase. SYN *malate* dehydrogenase.

6-py·ru·vo·yl·tet·ra·hy·drop·ter·in syn·thase (6-PTS). An enzyme that catalyzes a step in the synthesis of tetrahydrobiopterin; a deficiency of this enzyme will result in one form of hyperphenylalaninemia.

pyr·vin·i·um pam·o·ate (pir-vin′i-ŭm). 6-(dimethylamino)-2-[2-(2,5-dimethyl-1-phenylpyrrol-3-yl)-vinyl]-1-methylquinolinium 4,4′-methylenebis[3-hydroxy-2-naphthoate] (2:1); a highly effective drug used in the eradication of human pinworms. SYN viprynium embonate.

Pyth·i·um in·si·di·o·sum (pith′ē-ŭm in-sid′ē-um). A species of fungi found in water or wet soil, and a cause of hyphomycosis or pythiosis. SYN *Hyphomyces destruens.*

py·tho·gen·e·sis (pī-thō-jen′ĕ-sis). **1.** Origination from decaying matter. **2.** The causation of decay. [G. *pythō*, to decay, + *genesis*, origin]

py·tho·gen·ic, py·thog·e·nous (pī-thō-jen′ik, pī-thoj′ĕ-nŭs). Originating from filth or putrescence.

py·u·ria (pī-yū′rē-ă). Presence of pus in the urine when voided. [G. *pyon*, pus, + *ouron*, urine]

Q Symbol for coulomb; quantity; quaternary; glutamine; glutaminyl; pseudouridine; coenzyme Q; electric charge; the second product formed in an enzyme-catalyzed reaction.

Q̇ Symbol for blood flow. SEE flow (3). [quantity + an overdot denoting the time derivative]

Q_{10} Symbol for the increase in rate of a process produced by raising the temperature 10°C; rate of contraction of an excised heart approximately doubles for every 10°C (*i.e.*, $Q_{10} = 2$).

Q_O, Q_{O_2}. Symbols for oxygen consumption (1).

Q_{CO_2} Symbol for the microliters STPD of CO_2 given off per milligram of tissue per hour.

△ **-Q_6.** Symbol for ubiquinone-6.

△ **-Q_{10}.** Symbol for ubiquinone-10.

q 1. In cytogenetics, symbol for long arm of a chromosome (in contrast to p for the short arm). **2.** Abbreviation for [L.] quodque, each; every. **3.** Symbol for heat.

QALY Acronym for quality adjusted life years, an adjustment that allows for prevalence of activity limitation.

Q-band·ing. SEE Q-banding *stain*.

q.d. Abbreviation for L. *quaque die*, every day.

QF Abbreviation for quality *factor*, the same as relative biologic effectiveness in radiation protection.

Q-H_2 Symbol for ubiquinol.

q.h. Abbreviation for L. *quaque hora*, every hour.

q.i.d. Abbreviation for L. *quater in die*, four times a day.

q.l. Abbreviation for L. *quantum libet*, as much as desired.

QNB Abbreviation for quinuclidinyl benzilate.

Q.R. Abbreviation for [L] *quantum rectum*, however much is correct.

q.s. Abbreviation for L. *quantum sufficiat* or *satis*, as much as suffices.

quack (kwak). SYN charlatan. [Abbreviation of quacksalver, Dutch *quack*, to boast + *salf*, cream]

quack·ery (kwak'er-ē). SYN charlatanism.

qua·dran·gu·lar (kwah-drang'yū-lăr). Having four angles. [L. *quadrangularis*, fr. *quadrangulum*, quadrangle]

quad·rant (kwah'drant). One quarter of a circle. In anatomy, roughly circular areas are divided for descriptive purposes into q.'s. The abdomen is divided into right upper and lower, and left upper and lower q.'s by a horizontal and a vertical line intersecting at the umbilicus. Q.'s of the ocular fundus (superior and inferior nasal, superior and inferior temporal) are demarcated by a horizontal and a vertical line intersecting at the optic disk. The tympanic membrane is divided into anterosuperior, anteroinferior, posterosuperior, and posteroinferior q.'s by a line drawn across the diameter of the drum in the axis of the handle of the malleus and another intersecting the first at right angles at the umbo. [L. *quadrans*, a quarter]

quad·rant·an·o·pia (kwah'drant-an-op'ē-ă). Loss of vision in a quarter section of the visual field of one or both eyes; if bilateral, it may be homonymous or heteronymous, binasal or bitemporal, or crossed, *e.g.*, involving the upper quadrant in one eye and the lower quadrant in the other. SYN quadrantic hemianopia.

quad·rate (kwah'drāt). Having four equal sides; square. [L. *quadratus*, square]

△ **quadri-.** Four. [L. *quattuor*]

quad·ri·ba·sic (kwah-dri-bā'sik). Denoting an acid having four hydrogen atoms that are replaceable by atoms or radicals of a basic character.

quad·ri·ceps (kwah'dri-seps). Having four heads; denoting a muscle of the thigh, q. femoris muscle, and one of the calf, q. surae muscle, or the combined gastrocnemius (with two heads), soleus, and plantaris, more commonly called triceps surae muscle, the plantaris being counted as a separate muscle. [L. fr. quadri- + *caput*, head]

quad·ri·ceps·plas·ty (kwah-dri-seps'plas-tē). A corrective surgical procedure on the quadriceps femoris. [quadriceps + G. *plastos*, formed]

quad·ri·cus·pid (kwah-dri-kŭs'pid). SYN tetracuspid.

quad·ri·dig·i·tate (kwah'dri-dij'i-tāt). SYN tetradactyl. [quadri- + L. *digitus*, digit]

quad·ri·gem·i·nal (kwah'dri-jem'i-năl). Four-fold. [quadri- + L. *geminus*, twin]

quad·ri·ge·mi·num (kwah'dri-jem'i-nŭm). One of the quadrigeminal bodies.

quad·ri·ge·mi·nus (kwah-dri-jem'i-nŭs). SYN quadruplet. [L.]

quad·ri·ge·mi·ny (kwah'dri-jem'i-nē). SYN quadrigeminal *rhythm*.

quad·ri·pa·re·sis (kwah'dri-pă-rē'sis). SYN tetraparesis.

quad·ri·ple·gia (kwah'dri-plē'jē-ă). Paralysis of all four limbs. SYN tetraplegia. [quadri- + G. *plēgē*, stroke]

quad·ri·ple·gic (kwah'dri-plē'jik). Pertaining to or afflicted with quadriplegia. SYN tetraplegic.

quad·ri·po·lar (kwah'dri-pō'lăr). Having four poles.

quad·ri·sect (kwah'dri-sekt). To divide into four parts. SYN quartisect. [quadri- + L. *seco*, pp. *sectus*, to cut]

quad·ri·sec·tion (kwah'dri-sek'shŭn). Division into four parts.

quad·ri·tu·ber·cu·lar (kwah'dri-tū-ber'kyū-lăr). Having four tubercles or cusps, as a molar tooth. [quadri- + L. *tuberculum*, tubercle]

quad·ri·va·lent (kwah-dri-vā'lent). Having the combining power (valency) of four. SYN tetravalent.

quad·ru·ped (kwah'drū-ped). A four-footed animal. [L. *quattuor*, four, + *pes* (*ped*-), foot]

quad·rup·let (kwah'drŭp-let, kwă-drū'plet). One of four children born at one birth. SYN quadrigeminus. [L. *quadruplus*, four fold]

qua·lim·e·ter (kwah-lim'ĕ-ter). An obsolete device for estimating the degree of hardness of x-rays. [L. *qualis*, of what kind, + G. *metron*, measure]

qual·i·ty as·sur·ance. Programs of regular assessment of medical and nursing activities to evaluate the quality of medical care.

quan·ta (kwahn'tă). Plural of quantum. [L.]

quan·ti·le (kwon'til). Division of a distribution into equal, ordered subgroups; deciles are tenths, quartiles are quarters, quintiles are fifths, terciles are thirds, centiles are hundredths. SYN centile. [L. *quantum*, how much, + *-ilis*, adj. suffix]

Quant's sign. See under sign.

quan·tum, pl. **quan·ta** (kwahn'tŭm, -tă). **1.** A unit of radiant energy (ε) varying according to the frequency (ν) of the radiation. **2.** A certain definite amount. [L. how much]

q. rectum, SEE Q.R. [L. however much is correct]

q. satis, SEE q.s. [L. however much is enough]

q. sink, in radiological imaging, the stage at which statistical information reaches its lowest level because of a low photon flux.

q. sufficiat, SEE q.s. [L. however much is enough]

q. vis, SEE *q.v.*. [L. however much you wish]

quan·tum mot·tle. SEE quantum *mottle*.

quar·an·tine (kwar'an-tēn). **1.** A period (originally 40 days) of detention of vessels and their passengers coming from an area where an infectious disease prevails. **2.** To detain such vessels and their passengers until the incubation period of an infectious disease has passed. **3.** A place where such vessels and their passengers are detained. **4.** The isolation of a person with a known or possible contagious disease. [It. *quarantina* fr. L. *quadraginta*, forty]

quark (qwark). A fundamental particle believed to be the primary constituent of all mesons and baryons; q.'s have a charge that is a fraction of 1 electron charge and interact through electromagnetic and nuclear forces. Six varieties are thought to exist with the unusual names of up, down, strange, charmed, bottom, and top. [a word of indeterminate sense used by James Joyce in his novel *Finnegans Wake*]

quart (kwōrt). **1.** A measure of fluid capacity; the fourth part of a gallon; the equivalent of 0.9468 liter. An imperial q. contains about 20% more than the ordinary q., or 1.1359 liters. **2.** A dry measure holding a little more than the fluid measure. [L. *quartus,* fourth]

quar·tan (kwōr'tan). Recurring every fourth day, including the first day of an episode in the computation, *i.e.,* after a free interval of two days. [L. *quartanus,* relating to a fourth (thing)]

double q., denoting malaria infection with two independent groups of q. parasites, so that paroxysms occur on two successive days followed by one day without fever.

triple q., denoting malaria infection with three independent groups of q. parasites, so that a paroxysm occurs every day, resembling a double tertian or a quotidian fever.

quar·ter-crack (kwōr'ter-krak). SEE sand-crack.

quar·ti·sect (kwōr'ti-sekt). SYN quadrisect. [L. *quartus,* fourth, + *seco,* pp. *sectus,* to cut]

quartz (kwōrts). A crystalline form of silicon dioxide used in chemical apparatus and in optical and electric instruments.

qua·si·dom·i·nance (kwā-si-dom'i-nans). Simulation by a recessive trait of the pedigree of dominant inheritance (*i.e.,* recurrence in several generations) by repeated, and often occult, consanguineous matings. SYN false dominance.

qua·si·dom·i·nant (kwā-si-dom'i-nănt). Denoting a trait in an inbred pedigree that exhibits quasidominance.

quas·sa·tion (kwah-sā'shŭn). The breaking up of crude drug materials, such as bark and woody stems, into small pieces to facilitate extraction and other treatment. [L. *quassatio,* fr. *quasso,* pp. *-atus,* to shake violently, fr. *quatio,* to shake]

quas·sia (kwah'shē-ă). Bitterwood, the heartwood of *Picrasma excelsa* (*Picraena excelsa*), known as Jamaica q., or of *Quassia amara* (family Simarubaceae), known as Surinam q.; a bitter tonic; the infusion has been administered by enema in the treatment of threadworms. [*Quassi,* a resident of Surinam who used it as a tonic]

quater in die (kua'ter-in-dē-ā). SEE q.i.d. [L. four times a day]

qua·ter·na·ry (Q) (kwah'ter-nār-ē, kwah-ter'nĕ-rē). **1.** Denoting a chemical compound containing four elements; *e.g.,* NaHSO₄. Cf. quaternary *structure.* **2.** Fourth in a series. **3.** Relating to organic compounds in which some central atom is attached to four functional groups; applied to the usually trivalent nitrogen in its "onium" state, R_4N^+, "quaternary nitrogen." **4.** Referring to a level of structure of macromolecules in which more than one biopolymer is present. Cf. quaternary *structure.* [L. *quaternarius,,* fr. *quaterni,* four each, fr. *quattuor,* four, + *-arius,* adj. suffix]

Quatrefages de Breau, Jean L.A. de, French naturalist, 1810–1892. SEE Quatrefages' *angle.*

qua·ze·pam (kwā'zĕ-pam). 7-Chloro-5-(*o*-fluorophenyl)-1,3-dihydro-1-(2,2,2-trifluoroethyl)-2*H*-1,4-benzodiazepine-2-thione; a benzodiazepine derivative used as a sedative and hypnotic.

que·brach·ine (kē-brah'chēn). An alkaloid, $C_{21}H_{26}N_2O_3$, from quebracho and identical with yohimbine; formerly used in cardiac dyspnea.

que·bra·cho (kē-brah'chō). The dried bark of a genus of trees, *Aspidosperma quebrachoblanco* (family Apocynaceae); has been used as a respiratory stimulant in emphysema, dyspnea, and chronic bronchitis; the two chief alkaloids are aspidospermine and quebrachine. [Port. *quebrahacho,* fr. *quebrar,* to break, + *hacha,* axe, referring to the hardness of the wood]

Queckenstedt, Hans, German physician, 1876–1918. SEE Q.-Stookey *test.*

queen (kwēn). A female cat of breeding age.

quench·ing (kwench'ing). **1.** The process of extinguishing, removing, or diminishing a physical property such as heat or light; *e.g.,* the cooling of a hot metal rapidly by plunging it into water or oil. **2.** In beta liquid scintillation counting, the shifting of the energy spectrum from a true to a lower energy; it is caused by a variety of interfering materials in the counting solution, including foreign chemicals and coloring agents. **3.** The process of stopping a chemical or enzymatic reaction. [M. E. *quenchen,* fr. O.E. *ācwencan*]

fluorescence q., a technique used in investigations dealing with binding of antigens (haptens) by purified antibodies, applicable in cases in which the bound antigen (hapten) absorbs (quenches) light emitted during fluorescence of protein (antibody) excited by ultraviolet light.

Quénu, Eduard A.V.A., French surgeon and anatomist, 1852–1933. SEE Q.'s hemorrhoidal *plexus;* Q.-Muret *sign.*

quer·ce·tin (kwer'sē-tin). 3,3′,4′,5,7-pentahydroxyflavone; an aglycon of quercitrin, rutin, and other glycosides; occurs usually as the 3-rhamnoside; used in the treatment of abnormal capillary fragility. SYN meletin, sophoretin.

quer·cus (kwer'kŭs). The bark of *Quercus alba,* white oak or stone oak; formerly used as an astringent. [L. oak]

quer·u·lent (kwer'ŭ-lent). Denoting one who is ever suspicious, always opposing any suggestion, complaining of ill treatment and of being slighted or misunderstood, easily enraged, and dissatisfied; characteristic of paranoid personalities. [L. *querulus,* complaining, fr. *queror,* to complain]

Quervain, Fritz de. SEE de Quervain.

ques·tion·naire (kwes-chŭn-ār'). A list of questions submitted orally or in writing to obtain personal information or statistically useful data.

Holmes-Rahe q., a survey to measure in life change units the stressfulness of various life events such as an acute illness, bankruptcy, death of a loved one, etc.

Quetelet. Lambert Alphonse Jacques, 1796–1857. Belgian astronomer and mathematician.

Queyrat, Auguste, French dermatologist, *1872. SEE *erythroplasia* of Q.

Quick, Armand J., U.S. physician, 1894–1978. SEE Q.'s *method, test.*

quick (kwik). **1.** Pregnant with a child whose fetal movements are recognizable. **2.** A sensitive part, painful to touch. [A.S. *cwic,* living]

quick·en·ing (kwik'ĕn-ing). Signs of life felt by the mother as a result of the fetal movements, usually noted from 16 to 20 weeks of pregnancy. [A.S. *cwic,* living]

quick·lime (kwik'līm). Unslaked lime. SEE lime (2).

quick·sil·ver (kwik'sil'ver). SYN mercury.

qui·es·cent (kwi-es'ent). At rest or inactive.

quin-2. (2-[(2-bis-[carboxymethyl]aono-5-methoxyphenyl)-methyl-6- methoxy-8-bis[carboxymethyl]aminoquinoline); a fluorescent compound that binds Ca^{++} tightly. The wavelengths of light that cause fluorescence when Ca^{++} is bound are longer than the wavelengths that cause fluorescence when Ca^{++} is not bound. When excited at two different wavelengths, the ratio of the fluorescence intensities at the two wavelengths gives the ratio of the concentrations of bound to free Ca^{++} Free quin-2 concentration can be measured precisely, so free Ca^{++} concentration can be calculated precisely. Quin-2 may be injected into cells to measure moment-to-moment changes in intracellular Ca^{++} concentration. SEE ALSO aequorin, fura-2.

quin-, quino-. Root of quinoline and quinone, hence used in many names of substances containing these structures (*e.g.,* quinine, quinol).

qui·na (kē'nă, kwē'nă). SYN cinchona. [Sp., fr. Peruv. *quina* or *kina,* cinchona]

quin·a·crine hy·dro·chlo·ride (kwin'ă-krēn, -krin). An acridine derivative, $C_{23}H_{30}ClN_3O\cdot2HCl\cdot2H_2O$, used as an antimalarial that destroys the trophozoites of *Plasmodium vivax* and *P. falciparum,* but does not affect the gametocytes, sporozoites, or exoerythrocytic stage of parasites; also used as an anthelmintic. As a dihydrochloride, it is used as a stain in cytogenetics to demonstrate Y chromatin by fluorescent microscopy. Q. h. intercalates with DNA and also uncouples oxidative and photophosphorylation. SYN atebrine hydrochloride, mepacrine hydrochloride.

quin·al·dic ac·id (kwin-al'dik). quinoline-2-carboxylic acid; a product of L-tryptophan catabolism, via kynurenic acid, found in human urine. SYN quinaldinic acid.

quin·al·dine red (kwin'al-dēn). A styrene-quinolinium iodide; used as a pH indicator (turns red at pH 3.2) in a 1% ethanol solution.

quin·al·din·ic ac·id (kwin-al-din'ik). SYN quinaldic acid.

qui·na·qui·na (kē'nă-kē'nă, kwin'ă-kwin'ă). SYN cinchona. [a reduplication of Sp. *quina,* cinchona]

qui·nate (kwī'nāt, kwin'āt). A salt or ester of quinic acid.

q. **dehydrogenase,** an oxidoreductase catalyzing reaction of quinate and NAD+ to form 3-dehydroquinate and NADH.

quin·a·zo·lines (kwin-a-zōl'ēns). A class of alkaloids that are derived biosynthetically from anthranilic acid.

quince (kwints). The edible fruit of *Cydonia oblongata* (family Rosaceae); the seeds have demulcent properties.

Quincke, Heinrich I., German physician, 1842–1922. SEE Q.'s *disease, edema, pulse, puncture, sign.*

quin·es·tra·di·ol, quin·es·tra·dol (kwin'es-tră-dī'ol, kwin-es'tră-dol). 3-(Cyclopentyloxy)estra-1,3,5(10)-triene-16α,17β-diol; an estrogen.

quin·es·trol (kwin-es'trōl). The 3-cyclopentyl ether of ethinyl estradiol; used as the estrogenic component in oral contraceptive preparations; the compound is stored in fat and can be taken weekly; an estrogen.

quin·eth·a·zone (kwin-eth'ă-zōn). 7-Chloro-2-ethyl-1,2,3,4-tetrahydro-4-oxo-6-quinazolinesulfonamide; a diuretic and antihypertensive agent.

quin·ges·ta·nol ac·e·tate (kwin-jes'tă-nol). 3-(Cyclopentyloxy)-19-nor-17α-pregna-3,5-dien-20-yn-17-ol acetate; a progestational agent.

quin·hy·drone (kwin-hī'drōn). A mixture of equimolecular quantities of quinone and hydroquinone; used in pH determinations (q. electrode).

quin·ic ac·id (kwin'ik). L-quinic acid; 1,3,4,5-tetrahydroxycyclohexanecarboxylic acid; the (–)-isomer is an acid found in cinchona bark and elsewhere in plants; 5-dehydroquinic acid is an intermediate in the biosynthesis of L-phenylalanine, L-tyrosine, and L-tryptophan from carbohydrate precursors; q. a. forms a γ-lactone upon heating. SYN chinic acid, kinic acid.

quin·i·dine (kwin'i-dēn, -din). β-quinine; one of the alkaloids of cinchona, a stereoisomer of quinine (the C-9 epimer); used as an antimalarial; also used in the treatment of atrial fibrillation and flutter, and paroxysmal ventricular tachycardia. SYN conquinine.

q. **polygalacturonate,** a salt of quinidine that may be used in place of quinidine sulfate; antiarrhythmic agent. SEE q. sulfate. SEE ALSO quinidine.

q. **sulfate,** the salt of q. that is customarily administered as a cardiac antiarrhythmic agent. The drug depresses myocardial conduction, contraction, automaticity and contraction; it also by a direct effect impairs conduction through the atrioventricular node. Has vagolytic action that may increase heart rate. SEE ALSO quinidine.

qui·nine (kwī'nīn, -nēn, kwin'-īn, -ēn). $C_{20}H_{24}N_2O_2 3H_2O$; the most important of the alkaloids derived from cinchona; an antimalarial effective against the asexual and erythrocytic forms of the parasite, but having no effect on the exoerythrocytic (tissue) forms. It does not produce a radical cure of malaria produced by *Plasmodium vivax, P. malariae,* or *P. ovale,* but is used in the treatment of cerebral malaria and other severe attacks of malignant tertian malaria, and in malaria produced by chloroquine-resistant strains of *P. falciparum;* it is also used as an antipyretic, analgesic, sclerosing agent, stomachic, and oxytocic (occasionally), and in the treatment of atrial fibrillation, myotonia congenita, and other myopathies.

q. **bisulfate,** the acid sulfate of q., very soluble in water.

q. **carbacrylic resin,** SEE resin.

q. **ethylcarbonate,** an almost tasteless form of q. that is poorly absorbed from the intestinal tract.

q. **sulfate,** the most frequently prescribed salt of q.

q. **and urea hydrochloride,** sclerosing agent for treatment of internal hemorrhoids, hydrocele, and varicose veins, containing not less than 58% and not more than 65% of anhydrous q.

q. **urethan,** a mixture of urethan and q. hydrochloride; a sclerosing agent for the treatment of varicose veins.

qui·nin·ism (kwī'ni-nizm, kwin'i-). SYN cinchonism.

Quinlan's test. See under test.

⌂**quino-.** SEE quin-.

quin·o·cide hy·dro·chlo·ride (kwin'ō-sīd). 8-(4-Aminopentylamino)-6-methoxyquinoline hydrochloride; an antimalarial comparable to primaquine in effectiveness and scope.

quin·ol (kwin'ol). SYN hydroquinone.

quin·o·line (kwin'ō-lēn, -lin). **1.** benzo[b]pyridine; 1-benzazine; a volatile nitrogenous base obtained by the distillation of coal tar, bones, alkaloids, etc.; a basic structure of many dyes and drugs; also used as an antimalarial. SYN chinoleine, leucoline. **2.** A class of alkaloids base on the q. (1) structure.

quin·o·lin·ic ac·id (kwin-ō-lin'ik). 2,3-Pyridinedicarboxylic acid; a catabolite of L-tryptophan and a precursor of NAD+.

quin·o·lin·ol (kwin-ol'in-ol). SYN 8-hydroxyquinoline.

quin·o·li·zi·dines (kwin-ol-i-za-dēns). A class of alkaloids based on the quinolizidine (norlupinane) structure.

qui·nol·o·gy (kwin-ol'ō-jē). The botany, chemistry, pharmacology, and therapeutics of cinchona and its alkaloids. [Sp. *quina,* cinchona, + G. *logos,* study]

quin·o·lones (kwin'ō-lōnz). A class of synthetic broad spectrum antibacterial agents that exhibit bactericidal action.

qui·none (kwin'ōn, kwī'nōn). **1.** General name for aromatic compounds bearing two oxygens in place of two hydrogens, usually in the *para* position; the oxidation product of a hydroquinone. **2.** SYN 1,4-benzoquinone (1).

q. **reductase,** SYN NADPH dehydrogenase (quinone).

qui·no·vose (kwin'ō-vōs). SYN D-epirhamnose.

quin·que·dig·i·tate (kwin'kwē-dij'i-tāt). SYN pentadactyl. [L. *quinque,* five, + *digitus,* digit]

quin·que·tu·ber·cu·lar (kwin'kwĕ-tū-ber'kyū-lăr). Having five tubercles or cusps, as certain molar teeth. [L. *quinque,* five, + *tuberculum,* tubercle, dim. of *tuber,* a swelling]

quin·que·va·lent (kwin-kwĕ-vā'lent). SYN pentavalent. [L. *quinque,* five, + *valentia,* strength]

quin·qui·na (kwin-kwi'nă). SYN cinchona.

quin·sy (kwin'zē). Obsolete term for peritonsillar *abscess.* [M.E. *quinsie (quinesie),* a corruption of L. *cynanche,* sore throat]

lingual q., phlegmonous inflammation of the lingual tonsil and neighboring structures.

quin·tan (kwin'tan). Recurring every fifth day, including the first day of an episode in the computation, *i.e.,* after a free interval of three days. [L. *quintus,* fifth]

quin·tu·plet (kwin-tŭp'let). One of five children born at one birth. [L. *quintuplex,* fivefold]

qui·nuc·li·din·yl ben·zi·late (QNB) (kwin-ū'-kli-di-nil ben'-zil-āt). A highly potent anticholinergic agent exhibiting 50- to 100-fold greater potency over atropine in binding with and blocking muscarinic cholinergic receptors. Originally developed as a potential military incapacitating agent, it is currently extensively used as a radioactive agent (usually tritiated -H3 -QNB) to identify and label muscarinic receptors in pharmacologic studies.

quis·qua·late (kwiz'kwa-lāt). An agonist at glutamate receptors of the amino-3-hydroxy-5-methyl-isoxazole-4-propionic acid (AMPA) type. The anion formed when quisqualic acid is dissoled in water. SEE quisqualic acid.

quis·qual·ic ac·id (kwiz'kwa-lik). Excitatory amino acid (EAA) obtained from the seeds of *Quisqualis chinensis.* Used to identify a specific subset of non-N-methyl D-aspartate (NMDA) EAA receptor; has anthelmintic properties.

quit·tor (kwit'ŏr). A fistulous tract leading from the coronet to the lateral cartilage of the horse, due to an injury, followed by bacterial infection and later by massive necrosis of cartilage and other tissues; the necrotic process may involve the joint capsule. [ME. *quetaur,* a boiling]

quod·que (q). Each, every. [L.]

quo·tid·i·an (kwō-tid'ē-ăn). Daily; occurring every day. [L. *quotidianus,* daily, fr. *quot,* as many as, + *dies,* day]

quo·tient (kwo′shĕnt). The number of times one amount is contained in another. SEE ALSO index (2), ratio. [L. *quoties,* how often]

achievement q., a ratio, percentile rating, or related q. denoting the amount a child has learned in relation to peers of his or her age or level of education.

Ayala's q., SYN Ayala's *index.*

cognitive laterality q. (CLQ), test for difference in cognitive performance of left and right sides of the brain.

growth q., the fractional part or percentage of the entire food energy which is utilized for growth in the young animal.

intelligence q. (IQ), the psychologist's index of measured intelligence as one part of a two-part determination of intelligence, the other part being an index of adaptive behavior and including such criteria as school grades or work performance. IQ is a score, or similar quantitative index, used to denote a person's standing relative to his age peers on a test of general ability, ordinarily expressed as a ratio between the person's score on a given test and the score which the average individual of comparable age attained on the same test, the ratio being computed by the psychologist or determined from a table of age norms, such as the various Wechsler intelligence scales.

Meyerhof oxidation q., an index for the effect of oxygen on glycolysis and on fermentation (*i.e.,* on the Pasteur effect); equal to the rate of anaerobic fermentation minus the rate of aerobic respiration divided by the rate of oxygen uptake.

P/O q., SYN P/O *ratio.*

protein q., the number obtained by dividing the quantity of globulin of the blood plasma by the quantity of albumin.

respiratory q. (R.Q.), the steady state ratio of carbon dioxide produced by tissue metabolism to oxygen consumed in the same metabolism; for the whole body, normally about 0.82 under basal conditions; in the steady state, the respiratory q. is equal to the respiratory exchange ratio. SYN respiratory coefficient.

spinal q., SYN Ayala's *index.*

quot. op. sit. Abbreviation for *quoties opus sit,* as often as necessary. [L.]

q.v. Abbreviation for [L] *quantum vis,* as much as you wish.

♻ **Combining forms**	**[NA] Nomina Anatomica**
Word*Finder* **Multi-term entry finder** **Preceding letter A**	**[MIM] Mendelian Inheritance in Man**
A.D.A.M. Anatomy Plates **Between letters L and M**	☆ **Official alternate term**
Appendices: **Following letter Z**	☆**[NA] Official alternate Nomina Anatomica term**
SYN Synonym; Cf., compare	**High Profile Term**

R

ρ **1.** Rho, the 17th letter of the Greek alphabet. **2.** Symbol for population correlation coefficient.

R Abbreviation or symbol for molar gas *constant*; electrical resistance; radical (usually an alkyl or aryl group, *e.g.,* ROH is an alcohol, RNH_2 an amine); Réaumur; respiration; respiratory exchange *ratio*; roentgen; the remainder of a chemical formula; the calculated unit representing vascular resistance in the cardiovascular system; arginine; purine nucleoside; (in italics) one of two stereochemical designations in the Cahn, Ingold, and Prelog system; the third product formed in an enzyme-catalyzed reaction.

℞ Symbol for *recipe* in a prescription. SEE prescription (2).

R$_f$, R$_F$. Symbol denoting movement of a substance in paper chromatography *relative* to the solvent *front* (*i.e.,* retardation factor); equal to the migration distance of a substance divided by the migration distance of the solvent front.

r Abbreviation for racemic, occasionally used in naming compounds in place of the more common DL- or (±)-, as "r-alanine" (more often as the prefix rac-); roentgen; radius.

r. Symbol for correlation *coefficient.*

Ra Symbol for radium.

rab·bet·ing (rab′et-ing). Making congruous stepwise cuts on apposing bone surfaces for stability after impaction. [Fr. *raboter,* to plane]

rab·bit·pox (rab′it-poks). A virulent epidemic disease among laboratory rabbits caused by the rabbitpox virus, a member of the family Poxviridae; it does not apparently occur among wild rabbits. SYN rabbit plague.

rab·id. Relating to or suffering from rabies. [L. *rabidus,* raving, mad]

ra·bies (rā′bēz). Highly fatal infectious disease that may affect all species of warm-blooded animals, including humans, is transmitted by the bite of infected animals including dogs, cats, skunks, wolves, foxes, racoons and bats, and is caused by a neurotropic lyssavirus, a member of the family Rhabdoviridae, in the central nervous system and the salivary glands. The symptoms are characteristic of a profound disturbance of the nervous system, *e.g.,* excitement, aggressiveness, and madness, followed by paralysis and death. Characteristic cytoplasmic inclusion bodies (Negri bodies) found in many of the neurons are an aid to rapid laboratory diagnosis. SYN hydrophobia. [L. rage, fury, fr. *rabio,* to rave, to be mad]

dumb r., SYN paralytic r.

furious r., the form or stage of r. in which the animal is markedly hyperactive, characterized by periods of agitation, thrashing, running, snapping, or biting.

paralytic r., a form or stage of r. marked by paralytic symptoms. SYN dumb r.

ra·bi·form (rā′bi-fōrm). Resembling rabies.

△**rac-.** Prefix for racemic.

ra·ce·fem·ine (rā-sĕ-fem′ēn). *dl-threo-*α-Methyl-*N*-(1-methyl-2-phenoxyethyl)phenethylamine; used as a uterine relaxant for relief of postpartum pain.

rac·e·mase (rā′sē-mās). An enzyme capable of catalyzing racemization, *i.e.,* inversions of asymmetric groups; when more than one center of asymmetry is present, "epimerase" is used (*e.g.,* hydroxyproline, ribulose phosphate).

rac·e·mate (rā′sē-māt). A racemic compound, or the salt or ester of such a compound. SEE ALSO racemic.

ra·ceme (rā-sēm′). An optically inactive chemical compound. SEE ALSO racemic.

ra·ce·mic (r) (rā-sē′mik, -sem′ik). Denoting a mixture of optically active compounds that is itself optically inactive, being composed of an equal number of dextro- and levorotatory substances, which are separable. Those compounds internally compensated (*i.e.,* having an internal plane of symmetry), and therefore not separable into D and L (or + and −) forms, are termed "meso."

rac·e·mi·za·tion (rā′sē-mi-zā′shŭn, ras-mi-). Partial conversion of one enantiomorph into another (as an L-amino acid to the corresponding D-amino acid) so that the specific optical rotation is decreased, or even reduced to zero, in the resulting mixture.

rac·e·mose (ras′ĕ-mōs). Branching, with nodular terminations; resembling a bunch of grapes. [L. *racemosus,* full of clusters]

rac·e·phed·rine hy·dro·chlo·ride (rās-ĕ-fed′rin). *dl*-Ephedrine hydrochloride; a sympathomimetic drug with peripheral effects similar to those of epinephrine, and with the same actions and uses as ephedrine.

△**rachi-, rachio-.** The spine. [G. *rhachis,* spine, backbone]

ra·chi·al (rā′kē-ăl). SYN spinal.

ra·chi·cen·te·sis (rā-kē-sen-tē′sis). SYN lumbar *puncture.* [rachi- + G. *kentēsis,* puncture]

ra·chid·i·al (rā-kid′ē-ăl). SYN spinal.

ra·chid·i·an (rā-kid′ē-an). SYN spinal.

ra·chi·graph (rā′kē-graf). A graph for recording the curves of the vertebrae. [rachi- + G. *graphō,* to write]

ra·chil·y·sis (ră-kil′i-sis). Forcible correction of lateral curvature of the spine by lateral pressure against the convexity of the curve. [rachi- + G. *lysis,* a loosening]

△**rachio-.** SEE rachi-.

ra·chi·o·camp·sis (rā-kē-ō-kamp′sis). Curvature of the spine. SEE kyphosis, lordosis, scoliosis. [rachio- + G. *kampsis,* a bending]

ra·chi·o·cen·te·sis (rā-kē-ō-sen-tē′sis). SYN lumbar *puncture.* [rachio- + G. *kentēsis,* puncture]

ra·chi·och·y·sis (rā-kē-ok′i-sis). A subarachnoid effusion of fluid in the spinal canal. [rachio- + G. *chysis,* a pouring out]

ra·chi·om·e·ter (rā-kē-om′ĕ-ter). An instrument for measuring the curvature of the spine, natural or pathologic, of the spinal column. [rachio- + G. *metron,* measure]

ra·chi·op·a·gus (rā-kē-op′ă-gŭs). Conjoined twins united back to back as a result of fusion of their spinal columns. SEE conjoined *twins,* under *twin.* SYN rachipagus. [rachio- + G. *pagos,* something fixed]

ra·chi·op·a·thy (rā-kē-op′ă-thē). SYN spondylopathy. [rachio- + G. *pathos,* suffering]

ra·chi·o·ple·gia (rā′kē-ō-plē′jē-ă). SYN spinal *paralysis.* [rachio- + G. *plēgē,* stroke]

ra·chi·o·sco·li·o·sis (rā-kē-ō-skō-lē-ō′sis). SYN scoliosis.

ra·chi·o·tome (rā′kē-ō-tōm). A specially devised instrument for dividing the laminae of the vertebrae. SYN rachitome. [rachio- + G. *tomē,* incision]

ra·chi·ot·o·my (rā-kē-ot′ō-mē). SYN laminotomy. [rachio- + G. *tomē,* incision]

ra·chip·a·gus (ră-kip′ă-gŭs). SYN rachiopagus.

ra·chis, pl. **rach·i·des, ra·chis·es** (rā′kis, rā′ki-dēz, rak-). SYN vertebral *column.* [G. spine, backbone]

ra·chis·chi·sis (ră-kis′ki-sis). **1.** Embryologic failure of fusion of vertebral arches and neural tube with consequent exposure of neural tissue at surface; spina bifida cystica with myelocele or myeloschisis. **2.** Spinal dysraphism. [G. *rhachis,* spine, + *schisis,* division]

r. partia′lis, SYN merorachischisis.

r. tota′lis, SYN holorachischisis.

ra·chit·ic (ră-kit′ic). Relating to or suffering from rickets (rachitis). SYN rickety.

ra·chi·tis (ră-kī′tis). SYN rickets. [G. *rhachitis*]

r. feta′lis, congenital rickets. SYN r. intrauterina, r. uterina.

r. feta′lis annula′ris, congenital enlargement of the epiphyses of the long bones.

r. feta′lis micromel′ica, a congenital condition in which development of the long bones is deficient.

r. intrauteri′na, r. uteri′na, SYN r. fetalis.

r. tar′da, SYN osteomalacia.

ra·chi·tism (rak′i-tizm). A rachitic state or tendency.

rach·i·to·gen·ic (ră-kit-ō-jen'ik). Producing or causing rickets. [rachitis + G. *genesis,* production]

ra·chi·tome (rak'i-tōm). SYN rachiotome.

ra·chit·o·my (ră-kit'ŏ-mē). SYN laminectomy.

rad 1. The unit for the dose absorbed from ionizing radiation, equivalent to 100 ergs per gram of tissue; 100 rad = 1 Gy. **2.** Symbol for radian. **3.** Abbreviation for racemic.

ra·dar·ky·mog·ra·phy (rā'dar-kī-mog'ră-fē). An obsolete procedure involving the video tracking of heart motion by means of image intensification and closed circuit television during fluoroscopy; enabled cardiac motion to be measured by reproducible linear graphic tracing.

ra·dec·to·my (rā-dek'tō-mē). SYN root *amputation.* [L. *radix,* root, + G. *ektomē,* excision]

Radford, Edward P., Jr., U.S. physiologist, *1922. SEE R. *nomogram.*

ra·di·a·bil·i·ty (rā'dē-ă-bil'i-tē). The property of being radiable.

ra·di·a·ble (rā'dē-ă-bl). Capable of being penetrated or examined by rays, especially by x-rays.

ra·di·ad (rā'dē-ad). In a direction toward the radial side.

ra·di·al (rā'dē-ăl). **1.** Relating to the radius (bone of the forearm), to any structures named from it, or to the radial or lateral aspect of the upper limb as compared to the ulnar or medial aspect. SYN radialis [NA]. **2.** Relating to any radius. **3.** Radiating; diverging in all directions from any given center. SYN brachio- (2). [L. *radialis,* fr. *radius,* ray, lateral bone of the forearm]

ra·di·a·lis (rā-dē-ā'lis) [NA]. SYN radial (1). [Mod. L.]

ra·di·an (rad) (rā'dē-ăn). A supplementary SI unit of plane angle. [L. *radius,* ray]

ra·di·ant (rā'dē-ant). **1.** Giving out rays. **2.** A point from which light radiates to the eye.

ra·di·ate (rā'dē-āt). **1.** To spread out in all directions from a center. **2.** To emit radiation. [L. *radio,* pp. -*atus,* to shine]

ra·di·a·tio, pl. **ra·di·a·ti·o·nes** (rā-dē-ā'shē-ō, -shē-ō'nēz). In neuroanatomy, a term applied to any one of the thalamocortical fiber systems that together compose the corona radiata of the cerebral hemisphere's white matter (*e.g.,* optic radiation, acoustic radiation, etc.). SYN radiation (3). [L.]

r. acus'tica [NA], SYN acoustic *radiation.*

r. cor'poris callo'si [NA], SYN *radiation* of corpus callosum.

r. op'tica [NA], SYN optic *radiation.*

r. pyramida'lis, SYN pyramidal *radiation.*

ra·di·a·tion (rā'dē-ā'shŭn). **1.** The act or condition of diverging in all directions from a center. **2.** The sending forth of light, short radio waves, ultraviolet or x-rays, or any other rays for treatment or diagnosis or for other purpose. Cf. irradiation (2). **3.** SYN radiatio. **4.** A ray. **5.** Radiant energy or a radiant beam. [L. *radiatio,* fr. *radius,* ray, beam]

acoustic r., the fibers that pass from the medial geniculate body to the transverse temporal gyri of the cerebral cortex by way of the sublentiform part of the internal capsule. SYN radiatio acustica [NA].

alpha r., an emission of a nucleus of high kinetic energy from the nucleus of an atom undergoing radioactive decay or fission.

annihilation r., the r. resulting when a positron from beta positive decay comes to rest. It encounters an electron, and they annihilate each other and convert their rest mass into two 0.51-MeV gamma rays emitted in exactly opposite directions.

anterior thalamic r.'s, r.'s formed by fibers interconnecting, via the anterior limb of the internal capsule, the anterior and medial thalamic nuclei and the cerebral cortex of the frontal lobe (excluding the precentral gyrus bordering on the central sulcus).

background r., irradiation from environmental sources, including the earth's crust, the atmosphere, cosmic rays, and ingested radionuclides in the body.

> Natural sources account for the largest amount of radiation received by most people each year (average annual dose, 3.00 mSv), with medical and occupational sources accounting for only a fraction (on average, less than .60 mSv). It is currently believed that radon, a gas produced by radium decay within crustal rock, constitutes the major source of background radiation throughout many parts of the U.S. Radon buildup in inadequately ventilated homes may pose a long-term health hazard. The deleterious effects of background radiation, estimated as causing 1–6% of spontaneous genetic mutations, rise with dose.

beta r., radiant energy from a source of beta rays.

central thalamic r.'s, r.'s formed by fibers interconnecting, through the posterior limb of the internal capsule, the ventral lateral, ventral posterolateral and posteromedial, lateral dorsal, and lateral posterior nuclei and the precentral gyrus and parietal lobe of the cerebral cortex.

Cerenkov r., light given off by a transparent medium when a high energy particle speeds through it at a velocity greater than that of light in that medium.

characteristic r., monochromatic r. that is produced when an electron is ejected from an atom and another takes its place by jumping from another shell; the energy of the photon is the difference between that of the two shell positions. SYN characteristic emission.

r. of corpus callosum, the spreading out of the fibers of the corpus callosum in the centrum semiovale of each cerebral hemisphere. SYN radiatio corporis callosi [NA].

corpuscular r., r. consisting of streams of subatomic particles such as protons, electrons, neutrons, etc.

electromagnetic r., r. originating in a varying electromagnetic field; *e.g.,* long and short radio waves; light, visible and invisible; x-radiation and gamma rays.

gamma r., ionizing electromagnetic r. resulting from nuclear processes, such as radioactive decay or fission.

geniculocalcarine r., SYN optic r.

Gratiolet's r., SYN optic r.

heterogeneous r., r. consisting of different frequencies, various energies, or a variety of particles.

homogeneous r., r. consisting of a narrow band of frequencies, the same energy, or a single type of particle.

ionizing r., corpuscular (*e.g.,* neutrons, electrons) or electromagnetic (*e.g.,* gamma) r. of sufficient energy to ionize the irradiated material.

K-r., usually a very penetrating form of x-r. excited by cathode rays (high speed electrons) impinging upon a metal anode such as tungsten; the energy of the r. is a function of the binding energy of the K-shell electrons of the metal anode.

L-r., an x-r. of slight penetrating power excited by cathode rays (high speed electrons) impinging on a metal anode; the energy of the r. is a function of the binding energy of the L-shell electrons of the metal anode.

neutron r., an emission of neutrons from the nucleus of an atom by decay or fission.

occipitothalamic r., SYN optic r.

optic r., the massive, fanlike fiber system passing from the lateral geniculate body of the thalamus to the visual cortex (striate or calcarine cortex, area 17 of Brodmann); the fibers follow the retrolenticular and sublenticular limbs of the internal capsule into the corona radiata but they curve back along the lateral wall of the temporal and occipital horns of the lateral ventricle to the striate cortex on the medial surface and pole of the occipital lobe. SYN radiatio optica [NA], geniculocalcarine r., geniculocalcarine tract, Gratiolet's fibers, Gratiolet's r., occipitothalamic r., Wernicke's r.

posterior thalamic r.'s, r.'s formed by fibers interconnecting through the retrolenticular part of the posterior limb of the internal capsule, the pulvinar complex and lateral geniculate nucleus and the posterior parietal and occipital lobes of the cerebral cortex.

primary r., an incident x-ray beam.

pyramidal r., corticospinal fibers passing from the cortex into the pyramid. SYN radiatio pyramidalis.

scattered r., secondary r. emitted from the interaction of x-rays with matter; generally lower in energy, with a directional distribution which depends on the energy of the incident r. SYN secondary r.

secondary r., SYN scattered r.

Wernicke's r., SYN optic r.

rad·i·cal (rad'i-kăl). **1.** In chemistry, a group of elements or atoms usually passing intact from one compound to another, but usually incapable of prolonged existence in a free state (*e.g.,* methyl, CH₃); in chemical formulas, a r. is often distinguished by being enclosed in parentheses or brackets. **2.** Thorough or extensive; relating or directed to the extirpation of the root or cause of a morbid process; *e.g.,* a r. operation. **3.** Denoting treatment by extreme, drastic, or innovative measures, as opposed to conservative. **4.** SYN free r. [L. *radix* (*radic-*), root]

acid r., a r. formed from an acid by loss of one or more hydrogen ions; *e.g.,* SO_4^-, NO_3^-.

color r., SYN chromophore.

---

free r., a radical in its (usually transient) uncombined state; an atom or atom group carrying an unpaired electron and no charge; *e.g.,* hydroxyl (·Q:H) and methyl

$$\begin{pmatrix} & \text{H} & \\ \text{H:} & \ddot{\text{C}} & \\ & \text{H} & \end{pmatrix}$$

Free r.'s may be involved as short-lived, highly active intermediates in various reactions in living tissue, notably in photosynthesis. The free radical nitric oxide, NO·, plays an important role in vasodilation. SYN radical (4).

It has been theorized that these also act in human tissues to promote heart disease, cancer, Alzheimer's disease, Parkinson's disease, and rheumatoid arthritis. Free radicals may be introduced to the body (through smoking, inhaling environmental pollutants, or exposure to UV radiation), and also occur naturally within the body as a result of metabolic process. They interact readily with nearby molecules, and may thereby cause cellular damage (including to genetic material). Free radicals may be involved in atherosclerosis, promoting the formation of arterial plaque. Natural enzymes such as superoxide dismutase and peroxidase are thought to counteract free radicals, and there is evidence that vitamins C, E, and beta-carotene also exert an antioxidant effect. Perhaps because they contain large amounts of these antioxidant substances, diets high in whole grains and fresh fruit (see low-fat diets) help lower the risk not only of heart disease, but possibly also of cancer.

---

oxygen derived free r.'s, an atom or atom group having an unpaired electron on an oxygen atom, typically derived from molecular oxygen. For example, one-electron reduction of O_2 produces the superoxide radical, $\bar{O}_2$·; other examples include the hydroperoxyl radical (HOO·), the hydroxyl radical (HO·), and nitric oxide (NO·).

ra·di·ces (rā-dī'sēz). Plural of radix.

rad·i·cle (rad'i-kl). A rootlet or structure resembling one, as the *r.* of a *vein*, a minute veinlet joining with others to form a vein, or the *r.* of a *nerve*, a nerve fiber which joins others to form a nerve. [L. *radicula,* dim. of *radix,* root]

rad·i·cot·o·my (rad-i-kot'ō-mē). SYN rhizotomy. [L. *radix* (*radic-*), root, + G. *tomē,* incision]

radicul-. SEE radiculo-.

ra·dic·u·la (ră-dik'yū-lă). A spinal nerve root. [L. dim of *radix,* root]

ra·dic·u·lal·gia (ra-dik'yū-lal'jē-ă). Neuralgia due to irritation of the sensory root of a spinal nerve. [radicul- + G. *algos,* pain]

ra·dic·u·lar (ra-dik'yū-lăr). **1.** Relating to a radicle. **2.** Pertaining to the root of a tooth.

ra·dic·u·lec·to·my (ra-dik'yū-lek'tō-mē). SYN rhizotomy. [radicul- + G. *ektomē,* excision]

ra·dic·u·li·tis (ra-dik-yū-lī'tis). SYN radiculopathy. [radicul- + G. *-itis,* inflammation]

acute brachial r., SYN neuralgic *amyotrophy.*

radiculo-, radicul-. Radicle; radicular. [L. *radicula,* radicle, dim. of *radix,* root]

ra·dic·u·lo·gang·li·o·ni·tis (ra-dik'yū-lō-gang'glē-ō-nī'tis). Involvement of roots and ganglia.

ra·dic·u·lo·me·nin·go·my·e·li·tis (ra-dik'yū-lō-mĕ-ning'gō-mī-ĕ-lī'tis). SYN rhizomeningomyelitis.

ra·dic·u·lo·my·e·lop·a·thy (ra-dik'yū-lō-mī'ĕ-lop'ă-thē). SYN myeloradiculopathy.

ra·dic·u·lo·neu·rop·a·thy (ra-dik'yū-lō-nū-rop'ă-thē). Disease of the spinal nerve roots and nerves.

ra·dic·u·lop·a·thy (ra-dik'yū-lop'ă-thē). Disorder of the spinal nerve roots. SYN radiculitis. [radiculo- + G. *pathos,* suffering]

diabetic thoracic r., a type of diabetic neuropathy that affects primarily elderly patients with diabetes mellitus; clinically characterized by thoracic or abdominal pain, mainly anterior, but sometimes with radiation around the trunk from the midline; usually unilateral; may extend over several segments; probably due to ischemic injury of two or more contiguous roots; one type of diabetic polyradiculopathy.

ra·di·ec·to·my (rā-dē-ek'tō-mē). SYN root *amputation.* [L. *radix,* root, + G. *ektomē,* excision]

ra·dif·er·ous (rā-dif'er-ŭs). Containing radium.

ra·dii (rā'dē-ī). Plural of radius. [L.]

radio-. **1.** Radiation, chiefly (in medicine) gamma or x-ray. **2.** SYN radioactive. **3.** SYN radius. [L. *radius,* ray]

ra·di·o·ac·tive (rā'dē-ō-ak'tiv). Possessing radioactivity. SYN radio- (2).

ra·di·o·ac·tive cow. Colloquialism for radionuclide *generator.* SEE ALSO cow.

ra·di·o·ac·tiv·i·ty (rā'dē-ō-ak-tiv'i-tē). The property of some atomic nuclei of spontaneously emitting gamma rays or subatomic particles (alpha and beta rays).

artificial r., the r. of isotopes created by the bombardment of naturally occurring isotopes by subatomic particles, or high levels of x- or gamma radiation. SYN induced r.

induced r., SYN artificial r.

ra·di·o·au·to·gram (rā'dē-ō-aw'tō-gram). Older term for autoradiograph.

ra·di·o·au·tog·ra·phy (rā'dē-ō-aw-tog'ră-fē). SYN autoradiography.

ra·di·o·bi·cip·i·tal (rā'dē-ō-bī-sip'i-tăl). Relating to the radius and the biceps muscle.

ra·di·o·bi·ol·o·gy (rā'dē-ō-bī-ol'ō-jē). The study of the biological effects of ionizing radiation upon living tissue. Cf. radiopathology.

ra·di·o·cal·ci·um (rā'dē-ō-kal'sē-ŭm). A radioisotope of calcium, particularly calcium-45.

ra·di·o·car·bon (rā'dē-ō-kar'bŏn). A radioactive isotope of carbon; *e.g.,* ¹⁴C.

ra·di·o·car·di·o·gram (rā'dē-ō-kar'dē-ō-gram). A graphic record of the concentration of injected radioisotope within the cardiac chambers.

ra·di·o·car·di·og·ra·phy (rā'dē-ō-kar-dē-og'ră-fē). The technique of recording or interpreting radiocardiograms.

ra·di·o·car·pal (rā'dē-ō-kar'păl). **1.** Relating to the radius and the bones of the carpus. **2.** On the radial or lateral side of the carpus.

ra·di·o·ceph·al·pel·vim·e·try (rā'dē-ō-sef-ăl-pel-vim'ĕ-trē). SYN pelvimetry. [radio- + cephal- + pelvimetry]

ra·di·o·chem·is·try (rā'dē-ō-kem'is-trē). **1.** The science of using radionuclides to synthesize labeled compounds for biochemical or biological research, or radiopharmaceuticals for clinical diagnostic studies. **2.** The study of methods of labeling compounds with radionuclides.

ra·di·o·chlo·rine (rā'dē-ō-klōr'ēn). A radioactive isotope of chlorine, *e.g.,* ³⁶Cl.

ra·di·o·chol·an·gi·og·ra·phy (rā'dē-ō-kō-lan-jē-og'ră-fē). Cholangiography obtained by the intravenous administration of an excreted radiopharmaceutical. [radio- + cholangiography]

ra·di·o·cho·le·cys·tog·ra·phy (rā'dē-ō-kō-lē-sis-tog'ră-fē). Visualization of the gallbladder by scintigraphic means using a radiopharmaceutical such as technetium-99m labeled iminodiacetic acid derivative. [radio- + cholecysoghraphy]

ra·di·o·cinean·gi·o·car·di·og·ra·phy (rā′dē-ō-sin′ē-an′jē-ō-kar-dē-og′ră-fē). Scintigraphic motion picture of the passage of a radiopharmaceutical through the heart and great vessels. [radio- + cineangiography]

ra·di·o·cinean·gi·og·ra·phy (rā′dē-ō-sin′ē-an′jē-og′ră-fē). Scintigraphic motion pictures of the passage of a radiopharmaceutical through blood vessels.

ra·di·o·cin·e·ma·tog·ra·phy (rā′dē-ō-sǐ-nē-mă-tog′ră-fē). Taking a motion picture of the movements of organs or other structures as revealed by an x-ray fluoroscopic examination. [radio- + G. *kinēma*, motion, + *graphō*, to write]

ra·di·o·co·balt (rā′dē-ō-kō′balt). A radioactive isotope of cobalt; *e.g.,* ^{60}Co.

ra·di·o·cur·a·ble (rā′dē-ō-kyūr′ă-bl). Curable by irradiation therapy.

ra·di·o·dense (rā′dē-ō-dens). SYN radiopaque.

ra·di·o·den·si·ty (rā′dē-ō-den′si-tē). SYN radiopacity.

ra·di·o·der·ma·ti·tis (rā′dē-ō-der-mă-tī′tis). Dermatitis due to exposure to x-rays or gamma rays causing ionization of tissue water with changes resembling thermal injury. SYN radioepidermitis.

ra·di·o·di·ag·no·sis (rā′dē-ō-dī-ag-nō′sis). Diagnosis using x-rays; or, more broadly, diagnostic imaging, including radiology, ultrasound, and magnetic resonance.

ra·di·o·dig·i·tal (rā′dē-ō-dij′i-tăl). Relating to the fingers on the radial or lateral side of the hand.

ra·di·o·e·lec·tro·phys·i·ol·o·gram (ra′dē-ō-e-lek′trō-fiz-ē-ol′ō-gram). The record obtained by means of the radioelectrophysiolograph.

ra·di·o·e·lec·tro·phys·i·ol·o·graph (rā′dē-ō-ē-lek′trō-fiz-ē-ol′ō-graf). Formerly, an apparatus carried by a mobile individual by means of which changes in electrical potential from the brain or heart can be picked up and radio-transmitted to an electroencephalograph or an electrocardiograph. SEE telemeter.

ra·di·o·e·lec·tro·phys·i·o·log·ra·phy (rā′dē-ō-ē-lek′trō-fiz′ē-ō-log′ră-fē). Formerly, recording the changes in the electrical potential of the brain or heart by means of the radioelectrophysiolograph. SEE telemetry.

ra·di·o·el·e·ment (rā′dē-ō-el′ĕ-ment). Any element possessing radioactivity.

ra·di·o·ep·i·der·mi·tis (rā′dē-ō-ep′i-der-mī′tis). SYN radiodermatitis.

ra·di·o·ep·i·the·li·tis (rā′dē-ō-ep′i-thē-lī′tis). Destructive changes in epithelium produced by ionizing radiation.

ra·di·o·fre·quen·cy (rā′dē-ō-frē′kwen-sē). **1.** Radiant energy of a certain frequency range; *e.g.,* radio and television employ radiant energy having a frequency between 10^5–10^{11} Hz, while diagnostic x-rays have a frequency in the range of 3×10^{18} Hz. **2.** In magnetic resonance imaging, the energy applied to switch or create a gradient in the magnetic field.

ra·di·o·gal·li·um (rā′dē-ō-gal′ē-ŭm). Gallium that is radioactive. SEE gallium-67, gallium-68.

ra·di·o·gen·e·sis (rā′dē-ō-jen′ĕ-sis). The formation or production of radioactivity resulting from radioactive transformation or disintegration of radioactive substances. [radio- + G. *genesis*, production]

ra·di·o·gen·ic (rā′dē-ō-jen′ik). **1.** Producing rays of any sort, especially electromagnetic rays. **2.** Caused by x- or gamma rays.

ra·di·o·gen·ics (rā′dē-ō-jen′iks). The science of radiation.

ra·di·o·gold col·loid (rā′dē-ō-gōld kol′oyd). A radioactive isotope of gold emitting negative beta particles and gamma radiation, with a half-life of 2.7 days; formerly used for irradiation of closed serous cavities in the palliative treatment of ascites and pleural effusion due to metastatic malignancies, and for liver scans. SYN ^{198}Au colloid, colloidal radioactive gold.

ra·di·o·gram (rā′dē-ō-gram). Obsolete term for radiograph. [radio- + G. *gramma*, something written]

ra·di·o·graph (rā′dē-ō-graf). A negative image on photographic film made by exposure to x-rays or gamma rays that have passed through matter or tissue. SYN roentgenogram, roentgenograph. [radio- + G. *graphō*, to write]

bitewing r., intraoral dental film adapted to show the coronal portion and cervical third of the root of the teeth in near occlusion; especially useful in detecting interproximal caries and determining alveolar septal height.

cephalometric r., a radiographic view of the jaws and skull permitting measurement. SYN cephalogram.

decubitus r., a r. of a recumbent subject on his side, made in the frontal projection with a horizontal x-ray beam. SYN lateral decubitus r.

lateral decubitus r., SYN decubitus r.

lateral oblique r., a radiographic view of the mandible, revealing one side of the mandible from symphysis to condyle by displacing the other side upwards.

lateral ramus r., a radiographic view of the mandibular ramus and condyle.

lateral skull r., a true lateral projection r. of facial bones and calvarium, showing bone structures and air-containing passages.

maxillary sinus r., a radiographic frontal view of the maxillary sinuses, orbits, nasal structures and zygomas; permits direct comparison of the sides. SYN Waters' view r.

occlusal r., intraoral section film positioned on the occlusal plane and used in visualizing entire sections of the jaw; especially useful in exploring calcifications of the sublingual salivary glands.

panoramic r., a radiographic view of the maxillae and mandible extending from the left to the right glenoid fossae.

periapical r., a r. demonstrating tooth apices and surrounding structures in a particular intraoral area.

scout r., SYN scout *film.*

submental vertex r., SYN submentovertex r.

submentovertex r., a radiographic projection showing the base of the skull, positions of the mandibular condyles, and zygomatic arches. SYN base view, submental vertex r.

Towne projection r., SEE Towne *projection.*

transcranial r., a radiographic view of the temporomandibular articulation.

Trendelenburg r., r. of a subject tilted head downwards, usually in the decubitus position; used to detect small pleural effusions.

Waters' view r., SYN maxillary sinus r.

ra·di·og·raph·er (rā-dē-og′ră-fĕr). A technician trained to position patients and take radiographs or perform other radiodiagnostic procedures.

ra·di·og·ra·phy (rā′dē-og′ră-fē). Examination of any part of the body for diagnostic purposes by means of x-rays with the record of the findings usually impressed upon a photographic film. SYN roentgenography.

advanced multiple-beam equalization r. (AMBER), a variant of scanning equalization r. using several x-ray beams.

air-gap r., chest r. with a space (at least 10 inches) between the subject and film. Instead of using a grid, this method uses the geometry and x-ray absorption by the air to remove scattered radiation.

bedside r., SYN portable r.

computed r., r. using a solid-state imaging device, such as a photostimulable phosphorplate, and recovering, enhancing, and displaying the image using a digital computer.

digital r., computed radiography or computer processing of a digitized image from a conventional image-intensifier and video camera. SEE DSA.

electron r., radiographic imaging in which x-radiation incident on the receptor is converted to a latent charge image and subsequently recovered by a special printing process; advantages include wider latitude of exposure and greater sensitivity than conventional film-screen combinations. SEE xeroradiography, phosphor *plate.*

magnification r., r. using a microfocal x-ray tube and increased subject-film distance to provide geometric magnification of the subject without unacceptable loss of sharpness and resolution or

ra

an undesirable increase in radiation exposure caused by increasing the distance between the subject and the film.

mucosal relief r., radiographic technique showing fine detail of gastrointestinal mucosa after coating it with a barium suspension and distending the organ with air or gas released from an ingested powder.

portable r., making radiographic films of a patient confined to bed by taking a movable x-ray machine to the room. SYN bedside r.

scanning equalization r., an electronically enhanced method of radiography in which a small x-ray beam is scanned over the patient while its attenuation is measured, providing feedback to modulate beam intensity in order to equalize average x-ray film exposure.

sectional r., SYN tomography.

serial r., making several x-ray exposures of a single region over a period of time, as in angiography.

spot-film r., an x-ray of a localized region, usually under study by fluoroscopy.

ra·di·o·hu·mer·al (rā′dē-ō-hyū′mer-ăl). Relating to the radius and the humerus; denoting the articulation between them.

ra·di·o·im·mu·ni·ty (rā′dē-ō-i-myū′ni-tē). Lessened sensitivity to radiation.

ra·di·o·im·mu·no·as·say (RIA) (rā′dē-ō-im′u-nō-as′sā). An immunological (immunochemical) procedure that uses the competition between radioisotope-labeled antigen (hormone) or other substance and unlabeled antigen for antiserums, resulting in quantitation of the unlabeled antigen; any method for detecting or quantitating antigens or antibodies using radiolabeled reactants.

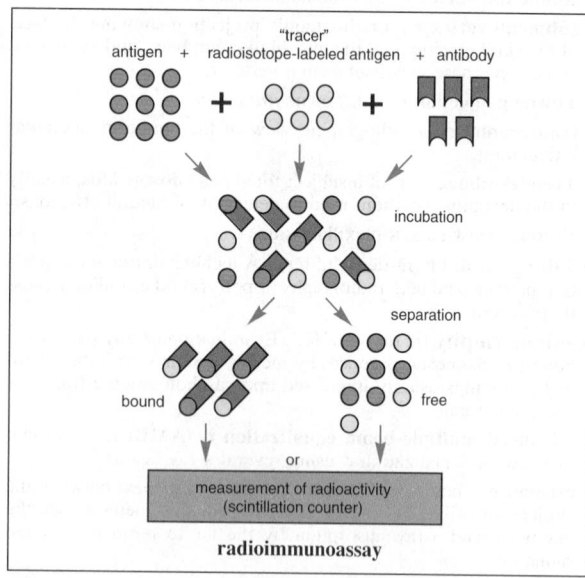

radioimmunoassay

ra·di·o·im·mu·no·dif·fu·sion (rā′dē-ō-im′yū-nō-di-fyū′zhŭn). A method for the study of antigen-antibody reactions by gel diffusion using radioisotope-labeled antigen or antibody.

ra·di·o·im·mu·no·elec·tro·pho·re·sis (rā′dē-ō-im′yū-nō-ē-lek′trō-fō-rē′sis). Immunoelectrophoresis in which the antigen or antibody is labeled with a radioisotope; e.g., in testing for insulin-binding antibodies by treating the test serum with radioactive iodine-labeled insulin, subjecting the mixture (antigen) to electrophoresis, precipitating the separated immunoglobulins with immunoglobulin-specific antiserum, and, then, with radiosensitive film (autoradiography), testing for bound insulin in the precipitates.

ra·di·o·im·mu·no·pre·cip·i·ta·tion (rā′dē-ō-im′yū-nō-prē-sip-i-tā′shŭn). Immunoprecipitation utilizing a radioisotope-labeled antibody or antigen.

ra·di·o·io·din·at·ed (rā′dē-ō-ī′ō-din-ā-ted). Treated or combined with radioiodine.

ra·di·o·i·o·dine (rā′dē-ō-i′ō-dīn). A radioactive isotope of iodine; e.g., ^{123}I.

ra·di·o·i·ron (rā′dē-ō-ī′ern). A radioactive isotope of iron; e.g., ^{59}Fe.

ra·di·o·i·so·tope (rā′dē-ō-ī′sō-tōp). An isotope that changes to a more stable state by emitting radiation.

ra·di·o·la·beled (rā′dē-ō-lā′bld). SEE tag (1).

ra·di·o·lead (rā′dē-ō-led′). A radioactive isotope of lead.

ra·di·o·le·sion (rā′dē-ō-lē′zhŭn). A lesion produced by ionizing radiation.

ra·di·o·li·gand (rā′dē-ō-lig′and). A molecule with a radionuclide tracer attached; usually used for radioimmunoassay procedures. [radio- + L. ligandus, that which is to be bound, fr. ligo, to bind]

ra·di·o·log·ic, ra·di·o·log·i·cal (rā-dē-ō-log′ik, -loj′i-kăl). Pertaining to radiology.

ra·di·ol·o·gist (rā-dē-ol′ō-jist). A physician trained in the diagnostic and/or therapeutic use of x-rays and radionuclides, radiation physics, and biology; a diagnostic r. would also be trained in diagnostic ultrasound and magnetic resonance imaging and applicable physics.

ra·di·ol·o·gy (rā-dē-ol′ō-jē). **1.** The science of high energy radiation and of the sources and the chemical, physical, and biologic effects of such radiation; the term usually refers to the diagnosis and treatment of disease. **2.** The scientific discipline of medical imaging using ionizing radiation, radionuclides, nuclear magnetic resonance, and ultrasound. [radio- + G. logos, study]

cardiovascular r., the clinical subspecialty of r. concerned with diagnosis and treatment of diseases of the vascular system.

chest r., the clinical subspecialty concerned with the diagnostic r. of diseases of the thorax, especially the heart or lungs.

interventional r., the clinical subspecialty that uses fluoroscopy, CT, and ultrasound to guide percutaneous procedures such as performing biopsies, draining fluids, inserting catheters, or dilating or stenting narrowed ducts or vessels.

pediatric r., the clinical subspecialty concerned with the radiological manifestations of diseases of children.

ra·di·o·lu·cen·cy (rā-dē-ō-lū′sen-sē). The state of being radiolucent.

ra·di·o·lu·cent (rā-dē-ō-lū′sent). Relatively penetrable by x-rays or other forms of radiation. Cf. radiopaque. [radio- + L. lucens, shining]

ra·di·o·lus (rā-dē′ō-lŭs). A probe or sound. [L. dim. of radius, spoke]

ra·di·om·e·ter (rā-dē-om′ĕ-ter). A device for determining the penetrative power of x-rays. SYN roentgenometer. [radio- + G. metron, measure]

ra·di·o·mi·crom·e·ter (rā′dē-ō-mī-krom′ĕ-ter). A sensitive thermopile designed for the measurement of minute changes in radiant energy.

ra·di·o·mi·met·ic (rā′dē-ō-mi-met′ik). Imitating the biologic effects of radiation, as in the case of chemicals such as nitrogen mustards. [radio- + G. mimētikos, imitative]

ra·di·o·mus·cu·lar (rā′dē-ō-mŭs′kyū-lăr). Relating to the radius and the neighboring muscles; denoting certain nerves and muscular branches of the radial artery.

ra·di·o·ne·cro·sis (rā′dē-ō-ne-krō′sis). Necrosis due to radiation; e.g., after excessive exposure to x- or gamma rays. SEE radiation burn.

ra·di·o·neu·ri·tis (rā′dē-ō-nū-rī′tis). Neuritis caused by prolonged or repeated exposure to x-rays or radium.

ra·di·o·ni·tro·gen (rā′dē-ō-nī′trō-jen). A radioactive isotope of nitrogen; e.g., ^{13}N.

ra·di·o·nu·clide (rā′dē-ō-nū′klīd). An isotope of artificial or natural origin that exhibits radioactivity.

Radionuclides serve as agents in nuclear medicine and genetic engineering, play a role in computer imaging for diagnosis and experiment, and account for a percentage of background radiation to which humans are exposed. In cancer therapy, radionuclides that localize to certain organs (e.g., radioactive iodine or gallium), deliver cytotoxic radiation doses to tumors. Similarly, radionuclides can be yoked to monoclonal antibodies engineered to attack specific populations of cancerous cells. In positron emission tomography, glucose molecules tagged with radionuclides are injected into the bloodstream. The gamma radiation emitted by the decay of the radionuclides reveals areas of active glucose uptake and thus offers a gauge of cell metabolism and function.

ra·di·o·pac·i·ty (rā′dē-ō-pas′i-tē). State of being radiopaque. SYN radiodensity.

ra·di·o·pal·mar (rā′dē-ō-pal′măr). Relating to the radial or lateral side of the palm.

ra·di·o·paque (rā-dē-ō-pāk′). Exhibiting relative opacity to, or impenetrability by, x-rays or any other form of radiation. Cf. radiolucent. SYN radiodense. [radio- + Fr. opaque fr. L. *opacus,* shady]

ra·di·o·pa·thol·o·gy (rā′dē-ō-path-ol′o-jē). A branch of radiology or pathology concerned with the effects of radiation on cells and tissues. Cf. radiobiology.

ra·di·o·pel·vim·e·try (rā′dē-ō-pel-vim′ĕ-trē). Radiographic measurement of the pelvis. SEE pelvimetry.

ra·di·o·phar·ma·ceu·ti·cal (rā′dē-ō-far-mă-sū′ti-kal). A radioactive chemical or pharmaceutical preparation, labeled with a radionuclide in tracer or therapeutic concentration, used as a diagnostic or therapeutic agent.

ra·di·o·pho·bia (rā′dē-ō-fō′bē-ă). Morbid fear of radiation, as from x-rays or nuclear energy. [radio- + G. *phobos,* fear]

ra·di·o·phos·pho·rus (rā′dē-ō-fos′fōr-ŭs). A radioactive isotope of phosphorus; *e.g.,* ^{32}P.

ra·di·o·pill (rā′dē-ō-pil). SYN radiotelemetering *capsule.*

ra·di·o·po·tas·si·um (rā′dē-ō-pō-tas′ē-ŭm). A radioactive isotope of potassium; *e.g.,* ^{40}K.

ra·di·o·re·ac·tion (rā′dē-ō-rē-ak′shŭn). A reaction of the body to radiation.

ra·di·o·re·cep·tor (rā′dē-ō-rē-sep′ter). **1.** A receptor that normally responds to radiant energy such as light or heat. **2.** A receptor used as a binding agent for unlabeled and radiolabeled analyte in a type of competitive binding assay called radioreceptor assay.

ra·di·o·re·sis·tant (rā′dē-ō-rē-zis′tant). Indicates cells or tissues that are less affected than average mammalian cells on exposure to radiation; when applied to neoplasms, indicates less susceptibility to damage from theurapeutic radiation than the surrounding host tissues.

ra·di·os·co·py (rā′dē-os′kŏ-pē). Archaic term for fluoroscopy. [radio- + G. *skopeō,* to view]

ra·di·o·sen·si·tive (rā′dē-ō-sen′si-tiv). Readily affected by radiation. Cf. radioresistant.

ra·di·o·sen·si·tiv·i·ty (rā′dē-ō-sen-si-tiv′i-tē). The condition of being readily affected by radiant energy.

ra·di·o·sen·si·ti·za·tion. The use of chemotherapy or other agents which increase the sensitivity of tissue to the effects or radiation therapy, usually by inhibiting cellular repair or increasing the percentage of cells in mitotic phases of the growth cycle.

ra·di·o·sen·si·tiz·er (rā′dē-ō-sen-si-tī′zĕr). A chemical substance that increases the radiosensitivity of tissues; restoring normal tissue oxygen tension to an anoxic region is also an effective r.

ra·di·o·so·di·um (rā′dē-ō-sō′dē-ŭm). A radioactive isotope of sodium; *e.g.,* ^{24}Na.

ra·di·o·ster·e·os·co·py (rā′dē-ō-ster-ē-os′kŏ-pē). Simultaneous viewing of two radiographs made in slightly different projections, usually with a device that reflects the image of one on each eye, allowing three-dimensional visualization of an object in relation to others. SEE stereoradiography, stereoscope. [radio- + G. *stereos,* solid, + *skopeō,* to view]

ra·di·o·stron·ti·um (rā′dē-ō-stron′tē-ŭm). A radioactive isotope of strontium; *e.g.,* ^{90}Sr.

ra·di·o·sul·fur (rā′dē-ō-sŭl′fŭr). A radioactive isotope of sulfur; *e.g.,* ^{35}S.

ra·di·o·sur·gery (rā′dē-ō-sŭr-gĕ-rē). Radiotherapy with a sharply delimited field, optimistically considered to be equivalent to resecting the irradiated region.

ra·di·o·te·lem·e·try (rā′dē-ō-tĕ-lem′ĕ-trē). SEE telemetry, biotelemetry.

ra·di·o·ther·a·peu·tic (rā′dē-ō-thār-ă-pyū′tik). Relating to radiotherapy or to radiotherapeutics.

ra·di·o·ther·a·peu·tics (rā′dē-ō-thār-ă-pyū′tiks). The study and use of radiotherapeutic agents.

ra·di·o·ther·a·pist (rā′dē-ō-thār′ă-pist). One who practices radiotherapy or is versed in radiotherapeutics. SYN radiation oncologist.

ra·di·o·ther·a·py (rā′dē-ō-thār′ă-pē). The medical specialty concerned with the use of electromagnetic or particulate radiation in the treatment of disease. SYN roentgenotherapy.

mantle r., r. with protection of uninvolved radiosensitive structures or organs.

ra·di·o·ther·my (rā′dē-ō-ther′mē). Diathermy effected by heat from radiant sources. [radio- + G. *thermē,* heat]

ra·di·o·thy·roid·ec·to·my (rā′dē-ō-thī′roy-dek-tō-mē). The destruction of thyroid tissue by administration of radioactive iodine.

ra·di·o·thy·rox·in (rā′dē-ō-thī-rok′sin). SYN radioactive *thyroxine.*

ra·di·o·tox·e·mia (rā′dē-ō-tok-sē′mē-ă). Radiation sickness caused by the products of disintegration produced by the action of x-rays or other forms of radioactivity and by the depletion of certain cells and enzyme systems from the organism. [radio- + G. *toxikon,* poison, + *haima,* blood]

ra·di·o·trac·er (rā′dē-ō-trā′sĕr). A radionuclide or radiolabeled chemical; a radioactive tracer.

ra·di·o·trans·par·ent (rā′dē-ō-trans-par′ent). Allowing relatively free transmission of radiant energy.

ra·di·o·trop·ic (rā′dē-ō-trop′ik). Affected by radiation. [radio- + G. *tropē,* a turning]

ra·di·o·ul·nar (rā′dē-ō-ŭl′năr). Relating to both radius and ulna.

ra·di·sec·to·my (rā-dē-ō-sek′tō-mē). SYN root *amputation.* [L. *radix,* root, + G. *ektomē,* excision]

ra·di·um (Ra) (rā′dē-ŭm). A metallic element, atomic no. 88, extracted in very minute quantities from pitchblende; ^{226}Ra, its longest lived isotope, is produced as an intermediate in the uranium series by the emission of an alpha particle from thorium-230 (ionium); ^{226}Ra emits alpha particles and gamma rays, breaking down to ^{222}Rn with a half-life of 1,599 years; chemically, it is an alkaline earth metal with properties similar to those of barium. Its therapeutic action is similar to that of x-rays, since the α emission is filtered out. [L. *radius,* ray]

ra·di·us, gen. and pl. **ra·di·i** (rā′dē-ŭs, rā′dē-ī). **1** [NA]. The lateral and shorter of the two bones of the forearm. **2.** A straight line passing from the center to the periphery of a circle. SYN radio- (3). [L. spoke of a wheel, rod, ray]

r. fix′us, a line passing from the hormion to the inion.

ra′dii len′tis [NA], 9 to 12 faint lines on the anterior and posterior surfaces of the lens that radiate from the poles toward the equator; they mark the lines along which the ends of lens fibers abut. SYN lens stars (1), lens sutures.

ra·dix (ray′diks). The hypothetical size of the birth cohort in a life table, commonly 1000 or 100,000.

ra·dix, gen. **ra·di·cis,** pl. **ra·di·ces** (rā′diks, rā-di′sis, rā′di-sēz or rā-dī′sēz) [NA]. **1.** SYN *root* of tooth. **2.** The hypothetical size of the birth cohort in a life table, commonly 1000 or 100,000. [L.]

r. ante′rior [NA], SYN ventral *root.*

r. ar′cus ver′tebrae, SYN *pedicle* of arch of vertebra.

r. bre′vis gan′glii cilia′ris, SYN parasympathetic *root* of ciliary ganglion.

r. clin′ica [NA], SYN clinical *root.*

r. cochlea′ris [NA], SYN cochlear *root* of VIII nerve.

ra′dices crania′les [NA], SYN cranial *root* of accessory nerve.

r. den′tis [NA], SYN *root* of tooth.

ra

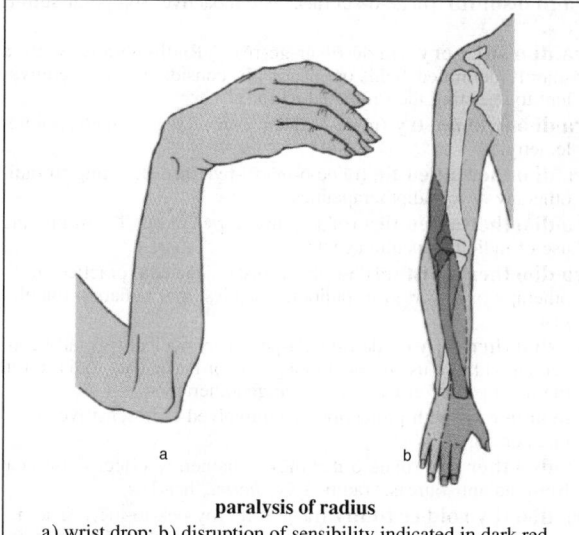

paralysis of radius
a) wrist drop; b) disruption of sensibility indicated in dark red

r. dorsa′lis, SYN dorsal *root.*

r. facia′lis [NA], SYN *nerve* of pterygoid canal.

r. infe′rior an′sae cervica′lis, SYN inferior *root* of ansa cervicalis.

r. infe′rior ner′vi vestibulocochlea′ris, SYN cochlear *root* of VIII nerve.

r. latera′lis ner′vi media′ni [NA], SYN lateral *root* of median nerve.

r. latera′lis trac′tus op′tici [NA], SYN lateral *root* of optic tract.

r. lin′guae [NA], SYN *root* of tongue.

r. lon′ga gan′glii cilia′ris, SYN sensory *root* of ciliary ganglion.

r. media′lis ner′vi media′ni [NA], SYN medial *root* of median nerve.

r. media′lis trac′tus op′tici [NA], SYN medial *root* of optic tract.

r. mesenter′ii [NA], SYN *root* of mesentery.

r. moto′ria [NA], ☆official alternate term for ventral *root.*

r. moto′ria ner′vi trigem′ini [NA], ☆official alternate term for motor *root* of trigeminal nerve.

r. na′si [NA], SYN *root* of nose.

r. nasocilia′ris [NA], ☆official alternate term for sensory *root* of ciliary ganglion.

r. ner′vi facia′lis, SYN *root* of facial nerve.

ra′dices ner′vi trigem′ini, SYN *roots* of trigeminal nerve, under *root.*

r. oculomoto′ria gan′glii cilia′ris [NA], ☆official alternate term for parasympathetic *root* of ciliary ganglion.

r. parasympath′ica gan′glii cilia′ris [NA], SYN parasympathetic *root* of ciliary ganglion.

r. pe′nis [NA], SYN *root* of penis.

r. pi′li, SYN hair *root.*

r. poste′rior [NA], SYN dorsal *root.*

r. pulmo′nis [NA], SYN *root* of lung.

r. senso′ria [NA], SYN dorsal *root.*

r. sensoria gan′glii cili′aris [NA], SYN sensory *root* of ciliary ganglion.

r. sensoria gan′glii pterygopalatini [NA], SYN ganglionic *branches* of maxillary nerve, under *branch.*

r. senso′ria ner′vi trigem′ini [NA], ☆official alternate term for sensory *root* of trigeminal nerve.

ra′dices spina′les nervi accessorii [NA], SYN spinal *root* of accessory nerve.

r. supe′rior an′sae cervica′lis, SYN superior *root* of ansa cervicalis.

r. supe′rior ner′vi vestibulocochlea′ris, SYN vestibular *root.*

r. sympath′ica gan′glii cilia′ris [NA], SYN sympathetic *root* of ciliary ganglion.

r. un′guis [NA], SYN *root* of nail.

r. ventra′lis, SYN ventral *root.*

r. vestibula′ris [NA], SYN vestibular *root.*

ra·don (Rn) (rā′don). A gaseous radioactive element, atomic no. 86, resulting from the breakdown of radium; of the isotopes with mass numbers between 198 and 228, only ^{222}Rn is medically significant as an alpha-emitter with a half-life of 3.8235 days; it is used in the treatment of certain malignancies. Poorly ventilated homes in some parts of the country accumulate a dangerous amount of naturally-occurring radon gas. [from radium]

Raeder, Georg Johann, Norwegian ophthalmologist, 1889–1956. SEE R.'s paratrigeminal *syndrome.*

raf·fi·nose (raf′i-nōs). A dextrorotatory trisaccharide, occurring in cotton seed and in the molasses of beet root, composed of D-galactose, D-glucose, and D-fructose and formed by transfer of D-galactose from UDP-D-galactose to sucrose; many seeds are rich in r. SYN gossypose, melitose, melitriose.

rage (rāj). Violent anger; a total discharge of the sympathetic portion of the autonomic nervous system. [Fr., fr. L. *rabies,* violent anger, fr. *rabo,* to rave]

sham r., a quasi-emotional state, characterized by manifestations of fear and anger upon trifling provocation; produced in animals by the removal of the cerebral cortex (decortication).

Rahe, Richard H., U.S. psychiatrist, *1936. SEE Holmes-R. *questionnaire.*

Rahn, Hermann, U.S. respiratory physiologist, *1912. SEE R.-Otis *sample.*

Rail·li·e·ti·na (rī-li-ě-tē′nă). A genus of tapeworms (family Davaineidae, order Cyclophyllidea), three species of which, *R. madagascariensis* or *R. demerariensis, R. asiatica,* and *R. formsana,* have been found in humans. However, the identification of many of these worms found in man has been questioned.

rail·li·e·ti·ni·a·sis (rī′li-ě-ti-nī′ă-sis). Infection of rodents and monkeys, and occasionally man, with tapeworms of the genus *Raillietina.*

Rainey, George, English anatomist, 1801–1884. SEE R.'s *corpuscles,* under *corpuscle.*

rale (rahl). Ambiguous term for an added sound heard on auscultation of breath sounds; used by some to denote rhonchus and by others for crepitation. [Fr. rattle]

amphoric r., sound heard through the stethoscope associated with the movement of fluid in a lung cavity communicating with a bronchus.

atelectatic r., transitory light crackling sound that disappears after deep breathing or coughing.

bubbling r., moist sound heard through the stethoscope as a result of air entering portions of lung tissue containing exudate and thus creating bubbles; sometimes associated with resolving pneumonia or small lung cavities.

cavernous r., a resonating, bubbling sound caused by air entering a cavity partly filled with fluid. SYN cavernous rhonchus.

clicking r., short, sticking sound usually associated with opening of small bronchi on deep breathing, sometimes heard in early pulmonary tuberculosis.

consonating r., a resonant r. produced in a bronchial tube and heard through consolidated lung tissue.

crackling r. (krak′ling), very fine sounds produced by fluid in very small airways in pneumonia or congestive heart *failure.*

crepitant r., a fine bubbling or crackling sound produced by air mixing with very thin secretions in the smaller bronchial tubes. SYN vesicular r.

dry r., a harsh or musical breath sound produced by a constriction in a bronchial tube or the presence of a viscid secretion narrowing the lumen.

gurgling r., coarse sound heard over large cavities or over trachea nearly filled with secretions.

guttural r., sound heard over the lung but resulting from upper airway obstruction.

metallic r., a r. of metallic quality caused by resonance in a large cavity.

moist r., a bubbling r. caused by air mixing with a fluid exudate in the bronchial tubes or a cavity.

mucous r., a bubbling r. heard on auscultation over bronchial tubes containing mucus.

palpable r., a vibration that can be felt accompanying a low-pitched, hard, musical, or sonorous r.

pleural r., SYN pleural *rub.*

sibilant r., a whistling sound caused by air moving through a viscid secretion narrowing the lumen of a bronchus. SYN whistling r.

Skoda's r., a r. in a bronchus heard through an area of consolidated tissue in pneumonia.

sonorous r., a cooing or snoring sound often produced by the vibration of a projecting mass of viscid secretion in a large bronchus.

subcrepitant r., a very fine crepitant r.

vesicular r., SYN crepitant r.

whistling r., SYN sibilant r.

ram. A male sheep of breeding age. [A.S.]

ra·mal (rā′măl). Relating to a ramus.

Raman, Sir Chandrasekhara V., Indian physicist and Nobel laureate, 1888–1970. SEE R. *effect, spectrum.*

Rambourg's stains. SEE Rambourg's chromic acid-phosphotungstic acid *stain,* Rambourg's periodic acid-chromic methenamine-silver *stain.*

ra·mex (rā′meks). Obsolete term for hernia, varicocele, or any scrotal tumor. [L. hernia; pl. blood vessels of the lungs, fr. *ramus,* a branch]

ra·mi (rā′mī). Plural of ramus. [L.]

ram·i·cot·o·my (ram-i-kot′ŏ-mē). SYN ramisection. [L. *ramus,* branch, + G. *tomē,* incision]

ram·i·fi·ca·tion (ram′i-fi-kā′shŭn). The process of dividing into a branchlike pattern.

ram·i·fy (ram′i-fī). To split into a branchlike pattern. [L. *ramus,* branch, + *facio,* to make]

ram·i·sec·tion (ram-i-sek′shŭn). Section of the rami communicantes of the sympathetic nervous system. SYN ramicotomy. [L. *ramus,* branch, + L. *sectio,* section]

ram·i·tis (ram-ī′tis). Inflammation of a ramus. [L. *ramus,* branch, + G. *-itis,* inflammation]

Ramón y Cajal, SEE Cajal.

ra·mose, ra·mous (rā′mōs, rā′mŭs). SYN branching. [L. *ramosus,* fr. *ramus,* a branch]

ramp. In electrical recording, a uniformly rising voltage or current. If reset to zero at regular intervals, it forms a sawtooth pattern used to provide the time sweep of a cathode ray oscilloscope beam; if reset to zero by a periodic event (*e.g.,* heart beats), the recorded height of the r.'s represents time between events.

Ramsay Hunt. SEE Hunt.

Ramsden, Jesse, English optician, 1735–1800. SEE R.'s *ocular.*

Ramstedt, Conrad, German surgeon, 1867–1963. SEE R. *operation;* Fredet-R. *operation.*

ram·u·lus, pl. **ram·u·li** (ram′yū-lŭs, -lī). A small branch or twig; one of the terminal divisions of a ramus. [L. dim. of *ramus,* a branch]

RAMUS

ra·mus, pl. **ra·mi** (rā′mŭs, rā′mī) [NA]. **1.** SYN branch. **2.** One of the primary divisions of a nerve or blood vessel. Arterial and nerve branches are also given under the major nerve or artery. SEE artery, nerve. **3.** A part of an irregularly shaped bone (less slender than a "process") that forms an angle with the main body (*e.g.,* ramus of mandible). **4.** One of the primary divisions of a cerebral sulcus. [L.]

r. acetabula′ris [NA], SYN acetabular *branch.*

r. acromia′lis arte′riae suprascapula′ris [NA], SYN acromial *branch* of suprascapular artery.

r. acromia′lis arte′riae thoracoacromia′lis [NA], SYN acromial *branch* of thoracoacromial artery.

ra′mi ad pon′tem [NA], ★official alternate term for pontine *arteries,* under *artery.*

ra′mi alveola′res superio′res anterio′res ner′vi infraorbita′lis [NA], SYN anterior superior alveolar *branches* of infraorbital nerve, under *branch.*

ra′mi alveola′res superio′res posterio′res ner′vi maxilla′ris [NA], SYN posterior superior alveolar *branches* of maxillary nerve, under *branch.*

r. alveola′ris supe′rior me′dius ner′vi infraorbita′lis [NA], SYN middle superior alveolar *branch* of infraorbital nerve.

r. anastomot′icus, SYN anastomotic *branch.* SEE ALSO communicating *branch.*

r. anastomot′icus arte′riae meninge′ae me′diae cum lacrima′li [NA], SYN anastomotic *branch* of middle meningeal artery to lacrimal artery.

r. ante′rior [NA], SYN anterior *branch.*

r. ante′rior ascen′dens [NA], SYN ascending anterior *branch.*

r. ante′rior descen′dens [NA], SYN descending anterior *branch.*

r. ante′rior latera′lis, the lateral anterior branch, the former name for the ascending anterior branch of the left pulmonary artery.

r. apica′lis [NA], SYN apical *branch.*

r. apica′lis lo′bi inferio′ris arte′riae pulmona′lis dex′trae [NA], SYN apical *branch* of inferior lobar branch of right pulmonary artery.

r. apicoposte′rior ve′nae pulmona′lis si′nistrae supe′rioris [NA], SYN apicoposterior *branch* of left superior pulmonary vein.

ra′mi articula′res [NA], SYN articular *branches,* under *branch.*

rami articulares arte′riae descenden′tis genicular′is [NA], SEE articular *branches,* under *branch.*

r. ascen′dens [NA], SYN ascending *branch.*

ra′mi atria′les [NA], SYN atrial *branches,* under *branch.*

ra′mi auricula′res anterio′res arte′riae tempora′lis superficia′lis [NA], SYN anterior auricular *branches* of superficial temporal artery, under *branch.*

r. auricula′ris arte′riae occipita′lis [NA], SYN auricular *branch* of occipital artery.

r. auricula′ris nervi va′gi [NA], SYN auricular *branch* of vagus nerve.

r. basa′lis ante′rior [NA], SYN anterior basal *branch.*

r. basa′lis latera′lis [NA], SYN lateral basal *branch.*

r. basa′lis media′lis [NA], SYN medial basal *branch* of pulmonary artery.

r. basa′lis poste′rior [NA], SYN posterior basal *branch.*

r. basalis tento′rii arte′riae caro′tidis inter′nae [NA], SYN basal tentorial *branch* of internal carotid artery.

ra′mi bronchia′les [NA], SYN bronchial *arteries,* under *artery.*

ra′mi bronchia′les segmento′rum [NA], SYN *branches* of segmental bronchi, under *branch.*

ra′mi bucca′les ner′vi facia′lis [NA], SYN buccal *branches* of facial nerve, under *branch.*

ra′mi calca′nei [NA], SYN calcaneal *arteries,* under *artery.*

ra′mi calca′nei latera′les ner′vi sura′lis [NA], SYN lateral calcaneal *branches* of sural nerve, under *branch.*

ra′mi calca′nei media′les ner′vi tibia′lis [NA], SYN medial calcaneal *branches* of tibial nerve, under *branch.*

r. calcari′nus arte′riae occipita′lis media′lis [NA], SYN calcarine *branch* of medial occipital artery.

ra′mi cap′sulae inter′nae [NA], the internal capsular branches, the branches of the anterior choroid artery to the internal capsule.

ra′mi capsula′res arte′riae rena′lis [NA], SYN capsular *branches* of renal artery, under *branch.*

ra′mi cardi′aci cervica′les inferio′res ner′vi va′gi [NA], SYN inferior cervical cardiac *branches* of vagus nerve, under *branch.*

ra′mi cardi′aci cervica′les superio′res ner′vi va′gi [NA], SYN superior cervical cardiac *branches* of vagus nerve, under *branch.*

ra′mi cardi′aci thora′cici ner′vi va′gi [NA], SYN thoracic cardiac *branches* of vagus nerve, under *branch*.

r. cardi′acus, obsolete term for medial basal *branch* of pulmonary artery.

ra′mi caroticotympan′ici, SYN caroticotympanic *arteries,* under *artery*.

r. carpa′lis dorsa′lis arte′riae radia′lis, SYN dorsal carpal *branch* of radial artery.

r. carpa′lis dorsa′lis arte′riae ulna′ris, SYN dorsal carpal *branch* of ulnar artery.

r. carpa′lis palma′ris arte′riae radia′lis, SYN palmar carpal *branch* of radial artery.

r. carpa′lis palma′ris arte′riae ulna′ris, SYN palmar carpal *branch* of ulnar artery.

r. car′peus dorsa′lis arte′riae radia′lis, SYN dorsal carpal *branch* of radial artery.

r. car′peus dorsa′lis arte′riae ulna′ris [NA], SYN dorsal carpal *branch* of ulnar artery.

r. car′peus palma′ris arte′riae radia′lis, SYN palmar carpal *branch* of radial artery.

r. car′peus palma′ris arte′riae ulna′ris, SYN palmar carpal *branch* of ulnar artery.

ra′mi cau′dae nu′clei cauda′ti [NA], branches to the tail of the caudate nucleus. **(1)** branches from either the anterior choroid or the posterior communicating artery, or both, to supply the tail of the caudate nucleus; **(2)** a branch from the middle cerebral artery to the tail of the caudate nucleus.

ra′mi cauda′ti [NA], SYN caudate *branches,* under *branch*.

ra′mi celi′aci ner′vi va′gi [NA], SYN celiac *branches* of vagus nerve, under *branch*.

ra′mi centra′les anteromedia′les [NA], SYN anteromedial central *branches,* under *branch*.

cephalic arterial rami, parietal branches of the sympathetic trunks conveying postsynaptic sympathetic fibers from the superior cervical ganglion to the carotid arteries for distribution within the head.

r. col′li ner′vi facia′lis [NA], SYN cervical *branch* of facial nerve.

r. cervicalis ner′vi facia′lis, ✫official alternate term for cervical *branch* of facial nerve.

r. chiasmat′icus [NA], the chiasmatic branch, a branch of the middle cerebral artery to the optic chiasm.

ra′mi choroi′dei [NA], SYN choroid *branches,* under *branch*.

r. choroi′dei posterio′res latera′les, lateral posterior choroid branches of posterior cerebral artery. SEE choroid *branches,* under *branch*.

r. choroi′dei posterio′res media′les, medial posterior choroid branches of posterior cerebral artery. SEE choroid *branches,* under *branch*.

r. choroi′dei ventric′uli latera′lis, lateral ventrical branch of anterior choroid artery. SEE choroid *branches,* under *branch*.

r. choroi′dei ventric′uli ter′tii, third ventricle choroid branch of anterior artery. SEE choroid *branches,* under *branch*.

r. choroi′dei ventric′uli quar′ti, fourth ventricle choroid branch of posterior inferior cerebellar artery. SEE choroid *branches,* under *branch*.

r. cingula′ris [NA], the cingular branch, a branch of the callosomarginal artery supplying the gyrus cinguli.

r. circumflex′us arte′riae corona′riae sinis′trae [NA], SYN circumflex *branch* of left coronary artery.

r. circumflex′us fibula′ris arte′riae tibia′lis posterio′ris [NA], SYN circumflex fibular *artery*.

r. clavicula′ris arte′riae thoracoacromia′lis [NA], SYN clavicular *branch* of thoracoacromial artery.

r. cli′vi [NA], the branch to the clivus, a branch of the cerebral part of the internal carotid artery supplying the clivus.

r. cochlea′ris arte′riae labyrin′thi [NA], SYN cochlear *branch* of labyrinthine artery.

r. collatera′lis arte′riarum intercosta′lium posterio′rum III–XI [NA], SYN collateral *branches* of posterior intercostal arteries 3–11, under *branch*.

r. commu′nicans, pl. **ra′mi communican′tes** [NA], SYN communicating *branch*.

r. commu′nicans arte′riae fibula′ris [NA], SYN communicating *branch* of peroneal artery.

r. commu′nicans arte′riae perone′ae, SYN communicating *branch* of peroneal artery.

r. commu′nicans cum chor′da tym′pani [NA], **(1)** SYN communicating *branch* of chorda tympani to lingual nerve. **(2)** SYN communicating *branch* of otic ganglion to chorda tympani.

r. commu′nicans cum ner′vo glossopharyn′geo [NA], **(1)** SYN communicating *branch* of facial nerve with glossopharyngeal nerve. **(2)** SYN communicating *branch* of glossopharyngeal nerve with auricular branch of vagus nerve.

r. commu′nicans fibula′ris ner′vi fibula′ris commu′nis [NA], SYN peroneal communicating *branch*.

r. commu′nicans gang′lii o′tici cum ner′vo auriculotempora′li [NA], SYN communicating *branch* of otic ganglion to auriculotemporal nerve.

r. commu′nicans gang′lii o′tici cum ner′vo pterygoi′deo media′li [NA], SYN communicating *branch* of otic ganglion with medial pterygoid nerve.

r. commu′nicans gang′lii o′tici cum ra′mo menin′geo nervi mandibularis [NA], SYN communicating *branch* of otic ganglion with meningeal branch of mandibular nerve.

r. commu′nicans ner′vi facia′lis cum plex′u tympan′ico [NA], SYN communicating *branch* of facial nerve with tympanic plexus.

r. commu′nicans ner′vi glossopharynge′i cum ra′mo auricula′ri ner′vi vaga′lis, SYN communicating *branch* of glossopharyngeal nerve with auricular branch of vagus nerve.

r. commu′nicans ner′vi lacrima′lis cum ner′vo zygomat′ico [NA], SYN communicating *branch* of lacrimal nerve with zygomatic nerve.

r. commu′nicans ner′vi laryn′gei recurren′tis cum ra′mo laryn′geo inter′no [NA], SYN communicating *branch* of superior laryngeal nerve with recurrent laryngeal nerve.

r. commu′nicans ner′vi laryn′gei superio′ris cum ner′vo laryn′geo recurrenti [NA], SYN communicating *branch* of superior laryngeal nerve with recurrent laryngeal nerve.

r. commu′nicans ner′vi media′ni cum ner′vo ulna′ri [NA], SYN communicating *branch* of median nerve with ulnar nerve.

r. commu′nicans ner′vi nasocilia′ris cum gan′glio cilia′ri [NA], SYN sensory *root* of ciliary ganglion.

r. commu′nicans perone′us ner′vi pero′nei commu′nis [NA], ✫official alternate term for peroneal communicating *branch*.

r. commu′nicans ulna′ris ner′vi radia′lis [NA], SYN ulnar communicating *branch* of superficial radial nerve.

ra′mi communican′tes gang′lii submandibula′ris cum ner′vo lingua′li [NA], SYN ganglionic *branches* of lingual nerve, under *branch*.

ra′mi communican′tes ner′vi auriculotempora′lis cum ner′vo facia′li [NA], SYN communicating *branches* of auriculotemporal nerve to facial nerve, under *branch*.

ra′mi communican′tes ner′vi lingua′lis cum ner′vo hypoglos′so [NA], SYN communicating *branches* of lingual nerve to hypoglossal nerve, under *branch*.

ra′mi communican′tes nervo′rum spina′lium [NA], SYN white rami communicantes.

communicating rami of spinal nerves, the communicating branches of spinal nerves, small bundles of nerve fibers connecting spinal nerves with sympathetic ganglia; the fibers passing from the ganglion to the spinal nerve are nonmyelinated and are called gray rami communicantes, those passing in the reverse direction are myelinated and are called white rami communicantes.

communicating rami of sympathetic trunk, SYN gray rami communicantes.

ra′mi cor′poris amygdaloi′dei [NA], the branches to the amygdaloid body, branches of the anterior choroid artery to the amygdaloid body.

r. cor′poris callo′si dorsa′lis [NA], the dorsal corpus callosal branches, branches of the medial occipital artery to the dorsum of the corpus callosum.

ra′mi cor′poris genicula′ti latera′lis [NA], the lateral geniculate body branches, branches of the anterior choroid artery to the lateral geniculate body.

r. costa′lis latera′lis arte′riae thora′cicae inter′nae [NA], SYN lateral costal *branch* of internal thoracic artery.

r. cricothyroi′deus [NA], SYN cricothyroid *artery*.

ra′mi cuta′nei anterio′res ner′vi femora′lis [NA], SYN anterior femoral cutaneous *nerves*, under *nerve*.

rami cuta′nei anteriores pectora′lis et abdomina′lis nervorum intercostalium [NA], SYN thoracoabdominal *nerves*, under *nerve*.

ra′mi cuta′nei cru′ris media′les ner′vi saphe′ni [NA], SYN medial crural cutaneous *branches* of saphenous nerve, under *branch*.

r. cuta′neus ante′rior ner′vi iliohypogas′trici [NA], SYN anterior cutaneous *branch* of iliohypogastric nerve.

r. cuta′neus ante′rior (pectora′lis et abdomina′lis) nervo′rum thoracico′rum [NA], SYN thoracoabdominal *nerves*, under *nerve*.

r. cuta′neus latera′lis [NA], SYN lateral cutaneous *branch*.

r. cuta′neus latera′lis ner′vi iliohypogas′trici [NA], lateral cutaneous branch of iliohypogastric nerve. SEE lateral cutaneous *branch*.

r. cuta′neus latera′lis ramor′um posterior′um arte′riae intercostal′ium [NA], lateral cutaneous branch of dorsal branch of posterior intercostal arteries. SEE lateral cutaneous *branch*.

r. cuta′neus media′lis [NA], SYN medial cutaneous *branch*.

r. cutaneus medialis rami dorsalis arteriarum intercostalium posteriorum III–XI [NA], medial cutaneous branch of dorsal branch of posterior intercostal arteries. SEE medial cutaneous *branch*.

r. cuta′neus media′lis ramor′um dorsalium nervo′rum thoracico′rum [NA], medial cutaneous branch of dorsal branch of thoracic nerves. SEE medial cutaneous *branch*.

r. cuta′neus ra′mi anterio′ris ner′vi obturato′rii [NA], SYN cutaneous *branch* of obturator nerve.

r. deltoi′deus [NA], SYN deltoid *branch*.

dental rami, SYN dental *branches*, under *branch*.

ra′mi denta′les [NA], SYN dental *branches*, under *branch*.

rami denta′les arte′riae alveola′ris inferio′ris [NA], dental branches of inferior alveolar artery. SEE dental *branches*, under *branch*.

rami denta′les arte′riae alveola′ris superio′ris posterio′ris [NA], dental branch of the posterior superior alveolar artery. SEE dental *branches*, under *branch*.

ra′mi denta′les inferio′res [NA], SYN inferior dental rami. SEE dental *branches*, under *branch*.

rami denta′les inferio′res plex′us denta′lis inferio′ris [NA], SYN inferior dental *branches* of inferior dental plexus, under *branch*.

ra′mi denta′les superio′res [NA], SYN superior dental rami.

rami denta′les superio′res plex′us denta′lis superio′ris [NA], SYN superior dental *branches* of superior dental plexus, under *branch*.

r. descen′dens [NA], SYN descending *branch*.

r. descen′dens arteri′ae circumflex′ae femo′ris latera′lis [NA], SYN descending *branch* of lateral circumflex femoral artery.

r. descen′dens arte′riae occipita′lis [NA], SYN descending *branch* of occipital artery.

r. dex′ter [NA], SYN right *branch*.

r. dex′ter arte′riae hepat′icae propri′ae [NA], SYN right hepatic *artery*.

r. dex′ter ve′nae por′tae hepa′tis [NA], SYN right *branch* of portal vein.

r. digas′tricus ner′vi facia′lis [NA], SYN digastric *branch* of facial nerve.

rami dorsa′les arte′riae intercosta′lis supre′mae [NA], SYN dorsal *branch* of the superior intercostal artery.

rami dorsa′les arte′riae subcosta′lis [NA], SYN dorsal *branch* of the subcostal artery.

ra′mi dorsa′les lin′guae arte′riae lingua′lis [NA], SYN dorsal lingual *branches* of lingual artery, under *branch*.

rami dorsa′les ner′vi ulna′ris [NA], SYN dorsal *branch* of the ulnar nerve.

r. dorsa′lis [NA], SYN dorsal primary r. of spinal nerve.

r. dorsa′lis arte′riae lumba′lium [NA], SYN dorsal *branch* of the lumbar artery.

r. dorsa′lis arte′riarum intercostal′ium posterior′um III–XI [NA], SYN dorsal *branch* of the posterior intercostal arteries 3–11.

r. dorsa′lis nervo′rum spina′lium [NA], SYN dorsal primary r. of spinal nerve.

r. dorsa′lis vena′rum intercostal′ium posterior′um IV–XI [NA], SYN dorsal *branch* of the posterior intercostal veins 4–11.

dorsal primary r. of spinal nerve, the smaller, posteriorly-directed major terminal branch (with the ventral primary r.) of all 31 pairs of mixed spinal nerves, formed at the intervertebral foramen and turning abruptly posteriorly to divide into lateral and medial branches, both of which will supply the deep (true) muscles of the back. The medial branch (rami medialis [NA]) of the dorsal primary r. also supplies articular branches to the zygopophyseal joints and the periosteum of the vertebral arch. In the neck and upper back, the medial branch continues through the deep and superficial back muscles to supply overlying skin; in the lower back, the lateral branch does this. Nomina Anatomica lists dorsal primary rami as "rami dorsales" for each group of spinal nerves: 1) cervical (nervorum cervicalium [NA]), 2) thoracic (nervorum thoracicorum [NA]), 3) lumbar (nervorum lumbalium [NA]), 4) sacral (nervorum sacralium [NA]), and 5) coccygeal (nervi coccygei [NA]). SYN r. dorsalis nervorum spinalium [NA], r. dorsalis [NA], rami posteriores nervorum spinalium⋆, dorsal branch (1), posterior primary division.

ra′mi duodena′les arte′riae pancreaticoduodena′lis superio′ris [NA], SYN duodoneal *branches* of superior pancreaticoduodenal artery, under *branch*.

ra′mi epiplo′icae, SYN epiploic *branches*, under *branch*.

ra′mi esophagea′les [NA], SYN esophageal *branches*, under *branch*.

ra′mi esophagea′les aor′tae thora′cicae [NA], SYN esophageal *branches* of the thoracic aorta, under *branch*.

ra′mi esophagea′les arte′riae gas′tricae sinis′trae [NA], SYN esophageal *branches* of the left gastric artery, under *branch*.

ra′mi esophagea′les arte′riae thyroi′deae inferio′ris [NA], SYN esophageal *branches* of the inferior thyroid artery, under *branch*.

ra′mi esopha′gei [NA], SYN esophageal *branches*, under *branch*.

ra′mi esopha′gei ner′vi laryn′gei recurren′tis [NA], SYN esophageal *branches* of the recurrent laryngeal nerve, under *branch*.

ra′mi esopha′gei ner′vi va′gi [NA], SYN esophageal *branches* of the vagus nerve, under *branch*.

r. externus nervi accessorii [NA], SYN spinal *root* of accessory nerve.

r. exter′nus ner′vi laryn′gei superio′ris [NA], SYN external *branch* of superior laryngeal nerve.

ra′mi faucia′les ner′vi lingua′lis [NA], ⋆official alternate term for faucial *branches* of lingual nerve, under *branch*.

r. femora′lis ner′vi genitofemora′lis [NA], SYN femoral *branch* of genitofemoral nerve.

r. fronta′lis anteromedia′lis [NA], anteromedial frontal branch of the callosomarginal artery.

r. fronta′lis arte′riae tempora′lis superficia′lis [NA], SYN frontal *branch* of superficial temporal artery.

r. fronta′lis interomedia′lis [NA], interomedial frontal branch of the callosomarginal artery.

r. fronta′lis posteromedia′lis [NA], posteromedial frontal branch of the callosomarginal artery.

rami gangli′i submandibula′ris [NA], SYN glandular *branches* of submandibular ganglion, under *branch*.

r. gang′lii trigemina′lis [NA], SYN ganglionic *branch* of internal carotid artery.

ra′mi gangliona′res [NA], ⋆official alternate term for ganglionic *branches* of maxillary nerve, under *branch*.

rami ganglio′nici ner′vi maxilla′ris [NA], SYN ganglionic *branches* of maxillary nerve, under *branch*.

ra

ra′mi gas′trici anterio′res ner′vi va′gi [NA], SYN gastric *branches* of anterior vagal trunk, under *branch.*

ra′mi gas′trici posterio′res ner′vi va′gi [NA], SYN gastric *branches* of posterior vagal *trunk,* under *branch.*

r. genita′lis ner′vi genitofemora′lis [NA], SYN genital *branch* of genitofemoral nerve.

ra′mi gingiva″les inferio′res plex′us denta′lis inferio′ris [NA], SYN inferior gingival *branches* of inferior dental plexus, under *branch.*

ra′mi gingiva″les superio′res plex′us denta′lis superio′ris [NA], SYN superior gingival *branches* of superior dental plexus, under *branch.*

ra′mi glandula′res [NA], SYN glandular *branches,* under *branch.*

r. glandulares anterior/lateralis/posterior arteriae thyroideae superioris [NA], SYN glandular *branches* of anterior/lateral/posterior branches of superior thyroid artery, under *branch.*

rami glandula′res arte′riae facia′lis [NA], SYN glandular *branches* of facial artery, under *branch.*

rami glandula′res arte′riae thyroi′deae inferio′ris [NA], SYN glandular *branches* of inferior thyroid artery, under *branch.*

rami glandular′es gang′lii submandibular′is [NA], SYN glandular *branches* of submandibular ganglion, under *branch.*

ra′mi glo′bi pal′lidi [NA], the branches to the globus pallidus, branches of the anterior choroid artery to the globus pallidus.

gray rami communicantes, short nerves arising from the lateral aspect of the sympathetic trunk conducting nonmyelinated postsynaptic sympathetic nerve fibers from the sympathetic trunk to the initial portions of all 31 pairs of ventral primary rami of spinal nerves for distribution by all parts (including the dorsal primary ramus) of the spinal nerve. The gray rami are the parietal branches of the sympathetic trunks since all postsynaptic fibers to be distributed to the body wall (including limbs) must pass through them. SYN communicating branches of sympathetic trunk, communicating rami of sympathetic trunk.

ra′mi hepat′ici ner′vi va′gi [NA], SYN hepatic *branches* of vagus nerve, under *branch.*

r. hypothalam′icus [NA], the hypothalamic branch, a branch of the middle cerebral artery to the hypothalamus.

r. ili′acus arte′riae iliolumba′lis [NA], SYN iliac *branch* of iliolumbar artery.

ra′mi intercosta′les anterio′res [NA], SYN anterior intercostal *arteries,* under *artery.*

r. infe′rior [NA], SYN inferior *branch.*

r. infe′rior arte′riae glute′ae superio′ris [NA], SYN inferior *branch* of superior gluteal artery.

inferior dental rami, inferior dental branches of inferior dental plexus. SYN rami dentales inferiores [NA].

ra′mi inferio′res ner′vi transver′si cervicalis [col′li] [NA], SYN inferior *branches* of transverse cervical nerve, under *branch.*

r. infe′rior ner′vi oculomoto′rii [NA], SYN inferior *branch* of oculomotor nerve.

r. infe′rior os′sis pu′bis [NA], SYN inferior *branch* of pubic bone.

r. infrahyoi′deus arte′riae thyroi′dea superio′ris [NA], SYN infrahyoid *branch* of superior thyroid artery.

r. infrapatella′ris ner′vi saphe′ni [NA], SYN infrapatellar *branch* of saphenous nerve.

ra′mi inguina′les arte′riae puden′dae exter′nae [NA], SYN inguinal *branches* of external pudendal arteries, under *branch.*

rami intercostal′is anterior′es arter′ia thora′cica inter′na, SYN anterior intercostal *arteries,* under *artery.*

ra′mi interganglionα′res [NA], SYN interganglionic rami.

interganglionic rami, the ganglionic branches, the nerve strands interconnecting the ganglia of the sympathetic trunk; they consist of pre- or postganglionic fibers passing to higher or lower levels of the trunk. SYN rami interganglionares [NA].

internal r. of accessory nerve, SYN internal *branch* of accessory nerve. SEE ALSO accessory *nerve.*

r. inter′nus ner′vi accesso′rii [NA], SYN internal *branch* of accessory nerve. SEE ALSO accessory *nerve.*

r. inter′nus ner′vi laryn′gei superio′ris [NA], SYN internal *branch* of superior laryngeal nerve.

ra′mi interventricula′res septa′les, SYN septal *branches,* under *branch.*

r. interventricula′ris poste′rior arte′riae corona′riae dex′trae [NA], SYN posterior interventricular *artery.*

r. interventricula′ris ante′rior arte′riae corona′riae sinis′trae [NA], SYN anterior interventricular *artery.*

ischial r., the branch of the ischial bone, formerly called inferior branch of the ischium; the portion of the bone that passes forward from the ischial tuberosity to join the inferior r. of the pubic bone, thus forming the ischiopubic r. SYN r. ossis ischii [NA].

ischiopubic r., the inferior r. of the pubis and the r. of the ischium continuous with it, forming the inferomedial boundary of the obturator foramen.

ra′mi isth′mi fau′cium ner′vi lingua′lis [NA], SYN faucial *branches* of lingual nerve, under *branch.*

ra′mi labia′les anterio′res arte′riae puden′dae exter′nae [NA], SYN anterior labial *arteries,* under *artery.*

ra′mi labia′les inferio′res ner′vi menta′lis [NA], SYN inferior labial *branches* of mental nerve, under *branch.*

ra′mi labia′les posterio′res arte′riae puden′dae inter′nae [NA], SYN posterior labial *arteries,* under *artery.*

ra′mi labia′les superio′res ner′vi infraorbita′lis [NA], SYN superior labial *branches* of infraorbital nerve, under *branch.*

ra′mi laryngopharyn′gei gang′lii cervica′lis superio′ris [NA], SYN laryngopharyngeal *branches* of superior cervical ganglion, under *branch.*

ra′mi latera′les [NA], SYN lateral *branches,* under *branch.*

rami latera′les arteria′rum centra′lium anterolatera′lium, lateral branch of anterolateral central arteries.

r. latera′lis duc′tus hepa′tici sinis′tri [NA], lateral branch left hepatic duct. SEE lateral *branches,* under *branch.*

rami latera′les ra′mi sinis′tri ve′nae por′tae hepa′tis [NA], lateral branch of left branch of portal vein. SEE lateral *branches,* under *branch.*

rami laterales ramorum dorsalium nervorum cervicalium/thoracalium/lumbalium/sac [NA], lateral branch of dorsal primary rami of spinal nerves. SEE lateral *branches,* under *branch.*

r. latera′lis ramor′um dorsa′lium nervo′rum thoracico′rum, lateral cutaneous branch of dorsal branch of thoracic nerves.

r. lateralis interventricularis anterioris arteriae coronariae sinistrae [NA], lateral branch of anterior interventricular artery. SEE lateral *branches,* under *branch.*

r. latera′lis ner′vi supraorbita′lis [NA], lateral branch of supraorbital nerve. SEE lateral *branches,* under *branch.*

r. latera′lis ramor′um dorsa′lium nervo′rum thoracico′rum, lateral cutaneous branch of dorsal branch of thoracic nerves.

r. lateralis ramorum lobaris medium arteriorum pulmonalium dextrorum [NA], lateral branch of middle lobe branch of right pulmonary artery. SEE lateral *branches,* under *branch.*

rami liena′les arte′riae liena′lis [NA], ☆official alternate term for splenic *branches* of splenic artery, under *branch.*

ra′mi lingua′les [NA], SYN lingual *branches,* under *branch.*

rami lingua′les ner′vi glossopharyn′gei [NA], lingual branch of glossopharyngeal nerve. SEE lingual *branches,* under *branch.*

rami lingua′les ner′vi hypoglos′si [NA], lingual branch of hypoglossal nerve. SEE lingual *branches,* under *branch.*

rami lingua′les ner′vi lingua′lis [NA], lingual branch of lingual nerve. SEE lingual *branches,* under *branch.*

r. lingua′lis [NA], SYN lingular *branch.*

r. lingula′ris infe′rior [NA], SYN inferior lingular *branch* of lingular branch of left pulmonary artery.

r. lingula′ris ner′vi facia′lis [NA], SYN lingual *branch* of facial nerve.

r. lingula′ris supe′rior [NA], SYN superior lingular *branch* of lingular branch of superior lobar left pulmonary artery.

r. lo′bi me′dii [NA], SYN middle lobe *branch.*

r. lobi medii arteriae pulmonalis dextrae [NA], middle lobe branch of right pulmonary artery. SEE middle lobe *branch.*

r. lo′bi me′dii ve′nae pulmona′lis dex′trae superio′ris [NA], middle lobe branch of right superior pulmonary vein. SEE middle lobe *branch.*

r. lumba′lis arte′riae iliolumba′lis [NA], SYN lumbar *branch* of iliolumbar artery.

ra′mi malleola′res latera′les [NA], SYN lateral malleolar *arteries*, under *artery*.

ra′mi malleola′res media′les [NA], SYN medial malleolar *arteries*, under *artery*.

ra′mi mamma′rii [NA], SEE lateral mammary *branches*, under *branch*, medial mammary *branches*, under *branch*.

ra′mi mamma′rii latera′les [NA], SYN lateral mammary *branches*, under *branch*.

rami mamma′rii latera′les arte′riae thora′cicae latera′lis [NA], SYN lateral mammary *branches* of lateral thoracic artery, under *branch*.

rami mamma′rii latera′les nervo′rum intercostal′ium, ☆official alternate term for lateral cutaneous *branches* of ventral primary ramus of thoracic spinal nerves, under *branch*.

rami mamma′rii latera′les ra′mi cuta′nei latera′lis nervo′rum thoracico′rum [NA], SYN lateral mammary *branches* of lateral cutaneous branches of thoracic spinal nerves, under *branch*.

rami mamma′rii latera′les ra′mi cuta′nei latera′lis nervo′rum intercosta′lium, ☆official alternate term for lateral mammary *branches* of lateral cutaneous branches of thoracic spinal nerves, under *branch*.

ra′mi mamma′rii media′les [NA], SYN medial mammary *branches*, under *branch*.

rami mammarii mediales rami cutanei anterioris nervorum intercostalium, medial mammary branches of anterior cutaneous branches of ventral primary rami of thoracic spinal nerves. SEE medial mammary *branches*, under *branch*.

rami mammarii mediales rami cutanei anterioris ramorum ventralium nervorum thoracicorum, medial mammary branches of anterior cutaneous branches of ventral primary rami of thoracic spinal nerves. SEE medial mammary *branches*, under *branch*.

rami mammarii mediales rami perforantis arteriae thoracicae internae [NA], medial mammary branches of perforating branches of internal thoracic artery. SEE medial mammary *branches*, under *branch*.

r. of mandible, the upturned perpendicular extremity of the mandible on either side; it gives attachment on its lateral surface to the masseter muscle. SYN r. mandibulae [NA].

r. mandib′ulae [NA], SYN r. of mandible.

r. margina′lis mandib′ulae ner′vi facia′lis [NA], SYN marginal mandibular *branch* of facial nerve.

r. margina′lis tento′rii arte′riae caroti′dis inter′nae [NA], SYN marginal tentorial *branch* of internal carotid artery.

ra′mi mastoi′dei arte′riae auricula′ris posterio′ris [NA], SYN mastoid *branches* of posterior auricular artery, under *branch*.

r. mastoi′deus arte′riae occipita′lis [NA], SYN mastoid *artery*.

r. mea′tus acu′s′tici inter′ni, ☆official alternate term for labyrinthine *artery*.

ra′mi media′les [NA], SYN medial *branches*, under *branch*.

rami media′les arteria′rum centra′lium anterolatera′lium [NA], medial branch of anterolateral central arteries. SEE medial *branches*, under *branch*.

rami media′les ra′mi sinis′tri ve′nae por′tae hepa′tis [NA], medial branch of left branch of portal vein. SEE medial *branches*, under *branch*.

r. media′lis duc′tus hepa′tici sinis′tri [NA], medial branch of left hepatic duct. SEE medial *branches*, under *branch*.

r. media′lis ner′vi supraorbita′lis [NA], medial branch of supraorbital nerve. SEE medial *branches*, under *branch*.

r. media′lis ra′mi loba′ris me′dii arterio′rum pulmona′lium dextro′rum [NA], medial branch of middle lobar branch of right pulmonary artery. SEE medial *branches*, under *branch*.

r. medialis ramorum dorsalium nervorum cervicalium/thoracicorum/lumbalium/sacralium [NA], medial branch of dorsal primary rami of spinal nerves. SEE medial *branches*, under *branch*.

ra′mi mediastina′les [NA], SYN mediastinal *branches*, under *branch*.

rami mediastina′les aor′tae thora′cicae [NA], SYN mediastinal *branches* of thoracic aorta, under *branch*.

rami mediastina′les arte′riae thora′cicae inter′nae [NA], SYN mediastinal *branches* of internal thoracic artery, under *branch*.

ra′mi medulla′res latera′les [NA], the lateral medullary branches, branches of the posterior inferior cerebellar artery to the lateral part of the medulla oblongata.

ra′mi medulla′res media′les [NA], the medial medullary branches, branches of the posterior inferior cerebellar artery to the medial part of the medulla oblongata.

r. membra′nae tym′pani ner′vi auriculotempora′lis [NA], SYN *branch* of auriculotemporal nerve to tympanic membrane.

rami meningei, SYN meningeal *branches*, under *branch*.

r. menin′geus accesso′rius arte′riae menin′geae me′diae [NA], SYN accessory meningeal *branch* of middle meningeal artery.

r. menin′geus ante′rior arte′riae vertebra′lis, meningeal branch of the vertebral artery.

r. menin′geus arte′riae carot′idis inter′nae, SYN meningeal *branch* of internal carotid artery.

r. menin′geus arte′riae occipita′lis [NA], SYN meningeal *branch* of occipital artery.

r. menin′geus me′dius ner′vi maxilla′ris [NA], SYN middle meningeal *branch* of maxillary nerve.

r. menin′geus ner′vi mandibula′ris [NA], SYN meningeal *branch* of mandibular nerve.

r. menin′geus ner′vi va′gi [NA], SYN meningeal *branch* of vagus nerve.

r. menin′geus nervo′rum spina′lium [NA], SYN meningeal *branch* of spinal nerves.

r. menin′geus poste′rior, the posterior meningeal branch of the vertebral artery.

ra′mi menta′les ner′vi menta′lis [NA], SYN mental *branches* of mental nerve, under *branch*.

ra′mi muscula′res [NA], SYN muscular *branches*, under *branch*.

r. mus′culi stylopharyn′gei ner′vi glossopharyn′gei [NA], SYN *branch* of glossopharyngeal nerve to stylopharyngeus muscle.

r. mylohyoi′deus arte′riae alveola′ris inferio′ris [NA], SYN mylohyoid *artery*.

ra′mi nasa′les exter′ni [NA], SYN external nasal *branches*, under *branch*.

rami nasa′les exter′ni ner′vi ethmoida′lis anterio′ris [NA], external nasal branch of nasociliary nerve; SEE external nasal *branches*, under *branch*.

rami nasa′les exter′ni ner′vi infraorbita′lis [NA], external nasal branch of infraorbital nerve; SEE external nasal *branches*, under *branch*.

ra′mi nasa′les inter′ni [NA], SYN internal nasal *branches*, under *branch*.

rami nasa′les inter′ni ner′vi ethmoida′lis anterio′ris [NA], internal nasal branch of nasociliary nerve. SEE internal nasal *branches*, under *branch*.

rami nasa′les inter′ni ner′vi infraorbita′lis [NA], internal nasal branch of infraorbital nerve. SEE internal nasal *branches*, under *branch*.

ra′mi nasa′les latera′les ner′vi ethmoida′lis anterio′ris [NA], SYN lateral nasal *branches* of anterior ethmoidal nerve, under *branch*.

ra′mi nasa′les media′les ner′vi ethmoida′lis anterio′ris [NA], SYN medial nasal *branches* of anterior ethmoidal nerve, under *branch*.

ra′mi nasa′les posterio′res inferio′res ner′vi palati′ni majo′ris [NA], SYN posterior inferior nasal *branches* of greater palatine nerve, under *branch*.

ra′mi nasa′les posterio′res superio′res latera′les gang′lii pterygopalati′ni [NA], SYN posterior superior lateral nasal *branches* of pterygopalatine ganglion, under *branch*.

ra′mi nasa′les posterio′res superio′res media′les gang′lii pterygopalati′ni [NA], SYN posterior superior medial nasal *branches* of pterygopalatine ganglion, under *branch*.

r. ner′vi oculomoto′rii arte′riae communican′tis posterio′ris [NA], the branch to the oculomotor nerve, a branch of the posterior communicating artery to the oculomotor nerve.

ra

r. no′di atrioventricula′ris [NA], SYN *artery* to atrioventricular node.

r. no′di sinuatria′lis arte′riae corona′ria dex′tra [NA], SYN *artery* to the sinuatrial (S-A) node.

ra′mi nucleo″rum hypothalamico′rum [NA], the branches to hypothalamic nuclei, branches of the anterior choroid artery to the nuclei of the hypothalamus.

r. obturato′rius arte′riae epigas′tricae inferio′ris [NA], SYN accessory obturator *artery*.

rami occipita′les arte′riae auricula′ris posterio′ris [NA], occipital branch of posterior auricular artery. SEE occipital *branch*.

rami occipita′les arte′riae occip′itis [NA], occipital branch of occipital artery. SEE occipital *branch*.

rami occipita′les ner′vi auricula′ris posterio′ris [NA], occipital branch posterior auricular nerve. SEE occipital *branch*.

r. occipita′lis [NA], SYN occipital *branch*.

r. occipitotempora′lis [NA], the occipitotemporal branch, a branch of the medial occipital artery to the occipital and temporal regions of the cerebral cortex.

ra′mi omenta′les [NA], SYN epiploic *branches*, under *branch*.

r. orbita′lis arte′riae menin′geae me′diae [NA], SYN orbital *branch* of middle meningeal artery.

r. orbita′lis gang′lii pterygopalati′ni [NA], SYN orbital *branch* of pterygopalatine ganglion, under *branch*.

r. orbitofronta′lis latera′lis [NA], SYN lateral frontobasal *artery*.

r. orbitofronta′lis media′lis [NA], SYN medial frontobasal *artery*.

r. os′sis is′chii [NA], SYN ischial r.

r. ova′ricus arte′riae uteri′nae [NA], SYN ovarian *branch* of uterine artery.

r. palma′ris ner′vi media′ni [NA], SYN palmar *branch* of median nerve.

r. palma′ris ner′vi ulna′ris [NA], SYN palmar *branch* of ulnar nerve.

r. palma′ris profun′dus arte′riae ulna′ris [NA], SYN deep palmar *branch* of ulnar artery.

r. palma′ris superficia′lis arte′riae radia′lis [NA], SYN superficial palmar *branch* of radial artery.

ra′mi palpebra′les ner′vi infratrochlea′ris [NA], SYN palpebral *branches* of infratrochlear nerve, under *branch*.

ra′mi pancreat′ici [NA], SYN pancreatic *branches*, under *branch*.

rami pancrea′tici arte′riae pancreaticoduodena′lis superio′ris [NA], pancreatic branch of superior pancreaticoduodenal arteries. SEE pancreatic *branches*, under *branch*.

rami pancrea′tici arte′riae sple′nicae [NA], pancreatic branch splenic artery. SEE pancreatic *branches*, under *branch*.

ra′mi parieta′les [NA], SYN parietal *branch*.

r. parietal′is arte′riae menin′geae me′diae [NA], SYN parietal *branch* of middle meningeal artery.

r. parietal′is arte′riae occipita′lis media′lis [NA], SYN parietal *branch* of medial occipital artery.

r. parietal′is arte′riae tempora′lis superficia′lis [NA], SYN parietal *branch* of superficial temporal artery.

r. pari′eto-occipita′lis [NA], parieto-occipital branch of medial occipital artery.

ra′mi parotid′ei [NA], SYN parotid *branches*, under *branch*.

r. parotid′ei arte′riae tempora′lis superficia′lis [NA], parotid branch of superficial temporal artery. SEE parotid *branches*, under *branch*.

rami parotid′ei ner′vi auriculotempora′lis [NA], parotid branch of auriculotemporal nerve. SEE parotid *branches*, under *branch*.

rami parotid′ei ve′nae facia′lis [NA], parotid branch of facial vein. SEE parotid *branches*, under *branch*.

ra′mi pectora′les arteri′ae thoracoacromia′lis [NA], SYN pectoral *branch* of thoracoacromial artery, under *branch*.

ra′mi peduncula′res [NA], the peduncular branches, branches of the posterior cerebral artery to the cerebral peduncles.

r. per′forans [NA], SYN perforating *branches*, under *branch*.

r. perfo′rans arte′riae fibula′ris [NA], SYN perforating *branch* of peroneal artery.

r. perforan′tes arte′riae thorac′icae inter′nae [NA], SYN perforating *branches* of internal thoracic artery, under *branch*.

r. perforan′tes arteria′rum metacarpa″lium palma′rium [NA], SYN perforating *branches* of palmar metacarpal arteries, under *branch*.

r. perforan′tes arteria′rum metatarsea′rum planta′rium [NA], SYN perforating *branches* of plantar metatarsal arteries, under *branch*.

ra′mi pericardi′aci aor′tae thora′cicae [NA], SYN pericardial *branch* of thoracic aorta, under *branch*.

r. pericardi′acus ner′vi phren′ici [NA], SYN pericardial *branch* of phrenic nerve.

ra′mi perinea′les ner′vi cuta′nei fem′oris posterio′ris [NA], SYN perineal *branches* of posterior femoral cutaneous nerve, under *branch*.

peroneal anastomotic r., SYN peroneal communicating *branch*.

r. petro′sus arte′riae menin′geae med′iae [NA], SYN petrosal *branch* of middle meningeal artery.

ra′mi pharyngea′les [NA], SYN pharyngeal *branches*, under *branch*.

rami pharyngea′les arte′riae pharyn′geae ascenden′tis [NA], SYN pharyngeal *branch* of the ascending pharyngeal artery.

rami pharyngea′les arte′riae thyroi′deae inferio′ris [NA], SYN pharyngeal *branch* of inferior thyroid artery.

rami pharyn′gei ner′vi glossopharyn′gei [NA], SYN pharyngeal *branch* of glossopharyngeal nerve.

rami pharyn′gei ner′vi va′gi [NA], SYN pharyngeal *branch* of vagus nerve.

r. pharyn′geus arte′riae cana′lis pterygoi′dei [NA], SYN pharyngeal *branch* of the artery of pterygoid canal.

r. pharyn′geus arte′riae palati′ni descen′dens [NA], SYN pharyngeal *branch* of descending palatine artery.

r. pharyn′geus gan′glii pterygopalati′ni [NA], SYN pharyngeal *branch* of pterygopalatine ganglion.

ra′mi phrenicoabdomina′les ner′vi phre′nici [NA], SYN phrenicoabdominal *branch* of phrenic nerve, under *branch*.

r. planta′ris profun′dus arte′riae dorsa′lis pe′dis [NA], SYN deep plantar *branch* of dorsalis pedis artery.

r. poste′rior arte′riae obturato′riae [NA], SYN posterior *branch* of obturator artery.

r. poste′rior arte′riae pancreaticoduodena′lis inferio′ris [NA], SYN posterior *branch* of inferior pancreaticoduodenal artery.

r. poste′rior arte′riae recurren′tis ulna′ris [NA], SYN posterior *branch* of recurrent ulnar artery.

r. poste′rior arte′riae rena′lis [NA], SYN posterior *branch* of renal artery.

r. poste′rior arte′riae thyroi′deae superio′ris [NA], SYN posterior *branch* of superior thyroid artery.

r. poste′rior ascen′dens [NA], SYN ascending posterior *branch*.

r. poste′rior descen′dens [NA], SYN descending posterior *branch*.

r. poste′rior duc′tus hepa′tici dex′tri [NA], SYN posterior *branch* of right hepatic duct.

rami posterio′res [NA], SYN posterior *branches*, under *branch*.

rami posterio′res nervo′rum spina′lium, ☆official alternate term for dorsal primary r. of spinal nerve.

r. poste′rior ner′vi auricula′ris mag′ni [NA], SYN posterior *branch* of great auricular nerve.

r. poste′rior ner′vi obturato′rii [NA], SYN posterior *branch* of obturator nerve.

r. poste′rior ra′mi dex′tri ve′nae por′tae hepa′tis [NA], SYN posterior *branch* of right branch of portal vein.

r. poste′rior sul′ci latera′lis cere′bri [NA], SYN posterior *branch* of lateral cerebral sulcus.

r. poste′rior ve′nae pulmona′lis dex′trae superio′ris [NA], SYN posterior *branch* of right superior pulmonary vein.

rami profun′di arte′riae circumflex′ae femo′ris media′lis [NA], SYN deep *branch* of the medial plantar artery.

rami profun′di arte′riae transver′sae cervi′cis [NA], SYN dorsal scapular *artery*.

r. profun′dus [NA], SYN deep *branch*.

r. profun′dus arte′riae circumflex′ae femo′ris media′lis [NA], SYN deep *branch* of the medial femoral circumflex artery.

r. profun′dus arte′ria scapula′ris descen′dens, SYN dorsal scapular *artery*.

r. profun′dus arte′riae transver′sae col′li [NA], SYN dorsal scapular *artery*.

r. profun′dus ner′vi plantar′is latera′lis [NA], SYN deep *branch* of the lateral plantar nerve.

r. profun′dus ner′vi radia′lis [NA], SYN anterior interosseous *nerve*.

r. profun′dus ner′vi ulna′ris [NA], SYN deep *branch* of the ulnar nerve.

ra′mi pterygoi″dei arte′riae maxilla′ris [NA], SYN pterygoid *branch* of maxillary artery, under *branch*.

pubic rami, SEE pubes.

r. pu′bicus arte′riae epigas′tricae inferio′ris [NA], SYN pubic *branch* of inferior epigastric artery.

r. pu′bicus arte′riae obturato′riae [NA], SYN pubic *branch* of obturator artery.

ra′mi pulmona″les systema′tis autono′mici [NA], SYN pulmonary *branch* of autonomic nervous system, under *branch*.

ra′mi radicula′res, ✩official alternate term for spinal *arteries*, under *artery*.

ra′mi rena′les ner′vi va′gi [NA], SYN renal *branch* of vagus nerve, under *branch*.

r. rena′lis ner′vi splanch′nici mino′ris [NA], SYN renal *branch* of lesser splanchnic *nerve*.

r. saphe′nus arte′riae descenden′tis genicula′ris [NA], SYN saphenous *branch* of descending genicular artery.

ra′mi scrota′les anterio′res arte′riae puden′dae exter′nae [NA], SYN anterior scrotal *branch* of external pudendal artery, under *branch*.

ra′mi scrota′les posterio′res arte′riae puden′dae inter′nae [NA], SYN posterior scrotal *branch* of internal pudendal artery, under *branch*.

ra′mi septa′les, rami interventricularis septales.

r. sinis′ter [NA], SYN left *branch*.

r. sinis′ter arte′riae hepat′icae pro′priae [NA], SYN left hepatic *artery*.

r. sinis′ter ve′nae por′tae hepa′tis [NA], left branch of hepatic portal vein.

r. si′nus carot′ici [NA], SYN carotid sinus *nerve*.

r. si′nus caverno′si [NA], the cavernous sinus branch, a branch of the cavernous part of the internal carotid artery supplying the walls of the cavernous sinus.

r. si′nus caverno′si arte′riae caro′tidis arte′riae [NA], SYN cavernous sinus *branch* of internal carotid artery.

ra′mi spina′les [NA], spinal branches (1) SYN spinal *arteries*, under *artery*. (2) veins draining the meninges and spinal cord, tributaries of the intervertebral veins.

ra′mi sple′nici arte′riae sple′nicae [NA], SYN splenic *branches* of splenic artery, under *branch*.

r. stape′dius arte′riae stylomastoi′deae [NA], SYN stapedial *branch* of stylomastoid artery.

ra′mi sterna′les arte′riae thora′cicae inter′nae [NA], SYN sternal *branches* of internal thoracic artery, under *branch*.

ra′mi ster′noclei′domastoi′dei arte′riae occipita′lis [NA], SYN sternocleidomastoid *branch* of occipital artery.

r. ster′noclei′domastoi′deus arte′riae thyroi′deae superio′ris [NA], SYN sternocleidomastoid *branch* of superior thyroid artery.

r. stylohyoi′deus ner′vi facia′lis [NA], SYN stylohyoid *branch* of facial nerve.

ra′mi subscapula′res arte′riae axilla′ris [NA], SYN subscapular *branches* of axillary artery, under *branch*.

ra′mi substan′tiae ni′grae [NA], the branches to the substantia nigra, the branches of the anterior choroid artery to the substantia nigra.

r. superficia′lis [NA], SYN superficial *branch*.

r. superficia′lis arte′riae glu′teae superio′ris [NA], SYN superficial *branch* of the superior gluteal artery.

r. superficia′lis arte′riae plantar′is media′lis [NA], SYN superficial *branch* of the medial plantar artery.

r. superficia′lis ner′vi plantar′is latera′lis [NA], SYN superficial *branch* of the lateral plantar nerve.

r. superficia′lis ner′vi radia′lis [NA], SYN superficial *branch* of the radial nerve.

r. superficia′lis ner′vi ulna′ris [NA], SYN superficial *branch* of the ulnar nerve.

r. supe′rior [NA], SYN superior *branch*. (2) SYN apical *branch*.

r. supe′rior arte′riae glu′teae superio′ris [NA], SYN superior *branch* of the superior gluteal artery.

superior dental rami, superior dental branches of superior dental plexus. SYN rami dentales superiores [NA].

r. superi′or ner′vi oculomoto′rii [NA], SYN superior *branch* of the oculomotor nerve.

r. supe′rior ner′vi transversa′lis cervica′lis (col′li) [NA], SYN superior *branch* of the transverse cervical nerve.

r. supe′rior os′sis pu′bis [NA], SYN superior pubic r.

superior pubic r., a bar of bone, triangular in section, which extends posterosuperiorly from the body of the pubis to form the superior boundary of the obturator foramen; developmentally, it contributes about one-fifth of the articular surface of the acetabulum. SYN r. superior ossis pubis [NA], superior branch of the pubic bone.

r. supe′rior ve′nae pulmona′lis dex′trae/sinis′trae inferio′ris [NA], SYN superior *branch* of the right and left inferior pulmonary veins.

r. suprahyoi′deus arte′riae lingua′lis [NA], SYN suprahyoid *branch* of lingual artery.

r. sympath′icus [sympatheti′cus] ad gang′lion submandibula′re, ✩official alternate term for sympathetic *branch* to submandibular ganglion.

ra′mi tempora′les anterio′res [NA], anterior temporal branches of lateral occipital artery, giving arterial supply to the cortex of the anterior part of the temporal lobe of the brain.

ra′mi tempora′les interme′dii media′les [NA], medial intermediate temporal branches of lateral occipital artery, giving arterial supply to the cortex of the intermediate and medial part of the temporal lobe of the brain.

ra′mi tempora′les ner′vi facia′lis [NA], SYN temporal *branch* of facial nerve, under *branch*.

ra′mi tempora′les posterio′res [NA], posterior temporal branches of lateral occipital artery giving arterial supply to the cortex of the posterior part of the temporal lobe of the brain.

ra′mi tempora′les superficia′les ner′vi auriculotempora′lis [NA], SYN superficial temporal *branch* of auriculotemporal nerve, under *branch*.

r. tentor′ii [NA], SYN tentorial *nerve*.

ra′mi thalam′ici [NA], branches of the posterior cerebral artery to the thalamus.

r. thalam′icus [NA], a branch of the middle cerebral artery to the thalamus.

ra′mi thy′mici [NA], SYN mediastinal *branches* of internal thoracic artery, under *branch*.

r. thyrohyoi′deus an′sae cervica′lis [NA], SYN *nerve* to thyrohyoid muscle.

r. tonsil′lae cerebel′lae [NA], the branch to the cerebellar tonsil, a branch from the posterior inferior cerebellar artery supplying the tonsil of the cerebellum.

ra′mi tonsilla′res ner′vi glossopharyn′gei [NA], SYN tonsillar *branch* of glossopharyngeal nerve, under *branch*.

r. tonsilla′ris arte′riae facia′lis [NA], SYN tonsillar *branch* of the facial artery.

ra′mi trachea′les [NA], SYN tracheal *branches*, under *branch*.

rami trachea′les arte′riae thyroi′deae inferio′ris [NA], tracheal branches of inferior thyroid artery. SEE tracheal *branches*, under *branch*.

rami trachea′les ner′vi laryn′gei recurren′tis [NA], tracheal branches of recurrent laryngeal nerve. SEE tracheal *branches*, under *branch*.

ra

ra′mi trac′tus op′tici [NA], the optic tract branches, branches of the anterior choroid artery to the optic tract.

r. transver′sus [NA], SYN transverse *branches*, under *branch*.

r. transver′sus arte′riae circumflex′ae femo′ris latera′lis [NA], transverse branches of lateral femoral circumflex artery. SEE transverse *branches*, under *branch*.

r. transver′sus arte′riae circumflex′ae femo′ris media′lis [NA], transverse branches of medial femoral circumflex artery SEE transverse *branches*, under *branch*.

r. tuba′rius [NA], SYN tubal *branch*.

r. tubari′us arte′riae ute′rinae [NA], SYN tubal *branch* of the uterine artery.

r. tuba′rius plex′us tympan′ici [NA], SYN tubal *branch* of the tympanic plexus.

ra′mi tu′beris cine′rei [NA], the branches of the anterior choroid artery to the tuber cinereum.

r. ulna′ris ner′vi cuta′nei antebra′chii media′lis [NA], SYN ulnar *branch* of medial antebrachial cutaneous nerve.

ra′mi ureter′ici [NA], SYN ureteric *branches*, under *branch*.

rami urete′rici arte′riae ovar′icae [NA], SYN ureteric *branches* of the ovarian artery, under *branch*.

rami urete′rici arte′riae rena′lis [NA], SYN ureteric *branches* of the renal artery, under *branch*.

rami urete′rici arte′riae testicula′ris [NA], SYN ureteric *branches* of the testicular artery, under *branch*.

rami urete′rici par′tis paten′tis arte′riae umbilica′le [NA], SYN ureteric *branches* of the patent part of umbilical artery, under *branch*.

ra′mi ventra′les nervo′rum cervica′lium [NA], SYN ventral primary rami of cervical spinal nerves. SEE ventral primary r. of spinal nerve.

ra′mi ventra′les nervo′rum lumba′lium [NA], SYN ventral primary rami of lumbar spinal nerves. SEE ventral primary r. of spinal nerve.

ra′mi ventra′les nervo′rum sacra′lium [NA], SYN ventral primary rami of sacral spinal nerves. SEE ventral primary r. of spinal nerve.

rami ventralis, SYN ventral *branch*.

r. ventra′lis ner′vi spina′lis [NA], SYN ventral primary r. of spinal nerve.

ventral primary rami of cervical spinal nerves, SEE ventral primary r. of spinal nerve. SYN rami ventrales nervorum cervicalium [NA].

ventral primary rami of lumbar spinal nerves, SEE ventral primary r. of spinal nerve. SYN rami ventrales nervorum lumbalium [NA].

ventral primary rami of sacral spinal nerves, SEE ventral primary r. of spinal nerve. SYN rami ventrales nervorum sacralium [NA].

ventral primary r. of spinal nerve, the larger, anterolaterally-directed major terminal branch (with the dorsal primary ramus) of all 31 pairs of mixed spinal nerves, formed at the intervertebral foramen. Most ventral primary rami, especially those involved in the innervation of the limbs, participate in the formation of the major nerve plexuses (cervical, brachial, and lumbosacral) and lose their identities. Most in the thoracic region, however, remain separate from adjacent rami to become the intercostal and subcostal nerves. Ventral primary rami provide innervation to the anterolateral body wall and trunk. Nomina Anatomica lists ventral primary rami as "rami ventrales" for each group of spinal nerves: 1) cervical (nervorum cervicalium [NA]), 2) thoracic (nervorum thoracicorum [NA]), 3) lumbar (nervorum lumbalium [NA]), 4) sacral (nervorum sacralium [NA])m, and 5) coccygeal (nervi coccygei [NA]). SYN r. ventralis nervi spinalis [NA], anterior primary division.

ra′mi vestibula′res arte′riae labyrin′thi [NA], vestibular branches of labyrinthine artery.

white rami communicantes, short nerves arising from the initial portion of the ventral primary rami of the thoracic and upper lumbar spinal nerves through which all presynaptic sympathetic nerve fibers must pass to reach the sympathetic trunks; also conveyed by the white rami communicans are visceral afferent (sensory) fibers which were conveyed to the sympathetic trunks

in splanchnic nerves. Most fibers conveyed by the white rami communicantes are myelinated. SYN rami communicantes nervorum spinalium [NA], communicating branches of spinal nerves.

ra′mi zygomat′ici ner′vi facia′lis [NA], SYN zygomatic *branch* of facial nerve, under *branch*.

r. zygomaticofacia′lis ner′vi zygoma′tici [NA], SYN zygomaticofacial *branch* of zygomatic nerve.

r. zygomaticotempora′lis ner′vi zygoma′tici [NA], SYN zygomaticotemporal *branch* of zygomatic nerve.

---

ra·my·cin (ră-mī′sin). SYN fusidic acid.

ran·cid (ran′sid). Having a disagreeable odor and taste, usually characterizing fat undergoing oxidation or bacterial decomposition to more volatile odoriferous substances. [L. *rancidus*, stinking, rank]

ran·cid·i·fy (ran-sid′i-fī). To make or become rancid.

ran·cid·i·ty (ran-sid′i-tē). The state of being rancid.

Rand, Gertrude, U.S. visual psychologist, 1886–1970. SEE Hardy-R.-Ritter *test*.

Rand, M.J. SEE Burn and R. *theory*.

Randall, Alexander, U.S. urologist, *1885. SEE R. stone *forceps*.

ran·dom (ran′dom). Governed by chance; used of a process in which the outcome is indeterminate but may assume any of set of values (the domain) with probabilities specifiable in advance. While the random process is widely used in probability theory, empirical justification for the term is more complicated. The minimum requirement is that repeated realization of the process will settle down to a stable distribution or, if not metrical, a stable set of frequencies if the trait is classifiable only. SEE random *mechanism*. [M.E. *randon*, speed, errancy, fr. O. Fr. *randir*, to run, fr. Germanic]

ran·dom·i·za·tion. Allocation of individuals to groups, *e.g.*, for experimental and control regimens, by chance.

Raney R. N.. Proprietary name for a finely powdered nickel catalyst made from Raney alloy by dissolving out the aluminum with alkali; used in the hydrogenation of organic substances. SYN Raney catalyst.

range (rānj). A statistical measure of the dispersion or variation of values determined by the endpoint values themselves or the difference between them; *e.g.*, in a group of children aged 6, 8, 9, 10, 13, and 16, the r. would be from 6 to 16 or, alternately, 10 (16 minus 6). [O.Fr. *rang*, line fr. Germanic]

therapeutic r., refers to either the dosage r. or blood plasma or serum concentration usually expected to achieve desired therapeutic effects. Some patients will require doses (or concentrations) above or below this r. Some patients will experience drug toxicity within this r.

ra·nine (rā′nīn). 1. Relating to the frog. 2. Relating to the undersurface of the tongue. [L. *rana*, a frog]

ra·ni·ti·dine (ră-nī′ti-dēn). *N*-[2-[[5-[(Dimethylamino)methyl]-furfuryl]thio]ethyl]-*N*′- methyl-2-nitro-1,1-ethenediamine; a histamine H_2 antagonist used in the treatment of duodenal and gastric ulcers, where it reduces hydrochloric acid secretion.

rank. 1. The ordinal position of an observation in the set of observations of which it is a member. 2. To order a set of observations according to their r.

Ranke, Johannes, German anthropologist and physician, 1836–1916. SEE R.'s *angle*.

Ranke, Karl E. von, German chemist, 1870–1926. SEE R.'s *formula*.

Rankin, Fred Wharton, U.S. surgeon, 1886–1954. SEE R.'s *clamp*.

Rankine, William J. McQ., Scottish physicist, 1820–1870. SEE R. *scale*.

Ransohoff, Joseph, U.S. surgeon, 1853–1921. SEE R.'s *sign*.

RANTES. A member of the interleukin-8 superfamily of cytokines. This cytokine is a selective chemoattractant for memory T lymphocytes and monocytes.

ran·u·la (ran′yū-lă). 1. Hypoglottis. 2. Any cystic tumor of the undersurface of the tongue or floor of the mouth, especially one of the floor of the mouth due to obstruction of the duct of the sublingual glands. SYN ptyalocele, ranine tumor, sialocele, sublingual cyst. [L. tadpole, dim. of *rana,* frog]

r. pancreat'ica, a cystic tumor caused by obstruction of the pancreatic duct.

ran·u·lar (ran'yū-lăr). Relating to a ranula.

Ranvier, Louis A., French pathologist, 1835–1922. SEE R.'s *crosses,* under *cross, disks,* under *disk, node, plexus, segment.*

RAO Abbreviation for right anterior oblique, a radiographic projection.

Raoult, François, M., French physicist, 1830–1899. SEE R.'s *law.*

RAPD Abbreviation for rapid analysis of polymorphic DNA.

rape (rāp). **1.** Sexual intercourse by force, duress, intimidation, or without legal consent (as with a minor). **2.** The performance of such an act. [L. *rapio,* to seize, to drag away]

rape·seed oil (rāp'sēd). The compressed oil from the seeds of *Brassica campestris* (family Cruciferae); used in the manufacture of soaps, margarine, and lubricants. [L. *rapa,* turnip]

ra·pha·nia (ră-fā'nē-ă). A spasmodic disease supposed to be due to poisoning by the seeds of *Rhaphanus rhaphanistrum,* the wild radish. SYN rhaphania.

ra·phe (rā'fē) [NA]. The line of union of two contiguous, bilaterally symmetrical structures. SYN rhaphe. [G. *rhaphē,* suture, seam]

amniotic r., the line of fusion of the amniotic folds over the embryo in reptiles, birds, and certain mammals.

r. anococcyg'ea, SYN anococcygeal *ligament.*

anogenital r., in the male embryo the line of closure of the genital folds and swellings extending from the anus to the tip of the penis; it is differentiated in the adult into three regions: perineal r., scrotal r., and penile r.

r. cor'poris callo'si, a slight anteroposterior furrow on the median line of the upper surface of the corpus callosum.

lateral palpebral r., a narrow fibrous band in the lateral part of the orbicularis oculi muscle formed by the interlacing of fibers passing through the upper and lower eyelids. SYN r. palpebralis lateralis [NA], palpebral r.

r. lin'guae, SYN median *groove* of tongue.

median longitudinal r. of tongue, SYN median *groove* of tongue.

r. medul'lae oblonga'tae [NA], the seamlike median zone of the medulla oblongata, marked by intercrossing fiber bundles among which lie scattered neuronal cell bodies.

r. nuclei, SEE *nuclei* raphes, under *nucleus.*

r. pala'ti [NA], SYN palatine r.

palatine r., a rather narrow, low elevation in the center of the hard palate that extends from the incisive papilla posteriorly over the entire length of the mucosa of the hard palate. SYN r. palati [NA], palatine ridge.

palpebral r., SYN lateral palpebral r.

r. palpebra'lis latera'lis [NA], SYN lateral palpebral r.

penile r., the continuation of the r. of the scrotum onto the underside of the penis. SYN r. penis [NA].

r. pe'nis [NA], SYN penile r.

perineal r., the central anteroposterior line of the perineum, most marked in the male, being continuous with the r. of the scrotum. SYN r. perinei [NA].

r. perine'i [NA], SYN perineal r.

pharyngeal r., the central line of the pharynx posteriorly where the muscular fibers meet and partly interlace. SYN r. pharyngis [NA].

r. pharyn'gis [NA], SYN pharyngeal r.

r. pon'tis [NA], the continuation of the r. medullae oblongatae into the pars dorsalis (or tegmentum) pontis.

pterygomandibular r., a tendinous thickening of the buccopharyngeal fascia, separating and giving origin to the buccinator muscle anteriorly and the superior constrictor of the pharynx posteriorly. SYN r. pterygomandibularis [NA], pterygomandibular ligament.

r. pterygomandibula'ris [NA], SYN pterygomandibular r.

r. ret'inae, the horizontal line separating the superior and inferi-

or portions of the temporal retina over which the retinal nerve fibers do not course.

scrotal r., a central line, like a cord, running over the scrotum from the anus to the root of the penis; it marks the position of the septum scroti. SYN r. scroti [NA], Vesling's line.

r. scro'ti [NA], SYN scrotal r.

Stilling's r., the transverse interdigitations of fiber bundles across the anterior median fissure of the medulla oblongata at the decussation of the pyramidal tracts.

Rapoport, Abraham, Canadian urologist, *1926. SEE R. *test.*

Rapoport, Samuel Mitja, Russian biochemist, *1912. SEE R.-Luebering *shunt.*

Rappaport clas·si·fi·ca·tion. See under classification.

rap·port (rap-ōr'). **1.** A feeling of relationship, especially when characterized by emotional affinity. **2.** A conscious feeling of harmonious accord, trust, empathy, and mutual responsiveness between two or more persons (*e.g.,* physician and patient) that fosters the therapeutic process. [Fr.]

rap·ture of the deep (rap'chūr). SEE nitrogen *narcosis* (2).

rar·e·fac·tion (rār-ĕ-fak'shŭn). The process of becoming light or less dense; the condition of being light; opposed to condensation. [L. *rarus,* thin, + *facio,* to make]

rar·e·fy (rār'ĕ-fī). To become light or less dense.

RAS Abbreviation for reticular activating *system.*

ra·sce·ta (ră-sē'tă). The transverse wrinkling on the anterior surface of the wrist. [Mod. L. *raseta,* fr. Ar. *rāhah,* palm of hand]

rash. Lay term for a cutaneous eruption. [O. Fr. *rasche,* skin eruption, fr. L. *rado,* pp. *rasus,* to scratch, scrape]

ammonia r., SYN diaper *dermatitis.*

antitoxin r., a cutaneous manifestation of serum sickness.

astacoid r., a massive exfoliation, sometimes occurring in malignant smallpox, the color of which resembles that of a boiled lobster.

black currant r., the cutaneous eruption of lentigines seen in xeroderma pigmentosum.

butterfly r., SYN butterfly (2).

caterpillar r., SYN caterpillar *dermatitis.*

crystal r., SYN miliaria crystallina.

diaper r., SYN diaper *dermatitis.*

drug r., SYN drug *eruption.*

heat r., SYN miliaria rubra.

hydatid r., a toxic eruption occasionally following the rupture of a hydatid cyst.

Murray Valley r., SYN epidemic *polyarthritis.*

napkin r., SYN diaper *dermatitis.*

nettle r., obsolete term for urticaria.

serum r., a cutaneous manifestation of serum sickness.

summer r., SYN miliaria rubra.

wildfire r., SYN miliaria rubra.

ra·sion (rā'zhŭn). The subdivision of a crude drug by a rasp to prepare it for extraction. [L. *rasio,* a scraping, fr. *rado,* pp. *rasus,* to scrape, shave]

Rasmussen, Fritz W., Danish physician, 1834–1881. SEE R.'s *aneurysm.*

Rasmussen, Grant L. American neuroanatomist, *1904. SEE *bundle* of Rasmussen.

ras·pa·to·ry (ras'pă-tōr-ē). A surgical instrument used to smooth the edges of a divided bone. [L. *raspatorium*]

RAST Acronym for radioallergosorbent *test.*

Rastelli, Gian C. SEE R.'s *operation, operation.*

rat. A rodent of the genus *Rattus* (family Muridae), involved in the spread of some diseases, including bubonic plague.

albino r.'s, r.'s with white fur and pink eyes; used extensively in laboratory experiments.

Wistar r.'s, an inbred strain of rats, homozygous at most loci, produced by strict brother-sister inbreeding over many generations to develop animals for research with the same general genetic composition. [*Wistar* Institute]

rate (rāt). A record of the measurement of an event or process in terms of its relation to some fixed standard; measurement is expressed as the ratio of one quantity to another (*e.g.*, velocity, distance per unit time). **2.** A measure of the frequency of an event in a defined population; the components of a r. are: the numerator (number of events); the denominator (population at risk of experiencing the event); the specified time in which the events occur; and usually a multiplier, a power of 10, which makes it possible to express the rate as a whole number rather than an awkward decimal. [L. *ratum,* a reckoning (see ratio)]

abortion r., the number of abortions per 1000 terminated pregnancies during a given period of time.

age-specific r., a r. for a specified age group, in which the numerator and denominator refer to the same age group.

attack r., a cumulative incidence rate used for particular groups observed for limited periods under special circumstances, such as during an epidemic.

average flow r., the flow r. determined by dividing the total volume of urine passed by the time of voiding.

basal metabolic r. (BMR), SYN basal *metabolism*.

baseline fetal heart r., the average heart r. for a particular fetus during the diastolic phase of uterine contractions.

birth r., a summary r. based on the number of live births in a population over a given period, usually one year; the numerator is the number of live births, the denominator is the midyear population.

case fatality r., the proportion of individuals contracting a disease that die of that disease.

concordance r., the proportion of a random sample of pairs that are concordant for a trait of interest. A high r. of concordance may be generated in several ways, many of which may result from irrelevant bias; but broadly it is taken as evidence of causal connection (*e.g.*, in the case of identical twins, a genetic component or in spouses of assortative mating).

critical r., a heart r. at which aberration or incomplete block will occur; a result of shortening of cycle length so that it barely includes the refractory period.

death r., an estimate of the proportion of the population that dies during a specified period, usually a year; the numerator is the number of people dying, the denominator is the number in the population, usually an estimate of the number at the mid-period. SYN crude death rate, mortality r.

erythrocyte sedimentation r. (ESR), the rate of settling of red blood cells in anticoagulated blood; increased r.'s are often associated with anemia or inflammatory states.

fatality r., the death r. observed in a designated series of persons affected by a simultaneous event such as a disaster.

fetal death r., the number of fetal deaths divided by the sum of live births and fetal deaths occurring in the same population during the same time period. SYN stillbirth r.

fetal heart r., in the fetus, the number of heart beats per minute, normally 120 to 160.

five year survival r., the proportion of patients still alive five years after a diagnosis or form of treatment is completed. Usually applied to statistics of survival of cancer patients, since after five years, recurrences are much less likely to occur.

general fertility r., a refined measure of fertility in a population; the numerator is the number of live births in a year, the denominator is the number of females of child-bearing age, usually defined as ages 15–44 (but increasingly recognized as extending to age 49).

glomerular filtration r. (GFR), the volume of water filtered out of the plasma through glomerular capillary walls into Bowman's capsules per unit time; it is considered to be equivalent to inulin clearance.

gross reproduction r., the average number of female children a woman would have if she survived to the end of her childbearing years and if, throughout that period, she were subject to a given set of age-specific fertility r.'s and a given sex ratio at birth; this r. provides a measure of the replacement fertility of a population in the absence of mortality.

growth r., absolute or relative growth increase, expressed per unit of time.

growth r. of population, a measure of population change in the

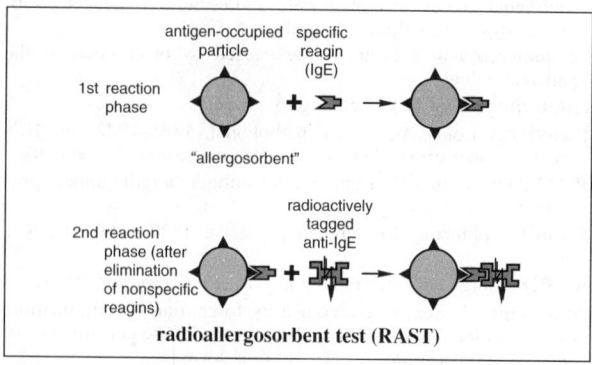

radioallergosorbent test (RAST)

absence of migration, comprising addition of newborns and subtraction of deaths; the result is known as the natural r. of increase of the population; it is the difference between the crude birth r. and the crude death r.

hazard r., theoretical measure of the risk of occurrence of an event, *e.g.*, death, new disease, at a point in time.

heart r., r. of the heart's beat, recorded as the number of beats per minute.

inception r., the r. at which new spells of illness or cases of a condition occur in a population.

incidence r., the r. at which new events occur in a population. The numerator is the number of new events occurring in a defined period; the denominator is the population at risk of experiencing the event during this period.

infant mortality r., a measure of the r. of deaths of liveborn infants before their first birthday; the numerator is the number of infants under one year of age born alive in a defined region during a calendar year who die before they are one year old; the denominator is the total number of live births; often quoted as a useful indicator of the level of health in a community.

initial r., SYN initial *velocity*.

lethality r., SYN mortality r.

maternal death r., the number of maternal deaths that occur as the direct result of the reproductive process per 100,000 live births. SEE rate. SEE ALSO maternal *death*.

mitotic r., the proportion of cells in a tissue that are undergoing mitosis, expressed as a mitotic index or, roughly, as the number of cells in mitosis in each microscopic high-power field in tissue sections.

morbidity r., the proportion of patients with a particular disease during a given year per given unit of population.

mortality r., SYN death r. SYN lethality r., mortality (2).

mutation r., the probability (or proportion) of progeny genes with a particular component of the genome not present in either biological parent; usually expressed as the number of mutants per generation occurring at one gene or locus.

neonatal mortality r., the number of deaths in the first 28 days of life divided by the number of live births occurring in the same population during the same period of time.

peak flow r., maximum urinary flow r. during voiding as measured by a uroflowmeter.

perinatal mortality r., the number of stillborn infants of 24 completed weeks or more plus the number of deaths occurring under 7 days of life divided by the number of stillborn infants of 24 weeks or more gestation plus all liveborn infants in the same population, regardless of the period of gestation.

pulse r., r. of the pulse as observed in an artery; recorded as beats per minute.

recurrence r., in genetic counseling, the risk that a future offspring will be affected given some specific set of relatives of whom at least one is already affected.

repetition r., the number of pulses per minute, describing an energy output*.g.,* ultrasound pulses in echocardiography rather than vascular pulses.

respiration r., frequency of breathing, recorded as the number of breaths per minute.

sedimentation r., the sinking velocity of blood cells, *i.e.,* the degree of rapidity with which the red cells sink in a mass of drawn blood.

shear r., the change in velocity of parallel planes in a flowing fluid separated by unit distance; its units expressed in seconds^{-1}.

slew r., in electronic pacemaker function, the maximum rate of change of an amplifier output voltage; important variable affecting heart function as controlled by an electronic pacemaker. Sensing circuits in the pacemaker often respond to the slew r. rather than to the absolute amplitude of the voltage pulse.

steady-state r., SYN steady-state *velocity.*

steroid metabolic clearance r. (MCR), a measure of the r. of metabolism of a given steroid within the body, usually expressed as liters of body fluid that contain the amount of steroid metabolized per day.

steroid production r., the total quantity of a given steroid formed in the body, usually expressed as milligrams per day; represents the sum of the glandular secretion of the steroid and extraglandular formation of it from various steroid precursors.

steroid secretory r., the r. of glandular secretion of a given steroid, usually expressed as milligrams per day; does not include any amount of the steroid that might be formed extraglandularly.

stillbirth r., SYN fetal death r.

voiding flow r., urinary flow as a function of time during micturition, as graphically recorded by a flow meter.

Rathke, Martin H., German anatomist, physiologist, and pathologist, 1793–1860. SEE R.'s *bundles,* under *bundle,* cleft *cyst, diverticulum, pocket, pouch,* pouch *tumor.*

ra·tio (ra′shē-ō). An expression of the relation of one quantity to another (*e.g.,* of a proportion or rate). SEE ALSO index (2), quotient. [L. *ratio* (*ration-*) a reckoning, reason, fr. *reor,* pp. *ratus,* to reckon, compute]

absolute terminal innervation r., the number of motor endplates divided by the number of terminal axons related to them.

accommodative convergence-accommodation r. (AC/A), the amount of convergence (measured in prism diopters of convergence) divided by the amount of accommodation (measured in diopters) required to direct both eyes upon an object.

A/G r., abbreviation for albumin-globulin r.

albumin-globulin r. (A/G r.), the r. of albumin to globulin in the serum or in the urine in kidney disease; the normal r. in the serum is approximately 1.55.

ALT:AST r., the r. of serum alanine aminotransferase to serum aspartate aminotransferase; elevated serum levels of both enzymes characterize hepatic disease; when both levels are abnormally elevated and the ALT:AST r. is greater than 1.0, severe hepatic necrosis or alcoholic hepatic disease is likely; when the r. is less than 1.0, an acute non-alcoholic hepatic condition is favored.

amylase-creatinine clearance r., a test for the diagnosis of acute pancreatitis; it is determined by measuring amylase and creatinine in serum and urine in apparently healthy individuals the renal clearance of amylase is less than 5% that of creatinine; in acute pancreatitis the r. is said to be greater than 0.05 or 5%.

body-weight r., body weight (in grams) divided by stature (in centimeters).

cardiothoracic r., the r. of the horizontal diameter of the heart to the inner diameter of the rib cage at its widest point as determined on a chest roentgenogram.

case fatality r., the mortality rate of a disease, usually expressed per 100 cases.

r. of decayed and filled surfaces (RDFS), an index of decayed and filled permanent surfaces per person, per full complement of 122 tooth surfaces.

r. of decayed and filled teeth (RDFT), an index of decayed and filled permanent teeth per person, per full complement of 28 teeth.

extraction r. (E), the fraction of a substance removed from the blood flowing through the kidney; it is calculated from the formula $(A - V)/A$, where A and V, respectively, are the concentrations of the substance in arterial and renal venous plasma.

fertility r., A measure of the fertility of a population based on

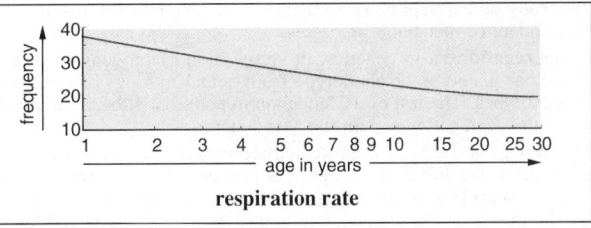

respiration rate

the female population in the child-bearing age-group, defined as ages 15-49 years.

flux r., the r. of the two unidirectional fluxes through a particular boundary layer or membrane.

functional terminal innervation r., the number of muscle fibers divided by the number of axons that innervate them.

grid r., in a radiographic scatter-absorbing grid, the r. of the height to the width of the gaps between lead strips; a higher grid r. removes more scattered radiation but requires more careful x-ray tube positioning to avoid grid cutoff of the primary radiation beam.

gyromagnetic r., in nuclear magnetic resonance, the r. of the magnetic dipole moment of the nucleus to the nuclear spin angular momentum; the gyromagnetic r. is a unique value for each type of nucleus. SYN magnetogyric r.

hand r., the r. of the length of the hand (measured on the dorsum from the styloid process of the ulna to the tip of the third finger) to the width across the knuckles.

IRI/G r., the r. of immunoreactive insulin to serum or plasma glucose; in hypoglycemic states a r. of less than 0.3 is usual with the exception of the hypoglycemia due to insulinoma, where the r. is often higher than 0.3.

K:A r., abbreviation for ketogenic-antiketogenic r.

ketogenic-antiketogenic r. (K:A r.), the proportion between substances that form ketones in the body and those that form D-glucose.

lecithin/sphingomyelin r. (L/S r.), a r. used to determine fetal pulmonary maturity, found by testing the amniotic fluid; when the lungs are mature, lecithin exceeds sphingomyelin by 2 to 1.

L/S r., abbreviation for lecithin/sphingomyelin r.

magnetogyric r. (mag′nĕ-tō-gȳ-rik), SYN gyromagnetic r.

mass-action r., the ratio of the product of all of the product concentrations divided by the product of all of the reactant concentrations of a particular reaction; when the reaction has been completed (*i.e.,* $t = \infty$), then this r. is equal to the equilibrium constant.

M:E r., the r. of myeloid to erythroid precursors in bone marrow; normally it varies from 2:1 to 4:1; an increased r. is found in infections, chronic myelogenous leukemia, or erythroid hypoplasia; a decreased r. may mean a depression of leukopoiesis or normoblastic hyperplasia depending on the overall cellularity of the bone marrow.

mendelian r., the r. of progeny with a particular phenotypes or genotypes expected in accordance with Mendel's law among the offspring of matings specified as to genotype or phenotype.

molecular weight r. (M_r), SYN molecular *weight.*

nuclear-cytoplasmic r., r. of volume of nucleus to volume of cytoplasm, fairly constant for a particular cell type and usually increased in malignant neoplasms.

nucleolar-nuclear r., r. of volume of nucleolus to volume of nucleus, usually increased in malignant neoplasms.

nutritive r., the ratio or proportion of digestible protein to digestible non-nitrogenous nutrients in a ration for livestock.

P/O r., a measure of oxidative phosphorylation; the r. of phosphate radicals esterified (forming adenosine 5′-triphosphate from adenosine 5′-diphosphate) to atoms of oxygen consumed by mitochondria; normally, the r. is 3 (starting from NADH). SYN P/O quotient.

respiratory exchange r., the r. of the net output of carbon dioxide to the simultaneous net uptake of oxygen at a given site, both expressed as moles or STPD volumes per unit time; in the steady state, respiratory exchange r. is equal to the respiratory quotient of metabolic processes.

segregation r., in genetics, the proportion of progeny of a particular genotype or phenotype from actual matings of specified genotypes. The test of a Mendelian hypothesis is the comparison of the segregation r. with the Mendelian r.

sex r., (1) the r. of male to female progeny at some specified stage of the life cycle, notably at conception (primary), at birth (secondary), or at any stage between birth and death (tertiary); **(2)** the r. of the numbers of males to females affected by a particular disease or trait.

signal-to-noise r., the relative intensity of a signal to the random variation in signal intensity, or noise; used to evaluate many imaging techniques and electronic systems.

standardized mortality r., the r. of the number of events observed in a population to the number that would be expected if the population had the same distribution as a standard or reference population.

systolic/diastolic r., a calculation from pulsed Doppler ultrasound determinations of blood flow velocities that reflects intrinsic resistance in an arterial blood vessel.

therapeutic r., the r. of the maximally tolerated dose of a drug to the minimal curative or effective dose; LD_{50} divided by ED_{50}.

variance r. (F), the distribution of the r. of two independent estimates of the same variance from a gaussian distribution based on samples of sizes $(n + 1)$ and $(m + 1)$ respectively. Estimates are usually based on one such sample analyzed in such a way as to make them independent *e.g.,* analysis of variance; and F may be used to test a null hypothesis that the observed differences among sample means is no greater than could readily be accounted for by chance.

ventilation/perfusion r. (V̇a/Q̇), the r. of alveolar ventilation to simultaneous alveolar capillary blood flow in any part of the lung; because both ventilation and perfusion are expressed per unit volume of tissue and per unit time, which cancel, the units become liters of gas per liter of blood.

zeta sedimentation r. (ZSR), the r. of the zetacrit to the hematocrit, normally 0.41 to 0.54 (41 to 54%); it is a sensitive indicator of the erythrocyte sedimentation rate (ESR) and, unlike the latter, is unaffected by anemia, which tends to elevate the ESR.

ra·tion·al (rash′ŭn-ăl). **1.** Pertaining to reasoning or to the higher thought processes; based on objective or scientific knowledge, in contrast to empirical (1). **2.** Influenced by reasoning rather than by emotion. **3.** Having the reasoning faculties; not delirious or comatose. [L. *rationalis,* fr. *ratio,* reason]

ra·tion·al·i·za·tion (ra-shŭn-ăl-i-zā′shŭn). A postulated psychoanalytic defense mechanism through which irrational behavior, motives, or feelings are made to appear reasonable. [L. *ratio,* reason]

Ratner. SEE Kurzrok-Ratner *test.*

rats·bane (rats′bān). SYN arsenic.

rat·tle·snake (rat′l-snāk). A member of the crotalid genera *Crotalus* and *Sistrurus,* characterized by possession of cuticular warning rattles at the tip of the tail.

Rat·tus (rat′ŭs). The rats, a genus of rodents, family Muridae. *R. rattus,* the black r., is the species most commonly responsible for transmitting plague to man by means of its flea, *Xenopsylla cheopis;* it is smaller and darker in color than the Norwegian, sewer, or brown rat (*Rattus norvegicus*) and has longer ears and tail. SEE rat.

Rau (Ravius, Raw), Johann J., Dutch anatomist, 1668–1719. SEE R.'s *process; processus* ravii.

Rauber, August A., German anatomist, 1841–1917. SEE R.'s *layer.*

Rauscher, F.J., 20th century U.S. oncologist. SEE R.'s *virus.*

Rau·wol·fia (row-wool′fē-ă, raw-, rah-). A genus of tropical trees and shrubs (family Apocynaceae). The powdered whole root of *R. serpentina* contains alkaloids that produce a sedative-antihypertensive-bradycrotic action; approximately 50% of the total activity is due to reserpine. [L. *Rauwolf,* German botanist, 16th century]

RAV Abbreviation for Rous-associated *virus.*

Ravius, SEE Rau.

ray (rā). **1.** A beam of light, heat, or other form of radiation. The r.'s from radium and other radioactive substances are produced by a spontaneous disintegration of the atom; they are electrically charged particles or electromagnetic waves of extremely short wavelength. **2.** A part or branch that extends radially from a structure. [L. *radius*]

actinic r., a light r. toward and beyond the violet end of the spectrum that acts upon a photographic plate and produces other chemical effects. SYN chemical r.

alpha r., SYN alpha *particle.*

anode r.'s, those originating in a gas discharge tube and moving in a direction opposite to that of cathode r.'s; made up of positively charged ions. SYN positive r.'s.

Becquerel r.'s, obsolete term for radiations given off by uranium and other radioactive substances; these include alpha, beta, and gamma r.'s.

beta r., SYN beta *particle.*

cathode r.'s, a stream of electrons emitted from the negative electrode (cathode) in a Crookes tube; their bombardment of the anode or the glass wall of the tube gives rise to x-r.'s.

chemical r., SYN actinic r.

cosmic r.'s, high velocity particles of enormous energies, bombarding earth from outer space; the "primary radiation" consists of protons and more complex atomic nuclei that, on striking the atmosphere, give rise to neutrons, mesons, and other less energetic "secondary radiation."

direct r.'s, SYN primary r.'s (2).

Dorno r.'s, the ultraviolet r.'s with wavelengths below 289 nm; those biologically active.

gamma r.'s, electromagnetic radiation emitted from radioactive substances; they are high energy x-r.'s, but originate from the nucleus rather than the orbital shell, and are not deflected by a magnet.

glass r.'s, those formed by cathode r.'s striking the wall of an x-ray tube.

grenz r. (grents), very soft x-r.'s, closely allied to the ultraviolet r.'s in their wavelength (i.e., long) and in their biologic action upon tissues; they are produced by a specially built vacuum tube with a hot cathode operating from a transformer delivering not more than 8 kw. [Ger. *Grenze,* borderline, boundary]

H r.'s, a stream of hydrogen nuclei; *i.e.,* protons.

hard r.'s, r.'s of short wavelength and great penetrability.

incident r., the r. that strikes the surface before reflection.

indirect r.'s, x-r.'s generated at a surface other than the anode target.

infrared r., SEE infrared.

intermediate r.'s, those between ultraviolet and x-r.'s. SYN W r.'s.

marginal r.'s, in geometric optics, those r.'s originating from the periphery.

medullary r., the center of the renal lobule, which has the shape of a small, steep pyramid, consisting of straight tubular parts; these may be either ascending or descending limbs of the nephronic loop or collecting tubules. SYN pars radiata lobuli corticalis renis [NA], Ferrein's pyramid, processus ferreini.

monochromatic r.'s, light r.'s or ionizing radiation of a very narrow band of wavelengths (ideally, of a single wavelength). Cf. photopeak, characteristic *radiation.*

Niewenglowski r.'s, radiation emitted from a phosphorescent body after exposure to sunlight.

parallel r.'s, r.'s parallel to the axis of an optical system.

paraxial r.'s, in geometric optics, those r.'s focused at the principal point.

positive r.'s, SYN anode r.'s.

primary r.'s, (1) cosmic r.'s in the form in which they first strike the atmosphere; **(2)** x-r.'s generated at the focal spot of the tube. SYN direct r.'s.

reflected r., a r. of light or other form of radiant energy which is thrown back from a nonpermeable or nonabsorbing surface; the r. which strikes the surface before reflection is the incident r.

roentgen r., SYN x-ray.

secondary r.'s, x-r.'s generated when primary x-r.'s impinge upon matter; scattered radiation.

soft r.'s, x-r.'s of relatively long wavelength and slight penetrability.

supersonic r.'s, r.'s with a wavelength higher than that perceptible to the human ear, above 20,000 Hz.

ultrasonic r.'s, SEE ultrasonic.

ultraviolet r.'s, SEE ultraviolet.

W r.'s, SYN intermediate r.'s.

x-r., SEE x-ray.

Rayer, Pierre F., French physician, 1793–1867. SEE R.'s *disease*.

rayl. Unit of acoustic impedance. 1 rayl = 1 kg × m^{-2} × sec^{-1}. [Baron *Rayleigh* (John W. Strutt), Eng. physicist]

Rayleigh, Lord John W.S., British physicist and Nobel laureate, 1842–1919. SEE R. *equation, test*.

Raynaud, Maurice, French physician, 1834–1881. SEE R.'s *syndrome, disease, phenomenon, sign*.

Rb Symbol for rubidium.

R-band·ing. SEE R-banding *stain*.

rbc, RBC Abbreviation for red blood *cell*; red blood count.

RBE Abbreviation used in radiation protection for relative biologic effectiveness; same as quality factor, QF.

RBF Abbreviation for renal blood flow. SEE effective renal blood *flow*.

R.C.P. Abbreviation for Royal College of Physicians (of England).

R.C.P.C.. Abbreviation for Royal College of Physicians.

R.C.P.(E), R.C.P.(Edin) Abbreviation for Royal College of Physicians (Edinburgh).

R.C.P.(I) Abbreviation for Royal College of Physicians (Ireland).

R.C.S. Abbreviation for Royal College of Surgeons (England).

R.C.S.C.. Abbreviation for Royal College of Surgeons of Canada.

R.C.S.(E), R.C.S.(Edin) Abbreviation for Royal College of Surgeons (Edinburgh).

R.C.S.(I) Abbreviation for Royal College of Surgeons (Ireland).

RCT. Abbreviation for randomized controlled *trial*.

R.D. Abbreviation for *reaction* of degeneration; registered dietician.

RDA Abbreviation for recommended daily *allowance*.

RDFS Abbreviation for *ratio* of decayed and filled surfaces.

RDFT Abbreviation for *ratio* of decayed and filled teeth.

R.D.H. Abbreviation for Registered Dental Hygienist.

R.E. Abbreviation for right eye.

Re Symbol for rhenium.

⟳re-. Prefix meaning again or backward. [L.]

re·act (rē-akt′). To take part in or to undergo a chemical reaction. [Mod. L. *reactus*]

re·ac·tance (X) (rē-ak′tans). The weakening of an alternating electric current by passage through a coil of wire or a condenser. SYN inductive resistance.

re·ac·tant (rē-ak′tant). A substance taking part in a chemical reaction.

acute phase r.'s, alpha and beta serum proteins whose concentrations increase or decrease in response to acute inflammation.

REACTION

---

re·ac·tion (rē-ak′shŭn). **1.** The response of a muscle or other living tissue or organism to a stimulus. **2.** The color change effected in litmus and certain other organic pigments by contact with substances such as acids or alkalies; also the property that such substances possess of producing this change. **3.** In chemistry, the intermolecular action of two or more substances upon

each other, whereby these substances are caused to disappear, new ones being formed in their place (chemical r.). **4.** In immunology, *in vivo* or *in vitro* action of antibody on specific antigen, with or without involvement of complement or other components of the immunological system. [L. *re-*, again, backward, + *actio*, action]

accelerated r., a response occurring in a shorter time than expected; the cutaneous manifestations occurring during the period between the second and tenth day following smallpox vaccination; because it is intermediate between a primary r. and an immediate r., it is regarded as evidence of some degree of resistance. SYN vaccinoid r.

acid r., (1) any test by which an acid r. is recognized such as the change of blue litmus paper to red; **(2)** an excess of hydrogen ions over hydroxide ions in aqueous solution indicated by a pH value less than 7 (at 22°C). Cf. dissociation *constant* of water.

acute phase r., refers to the changes in synthesis of certain proteins within the serum during an inflammatory response; this response provides rapid protection for the host against microorganisms via nonspecific defense mechanisms.

acute situational r., SYN stress r.

acute stress r., SYN anxiety r.

adverse r., any undesirable or unwanted consequence of a preventive, diagnostic, or therapeutic procedure or regimen.

alarm r., the various phenomena, *e.g.,* stimulated endocrine activity, which the body exhibits as an adaptive response to injury or stress; first phase of the general adaptation syndrome.

aldehyde r., the r. of the indole derivatives with aromatic aldehydes; *e.g.,* tryptophan and *p*-dimethylaminobenzaldehyde in H$_2$SO$_4$ give a red-violet color useful in assaying proteins for tryptophan content. SYN Ehrlich r.

alkaline r., (1) any test by which an alkaline r. is recognized, such as the change of red litmus paper to blue; **(2)** an excess of hydroxide ions over hydrogen ions in aqueous solution as indicated by a pH value greater than 7 (at 22°C). Cf. dissociation *constant* of water. SYN basic r.

allergic r., a local or general r. of an organism following contact with a specific allergen to which it has been previously exposed and sensitized; immunologic interaction of endogenous or exogenous antigen with antibody or sensitized lymphocytes gives rise to inflammation or tissue damage. Allergic r.'s are classified into four major types: type I, anaphylactic and IgE dependent; type II, cytotoxic; type III, immune-complex mediated; type IV, cellmediated (delayed). SYN hypersensitivity r.

amphoteric r., a double r. possessed by certain fluids which have a combination of acid and alkaline properties.

anamnestic r., augmented production of an antibody due to previous response of the subject to stimulus by the same antigen.

anaphylactic r. (an′a-fĭ-lak′tik), SYN anaphylaxis.

anaplerotic r., SEE anaplerotic.

antigen-antibody r. (AAR), the phenomenon, occurring *in vitro* or *in vivo*, of antibody combining with antigen of the type that stimulated the formation of the antibody, thereby resulting in agglutination, precipitation, complement fixation, greater susceptibility to ingestion and destruction by phagocytes, or neutralization of exotoxin. SEE ALSO skin *test*.

anxiety r., a psychological r. or experience involving the apprehension of danger accompanied by a feeling of dread and such physical symptoms as an increase in the rate of breathing, sweat-

⟳ **Combining forms**	**[NA] Nomina Anatomica**
Word*Finder*	**[MIM] Mendelian**
Multi-term entry finder	**Inheritance in Man**
Preceding letter A	
A.D.A.M. Anatomy Plates	☆ **Official alternate term**
Between letters L and M	
Appendices:	☆**[NA] Official alternate**
Following letter Z	**Nomina Anatomica term**
SYN Synonym; Cf., compare	**High Profile Term**

re

ing, and tachycardia, in the absence of a clearly identifiable fear stimulus; when chronic, it is called generalized anxiety *disorder*. SEE ALSO panic *attack*. SYN acute stress r.

Arias-Stella r., SYN Arias-Stella *phenomenon*.

arousal r., change in pattern of the brain waves when the subject is suddenly awakened and becomes alert.

Arthus r., (1) SYN Arthus *phenomenon*. **(2)** arthus-type r.'s, r.'s in man and other species that result from the same basic immunologic (allergic) mechanism which evokes, in the rabbit, the typical Arthus phenomenon. SEE ALSO immune complex *disease*.

Ascoli r., a method for confirming the diagnosis of anthrax by means of a precipitin r. which indicates the presence of heat-stable *Bacillus anthracis* antigen in the extracted tissue.

associative r., a secondary or side r.

basic r., SYN alkaline r.

Bence Jones r., the classic means of identifying Bence Jones protein, which precipitates when urine (from patients with this type of proteinuria) is gradually warmed to 45° to 70°C and redissolves as the urine is heated to near boiling; as the specimen cools, the Bence Jones protein precipitates in the indicated range of temperature, and redissolves as the temperature of the specimen becomes less than 30° to 35°C.

Berthelot r., the r. of ammonia with phenol-hypochlorite to give indophenol; the principle is used to analyze ammonia concentration in body fluids.

bi-bi r., a r. catalyzed by a single enzyme in which two substrates and two products are involved; the ping-pong mechanism may be involved in such a r. Cf. mechanism.

Bittorf's r., in cases of renal colic, pain radiating to the kidney upon squeezing the testicle or pressing the ovary.

biuret r., the formation of biuret ($NH_2CONHCONH_2$), which gives a violet color due to the r. of a polypeptide of more than three amino acids with $CuSO_4$ in strongly alkaline solution; dipeptides and amino acids (except histidine, serine, and threonine) do not so react; used for the detection and quantitation of polypeptides, or proteins, in biological fluids.

Bloch's r., SYN dopa r.

Bordet and Gengou r., SEE complement *fixation*.

Brunn r., the increased absorption of water through the skin of the frog when the animal is injected with pituitrin and immersed in water; one of the physiological reactions used to study and classify posterior pituitary polypeptides and their analogues.

Burchard-Liebermann r., a blue-green color produced by acetic anhydride with cholesterol (and other sterols) dissolved in chloroform, when a few drops of concentrated sulfuric acid are added. SEE Liebermann-Burchard *test*.

Cannizzaro's r., formation of an acid and an alcohol by the simultaneous oxidation of one aldehyde molecule and reduction of another; a dismutation: $2RCHO \rightarrow RCOOH + RCH_2OH$; when the aldehydes are not identical, this is referred to as a crossed Cannizzaro reaction.

capsular precipitation r., SYN quellung r. (2).

Carr-Price r., the r. of antimony trichloride with vitamin A to yield a brilliant blue color; this r. forms the basis of several quantitative techniques for the determination of vitamin A.

catalatic r., decomposition of H_2O_2 to O_2 and H_2O, as in the action of catalase; analogous to peroxidase r.

catastrophic r., the disorganized behavior that is the response to a severe shock or threatening situation with which the person cannot cope.

cell-mediated r., immunological r. of the delayed type, involving chiefly T lymphocytes, important in host defense against infection, in autoimmune diseases, and in transplant rejection. SEE ALSO skin *test*.

chain r., a self-perpetuating r. in which a product of one step in the r. itself serves to bring about the next step in the r., and so on. Cf. autocatalysis.

Chantemesse r., a conjunctival r., especially as applied to typhoid.

cholera-red r., a test for cholera vibrio whereby the addition of 3 or 4 drops of sulfuric acid (concentrated, chemically pure) to an 18-hour-old bouillon or peptone culture of the organism produces a color from rose-pink to claret.

chromaffin r., production of a yellow-brown to brown coloration in normal and abnormal cells containing epinephrine and norepinephrine, when fresh tissue slices are placed in a dichromate-chromate mixture overnight; useful for detection of pheochromocytoma (adrenal medulla) and other tumors which produce catecholamines.

circular r., in sensorimotor theory, the tendency of an organism to repeat novel experiences.

cocarde r., cockade r., SEE Römer's *test*.

colloidal gold r., a test (now obsolete) based on precipitation of cerebrospinal fluid protein when mixed with colloidal gold. Abnormalities in this reaction were observed in patients with syphilis, multiple *sclerosis*, poliomyelitis, and encephalitis.

complement-fixation r., SEE complement *fixation*.

consensual r., contraction of the pupil of the fellow eye in consensus with the pupil of the illuminated eye. SYN consensual light reflex, indirect pupillary r.

constitutional r., a generalized r. in contrast to a focal or local r.; in allergy the immediate or delayed response, following the introduction of an allergen, occurring at sites remote from that of injection.

conversion r., SYN conversion *hysteria*.

cross r., a specific r. between an antiserum and an antigen complex other than the antigen complex that evoked the various specific antibodies of the antiserum, due to at least one antigenic determinant that is included among the determinants of the other complex.

cutaneous r., SYN cutireaction.

cutaneous graft versus host r., an acute erythematous maculopapular r. with bulla formation in the most severe cases; chronic changes may resemble lichen planus or scleroderma.

cytotoxic r., an immunologic (allergic) r. in which noncytotropic IgG or IgM antibody combines with specific antigen on cell surfaces; the resulting complex initiates the activation of complement which causes cell lysis or other damage, or which, in the absence of complement, may lead to phagocytosis or may enhance T lymphocyte involvement.

Dale r., SEE Schultz-Dale r.

dark r., in photosynthesis, the fixation of CO_2 into carbohydrate, which is independent in place and time of the absorption of light.

decidual r., the cellular and vascular changes occurring in the endometrium at the time of implantation.

r. of degeneration (DR, R.D.), the electrical r. in a degenerated nerve and the muscles supplied by it; characterized by absence of response to both galvanic and faradic stimulus in the nerve and to faradic stimulus in the muscles; the muscles may still respond to galvanic stimulation, but the cathodal closing contraction is greater than the anodal closing contraction, the reverse of normal.

delayed r., a local or generalized response that begins 24 to 48 hours after exposure to an antigen. SEE cell-mediated r. SYN contact hypersensitivity (2), delayed hypersensitivity (2), late r., tuberculin-type hypersensitivity.

depot r., reddening of the skin at the point where the needle entered, in the subcutaneous tuberculin test.

depressive r., SYN depression.

dermotuberculin r., SYN Pirquet's *test*.

diazo r., the r. of diazotized sulfanilic acid with bilirubin to form azobilirubin, which forms the basis of quantitating the amount of bilirubin in biological fluids. SEE van den Bergh's *test*. SYN Ehrlich's diazo r.

digitonin r., the r. of naturally occurring steroids with 3β-hydroxyl groups with digitonin, a steroid glycoside, resulting in the formation of an insoluble precipitate; useful in determining the presence of cholesterol and ergosterol.

Dische r., the assay of DNA by means of the blue color formed with diphenylamine in acid (Dische reagent).

dissociative r., r. characterized by such dissociative behavior as amnesia, fugues, sleepwalking, and dream states.

dopa r., a dark staining observed in fresh tissue sections to which a solution of dopa has been applied, presumably due to the presence of dopa oxidase in the protoplasm of certain cells. SYN Bloch's r.

dystonic r., a state of abnormal tension or muscle tone, similar to dystonia, produced as a side effect of certain antipsychotic medication; a severe form, where the eyes appear to roll up into the head, is called oculogyric crisis.

early r., SYN immediate r.

echo r., SYN echolalia.

Ehrlich r., SYN aldehyde r.

Ehrlich's benzaldehyde r., a test for urobilinogen in the urine, by dissolving 2 g of dimethyl-*p*-aminobenzaldehyde in 100 ml of 5% hydrochloric acid and adding this reagent to urine; a red color in the cold indicates the presence of an excessive amount of urobilinogen.

Ehrlich's diazo r., SYN diazo r.

eosinopenic r., reduction in the numbers of circulating eosinophils by ACTH or by adrenal corticoids.

erythrophore r., a reddish coloration (nuptial coloration) caused in certain male fishes (bitterling) by the injection of the gonad hormone. SYN fish test.

eye-closure pupil r., a constriction of both pupils when an effort is made to close eyelids forcibly held apart. A variant of the pupil response to near vision. SYN Galassi's pupillary phenomenon, Gifford's reflex, lid-closure r., orbicularis phenomenon, orbicularis pupillary reflex, Piltz sign, Westphal's pupillary reflex, Westphal-Piltz phenomenon.

false-negative r., an erroneous or mistakenly negative response.

false-positive r., an erroneous or mistakenly positive response.

Fenton r., (1) the use of H_2O_2 and ferrous salts (Fenton's reagent) to oxidize α-hydroxy acids to α-keto acids or to convert 1,2-glycols to α-hydroxy aldehydes; **(2)** the formation of OH·, OH⁻, and Fe^{3+} from the nonenzymatic r. of Fe^{2+} with H_2O_2; a r. of importance in the oxidative stress in blood cells and various tissues.

Fernandez r., a delayed hypersensitivity lepromin r., similar to a tuberculin r., at the site of intradermal injection of Dharmendra antigen in a lepromin test.

ferric chloride r. of epinephrine, an intense emerald green color in a neutral or slightly acid solution of epinephrine when ferric chloride is added to it; a r. typical of catechols.

Feulgen r., SEE Feulgen *stain.*

fight or flight r., the theory advanced by Walter Cannon, that in the autonomic nervous system and the effectors connected with it, the organism in situations of danger requiring either fight or flight is provided with a check-and-drive mechanism that puts it in readiness to meet emergencies with undivided energy output. Also known as the emergency *theory.*

first-order r., a r. the rate of which is proportional to the concentration of the single substance undergoing change; radioactive decay is a first-order process, defined by the equation $-(dN/dt){=}kN$, where N is the number of atoms subject to decay (reaction), t is time, and k is the first-order decay (reaction) constant, *i.e.,* the fraction of all atoms decaying per unit of time. SEE ALSO decay *constant,* order.

fixation r., SEE complement *fixation.*

flocculation r., a form of precipitin r. in which precipitation occurs over a narrow range of antigen-antibody ratio, due chiefly to peculiarities of the antibody (precipitin).

focal r., a r. which occurs at the point of entrance of an infecting organism or of an injection, as in the Arthus phenomenon. SYN local r.

Folin's r., the r. of amino acids in alkaline solution with 1,2-naphthoquinone-4-sulfonate (Folin's reagent) to yield a red color; useful for quantitative assay. SYN Folin's reagent.

Forssman r., SYN Forssman antigen-antibody r.

Forssman antigen-antibody r., the combination of Forssman antibody with heterogenetic antigen of the Forssman type, as in the agglutination of sheep erythrocytes (which contain Forssman antigen) by serum from a person with infectious mononucleosis which contains Forssman antibody. SYN Forssman r.

fragment r., a r. used to assay the activity of peptidyl transferase.

Frei-Hoffmann r., SYN Frei *test.*

fright r., after section and degeneration of the facial nerve of an animal, the denervated facial muscles contract if the animal is frightened or becomes angry; due to the release of acetylcholine into the circulation.

fuchsinophil r., the property possessed by certain elements, when stained with acid fuchsin, of retaining the stain when treated with picric acid alcohol.

furfurol r., production of a red color on addition of furfurol to a solution of aniline.

galvanic skin r., SYN galvanic skin *response.*

gel diffusion r.'s, SYN gel diffusion precipitin *tests,* under *test.*

Gell and Coombs r.'s, SEE allergic r.

gemistocytic r., a r. to injury resulting in the proliferation of reactive, protoplastic, or gemistocytic astrocytes.

general adaptation r., SEE general adaptation *syndrome.*

Gerhardt's r., SYN Gerhardt's *test* for acetoacetic acid.

graft versus host r. (GVHR), clinical and histologic changes of graft versus host disease occurring in a specific organ.

group r., a r. with an agglutinin or other antibody that is common (though usually in varying concentrations) to an entire group of related bacteria, *e.g.,* the coli group.

Gruber's r., SYN Widal's r.

Gruber-Widal r., SYN Widal's r.

Günning's r., the formation of iodoform from acetone by iodine and ammonia in alcohol.

Haber-Weiss r., the reaction of superoxide ($O_2^{·-}$ with hydrogen peroxide to produce molecular oxygen (O_2), hydroxide radical (OH·), and OH⁻; often, iron catalyzed; a source of oxidative stress in blood cells and various tissues.

harlequin r., sudden blanching of the lower half of the body of an infant lying on its side, leaving the remaining half of the body the normal pink color.

heel-tap r., SEE heel *tap.*

hemoclastic r., hemolysis as observed in the laking of the blood.

Henle's r., dark brown staining of the medullary cells of the adrenal bodies when treated with the salts of chromium, the cortical cells remaining unstained.

Herxheimer's r., an inflammatory r. in syphilitic tissues (skin, mucous membrane, nervous system, or viscera) induced in certain cases by specific treatment with Salvarsan, mercury, or antibiotics; believed to be due to a rapid release of treponemal antigen with an associated allergic reaction in the patient. SYN Jarisch-Herxheimer r.

Hill r., that portion of the photosynthesis r. that involves the photolysis of water and the liberation of oxygen and does not include carbon dioxide fixation. It involves the addition of oxidants (quinones or ferricyanide) to chloroplasts; upon illumination, O_2 is evolved and the added oxidant is reduced.

homograft r., rejection of an allogenic graft by the host.

hunting r., an unusual r. of digital blood vessels exposed to cold; vasoconstriction is alternated with vasodilation in irregular repeated sequences, in an apparent hunting of equilibrium of skin temperature. SYN hunting phenomenon.

hypersensitivity r., SYN allergic r.

id r., an allergic manifestation of candidiasis, the dermatophytoses, and other mycoses characterized by itching, vesicular lesions that appear in response to circulating antigens at sites that are often far distant from the primary fungal lesion itself. SEE ALSO dermatophytid, -id (1).

r. of identity, SEE gel diffusion precipitin *tests* in two dimensions, under *test.*

immediate r., local or generalized response that begins within a few minutes to about an hour after exposure to an antigen to which the individual has been sensitized. SEE ALSO skin *test,* wheal-and-erythema r. SYN early r.

immediate hypersensitivity r., an immune response mediated by antibody, usually IgE, which occurs within minutes after a second encounter with an antigen, resulting in the release of histamine and subsequent swelling and vasodilation.

immune r., antigen-antibody r. indicating a certain degree of resistance, usually in reference to the 36- to 48-hour reaction in vaccination against smallpox; because the degree of resistance indicated by the r. is not true immunity and may disappear relatively rapidly there is a tendency to refer to the immune r. as an allergic r.

incompatible blood transfusion r., a syndrome due to intravascular hemolysis of transfused blood by serum antibodies of the recipient, which react with an antigen of the donor red cells; characterized by chills, fever (often with urticaria), backache or muscle cramps, hemoglobinemia, hemoglobinuria, and oliguria, which may result in acute renal failure, DIC, and death.

indirect pupillary r., SYN consensual r.

intracutaneous r., intradermal r., a r. following the injection of antigen into the skin of a sensitive subject, such as in the case of the tuberculin test.

iodate r. of epinephrine, a r. dependent upon the oxidation of epinephrine by iodine liberated from iodate, which is decomposed by the hormone; a faint pink color results.

iodine r. of epinephrine, a r. resulting from the oxidation of the hormone, a faint pink color appearing upon the addition of iodine.

irreversible r., a r. or response by the tissues to a pathogenic agent characterized by a permanent pathologic change.

Jaffe r., a bright orange-red complex resulting from the treatment of creatinine with alkaline picrate solution; the basis of most routine creatinine tests.

Jarisch-Herxheimer r., SYN Herxheimer's r.

Jolly's r., rapid loss of response to faradic stimulation of a muscle with the galvanic response and the power of voluntary contraction retained. SYN myasthenic r.

Kiliani-Fischer r., SEE Kiliani-Fischer *synthesis.*

late r., SYN delayed r.

lengthening r., in the decerebrate animal, the rather sudden relaxation with lengthening of the extensor muscles when a limb is passively flexed; associated with clasp-knife spasticity.

lepromin r., a delayed hypersensitivity r. at the site of an intradermal injection of a lepromin, such as the Dharmendra antigen or Mitsuda antigen, in a lepromin test; the r.'s, such as the Fernandez or Mitsuda r., are variable, occurring in 48 hours or three to five weeks, but are uniformly negative in lepromatous leprosy, borderline leprosy, and mid-borderline leprosy.

leukemoid r., SEE leukemoid reaction.

lid-closure r., SYN eye-closure pupil r.

Liebermann-Burchard r., SEE Burchard-Liebermann r.

local r., SYN focal r.

local anesthetic r., a toxic r. due to absorption of local anesthetic drug during regional anesthesia, ranging from drowsiness to convulsions and cardiovascular collapse.

Loewenthal's r., the agglutinative r. in relapsing fever.

Lohmann r., the r. catalyzed by creatine kinase.

magnet r., a r. seen in an animal deprived of its cerebellum; when the animal is placed upon its back and the head strongly flexed, the four limbs become flexed in all their joints. Due to stimulation of receptors in the deep layers of the skin, light pressure made upon a toe-pad with the finger causes reflex contraction of the limb extensors; the limb is thus pressed gently against the finger, and when the finger is withdrawn slightly, the experimenter has the sensation that his finger is raising the limb or drawing it out as by a magnet.

Marchi's r., failure of the myelin sheath of a nerve to blacken when submitted to the action of osmic acid.

Mazzotti r., SYN Mazzotti *test.*

Millon r., the r. of phenolic compounds (*e.g.,* tyrosine in protein) with $Hg(NO_3)_2$ in HNO_3 (and a trace of HNO_2) to give a red color.

miostagmin r., a physiochemical immunity test, designed by Ascoli, consisting in determination of the surface tension of an immune serum to which its specific antigen has been added, before and after incubation at 37°C for 2 hours; in a positive r. the surface tension, as measured by the stalagmometer, is lowered.

Mitsuda r., a delayed hypersensitivity lepromin r., in the form of erythematous papular nodules, at the site of intradermal injection of Mitsuda antigen in a lepromin test.

mixed agglutination r., immune agglutination in which the aggregates contain cells of two different kinds but with common antigenic determinants; when used to identify isoantigens, the test cells are exposed to appropriate isoantibody, washed, and then mixed with indicator erythrocytes that combine with free sites on the test cell-attached isoantibody. SYN mixed agglutination.

mixed lymphocyte culture r., SEE mixed lymphocyte culture *test.*

monomolecular r., a r. involving a single molecule (*e.g.,* decomposition, intramolecular rearrangement, intramolecular oxidation or reduction), even if a catalytic agent, such as acid or alkali, is present in large excess, on a molecular basis, or is not rate-determining; such r.'s are usually first-order r.'s. Cf. molecularity. SYN unimolecular r.

myasthenic r., SYN Jolly's r.

Nadi r., SYN peroxidase r.

near r., the pupillary constriction associated with a near vision effort, *i.e.,* with accommodation and convergence.

Neufeld r., SYN Neufeld capsular *swelling.*

neurotonic r., muscular contraction continuing well after cessation of stimulation.

neutral r., pH of 7.00; H^+ and OH^- ion concentrations equal at 10^{-7} M at 22°C. Cf. dissociation *constant* of water.

ninhydrin r., a test for proteins, peptones, peptides, and amino acids possessing free carboxyl and α-amino groups that is based upon the r. with triketohydrinene hydrate; a blue color r. is used to quantitate free amino acids (*e.g.,* after hydrolysis and separation of the amino acids of a protein). SYN triketohydrindene r.

nitritoid r., a severe r. resembling that following the administration of nitrites, sometimes following intravenous administration of arsphenamine or other drugs; consists of flushing of the face, edema of the tongue and lips, vomiting, profuse sweating, a fall in blood pressure, and sometimes death.

r. of nonidentity, SEE gel diffusion precipitin *tests* in two dimensions, under *test.*

nuclear r., the interaction of two atomic nuclei or of one such with a subatomic particle, or of the subatomic particles within an atomic nucleus, resulting in a change in the nature of the nuclei concerned or in the energy content of the nuclei or both, usually manifested by transmutation (accompanied by emission of alpha-, beta-, or gamma-rays) or by fission or fusion of the nuclei.

oxidase r., (1) the formation of indol blue when a blood smear containing myeloid leukocytes is treated with a mixture of α-naphthol and *p*-dimethylaniline sulfate; the myeloid leukocytes contain an oxidase that catalyzes this r., the lymphoid leukocytes do not; (2) in bacteriology, a r. that depends on the presence of certain oxidases in some bacteria that catalyze the transport of electrons between electron donors in the bacteria and an oxidation reduction dye, such as tetramethyl-*p*-phenylenediamine; the dye is reduced to a blue or black color.

oxidation-reduction r., SEE oxidation-reduction.

pain r., dilation of the pupil or any other involuntary act occurring in response to a stimulus causing sharp pain anywhere.

Pandy's r., a test to determine the presence of proteins (chiefly globulins) in the spinal fluid, by adding one drop of spinal fluid to 1 ml of solution (*e.g.,* carbolic acid crystals in distilled water, cresol, or pyrogallic acid); the r. varies from a faint turbidity to a dense "milky" precipitate according to the degree of protein content. SYN Pandy's test.

r. of partial identity, SEE gel diffusion precipitin *tests* in two dimensions, under *test.*

passive cutaneous anaphylactic r., SEE passive cutaneous *anaphylaxis.*

Paul's r., pus is rubbed into a scarification on a rabbit's eye; if the pus is from a variolous or vaccinal pustule a condition of epitheliosis develops in from 36 to 48 hours; the sputum of a smallpox patient is said to cause the same r. SYN Paul's test.

performic acid r., oxidative destruction of the ethylene double bond (–HC=CH–) which is converted to a Schiff-reactive double aldehyde; used to indicate the presence of unsaturated lipids, such as phospholipids and cerebrosides, as well as cystine-rich substances, such as keratin, in tissue sections.

periosteal r., radiographically detectable new subperiosteal bone formed as a r. to soft tissue or osseous disease.

peroxidase r., formation of indophenol blue by the action of an oxidizing enzyme present in certain cells and tissues when they are treated with a solution of α-naphthol and dimethylparaphenylenediamine; by this method, cells of the myelocyte series, which give a positive r., may be distinguished from those of the lymphocyte series, which give a negative r.; endothelial leukocytes give a variable r., probably positive when they have phagocytized the debris of myeloid cells. SYN Nadi r.

phosphoroclastic r., cleavage of C–C bonds that involves phosphate transfer but not, as in phosphorolysis, directly to one of the products; *e.g.,* the decomposition of pyruvate to acetate + CO_2, in which P_i is added to ADP to form ATP.

Pirquet's r., SYN Pirquet's *test*.

plasmal r., a histochemical technique that uses mercuric chloride to unmask the aldehyde group of acetalphosphatides and permit Schiff staining.

pleural r., thickening of the pleural stripe on chest radiographs, representing pleuritis, pleural effusion, or pleural fibrosis.

polymerase chain r. (PCR) (po-lim′er-ās), an enzymatic method for the repeated copying and amplification of the two strands of DNA of a particular gene sequence. It is widely used in the detection of HIV.

> In vivo, DNA polymerase facilitates the replication of DNA. During replication, a helical DNA molecule "unzips" and the polymerase moves along one strand mediating the addition of free nucleotides to form complementary base pairs with the nucleotides on the strand. The laboratory technique known as polymerase chain reaction exploits the capacity of DNA polymerase to assemble new DNA. The polymerase is added to a mixture of free nucleotides and primers. Primers are specially prepared units containing both RNA and DNA with a free terminus where the polymerase will react. The short sequence of DNA to be amplified is flanked by two primers. Once the reaction begins, the polymerase churns out multiple copies of the target sequence, which can then be recovered for analysis. PCR is used as a forensic tool, one which is more accurate by one or two magnitudes than DNA fingerprinting.

Porter-Silber r., the basis of the 17-hydroxycorticosteroid test; C-21 adrenocorticosteroids, which contain a dihydroxyacetone group at carbons 19, 20, and 21, react with phenylhydrazine.

Prausnitz-Küstner r., a test for the presence of immediate hypersensitivity in humans; test serum from an atopic individual is injected intradermally into a normal subject; the normal subject is challenged 24–48 hours later with the antigen suspected of causing the immediate hypersensitivity r. in the atopic individual. SYN P-K test.

precipitin r., SEE precipitin, precipitin *test*.

primary r., SYN vaccinia.

prozone r., SEE prozone.

psychogalvanic r., psychogalvanic skin r., SYN galvanic skin *response*.

quellung r., (1) SYN Neufeld capsular *swelling*. **(2)** if pneumococcal organisms, India ink, and specific antisera are mixed, the antibodies present in the sera will bind to the polysaccharide antigens of the pneumococcal capsule and the capsule will appear more opaque and swollen. This test will identify the organism as being pneumococci as well as the specific capsular types. SYN capsular precipitation r. [Ger. *Quellung,* swelling]

reversed Prausnitz-Küstner r., the appearance of an urticarial r. at the site of injection when serum containing reaginic antibody is injected into the skin of a person in whom the allergen is already present.

reversible r., a chemical r. that takes place in either direction *i.e.,* from the forward or reverse direction; ionization is such a r., as are r.'s involving racemases, isomerases, mutases, transferases, etc.

Sakaguchi r., guanidines in alkaline solution develop an intense red color when treated with α-naphthol and sodium hypochlorite; a qualitative test for arginine, free or in a protein.

Schardinger r., the reduction of methylene blue to methylene white by formaldehyde is rapidly catalyzed by fresh milk but not by boiled milk, the catalyzing agent being xanthine oxidase (Schardinger's enzyme); an example of oxidation in the absence of O_2 with an organic hydrogen acceptor (the dye).

Schultz r., SEE Schultz *stain*.

Schultz-Charlton r., the specific blanching of a scarlatinal rash at the site of intracutaneous injection of scarlatina antiserum. SYN Schultz-Charlton phenomenon.

Schultz-Dale r., the contraction of an excised intestinal loop (Schultz) or of an excised strip of virginal uterus (Dale) from a sensitized animal (guinea pig) which occurs when the tissue is exposed to the specific antigen.

serum r., SYN serum *sickness*.

shortening r., the adaptive shortening of the extensor muscles of the limb of a decerebrate animal when the limb is extended after it has been flexed. Cf. lengthening r.

Shwartzman r., SYN Shwartzman *phenomenon*.

skin r., SYN skin *test*.

specific r., the phenomena produced by an agent that is identical with or immunologically related to the one that has already caused an alteration in capacity of the tissue to react.

startle r., SYN startle *reflex* (1).

Straus r., a diagnostic test for glanders. Male guinea pigs are inoculated intraperitoneally with suspected material; if the glanders organism is present, it will usually set up a necrotizing inflammation in the scrotal sac within a few days and the specific organism can be confirmed bacteriologically.

stress r., an acute emotional r. related to extreme environmental stress. SYN acute situational r.

supporting r.'s, described by Magnus, who distinguished two types: **positive supporting r.'s,** consisting of those reflex muscular contractions whereby the body is supported against gravity; seen in an exaggerated form in the decerebrate animal; **negative supporting r.'s,** consisting of inhibition of the extensor muscles and unfixing of the joints which thus enable the limb to be flexed and moved into a new position. SYN supporting reflexes.

symptomatic r., an allergic response similar to the original one, but occurring after the use of a test or therapeutic dose of an allergen or atopen.

thermoprecipitin r., the throwing down of a precipitate on the application of heat, as in the case of proteinaceous urine.

***Treponema pallidum* immobilization r.,** SYN Treponema pallidum immobilization *test*.

triketohydrindene r., SYN ninhydrin r.

type III hypersensitivity r., SYN immune complex *disease*.

unimolecular r., SYN monomolecular r.

vaccinoid r., SYN accelerated r.

Voges-Proskauer r., a chemical r. used in testing for the production of acetyl methyl carbinol by various bacteria; potassium hydroxide is added to a 24-hour culture in a suitable medium and thoroughly mixed; the treated culture is exposed to air and is observed at intervals of 2, 12, and 24 hours; a positive r. consists of the development of an eosin-like pink color, due to the production of acetylmethylcarbinol, which in the presence of alkali and oxygen is oxidized to diacetyl.

Wassermann r. (W.r.), SYN Wassermann *test*.

Weidel's r., a r. showing the presence of xanthine; a solution of the suspected substance in chlorine water with a little nitric acid is evaporated in a water bath, and then exposed to the vapor of ammonia; the presence of xanthine is indicated when a red or purple color develops.

Weil-Felix r., SYN Weil-Felix *test*.

Weinberg's r., a complement fixation test of the presence of hydatid disease.

Wernicke's r., in hemianopsia, a r. due to damage of the optic tract, consisting in loss of pupillary constriction when the light is directed to the blind side of the retina; pupillary constriction is maintained when light stimulates the normal side. This sign

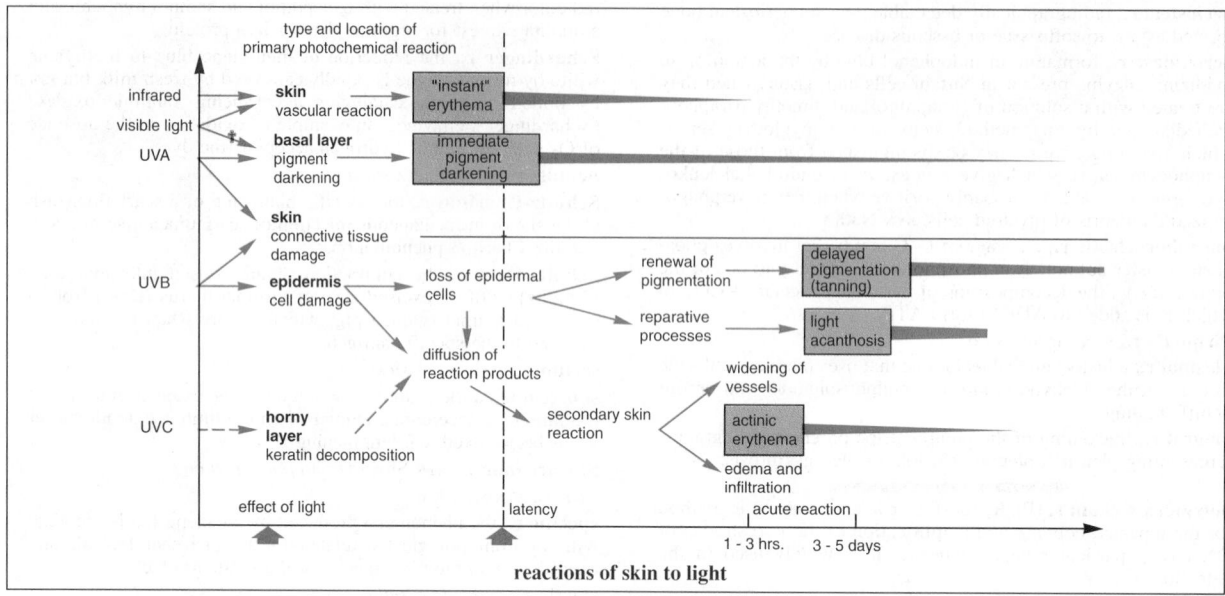

type and location of
primary photochemical reaction

infrared → **skin** vascular reaction → "instant" erythema

visible light
UVA → **basal layer** pigment darkening → immediate pigment darkening

skin connective tissue damage

UVB → **epidermis** cell damage → loss of epidermal cells → renewal of pigmentation → delayed pigmentation (tanning)

reparative processes → light acanthosis

diffusion of reaction products

widening of vessels

UVC → **horny layer** keratin decomposition → secondary skin reaction → actinic erythema

edema and infiltration

effect of light | latency | acute reaction

1 - 3 hrs.   3 - 5 days

reactions of skin to light

cannot be seen with a bright light because of intraocular scatter onto the seeing half of the retina. SYN Wernicke's sign.

wheal-and-erythema r., the characteristic immediate r. observed in the skin test; within 10 to 15 minutes after injection of antigen (allergen), an irregular, blanched, elevated wheal appears, surrounded by an area of erythema (flare). SYN wheal-and-flare r.

wheal-and-flare r., SYN wheal-and-erythema r.

white r., the response seen in many individuals after the skin is lightly stroked with a blunt instrument; it is attributed to capillary action.

whitegraft r., an immune r. to a tissue graft that results in failure of graft vascularization and ensuing rejection.

Widal's r., agglutination r. as applied to the diagnosis of typhoid. SYN Gruber's r., Gruber-Widal r.

xanthoprotein r., a qualitative test for proteins; a yellow product is formed by reacting proteins with hot, concentrated nitric acid.

Yorke's autolytic r., a test for paroxysmal hemoglobinuria; serum is placed in an ice chest and kept at 0°C for 5 to 7 minutes, then in an incubator at 37°C with erythrocytes for 1 hour, at which time, if the r. is positive, hemolysis occurs; if the serum is kept at 1°C for an hour and then placed in the incubator with erythrocytes there is little hemolysis.

zero-order r., a r. that proceeds at a particular rate independently of the concentration of the reactant or reactants.

Zimmermann r., a chemical r. between an alkaline solution of *meta*-dinitrobenzene and an active methylene group (carbon-16) of 17-ketosteroids; it is the basis of the 17-ketosteroid assay t.; more generally, a r. between methylene ketones and aromatic polynitro compounds in alkaline solutions. SYN Zimmermann test.

re·ac·ti·vate (rē-ak′ti-vāt). **1.** To render active again. **2.** In particular, of an inactivated immune serum to which normal serum (complement) is added.

re·ac·ti·va·tion (rē′ak-ti-vā′shŭn). **1.** Restoration of the lytic activity of an inactivated serum by means of the addition of complement. **2.** Restoration of activity in an inactivated enzyme.

re·ac·tiv·i·ty (rē-ak-tiv′i-tē). **1.** The property of reacting, chemically or in any other sense. **2.** The process of reacting.

read·ing frame. the grouping of nucleotides by threes into codons. SEE frame-shift *mutation.*

blocked r. f., a sequence of DNA that cannot be translated into a viable protein; usually due to the interruption by one or more termination codons. SYN closed r. f.

closed r. f., SYN blocked r. f.

open r. f., a gene presumed to code for a protein but for which no gene product has been identified; also known as unidentified r. f. SYN unidentified r. f.

unidentified r. f. (URF), SYN open r. f.

read·through (rēd′thrū). In molecular biology, transcription of a nucleic acid sequence beyond its normal termination sequence.

re·a·gent (rē-ā′jent). Any substance added to a solution of another substance to participate in a chemical reaction. [Mod. L. *reagens*]

amino acid r., a r. used in the identification and quantification of amino acids.

Benedict-Hopkins-Cole r., magnesium glyoxalate, made from a mixture of oxalic acid and magnesium, used for testing proteins for the presence of tryptophan.

biuret r., an alkaline solution of copper sulfate.

Cleland's r., SYN dithiothreitol.

diazo r., two solutions, one of sodium nitrite, the other of acidified sulfanilic acid, used in bringing about diazotization. SYN Ehrlich's diazo r.

Dische r., SEE Dische *reaction.*

Dische-Schwarz r., r. used in the colorimetric detection of RNA.

Drabkin's r., a solution used in the cyanmethemoglobin method of measuring hemoglobin. It consists of sodium bicarbonate, potassium cyanide, and potassium ferricyanide.

Dragendorff r., a r. used in the detection of alkaloids.

Edlefsen's r., an alkaline permanganate solution used in the determination of sugar in the urine.

Edman's r., SYN phenylisothiocyanate.

Ehrlich's diazo r., SYN diazo r.

Erdmann's r., a mixture of sulfuric and nitric acids, used in testing alkaloids.

Esbach's r., picric acid, citric acid, and water (in the proportions 1, 2, and 97) used for the detection of albumin in the urine.

Exton r., 50 g sulfosalicylic acid and 200g $Na_2SO_4 \cdot 10H_2O$ in a liter of water, used as a test for albumin.

Fehling's r., SYN Fehling's *solution.*

Folin's r., SYN Folin's *reaction.*

Fouchet's r., a 25% solution of trichloroacetic acid, containing 0.9% ferric chloride; a drop of the r. added at the surface line of barium chloride-impregnated filter paper which has been dipped in urine for 10 sec will give a green color if bilirubin is present. SEE ALSO Fouchet's *stain.*

Froehde's r., sodium molybdate 1, in strong sulfuric acid 1000; gives various color reactions with alkaloids.

Frohn's r., bismuth subnitrate (1.5) and water (20.0) heated to boiling, to which hydrochloric acid (10.0) and potassium iodide (7.0) are added; used to test for alkaloids and for sugar.

Girard's r., the hydrazine of betaine chloride, used to extract ketonic steroids by forming water-soluble hydrazones with them.

Günzberg's r., phloroglucin and vanillin used as a r. in Günzberg's test.

Hahn's oxine r., an alcoholic solution of 8-hydroxyquinoline used in the determination of zinc, aluminum, magnesium, etc.

Hammarsten's r., a mixture of 1 part 25% solution of nitric acid and 19 parts 25% solution of hydrochloric acid; the addition of a few drops to a mixture of 1 part of this r. and 4 parts alcohol will give a green color if bile is present.

Ilosvay r., sulfanilic acid 0.5, dissolved in dilute acetic acid 150, mixed with naphthylamine 1, and dissolved in boiling water 20; the blue sediment which forms is dissolved in dilute acetic acid 150; a few drops of this r. added to water, saliva, or other fluid to be tested will produce a red color if nitrites are present.

Kasten's fluorescent Schiff r.'s, fluorescent analogues of Schiff's r. which are fluorescent basic dyes lacking acidic side groups and containing one or more primary amine groups; used in cytochemical detection of DNA in Kasten's fluorescent Feulgen stain, polysaccharides in Kasten's fluorescent PAS stain, and proteins in the ninhydrin-Schiff stain; such analogues include acriflavine, auramine O, and flavophosphine N.

Lloyd's r., precipitated aluminum silicate, used in the determination of alkaloids.

Mandelin's r., a solution of ammonium vanadate in sulfuric acid, used in color tests for alkaloids.

Marme's r., a solution of potassium iodide and cadmium iodide used in testing for alkaloids.

Marquis' r., a solution of formaldehyde in sulfuric acid used in color tests for formaldehyde.

Mecke's r., a solution of selenous acid in sulfuric acid, used for color tests of alkaloids.

Meyer's r., a solution of phenolphthalein 0.032, in decinormal sodium hydroxide 21, with water (distilled from glass) sufficient to make 100; in the presence of minute traces of blood, the solution becomes purple or blue-red.

Millon's r., mercuric nitrate and nitric acid as used in the Millon reaction.

Nessler's r., a solution of potassium hydroxide, mercuric iodide, and potassium iodide; it yields a yellow color with ammonia (a brown precipitate with larger amounts) that can be used for quantitative assay.

Rosenthaler-Turk r., a solution of potassium arsenate in sulfuric acid used in obtaining color tests for various opium alkaloids.

Sanger's r., SYN fluoro-2,4-dinitrobenzene.

Schaer's r., an alcoholic or aqueous solution of chloral hydrate used as an extraction medium in investigations of alkaloids.

Scheibler's r., a solution of sodium tungstate in phosphoric acid used in tests for alkaloids.

Schiff's r., an aqueous solution of basic fuchsin or pararosaniline which is decolorized by sulfur dioxide, commonly prepared by addition of hydrochloric acid to a dye solution containing a metabisulphite or bisulphite salt; used for aldehydes and in histochemistry to detect polysaccharides, DNA, and proteins. SEE Feulgen *stain,* periodic acid-Schiff *stain,* ninhydrin-Schiff *stain* for proteins.

Scott-Wilson r., an alkaline solution of mercuric cyanide and silver nitrate used in the detection of acetone.

sulfhydryl r., r. that react with thiol groups, particularly those in proteins.

Sulkowitch's r., a r. for the detection of calcium in the urine, consisting of 2.5 g of oxalic acid, 2.5 g of ammonium oxalate, 5 cc of glacial acetic acid, and distilled water to make 150 cc; a milky precipitate of calcium oxalate is formed when the r. is added to urine that contains calcium.

Uffelmann's r., to a 2% solution of phenol in water is added to aqueous ferric chloride until the solution becomes violet in color; this turns lemon yellow in the presence of lactic acid, assumes an opaline tint in butyric acid, and is decolorized by hydrochloric acid.

Wurster's r., filter paper impregnated with tetramethyl-*p*-phenylenediamine, which turns blue in the presence of ozone or hydrogen peroxide.

re·a·gin (rē-ā′jin). **1.** Wolff-Eisner's term for antibody. **2.** Old term for the "Wassermann" antibody; not to be confused with the Prausnitz-Küstner antibody. **3.** Antibodies that mediate immediate hypersensitivity reactions (IgE in humans).

atopic r., SYN Prausnitz-Küstner *antibody.*

re·a·gin·ic (rē-ā-jin′ik). Pertaining to a reagin.

re·al·i·ty (rē-al′i-tē). That which exists objectively and in fact, and can be consensually validated. [L. *res,* thing, fact]

re·al·i·ty aware·ness. The ability to distinguish external objects as being different from oneself.

re·al·i·ty test·ing. See under testing.

ream·er (rē′mer). A rotating finishing or drilling tool used to shape or enlarge a hole. [A.S. *ryman,* to widen]

engine r., an engine-mounted spirally-bladed instrument, used for enlarging the root canals of teeth.

intramedullary r., a rasp used for shaping the intramedullary portion of the metaphysis prior to the insertion of an appliance or a prosthesis.

re·ar·range·ment (rē-a-rānj-ment). A restructuring; *e.g.,* in a molecule.

Amadori rearrangement, a rearrangement that occurs in cross-linking reactions seen in collagen and in protein glycosylations; *e.g.,* conversion of *N*-glycosides of aldoses to *N*-glycosides of the corresponding ketoses.

re·at·tach·ment (rē-ă-tach′ment). New epithelial or connective tissue attachment to the surface of a tooth that was surgically detached and not exposed to oral environment.

Réaumur, René A.F. de, French physicist, 1683–1757. SEE R. *scale.*

re·base (rē′bās). In dentistry, to refit a denture by replacing the denture base material without changing the occlusal relationship of the teeth. SEE ALSO reline.

re·breath·ing (rē-brēdh′ing). Inhalation of part or all of gases previously exhaled.

Rebuck skin win·dow tech·nique. See under technique.

RecA. An *Escherichia coli* protein that specifically recognizes single-stranded DNA and anneals it to a complementary sequence in a duplex which is homologous. This results in the displacement of the original complementary strand of the duplex.

re·cal·ci·fi·ca·tion (rē-kal′si-fi-kā′shŭn). Restoration to the tissues of lost calcium salts.

re·call (rē′kawl). The process of remembering thoughts, words, and actions of a past event in an attempt to recapture actual happenings.

Récamier, Joseph C.A., French gynecologist, 1774–1852. SEE R.'s *operation.*

re·ca·nal·i·za·tion (rē-kan′ăl-i-zā′shŭn). **1.** Restoration of a lumen in a blood vessel following thrombotic occlusion, by organization of the thrombus with formation of new channels. **2.** Spontaneous restoration of the continuity of the lumen of any occluded duct or tube, as with post-vasectomy r.

re

re·ca·pi·tu·la·tion (rē′kă-pit′yū-lā′shŭn). SEE recapitulation *theory.*

re·ceiv·er (rē-sē′ver). In chemistry, a vessel attached to a condenser to receive the product of distillation. [L. *receptor*, fr. *recipio,* to receive]

re·cep·tac·u·lum, pl. **re·cep·tac·u·la** (rē′sep-tak′yū-lŭm, -lă). A receptacle. SYN reservoir. [L. fr. *re-cipio,* pp. *-ceptus,* to receive, fr. *capio,* to take]

r. chy′li, SYN *cisterna* chyli.

r. gan′glii petro′si, SYN petrosal *fossula.*

r. pecquet′i, SYN *cisterna* chyli.

re·cep·tive. Sensitive or responsive to stimulus.

r. field, that part of the retina whose photoreceptors (rods and cones) pertain to a single optic nerve fiber. The response of a neuron to stimulation of its receptive field depends on the type of neuron and the part of the field that is illuminated; an "on-center" neuron is stimulated by light falling at the center of its r. field and inhibited by light falling at the periphery; an "off-center" neuron reacts in exactly the opposite fashion; that is, it is inhibited by light falling at the center of its receptive field. In either case, the net response depends on a complex switching action in the retina. When an entire receptive field is equally illuminated, the response of receptors at the center of the field predominates.

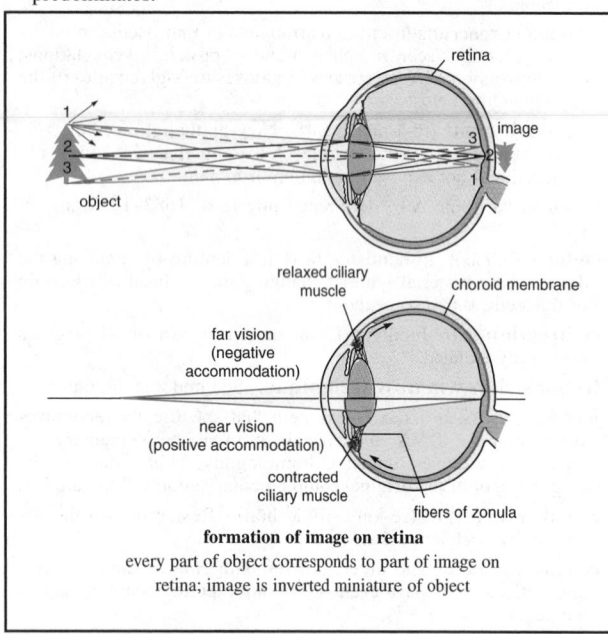

formation of image on retina
every part of object corresponds to part of image on
retina; image is inverted miniature of object

re·cep·to·ma (rē-sep-tō′mă). Obsolete term for chemodectoma.

re·cep·tor (rē-sep′tŏr, tōr). **1.** A structural protein molecule on the cell surface or within the cytoplasm that binds to a specific factor, such as a hormone, antigen, or neurotransmitter. **2.** C. Sherrington's term for any one of the various sensory nerve endings in the skin, deep tissues, viscera, and special sense organs. SYN ceptor. [L. receiver, fr. *recipio,* to receive]

adrenergic r.'s, reactive components of effector tissues, most of which are innervated by adrenergic postganglionic fibers of the sympathetic nervous system. Such r.'s can be activated by norepinephrine and/or epinephrine and by various adrenergic drugs; r. activation results in a change in effector tissue function, such as contraction of arteriolar muscles or relaxation of bronchial muscles; adrenergic r.'s are divided into α-r.'s and β-r.'s, on the basis of their response to various adrenergic activating and blocking agents. SYN adrenoceptor, adrenoreceptors.

α-adrenergic r.'s, adrenergic r.'s in effector tissues capable of selective activation and blockade by drugs; conceptually derived from the ability of certain agents, such as phenoxybenzamine, to block only some adrenergic r.'s and of other agents, such as methoxamine, to activate only the same adrenergic r.'s. Such r.'s

are designated as α-receptors. Their activation results in physiological responses such as increased peripheral vascular resistance, mydriasis, and contraction of pilomotor muscles.

β-adrenergic r.'s, adrenergic r.'s in effector tissues capable of selective activation and blockade by drugs; conceptually derived from the ability of certain agents, such as propranolol, to block only some adrenergic r.'s and of other agents, such as isoproterenol, to activate only the same adrenergic r.'s. Such r.'s are designated as β-receptors. Their activation results in physiological responses such as increases in cardiac rate and force of contraction (β_1), and relaxation of bronchial and vascular smooth muscle (β_2).

β-adrenergic receptors		
---		
the principal effects on organs of various β-receptor subtypes		
	organ	function of receptor
β_1 type	heart	increases heart rate, contractility, speed of conduction
	kidney	increases release of renin
	fatty tissue	increases lipolysis
β_2 type	bronchial passages, blood vessels, uterus	reduces tension of smooth muscle
	pancreas (β cells)	increases release of insulin
	liver, skeletal muscles	increases glycogenolysis
	fatty tissue	increases lipolysis

AMPA r., a type of glutamate r. that participates in excitatory neurotransmission and also binds α-amino-3-hydroxy-5-methyl-4-isoxazole propionic acid and acts as a cation channel. SYN quisqualate r.

ANP r.'s, cell surface r.'s for atrial natriuretic peptide that have a single transmembrane spanning element; these have integral kinase and guanylate cyclase domains.

ANP clearance r.'s, cell surface proteins that bind atrial natriuretic peptide and ANP fragments without initiating biological action.

asialoglycoprotein r., a surface r. found in hepatocytes that binds galactose-terminal glycoproteins; thus, this r. removes those proteins from circulation and they are in turn acted upon by hepatocyte lysosomes.

B cell antigen r.'s, in the primary immune response immunoglobulin D and monomeric immunoglobulin M are the B cell antigen r.'s. On memory B cells, other immunoglobulin molecules can serve as antigen r.'s.

cholinergic r.'s, chemical sites in effector cells or at synapses through which acetylcholine exerts its action.

Fc r., r.'s present on a variety of cells for the Fc fragment of immunoglobulins. These r.'s recognize immunoglobulins of the IgG and IgE class.

kainate r., a type of glutamate r. that participates in excitatory neurotransmission and also binds kainate and acts as a cation channel; injection of kainate causes death of neurons but preserves glial cells and axons.

laminin r., a r. found in many cell types that binds laminin and has a role in cell attachment and neurite outgrowth.

L-AP₄ r., a type of glutamate receptor that also binds a particular synthetic agonist and acts as a cation channel.

low-density lipoprotein r.'s, r.'s on the surface of cells, especially liver cells, which bind to low density lipoprotein and promote clearance of LDL from the plasma.

mannose-6-phosphate r.'s (MPR), r.'s in Golgi apparatus to which newly synthesized proteins that are destined to enter lysosomes bind.

metabotropic r., a type of r. that is linked to intracellular production of 1,2-diacylglycerol and inositol 1,4,5-trisphosphate. [metabolism + G. *tropē*, turning, inclination, + -ic]

muscarinic r.'s, membrane-bound proteins whose extracellular domain contains a recognition site for acetylcholine (ACh); combination of Ach with the r. initiates a physiologic change (slowing of heart rate, increased glandular secretory activity and stimulation of smooth muscle contractions); changes are observed after treatment with the mushroom alkaloid, muscarine. Muscarinic r.'s are to be distinguished from nicotinic r.'s.

nicotinic r.'s, a class of cholinergic r.'s on skeletal muscle cells that are linked to ion channels in the cell membrane.

nicotinic cholinergic r., a class of r.'s responsive to acetylcholine that also are activated by nicotine; ganglionic (including the adrenal medulla) and neuromuscular r.'s. Two classes exist: nicotinic- neuronal and nicotinic-muscular.

NMDA r., a type of glutamate r. that participates in excitatory neurotransmission and also binds *N*-methyl-D-aspartate; may be particularly involved in the cell damage observed in individuals with Huntington's disease.

opiate r.'s, regions of the brain which have the capacity to bind morphine; some, along the aqueduct of Sylvius and in the center median, are in areas related to pain, but others, as in the striatum, are not related.

quisqualate r., SYN AMPA r.

sensory r.'s, peripheral endings of afferent neurons.

stretch r.'s, r.'s that are sensitive to elongation, especially those in Golgi tendon organs and muscle spindles, but also those found in visceral organs such as the stomach, small intestine, and urinary bladder; these r.'s have the function of detecting elongation, and this distinguishes them from baroreceptors, which actually are activated by stretching of the wall of the blood vessel but whose function is to elicit central reflex mechanism reducing the arterial blood pressure.

T cell antigen r.'s, r.'s present on T cells that interact with both processed antigen and major histocompatibility antigens simultaneously.

re·cep·to·somes (rē-sep'tō-sōms). Vesicles that avoid lysosomes and deliver their contents to other intracellular sites.

re·cess (rē'ses). A small hollow or indentation. SYN recessus [NA]. [L. *recessus*]

anterior r., a circumscript deepening of the interpeduncular fossa in the direction of the mamillary bodies. SYN recessus anterior.

anterior r. of tympanic membrane, a slitlike space on the tympanic wall between the anterior malleolar fold and the tympanic membrane. SYN recessus membranae tympani anterior [NA], Tröltsch's pockets, Tröltsch's r.'s.

azygoesophageal r., the region below the azygos vein arch in which the right lung intrudes into the mediastinum between the heart and vertebral column, bordered on the left by the esophagus.

cecal r., SYN retrocecal r.

cerebellopontine r., the angle formed at the junction of cerebellum, pons, and medulla. SYN pontocerebellar r.

cochlear r., a small depression on the inner wall of the vestibule of the labyrinth at the portion of the pyramid of vestibule, between the two limbs into which the vestibular crest divides posteriorly; it is perforated by foramina giving passage to fibers which the cochlear branch of the vestibulocochlear nerve sends to the posterior extremity of the cochlear duct. SYN recessus cochlearis [NA], Reichert's cochlear r.

costodiaphragmatic r., the cleftlike extension of the pleural cavity between the diaphragm and the rib cage; pleural effusions collect here when in the upright position, and since the lung only partially enters, this is the site of thoracocentesis. SYN recessus costodiaphragmaticus [NA], phrenicocostal sinus.

costomediastinal r., the recess of the pleural cavity between the costal cartilages and the mediastinum. SYN recessus costomediastinalis [NA], costomediastinal sinus.

duodenojejunal r., SYN superior duodenal r.

elliptical r., an oval depression in the roof and inner wall of the vestibule of the labyrinth, lodging the utriculus. SYN recessus ellipticus [NA], fovea elliptica, fovea hemielliptica.

epitympanic r., the upper portion of the tympanic cavity above the tympanic membrane; it contains the head of the malleus and the body of the incus. SYN recessus epitympanicus [NA], attic, epitympanic space, epitympanum, Hyrtl's epitympanic r., tympanic attic.

hepatoenteric r., a peritoneal r. at the caudal end of the embryonic pneumatoenteric r.; it separates the developing liver and stomach.

hepatorenal r., the deep recess of the peritoneal cavity on the right side extending upward between the liver in front and the kidney and suprarenal behind; this is a gravity-dependent portion of the peritoneal cavity when in the supine position; fluids draining from the omental bursa drain here. SYN recessus hepatorenalis [NA], hepatorenal pouch, Morison's pouch.

Hyrtl's epitympanic r., SYN epitympanic r.

inferior duodenal r., the variable peritoneal recess which lies behind the inferior duodenal fold and along the ascending part of the duodenum. SYN recessus duodenalis inferior [NA], Gruber-Landzert fossa, inferior duodenal fossa.

inferior ileocecal r., a deep fossa sometimes found between the ileocecal fold, the mesoappendix, and the cecum. SYN recessus ileocecalis inferior [NA].

inferior omental r., a recess of the omental bursa extending between anterior and posterior layers of the great omentum. SYN recessus inferior omentalis [NA].

infundibular r., a funnel-shaped diverticulum leading from the anterior portion of the third ventricle down into the infundibulum of the hypophysis. SYN recessus infundibuli [NA], aditus ad infundibulum.

intersigmoid r., a triangular peritoneal recess behind and below the sigmoid colon created by the attachment of the sigmoid mesocolon ascending across the left psoas then turning sharply to descend into the pelvis; the left ureter (pars tecta ureterica) passes posterior to this recess. SYN recessus intersigmoideus [NA].

Jacquemet's r., a pouch of peritoneum between the gallbladder and the liver.

lateral r. of fourth ventricle, the narrow r. of the ventricle that extends laterally over, and down along the side of, the inferior cerebellar peduncle and the overlying cochlear nuclei; at its tip it opens by way of Luschka's foramen into the interopeduncular cistern of the subarachnoid space. By way of this r., part of the choroid plexus of the fourth ventricle protrudes into the subarachnoid space. SYN recessus lateralis ventriculi quarti [NA].

mesentericoparietal r., SYN parajejunal *fossa*.

optic r., a diverticulum extending forward from the anterior part of the third ventricle above the optic chiasm. SYN recessus opticus [NA].

pancreaticoenteric r., a r. of the embryonic peritoneal cavity that develops into the adult omental bursa.

paracolic r.'s, SYN paracolic *gutters*, under *gutter*.

paraduodenal r., an occasional recess in the peritoneum to the left of the terminal portion of the duodenum located behind a fold containing the inferior mesenteric vein. SYN recessus paraduodenalis [NA], fossa venosa, paraduodenal fossa.

parotid r., SYN parotid *space*.

pharyngeal r., a slitlike depression in the membranous (nonmuscular) pharyngeal wall extending posterior to the opening of the auditory (eustachian) tube. SYN recessus pharyngeus [NA], recessus infundibuliformis, Rosenmüller's fossa, Rosenmüller's r.

phrenicomediastinal r., the recess of the pleural cavity between the diaphragm and the mediastinum. SYN recessus phrenicomediastinalis [NA].

pineal r., a diverticulum from the posterior part of the third ventricle extending back between the posterior commissure and the habenular commissure. SYN recessus pinealis [NA].

piriform r., SYN piriform *fossa*.

pleural r.'s, three recesses of the pleural cavity, one behind the sternum and costal cartilages (costomediastinal r.), one between the diaphragm and chest wall (costodiaphragmatic r.), and one between the diaphragm and mediastinum (phrenicomediastinal r.). SYN recessus pleurales [NA], pleural sinuses.

pneumatoenteric r., pneumoenteric r., a r. of the embryonic celom between the right lung bud and the gut; it is normally largely obliterated before birth, leaving only the superior r. of the vestibule of the lesser peritoneal sac as a vestige.

pontocerebellar r., SYN cerebellopontine r.

posterior r., a deepening of the interpeduncular fossa toward the pons. SYN recessus posterior.

posterior r. of tympanic membrane, a narrow pocket in the tympanic wall between the posterior malleolar fold and the tympanic membrane. SYN recessus membranae tympani posterior [NA], Tröltsch's pockets, Tröltsch's r.'s.

Reichert's cochlear r., SYN cochlear r.

retrocecal r., one of several small pockets sometimes found extending alongside the right margin of the ascending colon near the cecum. SYN recessus retrocecalis [NA], cecal r.

retroduodenal r., a peritoneal recess occasionally found behind the third part of the duodenum, between it and the aorta. SYN recessus retroduodenalis [NA], infraduodenal fossa, retroduodenal fossa.

Rosenmüller's r., SYN pharyngeal r.

sacciform r., (1) an extension of the cavity of the distal radioulnar articulation proximad between the two bones; (2) an extension of the capsule of the elbow joint at the neck of the radius. SYN recessus sacciformis.

sphenoethmoidal r., a small cleftlike pocket of the nasal cavity above the superior concha into which the sphenoid sinuses drain. SYN recessus sphenoethmoidalis [NA].

spherical r., a rounded depression on the inner wall of the vestibule of the labyrinth, lodging the sacculus. SYN recessus sphericus [NA], fovea hemispherica, fovea spherica.

splenic r., the extension of the omental bursa toward the hilum of the spleen. SYN recessus splenicus [NA], recessus lienalis.

subhepatic r., the part of the peritoneal cavity between the visceral surface of the liver and the transverse colon. SYN recessus subhepaticus [NA].

subphrenic r.'s, the recesses in the peritoneal cavity between the anterior part of the liver and the diaphragm, separated into right and left by the falciform ligament. SYN recessus subphrenici [NA], suprahepatic spaces.

subpopliteal r., the extension of the cavity of the knee joint between the tendon of the popliteus and lateral condyle of the femur. SYN recessus subpopliteus [NA], bursa of popliteus.

superior azygoesophageal r., the region above the azygos vein arch in which the right lung is in contact with the esophagus.

superior duodenal r., a peritoneal recess extending upward behind the superior duodenal fold. SYN recessus duodenalis superior [NA], duodenojejunal fossa, duodenojejunal r., Jonnesco's fossa, superior duodenal fossa.

superior ileocecal r., a shallow pouch occasionally existing between the terminal ileum, the cecum, and the ileocolic artery when the latter is present. SYN recessus ileocecalis superior [NA].

superior r. of lesser peritoneal sac, SEE pneumatoenteric r.

superior omental r., a portion of the vestibule of the bursa omentalis that extends upward between the inferior vena cava and the esophagus. SYN recessus superior omentalis [NA].

superior r. of tympanic membrane, a space in the mucous membrane on the inner surface of the tympanic membrane between the flaccid part of the membrane and the neck of the malleus. SYN recessus membranae tympani superior [NA], Prussak's pouch, Prussak's space.

suprapineal r., a variable diverticulum from the posterior portion of the third ventricle of the brain, running backward some distance above and beyond the pineal r. SYN recessus suprapinealis [NA].

supratonsillar r., SYN supratonsillar *fossa*.

triangular r., an occasional evagination of the anterior wall of the third ventricle of the brain between the anterior commissure and the diverging pillars of the fornix. SYN recessus triangularis.

Tröltsch's r.'s, SYN anterior r. of tympanic membrane, posterior r. of tympanic membrane.

tubotympanic r., the dorsal portion of the embryonic first endodermal pharyngeal pouch; it develops into the middle ear cavity.

re·ces·sion (rē-sesh'ŭn). A withdrawal or retreating. SEE ALSO retraction. [L. *recessio* (see recessus)]

clitoral r., operative procedure to reduce the visual prominence of the clitoris that often occurs in females with congenital adrenal hyperplasia; distinct from clitoral amputation (clitorectomy) or clitoral reduction. SEE ALSO clitoroplasty.

gingival r., apical migration of the gingiva along the tooth surface, with exposure of the tooth surface. SYN gingival atrophy, gingival resorption.

tendon r., surgical displacement of the tendon of an eye muscle posterior to its anatomic insertion. SYN curb tenotomy.

re·ces·si·tiv·i·ty (rē'ses-i-tiv'i-tē). The state of being recessive (2).

re·ces·sive (rē-ses'iv). **1.** Drawing away; receding. **2.** In genetics, denoting a trait due to a particular allele that does not manifest itself in the presence of other alleles that generate traits dominant to it.

re·ces·sus, pl. **re·ces·sus** (rē-ses'ŭs) [NA]. SYN recess. [L. a withdrawing, a receding]

r. ante′rior, SYN anterior *recess*.

r. cochlea′ris [NA], SYN cochlear *recess*.

r. costodiaphragmat′icus [NA], SYN costodiaphragmatic *recess*.

r. costomediastina′lis [NA], SYN costomediastinal *recess*.

r. duodena′lis infe′rior [NA], SYN inferior duodenal *recess*.

r. duodena′lis supe′rior [NA], SYN superior duodenal *recess*.

r. ellip′ticus [NA], SYN elliptical *recess*.

r. epitympan′icus [NA], SYN epitympanic *recess*.

r. hepatorena′lis [NA], SYN hepatorenal *recess*.

r. ileoceca′lis infe′rior [NA], SYN inferior ileocecal *recess*.

r. ileoceca′lis supe′rior [NA], SYN superior ileocecal *recess*.

r. infe′rior omenta′lis [NA], SYN inferior omental *recess*.

r. infundib′uli [NA], SYN infundibular *recess*.

r. infundibulifor′mis, SYN pharyngeal *recess*.

r. intersigmoi′deus [NA], SYN intersigmoid *recess*.

r. latera′lis ventric′uli quar′ti [NA], SYN lateral *recess* of fourth ventricle.

r. liena′lis, SYN splenic *recess*.

r. membra′nae tym′pani ante′rior [NA], SYN anterior *recess* of tympanic membrane.

r. membra′nae tym′pani poste′rior [NA], SYN posterior *recess* of tympanic membrane.

r. membra′nae tym′pani supe′rior [NA], SYN superior *recess* of tympanic membrane.

r. op′ticus [NA], SYN optic *recess*.

r. paraduodena′lis [NA], SYN paraduodenal *recess*.

r. parotid′eus, SYN parotid *space*.

r. pharyn′geus [NA], SYN pharyngeal *recess*.

r. phrenicomediastina′lis [NA], SYN phrenicomediastinal *recess*.

r. pinea′lis [NA], SYN pineal *recess*.

r. pirifor′mis [NA], SYN piriform *fossa*.

r. pleura′les [NA], SYN pleural *recesses*, under *recess*.

r. poste′rior, SYN posterior *recess*.

r. retroceca′lis [NA], SYN retrocecal *recess*.

r. retroduodena′lis [NA], SYN retroduodenal *recess*.

r. saccifor′mis, SYN sacciform *recess*.

r. sphenoethmoida′lis [NA], SYN sphenoethmoidal *recess*.

r. spher′icus [NA], SYN spherical *recess*.

r. splenicus [NA], SYN splenic *recess*.

r. subhepat′icus [NA], SYN subhepatic *recess*.

r. subphren′ici [NA], SYN subphrenic *recesses*, under *recess*.

r. subpoplit′eus [NA], SYN subpopliteal *recess.*

r. supe′rior omenta′lis [NA], SYN superior omental *recess.*

r. suprapinea′lis [NA], SYN suprapineal *recess.*

r. triangula′ris, SYN triangular *recess.*

re·cid·i·va·tion (rē-sid-i-vā′shŭn). Relapse of a disease, a symptom, or a behavioral pattern such as an illegal activity for which one was previously imprisoned. [L. *recidivus,* falling back, recurring, fr. *re- cido,* to fall back]

re·cid·i·vism (rē-sid′i-vizm). The tendency of an individual toward recidivation. [L. *recidivus,* recurring]

re·cid·i·vist (rē-sid′i-vist). A person who tends toward recidivation.

rec·i·pe (res′i-pē). **1.** The superscription of a prescription, usually indicated by the sign ℞. **2.** A prescription or formula. [L. imperative *recipio,* to receive]

re·cip·i·ent (rē-sip′ē-ent). One who receives, as in blood transfusion or tissue or organ transplant. [L. *recipiens,* fr. *recipio,* to receive]

re·cip·i·o·mo·tor (rē-sip′ē-ō-mō′ter). Relating to the reception of motor stimuli. [L. *recipio,* to receive, + *motor,* mover]

re·cip·ro·ca·tion (rē-sip-rō-kā′shŭn). In prosthodontics, the means by which one part of an appliance is made to counter the effect created by another part. [L. *reciprocare,* pp. *reciprocatus,* to move back and forth]

Recklinghausen, Friedrich D. von, German histologist and pathologist, 1833–1910. SEE central R.'s disease type II; R. *disease* of bone, *disease* type I, *tumor;* von R. *disease.*

rec·li·na·tion (rek-li-nā′shŭn). Turning the cataractous lens over into the vitreous to displace it from the line of vision; distinguished from couching, in which the lens is simply depressed into the vitreous. [L. *reclino,* pp. *-atus,* to bend back]

rec·ol·lec·tion (rē-kŏ-lek′shŭn). In renal physiology, a technique in which a known fluid is infused into a renal tubule lumen at one point and collected for analysis by a second micropipette further downstream. [re- + L. *collectus,* pp. of *colligo,* to collect]

re·com·bi·nant (rē-kom′bi-nant). **1.** A progeny that has received chromosomal parts from different parental strains as a result of uncorrected crossing over. **2.** Pertaining to or denoting such organisms. **3.** In linkage analysis, the change of coupling phase at two loci during meiosis. If two syntenic, non-allelic genes are inherited from the same parent, they must be in coupling. An offspring that inherits only one of them is r. and indicates an odd number of cross-overs between the loci; an offspring that inherits neither or both is non-recombinant and may indicate an even number of cross-overs or none.

re·com·bi·nant DNA. Altered DNA resulting from the insertion into the chain, by chemical, enzymatic, or biological means, of a sequence (a whole or partial chain of DNA) not originally (biologically) present in that chain.

re·com·bi·na·tion (rē-kom-bi-nā′shŭn). The process of reuniting of parts that had become separated. **2.** The reversal of coupling phase in meiosis as gauged by the resulting phenotype. SEE ALSO recombinant.

genetic r., (1) the presence in progeny of combinations of genotypes and perhaps phenotypes, not present in either parent, resulting from crossing-over; (2) in microbial genetics, the inclusion of a chromosomal part or extrachromosomal element of one microbial strain in the chromosome of another; the interchange of chromosomal parts between different microbial strains.

site specific r., integration of foreign DNA into a particular site in the host genome.

re·con (rē′kon). Obsolete term for the smallest unit (corresponding to a single DNA nucleotide) of recombination or crossing-over between two homologous chromosomes.

re·con·sti·tu·tion (rē′kon-sti-tū′shŭn). **1.** The restitution or return to an original state of a substance, or combination of parts to make a whole. **2.** In the case of a lower organism, the restoration of a part of the body by regeneration.

re·con·struc·tion (rē-cŏn-strŭk′shŭn). The computerized synthesis of one or more two-dimensional images from a series of x-ray projections in computed tomography, or from a large number of measurements in magnetic resonance imaging; several methods are used; the earliest was back-projection, most common is 2D Fourier transformation.

rec·ord (rek′erd). **1.** In medicine, a chronologic written account that includes a patient's initial complaint(s) and medical history, the physician's physical findings, the results of diagnostic tests and procedures, and any therapeutic medications and/or procedures. **2.** In dentistry, a registration of desired jaw relations in a plastic material or on a device to permit these relationships to be transferred to an articulator. [M.E. *recorden,* fr. O.Fr. *recorder,* fr. L. *re-cordor,* to remember, fr. *re-,* back, again, + *cor,* heart]

anesthesia r., a written account of drugs administered, procedures undertaken, and physiologic responses during the course of surgical or obstetrical anesthesia.

face-bow r., a registration utilizing a face-bow of the position of the hinge axis and/or the condyles; the face-bow r. is used to orient the maxillary cast to the opening and closing axis of the articulator.

functional chew-in r., a r. of the natural chewing movements of the mandible made on an occlusion rim by teeth or scribing studs.

hospital r., the medical r. generated during a period of hospitalization, usually including written accounts of consultants' opinions, physician observations, as well as nurses' observations and treatments.

interocclusal r., a r. of the positional relationship of the teeth or jaws to each other, recorded by placing a plastic material which hardens (such as plaster of Paris, wax, etc.) between the occlusal surfaces of the rims or teeth; the hardened material serves as the r.; it may be registered in centric or eccentric positions, as **centric interocclusal r.,** a r. of centric jaw relation; **eccentric interocclusal r.,** a r. of jaw position in other than centric relation; **lateral interocclusal r.,** a r. of a lateral eccentric jaw position; and **protrusive interocclusal r.,** a r. of a protruded eccentric jaw position. SYN checkbite.

maxillomandibular r., (1) a r. of the relation of the mandible to the maxillae; (2) the act of recording the relation of the mandible to the maxillae. SYN biscuit bite, maxillomandibular registration.

medical r., SEE record (1).

occluding centric relation r., a registration of centric relation made at the established occlusal vertical dimension.

preextraction r., SYN preoperative r.

preoperative r., in dentistry, any r. made for the purpose of study or treatment planning. SEE ALSO diagnostic *cast.* SYN preextraction r.

problem-oriented r. (POR), a system of record keeping in which a list of the patient's problems is made and all history, physical findings, laboratory data, etc. pertinent to each problem are placed under that heading; especially useful for out-patient records of patients with multiple problems who are followed for long periods.

profile r., a registration or r. of the profile of a patient.

protrusive r., a registration of a forward position of the mandible with reference to the maxillae.

terminal jaw relation r., a r. of the relationship of the mandible to the maxillae made at the vertical relation of occlusion and at the centric position.

three-dimensional r., a maxillomandibular r. made at the occluding relation.

re·cord·ing (rē-kōrd′ing). Preserving the results of a study.

clinical r., SYN charting.

depth r., study of subcortical cerebral electrical activity after placing electrodes in these areas.

re·cov·er·y (rē-kŏv′er-ē). **1.** A getting back or regaining; recuperation. **2.** Emergence from general anesthesia. **3.** In nuclear magnetic resonance, refers to relaxation. [M.E., fr. O.Fr. *recoverer,* fr. L. *recupero,* to recover, get back, fr. *re-,* again, + *capio,* to take]

creep r., the time-dependent portion of the decrease in strain in a material or object following removal of the stress that has deformed it.

inversion r., a magnetic resonance pulse sequence in which a series of 180° magnetic field inversions is followed by a spin

re

echo sequence for signal detection; of note, during r., the longitudinal magnetization vector passes through zero.

short TI inversion r. (STIR), an inversion r. sequence that uses a short inversion time, about 100 ms., between 180° pulses; by proper selection of TI, the signal from water or fat can be suppressed.

spontaneous r., the return of the conditioned response, after apparent extinction, in the presence of the conditioned stimulus without the unconditioned stimulus also being present. SEE classical *conditioning.*

ultrasonic egg r., obtaining an egg for *in vitro* fertilization by means of an ultrasonically guided needle aspiration of ovarian follicles; may be performed transvesically or via the cul-de-sac.

re·cov·ery room. A hospital facility with special equipment and personnel for the immediate postoperative care of patients as they recover from anesthesia and surgery.

re·cru·des·cence (rē-krū-des′ens). Resumption of a morbid process or its symptoms after a period of remission. [L. *re-crudesco,* to become raw again, break out afresh, fr. *crudus,* raw, harsh]

re·cru·des·cent (rē-krū-des′ent). Becoming active again, relating to a recrudescence.

re·cruit·ment (rē-krūt′ment). **1.** A term used in the testing of hearing: the unequal reaction of the ear to equal steps of increasing intensity, measured in decibels, when such inequality of response results in a greater than normal increment of loudness. **2.** The bringing into activity of additional motor neurons and thus causing greater activity in response to increased duration of the stimulus applied to a given receptor or afferent nerve. SYN recruiting response. SEE ALSO irradiation. **3.** The adding of parallel channels of flow in any system. [Fr. *recrutement,* fr. L. *re-cresco,* pp. *-cretus,* to grow again]

△**rect-.** SEE recto-.

rec·tal (rek′tăl). Relating to the rectum.

rec·tal·gia (rek-tal′jē-ă). SYN proctalgia.

rec·tec·to·my (rek-tek′tō-mē). SYN proctectomy.

rec·ti·fi·er (rek′ti-fī-ĕr). An electronic device for converting alternating to direct voltage, part of the circuit of an x-ray machine. [Mediev.L. *rectifico,* to make right, fr. *rectus,* right + *facio* to make]

rec·ti·fy (rek′ti-fī). **1.** To correct. **2.** To purify or refine by distillation; usually implies repeated distillations. [L. *rectus,* right, straight]

rec·ti·tis (rek-tī′tis). SYN proctitis.

△**recto-, rect-.** The rectum. SEE ALSO procto-. [L. *rectum,* fr. *rectus,* straight]

rec·to·ab·dom·i·nal (rek′tō-ab-dom′i-năl). Relating to the rectum and the abdomen; denoting a bimanual method of examination with one hand on the abdominal wall and a finger of the other hand in the rectum.

rec·to·cele (rek′tō-sēl). SYN proctocele. [recto- + G. *kēlē,* tumor, hernia]

rec·toc·ly·sis (rek-tok′li-sis). SYN proctoclysis.

rec·to·coc·cyg·e·al (rek-tō-kok-sij′ē-ăl). Relating to the rectum and the coccyx.

rec·to·coc·cy·pexy (rek-tō-kok′si-pek-sē). SYN proctococcypexy.

rec·to·co·li·tis (rek′tō-kō-lī′tis). SYN coloproctitis.

rec·to·per·i·ne·al (rek′tō-per-i-nē′ăl). Relating to the rectum and perineum.

rec·to·per·i·ne·or·rha·phy (rek′tō-per-i-nē-ōr′a-fē). SYN proctoperineoplasty. [recto- + perineo- + G. *rhaphē,* a sewing]

rec·to·pexy (rek′tō-pek-sē). SYN proctopexy.

rec·to·pho·bia (rek-tō-fō′bē-ă). SYN proctophobia. [recto- + G. *phobos,* fear]

rec·to·plas·ty (rek′tō-plas-tē). SYN proctoplasty.

rec·tor·rha·phy (rek-tōr′ă-fē). SYN proctorrhaphy.

rec·to·scope (rek′tō-skōp). SYN proctoscope.

rec·tos·co·py (rek-tos′kŏ-pē). SYN proctoscopy.

rec·to·sig·moid (rek′tō-sig′moyd). The rectum and sigmoid colon considered as a unit; the term is also applied to the junction of the sigmoid colon and rectum.

rec·to·ste·no·sis (rek′tō-stĕ-nō′sis). SYN proctostenosis.

rec·tos·to·my (rek-tos′tō-mē). SYN proctostomy.

rec·to·tome (rek′tō-tōm). SYN proctotome.

rec·tot·o·my (rek-tot′ō-mē). SYN proctotomy.

rec·to·u·re·thral (rek-tō-yū-rē′thrăl). Relating to the rectum and the urethra.

rec·to·u·ter·ine (rek-tō-yū′ter-in). Relating to the rectum and the uterus.

rec·to·vag·i·nal (rek-tō-vaj′i-năl). Relating to the rectum and the vagina.

rec·to·ves·i·cal (rek-tō-ves′i-kăl). Relating to the rectum and the bladder.

rec·to·ves·tib·u·lar (rek′tō-ves-tib′yū-lăr). Relating to the rectum and the vestibule of the vagina.

rec·tum, pl. **rec·tums, rec·ta** (rek′tŭm, rek′tă) [NA]. The terminal portion of the digestive tube, extending from the rectosigmoid junction to the anal canal. (Perineal flexure). [L. *rectus,* straight, pp. of *rego,* to make straight]

re·cum·bent (rē-kŭm′bent). Leaning; reclining; lying down. [L. *recumbo,* to lie back, recline, fr. *re-,* back, + *cubo,* to lie]

re·cu·per·ate (rē-kū′per-āt). To undergo recuperation. [L. *recupero* (or *recip-*), pp. *-atus,* to take again, recover]

re·cu·per·a·tion (rē-kū-per-ā′shŭn). Recovery of or restoration to the normal state of health and function. [L. *recuperatio* (see recuperate)]

re·cur·rence (rē-kŭr′ens). **1.** A return of the symptoms, occurring as a phenomenon in the natural history of the disease, as seen in recurrent fever. **2.** SYN relapse. **3.** Appearance of a genetic trait in a genetic relative of a proband. [L. *re-curro,* to run back, recur]

re·cur·rent (rē-kŭr′ent). **1.** In anatomy, turning back on itself. **2.** Denoting symptoms or lesions reappearing after an intermission or remission.

re·cur·va·tion (rē-ker-vā′shŭn). A backward bending or flexure. [L. *re-curvus,* bent back]

red. One of the primary colors, occupying the lower extremity of the spectrum at the other end from violet. For individual red dyes, see specific name. [A.S. *reád*]

Red Cross. A red Geneva cross on a white background, an international sign to identify medical and other personnel caring for the sick and wounded and facilities devoted to their care in times of war, also the emblem of the American Red Cross.

re·dia, pl. **re·di·ae** (rē′dē-ă, -dē-ē). Intramolluscan development stage of a digenetic trematode, following the primary sporocyst stage, which forms after penetration of the snail tissues by the miracidium. Rediae are produced from cells within the sporocyst, are liberated from the latter, and develop in the tissues of the host snail as elongated, saclike, muscular organisms with a mouth and gut. The rediae may produce one or a number of additional generations in the snail, but they ultimately produce the final development stage, the cercaria. SEE ALSO sporocyst (1), miracidium. [F. *Redi,* Italian physician, 1626–1697]

re·dif·fer·en·ti·a·tion (rē-dif′er-en′shē-ā′shŭn). The return to a fully specialized condition for the performance of a particular function after a period of nonspecific activity.

re·din·te·gra·tion (rē′din-tĕ-grā′shŭn). **1.** The restoration of lost or injured parts. **2.** Restoration to health. **3.** The recalling of a whole experience on the basis only of some item or portion of the original stimulus or circumstances of the experience. [L. *red-integro,* pp. *-atus,* to make whole again, renew, fr. *integer,* untouched, entire]

Redlich, Emil, Austrian neurologist, 1866–1930. SEE Obersteiner-R. *line, zone.*

re·dox (red′oks). Contraction of oxidation-reduction. SEE oxidation-reduction *potential.*

re·dresse·ment for·cé (rĕ-dres-mon′ fōr-sā′). Straightening by force of a deformed part, as of knock-knee. [Fr.]

re·dress·ment (rē-dres′ment). **1.** Correction of a deformity; putting a part straight. **2.** A renewed dressing of a wound.

re·duce (rē-dūs′). **1.** To perform reduction (1). **2.** In chemistry, to initiate reduction (2). [L. *re-duco,* to lead back, restore, reduce]

re·duc·i·ble (rē-dūs′i-bl). Capable of being reduced.

re·duc·tant (rē-dŭk′tant). The substance that is oxidized in the course of reduction.

re·duc·tase (rē-dŭk′tās). An enzyme that catalyzes a reduction; since all enzymes catalyze reactions in either direction, any r. can, under the proper conditions, behave as an oxidase and vice versa, hence the term oxidoreductase. For individual r.'s, see the specific names. SYN reducing enzyme.

re·duc·tic ac·id (rē-dŭk′tik). 2,3-Dihydroxy-2-cyclopenten-1-one; a strong reducing product (antioxidant) formed in hot alkaline sugar solutions.

re·duc·tion (rē-dŭk′shŭn). **1.** The restoration, by surgical or manipulative procedures, of a part to its normal anatomical relation. SYN repositioning. **2.** In chemistry, a reaction involving a gain of one or more electrons by a substance, such as when iron passes from the ferric (3+) to the ferrous (2+) state, or when hydrogen is added to the double bond of an organic compound, or when an aldehyde is converted to an alcohol. [L. *reductio,* fr. *re-duco,* pp. *ductus,* to lead back]

r. of chromosomes, the process during meiosis whereby one member of each homologous pair of chromosomes is distributed to a sperm or ovum; the diploid set of chromosomes (46 in humans) is thus reduced to the haploid set in each gamete; union of the sperm and ovum then restores the diploid or somatic number in the one-cell zygote.

closed r. of fractures, r. by manipulation of bone, without incision in the skin.

r. en masse, r. of hernial sac and contents, so that intestinal obstruction is still present.

open r. of fractures, r. by manipulation of bone, after incision in skin and muscle over the site of the fracture.

selective r., a technique for intrauterine termination of one or more fetuses while leaving one or more fetuses undisturbed, usually in pregnancies with fetal anomalies or with multiple gestations.

tuberosity r., the surgical excision of excessive fibrous or bony tissue in the area of the maxillary tuberosity prior to the construction of prosthetic appliances.

re·dun·dan·cy (rē-dun′dăns-ē). Occurrence of linearly arranged, largely identical, repeated sequences of DNA.

terminal r., the condition in a viral chromosome in which identical genetic information occurs at each end of the chromosome.

re·du·pli·ca·tion (rē′dū′pli-kā′shŭn). **1.** A redoubling. **2.** A duplication or doubling, as of the sounds of the heart in certain morbid states or the presence of two instead of a normally single part. **3.** A fold or duplicature. [L. *reduplicatio,* fr. *re-,* again, + *duplico,* to double, fr. *duplex,* two-fold]

re·du·vid, re·du·vi·id (rē-dū′vĭd -vid). A member of the family Reduviidae.

Red·u·vi·i·dae (rē-dū-vī′i-dē). A family (order Hemiptera) of predatory insects, the assassin bugs, which attack animals and humans. It includes the subfamily Triatominae, the kissing or cone-nosed bugs, whose type genus *Triatoma* includes species that are vectors of *Trypanosoma cruzi.*

Reed, Dorothy M., U.S. pathologist, 1874–1964. SEE R. *cells,* under *cell;* R.-Sternberg *cells,* under *cell;* Sternberg-R. *cells,* under *cell.*

Reed, Walter, 1851–1902. U.S. Army surgeon, elucidated epidemiology of yellow fever.

reef·ing (rēf′ing). Surgically reducing the extent of a tissue by folding it and securing with sutures, as in plication.

stomach r., SYN gastroplication.

re·en·act·ment (rē-en-akt′ment). In psychodrama, the acting out of a past experience.

Reenstierna, John, Swedish dermatologist, *1882. SEE Ito-R. *test.*

re·en·try (rē-en′trē). Return of the same impulse into a zone of heart muscle that it has recently activated; sufficiently delayed that the zone is no longer refractory, as seen in most ectopic beats, reciprocal rhythms, and most tachycardias.

Rees, H. Maynard, 20th century U.S. physician. SEE R.-Ecker *fluid.*

Reese, Algernon B., U.S. ophthalmologist, 1896–1981. SEE Cogan-R. *syndrome.*

re·fect (rē-fekt′). To induce refection.

re·fec·tion (rē-fek′shŭn). A restoring to the normal state. [L. *refectio,* fr. *reficere,* to restore, fr. *re-* + *facio,* to do]

Refetoff, S. SEE R. *syndrome.*

re·fine (rē-fīn′). To free from impurities.

re·flect (rē-flekt′). **1.** To bend back. **2.** To throw back, as of radiant energy from a surface. **3.** To meditate; to think over a matter. **4.** To send back a motor impulse in response to a sensory stimulus. [L. *re- flecto,* pp. *-flexus,* to bend back]

re·flec·tion (rē-flek′shŭn). **1.** The act of reflecting. **2.** That which is reflected. **3.** In psychotherapy, a technique in which a patient's statements are repeated, restated, or rephrased in order that the patient will continue to explore and expound on emotionally significant content. [L. *reflexio,* a bending back]

re·flec·tor (rē-flek′ter). Any surface that reflects light, heat, or sound.

REFLEX

re·flex (rē′fleks). **1.** An involuntary reaction in response to a stimulus applied to the periphery and transmitted to the nervous centers in the brain or spinal cord. Most of the deep r.'s listed as subentries are stretch or myotatic r.'s, elicited by striking a tendon or bone, causing stretching, even slight, of the muscle which then contracts as a result of the stimulus applied to its proprioceptors. SEE ALSO phenomenon. **2.** A reflection. **3.** SYN consensual. [L. *reflexus,* pp. of *re-flecto,* to bend back]

the principal reflexes			
type	stimulus	effect	spinal segment
biceps tendon r.	percussion of finger resting on biceps tendon	flexion of elbow joint	C_5–C_6
periosteo-radial r.	tap near distal end of radius	flexion of elbow joint	C_5–C_6
pronator r.	tapping of volar surface of distal radius (with forearm in supination)	pronation of forearm	C_6–C_8
triceps r.	tap on triceps tendon directly over olecranon	extension of elbow joint	C_6–C_8
patellar r.	tap on the patellar tendon	extension of knee joint	L_2–L_4
Achilles r.	tap on the Achilles tendon	plantar flexion of foot	S_1–S_2

abdominal r.'s, contraction of the muscles of the abdominal wall upon stimulation of the skin (superficial a. r.'s) or tapping neighboring bony structures (deep a. r.'s). SYN supraumbilical r. (2).

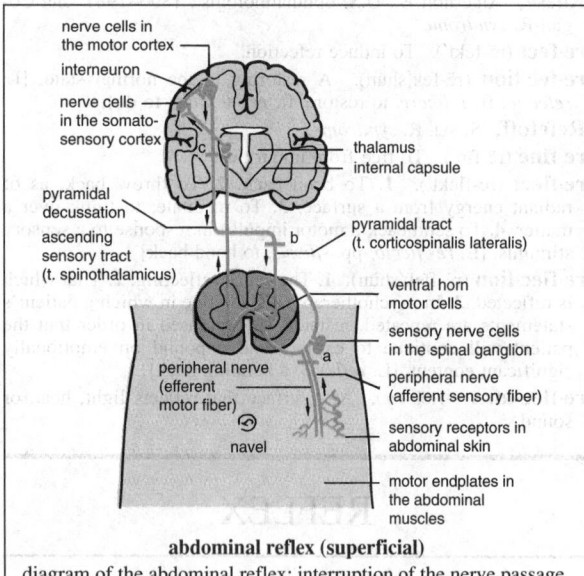

abdominal reflex (superficial)

diagram of the abdominal reflex: interruption of the nerve passage in the peripheral (a) and central (b, c) areas leads to hyporeflexia and areflexia, respectively

abdominocardiac r., mechanical stimulation (usually distention) of abdominal viscera causing changes (usually a slowing) in the heart rate or the occurrence of extrasystoles.

Abrams' heart r., a contraction of the myocardium when the skin of the precordial region is irritated.

accommodation r., increased convexity of the lens, due to contraction of the ciliary muscle and relaxation of the suspensory ligament, to maintain a distinct retinal image.

Achilles r., Achilles tendon r., a contraction of the calf muscles when the tendo calcaneus is sharply struck. SYN ankle jerk, ankle r., tendo Achillis r., triceps surae r.

acousticopalpebral r., SYN cochleopalpebral r.

acquired r., SYN conditioned r.

acromial r., contraction of the biceps muscle caused by a tap on the acromion or the coracoid process.

adductor r., contraction of the adductors of the thigh caused by tapping the tendon of the adductor magnus muscle while the thigh is abducted.

allied r.'s, r.'s which, acting toward a common purpose, can traverse the final common path together.

anal r., contraction of the internal sphincter gripping the finger passed into the rectum.

ankle r., SYN Achilles r.

antagonistic r.'s, r.'s which do not act toward a common purpose, and cannot together traverse the final common path.

aortic r., SYN cardiac depressor r.

aponeurotic r., plantar flexion of the foot and toes elicited by tapping the sole near its outer edge; has the same significance as the Rossolimo toe flexion r. Also called Guillain-Barré, Weingrow's, or sole tap r. SYN Guillain-Barré r., sole tap r., Weingrow's r.

Aschner-Dagnini r., SYN oculocardiac r.

Aschner's r., SYN oculocardiac r.

attitudinal r.'s, SYN statotonic r.'s.

auditory r., any r. occurring in response to a sound, *e.g.,* cochleopalpebral r.

auditory oculogyric r., rotation of the eyes toward the source of a sudden sound.

auricular r., a movement of the ears in animals in response to a sound; part of the investigatory r.

auriculopalpebral r., SYN Kisch's r.

auriculopressor r., peripheral vasoconstriction and a rise in blood pressure in response to a fall in pressure in the great veins. SYN Pavlov's r.

auropalpebral r., SYN cochleopalpebral r.

axon r., an effect brought about by the passage of the nerve impulses from a sensory ending to the effector organ along divisions of the nerve fiber without traversing a synapse, *e.g.,* as in the vasodilation resulting from stimulation of the skin or the irritation of the conjunctiva; the reaction occurs even when the nerve fiber has been sectioned and thus isolated from the nervous centers.

Babinski r., SYN Babinski's *sign* (1).

back of foot r., dorsum of foot r., SYN Mendel's instep r.

Bainbridge r., an increase in heart rate caused by a rise in pressure of the blood in the right atrium due to increased flow and/or pressure in the great veins at its entrance.

Barkman's r., contraction of the ipsilateral rectus muscle in response to a stimulus applied to the skin below a nipple.

basal joint r., opposition and adduction of the thumb with flexion at its metacarpophalangeal joint and extension at its interphalangeal joint, when firm passive flexion of the third, fourth, or fifth finger is made; the r. is present normally but is absent in pyramidal lesions. SYN finger-thumb r., Mayer's r.

Bechterew-Mendel r., percussion of the dorsum of the foot causes flexion of the toes; present in a pyramidal lesion. SYN dorsum pedis r., Mendel-Bechterew r.

behavior r., SYN conditioned r.

Benedek's r., plantar flexion of the foot by tapping the anterior margin of the lower part of the fibula, while the foot is slightly dorsiflexed.

Bezold-Jarisch r., a r. with afferent and efferent pathways in the vagus, originating in unidentified chemoreceptors in the heart and resulting in sinus bradycardia, hypotension, and probable peripheral vasodilation.

biceps r., contraction of the biceps muscle when its tendon is struck.

biceps femoris r., contraction of the biceps femoris upon tapping its lower part, just above its attachment to the head of the fibula, while the limb is partly flexed at hip and knee.

Bing's r., when the foot is passively dorsiflexed, plantar flexion occurs if any point on the ankle between the two malleoli is tapped.

bladder r., SYN micturition r.

body righting r.'s, r. effects upon the neck muscles which bring the head into the correct position in space caused by stimulation of pressoreceptors in the body wall by contact with the ground.

bone r., a r. excited by a stimulus applied to a bone.

brachioradial r., with the arm supinated to 45°, a tap near the lower end of the radius causes contraction of the brachioradial (supinator longus) muscle. SYN radioperiosteal r., styloradial r., supination r., supinator jerk, supinator r., supinator longus r.

Brain's r., SYN quadripedal extensor r.

bregmocardiac r., in infants, pressure upon the anterior fontanelle causing cardiac slowing.

Brissaud's r., tickling the sole causes a contraction of the tensor fasciae latae muscle, even when there is no responsive movement of the toes.

bulbocavernosus r., a sharp contraction of the bulbocavernosus and ischiocavernosus muscles when the glans penis is suddenly compressed or tapped.

bulbomimic r., in a case of coma from severe apoplexy, pressure on the eyeballs causes contraction of the facial muscles of expression on the side opposite to the lesion; if coma due to diabetes, uremia, or other toxic cause the r. is present on both sides. SYN facial r., Mondonesi's r.

Capps' r., obsolete eponym for vasomotor collapse at the time of crisis in pneumonia.

cardiac depressor r., a fall in blood pressure due to peripheral vasodilation and cardiac inhibition by stimulations of the terminations of a cardiac depressor nerve in the aortic arch and base of the heart. SYN aortic r., depressor r.

locations of neuronal cell bodies of the afferent and efferent limbs of representative reflexes

Reflex	Cell of Origin/ Afferent Limb	Cell of Origin/Efferent Limb	Functional Response
Abdominal	Dorsal root ganglia at spinal cord levels T_8–T_{11}	Ventral horn motor neurons at spinal cord levels T_6–T_{11}	Contraction of abdominal muscles with deflection of umbilicus toward stimulus
Achilles (ankle jerk)	Dorsal root ganglia at spinal cord levels L_5–S_1	Ventral horn motor neurons at spinal cord levels L_5–S_1	Contraction of the gastrocnemius and soleus muscles with plantar flexion of foot
Babinski (Babinski sign)	Dorsal root ganglia at spinal cord levels L_5–S_1 (usually only the latter)	Ventral horn motor neurons at spinal cord levels L_4–S_1	Dorsiflexion of the large toe and fanning of the other toes subsequent to a firm stroke on the bottom of the foot; considered indicative of CNS disease after about 14–15 months of age, suggesting damage in the corticospinal system
Carotid sinus	Inferior ganglion of the glosso-pharyngeal nerve	Preganglionic cells in the dorsal motor vagal nucleus, postganglionic cells in ganglia of heart that act on atrial muscle	Regulation of (arterial) blood pressure
Corneal (blink)	Trigeminal ganglion	Facial motor nucleus	Contraction of muscles of the eyelids and closure of the palpebral fissure in response to touching the cornea
Crossed extension	Dorsal root ganglia at about C_7–T_1 (for hand) and L_5–S_1 (for foot)	Contralateral ventral horn cells at about C_5–T_1 (for arm) and L_2–S_1 (for leg)	Extension of the extremity on the side opposite a noxious stimulus to help stabilize the body, works in concert with the withdrawal reflex
Flexor (withdrawal)	Dorsal root ganglia at about C_7–T_1 (for hand) and L_5–S_1 (for foot)	Ipsilateral ventral horn cells at about C_5–T_1 (for arm) and L_2–S_1 (for leg)	Sudden withdrawal of the extremity from a noxious stimulus
Gag	Inferior ganglion of glossopharyngeal and/ or vagus nerves	Bilateral cells in ambiguous nuclei	Constriction of pharyngeal muscles and elevation of the soft palate and uvula
Hoffmann (Hoffmann sign)	Dorsal root ganglia at spinal cord levels C_7–C_8	Ventral horn motor neurons at spinal cord levels C_7–T_1	Brisk flicking of the distal phalanx on the third digit produces a flexion of the thumb and first finger or thumb and all other fingers
Jaw (jaw jerk)	Mesencephalic nucleus of trigeminal nerve	Trigeminal motor nucleus	Bilateral contraction of temporal and masseter muscles in response to a slightly downward tap on the chin
Patellar (knee jerk)	Dorsal root ganglia at spinal cord levels L_2–L_4	Ventral horn motor neurons at spinal cord levels L_2–L_4	Contraction of quadriceps muscle with extension of the leg at the knee
Pupillary (light)	Ganglion cells in retina	Preganglionic cells in Edinger-Westphal nucleus, postganglionic cells in ciliary ganglion	Contraction of the sphincter pupillae muscles and decrease in the size of the pupil in response to light shone in eye; *direct reaction* is contraction of pupil ipsilateral to stimulus, *consensual reaction* is contraction of opposite pupil
Rooting	Trigeminal ganglion	Facial motor nucleus	Pursing of the lips and rotation of the mouth toward the source of the stimulus, elicited by rubbing corner of mouth or cheek, seen in infants during early months
Salivatory	Geniculate ganglion (CN VII) and inferior ganglion of glosso-pharyngeal and (possibly) vagus nerves	Preganglionic cells in superior salivatory nucleus (CN VII) and in inferior salivatory nucleus (CN IX), postganglionic cells in ganglia found in (or on) the sublingual and submandibular glands and the parotid gland	Vasodilation and increased secretions of salivary glands in response to food in oral cavity and consequent stimulation of taste receptors
Snout	Trigeminal ganglion	Facial motor nucleus	Pursing or puckering of the muscles around the mouth in response to a tap to the upper lip, usually considered indicative of damage in the corticospinal system
Swallowing	Inferior ganglia of glossopharyngeal and vagus nerves	Nucleus ambiguus for pharyngeal muscles, preganglionic cells in dorsal motor vagal nucleus and postganglionic cells in myenteric ganglia in the esophagus	Contraction of pharyngeal muscles, wave-like contractions of esophageal muscles, together move food through pharynx and into (and down) esophagus
Vomiting (pharyngeal)	Inferior ganglia of glossopharyngeal and vagus nerves	Nucleus ambiguus for constriction of pharyngeal muscles and closure of epiglottis; dorsal motor vagal nucleus supplies preganglionic fibers to postganglionic cells in esophagus and stomach; intermediolateral cell column at upper thoracic levels supplies preganglionic fibers to post-ganglionic cells in esophagus and stomach and pyloric sphincter; ventral horn motor neurons innervate skeletal muscles of abdominal wall	Vomiting; retrograde movement of stomach contents up the esophagus and into the oral cavity; closure of epiglottis prevents movement of vomitus into lungs, contraction of abdominal muscles assists emptying of stomach; the vomiting reflex is essentially a gag reflex that has spread wider in the neuraxis and influenced a wider range of visceral and somatic centers

☐ reflex related to brainstem and cranial nerves   ☐ reflex related to spinal cord   ▨ reflex with brainstem and spinal components

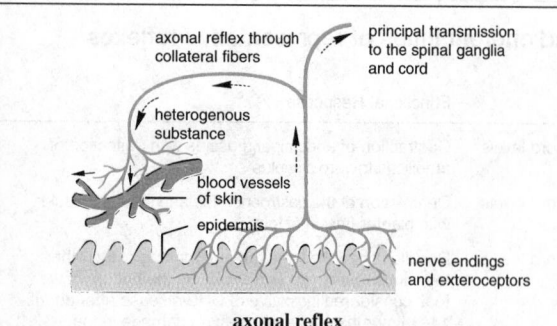

axonal reflex through collateral fibers

principal transmission to the spinal ganglia and cord

heterogenous substance

blood vessels of skin

epidermis

nerve endings and exteroceptors

axonal reflex

impulses from the pain sensors of the skin, in addition to their normal transmission to the spinal ganglion and cord, are transmitted in an antidromic direction to the blood vessels, through collateral fibers

carotid sinus r., a normal r. relating to the carotid sinus *syndrome*, which results from hypersensitivity or hyperactivation of the carotid sinus.

celiac plexus r., arterial hypotension coincident with surgical manipulations in the upper abdomen during general anesthesia.

cephalic r.'s, r.'s associated with the cranial nerves.

cephalopalpebral r., contraction of the orbicularis muscle elicited by tapping the vertex of the skull.

Chaddock r., SYN Chaddock *sign.*

chain r., a series of r.s, each serving as a stimulus for the next.

chin r., SYN jaw r.

Chodzko's r., contractions of several muscles of the shoulder girdle and arm when the manubrium sterni is percussed.

ciliospinal r., SYN pupillary-skin r.

clasping r., the strong flexion of the forelimbs of amphibia and certain other animals during the mating season when the chest or abdomen is stimulated; it is dependent upon the male sex hormone.

cochleo-orbicular r., SYN cochleopalpebral r.

cochleopalpebral r., a form of the wink r. in which there is a contraction, sometimes very slight, of the orbicularis palpebrarum muscle when a sudden noise is made close to the ear; it is absent in labyrinthine disease with total deafness. SYN acoustico-palpebral r., auropalpebral r., cochleo-orbicular r., startle r. (2).

cochleopupillary r., constriction of the pupil in response to a sudden loud sound. The normal response to such a stimulus is pupil dilation.

cochleostapedial r., contraction of the stapedius muscle in response to a loud sound; this is a protective r. which with the r. contraction of the tensor tympani reduces the amplitude of the vibrations of the tympanic membrane and ossicles.

conditioned r. (CR), a r. that is gradually developed by training and association through the frequent repetition of a definite stimulus. SEE conditioning. SYN acquired r., behavior r., trained r.

conjunctival r., closure of the eyes in response to irritation of the conjunctiva.

consensual light r., SYN consensual *reaction.*

contralateral r., SYN Brudzinski's *sign* (1).

convulsive r., an incoordinated r. in which muscles, even those opposing one another as in strychnine poisoning, contract.

coordinated r., a r. in which several muscles take part in the performance of a purposeful act.

corneal r., (1) a contraction of the eyelids when the cornea is lightly touched with a camel-hair pencil; SYN lid r. **(2)** reflection of light from the surface of the cornea.

costal arch r., contraction of the rectus abdominis muscle by tapping the costal margin inside the mammary line.

costopectoral r., SYN pectoral r.

cough r., the r. which mediates coughing in response to irritation of the larynx or tracheobronchial tree. SYN laryngeal r.

craniocardiac r., stimulation of nerve endings of certain cranial

nerves (*e.g.,* olfactory, ophthalmic branch of trigeminal), with resultant cardiac depressor r., manifested by bradycardia and hypotension, through the cardiac branch of the vagus.

cremasteric r., a drawing up of the scrotum and testicle of the same side when the skin over Scarpa's triangle or on the inner side of the thigh is scratched.

crossed r., a r. movement on one side of the body in response to a stimulus applied to the opposite side. SYN crossed jerk.

crossed adductor r., contraction of the adductors of the thigh and inward rotation of the limb elicited by tapping the sole. SYN crossed adductor jerk.

crossed extension r., extension of the contralateral hind limb when the paw of an animal is painfully stimulated or the central cut end of an afferent nerve, *e.g.,* the peroneal, is stimulated; sometimes occurs in humans upon tapping the skin.

crossed knee r., contraction of the contralateral quadriceps when a patellar r. is elicited. SYN crossed knee jerk.

crossed r. of pelvis, contraction of the contralateral adductors of the thigh upon tapping the anterior superior iliac spine. SYN crossed spino-adductor r.

crossed spino-adductor r., SYN crossed r. of pelvis.

cry r., a sudden unconscious cry, during sleep, in a child with hip disease, long bone fractures, or other painful conditions of the extremities, elicited by movement of muscles that have relaxed after prolonged muscle spasms.

cuboidodigital r., flexion of the toes on tapping over the cuboid bone; almost identical with Guillain-Barré r., and fundamentally similar to Rossolimo's r. SYN metatarsal r.

cutaneous r., wrinkling of the skin, caused by a cutaneous stimulus, due to contraction of arrectores pilorum muscles.

cutaneous pupil r., cutaneous-pupillary r., SYN pupillary-skin r.

darwinian r., the tendency of young infants to grasp a bar and hang suspended. Cf. grasping r.

deep r., an involuntary muscular contraction following percussion of a tendon or bone. SYN jerk (2).

deep abdominal r.'s, contraction of abdominal muscles elicited by stimulation, such as tapping a deep structure; *e.g.,* the costal margin. SEE ALSO Galant's r., upper abdominal periosteal r.

defense r., (1) SYN flexor r. **(2)** automatic reactions of an animal, *e.g.,* raising of hair or feathers, dilation of the pupils, or baring of claws, when alarmed.

deglutition r., SYN swallowing r.

Dejerine's r., SYN Dejerine's hand *phenomenon.*

delayed r., a r. in which a little time elapses between stimulus and response. SEE ALSO trace conditioned r.

depressor r., SYN cardiac depressor r.

diffused r., one of several r.'s occurring in association with the main r.

digital r., SYN Hoffmann's *sign* (2).

diving r., a r. by which immersing the face or body in water, especially cold water, tends to cause bradycardia and peripheral vasoconstriction; mean aortic pressure is little affected because the reduction in cardiac output tends to balance the increased peripheral resistance that reduces peripheral blood flow. Although relatively minor in most humans, the changes can be profound in some diving species of animal, *e.g.,* ducks and seals.

dorsal r., contraction of the muscles of the back elicited by cutaneous stimulation over the erector spinal muscle.

dorsum pedis r., SYN Bechterew-Mendel r.

elbow r., SYN triceps r.

enterogastric r., peristaltic contraction of the small intestine induced by the entrance of food into the stomach. SEE ALSO gastrocolic r.

epigastric r., a contraction of the upper portion of the rectus abdominis muscle when the skin of the epigastrium above is scratched. SYN supraumbilical r. (1).

erector-spinal r., a contraction of part of the erector spinae muscle following scratching of the skin on its outer border.

esophagosalivary r., salivation caused by irritation of the lower end of the esophagus, as by carcinoma. SYN Roger's r.

external oblique r., contraction of the external oblique and rectus abdominis muscles upon tapping the anterior and outer part of the lower thoracic wall.

eye r., SYN light r. (2).

eyeball compression r., SYN eyeball-heart r.

eyeball-heart r., slowing of the heart rate due to the vagal effects of compressing an eyeball. SYN eyeball compression r.

eye-closure r., SYN wink r.

facial r., SYN bulbomimic r.

faucial r., SYN gag r.

femoral r., scratching the skin of the upper part of the front of the thigh causes extension of the knee and flexion of the foot.

femoroabdominal r., contraction of the abdominal muscles upon stroking the inner aspect of the thigh; in association with the cremasteric r. SYN hypogastric r.

finger-thumb r., SYN basal joint r.

flexor r., flexion of ankle, knee, and hip when the foot is painfully stimulated; the crossed extension r. occurs in association with it. SYN defense r. (1), nociceptive r., withdrawal r.

forced grasping r., SYN grasping r.

front-tap r., contraction of the gastrocnemius muscle when the shin is struck. SYN periosteal r. (1).

fundus r., SYN light r. (2).

gag r., contact of a foreign body with the mucous membrane of the fauces causes retching or gagging. SYN faucial r.

Galant's r., a deep abdominal r. in which there is a contraction of the abdominal muscles on tapping the anterior superior iliac spine. SYN lower abdominal periosteal r.

galvanic skin r., SYN galvanic skin *response*.

gastrocolic r., a mass movement of the contents of the colon, frequently preceded by a similar movement in the small intestine, that sometimes occurs immediately following the entrance of food into the stomach.

gastroileac r., opening of the ileocolic valve induced by entrance of food into the stomach.

Geigel's r., in the female, a contraction of the muscular fibers at the upper edge of Poupart's ligament on gently stroking the inner side of the thigh; analogue of the cremasteric r. in males.

Gifford's r., SYN eye-closure pupil *reaction*.

gluteal r., contraction of the gluteal muscles following irritation of the skin of the buttocks.

Gordon r., dorsal flexion of the great toe produced by firm lateral pressure on the calf muscles. SYN paradoxical flexor r.

grasp r., SYN grasping r.

grasping r., an involuntary flexion of the fingers to tactile or tendon stimulation on the palm of the hand, producing an uncontrollable grasp; usually associated with frontal lobe lesions. Cf. darwinian r. SYN forced grasping r., grasp r.

great-toe r., SYN Babinski's *sign* (1).

Guillain-Barré r., SYN aponeurotic r.

gustatory-sudorific r., sweating, especially over the face, when chewing food. SEE ALSO auriculotemporal nerve *syndrome*.

H r., a monosynaptic r. consistently obtained in normal adults only by stimulating the tibial nerve, generally in the popliteal fossa, while recording from the gastrocnemius-soleus muscle group; similar to the Achilles r., except the neuromuscular spindles are bypassed; widely used in the EMG laboratory to diagnose S1 radiculopathies and polyneuropathies.

hepatojugular r., SEE hepatojugular *reflux*.

Hering-Breuer r., the effects of afferent impulses from the pulmonary vagi in the control of respiration, *e.g.,* inflation of the lungs arrests inspiration with expiration then ensuing, while deflation of the lungs brings on inspiration.

Hoffmann's r., SYN Hoffmann's *sign* (2).

hypochondrial r., a quick inspiration induced by sharp pressure beneath the costal margin.

hypogastric r., SYN femoroabdominal r.

inborn r., a r. such as breathing that is innate.

innate r., an unlearned or instinctive r. such as sucking, which is present at birth.

interscapular r., SYN scapular r.

intrinsic r., a r. muscular contraction elicited by the application

of a stimulus, usually stretching, to the muscle itself as opposed to a muscular contraction caused by an extrinsic stimulus, *e.g.,* skin, as in the abdominal skin r.'s.

inverted r., SYN paradoxical r.

inverted radial r., flexion of the fingers without flexion of the forearm, on tapping the lower end of the radius; regarded as indicating a lesion of the fifth cervical segment of the spinal cord.

investigatory r., SYN orienting r.

ipsilateral r., a r. in which the response occurs on the side of the body that is stimulated.

Jacobson's r., flexion of the fingers elicited by tapping the flexor tendons over the wrist joint or the lower end of the radius.

jaw r., a spasmodic contraction of the temporal muscles following a downward tap on the loosely hanging mandible. SYN chin jerk, chin r., jaw jerk, mandibular r., masseter r.

jaw-working r., SYN jaw-winking *syndrome*.

Joffroy's r., twitching of the glutei muscles when firm pressure is made on the nates, in cases of spastic paralysis. SYN hip phenomenon.

Kisch's r., closure of the eye in response to stimulation of the skin at the depth of the external auditory meatus. SYN auriculo-palpebral r.

knee r., SYN patellar r.

knee-jerk r., SYN patellar r.

labyrinthine r.'s, r.'s initiated through stimulation of receptors in the utricle or semicircular canals. SEE ALSO statotonic r.'s, statokinetic r., righting r.'s.

labyrinthine righting r.'s, stimulation of the proprioceptors of the labyrinth causes changes in tone of the neck muscles which bring the head into its natural position in space.

lacrimal r., discharge of tears when the conjunctiva is irritated.

lacrimo-gustatory r., chewing of food causing secretion of tears. SEE ALSO crocodile tears *syndrome*.

laryngeal r., SYN cough r.

laryngospastic r., SYN laryngospasm.

latent r., a r. which must be considered normal but which usually appears only under some pathologic circumstance that lowers its threshold.

laughter r., uncontrollable laughter excited by tickling.

let-down r., SYN milk-ejection r.

lid r., SYN corneal r. (1).

Liddell-Sherrington r., SYN myotatic r.

light r., (1) SYN pupillary r. **(2)** a red glow reflected from the fundus of the eye when a light is cast upon the retina, as in retinoscopy; SYN eye r., fundus r. **(3)** SYN *pyramid* of light.

lip r., a pouting movement of the lips provoked in young infants by tapping near the angle of the mouth.

lordosis r., adoption of a copulatory posture when touched on the back; exhibited by female animals of certain species but only during the time of estrus.

Lovén r., a reaction in which a local dilation of vessels accompanies a general vasoconstriction; *e.g.,* when the central end of an afferent nerve to an organ is suitably stimulated, its efferent vasomotor fibers remaining intact, a general rise in blood pressure occurs together with a dilation of the vessels of the organ.

lower abdominal periosteal r., SYN Galant's r.

magnet r., SEE magnet *reaction*.

mandibular r., SYN jaw r.

mass r., in cases of gross injury to the spinal cord, as the stage of r. activity follows the primary flaccidity of the shock, a condition arises in which a strong stimulus to any part of one of the paralyzed limbs will be followed by contraction of the hip, knee, and ankle of the same side and often, when the stimulus is applied to the middle line of the body, of both sides, as well as of the abdominal wall, and even evacuation of the bladder and sweating over an area corresponding to the level of the lesion.

masseter r., SYN jaw r.

Mayer's r., SYN basal joint r.

McCarthy's r.'s, (1) SYN spino-adductor r. **(2)** SYN supraorbital r.

mediopubic r., contraction of the adductors of the thigh upon tapping the pubic bone near the symphysis.

Mendel-Bechterew r., SYN Bechterew-Mendel r.

Mendel's instep r., the foot being firmly supported on its inner side, a sharp tap on the dorsal tendons causes extension of the second to the fifth toes. SYN back of foot r., dorsum of foot r.

metacarpohypothenar r., flexion of the little finger on tapping the dorsum of the hand; seen in pyramidal tract lesions and is similar to Starling's r.

metacarpothenar r., SYN thumb r.

metatarsal r., SYN cuboidodigital r.

micturition r., contraction of the walls of the bladder and relaxation of the trigone and urethral sphincter in response to a rise in pressure within the bladder; the r. can be voluntarily inhibited and the inhibition readily abolished to control micturition. SYN bladder r., urinary r., vesical r.

milk-ejection r., release of milk from the breast following tactile stimulation of the nipple; the afferent path is postulated to exist from the nipple to the hypothalamus; the efferent limb is represented by the neurohypophysial release of oxytocin into the systemic circulation; contraction of myoepithelial elements within the breast, caused by oxytocin, moves milk into the collecting ducts and toward the nipple. SYN let-down r., milk let-down r.

milk let-down r., SYN milk-ejection r.

Mondonesi's r., SYN bulbomimic r.

Moro r., SYN startle r. (1).

muscular r., SYN myotatic r.

myenteric r., contraction above and relaxation below a stimulated point in the intestine. SYN law of intestine.

myotatic r., tonic contraction of the muscles in response to a stretching force, due to stimulation of muscle proprioceptors. SYN Liddell-Sherrington r., muscular r., stretch r.

nasal r., sneezing caused by irritation of the nasal mucous membrane.

nasomental r., contraction of the mentalis muscle following a tap on the side of the nose.

near r., pupillary constriction with a near vision effort, with ocular convergence, or with accommodation; an associated reaction, not a true r.

neck r.'s, changes in position of the head cause alterations in tone of the neck muscles through stimulation of proprioceptors in the labyrinth which bring the head into its correct position in space; stimulation of proprioceptors in the neck muscles causes in turn r. movements of the limbs which bring the animal into the normal position in relation to the head.

nociceptive r., SYN flexor r.

nocifensor r., vascular dilation in a part surrounding an injury or in its neighborhood.

nose-bridge-lid r., SYN orbicularis oculi r.

nose-eye r., SYN orbicularis oculi r.

oculocardiac r., a decrease in pulse rate associated with traction on extraocular muscles or compression of the eyeball; especially sensitive in children; may produce asystolic cardiac arrest. SYN Aschner's phenomenon, Aschner's r., Aschner-Dagnini r., oculovagal r.

oculocephalic r., SYN oculocephalogyric r.

oculocephalogyric r., turning of the eyes and head toward the source of an auditory, visual, or other form of stimulation. SYN oculocephalic r.

oculovagal r., SYN oculocardiac r.

olecranon r., flexion of the forearm caused by tapping the olecranon. SYN paradoxical triceps r.

Oppenheim's r., extension of the toes induced by scratching of the inner side of the leg or by following sudden flexion of the thigh on the abdomen and the leg on the thigh; a sign of cerebral irritation.

optical righting r.'s, visual stimuli that enable an animal to maintain the correct position of the head in space, by bringing about movements of the muscles of the neck and limbs.

orbicularis oculi r., contraction of the orbicularis oculi muscles upon tapping the margin of the orbit, or the bridge or tip of the nose. SYN nose-bridge-lid r., nose-eye r.

orbicularis pupillary r., SYN eye-closure pupil *reaction.*

orienting r., an aspect of attending in which an organism's initial response to a change or to a novel stimulus is such that the organism becomes more sensitive to the stimulation; *e.g.,* dilation of the pupil of the eye in response to dim light. SYN investigatory r., orienting response.

palatal r., palatine r., swallowing r. induced by stimulation of the palate.

palmar r., flexion of the fingers following tickling of the palm.

palm-chin r., SYN palmomental r.

palmomental r., unilateral (sometimes bilateral) contraction of the mentalis and orbicularis oris muscles caused by a brisk scratch made on the palm of the ipsilateral hand. SYN palm-chin r.

parachute r., SYN startle r. (1).

paradoxical r., any r. in which the usual response is reversed or does not conform to the pattern characteristic of the particular r. SYN inverted r.

paradoxical extensor r., SYN Babinski's *sign* (1).

paradoxical flexor r., SYN Gordon r.

paradoxical patellar r., (1) a tap on the patellar tendon causes contraction of the adductor; (2) sudden passive extension of the leg causes a contraction of the extensor muscles of the leg.

paradoxical pupillary r., a pupillary response to light, the reverse of that expected; *e.g.,* contraction of the pupil in response to turning the lights off. SYN Flynn phenomenon, paradoxical pupillary phenomenon.

paradoxical triceps r., SYN olecranon r.

patellar r., a sudden contraction of the anterior muscles of the thigh, caused by a smart tap on the patellar tendon while the leg hangs loosely at a right angle with the thigh. SYN knee jerk, knee phenomenon, knee r., knee-jerk r., patellar tendon r., quadriceps r.

patellar tendon r., SYN patellar r.

patello-adductor r., crossed adduction of the leg on tapping the quadriceps tendon.

Pavlov's r., SYN auriculopressor r.

pectoral r., contraction of the pectoralis major muscle elicited by tapping the seventh rib between the anterior and the medial axillary lines while the arm is abducted; contraction of the deltoid and biceps may also occur. SYN costopectoral r.

Perez r., running a finger down the spine of an infant held supported in a prone position will normally cause the whole body to become extended.

pericardial r., a vagal r. seen during operations involving pericardial manipulation; characterized by signs of vagal stimulation (bradycardia and arterial hypotension).

periosteal r., (1) SYN front-tap r. (2) a muscular contraction in the arm following a tap on the radius or ulna.

pharyngeal r., (1) SYN swallowing r. (2) SYN vomiting r.

phasic r., a coordinated complex response such as the scratch r. in the spinal animal.

Phillipson's r., a contraction of the extensors of the knee when the extensors of the opposite knee are inhibited.

pilomotor r., contraction of the smooth muscle of the skin resulting in "gooseflesh" caused by mild application of a tactile stimulus or by local cooling.

plantar r., the response to tactile stimulation of the ball of the foot, normally plantar flexion of the toes; the pathologic response is Babinski's *sign* (1). SYN sole r.

plantar muscle r., SYN Rossolimo's r.

pneocardiac r., a modification in the blood pressure or heart rhythm caused by the inhalation of an irritating vapor.

pneopneic r., a modification of the respiratory rhythm caused by the inhalation of an irritating vapor.

postural r., responses that control the position of the trunk and extremities. SEE ALSO righting r.'s. SYN static r. (1).

pressoreceptor r., a normal r. related to the carotid sinus *syndrome.*

pronator r., SYN ulnar r.

proprioceptive r.'s, any r. brought about by stimulation of proprioceptors. SEE ALSO proprioceptor.

proprioceptive-oculocephalic r., SYN vestibular ocular r.

protective laryngeal r., closure of the glottis to prevent entry of foreign substances into the respiratory tract.

psychocardiac r., a change in the circulatory rate and subjective heart consciousness (often "thumping") resulting from a memory of, or a subconscious dream state recollection of, an emotional impression or experience.

psychogalvanic r., psychogalvanic skin r., SYN galvanic skin *response.*

pulmonocoronary r., r. constriction of the coronary arteries as a result of vagal stimuli arising in the lungs, as in pulmonary embolism.

pupillary r., change in diameter of the pupil as a reflex response to any type of stimulus; *e.g.,* constriction caused by light. SYN light r. (1).

pupillary-skin r., dilation of the pupil following scratching of the skin of the neck. SYN ciliospinal r., cutaneous pupil r., cutaneous-pupillary r., skin-pupillary r.

quadriceps r., SYN patellar r.

quadripedal extensor r., extension of the arm of a hemiplegic patient when turned prone as if on all fours. SYN Brain's r.

radial r., on tapping the lower end of the radius, flexion of the forearm occurs, and sometimes, on strong percussion, flexion of the fingers. SEE ALSO inverted radial r.

radiobicipital r., contraction of the biceps muscle which sometimes occurs in the elicitation of the brachioradial r.

radioperiosteal r., SYN brachioradial r.

rectal r., the entrance of fecal matter into the rectum from the sigmoid colon causes an impulse to defecate.

rectocardiac r., a parasympathetic r. producing bradycardia and hypotension upon stimulation of the pelvic nerve, the afferent limb being the sacral outflow of the parasympathetic division of the autonomic nervous system, and the efferent limb, the cardiac vagus; said to accompany proctologic examinations.

rectolaryngeal r., laryngeal spasm precipitated by stretching the anal sphincter.

red r., SYN *pyramid* of light.

Remak's r., plantar flexion of the first three toes and, sometimes, the foot with extension of the knee induced by stroking of the upper anterior surface of the thigh; it occurs when the conducting paths in the cord are interrupted.

renal r., anuria caused by injury to a remote part of the body or by disease or injury to one kidney or ureter.

righting r.'s, r.'s which through various receptors, in labyrinth, eyes, muscles, or skin, tend to bring an animal's body into its normal position in space and which resist any force acting to put it into a false position, *e.g.,* on its back. SEE ALSO body righting r.'s, labyrinthine righting r.'s, neck r.'s, optical righting r.'s. SYN static r. (2).

Roger's r., SYN esophagosalivary r.

rooting r., in infants, rubbing or scratching about the mouth causes a puckering of the lips.

Rossolimo's r., flicking the tops of the toes from the plantar surface causes flexion of the toes; a stretch r. of the flexors of the toes seen in lesions of the pyramidal tracts. SEE ALSO Starling's r. SYN plantar muscle r., Rossolimo's sign.

scapular r., contraction of the upper muscles of the back by stimulation between the scapulae. SYN interscapular r.

scapulohumeral r., contraction of muscles of the shoulder girdle and arm caused by tapping the lower part of the unilateral border of the scapula; the muscles which respond vary according to their degree of stretching at the time. SYN scapuloperiosteal r.

scapuloperiosteal r., SYN scapulohumeral r.

Schäffer's r., in cases of injury to the corticospinal tract, the great toe is dorsiflexed when the skin over the Achilles tendon is pinched.

scratch r. in dogs, stimulus applied to the skin of a saddle-shaped area of the back, sides, and flanks produces a scratching movement of the hind leg of the side stimulated.

semimembranosus r., semitendinosus r., contraction of these muscles by tapping in the region of the tuberosity of the tibia.

shot-silk r., SYN shot-silk *retina.*

sinus r., SEE carotid sinus *syndrome.*

skin r.'s, SYN skin-muscle r.'s.

skin-muscle r.'s, superficial or cutaneous r.'s, such as the superficial abdominal r.'s. SYN skin r.'s.

skin-pupillary r., SYN pupillary-skin r.

snapping r., SYN Hoffmann's *sign* (2).

snout r., pouting or pursing of the lips induced by light tapping of closed lips near the midline; seen in defective pyramidal innervation of facial musculature.

sole r., SYN plantar r.

sole tap r., SYN aponeurotic r.

spinal r., a r. arc involving the spinal cord. SEE reflex *arc.*

spino-adductor r., contraction of the adductors of the thigh upon tapping the spinal column. SYN McCarthy's r.'s (1).

Starling's r., tapping the volar surfaces of the fingers causes flexion of the fingers; analogous to Rossolimo's r., for the toes.

startle r., (1) the r. response of an infant (contraction of the limb and neck muscles) when allowed to drop a short distance through the air or startled by a sudden noise or jolt; SYN Moro r., parachute r., startle reaction. (2) SYN cochleopalpebral r.

static r., (1) SYN postural r. (2) SYN righting r.'s.

statokinetic r., a r. which, through stimulation of the receptors in the neck muscles and semicircular canals, brings about movements of the limbs and eyes appropriate to a given movement of the head in space.

statotonic r.'s, r.'s in which utricular receptors in the vestibular apparatus sense changes in the head's position in space in terms of linear acceleration and the earth's gravitational field while receptors in the neck muscles sense changes in the position of the head relative to the trunk; input from these receptors reflexly controls the tone of the limb muscles to maintain or regain the desired posture. SYN attitudinal r.'s.

stepping r., if the plantar surface of a hind foot of a dog is pressed gently, a movement of extension of the limb will follow, accompanied sometimes by flexion of the opposite hind limb.

sternobrachial r., contraction of the adductors of the arm when the sternum is tapped.

stretch r., SYN myotatic r.

Strümpell's r., stroking the abdomen or thigh causes flexion of the leg and adduction of the foot.

styloradial r., SYN brachioradial r.

suckling r., the r. liberation of prolactin from the anterior lobe of the hypophysis evoked by stimulation of nerves in the nipple during the act of suckling by the newborn animal.

superficial r., any r., *e.g.,* the abdominal or cremasteric r., which is elicited by stimulation of the skin.

supination r., SYN brachioradial r.

supinator r., supinator longus r., SYN brachioradial r.

supporting r.'s, SYN supporting *reactions,* under *reaction.*

supraorbital r., contraction of the orbicularis oculi muscle induced by tapping the supraorbital nerve. SYN McCarthy's r.'s (2), trigeminofacial r.

suprapatellar r., the patella rises when a tap is given on the quadriceps tendon above the patella.

supraumbilical r., (1) SYN epigastric r. (2) SYN abdominal r.'s.

swallowing r., the act of swallowing (second stage) induced by stimulation of the palate, fauces, or posterior pharyngeal wall. SYN deglutition r., pharyngeal r. (1).

synchronous r., subsidiary r. actions occurring in association with the main or leading r.

tapetal light r., the glow from the eyes of some animals in the dark when a light illuminates the retina; due to the reflection of the light from the tapetum, an iridescent layer (containing guanidine crystals) in the choroid.

tarsophalangeal r., extension of all the toes except the first, when the outer part of the tarsus is tapped; in certain cerebral diseases the reverse takes place, the toes being flexed.

tendo Achillis r., SYN Achilles r.

tendon r., a myotatic or deep r. in which the muscle stretch receptors are stimulated by percussing the tendon of a muscle.

re

thumb r., flexion of the thumb upon tapping the dorsum of the hand. SYN metacarpothenar r.

tonic r., the occurrence of an appreciable interval after the production of a r. before relaxation, *e.g.,* the leg remains up for a time after a knee jerk. SYN Gordon's symptom.

trace conditioned r., a conditioned r. established by applying the stimulus a short time before reinforcement; in the conditioned r. of the animal so prepared, the response occurs at the same interval of time after the application of the stimulus as during the period of training.

trained r., SYN conditioned r.

triceps r., a sudden contraction of the triceps muscle caused by a smart tap on its tendon while the forearm hangs loosely at a right angle with the arm. SYN elbow jerk, elbow r.

triceps surae r., SYN Achilles r.

trigeminofacial r., SYN supraorbital r.

trochanter r., contraction of the adductor muscles of the thigh elicited by a tap on the trochanter.

Trömner's r., a modified Rossolimo r. in which, with the fingers of the patient partially flexed, the tapping of the volar aspect of the tip of the middle or index finger causes flexion of all four fingers and thumb; seen in pyramidal tract lesions with moderate spasticity.

ulnar r., pronation and adduction of the hand caused by tapping the styloid process of the ulna. SYN pronator r.

unconditioned r., an instinctive r. not dependent on previous learning or experience.

upper abdominal periosteal r., percussing the lower margin of the costal cartilages in the nipple line causes a contraction of the ipsilateral abdominal muscles (inconstant).

urinary r., SYN micturition r.

utricular r.'s, SEE statotonic r.'s.

vagovagal r., bradycardia with arterial hypotension, often with supraventricular arrhythmias; ascribed to stimulation, especially mechanical, of afferent vagal pathways in the abdomen, thorax, or airway, the efferent arc being vagal cardioinhibitory fibers.

vasopressor r., vasoconstriction caused by stimulation of certain afferent fibers, *e.g.,* in vagus nerve.

venorespiratory r., stimulation of respiration and increased pulmonary ventilation in response to an increase in pressure in the right atrium.

vertebra prominens r., pressure upon the last cervical vertebra of an animal, especially of one whose labyrinths have been destroyed and the vestibular nuclei isolated, causes relaxation or reduced tone of all four limbs.

vesical r., SYN micturition r.

vestibular ocular r., SYN doll's eye *sign.* SYN proprioceptive-oculocephalic r.

vestibulospinal r., the influence of vestibular stimulation on body posture.

visceral traction r., laryngeal spasm precipitated during an operation by traction on the stomach, gallbladder, or appendiceal mesentery.

viscerogenic r., any of a number of r.'s, such as headache, cough, disturbed pulse, etc., caused by disordered conditions of any of the viscera.

visceromotor r., contraction of the muscles of the thorax or abdomen in response to a stimulus from one of the viscera therein.

visceropannicular r., contraction of the panniculus carnosus muscle in the cat and certain other animals, in response to a stimulus applied to an abdominal viscus; the center for the r. is in the spinal cord, the afferent pathway is the splanchnic nerves.

viscerosensory r., an area of pain or sensitivity to pressure in the external body wall due to disease of one of the viscera. SEE ALSO Head's *lines,* under *line.*

viscerotrophic r., a degenerative change in the skeletal soft tissues consequent upon a chronic inflammatory condition of any of the thoracic or abdominal viscera.

visual orbicularis r., contraction of the orbicularis oculi muscle caused by a sudden visual stimulus. SEE ALSO wink r.

vomiting r., vomiting (contraction of the abdominal muscles

with relaxation of the cardiac sphincter of the stomach and of the muscles of the throat) elicited by a variety of stimuli, especially one applied to the region of the fauces. SYN pharyngeal r. (2).

Weingrow's r., SYN aponeurotic r.

Westphal's pupillary r., SYN eye-closure pupil *reaction.*

white pupillary r., SYN leukocoria.

wink r., general term for r. closure of eyelids caused by any stimulus. SYN eye-closure r.

withdrawal r., SYN flexor r.

wrist clonus r., sudden extension of the wrist induces a sustained clonic movement.

---

re·flex·o·gen·ic (rē-flek-sō-jen′ik). Causing a reflex. SYN reflexogenous.

re·flex·og·e·nous (rē-flek-soj′ĕ-nŭs). SYN reflexogenic.

re·flex·o·graph (rē-flek′sō-graf). An instrument for graphically recording a reflex. [reflex + G. *graphō,* to write]

re·flex·ol·o·gy (rē-flek-sol′ō-jē). The study of reflexes. [reflex + G. *logos,* study]

re·flex·om·e·ter (rē-flek-som′ĕ-ter). An instrument for measuring the force necessary to excite a reflex. [reflex + G. *metron,* measure]

re·flex·o·phil, re·flex·o·phile (rē-flek′sō-fil, -fīl). Having exaggerated reflexes. [reflex + G. *phileō,* to love]

re·flex·o·ther·a·py (rē-flek′sō-thār′ă-pē). SYN reflex *therapy.*

re·flux (rē′flŭks). 1. A backward flow. SEE ALSO regurgitation. 2. In chemistry, to boil without loss of vapor because of the presence of a condenser that returns vapor as liquid. [L. *re-,* back, + *fluxus,* a flow]

abdominojugular r., SYN hepatojugular r.

esophageal r., gastroesophageal r., regurgitation of the contents of the stomach into the esophagus, possibly into the pharynx where they can be aspirated between the vocal cords and down into the trachea; symptoms of burning pain and acid taste result; pulmonary complications of aspiration are dependent upon the amount, content, and acidity of the aspirate.

hepatojugular r., an elevation of venous pressure visible in the jugular veins and measurable in the veins of the arm, produced in active or impending congestive heart failure by firm pressure with the flat hand over the abdomen. Often called hepatojugular reflex when pressure is exclusively over the liver. SYN abdominojugular r.

intrarenal r., urinary r. from renal pelvis and calices into the collecting ducts. This is seen as a blush of the renal pyramid on voiding cystourethrography. SYN pyelotubular r.

pyelotubular r., SYN intrarenal r.

ureterorenal r., backward flow of urine from ureter into renal pelvis.

vesicoureteral r., backward flow of urine from bladder into ureter.

re·for·mat (rē-for′mat). In computed tomography, when data from a series of contiguous transverse scan images are recombined to produce images in a different plane, such as sagittal or coronal.

re·fract (rē-frakt′). 1. To change the direction of a ray of light. 2. To detect an error of refraction and to correct it by means of lenses. [L. *refringo,* pp. *-fractus,* to break up]

re·frac·ta·ble (ri-frak′ta-bil). Subject to refraction. SYN refrangible.

re·frac·tion (rē-frak′shŭn). 1. The deflection of a ray of light when it passes from one medium into another of different optical density; in passing from a denser into a rarer medium it is deflected away from a line perpendicular to the surface of the refracting medium; in passing from a rarer to a denser medium it is bent toward this perpendicular line. 2. The act of determining the nature and degree of the refractive errors in the eye and correction of the same by lenses. SYN refringence. [L. *refractio* (see refract)]

double r., the property of having more than one refractive index according to the direction of the transmitted light. SYN birefringence.

dynamic r., r. of the eye during accommodation.

static r., r. without accommodation.

re·frac·tion·ist (rē-frak'shŭn-ist). A person trained to measure the refraction of the eye and to determine the proper corrective lenses.

re·frac·tion·om·e·ter (rē-frak-shŭn-om'ĕ-ter). SYN refractometer.

re·frac·tive (rē-frak'tiv). **1.** Pertaining to refraction. **2.** Having the power to refract. SYN refringent.

re·frac·tiv·i·ty (rē-frak-tiv'i-tē). Refractive power. SYN refringency.

re·frac·tom·e·ter (rē-frak-tom'ĕ-ter). An instrument for measuring the degree of refraction in translucent substances, especially the ocular media. SEE refractive *index.* SYN objective optometer, refractionometer. [refraction + G. *metron,* measure]

re·frac·tom·e·try (rē-frak-tom'ĕ-trē). **1.** Measurement of the refractive index. **2.** Use of a refractometer to determine the refractive error of the eye.

re·frac·to·ry (rē-frak'tōr-ē). **1.** Resistant to treatment, as of a disease. SYN intractable (1), obstinate (2). **2.** SYN obstinate (1). [L. *refractarius,* fr. *refringo,* pp. *-fractus,* to break in pieces]

re·frac·ture (rē-frak'chŭr). Breaking a bone that has united after a previous fracture. [re- + fracture]

re·fran·gi·ble (rē-fran'ji-bl). SYN refractable. [L. *refringo,* to break in pieces]

re·fresh (rē-fresh'). **1.** To renew; to cause to recuperate. **2.** To perform revivification (2). [O. Fr. *re-frescher*]

re·frig·er·ant (rē-frij'er-ănt). **1.** Cooling; reducing slight fever. **2.** An agent that gives a sensation of coolness or relieves feverishness. [L. *re-frigero,* pp. *-atus,* pr. p. *-ans,* to make cold, fr. *frigus (frigor-),* cold]

re·frig·er·a·tion (rē-frij-er-ā'shŭn). The act of cooling or reducing fever. [L. *refrigeratio* (see refrigerant)]

re·frin·gence (rē-frin'jens). SYN refraction.

re·frin·gen·cy (rē-frin'jen-sē). SYN refractivity.

re·frin·gent (rē-frin'jent). SYN refractive.

Refsum, Sigvald, Norwegian neurologist, *1907. SEE R.'s *disease, syndrome.*

re·fu·sion (rē-fū'zhŭn). Return of the circulation of blood which has been temporarily cut off by ligature of a limb. [L. *re-fundo,* pp. *-fusus,* to pour back]

re·gain·er (rē-gān'er). An appliance used in an attempt to regain space in the dental arches.

Regaud, Claude, French radiologist, 1870–1940. SEE R.'s *fixative;* residual *body* of R.

re·gen·er·ate (rē-jen'er-āt). To renew; to reproduce. [L. *regenero,* pp. *-atus,* to reproduce, fr. *genus (gener-),* birth, race]

re·gen·er·a·tion (rē'jen-er-ā'shŭn). **1.** Reproduction or reconstitution of a lost or injured part. SYN neogenesis. **2.** A form of asexual reproduction; *e.g.,* when a worm is divided into two or more parts, each segment is regenerated into a new individual. [L. *regeneratio* (see regenerate)]

aberrant r., misdirected regrowth of nerve fibers seen for example, after oculomotor nerve injury. SYN misdirection phenomenon.

reg·i·men (rej'i-men). A program, including drugs, which regulates aspects of one's life-style for a hygienic or therapeutic purpose; a program of treatment; sometimes mistakenly called regime. [L. direction, rule]

REGIO

re·gio, gen. **re·gi·o·nis,** pl. **re·gi·o·nes** (rē'jē-ō, -ō'nis, -ō'nēz) [NA]. SYN region. [L.]

regio'nes abdo'minis [NA], SYN abdominal *regions,* under *region.*

r. ana'lis [NA], SYN anal *triangle.*

r. antebrachia'lis ante'rior [NA], SYN anterior *region* of forearm.

r. antebrachia'lis poste'rior [NA], SYN posterior *region* of forearm.

r. axilla'ris [NA], SYN axillary *region.*

r. brachia'lis ante'rior [NA], SYN anterior *region* of arm.

r. brachia'lis poste'rior [NA], SYN posterior *region* of arm.

r. bucca'lis [NA], SYN buccal *region.*

r. calca'nea [NA], SYN calcaneal *region.*

regio'nes cap'itis [NA], SYN *regions* of head, under *region.*

r. carpa'lis ante'rior [NA], SYN anterior carpal *region.*

r. carpa'lis poste'rior [NA], SYN posterior carpal *region.*

regio'nes cervica'les [NA], SYN *regions* of neck, under *region.*

r. cervica'lis ante'rior, SYN anterior *triangle* of neck.

r. cervica'lis latera'lis, SYN posterior *triangle* of neck.

r. cervica'lis poste'rior, SYN posterior *region* of neck.

regio'nes cor'poris [NA], SYN *regions* of body, under *region.*

r. crura'lis ante'rior [NA], SYN anterior *region* of leg.

r. crura'lis poste'rior [NA], SYN posterior *region* of leg.

r. cubita'lis ante'rior [NA], SYN anterior *region* of elbow.

r. cubita'lis poste'rior [NA], SYN posterior *region* of elbow.

r. deltoi'dea [NA], SYN deltoid *region.*

regio'nes dorsa'les [NA], SYN *regions* of back, under *region.*

r. epigas'trica [NA], SYN epigastric *region.*

regio'nes facia'les [NA], SYN *regions* of face, under *region.*

r. femora'lis [NA], SYN femoral *region.*

r. femora'lis ante'rior, SYN anterior *region* of thigh.

r. femora'lis poste'rior, SYN posterior *region* of thigh.

r. fronta'lis cap'itis [NA], SYN frontal *region* of head.

r. ge'nus ante'rior [NA], SYN anterior knee *region.*

r. ge'nus poste'rior [NA], SYN posterior knee *region.*

r. glutea'lis [NA], SYN gluteal *region.*

r. hypochondri'aca [NA], SYN hypochondriac *region.*

r. infraclavicula'ris, SYN infraclavicular *fossa.*

r. inframamma'ria [NA], SYN inframammary *region.*

r. infraorbita'lis [NA], SYN infraorbital *region.*

r. infrascapula'ris [NA], SYN infrascapular *region.*

r. inguina'lis [NA], SYN inguinal *region.*

r. latera'lis [NA], SYN lateral *region.*

r. lumba'lis [NA], SYN lumbar *region.*

r. mamma'ria [NA], SYN mammary *region.*

regio'nes mem'bri inferio'ris [NA], SYN *regions* of lower limb, under *region.*

regio'nes mem'bri superio'ris [NA], SYN *regions* of upper limb, under *region.*

r. menta'lis [NA], SYN mental *region.*

r. nasa'lis [NA], SYN nasal *region.*

r. nucha'lis [NA], ☆official alternate term for posterior *region* of neck.

r. occipita'lis cap'itis [NA], SYN occipital *region* of head.

r. olfacto'ria tu'nicae muco'sae na'si [NA], SYN *region* of olfactory mucosa.

r. ora'lis [NA], SYN oral *region.*

r. orbita'lis [NA], SYN orbital *region.*

r. parieta'lis cap'itis [NA], SYN parietal *region.*

re

regio′nes pectora′les [NA], SYN *regions* of chest, under *region*.

r. pectora′lis [NA], SYN pectoral *region*.

r. perinea′lis [NA], SYN perineal *region*.

r. plantaris, ☆official alternate term for *sole* of foot.

r. presterna′lis [NA], SYN presternal *region*.

r. pu′bica [NA], SYN pubic *region*.

r. respirato′ria tu′nicae muco′sae na′si [NA], SYN *region* of respiratory mucosa.

r. sacra′lis [NA], SYN sacral *region*.

r. scapula′ris [NA], SYN scapular *region*.

r. sternocleidomastoi′dea [NA], SYN sternocleidomastoid *region*.

r. sura′lis [NA], SYN sural *region*, sural *region*.

r. talocrura′lis [NA], SYN ankle *region*.

r. tempora′lis cap′itis [NA], SYN temporal *region* of head.

r. umbilica′lis [NA], SYN umbilical *region*.

r. urogenita′lis [NA], SYN urogenital *triangle*.

r. vertebra′lis [NA], SYN vertebral *region*.

r. zygomat′ica [NA], SYN zygomatic *region*.

---

re·gion (rē′jŭn). **1.** An often arbitrarily limited portion of the surface of the body. SEE ALSO space, zone. **2.** A portion of the body having a special nervous or vascular supply, or a part of an organ having a special function. SEE ALSO area, space, spatium, zone. SYN regio [NA]. [L. *regio*]

abdominal r.'s, the topographical subdivisions of the abdomen; based on subdividing the abdomen by the transpyloric, interspinous and midclavicular planes; including the right and left hypochondriac, right and left lateral, right and left inguinal, and the unpaired epigastric, umbilical and pubic regions. SYN regiones abdominis [NA], abdominal zones.

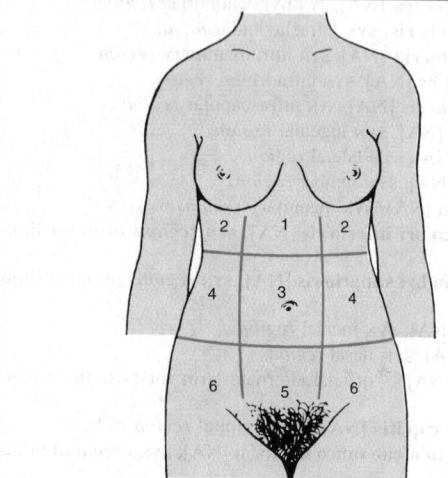

topography of abdominal regions
1) epigastric; 2) hypochondriac (right and left); 3) umbilical; 4) lateral (right and left); 5) pubic; and 6) inguinal (right and left)

anal r., SYN anal *triangle*.

ankle r., the region of the lower limb between the leg (crus) and the foot (pes). SYN regio talocruralis [NA].

anterior antebrachial r., SYN anterior r. of forearm.

anterior r. of arm, area between deltoid region superiorly and anterior region of elbow inferiorly. SYN facies brachialis anterior [NA], regio brachialis anterior [NA], anterior surface of arm, facies anterior brachii.

anterior brachial r., the anterior region of the arm.

anterior carpal r., the anterior part of the wrist. SYN regio carpalis anterior [NA].

anterior crural r., SYN anterior r. of leg.

anterior cubital r., SYN anterior r. of elbow.

anterior r. of elbow, the area in front of the elbow, including the cubital fossa. SYN facies cubitalis anterior [NA], regio cubitalis anterior [NA], anterior cubital r., anterior surface of elbow.

anterior r. of forearm, the area between the radial and ulnar borders of the forearm anteriorly. SYN facies antebrachialis anterior [NA], regio antebrachialis anterior [NA], anterior antebrachial r., anterior surface of forearm, facies anterior antebrachii.

anterior hypothalamic r., the rostral portion of the hypothalamus that includes preoptic, supraoptic, paraventricular and anterior hypothalamic nuclei; the hypothalamic structures located internally in the general area of the optic chiasm.

anterior knee r., the anterior region of the knee. SYN regio genus anterior [NA].

anterior r. of leg, the anterior surface of the inferior limb between the knee and the ankle. SYN facies cruralis anterior [NA], regio cruralis anterior [NA], anterior crural r., anterior surface of leg, facies anterior cruris.

anterior r. of neck, SYN anterior *triangle* of neck.

anterior r. of thigh, the front of the thigh, including the femoral triangle. SYN facies femoralis anterior☆ [NA], anterior surface of thigh, regio femoralis anterior.

axillary r., the region of the axilla, including the axillary fossa. SYN regio axillaris [NA].

r.'s of back, the topographical regions of the back of the trunk, including the vertebral r., sacral r., scapular r., infrascapular r., and lumbar r. SYN regiones dorsales [NA].

r.'s of body, the topographical divisions of the body. SYN regiones corporis [NA].

buccal r., the region of the cheek, corresponding approximately to the outlines of the underlying buccinator muscle. SYN regio buccalis [NA].

calcaneal r., the region of the heel. SYN regio calcanea [NA].

r.'s of chest, r. of chest, the topographic divisions of the chest: presternal, mammary, inframammary, and axillary. SEE pectoral r. SYN regiones pectorales [NA].

chromosomal r., that part of a chromosome defined either by anatomical details, notably banding, or by its linkages (linkage group).

complementarity determining r.'s, that part of an antibody or T cell receptor variable r. that binds with antigen or antigen/major histocompatibility molecule.

constant r., SEE immunoglobulin.

deltoid r., the lateral aspect of the shoulder demarcated by the outlines of the deltoid muscle. SYN regio deltoidea [NA].

dorsal hypothalamic r., the portion of the hypothalamus located immediately ventral to the hypothalamic sulcus; contains small nuclei, some of which are associated with the ansa lenticularis and the entopeduncular nucleus.

epigastric r., the region of the abdomen located between the costal margins and the subcostal plane. SYN epigastrium [NA], regio epigastrica [NA].

r.'s of face, the topographical subdivisions of the face, including nasal, oral, mental, orbital, infraorbital, buccal, and zygomatic. SYN regiones faciales [NA].

femoral r., the region of the thigh between hip and knee. SYN regio femoralis [NA].

frontal r. of head, the surface region of the head corresponding to the outlines of the frontal bone. SYN regio frontalis capitis [NA].

gluteal r., the region of the buttocks. SYN regio glutealis [NA].

r.'s of head, the topographical division of the cranium in relation to the bones of the cranial vault; the regions include frontal, parietal, occipital, and temporal. SYN regiones capitis [NA].

hinge r., (1) that part of a tRNA structure that is deformed, bending a "cloverleaf" (two-dimensional) model to form an "L" model (crystal form, as seen by electron microscopy); (2) in an immunoglobulin, a short sequence of amino acids that lies between two longer sequences and allows the latter to bend about the former.

hypervariable r.'s (hī-per′var-ĭ-a-ble), the r.'s of the immunoglobulin molecule that contain most of the residues involved in the antibody binding site.

hypochondriac r., the region on each side of the abdomen covered by the costal cartilages; it is lateral to the epigastric region. SYN regio hypochondriaca [NA], hypochondrium.

I r., that area of the H-2 complex of mice that contains Class II major histocompatibility complex genes.

iliac r., SYN inguinal r.

r.'s of inferior limb, SYN r.'s of lower limb.

inframammary r., the region of the chest inferior to the mammary gland. SYN regio inframammaria [NA].

infraorbital r., the region of the face below the orbit and alongside the nose on each side. SYN regio infraorbitalis [NA].

infrascapular r., the region of the back lateral to the vertebral region and below the scapula. SYN regio infrascapularis [NA].

inguinal r., the topographical area of the inferior abdomen related to the inguinal canal, lateral to the pubic region. SYN regio inguinalis [NA], groin (1), iliac r., inguen.

r. of interest, in computed tomography or other computerized imaging, an interactively selected portion of the image, whose individual or average pixel values can be displayed numerically.

intermediate hypothalamic r., the infundibular portion of the hypothalamus, includes the medial tuberal nuclei and portions of the dorsomedial, ventromedial, arcuate (infundibular), posterior and lateral hypothalamic nuclei; located internally in the general area of the infundibulum.

K r., carbons 9 and 10 of the phenanthrene ring system; thought by some to be the reactive spot in the various hydrocarbon carcinogens.

lateral r., the area of the abdomen on each side of the umbilical region between transpyloric plane and intertubercular or interspinous plane. SYN regio lateralis [NA].

lateral hypothalamic r., extends throughout most of the rostrocaudal extent of the hypothalamus lateral to the column of the fornix; includes lateral tuberal nuclei, tuberomamillary nuclei, and diffuse populations of cells. SYN lateral hypothalamic area.

lateral r. of neck, SYN posterior *triangle* of neck.

r.'s of lower limb, the topographic divisions of the lower limb: gluteal, thigh (or femoral), knee, leg (or crural), ankle, and foot. SYN regiones membri inferioris [NA], r.'s of inferior limb.

lumbar r., the region of the back lateral to the vertebral region and between the rib cage and the pelvis. SYN regio lumbalis [NA].

mammary r., the region of the breast. SYN regio mammaria [NA].

mental r., the region of the chin. SYN regio mentalis [NA].

nasal r., the region of the nose. SYN regio nasalis [NA].

r.'s of neck, the topographical subdivisions of the neck. SYN regiones cervicales [NA], neck (1).

nuchal region, SYN posterior r. of neck.

nucleolus organizer r., an arrangement of the DNA coding for the production of ribosomal RNA (rRNA).

occipital r. of head, the surface region of the head corresponding to the outlines of the occipital bone. SYN regio occipitalis capitis [NA].

r. of olfactory mucosa, the specialized olfactory receptive area that includes the upper one-third of the nasal septum and the lateral wall above the superior concha; it is lined with olfactory mucosa. SYN regio olfactoria tunicae mucosae nasi [NA], olfactory r. of tunica mucosa of nose, Schultze's membrane.

olfactory r. of tunica mucosa of nose, SYN r. of olfactory mucosa.

oral r., the region of the face including the lips and mouth. SYN regio oralis [NA].

orbital r., the region about the orbit. SYN regio orbitalis [NA].

parietal r., the surface region of the head corresponding to the outlines of the underlying parietal bone. SYN regio parietalis capitis [NA].

pectoral r., pectoral r.'s, the region of the chest demarcated by the outline of the pectoralis major muscle. SEE pectoral r., r.'s of chest. SYN regio pectoralis [NA].

perineal r., the r. at the lower end of the trunk, anterior to the sacral region and posterior to the pubic region between the thighs; it is divided into the anal triangle posteriorly and the urogenital triangle anteriorly. SYN regio perinealis [NA].

popliteal r., SYN popliteal *fossa.*

posterior antebrachial r., SYN posterior r. of forearm.

posterior r. of arm, the back of arm. SYN facies brachialis posterior [NA], regio brachialis posterior [NA], posterior brachial r., posterior surface of arm.

posterior brachial r., SYN posterior r. of arm.

posterior carpal r., the posterior part of the wrist. SYN regio carpalis posterior [NA].

posterior crural r., SYN posterior r. of leg.

posterior cubital r., SYN posterior r. of elbow.

posterior r. of elbow, the back of the elbow. SYN facies cubitalis posterior [NA], regio cubitalis posterior [NA], posterior cubital r., posterior surface of elbow.

posterior r. of forearm, the area between the radial and ulnar borders of the forearm posteriorly. SYN regio antebrachialis posterior [NA], facies antebrachialis posterior [NA], posterior antebrachial r., posterior surface of forearm.

posterior hypothalamic r., caudal portions of the hypothalamus located internally in the area of the mamillary body, includes medial, intermediate, and lateral mamillary nuclei and the posterior hypothalamic nuclei. SYN posterior hypothalamic area.

posterior knee r., the posterior region of the knee, including the popliteal fossa. SYN regio genus posterior [NA].

posterior r. of leg, the back of the leg. SYN regio cruralis posterior [NA], posterior crural r., posterior surface of leg.

posterior r. of neck, the back of neck, including the suboccipital region. SYN regio nuchalis [NA], nuchal region, posterior neck r., regio cervicalis posterior.

posterior neck r., SYN posterior r. of neck.

posterior r. of thigh, the back of the thigh. SYN facies femoralis posterior [NA], posterior surface of thigh, regio femoralis posterior.

preoptic r., the most anterior part of the hypothalamus surrounding the anterior or preoptic part of the third ventricle and including the lamina terminalis; containing the lateral and medial preoptic nucleus continuous caudally with, respectively, the lateral and anterior hypothalamic nucleus; rostrally the preoptic r. is continuous with the precommissural septum, laterally with the innominate substance. SYN preoptic area.

presternal r., the part of the chest over the sternum. SYN regio presternalis [NA].

presumptive r., in experimental embryology, an area of the blastula from which a specific tissue or organ may be expected to develop.

pretectal r., SYN pretectal *area.*

pubic r., the lower central region of the abdomen below the umbilical region. SYN hypogastrium [NA], regio pubica [NA].

r. of respiratory mucosa, the area commencing at the vestibule of the nose lined with respiratory mucosa; with the exception of the olfactory mucusa, it includes the entire nasal cavity. SYN regio respiratoria tunicae mucosae nasi [NA], respiratory r. of tunica mucosa of nose.

respiratory r. of tunica mucosa of nose, SYN r. of respiratory mucosa.

sacral r., the area of the back overlying the sacrum. SYN regio sacralis [NA].

scaffold-associated r.'s (SAR), sites in DNA that bind topoisomerase II and other scaffold proteins; found in introns.

scapular r., the area of the back corresponding to the outlines of the scapula. SYN regio scapularis [NA].

sternocleidomastoid r., the region overlying the sternocleidomastoid muscle, including the lesser supraclavicular fossa. SYN regio sternocleidomastoidea [NA].

suboccipital r., upper back of neck, inferior to occipital region of head and above the level of the second cervical vertebra; overlies (or includes, deeply) the suboccipital triangle.

r.'s of superior limb, SYN r.'s of upper limb.

sural r., the muscular swelling of the back of the leg below the knee, formed chiefly by the bellies of the gastrocnemius and soleus muscles. SYN regio suralis [NA], sura [NA], calf (1).

temporal r. of head, the surface region of the head corresponding approximately to the outlines of the temporal bone. SYN regio temporalis capitis [NA].

umbilical r., the central region of the abdomen about the umbilicus. SYN regio umbilicalis [NA].

r.'s of upper limb, the topographic divisions of the upper limb: deltoid, arm, elbow, forearm, carpal region, and hand. SYN regiones membri superioris [NA], r.'s of superior limb.

urogenital r., SYN urogenital *triangle.*

variable r., SEE immunoglobulin.

vertebral r., the central region of the back, corresponding to the underlying vertebral column. SYN regio vertebralis [NA].

Wernicke's r., SYN Wernicke's *center.*

zygomatic r., the region of the face outlined by the zygomatic bone; the prominence above the cheek. SYN regio zygomatica [NA].

re·gion·al (rē'jŭn-ăl). Relating to a region.

re·gi·o·nes (rē'jē-ō'nēz). Plural of regio. [L.]

reg·is·ter. The file of data concerning all cases of a specified condition, such as cancer, occurring in a defined population; the register is the actual document, the registry is the system of ongoing registration. [Mediev. L. *registrum,* fr. L.L. *re-gero,* pp. *re-gestum* to record]

reg·is·tra·tion (rej-is-trā'shŭn). In dentistry, a record.

maxillomandibular r., SYN maxillomandibular *record.*

tissue r., in dentistry, **(1)** the accurate r. of the shape of tissues under any condition by means of a suitable material; **(2)** an impression.

reg·is·try (rej'is-trē). **1.** An organization that lists professionals in certain fields. **2.** An agency for the collection of pathological material and related information and the organization of these materials for the purpose of study. **3.** An agency for the collection of data on individuals who have had a certain disease to allow follow-up and evaluation of response to therapy.

reg·nan·cy (reg'nan-sē). The briefest unit of experience; the unit composed of the total physiological processes occurring at a single moment, which constitute dominant configurations in the brain. A single process comprising part of the r. is referred to as a regnant process. [L. *regnant-, regnans,* pres. p. of *regno,* to rule]

re·gres·sion (rē-gresh'ŭn). **1.** A subsidence of symptoms. **2.** A relapse; a return of symptoms. **3.** Any retrograde movement or action. **4.** A return to a more primitive mode of behavior due to an inability to function adequately at a more adult level. **5.** The tendency for offspring of exceptional parents to possess characteristics closer to those of the general population. **6.** An unconscious defense mechanism by which there occurs a return to earlier patterns of adaptation. **7.** The distribution of one random variable given particular values of other variables relevant to it, *e.g.,* a formula for the distribution of weight as a function of height and chest circumference. The method was formulated by Galton in his study of quantitative genetics. [L. *re-gredior,* pp. *-gressus,* to go back]

phonemic r., a decrease in intelligibility of speech associated with an increase in loudness.

re·gres·sive (rē-gres'iv). Relating to or characterized by regression.

reg·u·la·tion (reg'yū-lā'shŭn). **1.** Control of the rate or manner in which a process progresses or a product is formed. **2.** In experimental embryology, the power of a pregastrula embryo to continue approximately normal development after a part or parts have been manipulated or destroyed. [L. *regula,* a rule]

enzyme r., control of the rate of a reaction catalyzed by an enzyme by some effector (*e.g.,* inhibitors or activators) or by alteration of some condition (*e.g.,* pH or ionic strength).

gene r., control of protein synthesis by means of activation or inhibition of that protein synthesis.

reg·u·la·tor (reg-yū-lā'tŏr). A substance or process that regulates another substance or process.

growth r.'s, substances that can alter the growth of a living organism.

reg·u·lon (reg'yū-lon). A set of structural genes, all with the same gene regulation, whose gene products are involved in the same reaction pathway.

re·gur·gi·tant (rē-ger'ji-tant). Regurgitating; flowing backward.

re·gur·gi·tate (rē-ger'ji-tāt). **1.** To flow backward. **2.** To expel the contents of the stomach in small amounts, short of vomiting. [L. *re-,* back, + *gurgito,* pp. *-atus,* to flood, fr. *gurges* (*gurgit-*), a whirlpool]

re·gur·gi·ta·tion (rē-ger'ji-tā'shŭn). **1.** A backward flow, as of blood through an incompetent valve of the heart. **2.** The return of gas or small amounts of food from the stomach. [L. *regurgitatio* (see regurgitate)]

aortic r., reflux of blood through an incompetent aortic valve into the left ventricle during ventricular diastole. SYN Corrigan's disease.

ischemic mitral r., a r. of the mitral valve caused by ischemic heart disease.

mitral r., reflux of blood through an incompetent mitral valve.

pulmonic r., incompetence of the pulmonic valve permitting retrograde flow.

valvular r., a leaky state of one or more of the cardiac valves, the valve not closing tightly and blood therefore regurgitating through it. SYN valvular incompetence, valvular insufficiency.

re·ha·bil·i·ta·tion (rē'hă-bil-i-tā'shŭn). Restoration, following disease, illness, or injury, of the ability to function in a normal or near normal manner. [L. *rehabilitare,* pp. *-tatus,* to make fit, fr. *re-* + *habilitas,* ability]

mouth r., restoration of the form and function of the masticatory apparatus to as nearly a normal condition as possible.

re·hears·al (rē-her'săl). A process associated with enhancing short-term and long-term memory wherein newly presented information, such as a name or a list of words, is repeated to oneself one or more times in order not to forget it.

Rehfuss, Martin E., U.S. physician, 1887–1964. SEE R. *method,* stomach *tube.*

re·hy·dra·tion (rē-hī-drā'shŭn). The return of water to a system after its loss.

Reichel, Friedrich P., German gynecologist and surgeon, 1858–1934. SEE R.-Pólya stomach *resection.*

Reichert, Karl B., German anatomist, 1811–1884. SEE R.'s *cartilage,* cochlear *recess;* R.-Meissl *number.*

Reid, Robert W., Scottish anatomist, 1851–1939. SEE R.'s base *line.*

Reifenstein, Edward C. Jr., U.S. endocrinologist, 1908–1975. SEE R.'s *syndrome.*

Reil, Johann C., German physician, neurologist, and histologist, 1759–1813. SEE R.'s *ansa, band, ribbon, triangle;* limiting *sulcus* of R.; circular *sulcus* of R.; *island* of R.

re·im·plan·ta·tion (rē'im-plan-tā'shŭn). SYN replantation.

re·in·fec·tion (rē-in-fek'shŭn). A second infection by the same microorganism, after recovery from or during the course of a primary infection.

re·in·force·ment (rē-in-fōrs'ment). **1.** An increase of force or strength; denoting specifically the increased sharpness of the patellar reflex when the patient at the same time closes the fist tightly or pulls against the flexed fingers or contracts some other set of muscles. SEE ALSO Jendrassik's *maneuver.* **2.** In dentistry, a structural addition or inclusion used to give additional strength in function; *e.g.,* bars in plastic denture base. **3.** In conditioning, the totality of the process in which the conditioned stimulus is followed by presentation of the unconditioned stimulus which, itself, elicits the response to be conditioned. SEE ALSO reinforcer, *schedules* of reinforcement, under *schedule,* classical *conditioning,* operant *conditioning.*

primary r., satisfaction of physiological needs or drives, such as that supplied by food or sleep.

secondary r., r. through something which, while it does not satisfy the need directly, has been associated with direct satisfaction of the need, such as the effect on behavior of a food or beer commercial on television.

re·in·forc·er (rē-in-fōrs′er). In conditioning, a pleasant or satisfaction-yielding (**positive r.**) or painful or unsatisfying (**negative r.**), stimulus, object, or stimulus event that is obtained upon the performance of a desired or predetermined operant. SEE ALSO reinforcement (3). SYN reward.

Reinke, Friedrich B., German anatomist, 1862–1919. SEE R. *crystalloids,* under *crystalloid.*

re·in·ner·va·tion (rē-in-ner-vā′shŭn). Restoration of nerve control of a paralyzed muscle or other effector organ by means of regrowth of nerve fibers, either spontaneously or after anastomosis.

re·in·oc·u·la·tion (rē′i-nok-yū-lā′shŭn). Reinfection by means of inoculation.

Reinsch, Adolf, German physician, 1862–1916. SEE R.'s *test.*

re·in·te·gra·tion (rē′in-tĕ-grā′shŭn). In the mental health professions, the return to well adjusted functioning following disturbances due to mental illness.

re·in·ver·sion (re-in-ver′shŭn). The correction, spontaneous or operative, of an inversion, as of the uterus.

Reisseisen, Franz D., German anatomist, 1773–1828. SEE R.'s *muscles,* under *muscle.*

Reissner, Ernst, German anatomist, 1824–1878. SEE R.'s *fiber, membrane.*

Reitan, Ralph M., U.S. psychologist, *1922. SEE Halstead-R. *battery.*

Reiter, Hans, German bacteriologist, 1881–1969. SEE R. *test;* R.'s *disease, syndrome;* Fiessinger-Leroy-R. *syndrome.*

re·jec·tion (rē-jek′shŭn). **1.** The immunological response to incompatibility in a transplanted organ. **2.** A refusal to accept, recognize, or grant; a denial. **3.** Elimination of small ultrasonic echoes from display. [L. *rejectio,* a throwing back]

accelerated r., a transplant r. manifested in less than three days.

acute r., SYN acute cellular r.

acute cellular r., graft r. which usually begins within 10 days after a graft has been transplanted into a genetically dissimilar host. Lesions at the site of the graft characteristically are infiltrated with large numbers of lymphocytes and macrophages which cause tissue damage. SEE primary r. SYN acute r.

allograft r. (al′lō-graft), the r. of tissue transplanted between two genetically different individuals of the same species. R. is caused by T lymphocytes responding to the foreign major histocompatibility complex of the graft. SYN homograft.

chronic r., a transplant r. occurring after a few or many months, mainly from persisting serum antibody action.

chronic allograft r., immunologically mediated damage to the allograft, typically a kidney allograft, manifested by diffuse interstitial fibrosis glomerular changes, typically membranous and sclerotic in nature, as well as intimal fibrosis of the blood vessels with tubular atrophy and loss of tubular structures.

first-set r., allograft transplantation between two organisms not previously sensitized to the graft tissue. Necrosis of the graft usually occurs within 10 days of transplantation.

hyperacute r., (1) a r. that usually develops in less than one hour from the implantation of a vascular graft; (2) a form of antibody-mediated, usually irreversible damage to a transplanted organ, particularly the kidney, manifested predominantly by diffuse thrombotic lesions, usually confined to the organ itself and only rarely disseminated; (3) for skin allograft rejection of this type, see white *graft.*

parental r., a child's denying, withholding, or unacceptance of affection or attention to or from a parent, or its obverse from a parent to or from a child.

primary r., a r. occurring more than seven days after transplantation, mainly from a cellular immune response.

second set r., an accelerated r. of a transplant that occurs when an individual has been previously sensitized to the graft.

re·ju·ve·nes·cence (rē-jū-vĕ-nes′ens). A renewal of youth; return of a cell or tissue to a state in which it was in an earlier stage of existence. [L. *re-,* again, + *juvenesco,* to grow young, fr. *juvenis,* a youth]

re·lapse (rē′laps). Return of the manifestations of a disease after

an interval of improvement. SYN recurrence (2). [L. *re-labor,* pp. *-lapsus,* to slide back]

re·laps·ing (rē-lap′sing). Recurring; said of a disease or its manifestations that returns in a new attack after an interval of improvement.

re·la·tion (rē-lā′shŭn). **1.** An association or connection between or among people or objects. SEE ALSO relationship. **2.** In dentistry, the mode of contact of teeth or the positional relationship of oral structures. [L. *relatio,* a bringing back]

acquired centric r., SEE centric jaw r.

acquired eccentric r., an eccentric r. that is assumed by habit in order to bring the teeth into occlusion.

buccolingual r., the position of a space or tooth in r. to the tongue and the cheek.

centric jaw r., centric r., (1) the most retruded physiologic r. of the mandible to the maxillae to and from which the individual can make lateral movements; it is a condition which can exist at various degrees of jaw separation, and it occurs around the terminal hinge axis; (2) the most posterior r. of the mandible to the maxillae at the established vertical r. SEE ALSO eccentric r. SYN median retruded r., median r.

dynamic r.'s, relative movements between two objects, *e.g.,* the relationship of the mandible to the maxillae.

eccentric r., any r. of the mandible to the maxillae other than centric r. SYN eccentric position.

intermaxillary r., SYN maxillomandibular r.

maxillomandibular r., any one of the many r.'s of the mandible to the maxillae, *e.g.,* centric jaw r., eccentric r. SYN intermaxillary r.

median retruded r., median r., SYN centric jaw r.

occluding r., the jaw r. at which the opposing teeth occlude.

protrusive r., the r. of the mandible to the maxillae when the lower jaw is thrust forward.

protrusive jaw r., a jaw r. resulting from a protrusion of the mandible.

rest r., the postural r. of the mandible to the maxillae when the patient is resting comfortably in the upright position and the condyles are in a neutral unstrained position in the glenoid fossa. SYN rest jaw r., unstrained jaw r.

rest jaw r., SYN rest r.

ridge r., the positional r. of the mandibular ridge to the maxillary ridge.

static r.'s, relationship between two parts that are not in motion.

unstrained jaw r., SYN rest r.

re·la·tion·ship (rē-lā′shŭn-ship). The state of being related, associated, or connected.

blood r., SYN consanguinity.

dose-response r., r. in which a change in the amount, intensity, or duration of exposure is associated with a change in risk of a specified outcome.

dual r.'s, r.'s in which a health service provider is concurrently participating in two or more role categories with a patient; such dual r.'s may be benign (as when both are members of the same social group) or exploitive (a sexual r.).

Haldane r., a mathematical r. between the equilibrium constant of an enzyme-catalyzed reaction and all of that enzyme's kinetic parameters (*e.g.,* V_{max} and K_m's).

hypnotic r., r. between hypnotizer, or hypnotist, and the hypnotized, or hypnotee.

object r., in the behavioral sciences, the emotional bond between an individual and another person (or between two groups), as opposed to the individual's (or group's) interest in him or herself (itself).

sadomasochistic r., a r. characterized by the complementary enjoyment of inflicting and suffering cruelty.

rel·a·tive bi·o·log·i·cal ef·fec·tive·ness. See under effectiveness.

re·lax (rē-laks′). **1.** To loosen; to slacken. **2.** To cause a movement of the bowels. [L. *re-laxo,* to loosen]

re·lax·ant (rē-lak′sănt). **1.** Relaxing; causing relaxation; reducing tension, especially muscular tension. **2.** An agent that reduces muscular tension or produces skeletal muscle paralysis, usually referred to as a muscle r.

depolarizing r., an agent, *e.g.,* succinylcholine, that induces depolarization of the motor endplate and so paralyzes skeletal muscle by a phase I block.

muscle r., a drug with the capacity to reduce muscle tone; may be either a peripherally acting muscle r. such as curare and act to produce blockade at the neuromuscular junction (and thus useful in surgery), or act as a centrally acting muscle r. exerting its effects within the brain and spinal cord to diminish muscle tone (and thus useful in muscle spasm or spasticity).

muscular r., an agent that relaxes striated muscle; includes drugs acting at the brain and/or spinal cord level or directly on muscle to decrease tone, as well as the neuromuscular r.'s.

neuromuscular r., an agent, *e.g.,* curare or succinylcholine, that produces relaxation of striated muscle by interruption of transmission of nervous impulses at the myoneural junction.

nondepolarizing r., an agent, *e.g.,* tubocurarine, that paralyzes skeletal muscle without depolarization of the motor endplate, as in phase II block.

smooth muscle r., an agent, such as an antispasmodic, bronchodilator, or vasodilator, that reduces the tension or tone of smooth (involuntary) muscle.

re·lax·a·tion (rē-lak-sā′shŭn). **1.** Loosening, lengthening, or lessening of tension in a muscle. **2.** In nuclear magnetic resonance, r. is the decay in magnetization of tissue after the direction of the surrounding magnetic field is changed; the different rates of r. for individual nuclei and tissues are used to provide contrast in imaging. [L. *relaxatio* (see relax)]

cardioesophageal r., r. of the lower esophageal sphincter which can allow reflux of acidic gastric contents into the lower esophagus, producing esophagitis.

isometric r., decrease in tension of a muscle while the length remains constant due to fixation of the ends.

isovolumetric r., SYN isovolumic r.

isovolumic r., that part of the cardiac cycle between the time of aortic valve closure and mitral opening, during which the ventricular muscle decreases its tension without lengthening so that ventricular volume remains unaltered; the heart is never precisely isovolumetric (vs. isovolumic) except during long diastoles with a midiastolic period of diastasis. SYN isovolumetric r.

longitudinal r., in nuclear magnetic resonance, the return of the magnetic dipoles of the hydrogen nuclei (magnetization vector) to equilibrium parallel to the magnetic field, after they have been flipped 90°; varies in rate in different tissues, taking up to 15 seconds for water. SEE TI. SYN spin-lattice r., spin-spin r.

spin-lattice r., SYN longitudinal r.

spin-spin r., SYN longitudinal r.

transverse r., in nuclear magnetic resonance, the rapid decay of the nuclear magnetization vector at right angles to the magnetic field after the 90° pulse is turned off; the signal is called free induction decay. SEE T2. Cf. longitudinal r.

re·lax·in (rē-lak′sin). A polypeptide hormone secreted by the corpora lutea of mammalian species during pregnancy. Facilitates the birth process by causing a softening and lengthening of the pubic symphysis and cervix; it also inhibits contraction of the uterus and may play a role in timing of parturition. SYN cervilaxin, ovarian hormone, releasin, uterine relaxing factor. [relax + -in]

re·learn·ing (rē-lern′ing). The process of regaining a skill or ability that has been partially or entirely lost; savings involved in r., as compared with original learning, give an index of the degree of retention.

re·leas·in. SYN relaxin.

re·li·a·bil·i·ty (rē-lī-ă-bil′i-tē). The degree of stability exhibitied when a measurement is repeated under identical conditions. SEE correlation *coefficient,* reliability *coefficient.* [M.E. *relien,* fr. O.Fr. *relier,* fr. L. *religo,* to bind]

equivalent form r., in psychology, the consistency of measurement based on the correlation between scores on two similar forms of the same test taken by the same individual. SEE ALSO reliability *coefficient.*

interjudge r., in psychology, the consistency of measurement obtained when different judges or examiners independently administer the same test to the same individual. SYN interrater r.

interrater r., SYN interjudge r.

test-retest r., in psychology, the consistency of measurement based on the correlation between test and retest scores for the same individual. SEE ALSO coefficient, reliability.

re·lief (rē-lēf′). **1.** Removal of pain or distress, physical or mental. **2.** In dentistry, reduction or elimination of pressure from a specific area under a denture base. SEE ALSO relief *area,* relief *chamber.* [see relieve]

re·lieve (rē-lēv′). To free wholly or partly from pain or discomfort, either physical or mental. [thru O. Fr. fr. L. *re-levo,* to lift up, lighten]

re·line (rē′līn′). In dentistry, to resurface the tissue side of a denture with new base material to make it fit more accurately. SEE ALSO rebase.

REM Acronym for rapid eye *movements,* under *movement;* reticular erythematous *mucinosis.*

rem Abbreviation for *roentgen*-equivalent-man. See entries under roentgen.

Remak, Ernst J., German neurologist, 1848–1911. SEE R.'s *reflex, sign.*

Remak, Robert, Polish-German anatomist and histologist, 1815–1865. SEE R.'s nuclear *division, fibers,* under *fiber, ganglia,* under *ganglion, plexus.*

re·me·di·a·ble (rē-mē′dē-ă-bl). Curable. [L. *remediabilis,* fr. *remedio,* to cure]

re·me·di·al (rē-mē′dē-ăl). Curative or acting as a remedy.

rem·e·dy (rem′ĕ-dē). An agent that cures disease or alleviates its symptoms. [L. *remedium,* fr. *re-,* again, + *medeor,* cure]

re·min·er·al·i·za·tion (rē′min′er-ăl-i-zā′shŭn). **1.** The return to the body or a local area of necessary mineral constituents lost through disease or dietary deficiencies; commonly used in referring to the content of calcium salts in bone. **2.** In dentistry, a process enhanced by the presence of fluoride whereby partially decalcified enamel, dentin, and cementum become recalcified by mineral replacement.

rem·i·nis·cence (rem-i-nis′sens). In the psychology of learning, an improvement in recall, over that shown on the last trial, of incompletely learned material after an interval without practice. [L. *reminiscentiae,* from *reminiscor,* to remember]

re·mis·sion (rē-mish′ŭn). **1.** Abatement or lessening in severity of the symptoms of a disease. **2.** The period during which such abatement occurs. [L. *remissio,* fr. *re-mitto,* pp. *-missus,* to send back, slacken, relax]

spontaneous r., in psychiatry and clinical psychology, disappearance of symptoms without formal treatment; causes of their disappearance are assumed to exist but are not known.

re·mit (rē-mit′). To become less severe for a time without absolutely ceasing. [see remission]

re·mit·tence (rē-mit′ens). A temporary amelioration, without actual cessation, of symptoms.

re·mit·tent (rē-mit′ent). Characterized by temporary periods of abatement of the symptoms of a disease.

rem·nant (rem′nant). Something remaining, a residue or vestige. [O. Fr., fr. *remaindre,* to remain, fr. L. *remaneo*]

re·mod·el·ing (rē-mod′el-ing). A cyclical process by which bone maintains a dynamic steady state through sequential resorption and formation of a small amount of bone at the same site; unlike the process of modeling, the size and shape of remodeled bone remain unchanged.

ren, gen. **re·nis,** pl. **re·nes** (ren, rē′nis, rē′nēz) [NA]. SYN kidney. [L.]

re·nal (rē′năl). SYN nephric.

re·nat·ur·a·tion (rē-nā-tyū-rā′shŭn). The conversion of a denatured and inactive macromolecule back to its natured and bioactive configuration.

ren·cu·lus (ren′kū-lŭs). **1.** SYN cortical *lobules* of kidney, under *lobule.* **2.** SYN reniculus (2).

Rendu, Henri J.L.M., French physician, 1844–1902. SEE R.-Osler-Weber *syndrome.*

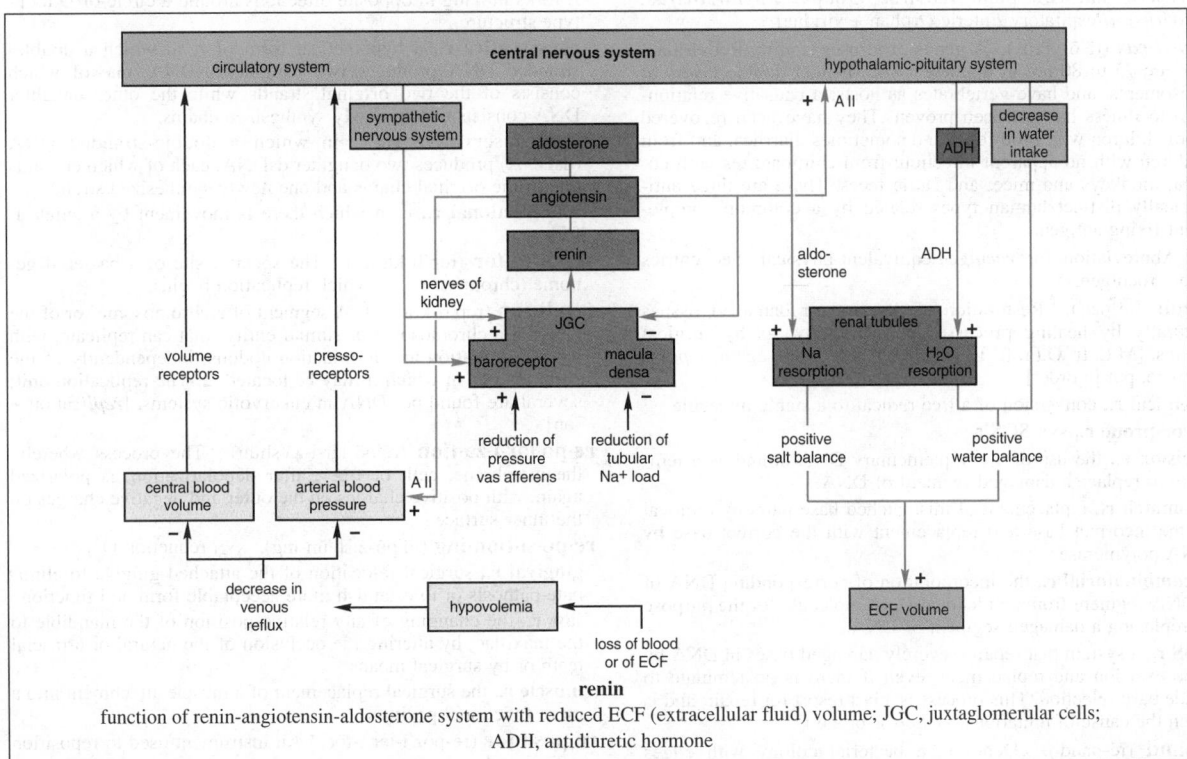

renin

function of renin-angiotensin-aldosterone system with reduced ECF (extracellular fluid) volume; JGC, juxtaglomerular cells; ADH, antidiuretic hormone

reni-. SEE reno-.

ren·i·cap·sule (ren'i-kap'sūl). The capsule of the kidney. [reni- + L. *capsula,* capsule]

ren·i·car·di·ac (ren'i-kar'dē-ak). SYN cardiorenal. [reni- + G. *kardia,* heart]

re·nic·u·lus, pl. **re·nic·u·li** (rĕ-nik'yū-lŭs, -lī). **1.** SYN cortical *lobules* of kidney, under *lobule.* **2.** A lobe of the human fetal kidney and that of some lower animals in which fibrous septa subdivide the organ. SYN renculus (2), renunculus (2). [L. dim. of *ren,* kidney]

re·ni·fleur (ren-i-fler'). A sniffer; one who is sexually excited by odors. [Fr.]

ren·i·form (ren'i-fōrm). SYN nephroid.

re·nin (rē'nin). A term originally used for a pressor substance obtained from rabbits' kidneys, now an enzyme that converts angiotensinogen to angiotensin I. SYN angiotensinogenase.

ren·i·por·tal (ren'i-pōr'tăl). **1.** Relating to the hilum of the kidney. **2.** Relating to the portal, or venous capillary circulation in the kidney. [reni- + L. *porta,* gate]

ren·nase (ren'ās). SYN chymosin.

ren·net (ren'et). SYN chymosin.

ren·nin (ren'in). SYN chymosin.

ren·nin·o·gen, ren·no·gen (rĕ-nin'ō-jen, ren'ō-jen). SYN prochymosin. [rennin + G. *-gen,* producing]

reno-, reni-. The kidney. SEE ALSO nephro-. [L. *ren*]

re·no·cu·ta·ne·ous (rē'nō-kyū-tā'nē-ŭs). Relating to the kidneys and the skin. [reno- + L. *cutis,* skin]

re·no·gas·tric (rē'nō-gas'trik). Relating to the kidneys and the stomach. [reno- + G. *gastēr,* stomach]

re·no·gen·ic (rē-nō-jen'ik). Originating in or from the kidney.

re·no·gram (rē'nō-gram). The assessment of renal function by external radiation detectors after the administration of a radiopharmaceutical that is filtered and excreted by the kidney. [reno- + G. *gramma,* something written]

re·nog·ra·phy (rē-nog'ră-fē). Radiography of the kidney.

re·no·in·tes·ti·nal (rē'nō-in-tes'ti-năl). Relating to the kidneys and the intestine.

re·no·meg·a·ly (rē'nō-meg'ă-lē). Enlargement of the kidney.

re·nop·a·thy (rē-nop'ă-thē). A rarely used term for nephropathy.

re·no·pri·val (rē-nō-prī'văl). Relating to, characterized by, or resulting from total loss of kidney function or from removal of all functioning renal tissue. [reno- + L. *privus,* deprived of]

re·no·pul·mo·nary (rē'nō-pŭl'mo-nār-ē). Relating to the kidneys and the lungs.

re·no·tro·phic (rē-nō-trof'ik). Relating to any agent influencing the growth or nutrition of the kidney or to the action of such an agent. SYN nephrotrophic, nephrotropic, renotropic. [reno- + G. *trophē,* nourishment]

re·no·tro·phin (rē-nō-trō'fin). An agent affecting the growth or nutrition of the kidney. SYN renotropin.

re·no·tro·pic (rē-nō-trop'ik). SYN renotrophic. [reno- + G. *tropē,* a turning]

re·no·tro·pin (rē-nō-trō'pin). SYN renotrophin.

re·no·vas·cu·lar (rē-nō-vas'kyū-ler). Pertaining to the blood vessels of the kidney, denoting especially disease of these vessels.

Renpenning, H., 20th century Canadian physician. SEE R.'s *syndrome.*

ren. sem. Abbreviation for [L.] *renovetur semel,* shall be renewed (only) once.

Renshaw, B., 20th century U.S. neurophysiologist. SEE R. *cells,* under *cell.*

re·nun·cu·lus (rē-nŭng'kyū-lŭs). **1.** SYN cortical *lobules* of kidney, under *lobule.* **2.** SYN reniculus (2). [L. dim. of *ren*]

Re·o·vir·i·dae (rē-ō-vir'i-dē). A family of double-stranded RNA viruses, some of which (*Reovirus*) previously were included with ECHO viruses, and others (*Orbivirus*), with arboviruses. Virions are 60 to 80 nm in diameter, usually naked, and ether-resistant; genomes contain double-stranded, segmented RNA (MW 10 to 16×10^6); capsids are of icosahedral symmetry with two layers of capsomeres. The family comprises six genera: *Reovirus, Orbivirus, Rotavirus,* cytoplasmic polyhedrosis virus group (*Cy-*

povirus), and two plant reovirus groups (*Phytoreovirus, Fijivirus*). [*R*espiratory *E*nteric *O*rphan + viridae]

Re·o·vi·rus (rē'ō-vī'rŭs). A genus of viruses (family Reoviridae) that are 75 to 80 nm in diameter, with distinct double layers of capsomeres, and have vertebrates as hosts; a causative relationship to illness has not been proven. They have been recovered from children with mild fever and sometimes diarrhea, and from children with no apparent infection; from chimpanzees with coryza; monkeys and mice; and cattle feces. There are three antigenically distinct human types related by a common complement-fixing antigen.

rep Abbreviation for *roentgen*-equivalent-physical. See entries under roentgen.

re·pair (rē-pār'). Restoration of diseased or damaged tissues naturally by healing processes or artificially, as by surgical means. [M.E.,fr. O.Fr.,fr. L. *re-paro*, fr. *re-*, back, again, + *paro*, prepare, put in order]

chemical r., conversion of a free radical to a stable molecule.

error-prone r., SYN SOS r.

excision r., the use of a complementary DNA strand as a template to replace a damaged segment of DNA.

mismatch r., replacement of mismatched base pairs by removal of the incorrect base and replacement with the correct base by DNA polymerase.

recombinatorial r., the incorporation of corresponding DNA of a DNA segment from an identical DNA molecule for the purpose of replacing a damaged segment of DNA.

SOS r., a system that repairs severely damaged bases in DNA by base excision and replacement, even if there is no template to guide base selection. This process is a last resort for repair, and is often the cause of mutations. SYN error-prone r.

re·pand (rē-pand'). Denoting a bacterial colony with edges marked by a series of slightly concave segments with angular projections at their points of union. [L. *repandus*, bent or turned back, fr. *re-*, back, + *pandus*, curved]

re·pel·lent (rē-pel'ent). 1. Capable of driving off or repelling; repulsive. 2. An agent that drives away or prevents annoyance or irritation by insect pests. 3. An astringent or other agent that reduces swelling. [L. *re-pello*, pp. *-pulsus*, to drive back]

rep·e·ti·tion-com·pul·sion (rep-e-tish'ŭn-kŏm-pŭl'shŭn). In psychoanalysis, the tendency to repeat earlier experiences or actions, in an unconscious effort to achieve belated mastery over them; a morbid need to repeat a particular behavior such as handwashing or repeated checking to see if the door is locked.

re·plant (rē'plant). 1. To perform replantation. 2. A part or organ so replaced or about to be so replaced.

re·plan·ta·tion (rē-plan-tā'shŭn). Replacement of an organ or part back in its original site and reestablishing its circulation. SYN reimplantation. [L. *re-*, again, + *planto*, pp. *-atus*, to plant, fr. *planta*, a sprout, slip]

intentional r., elective extraction of a tooth, obturation of the root canal(s), and replacement of the tooth into the alveolus.

re·ple·tion (rē-plē'shŭn). 1. SYN hypervolemia. 2. SYN plethora (2). [L. *repletio*, fr. *re-pleo*, pp. *-pletus*, to fill up]

rep·li·ca (rep'li-kă). A specimen for electron microscopic examination obtained by coating a crystalline array or other virus material with carbon; the mold (the r.) obtained after the viral material has been dissolved provides details of structure and arrangement. [It., fr. L.L. *re-plico*, to fold back]

rep·li·case (rep'li-kās). Descriptive term for RNA-directed RNA polymerase (EC 2.7.7.48) associated with replication of RNA viruses.

rep·li·cate (rep'li-kāt). 1. One of several identical processes or observations. 2. To repeat; to produce an exact copy.

rep·li·ca·tion (rep-li-kā'shŭn). 1. The execution of an experiment or study more than once so as to confirm the original findings, increase precision, and obtain a closer estimate of sampling error. 2. Autoreproduction, as in mitosis or cellular biology. SEE autoreproduction. 3. DNA-directed DNA synthesis. [L. *replicatio*, a reply, fr. *replico*, pp. *-atus*, to fold back]

bidirectional r., a situation in which DNA r. proceeds with two

r. forks moving in opposite directions around a circle or D loop-type structure.

conservative r., a hypothetical form of r. in which a double-stranded DNA produces two daughter dsDNA, one of which consists of the two original strands while the other daughter DNA consists of two newly synthesized chains.

semiconservative r., r. in which a double-stranded DNA (dsDNA) produces two daughter dsDNA, each of which contains one of the original chains and one newly synthesized strand.

unidirectional r., r. in which there is movement by a single r. fork.

rep·li·ca·tor (rep'li-kā-ter). The specific site of a bacterial genome (chromosome) at which replication begins.

rep·li·con (rep'li-kon). 1. A segment of a chromosome (or of the DNA of a chromosome or similar entity) that can replicate, with its own initiation and termination codons, independently of the chromosome in which it may be located. 2. The replication unit; several are found per DNA in eukaryotic systems. [*replic*ation + -*on*]

re·po·lar·i·za·tion (rē'pō-lăr-i-zā'shŭn). The process whereby the membrane, cell, or fiber, after depolarization, is polarized again, with positive charges on the outer and negative charges on the inner surface.

re·po·si·tion·ing (rē'pō-zish'ŭn-ing). SYN reduction (1).

gingival r., surgical relocation of the attached gingiva to eliminate pathosis or to establish more acceptable form and function.

jaw r., the changing of any relative position of the mandible to the maxillae, by altering the occlusion of the natural or artificial teeth or by surgical means.

muscle r., the surgical replacement of a muscle attachment into a more functional position.

re·pos·i·tor (rē-poz'i-ter, -tōr). An instrument used to reposition a displaced organ.

re·pressed (rē-prest'). Subjected to repression.

re·pres·sion (rē-presh'ŭn). 1. In psychotherapy, the active process or defense mechanism of keeping out and ejecting, banishing from consciousness, ideas or impulses that are unacceptable to it. 2. Decreased expression of some gene product. [L. *re-primo*, pp. *-pressus*, to press back, repress]

catabolite r., the decreased expression of an operon due to elevated levels of a catabolite of a biochemical pathway.

end product r., catabolite r. in which the catabolite is an end product of a particular pathway.

enzyme r., inhibition of enzyme synthesis by some metabolite.

primal r., r. of material never in conscious thought.

re·pres·sor (rē-pres'er). The product of a regulator or r. gene.

active r., a r. that combines directly with an operator gene to repress the operator and its structural genes, thus repressing protein synthesis; active r. may be repressed by an inducer, with resulting protein synthesis; a homeostatic mechanism for regulation of inducible enzyme systems.

inactive r., a r. that cannot combine with an operator gene until it has combined with a corepressor (usually a product of a protein pathway); after activation, the r. arrests production of the proteins controlled by the operator gene; a homeostatic mechanism for regulation of repressible enzyme systems. SYN aporepressor.

re·pro·duc·i·bil·i·ty (rē-prō-dus'i-bil'i-tē). 1. Ability to cause to exist again or to present again. 2. The ability to duplicate measurements over long periods of time by different laboratories.

re·pro·duc·tion (rē-prō-dŭk'shŭn). 1. The recall and presentation in the mind of the elements of a former impression. 2. The total process by which organisms produce offspring. SYN generation (1), procreation. [L. *re-*, again, + *pro-duco*, pp. *-ductus*, to lead forth, produce]

asexual r., r. other than by union of male and female sex cells. SYN agamogenesis, agamogony.

cytogenic r., r. by means of unicellular germ cells; includes both sexual r. and asexual r. by means of spores.

sexual r., r. by union of male and female gametes to form a zygote. SYN gamogenesis, syngenesis.

somatic r., asexual r. by fission or budding of somatic cells.

vegetative r., SEE asexual r.

re·pro·duc·tive (rē'prō-dŭk'tiv). Relating to reproduction.

rep·ti·lase (rep'til-as). An enzyme found in the venom of *Bothrops atrox* that clots fibrinogen by splitting off its fibrinopeptide. [reptile + -ase]

Rep·til·ia (rep-til'ē-ă). A class of vertebrates comprising the alligators, crocodiles, lizards, turtles, tortoises, and snakes. [L. *reptilis,* ntr. *-e,* creeping; ntr. as n., reptile]

re·pul·lu·la·tion (rē-pul-yū-lā'shŭn). Renewed germination; return of a morbid process or growth. [L. *re-,* again, + *pullulo,* pp. *-atus,* to sprout]

re·pul·sion (rē-pŭl'shŭn). **1.** The act of repelling or driving apart, in contrast to attraction. **2.** Strong dislike; aversion; repugnance. **3.** Coupling phase of genes at linked loci that are borne on opposite chromosomes. SEE coupling *phase.* [L. *re-pello,* pp. *-pulsus,* to drive back]

re·quire·ment (rē-kwīr'ment). **1.** Something needed. **2.** A condition.

minimum protein r., the age-dependent amount of protein required daily in the diet.

quantum r., the number of quanta of light absorbed required for the transformation of one molecule; the inverse of the quantum yield.

RES Abbreviation for reticuloendothelial *system.*

res·a·zu·rin (rē-saz'yū-rin). A blue compound, 7-hydroxy-3*H*-phenoxazin-3-one 10-oxide, used as a redox indicator in the reductase test of milk and also as a pH indicator (orange at 3.8, violet at 6.5).

res·cin·na·mine (rē-sin'ă-mēn, -min). 3,4,5-Trimethoxycinnamic acid ester of methyl reserpate; a purified ester alkaloid of the alseroxylon fraction of species of *Rauwolfia;* chemically and pharmacologically related to reserpine, with similar uses.

re·sect (rē-sekt'). **1.** To cut off, especially to cut off the articular ends of one or both bones forming a joint. **2.** To excise a segment of a part. [L. *re-seco,* pp. *sectus,* to cut off]

re·sect·a·ble (rē-sek'tă-bl). Amenable to resection.

re·sec·tion (rē-sek'shŭn). **1.** Removal of articular ends of one or both bones forming a joint. **2.** SYN excision (1).

gum r., SYN gingivectomy.

loop r., SYN loop *excision.*

Miles r., SYN Miles' *operation.*

muscle r., shortening of the tendon of the ocular muscle in strabismus.

Reichel-Pólya stomach r., retrocolic anastomosis of the full circumference of the open stomach to the jejunum.

root r., SYN apicoectomy.

scleral r., shortening of the outer coat of the eye in retinal separation.

transurethral r., endoscopic removal of the prostate gland or bladder lesions, usually for relief of prostatic obstruction or treatment of bladder malignancies.

wedge r., removal of a wedge-shaped portion of the ovary; used in the treatment of virilizing disorders of ovarian origin, such as the polycystic ovarian syndrome.

re·sec·to·scope (rē-sek'tō-skōp). A special endoscopic instrument for the transurethral electrosurgical removal of lesions involving the bladder, prostate gland, or urethra.

re·ser·pine (rē-ser'pēn, -pin). An ester alkaloid isolated from the root of certain species of *Rauwolfia;* it decreases the 5-hydroxytryptamine and catecholamine concentrations in the central nervous system and in peripheral tissues; used in conjunction with other hypotensive agents in the management of essential hypertension and is useful as a tranquilizer in psychotic states.

re·serve (rē-zerv'). Something available but held back for later use, as strength or carbohydrates. [L. *re-servo,* to keep back, reserve]

alkali r., the sum total of the basic ions (mainly bicarbonates) of the blood and other body fluids which, acting as buffers, maintain the normal pH of the blood.

breathing r., the difference between the pulmonary ventilation

reproduction							
asexual				sexual			
somatic		agamic		agamic		gamic	
poly-cytogen	mono-cytogen	mono-cytogen		mono-cytogen	mono-cytogen	dicytogen	
1	2	3	4	5	6	7	8

1. brood buds: e.g., echinococcus hyatid; fragmentation: e.g., actinomyces; 2. cell division, cell germination: e.g., protists, yeast; 3. mitoagamic: e.g., penicillium (gonidia); 4. meioagamic: e.g., mosses, ferns (spores); 5. meioagamic: e.g., basidiomycetes; 6. parthenogenesis: e.g., honey bee (♂); 7. mitogamic: e.g., mosses, ferns (gametes); 8. meiogamic: e.g., human beings, vertebrates

(*i.e.,* the volume of air breathed under ordinary resting conditions) and the maximum breathing capacity.

cardiac r., the work which the heart is able to perform beyond that required under the ordinary circumstances of daily life, depending upon the state of the myocardium and the degree to which, within physiologic limits, the cardiac muscle fibers can be stretched by the volume of blood reaching the heart during diastole.

res·er·voir (rez'ĕv-wor). SYN receptaculum. [Fr.]

r. of infection, living or nonliving material in or on which an infectious agent multiplies and/or develops and is dependent for its survival in nature.

Ommaya r., a plastic container placed in the subgaleal space which is connected to the lateral ventricle by tubing; it is used to instill medication into, or remove fluid from, the ventricle.

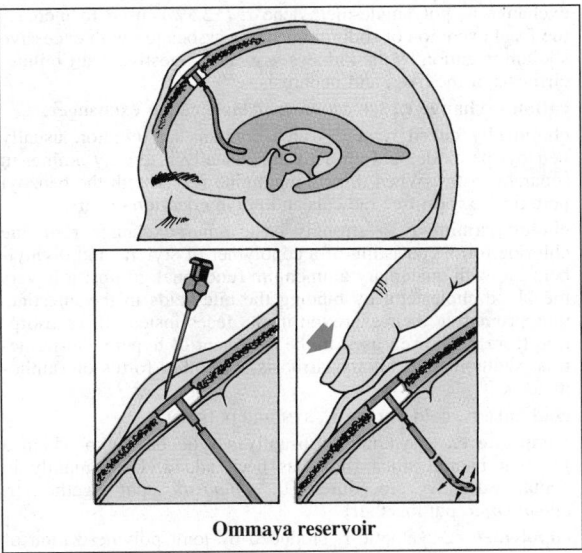

Ommaya reservoir

Pecquet's r., SYN *cisterna* chyli.

r. of spermatozoa, the site where spermatozoa are stored; the distal portion of the tail of the epididymis and the beginning of the ductus deferens.

vitelline r., SYN vitellarium.

re·set no·dus si·nu·a·tri·a·lis (rē'set nō'dŭs sī'nū-ă-trē-ā'lis). Reset of the sinoatrial node produced by premature depolarization (usually atrial) when the sum of the duration of the premature cycle and the return cycle is less than twice the spontaneous cycle length. Cf. nonreset nodus sinuatrialis.

res·i·dent (rez'i-dent). A house officer attached to a hospital for clinical training; formerly, one who actually resided in the hospital. SYN resident physician. [L. *resideo*, to reside]

re·sid·ua (rē-zid′yū-ă). Plural of residuum.

re·sid·u·al (rē-zid′yū-ăl). Relating to or of the nature of a residue.

res·i·due (rez′i-dū). That which remains after removal of one or more substances. SYN residuum. [L. *residuum*]

   day r., psychoanalytic term for a dream related to an experience of the previous day.

re·sid·u·um, pl. **re·sid·ua** (rē-zid′yū-ŭm, -yū-ă). SYN residue. [L. ntr. of *residuus*, left behind, remaining, fr. *re- sideo*, to sit back, remain behind]

re·sil·ience (rē-zil′yens). **1.** Energy (per unit of volume) released upon unloading. **2.** Springiness or elasticity. [L. *resilio*, to spring back, rebound]

res·in (rez′in). **1.** An amorphous brittle substance consisting of the hardened secretion of a number of plants, probably derived from a volatile oil and similar to a stearoptene. **2.** SYN rosin. **3.** A precipitate formed by the addition of water to certain tinctures. **4.** A broad term used to indicate organic substances insoluble in water; these monomers are named according to their chemical composition, physical structure, and means for activation or curing, *e.g.,* acrylic r., autopolymer r. [L. *resina*]

   acrylic r., a general term applied to a resinous material of the various esters of acrylic acid; used as a denture base material, for other dental restorations, and for trays.

   activated r., SYN autopolymer r.

   anion-exchange r., SEE anion exchange, anion exchanger.

   autopolymer r., autopolymerizing r., any r. that can be polymerized by chemical catalysis rather than by the application of heat; used in dentistry for dental restoration, denture repair, and impression trays. SYN activated r., cold cure r., cold-curing r., quick cure r., self-curing r.

   carbacrylamine r.'s, a mixture of the cation-exchange r.'s, carbacrylic r. and potassium carbacrylic r. (87.5%) and of the anion-exchange r., polyamine-methylene r. (12.5%), used to increase the fecal excretion of sodium in edema associated with excessive sodium retention by the kidneys, *e.g.,* in congestive heart failure, cirrhosis of the liver, and nephrosis.

   cation-exchange r., SEE cation exchange, cation exchanger.

   chemically cured r., a r. which contains an initiator, usually benzoyl peroxide, and an activator, usually a tertiary amine, in separate pastes. When mixed, the amine reacts with the benzoyl peroxide to form free radicals and polymerization occurs.

   cholestyramine r., a strongly basic anion-exchange r. in the chloride form, consisting of a copolymer of styrene and divinylbenzene with quaternary ammonium functional groups; it lowers the blood cholesterol by binding the bile acids in the intestine, thus promoting their excretion in the feces instead of reabsorption from the bowel; used in the treatment of hypercholesterolemia, xanthomatous biliary cirrhosis, and other forms of xanthomatosis.

   cold cure r., cold-curing r., SYN autopolymer r.

   composite r., a synthetic r. usually acrylic based, to which a glass or natural silica filter has been added. Used mainly in dental restorative procedures. [L. *compositus*, put together, fr. *compono*, to put together]

   copolymer r., synthetic r. produced by joint polymerization of two or more different monomers or polymers.

   cross-linked r., SYN cross-linked *polymer.*

   direct filling r., an autopolymerizing r. especially designed as a dental restorative material.

   dual-cure r., a r. which utilizes both light and chemical initiation to activate polymerization.

   epoxy r., any thermosetting r. based on the reactivity of epoxy; used as adhesives, protective coatings, and embedding media for electron microscopy.

   gum r., the dry exudate from a number of plants, consisting of a mixture of a gum and a r., the former soluble in water but not alcohol, the latter soluble in alcohol but not water.

   heat-curing r., r. that requires heat to initiate polymerization.

   Indian podophyllum r., r. obtained from *Podophyllum emodi;* a cathartic and cholagogue.

   ion-exchange r., SEE ion exchange, ion exchanger.

   ipomea r., r. obtained from the dried root of *Ipomoea orizabensis;* a cathartic. SEE ALSO scammony.

   jalap r., r. extracted from the dried tuberous root of *Exogonium purga;* a purgative.

   light-activated r., SYN light-cured r.

   light-cured r., a r. which uses visible or ultraviolet light to excite a photoinitiator which interacts with an amine to form free radicals and initiate polymerization. Used mainly in restorative dentistry. SYN light-activated r.

   melamine r., a plastic material mixed with plaster of Paris for casts. Such a cast is lighter and stronger than one made with plaster of Paris alone. SYN melamine formaldehyde.

   methacrylate r., polymerized methacrylic acid; a translucent plastic material, used for the manufacture of various medical appliances, surgical instruments, and seating components used in total joint replacement; it possesses the optical properties of fused quartz, and is readily molded when heated; formerly used in electron microscopy for embedding tissues, now superseded by epoxy r.'s.

   Podophyllum r., a r. extracted from the dried roots and rhizomes of *Podophyllum peltatum*, a perennial herb common in moist, shady situations in the eastern parts of Canada and the United States. The drug has been used by American Indians as a vermifuge and emetic. The chief constituents of the r. belong to the group of lignins, which are C_{118} compounds related biosynthetically to the flavonoids and derived by dimerization of two C_6-C_3 units. The most important ones present in podophyllum r. are podophyllotoxin (about 20%), β-peltatin (about 10%) and α-peltatin (about 5%). All three occur both free and as glucosides. The r. has been used as a purgative but has been replaced by milder agents. It is cytotoxic and used as a paint in the treatment of soft venereal and other warts.

   podophyllum r., a mixture of r.'s obtained from the dried rhizomes and roots of *Podophyllum peltatum* or *P. hexandrum;* used as a laxative. SYN May apple root, podophyllin, wild mandrake.

   polyamine-methylene r., a synthetic acid-binding r. used as a gastric antacid.

   polyester r., r. in which the polymers are insoluble in most organic solvents and are polymerized by light, heat, or oxygen; used in electron microscopy as a tissue embedding medium.

   quick cure r., SYN autopolymer r.

   quinine carbacrylic r., SYN azuresin.

   self-curing r., SYN autopolymer r.

res·in ac·ids. A class of organic compounds derived from various natural plant resins; diterpenes containing a phenanthrene ring system; *e.g.,* abietic acid, pimaric acid, ester gums. SYN resinic acids.

res·in·ates (rez′in-āts). Salts or esters of resin acids.

res·ines (rez′ēns). Esters of resin acids.

res·in·ic ac·ids. SYN resin acids.

res·in·oid (rez′i-noyd). **1.** A substance containing a resin or resembling one. **2.** An extract obtained by evaporating a tincture. **3.** Resembling rosin.

res·in·ols (rez′i-nols). Resin alcohols.

res·in·ous (rez′i-nŭs). Relating to or derived from a resin.

re·sis·tance (rē-zis′tans). **1.** A passive force exerted in opposition to another active force. **2.** The opposition in a conductor to the passage of a current of electricity, whereby there is a loss of energy and a production of heat; specifically, the potential difference in volts across the conductor per ampere of current flow; unit: ohm. Cf. impedance. **3.** The opposition to flow of a fluid through one or more passageways (*e.g.,* blood flow, respiratory gases in the tracheobronchial tree), analogous to (2); units are usually those of pressure difference per unit flow. Cf. impedance (2). **4.** In psychoanalysis, an individual's unconscious defense against bringing repressed thoughts to consciousness. **5.** The ability of red blood cells to resist hemolysis and to preserve their shape under varying degrees of osmotic pressure in the blood plasma. **6.** The natural or acquired ability of an organism to maintain its immunity to or to resist the effects of an antagonistic agent, *e.g.,* pathogenic microorganism, toxin, drug. [L. *re-sisto,* to stand back, withstand]

airway r., in physiology, the r. to flow of gases during ventilation due to obstruction or turbulent flow in the upper and lower airways; to be differentiated during inhalation from r. to inflation due to decreases in pulmonary or thoracic compliance.

bacteriophage r., r. of a bacterial mutant to infection by a bacteriophage to which the parent (wild type) strain is susceptible.

dicumarol r., a well-defined autosomal dominant resistance to it, over and above general variability in tolerance to the drug.

drug r., the capacity of disease-causing pathogens to withstand drugs previously toxic to them; achieved by spontaneous mutation or through selective pressure after exposure to the drug in question.

> Overprescription of antibiotics has contributed to the development of resistant strains as has massive dosing of food animals, generally through antibiotic-laced feed. (Resistant strains are then passed to humans by unsanitary kitchen practices or insufficient cooking.) Drug resistance has become a problem facing clinicians worldwide. Numerous strains of bacteria and parasites have developed resistance, including those causing bacterial pneumonia (*Streptococcus pneumoniae*), malaria (*Plasmodium falciparum*), tuberculosis (*Mycobacterium tuberculosis*), and gonorrhea (*Neisseria gonorrhoeae*). Resistant strains of streptococcal and staphylococcal bacteria have become prevalent in the U.S., particularly among children. Especially worrisome to public health officials is the spread of antibiotic-resistant tuberculosis since the mid-1980s. Throughout Southeast Asia, China, and Haiti, about 5% (and in places as many as 20%) of Mycobacterium strains are suspected to have developed resistance. In Miami and New York City, HIV patients have presented with tuberculosis that fails to respond to treatment with a single drug. Currently, a four-drug regimen is advised (isoniazid, rifampin, pyrazinamide, ethambutol), along with close monitoring to ensure that patients complete the therapy, since failure of previous patients to do so appears to be the principal manner in which resistant strains have arisen.

expiratory r., r. to flow of gas out of the lungs or the total r. to flow of gas during the expiratory phase of the respiratory cycle.

impact r., the ability of a lens for eyewear to withstand impact without shattering or breaking, *i.e.,* of a ⅜ -inch steel ball dropped 50 feet; criteria for determination of impact r. are specified by U.S. regulations.

inductive r., SYN reactance.

insulin r., diminished effectiveness of insulin in lowering blood sugar levels; arbitrarily defined as requiring 200 units or more of insulin per day to prevent hyperglycemia or ketosis; usually due to insulin binding by antibodies, but abnormalities in insulin receptors on cell surfaces also occur; associated with obesity, ketoacidosis, infection, and certain rare conditions.

multidrug r., the insensitivity of various tumors to a variety of chemically related anticancer drugs; mediated by a process of inactivating the drug or removing it from the target tumor cells.

mutual r., SYN antagonism.

peripheral r., SYN total peripheral r.

synaptic r., the ease or difficulty with which a nerve impulse can cross a synapse.

systemic vascular r., an index of arteriolar compliance or constriction throughout the body; equal to the blood pressure divided by the cardiac output.

thyrotropin r., an autosomal recessive disorder in which the thyrocytes are unresponsive to thyrotropin. Cf. pseudohypoparathyroidism.

total peripheral r. (TPR), the total r. to flow of blood in the systemic circuit; the quotient produced by dividing the mean arterial pressure by the cardiac minute-volume. SYN peripheral r.

---

biochemical mechanisms of bacterial resistance

1. enzymatic inactivation: penicillins, cephalosporins, aminoglycosides, chloramphenicol

2. reduced cell permeability: tetracyclines, sulfonamides

3. changes within the receptor (or its environment): streptomycin, rifampicin, sulfonamides

---

re·sis·tiv·i·ty (rē′zis-tiv′i-tē). A measure of a material's resistance to the passage of electrical current; the reciprocal of conductivity. [L. *re-sito,* to withstand]

re·sis·tor (rē-zis′ter, -tŏr). An element included in an electrical circuit to provide resistance to the flow of current.

res·o·lu·tion (rez-ō-lū′shŭn). **1.** The arrest of an inflammatory process without suppuration; the absorption or breaking down and removal of the products of inflammation or of a new growth. SEE line *pairs,* under *pair.* **2.** The optical ability to distinguish detail such as the separation of closely adjacent objects. SYN resolving power (3). [L. *resolutio,* a slackening, fr. *re-solvo,* pp. *-solutus,* to loosen, relax]

re·sol·vase (rē-sol-vas). A gene encoded by a transposon that can catalyze a second stage of transposition as well as participate in the regulation of its own expression. [resolve + -ase]

re·solve (rē-zolv′). To return or cause to return to the normal, particularly without suppuration, said of a phlegmon or other form of inflammation. [L. *resolvo,* to loosen]

re·sol·vent (rē-zol′vent). **1.** Causing resolution. **2.** An agent that arrests an inflammatory process or causes the absorption of a neoplasm.

res·o·nance (rez′ō-nans). **1.** Sympathetic or forced vibration of air in the cavities above, below, in front of, or behind a source of sound; in speech, modification of the quality (*e.g.,* tone) of a sound by the passage of air through the chambers of the nose, pharynx, and head, without increasing the intensity of the sound. **2.** The sound obtained on percussing a part that can vibrate freely. **3.** The intensification and hollow character of the voice sound obtained on auscultating over a cavity. **4.** In chemistry, the manner in which electrons or electric charges are distributed among the atoms in compounds that are planar and symmetrical, particularly those with conjugated (alternating) double bonds; the existence of r. in the latter case lowers the energy content and increases the stability of a compound. **5.** The natural or inherent frequency of any oscillating system. **6.** SYN resonant *frequency.* [L. *resonantia,* echo, fr. *re-sono,* to resound, to echo]

amphoric r., a percussion sound, like that produced by striking a large empty bottle, obtained by percussing over a pulmonary cavity. SYN cavernous r.

bandbox r., SYN vesiculotympanitic r.

bellmetal r., in cases of a large pulmonary cavity or of pneumothorax, a clear metallic sound obtained by striking a coin, held against the chest, by another coin, or by flicking the chest wall with one's fingernail; the sound is heard on auscultating the chest wall on the same side anteroposteriorly. SYN anvil sound, bell sound, coin test.

cavernous r., SYN amphoric r.

cracked-pot r., a peculiar sound, resembling that heard on striking a cracked pot, elicited on percussing over a pulmonary cavity that commmunicates with a bronchial tube, when the patient's mouth is open. SYN cracked-pot sound.

electron paramagnetic r. (EPR), SYN electron spin r.

electron spin r. (ESR), a spectrometric method, based on measurement of electron spins and magnetic moments, for detecting and estimating free radicals in reactions and in biological systems. SYN electron paramagnetic r.

hydatid r., a peculiar vibratile r. heard on auscultatory percussion over a hydatid cyst.

nuclear magnetic r. (NMR), the phenomenon in which certain atomic nuclei possessing a magnetic moment will precess around the axis of a strong external magnetic field, the frequency of precession (Larmor frequency) being specific for each nucleus and the strength of the magnetic field; spinning nuclei induce their own oscillating magnetic fields and therefore emit electromagnetic radiation that can produce a detectable signal at the Larmor frequency. NMR is used as a method of identifying covalent bonds and is applied clinically in magnetic resonance *imaging*.

skodaic r., a peculiar, high-pitched sound, less musical than that obtained over a cavity, elicited by percussion just above the level of a pleuritic effusion. SYN Skoda's sign, Skoda's tympany.

tympanitic r., SYN tympany.

vesicular r., the sound obtained on percussing over the normal lungs.

vesiculotympanitic r., a peculiar, partly tympanitic, partly vesicular sound, obtained on percussion in cases of pulmonary emphysema. SYN bandbox r., wooden r.

vocal r. (VR), the voice sounds as heard on auscultation of the chest.

wooden r., SYN vesiculotympanitic r.

res·o·na·tor (rez'ō-nā-ter). A device for employing inductance to create an electrical current of very high potential and small volume.

re·sorb (rē-sōrb'). To reabsorb; to absorb what has been excreted, as an exudate or pus. [L. *re-sorbeo,* to suck back]

res·or·cin (rē-zōr'sin). SYN resorcinol.

res·or·cin·ol (rē-zōr'si-nol). *m*-dihydroxybenzene; 1,3-benzenediol; used internally for the relief of nausea, asthma, whooping cough, and diarrhea, but chiefly as an external antiseptic in psoriasis, eczema, seborrhea, and ringworm; pyrocatechol and hydroquinone are isomers of r. SYN resorcin.

r. monoacetate, used externally in the treatment of acne, sycosis, and seborrhea.

r. phthalic anhydride, SYN fluorescein.

res·or·cin·ol·phtha·lein (rē-zōr'si-nol-thal'ē-in). SYN fluorescein.

r. sodium, SYN *fluorescein* sodium.

re·sorp·tion (rē-sōrp'shŭn). **1.** The act of resorbing. **2.** A loss of substance by lysis, or by physiologic or pathologic means.

bone r., the removal of osseous tissue.

gingival r., SYN gingival *recession*.

horizontal r., SYN horizontal *atrophy*.

internal r., a loss of tooth structure originating within the pulp cavity.

ridge r., a loss in the volume and size of the alveolar portion of the mandible or maxilla.

root r., dissolution of the root of a tooth; either external, with loss or blunting of the apical portion, or internal, with loss of dentin from the inside (pulpal) part of the root area.

res·pi·ra·ble (re-spīr'ă-bl, res'pĭ-ră-bl). Capable of being breathed.

res·pi·ra·tion (res-pi-rā'shŭn). **1.** A fundamental process of life, characteristic of both plants and animals, in which oxygen is used to oxidize organic fuel molecules, providing a source of energy as well as carbon dioxide and water. In green plants, photosynthesis is not considered r. **2.** SYN ventilation (2). [L. *respiratio,* fr. *re-spiro,* pp. *-atus,* to exhale, breathe]

abdominal r., breathing effected mainly by the action of the diaphragm.

aerobic r., a form of r. in which molecular oxygen is consumed and carbon dioxide and water are produced.

amphoric r., a sound like that made by blowing across the mouth of a bottle, heard on auscultation in some cases in which a large pulmonary cavity exists, or occasionally in pneumothorax.

anaerobic r., a form of r. in which molecular oxygen is not consumed; *e.g.,* nitrate r., sulfate r.

artificial r., SYN artificial *ventilation*.

assisted r., SYN assisted *ventilation*.

Biot's r., abrupt, irregular alternating periods of apnea with constant rate and depth of breathing, as that resulting from le-

sions due to increased intracranial pressure. SYN ataxic breathing, Biot's breathing, respiratory ataxia.

Biot's r., completely irregular breathing pattern, with continually variable rate and depth of breathing; results from lesions in the respiratory centers in the brainstem, extending from the dorsomedial medulla caudally to the obex.

bronchial r., a tubular blowing sound caused by the passage of air through a bronchus in an area of consolidated lung tissue.

bronchovesicular r., combined bronchial and vesicular r.

cavernous r., a hollow reverberating sound heard on auscultation over a cavity in the lung.

Cheyne-Stokes r., the pattern of breathing with gradual increase in depth and sometimes in rate to a maximum, followed by a decrease resulting in apnea; the cycles ordinarily are 30 seconds to 2 minutes in duration, with 5 to 30 seconds of apnea; seen with bilateral deep febrile hemisphere lesions, with metabolic encephalopathy and, characteristically in coma from affection of the nervous centers of respiration.

cogwheel r., the inspiratory sound being broken into two or three by silent intervals. SYN interrupted r., jerky r.

controlled r., SYN controlled *ventilation*.

costal r., SYN thoracic r.

diffusion r., maintenance of oxygenation during apnea by intratracheal insufflation of oxygen at high flow rates. SYN apneic oxygenation.

electrophrenic r., the rhythmical electrical stimulation of the phrenic nerve by an electrode applied to the skin at the motor points of the phrenic nerve; it is used in paralysis of the respiratory center resulting from acute bulbar poliomyelitis.

external r., the exchange of respiratory gases in the lungs as distinguished from internal or tissue r.

forced r., voluntary hyperventilation.

internal r., SYN tissue r.

interrupted r., SYN cogwheel r.

jerky r., SYN cogwheel r.

Kussmaul r., deep, rapid r. characteristic of diabetic or other causes of acidosis. SYN Kussmaul-Kien r.

Kussmaul-Kien r., SYN Kussmaul r.

labored r., difficult, usually deep, breathing in patients with cardiac or pulmonary disease or disease affecting nervous system control of ventilation.

mouth-to-mouth r., a method of artificial ventilation involving an overlap of the patient's mouth (and nose in small children) with the operator's mouth to inflate the patient's lungs by blowing, followed by an unassisted expiratory phase brought about by elastic recoil of the patient's chest and lungs; repeated 12 to 16 times a minute; where the nose is not covered by the operator's mouth, the nostrils must be closed by pinching.

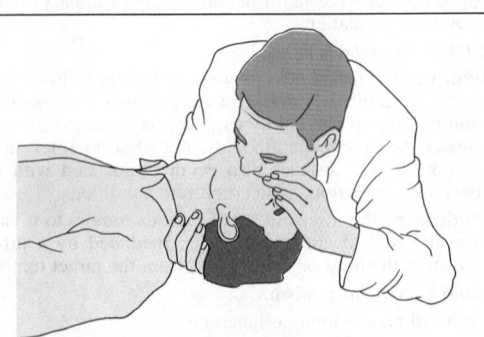

mouth-to-mouth respiration

tilt back head, closing nose of patient, and blow in (exhaled air); passive expiration by patient; frequency: 10-12 times per minute

nitrate r., the process of r. used by some anaerobic organisms, in which nitrate rather than molecular oxygen is used to oxidize organic molecules to obtain energy.

paradoxical r., deflation of the lung during inspiration and inflation of the lung during the phase of expiration; seen in the lung on the side of an open pneumothorax.

puerile r., an exaggeration of the normal respiratory sounds, heard in children and in adults after exertion.

stertorous r., harsh, noisy breathing usually heard in an comatous patient. SYN stertorous breathing.

sulfate r., the process of r. used by some anaerobic organisms, in which sulfate rather than molecular oxygen is used to oxidize organic molecules to obtain energy.

thoracic r., r. effected chiefly by the action of the intercostal and other muscles that raise the ribs, causing expansion of the chest. SYN costal r.

tissue r., the interchange of gases between the blood and the tissues. SYN internal r.

tubular r., high-pitched bronchial r.

vesicular r., the respiratory murmur heard on auscultating over the normal lung. SYN respiratory murmur, vesicular murmur.

vesiculocavernous r., cavernous r., due to the presence of a cavity, mingled with the vesicular murmur of the surrounding normal lung tissue.

res·pi·ra·tor (res′pi-rā-ter, -tōr). **1.** An appliance fitting over the mouth and nose, used for the purpose of excluding dust, smoke, or other irritants, or of otherwise altering the air before it enters the respiratory passages. SYN inhaler (1). **2.** An apparatus for administering artificial respiration, especially for a prolonged period, in cases of paralysis or inadequate spontaneous ventilation.

cuirass r., one of several types of r.'s producing alternating negative pressure about the thoracic cage; now rarely used.

Drinker r., a mechanical r. in which the body except the head is encased within a metal tank, which is sealed at the neck with an airtight gasket; artificial respiration is induced by making the air pressure inside negative. SYN iron lung, tank r.

pressure-controlled r., a r. that provides a predetermined pressure to gases during inhalation, the volume of gas moved being variable, depending upon resistance.

tank r., SYN Drinker r.

volume-controlled r., a r. that provides a predetermined volume of gases during inhalation, with the pressure required to move that volume remaining variable, depending upon resistance.

res·pi·ra·to·ry (res′pi-ră-tōr-ē, rĕ-spīr′ă-tōr-ē). Relating to respiration.

re·spire (rĕ-spīr′). **1.** To breathe. **2.** To consume oxygen and produce carbon dioxide by metabolism. [L. *respiro,* to breathe]

res·pi·rom·e·ter (res-pĭ-rom′ĕ-ter). **1.** An instrument for measuring the extent of the respiratory movements. **2.** An instrument for measuring oxygen consumption or carbon dioxide production, usually of an isolated tissue. [L. *respiro,* to breathe, + G. *metron,* measure]

Dräger r., an inferential meter to measure tidal and minute volume from the number of revolutions of a vane rotated by the gas stream as the latter passes through two lightweight lozenge-shaped meshing rotors.

Wright r., an inferential meter to measure tidal and minute volume from the number of revolutions of a vane rotated by the gas stream as the latter passes through 10 tangential slots in a cylindrical stator ring to turn a flat two-bladed rotor.

re·sponse (rē-spons′). **1.** The reaction of a muscle, nerve, gland, or other excitable tissue to a stimulus. **2.** Any act or behavior, or its constituents, that a living organism is capable of emitting. Reflexes are usually excluded because they are typically elicited by a specifiable (unconditioned or natural) stimulus rather than emitted under circumstances in which the stimulus was not specifiable. [L. *responsus,* an answer]

anamnestic r. (an′am-nes-tik), SYN secondary immune r. SEE immune r.

biphasic r., (1) two separate and distinct responses that are separated in time; (2) immediate reaction to an antigenic challenge followed by a recurrence of symptoms after an interval of quiescence.

booster r., SYN secondary immune r. SEE immune r.

conditioned r., a r. already in an individual's repertoire but

which, through repeated pairings with its natural stimulus, has been acquired or conditioned anew to a previously neutral or conditioned stimulus. SEE conditioning. Cf. unconditioned r.

Cushing r., SYN Cushing *phenomenon.*

depletion r., subnormal metabolic r. to trauma in a person whose physiologic processes are already depressed by disease.

early-phase r., prompt onset of symptoms following an antigenic stimulus.

evoked r., an alteration in the electrical activity of a region of the nervous system through which an incoming sensory stimulus is passing; may be somatosensory (SER), auditory (BAER), or visual (VER). SEE ALSO evoked *potential.*

flight or fight r., SEE emergency *theory.*

galvanic skin r. (GSR), a measure of changes in emotional arousal recorded by attaching electrodes to any part of the skin and recording changes in moment-to-moment perspiration and related autonomic nervous system activity. SYN galvanic skin reaction, galvanic skin reflex, psychogalvanic reaction, psychogalvanic skin reaction, psychogalvanic reflex, psychogalvanic skin reflex, psychogalvanic r., psychogalvanic skin r.

Henry-Gauer r., inhibition of antidiuretic hormone secretion due to a rise in atrial pressure which stimulates atrial stretch receptors.

immune r., (1) any r. of the immune system to an antigen including antibody production and/or cell-mediated immunity; **(2)** the r. of the immune system to an antigen (immunogen) that leads to the condition of induced sensitivity; the immune r. to the initial antigenic exposure (primary immune r.) is detectable, as a rule, only after a lag period of from several days to two weeks; the immune r. to a subsequent stimulus (secondary immune r.) by the same antigen is more rapid than in the case of the primary immune r.

isomorphic r., SYN Köbner's *phenomenon.*

late-phase r., recurrence of symptoms after an appreciable interval following challenge with an antigen; preceded by an initial early-phase r.

oculomotor r., widespread myogenic potential evoked by visual stimuli.

orienting r., SYN orienting *reflex.*

primary immune r., SEE immune r.

psychogalvanic r. (PGR), psychogalvanic skin r., SYN galvanic skin r.

recruiting r., SYN recruitment (2).

relaxation r., an integrated hypothalamic reaction resulting in decreased sympathetic nervous system activity which, physiologically and psychologically, is almost a mirror image of the body's r.'s to Cannon's emergency theory (flight or fight r.); can be self-induced through the use of techniques associated with transcendental meditation, yoga, and biofeedback. SEE ALSO emergency *theory.*

secondary immune r., SYN anamnestic r., booster r. SEE immune r.

sonomotor r., widespread myogenic potential evoked by click stimulation.

stringent r., the cellular response to amino acid starvation that reduces the amount of ribosomes to what can be employed under the nutrient conditions.

target r., SYN operant.

triple r., the triphasic r. to the firm stroking of the skin: Phase 1 is the sharply demarcated erythema that follows a momentary blanching of the skin, and is the result of release of histamine from the mast cells. Phase 2 is the intense red flare extending beyond the margins of the line of pressure but in the same configuration, and is the result of arteriolar dilation; also called axon flare because it is mediated by axon reflex. Phase 3 is the appearance of a line wheal in the configuration of the original stroking.

unconditioned r., a r., such as salivation, which is a part of the animal or human repertoire. Cf. conditioned r.

rest. 1. Quiet; repose. [A.S. *raest*] **2.** To repose; to cease from work. [A.S. *raestan*] **3.** A group of cells or a portion of fetal tissue that has become displaced and lies embedded in tissue of another character. [L. *restare,* to remain] **4.** In dentistry, an extension from a prosthesis that affords vertical support for a restoration.

adrenal r., SYN accessory *adrenal*.

bed r., maintenance of the recumbent position, in bed, to minimize activity and help recovery from disease; formerly used extensively in treatment of tuberculosis, myocardial infarction, and other diseases.

cingulum r., the rigid part of a removable partial denture supported by a prepared r. area on the cingulum of an anterior tooth or crown.

incisal r., the portion of a removable partial denture supported by an incisal edge.

lingual r., a metallic extension onto the lingual surface of a tooth to provide support or indirect retention for a removable partial denture.

Malassez' epithelial r.'s, epithelial remains of Hertwig's root sheath in the periodontal ligament.

Marchand's r., SYN Marchand's *adrenals*, under *adrenal*.

mesonephric r., SYN wolffian r.

occlusal r., a rigid extension of a removable partial denture onto the occlusal surface of a posterior tooth for support of the prosthesis.

precision r., a r. consisting of closely interlocking parts.

r.'s of Serres, remnants of dental lamina epithelium entrapped within the gingiva.

Walthard's cell r., a nest of epithelial cells occurring in the peritoneum of the uterine tubes or ovary; when neoplastic, possibly comprising one of the components of the Brenner tumor.

wolffian r., remnants of the wolffian duct in the female genital tract that give rise to cysts; *e.g.,* Gartner's cyst. SYN mesonephric r.

re·ste·no·sis (rē'sten-ō-sis). Recurrence of stenosis after corrective surgery on the heart valve; narrowing of a structure (usually a coronary artery) following the removal or reduction of a previous narrowing. [re-, + G. *stenōsis,* a narrowing]

res·ti·form (res'ti-fōrm). Ropelike; rope-shaped; referring to the restiform body, the larger (lateral) part of the inferior cerebellar peduncle; contains fibers from the spinal cord (spinocerebellar) and medulla (cuneo-, olivo-, reticulocerebellar, etc.) to cerebellum. [L. *restis,* rope, + *forma,* form]

rest·i·tope (res'ti-tōp). The part of the T cell receptor that associates with the class II major histocompatibility molecule. [*restriction* + *-tope*]

res·ti·tu·tion (res-ti-tū'shŭn). In obstetrics, the return of the rotated head of the fetus to its natural relation with the shoulders after its emergence from the vulva. [L. *restitutio,* act of restoring]

res·to·ra·tion (res-tō-rā'shŭn). In dentistry: **1.** A prosthetic r. or appliance; a broad term applied to any inlay, crown, bridge, partial denture, or complete denture which restores or replaces lost tooth structure, teeth, or oral tissues. **2.** A plug or stopping; any substance such as gold, amalgam, etc., used for restoring the portion missing from a tooth as a result of removing decay in the tooth. [L. *restauro,* pp. *-atus,* to restore, to repair]

acid-etched r., the r. of tooth structure with a resin after the surface of the tooth has been treated with an acid solution that etches the tooth surface, thereby increasing retention of the r.

combination r., a tooth r. of two or more materials applied in layers.

compound r., a r. of more than one surface of a tooth.

direct acrylic r., a direct resin r. of autopolymerizing acrylic.

direct composite resin r., SYN direct resin r.

direct resin r., a direct r. made by inserting a plastic mix of auto or light-polymerized resins in a cavity prepared in a tooth. SYN direct composite resin r.

overhanging r., a r. with excessive material at the junction of the r. margin and the tooth.

permanent r., a definitive r., in contradistinction to a temporary or provisional r.

root canal r., a gutta-percha, silver, or plastic cone that has been carried into a root canal, either alone or in conjunction with a cement, paste, or solvent, for the purpose of obturating the canal space.

silicate r.'s, r.'s of lost tooth structure made with silicate cement.

temporary r., a r. to be used for a limited period of time, in contradistinction to a permanent r.

re·stor·a·tive (re-stōr'ă-tiv). **1.** Renewing health and strength. **2.** An agent that promotes a renewal of health or strength. [L. *restauro,* to restore]

re·straint (re-strānt'). In hospital psychiatry, intervention to prevent an excited or violent patient from doing harm to himself or others; may involve the use of a camisole (straightjacket). [O. Fr. *restrainte*]

re·stric·tion (re-strik'shŭn). **1.** The process with which foreign DNA that has been introduced into a prokaryotic cell becomes ineffective. **2.** A limitation.

lactase r., an inherited trait in which there is low lactase activity and thus there is defective lactose intestinal metabolism. Cf. lactase *persistence*.

MHC r., T helper cells recognize an antigen that is presented with class II major histocompatibility antigens while T cytotoxic cells usually only recognize a processed antigen in conjunction with class I major histocompatibility antigens.

re·sus·ci·tate (rē-sŭs'i-tāt). To perform resuscitation. [L. *re-suscito,* to raise up again, revive]

re·sus·ci·ta·tion (rē-sŭs'i-tā'shŭn). Revival from potential or apparent death. [L. *resuscitatio*]

cardiopulmonary r. (CPR), restoration of cardiac output and pulmonary ventilation following cardiac arrest and apnea, using artificial respiration and manual closed chest compression or open chest cardiac massage.

mouth-to-mouth r., mouth-to-mouth respiration employed as part of emergency cardiopulmonary r.

re·sus·ci·ta·tor (rē-sŭs'i-tā-ter, -tŏr). Obsolete term for an apparatus that forces gas (usually O_2) into lungs to produce artificial ventilation.

re·tain·er (re-tān'er). Any type of clasp, attachment, or device used for the fixation or stabilization of a prosthesis; an appliance used to prevent the shifting of teeth following orthodontic treatment.

continuous bar r., a metal bar, usually resting on lingual surfaces of teeth, to aid in their stabilization and to act as indirect r.'s. SYN continuous clasp.

direct r., a clasp or attachment applied to an abutment tooth for the purpose of maintaining a removable appliance in position.

extracoronal r., a r. that depends upon contact with the outer circumference of the crown of a tooth for its retentive qualities.

Hawley r., a removable wire and acrylic palatal appliance used to retain or stabilize the teeth in their new position following orthodontic tooth movement; with modifications it can be used to move teeth as an active orthodontic appliance. SYN Hawley appliance.

indirect r., a part of a removable partial denture which assists the direct r.'s in preventing occlusal displacement of the distal extension bases by functioning through lever action on the opposite side of the fulcrum line.

intracoronal r., a r. that depends upon components placed within the crown portion of a tooth for its retentive qualities.

matrix r., a mechanical device designed to hold a matrix around a tooth during restorative procedures, usually by engaging the ends of the matrix band and drawing the band tight.

space r., SYN space *maintainer*.

re·tard·ate (rē-tahr'dāt). A mildly pejorative term, which is decreasing in usage, for a person who has mental retardation. [L. *retardo,* to delay, hinder]

re·tar·da·tion (rē-tahr-dā'shŭn). Slowness or limitation of development.

mental r., subaverage general intellectual functioning that originates during the developmental period and is associated with impairment in adaptive behavior. The American Association on Mental Deficiency lists eight medical classifications and five psychological classifications; the latter five replace the three former classifications of moron, imbecile, and idiot. Mental r. classification requires assignment of an index for performance relative to a person's peers on two interrelated criteria: measured intelligence (IQ) and overall socio-adaptive behavior (a judgmental rating of the individual's relative level of performance in school, at work, at home, and in the community). In general an IQ of 70 or below indicates mental retardation. (mild = 50/55-70; moderate= 35/40-50/55; severe = 20/25-35/40; profound = below 20/25); an IQ of 70-85 signifies borderline intellectual functioning. SYN amentia (1), mental deficiency, oligophrenia.

psychomotor r., slowed psychic activity or motor activity, or both.

viscoelastic r., a technique for the measurement of the molecular weight of large DNA molecules; the DNA is stretched by hydrodynamic shear forces and, when the molecules relax, the relaxation time is measured.

re·tard·er (rē-tar′der). An agent used to slow the chemical hardening of gypsum, resins, or impression materials used in dentistry.

retch. To make an involuntary effort to vomit. [A.S. *hraecan,* to hawk]

retch·ing. Gastric and esophageal movements of vomiting without expulsion of vomitus. SYN dry vomiting, vomiturition.

re·te, pl. **re·tia** (rē′tē; rē′shē-ă, -tē-ă) [NA]. **1.** SYN network (1). **2.** A structure composed of a fibrous network or mesh. [L. a net]

r. acromia′le [NA], SYN acromial arterial *network.*

r. arterio′sum [NA], SYN arteriolar *network.*

r. articula′re cu′biti [NA], SYN articular vascular *network* of elbow.

r. articula′re ge′nus [NA], SYN articular vascular *network* of knee.

r. calca′neum [NA], SYN calcaneal arterial *network.*

r. cana′lis hypoglos′si, SYN *plexus* of hypoglossal canal.

r. car′pi dorsa′le [NA], SYN dorsal carpal *network.*

r. car′pi poste′rius, SYN dorsal carpal *network.*

r. cuta′neum co′rii, the network of vessels parallel to the surface between the corium and the tela subcutanea.

r. foram′inis ova′lis, SYN venous *plexus* of foramen ovale.

Haller's r., r. hal′leri, SYN r. testis.

r. malleola′re latera′le [NA], SYN lateral malleolar *network.*

r. malleola′re media′le [NA], SYN medial malleolar *network.*

malpighian r., SYN malpighian *stratum.*

r. mirab′ile [NA], a vascular network interrupting the continuity of an artery or vein, such as occurs in the glomeruli of the kidney (arterial) or in the liver (venous).

r. ova′rii, a transient network of cells in the developing ovary; homologous to the r. testis.

r. patel′lae [NA], SYN patellar *network.*

r. subpapilla′re, the network of vessels between the papillary and reticular strata of the corium.

r. tes′tis [NA], the network of canals at the termination of the straight tubules in the mediastinum testis. SYN Haller's r., r. halleri.

r. vasculosum articula′re [NA], SYN articular vascular *network.*

r. veno′sum dorsa′le ma′nus [NA], SYN dorsal venous *network* of hand.

r. veno′sum dorsa′le pe′dis [NA], SYN dorsal venous *network* of foot.

r. veno′sum planta′re [NA], SYN plantar venous *network.*

re·ten·tion (rē-ten′shŭn). **1.** The keeping in the body of what normally belongs there, especially the retaining of food and drink in the stomach. **2.** The keeping in the body of what normally should be discharged, as urine or feces. **3.** Retaining that which has been learned so that it can be utilized later as in recall, recognition, or, if r. is partial, relearning. SEE ALSO memory. **4.** Resistance to dislodgement. **5.** In dentistry, a passive period following treatment when a patient is wearing an appliance or appliances to maintain or stabilize the teeth in the new position into which they have been moved. [L. *retentio,* a holding back]

denture r., the means by which dentures are held in position in the mouth.

direct r., r. obtained in a removable partial denture by the use of attachments or clasps which resist their removal from the abutment teeth.

indirect r., r. obtained in a removable partial denture through the use of indirect retainers.

partial denture r., the fixation of a removable partial denture by the use of clasps, indirect retainers, or precision attachments.

re·tia (rē′shē-ă, -tē-ă). Plural of rete. [L.]

re·ti·al (rē′shē-ăl). Relating to a rete.

⚠**reticul-.** SEE reticulo-.

re·tic·u·la (re-tik′yū-lă). Plural of reticulum. [L.]

re·tic·u·lar, re·tic·u·lated (re-tik′yū-lăr, -lāt-ed). Relating to a reticulum.

re·tic·u·la·tion (re-tik-yū-lā′shŭn). The presence or formation of a reticulum or network, such as that observed in the red blood cells during active regeneration of blood. Also used to describe a chest radiographic pattern. SEE reticulonodular *pattern.*

re·tic·u·lin (re-tik′yū-lin). Name given to the chemical substance of reticular fibers, which once were thought to be distinct from collagen by reason of their distinctive structure and staining properties but are now regarded as type III collagen (with its associated proteoglygans and structural glycoproteins).

re·tic·u·li·tis (re-tik′yū-lī′tis). Inflammation of the reticulum of ruminant animals. [reticul- + G. *-itis,* inflammation]

⚠**reticulo-, reticul-.** Reticulum; reticular. [L. *reticulum,* a small net, dim. of *rete,* a net]

re·tic·u·lo·cyte (re-tik′yū-lō-sīt). A young red blood cell with a network of precipitated basophilic substance representing residual polyribosomes, and occurring during the process of active blood regeneration. SEE ALSO erythroblast. SYN reticulated corpuscle, skein cell. [reticulo- + G. *kytos,* cell]

re·tic·u·lo·cy·to·pe·nia (re-tik′yū-lō-sī-tō-pē′nē-ă). Paucity of reticulocytes in the blood. SYN reticulopenia. [reticulocyte + G. *penia,* poverty]

re·tic·u·lo·cy·to·sis (re-tik′yū-lō-sī-tō′sis). An increase in the number of circulating reticulocytes above the normal, which is less than 1% of the total number of red blood cells; it occurs during active blood regeneration (stimulation of red bone marrow) and in certain anemias, especially congenital hemolytic anemia. [reticulocyte + G. *osis,* condition]

re·tic·u·lo·en·do·the·li·al (re-tik′yū-lō-en-dō-thē′lē-ăl). Denoting or referring to reticuloendothelium.

re·tic·u·lo·en·do·the·li·o·ma (re-tik′yū-lō-en′dō-thē-lē-ō′mă). Obsolete term for a localized reticulosis, or neoplasm derived from reticuloendothelial tissue. [reticuloendothelium + G. *-oma,* tumor]

re·tic·u·lo·en·do·the·li·o·sis (re-tik′yū-lō-en′dō-thē-lē-ō′sis). Obsolete term for proliferation of the reticuloendothelium in any of the organs or tissues. SEE ALSO reticulosis. [reticuloendothelium + G. *-osis,* condition]

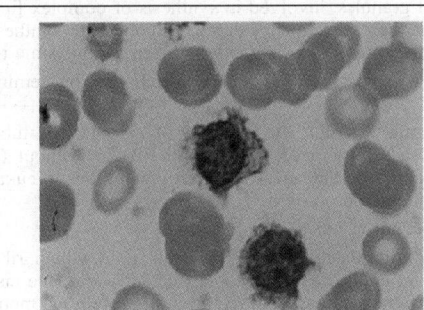

reticuloendotheliosis ("hairy" cells)

avian r., a leukosis-like disease of fowl caused by viruses of the avian type C retroviruses.

leukemic r., obsolete term for hairy cell *leukemia.*

re·tic·u·lo·en·do·the·li·um (re-tik′yū-lō-en-dō-thē′lē-ŭm). The cells making up the reticuloendothelial system. [reticulo- + endothelium]

re·tic·u·lo·his·ti·o·cy·to·ma (re-tik′yū-lō-his′tē-ō-sī-tō′mă). A solitary skin nodule composed of glycolipid-containing multinu-cleated large histiocytes; multiple lesions sometimes occur in association with arthritis. [reticulo- + histiocytoma]

re·tic·u·lo·his·ti·o·cy·to·sis (re-tik′yū-lō-his′tē-ō-sī-tō′sis). SEE reticulosis.

multicentric r., a rare disease in which cutaneous papules composed of histiocytes containing glycolipids are associated with polyarthritis, often leading to shortening of the fingers.

re·tic·u·loid (re-tik′yū-loyd). 1. Resembling a reticulosis. 2. A condition resembling reticulosis.

actinic r., chronic pruritic erythema beginning on sun-exposed areas in elderly males, with marked thickening and ridging of exposed skin simulating lymphoma; there is infiltration by atypical CD8-positive T lymphocytes. Occurs after several years.

re·tic·u·lo·pe·nia (re-tik′yū-lō-pē′nē-ă). SYN reticulocytopenia.

re·tic·u·lo·per·i·to·ni·tis. Inflammation of the reticulum and peritoneum of ruminant animals.

traumatic reticuloperitonitis, SYN traumatic *gastritis.*

re·tic·u·lo·sis (re-tik-yū-lō′sis). 1. An increase in histiocytes, monocytes, or other reticuloendothelial elements. 2. Obsolete term for lymphoma. [reticulo- + G. -osis, condition]

benign inoculation r., SYN cat-scratch *disease.*

histiocytic medullary r., obsolete term for histiocytic medullary r.

leukemic r., SYN monocytic *leukemia.*

lipomelanic r., SYN dermatopathic *lymphadenopathy.*

malignant midline r., obsolete term for polymorphic r.

midline malignant reticulosis r., SYN lethal midline *granuloma.*

pagetoid r., SYN Woringer-Kolopp *disease.*

polymorphic r., a necrotizing lymphoproliferative lesion with a predilection for the upper respiratory tract. Previously called lethal midline granuloma or malignant midline reticulosis. Treatment is irradiation.

re·tic·u·lo·spi·nal (re-tik-yū-lō-spī′năl). Pertaining to the reticulospinal *tract.*

re·tic·u·lot·o·my (rē-tik-yū-lot′ō-mē). Production of lesions in the reticular formation. [reticulo- + G. *tomē,* incision]

re·tic·u·lum, pl. **re·tic·u·la** (re-tik′yū-lŭm, -lă). 1. A fine network formed by cells, or formed of certain structures within cells or of connective tissue fibers between cells. 2. SYN neuroglia. 3. The second compartment of the stomach of a ruminant, a comparatively small chamber communicating with the rumen; sometimes called the honeycomb because of the characteristic structure of its wall. [L. dim of *rete,* a net]

agranular endoplasmic r., endoplasmic r. that is lacking in ribosomal granules; involved in synthesis of complex lipids and fatty acids, detoxification of drugs, carbohydrate synthesis, and sequestering of Ca++. SYN smooth-surfaced endoplasmic r.

Ebner′s r., a network of nucleated cells in the seminiferous tubules.

endoplasmic r. (ER), the network of cytoplasmic tubules or flattened sacs (cisternae) with (rough ER) or without (smooth ER) ribosomes on the surface of their membranes in eukaryotes. SYN endomembrane system.

Golgi internal r., SYN Golgi *apparatus.*

granular endoplasmic r., endoplasmic r. in which ribosomal granules are applied to the cytoplasmic surface of the cisternae; involved in the synthesis and secretion of protein via membrane-bound vesicles to the extracellular space. SYN chromidial substance, ergastoplasm, rough-surfaced endoplasmic r.

Kölliker′s r., SYN neuroglia.

rough-surfaced endoplasmic r., SYN granular endoplasmic r.

sarcoplasmic r., the endoplasmic r. of skeletal and cardiac muscle; the complex of vesicles, tubules, and cisternae forming a continuous structure around striated myofibrils, with a repetition of structure within each sarcomere.

smooth-surfaced endoplasmic r., SYN agranular endoplasmic r.

stellate r., a network of epithelial cells disposed in a fluid-filled

compartment in the center of the enamel organ between the outer and inner enamel epithelium.

trabecular r., the network of fibers (pectinate ligaments) at the iridocorneal angle between the anterior chamber of the eye and the venous sinus of the sclera; it contains spaces between the fibers that are involved in drainage of the aqueous humor, and is composed of two portions: the corneoscleral part, the part attached to the sclera, and the uveal part, the part attached to the iris. SYN r. trabeculare sclerae [NA], Gerlach′s valvula, Hueck′s ligament, ligamentum annulare bulbi, pectinate ligaments of iridocorneal angle, pillar of iris, trabecular meshwork, trabecular network, trabecular zone.

r. trabecula′re sclerae [NA], SYN trabecular r.

trans-Golgi r., that part of the Golgi apparatus that takes newly processed proteins and delivers them to secretory vesicles that will fuse with other biomembranes (*e.g.,* the plasma membrane).

ret·i·form (ret′i-fōrm). Resembling a net or network. [L. *rete,* network]

retin-. SEE retino-.

ret·i·na (ret′i-nă) [NA]. Grossly, the r. consists of three parts: optic part of retina, ciliary part of retina, and iridial part of retina. The optic part, the physiologic portion that receives the visual light rays, is further divided into two parts, pigmented part (pigment epithelium) and nervous part, which are arranged in the following layers: 1) pigment epithelium; 2) layer of rods and cones; 3) external limiting lamina, actually a row of junctional complexes; 4) external nuclear lamina; 5) external plexiform lamina; 6) internal nuclear lamina; 7) internal plexiform lamina; 8) ganglionic cell lamina; 9) lamina of nerve fibers; 10) internal limiting lamina. Layers 2 through 10 comprise the nervous part. At the posterior pole of the visual axis is the macula, in the center of which is the fovea, the area of acute vision. Here layers 6, 7, 8, and 9 and blood vessels are absent, and only elongated cones are present. About 3 mm medial to the fovea is the optic disk, where axons of the ganglionic cells converge to form the optic nerve. The ciliary and iridial parts of the r. are forward prolongations of the pigmented layer and a layer of supporting columnar or epithelial cells over the ciliary body and the posterior surface of the iris, respectively. SYN tunica interna bulbi [NA], nervous tunic of eyeball, optomeninx. [Mediev, L. prob. fr. L. *rete,* a net]

albedo r.′s, obsolete term for a white area of the retina due to edema or infarction.

coarctate r., obsolete term for a ringlike effusion of fluid between the choroid and r., giving the latter a funnel shape.

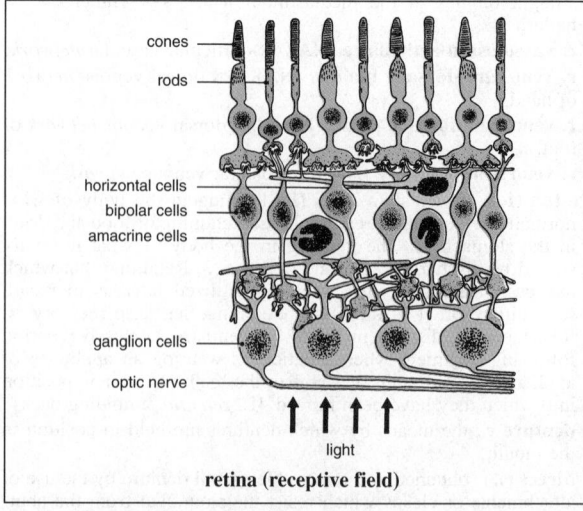

retina (receptive field)

detached r., SYN retinal *detachment*.

flecked r., an r. exhibiting fundus flavimaculatus, hereditary drusen, or fundus albipunctatus.

fleck r. of Kandori [MIM*228990], an autosomal-recessive disorder of the retinal pigment epithelium occurring among Japanese.

leopard r., SYN tessellated *fundus*.

shot-silk r., the appearance of numerous wavelike, glistening reflexes, like the shimmer of silk, observed sometimes in the r. of a young person. SYN shot-silk phenomenon, shot-silk reflex.

tigroid r., SYN tessellated *fundus*.

ret·i·nac·u·lum, gen. **ret·i·nac·u·li,** pl. **ret·i·nac·u·la** (ret-i-nak'yū-lŭm, -lī, -lă) [NA]. A frenum, or a retaining band or ligament. [L. a band, a halter, fr. *retineo,* to hold back]

antebrachial flexor r., thickening of distal antebrachial fascia just proximal to radiocarpal (wrist) joint. Continuous with extensor r. at margins of forearm. This structure is distinct from the transverse carpal *ligament,* commonly called "the flexor retinaculum," which forms the roof of the carpal tunnel. SYN flexor r. of forearm, palmar carpal ligament.

r. of articular capsule of hip, one of several longitudinal folds of the articular capsule of the hip joint reflected onto the femoral neck deep to which the retinacular branches of the medial femoral circumflex artery pass to reach the femoral head. SYN r. capsulae articularis coxae, Weitbrecht's fibers.

r. cap'sulae articula'ris cox'ae, SYN r. of articular capsule of hip.

caudal r., fibrous bands, remnants of the notochord, that extend from the skin to the coccyx, forming the coccygeal foveola. SYN r. caudale [NA], caudal ligament, ligamentum caudale.

r. cauda'le [NA], SYN caudal r.

r. cu'tis [NA], one of the numerous small fibrous strands that extend through the superficial fascia attaching the deep surface of the dermis to the underlying deep fascia determining the mobility of the skin over the deep structures; these are particularly well developed over the breast where they are known as suspensory ligaments of the breast; they are also well-developed, but short, in the palms and soles. SYN r. of skin.

extensor r., a strong fibrous band formed as a thickening of the antebrachial deep fascia, stretching obliquely across the back of the wrist, attaching deeply to ridges on the dorsal aspect of the radius, triquetral and pisiform bones, binding down the extensor tendons of the fingers and thumb. SYN r. extensorum [NA], dorsal carpal ligament, ligamentum carpi dorsale.

retinacula of extensor muscles, SEE inferior extensor r., superior extensor r.

r. extenso'rum [NA], SYN extensor r.

flexor r., SYN transverse carpal *ligament.*

flexor r. of forearm, SYN antebrachial flexor r.

flexor r. of lower limb, a wide band passing from the medial malleolus to the medial and upper border of the calcaneus and to the plantar surface as far as the navicular bone; it holds in place the tendons of the tibialis posterior, flexor digitorum longus, and flexor hallucis longus. SYN r. musculorum flexorum [NA], laciniate ligament, ligamentum laciniatum, r. of flexor muscles.

r. of flexor muscles, SYN flexor r. of lower limb.

r. flexo'rum [NA], SYN transverse carpal *ligament.*

inferior extensor r., a Y-shaped ligament restraining the extensor tendons of the foot distal to the ankle joint. SYN r. musculorum extensorum inferius [NA], cruciate ligament of leg, inferior r. of extensor muscles, ligamentum cruciatum cruris.

inferior r. of extensor muscles, SYN inferior extensor r.

lateral patellar r., part of the aponeurosis of the vastus lateralis muscle passing lateral to the patella to attach to the tibial tuberosity. SYN r. patellae laterale [NA].

medial patellar r., part of the aponeurosis of the vastus medialis muscle passing medial to the patella to attach to the medial condyle of the tibia, forming the anteromedial aspect of the fibrous capsule of the knee joint. SYN r. patellae mediale.

Morgagni's r., SYN *frenulum* of ileocecal valve.

r. musculo'rum extenso'rum infe'rius [NA], SYN inferior extensor r.

r. musculo'rum extenso'rum supe'rius [NA], SYN superior extensor r.

retinac'ula musculo'rum fibula'rium [NA], ✩ official alternate term for peroneal r., peroneal r.

r. musculo'rum flexo'rum [NA], SYN flexor r. of lower limb.

retinac'ula musculo'rum peroneo'rum [NA], SYN peroneal r.

retinacula of nail, fibrous attachments of the nail-bed to the underlying phalanx. SYN retinacula unguis [NA].

r. patel'lae latera'le [NA], SYN lateral patellar r.

r. patel'lae media'le, SYN medial patellar r.

patellar r., extensions of the aponeuroses of the vasti medialis and lateralis muscles which pass on each side of the patella, attaching to the margins of the patella and patellar ligament anteriorly, the collateral ligaments posteriorly and the tibial condyles distally; form the anteromedial and (with the fibrous expansion of the iliotibial tract) the anteromedial portions of the fibrous capsule of the knee. SEE lateral patellar r., medial patellar r.

peroneal r., superior and inferior fibrous bands retaining the tendons of the peroneus longus and brevis in position as they cross the lateral side of the ankle. SYN retinacula musculorum peroneorum [NA], retinacula musculorum fibularium✩ [NA], retinacula of peroneal muscles.

retinacula of peroneal muscles, SYN peroneal r.

r. of skin, SYN r. cutis.

superior extensor r., the ligament that binds down the extensor tendons proximal to the ankle joint; it is continuous with (a thickening of) the deep fascia of the leg. SYN r. musculorum extensorum superius [NA], ligamentum transversum cruris, superior r. of extensor muscles, transverse crural ligament, transverse ligament of leg.

superior r. of extensor muscles, SYN superior extensor r.

r. ten'dinum, a ligamentous structure to restrain tendons, such as the flexor or extensor retinacula, or the annular parts of the digital fibrous sheaths.

retinac'ula un'guis [NA], SYN retinacula of nail.

ret·i·nal. 1 (ret'i-năl). Relating to the retina. 2 (ret'i-nal). retinaldehyde; most commonly referring to the all-*trans* form.

r. dehydrogenase, an oxidoreductase catalyzing the interconversion of retinaldehyde and NAD^+ to retinoic acid and NADH; thus affecting growth and differentiation. SYN retinaldehyde dehydrogenase.

r. isomerase, an isomerase that catalyzes the *cis-trans*-interconversion of all-*trans*-retinal(dehyde) to 11-*cis*-retinal(dehyde); a part of the vision cycle. SYN retinaldehyde isomerase.

r. reductase, alcohol dehydrogenase $(NAD(P)^+)$.

11-*cis*-ret·i·nal. The isomer of retinaldehyde that can combine with opsin to form rhodopsin; it is formed from 11-*trans*-retinal by retinal isomerase. SYN neoretinal b.

***trans*-ret·i·nal.** SYN all-*trans*-retinal.

ret·i·nal·de·hyde (ret-i-nal'dĕ-hīd). Retinol oxidized to a terminal aldehyde; a carotene released (as all-*trans*-retinal(dehyde)) in

re

the bleaching of rhodopsin by light and the dissociation of opsin in the vision cycle. SYN retinene-1, retinene, vitamin A aldehyde.

r. dehydrogenase, SYN *retinal* dehydrogenase.

r. isomerase, SYN *retinal* isomerase.

r. reductase, alcohol dehydrogenase $(NAD(P))^+$.

ret·i·nec·to·my. A surgical excision of a piece of the retina.

ret·i·nene (ret'i-nēn). SYN retinaldehyde.

ret·i·nene-1. SYN retinaldehyde.

ret·i·nene-2. SYN dehydroretinaldehyde.

ret·i·ni·tis (ret-i-nī'tis). Inflammation of the retina. [retina + G. *-itis,* inflammation]

albuminuric r., SEE hypertensive *retinopathy.*

apoplectic r., obsolete term for the appearance of the retina after occlusion of the central retinal vein.

azotemic r., obsolete term for hypertensive *retinopathy.* SEE hypertensive *retinopathy.*

central angiospastic r., obsolete term for central serous *choroidopathy.*

circinate r., SEE circinate *retinopathy.*

diabetic r., SEE diabetic *retinopathy.*

exudative r., r. exudati′va, a chronic abnormality characterized by deposition of cholesterol and cholesterol esters in outer retinal layers and subretinal space. In adults, often preceded by uveitis; in children, often preceded by retinal vascular abnormalities. SYN Coats' disease.

gravidic r., obsolete term for toxemic *retinopathy* of pregnancy. SEE toxemic *retinopathy* of pregnancy.

leukemic r., SEE leukemic *retinopathy.*

metastatic r., purulent or septic r. resulting from the arrest of septic emboli in the retinal vessels. SYN purulent r., septic r.

r. pigmento′sa, a progressive abiotrophy of the neuroepithelium, with atrophy and pigmentary infiltration of the inner layers of the retina. There is abundant evidence of mendelian inheritance mostly as a dominant [MIM*180100] but also as a recessive or X-linked trait [MIM*268000, *312600, *312610]. SYN pigmentary retinopathy.

r. prolif′erans, SYN proliferative *retinopathy.*

punctate r., SEE *retinopathy* punctata albescens.

purulent r., SYN metastatic r.

recurrent central r., obsolete term for central serous *retinopathy.*

r. sclopeta′ria, a severe contusion lesion of the retina, as from a shot pellet or BB. [from *sclopetum,* a medieval handgun]

secondary r., r. that follows uveal inflammation.

septic r., SYN metastatic r.

serous r., edema of the retina; an inflammation of the inner layers of the retina. SYN simple r.

simple r., SYN serous r.

r. syphilit′ica, syphilitic r., r. often associated with syphilitic choroiditis, especially in congenital syphilis.

⌂**retino-, retin-.** The retina. [Med. L. *retina*]

ret·i·no·blas·to·ma (ret'i-nō-blas-tō'mă) [MIM*180200, MIM*180201, MIM*180202]. Malignant ocular neoplasm of childhood usually occurring before the third year of life, composed of primitive retinal small round cells with deeply staining nuclei and by elongate cells forming rosettes. In familial forms, the disease is commonly bilateral and multiple within an eye; in sporadic cases, rarely so. [retino- + G. *blastos,* germ, + *-oma,* tumor]

ret·i·no·cho·roid (ret'i-nō-kō'royd). SYN chorioretinal.

ret·i·no·cho·roid·i·tis (ret'i-nō-kō-roy-dī'tis). Inflammation of the retina extending to the choroid. SYN chorioretinitis, choroidoretinitis. [retinochoroid + G. *-itis,* inflammation]

bird shot r., bilateral diffuse retinal vasculitis with depigmentation of multiple areas of the choroid and retinal pigment epithelium posterior to the ocular equator, often with an associated papillitis or optic atrophy; vitiligo occurs occasionally.

r. juxtapapilla′ris, r. close to the optic disk. SYN Jensen's disease.

ret·i·no·di·al·y·sis (ret'i-nō-dī-al'i-sis). SYN *dialysis* retinae. [retino- + G. *dialysis,* separation]

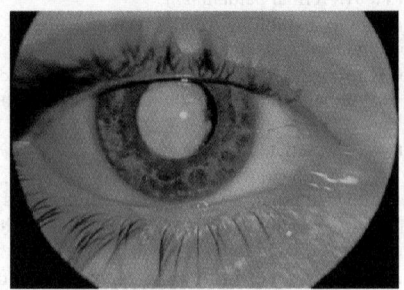

retinoblastoma
the tumor appears yellow in the pupil

ret·i·no·ic ac·id (ret-i-nō'ik). Vitamin A_1 acid; retinaldehyde in which the terminal –CHO has been oxidized to a –COOH; used topically in the treatment of acne; plays an important role in growth and differentiation. SYN vitamin A_1 acid.

13-*cis*-r. a., the retinoid most used in the United States to treat acne; it works by reducing sebum secretion. Use in pregnancy is contraindicated because of teratogenicity.

ret·i·noid (ret'i-noyd). **1.** Resembling a resin; resinous. [G. *rētinē,* resin, + *eidos,* resemblance] **2.** Resembling the retina. [Mediev. L. *retina*] **3.** In plural form, term used to describe the natural forms and synthetic analogs of retinol.

In experiments with rats, hamsters, and other animals, these vitamin A analogs have been shown to block carcinogenesis in a variety of epithelial tissues. Clinical trials have announced success of retinoid drugs in preventing actinic keratosis, bronchial metaplasia, cervical dysplasia, oral leukoplakia, tumors in the aerodigestive tract, and some skin cancers. Although the mechanism by which retinoids act is not fully understood, they may modulate gene expression and thereby slow or suppress the multistep process that leads to the creation, proliferation, and spread of cancerous cells.

ret·i·noids (ret'i-noydz). A class of keratolytic drugs derived from retinoic acid and used for treatment of severe acne and psoriasis.

ret·i·nol (ret'i-nol). vitamin A_1alcohol; 2,6,6-trimethyl-1-(9′-hydroxy-3′,7′-dimethylnona-1′,3′,5′,7′-tetraenyl)cyclohex-1-ene; a half-carotene bearing the β (or β-ionone) form of the cyclic end group and a CH_2OH at the C-15 position (numbering as in carotenoids) or 9′-position (numbering as a nonyl side chain on a cyclohexene ring); an intermediate in the vision cycle; it also plays a role in growth and differentiation. SEE ALSO dehydroretinol. SYN vitamin A_1 alcohol, vitamin A_1.

r. dehydrogenase, an oxidoreductase catalyzing interconversion of retinal and NADH to retinol and NAD^+.

11-*cis*-ret·i·nol. Retinol with *cis* configuration at the 11-position (carotenoid numbering) or 5′-position (retinol numbering) of the side chain; an intermediate in the vision cycle. SYN neoretinene B.

ret·i·no·pap·il·li·tis (ret'i-nō-pap-i-lī'tis). Inflammation of the retina extending to the optic disk.

r. of premature infants, SYN *retinopathy* of prematurity.

ret·i·nop·a·thy (ret-i-nop'ă-thē). Noninflammatory degenerative disease of the retina. [retino- + G. *pathos,* suffering]

arteriosclerotic r., r. distinguished by attenuated retinal arterioles with increased tortuosity, copper- or silver-wire appearance, perivascular sheathing, irregularity of lumen and scattered small hemorrhages, and small, sharp-edged deposits without surrounding edema.

central angiospastic r., SYN central serous *choroidopathy.*

central serous r., SYN central serous *choroidopathy.*

circinate r., a retinal degeneration marked by a girdle of sharply defined white exudates around an edematous macula; usually bilateral and typically affects the aged.

compression r., (1) SEE Berlin's *edema*. SEE traumatic r.

---

diabetic r., retinal changes occurring in diabetes of long duration, marked by hemorrhages, microaneurysms, and sharply defined waxy deposits, or by proliferative retinopathy. SYN fundus diabeticus.

> Progressive degeneration of retinal blood vessels is a consequence of diabetes mellitus. Blood leakage and fluid buildup from deteriorating and weakly formed new blood vessels initially cause macular edema. As the damage proliferates, scarring and sometimes retinal detachment result. Some 40% of diabetics manifest this condition to a degree. In the U.S. 5,000 go blind from it each year (worldwide, 30,000 to 40,000). With early diagnosis, the condition can be treated by laser photocoagulation, whereby leaking blood vessels are cauterized. Photocoagulation halts or retards retinopathy, and cuts the chance of blindness in half.

---

dysproteinemic r., retinal venous congestion due to increased blood viscosity in dysproteinemia.

eclamptic r., SYN toxemic r. of pregnancy.

electric r., SYN photoretinopathy.

external exudative r., SEE exudative *retinitis*.

gravidic r., SYN toxemic r. of pregnancy.

hypertensive r., a retinal condition occurring in accelerated vascular hypertension, marked by arteriolar constriction, flame-shaped hemorrhages, cotton-wool patches, star-figure edema at the macula, and papilledema.

Leber's idiopathic stellate r., SEE neuroretinitis.

leukemic r., appearance of the retina in all types of leukemia, characterized by engorgement and tortuosity of veins, scattered hemorrhages, and edema of the retina and disk.

lipemic r., a milkiness of the retinal vessels (lipemia retinalis) combined with hard-edged fatty exudates, seen in patients with diabetic acidosis and hyperlipemia.

macular r., SYN maculopathy.

pigmentary r., SYN *retinitis* pigmentosa.

r. of prematurity, abnormal replacement of the sensory retina by fibrous tissue and blood vessels, occurring mainly in premature infants having a birth weight of less than 1500 g who are placed in a high-oxygen environment. SYN retinopapillitis of premature infants, retrolental fibroplasia, Terry's syndrome.

proliferative r., neovascularization of the retina extending into the vitreous humor. SYN retinitis proliferans.

r. puncta′ta al′bescens, a disease in which both fundi show numerous white dots through the retina; causes night blindness.

Purtscher's r., transient traumatic retinal angiopathy due to a sudden rise in venous pressure, as in compression of the body from seat belt injury; ocular fundi show large white patches associated with the retinal veins about the disk or macula, hemorrhages, and retinal edema;thought to be due to fat embolism from bone marrow. SYN Purtscher's disease, transient r., traumatic r.

renal r., hypertensive r. associated with chronic glomerulonephritis or nephrosclerosis.

rubella r., peripheral pigmentary retinal changes in congenital rubella, not affecting visual function.

sickle cell r., a condition marked by dilation and tortuosity of retinal veins, and by microaneurysms and retinal hemorrhages; advanced stages may show neovascularization, vitreous hemorrhage, or retinal detachment.

solar r., SYN photoretinopathy.

toxemic r. of pregnancy, sudden angiospasm of retinal arterioles, later followed by retinal vascular signs of advanced hypertensive r.; vascular changes disappear rapidly after termination of the pregnancy. SYN eclamptic r., gravidic r.

toxic r., retinal changes due to prolonged administration of various drugs.

transient r., SYN Purtscher's r.

traumatic r., SYN Purtscher's r.

venous-stasis r., a uniocular retinopathy associated with occlusion of the central retinal vein; a nonischemic central retinal vein occlusion.

ret·i·no·pexy (ret′i-nō-pek′sē). A procedure to repair a detached retina by holding it in place; *e.g.,* by producing chorioretinal adhesions by freezing ("retinal cryopexy"). [retino- + G. *pēxis,* fixation]

fluid r., a procedure to repair a detached retina by holding it in place with a fluid that is heavier than vitreous fluid.

gas r., a retinal detachment repair in which the retina is held in place by an expandable gas. SYN pneumatic r.

pneumatic r., SYN gas r.

ret·i·no·pi·e·sis (ret′i-nō-pī-ē′sis). Repositioning a detached retina by pressing it into position by gas or fluid. SEE retinopexy. [retino- + G. *piesis,* pressure]

ret·i·nos·chi·sis (ret-i-nos′ki-sis). Degenerative splitting of the retina, with cyst formation between the two layers. [retino- + G. *schisis,* division]

juvenile r. [MIM*268100], r. occurring before 10 years of age and within the nerve-fiber layer, with frequent macular involvement; at first, the inner wall is a translucent veil-like membrane, but it becomes more dense and may render the retina white; autosomal recessive inheritance. There is a form of this condition in middle age that is X-linked [MIM*312700] and a rare autosomal dominant form [MIM*180270].

senile r., r. occurring most often in the elderly and affecting the outer plexiform layer; it begins in the extreme inferotemporal periphery and is not significantly progressive; vision usually is good.

ret·i·no·scope (ret′i-nō-skōp). An optical device used to illuminate a subject's retina during retinoscopy. [retino- + G. *skopeō,* to view]

luminous r., a portable optical device providing either a circular or linear (streak) beam of light.

reflecting r., a plane or concave mirror with a central perforation that allows the observer to see rays emerge from the subject's eye.

ret·i·nos·co·py (ret′i-nos′kŏ-pē). A method of determining errors of refraction by illuminating the retina and observing the rays of light emerging from the eye. SYN scotoscopy, shadow test, skiascopy. [retino- + G. *skopeō,* to view]

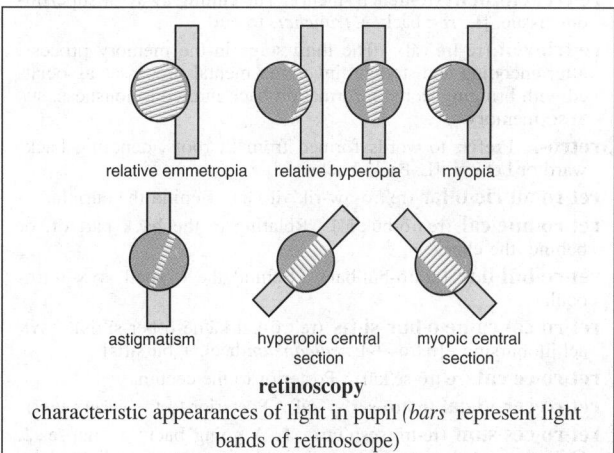

relative emmetropia   relative hyperopia   myopia

astigmatism   hyperopic central section   myopic central section

retinoscopy
characteristic appearances of light in pupil *(bars* represent light bands of retinoscope)

cylinder r., determination of spherical, astigmatic, and refractive error using cylindrical lenses.

fogging r., the method of reducing vision with convex lenses until accommodation is suspended; a static, noncycloplegic technique.

ret·i·not·o·my. A surgical incision through the retina.

ret·i·nyl phos·phate (ret′i-nil fos′fāt). The phosphoester of all-*trans* retinol; essential for the biosynthesis of certain glycoproteins needed for growth regulation and for mucous secretion.

ret·o·per·i·the·li·um (rē'to-per-i-thē'lē-ŭm). The reticular cells related to the reticular fiber network, as in the stroma of lymphatic tissue. [L. *rete,* net, + G. *peri,* around, + Mod. L. *thelium,* fr. G. *thēlē,* nipple]

re·tort (rē-tōrt'). **1.** A flasklike vessel with a long neck passing outward, once used in distilling. **2.** A small furnace. [Mediev. L. *retorta,* fem. pp. of *retorqueo,* pp. *-tortus,* to twist or bend back]

Re·tor·tam·o·nas (rē-tōr-tam'ō-nas). A genus of protozoan flagellates, one species of which, *R. intestinalis,* is found occasionally in the human intestine, although it is nonpathogenic and infrequently reported. [L. *re-torqueo,* to twist back, + G. *monas,* single, a unit]

ret·o·the·li·o·ma (ret'ō-thē-lē-ō'mă). Old term for a neoplasm derived from reticular cells of the reticuloendothelial system.

re·tract (rē-trakt'). To shrink, draw back, or pull apart. [L. *retraho,* pp. *-tractus,* a drawing back]

re·trac·tile (rē-trak'til). Retractable; capable of being drawn back.

re·trac·tion (rē-trak'shŭn). **1.** A shrinking, drawing back, or pulling apart. **2.** Posterior movement of teeth, usually with the aid of an orthodontic appliance. [L. *retractio,* a drawing back]

gingival r., (1) lateral movement of the gingival margin away from the tooth surface; may be indicative of underlying inflammation or pocket formation; **(2)** displacement of the marginal gingivae away from the tooth by mechanical, chemical, or surgical means.

mandibular r., a type of facial anomaly in which the gnathion lies posterior to the orbital plane.

re·trac·tor (rē-trak'ter, -tōr). **1.** An instrument for drawing aside the edges of a wound or for holding back structures adjacent to the operative field. **2.** A muscle that draws a part backward, *e.g.,* the middle part of the trapezius muscle is a r. of the scapula; the horizontal fibers of the temporalis muscle serve to retract the mandible.

re·trad (rē'trad). Backward; toward the back part; directed posteriorly. [L. *retro,* backward, + *ad,* to]

re·tra·hens au·rem, re·tra·hens au·ric·u·lam (rēt'ră-henz aw'rem, aw-rik'yū-lam). SEE posterior auricular *muscle.* [L. drawing back the ear, or auricle]

re·treat from re·al·i·ty. Substitution of imaginary satisfactions or fantasy for relations with the real world.

re·trench·ment (rē-trench'-ment). The cutting away of superfluous tissue. [F. *re-,* back, + *trancher,* to cut]

re·triev·al (rē-trē'văl). The third stage in the memory process, after encoding and storage, involving mental processes associated with bringing stored information back into consciousness. SEE ALSO memory.

⚕**retro-.** Prefix, to words formed from L. roots, denoting backward or behind. [L. back, backward]

ret·ro·au·ric·u·lar (re'trō-aw-rik'yū-lăr). Behind the auricle.

ret·ro·buc·cal (re'trō-bŭk'ăl). Relating to the back part of, or behind, the cheek.

ret·ro·bul·bar (re'trō-bŭl'bar). Behind the eyeball. SYN retroocular.

ret·ro·cal·ca·ne·o·bur·si·tis (re'trō-kal-kā'nē-ō-ber-sī'tis). SYN achillobursitis. [retro- + L. *calcaneum* heel, + bursitis]

ret·ro·ce·cal (re'trō-sē'kăl). Posterior to the cecum.

ret·ro·cer·vi·cal (re'trō-ser'vi-kăl). Posterior to the cervix uteri.

ret·ro·ces·sion (re-trō-sesh'ŭn). **1.** A going back; a relapse. **2.** Cessation of the external symptoms of a disease followed by signs of involvement of some internal organ or part. **3.** Denoting a position of the uterus or other organ farther back than is normal. [L. *retro-cedo,* pp. *-cessus,* to go back, retire]

ret·ro·clu·sion (re-trō-klū'zhŭn). A form of acupressure for the arrest of bleeding; the needle is passed through the tissues above the cut end of the artery, is turned around, and then is passed backward beneath the vessel to come out near the point of entrance. [retro- + L. *claudo* (*cludo*) to close]

ret·ro·co·lic (re'trō-kol'ik). Posterior to the colon. [retro- + G. *kolon,* colon]

ret·ro·col·lic (re'trō-kol'ik). Relating to the back of the neck; drawing back the head. [retro- + L. *collum,* neck]

ret·ro·col·lis (re-trō-kol'is). SYN retrocollic *spasm.*

ret·ro·con·duc·tion (re-trō-kon-dŭk'shŭn). SYN retrograde *conduction.*

ret·ro·cur·sive (re'trō-ker'siv). Running backward. [retro- + L. *cursus,* a running]

ret·ro·de·vi·a·tion (re'trō-dē-vē-ā'shŭn). A backward bending or inclining.

ret·ro·dis·place·ment (re'trō-dis-plās'ment). Any backward displacement, such as retroversion or retroflexion of the uterus.

ret·ro·e·soph·a·ge·al (re'trō-ē-sof'ă-jē'ăl). Posterior to the esophagus.

ret·ro·fil·ling (re-trō-fil'ing). Placement of a sealing material into the apical foramen of a dental root from the apical end.

ret·ro·flect·ed (re'trō-flek-ted). SYN retroflexed.

ret·ro·flec·tion (re-trō-flek'shŭn). SYN retroflexion.

ret·ro·flexed (re'trō-flekst). Bent backward or posteriorly. SYN retroflected. [retro- + L. *flecto,* pp. *flexus,* to bend]

ret·ro·flex·ion (re-trō-flek'shŭn). Backward bending, as of the uterus when the corpus is bent back, forming an angle with the cervix. SYN retroflection.

r. of iris, abnormal position of the iris on the ciliary body after severe concussion.

ret·ro·gnath·ic (re-trō-nath'ik). Denoting a state in which the mandible is located posterior to its normal position in relation to the maxillae.

ret·ro·gnath·ism (re-trō-nath'izm). A condition of facial disharmony in which one or both jaws are posterior to normal in their craniofacial relationships; usually used in reference to the mandible. [retro- + G. *gnathos,* jaw]

ret·ro·grade (ret'rō-grād). **1.** Moving backward. **2.** Degenerating; reversing the normal order of growth and development. [L. *retrogradus,* fr. retro- + *gradior,* to go]

ret·rog·ra·phy (re-trog'ră-fē). SYN mirror-writing. [retro- + G. *graphō,* to write]

ret·ro·gres·sion (re-trō-gresh'ŭn). SYN cataplasia. [L. *retrogressus* fr. *retrogradior,* to go backwards]

ret·ro·in·hi·bi·tion (re'trō-in-hi-bish'ŭn; DEF ABB: r.). SYN feedback *inhibition.*

ret·ro·i·rid·i·an (re'trō-i-rid'ē-an). Posterior to the iris.

ret·ro·jec·tion (re-trō-jek'shŭn). The washing out of a cavity by the backward flow of an injected fluid. [L. *retro,* backward, + *jacio,* to throw]

ret·ro·jec·tor (re'trō-jek-ter, -tōr). A form of syringe with long tubular attachment to the nozzle, used in retrojection.

ret·ro·len·tal (re'trō-len'tăl). Posterior to the lens of the eye. SYN retrolenticular (1).

ret·ro·len·tic·u·lar (re'trō-len-tik'yū-lăr). **1.** SYN retrolental. **2.** Behind the lentiform nucleus of the brain.

ret·ro·lin·gual (re'trō-ling'gwăl). Relating to the back part of the tongue; posterior to the tongue. [retro- + L. *lingua,* tongue]

ret·ro·mam·ma·ry (re'trō-mam'ă-rē). Posterior to the mamma.

ret·ro·man·dib·u·lar (re'trō-man-dib'yū-lăr). Posterior to the lower jaw. [retro- + L. *mandibula,* lower jaw]

ret·ro·mas·toid (re'trō-mas'toyd). Posterior to the mastoid process; relating to the posterior mastoid cells.

ret·ro·mo·lar (re-trō-mō'lăr). Distal (or posterior) to the last erupted (or present) molar tooth.

ret·ro·mor·pho·sis (re-trō-mōr'fō-sis, -mōr-fō'sis). SYN cataplasia. [retro- + G. *morphōsis,* process of forming]

ret·ro·na·sal (re'trō-nā'zăl). Posterior nasal; relating to the posterior nares.

ret·ro·oc·u·lar (re'trō-ok'yū-lăr). SYN retrobulbar.

ret·ro·per·i·to·ne·al (re'trō-per'i-tō-nē'ăl). External or posterior to the peritoneum.

ret·ro·per·i·to·ne·um (re'trō-per'i-tō-nē'ŭm). SYN retroperitoneal *space.* [retro- + peritoneum]

ret·ro·per·i·to·ni·tis (ret′rō-per-i-tō-nī′tis). Inflammation of the cellular tissue behind the peritoneum.

idiopathic fibrous r., SYN retroperitoneal *fibrosis*.

ret·ro·pha·ryn·ge·al (re′trō-fă-rin′jē-ăl). Posterior to the pharynx.

ret·ro·phar·ynx (re′trō-făr′ingks). The posterior part of the pharynx.

ret·ro·pla·cen·tal (re′trō-pla-sen′tăl). Behind the placenta.

ret·ro·pla·sia (ret-rō-plā′zē-ă). That state of cell or tissue in which activity is decreased below that considered normal; associated with retrogressive changes (*e.g.,* injury, degeneration, death, necrosis). [retro- + G. *plasis*, a molding]

ret·ro·posed (re′trō-pōzd). Denoting retroposition. [retro- + L. *pono*, pp. *positus*, to place]

ret·ro·po·si·tion (re′trō-pō-zish′ŭn). Simple backward displacement of a structure or organ, as the uterus, without inclination, bending, retroversion, or retroflexion. [retro- + L. *positio*, a placing]

ret·ro·pos·on (re-trō-pōs′on). A transposition of sequences in a DNA that does not originate in the DNA but, in an mRNA that is transcribed back into the genomic DNA by reverse transcription. [retro- + L. *pono*, pp. *positum*, to place, + -on]

ret·ro·pu·bic (re-trō-pyū′bik). Posterior to the pubic bone.

ret·ro·pul·sion (re-trō-pŭl′shŭn). **1.** An involuntary backward walking or running, occurring in patients with the parkinsonian syndrome. **2.** A pushing back of any part. [retro- + L. *pulsio*, a pushing, fr. *pello*, pp. *pulsus*, beat, drive]

ret·ro·spec·tion (re-trō-spek′shŭn). The act or process of surveying and reviewing the past. [retro- + L. *specto*, pp. *spectatus*, to look at]

ret·ro·spec·tive (re-trō-spek′tiv). Relating to retrospection.

ret·ro·spon·dy·lo·lis·the·sis (re′trō-spon′di-lō-lis-thē′sis). Slipping posteriorly of the body of a vertebra, bringing it out of line with the adjacent vertebrae. [retro- + G. *spondylos*, vertebra, + *olisthēsis*, a slipping]

ret·ro·ster·nal (re′trō-ster′năl). Posterior to the sternum.

ret·ro·ste·roid (re-trō-stēr′oyd, -ster′oyd). A term sometimes used to designate a steroid in which the orientations of the substituents at carbons-9 and -10 are the opposite of those of the reference or "parent" compound.

ret·ro·tar·sal (re′trō-tar′săl). Posterior to the tarsus, or edge of the eyelid.

ret·ro·u·ter·ine (re′trō-yū′ter-in). Posterior to the uterus.

ret·ro·ver·si·o·flex·ion (re-trō-ver′sē-ō-flek′shŭn, -ver′zhō-). Combined retroversion and retroflexion of the uterus.

ret·ro·ver·sion (re-trō-ver′zhŭn). **1.** A turning backward, as of the uterus. **2.** Condition in which the teeth are located in a more posterior position than is normal. [retro- + L. *verto*, pp. *versus*, to turn]

ret·ro·vert·ed (re′trō-ver-ted). Denoting retroversion.

Ret·ro·vir·i·dae (re-trō-vir′i-dē). A family of viruses resembling the orthomyxoviruses in size and shape, but structurally more complex; they possess RNA-dependent DNA polymerases (reverse transcriptases) and are grouped in three subfamilies: Oncovirinae (HTLV-I, HTLV-II RNA tumor viruses), Spumavirinae (foamy viruses), and Lentivirinae (HIV-like viruses, visna and related agents). Virions are about 100 nm in diameter, enveloped, and contain two identical molecules of positive sense, single-stranded RNA of high molecular weight (5 to 10×10^6); genomic RNA serves as a template for the synthesis of a complementary DNA, which may be integrated into the host DNA.

ret·ro·vi·rus (re′trō-vī′rŭs). Any virus of the family Retroviridae.

Retroviruses are potent disease agents (HIV belongs to this family), but they have also proven invaluable research tools in molecular biology. In 1979, molecular biologist Richard Mulligan used a genetically altered retrovirus to trigger the production of hemoglobin in vitro by monkey kidney cells. His technique for using retroviruses to import alien genes into cells has been widely adopted in the laboratory. Medical researchers have also explored retroviral transport as a means of gene therapy. A pioneer experiment was performed in 1990, when two patients with adenosine deaminase deficiency were treated with altered leukemia retroviruses. However, evidence exists that retroviruses may play a role in carcinogenesis, raising a question concerning the safety of their use in gene therapy. (See oncogene)

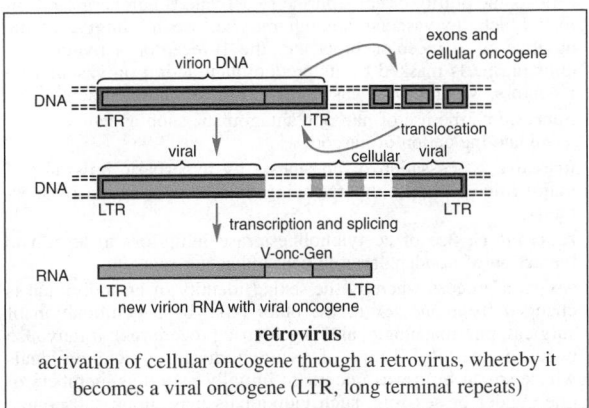

retrovirus

activation of cellular oncogene through a retrovirus, whereby it becomes a viral oncogene (LTR, long terminal repeats)

re·tru·sion (rē-trū′zhŭn). **1.** Retraction of the mandible from any given point. **2.** The backward movement of the mandible. [L. *retrudo*, pp. *-trusus*, to push back]

Rett, Andreas, 20th century Austrian pediatrician. SEE R.'s *syndrome*.

Retzius, Anders A., Swedish anatomist and anthropologist, 1796–1860. SEE R.'s *cavity*; *cavum* retzii; R.'s *fibers*, under *fiber*, *gyrus*, *ligament*, *space*, *veins*, under *vein*.

Retzius, Magnus G., Swedish anatomist and anthropologist, 1842–1919. SEE R.'s *striae*, under *stria*; *lines* of R., under *line*; R.'s *foramen*; calcification *lines* of R., under *line*; Key-R. *corpuscles*, under *corpuscle*; *foramen* of R.; *sheath* of Key and R.

re·u·ni·ent (rē-yū′nē-ent). Connecting; denoting the ductus reuniens. [L. *re-*, again, + *unio*, pp. *unitus*, to unite]

Reuss, August von, Austrian ophthalmologist, 1841–1924. SEE R.'s *formula*, color *tables*, under *table*, *test*.

re·vac·ci·na·tion (rē′vak-si-nā′shŭn). Vaccination of an individual previously successfully vaccinated.

re·vas·cu·lar·i·za·tion (rē-vas′kyū-lăr-i-zā′shŭn). Reestablishment of blood supply to a part.

re·ver·ber·a·tion (rē′vĕr-bĕ-rā′shŭn). Multiple echoes or reflections; in ultrasonography, an artifactual image caused by delay of an echo which has been reflected back and forward again before returning to the transducer.

Reverdin, Jacques L., Swiss surgeon, 1842–1929. SEE R. *graft*; R.'s *method*.

re·ver·sal (rē-ver′săl). **1.** A turning or changing to the opposite direction, as of a process, disease, symptom, or state. **2.** The changing of a dark line or a bright one of the spectrum into its

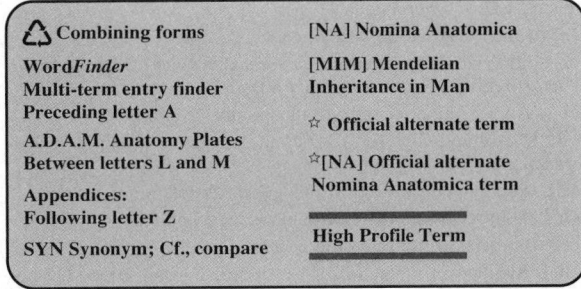

♻ **Combining forms**	**[NA] Nomina Anatomica**
Word*Finder*	**[MIM] Mendelian**
Multi-term entry finder	**Inheritance in Man**
Preceding letter A	
A.D.A.M. Anatomy Plates	☆ **Official alternate term**
Between letters L and M	
	☆**[NA] Official alternate**
Appendices:	**Nomina Anatomica term**
Following letter Z	
	High Profile Term
SYN Synonym; Cf., compare	

re

opposite. **3.** Denoting the difficulty of some persons in distinguishing the lower case printed or written letter *p* from *q* or *g*, *b* from *d*, or *s* from *z*. **4.** In psychoanalysis, the change of an instinct or affect into its opposite, as from love into hate. [L. *re-verto*, pp. *-versus*, to turn back or about]

adrenaline r., SYN epinephrine r.

epinephrine r., the fall in blood pressure produced by epinephrine when given following blockage of α-adrenergic receptors by an appropriate drug such as phenoxybenzamine; the vasodilation reflects the ability of epinephrine to activate β-adrenergic receptors which, in vascular smooth muscle, are inhibitory; in the absence of α-receptor blockade, the β-receptor activation by epinephrine is masked by its predominant action on vascular α-receptors, which causes vasoconstriction. SYN adrenaline r.

narcotic r., the use of narcotic antagonists, such as naloxone, to terminate the action of narcotics.

pressure r., cessation of anesthesia by hyperbaric pressure; of major importance in understanding the mode of action of anesthetics.

relaxant r., use of acetylcholinesterase inhibitors to terminate the action of nondepolarizing neuromuscular relaxants.

sex r., a process whereby the sexual identity of an individual is changed from one sex to the other (*e.g.,* by a combination of surgical, pharmacologic, and psychiatric procedures); it may also occur in the life history of pseudohermaphroditic individuals whose sex at birth was uncertain; initially reared as members of one gender or sex role, such individuals may, upon subsequent medical examination and advice, be reared thereafter as members of the opposite gender or sex role.

re·vers·i·ble (rē-ver'si-bl). Capable of reversal; said of diseases or chemical reactions.

re·ver·sion (rē-ver'zhŭn). **1.** The manifestation in an individual of certain characteristics, peculiar to a remote ancestor, which have been suppressed during one or more of the intermediate generations. **2.** The return to the original phenotype, either by reinstatement of the original genotype (true r.) or by a mutation at a site different from that of the first mutation which cancels the effect of the first mutation (suppressor mutation). [L. *reversio* (see reversal)]

re·ver·tant (rē-ver'tant). In microbial genetics, a mutant that has reverted to its former genotype (true reversion) or to the original phenotype by means of a suppressor mutation. [L. *re-vertans*, pros. p. of *re-verto*, to turn back]

Revilliod, Léon, Swiss physician, 1835–1919. SEE R.'s *sign*.

rev·i·ves·cence (re-vi-ves'ens). SYN revivification (1). [L. *re-vivesco*, to come to life again, fr. *vivo*, to live]

re·viv·i·fi·ca·tion (rē-viv'i-fi-kā'shŭn). **1.** Renewal of life and strength. SYN revivescence. **2.** Refreshening the edges of a wound by paring or scraping to promote healing. SYN vivification. [L. *re-*, again, + *vivo*, to live, + *facio*, to make]

re·vul·sion (rē-vŭl'shŭn). **1.** SYN counterirritation. **2.** SYN derivation (1). [L. *revulsio*, act of pulling away, fr. *re-vello*, pp. *-vulsus*, to pluck or pull away]

re·ward (rē-ward'). SYN reinforcer.

re·warm·ing (rē-warm'ing). Application of heat to correct hypothermia.

Rexed. Bror A., Swedish physician, scientist, and public servant, *1914. SEE *lamina* of Rexed.

Reye, Ralph Douglas Kenneth, 20th century Australian pathologist. SEE R.'s *syndrome*.

Reymond. SEE Du Bois-Reymond.

RF Abbreviation for releasing *factors*; rheumatoid *factors*, under *factor*; replicative *form*; reticular *formation*.

RFA Abbreviation for right frontoanterior position.

RFLP Abbreviation for restriction fragment length *polymorphism*.

RFP Abbreviation for right frontoposterior position.

RFT Abbreviation for right frontotransverse position.

RH Abbreviation for releasing *hormone*.

Rh 1. Symbol for rhodium. **2.** See Rh blood group, Blood Groups appendix.

Rha. Abbreviation for L-rhamnose.

rha·bar·ber·one (ra-bar'ber-ōn). SYN aloe-emodin.

△**rhabd-.** SEE rhabdo-.

rhabditiform. SEE rhabditiform *larva*.

Rhab·di·tis (rab-dī'tis). A genus of small nematodes (family Rhabditidae, order Rhabditida), some of which are free-living, others parasitic on plants and animals; by dwelling on decaying organic matter, including putrefying flesh, some species have been viewed as parasitic or incipient parasites. *R. strongyloides* may invade the skin of dogs, cattle, and rodents, causing dermatitis. [G. *rhabdos*, a rod]

R.-like, SEE rhabditiform *larva*.

△**rhabdo-, rhabd-.** Rod; rod-shaped (rhabdoid). [G. *rhabdos*]

rhab·do·cyte (rab'dō-sīt). Rarely used term for band cell or metamyelocyte. [rhabdo- + G. *kytos*, cell]

rhab·doid (rab'doyd). Rod-shaped. [rhabdo- + G. *eidos*, resemblance]

rhab·do·my·o·blast (rab-dō-mī'ō-blast). Large round, spindle-shaped, or strap-shaped cells with deeply eosinophilic fibrillar cytoplasm which may show cross striations; found in some rhabdomyosarcomas. [rhabdo- + G. *mys*, muscle, + *blastos*, germ]

rhab·do·my·ol·y·sis (rab'dō-mī-ol'i-sis). An acute, fulminating, potentially fatal disease of skeletal muscle that entails destruction of skeletal muscle as evidenced by myoglobinemia and myoglobinuria. [rhabdo- + G. *mys*, muscle, + *lysis*, loosening]

acute recurrent r. [MIM*268200], repeated paroxysmal attacks of muscle pain and weakness followed by passage of dark red-brown urine, diagnosed by demonstration of myoglobin in the urine; it is attributed to abnormal phosphorylase activity in skeletal muscle, but there may be more than one biological type; it is more common in males than females; the genetics is obscure. In some cases, at least, there is deficiency of palmitoyl transferase. SYN familial paroxysmal r.

exertional r., r. produced in susceptible individuals by muscular exercise.

familial paroxysmal r., SYN acute recurrent r.

idiopathic paroxysmal r., SYN myoglobinuria.

rhab·do·my·o·ma (rab'dō-mī-ō'mă). A benign neoplasm derived from striated muscle, occurring in the heart in children, probably as a hamartomatous process. [rhabdo- + G. *mys*, muscle, + *-oma*, tumor]

rhab·do·my·o·sar·co·ma (rab'dō-mī-ō-sar-kō'mă). A malignant neoplasm derived from skeletal (striated) muscle, occurring in children or, less commonly, in adults; classified as embryonal alveolar (composed of loose aggregates of small round cells), or pleomorphic (containing rhabdomyoblasts). SYN rhabdosarcoma. [rhabdo- + G. *mys*, muscle, + *sarkōma*, sarcoma]

embryonal r.'s, malignant neoplasms occurring in children, consisting of loose, spindle-celled tissue with rare cross-striations, and arising in many parts of the body in addition to skeletal muscles.

rhab·do·pho·bia (rab-dō-fō'bē-ă). Morbid fear of a rod (or switch) as an instrument of punishment. [rhabdo- + G. *phobos*, fear]

rhab·do·sar·co·ma (rab'dō-sar-kō'mă). SYN rhabdomyosarcoma.

rhab·do·sphinc·ter (rab'dō-sfingk'ter). A sphincter made up of striated musculature. SYN striated muscular sphincter. [rhabdo- + G. *sphinktēr*, sphincter]

Rhab·do·vir·i·dae (rab'dō-vir'i-dē). A family of rod- or bullet-shaped viruses of vertebrates, insects, and plants, including rabies virus and vesicular stomatitis virus (of cattle). Virions (60 to 400 by 60 to 85 nm), formed by budding from surface membranes of cells, are enveloped and ether-sensitive, with surface spikes to 10-nm long; nucleocapsids contain negative sense single-stranded RNA (MW 3 to 5×10^6) and are of helical symmetry. Two genera have been assigned names, *Vesiculovirus* and *Lyssavirus;* others are currently unnamed.

rhab·do·vi·rus (rab'dō-vī'rŭs). Any virus of the family Rhabdoviridae.

△**rhachi-.** For words so beginning, see rachi-.

rhag·a·des (rag′ă-dēz). Chaps, cracks, or fissures occurring at mucocutaneous junctions; seen in vitamin deficiency diseases and in congenital syphilis. [G. *rhagas,* pl. *rhagades,* a crack]

rha·gad·i·form (ră-gad′i-fŏrm). Resembling or characterized by rhagades. [G. *rhagas* (*rhagad-*), crack, + L. *forma,* shape]

-rhagia. SEE -rrhagia.

L-**rham·nose (Rha.)** (ram′nōs). A methylpentose present in a number of plant glycosides, free in poison sumac, in lipopolysaccharides of *Enterobacteriaceae,* and in rutinose (a disaccharide). SYN isodulcit.

rham·no·side (ram′nō-sīd). A glycoside of rhamnose.

rham·no·xan·thin (ram-nō-zan′thin). SYN frangulin.

Rhamnus (ram′nŭs). A genus of shrubs and trees (family Rhamnaceae). The bark and berries of *R. cathartica* are cathartic; *R. frangula* is the source of frangula; *R. purshiana* is the source of cascara sagrada. SYN buckthorn. [G. *rhamnos*]

rha·pha·nia (ră-fā′nē-ă). SYN raphania.

rha·phe (rā′fē). SYN raphe.

-rhaphy. SEE -rrhaphy.

rha·thy·mia (ră-thī′mē-ă). Rarely used term for outgoing, care-free behavior. [G. *rhathymeō,* to take a holiday, be relaxed]

rhe (rē). The absolute unit of fluidity, the reciprocal of the unit of viscosity. [G. *rheos,* a stream]

-rhea. SEE -rrhea.

rheg·ma (reg′mă). A rent or fissure. [G. breakage]

rheg·ma·tog·e·nous (reg-mă-toj′ĕ-nŭs). Arising from a bursting or fractionating of an organ. SEE rhegmatogenous retinal *detachment.* [G. *rhēgma,* breakage, + *-gen,* producing]

rhe·ic (rē′ik). Relating to rheum (rhubarb).

Rheinberg mi·cro·scope. See under microscope.

rhe·ni·um (Re) (rē′nē-ŭm). A metallic element of the platinum group; atomic wt. 186.207, atomic no. 75. [Mod. L., fr. L. *Rhenus,* Rhine river]

rheo-. Blood flow; electrical current. [G. *rheos,* stream, current, flow]

rhe·o·base (rē′ō-bās). The minimal strength of an electrical stimulus of indefinite duration that is able to cause excitation of a tissue, *e.g.,* muscle or nerve. SEE ALSO chronaxie. SYN galvanic threshold. [rheo- + G. *basis,* a base]

rhe·o·ba·sic (rē-ō-bā′sik). Pertaining to or having the characteristics of a rheobase.

rhe·o·car·di·og·ra·phy (rē′ō-kar-dē-og′ră-phē). Impedance plethysmography applied to the heart. [rheo- + cardiography]

rhe·o·chrys·i·din (rē-ō-kris′i-din). The 3-methyl ether of emodin.

rhe·o·en·ceph·a·lo·gram (rē′ō-en-sef′ă-lō-gram). Graphic registration of the changes in conductivity of tissue of the head caused by vascular factors.

rhe·o·en·ceph·a·log·ra·phy (rē′ō-en-sef-ă-log′ră-fē). The technique of measuring blood flow of the brain; commonly used to denote impedance r. which uses changes in electrical impedance and resistance as a measure of flow. [rheo- + encephalography]

rhe·o·gram (rē′ō-gram). A plot of the shear stress versus the shear rate for a fluid. [rheo- + G. *gramma,* something written]

rhe·ol·o·gist (rē-ol′ō-jist). A specialist in rheology.

rhe·ol·o·gy (rē-ol′ō-jē). The study of the deformation and flow of materials. [rheo- + G. *logos,* study]

rhe·om·e·ter (rē-om′ĕ-ter). 1. An instrument for measurement of the rheologic properties of materials, *e.g.,* of blood. 2. A galvanometer. [rheo- + G. *metron,* measure]

rhe·om·e·try (rē-om′ĕ-trē). Measurement of electrical current or blood flow.

rhe·o·pexy (rē′ō-pek-sē). A property of certain materials in which an increased rate of shear favors an increase in viscosity. [rheo- + G. *pēxis,* fixation]

rhe·o·stat (rē′ō-stat). A variable resistor used to adjust the current in an electrical circuit. [rheo- + G. *statos,* stationary]

rhe·os·to·sis (rē-os-tō′sis). A hypertrophying and condensing osteitis which tends to run in longitudinal streaks or columns, like wax drippings on a candle, and which involves a number of the long bones. SYN flowing hyperostosis, streak hyperostosis. [rheo- + G. *osteon,* bone, + *-osis,* condition]

rhe·o·tax·is (rē-ō-tak′sis). A form of positive barotaxis, in which a microorganism in a fluid is impelled to move against the current flow of its medium. [rheo- + G. *taxis,* orderly arrangement]

rhe·ot·ro·pism (rē-ot′rō-pizm). A movement contrary to the motion of a current, involving part of an organism, rather than the organism as a whole, as in rheotaxis. [rheo- + G. *tropos,* a turning]

rhes·to·cy·the·mia (res′tō-sī-thē′mē-ă). The presence of broken down red blood cells in the peripheral circulation. [G. *rhaiō,* to destroy, + *kytos,* a hollow (a cell), + *haima,* blood]

rhe·sus (rē′sŭs). Generic name for *Macaca mulatta.* [Mod. L., fr. L. *Rhesus,* G. *Rhesos,* a mythical king of Thrace]

rheum (rūm). A mucous or watery discharge. [G. *rheuma,* a flux]

rheu·ma·tal·gia (rū-mă-tal′jē-ă). Obsolete term for rheumatic pain. [G. *rheuma,* flux, + *algos,* pain]

rheu·mat·ic (rū-mat′ik). Relating to or characterized by rheumatism. SYN rheumatismal. [G. *rheumatikos,* subject to flux, fr. *rheuma,* flux]

rheu·ma·tid (rū′mă-tid). Rheumatic nodules or other eruptions which may accompany rheumatism. [G. *rheum,* flux, + -id (1)]

rheu·ma·tism (rū′mă-tizm). 1. Obsolete term for rheumatic *fever.* 2. Indefinite term applied to various conditions with pain or other symptoms of articular origin or related to other elements of the musculoskeletal system. [G. *rheumatismos,* rheuma, a flux]

important rheumatic diseases
A. diseases of rheumatic type in the strict sense: collagenoses
1. rheumatoid arthritis
2. disseminated (or systemic) lupus erythematosus
3. Sjögren's syndrome
4. mixed connective tissue disease
5. spondylarthritis ankylopoetica (Bechterew disease)
6. Reiter's syndrome
7. panarteriitis
8. scleroderma
9. polymyositis, etc.
B. infectious arthritis
C. concomitant arthritis
1. with infections (e.g., rheumatic fever)
2. with internal diseases
3. with metabolic or endocrine diseases
4. with tumors
5. with allergies, etc.
D. degenerative joint diseases (arthroses)
E. psoriatic arthritis

articular r., SYN arthritis.

cerebral r., central nervous system symptoms resulting from a rheumatic disease. Formerly seen primarily as a manifestation of rheumatic *fever,* now seen less frequently as a part of other diseases such as systemic *lupus* erythematosus. SEE ALSO Sydenham's *chorea.*

chronic r., a nonspecific disorder of the joints, slow in progress,

rh

producing a painful thickening and contraction of the fibrous structures, interfering with motion, and causing deformity.

gonorrheal r., an arthritis, often initally a polyarthritis, caused by systemic infection with the gonococcus.

r. of the heart, rheumatic cardiac valvular disease, most often of the mitral and aortic valves.

inflammatory r., rheumatoid arthritis or other cause of joint inflammation.

lumbar r., SYN lumbago.

Macleod's r., rheumatoid arthritis with abundant serous effusion in the affected joints.

muscular r., SYN fibrositis (2).

nodose r., (1) SYN rheumatoid *arthritis.* **(2)** an acute or subacute articular r., accompanied by the formation of nodules on the tendons, ligaments, and periosteum in the neighborhood of the affected joints.

subacute r., a mild but usually protracted form of acute rheumatic fever, often resistant to treatment.

tuberculous r., an inflammatory condition of the joints or fibrous tissues during the course of tuberculosis.

rheu·ma·tis·mal (rū-mă-tiz′măl). SYN rheumatic.

rheu·ma·to·ce·lis (rū′mă-tō-sē′lis). Rarely used term for Henoch-Schönlein *purpura.* [G. *rheuma,* flux, + *kēlis,* spot]

rheu·ma·toid (rū′mă-toyd). Resembling r. arthritis in one or more features. [G. *rheuma,* flux, + *eidos,* resemblance]

rheu·ma·tol·o·gist (rū-mă-tol′ō-jist). A specialist in rheumatology.

rheu·ma·tol·o·gy (rū-mă-tol′ō-jē). The medical specialty concerned with the study, diagnosis, and treatment of rheumatic conditions. [G. *rheuma,* flux, + *logos,* study]

rhex·is (rek′sis). Obsolete term for bursting or rupture of an organ or vessel. [G. *rhēxis,* rupture]

rhi·go·sis (ri-gō′sis). The perception of cold. [G. *rhigoō,* to be cold, + *-osis,* condition]

rhi·got·ic (ri-got′ik). Pertaining to rhigosis.

△**rhin-, rhino-.** The nose. [G. *rhis*]

rhi·nal (rī′năl). SYN nasal.

rhi·nal·gia (rī-nal′jē-ă). Pain in the nose. SYN rhinodynia. [rhin- + G. *algos,* pain]

rhi·nar·i·um, pl. **rhi·nar·ia** (rī-nā′rē-ŭm, -rē-ă). The area of hairless skin surrounding the nostrils in some mammals.

rhin·e·de·ma (rī′ne-dē′mă). Swelling of the nasal mucous membrane. [rhin- + G. *oidēma,* swelling]

rhin·en·ce·phal·ic (rī′nen-se-fal′ik). Relating to the rhinencephalon.

rhin·en·ceph·a·lon (rī′nen-sef′ă-lon). Collective term denoting the parts of the cerebral hemisphere directly related to the sense of smell: the olfactory bulb, olfactory peduncle (together still listed as the first cranial nerve or olfactory nerve despite the fact that they form part of the central nervous system), olfactory tubercle, and olfactory or piriform cortex including the cortical nucleus of the amygdala. The term originally also encompassed the hippocampus, the entire amygdala, and the fornicate gyrus, which are no longer believed to be specifically related to the sense of smell. SEE ALSO limbic *system.* SYN smell-brain. [rhin- + G. *enkephalos,* brain]

rhin·en·chy·sis (rī-nen′kī-sis). A nasal douche; washing out the nasal cavities. [rhin- + G. *enchysis,* a pouring in]

rhin·i·on (rin′ē-on). A craniometric point: the lower end of the internal suture. [G. *rhinion,* nostril, dim. of *rhis* (*rhin-*), nose]

rhi·nism (rī′nizm). SYN rhinolalia.

rhi·ni·tis (rī-nī′tis). Inflammation of the nasal mucous membrane. SYN nasal catarrh. [rhin- + G. *-itis,* inflammation]

acute r., an acute catarrhal inflammation of the mucous membrane of the nose, marked by sneezing, lacrimation, and a profuse secretion of watery mucus; usually associated with infection by one of the common cold viruses. SYN cold in the head, coryza.

allergic r., r. associated with hay fever.

atrophic r., chronic r. with thinning of the mucous membrane; often associated with crusts and foul-smelling discharge.

atrophic r. of swine, a disease manifested by atrophy, shrinkage,

and often almost complete disappearance of the turbinate bones, accompanied by distortion of the facial bones, sneezing, and stunting of the growth of young animals; caused principally by the bacterium *Bordetella bronchiseptica.*

r. caseo′sa, caseous r., a form of chronic r. in which the nasal cavities are more or less completely filled with an ill-smelling cheesy material.

chronic r., a protracted sluggish inflammation of the nasal mucous membrane; in the later stages the mucous membrane with its glands may be thickened (hypertrophic r.) or thinned (atrophic r.).

gangrenous r., SEE *cancrum* nasi.

hypertrophic r., chronic r. with permanent thickening of the mucous membrane.

inclusion body r., a respiratory disease of pigs caused by the cytomegalovirus porcine herpesvirus 2 and characterized by r. and conjunctivitis in young pigs.

r. medicamento′sa, inflammation of the nasal mucosa secondary to excessive or improper topical medication.

necrotic r. of pigs, an infection of the subcutaneous structures of the snout of swine which causes malformation of the face; it is frequently due to infection of wounds made for the insertion of metal rings to discourage or prevent the animal from rooting in the soil; *Fusobacterium necrophorum* plays an important role in this disease. SYN bullnose.

r. nervo′sa, SYN hay *fever.*

scrofulous r., tuberculous infection of the nasal mucous membrane.

r. sic′ca, a form of chronic r. with little or no secretion.

vasomotor r., congestion of nasal mucosa without infection or allergy.

△**rhino-.** SEE rhin-.

rhi·no·an·e·mom·e·ter (rī′nō-an-ĕ-mom′ĕ-ter). A variation of the pneumotachometer, used for measuring nasal air flow and nasal resistance to air flow. [rhino- + G. *anemos,* wind, + *metron,* measure]

rhi·no·can·thec·to·my (rī′nō-kan-thek′tō-mē). Obsolete term for excision of the inner canthus of the eye. [rhino- + G. *kanthos,* canthus, + *ektomē,* excision]

rhi·no·cele (rī′nō-sēl). Cavity (ventricle) of the rhinencephalon, the primitive olfactory part of the telencephalon. [rhino- + G. *koilia,* a hollow]

rhi·no·ceph·a·ly, rhi·no·ce·pha·lia (rī′nō-sef′ă-lē, -se-fā′lē-ă). Rhinencephaly; a form of cyclopia in which the nose is represented by a fleshy proboscis-like protuberance arising above the slitlike orbits, and the rhinencephalic lobes of the telencephalon are poorly developed with some tendency to become fused together. [rhino- + G. *kephalē,* head]

rhi·no·chei·lo·plas·ty, rhi·no·chi·lo·plas·ty (rī-nō-kī′lō-plas-tē). Plastic surgery of the nose and upper lip. [rhino- + G. *cheilos,* lip, + *plastos,* formed]

Rhi·no·clad·i·el·la (rī′nō-klad-ē-el′ă). A genus of dematiaceous (dark colored) fungi, characterized by acrotheca, that cause chromoblastomycosis. SEE ALSO *Phialophora.*

rhi·no·clei·sis (rī-nō-klī′sis). SYN rhinostenosis. [rhino- + G. *kleisis,* a closure]

rhi·no·dac·ry·o·lith (rī-nō-dak′rē-ō-lith). Obsolete term for a calculus in the nasolacrimal duct. [rhino- + G. *dakryon,* tear (duct), + *lithos,* stone]

rhi·no·dym·ia (rī-nō-dim′ē-ă). Duplication of the nose on an otherwise normal face. [rhino- + G. *-dymos,* fold]

rhi·no·dyn·ia (rī-nō-din′ē-ă). SYN rhinalgia. [rhino- + G. *odynē,* pain]

rhi·no·es·tro·sis (rī′nō-es-trō′sis). Infection of horses and donkeys, rarely humans, with larvae of the fly *Rhinoestrus purpureus;* human infection is usually benign and of short duration, limited to the first stage of the larva and resulting in a mild ophthalmomyiasis.

Rhi·no·es·trus pur·pu·re·us (rī-nō-es′trŭs pŭr-pū′rē-ŭs). A species of fly of the family Oestridae, the nasal botflies, that causes rhinoestrosis.

rhi·nog·e·nous (rī-noj′ĕ-nŭs). Originating in the nose. [rhino- + G. -*gen*, producing]

rhi·no·ky·phec·to·my (rī′nō-kī-fek′tō-mē). Obsolete term referring to plastic surgery for rhinokyphosis. [rhino- + G. *kyphōsis*, humped condition, + *ektomē*, excision]

rhi·no·ky·pho·sis (rī′nō-kī-fō′sis). A humpback deformity of the nose. [rhino- + G. *kyphōsis*, humped condition]

rhi·no·la·lia (rī′nō-lā′lē-ă). Nasalized speech. SYN rhinism, rhinophonia. [rhino- + G. *lalia*, talking]

r. aper′ta, abnormal speech attributable to inadequate velopharyngeal closure.

r. clau′sa, abnormal speech attributable to nasal obstruction.

rhi·no·lite (rī′nō-līt). SYN rhinolith.

rhi·no·lith (rī′nō-lith). A calcareous concretion in the nasal cavity often around an undetected foreign body. SYN nasal calculus, rhinolite. [rhino- + G. *lithos*, stone]

rhi·no·li·thi·a·sis (rī′nō-li-thī′ă-sis). The presence of a nasal calculus. [rhinolith + G. -*iasis*, condition]

rhi·no·log·ic (rī-nō-loj′ik). Relating to rhinology.

rhi·nol·o·gist (rī-nol′ō-jist). A specialist in diseases of the nose.

rhi·nol·o·gy (rī-nol′ō-jē). The branch of medical science concerned with the nose and its diseases. [rhino- + G. *logos*, study]

rhi·no·ma·nom·e·ter (rī′nō-mă-nom′ĕ-ter). A manometer used to determine the presence and amount of nasal obstruction, and the nasal air pressure and flow relationships. [rhino- + manometer]

rhi·no·ma·nom·e·try (rī′nō-mă-nom′ĕ-trē). **1.** The use of a rhinomanometer. **2.** The study and measurement of nasal air flow and pressures.

rhi·no·mu·cor·my·co·sis (rī′nō-myū′kōr-mī-kō′sis). SYN entomophthoramycosis. [rhino- + mucormycosis]

rhi·no·my·co·sis (rī′nō-mī-kō′sis). Fungus infection of the nasal mucous membranes. [rhino- + mycosis]

rhi·no·ne·cro·sis (rī′nō-ne-krō′sis). Necrosis of the bones of the nose. [rhino- + necrosis]

rhi·nop·a·thy (rī-nop′ă-thē). Disease of the nose. [rhino- + G. *pathos*, suffering]

rhi·no·pha·ryn·ge·al (rī′nō-fă-rin′jē-ăl). **1.** SYN nasopharyngeal. **2.** Relating to the rhinopharynx.

rhi·no·pha·ryn·go·lith (rī′nō-fă-ring′gō-lith). A concretion in the rhinopharynx. [rhinopharynx + G. *lithos*, stone]

rhi·no·phar·ynx (rī′nō-far′ingks). SYN nasopharynx. [rhino- + pharynx]

rhi·no·pho·nia (rī′nō-fō′nē-ă). SYN rhinolalia. [rhino- + G. *phōnē*, voice]

rhi·no·phy·co·my·co·sis (rī′nō-fī′cō-mī-kō′sis). SYN entomophthoramycosis.

rhi·no·phy·ma (rī′nō-fī′mă). Hypertrophy of the nose with follicular dilation, resulting from hyperplasia of sebaceous glands with fibrosis and increased vascularity. SYN brandy nose, copper nose, hammer nose, hypertrophic rosacea, potato nose, rum nose, rum-blossom, toper's nose. [rhino- + G. *phyma*, tumor, growth]

rhi·no·plas·ty (rī′nō-plas-tē). **1.** Repair of a defect of the nose with tissue taken from elsewhere. **2.** Plastic surgery to change the shape or size of the nose. [rhino- + G. *plastos*, formed]

English r., r. utilizing a flap from the cheek.

Indian r., r. utilizing a flap from the forehead. SYN Carpue's method, Indian method, Indian operation.

Italian r., Italian method r. utilizing a flap from the arm. SYN Italian method, Italian operation, tagliacotian operation.

Joseph r., obsolete term for reduction and reshaping of the nose.

rhi·no·pneu·mo·ni·tis (rī′nō-nū-mō-nī′tis). Inflammation of the mucous membranes of the nose and lung in animals. [rhino- + G. *pneumōn*, lung, + -*itis*, inflammation]

equine r., a mild respiratory disease of horses, caused by equine herpesvirus 4, a member of the Herpesviridae, and characterized by fever, serous rhinitis, and leukopenia, sometimes resulting in abortion in mares.

rhi·nor·rhea (rī-nō-rē′ă). A discharge from the nasal mucous membrane. [rhino- + G. *rhoia*, flow]

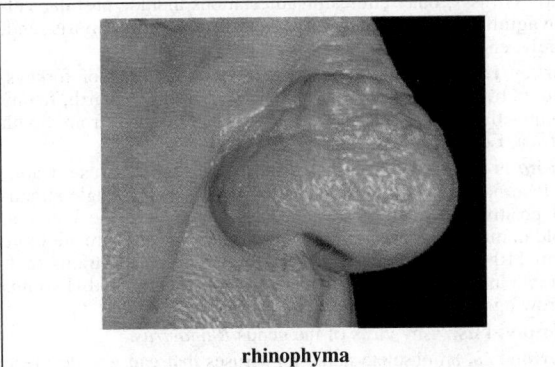

rhinophyma

cerebrospinal fluid r., a discharge of cerebrospinal fluid from the nose.

gustatory r., watery nasal discharge associated with stimulation of the sense of taste.

rhi·no·sal·pin·gi·tis (rī′nō-sal-pin-jī′tis). Inflammation of the mucous membrane of the nose and eustachian tube. [rhino- + G. *salpinx*, tube, + -*itis*, inflammation]

rhi·no·scle·ro·ma (rī′nō-sklē-rō′mă). A chronic granulomatous process involving the nose, upper lip, mouth, and upper air passages; starts usually as a growth of hard smooth nodules in the anterior nares which spreads backward into the pharynx, larynx, trachea, and even into the bronchi; it may involve the external auditory meatus and is believed to be due to a specific bacterium, possibly a strain of *Klebsiella*. [rhino- + G. *sklērōma*, an induration]

rhi·no·scope (rī′nō-skōp). A small mirror attached at a suitable angle to a rodlike handle, used in posterior rhinoscopy.

rhi·no·scop·ic (rī′nō-skop′ik). Relating to the rhinoscope or to rhinoscopy.

rhi·nos·co·py (rī-nos′kŏ-pē). Inspection of the nasal cavity. [rhino- + G. *skopeō*, to view]

anterior r., inspection of the anterior portion of the nasal cavity with or without the aid of a nasal speculum.

median r., inspection of the roof of the nasal cavity and openings of the posterior ethmoid cells and sphenoidal sinus by means of a long-bladed nasal speculum or nasopharyngoscope.

posterior r., inspection of the nasopharynx and posterior portion of the nasal cavity by means of the rhinoscope, or with a nasopharyngoscope. SEE ALSO nasopharyngoscopy.

rhi·no·spo·rid·i·o·sis (rī′nō-spō-rid-ē-ō′sis). Invasion of the nasal cavity by *Rhinosporidium seeberi*, resulting in a chronic granulomatous disease producing polyps or other forms of hyperplasia on mucous membranes; it is found in natives of North and South America, Pakistan, India, and Sri Lanka.

Rhi·no·spo·rid·i·um see·beri (rī′nōspō-rid′ē-ŭm sē-bē′rī). A fungal-like organism, of worldwide distribution and uncertain taxonomic position, found in certain vascular raspberry-like tumors of the septum nasi (rhinosporidiosis). [rhino- + G. *sporidion*, dim. of *sporos*, seed]

rhi·no·ste·no·sis (rī′nō-ste-nō′sis). Nasal obstruction. SYN rhinocleisis. [rhino- + G. *stenōsis*, a narrowing]

rhi·not·o·my (rī-not′ō-mē). **1.** Any cutting operation on the nose. **2.** Operative procedure in which the nose is incised along one side so that it may be turned away to provide full vision of the nasal passages for radical sinus operations. [rhino- + G. *tomē*, incision, cutting]

rhi·no·tra·che·i·tis (rī′nō-trā-kē-ī′tis). Inflammation of the nasal cavities and trachea. [rhino- + trachea + -*itis*, inflammation]

feline viral r., an acute upper respiratory tract infection of cats caused by the feline rhinotracheitis virus; it is frequently fatal in kittens but mild in adults, who sometimes become convalescent carriers of the virus.

infectious bovine r. (IBR), an infectious disease of cattle characterized by tracheitis, rhinitis, and fever, and caused by bovine herpesvirus 1; other clinical manifestations include pustular vulvovaginitis or balanoposthitis, abortion, conjunctivitis and, rarely, encephalitis.

turkey r., a disease of the upper respiratory tract of turkeys, caused by the turkey r. virus and characterized by catarrh, foamy conjunctivitis, and sinusitis; it has been reported from South Africa, Europe, and Israel.

Rhi·no·vi·rus (rī′nō-vī′rŭs). A genus of acid-labile viruses (family Picornaviridae) of worldwide distribution with a single-stranded positive sense RNA genome, associated with the common cold in man and foot-and-mouth disease in cattle. There are more than 110 antigenic types, formerly classified as M strains (culturable in rhesus monkey kidney and human cells) and H strains (growing only in cultures of human cells).

rhi·no·vi·rus. Any virus of the genus *Rhinovirus.*

bovine r.'s, an obsolete name for viruses that cause widespread subclinical and occasionally mild clinical respiratory diseases of calves in the United States and Europe.

equine r.'s, an obsolete name for viruses that cause inapparent as well as mild to relatively severe upper respiratory tract disease in the United States and Europe; most prevalent in breeding stables, and associated with high morbidity but negligible mortality; all equine isolates are related serologically to the original isolate.

Rhi·pi·ceph·a·lus (rī-pi-sef′ă-lŭs). A genus of inornate hard ticks (family Ixodidae) consisting of about 50 species, all of which are Old World except *R. sanguineus.* Eyes and festoons are present in both sexes; short palpi and ventral plates are present only in the male. The genus includes important vectors of diseases in humans and domestic animals. [G. *rhipis,* fan, + *kephalē,* head]

R. appendicula'tus, the brown ear tick, a species that transmits *Theileria parva parva,* the cause of East Coast fever, and *Theileria parva lawrencei,* the cause of Corridor disease, and *Theileria parva bovis,* the cause of Rhodesian malignant theileriosis.

R. evert'si, the red-legged or African red t., a vector of East Coast fever and of *Borrelia theileri.*

R. pulchel'lus, the yellow-backed or zebra tick; a vector of *Theileria taurotragi,* the cause of benign bovine theileriosis in Africa.

R. sanguin'eus, the brown dog tick, probably the most common and cosmopolitan species found on dogs in the U.S.; it may attack other animals but rarely attacks humans; it is a vector of Rocky Mountain spotted fever in Mexico, the major vector of canine babesiosis, transmits canine ehrlichiosis, and is a vector of the rickettsia of boutonneuse fever.

△**rhizo-.** Combining form denoting root. [G. *rhiza*]

rhi·zoid (rī′zoyd). **1.** Rootlike. **2.** Irregularly branching, like a root; denoting a form of bacterial growth. **3.** In fungi, the rootlike hyphae which arise at the nodes of the hyphae of *Rhizopus* species. [rhizo- + G. *eidos,* resemblance]

rhi·zome (rī′zōm). The creeping underground stem of plants such as iris, calamus, and sanguinaria. [G. *rhizōma,* mass of roots, fr. *rhiza,* root, + *-oma,* mass]

rhi·zo·me·lia (rī-zō-mē′lē-ă). **1.** Disproportion in the length of the most proximal segment of the limbs (upper arms and thighs). **2.** A disorder involving the shoulder and hip joint. [rhizo- + G. *melos,* limb]

rhi·zo·me·nin·go·my·e·li·tis (rī′zō-mĕ-ning′gō-mī-ĕ-lī′tis). Inflammation of the nerve roots, the meninges, and the spinal cord. SYN radiculomeningomyelitis. [rhizo- + G. *mēninx,* membrane, + *myelon,* marrow, + *-itis,* inflammation]

rhi·zo·plast (rī′zō-plast). A fine connection between the flagellum or blepharoplast and the nucleus of a protozoan. [rhizo- + G. *plastos,* formed]

Rhi·zop·o·da (rī-zō-pō′dă). A superclass in the subphylum Sarcodina that includes the amebae of humans, having pseudopodia of various forms but without axial filaments. SYN Rhizopodasida, Rhizopodea. [rhizo + G. *pous* (*pod*-), foot]

Rhi·zo·po·das·i·da (rī′zō-pō-das′i-dă). SYN Rhizopoda.

Rhi·zo·po·dea (rī-zō-pō′dē-ă). SYN Rhizopoda. [rhizo- + G. *pous* (*pod*-), foot]

rhi·zop·ter·in (rī-zop′ter-in). 10-formylpteroic acid; a folic acid

factor for certain bacteria. SYN SLR factor, *Streptococcus lactis* R factor.

Rhi·zo·pus (rī-zō′pŭs). A genus of fungi (class Zygomycetes, family Mucoraceae); some species cause zygomycosis in humans.

rhi·zot·o·my (rī-zot′ō-mē). Section of the spinal nerve roots for the relief of pain or spastic paralysis. SYN radicotomy, radiculectomy. [G. *rhiza,* root, + *tomē,* section]

anterior r., section of anterior spinal root.

facet r., a percutaneous radio frequency lysis of the innervation of a facet.

posterior r., section of posterior spinal root. SYN Dana's operation.

trigeminal r., division or section of a sensory root of the fifth cranial nerve, accomplished through a subtemporal (Frazier-Spiller operation), suboccipital (Dandy operation), or transtentorial approach. SYN retrogasserian neurectomy, retrogasserian neurotomy.

rho (ρ) (rō). **1.** 17th Letter of the Greek alphabet. **2.** Symbol for density. **3.** SEE rho *factor.*

△**rhod-.** SEE rhodo-.

rho·da·mine B (rō′dă-mēn, -min) [C.I. 45170]. A fluorescent red basic xanthene dye, tetraethylrhodamine chloride, used in histology as a contrasting stain to methylene blue and methyl green, and as a vital fluorochrome.

rho·da·nate (rō′dă-nāt). SYN thiocyanate.

rho·da·nese (rō′dă-nēz). SYN *thiosulfate* sulfurtransferase.

rho·dan·ic ac·id (rō-dan′ik). SYN thiocyanic acid.

rho·da·nile blue (rō′dă-nīl). A dye mixture, considered by some to be a salt of rhodamine B and Nile blue, used to stain keratinized epithelium (red) and fibroblasts (blue), as well as spermatozoa and normal and pathologic acidophilic, basophilic, and certain neutrophilic elements of cells and tissues; used as a substitute for hematoxylin and eosin.

rho·de·ose (rō′dē-ōs). SYN fucose.

rho·din (rō′din). A dihydroporphyrin derivative (the two additional hydrogens being at positions 17 and 18) of the type found in chlorophyll *b* and with a formyl group on position 7 rather than a methyl group.

rho·di·um (Rh) (rō′dē-ŭm). A metallic element, atomic no. 45, atomic wt. 102.90550. [Mod. L. fr. G. *rhodon,* a rose]

△**rhodo-, rhod-.** Rosy, red color. [G. *rhodon,* rose]

Rho·do·coc·cus (rō-dō-kok′us). A genus of rod-shaped, Gram-positive, partially acid-fast, aerobic bacteria found in soil and in the feces of herbivores. Some species are pathogenic for animals and human beings. The type species is *Rhodococcus rhodochrous.*

R. equi, a species causing bronchopneumonia and the formation of abscesses in the lungs of foals. It can cause bronchopneumonia in immunocompromised humans, especially those with AIDS. SYN *Corynebacterium equi.*

rho·do·gen·e·sis (rō′dō-jen′ĕ-sis). The production of rhodopsin by the combination of 11-*cis*-retinal and opsin in the dark. [rhodopsin + G. *genesis,* production]

rho·do·phy·lac·tic (rō′dō-fī-lak′tik). Relating to rhodophylaxis.

rho·do·phy·lax·is (rō′dō-fī-lak′sis). The action of the pigment cells of the choroid in preserving or facilitating the reproduction of rhodopsin. [rhodopsin + G. *phylaxis,* a guarding]

rho·dop·sin (rō-dop′sin). A red thermolabile protein, MW *ca.* 40,000, found in the external segments of the rods of the retina; it is bleached by the action of light, which converts it to opsin and all-*trans*-retinal, and is restored in the dark by rhodogenesis; the dominant protein in the plasma membrane of rod cells. SYN visual purple.

r. kinase, an enzyme that regulates r. function by phosphorylating activated r. at a number of sites; phosphorylated photoactivated r. binds to arrestin.

*meta-***rho·dop·sin I,** *meta-***rho·dop·sin II,** *meta-***rho·dop·sin III.** Precursors of opsin and all-*trans*-retinal, formed from lumirhodopsin in the visual cycle.

Rho·do·tor·u·la (rō-dō-tōr′yū-lă). A genus of yeasts, usually

rhythm				
		pacemaker disturbances	conduction disturbances	
nomotopic	single-beat	sinus extrasystole	atrial	sinoauricular block
	rhythm	sinus bradycardia sinus tachycardia sinus arrhythmia wandering pacemaker	atrioventricular	atrioventricular block (1st, 2nd, and 3rd degrees) Wenckebach period Möbitz block
heterotopic	single-beat	atrial extrasystole A-V nodal extrasystole ventricular extrasystole sinoatrial block	intraventricular	left branch block right branch block bundle branch block WPW-syndrome
	rhythm	A-V nodal rhythm ventricular rhythm supraventricular tachycardia A-V nodal tachycardia ventricular tachycardia atrial flutter ventricular flutter atrial fibrillation ventricular fibrillation	combined disturbances of impulse formation and conduction	

rh

pink to red and of questionable pathogenicity, which are generally introduced iatrogenically in prosthetic implants and into immunocompromised patients via intravenous catheters.

rhomb·en·ceph·a·lon (rom-ben-sef′ă-lon) [NA]. That part of the developing brain that is the most caudal of the three primary vesicles of the embryonic neural tube; secondarily divided into metencephalon and myelencephalon; the r. includes the pons, cerebellum, and medulla oblongata. SYN hindbrain vesicle, hindbrain. [rhombo- + G. *enkephalos*, brain]

rhom·bic (rom′bik). 1. SYN rhomboid. 2. Relating to the rhombencephalon.

♲rhombo-. Rhombic, rhomboid. [G. *rhombos*]

rhom·bo·at·loi·de·us. SEE *musculus* rhomboatloideus.

rhom·bo·cele (rom′bō-sēl). SYN rhomboidal *sinus*. [rhombo- + G. *koilia*, a hollow]

rhom·boid, rhom·boi·dal (rom′boyd, rom-boy′dăl). Resembling a rhomb; *i.e.*, an oblique parallelogram, but having unequal sides; in anatomy, denoting especially a ligament and two muscles. SYN rhombic (1). [rhombo- + G. *eidos*, appearance]

rhom·boi·de·us (rom-bō-id′ē-ŭs). SEE rhomboid minor *muscle*.

rhom·bo·mere. Segments of the developing neural tube in the rhombencephalon; nine rhombomeres appear in the developing human. [rhombencephalon + G. *meros*, part]

rhon·chal, rhon·chi·al (rong′kăl, rong′kē-ăl). Relating to or characteristic of a rhonchus.

rhon·chus, pl. **rhon·chi** (rong′kŭs, -kī). An added sound with a musical pitch occurring during inspiration or expiration, heard on auscultation of the chest, and caused by air passing through bronchi that are narrowed by inflammation, spasm of smooth muscle, or presence of mucus in the lumen; if low-pitched, it is called **sonorous r.**; if high-pitched, with a whistling or squeaky quality, **sibilant r.**. [L. fr. G. *rhenchos*, a snoring]

cavernous r., SYN cavernous *rale*.

rho·phe·o·cy·to·sis (rō′fē-ō-sī-tō′sis). Formation of vacuoles at a cell surface without prior formation of cytoplasmic projections, by which the cell appears to aspirate surrounding material. SEE ALSO pinocytosis. [G. *rhopheō*, to gulp down, or aspirate, + *kytos*, cell, + *-osis*, condition]

rhop·try, pl. **rhop·tries** (rōp′trē, -trēs). Electron-dense club-shaped, tubular or saccular organelles extending back from the anterior end of sporozoites and other stages of certain sporozoans in the subphylum Apicomplexa. SYN paired organelles, toxoneme. [G. *rhopalon*, club]

rho·ta·cism (rō′tă-sizm). Mispronunciation of the "r" sound. [G. *rhō*, the letter r]

rhu·barb (rū′barb). Any plant of the genus *Rheum* (family Polygonaceae), especially *R. rhaponticum*, garden rhubarb, and *R. officinale* or *R. palmatum;* the last two species or their hybrids, deprived of periderm tissues, dried, and powdered, are used for their astringent, tonic and laxative effects.

Rhus (rūs, rŭs). A genus of vines and shrubs (family Anacardiaceae) containing various species that are used for their ornamental foliage; formerly used in tanning. Certain poisonous species are classified as *Toxicodendron*. [L., fr. G. *rhous*, sumac]

rhy·pa·ria (rī-pā′rē-ă). SYN sordes. [G. filth, fr. *rhypos*, filth]

rhy·poph·a·gy (rī-pof′ă-jē). SYN coprophagia. [G. *rhypos*, filth, + *phagō*, to eat]

rhy·po·pho·bia (rī-pō-fō′bē-ă). An abnormal aversion to or morbid fear of dirt or filth. [G. *rhypos*, filth, + *phobos*, fear]

rhythm (rith′ŭm). 1. Measured time or motion; the regular alternation of two or more different or opposite states. 2. SYN rhythm *method*. 3. Regular occurrence of an electrical event in the electroencephalogram. SEE ALSO wave. 4. Sequential beating of the heart generated by a single beat or sequence of beats. [G. *rhythmos*]

agonal r., an idioventricular r., characterized by unusually wide and bizarre ventricular complexes, often seen in moribund patients.

alpha r., (1) a wave pattern in the encephalogram in the frequency band of 8 to 13 Hz; (2) the posterior dominant 8–13 Hz r. in the awake, relaxed person with closed eyes, that attenuates with eye opening. SYN alpha wave, Berger r.

atrioventricular junctional r., the cardiac r. when the heart is controlled by the A-V junction (including node); arising in the A-V junction, the impulse ascends to the atria and descends to the ventricles, each at varying speeds depending on site of the pacemaker. SYN A-V junctional r., nodal bradycardia, nodal r.

A-V junctional r., SYN atrioventricular junctional r.

basic electrical r. (BER), a slow wave of depolarization of smooth muscle from the fundus to the pylorus that coordinates gastric peristalsis and emptying.

Berger r., SYN alpha r.

beta r., a wave pattern in the electroencephalogram in the frequency band of 18 to 30 Hz. SYN beta wave.

bigeminal r., that cardiac r. when each beat of the dominant rhythm (sinus or other) is followed by a premature beat, with the result that the heartbeats occur in pairs (bigeminy). SYN coupled r.

cantering r., SYN gallop.

circadian r., SEE circadian.

circus r., SYN circus *movement.*

coronary nodal r., formerly applied by some authorities to the electrocardiographic pattern of normal upright P waves in leads I and II with a short P-R interval.

coronary sinus r., an ectopic atrial r. supposedly originating from a pacemaker at the mouth of the coronary sinus; recognized in the electrocardiogram by P-waves that are inverted in leads II, III, and a VI with a normal or prolonged P-R interval; an ectopic ("lower") atrial rhythm.

coupled r., SYN bigeminal r.

delta r., a wave pattern in the electroencephalogram in the frequency band of 1.5 to 4.0 Hz. SYN delta wave (2).

diurnal r., SEE diurnal.

ectopic r., any cardiac r. arising from a center other than the normal pacemaker, the sinus node.

escape r., three or more consecutive impulses at a rate not exceeding the upper limit of the inherent pacemaker; extreme range of impulse formation at the sinoatrial node is between 40 to 180 impulses per minute, that of the atrioventricular junction is normally 40 to 60 impulses per minute, and the normal rate of the ventricular myocardium (idioventricular rhythm) is 20 to 40 impulses per minute.

gallop r., SYN gallop.

idiojunctional r., SYN idionodal r.

idionodal r., an independent r., the ventricles being under control of the A-V node (A-V junction). SYN idiojunctional r.

idioventricular r., a slow independent ventricular r. under control of a ventricular center (which is, by definition, ectopic). SYN ventricular r.

junctional r., r.'s originating anywhere within the A-V junction. Formerly, "A-V nodal" or simply "nodal" r.'s.

nodal r., SYN atrioventricular junctional r.

pendulum r., SYN embryocardia.

quadrigeminal r., a cardiac arrhythmia in which the heartbeats are grouped in fours, each usually composed of one sinus beat followed by three extrasystoles, but a repetitive group of four of any composition is quadrigeminal. SYN quadrigeminy.

quadruple r., a quadruple cadence to the heart sounds due to the easy audibility of both third and fourth heart sounds, indicative of serious myocardial disease. SYN trainwheel r.

reciprocal r., a cardiac arrhythmia in which the impulse arising in the A-V junction descends to and activates the ventricles on one intrajunctional pathway and simultaneously ascends toward the atria in parallel pathways; before reaching the atria, however, the impulse is reflected downward and again activates the ventricles, producing an echo or reciprocal beat; recognized in the electrocardiogram by the presence of an inverted P wave in lead aVF and usually II sandwiched between two ventricular complexes aberrantly, both of which may be normal or one of which may be conducted.

reciprocating r., a cardiac arrhythmia initiated by an A-V junctional beat followed in turn by a reciprocal beat; the descending impulse of the reciprocal beat, before reaching the ventricles, is also reflected backward to the atria, but before reaching the atria is reflected downward again to the ventricles, so that there is both retrograde atrial activation and orthograde ventricular activation.

reversed reciprocal r., a cardiac arrhythmia in which a normal sinus impulse, before reaching the ventricles, is reflected backward to the atria; thus in the electrocardiogram a ventricular complex is sandwiched between a normal sinus P wave and a retrograde P wave; if the dysrhythmia continues, subsequent cycles are similar to those of reciprocating r.

sinus r., normal cardiac r. proceeding from the sinoatrial node.

systolic gallop r., obsolete term for extra sounds, usually clicks, heard during systole.

theta r., a wave pattern in the electroencephalogram in the frequency band of 4 to 7 Hz. SYN theta wave.

tic-tac r., SYN embryocardia.

trainwheel r., SYN quadruple r.

trigeminal r., a cardiac arrhythmia in which the beats are grouped in trios, usually composed of a sinus beat followed by two extrasystoles. SYN trigeminy.

triple r., a triple cadence to the heart sounds at any heart rate, due to the easy audibility of a third (usually) or fourth heart sound, or at faster rates a summation sound due to coincidence of the third and fourth heart sounds.

ultradian r., SEE ultradian.

ventricular r., SYN idioventricular r.

rhyt·i·dec·to·my (rit-i-dek′tō-mē). Elimination of wrinkles from, or reshaping of, the face by excising any excess skin and tightening the remainder; the so-called face-lift. SYN rhytidoplasty. [G. *rhytis (rhytid-),* a wrinkle]

rhyt·i·do·plas·ty (rit′i-dō-plas-tē). SYN rhytidectomy. [G. *rhytis,* a wrinkle, + *plastos,* formed]

rhyt·i·do·sis (rit-i-dō′sis). **1.** Wrinkling of the face to a degree disproportionate to age. **2.** Laxity and wrinkling of the cornea, an indication of approaching death. SYN rutidosis. [G. a wrinkling, fr. *rhytis,* a wrinkle, + *-osis,* condition]

r. retinae, retinal wrinkling.

RIA Abbreviation for radioimmunoassay.

Rib Symbol for ribose. SYN os costale [NA], costa (1).

rib. One of the twenty-four elongated curved bones forming the main portion of the bony wall of the chest. [A.S. *ribb*]

bicipital r., fusion of first thoracic r. with cervical vertebra.

bifid r., one in which the body bifurcates.

cervical r., a supernumerary rib articulating with a cervical vertebra, usually the seventh, but not reaching the sternum anteriorly. SEE ALSO cervical rib *syndrome.* SYN costa cervicalis [NA].

false r.'s, five lower ribs on either side that do not articulate with the sternum directly. SYN costae spuriae [NA], vertebrochondral r.'s.

floating r.'s, the two lower ribs on either side that are not attached anteriorly. SYN costae fluitantes [NA], costae fluctuantes, vertebral r.'s.

lumbar r., an occasional r. articulating with the transverse process of the first lumbar vertebra.

r. notching, a smooth defect in the lower border of one or more upper r.'s caused by enlarged intercostal collateral vessels, most often a sign of coarctation of the aorta.

slipping r., subluxation of a r. cartilage, with costochondral separation.

true r.'s, seven upper ribs on either side whose cartilages articulate directly with the sternum. SYN costae verae [NA], vertebrosternal r.'s.

vertebral r.'s, SYN floating r.'s.

vertebrochondral r.'s, SYN false r.'s.

vertebrosternal r.'s, SYN true r.'s.

△**rib-.** SEE ribo-.

ri·ba·vi·rin (rī′bă-vī-rin). 1-β-D-Ribofuranosyl-1,2,4-triazole-3-carboxamide; a synthetic nucleoside antiviral agent which, by its inhibitory effect on the synthesis of guanosine 5′-phosphate, inhibits both DNA and RNA synthesis.

α-ri·ba·zole (rī′bă-zōl). 1-α-D-ribofuranosyl-5,6-dimethylbenzimidazole; the benzimidazole nucleoside in vitamin B_{12}.

Ribbert, Moritz W.H., German pathologist, 1855–1920. SEE R.'s *theory.*

rib·bon (rib′ŏn). A ribbon-shaped structure. [M. E. *riban*]

Reil's r., SYN medial *lemniscus.*

Ribes, François, French physician, 1765–1845. SEE R.'s *ganglion.*

ri·bi·tol (rī′bi-tol). $HOCH_2(CHOH)_3CH_2OH$; reduction product of ribose (–CHO at position 1 of ribose reduced to –CH_2OH). SYN adonitol.

ri·bi·tyl (rī′bi-til). The radical of ribitol; a constituent of riboflavin.

△**ribo-.** **1.** Ribose. **2.** As an italicized prefix to the systematic name of a monosaccharide, *ribo-* indicates that the configuration of a set of three consecutive, but not necessarily contiguous, CHOH (or asymmetric) groups is that of ribose; *e.g.,* D-ribose, a trivial name, is D-*ribo*-pentose in systematic nomenclature. [German *Ribose*]

ri·bo·fla·vin, ri·bo·fla·vine (rī′bō-flā-vin). 7,8-dimethyl-10-ribitylisoalloxazine; a heat-stable factor of the vitamin B complex whose isoalloxazine nucleotides are coenzymes of the flavodehydrogenases. The daily human requirement is 1.7 mg for adult men and 1.3 mg for adult women, with a higher daily requirement during pregnancy and lactation; dietary sources include green vegetables, liver, kidneys, wheat germ, milk, eggs, cheese, and fish. SYN flavin (1), flavine, lactoflavin (2), vitamin B_2 (1).

r. kinase, a cytosolic enzyme catalyzing the formation of flavin mononucleotide (r. phosphate) from r., utilizing ATP as phosphorylating agent. SYN flavokinase.

methylol r., a mixture of methylol derivatives of r. formed by the action of formaldehyde on r. in weakly alkaline solution; it has the same action as r., but is preferred for parenteral administration.

ri·bo·fla·vin 5′-phos·phate. SYN *flavin* mononucleotide.

ri·bo·fu·ra·nose (rī-bō-fūr′ă-nōs). The 1,4 cyclic furan form of ribose.

9-β-D-ri·bo·fu·ran·o·syl·ad·e·nine (rī′bō-fūr-an′o-sil-ad′ĕ-nēn). SYN adenosine.

1-β-D-ri·bo·fu·ran·o·syl·cy·to·sine (rī′bō-fūr-an′o-sil-sī′tō-sēn). SYN cytidine.

9-β-D-ri·bo·fu·ran·o·syl·gua·nine (rī′bō-fūr-an′ō-sil-gwah′nēn). SYN guanosine.

9-β-ribofuranosylpurine. SYN nebularine.

ri·bo·fu·ran·o·syl·thy·mine (rī′bō-fūr-an′ō-sil-thī′mēn). SYN ribothymidine.

1-β-D-ri·bo·fu·ran·o·syl·u·ra·cil (rī′bō-fūr-an′ō-sil-yūr′ă-sil). SYN uridine.

ri·bo-2-hex·u·lose. SYN psicose.

ri·bo·nu·cle·ase (RNase) (rī-bō-nū′klē-ās). A transferase or phosphodiesterase that catalyzes the hydrolysis of ribonucleic acid. SEE ALSO ribonuclease (pancreatic), ribonuclease (*Bacillus subtilis*). SYN ribonucleinase.

RNase A, ribonuclease (pancreatic).

alkaline RNase, ribonuclease (pancreatic).

RNase alpha, an enzyme catalyzing endonucleolytic cleavage of O-methylated RNA yielding 5′-phosphomonoesters.

r. D (RNase D), an enzyme (endonuclease) that trims the extra 3′ nucleotides from immature tRNA.

Escherichia coli **RNase I,** SYN RNase T_2.

RNase I, ribonuclease (pancreatic).

RNase II [EC 3.1.13.1], an enzyme cleaving RNA exonucleolytically in the 3′ to 5′ direction, yielding 5′-phosphomononucleotides. SEE ALSO microbial RNase II.

RNase III, an enzyme catalyzing endonucleolytic cleavage of double-stranded RNA yielding 5′-phosphomonoesters.

microbial RNase II, SYN RNase T_2.

RNase N_1, SYN RNase T_1.

RNase N_2, SYN RNase T_2.

RNase P, an enzyme catalyzing the endonucleolytic cleavage tRNA precursors to yield 5′-phosphomonoesters.

r. P (RNase P), an enzyme (endonuclease) that trims the extra 5′ nucleotides from immature tRNA; a protein RNA complex.

pancreatic RNase, SEE ribonuclease (pancreatic).

plant RNase, SYN RNase T_2.

RNase T_1, a nuclease endonucleolytically cleaving ribonucleic acids at the 3′-5′ link of a guanosine 3′-phosphate residue, producing oligonucleotides terminating in this nucleotide; a transferase (endonuclease) in the first (cyclizing) step, a phosphodiesterase on the second (hydrolyzing) step. SYN guanyloribonuclease, RNase N_1.

RNase T_2, an enzyme endonucleolytically cleaving RNA to 3′-nucleotides with 2′,3′-cyclic nucleotides as intermediates. SYN *Escherichia coli* RNase I, microbial RNase II, plant RNase, RNase N_2.

RNase U_2, an enzyme endonucleolytically cleaving RNA to 3′-phospho-mono- and oligonucleotides ending in adenylate or guanylate residues with 2′,3′-cyclic phosphate intermediates.

RNase U_4, SYN yeast RNase.

yeast RNase, an enzyme catalyzing the exonucleolytic cleavage of RNA to yield 3′-phosphomononucleotides. SYN RNase U_4.

ri·bo·nu·cle·ase (*Ba·cil·lus sub·ti·lis*). **1.** Ribonuclease (*Azotobacter agilis*); ribonuclease (*Proteus mirabilis*); an enzyme catalyzing the endonucleolytic cleavage of RNA to yield 2′,3′-cyclic nucleotides. **2.** Ribonuclease T_1.

ri·bo·nu·cle·ase (pan·cre·at·ic). An enzyme that transfers the 3′-phosphate of a pyrimidine ribonucleotide residue in a polynucleotide from the 5′-position of the adjoining nucleotide to the 2′-position of the pyrimidine nucleotide itself (a transferase, endonuclease action), thus breaking the chain and forming a pyrimidine 2′,3′-cyclic phosphate, then (or independently) hydrolyzing this phosphodiester to leave a pyrimidine nucleoside 3′-phosphate residue (phosphodiesterase action); used in cytochemistry to selectively degrade and remove RNA as a control for staining of RNA.

ri·bo·nu·cle·ic ac·id (RNA) (rī′bō-nū-klē′ik). A macromolecule consisting of ribonucleoside residues connected by phosphate from the 3′-hydroxyl of one to the 5′-hydroxyl of the next nucleoside. RNA is found in all cells, in both nuclei and cytoplasm and in particulate and nonparticulate form, and also in many viruses; polynucleotides made *in vitro* are generally called such. Various RNA fractions are identified by location, form, or function.

acceptor RNA, SYN transfer RNA.

antisense RNA, the transcription product of the DNA antisense strand; it can play a role in the inhibition of translation. SEE ALSO antisense DNA.

chromosomal RNA, RNA associated with the chromosome (not mRNA, tRNA, or rRNA) that may have a role in transcription.

heterogeneous nuclear RNA (hnRNA), an ill-defined form of RNA, of high molecular weight, that never leaves the nucleus and is thought to be the precursor of messenger RNA.

informational RNA, SYN messenger RNA.

initiation tRNA, tRNA in prokaryotes containing a formyl-methionyl residue that initiates translation. SYN formyl-methionyl-tRNA, starter tRNA.

messenger RNA (mRNA), the RNA reflecting the exact nucleoside sequence of the genetically active DNA and carrying the "message" of the latter, coded in its sequence, to the cytoplasmic areas where protein is made in amino acid sequences specified by the mRNA, and hence primarily by the DNA; viral RNA's are considered to be natural messenger RNA's. SYN informational RNA, template RNA.

messenger-like RNA (mlRNA), SEE heterogeneous nuclear RNA.

nuclear RNA (nRNA), rNA found in nuclei, or associated with DNA, or with nuclear structures (nucleoli).

RNA polymerase, SEE nucleotidyltransferases.

ribosomal RNA, the RNA of ribosomes and polyribosomes.

small nuclear RNA (snRNA), small RNA, *i.e.,* about 90 to 300 nucleotides long in the nucleus believed to have a role in RNA processing and cellular architecture.

soluble RNA (sRNA), SYN transfer RNA. [soluble in molar salt]

starter tRNA, SYN initiation tRNA.

suppressor tRNA, the tRNA associated with a suppressor mutation.

template RNA, SYN messenger RNA.

transfer RNA (tRNA), short-chain RNA molecules present in cells in at least 20 varieties, each variety capable of combining with a specific amino acid (see aminoacyl-tRNA). By joining (through their anticodons) with particular spots (codons) along the messenger RNA molecule and carrying their amino acyl residues along, they lead to the formation of protein molecules with a specific amino acid arrangement—the one ultimately dictated by a segment of DNA in the chromosomes. Each tRNA has about 80 nucleotides (MW about 25,000); most of the 20 varieties occur in multiple "isoacceptor" forms, separable by chromatography. Further subvarieties exist in different strains of an organism, in subcellular organelles, in different metabolic states, etc. Cognate tRNA's are the tRNA's recognized by the specific amino acyl-tRNA synthetases. SYN acceptor RNA, soluble RNA.

ri·bo·nu·cle·i·nase (rī-bō-nū′klē-i-nās). SYN ribonuclease.

ri·bo·nu·cle·o·pro·tein (RNP) (rī'bō-nū'klē-ō-prō'tēn). A combination of ribonucleic acid and protein.

ri·bo·nu·cle·o·side (rī-bō-nū'klē-ō-sīd). A nucleoside in which the sugar component is ribose; the common r.'s of RNA are adenosine, cytidine, guanosine, and uridine.

ri·bo·nu·cle·o·tide (rī-bō-nū'klē-ō-tīd). A nucleotide (nucleoside phosphate) in which the sugar component is ribose; the major r.'s of RNA are adenylic acid, cytidylic acid, guanylic acid, and uridylic acid.

r. reductase, a protein complex that converts ribonucleotide diphosphates (NDPs) such as ADP and CDP to 2'-deoxyribonucleotide diphosphates (dNDPs) such as dADP and dCDP. This complex requires thioredoxin, thioredoxin reductase, and NADPH. It is crucial for DNA synthesis.

ri·bo·pho·rins (rī'-bō-for'inz). Ribosome receptor proteins that interact specifically with the large ribosomal subunit and aid in translocation of newly synthesized proteins across the endoplasmic reticulum. [*ribo*nucleic acid + G. *phoros,* carrying, + -in]

ri·bo·pyr·a·nose (rī-bō-pir'ă-nōs). The 1,5-cyclic form of ribose.

ri·bose (Rib) (rī'bōs). The pentose that, as the D-isomer, is present in ribonucleic acid; epimers of D-r. are D-arabinose, D-xylose, and L-lyxose.

ri·bose-5-phos·phate. Ribose phosphorylated on carbon-5; an intermediate in the pentose phosphate pathway.

r.-5-p. isomerase, an enzyme catalyzing interconversion of D-ribose 5-phosphate and D-ribulose 5-phosphate; of importance in ribose metabolism and in the pentose phosphate pathway. SYN phosphopentose isomerase, phosphoriboisomerase.

ri·bo·side (rī'bō-sīd). The product formed by replacement of the H of the C-1 OH of ribose by an alcohol residue (which may be another sugar); differs from ribosyl compounds and does not occur in ribonucleic acids, where the radical is a ribosyl (1-OH missing entirely). See structure for methyl β-D-ribofuranoside below.

ri·bo·some (rī'bō-sōm). A granule of ribonucleoprotein, 120 to 150 Å in diameter, that is the site of protein synthesis from aminoacyl-tRNAs as directed by mRNAs. SYN Palade granule.

ri·bo·su·ria (rī-bō-sū'rē-ă). The enhanced urinary excretion of D-ribose; commonly one manifestation of muscular dystrophy. [ribose + G. *ouron,* urine]

ri·bo·syl (rī'bō-sil). The radical formed by loss of the hemiacetal OH group from either of the two cyclic forms of ribose (yielding ribofuranosyl and ribopyranosyl compounds), by combination with an H of an –NH– or a –CH– group; the natural nucleosides are ribosyl compounds, not ribosides, as the bond between ribose and aglycon is C–N or C–C, not –C–O–X–.

ri·bo·syl·a·tion (rī-bō-sil-ā-shŭn). The covalent attachment of one or more ribosyl groups to a molecule (usually a macromolecule).

ADP r., covalent attachment of an ADP-ribosyl moiety to a macromolecule; *e.g.,* the action of diphtheria toxin.

1-ri·bo·syl·or·o·tate (rī'bō-sil-ōr'ō-tāt). SYN orotidine.

ri·bo·syl·pur·ine (rī'bō-sil-pyūr'ēn). SYN nebularine.

ri·bo·syl·thy·mi·dine. SYN ribothymidine.

ri·bo·thy·mi·dine (T, Thd) (rī-bō-thī'mi-dēn). 5-methyluridine; the ribosyl analog of thymidine (deoxyribosylthymine); a nucleoside found in small amounts in ribonucleic acids. SYN ribofuranosylthymine, ribosylthymidine.

ri·bo·thy·mi·dyl·ic ac·id (rTMP, TMP) (rī'bō-thī-mi-dil'ik). Ribothymidine 5'-phosphate; the ribose analog of thymidylic acid; a rare component of transfer RNAs.

ri·bo·tide (rī'bō-tīd). A corruption of riboside, by analogy with nucleoside-nucleotide, to mean ribonucleotide.

ri·bo·vi·rus (rī'bō-vī'rŭs). SYN RNA *virus.*

ri·bo·zyme (rī'bō-zīm). A nonprotein biocatalyst; several cleave precursors of tRNA to yield functional tRNAs; others act on rRNA; plays a key role in intron splicing events. SYN organic catalyst (1), RNA enzyme. [*ribo*nucleic acid + -zyme]

ri·bo·zyme (rī'bō-zōm). A catalytic type of RNA.

ri·bu·lose (rī'byū-lōs). D-*erythro*-Pentulose; D-adonose; D-

erythro-2-ketopentose; the 2-keto isomer of ribose. As the 5-phosphate, it participates in the pentose monophosphate shunt; as the 1,5-bisphosphate, it combines with CO_2 at the start of the photosynthetic process in green plants ("carbon dioxide trap"); D-r. is the epimer of D-xylulose.

ri·bu·lose-1,5-bis·phos·phate car·box·yl·ase. A dimerizing carboxy-lyase; an enzyme that catalyzes the addition of carbon dioxide to D-ribulose 1,5-bisphosphate and the hydrolysis of the addition product to two molecules of 3-D-phosphoglyceric acid, a key reaction in the fixation of CO_2 in photosynthesis. SYN carboxydismutase.

ri·bu·lose-phos·phate 3-ep·i·mer·ase. An enzyme catalyzing the reversible interconversion of D-xylulose 5-phosphate and its epimer, D-ribulose 5-phosphate; a step in the nonoxidative phase of the pentose phosphate pathway. SYN phosphoribulose epimerase.

Riccò, Annibale, Italian astrophysicist, 1844–1919. SEE R.'s *law.*

rice (rīs). The grain of *Oryza sativa* (family Gramineae), the rice plant; a food; also used, finely pulverized, as a dusting powder. [G. *oryza*]

Rich, Arnold R., U.S. pathologist, 1893–1968. SEE Hamman-R. *syndrome.*

Richard, Felix Adolphe, Paris surgeon, 1822–1872. SEE R.'s *fringes,* under *fringe.*

Richards, Barry Wyndham, 20th century English physician.

Richardson, John Clifford, Canadian neurologist, *1909. SEE Steele-R.-Olszewski *disease, syndrome.*

Richards-Rundle syn·drome. See under syndrome.

Richter, August G., German surgeon, 1742–1812. SEE R.'s *hernia;* R.-Monro *line;* Monro-R. *line.*

Richter, Maurice N., U.S. pathologist, *1897. SEE R.'s *syndrome.*

ri·cin (rī'sin, ris'in). A highly toxic lectin and hemagglutin occurring in the seeds (castor beans) of the castor oil plant, *Ricinus communis;* if eaten, acts as a violent irritant and may be fatal; an N-glycosidase that acts on the GOS subunit of rRNA.

ric·i·nism (ris'i-nizm). Poisoning by ingestion of toxic principles from seeds (castor beans) or leaves of the castor oil plant, *Ricinus communis.*

ric·in·o·le·ate (ris-i-nō'lē-āt). A salt of ricinoleic acid.

ric·in·o·le·ic ac·id (ris-i-nō-lē'ik, rī-si-). $C_{18}H_{34}O_3$; $[R – Z]$-12-hydroxy-9-octadecenoic acid; an unsaturated hydroxy acid present in castor oil.

Ric·i·nus (ris'i-nŭs). A genus of plants (family Euphorbiaceae) with one species, *R. communis,* the castor oil plant, the source of castor oil; the leaves are said to be a galactagogue. SYN castor bean. [L.]

rick·ets (rik'ets). A disease due to vitamin-D deficiency and characterized by overproduction and deficient calcification of osteoid tissue, with associated skeletal deformities, disturbances in growth, hypocalcemia, and sometimes tetany; usually accompanied by irritability, listlessness, and generalized muscular weakness; fractures are frequent. SYN infantile osteomalacia, juvenile osteomalacia, rachitis. [E. *wrick,* to twist]

acute r., SYN hemorrhagic r.

adult r., SYN osteomalacia.

celiac r., arrested growth, and osseous deformities associated with defective absorption of fat and calcium in celiac disease.

familial hypophosphatemic r., SYN vitamin D-resistant r.

hemorrhagic r., bone changes seen in infantile scurvy, consisting of subperiosteal hemorrhage and deficient osteoid tissue formation; often used to indicate simultaneous occurrence of r. and scurvy. SYN acute r.

hereditary hypophosphatemic r., with hypercalciuria, an inherited disorder in which there is a defect in renal tubular reabsorption.

late r., SYN osteomalacia.

refractory r., r. that does not respond to treatment with usual doses of vitamin D and adequate dietary calcium and phosphorus. Most often due to inherited renal tubular disorder *e.g.,* Fanconi syndrome.

renal r., a form of r. occurring in children in association with and apparently caused by renal disease with hyperphosphatemia. SYN pseudorickets, renal fibrocystic osteosis, renal infantilism, renal osteitis fibrosa.

scurvy r., SYN infantile *scurvy*.

vitamin D-resistant r., a group of disorders characterized by hypophosphatemic osteomalacia; heritable renal tubular disorders and abnormalities in vitamin-D metabolism occur in some patients. There is an autosomal dominant form [MIM*193100] and an X-linked form [MIM*307800]; neither is responsive to standard therapeutic doses of vitamin D, but they may respond to very large doses of phosphate and of vitamin D. There is also an autosomal recessive form [MIM*277440] which is apparently due to end organ insensitivity. SYN familial hypophosphatemic r.

Ricketts, Howard T., U.S. pathologist, 1871–1910. SEE *Rickettsia.*

Rick·ett·si·a (ri-ket′sē-ă). A genus of bacteria (order Rickettsiales) containing small (nonfilterable), often pleomorphic, coccoid to rod-shaped, Gram-negative organisms that usually occur intracytoplasmically in lice, fleas, ticks, and mites but do not grow in cell-free media; pathogenic species are parasitic in man and other animals, causing epidemic typhus, murine or endemic typhus, Rocky Mountain spotted fever, tsutsugamushi disease, rickettsialpox, and other diseases; type species is *R. prowazekii.* [Howard T. *Ricketts*]

R. ak′ari, a species causing human rickettsialpox; transmitted by the house mouse mite, *Liponyssoides sanguineus;* a mild febrile disease of 7 to 10 days is produced with an urban distribution in the northeastern U.S. and in wild or commensal rodents in the countries of the former USSR and Africa.

R. austral′is, a species causing a spotted fever, North Queensland tick typhus, clinically and serologically similar to the disease caused by the agent of rickettsialpox; *Ixodes holocyclus* and *I. tasmani* are probable vectors. Small marsupials are suspected reservoirs of this agent, which is found over much of coastal Queensland, especially in secondary scrub and savannah.

R. burnet′ii, former name for *Coxiella burnetii.*

R. canis, former name for *Ehrlichia canis.*

R. conorii, a widespread African species probably causing boutonneuse fever in humans, transmitted by various ticks, such as the dog tick *Rhipicephalis sanguineus,* as well as ticks serve as the reservoir of human infection.

R. mooseri, a species similar to *R. prowazekii* but with less variation in appearance; the resultant endemic typhus is milder and has a somewhat slower onset.

R. prowazek′ii, a species causing epidemic and recrudescent typhus, transmitted by body lice; type species of the genus *R.*

R. psi′ttaci, former name for *Chlamydia psittaci.*

R. ricketts′ii, the agent of Rocky Mountain spotted fever, South African tick-bite fever, São Paulo exanthematic typhus of Brazil, Tobia fever of Colombia, and spotted fevers of Minas Gerais and Mexico; transmitted by infected ixodid ticks, especially *Dermacentor andersoni* and *D. variabilis.*

R. ruminantium, former name for *Cowdria ruminantium.*

R. sennetsu, SYN *Ehrlichia sennetsu.*

R. sibir′ica, the agent of Siberian or North Asian tick typhus, transmitted by various ixodid ticks, which also serve as reservoirs, possibly aided by rodents and hares; the disease resembles Rocky Mountain spotted fever.

R. tsutsugamu′shi, a species causing tsutsugamushi disease and scrub typhus; transmitted by trombiculid mites.

R. ty′phi, a species causing murine or endemic typhus fever, transmitted by the rat flea.

rick·ett·si·al (ri-ket′sē-ăl). Pertaining to or caused by rickettsiae.

rick·ett·si·al·pox (ri-ket′sē-ăl-poks′). Infection with *Rickettsia akari,* which is spread by mites from reservoir in mice; a benign self-limited process first recognized in 1956 in the area of New York City called Kew Gardens, a few limited outbreaks observed elsewhere since. SYN Kew Gardens fever, mite-born typhus, vesicular rickettsiosis.

rick·ett·si·o·sis (ri-ket-sē-ō′sis). Infection with rickettsiae.

   vesicular r., SYN rickettsialpox.

rick·ett·si·o·stat·ic (ri-ket′sē-ō-stat′ik). An agent inhibitory to the growth of *Rickettsia.* [*Rickettsia* + G. *statikos,* bringing to a standstill]

rick·e·ty (rik′ĕ-tē). SYN rachitic.

Rickles, Norman H., U.S. oral pathologist, *1920. SEE R. *test.*

RID Abbreviation for radial *immunodiffusion.*

Rideal, Samuel, English chemist and bacteriologist, 1863–1929. SEE R.-Walker *coefficient, method.*

Ridell's op·er·a·tion. See under operation.

ridge (rij). **1.** A (usually rough) linear elevation. SEE ALSO crest. **2.** In dentistry, any linear elevation on the surface of a tooth. **3.** The remainder of the alveolar process and its soft tissue covering after the teeth are removed. [A. S. *hyrcg,* back, spine]

alveolar r., SYN alveolar *process.*

apical ectodermal r., the layer of surface ectodermal cells at the apex of the embryonic limb bud; considered to exert an inductive influence on the condensation of underlying mesenchyme.

basal r., (1) SYN alveolar *process.* (2) SYN *cingulum* of tooth.

bicipital r.'s, SYN *crest* of greater tubercle, *crest* of lesser tubercle.

buccocervical r., a convexity within the cervical third of the buccal surface of molars.

buccogingival r., a distinct r. on the buccal surface of a deciduous molar tooth, approximately 1.5 mm from the crown-root junction.

bulbar r., one of two spiral subendocardial thickenings in the embryonic bulbus cordis; when they fuse, they divide the bulbus into the aorta and pulmonary artery.

bulboventricular r., an elevation on the inner surface of the embryonic heart at four to five weeks; it indicates the division between the developing ventricles and the bulbus cordis.

dental r., the prominent border of a cusp or margin of a tooth.

epidermal r.'s, ridges of the epidermis of the palms and soles, where the sweat pores open. SYN cristae cutis [NA], skin r.'s.

epipericardial r., an elevation separating the developing pharyngeal region from the embryonic pericardium.

external oblique r., a horizontal bony crest on the external surface of the body of the mandible, inferior to the alveolar bone, marking the site of attachment of the buccinator muscle.

ganglion r., SYN neural *crest.*

genital r., SYN gonadal r.

gluteal r., SYN gluteal *tuberosity.*

gonadal r., an elevation of thickened mesothelium and underlying mesenchyme on the ventromedial border of the embryonic mesonephros; the primordial germ cells become embedded in it, establishing it as the primordium of the testis or ovary. SYN genital r.

interpapillary r.'s, SYN rete r.'s.

key r., SYN zygomaxillare.

lateral epicondylar r., SYN lateral supracondylar r.

lateral supracondylar r., the distal sharp portion of the lateral margin of the humerus. SYN crista supracondylaris lateralis [NA], lateral epicondylar crest, lateral epicondylar r., lateral supracondylar crest.

linguocervical r., SYN linguogingival r.

linguogingival r., a r. occurring on the lingual surface, near the cervix, of the incisor and cuspid teeth. SYN linguocervical r.

Mall's r.'s, rarely used eponym for pulmonary r.'s.

mammary r., bandlike thickening of ectoderm in the embryo extending on either side from just below the axilla to the inguinal region; in human embryos, the mammary glands arise from primordia in the thoracic part of the r., the balance of the r. disappearing; in some lower mammals which give birth to a litter of young, several milk glands develop along these lines. SYN mammary fold, milk line, milk r.

marginal r., SYN marginal *crest.*

medial epicondylar r., SYN medial supracondylar r.

medial supracondylar r., the distal sharp portion of the medial margin of the humerus. SYN crista supracondylaris medialis [NA], medial epicondylar crest, medial epicondylar r., medial supracondylar crest.

ri

mesonephric r., a r. which, in early human embryos, comprises the entire urogenital r.; however, later in development a more medial genital r., the potential gonad, is demarcated from it. SEE ALSO urogenital r. SYN mesonephric fold.

milk r., SYN mammary r.

mylohyoid r., SYN mylohyoid *line.*

nasal r., SYN *agger* nasi.

oblique r., a r. on the masticatory surface of an upper molar tooth from the mesiolingual to the distobuccal cusp.

oblique r. of trapezium, SYN *tubercle* of trapezium.

palatine r., SYN palatine *raphe.*

Passavant's r., SYN Passavant's *cushion.*

pectoral r., SYN *crest* of greater tubercle.

pharyngeal r., SYN palatopharyngeal *sphincter.*

primitive r., one of the paired r.'s on either side of the primitive groove.

pronator r., an oblique r. on the anterior surface of the ulna, giving attachment to the pronator quadratus muscle.

pterygoid r. of sphenoid bone, SYN infratemporal *crest.*

pulmonary r.'s, a pair of r.'s overlying the common cardinal veins and bulging from the lateral body wall into the embryonic celom; so called because they give early indication of where the pleuropericardial folds will develop.

residual r., that portion of the processus alveolaris remaining in the edentulous mouth following resorption of the section containing the alveoli.

rete r.'s, downward thickening of the epidermis between the dermal papillae; peg is a misnomer because the dermal papillae are cylindrical but the epidermal thickening between papillae is not. SYN interpapillary r.'s, rete pegs.

skin r.'s, SYN epidermal r.'s.

sphenoidal r.'s, sharp posterior margins of the lesser wings of the sphenoid bone which end medially in the anterior clinoid process; the sphenoidal r.'s demarcate the anterior cranial fossa from the lateral part of the middle cranial fossa.

superciliary r., SYN superciliary *arch.*

supplemental r., a r. on the surface of a tooth that is not normally present.

supraorbital r., SYN supraorbital *margin.*

taste r., one of the r.'s surrounding the vallate papillae of the tongue.

temporal r., SYN inferior temporal *line,* superior temporal *line.*

transverse r., SYN *crista* transversalis.

transverse palatine r., SYN transverse palatine *fold.*

trapezoid r., SYN trapezoid *line.*

triangular r., SYN *crista* triangularis.

urogenital r., one of the paired longitudinal r.'s developing in the dorsal body wall of the embryo on either side of the dorsal mesentery; the r. is formed at first by the growing mesonephros and later by the mesonephros and the gonad. SYN genital fold, wolffian r.

wolffian r., SYN urogenital r.

Ridley, Humphrey, English anatomist, 1653–1708. SEE R.'s *circle, sinus; circulus* venosus ridleyi.

Riedel, Bernhard M.C.L., German surgeon, 1846–1916. SEE R.'s *disease, lobe, struma, thyroiditis.*

Rieder, Hermann, German pathologist, 1858–1932. SEE R. *cells,* under *cell,* cell *leukemia;* R.'s *lymphocyte.*

Riegel, Franz, German physician, 1843–1904. SEE R.'s *pulse.*

Rieger, Herwigh, German ophthalmologist. SEE R.'s *anomaly, syndrome.*

Riehl, Gustav, Austrian dermatologist, 1855–1943. SEE R.'s *melanosis.*

RIF Abbreviation for resistance-inducing *factor.*

ri·fam·pi·cin (rif'am-pi-sin). SYN rifampin.

rif·am·pin (rif'am-pin). Rifaldazine; 3-[(4-methylpiperazinyl)-iminomethyl] rifamycin SV; an antibiotic antibacterial agent used in the treatment of tuberculosis; a powerful inducer of hepatic microsomal enzymes. SYN rifampicin.

rif·a·my·cin, rif·o·my·cin (rif-ă-mī'sin, rif-ō-). A complex an-

tibiotic, isolated from *Nocardia mediterranei,* that is active against *Mycobacterium tuberculosis* and *Staphylococcus aureus;* it is poorly absorbed from the gastrointestinal tract and often causes irritation and severe pain at the sites of injection.

Riga, Antonio, Italian physician, 1832–1919. SEE R.-Fede *disease.*

right-eyed (rīt-īd). SYN dextrocular.

right-foot·ed (rīt'fŭt-ed). SYN dextropedal.

right-hand·ed (rīt'hand-ed). Denoting the habitual or more skillful use of the right hand for writing and most manual operations. SYN dextral, dextromanual.

ri·gid·i·ty (ri-jid'i-tē). **1.** Stiffness or inflexibility. SYN rigor (1). **2.** In psychiatry and clinical psychology, an aspect of personality characterized by an individual's resistance to change. [L. *rigidus,* rigid, inflexible]

anatomic r., r. of the cervix uteri in labor, not due to any pathologic infiltration.

cadaveric r., SYN *rigor* mortis.

catatonic r., r. associated with catatonic psychotic states in which all muscles exhibit flexibilitas cerea.

cerebellar r., increased tone of the extensor muscles, related to injury of the vermis of the cerebellum.

clasp-knife r., SYN clasp-knife *spasticity.*

cogwheel r., a type of r. seen in parkinsonism in which the muscles respond with cogwheel-like jerks to the use of constant force in bending the limb.

decerebrate r., a postural change that occurs in some comatose patients, consisting of episodes of opisthotonos, rigid extension of the limbs, internal rotation of the upper extremities, and marked plantar flexion of the feet; produced by a variety of metabolic and structural brain disorders. SYN decerebrate state.

decorticate r., a unilateral or bilateral postural change, consisting of the upper extremities flexed and adducted and the lower extremities in rigid extension; due to structural lesions of the thalamus, internal capsule, or cerebral white matter. SYN decorticate state.

lead-pipe r., the plastic type of r. resembling that of a pipe of lead seen in certain forms of parkinsonism.

ocular r., the resistance offered by the eyeball to a change in intraocular volume; manifested as a change in intraocular pressure.

pathologic r., r. of the cervix uteri in labor, due to fibrosis, scarring, cancer, or other condition.

postmortem r., SYN *rigor* mortis.

scleral r., the resistance of the eye to changes in shape with changes in intraocular pressure.

rig·or (rig'er). **1.** SYN rigidity (1). **2.** SYN chill (2). [L. stiffness]

acid r., coagulation of muscle protein induced by acids.

calcium r., arrest of the heart in the fully contracted state as a result of poisoning with calcium.

heat r., coagulation of muscle protein induced by heat.

r. mor'tis, stiffening of the body, from 1 to 7 hours after death, from hardening of the muscular tissues in consequence of the coagulation of the myosinogen and paramyosinogen; it disappears after from 1 to 5 or 6 days, or when decomposition begins. SYN cadaveric rigidity, postmortem rigidity.

myocardial r. mortis, SYN ischemic *contracture* of the left ventricle.

Riley, Conrad M., U.S. pediatrician, *1913. SEE R.-Day *syndrome.*

Riley, Harris D., Jr., 20th century U.S. physician. SEE Smith-R. *syndrome.*

rim. A margin, border, or edge, usually circular in form.

bite r., SYN occlusion r.

occlusal r., SYN occlusion r.

occlusion r., occluding surfaces built on temporary or permanent denture bases for the purpose of making maxillomandibular relation records and for arranging teeth. SYN bite r., occlusal r., record r.

orbital r., the mostly sharp edge of the orbital opening which is the peripheral border of the base of the pyramid-shaped orbit.

The superior half of the orbital r. is the supraorbital margin; the inferior half is the infraorbital margin. The frontal, maxillary, and zygomatic bones contribute to the orbital r., which is generally strong to protect the orbital contents. Weak, potential fracture sites of the r. coincide with the sutures between the participating bones. SYN margin of orbit.

    record r., SYN occlusion r.

ri·ma, gen. and pl. **ri·mae** (rī′mă, rī′mē) [NA]. A slit or fissure, or narrow elongated opening between two symmetrical parts. [L. a slit]

    r. glot′tidis [NA], the interval between the true vocal cords. SYN glottis vera, r. vocalis, true glottis.

    r. o′ris [NA], the mouth slit; the aperture of the mouth. SYN oral fissure.

    r. palpebra′rum [NA], the lid slit, or fissure between the eye lids. SYN palpebral fissure.

    r. puden′di [NA], SYN pudendal *cleft.*

    r. respirato′ria, SYN r. vestibuli.

    r. vestib′uli [NA], the interval between the false vocal cords or vestibular folds. SYN false glottis, glottis spuria, r. respiratoria.

    r. voca′lis, SYN r. glottidis.

    r. vul′vae, SYN pudendal *cleft.*

ri·man·ta·dine (rĭ-man′tă-dēn). An antiviral agent resembling amantadine in its activity but seemingly with fewer central nervous system adverse reactions.

Rimini's test. See under test.

ri·mose (rī′mōs). Fissured; marked by cracks in all directions, like the crackle of porcelain. [L. *rimosus,* fr. *rima,* a fissure]

rim·u·la (rim′yū-lă). A minute slit or fissure. [L. dim. of *rima*]

rin·der·pest (rin′der-pest). An acute, highly contagious, disease caused by rinderpest virus of the genus *Morbillivirus* and characterized by severe necrotizing inflammation of the alimentary canal and severe diarrhea; all ruminants and pigs are susceptible but natural infection occurs commonly only in cattle and buffaloes, sometimes in epizootic proportions. SYN cattle plague. [Ger. *rinder,* cattle]

Rindfleisch, Georg E., German physician, 1836–1908. SEE R.'s *cells,* under *cell,* *folds,* under *fold.*

ring. **1.** A circular band surrounding a wide central opening; a ring-shaped or circular structure surrounding an opening or level area. **2.** In anatomy, annulus; sometimes anulus when used as an official alternate Nomina Anatomica term. **3.** The closed (*i.e.,* endless) chain of atoms in a cyclic compound; commonly used for "cyclic" or "cycle". **4.** A marginal growth on the upper surface of a broth culture of bacteria, adhering to the sides of the test tube in the form of a circle. SYN annulus [NA], anulus☆ [NA]. [A.S. *hring*]

    abdominal r., SYN deep inguinal r.

    amnion r., the r. formed by the attachment of the amnion to the umbilical cord at its point of emergence from the umbilicus.

    annuloplasty r., the dilated annulus is sutured, often to a prosthetic r., thereby reducing it to its normal systolic size.

    anterior limiting r., the periphery of the cornea marking the termination of Descemet's membrane and the anterior border of the trabecular meshwork; an important landmark in gonioscopy. SYN Schwalbe's r.

    Balbani r., an extremely large puff at a band of a polytene chromosome.

    Bandl's r., SYN pathologic retraction r.

    benzene r., the closed-chain arrangement of the carbon and hydrogen atoms in the benzene molecule. SEE ALSO cyclic *compound.*

    Bickel's r., SYN lymphoid r.

    Cannon's r., SYN Cannon's *point.*

    cardiac lymphatic r., SYN lymphatic r. of cardiac part of stomach.

    casting r., SYN refractory *flask.*

    choroidal r., a lightly pigmented crescent or r. adjacent to the optic disk.

    ciliary r., SYN orbiculus ciliaris.

    common tendinous r., a fibrous ring that surrounds the optic canal and the medial part of the superior orbital fissure; it gives origin to the four rectus muscles of the eye and is partially fused with the sheath of the optic nerve. SYN annulus tendineus communis [NA], Zinn's ligament, Zinn's r., Zinn's tendon.

    conjunctival r., a narrow ring at the junction of the periphery of the cornea with the conjunctiva. SYN annulus conjunctivae [NA].

    constriction r., **(1)** true spastic stricture of the uterine cavity resulting when a zone of muscle goes into local tetanic contraction and forms a tight constriction about some part of the fetus; **(2)** SYN amniotic *bands,* under *band.*

    crural r., SYN femoral r.

    deep inguinal r., the opening in the transversalis fascia through which the ductus deferens (or round ligament in the female) and gonadal vessels enter the inguinal canal. Located midway between anterior superior iliac spine and pubic tubercle, it is bounded medially by the lateral umbilical ligament (inferior epigastric vessels) and inferiorly by the inguinal ligament. Indirect inguinal hernias exit the abdominal cavity via the deep inguinal r. SYN annulus inguinalis profundus [NA], abdominal r., annulus abdominalis, internal inguinal r.

    Donders' r.'s, an obsolete term for the iridescent r.'s or haloes observed by a cloudy cornea due to acute glaucoma.

    external inguinal r., SYN superficial inguinal r.

    femoral r., the superior opening of the femoral canal, bounded anteriorly by the inguinal ligament, posteriorly by the pectineus muscle, medially by the lacunar ligament, and laterally by the femoral vein. Passageway by which many lymphatics from lower limb pass to abdomen. Accommodates enlargement of femoral vein in Valsalva maneuver. Often occupied by a lymph node (Cloquet's) and is the site of femoral hernias. SYN annulus femoralis [NA], crural r.

    fibrocartilaginous r. of tympanic membrane, the thickened portion of the circumference of the tympanic membrane that is fixed in the tympanic sulcus. SYN annulus fibrocartilagineus membranae tympani [NA], Gerlach's annular tendon.

    fibrous r., **(1)** SYN fibrous r. of heart. **(2)** SYN *annulus* fibrosus of intervertebral disc.

    fibrous r. of heart, one of four fibrous r.'s that surround atrioventricular and arterial orifices of the heart, providing attachment for the valve leaflets and maintaining patency of the orifice. As part of the fibrous skeleton of the heart, the fibrous r.'s also provide origin and insertion for the myocardium. SYN annulus fibrosus cordis [NA], annulus fibrosus (1) [NA], coronary tendon, fibrous r. (1), Lower's r.

    fibrous r. of intervertebral disc, SYN *annulus* fibrosus of intervertebral disc.

    Fleischer's r., an incomplete ring often present at the base of the keratoconus cone; it may be yellow or greenish from deposition of hemosiderin.

    Fleischer-Strumpell r., SYN Kayser-Fleischer r.

    Flieringa's r., a stainless steel r. sutured to the sclera to prevent collapse of the globe in difficult intraocular operations.

    glaucomatous r., SYN glaucomatous *halo* (1). SEE Donders' r.'s.

    Graefenberg r., obsolete term for a silver or silkworm gut r. designed for insertion into the uterine cavity as a means of contraception.

    greater r. of iris, the outer, broader of the two zones of the iris. SYN annulus iridis major.

    Imlach's r., that part of the inguinal canal which lodges the round ligament of the uterus.

    internal inguinal r., SYN deep inguinal r.

    r. of iris, either of two zones on the anterior surface of the iris, separated by a circular line concentric with the pupillary border. SYN annulus iridis.

    Kayser-Fleischer r., a greenish yellow pigmented r. encircling the cornea just within the corneoscleral margin, seen in hepatolenticular degeneration, due to copper deposited in Descemet's *membrane.* SYN Fleischer-Strumpell r.

    lesser r. of iris, the narrow inner zone of the iris. SYN annulus iridis minor.

    Liesegang r.'s, colored r.'s of precipitated silver chromate formed when a drop of concentrated silver nitrate is added to the surface of a gel (such as gelatin, agar, or silica gel) containing potassium dichromate.

Lower's r., SYN fibrous r. of heart.

lymphatic r. of cardiac part of stomach, a group of lymph nodes surrounding the cardia of the stomach. SYN annulus lymphaticus cardiae [NA], cardiac lymphatic r.

lymphoid r., the broken r. of lymphoid tissue, formed of the lingual, faucial, and pharyngeal tonsils. SYN Bickel's r., tonsillar r., Waldeyer's throat r.

neonatal r., SYN neonatal *line.*

pathologic retraction r., a constriction located at the junction of the thinned lower uterine segment with the thick retracted upper uterine segment, resulting from obstructed labor; this is one of the classic signs of threatened rupture of the uterus. SYN Bandl's r., Baudelocque's uterine circle, Scanzoni's second os.

physiologic retraction r., a ridge on the inner uterine surface at the boundary line between the upper and lower uterine segment that occurs in the course of normal labor.

polar r., a thickened, electron-dense ring at the anterior end of certain stages of the Apicomplexa; part of the apical complex characteristic of these sporozoans.

Schatzki's r., a contraction r. or incomplete mucosal diaphragm in the lower third of the esophagus which is occasionally symptomatic.

Schwalbe's r., SYN anterior limiting r.

scleral r., the appearance of the sclera adjacent to the optic disk when the retinal pigment epithelium does not extend to the optic nerve.

signet r., the early stage of trophozoite development of the malaria parasite in the red blood cell; the parasite cytoplasm stains blue around its circular margin, and the nucleus stains red in Romanowsky stains, while the central vacuole is clear, giving the ringlike appearance.

r. of Soemmerring, a mass of lenticular fibers enclosed between the anterior and posterior portion of the lenticular capsule, leaving the pupillary area relatively free.

subcutaneous r., SYN superficial inguinal r.

superficial inguinal r., the slit-like opening in the aponeurosis of the external oblique muscle of the abdominal wall through which the spermatic cord (round ligament in the female) and inguinal hernias emerge from the inguinal canal. SEE ALSO *aponeurosis* of external abdominal oblique muscle. SYN annulus inguinalis superficialis [NA], external inguinal r., subcutaneous r.

tonsillar r., SYN lymphoid r.

tracheal r., SYN tracheal *cartilages,* under *cartilage.*

tympanic r., in the fetus, a more or less complete bony ring at the medial end of the cartilaginous external acoustic meatus, to which is attached the tympanic membrane. SYN annulus tympanicus [NA], tympanic bone.

umbilical r., an opening in the linea alba through which pass the umbilical vessels in the fetus; in young embryos it is relatively nearer to the pubis, but gradually ascends to the center of the abdomen; it is closed in the adult, its site being indicated by the umbilicus or navel. SYN annulus umbilicalis [NA], canalis umbilicalis.

vascular r., anomalous arteries (aortic arches) congenitally encircling the trachea and esophagus, at times producing pressure symptoms.

Vieussens' r., SYN *limbus* fossae ovalis.

Vossius' lenticular r., a ring-shaped opacity found on the anterior lens capsule after contusion of the eye, due to pigment and blood.

Waldeyer's throat r., SYN lymphoid r.

Zinn's r., SYN common tendinous r.

ring·bone (ring′bōn). Exostoses involving either the first or second phalanx of the horse, sometimes differentiated into high and low r., usually found in the foreleg; lameness may or may not result.

false r., an exostosis on the middle or upper part of the long pastern bone in the horse.

Ringer, Sydney, English physiologist, 1835–1910. SEE R.'s in-

jection, *solution;* lactated R. *injection;* Krebs-R. *solution;* Locke-R. *solution.*

ring-knife (ring-nīf). A circular or oval ring with internal cutting edge, on the model of the carpenter's spoke-shave, for shaving off tumors in the nasal and other cavities. SYN spoke-shave.

ring·worm (ring′werm). SYN tinea.

r. of beard, SYN *tinea* barbae.

black-dot r., tinea capitis due most commonly to *Trichophyton tonsurans* or *T. violaceum.*

r. of body, SYN *tinea* corporis.

crusted r., SYN favus.

r. of foot, SYN *tinea* pedis.

r. of genitocrural region, SYN *tinea* cruris.

honeycomb r., SYN favus.

r. of nails, SYN onychomycosis.

Oriental r., SYN *tinea* imbricata.

r. of scalp, SYN *tinea* capitis.

scaly r., SYN *tinea* imbricata.

Tokelau r., SYN *tinea* imbricata. [*Tokelau* Islands in S. Pacific Ocean]

Rinne, Friedrich Heinrich A., German otologist, 1819–1868. SEE R.'s *test.*

Riolan, Jean, French anatomist and botanist, 1577–1657. SEE R.'s *anastomosis, arc, arcades,* under *arcade, bones,* under *bone, bouquet, muscle.*

ri·par·i·an (ri-pār′ē-an, rī-). Relating to a ripa; marginal.

Ripault, Louis H.A., French physician, 1807–1856. SEE R.'s *sign.*

rip·en·ing (rī′pen-ing). Denoting progressive oxidation of dye solutions, as in the r. of hematoxylin solutions to hematein or of methylene blue to azure dyes.

RISA Abbreviation for radioiodinated serum *albumin.*

risk. The probability that an event will occur.

attributable r., the rate of a disease or other outcome in exposed individuals that can be attributed to the exposure.

competing r., an event that removes a subject from being at r. for an outcome under investigation.

empiric r., r. that is based on empirical evidence alone, without any appeal to formal theory or surmise.

radiation r.'s, The r.'s to health posed by exposure to radiation. Exposure comes from both natural sources and from man-made ones (medical and occupational). SEE background *radiation.*

> Because any amount of radiation may cause cellular mutations, considerable effort has been made by government and independent researchers to establish exposure guidelines. In most cases, natural sources account for the bulk of received radiation, with artificial sources adding only a small percentage to the average annual dose. Public perception of the hazards of radiation is often at odds with scientific positions on the matter. In part, equivocal research results (as in attempts to assess the added cancer risk posed by mammograms) contribute to public fears. Some psychological studies have concluded that whether or not public fears of nuclear power plants and other radiation sources are justified, the added stress caused by such fears in itself constitutes a threat to health that should be addressed.

recurrence r., r. that a disease will occur elsewhere in a pedigree, given that at least one member of the pedigree (the proband) exhibits the disease.

relative r., the ratio of the r. of disease among those exposed to a r. factor, to the r. among those not exposed.

Risley, Samuel D., U.S. ophthalmologist, 1845–1920. SEE R.'s rotary *prism.*

ri·so·ri·us (ri-sōr′ē-ŭs). SEE risorius *muscle.* [L. *risor,* a laughter, fr. *rideo,* pp. *risus,* to laugh]

RIST Abbreviation for radioimmunosorbent *test.*

ris·to·ce·tin (ris-tō-sē′tin). An antibiotic produced by the fermentation of *Nocardia lurida,* comprising two substances; r. A and r. B; it is useful against staphylococcic and enterococcic infections refractory to other antibiotics.

ri·sus ca·ni·nus (rī′sŭs kā-nī′nŭs). The semblance of a grin caused by facial spasm especially in tetanus. SYN canine spasm, cynic spasm, risus sardonicus, sardonic grin, spasmus caninus, trismus sardonicus. [L. *risus,* laugh + *caninus,* doglike]

ri·sus sar·do·ni·cus (sar-don′i-kŭs). SYN risus caninus. [L. *risus,* laughter, + *sardonicus,* fr. G. *sardanios,* scornful, infl. by *sardonios,* Sardinian, ref. to effects of *Strychnos nux-vomica,* poisonous herb fr. Sardinia]

Ritgen, Ferdinand August Marie Franz von, German obstetrician, 1787–1867. SEE R.'s *maneuver.*

ri·to·drine (rī′tō-drēn). *erythro-p*-Hydroxy-α-{1-[(p-hydroxyphenethyl)amino]ethyl} benzyl alcohol; a sympathomimetic agent with β_2-adrenergic stimulant actions, used as a uterine relaxant.

Ritter, Johann W., German physicist, 1776–1810. SEE R.'s *law,* opening *tetanus;* R.-Rollet *phenomenon.*

rit·u·al (rich′ū-ăl). In psychiatry and psychology, any psychomotor activity (*e.g.,* morbid handwashing) sustained by an individual to relieve anxiety or forestall its development; typically seen in obsessive-compulsive neurosis. [L. *ritualis,* fr. *ritus,* rite]

ri·val·ry (rī′văl-rē). Competition between two or more individuals for the same object or goal. [L. *rivalis,* competitor, rival]

   binocular r., alteration in perception of portions of the visual field when the two eyes are simultaneously and rapidly exposed to targets containing dissimilar colors or borders.

   r. of retina, simultaneous excitation of corresponding retinal areas of each eye by stimuli that differ in size, color, shape, or luminance, making fusion impossible.

   sibling r., jealous competition among children, especially for the attention, affection, and esteem of their parents; by extension, a factor in both normal and abnormal competitiveness throughout life.

Riv·ea co·rym·bo·sa (riv′ē-ă kō-rim-bō′să). Mexican bindweed, a plant of the family Convulvulaceae, the seeds of which were used in ceremonies by Aztec Indians in Mexico and contain lysergic acid amide, isolysergic acid, lysergic acid monoethylamide, chanoclavine, and other indole alkaloids; several hundred seeds must be ingested to produce hallucinatory and euphoric effects. SYN morning glory (2).

Riverius. SEE Rivière.

Rivero-Carvallo, José Manuel, Mexican cardiologist, *1905. SEE Carvallo's *sign;* Rivero-Carvallo *effect.*

Rivers, William H., English physician, 1864–1922. SEE R.'s *cocktail.*

Rivière (Riverius), Lazare (Lazarus), French physician, 1589–1655. SEE R.'s *salt.*

Rivinus (Latin form of Bachmann). August Q., German anatomist, 1652–1723. SEE Rivinus' *canals,* under *canal,* Rivinus' *ducts,* under *duct,* Rivinus' *gland,* Rivinus' *incisure,* Rivinus' *membrane,* Rivinus' *notch.*

ri·vus la·cri·ma·lis (rī′vŭs lak-ri-mā′lis) [NA]. A space between the closed lids and the eyeball through which the tears flow to the punctum lacrimale. SYN Ferrein's canal. [L. *rivus,* stream, + Mediev. L. *lacrimalis,* fr. L. *lacrima,* a tear]

riz·i·form (riz′i-fōrm). Resembling rice grains. [Fr. *riz,* rice]

RLL Abbreviation for right lower lobe (of lung).

RLQ Abbreviation for right lower quadrant (of abdomen).

RMA Abbreviation for right mentoanterior position.

RML Abbreviation for right middle lobe (of lung).

RMP Abbreviation for right mentoposterior position.

RMT Abbreviation for right mentotransverse position.

RMV Abbreviation for respiratory minute *volume.*

R.N. Abbreviation for registered *nurse.*

Rn Symbol for radon.

RNA Abbreviation for ribonucleic acid. For terms bearing this abbreviation, see subentries under ribonucleic acid.

RNase Abbreviation for ribonuclease. For terms bearing this abbreviation, see subentries under ribonuclease.

RNase D Abbreviation for *ribonuclease* D.

RNase P Abbreviation for *ribonuclease* P.

RNA splic·ing. SYN splicing (2).

RNP Abbreviation for ribonucleoprotein.

ROA Abbreviation for right occipitoanterior position.

Roach, F. Ewing, U.S. prosthodontist, 1868–1960. SEE R. *clasp.*

Roaf's syn·drome. See under syndrome.

roar·ing (rōr′ing). A loud, rough, whistling or roaring sound emitted upon inspiration during active exercise by a horse that is suffering from laryngeal hemiplegia; caused by unilateral or bilateral paralysis of certain laryngeal muscles due to injury of the recurrent laryngeal nerve.

Robert, Heinrich, L.F., German gynecologist, 1814–1878. SEE R.'s *pelvis.*

Roberts, J.B., 20th century U.S. physician. SEE R. *syndrome.*

Robertshaw, Frank L., 20th century English anesthesiologist. SEE R. *tube.*

Robertson, Douglas Argyll, Scottish ophthalmologist, 1837–1909. SEE Argyll R. *pupil;* R. *pupil.*

Robin, Charles P., French physician, 1821–1885. SEE Virchow-R. *space.*

Robin, Pierre, French pediatrician, 1867–1950. SEE Pierre R. *syndrome.*

Robinson, Andrew, U.S. dermatologist, 1845–1924. SEE R.'s *disease.*

Robinson, Brian F., 20th century British cardiologist. SEE R. *index.*

Robinson, Robert A., U.S. orthopedic surgeon, *1914. SEE Smith-R. *operation.*

Robinson cath·e·ter. See under catheter.

Robison, Robert, English chemist, 1884–1941. SEE R. *ester,* ester *dehydrogenase;* R.-Embden *ester.*

Robles, Rudolfo (Valverde), Guatemalan dermatologist, 1878–1939.

ro·bot·ic (rō-bot′ik). Pertaining to or characteristic of a robot, an automatic mechanical device designed to duplicate a human function without direct human operation. [Czech *robot,* robot, fr. *robota,* drudgery, + -ic]

Robson. SEE Mayo-Robson.

ro·bust·ness (rō-bust′ness). In statistics, the degree to which the probability of drawing a wrong conclusion from the test result is not seriously affected by moderate departures from the assumptions implicit in the model on which the test is based. [L. *robustus,* hale, strong, fr. *robur,* oak, hard]

ROC Acronym for receiver operating *characteristic,* an analytic expression of accuracy. SEE ROC *curve.*

roc·cel·lin (rok′sel-in) [C.I. 15620]. SYN archil.

Ro·cha·li·maea (rō-chă-lī′mā-ă). A genus of bacteria (family Rickettsiaceae) closely resembling *Rickettsia* in staining properties, morphology, and mode of transmission between hosts. They usually reside in the extracellular environment in the arthropod host and can be cultivated in cell-free media. Related bacterium causes bacillary angiomatosis in immunocompromised humans, especially those with AIDS. The type species is *R. quintana.* [da Rocha-Lima, Brazilian microbiologist]

   R. henselae, a recently recognized species of the Rickettsiaceae family, causing bacillary angiomatosis and cat-scratch disease.

   R. quintana, a species that cause trench fever in humans. It is the type species of the genus *Rochalimaea.*

Rocher, Henri Gaston Louis, French surgeon, *1876. SEE R.'s *sign.*

rock oil (rok oyl). SYN petroleum.

rod. 1. A straight slender cylindrical structure or device. For surgical rods, see also under nail; pin. 2. The photosensitive, outward-directed process of a rhodopsin-containing r. cell in the external granular layer of the retina; many millions of such r.'s, together with the cones, form the photoreceptive layer of r.'s and cones. SYN rod cell of retina. [A.S. *rōd*]

   analyzing r., a device used with a surveyor to determine the

ro

relative positions of parallel surfaces and undercuts when designing removable partial dentures.

Auer r.'s, SYN Auer *bodies,* under *body.*

basal r., SYN costa (2).

Corti's r.'s, SYN pillar *cells,* under *cell.*

enamel r.'s, SYN *prismata* adamantina, under *prisma.*

germinal r., SYN sporozoite.

Maddox's r., a glass r., or a series of parallel glass r.'s, that converts the image of a light source into a streak of light perpendicular to the axis of the rod. The position of this streak in relation to the image of the light source seen by the fellow eye indicates the presence and amount of heterophoria.

Ro·den·tia (rō-den′shē-ă). The rodents; the largest order of placental mammals (class Eutheria), all possessing one pair of chisel-like upper incisors for gnawing and flat-crowned premolars and molars for grinding; it includes the mice, rats, guinea pigs, squirrels, beavers, and many more. [Mod. L., fr. L. *rodo,* pres. p. *rodens,* to gnaw]

ro·den·ti·cide (rō-den′ti-sīd). An agent lethal to rodents. [rodent + L. *caedo,* to kill]

ro·don·al·gia (rō-don-al′jē-ă). SYN erythromelalgia. [G. *rhodon,* rose, + *algos,* pain]

Roentgen, Wilhelm K., German physicist and Nobel laureate, 1845–1923. Discovered x-rays in November, 1895; awarded Nobel Prize in Physics in 1901 for his discovery. SEE roentgen; roentgen *ray.*

roent·gen (R, r) (rent′gen, rent′chen). The international unit of exposure dose for x-rays or gamma rays; that quantity of radiation that will produce in 1 cm of air at STP, or 0.001293 g of air, 2.08×10^9 ions of both signs, each totaling 1 electrostatic unit (e.s.u.) of charge; in the MKS system this is 2.58×10^{-4} coulombs per kg of air. [W. K. *Roentgen*]

r.-equivalent-man (rem), a unit of dose equivalent to that quantity of ionizing radiation of any type that produces in man the same biologic effect as one rad of x-rays or gamma rays; the number of rems is equal to the absorbed dose, measured in rads, multiplied by the quality factor of the radiation in question.100 rem = 1 Sv.

r.-equivalent-physical (rep), obsolete unit of measurement; that quantity of ionizing radiation of any kind which, upon absorption by living tissue, produces an energy gain per gram of tissue equivalent to that produced by 1 r. of x-rays or gamma-rays. SEE rad.

roent·gen·ky·mo·gram (rent′gen-kī′mō-gram). A record of the heart's movements taken with the roentgenkymograph.

roent·gen·ky·mo·graph (rent′gen-kī′mō-graf). An apparatus for recording the movements of the heart and great vessels or of the diaphragm on a single film. It consists of a lead sheet called the grid in which are cut horizontal or vertical slits, typically less than 1 mm wide, spaced 1–2 cm apart. During an x-ray exposure lasting as long as several cardiac or respiratory cycles, the grid or the film is moved vertically to record cardiac motion or horizontally for diaphragm motion.

roent·gen·ky·mog·ra·phy (rent′gen-kī-mog′ră-fē). An obsolete technique involving the recording of movements of the heart by means of the roentgenkymograph.

roent·gen·o·gram (rent′gen-ō-gram). SYN radiograph.

roent·gen·o·graph (rent′gen-ō-graf). SYN radiograph.

roent·gen·og·ra·phy (rent′ge-nog′ră-fē). SYN radiography.

roent·gen·ol·o·gist (rent′gen-ol′ō-jist). A person skilled in the diagnostic or therapeutic application of roentgen rays; a radiologist.

roent·gen·ol·o·gy (rent′gen-ol′ō-jē). The study of roentgen rays in all their applications. Radiology is the preferred term in the context of medical imaging.

roent·gen·om·e·ter (rent′ge-nom′ĕ-ter). SYN radiometer.

roent·gen·om·e·try (rent-ge-nom′ĕ-trē). Measurement of an administered therapeutic or diagnostic dose and the penetrating power of x-rays. SYN x-ray dosimetry.

roent·gen·o·scope (rent′gen-ō-scōp). SYN fluoroscope.

roent·gen·os·co·py (rent-gen-os′kŏ-pē). SYN fluoroscopy.

roent·gen·o·ther·a·py (rent′gen-ō-thār′ă-pē). SYN radiotherapy.

roeth·eln. SEE röteln.

Roger, Georges Henri, French physiologist, 1860–1946. SEE R.'s *reflex.*

Roger, Henri L., French physician, 1809–1891. SEE R.'s *disease, murmur; bruit* de R.; *maladie* de R.

Roger-Anderson pin fix·a·tion ap·pli·ance. See under appliance.

Rogers, Oscar H., U.S. physician, 1857–1941. SEE R.'s *sphygmomanometer.*

Rohr, Karl, Swiss embryologist and gynecologist, *1863. SEE R.'s *stria.*

Röhrer's in·dex. See under index.

Rokitansky, Karl Freiherr von, Austrian pathologist, 1804–1878. SEE R.'s *disease, hernia;* R.-Aschoff *sinuses,* under *sinus;* Mayer-R.-Küster-Hauser *syndrome.*

ro·lan·dic (rō-lan′dik). Relating to or described by Luigi Rolando.

Rolando, Luigi, Italian anatomist, 1773–1831. SEE R.'s *angle, area, cells,* under *cell, column;* rolandic *epilepsy;* R.'s *gelatinous substance, tubercle; fissure* of R.

role (rōl). The pattern of behavior that a person exhibits in relationship to significant persons in his or her life; it has its roots in childhood and is influenced by significant people with whom the person has or had primary relationships. [Fr.]

complementary r., a r. in which the behavior pattern conforms with the expectations and demands of other people.

gender r., the sex of a child assigned by a parent; when opposite to the child's anatomical sex (*e.g.,* due to genital ambiguity at birth or to the parents' strong wish for a child of the opposite sex), the basis is set for postpubertal dysfunctions. SEE sex r., sex *reversal.*

noncomplementary r., a r. that does not conform with the expectations and demands of other people.

sex r., the degree to which an individual acts out a stereotypical masculine or feminine r. in everyday behavior. Cf. gender r.

sick r., in medical sociology, the familially or culturally accepted behavior pattern or r. which one is permitted to exhibit during illness or disability, including sanctioned absence from school or work and a submissive, dependent relationship to family, health care personnel, and significant others.

role-play·ing. A psychotherapeutic method used in psychodrama to understand and treat emotional conflicts through the enactment or re-enactment of stressful interpersonal events. SEE psychodrama.

ro·li·tet·ra·cy·cline (rō′li-tet-ră-sī′klēn). N-(Pyrrolidinomethyl)-tetracycline; a more soluble and less irritating derivative of tetracycline; uses and effectiveness are similar to those of tetracycline, and it may be administered intravenously or intramuscularly, which makes it useful when oral administration of a tetracycline is impossible or impracticable.

roll (rōl). A mass or structure in the shape of a roll.

iliac r., a sausage-shaped, often painful, nonfluctuating mass, with convexity to the right, palpable in the left iliac fossa, due to induration of the walls of the sigmoid flexure.

scleral r., SYN scleral *spur.*

Roller, Christian F.W., German neurologist and psychiatrist, 1844–1978. SEE R.'s *nucleus.*

roll·er (rō′ler). SEE roller *bandage.*

Rolleston, Sir Humphry D., British physician, 1862–1944. SEE R.'s *rule.*

Rollet, Alexander, Austrian physiologist, 1834–1903. SEE R.'s *stroma;* Ritter-R. *phenomenon.*

Romaña, Cecilio, Argentinian physician in Brazil, *1899. SEE R.'s *sign.*

Romano, C., 20th century Italian physician. SEE Romano-Ward *syndrome.*

Romanowsky, Dimitri L., Russian physician, 1861–1921. SEE R.'s blood *stain.*

Romberg, Moritz H., German physician, 1795–1873. SEE R. *test;* R.'s *disease;* facial *hemiatrophy* of R.; R.'s *sign, symptom, syndrome, trophoneurosis;* R.-Howship *symptom.*

rom·berg·ism (rom′berg-izm). SYN Romberg's *sign.*

Römer, Paul H., German bacteriologist, 1876–1916. SEE R.'s *test.*

ron·geur (rawn-zhĕr′). A strong biting forceps for nipping away bone. [Fr. *ronger,* to gnaw]

Rønne, Henning K.T., Danish ophthalmologist, 1878–1947. SEE R.'s nasal *step.*

roof (rūf). A covering or rooflike structure; *e.g.,* a tectorium, tectum, tegmen, tegmentum, integument. [A.S. *hrōf*]

r. of fourth ventricle, SYN *tegmen* ventriculi quarti.

r. of mouth, SYN palate.

r. of orbit, formed by the orbital plate of the frontal bone and the lesser wing of the sphenoid bone, the optic canal opens at its posterior limit; an indentation, the fossa for the lacrimal gland, is located in the anterolateral part of the roof. SYN paries superior orbitae [NA], superior wall of orbit.

r. of skull, SYN calvaria.

r. of tympanic cavity, the superior wall, or roof, of the tympanic cavity, formed by the tegmen tympani of the temporal bone. SYN paries tegmentalis cavi tympani [NA], tegmental wall of middle ear.

r. of tympanum, SYN *tegmen* tympani.

roof·plate (rūf′plāt). SEE roof *plate.*

root (rūt). **1.** The primary or beginning portion of any part, as of a nerve at its origin from the brainstem or spinal cord. **2.** SYN r. of tooth. **3.** The descending underground portion of a plant; it absorbs water and nutrients, provides support, and stores nutrients. For r.'s of pharmacological significance not listed below, see specific names. [A.S. rot]

anatomical r., that portion of a tooth extending from the cervical line to its apical extremity.

anterior r., SYN ventral r.

clinical r., that portion of a tooth embedded in the investing structures; the portion of a tooth not visible in the oral cavity. SYN radix clinica [NA].

cochlear r. of vestibulocochlear nerve, SYN cochlear r. of VIII nerve.

cochlear r. of VIII nerve, one of the components of the vestibulocochlear nerve; it is made up of the central processes of the bipolar neurons which compose the spiral (cochlear) ganglion in the spiral canal of the modiolus of the bony cochlea; the cochlear r. enters the cranial cavity by passing in fascicles through the spiral foraminous tract at the bottom of the internal auditory meatus; it enters the brainstem through the pontomedullary groove, closely adhering to the caudoventral aspect of the vestibular r., and distributes its fibers to the ventral and dorsal cochlear nuclei in the floor of the lateral recess of the fourth ventricle. SYN radix cochlearis [NA], cochlear r. of vestibulocochlear nerve, inferior r. of vestibulocochlear nerve, radix inferior nervi vestibulocochlearis.

cranial r.'s, SYN cranial r. of accessory nerve.

cranial r. of accessory nerve, the r.'s of the accessory nerve which arise from the medulla; the nerve fibers of the cranial r. join the intracranial portion of the vagus nerve and are distributed to the pharyngeal plexus, providing the motor innervation of the soft palate (except the tensor veli palati) and the pharynx. SYN pars vagalis nervi accessorii [NA], radices craniales [NA], accessory portion of spinal accessory nerve, cranial r.'s, vagal part of accessory nerve, vagal part.

Culver's r., SYN leptandra.

dorsal r., the sensory root of a spinal nerve, having a dorsal r. ganglion containing the nerve cell bodies of the fibers conveyed by the root in its distal end. SYN radix posterior [NA], radix sensoria [NA], posterior r., radix dorsalis.

facial r., SYN *nerve* of pterygoid canal.

r. of facial nerve, fibers running from the facial motor nucleus upward to the facial colliculus where they curve around the abducens nucleus and then pass peripherally between the superior olive and sensory nucleus of the trigeminal, to emerge as the facial nerve from the pontomedullary groove. SYN radix nervi facialis.

r. of foot, SYN tarsus.

hair r., the part of a hair that is embedded in the hair follicle, its lower succulent extremity capping the dermal papilla pili in the deep bulbous portion of the follicle. SYN radix pili.

inferior r. of ansa cervicalis, fibers from the second and third cervical nerves that pass forward and downward along the internal jugular vein; they contribute to the ansa cervicalis and innervate the infrahyoid muscles. SYN descendens cervicalis, radix inferior ansae cervicalis.

inferior r. of vestibulocochlear nerve, SYN cochlear r. of VIII nerve.

lateral r. of median nerve, the part of the median nerve arising from the lateral cord of the brachial plexus. SYN radix lateralis nervi mediani [NA].

lateral r. of optic tract, the larger division of the posterior end of the optic tract that terminates in the lateral geniculate body. SYN radix lateralis tractus optici [NA].

long r. of ciliary ganglion, SYN sensory r. of ciliary ganglion.

r. of lung, all the structures entering or leaving the lung at the hilum, forming a pedicle invested with the pleura; includes the bronchi, pulmonary artery and veins, bronchial arteries and veins, lymphatics, and nerves. SYN radix pulmonis [NA].

May apple r., SYN podophyllum *resin.*

medial r. of median nerve, the part of the median nerve coming from the medial cord of the brachial plexus. SYN radix medialis nervi mediani [NA].

medial r. of optic tract, the smaller division of the posterior end of the optic tract that disappears under the medial geniculate body. SYN radix medialis tractus optici [NA].

r. of mesentery, the origin of the mesentery of the small intestine (jejunum and ileum) from the posterior parietal peritoneum; about 9 inches (23 cm.) in length, it extends from the duodenojejunal flexure (just to the left of the midline at the L_2 vertebral level) to the ileocecal junction (iliac fossa). SYN radix mesenterii [NA].

motor r., SYN ventral r.

motor r. of ciliary ganglion, SYN parasympathetic r. of ciliary ganglion.

motor r.'s of submandibular ganglion, SYN ganglionic *branches* of lingual nerve, under *branch.*

motor r. of trigeminal nerve, the smaller root of the trigeminal nerve, composed of fibers originating from the trigeminal motor nucleus and emerging from the pons medial to the much larger sensory root, to join the mandibular nerve; it carries motor and proprioceptive fibers to the muscles derived from the first bronchial (mandibular) arch, including the four muscles of mastication, plus the mylohyoid, anterior belly of the digastric, and the tensores tympani and veli palati. SYN radix motoria nervi trigemini [NA], masticator nerve, portio minor nervi trigemini.

r. of nail, the proximal end of the nail, concealed under a fold of skin. SYN radix unguis [NA].

nasociliary r., SYN sensory r. of ciliary ganglion.

nerve r., one of the two bundles of nerve fibers (dorsal and ventral r.'s) emerging from the spinal cord that join to form a single segmental (mixed) spinal nerve; some of the cranial nerves are similarly formed by the union of two r.'s, in particular the fifth or trigeminal nerve; in the case of the eighth cranial (vestibulocochlear) nerve, each of its two components (vestibular r. and cochlear r.) is referred to as a root even though they do not join each other and their central connections are distinctive; **conjoined nerve r.,** two adjacent nerve r.'s with the same common origin from the dura mater.

r. of nose, the upper least protruding portion of the external nose situated between the two orbits. SYN radix nasi [NA].

oculomotor r. of ciliary ganglion, SYN parasympathetic r. of ciliary ganglion.

olfactory r.'s, SYN olfactory *striae,* under *stria.*

r.'s of olfactory tract, lateral and medial, the two fiber bands that form the caudal continuation of the olfactory tract which, upon diverging, enclose the olfactory tubercle.

parasympathetic r. of ciliary ganglion, a branch of the oculomotor nerve supplying parasympathetic preganglionic nerve fibers to the ciliary ganglion. SYN radix parasympathica ganglii ciliaris [NA], radix oculomotoria ganglii ciliaris☆ [NA], motor r. of ciliary ganglion, oculomotor r. of ciliary ganglion, radix brevis ganglii ciliaris, short r. of ciliary ganglion.

r. of penis, the proximal attached part of the penis, including the two crura and the bulb. SYN radix penis [NA].

posterior r., SYN dorsal r.

sensory r. of ciliary ganglion, sensory fibers passing from the eyeball through the ciliary ganglion to their cell bodies in the trigeminal ganglion via the nasociliary nerve. SYN radix sensoria ganglii ciliaris [NA], ramus communicans nervi nasociliaris cum ganglio ciliari [NA], radix nasociliaris☆ [NA], long r. of ciliary ganglion, nasociliary r., radix longa ganglii ciliaris.

sensory r. of pterygopalatine ganglion, SYN ganglionic *branches* of maxillary nerve, under *branch.*

sensory r. of trigeminal nerve, the large sensory root of the trigeminal (or fifth cranial) nerve, extending from the semilunar ganglion into the pons through the middle cerebellar peduncle or brachium pontis, immediately lateral to the small motor r. SYN radix sensoria nervi trigemini☆ [NA], portio major nervi trigemini.

short r. of ciliary ganglion, SYN parasympathetic r. of ciliary ganglion.

spinal r. of accessory nerve, originates from the upper five or six cervical spinal segments, emerges from the lateral surface of the spinal cord and ascends through the foramen magnum to join the cranial root. SYN radices spinales nervi accessorii [NA], ramus externus nervi accessorii [NA], pars spinalis nervi accessorii☆, spinal part of accessory nerve.

superior r. of ansa cervicalis, the fibers that arise from the first and second cervical nerves, accompany the hypoglossal nerve, then branch off to meet the inferior root in the ansa cervicalis; they innervate the infrahyoid muscles. SYN descendens hypoglossi, descending branch of hypoglossal nerve, radix superior ansae cervicalis.

superior r. of vestibulocochlear nerve, SYN vestibular r.

sympathetic r. of ciliary ganglion, postganglionic fibers ,having cell bodies in the superior cervical ganglion, branching from the carotid plexus passing through the ciliary ganglion without synapse to reach the eyeball. SYN radix sympathica ganglii ciliaris [NA].

r. of tongue, the posterior attached portion of the tongue. SYN radix linguae [NA], base of tongue.

r. of tooth, that part of a tooth below the neck, covered by cementum rather than enamel, and attached by the periodontal ligament to the alveolar bone. SYN radix dentis [NA], radix (1) [NA], root (2).

r.'s of trigeminal nerve, collective term for the sensory r. of trigeminal nerve and motor r. of trigeminal nerve. SYN radices nervi trigemini.

tuberous r., a r. that is swollen for food storage; tuberous primary r.'s occur in aconite, beet, and carrot; tuberous secondary r.'s occur in plants of the Umbelliferae; and tuberous adventitious roots occur in jalap and sweet potato.

ventral r., the motor root of a spinal nerve. SYN radix anterior [NA], radix motoria☆ [NA], anterior r., motor r., radix ventralis.

vestibular r., SYN radix vestibularis [NA], radix superior nervi vestibulocochlearis, superior r. of vestibulocochlear nerve, vestibular r. of vestibulocochlear nerve.

vestibular r. of vestibulocochlear nerve, SYN vestibular r.

root·lets (rūt′lets). In neuroanatomy, nerve rootlets (fila radicularia). SEE filum.

root plan·ing (plān′ing). In dentistry, abrading of rough root surfaces to achieve a smooth surface.

ROP Abbreviation for right occipitoposterior position.

ro·pal·o·cy·to·sis (rō-pal′ō-sī-tō′sis). Formation of numerous processes of erythroid cells, which in ultrathin sections appear club-shaped, associated with cytoplasmic vesicles and found in some diseases of the blood. [G. *ropalon,* club, + *kytos,* cell, + *-osis,* condition]

Ropes test. See under test.

Rorschach, Hermann, Swiss psychiatrist, 1884–1922. SEE R. *test.*

Ro·sa (rō′ză). A genus of plants including the roses (family Rosaceae); several varieties are the sources of rose oil: *R. alba,* cottage rose; *R. centifolia,* the pale rose or cabbage rose (source of official rose oil); *R. damascena,* damask rose; and *R. gallica,* red rose or French rose. [L. rose]

ro·sa·cea (rō-zā′she-ă). Chronic vascular and follicular dilation involving the nose and contiguous portions of the cheeks; may vary from mild but persistent erythema to extensive hyperplasia of the sebaceous glands, seen especially in men as rhinophyma and by deep-seated papules and pustules; accompanied by telangiectasia at the affected erythematous sites. SYN acne erythematosa, acne rosacea. [L. *rosaceus,* rosy]

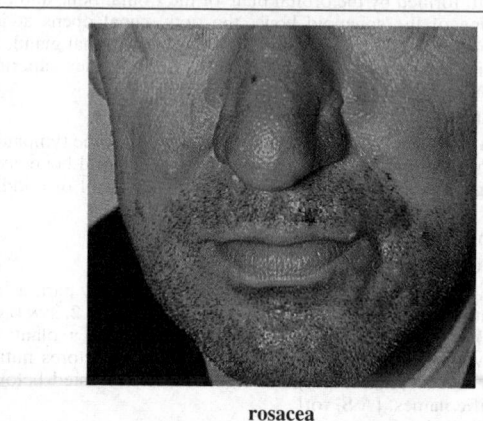

rosacea

granulomatous r., papular lesions in r., characterized microscopically by perifollicular granulomas with central necrosis and scattered giant cells. Lupus miliaris disseminatus faciei is probably a form of granulomatous r. SYN rosacea-like tuberculid, tuberculoid r.

hypertrophic r., SYN rhinophyma.

tuberculoid r., SYN granulomatous r.

ros·an·i·lin (rō-zan′i-lin) [C.I. 42510]. A tris(aminophenyl)-methyl compound; together with pararosanilin it is a component of basic fuchsin; also used as an antifungal agent.

ro·sap·ros·tol (rō′să-prost-ol). A prostaglandin analog with protective properties for the gastric mucosa. Similar to misoprostol and also used as an antiulcerative drug.

ro·sa·ry (rō′zer-ē). A beadlike arrangement or structure.

rachitic r., a row of beading at the junction of the ribs with their cartilages, often seen in rachitic children. SYN beading of the ribs.

Roscoe, Sir Henry E., British chemist, 1833–1915. SEE Bunsen-R. *law.*

Rose, Edmund, German physician, 1836–1914. SEE R.'s *position,* cephalic *tetanus.*

Rose, H.M., U.S. microbiologist, *1906. SEE R.-Waaler *test.*

rose (rōz). **1.** SYN erysipelas. **2.** The petals of *Rosa gallica,* collected before expanding; used for its agreeable odor. [L. *rosa*]

r. oil, a volatile oil from *Rosa centifolia;* used in perfumery and in ointments. SYN attar of rose.

rose ben·gal (rōz′ ben′gal) [C.I. 45440]. The sodium salt of tetraiodotetra-chlorfluorescein, $C_{20}H_2O_5I_4Cl_4Na_2$, used as a stain for bacteria, as a stain in the diagnosis of keratitis sicca, and in liver function tests.

Rose-Bradford kid·ney. See under kidney.

rose hips. The fruit or berries from wild rose bushes and in particular *Rosa canina, R. gallica, R. condita,* and *R. Rugosa,* (family Rosaceae). A rich source of vitamin C (ascorbic acid). SYN hipberries.

rose·mary oil (rōz′măr-ē). The volatile oil distilled with steam from the fresh flowering tops of *Rosmarinus officinalis* (family Labiatae); used as a flavoring and in perfumery.

Rosenbach, Ottomar, German physician, 1851–1907. SEE R.'s *disease, law, sign, test;* R.-Gmelin *test.*

Rosenmüller, Johann C., German anatomist, 1771–1820. SEE R.'s *fossa, gland, node, recess, valve; organ* of R.

Rosenthal, Curt, 20th century German psychiatrist. SEE Melkersson-R. *syndrome.*

Rosenthal, Friedrich C., German anatomist, 1780–1829. SEE R.'s *canal, vein;* basal *vein* of R.

Rosenthaler-Turk re·a·gent. See under reagent.

Rosenthal fi·ber. See under fiber.

ro·se·o·la (rō-zē′ō-lă). A symmetrical eruption of small closely aggregated patches of rose-red color. It is believed to be caused by human herpesvirus type 6. SEE ALSO *exanthema* subitum. SYN macular erythema. [Mod. L. dim. of L. *roseus,* rosy]

epidemic r., SYN rubella.

idiopathic r., r. not occurring as a symptom of a recognized general disease.

r. infan′tilis, r. infan′tum, SYN *exanthema* subitum.

syphilitic r., usually the first eruption of syphilis, occurring 6 to 12 weeks after the initial lesion. SYN erythematous syphilid, macular syphilid.

ro·se·o·lous (rō-zē′ō-lŭs). Relating to or resembling roseola.

Roser, Wilhelm, German surgeon, 1817–1888. SEE R.-Nélaton *line.*

ro·sette (rō-zet′). **1.** The quartan malarial parasite *Plasmodium malariae* in its segmented or mature phase. **2.** A grouping of cells characteristic of neoplasms of neuroblastic or neuroectodermal origin; a number of nuclei form a ring from which neurofibrils, which can be demonstrated by silver impregnation, extend to interlace in the center. **3.** Roselike coiling of the uterus among certain pseudophyllidean tapeworms, such as *Diphyllobothrium latum.* [Fr. a little rose]

E r. (ro-zet′), the adherence of erythrocytes to cells. Sheep erythrocytes will adhere spontaneously to human T cells, forming rosettes.

EAC r., indicates the presence of complement receptors. Erythrocytes (E) coated with antibody (A) and complement (C) are incubated with test cells. If the test cells have complement receptors, the EAC will adhere to these cells, forming rosettes.

Homer-Wright r.'s, pseudorosettes formed by the arrangement of tumor cells around an area of fibrillarity, evidence of neuroblastic differentiation in a medulloblastoma or primitive neuroectodermal tumor.

Wintersteiner r.'s, r.'s found only in retinal embryonic tumors, formed by a group of columnar cells with a peripheral basement membrane arranged in a radial manner around a central cavity, the spokes corresponding to the photoreceptors.

ros·in (roz′in). The solid resin obtained after steam distillation of crude balsam from *Pinus palustris* and from other species of *Pinus* (family Pinaceae); used in plasters to render them adhesive and also in ointments to render them locally stimulating. SYN colophony, resin (2).

p-ro·so·lic ac·id (rō-sol′ik). SYN aurin.

Ross, Sir George W., Canadian physician, 1841–1931. SEE R.-Jones *test.*

Ross, Sir Ronald, English physician and Nobel laureate, 1857–1932. SEE R. *cycle.*

Rossolimo, Grigoriy I., Russian neurologist, 1860–1928. SEE R.'s *reflex, sign.*

ros·tel·lum (ros-tel′ŭm). The anterior fixed or invertible portion of the scolex of a tapeworm, frequently provided with a row (or several rows) of hooks. [L. dim. of *rostrum,* a beak]

armed r., r. with one or more rows of hooks.

unarmed r., r. lacking hooks.

ros·trad (ros′trăd). **1.** In a direction toward any rostrum. **2.** Situated nearer a rostrum or the snout end of an organism in relation to a specific reference point; opposite of caudad (2). [L. *rostrum,* beak, + *-ad,* toward]

ros·tral (ros′trăl). Relating to any rostrum or anatomical structure resembling a beak. SYN rostralis [NA]. [L. *rostralis,* fr. *rostrum,* beak]

ros·tra·lis (ros′trā′lis) [NA]. SYN rostral, rostral. [L. fr. *rostrum,* beak]

ros·trate (ros′trāt). Having a beak or hook. [L. *rostratus*]

ros·tri·form (ros′tri-fōrm). Beak-shaped. [L. *rostrum,* beak]

ros·trum, pl. **ros·tra, ros·trums** (ros′trŭm, -tră) [NA]. Any beak-shaped structure. [L. a beak]

r. cor′poris callo′si [NA], SYN r. of corpus callosum.

r. of corpus callosum, beak of the corpus callosum, the recurved portion of the corpus callosum passing backward from the genu to the anterior commissure. SYN r. corporis callosi [NA].

r. sphenoida′le [NA], SYN r. of the sphenoid bone.

r. of the sphenoid bone, the anterior projecting part of the body of the sphenoid bone which articulates with the vomer. SYN r. sphenoidale [NA].

ROT Abbreviation for right occipitotransverse position.

rot. To decay or putrify. [A.S. *rotian*]

Barcoo r., SYN desert *sore.* [*Barcoo,* a river in S. Australia]

foot r., **(1)** in sheep and goats, a highly contagious bacterial disease caused by the interaction of *Bacteroides nodosus* and *Fusobacterium necrophorum,* and characterized by lameness and bidigital separation of the hoof corneum from the basal epithelium and derma; **(2)** in cattle, a complex of diseases characterized by lameness and associated with a foul-smelling necrotic process of the feet from which *F. necrophorum* can invariably be isolated.

pizzle r., SYN ulcerative *posthitis.*

sheath r., SYN ulcerative *posthitis.*

ro·tam·e·ter (rō-tam′ĕ-ter). A device for measuring the flow of gas or liquid; the fluid flowing up through a slightly tapered tube elevates a ball or other weight that partially obstructs the flow, until the wider cross-section allows that flow to pass around the floating obstruction. [L. *rota,* wheel, + G. *metron,* measure]

ro·ta·tion (rō-tā′shŭn). **1.** Turning or movement of a body round its axis. **2.** A recurrence in regular order of certain events, such as the symptoms of a periodic disease. [L. *rotatio,* fr. *roto,* pp. *rotatus,* to revolve, rotate]

intestinal r., SEE malrotation.

molecular r., one hundredth of the product of the specific r. of an optically active compound and its molecular weight.

optical r., the change in the plane of polarization of polarized light of a given wavelength upon passing through optically active substances; measured in terms of specific rotation by polarimetry, an important tool in chemical structural work, especially on carbohydrates.

specific optical r. ([α]), the arc through which the plane of polarized light is rotated by 1 gram of a substance per milliliter of water when the length of the light path through the solution is 1 decimeter, typically using light corresponding to the D line of sodium.

ro·ta·tor (rō-tā′ter, -tōr). A muscle by which a part can be turned circularly. SEE rotatores *muscles,* under *muscle.* [L. See rotation]

medial r., SYN intortor.

ro·ta·vi·rus (rō′tă-vī′rŭs). A group of RNA viruses (family Reoviridae) that are wheel-like in appearance and form a genus, *Rotavirus,* which includes the human gastroenteritis viruses (a major cause of infant diarrhea throughout the world), Nebraska calf scours virus, epizootic diarrhea virus of infant mice, and others. They are fastidious, and *in vitro* culture is difficult. SYN duovirus, gastroenteritis virus type B, infantile gastroenteritis virus, reovirus, reovirus-like agent. [L. *rota,* wheel, + virus]

Rotch, Thomas M., U.S. physician, 1848–1914. SEE R.'s *sign.*

röt·eln, roeth·eln (ruht′eln). SYN rubella. [Ger. little red spots, fr. *rot,* red, + *-el,* dim. suffix]

ro·te·none (rō′te-nōn). The principal insecticidal component of derris root, *Derris elliptica, D. malaccensis,* and other species of *D.,* and from *Lonchocarpus nicou* (family Leguminosae); used externally for the treatment of scabies and infestation with chiggers, and in veterinary medicine for follicular mange and infestation with lice, fleas, and ticks; an inhibitor of the respiratory chain.

Roth, Moritz, Swiss physician and pathologist, 1839–1914. SEE R.'s *spots,* under *spot; vas* aberrans of R.

Ro

Roth, Vladimir K., Russian neurologist, 1848–1916. SEE R.'s *disease;* R.-Bernhardt *disease;* Bernhardt-R. *syndrome.*

Roth. SEE Benedict-Roth *apparatus.*

Rothera, Arthur C.H., English biochemist, 1880–1915. SEE Rothera's nitroprusside *test.*

Roth·ia (roth'ē-ă). A genus of nonmotile, nonsporeforming, non-acid-fast, aerobic to facultatively anaerobic bacteria (family Actinomycetaceae) containing Gram-positive, coccoid, diphtheroid, or filamentous cells; metabolism is fermentative, and glucose fermentation yields primarily lactic acid but no propionic acid. These organisms are normal inhabitants of the human oral cavity and are opportunistic pathogens. The type species is *R. dentocariosa.* [G. D. *Roth*]

R. dentocariosa, rare cause of infective endocarditis in humans.

Rothmund, August von, German physician, 1830–1906. SEE R.'s *syndrome;* R.-Thomson *syndrome.*

Rotor, Arturo B., 20th century Philippine internist. SEE R.'s *syndrome.*

ro·to·sco·li·o·sis (rō'tō-skō-lē-ō'sis). Combined lateral and rotational deviation of the vertebral column. [L. *roto,* to rotate, + G. *skoliōsis,* crookedness]

ro·to·tome (rō'tō-tōm). A rotating cutting instrument used in arthroscopic surgery.

ro·tox·a·mine (rō-tok'să-mēn). (—)-2-[*p*-Chloro-α-(2-dimethylaminoethoxy)benzyl]pyridine; active isomer of carbinoxamine; an antihistaminic.

Rouget, Antoine D., 19th century French physiologist. SEE R.'s *bulb.*

Rouget, Charles M.B., French physiologist, 1824–1904. SEE R. *cell;* R.'s *muscle;* R.-Neumann *sheath.*

rough (rŭf). Not smooth; denoting the irregular, coarsely granular surface of a certain bacterial colony type.

rough·age (rŭf'ij). **1.** Anything in the diet, *e.g.,* bran, serving as a bulk stimulant of intestinal peristalsis. **2.** Hay or other coarse feed fed to cattle and other herbivores.

Roughton, Francis J.W., British scientist, 1899–1972. SEE R.-Scholander *apparatus, syringe.*

Rougnon de Magny, Nicholas F., French physician, 1727–1799. SEE Rougnon-Heberden *disease.*

rou·leau, pl. **rou·leaux** (roo-lō'). An aggregate of erythrocytes stacked like a pile of coins. R. formation commonly indicates an increase in plasma immunoglobulin. [Fr. spool, cylinder, fr. *rouler,* to roll, fr. L.L. *rotulo,* fr. *rota,* wheel]

round·worm (rownd'werm). A nematode member of the phylum Nematoda, commonly confined to the parasitic forms.

Rous, F. Peyton, U.S. pathologist and Nobel laureate, 1879–1970. SEE R. *sarcoma,* sarcoma *virus, tumor;* R.-associated *virus.*

Roussy, Gustave, French pathologist, 1874–1948. SEE R.-Lévy *disease, syndrome;* Dejerine-R. *syndrome.*

Rouviere, Henri, French anatomist and embryologist, *1875. SEE *node* of R.

Roux, César, Swiss surgeon, 1857–1934. SEE R.-en-Y *anastomosis, operation.*

Roux, Philibert J., French surgeon, 1780–1854. SEE R.'s *method.*

Roux, Pierre P.E., French bacteriologist, 1853–1933. SEE R. *spatula;* R.'s *stain.*

Rovsing, Niels T., Danish surgeon, 1862–1927. SEE R.'s *sign.*

Rowntree, Leonard G., U.S. physician, *1883. SEE R. and Geraghty *test.*

RPF Abbreviation for renal plasma flow. SEE effective renal plasma *flow.*

R.Ph. Abbreviation for Registered Pharmacist.

rpm Abbreviation for revolutions per minute.

RPO Abbreviation for right posterior oblique, a radiographic projection.

R.Q. Abbreviation for respiratory *quotient.*

△-rrhagia. Excessive or unusual discharge. [G. *rhēgnymi,* to burst forth]

△-rrhaphy. Surgical suturing. [G. *rhaphē,* suture]

△-rrhea. A flowing; a flux. [G. *rhoia,* a flow]

△-rrhoea. SEE -rrhea.

rRNA Abbreviation for ribosomal ribonucleic acid.

RSA Abbreviation for right sacroanterior position.

RSD Abbreviation for reflex sympathetic *dystrophy.*

RSP Abbreviation for right sacroposterior position.

RST Abbreviation for right sacrotransverse position.

RSV Abbreviation for Rous sarcoma *virus.*

RT, rt Abbreviation for room *temperature.*

RT₃ Symbol for reverse triiodothyronine.

rTMP Abbreviation for ribothymidylic acid.

RU-486. SYN mifepristone.

Ru Symbol for ruthenium.

rub (rŭb). Friction encountered in moving one body over another.

friction r., SYN friction *sound.*

pericardial r., pericardial friction r., SYN pericardial friction *sound.*

pleural r., friction rub sound caused by inflammation of the pleura. SYN pleural friction r., pleural rale.

pleural friction r., SYN pleural r.

pleuritic r., a friction sound produced by the rubbing together of the roughened surfaces of the costal and visceral pleurae.

Rubarth, Sven, Swedish veterinarian, *1905. SEE R.'s *disease,* disease *virus.*

rub·ber (rŭb'er). poly(*cis*-1,4-isoprene); the prepared inspissated milky juice of *Hevea brasiliensis* and other species of *Hevea* (family Euphorbiaceae), known in commerce as pure Para r.; used in the manufacture of various plasters, tissues, bandages, etc.

rub·ber po·lice·man. SEE policeman.

ru·be·an·ic ac·id (rū'bē-an-ik). Dithiooxamide, which forms complete dark greenish-black complexes with copper in alkaline ethanolic solution; used histochemically for demonstrating pathologic copper deposits, as in Wilson's disease; also reacts with cobalt and nickel.

ru·be·do (rū-bē'dō). A temporary redness of the skin. [L. redness, fr. *ruber,* red]

ru·be·fa·cient (rū-bē-fā'shent). **1.** Causing a reddening of the skin. **2.** A counterirritant that produces erythema when applied to the skin surface. [L. *rubi-facio,* fr. *ruber,* red, + *facio,* to make]

ru·be·fac·tion (rū-bē-fak'shŭn). Erythema of the skin caused by local application of a counterirritant. [see rubefacient]

ru·bel·la (rū-bel'ă). An acute exanthematous disease caused by rubella virus (*Rubivirus*), with enlargement of lymph nodes, but usually with little fever or constitutional reaction; a high incidence of birth defects in children results from maternal infection during the first several months of fetal life (congenital rubella syndrome). SYN epidemic roseola, German measles, röteln, roetheln, third disease, three-day measles. [L. *rubellus,* fem. *-a,* reddish, dim. of *ruber,* red]

ru·bel·lin (rū-bel'in). A cardiac glycoside with a digitalis-like action, obtained from *Urginia rubella* (family Liliaceae).

ru·be·o·la (rū-bē'ō-lă, -bē-ō'lă). A term used for measles; not to be confused with rubella. [Mod. L. dim. of *ruber,* red, reddish]

ru·be·o·sis (rū-bē-ō'sis). Reddish discoloration, as of the skin. [L. *ruber,* red, + G. *-osis,* condition]

r. i'ridis diabet'ica, neovascularization of the anterior surface of the iris in diabetes mellitus.

ru·be·ryth·ric ac·id (rū-ber'ē-thrik). See under acid.

ru·bes·cent (rū-bes'ent). Reddening. [L. *rubesco,* pr. p. *rubescens,* to become red]

ru·bid·i·um (Rb) (rū-bid'ē-ŭm). An alkali element, atomic no. 37, atomic wt. 85.4678; its salts have been used in medicine for the same purposes as the corresponding sodium or potassium salts. [L. *rubidus,* reddish, dark red, fr. *rubeo,* to be red]

ru·bid·o·my·cin (dau·no·ru·bi·cin) (rū-bid'ō-mī-sin). An antibiotic used as an antineoplastic; similar to doxorubicin in antitumor activity and in exhibiting cumulative cardiotoxicity.

Rubin, Isidor C., U.S. gynecologist, 1883–1958. SEE R. *test.*

ru·bin S, ru·bine (rū′bin, bēn) [C.I. 42685]. SYN acid *fuchsin*.

Rubinstein, Jack H., U.S. child psychiatrist and pediatrician, *1925. SEE R.-Taybi *syndrome*.

Ru·bi·vi·rus (rū′bi-vī′rŭs). A genus of viruses (family Togaviridae) that includes the rubella virus. [*rubel*la + virus]

Rubner, Max, German hygienist and biochemist, 1854–1932. SEE R.'s *laws* of growth, under *law, test.*

ru·bor (rū′bōr). Redness, as one of the four signs of inflammation (r., calor, dolor, tumor) enunciated by Celsus. [L.]

ru·bra·tox·in (rū-bră-tok′sin). A mycotoxin produced by *Penicillium rubrum* and *P. purpurogenum*, which form readily on cereal grains; responsible for outbreaks of toxicosis in the U.S.

ru·bre·dox·ins (rū-brĕ-dok′sinz). Ferredoxins without acid-labile sulfur and with the iron in a typical mercaptide coordination.

ru·bri·blast (rū′bri-blast). SYN pronormoblast. [L. *ruber*, red, + G. *blastos*, germ]

    pernicious anemia type r., SYN promegaloblast. SEE erythroblast.

rub·ric. Section or chapter heading, used with reference to groups of diseases, as in ICD. [M.E. *rubrike*, title or heading in red, fr. L. *ruber*, red]

ru·bri·cyte (rū′bri-sīt). Polychromatic normoblast. SEE erythroblast. [L. *ruber*, red, + *kytos*, cell]

ru·bro·spi·nal (rū′brō-spī′năl). Relating to the nerve fibers passing from the red nucleus to the spinal cord: the rubrospinal *tract*.

ruc·tus (rŭk′tŭs). SYN eructation. [L. fr. *ructo*, pp. *-atus*, to belch]

Rud, Einar, Danish physician, *1892. SEE R.'s *syndrome*.

ru·di·ment (rū′di-ment). **1.** An organ or structure that is incompletely developed. **2.** The first indication of a structure in the course of ontogeny. SYN rudimentum [NA]. [L. *rudimentum*, a beginning, fr. *rudis*, unformed]

ru·di·men·ta·ry (rū-di-men′tār-ē). Relating to a rudiment. SYN abortive (2).

ru·di·men·tum, pl. **ru·di·men·ta** (rū′di-men′tŭm, -tă) [NA]. SYN rudiment, rudiment. [L.]

    r. hippocam′pi, SEE *indusium* griseum.

Ruffini, Angelo, Italian histologist, 1864–1929. SEE R.'s *corpuscles*, under *corpuscle;* flower-spray *organ* of R.

ru·fous (rū′fŭs). SYN erythristic. [L. *rufus*, reddish]

ru·ga, pl. **ru·gae** (rū′gă, rū′gē) [NA]. A fold, ridge, or crease; a wrinkle. [L. a wrinkle]

    r. gas′trica, SYN rugae of stomach.

    r. palati′na, SYN transverse palatine *fold*.

    rugae of stomach, characteristic folds of the gastric mucosa, especially evident when the stomach is contracted. SYN plicae gastricae [NA], gastric folds, r. gastrica.

    rugae of vagina, a number of transverse ridges in the mucous membrane of the vagina. SYN rugae vaginales [NA].

    ru′gae vagina′les [NA], SYN rugae of vagina.

ru·gine (rū-zhēn′). **1.** SYN periosteal *elevator*. **2.** A raspatory. [Fr.]

ru·gi·tus (rū′ji-tŭs). A rumbling sound in the intestines. SEE ALSO borborygmus. [L. a roaring, fr. *rugio*, to roar]

ru·gose (rū′gōs). Marked by rugae; wrinkled. SYN rugous. [L. *rugosus*]

ru·gos·i·ty (rū-gos′i-tē). **1.** The state of being thrown into folds or wrinkles. **2.** A ruga.

ru·gous (rū′gŭs). SYN rugose.

RUL Abbreviation for right upper lobe (of lung).

rule (rūl). A criterion, standard, or guide governing a procedure, arrangement, action, etc. SEE ALSO law, principle, theorem. [O. Fr. *reule*, fr. L. *regula*, a guide, pattern]

    Abegg's r., the tendency of the sum of the maximum positive and maximum negative valence of a particular element to equal 8; *e.g.*, C may have a valence of +4 and −4, O of +6 and −2. Sometimes loosely stated as all atoms have the same number of valences, a consequence of the tendency of valence electron shells to be filled to 8.

    American Law Institute r., a test of criminal responsibility

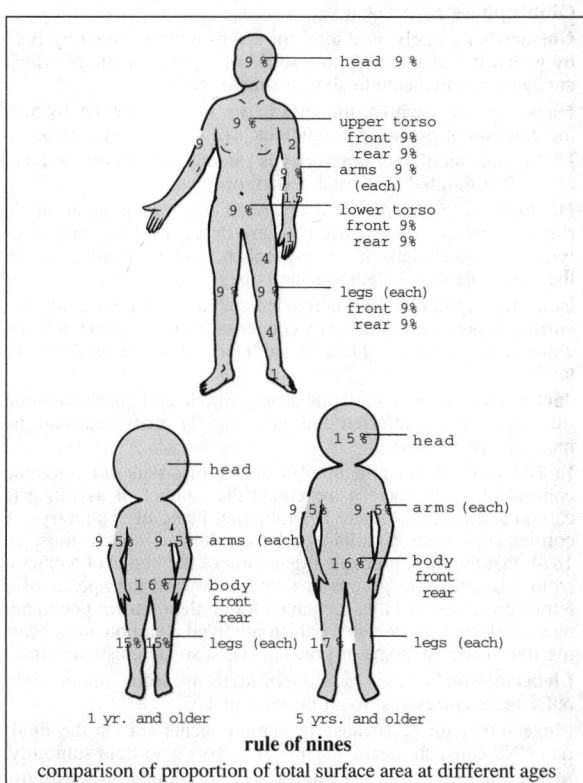

rule of nines
comparison of proportion of total surface area at diffferent ages

(1962): "a person is not responsible for criminal conduct if at the time of such conduct as a result of mental disease or defect he lacks substantial capacity either to appreciate the wrongfulness of his conduct or to conform his conduct to the requirements of law."

    r. of bigeminy, r. that a ventricular premature beat will follow the beat terminating a long cycle. Sudden prolongation of the ventricular cycle, by changing the refractoriness in the conduction system, causes a peripheral region of bidirectional block to become transiently unidirectional and thus opens potential pathways for reentry to occur.

    Chargaff's r., in DNA the number of adenine units equals the number of thymine units; likewise, the number of guanine units equals the number of cytosine units.

    Clark's weight r., an obsolete r. for an approximate child's dose, obtained by dividing the child's weight in pounds by 150 and multiplying the result by the adult dose.

    Cowling's r., an obsolete r. for a child's dose: that fraction of the adult dose obtained by dividing the age of the child at the nearest birthday by 24.

    Durham r., an American test of criminal responsibility (1954): "an accused is not criminally responsible if his unlawful act was the product of mental disease or mental defect."

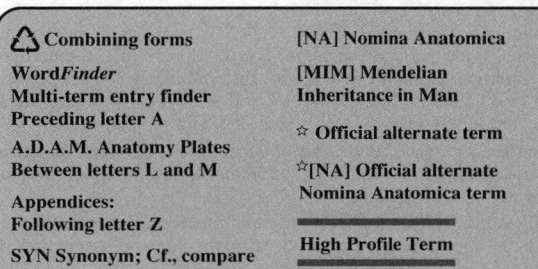

Combining forms	[NA] Nomina Anatomica
Word*Finder* **Multi-term entry finder** **Preceding letter A**	**[MIM] Mendelian** **Inheritance in Man**
A.D.A.M. Anatomy Plates **Between letters L and M**	☆ **Official alternate term**
Appendices: **Following letter Z**	☆**[NA] Official alternate** **Nomina Anatomica term**
SYN Synonym; Cf., compare	**High Profile Term**

ru

Gibb's phase r., SYN phase r.

Goriaew's r., rarely used term for a r. of a blood counting field by which it is marked off in a series of squares, some of which are again subdivided into sixteen smaller ones.

Haase's r., the length of the fetus in centimeters, divided by 5, is the duration of pregnancy in months, *i.e.,* the age of the fetus.

His' r., the duration of pregnancy is calculated from the first day of the first omitted menstrual period; obsolete.

Hückel's r., the number of depolarized electrons in an aromatic ring is equal to $4n + 2$ where n is zero or any positive integer; L-tyrosine, L-phenylalanine, L-tryptophan, and L-histidine (when the imidazole ring is deprotonated) obey this rule.

isoprene r., the classical, outmoded statement that naturally occurring terpenes are built up by condensation of isoprene units by either a 1-4 linkage ("head to tail") or a 4-4 linkage ("tail to tail").

Jackson's r., after an epileptic attack, simple and quasiautomatic functions are less affected and more rapidly recovered than the more complex ones.

Le Bel-van't Hoff r., the number of stereoisomers of an organic compound is 2^n where n represents the number of asymmetric carbon atoms (unless there is an internal plane of symmetry). A corollary of their simultaneously announced conclusions, in 1874, that the most probable orientation of the bonds of a carbon atom linked to four groups or atoms is toward the apexes of a tetrahedron, and that this accounted for all then-known phenomena of molecular asymmetry (which involved a carbon atom bearing four different atoms or groups). SEE ALSO stereoisomerism.

Liebermeister's r., in adult febrile tachycardia, about eight pulse beats correspond to an increase of 1°C.

Meyer-Overton r., because inhalation agents act via the lipid-rich CNS cells, anesthetic potency increases with lipid solubility.

M'Naghten r., the classic English test of criminal responsibility (1843): "to establish a defense on the ground of insanity, it must be clearly proved that, at the time of committing the act, the party accused was laboring under such a defect of reasoning, from disease of the mind, as not to know the nature and quality of the act he was doing, or if he did know it, that he did not know he was doing what was wrong."

Nägele's r., means of estimating date of delivery by counting back three months from the first day of the last menstrual period and adding seven days.

New Hampshire r., pioneering American test of criminal responsibility (1871): "if the [criminal] act was the offspring of insanity, a criminal intent did not produce it."

r. of nines, method used in calculating body surface area involved in burns whereby values of 9 or 18 percent of surface area are assigned to specific regions as follows: Head and neck, 9%; anterior thorax, 18%; posterior thorax, 18%; arms, 9% each; legs, 18% each; perineum 1%.

Ogino-Knaus r., the time in the menstrual period when conception is most likely to occur is at about midway between two menstrual periods; fertilization of the ovum is least likely just before or just after menstruation; the basis for the rhythm method of contraception.

r. of outlet, an obstetric r. for determining whether the pelvic outlet will permit the passage of a fetus; the sum of the posterior sagittal diameter and the transverse diameter of the outlet must equal at least 15 cm if a normal-sized baby is to pass.

phase r., an expression of the relationships existing between systems in equilibrium: $P + V = C + 2$, where P is the number of phases, V the variance or degrees of freedom, and C the number of components; it also follows that the variance is, $V = C + 2 - P$. For H_2O at its triple point, $V = 1 + 2 - 3 = 0$, *i.e.,* both temperature and pressure are fixed. SYN Gibb's phase r.

Prentice's r., each centimeter of decentration of a lens results in 1 prism diopter of deviation of light for each diopter of lens power.

Rolleston's r., the ideal adult systolic blood pressure is 100 plus half the age, whereas the maximal physiologic pressure is 100 plus the age; of historical interest.

Schütz r., the rate of an enzyme reaction is proportional to the

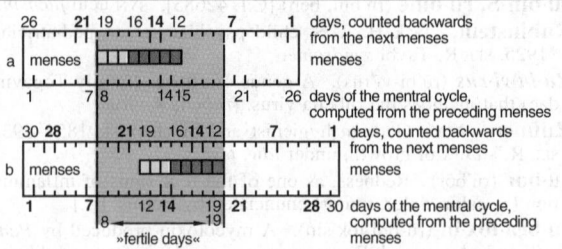

Ogino-Knaus rule

determination of fertile period by Ogino method, with cycles of from 26 to 30 days; yellow squares represent the maximum survival period of spermatozoa, blue squares the period during which ovulation is expected to take place; a) for a 26-day cycle, the fertile period is from day 8 to day 15; b) for a 30-day cycle, the fertile period is from day 8 to day 19

square root of the enzyme concentration; applied specifically to pepsin within a limited range. SYN Schütz' law.

Trusler's r. for pulmonary artery banding, a method that gives guidance as to the correct tightness of the band; the degree of banding for a complex congenital cardiac anomaly with bidirectional shunting less than that for simple ones.

Young's r., an obsolete r. to determine a child's dose: 12 is added to the child's age and the sum is divided by the age; the adult dose divided by the figure so obtained gives the proper dose.

rul·er (rū′ler). A calibrated strip for measuring plane surfaces.

isometric r., a calibrated scale for eliminating distortion in the measurement of plane surfaces.

rum (rŭm). A spirit distilled from the fermented juice of the sugar cane.

rum-blos·som (rŭm-blos′ŭm). SYN rhinophyma.

ru·men, pl. **ru·mi·na** (rū′men, rū′mi-nă). The largest compartment of the stomach of a cow or other ruminant. SYN paunch. [L. gullet, throat]

ru·men·i·tis (rū-mĕ-nī′tis). Inflammation of the rumen of ruminant animals. [rumen + G. *-itis,* inflammation]

ru·men·ot·o·my (rū-mĕ-not′ō-mē). Incision into the rumen. [rumen + G. *tomē,* incision]

ru·mi·nant (rū′mi-nănt). An animal that chews the cud, material regurgitated from the rumen for rechewing; *e.g.,* the sheep, cow, deer, or antelope.

ru·mi·na·tion (rū-mi-nā′shŭn). **1.** The physiologic process in ruminant animals in which coarse, hastily eaten food is regurgitated from the rumen, thoroughly rechewed, reduced to finer particles, mixed with saliva, and reswallowed. **2.** A disorder of infancy characterized by repeated regurgitation of food, with weight loss or failure to thrive, developing after a period of normal functioning. **3.** Periodic reconsideration of the same subject. [L. *ruminatio,* fr. *rumino,* to chew the cud, think over, fr. *rumen,* throat]

ru·mi·na·tive (rū′min-ă-tiv). Characterized by a preoccupation with certain thoughts and ideas.

ru·mi·no·re·tic·u·lum (rū′mi-nō-re-tik′yū-lŭm). The rumen and reticulum of the ruminant stomach taken together, since they freely communicate via the ruminoreticular orifice.

Rumpel, Theodor, German physician, 1862–1923. SEE R.-Leede *sign, test, phenomenon.*

run·a·round, run·round (rŭn′ă-rownd, rŭn′rownd). Colloquialism for paronychia.

Rundle. A.T., British physician. SEE Richards-Rundle *syndrome.*

Runeberg, Johan W., Finnish physician, 1843–1918. SEE R.'s *formula.*

run·off (rŭn′awf). Delayed part of the angiographic examination of a vascular bed, to show small artery patency.

runt (rŭnt). A stunted animal, occurring most frequently in species which give birth to large litters. [A.S.]

ru·pia (rū′pē-ă). **1.** Ulcers of late secondary syphilis, covered with yellowish or brown crusts that have been compared in their appearance to oyster shells. **2.** SYN yaws. **3.** Term occasionally used to designate a very scaly, heaped-up, and secondarily infected psoriatic lesion. [G. *rhypos,* filth]

    r. escharot′ica, SYN *dermatitis* gangrenosa infantum.

ru·pi·al (rū′pē-ăl). Relating to rupia.

ru·pi·oid (rū′pē-oyd). Resembling rupia. [G. *rhypos,* filth (rupia), + *eidos,* resemblance]

rup·ture (rŭp′chūr). **1.** SYN hernia. **2.** A solution of continuity or a tear; a break of any organ or other of the soft parts. [L. *ruptura,* a fracture (of limb or vein), fr. *rumpo,* pp. *ruptus,* to break]

RUQ Abbreviation for right upper quadrant (of abdomen).

Rushton, Martin, British pathologist. SEE R. *bodies.*

Russell, Albert L., U.S. dentist, *1905. SEE R.'s Periodontal Index.

Russell, Alexander, 20th century British pediatrician. SEE R.'s *syndrome;* Silver-R. *dwarfism, syndrome.*

Russell, G.F.M., 20th century English physician. SEE R.'s *sign.*

Russell, Hamilton, 20th century Australian surgeon. SEE R. *traction.*

Russell, James S. Risien, British physician, 1863–1939. SEE hooked *bundle* of R.; uncinate *bundle* of R.

Russell, Patrick, Irish physician in India, 1727–1805. SEE R.'s viper *venom, viper.*

Russell, William, Scottish physician, 1852–1940. SEE R. *bodies,* under *body.*

Russell, William James, English chemist, 1830–1909. SEE R. *effect.*

Russell's Per·i·o·don·tal In·dex. An index that estimates the degree of periodontal disease present in the mouth by measuring both bone loss around the teeth and gingival inflammation; used frequently in the epidemiological investigation of periodontal disease.

Rust, Johann N., German surgeon, 1775–1840. SEE R.'s *disease, phenomenon.*

rusts (rŭsts). Species of *Puccinia* and other microbes comprising important pathogens of plants, especially cereal grains; they are important allergens for humans when inhaled in large numbers, as in harvesting processes.

rut (rŭt). A period of sexual excitement in the males of certain mammals, such as deer, camels, and elephants, which occurs seasonally. It is only during this season that spermatogenesis occurs and the males will mate; in most mammalian males spermatogenesis is continuous and breeding occurs whenever the females will accept the males. Cf. estrus. [O. F. *ruit,* roaring of deer in the breeding season]

ru·the·ni·um (Ru) (rū-thē′nē-ŭm). A metallic element of the platinum group; atomic no. 44, atomic wt. 101.07; ^{106}Ru, with a half-life of 1.020 years, has been used in the treatment of certain eye problems. [Mediev. L. *Ruthenia,* Russia, where first obtained]

ru·the·ni·um red. Ammoniated r. r. oxychloride, Ru_3-$(NH_3)_{14}O_2Cl_6$, used in histology and electron microscopy as a stain for certain complex polysaccharides.

ruth·er·ford (rŭth′er-ferd). Obsolete term for a unit of radioactivity, representing that quantity of radioactive material in which a million disintegrations are taking place per second; 37 r. equal 1 mCi. SEE Becquerel. [Ernest *Rutherford,* British physicist and Nobel laureate, 1871–1937]

ru·ti·do·sis (rū-ti-dō′sis). SYN rhytidosis.

ru·tin (rū′tin). quercetin-3-rutinoside; quercetin-3-rhamnoglucoside; a flavonoid obtained from buckwheat, that causes decreased capillary fragility. SYN rutoside.

ru·tin·ose (rū′ti-nōs). 6-*O*-α-L-Rhamnosyl-D-glucose; a disaccharide of D-glucose and L-rhamnose, and a component of rutin.

ru·to·side (rū′tō-sīd). SYN rutin.

Ruysch, Frederik, Dutch anatomist, 1638–1731. SEE R.'s *membrane, muscle, tube, veins,* under *vein.*

RV Abbreviation for residual *volume.*

ry·an·o·dine (rī-an′ō-dēn). An alkaloid obtained from *Ryania speciosa* (family Flacourtiaceae). Has a disruptive effect on calcium storage in cardiac and skeletal muscle where it produces sustained contractions. Used as an insecticide.

rye smut (rī′ smŭt′). SYN ergot.

Ryle, John A., English physician, 1889–1950. SEE R.'s *tube.*

Ry

σ, Σ **1.** The 18th letter of the Greek alphabet, sigma. **2.** (σ) Symbol for reflection *coefficient*; standard *deviation*; a factor in prokaryotic RNA initiation; wavenumber; surface *tension*. **3.** (Σ) Summation of a series.

S 1. Abbreviation for sacral vertebra (S1 to S5); spherical or spherical *lens*; Svedberg *unit*. **2.** Symbol for siemens; sulfur; entropy in thermodynamics; substrate in the Michaelis-Menton mechanism; percentage saturation of hemoglobin (when followed by subscript O_2 or CO); serine; one of the two stereochemical designations (in italics) in the Cahn-Ingold-Prelog system. **3.** Designation of a rare human antigen (hemagglutinogen) related genetically to the MNSs blood group. See Blood Groups appendix.

^{35}**S** Symbol for sulfur-35.

S_1 Symbol for first heart *sound*.

S_2 Symbol for second heart *sound*.

S_3 Symbol for third heart *sound*.

S_4 Symbol for fourth heart *sound*.

S_7 SYN summation *gallop*.

S_f Symbol for flotation *constant*.

s Abbreviation of L. *sinister*, left; L. *semis*, half; second; as a subscript, denotes steady *state*.

s̄ Abbreviation for L. *sine*, without.

s Symbol for selection *coefficient*; sedimentation *coefficient*.

S-A Abbreviation for sinuatrial.

sab·a·dil·la (sab-ă-dil′ă). The seed of *Schoenocaulon officinale* (family Liliaceae), a plant of the shores of the Gulf of Mexico and Caribbean Sea; it yields cevadine, veratridine, and several other alkaloids; has been used externally as a parasiticide. SYN cevadilla. [Sp. *cevadilla*, ult. fr. L. *cibus*, food]

Sabin, Albert B., Polish-U.S. virologist, 1906–1993. SEE S. *vaccine*; S.-Feldman dye *test*.

Sabin-Feldman dye test. See under test.

Sabouraud, Raymond J.A., French dermatologist, 1864–1938. SEE S.'s *agar, pastils*, under *pastil*; S.-Noiré *instrument*.

sab·u·lous (sab′yū-lŭs). Sandy; gritty. [L. *sabulosus*, fr. *sabulum*, coarse sand]

sa·bur·ra (să-bŭr′ă). **1.** Foulness of the stomach or mouth resulting from decomposed food. **2.** SYN sordes. [L. sand]

sa·bur·ral (să-bŭr′ăl). Relating to saburra (1).

sac (sak). **1.** A pouch or bursa. SEE sacculus. **2.** An encysted abscess at the root of a tooth. **3.** The capsule of a tumor, or envelope of a cyst. SYN saccus [NA]. [L. *saccus*, a bag]

abdominal s., the part of the embryonic celom that becomes the abdominal cavity.

air s., SYN alveolar s.

allantoic s., the dilated distal portion of the allantois; it forms part of the placenta in many mammals.

alveolar s., (1) terminal dilation of the alveolar ducts that give rise to alveoli in the lung; a small air chamber in the pulmonary tissue from which the pulmonary alveoli project like bays and into which an alveolar duct opens; **(2)** in birds, air-containing extensions of bronchi that connect with bone cavities. SYN sacculus alveolaris [NA], air s.

amniotic s., SYN amnion.

anal s., a vesicular cutaneous invagination opening by a duct on each side of the anal canal in carnivores (best developed in skunks, but absent in some bears, the raccoon, kinkajou, coati, and sea otter), each lying between the external and internal anal sphincter muscles, which aid in emptying the contents. The s. stores odoriferous scent markers produced by glands that line its wall or duct; frequently the s. becomes impacted in the dog or cat, requiring manual emptying.

aneurysmal s., the dilated wall of an artery in a saccular aneurysm.

aortic s., in mammalian embryos, the endothelially lined dilation just distal to the truncus arteriosus; it is the primordial vascular channel from which the aortic arches arise and is homologous to the ventral aorta of gill-bearing vertebrates.

chorionic s., SYN chorion.

conjunctival s., the space bound by the conjunctival membrane between the palpebral and bulbar conjunctiva; into which the lacrimal fluid is secreted; it opens anteriorly between the eyelids. SYN saccus conjunctivae [NA].

cupular blind s., SYN cupular *cecum* of the cochlear duct.

dental s., the outer connective tissue envelope surrounding a developing tooth; also applied to the mesenchymal concentration that is the primordium of the s. SEE ALSO dental *follicle*.

endolymphatic s., the dilated blind extremity of the endolymphatic duct. SYN saccus endolymphaticus [NA], Böttcher's space, Cotunnius' space, sacculus endolymphaticus.

heart s., SYN pericardium.

hernial s., the peritoneal envelope of a hernia.

Hilton's s., SYN *saccule* of larynx.

lacrimal s., the upper portion of the nasolacrimal duct into which empty the two lacrimal canaliculi; empty. SYN saccus lacrimalis [NA], dacryocyst, sacculus lacrimalis, tear s.

lesser peritoneal s., SYN omental *bursa*.

lymph s.'s, the earliest lymphatic vessels formed in the embryo.

nasal s.'s, the deepened nasal pits that develop into the definitive nasal cavities.

omental s., SYN omental *bursa*.

preputial s., the space between the prepuce and the glans penis.

pudendal s., a pear-shaped encapsulated collection of connective tissue and fat in each labium majus. SYN Broca's pouch.

tear s., SYN lacrimal s.

tooth s., a capsule that encloses the developing tooth.

vestibular blind s., SYN vestibular *cecum* of the cochlear duct.

vitelline s., SYN yolk s.

yolk s., (1) in vertebrates with telolecithal eggs; the highly vascular layer of splanchnopleure surrounding the yolk of an embryo; **(2)** in humans and other mammals, the s. of extraembryonic membrane that is located ventral to the embryonic disk and, after formation of the gut tube, is connected to the midgut; by the second month of development, this connection has become the narrow yolk stalk; the yolk s. is the first hematopoietic organ of the embryo, and its vitelline circulation plays an important role in the early embryonic circulation; the s. is also the site of origin of the primordial germ cells. SYN umbilical vesicle, vesicula umbilicalis, vitelline s.

sac·brood (sak′brūd). A viral disease affecting the larvae of bees.

sac·cade (să-kād′). Rapid eye movement to redirect the line of sight. [Fr. *saccade*, sudden check of a horse]

sac·cad·ic (să-kad′ik). Jerky. SEE saccadic *movement*.

sac·cate (sak′āt). Relating to a sac. [L. *saccus*, sac]

△**sacchar-.** SEE saccharo-.

sac·cha·rase (sak′ă-rās). SYN β-fructofuranosidase.

sac·cha·rate (sak′ă-rāt). A salt or ester of saccharic acid.

sac·char·eph·i·dro·sis (sak-ar-ef-i-drō′sis). The presence of sugar in the sweat. [sacchar- + G. *ephidrōsis*, a slight perspiration]

△**sacchari-.** SEE saccharo-.

sac·char·ic (să-kar′ik). Relating to sugar.

sac·char·ic ac·id (sak′ă-rik). Term used to denote the class of dicarboxy sugar acids.

sac·cha·rides (sak′ă-rīdz). S. are classified as mono-, di-, tri-, and polysaccharides according to the number of monosaccharide groups composing them. SEE carbohydrates.

sac·cha·rif·er·ous (sak′ă-rif′er-ŭs). Producing sugar.

sac·char·i·fi·ca·tion (să-kar′i-fi-kā′shŭn). The process of saccharifying.

sac·char·i·fy (să-kar'i-fī). To convert starch or cellulose or other polysaccharides into sugar. [sacchari- + L. *facio,* to make]

sac·cha·rim·e·ter (sak-ă-rim'ĕ-ter). An instrument for determining the amount of sugar in a solution; it may be a polarimeter, a hygrometer, or a container in which the solution is fermented and the amount estimated by the volume of CO_2 produced. SYN saccharometer. [(sacchari- + G. *metron,* measure]

sac·cha·rin (sak'ă-rin). *o*-sulfobenzimide; 2,3-dihydro-3-oxobenzisosulfonazole; in dilute aqueous solution it is 300 to 500 times sweeter than sucrose; used as a sweetening agent (sugar substitute); s. sodium and s. calcium have the same use. SYN benzosulfimide.

sac·cha·rine (sak'ă-rēn, -rin, -rīn). Relating to sugar; sweet.

⌂**saccharo-, sacchar-, sacchari-.** Combining forms denoting sugar (saccharide). [G. *sakcharon,* sugar]

sac·cha·ro·gen am·y·lase (sak'ă-rō-jen). SYN β-amylase.

sac·cha·ro·lyt·ic (sak'ă-rō-lit'ik). Capable of hydrolyzing or otherwise breaking down a sugar molecule. [saccharo- + G. *lysis,* loosening]

sac·cha·ro·met·a·bol·ic (sak'ă-rō-met'ă-bol'ik). Relating to saccharometabolism.

sac·cha·ro·me·tab·o·lism (sak-ă-rō-mĕ-tab'ō-lizm). Metabolism of sugar; the process of utilization of sugar in cells.

sac·cha·rom·e·ter (sak-ă-rom'ĕ-ter). SYN saccharimeter.

Sac·cha·ro·my·ces (sak'ă-rō-mī'sēz). A genus of budding yeasts (family Saccharomycetaceae); an ascomycete. *S. cerevisiae* is used to produce brewer's yeast and ethanol. *S. cerevisiae* has been reported to cause paronychia in diabetics and immunocompromised patients. [saccharo- + G. *mykēs,* fungus]

Sac·cha·ro·my·ce·ta·ce·ae (sak'ă-rō-mī-sē-tā'sē-ē). The family of yeasts; that group of fungi comprising the ascomycetes which possess a predominantly unicellular thallus, reproduce asexually by budding, transverse division, or both, and produce ascospores in an ascus, originating from a zygote or pathogenetically from a single somatic cell. The term yeastlike fungus is often applied to fungi that are not known to form ascospores, but otherwise possess the characteristics of yeasts; such forms are properly placed with the Fungi Imperfecti unless methods of sexual reproduction are known; *e.g., Cryptococcus neoformans.*

Sac·cha·ro·my·ce·ta·les (sak'ă-rō-mī'sē-tā'lēz). SYN Endomycetales.

sac·cha·ro·pine (sak-ar'ō-pēn). $HOOC(CH_2)_2CH(COOH)NH(CH_2)_4CH(NH_2)COOH$; a derivative of α-ketoglutarate and L-lysine that is an intermediate in L-lysine catabolism; elevated in cases of saccharopinuria.

s. dehydrogenase, two enzymes that are used in the pathway of L-lysine catabolism; the first isoform catalyzes the reversible conversion of L-lysine, α-ketoglutarate, and NADH to s. and NAD^+; the other isoform reversibly catalyzes to conversion of s. and NAD^+ to L-glutamate, NADH, and L-α-aminoadipate δ-semialdehyde. A deficiency of one of these isoforms is associated with familial hyperlysinemia and saccharopinuria.

sac·cha·ro·pi·nu·ria (sak-ar'ō-pēn-ūr-ē-ă). Elevated levels of saccharopine in the urine; associated with a variant of familial hyperlysinuria.

sac·cha·ror·rhea (sak'ă-rō-rē'ă). Obsolete term for glycosuria. [saccharo- + G. *rhoia,* a flow]

sac·cha·rose (sak'ă-rōs). SYN sucrose.

sac·cha·ro·su·ria (sak'ă-rō-sū'rē-ă). Obsolete term denoting the excretion of saccharose in the urine. [saccharose + G. *ouron,* urine]

sac·cha·rum (sak'ă-rŭm). SYN sucrose. [Mod. L. fr. G. *sakcharon*]

s. canaden'se, SYN maple *sugar.*

s. lac'tis, SYN lactose.

sac·ci·form (sak'si-fŏrm). Pouched; sac-shaped. SYN saccular, sacculated. [L. *saccus,* sack, + *forma,* form]

sac·cu·lar (sak'yū-lăr). SYN sacciform.

sac·cu·lat·ed (sak'yū-lā'ted). SYN sacciform.

sac·cu·la·tion (sak'yū-lā'shŭn). **1.** A structure formed by a group of sacs. **2.** The formation of a sac or pouch.

s.'s of colon, SYN *haustra* of colon, under *haustrum.*

sac·cule (sak'yūl). SYN sacculus. [L. *sacculus*]

s. of larynx, a small diverticulum provided with mucous glands extending upward from the ventricle of the larynx between the vestibular fold and the lamina of the thyroid cartilage; it is a vestigial structure, being a much larger structure interdigitating with the neck musculature in some of the great apes where it serves as a resonating chamber. SYN sacculus laryngis [NA], appendix ventriculi laryngis, Hilton's sac, laryngeal pouch.

sac·cu·lo·co·chle·ar (sak'yū-lō-kok'lē-ăr). Relating to the sacculus and the membranous cochlea.

sac·cu·lus, pl. **sac·cu·li** (sak'yū-lŭs, -lī). **1** [NA]. The smaller of the two membranous sacs in the vestibule of the labyrinth, lying in the spherical recess; it is connected with the cochlear duct by a very short tube, the ductus reuniens, and with the utriculus by the beginning of the ductus endolymphaticus and the ductus utriculosaccularis that joins it. **2.** The immense bag-shaped structure formed by peptidoglycans as part of the cell wall of certain microorganisms. SYN saccule, s. proprius, s. vestibuli. [L. dim. of *saccus,* sac]

s. alveola'ris, pl. **sacculi alveola'res** [NA], SYN alveolar *sac.*

s. commu'nis, SYN utricle.

s. endolymphat'icus, SYN endolymphatic *sac.*

s. lacrima'lis, SYN lacrimal *sac.*

s. laryn'gis [NA], SYN *saccule* of larynx.

s. pro'prius, SYN sacculus.

s. vestib'uli, SYN sacculus.

sac·cus, pl. **sac·ci** (sak'ŭs, sak'sī) [NA]. SYN sac. [L. a bag, sack]

s. conjuncti'vae [NA], SYN conjunctival *sac.*

s. endolymphat'icus [NA], SYN endolymphatic *sac.*

s. lacrima'lis [NA], SYN lacrimal *sac.*

s. reu'niens, SYN *sinus* venosus.

s. vagina'lis, an embryonic peritoneal fossa indicating the site where the processus vaginalis peritonei extends through the anterior abdominal wall during descent of the testis.

Sachs, Bernard, U.S. neurologist, 1858–1944. SEE Tay-S. *disease.*

Sachs, Hans, German bacteriologist, 1877–1945. SEE S.-Georgi *test.*

Sachs, M. SEE S.'s *bacillus;* Ghon-S. *bacillus.*

Sachs, Maurice D., U.S. radiologist, *1909. SEE Hill-S. *lesion.*

Sacks, Benjamin, U.S. physician, 1896–1939. SEE Libman-S. *endocarditis, syndrome.*

⌂**sacr-.** SEE sacro-.

sa·crad (sā'krad). In the direction of the sacrum. [sacr- + L. *ad,* to]

sa·cral (sā'krăl). Relating to or in the neighborhood of the sacrum.

sa·cral·gia (sā-kral'jē-ă). Pain in the sacral region. SYN sacrodynia. [sacr- + G. *algos,* pain]

sa·cral·i·za·tion (sā'kral-i-zā'shŭn). Lumbar development of the first sacral vertebra.

sa·crec·to·my (sā-krek'tō-mē). Resection of a portion of the sacrum to facilitate an operation. SYN sacrotomy. [sacr- + G. *ektomē,* excision]

⌂**sacro-, sacr-.** Muscular substance; resemblance to flesh. [L. *os sacrum,* sacred bone]

sa·cro·coc·cyg·e·al (sā-krō-kok-sij'ē-ăl). Relating to both sacrum and coccyx.

sa·cro·coc·cyg·e·us (sā'krō-kok-si-jē'ŭs). SEE muscle.

sa·cro·dyn·ia (sā'krō-din'ē-ă). SYN sacralgia. [sacro- + G. *odynē,* pain]

sa·cro·il·i·ac (sā-krō-il'ē-ak). Relating to the sacrum and the ilium.

sa·cro·il·i·i·tis (sā'krō-il-ē-ī'tis). Inflammation of the sacroiliac joint.

sa·cro·lis·the·sis (sā'krō-lis'thē-sis). SYN spondylolisthesis. [sacro- + G. *olisthēsis,* a slipping and falling]

sa

sa·cro·lum·ba·lis (sā′krō-lŭm-bā′lis). The iliocostalis lumborum muscle.

sa·cro·lum·bar (sā′krō-lŭm′băr). SYN lumbosacral.

sa·cro·sci·at·ic (sā′krō-sī-at′ik). Relating to both sacrum and ischium.

sa·cro·spi·nal (sā′krō-spī′năl). Relating to the sacrum and the vertebral column above.

sa·crot·o·my (sā-krot′ō-mē). SYN sacrectomy. [sacro- + G. tomē, incision]

sa·cro·ver·te·bral (sā′krō-ver′tē-brăl). Relating to the sacrum and the vertebrae above.

sa·crum, pl. **sa·cra** (sā′krŭm, sā′kră) [NA]. The segment of the vertebral column forming part of the pelvis; a broad, slightly curved, spade-shaped bone, thick above, thinner below, closing in the pelvic girdle posteriorly; it is formed by the fusion of five originally separate sacral vertebrae; it articulates with the last lumbar vertebra, the coccyx, and the hip bone on either side. SYN os sacrum [NA], sacred bone, vertebra magna. [L. (lit. sacred bone), neuter of sacer (sacr-), sacred]

assimilation s., one which is composed of six segments, the last lumbar vertebra assuming the appearance of a sacral segment; or one which is composed of but four segments, the first sacral being free and having the characteristics of a lumbar vertebra.

SACT Abbreviation for sinoatrial conduction time.

SAD (sea·son·al af·fec·tive dis·or·der) Abbreviation for seasonal affective disorder.

sad·dle (sad′l). 1. A structure shaped like, or suggestive of, a seat or s. used in riding horseback. SYN sella. 2. SYN denture base.

Turkish s., SYN sella turcica.

sa·dism (sā′dizm, sad′izm). A form of perversion, often sexual in nature, in which a person finds pleasure in inflicting abuse and maltreatment. Cf. masochism. [Marquis de Sade, 1740–1814, confessedly addicted to the practice]

sa·dist (sā′dist, sad′ist). One who practices sadism.

sa·dis·tic (să-dis′tik). Pertaining to or characterized by sadism.

sa·do·mas·och·ism (sā-dō-mas′ō-kizm, sad-o-). A form of perversion marked by enjoyment of cruelty and/or humiliation in its received or active and/or dispensed and passive form. [sadism + masochism]

Saemisch, Edwin T., German ophthalmologist, 1833-1909. SEE S.'s section, ulcer.

Saenger, Alfred, German neurologist, 1860–1921. SEE S.'s sign.

Saenger, M., Prague obstetrician, 1853–1903. SEE S.'s macula, operation.

saf·flow·er (saf′low-er). SYN carthamus. [Ar. safrā, yellow]

saf·flow·er oil. An oil extracted from the seeds of Carthamus tinctorius, containing 74.5% linoleic acid and 6.6% saturated fatty acids; used in hypercholesteremia, myocardial infarction, and coronary insufficiency.

saf·fron (saf′ron). SYN crocus. [Ar. zafarān, fr. safrā, yellow]

saf·ra·nin O (saf′ră-nin) [C.I. 50240]. A mixture of dimethyl- and trimethylphenosafranin chloride, a basic red dye that exhibits orange metachromasia; used in histology as a nuclear stain, in microbiology as a counterstain in the Gram method, and to demonstrate enterochromaffin.

saf·ra·no·phil, saf·ra·no·phile (saf′ră-nō-fil, -fīl). Staining readily with safranin; denoting certain cells and tissues.

saf·role (saf′rōl). $C_{10}H_{10}O_2$; the methylene ether of allyl pyrocatechol; contained in oil of sassafras, oil of camphor, and various other volatile oils; it is obtained chiefly from oil of camphor by fractional distillation; used as a tonic and carminative; prolonged administration causes fatty degeneration.

sage (sāj). SYN salvia. [L. salvia, the sage plant, fr. salvus, safe]

sa·git·ta (saj′i-tă). SYN statoliths.

sag·it·tal (saj′i-tăl). Resembling an arrow; in the line of an arrow shot from a bow, i.e., in an anteroposterior direction. referring to a sagittal plane or direction. SYN sagittalis [NA]. [L. sagitta, an arrow]

sa·git·ta·lis (saj-i-tā′lis) [NA]. SYN sagittal. [L.]

Saint, Charles F.M., African surgeon, *1886. SEE S.'s triad.

Saint Anthony's fire (sānt anth-ō-nēz). 1. SYN ergotism. 2. Any of several inflammations or gangrenous conditions of the skin (e.g., erysipelas). [St. Anthony, Egyptian monk, about 250–350 A.D.]

Sakaguchi re·ac·tion. See under reaction.

Sakurai. Japanese ophthalmologist SEE Sakurai-Lisch nodule.

sal, pl. **sales** (sal, sal′ēz). SYN salt. [L.]

s. alem′broth, the product obtained by crystallization from a solution of equal parts of ammonium chloride and mercuric chloride. SYN salt of wisdom. [an alchemist's term of unknown origin]

s. ammo′niac, SYN ammonium chloride.

s. diuret′icum, SYN potassium acetate.

s. soda, SYN sodium carbonate.

s. vol′atile, SYN aromatic ammonia spirit.

Salah, M., 20th century Egyptian surgeon. SEE S.'s sternal puncture needle.

sal·bu·ta·mol (sal-byū′tă-mol). SYN albuterol.

sal·i·cin (sal′i-sin). Saligenin-β-D-glucopyranoside; a glucoside of o-hydroxybenzylalcohol, obtained from the bark of several species of Salix (willow) and Populus (poplar); s. is hydrolyzed to glucose and saligenin (salicyl alcohol); formerly used in rheumatoid arthritis.

sal·i·cyl (sal′i-sil). The acyl radical of salicylic acid.

s. aldehyde, o-hydroxybenzaldehyde; obtained from Spirea ulmaria (meadow sweet), and made synthetically; used as a diuretic and antiseptic, and in perfumery. SYN salicylic aldehyde.

sal·i·cyl·am·ide (sal-i-sil′ă-mīd). The amide of salicylic acid, o-hydroxybenzamide; an analgesic, antipyretic and antiarthritic, similar in action to aspirin.

sal·i·cyl·an·i·lide (sal′i-sil-an′i-līd). N-Phenylsalicylamide; an antifungal agent especially useful in the treatment of tinea capitis caused by Microsporum audouinii.

sa·lic·y·late (să-lis′i-lāt). 1. A salt or ester of salicylic acid. 2. To treat foodstuffs with salicylic acid as a preservative. SYN salicylize.

sa·lic·y·lat·ed (să-lis′i-lāt-ĕd). Treated by the addition of salicylic acid as a preservative.

sal·i·cyl·az·o·sul·fa·pyr·i·dine (sal′i-sil-az′ō-sūl-fă-pir′i-dēn). SYN sulfasalazine.

sal·i·cyl·ic ac·id (sal-i-sil′ik). o-Hydroxybenzoic acid; a component of aspirin, derived from salicin and made synthetically; used externally as a keratolytic agent, antiseptic, and fungicide.

sal·i·cyl·ic al·de·hyde (sal-i-sil′ik). SYN salicyl aldehyde.

sal·i·cyl·ism (sal′i-sil-izm). Poisoning by salicylic acid or any of its compounds.

sal·i·cyl·ize (sal′i-sil-īz). SYN salicylate (2).

sal·i·cyl·sal·i·cyl·ic ac·id (sal′i-sil-sal-i-sil′ik). SYN salsalate.

sal·i·cyl·sul·fon·ic ac·id (sal′i-sil-sŭl-fon′ik). SYN sulfosalicylic acid.

sal·i·cyl·u·ric ac·id (sal′i-sil-yūr′ik). The conjugation product of glycine with salicylic acid; excreted in urine after the administration of salicylic acid or some of its compounds.

sa·lient (sā′lē-ent, sāl′yent). 1. SYN projection. 2. In radiology, an obsolete term for projection. [L. salio, to leap or spring up]

pulmonary s., the middle of the three normal convexities along the left cardiac border on a chest radiograph. It is caused by the prominence of the main pulmonary artery.

sal·i·fi·a·ble (sal-i-fī′ă-bl). Capable of being made into salts; said of a base that combines with acids to make salts.

sal·i·fy (sal′i-fī). To convert into a salt.

sal·i·gen·in, sal·i·gen·ol (sal-i-jen′in, sal′i-jen-ol). obtained by the hydrolysis of salicin; a local anesthetic.

sa·lim·e·ter (să-lim′ĕ-ter). A hydrometer used to determine the specific gravity, or the concentration, of a saline solution.

sa·line (sā′lēn, -līn). 1. Relating to, of the nature of, or containing salt; salty. 2. A salt solution, usually sodium chloride. [L. salinus, salty, fr. sal, salt]

physiological s., an isotonic aqueous solution of salts, containing 0.9% sodium chloride.

sa·li·nom·e·ter (sal-i-nom′ĕ-ter). A hydrometer so calibrated as to give a direct reading of the percentage of a particular salt present in solution.

sa·li·va (să-lī′vă). A clear, tasteless, odorless, slightly acid (pH 6.8) viscid fluid, consisting of the secretion from the parotid, sublingual, and submandibular salivary glands and the mucous glands of the oral cavity; its function is to keep the mucous membrane of the mouth moist, to lubricate the food during mastication, and, in a measure, to convert starch into maltose, the latter action being effected by a diastatic enzyme, ptyalin. SYN spittle. [L. akin to G. *sialon*]

chorda s., the secretion of the submaxillary gland obtained by stimulation of the chorda tympani nerve.

ganglionic s., submaxillary s. obtained by direct irritation of the gland.

resting s., the s. found in the mouth in the intervals of food taking and mastication.

sympathetic s., submaxillary s. obtained by stimulation of the sympathetic fibers innervating the gland.

sal·i·vant (sal′i-vant). **1.** Causing a flow of saliva. **2.** An agent that increases the flow of saliva. SYN salivator.

sal·i·vary (sal′i-vār-ē). Relating to saliva. SYN sialic, sialine. [L. *salivarius*]

sal·i·vate (sal′i-vāt). To cause an excessive flow of saliva.

sal·i·va·tion (sal′i-vā′shŭn). SYN sialism.

sal·i·va·tor (sal′i-vā-ter). SYN salivant (2).

sa·li·vo·li·thi·a·sis (sa-lī′vō-li-thī′ă-sis). SYN sialolithiasis.

Salk, Jonas, U.S. immunologist, *1914. SEE S. vaccine.

Sal·mo·nel·la (sal′mō-nel′ă). A genus of aerobic to facultatively anaerobic bacteria (family Enterobacteriaceae) containing Gram-negative rods that are either motile or nonmotile; motile cells are peritrichous. These organisms do not liquefy gelatin or produce indole and vary in their production of hydrogen sulfide; they utilize citrate as a sole source of carbon; their metabolism is fermentative, producing acid and usually gas from glucose, but they do not attack lactose; most are aerogenic, but *S. typhi* never produces gas; they are pathogenic for humans and other animals. The type species is *S. choleraesuis*. [Daniel E. *Salmon*, U.S. pathologist, 1850–1914]

S. choleraesuis, a species that occurs in pigs, where it is an important secondary invader in the virus disease hog cholera, but does not occur as a natural pathogen in other animals; occasionally causes acute gastroenteritis and enteric fever in humans; it is the type species of the genus *S.*

S. enterit′idis, a widely distributed species that occurs in humans and in domestic and wild animals, especially rodents. SYN Gärtner's bacillus.

S. paratyphi A, an etiologic agent of enteric fever.

S. schottmül′leri, a species causing enteric fever in man; found rarely in cattle, sheep, swine, chickens, and lower primates. SYN Schottmueller's bacillus.

S. ty′phi, a species that causes typhoid fever in humans and is transmitted in contaminated water and food. SYN Eberth's bacillus, typhoid bacillus.

S. typhimu′rium, a species causing food poisoning in humans; it is a natural pathogen of all warm-blooded animals and is also found in snakes.

S. typho′sa, former name for *S. typhi.*

sal·mo·nel·lo·sis (sal′mō-nel-ō′sis). Infection with bacteria of the genus *Salmonella*. Patients with sickle cell anemia and compromised immune systems are particularly susceptible. [*Salmonella* + G. *-osis*, condition]

sal·ol (sal′ol). SYN *phenyl salicylate.*

△**salping-.** SEE salpingo-.

sal·pin·gec·to·my (sal-pin-jek′tō-me). Removal of the fallopian tube. SYN tubectomy. [salping- + G. *ektomē*, excision]

abdominal s., removal of one or both fallopian tubes through an abdominal incision. SYN celiosalpingectomy, laparosalpingectomy.

sal·pin·gem·phrax·is (sal′pin-jem-frak′sis). Obstruction of the

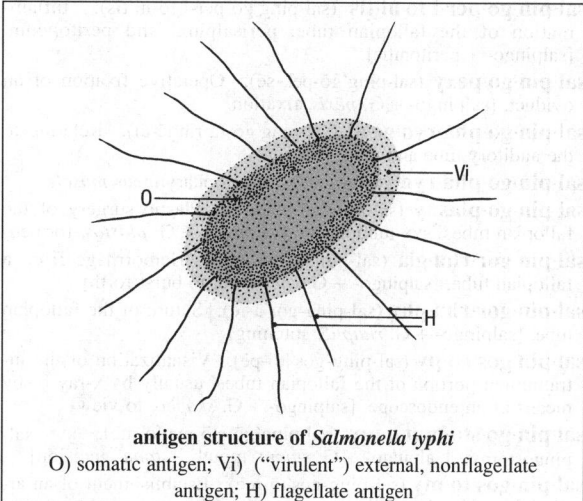

antigen structure of *Salmonella typhi*
O) somatic antigen; Vi) ("virulent") external, nonflagellate antigen; H) flagellate antigen

eustachian or the fallopian tube. [salping- + G. *emphraxis,* a stopping]

sal·pin·ges (sal-pin′jēz). Plural of salpinx.

sal·pin·gi·an (sal-pin′jē-ăn). Relating to the fallopian tube or to the auditory tube.

sal·pin·gi·o·ma (sal-pin-jē-ō′mă). Any tumor arising in the tissues of a fallopian tube. [salping- + G. *-oma,* tumor]

sal·pin·git·ic (sal-pin-jit′ik). Relating to salpingitis.

sal·pin·gi·tis (sal-pin-jī′tis). Inflammation of the fallopian or the eustachian tube. [salping- + G. *-itis,* inflammation]

chronic interstitial s., s. in which fibrosis or mononuclear cell infiltration involves all layers of the fallopian or eustachian tube. SYN pachysalpingitis.

foreign body s., s. in which giant cells form in the tissue, as a result of introduction of foreign material into the fallopian tube.

gonorrheal s., inflammation of the fallopian tube following acute gonorrheal infection.

s. isth′mica nodo′sa, a condition of the fallopian tube characterized by nodular thickening of the tunica muscularis of the isthmic portion of the tube enclosing gland-like or cystic duplications of the lumen. SYN adenosalpingitis.

pyogenic s., a form of acute s. usually occurring with puerperal infection.

△**salpingo-, salping-.** A tube (usually the fallopian or eustachian tubes). SEE ALSO tubo-. Cf. tubo-. [G. *salpinx,* trumpet (tube)]

sal·pin·go·cele (sal-ping′gō-sēl). Hernia of a fallopian tube. [salpingo- + G. *kēlē,* hernia]

sal·pin·go·cy·e·sis (sal-ping′gō-sī-ē′sis). SYN tubal *pregnancy.* [salpingo- + G. *kyēsis,* pregnancy]

sal·pin·gog·ra·phy (sal-ping-gog′ră-fē). Radiography of the fallopian tubes after the injection of radiopaque contrast medium. [salpingo- + G. *graphō,* to write]

sal·pin·gol·y·sis (sal-ping-gol′i-sis). Freeing the fallopian tube from adhesions. [salpingo- + G. *lysis,* loosening]

△**salpingo-oophor-, salpingo-oophoro-.** The fallopian tube and ovary. [salpingo- + Mod. L. *oophoron,* ovary, fr. G. *ōophoros,* egg-bearing]

sal·pin·go·o·o·pho·rec·to·my (sal-ping′gō-ō-of-ō-rek′tō-mē). Removal of the ovary and its fallopian tube. SYN salpingo-ovariectomy, tubo-ovariectomy.

abdominal s.-o., SYN laparosalpingo-oophorectomy.

sal·pin·go·o·o·pho·ri·tis (sal-ping′gō-ō-of-ō-rī′tis). Inflammation of both fallopian tube and ovary. SYN tubo-ovaritis.

sal·pin·go·o·oph·o·ro·cele (sal-ping′gō-ō-of′ō-rō-sēl). Hernia of both ovary and fallopian tube.

sal·pin·go·o·var·i·ec·to·my (sal-ping′gō-ō-var-ē-ek′tō-mē). SYN salpingo-oophorectomy.

sa

sal·pin·go·per·i·to·ni·tis (sal-ping'gō-per-i-tō-nī'tis). Inflammation of the fallopian tube, perisalpinx, and peritoneum. [salpingo- + peritonitis]

sal·pin·go·pexy (sal-ping'gō-pek-sē). Operative fixation of an oviduct. [salpingo- + G. *pēxis*, fixation]

sal·pin·go·pha·ryn·ge·al (sal-ping'gō-fă-rin'jē-ăl). Relating to the auditory tube and pharynx.

sal·pin·go·pha·ryn·ge·us. SEE salpingopharyngeus *muscle*.

sal·pin·go·plas·ty (sal-ping'gō-plas-tē). Plastic surgery of the fallopian tubes. SYN tuboplasty. [salpingo- + G. *plastos*, formed]

sal·pin·gor·rha·gia (sal-ping-gō-rā'jē-ă). Hemorrhage from a fallopian tube. [salpingo- + G. *rhēgnymi*, to burst forth]

sal·pin·gor·rha·phy (sal-ping-gōr'ă-fē). Suture of the fallopian tube. [salpingo- + G. *rhaphē*, stitching]

sal·pin·gos·co·py (sal-ping-gos'kō-pē). Visualization of the intraluminal portion of the fallopian tubes, usually by x-ray or by means of an endoscope. [salpingo- + G. *skopeō*, to view]

sal·pin·go·sto·mat·o·my (sal-ping'gō-stō-mat'ō-mē). SYN salpingostomy. [salpingo- + G. *stoma*, mouth, + *tomē*, incision]

sal·pin·gos·to·my (sal-ping-gos'tō-mē). Establishment of an artificial opening in a fallopian tube primarily as surgical treatment for an ectopic pregnancy. SYN salpingostomatomy. [salpingo- + G. *stoma*, mouth]

sal·pin·got·o·my (sal-ping-got'ō-mē). Incision into a fallopian tube. [salpingo- + G. *tomē*, incision]

  abdominal s., incision into the fallopian tube through an opening in the abdominal wall. SYN celiosalpingotomy, laparosalpingotomy.

sal·pinx, pl. **sal·pin·ges** (sal'pingks, sal-pin'jēz). **1** [NA]. ☆official alternate term for uterine *tube*. **2.** SYN auditory *tube*. [G. a trumpet (tube)]

  s. uteri′na [NA], SYN uterine *tube*.

sal·sa·late (sal'să-lāt). A combination of 2 molecules of salicylic acid in ester linkage. The compound is hydrolyzed during and after absorption to salicylic acid which, like other salicylates, exerts analgesic and anti-inflammatory effects. SYN salicylsalicylic acid.

salt. 1. A compound formed by the interaction of an acid and a base, the ionizable hydrogen atoms of the acid being replaced by the positive ion of the base. **2.** Sodium chloride, the prototypical s. **3.** A saline cathartic, especially magnesium sulfate, sodium sulfate, or Rochelle s.; often denoted by the plural, salts. SYN sal. [L. *sal*]

  acid s., a s. in which not all of the ionizable hydrogen of the acid is replaced by the electropositive element; *e.g.,* $NaHSO_4$, KH_2PO_4. SYN bisalt, protosalt.

  artificial Carlsbad s., a mixture of potassium sulfate, sodium chloride, sodium bicarbonate, and dried sodium sulfate; a laxative.

  artificial Kissingen s., a mixture of potassium chloride, sodium chloride, anhydrous magnesium sulfate, and sodium bicarbonate; an antacid and laxative.

  artificial Vichy s., a mixture of sodium bicarbonate, anhydrous magnesium sulfate, potassium carbonate, and sodium chloride; an antacid.

  basic s., a s. in which there are one or more hydroxyl ions not replaced by the electronegative element of an acid; *e.g.,* Fe-$(OH)_2Cl$.

  bile s.'s, the s. forms of bile acids; *e.g.,* taurocholate, glycocholate.

  bone s., SEE bone-salt.

  common s., SYN *sodium* chloride.

  diazonium s.'s, s.'s of a theoretical base R–N̄⁺≡N or R–N=NOH useful in histochemistry to demonstrate tissue phenols and aryl amines or with enzymatically released naphthols and naphthylamines to form the chromophore azo group –N=N–; diazonium s.'s contain only one R–N≡N group, tetrazonium s.'s contain two, and hexazonium s.'s contain three; examples include fast garnet GBC base and naphthol AS.

  double s., a s. in which two different positive ions are bonded to the same negative ion, or vice versa; *e.g.,* $NaKSO_4$.

  effervescent s.'s, preparations made by adding sodium bicarbonate and tartaric and citric acids to the active s.; when thrown into water the acids break up the sodium bicarbonate, setting free the carbonic acid gas.

  Epsom s.'s, SYN *magnesium* sulfate.

  Glauber's s., SYN *sodium* sulfate.

  hexazonium s.'s, diazonium s.'s that contain three azo groups.

  Reinecke s., an ammonium salt prepared by fusing ammonium thiocyanate with ammonium dichromate; dark red crystals; used in the detection and analysis of primary and secondary amines, including amino acids; also used as a reagent for mercury.

  Rivière's s., SYN *potassium* citrate.

  Rochelle s., SYN *potassium* sodium tartrate.

  Seignette's s., SYN *potassium* sodium tartrate.

  smelling s.'s, SYN aromatic ammonia *spirit*.

  table s., SYN *sodium* chloride.

  tetrazonium s.'s, diazonium s.'s that contain three azo groups.

  s. of wisdom, SYN *sal* alembroth.

sal·ta·tion (sal-tā'shŭn). A dancing or leaping, as in a disease (*e.g.,* chorea) or physiologic function (*e.g.,* saltatory conduction). [L. *saltatio,* fr. *salto,* pp. *-atus,* to dance, fr. *salio,* to leap]

sal·ta·to·ry (sal'tă-tōr-ē). Pertaining to, or characterized by, saltation.

Salter, Robert, 20th century Canadian orthopedist. SEE S.-Harris *classification* of epiphysial plate injuries.

Salter, Sir Samuel J.A., English dentist, 1825–1897. SEE S.'s incremental *lines,* under *line*.

salt·ing in (solt'ing). The increase in solubility (as observed for some proteins) by dilute salt solutions (as compared to pure water).

salt·ing out. The precipitation of a protein from its solution by saturation or partial saturation with such neutral salts as sodium chloride, magnesium sulfate, or ammonium sulfate.

salt·pe·ter (salt'pē-ter). SYN *potassium* nitrate.

  Chilean s., SYN *sodium* nitrate.

salt sub·sti·tute. A low-sodium food additive that tastes like salt, such as potassium chloride; useful as a dietary alternative to salt.

sa·lu·bri·ous (să-lū'brē-ŭs). Healthful, usually in reference to climate. [L. *salubris,* healthy, fr. *salus,* health]

sal·u·re·sis (sal-yū-rē'sis). Excretion of sodium in the urine. [L. *sal,* salt, + G. *ourēsis,* uresis (urination)]

sal·u·ret·ic (sal-yū-ret'ik). Facilitating the renal excretion of sodium.

Salus, Robert, Bohemian ophthalmologist, *1877.

sal·u·ta·ri·um (sal-yū-tār'ē-ŭm). SYN sanitarium. [L. *salutaris,* healthful, fr. *salus* (*salut*-), health]

sal·u·tary (sal'yū-tār-ē). Healthful; wholesome. [L. salutaris]

Sal·var·san (sal'var-san). Historic proprietary name for arsphenamine. [L. *salvare,* to preserve, + *sanitas,* health]

salve (sav). SYN ointment. [A.S. *sealf*]

sal·via (sal'vē-ă). The dried leaves of *Salvia officinalis* (family Labiatae), garden or meadow sage; it inhibits secretory activity, especially of the sweat glands, and was also used in bronchitis and inflammation of the throat. SYN sage. [L.]

Salzmann, Maximilian, German ophthalmologist, 1862–1954. SEE S.'s nodular corneal *degeneration*.

SAM Abbreviation for *S*-adenosyl-L-methionine.

sam·an·da·rine (sa-măn'da-rēn). A toxic alkaloid from salamanders; causes hemolysis.

sa·mar·i·um (Sm) (să-mār'ē-ŭm). A metallic element of the lanthanide group, atomic no. 62, atomic wt. 150.36. [bands indicating its presence first found in the spectrum of *samarskite,* a mineral named after Col. von Samarski, 19th century Russian mine official]

sam·bu·cus (sam-byū'kŭs). The dried flowers of *Sambucus canadensis* or *S. nigra* (family Caprifoliaceae), the common elder or black elder; slightly laxative. SYN elder, elder flowers. [L. an elder-tree]

sAMP Abbreviation for adenylosuccinic acid.

sam·ple. A specimen of a whole entity small enough to involve no threat or damage to the whole; an aliquot.

cluster s., each sampling unit is a group of individuals.

end-tidal s., a s. of the last gas expired in a normal expiration, ideally consisting only of alveolar gas.

Haldane-Priestley s., an approximation of alveolar gas obtained from the end of a sudden maximal expiration into a Haldane tube.

probability s., each individual in the s. has a known, generally equal, chance of being selected.

Rahn-Otis s., an approximation of alveolar gas continuously provided by a simple device that admits just the latter part of each expiration.

random s., a selection on the basis of chance of individuals or items in a population for research; selection is made in such a way that all members presumably have the same chance of being selected.

stratified s., a subset of a total population, defined by some objective criterion such as age or occupation, is sampled.

sam·ple. A selected subset of a population; a sample may be random or nonrandom (haphazard); representative or nonrepresentative. [M.E. *ensample*, fr. L. *exemplum*, example]

sam·pling. The policy of inferring the behavior of a whole batch by studying a fraction of it. [MF *essample*, from L. *exemplum*, taking out]

biological sampling, denotes sampling that can be taken without jeopardy to the whole organism (*e.g.,* for hematological or biochemical study). Because of the complexity of biological samples it is usually supposed that the source of the sample is thoroughly mixed and hence representative; this assumption is often not true *e.g.,* in genetic studies in mosaic patients.

chemical sampling, a sample that is obtained by whatever means is convenient and then purified of irrelevant elements before analysis; the assumption of thorough mixing is not necessary.

haphazard sampling, the assembly of data in an unprescribed and undefined fashion that allows no sound scientific inferences other than establishing the existence of types. (Finding even one unicorn in such a set would establish that unicorns can exist, but no inference about their prevalence could be made from it.) Cf. random *sample*.

random sampling, a selection of elements by a formal randomizing device for purposes of inference about a population of inference from that population in such a way that the probability of each possible outcome may be precisely specified in advance; the inferences are necessarily stochastic.

snowball sampling, a method whereby interview subjects for a statistical study are obtained from subjects already interviewed for that study.

> This technique is most often used with target populations made up of elusive or uncooperative subjects (e.g., IV drug users). Those subjects first contacted are asked to name acquaintances, who are then approached, interviewed, and asked for additional names. In this way, a sufficient number of subjects can be accumulated to give a study adequate power.

Sanarelli, Giuseppe, Italian bacteriologist, 1864–1940. SEE S. *phenomenon;* S.-Shwartzman *phenomenon.*

san·a·tive (san′ă-tiv). Having a tendency to heal. [L. *sano,* to cure, heal]

san·a·to·ri·um (san′ă-tōr′ē-ŭm). An institution for the treatment of chronic disorders and a place for recuperation under medical supervision. Cf. sanitarium. [Mod. L. neuter of *sanatorius,* curative, fr. *sano,* to cure, heal]

san·a·to·ry (san′ă-tōr-ē). Health-giving; conducive to health. [Mod. L. *sanatorius*]

Sanchez Salorio, Manuel, Spanish ophthalmologist, *1930. SEE Sanchez Salorio *syndrome.*

sand. The fine granular particles of quartz and other crystalline rocks, or a gritty material resembling s. [A.S.]

brain s., SYN *corpora* arenacea, under *corpus.*

hydatid s., the scoleces of *Echinococcus* tapeworms in the fluid within a primary or daughter hydatid cyst.

intestinal s., minute calculi or gritty material occurring in feces, composed of soaps, bile pigment, cholesterol, magnesium salts, succinic acid, etc.

urinary s., multiple small calculous particles passed in the urine of patients with nephrolithiasis; each particle is usually too small to cause significant symptoms or to be identified as a true calculus.

san·dal·wood oil (san′dăl-wŭd). SYN santal oil.

sand-crack (sand′krak). A crack or fissure in the hoof of the horse, occurring usually on the inside of the forefoot (quarter-crack) or in the forepart of the hindfoot (toe-crack); when the crack is deep enough to expose the sensitive laminae, or when it extends to the coronary band, lameness results.

sand·fly (sand′flī). A small, biting, dipterous midge of the genus *Phlebotomus* or *Lutzomyia;* a vector of leishmaniasis.

Sandhoff, K., contemporary German biochemist. SEE S.'s *disease.*

Sandison, J. Calvin, U.S. surgeon, *1899. SEE S.-Clark *chamber.*

Sandström, I., Swedish anatomist, 1852–1889. SEE S.'s *bodies,* under *body.*

sand·worm (sand′werm). Any of the various dog and cat hookworms whose larvae cause cutaneous larva migrans.

sane (sān). Denoting sanity. [L. *sanus*]

Sanfilippo, Sylvester J., 20th century U.S. pediatrician. SEE S.'s *syndrome.*

Sanger, Frederick, English biochemist and twice Nobel laureate, *1918. SEE S.'s *reagent;* S. *method.*

Sanger's re·a·gent. See under reagent.

△**sangui-, sanguin-, sanguino-.** Blood, bloody. [G. *sanguis*]

san·gui·fa·ci·ent (sang-gwi-fā′shent). SYN hemopoietic. [sangui- + L. *facio,* to make]

san·guif·er·ous (sang-gwif′er-ŭs). Conveying blood. SYN circulatory (2). [sangui- + L. *fero,* to carry]

san·gui·fi·ca·tion (sang′gwi-fi-kā′shŭn). SYN hemopoiesis. [sangui- + L. *facio,* to make]

san·guin·a·rine (sang-gwi-nā′rēn). An alkaloid obtained from the bloodroot plant, *Sanguinaria canadensis,* used to treat and remove dental plaque.

san·guine (sang′gwin). **1.** SYN plethoric. **2.** Formerly, denoting a temperament characterized by a light, fair complexion, full pulse, good digestion, optimistic outlook, and a quick but not lasting temper. SYN sanguineous (3). [L. *sanguineus*]

san·guin·e·ous (sang-gwin′ē-ŭs). **1.** Relating to blood; bloody. **2.** SYN plethoric. **3.** SYN sanguine (2). [L. *sanguineus*]

san·guin·o·lent (sang-gwin′ō-lent). Bloody; tinged with blood. [L. *sanguinolentus*]

san·gui·no·pu·ru·lent (sang′gwi-nō-pū′rū-lent). Denoting exudate or matter containing blood and pus. [sanguino- + L. *purulentus,* festering (suppurative), fr. *pus,* pus]

San·gui·su·ga (sang-gwi-sū′gă). Former name for *Hirudo.* [L. a leech, fr. *sanguis,* blood, + *sugo,* pp. *suctus,* to suck]

san·guiv·or·ous (sang-gwiv′er-ŭs). Bloodsucking, as applied to certain bats, leeches, insects, etc. [sangui- + L. *voro,* to devour]

sa·ni·es (sā′nē-ēz). A thin, blood-stained, purulent discharge. [L.]

sa·ni·o·pu·ru·lent (sā′nē-ō-pū′rū-lent). Characterized by bloody pus. [L. *sanies,* thin, bloody matter, + *purulentus,* festering (suppurative), fr. *pus,* pus]

sa·ni·o·se·rous (sā′nē-ō-sēr′ŭs). Characterized by blood-tinged serum.

sa·ni·ous (sā′nē-ŭs). Relating to sanies; ichorous and blood-stained.

san·i·tar·i·an (san-i-tār′ē-ăn). One who is skilled in sanitation and public health. [L. *sanitas,* health, fr. *sanus,* sound]

san·i·tar·i·um (san-i-tār′ē-ŭm). A health resort. Cf. sanatorium. SYN salutarium. [L. *sanitas,* health]

san·i·tary (san′i-tār-ē). Healthful; conducive to health; usually in reference to a clean environment. [L. *sanitus,* health]

san·i·ta·tion (san-i-tā'shŭn). Use of measures designed to promote health and prevent disease; development and establishment of conditions in the environment favorable to health. [L. *sanitas,* health]

san·i·ti·za·tion (san'i-ti-zā'shŭn). The process of making something sanitary.

san·i·ty (san'i-tē). Soundness of mind, emotions, and behavior; of a sound degree of mental health. [L. *sanitas,* health]

San Jose. SEE Maldonado-San Jose *stain.*

Sansom, Arthur E., English physician, 1838–1907. SEE S.'s *sign.*

Sanson, Louis J., French physician, 1790–1841. SEE S.'s *images,* under *image;* Purkinje-S. *images,* under *image.*

san·tal oil (san'tăl). A volatile oil distilled from the wood of *Santalum album* (family Santalaceae), a tree of India; formerly used in subacute bronchitis and in gonorrhea. SYN sandalwood oil.

Santini's boom·ing sound. See under sound.

san·to·nin (san'tō-nin). The inner anhydride or lactone of santoninic acid, obtained from santonica, the unexpanded flower heads of *Artemisia cina* and other species of *Artemisia* (family Compositae); has been used to effect expulsion of roundworms (*Ascaris lumbricoides*); and in the treatment of urinary incontinence. [G. *santonikon,* wormwood]

Santorini, Giandomenico (Giovanni Domenico), Italian anatomist, 1681–1737. SEE S.'s *canal, cartilage,* major *caruncle,* minor *caruncle, concha, duct, fissures,* under *fissure, incisures,* under *incisure, labyrinth, muscle, tubercle, vein; concha* santorini; *incisurae* santorini, under *incisura.*

sap. The juice or tissue fluid of a living organism.

cell s., contents of vacuoles.

nuclear s., SYN karyolymph.

sa·phe·na (să-fē'nă). SEE vein. [Med. L. attributed by some as derived fr. Ar. *safin,* standing; by others, fr. G. *saphēnēs,* manifest, clearly visible]

saph·e·nec·to·my (saf-ĕ-nek'tō-mē). Excision of a saphenous vein. [saphena + G. *ektomē,* excision]

sa·phe·nous (să-fē'nŭs). Relating to or associated with a saphenous vein; denoting a number of structures in the leg. [see saphena]

⚠**sapo-, sapon-.** Soap. [L. *sapo*]

sap·o·gen·in (să-poj'ĕ-nin). The aglycon of a saponin; one of a family of steroids of the spirostan type (a 16,22:22,26-diepoxycholestane).

sap·o·na·ceous (sap-ō-nā'shŭs). Soapy; relating to or resembling soap.

sap·o·na·tus (sap-ŏ-nā'tŭs). Mixed with soap. [L.]

sa·pon·i·fi·ca·tion (să-pon'i-fi-kā'shŭn). Conversion into soap, denoting the hydrolytic action of an alkali upon fat especially, on triacylglycerols; in histochemistry, s. is used to demethylate or reverse blockage of carboxylic acid groups, thus permitting basophilia to occur. [sapo- (*sapon-*) + L. *facio,* to make]

sa·pon·i·fy (să-pon'i-fī). To perform or undergo saponification.

sap·o·nins (sap'ō-ninz). Glycosides of plant origin characterized by properties of foaming in water and of lysing cells (as in hemolysis of erythrocytes when s. are injected into the bloodstream); powerful surfactants; many have antibiotic activities.

Sappey, Marie P.C., French anatomist, 1810–1896. SEE S.'s *fibers,* under *fiber, plexus, veins,* under *vein.*

sap·phism (saf'izm). SYN lesbianism. [*Sapphō,* homosexual Greek poet, queen of the island of Lesbos]

⚠**sapr-.** SEE sapro-.

sa·pre·mia (să-prē'mē-ă). SYN septicemia. [sapr- + G. *haima,* blood]

⚠**sapro-, sapr-.** Rotten, putrid, decayed. [G. *sapros*]

sap·robe (sap'rōb). An organism that lives upon dead organic material. This term is preferable to saprophyte, since bacteria and fungi are no longer regarded as plants. [sapro- + G. *bios,* life]

sa·pro·bic (sap-rō'bik). Pertaining to a saprobe.

sap·ro·don·tia (sap-rō-don'shē-ă). SYN dental *caries.* [sapro- + G. *odous,* tooth]

sap·ro·gen (sap'rō-jen). An organism living on dead organic matter and causing the decay thereof. [sapro- + G. *-gen,* producing]

sap·ro·gen·ic, sa·prog·e·nous (sap-rō-jen'ik, să-proj'ĕ-nŭs). Causing or resulting from decay.

sa·proph·i·lous (să-prof'i-lŭs). Thriving on decaying organic matter. [sapro- + G. *philos,* fond]

sap·ro·phyte (sap'rō-fīt). An organism that grows on dead organic matter, plant or animal. SEE saprobe. SYN necroparasite. [sapro- + G. *phyton,* plant]

facultative s., an organism, usually parasitic, that occasionally may live and grow as a s.

sap·ro·phyt·ic (sap-rō-fit'ik). Relating to a saprophyte.

sap·ro·zo·ic (sap-rō-zō'ik). Living in decaying organic matter; especially denoting certain protozoa. [sapro- + G. *zōikos,* relating to animals]

sap·ro·zo·o·no·sis (sap'rō-zō-ō-nō'sis). A zoonosis the agent of which requires both a vertebrate host and a nonanimal (food, soil, plant) reservoir or developmental site for completion of its cycle. Combination terms may be used, such as saprometazoonoses for fluke infections, when metacercariae encyst on plants, or saprocyclozoonoses for tick infestations, whose agents complete part of their life cycles in soil. [sapro- + G. *zōon,* animal, + *nosos,* disease]

SAR Abbreviation for scaffold-associated *regions,* under *region.*

Sar Abbreviation for sarcosine.

sar·al·a·sin ac·e·tate (sar-al'ă-sin). An angiotensin II antagonist used in the treatment of essential hypertension.

α-sar·cin (sar'sin). A fungal toxin that acts on the large subunit of rRNA and inactivates the ribosome.

Sar·ci·na (sar'si-nă). A genus of nonmotile, strictly anaerobic bacteria (family Micrococcaceae) containing Gram-positive cocci, 1.8 to 3.0 μm in diameter, which divide in three perpendicular planes, producing regular packets of eight or more cells. The metabolism of these chemoorganotrophic organisms is fermentative. Saprophytic and facultatively parasitic species occur. The type species is *S. ventriculi.* [L. *sarcina,* a pack, bundle, fr. *sarcio,* to mend, patch]

S. max'ima, a species from the hull or outer coat of cereal grains such as wheat, oat, rice, and rye, and from horse manure and soil.

S. ventric'uli, a species found in soil, mud, the contents of a diseased human stomach, rabbit and guinea pig stomach contents, and on the surfaces of cereal seeds; it is the type species of the genus S.

sar·cine (sar'sēn). **1.** Obsolete term for hypoxanthine. **2.** A packet of cocci of the genus *Sarcina.*

⚠**sarco-.** Combining form denoting muscular substance or a resemblance to flesh. [G. *sarx* (*sark-*), flesh]

sar·co·blast (sar'kō-blast). SYN myoblast. [sarco- + G. *blastos,* germ]

sar·co·cele (sar'kō-sēl). Obsolete term for a fleshy tumor or sarcoma of the testis. [sarco- + G. *kēlē,* tumor]

Sar·co·cys·tis (sar-kō-sis'tis). A genus of protozoan parasites, related to the sporozoan genera *Eimeria, Isospora,* and *Toxoplasma,* and placed in a distinct family, Sarcocystidae, but with the above genera in the same suborder, Eimeriina, within the subclass Coccidia, class Sporozoea, and phylum Apicomplexa. Tissue stages of *S.* are usually seen as thick-walled cylindrical or (often extremely large (1 cm or more) fusiform cysts (Miescher's tubes) in reptile, bird, or mammal striated muscles. Cysts are smooth in the house mouse form or with radial spines (cytophaneres) in sheep or rabbit cysts; contents may be compartmentalized by septa. Variably-shaped spores (Rainey's corpuscles) probably are peripheral rounded cells (sporoblasts, cytomeres) that divide to form mature "spores" (bradyzoites), motile bodies when released from the cyst; sexual stages have been described in tissue cultures. These parasites are abundant but rarely of pathogenic significance. [sarco- + G. *kystis,* bladder]

S. bovihominis, SYN *S. hominis.*

S. fusifor'mis, a species found in the striated and heart muscle of cattle and water buffalo.

S. hom'inis, a species now recognized as a two-host infection, with beef serving as the intermediate host source of infective tissue cysts to humans, as the final host. Gamogony and sporogony occur in mucosal cells of the human small intestine; cattle become infected from human feces contaminated with *S. hominis* sporocysts. SYN *S. bovihominis*.

S. lindeman'ni, a species described on rare occasions from the striated and heart muscles of humans, probably as an infection due to various species, possibly from domestic dogs or other final hosts from which infective oocysts or sporocysts were passed to man via water or direct exposure; in these instances man serves as an intermediate rather than a final host.

S. miescheria'na, a common species of worldwide distribution that is found in the striated and heart muscle of pigs; it is the type species of the genus *S.*

S. suihom'inis, a form of *S.* in which man serves as the final host, with the pig serving as intermediate host, the source of infected tissues to humans. The life cycle and moderate disease induced follow the pattern of *S. hominis*, though the disease appears to be somewhat more pathogenic. Human infection is widespread, having been reported in Europe, the Mediterranean area, northern and western Africa, Indonesia, and South America.

S. tenel'la, an extremely common species of worldwide distribution that is found in the striated and heart muscle of sheep and goats.

sar·co·cys·to·sis (sar′kō-sis-tō′sis). Infection with protozoan parasites of the genus *Sarcocystis*.

sar·code (sar′kōd). A term of historical interest (1835), applied to the protoplasm of protozoa before the term protoplasm was coined. [sarco- + G. *eidos,* resemblance]

Sar·co·di·na (sar′kō-dī′nă, -dē′nă). The amebae; a subphylum of protozoa in the phylum Sarcomastigophora, possessing pseudopodia or locomotive protoplasmic flow for movement. Includes forms that possess flagella during development and forms with an internal or external test or skeleton and others lacking such a structure; asexual reproduction occurs by fission, and sexual reproduction, if present, by flagellate or ameboid gametes; most species are free-living. [Mod. L. fr. G. *sarx,* flesh]

sar·cog·lia (sar-kog′lē-ă). The accumulation of neurolemma cells at the motor endplate. [sarco- + G. *glia,* glue]

sar·coid (sar′koyd). **1.** SYN sarcoidosis. **2.** Obsolete term for a tumor resembling a sarcoma. [sarco- + G. *eidos,* resemblance]

Boeck's s., SYN sarcoidosis.

Spiegler-Fendt s., SYN benign *lymphocytoma* cutis.

sar·coid·o·sis (sar-koy-dō′sis). A systemic granulomatous disease of unknown cause, especially involving the lungs with resulting fibrosis, but also involving lymph nodes, skin, liver, spleen, eyes, phalangeal bones, and parotid glands; granulomas are composed of epithelioid and multinucleated giant cells with little or no necrosis. SYN Besnier-Boeck-Schaumann disease, Besnier-Boeck-Schaumann syndrome, Boeck's disease, Boeck's sarcoid, sarcoid (1), Schaumann's syndrome. [sarcoid + G. *-osis,* condition]

hypercalcemic s., s. with hypercalcemia of unknown cause, not necessarily associated with detectable bone involvement by s.

sar·co·lem·ma (sar′kō-lem′ă). The plasma membrane of a muscle fiber; formerly, the delicate connective tissue of the endomysium was included under this term by some. SYN myolemma. [sarco- + G. *lemma,* husk]

sar·co·lem·mal, sar·co·lem·mic, sar·co·lem·mous (sar′kō-lem′ăl, -lem′ik, -lem′ŭs). Relating to the sarcolemma.

sar·col·o·gy (sar-kol′ō-jē). **1.** SYN myology. **2.** The anatomy of the soft parts, as distinguished from osteology. [sarco- + G. *logos,* study]

sar·co·ly·sine (sar-kō-lī′sēn). SYN merphalan.

sar·co·ma (sar-kō′mă). A connective tissue neoplasm, usually highly malignant, formed by proliferation of mesodermal cells. [G. *sarkōma,* a fleshy excrescence, fr. *sarx,* flesh, + *-oma,* tumor]

alveolar soft part s., a malignant tumor formed of a reticular stroma of connective tissue enclosing aggregates of large round or polygonal cells; occurs in subcutaneous and fibromuscular tissues.

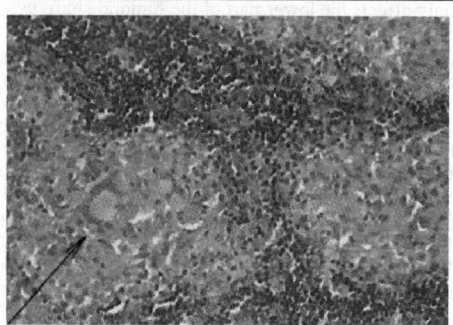

sarcoidosis
lymph nodes with epitheloid cell clusters and giant cells

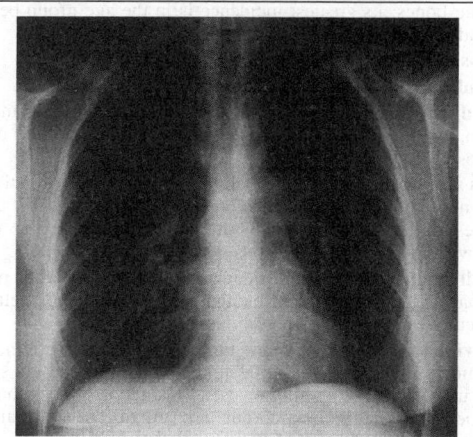

sarcoidosis (x-ray of thorax)
in otherwise normal lungs, the hila pulmonis are widened
on both sides

ameloblastic s., SYN ameloblastic *fibrosarcoma.*

angiolithic s., SYN psammomatous *meningioma.*

avian s., SYN Rous s.

botryoid s., a polypoid form of embryonal rhabdomyosarcoma which occurs in children, most frequently in the urogenital tract, characterized by the formation of grossly apparent grapelike clusters of neoplastic tissue that consist of rhabdomyoblasts, spindle, and stellate cells in a myxomatous stroma; neoplasms of this type grow relatively rapidly and are highly malignant.

endometrial stromal s., a term sometimes used for a relatively rare s. believed to be a form of endometriosis in which the lesions form multiple foci in the myometrium and in vascular spaces in other sites, and which consist of histologic and cytologic elements that resemble those of the endometrial stroma. SYN stromatosis.

Ewing's s., SYN Ewing's *tumor.*

fascicular s., SYN spindle cell s.

giant cell s., a malignant giant cell tumor of bone.

giant cell monstrocellular s. of Zülch, SYN gigantocellular *glioma.*

granulocytic s., a malignant tumor of immature myeloid cells, frequently subperiosteal, associated with or preceding granulocytic leukemia. SEE ALSO chloroma. SYN myeloid s.

immunoblastic s., obsolete term for immunoblastic *lymphoma.*

Jensen's s., a mouse tumor transmissible by inoculation.

juxtacortical osteogenic s., a form of osteogenic s. of relatively low malignancy, probably arising from the periosteum and initially involving cortical bone and adjacent connective tissue, which occurs in middle-aged as well as young adults and most commonly affects the lower part of the femoral shaft. SYN periosteal s.

Kaposi's s., a multifocal malignant neoplasm of primitive vasoformative tissue, occurring in the skin and sometimes in lymph nodes or viscera, consisting of spindle cells and irregular small vascular spaces frequently infiltrated by hemosiderin-pigmented macrophages and extravasated red cells; clinically manifested by cutaneous lesions consisting of reddish-purple to dark blue macules, plaques, or nodules; seen most commonly in men over 60 years of age and as an opportunistic disease in AIDS patients. SYN multiple idiopathic hemorrhagic s.

leukocytic s., SYN leukemia.

lymphatic s., obsolete term for lymphosarcoma.

medullary s., a soft, extremely vascular s.

multiple idiopathic hemorrhagic s., SYN Kaposi's s.

myelogenic s., s. originating in the bone marrow.

myeloid s., SYN granulocytic s.

osteogenic s., the most common and malignant of bone s.'s, which arises from bone-forming cells and affects chiefly the ends of long bones; its greatest incidence is in the age group between 10 and 25 years. SYN osteosarcoma.

periosteal s., SYN juxtacortical osteogenic s.

reticulum cell s., obsolete term for histiocytic *lymphoma*.

round cell s., old term for an undifferentiated malignant neoplasm, believed to be of mesenchymal origin, composed chiefly of closely packed round cells.

Rous s., a fibrosarcoma, originally observed in a Plymouth Rock hen, now thought to be an expression of infection by certain viruses of the avian leukosis-sarcoma complex in the family Retroviridae. SYN avian s., Rous tumor.

spindle cell s., a malignant neoplasm, believed to be of mesenchymal origin, composed of elongated, spindle-shaped cells. SYN fascicular s.

synovial s., a rare malignant tumor of synovial origin, most commonly involving the knee joint and composed of spindle cells usually enclosing slits or pseudoglandular spaces that may be lined by radially disposed epithelial-like cells. SYN malignant synovioma.

telangiectatic osteogenic s., a lytic cystic variant of osteogenic s. composed of aneurysmal blood-filled spaces lined by sarcoma cells producing osteoid.

Sar·co·mas·ti·goph·o·ra (sar'kō-mas-ti-gof'ŏ-ră). A phylum of the subkingdom Protozoa characterized by flagellae, pseudopodia, or both types of locomotory organelles; includes both the flagellates (subphylum Mastigophora) and the amebae (subphylum Sarcodina) in a single large assemblage. [sarco- + G. *mastix* (*mastig-*), whip, + *phoros,* to bear]

sar·co·ma·toid (sar-kō'mă-toyd). Resembling a sarcoma. [sarcoma + G. *eidos,* resemblance]

sar·co·ma·to·sis (sar'kō-mă-tō'sis). Occurrence of several sarcomatous growths on different parts of the body. [sarcoma + G. *-osis,* condition]

sar·com·a·tous (sar-kō'mă-tŭs). Relating to or of the nature of sarcoma.

sar·co·mere (sar'kō-mēr). The segment of a myofibril between two adjacent Z lines, representing the functional unit of striated muscle. [sarco- + G. *meros,* part]

sar·co·neme (sar'kō-nēm). SYN microneme. [sarco- + G. *nēma,* thread]

sar·co·plasm (sar'kō-plazm). The nonfibrillar cytoplasm of a muscle fiber. [sarco- + G. *plasma,* a thing formed]

sar·co·plas·mic (sar-kō-plaz'mik). Relating to sarcoplasm.

sar·co·plast (sar'kō-plast). SYN satellite *cell* of skeletal muscle. [sarco- + G. *plastos,* formed]

sar·co·poi·et·ic (sar'kō-poy-et'ik). Forming muscle. [sarco- + G. *poiēsis,* a making]

Sar·cop·syl·la pen·e·trans (sar-kō-sil'ă pen'ĕ-tranz). SYN *Tunga penetrans.*

Sar·cop·syl·li·dae (sar-kop-sil'li-dē). Older name for Tungidae. [sarco- + G. *psylla,* flea]

Sar·cop·tes sca·bi·ei (sar-kop'tēz skā'bē-ī). Formerly *Acarus*

scabiei, the itch mite, varieties of which are distributed worldwide and affect humans, horses, cattle, swine, sheep, dogs, cats, and many wild animals; serious and fatal infections are not uncommon in untreated animals. Although considered to belong to a single species, they do not readily pass from one host to another of a different animal species; transitory infections of this type do occur, however, especially from various animals to humans, and are spread by direct contact. The mite burrows into the skin and lays eggs within the burrow; intense itching and rash develop near the burrow in about a month. SEE scabies, mange. [sarco- + G. *koptō,* to cut; L. *scabies,* scurf]

sar·cop·tic (sar-kop'tik). Of, relating to, or caused by mites of the genus Sarcoptes or other members of the family Sarcoptidae.

sar·cop·tid (sar-kop'tid). Common name for members of the Sarcoptidae, a family of mites that includes the genera *Sarcoptes, Knemidokoptes,* and *Notoedres.*

sar·co·sine (Sar) (sar'kō-sēn). *N*-Methylglycine; an intermediate in the metabolism of choline; it can donate a methyl group to tetrahydrofolate, yielding N^5,N^{10}-methylenetetrahydrofolate; demethylation by s. dehydrogenase yields formaldehyde, glycine, and a reduced acceptor; elevated in certain inherited disorders.

s. dehydrogenase, an enzyme that cleaves s. using some acceptor to produce glycine, formaldehyde, and a reduced acceptor molecule; a deficiency of this enzyme will result in sarcosinemia.

sar·co·si·ne·mia (sar'kō-si-nē'mē-ă) [MIM*268900]. A disorder of amino acid metabolism due to deficiency of sarcosine dehydrogenase, causing the sarcosine level to rise in blood plasma and be excreted in the urine; affected infants fail to thrive, are irritable, may have muscle tremors, and have retarded motor and mental development; autosomal recessive inheritance. SYN hypersarcosinemia.

sar·co·sis (sar-kō'sis). **1.** An abnormal increase of flesh. **2.** A multiple growth of fleshy tumors. **3.** A diffuse sarcoma involving the whole of an organ. [G. *sarkōsis,* the growth of flesh, fr. *sarx,* flesh]

sar·co·some (sar'kō-sōm). **1.** Formerly, any granule in a muscle fiber. **2.** Now, sometimes used synonymously with myomitochondrion. [sarco- + G. *soma,* body]

sar·cos·to·sis (sar-kos-tō'sis). Ossification of muscular tissue. [sarco- + G. *osteon,* bone, + *-osis,* condition]

sar·cot·ic (sar-kot'ik). **1.** Relating to sarcosis. **2.** Causing an increase of flesh.

sar·co·trip·sy (sar'kō-trip-sē). Rarely used term for use of a crushing forceps to stop hemorrhage. [sarco- + G. *tripsis,* a rubbing]

sar·co·tu·bules (sar-kō-tū'būlz). The continuous system of membranous tubules in striated muscle that corresponds to the smooth endoplasmic reticulum of other cells.

sar·cous (sar'kŭs). Relating to muscular tissue; fleshy. [G. *sarx,* flesh]

sar·don·ic grin (sar-don'ik). SYN risus caninus.

sa·rin (zah-rēn'). Isopropyl methylphosphonofluoridate; a nerve poison similar to diisopropyl fluorophosphate and tetraethyl pyrophosphate; a very potent irreversible cholinesterase inhibitor and a more toxic nerve gas than tabun or soman. [Ger.]

sar·mas·sa·tion (sar-mă-sā'shŭn). Erotic squeezing, kneading, or caressing of female tissues and organs. [G. *sarx,* flesh, + *massō,* to knead]

sar·sa·pa·ril·la (sar'să-per-il'ă, sas-per-il'ă). The dried root of *Smilax aristolochiaefolia* (Mexican s.), *S. regelii* (Honduras s.), *S. febrifuga* (Ecuadorian s.), or of undetermined species of *Smilax* (family Liliaceae), a thorny vine widely distributed throughout the tropical and semitropical world; it has been used in psoriasis, gout, rheumatism, and syphilis, and popularly as a "blood purifier." [Sp. *zarza,* a bramble]

SART Abbreviation for sinoatrial recovery *time.*

sar·to·ri·us (sar-tōr'ē-ŭs). SEE sartorius *muscle.* [L. *sartor,* a tailor, the muscle being used in crossing the legs in the tailor's position, fr. *sarcio* pp. *sartus,* to patch, mend]

sas·sa·fras (sas'ă-fras). The dried bark of the root of *Sassafras albidum* (family Lauraceae), a tree of the eastern U.S.; a flavoring agent, diuretic, and diaphoretic; s. oil, a volatile oil obtained by distillation from the bark of *S. albidum* and *S. variifolium*, is used as a carminative, topical antiseptic, pediculicide, and flavoring agent.

sat Abbreviation for saturated.

sat·el·lite (sat′ĕ-līt). **1.** A minor structure accompanying a more important or larger one; *e.g.*, a vein accompanying an artery, or a small or secondary lesion adjacent to a larger one. **2.** The posterior member of a pair of gregarine gamonts in syzygy, several of which may be found in some species. SEE ALSO primite. [L. *satelles* (*sattelit-*), attendant]

chromosome s., a small chromosomal segment separated from the main body of the chromosome by a secondary constriction; in humans it is usually associated with the short arm of an acrocentric chromosome.

perineuronal s., an oligodendroglia cell surrounding the neuron.

sat·el·lit·o·sis (sat′ĕ-lī-tō′sis). **1.** A condition marked by an accumulation of neuroglia cells around the neurons of the central nervous system; often as a prelude to neuronophagia. **2.** The presence of satellite, smaller structures, or lesions, *e.g.*, metastic melanoma in the skin adjacent to the primary tumor, or lymphocytes in contact with a damaged keratinocyte in acute cutaneous graft versus host reaction. [L. *satelles* (*satellit-*), an attendant, + G. *-ōsis,* condition]

sa·ti·a·tion (sā-shē-ā′shŭn). The state produced by fulfillment of a specific need, such as hunger or thirst. [L. *satio,* pp. *-atus,* to fill, satisfy]

sat. sol., sat. soln. Abbreviation for saturated *solution.*

Sattler, Hubert, Austrian ophthalmologist, 1844–1928. SEE S.'s elastic *layer, veil.*

sat·u·rate (satch′ŭ-rāt). **1.** To impregnate to the greatest possible extent. **2.** To neutralize; to satisfy all the chemical affinities of a substance (as by converting all double bonds to single bonds). **3.** To dissolve a substance up to that concentration beyond which the addition of more results in two phases. [L. *saturo,* pp. *-atus,* to fill, fr. *satur,* sated]

sat·u·ra·tion (satch-ŭ-rā′shŭn). **1.** Impregnation of one substance by another to the greatest possible extent. **2.** Neutralization, as of an acid by an alkali. **3.** That concentration of a dissolved substance that cannot be exceeded. **4.** In optics, see saturated *color.* **5.** Filling of all the available sites on an enzyme molecule by its substrate, or on a hemoglobin molecule by oxygen (symbol S_{O_2}) or carbon monoxide (symbol S_{CO}). [L. *saturatio,* fr. *saturo,* to fill, fr. *satis,* enough]

secondary s., a technique of nitrous oxide anesthesia consisting of an abrupt curtailment of the oxygen in the inhaled mixture to produce a deep plane of anesthesia, following which oxygen is administered to correct hypoxia.

sat·ur·nine (sat′er-nīn). **1.** Relating to lead. **2.** Due to or symptomatic of lead poisoning. [Mediev. L. *saturninus,* fr. *saturnus,* lead, fr. L. *saturnus,* the god and planet Saturn]

sat·urn·ism (sat′er-nizm). SYN lead *poisoning.* [Mediev. L. *saturnus,* alchemical name for lead]

sat·y·ri·a·sis (sat-i-rī′ă-sis). satyromania; excessive sexual excitement and behavior in the male; the counterpart of nymphomania in the female. SYN satyrism. [G. *satyros,* a satyr]

sat·y·rism (sat′i-rizm). SYN satyriasis.

sau·cer·i·za·tion (saw′ser-i-zā′shŭn). Excavation of tissue to form a shallow depression, performed in wound treatment to facilitate drainage from infected areas. SYN craterization.

Saundby, Robert, English physician, 1849–1918. SEE S.'s *test.*

sau·ri·a·sis (saw-rī′ă-sis). SYN ichthyosis. [G. *sauros,* lizard, + *-iasis,* condition]

sau·ri·der·ma (saw-ri-der′mă). SYN ichthyosis. [G. *sauros,* lizard, + *derma,* skin]

sau·ri·o·sis (saw-ri-ō′sis). SYN ichthyosis. [G. *sauros,* lizard, + *-osis,* condition]

sau·ro·der·ma (saw′rō-der′mă). SYN ichthyosis. [G. *sauros,* lizard, + *derma,* skin]

Savage, Henry, English anatomist and gynecologist, 1810–1900. SEE S.'s perineal *body.*

saw. A metal operating instrument having an edge of sharp, toothlike projections, for dividing bone, cartilage, or plaster;

edges may be attached to a rigid band, a flexible wire or chain, or a motorized oscillator. [A.S. *saga*]

Gigli's s., a hand-held wire s. for use in craniotomy or pubiotomy.

Stryker s., a rapidly oscillating s. used for cutting bone or plaster casts; it cuts hard matter, but soft tissues give and thus are not injured.

sax·i·tox·in (sak-si-tok′sin). A potent neurotoxin found in shellfish, such as the mussel or the clam, produced by the dinoflagellate *Gonyaulax catenella*, which is ingested by the shellfish; the cause of cases of poisoning from eating California sea mussel (*Mytilus californianus*), the scallop, and the Alaskan butterclam (*Saxidomus giganteus*).

Sayre, George P., U.S. ophthalmologist, *1911. SEE Kearns-S. *syndrome.*

Sayre, Lewis A., U.S. surgeon, 1820–1900. SEE S.'s suspension *traction,* suspension *apparatus, jacket.*

Sb Symbol for antimony.

SBE Abbreviation for subacute bacterial *endocarditis.*

Sc Symbol for scandium.

s.c. Abbreviation for subcutaneous; subcutaneously.

scab (skab). A crust formed by coagulation of blood, pus, serum, or a combination of these, on the surface of an ulcer, erosion, or other type of wound. [A.S. *scaeb*]

scab·i·ci·dal (skā-bi-sī′dăl). Destructive to scabies mites.

scab·i·cide (skā′bi-sīd). An agent lethal to scabies mites. SYN scabieticide.

sca·bies (skā′bēz). **1.** An eruption due to the mite *Sarcoptes scabiei* var. *hominis;* the female of the species burrows into the skin, producing a vesicular eruption with intense pruritus between the fingers, on the male genitalia, buttocks, and elsewhere on the trunk and extremities. **2.** In animals, s. or scab is usually applied to cutaneous acariasis in sheep, which may be caused by *Sarcoptes, Psoroptes,* or *Chorioptes.* [L. *scabo,* to scratch]

Norwegian s., a severe form of s. with innumerable mites in thickened stratum corneum. SYN Norway itch.

sca·bi·et·i·cide (skā-bē-et′i-sīd). SYN scabicide.

sca·bi·ous (skā′bē-ŭs). Relating to or suffering from scabies.

sca·brit·i·es (skā-brish′i-ēz). Roughness of the skin. [L., fr. *scaber,* scurfy]

s. un′guium, thickening and distortion of the nails.

sca·la, pl. **sca·lae** (skā′lă, -lē) [NA]. One of the cavities of the cochlea winding spirally around the modiolus. [L. a stairway]

Löwenberg's s., SYN cochlear *duct.*

s. me′dia, SYN cochlear *duct.*

s. tym′pani [NA], the division of the spiral canal of the cochlea lying on the basal side of the spiral lamina.

s. vestib′uli [NA], the division of the spiral canal of the cochlea lying on the apical side of the spiral lamina and vestibular membrane. SYN vestibular canal.

scald (skawld). **1.** To burn by contact with a hot liquid or steam. **2.** The lesion resulting from such contact. **3.** SYN scall. [L. *excaldo,* to wash in hot water]

scald·ing (skawl′ding). A burning pain in urinating.

scale (skāl). **1.** A standardized test for measuring psychological, personality, or behavioral characteristics. SEE ALSO test. **2.** SYN squama. **3.** A small thin plate of horny epithelium, resembling a fish s., cast off from the skin. **4.** To desquamate. **5.** To remove tartar from the teeth. [L. *scala,* a stairway]

absolute s., obsolete term for Kelvin s.

activities of daily living s., a s. to score physical activity and its limitations, based on answers to simple questions about mobility, self-care, grooming, etc; widely used in geriatrics, rheumatology, etc.

adaptive behavior s.'s, a behavioral assessment device to quantify the levels of skills of mentally retarded and developmentally delayed individuals in interacting with the environment; consists of three developmentally related factors: 1) personal self-sufficiency, *e.g.,* eating, dressing; 2) community self-sufficiency, *e.g.,* shopping, communicating; 3) personal and social responsibility, *e.g.,* use of leisure time, job performance. SEE intelligence.

Ångström s., a table of wavelengths of a large number of light rays corresponding to as many Fraunhofer's lines in the spectrum.

Baumé s., a hydrometer s. for determining the specific gravity of liquids heavier and lighter than water, respectively: for liquids lighter than water, divide 140 by 130 plus the Baumé degree; for liquids heavier than water, divide 145 by 145 minus the Baumé degree.

Brazelton's Neonatal Behavioral Assessment s.'s, a s. used by obstetricians, pediatricians, and pediatric psychologists to assess the sensory, motor, emotional and physical development of the neonate, usually beginning at birth or in the first month of life.

Bayley s.'s of Infant Development, a psychological test used to measure the developmental progress of infants over the first two and one-half years of life; consists of three scales: mental, motor, and behavior record.

Binet s., a measure of intelligence designed for both children and adults.

Binet-Simon s., forerunner of individual intelligence tests, particularly the Stanford-Binet intelligence s., and sometimes referred to as the Binet s.

Cattell Infant Intelligence S., a standardized s. for assessment of the cognitive development of infants between the ages of 3 and 30 months.

Celsius s., a temperature s. that is based upon the triple point of water (defined to be 273.16 K) and assigned the value of 0.01°C; this has replaced the centigrade scale because the triple point of water can be more accurately measured than the ice point; although, for most practical purposes, the two s.'s are equivalent.

centigrade s., a thermometer s. in which there are 100 degrees between the freezing point of water (assigned the value of 0.0°C) and the boiling point of water at sea level; technically, supplanted by the Celsius s. Cf. Celsius s.

Charrière s., SYN French s.

Columbia Mental Maturity S., an individually administered intelligence test that provides an estimate of the intellectual ability of children; provides mental ages ranging from 3 to 12 years, and requires no verbal response and minimal motor response. [*Columbia University,* NY]

coma s., a clinical s. to assess impaired consciousness; assessment may include motor responsiveness, verbal performance, and eye opening, as in the Glasgow (Scotland) c.s., or the same three items and dysfunction of cranial nerves, as in the Maryland (U.S.) c.s.

digital gray s., SYN latitude.

Fahrenheit s., a thermometer s. in which the freezing point of water is 32°F and the boiling point of water 212°F; 0°F indicates the lowest temperature Fahrenheit could obtain by a mixture of ice and salt in 1724; °C = (5/9)(°F − 32).

French s. (Fr), a s. for grading sizes of sounds, tubules, and catheters as based on a measurement of ⅓ mm and equaling 1 fr on the scale (*e.g.,* 3 fr = 1 mm); grading to scale is carried out using a metal plate with holes ranging from ⅓ mm to 1 cm in diameter. SYN Charrière s.

Gaffky s., SYN Gaffky *table.*

gray s., SYN latitude. SEE gray-scale *ultrasonography.*

hardness s., a qualitative s. in which minerals are classified in order of their increasing hardness, based on the fact that the harder of two materials will scratch the softer and will not be scratched by it. The s. lists 15 substances: 1, talc; 2, gypsum; 3, calcite; 4, fluorite; 5, apatite; 6, orthoclase, periclase; 7, vitreous pure silica; 8, quartz, stellite; 9, topaz; 10, garnet; 11, tantalum carbide, fused zirconia; 12, fused alumina; 13, silicon carbide; 14, boron carbide; 15, diamond. SYN Mohs s.

homigrade s., a special thermometer s. in which 100° indicates the normal temperature of man (98.6°F, 37°C), 0° the freezing point, and 270° the boiling point (212°F, 100°C).

interval s., like a temperature s. in centigrade or Fahrenheit units, a s. on which the intervals are equal but which has an arbitrary zero point; *e.g.,* intelligence quotient values are values along an interval s.

Karnofsky s., a performance s. for rating a person's usual activi-

ties; used to evaluate a patient's progress after a therapeutic procedure.

Kelvin s., temperature scale in which the triple point of water is assigned the value of 273.16 K; °C = K − 273.15.

Leiter International Performance S., a nonverbal (performance) test for measuring intelligence which contains norms for each age between 2 and 18; originally developed as a method of assessing the comparative intellectual abilities of Caucasian, Chinese, and Japanese children, but now occasionally used for assessing slow learners and those who are blind, deaf, or verbally handicapped.

Likert s., a method of measuring attitudes that asks respondents to indicate their degree of agreement or disagreement with statements, according to a three- or five-point scoring system, *e.g.,* "strongly agree" "no opinion" or "strongly disagree."

masculinity-femininity s., any s. on a psychological test that assesses the relative masculinity or femininity of an individual; s.'s vary and may focus, for example, on basic identification with either sex or preference for a particular sex role.

Mohs s., SYN hardness s.

ordinal s., a s. that is based on classification of persons or things into ordered qualitative categories, such as socioeconomic status.

pH s., SYN Sörensen s.

Rahe-Holmes social readjustment rating s., a widely used s. in the social and behavioral sciences that assigns values to significant life events such as marriage, birth of offspring, bereavement, loss of job; such events correlate with emotional states.

Rankine s., a thermometer s. in which each degree Rankine (°Rank) is equal to the Fahrenheit but applied to the absolute temperature s. with its zero point at absolute zero; °Rank = °F + 459.67.

ratio s., a s. that involves physical units and demonstrates their relations.

Réaumur s., a thermometer s. in which each degree Réaumur (°R) is ⅟₈₀ of the temperature difference between the freezing point and boiling point of pure water at 1 atmosphere pressure, with 0°R set at the freezing point and 80°R set at the boiling point of water.

Shipley-Hartford s., a test of intellectual and conceptual aptitude. [*Hartford* Retreat, CT, where Shipley was employed]

Sörensen s., the negative logarithm of the hydrogen ion concentration, used as a s. for expressing acidity and alkalinity. SEE ALSO pH. SYN pH s.

Stanford-Binet intelligence s., a standardized test for the measurement of intelligence consisting of a series of questions, graded according to the intelligence of normal children at different ages, the answers to which indicate the mental age of the person tested; primarily used with children, but also contains norms for adults standardized against adult age levels rather than those of children, as formerly was the case. SYN Binet test.

Wechsler-Bellevue s., a measure of general intelligence superseded by the Wechsler adult intelligence s. and its subsequent revision. SEE ALSO Wechsler intelligence s.'s.

Wechsler intelligence s.'s, continuously revised and updated standardized s.'s for the measurement of general intelligence in preschool children (Wechsler preschool and primary s. of intelligence), in children (Wechsler intelligence s. for children), and in adults (Wechsler adult intelligence s., the successor to the Wechsler-Bellevue s.).

Zubrod s., a 5-point s. similar to the 10-point Karnofsky s.; both measure the performance status of a patient's ambulatory nature, from normal activity to total dependence on others for care. SEE ALSO Karnofsky s.

sca·le·ne (skā'lēn). **1.** Having sides of unequal length, said of a triangle so formed. **2.** One of several muscles so named. SEE scalenus anterior *muscle, musculus* scalenus anticus, scalenus medius *muscle,* scalenus minimus *muscle,* scalenus posterior *muscle, musculus* scalenus posticus. SYN scalenus. [G. *skalēnos,* uneven]

sca·le·nec·to·my (skā'lē-nek'tō-mē). Resection of the scalene muscles. [scalene + G. *ektomē,* excision]

sca·le·not·o·my (skā'lē-not'ō-mē). Division or section of the anterior scalene muscle. [scalene + G. *tomē,* incision]

sca·le·nus (skā-lē'nŭs). SYN scalene. [L.]

scal·er (skā'ler). **1.** An instrument for removing tartar from the teeth. **2.** A device for counting electrical impulses, as in the assay of radioactive materials.

hoe s., a hoe-shaped s. with a very short blade.

ultrasonic s., an ultrasonic instrument that uses high frequency vibration to remove adherent deposits from the teeth.

scal·ing (skā'ling). In dentistry, removal of accretions from the crowns and roots of teeth by use of special instruments.

scall (skawl). Any crusted or pustular scaly eruption or lesion of the skin or scalp, *e.g.,* favus. SYN scald (3). [Ice. *skalli,* bald-head]

milk s., SYN *crusta* lactea.

scal·lop·ing (skal'ō-ping). A series of indentations or erosions on a normally smooth margin of a structure.

scalp (skalp). The skin and subcutaneous tissue normally hair bearing covering the neuro-cranium. [M. E. fr. Scand. *skalpr,* sheath]

scal·pel (skal'pl). A knife used in surgical dissection. [L. *scalpellum;* dim. of *scalprum,* a knife]

plasma s., a s. that uses a fine high-temperature gas jet, instead of a blade, for cutting.

scal·pri·form (skal'pri-fōrm). Chisel-shaped. [L. *scalprum,* chisel, + *forma,* shape]

scal·prum (skal'prŭm). **1.** A large strong scalpel. **2.** A raspatory. [L. chisel, penknife, fr. *scalpo,* pp. *scalptus,* to carve]

scaly (skā'lē). SYN squamous.

scam·mo·ny (skam'ō-nē). The plant, *Convolvulus scammonia* (family Convolvulaceae), the dried root of which contains a cathartic resin. SEE ALSO ipomea. [G. *skammōnia*]

scan (skan). **1.** To survey by traversing with an active or passive sensing device. **2.** The image, record, or data obtained by scanning, usually identified by the technology or device employed; *e.g.,* CT s., radionuclide s., ultrasound s., etc. **3.** Abbreviated form of scintiscan, usually identified by the organ or structure examined; *e.g.,* brain s., bone s., etc.

duplex Doppler s., a method of visualizing and selectively assessing the flow patterns of peripheral arteries and veins using ultrasound imaging and pulsed Doppler.

EMI s., historically, the name commonly used for computed tomography of the head, the technique devised by Hounsfield, who was a scientist at EMI, an English electronics firm.

Meckel s., use of technetium-99m pertechnetate in a s. of the gastric mucosa to detect ectopic gastric mucosa in Meckel's diverticulum; the pertechnetate anion is secreted by epithelial cells in the gastric mucosa.

sector s., in ultrasonography, a system in which the transducer or transmitted ultrasound beam is rotated through an angle, resulting in a pie-shaped image.

ventilation-perfusion s., a lung function test, especially useful for pulmonary embolism, employing an inhaled radionuclide for ventilation and an intravenous radionuclide for perfusion; their respective distributions in the lung are recorded scintigraphically.

scan·di·um (Sc) (skan'dē-ŭm). A metallic element, atomic no. 21, atomic wt. 44.955910. [L. *Scandia,* Scandinavia, where discovered]

scan·ner (skan'er). A device or instrument that scans.

scan·ning (skan'ing). The act of imaging by traversing with an active or passive sensing device, often identified by the technology or device employed.

scan·o·gram (skan'ō-gram). A radiographic technique for showing true dimensions by moving a narrow orthogonal beam of x-rays along the length of the structure being measured, *e.g.,* the lower extremities. [scan- + G. *gramma,* something written]

Scanzoni, Friedrich W., German obstetrician, 1821–1891. SEE S.'s *maneuver,* second *os.*

sca·pha (skaf'ă, skā'fă) [NA]. **1** [na]. The longitudinal furrow between the helix and the antihelix of the auricle. SYN fossa of helix, scaphoid fossa (2). **2.** Obsolete term for scaphoid *fossa* (1). [L. fr. G. *skaphē,* skiff]

△scapho-. A scapha, scaphoid. [G. *skaphē,* skiff, boat]

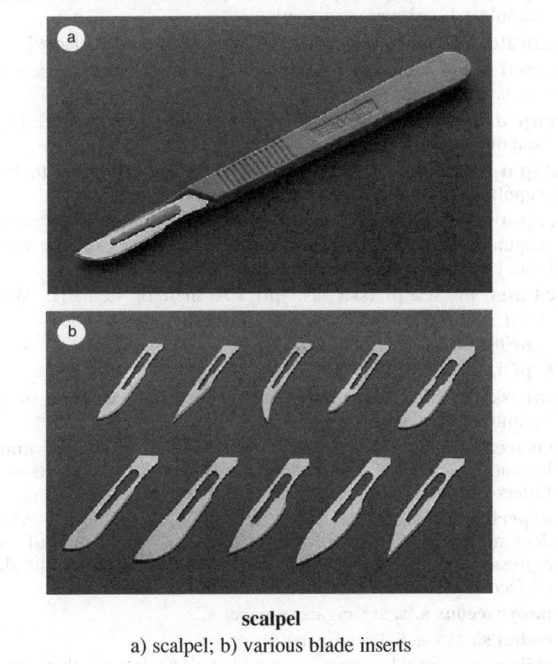

scalpel
a) scalpel; b) various blade inserts

scaph·o·ce·phal·ic (skaf-ō-se-fal'ik). Denoting or relating to scaphocephaly. SYN scaphocephalous, tectocephalic.

scaph·o·ceph·a·lism (skaf-ō-sef'ă-lizm). SYN scaphocephaly.

scaph·o·ceph·a·lous (skaf-ō-sef'ă-lŭs). SYN scaphocephalic.

scaph·o·ceph·a·ly (skaf-ō-sef'ă-lē). A form of craniosynostosis that results in a long, narrow head in which the parietal eminences are absent and frontal and occiptal protrusions are conspicuous; there may be a crest indicating the site of a prenatally closed sagittal suture; sometimes accompanied by mental retardation. SYN cymbocephaly, sagittal synostosis, scaphocephalism, tectocephaly. [scapho- + G. *kephalē,* head]

scaph·o·hy·dro·ceph·a·lus, scaph·o·hy·dro·ceph·a·ly (skaf'ō-hī'drō-sef'ă-lŭs, -lē). Occurrence of hydrocephalus in a scaphocephalic individual.

scaph·oid (skaf'oyd). Boat-shaped; hollowed. SEE scaphoid *bone.* SYN navicular. [scapho- + G. *eidos,* resemblance]

scap·u·la, gen. and pl. **scap·u·lae** (skap'yū-lă, -lē) [NA]. A large triangular flattened bone lying over the ribs, posteriorly on either side, articulating laterally with the clavicle at the acromioclavicular joint and the humerus at the glenohumeral joint. It forms a functional joint with the chest wall, the scapulothoracic joint. SYN blade bone, shoulder blade. [L. *scapulae,* the shoulder blades]

s. ala'ta, SYN winged s.

s. eleva'ta, SYN Sprengel's *deformity.*

scaphoid s., a s. in which the vertebral border below the level of the spine presents concavity instead of the normal convexity; the **scaphoid type of s.** (Graves) is a s. in which the vertebral border between the spine and the teres major process is either straight or tends toward concavity.

winged s., condition wherein the medial border of the scapula protrudes away from the thorax; the protrusion is posterior and lateral, as the scapula rotates out; caused by paralysis of the serratus anterior muscle. SYN s. alata.

scap·u·lal·gia (skap'yū-lal'jē-ă). Rarely used term meaning pain in the shoulder blades. SYN scapulodynia. [scapula + G. *algos,* pain]

scap·u·lar (skap'yū-lăr). Relating to the scapula.

scap·u·lary (skap'yū-lār-ē). A form of brace or suspender for keeping a belt or body bandage in place.

scap·u·lec·to·my (skap'yū-lek'tō-mē). Excision of the scapula. [scapula + G. *ektomē,* excision]

⬧ **scapulo-.** Scapula, scapular. [L. *scapulae,* shoulder blades]

scap·u·lo·cla·vic·u·lar (skap'yū-lō-klă-vik'yū-lăr). **1.** SYN acromioclavicular. **2.** SYN coracoclavicular.

scap·u·lo·dyn·ia (skap'yū-lō-din'ē-ă). SYN scapulalgia. [scapulo- + G. *odynē,* pain]

scap·u·lo·hu·mer·al (skap'yū-lō-hyū'mer-ăl). Relating to both scapula and humerus. SEE ALSO glenohumeral.

scap·u·lo·pexy (skap'yū-lō-pek-sē). Operative fixation of the scapula to the chest wall or to the spinous process of the vertebrae. [scapulo- + G. *pēxis,* fixation]

sca·pus, pl. **sca·pi** (skā'pŭs, -pī). A shaft or stem. [L. shaft, stalk]

s. pe'nis, SYN *body* of penis.

s. pi'li, SYN hair *shaft.*

scar (skar). The fibrous tissue replacing normal tissues destroyed by injury or disease. [G. *eschara,* scab]

cigarette-paper s.'s, atrophic s.'s in the skin at sites of minor lacerations over the knees, shins, and elbows of persons with Ehlers-Danlos syndrome. SYN papyraceous s.'s.

hypertrophic s., an elevated s. resembling a keloid but which does not spread into surrounding tissues, is rarely painful, and regresses spontaneously; collagen bundles run parallel to the skin surface.

papyraceous s.'s, SYN cigarette-paper s.'s.

radial s., SYN radial sclerosing *lesion.*

shilling s.'s, obsolete term for round, well healed s.'s that follow involution of rupial syphilids.

Scardino, Peter L., U.S. urologist, *1915. SEE S. vertical flap *pyeloplasty.*

Scarff, John E., U.S. neurosurgeon, *1898. SEE Stookey-S. *operation.*

scar·i·fi·ca·tion (skar-i-fi-kā'shŭn). The making of a number of superficial incisions in the skin. [L. *scarifico,* to scratch, fr. G. *skariphos,* a style for sketching]

scar·i·fi·ca·tor (skar'i-fi-kā-tŏr). An instrument for scarification, consisting of a number of concealed spring-projected cutting blades, set near together, that make superficial incisions in the skin.

scar·i·fy (skar'i-fī). To produce scarification.

scar·la·ti·na (skar'lă-tē'nă). An acute exanthematous disease, caused by infection with streptococcal organisms producing erythrogenic toxin, marked by fever and other constitutional disturbances, and a generalized eruption of closely aggregated points or small macules of a bright red color followed by desquamation in large scales, shreds, or sheets; mucous membrane of the mouth and fauces is usually also involved. SYN scarlet fever. [through It. fr. Mediev. L. *scarlatum,* scarlet, a scarlet cloth]

anginose s., s. angino'sa, a form of s. in which the throat affection is unusually severe. SYN Fothergill's disease (2).

s. hemorrhag'ica, a form of s. in which blood extravasates into the skin and mucous membranes, giving to the eruption a dusky hue; frequent bleeding from the nose and into the intestine also occurs.

s. la'tens, latent s., a form of s. in which the rash is absent, but other complications of streptococcal infection occur, such as acute nephritis.

s. malig'na, a severe scarlet fever in which the patient is quickly overcome with the intensity of the systemic intoxication.

s. rheumat'ica, SYN dengue.

s. sim'plex, a mild form of the disease.

scar·la·ti·nal (skar-lă-tē'năl). Relating to scarlatina.

scar·la·ti·nel·la (skar-lă-ti-nel'ă). SYN Filatov Dukes' *disease.* [dim. of *scarlatina*]

scar·la·ti·ni·form (skar-lă-tē'ni-fōrm, -tin'i-fōrm). Resembling scarlatina, denoting a rash. SYN scarlatinoid (1).

scar·la·ti·noid (skar-lă-tē'noyd, skar-lat'i-noyd). **1.** SYN scarlatiniform. **2.** SYN fourth *disease.* [scarlatina + G. *eidos,* resemblance]

scar·let (skar'let). Denoting a bright red color tending toward orange. [Mediev. L. *scarlatum,* scarlet cloth]

scar·let red [C.I. 26905]. *o*-Tolylazo-*o*-tolylazo-β-naphthol. An azo dye; a dark, brownish red powder, soluble in oils, fats, and chloroform, but insoluble in water; used in medicine as a vulnerary, in histology to stain fat in tissue sections and basic proteins at high pH, and in immunoelectrophoresis. SYN Biebrich scarlet red, medicinal scarlet red, scharlach red, Sudan IV.

scar·let red sul·fo·nate. An azo dye that has been used to stimulate healing of chronic superficial wounds and ulcers.

Scarpa, Antonio, Italian anatomist, orthopedist, and ophthalmologist, 1747–1832. SEE *canals* of S., under *canal;* S.'s *fascia, fluid, foramina,* under *foramen; fossa* scarpae major; S.'s *ganglion, habenula, hiatus, liquor, membrane, method, sheath, staphyloma, triangle.*

Scatchard, George, U.S. chemist and biochemist, 1892–1973. SEE S. *plot.*

sca·te·mia (skă-tē'mē-ă). Intestinal autointoxication. [scato- + G. *haima,* blood]

⬧ **scato-.** Feces. SEE ALSO copro-, sterco-. [G. *skōr (skat-),* excrement]

scat·o·log·ic (skat-ō-loj'ik). Pertaining to scatology.

sca·tol·o·gy (skă-tol'o-jē). **1.** The scientific study and analysis of feces, for physiologic and diagnostic purposes. SYN coprology. **2.** The study relating to the psychiatric aspects of excrement or excremental (anal) function. [scato- + G. *logos,* study]

sca·to·ma (ska-tō'mă). SYN coproma. [scato- + G. *-oma,* tumor]

sca·toph·a·gy (skă-tof'ă-jē). SYN coprophagia. [scato- + G. *phagō,* to eat]

sca·tos·co·py (skă-tos'kŏ-pē). Examination of the feces for purposes of diagnosis. [scato- + G. *skopeō,* to view]

scat·ter (skat'er). **1.** A change in direction of a photon or subatomic particle, as the result of a collision or interaction. **2.** The secondary radiation resulting from the interaction of primary radiation with matter.

Compton s., the mechanism of s. called the Compton effect scintillator.

liquid s., a liquid with the properties of a scintillator, in which the substance whose radioactivity is to be measured can be dissolved and placed in a well counter.

scat·ter·gram (skăt-er-gram). Graphical display of distribution of two variables in relation to each other. [scatter + G. *gramma,* something written]

scat·u·la (skat'yū-lă). A square pillbox. [Mediev. L. a rectangular figure whose width is one-tenth of its length]

Sced·os·por·i·um ap·i·o·sper·mum (sked-os-pōr'ē-ŭm ā-pē-os'per-mŭm). The imperfect state of the fungus *Pseudallescheria boydii,* one of the 16 species of true fungi that may cause mycetoma in humans. SYN *Monosporium apiospermum.*

sce·lal·gia (se-lal'jē-ă). Pain in the leg. [G. *skelos,* leg, + *algos,* pain]

scent (sent). SYN odor. [M.E., fr. O.Fr., fr. L. *sentio,* to feel]

Schacher, Polycarp G., German physician, 1674–1737. SEE S.'s *ganglion.*

Schaer's re·a·gent. See under reagent.

Schafer, Sir Edward A. Sharpey-, English physiologist and histologist, 1850–1935. SEE Schäfer's *method.*

Schäffer, Max, German neurologist, 1852–1923. SEE S.'s *reflex.*

Schaffer's test. See under test.

Schamberg, Jay F., U.S. dermatologist, 1870–1934. SEE S.'s *dermatitis.*

Schanz, Alfred, German orthopedic surgeon, 1868–1931. SEE S. *syndrome.*

Schapiro, Heinrich, Russian physician, 1852–1901. SEE S.'s *sign.*

Schardinger, Franz, 19th century Austrian scientist. SEE S. *dextrins,* under *dextrin, enzyme, reaction.*

schar·lach red (shar'lak). SYN scarlet red.

Schat·zki, Richard, U.S. radiologist, 1901–1992. SEE Schatzki's *ring.*

Schaudinn, Fritz R., German bacteriologist, 1871–1906. SEE S.'s *fixative.*

Schaumann, Jörgen, Swedish physician, 1879–1953. SEE S. *bodies,* under *body;* S.'s *lymphogranuloma, syndrome;* Besnier-Boeck-S. *disease, syndrome.*

Schaumberg, H.H., U.S. neuropathologist, *1912.

Schauta, Friedrich, Austrian gynecologist, 1849–1919. SEE S. vaginal *operation.*

Schede, Max, German surgeon, 1844–1902. SEE S.'s *clot, method.*

sched·ule (sked′jūl). A procedural plan for a proposed objective, especially the sequence and time allotted for each item or operation required for its completion. [L. *scheda,* fr. *scida,* a strip of papyrus, leaf of paper]
  s.'s of reinforcement, in the psychology of conditioning, established procedures or sequences for reinforcing operant behavior; *e.g.,* in a lever pressing situation, every displacement of the lever will bring a pellet of food or comparable reinforcer (**continuous reinforcement s.**), or the reinforcer will come at every 5 seconds, regardless of how many displacements occur earlier (**fixed-interval reinforcement s.**), at every 10th displacement (**fixed-ratio reinforcement s.**), or on an average of every 5 seconds (**variable-interval reinforcement s.**), or the reinforcer will come in a noncontinuous fashion in which less than 100% of the displacements bring a reinforcer (**intermittent reinforcement s.**).

Scheele, Karl W., Swedish chemist, 1742–1786. SEE S.'s *green.*

Scheibe's deaf·ness. See under deafness.

Scheibler's re·a·gent. See under reagent.

Scheie, Harold G., U.S. ophthalmologist, *1909. SEE S.'s *syndrome.*

Scheiner, Christoph, German physicist, 1575–1650. SEE S.'s *experiment.*

Schellong, Fritz, German physician, 1891–1953. SEE S. *test;* S.-Strisower *phenomenon.*

sche·ma, pl. **sche·ma·ta** (skē′mă, skē-mah′tă). **1.** A plan, outline, or arrangement. SYN scheme. **2.** In sensorimotor theory, the organized unit of cognitive experience. [G. *schēma,* shape, form]
  body s., SYN body *image.*

sche·mat·ic (skē-mat′ik). Made after a definite type of formula; representing in general, but not with absolute exactness; denoting an anatomical drawing or model. [G. *schēmatikos,* in outward show, fr. *schēma,* shape, form]

sche·mat·o·graph (skē-mat′ō-graf). An instrument for making a tracing in reduced size of the outline of the body. [G. *schēma,* form, + *graphō,* to write]

scheme (skēm). SYN schema (1).
  occlusal s., SYN occlusal *system.*

sche·mo·chromes (skē-mō-krōmz). SYN structural *color.*

Schenck, Benjamin R., U.S. surgeon, 1873–1920. SEE S.'s *disease.*

Scheuermann, Holger W., Danish surgeon, 1877–1960. SEE S.'s *disease.*

Schick, Bela, Austrian pediatrician in U.S., 1877–1967. SEE S. *method, test,* test *toxin.*

Schiff, Hugo, German chemist in Florence, 1834–1915. SEE S. *base;* S.'s *reagent;* Kasten's fluorescent S. *reagents,* under *reagent;* periodic acid-S. *stain;* ninhydrin-S. *stain* for proteins.

Schiff, Moritz, German physiologist, 1823–1896. SEE S.-Sherrington *phenomenon.*

Schilder, Paul Ferdinand, Austrian neurologist, 1886–1940.

Schiller, Walter, Austrian pathologist in U.S., 1887–1960. SEE S.'s *test.*

Schilling, Victor, German hematologist, 1883–1960. SEE S.'s *blood count,* band *cell, index;* S. *test,* type of monocytic *leukemia.*

schin·dy·le·sis (skin-dī-lē′sis) [NA]. SYN wedge-and-groove joint. [G. *schindylēsis,* splintering]

Schiötz, Hjalmar, Norwegian physician, 1850–1927. SEE S. *tonometer.*

Schirmer, Otto W.A., German ophthalmologist, 1864–1917. SEE S. *test.*

△**schisto-.** Cleft, division. SEE ALSO schizo-. [G. *schistos,* split]

schis·to·ce·lia (skis-tō-sē′lē-ă). Congenital fissure of the abdominal wall. [schisto- + G. *koilia,* a hollow]

schis·to·cor·mia (skis-tō-kōr′mē-ă). Congenital clefting of the trunk, the lower extremities of the fetus usually being imperfectly developed. SYN schistosomia. [schisto- + G. *kormos,* trunk of a tree]

schis·to·cys·tis (skis-tō-sis′tis). Fissure of the bladder. [schisto- + G. *kystis,* bladder]

schis·to·cyte (skis′tō-sīt). A variety of poikilocyte that owes its abnormal shape to fragmentation occurring as the cell flows through damaged small vessels. SYN schizocyte. [schisto- + G. *kytos,* cell]

schis·to·cy·to·sis (skis′tō-sī-tō′sis). The occurrence of many schistocytes in the blood. SYN schizocytosis.

schis·to·glos·sia (skis-tō-glos′ē-ă). Congenital fissure or cleft of the tongue. [schisto- + G. *glōssa,* tongue]

schis·to·me·lia (skis′tō-mel′ē-ă). Congenital cleft of a limb.

schis·tor·rha·chis (skis-tōr′ă-kis). SYN *spina* bifida. [schisto- + G. *rhachis,* spine]

Schis·to·so·ma (skis-tō-sō′mă). A genus of digenetic trematodes, including the important blood flukes of man and domestic animals, that cause schistosomiasis; characterized by elongate shape, by separate sexes with marked sexual dimorphism, by their unusual location in the smaller blood vessels of their host, and by utilization of water snails as intermediate hosts. [schisto- + G. *sōma,* body]
  S. bo′vis, a species infecting cattle, buffalo, sheep, goats, and wild ruminants in Africa, the Middle East, southern Europe, and Asia; characterized by long spindle-shaped eggs with a terminal spine.
  S. haemato′bium, the vesical blood fluke, a species with terminally spined eggs that occurs as a parasite in the portal system and mesenteric veins of the bladder (causing human schistosomiasis haematobium) and rectum; common in the Nile delta but is found along waterways, irrigation ditches, or streams throughout Africa and in parts of the Middle East; the intermediate host is *Bulinus truncatus* in Egypt; elsewhere, other snails of the subfamily Bulininae (*Bulinus, Physopsis, Pyrgophysa*) are involved.
  S. in′dicum, a species that occurs in the portal and mesenteric veins of cattle, sheep, goats, horses, and camels in Indo-Pakistan.
  S. intercala′tum, a blood fluke species related to *S. haematobium* locally distributed in Zaire and other areas of central Africa, causing mild dysentery and abdominal pains, with enlargement of the spleen and liver; a planorbid snail, *Bulinus (Physopis) africanus,* serves as the intermediate host.
  S. japon′icum, the Oriental or Japanese blood fluke, a species having eggs with small lateral spines, usually only a small knob; causes schistosomiasis japonica, with extensive pathology from encapsulation of the eggs, particularly in the liver, and is the most pathogenic of the three common schistosome species afflicting man, possibly owing to greater egg production per female worm; it is also the most intractable to treatment and the most difficult to control, as the intermediate hosts are amphibious snails (species of *Oncomelania,* family Hydrobiidae) that can leave the water to avoid molluscicides, and also because many other animals, such as pigs, oxen, cattle, and dogs, serve as reservoir hosts.
  S. malayensis, a member of the *S. japonicum* complex described from the rodent *Rattus muelleri* in peninsular Malaysia. The aquatic snail *Robertsiella kaporensis* and two other species of this genus were found to be naturally infected. *S. malayensis* is considered most closely related to *S. mekongi.* Human infections, based on serological evidence, were reported among the indigenous people of central peninsular Malaysia.
  S. manso′ni, a common species characterized by large eggs with a strong lateral spine and transmitted by planorbid snails of the genus *Biomphalaria;* causes schistosomiasis mansoni in man in Africa, parts of the Middle East, and West Indies, South America, and certain Caribbean islands.
  S. mat′theei, a species found in the portal and mesenteric veins

sc

of ruminants, primates (including man), zebra, and rodents in Africa.

S. mekon′gi, the Mekong schistosome, a species described from the Mekong delta near Khong Island in southern Laos and northern Cambodia. Infection rates are highest for ages 7 to 15; dogs appear to be the chief reservoir host; the intermediate host snail is the 3 mm-long operculid snail, *Tricula aperta.* Pathology is similar to but generally less severe than that of *S. japonicum.*

S. spinda′le, a species parasitic in the portal and mesenteric veins of ruminants, and occasionally horses and dogs, in Africa, Indo-Pakistan, and Southeast Asia.

schis·to·some (skis′tō-sōm). Common name for a member of the genus *Schistosoma.*

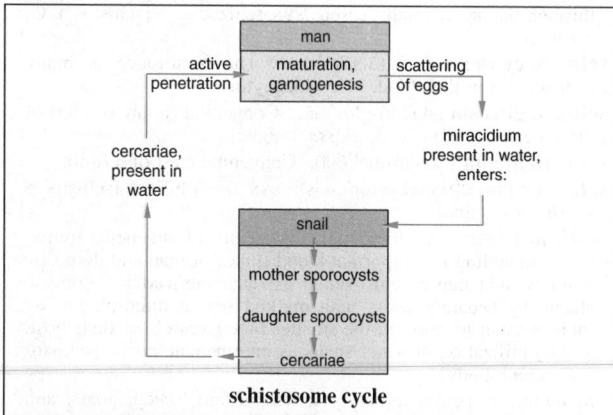

schistosome cycle

schis·to·so·mia (skis-tō-sō′mē-ă). SYN schistocormia. [schisto- + G. *sōma,* body]

schis·to·so·mi·a·sis (skis′tō-sō-mī′ă-sis). Infection with a species of *Schistosoma;* manifestations of this often chronic and debilitating disease vary with the infecting species but depend in large measure upon tissue reaction (granulation and fibrosis) to the eggs deposited in venules and in the hepatic portals, the latter resulting in portal hypertension and esophageal varices, as well as liver damage leading to cirrhosis. SEE tropical *diseases,* under *disease.* SEE ALSO schistosomal *dermatitis,* Symmers' clay pipestem *fibrosis.* SYN bilharziasis, bilharziosis, hemic distomiasis, snail fever.

Asiatic s., SYN s. japonica.

bladder s., SYN s. haematobium.

cutaneous s. japonica, SYN s. japonica.

ectopic s., a clinical form of s. that occurs outside of the normal site of parasitism (mesenteric vein or hepatic portals); may result from accidental blood-borne transport of schistosome eggs or, rarely, adult worms, to various unusual sites such as the skin, brain, or spinal cord.

s. haemato′bium, infection with *Schistosoma haematobium,* the eggs of which invade the urinary tract, causing cystitis and hematuria, and possibly an increased likelihood of bladder cancer. SYN bladder s., Egyptian hematuria, endemic hematuria, urinary s.

s. intercalatum, infection with *Schistosoma intercalatum;* occurs only in West Africa; few symptoms reported and no cases of hepatic fibrosis known.

intestinal s., SYN s. mansoni.

s. japon′ica, Japanese s., infection with *Schistosoma japonicum,* characterized by dysenteric symptoms, painful enlargement of the liver and spleen, dropsy, urticaria, and progressive anemia. SYN Asiatic s., cutaneous s. japonica, kabure itch, kabure, Katayama syndrome, Kinkiang fever, Oriental s., rice itch, urticarial fever, Yangtze Valley fever.

s. manso′ni, infection with *Schistosoma mansoni,* the eggs of which invade the wall of the large intestine and the liver, causing irritation, inflammation, and ultimately fibrosis. SYN intestinal s., Manson's disease, Manson's s.

Manson's s., SYN s. mansoni.

s. mekon′gi, infection with *Schistosoma mekongi,* which chiefly afflicts children in the Mekong delta, where it was discovered; the disease is similar to s. japonica.

Oriental s., SYN s. japonica.

pulmonary s., pulmonary manifestations of infection with *schistosoma,* usually *Schistosoma mansoni,* occurring when schistosomals, which form in the skin from the cercariae which have entered from infected water, migrate via the blood stream to the lungs, en route to the gastrointestinal tract and the portal vein; symptoms are usually limited to cough.

urinary s., SYN s. haematobium.

schis·to·som·u·lum, pl. **schis·to·som·u·la** (skis-tō-sō′myū-lŭm, -lă). The stage in the life cycle of a blood fluke of the genus *Schistosoma* immediately after penetration of the skin as a cercaria; marked by loss of the tail and gaining of physiological modifications allowing it to survive in a mammalian bloodstream.

schis·to·ster·nia (skis-tō-ster′nē-ă). SYN schistothorax. [schisto- + G. *sternon,* sternum]

schis·to·tho·rax (skis-tō-thōr′aks). Congenital cleft of the chest wall. SYN schistosternia. [schisto- + G. *thōrax,* thorax]

△ **schiz-.** SEE schizo-.

schiz·am·ni·on (skiz-am′nē-on). An amnion developing, as in the human embryo, by the formation of a cavity within the inner cell mass. [schiz- + amnion]

schiz·ax·on (skiz-ak′son). An axon divided into two branches. [schiz- + G. *axōn,* axis]

schiz·en·ceph·aly (skiz-en-sef′ă-lē). Abnormal divisions or clefts of the brain substance. [schiz- + G. *enkephalos,* brain]

△ **schizo-, schiz-.** Split, cleft, division; schizophrenia. SEE ALSO schisto-. [G. *schizō,* to split or cleave]

schiz·o·af·fec·tive (skiz′ō-ă-fek′tiv). Having an admixture of symptoms suggestive of both schizophrenia and affective (mood) disorder.

schiz·o·cyte (skiz′ō-sĭt). SYN schistocyte. [schizo- + G. *kytos,* cell]

schiz·o·cy·to·sis (skiz′ō-sī-tō′sis). SYN schistocytosis.

schiz·o·gen·e·sis (skiz-ō-jen′ĕ-sis). Reproduction by fission. SYN fissiparity, scissiparity. [schizo- + G. *genesis,* origin]

schi·zog·o·ny (ski-zog′ō-nē). Multiple fission in which the nucleus first divides and then the cell divides into as many parts as there are nuclei; called merogony if daughter cells are merozoites, sporogony if daughter cells are sporozoites, or gametogony if daughter cells are gametes. SYN agamocytogeny. [schizo- + G. *gonē,* generation]

schiz·o·gy·ria (skiz-ō-jī′rē-ă, -jir′ē-ă). Deformity of the cerebral convolutions marked by occasional interruptions of their continuity. [schizo- + G. *gyros,* circle (convolution)]

schiz·oid (skiz′oyd). Socially isolated, withdrawn, having few (if any) friends or social relationships; resembling the personality features characteristic of schizophrenia, but in a milder form. SEE ALSO schizoid *personality.* [schizo(phrenia), + G. *eidos,* resemblance]

schiz·oid·ism (skiz′oy-dizm). A schizoid state; the manifestation of schizoid tendencies.

schiz·o·my·cete (skiz′ō-mī-sēt). A member of the class Schizomycetes; a bacterium.

Schiz·o·my·ce·tes (skiz′ō-mī-sē′tēz). Naegeli's term for a class comprised of all the bacteria; a misnomer, since bacteria are generally not considered to be fungi. The bacteria are now classified in the kingdom Prokaryotae. SYN fission fungi. [schizo- + G. *mykēs,* fungus]

schiz·o·my·cet·ic (skiz-ō-mī-sē′tik). Relating to or caused by fission fungi (bacteria).

schiz·o·my·co·sis (skiz-ō-mī-kō′sis). Any schizomycetic or bacterial disease.

schiz·ont (skiz′ont). A sporozoan trophozoite (vegetative form) that reproduces by schizogony, producing a varied number of daughter trophozoites or merozoites. SEE ALSO meront, segmenter. SYN agamont, segmenting body. [schizo- + G. *ōn (ont-),* a being]

schi·zon·ti·cide (ski-zon'ti-sīd). An agent that kills schizonts. [schizont + L. *caedo*, to kill]

schiz·o·nych·ia (skiz-ō-nik'ē-ă). Splitting of the nails. [schizo- + G. *onyx*, nail]

schiz·o·pha·sia (skiz-ō-fā'zē-ă). The disordered speech (word salad) of the schizophrenic individual. [schizo- + G. *phasis*, speech]

schiz·o·phre·nia (skiz-ō-frē'nē-ă, skit'sō-). A term, coined by Bleuler, synonymous with and replacing dementia praecox; a common type of psychosis, characterized by a disorder in perception, content of thought, and thought processes (hallucinations and delusions), and extensive withdrawal of the individual's interest from other people and the outside world, and the investment of it in his own; now considered a group or spectrum of schizophrenic disorders rather than as a single entity, with distinction sometimes made between process s. and reactive s. Although there seem to be well-defined autosomal dominant forms [MIM*181500-*181510], in the absence of a well-defined mechanism (biochemical or at least psychopathologic model) such claims will continue to be taken with reservation. SYN depersonalization disorder. [schizo- + G. *phrēn*, mind]

> During the 1940s, schizophrenia was thought to be induced in children by family interactions. For a time, the focus was on the schizophrenia-causing (schizophrenogenic) mother, thought to be domineering and destructive of the child's psychosexual development. This hypothesis was abandoned when evidence failed to support it. Current theory views schizophrenia as brain-based, possibly involving abnormalities in neuronal networks and biochemical imbalances, which may be developmental or genetic. It remains the most prevalent of the psychoses, although men and women alike run only a 1% chance of developing the disorder in their lifetimes. Those who experience schizophrenic ideation for less than 6 months, on a one-time basis with full recovery of normal thought patterns, are said to be suffering from a schizophreniform disorder, which may or may not be related causally to other schizophrenias.

acute s., a disorder in which the symptoms of s. occur abruptly; they may subside or become chronic over time. SYN acute schizophrenic episode.

ambulatory s., a milder form of s. in which the patient is capable of maintaining himself or herself in society and need not be hospitalized.

catatonic s., s. characterized by marked disturbance, which may involve stupor, negativism, rigidity, excitement, or posturing; sometimes there is rapid alteration between the extremes of excitement and stupor. Associated features include stereotypic behavior, mannerisms, and waxy flexibility; mutism is particularly common.

childhood s., SYN infantile *autism*.

disorganized s., a severe form of s. characterized by the predominance of incoherence, blunted, inappropriate or silly affect, and the absence of systematized delusions. SYN hebephrenic s.

hebephrenic s., SYN disorganized s.

latent s., a preexisting susceptibility for developing overt s. under strong emotional stress.

paranoid s., s. characterized predominantly by delusions of persecution and megalomania.

process s., an obsolete term for those forms of severe schizophrenic disorders in which chronic and progressive biologic conditions in the brain are considered to be the primary cause and in which prognosis is poor as well, with insidious onset at a young age, as contrasted with reactive s.

pseudoneurotic s., s. in which the underlying psychotic process is masked by complaints ordinarily regarded as neurotic.

reactive s., those forms of severe schizophrenic disorders which are distinguished from process s. by their more acute onset, greater relation to environmental stress, and better prognosis.

residual s., blunted or inappropriate affect, social withdrawal, eccentric behavior, or loose associations, but without prominent psychotic symptoms, as the remains of former psychotic symptoms of s.

simple s., s. characterized by withdrawal, apathy, indifference, and impoverishment of human relationships without overt psychotic features.

schiz·o·phren·ic (skiz-ō-fren'ik, -frē'nik, skit-sō-). Relating to, characteristic of, or suffering from one of the schizophrenias.

schiz·o·the·mia (skiz-ō-thē'mē-ă). Rarely used term for repeated interruptions in a conversation by the speaker introducing other topics. [schizo- + G. *thema*, theme]

schiz·o·to·nia (skiz-ō-tō'nē-ă). Division of the distribution of tone in the muscles. [schizo- + G. *tonos*, tension, tone]

schiz·o·trich·ia (skiz-ō-trik'ē-ă). A splitting of the hairs at their ends. SYN scissura pilorum. [schizo- + G. *thrix*, hair]

Schiz·o·tryp·a·num cru·zi (skiz-ō-trī'pan-ŭm krū'zī). A distinct generic designation used for *Trypanosoma cruzi*, used frequently by workers in the endemic area of South American trypanosomiasis; also used as a subgeneric designation, *i.e., Trypanosoma (Schizotrypanum) cruzi*. [schizo- + G. *trypanon*, a borer, an auger]

schiz·o·zo·ite (skiz-ō-zō'īt). A merozoite prior to schizogony, as in the exoerythrocytic phase of the development of the *Plasmodium* agent after sporozoite invasion of the hepatocyte and before multiple division. [schizo- + G. *zōon*, animal]

schlamm·fie·ber (shlăm'fē-ber). Name given to an outbreak of leptospirosis near Breslau in Germany thought to have been due to infection with *Leptospira grippotyphosa*.

Schlatter, Carl, Swiss surgeon, 1864–1934. SEE Osgood-S. *disease*.

Schlemm, Friedrich, German anatomist, 1795–1858. SEE S.'s *canal*.

Schlesinger, Hermann, Austrian physician, 1868–1934. SEE S.'s *sign;* Pool-S. *sign*.

schlieren (schlēr'en). SEE schlieren *optics*.

Schmid, Rudi, Swiss-U.S. internist and biochemist, *1922. SEE McArdle-S.-Pearson *disease*.

Schmid, W. SEE S.-Fraccaro *syndrome*.

Schmidel, Kasimir C., German anatomist, 1718–1792. SEE S.'s *anastomoses*, under *anastomosis*.

Schmidt, Gerhard, U.S. biochemist, *1900. SEE S.-Thannhauser *method*.

Schmidt, Henry D., U.S. anatomist and pathologist, 1823–1888. SEE S.-Lanterman *clefts*, under *cleft*, *incisures*, under *incisure*.

Schmidt, Johann F.M., German laryngologist, 1838–1907. SEE S.'s *syndrome*.

Schmidt, Martin Benno, German physician, 1863–1949. SEE S.'s *syndrome*.

Schmorl, Christian G., German pathologist, 1861–1932. SEE S.'s *bacillus, nodule*, ferric-ferricyanide reduction *stain*, picrothionin *stain, jaundice*.

Schneider, C.V., German anatomist, 1614–1680. SEE schneiderian *membrane*.

Schneider, Franz C., German chemist, 1813–1897. SEE S.'s *carmine*.

Schneider, Kurt, 20th century German psychiatrist.

Schnei·der·sitz (shnī'der-zitz). A typical sitting position with legs crossed in front, exhibited by severely defective patients with phenylketonuria and resembling the position which was commonly attributed to tailors. [Ger.]

Scholander, Per F., Norwegian physiologist, 1905–1980. SEE S. *apparatus;* Roughton-S. *apparatus, syringe*.

Scholz, Willibald, German neurologist, *1889. SEE S.'s *disease*.

Schönbein, Christian F., German chemist, 1799–1868. SEE S.'s *test*.

Schönlein, Johann L., German physician, 1793–1864. SEE S.'s *disease, purpura;* Henoch-S. *purpura*.

school (skūl). A set of beliefs, teachings, methods, etc. [O. E. *scōl*]

biometrical s., a group of British geneticists, followers of Galton and Karl Pearson, whose approach to genetics was quantitative rather than enumerative.

dogmatic s., ancient Greek s. or tradition in medicine whose members were the successors to or followers of Hippocrates; they based their conceptions of disease upon the humoral theory and their practice upon experience and sound reasoning, and were comparatively free from fads, speculative theories, and dogma, which the term dogmatic falsely implies.

dynamic s., a group of theorists founded by Stahl, who professed the belief that all vital action is the result of an internal force independent of anything external to the body.

hippocratic s., the followers of the teachings of Hippocrates. SEE ALSO dogmatic s.

iatromathematical s., a group of academicians, of whom Descartes was one of the foremost proponents, who maintained that all physiologic processes were the result of physical laws. SYN mechanistic s.

mechanistic s., SYN iatromathematical s.

Schott, Theodor, 1850–1921, German physician in Bad Nauheim. SEE S. *treatment.*

Schottmueller, Hugo A.G., German physician, 1867–1936. SEE S.'s *bacillus, disease.*

schra·dan (schrā′dan). C₈H₂₄N₄O₃P₂; a potent irreversible organophosphate cholinesterase inhibitor used as an insecticide. It was prepared for potential use as a nerve gas. Poisoning produces a cholinergic crisis which can be fatal. SYN octamethyl pyrophosphoramide. [Gerhard *Schrader,* Ger. chemist, + -an]

Schreger, Christian H.T., German anatomist and chemist, 1768–1833. SEE S.'s *lines,* under *line;* Hunter-S. *bands,* under *band, lines,* under *line.*

Schridde, Hermann, German pathologist, *1875. SEE S.'s cancer *hairs,* under *hair.*

Schroeder, Karl L.E., German gynecologist, 1838–1887. SEE S.'s *operation.*

Schuchardt, Karl A., German surgeon, 1856–1901. SEE S.'s *operation.*

Schüffner, Wilhelm, German pathologist in Sumatra, 1867–1949. SEE S.'s *granules,* under *granule, dots,* under *dot.*

Schüller, Artur, Austrian neurologist, *1874. SEE S.'s *disease, phenomenon, syndrome;* Hand-S.-Christian *disease.*

Schüller, Karl H.L.A. Max, German surgeon, 1843–1907. SEE S.'s *ducts,* under *duct.*

Schultes, Johann. SEE Scultetus.

Schultz, Arthur R.H., German physician, *1890. SEE S. *reaction, stain.*

Schultz, Werner, German internist, 1878–1947. SEE S.-Charlton *phenomenon, reaction;* S.-Dale *reaction.*

Schultze, Bernhard, German obstetrician, 1827–1919. SEE S.'s *fold, mechanism, phantom, placenta.*

Schultze, Max J., German histologist and zoologist, 1825–1874. SEE S.'s *cells,* under *cell, membrane, sign;* comma *bundle* of S.; comma *tract* of S.

Schütz, Erich, German biochemist, *1902. SEE S.'s *law;* S. *rule.*

Schütz, Hugo, 19th century German anatomist. SEE S.'s *bundle.*

Schwabach, Dagobert, German otologist, 1846–1920. SEE S. *test.*

Schwalbe, Gustav A., German anatomist, 1844–1916. SEE S.'s *corpuscle, nucleus, ring, spaces,* under *space.*

Schwann, Theodor, German histologist and physiologist, 1810–1882. SEE S. *cells,* under *cell,* cell *unit;* S.'s white *substance;* sheath of S.

schwan·no·ma (shwah-nō′mă). A benign, encapsulated neoplasm in which the fundamental component is structurally identical to a syncytium of Schwann cells; the neoplastic cells proliferate within the endoneurium, and the perineurium forms the capsule. The neoplasm may originate from a peripheral or sympathetic nerve, or from various cranial nerves, particularly the eighth nerve; when the nerve is small, it is usually found (if at all) in the capsule of the neoplasm; if the nerve is large, the s. may develop within the sheath of the nerve, the fibers of which may then spread over the surface of the capsule as the neoplasm

enlarges. Microscopically, s.'s are composed of combinations of two cell types, Antoni types A and B (see below), either of which may be predominant in various examples of s.'s. SEE ALSO neurofibroma. SYN neurilemoma, neuroschwannoma. [Theodor *Schwann* + -oma]

acoustic s., a benign neoplasm of the intracranial segment of the eighth cranial nerve, producing cerebellar, lower cranial nerve, and brainstem signs and symptoms. SYN acoustic neuroma, cerebellopontine angle tumor, eighth nerve tumor.

schwan·no·sis (shwah-nō′sis). A non-neoplastic proliferation of Schwann cells in the perivascular spaces of the spinal cord; seen particularly in older patients, especially those with diabetes mellitus.

Schwartz, Henry, U.S. neurosurgeon, *1909. SEE S. *tractotomy.*

Schwartz, Oscar, U.S. pediatrician, *1919. SEE S. *syndrome.*

Schwartz. S., U.S. physician, born 1916, Research Professor of Medicine at the university of Minnesota.

Schweigger-Seidel, Franz, German physiologist, 1834–1871. SEE *sheath* of Schweigger-Seidel.

Schweninger, Ernst, German dermatologist, 1850–1924. SEE S.-Buzzi *anetoderma;* S.'s *method.*

sci·age (sē-ahzh′). A to-and-fro, sawlike movement of the hand in massage. [Fr. *scie,* saw]

sci·at·ic (sī-at′ik). **1.** Relating to or situated in the neighborhood of the ischium or hip. Ischial or sciatic. SYN ischiadic, ischial, ischiatic. **2.** Relating to sciatica. SYN ischiadicus [NA]. [Mediev. L. *sciaticus,* a corruption of G. *ischiadikos,* fr. *ischion,* the hip joint]

sci·at·i·ca (sī-at′i-kă). Pain in the lower back and hip radiating down the back of the thigh into the leg, initially attributed to sciatic nerve dysfunction (hence the term), but now known to usually be due to herniated lumbar disk compromising the L5 or S1 root. SYN Cotunnius disease, sciatic neuralgia, sciatic neuritis. [see sciatic]

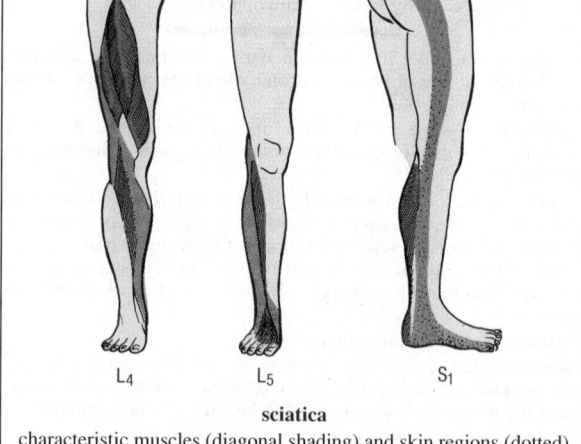

sciatica
characteristic muscles (diagonal shading) and skin regions (dotted) for nerve roots L₄, L₅ and S₁

SCID Abbreviation for severe combined *immunodeficiency.*

SCID mice Abbreviation for severe combined immunodeficient mice.

sci·ence (sī′ens). **1.** The branch of knowledge that produces theoretical explanations of natural phenomena based on experiments and observations. **2.** An area of such knowledge that is restricted to explaining a limited class of phenomena. [L. *scientia,* knowledge, fr. *scio,* to know]

scil·la (sil′ă). SYN squill. [G.]

scil·la·ren (sil′lă-ren). A mixture of glycosides, possessing digitalis-like actions, present in squill.

s. A, a crystalline steroidal glycoside, present in squill (*Scilla* *maritima*), that can be hydrolyzed to glucose and proscillaridin A; the latter can be hydrolyzed to rhamnose and the steroid aglycone scillaridin A; same actions and uses as digitalis glycosides. SYN transvaalin.

s. B, an amorphous glycosidal fraction obtained from squill, consisting of at least seven cardioactive glycosides: glucoscillaren A, scillipheoside, glucoscillipheoside, scillicryptoside, scilliglaucoside, scillicyanoside, and scillazuroside.

scil·lar·i·cide (sil'ar-ĭ-sīd). A toxic principle from squill used as a rodenticide.

scil·lir·o·side (sil'ir-ō-sīd). Glycoside from red squill, the red variety of *Urginea maritima* (family Liliaceae). Used as a rodenticide.

scin·ti·cis·tern·og·ra·phy (sin'ti-sis-tern-og'ră-fē). Cisternography performed with a radiopharmaceutical and recorded with a stationary imaging device.

scin·ti·gram (sin'ti-gram). SYN scintiscan. [L. *scintilla*, spark, + G. *gramma*, something written]

scin·ti·graph·ic (sin'ti-graf'ik). Relating to or obtained by scintigraphy.

scin·tig·ra·phy (sin-tig'ră-fē). A diagnostic procedure consisting of the administration of a radionuclide with an affinity for the organ or tissue of interest, followed by recording the distribution of the radioactivity with a stationary or scanning external scintillation camera. SEE gamma *camera*.

scin·til·la·scope (sin-til'ă-skōp). Obsolete term for scintillation *counter*. [L. *scintilla*, spark, + G. *skopeō*, to observe]

scin·til·la·tion (sin-ti-lā'shŭn). **1.** Flashing or sparkling; a subjective sensation as of sparks or flashes of light. **2.** In radiation measurement, the light produced by an ionizing event in a phosphor, as in a crystal or liquid scintillator. SEE ALSO scintillation *counter*. [L. *scintilla*, a spark]

scin·til·la·tor (sin'ti-lā-ter, -tōr). A substance that emits visible light when hit by a subatomic particle or x- or gamma ray. SEE ALSO scintillation *counter*.

scin·til·lom·e·ter (sin-ti-lom'ĕ-ter). SYN scintillation *counter*. [L. *scintilla*, spark, + G. *metron*, measure]

scin·ti·pho·to·graph (sin-ti-fō'tō-graf). The image obtained by scintiphotography. SEE ALSO scintiscan.

scin·ti·pho·tog·ra·phy (sin'ti-fō-tog'ră-fē). The process of obtaining a photographic recording of the distribution of an internally administered radiopharmaceutical with the use of a gamma camera. SYN scintography.

scin·ti·scan (sin'ti-skan). The record obtained by scintigraphy. SEE ALSO scan. SYN photoscan, scintigram.

scin·ti·scan·ner (sin'ti-skan'er). The apparatus used to make a scintiscan.

scint·og·ra·phy. SYN scintiphotography.

sci·on (sī'on). In experimental embryology, an embryonic tissue or part grafted to another embryo of the same or of another species. SEE ALSO chimera. [O. Fr. *sion*, shoot, sprig, fr. L. *seco*, to cut]

sci·os·o·phy (sī-os'ō-fē). Rarely used term for a system of beliefs that are claimed to be facts but are not supported by scientific data. [G. *skia*, shadow, + *sophia*, wisdom]

scir·rhen·can·this (skir-en-kan'this, sir-en-). Obsolete term for an indurated tumor of the lacrimal gland. [G. *skirrhos*, hard, a hard tumor, + *en*, in, + *kanthos*, canthus]

scir·rhos·i·ty (skir-os'i-tē, sir-). A scirrhous state or hardness of a tumor.

scir·rhous (skir'us, sir'). Hard; relating to a scirrhus.

scir·rhus (skir'ŭs, sir'). Obsolete term for any fibrous indurated area, especially an indurated carcinoma. [G. *skirrhos*, hard, a hard tumor]

scis·sion (sizh'ŭn). **1.** A separation, division, or splitting, as in fission. **2.** SYN cleavage (2). [L. *scissio*, fr. *scindo*, pp. *scissus*, to cleave]

scis·si·par·i·ty (sis-i-par'i-tē). SYN schizogenesis. [L. *scissio*, cleavage, + *pario*, to bring forth]

scis·sors (siz'erz). An instrument with two blades, moving on a

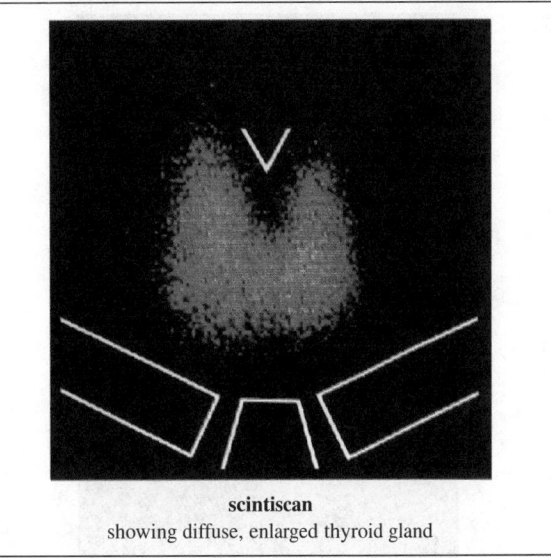

scintiscan
showing diffuse, enlarged thyroid gland

pivot, that cut against each other. SYN shears. [L. *scindo*, pp. *scissus*, to cut]

de Wecker's s., a small s. with sharp points for intraocular cutting of the iris and lens capsule.

Smellie's s., obsolete term for lance-pointed shears, with external cutting edges, used for fetal craniotomy.

scis·sors-shad·ow. A distorted image seen in mixed astigmatism by retinoscopy.

scis·su·ra, pl. **scis·su·rae** (si-sū'ră, -rē). **1.** Cleft or fissure. **2.** A splitting. SYN scissure. [L.]

s. pilo'rum, SYN schizotrichia.

scis·sure (sish'ūr). SYN scissura.

△scler-. SEE sclero-.

scle·ra, pl. **scle·ras, scler·ae** (sklēr'ă, -ăz, -ē) [NA]. A portion of the fibrous tunic forming the outer envelope of the eye, except for its anterior sixth, which is the cornea. SYN sclerotic coat, sclerotica, tunica albuginea oculi, tunica sclerotica. [Mod. L. fr. G. *sklēros*, hard]

blue s.,

scler·ad·e·ni·tis (sklēr'ad-ĕ-nī'tis). Inflammatory induration of a gland. [scler- + G. *adēn*, gland, + *-itis*, inflammation]

scle·ral (sklēr'ăl). Relating to the sclera. SYN sclerotic (2).

scle·ra·tog·e·nous (sklēr-ă-toj'ĕ-nŭs). SYN sclerogenous.

scle·rec·ta·sia (sklēr-ek-tā'zē-ă). Localized bulging of the sclera. SYN scleral ectasia. [scler- + G. *ektasis*, an extension]

partial s., partial protrusion of a portion of the sclera, typically seen in severe myopia. SEE staphyloma.

total s., uniform stretching of the entire sclera, typically seen in buphthalmos.

scle·rec·to·my (sklĕ-rek'tō-mē). **1.** Excision of a portion of the

sc

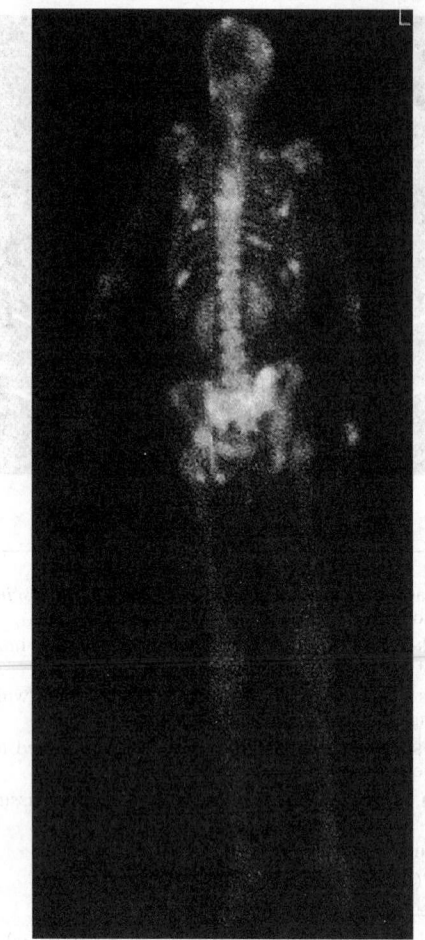

scintiphotography
multiple metastases in a patient with breast cancer

sclera. **2.** Removal of the fibrous adhesions formed in chronic otitis media. [scler- + G. *ektomē,* excision]

scle·re·de·ma (sklēr-e-dē′mă). Hard nonpitting edema of the skin of the dorsal aspect of the upper body and extremities, giving a waxy appearance and no sharp demarcation; seen in diabetics and in s. adultorum. [scler- + G. *oidēma,* a swelling (edema)]

s. adulto′rum, a benign spreading induration of the skin and subcutaneous tissue, possibly streptoccocal in origin, that may follow a febrile illness, with thickening of the skin by collagen and mucin deposit appearing first on the head and neck and extending over the trunk; a misnomer, because the disease is not restricted to adults. SYN Buschke's disease (1).

scle·re·ma (sklě-rē′mă). Induration of subcutaneous fat. [scler- + edema]

s. adipo′sum, SYN s. neonatorum.

s. neonato′rum, s. appearing at birth or in early infancy, usually in premature and hypothermic infants, as sharply demarcated and yellowish white indurated plaques that usually involve the cheeks, buttocks, shoulders, and calves; subcutaneous fat has a high proportion of saturated fatty acids; microscopically, there is thickening of interlobular fibrous tissue and formation of triglyceride crystals and foreign body giant cells; prognosis is poor for widespread lesions, but localized lesions may resolve slowly over a period of many months. SYN s. adiposum, Underwood's disease.

scle·ren·ceph·a·ly, scle·ren·ce·pha·lia (sklēr-en-sef′ă-lē, -en-

sě-fā′lē-ă). Sclerosis and shrinkage of the brain substance. [scler- + G. *enkephalos,* brain]

scle·ri·a·sis (sklě-rī′ă-sis). A diffuse, symmetrical scleroderma. [scler- + G. *-iasis,* condition]

scle·ri·tis (sklě-rī′tis). Inflammation of the sclera.

annular s., an often protracted inflammation of the anterior portion of the sclera, forming a ring around the corneoscleral limbus.

anterior s., inflammation of the sclera adjacent to the cornea.

brawny s., a gelatinous-appearing swelling surrounding the cornea with a tendency to involve the periphery of the cornea. SYN gelatinous s.

deep s., severe inflammation of the sclera, with involvement of the underlying uvea.

gelatinous s., SYN brawny s.

malignant s., progressive inflammation of the anterior sclera and adjacent choroid with associated uveitis.

necrotizing s., fibrinoid degeneration and necrosis of the sclera.

nodular s., firm, immobile, single or multiple areas of localized s.

posterior s., inflammation, often monocular, of the sclera adjacent to the optic nerve, with frequent extension to the retina and choroid.

⚠**sclero-, scler-.** Hardness (induration), sclerosis, relationship to sclera. [G. *sklēros,* hard]

scle·ro·at·ro·phy (sklēr-ō-at′rō-fē). SYN sclerotylosis.

scle·ro·blas·te·ma (sklēr-ō-blas-tē′mă). The embryonic tissue entering into the formation of bone. [sclero- + G. *blastēma,* sprout]

scle·ro·cho·roi·dal (sklēr-ō-kō-roy′dăl). Relating to both the sclera and the choroid.

scle·ro·cho·roid·i·tis (sklēr′ō-kō-roy-dī′tis). Inflammation of the sclera and choroid.

s. ante′rior, a secondary inflammation of the sclera by an extension of a process from the uvea.

s. poste′rior, SYN posterior *staphyloma.*

scle·ro·con·junc·ti·val (sklēr′ō-kon-jŭngk-tī′văl). Relating to the sclera and the conjunctiva.

scle·ro·cor·nea (sklēr-ō-kōr′nē-ă). **1.** The cornea and sclera regarded as forming together the hard outer coat of the eye, the fibrous tunic of the eye. **2.** A congenital anomaly in which the whole or part of the cornea is opaque and resembles the sclera; other ocular abnormalities are frequently present.

scle·ro·dac·ty·ly, scle·ro·dac·tyl·ia (sklēr-ō-dak′ti-lē, -dak-til′ē-ă). SYN acrosclerosis. [sclero- + G. *daktylos,* finger or toe]

scle·ro·der·ma (sklēr-ō-der′mă). Thickening and induration of the skin caused by new collagen formation, with atrophy of pilosebaceous follicles; either a manifestation of progressive systemic sclerosis or localized (morphea). SYN dermatosclerosis, sclerosis corii, sclerosis cutanea. [sclero- + G. *derma,* skin]

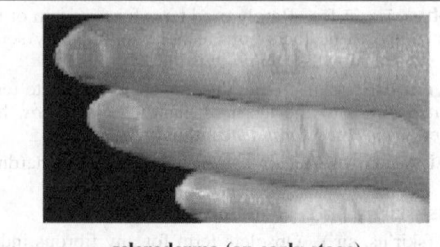

scleroderma (an early stage)

localized s., SYN morphea.

progressive familial s. [MIM*181750], a syndrome characterized by calcinosis cutis, Raynaud's phenomenon, sclerodactyly, and telangiectasia; usually due to s.; autosomal dominant form of progressive systemic sclerosis.

scle·ro·der·ma·ti·tis (sklēr′ō-der-mă-tī′tis). Inflammation and thickening of the skin. [sklero- + G. *derma,* skin + *-itis,* inflammation]

scle·ro·der·ma·tous (sklēr-ō-der′mă-tŭs). Marked by, or resembling, scleroderma.

scle·rog·e·nous, scle·ro·gen·ic (skle-roj′ĕ-nŭs, sklēr-ō-jen′ik). Producing hard or sclerotic tissue; causing sclerosis. SYN scleratogenous. [sclero- + G. *-gen,* producing]

scle·roid (sklēr′oyd). Indurated or sclerotic, of unusually firm texture, leathery, or of scar-like texture. SYN sclerosal, sclerous. [sclero- + G. *eidos,* resemblance]

scle·ro·i·ri·tis (sklēr′ō-ī-rī′tis). Inflammation of both sclera and iris.

scle·ro·ker·a·ti·tis (sklēr′ō-ker-ă-tī′tis). Inflammation of the sclera and cornea. [sclero- + G. *keras,* horn]

scle·ro·ker·a·to·i·ri·tis (sklēr-ō-ker′ă-tō-ī-rī′tis). Inflammation of sclera, cornea, and iris.

scle·ro·ma (skle-rō′mă). A circumscribed indurated focus of granulation tissue in the skin or mucous membrane. [G. *sklērōma,* an induration]

    respiratory s., rhinoscleroma in which the lesion involves the mucous membrane of the greater part or all of the upper respiratory tract.

scle·ro·ma·la·cia (sklēr′ō-mă-lā′shē-ă). Degenerative thinning of the sclera, occurring in persons with rheumatoid arthritis and other collagen disorders. [sclero- + G. *malakia,* a softening]

scle·ro·mere (sklēr′ō-mēr). 1. Any metamere of the skeleton, such as a vertebral segment. 2. Caudal half of a sclerotome. [sclero- + G. *meros,* part]

scle·rom·e·ter (sklē-rom′ĕ-ter). A device for determining the density or hardness of any substance. [sclero- + G. *metron,* measure]

scle·ro·myx·e·de·ma (sklēr′ō-mik-se-dē′mă). Generalized lichen myxedematosus with diffuse thickening of the skin underlying the papules. SYN Arndt-Gottron syndrome.

scle·ro·nych·ia (sklēr-ō-nik′ē-ă). Induration and thickening of the nails. [sclero- + G. *onyx,* nail, + *-ia,* condition]

scle·ro·o·o·pho·ri·tis (sklēr′ō-ō-of′ō-rī′tis). Inflammatory induration of the ovary. [sclero- + Mod. L. *oophoron,* ovary + G. *-itis,* inflammation]

scle·roph·thal·mia (sklēr-of-thal′mē-ă). An abnormality in which most of the normally transparent cornea resembles the opaque sclera. [sclero- + G. *ophthalmos,* eye]

scle·ro·plas·ty (sklēr′ō-plas-tē). Plastic surgery of the sclera. [sclero- + G. *plastos,* formed]

scle·ro·pro·tein (sklēr-ō-prō′tēn). SYN albuminoid (3). SEE ALSO fibrous *protein.*

scle·ro·sal (sklĕ-rō′săl). SYN scleroid.

scle·ro·sant (sklēr′ō-sant). An injectable irritant used to treat varices by producing thrombi in them.

scle·rose (sklĕ-rōz′). To harden; to undergo sclerosis.

scle·ro·sis, pl. **scle·ro·ses** (sklĕ-rō′sis, -sēz). 1. SYN induration (2). 2. In neuropathy, induration of nervous and other structures by a hyperplasia of the interstitial fibrous or glial connective tissue. [G. *sklērōsis,* hardness]

    Alzheimer's s., hyaline degeneration of the medium and smaller blood vessels of the brain.

    amyotrophic lateral s. (ALS), a disease of the motor tracts of the lateral columns and anterior horns of the spinal cord, causing progressive muscular atrophy, increased reflexes, fibrillary twitching, and spastic irritability of muscles; associated with a defect in superoxide dismutase. A number of cases are inherited as an autosomal dominant trait [MIM*105400]. This disorder affects adults, is 90–95% sporadic in nature, and is usually fatal within 2 to 4 years of onset. Variants include progressive spinal muscle atrophy, in which only a lower motor neuron component occurs, and progressive bulbar palsy, in which isolated or predominantly lower brainstem motor involvement is seen. SYN Aran-Duchenne disease, Charcot's disease, creeping palsy, Cruveilhier's disease, Duchenne-Aran disease, Lou Gehrig's disease, muscular trophoneurosis, progressive muscular atrophy, progressive spinal amyotrophy, wasting palsy, wasting paralysis.

arterial s., SYN arteriosclerosis.

arteriocapillary s., arteriosclerosis, especially of the finer vessels.

arteriolar s., SYN arteriolosclerosis.

bone s., SYN eburnation.

Canavan's s., SYN Canavan's *disease.*

central areolar choroidal s., SYN areolar *choroidopathy.*

combined s., SYN subacute combined *degeneration* of the spinal cord.

s. co′rii, SYN scleroderma.

s. cuta′nea, SYN scleroderma.

diffuse infantile familial s., SYN globoid cell *leukodystrophy.*

disseminated s., SYN multiple s.

endocardial s., **(1)** SYN endocardial *fibroelastosis* (1). **(2)** SYN endocardial *fibrosis.*

focal s., SYN multiple s.

glomerular s., SYN glomerulosclerosis.

hippocampal s., a loss of cortical neurons and a reactive astrocytosis in the hippocampal regions of some persons with epilepsy.

idiopathic hypercalcemic s. of infants, SEE idiopathic *hypercalcemia* of infants.

insular s., SYN multiple s.

laminar cortical s., a degeneration of nerve fibers in the corona radiata in a laminar pattern.

lateral spinal s., SYN primary lateral s.

lobar s., SYN Pick's *atrophy.*

mantle s., a common cerebral lesion in the palsied states of early life characterized by nodular cortical atrophy.

menstrual s., SYN physiologic s.

Mönckeberg's s., SYN Mönckeberg's *arteriosclerosis.*

multiple s. (MS), common demyelinating disorder of the central nervous system, causing patches of sclerosis (plaques) in the brain and spinal cord; occurs primarily in young adults, and has protean clinical manifestations, depending upon the location and size of the plaque; typical symptoms include visual loss, diplopia, nystagmus, dysarthria, weakness, paresthesias, bladder abnormalities, and mood alterations; characteristically, the plaques are "separated in time and space" and clinically the symptoms show exacerbations and remissions. SYN disseminated s., focal s., insular s.

nodular s., SYN atherosclerosis.

nuclear s., increased refractivity of the central portion of the lens of the eye. SEE nuclear *cataract.*

ovulational s., SYN physiologic s.

physiologic s., a slowly progressive s. in the walls of the ovarian arteries which commences after puberty. SYN menstrual s., ovulational s.

posterior s., SYN tabetic *neurosyphilis.*

posterior spinal s., SYN tabetic *neurosyphilis.*

primary lateral s., considered by many to be a subgroup of motor neuron disease; a slowly progressive degenerative disorder of the motor neurons of the cerebral cortex, resulting in widespread weakness on an upper motor neuron basis; spasticity, hyperreflexia, and Babinski signs are present, but not fasciculation potentials, nor any electrodiagnostic evidence of a lower motor neuron lesion. SYN lateral spinal s.

systemic s., a systemic disease characterized by formation of hyalinized and thickened collagenous fibrous tissue, with thickening of the skin and adhesion to underlying tissues (especially of the hands and face), dysphagia due to loss of peristalsis and submucosal fibrosis of the esophagus, dyspnea due to pulmonary fibrosis, myocardial fibrosis, and renal vascular changes resembling those of malignant hypertension; Raynaud's phenomenon, atrophy of the soft tissues, and osteoporosis of the distal phalanges (acrosclerosis), sometimes with gangrene at the ends of the digits, are common findings. The term progressive systemic s. is commonly used and is appropriate for cases with initially widespread skin involvement including the trunk. However, when skin involvement is limited to the distal extremities and face there is often prolonged delay in appearance of visceral manifestations.

tuberous s. [MIM*191100], phacomatosis characterized by the

sc

formation of multisystem hamartomas producing seizures, mental retardation, and skin nodules of the face, originally considered to be sebaceous adenomas but since shown to be angiofibromas; the cerebral and retinal lesions are glial nodules; other skin lesions are white macules, shagreen patches, and periungual fibromas; autosomal dominant inheritance with variable expression. SYN Bourneville's disease, epiloia.

unicellular s., a growth of fibrous tissue between and isolating the individual cells of a part.

valvular s., fibrosis, often with calcification of valves, considered to be an aging change and not due to primary valvular disease.

vascular s., SYN arteriosclerosis.

s. of white matter, SYN leukodystrophy.

scle·ro·ste·no·sis (sklēr-ō-ste-nō'sis). Induration and contraction of the tissues. [sclero- + G. *stenōsis*, a narrowing]

Scle·ros·to·ma (sklĕ-ros'tō-mă). A former generic name for strongyle (hookworm) nematodes and for trichostrongyle worms of horses; now replaced by other genera but still used as a collective term for this group. Species include *S. duodenale* (*Ancylostoma duodenale*) and *S. syngamus* (*Syngamus trachea*) [sclero- + G. *stoma*, mouth]

scle·ros·to·my (sklĕ-ros'tō-mē). Surgical perforation of the sclera, as for the relief of glaucoma. [sclero- + G. *stoma*, mouth]

scle·ro·ther·a·py (sklēr-ō-thār'ă-pē). Treatment involving the injection of a sclerosing solution into vessels or tissues. SYN sclerosing therapy.

scle·ro·thrix (sklēr'ō-thriks). Induration and brittleness of the hair. SYN sclerotrichia. [sclero- + G. *thrix*, hair]

scle·rot·ic (sklĕ-rot'ik). **1.** Relating to or characterized by sclerosis. **2.** SYN scleral.

scle·rot·i·ca (sklĕ-rot'i-kă). SYN sclera. [Mod. L. *scleroticus*, hard]

scle·ro·ti·um, pl. **scle·ro·tia** (sklĕ-rō'shē-ŭm, -shē-ă). **1.** In fungi, a variably sized resting body composed of a hardened mass of hyphae with or without host tissue, usually with a darkened rind, from which fruit bodies, stromata, conidiophores, or mycelia may develop. **2.** The hardened resting condition of the plasmodium of Myxomycetes.

scle·ro·tome (sklēr'ō-tōm). **1.** A knife used in sclerotomy. **2.** The group of mesenchymal cells emerging from the ventromedial part of a mesodermic somite and migrating toward the notochord. Sclerotomal cells from adjacent somites become merged in intersomitically located masses that are the primordia of the centra of the vertebrae. [sclero- + G. *tomē*, a cutting]

scle·rot·o·my (sklĕ-rot'ō-mē). An incision through the sclera. [sclero- + G. *tomē*, incision]

anterior s., incision into the anterior chamber of the eye.

posterior s., incision through the sclera into the vitreous humor.

scle·ro·trich·ia (sklēr-ō-trik'ē-ă). SYN sclerothrix.

scle·ro·ty·lo·sis (sklēr'ō-tī-lō'sis) [MIM*181600]. Atrophic fibrosis of the skin, hypoplasia of the nails, and palmoplantar keratoderma; associated with gastrointestinal cancer; autosomal dominant inheritance. SYN scleroatrophy. [sclero- + G. *tylōsis*, the process of becoming callous]

scle·rous (sklēr'ŭs). SYN scleroid. [G. *sklēros*, hard]

scol·e·ces (skō'le-sez). Plural of scolex.

sco·le·ci·a·sis (skō-lē-sī'ă-sis). Infection of the intestine by larvae of lepidopterans (moths and butterflies). [G. *skōlēx*, worm, + *-iasis*, condition]

sco·le·ci·form (skō-lē'si-fōrm). SYN scolecoid.

sco·le·coid (skō'lē-koyd). **1.** Resembling a tapeworm scolex. **2.** Wormlike. SEE ALSO lumbricoid (1), vermiform. SYN scoleciform. [G. *skōlēkoeidēs*, fr. *skōlēx*, worm, + *eidos*, appearance]

sco·le·col·o·gy (skō-lē-kol'ŏ-jē). SYN helminthology. [G. *skōlēx*, worm, + *logos*, study]

sco·lex, pl. **scol·e·ces, scol·i·ces** (skō'leks, skō'le-sēz, skō'li-sēz). The head or anterior end of a tapeworm attached by suckers, and frequently by rostellar hooks, to the wall of the intestine; it is formed within the hydatid cyst in *Echinococcus*, within a cysticercus in *Taenia*, a cysticercoid in *Hymenolepis*, or

by a plerocercoid, as in *Diphyllobothrium latum*. The form of the s. varies greatly, the most familiar being rounded or club-shaped with four circular muscular suckers and an armed or unarmed rostellum, or a spatulate flattened s. with a pair of slitlike suckers (bothria) and no rostellum, as in *Diphyllobothrium* and its allies. Other forms have complex leaflike, cup-shaped, or fimbriated shapes, or retractile, multiply spined proboscides. These varied forms characterize the orders of cestodes, which are particularly well developed as parasites of sharks and skates or rays. [G. *skōlēx*, a worm]

sco·li·o·ky·pho·sis (skō'lē-ō-kī-fō'sis). Lateral and posterior curvature of the spine. [G. *scolios*, curved, + *kyphōsis*, kyphosis]

sco·li·om·e·ter (skō-lē-om'ĕ-ter). An instrument for measuring curves, especially those in lateral curvature of the spine. [G. *skolios*, curved, + *metron*, measure]

sco·li·o·sis (skō-lē-ō'sis). Abnormal lateral curvature of the vertebral column. Depending on the etiology, there may be one curve, or primary and secondary compensatory curves; s. may be "fixed" as a result of muscle and/or bone deformity or "mobile" as a result of unequal muscle contraction. SYN rachioscoliosis. [G. *skoliōsis*, a crookedness]

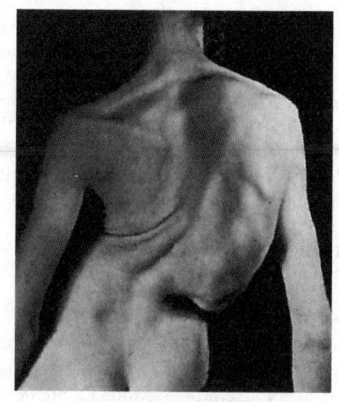

severe poliomyelitic scoliosis

coxitic s., s. in the lumbar spine resulting from tilting of the pelvis in a case of hip disease.

empyemic s., s. due to retraction of one side of the chest following an empyema.

habit s., s. supposedly due to habitual standing or sitting in an improper position.

myopathic s., lateral curvature due to weakness of the spinal muscles, as in poliomyelitis.

ocular s., ophthalmic s., s. supposed to be due to head tilting, caused by ophthalmological dysfunction.

osteopathic s., lateral curvature of the spine due to vertebral disease.

paralytic s., lateral curvature of the spine due to paralysis of spinal muscles.

rachitic s., s. occurring as a result of rickets.

sciatic s., s. caused by asymmetric spasm of spinal muscles usually associated with sciatica, usually presenting as a list toward one side.

static s., lateral curvature of the spine due to inequality in length of the legs.

sco·li·ot·ic (skō'lē-ot'ik). Relating to or suffering from scoliosis.

sco·li·o·tone (skō'lē-ō-tōn). An apparatus for stretching the spine and reducing the curve in scoliosis. [G. *skolios*, crooked, + *tonos*, tension]

Scol·o·pen·dra (skō-lō-pen'dră). A genus of centipedes characterized by 21 to 23 pairs of legs. Common U.S. species are *S. heros* (the western house centipede) and *S. morsitans*. [Mod. L., fr. G. *skōlopendra*, multipede]

s-cone. Short wavelength sensitive c. (blue c.).

scoop (skūp). A narrow, spoonlike instrument for extracting the contents of cavities or cysts. [A.S. *skopa*]

△**-scope.** Viewing, staring; an instrument for viewing but extended to include other methods of examination (*e.g.,* stethoscope). [G. *skopeō,* to view]

sco·pine (skō'pēn). Scopolamine less the tropic acid side chain, *i.e.,* 6,7-epoxytropine, or 6,7-epoxy-3-hydroxytropane.

sco·pol·a·mine (skō-pol'ă-mēn, -min). scopine tropate; an alkaloid found in the leaves and seeds of *Hyoscyamus niger, Duboisia myoproides, Scopolia japonica, Scopolia carniolica, Atropa belladonna,* and other solanaceous plants; the 6,7-epoxide of atropine, *i.e.,* 6,7-epoxytropine tropate. Exerts anticholinergic actions similar to atropine; thought to have greater central nervous system effects; useful in preventing motion sickness. SYN hyoscine.

s. hydrobromide, anticholinergic action is similar to that of atropine. SYN hyoscine hydrobromide.

s. methylbromide, a quaternary ammonium derivative of s.; used when spasmolytic or antisecretory effects are desired.

sco·po·lia (skō-pō'lē-ă). The dried rhizome and roots of *Scopolia carniolica* (family Solanaceae), a herb of Austria and neighboring countries of Europe; it resembles belladonna in pharmacologic action. [G.A. *Scopoli,* Italian naturalist, 1723–1788]

s. japon'ica, Japanese belladonna, the leaves, root, and seeds of which contain scopolamine.

sco·po·line (skō'pō-lēn). 3β,7β-Epoxy-1β*H*,5β *H*-tropan-6α-ol; a decomposition product of scopolamine, and an isomer of scopine, in that the epoxy and hydroxyl groups are in different locations.

sco·pom·e·ter (skō-pom'ĕ-ter). A device for determining the density of a precipitate by the degree of translucency of a fluid containing it. SEE ALSO nephelometer. [G. *skopeō,* to view, + *metron,* measure]

sco·po·mor·phi·nism (skō-pō-mōr'fi-nizm). Associated chronic addiction to scopolamine and morphine.

sco·po·phil·ia (skō-pō-fil'ē-ă). SYN voyeurism. [G. *skopeō,* to view, + *philos,* fond]

sco·po·pho·bia (skō-pō-fō'bē-ă). Morbid dread of being stared at. [G. *skopeō,* to view, + *phobos,* fear]

Scop·u·lar·i·op·sis (skō'pyū-lar-ē-op'sis). A genus of filamentous fungi rarely pathogenic for humans; several species have been implicated in onychomycosis, ulcerating granuloma, and other "mycotic" entities. *Penicillium*-like, it is common in nature and generally a contaminant in laboratory cultures of human tissues. [Mod. L. *scopula,* a small broom, + G. *opsis,* appearance]

△**-scopy.** An action or activity involving the use of in instrument for viewing. [G. *skopeō,* to view]

scor·bu·tic (skōr-byū'tik). Relating to, suffering from, or resembling scurvy (scorbutus).

scor·bu·ti·gen·ic (skōr-byū-ti-jen'ik). Scurvy-producing.

scor·bu·tus (skōr-byū'tŭs). SYN scurvy. [Mediev. L. form of Teutonic *schorbuyck,* scurvy]

scor·di·ne·ma (skōr'di-nē'mă). Heaviness of the head with yawning and stretching, occurring as a prodrome of an infectious disease. [G. *skordinēma,* yawning]

score (skōr). An evaluation, usually expressed numerically, of status, achievement, or condition in a given set of circumstances. [M. E. *scor,* notch, tally]

APACHE s., *A*cute *p*hysiology *a*nd *c*hronic *h*ealth *e*valuation. The most widely used method of assessing the severity of illness in acutely ill patients in intensive care units.

Apgar s., evaluation of a newborn infant's physical status by assigning numerical values (0 to 2) to each of 5 criteria: 1) heart rate, 2) respiratory effort, 3) muscle tone, 4) response stimulation, and 5) skin color; a score of 8 to 10 indicates the best possible condition.

Dubowitz s., a method of clinical assessment of gestational age in the newborn that includes neurological criteria for the infant's maturity and other physical criteria to determine the gestational age of the infant; useful from birth to 5 days of life.

Gleason's s., SEE Gleason's tumor *grade.*

Apgar score				
after 60 seconds	score	0	1	2
heart rate	....	absent	under 100	over 100
respiratory effort	....	absent	slow, irregular	good (screams)
muscle tone	....	limp	good in limbs	active movement
response stimulation	....	none	makes grimaces	coughing or sneezing
skin color	....	pale	rosy trunk, blue extremities	rosy
score	══════	(total points; 8–10 is normal)		

raw s., the actual s., measurement, or value obtained before any statistics are applied to it. Cf. standard s.

recovery s., a number expressing the condition of an infant at various stipulated intervals greater than 1 minute after birth and based on the same features assessed by the Apgar s. at 60 seconds after birth.

standard s., a statistically referenced or derived s. representing the deviation of a raw s. from its mean in standard deviation units.

symptom s., American Urological Association's scoring system to evaluate prostatic obstruction.

scor·pi·on (skōr'pē-on). A member of the order Scorpionida; includes the devil s., *Vejovis,* and the hairy s., *Hadrurus.* [G. *skorpios*]

Scor·pi·on·i·da (skōr-pē-on'i-dă). The scorpions; an order of venomous, predaceous, arachnid arthropods characterized by a distinctly segmented bony abdomen terminating in a sharply recurved stinging spine equipped with a poison gland; causes a severely painful but rarely fatal sting. North American genera include *Centruroides, Hadrurus,* and *Vejovis.* [Mod. L.]

△**scoto-.** Darkness. [G. *skotos*]

scot·o·chro·mo·gens (skō'tō-krō'mō-jenz). SYN group II *mycobacteria.* [scoto- + G. *chrōma,* color, + *-gen,* producing]

scot·o·graph (skō'tō-graf). **1.** An appliance for aiding one to write in straight lines in the dark or for aiding the blind to write, as used by the historian W.H. Prescott. **2.** An impression made on a photographic film by a radioactive substance without the intervention of any opaque object other than the screen of the film. SYN noctograph. [scoto- + G. *graphō,* to write]

sco·to·ma, pl. **sco·to·ma·ta** (skō-tō'mă, skō-tō'mă-tă). **1.** An isolated area of varying size and shape, within the visual field, in which vision is absent or depressed. **2.** A blind spot in psychological awareness. [G. *skotōma,* vertigo, fr. *skotos,* darkness]

absolute s., a s. in which there is no perception of light.

annular s., a circular s. surrounding the center of the field of vision. SEE ring s.

arcuate s., a s. extending from the blind spot and arching into the nasal field following the lines of retinal nerve fibers.

Bjerrum's s., a comet-shaped s., occurring in glaucoma, attached at the temporal end to the blind spot or separated from it by a narrow gap; the defect widens as it extends above and nasally curves around the fixation spot, and then extends downward to end exactly at the nasal horizontal meridian. SYN Bjerrum's sign, sickle s.

cecocentral s., a s. involving the optic disk area (blind spot) and the papillomacular fibers; there are three forms: 1) the cecocentral defect which extends from the blind spot toward or into the fixation area; 2) angioscotoma; 3) glaucomatous nerve-fiber bundle s., due to involvement of nerve-fiber bundles at the edge of the optic disk. SEE ALSO Bjerrum's s., Rønne's nasal *step.*

central s., a s. involving the fixation point.

color s., an area of depressed color vision in the visual field.

flittering s., SYN scintillating s.

glaucomatous nerve-fiber bundle s., SEE cecocentral s.

hemianopic s., a s. involving half of the central field.

mental s., absence of insight into, or inability to comprehend, items relative to a subject whose content is highly emotional to the individual. SYN blind spot (2).

negative s., a s. that is not ordinarily perceived, but is detected only on examination of the visual field.

paracentral s., a s. adjacent to the fixation point.

pericentral s., a s. that surrounds the fixation point more or less symmetrically.

peripheral s., a s. outside of the central 30 degrees of the visual field.

physiologic s., the negative s. in the visual field, corresponding to the optic disk. SYN blind spot (1).

positive s., a s. that is perceived as a black spot within the field of vision.

quadrantic s., a s. involving a quarter segment of the central visual field.

relative s., a s. in which there is visual depression but not complete loss of light perception.

ring s., an annular area of blindness in the visual field surrounding the fixation point in pigmentary degeneration of the retina and in glaucoma.

scintillating s., a localized area of blindness edged by brilliantly colored shimmering lights (teichopsia); usually a prodromal symptom of migraine. SEE ALSO fortification *spectrum*. SYN flittering s.

Seidel's s., a form of Bjerrum's s. SEE ALSO Seidel's *sign*.

sickle s., SYN Bjerrum's s.

zonular s., a curved s. not corresponding to the path of retinal nerve fibers.

sco·to·ma·ta (skō-tō′mă-tă). Plural of scotoma.

sco·tom·a·tous (skō-tō′mă-tŭs). Relating to scotoma.

sco·tom·e·ter (skō-tom′ĕ-ter). An instrument for determining the size, shape, and intensity of a scotoma.

sco·tom·e·try (skō-tom′ĕ-trē). The plotting and measuring of a scotoma. [scoto- + G. *metron*, measure]

scot·o·phil·ia (skō-tō-fil′ē-ă). SYN nyctophilia. [scoto- + G. *philos*, fond]

scot·o·pho·bia (skō-tō-fō′bē-ă). SYN nyctophobia. [scoto- + G. *phobos*, fear]

sco·to·pia (skō-tō′pē-ă). SYN scotopic *vision*. [scoto- + G. *opsis*, vision]

sco·top·ic (skō-tō′pik, -top′ik). Referring to low illumination to which the eye is dark-adapted. SEE scotopic *vision*.

sco·top·sin (skō-top′sin). The protein moiety of the pigment in the rods of the retina.

sco·tos·co·py (skō-tos′kŏ-pē). SYN retinoscopy. [scoto- + G. *skopeō*, to view]

Scott, Charles I., Jr., U.S. pediatrician, *1934. SEE Aarskog-S. *syndrome*.

Scott, H. William, U.S. surgeon, *1916. SEE S. *operation*.

Scott-Wilson, H., English scientist. SEE Scott-Wilson *reagent*.

scot·ty dog (scot′te dawg). The fancied appearance of the articular facets on oblique radiographs of the lumbar spine; the neck of the s. d. is the pars interarticularis, site of the most common defect in spondylolysis.

scours. Neonatal diarrhea in ruminants.

calf scours, a diarrheal disease of newborn calves caused by several different enteropathogens, particularly the bacterium *Escherichia coli;* two syndromes are recognized, acute disease characterized by dehydration and rapid death and subacute disease characterized by persistent diarrhea and emaciation.

scrape (skrāp). A specimen scraped from a lesion or specific site, for cytological examination. SEE ALSO smear.

scrap·ie (skrap′ē, skrā′pē). A communicable spongiform encephalopathy of the central nervous system of sheep and goats caused by a virus-like agent (classified as a prion) and characterized by a very long incubation period followed by pruritus, abnormalities of gait, and frequently death; it resembles Creutzfeldt-Jacob disease and kuru in humans. [from scraping by affected animals against objects to relieve itching]

scratch·es (skratch′ez). SYN grease *heel* (2).

screen (skrēn). **1.** A sheet of any substance used to shield an object from any influence, such as heat, light, x-rays, etc. **2.** A sheet upon which an image is projected. **3.** Formerly, to make a fluoroscopic examination. **4.** In psychoanalysis, concealment, as one image or memory concealing another. SEE ALSO screen *memory*. **5.** To examine, evaluate; to process a group to select or separate certain individuals from it. **6.** A thin layer of crystals that converts x-rays to light photons to expose film; used in a cassette to produce radiographic images on film. [Fr. *écran*]

Bjerrum s., SYN tangent s.

s.-film contact, the closeness and uniformity with which the x-ray film in a cassette lies against the s. (6). Image resolution is dependent on this closeness and uniformity of s.

fluorescent s., a s. coated with fluorescent crystals such as the calcium tungstate used in the fluoroscope.

Hess s., a s. used in the measurement of ocular deviation.

intensifying s., a s. (6) used in radiography.

rare-earth s., an intensifying s. (6) made of a rare-earth oxide phosphor, more efficient than calcium tungstate, especially at the higher kilovoltages used in modern radiography.

tangent s., a flat, usually black surface used to measure the central 30 degrees of the field of vision. SYN Bjerrum s.

vestibular s., a s. made of acrylic resin that covers the labial or buccal surfaces of one or both dental arches; used to treat oral habits and to stimulate tooth movement by using perioral muscle force.

screen·ing (skrēn′ing). **1.** To screen (5). **2.** Examination of a group of usually asymptomatic individuals to detect those with a high probability of having a given disease, typically by means of an inexpensive diagnostic test. **3.** In the mental health professions, initial patient evaluation that includes medical and psychiatric history, mental status evaluation, and diagnostic formulation to determine the patient's suitability for a particular treatment modality.

carrier s., indiscriminate examination of members of a population to detect heterozygotes for serious disorders and counsel about the risks of marriages with other carriers, and by antenatal diagnosis where a married couple are both carriers; often sacrifices precision to simplicity and is most effectively applied to populations known to be at high risk.

cytologic s., a s. for the detection of early disease, usually cancer, through microscopic examination of a cellular specimen by inspecting each cell and structure present, usually at ×100 magnification with a mechanical stage, so that all areas are screened; the findings are evaluated and significant abnormalities are flagged (*e.g.,* by dotting the cover slip) for further evaluation by a cytopathologist. This s. is usually performed by a cytotechnologist, but at times is done by automated machine prescreening.

familial s., s. directed at close relatives of probands with diseases that may lie latent, as in age-dependent dominant traits, or that may involve risk to progeny, as X-linked traits.

mass s., examination of a large population to detect the manifestation of a disease in order to initiate treatment or prevent spread, as part of a public health campaign.

multiphasic s., the routine use of multiple tests, usually biochemical, for the purpose of detecting disease at a preventable or curable stage.

neonatal s., testing of newborns for the detection of preventable or curable disease.

prenatal s., s. for the detection of fetal disease, usually by ultrasound examination or by testing amniotic fluid obtained by amniocentesis. Other s. techniques include testing maternal serum and placental biopsy.

screw (skrū). A helically grooved cylinder for fastening two objects together or for adjusting the position of an object resting on one end of the s.

afterloading s., a device for setting the length at which a contracting muscle encounters an afterload.

screw-worm (skrū′werm). The larva of the botfly, *Cochliomyia hominivorax,* and other similar forms that cause human and animal myiasis.

    primary s.-w., an obligatory s.-w. that can penetrate normal tissues and feed as a primary invader. The important myiasis flies of man that serve as p. s.-w.'s are *Cochliomyia hominivorax, Chrysomyia bezziana,* and *Wohlfahrtia magnifica.*

    secondary s.-w., an accidental or facultative s.-w. that enters a prior wound or suppurated condition and feeds on infected rather than intact tissues. Many blowflies are included, such as *Calliphora vicina, Phaenicia sericata, Phormia regina, Cochliomyia macellaria, Chrysomyia* species, and other fleshflies.

scribe (skrīb). **1.** To write, trace, or mark by making a line with a marker or pointed instrument, as in surveying a dental cast for a removable prosthesis. **2.** To form, by instrumentation, negative areas within a master cast to provide a positive beading in the framework of a removable partial denture, or the posterior palatal seal area for a complete denture. [L. *scribo,* pp. *scripto,* to write]

Scribner, Belding H., U.S. nephrologist, *1921. SEE S. *shunt.*

scro·bic·u·late (skrō-bik′yū-lāt). Pitted; marked with minute depressions. [L. *scrobiculus;* dim. of *scrobis,* a trench]

scro·bic·u·lus cor·dis (skrō-bik′yū-lŭs kōr′dis). SYN epigastric *fossa.* [L. pit or fossa of the heart]

scrof·u·la (skrof′yū-lă). Obsolete term for cervical tuberculous lymphadenitis. [L. *scrofulae* (pl. only), a glandular swelling, scrofula, fr. *scrofa,* a breeding sow]

scrof·u·lo·der·ma (skrof′yū-lō-der′mă). Tuberculosis resulting from extension into the skin from underlying atypical mycobacterial infection, most commonly of cervical lymph nodes. [scrofula + G. *derma,* skin]

    s. gummo′sa, a deep cutaneous tuberculous lesion.

    papular s., SYN *lichen* scrofulosorum.

    verrucous s., SYN *tuberculosis* cutis verrucosa.

scrof·u·lous (skrof′yū-lŭs). Relating to or suffering from scrofula.

scro·tal (skrō′tăl). Relating to the scrotum. SYN oscheal.

scro·tec·to·my (skrō-tek′tō-mē). Removal of all or part of scrotum. [scrotum, + G. *ektomē,* excision]

scro·ti·form (skrō′ti-fōrm). Having the shape or form of a scrotum.

scro·ti·tis (skrō-tī′tis). Inflammation of the scrotum.

scro·to·cele (skrō′tō-sēl). Obsolete term for scrotal *hernia.* [scrotum + G. *kēlē,* hernia]

scro·to·plas·ty (skrō′tō-plas-tē). Surgical reconstruction of the scrotum. SYN oscheoplasty. [scrotum + G. *plastos,* formed]

scro·tum, pl. **scro·ta, scro·tums** (skrō′tŭm, -tă, -tŭmz) [NA]. A musculocutaneous sac containing the testes; it is formed of skin, containing a network of nonstriated muscular fibers (the dartos or dartus fascia), which also forms the scrotal septum internally. SYN marsupium (1). [L.]

    lymph s., SYN *elephantiasis* scroti.

    watering-can s., urinary fistulas in scrotum and perineum, resulting from disease of the perineal urethra.

scru·ple (skrū′pl). An apothecaries' weight of 20 grains or one-third of a dram. [L. *scrupulus,* a small sharp stone, a weight, the 24th part of an ounce, a scruple, dim. of *scrupus,* a sharp stone]

SCUBA Acronym for *s*elf-contained *u*nderwater *b*reathing *a*pparatus.

Scultetus (Scul·tet), Originally Schultes, Johann, German surgeon, 1595–1645. SEE S.'s *bandage, position.*

scum (skŭm). A film of insoluble material that rises to the surface of a liquid, as in epistasis. [M.E.]

scurf (skerf). SYN dandruff. [A.S.]

scur·vy (sker′vē). A disease marked by inanition, debility, anemia, edema of the dependent parts, a spongy condition, sometimes with ulceration of the gums and hemorrhages into the skin and from the mucous membranes; due to a diet lacking vitamin C. SYN scorbutus, sea s. [fr. A. S. scurf]

    Alpine s., SYN pellagra.

---

origin	benign	malignant	relative frequency
germ cell		seminoma	45–55%
		embryonal carcinoma (MTU) teratocarcinoma (MTI) teratoma (TD)	25–35%
		choriocarcinoma (MTT) yolk-sac tumor	1–2%
stroma	Sertoli's cell adenoma	androblastoma Sertoli's cell tumor granulosa cell tumor	3–4%
other			< 1%

---

    hemorrhagic s., s. with extensive hemorrhages in gums, skin and other tissues, typical of severe stage of the disease.

    infantile s., osteopathia hemorrhagia infantum; a cachectic condition in infants, resulting from malnutrition and marked by pallor, fetid breath, coated tongue, diarrhea, and subperiosteal hemorrhages; probably a combination of s. and rickets due to combined deficiency of vitamins C and D. SYN Barlow's disease, Cheadle's disease, osteopathia hemorrhagica infantum, scurvy rickets.

    land s., formerly, s. occurring in people who had not been to sea.

    sea s., SYN scurvy.

scu·tate (skū′tāt). SYN scutiform.

scute (skūt). A thin lamina or plate. SYN scutum (1). [L. *scutum,* shield]

    tympanic s., the thin bony plate separating the epitympanic recess from the mastoid cells.

scu·ti·form (skū′ti-fōrm). Shield-shaped. SYN scutate. [L. *scutum,* shield, + *forma,* form]

Scu·tig·e·ra (skū-tij′er-ă). A genus of centipedes commonly found in the eastern U.S.; the eastern house centipede is a member of the species *S. cleopatra.* [L. *scutum,* an oblong shield]

scu·tu·lar (skū′tyū-lăr). Relating to a scutulum.

scu·tu·lum, pl. **scu·tu·la** (skū′tyū-lŭm, -lă; skū′chū-lŭm). A yellow saucer-shaped crust, the characteristic lesion of favus, consisting of a mass of hyphae and spores. [L. dim. of *scutum,* shield]

scu·tum, pl. **scu·ta** (skū′tŭm, -tă). **1.** SYN scute. **2.** In ixodid (hard) ticks, a plate that largely or entirely covers the dorsum of the male and forms an anterior shield behind the capitulum of the female or immature ticks. [L. shield]

scyb·a·la (sib′ă-lă). Plural of scybalum.

scyb·a·lous (sib′ă-lŭs). Relating to scybala.

scyb·a·lum, pl. **scyb·a·la** (sib′ă-lŭm, -lă). A hard round mass of inspissated feces. [G. *skybalon,* excrement]

scy·phi·form (sī′fi-fōrm). SYN scyphoid. [G. *skyphos,* goblet, cup, + L. *forma,* form]

scy·phoid (sī′foyd). Cup-shaped. SYN scyphiform. [G. *skyphos,* cup, + *eidos,* resemblance]

SD Abbreviation for streptodornase; standard *deviation.*

SDA Abbreviation for specific dynamic *action.*

SDS Abbreviation for *sodium* dodecyl sulfate.

Se Symbol for selenium.

seal (sēl). **1.** An airtight closure. **2.** To effect an airtight closure.

    border s., the contact of the denture border with the underlying or adjacent tissues to prevent the passage of air or other substances. SYN peripheral s.

    palatal s., SYN posterior palatal s.

    peripheral s., SYN border s.

posterior palatal s., the s. at the posterior border of a denture. SEE ALSO posterior palatal seal *area.* SYN palatal s., post dam, postdam, postpalatal s.

postpalatal s., SYN posterior palatal s.

velopharyngeal s., closure between the oral and nasopharyngeal cavities.

seal·ant (sē′lănt). A material used to effect an airtight closure.

dental s., SYN fissure s.

fissure s., a dental material usually made from interaction between bisphenol A and glycidyl methacrylate; such s.'s are used to seal nonfused, noncarious pits and fissures on surfaces of teeth. SYN dental s.

search·er (ser′cher). A form of sound used to determine the presence of a calculus in the bladder.

Seashore, Carl E., U.S. psychologist, 1866–1949. SEE S. *test.*

sea·sick·ness (sē′sik-nes). A form of motion sickness caused by the motion of a floating platform, such as a ship, boat, or raft. SYN mal de mer, naupathia, vomitus marinus.

sea·son (sē′zŏn). A particular phase of some slow cyclic phenomenon, especially the annual weather cycle.

mating s., the period during which an animal will mate, *i.e.,* the period during which estrus occurs.

seat (sēt). A surface against which an object may rest to gain support.

basal s., SYN denture foundation *area.*

rest s., SYN rest *area.*

seat·worm (sēt′werm). SYN pinworm.

△**seb-.** SEE sebo-.

se·ba·ceous (sē-bā′shŭs). Relating to sebum; oily; fatty. SYN sebaceus. [L. *sebaceus*]

se·ba·ceus (sē-bā′shŭs). SYN sebaceous. [L.]

seb·i·a·gog·ic (seb′ē-ă-goj′ik). SYN sebiferous. [sebi- + G. *agōgos,* leading]

se·bif·er·ous (sē-bif′er-ŭs). Producing sebaceous matter. SYN sebiagogic, sebiparous. [sebi- + L. *fero,* to bear]

Sebileau, Pierre, French anatomist, 1860–1953. SEE S.'s *hollow, muscle.*

se·bip·a·rous (sē-bip′ă-rŭs). SYN sebiferous. [sebi- + L. *pario,* to produce]

△**sebo-, seb-, sebi-.** Sebum, sebaceous. [L. *sebum,* suet, tallow]

seb·o·lith (seb′ō-lith). A concretion in a sebaceous follicle. [sebo- + G. *lithos,* stone]

seb·or·rhea (seb-ō-rē′ă). Overactivity of the sebaceous glands, resulting in an excessive amount of sebum. [sebo- + G. *rhoia,* a flow]

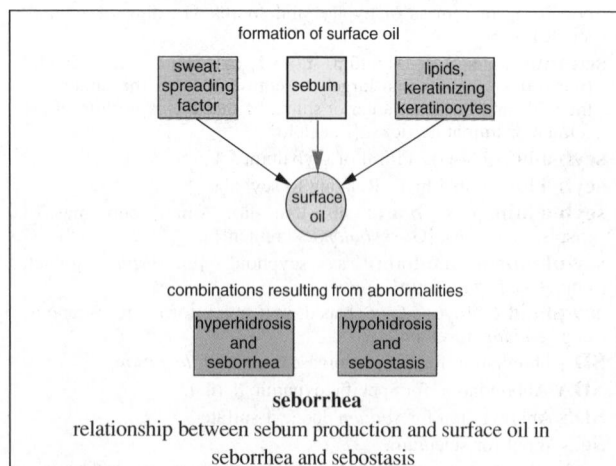

formation of surface oil

combinations resulting from abnormalities

seborrhea
relationship between sebum production and surface oil in seborrhea and sebostasis

s. adipo′sa, SYN s. oleosa.

s. cap′itis, s. of the scalp. SYN branny tetter (2).

s. ce′rea, waxy secretion of sebum.

concrete s., thick, oily crusts on scalp and eyebrows.

s. cor′poris, SYN seborrheic *dermatitis.*

eczematoid s., seborrheic eczema in which lesions have lost definition and have become confluent, usually as a result of trauma and overzealous use of soap and medication.

s. facie′i, s. of face, s. oleosa affecting especially the nose and forehead.

s. furfura′cea, SYN s. sicca (1).

s. ni′gra, a form of s. characterized by a pigmented secretion.

s. oleo′sa, a greasy condition of the skin due to excessive secretion of the sebaceous glands. SYN cutis unctuosa, hyperhidrosis oleosa, s. adiposa.

s. sic′ca, (1) an accumulation on the skin, especially the scalp, of dry scales; SYN s. furfuracea. **(2)** SYN dandruff.

s. squamo′sa neonato′rum, seborrheic dermatitis in infants.

seb·or·rhe·ic (seb-ō-rē′ik). Relating to seborrhea.

se·bum (sē′bŭm). The secretion of the sebaceous glands. [L. tallow]

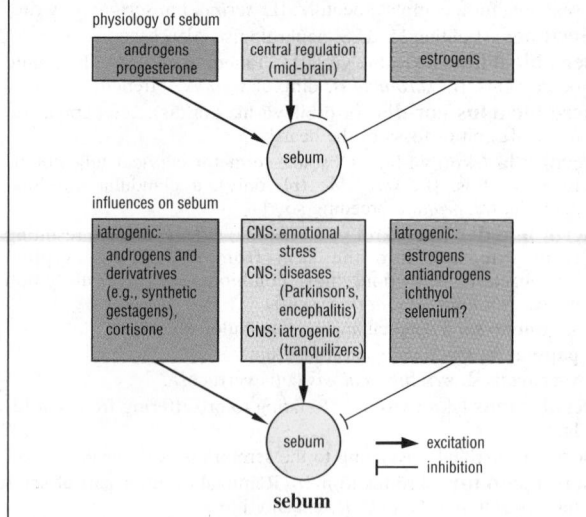

physiology of sebum

influences on sebum

sebum

s. cuta′neum, cutaneous fatty secretion.

s. preputia′le, SYN *smegma* preputii.

sec Abbreviation for second.

Se·cer·nen·tas·i·da (se-ser-nen-tas′i-dă). A class of nematodes possessing lateral canals opening into the excretory system and phasmids; it includes most of the familiar nematode parasites of humans and domestic animals, including the soil-borne nematodes, strongyles, and filiariae. SEE ALSO Adenophorasida. SYN Phasmidia, Secernentia. [L. *secerno,* to separate, hide]

Se·cer·nen·tia (se-ser-nen′shē-ă). SYN Secernentasida.

Seckel, Helmut P.G., German physician, *1900. SEE S. *dwarfism, syndrome.*

sec·o·bar·bi·tal (sē-kō-bar′bi-tahl). 5-Allyl-5-(1-methylbutyl)-barbituric acid; an obsolescent sedative and short-acting hypnotic; largely replaced by benzodiazepines.

sec·on·dar·ies (sek′ŏn-dār-ēz). **1.** SYN metastasis. **2.** The lesions of secondary syphilis.

se·cos·te·roid (sek′ō-stēr′oyd). A compound derived from a steroid in which there has been a ring cleavage. [L. *seco,* to cut, + steroid]

se·cre·ta (se-krē′tă). Secretions. [L. neuter pl. of *secretus,* pp. of *se-cerno,* to separate]

se·cre·ta·gogue (se-krē′tă-gog). An agent that promotes secretion; *e.g.,* acetylcholine, gastrin, secretin. SYN secretogogue. [secreta + G. *agōgos,* drawing forth]

Secrétan, H., Swiss surgeon, 1856–1916. SEE S.'s *syndrome.*

se·cre·tase (sē-krē′tās). A term used to describe a proteinase that acts on amyloid precursor protein to produce peptides that do not contain the entire amyloid β protein (a major constituent of the plaques found in Alzheimer's disease), are soluble, and do not precipitate to produce amyloid.

se·crete (se-krēt'). To elaborate or produce some physiologically active substance (*e.g.,* enzyme, hormone, metabolite) by a cell and to deliver it into blood, body cavity, or sap, either by direct diffusion, cellular exocytosis, or by means of a duct. [L. *secerno,* pp. *-cretus,* to separate]

se·cre·tin (se-krē'tin). A hormone, formed by the epithelial cells of the duodenum under the stimulus of acid contents from the stomach, that incites secretion of pancreatic juice; used as a diagnostic aid in the diagnosis of pancreatic exocrine disease and as an adjunct in obtaining desquamated pancreatic cells for cytological examination. SYN oxykrinin. [sectete + -in]

s. family, a class of hormones that are structurally and functionally similar to s.; *e.g.,* s., glucagon, gastric inhibitory polypeptide, vasoactive intestinal polypeptide, and glicentin.

se·cre·tion (se-krē'shŭn). **1.** Production by a cell or aggregation of cells (a gland) of a physiologically active substance and its movement out of the cell or organ in which it is formed. **2.** The solid, liquid, or gaseous product of cellular or glandular activity that is stored up in or utilized by the organism in which it is produced. Cf. excretion. [L. *se-cerno,* pp. *-cretus,* to separate]

cytocrine s., the transfer of secretory material from one cell to another, such as the transfer of melanin granules from melanocytes to epidermal cells.

external s., a substance formed by a cell and transported outside the cell walls as a means of ridding the cell of the substance or as a messenger to affect the function of other cells.

neurohumoral s., transmission of a nerve impulse across a synapse or to an end-organ by s. of a minute amount of a chemical transmitter such as acetylcholine.

se·cre·to·gogue (se-krē'tō-gog). SYN secretagogue.

se·cre·to·mo·tor, se·cre·to·mo·tory (se-krē'tō-mō'ter, -mō'ter-ē). Stimulating secretion. [secrete = *motor,* mover]

se·cre·tor (se-krē'ter, tōr). An individual whose bodily fluids (saliva, semen, vaginal secretions) contain a water-soluble form of the antigens of the ABO blood group. S.'s constitute 80% of the population. In forensic medicine, the examination of fluids has enhanced the ability of law enforcement officials to develop identifying information about perpetrators and narrow a field of suspects.

se·cre·to·ry (se-krēt'ĕ-rē, sē'krĕ-tōr-ē). Relating to secretion or the secretions.

sec·tile (sek'til, tīl). **1.** Capable of being cut or divided. **2.** Having the appearance of being divided. [L. *sectilis,* fr. *seco,* to cut]

sec·tio, pl. **sec·ti·o·nes** (sek'shē-ō, sek-shē-ō'nēz) [NA]. In anatomy, a subdivision or segment. [L.]

sec·tion (sek'shŭn). **1.** The act of cutting. **2.** A cut or division. **3.** A segment or part of any organ or structure delimited from the remainder. **4.** A cut surface. **5.** A thin slice of tissue, cells, microorganisms, or any material for examination under the microscope. SYN microscopic s. [L. *sectio,* a cutting, fr. *seco,* to cut]

abdominal s., SYN celiotomy.

attached cranial s., SYN attached *craniotomy.*

axial s., SYN transverse s.

cesarean s., incision through the abdominal wall and the uterus (abdominal hysterotomy) for extraction of the fetus.

classical cesarean s., a cesarean s. in which the uterus is entered through a vertical fundal incision.

coronal s., a cross section attained by slicing, actually or through imaging techniques, the body or any part of the body or any anatomic structure in the coronal or frontal plane, *i.e.,* in a vertical plane perpendicular to the median or sagittal plane. Since actual sectioning in the coronal plane results in an anterior and a posterior portion, an anatomical coronal section may be a two-dimensional view of the cut surface of the posterior aspect of the anterior portion, or of the anterior aspect of the posterior portion. SYN frontal s.

cross s., **(1)** a planar or two-dimensional view, diagram, or image of the internal structure of the body, part of the body, or any anatomic structure afforded by slicing, actually or through imag-

ing (radiographic, magnetic, or microscopic) techniques, the body or structure along a particular plane. Traditionally, "cross section" referred to views resulting from slicing at right angles to the longitudinal axis of the structure, but in contemporary use, the term is applied when the structure is sliced in any given plane; **(2)** the slice or section of a given thickness created by actual serial parallel cuts through a structure or by the application of imaging technique.

detached cranial s., SYN detached *craniotomy.*

diagonal s., SYN oblique s.

frontal s., SYN coronal s.

frozen s., a thin slice of tissue cut from a frozen specimen, often used for rapid microscopic diagnosis.

Latzko's cesarean s., a cesarean s. in which the uterus is entered by paravesical blunt dissection without entering the peritoneal cavity.

longitudinal s., a cross s. attained by slicing in any plane parallel to the long or vertical axis, actually or through imaging techniques, the body or any part of the body or anatomic structure. Longitudinal sections include, but are not limited to, median, sagittal, and coronal sections.

lower uterine segment cesarean s., a cesarean s. in which the uterus is entered in its lower segment by a transperitoneal approach.

median s., a cross s. attained by slicing in the median plane, actually or through imaging techniques, the body or any part of the body which occupies or crosses the median plane or by slicing any generally symmetrical anatomic structure, such as a finger or a cell, in its midline. Since actual sectioning the median plane results in a right and a left half, an anatomical median s. may be a two-dimensional view of the cut surface on the medial aspect of either half. SYN midsagittal s.

microscopic s., SYN section (5).

midsagittal s., SYN median s.

oblique s., a diagonal cross s. attained by slicing, actually or through imaging techniques, the body or any part of the body or anatomic structure, in any plane which does not parallel the longitudinal axis or intersect it at a right angle, *i.e.,* which is neither longitudinal (vertical) nor transverse (horizontal). SYN diagonal s.

parasagittal s., SYN sagittal s.

perineal s., any s. through the perineum, either lateral or median lithotomy or external urethrotomy.

pituitary stalk s., transection of the neurovascular connection between the hypothalamus and the pituitary gland.

Saemisch's s., procedure of transfixing the cornea beneath an ulcer and then cutting from within outward through the base.

sagittal s., a cross s. obtained by slicing, actually or through imaging techniques, the body or any part of the body, or any anatomic structure in the sagittal plane, *i.e.,* in a vertical plane parallels to the median plane. Since actual sectioning in the sagittal plane results in a right and a left portion, an anatomical sagittal section may be a two-dimensional view of the cut surface on the medial aspect of either portion. SYN parasagittal s.

serial s., one of a number of consecutive microscopic s.'s.

thin s., ultrathin s., a s. of tissue for electron microscopic examination; the specimen is fixed, typically in glutaraldehyde and/or in osmium tetroxide, embedded in a plastic resin, and sectioned at less than 0.1 μm in thickness with a glass or diamond knife in an ultramicrotome.

transverse s., a cross section obtained by slicing, actually or through imaging techniques, the body or any part of the body structure, in a horizontal plane, *i.e.,* a plane which intersects the longitudinal axis at a right angle. Since actual sectioning in the transverse plane results in an inferior and a superior portion, an anatomical transverse section may be a two-dimensional view of the cut surface on the inferior aspect of the superior portion, or of the superior aspect of the inferior portion. By convention, in medical imaging transverse sections demonstrate the former unless otherwise stated. SYN axial s.

sec·ti·o·nes (sek-shē-ō'nēz). Plural of sectio.

sec·tor·an·o·pia (sek'tŏr-an-ō'pē-ă). Loss of vision in a sector of the visual field. [sector + G. *an-* priv. + *opsis,* vision]

sec·to·ri·al (sek-tōr′ē-ăl). **1.** Relating to a sector. **2.** Cutting or adapted for cutting; denoting the carnassial or shearing molar and premolar teeth of carnivores. [L. *sector,* cutter]

se·cun·di·grav·i·da (sek′ŭn-di-grav′i-dă). SEE gravida.

se·cun·di·na, pl. **se·cun·di·nae** (sek-ŭn-dī′nă, -nē). SYN afterbirth. [L. *secundinae,* the afterbirth, fr. *secundus,* second]

se·cun·dines (sek′ŭn-dēnz). SYN afterbirth. [L. *secundinae,* the afterbirth]

se·cun·dip·a·ra (sek′ŭn-dip′ă-ră). SEE para.

se·date (sĕ-dāt′). To bring under the influence of a sedative. [L. *sedatus;* see sedation]

se·da·tion (sĕ-dā′shŭn). **1.** The act of calming, especially by the administration of a sedative. **2.** The state of being calm. [L. *sedatio,* to calm, allay]

sed·a·tive (sed′ă-tiv). **1.** Calming; quieting. **2.** A drug that quiets nervous excitement; designated according to the organ or system upon which specific action is exerted; *e.g.,* cardiac, cerebral, nervous, respiratory, spinal. [L. *sedativus;* see sedation]

differing effects of sedatives (I) and neuroleptics (II)	
I. (e.g., barbiturates, meprobamate, alcohol)	II. (e.g., phenothiazines, reserpine)
with increasing dosage:	antipsychotic effect
anxiolysis	easier arousal (when compared to I)
sedation	
anticonvulsant effect	extrapyramidal symptoms
ataxia	parkinsonism
agitation, confusion, loss of inhibition	dystonia
anesthesia	cramps
respiratory and circulatory depression (can be fatal)	effect upon autonomous nervous system (atropine-like, sympatholytic)
with chronic use:	
psychological and physical dependence	
development of tolerance	

se·dig·i·tate (se-dij′i-tāt). SYN sexdigitate. [L. *sex,* six, + *digitus,* digit]

sed·i·ment (sed′i-ment). **1.** Insoluble material that tends to sink to the bottom of a liquid, as in hypostasis. SYN sedimentum. **2.** To cause or effect the formation of a sediment or deposit, as in the case of centrifugation or ultracentrifugation. SYN sedimentate. [L. *sedimentum,* a settling, fr. *sedeo,* to sit, settle down]

sed·i·men·tate (sed′i-men-tāt). SYN sediment (2).

sed·i·men·ta·tion (sed′i-men-tā′shŭn). Formation of a sediment.

sed·i·men·ta·tor (sed′i-men-tā′ter, tōr). A centrifuge.

sed·i·men·tom·e·ter (sed′ĭ-men-tom′ĕ-ter). A photographic apparatus for the automatic recording of the blood sedimentation rate. [sediment + G. *metron,* measure]

sed·i·men·tum (sed-i-men′tŭm). SYN sediment (1). [L.]

  s. laterit′ium, SYN brickdust *deposit.*

se·do·hep·tu·lose (sē-dō-hep′tyū-lōs). A 2-ketoheptulose formed metabolically in the pentose monophosphate pathway as the 7-phosphate by condensation of D-xylulose 5-phosphate and D-ribose 5-phosphate, splitting out D-glyceraldehyde 3-phosphate; the unphosphorylated sugar is found in *Sedum* (stonecrop). SYN D-*altro*-2-heptulose.

seed (sēd). **1.** The reproductive body of a flowering plant; the mature ovule. SYN semen (2). **2.** In bacteriology, to inoculate a culture medium with microorganisms. [A.S. *soed*]

Seeligmüller, Otto L.G.A., German neurologist, 1837–1912. SEE S.'s *sign.*

Seessel, Albert, U.S. embryologist, 1850–1910. SEE S.'s *pocket, pouch.*

seg·ment. **1.** A section; a part of an organ or other structure delimited naturally, artificially, or by invagination from the remainder. SEE ALSO metamere. **2.** A territory of an organ having independent function, supply, or drainage. **3.** To divide and redivide into minute equal parts. SYN segmentum [NA]. [L. *segmentum,* fr. *seco,* to cut]

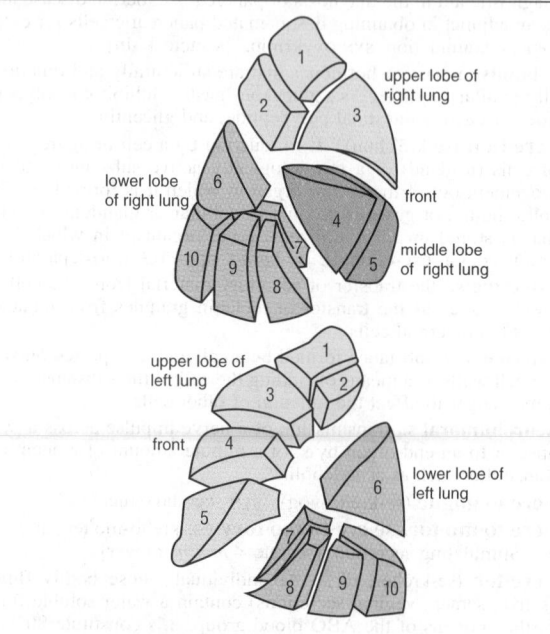

bronchopulmonary segments
viewed from either side:
1) apical segment (s.);
2) posterior s. (in left lung, 1 + 2 = apicoposterior s., formerly "apicobasal";
3) anterior s.;
4) lateral s. of right lung (for left lung, superior lingular s.);
5) medial s. of right lung (for left lung, inferior lingular s.);
6) apical s. (or superior);
7) medial basal s. (or cardiac s. of right lung; inconstant in left lung);
8) anterior basal s.;
9) lateral basal s.;
10) posterior basal s.

anterior s., a delimited part or section of an organ or other structure which lies in front of or ventral to the other similar parts or sections. 1) segmentum anterius (hepar) [NA]; the anterior or segment of the right lobe of the liver. 2) segmentum anterius (pulmo dexter et sinister) [NA]; [S 3]; the anterior segment of the superior lobe of the right and left lungs. 3) anterior segment of the eye; the intraocular segment of the eyeball occupied by the aqueous which lies in front of, and is separated from the vitreous-filled posterior segment by, the lens and zonule; it is subdivided by the iris into anterior and posterior chambers. SYN segmentum anterius.

anterior basal s., anterior basal segment of inferior lobe of right and left lung; lies between middle lobe and diaphragm. SYN segmentum basale anterius [NA].

anterior inferior s., anterior inferior segment of kidney. SYN segmentum anterius inferius [NA].

anterior ocular s., that portion of the eye comprising the cornea, iris, lens, and their associated chambers and adnexa.

anterior superior s., anterior superior segment of kidney. SYN segmentum anterius superius [NA].

apical s., (1) apical segment of the superior lobe of the right lung; **(2)** apical segment of the inferior lobe of the right and left lungs. SYN segmentum superius (2)★ [NA]. SYN segmentum superius (1) [NA], segmentum apicale, superior s. (2).

apicoposterior s., apicoposterior segment of superior lobe of left lung, composed of two segments and wedged between the anterior segment of the upper lobe and the oblique fissure. SYN segmentum apicoposterius [NA].

arterial s.'s of kidney, SYN renal s.'s.

bronchopulmonary s., the largest subdivision of a lobe of the lung; it is supplied by a direct tertiary (lobular) bronchus and a tertiary branch of the pulmonary artery; it is separated from adjacent segments by connective tissue septa. SYN segmentum bronchopulmonale [NA].

cardiac s., SYN medial basal s.

cervical s.'s of spinal cord, the eight cervical segments [C_1–C_8] of the spinal cord which give rise to the eight pairs of cervical spinal nerves and constitute the cervical part of the spinal cord. SYN segmenta medullae spinalis cervicalia.

coccygeal s.'s of spinal cord, the three coccygeal segments [Co_1–Co_3] of the spinal cord which give rise to the three pairs of coccygeal spinal nerves and constitute the coccygeal part of the spinal cord.

hepatic s.'s, territories of the liver with independent portobilioarterial distribution or independent venous drainage. The naming of segments in the NA is based upon the portobilioarterial distribution. SEE anterior s., lateral s., medial s., posterior s. SYN segmenta hepatis, s.'s of liver.

hepatic venous s.'s, SYN venous s.'s of liver.

inferior s., inferior segment of kidney, which typically consists of approximately the inferior third of the kidney viewed either anteriorly or posteriorly. SYN segmentum inferius [NA].

inferior lingular s., inferior lingular segment of superior lobe of left lung; between superior lingular segment and oblique fissure. SYN segmentum lingulare inferius [NA].

interannular s., SYN internodal s.

intermaxillary s., the primordial mass of tissue formed by the merging of the medial nasal prominences of the embryo; it contributes to the intermaxillary portion of the upper jaw, the prolabial portion of the upper lip, and the primary palate.

internodal s., the portion of a myelinated nerve fiber between two successive nodes. SYN interannular s., internode, Ranvier's s., segmentum internodale.

Lanterman's s.'s, the divisions of the nerve fiber between the Schmidt-Lanterman incisures.

lateral s., a delimited part or section of an organ or other structure which lies farthest to the left or right side of the other similar parts or sections. 1) segmentum laterale (hepar) [NA]; the lateral segment of the left lobe of the liver. 2) segmentum laterale (pulmo dexter) [NA]; [S 4]; the lateral segment of the middle lobe of the right lung. SYN segmentum laterale.

lateral basal s., lateral basal segment of inferior lobe of right and left lung; between anterior and posterior basal segments. SYN segmentum basale laterale [NA].

s.'s of liver, SYN hepatic s.'s.

lower uterine s., the inferior portion or isthmus of the uterus, the lower extremity of which joins with the cervical canal and, during pregnancy, expands to become the lower part of the uterine cavity.

lumbar s.'s of spinal cord, the five lumbar segments [L_1–L_5] of the spinal cord which give rise to the five pairs of lumbar spinal nerves and constitute the lumbar part of the spinal cord. SYN segmenta medullae spinalis lumbaria.

medial s., a delimited part or section of an organ or other structure which lies closer or closest to the midline than the other similar parts or sections. 1) segmentum mediale (hepar) [NA]; the medial segment of the left lobe of the liver. 2) segmentum mediale (pulmo dexter) [NA]; [S 5]; the medial segment of the middle lobe of the right lung. SYN segmentum mediale.

medial basal s., cardiac segment; medial basal segment of inferior lobe of right and left lung; can only be seen from medial and inferior surfaces since it does not reach lateral surface of lung. SYN segmentum basale mediale [NA], segmentum cardiacum★ [NA], cardiac s.

mesoblastic s., SYN somite.

neural s., SYN neuromere.

posterior s., a delimited part or section of an organ or other structure which lies in back of or dorsal to the other similar parts or sections; 1) segmentum posterius (hepar) [NA]; the posterior segment of the right lobe of the liver; 2) segmentum posterius (pulmo dexter) [NA]; [S 2]; the posterior segment of the superior lobe of the right lung; 3) segmentum posterius (ren) [NA]; the posterior segment of the kidney; 4) camera vitrea bulbi [NA]; vitreous camera; vitreous chamber of eye; the posterior intraocular segment of the eyeball occupied by the vitreous which lies behind the aqueous-filled anterior segment and is separated from it by the lens and zonule. SYN segmentum posterius.

posterior s. of eyeball, the large space between the lens and the retina; it is filled with the vitreous body. SYN camera vitrea bulbi [NA], vitreous camera, vitreous chamber of eye.

posterior basal s., posterior basal segment of inferior lobe of right and left lungs; lies adjacent to vertebral column below superior segment. SYN segmentum basale posterius [NA].

P-R s., that part of the electrocardiographic curve between the end of the P wave and the beginning of the QRS complex.

Ranvier's s., SYN internodal s.

renal s.'s, regions of the kidney supplied by end arteries branching from the renal arteries; they are named anterior inferior s., anterius superior s., inferior s. , posterior s., and superior s. SYN segmenta renalia [NA], arterial s.'s of kidney.

RST s., the part of the electrocardiogram between the QRS complex and the T wave. Virtually never distinct in normal hearts in which it forms the initial limb of the T wave without an agreed endpoint.

s.'s of spinal cord, portions of the spinal cord corresponding to the line of attachment of the roots of the individual spinal nerves. These are the cervical spinal cord segments [C_1–C_8]; the thoracic spinal cord segments [T_1–T_{12}]; the lumbar spinal cord segments [L_1–L_5]; the sacral spinal cord segments [S_1–S_5]; and the coccygeal spinal cord segments [Co_1–Co_3]. SYN segmenta medullae spinalis [NA].

s.'s of spleen, splenic territories receiving independent arterial supply or drained by independent roots of the splenic vein. SYN segmenta lienis.

S-T s., that part of the electrocardiographic tracing immediately following the QRS complex and merging into the T wave.

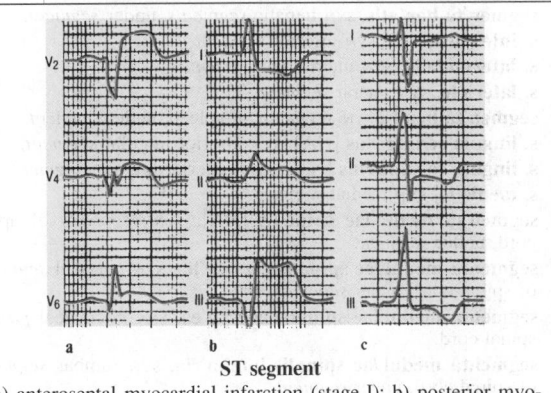

ST segment
a) anteroseptal myocardial infarction (stage I); b) posterior myocardial infarction (stage I); and c) hypertrophy of right side of heart

subapical s., an inconstant segment of the inferior lobe of the right and left lungs. SYN segmentum subapicale, segmentum subsuperius, subsuperior s.

subsuperior s., SYN subapical s.

se

superior s., (**1**) the uppermost segment of the kidney; (**2**) SYN apical s.

superior lingular s., superior lingular segment of the superior lobe of the left lung; lies above inferior lingular segment. SYN segmentum lingulare superius [NA].

sympathetic s., a divison of the sympathetic trunks based on the origins of the gray communicating branches.

upper uterine s., the main portion of the body of the gravid uterus, the contraction of which furnishes the chief force of expulsion in labor.

venous s.'s of the kidney, anatomical s.'s of the kidney drained by tributaries of the renal vein; not a true segmental distribution, since cross communication exists between the various tributaries within the kidney.

venous s.'s of liver, each of the four territories of the liver separately drained by the hepatic veins. SYN hepatic venous s.'s.

seg·men·ta (seg-men'tă). Plural of segmentum.

seg·men·tal (seg-men'tăl). Relating to a segment.

seg·men·ta·tion (seg'men-tā'shŭn). **1.** The act of dividing into segments; the state of being divided into segments. **2.** SYN cleavage (1).

seg·men·tec·to·my (seg-men-tek'tō-mē). Excision of a segment of any organ or gland.

seg·ment·er (seg'men-ter). A schizont; usually applied to the malaria parasite developing in a red blood cell after having undergone nuclear and cytoplasmic division, just before cell rupture and release of the merozoites.

Seg·men·ti·na (seg-men-tī'nă). A genus of freshwater pulmonate snails (family Planorbidae, subfamily Segmentininae); includes the species *S. hemisphaerula,* an important intermediate host of *Fasciolopsis buski.* [L. *segmentum,* fr. *seco,* to cut]

seg·men·tum, pl. **seg·men·ta** (seg-men'tŭm, -tă) [NA]. SYN segment. [L. segment]

s. ante'rius, SYN anterior *segment.*

s. ante'rius infe'rius [NA], SYN anterior inferior *segment.*

s. ante'rius supe'rius [NA], SYN anterior superior *segment.*

s. apica'le, SYN apical *segment.* (**2**) apical segment of the inferior lobe of the right and left lungs.

s. apicoposte'rius [NA], SYN apicoposterior *segment.*

s. basa'le ante'rius [NA], SYN anterior basal *segment.*

s. basa'le latera'le [NA], SYN lateral basal *segment.*

s. basa'le media'le [NA], SYN medial basal *segment.*

s. basa'le poste'rius [NA], SYN posterior basal *segment.*

s. bronchopulmona'le [NA], SYN bronchopulmonary *segment.*

s. cardi'acum [NA], ✩official alternate term for medial basal *segment.*

segmen'ta hep'atis, SYN hepatic *segments,* under *segment.*

s. infe'rius [NA], SYN inferior *segment.*

s. internoda'le, SYN internodal *segment.*

s. latera'le, SYN lateral *segment.*

segmen'ta lien'is, SYN *segments* of spleen, under *segment.*

s. lingula're infe'rius [NA], SYN inferior lingular *segment.*

s. lingula're supe'rius [NA], SYN superior lingular *segment.*

s. media'le, SYN medial *segment.*

segmen'ta medul'lae spina'lis [NA], SYN *segments* of spinal cord, under *segment.*

segmenta medul'lae spinalis cervica'lia, SYN cervical *segments* of spinal cord, under *segment.*

segmenta medul'lae spinalis coccyg'ea, SYN coccygeal *part of* spinal cord.

segmenta medul'lae spinalis lumba'ria, SYN lumbar *segments* of spinal cord, under *segment.*

segmenta medul'lae spinalis sacra'lia, SYN sacral *part of* spinal cord.

segmenta medul'lae spinalis thora'cica, SYN thoracic *part of* spinal cord.

s. poste'rius, SYN posterior *segment.*

segmen'ta rena'lia [NA], SYN renal *segments,* under *segment.*

s. subapica'le, SYN subapical *segment.*

s. subsupe'rius, SYN subapical *segment.*

s. supe'rius [NA], (**1**) SYN apical *segment.* (**2**) ✩official alternate term for apical *segment* (2).

seg·re·ga·tion (seg-rĕ-gā'shŭn). **1.** Removal of certain parts from a mass, *e.g.,* those with infectious diseases. **2.** Separation of contrasting characters in the offspring of heterozygotes. **3.** Separation of the paired state of genes, which occurs at the reduction division of meiosis; only one member of each somatic gene pair is normally included in each sperm or ovum; *e.g.,* an individual heterozygous for a gene pair, *Aa,* will form gametes half containing gene *A* and half containing gene *a.* **4.** Progressive restriction of potencies in the zygote to the following embryo. [L. *segrego,* pp. *-atus,* to set apart from the flock, separate]

seg·re·ga·tor (seg're-gā-ter, tōr). SYN separator (2).

Seidel, Erich, German ophthalmologist, 1882–1946. SEE S.'s *scotoma, sign.*

Seignette, Pierre, French apothecary, 1660–1719. SEE S.'s *salt.*

Seiler, Carl, Swiss laryngologist and anatomist in U.S., 1849–1905. SEE S.'s *cartilage.*

Seip, Martin, 20th century Scandinavian physician. SEE Lawrence-S. *syndrome.*

seis·mo·car·di·o·gram (sīz'mō-kar'dē-ō-gram). Recording of cardiac vibrations as they affect the entire body, by various techniques. [G. *seismos,* a shaking, + cardiogram]

seis·mo·ther·a·py (sīz-mō-thār'ă-pē). SYN vibratory *massage.* [G. *seismos,* a shaking, vibration]

sei·zure (sē'zher). **1.** An attack; the sudden onset of a disease or of certain symptoms. **2.** An epileptic attack. SYN convulsion (2). [O. Fr. *seisir,* to grasp, fr. Germanic]

absence s., a brief s. characterized by arrest of activity and occasionally clonic movements. There is loss of consciousness or slowing of thought. The EEG typically shows generalized spike wave discharges greater than 2.5 Hz. More prolonged absence seizures may have automatisms.

akinetic s., SYN atonic s.

anosognosic s.'s, SYN anosognosic *epilepsy.*

atonic s., s. characterized by sudden loss of muscle tone. SYN akinetic s.

atypical absence s., an absence s. associated with an EEG pattern of irregular or slow spike and wave at less than 2.5 Hz or paroxysmal fast activity on an abnormally slow background EEG.

audiogenic s., a reflex s. precipitated by loud noises, rare in humans. Audiogenic seizures in rodents are an animal model of epilepsy.

clonic s., a s. characterized by repetitive rhythmical jerking of all or part of the body.

complex partial s., a partial s. with impairment of consciousness without features of a generalized s. Complex partial s.'s are commonly associated with automatisms.

convulsive s., s. with clonic or tonic-clonic motor activity.

early s., a s. occurring within one week after craniocerebral trauma.

electrographic s., SYN subclinical s.

epileptic s., a s. that is caused by epilepsy.

febrile s., SYN febrile *convulsion.*

focal motor s., a simple partial s. with localized motor activity.

gelastic s., a s. characterized by laughing. This seizure type is often accompanied by hypothalamic lesions, such as hamartomas.

generalized s., s.'s characterized by generalized cerebral onset clinically and on EEG.

generalized tonic-clonic s., a generalized s. characterized by the sudden onset of tonic contraction of the muscles often associated with a cry or moan, and frequently resulting in a fall to the ground. The tonic phase of the s. gradually give way to clonic convulsive movements occurring bilaterally and synchronously before slowing and eventually stopping, followed by a variable period of unconsciousness and gradual recovery. SYN cryptogenic epilepsy, generalized tonic-clonic epilepsy, grand mal s., grand mal, idiopathic epilepsy (2), major epilepsy.

grand mal s., SYN generalized tonic-clonic s.

Jacksonian s., a s. originating in or near the rolandic neocortex, which clinically involves one part of the body; s. spread is accompanied by progressive spread to other parts of the body on the same side; may become generalized. SYN jacksonian epilepsy.

late s., a s. that occurs greater than one week after a craniocerebral trauma or CNS insult.

major motor s., a grand mal s. or other convulsive s.

minor motor s., old term for nonconvulsive s. seen in patients with secondary generalized epilepsies.

myoclonic s., s. associated with single or repetitive myoclonic jerks.

nonconvulsive s., a s. without clonic or tonic activity or other convulsive motor activity. SEE ALSO complex partial s., absence s.

nonepileptic s., any behavior that resembles a s., but is not epileptic, *i.e.,* not associated with abnormal cerebral EEG activity. SEE ALSO psychogenic s.

partial s., s. characterized by localized cerebral ictal onset. The symptoms experienced are dependent on the cortical area of ictal onset or seizure spread.

petit mal s., an absence s.

psychic s., a simple partial s. characterized by an attack of psychic phenomena such as a dreamy state, déjà vu, autonomic sensation or emotion; commonly, but not exclusively, associated with temporal lobe epilepsy.

psychogenic s., a clinical spell that resembles an epileptic s., but is not due to epilepsy. The EEG is normal during an attack, and the behavior is often related to psychiatric disturbance, such as a conversion disorder.

psychomotor s., SYN psychomotor *epilepsy.*

secondarily generalized tonic-clonic s., a generalized tonic-clonic s. that begins with a partial s. and evolves into a generalized tonic-clonic s.

simple partial s., a partial s. that is not associated with impairment of consciousness.

subclinical s., a s. detected by EEG, which has no clinical correlate, *i.e.,* an EEG seizure alone or an electrical seizure alone. SYN electrographic s.

tonic s., a s. characterized by increased muscle tone, usually generalized.

tonic-clonic s., a generalized tonic-clonic s.

versive s., a partial s. associated with head and eye deviation to one side.

se·junc·tion (sē-jŭngk′shŭn). Rarely used term for a separation; a breaking of continuity in the mental processes. [L. *se-jungo,* pp. *-junctus,* to disjoin]

se·la·pho·bia (sē-lă-fō′bē-ă). Rarely used term for a morbid fear of a flash of light. [G. *selas,* light, + *phobos,* fear]

Sel·din·ger, Sven Ivar, Swedish radiologist, *1921. SEE Seldinger *technique.*

se·lec·tins. Glycoproteins which are found on the surface of lymphocyte or endothelial cells which regulate the traffic patterns of lymphocytes. [L. *se-ligo,* pp. *se-lectum,* to sort, choose, + -in]

se·lec·tion (sĕ-lek′shŭn). The combined effect of the causes and consequences of genetic factors that determine the average number of progeny of a species that attain sexual maturity; phenotypes that are lethal early in life (*e.g.,* Tay-Sachs disease), that cause sterility (*e.g.,* Turner's syndrome), or that produce sterile progeny are selected against. When s. is used of individual pedigrees, other factors, notably variance of the number of progeny and number that survive to maturity, are important considerations; in large populations, these factors even out and the mean only is of importance. [L. *se-ligo,* to separate, select, fr. *se,* apart, + *lego,* to pick out]

artificial s., interference by man with natural s. by purposeful breeding of animals or plants of specific genotype or phenotype to produce a strain with desired characteristics; *e.g.,* breeding of dairy cattle for high milk production.

medical s., preservation, by medical care and treatment, of individuals of pathologic genotypes who would not otherwise reproduce, thus tending to increase the frequency of pathologic genes in the population; conversely, reduction of the frequency of path-

ologic genes by preventing reproduction of individuals of specified genotype by surgical sterilization or other means.

natural s., "survival of the fittest," the principle that in nature those individuals best able to adapt to their environment will survive and reproduce, while those less able will die without progeny; and the genes carried by the survivors will increase in frequency. This principle is heuristic rather than rigorous since it cannot be tested, the outcome being tautologous with the empirical definition of fitness.

sexual s., a form of natural s. in which, according to Darwin's theory, the male or female is attracted by certain characteristics, form, color, behavior, etc., in the opposite sex; thus modifications of a special nature are brought about in the species.

se·leg·i·line (sē-lej′e-lēn). A monoamine oxidase enzyme inhibitor; inhibits only the type B isozyme so that consuming tyramine-containing foods or beverages is less likely to induce hypertensive crisis in persons treated with selegiline than in persons treated with nonselective monoamine oxidase inhibitors. The drug is used in the treatment of Parkinson's disease. SYN deprenyl.

se·le·ne un·gui·um (sē-lē′nē ŭng′gwi-ŭm). SYN lunula (1). [G. *selēnē,* moon; gen. pl. of L. *unguis,* nail]

se·le·ni·um (Se) (sĕ-lē′nē-ŭm). A metallic element chemically similar to sulfur, atomic no. 34, atomic wt. 78.96; an essential trace element toxic in large quantities; required for glutathione peroxidase and a few other enzymes; ^{75}Se (half-life equal to 119.78 days) is used in scintography of the pancreas and parathyroid glands. [G. *selēnē,* moon]

s. sulfide, a mixture of crystalline s. monosulfide and solid solutions of s. and sulfur in an amorphous form, containing 52 to 55.5% Se; used in the treatment of seborrhea of the scalp or dandruff; it is applied to the scalp as a suspension.

se·le·no·cys·teine (sĕ-lē-nō-sis′tēn). Cysteine containing selenium in place of one sulfur atom, found in nature and, at least in part, responsible for certain curative effects of cysteine; present in certain bacterial formate dehydrogenases and glycine reductases.

se·len·o·dont (sĕ-lē′nō-dont). Denoting an animal, or man, having teeth, as the human molars, with longitudinal crescent-shaped ridges. [G. *selēnē,* moon, + *odous* (*odont-*), tooth]

se·le·no·me·thi·o·nine (sĕ-lē′nō-me-thī′ō-nēn). Methionine containing selenium in place of sulfur.

Se·le·no·mo·nas (sĕ-lē′nō-mō′nas). A genus of bacteria of uncertain taxonomic affiliation, containing curved to crescentic or helical, Gram-negative, strictly anaerobic rods that are motile with an active tumbling motion. Several flagella are present in a tuft, often near the center of the concave side. The type species, *S. sputigena,* is found in the human buccal cavity. [G. *selēnē,* moon, + *monas,* single (unit)]

self. 1. A sum of the attitudes, feelings, memories, traits, and behavioral predispositions that make up the personality. 2. The individual as represented in his or her own awareness and in his or her environment. 3. In immunology, an individual's autologous cell components as contrasted with non-s., or foreign, constituents; the basic mechanism underlying recognition of s. from non-s. is unknown, but serves to protect the host from an immunologic attack on his own antigenic constituents, as opposed to immune system destruction or elimination of foreign antigens.

subliminal s., the sum of the mental processes which take place without the conscious knowledge of the individual. SYN subconscious mind.

self-ac·cu·sa·tion. A common psychiatric symptom, encountered most characteristically in agitated depression.

self-a·naly·sis. SYN autoanalysis.

self-a·ware·ness. Realization of one's ongoing feeling and emotional experience; a major goal of all psychotherapy.

self-cen·tered·ness. SYN autosynnoia.

self-com·mit·ment. Voluntary mental hospitalization.

self-con·trol. 1. Self-regulation of one's behavior in accordance with personal beliefs, goals, attitudes and societal expectations. 2. Use by an individual of active coping strategies to deal with problem situations, in contrast to passive conditioning strategies which do things to the individual and require no action by the person.

self·dif·fer·en·ti·a·tion. Differentiation resulting from the action of intrinsic causes.

self·dis·cov·e·ry. In psychoanalysis, the freeing of the repressed ego in a person raised to be submissive to those around him.

self·ef·fi·ca·cy. An individual's estimate or personal judgment of his or her own ability to succeed in reaching a specific goal, *e.g.,* quitting smoking or losing weight or a more general goal, *e.g.,* continuing to remain at a prescribed weight level.

self·fer·til·i·za·tion. Fecundation of the ovules by the pollen of the same flower, or of the ova by the spermatozoa of the same animal in hermaphrodite forms; denoting an extreme type of inbreeding seen in certain plants and animal forms which produce both male and female gametes.

self·in·fec·tion. SYN autoinfection.

self·knowl·edge. SYN autognosis.

self·lim·it·ed. Denoting a disease that tends to cease after a definite period; *e.g.,* pneumonia.

self·love. SYN narcissism.

self·poi·son·ing. SYN autointoxication.

self·reg·u·la·tion. A three-stage strategy patients are taught to use in order to end risky health-associated behaviors such as smoking and overeating. 1. self-monitoring (self-observation), the first stage in self-regulation involves the individual's deliberately attending to and recording his or her own behavior; 2. self-evaluation, the second stage, in which the individual assesses what was learned by self-monitoring, such as how often and where one smokes, and uses those observational data to establish health goals or criteria; 3. self-reinforcement, the third stage, in which the individual rewards him/herself for each behavioral success on the road to that goal, thereby enhancing the chance of reaching it.

self·stim·u·la·tion. A technique for electrical stimulation of peripheral nerves, spinal cord, or brain by the patient himself to relieve pain.

Selivanoff, Feodor, Russian chemist, *1859. SEE S.'s *test.*

sel·la (sel'ă). SYN saddle (1). [L. saddle]

  empty s., a sella turcica, often enlarged, that contains no discernible pituitary gland; may be primarily due to an incompetent sellar diaphragm with compression of the pituitary gland by herniating arachnoid or secondarily due to surgery or radiotherapy.

  s. tur'cica [NA], a saddle-like bony prominence on the upper surface of the body of the sphenoid bone, constituting the middle part of the butterfly-shaped middle cranial fossa; it includes the tuberculum sellae anteriorly and the dorsum sellae posteriorly; with its covering of dura mater it constitutes the hypophysial fossa which accommodates the hypophysis or pituitary gland. SYN pars sellaris, Turkish saddle.

sel·lar (sel'ăr). Relating to the sella turcica.

Sellick, Brian A., 20th century British anesthetist. SEE S.'s *maneuver.*

Selye, Hans, Austrian endocrinologist in Canada, 1907–1982. SEE adaptation *syndrome* of S.

SEM Abbreviation for standard error of the *mean.*

se·man·tics (se-man'tiks). A branch of semiotics: **1.** The study of the significance and development of the meaning of words. **2.** The study concerned with the relations between signs and their referents; the relations between the signs of a system; and human behavioral reaction to signs, including unconscious attitudes, influences of social institutions, and epistemological and linguistic assumptions. [G. *sēmainō,* to show]

Sémélaigne, Georges, 20th century French pediatrician. SEE Debré-S. *syndrome;* Kocher-Debré-S. *syndrome.*

sem·el·in·ci·dent (sem-el-in'si-dent). An obsolete term that means happening once only; said of an infectious disease, one attack of which confers permanent immunity. [L. *semel,* once, + *incido,* to happen, fr. *cado,* to fall]

se·men, pl. **sem·i·na, se·mens** (sē'men, sē-mi'nă, sē'menz). **1** [NA]. The penile ejaculate; a thick, yellowish-white, viscid fluid containing spermatozoa; a mixture produced by secretions of the

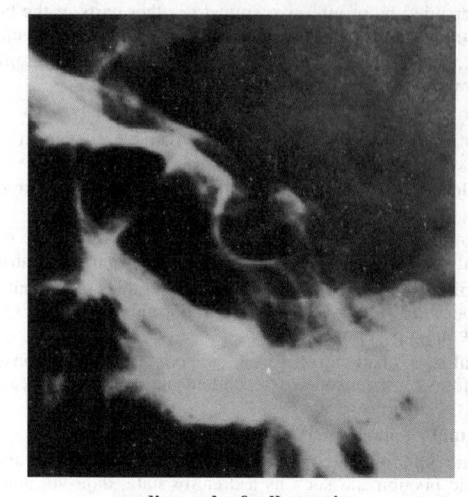

radiograph of sella turcica

testes, seminal vesicles, prostate, and bulbourethral glands. SYN sperm (2) [NA], seminal fluid. **2.** SYN seed (1). [L. *semen* (*semin*-), seed (of plants, men, animals)]

se·me·nu·ria (sē-mĕ-nū'rē-ă). The excretion of urine containing semen. SYN seminuria, spermaturia.

semi-. One-half; partly (properly used with words derived from L. roots). Cf. hemi-. [L. *semis,* half]

sem·i·al·de·hyde (sem-ē-al'dĕ-hīd). The monoaldehyde of a dicarboxylic acid, so called because half the COOH groups of the original acid are reduced to the aldehyde while the other half are unchanged; *e.g.,* glutamic acid γ-s., $OHC-CH_2CH_2CH(NH_3)^+-COO^-$. Many s.'s are intermediates in the biosynthesis and metabolic degradation of amino acids (*e.g.,* L-proline, L-lysine, L-glutamate).

sem·i·ca·nal (sem'ē-kă-nal'). A half canal; a deep groove on the edge of a bone which, uniting with a similar groove or part of an adjoining bone, forms a complete canal. SYN semicanalis.

  s. of auditory tube, the inferior division of the musculotubal canal which forms the bony part of the auditory (eustachian) tube. SYN semicanalis tubae auditivae [NA].

  s. for tensor tympani muscle, semicanal of the tensor muscle of the tympanum; the superior division of the canalis musculotubarius containing the tensor tympani muscle. SYN semicanalis musculi tensoris tympani [NA].

sem·i·ca·na·lis, pl. **sem·i·ca·na·les** (sem'ē-kă-nal'is, -ēz). SYN semicanal. [L.]

  s. mus'culi tensor'is tym'pani [NA], SYN *semicanal* for tensor tympani muscle.

  s. tu'bae auditi'vae [NA], SYN *semicanal* of auditory tube.

sem·i·car·ti·lag·i·nous (sem'ē-kar-ti-laj'i-nŭs). Composed partly of cartilage.

sem·i·cir·cu·lar (sem'ē-sir'kyū-lăr). Forming a half circle or an incomplete circle. SYN semiorbicular.

sem·i·co·ma. SEE semicomatose.

sem·i·com·a·tose. An imprecise term for a state of drowsiness and inaction, in which more than ordinary stimulation may be required to evoke a response, and the response may be delayed or incomplete. SYN semiconscious.

sem·i·con·duc·tor (sem'ē-kon-dŭk'ter). A metalloid, in one form or another, that conducts electricity more easily than a true nonmetal but less easily than a metal; *e.g.,* silicon, germanium.

sem·i·con·scious. SYN semicomatose.

sem·i·con·serv·a·tive. The process of replicating DNA in which the two strands remain intact, separate, are copied and one parental strand goes to each daughter cell.

sem·i·cris·ta (sem'ē-kris'tă). A small or imperfect ridge or crest. [semi- + L. *crista,* crest, tuft]

s. incisi'va, SYN nasal *crest.*

sem·i·de·cus·sa·tion (sem'ē-dē-kŭs-sā'shŭn). Incomplete decussation such as occurs in the human optic chiasm.

sem·i·flex·ion (sem-ē-flek'shŭn). The position of a joint or segment of a limb midway between extension and flexion.

sem·i·lu·nar (sem-ē-lū'năr). SYN lunar (2). [semi- + L. *luna,* moon]

sem·i·lu·na·re (sem-ē-lū-nā'rē). Obsolete term for lunate *bone.*

sem·i·lux·a·tion (sem-ē-lŭk-sā'shŭn). SYN subluxation.

sem·i·mem·bra·no·sus (sem'ē-mem-bră-nō'sŭs). SEE semimembranosus *muscle.*

sem·i·mem·bra·nous (sem'ē-mem'bră-nŭs). Consisting partly of membrane; denoting the semimembranosus muscle.

sem·i·nal (sem'i-năl). **1.** Relating to the semen. **2.** Original or influential of future developments.

sem·i·na·tion (sem-i-nā'shŭn). SYN insemination.

sem·i·nif·er·ous (sem'i-nif'er-ŭs). Carrying or conducting the semen; denoting the tubules of the testis. [L. *semen,* seed (semen) + *fero,* to carry]

sem·i·no·ma (sem-i-nō'mă). A radiosensitive malignant neoplasm usually arising from germ cells in the testis of young male adults which metastasizes to the paraortic lymph nodes; a counterpart of dysgerminoma of the ovary. [L. *semen,* seed (semen) + G. *-oma,* tumor]

spermacytic s., a relatively slow-growing, locally invasive type of testicular s. that does not metastasize and has no ovarian counterpart.

se·mi·no·ma·tous (sem-i-nō'mă-tŭs). Relating to a seminoma.

sem·i·nor·mal (N/2) (sem-ē-nōr'măl). Denoting a solution one-half the strength of a normal solution (0.5 N).

sem·i·nu·ria (sē-mi-nū'rē-ă). SYN semenuria.

se·mi·og·ra·phy, se·mei·og·ra·phy (sē-mē-og'ră-fē). Obsolete term for a treatise on symptomatology or a description of the symptoms of a disease. [G. *sēmeion,* sign, + *graphē,* a description]

se·mi·o·log·ic, se·mei·o·log·ic (sē'mē-ō-loj'ik). **1.** The general philosophical theory of signs and symbols in communication, having three branches: syntactics, semantics, and pragmatics. **2.** Obsolete term for symptomatic.

se·mi·ol·o·gy, se·mei·ol·o·gy (sē-mē-ol'ō-jē). Obsolete term for symptomatology. [G. *sēmeion,* sign, + *logos,* study]

sem·i·o·path·ic, se·mei·o·path·ic (sē'mē-ō-path'ik). Denoting the disordered use of symbols. [G. *sēmeion,* sign, + *pathos,* disease]

sem·i·or·bic·u·lar (sē-mē-ōr-bik'yū-lăr). SYN semicircular.

se·mi·o·sis, se·mei·o·sis (sē-mē-ō'sis) The mental or symbolic process in which something (*e.g.,* word, symbol, nonverbal cue) functions as a sign for the organism. [G. *sēmeiōsis,* fr. *sēmeion,* sign]

se·mi·ot·ic, se·mei·ot·ic (sē-mē-ot'ik, sem-ē-). **1.** Relating to semiotics. **2.** Relating to signs, linguistic or bodily. [G. *sēmeiō-tikos,* fr. *sēmeion,* sign]

se·mi·ot·ics, se·mei·ot·ics (sē-mē-ot'iks, sem-e-). **1.** The general philosophical theory of signs and symbols in communication, having three branches: syntactics, semantics, and pragmatics. **2.** Obsolete term for symptomatology. [see semiotic]

sem·i·pen·ni·form (sem'ē-pen'i-fōrm). Penniform on one side. SEE unipennate *muscle.*

sem·i·per·me·a·ble (sem-ē-per'mē-ă-bl). Freely permeable to water (or other solvent) but relatively impermeable to solutes. Depending on the context, it has been used to imply impermeability to all solutes except very small uncharged molecules (*e.g.,* a cell membrane), or merely impermeability to very large molecules such as proteins (*e.g.,* a capillary membrane).

sem·i·pla·cen·ta (sem'ē-pla-sen'tă). The type of placenta in ruminants, horse and pig, in which the maternal and fetal placentas do not grow together but can be easily separated without tearing; an apposed or contact placenta.

sem·i·pro·na·tion (sem'ē-prō-nā'shŭn). The attitude or assumption of a partly prone position, as in Sims' position.

sem·i·prone (sem-ē-prōn'). Denoting semipronation.

sem·i·qui·none (sem-ē-kwin'ōn). A free radical resulting from the removal of one hydrogen atom with its electron during the process of dehydrogenation of a hydroquinone to quinone or similar compound (*e.g.,* flavin mononucleotide).

sem·i·spi·nal (sem-ē-spī'năl). Half spinal; denoting muscles attached in part to the spinous processes of the vertebrae.

Sem·i·sul·co·spi·na (sem'ē-sŭl-kō-spī'nă). A genus of operculate snails (family Pleuroceriidae, subclass Prosobranchiata). An oriental form, *S. libertina,* is the first intermediate host of a number of trematodes, including *Paragonimus westermani.* [semi- + L. *sulcus,* a furrow + *spina,* thorn, spine]

sem·i·sul·cus (sem'ē-sŭl'kŭs). A slight groove on the edge of a bone or other structure, which, uniting with a similar groove on the corresponding adjoining structure, forms a complete sulcus.

sem·i·su·pi·na·tion (sem'ē-sū-pi-nā'shŭn). The attitude or assumption of a partly supine position.

sem·i·su·pine (sem-ē-sū-pīn'). Denoting semisupination.

sem·i·syn·thet·ic (sem'ē-sin-thet'ik). Describing the process of synthesizing a particular chemical utilizing a naturally occurring chemical as a starting material, thus obviating part of a total synthesis; *e.g.,* the conversion of cholesterol (obtained from a natural source) into a corticosteroid.

sem·i·sys·tem·at·ic name (sem'ē-sis-tě-mat'ik). A name of a chemical of which at least one part is systematic and at least one part is not (*i.e.,* is trivial). For example, calciferol includes the -ol suffix denoting an –OH radical, while calcifer-, which has no systematic meaning, is used only in this word. Cortisone contains the -one suffix, indicating a ketone group, but the rest of the term derives from cortex (adrenal). Hippuric acid (trivial) may be defined as *N*-benzoylglycine (semitrivial name); benzoyl is systematic for the C_6H_5-CO– radical, whereas glycine is the trivial name for α-aminoacetic (or 2-aminoethanoic, to be completely systematic) acid, and the *N* signifies that the benzoyl is attached to the nitrogen of glycine; from this, the structure C_6H_5-CO–NH–CH_2–COOH is uniquely defined. Many generic or nonproprietary names of drugs, including USAN names, hormones, etc., are semitrivial in this chemical sense, although often termed trivial names; distinction between trivial and semitrivial is not often made. SYN semitrivial name.

sem·i·ten·di·no·sus (sem'ē-ten-di-nō'sŭs). SYN semitendinous. [L.]

sem·i·ten·di·nous (sem'ē-ten'di-nŭs). Composed in part of tendon; denoting the semitendinosus muscle. SYN semitendinosus. [L. *semitendinosus*]

sem·i·ter·tian (sem-ē-ter'shē-ăn, -ter'shŭn). Partly tertian, partly quotidian; denoting a malarial fever in which two paroxysms occur on one day and one on the succeeding day.

sem·i·triv·i·al name (sem-ē-triv'ē-ăl). SYN semisystematic name.

sem·i·va·lent (sem-ē-vā'lent). Denoting the ability to form a one-electron bond.

Semon, Sir Felix, German laryngologist in Britain, 1849–1921. SEE S.'s *law;* Gerhardt-S. *law.*

Semon, Richard W., German biologist, 1859–1908. SEE S.-Hering *theory.*

Semple, Sir David, English physician, 1856–1937. SEE S. *vaccine.*

se·mus·tine. SYN methyl-CCNU.

Senear, Francis E., U.S. dermatologist, 1889–1958. SEE S.-Usher *disease, syndrome.*

Se·ne·cio (sě-nē'sē-ō, -shē-ō). **1.** A large genus of plants (family Compositae), many species of which contain alkaloids that produce hepatic necrosis. **2.** *Senecio aureus;* life-root; squaw-weed; ragwort; a common weed of the eastern U.S., formerly used in the treatment of amenorrhea and other menstrual irregularities. [L. a plant, groundsel, fr. *senecio,* an old man]

se·ne·ci·o·ic ac·id (sě-nē'si-ō-ik). $(CH_3)_2C=CH$—COOH; 3-Methyl-2-butenoic acid; 3,3-dimethylacrylic acid; methylcrotonic acid; a polymer precursor and a precursor of isoprenoid and terpene compounds; the acid component of binapacryl in which it is esterified with 4,6-dinitro-2-(1-methylpropyl)phenol; the coenzyme A derivative is an intermediate in L-leucine degradation; used as a fungicide and miticide.

se·ne·ci·o·sis (sĕ-nē-sē-ō′sis). Liver degeneration and necrosis caused by ingestion of plants of the genus *Senecio*, such as ragwort and groundsel; similar hepatotoxic properties have been observed after ingestion of some kinds of *Crotalaria* and *Heliotropium*.

sen·e·ga (sen′ē-gă). The dried root of *Polygala senega* (family Polygalaceae), a herb of eastern and central North America; an expectorant. SYN Seneca snakeroot. [*Seneca,* an Indian tribe]

se·nes·cence (se-nes′ens). The state of being old. [L. *senesco,* to grow old, fr. *senex,* old]

dental s., that condition of the teeth and associated structures in which there is deterioration due to normal or premature aging processes.

se·nes·cent (sē-nes′ent). Growing old.

Sengstaken, Robert W., U.S. neurosurgeon, *1923. SEE S.-Blakemore *tube.*

se·nile (sē′nīl, sen′īl). Relating to or characteristic of old age. [L. *senilis*]

se·nil·i·ty (se-nil′i-tē). Old age; a general term for a variety of mental disorders occurring in old age which consist of two broad categories, organic and psychological disorders. SYN anility. [see senile]

se·ni·um (sē′nē-ŭm). Rarely used term for old age; especially the debility of advanced age. [L. the feebleness of age, fr. *seneo,* to be old, feeble]

sen·na (sen′ă). The dried leaflets or legumes of *Cassia acutifolia* (Alexandrine s.) and *C. angustifolia* (Tinnevelly or Indian s.); a laxative. [Ar. *senā*]

sen·no·side A, sen·no·side B (sen′ō-sīdz). Two anthraquinone glucosides that are the laxative principles of senna.

sen·sate (sen′sāt). Able to perceive touch and other sensations; used in reference to patients who have had partial nerve or spinal cord injuries.

sen·sa·tion (sen-sā′shŭn). A feeling; the translation into consciousness of the effects of a stimulus exciting any of the organs of sense. [L. *sensatio,* perception, feeling, fr. *sentio,* to perceive, feel]

cincture s., SYN zonesthesia.

delayed s., a s. that is not perceived until the lapse of an appreciable interval following the application of the stimulus.

general s., a s. referred to the body as a whole rather than to any particular part.

girdle s., SYN zonesthesia.

objective s., a s. caused by a verifiable stimulus.

primary s., a s. that is the direct result of a stimulus.

referred s., a s. felt in one place in response to a stimulus applied in another. SYN reflex s., transferred s.

reflex s., SYN referred s.

special s., a s. referred to a stimulus produced by an external body and acting on any of the sense organs.

subjective s., a s. not readily referrable to a denotably verifiable stimulus.

transferred s., SYN referred s.

sense (sens). The faculty of perceiving any stimulus. [L. *sentio,* pp. *sensus,* to feel, to perceive]

color s., the ability to perceive variations in hue, luminosity, and saturation of light.

s. of equilibrium, the s. that makes possible a normal physiologic posture. SYN static s.

geometrical s., one or other of two directions along a curve in which something is moving *e.g.,* clockwise or counterclockwise.

joint s., SYN articular *sensibility.*

kinesthetic s., SYN myesthesia.

light s., the ability to perceive variations in the degree of light or brightness.

muscular s., SYN myesthesia.

obstacle s., the ability, often found in the blind, to avoid objects without visual warning.

position s., SYN posture s.

sensation			
modality of sensation	object of perception	nature of stimuli	receptor type
sense of sight	brightness, darkness, colors	electro-magnetic radiation 4000–7000 Å	photo-receptors
sense of temperature	cold, heat	electro-magnetic radiation 7000–9000 Å, convective heat transport	thermo-receptors
tactile sense of skin	pressure, touch	modification of mechano-receptors by solid objects or transmission of air-pressure changes	mechano-receptors
sense of hearing	sound frequencies		
statokinetic sense	absolute body position, speed of body, relative body position and movement of body parts and joints, sense of strength		
sense of smell	various odors	chemical substances	chemo-receptors
sense of taste	sour, salty, sweet, bitter	ions	
sense of pain	pain	mechanical tissue injury	nociceptors

posture s., the ability to recognize the position in which a limb is passively placed, with the eyes closed. SYN position s.

pressure s., the faculty of discriminating various degrees of pressure on the surface. SYN baresthesia, piesesthesia.

seventh s., SYN visceral s.

sixth s., SYN cenesthesia.

space s., the faculty of perceiving the relative positions of objects in the external world.

special s., one of the five senses related respectively to the organs of sight, hearing, smell, taste, and touch.

static s., SYN s. of equilibrium.

tactile s., SYN touch (1).

temperature s., SYN thermoesthesia.

thermal s., thermic s., SYN thermoesthesia.

time s., the faculty by which the passage of time is appreciated.

visceral s., the perception of the existence of the internal organs. SYN seventh s., splanchnesthesia, splanchnesthetic sensibility.

weight s., SYN weight s. SYN weight s.

sen·si·bil·i·ty (sen-si-bil′i-tē). The consciousness of sensation; the capability of perceiving sensible stimuli. [L. *sensibilitas*]

articular s., appreciation of sensation in joint surfaces. SYN arthresthesia, joint sense.

bone s., SYN pallesthesia.

cortical s., the integration of sensory stimuli by the cerebral cortex.

deep s., SYN bathyesthesia, myesthesia.

dissociation s., the loss of the pain and the thermal senses with preservation of tactile sensibility or vice versa.

electromuscular s., s. of muscular tissue to stimulation by electricity.

epicritic s., SEE epicritic.

mesoblastic s., SYN myesthesia.

pallesthetic s., SYN pallesthesia.

proprioceptive s., SEE proprioceptive.

protopathic s., SEE protopathic.

splanchnesthetic s., SYN visceral *sense*.

vibratory s., SYN pallesthesia.

sen·si·ble (sen′si-bl). **1.** Perceptible to the senses. **2.** Capable of sensation. **3.** SYN sensitive. **4.** Having reason or judgment; intelligent. [L. *sensibilis,* fr. *sentio,* to feel, perceive]

sen·sif·er·ous (sen-sif′er-ŭs). Conducting a sensation. [L. *sensus,* sense, + *fero,* to carry]

sen·sig·e·nous (sen-sij′e-nŭs). Giving rise to sensation. [L. *sensus,* sense, + G. *-gen,* to produce]

sen·sim·e·ter (sen-sim′ĕ-ter). An instrument that measures degrees of cutaneous sensation. [L. *sensus,* sense, + G. *metron,* measure]

sen·si·tive (sen′si-tiv). **1.** Capable of perceiving sensations. **2.** Responding to a stimulus. **3.** Acutely perceptive of interpersonal situations. **4.** One who is readily hypnotizable. **5.** Readily undergoing a chemical change, with but slight change in environmental conditions, as a s. reagent. **6.** In immunology, denoting: 1) a sensitized *antigen*; 2) a person (or animal) rendered susceptible to immunological reactions by previous exposure to the antigen concerned. SYN sensible (3).

sen·si·tiv·i·ty (sen-si-tiv′i-tē). **1.** The ability to appreciate by one or more of the senses. **2.** State of being sensitive. SYN esthesia (2). **3.** In clinical pathology and medical screening, the proportion of individuals with a positive test result for the disease that the test is intended to reveal, *i.e.,* true positive results as a proportion of the total of true positive and false negative results. Cf. specificity (2). [L. *sentio,* pp. *sensus,* to feel]

acquired s., SYN allergy (1).

analytical s., the degree of response to a change in concentration of analyte being measured in an assay; synonymous with the detection limit.

antibiotic s., microbial susceptibility to antibiotics. SEE ALSO antibiotic sensitivity *test,* minimal inhibitory *concentration.*

clinical s., test positivity in disease; ability of a test to correctly identify disease. SEE ALSO diagnostic s.

contrast s., in optics, the ability to discern the difference in brightness of adjacent areas; in radiology, allergic reaction to iodinated radiographic contrast medium.

diagnostic s., the probability (P) that, given the presence of disease (D), an abnormal test result (T) indicates the presence of disease; *i.e.,* P(T/D). SEE ALSO clinical s.

idiosyncratic s., a type I allergic reaction (atopic).

induced s., SYN allergy (1).

multiple chemical s., a symptom array of variable presentation attributed to recurrent exposure to known environmental toxins at dosages generally below levels established as harmful; complaints involve multiple organ systems. SYN environmental illness.

pacemaker s., the minimum cardiac activity required to consistently trigger a pulse generator.

photoallergic s., SEE photosensitization.

phototoxic s., SEE photosensitization.

primaquine s., nonimmunological inborn s. to primaquine, causing hemolysis on exposure to the drug, due to deficiency of glucose 6-phosphate dehydrogenase in red cells.

relative s., the s. of a medical screening test as determined by comparison with the same type of test; *e.g.,* s. of a new serological test relative to s. of an established serological test.

salt s., the tendency of certain bacterial suspensions to agglutinate spontaneously in physiological saline solution.

spectral s., the reciprocal of the amount of monochromatic radiation that produces a fixed response.

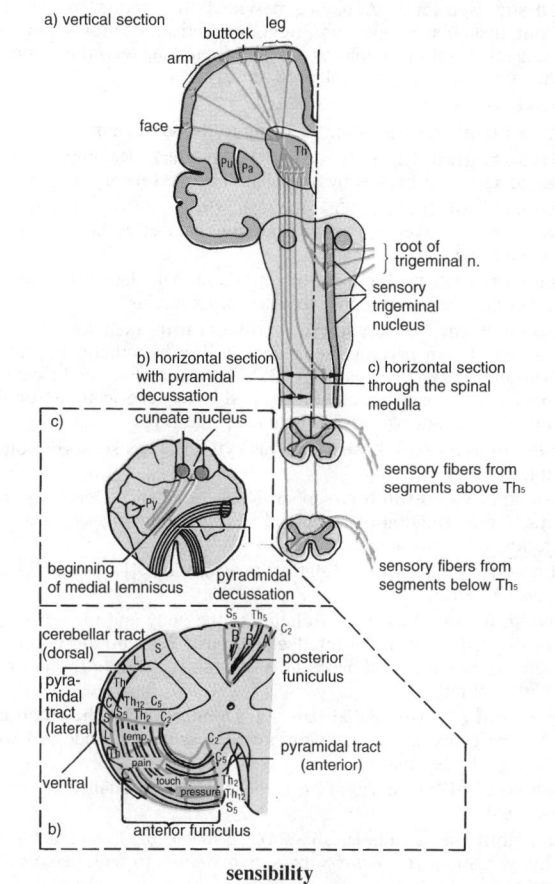

sensibility

ascending nervous system in vertical (a) and horizontal (b, c) sections with locations of pathways originating in thoracic, lumbar, and sacral regions of spinal cord

sen·si·ti·za·tion (sen′si-ti-zā′shŭn). Immunization, especially with reference to antigens (immunogens) not associated with infection; the induction of acquired sensitivity or of allergy.

autoerythrocyte s., SEE autoerythrocyte sensitization *syndrome.*

covert s., aversive conditioning or training to rid onself of an unwanted behavior during which the patient is taught to imagine unpleasant and related aversive consequences while engaging in the unwanted habit.

photodynamic s., the action by which certain substances, notably fluorescing dyes (acridine, eosin, methylene blue, rose bengal) absorb visible light and emit the energy at wavelengths that are deleterious to microbes or other organisms in the dye-containing suspension, or selectively destroy cancer cells sensitized by intravenous porphyrin and exposed to red laser light. SYN photosensitization (2).

sen·si·tize (sen′si-tīz). To render sensitive; to induce acquired sensitivity, to immunize. SEE ALSO sensitized *antigen.*

sen·si·tiz·er (sen′si-tīz-er). **1.** SYN antibody. **2.** A substance that causes dermatitis only after alteration (sensitization) of the skin by previous exposure to that substance.

sens·i·tom·e·try (sen-si-tom′ĕ-trē). In radiology, the procedure of measuring film response to radiation. [sensitivity + G. *metron,* measure]

sen·so·mo·bile (sen-sō-mō′bēl). Capable of movement in response to a stimulus.

sen·so·mo·bil·i·ty (sen-sō-mō-bil′i-tē). The state of being sensomobile.

sen·so·mo·tor (sen-sō-mō′ter). SYN sensorimotor.

sen·sor (sen′sŏr). A device designed to respond to physical stimuli such as temperature, light, magnetism, or movement, and transmit resulting impulses for interpretation, recording, movement, or operating control. [see sense]

△**sensori-.** Sensory. [L. *sensorius*]

sen·so·ri·al (sen-sōr′ē-ăl). Relating to the sensorium.

sen·so·ri·glan·du·lar (sen′sōr-i-glan′dyū-lăr). Relating to glandular secretion excited by stimulation of the sensory nerves.

sen·so·ri·mo·tor (sen′sōr-i-mō′ter). Both sensory and motor; denoting a mixed nerve with afferent and efferent fibers. SYN sensomotor.

sen·so·ri·mus·cu·lar (sen′sōr-i-mŭs′kyū-lăr). Denoting muscular contraction in response to a sensory stimulus.

sen·so·ri·um, pl. **sen·so·ria**, **sen·so·ri·ums** (sen-sōr′ē-ŭm, -ă, -ŭmz). **1.** An organ of sensation. **2.** The hypothetical "seat of sensation." SYN perceptorium. **3.** In human biology and psychology, consciousness; sometimes used as a generic term for the intellectual and cognitive functions. [Late L.]

sen·so·ri·vas·cu·lar (sen′sōr-i-vas′kyū-lăr). SYN sensorivasomotor.

sen·so·ri·vas·o·mo·tor (sen′sōr-i-vas-ō-mō′ter). Denoting contraction or dilation of the blood vessels occurring as a sensory reflex. SYN sensorivascular.

sen·so·ry (sen′sŏ-rē). Relating to sensation. [L. *sensorius,* fr. *sensus,* sense]

sen·su·al (sen′shū-ăl). **1.** Relating to the body and the senses, as distinguished from the intellect or spirit. **2.** Denoting bodily or sensory pleasure, not necessarily sexual. [L. *sensualis,* endowed with feeling]

sen·su·al·ism (sen′shū-ăl-izm). **1.** Domination by the emotions. **2.** Indulgence in sensory pleasures. [L. *sensualis,* endowed with feeling, fr. *sentio,* to feel]

sen·su·al·i·ty (sen-shŭ-al′i-tē). The state or quality of being sensual.

sen·tient (sen′shent, sen′shē-ent). Capable of, or characterized by, sensation. [L. *sentiens,* pres. p. of *sentio,* to feel, perceive]

sen·ti·ment (sen′ti-ment). **1.** Feeling or emotion in relation to one idea. **2.** A complex disposition or organization of a person with reference to a given object (a person, thing, or abstract idea) that makes the object what it is for him or her. [L. *sentio,* to feel]

sen·ti·sec·tion (sen-ti-sek′shŭn). Vivisection of an animal that is not anesthetized. [L. *sentio,* to feel, + *sectio,* a cutting]

sep·a·ra·tion (sep-ă-rā′shŭn). **1.** The act of keeping apart or dividing, or the state of being held apart. **2.** In dentistry, the process of gaining slight spaces between the teeth preparatory to treatment.

jaw s., the amount of space between the jaws at any degree of opening.

s. of retina, SYN retinal *detachment.*

sternochondral s., s. of the sternochondral articulation, especially of the 2nd to 7th ribs, which are true joints lined with synovial membranes.

s. of teeth, (1) loss of proximal contact of teeth; **(2)** in orthodontics, the creation of interproximal spaces for the fitting of an appliance.

sep·a·ra·tor (sep′er-ā-ter). **1.** That which divides or keeps apart two or more substances or prevents them from mingling. **2.** In dentistry, an instrument for forcing two teeth apart, so as to gain access to adjacent proximal walls. SYN segregator. [L. *se-paro,* pp. *-atus,* to separate, fr. *se,* apart, + *paro,* to prepare]

Se·pha·dex (sef′a-deks). Trade name for certain polydextrans used in column chromatography.

sep·sis, pl. **sep·ses** (sep′sis, -sēz). The presence of various pusforming and other pathogenic organisms, or their toxins, in the blood or tissues; septicemia is a common type of s. [G. *sēpsis,* putrefaction]

intestinal s., s. associated with autointoxication of intestinal origin.

s. len′ta, a slowly developing and more or less localized infection.

puerperal s., SYN puerperal *fever.*

△**sept-.** SEE septi-, septico-, septo-.

sep·ta (sep′tă). Plural of septum. [L.]

intra-alveolar septa, SYN interradicular *septa,* under *septum.*

sep·tal (sep′tăl). Relating to a septum.

sep·tan (sep′tăn). Denoting a malarial fever the paroxysms of which recur every seventh day, counting the day of the occurrence as the first day, *i.e.,* with a five-day asymptomatic interval. [L. *septem,* seven]

Sep·ta·ta (sep-tă′tă). A recently described member of the protozoan phylum Microspora found in the intestine of an immunocompromised individual. The species described is *S. intestinalis.*

sep·tate (sep′tāt). Having a septum; divided into compartments. [L. *saeptum,* septum]

sep·tec·to·my (sep-tek′tō-mē). Operative removal of the whole or a part of a septum, specifically of the nasal septum. [L. *saeptum,* septum, + G. *ektomē,* excision]

sep·te·mia (sep-tē′mē-ă). A rarely used term for septicemia.

△**septi-, sept-.** Seven. [L. *septem*]

sep·tic (sep′tik). Relating to or caused by sepsis.

sep·ti·ce·mia (sep-ti-sē′mē-ă). Systemic disease caused by the spread of microorganisms and their toxins via the circulating blood; formerly called "blood poisoning". SEE ALSO pyemia. SYN hematosepsis, sapremia, septic fever, septic intoxication. [G. *sēpsis,* putrefaction, + *haima,* blood]

causes of septicemia (figures obtained from blood cultures of 660 hospitalized patients)		
organism	count	%
Neisseria meningitidis	7	
Haemophilus influenzae	4	
Staphylococcus aureus	172	27
Staphylococcus epidermidis	11	2
Streptococcus pyogenes	16	3
Streptococcus viridans	37	6
Streptococcus faecalis	31	5
Streptococcus pneumoniae	28	4
Escherichia coli	125	19
Citrobacter	1	
Klebsiella, Enterobacter, Serratia	96	15
Proteus species	18	3
Salmonella typhi	4	
Salmonella enteritidis	12	2
Pseudomonas species	61	9
Acinetobacter calcoaceticus	13	2
Alcaligenes species	1	
nonfermenting Gram-negative bacteria	8	
Peptostreptococcus	2	
Bacteroides species	1	
Candida species	12	

acute fulminating meningococcal s., SYN Waterhouse-Friderichsen *syndrome.*

anthrax s., SYN anthracemia.

cryptogenic s., a form of s. in which no primary focus of infection can be found.

hemorrhagic s., a bacterial disease in animals caused by members of the genus *Pasteurella;* occurs in cattle, sheep, swine, rabbits, and fowls. SYN s. pluriformis.

metastasizing s., sepsis, with entry of microorganisms into the blood stream leading to abscess formation at a distance from the original site of infection.

morphine injector's s., blood stream infection in an individual who injects him or herself with narcotics, usually intravenously, due to bacterial contamination of equipment used. Seen more often with heroin and narcotics other than morphine.

plague s., infection with the plague organism, *Yersinia pestis,* with blood-stream infection.

s. pluriform'is, SYN hemorrhagic s.

puerperal s., a severe bloodstream infection resulting from an obstetric delivery or procedure.

typhoid s., typhoid during the phase when the organism can be cultured from the blood. SYN typhosepsis.

sep·ti·ce·mic (sep-ti-sē'mik). Relating to, suffering from, or resulting from septicemia.

⌂**septico-, septic-.** Sepsis, septic. [G. *sēptikos,* putrifying, fr. *sēpsis,* putrefaction]

sep·ti·co·py·e·mia (sep'ti-kō-pī-ē'mē-ă). Pyemia and septicemia occurring together.

sep·ti·co·py·e·mic (sep'ti-kō-pī-ē'mik). Relating to septicopyemia.

sep·ti·me·tri·tis (sep'ti-mĕ-trī'tis). Obsolete term for septic inflammation of the uterus. [G. *sēptikōs,* septic, + *mētra,* uterus, + *-itis,* inflammation]

sep·ti·va·lent (sep-ti-vā'lent, sep-tiv'ă-lent). Having a combining power (valency) of seven.

⌂**septo-, sept-.** Septum. [L. *saeptum*]

sep·to·der·mo·plas·ty (sep-tō-der'mō-plas-tē). Operation to graft squamous epithelium to replace the mucosa of the nasal septum, especially in cases of hereditary hemorrhagic telangiectasia. [septo- + dermo- + G. *plastos,* formed]

sep·to·mar·gi·nal (sep'tō-mar'ji-năl). Relating to the margin of a septum, or to both a septum and a margin.

sep·to·na·sal (sep'tō-nā'săl). Relating to the nasal septum.

sep·to·plas·ty (sep'tō-plas-tē). Operation to correct defects or deformities of the nasal septum, often by alteration or partial removal of supporting structures. [septo- + G. *plastos,* formed]

sep·to·rhi·no·plas·ty (sep-tō-rī'nō-plas-tē). Combined operation to repair defects or deformities of the nasal septum and of the external nasal pyramid. [septo- + G. *rhis,* nose, + *plastos,* formed]

sep·tos·to·my (sep-tos'tō-mē). Surgical creation of a septal defect. [septo- + G. *stoma,* mouth]

sep·tu·lum, pl. **sep·tu·la** (sep'tyū-lŭm, -lă). A minute septum. [Mod. L. dim. of *septum*]

s. tes'tis [NA], SYN septula of testis.

septula of testis, one of the trabeculae of the testis; imperfect septa and fibrous cords radiating toward the surface of the gland from the mediastinum testis. SYN s. testis [NA], trabecula testis.

SEPTUM

sep·tum, gen. **sep·ti,** pl. **sep·ta** (sep'tŭm, -tī, -tă). **1** [NA]. A thin wall dividing two cavities or masses of softer tissue. SEE septal *area,* transparent s. **2.** In fungi, a wall; usually a cross-wall in a hypha. [L. *saeptum,* a partition]

s. accesso'rium, an additional ridge forming the lower border of the limbus fossae ovalis.

alveolar s., SYN interalveolar s.

aortopulmonary s., the spiral s. which, during development, separates the truncus arteriosus into a ventral pulmonary trunk and dorsal aorta. SEE ALSO bulbar *ridge.*

atrioventricular s., the small part of the membranous s. of the heart just above the septal cusp of the tricuspid valve that separates the right atrium from the left ventricle. SYN s. atrioventriculare [NA], pars membranacea septi atriorum.

s. atrioventricula're [NA], SYN atrioventricular s.

s. of auditory tube, a very thin horizontal plate of bone forming two semicanals, the upper, smaller, for the tensor tympani muscle, the lower, larger for the auditory tube; its termination in the middle ear is the processus cochleariformis. SYN s. canalis musculotubarii [NA], s. of musculotubal canal, s. tubae.

Bigelow's s., SYN *calcar* femorale.

bony nasal s., the bones supporting the bony part of the nasal septum; these are the perpendicular plate of the ethmoid, the vomer, the sphenoidal rostrum, the crest of the nasal bones, the frontal spine, and the median crest formed by the apposition of the maxillary and palatine bones. SYN s. nasi osseum [NA].

bulbar s., obsolete term for spiral s.

s. bul'bi ure'thrae, a fibrous s. in the interior of the bulb of the penis which divides it into two hemispheres.

s. cana'lis musculotuba'rii [NA], SYN s. of auditory tube.

cartilaginous s., SYN nasal septal *cartilage.*

s. cervica'le interme'dium [NA], SYN intermediate cervical s.

s. clitor'idis, an incomplete fibrous s. between the corpora cavernosa of the clitoris. SYN s. corporum cavernosorum clitoridis [NA].

Cloquet's s., SYN femoral s.

comblike s., SYN pectiniform s.

s. cor'porum cavernoso'rum clitor'idis [NA], SYN s. clitoridis.

crural s., SYN femoral s.

distal spiral s., SEE spiral s.

endovenous s., s. endoveno'sum, a remnant of the primitive separation between veins which fused to form a definitive trunk, such as the trunk leading to the left common iliac and the left renal veins.

femoral s., the delicate fibrous membrane that closes the femoral ring at the base of the femoral canal. SYN s. femorale [NA], Cloquet's s., crural s.

s. femora'le [NA], SYN femoral s.

s. of frontal sinuses, the bony partition between the right and left frontal sinuses; it is often deflected to one side of the middle line. SYN s. sinuum frontalium [NA].

gingival s., SYN interdental *papilla.*

s. glan'dis [NA], SYN s. of glans penis.

s. of glans penis, a fibrous partition extending through the glans penis from the lower surface of the tunica albuginea to the urethra. SYN s. glandis [NA].

hanging s., the deformity caused by an abnormal width of the septal portion of the alar cartilages.

interalveolar s., (1) the tissue intervening between two adjacent pulmonary alveoli; it consists of a close-meshed capillary network covered on both surfaces by very thin alveolar epithelial cells; **(2)** one of the bony partitions between the tooth sockets. SYN s. interalveolare [NA], alveolar s., septal bone.

s. interalveola're, pl. **sep'ta interalveola'ria** [NA], SYN interalveolar s.

interatrial s., the wall between the atria of the heart. SEE ALSO s. primum, s. secundum. SYN s. interatriale [NA].

s. interatria'le [NA], SYN interatrial s.

interdental s., the bony portion separating two adjacent teeth in a dental arch.

interlobular s., the connective tissue between pulmonary lobules, usually containing a vein and lymphatics; seen radiographically when thickened as a Kerley B line.

intermediate cervical s., a thin s. composed of glia fiber and leptomeningeal connective tissue in the cervical spinal cord marking the border between the gracile fasciculi and cuneatus of the dorsal funiculus. SYN s. cervicale intermedium [NA].

s. interme'dium, old term for the s. of the atrioventricular canal of the embryonic heart formed by the fusion of the dorsal and ventral atrioventricular canal cushions.

intermuscular s., a term applied to aponeurotic sheets separating various muscles of the limbs; these are anterior and posterior

se

crural, lateral and medial femoral, lateral and medial humeral. SYN s. intermusculare [NA].

s. intermuscula're [NA], SYN intermuscular s.

interpulmonary s., SYN mediastinum (2).

interradicular septa, the bony partitions that project into the alveoli between the roots of the molar teeth. SYN septa interradicularia [NA], intra-alveolar septa.

sep'ta interradicula'ria [NA], SYN interradicular septa.

interventricular s., the wall between the ventricles of the heart. SYN s. interventriculare [NA], ventricular s.

s. interventricula're [NA], SYN interventricular s.

s. lin'guae [NA], SYN lingual s.

lingual s., the median vertical fibrous partition of the tongue merging posteriorly into the aponeurosis of the tongue. SYN s. linguae [NA], s. of tongue.

s. lu'cidum, SYN transparent s.

s. mediastina'le, SYN mediastinum (2).

s. membrana'ceum ventriculo'rum, SYN membranous *part* of interventricular septum.

membranous s., (1) SYN membranous *part* of nasal septum. **(2)** SYN membranous *part* of interventricular septum.

s. mo'bile na'si, SYN mobile *part* of nasal septum.

s. muscula're ventriculo'rum, SYN muscular *part* of interventricular septum of heart.

s. of musculotubal canal, SYN s. of auditory tube.

nasal s., the wall dividing the nasal cavity into halves; it is composed of a central supporting skeleton covered on each side by a mucous membrane. SYN s. nasi [NA].

s. na'si [NA], SYN nasal s.

s. na'si oss'eum [NA], SYN bony nasal s.

orbital s., a fibrous membrane attached to the margin of the orbit and extending into the lids, containing the orbital fat and constituting in great part the posterior fascia of the orbicularis oculi muscle. SYN s. orbitale [NA].

s. orbita'le [NA], SYN orbital s.

pectiniform s., s. pectinifor'me, the anterior portion of the s. penis which is broken by a number of slitlike perforations. SYN comblike s.

s. pellu'cidum [NA], SYN transparent s.

s. pe'nis [NA], the portion of the tunica albuginea incompletely separating the two corpora cavernosa of the penis.

placental septa, incomplete partitions between placental cotyledons; they are covered with trophoblast and contain a core of maternal tissue.

precommissural s., SEE septal *area*.

s. pri'mum, a crescentic s. in the embryonic heart that develops on the dorsocephalic wall of the originally single atrium and initiates its partitioning into right and left chambers; the tips of the s. grow toward and fuse with the atrioventricular canal cushions.

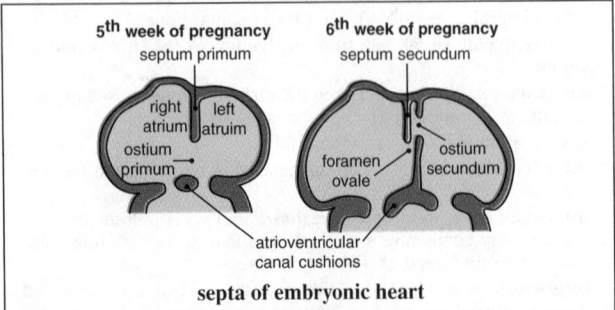

5th week of pregnancy   septum primum

6th week of pregnancy   septum secundum

right atrium | left atrium

ostium primum

foramen ovale | ostium secundum

atrioventricular canal cushions

septa of embryonic heart

proximal spiral s., SEE spiral s.

rectovaginal s., the fascial layer between the vagina and the lower part of the rectum. SYN s. rectovaginale [NA].

s. rectovagina'le [NA], SYN rectovaginal s.

rectovesical s., a fascial layer that extends superiorly from the central tendon of the perineum to the peritoneum between the prostate and rectum. SYN s. rectovesicale [NA], Denonvilliers' aponeurosis, rectovesical fascia, Tyrrell's fascia.

s. rectovesica'le [NA], SYN rectovesical s.

scrotal s., an incomplete wall of connective tissue and non-striated muscle (dartos fascia) dividing the scrotum into two sacs, each containing a testis. SYN s. scroti [NA].

s. scro'ti [NA], SYN scrotal s.

s. secun'dum, the second of two major septal structures involved in the partitioning of the atrium, developing later than the s. primum and located to the right of it; like the s. primum, it is crescentic, but its tips are directed toward the sinus venosus, and it is more heavily muscular; it remains an incomplete partition until after birth, with its unclosed area constituting the foramen ovale.

sinus s., a small fold forming the medial end of the valve of the inferior vena cava; it is developed from the dorsal wall of the embryonic sinus venosus.

s. sin'uum fronta'lium [NA], SYN s. of frontal sinuses.

s. sin'uum sphenoida'lium [NA], SYN s. of sphenoidal sinuses.

s. of sphenoidal sinuses, the bony partition between the two sphenoidal sinuses, often deflected to one side of the mid line. SYN s. sinuum sphenoidalium [NA].

spiral s., a s. dividing the embryonic bulbus cordis into pulmonary and aortic outflow tracts from the developing heart; the distal spiral s. is derived from the right and left endocardial cushions and so separates the pulmonary and aortic orifices; the proximal spiral s. is the portion of the s. that is incorporated into the membranous part of the interventricular s.

spiral bulbar s., SEE spiral s.

s. spu'rium, a s. in the right atrium of the embryonic heart formed by the right venous valve and its continuation onto the dorsocephalic wall of the atrium; in human embryos, it reaches its fullest development during the third month and then undergoes regression, taking no part in atrial partitioning (hence its designation as false); reduced portions persist as the valve of the inferior vena cava and the valve of the coronary sinus.

s. of testis, SYN *mediastinum* testis.

s. of tongue, SYN lingual s. SYN nucleus fibrosus linguae.

transparent s., a thin plate of brain tissue, containing nerve cells and numerous nerve fibers, that is stretched like a flat, vertical sheet between the column and body of fornix below, the corpus callosum above and anteriorly; it is usually fused in the median plane with its partner on the opposite side so as to form a thin, median partition between the left and right frontal horn of the lateral ventricles; in less than 10% of humans there is a blind, slitlike, fluid-filled space between the two transparent septa, the cavity of s. pellucidum. The transparent s. is continuous ventralward through the interval between the corpus callosum and the anterior commissure with the precommissural septum and subcallosal gyrus. SEE ALSO cavity of septum pellucidum, septal *area*. SYN s. pellucidum [NA], s. lucidum.

transverse s., (1) SYN ampullary *crest*. **(2)** the mesodermal mass separating the pericardial and peritoneal cavities; it is covered with mesothelium except where intimately associated with the liver, which originally develops within it; the s. is definitively incorporated into the diaphragm as the central tendon.

s. tu'bae, SYN s. of auditory tube.

urogenital s., the coronally placed ridge formed by the caudal portion of the urogenital ridges fusing in the midline of the embryo; it lies between the hindgut dorsally and the bladder ventrally.

urorectal s., in embryos, a partition dividing the cloaca into a dorsal, rectal portion and a ventral portion called the urogenital sinus; reaching the cloacal membrane at about the time of its disintegration, the urorectal s. divides the cloacal exit into an anal and a urogenital orifice. SYN urorectal fold.

ventricular s., SYN interventricular s.

se·que·la, pl. **se·que·lae** (sē-kwel'ă, sē-kwel'ē). A condition following as a consequence of a disease. [L. *sequela*, a sequel, fr. *sequor*, to follow]

se·quence (sē′kwens). The succession, or following, of one thing or event after another. [L. *sequor,* to follow]

Alu s.'s, in the human genome a repeated, relatively conserved s. of about 300 bp that often contains a cleavage site for the restriction enzyme AluI near the center; about 1 million copies in the human genome.

chi s., an octomeric s. of bases in DNA that participates in RecBC-mediated genetic recombination.

chi-s.'s, a specific DNA s. in bacterial genomes that allows for extensive genetic recombination.

coding s., the portion of DNA that codes for transcription of messenger RNA. SEE exon.

insertion s., discrete DNA s.'s of approximately 1000 nucleotides which are repeated at various sites on a bacterial chromosome, certain plasmids, and bacteriophages, which can move from one site to another on the chromosome, to another plasmid in the same bacterium, or to a bacteriophage.

intervening s., SYN intron.

leader s.'s, s.'s at the end of either nucleic acids (DNA and RNA) or proteins that must be processed off to allow for a specific function of the mature molecule.

long terminal repeat s.'s, regions of the RNA genome associated with regulation, integration, and expression of retroviruses.

monotonic s., a s. in which each value in a set is greater than the preceding value.

palindromic s., SEE palindrome.

regulatory s., any DNA s. that is responsible for the regulation of gene expression, such as promoters and operators.

Shine-Dalgarno s., a purine-rich, untranslated region of mRNA upstream from the initiation codon in prokaryotes; assists in aligning the mRNA on the ribosome.

termination s., SYN termination *codon.*

se·quence lad·der. The array of bands, made conspicuous by labeling, when DNA fragmented by endonucleases is subject to gel electrophoresis; corresponds to the nucleotide sequence.

se·quenc·ing (sē′kwens-ing). The determination of the sequence of subunits in a macromolecule.

dideoxy sequencing, a method of sequencing DNA using 2′,3′-dideoxyribonucleoside triphosphates.

Maxim-Gilbert sequencing, a method of sequencing DNA using dimethyl sulfate and hydrazinolysis.

se·quen·tial (sē-kwen′shăl). Occurring in sequence.

se·ques·ter (sē-kwes′ter). To separate off from the main mass of tissue.

se·ques·tra (sē-kwes′tră). Plural of sequestrum.

se·ques·tral (sē-kwes′trăl). Relating to a sequestrum.

se·ques·tra·tion (sē-kwes-trā′shŭn). **1.** Formation of a sequestrum. **2.** Loss of blood or of its fluid content into spaces within the body so that it is withdrawn from the circulating volume, resulting in hemodynamic impairment, hypovolemia, hypotension, and reduced venous return to the heart. [L. *sequestratio,* fr. *sequestro,* pp. *-atus,* to lay aside]

bronchopulmonary s., a congenital anomaly in which a mass of lung tissue becomes isolated, during development, from the rest of the lung; the bronchi in the mass are usually dilated or cystic and are not connected with the bronchial tree; it is supplied by a branch of the aorta.

se·ques·trec·to·my (sē-kwes-trek′tō-mē). Operative removal of a sequestrum. SYN sequestrotomy. [sequestrum + G. *ektomē,* excision]

se·ques·trot·o·my (sē-kwes-trot′ō-mē). SYN sequestrectomy. [sequestrum + G. *tomē, incision*]

se·ques·trum, pl. **se·ques·tra** (sē-kwes′trŭm, -tră). A piece of necrotic tissue, usually bone, that has become separated from the surrounding healthy tissue. [Mod. L. use of Mediev. L. *sequestrum,* something laid aside, fr. L. *sequestro,* to lay aside, separate]

primary s., a completely detached s.

se·quoi·o·sis (sē-kwoy-ō′sis). Extrinsic allergic alveolitis caused by inhalation of redwood sawdust containing spores of *Graphium, Pullularia, Aureobasidium,* and other fungi. [*Sequoia* (genus

name) for *Sequoah* (George Guess), Cherokee scholar, + G. *-osis,* condition]

SER Abbreviation for somatosensory evoked response. SEE ALSO evoked *response.*

Ser Symbol for serine and its radical.

se·ra (sēr′ă). Plural of serum.

ser·al·bu·min (sēr-al-byū′min). SYN serum *albumin.*

ser·en·dip·i·ty (ser-en-dip′i-tē). Accidental discovery; in science, finding one thing while looking for something else, as in Fleming's discovery of penicillin. [coined by Horace Walpole and relates to *The Three Princes of Serendip,* fr. alternate spelling of *Serendib,* ancient name for Sri Lanka]

Sergent, Emile, French physician, 1867–1943. SEE S.'s white *line;* Bernard-S. *syndrome.*

se·ries, pl. **se·ries** (sēr′ēz). **1.** A succession of similar objects following one another in space or time. **2.** In chemistry, a group of substances, either elements or compounds, having similar properties or differing from each other in composition by a constant ratio. [L. fr. *sero,* to join together]

aromatic s., all the compounds derived from benzene, or similar cyclic compounds that obey Hückel's rule, distinguished from those compounds that are acyclic or that contain rings that lack the conjugated double bond structure characteristic of benzene.

erythrocytic s., the cells in the various stages of development in the red bone marrow leading to the formation of the erythrocyte, *e.g.,* erythroblasts, normoblasts, erythrocytes.

fatty s., the alkanes; all the acyclic compounds in the methane, ethane, propane, etc., group, distinguished from the aromatic s.

granulocytic s., the cells in the several stages of development in the bone marrow leading to the mature granulocyte of the circulation, *e.g.,* myeloblasts, different stages of the myelocyte, granulocytes.

Hofmeister s., the series of cations Mg^{2+}, Ca^{2+}, Sr^{2+}, Ba^{2+}, Li^+, Na^+, K^+, Rb^+, Cs^+, and of anions citrate^{3-}, tartrate^{2-}, SO_4^{2-}, acetate$^-$, NO_3^-, ClO_3^-, I^-, CNS^- (among others), each series arranged in order of decreasing ability to: 1) precipitate the dispersed substance of lyophilic sols; 2) "salt out" organic substances (*e.g.,* aniline, ethyl acetate) from aqueous solutions; or 3) inhibit the swelling of gels. These effects, among other related ones, are ascribable to the abstraction and binding of water by these ions (*i.e.,* hydration), which also decreases in the orders given, so that (in the monovalent cation series) Li^+, with the smallest crystal radius, has the largest hydrated radius, and vice versa for Cs^+. SYN lyotropic s.

homologous s., a s. of organic compounds, the succeeding members of which differ from each other by the radical CH_2 (as in the fatty series).

lymphocytic s., lymphoid s., the cells at various states in the development in lymphoid tissue of the mature lymphocytes, *e.g.,* lymphoblasts, young lymphocytes, mature lymphocytes.

lyotropic s., SYN Hofmeister s.

myeloid s., the granulocytic and the erythrocytic s.

small bowel s., radiographic examination of the small intestine following the oral administration of contrast medium, usually barium sulfate. Cf. small bowel *enema.*

thrombocytic s., the cells of successive stages in thrombocytic (platelet) development in the bone marrow, *e.g.,* thromboblasts, thrombocytes.

Combining forms	[NA] Nomina Anatomica
Word*Finder* Multi-term entry finder Preceding letter A	[MIM] **Mendelian Inheritance in Man**
A.D.A.M. Anatomy Plates Between letters L and M	☆ **Official alternate term**
Appendices: Following letter Z	☆[NA] **Official alternate Nomina Anatomica term**
SYN Synonym; Cf., compare	**High Profile Term**

upper GI s., a radiographic contrast study of the esophagus, stomach, and duodenum.

ser·ine (S, Ser) (ser′ēn). 2-Amino-3-hydroxypropanoic acid; the L-isomer is one of the amino acids occurring in proteins.

s. deaminase, SYN *threonine* dehydratase.

s. dehydrase, SYN L-s. dehydratase.

L-s. dehydratase, L-Hydroxyamino acid dehydratase; a deaminating hydro-lyase converting L-serine to pyruvate and NH₃; a part of amino acid catabolism. SEE ALSO *threonine* dehydratase. SYN s. dehydratase.

s. diazoacetate, SYN azaserine.

s. sulfhydrase, SYN cystathionine β-synthase.

L-ser·ine de·hy·dra·tase. See under serine.

se·ri·o·graph (sēr′ē-ō-graf). An instrument for making a series of radiographs; used, *e.g.,* in cerebral angiography; an obsolete term for rapid film changes. [series + G. *graphō,* to write]

se·ri·og·ra·phy (ser-ē-og′ră-fē). The taking of a series of radiographs by means of the seriograph.

se·ri·os·co·py (ser-ē-os′kŏ-pē). Formerly, a series of radiographs of a region taken from different directional points and later combined. [series + G. *skopeō,* to view]

ser·i·scis·sion (ser-i-sish′ŭn). Rarely used term denoting division of the pedicle of a tumor or other tissue by a silk ligature. [L. *sericum,* silk, + *scissio,* a cleaving]

⌂**sero-.** Serum, serous. [L. *serum,* whey]

se·ro·co·li·tis (sēr′ō-kō-lī′tis). SYN pericolitis. [Mod. L. *serosa,* serous membrane, + colitis]

se·ro·con·ver·sion (sēr′ō-kon-ver′zhŭn). Development of detectable specific antibodies in the serum as a result of infection or immunization.

se·ro·cys·tic (ser-ō-sis′tik). Relating to one or more serous cysts.

se·ro·di·ag·no·sis (sēr′ō-dī-ag-nō′sis). Diagnosis by means of a reaction using blood serum or other serous fluids in the body (serologic tests).

se·ro·en·ter·i·tis (sēr′ō-en-ter-ī′tis). SYN perienteritis. [Mod. L. *serosa,* serous membrane, + enteritis]

se·ro·ep·i·de·mi·ol·o·gy (sēr′ō-ep-i-dē-mē-ol′ō-jē). Epidemiological study based on the detection of infection by serological testing.

se·ro·fast (sēr′ō-fast). SYN serum-fast.

se·ro·fi·brin·ous (sēr-ō-fī′bri-nŭs). Denoting an exudate composed of serum and fibrin.

se·ro·fi·brous (sēr-ō-fī′brŭs). Relating to a serous membrane and a fibrous tissue.

se·ro·log·ic (sēr-ō-loj′ik). Relating to serology.

se·rol·o·gy (sĕ-rol′ō-jē). The branch of science concerned with serum, especially with specific immune or lytic serums; to measure either antigens or antibodies in sera. [sero- + G. *logos,* study]

se·ro·ma (sē-rō′mă). A mass or tumefaction caused by the localized accumulation of serum within a tissue or organ. [sero- + G. *-oma,* tumor]

se·ro·mem·bra·nous (sēr′ō-mem′bră-nŭs). Relating to a serous membrane.

se·ro·mu·coid (sēr-ō-myū′koyd). General term for a mucoprotein (glycoprotein) from serum.

acid s., SYN orosomucoid.

se·ro·mu·cous (sēr-ō-myū′kŭs). Pertaining to a mixture of watery and mucinous material, such as that of certain glands.

ser·o·my·ot·o·my (se′rō-mī-ot′ō-mē). Incision in the wall of a hollow viscus that involves the serosa and muscularis but not the mucosa. [serosa 1. + G. *mys,* muscle, + *tomē,* a cutting]

se·ro·neg·a·tive (sēr-ō-neg′ă-tiv). Lacking an antibody of a specific type in serum; used to mean absence of prior infection with a specific agent (*e.g.,* rubella virus), disappearance of antibodies after treatment of a disease (*e.g.,* syphilis), or absence of antibody usually found in a given syndrome (*e.g.,* rheumatoid arthritis without rheumatoid factor).

se·ro·pos·i·tive (sēr-ō-poz′i-tiv). Containing antibody of a specific type in serum; used to indicate presence of immunological

evidence of a specific infection (*e.g.,* Lyme disease, syphilis) or presence of a diagnostically useful antibody (*e.g.,* rheumatoid arthritis with rheumatoid factor).

se·ro·pu·ru·lent (sēr′ō-pū′rū-lent). Composed of or containing both serum and pus; denoting a discharge of thin watery pus (seropus).

se·ro·pus (sēr′ō-pŭs). Purulent serum, *i.e.,* pus largely diluted with serum.

se·ro·re·ver·sion (sir-ō-rē-vur′zhŭn). A loss in serological reactivity; may be spontaneous or in response to therapy.

se·ro·sa (se-rō′să). **1.** The outermost coat or serous layer of a visceral structure that lies in the body cavities of abdomen or thorax; it consists of a surface layer of mesothelium reinforced by irregular fibroelastic connective tissue. SEE ALSO chorion. **2.** The outermost of the extraembryonic membranes that encloses the embryo and all its other membranes; it consists of somatopleure, *i.e.,* ectoderm reinforced by somatic mesoderm; the serosa of mammalian embryos is frequently called the trophoderm. SYN membrana serosa (2). SYN tunica serosa [NA], membrana serosa (1), serous coat, serous membrane, serous tunic. [fem. of Mod. L. *serosus,* serous]

s. of colon, serous coat of the colon; the visceral peritoneum of the large intestine. SYN tunica serosa coli [NA].

s. of gallbladder, serous coat of the gallbladder; the visceral peritoneum covering the portions of the gallbladder not in direct contact with the liver. SYN tunica serosa vesicae biliaris [NA], tunica serosa vesicae felleae★ [NA].

s. of liver, serous coat of the liver; peritoneal covering of the liver, enclosing almost all except for a triangular area on its posterior surface, (the "bare area of the liver") and a smaller area where the liver and gallbladder are in direct contact. SYN tunica serosa hepatis [NA].

s. of small intestine, serous coat of the small intestine; the peritoneal covering of the external surface of the small intestine. SYN tunica serosa intestini tenuis [NA].

s. of stomach, serous coat of the stomach; the visceral peritoneum covering the outer surface of the stomach. SYN tunica serosa gastrica [NA], tunica serosa ventriculi★ [NA].

s. of urinary bladder, serous coat of the urinary bladder; the visceral peritoneum covering the roof and lateral walls of the urinary bladder. SYN tunica serosa vesicae urinariae [NA].

s. of uterine tube, serous coat of the uterine tube; the visceral peritoneum forming the outer surface of the uterine tubes. SYN tunica serosa tubae uterinae [NA].

s. of uterus, serous coat of uterus; the visceral peritoneum covering the fundus and posterior body of the uterus. SYN tunica serosa uteri [NA].

se·ro·sa·mu·cin (se-rō-să-myū′sin). Mucoid material found in serous fluids, *e.g.,* in ascitic or synovial fluid.

se·ro·san·guin·e·ous (sēr′ō-sang-gwin′ē-ŭs). Denoting an exudate or a discharge composed of or containing serum and also blood.

se·ro·se·rous (sēr-ō-sēr′ŭs). **1.** Relating to two serous surfaces. **2.** Denoting a suture, as of the intestine, in which the edges of the wound are infolded so as to bring the two serous surfaces in apposition.

se·ro·si·tis (sēr-ō-sī′tis). Inflammation of a serous membrane.

infectious s., a contagious disease of young ducks and turkeys caused by the bacterium *Pasteurella anatipestifer* and characterized in ducks by ocular and nasal discharges, coughing and sneezing, and incoordination, and in turkeys by dyspnea, droopiness, lameness, and a twisted neck. SYN new duck disease.

multiple s., SYN polyserositis.

se·ros·i·ty (se-ros′i-tē). **1.** A serous fluid or a serum. **2.** The condition of being serous. **3.** The serous quality of a liquid.

se·ro·syn·o·vi·al (sēr′ō-si-nō′vē-ăl). Relating to serum and also synovia.

se·ro·syn·o·vi·tis (sēr′ō-sin-ō-vī′tis). Synovitis attended with a copious serous effusion.

se·ro·tax·is (sēr-ō-tak′sis). Edema of the skin induced by the application of a strong cutaneous irritant. [sero- + G. *taxis,* an arranging]

se·ro·ther·a·py (sēr-ō-thār'ă-pē). Treatment of an infectious disease by injection of an antitoxin or serum containing specific antibody. SYN serum therapy.

ser·o·ti·na (sēr'ō-tī'nă). SEE decidua. [L. fem. of *serotinus,* late]

se·ro·to·ner·gic (sēr-ō-tō-ner'jik, sĕr-). Related to the action of serotonin or its precursor L-tryptophan. [serotonin + G. *ergon,* work]

se·ro·to·nin (sēr-ō-tō'nin). 3-(2-aminoethyl)-5-indolol; a vasoconstrictor, liberated by the blood platelets, that inhibits gastric secretion and stimulates smooth muscle; present in relatively high concentrations in some areas of the central nervous system (hypothalamus, basal ganglia), and occurs in many peripheral tissues and cells and in carcinoid tumors. SYN 5-hydroxytryptamine, enteramine, thrombocytin, thrombotonin. [sero- + G. *tonos,* tone, tension, + -in]

se·ro·type (sēr'ō-tīp). SYN serovar.

  heterologous s. (het'ter-ō-log'ŭs), an antibody that was induced by one antigen and reacts with another antigen.

  homologous s. (hō'mō-log'ŭs), an antibody that was induced by a particular antigen and reacts with that antigen.

se·rous (sēr'ŭs). Relating to, containing, or producing serum or a substance having a watery consistency.

se·ro·vac·ci·na·tion (sēr'ō-vak-si-nā'shŭn). A process for producing mixed immunity by the injection of a serum, to secure passive immunity, and by vaccination with a modified or killed culture to acquire active immunity later.

se·ro·var (sēr'ō-var). A subdivision of a species or subspecies distinguishable from other strains therein on the basis of antigenic character. SYN serotype. [sero- + *variant*]

se·ro·zyme (sēr'ō-zīm). SYN prothrombin.

ser·pen·tar·ia (ser-pen-tā'rē-ă, -tar'ē-ă). The dried rhizome and roots of *Aristolochia serpentaria,* Virginia snakeroot, or of *A. reticulata,* Texas snakeroot (family Aristolochiaceae); a stomachic. SYN snakeroot. [L. snakeweed]

ser·pig·i·nous (ser-pij'i-nŭs). Creeping; denoting an ulcer or other cutaneous lesion that extends with an arciform border; the margin has a wavy or serpent-like border. [Mediev. L. *serpigo-(-gin),* ringworm, fr. L. *serpo,* to creep]

ser·pi·go (ser-pī'gō). **1.** SYN tinea. **2.** SYN herpes. **3.** Any creeping or serpiginous eruption. [Mediev. L. *serpigo (-gin),* ringworm, fr. L. *serpo,* to creep]

ser·pins. SYN serine protease *inhibitors,* under *inhibitor.* [*ser*ine *p*rotease *in*hibitor*s*]

ser·rate, ser·rat·ed (ser'āt, -ā'ted). Toothed. [L. *serratus,* fr. *serra,* a saw]

Ser·ra·tia (se-rā'shē-ă). A genus of motile, peritrichous, aerobic to facultatively anaerobic bacteria (family Enterobacteriaceae) which contain small, Gram-negative rods. Some strains are encapsulated. Many strains produce a pink, red, or magenta pigment; their metabolism is fermentative and they are saprophytic on decaying plant and animal materials. The type species is *S. marcescens.* [Serafino *Serrati,* 18th century Italian physicist]

  S. marces'cens, a species found in water, soil, milk, foods, and silkworms and other insects; hospital-acquired infection has been reported in patients with impaired immunity; it is the type species of the genus *S.*

ser·ra·tion (se-rā'shŭn). **1.** The state of being serrated or notched. **2.** Any one of the processes in a serrate or dentate formation. [L. *serra,* saw]

serre·fine (ser-e-fēn'). A small spring forceps used for approximating the edges of a wound or for temporarily closing an artery during an operation. [Fr.]

ser·re·no·eud (ser-e-no-ūd'). An instrument for tightening a ligature. [Fr. *serrer,* to press, + *noeud,* knot]

Serres, Antoine E.R.A., French anatomist, 1786–1868. SEE S.'s *angle, glands,* under *gland; rest's* of S., under *rest.*

ser·ru·late, ser·ru·lat·ed (ser'yū-lāt, -lā'ted). Finely serrate. [L. *serrula,* a small saw, dim. of *serra*]

Sertoli, Enrico, Italian histologist, 1842–1910. SEE S.'s *cells,* under *cell, columns,* under *column;* S. cell *tumor;* S.-cell-only *syndrome.*

ser·tra·line (ser'tră-lēn). An antidepressant which exhibits selectivity for the blockade of serotonin reuptake; similar to fluoxetine.

se·rum, pl. **se·rums, se·ra** (sēr'ŭm, -ŭmz, -ă). **1.** A clear watery fluid, especially that moistening the surface of serous membranes, or exuded in inflammation of any of those membranes. **2.** The fluid portion of the blood obtained after removal of the fibrin clot and blood cells, distinguished from the plasma in circulating blood. Sometimes used as a synonym for antiserum or antitoxin. [L. whey]

  anticomplementary s., s. that destroys or inactivates complement.

  antiepithelial s., an antiserum (cytotoxin) for epithelial cells.

  antilymphocyte s. (ALS), antiserum against lymphocytes, used to suppress rejection of grafts or organ transplants; when used in man, the globulin fraction of the heterologous s. (prepared in horse or other animals) is usually used in conjunction with other immunosuppressive agents (drugs or chemicals) and for a limited period of time. SYN antilymphocyte globulin.

  antirabies s., a sterile solution containing antibodies obtained from the blood s. or plasma of a healthy animal, or human, that has been immunized against rabies by means of vaccine; administered immediately after severe or multiple bites by domestic animals suspected to be rabid and in all wild animal bites, to be followed by a regimen of rabies vaccine.

  antireticular cytotoxic s., an antiserum specific for cells of the reticuloendothelial system.

  antitoxic s., an antitoxin.

  bacteriolytic s., an antiserum (bacteriolysin) that sensitizes a bacterium to the lytic action of complement.

  blood s., SEE serum (2).

  convalescent s., s. from patients recently recovered from a disease; useful in preventing or modifying by passive immunization the same disease in exposed susceptible individuals.

  Coombs' s., SYN antihuman *globulin.*

  dried human s., s. prepared by drying liquid human s. by freeze-drying or by any other method that will avoid denaturation of the proteins and will yield a product readily soluble in a quantity of water equal to the volume of liquid human s. from which it was prepared.

  foreign s., a s. derived from an animal and injected into an animal of another species or into humans.

  human s., SEE dried human s., normal human s.

  human measles immune s., obtained from the blood of a healthy person who has survived an attack of measles. SYN measles convalescent s.

  human pertussis immune s., the sterile s. prepared from the pooled blood of healthy adult human beings who have received repeated courses of phase I pertussis vaccine; administered intravenously or intramuscularly for the prophylaxis or treatment of whooping cough.

  human scarlet fever immune s., scarlet fever convalescent s., obtained from healthy persons who have survived an attack of scarlet fever.

  hyperimmune s., antisera with a high antibody titer produced by repeated injections of antigens.

  immune s., SYN antiserum.

  inactivated s., s. that has been heated 50°C for 30 minutes to destroy the lytic activity of complement.

  s. lactis, SYN whey.

  liquid human s., the pool of fluids separated from blood withdrawn from human subjects and allowed to clot in the absence of any anticoagulant; not more than 10 separate donations are pooled; the contributions from donors of A, O, and either B or AB groups are represented in approximately the ratio 9:9:2.

  measles convalescent s., SYN human measles immune s.

  muscle s., the fluid remaining after the coagulation of muscle plasma and the separation of myosin.

  nonimmune s., a s. from a subject that is not immune; a s. that is free of antibodies to a given antigen.

  normal s., a nonimmune s., usually with reference to a s. obtained prior to immunization.

se

normal horse s., the sterile and filtered s. of a healthy, unvaccinated horse.

normal human s., sterile s. obtained by pooling approximately equal amounts of the liquid portion of coagulated whole blood from eight or more persons who are free from any disease transmissible by transfusion.

polyvalent s., an antiserum obtained by inoculating an animal with several different antigens or species or strains of bacteria.

pooled s., pooled blood s., the mixed s. from a number of individuals.

salted s., SYN salted *plasma*.

specific s., a monovalent antiserum, *i.e.,* one obtained by inoculating an animal with one antigen or species or strain of bacteria.

thyrotoxic s., an antiserum obtained by injecting into animals the nucleoproteins of the thyroid gland.

truth s., colloquialism for a drug, such as amobarbital sodium or thiopental sodium, intravenously injected for the purpose of eliciting information from the subject under its influence; a misnomer because the subject's revelations may or may not be factually true, and its legal status and use is questionable.

se·rum·al (sēr'ŭm-ăl). Relating to or derived from serum.

se·rum-fast (ser'ŭm-fast). **1.** Pertaining to a serum in which there is little or no change in the titer of antibody, even under conditions of treatment or immunologic stimulation. **2.** Resistant to the destructive effect of sera. SYN serofast.

se·rum glu·tam·ic-ox·a·lo·ace·tic trans·am·i·nase (SGOT). SYN *aspartate* aminotransferase.

se·rum glu·tam·ic-py·ru·vic trans·am·i·nase (SGPT). SYN alanine aminotransferase.

ser·va·tion (ser-vā'shŭn). The use or function of an organ.

Servetus (Servet, Servide), Miguel, Spanish anatomist and theologian, 1511–1553. SEE S.'s *circulation*.

ser·vo·mech·a·nism (ser'vō-mek'ă-nizm). **1.** A control system using negative feedback to operate another system. **2.** A process that behaves as a self-regulatory device; *e.g.,* the reaction of the pupil to light. [L. *servus,* servant, + G. *mēchanē,* contrivance]

ser·yl (ser'il). A radical of serine.

ses·a·me (ses'ă-mē). Benne plant, an herb, *Sesamum indicum* (family Pedaliaceae), the seeds of which are used as a food, and which are the source of sesame oil. [G. *sēsamē,* sesame, an eastern leguminous plant]

s. oil, the refined fixed oil obtained from the seed of one or more cultivated varieties of *Sesamum indicum;* a solvent for intramuscular injections. SYN benne oil, gingili oil, teel oil.

ses·a·moid (ses'ă-moyd). **1.** Resembling in size or shape a grain of sesame. **2.** Denoting a sesamoid bone. [G. *sēsamoeidēs,* like sesame]

ses·a·moid·i·tis (ses-ă-moy-dī'tis). Inflammation of the proximal sesamoid bones in the horse.

⚠**sesqui-.** Prefix denoting ³⁄₂; at one time used in chemistry to indicate a ratio of 3 to 2 between the two parts of a compound (*e.g.,* sesquisulfide, sesquibasic), but presently used only for sesquihydrates and sesquiterpenes. [L.]

ses·qui·hy·drates (ses-kwi-hī'drāts). Compounds crystallizing with (nominally) 1.5 molecules of water.

ses·qui·ter·penes (ses-kwi-ter'pēnz). Compounds formed from three isoprene units; may be acyclic, mono-, di-, or tricyclic; synthesized from farnesylpyrophosphate (*e.g.,* trichothecin, nicin).

ses·sile (ses'il). Having a broad base of attachment; not pedunculated. [L. *sessilis,* low-growing, fr. *sedeo,* pp. *sessus,* to sit]

ses·ter·ter·penes (ses'ter-ter-pēnz). Compounds formed from five isoprene units; often have a tricyclic structure; formed from geranylfarnesylpyrophosphate (*e.g.,* cochliobolin B). [L. *sestertius,* two and one-half, fr. *semis,* half, + *tertius,* third, + terpene]

set. 1. A readiness to perceive or to respond in some way; an attitude which facilitates or predetermines an outcome; *e.g.,* prejudice or bigotry as a s. to respond negatively, independently of the merits of the stimulus. **2.** To reduce a fracture; *i.e.,* to bring the bones back into a normal position or alignment.

haploid s. (hap'loyd), the genetic content of a normal gamete in which every autosomal locus is represented by a single allele and either one full set of X-linked genes or one full set of Y-linked genes; the normal adult somatic cell contains two diploid s.

learning s., a readiness or predisposition to learn developed from previous learning experiences, as when an organism learns to solve each successive problem (of equal or increasing difficulty) in fewer trials.

postural s., an overall motor readiness to respond, as in a runner instructed to get set and on the mark.

se·ta, pl. **set·ae** (sē'tă, -tē). A bristle or a slender, stiff, bristle-like structure. SYN chaeta. [L. *saeta* or *seta,* a stiff hair or bristle]

se·ta·ceous (sē-tā'shŭs). **1.** Having bristles. **2.** Resembling a bristle. [L. *seta,* a bristle]

Se·tar·ia (sē-tā'rē-ă, -tar'ē-ă). A nematode genus of the family Stephanofilariidae (superfamily Filarioidea). Adults are long and thin, typically occur in the peritoneal cavity, and produce sheathed microfilariae in the blood that are transmitted to other hosts after cyclical development in appropriate mosquito hosts. They are parasitic in cattle or equines (wild or domestic) and generally are nonpathogenic, although occasionally young worms may wander into the anterior chamber of the eye. [L. *seta,* a bristle]

S. cer'vi, a species that occurs in the abdominal cavity of cattle, buffalo, bison, yak, and various deer, but rarely in sheep.

S. equi'na, a species that is a common parasite of horses and other equids in all parts of the world; they are slender whitish filaments, several inches in length, usually found free in the peritoneal cavity, but occasionally reported in the pleural cavity, lungs, scrotum, eye, and intestine.

se·ta·ri·a·sis (sē'tā-rē-ā'-sis). An infection with filarial parasites of the genus *Setaria,* usually of little pathogenic significance; aberrant migration in horses, sheep, and goats can lead to paralysis and blindness.

set·back (set'bak). A surgical operation for treatment of a bilateral cleft of the palate in which the premaxilla is moved posteriorly; the procedure is often accompanied by bone grafting.

se·tif·er·ous (sē-tif'er-ŭs). Bristly or having bristles. SYN setigerous. [L. *seta,* bristle, + *fero,* to carry]

se·tig·er·ous (sē-tij'er-ŭs). SYN setiferous. [L. *seta,* bristle, + *gero,* to bear]

se·ton (sē'tŏn). A wisp of threads, a strip of gauze, a length of wire, or other foreign material passed through the subcutaneous tissues or a cyst to form a sinus or fistula. [L. *seta,* bristle]

set·ting. Hardening, as of amalgam.

set-up. 1. The arrangement of teeth on a trial denture base. **2.** A procedure in dental case analysis involving cutting off and repositioning of teeth in the desired positions on a plaster cast.

se·vere com·bined im·mu·no·de·fi·cient mice (SCID mice). Mice that lack both T and B lymphocytes and are used for transplantation and study of human lymphoid tissues resulting in a SCID-human mouse chimera. SEE ALSO severe combined *immunodeficiency.*

Severinghaus, John W., U.S. physiologist and anesthesiologist, *1922. SEE S. *electrode.*

se·vo·flu·rane (sev-ō-flūr'ān). Fluoromethyl 2,2,2-trifluoro-1-(trifluoromethyl)ethyl ether; a halogenated ether for inhalation anesthesia.

se·vum (sē'vŭm). Suet or tallow. [L.]

sex (seks). **1.** The biological character or quality that distinguishes male and female from one another as expressed by analysis of the individual's gonadal, morphological (internal and external), chromosomal, and hormonal characteristics. Cf. gender. **2.** The physiological and psychological processes within an individual which prompt behavior related to procreation or erotic pleasure. [L. *sexus*]

safe s., sexual practices that limit the risk of transmitting or acquiring an infectious disease via exchanges of semen, blood, and other bodily fluids, *e.g.,* use of a condom, mutual masturbation, and avoidance of anal intercourse.

sex·dig·i·tate (seks-dij'i-tāt). Having six digits on one or both hands or feet. SYN sedigitate. [L. *sex,* six, + *digitus,* finger or toe]

sex·duc·tion (seks'dŭk-shŭn). SYN F *duction.*

sex·in·flu·enced. Denoting a class of genetic disorders in which the same genotype has differing manifestations in the two sexes; the variation may be rational (*e.g.*, breast cancer occurs less frequently in males) or have only empirical support (*e.g.*, pattern baldness behaves as a dominant trait in the male and as a recessive trait in the female). SEE ALSO sex-influenced *inheritance.*

sex·i·va·lent (sek-sǐ-vā′lent, sek-siv′ă-lent). Having a valence of six. [L. *sex*, six, + *valencia*, strength]

sex-lim·it·ed. Occurring in one sex only. SEE sex-limited *inheritance.*

sex-linked. SEE sex *linkage.*

sex·ol·o·gy (sek-sol′ō-jē). The study of all aspects of sex and, in particular, sexual behavior. [L. *sexus*, sex, + G. *logos*, study]

sex·tan (seks′tăn). Denoting a malarial fever the paroxysms of which recur every sixth day, counting the day of the episode as the first; *i.e.*, with a four-day asymptomatic interval. [L. *sextus*, sixth]

sex·u·al (sek′shū-ăl). **1.** Relating to sex; genital. **2.** A person as perceived by his or her s. attractiveness, tendencies, and overall sexuality. [L. *sexualis*, fr. *sexus*, sex]

sex·u·al·i·ty (sek-shū-al′i-tē). **1.** The sum of a person's sexual behaviors and tendencies, and the strength of such tendencies. **2.** One's degree of sexual attractiveness. **3.** The quality of having sexual functions or implications.

infantile s., in psychoanalytic personality theory, the concept concerning psychosexual development in infants and children; encompasses the overlapping oral, anal, and phallic phases during the first five years of life.

sex·u·al·i·za·tion (sek′shū-ăl-i-zā′shŭn). **1.** The state characterized by the presence of sexual energy or drive. **2.** The act of acquiring sexual energy or drive.

sex·u·al pref·er·ence. The biologic sex preferred in one's sexual partners.

Sézary, A., French dermatologist, 1880–1956. SEE S. *cell, erythroderma, syndrome.*

SFO Abbreviation for subfornical *organ.*

S.G.O. Abbreviation for Surgeon General's Office.

SGOT Abbreviation for serum glutamic-oxaloacetic transaminase.

SGPT Abbreviation for serum glutamic-pyruvic transaminase.

SH 1. Abbreviation for serum *hepatitis.* **2.** Abbreviation for sulfhydryl.

shad·ow (shad′ō). **1.** A surface area defined by the interception of light rays by a body. SEE ALSO density (3). **2.** In jungian psychology, the archetype consisting of collective animal instincts. **3.** SYN achromocyte.

acoustic s., sonographic appearance of reduced echo amplitude from regions lying beyond an attenuating object. Cf. acoustic *enhancement.*

Gumprecht's s.'s, SYN smudge *cells,* under *cell.*

hilar s., radiographic hilum of the lung; a composite radiographic shadow of the central pulmonary arteries and veins, with associated bronchial walls and lymph nodes, within the right or left lung.

Ponfick's s., SYN achromocyte.

radiographic parallel line s.'s, SYN tram *lines,* under *line.*

shad·ow-cast·ing. Deposition of a film of carbon or certain metals such as palladium, platinum, or chromium on a contoured microscopic object in order to allow the object to be seen in relief with the electron microscope or sometimes with the light microscope.

Shaffer, A., U.S. biochemist, 1881–1960. SEE S.-Hartmann *method.*

shaft. An elongated rodlike structure, as the part of a long bone between the epiphysial extremities. The shaft of a long bone, as distinguished from the epiphyses, or extremities, and apophyses, or outgrowths. SYN diaphysis [NA]. [A.S. *sceaft*]

s. of femur, the cylindrical shaft of the thigh bone. SYN corpus ossis femoris [NA], body of thigh bone, corpus femoris.

s. of fibula, the body of fibula; of the fibula elongated, rod-like

portion which accounts for most of its length. SYN corpus fibulae [NA].

hair s., the non-growing portion of a hair which protrudes from the skin, *i.e.,* from the follicle. SYN scapus pili.

s. of humerus, the elongated rod-like portion of the humerus between the surgical neck proximally and the emergence of the supracondylar ridges distally. SYN corpus humeri [NA].

s. of radius, the triangular body of the radius located between the expanded proximal and distal extremities of the bone. SYN corpus radii [NA].

s. of tibia, the triangular body of tibia between its expanded proximal and distal ends. SYN corpus tibiae [NA], body of tibia.

s. of ulna, the s. of the ulna between the proximal extremity and the head. SYN body of ulna.

shakes. The vernacular term for a paroxysm associated with an intermittent fever.

smelter's shakes, SYN smelter's *fever.*

shank. 1. The tibia; the shin; the leg. **2.** The portion of an instrument that connects the cutting or functional portion to a handle; with rotary tools, such as burrs and drills, the end that fits into the chuck. [A.S. *sceanca*]

shap·ing (shāp′ing). In operant conditioning, when the operant response is not in the organism's repertoire, a procedure in which the experimenter breaks down the response into those parts which appear most frequently, begins reinforcing them, and then slowly and successively withholds the reinforcer until more and more of the operant is emitted.

shark liv·er oil. Oil extracted from the livers of sharks, mainly of the species *Hypoprion brevirostris;* a rich source of vitamins A and D.

Sharpey, William, Scottish physiologist and histologist, 1802–1880. SEE S.'s *fibers,* under *fiber.*

Sharpey-Schäfer. SEE Schafer.

Shaver, Cecil Gordon, Canadian physician, *1901. SEE S.'s *disease.*

SHBG Abbreviation for sex hormone-binding *globulin.*

shear (shēr). The distortion of a body by two oppositely directed parallel forces. The distortion consists of a sliding over one another of imaginary planes (within the body) parallel to the planes of the forces. [A.S.]

shears (shērz). SYN scissors.

Liston's s., strong s. for cutting plaster of Paris bandages.

sheath (shēth). **1.** Any enveloping structure, such as the membranous covering of a muscle, nerve, or blood vessel. any sheathlike structure. SYN vagina (1). **2.** The prepuce of male animals, especially of the horse. **3.** A specially designed tubular instrument through which special obturators or cutting instruments can be passed, or through which blood clots, tissue fragments, calculi, etc. can be evacuated. **4.** A tube used as an orthodontic appliance, usually on molars. [A.S. *scaeth*]

axillary s., fibrous neurovascular s., formed as an extension of the prevertebral layer of deep cervical fascia through the cervicoaxillary canal, which enclosed the first part of the axillary artery, the axillary vein, and the brachial plexus.

carotid s., the dense fibrous investment of the carotid artery, internal jugular vein, and vagus nerve on each side of the neck, deep to the sternocleidomastoid muscle; the layers of cervical fascia blend with it. SYN vagina carotica [NA].

caudal s., a group of microtubules arranged cylindrically around the caudal pole of the nucleus in a developing spermatozoon.

common flexor s., the synovial sheath that surrounds the eight tendons of the superficial and deep flexors of the digits of the hand as they pass through the carpal canal; it is commonly continuous with the digital sheath of the little finger. SYN vagina communis musculorum flexorum [NA], ulnar bursa.

common peroneal tendon s., the sheath that surrounds the tendons of the peroneus longus and brevis muscles in their passage across the ankle. SYN vagina tendinum musculorum peroneorum communis [NA], vagina tendinum musculorum fibularium communis⁎.

crural s., SYN femoral s.

dentinal s., a layer of tissue relatively resistant to the action of acids, which forms the walls of the dentinal tubules. SYN Neumann's s.

dural s., an extension of the dura mater that ensheathes the roots of spinal nerves or, more particularly, the vagina externa nervi optici.

dural s. of optic nerve, SYN external s. of optic nerve.

enamel rod s., organic covering of the individual enamel rod.

external s. of optic nerve, the outer sheath around the optic nerve, continuous with the dura mater. SYN vagina externa nervi optici [NA], dural s. of optic nerve.

external root s., SEE root s.

s. of eyeball, SYN fascial s. of eyeball.

fascial s.'s of extraocular muscles, muscular s.; the part of the orbital s. that envelops the extraocular muscles; it is thin posteriorly but becomes thicker where it is continuous with the bulbar sheath; the fascial s.'s of the four rectus muscles are connected by an intermuscular membrane. SYN fascia muscularis musculorum bulbi [NA], fascia of extraocular muscles, muscular fascia of extraocular muscle.

fascial s. of eyeball, a condensation of connective tissue on the outer aspect of the sclera from which it is separated by a narrow cleftlike episcleral space; the sheath is attached to the sclera near the sclerocorneal junction and blends with the fascia of the extraocular muscles. SYN vagina bulbi [NA], capsula bulbi, eye capsule, fascia bulbi, s. of eyeball, Tenon's capsule, vagina oculi.

femoral s., the fascia enclosing the femoral vessels, formed by the transversalis fascia anteriorly and the iliac fascia posteriorly; two septa divide the s. into three compartments, the lateral of which contains the femoral artery and the femoral branch of the genitofemoral nerve, the middle the femoral vein, and the medial is the femoral canal. SYN crural s., infundibuliform s.

fenestrated s., a s. with a window cut in the tip or lateral convexity, through which special cutting instruments can be passed.

fibrous s.'s, SEE fibrous tendon s., fibrous digital s.'s of hand, fibrous digital s.'s of foot.

fibrous digital s.'s of foot, fibrous sheaths of the toes, the tubular fibrous layer enclosing the synovial sheath and the tendons of the long and short flexors of the toes and the flexor hallucis longus in the digits; they are composed of annular and cruciform parts. SYN vaginae fibrosae digitorum pedis [NA].

fibrous digital s.'s of hand, fibrous sheaths of the digits of the hand, the tubular fibrous layers that enclose the synovial sheaths and the superficial and deep flexor tendons and the tendon of the flexor pollicis longus in their passage along their respective digits; they are composed of annular and cruciform parts. SYN vaginae fibrosae digitorum manus [NA].

fibrous tendon s., fibrous sheath of a tendon. SYN vagina fibrosa tendinis [NA].

Henle's s., SYN endoneurium.

Hertwig's s., the merged outer and inner epithelial layers of the enamel organ which extends beyond the region of the anatomical crown and initiates formation of dentin in the root of a developing tooth; it atrophies as the root is formed, and any of the cells that persist are called Malassez' epithelial rests.

Huxley's s., SYN Huxley's *layer*.

infundibuliform s., SYN femoral s.

internal s. of optic nerve, the innermost sheath around the optic nerve, continuous with the leptomeninges (pia-arachnoid) and including a cerebrospinal fluid-filled intervaginal space, continuous with the subarachnoid space. SYN vagina interna nervi optici [NA].

internal root s., SEE root s.

intertubercular s., the extension of the synovial membrane of the shoulder joint downward in the intertubercular groove to surround the tendon of the long head of the biceps. SYN vagina intertubercularis.

s. of Key and Retzius, SYN endoneurium.

Mauthner's s., SYN axolemma.

medullary s., SYN myelin s.

microfilarial s., the membrane surrounding the embryos of certain blood-borne microfilariae, such as *Wuchereria, Brugia,* and

Loa of humans; thought to be derived from the vitelline membrane.

mitochondrial s., the spirally arranged mitochondria in the middle piece of a spermatozoon; may control movement of the tail.

mucous s. of tendon, SYN synovial tendon s.

myelin s., the lipoproteinaceous envelope in vertebrates surrounding most axons of more than 0.5-μm diameter; it consists of a double plasma membrane wound tightly around the axon in a variable number of turns, and supplied by oligodendroglia cells (in the brain and spinal cord) or Schwann cells (in peripheral nerves); unwound, the double membrane would appear as a sheetlike cell expansion that is empty of cytoplasm but for a few narrow cytoplasmic strands corresponding to apparent interruptions of the regular myelin structure, the incisures of Schmidt-Lanterman; the myelin s. of each axon is composed of a fairly regular longitudinal sequence of segments, each corresponding to the length of s. supplied by a single oligodendroglia or Schwann cell; in the short interval between each two neighboring segments, the nodes of Ranvier, the axon is unmyelinated even though enclosed by complex finger-like plasmatic expansions of the neighboring oligodendroglia or Schwann cells. SYN medullary s.

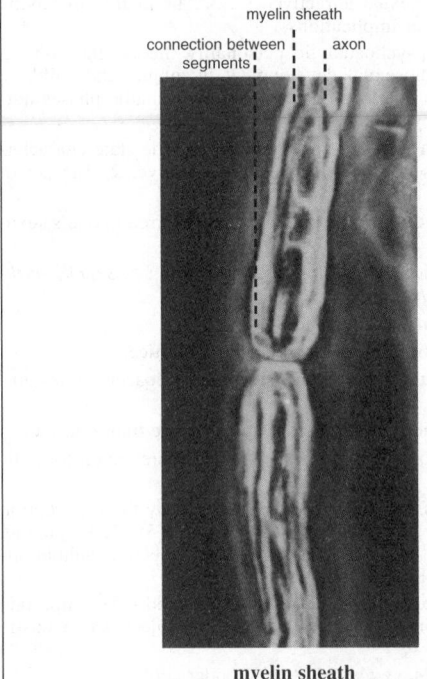

myelin sheath
connection between segments · · · axon

myelin sheath

Neumann's s., SYN dentinal s.

neurovascular s., fibrous tissue enveloping and binding together arteries, their accompanying veins (venae comitantes) and nerves which run together; often it is merely the adventitious tissue of the neurovascular structures, but may be highly developed as a distinct fascial layer (*e.g.,* in the case of the carotid or axillary s.'s).

notochordal s., the fibrous outer covering of the notochord.

parotid s., SYN parotid *fascia.*

plantar tendon s. of peroneus longus muscle, the synovial sheath surrounding the tendon of the peroneus longus in its course across the sole of the foot. SYN vagina tendinis musculi peronei longi plantaris [NA].

prostatic s., loose fibrous, partly vascular enclosure of the prostate and its dense (true) fibrous capsule; it is continuous inferiorly with the superior fascia of the urogenital diaphragm and posteriorly becomes part of the rectovesical septum; it contains the prostatic venous plexus.

rectus s., sheath of the rectus abdominis, formed by the aponeuroses of the three anterolateral muscles of the abdominal wall that split to enclose the rectus and fuse medially to form the linea alba; it consists of an anterior lamina and a posterior lamina, the latter being absent below the arcuate line. SEE ALSO *aponeurosis* of external abdominal oblique muscle, *aponeurosis* of internal abdominal oblique muscle. SYN vagina musculi recti abdominis [NA].

resectoscope s., an operative s. through which transurethral electroresection of bladder tumors or prostate gland can be performed.

root s., one of the epidermic layers of the hair follicle: external root s. is continuous with the stratum basale and stratum spinosum of the epidermis; internal root s. comprises the cuticle of the internal roots, Huxley's layer, and Henle's layer.

Rouget-Neumann s., the amorphous ground substance between an osteocyte and the lacunar or canalicular wall.

Scarpa's s., SYN cremasteric *fascia*.

s. of Schwann, SYN neurilemma.

s. of Schweigger-Seidel, SYN ellipsoid.

s. of styloid process, a crest of bone (edge of the tympanic portion of the temporal bone) running from the front and medial side of the mastoid process to the spine of the sphenoid; it splits to ensheath the base of the styloid process. SYN vagina processus styloidei [NA], vaginal process.

synovial s., SEE synovial tendon s., *vagina* synovialis trochleae, synovial s.'s of digits of hand, synovial s.'s of digits of foot.

synovial s.'s of digits of foot, similar in structure to the corresponding sheaths of the hand. SYN vaginae synoviales digitorum pedis [NA].

synovial s.'s of digits of hand, the synovial sheaths that enclose the flexor tendons of the fingers and line the inside of the fibrous tendon sheaths. SYN vaginae synoviales digitorum manus [NA].

synovial tendon s., a sheath of synovial membrane enveloping certain of the tendons; it contains a small amount of synovial fluid. SYN vagina synovialis tendinis [NA], mucous s. of tendon, theca tendinis, vagina mucosa tendinis, vaginal synovial membrane.

tail s., the protoplasmic envelope in the tail of a spermatozoon.

tendon s. of abductor pollicis longus and extensor pollicis brevis muscles, the synovial sheath lining the compartment of the extensor retinaculum that contains the abductor pollicis longus and extensor pollicis brevis tendons. SYN vagina tendinum musculorum abductoris longi et extensoris brevis pollicis [NA].

tendon s. of extensor carpi radialis muscles, the synovial sheath lining the compartment of the extensor retinaculum containing the tendons of the extensor carpi radialis longus and brevis muscles. SYN vagina tendinum musculorum extensorum carpi radialium [NA].

tendon s. of extensor carpi ulnaris muscle, the synovial sheath surrounding the tendon of the extensor carpi ulnaris in its course deep to the extensor retinaculum. SYN vagina tendinis musculi extensoris carpi ulnaris [NA], peritenon.

tendon s. of extensor digiti minimi muscle, the synovial sheath surrounding the tendon of the extensor digiti minimi in its passage deep to the extensor retinaculum. SYN vagina tendinis musculi extensoris digiti minimi [NA].

tendon s. of extensor digitorum and extensor indicis muscles, the synovial sheath that surrounds the four tendons of the extensor digitorum muscle and the tendon of the extensor indicis deep to the extensor retinaculum. SYN vagina tendinum musculorum extensoris digitorum et extensoris indicis [NA].

tendon s. of extensor digitorum longus muscle of foot, the synovial sheath that surrounds the tendons of the extensor digitorum longus muscle and the peroneus tertius in their passage across the ankle. SYN vagina tendinum musculi extensoris digitorum pedis longi [NA].

tendon s. of extensor hallucis longus muscle, the synovial sheath that surrounds the tendon of the extensor hallucis longus in its passage across the ankle. SYN vagina tendinis musculi extensoris hallucis longi [NA].

tendon s. of extensor pollicis longus muscle, the synovial sheath surrounding the extensor pollicis longus tendon in its passage deep to the extensor retinaculum. SYN vagina tendinis musculi extensoris pollicis longi [NA].

tendon s. of flexor carpi radialis muscle, the synovial sheath enclosing the tendon of the flexor carpi radialis as it crosses the wrist. SYN vagina tendinis musculi flexoris carpi radialis [NA].

tendon s. of flexor digitorum longus muscle of foot, the synovial sheath that envelops the flexor digitorum longus tendons as they pass into the foot deep to the flexor retinaculum. SYN vagina tendinum musculi flexoris digitorum pedis longi [NA].

tendon s. of flexor hallucis longus muscle, the synovial sheath that envelops the tendon of the flexor hallucis longus as it passes into the foot deep to the flexor retinaculum. SYN vagina tendinis musculi flexoris hallucis longi [NA].

tendon s. of flexor pollicis longus muscle, the synovial sheath that envelops the tendon of the flexor pollicis longus in its course through the carpal canal; it is continuous with the digital sheath of the thumb, the two generally being considered as one sheath. SYN vagina tendinis musculi flexoris pollicis longi [NA], radial bursa.

tendon s. of superior oblique muscle, the synovial sheath enclosing the tendon of the superior oblique muscle as it passes through the trochlea. SYN vagina tendinis musculi obliqui superioris [NA], synovial trochlear bursa, trochlear synovial bursa, vagina synovialis trochleae.

tendon s. of tibialis anterior muscle, the synovial sheath, deep to the extensor retinaculum, that surrounds the tendon of the tibialis anterior as it crosses the ankle. SYN vagina tendinis musculi tibialis anterioris [NA].

tendon s. of tibialis posterior muscle, the synovial sheath surrounding the tendon of the tibialis posterior as it passes into the foot deep to the flexor retinaculum. SYN vagina tendinis musculi tibialis posterioris [NA].

s. of thyroid gland, covering of the thyroid gland external to its capsule formed by a splitting of the pretracheal layer of deep cervical fascia at the gland's posterior border; the anterior lamina covers the gland anterolaterally, attaching to the arch of the cricoid cartilage superior to the isthmus of the gland (causing it to move with the trachea during elevation/depression of the larynx); the posterior lamina passes posterior to the esophagus to blend with the buccopharyngeal fascia; inferiorly, the sheath extends along the inferior thyroid veins to open into the superior mediastinum (hence, expansion of the thyroid, as by goiter, can take this direction).

vascular s.'s, fibrous envelopes ensheathing the arteries with their accompanying veins and sometimes nerves as well. SYN s.'s of vessels, vaginae vasorum.

s.'s of vessels, SYN vascular s.'s.

Waldeyer's s., the tubular space between the bladder wall and the intramural portion of the ureter as it courses obliquely through this structure; actually a space and not a true s. SYN Waldeyer's space.

Sheehan, H.L., 20th century British pathologist. SEE S.'s *syndrome*.

sheep-pox (shēp′poks). A highly contagious disease of sheep, chiefly in parts of Asia, Africa, the Middle East, and southern Europe, caused by the sheep-pox virus, a member of the family Poxviridae. SYN ovinia.

Sheldon, J.H., English pediatrician, 1920–1964. SEE Freeman-S. *syndrome*.

shelf. In anatomy, a structure resembling a shelf.

Blumer's s., SYN rectal s.

dental s., SYN dental *ledge*.

palatal s., a medially directed outgrowth of the embryonic maxilla; when fused with its opposite number it forms the secondary palate.

rectal s., a s. palpable by rectal examination, due to metastatic tumor cells gravitating from an abdominal cancer and growing in the rectovesical or rectouterine pouch. SYN Blumer's s.

vocal s., SYN vocal *fold*.

shell. An outer covering.

cytotrophoblastic s., the external layer of fetally derived trophoblastic cells on the maternal surface of the placenta.

sh

diffusion s., a small vessel made of a semipermeable membrane through which peptone, but not serum albumin, can pass; used in performing the Abderhalden test.

K s., the innermost electron orbit or shell; it can hold two electrons.

shel·lac (shĕ-lak′). A resinous excretion of an insect, *Laccifer (Tachardia) lacca* (family Coccidae). The insects suck the juice of various resiniferous Asiatic (chiefly Indian) trees and excrete and deposit "stick-lac." S. softens at a low temperature. It has many nonmedicinal uses and is also used to coat confections and tablets and in dental materials, *e.g.,* impression compound and denture base plates. SYN lacca.

Shemin, David, U.S. biochemist, *1911. SEE S. *cycle.*

Shenton, Edward W.H., English radiologist, 1872–1955. SEE S.'s *line.*

Shepherd, Francis J., Canadian surgeon, 1851–1929. SEE S.'s *fracture.*

Sherman, Henry C., U.S. biochemist, 1875–1955. SEE S. *unit;* S.-Bourquin *unit* of vitamin B₂; S.-Munsell *unit.*

Sherrington, Sir Charles, English physiologist and Nobel laureate, 1857–1952. SEE S. *phenomenon;* S.'s *law;* Schiff-S. *phenomenon;* Liddell-S. *reflex.*

shield (shēld). A protecting screen; lead sheet for protecting the operator and patient from x-rays. [A.S. *scild*]

embryonic s., a thickened area of the embryonic blastoderm from which the embryo develops.

nipple s., a cap or dome placed over the nipple to protect it during nursing.

oral s.'s, removable appliances used in orthodontic treatment, usually placed between the labial and buccal mucosa and the teeth.

shift. SYN change. SEE ALSO deviation.

antigenic s., mutation, *i.e.,* sudden change in molecular structure of RNA/DNA in microorganisms, especially viruses, which produces new strains of the microorganism; hosts previously exposed to other strains have little or no acquired immunity to the new strain; antigenic s. is believed to be the explanation for the occurrence of strains of microorganisms, such as the influenza virus, associated with large scale epidemics.

axis s., SYN axis *deviation.*

chemical s., dependence of the resonance frequency of a nucleus on the chemical binding of the atom or molecule in which it is contained. SEE chemical shift *artifact.*

chloride s., when CO_2 enters the blood from the tissues, it passes into the red blood cell and is converted by carbonate dehydratase to bicarbonate (HCO_3^-); HCO_3^- ion passes out into the plasma while Cl^- migrates into the red blood cell. Reverse changes occur in the lungs when CO_2 is eliminated from the blood. SYN Hamburger's phenomenon.

Doppler s., the magnitude of the frequency change in hertz when sound and observer are in relative motion away from or toward each other. SEE ALSO Doppler *effect.*

s. to the left, (1) a marked increase in the percentage of immature cells in the circulating blood, based on the premise in hematology that the bone marrow with its immature myeloid cells is on the left, while the circulating blood with its mature neutrophils is on the right; SYN deviation to the left. **(2)** SEE maturation *index.*

luteoplacental s., the change in site of production of the estrogen and progesterone essential for human pregnancy from the corpus luteum to the placenta; ovariectomy always terminates pregnancy in most mammals because their placentas never produce enough estrogen and progesterone, but, after the sixth week of pregnancy, a human placenta can produce enough of these hormones to prevent abortion despite ovariectomy.

phase s., in nuclear magnetic resonance, the change in phase caused by movement of the spins, which can be used to show fluid flow.

Purkinje s., SYN Purkinje's *phenomenon.*

s. to the right, (1) in a differential count of white blood cells in the peripheral blood, the absence of young and immature forms; SYN deviation to the right. **(2)** SEE maturation *index.*

threshold s., measurement of the degree of hearing loss or impairment in terms of a decibel s. from an individual's previous audiogram.

Shiga, Kiyoshi, Japanese bacteriologist, 1870–1957. SEE *Shigella;* S. *bacillus;* S.-Kruse *bacillus.*

Shi·gel·la (shē-gel′lă). A genus of nonmotile, aerobic to facultatively anaerobic bacteria (family Enterobacteriaceae) containing Gram-negative nonencapsulated rods. These organisms cannot use citrate as a sole source of carbon; their growth is inhibited by potassium cyanide and their metabolism is fermentative; they ferment glucose and other carbohydrates with the production of acid but not gas; lactose is ordinarily not fermented, although it is sometimes slowly attacked; the normal habitat is the intestinal tract of humans and of higher apes; all of the species produce dysentery. The type species is *S. dysenteriae.* [Kiyoshi *Shiga*]

S. boy′dii, a species found only in feces of symptomatic individuals; occurs in a low proportion of cases of bacillary dysentery.

S. dysenter′iae, a species causing dysentery in humans and in monkeys, found only in feces of symptomatic individuals; the type species of the genus *S.* SYN Shiga bacillus, Shiga-Kruse bacillus.

S. flexne′ri, a species found in the feces of symptomatic individuals and of convalescents or carriers; the most common cause of dysentery epidemics and sometimes of infantile gastroenteritis. Now known sometimes to be sexually transmitted through anal intercourse. SYN Flexner's bacillus, paradysentery bacillus.

S. son′nei, a species causing mild dysentery and also summer diarrhea in children. SYN Sonne bacillus.

shig·el·lo·sis (shig-ĕ-lō′sis). Bacillary dysentery caused by bacteria of the genus *Shigella,* often occurring in epidemic patterns; an opportunistic infection of person with AIDS.

shi·kim·ate de·hy·dro·gen·ase (shi-kim′āt). An oxidoreductase reversibly reacting 3-dehydroshikimic acid with NADPH acid to produce shikimic acid and NADP⁺ in L-phenylalanine and L-tyrosine biosynthesis.

shim (shim). In magnetic resonance imaging, fine adjustment of the magnetic field to improve uniformity; derived from its use in carpentry.

shin. SYN anterior *border* of tibia. [A.S. *scina*]

bucked s.'s, SYN sore s.'s.

saber s., the sharp-edged anteriorly convex tibia in congenital syphilis.

sore s.'s, a condition seen most frequently in young thoroughbred horses during early training, and characterized by periostitis of the dorsal surface of the third metacarpal or metatarsal bone. SYN bucked s.'s.

toasted s.'s, SYN *erythema* caloricum.

Shine. J., contemporary Australian molecular biologist.

shin·gles (shing′glz). SYN *herpes* zoster. [L. *cingulum,* girdle]

shin-splints. Tenderness and pain with induration and swelling of pretibial muscles, following athletic overexertion by the untrained; it may be a mild form of anterior tibial compartment syndrome.

ship. A structure resembling the hull of a ship.

Fabricius′ s., the outlines of the sphenoid, occipital, and frontal bones, from their fancied resemblance to the hull of a s.

Shipley, Walter C., U.S. psychiatrist, *1903. SEE S.-Hartford *scale.*

Shirodkar, N.V., Indian obstetrician and gynecologist, 1900–1971. SEE S. *operation.*

shiv·er. **1.** To shake or tremble, especially from cold. **2.** A tremor; a slight chill.

shiv·er·ing. **1.** Trembling from cold or fear. **2.** A spasmodic affection, resembling chorea, affecting the thigh muscles of the horse.

shoat (shōt). A young hog. SYN shote. [M.E. *shote*]

shock (shok). **1.** A sudden physical or mental disturbance. **2.** A state of profound mental and physical depression consequent upon severe physical injury or an emotional disturbance. **3.** The abnormally palpable impact, appreciated by a hand on the chest wall, of an accentuated heart sound. SEE diastolic s., systolic s. [Fr. *choc,* fr. Germanic]

anaphylactic s., a severe, often fatal form of s. characterized by smooth muscle contraction and capillary dilation initiated by cytotropic (IgE class) antibodies; typically an antibody-associated phenomenon that does not occur in sensitivities of the delayed kind (type IV allergic reaction). SEE ALSO anaphylaxis, serum *sickness.*

anaphylactoid s., a reaction that is similar to anaphylactic s., but which does not require the incubation period characteristic of induced sensitivity (anaphylaxis); it is unrelated to antigen-antibody reactions. SYN anaphylactoid crisis (1), pseudoanaphylactic s.

anesthetic s., s. produced by the administration of anesthetic drug(s), usually in relative overdosage.

break s., the s. produced by breaking a constant current passing through the body.

cardiac s., SYN cardiogenic s.

cardiogenic s., s. resulting from decline in cardiac output secondary to serious heart disease, usually myocardial infarction. SYN cardiac s.

chronic s., the state of peripheral circulatory insufficiency developing in elderly patients with a debilitating disease, *e.g.,* carcinoma; a subnormal blood volume makes the patient susceptible to hemorrhagic s. as a result of even a moderate blood loss such as may occur during an operation.

counter-s., SEE countershock.

cultural s., a form of stress associated with the beginning of an individual's assimilation into a new culture vastly different from that in which he or she was raised.

declamping s., SYN declamping *phenomenon.*

deferred s., delayed s., a state of s. coming on at a considerable interval after the receipt of the injury.

delirious s., SYN erethistic s.

diastolic s., the abnormally palpable impact, appreciated by a hand on the chest wall, of an accentuated third heart sound.

electric s., a sudden violent impression caused by the passage of a current of electricity through any portion of the body.

endotoxin s., s. induced by release of endotoxin from Gram-negative bacteria, especially by *Escherichia coli.*

erethistic s., traumatic or toxic delirium following s. SYN delirious s.

hemorrhagic s., hypovolemic s. resulting from acute hemorrhage, characterized by hypotension, tachycardia, pale, cold, and clammy skin, and oliguria.

histamine s., the s. state produced in animals by the injection of histamine; characterized by bronchiolar spasm in the guinea pig and constriction of hepatic veins in the dog.

hypovolemic s., s. caused by a reduction in volume of blood, as from hemorrhage or dehydration.

insulin s., severe hypoglycemia produced by administration of insulin, manifested by sweating, tremor, anxiety, vertigo, and diplopia, followed by delirium, convulsions, and collapse. SYN wet s.

irreversible s., s. that has progressed beyond the stage when it will respond to transfusion or other form of treatment, and recovery is impossible.

nitroid s., a syndrome resembling that produced by the administration of a large dose of a nitrite, sometimes caused by a too rapid intravenous injection of arsphenamine or some other drug; SEE nitritoid *reaction.*

oligemic s., s. associated with pronounced fall in blood volume, sometimes resulting from increased permeability of blood vessels.

osmotic s., a sudden change in the osmotic pressure to which a cell is subjected, usually in order to cause it to lyse and lose its contents.

primary s., s. mainly nervous in nature, from pain, anxiety, etc., which ensues almost immediately upon the receipt of a severe injury.

protein s., the systemic reaction following the parenteral administration of a protein.

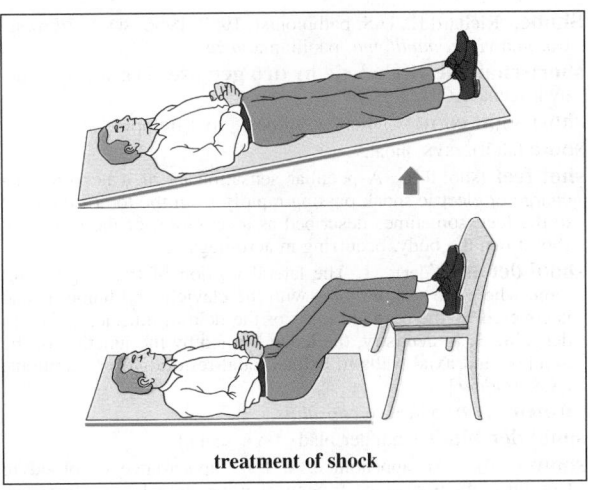

treatment of shock

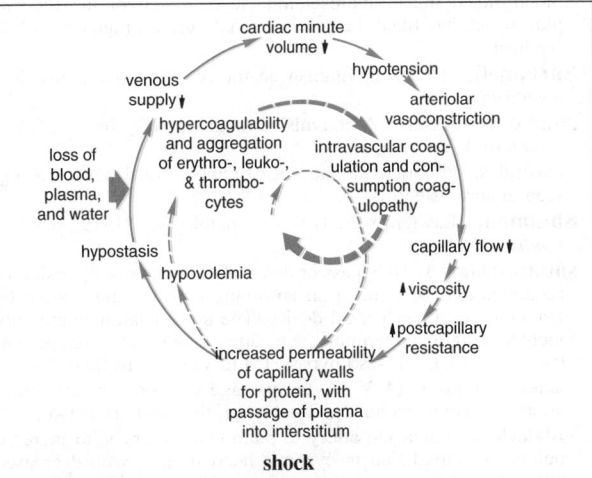

shock

pathogenesis of hypovolemic shock; *inner arrows* indicate etiology of shock in metabolic crises, endogenous and exogenous intoxications

pseudoanaphylactic s., SYN anaphylactoid s.

reversible s., s. that will respond to treatment and from which recovery is possible.

septic s., (1) s. associated with sepsis, usually associated with abdominal and pelvic infection complicating trauma or operations; **(2)** s. associated with septicemia caused by Gram-negative bacteria.

serum s., anaphylactic or anaphylactoid s. caused by the injection of antitoxic or other foreign serum.

shell s., SYN battle *fatigue.*

spinal s., transient depression or abolition of reflex activity below the level of an acute spinal cord injury or transection.

systolic s., the abnormally palpable impact, appreciated by a hand on the chest wall, of an accentuated first heart sound.

toxic s., SEE toxic shock *syndrome.*

vasogenic s., s. resulting from depressed activity of the higher vasomotor centers in the brain stem and the medulla, producing vasodilation without loss of fluid so that the container is disproportionately large. In oligemic s., blood volume is reduced; in both, return of venous blood is inadequate.

wet s., SYN insulin s.

Shone, John D., 20th century English cardiologist. SEE S.'s *anomaly, complex, syndrome.*

shook jong (shuk-yong′). SYN koro.

Shope, Richard E., U.S. pathologist, 1902–1966. SEE S. *fibroma*, fibroma *virus*, *papilloma*, papilloma *virus*.

short-chain ac·yl-CoA de·hy·dro·gen·ase. SEE *acyl-CoA* dehydrogenase (NADPH⁺).

short·sight·ed·ness (shŏrt′sīt-ed-nes). SYN myopia.

shote (shōt). SYN shoat.

shot-feel (shot′fēl). A peculiar sensation as of a nervous discharge or electric shock passing rapidly from the top of the head to the feet, sometimes described as a sensation of the rolling of shot down the body, occurring in acromegaly.

shoul·der (shŏl′der). **1.** The lateral portion of the scapular region, where the scapula joins with the clavicle and humerus and is covered by the rounded mass of the deltoid muscle. **2.** Shoulder joint. **3.** In dentistry, the ledge formed by the junction of the gingival and axial walls in extracoronal restorative preparations. [A.S. *sculder*]

frozen s., SYN adhesive *capsulitis*.

shoul·der blade (shŏl′der blād). SYN scapula.

show (shō). An appearance. **1.** First appearance of blood in beginning menstruation. **2.** Sign of impending labor, characterized by the discharge from the vagina of a small amount of blood-tinged mucus representing the extrusion of the mucous plug which has filled the cervical canal during pregnancy. [A.S. *sceáwe*]

Shrapnell, Henry J., English anatomist, 1761–1841. SEE S.'s *membrane*.

shud·der (shŭd′er). A convulsive or involuntary tremor. [M.E. *shodderen*]

carotid s., vibrations at the crest of the carotid pulse tracing, seen in aortic stenosis.

Shulman, Lawrence E., U.S. rheumatologist, *1919. SEE S.'s *syndrome*.

shunt (shŭnt). **1.** To bypass or divert. **2.** A bypass or diversion of accumulations of fluid to an absorbing or excreting system by fistulation or a mechanical device. The nomenclature commonly includes origin and terminus, *e.g.,* atriovenous, splenorenal, ventriculocisternal. SEE ALSO bypass. [M.E. *shunten,* to flinch]

arteriovenous s. (A-V s.), the passage of blood directly from arteries to veins, without going through the capillary network.

Blalock s., subclavian artery to pulmonary artery s. to increase pulmonary circulation in cyanotic heart disease with decreased pulmonary flow.

Blalock-Taussig s., a palliative subclavian artery to pulmonary artery anastomosis.

cavopulmonary s., SYN cavopulmonary *anastomosis*.

Denver s., leVeen-type s. with an implanted, valved, manually compressible chamber used to determine and maintain patency.

dialysis s., arteriovenous s. connecting the arterial and venous cannulas in arm or leg.

Dickens s., SYN pentose phosphate *pathway*.

distal splenorenal s., SYN Warren s.

Glenn s., SYN cavopulmonary *anastomosis*.

H s., a side-to-side s. between adjacent vessels which utilizes a connecting conduit. SYN H graft.

hexose monophosphate s., SYN pentose phosphate *pathway*.

jejunoileal s., SYN jejunoileal *bypass*.

left-to-right s., a diversion of blood from the left side of the heart to right (as through a septal defect), or from the systemic circulation to the pulmonary (as through a patent ductus arteriosus).

LeVeen s., a plastic tube used to transport ascitic fluid from the abdomen, via a jugular vein, to the superior vena cava.

mesocaval s., (1) anastomosis of the side of the superior mesenteric vein to the proximal end of the divided inferior vena cava, for control of portal hypertension; **(2)** h-shunt anastomosis of the inferior vena cava to the superior mesenteric vein, using a synthetic conduit or autologous vein.

pentose monophosphate s., SYN pentose phosphate *pathway*.

peritoneovenous s., a s., usually by a catheter, between the peritoneal cavity and the venous system.

portacaval s., (1) surgical anastomosis between portal and sys-

temic veins; **(2)** surgical anastomosis between the portal vein and the vena cava, as in an Eck fistula.

portasystemic s., a s. between any parts of the portal and systemic venous systems, including portacaval, mesocaval, splenorenal s.'s or spontaneously occurring s.'s.

Rapoport-Luebering s., part of the glycolytic pathway characteristic of human erythrocytes in which 2,3-bisphosphoglycerate (2,3-P_2Gri) is formed as an intermediate between 1,3-P_2Gri and 3-phosphoglycerate; 2,3-P_2Gri is an important regulator of the affinity of hemoglobin for oxygen.

renal-splenic venous s., SYN splenorenal s.

reversed s., right-to-left s. that had previously been a left-to-right s.; rarely the opposite.

right-to-left s., the passage of blood from the right side of the heart into the left (as through a septal defect), or from the pulmonary artery into the aorta (as through a patent ductus arteriosus); such a shunt can occur only when the pressure on the right side exceeds that in the left, as in advanced pulmonic stenosis, or when the pulmonary artery pressure exceeds aortic pressure, as in one form of Eisenmenger's syndrome or in tricuspid atresia.

Scribner s., connection of an artery, customarily the radial, to the cephalic vein via a short extracorporeal catheter.

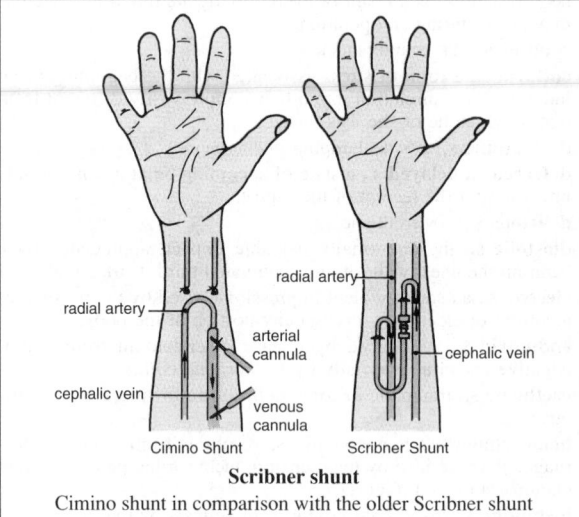

radial artery

radial artery

arterial cannula

cephalic vein

cephalic vein

venous cannula

Cimino Shunt

Scribner Shunt

Scribner shunt
Cimino shunt in comparison with the older Scribner shunt

splenorenal s., anastomosis of the splenic vein to the left renal vein, usually end-to-side, for control of portal hypertension. SYN renal-splenic venous s.

Torkildsen s., a ventriculocisternal s. SEE shunt (2).

transjugular intrahepatic portosystemic s. (TIPS), an interventional radiology procedure to relieve portal hypertension.

Warburg-Dickens-Horecker s., SYN pentose phosphate *pathway*.

Warburg-Lipmann-Dickens-Horecker s., SYN pentose phosphate *pathway*.

Warren s., anastomosis of the splenic end of the divided splenic vein to the left renal vein. SYN distal splenorenal s.

Waterston s., creation of a narrow (about 3 mm) opening between the ascending aorta and the subjacent right pulmonary artery to increase pulmonary circulation in cyanotic heart disease with decreased pulmonary flow.

shut·tle (shut′il). A going back and forth regularly; used in respect to certain transport processes across a biomembrane.

glycerophosphate shuttle, a mechanism for the transfer of reducing equivalents from the cytosol into the mitochondria; NADH is used to synthesize glycerol 3-phosphate in the cytosol; this compound is then transported into the mitochondria where it is converted to dihydroxyacetone phosphate (DHAP) using FAD;

DHAP then returns to the cytosol to complete the cycle; found in brain tissue, brown adipose tissue, and white muscle.

malate-aspartate shuttle, a mechanism for the transfer of NADH reducing equivalents from the cytosol into the mitochondria using two isozymes of malate dehydrogenase and aspartate transaminase.

Shwachman, Harry, U.S. pediatrician, 1910–1986. SEE Shwachman *syndrome.*

Shwachman syn·drome. See under syndrome.

Shwartzman, Gregory, Russian bacteriologist in U.S., 1896–1965. SEE S. *phenomenon, reaction;* generalized S. *phenomenon;* Sanarelli-S. *phenomenon.*

Shy, G. Milton, U.S. neurologist, 1919–1967. SEE S.-Drager *syndrome.*

Shy Abbreviation for 6-mercaptopurine.

SI Abbreviation for International System of Units (Système International d'Unités).

Si Symbol for silicon.

sI. Abbreviation for 6-mercaptopurine ribonucleoside (or 6-thioinosine).

Sia Abbreviation for sialic acids.

SIADH Abbreviation for *syndrome* of inappropriate secretion of antidiuretic hormone.

♻**sial-.** SEE sialo-.

si·a·la·den (sī-al′ă-den). A salivary gland. [sial- + G. *adēn,* gland]

si·al·ad·e·ni·tis (sī′al-ad-ĕ-nī′tis). Inflammation of a salivary gland. SYN sialoadenitis. [sial- + G. *adēn,* gland, + *-itis,* inflammation]

si·al·ad·en·on·cus (si′al-ad-ĕ-nong′kŭs). Old term for a neoplasm of salivary tissue. [sial- + G. *adēn,* gland, + *onkos,* bulk (tumor)]

si·al·ad·e·no·tro·pic (si′al-ad′ĕ-nō-trop′ik). Having an influence on the salivary glands. [sial- + G. *adēn,* gland, + *tropē,* a turning]

si·al·a·gogue (si-al′ă-gog). **1.** Promoting the flow of saliva. **2.** An agent having this action (*e.g.,* anticholinesterase agents). SYN ptyalagogue, sialogogue. [sial- + G. *agōgos,* drawing forth]

si·al·ec·ta·sis (si′ă-lek′tă-sis). Dilation of a salivary duct. SYN ptyalectasis. [sial- + G. *ektasis,* a stretching]

si·al·em·e·sis, si·al·e·me·sia (si′al-em′ē-sis, -ĕ-mē′zē-ă). Vomiting of saliva, or vomiting caused by or accompanying an excessive secretion of saliva. [sial- + G. *emesis,* vomiting]

si·al·ic (si-al′ik). SYN salivary.

si·al·ic ac·ids (Sia) (si-al′ik). Esters and other *N-* and *O-*acyl derivatives of neuraminic acid; radicals of s. a. are sialoyl, if the OH of the COOH is removed, and sialosyl, if the OH comes from the anomeric carbon (C-2) of the cyclic structure; *e.g., N-*acetylneuraminic acid.

si·al·i·dase (si-al′i-dās). An enzyme that cleaves terminal acylneuraminic residues from 2,3-, 2,6-, and 2,8 linkages in oligosaccharides, glycoproteins, or glycolipids; present as a surface antigen in myxoviruses; used in histochemistry to selectively remove sialomucins, as from bronchial mucous glands and the small intestine; a deficiency of this enzyme will result in sialidosis. SYN neuraminidase.

si·al·i·do·sis (si-al-i-dō′sis). SYN cherry-red spot myoclonus *syndrome.*

si·a·line (si′ă-lēn). SYN salivary.

si·a·lism, si·a·lis·mus (si′ă-lizm, si′ă-liz′mŭs). An excess secretion of saliva. SYN hygrostomia, ptyalism, salivation, sialorrhea, sialosis. [G. *sialismos*]

♻**sialo-, sial-.** Saliva, salivary glands. SEE ALSO ptyal-. Cf. ptyal-. [G. *sialon*]

si·a·lo·ad·e·nec·to·my (si′ă-lō-ad-ĕ-nek′tō-mē). Excision of a salivary gland. [sialo- + G. *adēn,* gland, + *ektomē,* excision]

si·a·lo·ad·e·ni·tis (si′ă-lō-ad-ĕ-ni′tis). SYN sialadenitis.

si·a·lo·ad·e·not·o·my (si′ă-lō-ad-ĕ-not′ŏ-mē). Incision of a salivary gland. [sialo- + G. *adēn,* gland, + *tomē,* incision]

si·a·lo·aer·oph·a·gy (si′ă-lō-ār-of′ă-jē). A habit of frequent swallowing whereby quantities of saliva and air are taken into

the stomach. SYN aerosialophagy. [sialo- + G. *aēr,* air, + *phagō,* to eat]

si·a·lo·an·gi·ec·ta·sis (si′ă-lō-an-jē-ek′tă-sis). Dilation of salivary ducts. [sialo- + G. *angeion,* vessel, + *ektasis,* a stretching]

si·a·lo·an·gi·i·tis (si′ă-lō-an-jē-i′tis). Inflammation of a salivary duct. [sialo- + G. *angeion,* vessel, + *-itis,* inflammation]

si·a·lo·cele (si′ă-lō-sēl). SYN ranula (2). [sialo- + G. *kēlē,* tumor]

si·a·lo·dac·ry·o·ad·e·ni·tis (si′al-ō-dak′rē-ō-ad-e- ni′tis). A disease of rats caused by the rat s. virus and characterized by a severe self-limiting inflammation and necrosis of the salivary and nasolacrimal glands.

si·a·lo·do·chi·tis (si′ă-lō-dō-ki′tis). Inflammation of the duct of a salivary gland. [sialo- + G. *dochē,* receptacle, + *-itis,* inflammation]

si·a·lo·do·cho·plas·ty (si′ă-lō-dō′kō-plas′tē). Repair of a salivary duct. [sialo- + G. *dochē,* receptacle, + *plassō,* to fashion]

si·a·log·e·nous (si′ă-loj′ĕ-nŭs). Producing saliva. SEE ALSO sialagogue. [sialo- + G. *-gen,* producing]

si·a·lo·glyc·o·sphin·go·lip·id. SYN ganglioside.

si·a·lo·gogue (si-al′ă-gog). SYN sialagogue.

si·a·lo·gram (si-al′ō-gram). The recorded display following sialography. [sialo- + G. *gramma,* a writing]

si·a·log·ra·phy (si-ă-log′ră-fē). Radiography of the salivary glands and ducts after the introduction of contrast medium into the ducts. SYN ptyalography. [sialo- + G. *graphō,* to write]

si·a·lo·lith (si′ă-lō-lith). A salivary calculus. SYN ptyalolith. [sialo- + G. *lithos,* stone]

si·a·lo·li·thi·a·sis (si′ă-lō-li-thi′ă-sis). The formation or presence of a salivary calculus. SYN ptyalolithiasis, salivolithiasis. [sialo-lith + G. *-iasis,* condition]

si·a·lo·li·thot·o·my (si′ă-lō-li-thot′ō-mē). Incision of a salivary duct or gland to remove a calculus. SYN ptyalolithotomy. [sialo-lith + G. *tomē,* incision]

si·al·o·met·a·pla·sia (si′ă-lō-met-ă-plā′zē-ă). Squamous metaplasia in the salivary ducts. [sialo- + metaplasia]

necrotizing s., squamous metaplasia of the salivary gland ducts and lobules, with ischemic necrosis of the salivary gland lobules; seen most frequently in the hard palate.

si·a·lom·e·try (si-ă-lom′ĕ-trē). A measurement of salivary secretion function, generally for a comparison of a denervated or diseased gland with its healthy counterpart. [sialo- + G. *metron,* measure]

si·a·lor·rhea (si′ă-lō-rē′ă). SYN sialism. [sialo- + G. *rhoia,* a flow]

si·a·los·che·sis (si′ă-los′kĕ-sis). Suppression of the secretion of saliva. [sialo- + G. *schesis,* retention]

si·a·lo·se·mi·ol·o·gy, si·a·lo·se·mei·ol·o·gy (si-ă-lō-sē-mē-ol′ō-jē). The study and analysis of saliva as an aid to diagnosis. [sialo- + G. *sēmeion,* sign, + *logos,* study]

si·a·lo·sis (si′ă-lō′sis). SYN sialism.

si·a·lo·ste·no·sis (si′ă-lō-ste-nō′sis). Stricture of a salivary duct. [sialo- + G. *stenōsis,* a narrowing]

sib. A member of a sibship.

sib·i·lant (sib′i-lănt). Hissing or whistling in character; denoting a form of rale. [L. *sibilans (-ant-),* pres. p. of *sibilo,* to hiss]

sib·i·lus (sib′i-lŭs). A sibilant rale. [L. a hissing]

sib·ling. Obsolete term for sib. [A. S. *sib,* relation, + *-ling,* diminutive]

sib·ship. 1. The reciprocal state between individuals who have the same pair of parents. **2.** All progeny of one pair of parents. [A.S. *sib,* relationship]

Sibson, Francis, English anatomist, 1814–1876. SEE S.'s *aponeurosis, fascia, groove, muscle,* aortic *vestibule.*

Sicard, Jean Anasthase, French physician, 1872-1929. SEE Collet-S. *syndrome.*

sic·cant (sik′ant). **1.** Drying; removing moisture from surrounding substances. **2.** A substance with such properties. SYN siccative. [L. *siccans (-ant-),* pres. p. of *sicco,* pp. *-atus,* to dry]

sic·ca·tive (sik′ă-tiv). SYN siccant.

si

sic·cha·sia (sĭ-kā′zē-ă). **1.** SYN nausea. **2.** Loathing for food. [G. *sikchasia*, loathing, fr. *sikchos*, squeamish]

sic·co·la·bile (sik-ō-lā′bil, -bĭl). Subject to alteration or destruction on drying. [L. *siccus*, dry, + *labilis*, perishable]

sic·co·sta·bile, sic·co·sta·ble (sik-ō-stā′bil; -bĭl, -bl). Not subject to alteration or destruction on drying. [L. *siccus*, dry, + *stabilis*, stable]

sick (sik). **1.** Unwell; suffering from disease. **2.** SYN nauseated. [A.S. *seóc*]

sick·le·mia (sik-lē′mē-ă). Presence of sickle- or crescent-shaped erythrocytes in peripheral blood; seen in sickle cell anemia and sickle cell trait.

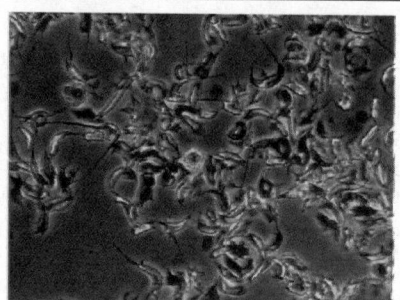

sicklemia
showing sickle cells by phase-contrast microscopy

sick·ling (sik′ling). Production of sickle-shaped erythrocytes in the circulation, as in sickle cell anemia.

sick·ness (sik′nes). SYN disease (1).

acute African sleeping s., SYN Rhodesian *trypanosomiasis.*

aerial s., SYN altitude s.

African horse s., a disease of horses and other equids in Africa, caused by an orbivirus, in the family Reoviridae, which is transmitted by biting gnats of several *Culicoides* species; the disease may be mild, subacute, or acute; in severe cases, death results from pulmonary edema.

African sleeping s., SEE Gambian *trypanosomiasis,* Rhodesian *trypanosomiasis.*

air s., a form of motion s. caused by flying in an airplane.

altitude s., (1) a syndrome caused by low inspired oxygen pressure (as at high altitude) and characterized by nausea, headache, dyspnea, malaise, and insomnia; in severe instances, pulmonary edema and adult respiratory distress syndrome can occur; SYN Acosta's disease, mountain s. (1), puna, soroche. (2) a similar disease in cattle, characterized by subcutaneous edema and congestive heart failure. SYN aerial s., altitude disease.

balloon s., a form of mountain s. occurring in someone as a result of ascent in a balloon.

black s., SYN visceral *leishmaniasis.*

bush s., anemia of sheep and cattle due to deficiency of cobalt.

caisson s., disease caused by rapid decompression. So named since it appeared in workers building tunnels or supports for bridges working in enclosed units under high atmospheric pressure to keep out surrounding water, called caissons. SEE decompression s.

car s., a form of motion s. caused by riding on a train or in an automobile or bus.

cave s., histoplasmosis acquired by inhalation of organism *Histoplasma capulatum* in caves (spelunking) or mine shafts containing bird roosts or bats, prime conditions for growth of the organisms.

chronic African sleeping s., SYN Gambian *trypanosomiasis.*

chronic mountain s., loss of high altitude tolerance after prolonged exposure (*e.g.*, by residence), characterized by extreme polycythemia, exaggerated hypoxemia, and reduced mental and physical capacity; relieved by descent. SYN altitude erythremia, chronic soroche, Monge's disease.

decompression s., a symptom complex caused by the escape from solution in the body fluids of nitrogen bubbles absorbed originally at high atmospheric pressure, as a result of abrupt reduction in atmospheric pressure (either rapid ascent to high altitude or return from a compressed-air environment); it is characterized by headache, pain in the arms, legs, joints, and epigastrium, itching of the skin, vertigo, dyspnea, coughing, choking, vomiting, weakness and sometimes paralysis, and severe peripheral circulatory collapse; bone infarcts can occur from bubbles in nutrient vessels leading to long-term consequences. SEE ALSO caisson s. SYN caisson disease, decompression disease, diver's palsy.

East African sleeping s., SYN Rhodesian *trypanosomiasis.*

falling s., SYN epilepsy.

green s., SYN chlorosis.

green tobacco s., an illness of tobacco harvest workers characterized by headache, dizziness and vomiting.

Indian s., SYN epidemic gangrenous *proctitis.*

Jamaican vomiting s., SYN ackee *poisoning.*

lambing s., SYN pregnancy *disease* of sheep.

laughing s., SEE pseudobulbar *paralysis.*

milk s., a disease of humans caused by ingesting contaminated milk from cows suffering from trembles; clinical manifestations include severe vomiting, labored breathing, delirium, convulsions, coma, and death; recovery from nonlethal illness is slow. SYN lactimorbus.

Monday morning s., SYN *azoturia* of horses.

morning s., the nausea and vomiting of early pregnancy. SYN nausea gravidarum.

motion s., the syndrome of pallor, nausea, weakness, and malaise, which may progress to vomiting and incapacitation, caused by stimulation of the semicircular canals during travel or motion as on a boat, plane, train, car, swing, or rotating amusement ride. SYN kinesia.

mountain s., (1) SYN altitude s. (1). (2) SYN brisket *disease.*

radiation s., a systemic condition caused by substantial wholebody irradiation, seen after nuclear explosions or accidents, rarely after radiotherapy. Manifestations depend on dose, ranging from anorexia, nausea, vomiting, and mild leukopenia, to thrombocytopenia with hemorrhage, severe leukopenia with infection, anemia, central nervous system damage, and death. SYN radiation poisoning.

railroad s., SYN transport *tetany.*

sea s., motion s. occurring in boat travellers.

serum s., an immune complex disease appearing some days (usually 1-2 weeks) after injection of a foreign serum or serum protein, with local and systemic reactions such as urticaria, fever, general lymphadenopathy, edema, arthritis, and occasionally albuminuria or severe nephritis; originally described in patients receiving serotherapy. SYN serum disease, serum reaction.

sleeping s., SEE Gambian *trypanosomiasis,* Rhodesian *trypanosomiasis.*

space s., dizziness as result of changes in inner ear resulting from absence of gravity. SYN physiologic vertigo.

spotted s., SYN pinta.

sweating s., an acute febrile disease of cattle in Africa caused by an epitheliotropic toxin produced by females of the tick *Hyalomma truncatum* and characterized by a profuse moist eczema and hyperemia of the skin and visible mucous membranes.

West African sleeping s., SYN Gambian *trypanosomiasis.*

side (sīd). One of the two lateral margins or surfaces of a body, midway between the front and back. [A.S. *síde*]

balancing s., in dentistry, the nonfunctioning s. from which the mandible moves during the working bite.

working s., in dentistry, the lateral segment of a dentition toward which the mandible is moved during occlusal function.

side·bones (sīd′bōnz). Ossification of the lateral cartilages of the horse's foot, seen most often in the forefeet of the heavier working breeds; exostoses often appear, and may be seen and palpated above the hoof line.

side ef·fect. A result of drug or other therapy in addition to or in extension of the desired therapeutic effect; usually but not necessarily, connoting an undesirable effect. Although technically the therapeutic effect carried beyond the desired limit (*e.g.,* a hemorrhage from an anticoagulant) is a s. e., the term more often refers to pharmacologic results of therapy unrelated to the usual objective (*e.g.,* a development of signs of Cushing's syndrome with steroid therapy).

sid·er·a·tion (sid-er-ā′shŭn). Any sudden attack, as of apoplexy. [L. *sideror,* pp. *sideratus,* to be blasted or palsied by a constellation, fr. *sidus* (*sider-*), a constellation, the heavens]

△**sidero-.** Iron. [G. *sidēros*]

sid·er·o·blast (sid′er-ō-blast). An erythroblast containing granules of ferritin stained by the Prussian blue reaction. [sidero- + G. *blastos,* germ]

sid·er·o·cyte (sid′er-ō-sīt). An erythrocyte containing granules of free iron, as detected by the Prussian blue reaction, in the blood of normal fetuses, where they constitute from 0.10 to 4.5% of the erythrocytes. [sidero- + G. *kytos,* cell]

sid·er·o·der·ma (sid′er-ō-der′mă). Brownish discoloration of the skin on the legs due to hemosiderin deposits. [sidero- + G. *derma,* skin]

sid·er·o·fi·bro·sis (sid′er-ō-fī-brō′sis). Fibrosis associated with small foci in which iron is deposited.

sid·er·og·en·ous (sid-er-oj′ĕ-nŭs). Iron-forming. [sidero- + G. *-gen,* producing]

sid·er·o·pe·nia (sid′er-ō-pē′nē-ă). An abnormally low level of serum iron. [sidero- + G. *penia,* poverty]

sid·er·o·pe·nic (sid′er-ō-pē′nik). Characterized by sideropenia.

sid·er·o·phage (sid′er-ō-fāj). SYN siderophore. [sidero- + G. *phagō,* to eat]

sid·er·o·phil, sid·er·o·phile (sid′er-ō-fil, -fīl). **1.** Absorbing iron. SYN siderophilous. **2.** A cell or tissue that contains iron. [sidero- + G. *philos,* fond]

sid·er·oph·i·lins (sid′er-ō-fil′in, -of′ĭ-lin). Nonheme, iron-binding proteins; there are three central classes of s.: transferrin (1) (in vertebrate blood), lactoferrin (in mammalian milk and other secretions), and conalbumin or ovotransferrin (avian blood and avian egg white).

sid·er·oph·i·lous (sid-er-of′i-lŭs). SYN siderophil (1).

sid·er·o·phone (sid′er-ō-fōn, sĭ-der′ō-fōn). Obsolete term for an electrical device for detecting a bit of iron in the eyeball, its presence causing the instrument to sound. [sidero- + G. *phōnē,* sound]

sid·er·o·phore (sid′er-ō-fōr). A large extravasated mononuclear phagocyte containing granules of hemosiderin, found in the sputum or in the lungs of individuals with longstanding pulmonary congestion from left ventricular failure. SEE ALSO heart failure *cells,* under *cell.* SYN siderophage. [sidero- + G. *phoros,* bearing]

sid·er·o·sil·i·co·sis (sid′er-ō-sil′i-kō′sis). Silicosis due to inhalation of dust containing iron and silica. SYN silicosiderosis. [sidero- + silicosis]

sid·er·o·sis (sid-er-ō′sis). **1.** A form of pneumoconiosis due to the presence of iron dust. **2.** Discoloration of any part by disposition of an iron pigment; usually called hemosiderosis. **3.** An excess of iron in the circulating blood. **4.** Degeneration of the retina, lens, and uvea as a result of the deposition of intraocular iron. [sidero- + G. *-osis,* condition]

pulmonary s., SYN *pneumoconiosis* siderotica.

sid·er·ot·ic (sid-er-ot′ik). Related to siderosis; pigmented by iron or containing an excess of iron.

SIDS Abbreviation for sudden infant death *syndrome.*

Siegert, Ferdinand, German pediatrician, 1865–1946. SEE S.'s *sign.*

Siegle, Emil, German otologist, 1833–1900. SEE S.'s *otoscope.*

Siemens, Hermann Werner, German dermatologist, 1891–1969. SEE Christ-S.-Touraine *syndrome.*

sie·mens (S) (sē′menz). The SI unit of electrical conductance; the conductance of a body with an electrical resistance of 1 ohm, allowing 1 ampere of current to flow per volt applied; equal to 1 mho. SYN mho. [Sir William *Siemens,* Ger. born British engineer, 1823–1883]

Siemerling, Ernst, German physician, 1857–1931.

side effects of drugs	
group I:	toxic reactions
	1. dose-related
	2. idiosyncratic
group II:	side effects or unexpected effects
	1. from specific drugs
	2. from specific pharmacodynamic groups
	3. from simultaneous administration of several drugs (combined effect)
group III:	reactions due to metabolic disturbance
	1. disorder of enzyme action
	2. other metabolic effects
group IV:	reactions caused by drug dependence
	1. psychological
	2. physical
group V:	reactions caused by sensitization
	1. allergic a) immediate b) accelerated c) delayed
	2. anaphylactic
	3. similar to allergy, through histamine release
group VI:	reactions caused by light
	1. phototoxicity
	2. photosensitivity
group VII:	teratogenic and embryotoxic reactions
	1. teratogenic effects
	2. embryotrophic toxicity
	3. perinatal toxicity
	4. selective neonatal toxicity
group VIII: biological reactions	

sieve (siv). A meshed or perforated device for separating fine particles from coarser ones. [O.E. *sive*]

molecular s., a gel-like material with pore sizes of such ranges as to exclude molecules above certain sizes; used in fractionating or purifying macromolecules.

sie·vert (Sv) (sē′vert). The SI unit of ionizing radiation effective dose, equal to the absorbed dose in gray, weighted for both the quality of radiation in question and the tissue response to that radiation. The unit is the joule per kilogram and 1 Sv = 100 rem. SEE effective *dose,* equivalent *dose.*

SIF Abbreviation for somatotropin release-inhibiting *factor.*

Sig. Abbreviation for L. *signa,* label, write, or *signetur,* let it be labeled.

Siggaard-Andersen, Ole, Danish clinical biochemist, *1932. SEE Siggaard-Andersen *nomogram.*

sigh (sī). **1.** An audible inspiration and expiration under the influence of some emotion. **2.** To perform such an act. [A.S. *sīcan*]

sight (sīt). The ability or faculty of seeing. SEE ALSO vision. [A.S. *gesihht*]

day s., SYN nyctalopia.

far s., SYN hyperopia.

long s., SYN hyperopia.

si

near s., SYN myopia.

night s., SYN hemeralopia.

second s., improved near vision in the aged as a result of increased refractivity of the nucleus of the lens causing myopia. SYN senile lenticular myopia.

short s., SYN myopia.

sig·ma (sig′mă). The 18th letter of the Greek alphabet, σ.

sig·ma·tism (sig′mă-tizm). SYN lisping. [G. *sigma,* the letter S]

sig·moid (sig′moyd). Resembling in outline the letter S or one of the forms of the Greek sigma. [G. *sigma,* the letter S, + *eidos,* resemblance]

△**sigmoid-.** SEE sigmoido-.

sig·moi·dec·to·my (sig-moy-dek′tō-mē). Excision of the sigmoid colon. [sigmoid- + G. *ektomē,* excision]

sig·moid·ic·i·ty (sig′moyd-i-sa-tē). Describing an S-shaped curve; *e.g.,* shape of enzyme-kinetic curves for enzymes displaying positive homotropic cooperativity.

sig·moid·i·tis (sig-moy-dī′tis). Inflammation of the sigmoid colon. [sigmoid- + G. *-itis,* inflammation]

△**sigmoido-, sigmoid-.** Sigmoid, usually the sigmoid colon. [G. *sigma,* the letter S, + *eidos,* resemblance]

sig·moi·do·pexy (sig-moy′dō-pek-sē). Operative attachment of the sigmoid colon to a firm structure to correct rectal prolapse. [sigmoido- + G. *pēxis,* fixation]

sig·moi·do·proc·tos·to·my (sig-moy′dō-prok-tos′tō-mē). Anastomosis between the sigmoid colon and the rectum. SYN sigmoidorectostomy. [sigmoido- + G. *prŏktos,* anus, + *stoma,* mouth]

sig·moi·do·rec·tos·to·my (sig-moy′dō-rek-tos′tō-mē). SYN sigmoidoproctostomy.

sig·moi·do·scope (sig-moy′dō-skōp). An endoscope for viewing the cavity of the sigmoid colon. SYN sigmoscope. [sigmoido- + G. *skopeō,* to view]

sig·moi·dos·co·py (sig′moy-dos′kŏ-pē). Inspection, through an endoscope, of the interior of the sigmoid colon.

sig·moi·dos·to·my (sig′moy-dos′tō-mē). Establishment of an artificial anus by opening into the sigmoid colon. [sigmoido- + G. *stoma,* mouth]

sig·moi·dot·o·my (sig′moy-dot′ō-mē). Surgical opening of the sigmoid. [sigmoido- + G. *tomē,* incision]

sig·mo·scope (sig′mō-skōp). SYN sigmoidoscope.

SIGN

sign (sīn). **1.** Any abnormality indicative of disease, discoverable on examination of the patient; an objective symptom of disease, in contrast to a symptom which is a subjective s. of disease. **2.** An abbreviation or symbol. **3.** In psychology, any object or artifact (stimulus) that represents a specific thing or conveys a specific idea to the person who perceives it. [L. *signum,* mark]

Aaron's s., in acute appendicitis, a referred pain or feeling of distress in the epigastrium or precordial region on continuous firm pressure over McBurney's point.

Abadie's s. of tabes dorsalis, insensibility to pressure over the tendo achillis.

Abrahams' s., an obsolete *s.*: **(1)** rales and other adventitious sounds, changes in the respiratory murmurs, and increase in the whispered sound can be heard on auscultation over the acromial end of the clavicle some time before they become audible at the apex; heard primarily in pulmonary tuberculosis affecting the apical portion of the lung; **(2)** a dull-flat note, *i.e.,* one between the normal dullness at the right apex and absolute flatness, heard on percussion in that region, indicating progress from incipient to advanced tuberculosis.

accessory s., a finding frequently but not consistently present in a disease. SYN assident s.

Allis' s., in fracture of the neck of the femur, the trochanter rides up, relaxing the fascia lata, so that the finger can be sunk deeply between the great trochanter and the iliac crest.

Amoss' s., in painful flexion of the spine, it is necessary to support a sitting position by extending the arms behind the torso with the weight placed on the hands.

Anghelescu's s., in vertebral tuberculosis, painful or impossible flexion of the spine when the patient attempts to rest weight on the heels and occiput.

antecedent s., SYN prodromic s.

assident s., SYN accessory s.

Auenbrugger's s., an epigastric prominence seen in cases of marked pericardial effusion.

Aufrecht's s., an obsolete s.: diminished breath sounds in the trachea just above the jugular notch, in cases of stenosis.

Babinski's s., (1) extension of the great toe and abduction of the other toes instead of the normal flexion reflex to plantar stimulation, considered indicative of pyramidal tract involvement ("positive" Babinski); SYN Babinski reflex, Babinski's phenomenon, great-toe reflex, paradoxical extensor reflex, toe phenomenon. **(2)** in hemiplegia, weakness of the platysma muscle on the affected side, as is evident in such actions as blowing or opening the mouth; **(3)** when the patient is lying upon his back, with arms crossed on the front of his chest, and attempts to assume the sitting posture, the thigh on the side of an *organic* paralysis is flexed and the heel raised, whereas the limb on the sound side remains flat; **(4)** in hemiplegia, the forearm on the affected side turns to a pronated position when placed in a position of supination.

Baccelli's s., an obsolete s.: good conduction of the whisper in nonpurulent pleural effusions. SYN aphonic pectoriloquy.

Ballance's s., the presence of a dull percussion note in both flanks, constant on the left side but shifting with change of position on the right, said to indicate ruptured spleen; the dullness is due to the presence of blood, fluid on the right side but coagulated on the left.

Bamberger's s., (1) jugular pulse in tricuspid insufficiency; **(2)** SYN allochiria. **(3)** dullness on percussion at the angle of the scapula, clearing up as the patient leans forward, indicating pericarditis with effusion.

bandage s., SYN Rumpel-Leede *test.*

Bárány's s., in cases of ear disease, in which the vestibule is healthy, injection into the external auditory canal of water below the body temperature (18°C or lower) will cause rotary nystagmus toward the opposite side; when the injected fluid is above the body temperature (41°C or higher) the nystagmus will be toward the injected side; if the labyrinth is diseased or nonfunctional there may be diminished or absent nystagmus.

Barré's s., if the hemiplegic is placed in the prone position with the limbs flexed at the knees, he is unable to maintain the flexed position on the side of the lesion but extends the leg.

Bassler's s., in chronic appendicitis, pinching the appendix between the thumb and the iliacus muscle causes sharp pain.

Bastedo's s., an obsolete s.: in chronic appendicitis, pain and tenderness in the right iliac fossa on inflation of the colon with air.

Battle's s., postauricular ecchymosis in cases of fracture of the base of the skull.

B6 bronchus s., in lung radiology, appearance of an air bronchogram of the superior segmental bronchus of the lower lobe because of segmental atelectasis or consolidation.

beak s., appearance of the distal esophagus, on a contrast esophagram, in achalasia; also used to describe the proximal pyloric canal on upper GI series in congenital pyloric stenosis.

Bechterew's s., paralysis of automatic facial movements, the power of voluntary movement being retained.

Beevor's s., with paralysis of the lower portions of the recti abdominis muscles the umbilicus moves upward.

Bezold's s., SYN Bezold's *symptom.*

Biederman's s., a dusky redness of the lower portion of the anterior pillars of the fauces in certain cases of syphilis.

Bielschowsky's s., in paralysis of a superior oblique muscle, tilting the head to the side of the involved eye causes that eye to rotate upward.

Biermer's s., SYN Gerhardt's s.

Biernacki's s., analgesia to percussion of the ulnar nerve in tabes dorsalis and dementia paralytica.

Biot's s., abnormal breathing pattern characterized by periods of apnea and periods in which several breaths of similar volume are taken; seen with increased intracranial pressure.

Biot's breathing s., irregular periods of apnea alternating with four or five deep breaths; seen with increased intracranial pressure.

Bird's s., the presence of a zone of dullness on percussion with absence of respiratory s.'s in hydatid cyst of the lung.

Bjerrum's s., SYN Bjerrum's *scotoma.*

blue dot s., a blue or black spot visible beneath the skin on the cranial aspect of testis or epididymis. This is a torsed testicular appendage and is usually quite tender.

Blumberg's s., pain felt upon sudden release of steadily applied pressure on a suspected area of the abdomen, indicative of peritonitis.

Bonhoeffer's s., loss of normal muscle tone in chorea.

Bozzolo's s., pulsating vessels in the nasal mucous membrane, noted occasionally in thoracic aneurysm.

Branham's s., bradycardia following compression or excision of an arteriovenous fistula.

Braxton Hicks s., irregular uterine contractions occurring after the third month of pregnancy.

Broadbent's s., a retraction of the thoracic wall, synchronous with cardiac systole, visible anywhere, but particularly in the left posterior axillary line; a s. of adherent pericardium.

Brockenbrough s., absolute decrease in pulse pressure of the beat immediately following a premature beat; a s. of idiopathic hypertrophic subaortic stenosis.

Brudzinski's s., (1) in meningitis, on passive flexion of the leg on one side, a similar movement occurs in the opposite leg; SYN contralateral reflex, contralateral s. **(2)** in meningitis, if the neck is passively flexed, flexion of the legs occurs. SYN neck s.

Bryant's s., in dislocation of the shoulder, an abnormal position of axillary folds occurs.

burning drops s., in certain cases of perforated gastric ulcer, a sensation as of drops of hot liquid falling into the abdominal cavity or as of a stream of intensely hot liquid being poured into the cavity.

calcium s., in chest radiography, displacement of the line of the calcified intima of the aorta away from its outer wall, a finding in a small percentage of cases of dissection of blood in the aortic media; the expression "displaced intimal calcification" is preferred to the listed term. SEE aortic *dissection.*

Calkins' s., the change of shape of the uterus from discoid to ovoid, indicating placental separation from the uterine wall.

Cantelli's s., SEE doll's eye s.

Carman's s., in gastric radiology, the appearance of a contrast-filled malignant ulcer, which does not extend beyond the line of the gastric wall as a benign ulcer would; also has a thick overhanging rim of tumor tissue.

Carnett's s., disappearance of abdominal tenderness to palpation when the anterior abdominal muscles are contracted, indicating pain of intra-abdominal origin; its persistence suggests a source in the abdominal wall, which is also indicated when tenderness is caused by gently pinching a fold of skin and fat between the thumb and forefinger.

Carvallo's s., an increase in the intensity of the pansystolic murmur of tricuspid regurgitation during or at the end of inspiration distinguishes tricuspid from mitral involvement.

Castellani-Low s., a fine tremor of the tongue observed in sleeping sickness.

Chaddock s., when the external malleolar skin area is irritated, extension of the great toe occurs in cases of organic disease of the corticospinal reflex paths. SYN Chaddock reflex, external malleolar s.

Chadwick's s., a bluish discoloration of the cervix and vagina, a s. of pregnancy.

chandelier s., colloquial term referring to severe pain elicited during pelvic examination of patients with pelvic inflammatory disease in which the patient responds by reaching upwards towards the ceiling for relief.

Chaussier's s., severe pain in the epigastrium, a prodrome of eclampsia; may be of central origin or caused by distention of the capsule of liver by hemorrhage.

Chvostek's s., facial irritability in tetany, unilateral spasm of the orbicularis oculi or oris muscle being excited by a slight tap over the facial nerve just anterior to the external auditory meatus. SYN Weiss' s.

Claybrook's s., in rupture of abdominal viscus, transmission of breath and heart sounds through the abdominal wall.

Cleemann's s., in fracture of the femur with overriding of the fragments, wrinkling of the skin occurs directly above the patella.

clenched fist s., in angina pectoris, pressing of the clenched fist against the chest to indicate the constricting, pressing quality of the pain.

Codman's s., in the absence of rotator cuff function, hunching of the shoulder occurs when the deltoid muscle contracts.

Collier's s., unilateral or bilateral lid retraction due to midbrain lesion; occurring at any age. SEE setting sun s., Epstein's s. SYN Collier's tucked lid s.

Collier's tucked lid s., SYN Collier's s.

colon cutoff s., radiographic s. of (usually) inflammatory disease preventing distention of the distal transverse colon.

Comby's s., an early s. of measles, consisting in thin whitish patches on the gums and buccal mucous membrane, formed of desquamating epithelial cells.

comet s., in chest radiology, the curved appearance of pulmonary arteries and veins associated with round atelectasis, fibrosis associated with organizing pleurisy. SYN comet tail s.

comet tail s., SYN comet s.

commemorative s., a phenomenon pointing to the previous existence of some disease other than the one present at the time.

Comolli's s., in cases of fracture of the scapula, a typical triangular cushion-like swelling appears, corresponding to the outline of the scapula.

contralateral s., SYN Brudzinski's s. (1).

conventional s.'s, s.'s that acquire their function through social (linguistic) custom; *e.g.,* words, mathematical symbols. SEE ALSO symbol (4).

Coopernail's s., in fracture of the pelvis, occurrence of ecchymosis of the perineum and scrotum, or labia.

Corrigan's s., a full hard pulse followed by a sudden collapse easily palpated and occurring in aortic regurgitation. SYN Corrigan's pulse.

Courvoisier's s., SYN Courvoisier's *law.*

Crichton-Browne's s., a slight tremor at the angles of the mouth and at the outer canthus of each eye in general paresis.

Cruveilhier-Baumgarten's s., a murmur over the umbilicus often in the presence of caput medusae, resulting from portal hypertension, usually with hepatic cirrhosis; recanalization of the umbilical vein with reverse blood flow from the liver into the abdominal wall veins creates the murmur.

Cullen's s., periumbilical darkening of the skin from blood, a s. of intraperitoneal hemorrhage, especially in ruptured ectopic pregnancy.

Dalrymple's s., retraction of the upper eyelid in Graves' disease, causing abnormal wideness of the palpebral fissure.

Dance's s., a slight retraction in the neighborhood of the right iliac fossa in some cases of intussusception.

Danforth's s., shoulder pain on inspiration, due to irritation of the diaphragm by a hemoperitoneum in ruptured ectopic pregnancy.

Darier's s., urtication on stroking of cutaneous lesions of urticaria pigmentosa (mastocytosis).

Dawbarn's s., pain of subacromial bursitis disappears when the arm is abducted.

Dejerine's s., aggravation of symptoms of radiculitis by the acts of coughing, sneezing, or straining to defecate.

Delbet's s., in a case of aneurysm of a main artery, efficient collateral circulation if the nutrition of the part below is well maintained, despite the fact that the pulse has disappeared.

de Musset's s., SYN Musset's s.

D'Éspine's s., an obsolete s.: **(1)** bronchophony over the spinous processes heard, at a lower level than in health, in pulmonary tuberculosis; **(2)** an echoed whisper following a spoken word, heard in the stethoscope placed over the seventh cervical or first or second dorsal spine, in cases of tuberculosis of the mediastinal glands.

dimple s., in dermatofibroma, dimpling elicited when the lesion is squeezed.

doll's eye s., reflex movement of the eyes in the opposite direction to that which the head is moved, *e.g.,* the eyes being lowered as the head is raised, and the reverse (Cantelli's sign); an indication of functional integrity of the brainstem tegmental pathways and cranial nerves involved in eye movement. SYN vestibular ocular reflex.

Dorendorf's s., fullness of one supraclavicular groove in aneurysm of the aortic arch.

double bubble s., in pediatric radiology, appearance of the dilated air-filled stomach and duodenal bulb, associated with duodenal atresia or web, less often midgut volvulus.

double track s., in pediatric radiology, a less common s. of congenital pyloric stenosis, when barium is caught between mucosal folds in the hypertrophied pylorus.

drawer s., in a knee examination, the forward or backward sliding of the tibia indicating laxity or tear of the anterior (forward slide) or posterior (backward slide) cruciate ligaments of the knee. SYN drawer test, Rocher's s.

drooping lily s., in urography, a s. of a double renal collecting system with an obstruction of the upper system depressing the opacified calyces of the lower system so they appear to droop.

Drummond's s., in certain cases of aortic aneurysm, a puffing sound, synchronous with cardiac systole, heard from the nostrils, when the mouth is closed.

Duchenne's s., falling in of the epigastrium during inspiration in paralysis of the diaphragm.

Dupuytren's s., (1) in congenital dislocation, free up and down movement of the head of the femur occurs upon intermittent traction; **(2)** a crackling sensation on pressure over the bone in certain cases of sarcoma.

Duroziez' s., SYN Duroziez' *murmur.*

Ebstein's s., in pericardial effusion, obtuseness of the cardiohepatic angle on percussion.

s. of edema of lower eyelid, swelling of the lower lid found in congestive failure, myxedema, or nephrosis.

Epstein's s., lid retraction in an infant giving it a frightened expression and a "wild glance." SEE setting sun s., Collier's s.

Erb s., (1) increased electric excitability of the muscles to the galvanic current, and frequently to the faradic, in tetany; **(2)** SYN Erb-Westphal s.

Erb-Westphal s., abolition of the patellar tendon reflex, in tabes and certain other diseases of the spinal cord, and occasionally also in brain disease. SYN Erb s. (2), Westphal's phenomenon, Westphal's s.

Erichsen's s., in sacroiliac disease, pain is felt when sudden pressure approximates the iliac bones; this s. is not present in hip disease.

Escherich's s., in hypoparathyroidism (latent tetany) tapping the skin at the angle of the mouth causes protrusion of the lips.

Ewart's s., in large pericardial effusions, an area of dullness with bronchial breathing and bronchophony below the angle of the left scapula. SYN Pins' s.

Ewing's s., (1) dullness on percussion to the inner side of the angle of the left scapula, denoting an accumulation of fluid in the pericardium behind the heart; **(2)** tenderness at the upper inner angle of the orbit at the point of attachment of the pulley of the superior oblique muscle, denoting closure of the outlet of the frontal sinus.

external malleolar s., SYN Chaddock s.

eyelash s., in a case of apparent unconsciousness due to functional disease, such as conversion hysteria, stroking the eyelashes will occasion movement of the lids, but no such reflex will occur

in case of severe organic brain lesion such as apoplexy, fracture of the skull, or other traumatism.

Faget's s., a slow pulse with an elevated temperature, often seen in yellow fever.

fan s., the spreading apart of the toes in the complete Babinski's sign.

Fischer's s., an obsolete s.: in tuberculosis of the mediastinal or peri-bronchial glands, after bending the patient's head as far back as possible, auscultation over the manubrium sterni will sometimes reveal a continuous loud murmur caused by the pressure of the enlarged glands on the large mediastinal vessels. SYN Fischer's symptom.

fissure s., in perfusion scintigraphy of the lungs, decreased uptake of radionuclide in the periphery of each lobe, making the fissures visible; caused by a variety of diseases and artifacts.

flag s., bands of discoloration of hair (reddish, blonde, or gray, depending on original color) resulting from fluctuations in nutrition characteristic of kwashiorkor and in diseases of protein depletion such as ulcerative colitis.

Forchheimer's s., the presence, in German measles, of a reddish maculopapular eruption on the soft palate.

Fothergill's s., in rectus sheath hematoma, the hematoma produces a mass that does not cross the midline and remains palpable when the rectus muscle is tense.

Friedreich's s., in adherent pericardium, sudden collapse of the previously distended veins of the neck at each diastole of the heart.

Froment's s., flexion of the distal phalanx of the thumb when a sheet of paper is held between the thumb and index finger in ulnar nerve palsy.

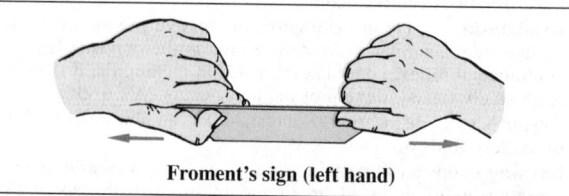

Froment's sign (left hand)

Gaenslen's s., pain on hyperextension of the hip with pelvis fixed by flexion of opposite hip; causes a torsion stress at the sacroiliac and lumbosacral joints.

Gauss' s., marked mobility of the uterus in the early weeks of pregnancy.

Gerhardt's s., complete bilateral paralysis of the adductor muscles of the larynx with severe inspiratory dyspnea. SYN Biermer's s.

Glasgow's s., a systolic murmur heard over the brachial artery in aneurysm of the aorta.

gloved-finger s., in chest radiology, the appearance of mucoid impaction of branching bronchi.

Goggia's s., the fibrillation of the biceps muscle, when pinched and tapped, is confined to a limited area in cases of debilitating disease, whereas in health it is general.

Goldstein's toe s., increased space between the great toe and its neighbor, seen in mongolism and occasionally in cretinism.

Goldthwait's s., in sprain of sacroiliac ligaments, flexion of hip with extended knee elicits pain in sacroiliac region; not now considered specific.

Goodell's s., softening of the cervix and vagina as being usually indicative of pregnancy.

Gordon's s., SYN finger *phenomenon.*

Gorlin's s., unusual ease in touching the tip of the nose with the tongue; seen in Ehlers-Danlos syndrome.

Graefe's s., in Grave's disease, lag of the upper eyelid as it follows the rotation of the eyeball downward. SYN von Graefe's s.

Grasset's s., normal contraction of the sternocleidomastoid muscle on the paralyzed side in cases of hemiplegia.

Grey Turner's s., local areas of discoloration about the umbilicus and in the region of the loins, in acute hemorrhagic pancreatitis and other causes of retroperitoneal hemorrhage.

Griesinger's s., erythema and edema over the posterior mastoid process resulting from septic thrombosis of the mastoid emissary vein and thrombophlebitis of the sigmoid sinus.

Grisolle's s., an obsolete s.; in smallpox, the continued presence and palpability of papules when the skin is stretched.

Grocco's s., (1) acute dilation of the heart following a muscular effort, described in Graves' disease; also occurring in various forms of myocardiopathy; **(2)** extension of the liver dullness several centimeters to the left of the midspinal line in cases of enlargement of that organ.

groove s., large, hard, fixed, and extremely tender lymph nodes in the groin above and below the inguinal ligament, with a groove along the ligament; characteristic of lymphogranuloma venereum.

Gunn's s., (1) compression of the underlying vein at arteriovenous crossings seen ophthalmoscopically in arteriolar sclerosis; **(2)** on alternate stimulation with light, the pupil of an eye with optic nerve transmission defect constricts poorly or even dilates when stimulated (a relative afferent pupillary defect). SYN Marcus Gunn's s.

Gunn's crossing s., retinal arteriovenous crossing with venous compression in hypertensive disease.

Guyon's s., (1) ballottement of the kidney in cases of nephroptosis, especially when there is also a renal tumor; **(2)** the hypoglossal nerve lies directly upon the external carotid artery, whereby this vessel may be distinguished from the internal carotid when ligation is necessary.

halo s., elevation of the subcutaneous fat layer over the fetal skull in a dead or dying fetus; said to be the most common radiologic sign of fetal death.

halo s. of hydrops, a discredited roentgenographic s. of fetal hydrops caused by scalp edema so that a definite corona surrounds the skull.

Hamman's s., a crunching, rasping sound, synchronous with heart beat, heard over the precordium and sometimes at a distance from the chest in mediastinal *emphysema.*

Hegar's s., softening and compressibility of the lower segment of the uterus in early pregnancy (about the seventh week) which, on bimanual examination, is felt by the finger in the vagina as though the neck and body of the uterus were separated, or connected by only a thin band of tissue.

Heim-Kreysig s., in adherent pericardium, an indrawing of the intercostal spaces, synchronous with the cardiac systole. SYN Kreysig's s.

Helbings' s., a malalignment of the Achilles tendon associated with a valgus deformity of the os calcis.

Hennebert's s., nystagmus produced by pressure applied to a sealed external auditory canal; may be seen in labyrinthine fistula or with intact tympanic membrane in syphilitic involvement of the otic capsule.

Higoumenakia s., sternoclavicular swelling in late congenital syphilis.

Hill's s., in aortic insufficiency, greater systolic blood pressure in the legs than in the arms; normal arterial systolic pressure in the leg is 10 to 20 mm of Hg above that in the arm, whereas in aortic insufficiency the difference may be 60 to 100 mm of Hg. SYN Hill's phenomenon.

Hoffmann's s., (1) in latent tetany mild mechanical stimulation of the trigeminal nerve causes severe pain; **(2)** flexion of the terminal phalanx of the thumb and of the second and third phalanges of one or more of the fingers when the volar surface of the terminal phalanx of the fingers is flicked. SYN digital reflex, Hoffmann's reflex, snapping reflex.

Hoagland's s., eyelid edema in infectious mononucleosis.

Homans' s., slight pain at the back of the knee or calf when the ankle is slowly and gently dorsiflexed (with the knee bent), indicative of incipient or established thrombosis in the veins of the leg.

Hoover's s.'s, (1) a person lying supine on a couch, when asked to raise one leg, involuntarily makes counterpressure with the heel of the other leg; if this leg is paralyzed, whatever muscular

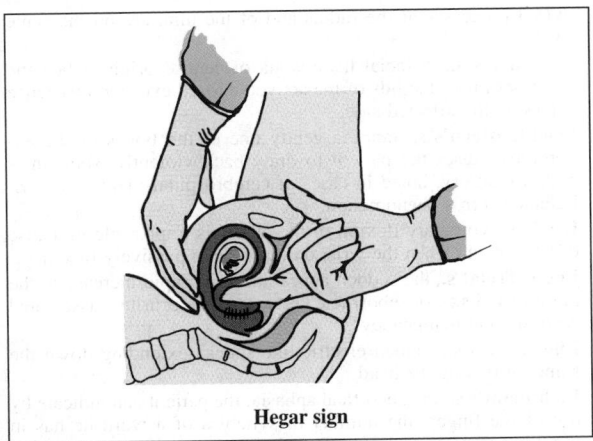

Hegar sign

power is preserved in it will be exerted in this way; or if the patient attempts to lift a paralyzed leg, counterpressure will be made with the other heel, whether any movement occurs in the paralyzed limb or not; not present in hysteria or malingering; **(2)** a modification in the movement of the costal margins during respiration, caused by a flattening of the diaphragm; suggestive of empyema or other intrathoracic condition causing a change in the contour of the diaphragm.

Hueter's s., in a case of fracture, the vibration expected on tapping the bone is not transmitted when tissue intervenes between the fractured parts of bone.

iconic s.'s, s.'s that acquire their function through similarity to what they signify; *e.g.,* a photograph as a s. of the person in the picture.

indexical s.'s, s.'s that acquire their function through a causal connection with what they signify; *e.g.,* smoke as a s. of fire.

inferior triangle s., in chest radiology, lateral displacement of the diaphragmatic pleura near the diaphragm, associated with collapse of the upper lobe, usually on the right side.

Jackson's s., during quiet respiration the movement of the paralyzed side of the chest may be greater than that of the opposite side, while in forced respiration the paralyzed side moves less than the other. [J. H. Jackson]

Joffroy's s., disorder of the arithmetical faculty (the person being unable to do simple sums in addition or multiplication) in the early stages of organic brain disease.

Keen's s., increased width at the malleoli in Pott's fracture.

Kehr's s., violent pain in the left shoulder in a case of rupture of the spleen.

Kernig's s., when the subject lies upon the back and the thigh is flexed to a right angle with the axis of the trunk, complete extension of the leg on the thigh is impossible; present in various forms of meningitis.

Kestenbaum's s., a decrease in the number of arterioles crossing optic disk margins as a s. of optic neuritis.

Kocher's s., in Graves' disease, on upward gaze, the globe lags behind the movement of the upper eyelid.

Kreysig's s., SYN Heim-Kreysig s.

Kussmaul's s., in constrictive pericarditis, a paradoxical increase in venous distention and pressure during inspiration; seen occasionally in effusive-constrictive pericarditis when tamponading pericardial fluid overlies a constricting epicarditis. SYN Kussmaul's symptom.

Lancisi's s., a large systolic jugular venous wave caused by tricuspid regurgitation replacing the normal negative systolic trough ("x" descent).

Landolfi's s., in aortic insufficiency, systolic contraction and diastolic dilation of the pupil.

Lasègue's s., when patient is supine with hip flexed, dorsiflexion of the ankle causing pain or muscle spasm in the posterior thigh indicates lumbar root or sciatic nerve irritation.

Laugier's s., in fracture of the lower portion of the radius, the styloid processes of the radius and of the ulna are on the same level.

Legendre's s., in facial hemiplegia of central origin, when the examiner raises the lids of the actively closed eyes the resistance is less on the affected side.

Leichtenstern's s., tapping gently one of the bones of the extremities causes the patient to draw back violently, sometimes with a loud cry; noted in cases of cerebrospinal meningitis. SYN Leichtenstern's phenomenon.

Leri's s., voluntary flexion of the elbow is impossible in a case of hemiplegia when the wrist on that side is passively flexed.

Leser-Trélat s., the sudden appearance and rapid increase in the number and size of seborrheic keratoses with pruritus; associated with internal malignancy.

Lhermitte's s., sudden electric-like shocks extending down the spine on flexing the head.

Lichtheim's s., in subcortical aphasia, the patient can indicate by use of the fingers the number of syllables of a word he has in mind but cannot speak. SYN Dejerine-Lichtheim phenomenon.

local s., the characteristic of a sensation that permits distinguishing it from another sensation by locating its position in space.

Lorenz' s., an obsolete s.: stiffness of the thoracic spine in early pulmonary tuberculosis.

Lovibond's profile s., SYN Lovibond's *angle*.

Ludloff's s., in traumatic separation of the epiphysis of the lesser trochanter: **(1)** swelling and ecchymosis appear at the base of Scarpa's triangle; **(2)** inability to raise the thigh in the sitting posture.

Macewen's s., percussion of the skull gives a cracked-pot sound in cases of hydrocephalus. SYN Macewen's symptom.

Magendie-Hertwig s., skew deviation of the eyes in acute cerebellar lesions. SYN Magendie-Hertwig syndrome.

Magnan's s., paresthesia in the psychosis of cocaine addicts, who imagine they have a foreign body, in the shape of a powder or fine sand, under the skin, and that it is constantly changing its position.

Magnus' s., an obsolete s.: after death, constriction of a limb or one of its segments is not followed by venous congestion of the distal part.

Mannkopf's s., acceleration of the pulse when a painful point is pressed upon.

Marañón's s., in Graves' disease, a vasomotor reaction following stimulation of the skin over the throat.

Marcus Gunn's s., SYN Gunn's s.

Masini's s., a marked degree of dorsal extension of the fingers on the metacarpals and of the toes on the metatarsals, noted in children with mental instability.

McBurney's s., tenderness at site two-thirds of the distance between the umbilicus and the anterior-superior iliac spine; seen in appendicitis.

Metenier's s., easy eversion of the upper eyelid in Ehlers-Danlos syndrome.

Mirchamp's s., a premonitory symptom of mumps; if a strongly flavored substance is placed on the tongue a painful reflex secretion of saliva occurs in the gland that is the seat of the incipient affection.

Möbius' s., impairment of ocular convergence in Graves' disease.

Mosler's s., tenderness over the sternum in a patient with acute myeloblastic anemia.

Muerhrcke's s., apparent leukonychia with white bands parallel to lanula of the nails, seen in hypoalbuminemia. SYN Muehrcke's bands.

Müller's s., in aortic insufficiency, rhythmical pulsatory movements of the uvula, synchronous with the heart's action; accompanied by swelling and redness of the velum palati and tonsils.

Munson's s., in keratoconus, the extra bowing of the lower eyelid caused by the misshapen cornea as the eye rotates downward.

Murphy's s., pain on palpation of the right subcostal area during inspiration frequently associated with acute cholecystitis.

Musset's s., in incompetence of the aortic valve, rhythmical nodding of the head, synchronous with the heart beat. SYN de Musset's s.

neck s., SYN Brudzinski's s. (2).

Néri's s., in hemiplegia, the knee bends spontaneously when the leg is passively extended.

Nikolsky's s., a peculiar vulnerability of the skin in pemphigus vulgaris; the apparently normal epidermis may be separated at the basal layer and rubbed off when pressed with a sliding motion.

objective s., a s. that is evident to the examiner.

s. of the orbicularis, in hemiplegia, inability to voluntarily close the eye on the paralyzed side except in conjunction with closure of the other eye. SYN Revilliod's s.

Osler's s., in acute bacterial endocarditis, circumscribed painful erythematous swellings, ranging in size from that of a pinhead to that of a pea, in the skin and subcutaneous tissues of the hands and feet.

Pastia's s., the presence of pink or red transverse lines at the bend of the elbow in the preeruptive stage of scarlatina; they persist through the eruptive stage and remain as pigmented lines after desquamation. SYN Thomson's s.

Payr's s., pain on pressure over the sole of the foot; a s. of thrombophlebitis.

Perez' s., rales audible over the upper part of the chest when the arms are alternately raised and lowered; common in cases of fibrous mediastinitis and also of aneurysm of the aortic arch.

Pfuhl's s., the pressure of pus within a subphrenic abscess rises during inspiration and falls during expiration, the reverse of what happens in the case of a purulent collection above the diaphragm; when the diaphragm is paralyzed this distinction is lost.

physical s., a s. that is observed or elicited by auscultation, percussion, or palpation.

Piltz s., SYN eye-closure pupil *reaction*.

Pins' s., SYN Ewart's s.

Pitres' s., **(1)** SYN haphalgesia. **(2)** diminished sensation in the testes and scrotum in tabes dorsalis.

placental s., slight endometrial oozing of blood which occurs in certain animals and sometimes in women at the time of implantation of the fertilized ovum; in women, if the blood appears externally it may be mistaken for a scanty menstrual period.

Pool-Schlesinger s., SYN Pool's *phenomenon* (1).

Potain's s., in dilation of the aorta, dullness on percussion extending from the manubrium sterni toward the second intercostal space and the third costal cartilage on the right, the upper limit extending from the base of the sternum in the segment of a circle to the right.

prodromic s., a s. that appears during the prodrome of a disease. SYN antecedent s.

pseudo-Graefe s., a lid retraction phenomenon similar to Graefe's s., but due to aberrant regeneration of fibers of the oculomotor nerve into the levator of the upper lid.

puddle s., a s. of free abdominal fluid: the patient assumes a position on all fours; one flank is percussed by repeated light flicking of constant intensity while a Bowles-type stethoscope is placed over the most dependent portion of the abdomen and gradually moved toward the flank opposite the percussion; a sharp increase in the intensity of the sound picked up by the stethoscope indicates the level of fluid.

pyramid s., any of the symptoms indicating a morbid condition of the pyramidal tracts, such as the Babinski or Gordon s., spastic spinal paralysis, foot clonus, etc.

Quant's s., a T-shaped depression in the occipital bone occurring in many cases of rickets, especially in infants lying constantly in bed with pressure on the occiput.

Quénu-Muret s., in aneurysm, well-maintained collateral circulation indicated by issue of blood when the main artery of the limb is compressed and a puncture is made at the periphery.

Quincke's s., SYN Quincke's *pulse*.

Ransohoff's s., yellow pigmentation in the umbilical region in rupture of the common bile duct.

Raynaud's s., SYN acrocyanosis.

Remak's s., dissociation of the sensations of touch and of pain in tabes dorsalis and polyneuritis.

reversed-three s., on an esophagram of a patient with coarctation of the aorta, the shape of the contrast-filled esophagus caused by the aortic arch (upper convexity) and post-stenotic dilatation (lower convexity); the cusp of the backwards 3 is at the level of the coarctation itself.

Revilliod's s., SYN s. of the orbicularis.

Ripault's s., a s. of death, consisting in a permanent change in the shape of the pupil produced by unilateral pressure on the eyeball.

Rocher's s., SYN drawer s.

Romaña's s., marked edema of one or both eyelids, usually a unilateral palpebral edema, thought to be a sensitization response to the bite of a triatomine bug infected with *Trypanosoma cruzi*, and a strong suggestion of acute Chagas' disease.

Romberg's s., with feet approximated, the patient stands with eyes open and then closed; if closing the eyes increases the unsteadiness, a loss of proprioceptive control is indicated, and the sign is positive. SYN Romberg test, Romberg's symptom (1), rombergism, station test.

Rosenbach's s., loss of the abdominal reflex in cases of acute inflammation of the viscera.

Rossolimo's s., SYN Rossolimo's *reflex.*

Rotch's s., in pericardial effusion, percussion dullness in the fifth intercostal space on the right.

Rovsing's s., pain at McBurney's point induced in cases of appendicitis, by pressure exerted over the descending colon.

Rumpel-Leede s., SYN Rumpel-Leede *test.*

Russell's s., abrasions and scars on the back of the hands of individuals with bulimia, usually due to manual attempts at self-induced vomiting.

Saenger's s., a lost light reflex of the pupil returns after a short time in the dark, noted in cerebral syphilis but absent in tabes dorsalis.

Sansom's s., in mitral stenosis, apparent duplication of the second heart sound.

Schapiro's s., in myocardial weakness, no slowing of the pulse occurs when the patient lies down.

Schlesinger's s., SYN Pool's *phenomenon* (1).

Schultze's s., in latent tetany, tapping the tongue causes its depression with a concave dorsum. SYN tongue phenomenon.

scimitar s., a curvilinear structure seen roentgenographically in the lung and associated with anomalous pulmonary venous drainage, suggesting the sickle shape, of a Turkish saber; also used to refer to the scalloped shape of the sacrum in spinal dysraphism with anterior meningocele.

Seeligmüller's s., contraction of the pupil on the affected side in facial neuralgia.

Seidel's s., a sickle-shaped scotoma appearing as an upward or downward extension of the blind spot.

sentinel loop s., in gastrointestinal radiology, dilatation of a segment of large or small intestine, indicative of localized ileus from nearby inflammation.

setting sun s., retraction of the upper lid without upgaze so that the iris seems to "set" below the lower lid; suggestive of neurologic damage in the newborn, but usually clears up without sequelae. SEE Collier's s., Epstein's s.

S s. of Golden, in pulmonary radiology, the combination of an atelectatic lobe and a central obstructing mass produces a concavity and a convexity, like the letter "S."

Shibley's s., on auscultation of the chest, the spoken sound "e" is heard as "ah" over an area of pulmonary consolidation or immediately above a pleural effusion.

Siegert's s., shortness and inward curvature of the terminal phalanges of the fifth fingers in Down's syndrome.

Signorelli's s., tenderness on pressure in the glenoid fossa in front of the mastoid process in meningitis.

silhouette s. of Felson, in pulmonary radiology, the obliteration of a normal air-soft tissue interface, such as the cardiac silhouette, when fluid fills the adjacent part of the lung.

Simon's s., in incipient meningitis in children, the movements of the diaphragm are dissociated from those of the thorax.

Skoda's s., SYN skodaic *resonance.*

Snellen's s., bruit heard on auscultation over the eye in a patient with Graves' *disease,* due to the hyperdynamic circulation.

spinal s., in pleurisy, the spinal muscles are in a state of tonic contraction on the affected side.

spine s., resistance to flexion of the spine in cases of meningitis.

Steinberg thumb s., in Marfan's syndrome, when the thumb is held across the palm of the same hand, it projects well beyond the ulnar surface of the hand.

Stellwag's s., infrequent and incomplete blinking in Graves' disease.

Sternberg's s., unilateral tenderness or discomfort on palpation of the shoulder girdle muscles in a patient with pleurisy on that side.

Stewart-Holmes s., in cerebellar disease, the inability to check a movement when passive resistance is suddenly released. SYN rebound phenomenon (1).

Stierlin's s., repeated emptying of the cecum, seen radiographically, with barium remaining in the terminal part of the ileum and in the transverse colon; due to irritation of the cecum, sometimes caused by tuberculous cecitis (typhilitis).

Straus' s., in facial paralysis, if an injection of pilocarpine is followed by sweating on the affected side later than on the other, the lesion is peripheral.

string s., in pediatric gastrointestinal radiology, the narrowed pyloric canal seen with congenital pyloric stenosis; also used to describe a narrowed segment in regional ileitis on small bowel series.

subjective s., a s. that is perceived only by the patient.

Sumner's s., a slight increase in tonus of the abdominal muscles, an early indication of inflammation of the appendix, stone in the kidney or ureter, or a twisted pedicle of an ovarian cyst; it is detected by exceedingly gentle palpation of the right or left iliac fossa.

superior triangle s., in chest radiology, widening of the superior mediastinum, usually on the right, associated with collapse of the lower lobe producing traction on the mediastinal pleura.

ten Horn's s., pain caused by gentle traction on the right spermatic cord, indicative of appendicitis.

Thomson's s., SYN Pastia's s.

Tinel's s. (DTP), a sensation of tingling, or of "pins and needles," felt in the distal extremity of a limb when percussion is made over the site of an injured nerve; it indicates a partial lesion or early regeneration in the nerve.

Toma's s., to distinguish between inflammatory and noninflammatory ascites: in inflammatory conditions of the peritoneum, the mesentery contracts, drawing the intestines over to the right side; consequently, when the patient lies on his back, tympany is elicited on the right side, dullness on the left.

Topolanski's s., congestion of the pericorneal region of the eye in Graves' disease.

Tournay s., SYN Tournay's *phenomenon.*

Traube's s., a double sound or murmur heard in auscultation over arteries (particularly the femoral arteries) in significant aortic regurgitation.

Trélat's s., an obsolete s.; the presence of disseminated yellowish spots in the neighborhood of tuberculous ulcers of the mouth; they are minute tubercles or miliary abscesses.

Trendelenburg's s., in congenital dislocation of the hip or in hip abductor weakness, the pelvis will sag on the side opposite to the dislocation when the hip and knee of the normal side is flexed; without dislocation or weakness, the pelvis will rise on the side of the flexed hip and knee.

Tresilian's s., a reddish prominence at the orifice of Stenson's duct, noted in mumps.

Trousseau's s., in latent tetany, the occurrence of carpopedal spasm accompanied by paresthesia elicited when the upper arm is compressed, as by a tourniquet or a blood pressure cuff.

Trunecek's s., palpable impulse of the subclavian artery near the point of origin of the sternomastoid muscle in cases of aortic sclerosis.

Uhthoff's s., SEE Uhthoff *symptom.*

Vierra's s., yellowing and canalization of the nail in fogo selvagem.

Vipond's s., a generalized adenopathy occurring during the period of incubation of various of the exanthemas of childhood, affording an early diagnostic s. in a case of known exposure.

vital s.'s, manifestation of breathing, heartbeat, and sustained blood pressure.

von Graefe's s., SYN Graefe's s.

Weber's s., SYN Weber's *syndrome.*

Weiss' s., SYN Chvostek's s.

Wernicke's s., SYN Wernicke's *reaction.*

Westermark's s., in chest radiography, an abrupt tapering of a vessel caused by pulmonary thromboembolic obstruction.

Westphal-Erb s.,

Westphal's s., SYN Erb-Westphal s.

Wilder's s., a slight twitch of the eyeball when changing its movement from abduction to adduction or the reverse, noted in Graves' disease.

Winterbottom's s., swelling of the posterior cervical lymph nodes, characteristic of early stages of African trypanosomiasis; useful for surveys or control of migrations from endemic areas of persons with preclinical infections.

wrist s., in Marfan's syndrome, when the wrist is gripped with the opposite hand, the thumb and fifth finger overlap appreciably.

sig·nal (sig′nal). **1.** Something that causes an action. **2.** The end product observed when a specific sequence of DNA or RNA is deleted by some method.

sig·na·ture (sig′nă-chūr, -tūr). The part of a prescription containing the directions to the patient. [Mediev. L. *signatura,* fr. L. *signum,* a sign, mark]

sig·nif·i·cant (sig-nif′i-kant). In statistics, denoting the reliability of a finding or, conversely, the probability of the finding being the result of chance (generally less than 5%). [L. *significo,* to make known, signify, fr. *signum,* sign, + *facio,* to make]

Signorelli, Angelo, Italian physician, 1876–1952. SEE S.'s *sign.*

sig·u·a·tera (sēg-wă-tā′ă). SEE ciguatera.

SIH Abbreviation for somatotropin release-inhibiting *hormone.*

Silber, Robert H., U.S. biochemist, *1915. SEE Porter-S. *chromogens,* under *chromogen, reaction,* chromogens *test.*

si·lent (sī′lent). Producing no detectable signs or symptoms, said of certain diseases or morbid processes.

sil·i·ca (sil′i-kă). SiO_2; the chief constituent of sand, hence of glass. SYN silicic anhydride, silicon dioxide. [Mod. L. fr. L. *silex* (*silic-*), flint]

s. gel, a precipitated form of silicic acid, used for adsorption of various gases.

sil·i·cate (sil′i-kāt). **1.** A salt of silicic acid. **2.** The term sometimes applied to dental restorations of synthetic porcelain.

sil·i·ca·to·sis (sil′i-kă-tō′sis). SYN silicosis.

si·li·ceous (si-lish′ŭs). Containing silica. SYN silicious.

si·lic·ic (si-lis′ik). Relating to silica or silicon.

si·lic·ic ac·id. $Si(OH)_4$; obtained in water as a colloid by treating silicates; precipitated s. a. is silica gel.

si·lic·ic an·hy·dride. SYN silica.

si·li·cious (si-lish′ŭs). SYN siliceous.

sil·i·co·an·thra·co·sis (sil′ĭ-kō-an′thră-kō- sis). A pneumoconiosis consisting of combination of silicosis and anthracosis, seen in hard coal miners.

sil·i·co·flu·o·ride (sil′i-kō-flūr′īd). A compound of silicon and fluorine with another element.

sil·i·con (Si) (sil′i-kon). A very abundant nonmetallic element, atomic no. 14, atomic wt. 28.0855, occurring in nature as silica and silicates; in pure form, used as a semiconductor and in solar batteries; also found in certain polysaccharide structures in mammary tissue. [L. *silex,* flint]

sil·i·con di·ox·ide. SYN silica.

colloidal s. d., a submicroscopic fumed silica prepared by the vapor-phase hydrolysis of a silicon compound; used as a tablet diluent and as a suspending and thickening agent.

sil·i·cone (sil′i-kōn). A polymer of organic silicon oxides, which may be a liquid, gel, or solid, depending on the extent of polymerization; formerly widely used in surgical implants, in intracorporeal tubes to conduct fluids, as dental impression material as a grease or sealing substance, as a coating on the inside of glass vessels for blood collection, and in various ophthalmological procedures.

> Approximately 2 million women in the U.S. have received breast implants since the 1960s, and it had been suggested that among them silicone leakage might cause, or worsen preexisting cases of, rheumatoid arthritis, systemic lupus, scleroderma, and other connective tissue ailments. As a result, silicone breast implants were banned in 1992 by the Food and Drug Administration. In 1994, manufacturers of the implants agreed in principle to establish a $4.2 billion fund for women possibly harmed by their products. However, a long- term study released the same year by researchers at the Mayo Clinic found no statistically significant increase in connective tissue disease among 749 women with implants who were tracked between 1964 and 1991. Their risk was equal to that of 1498 control subjects without implants. Silicone's role in immune disorders and multiple sclerosis, which also has been debated, has yet to be clinically evaluated.

s.-related disease problems, disease apparently resulting from release of silicone into the body, mainly due to the silicone envelope or filling of breast implants.

sil·i·co·pro·te·i·no·sis (sil′i-kō-prō′tē-i-nō′sis). An acute pulmonary disorder, radiographically and histologically similar to pulmonary alveolar proteinosis, resulting from relatively short exposure to high concentrations of silica dust; pulmonary symptoms are of rapid onset and the condition is invariably fatal.

sil·i·co·sid·er·o·sis (sil′i-kō-sid′er-ō′sis). SYN siderosilicosis.

sil·i·co·sis (sil-i-kō′sis). A form of pneumoconiosis resulting from occupational exposure to and inhalation of silica dust over a period of years; characterized by a slowly progressive fibrosis of the lungs, which may result in impairment of lung function; s. predisposes to pulmonary tuberculosis. SYN pneumosilicosis, silicatosis, stone-mason's disease. [L. *silex,* flint, + *-osis,* condition]

sil·i·co·tu·ber·cu·lo·sis (sil′i-kō-tū-ber-kyū-lō′sis). Silicosis associated with tuberculous pulmonary lesions.

si·li·qua oli·vae (sil′i-kwă ō-lī′vē). The arcuate fibers, which appear to encircle the inferior olive in the medulla oblongata. [L. the husk of the olive]

silk. The fibers or filaments obtained from the cocoon of the silkworm.

floss s., SYN dental *floss.*

surgical s., thread prepared from the cocoon filaments of glutinous gum which are spun by the mulberry silkworm *Bombyx mori;* used as suture material in 14 sizes from 0.025 mm to 1.016 mm in diameter and numbered accordingly from 7-0 to 7.

virgin s., an extremely fine ophthalmic suture material consisting of two to seven natural s. filaments bonded together by sericin, a natural adhesive.

Silver, Henry K., U.S. pediatrician, *1918. SEE S.-Russell *dwarfism, syndrome.*

sil·ver (Ag). L. argentum; a metallic element, atomic no. 47, atomic wt. 107.8682. Many salts have clinical applications. SYN argentum. [A.S. *seolfor*]

s. chloride, used in the preparation of antiseptic silver preparations.

colloidal s. iodide, an antiseptic used for treatment of inflammation of the mucous membranes.

s. fluoride, $AgF_2 \cdot H_2O$; an antiseptic.

fused s. nitrate, SYN toughened s. nitrate.

s. iodate, a reagent for the determination of chloride.

s. lactate, has been used as an astringent and antiseptic.

s. nitrate, an antiseptic and astringent; used externally, in solution, in the prevention of ophthalmia neonatorum (presently penicillin is often used); also used in the special staining of the nervous system, spirochetes, reticular fibers, Golgi apparatus, nucleolar organizer region, and calcium.

s. oxide, has been used in epilepsy and chorea; it is explosive when mixed with readily combustible substances.

s. picrate, an ionizable salt of s.; has been used in the treatment of trichomoniasis and moniliasis of the vagina.

strong s. protein, a compound of s. and protein containing not less than 7.5 and not more than 8.5% of s.; used externally as an antiseptic, devoid of astringent and nearly so of irritant properties.

s. sulfadiazine, the s. derivative of sulfadiazine, used externally as a topical antibacterial agent in preventing and treating infections in burns.

toughened s. nitrate, S. nitrate mixed with s. chloride and allowed to dry. Usually applied to the ends of small wooden applicator sticks or made available as pencils. These are used after wetting as a caustic chemical for the removal of warts. SYN fused s. nitrate, lunar caustic.

sil·ver im·preg·na·tion. Silver complexes employed to demonstrate reticulin in normal and diseased tissues, as well as neuroglia, neurofibrillae, argentaffin cells, and Golgi apparatus.

Silverman, Leslie, U.S. engineer, 1914–1966. SEE S.-Lilly *pneumotachograph.*

Silverman, William A., 20th century U.S. pediatrician. SEE Caffey-S. *syndrome.*

Silverskiöld, Nils G., Swedish orthopedist, 1888–1957. SEE S.'s *syndrome.*

sil·vol. SYN mild *silver* protein.

si·meth·i·cone (si-meth'i-kōn). A mixture of dimethyl polysiloxanes and silica gel; an antiflatulent.

si·mi·lia si·mi·li·bus cur·an·tur (si-mil'ē-ă si-mil'i-bŭs ker-an' ter). The homeopathic formula expressing the law of similars, the doctrine that any drug capable of producing morbid symptoms in the healthy will remove similar symptoms occurring as an expression of disease. Another reading of the formula, employed by Hahnemann, the founder of homeopathy, is *similia similibus curentur,* let likes be cured by likes. [L. likes are cured by likes]

si·mil·i·mum, si·mil·li·mum (si-mil'i-mŭm). In homeopathy, the remedy indicated in a certain case because the same drug, when given to a healthy person, will produce the symptom complex most nearly approaching that of the disease in question. [L. *simillimus,* most like, superl. of *similis,* like]

Simmonds, Morris, German physician, 1855–1925. SEE S.'s *disease.*

Simmons, J.S., U.S. bacteriologist, 1890–1954. SEE S.'s citrate *medium.*

Simon, Charles E., U.S. physician, 1866–1927. SEE S.'s *sign.*

Simon, Gustav, German surgeon, 1824–1876. SEE S.'s *position.*

Simon, Théodore, French physician, 1873–1961. SEE Binet-S. *scale.*

Simonart, Pierre J.C., Belgian obstetrician, 1817–1847. SEE S.'s *bands,* under *band, ligaments,* under *ligament, threads,* under *thread.*

Si·mo·nea fol·lic·u·lo·rum (si-mō'nē-ă fŏ-lik-yū-lōr'ŭm). SYN *Demodex folliculorum.*

Simons, Arthur, German physician, *1877. SEE S.'s *disease.*

Simonsiella (sī'mon-sē-el'ah). Genus of nonphotosynthetic, nonfruiting, Gram-negative, chemoorganotrophic, gliding bacteria that exist as multicellular filaments with the long axis of individual cells perpendicular to the long axis of the filament. The cells are flattened and curved to yield a convex-concave, crescent shaped symmetry. Isolated from the oral cavity of mammals. Type species is *Simonsiella muelleri.*

sim·ple (sim'pl). **1.** Not complex or compound. **2.** In anatomy, composed of a minimum number of parts. **3.** A medicinal herb. [L. *simplex*]

Sim·pli·fied Oral Hy·giene In·dex (OHI-S). An index that measures the current oral hygiene status based upon the amount of debris and calculus occurring on six representative tooth surfaces in the mouth; often used in field surveys of periodontal disease.

Simpson, Sir James Y., Scottish obstetrician, 1811–1870. SEE S. uterine *sound;* S.'s *forceps.*

Simpson, William, British civil engineer, †1917.

Sims, J. Marion, U.S. gynecologist, 1813–1883. SEE S.'s *position;* S. uterine *sound.*

sim·u·la·tion (sim-yū-lā'shŭn). Imitation; said of a disease or symptom that resembles another, or of the feigning of illness as in factitious illness or malingering; in radiation therapy, using a geometrically similar radiographic system or computer to plan the location of therapy ports. [L. *simulatio,* fr. *simulo,* pp. *-atus,* to imitate, fr. *similis,* like]

computer s., SYN computer *model.*

sim·u·la·tor (sim'yū-lā-ter, tōr). An apparatus designed to produce effects simulating those of specific environmental conditions; used in experimentation and training.

Sim·u·lium (si-myū'lē-ŭm). A genus of biting gnats or midges, the black flies, humpbacked flies, or buffalo gnats in the dipteran family Simuliidae. The aquatic larvae require swift-flowing streams or highly oxygenated waters for their development, a critical epidemiological factor in the role of these flies as disease vectors. In Central and South America, Mexico, and across central Africa, various species transmit *Onchocerca volvulus,* agent of human onchocerciasis; in North America, *Onchocerca gutturosa* and other onchocercid infections of cattle, horses, and various wild ruminants are transmitted by other black flies. SYN *Eusimulium.* [L. *simulo,* to simulate]

S. damno'sum, species that is an important vector of onchocerciasis in central Africa.

S. neav'ei, species that is an important vector of onchocerciasis in eastern Africa where its larvae and pupae are attached to the shells of crabs of the genus *Potamonantes.*

S. ochra'ceum, species that is a vector of human onchocerciasis in Central America.

S. orna'tum, species that is a vector of bovine onchocerciasis in Australia.

S. ruggle'si, species that is a vector of *Leucocytozoon simondi* in Canada and the northern U.S.

simultagnosia. SYN simultanagnosia.

si·mul·tan·ag·no·sia (sī-mŭl-tan-ag-nō'sē-ă). Inability to recognize multiple elements in a visual presentation, *i.e.,* one object or some elements of a scene can be appreciated but not the display as a whole. SYN simultagnosia. [simultaneous + agnosia]

SIMV Abbreviation for spontaneous intermittent mandatory *ventilation,* synchronized intermittent mandatory *ventilation.*

sim·va·sta·tin (sim'vă-sta-tin). A potent HMG-CoA reductase (the rate-limiting enzyme for cholesterol biosynthesis) inhibitor. Used for the treatment of hyperlipidemia; similar to lovastatin.

sin·ca·lide (sin'kă-līd). The C-terminal octapeptide of cholecystokinin; it causes smooth muscle contraction of the gallbladder and small intestine, relaxation of the choledoduodenal junction, and stimulates pancreatic and gastric secretions; also used as a diagnostic aid to retrieve bile for analysis.

⌂ **Combining forms**	**[NA] Nomina Anatomica**
Word*Finder* **Multi-term entry finder** **Preceding letter A**	**[MIM] Mendelian Inheritance in Man**
A.D.A.M. Anatomy Plates **Between letters L and M**	☆ **Official alternate term**
Appendices: **Following letter Z**	☆**[NA] Official alternate Nomina Anatomica term**
SYN Synonym; Cf., compare	**High Profile Term**

sin·cip·i·tal (sin-sip′i-tăl). Relating to the sinciput.

sin·ci·put, pl. **sin·cip·i·ta**, **sin·ci·puts** (sin′si-put, sin-sip′i-tă). The anterior part of the head just above and including the forehead. [L. half of the head]

SINES Abbreviation for short interspersed *elements*, under *element*.

sin·ew (sin′ū). SYN tendon. [A.S. *sinu*]

sin·gul·ta·tion (sing′gŭl-tā′shŭn). Hiccupping. SEE hiccup. [L. *singulto*, pp. *-atus*, to hiccup]

sin·gul·tous (sing-gŭl′tŭs). Relating to hiccups.

sin·gul·tus (sing-gŭl′tŭs). A hiccup. [L.]

sin·i·grase, sin·i·gri·nase (sin′i-grās, -gri-nās). SYN thioglucosidase.

sin·is·ter (si-nis′ter) [NA]. Left. [L.]

sin·is·trad (sin′is-trad, si-nis′trad). Toward the left side. [L. *sinister*, left, + *ad*, to]

sin·is·tral (sin′is-trăl, sĭ-nis′trăl). 1. Relating to the left side. SYN sinistrous. 2. Denoting a left-handed person.

sin·is·tral·i·ty (sin-is-tral′i-tē). The condition of being left-handed.

⌂**sinistro-.** Left, toward the left. [L. *sinister*]

sin·is·tro·car·dia (sin′is-trō-kar′dē-ă). Displacement of the heart beyond the normal position on the left side. [sinistro- + G. *kardia*, heart]

sin·is·tro·ce·re·bral (sin′is-trō-ser′ĕ-brăl). Relating to the left cerebral hemisphere. [sinistro- + L. *cerebrum*, brain]

sin·is·troc·u·lar (sin-is-trok′yū-lăr). Seldom-used term denoting one who prefers the left eye in monocular work, such as in the use of a microscope. Cf. dominant *eye*. [sinistro- + L. *oculus*, eye]

sin·is·tro·gy·ra·tion (sin′is-trō-jī-rā′shŭn). SYN sinistrotorsion. [sinistro- + L. *gyratio*, a turning around (gyration)]

sin·is·tro·man·u·al (sin′is-trō-man′yū-ăl). SYN left-handed. [sinistro- + L. *manus*, hand]

sin·is·trop·e·dal (sin-is-trop′ĕ-dăl). Denoting one who uses the left leg by preference. SYN left-footed. [sinistro- + L. *pes* (ped-), foot]

sin·is·tro·ro·ta·tion (sin′is-trō-rō-tā′shŭn). SYN sinistrotorsion.

sin·is·trorse (sin′is-trors). Turned or twisted to the left. [L. *sinistrorsus*, on the left side, fr. *sinister*, left, + *verto*, pp. *versus*, to turn]

sin·is·tro·tor·sion (sin′is-trō-tōr′shŭn). A turning or twisting to the left. SYN levorotation (2), levotorsion (1), sinistrogyration, sinistrorotation. [sinistro- + L. *torsio*, a twisting (torsion)]

sin·is·trous (sin′is-trŭs, si-nis′trŭs). SYN sinistral (1).

si·no·a·tri·al (sī′nō-ā′trē-ăl). SYN sinuatrial.

si·nog·ra·phy (sī-nog′ră-fē). Radiologic use of a contrast medium to opacify a sinus tract. [sinus + G. *graphō*, to write]

si·no·pul·mo·nary (sī′nō-pŭl′mŏ-nār-ē). Relating to the paranasal sinuses and the pulmonary airway.

si·no·vag·i·nal (sī-nō-vaj′i-năl). Relating to that part of the vagina derived from the urogenital sinus.

sin·ter. To heat a powdered substance without thoroughly melting it, causing it to fuse into a solid but porous mass. [Ger. dross, slag]

si·nu·a·tri·al (S-A) (sin′yū-ā′trē-ăl, sī′nū-). Relating to the sinus venosus and the right atrium of the heart. SYN sinoatrial.

SINUS

si·nus, pl. **si·nus**, **si·nus·es** (sī′nŭs, -ĕz). 1 [NA]. A channel for the passage of blood or lymph, without the coats of an ordinary vessel; *e.g.*, blood passages in the gravid uterus or those in the cerebral meninges. 2 [na]. A cavity or hollow space in bone or other tissue. 3 [NA]. A dilatation in a blood vessel. 4. A fistula or tract leading to a suppurating cavity. [L. *sinus*, cavity, channel, hollow]

s. a′lae par′vae, SYN sphenoparietal s.

anal sinuses, (1) the grooves between the anal columns; SYN Morgagni's s. (1). (2) pockets or crypts in the columnar zone of the anal canal between the anocutaneous line and the anorectal line; the sinuses give the mucosa a scalloped appearance. SYN s. anales [NA], anal crypts, Morgagni's crypts, rectal sinuses.

s. ana′les [NA], SYN anal sinuses.

anterior sinuses, SYN anterior ethmoidal air *cells*, under *cell*.

s. aor′tae [NA], SYN aortic s.

aortic s., the space between the superior aspect of each cusp of the aortic valve and the dilated portion of the wall of the ascending aorta, immediately above each cusp. SYN s. aortae [NA], Petit's s., Valsalva's s.

Arlt's s., an inconstant depression on the lower portion of the internal surface of the lacrimal sac.

barber's pilonidal s., pilonidal s. occurring in barbers, usually in the web between the fingers, due to the burying of exogenous hairs by the alternate loosening and tightening of tissues of the hand by the manipulation of scissors.

basilar s., SYN basilar *plexus*.

Breschet's s., SYN sphenoparietal s.

s. carot′icus [NA], SYN carotid s.

carotid s., a slight dilation of the common carotid artery at its bifurcation into external and internal carotids; it contains baroreceptors which, when stimulated, cause slowing of the heart, vasodilation, and a fall in blood pressure and is innervated primarily by the glossopharyngeal nerve. SYN s. caroticus [NA], carotid bulb.

s. caverno′sus [NA], SYN cavernous s.

cavernous s., a paired dural venous s. on either side of the sella turcica, the two being connected by anastomoses, the anterior and posterior intercavernous s., in front of and behind the hypophysis, respectively, making thus the circular s.; the cavernous s. is unique among dural venous sinuses in being trabeculated; coursing within the sinus are the internal carotid artery and the abducent nerve. SYN s. cavernosus [NA].

cerebral sinuses, SYN dural venous sinuses.

cervical s., in young mammalian embryos a depression in the nuchal region caudal to the hyoid arch, with the third and fourth branchial arches and ectodermal grooves in its floor; normally it is obliterated after the second month, but occasionally cervical fistulae persist as vestiges of it. SYN precervical s.

circular s., (1) dural venous formation which surrounds the hypophysis, composed of right and left cavernous sinuses and the intercavernous sinuses; SYN circulus venosus ridleyi, Ridley's circle. (2) a venous s. at the periphery of the placenta; (3) SYN s. venosus sclerae.

s. circula′ris, SYN s. venosus sclerae.

coccygeal s., a fistula opening in the region of the coccyx, being the result of incomplete closure of the caudal end of the neurenteric canal. SEE ALSO pilonidal s.

s. corona′rius [NA], SYN coronary s.

coronary s., a short trunk receiving most of the cardiac veins, beginning at the junction of the great cardiac vein and the oblique vein of the left atrium, running in the posterior part of the coronary sulcus and emptying into the right atrium between the inferior vena cava and the atrioventricular orifice. SYN s. coronarius [NA].

costomediastinal s., SYN costomediastinal *recess*.

cranial sinuses, SYN dural venous sinuses.

dermal s., a s. lined with epidermis and skin appendages extending from the skin to some deeper-lying structure, most frequently the spinal cord.

s. du′rae ma′tris [NA], SYN dural venous sinuses.

dural venous sinuses, endothelium-lined venous channels in the dura mater. SYN s. durae matris [NA], cerebral sinuses, cranial sinuses, sinuses of dura mater, venous sinuses.

sinuses of dura mater, SYN dural venous sinuses.

Englisch's s., SYN inferior petrosal s.

s. epididym′idis [NA], SYN s. of epididymis.

s. of epididymis, a narrow space between the body of the epididymis and the testis. SYN s. epididymidis [NA].

ethmoidal sinuses, ethmoidal air-cells; evaginations of the mucous membrane of the middle and superior meatuses of the nasal cavity into the ethmoidal labyrinth forming multiple small paranasal sinuses; they are subdivided into anterior, middle and posterior ethmoidal sinuses. SYN s. antra ethmoidalia.

s. ethmoida′les [NA], SYN ethmoid air *cells,* under *cell.*

s. ethmoidales anterio′res [NA], SYN anterior ethmoidal air *cells,* under *cell.*

s. ethmoidales me′diae [NA], SYN middle ethmoidal air *cells,* under *cell.*

s. ethmoidales posterio′res [NA], SYN posterior ethmoidal air *cells,* under *cell.*

frontal s., a hollow paranasal sinus formed on either side in the lower part of the squama of the frontal bone; it communicates by the ethmoidal infundibulum with the middle meatus of the nasal cavity of the same side. SYN s. frontalis [NA].

s. fronta′lis [NA], SYN frontal s.

Guérin's s., a cul-de-sac or diverticulum behind the valve of the navicular fossa.

Huguier's s., SYN *fossula* fenestrae vestibuli.

inferior longitudinal s., SYN inferior sagittal s.

inferior petrosal s., a paired dural venous s. running in the groove on the petrooccipital fissure connecting the cavernous s. with the superior bulb of the internal jugular vein. SYN s. petrosus inferior [NA], Englisch's s.

inferior sagittal s., an unpaired dural venous s. in the lower margin of the falx cerebri, running parallel to the superior sagittal s. and merging with the great cerebral vein to form the the straight s. SYN s. sagittalis inferior [NA], inferior longitudinal s.

s. intercaverno′si [NA], SYN intercavernous sinuses.

intercavernous sinuses, the anterior and posterior anastomoses between the cavernous s.'s, passing anterior and posterior to the hypophysis and forming, with the cavernous sinuses, the circular s. (1). SYN s. intercavernosi [NA], Ridley's s.

jugular s., s. jugula′ris, one of three enlargements of the jugular veins; the external jugular s. is between the two sets of valves; the internal jugular s.'s are at the origin (superior bulb) and near the termination (inferior bulb).

s. lactif′eri [NA], SYN lactiferous s.

lactiferous s., a circumscribed spindle-shaped dilation of the lactiferous duct just before it enters the nipple. In nursing mothers this dilatation stores a droplet of milk which is expressed by compression as the infant begins to suckle; this is thought to encourage continual suckling while the let-down reflex ensues. SYN s. lactiferi [NA], ampulla lactifera, ampulla of milk duct, lactiferous ampulla.

laryngeal s., SYN laryngeal *ventricle.*

s. laryn′geus, SYN laryngeal *ventricle.*

lateral s., SYN transverse s.

s. lie′nis [NA], SYN splenic s.

longitudinal s., SEE inferior sagittal s., superior sagittal s.

longitudinal vertebral venous s., large, plexiform veins forming portions of the anterior internal vertebral venous plexus lying on the posterior surfaces of the vertebral bodies on either side of the posterior longitudinal ligament. SYN s. vertebrales longitudinales.

Luschka's s., venous s. in the petrosquamous suture.

lymph s., SYN lymphatic s.

lymphatic s., the channels in a lymph node crossed by a reticulum of cells and fibers and bounded by littoral cells; there are subcapsular, trabecular, and medullary s.'s. SYN lymph s.

Maier's s., an infundibuliform depression on the internal surface of the lacrimal sac which receives the lacrimal canaliculi.

marginal sinuses of placenta, discontinuous venous lakes at the margin of the placenta.

mastoid sinuses, SYN mastoid air *cells,* under *cell.*

s. maxilla′ris [NA], SYN maxillary s.

maxillary s., the largest of the paranasal sinuses occupying the body of the maxilla, communicating with the middle meatus of the nose. SYN s. maxillaris [NA], antrum of Highmore, genyantrum, maxillary antrum.

Meyer's s., a small concavity in the floor of the external auditory canal near the membrana tympani.

middle ethmoidal sinuses, SYN middle ethmoidal air *cells,* under *cell.*

Morgagni's s., (1) SYN anal sinuses (1). **(2)** SYN prostatic *utricle.* **(3)** SYN laryngeal *ventricle.*

s. of nail, SYN s. unguis.

oblique pericardial s., the recess in the pericardial cavity posterior to the base of the heart bounded laterally by the pericardial reflections on the pulmonary veins and inferior vena cava, and posteriorly by the pericardium overlying the anterior aspect of the esophagus. SYN s. obliquus pericardii [NA], oblique s. of pericardium.

oblique s. of pericardium, SYN oblique pericardial s.

s. obli′quus pericar′dii [NA], SYN oblique pericardial s.

occipital s., an unpaired dural venous s. commencing at the confluence of the sinuses and passing downward in the base of the falx cerebelli to the foramen magnum. SYN s. occipitalis [NA].

s. occipita′lis [NA], SYN occipital s.

Palfyn's s., a space within the crista galli of the ethmoid described as communicating with the ethmoidal and frontal s.'s.

paranasal sinuses, the paired air-filled cavities in the bones of the face lined by mucous membrane continuous with that of the nasal cavity; these s.'s are the frontal, sphenoidal, maxillary, and ethmoidal. SYN s. paranasales [NA].

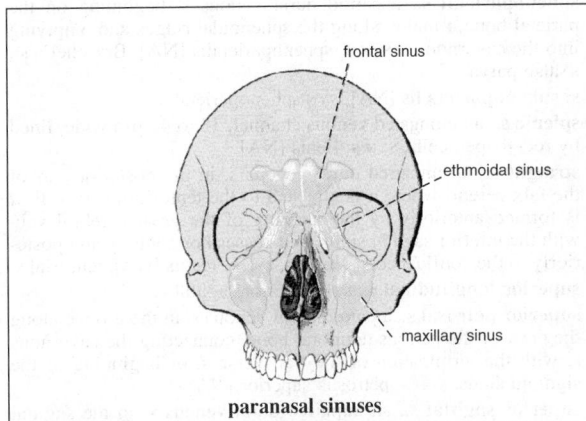

frontal sinus

ethmoidal sinus

maxillary sinus

paranasal sinuses

s. paranasa′les [NA], SYN paranasal sinuses.

parasinoidal sinuses, SYN lateral venous *lacunae,* under *lacuna.*

Petit's s., SYN aortic s.

petrosal s., SEE inferior petrosal s., superior petrosal s.

s. petro′sus infe′rior [NA], SYN inferior petrosal s.

s. petro′sus supe′rior [NA], SYN superior petrosal s.

phrenicocostal s., SYN costodiaphragmatic *recess.*

pilonidal s., a fistula or pit in the sacral region, communicating with the exterior, containing hair which may act as a foreign body producing chronic inflammation. SYN pilonidal fistula.

piriform s., SYN piriform *fossa.*

pleural sinuses, SYN pleural *recesses,* under *recess.*

s. pocula′ris, SYN prostatic *utricle.*

s. poste′rior [NA], a deep groove above the pyramidal eminence extending to the incudal fossa in the posterior wall of the tympanic cavity.

precervical s., SYN cervical s.

prostatic s., the groove on either side of the urethral crest in the prostatic part of the urethra into which the prostatic ducts open. SYN s. prostaticus [NA].

s. prostat′icus [NA], SYN prostatic s.

pulmonary sinuses, the space at the origin of the pulmonary trunk between the dilated wall of the vessel and each cusp of the pulmonic valve. SYN s. trunci pulmonalis [NA].

rectal sinuses, SYN anal sinuses.

s. rec′tus [NA], SYN straight s.

renal s., the cavity of the kidney, containing the calyces and pelvis of the ureter and the segmental vesels embedded within a fatty matrix. The renal sinuses cause the kidneys to appear hollow or C-shaped on cross section or medical imaging. SYN s. renalis [NA].

s. rena′lis [NA], SYN renal s.

s. reu′niens, obsolete term for s. venosus.

rhomboidal s., s. rhomboidalis, a dilation of the central canal of the spinal cord in the lumbar region. SYN rhombocele.

Ridley's s., SYN intercavernous sinuses.

Rokitansky-Aschoff sinuses, small outpocketings of the mucosa of the gallbladder which extend through the muscular layer; they may be congenital.

s. sagitta′lis infe′rior [NA], SYN inferior sagittal s.

s. sagitta′lis supe′rior [NA], SYN superior sagittal s.

sigmoid s., the S-shaped dural venous s. lying deep to the mastoid process of the temporal bone and immediately posterior to the petrous temporal bone; it is continuous with the transverse s. and empties into the internal jugular vein as it passes through the jugular foramen. SYN s. sigmoideus [NA].

s. sigmoi′deus [NA], SYN sigmoid s.

sphenoidal s., one of a pair of paranasal sinuses in the body of the sphenoid bone communicating with the upper posterior nasal cavity or spenoethmoidal recess. SYN s. sphenoidalis [NA].

s. sphenoida′lis [NA], SYN sphenoidal s.

sphenoparietal s., a paired dural venous s. beginning on the parietal bone, running along the sphenoidal ridges and emptying into the cavernous s. SYN s. sphenoparietalis [NA], Breschet's s., s. alae parvae.

s. sphenoparieta′lis [NA], SYN sphenoparietal s.

splenic s., an elongated venous channel, 12 to 40 μm wide, lined by rod-shaped cells. SYN s. lienis [NA].

straight s., an unpaired dural venous s. in the posterior part of the falx cerebri where it is attached to the tentorium cerebelli; it is formed anteriorly by the merging of the great cerebral vein with the inferior sagittal sinus, and passes horizontally and posteriorly to the confluence of sinuses. SYN s. rectus [NA], tentorial s.

superior longitudinal s., SYN superior sagittal s.

superior petrosal s., a paired dural venous s. in the groove along the crest of the petrous temporal bone, connecting the cavernous s. with the termination of the transverse s. or beginning of the sigmoid sinus. SYN s. petrosus superior [NA].

superior sagittal s., an unpaired dural venous s. in the sagittal groove, beginning at the foramen caecum and terminating at the confluence of sinuses where it merges with the straight sinus; receives the superior cerebral veins and has lateral extensions, the lateral venous lacunae. SYN s. sagittalis superior [NA], superior longitudinal s.

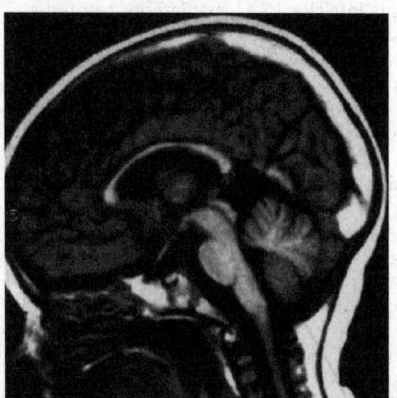

thrombosis of superior sagittal sinus (white contour in MRI)

tarsal s., a hollow or canal formed by the groove of the talus and

the interosseous groove of the calcaneus which is occupied by the interosseous talocalcaneal ligament. SYN s. tarsi [NA], tarsal canal.

s. tar′si [NA], SYN tarsal s.

tentorial s., SYN straight s.

terminal s., s. termina′lis, the vein bounding the area vasculosa in the blastoderm.

s. tonsilla′ris, SYN tonsillar *fossa*.

Tourtual's s., SYN supratonsillar *fossa*.

transverse s., a paired dural venous s. that drains the confluence of sinuses, running along the occipital attachment of the tentorium cerebelli and terminating in the sigmoid s. SYN s. transversus [NA], lateral s.

transverse pericardial s., a passage in the pericardial sac between the origins of the great vessels, *i.e.,* posterior to the intrapericardial portions of the pulmonary trunk and ascending aorta and anterior to the superior vena cava and superior to the atria; it is formed as a result of the flexure of the heart tube, partially approximating the great venous and arterial vessels. SYN s. transversus pericardii [NA], Theile's canal, transverse s. of pericardium.

transverse s. of pericardium, SYN transverse pericardial s.

s. transver′sus [NA], SYN transverse s.

s. transver′sus pericar′dii [NA], SYN transverse pericardial s.

s. trun′ci pulmona′lis [NA], SYN pulmonary sinuses.

s. tym′pani [NA], SYN tympanic s.

tympanic s., a depression in the tympanic cavity posterior to the tympanic promontory. SYN s. tympani [NA].

s. un′guis, the deep cleft housing the root of the nail. SYN s. of nail.

urogenital s., (1) the ventral part of the cloaca after its separation from the rectum by the growth of the urorectal septum; from it develops the lower part of the bladder in both sexes, the prostatic portion of the male urethra, and the urethra and vestibule in the female; (2) SYN persistent *cloaca*.

s. urogenita′lis, SYN persistent *cloaca*.

uterine s., a small irregular vascular channel in the endometrium, of a type that forms during pregnancy. SYN uterine sinusoid.

uteroplacental sinuses, irregular vascular spaces in the zone of the chorionic attachment to the decidua basalis.

Valsalva's s., SYN aortic s.

s. of the vena cava, the portion of the cavity of the right atrium of the heart that receives the blood from the venae cavae; it is separated from the rest of the atrium by the crista terminalis. SYN s. venarum cavarum [NA].

s. vena′rum cava′rum [NA], SYN s. of the vena cava.

s. veno′sus [NA], a cavity at the caudal end of the embryonic cardiac tube in which the veins from the intra- and extraembryonic circulatory arcs unite; in the course of development it forms the portion of the right atrium known in adult anatomy as the sinus of the vena cava. SYN s. saccus reuniens.

s. veno′sus scle′rae [NA], the vascular structure encircling the anterior chamber of the eye and through which the aqueous is returned to the blood circulation. SYN circular s. (3), Fontana's canal, Lauth's canal, Schlemm's canal, s. circularis, venous s. of sclera.

venous sinuses, SYN dural venous sinuses.

venous s. of sclera, SYN s. venosus sclerae.

s. vertebra′les longitudina′les, SYN longitudinal vertebral venous s.

si·nus·i·tis (sī-nŭ-sī′tis). Inflammation of the lining membrane of any sinus, especially of one of the paranasal sinuses. [sinus + G. *-itis,* inflammation]

frontal s., infection in one or both frontal sinuses.

infectious s. of turkeys, SEE chronic respiratory *disease*.

si·nus·oid (si′nŭ-soyd). 1. Resembling a sinus. 2. Sinusoidal capillary; a thin-walled terminal blood vessel having an irregular and larger caliber than an ordinary capillary; its endothelial cells have large gaps and the basal lamina is either discontinuous or absent. SYN sinusoidal capillary. [sinus + G. *eidos,* resemblance] uterine s., SYN uterine *sinus.*

si·nus·oi·dal (sī-nŭ-soy'dăl). Relating to a sinusoid.

si·nus·ot·o·my (sin-ŭ-sot'ŏ-mē). Incision into a sinus. [sinus + G. *tomē,* incision]

si op. sit Abbreviation for L. *si opus sit,* if needed.

si·phon (sī'fŏn). A tube bent into two unequal lengths, used to remove fluid from a cavity or vessel by atmospheric pressure. [G. *siphōn,* tube]

si·phon·age (sī'fŏn-ij). Emptying of the stomach or other cavity by means of a siphon.

Si·pho·na ir·ri·tans (sī-fō'nă ir'i-tanz). The horn fly, a blood-sucking muscoid fly that causes great irritation and annoyance to cattle, and transmits *Stephanofilaria stilesi.* [G. *siphōn,* tube]

Si·pho·nap·tera (sī-fō-nap'tĕ-ră). The fleas, an order of wingless insect ectoparasites highly adapted for survival in mammalian fur; they are flattened laterally, spined, and equipped with well-developed metathoracic legs for jumping. [G. *siphōn,* tube, + G. *a-* priv. + *pteron,* wing]

Siphovi·ri·dae (sif'ō-vī'rā-dā). Provisional name for a family of nonenveloped double-stranded DNA bacteriophages with long, noncontractile tails. [L. *sipho,* little tube, pipe, fr. G. *siphōn,* + virus]

Sipple, J.H., U.S. physician, *1930. SEE S.'s *syndrome.*

Sippy, Bertram W., U.S. physician, 1866–1924. SEE sippy *diet.*

si·ren·i·form (sī-ren'i-fŏrm). Denoting a malformation with the appearance of sirenomelia.

si·re·no·me·lia (sī'rĕ-nō-mē'lē-ă). Union of the legs with partial or complete fusion of the feet. SEE ALSO sympus. SYN mermaid deformity, symmelia. [L. *siren,* G. *seirēn,* a siren]

si·ri·a·sis (si-rī'ă-sis). SYN sunstroke. [G. *seiriasis,* from *seiriaō,* to be hot]

Siris, Evelyn, U.S. radiologist, *1914. SEE Coffin-S. *syndrome.*

sir·up (sir'ŭp). SYN syrup.

sis·mo·ther·a·py (sis-mō-thār'ă-pē). SYN vibratory *massage.* [G. *seismos,* a shaking, fr. *seiō,* fut. *seisō,* to shake]

sis·o·mi·cin sul·fate (sis-ō-mī'sin). $(C_{19}H_{37}N_5O_7)_2 \cdot 5H_2SO_4$; an antibiotic produced by *Micromonospora inyoensis* that has a spectrum of activity and application similar to that of gentamicin.

sis·ter. In Great Britain: **1.** The title of a head nurse in a public hospital or in a ward or the operating room of a hospital; **2.** Any registered nurse in private practice.

Sister Mary Joseph Dempsey, Superintendent at Saint Mary's hospital, Mayo Clinic, and surgical assistant to Dr. William Mayo, c. 1928, 1856–1929. SEE Sister Joseph's *nodule.*

Sistrunk, Walter Ellis, U.S. surgeon, 1880–1933. SEE S. *operation.*

site (sīt). A place or location. SYN situs. [L. *situs*]

acceptor s., the ribosomal binding s. for the aminoacyl-tRNA during protein synthesis.

acceptor splicing s., SYN right splicing *junction.*

active s., that portion of an enzyme molecule at which the actual reaction proceeds; considered to consist of one or more residues or atoms in a spatial arrangement that permits interaction with the substrate to effect the reaction of the latter.

allosteric s., postulated as the place on an enzyme, other than the active s., where a compound, which may be the ultimate product of the biosynthetic pathway involving the enzyme, may bind and influence the activity of the enzyme by changing the enzyme's conformation; the influence of CTP on aspartate carbamoyltransferase activity exemplifies the concept of an allosteric site on an allosteric protein.

antibody combining s., SYN paratope.

antigen-binding s., SYN paratope.

antigen-combining site, SEE paratope.

cleavage s., SYN restriction s.

combining s., SYN paratope.

fragile s. [MIM*136540-136670], a non-staining gap at a specific point on a chromosome, usually involving both chromatids, always at the same point on chromosomes of different cells from an individual or kindred; it results in *in vitro* production of acentric fragments, deleted chromosomes, or other chromosome anomalies; inherited as a dominant chromosome marker.

immunologically privileged s.'s, s.'s where allografts are not readily rejected, probably because these particular areas have poor lymphatic drainage.

ligand binding s., the s. on a protein's surface that binds a ligand; equivalent to the active s. if the ligand is the substrate of an enzyme.

privileged s., an anatomic area lacking lymphatic drainage, such as the brain, cornea, and hamster cheek pouch, in which heterologous tumors may grow because the host does not become sensitized.

receptor s., point of attachment of viruses, hormones, or other activators to cell membranes.

replication s., the *in vivo* s. on DNA of DNA replication.

restriction s., a s. in nucleic acid in which the bordering bases are of such a type as to leave them vulnerable to the cleaving action of an endonuclease. SYN cleavage s.

sequence-tagged s.'s (STSs), short stretches of DNA sequences that can be detected by use of the polymerase chain reaction.

switching s., the break point in a DNA sequence at which a gene segment unites with another gene segment, as in the production of the immunoglobulins.

△sito-. Food, grain. [G. *sitos, sition*]

si·to·stane (sī'tō-stān). SYN stigmastane.

β-si·tos·ter·ol (sī-tō-stēr'ol). stigmast-5-en-3β-ol; (24*R*)-24-ethyl-5-cholesten-3β-ol; an anticholesteremic. SYN cinchol.

si·to·tax·is (sī-tō-tak'sis). SYN sitotropism. [sito- + G. *taxis,* orderly arrangement]

si·to·tox·in (sī-tō-tok'sin). Any food poison, especially one developing in grain. [sito- + G. *toxikon,* poison]

si·to·tox·ism (sī-tō-tok'sizm). **1.** Poisoning by spoiled or fungous grain. **2.** Food poisoning in general. [sito- + G. *toxikon,* poison]

si·tot·ro·pism (sī-tot'rō-pizm). Turning of living cells to or away from food. SYN sitotaxis. [sito- + G. *tropē,* a turning]

sit·u·a·tion (sich-yū-ā'shŭn). The aggregate of biological, psychological, and sociological factors that affect an individual's behavioral pattern.

psychoanalytic s., the relationship, characteristically restricted to the therapist's office, between patient and therapist.

si·tus (sī'tŭs). SYN site. [L.]

s. inver'sus, reversal of position or location. SYN s. transversus.

s. inversus viscerum, a transposition of the viscera, *e.g.,* the liver developing on the left side or the heart on the right. SYN visceral inversion.

s. perver'sus, malposition of any viscus.

s. sol'itus, the normal visceral arrangement.

s. transver'sus, SYN s. inversus.

Siwe, Sture A., Swedish pediatrician, 1897–1966. SEE Letterer-S. *disease.*

siz·er (sī'zer). A cylinder of variable diameter, with rounded ends, used to measure the internal diameter of the bowel in preparation for stapling.

Sjögren, Henrik C., Swedish ophthalmologist, *1899. SEE S.'s *disease, syndrome;* Gougerot-S. *disease.*

Sjögren, Torsten, Swedish physician, 1859–1939. SEE S.-Larsson *syndrome;* Torsten S.'s *syndrome;* Marinesco-Sjögren *syndrome.*

Sjöqvist, O., Swedish neurosurgeon, 1901–1954. SEE S. *tractotomy.*

SK Abbreviation for streptokinase.

△skato-. Obsolete spelling of scato-.

skat·ole (skat'ōl). 3-Methyl-1*H*-indole, formed in the intestine by the bacterial decomposition of L-tryptophan and found in fecal matter, to which it imparts its characteristic odor.

skat·ox·yl (skă-tok'sil). 3-Hydroxymethylindole, formed in the intestine by the oxidation of skatole; some undergoes conjugation in the body with sulfuric or gluronic acids and is excreted in the urine in conjugated form.

skein (skān). The coiled threads of chromatin seen in the prophase of mitosis. [Gael. *sgeinnidh,* hempen thread]

choroid s., SYN choroid *glomus.*

skel·e·tal (skel′ĕ-tăl). Relating to the skeleton.

skel·e·tol·o·gy (skel-ĕ-tol′ō-jē). The branch of anatomy and of mechanics dealing with the skeleton.

skel·e·ton (skel′ĕ-tŏn). **1.** The bony framework of the body in vertebrates (endoskeleton) or the hard outer envelope of insects (exoskeleton or dermoskeleton). **2.** All the dry parts remaining after the destruction and removal of the soft parts; this includes ligaments and cartilages as well as bones. **3.** All the bones of the body taken collectively. **4.** A rigid or semi-rigid non-osseous structure which functions as the supporting framework of a particular sutructure. [G. *skeletos,* dried, ntr. *skeleton,* a mummy, a skeleton]

appendicular s., the bones of the limbs including the shoulder and pelvic girdles. SYN s. appendiculare [NA].

s. appendicula′re [NA], SYN appendicular s.

articulated s., mounted s., one with the various parts connected in such a way as to demonstrate normal relationships and allow motion between components as in the living body.

axial s., articulated bones of head and vertebral column, *i.e.,* head and trunk, as opposed to the appendicular skeleton, the articulated bones of the upper and lower limbs. SYN s. axiale [NA].

s. axia′le [NA], SYN axial s.

cardiac s., SYN fibrous s. of heart.

cardiac fibrous s., SYN fibrous s. of heart.

fibrous s. of heart, a complex framework of dense collagen forming four fibrous rings (annuli fibrosi), which surround the ostia of the valves, a right and left fibrous trigone, formed by connecting the rings, and the membranous portions of the interatrial and interventricular septa; it is found in association with the base of the ventricles, *i.e.,* at the level of the coronary sulcus; its functions include: 1) contributing reinforcement of the valvular ostia while providing attachment for the leaflets and cusps of the valves; 2) providing origin and insertion for the myocardium; and 3) serving as a sort of electrical "insulator," separating the electrically conducted impulses of the atria and ventricles and providing passage for the common atrioventricular bundle of conductive tissue through the right fibrous trigone and membranous interventricular septum. SYN cardiac fibrous s., cardiac s., s. of heart.

s. of free inferior limb, the bones of the lower limb except the hip bones, *i.e.,* all lower limb bones including and distal to the femur .

s. of free superior limb, the bones of the upper limb except the scapula and clavicle, *i.e.,* all upper limb bones including and distal to the humerus .

gill arch s., cartilages associated with the visceral portion of the embryonic mammalian chondrocranium, representing the gill arch (branchial) skeletons as seen in shark-type fishes; they are the primordia of Meckel's cartilage, the styloid, hyoid, cricoid, thyroid, and arytenoid cartilages, and the auditory ossicles. SEE ALSO branchial *arches,* under *arch.*

s. of heart, SYN fibrous s. of heart.

jaw s., SYN viscerocranium.

s. thoracicus, ☆official alternate term for thoracic *cage.*

visceral s., SYN visceroskeleton (2).

Skene, Alexander J.C., U.S. gynecologist, 1838–1900. SEE S.'s *glands,* under *gland, tubules,* under *tubule; ducts* of S. glands, under *duct.*

ske·nei·tis, ske·ni·tis (skē-nī′tis). Inflammation of Skene's glands.

skene·o·scope (skēn′ō-skōp). A form of endoscope for inspecting Skene's glands.

skew (skyū). In statistics, departure from symmetry of a frequency distribution.

△**skia-.** Shadow; superseded by radio-. [G. *skia*]

ski·as·co·py (skī-as′kŏ-pē). SYN retinoscopy.

Skillern, Penn Gaskell, U.S. surgeon, *1882. SEE S.'s *fracture.*

skin. The membranous protective covering of the body, consisting of the epidermis and corium (dermis). SYN cutis [NA]. [A.S. *scinn*]

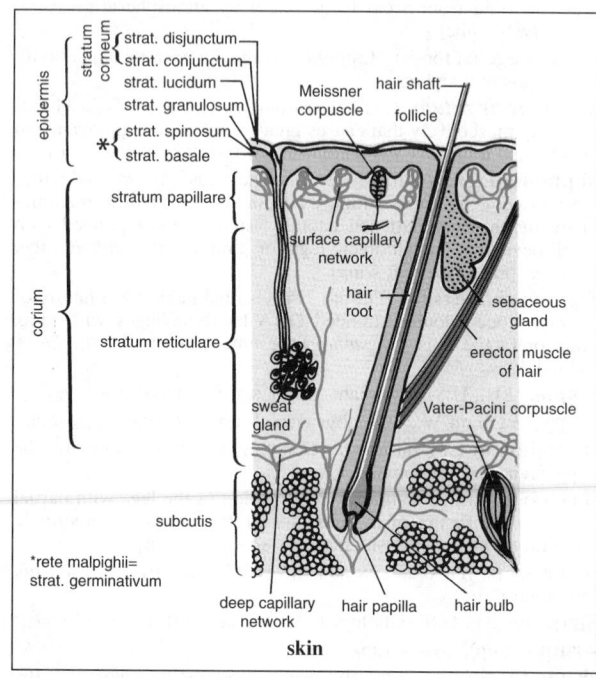

skin

diamond s., the appearance of the affected site in erysipeloid.

elastic s., SEE Ehlers-Danlos *syndrome.*

farmer's s., dry, wrinkled s. with presence of dry premalignant keratoses; observed most commonly in fair-skinned, blue-eyed persons who are exposed by occupation or sport to sunshine for prolonged periods and over many years. SYN golfer's s., sailor's s.

fish s., SYN ichthyosis.

glabrous s., s. that is normally devoid of hair.

glossy s., shiny atrophy of the s., usually of the hands, following nerve injury. SYN atrophoderma neuriticum.

golfer's s., SYN farmer's s.

hidden nail s., SYN eponychium (2).

loose s., SYN *cutis* laxa.

parchment s., parchment-like appearance of the s. caused by loss of underlying connective and elastic tissue, or by the relatively rapid and persistent loss of water from the horny layer.

piebald s., SYN piebaldness.

pig s., soft s. in which follicles are widely dilated; seen in pretibial myxedema.

porcupine s., SYN epidermolytic *hyperkeratosis.*

sailor's s., SYN farmer's s.

sex s., the s. of the genital regions of the *Macaca mulatta* and other primates which becomes hyperemic during estrus; at the same time the dermis becomes gelatinous and the epidermis thickened.

shagreen s., an oval-shaped nevoid plaque, skin-colored or occasionally pigmented, smooth or crinkled, appearing on the trunk or lower back in early childhood; sometimes seen with other signs of tuberous sclerosis. SYN shagreen patch.

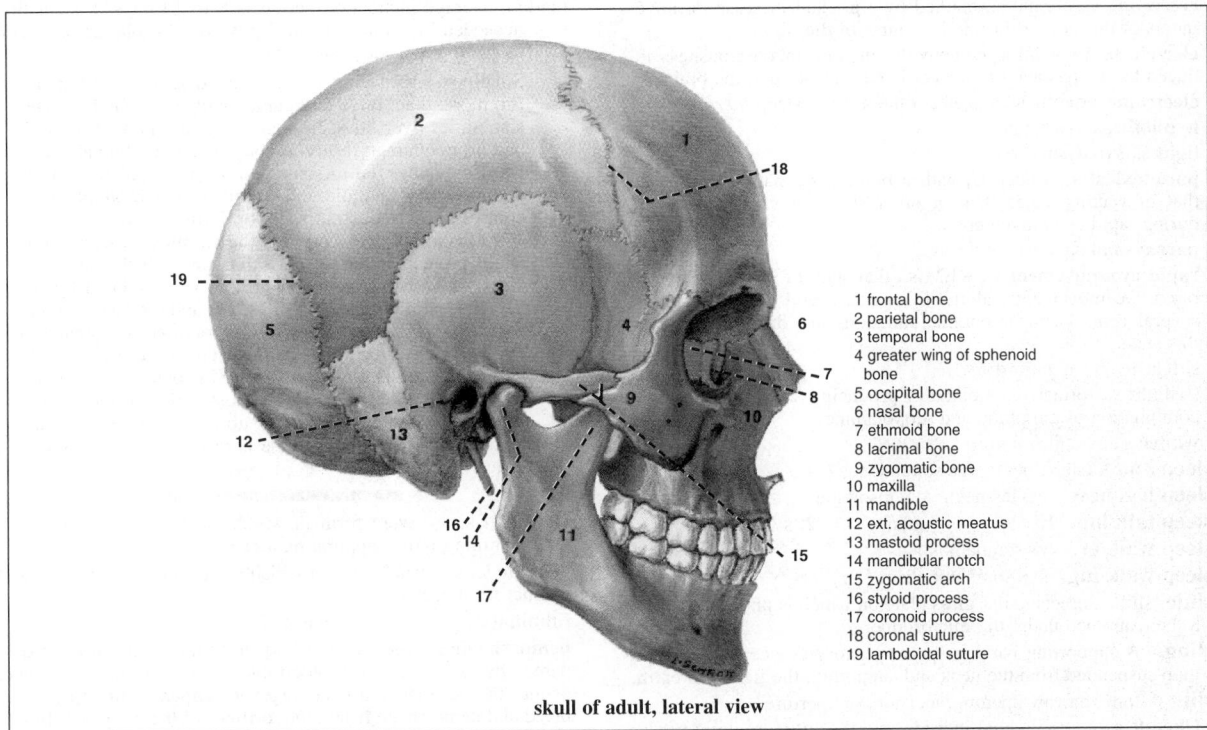

1 frontal bone
2 parietal bone
3 temporal bone
4 greater wing of sphenoid
  bone
5 occipital bone
6 nasal bone
7 ethmoid bone
8 lacrimal bone
9 zygomatic bone
10 maxilla
11 mandible
12 ext. acoustic meatus
13 mastoid process
14 mandibular notch
15 zygomatic arch
16 styloid process
17 coronoid process
18 coronal suture
19 lambdoidal suture

skull of adult, lateral view

sl

s. tag, SYN auricle of *atrium.*

s. of teeth, SYN enamel *cuticle.*

toad s., SYN phrynoderma.

yellow s., (1) SYN xanthochromia. **(2)** SYN xanthoderma (2).

Skinner, Burrhus F., U.S. psychologist, 1904–1990. SEE skinner-ian *conditioning;* S. *box.*

skin writ·ing. SYN dermatographism.

Sklowsky, E.L., 20th century German physician. SEE S. *symptom.*

Skoda, Joseph, Bohemian clinician in Vienna, 1805–1881. SEE skodaic *resonance;* S.'s *rale, sign, tympany.*

sko·da·ic (skō-dā'ik). Relating to Skoda.

skull (skŭl). The bones of the head collectively. In a more limited sense, the neurocranium, the bony brain-case containing the brain, excluding the bones of the face (viscero-cranium). SYN cranium [NA]. [Early Eng. *skulle,* a bowl]

cloverleaf s., SEE cloverleaf skull *syndrome.*

maplike s., various defects in the s., especially in the temporal bone, the anterior fossa, and orbits, forming irregular outlines resembling the national boundaries in an atlas.

natiform s. (na'tĭ-fōrm), palpable bony nodules on the surface of the skull in infants with congenital *syphilis.*

steeple s., tower s., SYN oxycephaly.

skull·cap (skŭl'kap). SYN calvaria.

sky blue (skī' blū'). A pigment mixture of cobaltous stannate and calcium sulfate; used biologically as an injection mass.

SL Abbreviation for spinal *length.*

sl Symbol for slyke.

slab-off. A process by which prism base-up is produced in the reading field of a spectacle lens through bicentric grinding.

slaf·ra·mine. An alkaloid produced by the fungus *Rhizoctonia leguminicola* which causes s. toxicosis in horses and cattle.

SLE Abbreviation for systemic *lupus* erythematosus.

sleep (slēp). A physiologic state of relative unconsciousness and inaction of the voluntary muscles, the need for which recurs periodically. The stages of sleep have been variously defined in terms of depth (light, deep), EEG characteristics (delta waves, synchronization), physiological characteristics (REM, NREM),

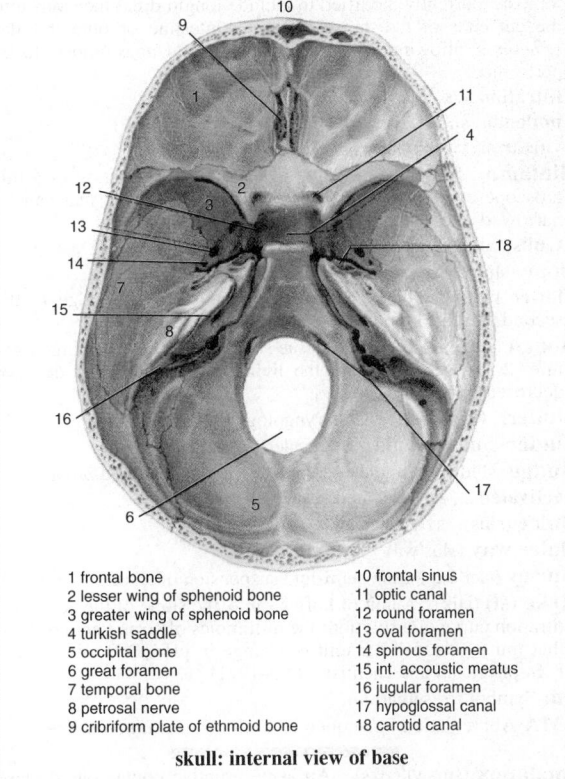

1 frontal bone	10 frontal sinus
2 lesser wing of sphenoid bone	11 optic canal
3 greater wing of sphenoid bone	12 round foramen
4 turkish saddle	13 oval foramen
5 occipital bone	14 spinous foramen
6 great foramen	15 int. accoustic meatus
7 temporal bone	16 jugular foramen
8 petrosal nerve	17 hypoglossal canal
9 cribriform plate of ethmoid bone	18 carotid canal

skull: internal view of base

and presumed anatomical level (pontine, mesencephalic, rhomb-encephalic, Rolandic, etc.). [A.S. *slaep*]

crescendo s., normal s., marked by a gradual increase in movements of the sleeper during the course of the night.

electric s., a condition of convulsions and unconsciousness induced by the passage of an electric current through the brain.

electrotherapeutic s., SEE electrotherapeutic sleep *therapy*.

hypnotic s., SYN hypnosis.

light s., SYN dysnystaxis.

paradoxical s., a deep s., with a brain wave pattern more like that of waking states than of other states of s., which occurs during rapid eye movement s.

paroxysmal s., SYN narcolepsy.

rapid eye movement s., REM s., that state of deep s. in which rapid eye movements, alert EEG pattern, and dreaming occur; several central and autonomic functions are distinctive during this state.

s. terror, SYN night-terrors.

twilight s., formerly a method of producing s. for delivery by a combination of morphine and scopolamine.

winter s., SYN hibernation.

sleep·i·ness (slēp'i-nes). SYN somnolence (1).

sleep·less·ness (slēp'les-nes). SYN insomnia.

sleep·talk·ing. 1. SYN somniloquence (1). **2.** SYN somniloquy.

sleep·walk·er. SYN somnambulist.

sleep·walk·ing. SYN somnambulism (1).

slide (slīd). A rectangular glass plate on which is placed an object to be examined under the microscope.

sling. A supporting bandage or suspensory device; especially a loop suspended from the neck and supporting the flexed forearm.

slit. A long, narrow opening, incision, or aperture.

Cheatle s., a longitudinal incision into the antimesenteric border of the small intestine, which when closed transversely creates a larger lumen than would be possible by simple end-to-end anastomosis; currently modified to include longitudinal incisions into the cut ends of the transected small intestine or other tubular structures, allowing a wide caliber elliptical anastomosis to be performed.

filtration s.'s, SYN slit *pores*, under *pore*.

pudendal s., SYN pudendal *cleft*.

vulvar s., SYN pudendal *cleft*.

slit·lamp. In ophthalmology, an instrument consisting of a microscope combined with a rectangular light source that can be narrowed into a slit. SYN biomicroscope, Gullstrand's s.

Gullstrand's s., SYN slitlamp.

slope (slōp). An inclination or slant.

lower ridge s., the s. of the mandibular residual ridge in the second and third molar as seen from the buccal side.

slough (slŭf). **1.** Necrosed tissue separated from the living structure. **2.** To separate from the living tissue, said of a dead or necrosed part. [M.E. *slughe*]

Sluder, Greenfield, U.S. laryngologist, 1865–1928.

Sluder's neu·ral·gia. See under neuralgia.

sludge (slŭdj). A muddy sediment. SEE ALSO sludged *blood*.

activated s., SEE activated sludge *method*.

sluice (slūs). SYN waterfall.

sluice·way (slūs'wā). SYN spillway.

slur·ry (sler'ē). A thin semifluid suspension of a solid in a liquid.

slyke (sl) (slīk). A unit of buffer value, the slope of the acid-base titration curve of a solution; the millimoles of strong acid or base that must be added per unit of change in pH. [D.D. Van *Slyke*, U.S. physician and chemist, 1883–1971]

Sm Symbol for samarium.

SMA Abbreviation for sequential multichannel *autoanalyzer*.

small·pox (smawl'poks). An acute eruptive contagious disease caused by a poxvirus (*Orthopoxvirus*, a member of the family Poxviridae) and marked at the onset by chills, high fever, backache, and headache; in from 2 to 5 days the constitutional symptoms subside and the eruption appears as papules which become umbilicated vesicles, develop into pustules, dry, and form scabs that on falling off, left a permanent marking of the skin (pock marks); average incubation period is 8 to 14 days. Vaccination has succeeded in eradicating smallpox. SYN variola major, variola. [E. *small pocks,* or pustules]

Smallpox was a universally dreaded scourge of humans for more than three millennia, with case fatality rates sometimes over 20%. In many ways a unique disease, it had no nonhuman reservoir species, and no human carriers. First subjected to some control by variolation in the tenth century in India and China, it was brought under control in the industrialized world after Edward Jenner's 1796 landmark discovery that the harmless cowpox virus could protect humans from infection with the smallpox virus. A global eradication project was initiated by the World Health Organization in 1966, and the last naturally occurring case of the disease was reported in Somalia in 1977. At the time this volume went to press, the only known reservoirs of the virus were in containment laboratories in Atlanta and Moscow; destruction of these laboratory stocks has been the subject of intense debate among scientists. The disease is now one of mainly historical interest.

confluent s., a severe form in which the lesions run into each other, forming large suppurating areas.

discrete s., the usual form in which the lesions are separate and distinct from each other.

fulminating s., SYN hemorrhagic s.

hemorrhagic s., a severe and frequently fatal form of s. accompanied by extravasation of blood into the skin in the early stage, or into the pustules at a later stage, accompanied often by nosebleed and hemorrhage from other orifices of the body. SYN fulminating s., variola hemorrhagica.

malignant s., SYN *variola* maligna.

modified s., varicelloid s., SYN varioloid (2).

West Indian s., SYN alastrim.

smear (smēr). A thin specimen for examination; it is usually prepared by spreading material uniformly onto a glass slide, fixing it, and staining it before examination.

	histology	cytology
	stratum corneum (superficial level)	superficial cells
	thickening zone	
	strat. spinosum superf. (intermediate level)	intermediary cells
	strat. spinosum profundum. (parabasal level)	parabasal cells
	stratum cylindricum (basal level)	basal cells

smear
relation between cells gathered by Pap smear and levels of vaginal epithelium

alimentary tract s., a group of cytologic specimens containing material from the mouth (oral s.), esophagus and stomach (gastric s.), duodenum (paraduodenal s.), and colon, obtained by specialized lavage techniques; used principally for the diagnosis of cancer of those areas.

bronchoscopic s., SYN lower respiratory tract s.

buccal s., a cytologic s. containing material obtained by scraping the lateral buccal mucosa above the dentate line, smearing, and fixing immediately; used principally for determining somatic sex as indicated by the presence of the sex chromocenter (Barr body).

cervical s., a generic name for different types of s.'s of the cervix uteri, *e.g.,* ectocervical, endocervical, pancervical; used principally for cervical screening.

colonic s., SEE alimentary tract s.

cul-de-sac s., a cytologic specimen of material obtained by aspirating the pouch of Douglas from the posterior vaginal fornix and prepared by smearing, centrifuging, or filtering; used principally for ovarian cancer.

cytologic s., a type of cytologic specimen made by smearing a sample (obtained by a variety of methods from a number of sites), then fixing it and staining it, usually with 95% ethyl alcohol and Papanicolaou stain. SYN cytosmear.

duodenal s., SEE alimentary tract s.

ectocervical s., a cytologic s. of material obtained from the ectocervix, usually by scraping; used principally for the diagnosis of late cervical cancers involving the ectocervix.

endocervical s., a cytologic s. of material obtained from the endocervical canal by swab, aspiration, or scraping; used principally for the detection of early cervical cancer.

endometrial s., a group of cytologic s.'s containing material obtained directly from the endometrium by aspiration, lavage, or brushing of the uterine cavity.

esophageal s., SEE alimentary tract s.

fast s., a cytologic smear containing material from the vaginal pool and pancervical scrapings, mixed and prepared on one microscopic slide, smeared, and fixed immediately; used principally for routine screening of ovaries, endometrium, cervix, vagina, and hormonal states.

FGT cytologic s., female genital tract cytologic s., any cytologic s. obtained from the female genital tract.

gastric s., SEE alimentary tract s.

lateral vaginal wall s., a cytologic s. containing material obtained by scraping the lateral wall of the vagina near the junction of its upper and middle third; used for cytohormonal evaluation.

lower respiratory tract s., a group of cytologic specimens containing material from the lower respiratory tract and consisting mainly of sputum (spontaneous, induced) and material obtained at bronchoscopy (aspirated, lavaged, brushed); used for cytologic study of cancer and other diseases of the lungs. SYN bronchoscopic s., sputum s.

oral s., SEE alimentary tract s.

pancervical s., a cytologic s. of material obtained from the endocervical canal, external os, and ectocervix by scraping these areas with a properly designed cervical spatula; used principally for early cervical cancer detection.

Pap s., a s. of vaginal or cervical cells obtained for cytological study. SYN Papanicolaou s.

Papanicolaou s., SYN Pap s.

sputum s., SYN lower respiratory tract s.

urinary s., a group of cytologic specimens containing processed urine obtained from bladder, ureters, or renal pelvis; used for cytologic study of cancer and other diseases of the urinary tract.

vaginal s., a s. of debris from the vaginal lumen of mammals, used to determine the stage of their reproductive cycle. It is most useful in subprimate mammals having short estrous cycles; nucleated epithelial cells and leukocytes prevail in the s. during diestrus and proestrus, and cornified cells during estrus.

VCE s., a cytologic s. of material obtained from the vagina, ectocervix, and endocervix, smeared separately (in that order) on one slide, and fixed immediately; used principally for the detection of cervical cancer and identification of the sites of diseases of those areas, and for hormonal evaluation.

smeg·ma (smeg′mă). A foul-smelling pasty accumulation of desquamated epidermal cells and sebum that has collected in moist areas of the genitalia. [G. unguent]

s. clitor′idis, the secretion of the apocrine glands of the clitoris, in combination with desquamating epithelial cells.

s. prepu′tii, whitish secretion that collects under the prepuce of the foreskin of the penis or of the clitoris; it is comprised chiefly of desquamating epithelial cells. SYN sebum preputiale.

smeg·ma·lith (smeg′mă-lith). A calcareous concretion in the smegma. [smegma + G. *lithos,* stone]

smell. 1. To scent; to perceive by means of the olfactory apparatus. **2.** SYN olfaction (1). **3.** SYN odor.

smell-brain (smel′brān). SYN rhinencephalon.

Smellie, William, English obstetrician, 1697–1763. SEE S.'s *scissors.*

Smith, David W., U.S. pediatrician, *1926. SEE S.-Lemli-Opitz *syndrome.*

Smith, G.W., U.S. neurosurgeon, 1917–1964. SEE S.-Robinson *operation.*

Smith, Henry, Irish born British military surgeon in India, 1862–1948. SEE S.'s *operation;* S.-Indian *operation.*

Smith, M.J.V., 20th century U.S. urologist.

Smith, Robert W., Irish surgeon, 1807–1873. SEE S.'s *fracture.*

Smith, Theobald, U.S. pathologist, 1859–1934. SEE Theobald S.'s *phenomenon.*

Smith, William R., 20th century U.S. physician. SEE S.-Riley *syndrome.*

Smith-Petersen, Marius N., U.S. surgeon, 1886–1953. SEE Smith-Petersen *nail.*

smog. Air pollution characterized by a hazy and often highly irritating atmosphere resulting from a mixture of fog with smoke and other air pollutants. [smoke + fog]

smut (smŭt). A fungus disease of cereal grains caused by species of *Ustilago* and characterized by dark brown or black masses of spores on the plants; *e.g.,* corn s. (*U. maydis*); loose s. of wheat (*U. nuda*)

Sn Symbol for tin.

¹¹³Sn Symbol for tin-113.

△sn-. Prefix meaning stereospecifically numbered; a system of numbering the glycerol carbon atoms in lipids, so that the locant numbers remain constant regardless of chemical substitutions, as opposed to systematic numbering.

snail (snāl). Common name for members of the class Gastropoda (phylum Mollusca). The freshwater pulmonate (nonoperculated, air-breathing) snails (subclass Pulmonata, order Basommatophora) include the majority of intermediate hosts of trematodes parasitic in humans and domestic birds and mammals, chiefly in the families Lymnaeidae and Planorbidae. The subclass Prosobranchiata, the operculate snails, includes the order Neogastropoda, which includes the venomous stinging cone snails (genus *Conus*), and the order Mesogastropoda, of which the family Hydrobiidae includes most of the medically important host snails. [M.E. *snaile*]

snake (snāk). An elongated, limbless, scaly reptile of the suborder Ophidia.

snake·root (snāk′rūt). SYN serpentaria.

Canada s., SYN *Asarum* canadense.

European s., SYN *Asarum* europaeum.

Seneca s., SYN senega.

Texas s., *Aristolochia reticulata*; botanical source of serpentaria.

Virginia s., *Aristolochia serpentaria;* botanical source of serpentaria.

snap. A click; a short sharp sound; said especially of cardiac sounds.

closing s., the accentuated first heart sound of mitral stenosis, related to closure of the abnormal valve.

opening s., a sharp, high-pitched click in early diastole, usually best heard between the cardiac apex and the lower left sternal border, related to opening of the abnormal valve in cases of mitral stenosis.

snare (snār). An instrument for removing polyps and other projections from a surface, especially within a cavity; it consists of a wire loop passed around the base of the tumor and gradually tightened. [A.S. *snear,* a cord]

cold s., an unheated s.

galvanocaustic s., hot s., a s. the wire of which is heated to a high temperature by an electric current.

SNE Abbreviation for subacute necrotizing *encephalomyelopathy*.

Sneddon, I.B., 20th century English dermatologist. SEE S.'s *syndrome;* S.-Wilkinson *disease.*

sneeze (snēz). **1.** To expel air from the nose and mouth by an involuntary spasmodic contraction of the muscles of expiration. **2.** An act of sneezing; a reflex excited by an irritation of the mucous membrane of the nose or, sometimes, by a bright light striking the eye. [A.S. *fneōsan*]

Snell, Simeon, English ophthalmologist, 1851–1909. SEE S.'s *law.*

Snellen, Hermann, Dutch ophthalmologist, 1834–1908. SEE S.'s *test types, sign.*

snore (snōr). **1.** A rough, rattling, inspiratory noise produced by vibration of the pendulous palate, or sometimes of the vocal cords, during sleep or coma. SEE ALSO stertor, rhonchus. **2.** To breathe noisily, or with a s. [A.S. *snora*]

snout (snowt). In veterinary anatomy, the rostral extremity of the face and rhinarium, frequently elongate and related to specialized feeding habits as in the gar, soft-shelled turtle, pig, etc. [M.E.]

snow (snō). SEE *carbon* dioxide snow.

snRNA Abbreviation for small nuclear RNA.

snuff (snŭf). **1.** To inhale forcibly through the nose. **2.** Finely powdered tobacco used by inhalation through the nose or applied to the gums. **3.** Any medicated powder applied by insufflation to the nasal mucous membrane. [echoic]

snuff-box (snŭf′boks). SEE anatomical snuffbox.

snuf·fles (snŭf′lz). Obstructed nasal respiration, especially in the newborn infant, sometimes due to congenital syphilis.

    rabbit s., acute inflammation of the upper nasal passages, usually associated with *Pasteurella* organisms; in outbreaks of s. in rabbitries there usually are some deaths from pneumonia.

Snyder, Marshall L., U.S. microbiologist, *1907. SEE S.'s *test.*

SOAP Acronym for *s*ubjective, *o*bjective, *a*ssessment, and *p*lan; used in problem-oriented records for organizing follow-up data, evaluation, and planning.

soap (sōp). The sodium or potassium salts of long chain fatty acids (*e.g.*, sodium stearate); used for cleansing purposes and as an excipient in the making of pills and suppositories. [A.S. *sape,* L. *sapo,* G. *sapōn*]

    animal s., s. made with sodium hydroxide and a purified animal fat consisting chiefly of stearin; used in pharmacy in the preparation of certain liniments. SYN curd s., domestic s., tallow s.

    Castile s., SYN hard s.

    curd s., domestic s., SYN animal s.

    green s., SYN medicinal soft s.

    hard s., a s. made with olive oil, or some other suitable oil or fat, and sodium hydroxide; used as a detergent, and in the form of a suppository or soapsuds enema for constipation; used also as an excipient in pills. SYN Castile s.

    insoluble s., s. made with a fatty acid and an earthy or metallic base (iron or calcium salts of fatty acids).

    marine s., a s. made of palm or coconut oil for use with sea water in which it is soluble. SYN salt water s.

    medicinal soft s., a s. made with vegetable oils, potassium hydroxide, oleic acid, glycerin, and purified water; used as a stimulant in chronic skin diseases. SYN green s., soft s.

    salt water s., SYN marine s.

    soft s., SYN medicinal soft s.

    soluble s., any s. made with potassium, sodium, or ammonium hydroxide: ordinary animal s., Castile s., green s., etc.

    superfatted s., a s. containing an excess (3 to 5%) of fat above that necessary to completely neutralize all the alkali; used in the manufacture of medicated s., and in the treatment of skin diseases.

    tallow s., SYN animal s.

soap·stone (sōp′stōn). SYN talc.

Soave, F., 20th century Italian pediatric surgeon. SEE S. *operation.*

so·cal·o·in (sō-kal′ō-in). $C_{15}H_{16}O_7$; an aloin obtained from aloes of the island of Socotra.

so·cia (sō′shē-ă). An ectopic, supernumerary, or accessory portion of an organ.

so·cial·i·za·tion (sō′shăl-i-zā′shŭn). **1.** The process of learning attitudes and interpersonal and interactional skills which are in conformity with the values of one's society. **2.** In a group therapy setting, a way of learning to effectively participate in the group. [L. *socius,* partner, companion]

so·cia pa·ro·ti·dis (sō′shē-ă pa-rot′i-dis). SYN accessory parotid *gland.* [L. companion of the parotid]

△**socio-.** Social, society. [L. *socius,* companion]

so·ci·o·cen·tric (sō′sē-ō-sen′trik). Outgoing; reactive to the social or cultural milieu. [socio- + L. *centrum,* center]

so·ci·o·cen·trism (sō′sē-ō-sen′trizm). Taking one's own social group as the standard by which others are measured.

so·ci·o·cosm (sō′sē-ō-kozm). The totality that includes human society, human thought, and the relationship of man to nature. [socio- + G. *kosmos,* universe]

so·ci·o·gen·e·sis (sō′sē-ō-jen′ĕ-sis). The origin of social behavior from past interpersonal experiences. [socio- + G. *genesis,* origin]

so·ci·o·gram (sō′sē-ō-gram). A diagrammatic representation of the valences and degrees of attractiveness and acceptance of each individual rated according to the interpersonal interactions between and among members of a group; a diagram in which group interactions are analyzed on the basis of mutual attractions or antipathies between group members. [socio- + G. *gramma,* something written]

so·ci·o·med·i·cal (sō′sē-ō-med′i-kăl). Pertaining to the relation of the practice of medicine to society.

so·ci·om·e·try (sō-sē-om′ĕ-trē). The study of interpersonal relationships in a group. [socio- + G. *metron,* measure]

so·ci·o·path (sō′sē-ō-path). Former designation for a person with an antisocial personality type of disorder. SEE ALSO antisocial *personality,* psychopath.

so·ci·op·a·thy (sō-sē-op′ă-thē). Obsolete term for the behavioral pattern exhibited by persons with an antisocial personality type of disorder. SEE ALSO personality *disorder.* [socio- + G. *pathos,* suffering]

sock·et (sok′et). **1.** The hollow part of a joint; the excavation in one bone of a joint which receives the articular end of the other bone. **2.** Any hollow or concavity into which another part fits, as the eye s. [thr. O. Fr. fr. L. *soccus,* a shoe, a sock]

    dry s., SYN alveoalgia.

    eye s., generally the orbit, although the true "socket" for the eyeball, into which a prosthetic eye would be inserted, is formed by the fascial sheath of the eyeball. SYN orbit.

    tooth s., a socket in the alveolar process of the maxilla or mandible, into which each tooth fits and is attached by means of the periodontal ligament. SYN alveolus dentalis [NA], alveolus (4) [NA].

SOD Abbreviation for superoxide dismutase.

so·da (sō′dă). SYN *sodium* carbonate. [It., possibly fr. Mediev. L. barilla plant]

    baking s., SYN *sodium* bicarbonate.

    caustic s., SYN *sodium* hydroxide.

    s. lime, a mixture of calcium and sodium hydroxides used to absorb carbon dioxide in situations in which rebreathing occurs; *e.g.,* in basal determinations or in certain types of anesthesia circuits.

    washing s., SYN *sodium* carbonate.

so·dic (sō′dik). Relating to or containing soda or sodium.

△**sodio-.** A compound containing sodium; as sodiocitrate, sodiotartrate, a citrate or tartrate of some element containing sodium in addition.

SODIUM

---

so·di·um (Na) (sō′dē-ŭm). A metallic element, atomic no. 11, atomic weight 22.989768; an alkali metal oxidizing readily in air or water; its salts are extensively used in medicine and industry. For organic s. salts not listed below, see under the name of the organic acid portion. SYN natrium. [Mod. L. fr. *soda*]

s. acetate, $CH_3COONa \cdot 3H_2O$; a systemic and urinary alkalizer, expectorant, and diuretic.

s. acid carbonate, SYN s. bicarbonate.

s. acid citrate, SYN s. citrate.

s. acid phosphate, SYN s. biphosphate.

s. alginate, SYN algin.

s. *p*-aminohippurate, used intravenously in renal function tests, to determine the renal plasma flow and the tubular excretion.

s. *p*-aminophenylarsonate, $h_2N–C_6H_4–AsO(OH)(ONa) \cdot 3H_2O$; a compound that was one of the first modern pentavalent arsenicals. SYN s. arsanilate.

s. aminosalicylate, $C_6H_3(p\text{-}NH_2)(o\text{-}OH)–COONa \cdot 2H_2O$; used for the same purposes as aminosalicylic acid.

s. antimonylgluconate, SYN stibogluconate sodium (2).

s. antimonyl tartrate, SYN *antimony* sodium tartrate.

s. arsanilate, SYN s. *p*-aminophenylarsonate.

s. ascorbate, same actions and uses as ascorbic acid; it is preferred for intramuscular administration.

s. aurothiomalate, SYN *gold* sodium thiomalate.

s. aurothiosulfate, SYN *gold* sodium thiosulfate.

s. benzoate, C_6H_5COONa; used in chronic and acute rheumatism and as a liver function test.

s. bicarbonate, $NaHCO_3$; used as a gastric and systemic antacid, to alkalize urine, and for washes of body cavities. SYN baking soda, s. acid carbonate, s. hydrogen carbonate.

s. biphosphate, $NaH_2PO_4 \cdot H_2O$; used to increase urinary acidity. SYN primary s. phosphate, s. acid phosphate, s. dihydrogen phosphate.

s. bisulfite, $NaHSO_3$; acid s. sulfite, used in gastric and intestinal fermentation, externally in the treatment of parasitic diseases, and as an antioxidant in certain injections (s. metabisulfite). SYN s. hydrogen sulfite, s. pyrosulfite.

s. borate, $Na_2B_4O_7 \cdot 10H_2O$; used in lotions, gargles, mouthwashes, and as a detergent. SYN borax, s. pyroborate, s. tetraborate.

s. bromide, $NaBr$; a hypnotic and sedative; used in epilepsy and other functional disorders of the nervous system.

s. cacodylate, $(CH_3)_2AsOONa \cdot 3H_2O$; used in anemia, leukemia, and malaria. SYN s. dimethylarsenate.

s. carbonate, $Na_2CO_3 \cdot 10H_2O$; used in the treatment of scaly skin diseases; otherwise rarely used in medicine because of its irritant action. SYN sal soda, soda, washing soda.

s. carboxymethyl cellulose, the s. salt of a polycarboxymethyl ether of cellulose; used as a laxative.

s. chloride, $NaCl$; the chief component of blood and other body fluids, and urine; used to make isotonic and physiological saline solutions, in the treatment of salt depletion, and topically for inflammatory lesions. SYN common salt, table salt.

s. citrate, $Na_3C_6H_5O_7 \cdot 2H_2O$; trisodium citrate; used as diuretic, antilithic, systemic and urinary alkalizer, expectorant, and anticoagulant (*in vitro*). SYN s. acid citrate.

s. citrate, acid, $C_6H_6O_7Na \cdot 1\frac{1}{2}H_2O$; disodium hydrogen citrate; same actions and uses as s. citrate; in addition, it may be used in solutions of glucose without producing caramelization of the latter during autoclaving.

s. cromoglycate, SYN cromolyn sodium.

s. dehydrocholate, a cholagogue; also used to determine circulation time.

s. diatrizoate, a water-soluble organic iodine compound formerly used for intravenous excretory urography and angiography.

dibasic s. phosphate, SYN s. phosphate.

s. dihydrogen phosphate, SYN s. biphosphate.

s. dimethylarsenate, SYN s. cacodylate.

s. dodecyl sulfate (SDS), a widely used detergent, identical with s. lauryl sulfate.

effervescent s. phosphate, exsiccated s. phosphate 200, s. bicar-

bonate 477, tartaric acid 252, and citric acid 162, mixed and passed through a sieve to make a granular salt.

exsiccated s. sulfite, anhydrous s. sulfite, used as a preservative in pharmaceutical preparations.

s. fluoride, used as a dental prophylactic in drinking water, and topically as a 2% solution applied on the teeth.

s. fluosilicate, SYN s. hexafluorosilicate.

s. folate, the s. salt of folic acid; action and uses are the same as those of folic acid, but it is preferred for parenteral administration. SYN s. pteroylglutamate.

s. fusidate, SYN fusidate sodium.

s. glycerophosphate, $C_3H_5(OH)_2PO_4Na$; has been used as a tonic.

s. hexafluorosilicate, Na_2SiF_6; used (in dilute solutions) as an antiseptic and deodorant, and for fluoridation of drinking water. SYN s. fluosilicate, s. silicofluoride.

s. hydrogen carbonate, SYN s. bicarbonate.

s. hydrogen sulfite, SYN s. bisulfite.

s. hydroxide, $NaOH$; used externally as a caustic. SYN caustic soda.

s. hypochlorite, strong oxidizer; explosive when anhydrous. Decomposes by absorbing carbon dioxide from the air. Liberates chlorine and oxygen; used in aqueous solution as a bleach and disinfectant. The active constituent of many household bleaches, *e.g.,* Clorox.

s. hypophosphite, $NaPH_2O_2 \cdot H_2O$; formerly used as a nerve tonic.

s. hyposulfite, SYN s. thiosulfate.

s. ichthyolsulfonate, an alterative and antiseptic.

s. indigotin disulfonate, SYN indigo carmine.

s. iodide, NaI; used as a source of iodine.

s. lactate, $C_3H_5NaO_3$; a systemic and urinary alkalizer.

s. lauryl sulfate, $CH_3(CH_2)_{10}CH_2OSO_3Na$; a surface-active agent of the anionic type.

s. levothyroxine, 3,3′,5,5′-tetraiodothyronine pentahydrate; s. salt of the natural isomer of thyroxine, a thyroid hormone. It is twice as effective as the racemic form. Used in the treatment of hypothyroidism in humans and animals and to treat lowered fertility in bulls and to stimulate lactation in animals.

s. liothyronine, s. L-triiodothyronine, the physiologically active isomer of triiodothyronine, twice as active as the racemic form; used in the treatment of thyroid deficiency syndromes.

s. metabisulfite, $Na_2S_2O_5$; used as an antioxidant in injectable solutions.

s. methicillin, SYN methicillin sodium.

s. methylarsonate, $Ch_3H_5O(ONa)_2 \cdot 5H_2O$; disodium monomethyl arsonate; formerly used in tuberculosis, chorea, and other affections in which the cacodylates were used.

s. nitrate, $NaNO_3$; formerly used for dysentery and as a diuretic. SYN Chilean saltpeter, cubic niter.

s. nitrite, $NaNO_2$; used to lower systemic blood pressure, to relieve local vasomotor spasms, especially in angina pectoris and Raynaud's disease, to relax bronchial and intestinal spasms, and as an antidote for cyanide poisoning.

s. nitroferricyanide, SYN s. nitroprusside.

s. nitroprusside, $(Na_2FeCCN)_5NO \cdot 5H_2O$; a rapidly acting and potent arterial and venous vasodilator used in hypertensive emergencies and administered intravenously. Acts in a manner similar to vasodilator nitrates and nitrites by donating nitric oxide which produces vasodilation; also used as a reagent for detection of organic compounds in the urine. SYN s. nitroferricyanide.

s. nucleate, s. nucleinate, s. salts of yeast acids, used in the treatment of anemias, rheumatism, and gout.

s. orthophosphate, SYN s. phosphate.

s. perborate, $NaBO_2H_2O_2 \cdot 3H_2O$; used in the extemporaneous preparation of hydrogen peroxide; a 2% solution is equivalent in germicidal action to 0.4% of hydrogen peroxide.

s. peroxide, Na_2O_2; used externally as a paste or soap in the treatment of comedones and acne.

s. phenolsulfonate, has been used in tonsillitis and as an intestinal antiseptic; has no antiseptic properties. SYN s. sulfocarbolate.

SO

s. phosphate, $Na_2HPO_4 \cdot H_2O$; a laxative. SYN dibasic s. phosphate, s. orthophosphate.

s. phosphate P 32, anionic radioactive phosphorus in the form of a solution of s. acid phosphate and s. basic phosphate; a beta emitter with a half-life of 14.3 days; after administration, highest concentrations are found in rapidly proliferating tissues; it is used in the treatment of polycythemia vera, chronic myelogenous leukemia, and osseous metastases. SEE ALSO chromic phosphate P 32 colloidal *suspension.*

s. polyanhydromannuronic acid sulfate, an anticoagulant drug prepared from alginic acid and having an action similar to that of heparin.

s. polystyrene sulfonate, a cationic exchange resin used in hyperpotassemia.

s. potassium tartrate, SYN *potassium* sodium tartrate.

pravastatin s., antihyperlipoproteinemic. An HMG-Co reductase inhibitor resembling lovastatin and simvastatin, which inhibits cholesterol formation.

primary s. phosphate, SYN s. biphosphate.

s. propionate, the s. salt of propionic acid; used for fungus infections of the skin, usually in combination with calcium propionate; used as a preservative.

s. psylliate, the s. salt of the liquid fatty acids of psyllium oil, prepared by dissolving the fatty acid in dilute s. hydroxide solution; used like morrhuate s. as a sclerosing agent in the treatment of varicose veins.

s. pteroylglutamate, SYN s. folate.

s. pyroborate, SYN s. borate.

s. pyrosulfite, SYN s. bisulfite.

s. rhodanate, SYN s. thiocyanate.

s. ricinoleate, s. ricinate, the s. salt of ricinoleic acid; a sclerosing agent similar in action to morrhuate s.

s. salicylate, an analgesic, antipyretic, and antirheumatic.

s. silicofluoride, SYN s. hexafluorosilicate.

sodium s., Na 99mTcO₄; a radiopharmaceutical used for brain, thyroid, and salivary gland scanning.

s. stearate, stearic acid sodium salt, used as a pharmaceutical adjuvant in ointments, creams, and suppositories.

s. sulfate, $Na_2SO_4 \cdot 10H_2O$; an ingredient of many of the natural laxative waters, and also used as a hydragogue cathartic. SYN Glauber's salt.

s. sulfite, $Na_2SO_3 \cdot 7H_2O$; has been used for the relief of intestinal fermentation, and externally for aphthous stomatitis.

s. sulfocarbolate, SYN s. phenolsulfonate.

s. sulfocyanate, SYN s. thiocyanate.

s. sulforicinate, s. sulforicinoleate, made by combining castor oil, sulfuric acid, and s. hydroxide and chloride; used as a solvent for iodine, iodoform, resorcinol, pyrogallol, and a number of other substances for external use.

s. tartrate, $Na_2C_4H_4O_6 \cdot 2H_2O$; a laxative.

s. taurocholate, the s. salt of taurocholic acid, extracted from the bile of carnivora; a cholagogue.

s. tetraborate, SYN s. borate.

s. tetradecyl sulfate, an anionic surface-active agent used for its wetting properties to enhance the surface action of certain antiseptic solutions; also used as a sclerosing agent similar to morrhuate s. in the treatment of varicose veins.

s. thiocyanate, NaSCN; used in the management of essential hypertension. SYN s. rhodanate, s. sulfocyanate.

s. thiosulfate, $Na_2S_2O_3 \cdot 5H_2O$; an antidote in cyanide poisoning in conjunction with s. nitrite; used as a prophylactic agent against ringworm infections in swimming pools and baths, and to measure the extracellular fluid volume of the body. SYN s. hyposulfite.

s. tungstoborate, used in electron microscopy as a negative stain.

---

so·di·um-24 (²⁴Na). The isotope of sodium with an atomic weight of 24, and a half-life of 14.96 hr; it emits beta and gamma rays, and is more easily prepared than the longer-lived, positron-emitting ²²Na (half-life, 2.605 yr). It is used to measure extracellular fluid by indicator dilution.

so·di·um group. The alkali metals: cesium, lithium, potassium, rubidium, and sodium.

so·do·ku (sō-dō'kū). SYN rat-bite *fever.* [Jap. rat poison]

sod·om·ist, sod·om·ite (sod'ŏ-mist, -mīt). One who practices sodomy. [G. *sodomitēs,* an inhabitant of the biblical city of Sodom, which was destroyed by fire because of the wickedness of its people]

sod·o·my (sod'ŏm-ē). A term denoting a number of sexual practices variously proscribed by law, especially bestiality, oral-genital contact, and anal intercourse. SYN buggery. [see sodomist]

Soemmerring, Samuel Thomas von, German anatomist, 1755–1830. SEE S.'s *ganglion, ligament, muscle, spot; ring* of S.

Soffer, Louis J., U.S. internist, *1904. SEE Sohval-S. *syndrome.*

soft·ware. The program or instructions for a computer.

Sohval, Arthur R., U.S. internist, *1904. SEE S.-Soffer *syndrome.*

so·ja (sō'yah). SYN soybean.

so·ko·sho (sō-kō'shō). SYN rat-bite *fever.* [Jap. *so,* rat, + *ko,* bite, + *sho,* malady]

sol. 1. A colloidal dispersion of a solid in a liquid. Cf. gel. **2.** Abbreviation for solution.

So·la·na·ce·ae (sō-lă-nā'sē-ē). A family of plants that includes the genus *Solanum* (nightshade) and some 84 other genera comprising 1,800 species, including the tomato and potato plants.

so·la·na·ceous (sō-lă-nā'shŭs, sol'ă-). Pertaining to plants of the family Solanaceae, or to drugs derived from them.

sol·a·no·chro·mene (sol'ă-nō-krō'mēn). SYN plastochromenol-8.

so·lap·sone (sō-lap'sōn). SYN solasulfone.

sol·a·sul·fone (sol-ă-sŭlf'ōn). tetrasodium 1,1′-[sulfonylbis(*p*-phenyleneimino)] bis [3-phenyl-1,3-propanedisulfonate]; a leprostatic agent. SYN solapsone.

sol·a·tion (sol-ā'shŭn). In colloidal chemistry, the transformation of a gel into a sol, as by melting gelatin.

sol·der (sod'er). **1.** A fusible alloy used to unite edges or surfaces of two pieces of metal of higher melting point; hard s.'s, usually containing gold or silver as their main constituent, are usually used in dentistry to connect noble metal alloys. **2.** To join two pieces of metal with such an alloy. [L. *solido,* to make solid, through Fr., various forms]

sole (sōl). The plantar surface or under part of the foot. SYN planta [NA], pelma. [A.S.]

s. of foot, the inferior aspect or bottom of the foot, much of which is in contact with the ground when standing; it is covered with hairless, usually nonpigmented skin that is especially thickened and provided with epidermal ridges over the weight-bearing areas. SYN planta pedis [NA], regio plantaris.

So·le·nog·ly·pha (sō-lĕ-nog'li-fă). A major category of snakes that includes the viper and rattlesnake families. [L., fr. G. *sōlēn,* pipe channel, + *glyphō,* to carve]

so·le·noid (sol'ĕ-noyd). A helical coil of wire energized electrically to produce a magnetic field, which induces a current in any conductor placed within or near the coil.

So·le·no·po·tes cap·il·la·tus (sō-lĕ-nop'ŏ-tēz kap-i-lā'tŭs). A sucking louse of cattle, called the little blue cattle louse in the U.S. and the tubercle-bearing louse in Australia. [G. *solen,* pipe, + *potos,* a drinking]

so·le·nop·sin A (sō-lĕ-nop'sin). *trans*-2-Methyl-6-*n*-undecylpiperidine; one of several, probably five, alkaloidal constituents present in the venom of the imported fire ant, *Solenopsis saevissima;* the venom has necrotoxic, hemolytic, insecticidal, and antibiotic properties.

so·le·us (sō-lē'ŭs). SEE soleus *muscle.* [Mod. L. fr. L. *solea,* a sandal, sole of the foot (of animals), fr. *solum,* bottom, floor, ground]

sol·id. 1. Firm; compact; not fluid; without interstices or cavities; not cancellous. **2.** A body that retains its form when not confined; one that is not fluid, neither liquid nor gaseous. [L. *solidus*]

sol·id·ism (sol'i-dizm). The theory propounded by Asclepiades and his followers that disease was due to an imbalance between solid particles (atoms) of the body and the spaces (pores) between them, a doctrine which opposed the humoral conception of Hippocrates. SYN methodism.

sol·id·ist (sol'i-dist). An adherent of the doctrine of solidism.

sol·id·is·tic (sol-i-dis'tik). Relating to solidism.

sol·i·dus (sol'i-dŭs). That line on a constitution diagram indicating the temperature below which all metal is solid.

sol·i·ped (sol'i-ped). A solid-hoofed animal such as the horse. [L. *solidus*, solid, + *pes*, foot]

sol·ip·sism (sō'lip-sizm, sol'ip-). A philosophical concept that whatever exists is a product of will and the ideas of the perceiving individual. [L. *solus*, alone, + *ipse*, self]

soln. Abbreviation for solution.

sol·u·bil·i·ty (sol-yū-bil'i-tē). The property of being soluble.

sol·u·ble (sol'yū-bl). Capable of being dissolved. [L. *solubilis*, fr. *solvo*, to dissolve]

so·lum (sō'lŭm). Bottom; the lowest part. [L.]

sol·ute (sol'yūt, sō'lūt). The dissolved substance in a solution. [L. *solutus*, dissolved, pp. of *solvo*, to dissolve]

so·lu·tio (sō-lū'shē-ō). SYN solution. [L.]

so·lu·tion (sol., soln.) (sō-lū'shŭn). **1.** The incorporation of a solid, a liquid, or a gas in a liquid or noncrystalline solid resulting in a homogeneous single phase. SEE dispersion, suspension. **2.** Generally, an aqueous s. of a nonvolatile substance. **3.** In the language of the Pharmacopeia, an aqueous s. of a nonvolatile substance is called a solution or liquor; an aqueous s. of a volatile substance is a water (aqua); an alcoholic s. of a nonvolatile substance is a tincture (tinctura); an alcoholic s. of a volatile substance is a spirit (spiritus); a s. in vinegar is a vinegar (acetum); a s. in glycerin is a glycerol (glyceritum); a s. in wine is a wine (vinum); a s. of sugar in water is a syrup (syrupus); a s. of a mucilaginous substance is a mucilage (mucilago); a s. of an alkaloid or metallic oxide in oleic acid is an oleate (oleatum). **4.** The termination of a disease by crisis. **5.** A break, cut, or laceration of the solid tissues. SEE s. of contiguity, s. of continuity. SYN solutio. [L. *solutio*]

acetic s., a vinegar.

amaranth s., a 1% s. of amaranth (trisodium naphthol sulfonic acid), a synthetic vivid red dye, stable in acid and intensified in sodium hydroxide s.; used as a red or pink colorant in liquid pharmaceuticals.

aqueous s., a s. containing water as the solvent; examples include lime water, rose water, saline s., and a large number of s.'s intended for intravenous administration.

Benedict's s., an aqueous solution of sodium citrate, sodium carbonate, and copper sulfate which changes from its normal blue color to orange, red, or yellow in the presence of a reducing sugar such as glucose. SEE ALSO Benedict's *test* for glucose.

Burow's s., a preparation of aluminium subacetate and glacial acetic acid, used for its antiseptic and astringent action on the skin.

chemical s., SEE solution (1).

colloidal s., a dispersoid, emulsoid, or suspensoid. SYN colloidal dispersion.

s. of contiguity, the breaking of contiguity; a dislocation or displacement of two normally contiguous parts.

s. of continuity, division of bones or soft parts that are normally continuous, as by a fracture, a laceration, or an incision. SYN dieresis.

Dakin's s., a bactericidal wound irrigant. SYN Dakin's fluid.

disclosing s., a s. that selectively stains all soft debris, pellicle, and bacterial plaque on teeth; used as an aid in identifying bacterial plaque after rinsing with water.

Earle's s., a tissue culture medium containing $CaCl_2$, $MgSO_4$, KCl, $NaHCO_3$, NaCl, $NaH_2PO_4·H_2O$, and glucose.

ethereal s., a s. of any substance in ether.

Fehling's s., an alkaline copper tartrate s. formerly used for detection of reducing sugars. SYN Fehling's reagent.

ferric and ammonium acetate s., a clear, aromatic, reddish-brown liquid which has been used in iron-deficiency anemia in animals and man; a source of iron. SYN Basham's mixture.

Fonio's s., a diluent with magnesium sulfate, used for stained smears of blood platelets.

Gallego's differentiating s., a dilute s. of formaldehyde and acetic acid used in a modified Gram stain to differentiate and enhance the basic fuchsin binding to Gram-negative microorganisms.

Gey's s., a salt s. usually used in combination with naturally occurring body substances (*e.g.*, blood serum, tissue extracts) and/or more complex chemically defined nutritive s.'s for culturing animal cells.

Hanks' s., a salt s. usually used in combination with naturally occurring body substances (*e.g.*, blood serum, tissue extracts) and/or more complex chemically defined nutritive s.'s for culturing animal cells; two variations contain $CaCl_2$, $MgSO_4·7H_2O$, KCl, KH_2PO_4, $NaHCO_3$, NaCl, $Na_2HPO_4·2H_2O$, and D-glucose.

Hartmann's s., SYN lactated Ringer's s.

Hartman's s., a s. used to desensitize dentin in dental operations; contains thymol, ethyl alcohol, and sulfuric ether.

Hayem's s., a blood diluent used prior to counting red blood cells.

Krebs-Ringer s., a modification of Ringer's s., prepared by mixing NaCl, KCl, $CaCl_2$, $MgSO_4$, and phosphate buffer, pH 7.4.

lactated Ringer's s., a s. containing NaCl, sodium lactate, $CaCl_2$(dihydrate), and KCl in distilled water; used for the same purposes as Ringer's s. SYN Hartmann's s.

Lange's s., a colloidal gold s. used to demonstrate protein abnormalities in spinal fluid. SEE Lange's *test*.

Locke-Ringer s., a s. containing NaCl, $CaCl_2$, KCl, $MgCl_2$, $NaHCO_3$, D-glucose, and water; used in the laboratory for physiological and pharmacological experiments.

Locke's s.'s, s.'s containing, in varying amounts, NaCl, $CaCl_2$, KCl, $NaHCO_3$, and D-glucose; used for irrigating mammalian heart and other tissues, in laboratory experiments; also used in combination with naturally occurring body substances (*e.g.*, blood serum, tissue extracts) and/or more complex chemically defined nutritive s.'s for culturing animal cells.

Lugol's iodine s., an iodine-potassium iodide s. used as an oxidizing agent, for removal of mercurial fixation artifacts, and also in histochemistry and to stain amebas.

molecular dispersed s., SYN dispersoid.

Monsel s., ferric subsulfate s. used to coagulate superficial bleeding such as that following skin biopsy.

normal s., SEE normal (3).

ophthalmic s.'s, sterile s.'s, free from foreign particles and suitably compounded and dispensed for instillation into the eye.

Ringer's s., **(1)** a s. resembling the blood serum in its salt constituents; it contains 8.6 g of NaCl, 0.3 g of KCl, and 0.33 g of $CaCl_2$ in each 1000 ml of distilled water; used topically for burns and wounds; **(2)** a salt s. usually used in combination with naturally occurring body substances (*e.g.*, blood serum, tissue extracts) and/or more complex chemically defined nutritive s.'s for culturing animal cells. SEE Ringer's *injection*.

saline s., **(1)** a s. of any salt; SYN salt s. **(2)** specifically, an isotonic sodium chloride s.; 0.85 to 0.9/100 ml water.

salt s., SYN saline s. (1).

saturated s. (sat. sol., sat. soln.), a s. that contains all of a substance capable of dissolving; a solution of a substance in equilibrium with an excess undissolved substance.

standard s., standardized s., a s. of known concentration, used as a standard of comparison or analysis.

supersaturated s., a s. containing more of the solid than the liquid would ordinarily dissolve; it is made by heating the solvent when the substance is added, and on cooling the latter is retained without precipitation; addition of a crystal or solid of any kind usually results in precipitation of the excess solute, leaving a saturated s.

test s., a s. of some reagent, in definite strength, used in chemical analysis or testing.

Tyrode's s., a modified Locke's s.; it contains 8 g of NaCl, 0.2 g of KCl, 0.2 g of $CaCl_2$, 0.1 g of $MgCl_2$, 0.05 g of NaH_2PO_4, 1 g

SO

of NaHCO₃, 1 g of D-glucose, and water to make 1000 ml; used to irrigate the peritoneal cavity, and in laboratory work.

volumetric s. (VS), a s. made by mixing measured volumes of the components.

Weigert's iodine s., an iodine-potassium iodide mixture used as a reagent to alter crystal and methyl violet so that they are retained by certain bacteria and fungi.

sol·vate (sol′vāt). A nonaqueous solution or dispersoid in which there is a noncovalent or easily reversible combination between solvent and solute, or dispersion means and disperse phase; when water is the solvent or dispersion medium, it is called a hydrate.

sol·va·tion (sol-vā′shŭn). Noncovalent or easily reversible combination of a solvent with solute, or of a dispersion means with the disperse phase; if the solvent is water, s. is called hydration. S. affects the size of ions in solution, thus Na⁺ is much larger in H₂O than in solid NaCl.

sol·vent. A liquid that holds another substance in solution, *i.e.,* dissolves it. [L. *solvens,* pres. p. of *solvo,* to dissolve]

amphiprotic s., a s. capable of acting as an acid or a base; *e.g.,* H₂O. SEE solvolysis. SEE solvolysis.

fat s.'s, organic liquids notable for their ability to dissolve lipids; usually, but not always, immiscible in water; *e.g.,* diethyl ether, carbon tetrachloride. SYN nonpolar s.'s.

nonpolar s.'s, SYN fat s.'s.

polar s.'s, s.'s that exhibit polar forces on solutes, due to high dipole moment, wide separation of charges, or tight association; *e.g.,* water, alcohols, acids.

universal s., a substance sought by the alchemists, and claimed by some to have been found, supposedly capable of dissolving all substances; sometimes, in a physiological sense, applied to water.

sol·vol·y·sis (sol-vol′i-sis). The reaction of a dissolved salt with the solvent to form an acid and a base; the (partial) reverse of neutralization. If the solvent is water, an amphiprotic solvent, s. is called hydrolysis.

so·ma (sō′mă). **1.** The axial part of the body, *i.e.,* head, neck, trunk, and tail, excluding the limbs. **2.** All of an organism with the exception of the germ cells. SEE ALSO body. **3.** The body of a nerve cell, from which axons, dendrites, etc. project. [G. *sōma,* body]

so·man (sō′man). Methylphosphonofluoridic acid 1,2,2-trimethylpropyl ester; an extremely potent cholinesterase inhibitor. SEE ALSO sarin, tabun.

so·mas·the·nia (sō-mas-the′nē-ă). SYN somatasthenia.

⌂**somat-.** SEE somato-.

so·ma·tag·no·sia (sō′mă-tag-nō′sē-ă). SYN somatotopagnosis. [somat- + G. *a-* priv. + *gnōsis,* recognition]

so·ma·tal·gia (sō-mă-tal′jē-ă). **1.** Pain in the body. **2.** Pain due to organic causes, as opposed to psychogenic pain. [somat- + G. *algos,* pain]

so·ma·tas·the·nia (sō′mă-tas-the′nē-ă). A condition of chronic physical weakness and fatigability. SYN somasthenia. [somat- + G. *astheneia,* weakness]

so·ma·tes·the·sia (sō′mă-tes-the′zē-ă). Bodily sensation, the conscious awareness of the body. SYN somesthesia. [somat- + G. *aisthēsis,* sensation]

so·mat·es·the·tic (sō′mat-es-thet′ik). Relating to somatesthesia.

so·mat·ic (sō-mat′ik). **1.** Relating to the soma or trunk, the wall of the body cavity, or the body in general. SYN parietal (2). **2.** Relating to or involving the skeleton or skeletal (voluntary) muscle and the innervation of the latter, as distinct from the viscera or visceral (involuntary) muscle and its (autonomic) innervation. SYN parietal (3). **3.** Relating to the vegetative, as distinguished from the generative, functions. [G. *sōmatikos,* bodily]

so·mat·i·co·splanch·nic (sō-mat-i-kō-splangk′nik). Relating to the body and the viscera. SYN somaticovisceral. [G. *sōmatikos,* relating to the body, + *splanchnikos,* relating to the viscera]

so·mat·i·co·vis·cer·al (sō-mat-i-kō-vis′er-ăl). SYN somaticosplanchnic.

so·ma·tist (sō′mă-tist). One who considers that neuroses and psychoses are manifestations of organic disease.

so·ma·ti·za·tion (sō′mat-i-zā′shŭn). The process by which psychological needs are expressed in physical symptoms; *e.g.,* the expression or conversion into physical symtoms of anxiety, or a wish for material gain associated with a legal action following and injury, or a related psychological need. SEE ALSO somatization *disorder.*

⌂**somato-, somat-, somatico-.** The body, bodily. [G. *sōma,* body]

so·ma·to·chrome (sō′mă-tō-krōm). Denoting the group of neurons or nerve cells in which there is an abundance of cytoplasm completely surrounding the nucleus. [somato- + G. *chrōma,* color]

so·ma·to·crin·in (sō′mă-tō-crin′in). Hypothalamic growth releasing hormone, GHRH. [somato- + G. *krinō,* to secrete, + -in]

so·ma·to·gen·ic (sō′mă-tō-jen′ik). **1.** Originating in the soma or body under the influence of external forces. **2.** Having origin in body cells. [somato- + G. *genesis,* origin]

so·ma·to·lib·er·in (sō′mă-tō-lib′er-in). A decapeptide released by the hypothalamus, which induces the release of human growth hormone (somatotropin). SYN growth hormone-releasing factor, growth hormone-releasing hormone, somatotropin-releasing factor, somatotropin-releasing hormone. [somatotropin + L. *libero,* to free, + -in]

so·ma·tol·o·gy (sō-mă-tol′ŏ-jē). The science concerned with the study of the body; includes both anatomy and physiology. [somato- + G. *logos,* study]

so·ma·to·mam·mo·tro·pin (sō′mă-tō-mam′ŏ-trō-pin). A peptide hormone, closely related to somatotropin in its biological properties, produced by the normal placenta and by certain neoplasms. [somato- + L. *mamma,* breast, + G. *tropē,* a turning, + -in]

human chorionic s. (HCS), SYN human placental *lactogen.*

so·ma·to·me·din (sō′mă-tō-mē′din). S. A is a peptide (MW of about 4,000), synthesized in the liver and probably in the kidney, that is capable of stimulating certain anabolic processes in bone and cartilage, such as synthesis of DNA, RNA, and protein (including chondromucoprotein), and the sulfation of mucopolysaccharides; secretion and/or biological activity of s. is known to be dependent on somatotropin. SEE ALSO insulin-like growth *factors,* under *factor.* SYN sulfation factor. [*somato,* tropin + *med*iator + -in]

so·ma·to·me·dins. SYN insulin-like growth *factors,* under *factor.*

so·ma·tom·e·try (sō-mă-tom′ě-trē). Classification of persons according to body form, and relation of the types to physiologic and psychologic characteristics. [somato- + G. *metron,* measure]

so·ma·top·a·gus (sō-mă-top′ă-gŭs). Conjoined twins united in their body regions. SEE conjoined *twins,* under *twin.* [somato- + G. *pagos,* something fixed]

so·ma·to·path·ic (sō′mă-tō-path′ik). Relating to bodily or organic illness, as distinguished from mental (psychologic) disorder. [somato- + G. *pathos,* suffering]

so·ma·top·a·thy (sō-mă-top′ă-the). Obsolete term for any disease of the body. [somato- + G. *pathos,* suffering]

so·ma·to·phre·nia (sō′mă-tō-frē′nē-ă). A tendency to imagine or exaggerate body ills. [somato- + G. *phrēn,* mind]

so·ma·to·plasm (sō′mă-tō-plazm, sō-mat′ō-). Aggregate of all the forms of specialized protoplasm entering into the composition of the body, other than germ plasm. [somato- + G. *plasma,* something formed]

so·ma·to·pleure (sō′mă-tō-plūr). Embryonic layer formed by association of the parietal layer of the lateral plate mesoderm with the ectoderm. [somato- + G. *pleura,* side]

so·ma·to·pros·thet·ics (sō′ma-tō-pros-thet′iks). The art and science of prosthetically replacing external parts of the body that are missing or deformed. [somato- + G. *prosthesis,* an addition]

so·ma·to·psy·chic (sō′mă-tō-sī′kik). Relating to the body-mind relationship; the study of the effects of the body upon the mind, as opposed to psychosomatic, which is mind on body. [somato- + G. *psychē,* soul]

so·ma·to·psy·cho·sis (sō′mă-tō-sī-kō′sis). An emotional disorder associated with an organic disease. [somato- + G. *psychōsis,* an animating]

so·ma·tos·co·py (sō-mă-tos′kŏ-pē). Examination of the body. [somato- + G. *skopeō*, to view]

so·ma·to·sen·so·ry (sō-mă-tō-sen′sō-rē). Sensation relating to the body's superficial and deep parts as contrasted to specialized senses such as sight.

so·ma·to·sex·u·al (sō′mă-tō-sek′shū-ăl). Denoting the somatic aspects of sexuality as distinguished from its psychosexual aspects.

so·ma·to·stat·in (sō′mă-tō-stat′in). A tetradecapeptide capable of inhibiting the release of somatotropin by the anterior lobe of the pituitary gland; s. has a short half-life; it also inhibits the release of insulin and gastrin. SYN growth hormone inhibiting hormone, somatotropin release-inhibiting factor, somatotropin release-inhibiting hormone. [somatotropin + G. *stasis*, a standing still, + -in]

so·ma·to·stat·i·no·ma (sō′mă-tō-stat-i-nō′mă). A somatostatin-secreting tumor of the pancreatic islets.

so·ma·to·ther·a·py (sō′mă-tō-thār′ă-pē). **1.** Therapy directed at physical disorders. **2.** In psychiatry, a variety of therapeutic interventions employing chemical or physical, as opposed to psychological, methods.

so·ma·to·top·ag·no·sis (sō′mă-tō-top′ag-nō′sis). The inability to identify any part of the body, either one's own or another's body. Cf. autotopagnosia. SYN somatagnosia. [somato- + top- + G. *a*- priv. + G. *gnōsis*, knowledge]

so·ma·to·top·ic (sō-mă-tō-top′ik). Relating to somatotopy.

so·ma·tot·o·py (sō-mă-tot′ō-pē). The topographic association of positional relationships of receptors in the body via respective nerve fibers to their terminal distribution in specific functional areas of the cerebral cortex; the continuation of these positional relationships in all stages of the ascent of nerve fibers through the central nervous system enables the brain and spinal cord to function on a basis of spatially designated units. [somato- + G. *topos*, place]

so·ma·to·tropes (sō-mă′tō-trōps). A subclass of pituitary acidophilic cells; site of synthesis of growth hormone.

so·ma·to·troph (sō′mă-tō-trof). A cell of the adenohypophysis that produces somatotropin.

so·ma·to·tro·phic (sō′mă-tō-trof′ik). SYN somatotropic. [somato- + G. *trophē*, nourishment]

so·ma·to·tro·pic (sō′mă-tō-trop′ik). Having a stimulating effect on body growth. SYN somatotrophic. [somato- + G. *tropē*, a turning]

so·ma·to·tro·pin (sō′mă-tō-trō′pin). A protein hormone of the anterior lobe of the pituitary, produced by the acidophil cells, that promotes body growth, fat mobilization, and inhibition of glucose utilization; diabetogenic when present in excess; a deficiency of s. is associated with a number of types of dwarfism (type III is an X-linked disorder). SYN growth hormone, pituitary growth hormone, somatotropic hormone. [for *somatotrophin*, fr. somato- + G. *trophē* nourishment; corrupted to -*tropin* and reanalyzed as fr. G. *tropē*, a turning]

so·ma·to·type (sō′mă-tō-tīp). **1.** The constitutional or body type of an individual. **2.** The particular constitutional or body type associated with a particular personality type.

so·ma·to·ty·pol·o·gy (sō′mă-tō-tī-pol′ō-jē). The study of somatotypes. [somato- + G. *typos*, form, + *logos*, study]

so·ma·trem (sō′mă-trem). *N*-L-Methionyl growth hormone (human); a purified polypeptide hormone, made by recombinant DNA techniques, that contains the identical sequence of 191 amino acids constituting naturally occurring somatotropin, plus an additional amino acid, methionine; used in long-term treatment of children deficient in somatotropin.

som·es·the·sia (sō-mes-thē′zē-ă). SYN somatesthesia.

so·mite (sō′mīt). One of the paired, metamerically arranged cell masses formed in the early embryonic paraxial mesoderm; commencing in the third or early fourth week in the region of the hindbrain, they develop in a caudal direction until 42 pairs are formed; their presence is considered evidence that metameric segmentation is a vertebrate characteristic. SYN mesoblastic segment. [G. *sōma*, body, + -*ite*]

occipital s., one of the four most rostral s.'s which become incorporated into the occipital region of the embryonic skull.

som·nam·bu·lance (som-nam′byū-lans). SYN somnambulism (1).

som·nam·bu·lism (som-nam′byū-lizm). **1.** A disorder of sleep involving complex motor acts which occurs primarily during the first third of the night but not during rapid eye movement sleep. SYN noctambulation, noctambulism, oneirodynia activa, sleep-walking, somnambulance. **2.** A form of hysteria in which purposeful behavior is forgotten. [L. *somnus*, sleep, + *ambulo*, to walk]

som·nam·bu·list (som-nam′byū-list). One who is subject to somnambulism (1). SYN sleepwalker.

som·ni·fa·cient (som-ni-fā′shent). SYN soporific (1). [L. *somnus*, sleep, + *facio*, to make]

som·nif·er·ous (som-nif′er-ŭs). SYN soporific (1). [L. *somnus*, sleep, + *fero*, to bring]

som·nif·ic (som-nif′ik). SYN soporific (1).

som·nif·u·gous (som-nif′yū-gŭs). Dispelling or resisting falling asleep. [L. *somnus*, sleep, + *fugo*, to put to flight]

som·nil·o·quence, som·nil·o·quism (som-nil′ō-kwens, -kwizm). **1.** Talking or muttering in one's sleep. SYN sleeptalking (1). **2.** SYN somniloquy. [L. *somnus*, sleep, + *loquor*, to talk]

som·nil·o·quist (som-nil′ō-kwist). A habitual sleep-talker.

som·nil·o·quy (som-nil′ō-kwē). Talking under the influence of hypnotic suggestion. SYN sleeptalking (2), somniloquence (2), somniloquism. [L. *somnus*, sleep, + *loquor*, to speak]

som·nip·a·thist (som-nip′ă-thist). One affected by or under the influence of somnipathy.

som·nip·a·thy (som-nip′ă-thē). **1.** Any disorder of sleep. **2.** SYN hypnotism (1). [L. *somnus*, sleep, + G. *pathos*, suffering]

som·no·cin·e·mat·o·graph (som′nō-sin-ĕ-mat′ō-graf). A device for recording the movements made by sleepers. [L. *somnos*, sleep, + G. *kinēma*, motion, + G. *graphō*, to write]

som·no·cin·e·ma·tog·ra·phy (som′nō-sin-ĕ-mă-tog′ră-fē). The process or technique of recording movements during sleep. SYN polycinematosomnography.

som·no·lence, som·no·len·cy (som′nō-lens, -len-sē). **1.** An inclination to sleep. SYN sleepiness. **2.** A condition of obtusion. SYN somnolentia (1). [L. *somnolentia*]

som·no·lent (som′nō-lent). **1.** Drowsy; sleepy; having an inclination to sleep. **2.** In a condition of incomplete sleep; semicomatose. [L. *somnus*, sleep]

som·no·len·tia (som-nō-len′shē-ă). **1.** SYN somnolence. **2.** SYN sleep *drunkenness*. [L.]

som·no·les·cent (som-nō-les′ent). Inclined to sleep; drowsy.

som·no·lism (som′nō-lizm). SYN hypnotism (1).

Somogyi, Michael, U.S. biochemist, 1883–1971. SEE S. *effect, method, unit*.

Sondermann, R., 20th century German ophthalmologist. SEE S.'s *canal*.

sone (sōn). A unit of loudness; a pure tone of 1000 Hz at 40 dB above the normal threshold of audibility has a loudness of 1 s. [L. *sonus*, sound]

son·ic (son′ik). Of, pertaining to, or determined by sound; *e.g.*, s. vibration. [L. *sonus*, sound]

son·i·cate (son′i-kāt). To expose a suspension of cells or microbes to the disruptive effect of the energy of high frequency sound waves.

son·i·ca·tion (son-i-kā′shŭn). The process of disrupting biologic materials by use of sound wave energy.

son·i·fi·ca·tion (son′i-fi-kā′shŭn). The production of sound, or of sound waves.

son·i·fi·er (son′i-fī-er). An instrument which produces sound waves, especially those of the frequencies used in sonification procedures.

son·i·fy (son′i-fī). To produce sound.

Sonne, Carl, Danish bacteriologist, 1882–1948. SEE S. *bacillus, dysentery*.

son·o·chem·is·try (son-ō-kem′is-trē). The branch of chemistry concerned with chemical changes caused by, or involving, sound, particularly ultrasound.

son·o·gram (son'ō-gram). SYN ultrasonogram. [L. *sonus,* sound, + G. *gramma,* a drawing]

son·o·graph (son'ō-graf). SYN ultrasonograph. [L. *sonus,* sound, + G. *graphō,* to write]

so·nog·ra·pher (sŏ-nog'ră-fer). SYN ultrasonographer.

so·nog·ra·phy (sŏ-nog'ră-fĭ). SYN ultrasonography. [L. *sonus,* sound. + G. *graphō,* to write]

son·o·lu·cent (son-o-lu'sent). In ultrasonography, containing few or no echoes; a misnomer for transonic or anechoic. SEE anechoic. [L. *sonus,* sound + L. *luceo,* to shine]

son·o·mic·rom·e·ter (son'ō-mī-krom'e-ter). An operatively implanted ultrasonic dimension gauge to measure the wall thickening and motion of the heart.

son·o·mo·tor (son-ō-mō'ter). Related to movements caused by sound. SEE sonomotor *response.*

so·phis·ti·cate (sō-fis'ti-kāt). To adulterate. [Mod. L. *sophisticare,* pp. *sophisticatus,* to alter deceptively, fr. G. *sophistikos,* deceitful]

soph·o·re·tin (sof-ŏ-rē'tin). SYN quercetin.

so·por (sō'pōr). An unnaturally deep sleep. [L.]

so·po·rif·er·ous (sō-pōr-if'er-ŭs, sop'ōr-). SYN soporific (1). [L. *soporifer,* fr. *sopor,* deep sleep, + *fero,* to bring]

so·po·rif·ic (sō-pōr-if'ik, sop'ōr-). **1.** Causing sleep. SYN somnifacient, somniferous, somnific, soporiferous. **2.** An agent that produces sleep. [L. *sopor,* deep sleep, + *facio,* to make]

sop·o·rose, so·po·rous (sō'pŏ-rōs, -rŭs). Relating to or causing an unnaturally deep sleep. [L. *sopor,* deep sleep]

sor·be·fa·cient (sor-bĕ-fā'shent). **1.** Causing absorption. **2.** An agent that causes or facilitates absorption. [L. *sorbeo,* to suck up, + *facio,* to make]

sor·bic ac·id (sor'bik). 2,4-Hexadienoic acid; obtained from berries of the mountain ash, *Sorbus aucuparia* (family Rosaceae), or prepared synthetically; it inhibits growth of yeast and mold and is nearly nontoxic to humans; used as a preservative.

sor·bin (sor'bin). SYN L-sorbose.

sor·bi·tan (sor'bi-tan). Sorbitol or sorbose and related compounds in ester combination with fatty acids, and with short oligo (ethylene oxide) side chains and an oleate terminus, to form detergents such as polysorbate 80.

sor·bite (sor'bīt). SYN sorbitol.

sor·bi·tol (sor'bi-tol). D-Sorbitol; D-glucitol; L-gulitol; a reduction product of glucose and sorbose found in the berries of the mountain ash, *Sorbus aucuparia* (family Rosaceae), and in many fruits and seaweeds. It has many industrial and pharmaceutical uses; medicinally, it is used as a diuretic and as a sweetening agent, and is almost completely metabolized (to CO_2 and H_2O); accumulates in type I diabetes mellitus; elevated levels can cause osmotic damage. SYN sorbite.

D-sor·bi·tol-6-phos·phate de·hy·dro·gen·ase. An oxidoreductase that catalyzes the interconversion of D-sorbitol 6-phosphate and NAD^+ to D-fructose 6-phosphate and NADH. A key step in fructose metabolism in the lens. SYN ketose reductase.

sor·bi·tose (sor'bi-tōs). SYN L-sorbose.

L-sor·bose (sor'bōs). A very sweet reducing, but not fermentable, 2-ketohexose obtained from the berries of the mountain ash, *Sorbus aucuparia* (family Rosaceae), and from sorbitol by fermentation with *Acetobacter suboxydans;* L-sorbose is epimeric with D-fructose and is used in the manufacture of vitamin C. SYN sorbin, sorbinose, sorbitose.

sor·des (sor'dēz). A dark brown or blackish crustlike collection on the lips, teeth, and gums of a person with dehydration associated with a chronic debilitating disease. SYN rhyparia, saburra (2). [L. fifth, fr. *sordeo,* to be foul]

sore (sōr). **1.** A wound, ulcer, or any open skin lesion. **2.** Painful; aching; tender. [A.S. *sār*]

bay s., SYN chiclero *ulcer.*

bed s., SEE bedsore.

canker s.'s, SYN aphtha (2).

cold s., colloquialism for *herpes* simplex.

Delhi s., SYN Oriental s.

desert s., any of a variety of chronic nonspecific cutaneous ulcers, most commonly on the shins, knees, hands, and forearms, and probably a variant of ecthyma, that occur in tropical and desert areas. SYN Barcoo rot, veldt s.

fungating s., a granulating chancroid.

hard s., SYN chancre.

Lahore s., SYN Oriental s.

Natal's s., lesion of cutaneous leishmaniasis.

Oriental s., SYN Oriental *ulcer.* SYN Delhi s., Lahore s.

pressure s., SYN decubitus *ulcer.*

soft s., SYN chancroid.

summer s.'s, SYN cutaneous *habronemiasis.*

tropical s., SYN cutaneous *leishmaniasis.*

tropical sore, SYN tropical *ulcer.*

veldt s., SYN desert s.

venereal s., SYN chancroid.

water s., SYN cutaneous *ancylostomiasis.*

sore·head (sōr'hed). SYN filarial *dermatosis.*

sore·mouth (sōr'mowth). SYN orf.

sore·muz·zle (sōr'mŭz-l). SYN bluetongue.

Sörensen, Sören P.L., Danish chemist, 1868–1939. SEE S. scale.

Soret, C., French radiologist, †1931. SEE S. *band;* S.'s *phenomenon.*

so·ro·che (sō-rō'chē). SYN altitude *sickness* (1). [Sp. (orig. ore, formerly attributed to toxic emanations of ores in mountains)]

chronic s., SYN chronic mountain *sickness.*

sorp·tion (sorp'shŭn). Adsorption or absorption.

Sorsby, Arnold, British ophthalmologist, *1900. SEE S.'s macular *degeneration, syndrome.*

s.o.s. Abbreviation for L. *si opus sit,* if needed.

so·ta·lol hy·dro·chlo·ride (sō'tă-lol). 4'-[1-Hydroxy-2-(isopropylamino)ethyl]methanesulfonanilide monohydrochloride; a β-receptor blocking agent with uses similar to those of propanolol; also possesses potassium blocking properties.

Sotos, J.F., U.S. pediatrician, *1927. SEE S.'s *syndrome.*

Sottas, Jules, French neurologist, 1866–1943. SEE Dejerine-S. *disease.*

souf·fle (sū'fl). A soft blowing sound heard on auscultation. [Fr. *souffler,* to blow]

cardiac s., a soft puffing heart murmur.

fetal s., a blowing murmur, synchronous with the fetal heart beat, sometimes only systolic and sometimes continuous, heard on auscultation over the pregnant uterus. SYN funic s., funicular s., umbilical s.

funic s., funicular s., SYN fetal s.

mammary s., a blowing murmur heard late in pregnancy and during lactation at the medial border of the breast, sometimes only systolic and sometimes continuous.

placental s., SYN uterine s.

umbilical s., SYN fetal s.

uterine s., a blowing sound, synchronous with the cardiac systole of the mother, heard on auscultation of the pregnant uterus. SYN placental s.

Soulier, Jean Pierre, French hematologist, *1915. SEE Bernard-S. *disease, syndrome.*

sound (sownd). **1.** The vibrations produced by a sounding body, transmitted by the air or other medium, and perceived by the internal ear. **2.** An elongated cylindrical, usually curved, instrument of metal, used for exploring the bladder or other cavities of the body, for dilating strictures of the urethra, esophagus, or other canal, for calibrating the lumen of a body cavity, or for detecting the presence of a foreign body in a body cavity. **3.** To explore or calibrate a cavity with a s. **4.** Whole; healthy; not diseased or injured.

after-s., SEE aftersound.

amphoric voice s., SEE amphoric *voice.*

anvil s., SYN bellmetal *resonance.*

atrial s., SYN fourth heart s.

auscultatory s., a rale, murmur, bruit, fremitus, or other s. heard on auscultation of the chest or abdomen.

bell s., SYN bellmetal *resonance*.

bowel s.'s, relatively high-pitched abdominal s.'s caused by propulsion of intestinal contents through the lower alimentary tract.

Campbell s., a miniature s. with a short round-tipped beak, especially curved for the deep urethra of the young male.

cannon s., SYN *bruit* de canon.

cardiac s., SYN heart s.'s.

cavernous voice s., SEE cavernous *voice*.

coconut s., a s. like that produced when a cracked coconut is tapped; it is elicited by percussing the skull of a patient with osteitis deformans.

cracked-pot s., SYN cracked-pot *resonance*.

Davis interlocking s., a s. comprised of two instruments with curved male and female tips, used to introduce a catheter into the bladder in the treatment of ruptured urethra; the male s. is introduced into the distal urethra via the meatus and the female s. is passed downward through the bladder neck into the proximal urethra via an open cystotomy; the ends of the two instruments are engaged, with the female s. guiding the male s. upward into the bladder; a catheter is then sutured to the tip of the male s. and withdrawn through the urethra to restore continuity of its lumen.

double-shock s., SYN *bruit* de rappel.

eddy s.'s, s.'s that punctuate the continuous murmur of patent ductus arteriosus, imparting to it a characteristic "uneven" quality.

ejection s.'s, click-like s.'s during ejection from a hypertensive aorta or pulmonary artery or associated with stenosis (particularly congenital) of the aortic or pulmonic valve.

first heart s. (S_1), occurs with ventricular systole and is mainly produced by closure of the atrioventricular valves.

fourth heart s. (S_4), the s. produced in late diastole in association with ventricular filling due to atrial systole and related to reduced ventricular compliance. It is a low frequency oscillation that may be normal at older ages owing to a physiologic decline in ventricular compliance but is nearly always abnormal at younger ages if it is of high intensity or palpable. It is common in ventricular hypertrophy, particularly with hypertension, and is almost invariable during acute myocardial infarction. Fourth heart s.'s may arise from the right or left ventricle or both. SYN atrial s.

friction s., the s., heard on auscultation, made by the rubbing of two opposed serous surfaces roughened by an inflammatory exudate, or, if chronic, by nonadhesive fibrosis. SYN friction murmur, friction rub.

gallop s., the abnormal third or fourth heart s. which, when added to the first and second s.'s, produces the triple cadence of gallop rhythm. SEE ALSO gallop.

heart s.'s, the noise made by muscle contraction and the closure of the heart valves during the cardiac cycle. SEE first heart s., second heart s., third heart s., fourth heart s. SYN cardiac s.'s, heart tones.

hippocratic succussion s., a splashing s. elicited by shaking a patient with hydro- or pyopneumothorax, the physician's ear being applied to the chest.

Jewett s., a short straight s. for dilating the anterior urethra.

Korotkoff s.'s, s.'s heard over an artery when pressure over it is reduced below systolic arterial pressure, as when blood pressure is determined by the auscultatory method.

Le Fort s., a curved s. threaded for a filiform bougie, used for dilation of urethral strictures in the male when small caliber or presence of false passages prevents safe passage of a standard s. or catheter.

McCrea s., a gently curved s. used to dilate the urethra in infants or children.

Mercier's s., a catheter the beak of which is short and bent almost at a right angle.

muscle s., a fine murmur heard on auscultation over the belly of a contracting muscle.

percussion s., any s. elicited on percussing over one of the cavities of the body.

pericardial friction s., a to-and-fro grating, rasping, or, rarely, creaking s. heard over the heart in some cases of pericarditis, due to rubbing of the inflamed pericardial surfaces as the heart contracts and relaxes; during normal sinus rhythm it is usually triphasic; during any rhythm it may be biphasic or uniphasic. SYN pericardial rub, pericardial friction rub.

pistol-shot s., s. created by lightly compressing an artery during aortic regurgitation; sometimes is audible without compression.

pistol-shot femoral s., a shotlike systolic s. heard over the femoral artery in high output states, especially aortic insufficiency; presumably due to sudden stretching of the elastic wall of the artery; pistol-shot s.'s may also be heard over other relatively large arteries, *e.g.,* brachial, radial.

posttussis suction s., a s. produced by the falling back of a drop of mucus or pus into a pulmonary cavity after the latter has been emptied by coughing.

respiratory s., a murmur, bruit, fremitus, rhonchus, or rale heard on auscultation over the lungs or any part of the respiratory tract.

sail s., a s., likened to the snapping of a sail; the abnormal first heart s. in some patients with Ebstein's anomaly.

Santini's booming s., a sonorous booming s. heard on auscultatory percussion of a hydatid cyst.

second heart s. (S_2), the second s. heard on auscultation of the heart; signifies the beginning of diastole and is due to closure of the semilunar valves. SYN second s.

second s., SYN second heart s.

Simpson uterine s., a slender flexible metal rod used to calibrate or dilate the cervical canal, or to hold the uterus in various positions during gynecologic surgery.

Sims uterine s., a slender flexible s. with a small projection about 7 cm from its tip, used to estimate the size and caliber of the uterine cavity.

splitting of heart s.'s, the production of major components of the first and second heart s.'s (rarely the third and fourth) due to contribution by the left-sided and right-sided valves; thus, the first heart s. would have a mitral and a tricuspid component and the second heart s. has an aortic and pulmonic component. The latter are best appreciated during respiration, with inspiration delaying the pulmonic component and producing an earlier aortic component.

succussion s., the noise made by fluid with overlying air when shaken, such as occurs with gastric dilatation or with fluid and air in a pleural cavity (hydropneumothorax).

tambour s., SYN *bruit* de tambour.

third heart s. (S_3), occurs in early diastole and corresponds with the end of the first phase of rapid ventricular filling; normal in children and younger people but abnormal in others. SYN third s.

third s., SYN third heart s.

tic-tac s.'s, SYN embryocardia.

to-and-fro s., doubling of an abnormal murmur usually in systole and diastole and formerly applied to pericardial rubs.

van Buren s., a standard s., available in several calibers, with a gently curved tip designed to follow the contour of the deep bulbous urethra in the male; used for urethral calibration or dilation.

waterwheel s., s. made by cardiac motion inducing splashes in the presence of fluid and air within the pericardial sac.

water-whistle s., a bubbling whistle heard on auscultation over a bronchial or pulmonary fistula.

Winternitz' s., a double-current catheter in which water at any desired temperature circulates.

xiphisternal crunching s., SEE Hamman's *sign*.

Southern, M.E., 20th century British biologist. SEE Southern blot *analysis*.

Southey, Reginald, English physician, 1835–1899. SEE S.'s *tubes*, under *tube*.

sow. A female hog of breeding age. [M.E.]

soy·a (soy′ă). SYN soybean. [Hind. *soyā,* fennel]

soy·bean (soy′bēn). The bean of the climbing herb *Glycine soja* or *G. hispida* (family Leguminosae); a bean rich in protein and containing little starch; it is the source of s. oil; s. flour is used in preparing a bread for diabetics, in feeding formulas for infants who are unable to tolerate cow's milk, and for adults allergic to cow's milk. SYN soja, soya. [Hind. *soyā*, fennel]

s. oil, obtained from s.'s by expression or solvent extraction; contains triglycerides of linoleic acid, oleic acid, linolenic acid, and saturated fatty acids; used as a food and in the manufacture of margarine and other food products.

SP1 Abbreviation for stimulatory *protein* 1.

sp. Abbreviation for subspecies; pl. form is spp.; L. *spiritus,* spirit.

spa (spah). A health resort, especially one where there are one or more mineral springs whose waters possess therapeutic properties. [*Spa,* a mineral spring health resort in Belgium]

SPACE

space (spās). Any demarcated portion of the body, either an area of the surface, a segment of the tissues, or a cavity. SEE ALSO area, region, zone. SYN spatium [NA]. [L. *spatium,* room, space]

alveolar dead s., the difference between physiologic dead s. and anatomical dead s.; it represents that part of the physiologic dead s. resulting from ventilation of relatively underperfused or nonperfused alveoli; it differs specifically in being placed so as to fill and empty in parallel with functional alveoli, rather than being interposed in the conducting tubes between functional alveoli and the external environment.

anatomical dead s., the volume of the conducting airways from the external environment (at the nose and mouth) down to the level at which inspired gas exchanges oxygen and carbon dioxide with pulmonary capillary blood; formerly presumed to extend down to the beginning of alveolar epithelium in the respiratory bronchioles, but more recent evidence indicates that effective gas exchange extends some distance up the thicker-walled conducting airways because of rapid longitudinal mixing. Cf. alveolar dead s., physiologic dead s. SYN anatomical airway.

antecubital s., SYN cubital *fossa.*

anterior clear s., SYN retrosternal s.

apical s., the s. between the alveolar wall and the apex of the root of a tooth where an alveolar abscess usually has its origin.

axillary s., SYN axilla.

Berger's s., the s. between the patellar fossa of the vitreous and the lens.

Bogros' s., SYN retroinguinal s.

Böttcher's s., SYN endolymphatic *sac.*

Bowman's s., SYN capsular s.

Burns' s., SYN suprasternal s.

capsular s., the slitlike s. between the visceral and parietal layers of the capsule of the renal corpuscle; it opens into the proximal tubule of the nephron at the neck of the tubule. SYN Bowman's s., filtration s.

cartilage s., SYN cartilage *lacuna.*

central palmar s., the more medial of the central palmar spaces, bounded medially by the hypothenar compartment; related distally to the synovial tendon sheaths of digits 3 and 4 and proximally to the common flexor sheath. SYN medial midpalmar s., middle palmar s.

Chassaignac's s., potential s. between the pectoralis major and the mammary gland.

Cloquet's s., a s. between the ciliary zonule and the vitreous body.

Colles' s., SYN superficial perineal s.

corneal s., one of the stellate s.'s between the lamellae of the cornea, each of which contains a cell or corneal corpuscle. SYN lacuna (4).

Cotunnius' s., SYN endolymphatic *sac.*

cranial epidural s., SYN *dura mater* of brain.

dead s., (1) a cavity, potential or real, remaining after the closure of a wound which is not obliterated by the operative technique; (2) SEE anatomical dead s., physiologic dead s.

deep perineal s., the region between the perineal membrane and the endopelvic fascia of the floor of the pelvis occupied by the membranous part of the urethra, the bulbourethral gland (in the male), the deep transverse perineal and sphincter urethrae muscles, and the dorsal nerve and artery of the penis or clitoris. SYN spatium perinei profundum [NA], deep perineal pouch.

denture s., (1) that portion of the oral cavity which is, or may be, occupied by maxillary and/or mandibular denture(s); (2) the s. between the residual ridges which is available for dentures. SEE ALSO interarch *distance.*

disk s., on radiographs of the spine, the radiolucent region between each pair of vertebral bodies.

Disse's s., SYN perisinusoidal s.

s. of Donders, the space between the dorsum of the tongue and the hard palate when the mandible is in rest position following the expiratory cycle of respiration.

epidural s., SYN epidural *cavity.*

episcleral s., the space between the fascial sheath of the eyeball and the sclera. SYN spatium episclerale [NA], interfascial s., spatium interfasciale, spatium intervaginale bulbi oculi, Tenon's s.

epitympanic s., SYN epitympanic *recess.*

filtration s., SYN capsular s.

Fontana's s.'s, SYN s.'s of iridocorneal angle.

freeway s., the s. between the occluding surfaces of the maxillary and mandibular teeth when the mandible is in physiologic resting position. SYN interocclusal clearance, interocclusal distance (2), interocclusal gap, interocclusal rest s. (2).

gingival s., SYN gingival *sulcus.*

haversian s.'s, s.'s in bone formed by the enlargement of haversian canals.

Henke's s., retropharyngeal s.

His' perivascular s., SYN Virchow-Robin s.

infraglottic s., SYN infraglottic *cavity.*

interalveolar s., SYN interarch *distance.*

intercostal s., an interval between the ribs, occupied by intercostal muscles, veins, arteries and nerves. SYN spatium intercostale [NA].

interfascial s., SYN episcleral s.

interglobular s., one of a number of irregularly branched spaces near the periphery of the dentin of the crown of a tooth, through which pass the ramifications of the tubules; they are caused by failure of calcification of the dentin. SYN spatium interglobulare [NA], interglobular s. of Owen.

interglobular s. of Owen, SYN interglobular s.

intermembrane s., the s. between the two membranes in a cell or organelle enclosed by a double biomembrane; *e.g.,* the space between the inner and outer membranes of the mitochondria; sometimes referred to as the external matrix.

interocclusal rest s., (1) SYN interocclusal *distance* (1). (2) SYN freeway s.

interosseous metacarpal s.'s, the s.'s between the metacarpal bones in the hand. SYN spatia interossea metacarpi [NA].

interosseous metatarsal s.'s, the s.'s between the metatarsal bones in the foot. SYN spatia interossea metatarsi [NA].

interpleural s., SYN mediastinum (2).

interproximal s., the s. between adjacent teeth in a dental arch; it is divided into the embrasure occlusal to the contact area, and the septal s. gingival to the contact area.

interradicular s., the s. between the roots of multirooted teeth.

interseptovalvular s., the interval in the developing embryonic heart between the septum primum and the left valve of the sinus venosus.

intersheath s.'s of optic nerve, SYN intervaginal s. of optic nerve.

intervaginal s. of optic nerve, the spaces within the internal sheath of the optic nerve, between the arachnoidal and pial layers, filled with cerebrospinal fluid and continuous with the subarachnoid space. SYN spatia intervaginalia nervi optici [NA], intersheath s.'s of optic nerve, Schwalbe's s.'s.

intervillous s.'s, the s.'s containing maternal blood, located between placenta villi; they are lined with syncytiotrophoblast.

intraretinal s., the potential cleft between the pigmented and neural layers of the retina; it represents the cavity of the embryonic optic vesicle; retinal detachment occurs by the opening of this space.

s.'s of iridocorneal angle, irregularly shaped endothelium-lined spaces within the trabecular reticulum, through which the aqueous filters to reach the sinus venosus sclerae. SYN spatia anguli iridocornealis [NA], ciliary canals, Fontana's s.'s.

Kiernan's s., interlobular s. in the liver.

Kretschmann's s., a slight depression in the epitympanic recess below the superior recess of tympanic membrane.

Kuhnt's s.'s, shallow diverticula or recesses between the ciliary body and ciliary zonule which open into the posterior chamber of the eye.

lateral central palmar s., the more lateral (radial) of the central palmar spaces, bounded laterally by the thenar compartment; related distally to the synovial tendon sheath of the index finger and proximally to the common flexor sheath. SYN lateral midpalmar s.

lateral midpalmar s., SYN lateral central palmar s.

lateral pharyngeal s., that part of the peripharyngeum s. located at the sides of the pharynx. SYN spatium lateropharyngeum [NA].

leeway s., the difference between the combined mesiodistal widths of the deciduous cuspids and molars and their successors.

lymph s., a s. in tissue or a vessel, filled with lymph.

Magendie's s.'s, s.'s between the pia and arachnoid at the level of the fissures of the brain.

Malacarne's s., SYN posterior perforated *substance*.

Meckel's s., SYN trigeminal *cave*.

medial midpalmar s., SYN central palmar s.

mediastinal s., SYN mediastinum (2).

medullary s., the central cavity and the cellular intervals between the trabeculae of bone, filled with marrow.

middle palmar s., SYN central palmar s.

midpalmar s., (1) either of the two central palmar s.'s (medial or lateral).

Mohrenheim's s., SYN infraclavicular *fossa*.

Nuel's s., an interval in the spiral organ (of Corti) between the outer pillar cells on one side and the phalangeal cells and hair cells on the other.

parapharyngeal s., SYN pharyngomaxillary s.

Parona's s., a s. between the pronator quadratus deep and the overlying flexor tendons of the forearm which is continuous through the carpal tunnel with the medial central palmar space.

parotid s., a deep hollow on the side at the sides of the face flanking the posterior aspect of the ramus of the mandible with its attached muscles which is occupied by the parotid gland; it is lined with fascial laminae (the parotid sheath) derived from the investing layer of deep cervical fascia; the structures bounding the s. collectively constitute the parotid bed. Surgeons operating in the area take advantage of the fact that the anteroposterior dimensions of the parotid s. increase with protrusion of the mandible. SYN parotid recess, recessus parotideus.

perforated s., SEE anterior perforated *substance*, posterior perforated *substance*.

perichoroid s., SYN perichoroidal s.

perichoroidal s., the interval between the choroid and the sclera filled by the loose meshes of the lamina fusca of sclera and the suprachoroid lamina. SYN spatium perichoroideale [NA], perichoroid s.

perilymphatic s., space between the bony and membranous portions of the labyrinth. SYN spatium perilymphaticum [NA], cisterna perilymphatica.

perineal s.'s, SEE deep perineal s., superficial perineal s.

perinuclear s., SYN *cisterna* caryothecae.

peripharyngeal s., the space, filled with loose areolar tissue, around the pharynx; it is divided into two portions, lateral pharyngeal s. and retropharyngeal s. SYN spatium peripharyngeum [NA].

periportal s. of Mall, a tissue s. between the limiting lamina and the portal canal in the liver.

perisinusoidal s., the potential extravascular s. between the liver sinusoids and liver parenchymal cells. SYN Disse's s.

perivitelline s., the s. between the vitelline membrane and the zona pellucida, appearing in an ovum immediately following fertilization.

personal s., a term used in the behavioral sciences to denote the physical area immediately surrounding an individual who is in proximity to one or more others, whether known or unknown, and which serves as a body buffer zone in such interpersonal transactions.

pharyngeal s., the area occupied by the pharynx (naso-, oro-, and laryngopharnynx). Not to be confused with the retropharyngeal s.

pharyngomaxillary s., the s. limited by the lateral wall of the pharynx, the cervical vertebrae, and the medial pterygoid muscle. SYN parapharyngeal s.

physiologic dead s. (V_D), the sum of anatomic and alveolar dead s.; the dead s. calculated when the carbon dioxide pressure in systemic arterial blood is used instead of that of alveolar gas in Bohr's equation; it is a virtual or apparent volume that takes into account the impairment of gas exchange because of uneven distributions of lung ventilation and perfusion.

plantar s., one of four areas between fascial layers in the foot, where pus may be confined when the foot is infected.

pleural s., SYN pleural *cavity*.

pneumatic s., any one of the paranasal sinuses.

Poiseuille's s., SYN still *layer*.

popliteal s., SYN popliteal *fossa*.

postpharyngeal s., SYN retropharyngeal s.

Proust's s., SYN rectovesical *pouch*.

Prussak's s., SYN superior *recess* of tympanic membrane.

pterygomandibular s., the area between the mandibular ramus and the pterygoid process of the sphenoid bone.

quadrangular s., musculotendinous formation providing passageway for the axillary nerve, posterior humeral circumflex artery and accompanying veins as they run from the axilla to the superior posterior arm; as the neurovascular structures enter the formation anteriorly, it is bounded superiorly by the shoulder joint, medially by the lateral border of subscapularis, laterally by the surgical neck of the humerus, and inferiorly by the tendon of latissimus dorsi; as the vessels exit the formation posteriorly, it is bounded superiorly by the teres minor, medially by the long head of the triceps, laterally by the lateral head of the triceps and inferiorly by the teres major muscle or tendon; as they emerge, most of the neurovascular structures run on the deep surface of the deltoid muscle, which they supply. SYN quadrilateral s.

quadrilateral s., SYN quadrangular s.

Reinke's s., the loose connective tissue in the superficial layer of the lamina propria of the vocal fold. Edema of this s. produces hoarseness in chronic smokers or in hypothyroidism.

respiratory dead s., that part of the respiratory tract or of a single breath which fails to exchange oxygen and carbon dioxide with pulmonary capillary blood; a nonspecific term which fails to distinguish between anatomical dead s. and physiologic dead s.

retroadductor s., potential s. between the adductor pollicis and first dorsal interosseous muscles.

retroinguinal s., a triangular s. between the peritoneum and the transversalis fascia, at the lower angle of which is the inguinal ligament; it contains the lower portion of the external iliac artery. SYN Bogros' s., spatium retroinguinale.

retromylohyoid s., the sulcus at the posterior end of the mylohyoid line.

retroperitoneal s., the space between the parietal peritoneum and the muscles and bones of the posterior abdominal wall. SYN spatium retroperitoneale [NA], retroperitoneum.

retropharyngeal s., that part of the peripharyngeal s. located posterior to the pharynx. SYN spatium retropharyngeum [NA], postpharyngeal s.

retropubic s., the area of loose connective tissue between the bladder with its related fascia and the pubis and anterior abdominal wall. SYN spatium retropubicum [NA], cavum retzii, Retzius' cavity, Retzius' s.

sp

retrosternal s., on lateral chest radiographs, the region dorsal to the sternum and ventral to the ascending aorta. SYN anterior clear s.

Retzius' s., SYN retropubic s.

Schwalbe's s.'s, SYN intervaginal s. of optic nerve.

subarachnoid s., the s. between the arachnoidea and pia mater, traversed by delicate fibrous trabeculae and filled with cerebrospinal fluid. Since the pia mater immediately adheres to the surface of the brain and spinal cord, the s. is greatly widened wherever the brain surface exhibits a deep depression (for example, between the cerebellum and medulla); such widenings are called cisternae. The large blood vessels supplying the brain and spinal cord lie in the subarachnoid s. SYN cavum subarachnoideum [NA], subarachnoid cavity.

subchorial s., the part of the placenta adjacently beneath the chorionic plate; it joins with irregular channels to form the marginal lakes. SYN subchorial lake.

subdural s., originally thought to be a narrow fluid-filled interval between the dural and arachnoid; now known to be an artificial s. created by the separation of the arachnoid from the dura as the result of trauma or some ongoing pathologic process; in the healthy state, the arachnoid is attached to the dura and a naturally occurring subdural s. is not present. SYN spatium subdurale [NA], cavum subdurale, subdural cavity, subdural cleavage, subdural cleft.

subgingival s., SYN gingival *sulcus.*

superficial perineal s., the superficial compartment of the perineum; the space bounded above by the perineal membrane (inferior fascia of the urogenital diaphragm) and below by the superficial perineal (Colles') fascia; it contains the root structure of the penis or clitoris and associated musculature, plus the superficial transverse perineal muscle and, in the female only, the greater vestibular glands. SYN spatium perinei superficiale [NA], Colles' s., superficial perineal pouch.

suprahepatic s.'s, SYN subphrenic *recesses,* under *recess.*

suprasternal s., a narrow interval between the deep and superficial layers of the cervical fascia above the manubrium of the sternum through which pass the anterior jugular veins. SYN Burns' s.

Tarin's s., SYN interpeduncular *cistern.*

Tenon's s., SYN episcleral s.

thenar s., SEE central palmar s.

Traube's semilunar s., a crescentic s. about 12 cm wide, bounded medially by the left border of the sternum, above by an oblique line from the sixth costal cartilage to the lower border of the eighth or ninth rib in the mid-axillary line and below by the costal margin; the percussion tone here is normally tympanitic, because of the underlying stomach, but is modified by pulmonary emphysema, a pleural effusion, or an enlarged spleen.

Trautmann's triangular s., the area of the temporal bone bounded by the sigmoid sinus, the superior petrosal sinus, and a tangent to the posterior semicircular canal.

vertebral epidural s., SEE *dura mater* of spinal cord.

Virchow-Robin s., a tunnel-like extension of the subarachnoid s. surrounding blood vessels that pass into the brain or spinal cord from the subarachnoid s.; the lining of the channel is composed of pia and glial feet of astrocytes; a continuation of the s. around capillaries and nerve cells probably does not occur. SYN His' perivascular s.

Waldeyer's s., SYN Waldeyer's *sheath.*

Westberg's s., the s. surrounding the origin of the aorta which is invested with the pericardium.

zonular s.'s, the spaces between the fibers of the ciliary zonule at the equator of the lens of the eye. SYN spatia zonularia [NA], Petit's canals.

---

spa·gyr·ic (spă-jir'ik). Relating to the paracelsian or alchemical system of medicine, which stressed the treatment of disease by various types of chemical substances. [G. *spaō,* to tear open, + *ageirō,* to collect]

spag·y·rist (spaj'ĭ-rist). A physician of the 16th century, a follower of the teachings of Paracelsus who believed in the essential

importance of chemical or alchemical knowledge in the understanding and treatment of disease.

spall (spawl). **1.** A fragment. **2.** To break up into fragments.

Spallanzani, Lazaro, Italian priest and scientist, 1729–1799. SEE S.'s *law.*

spall·a·tion (spaw-lā'shŭn). **1.** SYN fragmentation. **2.** Nuclear reaction in which nuclei, on being bombarded by high energy particles, liberate a number of protons and alpha particles. [M.E. *spalle,* fragment]

span. The amount, distance, or length between two points; the full extent or reach of anything.

memory s., the maximum number of items recalled after a single presentation (auditory or visual).

span·nungs-P (spahn'nŭngz). Prominent prolonged and high voltage P waves recorded in electrocardiograms (usually largest in lead II) of patients with hypertrophy of the right or both atria, particularly in those with congenital heart disease. SEE ALSO P-congenitale. [Ger. *Spannung,* tightening; stretching or straining, + P wave]

spar·ga·no·ma (spar-gă-nō'mă). A localized mass resulting from sparganosis.

spar·ga·no·sis (spar-gă-nō'sis). Infection with the plerocercoid or sparganum of a pseudophyllidean tapeworm, usually in a dermal sore resulting from application of infected flesh as a poultice; infection may also occur from ingestion of uncooked frog, snake, mammal, or bird intermediate or transport host bearing the spargana, but not from fish with *Diphyllobothrium* larvae, since s. is an infection with nonhuman pseudophyllidean tapeworms, usually species of *Spirometra.* S. may also develop from ingestion of water containing procercoid-infected *Cyclops.*

ocular s., infestation of the orbits with the sparganum of *Spirometra mansoni;* characterized by redness and edema of the eyelids, lacrimation, and blepharoptosis; acquired by application of infected raw frog flesh against the eye as a poultice.

spar·ga·num (spar'gă-nŭm). Originally described as a genus, but now restricted to the plerocercoid stage of certain tapeworms. [G. *sparganon,* a swathing band, fr. *spargō,* to swathe]

spar·te·ine (spar'tē-ēn, -tē-in). *l*-Sparteine; an alkaloid obtained from scoparius, *Cytisus scoparius* and *Lupinus luteus;* s. sulfate was used as an oxytocic drug. SYN lupinidine.

spasm (spazm). A sudden involuntary contraction of one or more muscle groups; includes cramps, contractures. SYN muscle s., spasmus. [G. *spasmos*]

s. of accommodation, excessive contraction of the ciliary muscle.

affect s.'s, rarely used term for spasmodic attacks of laughing, weeping, and screaming, accompanied by marked tachypnea.

anorectal s., SYN *proctalgia* fugax.

Bell's s., SYN facial *tic.*

cadaveric s., rigor mortis occurring irregularly in the different muscles, causing movements of the limbs.

canine s., SYN risus caninus.

carpopedal s., s. of the feet and hands observed in hyperventilation, calcium deprivation, and tetany: flexion of the hands at the wrists and of the fingers at the metacarpophalangeal joints and extension of the fingers at the phalangeal joints; the feet are dorsiflexed at the ankles and the toes plantar flexed. SYN carpopedal contraction.

clonic s., alternate involuntary contraction and relaxation of a muscle.

cynic s., SYN risus caninus.

dancing s., SYN saltatory s.

diffuse esophageal s., abnormal contraction of the muscular wall of the esophagus causing pain and dysphagia, often in response to regurgitation of acid gastric contents.

epidemic transient diaphragmatic s., SYN epidemic *pleurodynia.*

esophageal s., a disorder of the motility of the esophagus characterized by pain or forceful eructations after swallowing food. Esophageal muscle contractions are of excessive force and duration. Chest pain can be confused with symptoms of cardiac or other origin.

facial s., SYN facial *tic.*

functional s., SYN occupational *neurosis.*

habit s., SYN tic.

histrionic s., SYN facial *tic.*

infantile s., brief (1 to 3 seconds) muscular s.'s in infants with West's syndrome, which often appear as nodding or salaam s.'s. SYN salaam convulsions.

intention s., a spasmodic contraction of the muscles occurring when a voluntary movement is attempted.

masticatory s., involuntary convulsive muscular contraction affecting the muscles of mastication.

mimic s., SYN facial *tic.*

mobile s., a tonic s. occurring in spastic infantile hemiplegia on attempted movement.

muscle s., SYN spasm.

nictitating s., involuntary spasmodic winking. SYN spasmus nictitans, winking s.

nodding s., (1) in infants, a drop of the head on the chest due to loss of tone in the neck muscles as in epilepsia nutans, or to tonic spasm of anterior neck muscles as in West's syndrome; **(2)** in adults, a nodding of the head from clonic s.'s of the sternomastoid muscles. SYN salaam attack, salaam s., spasmus nutans (1).

occupational s., professional s., obsolete term for occupational dystonia.

phonic s., SYN *dysphonia* spastica.

progressive torsion s., SYN *dystonia* musculorum deformans.

retrocollic s., torticollis in which the s. affects the posterior neck muscles. SYN retrocollis.

rotatory s., SYN spasmodic *torticollis.*

salaam s., SYN nodding s.

saltatory s., a spasmodic affection of the muscles of the lower extremities. SYN Bamberger's disease (1), dancing s., Gowers disease (1).

sewing s., SYN seamstress's *cramp.*

synclonic s., clonic s. of two or more muscles.

tailor's s., SYN tailor's *cramp.*

tonic s., a continuous involuntary muscular contraction.

tonoclonic s., convulsive contraction of muscles.

tooth s.'s, infantile convulsions associated with teething.

torsion s., SYN dystonia.

vasomotor s., spasmodic contraction of the smaller arteries.

winking s., SYN nictitating s.

△**spasmo-.** Spasm. [G. *spasmos*]

spas·mod·ic (spaz-mod'ik). Relating to or marked by spasm. [G. *spasmōdes,* convulsive, fr. *spasmos,* + *eidos,* form]

spas·mo·gen (spaz'mō-jen). A substance causing contraction of smooth muscle; *e.g.,* histamine.

spas·mo·gen·ic (spaz-mō-jen'ik). Causing spasms. [spasmo- + G. *-gen,* producing]

spas·mol·o·gy (spaz-mol'ō-jē). Study of the nature, causation, and means of relief of spasms. [spasmo- + G. *logos,* study]

spas·mo·lyg·mus (spaz-mō-lig'mŭs). **1.** Spasmodic sobbing. **2.** Spasmodic hiccup. [spasmo- + G. *lygmos,* a sobbing, hiccup, fr. *lyzō,* to hiccup, sob]

spas·mol·y·sis (spaz-mol'i-sis). The arrest of a spasm or convulsion. [spasmo- + G. *lysis,* dissolution]

spas·mo·lyt·ic (spaz'mō-lit'ik). **1.** Relating to spasmolysis. **2.** Denoting a chemical agent that relieves smooth muscle spasms.

spas·mo·phil·ia (spaz-mō-fil'ē-ă). SYN latent *tetany.* [spasmo- + G. *phileō,* to love]

spas·mo·phil·ic (spaz-mō-fil'ik). Relating to spasmophilia.

spas·mus (spaz'mŭs). SYN spasm. [L. fr. G. *spasmos,* spasm]

s. cani'nus, SYN risus caninus.

s. coordina'tus, compulsive movements, such as imitative or mimic tics, festination, etc.

s. glot'tidis, SYN *laryngismus* stridulus.

s. nic'titans, SYN nictitating *spasm.*

s. nu'tans, (1) SYN nodding *spasm.* **(2)** a fine nystagmus, sometimes rotary, sometimes monocular, associated with head-nodding movements.

spas·tic (spas'tik). **1.** SYN hypertonic (1). **2.** Relating to spasm or to spasticity. [L. *spasticus,* fr. G. *spastikos,* drawing in]

spas·tic·i·ty (spas-tis'i-tē). A state of increased muscular tone with exaggeration of the tendon reflexes.

clasp-knife s., initial increased resistance to stretch of the extensor muscles of a joint that give way rather suddenly allowing the joint then to be easily flexed; the rigidity is due to an exaggeration of the stretch reflex. SEE ALSO lengthening *reaction.* SYN clasp-knife effect, clasp-knife rigidity.

spa·tia (spā'shē-ă). Plural of spatium. [L.]

spa·tial (spā'shăl). Relating to space or a space.

spa·ti·um, pl. **spa·tia** (spā'shē-ŭm, -shē-ă) [NA]. SYN space. [L.]

spa'tia an'guli iridocornea'lis [NA], SYN *spaces* of iridocorneal angle, under *space.*

s. episclera'le [NA], SYN episcleral *space.*

s. intercosta'le [NA], SYN intercostal *space.*

s. interfascia'le [NA], SYN episcleral *space.*

s. interglobula're, pl. **spa'tia interglobula'ria** [NA], SYN interglobular *space.*

spa'tia interos'sea metacar'pi [NA], SYN interosseous metacarpal *spaces,* under *space.*

spa'tia interos'sea metatar'si [NA], SYN interosseous metatarsal *spaces,* under *space.*

s. intervagina'le bulb'i oc'uli, SYN episcleral *space.*

spa'tia intervagina'lia ner'vi op'tici [NA], SYN intervaginal *space* of optic nerve.

s. lateropharyn'geum [NA], SYN lateral pharyngeal *space.* SEE ALSO retropharyngeal *space.*

s. perichoroidea'le [NA], SYN perichoroidal *space.*

s. perilymphat'icum [NA], SYN perilymphatic *space.*

s. perine'i profun'dum [NA], SYN deep perineal *space.*

s. perine'i superficia'le [NA], SYN superficial perineal *space.*

s. peripharyn'geum [NA], SYN peripharyngeal *space.*

s. retroinguina'le, SYN retroinguinal *space.*

s. retroperitonea'le [NA], SYN retroperitoneal *space.*

s. retropharyn'geum [NA], SYN retropharyngeal *space.* SEE ALSO lateral pharyngeal *space.*

s. retropu'bicum [NA], SYN retropubic *space.*

s. subdura'le [NA], SYN subdural *space.*

spa'tia zonula'ria [NA], SYN zonular *spaces,* under *space.*

spat·u·la (spach'ŭ-lă). A flat blade, like a knife blade but without a sharp edge, used in pharmacy for spreading plasters and ointments and as an aid to mixing ingredients with a mortar and pestle. [L. dim. of *spatha,* a broad, flat wooden instrument, fr. G. *spathē*]

Roux s., a very small nickeled steel s. used to transfer bits of infected material, such as diphtheritic membrane, to culture tubes.

spat·u·late (spach'ŭ-lāt). **1.** Shaped like a spatula. **2.** To manipulate or mix with a spatula. **3.** To incise the cut end of a tubular structure longitudinally and splay it open, to allow creation of an elliptical anastomosis of greater circumference than would be possible with conventional transverse or oblique (bevelled) end-to-end anastomoses. SYN spatulated.

spat·u·lat·ed (spach'ŭ-lāt-ed). SYN spatulate.

♻ **Combining forms**	**[NA]** Nomina Anatomica
Word*Finder* **Multi-term entry finder** Preceding letter A	**[MIM]** Mendelian **Inheritance in Man**
A.D.A.M. Anatomy Plates Between letters L and M	☆ **Official alternate term**
Appendices: **Following letter Z**	☆**[NA]** Official alternate Nomina Anatomica term
SYN Synonym; **Cf.,** compare	**High Profile Term**

spat·u·la·tion (spach′ŭ-lā′shŭn). Manipulation of material with a spatula.

Spatz, Hugo, German neurologist and psychiatrist, 1888–1969. SEE Hallervorden-S. *disease, syndrome.*

spav·in. A disease of the tarsal joints of the horse. [M.E. *spavayne,* swelling fr. O. Fr. *esparvain*]

blood s., a distention of the veins in the vicinity of the tarsus in a horse, due to pressure from the swelling of bog s. impeding the return flow of blood.

bog s., a chronic synovitis of the tibiotarsal joint in the horse resulting in distention of the joint capsule with fluid; it usually causes little or no lameness.

bone s., a rarefying osteitis involving the bones of the tarsus of the horse, usually those on the medial surface, resulting in exostoses and ankylosis.

spav·ined (spav′ind). Affected with spavin.

spay (spā). To remove the ovaries of an animal. [Gael. *spoth,* castrate, or G. *spadōn,* eunuch]

SPCA Abbreviation for serum prothrombin conversion *accelerator.*

spear·mint (spēr′mint). The leaves and flowering tops of *Mentha viridis* (green garden or lamb mint) or *M. cardiaca* (family Labiatae); a carminative and flavoring agent.

s. oil, the volatile oil, distilled with steam from the fresh overground parts of the flowering plant of *Mentha viridis* or *M. cardiaca,* a flavoring agent.

spe·cial·ist (spesh′ă-list). One who devotes professional attention to a particular specialty or subject area.

spe·cial·i·za·tion (spesh′ă-li-zā′shŭn). **1.** Professional attention limited to a particular specialty or subject area for study, research, and/or treatment. **2.** SYN differentiation (1).

spe·cial·ize (spesh′ă-līz). To engage in specialization (1).

spe·cial·ty (spesh′al-tē). The particular subject area or branch of medical science to which one devotes professional attention. [L. *specialitas* fr. *specialis,* special]

spe·ci·a·tion (spē-shē-ā′shŭn). The evolutionary process by which diverse species of animals or plants are formed from a common ancestral stock.

spe·cies, pl. **spe·cies** (spē′shēz). **1.** A biological division between the genus and a variety or the individual; a group of organisms that generally bear a close resemblance to one another in the more essential features of their organization, and breed effectively producing fertile progeny. **2.** A class of pharmaceutical preparations consisting of a mixture of dried plants, not pulverized, but in sufficiently fine division to be conveniently used in the making of extemporaneous decoctions or infusions, as a tea. [L. appearance, form, kind, fr. *specio,* to look at]

type s., the name of the single s. or of one of the s. of a genus or subgenus when the name of the genus or subgenus was originally validly published.

spe·cies-spe·cif·ic. Characteristic of a given species; serum that is produced by the injection of immunogens into an animal, and that acts only upon the cells, protein, etc., of a member of the same species as that from which the original antigen was obtained.

spe·cif·ic (spĕ-sif′ik). **1.** Relating to a species. SEE ALSO specific *epithet.* **2.** Relating to an individual infectious disease, one caused by a special microorganism. **3.** A remedy having a definite therapeutic action in relation to a particular disease or symptom, as quinine in relation to malaria. [L. *specificus* fr. *species + facio,* to make]

spec·i·fic·i·ty (spes-i-fis′i-tē). **1.** The condition or state of being specific, of having a fixed relation to a single cause or to a definite result; manifested in the relation of a disease to its pathogenic microorganism, of a reaction to a certain chemical union, or of an antibody to its antigen or the reverse. **2.** In clinical pathology and medical screening, the proportion of individuals with negative test results for the disease that the test is intended to reveal, *i.e.,* true negative results as a proportion of the total of true negative and false-positive results. Cf. sensitivity (2).

analytical s., freedom from interference by any element or compound other than the analyte.

diagnostic s., the probability (P) that, given the absence of disease (D), a normal test result (T) excludes disease; *i.e.,* P(T/D).

relative s., the s. of a medical screening test as determined by comparison with the same type of test (*e.g.,* s. of a new serological test relative to s. of an established serological test).

substrate s., the ability of an enzyme to recognize and bind its substrates, typically measured by the V_{max}/K_m or k_{cat}/K_m ratios.

spe·cif·ic optical ro·ta·tion ([α]). See under rotation.

spe·cil·lum, pl. **spe·cil·la** (spe-sil′ŭm, -lă). A probe or small sound. [L. a probe, fr. *specio,* to look at]

spec·i·men (spes′ĭ-men). A small part, or sample, of any substance or material obtained for testing. [L. fr. *specio,* to look at]

cytologic s., a s. obtainable by a variety of methods from many areas of the body, including the female genital tract, respiratory tract, urinary tract, alimentary tract, and body cavities; used for cytologic examination and diagnosis (*e.g.,* cytologic smears, filter preparations, centrifuged buttons).

SPECT Abbreviation for single photon emission computed *tomography.*

spec·ta·cles (spek′tĭ-klz). Lenses set in a frame that holds them in front of the eyes, used to correct errors of refraction or to protect the eyes. The parts of the s. are the *lenses;* the *bridge* between the lenses, resting on the nose; the *rims* or *frames,* encircling the lenses; the *sides* or *temples* that pass on either side of the head to the ears; the *bows,* the curved extremities of the temples; the *shoulders,* short bars attached to the rims or the lenses and jointed with the sides. SYN eyeglasses, glasses (1). [L. *specto,* pp. *-atus,* to watch, observe]

bifocal s., s. with bifocal lenses. SEE lens.

clerical s., SYN half-glass s.

divers' s., strongly convex lenses for clear vision underwater.

divided s., SYN Franklin s.

Franklin s., an early form of bifocal s. in which the lower half of the lens is for near vision, the upper half for distant vision. SYN divided s.

half-glass s., s., used for reading, in which the upper portion of the lenses are removed. SYN clerical s., pantoscopic s., pulpit s.

hemianopic s., s. with a prism or mirror to allow the individual with homonymous hemianopia to see objects in his blind half field.

lid crutch s., s. with little offsets of metal with smooth edges which engage above the upper eyelid and keep it raised above the pupil in cases of paralytic blepharoptosis. SYN Masselon's s.

Masselon's s., SYN lid crutch s.

orthoscopic s., convex lenses with base-in prisms for close work.

pantoscopic s., SYN half-glass s.

photochromic s., s. with lenses that darken on exposure to ultraviolet light.

protective s., s. which protect against ultraviolet or infrared rays or against mechanical injuries. SYN safety s.

pulpit s., SYN half-glass s.

safety s., SYN protective s.

stenopeic s., stenopaic s. (sten-ō-pā′ik), **(1)** opaque disks with narrow slits in the center allowing only a minimum amount of light to enter; used as a protection against snow blindness; **(2)** s. having opaque disks with multiple perforations used to aid vision in incipient cataract and in discrete opacities of the cornea; occasionally used as a substitute for corrective lenses or sunglasses.

telescopic s., magnifying s. obtained by using a convex objective lens and a concave eyepiece separated by the difference in their focal lengths.

spec·ti·no·my·cin hy·dro·chlo·ride (spek′ti-nō-mī′sin). Actinospectacin decahydro-4a,7,9-trihydroxy-2-methyl-6,8-bis-(methylamino)-4*H*-pyrano [2,3-*b*] [1,4]benzodioxin-4-one dihydrochloride; an antibiotic antibacterial agent.

spec·tra (spek′tră). Plural of spectrum. [L.]

spec·tral (spek′trăl). Relating to a spectrum.

spec·trin (spek'trin). A filamentous contractile protein that together with actin and other cytoskeleton proteins forms a network that gives the red blood cell membrane its shape and flexibility; a defect or deficiency of s. is associated with hereditary spherocytosis and hereditary elliptocytosis; the principal component of the membrane skeleton of red cells. It comprises two units, an alpha unit of molecular weight 240,000 [MIM*182860] and a beta unit of molecular weight 225,000 [MIM*182870].

spectro-. A spectrum. [L. *spectrum,* an image]

spec·tro·chem·is·try (spek'trō-kem'is-trē). The study of chemical substances and their identification by means of spectroscopy, *i.e.,* by light emitted or absorbed.

spec·tro·col·or·im·e·ter (spek'trō-kŏl-er-im'ĕ-ter). A colorimeter using a source of light from a selected portion of the spectrum, *i.e.,* of a selected wavelength.

spec·tro·flu·o·rom·e·ter (spek'trō-flŭr-om'ĕ-ter). An instrument for measuring the intensity and quality of fluorescence.

spec·tro·gram (spek'trō-gram). A graphic representation of a spectrum. [spectro- + G. *gramma,* something written]

spec·tro·graph (spek'trō-graf). An instrument used in spectography.

mass s., an instrument that subjects charged and accelerated ions (atomic or molecular) to a magnetic field that imparts a curved path that differs for each mass-to-charge ratio, thus separating individual species; used in detecting and assaying isotopic ratios and in molecular structure determinations.

spec·trog·ra·phy (spek-trog'ră-fē). The procedure of photographing or tracing a spectrum. [spectro- + G. *graphō,* to write]

spec·trom·e·ter (spek-trom'ĕ-ter). An instrument for determining the wavelength or energy of light or other electromagnetic emission. [spectro- + G. *metron,* measure]

spec·trom·e·try (spek-trom'ĕ-trē). The procedure of observing and measuring the wavelengths of light or other electromagnetic emissions.

clinical s., SYN biospectrometry.

spec·tro·pho·bia (spek-trō-fō'bē-ă). Morbid fear of mirrors or of one's mirrored image. [spectro- + G. *phobos,* fear]

spec·tro·pho·to·flu·o·rim·e·try (spek'trō-fō'tō-flŭr-im'ĕ-trē). Measurement of the intensity and quality of fluorescence by means of a spectrophotometer.

spec·tro·pho·tom·e·ter (spek'trō-fō-tom'ĕ-ter). An instrument for measuring the intensity of light of a definite wavelength transmitted by a substance or a solution, giving a quantitative measure of the amount of material in the solution absorbing the light; a colorimeter with a choice of wavelength and photometric measurement. [spectro- + photometer]

spec·tro·pho·tom·e·try (spek'trō-fō-tom'ĕ-trē). Analysis by means of a spectrophotometer.

atomic absorption s., determination of concentration by the ability of atoms to absorb radiant energy of specific wavelengths.

flame emission s., determination of the concentration of an element by measurement of light emitted when the element is excited by energy in the form of heat.

spec·tro·po·lar·im·e·ter (spek'trō-pō-lar-im'ĕ-ter). An instrument for measuring the rotation of the plane of polarized light of specific wavelength upon passage through a solution or translucent solid. [spectro- + polarimeter]

spec·tro·scope (spek'trō-skōp). An instrument for resolving light from any luminous body into its spectrum, and for the analysis of the spectrum so formed. It consists of a prism that refracts the light or a grating for diffraction of the light, an arrangement for rendering the rays parallel, and a telescope that magnifies the spectrum. [spectro- + G. *skopeō,* to view]

direct vision s., a s. consisting of a single tube containing a series of prisms; one end of the tube is placed in as close contact as possible with the substance to be examined while the observer places his eye at the opposite end; it can be used to make a spectroscopic examination of the blood *in vivo,* as in the ear lobe or web of the thumb.

spec·tro·scop·ic (spek-trō-skop'ik). Relating to or performed by means of a spectroscope.

spec·tros·co·py (spek-tros'kŏ-pē). Observation and study of spectra of absorbed or emitted light by means of a spectroscope.

clinical s., SYN biospectroscopy.

infrared s., the study of the specific absorption in the infrared region of the electromagnetic spectrum; used in the study of the chemical bonds within molecules.

magnetic resonance s., detection and measurement of the resonant spectra of molecular species in a tissue or sample.

spec·trum, pl. **spec·tra, spec·trums** (spek'trŭm, -ă, -ŭmz). **1.** The range of colors presented when white light is resolved into its constituent colors by being passed through a prism or through a diffraction grating: red, orange, yellow, green, blue, indigo, and violet, arranged in increasing frequency of vibration or decreasing wavelength. **2.** Figuratively, the range of pathogenic microorganisms against which an antibiotic or other antibacterial agent is active. **3.** The plot of intensity vs. wavelength of light emitted or absorbed by a substance, usually characteristic of the substance and used in qualitative and quantitative analysis. **4.** The range of wavelengths presented when a beam of radiant energy is subjected to dispersion and focused. [L. an image, fr. *specio,* to look at]

absorption s., the s. observed after light has passed through, and been partially absorbed by a solution or translucent substance; many molecular groupings have characteristic light absorption patterns, which can be used for detection and quantitative assay.

antimicrobial s., SEE spectrum (2).

broad s., a term indicating a broad range of activity of an antibiotic against a wide variety of microorganisms.

chromatic s., the continuum of colors that white light forms on passing through a prism or diffraction grating. SYN color s.

color s., SYN chromatic s.

continuous s., a s. in which there are no absorption bands or lines.

excitation s., fluorescence produced over a range of wavelengths of the exciting light.

fluorescence s., fluorescence evoked over a range of wavelengths when the excitation wavelength is at a maximum.

fortification s., the zigzag banding of light, resembling the walls of fortified medieval towns, that marks the margin of the scintillating scotoma of migraine. SYN fortification figures, telehopsias.

frequency s., the range of frequencies in a signal, used to describe the resolving power of an imaging system in radiology.

infrared s., the part of the invisible s. of wave length just longer than that of visible red light. SYN thermal s.

invisible s., the radiation lying on either side of visible light, *i.e.,* infrared and ultraviolet light.

Raman s., the characteristic array of light produced by the Raman effect.

thermal s., SYN infrared s.

toxin s., a figure in the form of a s. used by Ehrlich to represent the neutralizing power of antitoxin in the presence of toxin, toxone, etc.

ultraviolet s., the electromagnetic s. beyond the violet end of the visible s.

visible s., that part of electromagnetic radiation that is visible to the human eye; it extends from extreme red, 7606 Å (760.6 nm), to extreme violet, 3934 Å (393.4 nm).

wide s., SEE spectrum (3).

spec·u·lum, pl. **spec·u·la** (spek'yū-lŭm, -lă). An instrument for enlarging the opening of any canal or cavity in order to facilitate inspection of its interior. [L. a mirror, fr. *specio,* to look at]

bivalve s., a s. with two adjustable blades.

Cooke's s., a three-pronged s. for rectal examinations and operations.

duckbill s., a bivalve s., the blades of which are broad and flattened, resembling a duck's bill, used in inspection of the vagina and cervix.

eye s., an instrument for keeping the eyelids apart during inspection of or operation on the eye. SYN blepharostat.

Kelly's rectal s., a tubular s. with obturator for rectal examination.

sp

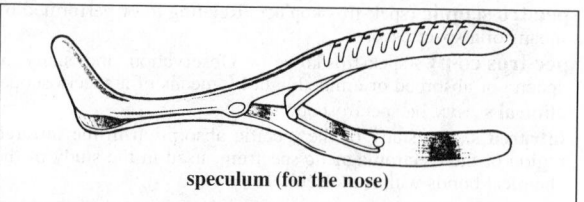

speculum (for the nose)

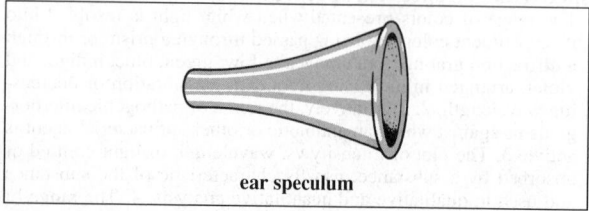

ear speculum

Pedersen's s., a narrow flat s. used in vaginas with a narrow introitus.

stop-s., a dilating s., as a s. of the eyelids, which is provided with a catch to prevent its being opened too wide.

Spee, Ferdinand Graf von, German embryologist, 1855–1937. SEE *curve* of S.

speech. Talk; the use of the voice in conveying ideas. [A.S. *spaec*]

alaryngeal s., a form of s. achieved after laryngectomy by using either an external vibratory source or the pharyngoesophageal segment as an internal vibratory source. Tracheoesophageal s. may be produced after laryngectomy by surgically diverting exhaled air to the pharynx by a permanently constructed tracheoesophageal fistula.

cerebellar s., an explosive type of utterance, with slurring of words.

clipped s., SYN scamping s.

echo s., SYN echolalia.

esophageal s., a technique for speaking following total laryngectomy; consists of swallowing air and regurgitating it, producing a vibration in the hypopharynx.

explosive s., loud, sudden s. related to injury of the nervous system. SYN logospasm (2).

helium s., the peculiar high-pitched, often unintelligible speech sounds produced when one breathes a mixture of up to 80 per cent helium and 20 per cent oxygen.

mirror s., a reversal of the order of syllables in a word, analogous to mirror writing.

scamping s., a form of lalling in which consonants or syllables that are difficult to pronounce are omitted. SYN clipped s.

scanning s., measured or metered, often slow s.

slurring s., slovenly articulation of the more difficult letter sounds.

spastic s., labored s. related to increased tone of muscles.

staccato s., an abrupt utterance, each syllable being enunciated separately; noted especially in multiple sclerosis. SYN syllabic s.

subvocal s., slight movements of the muscles of s. related to thinking but producing no sound.

syllabic s., SYN staccato s.

tracheoesophageal s., a form of alaryngeal s. obtained by a surgical technique which creates a shunt between trachea and esophagus, allowing pulmonary air to generate upper esophageal and pharyngeal mucosal vibrations as a substitute for vocal cord vibrations when the larynx is surgically removed.

speed (spēd). The magnitude of velocity without regard to direction. Cf. velocity.

spe·len·ceph·a·ly (spē-len-sef′ă-lē). SYN porencephaly. [*spēlaion,* cave, + *enkephalos,* brain]

Spens, Thomas, Scottish physician, 1764–1842. SEE S.'s *syndrome.*

sperm [NA]. **1.** SYN spermatozoon. **2.** SYN semen (1). [G. *sperma,* seed]

△**sperma-, spermato-, spermo-.** Semen, spermatozoa. [G. *sperma,* seed]

sper·ma·ce·ti (sper-mă-set′ē). A peculiar fatty, waxy substance, chiefly cetin (cetyl palmitate), obtained from the head of the sperm whale, *Physeter macrocephalus;* used to impart firmness to ointment bases. SYN cetaceum. [sperma- + G. *ketos,* whale]

sperm·ag·glu·ti·na·tion (sperm′ă-glū-ti-nā′shŭn). Agglutination of spermatozoa.

sperm-as·ter (sperm′as-ter). Cytocentrum with astral rays in the cytoplasm of an inseminated ovum; it is brought in by the penetrating spermatozoon and evolves into the mitotic spindle of the first cleavage division. [sperm + G. *astēr,* a star (aster)]

sper·mat·ic (sper-mat′ik). Relating to the sperm or semen.

sper·ma·tid (sper′mă-tid). A cell in a late stage of the development of the spermatozoon; it is a haploid cell derived from the secondary spermatocyte and evolves by spermiogenesis into a spermatozoon. SYN nematoblast. [spermat- + *-id* (2)]

sper·ma·tin (sper′mă-tin). Name proposed for an albuminoid in the seminal fluid.

△**spermato-.** SEE sperma-.

sper·ma·to·blast (sper′mă-tō-blast). SYN spermatogonium. [spermato- + G. *blastos,* germ]

sper·ma·to·cele (sper′mă-tō-sēl). Cyst of the epididymis containing spermatozoa. SYN spermatocyst. [spermato- + G. *kēlē,* tumor]

sper·ma·to·ci·dal (sper′mă-tō-sī′dăl). Destructive to spermatozoa. SYN spermicidal.

sper·ma·to·cide (sper′mă-tō-sīd). An agent destructive to spermatozoa. SYN spermicide. [spermato- + L. *caedo,* to kill]

sper·ma·to·cyst. SYN spermatocele.

sper·ma·to·cy·tal (sper-mă-tō-sī′tăl). Relating to spermatocytes.

sper·ma·to·cyte (sper′mă-tō-sīt). Parent cell of a spermatid, derived by mitotic division from a spermatogonium. [spermato- + G. *kytos,* cell]

primary s., the s. derived by a growth phase from a spermatogonium, and that undergoes the first division of meiosis.

secondary s., the s. derived from a primary s. by the first meiotic division; each secondary s. produces two spermatids by the second meiotic division.

sper·ma·to·cy·to·gen·e·sis (sper′mă-tō-sī′tō-jen′ĕ-sis). SYN spermatogenesis.

sper·ma·to·gen·e·sis (sper′mă-tō-jen′ĕ-sis). The entire process by which spermatogonial stem cells divide and differentiate into spermatozoa. SEE ALSO spermiogenesis. SYN spermatocytogenesis, spermatogeny. [spermato- + G. *genesis,* origin]

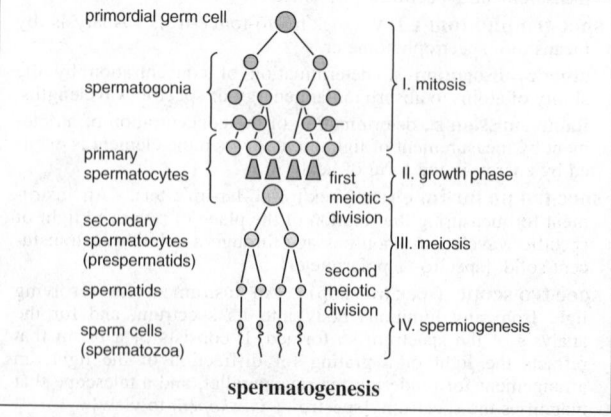

spermatogenesis

sper·ma·to·ge·net·ic (sper′mă-tō-jĕ-net′ik). SYN spermatogenic.

sper·ma·to·gen·ic (sper′mă-tō-jen′ik). Relating to spermatogenesis; sperm-producing. SYN spermatogenetic, spermatogenous, spermatopoietic (1).

sper·ma·tog·e·nous (sper-mă-toj′ĕ-nŭs). SYN spermatogenic.

sper·ma·tog·e·ny (sper-mă-toj′ĕ-nē). SYN spermatogenesis.

sper·ma·to·gone (sper′mă-tō-gōn). SYN spermatogonium.

sper·ma·to·go·ni·um (sper′mă-tō-gō′nē-ŭm). The primitive sperm cell derived by mitotic division from the germ cell; increasing several times in size, it becomes a primary spermatocyte. SEE ALSO spermatid. SYN spermatoblast, spermatogone. [spermato- + G. *gonē,* generation]

sper·ma·toid (sper′mă-tōid). **1.** Resembling a sperm, a sperm tail, or semen. **2.** A male or flagellated form of the malarial microparasite. [spermato + G. *eidos,* form]

sper·ma·tol·o·gy (sper-mă-tol′ō-jē). The branch of histology, physiology, and embryology concerned with sperm and/or seminal secretion. [spermato- + G. *logos,* study]

sper·ma·tol·y·sin (sper-mă-tol′i-sin). A specific lysin (antibody) formed in response to the repeated injection of spermatozoa.

sper·ma·tol·y·sis (sper-mă-tol′i-sis). Destruction, with dissolution, of the spermatozoa. SYN spermolysis. [spermato- + G. *lysis,* dissolution]

sper·ma·to·lyt·ic (sper′mă-tō-lit′ik). Relating to spermatolysis.

sper·ma·to·pho·bia (sper′mă-tō-fō′bē-ă). Morbid fear of spermatorrhea or loss of semen. [spermato- + G. *phobos,* fear]

sper·ma·to·phore (sper′mă-tō-fōr). A capsule containing spermatozoa; found in a number of invertebrates. [spermato- + G. *phoros,* bearing]

sper·ma·to·poi·et·ic (sper′mă-tō-poy-et′ik). **1.** SYN spermatogenic. **2.** Secreting semen. [spermato- + G. *poieō,* to make]

sper·ma·tor·rhea (sper′mă-tō-rē′ă). An involuntary discharge of semen, without orgasm. [spermato- + G. *rhoia,* a flow]

sper·ma·tox·in (sper-mă-tok′sin). A cytotoxic antibody specific for spermatozoa. SYN spermotoxin.

sper·ma·to·zoa (sper′mă-tō-zō′ă). Plural of spermatozoon.

sper·ma·to·zo·al, sper·ma·to·zo·an (sper′ma-tō-zō′ăl, -zō′ăn). Relating to spermatozoa.

sper·ma·to·zo·on, pl. **sper·ma·to·zoa** (sper′mă-tō-zō′on, -zō′ă). The male gamete or sex cell that contains the genetic information to be transmitted by the male, exhibits autokinesia, and is able to effect zygosis with an ovum. The human s. is composed of a head and a tail, the tail being divisible into a neck, a middle piece, a principal piece, and an end piece; the head, 4 to 6 μm in length, is a broadly oval, flattened body containing the nucleus; the tail is about 55 μm in length. SYN sperm (1) [NA], sperm cell. [G. *sperma,* seed, + *zōon,* animal]

sper·ma·tu·ria (sper-mă-tū′rē-ă). SYN semenuria.

sper·mia (sper′mē-ă). Plural of spermium.

sper·mi·ci·dal (sper-mi-sī′dăl). SYN spermatocidal.

sper·mi·cide (sper′mi-sīd). SYN spermatocide.

sper·mi·dine (sper′mi-dēn). NH₂(CH₂)₄NH(CH₂)₃NH₂; *N*-(3-Aminopropyl)butanediamine; a polyamine found with spermine in a wide variety of organisms and tissues; found in human sperm; important in cell and tissue growth.

sper·mi·duct (sper′mi-dŭkt). **1.** SYN *ductus* deferens. **2.** SYN ejaculatory *duct.*

sperm·ine (sper′mēn). NH₂(CH₂)₃NH(CH₂)₄NH(CH₂)₃NH₂; *N,N*′-bis(3-aminopropyl)-1,4-butanediamine; an essential growth factor in some bacteria; associated with nucleic acids in some viruses; found in human sperm; important in cell and tissue growth. SYN gerontine, musculamine, neuridine.

sper·mi·o·gen·e·sis (sper′mē-ō-jen′ĕ-sis). That segment of spermatogenesis during which immature spermatids become spermatozoa. [sperm- + G. *genesis,* origin]

sperm·ism (sper′mizm). The belief by preformationists that the male sex cell (sperm) contains a miniature preformed body called the homunculus.

sperm·ist. A preformationist who believed in the concept of spermism.

sper·mi·um, pl. **sper·mia** (sper′mē-ŭm, -ă). H.W.G. Waldeyer's term for the mature male germ cell or spermatozoon.

spermo-. SEE sperma-.

sper·mo·lith (sper′mō-lith). A concretion in the ductus deferens. [spermo- + G. *lithos,* stone]

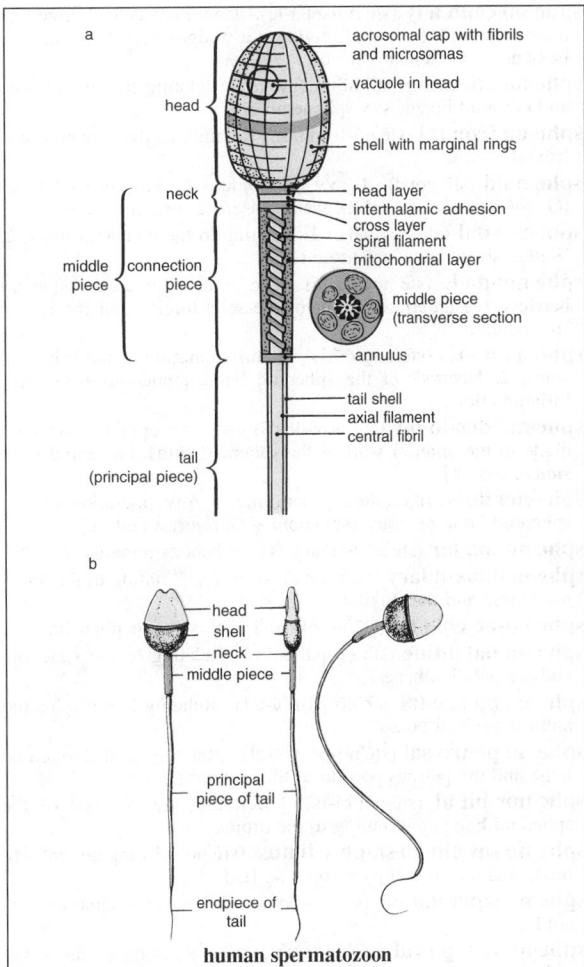

human spermatozoon

sper·mol·y·sis (sper-mol′i-sis). SYN spermatolysis.

sper·mo·tox·in (sper-mō-tok′sin). SYN spermatoxin.

SPF Abbreviation for sun protection *factor.*

sp. gr. Abbreviation for specific *gravity.*

sph. Abbreviation for spherical, or spherical *lens.*

sphac·e·late (sfas′ĕ-lāt). To become gangrenous or necrotic. [G. *sphakelos,* gangrene]

sphac·e·la·tion (sfas-ĕ-lā′shŭn). **1.** The process of becoming gangrenous or necrotic. **2.** Gangrene or necrosis. [G. *sphakelos,* gangrene]

sphac·el·ism (sfas′ĕ-lizm). The condition manifested by a sphacelus.

sphac·e·lo·der·ma (sfas′ĕ-lō-der′mă). Gangrene of the skin. [G. *sphakelos,* gangrene, + *derma,* skin]

sphac·e·lous (sfas′ĕ-lŭs). Sloughing, gangrenous, or necrotic.

sphac·e·lus (sfas′ĕ-lŭs). A mass of sloughing, gangrenous, or necrotic matter. [G. *sphakelos,* gangrene]

sphen·eth·moid (sfē-neth′moyd). SYN sphenoethmoid.

sphe·ni·on (sfē′nē-on). The tip of the sphenoidal angle of the parietal bone; a craniometric point. [Mod. L. fr. G. *sphēn,* wedge, + dim. *-iōn*]

△spheno-. Wedge, wedge-shaped; the sphenoid bone. [G. *sphēn,* wedge]

sphe·no·bas·i·lar (sfē′nō-bas′i-lăr). Relating to the sphenoid bone and the basilar process of the occipital bone. SYN spheno-occipital, sphenoccipital.

sphe·noc·cip·i·tal (sfē′nok-sip′i-tăl). SYN sphenobasilar.

sp

sphe·no·ceph·a·ly (sfē′nō-sef′ă-lē). Condition characterized by a deformation of the skull giving it a wedge-shaped appearance. [spheno- + G. *kephalē*, head]

sphe·no·eth·moid (sfē-nō-eth′moyd). Relating to the sphenoid and ethmoid bones. SYN sphenethmoid.

sphe·no·fron·tal (sfē′nō-fron′tăl). Relating to the sphenoid and frontal bones.

sphe·noid (sfē′noyd). 1. SYN sphenoidal. 2. SYN sphenoid *bone*. [G. *sphēnoeidēs*, fr. *sphēn*, wedge, + *eidos*, resemblance]

sphe·noi·dal (sfē-noy′dăl). 1. Relating to the sphenoid bone. 2. Wedge-shaped. SYN sphenoid (1).

sphe·noi·da·le (sfē-noy-dā′lē). The point of greatest convexity between the anterior contour of the sella turcica and the jugum sphenoidale.

sphe·noid·i·tis (sfē-noy-dī′tis). 1. Inflammation of the sphenoid sinus. 2. Necrosis of the sphenoid bone. [sphenoid + G. *-itis*, inflammation]

sphe·noi·dos·to·my (sfe-noy-dos′tō-mē). An operative opening made in the anterior wall of the sphenoid sinus. [sphenoid + G. *stoma*, mouth]

sphe·noi·dot·o·my (sfē′noy-dot′ō-mē). Any operation on the sphenoid bone or sinus. [sphenoid + G. *tomē*, a cutting]

sphe·no·ma·lar (sfē′nō-mā′lăr). SYN sphenozygomatic.

sphe·no·max·il·lary (sfē′nō-mak′si-lār-ē). Relating to the sphenoid bone and the maxilla.

sphe·no·oc·cip·i·tal (sfē′nō-ok-sip′i-tăl). SYN sphenobasilar.

sphe·no·pal·a·tine (sfē-nō-pal′ă-tīn). Relating to the sphenoid and the palatine bones.

sphe·no·pa·ri·e·tal (sfē′nō-pă-rī′ă-tăl). Relating to the sphenoid and the parietal bones.

sphe·no·pe·tro·sal (sfē′nō-pe-trō′săl). Relating to the sphenoid bone and the petrous portion of the temporal bone.

sphe·nor·bit·al (sfē-nōr′bi-tăl). Denoting the portions of the sphenoid bone contributing to the orbits.

sphe·no·sal·pin·go·staph·y·li·nus (sfē′nō-sal-ping′gō-staf-i-lī′ nŭs). SEE tensor veli palati *muscle*. [L.]

sphe·no·squa·mo·sal (sfē′nō-skwā-mō′săl). SYN squamosphenoid.

sphe·no·tem·po·ral (sfē′nō-tem′pŏ-răl). Relating to the sphenoid and the temporal bones.

sphe·not·ic (sfē-nō′tik). Relating to the sphenoid bone and the bony case of the ear. [spheno- + G. *ous*, ear]

sphe·no·tur·bi·nal (sfē′nō-ter′bi-năl). Denoting the concha sphenoidalis.

sphe·no·vo·mer·ine (sfē′nō-vō′mer-ēn, -īn). Relating to the sphenoid bone and the vomer.

sphe·no·zy·go·mat·ic (sfē′nō-zī-gō-mat′ik). Relating to the sphenoid and the zygomatic bones. SYN sphenomalar.

sphere (sfēr). A ball or globular body. [G. *sphaira*]
    attraction s., SYN astrosphere.
    Morgagni's s.'s, SYN Morgagni's *globules,* under *globule.*

sphe·res·the·sia (sfēr-es-thē′zē-ă). Rarely used term for *globus hystericus.* [G. *sphaira,* sphere, + *aisthēsis,* sensation]

spher·i·cal (sph.) (sfēr′i-kăl). Pertaining to, or shaped like, a sphere.

△ **sphero-.** Spherical, a sphere. [G. *sphaira,* globe]

sphe·ro·cyl·in·der (sfēr′ō-sil′in-der). SYN spherocylindrical *lens.*

sphe·ro·cyte (sfēr′ō-sīt). A small, spherical red blood cell. [sphero- + G. *kytos,* cell]

sphe·ro·cy·to·sis (sfēr′ō-sī-tō′sis). Presence of sphere-shaped red blood cells in the blood. [spherocyte + G. *-osis,* condition]
    hereditary s. [MIM*182900], a congenital defect of spectrin [MIM*182860] the main component of the erythrocyte cell membrane, which becomes abnormally permeable to sodium, resulting in thickened and almost spherical erythrocytes that are fragile and susceptible to spontaneous hemolysis, with decreased survival in the circulation; results in chronic anemia with reticulocytosis, episodes of mild jaundice due to hemolysis, and acute crises with gallstones, fever, and abdominal pain; symptomatolo-

gy is highly variable; autosomal dominant inheritance. However, as with elliptocytosis, there is an autosomal recessive form [MIM*270970]. SYN chronic acholuric jaundice, chronic familial icterus, chronic familial jaundice, congenital hemolytic icterus, congenital hemolytic jaundice, globe cell anemia, icterohemolytic anemia, spherocytic anemia.

sphe·roid, sphe·roi·dal (sfēr′oyd, sfir-; sfē-royd′ăl). Shaped like a sphere. [L. *spheroideus*]

sphe·rom·e·ter (sfēr-om′ě-ter). An instrument to determine the curvature of a sphere or a spherical lens. SEE Geneva lens measure. [sphero- + G. *metron,* measure]

sphe·ro·pha·ki·a (sfēr-ō-fā′kē-ă). A congenital bilateral aberration in which the lenses are small, spherical, and subject to subluxation; may occur as an independent anomaly or may be associated with the Weill-Marchesani syndrome. [sphero- + G. *phakos,* lens]

sphe·ro·plast (sfēr′ō-plast). A bacterial cell from which the rigid cell wall has been incompletely removed. The bacterium loses its characteristic shape and becomes round. [sphero- + G. *plastos,* formed]

sphe·ro·prism (sfēr′ō-prizm). A spherical lens decentered to produce a prismatic effect, or a combined spherical lens and prism.

sphe·ro·sper·mia (sfēr′ō-sper′mē-ă). Spheroid spermatozoa lacking an elongated tail, in contrast to the threadlike, tailed sperm of humans and other mammals (nematospermia). [sphero- + G. *sperma,* seed]

spher·ule (sfēr′ūl). 1. A small spherical structure. 2. A sporangial-like structure filled with endospores at maturity, produced within tissue and *in vitro* by *Coccidioides immitis.* [LL. *sphaerula,* dim. of L. *sphaera,* sphere, ball]

sphinc·ter (sfingk′ter). A muscle that encircles a duct, tube or orifice in such a way that its contraction constricts the lumen or orifice; it is the closing component of a pylorus (the outer component is the s. dilator). SYN musculus sphincter [NA], sphincter muscle. [G. *sphinktēr,* a band or lace]
    anatomical s., an accumulation of muscular circular fibers or specially arranged oblique fibers the function of which is to reduce partially or totally the lumen of a tube, the orifice of an organ, or the cavity of a viscus; the closing component of a pylorus.
    s. angula′ris, angular s., thickening of the circular muscular layer forming a proposed intermediate s. at the level of the angular notch of the stomach. While the thickening of the circular muscle may indicate the commencement of the pyloric antrum, true functional sphincteric activity distinct from the other peristaltic contractions of the stomach is not observed although some of these may in fact temporarily close off the antrum from the remainder of the stomach lumen. SYN antral s., midgastric transverse s., s. antri, s. intermedius, s. of antrum, s. of gastric antrum.
    s. a′ni, anal s., SEE external anal s., internal anal s.
    s. a′ni ter′tius, the third s. of the anorectum, a physiological s. at the sigmoidorectal junction.
    annular s., a short thickening of circular muscular fibers, similar to a ring; a ring-shaped s. as opposed to a segmental s.
    antral s., SYN s. angularis.
    s. an′tri, SYN s. angularis.
    s. of antrum, SYN s. angularis.
    artificial s., a s. produced by surgical procedures to reduce speed of flow in the digestive system or to maintain continence of the intestine.
    basal s., the thickening of the circular muscular coat at the base of the ileal papilla at the terminal ileum. SYN sphincteroid tract of ileum.
    bicanalicular s., a s. encircling two canals, such as the terminal portions of the common bile duct and the main pancreatic duct.
    Boyden's s., SYN s. of common bile duct.
    canalicular s., a s. located somewhere along the course of an organ, a tube, or a duct, as opposed to ostial s.
    choledochal s., SYN s. of common bile duct.
    colic s., one of the physiological s.'s of the colon.

s. of common bile duct, smooth muscle sphincter of the common bile duct immediately proximal to the hepatopancreatic ampulla; it is this sphincter that controls the flow of bile in the duodenum. SYN musculus sphincter ductus choledochi [NA], Boyden's s., choledochal s., sphincter muscle of common bile duct.

s. constric'tor car'diae, SYN inferior esophageal s.

duodenal s., one of the physiological s.'s described in the duodenum.

duodenojejunal s., the s. supposedly present at the duodenojejunal flexure.

external anal s., a fusiform ring of striated muscular fibers surrounding the anus, attached posteriorly to the coccyx and anteriorly to the central tendon of the perineum; it is subdivided, often indistinctly, into a subcutaneous part, a superficial part and a deep part for descriptive purposes. SYN musculus sphincter ani externus [NA], external sphincter muscle of anus.

external urethral s., SYN s. urethrae.

extrinsic s., a s. provided by circular muscular fibers extraneous to the organ.

first duodenal s., the s. supposedly located at the level of the aboral extremity of the duodenal bulb.

functional s., SYN physiological s.

s. of gastric antrum, SYN s. angularis.

Glisson's s., SYN s. of hepatopancreatic ampulla.

s. of hepatic flexure of colon, physiological s. at the level of the right colic flexure.

hepatopancreatic s., SYN s. of hepatopancreatic ampulla.

s. of hepatopancreatic ampulla, the smooth muscle sphincter of the hepatopancreatic ampulla within the duodenal papilla. SYN musculus sphincter ampullae hepatopancreaticae [NA], Glisson's s., hepatopancreatic s., Oddi's s.

Hyrtl's s., a band, generally incomplete, of circular muscular fibers in the rectum about 10 cm above the anus (upper rectal ampulla). SEE Nélaton's s.

ileal s., a thickening of circular musculature at the free margin of the ileal papilla. SYN ileocecocolic s., marginal s., operculum ilei, Varolius' s.

ileocecocolic s., SYN ileal s.

iliopelvic s., SYN midsigmoid s.

inferior esophageal s., a s. supposedly present at the esophagogastric junction; this is in fact an extrinsic sphincter formed by the surrounding musculature of the esophageal hiagus of the right crus of the diaphragm; causes a normally-occuring constriction at the esophagogastric junction observable with a barium swallow. SYN s. constrictor cardiae.

s. intermedius, SYN s. angularis.

internal anal s., a smooth muscle ring, formed by an increase of the circular fibers of the rectum, situated at the upper end of the anal canal, internal to the outer voluntary external anal sphincter. This sphincter is maximally-contracted when the rectal ampulla is "at rest" - empty or relaxed to accommodate a distending fecal mass. It is inhibited with filling of the ampulla, increased distension and peristalsis. SYN musculus sphincter ani internus [NA], internal sphincter muscle of anus.

internal urethral s., SYN s. vesicae.

intrinsic s., a thickening of the circular fibers of the muscular coat of an organ.

lower esophageal s. (LES), musculature of the gastroesophageal junction that is tonically active except during swallowing.

macroscopic s., a s. visible to the naked eye.

marginal s., SYN ileal s.

mediocolic s., a physiological s. located midway in the ascending colon.

microscopic s., a s. visible only under the microscope.

midgastric transverse s., SYN s. angularis.

midsigmoid s., the physiological s. midway in the sigmoid colon. SYN iliopelvic s.

myovascular s., a s. having a muscular and a vascular (usually venous) component. SEE myovenous s.

myovenous s., a s. having a muscular and a venous component, *e.g.,* at the pharyngoesophageal junction and anal canal.

Nélaton's s., SEE transverse rectal *folds,* under *fold.* SYN Nélaton's fibers.

O'Beirne's s., SYN rectosigmoid s.

s. oc'uli, SYN orbicularis oculi *muscle.*

Oddi's s., SYN s. of hepatopancreatic ampulla.

s. o'ris, SYN orbicularis oris *muscle.*

ostial s., a thickening of circular muscular fibers at the level of an orifice.

palatopharyngeal s., a constant band of the superior pharyngeal constrictor muscle which sweeps posteriorly from the anterolateral part of the superior surface of the palatine aponeurosis. It creates a visible ridge when the superior constrictor is contracted, meeting the elevated soft palate to seal off the pharyngeal isthmus during swallowing. SYN pharyngeal ridge, s. of the pharyngeal isthmus, velopharyngeal s.

pancreatic s., SYN s. of pancreatic duct.

s. of pancreatic duct, smooth muscle sphincter of the main pancreatic duct immediately proximal to the hepatoduodenal, ampulla. SYN musculus sphincter ductus pancreatici, pancreatic s., sphincter muscle of pancreatic duct.

pathologic s., a thickening of circular musculature caused by disease.

pelvirectal s., SYN rectosigmoid s.

s. of the pharyngeal isthmus, SYN palatopharyngeal s.

physiological s., a section of a tubular structure that acts as if it has a band of circular muscle to constrict it, although no such specialized structure can be found on morphological examination. SYN functional s., radiological s.

postpyloric s., the duodenal portion of the s. or closing mechanism of the gastroduodenal pylorus.

prepapillary s., a s. of duodenum described in the location oral to the major duodenal papilla.

preprostate urethral s., SYN s. vesicae.

prepyloric s., a band of circular muscular fibers in the wall of the stomach near the gastroduodenal pylorus.

proximal urethral s., SYN s. vesicae.

s. pupil'lae, a ring of smooth muscle fibers surrounding the pupillary border of the iris. SYN musculus sphincter pupillae [NA], sphincter muscle of pupil.

pyloric s., a thickening of the circular layer of the gastric musculature encircling the gastroduodenal junction. SYN musculus sphincter pylori [NA], sphincter muscle of pylorus.

radiological s., SYN physiological s.

rectosigmoid s., a circular band of muscular fibers at the rectosigmoid junction. SYN O'Beirne's s., O'Beirne's valve, pelvirectal s.

segmental s., a s. of a segment of an organ, a tube, or a canal, and longer than an annular s.

smooth muscular s., SYN lissosphincter.

striated muscular s., SYN rhabdosphincter.

superior esophageal s., SYN cricopharyngeus *muscle.* SEE inferior constrictor *muscle* of pharynx.

s. of third portion of duodenum, a physiological s. supposedly located at the horizontal (inferior) portion of the duodenum.

unicanalicular s., a s. limited to one visceral canal or tube.

s. ure'thrae, *origin,* ramus of pubis; *insertion,* with fellow in median raphe behind and in front of urethra; *action,* constricts membranous urethra; *nerve supply,* pudendal. SYN musculus sphincter urethrae [NA], external urethral s., Guthrie's muscle, musculus compressor urethrae, musculus constrictor urethrae, musculus sphincter urethrae membranaceae, sphincter muscle of urethra, Wilson's muscle (1).

s. vagi'nae, (1) SYN bulbocavernosus *muscle.* **(2)** SYN deep transverse perineal *muscle.*

Varolius' s., SYN ileal s.

velopharyngeal s., SYN palatopharyngeal s.

s. vesi'cae, the complete collar of smooth muscle cells of the neck of the urinary bladder which extend distally to surround the preprostatic sportion of the male urethra. There is not a comparable structure in the neck of the femoral bladder; the internal urethral s. may exist to prevent reflux of semen into bladder. SYN annulus urethralis, internal urethral s., musculus sphincter vesicae, preprostate urethral s., proximal urethral s., sphincter muscle of urinary bladder.

s. vesi'cae biliaris, the s. of the gallbladder, at the transition between the neck of the gallbladder and the cystic duct.

sphinc·ter·al (sfingk'ter-ăl). Relating to a sphincter. SYN sphincterial, sphincteric.

sphinc·ter·al·gia (sfing-ter-al'jē-ă). Pain in the sphincter ani muscles. [sphincter + G. *algos,* pain]

sphinc·ter·ec·to·my (sfingk-ter-ek'tō-mē). 1. Excision of a portion of the pupillary border of the iris. 2. Dissecting away any sphincter muscle. [sphincter + G. *ektomē,* excision]

sphinc·te·ri·al, sphinc·ter·ic (sfingk-tēr'ē-ăl, -ter-ik). SYN sphincteral.

sphinc·ter·is·mus (sfingk-ter-iz'mŭs). Spasmodic contraction of the sphincter ani muscles.

sphinc·ter·i·tis (sfingk'ter-ī'tis). Inflammation of any sphincter.

sphinc·ter·oid (sfingk'ter-oyd). Denoting similarity to a musculus sphincter. [sphincter + G. *eidos,* resemblance]

sphinc·ter·ol·y·sis (sfingk-ter-ol'i-sis). An operation for freeing the iris from the cornea in anterior synechia involving only the pupillary border. [sphincter, + G. *lysis,* loosening]

sphinc·ter·o·plas·ty (sfingk'ter-ō-plas-tē). Plastic surgery of any sphincter muscle. [sphincter + G. *plastos,* formed]

sphinc·ter·o·scope (sfingk'ter-ō-skōp). A speculum to facilitate inspection of the internal sphincter ani muscle. [sphincter + G. *skopeō,* to view]

sphinc·ter·os·co·py (sfingk'ter-os'kŏ-pē). Visual examination of a sphincter.

sphinc·ter·o·tome (sfingk'ter-ō-tōm). An instrument for incising a sphincter.

sphinc·ter·ot·o·my (sfingk-tĕ-rot'ō-mē). Incision or division of a sphincter muscle. [sphincter + G. *tomē,* incision]

external s., transurethral incision of external urethral sphincter.

transduodenal s., division of Oddi's sphincter; an operation to open the lower end of the common duct to remove impacted stones or to relieve spasm or stricture of the terminal bile and pancreatic ducts.

sphin·ga·nine (sfing'gă-nēn). Dihydrosphingosine; 2*D*- or D-*erythro*-2- or (2*S*,3*R*)-2-amino-1,3-octadecanediol; a constituent of the sphingolipids.

(4*E***)-sphin·gen·ine** (sfing'gen-ēn). SYN sphingosine.

sphing·ol (sfing'gol). SYN sphingosine.

sphin·go·lip·id (sfing'gō-lip-id). Any lipid containing a long-chain base like that of sphingosine (*e.g.,* ceramides, cerebrosides, gangliosides, sphingomyelins); a constituent of nerve tissue.

sphin·go·lip·i·do·sis (sfing'gō-lip-i-dō'sis). Collective designation for a variety of diseases characterized by abnormal sphingolipid metabolism, *e.g.,* gangliosidosis, Gaucher's disease, Niemann-Pick disease. SYN sphingolipodystrophy.

cerebral s., any one of a group of inherited diseases characterized by failure to thrive, hypertonicity, progressive spastic paralysis, loss of vision and occurrence of blindness, usually with macular degeneration and optic atrophy, convulsions, and mental deterioration; associated with abnormal storage of sphingomyelin and related lipids in the brain. Four types are recognized as clinically and enzymatically distinct: 1) **infantile type** (Tay-Sachs disease, G_{M2} gangliosidosis) due to a deficiency of hexosaminidase A; 2) **early juvenile type** (Jansky-Bielschowsky or Bielschowsky's disease); 3) **late juvenile type** (Spielmeyer-Vogt disease; Spielmeyer-Sjögren disease; Batten-Mayou disease; ceroid lipofuscinosis); and 4) **adult type** (Kufs disease). SYN cerebral lipidosis.

sphin·go·lip·o·dys·tro·phy (sfing'gō-lip-ō-dis'trō-fē). SYN sphingolipidosis.

sphin·go·my·e·li·nase (sfing'gō-mi'ĕ-li-nās). SYN sphingomyelin phosphodiesterase.

sphin·go·my·e·lin phos·pho·di·es·ter·ase (sfing'gō-mī'ĕ-lin). An enzyme catalyzing hydrolysis of sphingomyelin to *N*-acylsphingosine (a ceramide) and phosphocholine; a deficiency of this enzyme is associated with type I Niemann-Pick disease. SYN sphingomyelinase.

sphingolipidosis classified according to storage substance and corresponding enzyme defect (not all variants included)		
disease	storage substance	enzymes in question
Niemann-Pick disease (sphingo-myelinosis, type A)	sphingomyelin	sphingo-myelinase
Gaucher's disease	gluco-cerebroside	β-glucosidase
globoid cell leukodystrophy	galacto-cerebroside	cerebroside-β-galactosidase
metachromatic leukodystrophy	sulfatide	cerebroside-sulfatase, arylsulfatase A
Fabry disease	ceramide-trihexoside	α-galactosidase
gangliosidoses (see table)		

sphin·go·my·e·lins (sfing'gō-mī'ĕ-linz). A group of phospholipids, found in brain, spinal cord, kidney, and egg yolk, containing 1-phosphocholine (choline *O*-phosphate) combined with a ceramide (a long-chain fatty acid linked to the nitrogen of a long-chain base, such as sphingosine). SYN ceramide 1-phosphorylcholine, phosphosphingosides.

sphin·go·sine (sfing'gō-sēn). $CH_3(CH_2)_{12}CH=CHCH(O H)CH(NH_2)CH_2OH$; (4*E*)-Sphingenine (2*S*,3*R*,4*E*)-2-amino-4-octadecene-1,3-diol; the principal long-chain base found in sphingolipids. SYN (4*E*)-sphingenine, sphingol.

△**sphygm-.** SEE sphygmo-.

sphyg·mic (sfig'mik). Relating to the pulse.

△**sphyg·mo-, sphygm-.** Pulse. [G. *sphygmos*]

sphyg·mo·car·di·o·graph (sfig'mō-kar'dē-ō-graf). A polygraph recording both the heartbeat and the radial pulse. SYN sphygmocardioscope. [sphygmo- + G. *kardia,* heart, + *graphō,* to write]

sphyg·mo·car·di·o·scope (sfig'mō-kar'dē-ō-skōp). SYN sphygmocardiograph. [sphygmo- + G. *skopeō,* to view]

sphyg·mo·chron·o·graph (sfig'mō-kron'ō-graf). A modified sphygmograph that represents graphically the time relations between the beat of the heart and the pulse; one recording the character of the pulse as well as its rapidity. [sphygmo- + G. *chronos,* time, + *graphō,* to write]

sphyg·mo·gram (sfig'mō-gram). The graphic curve made by a sphygmograph. SYN pulse curve. [sphygmo- + G. *gramma,* something written]

sphyg·mo·graph (sfig'mō-graf). An instrument consisting of a lever, the short end of which rests on the radial artery at the wrist, its long end being provided with a stylet which records on a moving ribbon of smoked paper the excursions of the pulse. [sphygmo- + G. *graphō,* to write]

sphyg·mo·graph·ic (sfig-mō-graf'ik). Relating to or made by a sphygmograph; denoting the s. tracing, or sphygmogram.

sphyg·mog·ra·phy (sfig-mog'ră-fē). Use of the sphygmograph in recording the character of the pulse.

sphyg·moid (sfig'moyd). Pulselike; resembling the pulse. [sphygmo- + G. *eidos,* resemblance]

sphyg·mo·ma·nom·e·ter (sfig'mō-mă-nom'ĕ-ter). An instrument for measuring arterial blood pressure consisting of an inflatable cuff, inflating bulb, and a guage showing the blood pressure. SYN sphygmometer. [sphygmo- + G. *manos,* thin, scanty, + *metron,* measure]

Mosso's s., an apparatus for measuring the blood pressure in the digital arteries.

Riva-Rocci s., the original blood pressure apparatus first used to noninvasively measure arterial pressure.

Rogers' s., an s. with an aneroid barometer gauge.

sphyg·mo·ma·nom·e·try (sfig′mō-mă-nom′ĕ-trē). Determination of the blood pressure by means of a sphygmomanometer.

sphyg·mom·e·ter (sfig-mom′ĕ-ter). SYN sphygmomanometer.

sphyg·mo·met·ro·scope (sfig-mō-met′rō-skōp). An instrument for auscultating the pulse, used especially in the auscultatory method of reading the blood pressure, particularly the diastolic pressure. [sphygmo- + G. *metron*, measure, + *skopeō*, to view]

sphyg·mo·os·cil·lom·e·ter (sfig′mō-os′i-lom′ĕ-ter). An instrument resembling an aneroid sphygmomanometer used in the measurement of the systolic and diastolic blood pressure. [sphygmo- + L. *oscillo*, to swing, + G. *metron*, measure]

sphyg·mo·pal·pa·tion (sfig′mō-pal-pa′shŭn). Feeling the pulse. [sphygmo- + L. *palpatio*, palpation]

sphyg·mo·phone (sfig′mō-fōn). An instrument by which a sound is produced with each beat of the pulse. [sphygmo- + G. *phōnē*, sound]

sphyg·mo·scope (sfig′mō-skōp). An instrument by which the pulse beats are made visible by causing fluid to rise in a glass tube, by means of a mirror projecting a beam of light, or simply by a moving lever as in the sphygmograph. [sphygmo- + G. *skopeō*, to view]

Bishop's s., an instrument for measuring the blood pressure, with special reference to diastolic pressure; the tube is filled with a solution of cadmium borotungstate, and the scale is the reverse of that of a mercurial manometer, the pressure being made directly by the weight of the liquid and not by compressed air.

sphyg·mos·co·py (sfig-mos′kŏ-pē). Examination of the pulse. [sphygmo- + G. *skopeō*, to view]

sphyg·mo·sys·to·le (sfig-mō-sis′tō-lē). Obsolete term for that segment of the pulse wave corresponding to the cardiac systole. [sphygmo- + G. *systolē*, a contracting]

sphyg·mo·ton·o·graph (sfig-mō-tō′nō-graf). An instrument for recording graphically both the pulse and the blood pressure. [sphygmo- + G. *tonos*, tension, + *graphō*, to write]

sphyg·mo·to·nom·e·ter (sfig-mō-tō-nom′ĕ-ter). An instrument, like the sphygmotonograph, for determining the degree of blood pressure. [sphygmo- + G. *tonos*, tension, + *metron*, measure]

sphyg·mo·vis·co·sim·e·try (sfig-mō-vis-kō-sim′ĕ-trē). Measurement of the pressure and the viscosity of the blood.

spi·ca, pl. **spi·cae** (spī′kă, spī′kē). SEE bandage. [L. a point, an ear of grain]

spic·u·la (spik′yū-lă). Plural of spiculum. [L.]

spic·u·lar (spik′yū-lăr). Relating to or having spicules.

spic·ule (spik′yūl). A small needle-shaped body. [L. *spiculum*, dim. of *spica*, or *spicum*, a point]

spic·u·lum, pl. **spic·u·la** (spik′yū-lŭm, -lă). A spicule or small spike. [L.]

spi·der (spī′der). **1.** An arthropod of the order Araneida (subclass Arachnida) characterized by four pairs of legs, a cephalothorax, a globose smooth abdomen, and a complex of web-spinning spinnerets. Among the venomous s.'s found in the New World are the black widow s., *Latrodectus mactans;* red-legged widow s., *Latrodectus bishopi;* pruning s., or Peruvian tarantula, *Glyptocranium gasteracanthoides;* Chilean brown s., *Loxosceles laeta;* Peruvian brown s., *Loxosceles rufiper;* brown recluse s. of North America, *Loxosceles reclusus.* **2.** SYN spider *angioma.* **3.** An obstructive growth in the teat of a cow. [O. E. *spinnan*, to spin]

arterial s., SYN spider *angioma.*

vascular s., SYN spider *angioma.*

spi·der·burst (spī′der-berst). Radiating dull red capillary lines on the skin of the leg, usually without any visible or palpable varicose veins, but nevertheless due to deep-seated venous dilation; sometimes referred to as skyrocket capillary ectasis. [*spider*web + sun*burst*]

Spiegelberg, Otto, German gynecologist, 1830–1881. SEE S.'s *criteria,* under *criterion.*

Spieghel, Adrian van der. SEE Spigelius.

Spiegler, Eduard, Austrian dermatologist, 1860–1908. SEE S.-Fendt *pseudolymphoma, sarcoid.*

Spielmeyer, Walter, Munich neurologist, 1879–1935. SEE S.'s acute *swelling;* S.-Stock *disease;* S.-Vogt *disease.*

spi·ge·li·an (spī-jē′lē-an). Relating to or described by Spigelius.

Spigelius, Adrian (van der Spieghel), Flemish anatomist in Padua, 1578–1625. SEE spigelian *hernia;* S.'s *line, lobe.*

spike. 1. A brief electrical event of 3 to 25 msec that gives the appearance in the electroencephalogram of a rising and falling vertical line. **2.** In electrophoresis, a sharply angled upward deflection on a densitometric tracing.

ponto-geniculo-occipital s., EEG spikes during REM sleep that arise in the pons and pass to the lateral geniculate body and occipital cortex.

spill. An overflow; a scattering of fluid or finely divided matter.

cellular s., a dissemination of cells through the lymph or blood, thereby resulting in metastases or implantation of foreign tissue in any part or organ.

Spiller, William G., U. S. neurologist, 1864–1940. SEE Frazier-S. *operation.*

spill·way. A groove or channel through which food may pass from the occlusal surfaces of teeth during the masticatory process. SYN sluiceway.

spi·lo·ma (spī-lō′mă). SYN nevus. [G. *spilos,* spot, + *-oma,* tumor]

spi·lo·plax·ia (spī-lō-plak′sē-ă). A red spot observed in leprosy or pellagra. [G. *spilos,* spot, + *plax,* a plaque, plate]

spi·lus (spī′lŭs). SYN *nevus* spilus. [Mod. L. fr. G. *spilos,* a spot]

△**spin-.** SEE spino-.

spi·na, gen. and pl. **spi·nae** (spī′nă, -nē). **1** [NA]. SYN vertebral *column.* **2.** SYN vertebral *column.* [L. a thorn, the backbone, spine]

s. angula′ris, SYN sphenoidal *spine.*

s. bif′ida, embryologic failure of fusion of one or more vertebral arches; subtypes of spina bifida are based upon degree and pattern of deformity associated with neuroectoderm involvement. SYN hydrocele spinalis, schistorrhachis.

s. bif′ida aper′ta, SYN s. bifida cystica.

s. bif′ida cys′tica, s. bifida associated with a meningeal cyst (meningocele) or a cyst containing both meninges and spinal cord (meningomyelocele) or only spinal cord (myelocele). SYN s. bifida aperta, s. bifida manifesta.

s. bif′ida manifes′ta, SYN s. bifida cystica.

s. bif′ida occul′ta, s. bifida in which there is a spinal defect, but no protrusion of the cord or its membrane, although there is often some abnormality in their development.

s. dorsa′lis, SYN vertebral *column.*

s. fronta′lis, s, nasalis ossis frontalis.

s. hel′icis [NA], SYN *spine* of helix.

s. ili′aca ante′rior infe′rior [NA], SYN anterior inferior iliac *spine.*

s. ili′aca ante′rior supe′rior [NA], SYN anterior superior iliac *spine.*

s. ili′aca poste′rior infe′rior [NA], SYN posterior inferior iliac *spine.*

s. ili′aca poste′rior supe′rior [NA], SYN posterior superior iliac *spine.*

s. ischiad′ica [NA], SYN ischial *spine.*

s. mea′tus, SYN suprameatal *spine.*

s. menta′lis [NA], SYN mental *spine.*

s. nasa′lis ante′rior [NA], SYN anterior nasal *spine.*

s. nasa′lis os′sis fronta′lis [NA], SYN nasal *spine* of frontal bone.

s. nasa′lis poste′rior [NA], SYN posterior nasal *spine.*

s. os′sis sphenoida′lis [NA], SYN sphenoidal *spine.*

spi′nae palati′nae [NA], SYN palatine *spines,* under *spine.*

s. pe′dis, obsolete term for a hard or soft corn.

s. peronea′lis, SYN peroneal *trochlea* of calcaneus.

s. pu′bis, SYN pubic *tubercle.*

s. scap′ulae [NA], SYN *spine* of scapula.

sp

s. supramea′tica [NA], SYN suprameatal *spine*.

s. trochlea′ris [NA], SYN trochlear *spine*.

s. tympan′ica ma′jor [NA], SYN greater tympanic *spine*.

s. tympan′ica mi′nor [NA], SYN lesser tympanic *spine*.

s. vento′sa, a condition occasionally seen in tuberculosis or tuberculous dactylitis, in which there is absorption of bone bordering the medulla, with a new deposit under the periosteum, resulting in a change that is suggestive of bone being inflated with gas.

spin·a·cene (spin′ă-sēn). Obsolete term for squalene.

spi·nal (spī′năl). **1.** Relating to any spine or spinous process. **2.** Relating to the vertebral column. SYN rachial, rachidial, rachidian, spinalis. [L. *spinalis*]

spi·na·lis (spī-nā′lis). SYN spinal. [L.]

spi·nant (spī′nant). An agent increasing the reflex irritability of the spinal cord.

spi·nate (spī′nāt). Spined; having spines.

spin·dle (spin′dl). In anatomy and pathology, any fusiform cell or structure. [A.S.]

aortic s., a fusiform dilation of the aorta immediately beyond the isthmus. SYN His' s.

central s., a central group of microtubules (continuous fibers) that course uninterrupted, between the asters, in contrast to the microtubules attached to the individual chromosomes (s. fibers).

cleavage s., the s. formed during the cleavage of a zygote or its blastomeres.

His' s., SYN aortic s.

Krukenberg's s., a vertical fusiform area of melanin pigmentation on the posterior surface of the central cornea.

Kühne's s., SYN neuromuscular s.

mitotic s., the fusiform figure characteristic of a dividing cell; it consists of microtubules (s. fibers), some of which become attached to each chromosome at its centromere and appear to be involved in chromosomal movement; other microtubules (continuous fibers) pass from pole to pole. SYN nuclear s.

muscle s., SYN neuromuscular s.

neuromuscular s., a fusiform end organ in skeletal muscle in which afferent and a few efferent nerve fibers terminate; it contains from 3 to 10 striated muscle fibers (intrafusal fibers) that are much smaller than the ordinary muscle fibers, are separated from them by a capsule that encloses the organ, and are innervated by the thin axon of a gamma motoneuron (gamma motor fiber); the sensory endings that occur on the intrafusal fibers are either annulospiral or flower spray endings; this sensory end organ is particularly sensitive to passive stretch of the muscle in which it is enclosed. SYN Kühne's s., muscle s.

neurotendinous s., SYN Golgi tendon *organ*.

nuclear s., SYN mitotic s.

sleep s., the electroencephalographic record of 14-per-second bursts of wave frequency seen on EEG examination.

spine (spīn). **1.** A short, sharp, thornlike process of bone; a spinous process. **2.** SYN vertebral *column*. **3.** The bar or stay in a horse's hoof. [L. *spina*]

alar s., SYN sphenoidal s.

angular s., SYN sphenoidal s.

anterior inferior iliac s., spine on the anterior border of the ilium between the anterior superior iliac s. and the acetabulum; site of origin for the direct head of the rectus femoris muscle. SYN spina iliaca anterior inferior [NA].

anterior nasal s. (ANS), a pointed projection at the anterior extremity of the intermaxillary suture; the tip, as seen on a lateral cephalometric radiograph, is used as a cephalometric landmark. SYN spina nasalis anterior [NA].

anterior superior iliac s., the anterior extremity of the iliac crest, which provides attachment for the inguinal ligament and the sartorius muscle. SYN spina iliaca anterior superior [NA].

bamboo s., in radiology, the appearance of the thoracic or lumbar spine with ankylosing spondylitis.

cleft s., SEE *spina* bifida.

dendritic s.'s, variably long excrescences of nerve cell dendrites, varying in shape from small knobs to thornlike or filamentous processes, usually more numerous on distal dendrite arboriza-

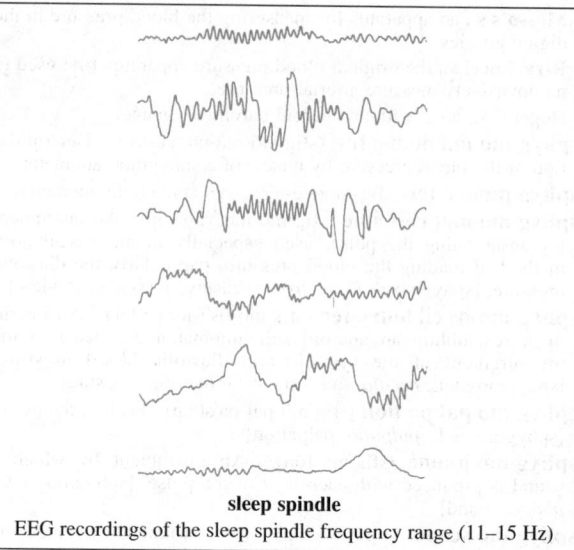

sleep spindle
EEG recordings of the sleep spindle frequency range (11–15 Hz)

tions than on the proximal part of dendritic trunks; they are a preferential site of synaptic axodendritic contact; sparse or absent in some types of nerve cells (motor neurons, the large cells of the globus pallidus, stellate cells of the cerebral cortex), exceedingly numerous in others such as the pyramidal cells of the cerebral cortex and the Purkinje cells of the cerebellar cortex. SYN dendritic thorns, gemmule (2).

dorsal s., SYN vertebral *column*.

greater tympanic s., the anterior edge of the tympanic notch (of Rivinus). SYN spina tympanica major [NA].

s. of helix, an anteriorly directed spine at the extremity of the crus of the helix of the auricle. SYN spina helicis [NA], apophysis helicis.

hemal s., the middle point on the underside of the hemal arch of the typical vertebra; considered by some to be represented by the sternum in humans.

Henle's s., SYN suprameatal s.

iliac s., SEE anterior inferior iliac s., anterior superior iliac s., posterior inferior iliac s., posterior superior iliac s.

ischiadic s., SYN ischial s.

ischial s., a pointed process from the posterior border of the ischium on a level with the lower border of the acetabulum; gives attachment to the sacrospinous ligament; the pudendal nerve passes dorsal to the ischial s., which is palpable per vagina or rectum, and thus is used as a target for the needle-tip in administering a pudendal nerve block. SYN spina ischiadica [NA], ischiadic s., sciatic s.

lesser tympanic s., the posterior edge of the tympanic notch (of Rivinus). SYN spina tympanica minor [NA].

meatal s., SYN suprameatal s.

mental s., a slight projection, sometimes two, in the middle line of the posterior surface of the body of the mandible, giving attachment to the geniohyoid muscle (below) and the genioglossus (above). SYN spina mentalis [NA], genial tubercle.

nasal s. of frontal bone, a projection from the center of the nasal part of the frontal bone, which lies between and articulates with the nasal bones and the perpendicular plate of the ethmoid. SYN spina nasalis ossis frontalis [NA].

neural s., the middle point of the neural arch of the typical vertebra, represented by the spinous process.

palatine s.'s, the longitudinal ridges along the palatine grooves on the inferior surface of the palatine process of the maxilla. SYN spinae palatinae [NA].

penis s.'s, epithelial excrescences on the glans of the p. of the guinea pig and cat; they are under the influence of the male hormone. SYN penis thorns.

poker s., stiff s. resulting from widespread joint immobility or overwhelming muscle spasm as might be evoked by an osteomyelitis of a vertebra or a rheumatoid spondylitis.

posterior inferior iliac s., spine at the inferior end of the posterior border of the ilium between the posterior superior iliac s. and the greater sciatic notch; it forms the upper margin of the latter. SYN spina iliaca posterior inferior [NA].

posterior nasal s., the sharp posterior extremity of the nasal crest of the hard palate. SYN spina nasalis posterior [NA], posterior palatine s.

posterior palatine s., SYN posterior nasal s.

posterior superior iliac s., the posterior extremity of the iliac crest, the uppermost point of attachment of the sacrotuberous and posterior sacroiliac ligaments; a readily apparent dimple occurs in the skin overlying the posterior superior iliac s. which is clinically useful as an indication of the level of the S-2 vertebra, the level of the inferior limit of the subarachnoid space. SYN spina iliaca posterior superior [NA].

pubic s., SYN pubic *tubercle.*

s. of scapula, the prominent triangular ridge on the dorsal aspect of the scapula, providing attachment for the trapezius and deltoid muscles and separating the supra- and infraspinous fossae. SYN spina scapulae [NA].

sciatic s., SYN ischial s.

sphenoidal s., a posterior and downward projection from the greater wing of the sphenoid bone on either side, located posterolateral to the foramen spinosum, so-named for its proximity to the sphenoidal s.; gives attachment to the sphenomandibular ligament. SYN processus spinosus [NA], spina ossis sphenoidalis [NA], alar s., angular s., spina angularis, spinous process (2).

Spix's s., SYN *lingula* of mandible.

suprameatal s., small bony prominence anterior to the supramastoid pit at the posterosuperior margin of the bony external acoustic meatus. SYN spina suprameatica [NA], Henle's s., meatal s., spina meatus.

thoracic s., the thoracic region of the vertebral column; the thoracic vertebrae as a whole; that part of the vertebral column which enters into the formation of the thorax.

trochlear s., a spicule of bone arising from the edge of the trochlear fovea, giving attachment to the pulley of the superior oblique muscle of the eyeball. SYN spina trochlearis [NA].

Spinelli, Pier G., Italian gynecologist, 1862–1929. SEE S. *operation.*

spi·nif·u·gal (spī-nif′yū-găl). Obsolete term for conducting in a direction away from the spinal cord; denoting the efferent fibers of the spinal nerves. [spine + L. *fugio,* to flee]

spi·nip·e·tal (spī-nip′ĕ-tăl). Obsolete term for conducting in a direction toward the spinal cord; denoting the afferent fibers of the spinal nerves. [spine + L. *peto,* to seek]

spinn·bar·keit (spin′bahr-kīt). The stringy, elastic character of cervical mucus during the ovulatory period; in contrast to other times in the menstrual cycle, cervical secretions at midcycle are clear, abundant, and of low viscosity. [Ger. *Spinnbarkeit,* visxosity, ability to form a thread]

△**spino-, spin-.** 1. The spine. 2. Spinous. [L. *spina*]

spi·no·bul·bar (spī′nō-bŭl′bar). SYN bulbospinal.

spi·no·cer·e·bel·lum (spī′nō-sār-ĕ-bel′ŭm). SYN paleocerebellum.

spi·no·col·lic·u·lar (spī′nō-col-ik′yū-lar). SYN spinotectal.

spi·no·cos·ta·lis (spī′nō-kos-tā′lis). The superior and inferior serratus posterior muscles regarded as one. [L.]

spi·no·gal·va·ni·za·tion (spī′nō-gal-van-i-zā′shŭn). Application of the constant electrical current to the spinal cord.

spi·no·gle·noid (spī′nō-glē′noyd). Relating to the spine and the glenoid cavity of the scapula.

spi·no·mus·cu·lar (spī′nō-mŭs′kyū-lăr). Relating to the spinal cord and the muscles supplied by the spinal nerves.

spi·no·neu·ral (spī-nō-nū′răl). Relating to the spinal cord and the nerves given off from it.

spi·nose (spī′nōs). SYN spinous.

spi·no·tec·tal (spī-nō-tek′tăl). Passing upward from the spinal cord to the tectum. SYN spinocollicular.

spi·no·trans·ver·sar·i·us (spī′nō-trans-ver-sār′ē-ŭs). The splenius and obliquus capitis major muscles regarded as one.

spi·nous (spī′nŭs). Relating to, shaped like, or having a spine or spines. SYN spinose.

spin·thar·i·con (spin-thăr′i-kon). A spark chamber device used to record the distribution of low energy emissions from radiopharmaceuticals administered internally, especially for thyroid scans using iodine-125. [G. *spinthēr,* spark]

spin·thar·i·scope (spin-thăr′i-skōp). SYN scintillation *counter.* [G. *spinthēr,* spark, + *skopeō,* to view]

spip·e·rone (spip′ĕ-rōn). 8-[3-(*p*-Fluorobenzoyl)propyl]-1-phenyl-1,3,8-triazaspiro[4.5]decan-4- one; an antipsychotic.

△**spir-.** SEE spiro-.

spi·ra·cle (spī′ră-kl, spir-). An aperture for breathing in arthropods and in sharks and related fishes. [L. *spiraculum,* fr. *spiro,* to breathe]

spi·rad·e·ni·tis (spī′rad-ĕ-nī′tis). SYN hidradenitis. [L. *spiro,* to breathe or perspire, + G. *adēn,* gland, + *-itis,* inflammation]

spi·rad·e·no·ma (spī-rad-ĕ-nō′mă). A benign tumor of sweat glands. [G. *speira,* coil, + adenoma]

eccrine s., a typically painful benign skin tumor composed of two cell types derived from the secretory part of eccrine sweat glands.

spi·ral (spī′răl). 1. Coiled; winding around a center like a watch spring; winding and ascending like a wire spring. 2. A structure in the shape of a coil. [Mediev. L. *spiralis,* fr. G. *speira,* a coil]

Curschmann's s.'s, spirally twisted masses of mucus occurring in the sputum in bronchial asthma.

s. of Tillaux, an imaginary line connecting the insertions of the recti muscles of the eye.

spir·a·my·cin (spir-ă-mī′sin). An antibiotic substance (almost identical to leucomycin) produced by *Streptomyces ambofaciens;* an antimicrobial agent.

spi·rem, spi·reme (spī′rem, spī′rēm). Term formerly applied to the first stage of mitosis (prophase) when extended chromosome filaments have the appearance of a loose ball of yarn, on the incorrect supposition that the filaments were continuous and later broke apart to form individual chromosomes. [G. *speirēma,* a coil 1]

spi·ril·la (spī-ril′ă). Plural of spirillum.

Spi·ril·la·ce·ae (spī-ri-lā′sē-ē). A family of usually motile, aerobic to facultatively anaerobic bacteria (order Pseudomonadales) containing Gram-negative, rod-shaped cells which are curved or spirally twisted. Motile cells contain a single polar flagellum or a tuft of polar flagella. These organisms are primarily water forms, although some are parasitic or pathogenic on humans and other higher animals. The type genus is *Spirillum.* [see *Spirillum*]

spi·ril·lar (spī-ril′ăr). S-shaped; referring to a bacterial cell with an S shape.

spi·ril·li·ci·dal (spī-ril-i-sī′dăl). Destructive to spirilla or spirochetes. [spirilla + L. *caedo,* to kill]

spi·ril·lo·sis (spī′ri-lō′sis). Any disease caused by the presence of spirilla in the blood or tissues.

Spi·ril·lum (spī-ril′ŭm). A genus of large (1.4 to 1.7 μm in diameter), rigid, helical, Gram-negative bacteria (family Spirillaceae) which are motile by means of bipolar fascicles of flagella. These freshwater organisms are obligately microaerophilic and chemoorganotrophic, possessing a strictly respiratory metabolism; they neither oxidize nor ferment carbohydrates. The type species is *S. volutans.* [Mod. L. dim. of L. *spira,* coil, fr. G. *speira*]

S. mi′nus, a species of uncertain taxonomic classification that causes a form of rat-bite fever (sodoku). This species has never been cultured.

S. volu′tans, a species found in fresh water; it is the type species of *S.*

spi·ril·lum, pl. **spi·ril·la** (spī-ril′ŭm, -ă). A member of the genus *Spirillum.*

Obermeier's s., SYN *Borrelia recurrentis.*

Vincent's s., the s. or spirochete found in association with

Vincent's bacillus. *Fusobacterium nucleatum* is frequently the only bacillus isolated.

spir·it (spir'it). **1.** An alcoholic liquor stronger than wine, obtained by distillation. **2.** Any distilled liquid. **3.** An alcoholic or hydroalcoholic solution of volatile substances; some s.'s are used as flavoring agents, others have medicinal value. SYN spiritus. [L. *spiritus,* a breathing, life soul, fr. *spiro,* to breathe]

ardent s.'s, brandy, whiskey, and other forms of distilled alcoholic liquors.

aromatic ammonia s., a hydroalcoholic solution containing approximately 2% ammonia and 4% ammonium carbonate and the aromatics: lemon oil, lavender oil, and myristica oil. Used mainly by inhalation to produce reflex stimulation in persons who have fainted or are at risk of syncope. SYN sal volatile, smelling salts.

industrial methylated s., methylated s., SYN denatured *alcohol.*

neutral s.'s, s.'s distilled from suitable raw materials, are 95% ethanol (v/v) that is, at least 190 proof when distilled. Used for blending with straight whiskey and for making gin, cordials, liqueurs, and vodka. SEE ALSO alcohol.

proof s., dilute alcohol, specific gravity 0.920, containing 49.5% by weight (57.27% by volume) of C_2H_5OH at 15.56°C. Originally in Great Britain it was the weakest alcohol that would permit ignition of gunpowder moistened with it. British proof s. has a specific gravity of 0.9198 and contains 49.2% C_2H_5OH by weight, or 57.1% by volume at the temperature of 10.56°C.

pyroligneous s., pyroxylic s., SYN *methyl* alcohol.

rectified s., SYN alcohol (2).

vital s.'s, in the galenical teachings, a vital essence or principle supposed to be generated from the air or pneuma in the left ventricle of the heart; carried in the blood to the brain, it was converted to animal s.'s which then flowed along the nerves to all parts of the body.

wine s., SYN alcohol (2).

wood s., SYN *methyl* alcohol.

spir·i·tu·ous (spir'i-chū-ŭs). Containing alcohol in large amount, denoting liquors.

spir·i·tus, gen. and pl. **spir·i·tus** (spir'i-tŭs). SYN spirit. [L.]

△**spiro-, spir-.** **1.** Coil, coil-shaped. [G. *speira*] **2.** Breathing. [L. *spiro,* to breathe]

Spi·ro·cer·ca lu·pi (spi-rō-ser'kă lū'pī). The esophageal worm of dogs and other carnivores, a red spiruroid nematode that occurs in nodules in the wall of the esophagus, stomach, and aorta of dogs, foxes, and wolves; intermediate hosts are various coprophagic beetles. Clinical symptoms occur only in very heavy infections, which are associated with esophageal carcinomata in dogs and with hypertrophic pulmonary osteoarthropathy. [L., fr. G. *speira,* coil, + G. *kerkos,* tail; L. *lupus,* wolf]

Spi·ro·chae·ta (spī'rō-kē'tă). A genus of motile bacteria (order Spirochaetales) containing presumably Gram-negative, flexible, undulating, spiral-shaped rods which may or may not possess flagelliform, tapering ends. The protoplast is spirally wound around an axial filament. No obvious periplast membrane or cross-striations occur. These organisms are motile by means of a creeping motion over the surfaces of supporting objects. They are not parasitic but are found free-living in fresh or sea water slime; they are commonly found in sewage and foul waters. At present the genus contains five species. The type species is *S. plicatilis.* [Mod. L. fr. G. *speira,* a coil, + *chaitē,* hair]

S. obermei'eri, SYN *Borrelia recurrentis.*

S. plicat'ilis, a very large species (sometimes as long as 200 μm) of bacteria; it is nonparasitic, so far as known; it is the type species of the genus *S.*

Spi·ro·chae·ta·ce·ae (spī-rō-kē-tā'sē-ē). A family of bacteria (order Spirochaetales) consisting of coarse, spiral cells, 30 to 50 μm in length and possessing definite protoplasmic structures. These organisms occur in stagnant, fresh, or salt water and in the intestinal tracts of bivalve molluscs. The type genus is *Spirochaeta.* [see *Spirochaeta*]

Spi·ro·chae·ta·les (spī-rō-kē-tā'lēz). An order of bacteria containing slender, flexuous cells, 6 to 500 μm in length, in the form of spirals with at least one complete turn. Some species may have an axial filament, a lateral crista, or ridge, or transverse striations. All of these organisms are motile, whirling or spinning about the long axis, thus driving the organism forward or backward. Free-living, saprophytic, and parasitic forms occur. The type family is Spirochaetaceae.

spi·ro·chet·al (spī-rō-kē'tăl). Relating to spirochetes, especially to infection with such organisms.

spi·ro·chete (spī'rō-kēt). A vernacular term used to refer to any member of the genus *Spirochaeta.*

spi·ro·chet·e·mia (spī'rō-kē-tē'mē-ă). Presence of spirochetes in the blood. [spirochete + G. *haima,* blood]

spi·ro·che·ti·cide (spī-rō-kē'tĭ-sīd). An agent destructive to spirochetes. [spirochete + L. *caedo,* to kill]

spi·ro·che·tol·y·sis (spī'rō-kē-tol'i-sis). Destruction of spirochetes, as by chemotherapy or by specific antibodies. [spirochete + G. *lysis,* a loosening]

spi·ro·che·to·sis (spī'rō-kē-tō'sis). Any disease caused by a spirochete.

avian s., a highly fatal bacterial disease of chickens, turkeys, pheasants, and other birds caused by *Borrelia anserina* and transmitted chiefly by the fowl tick, *Argas persicus.*

bronchopulmonary s., SYN hemorrhagic *bronchitis.*

spi·ro·che·tot·ic (spī'rō-kē-tot'ik). Relating to or marked by spirochetosis.

spi·ro·gram (spī'rō-gram). The tracing made by the spirograph.

spi·ro·graph (spī'rō-graf). A device for representing graphically the depth and rapidity of respiratory movements. [L. *spiro,* to breathe, + G. *graphō,* to write]

spi·ro·in·dex (spī'rō-in-deks). Vital capacity divided by the height of the individual.

spi·rom·e·ter (spī-rom'ĕ-ter). A gasometer used for measuring respiratory gases; usually understood to consist of a counterbalanced cylindrical bell sealed by dipping into a circular trough of water. In physiology, a gasometer is more commonly used for vessels of large capacity (*e.g.,* 100 liters), while a s. is more commonly used for small vessels (*e.g.,* 10 liters). [L. *spiro,* to breathe, + G. *metron,* measure]

chain-compensated s., a Tissot s. in which compensation for change in bell buoyancy is accomplished automatically by a suspending chain of correct mass per unit length.

Krogh s., a water-sealed s. in which the bell is a large, shallow, rectangular box rotating slightly around a horizontal axis extending along one edge, with an arm extending beyond that axis to a counterbalancing weight; comparable to a wedge s.

Tissot s., a very large water-sealed s. designed for accumulating expired gas over a long period of time; the counterbalancing of the bell (almost frictionless) is compensated for the bell's change in buoyancy as it emerges from the water, keeping the contained gas precisely at ambient atmospheric pressure.

wedge s., a waterless s. constructed of two large rectangular plates with edges connected by accordion-pleated rubber so that large changes in volume are accommodated by small changes in the acute angle of the wedge-shaped interior, sensed by an electrical transducer; designed for rapid response by reducing the acceleration of the moving parts.

Spi·ro·me·tra (spī-rō-mē'tră). A genus of pseudophyllid tapeworms. [G. *speira,* coil, + *mētra,* womb (uterus)]

S. manso'ni, a species of pseudophyllid tapeworms of wild and feral cats, the larval form of which (sparganum) may survive in human tissues; it has been commonly found in humans in the Orient, but is also reported from widely scattered areas elsewhere; infection of humans with the sparganum occurs from active migration of the larva from freshly split infected frogs used as a poultice for wounds, sore eyes (as in ocular sparganosis>), bruises, or ulcerations; it is also likely that humans may be infected with sparganum larvae from eating any vertebrate harboring these plerocercoids. SYN *Diphyllobothrium linguloides, Diphyllobothrium mansoni.*

S. mansonoi'des, a species of pseudophyllid tapeworms from North America, whose larva (sparganum) may be a cause of sparganosis of man in Florida and the Gulf States. SYN *Diphyllobothrium mansonoides.*

spi·rom·e·try (spī-rom'ĕ-trē). Making pulmonary measurements with a spirometer.

spi·ro·no·lac·tone (spī'rō-nō-lak'tōn). 3-(3-Oco-7α-acetylthio-17β-hydroxy-4-androsten-17α-yl)propionic acid-α-lactone; a diuretic agent that blocks the renal tubular actions of aldosterone. It increases the urinary excretion of sodium and chloride, decreases the excretion of potassium and ammonium, and reduces the titratable acidity of the urine; most effectively used to potentiate the natriuretic action and reduce the potassium excretion produced by other diuretics.

spi·ro·scope (spī'rō-skōp). A device for measuring the air capacity of the lungs. [L. *spiro*, to breathe, + G. *skopeō*, to view]

spi·ro·stan (spī'rō-stan). A 16,22:22,26-diepoxycholestane.

spi·ru·roid (spī'rū-royd). Common name for a member of the superfamily Spiruroidea.

Spi·ru·roi·dea (Spī-rū-roy'dē-ă). A superfamily of arthropod-borne nematode parasites of the alimentary tract, respiratory system, or orbital, nasal, or oral cavities of vertebrates. They are common and frequently pathogenic parasites of domestic mammals and birds, producing ulcerations from penetration of the anterior end of these spiny worms through the alimentary lining; includes the families Acuariidae, Gnathostomatidae, Rictulariidae, Seuratidae, Physalopteridae, Spiruridae, and Thelaziidae. [G. *speiroeidēs*, spiral]

spis·si·tude (spis'i-tūd). The state of being inspissated; the condition of a fluid thickened almost to a solid by evaporation or inspissation. [L. *spissitudo*, fr. *spissus*, thick]

spit·ting. SYN expectoration (2).

spit·tle (spit'l). SYN saliva. [A.S. *spätl*]

Spitz, 20th century U.S. pathologist. SEE S. *nevus*.

Spitzer, Alexander, Austrian anatomist, 1868–1943. SEE S.'s *theory*.

Spitzka, Edward C., U.S. neurologist, 1852–1914. SEE S.'s *nucleus*, marginal *tract*, marginal *zone; column* of S.-Lissauer.

Spix, Johann B., German anatomist, 1781–1826. SEE S.'s *spine*.

SPL Abbreviation for sound pressure *level*.

⟡**splanchn-.** SEE splanchno-.

splanch·nap·o·phys·i·al, splanch·nap·o·phys·e·al (splangk'nă-pō-fiz'ē-ăl). Relating to a splanchnapophysis.

splanch·na·poph·y·sis (splangk'nă-pof'i-sis). An apophysis of the typical vertebra, on the side opposite to the neural apophysis, or any bony process, giving attachment to a viscus or part of the alimentary tract. [splanchn- + G. *apophysis*, offshoot]

splanch·nec·to·pia (splangk-nek-tō'pē-ă). Displacement of any of the viscera. [splanchn- + G. *ektopos*, out of place]

splanch·nem·phrax·is (splangk-nem-frak'sis). Obsolete term for intestinal obstruction. [splanchn- + G. *emphraxis*, a stoppage]

splanch·nes·the·sia (splangk-nes-thē'zē-ă). SYN visceral *sense*. [splanch- + G. *aisthēsis*, sensation]

splanch·nic (splangk'nik). SYN visceral.

splanch·ni·cec·to·my (splangk-ni-sek'tō-mē). Resection of the splanchnic nerves and usually of the celiac ganglion as well. [splanchni- + G. *ektomē*, excision]

splanch·ni·cot·o·my (splangk-ni-kot'ō-mē). Section of a splanchnic nerve or nerves, a surgical procedure formerly used in the treatment of hypertension. [splanchni- + G. *tomē*, incision]

⟡**splanchno-, splanchn-, splanchni-.** The viscera. SEE ALSO viscero-. [G. *splanchnon*, viscus]

splanch·no·cele (splangk'nō-sēl). 1. The primitive body cavity or celom in the embryo. [G. *koilos*, hollow] 2. Hernia of any of the abdominal viscera. [G. *kēlē*, hernia]

splanch·no·cra·ni·um (splangk-nō-krā'nē-ŭm). SYN viscerocranium.

splanch·no·di·as·ta·sis (splangk'nō-dī-as'tă-sis). Obsolete term for splanchnectopia. [splanchno- + G. *diastasis*, separation]

splanch·nog·ra·phy (splangk-nog'ră-fē). A treatise on or description of the viscera. [splanchno- + G. *graphō*, to write]

splanch·no·lith (splangk'nō-lith). An intestinal calculus. [splanchno- + G. *lithos*, stone]

splanch·no·lo·gia (splangk'nō-lō'jē-ă) [NA]. SYN splanchnology, splanchnology.

splanch·nol·o·gy (splangk-nol'ŏ-jē). The branch of medical science dealing with the viscera. SYN splanchnologia [NA]. [splanchno- + G. *logos*, study]

splanch·no·meg·a·ly (splangk-nō-meg'ă-lē). SYN visceromegaly. [splanchno- + G. *megas*, large]

splanch·no·mic·ria (splangk-nō-mik'rē-ă). Condition in which the splanchnic organs are of smaller than normal size. [splanchno- + G. *mikros*, small]

splanch·nop·a·thy (splangk-nop'ă-thē). Any disease of the abdominal viscera. [splanchno- + G. *pathos*, disease]

splanch·no·pleu·ral (splangk-nō-plūr'ăl). SYN splanchnopleuric.

splanch·no·pleure (splangk'nō-plūr). The embryonic layer formed by association of the visceral layer of the lateral plate mesoderm with the endoderm. [splanchno- + G. *pleura*, side]

splanch·no·pleu·ric (splangk-nō-plūr'ik). Relating to the splanchnopleure. SYN splanchnopleural.

splanch·nop·to·sis, splanch·nop·to·sia (splangk'nō-tō'sis, -tō'sē-ă). SYN visceroptosis. [splanchno- + G. *ptōsis* a falling]

splanch·no·scle·ro·sis (splangk'nō-skle-rō'sis). Hardening, through connective tissue overgrowth, of any of the viscera. [splanchno- + G. *sklērōsis*, hardening]

splanch·no·skel·e·tal (splangk-nō-skel'ĕ-tăl). SYN visceroskeletal.

splanch·no·skel·e·ton (splangk-nō-skel'ĕ-tŏn). SYN visceroskeleton (2).

splanch·no·so·mat·ic (splangk'nō-sō-mat'ik). SYN viscerosomatic. [splanchno- + G. *sōma*, body]

splanch·not·o·my (splangk-not'ō-mē). Dissection of the viscera by incision. [splanchno- + G. *tomē*, incision]

splanch·no·tribe (splangk'nō-trīb). An instrument resembling a large angiotribe used for occluding the intestine temporarily, prior to resection. [splanchno- + G. *tribō*, to rub, bruise]

splay (splā). 1. To lay open the end of a tubular structure by making a longitudinal incision to increase its potential diameter. SEE ALSO spatulate. 2. The rounding of the corner on the graph relating rate of renal tubular secretion or reabsorption of a substance to its arterial plasma concentration, due primarily to the fact that some nephrons reach their tubular maximum before others do.

spleen (splēn). A large vascular lymphatic organ lying in the upper part of the abdominal cavity on the left side, between the stomach and diaphragm, composed of white and red pulp; the white consists of lymphatic nodules and diffuse lymphatic tissue; the red consists of venous sinusoids between which are splenic cords; the stroma of both red and white pulp is reticular fibers and cells. A framework of fibroelastic trabeculae extending from the capsule subdivides the structure into poorly defined lobules. It is a blood-forming organ in early life and later a storage organ for red corpuscles and platelets; because of the large number of macrophages, it also acts as a blood filter, both identifying and destroying effete erythrocytes. SYN splen [NA], lien⭑ [NA]. [G. *splēn*]

accessory s., one of the small globular masses of splenic tissue occasionally found in the region of the spleen, in one of the peritoneal folds or elsewhere. SYN splen accessorius [NA], lien accessorius, lien succenturiatus, lienculus, lienunculus, spleneolus, spleniculus, splenule, splenulus, splenunculus.

diffuse waxy s., a condition of amyloid degeneration of the s., affecting chiefly the extrasinusoidal tissue spaces of the pulp.

floating s., a s. that is palpable because of excessive mobility from a relaxed or lengthened pedicle rather than because of enlargement. SYN lien mobilis, movable s.

lardaceous s., SYN waxy s.

movable s., SYN floating s.

sago s., amyloidosis in the s. affecting chiefly the malpighian bodies.

sugar-coated s., hyaloserositis involving the s.

waxy s., amyloidosis of the s. SYN lardaceous s.

sp

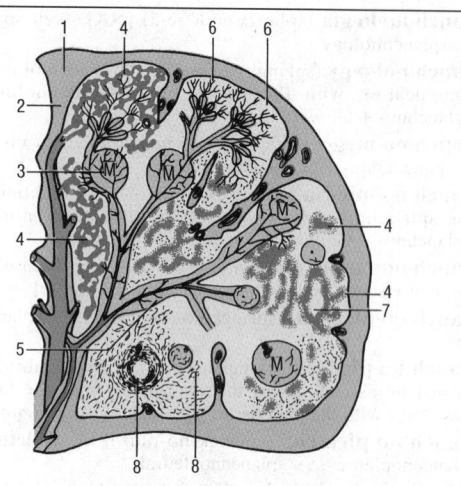

the spleen

1) fibrous envelope (capsula lienis); 2) trabeculae; 3) lymph follicle, with central artery and nodular capillaries; 4) venous sinusoids; 5) periarterial lymphatic sheath; 6) penicilli (arterial "twigs" and "tufts"); 7) splenic cord; and 8) reticular fibers

splen [NA]. SYN spleen. [G. *splen,* spleen]

s. accessorius [NA], SYN accessory *spleen.*

⌂**splen-.** SEE spleno-.

sple·nal·gia (splē-nal′jē-ă). A rarely used term for a painful condition of the spleen. SYN splenodynia. [splen- + G. *algos,* pain]

sple·nauxe (splē-nawk′sē). SYN splenomegaly. [splen- + G. *auxē,* increase]

Splendore, A., 20th century Italian physician. SEE S.-Hoeppli *phenomenon;* Lutz-S.-Almeida *disease.*

sple·nec·to·my (splē-nek′tō-mē). Removal of the spleen. [splen- + G. *ektomē,* excision]

sple·nec·to·pia, sple·nec·to·py (splen′ek-tō′pē-ă, splē-nek′tō-pē). **1.** Displacement of the spleen, as in a floating spleen. **2.** The presence of rests of splenic tissue, usually in the region of the spleen. [splen- + G. *ektopos,* out of place]

sple·nel·co·sis (splen-el-kō′sis). Abscess of the spleen. [splen- + G. *helkōsis,* ulceration]

sple·nem·phrax·is (splen-em-frak′sis). Congestion of the spleen. [splen- + G. *emphraxis,* stoppage]

sple·ne·o·lus (splē-nē′ō-lŭs). SYN accessory *spleen.* [Mod. L. dim. of G. *splēn*]

sple·net·ic (splē-net′ik). **1.** SYN splenic. **2.** Fretfully surly.

sple·ni·al (splē′nē-ăl). **1.** Relating to the splenium. **2.** Relating to a splenius muscle. [G. *splēnion,* bandage]

splen·ic (splen′ik). Relating to the spleen. SYN lienal, splenetic (1).

sple·ni·cu·lus (splen-ik′yū-lŭs). SYN accessory *spleen.* [Mod. L.]

splen·i·form (splen′i-fōrm, splē′ni-). SYN splenoid.

splen·i·ser·rate (splen′i-ser′āt). Relating to the splenius and serratus muscles.

sple·ni·tis (splē-nī′tis). Inflammation of the spleen. [splen- + G. *-itis,* inflammation]

sple·ni·um, pl. **sple·nia** (splē′nē-ŭm, -ă). **1.** A compress or bandage. **2** [NA]. A structure resembling a bandaged part. [Mod. L. fr. G. *splēnion,* bandage]

s. cor′poris callo′si [NA], SYN s. of corpus callosum. SYN tuber corporis callosi.

s. of corpus callosum, the thickened posterior extremity of the corpus callosum. SYN s. corporis callosi [NA].

sple·ni·us (splē′nē-ŭs). SEE splenius *muscle* of head, splenius *muscle* of neck. [Mod. L. fr. G. *splēnion,* a bandage]

♻**spleno-, splen-.** The spleen. [G. *splēn*]

sple·no·cele (splē′nō-sēl). **1.** SYN splenoma. **2.** A splenic hernia. [spleno- + G. *kēlē,* tumor, hernia]

sple·no·clei·sis (splē-nō-klī′sis). Inducing the formation of new fibrous tissue on the surface of the spleen by friction or wrapping with gauze. [spleno- + G. *kleisis,* closure]

sple·no·co·lic (splē′nō-kol′ik). Relating to the spleen and the colon; denoting a ligament or fold of peritoneum passing between the two viscera.

sple·no·dyn·ia (splē′nō-din′ē-ă). SYN splenalgia. [spleno- + G. *odynē,* pain]

sple·no·he·pa·to·meg·a·ly, sple·no·he·pa·to·me·ga·lia (splē′nō-hep′ă-tō-meg′ă-lē, -mě-gā′ē-ă). Enlargement of both spleen and liver. [spleno- + G. *hēpar,* liver, + *megas,* large]

sple·noid (splē′noyd). Resembling the spleen. SYN spleniform. [spleno- + G. *eidos,* resemblance]

sple·no·lym·phat·ic (splē′nō-lim-fat′ik). Relating to the spleen and the lymph nodes.

sple·no·ma (splē-nō′mă). General nonspecific term for an enlarged spleen. SYN splenocele (1), splenoncus. [spleno- + G. *-oma,* tumor]

sple·no·ma·la·cia (splē′nō-mă-lā′shē-ă). Softening of the spleen. [spleno- + G. *malakia,* softness]

sple·no·med·ul·lary (splē-nō-med′ŭ-lār-ē). SYN splenomyelogenous. [spleno- + L. *medulla,* marrow]

sple·no·meg·a·ly, sple·no·me·ga·lia (splē-nō-meg′ă-lē, -mě-gā′lē-ă). Enlargement of the spleen. SYN megalosplenia, splenauxe. [spleno- + G. *megas* (*megal-*), large]

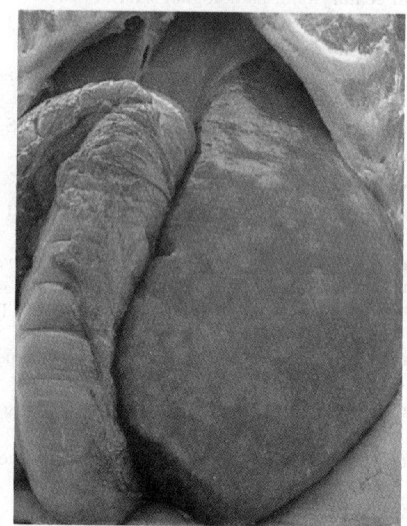

splenomegaly
due to granulocytic leukemia (weight of spleen: 9 lbs. 2 oz.)

congestive s., enlargement of the spleen due to passive congestion; sometimes used as a synonym for Banti's syndrome.

Egyptian s., term sometimes used as a synonym for schistosomiasis mansoni, although hepatomegaly and fibrosis are more consistently found than is an enlarged spleen.

hemolytic s., s. associated with congenital hemolytic jaundice.

hyperreactive malarious s., a syndrome characterized by persistent splenomegaly, exceptionally high serum IgM and malaria antibody levels, and hepatic sinusoidal lymphocytosis; believed to be a disturbance in the T-lymphocyte control of the humoral response to recurrent malaria. SYN tropical splenomegaly syndrome.

Niemann's s., enlargement of spleen occurring in Niemann-Pick disease.

tropical s., SYN visceral *leishmaniasis.*

sple·no·my·e·log·e·nous (splē'nō-mī-ĕ-loj'ĕ-nŭs). Originating in the spleen and bone marrow, denoting a form of leukemia. SYN lienomedullary, lienomyelogenous, splenomedullary. [spleno- + G. *myelos,* marrow, + *-gen,* producing]

sple·no·my·e·lo·ma·la·cia (splē'nō-mī'ĕ-lō-mă-lā'shē-ă). Pathologic softening of the spleen and bone marrow. [spleno- + G. *myelos,* marrow, + *malakia,* softness]

sple·non·cus (splē-nong'kŭs). SYN splenoma. [spleno- + G. *onkos,* mass]

sple·no·neph·ric (splē'nō-nef'rik). SYN splenorenal. [spleno- + G. *nephros,* kidney]

sple·no·pan·cre·at·ic (splē'nō-pan-krē-at'ik). Relating to the spleen and the pancreas. SYN lienopancreatic.

sple·nop·a·thy (splē-nop'ă-thē). Any disease of the spleen. [spleno- + G. *pathos,* suffering]

sple·no·pexy, sple·no·pex·ia (splē'nō-pek-sē, splē-nō-pek'sē-ă). Suturing in place an ectopic or floating spleen. SYN splenorrhaphy (2). [spleno- + G. *pēxis,* fixation]

sple·no·phren·ic (splē'nō-fren'ik). Relating to the spleen and the diaphragm; denoting a ligament or fold of peritoneum extending between the two structures. [spleno- + G. *phrēn,* diaphragm]

sple·no·por·to·gram (splē-nō-pōr'tō-gram). Radiographic record of the splenic and portal veins and their collaterals following direct injection of water-soluble contrast materials into the spleen.

sple·no·por·tog·ra·phy (splē'nō-pōr-tog'ră-fē). Introduction of radiopaque material into the spleen to obtain an x-ray visualization of the portal vessel of the portal circulation. SYN splenic portal venography. [spleno- + portography]

sple·nop·to·sis, sple·nop·to·sia (splē-nop-tō'sis, -tō'sē-ă). Downward displacement of the spleen, as in a floating spleen. [spleno- + G. *ptōsis,* falling]

sple·no·re·nal (splē'nō-rē'năl). Relating to the spleen and the kidney; denoting a ligament or fold of peritoneum extending between the two structures. SYN lienorenal, splenonephric.

sple·nor·rha·gia (splē'nō-rā'jē-ă). Hemorrhage from a ruptured spleen. [spleno- + G. *rhēgnymi,* to burst forth]

sple·nor·rha·phy (splē-nōr'ă-fē). 1. Suturing a ruptured spleen. 2. SYN splenopexy. [spleno- + G. *rhaphē,* suture]

sple·no·sis (splē-nō'sis). Implantation and subsequent growth of splenic tissue within the abdomen as a result of splenic rupture or iatrogenic injury.

sple·not·o·my (splē-not'ō-mē). 1. Anatomy or dissection of the spleen. 2. Surgical incision of the spleen. [spleno- + G. *tomē,* incision]

sple·no·tox·in (splē-nō-tok'sin). A cytotoxin specific for cells of the spleen. [spleno- + G. *toxikon,* poison]

splen·ule (splen'yūl). SYN accessory *spleen.* [Mod. L. *splenulus*]

splen·u·lus, pl. **splen·u·li** (splen'yū-lūs, -lī). SYN accessory *spleen.* [Mod. L. dim. of L. *splen,* spleen]

sple·nun·cu·lus, pl. **sple·nun·cu·li** (splē-nŭng'kyū-lŭs, -lī). SYN accessory *spleen.* [Mod. L. dim. of L. *splen,* spleen]

splice·o·some (splī'sē-ō-sōm). A specialized structure that participates in the removal of introns and resplicing of remaining exons of mRNA; in addition to the mRNA primary transcript, at least four small nuclear RNAs (snRNAs) and some proteins are involved. [splice + -some]

splic·ing (splīs'ing). 1. Attachment of one DNA molecule to another. SYN gene splicing. 2. Removal of introns from mRNA precursors and the reattachment or annealing of exons. SYN RNA splicing.

splint. 1. An appliance for preventing movement of a joint or for the fixation of displaced or movable parts. **2.** The s. bone, or fibula. [Middle Dutch *splinte*]

acid etch cemented s., a s. of heavy wire which is cemented to the labial surfaces of teeth with any of the acid etch cement techniques; used to stabilize traumatically displaced or periodontally diseased teeth.

active s., SYN dynamic s.

air s., a plastic s. inflated by air used to immobilize part or all of an extremity. SYN inflatable s.

airplane s., a complicated s. that holds the arm in abduction at about shoulder level with the forearm midway in flexion, generally with an axillary strut for support.

anchor s., a s. used for fracture of the jaw, with wires around teeth and a rod to hold it in place.

Anderson s., a skeletal traction s. with pins inserted into proximal and distal ends of a fracture; reduction is obtained by an external plate attached to the pins.

backboard s., a board s. with slots for fixation by straps; shorter ones are used for neck injuries, longer ones for back injuries.

Balkan s., SYN Balkan *frame.*

cap s., a plastic or metallic fracture appliance designed to cover the crowns of the teeth and usually cemented to them.

coaptation s., a short s. designed to prevent overriding of the ends of a fractured bone, usually supplemented by a longer s. to fix the entire limb.

contact s., a slotted plate, held by screws, used in the treatment of fracture of long bones.

Cramer wire s., SYN ladder s.

Denis Browne s., a light aluminum s. applied to the lateral aspect of the leg and foot; used for clubfoot.

dynamic s., a s. utilizing springs or elastic bands that aids in movements initiated by the patient by controlling the plane and range of motion. SYN active s., functional s. (1).

Essig s., a stainless steel wire passed labially and lingually around a segment of the dental arch and held in position by individual ligature wires around the contact areas of the teeth; used to stabilize fractured or repositioned teeth and the involved alveolar bone.

Frejka pillow s., a pillow s. used for abduction and flexion of the femurs in treatment of congenital hip dysplasia or dislocation in infants.

functional s., (1) SYN dynamic s. **(2)** the joining of two or more teeth into a rigid unit by means of fixed restorations that cover all or part of the abutment teeth.

Gunning s., a prosthesis fabricated from models of endentulous maxillary and mandibular arches in order to aid in reduction and fixation of a fracture.

Hodgen s., a suspension leg s. for fractures of the middle or lower end of the femur; it provides support for traction.

inflatable s., SYN air s.

interdental s., a s. for a fractured jaw, consisting of two metal or acrylic resin bands wired to the teeth of the upper and lower jaws, respectively, and then fastened together to keep the jaws immovable.

Kingsley s., a winged maxillary s. used to apply traction to reduce maxillary fractures as well as immobilize them by having the wings attached to a head appliance by elastics. SYN reverse Kingsley s.

labial s., an appliance of plastic, metal, or in combination, made to conform to the outer aspect of the dental arch and used in the management of jaw and facial injuries.

ladder s., a flexible s. consisting of two stout parallel wires with finer cross wires. SYN Cramer wire s.

lingual s., one similar to the labial s., but conforming to the inner aspect of the dental arch.

Liston's s., a long s. extending from the axilla to the sole of the foot.

plaster s., a s. constructed of bandages impregnated with plaster of Paris.

reverse Kingsley s., SYN Kingsley s.

Stader s., a s. used primarily in veterinary medicine; with metal pins through the proximal and distal segments of a long bone fracture, the fixation of the pins is maintained by the apparatus which is external to the limb.

surgical s., general term for a device used to maintain tissues in a new position following surgery.

Taylor's s., SYN Taylor's back *brace.*

Thomas s., a long leg s. extending from a ring at the hip to

sp

beyond the foot, allowing traction to a fractured leg, for emergencies and transportation.

Tobruk s., a Thomas s., applied and held in plaster with plaster of Paris dressings; a s. first used during World War II to immobilize the limb during hazardous conditions such as transport from small to large boats. [port of *Tobruk,* Libya]

wire s., a device to stabilize teeth loosened by accident or by a periodontal condition in the maxilla or mandible; a device to reduce and stabilize maxillary or mandibular fractures by applying it to both jaws and connecting it by intermaxillary wires or rubber bands.

splint·ing. 1. Application of a splint or treatment using a splint. **2.** In dentistry, the joining of two or more teeth into a rigid unit by means of fixed or removable restorations or appliances. **3.** Stiffening of a body part to avoid pain caused by movement of the part, as from a fracture.

splints. Exostoses occurring along the course of the small metacarpal and metatarsal bones of the horse. [see splint]

split·ting. In chemistry, the cleavage of a covalent bond, fragmenting the molecule involved.

spm Abbreviation for a gene that leads to *su*ppression and *m*utation of mutants that are unstable.

spo·dog·e·nous (spŏ-doj'ĕ-nŭs). Caused by waste material. [G. *spodos,* ashes, + *-gen,* producing]

spod·o·gram (spŏ'dō-gram). The pattern of ash residue formed by microincineration of a minute tissue specimen, usually a thin section. [G. *spodos,* ashes, + *gramma,* a drawing]

spo·dog·ra·phy (spŏ-dog'-ră-fē). SYN microincineration. [G. *spodos,* ashes, + *graphō,* to write]

spo·doph·o·rous (spŏ-dof'ō-rŭs). Removing or carrying off waste materials from the body. [G. *spodos,* ashes, + *phoros,* bearing]

spoke-shave (spōk' shāv). SYN ring-knife.

spon·da·ic (spon-dā'ik). Relating to spondee.

spon·dee (spon'dē). A bisyllabic word with generally equivalent stress on each of the two syllables; used in the testing of speech hearing. [Fr.]

△**spondyl-.** SEE spondylo-.

spon·dy·lal·gia (spon-di-lal'jē-ă). Pain in the spine. [spondyl- + G. *algos,* pain]

spon·dy·lar·thri·tis (spon'dil-ar-thrī'tis). Inflammation of the intervertebral articulations. [spondyl- + G. *arthron,* joint, + *-itis,* inflammation]

spon·dy·lar·throc·a·ce (spon-dil-ar-throk'ă-sē). **1.** SYN tuberculous *spondylitis.* **2.** SYN Rust's *disease.* [spondyl- + G. *arthron,* joint, + *kakē,* badness]

spon·dy·lit·ic (spon-di-lit'ik). Relating to spondylitis.

spon·dy·li·tis (spon-di-lī'tis). Inflammation of one or more of the vertebrae. [spondyl- + G. *-itis,* inflammation]

ankylosing s., arthritis of the spine, resembling rheumatoid arthritis, that may progress to bony ankylosis with lipping of vertebral margins; the disease is more common in the male often with the rheumatoid factor absent and the HLA antigen present. There is a striking association with the B27 tissue type and the strong familial aggregation suggest an important genetic factor, perhaps inherited as an autosomal dominant [MIM*106300]; the mechanism, however, remains obscure. SYN Marie-Strümpell disease, rheumatoid s., Strümpell-Marie disease.

s. defor'mans, arthritis and osteitis deformans involving the spinal column; marked by nodular deposits at the edges of the intervertebral disks with ossification of the ligaments and bony ankylosis of the intervertebral articulations, it results in a rounded kyphosis with rigidity. SYN Bechterew's disease, poker back, Strümpell's disease (1).

Kümmell's s., late posttraumatic collapse of a vertebral body.

rheumatoid s., SYN ankylosing s.

tuberculous s., tuberculous infection of the spine associated with a sharp angulation of the spine at the point of disease. SYN Pott's disease, spondylarthrocace (1), spondylocace (1), trachelocyrtosis, trachelokyphosis.

△**spondylo-, spondyl-.** The vertabrae. [G. *spondylos,* vertebra]

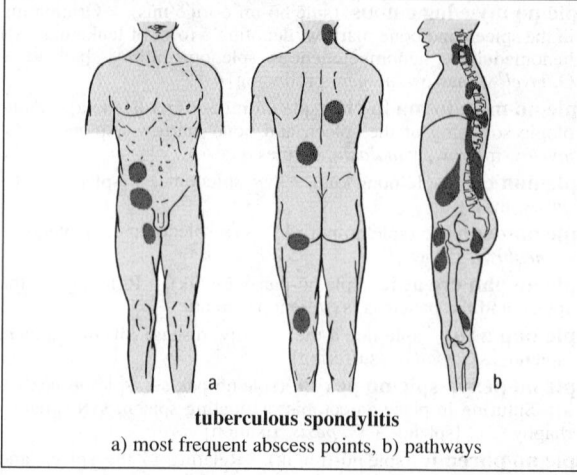

tuberculous spondylitis
a) most frequent abscess points, b) pathways

spon·dy·loc·a·ce (spon-di-lok'ă-sē). **1.** SYN tuberculous *spondylitis.* **2.** SYN Rust's *disease.* [spondylo- + G. *kakē,* badness]

spon·dy·lo·lis·the·sis (spon'di-lō-lis-thē'sis). Forward movement of the body of one of the lower lumbar vertebrae on the vertebra below it, or upon the sacrum. SYN sacrolisthesis, spondyloptosis. [spondylo- + G. *olisthēsis,* a slipping and falling]

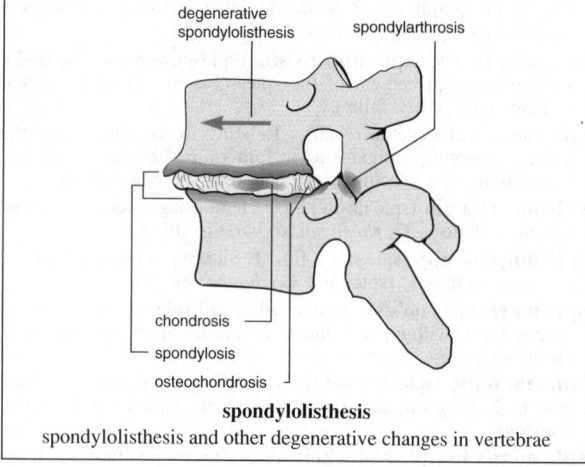

spondylolisthesis
spondylolisthesis and other degenerative changes in vertebrae

spon·dy·lo·lis·thet·ic (spon'di-lō-lis-thet'ik). Relating to or marked by spondylolisthesis.

spon·dy·lol·y·sis (spon-di-lol'i-sis). Degeneration or deficient development of the articulating part of a vertebra. [spondylo- + G. *lysis,* loosening]

spon·dy·lo·ma·la·cia (spon'di-lō-mă-lā'shē-ă). Softening of vertebrae with multiple collapsed vertebral bodies. [spondylo- + G. *malakia,* softness]

spon·dy·lop·a·thy (spon-di-lop'ă-thē). Any disease of the vertebrae or spinal column. SYN rachiopathy. [spondylo- + G. *pathos,* suffering]

spon·dy·lop·to·sis (spon'di-lō-tō'sis). SYN spondylolisthesis. [spondylo- + G. *ptōsis,* a falling]

spon·dy·lo·py·o·sis (spon'di-lō-pī-ō'sis). Suppurative inflammation of one or more of the vertebral bodies. [spondylo- + G. *pyōsis,* suppuration]

spon·dy·los·chi·sis (spon-di-los'ki-sis). Embryologic failure of fusion of vertebral arch. SEE *spina* bifida. [spondylo- + G. *schisis,* fissure]

spon·dy·lo·sis (spon-di-lō'sis). Ankylosis of the vertebra; often applied nonspecifically to any lesion of the spine of a degenerative nature. [G. *spondylos,* vertebra]

cervical s., s. affecting the cervical vertebrae, intervertebral discs, and surrounding soft tissue.

hyperostotic s., SYN diffuse idiopathic skeletal *hyperostosis.*

spon·dy·lo·syn·de·sis (spon'di-lō-sin-dē'sis). SYN spinal *fusion.* [spondylo- + G. *syndesis,* binding together]

spon·dy·lo·tho·rac·ic (spon'di-lō-thō-ras'ik). Relating to the vertebra and the thorax.

spon·dy·lot·o·my (spon-di-lot'ō-mē). SYN laminectomy. [spondylo- + G. *tomē,* incision]

spon·dyl·ous (spon'di-lŭs). Relating to a vertebra.

sponge (spŭnj). **1.** Absorbent material, such as gauze or prepared cotton, used to absorb fluids. **2.** A member of the phylum Porifera, the cellular endoskeleton of which is a source of commercial s.'s. SYN spongia. [G. *spongia*]

absorbable gelatin s., a sterile, absorbable, water-insoluble gelatin base s., used to control capillary bleeding in surgical operations; it is left *in situ* and is absorbed in from 4 to 6 weeks.

Bernays' s., a compressed disk of aseptic cotton that swells when moistened; used in packing cavities.

bronchoscopic s., a small fold of gauze used on a long applicator to apply medication or remove secretions through a bronchoscope.

compressed s., a s. is impregnated with thin mucilage of acacia, wrapped with twine to the desired shape, and then dried; used to dilate sinuses, the os uteri, etc. by absorbing moisture after insertion. SYN sponge tent.

contraceptive s., a resilient, hydrophilic s. of polyurethane foam impregnated with a spermicide; contraception is achieved by action of the spermicide.

spon·gia (spŭn'jē-ă). SYN sponge. [G.]

spon·gi·form (spŭn'ji-fōrm). SYN spongy.

⌂**spongio-.** Sponge, sponglike, spongy. [G. *spongia*]

spon·gi·o·blast (spŭn'jē-ō-blast). A neuroepithelial, filiform ependyma cell extending across the entire thickness of the wall of the brain or spinal cord, *i.e.,* from the internal to the external limiting membrane; become neuroglial and ependymal cells. SEE ALSO glioblast. [spongio- + G. *blastos,* germ]

spon·gi·o·blas·to·ma (spŭn'jē-ō-blas-tō'mă). **1.** A glioma consisting of cells (elongated, spindle-shaped, and sometimes pleomorphic, with one or two fibrillary processes) that resemble the embryonic spongioblasts, occurring normally around the neural canal of the human embryo; it grows relatively slowly, usually originating in the brainstem, optic chiasm, or infundibulum, and infiltrates adjacent structures or causes compression of the third and fourth ventricle. S.'s were formerly subclassified as s. polare and s. unipolare. **2.** Obsolete term for glioblastoma multiforme. [spongioblast + G. *-oma* tumor]

spon·gi·o·cyte (spŭn'jē-ō-sīt). **1.** A neuroglial cell. **2.** A cell in the zona fasciculata of the adrenal containing many droplets of lipid material which, after staining with hematoxylin and eosin, show pronounced vacuolization. [spongio- + G. *kytos,* cell]

spon·gi·oid (spŭn'jē-oyd). SYN spongy. [spongio- + G. *eidos,* resemblance]

spon·gi·ose (spŭn'jē-ōs). Resembling or characteristic of a sponge. [L. *spongiosus*]

spon·gi·o·sis (spŭn-jē-ō'sis). Inflammatory intercellular edema of the epidermis.

spon·gi·o·si·tis (spŭn-jē-ō-sī'tis). Inflammation of the corpus spongiosum, or corpus cavernosum urethrae.

spongy (spŭn'jē). Of spongelike texture or appearance. SYN spongiform, spongioid.

spon·ta·ne·ous (spon-tā'nē-ŭs). Without apparent cause; said of disease processes or remissions. [L. *spontaneus,* voluntary, capricious]

spoon (spūn). An instrument with a handle and a small bowl- or cup-shaped extremity. [A.S. *spōn,* chip]

cataract s., a small concave instrument for removing a cataractous lens.

Daviel's s., a small oval-shaped instrument for removing the remains of a cataract after discission.

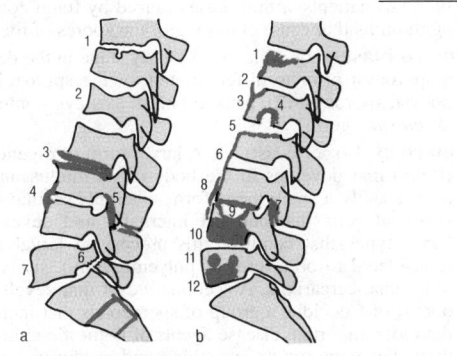

spondylopathy

a) *degenerative*: 1) Scheuermann's disease; 2) codfish vertebrae, in osteoporosis; 3) osteochondrosis; 4) hyperostotic spondylosis; 5) spondylarthrosis; 6,7) spondylolisthesis with spondylolysis

b) *infectious and neoplastic*: 1) vertebral TB (spondylitis); 2–7) Bechterew's disease (2, syndesmophyte; 3, periostosis; 4, spondylitis; 5, spondylodiscitis; 6, ankylosing syndesmophyte; 7, spondylarthritis; 8) "paradesmophytes" (e.g., in Reiter's syndrome); 9) infectious spondylodiscitis 10) myeloma; 11,12) osteoplastic and osteolytic foci

sharp s., an instrument with a small cup-shaped extremity having sharpened edges, used for scraping skin lesions.

Volkmann's s., a sharp s. for scraping away carious bone or other diseased tissue.

⌂**spor-.** SEE sporo-.

spo·rad·ic (spō-rad'ik). **1.** Denoting a temporal pattern of disease occurence in an animal or human population in which the disease occurs only rarely and without regularity. SEE endemic, epidemic, enzootic, epizootic. **2.** In the genetic context denotes a singleton or sport. Several quite different and disparate phenomena are covered by this term, including a new mutation; occult nonpaternity; the chance outcome for a recessive trait in two carrier parents with a small family; extreme variability in the expression of a gene; an environmental phenocopy; a multilocal genocopy, etc. No useful properties can be predicated of all members of this class; and the term is notionally useless. **3.** Occurring irregularly, haphazardly. [G. *sporadikos,* scattered]

spo·ra·din (spōr'ă-din). Gamont stage of a gregarine parasite after it has lost its epimerite or mucron.

spo·ran·gi·o·phore (spō-ran'jē-ō-fōr). In fungi, a specialized hypha that bears a sporangium at its tip. [sporangium + G. *phoros,* bearing]

spo·ran·gi·um, pl. **spo·ran·gia** (spō-ran'jē-ŭm, -ă). A saclike structure (a cell) within a fungus, in which asexual spores are borne by progressive cleavage. [L. fr. G. *sporos,* seed, + *angeion,* vessel]

spore (spōr). **1.** The asexual or sexual reproductive body of fungi or sporozoan protozoa. **2.** A cell of a plant lower in organization than the seed-bearing spermatophytic plants. **3.** A resistant form of certain species of bacteria. **4.** The highly modified reproductive body of certain protozoa, as in the phyla Microspora and Myxozoa. [G. *sporos,* seed]

black s., a degenerating malarial or other blood parasite in the body of the mosquito.

spo·ri·ci·dal (spōr-i-sī'dăl). Lethal to spores. [spori- + L. *caedo,* to kill]

spo·ri·cide (spōr'i-sīd). An agent that kills spores.

spo·rid·i·um, pl. **spo·rid·ia** (spō-rid'ē-ŭm, -ă). A protozoan spore; an embryonic protozoan organism. [Mod. L. dim., fr. G. *sporos,* seed]

⌂**sporo-, spori-, spor-.** Seed, spore. [G. *sporos*]

spo·ro·ag·glu·ti·na·tion (spōr'ō-ă-glū-ti-nā'shŭn). A diagnostic method in relation to the mycoses, based upon the fact that the blood of patients with diseases caused by fungi contains specific agglutinins that cause clumping of the spores of these organisms.

spo·ro·blast (spōr'ō-blast). An early stage in the development of a sporocyst prior to differentiation of the sporozoites. SEE ALSO oocyst, sporocyst (2), pansporoblast. SYN zygotomere. [sporo- + G. *blastos,* germ]

spo·ro·cyst (spōr'ō-sist). **1.** A larval form of digenetic trematode (fluke) that develops in the body of its molluscan intermediate host, usually a snail; the s. forms a simple saclike structure with germinal cells that bud off internally and develop into other larval types that continue this process of larval multiplication (considered to be a form of polyembryony). SEE ALSO miracidium, redia, cercaria. **2.** A secondary cyst that develops within the oocyst of Coccidia, a group of sporozoans that includes many of the most important disease agents of domestic animals and fowl; the s. develops from a sporoblast and produces within itself one or several sporozoites, the infective agents for infection and multiplication in the next host. [sporo- + G. *kystis,* bladder]

Spo·ro·cys·tin·ea (spōr'ō-sis-tin'ē-ă). In older classification schemes, a suborder of Coccidia in which the sporoblasts develop sporocysts. [sporo + G. *kystis,* bladder]

spo·ro·do·chi·um (spo-rō-dō'kē-ŭm). In fungi, a cushion-shaped stroma covered with conidiophores.

spo·ro·gen·e·sis (spōr-ō-jen'ĕ-sis). SYN sporogony. [sporo- + G. *genesis,* production]

spo·rog·e·nous (spŏ-roj'ĕ-nŭs). Relating to or involved in sporogony.

spo·rog·e·ny (spŏ-roj'ĕ-nē). SYN sporogony.

spo·rog·o·ny (spŏ-rog'ŏ-nē). The formation of sporozoites in sporozoan protozoa, a process of asexual division within the sporoblast, which becomes the sporocyst within an oocyst; follows fusion of gametes (gametogony) and zygote (sporont) formation. SYN sporogenesis, sporogeny. [sporo- + G. *goneia,* generation]

spo·ront (spōr'ont). The zygote stage within the oocyst wall in the life cycle of coccidia; gives rise to sporoblasts, which form sporocysts, within which the infective sporozoites are produced. [sporo- + G. *ōn (ont-),* being]

spo·ro·phore (spōr'ō-fōr). Any specialized hyphae in fungi that give rise to spores. [sporo- + G. *phoros,* bearing]

spo·ro·plasm (spōr'ō-plazm). The protoplasm of a spore. [sporo- + G. *plasma,* thing formed]

spo·ro·the·ca (spōr'o-the'ka). The envelope enclosing the minute needle-like spores of certain Sporozoea. [sporo- + G. *thēkē,* case]

Spo·ro·thrix (spōr'ō-thriks). A genus of dimorphic imperfect fungi, including the species *S. schenckii,* an organism of worldwide distribution and the causative agent of sporotrichosis in man and animals, which grows in soil or vegetation, especially in thorny bushes, and is acquired by man when infected thorns are introduced into subcutaneous tissues; at 37°C it grows as a yeast and parasitizes tissues as a yeast. [Mod. L., fr. G. *sporos,* seed, + *thrix,* hair]

spo·ro·tri·cho·sis (spōr'ō-tri-kō'sis). A chronic cutaneous mycosis spread by way of the lymphatics and caused by inoculation of *Sporothrix schenckii,* typically rare in tissue sections but rapidly growing in cultures. The disease may remain localized or may become generalized, involving bones, joints, lungs, and the central nervous system; lesions may be granulomatous or suppurative, ulcerative, or draining. SYN Schenck's disease.

Spo·ro·tri·chum (spŏ-rot'ri-kŭm). A genus of imperfect fungi (Hyphomycetes) that are usually common contaminants. [Mod. L. fr. G. *sporos,* seed, + *thrix,* hair]

spo·ro·zo·an (spōr-ō-zō'an). **1.** An individual organism of the class Sporozoea. SYN sporozoon. **2.** Relating to the Sporozoea.

Spo·ro·zo·as·i·da (spōr'ō-zō-as'i-dă). SYN Sporozoea.

Spor·o·zo·ea (spōr-ō-zō'ē-ă). A large class of protozoans (phylum Apicomplexa, subkingdom Protozoa) consisting of obligatory parasites with simple spores lacking polar filaments; cilia and flagella are absent (except for microgametes, found in some groups), and locomotion is by undulation, gliding, or body flexion; sexuality, when present, is by syngamy, forming oocysts

with infective sporozoites from sporogony. The class includes the gregarines and coccidia, the latter including many agents of human and animal disease, such as the plasmodia of malaria. SYN Sporozoasida, Telosporea. [Mod. L., fr. G. *sporos,* seed, + *zōon,* animal]

spo·ro·zo·ite (spōr-ō-zō'īt). One of the minute elongated bodies resulting from the repeated division of the oocyst during sporogony. In the case of the malarial parasite, it is the form that is concentrated in the salivary glands and introduced into the blood by the bite of a mosquito; it enters the liver cells (exoerythrocytic cycle), whose progeny, the merozoites, infect the red blood cells to initiate clinical malaria. SYN germinal rod, zoite, zygotoblast. [sporo- + G. *zōon,* animal]

spo·ro·zo·oid (spōr-ō-zō'oyd). Obsolete term for a falciform figure seen in certain cancerous tumors, formerly regarded by some as a sporozoan spore or sporozoite. [sporo- + G. *zōon,* animal, + *eidos,* resemblance]

spo·ro·zo·on (spōr-ō-zō'on). SYN sporozoan (1).

sport (spōrt). An organism varying in whole or in part, without apparent reason, from others of its type; this variation may be transmitted to the descendants or the latter may revert to the original type. [M.E. *disporte,* fr. O.Fr. *desport,* diversion]

spor·u·lar (spōr'yū-lăr). Relating to a spore or sporule.

spor·u·la·tion (spor'ū-lā'shŭn). The process by which yeasts undergo meiosis, and the meiotic products are encased in spore coats.

spor·ule (spōr'ūl). A spore; a small spore. [Mod. L. *sporula;* dim. of G. *sporos,* seed]

spot. **1.** SYN macula. **2.** To lose a slight amount of blood through the vagina.

acoustic s.'s, SEE *macula* of utricle, *macula* of saccule.

Bitot's s.'s, small, circumscribed, lusterless, grayish white, foamy, greasy, triangular deposits on the bulbar conjunctiva adjacent to the cornea in the area of the palpebral fissure of both eyes; occurs in vitamin A deficiency.

blind s., (1) SYN physiologic *scotoma.* (2) SYN mental *scotoma.* (3) SYN optic *disk.*

blood s.'s, hemorrhagic graafian follicles seen in ovaries of mice, caused by injection of urine of pregnant women; a positive result in the now obsolete Aschheim-Zondek test for pregnancy.

blue s., (1) SYN *macula* cerulea. (2) SYN mongolian s.

Brushfield's s.'s, light-colored condensations of the surface of the mid-iris; seen in Down syndrome.

cherry-red s., the ophthalmoscopic appearance of the normal choroid beneath the fovea centralis, appearing as a red s. surrounded by white retinal edema in central artery closure or lipid infiltration in sphingolipidosis. SYN Tay's cherry-red s.

corneal s., SYN *macula* corneae.

cotton-wool s.'s, SYN cotton-wool *patches,* under *patch.*

De Morgan's s.'s, SYN senile *hemangioma.*

Elschnig's s.'s, isolated choroidal bright yellow or red s.'s with black pigment flecks at their borders, seen ophthalmoscopically in advanced hypertensive retinopathy.

Filatov's s.'s, SYN Koplik's s.'s.

flame s.'s, hemorrhagic areas occurring in the nerve fiber layer of the retina.

focal s., the site of bombardment by electrons and emission of x-rays from the anode of an x-ray tube. SEE ALSO focal spot size.

Fordyce's s.'s, a condition marked by the presence of numerous small, yellowish white bodies or granules on the inner surface and vermilion border of the lips; histologically the lesions are ectopic sebaceous glands. SYN Fordyce's disease, Fordyce's granules, pseudocolloid of lips.

Fuchs' black s., an area of pigment proliferation in the macular region in degenerative myopia.

Graefe's s.'s, small areas over the vertebrae or near the supraorbital foramen, pressure upon which causes relaxation of blepharofacial spasm.

hot s., a region in a gene in which there is a putatively high rate of mutation; of the size of the region concerned, the readiness with which the mutation could be detected, and the possibility that selection against mutants at that point is less than against mutants elsewhere, all call for caution in making such claims.

hypnogenic s., a pressure-sensitive point on the body of certain susceptible persons, which, when pressed, causes the induction of sleep.

Koplik's s.'s, small red s.'s on the buccal mucous membrane, in the center of each of which may be seen, in a strong light, a minute bluish white speck; they occur early in measles (morbilli), before the skin eruption, and are regarded as a pathognomonic sign of the disease. SYN Filatov's s.'s.

liver s., SYN senile *lentigo*.

Mariotte's blind s., SYN optic *disk*.

milk s.'s, (1) white plaques of hyalinized fibrous tissue situated in the epicardium overlying the right ventricle of the heart where it is not covered by lung; SYN soldier's patches. **(2)** white macroscopic areas in the omentum, due to accumulation of macrophages and lymphocytes. SYN tache laiteuse (1).

mongolian s., any of a number of dark bluish or mulberry-colored rounded or oval s.'s on the sacral region due to the ectopic presence of scattered melanocytes in the dermis. These congenital lesions are frequent in black, native American, and Asian children from 2 to 12 years, after which time they gradually recede; they do not disappear on pressure and are sometimes mistaken for bruises from child abuse. SYN blue s. (2), mongolian macula.

mulberry s.'s, the abdominal eruption in typhus fever.

rose s.'s, characteristic exanthema of typhoid fever; 10–20 small pink papules on the lower trunk lasting a few days and leaving hyperpigmentation.

Roth's s.'s, a round white retina s. surrounded by hemorrhage in bacterial endocarditis, and in other retinal hemorrhagic conditions.

ruby s.'s, SYN senile *hemangioma*.

saccular s., SYN *macula* of saccule.

Soemmerring's s., SYN *macula* retinae.

spongy s., SYN vascular *zone*.

Tardieu's s.'s, SYN Tardieu's *ecchymoses*, under *ecchymosis*.

Tay's cherry-red s., SYN cherry-red s.

temperature s., one of a number of definitely arranged s.'s on the skin sensitive to heat and cold, but not to ordinary pressure or pain stimuli.

tendinous s., SYN *macula* albida.

Trousseau's s., SYN meningitic *streak*.

utricular s., SYN *macula* of utricle.

white s., SYN *macula* albida.

yellow s., SYN *macula* retinae.

spp. Plural of sp., abbreviation for species.

sprain (sprān). **1.** An injury to a ligament when the joint is carried through a range of motion greater than normal, but without dislocation or fracture. **2.** To cause a s. of a joint. SYN stremma.

spray (sprā). A jet of liquid in fine drops, coarser than a vapor; it is produced by forcing the liquid from the minute opening of an atomizer, mixed with air.

spread·er (spred′er). **1.** An instrument used to distribute a substance over a surface or area. **2.** A device for spacing or parting structures.

gutta-percha s., an instrument used in dentistry for condensing gutta-percha laterally in a root canal.

rib s., an instrument for widening the space between ribs in intrathoracic operations.

root canal s., a tapered instrument utilized for condensing root filling materials laterally.

Sprengel, Otto G.K., German surgeon, 1852–1915. SEE S.'s *deformity*.

sprout (sprowt). A structure resembling the s. of a plant.

syncytial s., SYN syncytial *knot*.

sprue (sprū). **1.** Primary intestinal malabsorption with steatorrhea. SYN cachexia aphthosa. **2.** In dentistry, wax or metal used to form the aperture(s) for molten metal to flow into a mold to make a casting; also, the metal that later fills the s. hole(s). [D. *spruw*]

celiac s., SYN celiac *disease*.

nontropical s., s. occurring in persons away from the tropics; usually called celiac disease; due to gluten-induced enteropathy.

tropical s., s. occurring in the tropics, often associated with enteric infection and nutritional deficiency, and frequently complicated by folate deficiency with macrocytic anemia. SYN tropical diarrhea.

sprue-form·er (sprū fōr′mer). The base to which the sprue (2) is attached while the wax pattern is being invested in a refractory investment in a casting flask; it is sometimes referred to as a crucible-former.

spud (spŭd). A triangular knife used for removing foreign bodies from the cornea.

Spu·ma·vir·i·nae (spū′mă-vir′i-nē). A subfamily of viruses (family Retroviridae) that includes the foamy viruses (agents) of primates and other mammals; in common with other retroviruses, they possess RNA-dependent DNA polymerases (reverse transcriptase). [L. *spuma*, foam]

Spu·ma·vi·rus (spū′mă-vī-rŭs). A virus genus encompassing a poorly characterized group of retroviruses that cause vacuolation (foaming) of cultured cells; a member of the subfamily Spumaviridae.

spur (sper). SYN calcar. [A.S. *spora*]

Fuchs' s., epithelial outgrowth of the dilator muscle of the pupil about midway in the breadth of the sphincter; part of the insertion of the dilator muscle onto the iris sphincter.

Grunert's s., epithelial outgrowth of the dilator muscle of the pupil at the junction of the iris and the ciliary body; part of the origin of the iris dilator muscle.

Michel's s., epithelial outgrowth of the dilator muscle of the pupil at the peripheral border of the sphincter; part of the insertion of the dilator muscle onto the iris sphincter.

Morand's s., SYN *calcar* avis.

scleral s., a ridge of the sclera at the internal scleral sulcus from which ciliary muscle fibers take origin. SYN scleral roll.

vascular s., partial septum between vessels (arteries and veins) at the level of fusion or branching at acute angle. SEE ALSO calcar (1).

spu·ri·ous (spū′rē-ŭs). False; not genuine. [L. *spurius*]

spu·tum, pl. **spu·ta** (spū′tŭm, -tă). **1.** Expectorated matter, especially mucus or mucopurulent matter expectorated in diseases of the air passages. SEE ALSO expectoration (1). **2.** An individual mass of such matter. [L. *sputum*, fr. *spuo*, pp. *sputus*, to spit]

s. aerogeno′sum, a green expectoration seen occasionally in jaundice, due to staining of the s. by bile pigments. SYN green s.

globular s., SYN nummular s.

green s., SYN s. aerogenosum.

nummular s., a thick, coherent mass expectorated in globular shape which does not run at the bottom of the cup but forms a discoid mass resembling a coin. SYN globular s.

prune-juice s., a thin reddish expectoration, characteristic of necrosis of lung tissue, usually by infection; due to hemorrhage caused by destruction of the lung parenchyma; sometimes seen with lung tumors. SYN prune-juice expectoration.

rusty s., a reddish brown, blood-stained expectoration characteristic of lobar pneumonococcal pneumonia.

SQ Abbreviation for subcutaneous.

squa·lene (skwā′lēn). A hexaisoprenoid (triterpenoid) hydrocarbon found in shark oil and in some plants; intermediate in the biosynthesis of cholesterol and other sterols and triterpenes.

s. epoxidase, an enzyme that catalyzes the conversion of s. to s. 2,3-oxide in the endoplasmic reticulum; a required step in order for cyclization to occur, resulting in the synthesis of the first sterol, lanosterol, in steroidogenesis; uses NADPH.

s. synthase, an enzyme that catalyzes the formation of s. from two molecules of farnesylpyrophosphate using NADPH and concomitant production of two molecules of pyrophosphate.

squa·ma, pl. **squa·mae** (skwā′mă, skwā′mē). **1.** A thin plate of bone. **2.** An epidermal scale. SYN scale (2), squame. [L. a scale]

frontal s., SYN squamous *part* of occipital bone.

s. fronta′lis [NA], SYN squamous *part* of frontal bone.

occipital s.,

s. occipita′lis, occipital s. [NA], SYN squamous *part* of occipital bone.

temporal s., SYN squamous *part* of temporal bone.

s. tempora′lis, SYN squamous *part* of temporal bone.

squa·mate (skwā′māt). SYN squamous.

squa·ma·ti·za·tion (skwā′mă-ti-zā′shŭn). Transformation of other types of cells into squamous cells.

squame (skwām). SYN squama.

△**squamo-.** Squama, squamous. [L. *squama*, a scale]

squa·mo·cel·lu·lar (skwā-mō-sel′yū-lăr). Relating to or having squamous epithelium.

squa·mo·co·lum·nar (skwā-mō-kol′ŭm-nar). Pertaining to the junction between a stratified squamous epithelial surface and one lined by columnar epithelium; *e.g.,* the cardia of the stomach or anus.

squa·mo·fron·tal (skwā′mō-frŏn′tăl). Relating to the squamous part of the frontal bone.

squa·mo·mas·toid (skwā′mō-mas′toyd). Relating to the squamous and petrous portions of the temporal bone.

squa·mo·oc·cip·i·tal (skwā′mō-ok-sip′i-tăl). Relating to the squamous portion of the occipital bone, developing partly in membrane and partly in cartilage.

squa·mo·pa·ri·e·tal (skwā′mō-pă-rī′ĕ-tăl). Relating to the parietal bone and the squamous portion of the temporal bone.

squa·mo·pe·tro·sal (skwā′mō-pĕ-trō′săl). SYN petrosquamosal, petrosquamosal.

squa·mo·sa, pl. **squa·mo·sae** (skwā-mō′să, -sē). The squamous parts of the frontal, occipital, or temporal bone, especially the latter. [L. *squamosus,* scaly, fr. *squama,* scale]

squa·mo·sal (skwā-mō′săl). Relating especially to the squamous part of the temporal bone.

squa·mo·sphe·noid (skwā′mō-sfē′noyd). Relating to the sphenoid bone and the squamous part of the temporal bone. SYN sphenosquamosal.

squa·mo·tem·po·ral (skwā′mō-tem′pŏ-răl). Relating to the squamous part of the temporal bone.

squa·mo·tym·pan·ic (skwa′mō-tim-man′ik). SYN tympanosquamosal.

squa·mous (skwā′mŭs). Relating to or covered with scales. SYN scaly, squamate. [L. *squamosus*]

squa·mo·zy·go·mat·ic (skwā′mō-zī-gō-mat′ik). Relating to the squamous part of the temporal bone and the zygomatic process of the temporal bone.

squar·rose, squar·rous (skwar′ōs, skwar′ŭs). Obsolete term for squamous. [L. *squarrosus*]

squill (skwil). The cut and dried fleshy inner scales of the bulb of the white variety of *Urginea maritima* (Mediterranean s.), or of *U. indica* (Indian s.) (family Liliaceae); the central portion of the bulb is excluded during its processing; s. contains cardiac glycosides (scillaren-A and scillaren-B) and scillaricide, a rodenticide. SYN scilla. [L. *squilla* or *scilla*]

squint (skwint). **1.** SYN strabismus. **2.** To suffer from strabismus.

convergent s., SYN esotropia.

divergent s., SYN exotropia.

external s., SYN exotropia.

internal s., SYN esotropia.

[85]Sr Abbreviation for strontium-85.

[87m]Sr Abbreviation for strontium-87m.

Sr Symbol for strontium.

[89]Sr Symbol for strontium-89.

[90]Sr Symbol for strontium-90.

SRF Abbreviation for somatotropin-releasing *factor*.

SRF-A Abbreviation for slow-reacting *factor* of anaphylaxis.

SRH Abbreviation for somatotropin-releasing *hormone*.

SRIF Abbreviation for somatotropin release-inhibiting *factor*.

sRNA Abbreviation for soluble RNA. See entries under ribonucleic acid.

S ro·ma·num (rō-mā′nŭm). Archaic term for sigmoid *colon*.

SRP Abbreviation for signal recognition *particle*.

SRS Abbreviation for slow-reacting *substance*.

SRS-A Abbreviation for slow-reacting *substance* of anaphylaxis.

ss Abbreviation for single-stranded, steady *state*.

SSPE Abbreviation for subacute sclerosing *panencephalitis*.

SSS Abbreviation for soluble specific *substance*.

stab. To pierce with a pointed instrument, as a knife or dagger. [Gael. *stob*]

sta·bi·late (stā′bi-lāt). A sample of organisms preserved alive on a single occasion.

sta·bile (stā′bīl, -bil). Steady; fixed; denoting: 1) certain constituents of serum unaffected by ordinary degrees of heat; 2) an electrode held steadily on a part during the passage of an electric current. Cf. labile. [L. *stabilis*]

stab·i·lim·e·ter (stā-bi-lim′ĕ-ter). An instrument to measure the sway of the body when standing with feet together and usually with eyes closed. [L. *stabilitas,* firmness, + G. *metron,* measure]

sta·bil·i·ty (stă-bil′i-tē). The condition of being stable or resistant to change.

denture s., the quality of a denture to be firm, steady, constant, and resist change of position when functional forces are applied. SYN stabilization (2).

detrusor s., a detrusor that accommodates increasing bladder volume without significant increase in detrusor pressure and without involuntary detrusor contraction.

dimensional s., the property of a material to retain its size and form.

endemic s., a situation in which all factors influencing disease occurrence are relatively stable, resulting in little fluctuation in disease incidence over time; changes in one or more of these factors (*e.g.,* reduction in proportion of individuals with immunity from exposure to infectious agent) can lead to an unstable situation in which major disease outbreaks occur. SYN enzootic s.

enzootic s., SYN endemic s.

suspension s., a very slow sedimentation rate.

sta·bi·li·za·tion (stā′bĭ-li-zā′shŭn). **1.** The accomplishment of a stable state. **2.** SYN denture *stability*.

sta·bi·liz·er (stā′bĭ-līz-zer). **1.** That which renders something else more stable. **2.** An agent that retards the effect of an accelerator, thus preserving a chemical equilibrium. **3.** A part possessing the quality of rigidity or creating rigidity when added to another part.

endodontic s., a pin implant passing through the apex of a tooth from its root canal and extending well into the underlying bone to provide immobilization of periodontally involved teeth.

sta·ble (stā′bl). Steady; not varying; resistant to change. SEE ALSO stabile.

stach·y·bot·ry·o·tox·i·co·sis (stak-ē-bot′rē-ō-tok-si-kō′sis). A type of mycotoxicosis seen in horses and cattle following ingestion of hay and fodder overgrown by the fungus *Stachybotrys atra;* may also occur in persons exposed to hay either by inhalation or by absorbing the toxin through the skin, and is manifested by skin rash, pharyngitis, and mild leukopenia.

stach·y·drine (stak′i-drēn). *N*-methylproline methylbetaine; the betaine of L-proline found in alfalfa, chrysanthemum, and citrus plants.

stach·y·ose (stak′ē-ōs). A raffinosegalactopyranoside; a tetrasaccharide that yields D-glucose, D-fructose, and 2 mol of D-galactose upon hydrolysis; present in certain tubers and other plant tissues.

stac·tom·e·ter (stak-tom′ĕ-ter). SYN stalagmometer. [G. *staktos,* dropping, fr. *stazō,* to let fall by drops, + *metron,* measure]

Stader, Otto, U.S. veterinary surgeon, *1894. SEE S. *splint*.

Staderini, Rutilio, 19th century Italian neuroanatomist. SEE S.'s *nucleus*.

sta·di·om·e·ter (stā-dē-om′ĕ-ter). An instrument for measuring standing or sitting height. [L. *stadium,* fr. G. *stadion,* a fixed length, + G. *metron,* measure]

sta·di·um, pl. **sta·dia** (stā′dē-ŭm, -dē-ă). Obsolete term for a stage in the course of a disease, especially of an acute pyretic disease. [L. fr. G. *stadion,* a fixed standard length]

staff. **1.** A specific group of workers. **2.** SYN director (1). [A.S. *staef*]

attending s., physicians and surgeons who are members of a hospital s. and regularly attend their patients at the hospital; may also supervise and teach house s., fellows, and medical students.

consulting s., specialists affiliated with a hospital who serve in an advisory capacity to the attending s.

house s., physicians and surgeons in specialty training at a hospital who care for the patients under the direction and responsibility of the attending s.

staff of Aes·cu·la·pi·us. A rod with only one serpent encircling it and without wings; symbol of medicine and emblem of the American Medical Association, Royal Army Medical Corps (Britain), and Royal Canadian Medical Corps. SEE ALSO caduceus. [L. *Aesculapius,* G. *Asklēpios,* god of medicine]

Stafne, Edward C., U.S. oral pathologist, *1894. SEE S. bone *cyst.*

stage (stāj). **1.** A period in the course of a disease; a description of the extent of involvement of a disease process or the status of a patient with a specific disease, as of the distribution and extent of dissemination of a malignant neoplastic disease; also, the act of determining the s. of a disease, especially cancer. SEE ALSO period. **2.** The part of a microscope on which the microslide bears the object to be examined. **3.** A particular step, phase, or position in a developmental process. For psychosexual stages, see entries under phase. [M.E. thr. O. Fr. *estage,* standing-place, fr. L. *sto,* pp. *status,* to stand]

algid s., the s. of collapse in cholera.

Arneth s.'s, a differential grouping of polymorphonuclear neutrophils in accordance with the number of lobes in their nuclei, *i.e.,* cells with 1, 2, 3, 4, or 5 (or more) lobes are designated, respectively, as class I, II, and so on. SEE ALSO Arneth *formula.*

bell s., third s. of tooth development, wherein the cells form the inner enamel epithelium, the stratum intermedium, the stellate reticulum, and the outer enamel epithelium; the enamel organ assumes a bell shape.

bud s., first s. of tooth development; development of the primordia of the enamel organs, the tooth buds.

cap s., second s. of tooth development wherein there is development of the inner and outer enamel epithelium.

cold s., the s. of chill in a malarial paroxysm.

defervescent s., SEE defervescence.

end s., the late, fully developed phase of a disease; *e.g.,* in endstage renal disease, a shrunken and scarred kidney that may result from a variety of chronic diseases that have become indistinguishable in their effect on the kidney.

eruptive s., the stage of an exanthematous illness in which the rash appears.

exoerythrocytic s., developmental s. of the malaria parasite (*Plasmodium*) in liver parenchyma cells of the vertebrate host before erythrocytes are invaded. The initial generation produces cryptozoites, the next generation metacryptozoites; reinfection of liver cells from blood cells apparently does not occur. Delayed development of the sporozoite (hypnozoite) of *Plasmodium vivax* and *P. ovale* appears to be responsible for malarial relapse that may occur with these disease agents.

genital s., referring to the psychic organization derived from, and characteristic of, the Freudian genital period of the infant's psychosocial organization. SEE genitality. SEE ALSO anality, orality.

imperfect s., a mycological term used to describe the asexual life cycle phase of a fungus. SEE anamorph.

incubative s., SYN incubation *period* (1). SYN latent s., prodromal s., s. of invasion.

intuitive s., in psychology, a s. of development, usually occurring between 4 and 7 years of age, in which a child's thought processes are determined by the most prominent aspects of the stimuli to which he or she is exposed, rather than by some form of logical thought.

s. of invasion, SYN incubative s.

s.'s of labor, SEE labor.

latent s., SYN incubative s.

perfect s., a mycological term used to describe the sexual life

cycle phase of a fungus in which spores are formed after nuclear fusion. SYN teleomorph.

preconceptual s., in psychology, the s. of development in an infant's life, prior to actual conceptual thinking, in which sensorimotor activity predominates.

prodromal s., SYN incubative s.

resting s., the quiescent s. of a cell or its nucleus in which no karyokinetic changes are taking place. SYN vegetative s.

Tanner s., a s. of puberty in the Tanner growth chart, based on pubic hair growth, development of genitalia in boys, and breast development in girls.

trypanosome s., SEE trypomastigote.

tumor s., the extent of the spread of a malignant neoplasm from its site of origin. SEE ALSO TNM *staging.*

vegetative s., SYN resting s.

stag·ger (stag'er). To walk unsteadily; to reel.

stag·gers (stag'erz). **1.** A form of decompression sickness in which vertigo, mental confusion, and muscular weakness are the chief symptoms. **2.** A disease in sheep, marked by swaying and uncertain gait, caused by the presence of the larva of the tapeworm *Multiceps multiceps* in the brain, or by other cerebral lesions. SYN gid.

blind s., subacute selenium poisoning in animals.

bracken s., a condition occurring in horses as a result of eating bracken; characterized by locomotor incoordination; due to thiamin deficiency (bracken contains thiaminase).

stag·ing (stāj'ing). **1.** The determination or classification of distinct phases or periods in the course of a disease or pathological process. **2.** The determination of the specific extent of a disease process in an individual patient.

Jewett and Strong s., s. of bladder carcinoma: O, noninvasive; A, with submucosal invasion; B, with muscle invasion; C, with invasion of perivascular fat; D, with lymph node metastasis.

TNM s., a system of clinicopathologic evaluation of tumors based on the extent of tumor involvement at the primary site (T, followed by a number indicating size and depth of invasion), and lymph node involvement (N) and metastasis (M) each followed by a number starting at 0 for no evident metastasis; numbers used depend on the organ involved and influence the prognosis and choice of treatment.

stag·na·tion (stag-nā'shŭn). Retardation or cessation of flow of blood in the vessels, as in passive congestion; marked slowing or accumulation in any part of a normally circulating fluid. [L. *stagnum,* a pool]

Stahl, Friedrich K., German physician, 1811–1873. SEE S.'s *ear.*

Stahl, George E., German physician and chemist, 1660–1734. He promulgated the phlogiston theory. SEE phlogiston.

Stähli, Jean, Swiss ophthalmologist, *1890. SEE Hudson-S. *line.*

STAIN

stain (stān). **1.** To discolor. **2.** To color; to dye. **3.** A discoloration. **4.** A dye used in histologic and bacteriologic technique. **5.** A procedure in which a dye or combination of dyes and reagents

st

Combining forms	[NA] Nomina Anatomica
Word*Finder* Multi-term entry finder Preceding letter A	[MIM] Mendelian Inheritance in Man
A.D.A.M. Anatomy Plates Between letters L and M	☆ Official alternate term
Appendices: Following letter Z	☆[NA] Official alternate Nomina Anatomica term
SYN Synonym; Cf., compare	High Profile Term

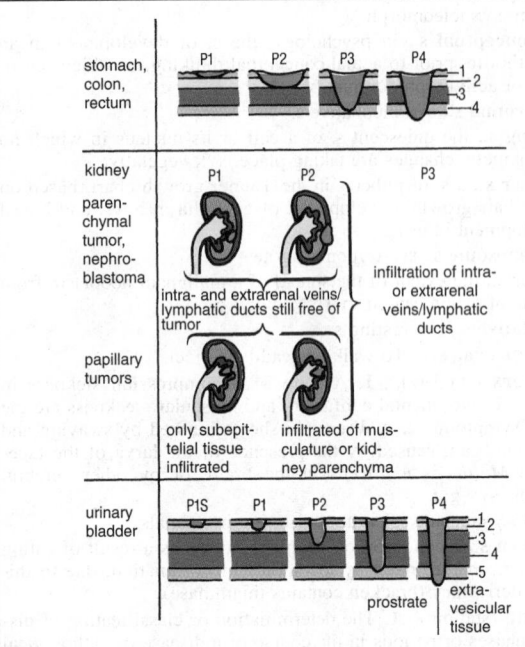

staging

pathological staging (p-staging) of neoplasms of digestive tract, kidney, and bladder [levels of *digestive tract:* 1) mucosa; 2) submucosa; 3) muscularis propria; 4) subserosa; *urinary bladder:* 1) epithelium; 2) tunica propria; 3) internal half of musculature; 4) external half of musculature; 5) adventitia]

TNM staging			
T — primary tumor			
TX	primary tumor cannot be judged		
TO	no basis for primary tumor		
Tis	carcinoma/tumor in situ		
T1, T2, T3, T4 increasing sizes and/or extent of primary tumor invasion			
N — regional lymph nodes			
NX	regional lymph nodes cannot be judged		
NO	no regional lymph node metastases		
N1, N2, N3 increasing invasion of regional lymph nodes			
M — metastasis			
MX	existence of metastases cannot be judged		
MO	no metastases		
M1	metastases present		
	the category M1 can be subdivided as follows:		
lung	PUL	marrow	MAR
bone	OSS	rib	PLE
liver	HEP	peritoneum	PER
brain	BRA	skin	SKI
lymph nodes	LYM	other organs	OTH
R — residual tumor (postoperative)			
RO	no residual tumor		
R1	microscopic residual tumor		
R2	macroscopic residual tumor		
G — histopathologic differentiation grade (grading)			
GX	differentiation grade cannot be determined		
G1	well-differentiated		
G2	moderately differentiated		
G3	poorly differentiated		
G4	undifferentiated		

is used to color the constituents of cells and tissues. For individual dyes or staining substances, see the specific names. [M.E. *steinen*]

Abbott's s. for spores, spores are stained blue with alkaline methylene blue; bodies of the bacilli become pink with eosin counterstain.

aceto-orcein s., a s. used for chromosomes in air-dried or squashed cytologic material.

acid s., a dye in which the anion is the colored component of the dye molecule, *e.g.,* sodium eosinate (eosin).

Ag-AS s., SYN silver-ammoniacal silver s.

Albert's s., a s. for diphtheria bacilli and their metachromatic granules; contains toluidine blue, methyl green, glacial acetic acid, alcohol, and distilled water.

Altmann's anilin-acid fuchsin s., a mixture of picric acid, anilin, and acid fuchsin which stains mitochondria crimson against a yellow background.

auramine O fluorescent s., a rapid and accurate technique for *Mycobacterium tuberculosis,* using auramine O-phenol and a methylene blue counterstain.

basic s., a dye in which the cation is the colored component of the dye molecule that binds to anionic groups of nucleic acids ($PO_4\equiv$) or acidic mucopolysaccharides (*e.g.,* chondroitin sulfate).

basic fuchsin-methylene blue s., a s. for intact epoxy sections; semi-thick sections of plastic-embedded tissues have nuclei stained purple; collagen, elastic lamina, and connective tissue are stained blue; mitochondria, myelin, and lipid droplets are stained red; cytoplasm, smooth muscle cells, axoplasm, and chondroblasts are stained pink.

Bauer's chromic acid leucofuchsin s., a s. for glycogen and fungi utilizing chromic acid as an oxidizing agent of polysaccharides, followed by Schiff's reagent; glycogen and fungi cell walls appear deep red.

Becker's s. for spirochetes, a s. applied to thin films fixed in formaldehyde-acetic acid; preparations are treated successively with tannin, carbolic acid, and carbol fuchsin.

Bennhold's Congo red s., an amyloid s. useful for amyloid detection in pathologic tissue; gives red staining of amyloid; also induces green birefringence to amyloid under polarized light.

Berg's s., a method for staining spermatozoa, utilizing a carbolfuchsin solution followed by dilute acetic acid and methylene blue; spermatozoa are stained a brilliant red and most other structures appear blue to purple.

Best's carmine s., a method for the demonstration of glycogen in tissues.

Bielschowsky's s., a method of treating tissues with silver nitrate to demonstrate reticular fibers, neurofibrils, axons, and dendrites.

Biondi-Heidenhain s., an obsolete s. for spirochetes, using acid fuchsin and orange G.

Birch-Hirschfeld s., an obsolete s. for demonstrating amyloid, using Bismarck brown and crystal violet; amyloid is usually stained a bright ruby red, whereas the cytoplasm of cells is not stained and nuclei are brown.

Bodian's copper-PROTARGOL **s.,** a s. employing a silver proteinate complex (PROTARGOL) to demonstrate axis cylinders and neurofibrils.

Borrel's blue s., a s. for demonstrating spirochetes, treponemes, and Borrelia organisms, using silver oxide (prepared by means of mixing solutions of silver nitrate and sodium bicarbonate) and methylene blue.

Bowie's s., a s. for juxtaglomerular granules in which the kidney sections are stained in a mixture of Biebrich scarlet red and ethyl violet; juxtaglomerular granules and elastic fibers are stained a deep purple, erythrocytes are amber, and background tissue appears in shades of red.

Brown-Brenn s., a method for differential staining of Gram-positive and Gram-negative bacteria in tissue sections; it utilizes a modified Gram s. of crystal violet, Gram's iodine, and basic fuchsin.

Cajal's astrocyte s., a method for demonstrating astrocytes by impregnation in a solution containing gold chloride and mercuric chloride.

carbol-thionin s., a s. useful for demonstrating typhoid bacilli in films and sections, and for Nissl substance.

C-banding s., a selective chromosome banding s. used in human cytogenetics, employing Giemsa s. after most of the DNA is denatured or extracted by treatment with alkali, acid, salt, or heat; only heterochromatic regions close to the centromeres and rich in satellite DNA stain, with the exception of the Y chromosome whose long arm usually stains throughout. SYN centromere banding s.

centromere banding s., SYN C-banding s.

chromate s. for lead, a method in which tissues preserved in chromate-containing fixatives, such as Regaud's or Orth's fixatives, precipitate lead as yellow lead chromate crystals; formalin-fixed sections are treated with potassium chromate acidified with acetic acid.

chrome alum hematoxylin-phloxine s., a s. used to demonstrate pancreatic islet cells; alpha cells appear red, beta cells blue or unstained.

Ciaccio's s., a method for demonstrating complex insoluble intra-cellular lipids using fixation in a formalin-dichromate solution, embedding in paraffin, staining with Sudan III or IV, and examination in aqueous mountant.

contrast s., a dye used to color one portion of a tissue or cell which remained unaffected when the other part was stained by a dye of different color. SYN differential s.

Da Fano's s., a silver s. that produces a blackening of Golgi elements after tissues are fixed in a mixture of nitrate and formalin.

Dane's s., a s. for prekeratin, keratin, and mucin which employs hemalum, phloxine, Alcian blue, and orange G; nuclei appear orange to brown, acid mucopolysaccharides pale blue, and keratins orange to red-orange.

DAPI s., a sensitive fluorescent probe for DNA, 4'6-diamidino-2-phenylindole·2HCl, used in fluorescence microscopy to detect DNA in yeast mitochondria, chloroplasts, viruses, mycoplasma, and chromosomes; DNA is visualized in vitally stained living cells and after cells are fixed in formaldehyde.

diazo s. for argentaffin granules, in enterochromaffin cells, a variety of diazonium salts are used to blacken the cells.

Dieterle's s., s. used to demonstrate spirochetes and Leishman-Donovan bodies; employs silver nitrate and uranium nitrate.

differential s., SYN contrast s.

double s., a mixture of two dyes, each of which stains different portions of a tissue or cell.

Ehrlich's acid hematoxylin s., an alum type of hematoxylin s. used as a regressive staining method for nuclei, followed by differentiation to required staining intensity; the solution may be allowed to ripen naturally in sunlight or partially oxidized with sodium iodate.

Ehrlich's aniline crystal violet s., a s. for Gram-positive bacteria.

Ehrlich's triacid s., a differential leukocytic s. comprised of saturated solutions of orange G, acid fuchsin, and methyl green.

Ehrlich's triple s., a mixture of indulin, eosin Y, and aurantia.

Einarson's gallocyanin-chrome alum s., a method for staining both RNA and DNA a deep blue; with proper controls, nucleic acid content of stained cells and nuclei may be estimated by cytophotometry; also useful for Nissl substance.

Eranko's fluorescence s., exposure of frozen sections to formaldehyde which produces a strong yellow-green fluorescence from cells containing norepinephrine.

Feulgen s., a selective cytochemical reaction for DNA in which sections or cells are first hydrolyzed with hydrochloric acid to produce apurinic acid and then are stained with Schiff's reagent to produce magenta-stained nuclei; generally the concentration of DNA in nucleoli and mitochondria is too low to permit detection by this s. SEE ALSO Kasten's fluorescent Feulgen s.

Field's rapid s., a s. to permit rapid positive diagnosis of malaria in endemic areas by using thick films; it employs methylene blue and azure B in a phosphate buffer, with the preparation counterstained by eosin in a phosphate buffer.

Fink-Heimer s., a method used for histologic demonstration of degenerating nerve fibers and terminals of the central nervous system (black on a yellow background).

Flemming's triple s., a s. comprised of safranin, methyl violet, and orange G.

fluorescence plus Giemsa s., a s. used to demonstrate sister chromatid exchange; cells are grown in 5-bromodeoxyuridine, followed by chromosome preparation, staining in HOECHST 33258, exposure to light, and staining in Giemsa; chromosomes exhibit a "harlequin" appearance.

fluorescent s., a s. or staining procedure using a fluorescent dye or substance that will combine selectively with certain tissue components and that will then fluoresce upon irradiation with ultraviolet or violet-blue light.

Fontana-Masson silver s., SYN Masson-Fontana ammoniacal silver s.

Fontana's s., a traditional method for silver-impregnation of treponemes and other spirochetal forms.

Foot's reticulin impregnation s., a silver s. in which reticulin stains black and collagen stains golden brown; sections are floated on the surface of solutions to avoid contamination with silver debris.

Fouchet's s., fouchet's reagent employed to demonstrate bile pigments; paraffin sections are used for conjugated bile pigments, frozen sections for unconjugated ones.

Fraser-Lendrum s. for fibrin, a multistaining procedure after Zenker's fixative in which fibrin, keratin, and some cytoplasmic granules appear red, erythrocytes appear orange, and collagen appears green.

Friedländer's s. for capsules, an obsolete s. employing gentian violet.

G-banding s., a unique chromosome staining technique, used in human cytogenetics to identify individual chromosomes, which produces characteristic bands; it utilizes acetic acid fixation, air drying, denaturing chromosomes mildly with proteolytic enzymes, salts, heat, detergents, or urea, and finally Giemsa s.; chromosome bands appear similar to those fluorochromed by Q-banding s. SYN Giemsa chromosome banding s.

Giemsa s., compound of methylene blue-eosin and methylene blue used for demonstrating Negri bodies, *Tunga* species, spirochetes and protozoans, and differential staining of blood smears; also used for chromosomes, sometimes after hydrolyzing the cytologic preparation in hot hydrochloric acid, and for showing chromosome G bands; often used in glycerol-methanol buffer solution.

Giemsa chromosome banding s., SYN G-banding s.

Glenner-Lillie s. for pituitary, a modification of Mann's methyl blue-eosin s. which changes the dye proportions, buffering the dye mixture, and staining at 60°C; basophils are stained blue to black, acidophils are dark red, chromophobe granules are gray to pink, and erythrocytes are orange; with modification, the method is also useful for enterochromaffin cells, goblet cells, Paneth cells, and pancreatic islet cells.

Golgi's s., any of several methods for staining nerve cells, nerve fibers, and neuroglia using fixation and hardening in formalin-osmic-dichromate combinations for various times, followed by impregnation in silver nitrate.

Gomori-Jones periodic acid-methenamine-silver s., a staining method using methenamine silver, periodic acid, gold chloride, hematoxylin, and eosin to delineate basement membrane, reticulin, collagen, and nuclei; used in renal histopathology. SEE ALSO Rambourg's periodic acid-chromic methenamine-silver s.

Gomori's aldehyde fuchsin s., a s. used to demonstrate beta cells of the pancreas, storage form of thyrotrophic hormone in beta cells of the anterior pituitary, hypophyseal neurosecretory substance, mast cells, granules, elastic fibers, sulfated mucins, and gastric chief cells.

Gomori's chrome alum hematoxylin-phloxine s., a technique used to demonstrate cytoplasmic granules, after Bouin's or formalin-Zenker fixatives, using oxidized hematoxylin plus phloxine; in the pancreas, beta cells are blue, alpha and delta cells are red, and zymogen granules are red to unstained; in the pituitary, alpha cells are pink, beta cells and chromophobes are gray-blue, and nuclei are purple to blue.

Gomori's methenamine-silver s.'s (GMS), GMS s., techniques for 1) *argentaffin cells:* a method using a methenamine-silver solution in combination with gold chloride, sodium thiosulphate, and safranin O; argentaffin granules appear brown-black against a green background; 2) *urates:* warm sections are treated directly with a hot methenamine-silver solution to produce a blackening of urates; 3) *fungi:* see Grocott-Gomori methenamine-silver s.; 4) *melanin,* which reduces silver nitrate.

Gomori's nonspecific acid phosphatase s., a method in which formalin-fixed frozen sections are incubated in a substrate containing sodium β-glycerophosphate and lead nitrate at pH 5.0; the insoluble lead phosphate produced is treated with ammonium sulfide to give a black lead sulfide.

Gomori's nonspecific alkaline phosphatase s., a calcium-cobalt sulfide method using frozen sections or cold acetone- or formalin-fixed paraffin sections, plus sodium β-glycerophosphate as a substrate at pH 9.0 to 9.5 with Mg^{++} as activator; calcium ions precipitate the liberated phosphate, cobalt salt replaces the calcium phosphate, and ammonium sulfide converts the product to a black cobalt sulfide.

Gomori's one-step trichrome s., a connective tissue s. that uses hematoxylin and a dye mixture containing chromotrope 2R and light green or aniline blue; muscle fibers appear red, collagen is green (or blue if aniline blue is used), and nuclei are blue to black.

Gomori's silver impregnation s., a reliable method for reticulin, as an aid in the diagnosis of neoplasm and early cirrhosis of the liver; the staining solution employs silver nitrate, potassium hydroxide, and ammonia water carefully prepared to avoid having silver precipitate.

Goodpasture's s., a s. for Gram-negative bacteria, using aniline fuchsin.

Gordon and Sweet s., a s. for reticulin, using acidified potassium permanganate, oxalic acid, iron alum, silver nitrate, formaldehyde, gold chloride, and sodium thiosulfate.

Gram's s., a method for differential staining of bacteria; smears are fixed by flaming, stained in a solution of crystal violet, treated with iodine solution, rinsed, decolorized, and then counterstained with safranin O; Gram-positive organisms stain purple black and Gram-negative organisms stain pink; useful in bacterial taxonomy and identification, and also in indicating fundamental differences in cell wall structure.

green s., a deposit, produced by chromogenic bacteria, found on the cervicolabial portions of the teeth, usually in children. SEE ALSO acquired *pellicle.*

Gridley's s., a silver staining method for reticulum.

Gridley's s. for fungi, a method for fixed tissue sections based on Bauer's chromic acid leucofuchsin s. with the addition of Gomori's aldehyde fuchsin s. and metanil yellow as counterstains; against a yellow background, hyphae, conidia, yeast capsules, elastin, and mucin appear in different shades of blue to purple.

Grocott-Gomori methenamine-silver s., a modification of Gomori's methenamine-silver s. for fungi in which sections are pretreated with chromic acid before addition of the methenamine-silver solution and then counterstained with light green to demonstrate black-brown fungi against a pale green background.

Hale's colloidal iron s., a s. used to distinguish acid mucopolysaccharides such as hyaluronic acid; may be combined with PAS to also visualize carbohydrate-containing proteins and glycoproteins.

Heidenhain's azan s., a technique using azocarmine B or G followed by aniline blue to stain nuclei and erythrocytes red, muscle orange, glia fibrils reddish, mucin blue, and collagen and reticulum dark blue. [*azo*carmine + *an*iline blue]

Heidenhain's iron hematoxylin s., an iron alum hematoxylin s. used for staining muscle striations and mitotic structures blue-black.

hematoxylin and eosin s., probably the most generally useful of all staining methods for tissues; nuclei are stained a deep blue-black with hematoxylin, and cytoplasm is stained pink after counterstaining with eosin, usually in water.

hematoxylin-malachite green-basic fuchsin s., a s. for epoxy resin-extracted sections; semi-thick sections have their plastic dissolved out and the residual tissue is stained sequentially with the various dyes; nuclei and astrocytes are purplish-pink and myelin, lipid droplets, nucleoli, and oligodendrocytes are bright blue-green.

hematoxylin-phloxine B s., a s. for intact epoxy sections; semi-thick sections of plastic-embedded tissues have the following structures stained blue to black; chromatin, nucleoli, basophilic cytoplasm, mitochondria, plasma and nuclear membranes, anisotropic myofibrils, mast cell granules, and elastic membranes of blood vessels; appearing pink to red are collagen fibrils, reticulum, goblet cell mucins, hyalin cartilage matrix, stereocilia, cytoplasm, and erythrocytes; fat droplets and perichondrocyte matrix are green.

Hirsch-Peiffer s., a s. used for cytologic demonstration staining of metachromatic leukodystrophy; excess sulfatides stain metachromatically (golden brown) with cresyl violet in acetic acid.

Hiss' s., a s. for demonstrating the capsules of microorganisms, using gentian violet or basic fuchsin followed by a copper sulphate wash.

Holmes' s., a silver nitrate staining method for nerve fibers.

Hortega's neuroglia s., one of several silver carbonate methods to demonstrate astrocytes, oligodendroglia, and microglia.

Hucker-Conn s., a crystal violet-ammonium oxalate mixture used in Gram's stain.

immunofluorescent s., s. resulting from combination of fluorescent antibody with antigen specific for the antibody portion of the fluorochrome conjugate.

India ink capsule s., a negative s. for crystal bacteria in which cells appear purple (Gram's crystal violet) and the capsules appear clear against a dark background.

intravital s., a s. which is taken up by living cells after parenteral administration, *e.g.,* intravenously or subcutaneously.

iodine s., a s. to detect amyloid, cellulose, chitin, starch, carotenes, and glycogen, and to stain amebas by virtue of their glycogen; feces and other wet preparations are stained directly with Lugol's iodine solution; smears are treated with Schaudinn's fixative and then stained with alcoholic iodine, followed by Heidenhain's iron hematoxylin.

Jenner's s., a methylene blue eosinate similar to Wright's s. but differing in not using polychromed methylene blue; used for staining of blood smears.

Kasten's fluorescent Feulgen s., a fluorescent modification of the Feulgen s., utilizing any one of a variety of fluorescent basic dyes to which SO_2 is added; the brilliant fluorescence makes this method unusually sensitive and adaptable to cytofluorometric quantification of DNA.

Kasten's fluorescent PAS s., a fluorescent modification of the periodic acid Schiff s. for polysaccharides which uses one of Kasten's fluorescent Schiff reagents.

Kinyoun s., a method for demonstrating acid-fast microorganisms, using carbol fuchsin, acid alcohol, and methylene blue; acid-fast microorganisms appear red against a blue background.

Kleihauer s., a combination of aniline blue and Biebrich scarlet red used for detection of fetal cells in the maternal blood.

Klinger-Ludwig acid-thionin s. for sex chromatin, a method using a preliminary acid treatment on buccal smears, prior to staining with buffered thionin, to differentiate Barr body.

Klüver-Barrera Luxol fast blue s., in combination with cresyl violet, a s. useful for demonstrating myelin and Nissl substance.

Kossa s., SYN von Kossa s.

Kronecker's s., a 5% sodium chloride s. rendered faintly alkaline with sodium carbonate, used in the examination of fresh tissues under the microscope.

Laquer's s. for alcoholic hyalin, a combination of Altmann's aniline-acid fuchsin s. with a Masson trichrome s. which, on a gray-brown background, stains alcoholic hyalin red, collagen green, and nuclei brown.

lead hydroxide s., a s. for electron microscopy; after aldehyde fixation, alkaline lead hydroxide preferentially stains RNA, but after OsO_4 fixation, it reacts largely with osmium in tissues to give a general s.; in addition to binding to cytomembranes, it also stains carbohydrates (*e.g.,* glycogen).

Leishman's s., a polychromed eosin-methylene blue s. used in the examination of blood films.

Lendrum's phloxine-tartrazine s., a s. for demonstrating acidophilic inclusion bodies, which appear red on a yellow background; nuclei stain blue, but Negri bodies do not stain.

Lepehne-Pickworth s., a staining technique for hemoglobin and other heme-containing substances in cryostat or frozen sections, which utilizes the presence of tissue peroxidase to oxidize benzidine to a blue quinhydrone.

Levaditi s., a silver nitrate s. for blackening spirochetes in tissue sections.

Lillie's allochrome connective tissue s., a procedure using PAS, hematoxylin, picric acid, and methyl blue; used for distinction between basement membrane and reticulin, and for demonstration of arteriosclerotic lesions.

Lillie's azure-eosin s., a s. in which an azure eosinate solution is used to s. bacteria and rickettsiae in tissues.

Lillie's ferrous iron s., a method using potassium ferrocyanide in acetic acid which demonstrates melanins as a deep green color; lipofuscins and heme pigments are unreactive.

Lillie's sulfuric acid Nile blue s., a technique for showing fatty acids when present in high concentrations.

Lison-Dunn s., a technique using leuco patent blue V and hydrogen peroxidase to demonstrate hemoglobin peroxidase on time sections and smears.

Loeffler's s., a s. for flagella; the specimen is treated with a mixture of ferrous sulfate, tannic acid, and alcoholic fuchsin, then stained with aniline-water fuchsin or gentian violet made alkaline with sodium hydroxide solution.

Loeffler's caustic s., a s. for flagella, utilizing an aqueous solution of tannin and ferrous sulfate with the addition of an alcoholic fuchsin s.

Luna-Ishak s., a staining method using celestine blue and acid fuchsin in which bile canaliculi s. pink to red.

Macchiavello's s., a basic fuchsin-citric acid-methylene blue sequence in smears which produces red staining of rickettsiae and inclusion bodies, with nuclei staining blue.

MacNeal's tetrachrome blood s., a s. for blood smears comprised of a mixture of methylene blue, azure A, methylene violet, and eosin Y.

malarial pigment s., a s. using phloxine-toluidine blue O sequence; malarial pigment and nuclei are bluish, erythrocytes and cytoplasm are red to orange; found in phagocytic cells of the reticuloendothelial system.

Maldonado-San Jose s., a staining method for staining pancreatic islet cells, using a phloxine-azure B-hematoxylin sequence; alpha cells are purple, beta cells are violet-blue, delta cells are light blue, and exocrine cells are grayish blue with red secretion granules.

Mallory's s. for actinomyces, a s. using alum hematoxylin, followed by eosin; immersion in Ehrlich's aniline crystal violet s., and Weigert's iodine solution; mycelia stain blue and clubs stain red.

Mallory's aniline blue s., SYN Mallory's trichrome s.

Mallory's collagen s., one of a number of staining methods using phosphomolybdic or phosphotungstic acid with an acid stain, such as aniline blue, or with hematoxylin for connective tissue staining.

Mallory's s. for hemofuchsin, sections are stained sequentially in alum hematoxylin and basic fuchsin; the lipofuchsin-like pigment and ceroid stain bright red, nuclei stain blue, while melanin and hemosiderin appear unstained in their natural browns.

Mallory's iodine s., amyloid appears red-brown after Gram's iodine, then violet and blue after flooding with dilute sulfuric acid.

Mallory's phloxine s., a technique based on retention of phloxine by hyaline after overstaining and then decolorizing with lithium carbonate, used in combination with alum hematoxylin to give nuclear staining; hyaline appears red, older hyaline is pink to colorless, amyloid is pale pink, and nuclei are blue-black.

Mallory's phosphotungstic acid hematoxylin s., SYN phosphotungstic acid *hematoxylin.*

Mallory's trichrome s., a method especially suitable for studying connective tissue; sections are stained in acid fuchsin, aniline blue-orange G solution, and phosphotungstic acid; fibrils of collagen are blue, fibroglia, neuroglia, and muscle fibers are red, and fibrils of elastin are pink or yellow. SYN Mallory's aniline blue s., Mallory's triple s.

Mallory's triple s., SYN Mallory's trichrome s.

Mann's methyl blue-eosin s., a s. useful for anterior pituitary and viral inclusion bodies; a mixture of the two dyes stains alpha cell granules red, beta cell granules dark blue, chromophobes gray to pink, colloid red, erythrocytes orange-red, and collagen fibers blue; this method is also useful for enterochromaffin, goblet, Paneth, and pancreatic islet cells; Negri bodies appear red while their nuclei and central granules are blue.

Marchi's s., a staining method in which the specimen is hardened for 8 to 10 days in a modified Müller's fixative, followed by immersion for 1 to 3 weeks in the same with the addition of osmic acid; fat and degenerating nerve fibers stain black.

Masson-Fontana ammoniacal silver s., a s. used to demonstrate melanin and argentaffin granules. SYN Fontana-Masson silver s.

Masson's argentaffin s., a s. used to stain enterochromaffin granules brown-black.

Masson's trichrome s., original composition for multicolored tissue preparations included Ponceau de xylidine, acid fuchsin, iron alum hematoxylin, and either aniline blue or fast green FCF; chromatin stains black, cytoplasm is in shades of red, granules of eosinophils and mast cells are deep red, erythrocytes are black, elastic fibers are red, and collagen fibers and mucus are dark blue (aniline blue) or green (fast green FCF); modifications substitute other dyes, such as Biebrich scarlet red and wool green S.

Maximow's s. for bone marrow, an alum-hematoxylin and azure II-eosin s. used to distinguish granulated leukocytes, mast cells, and cartilage.

Mayer's hemalum s., a progressive nuclear s. also used as a counterstain.

Mayer's mucicarmine s., SEE mucicarmine.

Mayer's mucihematein s., SEE mucihematein.

May-Grünwald s., a German equivalent of Jenner's s., used for blood staining and in cytology; often used in combination with Giemsa s.; valuable in demonstrating parasitic flagellates.

metachromatic s., a s., such as methylene blue, thionin, or azure A, that has the ability to produce different colors with various histological or cytological structures.

methyl green-pyronin s., a staining method useful for identification of plasma cells which are intensely pyroninophilic; a mixture of a green and a red dye that has the property of staining highly polymerized nucleic acid (DNA) green and low molecular weight nucleic acids (RNA) red. SEE Unna-Pappenheim s.

Mowry's colloidal iron s., a s. used for demonstrating acid mucopolysaccharides.

MSB trichrome s., a s. for fibrin using martius yellow, brilliant crystal scarlet 6R, and soluble blue; fibrin is selectively stained red and connective tissue appears blue.

multiple s., a mixture of several dyes each having an independent selective action on one or more portions of the tissue.

Nakanishi's s., a method for vital staining of bacteria in which a slide is treated with hot methylene blue solution until it acquires a sky-blue color, after which a drop of an emulsion of the bacteria is put on the cover glass and the latter laid on the slide; the bacteria are stained differentially, some parts more intensely than others.

Nauta's s., a s. for degenerating axons in which they stain with silver and appear as fragmented and swollen fibers.

negative s., s. forming an opaque or colored background against which the object to be demonstrated appears as a translucent or colorless area; in electron microscopy, an electron opaque material, such as phosphotungstic acid or sodium phosphotungstate, is used to give detail as to surface structure.

Neisser's s., a s. for the polar nuclei of the diphtheria bacillus which uses a mixture of methylene blue and crystal violet.

neutral s., a compound of an acid s. and a basic s., such as the eosinate of methylene blue, in which the anion and cation each contains a chromophore group. SYN salt dye.

Nicolle's s. for capsules, s. in a mixture of a saturated solution of gentian violet in alcohol-phenol.

ninhydrin-Schiff s. for proteins, proteins are revealed by using ninhydrin or alloxan to produce aldehydes from primary aliphatic amines by oxidative deamination; the aldehydes are shown by reaction with Schiff's reagent.

Nissl's s., (1) a method for staining nerve cells with basic fuchsin; (2) a method for staining aggregates of rough endoplasmic reticulum and ribosomes in neuronal cell bodies and dendrites with basic dyes such as cresyl violet (or cresyl echt violet), thionine, toluidin blue O, or methylene blue.

Noble's s., a basic fuchsin-orange G staining technique for detection of viral inclusion bodies in fixed tissues.

nuclear s., a s. for cell nuclei, usually based on the binding of a basic dye to DNA or nucleohistone.

Orth's s., a lithium carmine s. for nerve cells and their processes.

Padykula-Herman s. for myosin ATPase, a technique similar to that of Gomori's nonspecific alkaline phosphatase s., except that incubation is carried out with ATP as the substrate at pH 9.4 in the absence of Mg^{++}; enzyme activity is demonstrated as blackened deposits in the A band of striated muscle sarcomeres; control tissue sections lacking substrate and containing sulfhydryl inhibitors are necessary.

Paget-Eccleston s., an aldehyde-thionin-PAS-orange G staining technique modified to identify seven different cell types in the anterior pituitary gland.

panoptic s., a s. in which a Romanowsky-type s. is combined with another s.; such a combination improves the staining of cytoplasmic granules and other bodies.

Papanicolaou s., a multichromatic s. used principally on exfoliated cytologic specimens and based on aqueous hematoxylin with multiple counterstaining dyes in 95% ethyl alcohol, giving great transparency and delicacy of detail; important in cancer screening, especially of gynecologic smears.

Pappenheim's s., a method for differentiating tubercle and smegma bacilli; the preparation is stained with hot carbol-fuchsin solution, then treated with an alcoholic solution of rosolic acid and methylene blue to which glycerin is added; tubercle bacilli are stained bright red, but smegma bacilli are decolorized.

paracarmine s., a staining fluid consisting of a solution of calcium chloride and carminic acid in 75% alcohol.

PAS s., SYN periodic acid-Schiff s.

periodic acid-Schiff s. (PAS), a tissue-staining procedure in which 1,2-glycol groupings are first oxidized with periodic acid to aldehydes, which then react with the sulfite leucofuchsin reagent of Schiff, and become colored red-violet; strong staining occurs with polysaccharides, such as glycogen, and mucopolysaccharides of epithelial mucins, basement membranes, and connective tissue. SYN PAS s.

Perls' Prussian blue s., a s. for ferric iron as in hemosiderins, using potassium ferrocyanide in acetic acid or dilute hydrochloric acid followed by a red counterstain such as safranin O or neutral red; various hemosiderins and most mineral irons give a blue-green reaction, while nuclei stain red.

peroxidase s., a method for demonstrating peroxidase granules in some neutrophils and in eosinophils; the enzyme promotes the oxidation of benzidine by hydrogen peroxide; tissues treated with horseradish peroxidase can also have the enzyme detected in the electron microscope.

phosphotungstic acid s., the first general s. used for electron microscopy; a selective s. for extracellular components such as elastin, collagen, and basement membrane mucopolysaccharides; it can be followed by uranyl acetate or lead. SYN PTA s.

picrocarmine s., a red crystalline powder derived from a solution of carmine, ammonia, and picric acid which is evaporated, leaving the powder (soluble in water); it produces excellent staining of keratohyaline granules.

picro-Mallory trichrome s., a modification of Mallory's trichrome s. that involves the addition of picric acid.

picronigrosin s., a solution of nigrosin in picric acid, used for staining connective tissue.

plasma s., plasmatic s., plasmic s., a s. whose principal affinity is for the cytoplasm of cells.

plastic section s., (1) for electron microscopy, a s. (*e.g.,* osmic acid, PTA, potassium permanganate) used on thin sections of plastic-embedded tissues, utilizing differential attachment of heavy atoms to various cellular and tissue structures so that electrons will be absorbed and scattered by these structures to produce an image; to achieve differential staining, the s. must penetrate nonwettable plastic embedments; (2) for light microscopy, a s. (*e.g.,* alkaline toluidine blue, silver methenamine) used on plastic-embedded tissues to attain higher resolution and more detail than normally possible; semi-thick (0.5-1.5 µm) sections are particularly useful in renal pathology, especially in combination with the phase microscope.

port-wine s., SYN *nevus* flammeus.

positive s., direct binding of a dye with a tissue component to produce contrast; in electron microscopy, heavy metals like uranyl and lead salts are used to bind to selective cell constituents to produce increased density to the electron beam, *i.e.,* contrast.

Prussian blue s., a s. employing acid potassium ferrocyanide to demonstrate iron, as in siderocytes.

PTA s., SYN phosphotungstic acid s.

Puchtler-Sweat s. for basement membranes, a staining method using resorcin-fuchsin and nuclear fast red solutions after Carnoy's fixative; basement membranes are gray to black and nuclei pink to red.

Puchtler-Sweat s. for hemoglobin and hemosiderin, a complex staining method in which, on a yellow background, hemoglobin is stained red, hemosiderin blue to green and elastic fibers are pink.

Q-banding s., a fluorescent s. for chromosomes which produces specific banding patterns for each pair of homologous chromosomes; the acridine dye derivative, quinacrine hydrochloride, or other derivatives like quinacrine mustard dihydrochloride produces a green-yellow fluorescence at pH 4.5 in chromosome segments rich in constitutive heterochromatin with deoxyadenylate-deoxythymidilate (A-T) bases of DNA; centromeric regions of human chromosomes 3, 4, and 13 are specifically stained, as are satellites of some acrocentric chromosomes and the end of the long arm of the Y chromosome; banding patterns are similar to those obtained with G-banding stain; similar fluorescent s. results are seen with the antibiotics adriamycin and daunomycin, as well as the tertiary dyes butyl proflavine and DAPI, and the bisbenzimidazole dye HOECHST 33258. SYN quinacrine chromosome banding s.

quinacrine chromosome banding s., SYN Q-banding s.

Rambourg's chromic acid-phosphotungstic acid s., a s. for glycoproteins, used with an electron microscope, with which ultrathin tissue sections reveal complex carbohydrates in the same locations as shown by Rambourg's periodic acid-chromic methenamine-silver s.

Rambourg's periodic acid-chromic methenamine-silver s., a s. for glycoproteins, used with an electron microscope, adapted from the Gomori-Jones periodic acid-methenamine-silver s.; it produces silver deposits in mature saccules of the Golgi apparatus, lysosomal vesicles, cell coat, and basement membranes.

R-banding s., a reverse Giemsa chromosome banding method that produces bands complementary to G-bands; induced by treatment with high temperature, low pH, or acridine orange staining; often used together with G-banding on human karyotype to determine whether there are deletions.

Romanowsky's blood s., prototype of the eosin-methylene blue s.'s for blood smears, using aqueous solutions made of a mixture of methylene blue (saturated) and eosin. Romanowsky-type s.'s depend for their action on compounds formed by interaction of methylene blue and eosin; most are of no value if water is present in the alcohol because neutral dyes become precipitated.

Roux's s., a double s. for diphtheria bacilli which employs crystal violet or dahlia and methyl green.

Schaeffer-Fulton s., a s. for bacterial spores using malachite green and safranin so that bacterial bodies are red to pink and spores are green.

Schmorl's ferric-ferricyanide reduction s., a s. to test for reducing substances in tissues, including melanin, argentaffin granules, thyroid colloid, keratin, keratohyalin, and lipofuscin pigments; ferricyanide is converted into ferrocyanide which is converted to insoluble Prussian blue in the presence of ferric ions.

Schmorl's picrothionin s., a s. for compact bone which employs thionin and picric acid solutions to produce blue to blue-black staining of bone canaliculi and cells; bone matrix is yellowish and cartilage ground substance is purple.

Schultz s., a s. for cholesterol; a relatively specific but insensitive histochemical test for cholesterol and cholesterol esters in which frozen sections of formalin-fixed tissues are oxidized in iron alum, hydrogen peroxide, or sodium iodate, then treated with sulfuric acid to give a blue-green to red color in a positive reaction; the presence of glycerol inhibits the reaction.

selective s., a s. that colors one portion of a tissue or cell exclusively or more deeply than the remaining portions.

silver s., any of a variety of s.'s (*e.g.,* Bielschowsky's, Gomori's silver, impregnation s.'s) which employ alkaline silver nitrate solutions to stain connective tissue fibers (reticulin, collagen), calcium salt deposits, spirochaetes, neurological tissue, and nucleolar organizer regions.

silver-ammoniacal silver s., a s. for the acid protein component of nucleolar regions which are active or which were transcriptionally active in the preceding interphase; uses silver nitrate, ammoniacal silver, and formalin. SYN Ag-AS s.

silver protein s., a silver proteinate complex used in staining nerve fibers, nerve endings, and flagellate protozoa; also used to demonstrate phagocytosis in living animals by the cells of the reticuloendothelial system.

Stirling's modification of Gram's s., a stable aniline-crystal violet s.

supravital s., a procedure in which living tissue is removed from the body and cells are placed in a nontoxic dye solution so that their vital processes may be studied.

Taenzer's s., an orcein solution used for staining elastic tissue. SYN Unna-Taenzer s.

Takayama's s., a s. containing pyridine, sodium hydrate, and dextrose; used for identification of blood stains; a drop added to a suspected blood stain results in the formation of hemochromogen crystals.

telomeric R-banding s., a modified R-banding s. in which the telomeres become strongly stained and faint R-banding still occurs over the rest of the chromosomes; uses air-dried slides, aging for several days, and staining in hot phosphate-buffered Giemsa s.

thioflavine T s., a s. employed to detect amyloid, which induces specific yellow fluorescence; tissue sections are first put in alum-hematoxylin to quench nuclear fluorescence and then stained in thioflavine T.

Tizzoni's s., a s. used as a test for iron in tissue; the tissue is treated with a solution of potassium ferrocyanide and then with dilute hydrochloric acid; a blue coloration indicates the presence of iron.

Toison's s., a blood diluent and leukocyte stain containing methyl violet, sodium chloride, sodium sulfate, and glycerin; also used for erythrocyte counts.

trichrome s., staining combinations which usually contain three dyes of contrasting colors selected to stain connective tissue, muscle, cytoplasm, and nuclei in bright colors; generally, tissue sections are first dyed in iron hematoxylin before being treated with the other dyes.

trypsin G-banding s., SEE G-banding s.

Unna-Pappenheim s., a contrast s. consisting of a methyl green-pyronin solution; originally used for gonococci, but later used to detect RNA and DNA in tissue sections; RNA is stained red and

DNA appears green; used to demonstrate plasma cells during chronic inflammation. SEE methyl green-pyronin s.

Unna's s., (1) an alkaline methylene blue s. for plasma cells; (2) a polychrome methylene blue s. with which mast cells are stained red (metachromatic).

Unna-Taenzer s., SYN Taenzer's s.

uranyl acetate s., a s. used in electron microscopy; uranyl acetate binds specifically to nucleic acids but selectively tends to be abolished by osmium fixation; proteins are well stained, but cytomembranes are poorly stained.

urate crystals s., a s. using silver methenamine to detect crystals, which polarize light in contrast with calcium crystals; useful in diagnosing gout and kidney infarcts resulting from uric acid build-up.

van Ermengen's s., a method for staining flagella which utilizes glacial acetic acid, osmic acid, tannic acid, silver nitrate, gallic acid, and potassium acetate.

van Gieson's s., a mixture of acid fuchsin in saturated picric acid solution, used in collagen staining.

Verhoeff's elastic tissue s., a s. for tissue sections in which a mixture of hematoxylin, ferric chloride, and Lugol's iodine solution is used; tissue may be counterstained, if desired, with eosin or van Gieson's s.; elastic fibers and nuclei appear blue-black to black while collagen and other components are shades of pink to red.

vital s., a s. applied to cells or parts of cells while they are still living.

von Kossa s., a s. for calcium in mineralized tissue, utilizing a silver nitrate solution followed by sodium thiosulfate; calcified bone but not osteoid is stained brown to black. SYN Kossa s.

Wachstein-Meissel s. for calcium-magnesium-ATPase, a method similar to that of Gomori's nonspecific acid phosphatase s., except that incubation is carried out with ATP as substrate at neutral pH; enzyme activity is generally demonstrated at cell membranes.

Warthin-Starry silver s., a s. for spirochetes in which preparations are incubated in 1% silver nitrate solution followed by a developer.

Weigert-Gram s., a s. for bacteria in tissues in which sections are stained in alum-hematoxylin, then in eosin, aniline methyl violet, and Lugol's solution.

Weigert's s. for actinomyces, a staining method using immersion in a dark red orsellin solution in alcohol, then staining in crystal-violet solution. SEE ALSO iron *hematoxylin.*

Weigert's s. for elastin, a staining solution of fuchsin, resorcin, and ferric chloride; elastic fibers stain blue-black.

Weigert's s. for fibrin, a staining method using solutions of aniline-crystal violet and iodine-potassium iodide, then decolorizing in aniline oil and xylol; the fibrin is stained dark blue.

Weigert's iron hematoxylin s., a nuclear staining solution containing hematoxylin, ferric chloride, and hydrochloric acid; useful in combination with von Gieson's s., especially for demonstrating connective tissue elements or *Entamoeba histolytica* in sections.

Weigert's s. for myelin, a staining method using ferric chloride and hematoxylin; myelin stains deep blue, degenerated portions a light yellowish color.

Weigert's s. for neuroglia, a complicated process in which the final treatment is like that for staining fibrin; neuroglia and nuclei stain blue.

Wilder's s. for reticulum, a silver impregnation technique in which reticulum appears as black, well-defined fibers without beading and with a relatively clear background.

Williams' s., a s. for Negri bodies which utilizes picric acid, fuchsin, and methylene blue; Negri bodies are magenta, granules and nerve cells blue, and erythrocytes yellowish.

Wright's s., a staining mixture of eosinates of polychromed methylene blue used in staining of blood smears.

Ziehl-Neelsen s., a method for staining acid-fast bacteria using Ziehl's s., decolorizing in acid alcohol, and counterstaining with methylene blue; acid-fast organisms appear red, other tissue elements light blue; a modification of this s. is also used for *Actinomycetes* and *Brucella.*

st

Ziehl's s., a carbol-fuchsin solution of phenol and basic fuchsin used to demonstrate bacteria and cell nuclei.

---

stain·ing (stān'ing). **1.** The act of applying a stain. SEE ALSO stain. **2.** In dentistry, modification of the color of the tooth or denture base.

progressive s., a procedure in which s. is continued until the desired intensity of coloring of tissue elements is attained.

regressive s., a type of s. in which tissues are overstained and the excess dye is then removed selectively until the desired intensity is obtained.

stains-all (stainz'awl). 4,5,4′,5′-Dibenzo-3,3′-diethyl-9-methylthiocarbocyanine bromide; a dye that stains phosphoproteins blue, proteins red, nucleic acids purple, and mucoproteins and mucopolysaccharides various colors on acrylamide gels; also used on tissue sections.

stair·case (stār'kās). A series of reactions that follow one another in progressively increasing or decreasing intensity, so that a chart shows a continuous rise or fall. SEE treppe.

stal·ag·mom·e·ter (stal-ă-gom'ĕ-ter). An instrument for determining exactly the number of drops in a given quantity of liquid; used as a measure of the surface tension of a fluid (the lower the tension, the smaller the drops and, consequently, the more numerous in a given quantity of the fluid). SYN stactometer. [G. *stalagma,* a drop, + *metron,* measure]

stalk (stawk). A narrowed connection with a structure or organ.

allantoic s., the narrow connection between the intraembryonic portion of the allantois and the extraembryonic allantoic vesicle.

body s., the extraembryonic precursor of the connecting s. or umbilical cord by which the embryo is attached to its trophoblastic chorion. SYN connecting s.

connecting s., SYN body s.

s. of epiglottis, the lower end or pedicle of the cartilage of the epiglottis, attached to the superior notch of the thyroid cartilage. SYN petiolus epiglottidis [NA].

infundibular s., SYN infundibular *stem.*

optic s., the constricted proximal portion of the optic vesicle in the embryo; it develops into the optic nerve.

pineal s., the attachment of the pineal body to the roof of the third ventricle; it contains the pineal recess of the third ventricle.

pituitary s., a process comprising the tuberal part investing the infundibular stem that attaches the hypophysis to the tuber cinereum at the base of the brain.

yolk s., the narrowed connection between the intraembryonic gut and the yolk sac; its walls are splanchnopleure. SYN umbilical duct, vitelline duct, vitellointestinal duct.

stal·tic (stawl'tik). SYN styptic. [G. *staltikos,* contractile]

stam·mer (stam'er). **1.** To hesitate in speech, halt, repeat, and mispronounce, by reason of embarrassment, agitation, unfamiliarity with the subject, or as yet unidentified physiologic causes. Cf. stutter. **2.** To mispronounce or transpose certain consonants in speech. [A.S. *stamur*]

stam·mer·ing (stam'er-ing). **1.** A speech disorder characterized by hesitation and repetition of words, or by mispronunciation or transposition of certain consonants, especially *l*, *r*, and *s*. **2.** Sounds other than speech, that are similar to stammering. SYN paralalia literalis, psellism.

s. of the bladder, SYN urinary *stuttering.*

Stam·no·so·ma (stam-nō-sō'mă). A genus of flukes of the family Heterophyidae, identical with *Centrocestus*. Two species, *S. armatum* and *S. formosanum,* have been described as sometimes infecting humans. [G. *stamnos,* a jar, + *sōma,* body]

stan·dard (stan'dard). **1.** Something that serves as a basis for comparison; a technical specification or written report by experts. **2.** SEE standard *substance*. [M.E., fr. O.Fr. *estandard,* rallying place, fr. Frankish *standan,* to stand, + *hard,* hard, fast]

stan·dard·i·za·tion (stan'dard-i-zā'shŭn). **1.** The making of a solution of definite strength so that it may be used for comparison and in tests. **2.** Making any drug or other preparation conform to the type or standard. **3.** A set of techniques used to remove as far as possible the effects of differences in the age or other confounding variables when comparing two or more populations.

s. of a test, in psychology, the following of definite procedures for administering, scoring, evaluating, and reporting the results of a new test which is under development.

stand·still. Cessation of activity.

atrial s., cessation of atrial contractions, marked by absence of atrial waves in the electrocardiogram. SYN auricular s.

auricular s., SYN atrial s.

cardiac s., SYN asystole.

sinus s., cessation of sinus node activity, marked by absence of normal P waves in the electrocardiogram.

ventricular s., cessation of ventricular contractions, marked by absence of ventricular complexes in the electrocardiogram.

Stanley, Edward, English surgeon, 1793–1862. SEE S.'s cervical *ligaments,* under *ligament.*

Stanley Way. SEE Way.

stan·nic (stan'ik). Relating to tin, especially when in combination in its higher valency. [L. *stannum,* tin]

stan·nic chlo·ride. $SnCl_4$; a fuming liquid (fuming spirit of Libavius), specific gravity 2.23, boiling point 115°C, that forms several hydrates; the pentahydrate (butter of tin) is used for mordanting and "loading" or "weighting" silk.

stan·nic ox·ide. SnO_2; used in industry; it is a cause of pneumoconiosis. SYN tin oxide.

Stannius, Herman F., German biologist, 1808–1883. SEE S. *ligature.*

stan·nous (stan'ŭs). Relating to tin, especially when in combination in its lower valency. [L. *stannum,* tin]

stan·nous flu·o·ride. A preparation containing not less than 71.2% of stannous tin and not less than 22.3% nor more than 25.5% of fluoride; used as a prophylactic against caries in dentistry.

stan·num (stan'ŭm). SYN tin. [L.]

stan·o·lone (stan'ŏ-lōn). 17β-hydroxy-5α-androstane-3-one; an androgen with the same actions and uses as testosterone; used for its anabolic and tumor-suppressing effects, specifically, in carcinoma of the breast. SYN dihydrotestosterone.

stan·o·zo·lol (stan-ō'zō-lol, -lōl). Androstanozole; stanozol, 17α-methyl-5α-androstan-17β-ol carrying a pyrazole ring (=CH–NH–N=) attached to C-2 and C-3 (see steroids for androstane structure). A semisynthetic, orally effective anabolic agent.

sta·pe·dec·to·my (stā-pĕ-dek'tō-mē). Operation to remove the stapes footplate in whole or part with replacement of the stapes superstructure (crura) by metal or plastic prosthesis; used for otosclerosis with stapes fixation to overcome a conductive hearing loss. [stapes + G. *ektomē,* excision]

sta·pe·di·al (stā-pē'dē-ăl). Relating to the stapes.

sta·pe·di·o·te·not·o·my (stā-pē'dē-ō-tē-not'ŏ-mē). Division of the tendon of the stapedius muscle. [stapedius + G. *tenōn,* tendon, + *tomē,* incision]

sta·pe·di·o·ves·tib·u·lar (stā-pē'dē-ō-ves-tib'yū-lăr). Relating to the stapes and the vestibule of the ear.

sta·pe·di·us, pl. **sta·pe·dii** (stā-pē'dē-ŭs, stā-pē'dē-ī). SYN stapedius *muscle.* [Mod. L.]

sta·pes, pl. **sta·pes, sta·pe·des** (stā'pēz, stā'pē-dēz) [NA]. The smallest of the three auditory ossicles; its base, or footpiece, fits into the vestibular (oval) window, while its head is articulated with the lenticular process of the long limb of the incus. SYN stirrup. [Mod. L. stirrup]

△**staphyl-.** SEE staphylo-.

staph·y·lec·to·my (staf-i-lek'tō-mē). SYN uvulectomy. [staphyl- + G. *ektomē,* excision]

staph·yl·e·de·ma (staf'il-e-dē'mă). Edema of the uvula. [staphyl- + G. *oidēma,* swelling (edema)]

staph·y·line (staf'i-līn, -lēn). SYN botryoid.

sta·phyl·i·on (stă-fil'ē-on). The midpoint of the posterior edge of the hard palate; a craniometric point. SEE ALSO posterior nasal spine. [G. dim. of *staphylē,* a bunch of grapes]

△**staphylo-, staphyl-.** Resemblance to a grape or a bunch of grapes, hence relating usually to staphylococci or, in obsolescent image, to the uvula palatina. SEE ALSO uvulo-. [G. *staphylē*, a bunch of grapes]

staph·y·lo·coc·cal (staf'i-lō-kok'ăl). Relating to or caused by any organism of the genus *Staphylococcus*.

staph·y·lo·coc·ce·mia (staf'i-lō-kok-sē'mē-ă). The presence of staphylococci in the circulating blood. SYN staphylohemia. [staphylo- + G. *haima*, blood]

staph·y·lo·coc·ci (staf'i-lō-kok'sī). Plural of staphylococcus.

staph·y·lo·coc·cia (staf'i-lō-kok'sē-ă). Any staphylococcic infection.

staph·y·lo·coc·cic (staf'i-lō-kok'sik). Relating to or caused by any species of *Staphylococcus*.

staph·y·lo·coc·col·y·sin (staf'i-lō-kŏ-kol'i-sin). SYN staphylolysin.

staph·y·lo·coc·col·y·sis (staf'i-lō-kŏ-kol'i-sis). Lysis or destruction of staphylococci. [staphylo- + G. *lysis*, dissolution]

staph·y·lo·coc·co·sis, pl. **staph·y·lo·coc·co·ses** (staf'i-lō-kok-ō'sis, -sēz). Infection by species of the bacterium *Staphylococcus*.

Sta·phy·lo·coc·cus (staf'i-lō-kok'ŭs). A genus of nonmotile, nonsporeforming, aerobic to facultatively anaerobic bacteria (family Micrococcaceae) containing Gram-positive, spherical cells, 0.5 to 1.5 μm in diameter, which divide in more than one plane to form irregular clusters. These organisms are chemoorganotrophic, and their metabolism is respiratory and fermentative. Under anaerobic conditions, lactic acid is produced from glucose; under aerobic conditions, acetic acid and small amounts of CO_2 are produced. Coagulase-positive strains produce a variety of toxins and are therefore potentially pathogenic and may cause food poisoning. These organisms are usually susceptible to antibiotics such as the β-lactam and macrolide antibiotics, tetracyclines, novobiocin, and chloramphenicol but are resistant to polymyxin and polyenes. They are susceptible to antibacterials such as phenols and their derivatives, surface-active compounds, salicylanilides, carbanilides, and halogens (chlorine and iodine) and their derivatives, such as chloramines and iodophors. They are found on the skin, in skin glands, on the nasal and other mucous membranes of warm-blooded animals, and in a variety of food products. The type species is *S. aureus*. [staphylo- + G. *kokkos*, a berry]

S. au′reus, a common species found especially on nasal mucous membrane and skin (hair follicles); it causes furunculosis, cellulitis, pyemia, pneumonia, osteomyelitis, endocarditis, suppuration of wounds, other infections, and food poisoning; also a cause of infection in burn patients. Humans are the chief reservoir. The type species of the genus *S.* SYN *S. pyogenes aureus*.

S. epider′midis, a species, originally found in small stitch abscesses and other skin wounds, which occurs on parasitic skin and mucous membranes of man and other animals; it is parasitic rather than pathogenic.

S. haemolyticus, coagulase-negative staphylococcus indigenous to human and mammalian hosts.

S. hominis, coagulase-negative staphylococcus indigenous to human and mammalian hosts.

S. hyi′cus, a species whose porcine subspecies are opportunistic pathogens associated with epidermites such as greasy pig disease.

S. pyog′enes al′bus, a name formerly applied to the organisms which are now regarded as the mutants of *S. aureus* which form white colonies.

S. pyog′enes au′reus, SYN *S. aureus*.

S. saprophyticus, a genus that causes urinary tract infections.

S. simulans, coagulase-negative staphylococcus indigenous to human and mammalian hosts.

staph·y·lo·coc·cus, pl. **staph·y·lo·coc·ci** (staf'i-lō-kok'ŭs, kok' sī). A vernacular term used to refer to any member of the genus *Staphylococcus*.

staph·y·lo·der·ma (staf'i-lō-der'mă). Pyoderma due to staphylococci. [staphylo- + G. *derma*, skin]

staph·y·lo·der·ma·ti·tis (staf'i-lō-der-mă-tī'tis). Inflammation of the skin due to the action of staphylococci.

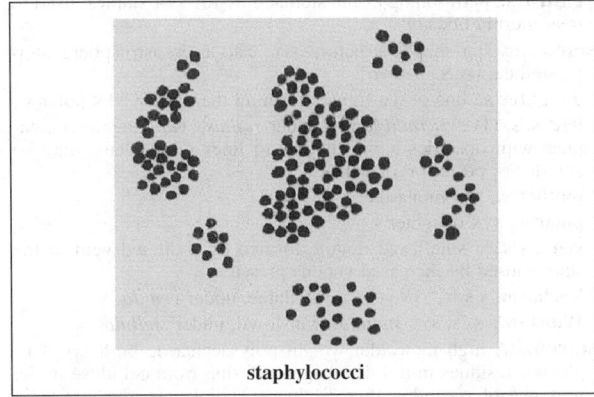

staphylococci

staph·y·lo·di·al·y·sis (staf'i-lō-dī-al'i-sis). SYN uvuloptosis. [staphylo- + G. *dialysis*, a separation]

staph·y·lo·he·mia (staf'i-lō-hē'mē-ă). SYN staphylococcemia.

staph·y·lo·he·mo·ly·sin (staf'i-lō-hē-mol'i-sin). A mixture of hemolysins (alpha, beta, gamma, and delta), included in staphylococcal exotoxin; the α hemolysin has a marked effect on vascular muscle.

staph·y·lo·ki·nase (staf'i-lō-kī'nās). A microbial metalloenzyme from *Staphylococcus aureus*, with action similar to that of urokinase and streptokinase, that can convert plasminogen to plasmin but requires Ca^{2+}; separated in forms A, B, and C.

staph·y·lol·y·sin (staf-i-lol'i-sin). **1.** A hemolysin elaborated by a staphylococcus. **2.** An antibody causing lysis of staphylococci. SYN staphylococcolysin.

staph·y·lo·ma (staf-i-lō'mă). A bulging of the cornea or sclera containing uveal tissue. [staphylo- + G. *-ōma*, tumor]

annular s., a s. extending around the periphery of the cornea.

anterior s., a bulging near the anterior pole of the eyeball. SYN corneal s.

ciliary s., scleral s. occurring in the region of the ciliary body.

corneal s., SYN anterior s.

equatorial s., a s. occurring in the area of exit of the vortex veins. SYN scleral s.

intercalary s., a scleral s. occurring between the insertion of the ciliary body and the root of the iris.

posterior s., a bulging near the posterior pole of the eyeball due to degenerative changes in severe myopia. SYN Scarpa's s., sclerochoroiditis posterior.

Scarpa's s., SYN posterior s.

scleral s., SYN equatorial s.

uveal s., seldom-used term for protrusion of the iris through a rupture of the sclera.

staph·y·lom·a·tous (staf-i-lō'mă-tŭs). Relating to or marked by staphyloma.

staph·y·lo·phar·yn·gor·rha·phy (staf'i-lō-far-in-gōr'ă-fē). Surgical repair of defects in the uvula or soft palate and the pharynx. SYN palatopharyngorrhaphy. [staphylo- + pharynx + G. *rhaphē*, suture]

staph·y·lo·plas·ty (staf'i-lō-plas-tē). SYN palatoplasty. [staphylo- + G. *plassō*, to form]

staph·y·lo·ple·gia (staf'i-lō-plē'jē-ă). SYN palatoplegia.

staph·y·lop·to·sis (staf'i-lop-tō'sis). SYN uvuloptosis. [staphylo- + G. *ptōsis*, a falling]

staph·y·lor·rha·phy (staf-i-lōr'ă-fē). SYN palatorrhaphy. [staphylo- + G. *rhaphē*, suture]

staph·y·lo·tox·in (staf'i-lō-tok'sin). The toxin elaborated by any species of *Staphylococcus*. SEE ALSO staphylohemolysin. [staphylo- + G. *toxikon*, poison]

sta·pling (stāp'ling). Use of a stapling device that unites two tissues, such as the two ends of bowel, by applying a row or circle of staples.

gastric s., partitioning of the stomach by rows of staples; used to treat morbid obesity.

star. Any star-shaped structure. SEE ALSO aster, astrosphere, stella, stellula. [A.S. *steorra*]

daughter s., one of the figures forming the diaster. SYN polar s.

lens s.'s, (1) SYN *radii* lentis, under *radius*. **(2)** congenital cataracts with opacities along the suture lines of the lens; may be anterior or posterior, or both.

mother s., SYN monaster.

polar s., SYN daughter s.

venous s., a small, red nodule formed by a dilated vein in the skin; caused by increased venous pressure.

Verheyen's s.'s, SYN *venulae* stellatae, under *venula*.

Winslow's s.'s, SYN *stellulae* winslowii, under *stellula*.

starch. A high molecular-weight polysaccharide built up of D-glucose residues in α-1,4 linkage, differing from cellulose in the presence of α- rather than β-glucoside linkages, that exists in most plant tissues; converted into dextrin when subjected to the action of dry heat, and into dextrin and D-glucose by amylases and glucoamylases in saliva and pancreatic juice; used as a dusting powder, an emollient, and an ingredient in medicinal tablets, and is an important raw material for the manufacture of alcohol, acetone, *n*-butanol, lactic acid, citric acid, glycerine, and gluconic acid by fermentation; chief storage carbohydrate in most higher plants. SYN amylum. [A.S. *stearc*, strong]

animal s., SYN glycogen.

liver s., SYN glycogen.

moss s., SYN lichenin.

soluble s., a high-molecular-weight, water-soluble dextrin produced by the partial acid hydrolysis of s.; useful in iodimetry, as it gives an easily visible purple-black end point in the presence of free iodine.

starch·eat·ing. SYN amylophagia.

stare (stār). **1.** To look intently or fixedly. **2.** An intent gaze. [A.S. *starian*]

postbasic s., obsolete term for the appearance of a child with a posterior basic meningitis, due to retraction of the upper eyelid (Collier's sign) and downward rotation of the eye.

Stargardt, Karl, German ophthalmologist, 1875–1927. SEE S.'s *disease*.

Starling, Ernest H., English physiologist, 1866–1927. SEE S.'s *curve, hypothesis, law, reflex*; Frank-S. *curve*.

Starr, Albert, U.S. physician, *1926. SEE Starr-Edwards *valve*.

Starry. SEE Warthin-Starry silver *stain*.

start·er (start'er). SYN primer (1).

star·va·tion (star-vā'shŭn). Lengthy and continuous deprivation of food.

starve. 1. To suffer from lack of food. **2.** To deprive of food so as to cause suffering or death. **3.** Formerly, to die of cold. [A.S. *steorfan*, to die]

Stas, Jean-Servais, Belgian chemist, 1813–1891. SEE S.-Otto *method*.

stas·i·mor·phia (stas-i-mōr'fē-ă). Deformity due to arrested development. [G. *stasis*, a standing still, + *morphē*, shape]

sta·sis, pl. **sta·ses** (stā'sis, stas'is; -ēz). Stagnation of the blood or other fluids. [G. a standing still]

intestinal s., SYN enterostasis.

papillary s., obsolete term for papilledema.

pressure s., SYN traumatic *asphyxia*.

venous s., congestion and slowing of circulation in veins due to blockage by either obstruction or high pressure in the venous system, usually best seen in the feet and legs.

stat. Abbreviation for L. *statim*, at once, immediately.

△**stat-.** Prefix applied to electrical units in the CGS-electrostatic system to distinguish them from units in the CGS-electromagnetic system (prefix ab-) and those in the metric system or SI system (no prefix).

△**-stat.** An agent intended to keep something from changing or moving. [G. *statēs*, stationary]

stat·am·pere (stat-am'pēr). The electrostatic unit of current; the flow of 1 electrostatic unit of charge (1 statcoulomb) per second; equal to 3.335641×10^{-10} ampere. [G. *statos*, standing (stationary), + ampere]

stat·cou·lomb (stat-kū'lom). The electrostatic unit of charge, such that two objects, each carrying such a charge and separated (center to center) by 1 cm in a vacuum, will repel each other with a force of 1 dyne (or 10^{-5} newton); equal to 3.335641×10^{-10} coulomb. [G. *statos*, standing (stationary), + coulomb]

state (stāt). A condition, situation, or status. [L. *status*, condition, state]

absent s., SYN dreamy s.

activated s., SYN excited s.

anxiety tension s., a milder form of an anxiety disorder. SEE anxiety *disorders*, under *disorder*.

apallic s., (1) diffuse, bilateral cerebral cortical degeneration caused by head injury, anoxia, or encephalitis; **(2)** a state of persistent unresponsiveness, such as akinetic mutism, caused by brain damage. SEE ALSO vegetative. SYN apallic syndrome, apallic.

carrier s., the s. of being a carrier of pathogenic organisms; *i.e.,* one who is infected but free of disease.

central excitatory s., the building up of excitatory influences produced by individual impulses finally causes firing of the next neuron.

convulsive s., SYN epilepsy.

decerebrate s., SYN decerebrate *rigidity*.

decorticate s., SYN decorticate *rigidity*.

dreamy s., the semiconscious s. associated with an epileptic attack. SYN absent s.

eunuchoid s., an imprecisely delineated condition of a male manifesting signs of inadequate androgen secretion during adolescent growth, regardless of the cause; usually referring to long legs, short trunk, and boyish beardless faces.

excited s., the condition of an atom or molecule after absorbing energy, which may be the result of exposure to light, electricity, elevated temperature, or a chemical reaction; such activation may be a necessary prelude to a chemical reaction or to the emission of light. SYN activated s.

ground s., the normal, inactivated s. of an atom from which, on activation, the singlet, triplet, and other excited s.'s are derived.

hypnoid s., a drowsy or sleeplike s. artificially induced by a hypnotist in individuals of higher than average levels of suggestibility. SEE hypnosis.

hypnotic s., SYN hypnosis.

hypometabolic s., a rare s. of reduced metabolism with symptoms resembling hypothyroidism but with some tests for thyroid gland function normal; also used to describe the reduced metabolic activity seen in true hypothyroidism.

imperfect s., in fungi, the s. or stage at which only asexual spores such as conidia are formed; most such species are classified as Deuteromycetes (Fungi Imperfecti).

lacunar s., the presence of lacunes in the brain. One of the major factors underlying cerebrovascular disease; high correlation with hypertension and atherosclerosis. Symptomatic forms include pure motor hemiplegia and pure hemisensory syndrome; multiple lacunar infarcts are the most common cause of pseudobulbar palsy.

local excitatory s., increased irritability of a nerve fiber or muscle fiber which is produced by an ineffective electrical stimulus; summation of the stimuli may occur, resulting in a propagated impulse if two or more subliminal stimuli are applied in rapid succession.

multiple ego s.'s, various psychological organizational s.'s reflecting different personas or life experiences.

perfect s., in fungi, that portion of the life cycle in which spores are formed after nuclear fusion.

post-steady s., any period of time, particularly in an enzyme-catalyzed reaction, after the steady-state interval; *e.g.,* when the rate of product formation is declining in an enzyme-catalyzed reaction.

pre-steady s., those conditions and the time interval prior to establishment of steady s.

refractory s., subnormal excitability immediately following a response to previous excitation; the s. is divided into absolute and relative phases.

singlet s., a transient, excited s. of a molecule (*e.g.,* of chlorophyll, upon absorbing light) that can release energy as heat or light (fluorescence) and thus return to the initial (ground) s.; it may alternatively assume a slightly more stable, but still excited s. (triplet s.), with an electron still dislocated as before but with reversed spin.

steady s. (ss, s), (1) a s. obtained in moderate muscular exercise, when the removal of lactic acid by oxidation keeps pace with its production, the oxygen supply being adequate, and the muscles do not go into debt for oxygen; **(2)** any condition in which the formation or introduction of substances just keeps pace with their destruction or removal so that all volumes, concentrations, pressures, and flows remain constant; **(3)** in enzyme kinetics, conditions such that the rate of change in the concentration of any enzyme species (*e.g.,* free enzyme or the enzyme-substrate binary complex) is zero or much less than the rate of formation of product. [often subscript s or ss]

triplet s., a second excited s. of a molecule (*e.g.,* chlorophyll) produced by absorption of light to produce the singlet s., then loss of some energy (fluorescence) to arrive at the longer-lived triplet s. The molecule may remain sufficiently long in the triplet s. for a second activating light quantum to be effective in producing a "second triplet" s., obviously at still a higher level of excitation, hence reactivity. Alternatively, it may lose the triplet s. energy directly and return to the ground s.

twilight s., a condition of disordered consciousness during which actions may be performed without the conscious volition of the individual and with no memory of such actions. Cf. somnambulic *epilepsy.*

stat·far·ad (stat-fa′rad). An electrostatic unit of capacitance, equal to 1.112650×10^{-12} farad.

stat·hen·ry (stat-hen′rē). An electrostatic unit of inductance, equal to 8.987552×10^{11} henries.

stath·mo·ki·ne·sis (stath′mō-ki-nē′sis). Condition of arrested mitosis after treatment with an agent, such as colchicine, which effectively alters the mitotic spindle to prevent typical rearrangement of the chromosomes preceding cell division. [G. *stathmos,* standing place, + *kinēsis,* motion]

sta·tim (stā′tim). At once; immediately. [L.]

stat·ins. SYN releasing *factors.*

sta·tion. The degree of descent of the presenting part of the fetus through the maternal pelvis, as measured in relation to the ischial spines of the maternal pelvis.

sta·tis·ti·cal sig·nif·i·cance. Statistical methods allow an estimate to be made of the probability of the observed degree of association between variables, and from this the statistical significance can be expressed, commonly in terms of the P value.

sta·tis·tics (stă-tis′tiks). **1.** A collection of numerical values, items of information, or other facts which are numerically grouped into definite classes and subject to analysis, particularly analysis of the probability that the resulting empirical findings are due to chance. **2.** The science and art of collecting, summarizing and analyzing data that are subject to random variation.

descriptive s., numerical values such as mean, median, and mode which describe the chief features of a group of scores, without regard to a larger population.

inferential s., s. from which an inference is made about the nature of a population; the purpose is to generalize about the population, based upon data from the sample selected from the population.

vital s., systematically tabulated information concerning births, marriages, divorces, separations, and deaths, based on the numbers of official registrations of these vital events; the branch of s. concerned with such data.

stat·o·a·cou·stic (stat′ō-ă-kū′stik). Relating to equilibrium and hearing. SYN vestibulocochlear (2). [G. *statos,* standing, + *akoustikos,* acoustic]

stat·o·co·nia, sing. **stat·o·co·ni·um** (stat′ō-kō′nē-ă, -nē-ŭm) [NA]. SYN statoliths. [L. fr. G. *statos,* standing, *konis,* dust]

stat·o·ki·net·ic (stat′ō-ki-net′ik). Pertaining to statokinetics.

stat·o·ki·net·ics (stat′ō-ki-net′iks). The adjustment made by the body in motion to maintain stable equilibrium. [G. *statos,* standing, + *kinēsis,* movement]

stat·o·liths (stat′ŏ-liths). Crystalline particles of calcium carbonate and a protein adhering to the gelatinous membrane of the maculae of the utricle and saccule. SYN statoconia [NA], ear crystals, otoconia, otoliths, otolites, sagitta. [G. *statos,* standing, + *lithos,* stone]

sta·tom·e·ter (stă-tom′ĕ-ter). SYN exophthalmometer. [G. *statos,* standing, + *metron,* measure]

stat·o·sphere (stat′ō-sfēr). SYN centrosphere.

stat·ure (statch′er). The height of a person. [L. *statura,* fr. *statuo,* pp. *statutus,* to cause to stand]

sta·tus (stā′tŭs, stat′ŭs). A state or condition. [L. a way of standing]

s. angino′sus, prolonged angina pectoris refractory to treatment.

s. arthrit′icus, obsolete term for gouty diathesis or predisposition.

s. asthmat′icus, a condition of severe, prolonged asthma.

s. cholera′icus, the cold stage of shock and depression in cholera, due to fluid and electrolyte loss and resulting hypovolemia; characterized by weak pulse, cold clammy skin, confusion, and depression.

s. chore′icus, a very severe form of chorea in which the persistence of the movements prevents sleep and the patient may die of exhaustion.

s. convul′sivus, SYN epilepsy.

s. cribro′sus, a condition marked by dilations of the perivascular spaces in the brain.

s. crit′icus, a very severe and persistent form of crisis in tabes dorsalis.

s. dysmyelinisa′tus, SYN Hallervorden-Spatz *syndrome.*

s. dysra′phicus, a condition in which there is failure of fusion of midline structures; related to syringomyelia and perhaps to Marfan's syndrome or arachnodactyly. SYN arrhaphia.

s. epilep′ticus, repeated seizure or a seizure prolonged for at least 30 minutes; may be convulsive (tonic-clonic), nonconvulsive (absence or complex partial) or partial (epilepsia partialis continuans) or subclinical (electrographic status epilepticus).

s. hemicra′nicus, a condition in which attacks of migraine succeed each other with such short intervals as to be almost continuous.

s. hypnot′icus, rarely used term for hypnosis.

s. lacuna′ris, a condition, occurring in cerebral arteriosclerosis, in which there are numerous small areas of degeneration in the brain.

s. lymphat′icus, SYN s. thymicolymphaticus.

s. marmora′tus, a congenital condition due to maldevelopment of the corpus striatum associated with choreoathetosis, in which the striate nuclei have a marblelike appearance caused by altered myelination.

s. nervo′sus, SYN s. typhosus.

s. prae′sens, obsolete term for the part of the history of a case describing the condition of the patient at the time when he comes under observation.

s. rap′tus, rarely used term for ecstasy.

s. spongio′sus, multiple fluid-filled spaces of microscopic size in the cerebral white matter; seen in certain hypoxic, toxic, and metabolic diseases.

s. ster′nuens, a state of continual sneezing.

s. thymicolymphat′icus, old term for a syndrome of supposed enlargement of the thymus and lymph nodes in infants and young children, formerly believed to be associated with unexplained sudden death; it was also erroneously believed that pressure of the thymus on the trachea might cause death during anesthesia. Prominence of these structures is now considered normal in young children, including those who have died suddenly without preceding illnesses that might lead to atrophy of lymphoid tissue. SEE ALSO sudden infant death *syndrome.* SYN s. lymphaticus, s. thymicus.

s. thy′micus, SYN s. thymicolymphaticus.

s. typho′sus, rarely used term for an erethistic or typhoidal state. SYN s. nervosus.

st

s. vertigino'sus, a condition in which attacks of vertigo occur in rapid succession. SYN chronic vertigo.

stat·u·vo·lence (stat-yū-vō′lens, stă-tū′vō-lens). SYN autohypnosis. [status (hypnoticus) + L. *volens,* pres. p. of *volo,* to wish]

sta·tu·vo·lent (stat-yū-vō′lent). Relating to or capable of statuvolence.

stat·volt (stat′vōlt). An electrostatic unit of potential or electromotive force, equal to 299.7925 volts. [G. *statos,* standing (stationary), + volt]

Staub, Hans, Swiss internist, *1890. SEE S.-Traugott *effect, phenomenon.*

stau·ri·on (staw′rē-on). A craniometric point at the intersection of the median and transverse palatine sutures. [G. dim. of *stauros,* cross]

STD Abbreviation for sexually transmitted *disease.*

steal (stēl). Diversion of blood via alternate routes or reversed flow, from a vascularized tissue to one deprived by proximal arterial obstruction. [M.E. *stelen,* fr. A.S. *stelan*]

coronary s., a s. caused by anomalous origin of the coronary artery from the pulmonary artery.

iliac s., the decrease in flow in one common iliac artery when an occlusion of the other common iliac artery is released.

renal-splanchnic s., diversion of blood from the right renal artery via the inferior adrenal branch into splanchnic collaterals distal to a stenosis of the celiac axis.

subclavian s., obstruction of the subclavian artery proximal to the origin of the vertebral artery; blood flow through the vertebral artery is reversed and the subclavian artery thus "steals" cerebral blood, causing symptoms of vertebrobasilar insufficiency (subclavian steal syndrome); manifest during vigorous use of an upper extremity.

ste·ap·sin (stē-ap′sin). SYN *triacylglycerol* lipase.

⚠**stear-.** SEE stearo-.

ste·a·ral (stē′ă-răl). octadecanal(dehyde); the aldehyde of stearic acid. SYN stearaldehyde.

ste·a·ral·de·hyde (stē-ă-ral′dĕ-hīd). SYN stearal.

ste·a·rate (stē′ă-rāt). A salt of stearic acid.

ste·ar·ic ac·id (stē′ă-rik). $CH_3-(CH_2)_6COOH$; *n*-Octadecanoic acid; one of the most abundant fatty acids found in animal lipids; used in pharmaceutical preparations, ointments, soaps, and suppositories.

ste·a·rin (stē′ă-rin). tristearoylglycerol; the "triglyceride" of stearic acid present in solid animal fats and in some vegetable fats; source of stearic acid; commercial s. also contains some palmitic acid. SYN tristearin.

Stearns, A. Warren, U.S. physician, 1885–1959. SEE S. alcoholic *amentia.*

⚠**stearo-, stear-.** Combining form denoting fat. SEE ALSO steato-. [G. *stear,* tallow]

ste·ar·rhea (stē-ă-rē′ă). SYN steatorrhea.

ste·a·ryl al·co·hol (stē′ă-ril). Octadecyl alcohol; octadecanol; an ingredient of hydrophilic ointment and hydrophilic petrolatum; also used in the preparation of creams.

ste·a·ryl-CoA, ste·a·ryl-co·en·zyme A (stēr′il). The coenzyme A thioester of stearic acid; precursor to oleic acid and, in the brain, the C_{22} and C_{24} fatty acids present in sphingomyelins; in the brain, use of s-CoA increases during myelination.

s-CoA desaturase, a protein complex that is key in the synthesis of unsaturated fatty acids; it introduces a double bond at Δ^9; high dietary levels of unsaturated fatty acids decrease this enzyme's activity in the liver; a number of agents will induce this enzyme (*e.g.,* insulin, hydrocortisone, and triiodothyronine).

ste·a·tite (stē′ă-tīt). Talc in the form of a mass.

ste·a·ti·tis (stē-ă-tī′tis). **1.** Inflammation of adipose tissue. **2.** A disease of young mink characterized by a brownish yellow discoloration of the adipose tissues; believed to be caused by feeding diets containing too much unsaturated fatty acid and too little vitamin E. [G. *stear* (*steat-*), tallow, + *-itis,* inflammation]

⚠**steato-.** Combining form denoting fat. SEE stearo-. [G. *stear* (*steat-*), tallow]

ste·a·to·cys·to·ma (stē′ă-tō-sis-tō′mă). A cyst with sebaceous gland cells in its wall.

s. mul'tiplex, widespread, multiple, thin-walled cysts of the skin that are lined by squamous epithelium, including lobules of sebaceous cells.

ste·a·to·gen·e·sis (stē′ă-tō-jen′ĕ-sis). Biosynthesis of lipids. The term is used specifically to designate lipid accumulation in the testes of nonmammalian vertebrates on completion of spermatogenesis in the breeding period. [steato- + G. *genesis,* production]

ste·a·tol·y·sis (stē-ă-tol′i-sis). The hydrolysis or emulsion of fat in the process of digestion. [steato- + G. *lysis,* dissolution]

ste·a·to·ly·tic (stē-ă-tō-lit′ik). Relating to steatolysis.

ste·a·to·ne·cro·sis (stē′ă-tō-ne-krō′sis). SYN fat *necrosis.* [steato- + G. *nekrōsis,* death]

ste·a·to·py·ga, ste·a·to·py·gia (stē′ă-tō-pī′gă, -pij′ē-ă). Excessive accumulation of fat on the buttocks. [steato- + G. *pygē,* buttocks]

ste·a·to·py·gous (stē-ă-top′ă-gŭs). Having excessively fat buttocks.

ste·a·tor·rhea (stē-at′ō-rē-a). The excretion of unabsorbed lipids with the stool; an absence of bile acids will increase s.

ste·a·tor·rhea (stē′ă-tō-rē′ă). Passage of fat in large amounts in the feces, due to failure to digest and absorb it; occurs in pancreatic disease and the malabsorption syndromes. SYN fat indigestion. SYN stearrhea. [steato- + G. *rhoia,* a flow]

biliary s., s. due to the absence of bile from the intestine; usually accompanied by jaundice.

intestinal s., s. due to malabsorption resulting from intestinal disease. SEE ALSO sprue, celiac *disease.*

pancreatic s., s. due to the absence of pancreatic juice from the intestine.

ste·a·to·sis (stē-ă-tō′sis). **1.** SYN adiposis. **2.** SYN fatty *degeneration.* [steato- + G. *-osis,* condition]

s. cardiaca (stē-ă-tō′sis kar′dē-ā-kă), excessive fat on the pericardium and invading the cardiac muscle.

s. cor'dis, fatty degeneration of the heart.

hepatic s., SYN fatty *liver.*

ste·a·to·zo·on (stē′ă-tō-zō′on). Common name for *Demodex folliculorum.* [steato- + G. *zōon,* animal]

Steele, John C., Canadian neurologist, fl. 1951–1968. SEE S.-Richardson-Olszewski *disease, syndrome.*

Steell, Graham, British physician, 1851–1942. SEE Graham Steell's *murmur.*

Steenbock, Harry, U.S. physiologist and chemist, 1886–1967. SEE S. *unit.*

ste·ge (stē′gē). The internal pillar of Corti's organ. [G. *stegos,* roof, a house]

steg·no·sis (steg-nō′sis). **1.** A stoppage of any of the secretions or excretions. **2.** A constriction or stenosis. [G. stoppage]

steg·not·ic (steg-not′ik). **1.** Astringent or constipating. **2.** An astringent or constipating agent.

Stein, Irving F., U.S. gynecologist, *1887. SEE S.-Leventhal *syndrome.*

Stein, Stanislav A.F. von, Russian otologist, *1855. SEE S.'s *test.*

Steinberg, I. SEE S. thumb *sign.*

Steinbrinck, W., 20th century Germany physician. SEE Chédiak-S.-Higashi *anomaly, syndrome.*

Steinert, Hans, German physician, *1875. SEE S.'s *disease.*

Steinmann, Fritz, Swiss surgeon, 1872–1932. SEE S. *pin.*

STEL Abbreviation for short-term exposure *limit.*

stel·la, pl. **stel·lae** (stel′ă, -ē). A star or star-shaped figure. [Mod. L.]

s. len'tis hyaloi'dea, the posterior pole of the lens. SEE *radii* lentis, under *radius.*

s. len'tis irid'ica, the anterior pole of the lens. SEE *radii* lentis, under *radius.*

stel·late (stel′āt). Star-shaped. [L. *stella,* a star]

stel·lec·to·my (stel-ek′tō-mē). Stellate ganglionectomy.

stel·lu·la, pl. **stel·lu·lae** (stel′yū-lă, -lē). A small star or star-shaped figure. [L. dim. of *stella,* star]

stel′lulae vasculo′sae, SYN stellulae winslowii.

stel′lulae verheyen′ii, SYN *venulae* stellatae, under *venula.*

stel′lulae winslo′wii, capillary whorls in the lamina choroidoca-pillaris from which arise the venae vorticosae. SYN stellulae vasculosae, Winslow's stars.

Stellwag, Carl von C., Austrian ophthalmologist, 1823–1904. SEE S.'s *sign.*

stem. A supporting structure similar to the stalk of a plant.

brain s., SEE brainstem.

infundibular s., the neural component of the pituitary stalk that contains nerve tracts passing from the hypothalamus to the pars nervosa. SYN infundibular stalk.

sten. A statistical term which uses the standard deviation to convert data into standardized scores which define 10 steps along a normal distribution, with five steps on either side of the mean.

Stender, Wilhelm P., 19th century Leipzig manufacturer of scientific apparatus. SEE S. *dish.*

Stenger test. See under test.

ste·ni·on (sten′ē-on). The termination in either temporal fossa of the shortest transverse diameter of the skull; a craniometric point. [G. *stenos,* narrow, + dim. *-iōn*]

Steno. SEE Stensen.

steno-. Narrowness, constriction; opposite of eury-. [G. *stenos,* narrow]

sten·o·breg·mat·ic (sten′ō-breg-mat′ik). Denoting a skull narrow anteriorly, at the part where the bregma is. [steno- + G. *bregma*]

sten·o·car·dia (sten-ō-kar′dē-ă). SYN *angina* pectoris. [steno- + G. *kardia,* heart]

sten·o·ce·pha·lia (sten-ō-se-fā′lē-ă). SYN stenocephaly.

sten·o·ceph·a·lous, sten·o·ce·phal·ic (sten-ō-sef′ă-lŭs, -se-fal′ik). Pertaining to, or characterized by, stenocephaly.

sten·o·ceph·a·ly (sten-ō-sef′ă-lē). Marked narrowness of the head. SYN stenocephalia. [steno- + G. *kephalē,* head]

sten·o·cho·ria (sten-ō-kō′rē-ă). Abnormal contraction of any canal or orifice, especially of the lacrimal ducts. [G. *stenochōria,* narrowness, fr. steno- + *chōra,* place, room]

sten·o·com·pres·sor (sten′ō-kom-pres′er, ōr). An instrument for compressing the ducts of the parotid glands (Stensen's duct) in order to keep back the saliva during dental operations.

sten·o·crot·a·phy, sten·o·cro·ta·phia (sten′ō-krot′ă-fē, -krō-tā′fē-ă). Narrowness of the skull in the temporal region; the condition of a stenobregmate skull. [steno- + G. *krotaphos,* temple]

Stenon. SEE Stensen. [*Stenonius,* Latin form of Stensen]

sten·o·pe·ic, sten·o·pa·ic (stĕn-ō-pē′ik, sten-ō-pā′ik). Provided with a narrow opening or slit, as in s. spectacles. [steno- + G. *opē,* opening]

ste·no·sal (ste-nō′săl). SYN stenotic.

ste·nosed (sten′ōzd). Narrowed; contracted: strictured.

ste·no·sis, pl. **ste·no·ses** (ste-nō′sis, -sēz). A stricture of any canal; especially, a narrowing of one of the cardiac valves. [G. *stenōsis,* a narrowing]

aortic s., pathologic narrowing of the aortic valve orifice.

buttonhole s., extreme narrowing, usually of the mitral valve.

calcific nodular aortic s., most common type of aortic s., occurring usually in elderly men, in which the cusps contain calcified fibrous nodules on both surfaces; the causes include rheumatic fever, atherosclerosis, age-related degeneration, and congenitally bicuspid aortic valve.

congenital pyloric s., SYN hypertrophic pyloric s.

coronary ostial s., narrowing of the mouths of the coronary arteries as a result of syphilitic aortitis or atherosclerosis.

Dittrich's s., SYN infundibular s.

double aortic s., subaortic s. associated with s. of the valve itself, both lesions being congenital.

fish-mouth mitral s., extreme mitral s.

hypertrophic pyloric s., muscular hypertrophy of the pyloric sphincter, associated with projectile vomiting appearing in the

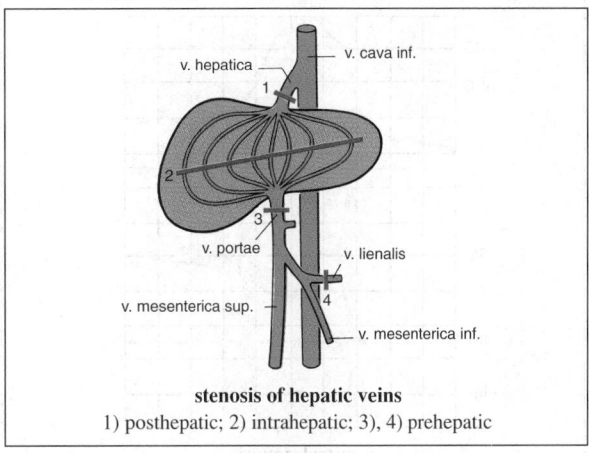

stenosis of hepatic veins
1) posthepatic; 2) intrahepatic; 3), 4) prehepatic

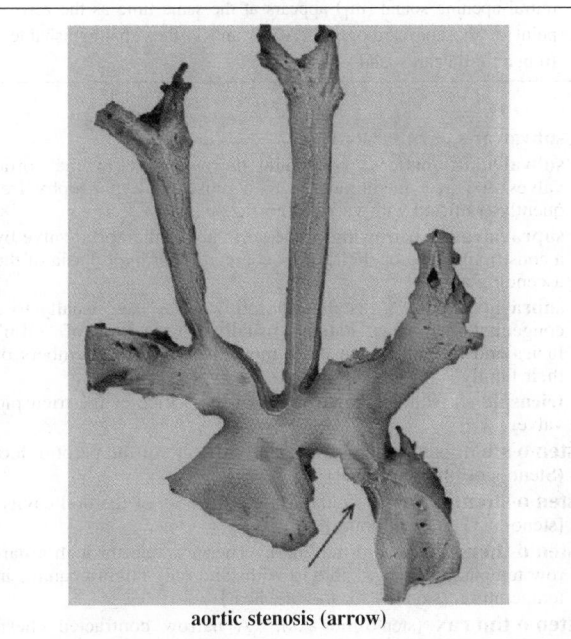

aortic stenosis (arrow)

second or third week of life, usually in males. SYN congenital pyloric s.

idiopathic hypertrophic subaortic s., left ventricular outflow obstruction due to hypertrophy, usually congenital, of the ventricular septum. SYN muscular subaortic s.

infundibular s., narrowing of the outflow tract of the right ventricle below the pulmonic valve; may be due to a localized fibrous diaphragm just below the valve or, more commonly, to a long narrow fibromuscular channel. SYN Dittrich's s.

laryngeal s., narrowing or stricture of any or all areas of the larynx; may be congenital or acquired.

mitral s. (MS), pathologic narrowing of the orifice of the mitral valve.

muscular subaortic s., SYN idiopathic hypertrophic subaortic s.

pulmonary s., narrowing of the opening into the pulmonary artery from the right ventricle.

pyloric s., narrowing of the gastric pylorus, especially by congenital muscular hypertrophy or scarring resulting from a peptic ulcer. SEE ALSO hypertrophic pyloric s.

subaortic s., congenital narrowing of the outflow tract of the left ventricle by a ring of fibrous tissue or by hypertrophy of the muscular septum below the aortic valve. SYN subvalvar s.

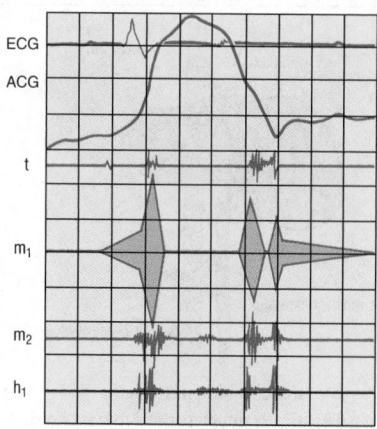

mitral stenosis

phonocardiogram of mitral valve stenosis with sinus rhythm; mitral-opening sound (m₁) appears at the same time as the zero-point of the apexcardiogram (ACG) and is thus distinguishable from a third heart sound

subvalvar s., SYN subaortic s.

subvalvular aortic s., congenital narrowing below the aortic valves due to a membrane or to a muscular hypertrophy frequently confused with valvular aortic stenosis.

supravalvar s., narrowing of the aorta above the aortic valve by a constricting ring or shelf, or by coarctation or hypoplasia of the ascending aorta.

supravalvular s., s. distal to the aortic valve due usually to a congenital membrane. Patients usually have a kind of "elfin" facies and resemble each other more than they do members of their family.

tricuspid s., pathologic narrowing of the orifice of the tricuspid valve.

sten·o·ste·no·sis (sten′ō-stĕ-nō′sis). Stricture of the parotid duct (Steno's or Stensen's duct).

sten·o·sto·mia (sten-ō-stō′mē-ă). Narrowness of the oral cavity. [steno- + G. *stoma*, mouth]

sten·o·ther·mal (sten-ō-ther′măl). Thermostable through a narrow temperature range; able to withstand only slight changes in temperature. [steno- + G. *thermē*, heat]

sten·o·tho·rax (sten′ō-thōr′aks). A narrow contracted chest. [steno- + thorax]

ste·not·ic (ste-not′ik). Narrowed; affected with stenosis. SYN stenosal.

sten·ox·e·nous (sten-ok′sĕ-nŭs). Denoting a parasite with a narrow host range; *e.g., Eimeria* (among the Coccidia), hookworm, biting and sucking lice. [steno- + G. *xenos*, a stranger, foreigner]

Stensen (Steno, Stenon, Stenonius). Niels (Nicholaus), Danish anatomist, 1638–1686. SEE Stensen's *duct,* Stensen's *experiment,* Stensen's *foramen,* Stensen's *plexus,* Stensen's *veins,* under vein.

Stent, C., English dentist, †1901. SEE stent; S. *graft.*

stent. 1. Device used to maintain a bodily orifice or cavity during skin grafting, or to immobilize a skin graft after placement. **2.** Slender thread, rod, or catheter, lying within the lumen of tubular structures, used to provide support during or after their anastomosis, or to assure patency of an intact but contracted lumen. [C. *Stent*]

Stenvers pro·jec·tion. See under projection.

Stenvers view. See under view.

step. 1. In dentistry, a dove-tailed or similarly shaped projection of a cavity prepared in a tooth into a surface perpendicular to the main part of the cavity for the purpose of preventing displacement of the restoration (filling) by the force of mastication. **2.** A change in direction resembling a stair-step in a line, a surface, or the construction of a solid body.

Krönig's s.'s, extension of the lower part of the right border of absolute cardiac dullness in hypertrophy of the right heart.

Rǿnne's nasal s., a nasal visual field defect with one margin corresponding to the retinal horizontal medium; seen in glaucoma.

ste·pha·ni·al (ste-fā′nē-ăl). Pertaining to the stephanion.

ste·pha·ni·on (ste-fā′nē-on). A craniometric point where the coronal suture intersects the inferior temporal line. [G. dim. of *stephanos,* crown]

ste·pha·no·fi·la·ri·a·sis (stef′a-nō-fil-a-rī′a-sis). nfection with filarial parasites of the genus *Stephanofilaria,* a genus of small filiarial worms (less than 6 mm) causing subcutanneous lesions in cattle and other large grazing mammals.

Ste·pha·no·fi·la·ria sti·le·si (stef′ă-nō-fi-lar′ē-ă stī-le′sī). A skin-infecting species of filaria parasitic in cattle and transmitted by the horn fly, *Haematobia irritans;* the only species known to occur in the U.S.; characterized by a row of spines behind the mouth of the adult worm, which is 6 to 8 mm in the female, 2 to 3 mm in the male. Both adults and larvae are found in granulomatous skin lesions in cattle, usually on the underside of the abdomen. [G. *stephanos,* crown, + filaria]

Steph·a·nu·rus den·ta·tus (stef-ă-nū′rŭs den-tā′tŭs). The kidney worm or lard worm of swine, a strongyle nematode parasite species that also occurs, though rarely, in the liver of cattle. Adult worms in swine live in the perirenal fat, the kidney pelvis, or as erratic forms in many other locations. Eggs are passed through the urine and infection is direct, by ingestion of infective larvae or by skin infection, or indirect, by ingestion of earthworms in which the larvae can survive. [G. *stephanos,* crown, + *oura,* tail]

step·page (step′aj). SYN steppage *gait.* [Fr.]

ste·ra·di·an (stĕ-rā′dē-ăn). The unit of solid angle; the solid angle that encloses an area on the surface of a sphere equivalent to the square of the radius of the sphere. [G. *stereos,* solid, + *radion,* radius]

ster·ane (ster′ān, stēr′ān). The hypothetical parent molecule for any steroid hormone; a saturated hydrocarbon compound that contains no oxygen. The name was originally conceived to achieve forms of systematic nomenclature, but is now supplanted by the fundamental variants: gonane, estrane, androstane, norandrostane (etiane), cholane, cholestane, ergostane, and stigmastane. SEE ALSO steroids.

△**sterco-.** Feces. SEE ALSO copro-, scato-. [L. *stercus,* excrement]

ster·co·bi·lin (ster′kō-bī′lin, -bil′in). A brown degradation product of hemoglobin, present in the feces. SEE ALSO bilirubinoids.

*l-***ster·co·bi·lin·o·gen** (ster′kō-bī-lin′ō-jen). Reduction product of *l*-urobilinogen, precursor of *l*-stercobilin in the final stages of bilirubin metabolism; excreted in feces, wherein it is oxidized to stercobilin. SEE ALSO bilirubinoids.

ster·co·lith (ster′kō-lith). SYN coprolith. [sterco- + G. *lithos,* stone]

ster·co·ra·ceous (ster-kō-rā′shŭs). Relating to or containing feces. SYN stercoral, stercorous.

ster·co·ral (ster′kō-răl). SYN stercoraceous.

ster·co·rin (ster′kō-rin). SYN coprosterol.

ster·co·ro·ma (ster-kō-rō′mă). SYN coproma. [sterco- + G. *-oma,* tumor]

ster·co·rous (ster′kō-rŭs). SYN stercoraceous.

ster·cus (ster′kŭs). SYN feces. [L. feces, excrement]

stere (stēr, stär). A measure of capacity; equivalent to a cubic meter or a kiloliter; equal to 1.307951 cubic yards. [Fr. fr. G. *stereos,* solid]

△**stereo-. 1.** A solid, a solid condition or state. **2.** Spatial qualities, three-dimensionality. [G. *stereos,* solid]

ster·e·o·ag·no·sis (ster′ē-ō-ag-nō′sis). SYN tactile *agnosia.*

ster·e·o·an·es·the·sia (ster′ē-ō-an-es-thē′zē-ă). SYN tactile *agnosia.* [stereo- + G. *an-* priv. + *aisthēsis,* sensation]

ster·e·o·ar·throl·y·sis (ster′ē-ō-ar-throl′i-sis). Production of a new joint with mobility in cases of bony ankylosis. [stereo- + G. *arthron,* joint, + *lysis,* loosening]

ster·e·o·cam·pim·e·ter (ster′ē-ō-kam-pim′ĕ-ter). An apparatus for studying the central visual fields while the fellow eye holds fixation. [stereo- + L. *campus*, field, + G. *metron*, measure]

ster·e·o·chem·i·cal (ster′ē-ō-kem′i-kăl). Relating to stereochemistry.

ster·e·o·chem·is·try (ster-ē-ō-kem′is-trē). The branch of chemistry concerned with the spatial three-dimensional relations of atoms in molecules, *i.e.*, the positions the atoms in a compound bear in relation to one another in space.

ster·e·o·cil·i·um, pl. **ster·e·o·cil·ia** (ster′ē-ō-sil′ē-ŭm, -ă). A nonmotile cilium or long microvillus. [stereo- + L. *cilium*, eyelid]

ster·e·o·cin·e·flu·o·rog·ra·phy (ster′ē-ō-sin′ē-flŭr-og′ră-fē). Obsolete practice of recording on motion picture film the images obtained by stereoscopic fluoroscopy; three-dimensional views are obtained.

ster·e·o·col·po·gram (ster′ē-ō-kol′pō-gram). Picture taken with the stereocolposcope.

ster·e·o·col·po·scope (ster′ē-ō-kol′pō-skōp). Instrument that provides the observer with a magnified three-dimensional gross inspection of the vagina and cervix. [stereo- + G. *kolpos*, a hollow (vagina), *skopeō*, to view]

ster·e·o·e·lec·tro·en·ceph·a·log·ra·phy (ster-ē-ō-ē-lek′trō-en-sef-ă-log′ră-fē). Recording of electrical activity in three planes of the brain, *i.e.*, with surface and depth electrodes.

ster·e·o·en·ceph·a·lom·e·try (ster′ē-ō-en-sef′ă-lom′ē-trē). The localization of brain structures by use of three-dimensional coordinates.

ster·e·o·en·ceph·a·lot·o·my (ster′ē-ō-en-sef′ă-lot′ō-mē). SYN stereotaxy. [stereo- + G. *encephalos*, brain, + *tomē*, a cutting]

ster·e·og·no·sis (ster′ē-og′nō′sis). The appreciation of the form of an object by means of touch. [stereo- + G. *gnōsis*, knowledge]

ster·e·og·nos·tic (ster′ē-og-nos′tik). Relating to stereognosis.

ster·e·o·gram (ster′ē-ō-gram). A stereoscopic radiographic image of a pair.

ster·e·o·graph (ster′ē-ō-graf). A stereoscopic x-ray apparatus.

ster·e·og·ra·phy (ster′ē-og′ră-fē). SYN stereoradiography.

ster·e·o·i·so·mer (ster′ē-ō-ī′sō-mer). A molecule containing the same number and kind of atom groupings as another but in a different arrangement in space; the stereoisomers are not interconvertible unless bonds are broken and reformed; by virtue of which it exhibits different optical properties; *e.g.*, as between D and L amino acids, 5α and 5β steroids. Cf. isomer. [stereo- + G. *isos*, equal, + *meros*, part]

ster·e·o·i·so·mer·ic (ster′ē-ō-ī-sō-mer′ik). Relating to stereoisomerism.

ster·e·o·i·som·er·ism (ster′ē-ō-ī-som′er-izm). Molecular asymmetry, isomerism involving different spatial arrangements of the same groups (*e.g.*, androsterone and isoandrosterone, differing only in that one has a 3α OH, the other a 3β OH). SEE ALSO stereoisomer, Le Bel-van't Hoff *rule*. SYN stereochemical isomerism.

ster·e·ol·o·gy (ster′ē-ol′ō-jē). A study of the three-dimensional aspects of a cell or microscopic structure. [stereo- + G. *logos*, study]

ster·e·om·e·ter (ster-ē-om′ē-ter). An instrument used in stereometry. [stereo- + G. *metron*, measure]

ster·e·om·e·try (ster-ē-om′ē-trē). **1.** Measurement of a solid object or the cubic capacity of a vessel. **2.** Determination of the specific gravity of a liquid.

ster·e·o·or·thop·ter (ster′ē-ō-ōr-thop′ter). A type of stereoscope used in visual training. [stereo- + G. *orthos*, straight, + *optikos*, optical]

ster·e·op·a·thy (ster-ē-op′ă-thē). Persistent stereotyped thinking.

ster·e·o·phan·to·scope (ster′ē-ō-fan′tō-skōp). An obsolete term for a stereophoroscope with rotating disks of different colors instead of pictures. [stereo- + G. *phantos*, visible, + *skopeō*, to view]

ster·e·o·pho·rom·e·ter (ster′ē-ō-fō-rom′ē-ter). A phorometer with a stereoscopic attachment.

ster·e·o·phor·o·scope (ster′ē-ō-fōr′ō-skōp). Obsolete term for a

stereoscope producing images having apparent motion. [stereo- + G. *phoros*, bearing, *skopeō*, to view]

ster·e·o·pho·to·mi·cro·graph (ster′ē-ō-fō′tō-mī′krō-graf). A stereoscopic photomicrograph that, when viewed with a stereoscope, appears three-dimensional.

ster·e·op·sis (ster-ē-op′sis). SYN stereoscopic *vision*. [stereo- + G. *opsis*, vision]

ster·e·o·ra·di·og·ra·phy (ster′ē-ō-rā-dē-og′ră-fē). Preparation of a pair of radiographs with appropriate shift of the x-ray tube or film so that the images can be viewed stereoscopically to give a three-dimensional appearance. SYN stereography, stereoroentgenography.

ster·e·o·roent·gen·og·ra·phy (ster′ē-ō-rent′gen-og′ră-fē). SYN stereoradiography.

ster·e·o·scope (ster′ē-ō-skōp). An instrument producing two horizontally separated images of the same object, providing a single image with an appearance of depth. [stereo- + G. *skopeō*, to view]

ster·e·o·scop·ic (ster′ē-ō-skop′ik). Relating to a stereoscope, or giving the appearance of three dimensions.

ster·e·os·co·py (ster-ē-os′kŏ-pē). **1.** An optical technique by which two images of the same object are blended into one, giving a three-dimensional appearance to the single image. **2.** SEE radiostereoscopy.

ster·e·o·se·lec·tive (ster′ē-ō-sě-lek′tiv). As applied to a reaction, denoting a process in which of two or more possible stereoisomeric products only one predominates; a s. process is not necessarily stereospecific.

ster·e·o·spe·cif·ic (ster′ē-ō-spě-sif′ik). As applied to a reaction, denoting a process in which stereoisomerically different starting materials give rise to stereoisomerically different products; a s. process is thus necessarily stereoselective, but not all stereoselective processes are s.

ster·e·o·tac·tic, ster·e·o·tax·ic (ster′ē-ō-tak′tik, -tak′sik). Relating to stereotaxis or stereotaxy.

ster·e·o·tax·is (ster′ē-ō-tak′sis). **1.** Three-dimensional arrangement. **2.** Stereotropism, but applied more exactly where the organism as a whole, rather than a part only, reacts. **3.** SYN stereotaxy. [stereo- + G. *taxis*, orderly arrangement]

ster·e·o·taxy (ster′ē-ō-tak′sē). A precise method of destroying deep-seated brain structures located by use of three-dimensional coordinates. SYN stereoencephalotomy, stereotactic surgery, stereotaxic surgery, stereotaxis (3).

ster·e·o·tro·pic (ster′ē-ō-trop′ik). Relating to or exhibiting stereotropism.

ster·e·ot·ro·pism (ster′ē-ot′rō-pizm). Growth or movement of a plant or animal toward (**positive s.**) or away from (**negative s.**) a solid body, usually applied where a part of the organism rather than the whole reacts. [stereo- + G. *tropos*, a turning]

ster·e·o·typy (ster′ē-ō-tī-pē). **1.** Maintenance of one attitude for a long period. **2.** Constant repetition of certain meaningless gestures or movements, as in certain forms of schizophrenia. [stereo- + G. *typos*, impression, type]

oral s., SYN verbigeration.

ste·ric (ster′ik, stēr-). Pertaining to stereochemistry.

s. hindrance, interference with or inhibition of a seemingly feasible reaction (usually synthetic) because the size of one or another reactant prevents approach to the required interatomic distance.

ster·id (ster′id, stēr-). SYN steroid (2).

ste·rig·ma, pl. **ste·rig·ma·ta** (ste-rig′mă, -mă-tă). A slender, pointed structure arising from a basidium upon which a basidiospore will develop. [G. *stērigma*, a support]

ster·ile (ster′il). Relating to or characterized by sterility. [L. *sterilis*, barren]

ste·ril·i·ty (stě-ril′i-tē). **1.** In general, the incapability of fertilization or reproduction. SEE female s., male s. **2.** Condition of being aseptic, or free from all living microorganisms and their spores. [L. *sterilitas*]

aspermatogenic s., s. due to a failure to produce living spermatozoa.

dysspermatogenic s., male s. due to some abnormality in production of spermatozoa.

female s., the inability of the female to conceive, due to inadequacy in structure or function of the genital organs. SYN infecundity.

male s., the inability of the male to fertilize the ovum; it may or may not be associated with impotence.

normospermatogenic s., male s. due to some cause other than failure to produce live, normal spermatozoa, *e.g.,* blockage of the seminiferous passages.

ster·il·i·za·tion (ster′ĭ-li-zā′shŭn). **1.** The act or process by which an individual is rendered incapable of fertilization or reproduction, as by vasectomy, partial salpingectomy, or castration. **2.** The destruction of all microorganisms in or about an object, as by steam (flowing or pressurized), chemical agents (alcohol, phenol, heavy metals, ethylene oxide gas) high-velocity electron bombardment, ultraviolet light radiation.

discontinuous s., SYN fractional s.

fractional s., exposure to a temperature of 100°C (flowing steam) for a definite period, usually an hour, on each of several days; at each heating the developed bacteria are destroyed; spores, which are unaffected, germinate during the intervening periods and are subsequently destroyed. SYN discontinuous s., intermittent s., tyndallization.

intermittent s., SYN fractional s.

ster·il·ize (ster′ĭ-līz). To produce sterility.

ster·il·iz·er (ster′i-lī-zer). An apparatus for rendering objects sterile.

glass bead s., a s. for endodontic equipment; the heat is transmitted to the instruments, absorbent points, or cotton pellets by means of glass beads.

hot salt s., a s. for endodontic equipment in which table salt is heated in a container at 218 to 246°C; the dry heat is transmitted to root canal instruments, absorbent points, or cotton pellets for their rapid (5 to 10 seconds) sterilization.

Stern, Heinrich, U.S. physician, 1868–1918. SEE S.'s *posture.*

⌂**stern-.** SEE sterno-.

ster·na (ster′nă). Plural of sternum.

ster·nad (ster′nad). In a direction toward the sternum.

ster·nal (ster′năl). Relating to the sternum.

ster·nal·gia (ster-nal′jē-ă). Pain in the sternum or the sternal region. SYN sternodynia. [stern- + G. *algos,* pain]

ster·na·lis (ster-nā′lis). SEE sternalis *muscle.*

Sternberg, George M., U.S. bacteriologist, 1838–1915. SEE S. *cells,* under *cell;* S.-Reed *cells,* under *cell;* Reed-S. *cells,* under *cell.*

ster·ne·bra, pl. **ster·ne·brae** (ster′nē-bră, -brē). One of the four segments of the primordial sternum of the embryo by the fusion of which the body of the adult sternum is formed. [Mod. L. fr. stern(um) + (vert)ebra]

ster·nen. Relating to the sternum independent of any other structures. [stern- + G. *en,* in]

⌂**sterno-, stern-.** The sternum, sternal. [G. *sternon,* chest]

ster·no·chon·dro·sca·pu·la·ris (ster′nō-kon′drō-skap-yū-lā′ris). SEE sternochondroscapular *muscle.* [Mod. L.]

ster·no·cla·vic·u·lar (ster′nō-kla-vik′yū-lăr). Relating to the sternum and the clavicle.

ster·no·cla·vi·cu·la·ris (ster′nō-kla-vik′yū-lā′ris). SEE sternoclavicular *muscle.*

ster·no·clei·dal (ster′nō-klī′dăl). Relating to the sternum and the clavicle. [sterno- + G. *kleis,* key (clavicle)]

ster·no·clei·do·mas·toid (ster′nō-klī′dō-mas′toyd). Relating to sternum, clavicle, and mastoid process.

ster·no·clei·do·mas·toi·de·us (ster′nō-klī′dō-mas-tō-id′-ē-ŭs). SEE sternocleidomastoid *muscle.* [Mod. L.]

ster·no·cos·tal (ster′nō-kos′tăl). Relating to the sternum and the ribs. [L. *costa,* rib]

ster·no·dyn·ia (ster-nō-din′ē-ă). SYN sternalgia. [sterno- + G. *odynē,* pain]

ster·no·fas·ci·a·lis (ster′nō-fash-ē-ā′lis). SEE *musculus* sternofascialis.

ster·no·glos·sal (ster-nō-glos′ăl). Denoting muscular fibers that occasionally pass from the sternohyoid muscle to join the hyoglossal muscle.

ster·no·hy·oi·de·us (ster′nō-hī-oyd′ē-ŭs). SEE sternohyoid *muscle.* [Mod. L.]

ster·noid (ster′noyd). Resembling the sternum. [sterno- + G. *eidos,* resemblance]

ster·no·mas·toid (ster′nō-mas′toyd). Relating to the sternum and the mastoid process of the temporal bone; applied to the sternocleidomastoid muscle.

ster·no·pa·gia (ster-nō-pā′jē-ă). Condition shown by conjoined twins united at the sterna or more extensively at the ventral walls of the chest. SEE conjoined *twins,* under *twin.* [sterno- + G. *pagos,* something fixed]

ster·no·per·i·car·di·al (ster′nō-per′i-kar′dē-ăl). Relating to the sternum and the pericardium.

ster·nos·chi·sis (ster-nos′ki-sis). Congenital cleft of the sternum. [sterno- + G. *schisis,* a cleaving]

ster·no·thy·roi·de·us (ster′nō-thī′royd′ē-ŭs). SEE sternothyroid *muscle.* [Mod. L.]

ster·not·o·my (ster-not′ō-mē). Incision into or through the sternum. [sterno- + G. *tomē,* incision]

median s., incision through the midline of the sternum usually used to gain access to the heart, mediastinal structures, and great vessels.

ster·no·tra·che·al (ster′nō-trā′kē-ăl). Relating to the sternum and the trachea.

ster·no·try·pe·sis (ster′nō-trī-pē′sis). Trephining of the sternum. [sterno- + G. *trypēsis,* a boring]

ster·no·ver·te·bral (ster′nō-ver′tĕ-brăl). Relating to the sternum and the vertebrae; denoting the true ribs, or the seven upper ribs on either side, which articulate with the vertebrae and with the sternum. SYN vertebrosternal.

ster·num, gen. **ster·ni,** pl. **ster·na** (ster′nŭm, -nī, -nă) [NA]. A long flat bone, articulating with the cartilages of the first seven ribs and with the clavicle, forming the middle part of the anterior wall of the thorax; it consists of three portions: the corpus or body, the manubrium, and the xiphoid process. SYN breast bone. [Mod. L. fr. G. *sternon,* the chest]

ster·nu·ta·tion (ster′nū-tā′shŭn). The act of sneezing. [L. *sternutatio,* fr. *sternuo (sternuto),* pp. *sternutatus,* to sneeze]

ster·nu·ta·tor (ster′nū-tā-ter, -tōr). A substance, such as a gas, that induces sneezing. SYN sneezing gas.

ster·nu·ta·to·ry (ster-nū′tă-tōr-ē). **1.** Causing sneezing. **2.** An agent that provokes sneezing. SYN ptarmic.

ste·roid (stēr′oyd, ster′oyd). **1.** Pertaining to the steroids. SYN steroidal. Cf. steroids. **2.** One of the steroids. SYN sterid. **3.** Generic designation for compounds closely related in structure to the steroids, such as sterols, bile acids, cardiac glycosides, and precursors of the D vitamins.

anabolic s., a s. compound with the capacity to increase muscle mass; compounds with androgenic properties which increase muscle mass and are used in the treatment of emaciation. Sometimes used by athletes in an effort to increase muscle size, strength, and endurance. Examples include methyltestosterone, nandrolone, methandrostenolone, and stanozolol.

s. hydroxylases, SYN s. monooxygenases.

s. 21-monooxygenase, an enzyme catalyzing the reaction of a steroid, O_2, and some reduced compound to produce water, the oxidized compound, and a 21-hydroxysteroid; a deficiency of this enzyme results in decreased cortisol synthesis, of which there are three types (salt-wasting, simple virilizing, and nonclassical).

s. monooxygenases, enzymes catalyzing addition of hydroxyl groups to the s. rings utilizing O_2; differentiated into, for example, s. 11β-monooxygenase, s. 17α-monooxygenase, and s. 21-monooxygenase, in accordance with the position of the catalytically introduced hydroxyl group. SYN s. hydroxylases.

s. 5α-reductase, an enzyme that uses NADPH to reduce certain steroids (*e.g.,* the conversion of testosterone to dihydrotestosterone a deficiency of this enzyme is associated with a form of male pseudohermaphroditism in which genetic males have male genitals as well as female external genitalia.

s. sulfatase deficiency, SYN X-linked *ichthyosis.*

ste·roi·dal (stēr′oy-dăl, ster′). SYN steroid (1).

ste·roi·do·gen·e·sis (stēr′oy-dō-jen′ĕ-sis, ster′). The formation of steroids; commonly referring to the biological synthesis of steroid hormones, but not to the production of such compounds in a chemical laboratory. [steroid + G. *genesis,* production]

ste·roids (stēr′oydz, ster-). A large family of chemical substances, comprising many hormones, body constituents, and drugs, each containing the tetracyclic cyclopenta[*a*]phenanthrene skeleton. Formula I of the accompanying page of structures shows the numbering and lettering of the rings, which are retained even if, in a given compound, any of the atoms shown are absent or involved in ring closures, or if rings are expanded ("homo," see below) or contracted ("nor," see below). Stereoisomerism among s. is not only common but of critical biological significance, and the isomeric groups are usually represented as shown in II. The conventions are that the nucleus is presented as if projected onto the plane of the paper, with groups then lying above that plane being denoted by thickened bonds and called β, those then lying below that plane by broken bonds and called α; the letter ξ indicates unknown or unspecified orientation. Depending on the situation at C-5, the molecule is sometimes represented in perspective as in III and IV; 5α, 5β, or 5ξ should be included in the name. Unless otherwise stated, it is assumed that atoms or groups attached to the other ring-junctions (8, 9, 10, 13, 14) are as in II, *i.e.,* 8β, 9α, 10β, 13β, 14α.

The principal classes of steroids, with the names for the unsubstituted, saturated hydrocarbon forms that are clearly related to physiological functions or sources are: 1) gonanes (in which the methyl group in formula II, C-18 and C-19, have been replaced by H), 2) estranes (in which the C-19 methyl groups in formula II has been replaced by H), 3) androstanes (equivalent to formula II), 4) norandrostanes (in which one of the methyl groups, typically C-18, has been replaced by H), 5) cholanes (formula II with $-CH(CH_3)(CH_2)_2CH_3$ bonded to C-17), 6) cholestanes (with $-CH(CH_3)(CH_2)_3CH(CH_3)_2$ at C-17, 7) ergostanes (with $-CH(CH_3)(CH_2)_2CH(CH_3)CH(CH_3)_2$ at C-17), and 8) stigmastanes (with $-CH(CH_3)(CH_2)_2CH(CH_2CHCH_3)CH(CH_3)_2$ at C-17). In addition, each of the classes can be in a 5α- or 5β-series.

The steroid derivatives known as cardanolides are androstanes with a 5-membered lactone linked to C-17. The squill-toad poisons known as the bufanolides are androstanes with a 6-membered lactone linked to C-17. Spirostans and furostans (the basic structures of many "genins," including the sapogenins) are androstanes having certain cyclic ether moieties.

The natural and synthetic derivatives are named by adding conventional chemical prefixes and suffixes for substituents; *e.g.,* -ol for a hydroxyl group, -on(e) for a keto group, -al for an aldehyde group. "Nor" indicates loss of a $-CH_2-$ group; "homo," the addition of a $-CH_2-$ group; each is preceded by the letter indicating which ring is contracted or expanded, respectively, or, in the case where the $-CH_2-$ is lost from a methyl group, the number of the carbon atom lost. "Seco" indicates fission of a ring with addition of hydrogen atoms at the positions indicated by numerals preceding the term. Unsaturation is denoted, as usual, by substituting appropriate terms, *e.g.,* -en(e), -yn(e), -adien(e), for the -ane or -an parts of the hydrocarbon or parent class names, with numerals indicating locations of the unsaturated bonds. The locations of double bonds are specified by the lower of the two (consecutive) numbers of the carbon atoms involved. When a double bond is formed between two nonconsecutive carbon atoms, the second is indicated in parentheses after the first; *e.g.,* estriol and the estradiols possess three double bonds, between C-1 and C-2, between C-3 and C-4, and between C-5 and C-10, respectively.

Steroid alkaloids may be named from the steroid parent, as above, or from trivial family names usually ending in -anine if the steroid is saturated or in -enine, -adienine, etc., if it is not saturated (*e.g.,* conanine, tomatanine).

ste·rol (stēr′ol). A steroid with one OH (alcohol) group; the

systematic names contain either the prefix hydroxy- or the suffix -ol, *e.g.,* cholesterol, ergosterol.

ster·tor (ster′tōr). A noisy inspiration occurring in coma or deep sleep, sometimes due to obstruction of the larynx or upper airways. [L. *sterto,* to snore].

hen-cluck s., a breath sound like the clucking of a hen, sometimes heard in cases of postpharyngeal abscess.

ster·to·rous (ster′tōr-ŭs). Relating to or characterized by stertor or snoring.

△**steth-.** SEE stetho-.

ste·thal·gia (ste-thal′jē-ă). Pain in the chest. [steth- + G. *algos,* pain]

steth·ar·te·ri·tis (steth′ar-ter-ī′tis). Inflammation of the aorta or other arteries in the chest. [steth- + L. *arteria,* artery, + G. *-itis,* inflammation]

△**stetho-, steth-.** Combining forms denoting the chest. the chest. [G. *stēthos*]

steth·o·cyr·to·graph (steth′ō-ser′tō-graf). An apparatus for measuring and recording the curvatures of the thorax. SYN stethokyrtograph. [stetho- + G. *kyrtos,* bent, + *graphō,* to write]

steth·o·cyr·tom·e·ter (steth′ō-ser-tom′ĕ-ter). An instrument for measuring curvature or deformity of the vertebral column in kyphosis. [stetho- + G. *kyrtos,* bent, + *metron,* measure]

steth·o·go·ni·om·e·ter (steth′ō-gō-nē-om′ĕ-ter). An apparatus for measuring the curvatures of the thorax. [stetho- + G. *gōnia,* angle, + *metron,* measure]

steth·o·graph (steth′ō-graf). An apparatus for recording the respiratory movements of the chest. [stetho- + G. *graphō,* to write]

steth·o·kyr·to·graph (steth′ō-ker′tō-graf). SYN stethocyrtograph.

steth·o·my·i·tis (steth′ō-mī-ī′tis). Inflammation of the muscles of the chest wall. SYN stethomyositis. [stetho- + G. *mys,* muscle, + *-itis,* inflammation]

steth·o·my·o·si·tis (steth′ō-mī-ō-sī′tis). SYN stethomyitis.

steth·o·pa·ral·y·sis (steth′ō-pă-ral′i-sis). Paralysis of the respiratory muscles.

steth·o·scope (steth′ō-skōp). An instrument originally devised by Laennec for aid in hearing the respiratory and cardiac sounds in the chest, but now modified in various ways and used in auscultation of any of vascular or other sounds anywhere in the body. [stetho- + G. *skopeō,* to view]

binaural s., a s. in which the two ear pieces connect with a single bell.

Bowles type s., a s. in which the chest piece is a shallow metal cup about 4.5 cm. in diameter, the mouth of which is covered by a hard rubber or celluloid diaphragm.

differential s., a s. having two chest pieces so that two sounds in different parts of the chest may be heard simultaneously and compared.

steth·o·scop·ic (steth-ō-skop′ik). **1.** Relating to or effected by means of a stethoscope. **2.** Relating to an examination of the chest.

ste·thos·co·py (stĕ-thos′kŏ-pē). **1.** Examination of the chest by means of auscultation, either mediate or immediate, and percussion. **2.** Mediate auscultation with the stethoscope.

steth·o·spasm (steth′ō-spazm). Spasm of the chest.

Stevens, Albert M., U.S. pediatrician, 1884–1945. SEE S.-Johnson *syndrome.*

Stewart, Fred Waldorf, U.S. physician, *1894. SEE S.-Treves *syndrome.*

Stewart, George N., Canadian-U.S. scientist, 1860–1930. SEE S.'s *test;* Stewart-Hamilton *method.*

Stewart, R.M., 20th century English neurologist. SEE S.-Morel *syndrome.*

Stewart, Thomas Grainger, 20th century English neurologist, 1877–1957. SEE S.-Holmes *sign.*

STH Abbreviation for somatotropic *hormone.*

sthe·ni·a (sthē′nē-ă). A condition of activity and apparent force, as in an acute sthenic fever. [G. *sthenos,* strength, + *-ia,* condition]

sthen·ic (sthen′ik). Active; marked by sthenia; said of a fever with strong bounding pulse, high temperature, and active delirium.

⌂stheno-. Strength, force, power. [G. *sthenos*]

sthe·nom·e·ter (sthĕ-nom′ĕ-ter). An instrument for measuring muscular strength. [stheno- + G. *metron,* measure]

sthe·nom·e·try (sthĕ-nom′ĕ-trē). The measurement of muscular strength. [stheno- + G. *metrin,* to measure]

stib·a·mine glu·co·side (stib′ă-mēn). A nitrogen glycoside of sodium *p*-aminobenzenestibonate; A pentavalent antimony compound; has been used in leishmaniasis (kala azar) and certain other tropical diseases, but is no longer marketed.

stib·e·nyl (stib′ĕ-nil). Sodium 4-acetamidobenzenestibonate; the first pentavalent antimonial used in the treatment of leishmaniasis (kala azar).

stib·i·al·ism (stib′ē-ă-lizm). Chronic antimonial poisoning. [L. *stibium,* antimony]

stib·i·a·ted (stib′ē-ā-ted). Impregnated with or containing antimony.

stib·i·a·tion (stib-ē-ā′shŭn). Impregnation with antimony.

stib·i·um (stib′ē-ŭm). SYN antimony. [L. fr. G. *stibi*]

stib·o·cap·tate (stib-ō-kap′tāt). SYN *antimony* dimercaptosuccinate.

stib·o·glu·co·nate so·di·um (stib-ō-glū′kŏ-nāt). **1.** pentavalent sodium stibogluconate; pentavalent sodium stibogluconate, used in the treatment of all types of leishmaniasis; toxic effects are frequent. SYN antimony sodium gluconate. **2.** trivalent sodium stibogluconate; trivalent antimony sodium gluconate, used in the treatment of schistosomiasis; toxic effects are frequent. SYN sodium antimonylgluconate.

sti·bo·ni·um (sti-bō′nē-ŭm). The hypothetical radical, SbH₄⁺, analogous to ammonium.

stib·o·phen (stib′ō-fen). Pentasodium bis[4,5-dihydroxybenz-1,3-disulfonate]antimonate; an organic trivalent antimony compound, used in the treatment of schistosomiasis, filariasis, leishmaniasis, and lymphogranuloma inguinale.

stich·o·chrome (stik′ō-krōm). Denoting a nerve cell in which the chromophil substance, or stainable material, is arranged in roughly parallel rows or lines. [G. *stichos,* a row, + *chrōma,* color]

Sticker, Georg, German physician, 1860–1960. SEE S.'s *disease.*

Stickler, Gunnar B., 20th century U.S. physician. SEE S.'s *syndrome.*

Stieda, Alfred, German surgeon, 1869–1945. SEE Pellegrini-S. *disease.*

Stieda, Ludwig, German anatomist, 1837–1918. SEE S.'s *process.*

Stierlin, Eduard, German surgeon, 1878–1919. SEE S.'s *sign.*

sti·fle (stī′fl). SYN stifle *joint.*

stig·ma, pl. **stig·mas, stig·ma·ta** (stig′mă, -mă-tă). **1.** Visible evidence of a disease. **2.** SYN follicular s. **3.** Any spot or blemish on the skin. **4.** A bleeding spot on the skin, which is considered a manifestation of conversion hysteria. **5.** The orange pigmented eyespot of certain chlorophyll-bearing protozoa, such as *Euglena viridis,* which serves as a light filter by absorbing certain wavelengths. **6.** A mark of shame or discredit. [G. a mark. fr. *stizō,* to prick]

follicular s., the point where the graafian follicle is about to rupture on the surface of the ovary. SYN macula pellucida, stigma (2).

malpighian stigmas, the points of entrance of the smaller veins into the larger veins of the spleen.

s. ventric′uli, one of a number of miliary ecchymoses of the gastric mucosa.

stig·mas·tane (stig-mas′tān). The parent substance of sitosterol. SYN sitostane.

stig·ma·ta (stig′mă-tă). Alternative plural of stigma.

stig·ma·ta may·dis (stig′mă-tă mā′dis). SYN zea.

stig·mat·ic (stig-mat′ik). Relating to or marked by a stigma.

stig·ma·tism (stig′mă-tizm). The condition of having a stigma. SYN stigmatization (1).

stig·ma·ti·za·tion (stig′mă-ti-zā′shŭn). **1.** SYN stigmatism. **2.** Production of stigmas, especially of a hysterical nature. **3.** Debasement of a person by attributing a negatively toned characteristic or other stigma to him or her.

stil·bam·i·dine (stil-bam′i-dēn). Stilbene-4,4′-dicarbonamidine; a compound used in the treatment of leishmaniasis (kala azar), in infections due to *Blastomyces dermatitidis,* and in actinomycosis; also used in multiple myeloma for the relief of bone pain.

stil·baz·i·um io·dide (stil-baz′ē-ŭm). 1-Ethyl-2,6-bis[(*p*-pyrrolidinylstyryl)]pyridinium iodide; an anthelmintic.

stil·bene (stil′bēn). **1.** C₆H₅CH=CHC₆H₅; α,β-Diphenylethylene; an unsaturated hydrocarbon, the nucleus of stilbestrol and other synthetic estrogenic compounds. **2.** A class of compounds based on s. (1).

stil·bes·trol (stil-bes′trol). SYN diethylstilbestrol.

Stiles, Walter, English physicist, *1901. SEE S.-Crawford *effect.*

sti·let, sti·lette (stī′let, stī-let′). SEE stylet.

Still, Sir George F., English physician, 1868–1941. SEE S.'s *disease, murmur;* S.-Chauffard *syndrome.*

still·birth (stil′berth). The birth of an infant who has died prior to delivery.

still·born (stil′bōrn). Born dead; denoting an infant dead at birth.

Stilling, Benedict, German anatomist, 1810–1879. SEE S.'s *canal, column, nucleus, raphe,* gelatinous *substance.*

Stilling, Jakob, German ophthalmologist, 1842–1915. SEE S. color *tables,* under *table.*

sti·lus (stī′lŭs). SEE stylus.

stim·u·lant (stim′yū-lănt). **1.** Stimulating; exciting to action. **2.** An agent that arouses organic activity, strengthens the action of the heart, increases vitality, and promotes a sense of well-being; classified according to the parts upon which they chiefly act: cardiac, respiratory, gastric, hepatic, cerebral, spinal, vascular, genital, etc. SYN excitor, stimulator. SEE ALSO stimulus. SYN excitant. [L. *stimulans,* pres. p. of *stimulo,* pp. *-atus,* to goad, incite, fr. *stimulus,* a goad]

diffusible s., a s. that produces a rapid but temporary effect.

general s., a s. that affects the entire body.

local s., a s. whose action is confined to the part to which it is applied.

stim·u·la·tion (stim-yū-lā′shŭn). **1.** Arousal of the body or any of its parts or organs to increased functional activity. **2.** The condition of being stimulated. **3.** In neurophysiology, the application of a stimulus to a responsive structure, such as a nerve or muscle, regardless of whether the strength of the stimulus is sufficient to produce excitation. [see stimulant]

dorsal column s., electrical s., either percutaneously or by direct application of electrodes to the dorsal columns of the spinal cord.

Ganzfeld s., illumination of the entire retina in the electroretinogram. [Ger. *Ganzfeld,* whole field]

percutaneous s., electrical s. of the peripheral nerves or spinal cord by the application of electrodes to the skin.

photic s., the use of a flickering light at various frequencies to influence the pattern of the occipital electroencephalogram and also to activate latent abnormalities.

stim·u·la·tor (stim′yū-lā-ter, -tōr). SYN stimulant (2).

long-acting thyroid s. (LATS), a substance, found in the blood of some hyperthyroid patients, that exerts a prolonged stimulatory effect on the thyroid gland; associated in plasma with the IgG (7S γ-globulin) fraction and seems to be an antibody or, perhaps, an immune complex.

stim·u·lus, pl. **stim·u·li** (stim′yū-lŭs, -lī). **1.** A stimulant. **2.** That which can elicit or evoke action (response) in a muscle, nerve, gland or other excitable tissue, or cause an augmenting action upon any function or metabolic process. [L. a goad]

adequate s., a s. to which a particular receptor responds effectively and that gives rise to a characteristic sensation; *e.g.,* light and sound waves that stimulate, respectively, visual and auditory receptors.

aversive s., a noxious stimulus such as an electric shock used in aversive *training* or conditioning. SEE ALSO aversive *training.*

conditioned s., (1) a s. applied to one of the sense organs (*e.g.,* receptors of vision, hearing, touch) which are an essential and integral part of the neural mechanism underlying a conditioned reflex; SEE classical *conditioning,* higher order *conditioning.* (2) a neutral s., when paired with the unconditioned s. in simultaneous presentation to an organism, capable of eliciting a given response.

discriminant s., a s. which can be differentiated from all other s. in the environment because it has been, and continues to serve as, an indicator of a potential reinforcer.

heterologous s., a s. that acts upon any part of the sensory apparatus or nerve tract.

heterotopic s., any electrical activation from an abnormal locus.

homologous s., a s. that acts only on the nerve terminations in a special sense organ.

inadequate s., a s. too weak to evoke a response. SYN subliminal s., subthreshold s.

liminal s., SYN threshold s.

maximal s., a s. strong enough to evoke a maximal response.

square wave stimuli, electrical stimulation in which the intensity of the current is brought suddenly to a given level and maintained at that level until it suddenly is cut off; this type of s. is particularly useful in obtaining a strength-duration curve.

subliminal s., SYN inadequate s.

subthreshold s., SYN inadequate s.

supramaximal s., a s. having strength significantly above that required to activate all of the nerve or muscle fibers in contact with the electrode; used when response of all the fibers is desired.

threshold s., a s. of threshold strength, *i.e.,* one just strong enough to excite. SEE ALSO adequate s. SYN liminal s.

train-of-four s., a method for measuring magnitude and type of neuromuscular blockade, based upon the ratio of the amplitude of the fourth evoked mechanical response to the first one, when four supramaximal 2-Hz electrical currents are applied for 2 seconds to a peripheral motor nerve.

unconditioned s., a s. that elicits an unconditioned response; *e.g.,* food is an unconditioned s. for salivation, which in turn is an unconditioned response in a hungry animal. SEE classical *conditioning.*

stim·u·lus word. The word used in association tests to evoke a response.

sting. 1. Sharp momentary pain, most commonly produced by the puncture of the skin by many species of arthropods, including hexapods, myriapods, and arachnids; can also be produced by jellyfish, sea urchins, sponges, mollusks, and several species of venomous fish, such as the stingray, toadfish, rabbitfish, and catfish. SEE ALSO bites. **2.** The venom apparatus of a stinging animal, consisting of a chitinous spicule or bony spine and a venom gland or sac. **3.** To introduce (or the process of introducing) a venom by stinging. [O.E. *stingan*]

sting·ers (sting′erz). SYN burners.

stink weed. SYN *Datura stramonium.*

stip·pling (stip′ling). **1.** A speckling of a blood cell or other structure with fine dots when exposed to the action of a basic stain, due to the presence of free basophil granules in the cell protoplasm. SYN punctate basophilia. **2.** An orange peel appearance of the attached gingiva. **3.** A roughening of the surfaces of a denture base to stimulate natural gingival s.

geographic s. of nails, regularly arranged longitudinal s. found commonly in psoriasis and occasionally in alopecia areata. SEE ALSO nail *pits,* under *pit.*

Ziemann's s., SYN Ziemann's *dots,* under *dot.*

STIR Acronym for short TI inversion *recovery.*

Stirling, William, British histologist and physiologist, 1851–1932. SEE S.'s modification of Gram's *stain.*

stir·rup (ster′ŭp, stir′ŭp). SYN stapes. [A.S. *stīrāp*]

stitch. 1. A sharp sticking pain of momentary duration. **2.** A single suture. **3.** SYN suture (2). [A.S. *stice,* a pricking]

STM Abbreviation for short-term *memory.*

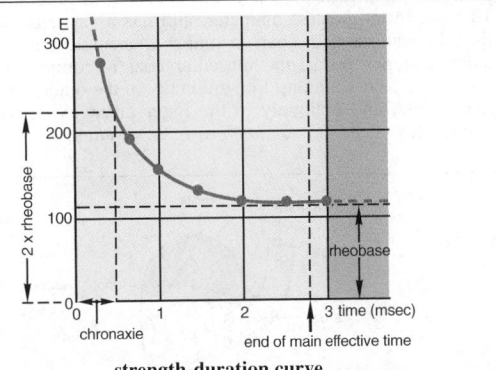

strength-duration curve
various durations of stimuli (*horizontal axis*) and corresponding threshold stimuli (*vertical axis*)

Stock, Wolfgang, German ophthalmologist, 1874–1956. SEE Spielmeyer-S. *disease.*

stock (stok). All the populations of organisms derived from an isolate without any implication of homogeneity or characterization. [A.S. *stoc*]

Stocker, Frederick William, U.S. ophthalmologist, 1893–1974. SEE S.'s *line.*

stock·ing (stok′ing). Edema of the leg in the horse.

Stoerk, Karl, Austrian laryngologist, 1832–1899. SEE S.'s *blennorrhea.*

Stoffel, Adolf, German orthopedic surgeon, 1880–1937. SEE S.'s *operation.*

stoi·chi·ol·o·gy (stoy-kē-ol′-ō-jē). The science concerned with the elements or principles in any branch of knowledge, especially in chemistry, cytology, or histology. [G. *stoicheion,* element (lit. one of a row), fr. *stoichos,* a row, + *logos,* study]

stoi·chi·o·met·ric (stoy′kē-ō-met′rik). Pertaining to stoichiometry.

stoi·chi·om·e·try (stoy-kē-om′ĕ-trē). Determination of the relative quantities of the substances concerned in any chemical reaction; *e.g.,* with the laws of definite proportions in chemistry, as in the molar proportions in a reaction. [G. *stoicheion,* element, + *metron,* measure]

stoke (stōk). A unit of kinematic viscosity, that of a fluid with a viscosity of 1 poise and a density of 1 g/ml; equal to 10^{-4} square meter per second. [Sir George Gabriel *Stokes*]

Stokes, Sir George Gabriel, British physicist and mathematician, 1819–1903. SEE stoke; S.'s *law* (2), *law* (3).

Stokes, William, Irish physician, 1804–1878. SEE S.'s *law* (1); Cheyne-S. *psychosis, respiration;* S.-Adams *disease;* Adams-S. *disease;* Morgagni-Adams-S. *syndrome.*

Stokes, Sir William, Irish surgeon, 1839–1900. SEE S. *amputation;* Gritti-S. *amputation.*

sto·lon (stō′lon). A runner or connective aerial hypha that forms a cluster of rhizoids when it touches the substrate, and then sends out other runners to produce the aerial mycelium and sporangiosphores typical of *Rhizopus.* [L. *stolō,* branch, shoot, twig]

△**stom-.** SEE stomato-.

sto·ma, pl. **sto·mas, sto·ma·ta** (stō′mă, stō′maz, stō′mă-tă). **1.** A minute opening or pore. **2.** An artificial opening between two cavities or canals, or between such and the surface of the body. [G. a mouth]

Fuchs' stomas, small depression on the surface of the iris near the margin of the pupil.

loop s., a specialized s. of intestine or ureter by which a loop of the hollow viscus is brought through an opening in the abdominal wall, with an opening created in the apex of the viscus to allow egress of its contents.

stom·ach (stŭm′ŭk). A large irregularly piriform sac between the esophagus and the small intestine, lying just beneath the diaphragm; when distended it is 25 to 28 cm in length and 10 to 10.5 cm in its greatest diameter, and has a capacity of about 1 liter. Its wall has four coats or tunics: mucous, submucous, muscular, and peritoneal; the muscular coat is composed of three layers, the fibers running longitudinally in the outer, circularly in the middle, and obliquely in the inner layer. SYN gaster [NA], ventriculus (1)✶. [G. *stomachos*, L. *stomachus*]

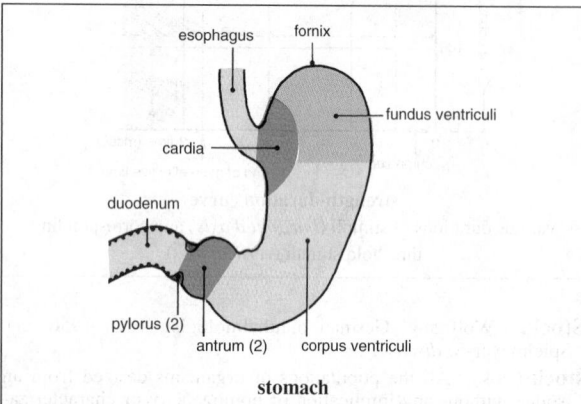

esophagus
fornix
fundus ventriculi
cardia
duodenum
pylorus (2)
antrum (2)
corpus ventriculi

stomach

bilocular s., SYN hourglass s.

s. bubble, the gas in the fundus of the s. seen on an upright radiograph.

cascade s., a radiographic description: when contrast material is swallowed while the patient is in the upright position, the gastric fundus acts as a reservoir until contrast overflows (cascades) into the antrum; a normal variant in a horizontal s.

drain-trap s., SYN water-trap s.

hourglass s., a condition in which there is a central constriction of the wall of the s. dividing it into two cavities, cardiac and pyloric. SYN bilocular s., ectasia ventriculi paradoxa.

leather-bottle s., marked thickening and rigidity of the s. wall, with reduced capacity of the lumen although often without obstruction; nearly always due to scirrhous carcinoma, as in linitis plastica. SYN sclerotic s.

miniature s., SYN Pavlov *pouch*.

Pavlov s., SYN Pavlov *pouch*.

powdered s., the dried and powdered defatted wall of the s. of the hog, *Sus scrofa;* it contains thermolabile factors including native vitamin B_{12} and intrinsic factor; has been used in the treatment of pernicious anemia.

sclerotic s., SYN leather-bottle s.

thoracic s., a condition in which part or all of the s. is contained within the thorax; a variant of hiatal hernia.

trifid s., a condition in which the s. is divided by two constrictions into three pouches.

wallet s., a form of dilated s. in which there is a general baglike distention, the antrum and fundus being indistinguishable.

water-trap s., a ptotic and dilated s., having a relatively high (though normally placed) pyloric outlet which is held up by the gastrohepatic ligament. SYN drain-trap s.

stom·ach·al (stŭm′ă-kăl). Relating to the stomach. SYN stomachic (1).

stom·a·chal·gia (stŭm-ă-kal′jē-ă). Obsolete term for stomach *ache*. [stomach + G. *algos*, pain]

sto·mach·ic (stō′mak′ik). **1.** SYN stomachal. **2.** An agent that improves appetite and digestion.

stom·a·cho·dyn·ia (stŭm′ă-kō-din′ē-ă). Obsolete term for stomach *ache*. [stomach + G. *odynē*, pain]

sto·mal (stō′măl). Relating to a stoma.

△**stomat-.** SEE stomato-.

sto·ma·ta (stō′mă-tă). Alternate plural of stoma.

sto·ma·tal (stō′mă-tăl). Relating to a stoma.

sto·ma·tal·gia (stō-mă-tal′jē-ă). Pain in the mouth. SYN stomatodynia. [stomat- + G. *algos*, pain]

sto·mat·ic (stō-mat′ik). Relating to the mouth; oral.

sto·ma·ti·tis (stō-mă-tī′tis). Inflammation of the mucous membrane of the mouth. [stomat- + G. *-itis*, inflammation]

angular s., SYN angular *cheilitis*.

aphthous s., SYN aphtha (2).

bovine papular s., a *Parapoxvirus* infection of cattle causing oral lesions. SYN s. papulosa.

epidemic s., contagious mouth infection, usually due to Group A Coxsackievirus. SEE ALSO herpangina.

fusospirochetal s., infection of the mouth with spirochetal organisms, usually in association with other anaerobes. SEE ALSO Vincent's *angina*.

gangrenous s., s. characterized by necrosis of oral tissue. SEE noma.

gonococcal s., inflammatory and ulcerative oral lesions resulting from infection with *Neisseria gonorrhoeae;* usually primary as a result of oral-genital contact, but occasionally is the result of gonococcemia.

lead s., oral manifestation of lead poisoning consisting of a bluish-black line following the contours of the marginal gingiva where lead sulfide has precipitated due to the inflamed environment.

s. medicamento′sa, inflammatory alterations of the oral mucosa associated with a systemic drug allergy; lesions may consist of erythema, vesicles, bullae, ulcerations, or angioneurotic edema.

mercurial s., alterations of the oral mucosa arising from chronic mercury poisoning; may consist of mucosal erythema and edema, ulceration, and deposition of mercurial sulfide in inflamed tissues, resulting in oral pigmentation resembling that of lead s.

nicotine s., heat stimulated lesions, usually on the palate, that begin with erythema and progress to multiple white papules with a red dot in the center. The red dot represents a dilated, inflamed salivary duct orifice.

s. papulo′sa, SYN bovine papular s.

primary herpetic s., first infection of oral tissues with herpes simplex virus; characterized by gingival inflammation, vesicles, and ulcers.

recurrent aphthous s., SYN aphtha (2).

recurrent herpetic s., reactivation of herpes simplex virus infection, characterized by vesicles and ulceration limited to the hard palate and attached gingiva.

recurrent ulcerative s., SYN aphtha (2).

ulcerative s., SYN aphtha (2).

vesicular s., a vesicular disease of horses, cattle, swine, and occasionally man caused by a vesiculovirus (vesicular stomatitis virus); in horses and cattle the disease usually causes mouth vesicles which, in cattle, cannot be differentiated clinically from those of foot-and-mouth disease.

△**stomato-, stom-, stomat-.** Mouth. [G. *stoma*]

sto·ma·to·cyte (stō′mă-tō-sīt). A red blood cell that exhibits a slit or mouth-shaped pallor rather than a central one on air-dried smears; *e.g.,* Rh null cells. [stomato- + G. *kytos*, cell]

sto·ma·to·cy·to·sis (stō′mă-tō-sī-tō′sis). A hereditary deformation of red blood cells, which are swollen and cup-shaped, causing congenital hemolytic anemia. SEE ALSO Rh null *syndrome*.

sto·ma·to·de·um (stō′mă-tō-dē′ŭm). SYN stomodeum (1).

sto·ma·to·dyn·ia (stō′mă-tō-din′ē-ă). SYN stomatalgia. [stomato- + G. *odynē*, pain]

sto·ma·to·dys·o·dia (stō′mă-tō-di-sō′dē-ă). SYN halitosis. [stomato- + G. *dysōdia*, bad odor]

sto·ma·to·gnath·ic (stō′mă-tog-nath′ik). Pertaining to the physiology of the mouth. [stomato- + G. *gnathos*, jaw]

sto·ma·to·log·ic (stō′mă-tō-loj′ik). Relating to stomatology.

sto·ma·tol·o·gist (stō-mă-tol′ŏ-jist). A specialist in diseases of oral cavity, membranes, and tissues.

sto·ma·tol·o·gy (stō-mă-tol′ŏ-jē). The study of the structures, functions, and diseases of the mouth. [stomato- + G. *logos*, study]

sto·ma·to·ma·la·cia (stō′mă-tō-mă-lā′shē-ă). Pathologic softening of any of the structures of the mouth. [stomato- + G. *malakia*, softness]

sto·ma·to·my·co·sis (stō′mă-tō-mī-kō′sis). Disease of the mouth due to the presence of a fungus. [stomato- + G. *mykēs*, fungus, + *-osis*, condition]

sto·ma·to·ne·cro·sis (stō′mă-tō-ně-krō′sis). SYN noma. [stomato- + G. *nekrōsis*, death]

sto·ma·to·no·ma (stō′mă-tō-nō′mă). SYN noma. [stomato- + G. *nomē*, a spreading (sore)]

sto·ma·top·a·thy (stō-mă-top′ă-thē). Any disease of the oral cavity. SYN stomatosis. [stomato- + G. *pathos*, suffering]

sto·ma·to·plas·tic (stō′mă-tō-plas′tik). Relating to stomatoplasty.

sto·ma·to·plas·ty (stō′mă-tō-plas-tē). Plastic surgery of the mouth. [stomato- + G. *plastos*, formed]

sto·ma·tor·rha·gia (stō′mă-tō-rā′jē-ă). Bleeding from the gums or other part of the oral cavity. [stomato- + G. *rhēgnymi*, to burst forth]

sto·ma·to·scope (stō′mă-tō-skōp). An apparatus for illuminating the interior of the mouth to facilitate examination. [stomato- + G. *skopeō*, to view]

sto·ma·to·sis (stō-mă-tō′sis). SYN stomatopathy. [stomato- + G. *-osis*, condition]

sto·mi·on (stō′mē-on). The median point of the oral slit when the lips are closed.

sto·mo·ceph·a·lus (stō′mō-sef′ă-lŭs). Malformed individual with an undeveloped jaw and a snoutlike mouth; likely to be combined with an ethmocephalic type of cyclopia. [G. *stoma*, mouth, + *kephalē*, head]

sto·mo·de·al (stō′mō-dē′ăl). Relating to a stomodeum.

sto·mo·de·um (stō-mō-dē′ŭm). **1.** A midline ectodermal depression ventral to the embryonic brain and surrounded by the mandibular arch; when the buccopharyngeal membrane disappears it becomes continuous with the foregut and forms the mouth. SYN stomatodeum. **2.** The anterior portion of the insect alimentary canal, consisting of mouth, buccal cavity, pharynx, esophagus, crop (frequently a diverticulum), and the proventriculus. [Mod. L. fr. G. *stoma*, mouth, + *hodaios*, on the way, fr. *hodos*, a way]

Sto·mox·ys cal·ci·trans (stō-mok′sis kal′si-tranz). The stable fly, a species of biting fly, resembling in size and general appearance the common housefly, which is an annoying pest of humans and domestic animals worldwide and is implicated in the mechanical transmission of diseases such as trypanosomiasis, anthrax, and equine infectious anemia. It is especially important in the spread of surra by transmitting *Trypanosoma evansi*, and also serves as intermediate host for *Habronema*, and for the deer filaria, *Setaria cervi*. [Mod. L., fr. C. *stoma*, mouth, + *oxys*, sharp; L. pres. p. of *calcitro*, to kick, fr. *calx*, the heel]

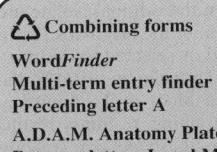**-stomy.** Artificial or surgical opening. SEE stomato-. [G. *stoma*, mouth]

stone (stōn). **1.** SYN calculus. **2.** An English unit of weight of the human body, equal to 14 pounds. [A.S. *stān*]

artificial s., a specially calcined gypsum derivative similar to plaster of Paris, but stronger, because the grains are nonporous.

bladder s.'s, urinary tract calculi that are symptomatic and may form in bladder. Throughout most of the history of humans, this was the predominant form of anuary stone disease, mentioned in the Hippocratic oath, and giving rise to the common ancient surgical procedure lithotomy. In much of the world, bladder s. disease has become uncommon and renal and ureteral s.'s (which are probably of different origins) have become more common. Bladder s.'s are now typically seen in patients with neurogenic bladders, urinary tract reconstruction, or infravesical obstruction. SYN bladder calculi.

philosopher's s., a s. sought by the alchemists of the Middle Ages which was supposedly able to transmute base metals into gold, to make precious s.'s, and to cure all ills, and thus confer longevity; it was also believed to be a universal solvent.

pulp s., SYN endolith.

skin s.'s, SYN *calcinosis* cutis.

tear s., SYN dacryolith.

vein s., SYN phlebolith.

Stookey, Byron, U.S. neurosurgeon, 1887–1966. SEE S.-Scarff *operation*; Queckenstedt-S. *test*.

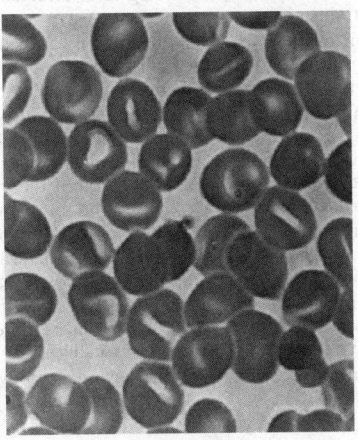

stomatocytosis

stool (stūl). **1.** A discharging of the bowels. **2.** The matter discharged at one movement of the bowels. SYN evacuation (2). SYN motion (3), movement (2). [A.S. *stōl*, seat]

butter s.'s, fatty s.'s, occurring especially in steatorrhea.

fatty s., a s. containing excessive amounts of fat.

rice-water s., a watery fluid containing whitish flocculi, discharged from the bowel in cholera and occasionally in other cases of serous diarrhea.

spinach s.'s, dark greenish porridge-like s.'s, resembling chopped spinach.

Trélat's s.'s, glairy s.'s streaked with blood, occurring in proctitis.

stops. Bends in, or wires soldered to, an archwire to limit passage through a bracket or tube.

stor·age (stōr′ij). The second stage in the memory process, following encoding and preceding retrieval, involving mental processes associated with retention of stimuli that have been registered and modified by encoding. SEE memory.

sto·rax (stōr′aks). A liquid balsam obtained from the wood and inner bark of *Liquidamber orientalis*, a tree of Asia Minor, or *L. styraciflua* (family Hamamelidaceae); has been used in the treatment of chronic inflammation of the mucous membranes, and externally for scabies. SYN styrax. [G. *styrax*, a sweet-smelling gum]

sto·ri·form (stōr′i-fōrm). Having a cartwheel pattern, as of spindle cells with elongated nuclei radiating from a center. [L. *storea*, woven mat, + *-formis*, form]

storm (stōrm). An exacerbation of symptoms or a crisis in the course of a disease.

thyroid s., SYN thyrotoxic *crisis*.

Stout's wir·ing. See under wiring.

STPD Symbol indicating that a gas volume has been expressed as if it were at standard temperature (0°C), standard pressure (760 mm Hg absolute), dry; under these conditions a mole of gas occupies 22.4 liters.

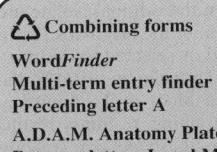**Combining forms**	**[NA] Nomina Anatomica**
Word*Finder* **Multi-term entry finder** **Preceding letter A**	**[MIM] Mendelian Inheritance in Man**
A.D.A.M. Anatomy Plates **Between letters L and M**	☆ **Official alternate term**
Appendices: **Following letter Z**	☆**[NA] Official alternate Nomina Anatomica term**
SYN Synonym; Cf., compare	**High Profile Term**

stra·bis·mal (stra-biz′măl). Relating to or affected with strabismus. SYN strabismic.

stra·bis·mol·o·gist (stra-biz-mol′ah-jist). A physician subspecializing in pediatric ophthalmology with an emphasis on the management of strabismus and amblyopia.

stra·bis·mom·e·ter (stra-biz-mom′ĕ-ter). An obsolete instrument having a plate with the upper margin curved, to conform with the lower lid, and marked in millimeters or fractions of an inch, used to measure the lateral deviation of the eye in strabismus. [G. *strabismos*, a squinting, + *metron*, measure]

stra·bis·mus (stra-biz′mŭs). A manifest lack of parallelism of the visual axes of the eyes. SYN crossed eyes, heterotropia, heterotropy, squint (1). [Mod. L., fr. G. *strabismos*, a squinting]

A-s., (1) s. in which esotropia is more marked in looking upward than downward; (2) s. in which exotropia is more marked on looking downward than upward. SYN A-pattern s.

accommodative s., s. in which the severity of deviation varies with accommodation.

alternate day s., SYN cyclic *esotropia*.

alternating s., a form of s. in which either eye fixes.

A-pattern s., SYN A-s.

comitant s., a condition in which the degree of s. is the same in all directions of gaze. SYN concomitant s.

concomitant s., SYN comitant s.

convergent s., SYN esotropia.

cyclic s., a s. that appears and disappears in rhythym, most frequently at 48-hour intervals.

s. deor′sum ver′gens, obsolete term for vertical s. in which the visual axis of one eye deviates downward.

divergent s., SYN exotropia.

external s., obsolete term for exotropia.

incomitant s., SYN paralytic s.

internal s., obsolete term for esotropia

kinetic s., s. due to spasm of an extraocular muscle.

manifest s., evident deviation of one eye or the other; may be alternating or monocular.

mechanical s., s. due to restriction of action of the ocular muscle within the orbit.

monocular s., obsolete term for s. in which one eye habitually deviates.

paralytic s., s. due to weakness of an ocular muscle or muscles. SYN incomitant s.

s. sur′sum ver′gens, an obsolete term for a vertical s. in which the visual axis of one eye deviates upward.

vertical s., a form of s. in which the visual axis of one eye deviates upward (s. sursum vergens) or downward (s. deorsum vergens).

X-s., s. in which exotropia is more marked when looking upward or downward than when looking straight ahead.

strab·o·tome (strab′ŏ-tōm). An obsolete instrument for use in a strabotomy.

stra·bot·o·my (stra-bot′ŏ-mē). Obsolete term for division of one or more of the ocular muscles or their tendons for the correction of squint. [G. *strabismos*, strabismus, + *tomē*, a cutting]

straight sem·i·nif·er·ous tu·bule. See under tubule.

strain (strān). 1. A population of homogeneous organisms possessing a set of defined characters; in bacteriology, the set of descendants that retains the characteristics of the ancestor; members of a s. that subsequently differ from the original isolate are regarded as belonging either to a substrain of the original s., or to a new s. 2. Specific host cell(s) designed or selected to optimize production of recombinant products. 3. To make an effort to the limit of one's strength. [L. *stringere*, to bind] 4. To injure by overuse or improper use. 5. An act of straining. 6. Injury resulting from s. or overuse. 7. The change in shape that a body undergoes when acted upon by an external force. 8. To filter; to percolate. [A.S. *stryand; streōnan*, to beget]

auxotrophic s.'s, s.'s which are derived from the prototrophic s. but which require extra growth factors.

carrier s., a bacterial s. that is contaminated with a bacteriophage of low infectivity. SYN pseudolysogenic s.

cell s., in tissue culture, cells derived from a single cell (clone) and possessing a specific feature such as a marker chromosome, antigen, or resistance to a virus.

congenic s., an inbred s. of animals produced by continued crossing of a gene of one line onto another inbred (isogenic) line.

HFR s., Hfr s., a s., or clone, in which a conjugative plasmid (such as an F′), integrated in the bacterial genome, is instrumental in the transfer (along with plasmid DNA) of integrated bacterial DNA in a sequential manner to a suitable recipient. [*high frequency of recombination*]

hypothetical mean s. (HMS), a hypothetical s. that possesses the characteristics of a calculated mean organism.

isogenic s., a s. of animals inbred for many generations and with high probability homozygous for certain specified genes.

lysogenic s., a s. of bacterium that is infected with a temporate bacteriophage. SEE lysogeny.

neotype s., a s. accepted by international agreement to replace a type s. which is no longer in existence or to serve as the type s. if a type s. was not designated and if no s. exists which can be designated as the type. SYN neotype culture.

prototrophic s.'s, s.'s that have the same nutritional requirements as the wild-type s.

pseudolysogenic s., SYN carrier s.

recombinant s., SEE recombinant (1).

stock s., a bacterial or other microbial s. that has been maintained under laboratory conditions as representative of its type.

type s., the nomenclatural type of a species or subspecies.

wild-type s., a s. found in nature or a standard s. SEE ALSO auxotrophic s.'s, prototrophic s.'s.

strains. Specific host cells designed or selected to optimize production of recombinant products.

strait (strāt). A narrow passageway. **inferior s.**, *apertura* pelvis superior; **superior s.**, *apertura* pelvis superior. [M.E. *streit* thr. O. Fr. fr. L. *strictus*, drawn together, tight]

strait·jack·et (strāt′jak-et). A garment-like device with long sleeves that can be secured to restrain a violently disturbed person. SYN camisole.

stra·mo·ni·um (stra-mō′nē-ŭm). The dried leaves and flowering or fruiting tops with branches of *Datura stramonium* or *D. tatula* (family Solanaceae), a herb abounding in temperate and subtropical countries; it contains an alkaloid, daturine, identical with hyoscyamine. It is an antispasmodic and has been used in the treatment of asthma and parkinsonism; when abused or taken inadvertently, it may cause an atropine-like toxic psychosis. [Mod. L.]

strand. In microbiology, a filamentous or threadlike structure.

anticoding s., the s. of duplex DNA which is used as a template for the synthesis of mRNA. SYN antisense s.

antiparallel s., a macromolecular s. that is oriented in the opposite direction of a neighboring s.

antisense s., SYN anticoding s.

coding s., the s. of duplex DNA that has the same sequence as the mRNA (except that mRNA contains ribonucleotides instead of deoxyribonucleotides). SYN sense s.

complementary s., SEE replicative *form.*

sense s., SYN coding s.

viral s., SEE replicative *form.*

Strandberg, James Victor., Swedish dermatologist, *1883. SEE Grönblad-S. *syndrome.*

stran·gal·es·the·sia (strang′gal-es-thē′zē-ă). SYN zonesthesia. [G. *strangalē*, halter, + *aisthēsis*, sensation]

stran·gle (strang′gl). To suffocate; to choke; to compress the trachea so as to prevent sufficient passage of air. [G. *strangaloō*, to choke, fr. *strangalē*, a halter]

stran·gles (strang′glz). An acute infectious bacterial disease in the horse, marked by mucopurulent nasal discharge and edematous and hemorrhagic nasal and pharyngeal respiratory passages with enlargement and suppuration of associated lymph nodes; it is caused by *Streptococcus equi* and affects chiefly horses under the age of five years.

stran·gu·lat·ed (strang′gyū-lā-ted). Constricted so as to prevent sufficient passage of air, as through the trachea, or to cut off venous return and/or arterial airflow, as in the case of a hernia. [L. *strangulo,* pp. *-atus,* to choke, fr. G. *strangaloō,* to choke (strangle)]

stran·gu·la·tion (strang'gyū-lā'shŭn). The act of strangulating or the condition of being strangulated, in any sense.

stran·gu·ry (strang'gyū-rē). Difficulty in micturition, the urine being passed drop by drop with pain and tenesmus. [G. *stranx* (*strang-*), something squeezed out, a drop, + *ouron,* urine]

strap. 1. A strip of adhesive plaster. **2.** To apply overlapping strips of adhesive plaster. [A.S. *stropp*]

Strassburg, Gustav A., German physiologist, *1848. SEE S.'s *test.*

Strassman, Paul F., German gynecologist, 1866–1938. SEE S.'s *phenomenon.*

stra·ta (strā'tă, strat'ă). Plural of stratum.

strat·i·fi·ca·tion (strat'i-fi-kā'shŭn). The process or result of separating a sample into subsamples according to specified criteria such as age or occupational groups. [L. *stratum,* layer, + *facio,* to make]

strat·i·fied (strat'i-fīd). Arranged in the form of layers or strata.

stra·tig·ra·phy (stra-tig'ră-fē). SYN tomography. [L. *stratum,* layer, + G. *graphē,* a writing]

STRATUM

stra·tum, gen. **stra·ti,** pl. **stra·ta** (strat'ŭm, tă; strā'tŭm; tī). One of the layers of differentiated tissue, the aggregate of which forms any given structure, such as the retina or the skin. SEE ALSO lamina, layer. [L. *sterno,* pp. *stratus,* to spread out, strew, ntr. of pp. as noun, *stratum,* a bed cover, layer]

s. aculea'tum, obsolete term for s. spinosum.

s. al'bum profun'dum, SYN deep gray *layer* of superior colliculus.

s. basa'le, (1) the outermost layer of the endometrium which undergoes only minimal changes during the menstrual cycle; SYN basal layer. **(2)** SYN s. basale epidermidis.

s. basa'le epider'midis, the deepest layer of the epidermis, composed of dividing stem cells and anchoring cells. SYN basal cell layer, columnar layer, germinative layer, palisade layer, s. basale (2), s. cylindricum, s. germinativum.

s. cerebra'le ret'inae, SYN cerebral *layer* of retina.

s. cine'reum collic'uli superio'ris, SYN gray *layer* of superior colliculus.

s. circula're membra'nae tym'pani, circular fibers deep to the radiate layer of the membrane that are more abundant near the periphery; not present in the pars flaccida. SYN circular layer of tympanic membrane.

s. circula're tu'nicae [NA], SYN circular *layer* of muscular coat.

s. circulare tunicae muscularis coli, circular layer of muscular coat of colon.

s. circulare tunicae muscularis gastricae [NA], SYN circular *layer* of muscular coat.

s. circula're tu'nicae muscula'ris intesti'ni ten'uis [NA], circular layer of muscular coat of small intestine.

s. circula're tu'nicae muscula'ris rec'ti [NA], circular layer of muscular coat of rectum.

s. circula're tu'nicae muscula'ris ventric'uli, circular layer of muscular coat of stomach.

s. compac'tum, the superficial layer of decidual tissue in the pregnant uterus, in which the interglandular tissue preponderates. SYN compacta.

s. cor'neum epider'midis, the outer layer of the epidermis, consisting of several layers of flat keratinized non-nucleated cells. SYN corneal layer of epidermis, horny layer of epidermis.

s. cor'neum un'guis, the outer, horny layer of the nail. SYN cornified layer of nail, horny layer of nail.

s. cuta'neum membra'nae tym'pani, the thin layer of skin on

the external surface of the tympanic membrane. SYN cutaneous layer of tympanic membrane.

s. cylin'dricum, SYN s. basale epidermidis.

s. disjunc'tum, the layer of partly detached cells on the free surface of the s. corneum, as seen in sections under the microscope; an artifact of fixation.

s. fibro'sum [NA], SYN fibrous articular *capsule,* fibrous *capsule.*

s. functiona'le, the endometrium except for the s. basale; formerly believed to be lost during menstruation but now considered to be only partially disrupted.

s. gangliona're ner'vi op'tici, SYN ganglionic *layer* of optic nerve.

s. gangliona're ret'inae, SYN ganglionic *layer* of retina.

s. ganglio'sum cerebel'li, SYN piriform neuron *layer.*

s. germinati'vum, SYN s. basale epidermidis.

s. germinati'vum un'guis, the deeper layer of the nail that is continuous with the s. germinativum of the surrounding skin and from which the nail plate is continuously formed. SYN germinative layer of nail.

s. granulo'sum cerebel'li [NA], SYN granular *layer* of cerebellum.

s. granulo'sum epider'midis [NA], SYN granular *layer* of epidermis.

s. granulo'sum follic'uli ova'rici vesiculo'si, the layer of small cells that forms the wall of an ovarian follicle. SYN granular layer of a vesicular ovarian follicle, granulosa, membrana granulosa, s. granulosum ovarii.

s. granulo'sum ova'rii, SYN s. granulosum folliculi ovarici vesiculosi.

s. gris'eum collic'uli superio'ris [NA], SYN gray *layer* of superior colliculus.

s. gris'eum me'dium, SEE gray *layer* of superior colliculus.

s. gris'eum profun'dum, SEE gray *layer* of superior colliculus.

s. gris'eum superficia'le, SEE gray *layer* of superior colliculus.

s. interoliva're lemnis'ci, the medial region of the medulla oblongata between the left and right olivary nucleus, traversed longitudinally by the left and right medial lemniscus, and transversely by the decussating olivocerebellar fibers.

s. lemnis'ci, a largely fibrous (hence whitish) layer of the superior colliculus separating the middle gray layer of superior colliculus from the deep gray layer of superior colliculus and containing, among others, fibers from the spinal and trigeminal lemnisci. SYN fillet layer.

s. longitudinale tunicae muscularis [NA], SYN longitudinal *layer* of muscular coat.

s. longitudina'le tu'nicae muscula'ris co'li [NA], longitudinal layer of the muscular tunic of the colon.

s. longitudinale tunicae muscularis gastricae [NA], SYN longitudinal *layer* of muscular coat.

s. longitudina'le tu'nicae muscula'ris intesti'ni ten'uis [NA], longitudinal layer of muscular coat of small intestine.

s. longitudina'le tu'nicae muscula'ris rec'ti [NA], longitudinal layer of muscular coat of rectum.

s. longitudina'le tu'nicae muscula'ris ventric'uli [NA], longitudinal layer of muscular coat of stomach.

s. lu'cidum, a layer of lightly staining corneocytes in the deepest level of the s. corneum; found primarily in the thick epidermis of the palmar and plantar skin. SYN clear layer of epidermis.

malpighian s., the living layer of the epidermis comprising the s. basale, s. spinosum, and s. granulosum. SYN malpighian layer, malpighian rete.

s. molecula're, SYN molecular *layer.*

s. molecula're cerebel'li [NA], SYN molecular *layer* of cerebellum.

s. molecula're ret'inae, SYN molecular *layer* of retina.

s. neuroepithelia'le ret'inae, SYN neuroepithelial *layer* of retina.

s. neurono'rum pirifor'mium [NA], SYN piriform neuron *layer.*

s. nuclea're exter'num et inter'num ret'inae, SYN nuclear *layers* of retina, under *layer.*

s. nuclea're exter'num ret'inae, SYN neuroepithelial *layer* of retina.

s. nuclea're inter'num ret'inae, SYN ganglionic *layer* of retina.

s. op'ticum, SYN optic *layer.*

s. papilla're cor'ii, the more superficial layer of the corium whose papillae interdigitate with the epidermis. SYN corpus papillare, papillary layer.

s. pigmen'ti bul'bi, SYN pigmented *layer* of retina.

s. pigmen'ti cor'poris cilia'ris, the continuation of the pigment layer of the retina onto the posterior aspect of the ciliary body. SYN pigmented layer of ciliary body.

s. pigmen'ti i'ridis, the double layer of pigmented epithelium on the posterior surface of the iris. SYN pigmented layer of iris.

s. pigmen'ti ret'inae, SYN pigmented *layer* of retina.

s. plexifor'me exter'num et inter'num ret'inae, SYN plexiform *layers* of retina, under *layer.*

s. radia'tum membra'nae tym'pani, the connective tissue layer of the tympanic membrane beneath the stratum cutaneum, the fibers of which radiate from the manubrium of the malleus to the peripheral fibrocartilaginous ring of the membrane; absent from the pars flaccida. SYN radiate layer of tympanic membrane.

s. reticula're co'rii, the thicker deep layer of the corium consisting of dense irregularly arranged connective tissue. SYN reticular layer of corium, s. reticulare cutis, tunica propria corii.

s. reticula're cu'tis, SYN s. reticulare corii.

s. spino'sum epider'midis, the layer of polyhedral cells in the epidermis; shrinkage artifacts and adhesion of these cells at their desmosomal junctions gives a spiny or prickly appearance. SYN prickle cell layer, spinous layer.

s. spongio'sum, the middle layer of the endometrium formed chiefly of dilated glandular structures; it is flanked by the compacta on the luminal side and the basalis on the myometrial side.

s. subcuta'neum, SYN superficial *fascia.*

s. synovia'le [NA], SYN synovial *membrane,* synovial *membrane.*

s. zona'le [NA], SYN zonular *layer.*

Straus, Isidore, French physician, 1845–1896. SEE S. *reaction;* S.'s *sign.*

Strauss, Lotte, U.S. pathologist, *1913. SEE Churg-S. *syndrome.*

Sträussler. SEE Gerstmann-Sträussler *syndrome.*

streak (strēk). A line, stria, or stripe, especially one that is indistinct or evanescent. [A.S. *strica*]

germinal s., SYN primitive s.

gonadal s., a form of aplasia in which the ovary is replaced by a functionless tissue, as found in Turner's syndrome. SYN streak gonad.

Knapp's s.'s, SYN *angioid* streaks.

meningitic s., a line of redness resulting from drawing a point across the skin, especially notable in cases of meningitis. SYN tache cérébrale, tache méningéale, Trousseau's spot.

Moore's lightning s.'s, photopsia manifested by vertical flashes of light, seen usually on the temporal side of the affected eye, caused by the involutional shrinkage of vitreous humor.

primitive s., an ectodermal ridge in the midline at the caudal end of the embryonic disk from which arises the intraembryonic mesoderm; achieved by inward and then lateral migration of cells; in human embryos, it appears on day 15 and gives a cephalocaudal axis to the developing embryo. SYN germinal s.

stream (strēm). SYN flumen.

hair s.'s, the curved lines along which the hairs are arranged on the head and various parts of the body, especially noticeable in the fetus. SYN flumina pilorum [NA].

stream·ing (strēm'ing). SEE streaming *movement.*

streb·lo·dac·ty·ly (streb-lō-dak'ti-lē). SYN camptodactyly. [G. *streblos,* twisted, + *daktylos,* finger]

Streeter, George L., U.S. embryologist, 1873–1948. SEE S.'s *bands,* under *band,* developmental horizon(s).

Streeter's developmental ho·ri·zon(s). A term borrowed from geology and archeology by Streeter to define 23 developmental stages in young human embryos, from fertilization through the first 2 months; each horizon spanned 2 to 3 days and emphasized specific anatomic characteristics, to avoid discrepan-

cies in the determination of age and body dimensions. [G.L. Streeter]

Streiff, Enrico Bernard, Swiss ophthalmologist, *1908.. SEE Hallermann-S. *syndrome;* Hallermann-S.-François *syndrome.*

strem·ma (strem'ă). SYN sprain. [G. a twist, fr. *strephō,* to twist]

strength. **1.** The quality of being strong or powerful. **2.** The degree of intensity. **3.** The property of materials by which they endure the application of force without yielding or breaking.

associative s., in psychology, the s. of a stimulus response linkage as measured by the frequency with which a stimulus elicits a particular response. SEE conditioning.

biting s., SYN *force* of mastication.

compressive s., tensile s., except that the stress is in compression.

fatigue s., the stress level below which a particular component will survive an indefinite number of load cycles (typically about 50% of the ultimate s. of the component).

ionic s. (I), symbolized as $\Gamma/2$ or I and set equal to $0.5\Sigma m_i z_i^2$, where m_i equals the molar concentration and z_i the charge of each ion present in solution; if molar concentrations (c_i) are used instead of molality (and the solution is dilute), then $I = 0.5(1/\rho_o)\Sigma c_i z_i^2$ where ρ_o is the density of the solvent; a number of biochemically important events (*e.g.*, protein solubility and rates of enzyme action) vary with the ionic s. of a solution.

tensile s., the maximum tensile stress or load that a material is capable of sustaining; usually expressed in pounds per square inch.

ultimate s., the maximum stress achieved prior to failure of a component on a single application of the load.

yield s., the amount of stress at which a permanent (plastic) deformation in a component becomes measurable (usually taken as 0.2% permanent strain).

streph·o·sym·bo·lia (stref'ō-sim-bō'lē-ă). **1.** Generally, the perception of objects reversed as if in a mirror. **2.** Specifically, difficulty in distinguishing written or printed letters that extend in opposite directions but are otherwise similar, such as *p* and *d,* or related kinds of mirror reversal. [G. *strephō,* to turn, + *symbolon,* a mark or sign]

stre·pi·tus (strep'i-tŭs). Rarely used term for a noise, usually an auscultatory sound. [L.]

strep·ti·ce·mia (strep-ti-sē'mē-ă). SYN streptococcemia.

strep·ti·dine (strep'ti-dēn). SYN streptomycin.

△**strepto-.** Curved or twisted (usually relating to organisms thus described). [G. *streptos,* twisted, fr. *strephō,* to twist]

Strep·to·ba·cil·lus (strep-tō-ba-sil'ŭs). A genus of nonmotile, nonsporeforming, aerobic to facultatively anaerobic bacteria (family Bacteroidaceae) containing Gram-negative, pleomorphic cells which vary from short rods to long, interwoven filaments which have a tendency to fragment into chains of bacillary and coccobacillary elements. These organisms are parasitic to pathogenic for rats, mice, and other mammals. The type species is *S. moniliformis.* [strepto- + bacillus]

S. monilifor'mis, a species commonly found as an inhabitant of the nasopharynx of rats; it occurs as the etiologic agent of an epizootic septic polyarthritis in mice and of one type of rat-bite fever; it is the type species of the genus *S.*

strep·to·bi·o·sa·mine (strep'tō-bī-ō'să-mēn). A methylamino disaccharide (streptose + *N*-methyl-L-glucosamine), with the oxygen link between C-2 of streptose and C-1 of the glucosamine; with streptidine, it forms streptomycin.

strep·to·bi·ose (strep-tō-bī'ōs). Old term for streptose.

strep·to·cer·ci·a·sis (strep'tō-ser-kī'ă-sis). Infection of man and higher primates with the nematode *Mansonella streptocerca.*

strep·to·coc·cal (strep'tō-kok'ăl). Relating to or caused by any organism of the genus *Streptococcus.*

strep·to·coc·ce·mia (strep'tō-kok-sē'-mē-ă). The presence of streptococci in the blood. SYN strepticemia, streptosepticemia. [streptococcus + G. *haima,* blood]

strep·to·coc·ci (strep'tō-kok'sī). Plural of streptococcus.

strep·to·coc·cic (strep'tō-kok'sik). Relating to or caused by any organism of the genus *Streptococcus.*

strep·to·coc·co·sis (strep'tō-kŏ-kō'sis). Any streptococcal infection.

Strep·to·coc·cus (strep-tō-kok'ŭs). A genus of nonmotile (with few exceptions), nonsporeforming, aerobic to facultatively anaerobic bacteria (family Lactobacillaceae) containing Gram-positive, spherical or ovoid cells which occur in pairs or short or long chains. Dextrorotatory lactic acid is the main product of carbohydrate fermentation. These organisms occur regularly in the mouth and intestines of humans and other animals, in dairy and other food products, and in fermenting plant juices. Some species are pathogenic. The type species is *S. pyogenes*. [strepto- + G. *kokkos*, berry (coccus)]

S. acidomin'imus, a species found in the bovine vagina and on the skin of calves.

S. agalac'tiae, a species found in the milk and tissues from udders of cows with mastitis; also reported to be associated with a variety of human infections, especially those of the urogenital tract.

S. angino'sus, a species found in the human throat, sinuses, abscesses, vagina, skin, and feces; this organism has been associated with glomerular nephritis and various types of mild respiratory diseases.

S. bo'vis, a species found in the bovine alimentary tract; this organism may also be found in blood and heart lesions in cases of subacute endocarditis.

S. dur'ans, a species found in dried milk powder and in the intestines of humans and other animals.

S. dysgalac'tiae, a species causing acute mastitis in cattle.

S. e'qui, a species causing strangles in horses.

S. equi'nus, a species that is the predominant organism in the intestines of horses.

S. equi subsp. *zooepidem'icus,* a species causing mastitis in cattle.

S. faeca'lis, a species found in human feces and in the intestines of many warm-blooded animals; occasionally found in urinary infections and in blood and heart lesions in cases of subacute endocarditis; associated with European foul brood of bees and with mild outbreaks of food poisoning.

S. lac'tis, a species found commonly as a contaminant in milk and dairy products; a common cause of the souring and coagulation of milk; some strains produce nisin, a powerful antibiotic that inhibits the growth of many other Gram-positive organisms.

S. mi'tis, a species found in the human mouth, throat, and nasopharynx; ordinarily, it is not considered to be pathogenic, but this organism may be recovered from ulcerated teeth and sinuses and from blood and heart lesions in cases of subacute endocarditis.

S. mu'tans, a species associated with the production of dental caries in humans and in some other animals and with subacute endocarditis.

S. pneumo'niae, a species of Gram-positive, lancet-shaped diplococci frequently occurring in chains; cells are readily lysed by bile salts. Virulent forms are enclosed in type-specific polysaccharide capsules, the basis for an effective vaccine. Normal inhabitants of the respiratory tract, and perhaps the most common cause of lobar pneumonia, they are relatively common causative agents of meningitis, sinusitis, and other infections. It is the type species of the genus *Diplococcus*. SYN Fraenkel's pneumococcus, Fraenkel-Weichselbaum pneumococcus, pneumococcus, pneumonococcus.

S. pyog'enes, a species found in the human mouth, throat, and respiratory tract and in inflammatory exudates, bloodstream, and lesions in human diseases; it is sometimes found in the udders of cows and in dust from sickrooms, hospital wards, schools, theaters, and other public places; it causes the formation of pus or even fatal septicemias. There is also a specific somatic antigen (M protein) for each of the approximately 85 types. It is the type species of the genus *S*.

S. saliva'rius, a species found in the human mouth, throat, and nasopharynx.

S. san'guis, a species originally found in the so-called vegetation on heart valves from cases of subacute bacterial endocarditis; occasionally found in infected sinuses and teeth and in house dust.

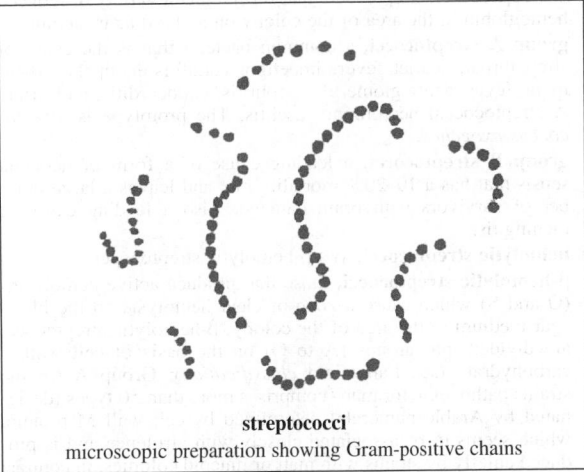

streptococci
microscopic preparation showing Gram-positive chains

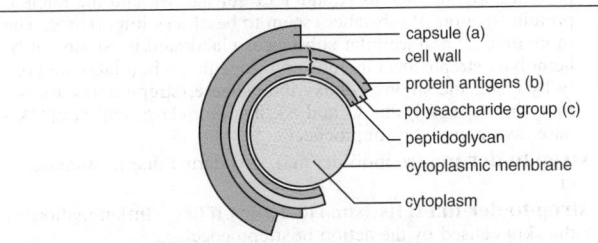

antigenic structure of *Streptococcus* cell
a) hyaluronic acid; b) protein antigens M, T, and R; c) group-specific polysaccharide group A streptococci contain rhamnose-*N*-acetyl-glucosamine)

Labels: capsule (a); cell wall; protein antigens (b); polysaccharide group (c); peptidoglycan; cytoplasmic membrane; cytoplasm

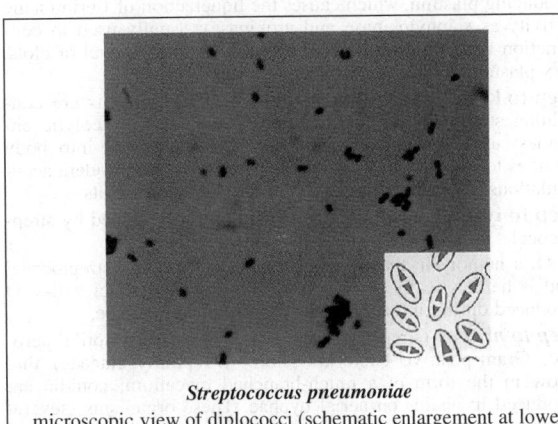

Streptococcus pneumoniae
microscopic view of diplococci (schematic enlargement at lower right)

S. u'beris, a species causing mastitis in cattle.

S. vir'idans, a name applied not to a distinct species but rather to the group of α-hemolytic streptococci as a whole; viridans streptococci have been isolated from the mouth and intestines of humans, the intestines of horses, the milk and feces of cows, milk and milk products, and the sputum and lungs in cases of primary atypical pneumonia.

S. zooepide'micus, former name for *S. equi* subsp. *zooepidemicus.*

strep·to·coc·cus, pl. **strep·to·coc·ci** (strep'tō-kok'ŭs, -kok'sī). A term used to refer to any member of the genus *Streptococcus*.

st

α-streptococci, streptococci that form a green variety of reduced hemoglobin in the area of the colony on a blood agar medium.

group A streptococci, a common bacteria that is the cause of strep throat, scarlet fever, impetigo, cellulitis-erysipelas, rheumatic fever, acute glomerular nephritis, endocarditis, and group A streptococcal necrotizing fasciitis. The prototype is *Streptococcus pyogenes.*

group B streptococci, a leading cause of a form of neonatal sepsis that has a 10–20% mortality rate and leaves a large number of survivors with brain damage. Also a leading cause of meningitis.

hemolytic streptococci, SYN β-hemolytic streptococci.

β-hemolytic streptococci, those that produce active hemolysins (O and S) which cause a zone of clear hemolysis on the blood agar medium in the area of the colony; β-hemolytic streptococci are divided into groups (A to O) on the basis of cell wall C carbohydrate (see Lancefield *classification*); Group A (in the strains pathogenic for man) comprises more than 50 types (designated by Arabic numerals) determined by cell wall M protein, which seems to be associated closely with virulence and is produced chiefly by strains with matt or mucoid colonies, in contrast to nonvirulent, glossy colony-producing strains; other surface protein antigens such as R and T (T substance) and the nucleoprotein fraction (P substance) seem to be of less importance. The more than 20 extracellular substances elaborated by strains of β-hemolytic streptococci include erythrogenic toxin (elaborated only by lysogenic strains), deoxyribonuclease (streptodornase), hemolysins (streptolysins O and S), hyaluronidase, and streptokinase. SYN hemolytic streptococci.

strep·to·der·ma (strep-tō-der′mă). Pyoderma due to streptococci.

strep·to·der·ma·ti·tis (strep′tō-der-mă-tī′tis). Inflammation of the skin caused by the action of streptococci.

strep·to·dor·nase (SD) (strep-tō-dōr′nās). A "dornase" (deoxyribonuclease) obtained from streptococci; used with streptokinase to facilitate drainage in septic surgical conditions.

strep·to·fu·ra·nose (strep-tō-fūr′ă-nōs). SYN streptose.

strep·to·ki·nase (SK) (strep-tō-kī′nās). An extracellular metalloenzyme from hemolytic streptococci that cleaves plasminogen, producing plasmin, which causes the liquefaction of fibrin (same activity as staphylokinase and urokinase); usually used in conjunction with streptodornase; thus, used in the removal of clots. SYN plasminokinase, streptococcal fibrinolysin.

strep·to·ki·nase-strep·to·dor·nase. A purified mixture containing streptokinase, streptodornase, and other proteolytic enzymes; used by topical application or by injection into body cavities to remove clotted blood and fibrinous and purulent accumulations of exudate; thus, used in the removal of clots.

strep·to·ly·sin (strep-tol′i-sin). A hemolysin produced by streptococci.

s. O, a hemolysin that is produced by β-hemolytic streptococci and is hemolytically active only in the reduced state; anti-s. O produced during infection is of diagnostic significance.

Strep·to·my·ces (strep-tō-mī′sēz). A genus of nonmotile, aerobic, Gram-positive bacteria (family Streptomycetaceae) that grow in the form of a much-branched mycelium; conidia are produced in chains on aerial hyphae. These organisms (several hundred species in the genus) are predominantly saprophytic soil forms; some are parasitic on plants or animals; many produce antibiotics. The type species is *S. albus.* [strepto- + G. *mykēs,* fungus]

S. al′bus, a species found in dust, soil, grains, and straw; some strains produce actinomycetin; others produce thiolutin or endomycin; it is the type species of the genus *S.*

S. gibso′nii, a species found in human infections. SYN *Nocardia gibsonii.*

S. somalien′sis, a species that causes Bouffardi's white mycetoma.

Strep·to·my·ce·ta·ce·ae (strep′tō-mī-sĕ-tā′sē-ē). A family of aerobic Gram-positive bacteria (order Actinomycetales) that produce a vegetative mycelium which does not fragment into bacillary or coccoid forms; they produce conidia which are borne on sporophores. These organisms occur primarily in the soil; some

are thermophiles found in rotting manure, a few are parasitic, and many produce antibiotics. The type genus is *Streptomyces.*

strep·to·my·cete (strep′tō-mī′sēt). A term used to refer to a member of the genus *Streptomyces;* it is sometimes improperly used to refer to any member of the family Streptomycetaceae.

strep·to·my·cin (strep-tō-mī′sin). An antibiotic agent obtained from *Streptomyces griseus* that is active against the tubercle bacillus and a large number of Gram-positive and Gram-negative bacteria; also used in the form of dihydrostreptomycin (aldehyde of s. reduced to CH_2OH). It is a glucoside and contains streptidine and streptobiosamine linked by an oxygen bridge between C-4 of the inositol residue and C-1 of the streptose residue; s. B has a mannose residue attached to the glucosamine and is a natural product, with less activity than s. A. It is used virtually exclusively in the treatment of tuberculosis; toxicity includes eighth cranial nerve damage leading to deafness and/or vestibular dysfunction. SYN streptidine, streptomycin A.

strep·to·my·cin A. SYN streptomycin.

strep·to·my·co·sis (strep′tō-mī-kō′sis). Old term for streptococcemia. [strepto- + G. *mykēs,* fungus, + -*osis,* condition]

strep·to·ni·vi·cin (strep′tō-ni-vī′sin). SYN novobiocin.

strep·tose (strep′tōs). 5-deoxy-3-*C*-formyl-L-lyxose; an unusual L-pentose that is a component of streptobiosamine, hence of streptomycin. SYN streptofuranose.

strep·to·sep·ti·ce·mia (strep′tō-sep-ti-sē′mē-ă). SYN streptococcemia.

strep·to·thri·cho·sis (strep′tō-thri-kō′sis). SYN dermatophilosis.

strep·to·tri·chi·a·sis (strep′tō-tri-kī′ă-sis). SYN dermatophilosis.

strep·to·tri·cho·sis (strep′tō-tri-kō′sis). SYN dermatophilosis.

strep·to·zo·cin (strep-tō-zō′sin). 2-Deoxy-2-(3-methyl-3-nitrosoureido)-D-glucopyranose; an antineoplastic agent used in the treatment of metastatic islet-cell carcinoma of the pancreas.

stress (stres). **1.** Reactions of the body to forces of a deleterious nature, infections, and various abnormal states that tend to disturb its normal physiologic equilibrium (homeostasis). **2.** In dentistry, the forces set up in teeth, their supporting structures, and structures restoring or replacing teeth as a result of the force of mastication. **3.** The force or pressure applied or exerted between portions of a body or bodies, generally expressed in pounds per square inch. **4.** In rheology, the force in a material transmitted per unit area to adjacent layers. **5.** In psychology, a physical or psychological stimulus such as very high heat, public criticism, or another noxious agent or experience which, when impinging upon an individual, produces psychological strain or disequilibrium. [L. *strictus,* tight, fr. *stringo,* to draw together]

life s., events or experiences that produce severe strain, *e.g.,* failure on the job, marital separation, loss of a love object.

shear s., the force acting in shear flow expressed per unit area; units in the CGS system: dynes/cm².

tensile s., a s. acting on a body per unit cross-sectional area so as to elongate the body.

yield s., the critical s. that must be applied to a material before it begins to flow, as in a Bingham plastic.

stress break·er. A device that relieves the abutment teeth, to which a fixed or removable partial denture is attached, of all or part of the forces generated by occlusal function.

stress ris·er. A mechanical defect, such as a hole, in bone or other materials that concentrates stress in the area.

stress shield·ing. Osteopenia occurring in bone as the result of removal of normal stress from the bone by an implant.

stretch·er. A litter, usually a sheet of canvas stretched to a frame with four handles, used for transporting the sick or injured. [A.S. *streccan,* to stretch]

stri·a, gen. and pl. **stri·ae** (strī′ă, strī′ē). **1.** A stripe, band, streak, or line, distinguished by color, texture, depression, or elevation from the tissue in which it is found. SYN striation (1). **2.** SYN striae cutis distensae. [L. channel, furrow]

acoustic striae, SYN medullary striae of fourth ventricle.

stri′ae atroph′icae, SYN striae cutis distensae.

auditory striae, SYN medullary striae of fourth ventricle.

brown striae, SYN Retzius' striae.

stri′ae cilia′res, shallow radial grooves on the surface of the orbiculus ciliaris extending from the teeth of the ora serrata and leading into the valleys between the ciliary processes.

stri′ae cu′tis disten′sae, bands of thin wrinkled skin, initially red but becoming purple and white, which occur commonly on the abdomen, buttocks, and thighs at puberty and/or during and following pregnancy, and result from atrophy of the dermis and overextension of the skin; also associated with ascites and Cushing's syndrome. SYN atrophoderma striatum, lineae albicantes, lineae atrophicae, linear atrophy, stretch marks, stria (2), striae atrophicae, striate atrophy of skin, traction atrophy, vergeture.

diagonalis s., SEE Broca's diagonal *band.*

s. for′nicis, SYN medullary s. of thalamus.

Gennari's s., SYN *line* of Gennari.

stri′ae gravida′rum, striae cutis distensae related to pregnancy.

Knapp's striae, SYN *angioid* streaks.

stri′ae lanci′si, the lateral longitudinal s. and the medial longitudinal s.

Langhans' s., fibrinoid that accumulates on the chorionic plate between the bases of placental villi during the first half of pregnancy.

lateral longitudinal s., a thin longitudinal band of nerve fibers accompanied by gray matter, near each outer edge of the upper surface of the corpus callosum under cover of the cingulate gyrus. SYN s. longitudinalis lateralis [NA], s. tecta, tectal s.

s. longitudina′lis latera′lis [NA], SYN lateral longitudinal s.

s. longitudina′lis media′lis [NA], SYN medial longitudinal s.

s. mallea′ris [NA], a bright line seen through the membrana tympani, produced by the attachment of the manubrium of the malleus. SYN mallear stripe.

medial longitudinal s., a thin longitudinal band of nerve fibers accompanied by gray matter, running along the surface of the corpus callosum on either side of the median line. Together with the lateral longitudinal s. it forms part of a thin layer of gray matter on the dorsal surface of the corpus callosum, the indusium griseum, a rudimentary component of the hippocampus. SYN s. longitudinalis medialis [NA].

stri′ae medulla′res ventric′uli quar′ti [NA], SYN medullary striae of fourth ventricle.

s. medulla′ris thal′ami [NA], SYN medullary s. of thalamus.

medullary striae of fourth ventricle, slender fascicles of fibers extending transversally below the ependymal floor of the ventricle from the median sulcus to enter the inferior cerebellar peduncle. They arise from the arcuate nuclei on the ventral surface of the medullary pyramid. SYN striae medullares ventriculi quarti [NA], acoustic striae, auditory striae, Bergmann's cords, medullary teniae, teniae acusticae.

medullary s. of thalamus, a narrow, compact fiber bundle that extends along the line of attachment of the roof of the third ventricle to the thalamus on each side and terminates posteriorly in the habenular nucleus. It is composed of fibers originating in the septal area, the anterior perforated substance, the lateral preoptic nucleus, and the medial segment of the globus pallidus. SYN s. medullaris thalami [NA], s. fornicis, s. ventriculi tertii.

s. na′si transver′sa, a single deep horizontal groove at the level of the alae, with no associated defects. SYN transverse nasal groove.

Nitabuch's s., SYN Nitabuch's *membrane.*

stri′ae olfacto′riae [NA], SYN olfactory striae.

olfactory striae, three distinct fiber bands (s. medialis, s. intermedia, s. lateralis) that caudally extend the olfactory tract beyond its attachment to the olfactory trigone. The medial s. curves dorsally into the tenia tecta; the intermediate, often barely visible, extends straight back and terminates in the olfactory tubercle; the lateral olfactory s., the largest of the three, passes along the lateral side of the olfactory tubercle, curving laterally as far as the limen insulae, then sharply medially to reach the uncus of the parahippocampal gyrus where it terminates in the plexiform layer of the olfactory cortex. SEE ALSO medial longitudinal s. SYN striae olfactoriae [NA], olfactory roots.

stri′ae paral′lelae, SYN Retzius' striae.

striae ret′inae, concentric lines on the surface of an abnormal retina.

striae retinae, SYN Paton's *lines,* under *line.*

Retzius' striae, dark concentric lines crossing the enamel prisms of the teeth, seen in axial cross sections of the enamel. SYN brown striae, striae parallelae.

Rohr's s., layer of fibrinoid in the intervillous spaces of the placenta.

s. spino′sa, a faint groove occasionally caused by the chorda tympani nerve on the spine of the sphenoid. SYN Lucas' groove, sulcus spinosus.

s. tec′ta, SYN lateral longitudinal s.

tectal s., SYN lateral longitudinal s.

terminal s., a slender, compact fiber bundle that connects the amygdala (amygdaloid body) with the hypothalamus and other basal forebrain regions. Originating from the amygdala, the bundle passes first caudalward in the roof of the temporal horn of the lateral ventricle; it follows the medial side of the caudate nucleus forward in the floor of the ventricle's central part (or body) until it reaches the interventricular foramen, in the posterior wall of which it curves steeply down to enter the hypothalamus, with fibers passing both rostral and caudal to the anterior commissure. Coursing caudalward in the medial part of the hypothalamus, the bundle terminates in the anterior and ventromedial hypothalamic nuclei. SYN s. terminalis [NA], Foville's fasciculus, Tarin's tenia, tenia semicircularis.

s. termina′lis [NA], SYN terminal s.

s. vascularis of cochlea, the stratified epithelium lining the upper part of the ligamentum spirale cochleae; it is penetrated by capillaries and is believed to be the site of production of endolymph. SYN s. vascularis ductus cochlearis [NA], psalterial cord, vascular stripe.

s. vascula′ris duc′tus cochlea′ris [NA], SYN s. vascularis of cochlea.

s. ventric′uli ter′tii, SYN medullary s. of thalamus.

Wickham's striae, fine whitish lines, having a network arrangement, on the surface of lichen planus papules.

striae of Zahn, SYN *lines* of Zahn, under *line.*

stri·a·tal (strī′ā-tăl). Relating to the corpus striatum.

stri·ate (strī′āt). Striped; marked by striae. [L. *striatus,* furrowed]

stri·a·tion (strī-ā′shŭn). **1.** SYN stria (1). **2.** A striate appearance. **3.** The act of streaking or making striae.

basal s.'s, the vertical infranuclear s.'s due to the infolded plasma membrane and mitochondria; they are seen in kidney tubules and certain intralobular salivary ducts.

tabby cat s.'s, SYN tigroid s.

tigroid s., linear whitish or yellowish markings on the fatty degenerated heart muscle. SYN tabby cat s.

stri·a·to·ni·gral (strī-ā-tō-nī′grăl). Referring to the efferent connection of the striatum with the *substantia* nigra.

stri·a·tum (strī-ā′tŭm). Collective name for the caudate nucleus and putamen which together with the globus pallidus or pallidum form the striate body. [L. neut. of *striatus,* furrowed]

stric·ture (strik′chūr). A circumscribed narrowing or stenosis of a hollow structure, usually consisting of cicatricial contracture or deposition of abnormal tissue. [L. *strictura,* fr. *stringo,* pp. *strictus,* to draw tight, bind]

anastomotic s., narrowing, usually by scarring, of an anastomotic suture line.

annular s., a ringlike constriction encircling the wall of a canal.

bridle s., narrowing of a canal by a band of tissue stretching across part of its lumen.

contractile s., SYN recurrent s.

functional s., SYN spasmodic s.

Hunner's s., bladder s. produced by interstitial cystitis (Hunner's ulcer).

organic s., a s. due to the presence of cicatricial or other new tissue, not spasmodic. SYN permanent s.

permanent s., SYN organic s.

recurrent s., a s. due to the presence of contractile tissue which may be dilated but soon returns. SYN contractile s.

spasmodic s., a s. due to localized spasm of muscular fibers in the wall of the canal. SYN functional s., temporary s.

st

temporary s., SYN spasmodic s.

urethral s., a stenosing lesion of the urethra, due usually to inflammation or to iatrogenic instrumentation and resulting in reduction of urethral caliber which may be focal or may involve virtually the entire length of the urethra.

stric·tur·o·plas·ty (strik′chur-plas′tē). Surgical procedure for widening a structured segment of intestine that involves incision and closure in opposing directions. [stricture + G. *plastos*, formed]

stric·tur·o·tome (strik′chūr-ō-tōm). A stricture knife; an instrument for use in dividing a stricture.

stric·tur·ot·o·my (strik-chūr-ot′ō-mē). Surgical opening or division of a stricture. [stricture + G. *tomē*, incision]

stri·dent (strī′dent). Creaking; grating; harsh-sounding; denoting an auscultatory sound or rale. [L. *stridens*, pres. p. of *strideo*, to creak]

stri·dor (strī′dōr). A high-pitched, noisy respiration, like the blowing of the wind; a sign of respiratory obstruction, especially in the trachea or larynx. [L. a harsh, creaking sound]

congenital s., crowing inspiration occurring at birth or within the first few months of life; sometimes without apparent cause and sometimes due to abnormal flaccidity of epiglottis or arytenoids. SYN laryngeal s.

s. den′tium, grinding of the teeth.

expiratory s., a singing sound due to the semi-approximated vocal folds offering resistance to the escape of air.

inspiratory s., a crowing sound during the inspiratory phase of respiration due to pathology involving the epiglottis or larynx.

laryngeal s., SYN congenital s.

s. serrat′icus, a rough grating like the sound of a saw.

strid·u·lous (strid′yū-lŭs). Having a shrill or creaking sound. [L. *stridulus*, fr. *strideo*, to creak, to hiss]

string. A slender cord or cordlike structure.

auditory s.'s, bundles of parallel filaments in the zona pectinata of the lamina basilaris of the cochlea; the length of the s.'s varies from 64 μm in the basal coil to 480 μm in the apex.

string·halt (string′halt). Myoclonic affliction of one or both hindlimbs in the horse seen as spasmodic overflexion of the joints.

strip. 1. To express the contents from a collapsible tube or canal, such as the urethra, by running the finger along it. SYN milk (4). **2.** Subcutaneous excision of a vein in its longitudinal axis, performed with a stripper. **3.** Any narrow piece, relatively long and of uniform width. [A.S. *strypan*, to rob]

abrasive s., a ribbon-like piece of linen on one side of which is bonded abrasive particles; used in dentistry for contouring and polishing proximal surfaces of restorations.

amalgam s., a linen s. without abrasive used to smooth proximal contours of newly placed amalgam restorations.

celluloid s., a clear plastic s. used as a matrix when inserting a silicate cement or acrylic resin cement in proximal cavity preparations of anterior teeth.

lightning s., a s. of metal with abrasive on one side, used to open rough or improper contacts of proximal restorations.

stripe (strīp). **1.** In anatomy, a streak, line, band, or stria. **2.** In radiography, a linear opacity differing in density from the adjacent parts of the image; usually represents the tangential image of a planar structure such as the pleura or peritoneum. SEE ALSO psoas *margin*. [M.E.]

s. of Gennari, SYN *line* of Gennari.

Hensen's s., a band on the undersurface of the membrana tectoria of the cochlear duct.

mallear s., SYN *stria mallearis*.

Mees' s.'s, SYN Mees' *lines*, under *line*.

pleural s., on a chest radiograph, the soft tissue s. between the opacity of the aerated lung and that of the cortex of the rib.

tracheal wall s., on a chest radiograph, the linear opacity between air in the trachea and in the right upper lobe.

vascular s., SYN *stria vascularis* of cochlea.

Strisower. SEE Schellong-Strisower *phenomenon*.

stro·bi·la, pl. **stro·bi·lae** (strō′bi-lă, -lē). A chain of segments, less the scolex and unsegmented neck portion, of a tapeworm; in the monozoic tapeworms (subclass Cestodaria and some members of the subclass Cestoda), it may consist of a single proglottid. [G. *stobile*, a twist of lint]

strob·i·lo·cer·cus (strō′bi-lō-ser′kŭs). A taenioid tapeworm larva of the cysticercus type, but with a conspicuous segmented neck, small terminal bladder, and everted scolex; the larval form of *Taenia taeniaeformis*, called *Cysticercus fasciolaris*. [G. *strobile*, a twist of lint, + *kerkos*, tail]

strob·i·loid (strō′bi-loyd). Resembling a chain of segments of a tapeworm. [G. *strobile*, strobile, + *eidos*, resemblance]

stro·bo·scope (strō′bō-skōp). An electronic instrument that produces intermittent light flashes of controlled frequency; used to influence electrical activity of the cerebral cortex.

stro·bo·scop·ic (strō-bō-skop′ik). Pertaining to the illusion of motion, retarded or accelerated, produced by visual images observed intermittently in rapid succession. [G. *strobos*, a twisting around, fr. *strephō*, to twist, + *skopeō*, to view]

Stroganoff, Vasili V., Russian obstetrician, 1857–1938. SEE S.'s *method*.

stroke (strōk). **1.** Term denoting the sudden development of focal neurological deficits usually related to impaired cerebral blood; more appropriate terms indicate the nature of the disturbance; *e.g.,* thrombosis, hemorrhage, or embolism. **2.** A pulsation. **3.** To pass the hand or any instrument gently over a surface. SEE ALSO stroking. **4.** A gliding movement over a surface. [A.S. *strāc*]

heart s., (1) impact of the apex of the heart against the wall of the chest; (2) SYN *angina* pectoris.

heat s., SEE heatstroke.

spinal s., abrupt onset of focal spinal cord dysfunction caused by a disturbance in its blood supply.

sun s., SEE sunstroke.

strok·ing (strōk′ing). The nonverbal fondling and nurturance accorded infants or the nonverbal and verbal forms of acceptance, reassurance, and positive reinforcement accorded to children and adults either by an individual to himself or herself or to another person in order to satisfy a basic biopsychological need of all developing humans; various psychopathological conditions are believed to result when such s. is absent or faulty.

stro·ma, pl. **stro·ma·ta** (strō′mă, strō′mă-tă) [NA]. **1.** The framework, usually of connective tissue, of an organ, gland, or other structure, as distinguished from the parenchyma or specific substance of the part. **2.** Aqueous phase of chloroplasts; *i.e.,* chloroplast matrix. **3.** Archaic term for mitochondrial matrix. [G. *strōma*, bed]

s. glan′dulae thyroi′deae [NA], SYN s. of thyroid gland.

s. i′ridis [NA], SYN s. of iris.

s. of iris, the delicate vascular connective tissue that lies between the anterior surface of the iris and the pars iridica retinae. SYN s. iridis [NA].

lymphatic s., the network of reticular fibers and associated reticular cells of lymphatic tissue.

nerve s., the connective tissue supporting structures of peripheral nerve fibers, consisting of endoneurium, perineurium, and epineurium.

s. ova′rii [NA], SYN s. of ovary.

s. of ovary, the fibrous tissue of the medulla of the ovary. SYN s. ovarii [NA].

Rollet's s., the colorless s. of the red blood cells.

s. of thyroid gland, the connective tissue that supports the lobules and follicles of the thyroid gland. SYN s. glandulae thyroideae [NA].

s. of vitreous, the delicate framework of the vitreous body embedded in or enclosing the vitrous humor. SYN s. vitreum [NA].

s. vit′reum [NA], SYN s. of vitreous.

stro·mal (strō′măl). Stromatic; relating to the stroma of an organ or other structure. SYN stromic.

stro·ma·tin (strō′mă-tin). An insoluble protein in the stroma of erythrocytes.

stro·ma·tol·y·sis (strō-mă-tol′i-sis). Destruction of the enveloping membrane of a cell, such as a red blood cell. [stroma + G. *lysis*, dissolution]

stro·ma·to·sis (strō-mă-tō'sis). SYN endometrial stromal *sarcoma*.

stro·muhr (strōm'ūr). An instrument for measuring the quantity of blood that flows per unit of time through a blood vessel. [Ger. *Strom*, stream, + *Uhr*, clock]

Ludwig's s., one of the first devices for measuring flow in blood vessels.

thermo-s., SEE thermostromuhr.

Strong, Edward K., Jr., U.S. psychologist, *1884. SEE S. vocational interest *test*.

strong. SEE Jewett and Strong *staging*.

stron·gyle (stron'jil). Common name for members of the family Strongylidae. [G. *strongylos*, round]

Stron·gyl·i·dae (stron-jil'i-dē). A family of parasitic nematode worms (order Strongyloidea) including the genera *Strongylus* and *Oesophagostomum*. [see *Strongyloides*]

Stron·gy·loi·dea (stron-ji-loy'dē-ă). A superfamily of strongyle nematode parasites including the genera *Ancyclostoma*, *Necator*, *Ostertagia*, *Haemonchus*, and *Strongylus*, as well as the gapeworms of fowl, the lungworms of carnivores, and some of the most important helminth pathogens of man and domestic animals. [see *Strongyloides*]

Stron·gy·loi·des (stron-ji-loy'dēz). The threadworm, a genus of small nematode parasites (superfamily Rhabditoidea), commonly found in the small intestine of mammals (particularly ruminants), that are characterized by an unusual life cycle that involves one or several generations of free-living adult worms. Human infection is chiefly by *S. stercoralis*, the small roundworm of man, widespread in all tropical regions, or by *S. fuelleborni*, a parasite of non-human primates in African and Asian tropics and of humans in African tropics. The subspecies *S. F. kellyi* occurs in New Guinea where it causes widespread infection. Fatal infection in 2-month-old infants, possibly infected by transmammary transmission, produces the condition known locally as swollen belly disease or swollen belly syndrome, which causes grossly distended abdomens, invariably fatal in these infants. Other species include *S. papillosus* in cattle, sheep, and goats, and *S. ransomi* in swine. [G. *strongylos*, round, + *eidos*, resemblance]

stron·gy·loi·di·a·sis (stron'ji-loy-dī'ă-sis). Infection with soil-borne nematodes of the genus *Strongyloides*, considered to be a parthenogenetic parasitic female. Larvae passed to the soil develop through 4 larval instars to form free-living adults or develop from first and second free-living stages into infective third stage strongyliform or filariform larvae, which penetrate the skin or enter the buccal mucosa via drinking water. Infection can occur by larvae of a new generation developed in the soil (indirect cycle), by infective larvae developed without an intervening adult stage (direct cycle), or by larvae that develop directly in the feces within the intestine of the host, penetrate the mucosa, and pass by blood-lung migration back to the intestine (autoreinfection); most serious human infections and nearly all fatalities result from autoreinfection, which commonly follow immunosuppression by steroids, ACTH, or other immunosuppressive agents. Autoreinfection also may develop in patients with AIDS. SYN strongyloidosis.

stron·gy·lo·sis (stron-ji-lō'sis). Disease caused by infection with a species of the nematode *Strongylus*; effects may be extreme from worm-caused lesions, nodules, and aneurysms.

Stron·gy·lus (stron'ji-lŭs). The palisade worm, a genus of large strongyle nematodes (subfamily Strongylinae, family Strongylidae) parasitic in horses and other equids, and the cause of strongylosis. [G. *strongylos*, round]

S. asi'ni, a species that occurs in the large intestine of the ass and other wild equids.

S. edenta'tus, a bloodsucking species occurring in the cecum and colon of the horse, ass, mule, and zebra.

S. equi'nus, a cosmopolitan bloodsucking species found in the cecum and (rarely) colon of horses and other equids.

S. radia'tus, SYN *Cooperia oncophora*.

S. ventrico'sus, SYN *Cooperia oncophora*.

S. vulga'ris, a bloodsucking species found chiefly in the cecum

of horses and other equids; in the course of their migration, larvae commonly lodge in the wall of the posterior aorta, causing wall damage and the development of verminous aneurysms in this vessel, especially in the anterior mesenteric arteries.

stron·ti·um (Sr) (stron'shē-ŭm). A metallic element, atomic no. 38, atomic wt. 87.62; one of the alkaline earth series and similar to calcium in chemical and biological properties. Various salts of s. are used therapeutically for their anions; *e.g.,* s. bromide, iodide, lactate. [*Strontian*, a town in Scotland]

stron·ti·um-85 (^{85}Sr). A radioactive strontium isotope with a half-life of 64.84 days; used in bone imaging.

stron·ti·um-87m (^{87m}Sr). A radioactive strontium isotope with a half-life of 2.80 hours; used in bone imaging.

stron·ti·um-89 (^{89}Sr). A radioactive strontium isotope; a beta emitter with half-life of 50.52 days; used as a tracer in studies of strontium absorption by the body, strontium incorporation in bone, etc.

stron·ti·um-90 (^{90}Sr). A radioactive strontium isotope; a beta emitter with half-life of 29.1 years; a major component (about 5%) of the uranium fission products; it is incorporated into bone tissue where turnover is slow; used in the therapy of certain eye conditions (*e.g.,* pterygia, traumatic corneal ulceration, etc.).

stro·phan·thin (strō-fan'thin). K-strophanthin; a glycoside or mixture of glycosides from *Strophanthus kombé;* a cardiac tonic, like ouabain (G-s.); extremely toxic.

Stro·phan·thus (strō-fan'thŭs). A genus of vines of east Africa (family Apocynaceae); the dried ripe seeds of *S. kombé* or *S. hispidus* contain the cardiac glycoside strophanthin, and were used as an arrow poison; the seeds of *S. gratus* are the botanical source of ouabain. [G. *strophos*, a twisted cord, + *anthos*, flower]

stroph·o·ceph·a·ly (strof-ō-sef'ă-lē). Condition characterized by a congenitally distorted head and face, in which there is a tendency toward cyclopia and malformation of the oral region. [G. *strophē*, a twist, + *kephalē*, head]

stroph·o·so·mia (strof-ō-sō'mē-ă). Severe form of a congenital ventral fissure, extremely rare in humans. [G. *strophē*, a twist, + *sōma*, body]

stroph·u·lus (strof'yū-lŭs). SYN *miliaria* rubra. [Mod. L. dim. of G. *strophus*, colic]

s. can'didus, a form of s. in which the papules are colorless and shining.

s. intertinc'tus, a form of s. marked by an eruption of itching papules. SYN s. pruriginosus.

s. prurigino'sus, SYN s. intertinctus.

Stroud, Bert B., 19th century U.S. physiologist, anatomist, and zoologist. SEE S.'s pectinated *area*.

struck (strŭk). A bacterial disease of adult sheep in Britain caused by *Clostridium perfringens* type C.

struc·tur·al (strŭk'chūr-ăl). Relating to the structure of a part; having a structure. SYN anatomical (2).

struc·tur·al·ism (strŭk'chūr-ăl-izm.). A branch of psychology interested in the basic structure and elements of consciousness.

struc·ture (strŭk'chūr). **1.** The arrangement of the details of a part; the manner of formation of a part. **2.** A tissue or formation made up of different but related parts. **3.** In chemistry, the specific connections of the atoms in a given molecule. [L. *structura*, fr. *struo*, pp. *structus*, to build]

brush heap s., haphazard interlocking of fibrils in a gel or hydrocolloid impression material.

chi s., a joint between two DNA duplex molecules. SEE ALSO chi *sequence*.

cointegrate s., a s. of DNA produced by the fusion of two replicons, one possessing a transposon.

complementary s.'s, s.'s that define one another; *e.g.,* the two strands of duplex DNA.

crystal s., the arrangement in space and the interatomic distances and angles of the atoms in crystals, usually determined by x-ray diffraction measurements.

denture-supporting s.'s, the tissues, teeth, and/or residual ridges, which serve as the foundation for removable partial or complete dentures.

fine s., SYN ultrastructure.

st

gel s., brush heap s. of fibrils giving firmness to hydrocolloids.

Holliday s., SYN Holliday *junction.*

primary s., in a macromolecule, the sequence of sub-units that make up that macromolecule; *e.g.,* the amino acid sequence of a protein.

quaternary s., the three-dimensional arrangement and constitution of a multimeric (*i.e.,* a substance containing more than one biopolymer) macromolecule; *e.g.,* the $\alpha_2\beta_2$ tetramer of hemoglobin A.

secondary s., the localized arrangement in space of regions of a biopolymer; often these types of s.'s are regular and recurring along one dimension; *e.g.,* the α-helix often found in proteins.

tertiary s., the three-dimensional configuration of a biopolymer.

tuboreticular s., tubules 20–30 nm in length that lie within cisterns of smooth endoplasmic reticulum; observed in connective tissue diseases such as SLE, and in various cancers and virus infections.

stru·ma, pl. **stru·mae** (strū′mă, -mē). **1.** SYN goiter. **2.** Formerly, any enlargement of a tissue. [L. a scrofulous tumor, fr. *struo,* to pile up, build]

s. aberra′ta, SYN aberrant *goiter.*

s. colloi′des, SYN colloid *goiter.*

Hashimoto's s., SYN Hashimoto's *thyroiditis.*

ligneous s., SYN Riedel's *thyroiditis.*

s. lymphomato′sa, SYN Hashimoto's *thyroiditis.*

s. malig′na, obsolete term for cancer of the thyroid gland.

s. medicamento′sa, goiter due to the use of some therapeutic agent.

s. ova′rii, a rare ovarian tumor, regarded as teratomatous, in which thyroid tissue has surpassed the other elements; occasionally associated with hyperthyroidism.

Riedel's s., SYN Riedel's *thyroiditis.*

stru·mec·to·my (strū-mek′tō-mē). Surgical removal of all or a portion of a goitrous tumor. [struma + G. *ektomē,* excision]

median s., removal of a median goiter or an enlarged isthmus of the thyroid gland.

stru·mi·form (strū′mi-fōrm). Resembling a goiter. [struma + L. *forma,* form]

stru·mi·tis (strū-mī′tis). Inflammation, with swelling, of the thyroid gland. SEE ALSO thyroiditis. [struma + G. *-itis,* inflammation]

stru·mous (strū′mŭs). Denoting or characteristic of a struma.

Strümpell, Ernst Adolf von, German physician, 1853–1925. SEE S.'s *disease, phenomenon, reflex;* Fleischer-Strumpell *ring;* S.-Marie *disease;* Marie-S. *disease;* S.-Westphal *disease;* Westphal-S. *pseudosclerosis.*

stru·vite (strū′vīt). MgNH₄PO₄·6H₂; a; the hexahydrate of magnesium ammonium phosphate; found in some renal calculi. Cf. bobierrite, newberyite. [H. C. G. von *Struve,* Russian diplomat + -ite 4]

strych·nine (strik′nin, -nēn, -nīn). +L $C_{21}H_{22}N_2O_2$; an alkaloid from *Strychnos nux-vomica;* colorless crystals of intensely bitter taste, nearly insoluble in water. It stimulates all parts of the central nervous system, and was used as a stomachic, an antidote for depressant poisons, and in the treatment of myocarditis. S. blocks the inhibitory neurotransmitter, glycine, and thus can cause convulsions. The formerly used salts of s. are s. hydrochloride, s. phosphate, and s. sulfate. It is a potent chemical capable of producing acute or chronic poisoning of humans or animals.

strych·nin·ism (strik′nin-izm). Chronic strychnine poisoning, the symptoms being those that arise from central nervous system stimulation; the first signs are tremors and twitching, progressing to severe convulsions and respiratory arrest.

Strych·nos (strik′nos). A genus of tropical shrubs or trees (family Loganiaceae); most South American species contain chiefly quaternary neuromuscular blocking alkaloids, *e.g.,* curare; the African, Asiatic, and Australian species contain tertiary strychnine-like alkaloids (*e.g.,* strychnine, brucine, and yohimbine-type alkaloids). [G. nightshade]

Stryker, Garold V., U.S. pathologist, *1896. SEE S.-Halbeisen *syndrome.*

Stryker, Homer H., U.S. orthopedic surgeon. SEE S. *frame, saw.*

STSs Abbreviation for sequence-tagged *sites,* under *site.*

Stuart. Surname of the patient in whom the S. or Stuart-Prower *factor* was first discovered.

Stu·dent. Pseudonym for William Sealy Gosset, British statistician, and chemist, 1876–1937. SEE Student's *t test.*

study (stŭd′ē). Research, detailed examination, and/or analysis of an organism, object, or phenomena. [L. *studium,* study, inquiry]

analytic s., in epidemiology, a s. designed to examine associations, commonly putative or hypothesized causal relationships; usually concerned with identifying or measuring the effects of risk factors or with the health effects of specific exposures.

blind s., a s. in which the experimenter is unaware of which group is subject to which procedure.

case control s., an epidemiological method that begins by identifying persons with the disease or condition of interest (the cases) and compares their past history of exposure to identified or suspected risk factors with the past history of similar exposures among persons who resemble the cases but do not have the disease or condition of interest (the controls).

cohort s., a s. using epidemiological methods, such as a clinical trial, in which a cohort with a particular attribute (*e.g.,* smokers, recipients of a drug) is followed prospectively and compared for some outcome (*e.g.,* disease, cure) with another cohort not possessing the attribute.

cross-over s., a s. in which the subject is switched from the experimental to the control procedure (or vice versa).

cross-sectional s., a s. in which groups of individuals of different types are composed into one large sample and studied at only a single point in time (*e.g.,* a survey of all voters regardless of age, religion, gender, or geographic location are sampled in one day). SYN synchronic s. (1).

diachronic s., a s. of the natural course of a life or disorder in which a cohort of subjects is serially observed over a period of time and no assumptions need be made about the stability of the system. SYN longitudinal s.

double blind s., a s. in which neither the experimenter nor any other assessor of the results, including patients, know which group is subject to which procedure, thus helping assure that the biases or expectations of either will not influence the results.

follow-up s., (2) study in which persons exposed to risk or given a designated preventive or therapeutic regimen are observed over a period or at intervals to determine the outcome of the exposure or regimen.

Framingham Heart S., ongoing epidemiologic study of a cohort of over 5,000 of the population of Framingham, MA conducted since 1949 under the auspices of the National Institutes of Health and Boston University.

longitudinal s., SYN diachronic s.

multivariate s.'s, the use of statistical techniques for the simultaneous investigations of the influence of several variables.

synchronic s., (1) SYN cross-sectional s.

stump (stŭmp). **1.** The extremity of a limb left after amputation. **2.** The pedicle remaining after removal of the tumor attached to it. [M.e. *stumpe*]

stun (stŭn). To stupefy; to render unconscious by cerebral trauma. [A.S. *stunian,* to make a loud noise]

stupe (stūp). A compress or cloth wrung out of hot water, usually impregnated with turpentine or other irritant, applied to the surface to produce counterirritation. [L. *stupa,* oakum, tow]

stu·pe·fa·cient (stū-pĕ-fā′shent). Causing stupor. SYN stupefactive. [L. *stupefacio*]

stu·por (stū′per). A state of impaired consciousness in which the individual shows a marked diminution in reactivity to environmental stimuli; only continual stimulation arouses the individual. [L. fr. *stupeo,* to be stunned]

benign s., a stuporous syndrome from which recovery is the rule, as opposed to malignant s. SYN depressive s.

catatonic s., s. associated with catatonia.

depressive s., SYN benign s.

malignant s., a stuporous condition from which recovery is infrequent, as opposed to benign s.

stu·por·ous (stū′per-ŭs). Relating to or marked by stupor. SYN carotic.

Sturge, William A., English physician, 1850–1919. SEE S.-Weber *syndrome, disease.*

Sturm, Johann C., 1635–1703. SEE S.'s *conoid, interval.*

Sturmdorf, A., U.S. gynecologist, 1861–1934. SEE S.'s *operation.*

stut·ter (stŭt′er). To enunciate certain words with difficulty and with frequent halting and repetition of the initial consonant of a word or syllable. [frequentative of *stut,* from Goth. *stautan,* to strike]

stut·ter·ing (stŭt′er-ing). A phonatory or articulatory disorder, characteristically beginning in childhood, with intense anxiety about the efficiency of oral communications, and characterized by hesitations, repetitions, and prolongations of sounds and syllables, interjections, broken words, circumlocutions, and words produced with excess tension. SYN logospasm (1).

urinary s., frequent involuntary interruption occurring during the act of urination. SYN stammering of the bladder.

sty, stye, pl. **sties, styes** (stī, stīz). SYN *hordeolum* externum.

meibomian s., SYN *hordeolum* internum.

zeisian s., inflammation of one of Zeis' glands.

style (stīl). SYN stylet.

sty·let, sty·lette (stī′let, stī-let′). 1. A flexible metallic rod inserted in the lumen of a flexible catheter to stiffen it and give it form during its passage. 2. A slender probe. SYN style, stylus (3), stilus. [It. *stilletto,* a dagger; dim. of L. *stilus* or *stylus,* a stake, a pen]

endotracheal s., a rod of malleable metal used to maintain the desired curve of a tracheal tube for its insertion into the trachea.

sty·li·form (stī′li-fōrm). SYN styloid. [L. *stilus* (*stylus*), a stake, + *forma,* form]

△**stylo-.** Styloid (specifically the styloid process of the temporal bone). [G. *stylos,* pillar, post]

sty·lo·au·ri·cu·la·ris (stī′lō-aw-rik-yū-lā′ris). SEE styloauricular *muscle.*

sty·lo·glos·sus (stī′lō-glos′ŭs). Relating to the styloid process and the tongue. SEE styloglossus *muscle.*

sty·lo·hy·al (stī-lō-hī′ăl). Relating to the styloid process of the temporal bone and to the hyoid bone. SYN stylohyoid (1).

sty·lo·hy·oid (stī-lō-hī′oyd). 1. SYN stylohyal. 2. Relating to the stylohyoid muscle.

sty·loid (stī′loyd). Peg-shaped; denoting one of several slender bony processes. SEE styloid *process* of third metacarpal bone, styloid *process* of temporal bone, styloid *process* of radius, styloid *process* of ulna. SYN styliform. [stylo- + G. *eidos,* resemblance]

sty·loi·di·tis (stī-loy-dī′tis). Inflammation of a styloid process.

sty·lo·la·ryn·ge·us (stī′lō-lar-in-jē′ŭs). SEE *musculus* stylolaryngeus.

sty·lo·man·dib·u·lar (stī′lō-man-dib′yū-lăr). Relating to the styloid process of the temporal bone and the mandible; denoting the stylomandibular ligament. SYN stylomaxillary.

sty·lo·mas·toid (stī′lō-mas′toyd). Relating to the styloid and the mastoid processes of the temporal bone; denoting especially a small artery and a foramen.

sty·lo·max·il·lary (stī′lō-mak′si-lăr-ē). SYN stylomandibular.

sty·lo·pha·ryn·ge·us (stī′lō-far-in-jē′ŭs). SEE stylopharyngeus *muscle.*

sty·lo·po·di·um (stī-lō-pō′dē-ŭm). The proximal intermediate segment of the limb skeleton, the humerus and the femur, in the embryo. [stylo- + G. *podion,* small foot]

sty·lo·staph·y·line (stī-lō-staf′i-līn). Relating to the styloid process of the temporal bone and the uvula.

sty·los·te·o·phyte (stī-los′tē-ō-fīt). A peg-shaped bony outgrowth. [G. *stylos,* post, + *osteon,* bone, + *phyton,* growth]

Sty·lo·vir·i·dae (stī-lō-vir′i-dē). Provisional name for a family of bacterial viruses with long, noncontractile tails and isometric or elongated heads, containing double-stranded DNA (MW 25 to 79 × 10⁶); includes the λ temperate phage group and probably other genera. [G. *stylos,* pillar, column]

sty·lus, sti·lus (stī′lŭs, stī′lŭs). 1. Any pencil-shaped structure. 2. A pencil-shaped medicinal preparation for external application; *e.g.,* a medicated bougie, or a pencil or stick of silver nitrate or other caustic. 3. SYN stylet. [L. *stilus* or *stylus,* a stake or pen]

stype (stīp). A tampon. [G. *stypē,* tow]

styp·tic (stip′tik). 1. Having an astringent or hemostatic effect. 2. An astringent hemostatic agent used topically to stop bleeding. SYN hemostyptic. SYN staltic. [G. *styptikos,* astringent]

styr·a·mate (stī′ră-māt). Carbamic acid β-hydroxyphenethyl ester; an orally effective skeletal muscle relaxant with a relatively long duration of action.

sty·rax (stī′raks). SYN storax.

sty·rene (stī′rēn). $C_6H_5CH=CH_2$; phenylethylene; the monomer from which polystyrenes, plastics, and synthetic rubber are made; together with divinylbenzene (for cross-linking), it is the basis of many synthetic ion exchangers. SYN cinnamene, ethenylbenzene, styrol, vinylbenzene.

sty·rol (stī′rol). SYN styrene.

sty·rone (stī′rōn). $C_9H_{10}O$; obtained from storax by distillation with potassium hydroxide; used as a deodorant in 12% glycerin solution, and as a decolorizing agent in histology. SYN cinnamic alcohol.

△**sub-.** Prefix, to words formed from L. roots, denoting beneath, less than the normal or typical, inferior. Cf. hypo-. [L. *sub,* under]

sub·ab·dom·i·nal (sŭb-ab-dom′i-năl). Below the abdomen.

sub·ab·dom·i·no·per·i·to·ne·al (sŭb-ab-dom′i-nō-per-i-tō-nē′ăl). Beneath the abdominal, as distinguished from the pelvic, peritoneum. SYN subperitoneoabdominal.

sub·ac·e·tate (sŭb-as′ĕ-tāt). A mixture or complex of a base and its acetate.

sub·a·cro·mi·al (sŭb-ă-krō′mē-ăl). Beneath the acromion process.

sub·a·cute (sŭb-ă-kyūt′). Between acute and chronic; denoting the course of a disease of moderate duration or severity.

sub·al·i·men·ta·tion (sŭb′al-i-men-tā′shŭn). A condition of insufficient nourishment. SYN hypoalimentation.

sub·a·nal (sŭb-ā′năl). Below the anus.

sub·a·or·tic (sŭb′ā-ōr′tik). Below the aorta.

sub·ap·i·cal (sŭb-ap′i-kăl). Below the apex of any part.

sub·ap·o·neu·rot·ic (sŭb-ap-ō-nū-rot′ik). Beneath an aponeurosis.

sub·a·rach·noid (sŭb-ă-rak′noyd). Underneath the arachnoid membrane.

sub·ar·cu·ate (sŭb-ar′kyū-āt). Slightly arcuate or bowed.

sub·a·re·o·lar (sŭb-ā-rē′ō-lăr). Beneath an areola; especially the areola of the mamma.

sub·as·trag·a·lar (sŭb-as-trag′ă-lăr). Beneath the calcaneus (astragalus).

sub·a·tom·ic (sŭb-ă-tom′ik). Pertaining to particles making up the intra-atomic structure; *e.g.,* protons, electrons, neutrons.

sub·au·ral (sŭb-aw′răl). Below the ear.

sub·au·ric·u·lar (sŭb-aw-rik′yū-lăr). Below an auricle; especially the concha or pinna of the ear.

sub·ax·i·al (sŭb-ak′sē-ăl). Below the axis of the body or any part.

sub·ax·il·lary (sŭb-ak′si-lăr-ē). Below the axillary fossa. SYN infra-axillary.

sub·bas·al (sŭb-bā′săl). Beneath any base or basal membrane.

sub·brach·y·ce·phal·ic (sŭb-brak-ē-se-fal′ik). Slightly brachycephalic; having a cephalic index of 80.01 to 83.33.

sub·cal·ca·rine (sŭb-kal′kă-rīn). Below the calcarine fissure; denoting the lingual gyrus.

sub·cal·lo·sal (sŭb-ka-lō′săl). Below the corpus callosum; denoting either the subcallosal gyrus or the fasciculus.

sub·cap·su·lar (sŭb-kap′sū-lăr). Beneath any capsule.

su

sub·car·bon·ate (sŭb-kar′bon-āt). A mixture or complex of a base and its carbonate.

sub·car·di·nal (sŭb-kar′di-năl). Lying ventral to the anterior or posterior cardinal veins in the embryo.

sub·car·ti·lag·i·nous (sŭb′kar-ti-laj′i-nŭs). **1.** Partly cartilaginous. **2.** Beneath a cartilage.

sub·ce·cal (sŭb-sē′kăl). Below the cecum; denoting a fossa.

sub·cel·lu·lar (sŭb-sel′yū-lăr). SYN noncellular (1).

sub·cep·tion (sŭb-sep′shŭn). Subliminal perception as in the reaction to a stimulus not fully perceived. SEE subliminal. [sub- + L. -ceptum, perceived]

sub·chlo·ride (sŭb-klōr′īd). The chloride of a series that contains proportionally the greatest amount of the other element in the compound; e.g., s. of mercury is Hg_2Cl_2, whereas chloride or perchloride of mercury is $HgCl_2$.

sub·chon·dral (sŭb-kon′drăl). Beneath or below the cartilages of the ribs.

sub·cho·ri·on·ic (sŭb′kō-rē-on′ik). Beneath the chorion.

sub·cho·roi·dal (sŭb-kō-roy′dăl). Beneath the choroid coat of the eye.

sub·class (sŭb′klas). In biologic classification, a division between class and order.

sub·cla·vi·an (sŭb-klā′vē-an). **1.** Beneath the clavicle. SYN infraclavicular. **2.** Pertaining to the s. artery or vein.

sub·cla·vic·u·lar (sŭb-kla-vik′yū-lăr). Pertaining to the region beneath the clavicle.

sub·cla·vi·us (sŭb-klā′vē-ŭs). SEE subclavius muscle.

sub·clin·i·cal (sŭb-klin′i-kăl). Denoting the presence of a disease without manifest symptoms; may be an early stage in the evolution of a disease.

sub·clon·ing (sŭb′klōn-ing). The process by which a DNA clone is cleaved into smaller pieces and recloned; analysis of overlapping regions of these smaller DNA fragments can confirm the entire sequence of the original DNA clone.

sub·col·lat·er·al (sŭb-kŏ-lat′er-ăl). Below the collateral fissure; denoting a cerebral convolution, or gyrus.

sub·con·junc·ti·val (sŭb′kon-jŭnk-tī′văl). Beneath the conjunctiva.

sub·con·junc·ti·vi·tis (sŭb′kon-jŭnk-ti-vī′tis). SYN episcleritis periodica fugax.

sub·con·scious (sŭb-kon′shŭs). **1.** Not wholly conscious. **2.** Denoting an idea or impression which is present in the mind, but of which there is at the time no conscious knowledge or realization.

sub·con·scious·ness (sŭb-kon′shŭs-nes). **1.** Partial unconsciousness. **2.** The state in which mental processes take place without the conscious perception of the individual.

sub·cor·a·coid (sŭb-kōr′ă-koyd). Beneath the coracoid process.

sub·cor·tex (sŭb-kōr′teks). Any part of the brain lying below the cerebral cortex, and not itself organized as cortex.

sub·cor·ti·cal (sŭb-kōr′ti-kăl). Relating to the subcortex; beneath the cerebral cortex.

sub·cos·tal (sŭb-kos′tăl). **1.** Beneath a rib or the ribs. SYN infracostal. **2.** Denoting certain arteries, veins, and nerves.

sub·cos·tal·gia (sŭb-kos-tal′jē-ă). Pain in the subcostal region. [subcostal + G. algos, pain]

sub·cos·to·ster·nal (sŭb-kos′tō-ster′năl). Below or beneath the ribs and sternum.

sub·cra·ni·al (sŭb-krā′nē-ăl). Beneath or below the cranium.

sub·crep·i·tant (sub-krep′i-tănt). Nearly, but not frankly, crepitant; denoting a rale.

sub·crep·i·ta·tion (sŭb′krep-i-tā′shŭn). **1.** The presence of subcrepitant rales. **2.** A sound approaching crepitation in character.

sub·cru·ra·lis (-krū-rā′lis). SYN articularis genu muscle.

sub·cru·re·us (sŭb-krū-rē-ŭs). SYN articularis genu muscle. [sub- + L. crus, leg]

sub·cul·ture (sŭb-kŭl′chūr). **1.** A culture made by transferring to a fresh medium microorganisms from a previous culture; a method used to prolong the life of a particular strain where there is a tendency to degeneration in older cultures. **2.** To make a fresh culture with material obtained from a previous one.

sub·cu·ra·tive (sŭb-kyūr′ă-tiv). Denoting a dose less than that necessary for a curative effect.

sub·cu·ta·ne·ous (s.c., SQ) (sŭb-kyū-tā′nē-ŭs). Beneath the skin. SYN hypodermic (1), subdermic, subintegumental, subtegumental. [sub- + L. cutis, skin]

sub·cu·tic·u·lar (sŭb-kyū-tik′yū-lăr). Beneath the cuticle or epidermis. SYN subepidermal, subepidermic.

sub·cu·tis (sŭb-kyū′tis). SYN superficial fascia.

sub·de·lir·i·um (sŭb-dē-lir′ē-ŭm). Slight or not continuous delirium.

sub·del·toid (sŭb-del′toyd). Beneath the deltoid muscle; denoting a bursa.

sub·den·tal (sŭb-den′tăl). Beneath the roots of the teeth.

sub·der·mic (sŭb-der′mik). SYN subcutaneous.

sub·di·a·phrag·mat·ic (sŭb′dī-ă-frag-mat′ik). Beneath the diaphragm. SYN infradiaphragmatic, subphrenic.

sub·dor·sal (sŭb-dōr′săl). Below the dorsal region.

sub·duce, sub·duct (sŭb-dūs′, sŭb-dŭkt′). To pull or draw downward. [L. sub-duco, pp. -ductus, to lead away]

sub·du·ral (sŭb-dū′răl). Beneath the dura mater or between it and the arachnoid. SEE spatium subdurale.

sub·en·do·car·di·al (sŭb-en-dō-kar′dē-ăl). Beneath the endocardium.

sub·en·do·the·li·al (sŭb′en-dō-thē′lē-ăl). Beneath the endothelium.

sub·en·do·the·li·um (sŭb′en-dō-thē′lē-ŭm). The connective tissue between the endothelium and inner elastic membrane in the intima of arteries.

sub·en·dy·mal (sŭb-en′di-măl). Beneath the endyma, or ependyma. SYN subependymal.

sub·ep·en·dy·mo·ma (sŭb-ep-en-di-mō′mă). Discrete lobulated ependymal nodules in the walls of the anterior third or posterior fourth ventricles commonly found at autopsy.

sub·ep·i·der·mal, sub·ep·i·der·mic (sŭb′ep-i-der′măl, -der′mik). SYN subcuticular.

sub·ep·i·the·li·al (sŭb′ep-i-thē′lē-ăl). Beneath the epithelium.

sub·ep·i·the·li·um (sŭb′ep-i-thē′lē-ŭm). Any structure beneath the epithelium.

sub·e·ric ac·id (sū-ber′ik). HOOC–$(CH_2)_6$–COOH; used in plastics and in the cross-linking of biopolymers; found in the urine as a product of ω-oxidation of fatty acids. SYN octandioic acid. [L. suber, cork oak, + -ic]

su·ber·o·sis (sū-ber-ō′sis). Extrinsic allergic alveolitis caused by inhalation of mold spores from contaminated cork. [L. suber, cork, + G. -osis, condition]

sub·fam·i·ly (sŭb-fam′i-lē). In biologic classification, a division between family and tribe or between family and genus.

sub·fas·cial (sŭb-fash′ē-ăl). Beneath a fascia.

sub·fer·til·i·ty (sŭb-fer-til′i-tē). Less than normal capacity for reproduction.

sub·fis·sure (sŭb-fish′er). A cerebral fissure beneath the surface, concealed by overlapping convolutions.

sub·fo·li·um (sŭb-fō′lē-ŭm). A secondary division of a cerebellar folium.

sub·gal·late (sŭb-gal′āt). Partially neutralized gallic acid; a basic gallate, such as bismuth s.

sub·gem·mal (sŭb-jem′ăl). Below a gemma or bud (e.g., a taste bud).

sub·ge·nus (sŭb-jē′nŭs). In biologic classification, a division between genus and species.

sub·gin·gi·val (sŭb-jin′ji-văl). Below the gingival margin.

sub·gle·noid (sŭb-glē′noyd). SYN infraglenoid.

sub·glos·sal (sŭb-glos′ăl). Below or beneath the tongue. SYN sublingual.

sub·glot·tic (sŭb-glot′ik). SYN infraglottic.

sub·gran·u·lar (sŭb-gran′yū-lăr). Slightly granular.

sub·grun·da·tion (sŭb-grŭn-dā′shŭn). The depression of one fragment of a broken cranial bone below the other. [sub- + A.S. grund, bottom, foundation]

sub·he·pat·ic (sŭb-he-pat'ik). Below the liver. SYN infrahepatic.

sub·hy·a·loid (sŭb-hī'ă-loyd). Beneath, on the vitreous side of, the hyaloid (vitreous) membrane.

sub·hy·oid, sub·hy·oid·e·an (sŭb-hī'oyd, sŭb-hī-oyd'ē-an). SYN infrahyoid.

sub·ic·ter·ic (sŭb-ik'ter-ik). Slightly elevated serum bilirubin without clinical evidence of jaundice. [sub- + G. *ikterikos,* jaundiced]

su·bic·u·lar (sū-bik'yū-lăr, sŭ-bik'). Relating to the subiculum.

su·bic·u·lum, pl. **su·bic·u·la** (sū-bik'yū-lŭm, sŭ-bik'; -lă). **1.** A support or prop. **2.** The zone of transition between the parahippocampal gyrus and Ammon's horn of the hippocampus. [L. dim. of *subex,* support]

s. promonto'rii [NA], support of the promontory; a bony ridge bounding the fossula fenestrae cochleae posteriorly. SYN ponticulus promontorii.

sub·il·i·ac (sŭb-il'ē-ak). **1.** Below the ilium. **2.** Relating to the subilium.

sub·il·i·um (sŭb-il'ē-ŭm). The portion of the ilium contributing to the acetabulum.

sub·in·fec·tion (sŭb-in-fek'shŭn). A secondary infection occurring in one exposed to and successfully resisting an epidemic of another infectious disease.

sub·in·flam·ma·to·ry (sŭb-in-flam'ă-tō-rē). Denoting a slightly inflammatory irritation of the tissues.

sub·in·teg·u·men·tal (sŭb'in-teg-yū-men'tăl). SYN subcutaneous.

sub·in·ti·mal (sŭb-in'ti-măl). Beneath the intima.

sub·in·trant (sŭb-in'trant). SYN proleptic. [L. *sub-intro,* pres. p. *-ans,* to enter by stealth]

sub·in·vo·lu·tion (sŭb-in-vō-lū'shŭn). Arrest of the normal involution of the uterus following childbirth with the organ remaining abnormally large.

sub·i·o·dide (sŭb-ī'ō-dīd). That one of a series of iodine compounds with a given cation containing the least iodine; analogous to subchloride.

sub·ja·cent (sŭb-jā'sent). Below or beneath another part. [L. *sub-jaceo,* to lie under]

sub·ject (sŭb'jekt). A person or organism that is the object of research, treatment, experimentation, or dissection. [L. *subjectus,* lying beneath]

sub·jec·tive (sŭb-jek'tiv). **1.** Perceived by the individual only and not evident to the examiner; said of certain symptoms, such as pain. **2.** Colored by one's personal beliefs and attitudes. Cf. objective (2). [L. *subjectivus,* fr. *subjicio,* to throw under]

sub·jec·tive as·sess·ment da·ta. Those facts that are observable and measurable by the nurse.

sub·ju·gal (sŭb-jū'găl). Below the zygomatic (jugal) bone.

sub·king·dom (sŭb-king'dom). In biologic classification, a division between kingdom and phylum.

sub·la·tion (sŭb-lā'shŭn). Detachment, elevation, or removal of a part. [L. *sublatio,* a lifting up]

sub·le·thal (sŭb-lē'thăl). Not quite lethal.

sub·leu·ke·mia (sŭb-lū-kē'mē-ă). SYN subleukemic *leukemia.*

sub·li·mate (sŭb'lim-āt). **1.** To perform or accomplish sublimation. **2.** Any substance that has been submitted to sublimation. [L. *sublimo,* pp. *-atus,* to raise on high, fr. *sublimis,* high]

corrosive s., SYN mercuric chloride.

sub·li·ma·tion (sŭb-lim-ā'shŭn). **1.** The process of converting a solid into a gas without passing through a liquid state; analogous to distillation. **2.** In psychoanalysis, an unconscious defense mechanism in which unacceptable instinctual drives and wishes are modified into more personally and socially acceptable channels.

sub·lime (sŭb-līm'). **1.** To sublimate. **2.** To undergo a process of sublimation.

sub·lim·i·nal (sŭb-lim'i-năl). Below the threshold of perception or excitation; below the limit or threshold of consciousness. [sub- + L. *limen (limin-),* threshold]

sub·li·mis (sŭb-lī'mis). **1.** At the top. **2.** SYN superficialis. [L.]

sub·lin·gual (sŭb-ling'gwăl). SYN subglossal.

sub·lob·u·lar (sŭb-lob'yū-lăr). Beneath a lobule, as of the liver.

sub·lum·bar (sŭb-lŭm'băr). Below the lumbar region.

sub·lu·mi·nal (sŭb-lū'mi-năl). Below or beneath the structure facing the lumen of an organ.

sub·lux·a·tion (sŭb-lŭk-sā'shŭn). An incomplete luxation or dislocation; though a relationship is altered, contact between joint surfaces remains. SYN semiluxation. [sub- + L. *locatio,* luxation (dislocation)]

sub·lym·phe·mia (sŭb-lim-fē'mē-ă). A blood state in which there is a great increase in the proportion of lymphocytes although the total number of white cells is normal. [sub- + L. *lympha,* lymph, + G. *haima,* blood]

sub·mam·ma·ry (sŭb-mam'ă-rē). **1.** Deep to the mammary gland. **2.** SYN inframammary.

sub·man·dib·u·lar (sŭb-man-dib'yū-lăr). Beneath the mandible or lower jaw. SYN inframandibular, submaxillary (2).

sub·mar·gin·al (sŭb-mar'ji-năl). Near the margin of any part.

sub·max·il·la (sŭb-mak-sil'ă). SYN mandible.

sub·max·il·lary (sŭb-mak'si-lār-ē). **1.** SYN mandibular. **2.** SYN submandibular.

sub·me·di·al, sub·me·di·an (sŭb-mē'dē-ăl, sŭb-mē'dē-an). Almost, but not exactly in the middle.

sub·mem·bra·nous (sŭb-mem'bră-nŭs). Partly or nearly membranous.

sub·men·tal (sŭb-men'tăl). Beneath the chin.

sub·merged (sŭb-merjd'). In dentistry, describing a field of operation covered by saliva.

sub·met·a·cen·tric (sŭb'met-ă-sen'trik). SEE submetacentric *chromosome.*

sub·mi·cron·ic (sŭb-mī-kron'ik). Smaller than 1 micron in size.

sub·mi·cro·scop·ic (sŭb'mī-krō-skop'ik). Too minute to be visible with a light microscope. SYN amicroscopic, ultramicroscopic.

sub·mor·phous (sŭb-mōr'fŭs). Neither definitely amorphous nor definitely crystalline, denoting the structure of certain calculi.

sub·mu·co·sa (sŭb-mū-kō'să). A layer of tissue beneath a mucous membrane. the layer of connective tissue beneath the tunica mucosa. SYN tela submucosa [NA], tunica submucosa.

sub·mu·cous (sŭb-myū'kŭs). Beneath a mucous membrane.

sub·nar·co·tic (sŭb-nar-kot'ik). Slightly narcotic.

sub·na·sal (sŭb-nā'săl). Under the nose.

sub·na·si·on (sŭb-nā'zē-on). The point of the angle between the septum of the nose and the surface of the upper lip.

sub·neu·ral (sŭb-nū'răl). Below the neural axis.

sub·ni·trate (sŭb-nī'trāt). A basic nitrate; a salt of nitric acid having one or more atoms of the base still capable of combining with the acid.

sub·nor·mal (sŭb-nōr'măl). Below the normal standard of some quality.

sub·nor·mal·i·ty (sŭb-nōr-mal'i-tē). A subnormal state or condition.

sub·no·to·chor·dal. Lying beneath the notochord.

sub·nu·cle·us (sŭb-nū'klē-ŭs). A secondary nucleus.

sub·oc·cip·i·tal (sŭb-ok-sip'i-tăl). Below the occiput or the occipital bone.

sub·op·ti·mal (sŭb-op'ti-măl). Below or less than the optimum.

sub·or·bit·al (sŭb-ōr'bi-tăl). SYN infraorbital.

sub·or·der (sŭb-ōr'der). In biologic classification, a division between order and family.

sub·ox·i·da·tion (sŭb'oks-i-dā'shŭn). Deficient oxidation.

sub·ox·ide (sŭb-ok'sīd). That one of a series of oxides containing the least oxygen. SYN protoxide.

sub·pap·u·lar (sŭb-pap'yū-lăr). Denoting the eruption of few and scattered papules, in which the lesions are very slightly elevated, being scarcely more than macules.

sub·pa·ri·e·tal (sŭb-pa-rī'ĕ-tăl). Below or beneath any structure called parietal: bone, lobe, layer of a serous membrane, etc.

su

sub·pa·tel·lar (sŭb-pa-tel'ăr). **1.** Deep to the patella. **2.** SYN infrapatellar.

sub·pec·to·ral (sŭb-pek'tŏ-răl). Beneath the pectoralis muscle.

sub·pel·vi·per·i·to·ne·al (sŭb-pel'vi-per-i-tō-nē'ăl). Beneath the pelvic, as distinguished from the abdominal, peritoneum. SYN subperitoneopelvic.

sub·per·i·car·di·al (sŭb-per-i-kar'dē-ăl). Beneath the pericardium.

sub·per·i·os·te·al (sŭb-per-ē-os'tē-ăl). Beneath the periosteum.

sub·per·i·to·ne·al (sŭb-per-i-tō-nē'ăl). Beneath the peritoneum.

sub·per·i·to·ne·o·ab·dom·i·nal (sŭb-per-i-tō-nē'ō-ab-dom'i-năl). SYN subabdominoperitoneal.

sub·per·i·to·ne·o·pel·vic (sŭb-per-i-tō-nē'ō-pel'vik). SYN subpelviperitoneal.

sub·pe·tro·sal (sŭb-pe-trō'săl). **1.** Denoting the inferior petrosal. **2.** Denoting a dural venous sinus.

sub·pha·ryn·ge·al (sŭb-fă-rin'jē-ăl). Below the pharynx.

sub·phren·ic (sŭb-fren'ik). SYN subdiaphragmatic.

sub·phy·lum (sŭb-fī'lŭm). In biologic classification, a division between phylum and class.

sub·pi·al (sŭb-pī'ăl). Beneath the pia mater.

sub·pla·cen·tal (sŭb-pla-sen'tăl). Beneath the placenta; denoting the decidua basalis.

sub·pleu·ral (sŭb-plu'răl). Beneath the pleura.

sub·plex·al (sŭb-plek'săl). Below or beneath any plexus.

sub·pre·pu·tial (sŭb-prē-pyū'shē-ăl). Beneath the prepuce.

sub·pu·bic (sŭb-pyū'bik). Beneath the pubic arch; denoting a ligament, arcuate pubic ligament, connecting the two pubic bones below the arch.

sub·pul·mo·nary (sŭb-pŭl'mŏ-nār-ē). Below the lungs.

sub·py·ram·i·dal (sūb-pi-ram'i-dăl). **1.** Below any pyramid; denoting especially the tympanic sinus. **2.** Nearly pyramidal in shape.

sub·ret·i·nal (sŭb-ret'i-năl). **1.** Between the sensory retina and the retinal pigment epithelium. **2.** Between the retinal pigment epithelium and the choroid.

sub·salt (sŭb'salt). A basic salt; a salt in which the base has not been completely neutralized by the acid.

sub·sar·to·ri·al (sŭb-sar-tō'rē-ăl). Beneath the sartorius muscle; denoting a nerve plexus and a fascia.

sub·scap·u·lar (sŭb-skap'yŭ-lăr). **1.** Deep to the scapula. **2.** SYN infrascapular.

sub·scap·u·la·ris (sŭb-skap-yū-lā'ris). SEE subscapularis *muscle*.

sub·scle·ral (sŭb-sklē'răl). Beneath the sclera of the eye, *i.e.*, on the choroidal side of this layer. SYN subsclerotic (1).

sub·scle·rot·ic (sŭb-skle-rot'ik). **1.** SYN subscleral. **2.** Partly or slightly sclerotic or sclerosed.

sub·scrip·tion (sŭb-skrip'shŭn). The part of a prescription preceding the signature, in which are the directions for compounding. [L. *subscriptio,* fr. *subscribo,* pp. *-scriptus,* to write under, subscribe]

sub·se·rous, sub·se·ro·sal (sŭb-sē'rŭs, sŭb-se-rō'săl). Beneath a serous membrane.

sub·sib·i·lant (sŭb-sib'i-lănt). Rarely used term denoting a rale with a quality between blowing and whistling.

sub·si·dence (sŭb-sī'dens). Sinking or settling in bone, as of a prosthetic component of a total joint implant.

sub·spi·na·le (sŭb-spi-nā'lē). In cephalometrics, the most posterior midline point on the premaxilla between the anterior nasal spine and the prosthion. SYN point A.

sub·spi·nous (sŭb-spī'nŭs). **1.** SYN infraspinous. **2.** Tendency to spininess.

sub·stage (sŭb'stāj). An attachment to a microscope, below the stage, supporting the condenser or other accessory.

sub·stance (sŭb'stans). Stuff; material. SYN substantia [NA], matter. [L. *substantia,* essence, material, fr. *sub- sto,* to stand under, be present]

alpha s., SYN reticular s. (1).

anterior perforated s., a region at the base of the brain through which numerous small branches of the anterior and middle cerebral arteries (lenticulostriate arteries) enter the depth of the cerebral hemisphere; it is bordered medially by the optic chasm and anterior half of the optic tract, rostrally and laterally by the lateral olfactory stria; its anteromedial part corresponds to the olfactory tubercle. SYN substantia perforata anterior [NA], locus perforatus anticus, olfactory area.

autacoid s. (aw-tă'-koyd), a s. formed metabolically by one set of cells, which alters the function of other cells. (This term is sometimes used in place of the term hormone.)

bacteriotropic s., opsonin or other s. that alters bacterial cells in such a manner that they are more susceptible to phagocytic action.

basophil s., SYN Nissl s.

basophilic s., SYN Nissl s.

blood group s., SYN blood group *antigen.*

blood group-specific s.'s A and B, solution of complexes of polysaccharides and amino acids that reduces the titer of anti-A and anti-B isoagglutinins in serum from group O persons; used to render group O blood reasonably safe for transfusion into persons of group A, B, or AB, but does not affect any incompatibility that results from various other factors, such as Rh.

central gray s., (1) in general: the predominantly small-celled gray matter adjoining or surrounding the central canal of the spinal cord and the third and fourth ventricles of the brainstem; (2) in particular: the thick sleeve of gray matter surrounding the cerebral sylvian aqueduct in the midbrain, rostrally continuous with the posterior nucleus of the hypothalamus; in sections stained for myelin it stands out from the adjoining tectum and tegmentum by the poverty of its myelinated fibers. SYN substantia grisea centralis [NA].

central and lateral intermediate s., the central gray matter of the spinal cord surrounding the central canal. SYN substantia intermedia centralis et lateralis [NA], anterior gray column, Stilling's gelatinous s., substantia gelatinosa centralis.

chromidial s., SYN granular endoplasmic *reticulum.*

chromophil s., SYN Nissl s.

compact s., SYN compact *bone.*

controlled s., a s. subject to the Controlled Substances Act (1970), which regulates the prescribing and dispensing, as well as the manufacturing, storage, sale, or distribution of s.'s assigned to five schedules according to their 1) potential for or evidence of abuse, 2) potential for psychic or physiologic dependence, 3) contributing a public health risk, 4) harmful pharmacologic effect, or 5) role as a precursor of other controlled s.'s.

cortical s., SYN cortical *bone.*

exophthalmos-producing s. (EPS), a factor found in crude extract of pituitary tissue that produced exophthalmos in laboratory animals (especially fish). Its existence and role in producing exophthalmopathy in Graves' *disease* is questioned.

filar s., SYN reticular s. (1).

gelatinous s., the apical part of the posterior horn (dorsal horn; posterior gray column) of the spinal cord's gray matter, composed largely of very small nerve cells; its gelatinous appearance is due to its very low content of myelinated nerve fibers. SYN substantia gelatinosa [NA], Rolando's gelatinous s., Rolando's s.

glandular s. of prostate, the glandular tissue of the prostate as distinct from the stroma and capsule. SYN substantia glandularis prostatae.

gray s., SYN gray *matter.*

ground s., the amorphous material in which structural elements occur; in connective tissue, it is composed of proteoglycans, plasma constituents, metabolites, water, and ions present between cells and fibers. SYN substantia fundamentalis.

H s., designation given by Sir Thomas Lewis to a diffusible s. in skin, indistinguishable in action from histamine, that is liberated by injury and causes the triple response. SYN released s.

innominate s., the region of the forebrain that lies ventral to the anterior half or so of the lentiform nucleus, extending in the frontal plane from the lateral preopticohypothalamic zone laterally over the optic tract to the amygdala (amygdaloid body); rostrally it tapers off over the dorsal border of the olfactory tubercle, caudally it ends where the internal capsule reaches the surface to form the cerebral peduncle or pes pedunculi. Notable among its polymorphic cell population is the large-celled basal nucleus of Meynert. These magnocellular elements within the s. i. are present in the medial septum and the diagonal band of Broca, but occur in largest numbers ventral to the globus pallidus. Histochemical evidence indicates that magnocellular elements distribute cholinergic fibers widely in the cerebral cortex and that these cells undergo selective degeneration in Alzheimer's disease. SYN substantia innominata.

interspongioplastic s., obsolete term for cytochylema.

Kendall's s., SYN Kendall's *compounds*, under *compound*.

s. of lens of eye, that which constitutes the lens of the eye, composed of a nucleus and a cortex and covered by an epithelium. SYN substantia lentis [NA].

medullary s., (1) the lipid material present in the myelin sheath of nerve fibers; SYN Schwann's white s. **(2)** medulla of bones and other organs. SYN substantia medullaris (2).

müllerian inhibiting s. (MIS), a 535 amino acid glycoprotein secreted by the Sertoli cells of the testis. It is related to inhibin. SYN müllerian inhibiting factor.

muscular s. of prostate, the smooth muscle in the stroma of the prostate. SYN substantia muscularis prostatae [NA], musculus prostaticus.

neurosecretory s., the secretion of nerve cell bodies located in the hypothalamus; the s. is transported by way of hypothalamo-hypophysial tract fibers into the neurohypophysis where the terminals of the nerve fibers contain the secretion. As seen in the fibers and terminals with a light microscope, the s. appears as Herring bodies or hyaline bodies of the pituitary (see under body). SEE hyaline *bodies* of pituitary, under *body*.

Nissl s., the material consisting of granular endoplasmic reticulum and ribosomes that occurs in nerve cell bodies and dendrites. SYN basophil s., basophilic s., chromophil s., Nissl bodies, Nissl granules, substantia basophilia, tigroid bodies, tigroid s.

s. P, a peptide neurotransmitter composed of eleven amino acid residues (with the carboxyl group amidated), normally present in minute quantities in the nervous system and intestines of man and various animals and found in inflamed tissue, that is primarily involved in pain transmission and is one of the most potent compounds affecting smooth muscle (dilation of blood vessels and contraction of intestine) and thus presumed to play a role in inflammation.

posterior perforated s., the bottom of the interpeduncular fossa at the base of the midbrain, extending from the anterior border of the pons forward to the mamillary bodies, and containing numerous openings for the passage of perforating branches of the posterior cerebral arteries. SYN substantia perforata posterior [NA], locus perforatus posticus, Malacarne's space.

pressor s., SYN pressor *base*.

proper s., SEE substantia *propria* of cornea, *substantia* propria membranae tympani, *substantia* propria sclerae.

Reichstein's s., one of several steroids; *e.g.,* Reichstein's s. F (cortisone), Reichstein's s. H (corticosterone), Reichstein's s. M (cortisol), Reichstein's s. Q (cortexone), and Reichstein's s. S (cortexolone). SYN Reichstein's compound.

released s., SYN H s.

reticular s., (1) a filamentous plasmatic material, beaded with granules, demonstrable by means of vital staining in the immature red blood cells; SYN alpha s., filar mass, filar s., substantia reticularis (1), substantia reticulofilamentosa. **(2)** SYN reticular *formation.*

Rolando's gelatinous s., Rolando's s., SYN gelatinous s.

Schwann's white s., SYN medullary s. (1).

sensitizing s., SYN complement-fixing *antibody.*

slow-reacting s. (SRS), slow-reacting s. of anaphylaxis (SRS-A), a leukotriene of low molecular weight which is released in anaphylactic shock and produces slower and more prolonged contraction of muscle than does histamine; it is active in the presence of antihistamines (but not epinephrine) and seems not to occur preformed in mast cells, but as a result of an antigen-antibody reaction on the granules. Cf. peptidyl *leukotrienes.*

soluble specific s. (SSS), SYN specific capsular s.

specific capsular s., a soluble type-specific polysaccharide pro-

duced during active growth of virulent pneumococci composing a large part of the capsule. SYN pneumococcal polysaccharide, soluble specific s., specific soluble polysaccharide, specific soluble sugar.

spongy s., SYN *substantia* spongiosa.

standard s., a pure, authentic s. used for identification purposes.

Stilling's gelatinous s., SYN central and lateral intermediate s.

threshold s., any material (*e.g.,* glucose) that is excreted in the urine only when its plasma concentration exceeds a certain value, termed its threshold. SYN threshold body.

tigroid s., SYN Nissl s.

vasodepressor s., an incompletely characterized chemical, apparently produced during liver damage, that tends to decrease vascular pressures and relax arterial walls.

white s., SYN white *matter.*

zymoplastic s., SYN thromboplastin.

sub·stan·tia, pl. **sub·stan·ti·ae** (sŭb-stan'shē-ă, -shē-ē) [NA]. SYN substance. [L.]

s. adamanti′na, SYN enamel.

s. al′ba [NA], SYN white *matter.*

s. basophi′lia, SYN Nissl *substance.*

s. cine′rea, SYN gray *matter.*

s. compac′ta [NA], SYN compact *bone.*

s. compac′ta os′sium, SYN compact *bone.*

s. cortica′lis [NA], SYN cortical *bone.*

s. ebur′nea, SYN dentin.

s. ferrugin′ea [NA], SYN *locus* ceruleus.

s. fundamenta′lis, SYN ground *substance.*

s. gelatino′sa [NA], SYN gelatinous *substance.*

s. gelatino′sa centra′lis, SYN central and lateral intermediate *substance.*

s. glandula′ris pros′tatae, SYN glandular *substance* of prostate.

s. gris′ea [NA], SYN gray *matter.*

s. gris′ea centra′lis [NA], SYN central gray *substance.*

s. innomina′ta, SYN innominate *substance.*

s. interme′dia centra′lis et latera′lis [NA], SYN central and lateral intermediate *substance.*

s. len′tis [NA], SYN *substance* of lens of eye.

s. medulla′ris, (1) SYN medulla. **(2)** SYN medullary *substance.*

s. muscula′ris prosta′tae [NA], SYN muscular *substance* of prostate.

s. ni′gra [NA], a large cell mass, crescentic on transverse section, extending forward over the dorsal surface of the crus cerebri from the rostral border of the pons into the subthalamic region; it is composed of a dorsal stratum of closely spaced pigmented (*i.e.,* melanin-containing) cells, the pars compacta, and a larger ventral region of widely scattered cells, the pars reticulata; the pars compacta in particular includes numerous cells that project forward to the striatum (caudate nucleus and putamen) and contain dopamine, which acts as the transmitter substance at their synaptic endings; other, apparently non-dopaminergic cells of the s. nigra project to a rostral part of the ventral nucleus of thalmus, the middle layers of the superior colliculus and to restricted parts of the reticular formation of the midbrain; the nigrostriatal projection is reciprocated by a massive striatonigral fiber system with multiple neurotransmitters, chief among which is γ-aminobutyric acid (GABA); s. n. receives smaller afferent projections from the subthalamic nucleus, the lateral segment of the globus pallidus, the dorsal nucleus of the raphe and the pedunculopontine nucleus of the midbrain. The pars reticulata forms part of the output system for the striate body. The s. n. is involved in the metabolic disturbances associated with Parkinson's disease and Huntington's disease. SYN locus niger, nucleus niger, Soemmerring's ganglion.

s. os′sea den′tis, SYN cementum.

s. perfora′ta ante′rior [NA], SYN anterior perforated *substance.*

s. perfora′ta poste′rior [NA], SYN posterior perforated *substance.*

s. pro′pria cor′neae [NA], SYN substantia *propria* of cornea.

s. pro′pria membra′nae tym′pani, proper substance of tympanic membrane, the layer of radial and circular collagenous fibers of the tympanic membrane.

s. pro′pria scle′rae [NA], proper substance of the sclera, the dense white fibrous tissue arranged in interlacing bundles that forms the main mass of the sclera, continuous anteriorly with the substantia propria corneae.

s. reticula′ris, (1) SYN reticular *substance* (1). **(2)** SYN reticular *formation*.

s. reticulofilamento′sa, SYN reticular *substance* (1).

s. spongio′sa [NA], bone in which the spicules or trabeculae form a three-dimensional latticework (cancellus) with the interstices filled with embryonal connective tissue or bone marrow. SYN s. trabecularis [NA], cancellous bone, spongy bone (1), spongy substance, trabecular bone.

s. trabecula′ris [NA], SYN s. spongiosa.

s. vit′rea, SYN enamel.

sub·ster·nal (sŭb-ster′năl). **1.** Deep to the sternum. **2.** SYN infrasternal.

sub·ster·no·mas·toid (sŭb-ster′nō-mas′toyd). Beneath the sternomastoid muscle; denoting a group of deep cervical lymph nodes.

sub·sti·tute (sŭb′sti-tūt). **1.** Anything that takes the place of another. **2.** In psychology, a surrogate.

blood s., any material (*e.g.,* human plasma, serum albumin, or a solution of such substances as dextran) used for transfusion in hemorrhage and shock.

plasma s., a solution of a substance (*e.g.,* dextran) used for transfusion in hemorrhage or shock as a s. for plasma. SYN plasma expander.

volume s., infusion of cell-free or volume-expanding fluids such as dextran for replacement of fluid lost from the circulation as part of the prevention or treatment of circulatory shock.

sub·sti·tu·tion (sŭb-sti-tū′shŭn). **1.** In chemistry, the replacement of an atom or group in a compound by another atom or group (*e.g.,* s. of H by Cl in CH$_4$ to give CH$_3$Cl). **2.** In psychoanalysis, an unconscious defense mechanism by which an unacceptable or unattainable goal, object, or emotion is replaced by one that is more acceptable or attainable; the process is more acute and direct, and less subtle, than sublimation. [L. *substitutio,* to put in place of another]

stimulus s., SYN classical *conditioning.*

symptom s., an unconscious psychological process by which a repressed impulse is indirectly manifested through a particular symptom, *e.g.,* anxiety, compulsion, depression, hallucination, obsession. SYN symptom formation.

sub·strate (S) (sŭb′strāt). **1.** The substance acted upon and changed by an enzyme; the reactant considered to be attacked in a chemical reaction. **2.** The base on which an organism lives or grows; *e.g.,* the s. on which microorganisms and cells grow in cell culture. [L. *sub-sterno,* pp. *-stratus,* to spread under]

suicide s., a competitive inhibitor that is converted to an irreversible inhibitor at the active site of the enzyme. SYN mechanism-based inhibitor.

sub·stra·tum (sŭb-strā′tŭm). Any layer or stratum lying beneath another. [L. see substrate]

sub·struc·ture (sŭb-strŭk′chŭr). A tissue or structure wholly or partly beneath the surface.

implant denture s., the metal framework which is placed beneath the soft tissues in contact with, or embedded into, bone for the purpose of supporting an implant denture superstructure.

sub·sul·fate (sŭb-sŭl′fāt). A basic sulfate; a sulfate that contains some base unneutralized and still capable of combining with the acid.

sub·sul·tus (sŭb-sŭl′tŭs). A twitching or jerking. [L. *subsilio,* pp. *-sultus,* to leap up, fr. *salio,* to leap]

s. clo′nus, SYN s. tendinum.

s. ten′dinum, a twitching of the tendons, especially noticeable at the wrist, occurring in low fevers. SYN s. clonus, tremor tendinum.

sub·tar·sal (sŭb-tar′săl). Below the tarsus.

sub·teg·u·men·tal (sŭb′teg-yū-men′tăl). SYN subcutaneous.

sub·ten·to·ri·al (sŭb-ten-tō′rē-ăl). Beneath the tentorium cerebelli.

sub·ter·mi·nal (sŭb-ter′mi-năl). Situated near the end or extremity of an oval or rod-shaped body.

sub·te·tan·ic (sŭb-te-tan′ik). Denoting tonic muscular spasms or convulsions that are not entirely sustained but have brief remissions.

sub·tha·lam·ic (sŭb-thă-lam′ik). Related to the subthalamus region or to the subthalamic nucleus.

sub·thal·a·mus (sŭb-thal′ă-mŭs). That part of the diencephalon that lies wedged between the thalamus on the dorsal side and the cerebral peduncle ventrally, lateral to the dorsal half of the hypothalamus from which it cannot be sharply delineated. It is composed of the subthalamic nucleus (corpus luysi), the zona incerta, and the fields of Forel; laterally it expands in a winglike fashion into the reticular nucleus of the thalamus; caudally it is continuous with the midbrain tegmentum.

sub·thy·roid·e·us (sŭb-thī-royd′ē-ŭs). A muscular bundle formed of fibers derived from the thyroarytenoid and vocalis muscles.

sub·til·i·sin (sŭb-ti-lī′sin). A proteinase formed by *Bacillus subtilis* and other species, similar to the serine proteinases of other molds and bacteria; it catalyzes the hydrolysis of a few specific peptide bonds in certain proteins, converting chymotrypsinogen to chymotrypsin and ovalbumin to plakalbumin in this manner, and cleaves pancreatic ribonuclease into S-peptide and S-protein. SYN subtilopeptidase.

sub·ti·lo·pep·ti·dase (sŭb′ti-lō-pep′ti-dās). SYN subtilisin.

sub·trac·tion (sŭb-trak′shŭn). A technique used to enhance detectability of opacified anatomic structures on radiographic or scintigraphic images; a negative of an image made before introduction of contrast medium or radionuclide is photographically or electronically removed from a later image; commonly used in cerebral angiography. SEE ALSO digital subtraction *angiography,* mask.

sub·tra·pe·zi·al (sŭb-tra-pē′zē-ăl). Beneath the trapezius muscle; denoting a nerve plexus.

sub·tribe (sŭb-trīb). In biologic classification, a division between tribe and genus.

sub·tro·chan·ter·ic (sŭb-trō-kan-ter′ik). Below any trochanter.

sub·troch·le·ar (sŭb-trok′lē-ar). Below any trochlea.

sub·tu·ber·al (sŭb-tū′ber-ăl). Lying below any tuber.

sub·tym·pan·ic (sŭb-tim-pan′ik). Below the tympanic cavity.

sub·um·bil·i·cal (sŭb-ŭm-bil′i-kăl). SYN infraumbilical.

sub·un·gual, sub·un·gui·al (sŭb-ŭng′gwăl, sŭb-ŭng′gwi-ăl). Beneath the finger or toe nail. SYN hyponychial (1). [L. *unguis,* nail]

sub·u·nit (sŭb′ū-nit). A unit that forms a distinct part of a larger structure. SEE ALSO monomer. **2.** The single protein or polypeptide chain that can be separated from an oligomer protein without cleaving covalent bonds other than disulfide bridges between cysteinyl residues. **3.** A single biopolymer separated from a larger multimeric structure.

sub·u·re·thral (sŭb-yū-rē′thrăl). Beneath the male or female urethra.

sub·vag·i·nal (sŭb-vaj′i-năl). **1.** Below the vagina. **2.** On the inner side of any tubular membrane serving as a sheath.

sub·val·var, sub·val·vu·lar (sŭb-val′văr, sŭb-val′vyū-lăr). Below any valve.

sub·ver·te·bral (sŭb-ver′tĕ-brăl). Beneath, or on the ventral side, of a vertebra or the vertebral column.

sub·vir·ile (sŭb-vir′il). Deficient in virility.

sub·vit·ri·nal (sŭb-vit′ri-năl). Beneath the vitreous body.

sub·vo·lu·tion (sŭb-vō-lū′shŭn). Obsolete term for turning over a flap of mucous membrane, as in the operation for pterygium, to prevent adhesion. [L. *sub,* under, + *volvo,* pp. *volutus,* to turn]

sub·wak·ing (sŭb-wāk′ing). Denoting the mental state between sleeping and waking.

sub·zon·al (sŭb-zō′năl). Below or beneath any zona or zone, such as the zona radiata or zona pellucida.

sub·zy·go·mat·ic (sŭb-zī-gō-mat′ik). Below or beneath the zygomatic bone or arch.

suc·ca·gogue (sŭk′ă-gog). **1.** Stimulating the flow of juice. **2.** An agent having such an effect. [L. *succus,* juice, + G. *agōgos,* leading]

suc·ce·da·ne·ous (sŭk-sē-dā′nē-ŭs). **1.** Relating to a succedaneum. **2.** Relating to the permanent or second teeth that replace the deciduous or primary teeth. [see succedaneum]

suc·ce·da·ne·um (sŭk-sē-dā′nē-ŭm). A substitute; a drug or any therapeutic agent that has the properties of and can be used in place of another. [L. *succedaneus,* following after, substituting, fr. *suc-cedo,* to follow, to take the place of, fr. *sub,* under, + *cedo,* to go]

suc·cen·tu·ri·ate (sŭk-sen-tyū′rē-āt). In anatomy, substituting for, or accessory to, some organ. [L. *suc-centurio,* pp. *-atus,* to substitute]

suc·ci·nate (sŭk′si-nāt). A salt of succinic acid.

active s., SYN succinyl-coenzyme A.

s. dehydrogenase, a flavoenzyme that catalyzes the removal of hydrogen from succinic acid and converts it into fumaric acid; *e.g.,* s. + FAD $\leftrightarrow$ fumarate + FADH$_2$; this complex is a part of the tricarboxylic acid cycle. SYN fumarate reductase (NADH), fumaric hydrogenase.

suc·ci·nate sem·i·al·de·hyde (sŭk′sin-āt sem-ē-ăl-dē′-hīd). $^-$OOC–CH$_2$–CH$_2$–CHO; an intermediate in the catabolism of γ-aminobutyrate.

s. s. dehydrogenase, an enzyme that catalyzes the reaction of s. s. and either NAD$^+$ or NADP$^+$ to form succinate and NADH (or NADPH); a deficiency of this enzyme is associated with 4-hydroxybutyric aciduria.

suc·cin·ic ac·id (sŭk-sin′ik). HOOC(CH$_2$)$_2$COOH; 1,4-Butanedioic acid; ethylenedicarboxylic acid; an intermediate in the tricarboxylic acid cycle; several of its salts have been variously used in medicine.

suc·cin·ic thi·o·ki·nase. SYN *succinyl-CoA* synthetase.

suc·cin·i·mide (suk′sin-ă-mīd). Chemical class of drugs from which the antiepileptic agents ethosuximide, methsuximide, and phensuximide are derived. Unsubstituted s. has been used as an antiurolithic.

suc·ci·nyl·ac·e·tone (sŭk′sin-il-ăs′e-tōn). A minor metabolite that is elevated in individuals with tyrosinemia IA.

N-suc·cin·yl·ad·en·yl·ic ac·id (sŭk-sin-il-ăd-ē-nil′ik). SYN adenylosuccinic acid.

suc·ci·nyl·cho·line (sŭk′si-nil-kō′lēn). A neuromuscular relaxant with short duration of action which characteristically first depolarizes the motor endplate (phase I block) but which is often later associated with a curare-like, nondepolarizing neuromuscular block (phase II block); used to produce relaxation for tracheal intubation and during surgical anesthesia. SYN diacetylcholine.

suc·ci·nyl-CoA (sŭk′sin-il). SYN succinyl-coenzyme A.

s.-CoA synthetase, (1) a ligase reversibly reacting succinate and CoA with ATP to produce ADP, inorganic phosphate, and succinyl-CoA; **(2)** a similar synthetase, but one able to use itaconate as well as succinate and GTP (or ITP) in place of ATP; a part of the tricarboxylic acid cycle. SYN succinic thiokinase, succinyl-CoA ligase.

suc·ci·nyl-CoA li·gase. SYN *succinyl-CoA* synthetase.

suc·ci·nyl-CoA syn·the·tase. See under succinyl-CoA.

suc·ci·nyl-co·en·zyme A (sŭk′si-nil-kō-en′zīm ā). The condensation product of succinic acid and CoA; one of the intermediates of the tricarboxylic acid cycle and a precursor in the synthesis of heme. SYN active succinate, succinyl-CoA.

suc·ci·nyl·di·cho·line (sŭk′si-nil-dī-kō′lēn). Succinylcholine chloride.

***O*-suc·ci·nyl·ho·mo·ser·ine (thi·ol)-ly·ase** (sŭk′si-nil-hō′mō-ser′ēn). An enzyme catalyzing the reaction between cystathionine and succinate to form L-cysteine and *O*-succinyl-L-homoserine. SYN cystathionine γ-synthase.

suc·ci·nyl·sul·fa·thi·a·zole (sŭk′si-nil-sŭl′fă-thī′ă-zōl). 4′-(2-Thiazolylsulfamoyl)succinanilic acid; the most effective of the

poorly absorbed bacteriostatic sulfonamides used for sterilization of the intestinal tract.

suc·ci·sul·fone im·i·no·di·eth·a·nol (sŭk-si-sŭl′fōn im′i-nō-dī-eth′ă-nol). 4′-Sulfanilylsuccinanilic acid 2,2′-iminodiethanol salt; an antimicrobial agent.

suc·cor·rhea (sŭk-ō-rē′ă). An abnormal increase in the secretion of a digestive fluid. [L. *succus,* juice, + G. *rhoia,* a flow]

suc·cu·bus (sŭk′yū-bŭs). A demon, in female form, believed to have sexual intercourse with a man during sleep. Cf. incubus. [L. *succubo,* to lie under]

suc·cus, gen. and pl. **suc·ci** (sŭk′ŭs, sŭk′sī). **1.** Obsolete term for the fluid constituents of the body tissues. **2.** Obsolete term for a fluid secretion, especially the digestive fluid. **3.** Formerly, a pharmacopeial preparation obtained by expressing the juice of a plant and adding to it sufficient alcohol (1 part to 3 of juice) to preserve it. SEE ALSO juice. [L.]

suc·cuss (sŭ-kŭs′). To make succussion.

suc·cus·sion (sŭ-kŭsh′ŭn). A diagnostic procedure that consists in shaking the body so as to elicit a splashing sound in a cavity containing both gas and fluid. [L. *sucussio,* fr. *suc-cutio* (*subc-*), pp. *-cussus,* to shake up, fr. *quatio,* to shake]

hippocratic s., a splashing noise produced by shaking the body when there is gas or air and fluid in the stomach or intestine, or free in the peritoneum, thorax, and, rarely, the pericardium.

suck (sŭk). **1.** To draw a fluid through a tube by exhausting the air in front. **2.** To draw a fluid into the mouth; specifically, to draw milk from the breast. [A.S. *sūcan*]

suck·le (sŭk′l). **1.** To nurse; to feed by milk from the breast. **2.** To suck; to draw sustenance from the breast.

Sucquet, J.P., French anatomist, 1840–1870. SEE S.'s *anastomoses,* under *anastomosis, canals,* under *canal;* S.-Hoyer *anastomoses,* under *anastomosis, canals,* under *canal.*

su·cral·fate (sū-kral′fāt). Sucrose octakis (hydrogen sulfate) aluminum complex; a polysaccharide with antipeptic activity, used to treat duodenal ulcers.

su·crase (sū′krās). SYN sucrose α-D-glucohydrolase.

su·crate (sū′krāt). A compound of sucrose.

su·crose (sū′krōs). A nonreducing disaccharide made up of D-glucose and D-fructose obtained from sugar cane, *Saccharum officinarum* (family Gramineae), from several species of sorghum, and from the sugar beet, *Beta vulgaris* (family Chenopodiaceae); the common sweetener, used in pharmacy in the manufacture of syrup, confections, etc. SYN saccharose, saccharum.

s. octaacetate, an alcohol denaturant.

su·crose α-D-glu·co·hy·dro·lase. An enzyme hydrolyzing sucrose and maltose; in a complex with isomaltase; hence, hydrolyzes both sucrose and isomaltose; found in the intestinal mucosa; a deficiency of this enzyme results in defective digestion of sucrose and linear α1,4-glucans. SYN sucrase.

su·cro·se·mia (sū-krō-sē′mē-ă). The presence of sucrose in the blood. [sucrose + G. *haima,* blood]

su·cro·su·ria (sū-krō-sū′rē-ă). The excretion of sucrose in the urine. [sucrose + G. *ouron,* urine]

suc·tion (sŭk′shŭn). The act or process of sucking. SEE ALSO aspiration (1), aspiration (2). [L. *sugo,* pp. *suctus,* to suck]

posttussive s., a s. sound heard on auscultation over a pulmonary cavity at the end of a cough.

Wangensteen s., a modified siphon that maintains constant negative pressure, used with a duodenal tube for the relief of gastric and intestinal distention. SYN Wangensteen tube.

suc·to·ri·al (sŭk-tō′rē-ăl). Relating to suction, or the act of sucking; adapted for sucking.

su·da·men, pl. **su·dam·i·na** (sū-dā′men, -dam′i-nă). A minute vesicle due to retention of fluid in a sweat follicle, or in the epidermis. [Mod. L., fr. L. *sudo,* to sweat]

su·dam·i·na (sū-dam′i-nă). **1.** Plural of sudamen. **2.** SYN *miliaria crystallina.*

su·dam·i·nal (sū-dam′i-năl). Relating to sudamina.

Su·dan III [C.I. 26100]. A red stain, (C$_6$H$_5$)N=N(C$_6$H$_4$)N=N(C$_{10}$H$_6$)OH, used for neutral fat in histologic technique; it also stains the fatty envelope of the tubercle bacillus. SYN Sudan red III.

Su·dan IV [C.I. 26105]. SYN scarlet red.

Su·dan black B [C.I. 26150]. A diazo dye, $C_{29}H_{24}N_6$, used as a stain for fats.

Su·dan brown [C.I. 12020]. A brown stain, $(C_{10}H_7)N=N(C_{10}H_6)OH$, derived from α-naphthylamine and used as a stain for fats.

su·dan·o·phil·ia (sū-dan-ō-fil′ē-ă). **1.** Affinity for an oil-soluble or Sudan dye. **2.** A condition in which leukocytes contain minute fat droplets that take a brilliant red stain when treated with 0.2% Sudan III and 0.1% cresyl blue in absolute alcohol.

su·dan·o·phil·ic (sū-dan-ō-fil′ik). Staining easily with Sudan dyes, usually referring to lipids in tissues.

su·dan·o·pho·bic (sū-dan-ō-fō′bik). Denoting tissue that fails to stain with a Sudan or fat-soluble dye.

Su·dan red III. SYN Sudan III.

Su·dan yel·low. Metadioxyazobenzene; a yellow stain for fats.

su·da·tion (sū-dā′shŭn). SYN perspiration (1). [L. *sudatio*, fr. *sudo*, pp. *-atus*, to sweat]

Sudeck, Paul H.M., German surgeon, 1866–1938. SEE S.'s *atrophy*, critical *point*, *syndrome*.

su·do·mo·tor (sū-dō-mō′ter). Denoting the autonomic (sympathetic) nerves that stimulate the sweat glands to activity. [L. *sudor*, sweat, + *motor*, mover]

su·dor (sū′dōr). SYN perspiration (3). [L.]

    s. sanguin′eus, SYN hematidrosis.

    s. urino′sus, SYN uridrosis.

△**sudor-.** Sweat, perspiration. [L. *sudor*]

su·dor·al (sū′dōr-ăl). Relating to perspiration.

su·dor an·gli·cus (sū′dōr ang′lĭ-cŭs). SYN English sweating *disease*.

su·do·re·sis (sū-dō-rē′sis). Profuse sweating. [sudor- + G. *-ēsis*, condition]

su·do·rif·er·ous (sū-dō-rif′er-ŭs). Carrying or producing sweat. [sudor- + L. *fero*, to bear]

su·do·rif·ic (sū-dō-rif′ik). Causing sweat. [sudor- + L. *facio*, to make]

su·dor·i·ker·a·to·sis (sū′dōr-i-ker-ă-tō′sis). Keratosis of the sudoriferous ducts.

su·do·rip·a·rous (sū-dō-rip′ă-rŭs). Secreting sweat. [sudor- + L. *pario*, to produce]

su·do·rom·e·ter (sū-dō-rom′ĕ-ter). An instrument for measuring the amount of perspiration. [sudor- + G. *metron*, measure]

su·dor·rhea (sū-dō-rē′ă). SYN hyperhidrosis. [sudor- + G. *rhoia*, a flow]

su·et (sū′et). The hard fat around the kidneys of cattle and sheep; when rendered it yields tallow.

    prepared s., the internal fat of the abdomen of the sheep, *Ovis aries*, purified by melting and straining; used in pharmacy in making ointments. SYN prepared mutton tallow.

su·fen·ta·nil cit·rate (sū-fen′tă-nil). *N*-[4-(Methoxymethyl)-1-[2-(2-thienyl)ethyl]-4-p iperidyl]proprionanilide; an injectable narcotic with short duration of effect resembling fentanil; used in "balanced anesthesia".

suf·fo·cate (sŭf′ō-kāt). **1.** To impede respiration; to asphyxiate. **2.** To be unable to breathe; to suffer from asphyxiation. [L. *suffoco (subf-)*, pp. *-atus*, to choke, strangle]

suf·fo·ca·tion (sŭf-ō-kā′shŭn). The act or condition of suffocating or of asphyxiation.

suf·fu·sion (sŭ-fyū′zhŭn). **1.** The act of pouring a fluid over the body. **2.** A reddening of the surface. **3.** The condition of being wet with a fluid. **4.** SYN extravasate (2). [L. *suffusio*, fr. *suffundo (subf-)*, to pour out]

sug·ar (shu-ger). One of the sugars; *q.v.*, pharmaceutical forms are compressible s. and confectioner's s. SEE ALSO sugars. [G. *sakcharon*; L. *saccharum*]

    amino s.'s, s.'s in which a hydroxyl group has been replaced with an amino group; *e.g.*, D-glucosamine.

    beechwood s., D-xylose. SEE xylose.

    beet s., D-sucrose. SEE sucrose.

    blood s., SEE D-glucose.

    brain s., D-galactose. SEE galactose.

    cane s., D-sucrose. SEE sucrose.

    corn s., SEE D-glucose.

    deoxy s., a s. containing fewer oxygen atoms than carbon atoms and in which, consequently, one or more carbons in the molecule lack an attached hydroxyl group. SYN desoxy sugar.

    fruit s., D-fructose. SEE fructose.

    gelatin s., SYN glycine.

    grape s., SEE D-glucose.

    invert s., a mixture of equal parts of D-glucose and D-fructose produced by hydrolysis of sucrose (inversion).

    s. of lead, SYN *lead* acetate.

    malt s., SYN maltose.

    manna s., SYN mannitol.

    maple s., sucrose extracted from the sap of the sugar maple, *Acer saccharinum*. SYN saccharum canadense.

    milk s., SYN lactose.

    oil s., SYN oleosaccharum.

    pectin s., D-arabinose. SEE arabinose.

    reducing s., a s., such as glucose in the urine, that has the property of reducing various inorganic ions, notably cupric ion to cuprous ion.

    specific soluble s., SYN specific capsular *substance*.

    starch s., SEE D-glucose.

    wood s., D-xylose. SEE xylose.

sug·ar ac·ids. Acids, such as gluconic, glycuronic, and saccharic acid, produced by the oxidation of glucose.

sug·ar al·co·hol. The polyalcohol resulting from the reduction of the carbonyl group in a monosaccharide to a hydroxyl group.

sug·ar al·de·hyde. A sugar that contains an internal acetal.

sug·ars (shug′erz). Those carbohydrates (saccharides) having the general composition $(CH_2O)_n$ and simple derivatives thereof. Although the simple monomeric s. (glycoses) are often written as polyhydroxy aldehydes or ketones, *e.g.*, $HOCH_2$–$(CHOH)_4$–CHO for aldohexoses (*e.g.*, glucose) or $HOCH_2$–$(CHOH)_3$–CO–CH_2OH for 2-ketoses (*e.g.*, fructose), cyclization can give rise to varied structures as described below. S. are generally identifiable by the ending -ose or, if in combination with a nonsugar (aglycon), -oside or -osyl. S. especially D-glucose, are the chief source of energy, by oxidation, in nature, and they and their derivatives (*e.g.*, D-glucosamine, D-glucuronic acid), in polymeric form, are major constituents of mucoproteins, bacterial cell walls, and plant structural material (*e.g.*, cellulose). S. are often found in combination with steroids (steroid glycosides) and other aglycons.

Fischer projection formulas of s., representations, by projection, of cyclic s., or derivatives thereof, in which the carbon chain is depicted vertically. The lowest-numbered asymmetric carbon atom (C-1 in aldoses; C-2 in 2-ketoses, *e.g.*, fructose) is drawn at the top, and the rest of the carbon atoms of the chain are drawn in sequence below the top carbon atom. For each carbon atom, depicted in projection as lying in the plane of the paper, the carbon-to-carbon bond(s), which actually point away from the viewer, are drawn as vertical lines. The left-hand and right-hand bonds of each carbon atom, which actually point toward the viewer, are, in projection, depicted as horizontal lines.

The conventions for the Fischer formulas of cyclic s. are as follows: 1) If the highest-numbered asymmetric carbon atom has its OH (or its replacement) lying to the right, as is the 2-OH of D-glyceraldehyde, the sugar has the D configuration; if the OH is to the left, the sugar has the L configuration. 2) On the anomeric carbon atom (C-1 in the aldoses; C-2 in the 2-ketoses), an OH or substituted OH that lies to the right, with the OH of the highest-numbered asymmetric carbon atom also to the right is defined to be α; if it is to the left, with the OH of the highest-numbered carbon atom still to the right, it is β; the reverse applies if the latter OH is to the left. 3) The orientation of a terminal CH_2OH group in the aldoses carries no configurational significance, as it contains no asymmetric carbon atom.

Haworth conformational formulas of cyclic s., for the pyranoses, these depict those shapes (conformations) on which none, one, or two ring-atoms lie outside the plane of the ring. If there are two such atoms *para* to each other, they can lie 1) on opposite sides of the plane (*trans*), giving chair forms, or 2) on the same side of the plane (*cis*), giving boat forms. For β-D-ribopyranose, the two chair forms ($^4C_1$ and $^1C_4$) are depicted.

Similarly, there are six boat conformations. If the two (*trans*) exoplanar atoms are *meta* to each other, the conformation is a skew form; if the two atoms are *ortho* to each other, the conformation is a half-chair form.

For the furanoses, the envelope conformations have one ring-atom exoplanar. If there are three adjacent, coplanar ring-atoms (the two exoplanar ring-atoms on opposite sides of the plane), the conformations are twist forms.

Haworth perspective formulas of cyclic s., perspective representations of furanose or pyranose structures as pentagons or hexagons, respectively, with the connecting bonds so shaded as to make them appear as though the plane of the ring is at an angle of 30° to the plane of the paper, and the bonds to H and OH are at right angles to the plane of the ring. These formulas depict the planar conformation, a situation not usually met. Other conformational formulas, *e.g.*, Haworth conformational formulas of cyclic s., attempt to depict the many deviations from planarity.

The basic conventions in Haworth formulas of cyclic s. (cyclic glycoses) are as follows: 1) The lowest-numbered asymmetric ring-carbon atom is depicted at the right. 2) If the highest-numbered asymmetric carbon atom is D, the sugar is D; the formula of an L-glycose may be derived from that of its D-isomer by reversing the up or down direction of all groups attached to the ring-carbon atoms. 3) If the hydroxyl group attached to the anomeric carbon (C-1 in aldoses; C-2 in 2-ketoses) is below the plane of the ring of a D-glycose, it is α; if above, it is β; the reverse applies if the sugar is L. SEE ALSO Fischer projection formulas of s.

sug·gest·i·bil·i·ty (sŭg-jes′tĭ-bil′i-tē). Responsiveness or susceptibility to a psychological process such as a hypnotic command whereby an idea is induced into, or adopted by, an individual without argument, command, or coercion. SYN sympathism.

sug·gest·i·ble (sŭg-jes′tĭ-bl). Susceptible to suggestion.

sug·ges·tion (sŭg-jes′chŭn). The implanting of an idea in the mind of another by some word or act on one's part; the subject's conduct or physical condition being influenced to some degree by the implanted idea. SEE ALSO autosuggestion. [L. *sug-gero* (*subg-*), pp. *-gestus,* to bring under, supply]

posthypnotic s., s. given to a subject who is under hypnosis for certain actions to be performed after he or she is "awakened" from the hypnotic trance.

sug·ges·tive (sŭg-jes′tiv). Relating to suggestion.

sug·gil·la·tion (sŭg-ji-lā′shŭn, sŭj-i-). A bruise or livedo. SEE ALSO contusion. [L. *sugillo,* pp. *-atus,* to beat black and blue]

postmortem s., SYN postmortem *livedo.*

Sugiura, M., 20th century Japanese surgeon. SEE S. *procedure.*

SUI. Abbreviation for stress urinary *incontinence.*

su·i·cide (sū′i-sīd). **1.** The act of taking one's own life. **2.** A person who commits such an act. [L. *sui,* self, + *caedo,* to kill]

sui·cid·ol·o·gy (sū′i-sī-dol′ō-jē). A branch of the behavioral sciences devoted to the study of the nature, causes, and prevention of suicide. [suicide + G. *logos,* study]

su·int (swint). The natural grease in sheep's wool, from which the official wool fat (anhydrous lanolin) is extracted. [Fr. wool-grease]

suit (sūt). An outer garment designed for protection against specific environmental conditions.

anti-G s., a garment with bladders that expand to apply external pressure to the abdomen and lower extremities during positive G maneuvers in flight or on a human centrifuge; the anti-G s. is worn to prevent the pooling of blood and serves to increase the wearer's ability to withstand exposure to higher G forces.

sul·bac·tam (sŭl-bak′tam). A β-lactamase inhibitor with weak antibacterial action; when used in conjunction with penicillins (*e.g.*, ampicillin) with little β-lactamase inhibiting action, it greatly increases their effectiveness against organisms which would ordinarily not be susceptible.

sul·bac·tam (sul′bak-tam). A semisynthetic β-lactamase inhibitor resembling clavulanic acid in its action; used in combination with β-lactam antibiotics such as aminopenicillins and cephalosporins as antibacterial agents.

sul·ben·tine (sŭl-ben′tēn). SYN dibenzthione.

sul·cal (sŭl′kăl). Relating to a sulcus.

sul·cate (sŭl′kāt). Grooved; furrowed; marked by a sulcus or sulci.

sul·ci·form (sŭl′si-fōm). Having the form of a groove or sulcus.

sul·cu·lus, pl. **sul·cu·li** (sŭl′kŭ-lŭs, -lī). A small sulcus. [Mod. L. dim. of L. *sulcus,* furrow]

SULCUS

---

sul·cus, gen. and pl. **sul·ci** (sūl′kŭs, sŭl′sī). **1** [NA]. One of the grooves or furrows on the surface of the brain, bounding the several convolutions or gyri; a fissure. SEE ALSO fissure. **2** [NA]. Any long narrow groove, furrow, or slight depression. SEE ALSO groove. **3.** A groove or depression in the oral cavity or on the surface of a tooth. [L. a furrow or ditch]

alveolobuccal s., SYN alveolobuccal *groove.*

alveololabial s., SYN alveololabial *groove.*

alveololingual s., SYN alveololingual *groove.*

s. ampulla′ris [NA], SYN ampullary s.

ampullary s., the groove on the external surface of the ampulla of each semicircular duct where the nerve enters the crista ampullaris. SYN s. ampullaris [NA].

s. angula′ris, SYN angular *notch.*

anterior intermediate s., a furrow occasionally seen in the adult between the anterior median fissure and the anterior lateral s. of the spinal cord but usually present only in the fetus. It indicates the lateral border of the anterior corticospinal fasciculus. SYN anterior intermediate groove, s. intermedius anterior.

anterior parolfactory s., a fissure marking the anterior border of the parolfactory area. SYN s. parolfactorius anterior.

anterolateral s., an indistinct furrow on the ventral surface of the spinal cord and medulla oblongata, on either side marking the line of exit of the anterior nerve roots. SYN s. lateralis anterior [NA], anterolateral groove.

s. anthel′icis transver′sus [NA], SYN transverse anthelicine *groove.*

aortic s., a broad deep groove on the medial aspect of the left lung above and behind the hilum receiving the arch of the aorta and the thoracic aorta. SYN sulcus aorticus.

s. arte′riae occipita′lis [NA], SYN occipital *groove.*

s. arte′riae tempora′lis me′diae [NA], SYN *groove* for middle temporal artery.

s. arte′riae vertebra′lis [NA], SYN *groove* for vertebral artery.

sul′ci arterio′si [NA], SYN arterial *grooves,* under *groove.*

atrioventricular s., SYN coronary *groove.*

s. auric′ulae ante′rior, SYN anterior *notch* of ear.

s. auric′ulae poste′rior [NA], SYN posterior auricular *groove.*

basilar s., SYN basilar pontine s.

s. basila′ris pon′tis [NA], SYN basilar pontine s.

basilar pontine s., a median groove on the ventral surface of the pons varolii in which lies the basilar artery. SYN s. basilaris pontis [NA], basilar s.

s. bicipita′lis latera′lis [NA], SYN lateral bicipital *groove.*

s. bicipita′lis media′lis [NA], SYN medial bicipital *groove.*

calcaneal s., SYN interosseous *groove* of calcaneus.

s. calca′nei [NA], SYN interosseous *groove* of calcaneus.

calcarine s., a deep fissure on the medial aspect of the cerebral cortex, extending on an arched line from the isthmus of the fornicate gyrus back to the occipital pole, marking the border between the lingual gyrus below and the cuneus above it. The cortex in the depth of the sulcus corresponds to the horizontal meridian of the contralateral half of the visual field. SYN s.

su

calcarinus [NA], calcarine fissure, fissura calcarina, posthippo-campal fissure.

s. calcari′nus [NA], SYN calcarine s.

callosal s., SYN s. of corpus callosum.

callosomarginal s., SYN cingulate s.

s. callosomargina′lis, SYN cingulate s.

s. carot′icus [NA], SYN carotid *groove*.

carotid s., SYN carotid *groove*.

s. car′pi [NA], SYN carpal *groove*.

central s., a double-S-shaped fissure extending obliquely upward and backward on the lateral surface of each cerebral hemisphere at the boundary between frontal and parietal lobes. SYN s. centralis [NA], fissure of Rolando.

s. centra′lis [NA], SYN central s.

cerebellar sulci, grooves between the folia cerebelli; commonly called fissures in cerebellum.

cerebral sulci, the grooves between the cerebral gyri or convolutions. SYN sulci cerebri [NA].

sul′ci cer′ebri [NA], SYN cerebral sulci.

chiasmatic s., SYN chiasmatic *groove*.

cingulate s., a fissure on the mesial surface of the cerebral hemisphere, bounding the upper surface of the cingulate gyrus (callosal convolution); the anterior portion is called the pars subfrontalis; the posterior portion which curves up to the supero-medial margin of the hemisphere and borders the paracentral lobule posteriorly, the pars marginalis. SYN s. cinguli [NA], callosomarginal fissure, callosomarginal s., s. callosomarginalis, s. of cingulum.

s. cin′guli [NA], SYN cingulate s.

s. of cingulum, SYN cingulate s.

circular s. of insula, a semicircular fissure demarcating the insula from the opercula above, below, and behind. SYN s. circularis insulae [NA], circular s. of Reil, limiting s. of Reil.

s. circula′ris in′sulae [NA], SYN circular s. of insula.

circular s. of Reil, SYN circular s. of insula.

collateral s., a long, deep sagittal fissure on the undersurface of the temporal lobe, marking the border between the fusiform gyrus laterally and the hippocampal and lingual gyri medially; the great depth of the collateral s. results in a bulging of the floor of the occipital and temporal horn of the lateral ventricle, the collateral eminence. SYN s. collateralis [NA], s. occipitotemporalis [NA], collateral fissure, fissura collateralis, occipitotemporal s.

s. collatera′lis [NA], SYN collateral s.

s. corona′rius [NA], SYN coronary *groove*.

coronary s., SYN coronary *groove*.

s. cor′poris callo′si [NA], SYN s. of corpus callosum.

s. of corpus callosum, the fissure between the corpus callosum and the cingulate gyrus. SYN s. corporis callosi [NA], callosal s.

s. cos′tae [NA], SYN costal *groove*.

s. costae arte′riae subcla′viae [NA], SYN costal *groove* for subclavian artery.

costophrenic s., the recess between the ribs and the lateral-most portion of the diaphragm, partially occupied by the most caudal part of the lung; seen on radiographs as the costophrenic angle.

s. cru′ris heli′cis [NA], SYN *groove* of crus of the helix.

sul′ci cu′tis [NA], SYN skin *furrows*, under *furrow*.

s. ethmoida′lis [NA], SYN ethmoidal *groove*.

external spiral s., a concavity in the outer wall of the cochlear duct between the prominentia spiralis and the spiral organ. SYN s. spiralis externus [NA].

fimbriodentate s., a shallow groove between the fimbria and the dentate gyrus of the hippocampus. SYN s. fimbriodentatus.

s. fimbriodenta′tus, SYN fimbriodentate s.

s. fronta′lis infe′rior [NA], SYN inferior frontal s.

s. fronta′lis me′dius, SYN middle frontal s.

s. fronta′lis supe′rior [NA], SYN superior frontal s.

s. frontomargina′lis, SEE middle frontal s.

gingival s., the space between the surface of the tooth and the free gingiva. SYN s. gingivalis [NA], gingival crevice, gingival space, subgingival space.

s. gingiva′lis [NA], SYN gingival s.

gingivobuccal s., SYN alveolobuccal *groove*.

gingivolabial s., SYN alveololabial *groove*.

gingivolingual s., SYN alveololingual *groove*.

s. glu′teus [NA], SYN gluteal *fold*.

s. for greater palatine nerve, SYN greater palatine *groove*.

habenular s., a small groove located between the habenular trigone and the adjacent dorsal thalamus.

s. ham′uli pterygoi′dei [NA], SYN *groove* of pterygoid hamulus.

hippocampal s., a shallow groove between the dentate gyrus and the parahippocampal gyrus; the remains of a fissure extending deep into the hippocampus between Ammon's horn and the dentate gyrus which becomes obliterated during fetal development. SYN s. hippocampi [NA], dentate fissure, fissura dentata, fissura hippocampi, hippocampal fissure.

s. hippocam′pi [NA], SYN hippocampal s.

hypothalamic s., a groove in the lateral wall of the third ventricle on either side leading from the interventricular foramen to the aditus ad aqueductum cerebri; the s.-demarcated boundary between dorsal thalamus and hypothalamus. SYN s. hypothalamicus [NA], Monro's s.

s. hypothalam′icus [NA], SYN hypothalamic s.

inferior frontal s., a sagittal fissure on the lateral convex surface of each frontal lobe of the cerebrum demarcating the middle from the inferior frontal gyrus. SYN s. frontalis inferior [NA].

inferior petrosal s., SYN *groove* for inferior petrosal sinus.

inferior temporal s., the s. on the basal aspect of the temporal lobe that separates the fusiform gyrus from the inferior temporal gyrus on its lateral side. SYN s. temporalis inferior [NA], Clevenger's fissure.

s. infraorbita′lis [NA], SYN infraorbital *groove*.

infrapalpebral s., the hollow or furrow below the lower eyelid. SYN s. infrapalpebralis.

s. infrapalpebra′lis, SYN infrapalpebral s.

s. interme′dius ante′rior, SYN anterior intermediate s.

s. interme′dius poste′rior [NA], SYN posterior intermediate s.

internal spiral s., a concavity in the floor of the cochlear duct formed by the overhanging labium vestibulare. SYN s. spiralis internus [NA].

interparietal s., SYN intraparietal s.

intertubercular s., SYN intertubercular *groove*.

s. intertubercula′ris [NA], SYN intertubercular *groove*.

s. interventricula′ris ante′rior [NA], SYN anterior interventricular *groove*.

s. interventricula′ris cor′dis, SEE anterior interventricular *groove*, posterior interventricular *groove*.

s. interventricula′ris poste′rior [NA], SYN posterior interventricular *groove*.

intragracile s., a fissure between the gracilis minor and gracilis posterior lobuli of the cerebellum. SYN s. intragracilis.

s. intragra′cilis, SYN intragracile s.

intraparietal s., a horizontal s. extending back from the postcentral s. over some distance, then dividing perpendicularly into two branches so as to form, with the postcentral s., a figure H. It divides the parietal lobe into superior and inferior parietal lobules. SYN s. intraparietalis [NA], interparietal s., intraparietal s. of Turner, Turner's s.

s. intraparieta′lis [NA], SYN intraparietal s.

intraparietal s. of Turner, SYN intraparietal s.

labial s., a furrow between the developing lip and gum. SYN labiodental s., lip s., primary labial groove.

labiodental s., SYN labial s.

s. lacrima′lis [NA], SYN lacrimal *groove*.

lateral cerebral s., the deepest and most prominent of the cortical fissures, extending from the anterior perforated substance first laterally at the deep incisure between the frontal and temporal lobes, then back and slightly upward over the lateral aspect of the cerebral hemisphere, with the superior temporal gyrus as its lower bank, the insula forming its greatly expanded floor. Two short side branches, the ramus anterior and ramus ascendens, divide the inferior frontal gyrus into an orbital part, triangular part, and opercular part. SYN s. lateralis cerebri [NA], fissura cerebri lateralis, lateral cerebral fissure, sylvian fissure, fissure of Sylvius.

s. latera′lis ante′rior [NA], SYN anterolateral s.

s. latera′lis cer′ebri [NA], SYN lateral cerebral s.

s. latera′lis poste′rior [NA], SYN posterolateral s.

lateral occipital s., one of several variable sulci on the lateral aspect of the occipital lobe of each cerebral hemisphere, bounding the lateral occipital convolutions. SYN s. occipitalis lateralis.

s. lim′itans [NA], SYN limiting s.

s. lim′itans fos′sae rhomboi′deae [NA], SYN limiting s. of rhomboid fossa.

limiting s., the medial longitudinal groove on the inner surface of the neural tube separating the alar and basal plates. SYN s. limitans [NA].

limiting s. of Reil, SYN circular s. of insula.

limiting s. of rhomboid fossa, a lateral groove running the whole length of the floor of the rhomboid fossa on either side of the midline, representing the remains of the s. demarcating the alar (dorsal) from the basal (ventral) plate of the embryonic rhombencephalon. SYN s. limitans fossae rhomboideae [NA].

lip s., SYN labial s.

longitudinal s. of heart, SEE anterior interventricular *groove*, posterior interventricular *groove*.

lunate s., SYN lunate cerebral s.

lunate cerebral s., a small, inconstant semilunar groove on the cortical convexity near the occipital pole, marking the anterior border of the striate cortex (area 17) and considered homologous with the major s. of the same name that is a more constant feature of the cerebral cortex in monkeys and apes. SYN s. lunatus cerebri [NA], ape fissure, lunate fissure, lunate s., simian fissure.

s. luna′tus cer′ebri [NA], SYN lunate cerebral s.

malleolar s., SYN *groove* for tibialis posterior tendon.

s. malleola′ris [NA], SYN *groove* for tibialis posterior tendon.

s. ma′tricis un′guis, the cutaneous furrow in which the lateral border of the nail is situated. SYN groove of nail matrix, vallecula unguis.

medial s. of crus cerebri, a groove in the lateral wall of the interpeduncular fossa of the midbrain from which the rootlets of the oculomotor nerve emerge. SYN s. medialis cruris cerebri [NA], s. nervi oculomotorii, s. of the oculomotor nerve.

s. media′lis cru′ris cer′ebri [NA], SYN medial s. of crus cerebri.

median s. of fourth ventricle, the shallow midline groove in the floor of the ventricle. SYN s. medianus ventriculi quarti [NA].

median frontal s., SYN middle frontal s.

s. media′nus lin′guae [NA], SYN median *groove* of tongue.

s. media′nus poste′rior medul′lae oblonga′tae [NA], SYN posterior median s. of medulla oblongata.

s. media′nus poste′rior medul′lae spina′lis [NA], SYN posterior median s. of spinal cord.

s. media′nus ventric′uli quar′ti [NA], SYN median s. of fourth ventricle.

mentolabial s., the indistinct line separating the lower lip from the chin. SYN mentolabial furrow, s. mentolabialis.

s. mentolabia′lis, SYN mentolabial s.

middle frontal s., a relatively shallow sagittal fissure of the brain dividing the middle frontal convolution into an upper and lower part; this s. is found only in humans and anthropoid apes; at its anterior extremity it bifurcates, the two branches spreading out laterally and constituting the frontomarginal s. SYN median frontal s., s. frontalis medius.

middle temporal s., the s. between the middle temporal gyrus and inferior temporal gyrus. SYN s. temporalis medius.

s. for middle temporal artery, SYN *groove* for middle temporal artery.

Monro's s., SYN hypothalamic s.

s. mus′culi subcla′vii [NA], SYN subclavian *groove*.

s. mylohyoi′deus [NA], SYN mylohyoid *groove*.

s. nasolabia′lis, SYN nasolabial *groove*.

s. ner′vi oculomoto′rii, SYN medial s. of crus cerebri.

s. ner′vi petro′si majo′ris [NA], SYN *groove* of greater petrosal nerve.

s. ner′vi petro′si mino′ris [NA], SYN *groove* of lesser petrosal nerve.

s. ner′vi radia′lis [NA], SYN *groove* for radial nerve.

s. ner′vi spina′lis [NA], SYN *groove* for spinal nerve.

s. ner′vi ulna′ris [NA], SYN *groove* for ulnar nerve.

nymphocaruncular s., a groove between the labium minor and the border of the remains of the hymen, in which is the opening of the duct of the greater vestibular gland on either side. SYN nymphohymenal s., s. nymphocaruncularis.

s. nymphocaruncula′ris, SYN nymphocaruncular s.

nymphohymenal s., SYN nymphocaruncular s.

s. obturato′rius [NA], SYN obturator *groove*.

s. of occipital artery, SYN occipital *groove*.

s. occipita′lis latera′lis, SYN lateral occipital s.

s. occipita′lis supe′rior, SYN superior occipital s.

s. occipita′lis transver′sus [NA], SYN transverse occipital s.

occipitotemporal s., SYN collateral s.

s. occipitotempora′lis [NA], SYN collateral s.

s. of the oculomotor nerve, SYN medial s. of crus cerebri.

s. olfacto′rius [NA], SYN olfactory s.

s. olfacto′rius cavum na′si [NA], SYN olfactory s. of nasal cavity.

olfactory s., the sagittal s. on the inferior or orbital surface of each frontal lobe of the cerebrum, demarcating the straight gyrus from the orbital gyri, and covered on the orbital surface by the olfactory bulb and tract. SYN s. olfactorius [NA], olfactory groove.

olfactory s. of nasal cavity, the narrow groove in the nasal cavity above the agger nasi that leads from the atrium to the olfactory area. SYN s. olfactorius cavum nasi [NA].

orbital sulci, a number of irregularly disposed, variable sulci dividing the inferior or orbital surface of each frontal lobe of the cerebrum into the orbital gyri. SYN sulci orbitales [NA].

sul′ci orbita′les [NA], SYN orbital sulci.

s. palati′nus, pl. **sul′ci palati′ni** [NA], SYN palatine *groove*.

s. palati′nus ma′jor [NA], SYN greater palatine *groove*.

s. palatovagina′lis [NA], SYN palatovaginal *groove*.

sul′ci paraco′lici [NA], SYN paracolic *gutters*, under *gutter*.

paraglenoid s., SYN preauricular *groove*.

s. paraglenoida′lis, SYN preauricular *groove*.

parieto-occipital s., a very deep, almost vertically oriented fissure on the medial surface of the cerebral cortex, marking the border between the parietal lobe and the cuneus of the occipital lobe; its lower part curves forward and fuses with the anterior extent of the calcarine fissure (sulcus calcarinus); the great depth of this combined fissure causes a bulge in the medial wall of the occipital horn of the lateral ventricle, the calcar avis. SYN s. parieto-occipitalis [NA], fissura parietooccipitalis, parieto-occipital fissure.

s. parieto-occipita′lis [NA], SYN parieto-occipital s.

s. parolfacto′rius ante′rior, SYN anterior parolfactory s.

s. parolfacto′rius poste′rior, SYN posterior parolfactory s.

periconchal s., SYN *fossa* of anthelix.

s. poplit′eus, SYN popliteal *groove*.

---

su

postcentral s., the s. that demarcates the postcentral gyrus from the superior and inferior parietal lobules. SYN s. postcentralis [NA].

s. postcentra'lis [NA], SYN postcentral s.

posterior intermediate s., a longitudinal furrow between the posterior median and the posterolateral sulci of the spinal cord in the cervical region, marking the gracile fasciculus from the cuneate fasciculus. SYN s. intermedius posterior [NA], posterior intermediate groove.

posterior median s. of medulla oblongata, the longitudinal groove marking the posterior midline of the medulla oblongata; continuous below with the posterior median s. of the spinal cord. SYN s. medianus posterior medullae oblongatae [NA], posterior median fissure of the medulla oblongata.

posterior median s. of spinal cord, a shallow furrow in the median line of the posterior surface of the spinal cord. SYN s. medianus posterior medullae spinalis [NA], posterior median fissure of spinal cord.

posterior parolfactory s., a shallow groove on the medial surface of the hemisphere demarcating the subcallosal gyrus or precommissural septum from the parolfactory area. SYN s. parolfactorius posterior.

posterolateral s., a longitudinal furrow on either side of the posterior median s. of the spinal cord marking the line of entrance of the posterior nerve roots. SYN s. lateralis posterior [NA], posterolateral groove.

preauricular s., SYN preauricular groove.

precentral s., an interrupted fissure anterior to and in general parallel with the central s., marking the anterior border of the precentral gyrus. SYN s. precentralis [NA], s. verticalis.

s. precentra'lis [NA], SYN precentral s.

prechiasmatic s., SYN chiasmatic groove.

s. prechias'matis [NA], SYN chiasmatic groove.

s. promonto'rii cavitatis tympanicae [NA], SYN s. of promontory of tympanic cavity.

s. of promontory of tympanic cavity, a narrow branched groove running vertically over the surface of the promontory in the middle ear, lodging the tympanic plexus. SYN s. promontorii cavitatis tympanicae [NA].

s. of pterygoid hamulus, SYN groove of pterygoid hamulus.

s. pterygopalati'nus, SYN greater palatine groove.

s. pulmona'lis [NA], SYN paravertebral gutter.

pulmonary s., SYN paravertebral gutter.

rhinal s., the shallow rostral continuation of the collateral s. that delimits the rostral part of the parahippocampal gyrus from the fusiform or lateral occipitotemporal gyrus. One of the oldest sulci of the pallium, it marks the border between the neocortex and the allocortical (olfactory). SYN s. rhinalis [NA], rhinal fissure.

s. rhina'lis [NA], SYN rhinal s.

sagittal s., SYN groove for superior sagittal sinus.

s. of sclera, SYN scleral s.

s. scle'rae [NA], SYN scleral s.

scleral s., a slight groove on the external surface of the eyeball indicating the line of union of the sclera and cornea or limbus of cornea. SYN s. sclerae [NA], s. of sclera.

sigmoid s., SYN groove for sigmoid sinus.

s. si'nus petro'si inferio'ris [NA], SYN groove for inferior petrosal sinus.

s. si'nus petro'si superio'ris [NA], SYN groove for superior petrosal sinus.

s. si'nus sagitta'lis superio'ris [NA], SYN groove for superior sagittal sinus.

s. si'nus sigmoi'dei [NA], SYN groove for sigmoid sinus.

s. si'nus transver'si [NA], SYN groove for transverse sinus.

s. spino'sus, SYN stria spinosa.

s. spira'lis exter'nus [NA], SYN external spiral s.

s. spira'lis inter'nus [NA], SYN internal spiral s.

subclavian s., SYN subclavian groove.

s. subclavia'nus, SYN subclavian groove.

s. subcla'vius, SYN groove of lung for subclavian artery.

subparietal s., a s. continuing the direction of the cingulate s. from where the marginal part of that fissure bends upward; it forms the upper boundary of the posterior portion of the cingulate gyrus. SYN s. subparietalis [NA].

s. subparieta'lis [NA], SYN subparietal s.

superior frontal s., a sagittal fissure on the superior surface of each frontal lobe of the cerebrum starting from the precentral s.; it forms the lateral boundary of the superior frontal convolution. SYN s. frontalis superior [NA].

superior longitudinal s., SYN groove for superior sagittal sinus.

superior occipital s., one of several small and variable sulci bordering the superior occipital gyri on the upper aspect of the occipital lobe of the cerebrum. SYN s. occipitalis superior.

superior petrosal s., SYN groove for superior petrosal sinus.

superior temporal s., the longitudinal s. that separates the superior and middle temporal gyri. SYN s. temporalis superior [NA], superior temporal fissure.

supra-acetabular s., SYN supra-acetabular groove.

s. supra-acetabula'ris [NA], SYN supra-acetabular groove.

talar s., SYN interosseous groove of talus.

s. ta'li [NA], SYN interosseous groove of talus.

sul'ci tempora'les transver'si [NA], SYN transverse temporal sulci.

s. tempora'lis infe'rior [NA], SYN inferior temporal s.

s. tempora'lis me'dius, SYN middle temporal s.

s. tempora'lis supe'rior [NA], SYN superior temporal s.

s. ten'dinis mus'culi fibula'ris lon'gi [NA], ✶official alternate term for groove for tendon of peroneus longus muscle.

s. ten'dinis mus'culi flexo'ris hal'lucis lon'gi [NA], SYN groove for tendon of flexor hallucis longus.

s. ten'dinis mus'culi perone'i lon'gi [NA], SYN groove for tendon of peroneus longus muscle. (2) the groove distal to the tuberosity of the cuboid bone.

terminal s., SYN s. terminalis.

s. termina'lis [NA], (1) s. terminalis linguae [NA]; a V-shaped groove, with apex pointing backward, on the surface of the tongue, marking the separation between the oral, or horizontal, and the pharyngeal, or vertical, parts; (2) s. terminalis atrii dextri [NA]; a groove on the surface of the right atrium of the heart, marking the junction of the primitive sinus venosus with the atrium. SYN terminal s.

tonsillolingual s., the space between the palatine tonsil and the tongue.

transverse occipital s., the posterior, vertical limb of the intraparietal s. SYN s. occipitalis transversus [NA].

s. for transverse sinus, SYN groove for transverse sinus.

transverse temporal sulci, the shallow sulci that demarcate the transverse temporal gyri on the opercular surface of the superior temporal gyrus. SYN sulci temporales transversi [NA].

s. tu'bae auditi'vae [NA], SYN groove for auditory tube.

Turner's s., SYN intraparietal s.

s. tympan'icus [NA], SYN tympanic groove.

s. for vena cava, SYN groove for inferior venae cava.

s. ve'nae ca'vae [NA], SYN groove for inferior venae cava.

s. ve'nae ca'vae crania'lis [NA], SYN groove for superior vena cava.

s. ve'nae subcla'viae [NA], SYN groove for subclavian vein.

s. ve'nae umbilica'lis [NA], SYN sulcus of umbilical vein.

sul'ci veno'si [NA], SYN venous grooves, under groove.

s. ventra'lis, SYN anterior median fissure of spinal cord.

s. for vertebral artery, SYN groove for vertebral artery.

s. vertica'lis, SYN precentral s.

vomeral s., SYN vomeral groove.

s. vomera'lis [NA], SYN vomeral groove, vomeral groove.

s. vo'meris [NA], SYN vomeral groove.

s. vomerovagina'lis [NA], SYN vomerovaginal groove.

△**sulf-, sulfo-.** **1.** Prefix denoting that the compound to the name of which it is attached contains a sulfur atom. This spelling (rather than sulph-, sulpho-) is preferred by the American Chemical Society and has been adopted by the USP and NF, but not by the BP. **2.** Prefix form of sulfonic acid or sulfonate.

sul·fa (sŭl'fă). Denoting the sulfa drugs, or sulfonamides.

sul·fa·benz·am·ide (sŭl-fă-ben'ză-mīd). An antimicrobial of the sulfonamide group. SYN *N*-sulfanilylbenzamide.

sul·fa·cet·a·mide (sŭl-fă-set'ă-mīd). An antibacterial agent of the sulfonamide group, primarily used topically; s. sodium has the same uses as s. and also is used locally for eye infections and for prevention of gonorrheal ophthalmia in newborn infants. SYN *N*-sulfanilylacetamide.

sulf·ac·id (sŭlf-as'id). SYN thioacid.

sul·fa·cy·tine (sŭl-fă-sī'tēn). A sulfonamide used as an oral antibiotic in the treatment of urinary tract infections.

sul·fa·di·a·zine (sŭl-fă-dī'ă-zēn). N^1-2-Pyrimidinylsulfanilamide; one of a group of diazine derivatives of sulfanilamide, the pyrimidine analogue of sulfapyridine and sulfathiazole; one of the components of the triple sulfonamide mixture. It is an inhibitor of bacterial folic acid synthesis, which has been highly effective against pneumococcal, staphylococcal, and streptococcal infections, against infections with *Escherichia coli* and *Klebsiella pneumoniae*, and in acute gonococcal arthritis; s. sodium has the same uses.

sul·fa·di·me·thox·ine (sŭl'fă-dī-mě-thok'sēn). 2,4-Dimethoxy-6-sulfanilamide-1,3-diazine; a long-acting sulfonamide that is rapidly absorbed after oral administration and is slowly excreted by the kidney; it accumulates in the tissue and requires lower doses to attain effective tissue concentrations than do the other sulfonamides.

sul·fa·dim·i·dine (sŭl-fă-dim'i-dēn). SYN sulfamethazine.

sul·fa·dox·ine (sŭl-fă-dok'sēn). N^1-(5,6-dimethoxy-4-pyrimidyl)sulfanilamide; a long-acting sulfonamide, used with quinine and pyrimethamine to reduce the relapse rate of malaria. SYN sulformethoxine.

sul·fa·eth·i·dole (sŭl-fă-eth'i-dōl). N^1-(5-Ethyl-1,3,4-thiadiazole-2-yl)sulfanilamide; a sulfonamide used in the treatment of systemic and urinary tract infections.

sul·fa·fur·a·zole (sŭl-fă-fyūr'ă-zōl). SYN sulfisoxazole.

sul·fa·gua·ni·dine (sŭl-fă-gwahn'i-dēn). N^1-amidinosulfanilamide; the guanidine derivative of sulfanilamide. It is poorly absorbed from the gastroenteric tract; useful for bacterial infections of the lower intestinal tract and for preoperative sterilization of the intestinal tract; a goitrogen. SYN sulfaguine.

sul·fa·guine. SYN sulfaguanidine.

sul·fa·lene (sŭl'fă-lēn). N^1-(3-Methoxy-2-pyrimidyl)-sulfanilamide; a very long-acting sulfonamide that enhances, as do other sulfonamides and sulfones, the effectiveness of antimalarial agents such as pyrimethamine, chloroguanide, or cycloguanil.

sul·fa·mer·a·zine (sŭl-fă-mer'ă-zēn). N^1-(4-Methyl-2-pyrimidinyl)sulfanilamide; an antibacterial agent; one of the components of the triple sulfonamide mixture.

sul·fa·me·ter (sŭlf'ă-mē-ter). 2-(4-aminobenzenesulfon-amido)-5-methoxypyrimidine; a slowly excreted sulfonamide once used in the treatment of acute and chronic urinary tract infections. SYN sulfamethoxydiazine.

sul·fa·meth·a·zine (sŭl-fă-meth'ă-zēn). N^1-(4,6-dimethyl-2-pyrimidinyl)sulfanilamide; an antibacterial agent; one of the components of the triple sulfonamide mixture. SYN sulfadimidine.

sul·fa·meth·i·zole (sŭl-fă-meth'i-zōl). N^1-(5-Methyl-1,3,4-thiadiazol-2-yl)sulfanilamide; a sulfonamide useful for the treatment of urinary tract infection, because of its high solubility.

sul·fa·meth·ox·a·zole (sŭl'fă-meth-ok'să-zōl). N^1-(5-Methyl-3-isoxazoyl)sulfanilamide; a sulfonamide related chemically to sulfisoxazole, with a similar antibacterial spectrum, but a slower rate of absorption from the gastrointestinal tract and urinary excretion.

sul·fa·me·thox·y·di·a·zine (sŭl'fă-me-thok'si-dī'ă-zēn). SYN sulfameter.

sul·fa·me·thox·y·py·rid·a·zine (sŭl'fă-me-thok'si-pi-rid'ă-zēn). A long-acting sulfonamide that requires a single daily dose for maintaining effective tissue concentrations. S. acetyl is a prepa-

ration well suited for pediatric use because it is tasteless; it is also used to enhance the actions of quinine and other suppressants in the chemoprophylaxis of malaria.

sul·fa·mox·ole (sŭl-fă-mok'sōl). Sulfadimethyloxazole; N^1-(4,5-dimethyl-2-oxazolyl)sulfanilamide; an antimicrobial agent of the sulfonamide group.

***p*-sul·fa·myl·ac·e·tan·il·ide** (sŭl'fă-mil-as-e-tan'il-īd). SYN N^4-acetylsulfanilamide.

sul·fa·nil·a·mide (sŭl-fă-nil'ă-mīd). *p*-Aminobenzenesulfonamide; the first sulfonamide used for its chemotherapeutic effect in infections caused by some β-hemolytic streptococci, meningococci, gonococci, *Clostridium welchii*, and in certain infections of the urinary tract, especially those due to *Escherichia coli* and *Proteus vulgaris;* less effective than sulfapyridine in the treatment of pneumococcic, staphylococcic, and *Klebsiella pneumoniae* infections. Toxic manifestations include acidosis, cyanosis, hemolytic anemia, and agranulocytosis.

***N*-sul·fan·i·lyl·a·cet·a·mide** (sŭl-fan'i-lil-ă-set'ă-mīd). SYN sulfacetamide.

***N*-sul·fan·i·lyl·benz·a·mide** (sŭl-fan'i-lil-ben'ză-mīd). SYN sulfabenzamide.

sul·fa·ni·tran (sŭl-fă-nī'tran). 4'-[(*p*-Nitrophenyl)sulfamoyl]-acetanilide; an antimicrobial agent of the sulfonamide group.

sul·fa·per·in (sŭl'fă-per-in). N'-(5-methyl-2-pyrimidinyl)-sulfanilamide; an antimicrobial agent of the sulfonamide group. SYN isosulfamerazine.

sul·fa·phen·a·zole (sŭl-fă-fen'ă-zōl). A long-acting sulfonamide that is rapidly absorbed after oral administration; one dose is sufficient to maintain effective tissue concentration for 24 hours.

sul·fa·pyr·a·zine (sŭl-fă-pir'ă-zēn). N^1-2-Pyrazinylsulfanilamide; an antibacterial agent of the sulfonamide group.

sul·fa·pyr·i·dine (sŭl-fă-pir'i-dēn). An antibacterial agent of the sulfonamide group.

sul·fa·sal·a·zine (sŭl-fă-sal'ă-zēn). 5-[*p*-(2-pyridylsulfamyl)-phenylazo]salicylic acid; a sulfonamide (acid-azosulfa compound) with a marked affinity for connective tissues, especially for those rich in elastin, used in chronic ulcerative colitis; it is broken down in the body to amino salicylic acid and sulfapyridine. SYN salicylazosulfapyridine.

sul·fa·tase (sŭl'fă-tās). **1.** Trivial name for enzymes in EC group 3.1.6, the sulfuric ester hydrolases, which catalyze the hydrolysis of sulfuric esters (sulfates) to the corresponding alcohols plus inorganic sulfate; includes aryl-, sterol, glycol-, chondroitin, choline-, cellulose, cerebroside, and chondro- sulfatases. **2.** SYN arylsulfatase.

multiple s. deficiency, an inherited disorder (autosomal recessive) in which there is a failure to hydrolyze sulfatides and sulfated mucopolysaccharides; this failure leads to their accumulation in neural and extraneural tissues causing demyelination, sulfatiduria, facial and skeletal dysmorphism, etc.

sul·fate (sŭl'fāt). A salt or ester of sulfuric acid.

acid s., SYN bisulfate.

active s., SYN adenosine 3'-phosphate 5'-phosphosulfate.

s. adenylyltransferase, an enzyme that catalyzes a step in the pathway for the synthesis of active sulfate; the enzyme reacts ATP with s. to produce pyrophosphate and adenosine 5'-phosphosulfate (APS). SYN ATP sulfurylase.

codeine s., a water-soluble salt of codeine, often used in solid pharmaceutical dosage forms. Also used in cough preparations, where the drug suppresses the cough reflex.

dermatan s., an anticoagulant with properties similar to heparin and sharing with heparin a sulfated mucopolysaccharide structure; a repeating polymer of L-iduronic acid and *N*-acetyl-D-galactosamine. *O*-sulfation of iduronic acid residues at the C-2 position and of galactosamine residues at the C-4 and C-6 positions occurs to a variable extent. SYN chondroitin sulfate B.

iron s., a soluble iron salt frequently used as an iron supplement in tablets and liquid preparations. SYN ferrous sulfate.

polysaccharide s. esters, s. esters of polysaccharides often found in cell walls.

sul·fa·thi·a·zole (sŭl-fă-thī'ă-zōl). 2-Sulfanilylaminothiazole; 2-

(*p*-aminobenzenesulfonamido)thiazole; an antibacterial agent of the sulfonamide group.

sul·fa·ti·dates (sŭl'fă-ti-dāts). SYN sulfatides.

sul·fa·tides (sŭl'fă-tīdz). Cerebroside sulfuric esters containing one or more sulfate groups in the sugar portion of the molecule. SYN sulfatidates.

sul·fa·ti·do·sis (sŭl'fă-ti-dō'sis) [MIM*272200]. A combination of metachromatic leukodystrophy and mucopolysaccharidosis caused by deficiency of sulfatase enzymes such as arylsulfatases A, B, and C, and steroid sulfatases; characterized by coarse facial features, ichthyosis, hepatosplenomegaly, and skeletal abnormalities, with increased urinary excretion of dermatan and heparan sulfates. SEE ALSO metachromatic *leukodystrophy*.

sul·fa·tion (sŭl-fā'shŭn). Addition of sulfate groups as esters to preexisting molecules.

sulf·he·mo·glo·bin (sŭlf-hē'mō-glō-bin). SYN sulfmethemoglobin.

sulf·he·mo·glo·bi·ne·mia (sŭlf-hē'mō-glō-bi-nē'mē-ă). A morbid condition due to the presence of sulfhemoglobin in the blood; it is marked by a persistent cyanosis, but the blood count does not reveal any special abnormality in that fluid; it is thought to be caused by the action of hydrogen sulfide absorbed from the intestine.

sulf·hy·drate (sŭlf-hī'drāt). A compound (hydrosulfide) containing the ion HS⁻. SYN sulfohydrate.

sulf·hy·dryl (SH) (sŭlf-hī'dril). The radical –SH; contained in glutathione, cysteine, coenzyme A, lipoamide (all in the reduced state), and in mercaptans (R–SH). SYN thiel.

sul·fide (sŭl'fīd). A compound of sulfur in which the sulfur has a valence of –2; *e.g.*, Na₂S, HgS; also, a thioether (*i.e.*, R–S–R′, such as lanthionine). SYN sulfuret.

sul·fi·ki·nase (sŭl'fō-kīn'ās). SYN sulfotransferase.

sul·fin·di·got·ic ac·id (sŭl'fin-dī-got'ik). C₈H₅NOSO₃; formed by the action of sulfuric acid on indigo, a reaction that also yields indigo carmine.

sul·fin·py·ra·zone (sŭl-fin-pir'ă-zōn). 1,2-Diphenyl-4-(2-phenylsulfinylethyl)pyrazolidine-3,5-dione; an analgesic and uricosuric agent, useful in gout, that promotes the excretion of uric acid, probably by interfering with the tubular reabsorption of uric acid.

β-sul·fi·nyl·py·ru·vic ac·id (sŭl'fi-nil-pī-rū'vik). HO₂S–CH₂–CO–COOH, an intermediate product of L-cysteine catabolism in mammalian tissue.

sul·fi·so·mi·dine (sŭl-fi-sō'mi-dēn). N^1-(2,6-Dimethyl-4-pyrimidinyl)sulfanilamide; the structural isomer of sulfamethazine, used in the treatment of systemic and urinary tract infections.

sul·fi·sox·a·zole (sŭl-fi-sok'să-zōl). N^1-(3,4-dimethyl-5-isoxazolyl)sulfanilamide; a sulfonamide used chiefly in bacterial infections of the urinary tract. SYN sulfafurazole.

s. diolamine, the 2,2′-iminodiethanol salt of s.; used for intravenous, subcutaneous, or intramuscular administration.

sul·fite (sŭl'fīt). A salt of sulfurous acid; elevated in cases of molybdenum cofactor deficiency.

s. dehydrogenase, an oxidoreductase catalyzing the reaction of sulfite with 2 ferricytochrome *c* and water to sulfate and 2-ferrocytochrome *c*.

s. oxidase, a liver oxidoreductase (hemoprotein) catalyzing the reaction of inorganic sulfite ion with O₂ and water to produce sulfate ion and H₂O₂; a lower activity of this enzyme is observed in cases of molybdenum cofactor deficiency.

s. reductase, oxidoreductase catalyzing reduction of sulfite to H₂S using some reduced acceptor.

sul·fi·tu·ria (sŭlf'ĭt-ūr-ē-ă). Elevated levels of sulfites in the urine.

sulf·met·he·mo·glo·bin (sŭlf-met-hē'mō-glō-bin). The complex formed by H₂S (or sulfides) and ferric ion in methemoglobin. SYN sulfhemoglobin.

△**sulfo-.** SEE sulf-.

sul·fo·ac·id (sŭl'fō-as-id). **1.** SYN thioacid. **2.** SYN sulfonic acid.

3-sul·fo·al·a·nine (sŭl-fō-al'ă-nēn). SYN cysteic acid.

sul·fo·bro·mo·phtha·lein so·di·um (sŭl'fō-brō-mō-thal'ē-in). A triphenylmethane derivative excreted by the liver, used in testing hepatic function, particularly of the reticuloendothelial cells. SYN bromosulfophthalein, bromsulfophthalein.

sul·fo·cy·a·nate (sul-fō-sī'ă-nāt). SYN thiocyanate.

sul·fo·cy·an·ic ac·id (sŭl-fō-sī-an'ik). SYN thiocyanic acid.

*S***-sul·fo·cys·teine** (sŭl-fō-sis'tē-ēn). A sulfated derivative of cysteine that is elevated in individuals with a molybdenum cofactor deficiency.

3-sul·fo·ga·lac·to·syl·cer·a·mide (sŭl'fō-kīn-ās). A sulfatide that accumulates in individuals with metachromatic leukodystrophy.

sul·fo·gel (sŭl'fō-jel). A hydrogel with sulfuric acid instead of water as the dispersion means.

sul·fo·hy·drate (sŭl-fō-hī'drāt). SYN sulfhydrate.

sul·fo·ki·nase. SYN sulfotransferase.

sul·fol·y·sis (sul-fol'i-sis). Lysis brought on or accelerated by sulfuric acid.

sul·fo·mu·cin (sul-fō-myū'sin). A mucin containing sulfuric esters in its mucopolysaccharides or glycoproteins.

sul·fo·myx·in so·di·um (sŭl-fō-mik'sin). A mixture of sulfomethylated polymyxin B and sodium bisulfite; an antibacterial agent.

sul·fon·a·mides (sul-fon'ă-mīdz). The sulfa drugs, a group of bacteriostatic drugs containing the sulfanilamide group (sulfanilamide, sulfapyridine, sulfathiazole, sulfadiazine, and other sulfanilamide derivatives).

sul·fo·nate (sŭl'fō-nāt). A salt or ester of sulfonic acid.

sul·fone (sul-fōn). A compound of the general structure R′–SO₂–R″.

sul·fon·ic ac·id (sul-fon'ik). Any of the compounds in which a hydrogen atom of a CH group is replaced by the s. a. group, –SO₃H; general formula: R–SO₃H. SYN sulfoacid (2).

sul·fo·ni·um salts (sŭl-fō'nē-um). Compounds containing sulfur covalently linked to three moieties; *e.g.*, RS⁺(R′)R‴, such as *S*-adenosyl-L-methionine.

sul·fo·nyl·u·re·as (sŭl'fō-nil-yū-rē'ăz). Derivatives of isopropylthiodiazylsulfanilamide, chemically related to the sulfonamides, which possess hypoglycemic action. Belonging to this series are acetohexamide, azepinamide, chlorpropamide, fluphenmepramide, glymidine, hydroxyhexamide, heptolamide, indylamide, thiohexamide, tolazamide, and tolbutamide.

sul·fo·pro·tein (sŭl-fō-prō'tēn). A protein molecule containing sulfate groups.

6-sul·fo·qui·no·vo·syl di·ac·yl·glyc·er·ol (sŭl'fō-kwī'nō-vō-sil, -kwin'ō). Quinovose containing an SO₃H on C-6 and a doubly substituted glycerol on C-1; the sulfolipid occurring in all photosynthetic tissues.

sul·fo·rho·da·mine B (sŭl-fō-rō'dă-mēn) [C.I. 45100]. C₂₇H₂₉N₂O₇S₂Na; a xanthene dye derivative, a fluorochrome used for tagging proteins by a sulfamido condensation; employed in immuno-fluorescence alone or in combination with fluorescein isothiocyanate for the simultaneous microscopic detection of two antigens in contrasting red and green colors. SYN lissamine rhodamine B 200.

sul·for·me·thox·ine (sŭl'fōr-me-thok'sēn). SYN sulfadoxine.

sul·fo·sal·i·cyl·ic ac·id (sŭl'fō-sal-i-sil'ik). HOC₆H₃(CO₂H)SO₃H; 3-carboxy-4-hydroxybenzenesulfonic acid; used as a test for albumin and ferric ion. SYN salicylsulfonic acid.

sul·fo·sol (sŭl'fō-sol). A hydrosol with sulfuric acid instead of water as the dispersion means.

sul·fo·trans·fer·ase (sŭl-fō-trans'fer-ās). Generic term for enzymes in EC sub-subclass 2.8.2 catalyzing the transfer of a sulfate group from 3′-phosphoadenylyl sulfate (active sulfate) to the hydroxyl group of an acceptor, producing the sulfated derivative and 3′-phosphoadenosine 5′-phosphate. SYN sulfikinase, sulfokinase.

sulf·ox·ide (sŭl-fok'sīd). The sulfur analog of a ketone, R′–SO–R″.

sulf·ox·one so·di·um (sŭl-fok'sōn). Disodium sulfonyl-*bis*(*p*-phenyleneimino)dimethanesulfinate; an antileprotic.

sul·fur (S) (sŭl′fer). An element, atomic no. 16, atomic wt. 32.066, that combines with oxygen to form s. dioxide (SO_2) and s. trioxide (SO_3), and these with water to make strong acids, and with many metals and nonmetallic elements to form sulfides; mildly laxative; has been used to treat rheumatism, gout, and bronchitis, and externally in the treatment of skin diseases. SYN brimstone. [L. *sulfur*, brimstone, sulfur]

s. dioxide, SO_2; a colorless, nonflammable gas with a strong, suffocating odor; a powerful reducing agent used to prevent oxidative deterioration of food and medicinal products. SEE ALSO sulfurous acid. SYN sulfurous oxide.

s. iodide, has been used in the treatment of certain skin diseases.

liver of s., SYN sulfurated *potash.*

precipitated s., sublimed s. boiled with lime water, the lime being removed from the precipitate by washing with diluted hydrochloric acid; used in preparing s. ointment and in the treatment of various skin disorders. SYN lac sulfuris, milk of sulfur.

roll s., sublimed s. melted and cast in cylindrical molds; sometimes called brimstone.

soft s., an allotropic form obtained by dropping very hot melted s. into water; it is then temporarily of a viscid or waxy consistency.

sublimed s., used in preparing s. ointment and in the treatment of various skin disorders. SYN flowers of sulfur.

s. trioxide, SO_3; forms sulfuric acid, H_2SO_4, by its reaction with water. SYN sulfuric oxide.

vegetable s., SYN lycopodium.

washed s., sublimed s. macerated in diluted ammonia water to remove the free acid; same therapeutic uses as sublimed s.

wettable s., s. prepared from calcium polysulfide solution containing a protective colloid such as casein; it is easily dispersed and suspended in water.

sul·fur-35 (^{35}S). A radioactive sulfur isotope; a beta emitter with a half-life of 87.2 days; used as a tracer in the study of metabolism of cysteine, cystine, methionine, etc.; also used to estimate, with labeled sulfate, extracellular fluid volumes.

sul·fu·ret (sŭl′fer-et). SYN sulfide.

sul·fur group. The elements sulfur, selenium, and tellurium; they form dibasic acids with hydrogen, and their oxyacids are also dibasic.

sul·fu·ric ac·id (sŭl-fyūr′ik). H_2SO_4; a colorless, nearly odorless, heavy, oily, corrosive liquid containing 96% of the absolute acid; used occasionally as a caustic. SYN oil of vitriol.

fuming s. a., SYN Nordhausen s. a.

Nordhausen s. a., s. a. containing sulfurous acid gas in solution. SYN fuming s. a. [named for *Nordhausen*, a town in Saxony where it was first prepared]

sul·fu·ric ether (sul-fyūr′ik). SYN diethyl ether.

sul·fu·ric ox·ide. SYN *sulfur* trioxide.

sul·fu·rous (sŭl′fŭr-ŭs). Designating a sulfur compound in which sulfur has a valence of +4 as contrasted to sulfuric compounds in which sulfur has a valence of +6, or sulfides (−2).

sul·fu·rous ac·id. H_2SO_3; a solution of about 6% sulfur dioxide in water; used chiefly as a disinfectant and bleaching agent, and occasionally as a spray in tonsillitis; it has been used externally for its parasiticidal effect in various skin diseases.

sul·fu·rous ox·ide. SYN *sulfur* dioxide.

sul·fur·yl (sŭl′fŭr-il). The bivalent radical, $-SO_2-$.

sul·fy·drate (sŭl-fī′drăt). A compound of SH^-.

sul·in·dac (sŭl-in′dak). *cis*-5-Fluoro-2-methyl-1-[(*p*-methylsulfinyl]benzylidene)]indene-3-acetic acid; a nonsteroidal anti-inflammatory agent with analgesic and antipyretic actions. S. is a prodrug which is reduced to an active drug.

sul·i·so·ben·zone (sū-lī′sō-ben′zōn). 5-Benzoyl-4-hydroxy-2-methoxybenzene sulfonic acid; a sunscreen agent.

Sulkowitch, Hirsh W., U.S. physician, *1906. SEE S.'s *reagent.*

△**sulph-, sulpho-.** SEE sulf-.

sul·pir·ide (sŭl′pir-īd). *N*-[(1-Ethyl-2-pyrrolidinyl)methyl]-5-sulfamoyl-*o*-anisamide; an antidepressant.

sul·thi·ame (sŭl-thi′ăm). *p*-Tetrahydro-2*H*-1,2-thiazin-2-yl)-benzenenesulfonamide, *S,S*-dioxide; an anticonvulsant used in the treatment of temporal lobe epilepsy and grand mal with psychomotor seizures; may cause ataxia, paresthesias, and psychotic episodes.

Sulzberger, Marion B., U.S. dermatologist, 1895–1983. SEE Bloch-S. *disease;* syndrome; S.-Garbe *disease, syndrome.*

sum·ma·tion (sŭm-ā′shŭn). The aggregation of a number of similar neural impulses or stimuli. [Mediev. L. *summatio,* fr. *summo,* pp. *-atus,* to sum up, fr. L. *summa,* sum]

s. of stimuli, cumulative muscular or neural effects produced by the frequent repetition of stimuli.

Sumner, F.W., 20th century British surgeon. SEE S.'s *sign.*

sun·burn (sŭn′bern). Erythema with or without blistering caused by exposure to critical amounts of ultraviolet light, usually within the range of 260 to 320 nm in sunlight (UVB). SYN erythema solare.

sun·down·ing (sŭn′down-ing). The onset or exacerbation of delirium during the evening or night with improvement or disappearance during the day; most often seen in mid and later stages of dementing disorders, such as Alzheimer's disease.

sun·flow·er seed oil (sŭn′flow-er). Oil from the seeds of *Helianthus annuus* (family Compositae); the glycerides consist mainly of the mixed triglycerides, each containing one or two linoleic acid radicals; used as a food, and in dietary supplements.

sun·screen (sŭn′skrēn). A topical product that protects the skin from ultraviolet-induced erythema and resists washing off; its use also reduces formation of solar keratoses and may prevent ultraviolet-B-induced skin cancer and wrinkling.

sun·stroke (sŭn′strōk). A form of heatstroke resulting from undue exposure to the sun's rays, probably caused by the action of actinic rays combined with high temperature; symptoms are those of heatstroke, but often without fever. SYN heliosis, ictus solis, insolation (2), siriasis, solar fever (2).

△**super-.** (Properly prefixed to words of L. derivation) denoting in excess, above, superior, or in the upper part of; often the same usage as L. *supra-*. Cf. hyper-. [L. *super,* above, beyond]

su·per·ab·duc·tion (sū-per-ab-dŭk′shŭn). Abduction of a limb beyond the normal limit.

su·per·a·cid·i·ty (sū′per-a-sid′i-tē). An excess of acid; excessive acidity.

su·per·a·cro·mi·al (sū-per-ă-krō′mē-ăl). Above the acromion process. SYN supra-acromial.

su·per·ac·tiv·i·ty (sū-per-ak-tiv′i-tē). Abnormally great activity. SYN hyperactivity (1).

su·per·a·cute (sū′per-ă-kyūt′). Extremely acute; marked by extreme severity of symptoms and rapid progress, as of the course of a disease.

su·per·a·li·men·ta·tion (sū′per-al′i-men-tā′shŭn). SYN hyperalimentation.

su·per·a·nal (sū-per-ā′năl). SYN supra-anal.

su·per·an·ti·gen. An antigen that interacts with the T cell receptor in a domain outside of the antigen recognition site. This type of interaction induces the activation of larger numbers of T cells compared to antigens that are presented in the antigen recognition site. SEE ALSO antigen.

su·per·cil·i·ary (sū-per-sil′ē-ār-ē). Relating to or in the region of the eyebrow. SYN supraciliary.

su·per·cil·i·um, pl. **su·per·cil·i·a** (sū′per-sil′ē-ŭm, -ă) [NA]. **1.** SYN eyebrow. **2.** An individual hair of the eyebrow. [L. fr. *super,* above, + *cilium,* eyelid]

su·per·coil·ing. SYN superhelicity.

su·per·di·crot·ic (sū-per-dī-krot′ik). SYN hyperdicrotic.

su·per·dis·ten·tion (sū′per-dis-ten′shŭn). SYN hyperdistention.

su·per·duct (sūper-dŭkt). To elevate or draw upward. [L. *super-duco,* pp. *-ductus,* to lead over]

su·per·e·go (sū-per-ē′gō). In psychoanalysis, one of the three components of the psychic apparatus in the freudian structural framework, the other two being the ego and the id. It is an outgrowth of the ego that has identified itself unconsciously with important persons, such as parents, from early life, and which results from incorporating the values and wishes of these persons and subsequently societal norms as part of one's own standards to form the "conscience."

su·per·e·rup·tion. Movement of a tooth beyond the normal plane of occlusion due to the loss of its antagonist(s).

su·per·ex·ci·ta·tion (sū'per-ek-sī-tā'shŭn). **1.** The act of exciting or stimulating unduly. **2.** A condition of extreme excitement or stimulation.

su·per·ex·ten·sion (sū-per-eks-ten'shŭn). SYN hyperextension.

su·per·fat·ted (sū'per-fat'ed). With additional fat added, as in the case of soap.

su·per·fe·ta·tion (sū'per-fe-tā'shŭn). The presence of two fetuses of different ages, not twins, in the uterus, due to the impregnation of two ova liberated at successive periods of ovulation; an obsolete concept. SYN hypercyesis, hypercyesia, multifetation, superimpregnation.

su·per·fi·cial (sū-per-fish'ăl). **1.** Cursory; not thorough. **2.** Pertaining to or situated near the surface. **3.** SYN superficialis. [L. *superficialis,* fr. *superficies,* surface]

su·per·fi·ci·a·lis (sū'per-fish-ē-ā'lis) [NA]. Situated nearer the surface of the body in relation to a specific reference point. Cf. profundus. SYN sublimis (2), superficial (3). [L.]

s. vo'lae, SYN superficial palmar *branch* of radial artery.

su·per·fi·cies (su-per-fish'ĭ-ēz). Outer surface; facies. [L. the top surface, fr. *super,* above, + *facies,* figure, form]

su·per·flex·ion (sū-per-flek'shŭn). SYN hyperflexion.

su·per·fuse (sū-per-fyūs'). To flush a fluid over the top of a tissue. Cf. perfuse, perifuse.

su·per·fu·sion (sū-per-fyū'zhŭn). The act of superfusing.

su·per·gen·u·al (sū-per-jen'yū-ăl). Above the knee or any genu.

su·per·hel·i·ci·ty (sū'per-hē-li'si-tē). Referring to native duplex DNA structure in which there is further twisting or coiling of the double helix. SYN supercoiling.

su·per·im·preg·na·tion (sū'per-im-preg-nā'shŭn). SYN superfetation.

su·per·in·duce (sū'per-in-dūs). To induce or bring on in addition to something already existing.

su·per·in·fec·tion (sū'per-in-fek'shŭn). A new infection in addition to one already present.

su·per·in·vo·lu·tion (sū'per-in-vō-lū'shŭn). An extreme reduction in size of the uterus, after childbirth, below the normal size of the nongravid organ. SYN hyperinvolution.

su·pe·ri·or (sū-pēr'ē-ōr). **1.** Situated above or directed upward. **2** [NA]. In human anatomy, situated nearer the vertex of the head in relation to a specific reference point; opposite of inferior. SYN cranial (2). [L. comparative of *superus,* above]

su·per·lac·ta·tion (sū'per-lak-tā'shŭn). The continuance of lactation beyond the normal period. SYN hyperlactation.

su·per·lig·a·men (sū-per-lig'ă-men). A retentive dressing; a bandage retaining a surgical dressing in place. [L. *ligamen,* bandage]

su·per·me·di·al (sū-per-mē'dē-ăl). Above the middle of any part.

su·per·mo·til·i·ty (sū'per-mō-til'i-tē). SYN hyperkinesis.

su·per·na·tant (sū-per-nā'tănt). SEE supernatant *fluid.* [super- + L. *natare,* to swim]

su·per·nu·mer·ary (sū-per-nū'mer-ār-ē). Exceeding the normal number. SYN epactal. [super- + L. *numerus,* number]

su·per·nu·tri·tion (sū'per-nū-trish'ŭn). Overeating leading to obesity. SYN hypernutrition.

su·per·o·lat·er·al (sū-per-ō-lat'er-ăl). At the side and above.

su·per·ov·u·la·tion (sū'per-ō-vyū-lā'shŭn). Ovulation of a greater than normal number of ova; usually the result of the administration of exogenous gonadotropins.

su·per·ox·ide (sū-per-oks'īd). An oxygen free radical, O_2^-, which is toxic to cells.

s. dismutase (SOD), an enzyme that the dismutation reaction, $2O_2^- + 2H^+ \rightarrow H_2O_2 + O_2$; there are three isozymes of SOD: an extracellular form (ECSOD) that contains copper and zinc, a cytoplasmic form that also contains copper and zinc, and a mito-

chondrial form that contains manganese; a deficiency of SOD is associated with amyotrophic lateral sclerosis.

su·per·par·a·site (sū-per-par'ă-sīt). A member of a large population of parasites living on a host, usually a parasitic hymenopteran larva in its insect host. SEE ALSO parasitoid.

su·per·par·a·sit·ism (sū-per-par'ă-si-tizm). **1.** Association between parasitic Hymenoptera and their insect hosts. **2.** An excess of parasites of the same species in a host, overtaxing the defense mechanism to the degree that disease or death results, in contrast to multiple parasitism.

su·per·pe·tro·sal (sū-per-pe-trō'săl). Above or at the upper part of the petrous portion of the temporal bone.

su·per·pig·men·ta·tion (sū'per-pig-men-tā'shŭn). SYN hyperpigmentation.

su·per·sat·u·rate (sū-per-sach'ŭ-rāt). To make a solution hold more of a salt or other substance in solution than it will dissolve when in equilibrium with that salt in the solid phase; such solutions are usually unstable with respect to precipitating the excess salt or substance and becoming saturated.

su·per·scrip·tion (sū'per-skrip'shŭn). The beginning of a prescription, consisting of the injunction, *recipe,* take, usually denoted by the sign ℞. [L. *super-scribo,* pp. *-scriptus,* to write upon or over]

su·per·son·ic (sū'per-son'ik). **1.** Pertaining to or characterized by a speed greater than the speed of sound. SEE ALSO hypersonic. **2.** Pertaining to sound vibrations of high frequency, above the level of human audibility. SEE ALSO ultrasonic. [super- + L. *sonus,* sound]

su·per·struc·ture (sū-per-strŭk'chūr). A structure above the surface.

implant denture s., the denture which is retained and stabilized by the implant denture substructure.

su·per·ten·sion (sū-per-ten'shŭn). Extreme tension; incorrectly used as a synonym of high blood pressure, or hyperpiesis.

su·per·volt·age (sū'per-vol'tij). In radiation therapy, a descriptor for high energy radiation above one thousand volts.

su·pi·nate (sū'pi-nāt). **1.** To assume, or to be placed in, a supine (face upward) position. **2.** To perform supination of the forearm or of the foot. [L. *supino,* pp. *-atus,* to bend backwards, place on back, fr. *supinus,* supine]

su·pi·na·tion (sū'pi-nā'shŭn). The condition of being supine; the act of assuming or of being placed in a supine position.

s. of the foot, inversion and abduction of the foot, causing an elevation of the medial edge.

s. of the forearm, rotation of the forearm in such a way that the palm of the hand faces foreward when the arm is in the anatomical position, or upward when the arm is extended at a right angle to the body.

su·pi·na·tor (sū'pi-nā-ter, -tōr). A muscle that produces supination of the forearm. SEE supinator *muscle,* biceps brachii *muscle.*

su·pine (sū-pīn'). **1.** Denoting the body when lying face upward. **2.** Supination of the forearm or of the foot. [L. *supinus*]

su·pine. Body position when lying on the back with the face up.

sup·pe·da·ni·um, pl. **sup·pe·da·nia** (sŭp-ĕ-dā'nē-ŭm, -ă). An application to the sole of the foot. [Late L., a footstool, fr. L. *sub,* beneath, + *pes,* foot]

sup·port (sŭ-pōrt'). **1.** SYN supporter. **2.** In dentistry, a term used to denote resistance to vertical components of masticatory force. [L. *supporto,* to carry]

sup·port·er (sŭ-pōrt'er). An apparatus intended to hold in place a dependent or pendulous part, prolapsed organ, or joint. SYN support (1). [see support]

sup·pos·i·to·ry (sŭ-poz'i-tōr-ē). A small solid body shaped for ready introduction into one of the orifices of the body other than the oral cavity (*e.g.,* rectum, urethra, vagina), made of a substance, usually medicated, which is solid at ordinary temperatures but melts at body temperature. S. bases usually used are theobroma oil, glycerinated gelatin, hydrogenated vegetable oils, mixtures of polyethylene glycols of various molecular weights, and fatty acid esters of polyethylene glycol. [L. *suppositorium,* fr. *suppositorius,* placed underneath]

glycerin s., a conical translucent dosage form for rectal administration intended for the relief of constipation; frequently used in young children. Contains glycerin and a stiffening agent such as sodium stearate (a soap). Action is produced by lubrication, water retention, and local irritation.

sup·pres·sion (sŭ-presh′ŭn). **1.** Deliberately excluding from conscious thought. Cf. repression. **2.** Arrest of the secretion of a fluid, such as urine or bile. Cf. retention (2). **3.** Checking of an abnormal flow or discharge, as in s. of a hemorrhage. **4.** The effect of a second, mutation which overwrites a phenotypic change caused by a previous mutation at a different point on the chromosome. SEE epistasis. **5.** Inhibition of vision in one eye when dissimilar images fall on corresponding retinal points. [L. *sub-primo* (*subp-*), pp. *-pressus*, to press down]

immune s., s. of the immune response by some compound or agent.

intergenic s., SEE suppressor *mutations*, under *mutation*.

intragenic s., SEE suppressor *mutations*, under *mutation*.

sup·pres·sor (sŭ-pres′ōr). A compound that suppresses the effects of mutation or suppresses what would be a normal course of events.

amber s., a mutant gene that codes for a tRNA whose anticodon has been altered so that the altered tRNA responds to UAG codons as well.

sup·pu·rant (sŭp′yūr-ant). **1.** Causing or inducing suppuration. **2.** An agent with this action. [L. *suppurans*, causing suppuration]

sup·pu·rate (sŭp′yŭr-āt). To form pus. [L. *sup-puro* (*subp-*), pp. *-atus*, to form *pus* (*pur*), pus]

sup·pu·ra·tion (sŭp′yŭ-rā′shŭn). The formation of pus. SYN pyesis, pyogenesis, pyopoiesis, pyosis. [L. *suppuratio* (see suppurate)]

sup·pu·ra·tive (sŭp′yŭr-ă-tiv). Forming pus.

△**supra-.** A position above the part indicated by the word to which it is joined; in this sense, the same as super-; opposite of infra-. [L. *supra*, on the upper side]

su·pra-a·cro·mi·al (sū-pră-ă-krō′mē-ăl). SYN superacromial.

su·pra-a·nal (sū-pră-ā′năl). Above the anus. SYN superanal.

su·pra-au·ric·u·lar (sū-pră-aw-rik′yū-lăr). Above the auricle or pinna of the ear.

su·pra-ax·il·lary (sū′pră-ak′si-lār′ē). Above the axilla.

su·pra·buc·cal (sū-pră-bŭk′ăl). Above the cheek.

su·pra·bulge (sū′pră-bŭlj). The portion of the crown of a tooth that converges toward the occlusal surface of the tooth.

su·pra·car·di·nal (sū-pră-kar′di-năl). Lying dorsal to the anterior or posterior cardinal veins in the embryo.

su·pra·cer·e·bel·lar (sū-pră-ser-ĕ-bel′ar). On or above the surface of the cerebellum.

su·pra·ce·re·bral (sū-pră-ser′ĕ-brăl, -sĕ-rē′brăl). On or above the surface of the cerebrum.

su·pra·cho·roid (sū-pră-kō′royd). On the outer side of the choroid of the eye.

su·pra·cho·roi·dea (sū′pră-kō-roy′dē-ă). SYN suprachoroid *lamina*.

su·pra·cil·i·ary (sū-pră-sil′ē-ār-ē). SYN superciliary.

su·pra·cla·vic·u·lar (sū-pră-kla-vik′yū-lăr). Above the clavicle, denoting some cutaneous nerves.

su·pra·cla·vic·u·lar·is (sū′pră-kla-vik′yū-lār′is). SEE supraclavicular *muscle*.

su·pra·con·dy·lar (sū-pră-kon′di-lăr). Above a condyle. SYN supracondyloid.

su·pra·cos·tal (sū-pră-kos′tăl). Above the ribs.

su·pra·cot·y·loid (sū-pră-kot′i-loyd). Above the cotyloid cavity, or acetabulum.

su·pra·cris·tal (sū-pră-kris′tăl). Above a crest or ridge; specifically used to denote a line or plane across the summits of the iliac crests.

su·pra·di·a·phrag·mat·ic (sū-pră-dī-ă-frag-mat′ik). Above the diaphragm.

su·pra·duc·tion (sū-pră-dŭk′shŭn). The upward rotation of one eye. SYN sursumduction.

su·pra·ep·i·con·dy·lar (sū-pră-ep′i-kon′di-lăr). Above an epicondyle.

su·pra·gle·noid (sū-pră-glē′noyd). Above the glenoid cavity or fossa.

su·pra·glot·tic (sū-pră-glot′ik). Above the glottis.

su·pra·he·pat·ic (sū-pră-he-pat′ik). Above the liver.

su·pra·hy·oid (sū-pră-hī′oyd). Above the hyoid bone, denoting, among other things, a group of muscles.

su·pra·in·gui·nal (sū-pră-ing′gwin-ăl). Above the inguinal region, or groin.

su·pra·in·tes·ti·nal (sū-pră-in-tes′ti-năl). Above the intestine.

su·pra·lim·i·nal (sū-pră-lim′i-năl). More than just perceptible; above the threshhold for conscious awareness. Cf. subliminal. [supra- + L. *limen*, threshold]

su·pra·lum·bar (sū-pră-lŭm′bar). Above the lumbar region.

su·pra·mal·le·o·lar (sū-pră-mal-ē-ō-lăr). Above a malleolus.

su·pra·mam·ma·ry (sū-pră-mam′ă-rē). Above the mammary gland.

su·pra·man·dib·u·lar (sū-pră-man-dib′yū-lăr). Above the mandible.

su·pra·mar·gin·al (sū-pră-mar′jin-ăl). Above any margin; denoting especially the s. gyrus.

su·pra·mas·toid (sū-pră-mas′toyd). Above the mastoid process of the temporal bone.

su·pra·max·il·la (sū′pră-mak-sil′ă). Obsolete term for maxilla.

su·pra·max·il·lary (sū-pră-mak′si-lār-ē). Above the maxilla.

su·pra·men·tal (sū-pră-men′tăl). Above the chin.

su·pra·men·ta·le (sū′pră-men-tā′lē). In cephalometrics, the most posterior midline point, above the chin, on the mandibula between the infradentale and the pogonion. SYN point B. [supra- + L. *mentum*, chin]

su·pra·na·sal (sū-pră-nā′săl). Above the nose.

su·pra·neu·ral (sū-pră-nū′răl). Above the neural axis.

su·pra·nu·cle·ar (sū-pră-nū′klē-er). Above (cranial to) the level of the motor neurons of the spinal or cranial nerves; the pathways the suprasegmental nerve fibers follow to reach the motor cell bodies in the brainstem; as used in clinical neurology, s. indicates disorders of movement caused by destruction or functional impairment of brain structures other than the motor neurons, such as the motor cortex, pyramidal tract, or striate body; *e.g.*, supranuclear palsy, as distinguished from the nuclear (or flaccid, or "lower motor neuron") paralysis that results from destruction or functional impairment of the motor neurons or their axons in a peripheral nerve.

su·pra·oc·clu·sion (sū′pră-ō-klū′zhŭn). An occlusal relationship in which a tooth extends beyond the occlusal plane.

su·pra·or·bit·al (sū-pră-ōr′bi-tăl). Above the orbit, either on the face or within the cranium; denoting numerous structures. SEE canal, foramen, notch, nerve.

su·pra·or·bi·to·me·a·tal (soo′pra-or-bit-ō-mē-at′al). Above or at the top of both the orbit and the external acoustic meatus; denotes a line or plane.

su·pra·pa·tel·lar (sū-pră-pă-tel′ăr). Above the patella, denoting especially a bursa.

su·pra·pel·vic (sū-pră-pel′vik). Above the pelvis.

su·pra·phys·i·o·log·ic, su·pra·phys·i·o·log·i·cal (sū′pră-fiz-ē-ō-loj′ik, -loj′i-kăl). Denoting any dose (of a chemical agent that either is or mimics a hormone, neurotransmitter, or other naturally occurring agent) that is larger or more potent than would occur naturally, or the effects of such a dose. Cf. homeopathic (2), pharmacologic (2), physiologic (4).

su·pra·pu·bic (sū-pră-pyū′bik). Above the pubic bone.

su·pra·re·nal (sū′pră-rē′năl). **1.** Above the kidney. SYN surrenal. **2.** Pertaining to the suprarenal glands. [supra- + L. *ren*, kidney]

△ Combining forms	[NA] Nomina Anatomica
Word*Finder* **Multi-term entry finder** Preceding letter A	[MIM] Mendelian Inheritance in Man
A.D.A.M. Anatomy Plates Between letters L and M	☆ Official alternate term
Appendices: Following letter Z	☆[NA] Official alternate Nomina Anatomica term
SYN Synonym; Cf., compare	**High Profile Term**

su·pra·scap·u·lar (sū-pră-skap′yū-lăr). Above the scapula, denoting especially an artery, vein and nerve.

su·pra·scle·ral (sū-pră-sklēr′ăl). On the outer side of the sclera, denoting the s. or perisclerotic space between the sclera and the fascia bulbi.

su·pra·sel·lar (sū-pră-sel′ăr). Above or over the sella turcica.

su·pra·spi·nal (sū-pră-spī′năl). Above the vertebral column or any spine.

su·pra·spi·na·lis (sū-pră-spi-nā′lis). SEE supraspinalis *muscle*.

su·pra·spi·na·tus (sū-pră-spī-nā′tŭs). SEE supraspinatus *muscle*.

su·pra·spi·nous (sū-pră-spī′nŭs). Above any spine; especially above one or more of the vertebral spines (*e.g.*, supraspinous ligament) or the spine of the scapula.

su·pra·sta·pe·di·al (sū-pră-sta-pēd′ē-ăl). Above the stapes.

su·pra·ster·nal (sū-pră-ster′năl). Above the sternum.

su·pra·syl·vi·an (sūp-ră-sil′vē-an). Above the fissure of Sylvius or lateral cerebral sulcus.

su·pra·sym·phys·ary (sū-pră-sim-phiz′ă-rē). Above the pubic symphysis.

su·pra·tem·po·ral (sū-pră-tem′pŏ-răl). Above the temporal region.

su·pra·ten·to·ri·al (sū′pră-ten-tōr′ē-ăl). Denoting cranial contents located above the tentorium cerebelli.

su·pra·tho·rac·ic (sū-pră-thō-ras′ik). Above or in the upper part of the thorax.

su·pra·ton·sil·lar (sū-pră-ton′si-lăr). Above the tonsil; denoting a recess above and slightly back of the tonsil.

su·pra·troch·le·ar (sū-pră-trok′lē-ăr). Above a trochlea, denoting a nerve.

su·pra·tur·bi·nal (sū-pră-ter′bi-năl). SYN supreme nasal *concha*.

su·pra·tym·pan·ic (sū-pră-tim-pan′ik). Above the tympanic cavity.

su·pra·vag·i·nal (sū-pră-vaj′i-năl). Above the vagina, or above any sheath.

su·pra·val·var (sū-pră-val′văr). Above the valves, either pulmonary or aortic. SYN supravalvular.

su·pra·ven·tric·u·lar (sū-pră-ven-trik′yū-lăr). Above the ventricles; especially applied to rhythms originating from centers proximal to the ventricles, namely in the atrium, A-V node, or A-V junction, in contrast to rhythms arising in the ventricles themselves.

su·pra·ver·gence (sū-pră-ver′jens). Obsolete term for upward rotation of an eye. [supra- + L. *vergo*, to incline or turn]

su·pra·ver·sion (sū-pră-ver′zhŭn). **1.** A turning (version) upward. **2.** In dentistry, the position of a tooth when it is out of the line of occlusion in an occlusal direction; a deep overbite. **3.** In ophthalmology, binocular conjugate rotation upward. [supra- + L. *verto*, pp. *versus*, to turn]

su·pro·fen (sū-prō′fen). *p*-2-Thenoylhydratropic acid; a nonsteroidal anti-inflammatory agent with antipyretic and analgesic properties; similar to ibuprofen.

su·ra (sū′ră) [NA]. SYN sural *region*. [L.]

su·ral (sū′răl). Relating to the calf of the leg.

sur·al·i·men·ta·tion (ser-al′i-men-tā′shŭn). SYN hyperalimentation. [Fr. *sur*, fr. L. *super*, above]

sur·a·min so·di·um (sū′ră-min). $C_{51}H_{34}N_6O_{23}S_6Na_6$; a complex derivative of urea; used in the treatment of trypanosomiasis, onchocerciasis, and pemphigus.

sur·face (ser′făs). The outer part of any solid. SYN face (2), facies (2). [F. fr. L. *superficius*, see superficial]

acromial articular s. of clavicle, a small oval facet on the lateral end of the clavicle for articulation with the acromion. SYN facies articularis acromialis claviculae [NA], acromial articular facies of clavicle.

anterior s., the surface of a structure or part of the body that faces forward. The NA recognizes an anterior surface (facies anterior ...) without qualification on the following structures: pancreas (... pancreatis [NA]); patella (... patellae [NA]); prostate (... prostatae [NA]); radius (... radii [NA]); suprarenal gland (...

glandulae suprarenalis [NA]); ulna (... ulnae [NA]). SYN facies anterior [NA].

anterior s. of arm, SYN anterior *region* of arm.

anterior articular s. of dens, the curved articular facet on the anterior aspect of the dens of the axis that articulates with the facet for the dens of the axis anterior arch of the atlas. SYN facies articularis anterior dentis [NA].

anterior s. of cornea, the external surface of the cornea. SYN facies anterior corneae [NA].

anterior s. of elbow, SYN anterior *region* of elbow.

anterior s. of eyelids, SYN *facies* anterior palpebrarum.

anterior s. of forearm, SYN anterior *region* of forearm.

anterior s. of iris, the anterior surface of the iris of the eye. SYN facies anterior iridis [NA].

anterior s. of kidney, the anterior surface of the kidney. SYN facies anterior renis [NA].

anterior s. of leg, SYN anterior *region* of leg.

anterior s. of lens, the anterior surface of the lens of the eye. SYN facies anterior lentis [NA].

anterior s. of lower limb, the anterior surface of the inferior limb. SYN facies anterior membri inferioris.

anterior s. of maxilla, the surface of the maxilla below the orbit and lateral to the nasal aperture. SYN facies anterior corporis maxillae [NA].

anterior s. of pancreas, the anterior surface of the pancreas. SYN facies anterior pancreatis [NA].

anterior s. of patella, the anterior surface of the patella. SYN facies anterior patellae [NA].

anterior s. of petrous part of temporal bone, the surface of the petrous part of the temporal bone contributing to the floor of the middle cranial fossa. SYN facies anterior partis petrosae ossis temporalis [NA].

anterior s. of prostate, the anterior surface of the prostate. SYN facies anterior prostatae [NA].

anterior s. of radius, the anterior surface of the radius. SYN facies anterior radii [NA].

anterior s. of suprarenal gland, the anterior surface of the suprarenal gland. SYN facies anterior glandulae suprarenalis [NA].

anterior s. of thigh, SYN anterior *region* of thigh.

anterior talar articular s. of calcaneus, underlies the head of the talus and contributes to the talocalcaneonavicular joint. SYN facies articularis talaris anterior calcanei [NA].

anterior s. of ulna, the anterior surface of the ulna. SYN facies anterior ulnae [NA].

anterolateral s. of shaft of humerus, the surface of the humerus lateral to the intertubercular groove. SYN facies anterior lateralis corporis humeri [NA], facies anterolateralis corporis humeri★ [NA].

anteromedial s. of shaft of humerus, the surface of the humerus between the anterior and medial borders of the bone. SYN facies anterior medialis corporis humeri [NA], facies anteromedialis corporis humeri★ [NA].

articular s., any articular surface. SYN facies articularis [NA].

articular s. of acromion, a small oval facet on the medial border of the acromion for articulation with the lateral end of the clavicle. SYN facies articularis acromii [NA].

articular s. of arytenoid cartilage, the oval surface on the undersurface of the muscular process of the arytenoid for articulation with the cricoid cartilage. SYN facies articularis cartilaginis arytenoideae [NA].

articular s. of head of fibula, the flat circular surface on the head of the fibula for articulation with the corresponding facet on the lateral condyle of the tibia. SYN facies articularis capitis fibulae [NA].

articular s. of head of rib, an articular surface on the head of a rib that articulates with the body of a vertebra. SYN facies articularis capitis costae [NA].

articular s. of patella, the posterior surface of the patella, covered with hyaline cartilage and subdivided by a vertical ridge into a larger lateral and a smaller medial surface for articulation with the corresponding condyles of the femur. SYN facies articularis patellae [NA].

articular s. of temporal bone, the smooth portion of the mandibular articular fossa and eminence of the temporal bone that articulates with the disk of the temporomandibular joint. SYN facies articularis ossis temporalis [NA].

articular s. of tubercle of rib, an oval facet on the inferomedial part of the tubercle of a rib for articulation with a facet on the transverse process of a vertebra. SYN facies articularis tuberculi costae [NA].

arytenoidal articular s. of cricoid, one of two oval facets on the superiorelateral margin of the cricoid lamina for articulation with the arytenoid cartilages. SYN facies articularis arytenoidea cricoideae [NA].

auricular s. of ilium, the irregular, L-shaped articular surface on the medial aspect of the ilium that articulates with the sacrum. SYN facies auricularis ossis ilii [NA].

auricular s. of sacrum, the rough articular surface on the lateral aspect of the sacrum that articulates with the ilium on each side. SYN facies auricularis ossis sacri [NA].

axial s., the s. of a tooth parallel with its long axis; the axial s.'s are the vestibular (labial or buccal), lingual, and contact (mesial or distal).

balancing occlusal s., SYN balancing *contact.*

basal s., the s. of the denture of which the detail is determined by the impression and which rests upon the basal seat.

buccal s., (1) SYN vestibular s. of tooth. **(2)** the mucosa of the cheek; **(3)** in prosthodontics, the side of a denture adjacent to the cheek.

calcaneal articular s. of talus, one of three articular surfaces on the talus for union with the calcaneus: facies articularis calcanea anterior tali, facies articularis calcanea media tali, and facies articularis calcanea posterior tali. SYN facies articularis calcanea tali [NA].

carpal articular s. of radius, the biconcave distal surface of the radius for articulation with the scaphoid bone laterally and the lunate medially. SYN facies articularis carpi radii [NA].

cerebral s., the internal s. of certain cranial bones; they are the greater wing of the sphenoid and the squamous part of the temporal bone. SYN facies cerebralis.

colic s. of spleen, the surface of the spleen in contact with the colon. SYN facies colica splenis [NA].

contact s. of tooth, the surface of a tooth that faces an adjacent tooth in the dental arch; the contact surface that is closest to the anterior midline of the dental arch is the mesial s. of a tooth; that farthest is the distal s. SYN facies approximalis dentis [NA], facies contactus dentis.

costal s., the surface of certain structures that face the ribs; they are the lungs and the scapula. SYN facies costalis [NA].

costal s. of lung, the surface of each lung that lies in contact with the costal pleura. SYN facies costalis pulmonis [NA].

costal s. of scapula, the concave aspect of the body of the scapula that faces the thorax and that principally lodges the subscapularis muscle. SYN facies costalis scapulae [NA].

cuboidal articular s. of calcaneus, the saddle-shaped surface on the anterior end of the calcaneus for articulation with the cuboid bone. SYN facies articularis cuboidea calcanei [NA].

denture basal s., SYN denture foundation s.

denture foundation s., that portion of the s. of a denture which has its contour determined by the impression and bears the greater part of the occlusal load. SYN denture basal s.

denture impression s., that portion of the s. of a denture which has its contour determined by the impression; it includes the borders of the denture and extends to the polished s.

denture occlusal s., that portion of the s. of a denture that makes contact or near contact with the corresponding s. of an opposing denture or tooth. SYN facies occlusalis dentis [NA], facies masticatoria, grinding s., masticating s., masticatory s., occlusal s. (2).

denture polished s., that portion of the denture which extends in an occlusal direction from the border of the denture and includes the palatal s.; it is the part of the denture base which is usually polished and includes the buccal and lingual s.'s of the teeth.

diaphragmatic s., the surface of an organ in contact with the diaphragm, as of the heart, liver, lungs, and spleen. SYN facies diaphragmatica [NA].

distal s. of tooth, the contact surface of a tooth that is directed away from the median plane of the dental arch; opposite to the mesial s. of a tooth. SYN facies distalis dentis [NA].

dorsal s., the dorsal surface of a structure such as the sacrum and the scapula. SYN facies dorsalis [NA].

dorsal s. of digit, the dorsal surface of a finger or toe. SYN facies digitalis dorsalis [NA].

dorsal s. of sacrum, the posterosuperior aspect of the sacrum marked by a median and two lateral sacral crests between which four dorsal sacral foramina are located on each side. SYN facies dorsalis ossis sacri [NA].

dorsal s. of scapula, the outer aspect of the body of the scapula, subdivided by the prominent spine of the scapula into a smaller supraspinous fossa and a larger infraspinous fossa. SYN facies dorsalis scapulae [NA].

external s., the outer convex surface of either the frontal or the parietal bone. SYN facies externa [NA].

external s. of frontal bone, the convex outer surface of the frontal bone. SYN facies externa ossis frontalis [NA].

external s. of parietal bone, the convex outer surface of the parietal bone. SYN facies externa ossis parietalis [NA].

facial s. of tooth, SYN vestibular s. of tooth.

fibular articular s. of tibia, the flat circular articular facet on the inferior and lateral aspect of the lateral condyle of the tibia for articulation with the head of the fibula. SYN facies articularis fibularis tibiae [NA].

gastric s. of spleen, the surface of the spleen in contact with the stomach. SYN facies gastrica splenis [NA].

glenoid s., SYN mandibular *fossa.*

gluteal s. of ilium, the external surface of the wing of the ilium marked by the anterior, posterior and inferior gluteal lines that separate the origins of the gluteal muscles. SYN facies glutea ossis ilii [NA].

grinding s., SYN denture occlusal s.

incisal s., SYN incisal *edge.*

inferior articular s. of tibia, the quadrilateral surface on the distal end of the tibia for articulation with the talus; it is concave anteroposteriorly and broader anteriorly. SYN facies articularis inferior tibiae [NA].

inferior s. of cerebellar hemisphere, it rests in the posterior cranial fossa and overlies the medulla; it includes the semilunaris inferior, biventer lobule, cerebellar tonsil, and flocculus. SYN facies inferior hemispherii cerebelli [NA].

inferior cerebral s., SYN *base* of brain.

inferior s. of pancreas, the surface of the body of the pancreas that faces downward. SYN facies inferior pancreatis [NA].

inferior s. of petrous part of temporal bone, inferior surface of petrous part of temporal bone; the portion of the petrous part of the temporal bone that contributes to the external base of the skull. SYN facies inferior partis petrosae ossis temporalis [NA].

inferior s. of tongue, the surface of the tongue that faces the floor of the oral cavity, its mucosa being thin, smooth and devoid of papillae. SYN facies inferior linguae [NA].

inferolateral s. of prostate, the surface of the prostate facing the body of the pubis and the pelvic diaphragm. SYN facies inferolateralis prostatae [NA].

infratemporal s. of maxilla, the convex posterolateral surface of the body of the maxilla that form the anterior wall of the infratemporal fossa. SYN facies infratemporalis maxillae [NA].

interlobar s.'s of lung, the pulmonary surfaces in the interlobar fissures of the lung. SYN facies interlobares pulmonis [NA].

internal s., the internal concave surface of either the frontal or the parietal bone. SYN facies interna [NA].

internal s. of frontal bone, the surface of the frontal bone that contributes to the wall of the cranial cavity. SYN facies interna ossis frontalis [NA].

internal s. of parietal bone, the concave surface of the parietal bone forming part of the wall of the cranial cavity. SYN facies interna ossis parietalis [NA].

intestinal s. of uterus, the posterosuperior surface of the uterus

su

with which loops of intestine come in contact. SYN facies intestinalis uteri [NA].

labial s., SYN vestibular s. of tooth.

lateral s., the surface of a part of the body that faces away from the midline. The NA recognizes a lateral surface on the following structures: fibula; ovary; radius; testis; tibia; zygomatic bone. SYN facies lateralis [NA].

lateral s. of arm, the lateral surface of the arm. SYN facies lateralis brachii.

lateral s. of fibula, the lateral surface of the fibula. SYN facies lateralis fibulae [NA].

lateral s. of finger, the lateral surface of a finger. SYN facies lateralis digiti manus.

lateral s. of leg, the lateral surface of the part of the inferior limb between the knee and the ankle. SYN facies lateralis cruris.

lateral s. of lower limb, the lateral surface of the inferior limb. SYN facies lateralis membri inferioris.

lateral malleolar s. of talus, that surface of the trochlea of the talus that articulates with the lateral malleolus of the fibula. SYN facies malleolaris lateralis tali [NA].

lateral s. of ovary, the surface of the ovary facing the pelvic wall. SYN facies lateralis ovarii [NA].

lateral s. of testis, the laterally directed surface of the testis. SYN facies lateralis testis [NA].

lateral s. of tibia, the laterally directed surface of the tibia. SYN facies lateralis tibiae [NA].

lateral s. of toe, the lateral surface of a toe. SYN facies lateralis digiti pedis.

lateral s. of zygomatic bone, the lateral surface of the zygomatic bone. SYN facies lateralis ossis zygomatici [NA].

lingual s. of tooth, the surface of a tooth that faces the tongue; opposite to the s. vestibulum dentis. SYN facies lingualis dentis [NA].

lunate s. of acetabulum, the curved articular surface that surrounds the acetabular fossa and articulates with the head of the femur. SYN facies lunata acetabuli [NA].

malleolar articular s. of fibula, the surface on the medial aspect of the lateral malleolus that articulates with the talus. SYN facies articularis malleoli fibulae [NA].

malleolar articular s. of tibia, the articular facet on the lateral surface of the medial malleolus for articulation with the side of the talus; it is continuous with the inferior articular surface of the tibia. SYN facies articularis malleoli tibiae [NA].

masticating s., SYN denture occlusal s.

masticatory s., SYN denture occlusal s.

maxillary s. of greater wing of sphenoid bone, aBCXYZ SYN facies maxillaris alae majoris.

maxillary s. of palatine bone, the lateral surface of the perpendicular plate of the palatine bone; SYN facies maxillaris ossis palatini [NA].

medial s., the surface of a part of the body that faces toward the midline. The NA recognizes a medial surface on the following structures: arytenoid cartilage; fibula; lung; ovary; testis; tibia; ulna. SYN facies medialis [NA].

medial s. of arytenoid cartilage, SYN *facies* medialis cartilaginis arytenoideae.

medial cerebral s., SYN medial s. of cerebral hemisphere.

medial s. of cerebral hemisphere, it faces, above as well as anterior and posterior to the corpus callosum, the falx cerebri; below it are the mesencephalon and the dura-covered medial wall of the middle cranial fossa. SYN facies medialis cerebri [NA], medial cerebral s.

medial s. of fibula, SYN *facies* medialis fibulae.

medial s. of lung, it consists of a vertebral part and a mediastinal part. SEE ALSO mediastinal s. of lung. SYN facies medialis pulmonis.

medial malleolar s. of talus, the surface of the trochlea of the talus that articulates with the medial malleolus of the tibia. SYN facies malleolaris medialis tali [NA].

medial s. of ovary, the surface of the ovary that faces the pelvic cavity. SYN facies medialis ovarii [NA].

medial s. of testis, SYN *facies* medialis testis.

medial s. of tibia, SYN *facies* medialis tibiae.

medial s. of toes, the medial surface of a toe. SYN facies medialis digiti pedis.

medial s. of ulna, SYN *facies* medialis ulnae.

mediastinal s. of lung, the part of the medial surface of a lung in contact with the mediastinum. SYN pars mediastinalis pulmonis [NA], facies mediastinalis pulmonis, mediastinal part of lung.

mesial s. of tooth, the contact surface of a tooth that is directed toward the median plane of the dental arch; opposite to the s. distalis dentis. SYN facies mesialis dentis [NA].

middle talar articular s. of calcaneus, underlies the head of the talus and contributes to the talocalcaneonavicular joint. SYN facies articularis talaris media calcanei [NA].

nasal s. of maxilla, the surface of the maxilla that forms part of the lateral nasal wall with a large defect (maxillary hiatus) posteriorly and the lacrimal sulcus in its midportion. SYN facies nasalis maxillae [NA].

nasal s. of palatine bone, (1) the nasal surface of the perpendicular lamina of the palatine bone that forms part of the lateral wall of the nasal cavity; (2) the nasal surface of the horizontal lamina of the palatine bone that forms part of the floor of the nasal cavity. SYN facies nasalis ossis palatini [NA].

navicular articular s. of talus, the large convex surface on the head of the talus for articulation with the navicular bone. SYN facies articularis navicularis tali [NA].

occlusal s., (1) the surface of a tooth that occludes with or contacts an opposing surface of a tooth in the opposing jaw; (2) SYN denture occlusal s.

orbital s., the surface of a bone which contributes to the walls of the orbit. The NA recognizes an orbital surface on the following bones: greater wing of the sphenoid bone; the maxilla; the frontal bone; the zygomatic bone. SYN facies orbitalis [NA].

palatine s. of horizontal plate of palatine bone, the inferior surface of the horizontal plate of the palatine bone. SYN facies palatina laminae horizontalis ossis palatini [NA].

palmar s. of fingers, the flat of the fingers; the flexor or anterior s. of the fingers. SYN facies digitalis ventralis [NA], facies digitalis palmaris☆ [NA], ventral s. of digit.

patellar s. of femur, the groove formed anteriorly between the anterosuperior portions of the femoral condyles that accommodates the patella. SYN facies patellaris femoris [NA], trochlea femoris.

pelvic s. of sacrum, the surface of the sacrum that faces downward and forward forming part of the posterior wall of the pelvic cavity. SYN facies pelvina ossis sacri [NA].

plantar s. of toe, SYN facies digitalis plantaris [NA].

popliteal s. of femur, the posterior surface of the lower end of the femur between the diverging lips of the linea aspera. SYN facies poplitea femoris [NA], planum popliteum, popliteal plane of femur.

posterior s., the surface of a part of the body that faces toward the posterior part of the body. The NA recognizes a posterior surface without qualification on the following structures: arm; arytenoid cartilage; cornea; eyelid; fibula; humerus; iris; kidney; leg; pancreas; prostate; radius; suprarenal gland; ulna. SYN facies posterior [NA].

posterior s. of arm, SYN posterior *region* of arm.

posterior articular s. of dens, the facet on the posterior surface of the dens of the axis that articulates with the transverse ligament of the atlas. SYN facies articularis posterior dentis [NA].

posterior s. of arytenoid cartilage, aBCXYZ

posterior s. of cornea, the posterior surface of the cornea. SYN facies posterior corneae [NA].

posterior s. of elbow, SYN posterior *region* of elbow.

posterior s. of eyelids, the internal surface of the eyelids, covered with conjunctiva. SYN facies posterior palpebrarum [NA].

posterior s. of fibula, the posterior surface of the fibula. SYN facies posterior fibulae [NA].

posterior s. of forearm, SYN posterior *region* of forearm.

posterior s. of iris, the posterior surface of the iris. SYN facies posterior iridis [NA].

posterior s. of kidney, the posterior surface of the kidney. SYN facies posterior renis [NA].

posterior s. of leg, SYN posterior *region* of leg. SYN facies cruralis posterior [NA], cruralis posterior, facies posterior cruris.

posterior s. of lens, the posterior surface of the lens of the eye. SYN facies posterior lentis [NA].

posterior s. of lower limb, the posterior surface of the inferior limb. SYN facies posterior membri inferioris.

posterior s. of pancreas, the posterior surface of the pancreas. SYN facies posterior pancreatis [NA].

posterior s. of petrous part of temporal bone, the surface of the petrous part of the temporal bone that contributes to the posterior cranial fossa. SYN facies posterior partis petrosae ossis temporalis [NA].

posterior s. of prostate, the posterior surface of the prostate. SYN facies posterior prostatae [NA].

posterior s. of radius, the posterior surface of the radius. SYN facies posterior radii [NA].

posterior s. of shaft of humerus, the posterior surface of the humerus. SYN facies posterior corporis humeri [NA].

posterior s. of suprarenal gland, the posterior surface of the suprarenal gland. SYN facies posterior glandulae suprarenalis [NA].

posterior talar articular s. of calcaneus, articulates with talus (subtalar joint) posterior to sinus tarsi. SYN facies articularis talaris posterior calcanei.

posterior s. of thigh, SYN posterior *region* of thigh.

posterior s. of tibia, the posterior surface of the tibia. SYN facies posterior tibiae [NA].

posterior s. of ulna, the posterior surface of the ulna. SYN facies posterior ulnae [NA].

pulmonary s. of heart, the lateral surface of the heart, directed toward the lungs; on the left it is principally the left ventricular wall; on the right it is the right atrial wall and the upper part of the right ventricular wall. SYN facies pulmonalis cordis [NA].

renal s. of spleen, the surface of the spleen in contact with the left kidney. SYN facies renalis lienis, facies renalis splenis.

renal s. of suprarenal gland, surface of suprarenal gland in contact with the kidney.

renal s. of the suprarenal gland, SYN *facies* renalis glandulae suprarenalis.

sacropelvic s. of ilium, the medial surface of the ilium behind and below the iliac fossa; it includes the iliac tuberosity, the auricular surface and the smooth pelvic surface below and in front of the auricular surface. SYN facies sacropelvina ossis ilii [NA].

sternal articular s. of clavicle, the oval surface on the sternal end of the clavicle that articulates with the fibrocartilaginous disk of the sternoclavicular joint. SYN facies articularis sternalis claviculae [NA].

sternocostal s. of heart, the anterior aspect of the heart, formed mostly by the right ventricle and to a lesser extent the left ventricle. SYN facies sternocostalis cordis [NA].

subocclusal s., a portion of the occlusal s. of a tooth which is below the level of the occluding portion of the tooth.

superior articular s. of tibia, the articular surface on the proximal end of the tibia that is divided into medial and lateral portions for articulation with the condyles of the femur. SYN facies articularis superior tibiae [NA].

superior s. of cerebellar hemisphere, it lies against the under surface of the tentorium and includes the ala lobuli centralis, quadrangular lobule, simple lobule, and superior semilunar lobule. SYN facies superior hemispherii cerebelli [NA].

superior s. of talus, the surface of the trochlea of the talus in contact with the inferior articular surface of the tibia. SYN facies superior tali [NA].

superolateral cerebral s., SYN superolateral s. of cerebrum.

superolateral s. of cerebrum, the aspect of the cerebral hemisphere that lies in contact with the flat bones of the skull; it includes parts of the frontal, parietal, temporal, and occipital lobes. SYN facies superolateralis cerebri [NA], cortical convexity, superolateral cerebral s.

symphysial s. of pubis, SYN *facies* symphysialis.

talar articular s. of calcaneus, any of the three facets of the calcaneus that articulate with the overlying talus; the talar articular surface anterior and middle talar articular surface contribute to the talocalcaneonavicular joint and are separated by the tarsal sinus from the posterior talar articular surface which enters into the subtalar joint. SYN facies articularis talaris calcanei [NA].

temporal s., the surface of a bone which contributes to the temporal fossa, namely, the greater wing of the sphenoid, the squamous part of the temporal, frontal and zygomatic bones. SYN facies temporalis [NA].

tentorial s., those areas of the occipital lobe (inferior aspect) and the cerebellum (superior aspect) that are apposed to the superior and inferior s.'s, respectively, of the tentorium cerebelli.

thyroidal articular s. of cricoid, one of two small circular facets on the lateral surface of the cricoid cartilage near the inferior margin of the junction of the arch and lamina for articulation with the inferior horns of the thyroid cartilage. SYN facies articularis thyroidea cricoideae [NA].

urethral s. of penis, the surface of the penis opposite to the dorsum penis. SYN facies urethralis penis [NA].

ventral s. of digit, SYN palmar s. of fingers.

vesical s. of uterus, the surface of the uterus facing the bladder and separated from it by the uterovesical pouch of peritoneum. SYN facies vesicalis uteri [NA].

vestibular s. of tooth, the surface of a tooth that faces the buccal or labial mucosa of vestibule of the mouth; opposite to the lingual s. of tooth. SYN facies vestibularis dentis [NA], facies facialis dentis [NA], buccal s. (1), facial s. of tooth, facies buccalis, facies labialis, labial s.

visceral s. of liver, the posteroinferior surface of the liver that faces adjacent abdominal organs; the porta hepatis and gallbladder are located on this surface. SYN facies visceralis hepatis [NA].

visceral s. of the spleen, the surface of the spleen in contact with adjacent viscera. SYN facies visceralis splenis [NA].

working occlusal s.'s, the s.'s of teeth upon which mastication can occur.

sur·face-ac·tive (ser′făs-ak′tiv). Indicating the property of certain agents of altering the physicochemical nature of surfaces and interfaces, bringing about lowering of interfacial tension; they usually possess both lipophilic and hydrophilic groups. SEE ALSO surfactant.

sur·fac·tant (ser-fak′tănt). 1. A surface-active agent, including substances commonly referred to as wetting agents, surface tension depressants, detergents, dispersing agents, emulsifiers, quaternary ammonium antiseptics, etc. 2. Those surface-active agents forming a monomolecular layer over pulmonary alveolar surfaces; lipoproteins that include lecithins and sphygomyelins that stabilize alveolar volume by reducing surface tension and altering the relationship between surface tension and surface area. [*surface active agent*]

nonionic s., a s. without a charged moiety.

zwitterionic s., a dipolar s.

sur·geon (ser′jŭn). 1. A physician who treats disease, injury, and deformity by operation or manipulation. 2. In England, formerly a practitioner without a degree of M.D. but with the license of the Royal College of Surgeons. [G. *cheirougos*; L. *chirurgus*]

attending s., a surgical member of the attending staff of a hospital.

dental s., a general practitioner of dentistry; a dentist with the D.D.S. or D.M.D. degree.

house s., the senior member of the surgical house staff responsible for the execution of the orders of the attending s., and who also substitutes when the latter is absent.

oral s., a dentist who specializes in oral surgery.

sur·geon gen·er·al (ser′jŭn-jen′ĕ-răl). The chief medical officer in the U.S. Army, Navy, Air Force, or Public Health Service. In some foreign military services any member of the medical corps who has the rank of general, not necessarily the chief medical officer.

sur·gery (ser′jer-ē). 1. The branch of medicine concerned with the treatment of disease, injury, and deformity by operation or

su

manipulation. **2.** The performance or procedures of an operation. [L. *chirurgia;* G. *cheir,* hand, + *ergon,* work]

ambulatory s., operative procedures performed on patients who are admitted to and discharged from a hospital on the same day.

aseptic s., the performance of an operation with sterilized hands, instruments, etc., and utilizing precautions against the introduction of infectious microorganisms from without.

closed s., s. without incision into skin, *e.g.,* reduction of a fracture or dislocation.

cosmetic s., s. in which the principal purpose is to improve the appearance, usually with the connotation that the improvement sought is beyond the normal appearance, and its acceptable variations, for the age and the ethnic origin of the patient. SYN esthetic s.

craniofacial s., simultaneous s. on the cranium and facial bones.

esthetic s., SYN cosmetic s.

featural s., rarely used term for plastic s. of the face, for correction or improvement of appearance.

keratorefractive s., SYN refractive *keratoplasty.*

laparoscopic s., operative procedure performed using minimally invasive surgical technique for exposure that avoids traditional incision. Visualization is achieved using a fiber optic instrument, usually attached to a video camera.

laparoscopically assisted s., operative procedure performed using combined laparoscopic and open techniques; most commonly applied to colon or small intestinal resections with anastomosis.

major s., SEE major *operation.*

microscopically controlled s., SYN Mohs' *chemosurgery.*

minimally invasive s., operative procedure performed in a manner derived to result in the smallest possible incision or no incision at all; includes laparoscopic, laparoscopically assisted, thoracoscopic, and endoscopic surgical procedures.

minor s., SEE minor *operation.*

Mohs' s., SYN Mohs' *chemosurgery.*

Mohs' micrographic s., SYN Mohs' *chemosurgery.*

open heart s., operative procedure(s) performed on or within the exposed heart, usually with cardiopulmonary bypass (as opposed to closed heart surgery).

oral s., the branch of dentistry concerned with the diagnosis and surgical and adjunctive treatment of diseases, injuries, and deformities of the oral and maxillofacial region.

orthognathic s., SYN surgical *orthodontics.*

orthopaedic s., the branch of s. that embraces the treatment of acute and chronic disorders of the musculoskeletal system, including injuries, diseases, dysfunction and deformities (orig. deformities in children) in the extremities and spine. SEE ALSO orthopaedics.

plastic s., the surgical specialty or procedure concerned with the restoration, construction, reconstruction, or improvement in the shape and appearance of body structures that are missing, defective, damaged, or misshapen.

reconstructive s., SEE plastic s.

stereotactic s., SYN stereotaxy.

thoracoscopic s., s. done using one or more endoscopic instruments.

transsexual s., procedures designed to alter a patient's external sexual characteristics so that they resemble those of the other sex.

video-assisted thoracic s. (VATS), a less morbid alternative to "open" thoracotomy that employs cameras, optic systems, percutaneous stapling devices, and assorted endoscopic graspers, retractors, and forceps. Also called video thoracoscopic surgery, it can be selectively applied to various pulmonary, pleural, and pericardial lesions.

sur·gi·cal (ser'ji-kăl). Relating to surgery.

sur·ra (ser'ă). A protozoal disease of camels, horses, mules, dogs, cattle, and other mammals in Africa, Asia, and Central and South America, caused by *Trypanosoma evansi;* infection is generally by mechanical transmission by a bloodsucking species of *Stomoxys* or *Tabanus.* SEE ALSO murrina. [East Indian name]

sur·re·nal (ser-rē'năl). SYN suprarenal (1).

sur·ro·gate (ser'ŏ-gāt). **1.** A person who functions in another's

life as a substitute for some third person such as a relative who assumes the nurturing and other responsibilities of the absent parent. **2.** A person who reminds one of another person so that one uses the first as an emotional substitute for the second. [L. *surrogo,* to put in another's place]

mother s., one who substitutes for or takes the place of the mother.

sur·sa·nure (ser-sā'nūr). A superficially healed ulcer, with pus beneath the surface. [Fr., fr. L. *super,* over, + *sanus,* healthy]

sur·sum·duc·tion (ser-sŭm-dŭk'shŭn). SYN supraduction. [L. *sursum,* upward, + *duco,* pp. -*ductus,* to draw]

sur·sum·ver·sion (ser-sŭm-ver'zhŭn). The act of rotating the eyes upward. [L. *sursum,* upward, + *verto,* pp. *versus,* to turn]

sur·veil·lance (ser-vā'lans). **1.** The collection, collation, analysis, and dissemination of data; a type of observational study that involves continuous monitoring of disease occurrence within a population. **2.** Ongoing scrutiny, generally using methods distinguished by practicability, uniformity, rapidity, rather than complete accuracy. [Fr. *surveiller,* to watch over, fr. L. *super-* + *vigilo,* to watch]

> Surveillance does not aim for accuracy or completeness; rather it is designed to provide practical and uniform results in a timely fashion, so that trends can be spotted and appropriate action taken. Such action might include further investigation of some aspect of an unfolding phenomenon, or even intervention. Surveillance is employed frequently in the monitoring of disease or factors influencing disease. The data being analyzed and interpreted may include 1) mortality and morbidity reports based on death certificates, hospital records, or general practice sentinels or notifications; 2) laboratory test results; 3) disease outbreak reports; 4) vaccine utilization-uptake and side effects; 5) reports of work- or school-related absences due to illness; (6) biological changes in known agents, vectors, or reservoirs of disease.

immune s., A theory that the immune system destroys tumor cells which are constantly arising during the life of the individual. SYN immunological s.

immunological s., SYN immune s.

post-marketing s., procedure implemented after a drug has been licensed for public use, designed to provide information on use and on occurrence of side effects, adverse effects, etc.

sur·vey (ser'vā). **1.** An investigation in which information is systematically collected but in which the experimental method is not used. **2.** a comprehensive examination or group of examinations to screen for one or more findings. **3.** a series of questions administered to a sample of individuals in a population. [O.Fr. *surveeir,* fr. Mediev.L. *supervideo,* fr. *super,* over, + *video,* to see]

field s., the planned collection of data among noninstitutionalized persons in the general population.

skeletal s., radiographic examination of all or selected parts of the skeleton, as for occult fractures, metastases, etc.

sur·vey·ing (ser-vā'ing). In dentistry, the procedure of locating and delineating the contour and position of the abutment teeth and associated structures before designing a removable partial denture.

sur·vey·or (ser-vā'er, ōr). In dentistry, the instrument used in surveying.

sur·viv·al (ser-vī'văl). Continued existence; persistence of life.

sus·cep·ti·bil·i·ty (su-sep-ti-bil'i-tē). **1.** Likelihood of an individual to develop ill effects from an external agent, such as *Mycobacterium tuberculosis,* high altitude, or ambient temperature. **2.** In magnetic resonance imaging, the loss of magnetization signal caused by rapid phase dispersion because of marked local inhomogeneity of the magnetic field, as with the multiple air-soft tissue interfaces in the lung; s. measurement can estimate calcium content in trabecular bone.

sus·pen·sion (sŭs-pen'shŭn). **1.** A temporary interruption of any function. **2.** A hanging from a support, as used in the treatment of spinal curvatures or during the application of a plaster jacket. **3.**

Fixation of an organ, such as the uterus, to other tissue for support. **4.** The dispersion through a liquid of a solid in finely divided particles of a size large enough to be detected by purely optical means; if the particles are too small to be seen by microscope but still large enough to scatter light (Tyndall phenomenon), they will remain dispersed indefinitely and are then called a colloidal s. SYN coarse dispersion. **5.** A class of pharmacopeial preparations of finely divided, undissolved drugs (*e.g.,* powders for s.) dispersed in liquid vehicles for oral or parenteral use. [L. *suspensio,* fr. *sus-pendo,* pp. *-pensus,* to hang up, suspend]

amorphous insulin zinc s., SYN prompt insulin zinc s.

chromic phosphate P 32 colloidal s., a pure β-emitting colloidal, nonabsorbable radiopharmaceutical administered into body cavities such as the pleural or peritoneal spaces to control malignant effusions. SEE ALSO *sodium* phosphate P 32.

Coffey s., an operative technique following partial excision of the cornu, as in salpingectomy, whereby the broad and the round ligament are sutured over the cornual wound to restore continuity of the peritoneum and to suspend the uterus on the operated side.

crystalline insulin zinc s., SYN extended insulin zinc s.

extended insulin zinc s., a long-acting insulin s., obtained from beef, with an approximate time of onset of 7 hours and a duration of action of 36 hours. SYN crystalline insulin zinc s.

insulin zinc s., a sterile buffered s. with zinc chloride, containing 40 or 80 units per ml; the solid phase of the s. consists of a mixture of 7 parts of crystalline insulin and 3 parts of amorphous insulin. SYN lente insulin.

magnesia and alumina oral s., a mixture of magnesium hydroxide and variable amounts of aluminum oxide; used as an antacid.

prompt insulin zinc s., sterile s. of insulin in buffered water for injection, modified by the addition of zinc chloride such that the solid phase of the s. is amorphous; it contains 40 or 80 units per ml; the duration of action is equivalent to that of insulin injection. SYN amorphous insulin zinc s., semilente insulin.

sus·pen·soid (sŭs-pen′soyd). A colloidal solution in which the disperse particles are solid and lyophobe or hydrophobe, and are therefore sharply demarcated from the fluid in which they are suspended. SYN hydrophobic colloid, lyophobic colloid, suspension colloid. [suspension + G. *eidos,* resemblance]

sus·pen·so·ry (sŭs-pen′sŏ-rē). **1.** Suspending; supporting; denoting a ligament, a muscle, or other structure that keeps an organ or other part in place. **2.** A supporter applied to uplift a dependent part, such as the scrotum or a pendulous breast.

sus·ten·tac·u·lar (sŭs-ten-tak′yū-lăr). Relating to a sustentaculum; supporting.

sus·ten·tac·u·lum, pl. **sus·ten·tac·u·la** (sŭs′ten-tak′yū-lŭm, -lă) [NA]. A structure that serves as a stay or support to another. [L. a prop, fr. *sustento,* to hold upright]

s. li′enis, SYN splenorenal *ligament.*

s. ta′li [NA], support of the talus, a bracket-like lateral projection from the medial surface of the calcaneus, the upper surface of which presents a facet for articulation with the talus.

su·sur·rus (sŭ-ser′ŭs). SYN murmur (1). [L.]

s. au′rium, murmur in the ear.

Sutter blood group. See Blood Groups appendix.

Sutton, Richard L., U.S. dermatologist, 1878–1952. SEE S.'s *disease* (1), *nevus.*

Sutton, Richard L., Jr., U.S. dermatologist, *1908. SEE S.'s *disease* (2), *ulcer.*

SUTURA

su·tu·ra, pl. **su·tu·rae** (sū′tū′ră, -rē) [NA]. SYN suture. [L. a sewing, a suture, fr. *suo,* pp. *sutus,* to sew]

s. corona′lis [NA], SYN coronal *suture.*

sutu′rae cra′nii [NA], SYN cranial *sutures,* under *suture.*

s. ethmoidolacrima′lis [NA], SYN ethmoidolacrimal *suture.*

s. ethmoidomaxilla′ris [NA], SYN ethmoidomaxillary *suture.*

s. fronta′lis [NA], SYN frontal *suture.*

s. frontoethmoida′lis [NA], SYN frontoethmoidal *suture.*

s. frontolacrima′lis [NA], SYN frontolacrimal *suture.*

s. frontomaxilla′ris [NA], SYN frontomaxillary *suture.*

s. frontonasa′lis [NA], SYN frontonasal *suture.*

s. frontozygomat′ica [NA], SYN frontozygomatic *suture.*

s. inci′siva [NA], SYN incisive *suture.*

s. infraorbita′lis, SYN infraorbital *suture.*

s. intermaxilla′ris [NA], SYN intermaxillary *suture.*

s. internasa′lis [NA], SYN internasal *suture.*

s. interparieta′lis, SYN sagittal *suture.*

s. lacrimoconcha′lis [NA], SYN lacrimoconchal *suture.*

s. lacrimomaxilla′ris [NA], SYN lacrimomaxillary *suture.*

s. lambdoi′dea [NA], SYN lambdoid *suture.*

s. meto′pica [NA], SYN metopic *suture.*

s. nasofronta′lis, SYN frontonasal *suture.*

s. nasomaxilla′ris [NA], SYN nasomaxillary *suture.*

s. no′tha (nō′tă), SYN false *suture.* [G. fem. of *nothos,* spurious]

s. occipitomastoi′dea [NA], SYN occipitomastoid *suture.*

s. palati′na media′na [NA], SYN median palatine *suture.*

s. palati′na transver′sa [NA], SYN transverse palatine *suture.*

s. palatoethmoida′lis [NA], SYN palatoethmoidal *suture.*

s. palatomaxilla′ris [NA], SYN palatomaxillary *suture.*

s. parietomastoi′dea [NA], SYN parietomastoid *suture.*

s. pla′na [NA], SYN plane *suture.*

s. sagitta′lis [NA], SYN sagittal *suture.*

s. serra′ta [NA], SYN serrate *suture.*

s. sphenoethmoida′lis [NA], SYN sphenoethmoidal *suture.*

s. sphenofronta′lis [NA], SYN sphenofrontal *suture.*

s. sphenomaxilla′ris [NA], SYN sphenomaxillary *suture.*

s. spheno-orbita′lis, SYN spheno-orbital *suture.*

s. sphenoparieta′lis [NA], SYN sphenoparietal *suture.*

s. sphenosquamo′sa [NA], SYN sphenosquamous *suture.*

s. sphenovomeria′na [NA], SYN sphenovomerine *suture.*

s. sphenozygoma′tica [NA], SYN sphenozygomatic *suture.*

s. squamo′sa [NA], **(1)** SYN squamous *suture.* **(2)** SYN squamoparietal *suture.*

s. squamosomastoi′dea [NA], SYN squamomastoid *suture.*

s. temporozygomat′ica [NA], SYN zygomaticotemporal *suture.*

s. zygomaticofronta′lis, SYN frontozygomatic *suture.*

s. zygomaticomaxilla′ris [NA], SYN zygomaticomaxillary *suture.*

s. zygomaticotempora′lis, SYN zygomaticotemporal *suture.*

su·tur·al (sū′chūr-ăl). Relating to a suture in any sense.

SUTURE

su·ture (sū′chūr). **1.** A form of fibrous joint in which two bones formed in membrane are united by a fibrous membrane continuous with the periosteum. **2.** To unite two surfaces by sewing. SYN stitch (3). **3.** The material (silk thread, wire, catgut, etc.) with which two surfaces are kept in apposition. **4.** The seam so formed, a surgical s. SYN sutura [NA], suture joint. [L. *sutura,* a seam]

absorbable surgical s., a surgical s. material prepared from a substance that can be digested by body tissues and is therefore not permanent; it is available in various diameters and tensile strengths, and can be treated to modify its resistance to absorption and be impregnated with antimicrobial agents.

Albert's s., a modified Czerny s., the first row of stitches passing through the entire thickness of the wall of the gut.

apposition s., a s. of the skin only. SYN coaptation s.

approximation s., a s. that pulls together the deep tissues.

atraumatic s., a s. swaged onto the end of an eyeless needle.

blanket s., a continuous lock-stitch used to approximate the skin of a wound.

bridle s., a s. passed through the superior rectus muscle to rotate the globe downward in eye surgery.

Bunnell's s., a method of tenorrhaphy using a pull-out wire affixed to buttons.

buried s., any s. placed entirely below the surface of the skin.

button s., a s. in which the threads are passed through the holes of a button and then tied; used to reduce the danger of the threads cutting through the flesh.

catgut s., SEE catgut.

coaptation s., SYN apposition s.

cobbler's s., SYN doubly armed s.

Connell's s., a continuous s. used for inverting the gastric or intestinal walls in performing an anastomosis.

continuous s., an uninterrupted series of stitches using one s.; the stitching is fastened at each end by a knot. SYN spiral s., uninterrupted s.

control release s., eyeless suture with thread attached to needle such that the two separate when tension is applied to the thread.

coronal s., the line of junction of the frontal with the two parietal bones of the skull. SYN sutura coronalis [NA].

cranial s.'s, the sutures between the bones of the skull. SYN suturae cranii [NA].

Cushing's s., a running horizontal mattress s. used to approximate two adjacent surfaces.

Czerny-Lembert s., an intestinal s. in two rows combining the Czerny s. (first) and the Lembert s. (second).

Czerny's s., the first row of the Czerny-Lembert intestinal s.; the needle enters the serosa and passes out through the submucosa or muscularis, and then enters the submucosa or muscularis of the opposite side and emerges from the serosa.

delayed s., a suturing of a wound after an interval of days.

dentate s., SYN serrate s.

doubly armed s., a s. with a needle attached at both ends. SYN cobbler's s.

Dupuytren's s., a continuous Lembert s.

end-on mattress s., a vertical mattress s. used for exact skin approximation.

ethmoidolacrimal s., the line of union of the orbital plate of the ethmoid and the posterior margin of the lacrimal bone. SYN sutura ethmoidolacrimalis [NA].

ethmoidomaxillary s., line of apposition of the orbital surface of the body of the maxilla with the orbital plate of the ethmoid bone. SYN sutura ethmoidomaxillaris [NA].

Faden s., a s. placed between an ocular rectus muscle and the posterior sclera to limit excessive action of the eyeball. [Ger. *Faden,* thread, twine]

false s., one whose opposing margins are smooth or present only a few ill-defined projections. SYN sutura notha.

far-and-near s., a s. utilizing alternate near and far stitches, used to approximate fascial edges.

figure-of-8 s., a s. utilizing criss-cross stitches, used to approximate fascial edges or the musculofascial and outer layers of an abdominal wound.

frontal s., the suture between the two halves of the frontal bone, usually obliterated by about the sixth year; if persistent it is called a metropic s. SYN sutura frontalis [NA].

frontoethmoidal s., line of union between the cribriform plate of the ethmoid and the orbital plate and posterior margin of the nasal process of the frontal bone. SYN sutura frontoethmoidalis [NA].

frontolacrimal s., line of union between the upper margin of the lacrimal and the orbital plate of the frontal bone. SYN sutura frontolacrimalis [NA].

frontomaxillary s., articulation of the frontal process of the maxilla with the frontal bone. SYN sutura frontomaxillaris [NA].

frontonasal s., line of union of the frontal and of the two nasal bones. SYN sutura frontonasalis [NA], sutura nasofrontalis.

frontozygomatic s., line of union between the zygomatic process of the frontal and the frontal process of the zygomatic bone. SYN sutura frontozygomatica [NA], sutura zygomaticofrontalis.

Frost s., intermarginal s. between the eyelids to protect the cornea.

Gély's s., a cobbler's s. used in closing intestinal wounds.

glover's s., a continuous s. in which each stitch is passed through the loop of the preceding one.

Gould's s., an intestinal mattress s. in which each loop is invaginated in such a way that the tissue at the loop is bulged out, becoming convex instead of concave.

Gussenbauer's s., a figure-of-8 s. for the intestine, resembling the Czerny-Lembert s. but not including the mucous membrane.

Halsted's s., a s. placed through the subcuticular fascia; used for exact skin approximation.

harmonic s., SYN plane s.

implanted s., passage of a pin through each lip of the wound parallel to the line of incision, the pins then being looped together with s.'s.

incisive s., line of union of the two portions of the maxilla (pre- and postmaxilla); it is present at birth but may persist into old age. SYN sutura incisiva [NA], premaxillary s.

infraorbital s., an inconstant suture running from the infraorbital foramen to the infraorbital groove. SYN sutura infraorbitalis.

intermaxillary s., the line of union of the two maxillae. SYN sutura intermaxillaris [NA].

internasal s., line of union between the two nasal bones. SYN sutura internasalis [NA].

interparietal s., SYN sagittal s.

interrupted s., a single stitch fixed by tying ends together.

Jobert de Lamballe's s., an interrupted intestinal s., used for invaginating the margins of the intestines in circular enterorrhaphy.

lacrimoconchal s., line of union of the lacrimal bone with the inferior nasal concha. SYN sutura lacrimoconchalis [NA].

lacrimomaxillary s., line of union, on the medial wall of the orbit, between the anterior and inferior margin of the lacrimal bone and the maxilla. SYN sutura lacrimomaxillaris [NA].

lambdoid s., line of union between the occipital and the parietal bones. SYN sutura lambdoidea [NA].

Lembert s., the second row of the Czerny-Lembert intestinal s.; an inverting s. for intestinal surgery, used either as a continuous s. or interrupted s., producing serosal apposition and including the collagenous submucosal layer but not entering the lumen of the intestine.

lens s.'s, SYN *radii* lentis, under *radius.*

mattress s., a s. utilizing a double stitch that forms a loop about the tissue on both sides of a wound, producing eversion of the edges when tied. SYN quilted s.

median palatine s., line of union between the horizontal plates of the palatine bones, continuing the intermaxillary suture posteriorly. SYN sutura palatina mediana [NA].

metopic s., a persistent frontal suture, sometimes discernible a short distance above s. frontonasalis. SYN sutura metopica [NA].

nasomaxillary s., line of union of the lateral margin of the nasal bone with the frontal process of the maxilla. SYN sutura nasomaxillaris [NA].

nerve s., SYN neurorrhaphy.

neurocentral s., SYN neurocentral *synchondrosis.*

nonabsorbable surgical s., surgical s. material that is relatively unaffected by the biological activities of the body tissues and is therefore permanent unless removed; *e.g.,* stainless steel, silk, cotton, nylon, and other synthetic materials.

occipitomastoid s., continuation of the lambdoid suture between the posterior border of the petrous portion of the temporal bone and the occipital. SYN sutura occipitomastoidea [NA].

palatoethmoidal s., line of junction of the orbital process of the palatine bone and the orbital plate of the ethmoid. SYN sutura palatoethmoidalis [NA].

palatomaxillary s., line of union, in the floor of the orbit, between the orbital process of the palatine bone and the orbital surface of the maxilla. SYN sutura palatomaxillaris [NA].

Pancoast's s., in plastic surgery, union of two edges by a tongue-and-groove arrangement.

Paré's s., the approximation of the edges of a wound by pasting

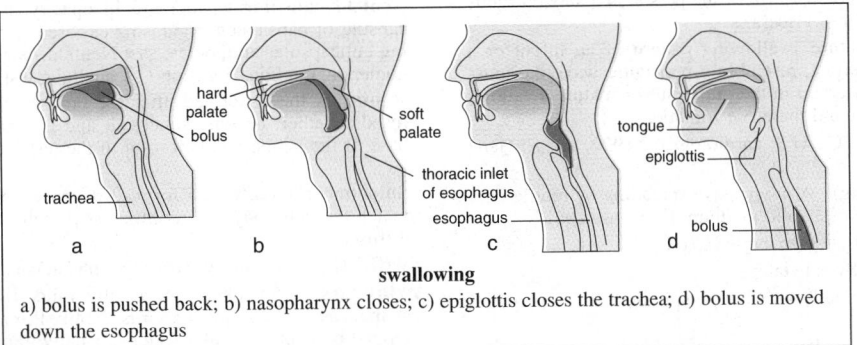

swallowing

a) bolus is pushed back; b) nasopharynx closes; c) epiglottis closes the trachea; d) bolus is moved down the esophagus

strips of cloth to the surface and stitching them instead of the skin.

parietomastoid s., articulation of the posterior inferior angle of the parietal with the mastoid process of the temporal bone. SYN sutura parietomastoidea [NA].

Parker-Kerr s., a continuous inverting s. used to close an open end of intestine.

petrosquamous s., SEE petrosquamous *fissure.*

plane s., a simple firm apposition of two smooth surfaces of bones, without overlap, as seen in the lacrimomaxillary suture. SYN sutura plana [NA], harmonia, harmonic s.

pledgetted s., a s. supported by a small piece of cloth or tissue so that the suture will tear through the tissue.

premaxillary s., SYN incisive s.

purse-string s., a continuous s. placed in a circular manner either for inversion (as for an appendiceal stump) or closure (as for a hernia).

quilted s., SYN mattress s.

relaxation s., a s. so arranged that it may be loosened if the tension of the wound becomes excessive.

retention s., a heavy reinforcing s. placed deep within the muscles and fasciae of the abdominal wall to relieve tension on the primary s. line and thus obviate postoperative wound disruption. SYN tension s.

sagittal s., line of union between the two parietal bones. SYN sutura sagittalis [NA], interparietal s., sutura interparietalis.

secondary s., delayed closure of a wound.

serrate s., one whose opposing margins present deep sawlike indentations, as most of the sagittal suture. SYN sutura serrata [NA], dentate s.

shotted s., a s. in which the ends are fastened by passing through a split shot (a partially divided lead pellet) which is then compressed.

sphenoethmoidal s., line of union between the crest of the sphenoid bone and the perpendicular and cribriform plates of the ethmoid. SYN sutura sphenoethmoidalis [NA].

sphenofrontal s., line of union between the orbital plate of the frontal and the lesser wings of the sphenoid on either side. SYN sutura sphenofrontalis [NA].

sphenomaxillary s., an inconstant suture between the pterygoid process of the sphenoid bone and the body of the maxilla. SYN sutura sphenomaxillaris [NA].

spheno-occipital s., SYN spheno-occipital *synchondrosis.*

spheno-orbital s., articulation between the orbital process of the palatine bone and the outer surface of the body of the sphenoid. SYN sutura spheno-orbitalis.

sphenoparietal s., line of union of the lower border of the parietal with the upper edge of the greater wing of the sphenoid. SYN sutura sphenoparietalis [NA].

sphenosquamous s., articulation of the greater wing of the sphenoid with the squamous portion of the temporal bone. SYN sutura sphenosquamosa [NA].

sphenovomerine s., the line of union of the vaginal process of the sphenoid with the wing of the vomer. SYN sutura sphenovomeriana [NA].

sphenozygomatic s., junction of the zygomatic bone and greater wing of the sphenoid. SYN sutura sphenozygomatica [NA].

spiral s., SYN continuous s.

squamomastoid s., line of union of the squamous and petrous portions of the temporal bone during development; it sometimes persists in the region of the mastoid process. SYN sutura squamosomastoidea [NA].

squamoparietal s., the articulation of the parietal with the squamous portion of the temporal bone. SYN sutura squamosa (2) [NA].

squamous s., a scalelike suture, one whose opposing margins are scalelike and overlapping; SYN sutura squamosa (1) [NA].

subcuticular s., SEE Halsted's s.

temporozygomatic s., SYN zygomaticotemporal s.

tendon s., SYN tenorrhaphy.

tension s., SYN retention s.

transfixion s., (1) a criss-cross stitch so placed as to control bleeding from a tissue surface or small vessel when tied; **(2)** a s. used to fix the columella to the nasal septum.

transverse palatine s., line of union of the palatine processes of the maxillae with the horizontal plates of the palatine bones. SYN sutura palatina transversa [NA].

tympanomastoid s., SYN tympanomastoid *fissure.*

uninterrupted s., SYN continuous s.

wedge-and-groove s., SYN wedge-and-groove *joint.*

zygomaticomaxillary s., articulation of the zygomatic bone with the zygomatic process of the maxilla. SYN sutura zygomaticomaxillaris [NA].

zygomaticotemporal s., line of junction of the zygomatic process of the temporal and the temporal process of the zygomatic bone. SYN sutura temporozygomatica [NA], sutura zygomaticotemporalis, temporozygomatic s.

---

su·tur·ec·to·my (sū-chūr-ek′tō-mē). Removal of cranial suture.

Suzanne, Jean G., French physician, *1859. SEE S.'s gland.

SV Abbreviation for simian *virus,* numbered serially; *e.g.,* SV1.

SV40 Symbol for simian vacuolating *virus* No. 40.

Sv Abbreviation for sievert.

Svedberg, Theodor, Swedish chemist and Nobel laureate, 1884–1971. SEE S. *equation,* of flotation, *unit.*

Svedberg of flo·ta·tion. SYN flotation *constant.*

swab (swob). A wad of cotton, gauze, or other absorbent material attached to the end of a stick or clamp, used for applying or removing a substance from a surface.

swage (swāj). **1.** To fuse suture thread to suture needles. **2.** To shape metal by hammering or adapting it onto a die, often by using a counterdie. [Old F. *souage*]

swal·low (swawl′ō). To pass anything through the fauces, pharynx, and esophagus into the stomach; to perform deglutition. [A.S. *swelgan*]

gastrografin s., esophagram or upper GI series using water-soluble iodinated contrast medium. SYN hypaque s.

hypaque s., SYN gastrografin s.

somatic s., a swallowing pattern with muscular contractions which appear to be under control of the person at a subconscious level; distinguished from visceral s.

visceral s., the immature swallowing pattern of an infant or a person with tongue thrust, resembling peristaltic wavelike muscular contractions observed in the gut; adult or mature swallowing is more volitional and therefore somatic.

Swan, Harold James C., U.S. cardiologist, *1922. SEE S.-Ganz *catheter*.

swarm·ing (swôrm'ing). A progressive spreading by motile bacteria over the surface of a solid medium. [A.S. *swearm*]

sway·back (swā'bak). SYN enzootic *ataxia*.

Sweat. SEE Puchtler-Sweat stains.

sweat (swet). **1.** Especially sensible perspiration. **2.** To perspire. [A.S. *swāt*]

colliquative s., profuse clammy s.

night s.'s, profuse sweating at night, occurring in pulmonary tuberculosis and other chronic debilitating affections with low-grade fever.

red s., reddening of s., especially in the axilla, due to pigment produced by *Streptomyces roseofulvis* . SEE ALSO chromidrosis.

sweat·ing (swet'ing). SYN perspiration (1).

Swediauer, Francois X., Austrian physician, 1748–1824. SEE S.'s *disease*.

sweeney (swē'nē). Disuse or neurogenic atrophy of the supraspinatus and infraspinatus muscles in horses.

sweep (swēp). The travel of the beam of a cathode ray oscilloscope from left to right, representing the time axis, produced by an artificially generated sawtooth voltage.

Sweet, Robert Douglas, 20th century English dermatologist. SEE S.'s *disease*.

Sweet. SEE Gordon and Sweet *stain*.

swell·head (swel'hed). **1.** SYN lecheguilla *poisoning*. **2.** In turkeys, distention of the sinuses due to accumulation of exudate in infectious sinusitis.

swell·ing (swel'ing). **1.** An enlargement, *e.g.,* a protuberance or tumor. **2.** In embryology, a primordial elevation that develops into a fold, ridge, or process.

albuminous s., SYN cloudy s.

arytenoid s., paired primordial elevations, on either side of the embryonic larynx, within which the arytenoid cartilages are formed.

brain s., a pathologic entity, localized or generalized, characterized by an increase in bulk of brain tissue, due to expansion of the intravascular (congestion) or extravascular (edema) compartments that may coexist or may occur separately and be clinically indistinguishable; clinical manifestations depend on disturbed neuronal function due to local s., shifting of intracranial structures, and the effects of intracranial hypertension or circulatory disturbance.

Calabar s., SYN loiasis.

cloudy s., s. of cells due to injury to the membranes affecting ionic transfer; causes an accumulation of intracellular water. SYN albuminous s., granular degeneration, hydropic degeneration, parenchymatous degeneration.

fugitive s., SYN loiasis.

genital s.'s, paired primordial elevations flanking the genital tubercle and the urogenital orifice of the embryo; they develop into the labioscrotal folds, which become the labia majora in the female and unite to form the scrotal pouch of the male. SYN labioscrotal s.'s.

hunger s., starvation edema caused by many factors, primarily reduced serum albumin.

labial s., the female embryonic genital s. which elongates to become the definitive labium majus. SEE ALSO genital s.'s.

labioscrotal s.'s, SYN genital s.'s.

lateral lingual s.'s, in the embryo, paired oval elevations that appear in the floor of the mouth at mandibular arch level; the primordial elevations, composed of mesenchyme covered by ectoderm of stomodeal origin, merge to form the greater part of the anterior two thirds of the tongue.

levator s., SYN levator *cushion*.

Neufeld capsular s., increase in opacity and visibility of the capsule of capsulated organisms exposed to specific agglutinating anticapsular antibodies. SYN Neufeld reaction, quellung phenomenon, quellung reaction (1), quellung test.

scrotal s., the s. formed after the embryonic genital s.'s have fused together, become spherical, and migrated caudally to the base of the penis; just before birth the testis comes to lie within it.

Spielmeyer's acute s., a form of degeneration of nerve cells in which the cell body and its processes swell and stain palely and diffusely.

Swift, H., 20th century Australian physician. SEE S.'s *disease*.

swine·pox (swīn'poks). A usually mild disease occurring in swine, caused by swinepox virus (family Poxviridae) and characterized by papulopustular lesions; usually transmitted by lice.

switch·ing (swich'ing). **1.** Making a shift or exchange. **2.** The movement of a defined region of DNA within a genome.

class s., a change in the expression of the C region of an immunoglobulin heavy chain.

Swyer, Paul R., U.S. pediatrician, *1921. SEE Swyer-James *syndrome*; S.-James-MacLeod *syndrome*.

sy·co·ma (sī-kō'mă). **1.** A pendulous figlike growth. **2.** A large soft wart. [G. *sykōma*, fr. *sykon*, fig, + *-oma*, tumor]

sy·co·si·form (sī-kō'si-fōrm). Resembling sycosis.

sy·co·sis (sī-kō'sis). A pustular folliculitis, particularly of the bearded area. SYN ficosis, mentagra. [G. *sykōsis*, fr. *sykōn*, fig, + *-osis*, condition]

s. frambesifor'mis, SYN acne *keloid*.

lupoid s., a papular or pustular inflammation of the hair follicles of the beard, followed by punctuate scarring and loss of the hair. SYN ulerythema sycosiforme.

s. nu'chae necroti'sans, acne keloid on the back of the neck at the hairline.

Sydenham, Thomas, English physician, 1624–1689. SEE S.'s *chorea, disease*.

Sydney crease. See under crease.

Sydney line. See under line.

syl·la·ble-stum·bling (sil'ă-bl stŭm'bling). A form of stuttering in which the patient halts before certain syllables that he finds difficult to enunciate. SYN dyssyllabia. [L. *syllabē*, several letters or sounds taken together]

syl·vat·ic (sil-vat'ik). Occurring in or affecting wild animals. [L. *silva*, woods]

Sylvest, Ejnar, Norwegian physician, 1880–1931. SEE S.'s *disease*.

syl·vi·an (sil'vē-an). Relating to Franciscus or Jacobus Sylvius or to any of the structures described by either of them.

Sylvius (Dubois, de le Boë). Le Böe, Franciscus (François), Dutch physician, anatomist, and physiologist, 1614–1672. SEE sylvian *angle*, sylvian *aqueduct*, sylvian *fissure*, sylvian *line*, sylvian *point*, sylvian *valve*, sylvian *ventricle*, fossa of Sylvius, *vallecula* sylvii.

Sylvius (Dubois). Jacobus (Jacques), French anatomist, 1478–1555. SEE *caro* quadrata sylvii, *os* sylvii.

△**sym-.** SEE syn-.

sym·bal·lo·phone (sim-bal'ō-fōn). A stethoscope having two chest pieces, designed to lateralize sound and produce a stereophonic effect. [G. *symballō*, to throw together, + *phōnē*, sound]

sym·bi·on, sym·bi·ont (sim'bē-on, -ont). An organism associated with another in symbiosis. SYN mutualist, symbiote. [G. *symbion*, neut. of *symbiōs, living together*]

sym·bi·o·sis (sim-bē-ō'sis). **1.** The biological association of two or more species to their mutual benefit. Cf. commensalism, mutualistic s., parasitism. **2.** The mutual cooperation or interdependence of two persons, as mother and infant, or husband and wife; sometimes used to denote excessive or pathological interdependence of two persons. [G. *symbiōsis*, state of living together, fr. sym- + *bios*, life, + *-osis*, condition]

dyadic s., s. between a child and one parent.

mutualistic s., s. in which all partners obtain an advantage.

triadic s., s. between a child and both parents.

sym·bi·ote (sim′bē-ōt). SYN symbion.

sym·bi·ot·ic (sim-bē-ot′ik). Relating to symbiosis.

sym·bleph·a·ron (sim-blef′ă-ron). Adhesion of one or both eyelids to the eyeball, partial or complete, resulting from burns or other trauma but rarely congenital. SYN atretoblepharia. [sym- + G. *blepharon*, eyelid]

anterior s., union between the lid and eyeball by a fibrous band not involving the fornix.

posterior s., adhesion between the eyeball and eyelid involving the fornix.

sym·bleph·a·rop·te·ryg·i·um (sim-blef′ă-rō-tĕ-rij′ē-ŭm). Obsolete term for adhesion of the eyelid to the eyeball. [symblepharon + pterygium]

sym·bol (sim′bŏl). **1.** A conventional sign serving as an abbreviation. **2.** In chemistry, an abbreviation of the name of an element, radical, or compound, expressing in chemical formulas one atom or molecule of that element (*e.g.,* H and O in H_2O); in biochemistry, an abbreviation of trivial names of molecules used primarily in combination with other similar s.'s to construct larger assemblies (*e.g.,* Gly for glycine, Ado for adenosine, Glc for glucose). **3.** In psychoanalysis, an object or action that is interpreted to represent some repressed or unconscious desire, often sexual. **4.** A philosophical-linguistic sign. SEE ALSO conventional *signs,* under *sign.* [G. *symbolon*, a mark or sign, fr. *sym-ballō*, to throw together]

sym·bo·lia (sim-bō′lē-ă). The capability of recognizing the form and nature of an object by touch. [G. *symbolon*, a mark or sign]

sym·bol·ism (sim′bō-lizm). **1.** In psychoanalysis, the process involved in the disguised representation in consciousness of unconscious or repressed contents or events. **2.** A mental state in which everything that happens is regarded by the individual as symbolic of his own thoughts. **3.** The description of the emotional life and experiences in abstract terms.

sym·bol·i·za·tion (sim′bō-li-zā′shŭn). An unconscious mental mechanism whereby one object or idea is represented by another.

sym·brach·y·dac·ty·ly (sim-brak′i-dak′ti-lē). Condition in which abnormally short fingers are joined or webbed in their proximal portions. [sym- + G. *brachys*, short, + *daktylos*, finger]

Syme, James, Scottish surgeon, 1799–1870. SEE S.'s *amputation, operation.*

Symington, Johnson, Scottish anatomist, 1851–1924. SEE S.'s anococcygeal *body.*

sym·me·lia (si-mē′lē-ă). SYN sirenomelia. [sym- + G. *melos*, limb]

Symmers, Douglas, U.S. pathologist, 1879–1952. SEE Brill-S. *disease.*

Symmers, W. St. C., British pathologist, 1863–1937. SEE S.'s clay pipestem *fibrosis.*

sym·me·try (sim′ĕ-trē). Equality or correspondence in form of parts distributed around a center or an axis, at the extremities or poles, or on the opposite sides of any body. [G. *symmetria*, fr. sym- + *metron*, measure]

inverse s., correspondence of the right or left side of an asymmetrical individual to the left or right side of another.

⌂**sympath-, sympatheto-, sympathico-, sympatho-.** The sympathetic part of the autonomic nervous system. [see sympathetic]

sym·pa·thec·to·my (sim-pă-thek′tō-mē). Excision of a segment of a sympathetic nerve or of one or more sympathetic ganglia. SYN sympathetectomy, sympathicectomy. [sympath- + G. *ektomē*, excision]

chemical s., destruction of the periarterial sympathetic nerves, as in Doppler's operation, by a corrosive such as phenol.

periarterial s., sympathetic denervation by arterial decortication. SYN histonectomy, Leriche's operation.

presacral s., SYN presacral *neurectomy.*

sym·pa·thet·ic (sim-pă-thet′ik). **1.** Relating to or exhibiting sympathy. **2.** Denoting the sympathetic part of the autonomic nervous system. SYN sympathic. [G. *sympathētikos*, fr. *sympatheō*, to feel with, sympathize, fr. *syn*, with, + *pathos*, suffering]

sym·pa·thet·o·blast (sim-pă-thet′ō-blast). SYN sympathoblast.

sym·pa·thet·o·blas·to·ma (sim-pă-thet′ō-blas-tō′mă). Obsolete term for neuroma.

sym·pa·thic (sim-path′ik). SYN sympathetic.

sym·path·i·cec·to·my (sim-path′i-sek′tō-mē). SYN sympathectomy.

⌂**sympathico-.** SEE sympath-.

sym·path·i·co·blast (sim-path′i-kō-blast). SYN sympathoblast.

sym·path·i·co·blas·to·ma (sim-path′i-kō-blas-tō′mă). Obsolete term for neuroma.

sym·path·i·co·go·ni·o·ma (sim-path′i-kō-gō-nē-ō′mă). Obsolete term for neuroma.

sym·path·i·co·lyt·ic (sim-path′i-kō-lit′ik). SYN sympatholytic.

sym·path·i·co·mi·met·ic (sim-path′i-kō-mi-met′ik). SYN sympathomimetic.

sym·path·i·co·neu·ri·tis (sim-path′i-kō-nū-rī′tis). Inflammation of the autonomic nerves.

sym·path·i·cop·a·thy (sim-path-i-kop′ă-thē). A disease resulting from a disorder of the autonomic nervous system. [sympathico- + G. *pathos*, suffering]

sym·path·i·co·to·nia (sim-path′i-kō-tō′nē-ă). A condition in which there is increased tonus of the sympathetic system and a marked tendency to vascular spasm and high blood pressure; opposed to vagotonia. [sympathico- + G. *tonos*, tone, tension]

sym·path·i·co·ton·ic (sim-path′i-kō-ton′ik). Relating to or characterized by sympathicotonia.

sym·path·i·co·trip·sy (sim-path′i-kō-trip′sē). Operation of crushing the sympathetic ganglion. [sympathico- + G. *tripsis*, a rubbing]

sym·path·i·co·tro·pic (sim-path′i-kō-trop′ik). Having a special affinity for the sympathetic nervous system. [sympathico- + G. *tropikos*, inclined, fr. *tropē*, a turning]

sym·pa·thin (sim′pă-thin). The substance diffusing into circulation from sympathetic nerve terminals when they are active. The term was introduced by W. B. Cannon, who thought that this substance differed from the mediator produced by the nerve ending (now known to be incorrect); the mediator itself (norepinephrine) diffuses into circulation. SYN sympathetic hormone.

sym·pa·thism (sim′pă-thizm). SYN suggestibility. [G. *sympatheia*, sympathy]

sym·pa·thist (sim′pă-thist). Obsolete term for one susceptible to suggestibility.

sym·pa·thiz·er (sim′pă-thī-zer). **1.** An eye affected with sympathetic ophthalmia. **2.** One who exhibits sympathy.

⌂**sympatho-.** SEE sympath-.

sym·pa·tho·ad·re·nal (sim′pă-thō-ă-drē′năl). Relating to the sympathetic part of the autonomic nervous system and the medulla of the adrenal gland, as the postganglionic neurons.

sym·pa·tho·blast (sim′pă-thō-blast). A primitive cell derived from the neural crest glia; with the pheochromoblasts, s.'s enter into the formation of the adrenal medulla and sympathetic ganglia. SYN sympathetoblast, sympathicoblast. [sympatho- + G. *blastos*, germ]

sym·pa·tho·blas·to·ma (sim′pă-thō-blas-tō′mă). Obsolete term for neuroblastoma. [sympathoblast + G. *-oma*, tumor]

sym·pa·tho·go·nia (sim′pă-thō-gō′nē-ă). The completely undifferentiated cells of the sympathetic nervous system. [sympatho- + G. *gonē*, seed]

sym·pa·tho·go·ni·o·ma (sim′pă-thō-gō-nē-ō′mă). Obsolete term for neuroblastoma. [sympathogonia + G. *-ōma*, tumor]

sym·pa·tho·lyt·ic (sim′pă-thō-lit′ik). Denoting antagonism to or inhibition of adrenergic nerve activity. SEE ALSO adrenergic blocking *agent,* antiadrenergic. SYN sympathicolytic. [sympatho- + G. *lysis*, a loosening]

sym·pa·tho·mi·met·ic (sim′pă-thō-mi-met′ik). Denoting mimicking of action of the sympathetic system. SEE ALSO adrenomimetic. SYN sympathicomimetic. [sympatho- + G. *mimikos*, imitating]

sym·pa·tho·mi·met·ic amines. A broad class of chemicals which mimic the actions of activation of the sympathetic nervous system and have an amine (usually β-phenyl-ethylamine) basic structure; examples include isoproterenol, amphetamine, ephedrine, and phenylephrine.

sym·pa·thy (sim′pă-thē). **1.** The mutual relation, physiologic or pathologic, between two organs, systems, or parts of the body. **2.** Mental contagion, as seen in mass hysteria or in the yawning induced by seeing another person yawn. **3.** An expressed sensitive appreciation or emotional concern for and sharing of the mental and emotional state of another person. Cf. empathy (1). [G. *sympatheia,* fr. sym- + *pathos,* suffering]

sym·per·i·to·ne·al (sim′per-i-tō-nē′ăl). Relating to the surgical induction of adhesion between two portions of the peritoneum.

sym·pex·is (sim-pek′sis). A term proposed by R.P. Heidenhain to denote the deposition of red blood cells according to the laws of surface tension. [G. concretion]

sym·pha·lan·gism, sym·pha·lan·gy (sim-fal′an-jizm, sim-fal′an-jē). **1.** SYN syndactyly. **2.** Ankylosis of the finger or toe joints. [sym- + phalanx]

sym·phys·i·al, sym·phys·e·al (sim-fiz′ē-ăl). Grown together; relating to a symphysis; fused. SYN symphysic.

sym·phys·ic (sim-fiz′ik). SYN symphysial.

sym·phys·i·on (sim-fiz′ē-on). A craniometric point, the most anterior point of the alveolar process of the mandible.

sym·phys·i·o·tome, sym·phys·e·o·tome (sim-fiz′ē-ō-tōm). Instrument for use in symphysiotomy.

sym·phys·i·ot·o·my, sym·phys·e·ot·o·my (sim-fiz-ē-ot′ō-mē). Division of the pubic joint to increase the capacity of a contracted pelvis sufficiently to permit passage of a living child. SYN pelviotomy (1), pelvitomy, synchondrotomy. [symphysis + G. *tomē,* incision]

sym·phy·sis, gen. **sym·phy·ses** (sim′fi-sis, -sēz). **1** [NA]. Form of cartilaginous joint in which union between two bones is effected by means of fibrocartilage. SYN amphiarthrosis. **2.** A union, meeting point, or commissure of any two structures. **3.** A pathologic adhesion or growing together. [G. a growing together]
  cardiac s., adhesion between the parietal and visceral layers of the pericardium.
  intervertebral s., the union between adjacent vertebral bodies composed of the nucleus pulposus, annular ligament, and the anterior and posterior longitudinal ligaments. SYN s. intervertebralis [NA].
  s. intervertebra′lis [NA], SYN intervertebral s.
  s. mandib′ulae, SYN mental s.
  manubriosternal s., the later union, by fibrocartilage, of the manubrium and the body of the sternum; it begins as a synchondrosis and becomes a symphysis, occasionally fusing to become a synostosis. SYN s. manubriosternalis [NA], sternomanubrial junction.
  s. manubriosterna′lis [NA], SYN manubriosternal s.
  mental s., the fibrocartilaginous union of the two halves of the mandible in the fetus; it becomes an osseous union during the first year. SYN s. mandibulae, s. mentalis, s. menti.
  s. menta′lis, SYN mental s.
  s. men′ti, SYN mental s.
  pubic s., the firm fibrocartilaginous joint between the two pubic bones. SYN s. pubica [NA], symphysis pubis.
  s. pu′bica [NA], SYN pubic s.
  s. sacrococcyg′ea, SYN sacrococcygeal *joint.*

sym·plas·mat·ic (sim-plaz-mat′ik). Relating to the union of protoplasm as in giant cell formation. [G. *sym- plassō,* to mold together]

sym·plast (sim′plast). A multinucleated cell that has formed by fusion of separate cells. [sym- + G. *plastos,* formed]

sym·po·dia (sim-pō′dē-ă). Condition characterized by union of the feet. SEE ALSO sirenomelia, sympus. [sym- + G. *pous,* foot]

sym·port (sim′pōrt). Coupled transport of two different molecules or ions through a membrane in the same direction by a common carrier mechanism (symporter). Cf. antiport, uniport. [sym- + L. *porto,* to carry]

sym·port·er (sim-pōrt′er). The protein responsible for mediating symport.

symp·tom (simp′tŏm). Any morbid phenomenon or departure from the normal in structure, function, or sensation, experienced by the patient and indicative of disease. SEE ALSO phenomenon (1), reflex (1), sign (1), syndrome. [G. *symptōma*]
  abstinence s.'s, SYN withdrawal s.'s.
  accessory s., a s. that usually but not always accompanies a certain disease, as distinguished from a pathognomonic s. SYN assident s., concomitant s.
  accidental s., any morbid phenomenon coincidentally occurring in the course of a disease, but having no relation with it.
  assident s., SYN accessory s.
  Baumès s., pain behind the sternum in angina pectoris.
  Bezold's s., inflammatory edema at the tip of the mastoid process in mastoiditis. SYN Bezold's sign.
  Bolognini's s., a feeling of crepitation on gradually increasing pressure on the abdomen in cases of measles.
  cardinal s., the primary or major s. of diagnostic importance.
  concomitant s., SYN accessory s.
  constitutional s., a s. indicating a systemic effect of a disease; *e.g.,* weight loss.
  deficiency s., manifestation of a lack, in varying degrees, of some substance (*e.g.,* hormone, enzyme, vitamin) necessary for normal structure and/or function of an organism.
  Demarquay's s., absence of elevation of the larynx during deglutition, said to indicate syphilitic induration of the trachea.
  Epstein's s., SEE Epstein's *sign.*
  equivocal s., a s. that points definitely to no special disease, being associated with any one of a number of morbid states, or whose presence is uncertain or indefinite.
  first rank s.'s (FRS), SYN Schneider's first rank s.'s.
  Fischer's s., SYN Fischer's *sign.*
  Frenkel's s., lowered muscular tonus in tabetic neurosyphilis.
  Gordon's s., SYN tonic *reflex.*
  Griesinger's s., edema of the superficial tissues at the tip of the mastoid process in cases of thrombosis of the sigmoid sinus.
  Haenel's s., absence of sensation on pressure of the eyeball in tabes.
  incarceration s., SYN Dietl's *crisis.*
  induced s., a s. excited by a drug, exercise, or other means, often intentionally for diagnostic purposes.
  Kerandel's s., deep-seated hyperesthesia observed in cases of sleeping sickness.
  Kussmaul's s., SYN Kussmaul's *sign.*
  local s., a s. of limited extent, caused by disease of a particular organ or part.
  localizing s., a s. indicating clearly the seat of the morbid process.
  Macewen's s., SYN Macewen's *sign.*
  objective s., a s. that is evident to the observer.
  Oehler's s., a sudden pallor and coldness in the arm with slight disability, occurring on lifting of a heavy weight.
  pathognomonic s., a s. that, when present, points unmistakably to the presence of a certain definite disease.
  Pratt's s., rigidity in the muscles of an injured limb, which precedes the occurrence of gangrene.
  presenting s., the complaint offered by the patient as the main reason for seeking medical care; usually synonymous with chief *complaint.*
  rainbow s., SYN glaucomatous *halo* (2).
  reflex s., a disturbance of sensation or function in an organ or part more or less remote from the morbid condition giving rise to it; *e.g.,* muscle spasm due to joint inflammation. SYN sympathetic s.
  Romberg-Howship s., in cases of incarcerated obturator hernia; lancinating pains along the inner side of the thigh to the knee, or down the leg to the foot; caused by compression of the obturator nerve. SYN Romberg's s. (2).
  Romberg's s., (1) SYN Romberg's *sign.* **(2)** SYN Romberg-Howship s.
  schneiderian first rank s.'s, SYN Schneider's first rank s.'s.
  Schneider's first rank s.'s, those s.'s that, when present, indi-

cate that the diagnosis of schizophrenia is likely, provided that organic or toxic etiology is ruled out: delusion of control, thought broadcasting, thought withdrawal, thought insertion, hearing one's thoughts spoken aloud, auditory hallucinations that comment on one's behavior, and auditory hallucinations in which two voices carry on a conversation. SYN first rank s.'s, schneiderian first rank s.'s.

Sklowsky s., the rupture of a varicella vesicle on very slight pressure with the finger, greater pressure being necessary to break the vesicles of smallpox, herpes, or other affections.

subjective s., a s. apparent only to the patient.

sympathetic s., SYN reflex s.

Trendelenburg's s., a waddling gait in paresis of the gluteal muscles, as in progressive muscular dystrophy.

Uhthoff s., a transient temperature-dependent numbness, weakness, or loss of vision. Conduction stops in any nerve if the temperature gets too high. In a damaged nerve, *e.g.,* by demyelinization, this shutdown temperature is lowered, and may approach normal body temperature. Transient neurological dysfunction may then appear with a hot shower, exercise, or fever. SYN Uhthoff syndrome.

Wartenberg's s., (1) intense pruritus of the tip of the nose and nostrils in cases of cerebral tumor; **(2)** flexion of the thumb when the patient attempts to flex the four fingers against resistance, a "pyramid sign".

withdrawal s.'s, a group of morbid s.'s, predominantly erethistic, occurring in an addict who is deprived of his accustomed dose of the addicting agent. SYN abstinence s.'s.

symp·to·mat·ic (simp-tō-mat'ik). Indicative; relating to or constituting the aggregate of symptoms of a disease.

symp·tom·a·tol·o·gy (simp'tō-mă-tol'ō-jē). **1.** The science of the symptoms of disease, their production, and the indications they furnish. **2.** The aggregate of symptoms of a disease. [symptom + G. *logos,* study]

symp·to·mat·o·lyt·ic (simp'tō-mat-ō-lit'ik). Removing symptoms. SYN symptomolytic. [symptom + G. *lytikos,* dissolving]

symp·to·sis (sim-tō'sis). A localized or general wasting of the body. [G. a falling together, collapse, fr. *syn,* together, + *ptōsis,* a falling]

sym·pus (sim'pŭs). A sirenomelus in which the fusion of the legs has extended to involve the feet. [G. *sympous,* fr. sym- + *pous,* foot]

s. a′pus, a sirenomelus without feet.

s. di′pus, a sirenomelus with both feet more or less distinct.

s. mo′nopus, a sirenomelus with but one foot externally visible.

Syms, Parker, U.S. surgeon, 1860–1933. SEE S. *tractor.*

syn-. (Properly prefixed to words of G. derivation) indicating together, with, joined; appears as sym- before b, p, ph, or m; corresponds to L. *con-.* [G. *syn,* with, together]

syn·a·del·phus (sin-ă-del'fŭs). Conjoined twins with single head, partially united trunk, and four upper and four lower limbs. SEE conjoined *twins,* under *twin.* [syn- + G. *adelphos,* brother]

syn·al·gia (si-nal'jē-ă). SYN referred *pain.* [syn- + G. *algos,* pain]

syn·al·gic (sin-al'jik). Relating to or marked by referred pain.

syn·a·nas·to·mo·sis (sin'an-as-tō-mō'sis). An anastomosis between several blood vessels.

syn·an·dro·gen·ic (sin'an-drō-jen'ik). Relating to any agent or condition that enhances the effects of androgens.

sy·nan·them, syn·an·the·ma (si-nan'them, sin'an-thē'mă). An exanthem consisting of several different forms of eruption. [G. *syn- antheō,* to blossom together]

sy·naph·o·cep·tors (si-naf-ō-sep'terz). Receptors stimulated by direct contact. [G. *synaphe,* contact, + L. *recipio,* to receive]

syn·apse, pl. **syn·aps·es** (sin'aps, sĭ-naps'; sĭ-nap'sēz). The functional membrane-to-membrane contact of the nerve cell with another nerve cell, an effector (muscle, gland) cell, or a sensory receptor cell. The s. subserves the transmission of nerve impulses, commonly from a variably large (1 to 12 μm), generally knob-shaped or club-shaped axon terminal (the presynaptic element) to the circumscript patch of the receiving cell's plasma membrane (the postsynaptic element) on which the s. occurs. In most cases the impulse is transmitted by means of a chemical

transmitter substance (such as acetylcholine, γ-aminobutyric acid, dopamine, norepinephrine) released into a synaptic cleft (15 to 50 nm wide) that separates the presynaptic from the postsynaptic membrane; the transmitter is stored in quantal form in synaptic vesicles: round or ellipsoid, membrane-bound vacuoles (10 to 50 nm in diameter) in the presynaptic element. In other s.'s transmission takes place by direct propagation of the bioelectrical potential from the presynaptic to the postsynaptic membrane; in such electrotonic s.'s ("gap junctions"), the synaptic cleft is no more than about 2 nm wide. In most cases, synaptic transmission takes place in only one direction ("dynamic polarity" of the s.), but in some s.'s synaptic vesicles occur on both sides of the synaptic cleft, suggesting the possibility of reciprocal chemical transmission. [syn- + G. *hapto,* to clasp]

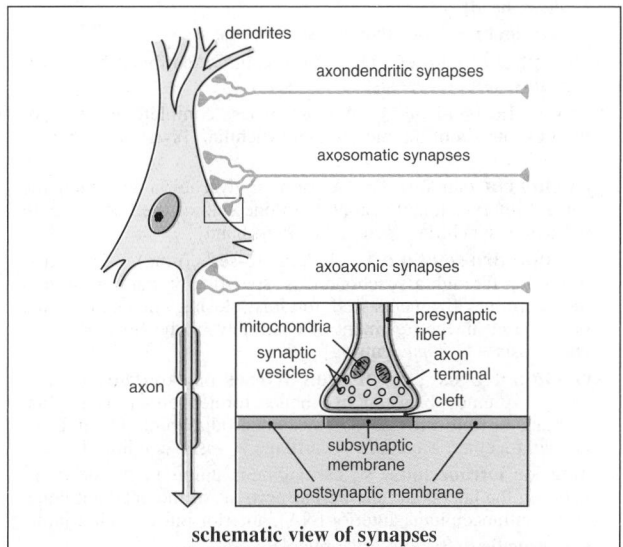

dendrites
axondendritic synapses
axosomatic synapses
axoaxonic synapses
axon
mitochondria
synaptic vesicles
presynaptic fiber
axon terminal
cleft
subsynaptic membrane
postsynaptic membrane

schematic view of synapses

axoaxonic s., the synaptic junction between an axon terminal of one neuron and either the initial axon segment or an axon terminal of another nerve cell.

axodendritic s., the synaptic contact between an axon terminal of one nerve cell and a dendrite of another nerve cell.

axosomatic s., the synaptic junction of an axon terminal of one nerve cell to the cell body of another nerve cell. SYN pericorpuscular s.

electrotonic s., SYN gap *junction.* SEE ALSO synapse.

pericorpuscular s., SYN axosomatic s.

syn·ap·sin I (si-nap'sin). A fibrous phosphoprotein that links synaptic vesicles together in the axon terminal; s. I is a substrate for certain kinases; phosphorylation of s. I allows release of neurotransmitters.

syn·ap·sis (si-nap'sis). The point-for-point pairing of homologous chromosomes during the prophase of meiosis. SYN synaptic phase. [G. a connection, junction]

syn·ap·tic (si-nap'tik). **1.** Relating to a synapse. **2.** Relating to synapsis.

syn·ap·tol·o·gy (sin'ap-tol'ō-jē). Study of the synapse.

syn·ap·to·phys·in (si-nap'tō-fī'sin). An integral membrane protein found in many types of active neurons; believed to form a hexamer that forms an ion channel and is involved in the uptake of neurotransmitters; s. is found in the membrane only after stimulation of the neurons.

syn·ap·to·some (si-nap'tō-sōm). Membrane-bound sac containing synaptic vesicles that breaks away from axon terminals when brain tissue is homogenized under controlled conditions; such particles can be separated from other subcellular particles by differential and density gradient centrifugation. [synapse + G. *sōma,* body]

syn·ar·thro·dia (sin'ar-thrō'dē-ă). SYN fibrous *joint.*

syn·ar·thro·di·al (sin-ar-thrō'dē-ăl). Relating to synarthrosis; denoting an articulation without a joint cavity.

syn·ar·thro·phy·sis (sin-ar-thrō-fī′sis). The process of ankylosis. [syn- + G. *arthron,* joint, + *physis,* growth]

syn·ar·thro·sis, pl. **syn·ar·thro·ses** (sin′ar-thrō′sis, -sēz). In the BNA, this class of joints has included those that in the NA are classified as articulatio fibrosa (fibrous joints) and articulatio cartilaginis (cartilagenous joints). SEE articulatio. [G. fr. *syn,* together, + *arthrōsis,* articulation]

syn·can·thus (sin-kan′thŭs). Adhesion of the eyeball to orbital structures. [syn- + L. *canthus,* wheel]

syn·car·y·on (sin-kar′ē-on). SYN synkaryon.

syn·ceph·a·lus (sin-sef′ă-lŭs). Conjoined twins having a single head with two bodies. SEE conjoined *twins,* under *twin.* Cf. craniopagus, janiceps. SYN monocephalus, monocranius. [syn- + G. *kephalē,* head]

s. asymmet′ros, SYN *janiceps* asymmetrus.

syn·ceph·a·ly (sin-sef′ă-lē). The condition exhibited by a syncephalus. SYN prozygosis.

syn·chei·lia (sin-kī′lē-ă). A more or less complete adhesion of the lips; atresia of the mouth. SYN synchilia. [syn- + G. *cheilos,* lip]

syn·chei·ria (sin-kī′rē-ă). A form of dyscheiria in which the subject refers a stimulus applied to one side of the body to both sides. SYN synchiria. [syn- + G. *cheir,* hand]

syn·chon·dro·se·ot·o·my (sin-kon′drō-sē-ot′ō-mē). Operation of cutting through a synchondrosis; specifically, cutting through the sacroiliac ligaments and forcibly closing the arch of the pubes; used in the treatment of exstrophy of the bladder. [synchondrosis + G. *tomē,* cutting]

syn·chon·dro·sis, pl. **syn·chon·dro·ses** (sin′kon-drō′sis, -sēz) [NA]. A union between two bones formed either by hyaline cartilage or fibrocartilage. SYN synchondrodial joint. [Mod. L. fr. G. *syn,* together, + *chondros,* cartilage, + *-osis,* condition]

anterior intraoccipital s., cartilaginous union in the newborn between the lateral and the basilar portions of the occipital bone. SYN s. intraoccipitalis anterior [NA], anterior intraoccipital joint.

s. arycornicula′ta, SYN arycorniculate s.

arycorniculate s., the junction of the corniculate cartilage (of Santorini) with the arytenoid. SYN s. arycorniculata.

cranial synchondroses, the cartilaginous joints of the skull; these include sphenoethmoidal s., spheno-occipital s., sphenopetrosa s., petro-occipital s., anterior intraoccipital and posterior intraoccipital s. SYN synchondroses cranii [NA].

synchondro′ses cra′nii [NA], SYN cranial synchondroses.

s. epiphy′seos, SYN epiphysial *line.*

synchondroses intersternebra′les, persisting cartilages uniting the bony elements of the sternum, as in some domestic animals such as the dog. SYN intersternebral joints.

s. intraoccipita′lis ante′rior [NA], SYN anterior intraoccipital s.

s. intraoccipita′lis poste′rior [NA], SYN posterior intraoccipital s.

s. manubriosterna′lis [NA], SYN manubriosternal *joint.*

neurocentral s., the cartilaginous union on either side between the body and arch of a vertebra in the young child. SYN neurocentral joint, neurocentral suture.

s. petro-occipita′lis [NA], SYN petro-occipital *joint.*

posterior intraoccipital s., cartilaginous union between the squamous and lateral parts of the occipital bone in the newborn. SYN s. intraoccipitalis posterior [NA], Budin's obstetrical joint, posterior intraoccipital joint.

sphenoethmoidal s., cartilaginous union between the body of the sphenoid and the posterior part of the ethmoidal labyrinth. SYN s. sphenoethmoidalis [NA].

s. sphenoethmoida′lis [NA], SYN sphenoethmoidal s.

spheno-occipital s., cartilaginous union between the body of the sphenoid and the basilar portion of the occipital; it fuses by the twentieth year; incorrectly called spheno-occipital suture. SYN s. spheno-occipitalis [NA], spheno-occipital joint, spheno-occipital suture.

s. spheno-occipita′lis [NA], SYN spheno-occipital s.

s. sphenopetro′sa [NA], SYN sphenopetrosal s.

sphenopetrosal s., sphenopetrous s., fibrocartilage filling the sphenopetrosal fissure. SYN s. sphenopetrosa [NA].

sternal synchondroses, the cartilaginous junctions between the body of the sternum and the manubrium, and the xiphoid process; in domestic animals, there may be several, *e.g.,* s. manubriosternalis, s. intersternebralis, and s. xiphosternalis. SYN synchondroses sternales [NA], sternal joints.

synchondro′ses sterna′les [NA], SYN sternal synchondroses.

s. xiphosterna′lis [NA], SYN xiphisternal *joint.*

syn·chon·dro·to·my (sin-kon-drot′ō-mē). SYN symphysiotomy.

syn·cho·ri·al (sin-kōr′ē-ăl). Relating to fused chorions as are found in multiple-fetus pregnancies. [syn- + chorion]

syn·chro·nia (sin-krō′nē-ă). **1.** SYN synchronism. **2.** Origin, development, involution, or functioning of tissues or organs at the usual time for such an event. Cf. heterochronia. [syn- + G. *chronos,* time]

syn·chron·ic (sin′krŏn-ik). Referring to the study of the natural history of a disease by its state and distribution in a population at one time. The inferences about longitudinal course from such a study are warranted only under special conditions, notably that the longitudinal course of the disease is itself unchanging and that subjects in the sample are a representative sample of the survivors.

syn·chro·nism (sin′krō-nizm). Occurrence of two or more events at the same time; the condition of being simultaneous. SYN synchronia (1). [syn- + G. *chronos,* time]

syn·chro·nous (sin′krō-nŭs). Occurring simultaneously. SYN homochronous (1). [G. *synchronos*]

syn·chro·ny (sin′krō-nē). The simultaneous appearance of two separate events. [syn- + G. *chronos,* time]

bilateral s., electroencephalographic activity that is recorded over both hemispheres simultaneously; usually used in reference to spike and wave activity.

syn·chro·tron (sin′krō-tron). A machine for generating high speed electrons or protons, as for nuclear studies.

syn·chy·sis (sin′kĭ-sis). Collapse of the collagenous framework of the vitreous humor, with liquefaction of the vitreous body. [G. a mixing together, fr. syn- + *chysis,* a pouring]

s. scintil′lans, an appearance of glistening spots in the eye, due to cholesterol crystals floating in a fluid vitreous.

syn·ci·ne·sis (sin-si-nē′sis). SYN synkinesis.

syn·cli·nal (sin′klĭ-năl). Denoting two structures inclined one toward the other. [G. *syn- klinō,* to incline together]

syn·clit·ic (sin-klit′ik). Relating to or marked by synclitism.

syn·cli·tism (sin′kli-tizm). Condition of parallelism between the planes of the fetal head and of the pelvis, respectively. [G. *synklinō,* to incline together]

syn·clo·nus (sin′klō-nŭs). Clonic spasm or tremor of several muscles. [syn- + G. *klonos,* tumult]

syn·co·pal (sin′kō-păl). Relating to syncope. SYN syncopic.

syn·co·pe (sin′kŏ-pē). Loss of consciousness and postural tone caused by diminished cerebral blood flow. [G. *synkopē,* a cutting short, a swoon]

Adams-Stokes s., s. due to complete atrioventricular block.

cardiac s., fainting with unconsciousness of any cardiac cause.

carotid sinus s., s. resulting from overactivity of the carotid sinus; attacks may be spontaneous or produced by pressure on a sensitive carotid sinus.

hysterical s., fainting due to, or to avoid, emotional stress.

laryngeal s., a paroxysmal neurosis characterized by attacks of coughing, with unusual sensations, as of tickling, in the throat, followed by a brief period of unconsciousness.

local s., limited numbness in a part, especially of the fingers; one of the symptoms, usually associated with local asphyxia, of Raynaud's disease.

micturition s., s. occurring in association with the act of emptying the bladder.

postural s., s. upon assuming an upright position; caused by failure of normal vasoconstrictive mechanisms.

swallow s., faintness or unconsciousness upon swallowing. This is nearly always due to excessive vagal effect on the heart that may already have bradycardia or atrioventricular block.

tussive s., fainting as a result of a coughing spell, caused by persistent increased intrathoracic pressure diminishing venous return to the heart, thus lowering cardiac output; most often occurs in heavy-set male smokers who have chronic bronchitis. SYN Charcot's vertigo, laryngeal vertigo.

vasodepressor s., faintness or loss of consciousness due to reflex reduction in blood pressure. SYN vasovagal s.

vasovagal s., SYN vasodepressor s.

syn·cop·ic (sin-kop'ik). SYN syncopal.

syn·cre·tio (sin-krē'shē-ō). Development of adhesion between inflamed opposing surfaces. [Mod. L., fr. G. *synkrētizō*, to unite the Cretan cities, reanalyzed as fr. syn- + L. *cresco*, pp. *cretum,* to grow]

syn·cy·a·nin (sin-sī'ă-nin). A blue pigment produced by *Pseudomonas syncyanea.*

syn·cy·tial (sin-sish'ăl, -sish'ē-ăl, -sit'ē-ăl). Relating to a syncytium.

syn·cy·ti·o·tro·pho·blast (sin-sish'ē-ō-trō'fō-blast). The syncytial outer layer of the trophoblast; site of synthesis of human chorionic gonadotropin. SEE ALSO trophoblast. SYN placental plasmodium, plasmodial trophoblast, plasmodiotrophoblast, syncytial trophoblast, syntrophoblast. [syncytium + trophoblast]

syn·cy·ti·um, pl. **syn·cy·tia** (sin-sish'ē-ŭm, -ă; -sit'ē-ŭm). A multinucleated protoplasmic mass formed by the secondary union of originally separate cells. [Mod. L. fr. syn- + G. *kytos,* cell]

syn·dac·tyl, syn·dac·tyle (sin-dak'til, -dak'tīl). SYN syndactylous.

syn·dac·tyl·ia, syn·dac·ty·lism (sin-dak-til'ē-ă, -dak'ti-lizm). SYN syndactyly.

syn·dac·ty·lous (sin-dak'ti-lŭs). Having fused or webbed fingers or toes. SYN syndactyl, syndactyle.

syn·dac·ty·ly (sin-dak'ti-lē). Any degree of webbing or fusion of fingers or toes, involving soft parts only or including bone structure; usually autosomal dominant inheritance. SYN symphalangism (1), symphalangy, syndactylia, syndactylism. [syn- + G. *daktylos,* finger or toe]

syn·dein (sin-dē'in). SYN ankyrin. [G. *syndeō,* to bind together, + -in]

syn·de·sis (sin-dē'sis). SYN arthrodesis. [syn- + G. *desis,* a binding]

♻ **syndesm-.** SEE syndesmo-.

syn·des·mec·to·my (sin-dez-mek'tō-mē). Cutting away a section of a ligament. [syndesm- + G. *ektomē,* excision]

syn·des·mec·to·pia (sin-dez-mek-tō'pē-ă). Displacement of a ligament. [syndesm- + G. *ektopos,* out of place]

syn·des·mi·tis (sin-dez-mī'tis). Inflammation of a ligament. [syndesm- + G. *-itis,* inflammation]

s. metatar'sea, inflammation of the metatarsal ligaments.

♻ **syndesmo-, syndesm-.** Ligament, ligamentous. [G. *syndesmos,* a fastening, fr. *syndeō,* to bind]

syn·des·mo·cho·ri·al (sin-dez-mō-kōr'ē-ăl). Relating to the placenta in ruminant animals. SEE syndesmochorial *placenta.* [syndesmo- + G. *chorion,* membrane]

syn·des·mo·di·al (sin-des-mō'dē-ăl). SYN syndesmotic.

syn·des·mog·ra·phy (sin-dez-mog'ră-fē). A treatise on or description of the ligaments. [syndesmo- + G. *graphō,* to write]

syn·des·mo·lo·gia (sin-dez'mō-lō'jē-ă). SYN arthrology.

syn·des·mol·o·gy (sin-dez-mol'ŏ-jē). SYN arthrology. [syndesmo- + G. *logos,* study]

syn·des·mo·pexy (sin-dez'mō-pek-sē). The joining of two ligaments, or attachment of a ligament in a new place. [syndesmo- + G. *pēxis,* fixation]

syn·des·mo·phyte (sin-dez'mō-fīt). An osseous excrescence attached to a ligament. [syndesmo- + G. *phyton,* plant]

syn·des·mo·plas·ty (sin-dez'mō-plas-tē). Rarely used term for plastic surgery of a ligament. [syndesmo- + G. *plastos,* formed]

syn·des·mor·rha·phy (sin-dez-mōr'ă-fē). Suture of ligaments. [syndesmo- + G. *rhaphē,* suture]

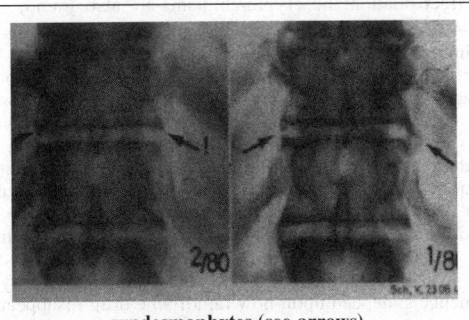
syndesmophytes (see arrows)

syn·des·mo·sis, pl. **syn·des·mo·ses** (sin'dez-mō'sis, -sēz) [NA]. A form of fibrous joint in which opposing surfaces that are relatively far apart are united by ligaments; *e.g.,* the union of the styloid process of the temporal bone and the hyoid bone via the stylohyoid ligament, and the union between the distal ends of the tibia and fibula. SYN syndesmodial joint, syndesmotic joint. [syndesmo- + G. *-osis,* condition]

radioulnar s., the fibrous union of the radius and ulna consisting of the oblique cord and the interosseous membrane. SYN s. radioulnaris [NA], middle radioulnar joint.

s. radioulna'ris [NA], SYN radioulnar s.

tibiofibular s., the fibrous union of the tibia and fibula consisting of the interosseous membrane and the anterior, interosseous and posterior tibiofibular ligaments at the distal extremities of the bones. SYN s. tibiofibularis [NA], distal tibiofibular joint, inferior tibiofibular joint, tibiofibular articulation (2).

s. tibiofibula'ris [NA], SYN tibiofibular s.

s. tympanostape'dia [NA], SYN tympanostapedial *junction,* tympanostapedial s.

tympanostapedial s., aBCXYZ SYN s. tympanostapedia [NA].

syn·des·mot·ic (sin-des-mot'ik). Relating to syndesmosis. SYN syndesmodial.

syn·des·mot·o·my (sin-dez-mot'ō-mē). Surgical division of a ligament. [syndesmo- + G. *tomē,* incision]

SYNDROME

syn·drome (sin'drōm). The aggregate of signs and symptoms associated with any morbid process, and constituting together the picture of the disease. SEE ALSO disease. [G. *syndromē,* a running together, tumultuous concourse; (in med.) a concurrence of symptoms, fr. *syn,* together, + *dromos,* a running]

Aarskog-Scott s., SYN faciodigitogenital *dysplasia.*

abdominal muscle deficiency s. [MIM*100100, MIM*264140], congenital absence (partial or complete) of abdominal muscles, in which the outline of the intestines is visible through the protruding abdominal wall; in males, genitourinary anomalies (uri-

---

♻ **Combining forms**	[NA] Nomina Anatomica
Word*Finder* Multi-term entry finder Preceding letter A	[MIM] Mendelian Inheritance in Man
A.D.A.M. Anatomy Plates Between letters L and M	☆ Official alternate term
Appendices: Following letter Z	☆[NA] Official alternate Nomina Anatomica term
SYN Synonym; Cf., compare	High Profile Term

sy

nary tract dilation and cryptorchidism) are also found; genetics unclear.

abstinence s., a constellation of physiologic changes undergone by persons or animals who have become physically dependent on a drug or chemical due to prolonged use at elevated doses, but who are abruptly deprived of that substance. The abstinence s. varies with the drug to which dependence has developed. Generally the effects observed are in an opposite direction from those produced by the drug; *e.g.,* the withdrawal s. from central nervous system depressants such as barbiturates and benzodiazepines consists of insomnia, restlessness, tremulousness, hallucinations, and, in the extreme, tonic-clonic convulsions which may prove fatal. The onset time and severity of the abstinence s. depend upon how rapidly the drug disappears from the body.

Achard s. [MIM*100700], arachnodactyly with small receding mandible, broad skull, and joint laxity limited to the hands and feet; genetics unclear.

Achard-Thiers s., one form of a virilizing disorder of adrenocortical origin in women, characterized by masculinization and menstrual disorders in association with manifestations of diabetes mellitus, such as glucosuria.

Achenbach s., hematoma of the finger pad with accompanying edema; of unknown cause in the absence of disturbances in blood coagulation mechanisms.

acquired immunodeficiency s., SYN AIDS.

acrofacial s., SYN acrofacial *dysostosis.*

acroparesthesia s., abnormal sensation such as numbness and tingling in the hands, usually in middle-aged women; classic symptom of carpal tunnel syndrome.

acute organic brain s., SYN organic brain s.

acute radiation s., a s. caused by exposure of the body to large amounts of radiation, (*e.g.,* from certain forms of therapy, accidents, and nuclear explosions; it is divided into three major forms which are, in ascending order of severity, the hematogic, gastrointestinal, and central nervous system-cardiovascular forms; its clinical manifestations are divided into prodromal, latent, overt, and recovery stages.

Adams-Stokes s., a s. characterized by slow or absent pulse, vertigo, syncope, convulsions, and sometimes Cheyne-Stokes respiration; usually as a result of advanced A-V block or sick sinus syndrome. SYN Adams-Stokes disease, Morgagni's disease, Morgagni-Adams-Stokes s., Spens' s., Stokes-Adams disease, Stokes-Adams s.

adaptation s. of Selye, general nonspecific adaptation of the organism in response to specific stimuli which trigger a cycle of extensive physiological changes in the endocrine and other organ systems due to prolonged and intense stress. SEE general adaptation s.

addisonian s., SYN chronic adrenocortical *insufficiency.*

adherence s., restriction action of an ocular muscle owing to adhesions between the muscle and its fascial sheath.

Adie s. [MIM*100300], an idiopathic postganglionic denervation of the parasympathetically innervated intraocular muscles, usually complicated by signs of aberrant regeneration of these nerves: a weak light reaction with segmental palsy of iris sphincter, a strong slow near response. Deep tendon reflexes are often asymmetrically reduced. SEE ALSO tonic *pupil.* SYN Adie's pupil, Holmes-Adie pupil, Holmes-Adie s., pupillotonic pseudotabes.

adiposogenital s., SYN *dystrophia* adiposogenitalis.

adrenal cortical s., an inexact (and obsolete) term that has been applied to Cushing's s., Addison's disease, or the adrenogenital s.

adrenal virilizing s., SYN adrenal *virilism.*

adrenogenital s., generic designation for a group of disorders caused by adrenocortical hyperplasia or malignant tumors and characterized by masculinization of women, feminization of men, or precocious sexual development of children; representative of excessive or abnormal secretory patterns of adrenocortical steroids, especially those with androgenic or estrogenic effects.

adult respiratory distress s. (ARDS), acute lung injury from a variety of causes, characterized by interstitial and/or alveolar edema and hemorrhage as well as perivascular pulmonary edema

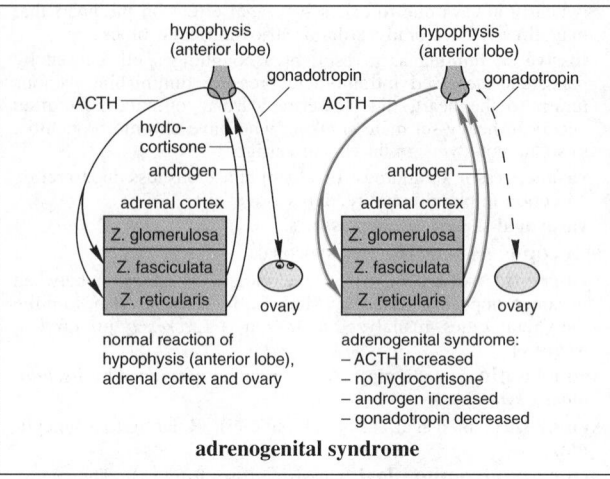

adrenogenital syndrome

associated with hyaline membrane, proliferation of collagen fibers, and swollen epithelium with increased pinocytosis. SYN wet lung (2), white lung.

afferent loop s., acute or chronic obstruction of the duodenum and jejunum proximal to the gastrojejunostomy performed in a Billroth II type gastrectomy; a distended afferent loop causes symptoms of pain and fullness. SYN gastrojejunal loop obstruction s.

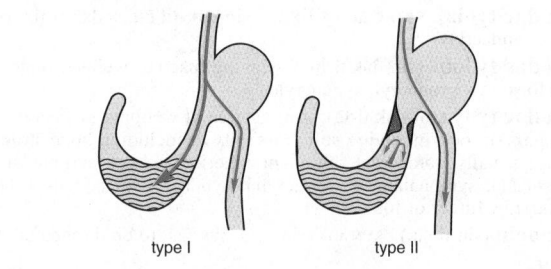

afferent loop syndrome

in *type I,* misplaced anastomosis favors filling of the loop; in *type II,* drainage of the loop is hindered

aglossia-adactylia s. [MIM*103300], congenital absence or hypoplasia of the tongue, associated with absence of the digits.

Ahumada-Del Castillo s., unphysiological lactation and amenorrhea not following pregnancy characterized by hyperprolactinemia and a pituitary adenoma. SYN Argonz-Del Castillo s.

Aicardi's s. [MIM*304050], agenesis of the corpus collosum with infantile spasms in female babies.

Albright's s., (1) SYN McCune-Albright s. **(2)** SYN Albright's hereditary *osteodystrophy.*

alcohol amnestic s., an amnestic s. resulting from alcoholism; alcoholic "blackouts." Cf. Korsakoff's s.

Aldrich s., SYN Wiskott-Aldrich s.

Alezzandrini's s., a rare s. appearing in adolescents and young adults, characterized by unilateral degenerative retinitis, followed by ipsilateral poliosis and facial vitiligo, and occasionally bilateral perceptive deafness.

Alice in Wonderland s., the illusion of dreams, feelings of levitation, and alteration in the sense of the passage of time, sometimes associated with migraine, epilepsy, and various diseases of the parietal lobe of the brain.

Allen-Masters s., pelvic pain resulting from an old laceration of the broad ligament received during delivery.

Alport's s., progressive microscopic hematuria leading to chronic renal failure earlier in males, accompanied by defects such as sensorineural hearing loss, lenticonus, and maculopathy; autosomal dominant [MIM*153640 and 153650], autosomal recessive

[MIM*203800], and X-linked [MIM*301050 and *303630] forms known.

Alström's s. [MIM*203800], retinal degeneration with nystagmus and loss of central vision, associated with obesity in childhood; sensorineural hearing loss and diabetes mellitus usually occur after age 10; autosomal recessive inheritance.

amenorrhea-galactorrhea s., unphysiologic lactation from endocrinological causes or from a pituitary tumor.

amnestic s., (1) SYN Korsakoff's s. (2) an organic brain s. with short term (but not immediate) memory disturbance, regardless of the etiology.

amniotic fluid s., pulmonary embolic phenomena thought to be due to infusion of amniotic fluid containing epithelial squames into maternal blood vessels; shock ensues and sudden death may occur.

Amsterdam s., SYN de Lange s. [*Amsterdam,* the Netherlands]

androgen resistance s.'s, a class of disorders associated with 5α-steroid reductase deficiency, testicular feminization, and related disorders. Cf. *steroid* 5α-reductase, Reifenstein's s., infertile male s., testicular feminization s.

Angelman s., microdeletion of 15 q-13, of maternal origin, resulting in mental retardation, ataxia, paroxysms of laughter, seizures, characteristic facies, and minimal speech. SEE Prader-Willi s.

Angelucci's s., extreme excitability, vasomotor disturbances, and palpitation associated with vernal conjunctivitis.

angio-osteohypertrophy s., SYN Klippel-Trenaunay-Weber s.

ankyloglossia superior s., a congenital condition in which the tongue adheres to the hard palate; no evidence of genetic factors.

anorectal s., soreness, burning, itching, or other irritation of the rectum together with redness about the anus, and sometimes accompanied by diarrhea, occurring as a toxic effect of the oral administration of certain broad spectrum antibiotics.

anterior chamber cleavage s. [MIM*261540], a congenital disorder originating from faulty separation of embryonic structures; it results in bilateral central corneal opacities, with an anterior ring attachment of the iridic pupillary border and anterior polar cataracts; associated with short-limbed dwarfism; autosomal dominant inheritance. SEE iridocorneal endothelial s. SYN Peters' anomaly.

anterior tibial compartment s., ischemic necrosis of the muscles of the anterior tibial compartment of the leg, presumed due to compression of arteries by swollen muscles following unaccustomed exertion.

antibody deficiency s., any of a group of disorders associated with a defective antibody production due to defects in the B-type lymphocyte system or in T-type lymphocytes; chief manifestation is an increased susceptibility to infection by various microorganisms. SEE agammaglobulinemia, hypogammaglobulinemia, immunodeficiency. SYN antibody deficiency disease.

Anton's s., in cortical blindness, lack of awareness of being blind.

anxiety s., the constellation of autonomic nervous system signs and symptoms accompanying the apprehension of danger and dread. SEE anxiety.

aortic arch s., atheromatous and/or thrombotic obliteration of the branches of the arch of the aorta leading to diminished or absent pulses in the neck and arms. SEE ALSO Takayasu's *arteritis,* reversed *coarctation.* SYN Martorell's s.

apallic s., SYN apallic *state.*

Apert's s., SYN acrocephalosyndactyly.

s. of approximate relevant answers, SYN Ganser's s.

Argonz-Del Castillo s., SYN Ahumada-Del Castillo s.

Arndt-Gottron s., SYN scleromyxedema.

Arnold-Chiari s., SYN Arnold-Chiari *malformation.*

arterial thoracic outlet s., a rare disorder due to compression of the subclavian artery (with resultant poststenotic dilation) by a fully formed cervical rib; thrombi form in the dilated distal arterial segment, and distal limb ischemia may occur due to thromboembolic events.

Ascher's s. [MIM*109900], a condition in which a congenital double lip is associated with blepharochalasis and nontoxic thyroid gland enlargement.

Asherman's s., synechiae within the endometrial cavity, often causing amenorrhea and infertility.

asplenia s., s. seen in patients who had no functional spleen, either due to surgical removal of disease (*e.g.,* sickle cell anemia); includes increased susceptibility to bacterial infection, especially pneumococcal infection.

ataxia telangiectasia s., SYN *ataxia* telangiectasia.

auriculotemporal nerve s., localized flushing and sweating of the ear and cheek in response to eating. SYN Frey's s., gustatory sweating s.

autoerythrocyte sensitization s., a condition, usually occurring in women, in which the individual bruises easily (purpura simplex) and the ecchymoses tend to enlarge and involve adjacent tissues, resulting in pain in the affected parts; so-called because similar lesions are produced by inoculation of the individual's blood or various components of red blood cells and it is thought to be a form of localized autosensitization, although no specific antibodies have been demonstrable; in some individuals, there seems to be a psychogenic mechanism. SYN Gardner-Diamond s., psychogenic purpura.

Avellis' s., unilateral paralysis of the larynx and velum palati, with contralateral loss of pain and temperature sensibility in the parts below. SYN jugular foramen s.

A-V strabismus s., strabismus in which the angle of deviation is more marked on looking upward or downward. SEE ALSO A-*esotropia,* V-*esotropia,* A-*exotropia,* V-*exotropia.*

Ayerza's s., sclerosis of the pulmonary arteries in chronic cor pulmonale; associated with severe cyanosis, it is a condition resembling polycythemia vera but resulting from primary pulmonary arteriosclerosis or primary pulmonary hypertension and characterized by plexiform lesions of arterioles. SYN Ayerza's disease, cardiopathia nigra, plexogenic pulmonary arteriopathy.

Babinski's s., the combination of cardiac, arterial, and central nervous system manifestations of late *syphilis.*

baby bottle s., SYN nursing bottle *caries.*

Balint's s., an entity characterized by optic *ataxia* and simultanagnosia. This difficulty in applying the visual system to a visual task is usually due to damage to the superior temporal-occipital areas in both hemispheres.

Bamberger-Marie s., SYN hypertrophic pulmonary *osteoarthropathy.*

Bannwarth's s., neurologic manifestations of Lyme disease, also called chronic lymphocytic meningitis and tick-borne meningo-polyneuritis.

Banti's s., chronic congestive splenomegaly that occurs primarily in children as a sequel to hypertension in the portal or splenic veins, usually as a result of thrombosis of the veins; anemia, splenomegaly, and irregular episodes of gastrointestinal bleeding are usually observed, with ascites, jaundice, leukopenia, and thrombocytopenia developing in various conbinations. SYN Banti's disease, splenic anemia.

Bardet-Biedl s. [MIM*209900], mental retardation, pigmentary retinopathy, polydactyly, obesity, and hypogenitalism; recessive inheritance. SEE ALSO Laurence-Moon-Biedl s.

bare lymphocyte s., absence of HLA antigens on peripheral mononuclear cells, which may result in immunodeficiency.

Barlow s. [MIM*157700], late apical systolic murmur or (so-called "mid-late") systolic click, or both, due to massive billowing of the anterior and/or posterior (mural) mitral valvular leaflet into the left atrial cavity (also, floppy valve s.); electrocardiographically, ST-T changes in a posteroinferior distribution resembling those of myocardial ischemia often coexist for unknown reasons; rhythm disturbances may coexist with this s. without demonstrable pathogenetic relationship.

Barrett's s., chronic peptic ulceration of the lower esophagus, which is lined by columnar epithelium, resembling the mucosa of the gastric cardia, acquired as a result of long-standing chronic esophagitis; esophageal stricture with reflux, and adenocarcinoma, also have been reported. SYN Barrett's esophagus.

Bart's s. [MIM*132000], a form of epidermolysis bullosa with blistering of the extremities and intertriginous areas, erosions of the mouth, and deformed nails; probably autosomal dominant;

sy

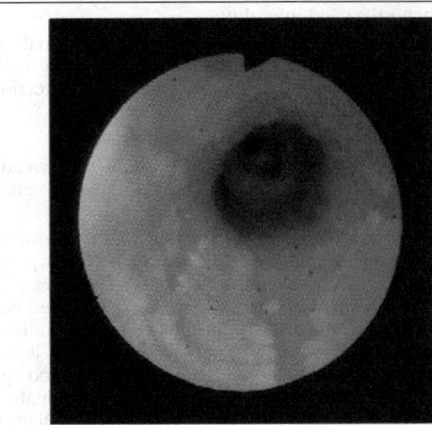

Barrett syndrome
endoscopic view of the mucosa of the esophageal-gastric region

there is often spontaneous improvement with no residual scarring.

Bartter's s. [MIM*241200], primary juxtaglomerular cell hyperplasia with secondary hyperaldosteronism, reported in children with hypokalemic alkalosis and elevated renin or angiotensin levels; however, the blood pressure is low or normal, edema is absent, and growth is usually retarded; recessive inheritance.

basal cell nevus s. [MIM*109400], a s. of myriad basal cell nevi with development of basal cell carcinomas in adult life, odontogenic keratocysts, erythematous pitting of the palms and soles, calcification of the cerebral falx, and frequently skeletal anomalies, particularly ribs that are bifid or broadened anteriorly; autosomal dominant inheritance. SYN Gorlin's s.

Basan's s., ectodermal dysplasia with hypotrichosis, hypohidrosis, defective teeth, and unusual dermatoglyphics.

Bassen-Kornzweig s., SYN abetalipoproteinemia.

battered child s., the clinical presentation of child abuse: various injuries to the skeleton, soft tissues, or organs of a child sustained as a result of repeated mistreatment or beating, usually by an individual responsible for the child's care.

battered spouse s., physical, psychological, and emotional injuries in a person subjected to abuse by a spouse or domestic partner; usually associated with alcoholism in the abusing spouse.

Bauer's s., aortitis and aortic endocarditis as a little recognized manifestation of rheumatoid arthritis.

Bazex's s., erythematous to plum-colored scaly acral skin lesions, paronychia, and nail dysplasia; associated with cancer of the upper respiratory or upper alimentary tract. SYN paraneoplastic acrokeratosis.

Beckwith-Wiedemann s. [MIM*130650], exomphalos, macroglossia, and gigantism, often with neonatal hypoglycemia; autosomal recessive inheritance. SYN EMG s.

Behçet's s. [MIM*109650], a s. characterized by simultaneously or successively occurring recurrent attacks of genital and oral ulcerations (aphthae) and uveitis or iridocyclitis with hypopyon, often with arthritis; a phase of a generalized disorder, occurring more often in men than in women, with variable manifestations, including dermatitis, erythema nodosum, thrombophlebitis, and cerebral involvement. SYN Behçet's disease, cutaneomucouveal s., iridocyclitis septica, oculobuccogenital s., recurrent hypopyon, triple symptom complex, uveo-encephalitic s.

Behr's s. [MIM*210000], adult or presenile form of heredomacular degeneration. SYN Behr's disease.

Benedikt's s., hemiplegia with clonic spasm or tremor and oculomotor paralysis on the opposite side.

Beradinelli's s., accelerated growth, lipodystrophy with muscular hypertrophy, hepatomegaly, and lipemia.

Bernard-Horner s., SYN Horner's s.

Bernard-Sergent s., SYN acute adrenocortical *insufficiency.*

Bernard-Soulier s., a coagulation disorder characterized by thrombocytopenia, giant platelets, and a bleeding tendency.

Bernhardt-Roth s., SYN *meralgia* paraesthetica.

Bernheim's s., systemic congestion resembling the consequences of right heart failure (enlarged liver, distended neck veins, and edema) without pulmonary congestion in subjects with left ventricular enlargement from any cause; reduction in the size of the right ventricular cavity is found by contrast imaging or echocardiography or at postmortem due to encroachment by the hypertrophied or aneurysmal ventricular septum.

Besnier-Boeck-Schaumann s., SYN sarcoidosis.

Beuren s., supravalvular aortic stenosis with multiple areas of peripheral pulmonary arterial stenosis, mental retardation, and dental anomalies.

Biemond s. [MIM*210350], iris coloboma, mental retardation, obesity, hypogenitalism, and postaxial polydactyly; a recessive inheritance disorder resembling Laurence-Moon and Bardet-Biedel s.'s.

billowing mitral valve s., SYN mitral valve prolapse s.

Bjornstad's s. [mim*262000], pili torti associated with sensorineural hearing loss, the severity of distortion and brittleness of the hair correlated with the degree of deafness; autosomal dominant inheritance.

Blatin's s., SYN hydatid *thrill.*

blind loop s., stagnation of intestinal contents with bacterial overgrowth producing substances that interfere with absorption of fat, vitamins, and other nutrients, usually occurring in the small intestine following operations that produce a blind loop or pouch.

Bloch-Sulzberger s., SYN *incontinentia* pigmenti.

Bloom's s. [MIM*210900], congenital telangiectatic erythema, primarily in butterfly distribution, of the face and occasionally of the hands and forearms, with sensitivity of skin lesions and dwarfism with normal body proportions except for a narrow face and dolichocephalic skull; chromosomes are excessively fragile; autosomal recessive inheritance.

blue toe s., progressive tissue injury or gangrene from microthromboembolism in the presence of palpable pedal pulses.

Boerhaave's s., spontaneous rupture of the lower esophagus, a variant of Mallory-Weiss s.

Bonnier's s., a s. due to a lesion of Deiters nucleus and its connection; the symptoms include ocular disturbances (*e.g.,* paralysis of accommodation, nystagmus, diplopia), as well as deafness, nausea, thirst, anorexia, and symptoms referable to the involvement of the vagus centers.

Böök s. [MIM*112300], premolar aplasia, hyperhidrosis, and premature canities; autosomal dominant trait.

Börjeson-Forssman-Lehmann s. [MIM*301900], a condition characterized by mental deficiency, epilepsy, hypogonadism, hypometabolism, obesity, and narrow palpebral fissures; X-linked recessive inheritance.

bowel bypass s., fever, chills, malaise, and inflammatory cutaneous papules and pustules on the extremities and upper trunk, sometimes with polyarthralgia, with recurrent symptoms following bowel bypass surgery.

bradytachycardia s. (brā′dē-tă-kē-car′dē-ă), alternate rapid and slow cardiac rates that may represent any rhythm disturbances in any combination usually related to sinus node disease. SYN tachybradycardia s.

Briquet's s., a chronic but fluctuating mental disorder, usually of young women, characterized by frequent complaints of physical illness involving multiple organ systems simultaneously.

Brissaud-Marie s., unilateral spasm of the tongue and lips, of hysterical nature.

Brock's s., SYN middle lobe s.

Brown's s., SYN tendon sheath s.

Brown-Séquard's s., s. with unilateral spinal cord lesions, proprioception loss and weakness occur ipsilateral to the lesion, while pain and temperature loss occur contralateral. SYN Brown-Séquard's paralysis.

Brugsch's s., SYN pachydermoperiostosis.

Budd-Chiari s., SYN Chiari's s.

Budd's s., SYN Chiari's s.

Bürger-Grütz s., SYN type I familial *hyperlipoproteinemia.*

burner s., multiple episodes of upper extremity burning pain, sometimes accompanied by shoulder girdle weakness, experienced during contact sports, especially football, with each forceful blow to the head or shoulder; attributed to an upper trunk brachial plexopathy.

Burnett's s., SYN milk-alkali s.

burning foot s., a disorder observed in prisoners-of-war in World War II, now believed to be due to a pantothenate deficiency.

burning vulva s., persistent vulvodynia in which a physical cause has not been identified.

Buschke-Ollendorf s., SYN osteodermatopoikilosis.

Caffey-Kempe s., SEE battered child s.

Caffey's s., SYN infantile cortical *hyperostosis.*

Caffey-Silverman s., SYN infantile cortical *hyperostosis.*

camptomelic s., also associated with flat facies, short vertebrae, hypoplastic scapula, and bowed tibia. SYN osteochondrodysplasia.

Capgras' s., the delusional belief that a person (or persons) close to the schizophrenic patient has been substituted for by one or more impostors; may have an organic etiology. SYN Capgras' phenomenon, illusion of doubles.

Caplan's s., intrapulmonary nodules, histologically similar to subcutaneous rheumatoid nodules, associated with rheumatoid arthritis and pneumoconiosis in coal workers. SYN Caplan's nodules.

carbonic anhydrase II deficiency s., an inherited deficiency of carbonic anhydrase II that results in osteopetrosis and metabolic acidosis. SYN osteopetrosis with renal tubular acidosis.

carcinoid s., a combination of symptoms and lesions usually produced by the release of serotonin from carcinoid tumors of the gastrointestinal tract that have metastasized to the liver; consists of irregular mottled blushing, flat angiomas of the skin, acquired tricuspid and pulmonary stenosis often with regurgitation, occasionally with some minor involvement of valves on the left side of the heart, diarrhea, bronchial spasm, mental aberration, and excretion of large quantities of 5-hydroxyindoleacetic acid. SYN malignant carcinoid s., metastatic carcinoid s.

cardiofacial s., (1) transient or persistent unilateral partial lower facial paresis accompanying some congenital heart disease. **(2)** a group of syndromes characterized by congenital cardiovascular, bone, soft tissue, and facial abnormalities. Examples include Rubinstein-Taybi s., Noonan's s. and Williams' s. SYN Williams' s.

Caroli's s., congenital malformation of the bile ducts leading to formation of multifocal dilatations and cysts.

carotid sinus s., stimulation of a hyperactive carotid sinus, causing a marked fall in blood pressure due to vasodilation, cardiac slowing, or both; syncope with or without convulsions or A-V block may occur. SYN Charcot-Weiss-Baker s.

carpal tunnel s., the most common nerve entrapment s., characterized by nocturnal hand paresthesia and pain, and sometimes sensory loss and wasting in the median hand distribution; affects women more than men and is often bilateral; caused by entrapment of the median nerve at the wrist, within the carpal tunnel.

Carpenter's s., (1) the association of primary hypothyroidism, primary adrenocortical insufficiency, and diabetes mellitus. [C. C. J. Carpenter] **(2)** SYN acrocephalopolysyndactyly. [G. Carpenter]

cataract-oligophrenia s., SYN Marinesco-Garland s.

cat's cry s., SYN cri-du-chat s.

cat's-eye s. [MIM*115470], iris colobomas (resembling the vertical pupils of a cat) and anal atresia, associated with an additional acrocentric chromosome; other malformations and mental retardation may be present. SYN Schmid-Fraccaro s.

cauda equina s., dull pain in upper sacral region with anesthesia or analgesia in buttocks, genitalia, or thigh; accompanied by disturbed bowel and bladder function.

cavernous sinus s., a s. caused by thrombosis of the cavernous intracranial sinus characterized by edema of eyelids and conjunctivae, and paralysis of the third, fourth and sixth nerves.

Ceelen-Gellerstedt s., SYN idiopathic pulmonary *hemosiderosis.*

celiac s., SYN celiac *disease.*

cellular immunity deficiency s., a s. marked by increased susceptibility to infection, especially to viral infection, associated with defective functioning of the mechanism responsible for acquired immunity of the cell-mediated kind. SEE ALSO immunodeficiency.

central cord s., quadriparesis most severely involving the distal upper extremities, with or without sensory loss and bladder dysfunction, usually due to ischemia from osteophytic or traumatic compression of the central part of the cervical spinal cord and/or artery.

cerebellar s., the signs and symptoms of cerebellar deficiency: dysmetria, dysarthria, asynergia, nystagmus, ataxia, staggering gait, and adiadochokinesia.

cerebellomedullary malformation s., SYN Arnold-Chiari *malformation.*

cerebellopontine angle s., a s. due most commonly to an acoustic tumor in the region between the cerebellum and pons, and marked by ataxia, nystagmus, tinnitus, deafness, disturbances of labyrinth function, and involvement of any of the cranial nerves, fifth, sixth, seventh, ninth, or tenth.

cerebrohepatorenal s. [MIM*214100, MIM*211410], a neonatal s. characterized by muscular hypotonia, incomplete myelinization of nervous tissue, craniofacial malformations, hepatomegaly, and small glomerular cysts of the kidney; there is a perturbation in peroxisomes; autosomal recessive inheritance. SYN Zellweger s.

cervical compression s., SYN cervical disc s.

cervical disc s., pain, paresthesias, and sometimes weakness in the area of the distribution of one or more cervical roots, due to pressure of a protruded cervical intervertebral disc. SYN cervical compression s.

cervical fusion s., SYN Klippel-Feil s.

cervical rib s., indefinite term, equally applicable to two different syndromes: 1) arterial thoracic outlet s. in which the subclavian artery is compromised by a fully formed cervical rib, and 2) true neurogenic thoracic outlet s. in which the proximal lower trunk of the brachial plexus is compromised by a translucent band extending from a rudimentary cervical rib to the first rib.

cervical rib and band s., SYN true neurogenic thoracic outlet syndrome.

cervical tension s., SYN posttraumatic neck s.

cervico-oculo-acoustic s. [MIM*314600], a congenital short neck associated with paralysis of the external ocular muscles and with perceptive deafness; occurs in girls. SYN Wildervanck s.

Cestan-Chenais s., contralateral hemiplegia, hemianesthesia, and loss of pain and temperature sensibility, with ipsilateral hemiasynergia and lateropulsion, paralysis of the larynx and soft palate, enophthalmia, miosis, and ptosis, due to lesions of the brain stem.

chancriform s., an ulcerative lesion at the site of primary infection by microorganisms, with regional lymph node enlargement; it occurs not only in chancroid infections but also in various bacterial and fungal infections.

Chandler s., iris atrophy with corneal edema. SYN iridocorneal syndrome.

Charcot's s., SYN intermittent *claudication.*

Charcot-Weiss-Baker s., SYN carotid sinus s.

Chauffard's s., the symptoms of Still's disease in one suffering from bovine or other nonhuman form of tuberculosis. SYN Still-Chauffard s.

Chédiak-Steinbrinck-Higashi s. [MIM*214500, MIM*214450], abnormalities of granulation and nuclear structure of all types of leukocytes with malformation of peroxidase-positive granules, cytoplasmic inclusions, and Döhle bodies, often with hepatosplenomegaly, lymphadenopathy, anemia, thrombocytopenia, roentgenologic changes of bones, lungs and heart, skin and psychomotor abnormalities, and susceptibility to infection, usually resulting in death in childhood; occurs in mink, cattle, and mice, as well as man; autosomal recessive inheritance. SYN Béguez César disease, Chédiak-Higashi disease, Chédiak-Steinbrinck-Higashi anomaly.

sy

Cheney s., acro-osteolysis with osteoporosis and changes in the skull and mandible.

cherry-red spot myoclonus s., a neuronal storage disorder in children characterized by a cherry red spot at the macula, progressive myoclonus, and easily controlled seizures; the result of sialidase deficiency. Type 1 is characterized by normal body habitus, cherry red macula, myoclonus, and normal β-galactosidase levels; type 2 by short stature, bony abnormalities, and deficient β-galactosidase. SYN sialidosis.

Chiari-Budd s., SYN Chiari's s.

Chiari-Frommel s., unphysiological lactation and amenorrhea following pregnancy, but not caused by infant's nursing; characterized by hyperprolactinemia and a pituitary adenoma.

Chiari II s., elongation of medulla and cerebellar tonsils and vermis with displacement through the foramen magnum into the upper spinal canal; often associated with other cerebral anomalies.

Chiari's s., thrombosis of the hepatic vein with great enlargement of the liver and extensive development of collateral vessels, intractable ascites, and severe portal hypertension. SYN Budd's s., Budd-Chiari s., Chiari's disease, Chiari-Budd s., Rokitansky's disease (2).

chiasma s., a s. characterized by a bitemporal visual field defect and optic nerve atrophy due to a lesion in or about the chiasm.

Chilaiditi's s., interposition of the colon between the liver and the diaphragm.

CHILD s., congenital *h*emidysplasia with *i*chthyosiform erythroderma and *l*imb *d*efects.

Chinese restaurant s., development of chest pain, feelings of facial pressure, and sensation of burning over variable portions of the body surface after ingestion of food containing monosodium L-glutamate (MSG) by persons sensitive to this food additive.

Chotzen's s. [MIM*101400], characterized by syndactyly as well as mild mental retardation, hypertelorism, and sometimes, ptosis; autosomal dominant inheritance. SEE ALSO type III *acrocephalosyndactyly*.

Christian's s., SYN Hand-Schüller-Christian *disease*.

Christ-Siemens-Touraine s., SYN anhidrotic ectodermal *dysplasia*.

chromosomal s., general designation for s.'s due to chromosomal aberrations; typically associated with mental retardation and multiple congenital anomalies.

chromosomal instability s.'s, chromosomal breakage s.'s, a group of mendelian conditions associated with chromosomal instability and breakage *in vitro*, they often manifest an increased tendency to certain types of malignancies. SEE Bloom's s., fragile X s., *xeroderma* pigmentosum.

chronic hyperventilation s., reduced CO_2 content of the blood (hypocapnia) as a result of hyperventilation of prolonged duration; may occur in anxiety states and in some chronic organic, usually cardiovascular, disease; alkalemia, paresthesia, and tetany may occur.

Churg-Strauss s., asthma, fever, eosinophilia, and varied symptoms and signs of vasculitis, primarily affecting small arteries, with vascular and extravascular granulomas. SYN allergic granulomatosis, allergic granulomatous angiitis.

Clarke-Hadfield s., SYN cystic *fibrosis*.

classic cervical rib s., SYN true neurogenic thoracic outlet syndrome.

Claude's s., midbrain s. with oculomotor palsy on the side of the lesion and incoordination on the opposite side.

click s., a syndrome, particularly of the atrioventricular valves, in which systole causes a sudden tensing of a scallop of a valve or an entire cusp producing the auscultatory click. SYN valvular prolapse.

climacteric s., SYN menopausal s.

cloverleaf skull s. [MIM*148800], intrauterine bone dysplasia and synostosis of the coronal and lambdoid sutures producing a trilobar head shape, with various craniofacial and long-bone anomalies; the condition is sporadic; no evidence to suggest a genetic cause.

Cobb s., cutaneous angiomas, usually in a dermatomal distribution on the trunk, associated with vascular abnormality of the spinal cord and resulting neurologic symptoms. SYN cutaneomeningospinal angiomatosis.

Cockayne's s. [MIM*216400, MIM*216410, MIM*216411], dwarfism, precociously senile appearance, pigmentary degeneration of the retina, optic atrophy, deafness, sensitivity to sunlight, and mental retardation; autosomal recessive inheritance. There is a variant with early onset [MIM*216410]. SYN Cockayne's disease.

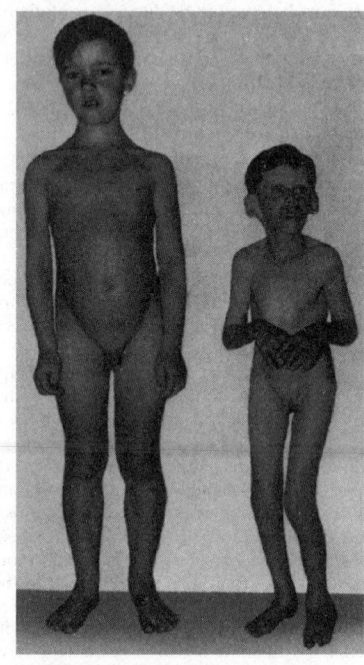

Cockayne syndrome
dwarfism and bodily posture in Cockayne syndrome (10 3/4 yr. old patient, next to a healthy boy of the same age)

Coffin-Lowry s., SYN Coffin-Siris s.

Coffin-Siris s. [MIM*135900], mental retardation with wide bulbous (pugilistic) nose, low nasal bridge, moderate hirsutism, and digital anomalies with nail hypoplasia (especially of the fifth fingers); the full s. occurs only in males, but female relatives may have abnormal fingers and mild mental retardation; X-linked inheritance, incompletely recessive. SYN Coffin-Lowry s.

Cogan-Reese s., SYN iridocorneal endothelial s.

Cogan's s., SYN oculovestibulo-auditory s.

Collet-Sicard s., unilateral lesions of the ninth, tenth, eleventh, and twelfth cranial nerves producing Vernet syndrome and paralysis of the tongue on the same side.

combined immunodeficiency s., a serious primary immunodeficiency affecting both T and B cells.

compartmental s., a condition in which increased pressure in a confined anatomical space adversely affects the circulation and threatens the function and viability of the tissues therein.

compression s., SYN crush s.

congenital rubella s., fetal infection with rubella virus during the first trimester of pregnancy resulting in a series of congenital abnormalities including heart disease, deafness, and blindness.

Conn's s., SYN primary *aldosteronism*.

Cornelia de Lange s., SYN de Lange s.

corpus luteum deficiency s., functional disturbances caused by insufficient ovarian luteinization; reflected by inadequate luteal phase endometrial response.

Costen's s., a symptom complex of loss of hearing, otalgia, tinnitus, dizziness, headache, and burning sensation of the throat, tongue, and side of the nose; originally attributed to temporomandibular joint dysfunction resulting from occlusal disharmony, but currently recognized as not being well founded on anatomic and physiologic principles.

costochondral s., pain in the chest with tenderness over one or more costochondral junctions.

costoclavicular s., one of the forerunners of thoracic outlet syndrome, in which the subclavian artery and vein and, on later reports, the brachial plexus, was thought to be compressed between the clavicle and normal first rib, with the assumption of certain body postures, *e.g.,* the military brace position.

Cotard's s., psychotic depression involving delusion of the existence of one's body, along with ideas of negation and suicidal impulses.

Crandall's s., pili torti and hearing defects associated with hypogonadism; a sex-linked trait in which there is a deficiency of luteinizing and of growth hormone. SEE ALSO Bjornstad's s.

CREST s., a variant of scleroderma characterized by *c*alcinosis, *R*aynaud's phenomenon, *e*sophageal motility disorders, *s*clerodactyly, and *t*elangiectasia.

cri-du-chat s., cri du chat s., cat-cry s., a disorder due to deletion of the short arm of chromosome 5, characterized by microcephaly, hypertelorism, antimongoloid palpebral fissures, epicanthal folds, micrognathia, strabismus, mental and physical retardation, and a characteristic high-pitched catlike whine. SYN cat's cry s., Lejeune s.

Crigler-Najjar s. [MIM*218800], a rare defect in ability to form bilirubin glucuronide due to deficiency of bilirubin-glucuronide glucuronosyltransferase; characterized by familial nonhemolytic jaundice and, in its severe form, by irreversible brain damage in infancy that resembles kernicterus and may be fatal; autosomal recessive inheritance. There is also an autosomal dominant form that may be identical with Gilbert's s. SYN Crigler-Najjar disease.

crocodile tears s., a flow of tears, usually unilateral, upon eating or the anticipation of eating; this happens when nerve fibers originally destined for a salivary gland are damaged and regrow, aberrantly, into the lacrimal gland.

Cronkhite-Canada s. [MIM*175500], a sporadically occurring s. of gastrointestinal polyps with diffuse alopecia and nail dystrophy; probably not genetic.

Crouzon's s., SYN craniofacial *dysostosis.*

crush s., the shocklike state that follows release of a limb or limbs or the trunk and pelvis after a prolonged period of compression, as by a heavy weight; characterized by suppression of urine, probably the result of damage to the renal tubules by myoglobin from the damaged muscles. SYN compression s.

Cruveilhier-Baumgarten s., cirrhosis of the liver with patent umbilical or paraumbilical veins and varicose periumbilical veins (caput medusae). SYN Cruveilhier-Baumgarten disease.

cryptophthalmus s., SYN Fraser's s.

Cushing's s., a disorder resulting from increased adrenocortical secretion of cortisol (giving clinical picture of Cushing's *disease*), due to any one of several sources: ACTH-dependent adrenocortical hyperplasia or tumor, ectopic ACTH-secreting tumor, or excessive administrations of steroids; characterized by trunkal obesity, moon face, acne, abdominal striae, hypertension, decreased carbohydrate tolerance, protein catabolism, psychiatric disturbances, and osteoporosis, amenorrhea, and hirsutism in females; when associated with an ACTH producing adenoma, called Cushing's disease. SYN Cushing's basophilism, pituitary basophilism.

Cushing's s. medicamentosus, a variable number of the signs and symptoms of Cushing's s.; produced by the chronic administration of large doses of any steroid that is a potent glucocorticoid.

cutaneomucouveal s., SYN Behçet's s.

DaCosta's s., SYN neurocirculatory *asthenia.*

Dandy-Walker s. [MIM*304340], developmental anomaly of the fourth ventricle associated with atresia of the foramina of Luschka and Magendie that results in cerebellar hypoplasia, hydrocephalus, and posterior fossa cyst formation.

dead fetus s., s. characterized by lengthy intrauterine retention of a dead fetus usually greater than 4 weeks with development of

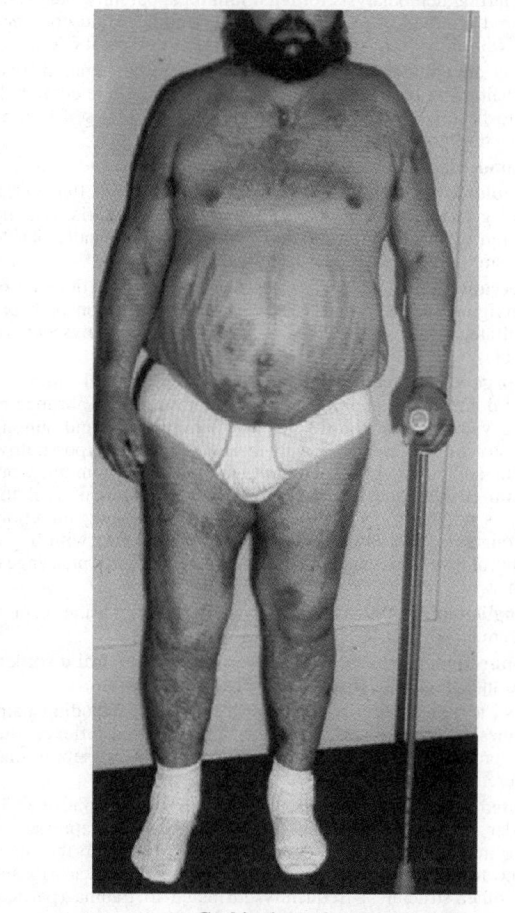

Cushing's syndrome
note abdominal obesity and striae

hypofibrinogenemia and occasionally disseminated intravascular coagulopathy.

Debré-Sémélaigne s., SYN Kocher-Debré-Sémélaigne s.

de Clerambault s., erotomania accompanied by the delusional belief that a certain person is in love with you.

Degos' s., SYN malignant atrophic *papulosis.*

Dejerine-Roussy s., SYN thalamic s.

de Lange s. [MIM 122470], a congenital anomaly characterized by impaired development, mental retardation, characteristic facies with snyophrys and hairline well down on forehead, depressed bridge of nose with uptilted tip of nose, small head with low-set ears, and flat spadelike hands with simian crease and short tapering fingers. SYN Amsterdam s., Cornelia de Lange s.

Del Castillo s., SYN Sertoli-cell-only s.

de Morsier's s., SYN septo-optic *dysplasia.*

dengue shock s., dengue fever of grade III or IV severity.

depersonalization s., SYN depersonalization.

depressive s., SYN depression.

dermatitis-arthritis-tenosynovitis s., disseminated infection with *Neisseria gonorrhoeae,* causing skin lesions (often pustular or necrotic), plus synovitis of major joints (such as knee, ankle, elbow), and tendon sheaths.

De Sanctis-Cacchione s. [MIM*278800], xeroderma pigmentosum with mental deficiency, dwarfism, and gonadal hypoplasia; recessive inheritance.

De Toni-Fanconi s., SYN cystinosis.

s. of deviously relevant answers, SYN Ganser's s.

dialysis disequilibrium s., nausea, vomiting, and hypertension, occasionally with convulsions, developing within several hours after starting hemodialysis for renal failure; apparently caused by too rapid removal of urea from the extracellular fluid compartment, with movement of water into cells, and cerebral edema.

dialysis encephalopathy s., a progressive, often fatal, diffuse encephalopathy occurring in a few patients on chronic hemodialysis; to be differentiated from the relatively acute, self-limited dialysis disequilibrium s. SYN dialysis dementia.

Diamond-Blackfan s., SYN congenital hypoplastic *anemia.*

diencephalic s. of infancy, profound emaciation after initial normal growth, locomotor hyperactivity and euphoria, usually with skin pallor, hypotension and hypoglycemia; usually due to neoplasm involving the anterior hypothalamus.

Di Ferrante s. [MIM*253230], associated with a deficiency of *N*-acetylglucosamine 6-sulfatase and urinary excretion of heparan sulfate and keratan sulfate. SYN type VIII mucopolysaccharidosis (1).

DiGeorge s., a condition arising from developmental failure of the third and fourth pharyngeal pouches, resulting in absence or underdevelopment of the thymus and parathyroid gland, among other structures; associated with facial deformity, hypoparathyroidism, and deficiency in cellular (T-lymphocyte) immunity, but humoral (B-lymphocyte) immunity is normal; ordinarily, if the tetany is not fatal, death ensues from overwhelming infection. SYN congenital aplasia of thymus, immunodeficiency with hypoparathyroidism, pharyngeal pouch s., third and fourth pharyngeal pouch s.

Di Guglielmo's s. [MIM*133180], eponym for the acute form of erythremic *myelosis.*

disconnection s., general term for various neurological disorders due to interruption of fiber pathways of the cerebrum.

disk s., a constellation of symptoms and signs, including pain, paresthesias, sensory loss, weakness, and impaired reflexes, due to a compressive radiculopathy caused by intervertebral disk pressure.

disputed neurogenic thoracic outlet s., a highly controversial disorder in which the brachial plexus is reputedly repressed at one or more sites along its course, particularly within the interscalene triangle, and between the normal first thoracic rib and some other structures; frequently attributed to trauma (particularly automobile accidents, and most often diagnosed in young to middle-aged women; no characteristic clinical presentation, although forequarter pain is characteristic; no definite objective findings are present, and no undisputed ancillary diagnostic studies are available.

Donohue's s., SYN leprechaunism.

Doose s., a rare familial type of primary, generalized myoclonic astatic epilepsy characterized by 2 to 3 or 4 to 6 Hz spike and wave complexes in the EEG; the condition usually responds to medication.

Dorfman-Chanarin s. [MIM*275630], congenital ichthyosis, leukocyte vacuoles, and variable involvement of other organ systems. SYN neutral lipid storage disease.

Down's s., a chromosomal dysgenesis syndrome consisting of a variable constellation of abnormalities caused by triplication or translocation of chromosome 21. The abnormalities include mental retardation, retarded growth, flat hypoplastic face with short nose, prominent epicanthic skin folds, small low-set ears with prominent antihelix, fissured and thickened tongue, laxness of joint ligaments, pelvic dysplasia, broad hands and feet, stubby fingers, and transverse palmar crease. Lenticular opacities and heart disease are common. The incidence of leukemia is increased and Alzheimer's disease is almost inevitable by age 40. SYN trisomy 21 s.

Dressler's s., SYN pericarditis.

dry eye s., SYN *keratoconjunctivitis* sicca.

Duane's s., SYN retraction s.

Dubin-Johnson s. [MIM*237500], autosomal recessive, inherited defect in hepatic excretory function characterized by levels of serum bilirubin up to about 6 mg/dL, over half of which is conjugated, and excretion of abnormal proportions of coproporphyrin I in urine. There is also retention of a dark pigment in the hepatocytes that is derived either from melanin or catecholamines, but otherwise liver histology is normal. Oral cholecysto-

Down's Syndrome: frequency of some bodily symptoms		
order of relative frequency	feature	percentage of cases with feature
1	retarded development	99%
2	mongoloid face	90%
3	palpebral fissure	86.5%
4	brachycephaly	75%
5	clinodactyly V	50–70%
6	epicanthus	67%
7	open mouth	65%
8	transverse palmar crease	59%
9	gap between 1st and 2nd toes	53%
10	flat, short nose	53%
11	lingua scrotalis	51%
12	Brushfield's spots	50%
13	ear muscle dysplasia	50%
14	macroglossia	41%
15	inborn heart defects	40–60%
16	muscular hypotonia	31%
17	brachydactyly	29%
18	strabismus	14–23%

gram fails to visualize the gall bladder, and excretion of bromosulfothalein by the liver is abnormal. The basic defect is apparently in canalicular transport. No therapy is necessary. SYN chronic idiopathic jaundice.

Dubreuil-Chambardel s., simultaneous caries of the upper incisor teeth occurring in either sex between the ages of 14 and 17; after an interval of varying length the other teeth also become involved.

Duchenne's s., subacute or chronic anterior spinal paralysis combined with multiple neuritis.

dumping s., the s. that occurs after eating, most often seen in patients with shunts of the upper alimentary canal; characterized by flushing, sweating, dizziness, weakness, and vasomotor collapse, occasionally with pain and headache; results from rapid passage of large amounts of food into the small intestine, with an osmotic effect removing fluid from plasma and causing hypovolemia. SYN postgastrectomy s.

Dyggve-Melchior-Clausen s. [MIM*223800], an osteochondrodysplasia that clinically resembles Morquio's s., but without excretion of mucopolysaccharides; characterized by mental retardation, short stature, progressive sternal bulging, flattening of vertebral bodies and iliac crests, shortening of metacarpals, and changes in long bones; autosomal recessive inheritance, but there is an X-linked form [MIM*304950].

dyskinesia (dis-ki-nē′zē-ă), clearance of mucus is sluggish and bronchiectasis is prevalent and intractable. There is evidence that the defect lies in dynein, a protein in the cilia. The pattern of inheritance is apparently autosomal recessive [MIM*242650] however multiple versions may exist.

dysmnesic s., SYN Korsakoff's s.

dysplastic nevus s. [MIM*155600], clinically atypical nevi (usually exceeding 5 mm in diameter and having variable pigmentation and ill defined borders) with an increased risk for development of cutaneous malignant melanoma; biopsies show melanocytic dysplasia; such nevi are very numerous in familial dysplastic nevus s. with hereditary melanoma, but histologically identical sporadic nevi also occur that appear to be clinically benign. Autosomal dominant.

Eagle s., facial pain due to an elongated styloid process.

Eagle-Barrett s., SYN prune belly s.

Eaton-Lambert s., SYN Lambert-Eaton s.

ectopic ACTH s., the association of Cushing's s. with a nonpituitary neoplasm, usually a lung carcinoma that produces ACTH.

ectrodactyly-ectodermal dysplasia-clefting s., an autosomal recessive disorder resulting in defects of hands and feet; the ectodermal dysplasia causes fair skin, anodontia, and cleft palate.

Edwards' s., SYN trisomy 18 s.

effort s., SYN neurocirculatory *asthenia.*

egg drop s., a disease of chickens caused by an adenovirus and characterized by production of soft-shelled and shell-less eggs in apparently healthy birds.

egg-white s., dermatitis, loss of hair, and loss of muscle coordination, produced in rats by diets containing large amounts of raw egg white, the avidin of which combines with biotin producing a deficiency of the latter. SYN egg-white injury.

Ehlers-Danlos s. [MIM*130000-130080, 225330, 225400,], a group of inherited generalized connective tissue diseases characterized by overelasticity and friability of the skin, hypermobility of the joints, and fragility of the cutaneous blood vessels and sometimes large arteries, due to deficient quality or quantity of collagen; the most common is inherited as an autosomal dominant trait; some recessive cases have hydroxylysine-deficient collagen due to deficiency of collagen lysyl hydroxylase, and two tentatively ascribed to X-linked inheritance.

Eisenlohr's s., numbness and weakness in the extremities, paralysis of the lips, tongue, and palate, and dysarthria.

Eisenmenger's s., cardiac failure with significant right to left shunt producing cyanosis due to higher pressure on the right side of the shunt. Usually due to the Eisenmenger complex, a ventricular septal defect with right ventricular hypertrophy, severe pulmonary hypertension, and frequent straddling of the defect by a misplaced aortic root.

Ekbom s., SYN restless legs s.

Ellis-van Creveld s., SYN chondroectodermal *dysplasia.*

E-M s., SYN eosinophilia-myalgia s.

EMG s., SYN Beckwith-Wiedemann s.

encephalotrigeminal vascular s., angiomatosis of the brain accompanied by nevi in the trigeminal area. SEE ALSO Sturge-Weber s.

eosinophilia-myalgia s., a probable autoimmune disorder precipitated by contaminated L-tryptophan tablets, and characterized by fatigue, low-grade fever, myalgias, muscle tenderness and cramps, weakness, paresthesias of the extremities, and skin indurations; marked eosinophilia is noted on peripheral blood studies, serum aldolase increased and biopsies of peripheral nerve, muscle, skin, and fascia show microangiopathy and inflammation in connective tissue. SYN E-M s.

episodic dyscontrol s., SYN intermittent explosive *disorder.*

erythrodysesthesia s., tingling sensation of the palms and soles, progressing to severe pain and tenderness with erythema and edema; caused by continuous infusion therapy.

euthyroid sick s. (yū-thī′royd), abnormalities in levels of hormones and function tests related to the thyroid gland occurring in patients with severe systemic disease. Thyroid function is actually normal in these patients, and it is uncertain whether treatment of these abnormalities would be beneficial. SYN sick euthyroid s.

Evans' s., acquired hemolytic anemia and thrombocytopenia.

exfoliation s., a condition, often leading to glaucoma, in which deposits on the surface of the lens resemble exfoliation of the lens capsule. SEE ALSO *pseudoexfoliation* of lens capsule.

extrapyramidal s., abnormalities of movement related to injury of motor pathways other than the pyramidal tract.

Faber's s., SYN achlorhydric *anemia.*

familial aortic ectasia s., the concurrence as an autosomal dominant trait of bicuspid aortic valve often with premature calcification, ectasia and dissection of the aorta and, rarely, coarctation of the aorta. Superficially resembles the Marfan's s. SYN familial aortic ectasia.

familial chylomicronemia s., an inherited disorder resulting in accumulation of chylomicrons as well as triacylglycerols. SEE ALSO chylomicronemia.

Fanconi's s. [MIM*227650 to 227660], **(1)** SYN Fanconi's *anemia.* **(2)** a group of conditions with characteristic disorders of renal tubular function, which may be classified as: 1) cystinosis, an autosomal recessive disease of early childhood; 2) adult Fanconi s., a rare hereditary form, probably due to a recessive gene different from that found in cystinosis, characterized by the tubular malfunction seen in cystinosis and by osteomalacia, but without cystine deposit in tissues; 3) acquired Fanconi s., which may be associated with multiple myeloma or may result from chemical poisoning, injury, or persisting damage of proximal tubular epithelium due to various causes, leading to multiple defects of tubular function.

Farber's s. [MIM*228000], SYN disseminated *lipogranulomatosis.*

fatty liver s., a noninfectious disease of chickens characterized by enlarged fat-infiltrated livers.

Favre-Racouchot s., periorbital and malar open comedones, often with marked solar elastosis.

feline urolithiasis s., SYN feline urological s.

feline urological s., a common disease of cats where development of urinary calculi produce urethral obstruction in males and cystitis and urethritis in females. SYN feline urolithiasis s.

Felty's s., rheumatoid arthritis with splenomegaly and leukopenia.

female urethral s., SYN urethral s.

fetal alcohol s., a specific pattern of fetal malformation with growth deficiency, craniofacial anomalies, and limb defects, found among offspring of mothers who are chronic alcoholics; mental retardation is often demonstrated later.

fetal aspiration s., a s. resulting from uterine aspiration of amniotic fluid and meconium by the fetus, usually caused by hypoxia and often leading to aspiration pneumonia.

fetal face s., a s. of facies resembling an early fetus with short forearms, and genital hypoplasia at birth, but without evidence of achondroplasia; leads to dwarfism without mental retardation. SYN Robinow's s.

fetal hydantoin s., a fetal s. resulting from maternal ingestion of hydantoin analogues (*e.g.,* phenytoin), characterized by growth deficiency, mental deficiency, dysmorphic facies, cleft palate and/or lip, cardiac defects, and abnormal genitalia.

fetal trimethadione s., a fetal s. resulting from maternal ingestion of trimethadione during the early weeks of pregnancy and characterized by developmental delay, V-shaped eyebrows, epicanthus, low-set ears with anteriorly folded helix, palatal anomaly, and irregular teeth.

fetal warfarin s., fetal bleeding, nasal hypoplasia, optic atrophy, and fetal death resulting from administration of warfarin to the pregnant patient.

fibrinogen-fibrin conversion s., a s. characterized by hypofibrinogenemia with incoagulable blood; it may be seen in abruptio placentae, prolonged retention of a dead fetus in an Rh-isosensitized mother, hemolytic blood reactions, bilateral renal cortical necrosis, and cases of trauma.

Fiessinger-Leroy-Reiter s., SYN Reiter's s.

Figueira's s., weakness of the neck muscles with slight spasticity of the muscles of the lower extremities and increased tendon reflexes; supposed to be an attenuated sporadic form of acute poliomyelitis.

first arch s., generic term including s.'s of malformations involving derivatives of the first branchial arch, with or without associated malformations; includes mandibulofacial dysostosis, micrognathia with peromelia, otomandibular dysostosis, acrofacial dysostosis, and others.

Fisher's s., a s. characterized by ophthalmoplegia, ataxia, and areflexia; a form of polyneuroradiculitis.

Fitz-Hugh and Curtis s., perihepatitis in women with a history of gonococcal or chlamydial salpingitis.

flashing pain s. [MIM*190400], sudden, intermittent, and severe brief episodes of pain, without apparent cause, in the distribution of a spinal dermatome; resembles in character the pain of tic douloureux. Cf. *tic* douloureux.

flecked retina s. [MIM*228980], hereditary retinal disorder with abnormal transmission of fluorescence through the retinal pigment epithelium on angiography.

floppy valve s., retrograde slippage of degenerating mitral or tricuspid valve leaflets into the valve's orifice beyond the point of closure during systole of the left ventricle; a feature of Barlow's s.

Flynn-Aird s. [MIM*136300], a familial s. characterized by muscle wasting, ataxia, dementia, skin atrophy, and ocular anomalies.

Foix-Alajouanine s., thrombophlebitis of spinal veins resulting in a subacute ascending painful flaccid paralysis from necrotic myelitis.

Foix-Cavany-Marie s., constellation of facio-pharyngo-glosso-masticatory diplegia with automatic voluntary dissociation without associated dementia or forced laughing or crying usually caused by bilateral large artery infarcts of the opercular cortex.

folded-lung s., collapse of part of the lung caught between shrinking fibrous pleura scars, sometimes resulting from pleural asbestosis. SYN round atelectasis.

Forbes-Albright s., pituitary tumor in a patient without acromegaly, which secretes excessive amounts of prolactin (LTH) and produces persistent lactation.

Foster Kennedy's s., SYN Kennedy's s.

Foville's s., a form of alternating hemiplegia characterized by abducens paralysis on one side, paralysis of the extremities on the other.

fragile X s., SEE fragile X *chromosome.*

Fraley s., dilation of the upper pole renal calices due to stenosis of the upper infundibulum, usually caused by compression from vessels supplying the upper and middle segments of the kidney.

Franceschetti-Jadassohn s., SYN Naegeli s.

Franceschetti's s., mandibulofacial *dysostosis,* when complete or nearly complete.

Fraser's s. [MIM*219000], an association of cryptophthalmus with multiple anomalies, including middle and outer ear malformations, cleft palate, laryngeal deformity, displacement of umbilicus and nipples, digital malformations, separation of symphysis pubis, maldevelopment of kidneys, and masculinization of genitalia in females; autosomal recessive inheritance. SYN cryptophthalmus s.

Freeman-Sheldon s., SYN craniocarpotarsal *dystrophy.*

Frenkel's anterior ocular traumatic s., an obsolete term for traumatic iridoplegia, which consists of mydriasis, hyphema, small iris tears near the pupil, discrete punctate opacities of the lens, and occasionally iridodialysis.

Frey's s., SYN auriculotemporal nerve s.

Friderichsen-Waterhouse s., SYN Waterhouse-Friderichsen s.

Fröhlich's s., dystrophia adiposogenitalis, originally involving an adenohypophysial tumor. SYN Launois-Cléret s.

Froin's s., an alteration in the cerebrospinal fluid, which is yellowish and coagulates spontaneously in a few seconds after withdrawal, owing to its greatly increased protein (albumin and globulin) content; noted in loculated portions of the subarachnoid space isolated from spinal fluid circulation by an inflammatory or neoplastic obstruction. SYN loculation s.

Fuchs' s. [MIM*136800], a s. characterized by heterochromia of the iris, iridocyclitis, keratic precipitates, and cataract. SYN Fuchs' heterochromic cyclitis.

functional prepubertal castration s., a s. characterized by the absence of testes from the scrotum but in their place mesonephric duct derivatives, pronounced gynecomastia and eunuchoid habitus, and increased urinary excretion of gonadotrophins.

G s. [MIM*145410], a s. of characteristic facies associated with hypospadias, ventral curvature of the penis, and dysphagia. Apparently the same as the BBB syndrome of Opritz et al. Autosomal dominant inheritance. [first letter of surname of affected person reported]

Gaisböck's s., SYN *polycythemia* hypertonica.

Ganser's s., a psychotic-like condition, without the symptoms and signs of a traditional psychosis, occurring typically in prisoners who feign insanity; *e.g.,* such a person, when asked to multiply 6 by 4, will give 23 as the answer, or he will call a key a

lock. SEE malingering, factitious *disorder.* SYN nonsense s., s. of approximate relevant answers, s. of deviously relevant answers.

Gardner-Diamond s., SYN autoerythrocyte sensitization s.

Gardner's s. [MIM*175100-006], multiple polyposis predisposing to carcinoma of the colon; also multiple tumors, osteomas of the skull, epidermoid cysts, and fibromas; autosomal dominant inheritance.

gastrocardiac s., disturbances of the heart's action due to faulty action of the digestive system, especially of the stomach.

gastrojejunal loop obstruction s., SYN afferent loop s.

gay bowel s., gastrointestinal discomfort experienced by homosexual males; includes abdominal pain, cramps, bloating, flatulence, nausea, vomiting, or diarrhea caused by enteric bacteria, viruses, fungi, zooparasites, or trauma.

Gélineau's s., SYN narcolepsy.

gender dysphoria s., a s. in which an individual experiences marked personal stress due to feelings that despite having the genitalia and secondary sexual characteristics of one gender there is a sense of compatibility and greater belonging to the other gender class; one may undergo surgery to reconstruct anatomy to that of the other gender.

general adaptation s., a s. introduced by Hans Selye to describe marked physiological changes in various organ systems of the body, especially the pituitary-endocrine system, as a result of exposure to prolonged physical or psychological stress, with the bodily changes progressing through three stages that the author described as the alarm reaction, resistance, and finally exhaustion.

Gerstmann s., finger agnosia, agraphia, confusion of laterality of body, and acalculia; caused by lesions between the occipital area and the angular gyrus.

Gerstmann-Sträussler s., a more chronic cerebellar form of spongiform encephalopathy.

Gianotti-Crosti s., a cutaneous manifestation of hepatitis B infection occurring in young children; an exanthem comprised of dusky papules on the legs, buttocks, and extensors of the arms; it lasts 2 to 8 weeks and is associated with adenopathy and malaise. SYN papular acrodermatitis of childhood.

Gilbert's s., SYN familial nonhemolytic *jaundice.*

Gilles de la Tourette's s. [MIM*137580], SYN Tourette s.

glucagonoma s., necrolytic migratory erythema or intertriginous and periorificial dermatitis, stomatitis, anemia, weight loss, and hyperglycemia resulting from glucagon-secreting pancreatic islet cell tumors.

Goldenhar's s. [MIM*257700], SYN oculoauriculovertebral *dysplasia.*

gold-myokymia s., the symptom complex of widespread myokymia, muscle aching, and autonomic disturbances (excess sweating; orthostatic hypotension) that can result from gold therapy.

Goltz s., SYN focal dermal *hypoplasia.*

Goodman's s., SYN acrocephalopolysyndactyly.

Goodpasture's s. [MIM*233450], glomerulonephritis of the anti-basement membrane type associated with or preceded by hemoptysis; the nephritis usually progresses rapidly to produce death from renal failure, and the lungs at autopsy show extensive hemosiderosis or recent hemorrhage.

Gopalan's s., severe discomfort of the feet associated with elevated skin temperature and excessive sweating.

Gorlin-Chaudhry-Moss s. [MIM*233500], craniofacial dysostosis, patent ductus arteriosus, hypertrichosis, hypoplasia of labia majora, and dental and ocular abnormalities; sporadic, and no basic mechanism is proposed. SEE ALSO Weill-Marchesani s.

Gorlin's s., SYN basal cell nevus s.

Gorman's s., hemangiomatosis of the skeletal system with or without involvement of the overlying skin, resulting in osteolysis and fibrous replacement of bone.

Gougerot-Carteaud s., SYN confluent and reticulate *papillomatosis.*

Gowers' s., s. consisting of palpitation, chest pain, respiratory difficulties, and disturbances in gastric motility; once attributed to vagal stimulation, now considered psychogenic (anxiety neurosis). SYN vagal attack, vasovagal attack.

gracilis s., osteonecrosis of the pubic bone following trauma.

Gradenigo's s., petrositis with abducens paralysis and pain in the temporal region, due to localized meningitis involving the fifth and sixth nerves.

Graham Little s., SYN *lichen* planopilaris.

gray s., gray baby s., gray appearance of an infant at birth and during the neonatal period which can be caused by transplacental toxic effects of the drug chloramphenicol taken by the mother during late pregnancy; the s. may be fatal.

gray collie s., SYN cyclic *hematopoiesis*.

Greig's s., SYN ocular *hypertelorism*.

Grönblad-Strandberg s., angioid streaks of the retina together with pseudoxanthoma elasticum of the skin.

Gubler's s., a form of alternating hemiplegia characterized by contralateral hemiplegia and ipsilateral facial paralysis. SYN Gubler's paralysis, Millard-Gubler s.

Gulf War s., a term often but inappropriately applied to various health problems experienced by US military personnel after serving in the Persian Gulf conflict of 1991; symptoms of fatigue, musculoskeletal pain, headaches, dyspnea, memory loss, and diarrhea have been reported, but an NIH panel has concluded that evidence of a specific syndrome is lacking. SYN Persian Gulf s.

Guillain-Barré s., SYN acute idiopathic *polyneuritis*.

Gunn's s., SYN jaw-winking s.

gustatory sweating s., SYN auriculotemporal nerve s.

Haber's s., a permanent flushing and telangiectasia of the cheeks, nose, forehead, and chin, with prominent follicular openings, small papules with scaling, and minute pitted areas; occasionally accompanied by scaly and keratotic lesions of the trunk.

Hallermann-Streiff s., SYN *dyscephalia* mandibulo-oculofacialis.

Hallermann-Streiff-François s., SYN *dyscephalia* mandibulo-oculofacialis.

Hallervorden s., SYN Hallervorden-Spatz s.

Hallervorden-Spatz s., a disorder characterized by dystonia with other extrapyramidal dysfunctions appearing in the first two decades of life; associated with large amounts of iron in the globus pallidus and substantia nigra. SYN Hallervorden s., Hallervorden-Spatz disease, status dysmyelinisatus.

Hallgren's s., vestibulocerebellar ataxia, pigmentary retinal dystrophy, congenital deafness, and cataract.

Hamman-Rich s., SYN usual interstitial *pneumonia* of Liebow.

Hamman's s., spontaneous mediastinal emphysema, resulting from rupture of alveoli. SYN Hamman's disease.

hand-and-foot s., recurrent painful swelling of the hands and feet occurring in infants and young children with sickle cell anemia. SYN sickle cell dactylitis.

Hanhart's s., SYN *micrognathia* with peromelia.

happy puppet s. [MIM*234400], a s. characterized by mental retardation, ataxia, hypotonia, epileptic seizures, easily provoked and prolonged spasms of laughter, prognathism, and an open-mouthed expression.

Harada's s., bilateral retinal edema, uveitis, choroiditis, and retinal detachment, with temporary or permanent deafness, graying of the hair (poliosis), and alopecia; related to the Vogt-Koyanagi s. and sympathetic ophthalmia. SYN Harada's disease, uveoencephalitis, uveomeningitis s.

Harris s., excessive insulin production with hypoglycemia, hunger, jitteriness, tachycardia, and flushing occurring in conditions such as functional disorders of the pancreas, hyperplasia of the islets of Langerhans, or insulinoma.

Hartnup s., SYN Hartnup *disease.*

Hayem-Widal s., obsolete term for acquired hemolytic *icterus*. SYN Widal's s.

head-bobbing doll s., bobbing motion of the head usually due to cysts in or about the third ventricle.

Hegglin's s., dissociation between electromechanical systole (Q-SII interval) and electrical systole (Q-T interval) so that the second heart tone (SII) is recorded before the end of the T wave; described by Hegglin as an energy-dynamic cardiac insufficiency during diabetic coma and other metabolic disorders.

HELLP s., type of severe preeclampsia involving *h*emolysis, *e*levated *l*iver function, and *l*ow *p*latelets.

Helweg-Larssen s. [MIM*125050], familial anhidrosis present from birth with neurolabyrinthitis developing in the fourth or fifth decade.

hemangioma-thrombocytopenia s., SYN Kasabach-Merritt s.

hemolytic uremic s., hemolytic anemia and thrombocytopenia occurring with acute renal failure. In children, characterized by sudden onset of gastrointestinal bleeding, hematuria, oliguria, and microangiopathic hemolytic anemia; in adults, associated with complications of pregnancy following normal delivery, or associated with oral contraceptive use or with infection.

Henoch-Schönlein s., SYN Henoch-Schönlein *purpura*.

hepatorenal s., hepatonephoric s., the occurrence of acute renal failure in patients with disease of the liver or biliary tract, apparently due to decreased renal blood flow; conditions that damage both organs, such as carbon tetrachloride poisoning and leptospirosis.

Herlitz s., SYN *epidermolysis* bullosa lethalis.

Hermansky-Pudlak s. type VI, SYN oculocutaneous *albinism*.

Hermansky-Pudlak s., a form of oculocutaneous albinism (autosomal recessive) with accumulation of ceroid in lysosomes with restrictive lung disease, granulomatous colitis, kidney failure, cardiomyopathy, and storage pool-deficient platelets.

Herrmann's s. [MIM*172500], a nervous system disorder beginning in late childhood or early adolescence, with photomyoclonus and hearing loss followed by diabetes mellitus, progressive dementia, pyelonephritis, and glomerulonephritis; progressive sensorineural hearing loss is of later onset; dominant inheritance.

Hinman s., SYN nonneurogenic neurogenic *bladder*.

Hirschowitz s., acanthosis nigricans associated with hypovitaminosis; responds well to topical retinoic acid therapy.

holiday s., regression, development of diffuse anxiety, feelings of helplessness, irritability, and depression; said to occur in certain psychoanalytic patients before Thanksgiving and continuing into the Christmas holiday season, ending a few days after January 1.

holiday heart s., arrhythmias of the heart, sometimes apparent after a vacation or weekend away from work, following excessive alcohol consumption; usually transient.

Holmes-Adie s., SYN Adie s.

Holt-Oram s. [MIM*142900], atrial septal defect in association with finger-like or absent thumb and other deformities of the forearm; autosomal dominant inheritance.

Horner's s., ptosis, miosis, and anhidrosis on the side of the sympathetic palsy. The enophthalmos is more apparent than real. The affected pupil is visibly slow to dilate in dim light; due to a lesion of the cervical sympathetic chain or its central pathways. SYN Bernard-Horner s., ptosis sympathetica.

Houssay s., the amelioration of diabetes mellitus by a destructive lesion in, or surgical removal of, the pituitary gland.

Hughes-Stovin s., s. characterized by aneurysms of the large and small pulmonary artery and thrombosis of peripheral veins and dural sinuses.

Hunt's s. [MIM*159700], **(1)** an intention tremor beginning in one extremity, gradually increasing in intensity, and subsequently involving other parts of the body; SYN progressive cerebellar tremor. **(2)** facial paralysis, otalgia, and herpes zoster resulting from viral infection of the seventh cranial nerve and geniculate ganglion; **(3)** a form of juvenile paralysis agitans associated with primary atrophy of the pallidal system. SYN paleostriatal s., pallidal s. SYN Ramsay Hunt's s. (1).

Hunter's s. [MIM*309900], an error of mucopolysaccharide metabolism characterized by deficiency of iduronate sulfatase, with excretion of dermatan sulfate and heparan sulfate in the urine; clinically similar to Hurler's s. but distinguished by less severe skeletal changes, no corneal clouding, and X-linked recessive inheritance. SYN type II mucopolysaccharidosis.

Hurler's s. [MIM*252800], mucopolysaccharidosis in which there is a deficiency of α-L-iduronidase, an accumulation of an abnormal intracellular material, and excretion of dermatan sulfate and heparan sulfate in the urine; with severe abnormality in development of skeletal cartilage and bone, with dwarfism, ky-

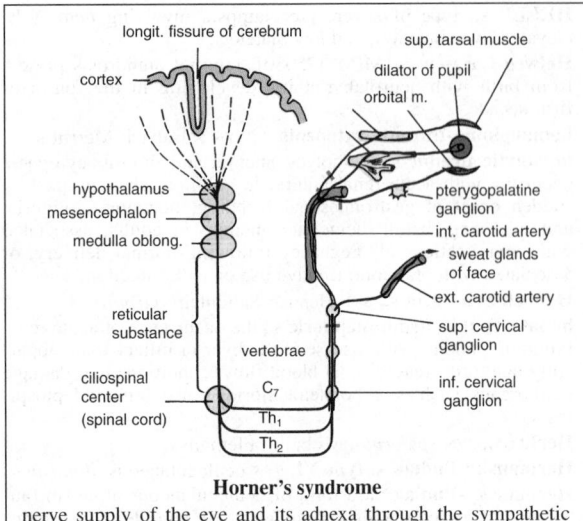

Horner's syndrome

nerve supply of the eye and its adnexa through the sympathetic nerve; A,B,C, and D indicate possibe points of interruption

phosis, deformed limbs, limitation of joint motion, spadelike hand, corneal clouding, hepatosplenomegaly, mental retardation, and gargoyle-like facies; autosomal recessive inheritance. SEE ALSO mucolipidosis. SYN dysostosis multiplex, Hurler's disease, lipochondrodystrophy, Pfaundler-Hurler s., type IH mucopolysaccharidosis.

Hurler-Scheie s., a phenotypic intermediate between Hurler s. and Scheie s.; a deficiency of α-L-iduronidase. SYN type I H/S mucopolysaccharidosis.

Hutchinson-Gilford s., SYN progeria.

Hutchison s., adrenal neuroblastoma of infants with metastasis to the orbit; at one time erroneously believed to arise predominantly from the left adrenal gland. SEE ALSO Pepper s.

hyaline membrane s., SYN hyaline membrane *disease* of the newborn.

hydralazine s., a s. simulating systemic lupus erythematosus, occurring during protracted therapy of hypertension with hydralazine.

17-hydroxylase deficiency s. [MIM*202110], congenital deficiency of adrenocortical, and possibly ovarian, steroid C-17α hydroxylase; the resulting excessive secretion of corticosterone and deoxycorticosterone produces hypertension and hypokalemic alkalosis; absence of aldosterone secretion in such patients may indicate a multiple enzymic deficiency.

hyperabduction s., pain running down the arm, numbness, paresthesias, and erythema, with weakness of the hands; due to abduction of the arm for a prolonged period (*e.g.,* during sleep or necessitated by occupation) which stretches the axillary vessels and the nerves of the brachial plexus. SYN subcoracoid-pectoralis minor tendon s., Wright's s.

hyperactive child s., SYN attention deficit hyperactivity *disorder.*

hypereosinophilic s., persistent peripheral eosinophilia with later infiltration into bone marrow, heart, and other organ systems; accompanied by nocturnal sweating, coughing, anorexia and weight loss, itching and various skin lesions, and symptoms of Löffler's endocarditis.

hyperimmunoglobulin E s., an immunodeficiency disorder characterized by high levels of plasma IgE concentrations, a leukocyte chemotactic defect, and recurrent staphylococcal infections of the skin, upper respiratory tract, and other sites. SYN Job s.

hyperkinetic s., a condition marked by pathologically excessive energy seen sometimes in young children with brain injury, mental illness, and attention deficit disorder, and in epileptics; hypermotility and emotional instability are the chief characteristics; distractibility, inattention, and lack of shyness and of fear are common accompaniments.

hyperkinetic heart s., loosely, a syndrome in which the heart appears to be "overworking", *i.e.,* beating excessively fast and/or causing subjective awareness of continual cardiac activity.

hyperornithinemia-hyperammonemia-hypercitrullinuria s., a rare inherited disorder in which there is impaired ornithine transport into the mitochondria. SEE ALSO lysinuric protein *intolerance.*

hypersensitive xiphoid s., abnormal tenderness of the xiphoid, often associated with spontaneous pains in the chest, upper abdomen, and shoulders.

hyperventilation s., SEE chronic hyperventilation s.

hyperviscosity s., a s. resulting from increased viscosity of the blood; an increase in serum proteins may be associated with bleeding from mucous membranes, retinopathy, and neurological symptoms, and is sometimes seen in Waldenström's macroglobulinemia and in multiple myeloma; an increased viscosity secondary to polycythemia may be associated with organ congestion and decreased capillary perfusion.

hypometabolic s., a clinical situation suggesting hypothyroidism or myxedema, in which some tests of thyroid function may be normal and the gland is not obviously atrophic or diseased; indicative of a lack of sensitivity of peripheral tissues to thyroid hormone.

hypoparathyroidism s., a s. characterized by fatigue, muscular weakness, paresthesia and cramps of the extremities, tetany, and laryngeal stridor; due to hypocalcemia resulting from a lack of parathyroid hormone; may be idiopathic, postoperative, or caused by organic lesions of the parathyroids.

hypophysial s., SYN *dystrophia* adiposogenitalis.

hypophysio-sphenoidal s., neoplastic invasion of the base of the skull in the region of the sphenoidal sinus, often with destruction of the dorsum sellae.

hypoplastic left heart s. [MIM*241550], association of underdevelopment of the left heart chambers with atresia or stenosis of the aortic and/or mitral valve and hypoplasia of the ascending aorta.

Imerslünd-Grasbeck s., enterocyte cobalamin malabsorption.

immotile cilia s. [MIM*242650], an inherited disorder characterized by recurrent sinopulmonary infections, reduced fertility in women, and sterility in men due to the inability of ciliated structures to beat effectively because of the absence of one or both dynein arms. Cf. Kartagener's s.

immunodeficiency s., an immunological deficiency or disorder, of which the chief symptom is an increased susceptibility to infection, the pattern of susceptibility being dependent upon the kind of deficiency. SEE ALSO immunodeficiency.

s. of inappropriate secretion of antidiuretic hormone (SIADH), continued secretion of antidiuretic hormone despite low serum osmolality and expanded extracellular volume.

indifference to pain s., congenital insensitivity to pain, possibly due to an absence of organized nerve endings in the skin.

infertile male s., an inherited disorder of the androgen receptor protein resulting in defective androgen activity. SEE ALSO Reifenstein's s.

internal capsule s., hemianopsia with contralateral hemianesthesia of the face.

inversed jaw-winking s., when there are supranuclear lesions of the trigeminal nerve, touching the cornea may produce a brisk movement of the mandible to the opposite side.

iridocorneal endothelial s., s. of glaucoma, iris atrophy, decreased corneal endothelium, anterior peripheral synechia, and multiple iris nodules. SYN Cogan-Reese s., iris-nevus s.

iridocorneal syndrome, SYN Chandler s.

iris-nevus s., SYN iridocorneal endothelial s.

Irvine-Gass s., macular edema, aphakia, and vitreous humor adherent to incision for cataract extraction.

Isaac's s., a rare sporadic disorder of unknown etiology with onset usually in late childhood or early adulthood, characterized by intermittent or continuous involuntary muscle contractions, producing "stiffness" or "clumsiness" and accompanied by increased sweating, increased skin temperature, fasciculations, and myokymia. If facial, pharyngeal, or laryngeal muscles are involved, dysphasia and respiratory obstruction can occur. Muscle abnormalities persist during sleep and general anesthesia, but are blocked by curare, indicating site of lesion is peripheral nerve.

Ivemark's s. [MIM*208530], a possibly heritable disorder in which organs of the left side of the body are a mirror image of their counterpart on the right side (*e.g.,* normal asymmetry of the lungs is lost and the left lung has three lobes); splenic agenesis and cardiac malformations are associated.

Jadassohn-Lewandowski s., SYN *pachyonychia* congenita.

Jahnke's s., sturge-Weber s. without glaucoma.

jaw-winking s. [MIM*154600], an increase in the width of the eye lids during chewing, sometimes with a rhythmic elevation of the upper lid when the mouth is open and ptosis when the mouth is closed. SYN Gunn phenomenon, Gunn's s., jaw-winking phenomenon, jaw-working reflex, Marcus Gunn phenomenon, Marcus Gunn s.

Jeghers-Peutz s., SYN Peutz-Jeghers s.

Jervell and Lange-Nielsen s., a prolonged Q-T interval recorded in the electrocardiogram of certain congenitally deaf children subject to attacks of unconsciousness resulting from Adams-Stokes seizures and ventricular fibrillation; autosomal recessive inheritance. SYN surdocardiac s.

Jeune's s., SYN asphyxiating thoracic *dysplasia.*

Job s., SYN hyperimmunoglobulin E s. [*Job,* biblical char.]

Joubert's s. [MIM*213300], agenesis of the cerebellar vermis, characterized clinically by attacks of tachypnea or prolonged apnea, abnormal eye movements, ataxia, and mental retardation.

jugular foramen s., SYN Avellis' s. **(2)** the depression in the anterior part of the neck just superior to the jugular notch of the manubrium sterni.

Kallmann's s., SYN *hypogonadism* with anosmia.

Kanner's s., SYN infantile *autism.*

Kartagener's s. [MIM*244400], complete situs inversus associated with bronchiectasis and chronic sinusitis associated with ciliary dysmotility and impaired ciliary mucous transport in the respiratory epithelium; autosomal recessive inheritance with variable penetrance. The mechanism of the reversal of laterality remains an enigma, but it appears to be strictly an abolition (indifference) of laterality rather than a true reversal. SEE ALSO immotile cilia s. SYN Kartagener's triad, Zivert s.

Kasabach-Merritt s., capillary hemangioma associated with thrombocytopenic purpura; bleeding commonly develops in the first year of life. SYN hemangioma-thrombocytopenia s.

Katayama s., SYN *schistosomiasis* japonica.

Kawasaki's s., SYN mucocutaneous lymph node s.

Kearns-Sayre s. [MIM*165100], a form of chronic progressive external ophthalmoplegia with associated cardiac conduction defects, short stature, and hearing loss; a sporadically ocurring mitochondrial myopathy presenting in childhood.

Kennedy's s., ipsilateral optic atrophy with central scotoma and contralateral choked disk or papilledema, caused by a meningioma of the ipsilateral optic nerve. SYN Foster Kennedy's s.

Key-Gaskell s., SYN canine *dysautonomia.*

Kimmelstiel-Wilson s., nephrotic syndrome and hypertension in diabetics, associated with diabetic glomerulosclerosis. SYN Kimmelstiel-Wilson disease.

Kleine-Levin s. [MIM*148840], a rare form of periodic hypersomnia associated with bulimia, occurring in males aged 10 to 25 years, characterized by periods of ravenous appetite alternating with prolonged sleep (as long as 18 hours), along with behavioral disturbances, impaired thought processes, and hallucinations; acute illness or fatigue may precede an episode, which may occur as often as several times a year.

Klinefelter's s., a chromosomal anomaly with chromosome count 47, XXY sex chromosome constitution; buccal and other cells are usually sex chromatin-positive; patients are male in development but have seminiferous tubule dysgenesis, elevated urinary gonadotropins, variable gynecomastia, and eunuchoid habitus; some patients are chromosomal mosaics, with two or more cell lines of different chromosome constitution; the male tortoise-shell cat (calico cat) is an animal model. SYN XXY s.

Klippel-Feil s. [MIM*148900], a congenital defect manifested as a short neck, extensive fusion of the cervical vertebrae, and abnormalities of the brainstem and cerebellum. SYN cervical fusion s.

Klippel-Trenaunay-Weber s. [MIM*149000], an anomaly of the extremity in which there is a combination of angiomatosis and anomalous development of the underlying bone and muscle, sometimes associated with localized gigantism. SYN angio-osteohypertrophy s., congenital dysplastic angiectasia, hemangiectatic hypertrophy.

Dejerine-Klumpke s., SYN Klumpke *palsy.*

Klüver-Bucy s., a s. characterized by psychic blindness or hyperreactivity to visual stimuli, increased oral and sexual activity, and depressed drive and emotional reactions; reported in monkeys after bilateral temporal lobe ablation, but rarely reported in humans.

Kniest s. [MIM*156550, 245190, 245160], a type of metatropic dwarfism with short limbs, round face with central depression, enlargement and stiffness of joints, contracture of fingers, and often cleft palate, scoliosis, retinal detachment and myopia, and deafness; autosomal dominant inheritance.

Kocher-Debré-Sémélaigne s., autosomal recessive inherited athyrotic cretinism associated with muscular pseudohypertrophy. SYN Debré-Sémélaigne s.

Koenig's s., alternating attacks of constipation and diarrhea, with colic, meteorism, and gurgling in the right iliac fossa, said to be symptomatic of cecal tuberculosis.

Koerber-Salus-Elschnig s., SYN convergence-retraction *nystagmus.*

Kohlmeier-Degos s., vascular occlusive disorder predominantly involving the small arteries of the skin and bowel with about one-fifth of patients having central nervous system symptoms secondary to arterial fibrosis and thrombosis.

Korsakoff's s., an alcohol amnestic s. characterized by confusion and severe impairment of memory, especially for recent events, for which the patient compensates by confabulation; typically encountered in chronic alcoholics; delirium tremens may precede the s., and Wernicke's s. often coexists; the precise pathogenesis is uncertain, but direct toxic effects of alcohol are probably less important than severe nutritional deficiencies often associated with chronic alcoholism. SYN amnestic psychosis, amnestic s. (1), dysmnesic psychosis, dysmnesic s., Korsakoff's psychosis, polyneuritic psychosis.

Kostmann's s., severe infantile agranulocytosis, an inherited disorder of infancy characterized by severe, recurrent infections, and neutropenia.

Kuskokwim s., congenital joint contractures resembling arthrogryposis, found in Eskimos of the Kuskokwim River delta in Alaska.

Laband's s. [MIM*135500 and 135300], fibromatosis of the gingivae associated with hypoplasia of the distal phalanges, nail dysplasia, joint hypermotility, and sometimes hepatosplenomegaly; autosomal dominant inheritance.

Labbé's neurocirculatory s., an anxiety neurosis that may occur in Basedow's disease but may be associated with tachycardia and exophthalmos without increase of basal metabolic rate or other evidence of hyperthyroidism.

LAMB s. [MIM*160980], the concurrence of lentigines, atrial myxoma, mucocutaneous myxomas, and blue nevi. SEE ALSO NAME s.

Lambert-Eaton s. (LES), progressive proximal muscle weakness in patients with carcinoma, in the absence of dermatomyositis or polymyositis; caused by antibodies directed against motor-nerve axon terminals. SEE myasthenic s. SYN carcinomatous myopathy, Eaton-Lambert s., Lambert's s.

Lambert's s., SYN Lambert-Eaton s.

Landau-Kleffner s., childhood generalized and psychomotor seizures associated with acquired aphasia; multifocal spikes and spike and wave discharges in the electroencephalogram. SYN acquired epileptic aphasia.

Landry s., SYN acute idiopathic *polyneuritis.*

Landry-Guillain-Barré s., SYN acute idiopathic *polyneuritis.*

Larsen's s., a s. characterized by multiple congenital dislocations with osseous anomalies, including characteristic flattened facies and cleft soft palate.

Lasègue's s., in conversion hysteria, inability to move an anesthetic limb, except under control of the sight.

lateral medullary s., SYN posterior inferior cerebellar artery s.

Launois-Bensaude s., SYN multiple symmetric *lipomatosis*.

Launois-Cléret s., SYN Fröhlich's s.

Laurence-Moon-Biedl s. [MIM*245800], mental retardation, pigmentary retinopathy, hypogenitalism, and spastic paraplegia; recessive inheritance.

Lawrence-Seip s., SYN lipoatrophy.

Lejeune s., SYN cri-du-chat s.

Lenègre's s., isolated damage of the cardiac conduction system as a result of a sclerodegenerative lesion; characterized ordinarily as idiopathic fibrosis of the atrioventricular nodal, His bundle, or bundle branches with corresponding conduction block(s). SYN Lenègre's disease.

Lennox s., SYN Lennox-Gastaut s.

Lennox-Gastaut s., a generalized myoclonic astatic epilepsy in children, with mental retardation, resulting from various cerebral afflictions such as perinatal hypoxia, cerebral hemorrhage, encephalitides, maldevelopment or metabolic disorders of the brain; characterized by multiple seizure types (generalized tonic, atonic, myoclonic, tonic-clonic, and atypical absence) and background slowing and slow spike and wave pattern on EEG; patients are usually mentally retarded or developmentally delayed. SYN Lennox s.

LEOPARD s., s. consisting of *l*entigines (multiple), *e*lectrocardiographic abnormalities, *o*cular hypertelorism, *p*ulmonary stenosis, *a*bnormalities of genitalia, *r*etardation of growth, and *d*eafness (sensorineural). An autosomal dominant hereditary disorder. SYN multiple lentigines s.

Leriche's s., aortoiliac occlusive *disease* producing distal ischemic symptoms and signs.

Leri-Weill s., SYN dyschondrosteosis.

Lermoyez' s., increasing deafness, interrupted by a sudden attack of dizziness, after which the hearing improves. SYN labyrinthine angiospasm.

Lesch-Nyhan s. [MIM*308000 several kinds], a disorder, associated with failure to form hypoxanthine phosphoribosyltransferase, characterized by hyperuricemia and uric acid urolithiasis, choreoathetosis, mental retardation, spastic cerebral palsy, and self-mutilation of fingers and lips by biting; X-linked recessive inheritance.

Lev's s., bundle branch block in a patient with normal myocardium and normal coronary arteries resulting from fibrosis or calcification including the conducting system; affects the membranous septum, the apex of the muscular septum, and often the mitral and aortic valve rings. SYN Lev's disease.

Libman-Sacks s., SYN Libman-Sacks *endocarditis*.

Li-Fraumeni cancer s. [MIM*151623 and 191170], familial breast cancer in young women, with soft-tissue sarcomas in children and other cancers in close relatives.

Lignac-Fanconi s., SYN cystinosis.

liver kidney s., severe loss of both liver and kidney function, seen in a variety of diseases, often with fatal outcome. Seen particularly in late-stage liver failure due to cirrhosis or hepatitis, and in several viral infections.

locked-in s., basis pontis infarct resulting in tetraplegia, horizontal ophthalmoplegia, dysphagia, and facial diplegia with preserved consciousness; caused by basilar artery occlusion. SYN pseudocoma.

loculation s., SYN Froin's s.

Löffler's s., (1) SYN simple pulmonary *eosinophilia*. **(2)** SYN Löffler's *endocarditis*.

Lorain-Lévi s., SYN pituitary *dwarfism*.

Louis-Bar s., SYN *ataxia* telangiectasia.

Lowe's s., SYN oculocerebrorenal s.

Lowe-Terrey-MacLachlan s., SYN oculocerebrorenal s.

Lown-Ganong-Levine s., electrocardiographic s. of a short P-R interval with normal duration of the QRS complex; it lacks the slurred delta wave of the Wolff-Parkinson-White s., but resem-

bles it in its frequent association with paroxysmal tachycardia which qualifies it as a s.; otherwise short P-R may occur in otherwise normal individuals.

low salt s., low sodium s., a s. resulting from salt restriction and use of diuretics in treatment of congestive heart failure and hypertension, characterized by weakness, drowsiness, muscle cramps, and a reduction in glomerular filtration with consequent nitrogen retention, renal failure, and sometimes death; occurs also in cirrhosis of the liver with ascites and in adrenal insufficiency. SYN salt depletion s.

lupus-like s., a clinical s. resembling that of systemic *lupus* erythematosus, but due to some other cause.

Lutembacher's s., a congenital cardiac abnormality consisting of a defect of the interatrial septum, mitral stenosis, and enlarged right atrium.

Lyell's s., SYN toxic epidermal *necrolysis*.

Macleod's s., SYN unilateral lobar *emphysema*.

Mad Hatter s., gastrointestinal and central nervous system manifestations of chronic mercury poisoning, including stomatitis, diarrhea, ataxia, tremor, hyperreflexia, sensorineural impairment, and emotional instability; previously seen in workers in lead manufacturing who put mercury-containing materials in their mouths to make them more pliable. [fr. char. in *Alice in Wonderland*]

Maffucci's s. [MIM*166000], enchondromatosis with multiple cavernous hemangiomas. SYN dyschondroplasia with hemangiomas.

Magendie-Hertwig s., SYN Magendie-Hertwig *sign*.

malabsorption s., a state characterized by diverse features such as diarrhea, weakness, edema, lassitude, weight loss, poor appetite, protuberant abdomen, pallor, bleeding tendencies, paresthesias, muscle cramps, etc., caused by any of several conditions in which there is ineffective absorption of nutrients, *e.g.*, sprue, gluten-induced enteropathy, gastroileostomy, tuberculosis, and certain fistulas.

malignant carcinoid s., SYN carcinoid s.

malignant mole s. [MIM*155600], irregularly shaped, variously colored, distinctively melanocytic, 5 to 10 mm nevi occurring in large numbers (to over 100) primarily on the trunk and extremities, with a high risk of malignancy reported in several members and three generations of a family.

Mallory-Weiss s., laceration of the lower end of the esophagus associated with bleeding, or penetration into the mediastinum, with subsequent mediastinitis; caused usually by severe retching and vomiting.

mandibulofacial dysotosis s., SYN mandibulofacial *dysostosis*.

mandibulo-oculofacial s., SYN *dyscephalia* mandibulo-oculofacialis.

Marañón's s., a s. characterized by ovarian insufficiency, scoliosis, and flat-feet.

Marchiafava-Micheli s., SYN paroxysmal nocturnal *hemoglobinuria*.

Marcus Gunn s., SYN jaw-winking s.

Marfan's s. [MIM*154700], a s. of congenital changes in the mesodermal and ectodermal tissues, skeletal changes (arachnodactyly, long limbs, laxness of joints), ectopia lentis, and vascular defects (particularly aneurysm of the aorta, dissecting or diffuse); iris transillumination is marked due to a deficiency of posterior epithelium pigment; autosomal dominant inheritance. SYN Marfan's disease.

Marie-Robinson s., insomnia and mild melancholia associated with alimentary levulosuria.

Marinesco-Garland s. [MIM*268800], a rare neurologic disorder characterized by cerebellolental degeneration with mental retardation; autosomal recessive inheritance. SYN cataract-oligophrenia s., Marinesco-Sjögren syndrome, Torsten Sjögren's s.

Maroteaux-Lamy s. [MIM*253200], an error of mucopolysaccharide metabolism characterized by excretion of dermatan sulfate in the urine, growth retardation, lumbar kyphosis, sternal protrusion, genu valgum, usually hepatosplenomegaly, and no mental retardation; onset occurs after two years of age; autosomal recessive inheritance. SYN polydystrophic dwarfism, type VI mucopolysaccharidosis.

Marshall s. [MIM*154780], s. of mid-face hypoplasia, cataract, sensorineural hearing loss, and hypohidrosis. It is disputed whether this s. is distinct from Stickler's s.

Martorell's s., SYN aortic arch s.

MASS s., a s. closely resembling both the Marfan's s. and the Barlow s. However, no dislocation of the lenses or aneurysmal changes occur in the aorta, and the mitral valve prolapse is by no means invariable. At present it has been assigned no separate MIM number, but shares that of the Barlow s. [MIM*157700]. [*m*itral valve prolapse, *a*ortic anomalies, *s*keletal changes, and *s*kin changes.]

massive bowel resection s., malabsorption following extensive resection of the bowel, particularly the small intestine, characterized by diarrhea, steatorrhea, hypoproteinemia, and malnutrition.

maternal deprivation s., a failure to thrive seen in infants and young children and exhibited as a constellation of physical signs, symptoms, and behaviors, usually associated with maternal loss, absence or neglect, and characterized by lack of responsiveness to the environment and often depression.

Mauriac's s., dwarfism with obesity and hepatosplenomegaly in children with poorly controlled diabetes mellitus.

Mayer-Rokitansky-Küster-Hauser s., primary amenorrhea, absence of vagina, or presence of a short vaginal pouch, and absence of the uterus with normal karyotype and ovaries. SYN Rokitansky-Küster-Hauser s.

May-White s., progressive myoclonus epilepsy with lipomas, deafness, and ataxia; probably a familial form of mitochondrial encephalomyopathy.

McArdle's s., SYN type 5 *glycogenosis*.

McCune-Albright s., polyostotic fibrous dysplasia with irregular brown patches of cutaneous pigmentation and endocrine dysfunction, especially precocious puberty in girls. SEE ALSO pseudohypoparathyroidism. SYN Albright's disease, Albright's s. (1).

Meadows' s., cardiomyopathy developing during pregnancy or the puerperium.

Meckel s., SYN dysencephalia splanchnocystica.

Meckel-Gruber s., SYN dysencephalia splanchnocystica.

meconium blockage s., low intestinal obstruction in newborn infants resulting from blockage of meconium.

megacystic s., a combination of a large smooth thin-walled bladder, vesicoureteral regurgitation, and dilated ureters.

megacystitis-megaureter s., radiologic findings of a large capacity, thin-walled bladder and massive vesicoureteral reflux, without obstruction or underlying neuropathy or dysfunctional voiding.

megacystitis-microcolon-intestinal hypoperistalsis s., a rare condition characterized by abdominal distention, lax abdominal musculature, incomplete intestinal rotation, and deficient intestinal peristalsis. A large bladder and often vesicoureteral reflux are seen. Typically affects female neonates and usually fatal in first year of life.

Meigs' s., fibromyoma of the ovary associated with hydroperitoneum and hydrothorax.

Melkersson-Rosenthal s. [MIM*155900], cheilitis granulomatosum, fissured tongue, and facial nerve paralysis.

Melnick-Needles s., SYN osteodysplasty.

Mendelson's s., pulmonary disorders resulting from aspiration of gastric contents into the lungs following vomiting or regurgitation in obstetrical patients.

Ménétrier's s., SYN Ménétrier's *disease*.

Ménière's s., SYN Ménière's *disease*.

Menkes' s., SYN kinky-hair *disease*.

menopausal s., recurring symptoms experienced by some women during the climacteric period; they include hot flashes, chills, headache, irritability, and depression. SYN climacteric s.

metastatic carcinoid s., SYN carcinoid s.

methionine malabsorption s., an inherited disorder in which there is an inability to absorb L-methionine from the gut.

Meyenburg-Altherr-Uehlinger s., SYN relapsing *polychondritis*.

Meyer-Betz s., SYN myoglobinuria.

middle lobe s., atelectasis with chronic pneumonitis of the middle lobe of the (right) lung, due to compression of the middle lobe bronchus, usually by enlarged lymph nodes, which may be tuberculous; chief symptoms are chronic cough, wheezing, recurrent respiratory infections, hemoptysis, chest pain, malaise, easy fatigability, and loss of weight; sometimes confused with interlobar accumulation of fluid in the lateral x-ray view. SYN Brock's s.

Mikulicz' s., the symptoms characteristic of Mikulicz' disease occurring as a complication of some other disease, such as lymphoma, leukemia, or uveoparotid fever.

milk-alkali s., a chronic disorder of the kidneys, reversible in its early stages, induced by ingestion of large amounts of calcium and alkali in the therapy of peptic ulcer; can progress to renal failure. SYN Burnett's s.

Milkman's s., osteomalacia with multiple pseudofractures, usually bilateral and symmetrical, may develop true pathologic fractures.

Millard-Gubler s., SYN Gubler's s.

minimal-change nephrotic s., nephrotic s. with minimal glomerular changes, occurring most frequently in children, marked by edema, albuminuria, and an increase in cholesterol in the blood, but otherwise with fairly good renal function; tubular epithelium is vacuolated by cholesterol droplets, but the glomeruli show only that the foot processes of the glomerular epithelial cells are fused, probably secondary to the proteinuria; the cause of the increased glomerular permeability to plasma protein is unknown.

Mirizzi's s., benign obstruction of the hepatic ducts due to spasm and/or fibrous scarring of surrounding connective tissue; often associated with a stone in the cystic duct and chronic cholecystitis.

mitral valve prolapse s., the clinical constellation of findings with or without symptoms due to prolapse of the mitral valve: a nonejection systolic click accentuated in the standing posture, sometimes multiple, sometimes with mitral regurgitation occurring relatively late in systole, and accompanied by echocardiographic evidence of the mitral valve prolapse, usually with thickened leaflets of the valve. Symptoms are nonspecific and may include vague chest pains and dyspnea on exertion. SYN billowing mitral valve s.

Möbius' s. [MIM*157900], a developmental bilateral facial paralysis usually associated with oculomotor or other neurological disorders. SYN congenital facial diplegia.

Mohr's s., autosomal recessive, OFD, oral-facial-digital s.

Monakow's s., contralateral hemiplegia, hemianesthesia, and homonomous hemianopsia due to occlusion of the anterior choroidal artery.

Morgagni-Adams-Stokes s., SYN Adams-Stokes s.

Morgagni's s. [MIM*144800], hyperostosis frontalis interna in elderly women, with obesity and neuropsychiatric disorders of uncertain cause; at least sometimes familial. SYN metabolic craniopathy, Stewart-Morel s.

morning glory s. [MIM*120330], a funnel-shaped hypoplastic optic nerve with a dot of white tissue at its center; surrounded by an elevated anulus of chorioretinal pigment.

Morquio's s. [MIM*253000], an error of mucopolysaccharide metabolism with excretion of keratan sulfate in urine; characterized by severe skeletal defects with short stature, severe deformity of spine and thorax, long bones with irregular epiphyses but with shafts of normal length, enlarged joints, flaccid ligaments, and waddling gait; autosomal recessive inheritance; type IV A mucopolysaccharidosis is due to an absence of galactose-1-sulfatase, while type IV B is due to a deficiency of a β-galactosidase. SYN Brailsford-Morquio disease, Morquio's disease, Morquio-Ullrich disease, type IVA, B mucopolysaccharidosis.

Morton's s., congenital shortening of the first metatarsal causing metatarsalgia.

Mounier-Kuhn s., SYN tracheobronchomegaly.

Mucha-Habermann s., SYN *pityriasis* lichenoides et varioliformis acuta.

Muckle-Wells s. [MIM*191900], a s. characterized by familial amyloidosis, notably involving the kidneys, progressive hearing loss of neural origin and unknown cause, and periods of febrile urticaria associated with pain in joints and muscles of the extremities; autosomal dominant inheritance.

mucocutaneous lymph node s., a polymorphous erythematous febrile, sometimes epidemic, disease of unknown etiology occurring in children, especially under two years of age; accompanied by conjunctivitis, pharyngitis, strawberry tongue, cervical lymphadenopathy, occasionally fatal arteritis with coronary artery aneurysm formation, and characteristic desquamation of perineum, fingers, and toes. SYN Kawasaki's disease, Kawasaki's s.

Muir-Torre s., SYN Torre's s.

multiple endocrine deficiency s., acquired deficiency of the function of several endocrine glands, usually on an auto-immune basis. SYN multiple glandular deficiency s.

multiple glandular deficiency s., SYN multiple endocrine deficiency s.

multiple hamartoma s., SYN Cowden's *disease.*

multiple lentigines s., SYN LEOPARD s.

multiple mucosal neuroma s., multiple submucosal neuromas or neurofibromas of the tongue, lips, and eyelids in young persons; sometimes associated with tumors of the thyroid or adrenal medulla, or with subcutaneous neurofibromatosis.

Munchausen s., repeated fabrication of clinically convincing simulations of disease for the purpose of gaining medical attention; a term referring to patients who wander from hospital to hospital feigning acute medical or surgical illness and giving false and fanciful information about their medical and social background for no apparent reason other than to gain attention. SEE factitious *disorder.*

Munchausen s. by proxy, a form of child maltreatment or abuse inflicted by a caretaker (usually the mother) with fabrications of symptoms and/or induction of signs of disease, leading to unnecessary investigations and interventions, with occasional serious health consequences, including death of the child.

Münchhausen s., SEE Munchausen s.

myasthenic s. (MS), a disorder of neuromuscular transmission marked primarily by limb and girdle weakness, absent deep tendon reflexes, dry mouth, and impotence; due to an immunological disorder; often, especially in males, a paraneoplastic syndrome linked to small cell carcinoma of the lung. SYN Lambert-Eaton s.

myeloproliferative s.'s [MIM*159595], a group of conditions that result from a disorder in the rate of formation of cells of the bone marrow, including chronic granulocytic leukemia, erythremia, myelosclerosis, panmyelosis, and erythremic myelosis and erythroleukemia.

myofacial pain-dysfunction s., dysfunction of the masticatory apparatus related to spasm of the muscles of mastication precipitated by occlusal dysharmony or alteration in vertical dimension of the jaws, and exacerbated by emotional stress; characterized by pain in the preauricular region, muscle tenderness, popping noise in the temporomandibular joint, and limitation of jaw motion. SYN temporomandibular joint pain-dysfunction s.

myofascial s., irritation of the muscles and fascia of the back and neck causing acute and chronic pain not associated with any neurological or bony evidence of disease; presumed to arise primarily from poorly understood changes in the muscle and fascia themselves.

Naegeli s. [MIM*161000], reticular skin pigmentation, diminished sweating, hypodontia, and hyperkeratosis of the palms and soles; may be confused with *incontinentia* pigmenti but is as common in males as in females; autosomal dominant inheritance. SYN Franceschetti-Jadassohn s.

Naffziger s., scalenus-anticus s.

nail-patella s. [MIM*101200], a congenital skeletal disorder characterized by hypoplasia of the patella, iliac horns, dysplasia of the fingernails and toenails, and thickening of the glomerular lamina densa; the lower ends of the femur have a shape very similar to Erlenmeyer flask deformity; autosomal dominant inheritance.

NAME s., the concurrence of nevi, atrial myxoma, myxoid neurofibromas, and ephilides.

Nelson s., a s. of hyperpigmentation, third nerve damage, and enlarging sella turcica caused by pituitary adenomas presumably present before adrenalectomy for Cushing's s. but enlarging and symptomatic afterward. SYN postadrenalectomy s.

nephritic s., the clinical symptoms of acute glomerulonephritis, particularly hematuria, hypertension, and renal failure.

nephrotic s., a clinical state characterized by edema, albuminuria, decreased plasma albumin, doubly refractile bodies in the urine, and usually increased blood cholesterol; lipid droplets may be present in the cells of the renal tubules, but the basic lesion is increased permeability of the glomerular capillary basement membranes, of unknown cause or resulting from glomerulonephritis, diabetic glomerulosclerosis, systemic lupus erythematosus, amyloidosis, renal vein thrombosis, or hypersensitivity to various toxic agents. SYN nephrosis (3).

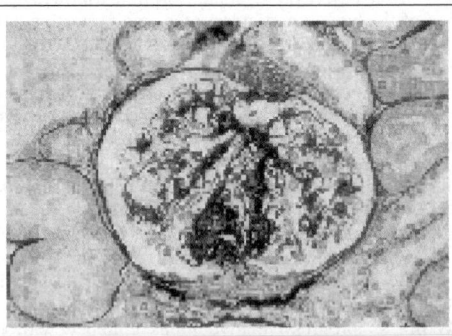

nephrotic syndrome (histology)
sclerosis with many fibers and few nuclei; fusion with
Bowman's capsule

Netherton's s. [MIM*256500], congenital ichthyosiform erythroderma or ichthyosis linearis circumscripta associated with bamboo hair, and irregularly with atopy, urticaria, intermittent aminoaciduria, and mental retardation; probably an autosomal recessive trait that frequently resolves or improves in adolescence.

neural crest s., s. consisting of loss of pain sensibility, autonomic dysfunction, pupillary abnormalities, neurogenic anhidrosis, vasomotor instability, aplasia of dental enamel, meningeal thickening, hyperflexion, and a degree of albinism; may reflect developmental abnormalities of the neural crest.

neurocutaneous s., the occurrence of nevi and sometimes various skeletal deformities with symptoms pointing to gliosis or abiotrophy of the central nervous system.

neuroleptic malignant s., hyperthermia with extrapyramidal and autonomic disturbances which may result in death, following the use of neuroleptic agents.

Nezelof s., SYN cellular *immunodeficiency* with abnormal immunoglobulin synthesis.

Nieden's s., multiple telangiectasis of the face, forearms, and hands, with cataract and aortic stenosis.

Noack's s., SYN acrocephalopolysyndactyly.

nonsense s., SYN Ganser's s.

Noonan's s. [MIM*163950, MIM*163955], the male phenotype of Turner's s., characterized by congenital heart disease, especially pulmonary stenosis, pigeon breast, webbing of the neck, antimongoloid slanting of the palpebrae, and other less regular minor features; autosomal dominant inheritance. It is equally common in males and in females; hence the alternative designation "Male Turner's s." (because of its similarity to the XO karyotype) is confusing.

Nothnagel's s., dizziness, staggering, and rolling gait, with irregular forms of oculomotor paralysis and often nystagmus, seen in cases of tumor of the midbrain.

nystagmus blockage s., strabismus with eyes and head in a position to minimize associated nystagmus.

OAV s., SYN oculoauriculovertebral *dysplasia.*

occipital horn s., an X-linked recessive disorder in which there is defective biliary excretion of copper resulting in a deficiency of lysyl oxidase causing skin and joint laxity.

ocular-mucous membrane s., Stevens-Johnson s. with associated ocular lesions (conjunctivitis, panophthalmitis, iritis), oral lesions (bullae, erosions, superficial ulcers), and genital lesions (urethritis, balanitis circinata, blebs).

oculobuccogenital s., SYN Behçet's s.

oculocerebrorenal s., a congenital s. with hydrophthalmia, cataracts, mental retardation, aminoaciduria, reduced ammonia production by the kidney, and vitamin D-resistant rickets; X-linked recessive inheritance. SYN Lowe's s., Lowe-Terrey-MacLachlan s.

oculocutaneous s., SYN Vogt-Koyanagi s.

oculomandibulofacial s., SYN *dyscephalia* mandibulo-oculofacialis.

oculopharyngeal s. [MIM*106310], a myopathic disorder with a slowly progressive blepharoptosis and dysphagia, beginning late in life; autosomal dominant inheritance; there is also a similar autosomal dominant trait.

oculovertebral s., SYN oculovertebral *dysplasia*.

oculovestibulo-auditory s., a nonsyphilitic interstitial keratitis characterized by an abrupt onset with vertigo and tinnitus followed by deafness; about 50% of patients have an associated systemic disease, most commonly polyarteritis nodosa. SYN Cogan's s.

OFD s., SYN orodigitofacial *dysostosis*.

Ogilvie's s., pseudo-obstruction believed to be the result of motility disturbance involving the large or small intestine but without physical obstruction.

Omenn's s. [MIM*267700], a rapidly fatal autosomal recessive immunodeficiency disease characterized by erythroderma, diarrhea, repeated infections, hepatosplenomegaly, and leukocytosis with eosinophilia.

Oppenheim's s., SYN *amyotonia* congenita (1).

orbital s., an obsolete term referring to neoplastic tissue formation involving the apex of the orbit, causing ophthalmoplegia and optic nerve atrophy.

organic brain s., a constellation of behavioral or psychological signs and symptoms including problems with attention, concentration, memory, confusion, anxiety, and depression caused by transient or permanent dysfunction of the brain. SYN acute organic brain s., OBS, organic mental s.

organic mental s. (OMS), SYN organic brain s.

organic mood s., s. attributed to an organic factor characterized by either depressive or manic mood. SEE bipolar *disorder*. SEE ALSO bipolar *disorder*.

orofaciodigital s., SYN orodigitofacial *dysostosis*.

osteomyelofibrotic s., SYN myelofibrosis.

Ostrum-Furst s., congenital synostosis of the neck.

Othello s., a delusional belief in the infidelity of one's spouse. [*Othello*, Shakespearian char.]

otomandibular s., SYN otomandibular *dysostosis*.

otopalatodigital s. [MIM*311300], conduction deafness and cleft palate with broad nasal root and frontal bossing, wide spacing of toes, broad thumbs and great toes, and often other signs of generalized bone dysplasia; X-linked recessive inheritance.

ovarian vein s., ureteral obstruction due to compression by enlarged ovarian vein, usually right side and during pregnancy.

pacemaker s., the occurrence of symptoms relating to the loss of atrial-ventricular synchrony in ventricularly paced patients, or symptoms caused by inadequate timing of atrial and ventricular contractions in paced patients.

pachydermoperiostosis s., SEE pachydermoperiostosis.

Paget-von Schrötter s., stress thrombosis or spontaneous thrombosis of the subclavian or axillary vein; a thoracic-outlet syndrome. SYN effort-induced thrombosis.

painful-bruising s., an intense inflammatory reaction to slight extravasation of blood, due to an allergic sensitivity to red blood cells; more commonly seen in adult women.

paleostriatal s., SYN Hunt's s. (3).

pallidal s., SYN Hunt's s. (3).

Pancoast s., lower trunk brachial plexopathy and Horner s. due to malignant tumor in the region of the superior pulmonary sulcus.

papillary muscle s., SYN papillary muscle *dysfunction*.

Papillon-Léage and Psaume s., SYN orodigitofacial *dysostosis*.

Papillon-Lefèvre s. [MIM*245000], a congenital hyperkeratosis of the palms and soles, with progessive destruction of alveolar bone about the deciduous and permanent teeth beginning as early as 2 years of age, and also with premature exfoliation of teeth; autosomal recessive inheritance.

paraneoplastic s., a s. directly resulting from a malignant neoplasm, but not resulting from the presence of tumor cells in the affected parts.

Parinaud's s., paralysis of conjugate upward gaze with a lesion at the level of the superior colliculi; Bell's phenomenon is present. SYN Parinaud's ophthalmoplegia.

Parinaud's oculoglandular s., unilateral conjunctival granuloma with preauricular adenopathy in tularemia, chancre, and tuberculosis.

Parsonage-Turner s., SYN neuralgic *amyotrophy*.

Patau's s., SYN trisomy 13 s.

Paterson-Brown-Kelly s., SYN tendon sheath s.

Paterson-Kelly s., SYN Plummer-Vinson s.

pathologic startle s.'s, a group of disorders characterized by markedly exaggerated startle reflex and other exaggerated stimulus-induced responses. Includes hyperexplexia and probably latah and the jumping Frenchman of Maine s.

Pellizzi's s., SYN *macrogenitosomia* praecox.

Pendred's s. [MIM*274600], a type of familial goiter; congenital nerve deafness with goiter (usually small) due to defective organic binding of iodine in the thyroid; afflicted individuals are usually euthyroid; autosomal recessive inheritance.

Pepper s., obsolete eponym for neuroblastoma of the adrenal gland with metastases in the liver; formerly believed to occur more frequently when the primary tumor was in the right adrenal, whereas tumors of the left adrenal tended to metastasize to the skull (Hutchison's syndrome).

pericolic membrane s., a symptom complex simulating chronic appendicitis, caused by congenital constricting pericolic membranes.

Persian Gulf s., SYN Gulf War s.

persistent müllerian duct s., familial disorder with presence of fallopian tube, uterus, and testis in a male. Deficient müllerian inhibitory substance secondary to Sertoli cell defect. SYN hernia uteri inguinale.

pertussis s., SYN pertussis.

pertussis-like s., a syndrome characterized by severe episodes of coughing resembling whooping *cough* (pertussis).

petrosphenoidal s., neoplastic infiltration of the apex of the petrous bone and the anterior part of the foramen lacerum.

Peutz-Jeghers s. [MIM*175200], generalized hamartomatous multiple polyposis of the intestinal tract, consistently involving the jejunum, associated with melanin spots of the lips, buccal mucosa, and fingers; autosomal dominant inheritance. SYN Jeghers-Peutz s., Peutz's s.

Peutz's s., SYN Peutz-Jeghers s.

Pfaundler-Hurler s., SYN Hurler's s.

Pfeiffer's s. [MIM*101600], SYN type V *acrocephalosyndactyly*.

pharyngeal pouch s., SYN DiGeorge s.

phospholipid s., the combination of antiphospholipid antibodies and the presence of either arterial or venous occlusive events such as thrombosis.

Picchini's s., a form of polyserositis involving the three great serosae in contact with the diaphragm, sometimes also the meninges, tunica vaginalis testis, synovial sheaths, and bursae, caused by the presence of a trypanosome. SYN Picchini.

Pick's s., SYN Pick's *disease*.

pickwickian s., a combination of severe, grotesque obesity, somnolence, and general debility, theoretically resulting from hypoventilation induced by the obesity; hypercapnia, pulmonary hypertension and cor pulmonale can result. [after the "fat boy" in Dickens' *Pickwick Papers*]

Pierre Robin s. [MIM*261800], micrognathia and abnormal smallness of the tongue, often with cleft palate, severe myopia,

sy

congenital glaucoma, and retinal detachment; weak evidence of autosomal recessive inheritance. SYN Robin's s.

Pins' s., dullness, diminution of vocal fremitus and of the vesicular murmur, and a slight distant blowing sound, heard in the posteroinferior region of the chest on the left side, in cases of pericardial effusion; there is sometimes also a fine rale in this region, but all the adventitious auscultatory signs disappear when the patient assumes the genupectoral position.

placental dysfunction s., fetal malnutrition and hypoxia resulting from impaired transfer of oxygen and various nutritive materials from mother to fetus.

Plummer-Vinson s., iron deficiency anemia, dysphagia, esophageal web, and atrophic glossitis. SYN Paterson-Kelly s., sideropenic dysphagia.

POEMS s., a condition characterized by *p*olyneuropathy, *o*rganomegaly, *e*ndocrinopathy, *m*onoclonal gammopathy, and *s*kin changes.

Poland's s., an anomaly consisting of absence of the pectoralis major and minor muscles, ipsilateral breast hypoplasia, and absence of two to four rib segments.

polycystic ovary s. [MIM*184700], a condition commonly characterized by hirsutism, obesity, menstrual abnormalities, infertility, and enlarged ovaries; thought to reflect excessive androgen secretion of ovarian origin. SYN sclerocystic disease of the ovary, Stein-Leventhal s.

polyendocrine deficiency s., polyglandular deficiency s., associated pathologic dysfunction of several endocrine glands, as in Schmidt's s.

polysplenia s., SYN bilateral *left-sidedness*.

popliteal entrapment s., a crush s. resulting from compression of the popliteal artery and impairment of its blood flow by structures of the popliteal space.

porcine stress s., SYN malignant *hyperthermia*.

postadrenalectomy s., SYN Nelson s.

postcardiotomy s., SYN postpericardiotomy s.

postcholecystectomy s., the persistence of signs and symptoms that led to removal of the gallbladder, as a sequel to cholecystectomy.

postcommissurotomy s., SYN postpericardiotomy s.

postconcussion s., SEE posttraumatic s.

posterior inferior cerebellar artery s., a s. due usually to thrombosis, characterized by dysarthria, dysphagia, staggering gait, and vertigo, and marked by hypotonia, incoordination of voluntary movement, nystagmus, Horner's s. on the ipsilateral side, and loss of pain and temperature senses on the side of the body opposite to the lesion. SYN lateral medullary s., Wallenberg's s.

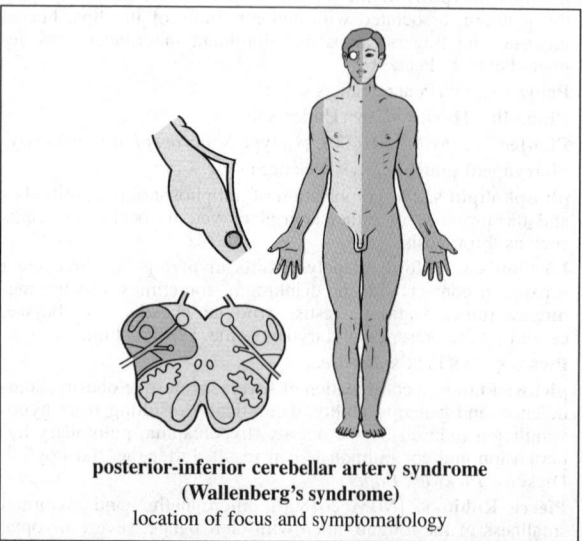

**posterior-inferior cerebellar artery syndrome
(Wallenberg's syndrome)**
location of focus and symptomatology

postgastrectomy s., SYN dumping s.

postmaturity s., gestation extending 43 weeks or longer; sometimes associated with fetal dysmaturity.

postmyocardial infarction s., a complication developing several days to several weeks after myocardial infarction; its clinical features are fever, leukocytosis, chest pain, and evidence of pericarditis, sometimes with pleurisy and pneumonitis, with a strong tendency to recurrence; probably of immunopathogenetic origin.

postpartum pituitary necrosis s., SYN Sheehan's s.

postpericardiotomy s., pericarditis, with or without fever and often in repeated episodes, weeks to months after cardiac surgery. SYN postcardiotomy s., postcommissurotomy s.

postphlebitic s., a state characterized by edema, pain, stasis dermatitis, cellulitis, and varicose veins, and ending in ulceration of the lower leg, developing as a sequel to deep venous thrombosis of the lower extremity.

postrubella s., a group of congenital defects resulting from maternal rubella during the first trimester of pregnancy and including microphthalmos, cataracts, deafness, mental retardation, patent ductus arteriosus, and pulmonary artery stenosis.

postthrombotic s., a s. that follows a vascular thrombosis. Term is usually used to indicate difficulties, such as persistent edema, following venous thrombosis.

posttraumatic s., a clinical disorder that often follows head injury, characterized by headache, dizziness, neurasthenia, hypersensitivity to stimuli, and diminished concentration. SYN traumatic neurasthenia.

posttraumatic neck s., a clinical complex of pain, tenderness, tight neck musculature, vasomotor instability, and ill-defined symptoms such as dizziness and blurred vision as the result of trauma to the neck. Also variously termed occipital or suboccipital neuralgia or neuritis; cervical tension s.; cervical myospasm, myositis, or fibrositis. SYN cervical fibrositis, cervical tension s.

posttraumatic stress s., a disorder appearing after a physically or psychologically traumatic event outside the range of usual human experience, (*e.g.,* a serious threat to one's life or seeing a loved one killed), characterized by symptoms of re-experiencing the event, numbing of responsiveness to the environment, exaggerated startle response, guilt feelings, impairment of memory, and difficulties in concentration and sleep.

Potter's s., renal agenesis with hypoplastic lungs and associated neonatal respiratory distress, hemodynamic instability, acidosis, cyanosis, edema, and characteristic (Potter's) facies; death usually occurs from respiratory insufficiency, which develops before uremia.

Prader-Willi s. [MIM*176270], a congenital s. of unknown etiology characterized by short stature, mental retardation, polyphagia with marked obesity, and sexual infantilism; initially severe muscular hypotonia and poor responsiveness to external stimuli decrease with age; a small deletion is demonstrable in chromosome 15.

precordial catch s., a benign s. of uncertain origin, characterized by sharp, sudden pain in the region of the cardiac apex on inspiration, yet usually relieved by forcing a deeper breath; tenderness is absent.

preexcitation s., SYN Wolff-Parkinson-White s.

preinfarction s., abrupt development of angina pectoris or worsening of existing angina by increases in its frequency or severity; sometimes heralds myocardial infarction.

premature senility s., SYN progeria.

premenstrual s. (PMS), in women of reproductive age, the regular monthly experience of physiological and emotional distress, usually during the several days preceding menses; characterized by nervousness, depression, fluid retention, and weight gain. SYN late luteal phase dysphoric disorder, menstrual molimina, premenstrual tension s., premenstrual tension.

PMS affects about one-third of menstruating women between ages 25 and 40, and some amenorrheic women as well. Its symptoms may only partly be relieved by over-the-counter medications. In extreme cases, progesterone appears effective. Reducing caffeine and salt intake may lessen associated nervousness and depression, and regular exercise and diets high in complex carbohydrates may help minimize the severity of episodes. Before being listed in the revised edition of the DSM-III, PMS became a subject of debate among feminists who believed that it did not qualify as a true disorder. PMS has been used as a successful defense in a murder trial in the U.K.

premenstrual salivary s., glandular abnormalities occurring prior to the onset of menses, including swelling of the breast tissues and enlargement of the salivary glands.

premenstrual tension s., SYN premenstrual s.

premotor s., hemiplegia with spasticity, Rossolimo's reflex, but not the Babinski sign, together with forced grasping and vasomotor disturbances.

Proteus s., a sporadic disorder of possible genetic origin, having a variable and changing phenotype; characterized by grossly enlarged hands and feet, distorted abnormal growth, and gigantism of the head; often confused with neurofibromatosis type I. SYN elephant man's disease.

prune belly s., a s. of deficient abdominal muscle, undescended testes, large hypotonic bladder and dilated, tortuous ureters. SYN Eagle-Barrett s.

psychogenic nocturnal polydipsia s., PNP s., emotionally induced excessive water drinking at night.

pterygium s. [MIM*178110, *265000, *312150], webbing of the neck, antecubital fossae, and popliteal fossae with flexion deformities of the extremities and anomalies of the vertebrae; observed in pseudo-Turner's s. and Turner's s.; mendelian inheritance of all these kinds.

pulmonary dysmaturity s., a respiratory disorder occurring in small, premature infants who are incapable of normal pulmonary ventilation and who often die of hypoxia after an illness of 6 to 8 weeks; the lungs contain widespread focal emphysematous blebs and the parenchyma has thickened alveolar walls; diagnosed principally on the basis of the clinical history, chest radiographic findings, and the findings at autopsy, which must include the absence of pathological changes characteristic of other pulmonary disorders commonly encountered in this age group. SYN Wilson-Mikity s.

punchdrunk s., a condition seen in boxers, often years after their retirement, and presumably caused by repeated cerebral injury, characterized by weakness in the lower limbs, unsteadiness of gait, slowness of muscular movements, tremors of hands, dysarthria, and slow cerebration.

Putnam-Dana s., SYN subacute combined *degeneration* of the spinal cord.

radial aplasia-thrombocytopenia s., thrombocytopenia-absent radius s.

radicular s., a group of symptoms resulting from any interference with the intradural portion of one or more spinal nerve roots; the chief symptoms are pain, paresthesia, hypesthesia, or hyperesthesia, motor, trophic, and reflex disturbances.

Raeder's paratrigeminal s., a postganglionic Horner's s. associated with trigeminal nerve dysfunction caused by involvement of the carotid sympathetic plexus, near Mechel' cave.

Ramsay Hunt's s., (1) SYN Hunt's s. **(2)** SYN *herpes* zoster oticus.

Raynaud's s., idiopathic paroxysmal bilateral cyanosis of the digits due to arterial and arteriolar contraction; caused by cold or emotion. SEE ALSO Raynaud's *phenomenon.* SYN Raynaud's disease, symmetric asphyxia.

Refetoff s., a condition characterized by goiter and elevated serum level of thyroid hormones without manifestations of thyrotoxicosis, due to target organ unresponsiveness to thyroid hormones.

Refsum's s., SYN Refsum's *disease.*

Reifenstein's s. [MIM*312300, *313700], partial androgen sensitivity; a familial form of male pseudohermaphroditism characterized by varying degrees of ambiguous genitalia or hypospadias, postpubertal development of gynecomastia, and infertility associated with seminiferous tubular sclerosis; cryptorchidism may be present, and Leydig cell hypofunction may lead to impo-

tence in later years; chromosomal studies are usually normal; X-linked recessive or autosomal dominant male-linked trait.

Reiter's s., the association of urethritis, iridocyclitis, mucocutaneous lesions, and arthritis, sometimes with diarrhea; one or more of these conditions may recur at intervals of months or years, but the arthritis may be persistent. SYN Fiessinger-Leroy-Reiter s., Reiter's disease.

REM s., a reticular erythematous dermatitis of the upper trunk, more common in women, in which there is perivascular infiltrate of lymphocytes, few plasma cells, and upper dermal deposits of mucin; worsens on exposure to ultraviolet light. SYN reticular erythematous mucinosis.

Rendu-Osler-Weber s., SYN hereditary hemorrhagic *telangiectasia.*

Renpenning's s. [MIM*309500], x-linked mental retardation with short stature and microcephaly not associated with the fragile X chromosome and occurring more frequently in males, although some females may also be affected.

residual ovary s., the development of a pelvic mass, pelvic pain, and occasionally dyspareunia following hysterectomy without removal of both ovaries.

resistant ovary s., SYN Savage s.

respiratory distress s. of the newborn, SYN hyaline membrane *disease* of the newborn.

restless legs s., a sense of indescribable uneasiness, twitching, or restlessness that occurs in the legs after going to bed, frequently leading to insomnia, which may be relieved temporarily by walking about; thought to be caused by inadequate circulation or as a side effect of antipsychotic medication. SEE ALSO akathisia. SYN Ekbom s., restless legs.

retraction s., a retraction of the globe and pseudoptosis on attempted adduction; due to co-innervation of the horizontal recti. Sometimes there is an inability to abduct the affected eye (type 1), or adduct the affected eye (type 2), or both (type 3). SYN Duane's s.

Rett's s. [MIM*312750], a progressive s. of autism, dementia, ataxia, and purposeless hand movements; associated with hyperammonemia, principally in girls.

Reye's s., an acquired encephalopathy of young children that follows an acute febrile illness, usually influenza or varicella infection; characterized by recurrent vomiting, agitation, and lethargy, which may lead to coma with intracranial hypertension; ammonia and serum transaminases are elevated; death may result from edema of the brain and resulting cerebral herniation.

Rh null s. [MIM*269150], a lack of all Rh antigens, compensated hemolytic anemia, and stomatocytosis.

Richards-Rundle s. [MIM*245100], a nervous system disorder beginning in early childhood with congenital severe, progressive sensorineural hearing loss, ataxia, muscle wasting nystagmus, absent deep tendon reflexes, mental retardation, and failure to develop secondary sexual characteristics; autosomal recessive inheritance.

Richter's s., a high-grade lymphoma developing during the course of chronic lymphocytic leukemia; associated with cachexia, pyrexia, dysproteinemia, and lymphomas with multinucleated tumor cells.

Rieger's s. [MIM*180500], iridocorneal mesodermal dysgenesis combined with hypodontia or anodontia and maxillary hypoplasia; autosomal dominant; there is a delayed sexual development and hypothyroidism; there is a deficiency in human growth hormone

right ovarian vein s., a condition characterized by intermittent abdominal pain due to ureteral compression by the right ovarian vein, occurring with most frequency on the right side, and thought to be due to aberrant crossing of the right ovarian vein over the ureter, generally at the level of the first sacral vertebra; dilation of the ovarian vein during pregnancy and unilateral ptosis of the kidney are thought to be contributing factors leading to intermittent ureteral obstruction and recurring bouts of pain and pyelonephritis.

Riley-Day s., SYN familial *dysautonomia.*

Roaf's s., a nonhereditary craniofacial-skeletal disorder characterized by congenital or early retinal detachment, cataracts, myopia, shortened long bones, and mental retardation; sensorineural progressive hearing loss is of later onset.

Roberts s. [MIM*268304], phocomelia or lesser degrees of hypomelia, microbrachycephaly, midfacial defect, prenatal growth deficiency, and cryptorchidism; autosomal recessive inheritance.

Robinow's s., SYN fetal face s.

Robin's s., SYN Pierre Robin s.

Rokitansky-Küster-Hauser s., SYN Mayer-Rokitansky-Küster-Hauser s.

Romano-Ward s. [MIM*192500], a prolonged Q-T interval in the electrocardiogram in children subject to attacks of unconsciousness that result from ventricular arrhythmias including ventricular fibrillation; autosomal dominant inheritance. Cf. Jervell and Lange-Nielsen s. SYN Ward-Romano s.

Romberg's s., SYN facial *hemiatrophy*.

Rothmund's s. [MIM*268400], atrophy, pigmentation, and telangiectasia of the skin, usually with juvenile cataract, saddle nose, congenital bone defects, disturbance of hair growth, hypogonadism; autosomal recessive inheritance. SYN poikiloderma atrophicans and cataract, poikiloderma congenitale, Rothmund-Thomson s.

Rothmund-Thomson s., SYN Rothmund's s.

Rotor's s., jaundice appearing in childhood due to impaired biliary excretion; most of the plasma bilirubin is conjugated, liver fraction tests are usually normal, and there is no hepatic pigmentation.

Roussy-Lévy s., SYN Roussy-Lévy *disease*.

Rubinstein-Taybi s. [MIM*180849], mental retardation, broad thumb and great toe, antimongoloid slant to the eyes, thin and beaked nose, prominent forehead, low-set ears, high arched palate, and cardiac anomaly; may be submicroscopic chromosomal defect.

Rud's s. [MIM*308200], ichthyosiform erythroderma associated with acanthosis nigricans, dwarfism, hypogonadism, and epilepsy; mostly sporadic, but may be an X-linked recessive trait.

runting s. (run'ting), if newborn mice are thymectomized, they do not gain weight and their lymphoid tissue atrophies. SYN wasting s. (1).

Russell's s., failure of infants and young children to thrive due to suprasellar lesions, commonly astrocytomas of the anterior third ventricle; although the growth hormone may be elevated, the child is emaciated and has loss of body fat. SEE ALSO pseudohydrocephaly.

Saethre-Chotzen s., SYN type III *acrocephalosyndactyly*.

Sakati-Nyhan s., SYN acrocephalopolysyndactyly.

salt depletion s., SYN low salt s.

salt-losing s., SYN salt-losing *nephritis*.

Samter's s., a triad of asthma, nasal polyps, and aspirin intolerance.

Sanchez Salorio s., a s. characterized by retinal pigmentary dystrophy, cataract, hypotrichosis of the lashes, mental deficiencies, and retarded somatic development.

Sanfilippo's s. [MIM*252900-*252960], an error of the mucopolysaccharide metabolism, with excretion of large amounts of heparan sulfate in the urine and severe mental retardation with hepatomegaly; skeleton may be normal or may present mild changes similar to those in Hurler's s.; several different types (A, B, C, and D) have been identified according to the enzyme deficiency; autosomal recessive inheritance. SYN type III mucopolysaccharidosis.

Savage s., obsolete term for amenorrhea associated with hypergonadotrophism and normal ovarian follicles. SYN resistant ovary s. [after the surname of the first reported patient]

scalded skin s., SEE staphylococcal scalded skin s.

scalenus anterior s., one of the precursors of disputed neurogenic thoracic outlet s.; a popular cause for upper extremity discomfort in the late 1930s and 1940s, based on the unproven concept that the lower trunk and brachial plexus and subclavian artery could be compressed in the intrascalene triangle by hypertrophic scalenus anticus muscle, the compression in turn affecting the nerves to it and setting up a vicious circle; this concept was essentially abandoned in the 1950s, when real causes, such as cervical radiculopathy and carpal tunnel syndrome, for upper extremity symptoms were appreciated, but resurrected in the 1980s, without attribution, as etiology for upper plexus type of disputed neurologic thoracic outlet syndrome.

scapulocostal s., pain of insidious development in the upper or posterior part of the shoulder radiating into the neck and occiput, down the arm, or around the chest; there may be numbness or tingling in the fingers; attributed to an alteration from the normal relationship between the scapula and posterior wall of the thorax.

Schanz s., spinal muscle weakness, marked by quick fatigue, pain on pressure over the spinous processes, pain produced by the prone position, and a tendency to curvature of the spine.

Schaumann's s., SYN sarcoidosis.

Scheie's s. [MIM*252800], related to Hurler's s.,perhaps an allele; characterized by α-L-iduronidase deficiency, corneal clouding, deformity of the hands, aortic valve involvement, and normal intelligence; autosomal rescessive. SYN type IS mucopolysaccharidosis.

Schmid-Fraccaro s., SYN cat's-eye s.

Schmidt's s., (1) unilateral paralysis of a vocal cord, the velum palati, trapezius, and sternocleidomastoid. [J. F. M. Schmidt] **(2)** the association of primary hypothyroidism, primary adrenocortical insufficiency, and insulin-dependent diabetes mellitus. [M. B. Schmidt]

Schönlein-Henoch s., SYN Henoch-Schönlein *purpura*.

Schüller's s., SYN Hand-Schüller-Christian *disease*.

Schwartz s. [MIM*255800], a congenital disorder characterized by myotonic myopathy, dystrophy of epiphyseal cartilages resulting in dwarfism, joint contractures, blepharophimosis, and characteristic facies; autosomal recessive inheritance.

Seckel s. [MIM*210600], an autosomal recessive disorder characterized by low birth weight, dwarfism, microcephaly, large eyes, beaked nose, receding mandible, and moderate mental retardation. SYN Seckel dwarfism.

Secrétan's s., factitious, traumatic, recurrent edema or hemorrhage of the dorsum of the hand.

Senear-Usher s., SYN *pemphigus* erythematosus.

Sertoli-cell-only s. [MIM*305700], the absence from the seminiferous tubules of the testes of germinal epithelium, Sertoli cells alone being present; there is sterility due to azoospermia but no other sexual abnormality, Leydig cells are normal, and the output of gonadotrophins in the urine is increased; probably represents one form of seminiferous tubule dysgenesis. SYN Del Castillo s.

Sézary s., exfoliative dermatitis with intense pruritus, resulting from cutaneous infiltration by atypical mononuclear cells (T lymphocytes with markedly convoluted or cerebriform nuclei) also found in the peripheral blood, and associated with alopecia, edema, and nail and pigmentary changes; a variant of mycosis fungoides. SYN Sézary erythroderma.

Sheehan's s., hypopituitarism arising from a severe circulatory collapse postpartum, with resultant pituitary necrosis. SYN postpartum pituitary necrosis s., thyrohypophysial s.

Shone's s., the association of obstructive lesions of the mitral valve complex, including supravalvular ring and parachute mitral valve, with left ventricular outflow obstruction and coarctation of the aorta.

short-bowel s., malabsorption and maldigestion resulting from disease or resection of large portions of the small intestine.

shoulder-girdle s., SYN neuralgic *amyotrophy*.

shoulder-hand s., SYN reflex sympathetic *dystrophy*.

Shulman's s., SYN eosinophilic *fasciitis*.

Shwachman s. [MIM*260400], an inherited disorder, autosomal recessive, characterized by sinusitis and bronchiectasis with pancreatic insufficiency, resulting in malnutrition; associated with neutropenia and defect in neutrophile chemotaxis, short stature, and bone abnormalities.

Shy-Drager s. [MIM*146500], a progressive disorder involving the autonomic system, characterized by hypotension, external ophthalmoplegia, iris atrophy, incontinence, anhidrosis, impotence, tremor, and muscle wasting.

sicca s., SYN Sjögren's s.

sick building s., a s. of nonspecific symptoms including fatigue, headache, dry eyes and throat, and nasal problems, occurring mostly in office workers; attributed to low-level exposures to substances used in building and interior construction; most symptoms lessen during off-work periods.

sick euthyroid s., SYN euthyroid sick s.

sick sinus s. [MIM*182190], symptoms ranging from dizziness to unconsciousness due to chaotic or absent atrial activity often with bradycardia alternating with tachycardia, recurring ectopic beats including escape beats, and runs of supraventricular and ventricular arrhythmias.

Silver-Russell s. [MIM*270050], a disorder characterized by low birth weight, late closure of the anterior fontanel, bilateral bodily asymmetry, clinodactyly of the fifth fingers, triangular facies, and carp mouth; little useful genetic evidence. SYN Silver-Russell dwarfism.

Silverskiöld's s., a type of osteochondrodystrophy with only slight vertebral changes but with shortened and curved long bones of the extremities.

sinus venosus s., the association of partial anomalous, pulmonary-venous connection, and a small venosus ASD.

Sipple's s. [MIM*171400], pheochromocytoma, medullary carcinoma of the thyroid, and neural tumors; autosomal dominant inheritance. SYN multiple endocrine neoplasia, type 2.

Sjögren-Larsson s. [MIM*270200], congenital ichthyosis in association with oligophrenia and spastic paraplegia; autosomal recessive inheritance.

Sjögren's s., keratoconjunctivitis sicca, dryness of mucous membranes, telangiectasias or purpuric spots on the face, and bilateral parotid enlargement, seen in menopausal woman, and often associated with rheumatoid arthritis, Raynaud's phenomenon, and dental caries; there are changes in the lacrimal and salivary glands resembling those of Mikulicz' disease. SYN Gougerot-Sjögren disease, sicca s., Sjögren's disease. [H. S. C. Sjögren]

sleep apnea s., a disorder characterized by multiple episodes of partial or complete cessation of respiration during sleep.

sleep phase delay s., a disorder in which the circadian rhythm of sleep and waking falls into a delayed but stable relationship with external time cues of day and night.

SLE-like s., a disease with manifestations suggestive of systemic *lupus* erythematosus, without meeting diagnostic criteria for that disease; sometimes used for drug-induced lupus.

slit ventricle s., in shunt dependent patients, a state characterized by intermittent or chronic headaches, small ventricles, and slow reflux of the valve mechanism.

Sly s., an autosomal recessive disorder due to a deficiency of a β-glucuronidase; defective lysosomal degradation of dermatan sulfate, heparan sulfate, and chondroitin sulfate; cellular function disrupted in most tissues. SYN type VII mucopolysaccharidosis, type VIII mucopolysaccharidosis.

Smith-Lemli-Opitz s. [MIM*270400], mental retardation, small stature, anteverted nostrils, ptosis, male genital anomalies, and syndactyly of the second and third toes, often in breech-born babies with delayed fetal activity; inherited as an autosomal recessive trait.

Smith-Riley s., multiple hemangiomas, macrocephaly, and blurred optic disks; angiomas appear at birth or later, and enlarge and multiply.

Sneddon's s., a cerebral arteriopathy of unknown etiology, characterized by noninflammatory intimal hyperplasia of medium-sized vessels associated with diffuse cutaneous livedo reticularis.

Sohval-Soffer s. [MIM 307500 and MIM 307300], hypogonadism, gynecomastia, skeletal anomalies, and mental retardation without chromosomal abnormality.

Sorsby's s., congenital macular coloboma and apical dystrophy of the extremities.

Sotos' s. [MIM*117550], cerebral gigantism and generalized large muscles in childhood, with mental retardation and defective coordination; of unknown etiology. Most cases have been sporadic, perhaps new dominant mutations with low fitness, but there is one set of concordant identical twins on record.

space adaptation s., alterations in normal physiology that occur during prolonged exposure to weightlessness, unless preventive measures are taken. Characterized by muscle atrophy, loss of mineral from bones, cardiovascular changes, etc.

spastic s. in cattle, a disease of the nervous system manifested

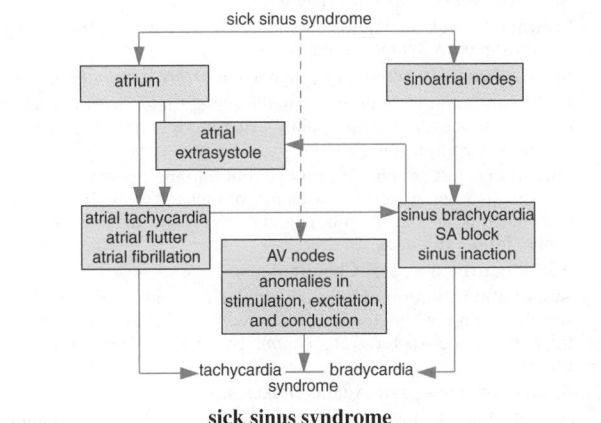

sick sinus syndrome
schematic diagram of pathogenesis of sick sinus syndrome showing tachy- and bradycardial anomalies

by spastic contractions of the muscles of one or both hind legs, most common in old bulls; the cramps usually become more frequent and severe, eventually resulting in decreasing the usefulness of the animal.

Spens' s., SYN Adams-Stokes s.

splenic flexure s., symptoms of pain, gas, bloating, a sense of fullness experienced in the left upper abdominal quadrant, sometimes beneath the ribs, in some instances radiating upward, and in some instances producing anterior chest pain central or predominantly on the left. It may be induced experimentally by the introduction and trapping of air in the splenic flexure.

staphylococcal scalded skin s., a disease affecting infants in which large areas of skin peel off, as in a second-degree burn, as a result of upper respiratory staphylococcal infection even though the skin lesions are sterile; the level of skin separation is subcorneal, unlike a burn or the clinically similar toxic epidermal necrolysis which occurs in children and adults and which involves subepidermal cleavage. SYN Lyell's disease.

Stauffer's s., elevation of liver function tests, in the absence of metastatic disease, due to cholestasis in renal cell cancer patients.

Steele-Richardson-Olszewski s., SYN progressive supranuclear *palsy.*

Stein-Leventhal s., SYN polycystic ovary s.

steroid withdrawal s., a condition exhibited by persons who previously had been receiving large therapeutic doses of glucocorticoid hormones for long periods of time; pituitary-adrenocortical insufficiency is manifested, particularly during stress, for as long as a year or more thereafter and varying degrees of emotional disturbance may be exhibited.

Stevens-Johnson s., a bullous form of erythema multiforme which may be extensive, involving the mucous membranes and large areas of the body; it may produce serious subjective symptoms and may have a fatal termination. SEE ALSO ocular-mucous membrane s. SYN ectodermosis erosiva pluriorificialis, erythema multiforme bullosum, erythema multiforme exudativum, erythema multiforme major.

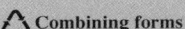

Combining forms	[NA] Nomina Anatomica
Word*Finder* **Multi-term entry finder** **Preceding letter A**	[MIM] Mendelian **Inheritance in Man**
A.D.A.M. Anatomy Plates **Between letters L and M**	☆ **Official alternate term**
Appendices: **Following letter Z**	☆[NA] **Official alternate Nomina Anatomica term**
SYN **Synonym; Cf., compare**	**High Profile Term**

Stewart-Morel s., SYN Morgagni's s.

Stewart-Treves s., angiosarcoma arising in arms affected by postmastectomy lymphedema.

Stickler's s., SYN hereditary progressive *arthro-ophthalmopathy*.

stiff heart s., any condition, usually acute, that causes the heart to be restricted in diastole mainly affecting the ventricles and at one time a complication of cardiac surgery.

stiff-man s., a chronic, progressive, but variable, central nervous system disorder of unknown cause, associated with fluctuating painful muscle spasm and rigidity involving muscles of the limbs, trunk, and neck.

Still-Chauffard s., SYN Chauffard's s.

Stockholm s., a form of bonding between a captive and captor in which the captive begins to identify with, and may even sympathize with, the captor. [*Stockholm,* Sweden, where early case reported]

Stokes-Adams s., SYN Adams-Stokes s.

straight back s., loss of the normal concavity of the thoracolumbar spine with a narrowed anteroposterior chest dimension, resulting compression of the heart between spine and sternum, and consequent prominent precordial pulsations, an ejection murmur, and radiologic evidence of a widened cardiac silhouette (pancaked heart).

Stryker-Halbeisen s., reddish, scaling, macular eruption on the head and upper trunk due to vitamin B complex deficiency; associated with macrocytic anemia.

Sturge-Kalischer-Weber s., SYN Sturge-Weber s.

Sturge-Weber s. [MIM*185300], in full, a triad of 1) congenital cutaneous angioma (flame nevus) in the distribution of the trigeminal nerve, usually unilateral; 2) homolateral meningeal angioma with intracranial calcification and neurologic signs; and 3) angioma of the choroid, often with secondary glaucoma. SEE ALSO encephalotrigeminal vascular s. SYN cephalotrigeminal angiomatosis, encephalotrigeminal angiomatosis, Sturge-Kalischer-Weber s., Sturge-Weber disease.

subclavian steal s., symptoms of vertebrobasilar insufficiency resulting from subclavian steal.

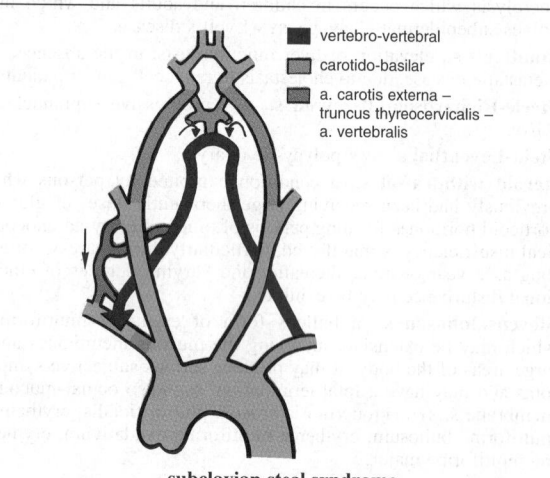

vertebro-vertebral

carotido-basilar

a. carotis externa – truncus thyreocervicalis – a. vertebralis

subclavian steal syndrome

schematic representation of detoured circulation when the subclavian artery and the beginning of the common carotid artery (shown in red) are blocked

subcoracoid-pectoralis minor tendon s., SYN hyperabduction s.

sudden infant death s. (SIDS), abrupt and inexplicable death of an apparently healthy infant; various theories have been advanced to explain such deaths (*e.g.,* sleep-induced apnea, laryngospasm, overwhelming infectious disease) but none has been generally accepted or demonstrated at autopsy. SYN cot death, crib death.

Sudeck's s., SYN Sudeck's *atrophy*.

Sulzberger-Garbe s., SYN Sulzberger-Garbe *disease*.

sump s., a complication of side-to-side choledochoduodenostomy in which the lower end of the common bile duct at times acts as a diverticulum, resulting in stasis, trapping of food particles, and infection.

superior cerebellar artery s., s. due to thrombosis of the superior cerebellar artery which supplies the spinothalamic tract and the superior cerebellar peduncle; there is incoordination in performing skilled movements, with loss of pain and temperature senses on the side of the face and body opposite to that of the lesion.

superior mesenteric artery s., partial or complete block of the superior mesenteric artery, with pain, vomiting, blood in the stool and/or vomitus, and abdominal distention with characteristic radiologic appearance (thumbprinting); often culminates in bowel infarction. SYN Wilkie's disease.

superior vena cava s., obstruction of the superior vena cava or its main tributaries by benign or malignant lesions, causing edema and engorgement of the vessels of the face, neck, and arms, nonproductive cough, and dyspnea; bluish looking venous stars may be found in the early phases, overlying the large veins to which they are tributary, but they tend to diminish in size and disappear after collateral circulation has been reestablished.

supine hypotensive s., in the supine pregnant woman at or near term, maternal hypotension; maternal hypotension is due to obstruction by the gravid uterus of the inferior vena cava with resulting decrease in venous return to the heart; fetal hypoxia is due to maternal hypotension and obstruction of the maternal aorta by the gravid uterus with resulting decrease in placental perfusion.

supraspinatus s., pain on abduction of the shoulder and tenderness upon deep pressure over the supraspinatus tendon; due to pressure of an injured tendon or inflamed subacromial bursa coming into contact or pressing upon the overlying acromial process when the arm is abducted within an arc of 60° to 120°.

supravalvar aortic stenosis s. [MIM*185500], supravalvar aortic stenosis (usually membranous) sometimes associated with pulmonary valvular or peripheral arterial stenosis but with normal facies and mentality; autosomal dominant inheritance. Cf. Williams s.

supravalvar aortic stenosis-infantile hypercalcemia s. [MIM* 194050], supravalvar aortic stenosis associated with elfin facies, mental retardation, and hypercalcemia; usually sporadic; perhaps an irregular dominant trait.

surdocardiac s., SYN Jervell and Lange-Nielsen s.

sweaty feet s., SYN isovaleric acidemia.

swollen belly s., SYN swollen belly *disease*.

swollen head s., a disease of chickens caused by the turkey rhinotracheitis virus.

Swyer-James s., (1) SYN unilateral lobar *emphysema*. **(2)** hyperlucency of one lung from obliterating bronchiolitis, usually caused by adenovirus infection in childhood, with decreased size and vascularity of the lung; distinguished from other causes of unilateral hyperlucency by demosntration of air trapping without central obstruction. SYN Swyer-James-MacLeod s.

Swyer-James-MacLeod s., SYN Swyer-James s.

tachybradycardia s., SYN bradytachycardia s.

tachycardia-bradycardia s., alternating periods of slow and rapid heart beat; often associated with disturbances of both sinoatrial and atrioventricular conduction. SEE ALSO sick sinus s.

Takayasu's s., SYN Takayasu's *arteritis*.

Tapia's s., unilateral paralysis of the larynx, the velum palati, and the tongue, with atrophy of the latter.

tarsal tunnel s., s. produced by entrapment neuropathy of terminal branches of posterior tibial nerve (medial plantar, lateral plantar, and calcanial nerves) at the ankle.

Taussig-Bing s., complete transposition of the aorta, which arises from the right ventricle, with a left sided pulmonary artery overriding the left ventricle, and with high ventricular septal defect, right ventricular hypertrophy, anteriorly situated aorta, and posteriorly situated pulmonary artery. SYN Taussig-Bing disease.

tegmental s., a s. usually caused by a vascular lesion in the tegmentum; marked by contralateral hemiplegia and ipsilateral ocular paresis.

temporomandibular s., those various symptoms of discomfort, pain, or pathosis stated to be caused by loss of vertical dimension, lack of posterior occlusion, or other malocclusion, trismus, muscle tremor, arthritis, or direct trauma to the temporomandibular joint.

temporomandibular joint pain-dysfunction s., SYN myofacial pain-dysfunction s.

tendon sheath s., limited elevation of the eye in adduction, appearing clinically as a paresis of the inferior oblique muscle, due to fascia contracting the superior oblique muscle on the same side. SYN Brown's s., Paterson-Brown-Kelly s.

Terry's s., SYN *retinopathy* of prematurity.

testicular feminization s. [MIM*313700], a type of male pseudohermaphroditism characterized by female external genitalia (may be ambiguous if the s. is incomplete), incompletely developed vagina often with rudimentary uterus and fallopian tubes, female habitus at puberty but with scanty or absent axillary and pubic hair and amenorrhea, and testes present within the abdomen or in the inguinal canals or labia majora; epididymis and vas deferens are usually present; androgens and estrogens are formed, but target tissues are largely unresponsive to androgens; individuals are sex chromatin-negative and have a normal male karyotype; X-linked recessive inheritance; there is a defect in the androgen receptor protein.

tethered cord s., abnormal low positioning (below the L_2 vertebrae) of the distal spinal cord (conus medullaris) by the filum terminale. May be associated with incontinence, progressive motor and sensory impairment in the legs, pain, and scoliosis.

thalamic s., a s. produced by infarction of the postero-inferior thalamus causing transient hemiparesis, severe loss of superficial and deep sensation with preservation of crude pain in the hypalgic limbs which frequently have vasomotor or trophic disturbances. SYN Dejerine-Roussy s.

Thiemann's s., avascular necrosis of the epiphyses of phalanges of fingers or toes, usually familial, beginning in childhood or adolescence, leading to deformity of fingers; also called familial arthropathy of the fingers or toes. SYN Thiemann's disease.

third and fourth pharyngeal pouch s., SYN DiGeorge s.

thoracic outlet s. (TOS), collective title for a number of conditions attributed to compromise of blood vessels or nerve fibers (brachial plexus) at any point between the base of the neck and the axilla; formerly classified on the basis of presumed injurious structure or mechanism, *i.e.,* scalenus anticus syndrome, hyperabduction syndrome, costoclavicular syndrome; currently classified on the basis of the structure known or presumed to be compromised, and divided into two main groups: vascular and neurologic (simultaneous compromise of both neural and vascular structures is rare); vascular subdivisions include arterial and venous, while neurological subdivisions include true and disputed.

Thorn's s., SYN salt-losing *nephritis*.

thrombocytopenia-absent radius s., TAR s. [MIM*270400], congenital absence of the radius associated with thrombocytopenia that is symptomatic in infancy but later improves; congenital heart disease and renal anomalies occur in some cases; autosomal recessive inheritance.

thrombopathic s., a nondescript term to describe any of a number of bleeding diseases in which clot formation is deficient rather than those in which there is an organic fault of the blood vessels.

thyrohypophysial s., SYN Sheehan's s.

Tietze's s., inflammation and painful, tender nonsuppurative swelling of a costochondral junction. SYN peristernal perichondritis.

Tolosa-Hunt s., cavernous sinus s. produced by an idiopathic granuloma.

tooth-and-nail s. [MIM*189500], hypodontia associated with absent or very small nails at birth. Common among Dutch Mennonites in Canada.

TORCH s., a group of infections with similar clinical manifestations, although symptoms may vary in degree and time of appearance: *t*oxoplasmosis, *o*ther infections, *r*ubella, *c*ytomegalovirus infection, and *h*erpes simplex. These infections might be associated with underlying HIV infection.

Tornwaldt's s., nasopharyngeal discharge, occipital headache, and stiffness of posterior cervical muscles, with halitosis due to chronic infection of the pharyngeal bursa.

Torre's s., multiple sebaceous gland neoplasms associated with multiple visceral malignancies. SYN Muir-Torre s.

Torsten Sjögren's s., SYN Marinesco-Garland s.

Tourette s., a tic disorder appearing in childhood, characterized by multiple motor tics and vocal tics present for more than one year. Obsessive-compulsive behavior, attention-deficit disorder, and other psychiatric disorders may be associated; coprolalia and echolalia rarely occur; autosomal dominant inheritance. SYN Gilles de la Tourette's disease, Gilles de la Tourette's s., Tourette's disease.

toxic shock s. (TSS), infection with toxin-producing staphylococci, occurring most often in the vagina of menstruating women using superabsorbent tampons and characterized by high fever, vomiting, diarrhea, a scarlatiniform rash followed by desquamation, and decreasing blood pressure and shock, which can result in death; hyperemia of the conjunctival, oropharyngeal, and vaginal mucous membranes also occurs.

transplant lung s., a s. associated with fever and diffuse bilateral pulmonary infiltration mainly at the base or at the hilum of the lung; can accompany rejection of an organ (kidney) transplant or follow a reduction in dosage of an immunosuppressive drug.

transurethral resection s., absorption of glycine from irrigation solution during TUR that the liver cannot metabolize, resulting in increased serum ammonia. SYN TUR s.

Treacher Collins' s. [MIM*154500], mandibulofacial *dysostosis,* when limited to the orbit and malar region.

trichorhinophalangeal s., a condition characterized by sparse fine hair, broad nose with a long philtrum, swollen middle phalanges with cone-shaped epiphyses, and growth retardation. There seems to be at least three similar disorders, two dominant [MIM*150230, 190350] and one recessive [MIM*275500].

triple X s., in principle, the phenotypic features characteristic of trisomy of the X chromosome. Original observations (made in mental institutions) were seriously biased and the phenotypic changes spurious; now, even the remaining claim, that there is mild mental retardation, is suspect. The outstanding feature of the s. is the occurence of twin Barr bodies in a typical cell.

trisomy 8 s., craniofacial dysmorphia, short wide neck but narrow cylindrical trunk, and multiple joint and digital defects.

trisomy 13 s., a s. that is usually fatal within two years; characterized by mental retardation and malformed ears in all patients, and in most patients cleft lip or palate, microphthalmia or coloboma, small mandible, polydactyly, cardiac defects, convulsions, renal anomalies, umbilical hernia, malrotation of intestines, and dermatoglyphic anomalies. SYN Patau's s., trisomy D s.

trisomy 18 s., a s. that is usually fatal within two to three years; characterized by mental retardation, abnormal skull shape, low-set and malformed ears, small mandible, cardiac defects, short sternum, diaphragmatic or inguinal hernia, Meckel's diverticulum, abnormal flexion of fingers, and dermatoglyphic anomalies. SYN Edwards' s.

trisomy 20 s., profound mental retardation with coarse facies, macrostomia and macroglossia, minor anomalies of the ears, pigmentary dysplasia of the skin, dorsal kyphoscoliosis, and other skeletal defects.

trisomy 21 s., SYN Down's s.

trisomy C s., trisomy for any chromosome of group C, numbers 6 through 12, most often number 8.

trisomy D s., SYN trisomy 13 s.

trochanteric s., tendonitis and bursitis around the trochanter major.

tropical splenomegaly s., SYN hyperreactive malarious *splenomegaly.*

Trousseau's s., **(1)** SYN gastric *vertigo.* **(2)** thrombophlebitis migrans associated with visceral cancer.

true neurogenic thoracic outlet syndrome, very chronic axon loss brachial plexopathy, caused by compromise of the lower trunk fibers by a congenital band extending from a rudimentary cervical rib to the first thoracic rib; rare disorder, found mostly in young to middle-aged women, that presents with unilateral hand wasting and weakness, particularly involving the lateral thenar eminence; sometimes accompanied by intermittent discomfort along the medial forearm and hand. SYN cervical rib and band s., classic cervical rib s.

tumor lysis s., hyperphosphatemia, hypocalcemia, hyperkalemia, and hyperuricemia following induction chemotherapy of malignant neoplasms; believed to be due to the release of intracellular products by cell lysis.

TUR s., SYN transurethral resection s.

Turcot s. [MIM*276300], a rare and perhaps distinct form of multiple intestinal polyposis in which brain tumors are present; probably autosomal recessive trait.

Turner's s., a s. with chromosome count 45 and only one X chromosome; buccal and other cells are usually sex chromatin-negative; anomalies include dwarfism, webbed neck, valgus of elbows, pigeon chest, infantile sexual development, and amenorrhea; the ovary has no primordial follicles and may be represented only by a fibrous streak; some individuals are chromosomal mosaic, with two or more cell lines of different chromosome constitution; seen in many animal species, in the meadow vole it is the normal female state. SYN XO s.

twiddler's s., condition in which a cardiac pacemaker wire is pulled out of position in the heart with rotation of the subcutaneous pacemaker by the patient's "twiddling."

Uhthoff s., SYN Uhthoff *symptom.*

Ullmann's s., a systemic angiomatosis due to multiple arteriovenous malformations.

Ulysses s., the ill effects of extensive diagnostic investigations conducted because of a false-positive result in the course of routine laboratory screening. [L. *Ulysses,* fr. G. *Odysseus,* myth. char.]

unroofed coronary sinus s., a spectrum of cardiac anomalies in which part or all of the common wall between the coronary sinus and the left atrium is absent.

urethral s., a condition of no certain etiology, characterized by urinary frequency, urgency, dysuria in the absence of specific infection, obstruction, or dysfunction. Suprapubic pain, hesitancy, and back pain may also occur. Usually seen in females. SYN female urethral s.

Usher's s. [MIM*276900 and *270901], autosomal recessive inheritance; the two forms are distinguishable only by linkage data; causing sensorineural heraring loss and retinitis pigmentosa.

uveocutaneous s., SYN Vogt-Koyanagi s.

uveo-encephalitic s., SYN Behçet's s.

uveomeningitis s., SYN Harada's s.

VACTERL s., abnormalities of *v*ertebrae, *a*nus, *c*ardiovascular *t*ree, *t*rachea, *e*sophagus, *r*enal system, and *l*imb buds associated with administration of sex steroids during early pregnancy.

van Buchem's s. [MIM*239100], an inherited skeletal dysplasia, with mandibular enlargement and thickening of the diaphyses and calvaria, and increased serum alkaline phosphatase; autosomal recessive inheritance. SYN generalized cortical hyperostosis.

van der Hoeve's s., a subtype of *osteogenesis* imperfecta in which progressive conductive hearing loss begins in childhood because of stapedial fixation.

vanished testis s., absence of both testes in a male with normal chromosomes (XY) and otherwise normal genitalia at birth and during childhood. Testes were present in at least the first trimester of gestation, but vanished sometime thereafter.

vanishing lung s., progressive decrease of radiographic opacity of the lung caused by accelerated development of emphysema or rapid cystic destruction of the lung from infection.

vasculocardiac s. of hyperserotonemia, obsolete term for carcinoid s.

vasovagal s., SYN vagal *attack.*

Verner-Morrison s., watery diarrhea, hypokalemia, and achlorhydria associated with secretion of vasoactive intestinal polypeptide by a pancreatic islet-cell tumor in the absence of gastric hypersecretion. SYN WDHA s.

Vernet's s., a s. characterized by paralysis of the motor components of the glossopharyngeal, vagus, and accessory cranial nerves as they lie in the posterior fossa; it is most commonly the result of head injury.

vertical retraction s., SEE retraction s.

vibration s., tingling, numbness, and blanching of the fingers resulting from use of hand-held vibration tools; may persist without further exposure to vibration.

virus-associated hemophagocytic s., a s. closely resembling malignant histiocytosis but potentially reversible, following a herpes group virus infection such as by the Epstein-Barr virus.

vitreoretinal choroidopathy s. [MIM*193220], an ocular condition characterized by peripheral pigmentary retinopathy, retinal vascular abnormalities, vitreous opacities, choroidal atrophy, and presenile cataracts; autosomal dominant inheritance.

vitreoretinal traction s., traction on the internal limiting membrane of the retina by adherent vitreous fibrils in vitreous humor detachment.

Vogt s., SYN double *athetosis.* [Cécile and Oscar Vogt]

Vogt-Koyanagi s., bilateral uveitis with iritis and glaucoma, premature graying of the hair, and alopecia, vitiligo, and dysacusia; related to Harada's s. and sympathetic ophthalmia. SYN oculocutaneous s., uveocutaneous s.

Vohwinkel s., SYN mutilating *keratoderma.*

von Hippel-Lindau s., a type of phacomatosis, consisting of hemangiomas of the retina, which may be multiple and bilateral, associated with hemangiomas or hemangioblastomas primarily of the cerebellum and walls of the fourth ventricle, occasionally involving the spinal cord; sometimes associated with cysts or hamartomas of kidney, adrenal, or other organs; autosomal dominant inheritance. SYN cerebroretinal angiomatosis, Lindau's disease.

vulnerable child s., a reaction characterized by disturbance in psychosocial development, often occurring in children whose parents expect them to die prematurely.

Waardenburg s. [MIM*193500, MIM*193510], Autosomal dominant disorder characterized by lateral dystopia of medial canthi and lacrimal puncta, increased width of the root of the nose, heterochromia or hypochromia iridis, cochlear deafness, white forelock, and synophrys.

Wagner's s., SYN hyaloideoretinal *degeneration.*

Waldenström's s., SYN Waldenström's *macroglobulinemia.*

Wallenberg's s., SYN posterior inferior cerebellar artery s.

Ward-Romano s., SYN Romano-Ward s.

wasting s., (1) SYN runting s. **(2)** a condition of 10% weight loss in conjunction with diarrhea or fever lasting over one month. Associated with AIDS.

Waterhouse-Friderichsen s., a condition occurring mainly in children under 10 years of age, characterized by vomiting, diarrhea, extensive purpura, cyanosis, toniclonic convulsions, and circulatory collapse, usually with meningitis and hemorrhage into the adrenal glands. SYN acute fulminating meningococcal septicemia, Friderichsen-Waterhouse s.

WDHA s., SYN Verner-Morrison s. [*w*atery *d*iarrhea, *h*ypokalemia, *a*chlorhydria]

weaving s., a behavioral disorder of caged or confined animals where the animal stands in one position but weaves from side to side or rocks back and forth.

Weber-Cockayne s. [MIM*131800], *epidermolysis* bullosa of the hands and feet.

Weber's s., midbrain tegmentum lesion characterized by ipsilateral oculomotor nerve paresis and contralateral paralysis of the extremities, face, and tongue. SYN Weber's sign.

Weill-Marchesani s. [MIM*277600], ectopia lentis (lens abnormally round and small), short stature, and brachydactyly; recessive autosomal inheritance.

Wells' s., recurrent cellulitis followed by brawny edematous skin lesions, or a less acute presentation of papular, annular, or gyrate skin lesions which are sometimes urticarial; affected skin and subcutis are heavily infiltrated by eosinophils and histiocytes, with scattered small necrotic foci (flame figures) of varied etiology; sometimes follows an arthropod bite. SYN eosinophilic cellulitis.

Werner's s. [MIM*277700], a disorder consisting of scleroderma-like skin changes, bilateral juvenile cataracts, progeria, hypogonadism, and diabetes mellitus; autosomal recessive inheritance.

Wernicke-Korsakoff s., the coexistence of Wernicke's and Korsakoff's s.'s.

Wernicke's s., a condition frequently encountered in chronic alcoholics, largely due to thiamin deficiency and characterized by disturbances in ocular motility, pupillary alterations, nystagmus, and ataxia with tremors; an organic-toxic psychosis is often an associated finding, and Korsakoff's s. often coexists; characteristic cellular pathology found in several areas of the brain. SYN superior hemorrhagic polioencephalitis, Wernicke's disease, Wernicke's encephalopathy.

West's s., an encephalopathy in infancy characterized by infantile spasms, arrest of psychomotor development, and hypsarrhythmia.

Weyers-Thier s., SYN oculovertebral *dysplasia*.

whistling face s., SYN craniocarpotarsal *dystrophy*.

white-out s., a psychosis which occurs in Arctic explorers or others similarly exposed to the stimulus deprivation of a snow-clad environment. SEE ALSO sensory *deprivation*.

Widal's s., SYN Hayem-Widal s.

Wildervanck s., SYN cervico-oculo-acoustic s.

Williams s., a congenital disorder characterized by mental deficiency, mild growth deficiency, elfin facies, supravalvular aortic stenosis, and, occasionally, elevated blood calcium; may be associated with hypersensitivity to vitamin D or excess ingestion of the vitamin during pregnancy. Cf. idiopathic *hypercalcemia* of infants.

Williams' s., SYN cardiofacial s.

Williams-Beurer s., SYN idiopathic *hypercalcemia* of infants.

Wilson-Mikity s., SYN pulmonary dysmaturity s.

Wilson's s., SYN Wilson's *disease* (1).

Wiskott-Aldrich s. [MIM*301000], an X-linked immunodeficiency disorder occurring in male children and characterized by thrombocytopenia, eczema, melena, and susceptibility to recurrent bacterial infections; death occurs from severe hemorrhage or overwhelming infection. SYN Aldrich s.

Wissler's s., high intermittent fever, irregularly recurring macular and maculo-papular eruption of the face, chest and limbs, leukocytosis, arthralgia, occasionally eosinophilia, and raised erythrocyte sedimentation rate; occurs in children and adolescents, with varying duration.

withdrawal s., the development of a substance-specific s. that follows the cessation of, or reduction in, intake of a psychoactive substance that the person previously used regularly; *e.g.,* clinical syndrome of disorientation, perceptual disturbance, and psychomotor agitation following the cessation of chronic use of excessive quantities of alcohol is termed alcohol withdrawal syndrome. The s. that develops varies according to the psychoactive substance used. Common symptoms include anxiety, restlessness, irritability, insomnia, and impaired attention. SEE ALSO abstinence s.

Wolff-Parkinson-White s. [MIM*194200], an electrocardiographic pattern sometimes associated with paroxysmal tachycardia; it consists of short P-R interval (usually 0.1 second or less; occasionally normal) together with a prolonged QRS complex with a slurred initial component (delta wave). SYN preexcitation s.

Wright's s., SYN hyperabduction s.

Wyburn-Mason s., arteriovenous malformation on the cerebral cortex, retinal arteriovenous angioma and facial nevus, usually occurring in mentally retarded individuals.

XO s., SYN Turner's s.

XXY s., SYN Klinefelter's s.

XYY s., a chromosomal anomaly with chromosome count 47, with a supernumerary Y chromosome; controversial evidence associates tallness, aggressiveness, and acne with this condition.

yellow nail s., SYN yellow *nail*.

Young s., obstructive azoospermia and chronic sinopulmonary infections.

Zellweger s., SYN cerebrohepatorenal s.

Zieve's s., transient jaundice, hemolytic anemia, and hyperlipemia associated with acute alcoholism in patients with cirrhosis or a fatty liver.

Zivert s., SYN Kartagener's s.

Zollinger-Ellison s. [MIM*131100], peptic ulceration with gastric hypersecretion and non-beta cell tumor of the pancreatic islets, sometimes associated with familial polyendocrine adenomatosis.

---

syn·drom·ic (sin-drom'ik, -drō'mik). Relating to a syndrome.

syn·ech·ia, pl. **syn·ech·i·ae** (si-nek'ē-ă, -kē-ē; si-nē'kē-ă). Any adhesion; specifically, anterior or posterior s. [G. *synecheia,* continuity, fr. *syn,* together, + *echō,* to have, hold]
  annular s., adhesion of the entire pupillary margin of the iris to the capsule of the lens.
  anterior s., adhesion of the iris to the cornea.
  s. pericar'dii, SYN concretio cordis.
  peripheral anterior s., SYN goniosynechia.
  posterior s., adhesion of the iris to the capsule of the lens.
  total s., adhesion of the entire surface of the iris to the lens capsule.

syn·ech·i·ot·o·my (si-nek'ē-ot'ō-mē). Division of the adhesions in synechia. [synechia + G. *tomē,* incision]

syn·ech·o·tome (si-nek'ō-tōm). A small knife for use in synechiotomy.

syn·ec·ten·ter·ot·o·my (si-nek'ten-ter-ot'ō-mē). Division of intestinal adhesions. [G. *synektos,* held together (see synechia), + *enteron,* intestine, + *tomē,* incision]

syn·en·ceph·a·lo·cele (sin-en-sef'ă-lō-sēl). Protrusion of brain substance through a defect in the skull, with adhesions preventing reduction. [syn- + G. *enkephalos,* brain, + *kēlē,* hernia]

syn·er·e·sis (si-ner'ĕ-sis). 1. The contraction of a gel, *e.g.,* a blood clot, by which part of the dispersion medium is squeezed out. 2. Degeneration of the vitreous humor with loss of gel consistency to become partially or completely fluid. [G. *synairesis,* a taking or drawing together]

syn·er·get·ic (sin-er-jet'ik). SYN synergistic.

syn·er·gia (si-ner'jē-ă). SYN synergism.

syn·er·gic (si-ner'jik). SYN synergistic.

syn·er·gism (sin'er-jizm). Coordinated or correlated action of two or more structures, agents, or physiologic processes so that the combined action is greater than the sum of each acting separately. Cf. antagonism. SYN synergia, synergistic effect, synergy. [G. *synergia,* fr. *syn,* together, + *ergon,* work]

syn·er·gist (sin'er-jist). A structure, agent, or physiologic process that aids the action of another. Cf. antagonist.

syn·er·gis·tic (sin-er-jis'tik). 1. Pertaining to synergism. 2. Denoting a synergist. SYN synergetic, synergic.

syn·er·gy (sin'er-jē). SYN synergism.

syn·es·the·sia (sin-es-thē'zē-ă). A condition in which a stimulus, in addition to exciting the usual and normally located sensation, gives rise to a subjective sensation of different character or localization; *e.g.,* color hearing, color taste. [syn- + G. *aisthēsis,* sensation]
  s. al'gica, SYN synesthesialgia.

syn·es·the·si·al·gia (sin'es-thē-zē-al'jē-ă). Painful synesthesia. SYN synesthesia algica.

Syn·gam·i·dae (sin-gam'i-dē). A family of nematodes (order Strongyloidea) parasitic in the respiratory system of birds and mammals. [see *Syngamus*]

Syn·ga·mus (sin'gă-mŭs). A genus of moderate-sized, blood-sucking, strongyle nematodes (family Syngamidae) that live in the bronchi and tracheae of birds, and are especially important parasites of gallinaceous birds. They are called gapeworms because the host often gapes with open mouth due to the presence of the worms in the throat, or forked worms because the male is permanently attached to the midregion of the female, where the bursa of the male is clasped over the female vulva. [syn- + G. *gamos,* marriage]

Sy

S. tra'chea, a worldwide parasite of the trachea of domestic fowl and many wild birds, causing gapes.

syn·ga·my (sin'gă-mē). Conjugation of the gametes in fertilization. [syn- + G. *gamos,* marriage]

syn·ge·ne·ic (sin'jĕ-nē'ik). Relating to genetically identical individuals. SYN isogeneic, isogenic, isologous, isoplastic, syngenic. [G. *syngenēs,* congenital]

syn·ge·ne·si·o·plas·ty (sin-jĕ-nē'zē-ō-plas-tē). Plastic surgery involving syngenesiotransplantation. [syn- + G. *genesis,* origin, + *plastos,* formed]

syn·ge·ne·si·o·trans·plan·ta·tion (sin-jĕ-nē'zē-ō-trans-plan-tā' shŭn). Transplantation in which the donor and recipient of a graft are closely related, *e.g.,* parent and child or siblings. [syn- + G. *genesis,* origin, + transplantation]

syn·gen·e·sis (sin-jen'ĕ-sis). SYN sexual *reproduction.* [syn- + G. *genesis,* origin]

syn·ge·net·ic (sin-jĕ-net'ik). Relating to syngenesis.

syn·gen·ic (sin-jen'ik). SYN syngeneic.

syn·gna·thia (sin-nath'ē-ă). Congenital adhesion of the maxilla and mandible by fibrous bands. [syn- + G. *gnathos,* jaw]

syn·graft (sin'graft). A tissue or organ transplanted between genetically identical individuals. SYN isogeneic graft, isograft, isologous graft, isoplastic graft, syngeneic graft.

syn·i·dro·sis (sin-i-drō'sis). A condition in which excessive sweating is part of the clinical manifestation. [syn- + G. *hidrosis,* sweating]

syn·i·ze·sis (sin-i-zē'sis). 1. Closure or obliteration of the pupil. 2. The massing of chromatin at one side of the nucleus that occurs usually at the beginning of synapsis. [G. collapse]

syn·kar·y·on (sin-kar'ē-on). The nucleus formed by the fusion of the two pronuclei in karyogamy. SYN syncaryon. [syn- + G. *karyon,* kernel (nucleus)]

syn·ki·ne·sis (sin-ki-nē'sis). Involuntary movement accompanying a voluntary one, as the movement of a closed eye following that of the uncovered one, or the movement occurring in a paralyzed muscle accompanying motion in another part. SYN syncinesis. [syn- + G. *kinēsis,* movement]

syn·ki·net·ic (sin-ki-net'ik). Relating to or marked by synkinesis.

syn·ne·ma·tin B (sin-ĕ-mā'tin, si-nē'mă-tin). SYN *cephalosporin* N.

syn·o·nych·ia (sin-ō-nik'ē-ă). Fusion of two or more nails of the digits, as in syndactyly. [sin- + G. *onyx* (*onych-*), nail]

syn·o·nym (sin'ō-nim). In biologic nomenclature, a term used to denote one of two or more names for the same species or taxonomic group (taxon).

objective s.'s, different names for the same organism, based on one and the same nomenclatural type, as when a species is transferred from one genus to another (*e.g.,* the transfer of *Diplococcus pneumoniae* to the genus *Streptococcus* as *Streptococcus pneumoniae*), in contrast to subjective s.'s.

senior s., the earliest published of two or more available names for the same organism, usually used as the correct name (law of priority).

subjective s.'s, different names, based on different nomenclatural types, for organisms that were originally regarded as different but were later considered to be identical, or nearly so, as a matter of personal opinion, in contrast to objective s.'s.

syn·oph'rys (sin-of'ris). Hypertrophy and fusion of the eyebrows. [syn- + G. *ophrys,* eyebrow]

syn·oph·thal·mia (sin-of-thal'mē-ă). SYN cyclopia. [syn- + G. *ophthalmos,* eye]

syn·op·to·phore (sin-op'tō-fōr). A modified form of Wheatstone stereoscope used in orthoptic training. [syn- + G. *ōps,* eye, + *phoros,* bearing]

syn·or·chi·dism, syn·or·chism (sin-ōr'ki-dizm, sin-ōr'kizm). Congenital fusion of the testes in the abdomen or scrotum. [syn- + G. *orchis,* testis]

syn·os·che·os (sin-os'kē-os). Partial or complete adhesion of the penis and scrotum, a malformation in hermaphroditism. [syn- + G. *oschē,* scrotum]

syn·os·te·ol·o·gy (sin-os'tē-ol'ō-jē). SYN arthrology. [syn- + G. *osteon,* bone, + *logos,* study]

syn·os·te·o·sis (sin-os-tē-ō'sis). SYN synostosis.

syn·os·to·sis (sin-os-tō'sis). Osseous union between the bones forming a joint. SYN bony ankylosis, synosteosis, true ankylosis. [syn- + G. *osteon,* bone, + *-osis,* condition]

sagittal s., SYN scaphocephaly.

tribasilar s., fusion in early life of the three bones at the base of the skull, resulting in interference with the development of the brain.

syn·os·tot·ic (sin-os-tot'ik). Relating to synostosis.

sy·no·tia (si-nō'shē-ă). Fusion or abnormal approximation of the lobes of the ears in otocephaly. [syn- + G. *ous,* ear]

syn·o·vec·to·my (sin-ō-vek'tō-mē). Excision of a portion or all of the synovial membrane of a joint. SYN villusectomy. [synovia + G. *ektomē,* excision]

syn·o·via (si-nō'vē-ă) [NA]. SYN synovial *fluid.* [Mod. L., a word coined by Paracelsus, fr. G. *syn,* together, + *ōon* (L. *ovum,* egg]

syn·o·vi·al (si-nō'vē-ăl). 1. Relating to, containing, or consisting of synovia. 2. Relating to the membrana synovialis.

syn·o·vi·o·ma (si-nō-vē-ō'mă). A tumor of synovial origin involving joint or tendon sheath. [synovium + G. *-oma,* tumor]

malignant s., SYN synovial *sarcoma.*

syn·o·vip·a·rous (sin'ō-vip'ă-rŭs). Producing synovia. [synovia + L. *pario,* to produce]

syn·o·vi·tis (sin-ō-vī'tis). Inflammation of a synovial membrane, especially that of a joint; in general, when unqualified, the same as arthritis. [synovia + G. *-itis,* inflammation]

bursal s., SYN bursitis.

chronic hemorrhagic villous s., SYN pigmented villonodular s.

dry s., s. with little serous or purulent effusion. SYN s. sicca.

filarial s., synovial inflammation often followed by fibrotic ankylosis due to microfilariae in the joint.

infectious s., a disease of chickens and turkeys caused by the bacterium *Mycoplasma synoviae* and characterized by lameness with swollen hocks and foot pads.

pigmented villonodular s., diffuse outgrowths of synovial membrane of a joint, usually the knee, composed of synovial villi and fibrous nodules infiltrated by hemosiderin- and lipid-containing macrophages and multinucleated giant cells; the condition may be inflammatory, although recurrence is likely to follow incomplete removal. SYN chronic hemorrhagic villous s.

purulent s., SYN suppurative *arthritis.*

serous s., s. with a large effusion of nonpurulent fluid.

s. sic'ca, SYN dry s.

suppurative s., SYN suppurative *arthritis.*

tendinous s., SYN tenosynovitis.

vaginal s., SYN tenosynovitis.

syn·o·vi·um (si-nō'vē-ŭm). SYN synovial *membrane.*

syn·pol·y·dac·ty·ly (sin'pol-ē-dak'ti-lē). Associated syndactyly and polydactyly.

syn·tac·tics (sin-tak'tiks). A branch of semiotics concerned with the formal relations between signs, in abstraction from their meaning and their interpreters. [syn- + G. *taxis,* order]

syn·tal·i·ty (sin-tal'i-tē). The consistent and predictable behavior of a social group. [prob. telescoped from syn- + mentality]

syn·tec·tic (sin-tek'tik). Pertaining to or marked by syntexis.

syn·ten·ic (sin-ten'ik). Pertaining to synteny.

syn·te·ny (sin'ten-ē). The relationship between two genetic loci (not genes) represented on the same chromosomal pair or (for haploid chromosomes) on the same chromosome; an anatomic rather than a segregational relationship. [syn- + G. *tainia,* ribbon]

syn·tex·is (sin-tek'sis). Emaciation or wasting. [G. *syn-tēxis,* a melting together]

syn·thase (sin'thās). Trivial name used in Enzyme Commission Report for a lyase reaction going in the reverse direction (NTP-independent). For individual s.'s, see the specific names. SEE ALSO synthetase.

syn·ther·mal (sin-ther′măl). Having the same temperature. [syn- + G. *thermē,* heat]

syn·the·sis, pl. **syn·the·ses** (sin′thĕ-sis, -sēz). **1.** A building up, putting together, composition. **2.** In chemistry, the formation of compounds by the union of simpler compounds or elements. **3.** Stage in the cell *cycle* in which DNA is synthesized as a preliminary to cell division. [G. fr. *syn,* together, + *thesis,* a placing, arranging]

s. of continuity, healing of the edges of a wound or fracture.

enzymatic s., s. by enzymes. SEE biosynthesis.

Kiliani-Fischer s., a synthetic procedure for the extension of the carbon atom chain of aldoses by treatment with cyanide; hydrolysis of the cyanohydrins followed by reduction of the lactone yields the homologous aldose; with this method, D-glucose and D-mannose can be synthesized from D-arabinose.

Merrifield s., the s. of peptides and proteins via an automated system on carrier polymers.

protein s., the process in which individual amino acids, whether of exogenous or endogenous origin, are connected to each other in peptide linkage in a specific order dictated by the sequence of nucleotides in DNA; this governing sequence is conveyed to the synthesizing apparatus in the ribosomes by mRNA, formed by base-pairing on the DNA template.

syn·the·size (sin′thĕ-sīz). To make something by synthesis, *i.e.,* synthetically.

syn·the·tase (sin′thĕ-tās). An enzyme catalyzing the synthesis of a specific substance. S. is limited, in the Enzyme Commission Report, to use as a trivial name for the ligases (EC class 6), which in turn are those synthesizing enzymes that require the cleavage of a pyrophosphate linkage in ATP or a similar compound. Reversal of lyase (EC class 4) reactions, producing a synthesis, is indicated (in trivial names) by synthase; such reactions do not involve pyrophosphate cleavage. For individual s.'s, see the specific names.

syn·thet·ic (sin-thet′ik). Relating to or made by synthesis.

syn·tho·rax (sin-thōr′aks). SYN thoracopagus.

syn·ton·ic (sin-ton′ik). Having even tone or temperament; a personality trait characterized by a high degree of emotional responsiveness to the environment. [G. *syntonos,* in harmony, fr. *syn,* together, + *tonos,* tone]

syn·tro·phism (sin′trō-fizm). State of mutual dependence, with reference to food supply, of organs or cells of a plant or an animal. [syn- + G. *trophē,* nourishment]

syn·tro·pho·blast (sin-trō′fō-blast, -trof′ō-). SYN syncytiotrophoblast.

syn·tro·pic (sin-trop′ik). Relating to syntropy.

syn·tro·py (sin′trō-pē). **1.** The tendency sometimes seen in two diseases to coalesce into one. **2.** The state of harmonious association with others. **3.** In anatomy, a number of similar structures inclined in one general direction; *e.g.,* the spinous processes of a series of vertebrae, the ribs. [syn- + G. *tropē,* a turning]

inverse s., a situation in which the presence of one disease tends to decrease the possibility of another.

syn·zyme (sin′zīm). A synthetic macromolecule having enzymatic activity. SYN enzyme analog.

Sy·pha·cia (si-fā′shē-ă). Genus of oxyurid nematode pinworms of rodents; *S. obvelata* is the common cecal pinworm of mice, and *S. muris,* of rats. SEE ALSO *Aspiculuris tetraptera.* [fr. L. *siphon,* tube]

⌂**syphil-.** SEE syphilo-.

syph·i·le·mia (sif-i-lē′mē-ă). A state in which the specific organism, *Treponema pallidum,* is present in the bloodstream. [syphilis + G. *haima,* blood]

syph·i·lid (sif′i-lid). Any of the several kinds of cutaneous and mucous membrane lesions of secondary and tertiary syphilis, but most commonly denoting the former. SYN syphiloderm, syphiloderma. [syphilis + *-id* (1)]

acneform s., SYN pustular s.

acuminate papular s., SYN follicular s.

annular s., cutaneous lesions of secondary syphilis in which the papules form annular lesions with raised papular borders and clear central portions.

bullous s., a rare manifestation of congenital syphilis. SYN pemphigoid s.

corymbose s., a secondary syphilitic eruption consisting of a large central papule surrounded by a more or less complete ring of smaller papules.

ecthymatous s., SYN pustular s.

erythematous s., SYN syphilitic *roseola.*

flat papular s., SYN lenticular s.

follicular s., secondary eruption of small follicular papules, usually appearing as groups of lesions. SYN acuminate papular s., lichen syphiliticus, miliary papular s.

frambesiform s., SYN rupial s.

gummatous s., SYN gumma.

impetiginous s., SYN pustular s.

lenticular s., eruption of flattened, dull reddish papules, 5 mm to 1 cm in diameter, occurring in secondary syphilis. SYN flat papular s.

macular s., SYN syphilitic *roseola.*

miliary papular s., SYN follicular s.

nodular s., SYN gumma.

nummular s., flat, disk-shaped papules of secondary syphilis.

palmar s., dull red papules in the palms, occurring in secondary syphilis.

papular s., SEE follicular s., lenticular s.

papulosquamous s., scaling papules of secondary syphilis.

pemphigoid s., SYN bullous s.

pigmentary s., lesions of secondary syphilis consisting of rounded white macules on the trunk.

plantar s., dull red papules on the soles in secondary syphilis.

pustular s., a type of pustular eruption occurring in secondary syphilis. SYN acne syphilitica, acneform s., ecthymatous s., impetiginous s., varioliform s.

rupial s., lesions that appear granulomatous and crusted, resembling those of yaws. SYN frambesiform s.

secondary s., a syphilitic skin lesion characteristic of the second stage of the disease.

tertiary s., a syphilitic skin lesion characteristic of the third stage of the disease.

varioliform s., SYN pustular s.

syph·i·lim·e·try (sif-i-lim′ĕ-trē). A test designed to determine intensity of syphilitic infection, *e.g.,* titered serologic test. [syphilis + G. *metron,* measure]

syph·i·li·on·thus (sif′i-li-on′thŭs). A copper-colored syphilid with branny scales. [syphilid + G. *ionthos,* acne of adolescence]

syph·i·lis (sif′i-lis). An acute and chronic infectious disease caused by *Treponema pallidum* and transmitted by direct contact, usually through sexual intercourse. After an incubation period of 12 to 30 days, the first symptom is a chancre, followed by slight fever and other constitutional symptoms (*primary s.*), followed by a skin eruption of various appearances with mucous patches and generalized lymphadenopathy (*secondary s.*), and subsequently by the formation of gummas, cellular infiltration, and functional abnormalities usually resulting from cardiovascular and central nervous system lesions (*tertiary s.*). SYN lues venerea, malum venereum. [Mod. L. *syphilis* (syphilid-), (?) fr. a poem, *Syphilis sive Morbus Gallicus,* by Fracastorius, *Syphilus* being a shepherd and principal char.]

cardiovascular s., involvement of the cardiovascular system seen in late s., usually resulting in aortitis, aneurysm formation, and aortic valvular insufficiency.

congenital s., s. acquired by the fetus *in utero,* thus present at birth. SYN hereditary s., s. hereditaria.

s. d'emblée (dom-blā′), s. occurring without an initial sore. [Fr. right away]

early s., primary, secondary, or early latent s., before any tertiary manifestations have appeared.

early latent s., infection with *Treponema pallidum,* the organism of syphilis, after the primary and secondary phases have subsided, during the first year after infection, before any manifestations of tertiary syphilis have appeared.

endemic s., SYN nonvenereal s.

sy

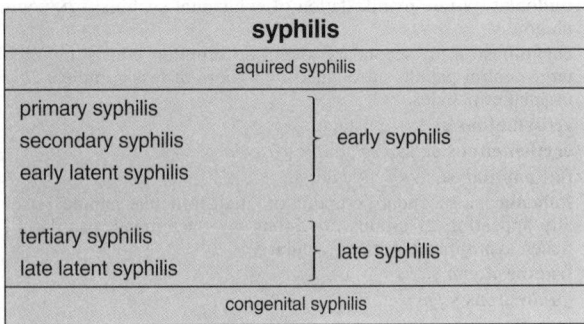

syphilis	
aquired syphilis	
primary syphilis secondary syphilis early latent syphilis	early syphilis
tertiary syphilis late latent syphilis	late syphilis
congenital syphilis	

equine s., SYN dourine.

s. heredita′ria, SYN congenital s.

hereditary s., SYN congenital s.

s. heredita′ria tar′da, s., believed to be congenital, but not manifesting itself until several years after birth.

late s., involvement of the cardiovascular or central nervous system, or the development of a gumma in any organ, due to infection with *Treponema pallidum;* usually several years to 2–3 decades after the initial infection. SYN tertiary s.

late benign s., late s., manifested by serologic evidence of infection, but without any clinical manifestations.

late latent s., Usually infectious in pregnant women only, who may pass the infection on to the fetus.

latent s., infection with *Treponema pallidum*, after the manifestations of primary and secondary s. have subsided (or were never noticed), before any manifestations of tertiary s. have appeared.

meningovascular s., a rare manifestation of secondary or tertiary s. characterized by mild, nonsuppurative, chronic inflammation of the leptomeninges and an intracranial or spinal angiitis.

nonvenereal s., s. caused by organisms closely related to *Treponema pallidum;* spread by personal, but not necessarily venereal, contact; usually acquired in childhood, most common in areas of provery and overcrowding; rare in the United States; includes yaws, pinta and bejel. SYN endemic s.

primary s., the first stage of s. SEE syphilis.

quaternary s., SYN parasyphilis.

secondary s., the second stage of s. SEE syphilis. SYN mesosyphilis.

tertiary s., SYN late s.

syph·i·lit·ic (sif-i-lit′ik). Relating to, caused by, or suffering from syphilis. SYN luetic.

⌂**syphilo-, syphil-, syphili-.** Syphilis. [see syphilis]

syph·i·lo·derm, syph·i·lo·der·ma (sif′i-lō-derm, -der′mă). SYN syphilid. [syphilo- + G. *derma,* skin]

syph·i·loid (sif′i-loyd). Resembling syphilis. [syphilo- + G. *eidos,* resemblance]

syph·i·lol·o·gist (sif-i-lol′o-jist). One who specializes in the study, diagnosis, and treatment of syphilis.

syph·i·lol·o·gy (sif-i-lol′ō-jē). The branch of medical science concerned with the origin, prevention, and treatment of syphilis. [syphilo- + G. *logos,* study]

syph·i·lo·ma (sif-i-lō′mă). SYN gumma. [syphilo- + G. *-oma,* tumor]

s. of Fournier, SYN Fournier's *disease.*

syph·i·lom·a·tous (sif-i-lō′mă-tŭs). SYN gummatous.

syr Abbreviation of Mod. L. *syrupus,* syrup.

sy·rig·mus (sĭ-rig′mŭs). SYN *tinnitus* aurium. [L. fr. G. *syrigmos,* a hissing]

⌂**syring-.** SEE syringo-.

syr·ing·ad·e·no·ma (sir′ing-ad-ĕ-nō′mă). A benign sweat gland tumor showing glandular differentiation typical of secretory cells. SYN syringoadenoma. [syring- + G. *adēn,* gland, + *-oma,* tumor]

syr·ing·ad·e·no·sus (sir′ing-ad-ĕ-nō′sŭs). Relating to the sweat glands. [L. fr. syring- + G. *adēn,* gland]

sy·ringe (sĭ-rinj′, sir′inj). An instrument used for injecting or withdrawing fluids. [G. *syrinx,* pipe or tube]

air s., SYN chip s.

chip s., a tapered metal tube through which air is forced from a rubber bulb or pressure tank to blow debris from, or to dry, a cavity in preparing teeth for restoration. SYN air s.

control s., a type of Luer-Lok s. with thumb and finger rings attached to the proximal end of the barrel and to the tip of the plunger, allowing operation of the s. with one hand. SYN ring s.

Davidson s., a rubber tube, armed with an appropriate nozzle, intersected with a compressible bulb, with valves so arranged that compression forces the fluid, into which one end of the tube is inserted, forward to the nozzle end.

dental s., a breech-loading metal cartridge s. into which fits a hermetically sealed glass cartridge containing the anesthetic solution.

fountain s., an apparatus consisting of a reservoir for holding fluid, to the bottom of which is attached a tube with a suitable nozzle; used for vaginal or rectal injections, irrigating wounds, etc., the force of the flow being regulated by the height of the reservoir above the point of discharge.

hypodermic s., a small s. with a barrel (which may be calibrated), perfectly matched plunger, and tip; used with a hollow needle for subcutaneous injections and for aspiration. SYN hypodermic (3).

Luer s., a glass s. with a metal tip and locking device to secure the needle; used for hypodermic and intravenous purposes. SYN Luer-Lok s.

Luer-Lok s., SYN Luer s.

Neisser's s., a urethral s. used in treatment of gonococcal urethritis.

probe s., a s. with an olive-shaped tip, used in treatment of diseases of the lacrimal passages.

ring s., SYN control s.

Roughton-Scholander s., SYN Roughton-Scholander *apparatus.*

rubber-bulb s., a s. with a hollow rubber bulb and cannula provided with a check valve, used to obtain a jet of air or water.

sy·rin·ge·al (sĭ-rin′jē-ăl). Relating to a syrinx.

sy·rin·gec·to·my (si-rin-jek′tō-mē). SYN fistulectomy. [syring- + G. *ektomē,* excision]

sy·rin·gi·tis (si-rin-jī′tis). Inflammation of the eustachian tube. [syring- + G. *-itis,* inflammation]

⌂**syringo-, syring-.** A syrinx; syringeal. [G. *syrinx,* pipe or tube]

sy·rin·go·ad·e·no·ma (sĭ-ring′gō-ad-ĕ-nō′mă). SYN syringadenoma.

sy·rin·go·bul·bia (sĭ-ring′gō-bŭl′bē-ă). A fluid-filled cavity of the brainstem, analogous to syringomyelia. [syringo- + L. *bulbus,* bulb (medulla oblongata)]

sy·rin·go·car·ci·no·ma (sĭ-ring′gō-kar-si-nō′mă). A malignant epithelial neoplasm which has undergone cystic change (cystic carcinoma). [syringo- + carcinoma]

sy·rin·go·cele (sĭ-ring′gō-sēl). 1. SYN central *canal.* 2. A meningomyelocele in which there is a cavity in the ectopic spinal cord. [syringo- + G. *koilia,* a hollow]

sy·rin·go·cys·tad·e·no·ma (sĭ-ring′gō-sis-tad-ĕ-nō′mă). A cystic benign sweat gland tumor. [syringo- + cystadenoma]

s. papillif′erum, a s. characterized by numerous finger-like projections of proliferated neoplastic epithelial cells in two layers on a stromal core of fibrous connective tissue infiltrated by plasma cells occurring singly or as part of a nevus sebaceus.

sy·rin·go·cys·to·ma (sĭ-ring′gō-sis-tō′mă). SYN hidrocystoma. [syringo- + cystoma]

sy·rin·go·en·ceph·a·lo·my·e·lia (sĭ-ring′gō-en-sef′ă-lō-mī-ē′lē-ă). A tubular cavity involving both brain and spinal cord and etiologically unrelated to vascular insufficiency. [syringo- + G. *enkephalos,* brain, + *myelos,* marrow]

sy·rin·goid (sĭ-ring′goyd). Resembling a tube or fistula. [syringo- + G. *eidos,* resemblance]

sy·rin·go·ma (si-ring-gō′mă). A benign, often multiple, sometimes eruptive benign, neoplasm of the sweat gland ducts composed of very small round cysts. [syringo- + G. *-ōma,* tumor]

chondroid s., a benign tumor of sweat glands with a mucoid stroma showing cartilaginous metaplasia. SYN mixed tumor of skin.

sy·rin·go·me·nin·go·cele (sĭ-ring′gō-mĕ-ning′gō-sēl). A form of spina bifida in which the dorsal sac consists chiefly of membranes, with very little cord substance, enclosing a cavity that communicates with a syringomyelic cavity. [syringo- + meningocele]

sy·rin·go·my·e·lia (sĭ-ring′gō-mī-ē′lē-ă). The presence in the spinal cord of longitudinal cavities lined by dense, gliogenous tissue, which are not caused by vascular insufficiency. S. is marked clinically by pain and paresthesia, followed by muscular atrophy of the hands and analgesia with thermoanesthesia of the hands and arms, but with the tactile sense preserved; later marked by painless whitlows, spastic paralysis in the lower extremities, and scoliosis of the lumbar spine. Some cases are associated with low grade astrocytomas or vascular malformations of the spinal cord. SYN hydrosyringomyelia, Morvan's disease, myelosyringosis, syringomyelus. [syringo- + G. *myelos,* marrow]

sy·rin·go·my·e·lo·cele (sĭ-ring′gō-mī′e-lō-sēl). A form of spina bifida, consisting in a protrusion of the membranes and spinal cord through a dorsal defect in the vertebral column, the fluid of the syrinx of the cord being increased and expanding the cord tissue into a thin-walled sac which then expands through the vertebral defect. [syringo- + myelocele]

sy·rin·go·my·e·lus (sĭ-ring′gō-mī′ĕ-lŭs). SYN syringomyelia. [syringo- + G. *myelos,* marrow]

sy·rin·go·pon·tia (sĭ-ring′gō-pon′shē-ă). A condition of cavity formation in the pons, of the same nature as syringomyelia. [syringo- + L. *pons,* bridge]

sy·rin·go·tome (sĭ-rin′gō-tōm). SYN fistulatome.

sy·rin·got·o·my (si-rin-got′ō-mē). SYN fistulotomy.

syr·inx, pl. **sy·ring·es** (sir′ingks, sĭ-rin′jēz). **1.** A rarely used synonym for fistula. **2.** A pathologic tube-shaped cavity in the brain or spinal cord. **3.** The lower part of the bird trachea, which produces vocal sounds. [G. a tube, pipe]

sy·ro·sing·o·pine (sir-ō-sin′gō-pēn). Carbethoxysyringoyl methyl reserpate; prepared from reserpine by hydrolysis and reesterification; an antihypertensive agent with actions similar to those of reserpine.

syr·up (ser′ŭp, sir′ŭp). **1.** Refined molasses; the uncrystallizable saccharine solution left after the refining of sugar. **2.** Any sweet fluid; a solution of sugar in water in any proportion. **3.** A liquid preparation of medicinal or flavoring substances in a concentrated aqueous solution of a sugar, usually sucrose; other polyols, such as glycerin or sorbitol, may be present to retard crystallization of sucrose or to increase the solubility of added ingredients. When the s. contains a medicinal substance, it is termed a medicated s.; although a syrup tends (due to its very high [approximately 85 percent] sucrose content) to resist mold or bacterial contamination, a s. may contain antimicrobial agents to prevent bacterial and mold growth. SYN sirup, syrupus. [Mod. L. *syrupus,* fr. Ar. *sharāb*]

ipecac s., a sweetened liquid medicinal preparation containing powdered ipecac extract, which contains the alkaloids emetine and cephaline; used as an emetic in certain cases of poisoning and (at lower doses) as an expectorant.

syr·u·pus (sir′ŭ-pŭs). SYN syrup. [Mod. L.]

syr·upy (ser′ŭ-pē, sir′). Relating to syrup; of the consistency of syrup.

sys·sar·co·sic (sis′ar-kō′sik). SYN syssarcotic.

sys·sar·co·sis (sis′ar-kō′sis). A muscular articulation; Union of bones by muscle; *e.g.,* in man, the muscular connections of the patella. [G. *syssarkōsis,* a being overgrown with flesh, fr. *syn,* with, + *sarx,* flesh]

sys·sar·cot·ic (sis′ar-kot′ik). Relating to or characterized by syssarcosis. SYN syssarcosic.

sys·tal·tic (sis-tahl′tik, -tal′tik). Obsolete term for pulsating; al-

ternately contracting and dilating; denoting the action of the heart. [G. *systaltikos,* contractile]

SYSTEM

sys·tem (sis′tĕm). **1.** A consistent and complex whole made up of correlated and semi-independent parts. A complex of anatomical structures functionally related. **2.** The entire organism seen as a complex organization of parts. **3.** Any complex of structures anatomically related (*e.g.,* vascular s.) or functionally related (*e.g.,* digestive s.). **4.** A scheme of medical theory. SEE ALSO apparatus, classification, system. **5.** S. followed by one or more letters denotes specific amino acid transporters; s. N is a sodium-dependent transporter specific for amino acids such as L-glutamine, L-asparagine, and L-histidine; s. y⁺ is a sodium-independent transporter of cationic amino acids. SYN systema [NA]. [G. *systēma,* an organized whole]

absolute s. of units, a s. based on absolute units accepted as being fundamental (length, mass, time) and from which other units (force, energy or work, power) are derived; such s.'s in common use are the foot-pound-second, centimeter-gram-second, and meter-kilogram-second s.'s.

absorbent s., SYN lymphatic s.

alimentary s., SYN digestive s.

anterolateral s., a composite bundle of fibers, located in the ventrolateral part of the lateral funiculus, containing spinothalamic, spinohypothalamic, spinoreticular, and spinomesencephalic (spinotectal, spinal to periaqueductal grey, etc.) fibers; occupies the combined areas of the spinal white matter historically divided into anterior and lateral spinothalamic tracts; located in white matter ventral to the denticulate ligament, hence the anatomical basis for the anterolateral cordotomy; concerned with the transmission of nociceptive and thermal information and with crude (nondiscriminative) touch.

arch-loop-whorl s. (A.L.W.), SEE Galton's system of classification of *fingerprints,* under *fingerprint.*

association s., groups or tracts of nerve fibers interconnecting different regions of one and the same major subdivision of the central nervous system, such as the various areas of the cerebral cortex or the various segments of the spinal cord.

autonomic nervous s., that part of the nervous system which represents the motor innervation of smooth muscle, cardiac muscle, and gland cells. It consists of two physiologically and anatomically distinct, mutually antagonistic components: the sympathetic and parasympathetic parts. In both of these parts the pathway of innervation consists of a synaptic sequence of two motor neurons, one of which lies in the spinal cord or brainstem as the preganglionic neuron, the thin but myelinated axon of which (preganglionic or B fiber) emerges with an outgoing spinal or cranial nerve and synapses with one or more of the postganglionic (or, more strictly, ganglionic) neurons composing the autonomic ganglia; the unmyelinated postganglionic fibers in turn innervate the smooth muscle, cardiac muscle, or gland cells. The preganglionic neurons of the sympathetic part lie in the intermediolateral cell column of the thoracic and upper two lumbar segments of the spinal gray matter; those of the parasympathetic part compose the visceral motor (visceral efferent) nuclei of the brainstem as well as the lateral column of the second to fourth sacral segments of the spinal cord. The ganglia of the sympathetic part are the paravertebral ganglia of the sympathetic trunk and the prevertebral or collateral ganglia; those of the parasympathetic part lie either near the organ to be innervated or as intramural ganglia within the organ itself except in the head, where there are four discrete parasympathetic ganglia (ciliary, otic, pterygopalatine, and submandibular). Impulse transmission from preganglionic to postganglionic neuron is mediated by acetylcholine in both the sympathetic and parasympathetic parts; transmission from the postganglionic fiber to the visceral effector tissues is classically said to be by acetylcholine in the parasympathetic part and by noradrenalin in the sympathetic part; recent evidence suggests the existence of further noncholinergic, nonadrenergic classes of postganglionic fibers. SYN pars autonomica [NA], systema nervosum autonomicum✩ [NA], autonomic part, involuntary nervous s., vegetative nervous s., visceral nervous s.

autonomic nervous system		
organ	function of sympathetic nervous system	function of parasympathetic nervous system
eye	pupil dilation, contraction of ciliary muscle for accomodation	constriction of pupil
lacrimal gland	slight or no effect	secretion
salivary glands	thick, viscous secretion	abundant, watery secretion
heart	increase of rate and strength of heartbeats, dilation of coronary vessels (indirectly?), reduction of conduction time	slowing of beats, contraction of coronary vessels (indirectly?), increase of conduction time
lungs	bronchodilation, inhibition of secretion	bronchial constriction, stimulation of secretion
digestive tract	peristaltic inhibition, vasoconstriction	stimulation of peristalsis and secretion
liver and gall bladder	release of glucose	excretion of bile
adrenal medulla	secretion of adrenaline	no connection
kidney	vasoconstriction, inhibition of urine formation	no effect(?)
bladder	retention of urine	release of urine
genitalia	ejaculation	penile and clitoral erections
sweat glands	secretion	no connection
peripheral blood vessels	constriction	no connection, apart from dilation in the genital area
skeletal muscle	constriction	dilation

Bethesda s., recent classification for categorizing cervical Papanicolaou smears. [*Bethesda*, Maryland, site of NIH]
blood group s.'s, see Blood Groups appendix.
blood-vascular s., SYN cardiovascular s.
bulbosacral s., SYN parasympathetic *part.*
cardiovascular s., the heart and blood vessels considered as a whole. SYN blood-vascular s.
caudal neurosecretory s., urohypophysis.
centimeter-gram-second s. (CGS, cgs), the scientific s. of expressing the fundamental physical units of length, mass, and time, and those units derived from them, in centimeters, grams, and seconds; currently being replaced by the International System of Units based on the meter, kilogram, and second.
central nervous s. (CNS), the brain and the spinal cord. SYN pars centralis [NA], systema nervosum centrale✩ [NA].

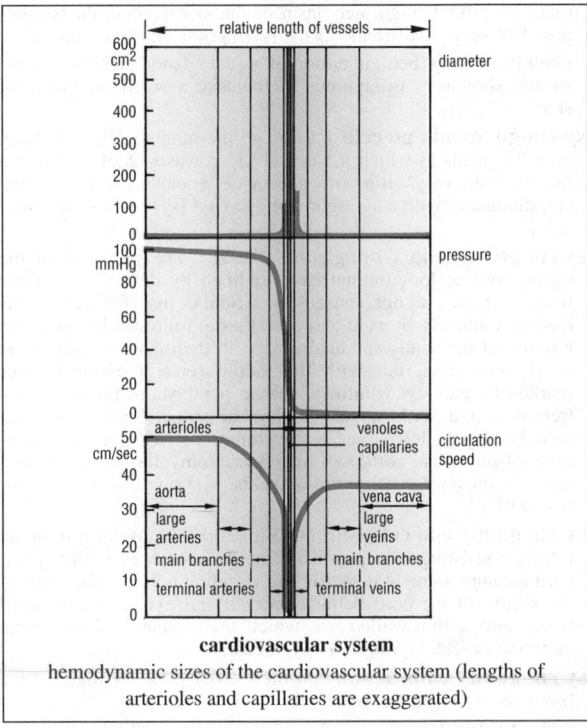

cardiovascular system
hemodynamic sizes of the cardiovascular system (lengths of arterioles and capillaries are exaggerated)

cerebrospinal s., the combined central nervous s. and peripheral nervous s.
charge transfer s., SYN charge transfer *complex.*
chromaffin s., the cells of the body that stain with chromium salts and occur in the medullary portion of the adrenal body, paraganglia, and in relation to certain sympathetic nerves.
circulatory s., SYN vascular s.
closed s., a s. in which there is no exchange of material, energy, or information with the environment.
colloid s., a combination of the two phases, internal and external, of a colloid solution; the various s.'s are: gas + liquid (foam); gas + solid (meerschaum); liquid + gas (fog); solid + gas (smoke); solid + liquid (sol); liquid + solid (gel); liquid + liquid (emulsion); solid + solid (colored glass).
complement s., a group of more than 20 serum proteins, some of which can be serially activated and participate in a cascade resulting in cell lysis.
conducting s. of heart, the s. of atypical cardiac muscle fibers comprising the sinoatrial node, internodal tracts, atrioventricular node and bundle, the bundle branches, and their terminal ramifications into the Purkinje network; sometimes also called cardionector.
craniosacral s., SYN parasympathetic *part.*
cytochrome s., SYN respiratory *chain.*
dermal s., dermoid s., the skin and its appendages, the nails and hair.
digestive s., the digestive tract from the mouth to the anus with all its associated glands and organs. SYN systema alimentarium✩, alimentary apparatus, alimentary s., systema digestorium.
ecological s., SYN ecosystem.
electron-transport s., SYN respiratory *chain.*
endocrine s., collective designation for those tissues capable of secreting hormones.
endomembrane s., SYN endoplasmic *reticulum.*
esthesiodic s., a s. of neurons and fiber tracts in the spinal cord and brain subserving sensation.
exterofective s., name applied by Cannon to the somatic nervous s. as opposed to the interofective or autonomic s.
extrapyramidal motor s., literally: all of the brain structures

affecting bodily (somatic) movement, excluding the motor neurons, the motor cortex, and the pyramidal (corticobulbar and corticospinal) tract. Despite its very wide literal connotation, the term is commonly used to denote in particular the striate body (basal ganglia), its associated structures (substantia nigra; subthalamic nucleus), and its descending connections with the midbrain.

feedback s., (1) a complex of neuronal circuits whereby a part of the efferent path returns to the input to modulate its activity, thus acting as a governor on the s.; **(2)** SEE feedback.

foot-pound-second s. (FPS, fps), a s. of absolute units based on the foot, pound, and second.

gamma motor s., SYN gamma *loop.*

genital s., the complex s. consisting of the male or female gonads, associated ducts, and external genitalia dedicated to the function of reproducing the species. SYN reproductive s.

genitourinary s., SYN urogenital s.

glandular s., all the glands of the body collectively.

haversian s., SYN osteon.

hematopoietic s., the blood-making organs; in the embryo at different ages these are the yolk sac, liver, thymus, spleen, lymph nodes, and bone marrow; after birth they are principally the bone marrow, spleen, thymus, and lymph nodes.

hepatic portal s., a venous portal s. in which the portal vein receives blood via its tributaries from the capillaries of most of the abdominal viscera and drains it into the hepatic sinusoids.

heterogeneous s., in chemistry, a s. that contains various distinct and mechanically separable parts or phases; *e.g.,* a suspension or an emulsion.

hexaxial reference s., the figure resulting if the lines of derivation of the unipolar limb leads of the electrocardiogram are added to the triaxial reference s.

His-Tawara s., the complex s. of interlacing Purkinje fibers within the ventricular myocardium. SEE ALSO conducting s. of heart.

homogeneous s., in chemistry, a s. whose parts cannot be mechanically separated, and is therefore uniform throughout and possesses in every part identically physical properties; *e.g.,* a solution of sodium chloride in water.

hypophyseoportal s. (hī'pō-fiz'ē-ō- por'tal), SYN portal hypophysial *circulation.*

hypophysial portal s., SYN portal hypophysial *circulation.*

hypophysioportal s., SYN portal hypophysial *circulation.*

hypothalamohypophysial portal s., SYN portal hypophysial *circulation.*

hypothalamohypophysial portal s., SYN renal portal s.

hypoxia warning s., a device designed to produce an audio or visual signal at a predetermined level of oxygen partial pressure; ideally, the system would warn of impending hypoxia in time for corrective action to be taken.

immune s., an intricate complex of interrelated cellular, molecular, and genetic components which provides a defense (immune response) against foreign organisms or substances and aberrant native cells.

indicator s., in *in vitro* immunological tests, a combination of reagents used to determine the degree to which immunological reagents have combined (*e.g.,* sensitized erythrocytes in complement-fixation tests; enzyme and substrate in enzyme-linked immunosorbent assays).

information s., combination of vital and health statistical data from multiple sources, used to derive information and make decisions about the health needs, health resources, costs, use, and outcome of health care.

integumentary s., the skin, hair, and nails; derived from ectoderm and subjacent mesoderm.

intermediary s., SYN interstitial *lamella.*

International S. of Units, SEE International System of Units.

interofective s., term applied by W. Cannon to the autonomic nervous s. as opposed to the somatic nervous s. or exterofective s.

involuntary nervous s., SYN autonomic nervous s.

kallikrein s., a blood serum s., the activity of which is initiated

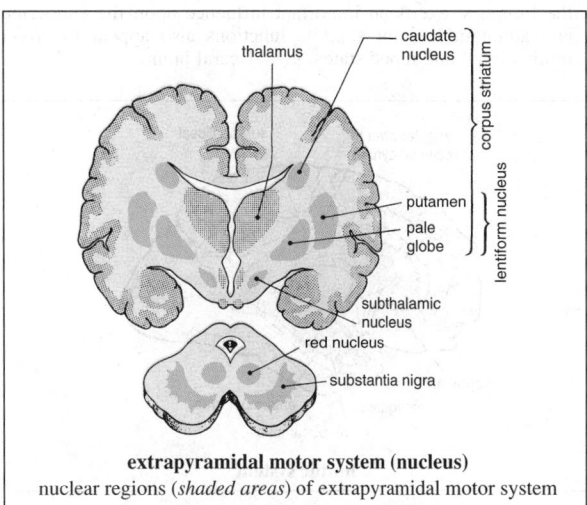

extrapyramidal motor system (nucleus)
nuclear regions (*shaded areas*) of extrapyramidal motor system

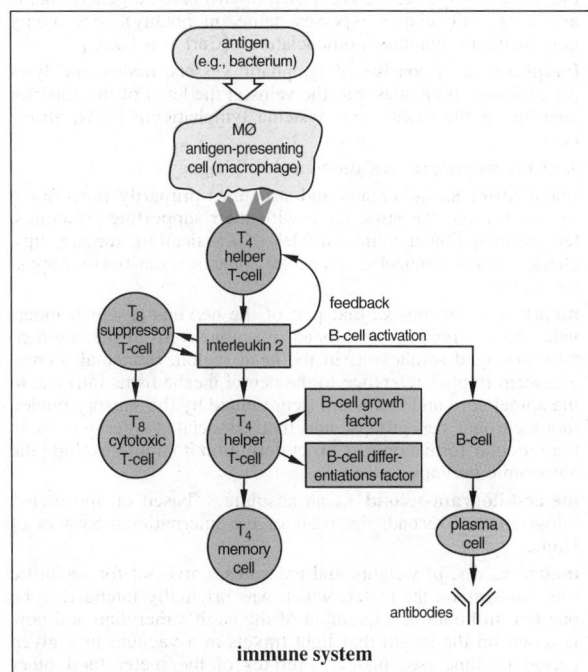

immune system

by factor XII (Hageman factor) leading to the production of prekallikrein activator and then to kallikrein which, after activation by plasmin, splits bradykinin from kininogen.

kinetic s., (1) a term proposed by G.W. Crile to denote the chain of organs through which latent energy is transformed into motion and heat: it includes the brain, the thyroid, the adrenals, the liver, the pancreas, and the muscles; **(2)** that part of the neuromuscular s. whereby active movements are effected; distinguished from the static s.

lateral line s., a series of sense organs that detect pressure or vibrations along the head and side of cyclostomes, fishes, and some amphibians.

limbic s., collective term denoting a heterogeneous array of brain structures at or near the edge (limbus) of the medial wall of the cerebral hemisphere, in particular the hippocampus, amygdala, and fornicate gyrus; the term is often used so as to include also the interconnections of these structures, as well as their connections with the septal area, the hypothalamus, and a medial zone of mesencephalic tegmentum. By way of the latter connections, the limbic s. exerts an important influence upon the endocrine and autonomic motor s.'s; its functions also appear to affect motivational and mood states. SYN visceral brain.

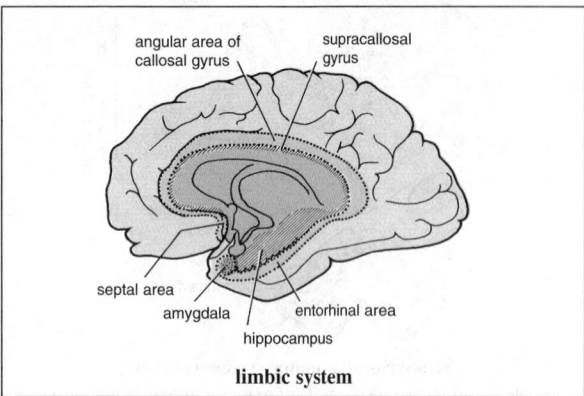

limbic system

linnaean s. of nomenclature, the s. of nomenclature in which the names of species are composed of two parts, a generic name and a specific epithet (species name, in botany). SYN binary nomenclature, binomial nomenclature. [Carl von *Linné*]

lymphatic s., it consists of lymphatic vessels, nodes, and lymphoid tissue; it empties into the veins at the level of the superior aperture of the thorax. SYN systema lymphaticum [NA], absorbent s.

s. of macrophages, SYN mononuclear phagocyte s.

masticatory s., the organs and structures primarily functioning in mastication: the jaws, teeth with their supporting structures, temporomandibular joint, muscles of mastication, tongue, lips, cheeks, and oral mucosa. SYN dental apparatus, masticatory apparatus (1).

metameric nervous s., that part of the nervous s. which innervates body structures developed in ontogeny from the segmentally arranged somites or, in the head region, branchial arches. The term implies reference to the neural mechanisms intrinsic to the spinal cord and brainstem (represented by the sensory nuclei, motoneuronal cell groups, and their associated interneurons in the reticular formation); by strict definition it should exclude the autonomic nervous system.

meter-kilogram-second s., an absolute s. based on the meter, kilogram, and second; the basis of the International System of Units.

metric s., a s. of weights and measures, universal for scientific use, based upon the meter, which was originally intended to be one ten-millionth of a quadrant of the earth's meridian and now is based on the length that light travels in a vacuum in a given period of time (see meter). Prefixes of the meter (and other standards) reflect either fractions or multiples of the meter and are identical to the International System of Units (see International System of Units). The unit of weight is the gram, which is the weight of one cubic centimeter of water, equivalent to 15.432358 grains. The unit of volume is the liter or one cubic decimeter, equal to 1.056688 U.S. liquid quarts; a cubic centimeter is about 16.23073 U.S. minims.

mononuclear phagocyte s. (MPS), a widely distributed collection of both free and fixed macrophages derived from bone marrow precursor cells by way of monocytes; their substantial phagocytic activity is mediated by immunoglobulin and the serum complement system. In both connective and lymphoid tissue, they may occur as free and fixed macrophages; in the sinusoids of the liver, as Kupffer cells; in the lung, as alveolar macrophages; and in the nervous system, as microglia. SYN s. of macrophages.

muscular s., all the muscles of the body collectively.

nervous s., the entire nerve apparatus, composed of a central part, the brain and spinal cord, and a peripheral part, the cranial and spinal nerves, autonomic ganglia, and plexuses. SYN systema nervosum [NA].

mononuclear phagocyte system (MPS)	
cells	location
precursor cell ↓	marrow
promonocyte ↓	marrow
monocyte ↓	marrow, blood
macrophages	connective tissue (histiocytes), liver (Kupffer cells), lungs (alveolar macrophages), spleen (free and fixed macrophages), marrow (macrophages), serous cavities (pleural and peritoneal macrophages), bone (osteoclasts)?, CNS (microglia)?

neuromuscular s., the muscles of the body collectively and the nerves supplying them.

nonspecific s., SYN reticular activating s.

occlusal s., the form or design and arrangement of the occlusal and incisal units of a dentition or the teeth on a denture. SYN occlusal scheme.

oculomotor s., that part of the central nervous s. having to do with eye movements; it is composed of pathways connecting various regions of the cerebrum, brainstem, and ocular nuclei, utilizing multisynaptic articulations.

open s., a s. in which there is a continual exchange of material, energy, and information with the environment.

O-R s., abbreviation for oxidation-reduction s.

oxidation-reduction s. (O-R s.), an enzyme s. in the tissues by which oxidation and reduction proceed simultaneously through the transference of hydrogen or of one or more electrons from one metabolite to another. SEE ALSO oxidation-reduction. SYN redox s.

parasympathetic nervous s., SEE parasympathetic *part*, autonomic nervous s.

pedal s., efferent fibers connecting the forebrain with more caudal structures.

periodic s., the arrangement of the chemical elements in a definite order as indicated by their respective atomic numbers in such a way that groups of elements with similar chemical properties (similar valence shell electron number) are grouped together. SEE Mendeléeff's *law*.

peripheral nervous s., the peripheral part of the nervous system external to the brain and spinal cord from their roots to their peripheral terminations. This includes the ganglia, both sensory and autonomic and any plexuses through which the nerve fibers run. SEE ALSO autonomic nervous s. SYN pars peripherica [NA], systema nervosum periphericum☆ [NA], peripheral part.

Pinel's s., the abolition of forcible restraint in the treatment of the mental hospital patient.

portal s., a s. of vessels in which blood, after passing through one capillary bed, is conveyed through a second capillary network, as in the hepatic portal system in which blood from the intestines passes through the liver sinusoids.

pressoreceptor s., the pressoreceptive areas which with their afferent fibers and connections with the autonomic system react to a rise in arterial blood pressure and serve to buffer it by inhibiting the heart rate and vascular tone. SEE ALSO baroreceptor.

projection s., the s. of axons carrying stimuli from one portion of the nervous system to other portions.

properdin s., an immunological s. that is the alternative pathway for complement, composed of several distinct proteins that react in a serial manner and activate C3 (third component of complement), seemingly without utilizing components C1, C4, and C2; in addition to properdin, the s. includes properdin factors A (native C3), B (C3 proactivator), D (C3 proactivator convertase), and perhaps at least one other, E; the s. can be activated, in the absence of specific antibody, by bacterial endotoxins, by a variety of polysaccharides and lipopolysaccharides, and by a component of cobra venom.

Purkinje s., terminal ramifications in the ventricles of the specialized conducting s. of the heart.

redox s., SYN oxidation-reduction s.

renal portal s., an arterial portal s., in which efferent glomerular arterioles receive blood from the capillaries of the renal glomeruli and carry it to the peritubular capillary plexus surrounding the proximal and distal convoluted tubules. SYN hypothalamohypophysial portal s.

renin-angiotensin s., a selective regulator of the aldosterone biosynthetic pathway that acts by increasing aldosterone production and sodium retention as a result of volume depletion, with resulting increased renin production in the kidney and conversion of angiotensin I in the plasma to angiotensin II.

renin-angiotensin-aldosterone s., the hormones, renin, angiotensin, and aldosterone work together to regulate blood pressure. A sustained fall in blood pressure cuases the kidney to release renin. This is converted to angiotensin in the circulation. Angiotensin then raises blood pressure directly by arteriolar constriction and stimulates adrenal gland to produce aldosterone which promotes sodium and water retention by kidney, such that blood volume and blood pressure increase.

reproductive s., SYN genital s.

respiratory s., all the air passages from the nose to the pulmonary alveoli. SYN apparatus respiratorius [NA], systema respiratorium☆ [NA], respiratory apparatus.

reticular activating s. (RAS), a physiological term denoting that part of the brainstem reticular formation that plays a central role in the organism's bodily and behavorial alertness; it extends as a diffusely organized neural apparatus through the central region of the brainstem into the subthalamus and the intralaminar nuclei of the thalamus; by its ascending connections it affects the function of the cerebral cortex in the sense of behavioral responsiveness; its descending (reticulospinal) connections transmit its activating influence upon bodily posture and reflex mechanisms (*e.g.,* muscle tonus), in part by way of the gamma motor neurons. SEE ALSO reticular *formation*. SYN nonspecific s.

reticuloendothelial s. (RES), a collection of putative macrophages, first described by Aschoff, which included most of the true macrophages (now classified under the mononuclear phagocytic s.) as well as cells lining the sinusoids of the spleen, lymph nodes, and bone marrow, and the fibroblastic reticular cells of hematopoietic tissues; all of these latter cells are only weakly phagocytic and are not true macrophages. The term persists in the literature and is often equated with the mononuclear phagocytic s.

second signaling s., pavlovian term for speech in which words are considered to be the "second signals" capable of producing conditioned responses.

skeletal s., the bones and cartilages of the body. SYN systema skeletale [NA].

somesthetic s., sensory data derived from skin, muscles, and body organs in contrast to that derived from the five special senses.

static s., that part of the neuromuscular s. whereby the animal organism is maintained in posture and equilibrium, and counteracts the forces of gravity and atmospheric pressure; distinguished from the kinetic s. (2).

stomatognathic s., all of the structures involved in speech and in the receiving, mastication, and deglutition of food. SEE ALSO masticatory s. SYN masticatory apparatus (2).

sympathetic nervous s., (1) originally, the entire autonomic nervous s.; **(2)** the sympathetic part of the nervous system. SEE ALSO autonomic nervous s. SYN pars sympathica [NA], sympathetic part.

T s., the transverse tubules that are continuous with the sarcolemma in skeletal and cardiac muscle fibers.

thoracolumbar s., SEE autonomic nervous s., sympathetic *part.*

triaxial reference s., the figure resulting from rearranging the lines of derivation of the three standard limb leads of the electrocardiogram (as represented in Einthoven's triangle) so that, instead of forming the sides of an equilateral triangle, they bisect one another. SYN Dieuaide diagram.

urinary s., SYN urogenital s.

urogenital s., includes all the organs concerned in reproduction and in the formation and voidance of the urine. SYN apparatus urogenitalis [NA], systema urogenitale☆ [NA], genitourinary apparatus, genitourinary s., urinary apparatus, urinary s., urogenital apparatus.

uropoietic s., the kidneys, ureters, bladder, and urethra, considered as a s. for the secretion and excretion of urine.

vascular s., the cardiovascular and lymphatic s.'s collectively. SYN circulatory s.

vegetative nervous s., SYN autonomic nervous s.

vertebral-basilar s., the arterial complex comprising the two vertebral arteries joining to form the basilar artery, and their immediate branches.

vertebral venous s., any of four interconnected venous networks surrounding the vertebral column; anterior external vertebral venous plexus, the small s. around the vertebral bodies; posterior external vertebral venous plexus, the extensive s. around the vertebral processes; anterior internal vertebral venous plexus, the s. running the length of the vertebral canal anterior to the dura; posterior internal vertebral venous plexus, the s. running the length of the vertebral canal posterior to the dura; the latter two constitute the epidural venous plexus. SYN plexus venosus vertebralis [NA], Batson's plexus, vertebral venous plexus.

visceral nervous s., SYN autonomic nervous s.

Zaffaroni s., a chromatographic s. for the separation of steroids.

---

sys·te·ma (sis'tē'mă) [NA]. SYN system. SEE ALSO system, apparatus. [L. fr. G. *systēma*]

s. alimentarium, ☆official alternate term for digestive *system.*

s. digesto′rium, SYN digestive *system,* digestive *system.*

s. lymphat′icum [NA], SYN lymphatic *system.*

s. nervo′sum [NA], SYN nervous *system.*

s. nervo′sum autonom′icum [NA], ☆official alternate term for autonomic nervous *system.*

s. nervo′sum centra′le [NA], ☆official alternate term for central nervous *system,* central nervous *system.*

s. nervo′sum peripher′icum [NA], ☆official alternate term for peripheral nervous *system.*

s. respirato′rium [NA], ☆official alternate term for respiratory *system.*

s. skeleta′le [NA], SYN skeletal *system.*

s. urogenita′le [NA], ☆official alternate term for urogenital *system.*

sys·tem·at·ic (sis'tĕ-mat'ik). Relating to a system in any sense; arranged according to a system.

sys·tem·at·ic name. As applied to chemical substances, a s. n. is composed of specially coined or selected words or syllables, each of which has a precisely defined chemical structural meaning, so that the structure may be derived from the name. Water (trivial name) is hydrogen oxide (systematic). The s. n. of histamine (a semisystematic name) is imidazolethylamine, which indicates that a radical of imidazole replaces one hydrogen atom of ethylamine, which in turn is an ethyl group attached to an amine group. Dimethyl sulfoxide states that two methyl radicals are attached to a sulfur atom that holds an oxygen atom. Carbolic acid (trivial name) or phenol (semisystematic name) are, systematically, phenyl hydroxide or hydroxybenzene. SEE ALSO semisystematic name.

sys·tem·a·ti·za·tion (sis-tĕ-mat'i-zā'shŭn, sis-tem'ă-ti-). The arrangement of ideas into orderly sequence.

Sys·tème In·ter·na·tion·al d'Un·i·tés. SEE International System of Units.

sys·tem·ic (sis-tem'ik). Relating to a system; specifically somatic, relating to the entire organism as distinguished from any of its individual parts.

sys·te·moid (sis'tĕ-moyd). Resembling a system; denoting a tumor of complex structure resembling an organ.

sys·to·le (sis'tō-lē). Contraction of the heart, especially of the

female urogenital system

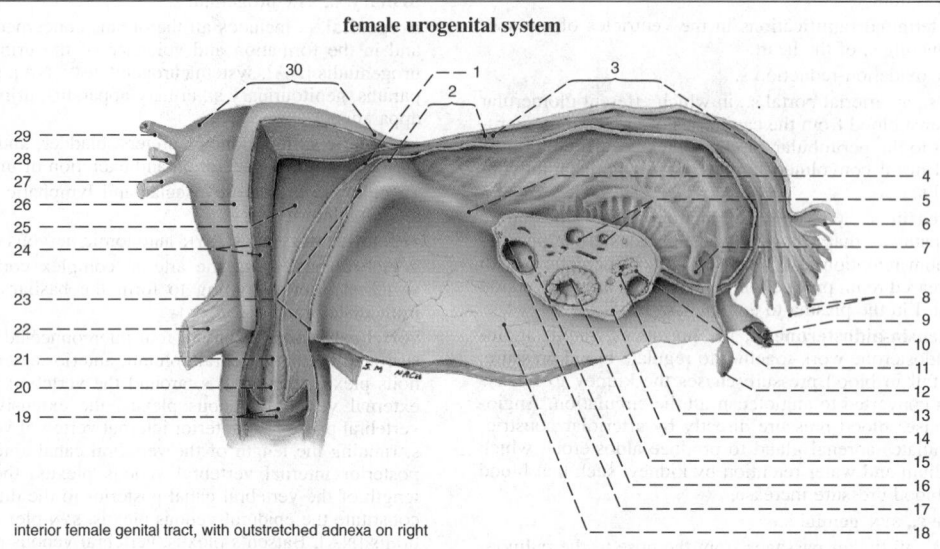

interior female genital tract, with outstretched adnexa on right

right side of uterus open from dorsal surface, as is portio region of vagina and right fallopian tube; right ovary is in frontal cross-section

fallopian tube
1 part of uterine tube
2 isthmus of uterine tube
3 ampulla of uterine tube
4 ovarian ligament
6 infundibulum of uterine tube
   (with ovarian extremity of oviduct)
7 ovarian fimbria
8 fimbriae of uterine tube
9 ovarian vein
10 ovarian artery
12 stalked hydatid
18 broad ligament of uterus

ovary
5 primary ovarian follicles
11 tubal extremity
13 corpus albicans
   (atretic corpus luteum)
14 stroma of ovary
15 corpus luteum
16 vesicular ovarian follicle
17 uterine extremity

uterus
19 mouth of womb (in nullipara, dimple-
   shaped; after birthing, slot-shaped)
20 vaginal part of uterine cervix
21 cervical canal
22 sacrouterine ligament
23 body of uterus
24 myometrium
25 uterine cavity, endometrium
26 perimetrium
27 ovarian ligament
28 round uterine ligament
29 uterine tube
30 fundus of uterus

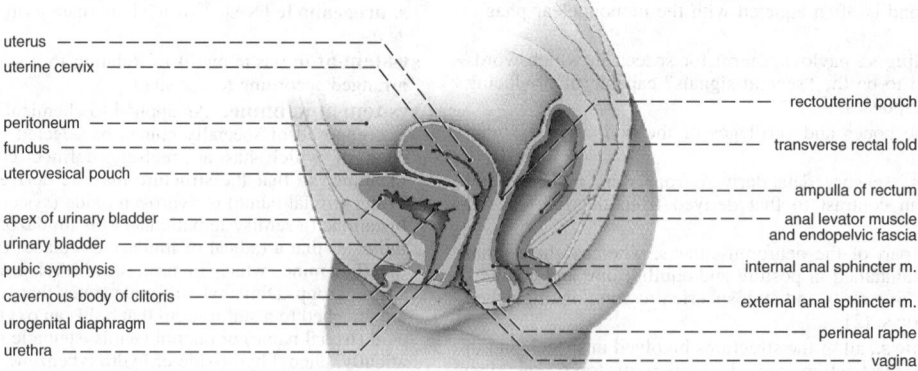

uterus
uterine cervix

peritoneum
fundus
uterovesical pouch

apex of urinary bladder
urinary bladder
pubic symphysis
cavernous body of clitoris
urogenital diaphragm
urethra

rectouterine pouch
transverse rectal fold
ampulla of rectum
anal levator muscle
and endopelvic fascia
internal anal sphincter m.
external anal sphincter m.
perineal raphe
vagina

female urogenital tract
sagittal view of female pelvis (schematic)

male urogenital system

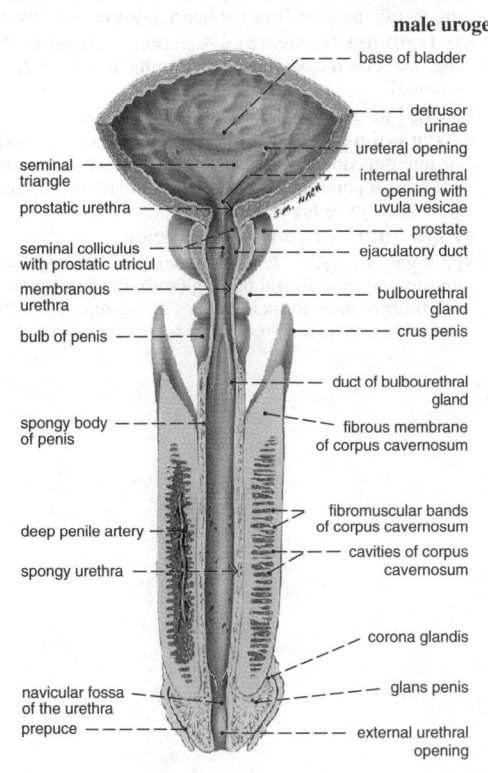

base of bladder
detrusor urinae
ureteral opening
internal urethral opening with uvula vesicae
seminal triangle
prostatic urethra
prostate
seminal colliculus with prostatic utricul
ejaculatory duct
membranous urethra
bulbourethral gland
bulb of penis
crus penis
duct of bulbourethral gland
spongy body of penis
fibrous membrane of corpus cavernosum
deep penile artery
fibromuscular bands of corpus cavernosum
spongy urethra
cavities of corpus cavernosum
corona glandis
navicular fossa of the urethra
glans penis
prepuce
external urethral opening

base of bladder and urethra in longitudinal section (skin of penis removed as far as prepuce)

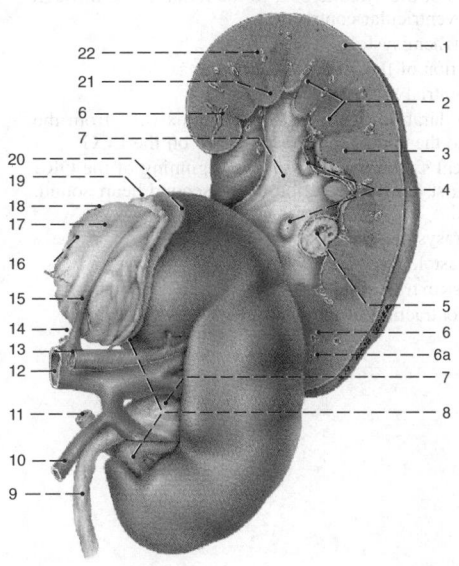

ventral view of left kidney and adrenal gland and frontal cross-section of adult left kidney

kidney

1 renal cortex
2 renal medulla, renal pyramid
3 renal column
4 cribriform area
5 fat body of renal artery
6 interlobar artery
6a arcuate artery
7 renal pelvis
8 renal hilum
9 left ureter
10 left testicular vein

11 posterior branch of renal artery
12 renal vein
13 anterior branch of renal artery
14 inferior suprarenal artery
15 suprarenal vein
16 middle suprarenal arteries
17 suprarenal gland
18 superior suprarenal arteries
19 perirenal fat
20 fibrous capsule of the kidney
21 base of renal pyramid; renal medulla
22 renal papilla

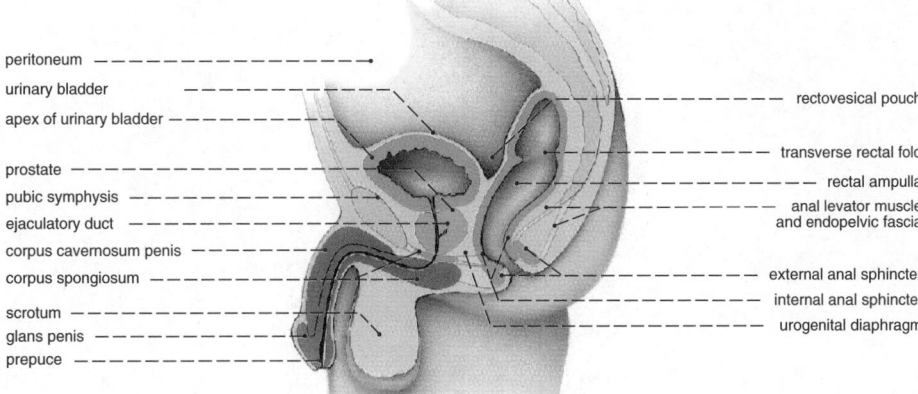

peritoneum
urinary bladder
apex of urinary bladder
prostate
pubic symphysis
ejaculatory duct
corpus cavernosum penis
corpus spongiosum
scrotum
glans penis
prepuce

rectovesical pouch
transverse rectal fold
rectal ampulla
anal levator muscle and endopelvic fascia
external anal sphincter
internal anal sphincter
urogenital diaphragm

male urogenital tract
sagittal view of male pelvis (schematic)

ventricles, by which the blood is driven through the aorta and pulmonary artery to traverse the systemic and pulmonary circulations, respectively; its occurrence is indicated physically by the first sound of the heart heard on auscultation, by the palpable apex beat, and by the arterial pulse. [G. *systolē,* a contracting]

aborted s., a loss of the systolic beat in the radial pulse through weakness of the ventricular contraction.

s. alter′nans, SYN hemisystole.

atrial s., contraction of the atria. SYN auricular s.

auricular s., SYN atrial s.

electrical s., the duration of the QRS-T complex (*i.e.,* from the earliest q-wave to the end of the latest T wave on the ECG.

electromechanical s., the period from the beginning of the QRS complex to the first (aortic) vibration of the second heart sound. SYN Q-S$_2$ interval.

extra-s., SEE extrasystole.

late s., SYN prediastole.

premature s., SYN extrasystole.

ventricular s., contraction of the ventricles.

sys·tol·ic (sis-tol′ik). Relating to, or occurring during cardiac systole.

sys·to·lom·e·ter (sis′tō-lom′ĕ-ter). **1.** An apparatus for determining the force of the cardiac contraction. **2.** An instrument for analyzing the sounds of the heart. [systole + G. *metron,* measure]

sys·trem·ma (sis-trem′ă). A muscular cramp in the calf of the leg, the contracted muscles forming a hard ball. [G. anything twisted]

sy·zyg·i·al (si-zij′ē-ăl). Relating to syzygy.

sy·zyg·i·ol·o·gy (si-zij′ē-ol′ō-jē). The study of interrelationships, or interdependencies, especially of the whole, as opposed to the study of separate parts or isolated functions. [G. *syzygios,* yoked (see syzygy), + *logos,* study]

sy·zyg·i·um (si-zij′ē-ŭm). SYN syzygy.

syz·y·gy (siz′i-jē). **1.** The association of gregarine protozoans end-to-end or in lateral pairing (without sexual fusion). **2.** Pairing of chromosomes in meiosis. SYN syzygium. [G. *syzygios,* yoked, bound together, fr. *syn,* together, + *zygon,* a yoke]

τ Tau, 19th letter of the Greek alphabet; symbol for relaxation *time*.

θ, Θ Theta, 8th letter in the Greek alphabet; symbol for angle.

T 1. Symbol for ribothymidine; tension (T+, increased tension; T–, diminished tension); tera-; tesla, the unit of magnetic field strength; tritium; threonine; torque; transmittance. **2.** As a subscript, refers to tidal *volume*. **3.** Abbreviation for thoracic vertebra (T1 to T12); tocopherol. **4.** Symbol for Tesla, the unit of magnetic field strength.

α-T. Symbol for α-tocopherol.

β-T. Symbol for β-tocopherol.

γ-T. Symbol for γ-tocopherol.

T1. In magnetic resonance, the time for 63% of longitudinal relaxation to occur; the value is a function of magnetic field strength and the chemical environment of the hydrogen nucleus; for protons in fat and in water, in a 1.5T magnet, about 250 msec and 3000 msec respectively. A T1-weighted image will have a bright fat signal.

T2. In magnetic resonance, the time for 63% of transverse relaxation to occur; the value is a function of magnetic field strength and the chemical environment of the hydrogen nucleus; for protons in fat and in water, in a 1.5T magnet, about 60 msec and 250 msec respectively. A T2-weighted image will have a bright water signal.

2,4,5-T Abbreviation for (2,4,5-trichlorophenoxy) acetic acid.

T Symbol for absolute *temperature* (kelvin).

T_m Symbol for *temperature* midpoint (kelvin); melting *point*.

T_3 Symbol for 3,5,3′-triiodothyronine.

T_4 Symbol for thyroxine.

t Abbreviation for metric ton; time.

t Symbol for temperature (Celsius); tritium.

t_m Symbol for *temperature* midpoint (Celsius).

Ta Symbol for tantalum.

tab·a·nid (tab′ă-nid). Common name for flies of the family Tabanidae. [L. *tabanus,* gadfly]

Ta·ban·i·dae (tă-ban′i-dē). A family of bloodsucking flies that includes the genera *Tabanus* (horsefly) and *Chrysops* (deerfly and mango fly), which are involved in transmission of several blood-borne parasites. [L. *tabanus,* gadfly]

Ta·ba·nus (tă-bā′nŭs). The gadflies and horseflies; a genus of biting flies, some species of which transmit surra, infectious equine anemia, anthrax, and other diseases. [L. a gadfly]

ta·bar·dil·lo (tah-bar-dē′yō). Mexican term for typhus. [Sp., fr. L.L. *tabardilii,* pustules]

ta·ba·tière an·a·to·mique (tab-ah-tē-ār′ an-ah-to-mēk′). SYN anatomical snuffbox. [Fr. snuffbox]

ta·bel·la, pl. **ta·bel·lae** (tă-bel′lă, -lē). A medicated tablet or lozenge. [L. dim. of *tabula,* tablet]

ta·bes (tā′bēz). Progressive wasting or emaciation. [L. a wasting away]

t. diabet′ica, diabetic neuropathy, especially affecting the motor nerves of the lower extremities, marked by muscular atrophy and a steppage gait.

t. dorsa′lis, SYN tabetic *neurosyphilis.*

t. ergot′ica, ataxia, amyotrophy, and neuralgic pain seen in ergot intoxication.

t. infan′tum, t. in infants with congenital syphilis.

t. mesenter′ica, tuberculosis of the mesenteric and retroperitoneal lymph nodes.

peripheral t., SYN pseudotabes.

t. spasmod′ica, SYN spastic *diplegia.*

t. spina′lis, SYN tabetic *neurosyphilis.*

ta·bes·cence (ta-bes′ens). The state of progressive wasting away.

ta·bes·cent (ta-bes′ent). Characteristic of tabes. [L. *tabesco,* to waste away, fr. *tabes,* a wasting away]

ta·bet·ic (ta-bet′ik). Relating to or suffering from tabes, especially tabes dorsalis. SYN tabic, tabid.

ta·bet·i·form (ta-bet′i-fōrm). Resembling tabes, especially tabes dorsalis. [irreg. formed fr. L. *tabes,* a wasting, + *forma,* form]

tab·ic (tab′ik). SYN tabetic.

tab·id. SYN tabetic. [L. *tabidus,* wasting away]

tab·la·ture (tab-lă-chūr). The state of division of the cranial bones into two plates separated by the diploë. [L. *tabula,* tablet]

ta·ble (tā′bl). **1.** One of the two plates or laminae, separated by the diploë, into which the cranial bones are divided. **2.** An arrangement of data in parallel columns, showing the essential facts in a readily appreciable form. [L. *tabula*]

Aub-DuBois t., t. of basal metabolic rates in calories per square meter of body surface per hour or day for different ages.

contingency t., a tabular cross-classification of data such that subcategories of one characteristic are indicated in rows (horizontally) and subcategories of another are indicated in columns (vertically).

examining t., a t. on which the patient lies during a medical examination.

Gaffky t., a numerical rating for the classification of tuberculosis according to the number of tubercle bacilli in the sputum, ranging from 1 (one to four organisms in the whole preparation) to 9 (an average of 100 per field). SYN Gaffky scale.

inner t. of skull, the inner compact layer of the cranial bones. SYN lamina interna cranii [NA].

life t., a representation of the probable years of survivorship of a defined population of subjects; since survivorship is changed by new methods of prevention or treatment, a diachronic study is commonly used because the main interest lies in the composite structure of the current population. (In the summarizing technique used to describe the pattern of mortality and survival in a population, survivors to age *x* are denoted by the symbol l*x* and the expectation of life at age *x* is denoted by the symbol *x*.)

occlusal t., the occlusal or grinding surfaces of the bicuspid and molar teeth.

operating t., a t. on which the patient lies during a surgical operation.

outer t. of skull, the outer compact layer of the cranial bones. SYN lamina externa cranii [NA].

Reuss' color t.'s, obsolete charts in which colored letters are printed on colored backgrounds in such combination that some of them are invisible to a person with deficient color vision. SYN Stilling color t.'s.

Stilling color t.'s, SYN Reuss' color t.'s.

tilt t., a t. with a top capable of being rotated on its transverse axis so that a patient lying upon it can be brought into the erect position as desired; used in experimental investigation and in physical therapy.

vitreous t., the inner t. of one of the cranial bones; it is more compact and harder than the outer t. SYN lamina internal ossium cranii.

ta·ble·spoon (tā′bl-spūn). A large spoon, used as a measure of the dose of a medicine, equivalent to about 4 fluidrams or ½ fluidounce or 15 ml.

tab·let. A solid dosage form containing medicinal substances with or without suitable diluents; it may vary in shape, size, and weight, and may be classed according to the method of manufacture, as molded t. and compressed t. SYN tabule. [Fr. *tablette,* L. *tabula*]

buccal t., usually a small, flat t. intended to be inserted in the buccal pouch, where the active ingredient is absorbed directly through the oral mucosa; such a t. dissolves or erodes slowly.

compressed t., a t. prepared, usually as a large-scale production, by means of great pressure; most compressed t.'s consist of the active ingredient and a diluent, binder, disintegrator, and lubricant.

dispensing t., a t. prepared by molding or by compression; used

ta

by the dispensing pharmacist to obtain certain potent substances in a convenient form for accurate compounding.

enteric coated t., an oral dosage form in which a t. is coated with a material to prevent or minimize dissolution in the stomach but allow dissolution in the small intestine. This type of formulation either protects the stomach from a potentially irritating drug (*e.g.,* aspirin) or protects the drug (*e.g.,* erythromycin) from partial degradation in the acidic environment of the stomach.

hypodermic t., a compressed or molded t. that dissolves completely in water to form an injectable solution.

prolonged action t., repeat action t., SYN sustained action t.

sublingual t., usually a small, flat t. intended to be inserted beneath the tongue, where the active ingredient is absorbed directly through the oral mucosa; such a t. (*e.g.,* nitroglyerine)-dissolves very promptly.

sustained action t., sustained release t., a drug product formulation that provides the required dosage initially and then maintains or repeats it at desired intervals. SYN prolonged action t., repeat action t.

t. triturate, a small, usually cylindrical, molded or compressed disk of varying size, containing a diluent usually consisting of dextrose (glucose) or of a mixture of lactose and powdered sucrose and a moistening agent or excipient, such as dilute alcohol.

ta·boo, ta·bu (tă-bū′). Restricted, prohibited, or forbidden; set apart for religious or ceremonial purposes. [Tongan, set apart]

ta·bo·pa·re·sis (tā′bō-pă-rē′sis, -par′ē-sis). A condition in which the symptoms of tabes dorsalis and general paresis are associated.

tab·u·lar (tab′yū-lăr). **1.** Tablelike. **2.** Arranged in the form of a table (2). [L. *tabularis,* fr. *tabula,* table]

tab·ule (tab′yūl). SYN tablet. [L. *tabula*]

ta·bun (tā′bŭn). Dimethylphosphoramidocyanidic acid, ethyl ester; an extremely potent cholinesterase inhibitor; the lethal dose for man is believed to be as low as 0.01 mg per kg; median lethal dosage (respiratory) is about 40 mg. min/m³ for resting men.

Tac (tak) A 55 kD polypeptide that is the one of the two chains that comprise the IL-2 receptor.

tache (tash). A circumscribed discoloration of the skin or mucous membrane, such as a macule or freckle. [Fr. spot]

t. blanche, SYN *macula* albida.

t. bleuâtre, SYN *macula* cerulea.

t. cérébrale, SYN meningitic *streak.*

t. laiteuse, (1) SYN milk *spots,* under *spot.* **(2)** SYN *macula* albida. [Fr., milky spot]

t. méningéale, SYN meningitic *streak.*

t. noire, a necrotic area covered with black crust (eschar), characteristic of the tick bite lesion in certain tick-borne diseases.

t. spina′le, a trophic bulla forming on the skin in certain cases of disease of the spinal cord.

ta·chet·ic (tă-ket′ik). Marked by bluish or brownish spots. [Fr. *tache,* spot]

ta·chis·tes·the·sia (tă-kis′tes-thē′zē-ă). An obsolete term for recognition of light flicker. [G. *tachistos,* very rapid, from *tachys,* rapid, + *aesthēsis,* perception]

ta·chis·to·scope (tă-kis′tō-skōp). An instrument to determine the shortest time an object must be exposed in order to be perceived. [G. *tachistos,* very rapid, fr. *tachys,* rapid, + *skopeō,* to view]

tach·o·gram (tak′ō-gram). Record made by a tachometer. [G. *tachos,* speed, + *gramma,* mark]

tach·o·graph (tak′ō-graf). A tachometer designed to provide a continuous record of speed or rate. [G. *tachos,* speed, + *graphō,* to write]

ta·chog·ra·phy (tă-kog′ră-fē). The recording of speed or rate. [G. *tachos,* speed, + *graphō,* to write]

ta·chom·e·ter (tă-kom′ĕ-ter). An instrument for measuring speed or rate; *e.g.,* revolutions of a shaft, heart rate (cardiotachometer), arterial blood flow (hemotachometer), respiratory gas flow (pneumotachometer). [G. *tachos,* speed, + *metron,* measure]

△**tachy-.** Rapid. [G. *tachys,* quick,]

tach·y·ar·rhyth·mia (tak′ē-ă-ridh′mē-ă). Any disturbance of the heart's rhythm, regular or irregular, resulting by convention in a rate over 100 beats per minute during physical examination. [tachy- + G. *a-* priv. + *rhythmos,* rhythm]

tach·y·aux·e·sis (tak′ē-awk-sē′sis). Type of growth in which a part grows more rapidly than the whole. [tachy- + G. *auxō,* to increase]

tach·y·car·dia (tak′i-kar′dē-ă). Rapid beating of the heart, conventionally applied to rates over 100 per minute. SYN polycardia, tachyrhythmia, tachysystole. [tachy- + G. *kardia,* heart]

atrial t., paroxysmal t. originating in an ectopic focus in the atrium. SYN auricular t.

atrial chaotic t., multifocal origin of tachycardia within the atrium; often confused with atrial fibrillation during physical examination.

atrioventricular junctional t., t. originating in the A-V junction. SYN A-V junctional t., nodal t.

auricular t., SYN atrial t.

A-V junctional t., SYN atrioventricular junctional t.

bidirectional ventricular t., ventricular t. in which the QRS complexes in the electrocardiogram are alternately mainly positive and mainly negative; many such cases may represent ventricular t. with alternating forms of aberrant ventricular conduction.

Coumel's t., a persistent junctional reciprocating t. that usually uses a slowly conducting posteroseptal pathway for the retrograde journey.

double t., the simultaneous t. of two ectopic pacemakers, *e.g.,* atrial and junctional t.

ectopic t., a t. originating in a focus other than the sinus node, *e.g.,* atrial, A-V junctional, or ventricular t.

t. en salves, short runs of paroxysmal t. of the Gallavardin type. Cf. Gallavardin's *phenomenon.* [Fr. *tachycardia in salvos*]

essential t., persistent rapid action of the heart due to no discoverable organic lesion.

t. exophthal′mica, rapid heart action occurring as one of the symptoms of exophthalmic goiter.

fetal t., a fetal heart rate of 160 or more beats per minute.

junctional t., supraventricular t. arising from the atrioventricular junction (formerly called nodal t.).

nodal t., SYN atrioventricular junctional t.

orthostatic t., increased heart rate on assuming the erect posture.

paroxysmal t., recurrent attacks of t., with abrupt onset and often also abrupt termination, originating from an ectopic focus which may be atrial, A-V junctional, or ventricular.

reflex t., increased heart rate in response to some stimulus conveyed through the cardiac nerves.

sinus t., t. originating in the sinus node.

supraventricular t., rapid heart rate due to a pacemaker anywhere above the ventricular level, *i.e.,* sinus node, atrium, atrioventricular junction. The QRS complexes are always narrow unless there is rate related aberrancy or preexisting intraventricular conduction delay.

ventricular t., paroxysmal t. originating in an ectopic focus in the ventricle. SEE ALSO torsade de pointes.

tach·y·car·di·ac (tak-i-kar′dē-ak). Relating to or suffering from excessively rapid action of the heart.

tach·y·car·dic (tar-i-kar′dik). Relating to rapid heart rate.

tach·y·crot·ic (tak′i-krot′ik). Relating to, causing, or characterized by a rapid pulse. [tachy- + G. *krotos,* a striking]

tach·y·ki·nin (tak-ē-kī′nin). Any member of a group of polypeptides, widely scattered in vertebrate and invertebrate tissues, that have in common four of the five terminal amino acids: Phe-Xaa-Gly-Leu-Met-NH₂; pharmacologically, they all cause hypotension in mammals, contraction of gut and bladder smooth muscle, and secretion of saliva. [G. *tachys,* swift, + *kineō,* to move, + *-in*]

tach·y·la·lia (tak-i-lā′lē-ă). Rarely used term for tachylogia. [tachy- + G. *lalia,* talking]

tach·y·lo·gia (tak-ĭ-lō′jē-ă). Rarely used term for rapid or voluble speech. SYN tachyphasia, tachyphemia, tachyphrasia. [tachy- + G. *logos,* word]

tach·y·pac·ing (tak′ĭ-pā′sing). Rapid pacing of the heart by an artificial electronic pacemaker operating faster than the basic cardiac rate.

tach·y·pha·gia (tak-i-fā′jē-ă). Rarely used term for rapid eating; bolting of food. [tachy- + G. *phagō*, to eat]

tach·y·pha·sia (tak-i-fā′zē-ă). SYN tachylogia. [tachy- + G. *phasis*, speaking]

tach·y·phe·mia (tak-ĭ-fē′mē-ă). SYN tachylogia. [tachy- + G. *phēmē*, speech]

tach·y·phra·sia (tak-ĭ-frā′zē-ă). SYN tachylogia. [tachy- + G. *phrasis*, speaking]

tach·y·phy·lax·is (tak′i-fĭ-lak′sis). Rapid appearance of progressive decrease in response following repetitive administration of a pharmacologically or physiologically active substance. [tachy- + G. *phylaxis*, protection]

tach·yp·nea (tak-ip-nē′ă). Rapid breathing. SYN polypnea. [tachy- + G. *pnoē* (*pnoiē*), breathing]

tach·y·rhyth·mia (tak-i-ridh′mē-ă). SYN tachycardia. [tachy- + G. *rhythmos*, rhythm]

ta·chys·ter·ol (tă-kis′ter-ōl). Sterol(s) formed by ultraviolet irradiation of any 5,7-diene-3β-sterol, which breaks the 9,10 bond, but usually from either or both of ergosterol and lumisterol to produce t.$_2$ (ertacalciol, (6*E*,22*E*)-9,10-secoergosta-5(10),6,8,22-tetraen-3β-ol) and from 7-dehydrocholesterol to produce t.$_3$ (tacalciol,(6*E*,3*S*)-9,10-secocholesta-5(10),6,8-trien-3β-ol). When reduced to the 5,7-diene (or 5,7,22-triene) form, dihydrotachysterol$_3$ (10,19-dihydrocalciol) or dihydrotachysterol$_2$ (10,19-dihydroercalciol), antirachitic action appears. This property has been of therapeutic interest, but t. is being replaced by the true vitamin D hormone (calcitriol) and its derivatives.

tach·y·sys·to·le (tak-i-sis′tō-lē). SYN tachycardia. [tachy- + G. *systolē*, contracting]

tach·y·zo·ite (tak-ĭ-zō′īt). A rapidly multiplying stage in the development of the tissue phase of certain coccidial infections, as in *Toxoplasma gondii* development in acute infections of toxoplasmosis. [tachy- + G. *zōon*, animal]

tac·rine (tak′rēn). 9-Amino-1,2,3,4-tetrahydroacridine; an anticholinesterase agent with nonspecific central nervous system stimulatory effects; has been used in early stages of Alzheimer's disease.

tac·tile (tak′til). Relating to touch or to the sense of touch. [L. *tactilis*, fr. *tango*, pp. *tactus*, to touch]

tac·tion (tak′shŭn). 1. The sense of touch. 2. The act of touching. [L. *tactio*, fr. *tango*, pp. *tactus*, to touch]

tac·tom·e·ter (tak-tom′ĕ-ter). SYN esthesiometer. [L. *tactus*, touch, + G. *metron*, measure]

tac·tor (tak′tăr, -tōr). A tactile end organ. [L. one who or that which touches]

tac·tu·al (tak′chūl). Relating to or caused by touch.

TAD Acronym for transient acantholytic *dermatosis*.

Tae·nia (tē′nē-ă). A genus of cestodes that formerly included most of the tapeworms, but is now restricted to those species infecting carnivores with cysticercus found in tissues of various herbivores, rodents, and other animals of prey. SEE ALSO tapeworm. [see taenia]

T. africa′na, a tapeworm found in native Africans, the cysticercus of which is unknown.

T. arma′ta, SYN *T. solium*.

T. crassic′ollis, SYN *T. taeniaeformis*.

T. demerarien′sis, former name for *Davainea madagascariensis*.

T. denta′ta, SYN *T. solium*.

T. equi′na, SYN *Anoplocephala perfoliata*.

T. hom′inis, unusual form of *T. saginata*.

T. hydatig′ena, a tapeworm of dogs, cats, wolves, foxes, and other carnivores; the larva is known as *Cysticercus tenuicollis*.

T. madagascarien′sis, former name for *Davainea madagascariensis*.

T. min′ima, former name for *Hymenolepis nana*.

T. o′vis, a tapeworm of dogs and foxes whose larval form is found in the muscles of sheep; heavy larval infections in sheep can have severe economic consequences due to condemnation of carcasses at meat inspection.

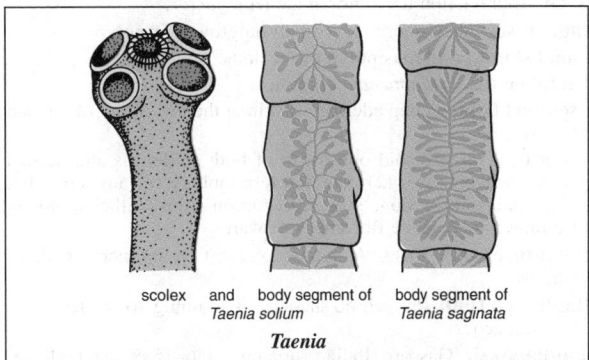

scolex and body segment of body segment of
Taenia solium *Taenia saginata*
Taenia

T. philippi′na, atypical form of *T. saginata*.

T. pisifor′mis, a common tapeworm of dogs, foxes, and other carnivores; the larval form is *Cysticercus pisiformis*.

T. quadriloba′ta, SYN *Anoplocephala perfoliata*.

T. sagina′ta, the beef, hookless, or unarmed tapeworm of humans, acquired by eating insufficiently cooked flesh of cattle infected with *Cysticercus bovis*.

T. so′lium, the pork, armed, or solitary tapeworm of man, acquired by eating insufficiently cooked pork infected with *Cysticercus cellulosae;* hatching of ova within the human intestine may result in establishment of cysticerci in human tissues, resulting in cysticercosis. SYN *T. armata*, *T. dentata*.

T. taeniaefor′mis, one of the common tapeworms of household cats; the larval form is called *Cysticercus fasciolaris*. SYN *Hydatigera taeniaeformis*, *T. crassicollis*.

tae·nia (tē′nē-ă). 1. A coiled bandlike anatomical structure. SEE tenia (1). 2. Common name for a tapeworm, especially of the genus *Taenia*. SYN tenia (2). [L., fr. G. *tainia*, band, tape, a tapeworm]

Tae·ni·a·rhyn·chus (tē′nē-ă-ring′kŭs). A genus established for the *Taenia* species having a rudimentary rostellum but lacking the rostellar hooklets typical of *Taenia*. The best known example is *Taeniarhynchus saginatus*, but the older name, *Taenia saginata*, is more commonly used. [G. *tainia*, band, + *rhynchos*, snout]

tae·ni·a·sis (tē-nē-ī′ă-sis). Infection with cestodes of the genus *Taenia*.

tae·ni·id (tē-nē′id). Common name for a member of the family Taeniidae.

Tae·ni·i·dae (tē-nē′i-dē). A family of parasitic cestodes (order Cyclophyllidea) that includes the genera *Taenia*, *Taeniarhynchus*, *Multiceps*, and *Echinococcus*.

tae·ni·oid (tē′nē-oyd). Denoting members of the genus *Taenia*.

Tae·ni·o·rhyn·chus (tē-nē-ō-ring′kŭs). A genus and subgenus of mosquitoes now considered synonymous with *Mansonia*. [G. *tainia*, band, + *rhynchos*, snout]

Taenzer, Paul R., German dermatologist, 1858–1919. SEE T.'s *stain;* Unna-T. *stain*.

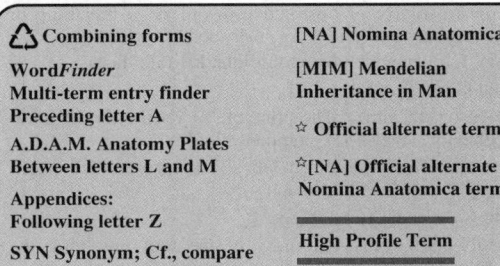

♻ **Combining forms**	**[NA] Nomina Anatomica**
Word*Finder* **Multi-term entry finder** Preceding letter A	**[MIM] Mendelian Inheritance in Man**
A.D.A.M. Anatomy Plates Between letters L and M	☆ **Official alternate term**
Appendices: Following letter Z	☆**[NA] Official alternate Nomina Anatomica term**
SYN Synonym; Cf., compare	**High Profile Term**

Ta

TAF Abbreviation for tumor angiogenic *factor*.

tag. **1.** SEE label, tracer. **2.** A small outgrowth or polyp.

anal skin t., a fibrous polyp of the anus.

epiploic t.'s, SYN *appendix* epiploica.

sentinel t., projecting edematous skin at the lower end of an anal fissure.

skin t., (1) a polypoid outgrowth of both epidermis and dermal fibrovascular tissue; **(2)** common terminology for any small benign cutaneous lesion. SYN acrochordon, fibroepithelial polyp, fibroma molle, senile fibroma, soft wart.

tag·a·tose (tag′ă-tōs). A ketohexose; D-t. is epimeric with D-fructose.

tag·li·a·co·ti·an (tal-yah-cō′shē-an). Pertaining to or described by Tagliacozzi.

Tagliacozzi, Gaspare, Italian surgeon, 1546–1599. SEE tagliacotian *operation.*

tail (tāl). **1.** Any tail, or tail-like structure, or tapering or elongated extremity of an organ or other part. **2.** In veterinary anatomy, a free appendage representing the caudal end of the vertebral column; covered by skin and hair, feathers, or scales. SYN cauda [NA]. [A.S. *taegl*]

t. of caudate nucleus, the elongated posterior extension of the caudate nucleus that parallels the body and inferior horn of the lateral ventricle. SYN cauda nuclei caudati [NA], cauda striati.

t. of dentate gyrus, SYN uncus *band* of Giacomini.

t. of epididymis, the inferior part of the epididymis that leads into the ductus deferens; part of the reservoir of spermatozoa. SYN cauda epididymidis [NA], cauda epididymis, globus minor.

t. of helix, a flattened process terminating the cartilage of the helix of the ear, posteriorly and inferiorly. SYN cauda helicis [NA].

t. of pancreas, the left extremity of the pancreas within the lienorenal ligament. SYN cauda pancreatis [NA].

tail·gut (tāl′gŭt). SYN postanal *gut*.

Tait, Robert L., English gynecologist, 1845–1899. SEE T.'s *law*.

Ta·ka·di·as·tase (tă′kă-dī′as-tās). SYN α-amylase.

Takahara, Shigeo, 20th century Japanese otolaryngologist. SEE T.'s *disease*.

Takayama, Masao, Japanese physician, *1872. SEE T.'s *stain*.

Takayasu (Takayashu). Michishige, Japanese ophthalmologist, *1872. SEE Takayasu's *arteritis*, Takayasu's *disease*, Takayasu's *syndrome*.

take (tāk). A successful grafting operation or vaccination.

ta·lal·gia (tă-lal′jē-ă). Pain in the ankle. [L. *talus,* ankle, G. *algos,* pain]

ta·lar (tā′lăr). Relating to the talus.

Talbot, William Henry Fox, British scientist, 1800–1877. SEE Plateau-T. *law*.

tal·bu·tal (tal′byū-tăl). 5-Allyl-5-*sec*-butylbarbituric acid; a short-acting hypnotic and sedative.

talc (tălk). Native hydrous magnesium silicate, sometimes containing small proportions of aluminum silicate, purified by boiling powdered t. with hydrochloric acid in water; used in pharmacy as a filter aid, as a dusting powder, and in cosmetic preparations. SYN French chalk, soapstone, talcum. [Ar. *talq*]

tal·co·sis (tal-kō′sis). A pulmonary disorder related to silicosis, occurring in workers exposed to talc mixed with silicates; characterized by restrictive or obstructive disorders of breathing or the two in combination. [talc + G. -osis, condition]

pulmonary t., pneumoconiosis from inhaling talc dusts.

tal·cum (tal′kŭm). SYN talc. [L.]

tal·i·on (tal′ē-on, tal′yŭn). The principle of retribution in intrapsychic behavior. [Welsh *tal,* compensation]

tal·i·on dread. The symbolic anxieties that represent the unconscious dread of penalties for an act.

tal·i·ped·ic (tal-i-ped′ik). Clubfooted.

tal·i·pes (tal′i-pēz). Any deformity of the foot involving the talus. [L. *talus,* ankle, + *pes,* foot]

t. arcua′tus, SYN t. cavus.

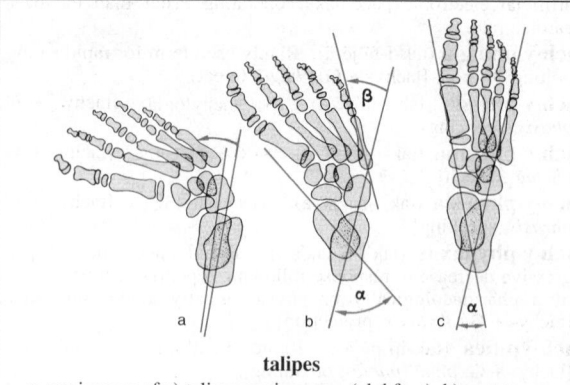

talipes
x-ray images of a) talipes equinovarus (clubfoot), b) metatarsus varus (intoe), c) normal foot

t. calcaneoval′gus, t. calcaneus and t. valgus combined; the foot is dorsiflexed, everted, and abducted. SEE clubfoot.

t. calcaneova′rus, t. calcaneus and t. varus combined; the foot is dorsiflexed, inverted, and adducted. SEE clubfoot.

t. calca′neus, a deformity due to weakness or absence of the calf muscles, in which the axis of the calcaneus becomes vertically oriented; commonly seen in poliomyelitis. SYN calcaneus (2).

t. ca′vus, an exaggeration of the normal arch of the foot. SYN contracted foot (1), pes cavus, t. arcuatus, t. plantaris.

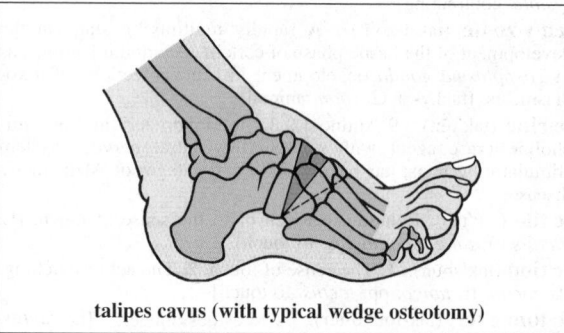

talipes cavus (with typical wedge osteotomy)

t. equinoval′gus, t. equinus and t. valgus combined; the foot is plantarflexed, everted, and abducted. SEE clubfoot. SYN equinovalgus, pes equinovalgus.

t. equinova′rus, t. equinus and t. varus combined; the foot is plantarflexed, inverted, and adducted. SEE clubfoot. SYN clubfoot, equinovarus, pes equinovarus.

t. equi′nus, permanent extension of the foot so that only the ball rests on the ground; it is commonly combined with t. varus.

t. planta′ris, SYN t. cavus.

t. pla′nus, SYN *pes* planus.

t. spasmod′icus, a temporary distortion of the foot, usually t. equinus, due to muscular spasm.

t. transversopla′nus, SYN *metatarsus* latus.

t. val′gus, permanent eversion of the foot, the inner side alone of the sole resting on the ground; it is usually combined with a breaking down of the plantar arch. SYN pes abductus, pes pronatus, pes valgus.

t. va′rus, inversion of the foot, the outer side of the sole only touching the ground; usually some degree of t. equinus is associated with it, and often t. cavus. SYN pes adductus, pes varus.

tal·i·pom·a·nus (tal-ĭ-pom′ă-nŭs, -pō-mā′nŭs). Archaic term for clubhand. [Mod. L. *talipes* + *manus,* hand]

tal·low (tal′ō). The rendered fat from mutton suet.

prepared mutton t., SYN prepared *suet*.

△**talo-**. The talus. [L. *talus,* ankle, ankle bone]

ta·lo·cal·ca·ne·al, ta·lo·cal·ca·ne·an (tā-lō-kal-kā′nē-ăl, tā-lō-kal-kā′nē-an). Relating to the talus and the calcaneus.

ta·lo·cru·ral (tā′lō-krū′răl). Relating to the talus and the bones of the leg; denoting the ankle joint.

ta·lo·fib·u·lar (tă′lō-fib′yū-lăr). Relating to the talus and the fibula.

tal·on. The caudally directed digit on the foot, particularly of a bird of prey. [Mediev. L. *talo,* claw of a bird]

ta·lo·na·vic·u·lar (tă′lō-nă-vik′yū-lăr). Relating to the talus and the navicular bone. SYN astragaloscaphoid, taloscaphoid.

ta·lo·scaph·oid (tă′lō-skaf′oyd). SYN talonavicular.

tal·ose (tal′ōs). An aldohexose, isomeric with glucose; D-t. is epimeric with D-galactose.

ta·lo·tib·i·al (tă′lō-tib′ē-ăl). Relating to the talus and the tibia.

ta·lus, gen. **ta·li** (tā′lŭs, -lī) [NA]. The bone of the foot that articulates with the tibia and fibula to form the ankle joint. SYN ankle bone, ankle (3). [L. ankle bone, heel]

tam·a·rind (tam′ă-rind). The pulp of the fruit of *Tamarindus indica* (family Leguminosae), a large tree of India; mildly laxative. [Mediev. L. fr. Ar. *tamr*]

tam·bour (tahm-bur′). The recording part of a graphic apparatus, such as a sphygmograph, consisting of a membrane stretched across the open end of a cylinder and the recording styile attached to it. [Fr. drum]

Tamm, Igor, U.S. virologist, *1922. SEE T.-Horsfall *mucoprotein, protein.*

ta·mox·i·fen cit·rate (tă-mok′si-fen). (Z)-2-[p-(1,2-Diphenyl-1-butenyl)phenoxy]-N,N-dimethylethylamine citrate (1:1); an antiestrogen agent used in the treatment of breast cancer.

tam·pon. 1. A cylinder or ball of cotton-wool, gauze, or other loose substance; used as a plug or pack in a canal or cavity to restrain hemorrhage, absorb secretions, or maintain a displaced organ in position. 2. To insert such a plug or pack. [O. Fr.]

Corner's t., a plug of omentum stuffed into a wound of the stomach or intestine as a temporary t.

tam·pon·ade, tam·pon·age (tam-pŏ-nād′, tam′pŏ-nij). The insertion of a tampon.

cardiac t., compression of the heart due to critically increased volume of fluid in the pericardium. SYN heart t.

chronic t., cardiac compression over long periods due to pathologically increased fluid in the pericardial sac.

heart t., SYN cardiac t.

tam·pon·ing, tam·pon·ment (tam′pon-ing, tam-pon′ment). The act of inserting a tampon.

ta·nace·tol, tan·a·ce·tone (ta-nās′tol, tan-ă-sē′tōn). SYN thujone.

tan·dem (tan′dem). Term used to describe multiple copies of the same sequence in a polynucleic acid that lie adjacent to one another.

tan·gen·ti·al·i·ty (tan-jen′shē-al′i-tē). A disturbance in the associative thought process in which one tends to digress readily from one topic under discussion to other topics which arise in the course of associations; observed in bipolar disorder and schizophrenia and certain types of organic brain disorders. Cf. circumstantiality. [off on a tangent, fr. L. *tango,* to touch]

tan·gle (tang′l). A small irregular knot.

neurofibrillary t., intraneuronal accumulations of helical filaments that assume twisted contorted patterns; found in cells of the hippocampus and cerebral cortex in individuals with Alzheimer disease.

tank. A device made to receive and/or hold liquids.

Hubbard t., a large t., usually filled with warm water, used for therapeutic exercises in a program of physiotherapy.

tan·nase (tan′ās). Tannin acyl-hydrolase, an enzyme produced in cultures of *Penicillium glaucum* and found in certain tannin-forming plants; it hydrolyzes digallate to gallate, and also acts on ester links in other tannins.

tan·nate (tan′āt). A salt of tannic acid.

Tanner growth chart. See under chart.

Tanner stage. See under stage.

tan·nic (tan′ik). Relating to tan (tan-bark) or to tannin.

tan·nic ac·id. A tannin, $C_{76}H_{52}O_{46}$, that occurs in many plants, particularly in the bark of oaks and other members of the Fagaceae; used as a styptic and astringent, and in the treatment of diarrhea; available also as tannic acid glycerite. Sometimes used synonymously with tannin.

tan·nin (tan′in). Any one of a group of complex nonuniform plant constituents that can be classified into hydrolyzable t.'s (esters of a sugar, usually glucose, and one or several trihydroxybenzenecarboxylic acids) and condensed t.'s (derivatives of flavonols). T.'s are used in tanning, dyeing, photography, and as clarifying agents for beer and wine. Sometimes used synonymously with tannic acid; they form black stains in the presence of iron.

tan·nyl·ac·e·tate (tan-il-as′ĕ-tāt). SYN acetyltannic acid.

tan·ta·lum (Ta) (tan′tă-lŭm). A heavy metal of the vanadium group, atomic no. 73, atomic wt. 180.9479; used in surgical prostheses because of its noncorrosive properties. [G. mythical king of Lydia *Tantalus*]

tan·trum (tan′trŭm). A fit of bad temper, especially in children.

tan·y·cyte (tan′i-sīt). A variety of ependymal cell found principally in the walls of the third ventricle of the brain; the t.'s may have branched or unbranched processes, some of which end on capillaries or neurons.

tan·y·pho·nia (tan-i-fō′nē-ă). A thin, weak voice resulting from tension of vocal muscles. [G. *tanyō,* to stretch, + *phonē,* sound]

tap. 1. To withdraw fluid from a cavity by means of a trocar and cannula, hollow needle, or catheter. 2. To strike lightly with the finger or a hammerlike instrument in percussion or to elicit a tendon reflex. 3. A light blow. 4. An East Indian fever of undetermined nature. 5. An instrument to cut threads in a hole in bone prior to inserting a screw. [M.E. *tappe,* fr. A.S. *taeppa*]

heel t., a reflex movement of the toes when the heel is tapped, present in multiple sclerosis and other diseases of the pyramidal tract.

mitral t., the palpable equivalent of the opening snap of the mitral valve.

pericardial t., SYN pericardicentesis.

spinal t., SYN lumbar *puncture.*

tape (tāp). A thin flat strip of fascia or tendon, or of synthetic material, used as a tie or suture. [A.S. *taeppe*]

adhesive t., fabric or film evenly coated on one side with a pressure-sensitive adhesive mixture.

ta·pe·to·cho·roi·dal (tă-pē′tō-kō-roy′dăl). Relating to the tapetum and the choroid.

ta·pe·to·ret·i·nal (tă-pē′tō-ret′i-năl). Relating to the retinal pigment epithelium and the sensory retina.

ta·pe·to·ret·in·op·a·thy (tă-pē′tō-ret-in-op′ă-thē). Hereditary degeneration of the sensory retina and pigmentary epithelium; seen in pigmentary retinopathy, choroideremia, gyrate atrophy, congenital nyctalopia, congenital amaurosis, and heredomacular degeneration. [tapetum + retinopathy]

ta·pe·tum, pl. **ta·pe·ta** (tă-pē′tŭm, -tă). 1. In general, any membranous layer or covering. 2. In neuroanatomy, a thin sheet of fibers in the lateral wall of the temporal and occipital horns of the lateral ventricle, continuous with the corpus callosum. SYN Fielding's membrane, membrana versicolor. 3. A dense layer in

△ **Combining forms**	**[NA]** Nomina Anatomica
Word*Finder* Multi-term entry finder Preceding letter A	**[MIM]** Mendelian Inheritance in Man
A.D.A.M. Anatomy Plates Between letters L and M	☆ **Official alternate term**
Appendices: Following letter Z	☆**[NA]** Official alternate Nomina Anatomica term
SYN Synonym; Cf., compare	**High Profile Term**

ta

the choroidea of the eye of many mammalian species, including the cat and dog but not humans, that forms a discrete or diffuse area of reflective cells, rodlets, and fibers; its strong light-reflecting properties cause the metallic hue and light-glow of such eyes in the dark. [L. *tapeta,* a carpet]

t. alve′oli, SYN periodontal *ligament.*

t. ni′grum, SYN pigmented *layer* of retina.

t. oc′uli, SYN pigmented *layer* of retina.

tape·worm (tāp′werm). An intestinal parasitic worm, adults of which are found in the intestine of vertebrates; the term is commonly restricted to members of the class Cestoidea. T.'s consist of a scolex, variously equipped with spined or sucking structures by which the worm is attached to the intestinal wall of the host, and strobila having several to many proglottids that lack a digestive tract at any stage of development. The ovum, entering the intestine of an appropriate intermediate host, hatches and the hexacanth penetrates the gut wall and develops into a specific larval form (*e.g.,* cysticercoid, cysticercus, hydatid, strobilocercus), which develops into an adult when the intermediate host is ingested by the proper final host. A three-host cycle with a swimming coracidium, procercoid and plerocercoid (sparganum) larva, and adult intestinal worm is found in aquatic life cycles, as in *Diphyllobothrium latum* (broad fish t.) and other pseudophyllid cestodes. Other important species of t. are *Echinococcus granulosus* (hydatid t.), *Hymenolepis nana* or *H. nana* var. *fraterna* (dwarf or dwarf mouse t.), *Taenia saginata* (beef, hookless, or unarmed t.), *T. solium* (armed, pork, or solitary t.), and *Thysanosoma actinoides* (fringed t. of sheep).

taph·o·phil·ia (taf-ō-fil′ē-ă). Morbid attraction for graves. [G. *taphos,* grave, + *phileō,* to love]

taph·o·pho·bia (taf-ō-fō′bē-ă). Morbid fear of being buried alive. [G. *taphos,* the grave, + *phobos,* fear]

Tapia, Antonio, Spanish otolaryngologist, 1875–1950. SEE T.'s *syndrome.*

tap·i·no·ce·phal·ic (tap′i-nō-sĕ-fal′ik, tă-pī′nō-). Having a low flat head; relating to tapinocephaly.

tap·i·no·ceph·a·ly (tă-pi-nō-sef′ă-lē). A condition of flat head in which the skull has a vertical index below 72; similar to chamecephaly. [G. *tapeinos,* low, + *kephalē,* head]

tap·i·o·ca (tap′ē-ō′kă). A starch from the root of *Janipha manihot* and other species of *J.* (family Euphorbiaceae), plants of tropical America; an easily digested starch, free of irritant properties. SYN cassava starch. [Braz. *tipioca*]

ta·pote·ment (tă-pot-mawn′). A massage movement consisting in striking with the side of the hand, usually with partly flexed fingers. SYN tapping (1). [Fr. fr. *tapoter,* to tap]

tap·ping (tap′ing). **1.** SYN tapotement. **2.** SYN paracentesis.

TAR Acronym for thrombocytopenia and absent radius. SEE thrombocytopenia-absent radius *syndrome.*

tar. A thick, semisolid, blackish brown mass, of complex hydrocarbon composition, obtained by the destructive distillation of carbonaceous materials. For individual t.'s, see specific names.

rectified t. oil, a volatile oil distilled from pine t.; used externally in the treatment of skin diseases such as eczema and psoriasis.

tar·an·tism (tar′an-tizm). A form of mass hysteria which originated in Taranto, Italy, in the late Middle Ages as a dancing mania to cure the madness allegedly caused by the bite of a tarantula.

ta·ran·tu·la (tă-ran′chū-lă). A very large, hairy spider, considered highly venomous and often greatly feared; the bite, however, is usually no more harmful than a bee sting, and the creature is relatively inoffensive. [see tarantism]

American t., *Eurypelma hentzii,* the Arkansas t.; although greatly feared, its bite is relatively uncommon and harmless to humans.

black t., *Sericopelma communis,* a large black t. of Panama and the Canal Zone, whose bite is poisonous, although the effect is localized.

European t., *Lycosa tarentula,* the large European wolf spider or true t. Its bite was once believed to cause madness, which inspired frenzied contortions and dancing to rid the body of the

venom, though the bite is, in fact, harmless, as is that of most of the large, hairy "tarantula spiders" of the tropics.

Peruvian t., pruning spider, *Glyptocranium gasteracanthoides,* a poisonous Peruvian spider whose bite causes local gangrene, hematuria, and neurotoxic symptoms.

ta·rax·a·cum (tă-rak′să-kŭm). The dried rhizome and root of *Taraxacum officinale* (family Compositae), the dandelion, a wild plant of wide distribution throughout the temperate regions of the northern hemisphere; a tonic and hepatic stimulant. [Mod. L. fr. Ar. *tarakshagūn,* wild chicory]

Tardieu, Auguste A., French physician, 1818–1879. SEE T.'s *ecchymoses,* under *ecchymosis, petechiae,* under *petechiae, spots,* under *spot.*

tar·dive (tar′div). Late; tardy.

cyanose t., cyanosis due to right to left shunt in congenital heart disease appearing only after cardiac failure. SYN late cyanosis, tardive cyanosis.

tar·get (tar′get). **1.** An object fixed as goal or point of examination. **2.** In the ophthalmometer, the mire. **3.** SYN target *organ.* **4.** Anode of an x-ray tube. SEE ALSO x-ray. [It. *targhetta,* a small shield]

tar·get·ing (tar′get-ing). The process of having proteins contain certain signals such that the proteins are directed specifically towards certain cellular locations, *e.g.,* the lysosome. Cf. processing.

Tarin (Tarini, Tarinus), Pierre, French anatomist, 1725–1761. SEE T.'s *space, tenia, valve; valvula* semilunaris tarini; *velum* tarini.

ta·rir·ic ac·id (tă-rī′rik). An 18-carbon acid, $CH_3(CH_2)_{10}$-$C{\equiv}C(CH_2)_4COOH$, notable for the presence of a triple bond.

Tarlov, Isadore Max, U. S. surgeon, *1905. SEE T.'s *cyst.*

Tarnier, Étienne Stephane, French obstetrician, 1828–1897. SEE T.'s *forceps.*

tar·ra·gon oil (tar′ă-gon). A volatile oil distilled from the leaves of *Artemisia dranculus* (family Compositae); a flavoring. SYN estragon oil.

△tars-. SEE tarso-.

tars·ad·e·ni·tis (tar′sad-ĕ-nī′tis). An obsolete term for inflammation of the tarsal borders of the eyelids and meibomian glands. [tarsus + G. *adēn,* gland, + *-itis,* inflammation]

tar·sal (tar′săl). Relating to a tarsus in any sense.

tar·sa·le, pl. **tar·sa·lia** (tar-sā′lē, tar-sā′lē-ă). Any tarsal bone. [Mod. L. fr. G. *tarsos,* sole of the foot]

tars·al·gia (tar-sal′jē-ă). SYN podalgia. [tarsus + G. *algos,* pain]

tar·sa·lis (tar-sā′lis). SEE inferior tarsal *muscle,* superior tarsal *muscle.*

tars·ec·to·my (tar-sek′tō-mē). Excision of the tarsus of the foot or of a segment of the tarsus of an eyelid. [tarsus + G. *ektomē,* excision]

tar·sec·to·pia, tar·sec·to·py (tar-sek-tō′pē-ă, -sek′tō-pē). Subluxation of one or more tarsal bones. [tarsus + G. *ektopos,* out of place]

tar·sen. Within the tarsus; relating to the tarsus independent of other structures. [tarsus + G. *en,* in]

tar·si·tis (tar-sī′tis). **1.** Inflammation of the tarsus of the foot. **2.** Inflammation of the tarsal border of an eyelid.

△tarso-, tars-. A tarsus. [See tarsus]

tar·so·chi·lo·plas·ty (tar-sō-kī′lō-plas-tē). Obsolete term for a blepharoplasty of the tarsal margin of the eyelid. [tarso- + G. *cheilos,* lip, + *plassō,* to form]

tar·so·cla·sia, tar·soc·la·sis (tar-sō-klā′zē-ă, tar-sok′lă-sis). Instrumental fracture of the tarsus, for the correction of talipes equinovarus. [tarso- + G. *klasis,* a breaking]

tar·so·ma·la·cia (tar′sō-mă-lā′shē-ă). Softening of the tarsal cartilages of the eyelids. [tarso- + G. *malakia,* softness]

tar·so·meg·a·ly (tar-sō-meg′ă-lē). A congenital maldevelopment and overgrowth of a tarsal or carpal bone. SYN dysplasia epiphysialis hemimelia. [tarso- + G. *megas,* large]

tar·so·met·a·tar·sal (tar-sō-met′ă-tar′săl). Relating to the tarsal and metatarsal bones; denoting the articulations between the two sets of bones, and the ligaments in relation thereto.

tar·so·met·a·tar·sus (tar′sō-met-ă-tar′sŭs). The lowermost long bone or shank in the leg of a bird; the distal tarsal elements fuse with the metatarsals, resulting in a compound bone unlike that in mammals.

tar·so·or·bit·al (tar′sō-ōr′bi-tăl). Relating to the eyelids and the orbit.

tar·so·pha·lan·ge·al (tar-sō-fă-lan′jē-ăl). Relating to the tarsus and the phalanges.

tar·so·phy·ma (tar-sō-fī′mă). An obsolete word for a tarsal tumor. [tarso- + G. *phyma,* a tumor, boil]

tar·sor·rha·phy (tar-sōr′ă-fē). The suturing together of the eyelid margins, partially or completely, to shorten the palpebral fissure or to protect the cornea in keratitis or in paralysis of the orbicularis oculi muscle. [tarso- + G. *rhaphē,* suture]

tar·so·tar·sal (tar′sō-tar′săl). SYN intertarsal.

tar·so·tib·i·al (tar′sō-tib′ē-al). SYN tibiotarsal.

tar·sot·o·my (tar-sot′ŏ-mē). **1.** Incision of the tarsal cartilage of an eyelid. **2.** Any operation on the tarsus of the foot. [tarso- + G. *tomē,* incision]

tar·sus, gen. and pl. **tar·si** (tar′sŭs, -sī) [NA]. **1.** As a division of the skeleton, the seven tarsal bones of the instep. SEE tarsal *bones,* under *bone.* **2.** The fibrous plates giving solidity and form to the edges of the eyelids; often erroneously called tarsal or ciliary cartilages. SYN root of foot. [G. *tarsos,* a flat surface, sole of the foot, edge of eyelid]
t. infe′rior [NA], SYN inferior t.
inferior t., the fibrous plate in the lower eyelid. SYN t. inferior [NA].
t. supe′rior [NA], SYN superior t.
superior t., the fibrous plate in the upper eyelid. SYN t. superior [NA].

tar·tar (tar′tăr). **1.** A crust on the interior of wine casks, consisting essentially of potassium bitartrate. **2.** A white, brown, or yellow-brown deposit at or below the gingival margin of teeth, chiefly hydroxyapatite in an organic matrix. SYN dental calculus (2). [Mediev. L. *tartarum,* ult. etym. unknown]
cream of t., SYN *potassium* bitartrate.
t. emetic, SYN *antimony* potassium tartrate.
soluble t., SYN *potassium* tartrate.

tar·tar·ic ac·id (tar-tar′ik). HOOC–CHOH–CHOH–COOH; Dihydroxysuccinic acid; made from crude tartar; a laxative and refrigerant; used in the manufacture of various effervescing powders, tablets, and granules.

tar·trate (tar′trāt). A salt of tartaric acid.
acid t., a salt of tartaric acid which contains an acid group still capable of combining with a base; *e.g.,* bitartrate.
normal t., t. that contains no uncombined acid groups.

tar·trat·ed (tar′trāt-ed). Combined with or containing tartar or tartaric acid.

tar·tra·zine (tar′tră-zēn) [C.I. 19140]. A yellow acid dye, $C_{16}H_9N_4O_9S_2Na_3$, used in place of orange G in a variant of Mallory's aniline blue stain for collagen and cellular inclusion bodies. SYN hydrazine yellow.

taste (tāst). **1.** To perceive through the medium of the gustatory nerves. **2.** The sensation produced by a suitable stimulus applied to the gustatory nerve endings in the tongue. [It. *tastare;* L. *tango,* to touch]
after-t., SEE aftertaste.
color t., a form of synesthesia in which the color sense and t. are associated, with stimulation of either sense inducing a subjective sensation in the associated sense. SYN pseudogeusesthesia.
franklinic t., a metallic or sour t. produced by the application of static electricity to the tongue. SYN voltaic t.
voltaic t., SYN franklinic t.

TAT Abbreviation for thematic apperception *test.*

tat·too (tă-tū′). **1.** A deliberate decorative implanting or injecting of indelible pigments into the skin or the tinctorial effect of accidental implantation. **2.** To produce such an effect. [Tahiti, *tatu*]

amalgam t., a bluish-black or gray macular lesion of the oral mucous membrane caused by accidental implantation of silver amalgam into the tissue during tooth restoration or extraction.

tau (τ). **1.** 19th Letter of the Greek alphabet. **2.** Symbol for tele; relaxation time. **3.** A protein that associates with microtubules and other elements of the cytoskeleton; t. accelerates tubulin polymerization and stabilizes microtubules; t. is also found in the plaque observed in individuals with Alzheimer's disease.

tau·rine (taw′rin, -rēn). **1.** $NH_2CH_2CH_2SO_3H$; an amino sulfonic acid, synthesized from L-cysteine and used in a number of roles, including in the synthesis of certain bile salts. **2.** Of or pertaining to a bull. [L. *taurinus,* of bulls, fr. *taurus,* bull, + suffix -*inus,* pertaining to]

tau·ro·cho·late (taw-rō-kō′lāt). A salt of taurocholic acid.

tau·ro·cho·lic ac·id (taw-rō-kō′lik). cholyltaurine; *N*-choloyltaurine; a compound of cholic acid and taurine, involving the carboxyl group of the former and the amino of the latter; a common bile salt in carnivores. SYN cholaic acid.

tau·ro·don·tism (taw-rō-don′tizm). A developmental anomaly involving molar teeth in which the bifurcation or trifurcation of the roots is very near the apex, resulting in an abnormally large and long pulp chamber with exceedingly short pulp canals. [L. *taurus,* bull, + G. *odous,* tooth]

Taussig, Helen B., U.S. pediatrician, *1898. SEE T.-Bing *disease, syndrome;* Blalock-T. *operation, shunt.*

tau·to·me·ni·al (taw-tō-mē′nē-ăl). Relating to the same menstrual period. [G. *tautos,* the same, + *mēn,* month]

tau·to·mer·ic (taw-tō-mer′ik). **1.** Relating to the same part. **2.** Relating to or marked by tautomerism. [G. *tautos,* the same, + *meros,* part]

tau·tom·er·ism (taw-tom′er-izm). A phenomenon in which a chemical compound exists in two forms of different structure (isomers) in equilibrium, the two forms differing, usually, in the position of a hydrogen atom; *e.g.,* keto-enol t., $R–CH_2–C(O)–R'$ $\leftrightarrow R–CH=C(OH)–R'$. [G. *tautos,* the same, + *meros,* part]

Tawara, K. Sunao, Japanese pathologist, 1873–1952. SEE T.'s *node;* His-T. *system; node* of Aschoff and T.

taxa (tak′să). Plural of taxon.

tax·is (tak′sis). **1.** Reduction of a hernia or of a dislocation of any part by means of manipulation. **2.** Systematic classification or orderly arrangement. **3.** The reaction of protoplasm to a stimulus, by virtue of which animals and plants are led to move or act in certain definite ways in relation to their environment; the various kinds of t. are designated by a prefix denoting the stimulus governing them; *e.g.,* chemotaxis, electrotaxis, thermotaxis. [G. orderly arrangement]
bipolar t., obsolete term for repositioning of a retroverted uterus by making traction on the cervix in the vagina, and pushing up the fundus by the finger in the rectum.
negative t., the repulsion of protoplasm away from a stimulus.
positive t., the attraction of protoplasm toward a stimulus.

Tax·ol (taks′ol). Trade name of paclitaxel; a complex alkaloid extracted from the Pacific yew *Taxus brevifolia* family (family Taxaceae). Active anticancer agent effective particularly in ovarian cancer. Acts on microtubules to promote assembly, produce overgrowth, and thus disrupt cellular proliferation. Tool in study of structure and function of microtubules; antineoplastic.

tax·on, pl. **taxa** (tak′son, tak′să). The name given to a particular level or grouping in a systematic classification of living things or organisms (taxonomy). [G. *taxis,* order, arrangement, + -*on*]

tax·o·nom·ic (tak-sō-nom′ik). Relating to taxonomy.

tax·on·o·my (tak-sawn′ŏ-mē). The systematic classification of living things or organisms. Kingdoms of living organisms are divided into groups (taxa) to show degrees of similarity or presumed evolutionary relationships, with the higher categories being larger, more inclusive, and more broadly defined, the lower categories being more restricted, with fewer species more closely related. The divisions below kingdom are, in descending order: phylum, class, order, family, genus, species, and subspecies (variety). Infra- and supra- or sub- and super- categories can be used when needed; additional categories, such as tribe, section, level,

ta

group, etc., are also used. [G. *taxis,* orderly arrangement, + *nomos,* law]

taxonomy	
sample taxonomic classification of *Leptospira interrogans*	
kingdom	Procaryotae
phylum	Gracilicutes
class	Scotobacteria
order	Spirochaetales
family	Leptospiraceae
genus	*Leptospira*
species	*Leptospira interrogans*
subspecies serovar	e.g., *Leptospira interrogans* icterohemorrhagiae

chemical t., an approach to the classification of organisms based on the distribution of natural products.

numerical t., an approach to the classification of organisms that strives for objectivity, wherein characters of organisms are given equal weight (adansonian classification) and the relationships of the organisms are numerically determined, usually by computer.

Tay, Warren, English physician, 1843–1927. SEE T.'s cherry-red *spot;* T.-Sachs *disease.*

Taybi, Hooshang, U.S. pediatrician and radiologist, *1919. SEE Rubinstein-T. *syndrome.*

Taylor, Charles F., U.S. orthopedic surgeon, 1827–1899. SEE T.'s back *brace, apparatus, splint.*

Taylor, Robert W., U.S. dermatologist, 1842–1908. SEE T.'s *disease.*

TB Colloquial abbreviation for tuberculosis.

Tb Symbol for terbium.

TBG Abbreviation for thyroxine-binding *globulin.*

tBoc Abbreviation for *tert*-butyloxycarbonyl.

TBP Abbreviation for thyroxine-binding *protein.*

TBPA Abbreviation for thyroxine-binding *prealbumin.*

TBV Abbreviation for total blood volume.

TBW Abbreviation for total body *water.*

Tc. Abbreviation for T cytotoxic *cells,* under *cell.*

Tc Symbol for technetium.

^{99}Tc. Symbol for technetium-99.

^{99m}Tc. Symbol for technetium-99m.

2,3,7,8-TCDD. Abbreviation for 2,3,7,8-tetrachlorodibenzo-[*b,e*]-[*1,4*]dioxin. SEE dioxin (3).

TCG Abbreviation for time compensation *gain.*

TCID$_{50}$, TCD$_{50}$ Abbreviation for tissue culture infectious *dose.*

TDF Abbreviation for testis-determining *factor.*

TDP Abbreviation for ribothymidine 5'-diphosphate. The thymidine analog is dTDP.

TE. In magnetic resonance spin echo pulse sequences, the time to echo, when the magnetization signal is sampled.

Te 1. In electrodiagnosis, abbreviation denoting tetanic contraction. **2.** Symbol for tellurium.

tea (tē). **1.** The dried leaves of various genera of the family Theaceae, including *Thea* (*T. senensis*), *Camellia,* and *Gordonia,* a shrub indigenous to China, southern and southeastern Asia, and Japan. Its chief constituent, upon which its stimulating action largely depends, is the alkaloid caffeine, which is present in the amount of 1% to 4%. **2.** The infusion made by pouring boiling water upon t. leaves. **3.** Any infusion or decoction made extemporaneously. SEE ALSO species (2). SYN thea. [Chinese (Amoy dial.) *t'e,* Mod. L. *thea*]

Hottentot t., SYN buchu.

Jesuit t., Mexican t., SYN chenopodium.

Paraguay t., SYN maté.

Teale, Thomas P., English surgeon, 1801–1868. SEE T.'s *amputation.*

tear (tēr). The fluid secreted by the lacrimal glands by means of which the conjunctiva and cornea are kept moist. [A.S. *teár*]

artificial t.'s, mixtures of fluid compounds to substitute for naturally produced t.'s.

crocodile t.'s, SEE crocodile tears *syndrome.*

tear (tār). A discontinuity in substance of a structure. Cf. laceration.

bucket-handle t., a t. in the central part of a semilunar cartilage.

Mallory-Weiss t., SYN Mallory-Weiss *lesion.*

tear·ing (tēr'ing). SYN epiphora.

tease (tēz). To separate the structural parts of a tissue by means of a needle, in order to prepare it for microscopic examination. [A. S. *taesan*]

tea·spoon (tē'spūn). A small spoon, holding about 1 dram (or about 5 ml) liquid; used as a measure in the dosage of fluid medicines.

teat (tēt). **1.** SYN nipple. **2.** SYN breast. **3.** SYN papilla. [A.S. *tit*]

teb·u·tate (teb'yū-tāt). USAN-approved contraction for tertiary butylacetate, $(CH_3)_3C–CH_2–CO_2^-$.

tech·ne·ti·um (Tc) (tek-nē'shē-um). An artificial radioactive element, atomic no. 43, atomic wt. 99, produced in 1937 by bombardment of molybdenum by deuterons; also a product of the fission of ^{235}U; used extensively as a radiographic tracer in imaging studies of internal organs. [G. *technetos,* artificial]

tech·ne·ti·um-99 (^{99}Tc). A radioisotope of technetium which is the decay product of technetium-99m and has a weak beta emission and a physical half-life of 213,000 years.

tech·ne·ti·um-99m (^{99m}Tc). A radioisotope of technetium which decays by isomeric transition, emitting an essentially monoenergetic gamma ray of 142 keV with a half-life of 6.01 hr. It is usually obtained from a radionuclide generator of molybdenum-99 and is used to prepare radiopharmaceuticals for scanning the brain, parotid, thyroid, lungs, blood pool, liver, heart, spleen, kidney, lacrimal drainage apparatus, bone, and bone marrow.

^{99m}Tc diphosphonate, a radionuclide complex used for bone scans.

^{99m}Tc-DPTA, a radionuclide chelate complex used for renal imaging and function testing.

^{99m}Tc sulfur colloid, a particulate radionuclide complex taken up by the reticuloendothelial system; used for imaging the liver and spleen.

tech·nic (tek-nik'). SYN technique.

tech·ni·cal (tek'ni-kăl). **1.** Relating to technique. **2.** Pertaining to some particular art, science, or trade. **3.** In connection with a chemical substance, denoting that the substance contains appreciable quantities of impurities.

tech·ni·cian (tek-nish'ŭn). SYN technologist. [G. *technē,* an art]

tech·nique (tek-nēk'). The manner of performance, or the details, of any surgical operation, experiment, or mechanical act. SEE ALSO method, operation, procedure. SYN technic. [Fr., fr. G. *technikos,* relating to *technē,* art, skill]

airbrasive t., a method of grinding, cutting tooth structure, or roughening the natural tooth surface or the surface of a restoration, by means of a device utilizing a gas-impelled jet of fine Al_2O_3 particles which, after striking the tooth, are removed by an aspirator. SEE ALSO microetching t.

air-gap t., chest radiography performed using a space between the subject and film instead of a grid to absorb scattered radiation; usually requires a target-film distance of 10 feet.

atrial-well t., an obsolete semi-closed surgical t. for repairing atrial septal defects and other cardiac abnormalities.

Barcroft-Warburg t., SEE Warburg's *apparatus.*

Begg light wire differential force t., SEE light wire *appliance.*

cellulose tape t., use of a piece of transparent cellulose tape applied to a glass slide to obtain perianal samples for identification of pinworm eggs.

direct t., SYN direct *method* for making inlays.

Ficoll-Hypaque t., a density-gradient centrifugation t. for separating lymphocytes from other formed elements in the blood; the sample is layered onto a Ficoll-sodium metrizoate gradient of specific density; following centrifugation, lymphocytes are collected from the plasma-Ficoll interface.

flicker fusion frequency t., SYN flicker *perimetry.*

fluorescent antibody t., a t. used to test for antigen with a fluorescent antibody, usually performed by one of two methods: *direct,* in which immunoglobulin (antibody) conjugated with a fluorescent dye is added to tissue and combines with specific antigen (microbe, or other), the resulting antigen-antibody complex being located by fluorescence microscopy, or *indirect,* in which unlabeled immunoglobulin (antibody) is added to tissue and combines with specific antigen, after which the antigen-antibody complex may be labeled with fluorescein-conjugated anti-immunoglobulin antibody, the resulting triple complex then being located by fluorescence microscopy.

flush t., a t. for determining the systolic blood pressure in infants; the elevated limb is "milked" of blood from the hand or foot proximally; the blood pressure cuff is then inflated above the likely systolic pressure and the limb lowered; the cuff pressure is then gradually released until the blanched limb flushes.

Hampton t., obsolete term for atraumatic, nonpalpation, fluoroscopic examination of the upper gastrointestinal tract in peptic ulcer disease with acute hemorrhage.

Hartel t., a method of reaching the gasserian ganglion by passing a needle from the mouth, inserting it about the level of the upper midmolar tooth, and passing it inward until the point reaches the bone in front and to the outer side of the foramen ovale, allowing an alcohol injection to be made for the relief of trigeminal neuralgia.

high-kV t., chest radiography using a kilovoltage of at least 125 kVp, usually 140–150 kVp, to reduce patient dose and increase latitude.

indirect t., SYN indirect *method* for making inlays.

Jerne t. (jern), a t. for measuring immunocompetence by quantitating the number of splenic antibody-forming cells found in a mouse that has been sensitized to sheep erythrocytes. The number of plaques formed correlates with the number of splenic antibody-forming cells.

Judkins t., a method of selective coronary artery catheterization utilizing the standard Seldinger t. through a percutaneous femoral artery puncture.

long cone t., the use of a cone distance of 14 inches or more in making oral roentgenographs.

McGoon's t., plastic reconstruction of an incompetent mitral valve, when the incompetence is due to rupture of chordae to the posterior leaflet, by plication of the redundant leaflet.

Merendino's t., plastic reconstruction of an incompetent mitral valve using heavy silk sutures to narrow the annulus in the region of the medial commissure.

microetching t., a method of roughening the surface of a natural tooth or a dental restoration utilizing a gas-impelled jet of fine abrasive. It enhances the attachment of resin cements or restorative materials to the surface. SEE ALSO airbrasive t.

Mohs' fresh tissue chemosurgery t., chemosurgery in which superficial cancers are excised after fixation *in vivo.*

Ouchterlony t., a t. in which both reaction partners (antigen and antibody) are allowed to diffuse to each other in a gel in a precipitation reaction.

PAP t., an unlabeled antibody peroxidase method which reacts both with the rabbit antihorseradish peroxidase antibody and free horseradish peroxidase to form a soluble complex of peroxidase antiperoxidase or PAP; a uniquely sensitive immunohistochemical method that is applicable to paraffin-embedded tissues.

rebreathing t., use of a breathing or anesthesia circuit in which exhaled air is subsequently inhaled either with or without absorption of CO_2 from the exhaled air.

Rebuck skin window t., an *in vivo* test of the inflammatory response in which the skin is abraded and a slide applied to the abraded area to permit visualization of leukocyte mobilization.

sealed jar t., a t. for producing suspended animation in small

experimental animals, consisting of sealing the animal in a jar which is then refrigerated.

Seldinger t., a method of percutaneous insertion of a catheter into a blood vessel or space, such as an abscess cavity: a needle is used to puncture the structure and a guide wire is threaded through the needle; when the needle is withdrawn, a catheter is threaded over the wire; the wire is then withdrawn, leaving the catheter in place.

sterile insect t., a t. used to control or eradicate insect pests or vectors, utilizing induction by irradiation of dominant lethality in the chromosomes of the released insects.

washed field t., the cutting of cavity preparations in teeth utilizing a constant irrigant which is immediately removed from the mouth by means of a vacuum device.

tech·no·cau·sis (tek-nō-kaw'sis). SYN actual *cautery.* [G. *technē,* art, + *kausis,* a burning]

tech·nol·o·gist (tek-nol'ŏ-jist). One trained in and using the techniques of a profession, art, or science. SYN technician.

tech·nol·o·gy (tek-nol'ō-jē). The knowledge and use of the techniques of a profession, art, or science. [G. *technē,* an art, + *logos,* study]

assisted reproductive t., originally, a range of techniques for manipulating eggs and sperm in order to overcome infertility. Encompasses drug treatments to stimulate ovulation; surgical methods for removing eggs (*e.g.,* laparoscopy and ultrasound-guided transvaginal aspiration) and for reimplanting embryos (*e.g.,* zygot intrafallopian transfer (or ZIFT); in vitro and in vivo fertilization (*e.g.,* artificial insemination and gamete intrafallopian transfer (or GIFT); ex utero and in utero fetal surgery; as well as laboratory regimes for freezing and screening sperm and embryos, and micromanipulating and cloning embryos. SEE eugenics.

The field's first major success came in 1978 with the birth of "test-tube baby" Louise Brown, engineered by Steptoe, Edwards, et al., of England. As the technologies spread, they increasingly are being employed for purposes beyond infertility, i.e., to reduce the risk of, or avoid passing on, hereditary disease and to select for infant sex. Further uses that would aim at improving the "quality" of offspring have been widely discussed and raise profound legal and ethical questions.

tec·lo·thi·a·zide (tek-lō-thī'ă-zīd). SYN tetrachlormethiazide.

tec·tal (tek'tăl). Relating to a tectum.

tec·ti·form (tek'ti-fōrm). Roof-shaped.

Tec·ti·vi·ri·dae (tek'tē-vī'rā-dā). Provisional name for a family of nonenveloped double-stranded DNA bacteriophages that have double capsids. [L. *tectum,* roof, covering, + virus]

tec·to·ce·phal·ic (tek'tō-sĕ-fal'ik). SYN scaphocephalic. [L. *tectum,* roof, + G. *kephalē,* head]

tec·to·ceph·a·ly (tek'tō-sef'ă-lē). SYN scaphocephaly.

tec·tol·o·gy (tek-tol'ō-jē). Structural morphology. [G. *tektōn,* builder, + *-logia*]

tec·ton·ic (tek-ton'ik). **1.** Relating to variations in structure in the eye, particularly the cornea. **2.** Obsolete term denoting plastic surgery or the restoration of lost parts by grafting. [G. *tektonikos,* relating to building]

tec·to·ri·al (tek-tōr'ē-ăl). Relating to or characteristic of a tectorium.

tec·to·ri·um (tek-tōr'ē-ŭm). **1.** An overlaying structure. **2.** SYN tectorial *membrane* of cochlear duct. [L. an overlaying surface (plaster, stucco), fr. *tego,* pp. *tectus,* to cover]

tec·to·spi·nal (tek-tō-spī'năl). Denoting nerve fibers passing from the mesencephalic tectum to the spinal cord.

tec·tum, pl. **tec·ta** (tek'tŭm, tek'tă) [NA]. Any rooflike covering or structure. [L. roof, roofed structure, fr. *tego,* pp. *tectus,* to cover]

t. mesenceph'ali [NA], SYN *lamina* of mesencephalic tectum.

TEDD Abbreviation for total end-diastolic *diameter.*

teel oil (tēl). SYN *sesame* oil.

teeth (tēth). Plural of tooth.

teeth·ing (tē'thing). Eruption or "cutting" of the teeth, especially of the deciduous teeth. SYN odontiasis.

tef·lu·rane (tef'lū-rān). 2-Bromo-1,1,1,2-tetrafluoroethane; a nonexplosive and nonflammable inhalation anesthetic of moderate potency.

teg·men, gen. **teg·mi·nis**, pl. **teg·mi·na** (teg'men, -mi-nis, -mi-nă) [NA]. A structure that covers or roofs over a part. [L. a covering, fr. *tego,* to cover]

t. cru′ris, old term for *tegmentum* mesencephali.

t. mastoi′deum, the lamina of bone roofing over the mastoid cells.

t. tym′pani [NA], the roof of the middle ear, formed by the thinned anterior surface of the petrous portion of the temporal bone. Its anterior edge is inserted into the petrosquamous fissure so that it can be seen as a wedge of bone subdividing that fissure into a squamo tympanic and a petrotympanic fissure. SYN roof of tympanum.

t. ventric′uli quar′ti [NA], roof of fourth ventricle, formed in its upper part by the superior medullary velum stretching between the two brachia conjunctiva (superior cerebellar peduncles), in its lower part by the inferior medullary velum composed of the choroid membrane and choroid plexus of the fourth ventricle. SYN roof of fourth ventricle.

teg·men·tal (teg-men′tăl). Relating to, characteristic of, or placed or oriented toward a tegmentum or tegmen.

teg·men·tot·o·my (teg-men-tot′ō-mē). Production of lesions in the reticular formation of the midbrain tegmentum. [tegmentum + G. *tomē,* incision]

teg·men·tum, pl. **teg·men·ta** (teg-men′tŭm, -tă) [NA]. **1.** A covering structure. **2.** SYN mesencephalic t. [L. covering structure, fr. *tego,* to cover]

t. mesenceph′ali [NA], SYN mesencephalic t.

mesencephalic t., that major part of the substance of the mesencephalon or midbrain that extends from the substantia nigra to the level of the cerebral aqueduct. SYN t. mesencephali [NA], tegmentum (2) [NA], midbrain t.

midbrain t., SYN mesencephalic t.

t. of pons, SYN dorsal *part* of pons.

t. rhombenceph′ali [NA], SYN rhombencephalic t.

rhombencephalic t., the portion of the pons continuous with the mesencephalic t.; it consists of reticular formation, tracts, and cranial nerve nuclei, and forms the dorsal part of the pons (pars dorsalis pontis). SYN t. rhombencephali [NA], t. of rhombencephalon.

t. of rhombencephalon, SYN rhombencephalic t.

teg·u·ment (teg′yū-ment). **1.** SYN integument. **2.** SYN integument (2). [L. *tegumentum,* a collat. form of *tegmentum*]

teg·u·men·tal, teg·u·men·ta·ry (teg-yū-men′tăl, teg-yū-ment-ă-rē). Relating to the integument.

Teichmann, Ludwig, German histologist, 1823–1895. SEE T.'s *crystals,* under *crystal.*

tei·cho·ic ac·ids (tī-kō′ik). One of two classes (the other being the muramic acids or mucopeptides) of polymers constituting the cell walls of Gram-positive bacteria, but also found intracellularly; linear polymers of a polyol (ribitol phosphate or glycerol phosphate) carrying D-alanyl residues esterified to OH groups and glycosidically linked sugars.

tei·chop·sia (tī-kop′sē-ă). The jagged, shimmering visual sensation resembling the fortifications of a walled medieval town; the scintillating scotoma of migraine. [G. *teichos,* wall, + *opsis,* vision]

⌂**tel-, tele-, telo-.** Distance, end, other end. [G. *tēle,* distant, *telos,* end]

te·la, gen. and pl. **te·lae** (tē′lă, tē′lē). **1.** Any thin weblike structure. **2.** A tissue; especially one of delicate formation. [L. a web]

t. choroi′dea, that portion of the pia mater that covers the ependymal roof or, in the case of the lateral ventricle, medial wall of a cerebral ventricle.

t. choroi′dea inferior, SYN choroid t. of fourth ventricle.

t. choroi′dea superior, SYN choroid t. of third ventricle.

t. choroi′dea ventric′uli quar′ti [NA], SYN choroid t. of fourth ventricle.

t. choroi′dea ventric′uli ter′tii [NA], SYN choroid t. of third ventricle.

choroid t. of fourth ventricle, the sheet of pia mater covering the lower part of the ependymal roof of the fourth ventricle. SYN t. choroidea ventriculi quarti [NA], t. choroidea inferior.

choroid t. of third ventricle, a double fold of pia mater, enclosing subarachnoid trabeculae, between the fornix above and the epithelial roof of the third ventricle and the thalami below; at each lateral margin is a vascular fringe projecting into the choroidal fissure of the lateral ventricle; on its undersurface are several small vascular projections filling the folds of the ependymal roof of the third ventricle. SYN t. choroidea ventriculi tertii [NA], t. choroidea superior, triangular lamella, velum interpositum, velum triangulare.

t. conjuncti′va, SYN connective *tissue.*

t. elas′tica, SYN elastic *tissue.*

t. subcuta′nea [NA], SYN superficial *fascia.*

t. submuco′sa [NA], SYN submucosa.

t. submuco′sa pharyn′gis, SYN pharyngobasilar *fascia.*

t. subsero′sa [NA], SYN subserous *layer.*

t. vasculo′sa, SYN choroid *plexus.*

Te·la·dor·sa·gia dav·ti·ani (tē′lă-dōr-sā′jē-ă dav-shē-ān′ī). One of the medium stomach worm species (family Trichostrongylidae) of sheep, goats, and deer occurring in the abomasum; it is similar to *Ostertagia trifurcata.* [tele- + L. *dorsum,* back]

tel·al·gia (tel-al′jē-ă). SYN referred *pain.* [G. *tēle,* distant, + *algos,* pain]

tel·an·gi·ec·ta·sia (tel-an′jē-ek-tā′zē-ă). Dilation of the previously existing small or terminal vessels of a part. [G. *telos,* end, + *angeion,* vessel, + *ektasis,* a stretching out]

cephalo-oculocutaneous t., an angioma involving the skin of the face, orbit, meninges, and brain. SEE ALSO Sturge-Weber *syndrome.*

essential t., (1) localized capillary dilation of undetermined origin; **(2)** SYN *angioma* serpiginosum.

hereditary hemorrhagic t. [MIM*187300], a disease with onset usually after puberty, marked by multiple small telangiectases and dilated venules that develop slowly on the skin and mucous membranes; the face, lips, tongue, nasopharynx, and intestinal mucosa are frequent sites, and recurrent bleeding may occur; autosomal dominant inheritance. SYN Rendu-Osler-Weber syndrome.

t. lymphat′ica, SYN lymphangiectasis.

t. macula′ris erupti′va per′stans, a disseminated eruption of telangiectases associated with erythematous and edematous macules.

primary t., SYN *angioma* serpiginosum.

secondary t., t. related to a known cause of prolonged dermal vascular dilatation such as sunlight, varicose veins, and connective tissue diseases; often associated with atrophy of the skin.

spider t., SYN spider *angioma.*

t. verruco′sa, SYN angiokeratoma.

tel·an·gi·ec·ta·sis, pl. **tel·an·gi·ec·ta·ses** (tel-an′jē-ek′tă-sis, -sēz). A lesion formed by a dilated capillary or terminal artery, most commonly on the skin. SEE telangiectasia.

tel·an·gi·ec·tat·ic (tel-an′jē-ek-tat′ik). Relating to or marked by telangiectasia.

tel·an·gi·ec·to·des (tel-an′jē-ek-tō′dēz). A term used to qualify highly vascular tumors. [telangiectasis + G. *-ōdēs,* fr. *eidos,* resemblance]

tel·an·gi·o·ma (tel-an′jē-ō′mă). Angioma due to dilation of the capillaries or terminal arterioles.

tel·an·gi·on (tel-an′jē-on). One of the terminal arterioles or a capillary vessel. SYN trichangion. [G. *telos,* end, + *angeion,* vessel]

tel·an·gi·o·sis (tel′an-jē-ō′sis). Any disease of the capillaries and terminal arterioles.

tele (tel′ē). Referring to the nitrogen atom of the imidazole ring of histidine that is the farthest from the β-carbon. Cf. *pros*. [G. far]

△**tele-.** SEE tel-.

tel·e·can·thus (tel-ĕ-kan'thŭs). Increased distance between the medial canthi of the eyelids. SYN canthal hypertelorism. [G. *tēle,* distant, + *kanthos,* canthus]

tel·e·car·di·o·gram (tel-ĕ-kar'dē-ō-gram). SYN telelectrocardiogram.

tel·e·car·di·o·phone (tel-ĕ-kar'dē-ō-fōn). A specially constructed stethoscope by means of which heart sounds can be heard by listeners at a distance from the patient. [G. *tēle,* distant, + *kardia,* heart, + *phōnē,* sound]

tel·e·co·balt (tel'ĕ-kō'bawlt). Teletherapy using radioactive cobalt as the source.

tel·e·di·ag·no·sis (tel'ĕ-dī-ag-nō'sis). Detection of a disease by evaluation of data transmitted to a receiving station, a process normally involving patient-monitoring instruments and a transfer link to a diagnostic center at some distance from the patient.

tel·e·di·a·stol·ic (tel'ĕ-dī-ă-stol'ik). Pertaining to or occurring toward the end of ventricular diastole. [G. *telos,* end, + *diastolē,* dilation]

tel·e·lec·tro·car·di·o·gram (tel'ē-lek-trō-kar'dē-ō-gram). An electrocardiogram recorded at a distance from the subject being tested; *e.g.,* the electrocardiogram obtained through telemetry, or, as with a galvanometer in the laboratory, being connected by a wire with the patient in another room. SYN telecardiogram. [G. *tēle,* distant, + electrocardiogram]

te·lem·e·ter (tĕ-lem'ĕ-ter). An electronic instrument that senses and measures a quantity, then transmits radio signals to a distant station for recording and interpretation. [G. *tēle,* distant, + *metron,* measure]

te·lem·e·try (tĕ-lem'ĕ-trē). The science of measuring a quantity, transmitting the results by radio signals to a distant station, and there interpreting, indicating, and/or recording the results. SEE ALSO biotelemetry.

  cardiac t., transmission of cardiac signals (electric or pressure derived) to a receiving location where they are displayed for monitoring.

tel·en·ce·phal·ic (tel'en-se-fal'ik). Relating to the telencephalon or endbrain.

tel·en·ceph·al·i·za·tion (tel-en-sef'ăl-i-zā'shŭn). SYN corticalization.

tel·en·ceph·a·lon (tel-en-sef'ă-lon) [NA]. The anterior division of the prosencephalon, which develops into the olfactory lobes, the cortex of the cerebral hemispheres, and the subcortical telencephalic nuclei, and the basal ganglia (nuclei), particularly the striatum and the amygdala. SYN endbrain. [G. *telos,* end, + *enkephalos,* brain]

te·le·ol·o·gy (tel-ē-ol'ō-jē). The philosophical doctrine according to which events, especially in biology, are explained in part by reference to final causes or end goals; the doctrine that goals or end states have a causal influence on present events and that the future as well as the past affect the present. [G. *telos,* end, + *logos,* study]

tel·e·o·mi·to·sis (tel'ē-ō-mī-tō'sis). A completed mitosis. [G. *teleos,* complete, + mitosis]

tel·e·o·morph (tel'ē-ō-morf). A reproductive structure of a fungus that is a result of plasmogamy and nuclear recombination; sexual state (sexual reproduction). SYN perfect stage.

tel·e·o·nom·ic (tel'ē-ō-nom'ik). 1. Pertaining to teleonomy. 2. In psychology, pertaining to those patterns of behavior that are a function of an inferred purpose or motive; *e.g.,* a child's behavior pattern may be classified teleonomically by an observer as attention-getting.

tel·e·on·o·my (tel-ē-on'ō-mē). The doctrine that life is characterized by endowment with a project or purpose; *i.e.,* the existence in an organism of a structure or function implies that it has had evolutionary survival value. [G. *telos,* end, + *nomos,* law]

tel·e·op·sia (tel-ē-op'sē-ă). An error in judging the distance of objects arising from lesions in the parietal temporal region. [G. *tēle,* distant, + *opsis,* vision]

tel·e·or·gan·ic (tel'ē-ōr-gan'ik). Manifesting life. [G. *teleos,* complete, + *organikos,* organic]

tel·e·ost (tel'ē-ost). One of the bony or true fishes. [G. *teleos,* complete, perfect, + *osteon,* bone]

tel·e·path·ine (tel-ĕ-path'ēn). SYN harmine.

te·lep·a·thy (tĕ-lep'ă-thē). Transmittal and reception of thoughts by means other than through the normal senses, as a form of extrasensory perception. SYN extrasensory thought transference, mind-reading. [G. *tēle,* distant, + *pathos,* feeling]

tel·e·ra·di·og·ra·phy (tel-ĕ-rā-dē-og'ră-fē). Radiography with the x-ray tube positioned about 2 m from the film thereby securing practical parallelism of the x-rays to minimize geometric distortion; the standard configuration for chest radiography. Cf. air-gap *technique.* SYN teleroentgenography. [G. *tēle,* distant, + radiography]

tel·e·ra·di·ol·o·gy (tel-ĕ-rā-dē-ol'-ō-jē). The interpretation of digitized diagnostic images transmitted by modem over telephone lines. [tele- + radiology]

tel·e·ra·di·um (tel'ĕ-rā'dē-ŭm). SEE teleradium *therapy.*

tel·e·re·cep·tor (tel'ĕ-rē-sep'ter, -tōr). An organ, such as the eye, that can receive sense stimuli from a distance.

tel·er·gy (tel'er-jē). SYN automatism. [G. *tēle,* far off, + *ergon,* work]

tel·e·roent·gen·og·ra·phy (tel'ĕ-rent-gen-og'ră-fē). SYN teleradiography.

tel·e·roent·gen·ther·a·py (tel'ĕ-rent'gen-thār'ă-pē). SYN teletherapy.

tel·e·sis (tel-ē'sis). A goal to be attained by planned conduct. [G. *telos,* end, + *-osis,* condition]

tel·e·sys·tol·ic (tel'ĕ-sis-tol'ik). Relating to the end of ventricular systole. [G. *telos,* end, + *systolē,* a contracting]

tel·e·tac·tor (tel-ĕ-tak'ter). An instrument to transmit sound waves to the skin. [G. *telos,* end, + L. *tactus,* touch]

tel·e·ther·a·py (tel-ĕ-thār'ă-pē). Radiation therapy administered with the source at a distance from the body. Cf. interstitial *therapy.* SYN teleroentgentherapy. [G. *tēle,* distant, + *therapeia,* treatment]

TeLinde, Richard W., U.S. gynecologist, *1894. SEE T. *operation.*

tel·lu·ric (tĕ-lūr'ik). 1. Relating to or originating in the earth. 2. Relating to the element tellurium, especially in its 6+ valence state. [L. *tellus* (*tellur-*), the earth]

tel·lu·rism (tel'ū-rizm). The alleged influence of soil emanations in producing disease. [L. *tellus* (*tellur-*), the earth]

tel·lu·ri·um (Te) (tel-ū'rē-ŭm). A rare semimetallic element, atomic no. 52, atomic wt. 127.60, belonging to the sulfur group. [L. *tellus* (*tellur-*), the earth]

△**telo-.** SEE tel-.

tel·o·den·dron (tel-ō-den'dron). An anomalous term that refers to the terminal arborization of an axon. SYN end-brush. [G. *telos,* end, + *dendron,* tree]

tel·o·gen (tel'ō-jen). Resting phase of hair cycle. [G. *telos,* end, + *-gen,* producing]

te·log·lia (tĕ-log'lē-ă). Accumulation of neurolemmal cells at the myoneural junction. [G. *telos,* end, + *glia,* glue]

tel·og·no·sis (tel-og-nō'sis). Obsolete term denoting diagnosis by means of radiographs or other diagnostic tests transmitted by telephone or radio. SEE teleradiology. [G. *tēle,* distant, + *gnōsis,* a knowing]

tel·o·ki·ne·sia (tel'ō-ki-nē'zē-ă). SYN telophase. [G. *telos,* end, + *kinēsis,* movement]

tel·o·lec·i·thal (tel-ō-les'i-thăl). Denoting an ovum in which a large amount of deuteroplasm accumulates at the vegetative pole, as in the eggs of birds and reptiles. [G. *telos,* end, + G. *lekithos,* yolk]

tel·o·me·rase (tel-ō'mer-ās). A protein that is believed to participate in the repair of telomere regions of chromosomes.

tel·o·mere (tel'ō-mēr). The distal end of a chromosome arm; telomeres undergo dramatic changes during the progression of cancer. [G. *telos,* end, + *meros,* part]

tel·o·pep·tide (tel-ō-pep′tīd). A peptide covalently bound in or on a protein, protruding therefrom and therefore subject to enzyme attack and maturation modification or cross-linking, and conferring immunogenic specificity.

tel·o·phase (tel′ō-fāz). The final stage of mitosis or meiosis that begins when migration of chromosomes to the poles of the cell has been completed; the chromosomes progressively lengthen while the nuclear membranes of the two daughter nuclei are reconstructed and a cell membrane at the equator complete the separation of the two daughter cells. SYN telokinesia. [G. *telos,* end, + *phasis,* appearance]

Te·lo·spo·rea (tel-ō-spō′rē-ă). SYN Sporozoea.

Te·lo·spo·rid·ia (tel′ō-spō-rid′ē-ă). A former order of Sporozoea. [G. *telos,* end, + *sporos,* seed]

tel·o·tism (tel′ō-tizm). The perfect performance of a function, as that of sight or hearing. [G. *telos,* end]

TEM Abbreviation for triethylenemelamine.

te·maz·e·pam (te-maz′ĕ-pam). A benzodiazepine sedative-hypnotic primarily used to relieve insomnia.

tem·per. 1. Disposition; in general, any characteristic or particular state of mind. SYN temperament (2). **2.** A display of irritation or anger. SEE tantrum. **3.** To treat metal by application of heat, as in annealing or quenching.

tem·per·a·ment (tem′per-ă-ment). **1.** The psychological and biological organization peculiar to the individual, including one's character or personality predispositions, which influence the manner of thought and action and general views of life. **2.** SYN temper (1). [L. *temperamentum,* proper measure, moderation, disposition]

tem·per·ance (tem′per-ans). Moderation in all things; especially, abstinence from the use of alcoholic beverages. [L. *temperantia,* moderation]

tem·per·ate (tem′per-ăt). Moderate; restrained in the indulgence of any appetite or activity.

tem·per·a·ture (tem′per-ă-chŭr). The sensible intensity of heat of any substance; the manifestation of the average kinetic energy of the molecules making up a substance due to heat agitation. SEE ALSO scale. [L. *temperatura,* due measure, temperature, fr. *tempero,* to proportion duly]

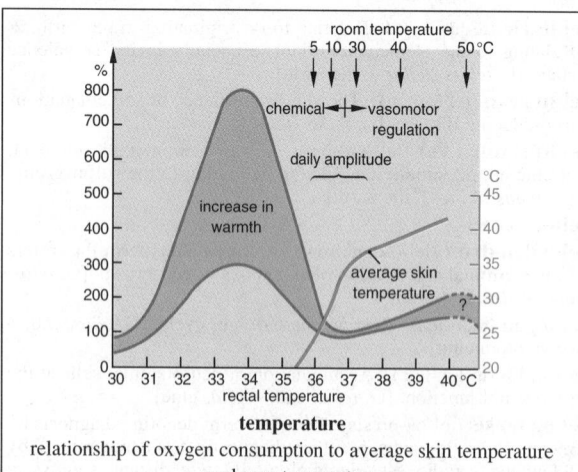

temperature

relationship of oxygen consumption to average skin temperature and core temperature

absolute t. (*T*), t. reckoned in Kelvins from absolute zero.

basal body t., the t. at rest, usually obtained on arising in the morning, without any influences that might increase it; gives indirect evidence of ovulation.

critical t., the t. of a gas above which it is no longer possible by use of any pressure, however great, to convert it into a liquid.

denaturation t. of DNA, that t. at which, under a given set of conditions, double-stranded DNA is changed (50%) to single-stranded DNA; under standard conditions, the base composition of the DNA can be estimated from the denaturation t., since the

temperature differences (°C) in the human body			
difference from rectal temperature		difference from femoral artery	
sternal marrow	−2.5	subclavial vein	−0.35
mouth	−0.4	superior vena cava	−0.1
esophagus	−0.25	inferior vena cava	±0
aorta	−0.25	right ventricle	±0
stomach	±0	pulmonary artery	±0
liver	±0	jugular vein	+0.25
hypothalamus	+0.3	hepatic vein	+0.25
uterus	+0.3	rectum (deep)	+0.25

greater the denaturation t., the greater the guanine-plus-cytosine content (*i.e.,* GC content) of the DNA. SYN melting t. of DNA.

effective t., a comfort index or scale which takes into account the t. of air, its moisture content, and movement.

equivalent t., the t. of a thermally uniform enclosure in which, under still air conditions, a "sizable" black body loses heat at the same rate as in the nonuniform environment.

eutectic t., the t. at which a eutectic mixture becomes fluid (melts).

fusion t. (wire method), the recorded t. at which a 20-gauge metal wire will collapse under a 3-ounce load; the recorded t. at which porcelain becomes glazed.

maximum t., in bacteriology, denoting a t. above which growth will not take place.

mean t., the average atmospheric t. in any locality for a designated period of time, as a month or a year.

melting t., SYN t. midpoint.

melting t. of DNA, SYN denaturation t. of DNA.

t. midpoint (T_m, t_m), the midpoint in the change in optical properties (absorbance, rotation) of a structured polymer (*e.g.,* DNA) with increasing t. SYN melting t.

minimum t., in bacteriology, denoting a t. below which growth will not take place.

optimum t., the t. at which any operation, such as the culture of any special microorganism, is best carried on.

room t. (RT, rt), the ordinary t. (65° to slightly less than 80°F, 18.3° to 26.7° C) of the atmosphere in the laboratory; a culture kept at room t. is one kept in the laboratory, not in an incubator.

sensible t., the atmospheric t. as felt by the individual, supposed to be that recorded by the wet-bulb thermometer.

standard t., a t. of 0°C or 273.15° absolute (Kelvin).

tem·plate (tem′plăt). **1.** A pattern or guide that determines the shape of a substance. **2.** Metaphorically, the specifying nature of a macromolecule, usually a nucleic acid or polynucleotide, with respect to the primary structure of the nucleic acid or polynucleotide or protein made from it *in vivo* or *in vitro*. **3.** In dentistry, a curved or flat plate utilized as an aid in setting teeth. **4.** An outline used to trace teeth, bones, or soft tissue in order to standardize their form. **5.** A pattern or guide that determines the specificity of antibody globulins. [Fr. *templet,* temple of a loom, fr. L. *templum,* small timber]

surgical t., (1) a thin, transparent, resin base shaped to duplicate the form of the impression surface of an immediate denture, used as a guide for surgically shaping the alveolar process to fit an immediate denture; (2) a guide for various osteotomy procedures; (3) a guide for duplicating size and shape for an autogenic (free) gingival graft.

tem·ple (tem′pl). **1.** The area of the temporal fossa on the side of the head above the zygomatic arch. **2.** The part of a spectacle frame passing from the rim backward over the ear. [L. *tempus* (*tempor-*), time, the temple]

tem·po·la·bile (tem-pō-lā′bil, -bīl). Undergoing spontaneous change or destruction during the passage of time. [L. *tempus,* time, + *labilis,* perishable]

tem·po·ra (tem'pŏ-ră). The temples. [L. pl. of *tempus*]

tem·po·ral (tem'pŏ-răl). **1.** Relating to time; limited in time; temporary. **2.** Relating to the temple. SEE temporal *region* of head. [L. *temporalis*, fr. *tempus* (*tempor-*), time, temple]

tem·po·ra·lis (tem-pŏ-rā'lis). SEE temporalis *muscle*. [L.]

△**temporo-.** Temporal (2). [L. *temporalis*, temporal]

tem·po·ro·au·ric·u·lar (tem'pŏ-rō-aw-rik'yū-lăr). Relating to the temporal region and the auricle.

tem·po·ro·hy·oid (tem'pŏ-rō-hī'oyd). Relating to the temporal and the hyoid bones or regions.

tem·po·ro·ma·lar (tem'pŏ-rō-mā'lăr). SYN temporozygomatic.

tem·po·ro·man·dib·u·lar (tem'pŏ-rō-man-dib'yū-lăr). Relating to the temporal bone and the mandible; denoting the joint of the lower jaw. SYN temporomaxillary (2).

tem·po·ro·max·il·lary (tem'pŏ-rō-mak'si-lār'ē). **1.** Relating to the regions of the temporal and maxillary bones. **2.** SYN temporomandibular.

tem·po·ro·oc·cip·i·tal (tem'pŏ-rō-ok-sip'i-tăl). Relating to the temporal and the occipital bones or regions.

tem·po·ro·pa·ri·e·tal (tem'pŏ-rō-pă-rī'ĕ-tăl). Relating to the temporal and the parietal bones or regions.

tem·po·ro·pon·tine (tem-pŏ-rō-pon'tīn). Referring to the projection fibers from the temporal lobe of the cerebral cortex to the basilar part of the pons.

tem·po·ro·sphe·noid (tem'pŏ-rō-sfē'noyd). Relating to the temporal and sphenoid bones.

tem·po·ro·zy·go·mat·ic (tem'pŏ-rō-zī'gō-mat'ik). Relating to the temporal and zygomatic bones or regions. SYN temporomalar.

tem·po·sta·bile, tem·po·sta·ble (tem-pō-stā'bil, -stā'bl). Not subject to spontaneous alteration or destruction. [L. *tempus*, time + *stabilis*, stable]

temps utile (temp' ū-tēl'). SYN utilization *time*. [Fr. service or utilization time]

tem·pus, gen. **tem·po·ris**, pl. **tem·po·ra** (tem'pŭs, -pŏ-ris, -pŏ-ră). **1.** The temple. **2.** SYN time. [L. time]

TEN Abbreviation for toxic epidermal *necrolysis*.

te·na·cious (tĕ-nā'shŭs). Sticky; denoting tenacity. [L. *tenax* (*tenac-*), fr. *teneo*, to hold]

te·nac·i·ty (tĕ-nas'i-tē). Adhesiveness; the character or property of holding fast. [L. *tenacitas*, fr. *teneo*, to hold]

cellular t., the inherent property of all cells to persist in a given form or direction of activity.

te·nac·u·lum, pl. **te·nac·u·la** (tĕ-nak'yū-lŭm, -lă). A surgical clamp designed to hold or grasp tissue during dissection. [L. a holder, fr. *teneo*, to hold]

tenac'ula ten'dinum, a tendinous restraining structure, such as an extensor or flexor retinaculum; historically applied to the vincula of tendon which are not however, restraining structures.

te·nal·gia (te-nal'jē-ă). Pain referred to a tendon. SYN tenodynia, tenontodynia. [G. *tenōn*, tendon, + *algos*, pain]

t. crep'itans, SYN tenosynovitis crepitans.

ten·as·cin (ten-as'sin). A protein that is present in the mesenchyme that surrounds epithelia in organs undergoing development in embryos; believed to participate in inducing differentiation of epithelia.

ten·der. Sensitive or painful as a result of pressure or contact that is not sufficent to cause discomfort in normal tissues. [L. *tener*, soft, delicate]

ten·der·ness (ten'der-nes). The condition of being tender.

pencil t., strictly localized t., elicited by pressure with the rubber tip of a pencil, *e.g.,* in cases of incomplete or subperiosteal fracture.

rebound t., t. felt when pressure, particularly pressure on the abdomen, is suddenly released.

ten·di·ni·tis (ten-di-nī'tis). SYN tendonitis.

ten·di·no·plas·ty (ten'din-ō-plas-tē). SYN tenontoplasty. [Mediev. L. *tendo* (*tendin-*), tendon, + G. *plastos,* formed]

ten·di·no·su·ture (ten'di-nō-sū'chŭr). SYN tenorrhaphy.

ten·di·nous (ten'di-nŭs). Relating to, composed of, or resembling a tendon.

ten·do, gen. **ten·di·nis**, pl. **ten·di·nes** (ten'dō, -di-nis, -di-nēz) [NA]. SYN tendon. For histological description, see tendon. [Mediev. L., fr. L. *tendo,* to stretch out, extend]

t. Achil'lis [NA], ⋆official alternate term for t. calcaneus, t. calcaneus.

t. calca'neus [NA], the tendon of insertion of the triceps surae (gastrocnemius and soleus) into the tuberosity of the calcaneus. SYN t. Achillis⋆ [NA], Achilles tendon, calcanean tendon, chorda magna, heel tendon.

t. calca'neus commu'nis, SEE hamstring (2).

t. conjuncti'vus [NA], ⋆official alternate term for conjoint *tendon.*

t. cricoesopha'geus [NA], SYN cricoesophageal *tendon.*

t. oc'uli, SYN medial palpebral *ligament.*

t. palpebra'rum, SYN medial palpebral *ligament.*

△**tendo-.** A tendon. SEE ALSO teno-. [L. *tendo*]

ten·dol·y·sis (ten-dol'i-sis). Release of a tendon from adhesions. SYN tenolysis. [tendo- + G. *lysis,* dissolution]

ten·do·mu·cin, ten·do·mu·coid (ten-dō-myū'sin, -myū'koyd). A form of mucin found in tendons.

ten·don (ten'dŏn). A fibrous cord or band of variable length that connects a muscle with its bony attachment or other structure; it may unite with the muscle at its extremity or may run along the side or in the center of the muscle for a longer or shorter distance, receiving the muscular fibers along its lateral border. It consists of fascicles of very densely arranged, almost parallel collagenous fibers, rows of elongated fibrocytes, and a minimum of ground substance. For gross anatomical description, see tendo. SYN tendo [NA], sinew. [L. *tendo*]

Achilles t., SYN *tendo* calcaneus.

bowed t., a condition caused by severe strain of the digital flexor tendons, the outer osseus (suspensory ligament), or the accessory ligament (distal cheek ligament) of the horse's limb and characterized by swelling, pain, and lameness; it occurs most frequently in race horses under stress of running.

calcanean t., SYN *tendo* calcaneus.

central t. of diaphragm, a three-lobed fibrous sheet occupying the center of the diaphragm. SYN centrum tendineum diaphragmatis [NA], trefoil t.

central t. of perineum, the fibromuscular mass between the anal canal and the urogenital diaphragm in the median plane; midline episiotomies extend into this structure. SYN centrum tendineum perinei [NA], perineal body, Savage's perineal body.

conjoined t., SYN conjoint t.

conjoint t., common t. of insertion of the transversus and obliquus internus muscles into the crest and spine of the pubis and iliopectineal line; it is frequently muscular rather than aponeurotic and may be poorly developed; forms posterior wall of medial inguinal canal. SEE ALSO *aponeurosis* of internal abdominal oblique muscle. SYN falx inguinalis [NA], tendo conjunctivus⋆ [NA], conjoined t., falx aponeurotica, inguinal aponeurotic fold.

contracted t., a condition of young horses in which the flexor t.'s of the leg are shortened.

coronary t., SYN fibrous *ring* of heart.

cricoesophageal t., longitudinal fiber of the esophagus that attaches to the posterior aspect of the cricoid cartilage of the larynx. SYN tendo cricoesophageus [NA], Gillette's suspensory ligament, suspensory ligament of esophagus.

Gerlach's annular t., SYN fibrocartilaginous *ring* of tympanic membrane.

hamstring t., SEE hamstring.

heel t., SYN *tendo* calcaneus.

slipped t., SEE perosis.

Todaro's t., an inconstant tendinous structure that extends from the right fibrous trigone of the heart toward the valve of the inferior vena cava.

trefoil t., SYN central t. of diaphragm.

Zinn's t., SYN common tendinous *ring.*

ten·don·i·tis (ten-dō-nī'tis). Inflammation of a tendon. SYN tendinitis, tenonitis (2), tenontitis, tenositis.

ten·doph·o·ny (ten-dof'ō-nē). SYN tenophony.

ten·do·plas·ty (ten′dō-plas-tē). SYN tenontoplasty.

ten·do·syn·o·vi·tis (ten′dō-si-nō-vī′tis). SYN tenosynovitis.

ten·dot·o·my (ten-dot′ō-mē). SYN tenotomy.

ten·do·vag·i·nal (ten-dō-vaj′i-năl). Relating to a tendon and its sheath. [tendo- + L. *vagina*, sheath]

ten·do·vag·i·ni·tis (ten′dō-vaj-i-nī′tis). SYN tenosynovitis. [tendo- + L. *vagina*, sheath, + G. *-itis*, inflammation]
radial styloid t., SYN de Quervain's *disease.*

te·nec·to·my (tĕ-nek′tō-mē). Resection of part of a tendon. SYN tenonectomy. [G. *tenōn*, tendon, + *ektomē*, excision]

te·nes·mic (tĕ-nez′mik). Relating to or marked by tenesmus.

te·nes·mus (te-nez′mŭs). A painful spasm of the anal sphincter with an urgent desire to evacuate the bowel or bladder, involuntary straining, and the passage of little fecal matter or urine. [G. *teinesmos*, ineffectual effort to defecate, fr. *teinō*, to stretch]

ten Horn, C., Dutch surgeon. SEE t. H.'s *sign.*

te·nia, pl. **te·ni·ae** (tē′nē-ă, tē′nē-ē). 1. Any anatomical bandlike structure. 2. SYN taenia (2). [L. fr. G. *tainia*, band, tape, a tapeworm]
te′niae acus′ticae, SYN medullary *striae* of fourth ventricle, under *stria.*
t. choroi′dea [NA], the somewhat thickened line along which a choroid membrane or plexus is attached to the rim of a brain ventricle. SYN t. telae [NA].
te′niae co′li [NA], the three bands in which the longitudinal muscular fibers of the large intestine, except the rectum, are collected; these are the mesocolic t., situated at the place corresponding to the mesenteric attachment; the free t., opposite the mesocolic t.; and the omental t., at the place corresponding to the site of adhesion of the greater omentum to the transverse colon. SYN bands of colon, colic teniae, teniae of Valsalva.
colic teniae, SYN teniae coli.
t. fim′briae, SYN t. fornicis.
t. for′nicis [NA], the line of attachment of the choroid plexus of the lateral ventricle to the fornix. SYN t. fimbriae, t. of the fornix.
t. of the fornix, SYN t. fornicis.
t. of fourth ventricle, SYN t. ventriculi quarti.
free t., SEE teniae coli. SYN t. libera [NA].
t. hippocam′pi, SYN *fimbria* hippocampi.
t. lib′era [NA], SYN free t. SEE teniae coli.
medullary teniae, SYN medullary *striae* of fourth ventricle, under *stria.*
mesocolic t., SEE teniae coli. SYN t. mesocolica [NA].
t. mesocol′ica [NA], SYN mesocolic t. SEE teniae coli.
omental t., SEE teniae coli. SYN t. omentalis [NA].
t. omenta′lis [NA], SYN omental t. SEE teniae coli.
t. semicircula′ris, SYN terminal *stria.*
Tarin's t., SYN terminal *stria.*
t. tec′ta, SEE *indusium* griseum.
t. te′lae [NA], SYN t. choroidea.
t. termina′lis, SYN *crista* terminalis.
t. thal′ami [NA], the sharp edge or angle between the superior and medial surface of the thalamus on either side; to it is attached the epithelial lamina forming the roof of the third ventricle. SYN t. ventriculi tertii, thalamic t.
thalamic t., SYN t. thalami.
teniae of Valsalva, SYN teniae coli.
t. ventric′uli quar′ti [NA], the line of attachment of the choroid roof to the rim of the fourth ventricle. SYN t. of fourth ventricle.
t. ventric′uli ter′tii, SYN t. thalami.

te·ni·a·cide (tē′nē-ă-sīd). An agent destructive to tapeworms. SYN tenicide. [L. *taenia*, tapeworm, + *caedo*, to kill]

te·ni·a·fuge (tē′nē-ă-fūj). An agent that causes the expulsion of tapeworms. SYN tenifuge. [L. *taenia*, tapeworm, + *fugo*, to put to flight]

ten·i·al (ten′ē-ăl). 1. Relating to a tapeworm. 2. Relating to one of the structures called tenia.

te·ni·a·sis (te-nī′ă-sis). Presence of a tapeworm in the intestine.
somatic t., invasion of the body by the cysticercus of a tenioid worm.

ten·i·cide (ten′i-sīd). SYN teniacide.

ten·i·form (ten′i-fōrm). SYN tenioid.

te·nif·u·gal (te-nif′yū-găl). Having the power to expel tapeworms.

ten·i·fuge (ten′i-fyūj). SYN teniafuge.

te·ni·oid (tē′nē-oyd). 1. Band-shaped; ribbon-shaped. 2. Resembling a tapeworm. SYN teniform. [G. *tainia*, a tape, + *eidos*, resemblance]

te·ni·o·la (tē-nī′ō-lă). A slender tenia or bandlike structure. [L. dim. of *taenia*, ribbon]
t. cor′poris callo′si, SYN rostral *lamina.*

⚠**teno-, tenon-, tenont-, tenonto-.** Tendon. SEE ALSO tendo-. [G. *tenōn*]

te·no·de·sis (tĕ-nod′ē-sis, ten′ō-dē′sis). Stabilizing a joint by anchoring the tendons which move that joint. [teno- + G. *desis*, a binding]

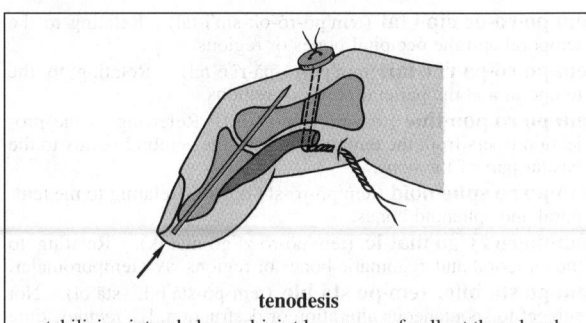

tenodesis
stabilizing interphalangeal joint by means of pullout thread and temporary arthrodesis with Kirschner wire

ten·o·dyn·ia (ten-ō-din′ĕă). SYN tenalgia. [teno- + G. *odynē*, pain]

ten·o·fi·bril (ten-ō-fī′bril). SYN tonofibril. [teno- + Mod. L. *fibrilla*, a small fiber]

ten·ol·y·sis (ten-ol′i-sis). SYN tendolysis.

ten·o·my·o·plas·ty (ten-ō-mī′ō-plas-tē). SYN tenontomyoplasty.

ten·o·my·ot·o·my (ten-ō-mī-ot′ō-mē). SYN myotenotomy.

Tenon, Jacques R., French pathologist and oculist, 1724–1816. SEE T.'s *capsule, space.*

⚠**tenon-.** SEE teno-.

ten·o·nec·to·my (ten-ō-nek′tō-mē). SYN tenectomy. [tenon- + G. *ektomē*, excision]

ten·o·ni·tis (ten-ō-nī′tis). 1. Inflammation of Tenon's capsule or the connective tissue within Tenon's space. 2. SYN tendonitis. [tenont- + G. *-itis*, inflammation]

ten·on·ti·tis (ten′on-tī′tis). SYN tendonitis. [tenont- + G. *-itis*, inflammation]

⚠**tenonto-.** SEE teno-.

te·non·to·dyn·ia (te-non′tō-din′ē-ă). SYN tenalgia.

te·non·tog·ra·phy (ten′on-tog′ră-fē). A treatise on or description of the tendons. [tenonto- + G. *graphē*, description]

te·non·to·lem·mi·tis (te-non′tō-lĕ-mī′tis). SYN tenosynovitis. [tenonto- + G. *lemma*, husk, + *-itis*]

te·non·tol·o·gy (ten′on-tol′ŏ-jē). The branch of science that has to do with the tendons. [tenonto- + G. *logos*, study]

te·non·to·my·o·plas·ty (te-non′tō-mī′ō-plas-tē). A combined tenontoplasty and myoplasty, used in the radical correction of a hernia. SYN tenomyoplasty. [tenonto- + G. *mys*, muscle, + *plastos*, formed]

te·non·to·my·ot·o·my (te-non′tō-mī-ot′ō-mē). SYN myotenotomy.

te·non·to·plas·tic (te-non′tō-plas-tik). Relating to tenontoplasty.

te·non·to·plas·ty (te-non′tō-plas-tē). Reparative or plastic surgery of the tendons. SYN tendinoplasty, tendoplasty, tenoplasty. [tenonto- + G. *plastos*, formed]

te·non·to·the·ci·tis (te-non'tō-thē-sī'tis). SYN tenosynovitis. [tenonto- + G. *thēkē*, case, box, + *-itis*]

te·noph·o·ny (te-nof'ō-nē). A heart murmur assumed to be due to an abnormal condition of the chordae tendineae. SYN tendophony. [teno- + G. *phōnē*, sound]

ten·o·phyte (ten'ō-fīt). Bony or cartilaginous growth in or on a tendon. [teno- + G. *phyton*, plant]

ten·o·plas·tic (ten-ō-plas'tik). Relating to tenoplasty.

ten·o·plas·ty (ten'ō-plas-tē). SYN tenontoplasty.

ten·o·re·cep·tor (ten'ō-rē-sep'ter, -tōr). A receptor in a tendon, activated by increased tension.

te·nor·rha·phy (te-nōr'ă-fē). Suture of the divided ends of a tendon. SYN tendinosuture, tendon suture, tenosuture. [teno- + G. *rhaphē*, suture]

ten·o·si·tis (ten-ō-sī'tis). SYN tendonitis.

ten·os·to·sis (ten-os-tō'sis). Ossification of a tendon. [teno- + G. *osteon*, bone, + *-osis*, condition]

ten·o·sus·pen·sion (ten'ō-sŭs-pen'shŭn). Using a tendon as a suspensory ligament, sometimes as a free graft or in continuity.

ten·o·su·ture (ten-ō-sū'chūr). SYN tenorrhaphy.

ten·o·syn·o·vec·to·my (ten'ō-sin-ō-vek'tō-mē). Excision of a tendon sheath. [teno- + synovia + G. *ektomē*, excision]

ten·o·syn·o·vi·tis (ten'ō-sin-ō-vī'tis). Inflammation of a tendon and its enveloping sheath. SYN tendinous synovitis, tendosynovitis, tendovaginitis, tenontolemmitis, tenontothecitis, tenovaginitis, vaginal synovitis. [teno- + synovia + G. *-itis*, inflammation]

t. crep'itans, inflammation of a tendon sheath in which movement of the tendon is accompanied by a cracking sound. SYN tenalgia crepitans.

localized nodular t., SYN giant cell *tumor* of tendon sheath.

villonodular pigmented t., SYN villous t.

villous t., a condition resembling pigmented villonodular synovitis but arising in periarticular soft tissue rather than in joint synovia; occurs most commonly in the hands. SYN villonodular pigmented t.

te·not·o·my (te-not'ō-mē). The surgical division of a tendon for relief of a deformity caused by congenital or acquired shortening of a muscle, as in clubfoot or strabismus. SYN tendotomy. [teno- + G. *tomē*, incision]

curb t., SYN tendon *recession*.

graduated t., partial incisions of the tendon of an eye muscle for correction of strabismus.

subcutaneous t., division of a tendon by means of a small pointed knife introduced through skin and subcutaneous tissue without an open operation.

ten·o·vag·i·ni·tis (ten'ō-vaj-i-nī'tis). SYN tenosynovitis. [teno- + L. *vagina*, sheath, + G. *-itis*, inflammation]

tense (tens). Tight, rigid, or strained; characterized by anxiety and psychological strain. [L. *tensus*, pp. of *tendo*, to stretch]

ten·si·om·e·ter (ten-sē-om'ĕ-ter). A device for measuring tension. [L. *tensio*, tension, + G. *metron*, measure]

ten·sion (ten'shŭn). **1.** The act of stretching. **2.** The condition of being stretched or tense, or a stretching or pulling force. **3.** The partial pressure of a gas, especially that of a gas dissolved in a liquid such as blood. **4.** Mental, emotional, or nervous strain; strained relations or barely controlled hostility between persons or groups. [L. *tensio*, fr. *tendo*, pp. *tensus*, to stretch]

arterial t., the blood pressure within an artery.

interfacial surface t., the t. or resistance to separation possessed by the film of liquid between two well-adapted surfaces, as of the thin film of saliva between the denture base and the tissues.

ocular t. (Tn), resistance of the tunics of the eye to deformation; it can be estimated digitally or measured by means of a tonometer.

premenstrual t., SYN premenstrual *syndrome*.

surface t. (γ, σ), the expression of intermolecular attraction at the surface of a liquid, in contact with air or another gas, a solid, or another immiscible liquid, tending to pull the molecules of the liquid inward from the surface; dimensional formula: mt^{-2}.

tissue t., a theoretical condition of equilibrium or balance between the tissues and cells whereby overaction of any part is restrained by the pull of the mass.

ten·sor, pl. **ten·so·res** (ten'sōr, ten-sō'rēz). A muscle the function of which is to render a part firm and tense. [Mod. L. fr. L. *tendo,* pp. *tensus,* to stretch]

tent. 1. Canopy used in various types of inhalation therapy to control humidity and concentration of oxygen in inspired air. **2.** Cylinder of some material, usually absorbent, introduced into a canal or sinus to maintain its patency or to dilate it. **3.** To elevate or pick up a segment of skin, fascia, or tissue at a given point, giving it the appearance of a t. [L. *tendo,* pp. *tensus,* to stretch]

oxygen t., a transparent enclosure, suspended over the bed and enclosing the patient, used to supply a high concentration of oxygen.

sponge t., SYN compressed *sponge.*

ten·ta·cle (ten'tă-kl). A slender process for feeling, prehension, or locomotion in invertebrates. [Mod. L. *tentaculum,* a feeler, fr. *tento,* to feel]

ten·to·ri·al (ten-tō'rē-ăl). Relating to a tentorium.

ten·to·ri·um, pl. **ten·to·ria** (ten-tō'rē-ŭm, -rē-ă) [NA]. A membranous cover or horizontal partition. [L. tent, fr. *tendo,* to stretch]

t. cerebel'li [NA], a strong fold of dura mater roofing over the posterior cranial fossa with an anterior median opening, the tentorial notch, through which the midbrain passes; the t. cerebelli is attached along the midline to the falx cerebri and separates the cerebellum from the basal surface of the occipital and temporal lobes of the cerebral hemisphere.

t. of hypophysis, SYN *diaphragm* of sella.

TEPA Abbreviation for triethylenephosphoramide.

teph·ro·ma·la·cia (tef'rō-mă-lā'shē-ă). Softening of the gray matter of the brain or spinal cord. [G. *tephros,* ashen-gray, + *malakia,* softness]

teph·ry·lom·e·ter (tef-ri-lom'ĕ-ter). An instrument for measuring the thickness of the cerebral cortex; it consists of a graduated tube of thin glass which is inserted into the brain substance, so the depth of the gray matter can be read off on the scale. [G. *tephros,* ashen, + *hylē,* stuff, + *metron,* measure]

TEPP Abbreviation for tetraethyl pyrophosphate.

tep·ro·tide (tē'prō-tīd). 2-L-tryptophan-3-de-L-leucine-4-de-L-proline-8-L-glutamine-bradykinin-potentiator B; a nonapeptide in which glycine is replaced by tryptophan, leucine and the first proline are missing, and the lysine is replaced by glutamine; an angiotensin-converting enzyme inhibitor. SYN bradykinin-potentiating peptide.

⌂**tera- (T). 1.** Prefix used in the SI and metric systems to signify one trillion. **2.** Combining form denoting a teras. SEE ALSO terato- . [G. *teras,* monster]

ter·as, pl. **ter·a·ta** (ter'as, ter'ă-tă). Fetus with deficient, redundant, misplaced, or grossly misshapen parts. [G.]

ter·at·ic (ter-at'ik). Relating to a teras.

ter·a·tism (ter'ă-tizm). SYN teratosis. [G. *teratisma,* fr. *teras*]

⌂**terato-.** A teras. SEE ALSO tera- (2). [G. *teras,* monster]

ter·a·to·blas·to·ma. A tumor containing embryonic tissue differing from a teratoma in that not all germ layers are present.

ter·a·to·car·ci·no·ma (ter'ă-tō-kar-si-nō'mă). **1.** A malignant teratoma, occurring most commonly in the testis. **2.** A malignant epithelial tumor arising in a teratoma.

te·rat·o·gen (ter'ă-tō-jen). A drug or other agent that causes abnormal fetal development. [terato- + G. *-gen,* producing]

ter·a·to·gen·e·sis (ter'ă-tō-jen'ē-sis). The origin or mode of production of a malformed fetus; the disturbed growth processes involved in the production of a malformed neonate. [terato- + G. *genesis,* origin]

ter·a·to·gen·ic, ter·a·to·ge·net·ic (ter'ă-tō-jen'ik, -jĕ-net'ik). **1.** Relating to teratogenesis. **2.** Causing abnormal embryonic development.

ter·a·to·ge·nic·i·ty (ter'ă-tō-jĕ-nis'i-tē). The property or capability of producing fetal malformation. [terato- + G. *genesis,* generation]

ter·a·toid (ter′ă-toyd). Resembling a teras. [G. *teratōdēs,* fr. *teras* (*terat-*), monster, + *eidos,* resemblance]

ter·a·to·log·ic (ter′ă-tō-loj′ik). Relating to teratology.

ter·a·tol·o·gy (ter-ă-tol′ō-jē). The branch of science concerned with the production, development, anatomy, and classification of malformed fetuses. SEE ALSO dysmorphology. [terato- + G. *logos,* study]

ter·a·to·ma (ter-ă-tō′mă). A neoplasm composed of multiple tissues, including tissues not normally found in the organ in which it arises. T.'s occur most frequently in the ovary, where they are usually benign and form dermoid cysts; in the testis, where they are usually malignant; and, uncommonly, in other sites, especially the midline of the body. SYN teratoid tumor. [terato- + G. *-oma,* tumor]

t. or′bitae, SYN orbitopagus.

sacrococcygeal t., found in the region of the primitive pit and node. Most common tumor in the newborn period.

triphyllomatous t., a t. composed of tissues derived from all three germ layers, *i.e.,* a teratoma. SYN tridermoma.

ter·a·tom·a·tous (ter′ă-tō′mă-tŭs). Relating to or of the nature of a teratoma.

ter·a·to·pho·bia (ter′ă-tō-fō′bē-ă). Morbid fear of carrying and giving birth to a malformed infant. [terato- + G. *phobos,* fear]

ter·a·to·sis (ter′ă-tō′sis). An anomaly producing a teras. SYN teratism. [terato- + G. *-osis,* condition]

atresic t., a t. in which any of the normal orifices, such as the nares, mouth, anus, or vagina, is imperforate.

ceasmic t., a t. in which there is a failure of the lateral halves of a part to unite, as in cleft palate.

ectogenic t., a t. in which there is a deficiency of parts.

ectopic t., a t. in which the organs or other parts are misplaced.

hypergenic t., a t. in which there is a redundancy of parts.

symphysic t., a t. in which there is a fusion of normally separated parts.

ter·a·to·sper·mia (ter′ă-tō-sper′mē-ă). Condition characterized by the presence of malformed spermatozoa in the semen. [terato- + G. *sperma,* seed]

te·ra·zo·sin hy·dro·chlo·ride (tĕ-rā′zō-sin). 1-(4-Amino-6,7-dimethoxy-2-quinazolinyl)-4-(tetrahydro-2-furoyl)piperazine monohydrochloride dihydrate; a peripherally acting antiadrenergic used to treat hypertension.

ter·bi·um (Tb) (ter′bē-ŭm). A metallic element of the lanthanide or rare earth series, atomic no. 65, atomic wt. 158.92534. [fr. *Ytterby,* a village in Sweden]

ter·bu·ta·line sul·fate (ter-byū′tă-lēn). α-[(*tert*-Butylamino)methyl]-3,5-dihydroxybenzyl alcohol sulfate; a sympathomimetic drug with relatively selective B₂ agonistic activity, used principally as a bronchodilator.

ter·e·bene (ter′ĕ-bēn). A thin colorless liquid of an aromatic odor and taste, a mixture of terpene hydrocarbons, chiefly dipentene and terpinene, obtained from oil of turpentine; used as an expectorant and in cystitis and urethritis.

ter·e·bin·thi·nate (ter-ĕ-bin′thĭ-nāt). 1. Containing or impregnated with turpentine. 2. A preparation containing turpentine. SYN terebinthine. [G. *terebinthos,* the terebinth or turpentine-tree]

ter·e·bin·thine (ter-ĕ-bin′thin). SYN terebinthinate.

ter·e·bin·thin·ism (ter-ĕ-bin′thin-izm). SYN turpentine *poisoning.*

ter·e·brant, ter·e·brat·ing (ter′ĕ-brant, -brā-ting). Boring; piercing; used figuratively, as in the term t. pain. [L. *terebro,* pp. *-atus,* to bore, fr. *terebra,* an auger]

ter·e·bra·tion (ter-ĕ-brā′shŭn). 1. The act of boring, or of trephining. 2. A boring, piercing pain. [L. *terebro,* to bore, fr. *terebra,* an auger]

te·res, gen. **ter·e·tis,** pl. **ter·e·tes** (ter′ēz, -tēr-; ter′ĕ-tis; ter′ĕ-tēz). Round and long; denoting certain muscles and ligaments. [L. round, smooth, fr. *tero,* to rub]

ter·fen·a·dine (ter-fen′ă-dēn). α-(*p-tert*-Butylphenyl)-4-(hydroxydiphenyl methyl)-1-piperidinebutanol; an antihistamine used to treat a variety of allergic conditions; reputed to have less sedative effects than other antihistamines.

ter·gal (ter′găl). SYN dorsal (1). [L. *tergum,* back]

ter·gum (ter′gŭm). SYN dorsum. [L.]

term. 1. A definite or limited period. 2. A name or descriptive word or phrase. SEE ALSO terminus, term *infant.* [L. *terminus,* a limit, an end]

ter·mi·nad (ter′mi-nad). Toward the terminus.

ter·mi·nal (ter′mi-năl). 1. Relating to the end; final. 2. Relating to the extremity or end of any body; *e.g.,* the end of a biopolymer. 3. A termination, extremity, end, or ending. [L. *terminus,* a boundary, limit]

amino t., SEE amino-terminal.

axon t.'s, the somewhat enlarged, often club-shaped endings by which axons make synaptic contacts with other nerve cells or with effector cells (muscle or gland cells). As isolated, by homogenizing brain or spinal cord, they contain acetylcholine and the related enzymes. T.'s contain neurotransmitters of various kinds, sometimes more than one. These can be demonstrated by chemical analysis and immunocytochemical methods. SEE ALSO synapse. SYN axonal terminal boutons, end-feet, neuropodia, pieds terminaux, synaptic boutons, synaptic endings, synaptic t.'s, terminal boutons, bouton terminaux.

carboxy t., SEE C-*terminus.*

synaptic t.'s, SYN axon t.'s.

ter·mi·nal de·ox·y·nu·cle·o·ti·dyl trans·fer·ase (dē-ok′sē-nū′klē-ō-tī-dil-trans′fer-ās). SYN DNA nucleotidylexotransferase.

ter·mi·na·tio, pl. **ter·mi·na·ti·o·nes** (ter′mi-nā′shē-ō, -ō′nēz) [NA]. SYN termination. SEE ALSO ending. [L.]

terminatio′nes nervo′rum li′berae [NA], SYN free nerve *endings,* under *ending.*

ter·mi·na·tion (ter′mi-nā′shŭn). An end or ending. A termination or ending, particularly a nerve ending. SEE termination, ending. SYN terminatio [NA]. [L. *terminatio*]

ter·mi·na·ti·o·nes (ter-mi-nā-shē-ō′nēz). Plural of terminatio. [L.]

ter·mi·nus, pl. **ter·mi·ni** (ter′mi-nŭs, -nī). A boundary or limit. [L.]

C-t., the end of a peptide or protein having a free carboxyl (–COOH) group.

ter′mini genera′les [NA], general terms; words that are of general use in descriptive anatomy.

N-t., SEE amino-terminal.

ter·mo·lec·u·lar (ter-mō-lek′ū-lar). Denoting three molecules; *e.g.,* a termolecular reaction requires three molecules to come together in order for the reaction to occur. [L. *ter,* thrice, + molecular]

ter·mone (ter′mōn). A type of ectohormone, secreted by some invertebrate organisms, that stimulates gametogenesis. [L. *ter,* thrice, threefold, + hormone]

ter·na·ry (ter′nār-ē). Denoting or comprised of three compounds, elements, molecules, etc. [L. *ternarius,* of three]

ter·ox·ide (ter-ok′sīd). SYN trioxide.

ter·pene (ter′pēn). One of a class of hydrocarbons with an empirical formula of $C_{10}H_{16}$, occurring in essential oils and resins. Acyclic t.'s may be regarded as isomers and polymers of isoprene units; cyclic forms include menthane, bornane, and camphene. T.'s containing 15, 20, 30, 40, etc., carbon atoms are called sesquiterpenes, diterpenes, triterpenes, tetraterpenes, etc.

p-**ter·phen·yl** (ter-fen′il). C_6H_5–C_6H_4–C_6H_5; useful as a scintillator in scintillation.

ter·pin. Dipenteneglycol; *p*-menthane-1,8-diol; a cyclic terpene alcohol, $C_{10}H_{18}(OH)_2$, obtained by the action of nitric acid and dilute sulfuric acid on pine oil.

t. hydrate, a monohydrate of terpin; an expectorant. SYN terpinol.

ter·pin·e·ol (ter-pin′ē-ol). *p*-Menth-1-en-8-ol; an unsaturated alcoholic terpene obtained by heating terpin hydrate with diluted phosphoric acid; an active antiseptic and a perfume.

ter·pi·nol (ter′pin-ol). SYN *terpin* hydrate.

ter·race (ter′as). To suture in several rows, in closing a wound through a considerable thickness of tissue. [thr. O. Fr. fr. L. *terra,* earth]

ter·ra ja·pon·i·ca (ter'ră jă-pon'i-kă). SEE gambir.

Terrey, Mary, 20th century U.S. physician. SEE Lowe-T.-MacLachlan *syndrome.*

Terrien, Louis-Felix, French surgeon, 1837–1908. SEE T.'s *valve,* marginal *degeneration.*

ter·ri·to·ri·al·i·ty (ter'i-tōr-ē-al'i-tē). **1.** The tendency of individuals or groups to defend a particular domain or sphere of interest or influence. **2.** The tendency of an individual animal to define a finite space as his own habitat from which he will fight off trespassing animals of his own species.

Terry, Theodore L., U.S. ophthalmologist, 1899–1946. SEE T.'s *syndrome.*

Terry's nails. See under nail.

Terson, Albert, French ophthalmologist, 1867–1935. SEE T.'s *glands,* under *gland.*

ter·tian (ter'shăn). Recurring every third day, counting the day of an episode as the first; actually, occurring every 48 hours or every other day. [L. *tertianus,* fr. *tertius,* third]

double t., denoting malarial infections with two different sets of organisms producing daily paroxysms. SEE ALSO quotidian *malaria.*

ter·ti·a·rism, ter·ti·a·ris·mus (ter'shē-ă-rizm, -riz'mŭs). All the symptoms of the tertiary stage of syphilis taken collectively.

TESD Abbreviation for total end-systolic *diameter.*

Tesla, Nikola, Serbian-American electrical engineer, 1856–1943. SEE tesla; T. *current.*

tesla (T) (tes'lă). In the SI system, the unit of magnetic flux density expressed as kg sec^{-2} A^{-1}; equal to one weber per square meter. [N. *Tesla*]

tes·sel·lat·ed (tes'ĕ-lāt-ed). Made up of small squares; checkered. [L. *tessella,* a small square stone]

Tessier (tes'ē-ā), 20th century French physician. SEE Tessier *classification.*

TEST

test. 1. To prove; to try a substance; to determine the chemical nature of a substance by means of reagents. **2.** A method of examination, as to determine the presence or absence of a definite disease or of some substance in any of the fluids, tissues, or excretions of the body, or to determine the presence or degree of a psychological or behavioral trait. **3.** A reagent used in making a t. **4.** SEE testa (2). SEE ALSO assay, reaction, reagent, scale, stain. [L. *testum,* an earthen vessel]

acetone t., a t. for ketonuria; the suspected urine is shaken up with a few drops of sodium nitroprusside, and strong ammonia water is then gently poured over the mixture; if acetone is present, a magenta ring forms at the line of contact; tablets containing sodium nitroprusside and alkali are now more commonly used.

achievement t., a standardized t. used to measure acquired learning, *e.g.,* competence in a specific subject area such as reading or arithmetic, in contrast to an intelligence t. which is a useful index of potential ability or learning.

acidified serum t., lysis of the patient's red cells in acidified fresh serum, specific for paroxysmal nocturnal hemoglobinuria. SYN Ham's t.

acid perfusion t., SYN Bernstein t.

acid phosphatase t. for semen, a screening t. for semen by determining acid phosphatase content; because seminal fluid contains high concentrations of acid phosphatase, while other body fluids and extraneous foreign materials have very low concentrations, high values of acid phosphatase on vaginal aspirate or lavage, or on wash fluid from stains, render positive identification of semen, even if the male is aspermic.

acid reflux t., a t. to detect gastroesophageal reflux by monitoring esophageal pH by an electrode in the distal esophagus either basally or after acid is instilled into the stomach.

ACTH stimulation t., a t. for adrenal cortical function; ACTH administered by continuous intravenous infusion, or intramuscularly, evokes an increase in plasma cortisol in normal persons; in adrenal cortical insufficiency, the expected increase in plasma cortisol is limited or nonexistent.

Addis t., SEE Addis *count.*

adhesion t., the diagnostic application of the immune adhesion phenomenon. SYN erythrocyte adherence t., immune adhesion t., red cell adherence t.

Adler's t., SYN benzidine t.

Adson's t., a t. for thoracic outlet syndrome; the patient is seated, with head extended and turned to the side of the lesion; with deep inspiration there is a diminution or total loss of radial pulse on the affected side. Not all patients with a positive Adson's test have thoracic outlet syndrome. SYN Adson maneuver.

agglutination t., any of a variety of t.'s that are dependent on the clumping of cells, microorganisms, or particles when mixed with specific antiserum.

Albarran's t., a t. for renal insufficiency wherein the drinking of large quantities of water will cause a proportionate increase in the volume of urine if the kidneys are sound, but not if the epithelium of the secreting tubules is damaged. SYN polyuria t.

alkali denaturation t., a t. for hemoglobin F (Hb F), based on the fact that hemoglobins, with the exception of Hb F, are denatured by alkali to alkaline hematin; the t. is sensitive to 2% or more Hb F.

Allen-Doisy t., a t. for estrogenic activity; the material to be investigated is injected repeatedly into immature or spayed rats or mice; the disappearance of leukocytes from the vaginal smear and the appearance of cornified cells constitutes a positive reaction.

Allen's t., (1) for phenol: upon the addition of 5 or 6 drops of hydrochloric acid and then 1 of nitric acid to the suspected fluid, a red color develops; [A.H. Allen] **(2)** for strychnine: fluid is extracted with ether, which is then evaporated by means of "drop-by-drop" pipetting into a warmed porcelain dish or crucible; the residue is treated with a small bit of manganese dioxide and dilute sulfuric acid; a red-blue or violet color develops if strychnine is present. [A.H. Allen] **(3)** a t. for radial or ulnar patency; either the radial or ulnar artery is digitally compressed by the examiner after blood has been forced out of the hand by clenching it into a fist; failure of the blood to diffuse into the hand when opened indicates that the artery not compressed is occluded. [Edgar Van Nuys Allen]

Almén's t. for blood, glacial acetic acid, gum guaiac solution, and hydrogen peroxide are added to an aqueous suspension of the suspected stain; if occult blood or blood pigment is present, a blue color develops. SYN guaiac t., Schönbein's t., van Deen's t.

Alpha t.'s, a set of paper and pencil-administered mental t.'s first used in the United States Army in 1917–1918 to determine the mental ability of literate recruits; the set includes 8 different types of t.'s: *i.e.,* directions, arithmetical problems, practical judgement, synonyms and antonyms, disarrayed sentences, number series completions, analogies, and information; they are designed especially for testing large groups of individuals simultaneously, and for rapid machine scoring; distinguished from the Army Beta t.'s, a complementary set for administration to recruits who could not read or write English, in which the instructions are given in signs and the t. material is pictorial. SEE Beta t.'s. SYN Army Alpha t.

alternate binaural loudness balance t., ABLB t., a t. for recruitment in one ear; the comparison of relative loudness of a series of intensities presented alternately to either ear.

alternate cover t., a t. to detect phoria or strabismus; attention is directed to a small fixation object, and one eye is covered for several seconds; then the cover is moved quickly to the other eye; if the eye moves when it is uncovered, a strabismus or phoria is present.

alternating light t., t. to detect a relative afferent defect in one eye by watching pupillary movements. With the patient fixing in the distance, the light is held on each eye for about a second, and quickly moved to the other eye. Assuming no defect of the innervation to the iris sphincter in one eye (which would produce an anisocoria in light), the eye with the weaker light response has a relative afferent pupillary defect. This asymmetry of pupillo-motor input can be estimated by holding neutral density filters in front of the better eye until the pupillary responses of the two eyes are balanced. SYN swinging light t.

Ames t., a screening t. for possible carcinogens using strains of *Salmonella typhinium* that are unable to synthesize histidine; if the test substance produces mutations that regain the ability to synthesize histidine, the substance is carcinogenic. SYN Ames assay.

Amsler t., projection of a visual field defect onto an Amsler chart.

Anderson-Collip t., a procedure for evaluating the thyrotropic activity of an extract of the anterior lobe of the pituitary gland, as indicated by an increased basal metabolic rate or histologic evidence of stimulation of the thyroid gland in a hypophysectomized rat injected with the t. extract.

Anderson and Goldberger t., a t. for typhus in which the patient's blood is injected into a guinea pig's peritoneal cavity. In typhus a typical temperature curve will be observed.

anoxemia t., a t. for coronary insufficiency; the patient breathes a mixture of 10% oxygen and 90% nitrogen; if anginal pain or electrocardiographic abnormalities are induced, the t. is positive. SYN hypoxemia t.

antibiotic sensitivity t., the *in vitro* testing of bacterial cultures with antibiotics to determine susceptibility of bacteria to antibiotic therapy.

antiglobulin t., SYN Coombs' t.

antihuman globulin t., SEE Coombs' t.

antithrombin t., a procedure for estimating the inhibitory effect of a defibrinated specimen of plasma on the action of thrombin in converting fibrinogen to fibrin.

Apt t., a t. for identifying fetal blood by the addition of sodium hydroxide and water to a specimen.

aptitude t., an occupation-oriented intelligence t. used to evaluate a person's abilities, talents, and skills; particularly valuable in vocational counseling.

Army Alpha t., SYN Alpha t.'s.

Army Beta t.'s, SYN Beta t.'s.

Army General Classification T., a selection screening t. of overall intellectual ability administered to entering army recruits for use in determining qualifications for entry into one of the wide range of positions to which each individual is assigned at the end of basic training.

Aschheim-Zondek t., an obsolete t. for pregnancy; repeated injections of small quantities of urine voided during the first months of pregnancy produce in infantile mice, within 100 hours, minute intrafollicular ovarian hemorrhages, and the development of lutein cells. SYN A.-Z. t., Zondek-Aschheim t.

Ascoli's t., a precipitin t. for anthrax using a tissue extract and anthrax antiserum.

ascorbate-cyanide t., a t. for glucose 6-phosphate-deficient red blood cells; blood is incubated with sodium cyanide and ascorbate; the hydrogen peroxide generated is free to oxidize hemoglobin to methemoglobin, since cyanide inhibits catalase; a brown color is produced more rapidly in glucose 6-phosphate-deficient cells.

association t., a word (stimulus word) is spoken to the subject, who is to reply immediately with another word (reaction word) suggested by the first; used as a diagnostic aid in psychiatry and psychology, clues being given by the length of time (association time) between the stimulus and reaction words, and also by the nature of the reaction words.

Astwood's t., SYN metrotrophic t.

atropine t., SYN Dehio's t.

augmented histamine t., SYN histamine t.

aussage t. (ows'zah-gǎ), a t. of ability to reproduce correctly something that has been seen for a brief interval. [Ger. *Aussage*, a declaration]

autohemolysis t., when sterile defibrinated blood is incubated at 37°C, normal red blood cells hemolyze slowly; cells with membrane or metabolic defects do so to a greater extent.

A.-Z. t., SYN Aschheim-Zondek t.

Bachman t., a skin t. for trichinosis in which an extract of *Trichinella* larvae is suspended in saline and injected intradermally. An immediate wheal-and-flare reaction or a delayed response indicates infection.

Bachman-Pettit t., a modification of Kober's t. for the detection of estradiol and similar estrogenic hormones in the urine.

Bagolini t., a t. for retinal correspondence with the subject observing a figure through two striated lenses.

BALB t., SYN binaural alternate loudness balance t.

Bárány's caloric t., a t. for vestibular function, made by irrigating the external auditory meatus with either hot or cold water; this normally causes stimulation of the vestibular apparatus, resulting in nystagmus and past-pointing; in vestibular disease, the response may be reduced or absent. SYN caloric t., nystagmus t.

BEI t., SYN butanol-extractable iodine t.

belt t., an obsolete t.: firm upward pressure on the lower part of the abdomen will remove the feeling of discomfort in cases of enteroptosia.

Bender gestalt t., a psychological t. used by neurologists and clinical psychologists to measure a person's ability to visually copy a set of geometric designs; useful for measuring visuospatial and visuomotor coordination to detect brain damage. SYN Bender Visual Motor Gestalt t.

Bender Visual Motor Gestalt t., SYN Bender gestalt t.

Benedict's t. for glucose, a copper-reduction t. for glucose in the urine, which involves thiocyanate in addition to copper sulfate for qualitative or quantitative use.

bentiromide t., a t. of pancreatic exocrine function that does not require duodenal intubation: orally administered bentiromide is cleaved by chymotrypsin within the lumen of the small intestine, releasing *p*-aminobenzoic acid which is absorbed and excreted in the urine; diminished urinary excretion of *p*-aminobenzoic acid suggests pancreatic insufficiency.

bentonite flocculation t., a flocculation t. for rheumatoid arthritis in which sensitized bentonite particles are added to inactivated serum; the t. is positive if half of the particles are clumped while the other half remain in suspension.

benzidine t., a t. for blood; the suspected fluid is treated with glacial acetic acid and ether, and the latter is then decanted and treated with hydrogen peroxide and a solution of benzidine in acetic acid; the presence of blood is indicated by a bluish color turning to purple. SYN Adler's t.

Bernstein t., a t. to establish that substernal pain is due to reflux esophagitis, performed by instillation of a weak hydrochloric acid solution directly into the lower esophagus; symptoms disappear when the acid solution is replaced by normal saline solution. SYN acid perfusion t.

Berson t., a t. of thyroid clearance of ^{131}I from the plasma by the thyroid gland.

Beta t.'s, a set of pictorially administered mental t.'s first used in the United States Army in 1917–1918 to determine the relative mental ability of recruits who were illiterate or deficient in reading and writing English, the instructions being given in signs and the t. material's pictorial in characters; distinguished from the Army Alpha t., which were administered at the same time to literate recruits. SYN Army Beta t.'s.

Betke-Kleihauer t., a slide t. for the presence of fetal red blood cells among those of the mother; hemoglobins other than Hb F are eluted from the red blood cells on an air-dried blood film by a buffer of pH 3.3.

Bettendorff's t., a t. for arsenic; after mixing the suspected fluid with hydrochloric acid a solution of stannous chloride is added; when a piece of tin foil is then added, a brown precipitate forms.

Bial's t., a t. for pentoses with orcinol. SYN orcinol t.

bile acid tolerance t., a sensitive t. of hepatic dysfunction; following oral administration of labeled or unlabeled bile acid, the measured fractional disappearance rate or 10-minute retention is measured.

bile esculin t., a biochemical t. used in characterizing group *O* streptococci, based on the ability of organisms to grow in a medium containing bile and to hydrolyze esculin.

bile solubility t., a procedure that differentiates *Streptococcus* *pneumoniae* from other α-hemolytic streptococci by demonstrating its susceptibility to lysis in the presence of bile.

binaural alternate loudness balance t., a t. for recruitment in one ear; the comparison of relative loudness of a series of intensities presented alternately to either ear. SYN BALB t.

Binet t., SYN Stanford-Binet intelligence *scale.*

Binz' t., a qualitative t. for the presence of quinine in the urine; a precipitate is formed on the addition of an aqueous solution of iodine and potassium iodide if quinine is present.

biuret t., a t. for the determination of serum proteins, based on the reaction of an alkaline copper reagent with substances containing two or more peptide bonds to produce a violet-blue color.

blind t., a method of testing in which an independent observer records the results of any t., drug, placebo, or procedure without knowing the identity of the samples or what result might be expected.

block design t., a performance t. using colored blocks which the individual must use to match pictured designs; one of the subtests of the Wechsler intelligence scales.

Bonney t., SYN Marshall t.

breath analysis t., (1) a t. of hepatic and intestinal absorptive function; aminopyrine labeled with radioactive carbon is administered orally; expired $^{14}CO_2$ is a measure of aminopyrine absorption and its metabolism in the liver; **(2)** a measurement of the amount of $^{14}CO_2$ exhaled after an oral dose of ^{14}C-O-xylose; **(3)** a measurement of exhaled hydrogen gas following an oral dose of lactose as a t. of lactose deficiency.

breath-holding t., a rough index of cardiopulmonary reserve measured by the length of time that a subject can voluntarily stop breathing; normal duration is 30 seconds or more; diminished cardiac or pulmonary reserve is indicated by a duration of 20 seconds or less.

Brigg's t., a t. using the reduction of molybdate to follow the excretion of homogentisic acid.

bromphenol t., a colorimetric t. for measurement of protein, albumin, and globulin in the urine by use of reagent strips.

bromsulphalein t., obsolete t. for liver function (hepatic excretory capacity) in which a known amount of dye, usually 5 mg/kg of body weight, is injected intravenously; subsequently (usually after 45 minutes elapsed time), the amount of dye remaining in the serum is measured; a concentration of 0.4 mg or less of bromsulphalein per 100 ml of serum or less than 4% of the injected dye is considered normal; bromsulphalein retention may follow decreased hepatic blood flow or biliary obstruction as well as hepatic cell damage. SYN BSP t.

BSP t., SYN bromsulphalein t.

butanol-extractable iodine t., an obsolete t. for thyroid function, applicable in patients who have received large amounts of iodine or iodized products. SYN BEI t.

California psychological inventory t., a personality inventory, used with normal persons, in which emphasis is upon social interaction variables.

Calmette t., conjunctival reaction to tuberculin.

caloric t., SYN Bárány's caloric t.

CAMP t., a t. to identify Group B β-streptococci based on their formation of a substance (CAMP factor) that enlarges the area of hemolysis formed by streptococcal β-hemolysin. [*C*hristie, *At*kins, and *M*unch-*P*etersen, developers of the t.]

cancer antigen 125 t. (CA125), t. for cell-surface antigen found on derivatives of coelomic epithelium. Elevated levels of this antigen are associated with ovarian malignancy and benign pelvic disease such as endometriosis.

capillary fragility t., a tourniquet t. used to determine presence of vitamin C deficiency or thrombocytopenia; a circle 2.5 cm in diameter, the upper edge of which is 4 cm below the crease of the elbow, is drawn on the inner aspect of the forearm, pressure midway between the systolic and diastolic blood pressure is applied above the elbow for 15 minutes, and a count of petechiae within the circle is made: 10, normal; 10 to 20, marginal zone; over 20, abnormal. SEE ALSO Rumpel-Leede t. SYN capillary resistance t., vitamin C t.

capillary resistance t., SYN capillary fragility t.

capon-comb-growth t., SYN comb-growth t.

carbohydrate utilization t., a t. for the definitive identification of clinically important yeasts and yeastlike organisms.

carotid sinus t., stimulation of one carotid sinus (never both) to produce reflex effects that may slow the heart, reduce the systolic blood pressure or both for diagnostic or, in the case of certain arrhythmias, therapeutic purposes.

Carr-Price t., a quantitative t. for vitamin A based on the reaction with antimony trichloride in chloroform.

Casoni intradermal t., a t. for hydatid disease in which hydatid fluid is injected intracutaneously; immediate or delayed wheal and flare reaction is positive. SYN Casoni skin t.

Casoni skin t., SYN Casoni intradermal t.

CF t., SYN complement *fixation.*

Chick-Martin t., a method of testing the *in vitro* efficiency of a bactericidal agent; a standard culture of *Salmonella typhi* which has been added to a fixed amount of sterilized feces or yeast is tested for a fixed period (30 minutes), against various concentrations of phenol solution and various concentrations of the disinfectant; the result is expressed as a ratio: the phenol coefficient, which is the highest dilution of the disinfectant under t. at which the bacteria are killed, divided by the highest dilution of phenol which sterilizes the solution in the same length of time.

chi-square t. (kī), a statistical method of assessing the significance of a difference, as when the data from two or more samples is represented by a discrete number such as the numbers of females and males attending each of two colleges. SYN x^2 t.

cis/trans t., a t. on the relative configuration on expression of two mutations.

Clauberg t., a t. for progestational activity; immature rabbits are treated with 8 daily injections of estrogen and then given 5 daily injections of the t. substance; the amount required to produce definite progestational changes in the endometrium is taken as the unit; it is equivalent to 0.75 mg of progesterone.

clomiphene t., a t. of pituitary gonadotropin reserve using clomiphene.

coccidioidin t., an intracutaneous t. for determining the presence of infection with the fungus *Coccidioides immitis;* a reaction of delayed hypersensitivity indicates a positive t. and is interpreted as meaning past or present infection with the fungus.

cock's comb t., SYN comb-growth t.

coin t., SYN bellmetal *resonance.*

cold bend t., a t. of the ability of a wire to be shaped; performed by counting the number of times a wire can be bent to a right angle and reversed at the same point before breaking; important in establishing specifications for orthodontic wires.

cold pressor t., a cardiocirculatory challenge conventionally performed by immersing one hand in ice cold water for two or more minutes (as tolerated) to acutely raise the blood pressure, thus imposing resistance to ejection of blood from the left ventricle into the systemic arterial system and consequently acutely increased afterload (afterload = increased left ventricular wall stress). SYN Hines-Brown t.

colloidal gold t., SEE Lange's t.

colorimetric caries susceptibility t., SYN Snyder's t.

comb-growth t., a t. for androgenic activity, based upon the stimulation of comb growth in capons (castrated cockerels) or immature roosters. SYN capon-comb-growth t., cock's comb t.

complement-fixation t., an immunological t. for determining the presence of a particular antigen or antibody when one of the two is known to be present, based on the fact that complement is "fixed" in the presence of antigen and its specific antibody. SEE ALSO Bordet-Gengou *phenomenon.*

contraction stress t., a t. used to evaluate fetal well-being by inducing contractions and analyzing the fetal heart rate response.

Coombs' t., a t. for antibodies, the so-called anti-human globulin t. using either the direct or indirect Coombs' t.'s. SYN antiglobulin t.

Corner-Allen t., a t. for progestational activity; adult female rabbits are mated during estrus and spayed 18 hours later; the t. substance is injected subcutaneously on 5 successive days; the minimal amount required to produce complete progestational proliferation of the endometrium is taken as a unit, equivalent to 1.25 mg of progesterone.

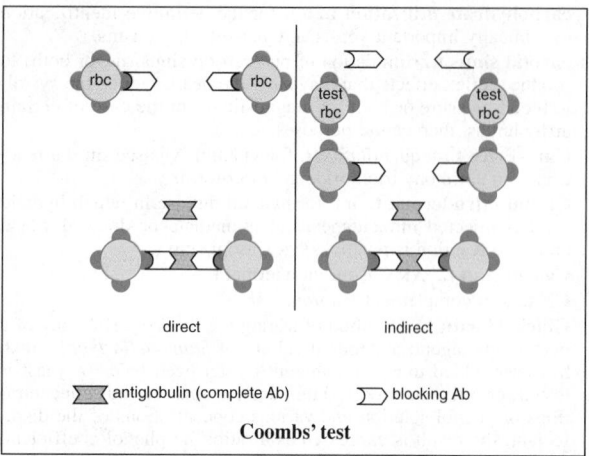

direct indirect

▨ antiglobulin (complete Ab) ◻ blocking Ab

Coombs' test

cover t., a t. used for objective demonstration of ocular deviation in strabismus; may be performed by two methods: the cover-uncover t. and the alternate cover t.

cover-uncover t., a t. to detect strabismus; the patient's attention is directed to a small fixation object, one eye is covered and after a few seconds, uncovered; if the uncovered eye moves to see the picture, strabismus is present.

CO₂-withdrawal seizure t., utilization of hyperventilation to demonstrate abnormalities in the brain waves or even to precipitate a convulsion.

Crampton t., a test for physical condition and resistance; a record is made of the pulse and the blood pressure in the recumbent and in the standing position, and the difference is graded from the theoretical perfection of 100 (seldom attained) downward (a reading of 75 is considered excellent, 65 poor); high values indicate a good physical resistance but low ones indicate weakness and a liability to shock after an operation.

t.'s of criminal responsibility, in forensic psychiatry, legal precedents upon which are based decisions concerning insanity in criminals. SEE ALSO American Law Institute *rule*, Durham *rule*, M'Naghten *rule*, New Hampshire *rule*.

cutaneous t., SYN skin t.

cutaneous tuberculin t., SEE tuberculin t.

cutireaction t., SYN skin t.

cyanide-nitroprusside t., a qualitative t. for diagnosis of cystinuria; the addition of fresh sodium cyanide formed by sodium nitroprusside to a sample of urine gives rise to a stable red-purple color in the presence of cystine.

cytotropic antibody t., a rosette t. for macrophage cytotropic antibody: monolayers of macrophages are exposed first to antibody cytotropic for macrophages, then to the antigen (for which the antibody is specific), and indicator sheep erythrocytes; if the antibody is specific for sheep erythrocytes, the latter will form a rosette around the macrophages directly, but if not, and the antigen is soluble, the antigen must be coupled to the sheep erythrocytes by an agent such as bis-diazotized benzidine.

DA pregnancy t., direct agglutination latex t. for pregnancy. SEE immunologic pregnancy t.

Day's t., a t. for blood by adding to the suspected fluid, or the washing of a suspected stain, tincture of guaiac and then hydrogen peroxide; the presence of blood results in a blue color.

d-dimer t., t. that detects the cross-linked fibrin degradation fragment, D-dimer. Elevations in this fragment are seen in primary and secondary fibrinolysis, during thrombolytic or defibrination therapy with tissue plasminogen activator, as a result of thrombotic disease, such as deep-vein thrombosis, pulmonary embolism or DIC, in vasoocclusive crisis of sickle cell anemia, in malignancies, and in surgery.

Dehio's t., if an injection of atropine relieves bradycardia, the condition is due to action of the vagus; if it does not, the condition may be due to an affection of the heart itself. SYN atropine t.

dehydrocholate t., a method of determining the speed of the

blood circulation; a solution of sodium dehydrocholate is injected intravenously, and the time that elapses before a bitter taste is noted in the mouth is recorded; the average of this time is normally about 13 seconds.

Denver Developmental Screening T., a scale used by psychologists and pediatricians to assess the developmental, intellectual, motor, and social maturity of children at any age level from birth to adolescence.

dexamethasone suppression t., a t. for the detection and diagnosis of Cushing's syndrome; following administration of 1.0 mg of dexamethasone at 11 p.m., normal persons suppress plasma cortisol to low levels; patients with Cushing's syndrome do not. Higher dose regimens distinguish between Cushing's syndrome due to tumor and due to hyperplasia.

Dick t., an intracutaneous t. of susceptibility to the erythrogenic toxin of *Streptococcus pyogenes* responsible for the rash and other manifestations of scarlet fever. SYN Dick method.

differential renal function t., SYN differential ureteral catheterization t.

differential ureteral catheterization t., a study performed to determine various functional parameters of one kidney compared to the contralateral kidney; ureteral catheters are inserted at cystoscopy into the ureter or renal pelvis bilaterally, and simultaneous measurements are made of urine flow rate, insulin, or PAH (if infused), endogenous creatinine, or various urinary solutes. SYN differential renal function t., split renal function t.

dinitrophenylhydrazine t., a screening t. for maple syrup urine disease; the addition of 2,4-dinitrophenylhydrazine in HCl to urine gives a chalky white precipitate in the presence of ketoacids.

direct Coombs' t., a t. for detecting sensitized erythrocytes in erythroblastosis fetalis and in cases of acquired immune hemolytic anemia: the patient's erythrocytes are washed with saline to remove serum and unattached antibody protein, then incubated with Coombs' anti-human globulin (usually serum from a rabbit or goat previously immunized with human globulin); after incubation, the system is centrifuged and examined for agglutination, which indicates the presence of so-called incomplete or univalent antibodies on the surface of the erythrocytes.

direct fluorescent antibody t., SEE fluorescent antibody *technique*.

discontinuation t., a t. to determine whether a certain drug is responsible for a reaction by observation of a remission of symptoms following cessation of its use.

Doerfler-Stewart t., examination of the patient's ability to respond to spondee words in the presence of a masking noise of the saw-tooth type; used especially in differentiating between functional and organic hearing loss. SYN D-S t.

double (gel) diffusion precipitin t. in one dimension, SEE gel diffusion precipitin t.'s in one dimension.

double (gel) diffusion precipitin t. in two dimensions, SEE gel diffusion precipitin t.'s in two dimensions.

Dragendorff's t., a qualitative t. for bile; a play of colors is produced by adding a drop of nitric acid to white filter paper or unglazed porcelain, moistened with a fluid containing bile pigments. The t. is essentially the same as Gmelin's t. for bile in urine.

drawer t., SYN drawer *sign*.

D-S t., SYN Doerfler-Stewart t.

Ducrey t., an intradermal t., using inactivated *Haemophilus ducreyi*, for diagnosis of chancroid; a positive delayed reaction is indicative of present or past infection; false-positive results occur. SYN Ito-Reenstierna t.

Dugas' t., in the case of an injured shoulder, if the elbow cannot be made to touch the chest while the hand rests on the opposite shoulder, the injury is a dislocation and not a fracture of the humerus.

Duke bleeding time t., a bleeding time t. in which an incision is made in the earlobe and the time until bleeding stops is measured.

dye exclusion t., a t. to determine cell viability in which a dilute solution of certain dyes (*e.g.,* trypan blue, eosin Y, nigrosin, Alcian blue) is mixed with a suspension of live cells; cells that exclude dye are considered to be alive while cells that stain are considered dead; it is not always an accurate t. because it indicates only the structural integrity of the cell membrane.

Ebbinghaus t., a psychological t. in which the patient is asked to complete certain sentences from which several words have been left out.

Ellsworth-Howard t., measurement of serum and urinary phosphorus after intravenous administration of parathyroid extract; used in the diagnosis of pseudohypoparathyroidism.

E-rosette t., a t. to identify T lymphocytes by mixing purified blood lymphocytes with serum and sheep erythrocytes; rosettes of erythrocytes form around human T lymphocytes on incubation.

erythrocyte adherence t., SYN adhesion t.

erythrocyte fragility t., SYN fragility t.

ether t., an obsolete t. to determine arm-to-lung circulation time; diluted ether is injected intravenously and the end point taken when the subject coughs or tastes ether or the observer smells ether on the subject's breath.

exercise t., any t. utilizing exercise to determine the patient's solidus responses and/or physical condition.

Farnsworth-Munsell color t., a t. for color perception; the task is to arrange 84 color disks (in four separate racks of 20–22 disks) in a sequence with minimal separation of hue between adjacent disks.

fern t., (1) a t. for estrogenic activity; cervical mucus smears form a fern pattern at those times when estrogen secretion is elevated, as at the time of ovulation; **(2)** a t. to detect ruptured amniotic membranes.

ferric chloride t., a qualitative t. for the detection of phenylketonuria; the addition of ferric chloride to urine gives rise to a blue-green color in the presence of phenylketonuria.

Fevold t., a t. for relaxin; based on the degree of relaxation of the pelvic ligaments of the guinea pig upon injection of extracts of the corpus luteum.

Finckh t., a psychological t. in which the patient is asked to explain certain proverbial expressions, such as "burn the candle at both ends," "the early bird catches the worm," etc.

finger-nose t., a t. of voluntary eye-motor coordination of the upper limb(s); the subject is asked to slowly touch the tip of his nose with his extended index finger; assesses cerebellar function.

finger-to-finger t., a t. for coordination and position sense of the upper limbs; the subject is asked to approximate the ends of his index fingers; assesses cerebellar function.

fish t., SYN erythrophore *reaction.*

Fishberg concentration t., a t. of renal water conservation; after overnight fluid deprivation, morning urine samples are collected and specific gravity is measured.

Fisher's exact t., the t. for association in a two-by-two table that is based on the exact distribution of the frequencies within the table.

fistula t., compression or rarefaction of the air in the external auditory canal excites nystagmus when there is an erosion of the otic capsule, so long as the labyrinth is still capable of functioning.

FIT t., SYN fusion-inferred threshold t.

Fleitmann's t., a t. for arsenic; hydrogen is generated in a t. tube containing the suspected fluid; the fluid is heated and a piece of filter paper moistened with silver nitrate solution is held over the top; if arsenic is present, the moistened paper is blackened.

flocculation t., SEE flocculation *reaction.*

fluorescein instillation t., a t. for patency of the lacrimal system; fluorescein instilled in the conjunctival sac can be recovered from the inferior nasal meatus. SYN Jones' t.

fluorescein string t., a string t. used to determine location of a bleeding intestinal lesion in which fluorescein is given intravenously to determine gastrointestinal hemorrhage; if the string fluoresces after removal, it has been contaminated by blood that has appeared since injection of the fluorescein; used to determine location of bleeding lesion.

fluorescent antinuclear antibody t., FANA t., a t. for antinuclear antibody components; used, in particular, for the diagnosis of collagen-vascular diseases.

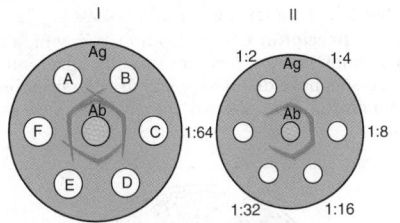

I: two-dimensional immunodiffusion, or Ouchterlony test; between A and B, cross-phenomena *and* idenity reaction (that is, two different Ag [antigen] determinants); between B and C and between D and E, *only* idenity reaction (through various additional determinants); between E and F, *only* cross-phenomena, or complete Ag heterogeneity
II: modification of Ouchterlony technique (rosette test) for semiquantitative precipitin determination

fluorescent treponemal antibody-absorption t., a sensitive and specific serologic t. for syphilis using a suspension of the Nichols strain of *Treponema pallidum* as antigen; the presence or absence of antibody in the patient's serum is indicated by an indirect fluorescent antibody technique. SYN FTA-ABS t.

foam stability t., a t. for fetal pulmonary maturity, determined by the ability of pulmonary surfactant in amniotic fluid to generate stable foam in the presence of ethanol after mechanical agitation. SYN shake t.

Folin-Looney t., a t. for tyrosine that gives a blue color in alkaline solution with a reagent consisting of sodium tungstate, phosphomolybdic acid, and phosphoric acid.

Folin's t., (1) a quantitative t. for uric acid by means of the color produced with phosphotungstic acid and a base; **(2)** a quantitative t. for urea; the urea is decomposed by boiling with magnesium chloride, and the freed ammonia is measured.

Fosdick-Hansen-Epple t., a t. for determining dental caries activity based on a solution of powdered human enamel in a saliva-glucose-enamel mixture.

Foshay t., an intradermal t. for cat-scratch disease or tularemia, using material prepared from suppurative lymph nodes of persons known to have had the disease.

fragility t., a t. that measures the resistance of erythrocytes to hemolysis in hypotonic saline solutions; erythrocytes to be tested are added to varying concentrations of saline (usually ranging from 0.85 to 0.10% sodium chloride with 0.05% increments), and beginning and complete hemolysis are measured; normal erythrocytes show initial hemolysis at concentrations of 0.45 to 0.39% and complete hemolysis at 0.33 to 0.30%; in hereditary spherocytosis the fragility of the erythrocytes is markedly increased, whereas in thalassemia, sickle cell anemia, and obstructive jaundice the fragility of the erythrocytes is usually reduced. SYN erythrocyte fragility t.

Frei t., an intracutaneous diagnostic t. for lymphogranuloma venereum: the Frei antigen is usually a sterile preparation of inactivated chlamydiae from domestic fowl; a positive delayed type reaction is not diagnostically specific for lymphogranuloma venereum and is rarely used. SYN Frei-Hoffmann reaction.

Fridenberg's stigometric card t., an obsolete t. of vision and accommodation for illiterates, using a card containing a series of dots and squares of graduated size, to be counted at various distances.

FTA-ABS t., SYN fluorescent treponemal antibody-absorption t.

fusion-inferred threshold t., employment of the phenomenon of cerebral fusion of binaural sounds to substitute for conventional masking in hearing testing. SYN FIT t.

Gaddum and Schild t., a sensitive method for identification of epinephrine in tissue or other material, based on the fluorescence of epinephrine exposed to ultraviolet light in the presence of alkali and oxygen; sensitivity ranges from 1:50 to 1:100 million.

galactose tolerance t., a liver function t., based on the ability of the liver to convert galactose to glycogen, measured by the rate of excretion of galactose following ingestion or intravenous injection of a known amount; normally, less than 3 g appear in the urine within 5 hours after the ingestion of 40 g.

gel diffusion precipitin t.'s, precipitin t.'s in which the immune precipitate forms in a gel medium (usually agar) into which one or both reactants have diffused; generally classified in two types, in one dimension, and in two dimensions. SYN gel diffusion reactions.

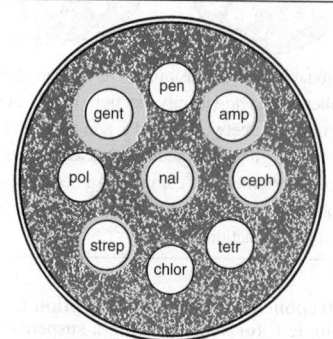

gel diffusion precipitin tests

pen = penicillin G; amp = ampicillin; cef = cephalothin; tetr = tetracycline; chlor = chloramphenicol; strep = streptomycin; pol = polymyxin B; gent = gentamicin; nal = nalidixic acid

gel diffusion precipitin t.'s in one dimension, precipitin t.'s in which antigen solution and antibody incorporated in agar are layered in tubes, permitting effective diffusion in the vertical dimension; the antibody-containing agar may be overlaid directly with antigen solution (*single (gel) diffusion in one dimension*).

gel diffusion precipitin t.'s in two dimensions, precipitin t.'s made in a layer of agar that permits radial diffusion, in both of the horizontal dimensions, of one or both reactants. *Double (gel) diffusion in two dimensions* (Ouchterlony test, technique, or method) incorporates antigen and antibody solutions placed in separate wells in a sheet of plain agar, permitting radial diffusion of both reactants; this method is widely used to determine antigenic relationships; the bands of precipitate that form where the reactants meet in optimal concentration are of three patterns, referred to as reaction of identity, reaction of partial identity (cross-reaction), and reaction of nonidentity.

Gellé t., a vibrating tuning fork is applied over the mastoid process; if it is heard, the air in the external auditory canal is compressed, by means of a rubber tube inserted into the canal and a hand bulb, thereby fixing the stapes in the oval window, and the sound ceases to be heard, but is again perceived if the air pressure is removed; a t. of the mobility of the ossicles.

Geraghty's t., SYN phenolsulfonphthalein t.

Gerhardt's t. for acetoacetic acid, in fresh urine a red color develops upon addition of FeCl₃; no color develops if the urine has first been boiled; this t. has low specificity and sensitivity. SYN Gerhardt's reaction.

Gerhardt's t. for urobilin in the urine, the urobilin is extracted with chloroform and then treated with iodine and potassium hydrate, a fluorescent green color being produced.

germ tube t., a t. for the identification of *Candida albicans;* after a 3-hr incubation in serum, an inoculum of *Candida* develops tubelike appendages.

glucose oxidase paper strip t., a qualitative t. for glucose in the urine, in which glucose is oxidized to gluconic acid by glucose oxidase; a specific t., unless ascorbic acid is present.

glucose tolerance t., a t. for diabetes, based upon the ability of the normal liver to absorb and store excessive amounts of glucose as glycogen; following ingestion of 75 g of glucose, the fasting blood sugar promptly rises and then falls to normal within 2 hours, but in a diabetic patient the increase is greater and the return to normal unusually prolonged.

Gmelin's t., a t. for bile in the urine or other body fluid; nitric acid, with a little nitrous acid, is cautiously added to a few milliliters of the material to be tested; if bile (bilirubin) is present, it is oxidized to varying degrees, thereby resulting in disklike zones that are (from the interface outward) yellow, red, violet, blue, and green; development of green and violet layers is essential to the validity of the t. SYN Rosenbach-Gmelin t.

Gofman t., a t. for various serum lipoproteins that contain cholesterol, as an index of the tendency to the development of atheromatous lesions and arteriosclerosis; the t. is based on the differential flotation of molecules of various sizes when the serum is treated in an ultracentrifuge.

Goldscheider's t., determination of the temperature sense by touching the skin with a sharp-pointed metallic rod, heated to varying degrees.

gold sol t., SYN Lange's t.

Goodenough draw-a-man t., a brief t. for assessing an individual's level of intelligence based on how accurately drawn and how many elements are included when a child or adult is given a pencil and sheet of white paper and asked to draw a man, the best man he or she is able to draw. Also called the Goodenough draw-a-person t. and, in its current form, the Goodenough-Harris drawing t.

goodness of fit t., a statistical t. of the hypothesis that data have been randomly sampled or generated from a population that follows a particular theoretical distribution.

Göthlin's t., a capillary fragility t. to determine the presence or absence of scurvy.

Graham-Cole t., SYN cholecystography.

group t., in psychology, a t. designed to be administered to more than one individual at a time; *e.g.,* scholastic achievement t., medical college admissions t.

guaiac t., SYN Almén's t. for blood.

Günzberg's t., a t. for hydrochloric acid utilizing phloroglucin vanillin (Gunzberg's reagent), with which a bright red color is produced in the presence of the acid.

Guthrie t., bacterial inhibition assay for direct measurement of serum phenylalanine; in widespread use for detection of phenylketonuria in the newborn.

Gutzeit's t., a t. for arsenic; a piece of zinc and a little sulfuric acid are added to the suspected liquid which is then boiled; a bit of filter paper with a silver nitrate solution is held in the vapor and will turn yellow if arsenic is present.

Ham's t., SYN acidified serum t.

Hardy-Rand-Ritter t., a t. for color vision deficiency using pseudoisochromatic cards. These excellent cards have not been reprinted by the American Optical Co. since the plates were accidentally destroyed in 1965.

Harrington-Flocks t., a rapid screening t. for visual field defects; patterns are viewed tachistoscopically, and the patterns are visible only when illuminated by a flash of ultraviolet light. Not available since 1970.

Harris t., SYN Harris and Ray t.

Harris and Ray t., a t. for vitamin C in the urine; a microtitration t. of the urine against a known amount of 0.05% aqueous solution of the dye 2,6-dichloroindophenol in 10% acetic acid (usually 0.05 ml of dye is used, roughly equivalent to 0.025 mg of ascorbic acid). SYN Harris t.

head-dropping t., a t. used in the diagnosis of disease of the extrapyramidal or striatal system (*e.g.,* parkinsonism, Wilson's disease); with the patient supine, relaxed, and his attention diverted, the examiner briskly lifts the patient's head with the right hand and then allows it to drop upon the palm of his left hand; the head of a normal person drops suddenly like a dead weight, whereas, in striatal disease the head falls slowly, gently, and almost hesitantly.

heat coagulation t., a t. for measurement of protein in urine; albumin and globulin are coagulated by heat at an acid pH, and the amount of turbidity present provides a qualitative estimation of the degree of proteinuria.

heat instability t., a t. for the presence of unstable hemoglobins; fresh red blood cells lysed in distilled water develop a precipitate within one hour at 50°C if unstable hemoglobin is present.

heel-tap t., SEE heel *tap.*

heel-to-knee-to-toe t., SYN heel-to-shin t.

heel-to-shin t., a test of lower limb coordination and position sense; the subject places the heel of one foot on the opposite knee and then slides it distally along the shin to the opposite side. SYN heel-to-knee-to-toe t.

Heinz body t., a t. for glucose 6-phosphate dehydrogenase-deficient red blood cells; an oxidant (acetylphenylhydrazine) is added to blood; after incubation at 37°C, glucose 6-phosphate dehydrogenase-deficient samples exhibit more than 30% Heinz bodies.

hemadsorption virus t., a method for detecting hemagglutinating viruses that is based on adherence of erythrocytes to infected cells.

hemagglutination t., a sensitive t. to meausre certain antigens, antibodies, or viruses, using their ability to agglutinate certain erythrocytes.

hemoccult t., a qualitative t. for occult blood in stool based upon detecting the peroxidase activity of hemoglobin; a t. kit can be used at home and the specimen mailed to a laboratory for evaluation.

Hering's t., a t. of binocular vision; the subject looks through an apparatus having at its farther end a thread near which a small sphere is dropped; with binocular vision the observer recognizes the location of the sphere in front of or behind the thread; with monocular vision this is not possible.

Hershberg t., a t. for anabolic steroids in which castrated male rats are treated with the substance being tested.

Hess' t., SYN Rumpel-Leede t.

Hines-Brown t., SYN cold pressor t.

Hinton t., a formerly widely used precipitin (flocculation) t. for syphilis in which the "antigen" consisted of glycerol, cholesterol, and beef heart extract.

Histalog t., a t. for measurement of maximal production of gastric acidity or anacidity; it is similar to the histamine t., but uses Histalog (betazole hydrochloride), an analogue of histamine. SYN maximal Histalog t.

histamine t., a t. for maximal production of gastric acidity or anacidity; after preliminary administration of an antihistamine, histamine acid phosphate is injected subcutaneously in a dose of 0.04 mg/kg of body weight, followed by analysis of gastric contents. SEE ALSO Histalog t. SYN augmented histamine t.

histoplasmin-latex t., a passive agglutination t. for histoplasmosis; latex particles, sensitized with antigen extracted from *Histoplasma capsulatum*, are used in a flocculation reaction with the patient's serum.

Hollander t., SYN insulin hypoglycemia t.

Holmgren's wool t., a t. for color blindness, in which the subject matches variously colored skeins of wool.

homovanillic acid t., a t. for homovanillic acid based upon the fact that dopamine is present in sympathetic nervous tissue as precursor of norepinephrine; since norepinephrine has a metabolic pathway which yields homovanillic acid, tumors such as neuroblastomas and ganglioneuromas may cause elevations of urinary dopamine and homovanillic acid. SYN HVA t.

Hooker-Forbes t., a t. for compounds with progestational activity; such compounds cause hypertrophy of the stromal nuclei of the endometrium in uteri obtained from spayed mice; a sensitive t. capable of detecting 0.0002 μg of progesterone.

Howard t., a differential ureteral catheterization t. performed by the insertion of bilateral ureteral catheters to measure simultaneous urinary volume and sodium concentration in patients with suspected renovascular hypertension.

Huhner t., determination of sperm quantity and motility in specimens obtained from the cervical canal following coitus, performed around the time of ovulation.

HVA t., SYN homovanillic acid t.

17-hydroxycorticosteroid t., a t., dependent on the Porter-Silber reaction, that is used as a measure of adrenocortical function and is performed on urine. Low values are seen in Addison's disease and hypopituitarism; high values are seen in Cushing's syndrome and extreme stress. SYN 17-OH-corticoids t., Porter-Silber chromogens t.

hyperventilation t., producing respiratory alkalosis by over-breathing to 1) produce clinical abnormalities, *e.g.,* tetany seizures; 2) cause EEG abnormalities; 3) cause EMG abnormalities.

hypoxemia t., SYN anoxemia t.

immune adhesion t., SYN adhesion t.

immunologic pregnancy t., a general term for t.'s for detection of increased human chorionic gonadotropin in plasma or urine by immunologic techniques including latex particle agglutination, hemagglutination inhibition, radioimmunoassay, and radioreceptor assays.

indirect t., SEE Prausnitz-Küstner *reaction*.

indirect Coombs' t., a t. routinely performed in cross-matching blood or in the investigation of transfusion reaction: t. for patient's serum is incubated with a suspension of donor erythrocytes; if specific antibodies are present, they become attached to the antigen in donor's cells; after a washing with saline, Coombs' antihuman globulin is added; agglutination at this point indicates that antibodies present in the original t. serum had indeed become attached to donor erythrocytes.

indirect fluorescent antibody t., SEE fluorescent antibody *technique*.

indirect hemagglutination t., SYN passive *hemagglutination*.

indole t., a t. used to identify members of the *Enterobacteriaceae* family and other Gram-negative bacilli, based on the ability of the organisms to produce indole from tryptophan.

inkblot t., SYN Rorschach t.

insulin hypoglycemia t., a t. to determine the completeness of vagotomy for peptic ulcer; after the surgical procedure is performed, insulin is administered to cause hypoglycemia; if vagotomy is complete, the acid output from the stomach following administration of insulin is less than that before insulin administration; if the reverse if true, incomplete vagotomy is likely. SYN Hollander t.

intelligence t., a t., using well researched items and involving a systematic method of administration and scoring, used to assess an individual's general aptitude or level of potential competence, in contrast to an achievement t.

iodine t., a t. for detecting the presence of starch based on its reaction with iodine.

Ishihara t., a t. for color vision deficiency that utilizes a series of pseudoisochromatic plates on which numbers or letters are printed in dots of primary colors surrounded by dots of other colors; the figures are discernable by individuals with normal color vision.

isopropanol precipitation t., a t. using the principle that the internal bonds of hemoglobin are weakened by nonpolar solvents; thus, unstable hemoglobins will precipitate more rapidly than other hemoglobins in isopropanol.

Ito-Reenstierna t., SYN Ducrey t.

^{131}I uptake t., a t. of thyroid function in which ^{131}I-iodide is given orally; after 24 hours, the amount present in the thyroid gland is measured and compared with normal values. SYN radioactive iodide uptake t., RAI t.

Ivy bleeding time t., a bleeding time t. in which a sphygmomanometer is inflated to 40 mm Hg around the upper arm, a 5-mm deep incision is made on the flexor surface of the forearm, and the time is measured to cessation of bleeding.

Jacquemin's t., a t. for phenol; to the suspected fluid an equal amount of aniline is added, and, after thorough admixture, a little solution of sodium hypochlorite; if phenol is present the fluid becomes blue.

Jaffe's t., (1) a qualitative t. for the presence of indicanuria; after an equal amount of HCl is added to the urine, the further addition of chloroform and $CaCl_2$ gives rise to blue or purple chloroform droplets which sink to the bottom if indican is present; **(2)** a quantitative t. for creatinine based on its reaction with alkaline picrate.

Janet's t., a t. for functional or organic anesthesia; the patient (with eyes closed) is told to say "yes" or "no" when he feels or does not feel the touch of the examiner's finger; in the case of functional anesthesia he may say "no" when an anesthetic area is touched, but will say nothing, being unaware that he is touched, in cases of organic anesthesia.

Jolles' t., a t. for bile; a precipitate is obtained by agitation with chloroform, a solution of barium chloride, and hydrochloric acid; the precipitate is removed, and the addition of a drop or two of sulfuric acid will produce a play of color if bile pigments are present.

Jones' t., SYN fluorescein instillation t.

Katayama's t., a qualitative colorimetric t. for the presence of carboxyhemoglobin in the blood.

ketogenic corticoids t., SYN 17-ketogenic steroid assay t.

17-ketogenic steroid assay t., a colorimetric t., based on the Zimmermann reaction, which indicates metabolites or adrenal and testicular steroids excreted as 17-ketones in the urine; increased values are most striking in adrenocortical tumors, decreased values in Addison's disease or in panhypopituitarism. SYN ketogenic corticoids t.

Kirby-Bauer t., a standardized t. for microbiological susceptibility performed by transferring a standardized pure culture of the organism of interest onto a sensitivity plate (Petri dish with Mueller-Hinton *agar*) and observing growth in the presence of disks containing antibiotics.

Knoop hardness t., SEE Knoop hardness *number*.

Kober t., a t. for naturally occurring estrogens, based upon the production of a pink color (absorption maximum: 520 mμ) when an estrogen is heated in a mixture of phenol and sulfuric acid.

Kolmer t., a former standard quantitative method for the Wassermann t., with numerous modifications (especially as to antigen).

Korotkoff's t., a t. of collateral circulation; while the artery above an aneurysm is compressed, the blood pressure in the distal circulation is estimated; if it is fairly high, the collateral circulation is good.

Kurzrok-Ratner t., a t. for estrogens in the urine; the urine is extracted with ethyl acetate and, after purification, the extract is subjected to bioassay as in the Allen-Doisy t.

Kveim t., an intradermal t. for the detection of sarcoidosis, done by injecting Kveim antigen (obtained from spleens of persons with sarcoidosis) and examining skin biopsies after three and six weeks; a positive t. is indicated by typical nodules showing evidence of sarcoid tissue. SYN Kveim-Stilzbach t., Nickerson-Kveim t.

Kveim-Stilzbach t., SYN Kveim t.

Lachman t., a maneuver to detect deficiency of the anterior cruciate ligament; with the knee flexed 20 to 30 degrees, the tibia is displaced anteriorly relative to the femur; a soft endpoint or greater than 4 millimeters of displacement is positive (abnormal).

Landsteiner-Donath t., SEE Donath-Landsteiner *phenomenon*.

Lange's t., an obsolete, nonspecific t. for altered proteins in spinal fluid. As originally used by Lange in 1912, the t. was thought to be specific for neurosyphilis; however, this proved to be incorrect. Dilutions of spinal fluid are made in saline and to these a colloidal gold solution is added; if altered proteins are present, there is a color change or precipitate formed. At present, its chief use is to demonstrate cerebrospinal fluid protein abnormalities in multiple sclerosis. SYN gold sol t., Zsigmondy's t.

latex agglutination t., a passive agglutination t. in which antigen is adsorbed onto latex particles which then clump in the presence of antibody specific for the adsorbed antigen. SYN latex fixation t.

latex fixation t., SYN latex agglutination t.

LE cell t., *in vitro* incubation of blood or bone marrow of patients with systemic lupus erythematosus, or action of their serum on normal leukocytes, causes formation of characteristic LE cells. SYN lupus erythematosus cell t.

Legal's t., a t. for acetone; the urine is rendered alkaline by a few drops of a solution of potassium hydroxide, and to this are added 2 or 3 drops of a freshly prepared 10% solution of sodium nitroprusside; it is colored red, then yellow; then a few drops of acetic acid are trickled down the side of the t. tube and at the line of junction of the two fluids is formed a carmine or purple ring.

leishmanin t. (lēsh'man-in), a delayed hypersensitivity t. for cutaneous leishmaniasis; a positive t. when granulomatous induration exceeds 5 min after 2–3 days at the intradermal injection site of a suspension of leishmanias in phenol. SYN Montenegro t. [leishmania + suffix -*in*, component, derivative]

lepromin t., a t. utilizing an intradermal injection of a lepromin, such as the Dharmendra antigen or Mitsuda antigen, to classify the stage of leprosy based on the lepromin reaction, such as the Fernandez reaction or Mitsuda reaction; it differentiates tuberculoid leprosy, in which there is a positive delayed reaction at the injection site, from lepromatous leprosy, in which there is no reaction (*i.e.,* a negative t. result) despite the active malignant *Mycobacterium leprae* infection; the t. is not diagnostic, since normal uninfected persons may react.

leukocyte adherence assay t., a t. to detect the ability of leukocytes to adhere to bacteria, performed *in vitro* using nylon fibers to measure adherence.

leukocyte bactericidal assay t., a t. of leukocytes to determine their ability to kill a culture of live bacteria.

Liebermann-Burchard t., a colorimetric t. for unsaturated sterols, notably cholesterol; a blue-green color develops when such substances are added to acetic anhydride and sulfuric acid in chloroform.

limulus lysate t., a t. for the rapid detection of Gram-negative bacterial meningitis; Gram-negative endotoxin induces gel formation of *Limulus polyphemus* (horseshoe crab) lysates.

line t., a t. for rickets, based on observation of the lines of calcification in the growing ends of rachitic long bones in rats given vitamin D preparations under standard t. conditions; used in biological assay of vitamin D by the USP.

lipase t., a diagnostic t. based on the measurement of lipase in blood and urine as an indicator of pancreatic disease.

Lombard voice-reflex t., the observation of fluctuations in the intensity of a patient's voice when a masking noise is increased or decreased; a t. useful in assessing functional hearing loss.

Lücke's t., a t. for hippuric acid; hot nitric acid is added to the urine and evaporated to dryness; the presence of hippuric acid is indicated by an odor of nitrobenzol upon further heating.

lupus band t., a direct immunofluorescent technique for demonstrating a band of immunoglobulins at the dermal-epidermal junction of the skin of patients with lupus erythematosus.

lupus erythematosus cell t., SYN LE cell t.

Machado-Guerreiro t., a complement-fixation t. for infection with *Trypanosoma cruzi*.

Maclagan's t., SYN thymol turbidity t.

Maclagan's thymol turbidity t., SYN thymol turbidity t.

macrophage migration inhibition t., SYN migration inhibitory factor t.

Mantel-Haenszel t., a summary chi-square t. developed by Mantel and Haenszel for stratified data, used when controlling for confounding.

Mantoux t., SEE tuberculin t.

Marshall t., manual deviation of bladder neck during strain or cough to ascertain presence of stress urinary incontinence. SYN Bonney t., Marshall-Marchetti t.

Marshall-Marchetti t., SYN Marshall t.

Master t., an early and long-used exercise challenge to identify ischemic heart disease using a pair of nine inch steps with a platform on top, the number of trips by the patient arbitrarily chosen and related to age and body weight. SEE ALSO two-step exercise t. SYN Master's two-step exercise t.

Master's two-step exercise t., SYN Master t.

Mauthner's t., an obsolete t. for color perception similar to Holmgren's, but made with vials filled with pigments instead of with skeins of wool.

maximal Histalog t., SYN Histalog t.

Mazzotti t., a t. for onchocerciasis using an oral t. dose of diethylcarbamazine (50 or 100 mg), resulting in the appearance of an acute rash in 2 to 24 hours from death of microfilariae in the skin. SYN Mazzotti reaction.

McMurray t., rotation of the tibia on the femur to determine injury to meniscal structures.

McNemar's t., a form of chi-square t. for matched paired data.

McPhail's t., a t. for progesterone and like substances; immature female rabbits are treated with 150 IU of estrone over a period of 6 days; the t. material is then given in five daily subcutaneous doses; progestational proliferation of the endometrium is noted and the results estimated according to a scale from 0 to ++++;

the amount required to produce an average (++) response is taken as a unit, equivalent to 0.25 mg of progesterone.

Meinicke t., the first successful application (1917–1918) of immune precipitation to diagnosis of syphilis, now obsolete.

Meltzer-Lyon t., a t. used in diagnosis of gallbladder conditions: 25 ml of a 25% solution of magnesium sulfate are delivered into the region of the sphincter of Oddi through a duodenal tube, causing contraction of the gallbladder, relaxation of the sphincter, and the expulsion of bile from the common duct and gallbladder; bile from the common duct is relatively pale and is expelled first, that from the gallbladder follows; samples aspirated from the tube are examined for pus cells, pigment granules, epithelial cells, cholesterol, etc.

metabisulfite t., a t. for sickle cell hemoglobin (Hb S); deoxygenation of cells containing Hb S is enhanced by addition of sodium metabisulfite to the blood, causing sickling visible on a slide; certain other abnormal hemoglobins (Hb C$_{Harlem}$ and Hb I) also sickle in this t.

3-methoxy-4-hydroxymandelic acid t., SYN vanillylmandelic acid t.

metrotrophic t., a t. for the assay of estrogenic substances; immature female rats (25 to 49 g) are injected subcutaneously with the hormone and killed after 6 hours, when the increase in uterine weight (due largely to imbibation of water) is taken as the criterion of estrogenic activity. SYN Astwood's t.

MHA-TP t., SYN microhemagglutination-Treponema pallidum t.

microhemagglutination-Treponema pallidum t., a microtiter version of the Treponema pallidum hemagglutination t. SYN MHA-TP t.

microprecipitation t., a precipitation t. in which reduced quantities of t. reagents are used.

migration inhibition t., SYN migration inhibitory factor t.

migration inhibitory factor t., a t. which measures the presence of migration inhibitory factor. Usually peritoneal macrophages are placed in a capillary tube in the presence or absence of supernatants from activated T cells. If MIF is present, the migration of monocyte/macrophages is reduced. SYN macrophage migration inhibition t., migration inhibition t.

milk-ring t., a special form of agglutination t. done on the pooled milk of many cows, usually entire herds, for the detection of herds containing individuals infected with bovine brucellosis.

Millon Clinical Multiaxial Inventory t., a paper and pencil test, consisting of 20 clinical scales derived from 175 self-descriptive statements, and developed in 1977 for use in the assessment of psychopathology and the more enduring patterns of personality; specifically designed to correspond with some of the disorders of personality included in the Diagnostic and Statistical Manual of Mental Disorders used in diagnosis by mental health professionals. SYN Millon clinical multiaxial inventory.

Millon-Nasse t., a t. for protein, the tyrosine of which reacts with nitrite after a brief treatment with mercuric ion in acid to give a color.

Minnesota multiphasic personality inventory t. (MMPI), a questionnaire type of psychological test for ages 16 and over, with 550 true-false statements coded in 4 validity and 10 personality scales which may be administered in both an individual or group format. SYN Minnesota Multiphasic Personality Inventory.

mixed agglutination t., SEE mixed agglutination *reaction.*

mixed lymphocyte culture t., a t. for histocompatibility of HL-A antigens in which donor and recipient lymphocytes are mixed in culture; the degree of incompatibility is indicated by the number of cells that have undergone transformation and mitosis, or by the uptake of radioactive isotope-labeled thymidine. SYN MLC t.

MLC t., SYN mixed lymphocyte culture t.

Molisch's t., a color t. for sugar, which condenses with α-naphthol or thymol in the presence of strong sulfuric acid, which converts the sugar to furfural derivatives.

Moloney t., a t. to detect a high degree of sensitivity to diphtheria toxoid; more than a minimal local reaction to diluted ¹⁄₂₀) toxoid given intradermally indicates that prophylactic toxoid should be inoculated in fractional doses at suitable intervals.

Montenegro t., SYN leishmanin t.

Mörner's t., (1) for cysteine, which gives a brilliant purple color with sodium nitroprusside; (2) for tyrosine, which gives a green color on boiling with sulfuric acid containing formaldehyde.

Moschcowitz t., demonstration of lower limb ischemia by occlusion of the arterial circulation for five minutes with a tourniquet or Esmarch bandage. Following release, skin color normally will return in a few seconds; with arterial obstruction (*e.g.,* arteriosclerotic) color returns more slowly.

Mosenthal t., an infrequently used t. to evaluate renal concentrating ability by measuring the density of urine every two hours during the ingestion of a controlled diet.

motility t., a t. based on microscopic observation or on the spread of growth in soft agar, used to determine if a microorganism is motile.

Motulsky dye reduction t., a t. for glucose 6-phosphate dehydrogenase deficiency in the blood, using a mixture of brilliant cresyl blue, glucose 6-phosphate, and NADP.

mucin clot t., a t. that reflects the polymerization of synovial fluid hyaluronate; a few drops of synovial fluid added to acetic acid form a clot; poor clot formation occurs in a variety of inflammatory conditions including septic arthritis, gouty arthritis, and rheumatoid arthritis. SYN Ropes t.

Mulder's t., SEE xanthoprotein *reaction.*

multiple puncture tuberculin t., a kind of tine t. SEE tuberculin t.

multiple sleep latency t., a t. of the propensity to fall asleep, done by performing polysomnography during multiple brief opportunities to sleep.

mumps sensitivity t., a skin t. for sensitivity to mumps, in which inactivated mumps virus is used as antigen.

Nagel's t., a t. for color vision in which the observer determines the relative amounts of red and green necessary to match spectral yellow; an instrument called Nagel's anomaloscope is used.

NBT t., abbreviation for nitroblue tetrazolium t.

neutralization t., SYN protection t.

niacin t., a t. of the ability of mycobacteria to elaborate niacin; used to distinguish different strains.

Nickerson-Kveim t., SYN Kveim t.

nitroblue tetrazolium t. (NBT t.), a t. to detect the phagocytic ability of polymorphonuclear leukocytes by measuring the capacity of the oxygen-dependent leukocytic bactericidal system.

nitroprusside t., a qualitative t. for cystinuria; following the addition of sodium cyanide to the urine, the further addition of nitroprusside produces a red-purple color if the cyanide has reduced any cystine present to cysteine.

nonstress t., a t. to evaluate fetal well-being by evaluating fetal heart rate response to fetal movement; a reactive nonstress t. is fetal heart rate accelerations in response to fetal movement.

nystagmus t., SYN Bárány's caloric t.

Obermayer's t., a t. for indican; solids in the urine are precipitated by means of a 20% solution of acetate of lead and then filtered, and to the filtrate is added fuming hydrochloric acid containing a small amount of ferric chloride solution; if indican is present, the addition of chloroform causes the formation of indigo, indicated by the blue color.

17-OH-corticoids t., SYN 17-hydroxycorticosteroid t.

oral lactose tolerance t., a t. for lactose deficiency; the plasma

---

♻ **Combining forms**

Word*Finder*
Multi-term entry finder
Preceding letter A

A.D.A.M. Anatomy Plates
Between letters L and M

Appendices:
Following letter Z

SYN Synonym; Cf., compare

[NA] Nomina Anatomica

[MIM] Mendelian
Inheritance in Man

☆ **Official alternate term**

☆**[NA] Official alternate**
Nomina Anatomica term

─────────────

High Profile Term

glucose response to an oral lactose load is measured as in the (oral) glucose tolerance t.

orcinol t., SYN Bial's t.

Ouchterlony t., double (gel) diffusion t. in two dimensions. SEE gel diffusion precipitin t.'s in two dimensions. SYN Ouchterlony method.

oxidase t., a colon t. for the presence of intracellular cytochrome oxidase based on the reaction with p-phenylenediamine; aids in the identification of *Neisseria* species and Pseudomonadaceae.

Pachon's t., in a case of aneurysm, determination of the collateral circulation by estimation of the blood pressure.

Palmer acid t. for peptic ulcer, in duodenal ulcer, the administration of acid by duodenal tube causes severe pain.

palmin t., palmitin t., a t. of pancreatic efficiency, based upon the fact that the presence of fat in the stomach causes the pylorus to open and admit the pancreatic juice; this splits the palmin so that an examination of the stomach contents, after a t. meal containing palmin, will reveal the presence of fatty acids.

pancreozymin-secretin t., SEE secretin t.

Pandy's t., SYN Pandy's *reaction.*

Pap t., microscopic examination of cells exfoliated or scraped from a mucosal surface after staining with Papanicolaou's stain; used especially for detection of cancer of the uterine cervix. SYN Papanicolaou smear t.

Papanicolaou smear t., SYN Pap t.

parallax t., measurement of the deviation in strabismus by the alternate cover t. combined with neutralization of the deviation using prisms.

parametric t., a statistical t. that depends on an assumption about the distribution of the data, *e.g.,* that the data are normally distributed.

passive cutaneous anaphylaxis t. (an′ă-fĭ-lak′sis), an animal is injected intradermally with antibody (usually IgE) and subsequently challenged intravenously with a mixture of antigen and Evans blue dye 24–48 hours later. A dark blue area indicates a positive reaction due to the leakage of the dye at the site of antigen-antibody reactions.

patch t., a t. of skin sensitiveness: a small piece of paper, tape, or a cup, wet with CøOnon-irritating diluted t. fluid, is applied to skin of the upper back or upper outer arm and after 48 hours the area previously covered is compared with the uncovered surface; an erythematous reaction with vesicles occurs if the substance causes contact allergy. SEE ALSO photo-patch t.

Patrick's t., a t. to determine the presence or absence of sacroiliac disease; with the patient supine, the hip and knee are flexed and the external malleolus is placed above the patella of the opposite leg; this can ordinarily be done without pain, but, on depressing the knee, pain is promptly elicited in sacroiliac disease.

Paul-Bunnell t., t. for detection of heterophil antibodies in infectious mononucleosis. SEE Forssman *antigen.*

Paul's t., SYN Paul's *reaction.*

PBI t., SYN protein-bound iodine t.

pentagastrin t., an alternative to histamine for stimulation of acid secretion in gastric analysis.

performance t., a t., such as five of the eleven Wechsler adult intelligence scale subtests, requiring little or no verbal instruction from the examiner and virtually no verbal response by the examinee.

Perls' t., a t. for hemosiderin, utilizing Perls' Prussian blue *stain.*

personality t., any of the category of psychological t.'s designed to t. the characteristics of the personality, emotional status, mental disorder, etc., in contrast to an intelligence t.

Perthes' t., a t. for patency of deep femoral vein; with the patient standing, a tourniquet is applied above the knee; after walking, if deep circulation is competent, the superficial varicosities remain unchanged and legs become painful.

phenolsulfonphthalein t., obsolete t. for renal function; after the patient has drunk a glass or two of water, 1 ml of a 0.6% solution of dye is injected hypodermically; the time between this injection and the appearance of a pink tinge in the urine as it falls into an alkaline solution is noted; the amount excreted in each of the

next 2 hours is then estimated colorimetrically. SYN Geraghty's t., phthalein t., red t., Rowntree and Geraghty t.

phentolamine t., a t. for pheochromocytoma; intravenous administration of phentolamine (5 mg) reduces hypertension due to a pheochromocytoma but not that due to other causes, *e.g.,* essential hypertension; the blood pressure is raised by the drug in the latter form of hypertension.

photo-patch t., a t. of contact photosensitization: after application of a patch with the suspected sensitizer for 48 hours to two sites, if there is no reaction one area is exposed to a weak erythema dose of sunlight or ultraviolet light; if positive, a more severe reaction with vesiculation develops at the exposed patch area than the nonexposed skin patch site.

photostress t., measurement of visual acuity before and after exposure of the eyes to intense light.

phrenic pressure t., pressure is made on the phrenic nerve on each side, above the clavicles where the nerve passes over the scalenus anticus muscle; if pain is felt and the patient inclines his head to the painful side, the problem is in the pleural space; if his head does not incline to one side, the problem is in the abdominal cavity.

phthalein t., SYN phenolsulfonphthalein t.

Pirquet's t., a cutaneous tuberculin t. SEE tuberculin t. SYN dermotuberculin reaction, Pirquet's reaction.

pivot shift t., a maneuver to detect a deficiency of the anterior cruciate ligament of the knee; when the knee is extended, a sudden subluxation of the lateral tibial condyle upon the distal femur is positive.

P-K t., SYN Prausnitz-Küstner *reaction.*

plasmacrit t., a serologic screening method used as an aid in the diagnosis of syphilis; after only a few drops of heparinized blood (obtained from a pricked finger) are collected in a special capillary tube, the capillary tube is centrifugated in order to collect plasma, which is then mixed with a 0.01-ml drop of antigen (cardiolipin previously treated with choline chloride as an anti-inhibitor, in order to avoid falsely negative results that may occur with nonheated plasma or serum). After mechanically agitating the antigen-plasma mixture for 4 min, the presence or absence of flocculation is observed. A positive result should not be regarded as conclusively diagnostic, but a negative result excludes the likelihood of syphilis.

platelet aggregation t., a t. of the ability of platelets to adhere to each other and hence form a hemostatic plug to prevent bleeding; failure to aggregate occurs in several conditions, *e.g.,* thrombasthenia, Von Willebrand's disease, and following administration of aspirin, phenylbutazone, and indomethacin; the t. is conducted by quantitating the decrease in turbidity that occurs in platelet-rich plasma following the *in vitro* addition of one or several platelet-aggregating agents (*e.g.,* ADP, epinephrine, or serotonin).

polyuria t., SYN Albarran's t.

Porges-Meier t., an early flocculation t. for syphilis; of significance in having introduced as antigens acetone-insoluble, alcohol-soluble fractions of tissue, and lecithin.

Porter-Silber chromogens t., SYN 17-hydroxycorticosteroid t.

P and P t., SYN prothrombin and proconvertin t.

precipitation t., SYN precipitin t.

precipitin t., an *in vitro* t. in which antigen is in soluble form and precipitates when it combines with added specific antibody in the presence of an electrolyte. SEE ALSO gel diffusion precipitin t.'s, ring precipitin t. SYN precipitation t.

prism cover t., measurement of the deviation in strabismus by the alternate cover t. combined with neutralization for the deviation using prisms.

prism vergence t., measurement of the amplitude of fusion by placing prisms of gradually increasing power in the direction tested until diplopia occurs.

projective t., a loosely structured psychological t. containing many ambiguous stimuli that require the subject to reveal his own feelings, personality, or psychopathology in response to them; *e.g.,* Rorschach t., thematic apperception t.

protection t., a t. to determine the antimicrobial activity of a serum by inoculating a susceptible animal with a mixture of the serum and the virus or other microbe being tested. SYN neutralization t.

protein-bound iodine t., a formerly used t. of thyroid function in which serum protein-bound iodine is measured to provide an estimate of hormone bound to protein in peripheral blood. SYN PBI t.

prothrombin t., a quantitative t. for prothrombin in the blood based on the clotting time of oxalated blood plasma in the presence of thromboplastin and calcium chloride; measures the integrity of the extrinsic and common pathways of coagulation. SEE ALSO prothrombin *time*. SYN Quick's method, Quick's t.

prothrombin and proconvertin t., a t. formerly used by some to control anticoagulant therapy with bishydroxycoumarin and indandione drugs. SYN P and P t.

provocative t., any procedure in which a suspected pathophysiological abnormality is deliberately induced by manipulating conditions known to provoke the abnormality.

provocative Wassermann t., an obsolete t. of historical interest only; the use of the Wassermann test from one or two days to one or two weeks after the administration of arsphenamine or neoarsphenamine; the result may then be positive when before the giving of arsphenamine it was negative.

psychological t.'s, t.'s designed to measure a person's achievements, intelligence, neuropsychological functions, skills, personality, or individual and occupational characteristics, or potentialities. SEE ALSO scale.

psychomotor t.'s, psychological t.'s which, although based on other psychological processes (*e.g.,* sensory, perceptual), require a motor reaction such as copying designs, building blocks, or manipulating controls.

pulp t., SYN vitality t.

Q tip t., a t. for determining the mobility of the urethra.

Queckenstedt-Stookey t., compression of the jugular vein in a healthy person causes an increase in the pressure of the spinal fluid in the lumbar region within 10 to 12 seconds, and an equally rapid fall to normal on release of the pressure on the vein; when there is a block of subarachnoid channels, compression of the vein causes little or no increase of pressure in the cerebrospinal fluid.

quellung t., SYN Neufeld capsular *swelling*.

Quick's t., SYN prothrombin t.

quinine carbacrylic resin t., a t. for gastric anacidity. SEE quinine carbacrylic *resin*.

Quinlan's t., a t. for bile; when a thin layer of bile is examined through a spectroscope, absorption lines appear in the violet.

radioactive iodide uptake t., SYN ^{131}I uptake t.

radioallergosorbent t. (RAST), a radioimmunoassay t. to detect IgE-bound allergens responsible for tissue hypersensitivity: the allergen is bound to insoluble material and the patient's serum is reacted with this conjugate; if the serum contains antibody to the allergen, it will be complexed to the allergen.

radioimmunosorbent t. (RIST), a competition t., performed *in vitro,* used to measure IgE specific for a particular antigen. Known amounts of radiolabeled IgE compete with the patient's unlabeled IgE to bind to a surface coated with anti-IgE. The reduction in radiolabeled IgE due to the presence of IgE in the patient's serum can be determined by comparison to known IgE standards; thus, the amount of the patient's total serum IgE can be determined.

RAI t., SYN ^{131}I uptake t.

rapid plasma reagin t., a group of serologic t.'s for syphilis in which unheated serum or plasma is reacted with a standard t. antigen containing charcoal particles; positive t.'s yield a flocculation. A modification, called the RPR (circle) card t., is widely used as a screening t. SYN RPR t.

Rapoport t., a differential ureteral catheterization t. used to evaluate suspected renovascular hypertension; urine specimens from each kidney are obtained by bilateral ureteral catheterization, and the tubular rejection fraction ratio is determined by measuring concentrations of sodium and creatinine in the urine from each kidney.

Rayleigh t., SYN Rayleigh *equation*.

red t., SYN phenolsulfonphthalein t.

red cell adherence t., SYN adhesion t.

Reinsch's t., a t. for arsenic in which a strip of copper is placed in the suspected fluid, which is then acidulated with hydrochloric acid and boiled; if arsenic is present a gray deposit occurs on the copper, and this deposit on heating is sublimated and deposited as a crystalline layer on a piece of glass held above the copper strip.

Reiter t., a complement-fixation t. for syphilis using as antigen material prepared from the Reiter strain of *Treponema pallidum;* the t. has been largely replaced in laboratory medicine by the fluorescent treponemal antibody-absorption (FTA-ABS) t.

resorcinol t., a t. for fructosuria; fresh urine treated with resorcinol in acid gives a red precipitate in the presence of fructose; the precipitate should form a red solution in ethanol. SYN Selivanoff's t.

Reuss' t., a t. for atropine; the addition of oxidizing agents and sulfuric acid to a liquid containing atropine produces an odor of orange-flowers and roses.

Rh blocking t., a t. for nonagglutinating Rh antibodies: an Rh agglutination t. is first carried out; if the t. for Rh agglutinins is negative, then 1 drop of anti-Rh$_0$ agglutinating serum of moderate titer is mixed with the patient's serum containing Rh-positive t. cells; if after incubating for from 1 to 2 hr at 37°C no agglutination occurs, Rh$_0$-blocking antibodies are assumed to be present in the patient's serum.

Rickles t., a colorimetric t. for predicting dental caries activity by incubating saliva in sucrose and determining pH changes.

Rimini's t., a t. for formaldehyde in urine, milk, and other fluids, by the use of dilute solution of phenylhydrazine hydrochloride, sodium nitroprusside, and sodium hydroxide.

ring t., SYN ring precipitin t.

ring precipitin t., a precipitin t. in which antigen solution is carefully layered over antibody solution in a tube; as diffusion proceeds, a disk of precipitate forms where the antibody ratio is optimal. SYN ring t.

Rinne's t., (1) as a positive t.: a vibrating tuning fork is held in contact with the skull (usually the mastoid process) until the sound is lost, its prongs are then brought close to the auditory orifice when, if the hearing is normal, a faint sound will again be heard; **(2)** as a negative t.: a vibrating tuning fork is heard longer and louder when in contact with the skull than when held near the auditory orifice, indicating some disorder of the sound conducting apparatus.

Romberg t., SYN Romberg's *sign.*

Römer's t., a t. of historical interest: tuberculin, either pure or diluted, is injected intracutaneously into a guinea pig; if the animal is tuberculous, a large papule with a necrotic hemorrhagic center appears in about 24 hours (cocarde or cockade reaction).

Ropes t., SYN mucin clot t.

Rorschach t., a projective psychological t. in which the subject reveals his or her attitudes, emotions, and personality by reporting what is seen in each of 10 inkblot pictures. SYN inkblot t.

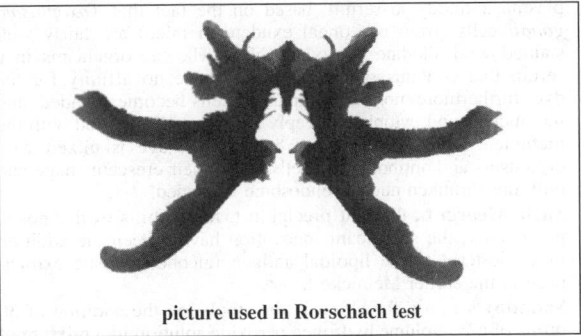

picture used in Rorschach test

rose bengal radioactive (^{131}I) t., a t. of liver function used as a means of measuring hepatic blood flow and for scintillation scanning of the liver to determine size and contour of the liver, or the presence of space-occupying masses in the liver.

Rosenbach-Gmelin t., SYN Gmelin's t.

Rosenbach's t., a t. for bile in the urine; the suspected urine is passed several times through the same filter paper, which is then dried and touched with a drop of slightly fuming nitric acid; the presence of bile is indicated by the resulting play of colors characteristic of the bile pigments (a yellow spot surrounded by rings of red, violet, blue, and green).

rosette t., a t. for rosette-forming cells (T-lymphocytes) in which these cells and sheep erythrocytes, are incubated and centrifuged lightly, then examined under a microscope for rosette formation or adherence of erythrocytes to T lymphocytes.

Rose-Waaler t., a t. of historical interest: when sheep red cells are suspended in a concentration of antiserum to sheep red cells which is too low to cause agglutination, the addition of serum from a patient with rheumatoid arthritis will cause agglutination.

Ross-Jones t., a t. for an excess of globulin in the cerebrospinal fluid; 1 ml of cerebrospinal fluid is carefully floated over 2 ml of a concentrated ammonium sulfate solution; if globulin is present in excess, a fine white ring appears at the line of junction in about 3 min.

Rothera's nitroprusside t., a t. for ketone bodies; 5 ml of fresh urine are saturated with solid ammonium sulfate and mixed with 10 drops of freshly prepared 2% sodium nitroprusside solution, which is then mixed with 10 drops of concentrated ammonia water and allowed to stand for 15 min; the presence of acetoacetic acid, or of larger concentrations of acetone, is indicated by the development of a blue-purple color.

Rowntree and Geraghty t., SYN phenolsulfonphthalein t.

RPR t., SYN rapid plasma reagin t.

rubella HI t., a hemagglutination inhibition (HI) t. for rubella, often performed routinely as part of a prenatal workup of the pregnant woman; the presence of any detectable HI titer in the absence of disease indicates previous infection and immunity to reinfection; if HI antibody is undetected, the patient is considered potentially susceptible and is followed accordingly. SEE ALSO hemagglutination *inhibition*.

Rubin t., an obsolete t. of patency of the fallopian tubes; a cannula is introduced into the cervix uteri, and carbon dioxide gas is passed through the cannula by means of a syringe with manometer attachment; if the tubes are patent, the escape of gas into the abdominal cavity is evidenced by a high-pitched bubbling sound heard on auscultation over the lower abdomen, or free gas under the diaphragm can be demonstrated by x-ray.

Rubner's t., a t. for lactose or glucose in the urine; lead acetate is added to the suspected urine which is then filtered; ammonia is added until a permanent precipitate is formed; if lactose is present, the precipitate will take on a pink to red color when the fluid is heated; if there is glucose, the color will be yellow to brown.

Rumpel-Leede t., a tourniquet t. for capillary fragility, often positive in the presence of severe thrombocytopenia. SEE ALSO capillary fragility t. SYN bandage sign, Hess' t., Rumpel-Leede sign.

Sabin-Feldman dye t., a method for the detection of anti-toxoplasma antibody in serum, based on the fact that *Toxoplasma gondii* cells (from peritoneal exudate in mice) are fairly well stained with alkaline methylene blue, whereas organisms in a serum that contains specific antibody have no affinity for the dye; furthermore, normal toxoplasma cells become rounded, and the nucleus and cytoplasm deeply stained, when treated with the methylene blue; on the other hand, when dye is mixed with organisms and antibody, the cells retain their crescent shape and only the shrunken nuclear endosome is stained.

Sachs-Georgi t., the first precipitin t. for syphilis of diagnostic practicality, the significant innovation having been the addition of cholesterol to the lipoidal antigen (alcoholic tissue extract) used in the earlier Meinicke t.

Saundby's t., a t. for blood in the stools; on the addition of 30 drops of a 20-volume hydrogen peroxide solution to a mixture of 10 drops of a saturated benzidine solution and a small quantity of feces in a test tube, a persistent dark blue color denotes the presence of blood.

scarification t., a t., *e.g.,* Pirquet's t., in which a material is pricked or scratched into the skin.

Schaffer's t., a t. for nitrites in the urine; urine is decolorized with animal charcoal and then 4 ml of a 10% solution of acetic acid and 3 drops of a 5% solution of potassium ferrocyanide are added; if nitrites are present, an intense yellow color will be produced.

Schellong t., a t. for circulatory function; the subject is required to stand for 10 to 20 minutes, during which time the blood pressure is measured continuously; a fall of systolic pressure of 20 mm Hg or more indicates poor circulatory function.

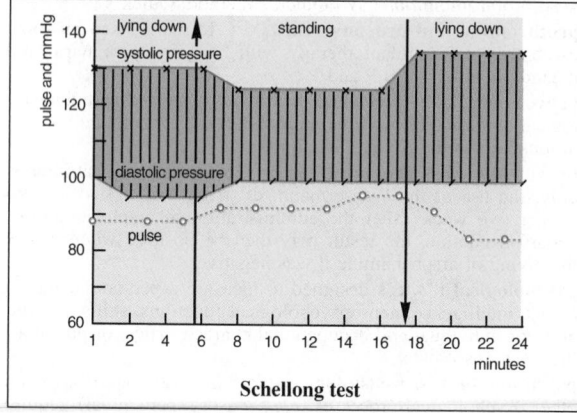

Schellong test

Schick t., a t. for susceptibility to *Corynebacterium diphtheriae* toxin: 0.1 ml of Schick test toxin is injected into the skin of one forearm (test site) and the same quantity of the same, but heat-inactivated, material into the skin of the other forearm (control site); individuals with toxin-neutralizing antibodies either will have no reaction at either injection site (negative test) or may have a pseudoreaction due to antibodies for substances (antigens) in the test materials other than diphtheria toxin; individuals lacking toxin-neutralizing antibodies may have a positive reaction, which consists of an area of redness appearing 24 to 36 hours at the test site only and persisting for 4 to 5 days. SYN Schick method.

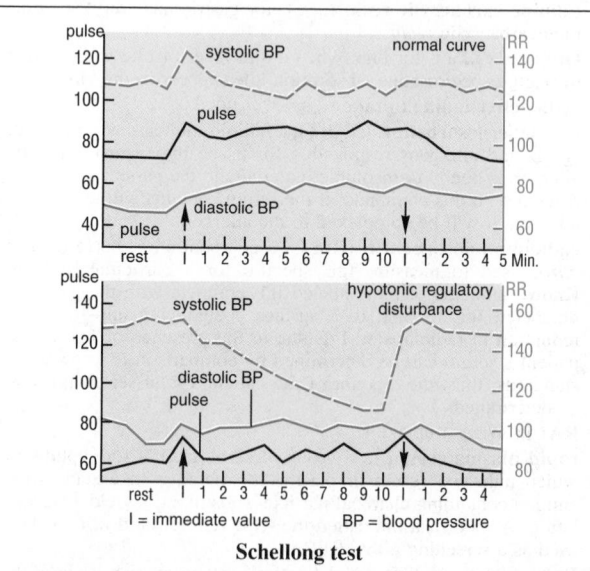

Schellong test

Schiller's t., a t. for nonglycogen-containing areas of the portio vaginalis of the cervix, which may be the site of early carcinoma; such areas fail to stain dark brown with iodine solution; loss of glycogen due to erosion and other benign conditions may also give a positive result.

Schilling t., a procedure for determining the amount of vitamin

B_{12} excreted in the urine using cyanocobalamin tagged with a radioisotope of cobalt.

Schirmer t., a t. for tear production using a strip of filter paper; a measurement of basal and reflex lacrimal gland function.

Schönbein's t., SYN Almén's t. for blood.

Schwabach t., a series of five tuning forks of different tones is used and the number of seconds is noted in which the patient can hear each by air and bone conduction.

scratch t., a form of skin t. in which antigen is applied through a scratch in the skin.

screening t., any testing procedure designed to separate people or objects according to a fixed characteristic or property.

Seashore t., a t. in which the individual must discriminate between two sounds; or in which the sense of pitch, intensity, rhythm, and other components of innate musical ability can be measured. SEE Halstead-Reitan *battery*.

secretin t., a t. of pancreatic exocrine function, variably performed and standardized, in which the bicarbonate, amylase, and volume of the duodenal aspirate are measured after intravenous administration of secretin.

Selivanoff's t., SYN resorcinol t.

shadow t., SYN retinoscopy.

shake t., SYN foam stability t.

sickle cell t., in an anaerobic wet preparation containing equal amounts of blood and 2% sodium bisulfite, erythrocytes containing hemoglobin S undergo a change in shape to a sickle cell form; the number of sickled red cells per 1000 red blood cells is determined, and expressed as a percentage.

single (gel) diffusion precipitin t. in one dimension, SEE gel diffusion precipitin t.'s in one dimension.

single (gel) diffusion precipitin t. in two dimensions, SEE gel diffusion precipitin t.'s in two dimensions.

SISI t., the sounding of a tone 20 dB above threshold, followed by a series of 200-msec tones 1 dB louder; perception of these is indicative of cochlear damage. SYN small increment sensitivity index t.

situational t., in psychology and psychiatry, a t. situation in which a subject is observed as he or she performs a task or an actual sample of the job or role to be performed; *e.g.,* a test used to select individuals for the Office of Strategic Services during the Second World War and for managerial positions today.

skin t., a method for determining induced sensitivity (allergy) by applying an antigen (allergen) to, or inoculating it into, the skin; induced sensitivity (allergy) to the specific antigen is indicated by an inflammatory reaction of one of two general kinds: 1) immediate, appears in minutes to an hour or so and in general is dependent upon circulating immunoglobulins (antibodies); 2) delayed, appears in 12 to 48 hours and is not dependent upon these soluble substances but upon cellular response and infiltration. SYN cutaneous t., cutireaction t., skin reaction.

skin-puncture t., t. for Behçet's syndrome; after pricking the skin with a sterile needle, pustulation follows within 24 hours, owing to the dermal sensitivity in this disease.

small increment sensitivity index t., SYN SISI t.

sniff t., at fluoroscopy, a t. for diaphragmatic function; paradoxical motion of a hemidiaphragm when a patient sniffs vigorously shows phrenic nerve paralysis or paresis of the hemidiaphragm. If rapid upward movement of the diaphragm occurs on brisk sniffing in the supine position, it is highly suggestive of paralysis of the diaphragm.

Snyder's t., a colorimetric t. for determining dental caries activity or susceptibility based on the rate of acid production by acidogenic oral microorganisms (*e.g.,* lactobacillus) in a glucose medium, using bromcresol green as the indicator, and producing a color change from green to yellow. SYN colorimetric caries susceptibility t.

solubility t., a screening t. for sickle cell hemoglobin (Hb S), which is reduced by dithionite and is insoluble in concentrated inorganic buffer; addition of blood showing Hb S to buffer and dithionite causes opacity of the solution.

spironolactone t., administration of spironolactone (400 mg orally) for 4 consecutive days: an increase in serum potassium during the t., and a decrease afterward, strongly suggest primary aldosteronism.

split renal function t., SYN differential ureteral catheterization t.

spot t. for infectious mononucleosis, a slide t. widely used for the diagnosis of infectious mononucleosis, based on the principle that the heterophil antibodies that occur in the serum of patients with infectious mononucleosis are absorbed by beef red cells but not by guinea pig kidney cells; thus, when horse red cells (which provoke heterophil antibodies) are mixed with patient serum and agglutination occurs in the presence of beef red cells, the presumptive diagnosis is infectious mononucleosis.

standard serologic t.'s for syphilis, STS for syphilis, nontreponemal antigen t.'s giving presumptive but not conclusive evidence of syphilis, including the Wassermann and VDRL t.'s.

standing t., a t. for the effect of a hypotensive drug, carried out by the patient: after taking the drug, he stands perfectly still for one minute commencing from the time that the maximal action of the drug should be manifested; if the dose is adequate, the patient should experience a slight hypotensive reaction.

standing plasma t., if plasma is stored at 4°C upright in a t. tube, chylomicrons will float to the top and form a creamy layer.

starch-iodine t., a t. for sweating in which iodine in oil is painted on the skin, followed by dusting with a starch powder which turns blue-black in the presence of iodine and moisture.

station t., SYN Romberg's *sign*.

Stein's t., in cases of labyrinthine disease the patient is unable to stand or to hop on one foot with his eyes shut.

Stenger t., a test for detecting simulation of unilateral deafness.

Stewart's t., estimation of the amount of collateral circulation, in case of an aneurysm of the main artery of a limb, by means of a calorimeter.

Strassburg's t., a t. for bile in the urine; albumin, if present, is precipitated, then cane sugar is added and filter paper is dipped in the fluid and dried; if bile pigments are present in the urine, sulfuric acid will turn the filter paper a reddish violet.

stress t., any cardiac challenge, physical, pharmacologic, or mental delivered under monitored conditions. Most commonly this is exercise, the most common monitor being electrocardiography although any other graphic technique, including cardiac catheterization, may be applied.

string t., (1) a t. to locate gastrointestinal hemorrhage; a string is repeatedly swallowed and removed, each time allowing the string to go further down the gut until blood is encountered; **(2)** a procedure to obtain a specimen of duodenal juices; a weighted string is swallowed, withdrawn after four hours, and the duodenal secretions extracted from the string for examination.

Strong vocational interest t., a t. that matches an individual's specific likes, dislikes, and interests to those characteristic of persons working in each of a number of vocations.

Student's *t* t., a statistical method analogous to the calculation of the normal deviation; the formula is $t = (x- x)/s$, where the numerator is the deviation from the mean, and the denominator is the standard deviation for sample sizes of less than 30 cases.

Stypven time t., a t. measuring the clotting time of plasma after addition of Russell's viper *venom*, useful in evaluating patients with deficiencies in factor X. [Trade name [*styp*tic + *ven*om]

sucrose hemolysis t., isotonic sucrose promotes binding of complement to red blood cells; in paroxysmal nocturnal hemoglobinuria a proportion of the cells is sensitive to complement-mediated lysis, and hemolysis ensues.

sulfosalicylic acid turbidity t., a t. for measurement of protein in the urine; sulfosalicylic acid precipitates protein in the urine with a turbidity that is approximately proportional to the concentration of protein in a solution.

sweat t., a t. for cystic fibrosis of the pancreas in which electrolytes are measured in collected sweat; sodium chloride concentration above 50 mEq/l (children) or 60 mEq/l (adults) is positive.

sweating t., a t. for locating the level of a lesion in the spinal cord; when the body is heated or the patient is given a diaphoretic, sweat secretion is absent below the level of the lesion.

swimming t., a t. for activity of adrenal cortical preparations; two days after adrenalectomy, rats are placed in water and the time during which they can swim is recorded; they are then injected with the material to be tested; the response is termed "positive" if the swimming time is doubled.

swinging light t., SYN alternating light t.

swordfish t., a rarely used t. for androgenic activity, based upon the fact that androgens cause the development of the sword, a male structure, in female swordfish (*Xiphophorus helleri*) SYN Xiphophorus t.

t **t.,** a t. that uses a statistic which under the null hypothesis has the *t* distribution, to test whether two means differ significantly.

Tactual Performance T., SYN Halstead-Reitan *battery.*

thematic apperception t. (TAT), a projective psychological t. in which the subject is asked to tell a story about standard ambiguous pictures depicting life-situations to reveal his or her own attitudes and feelings.

thermostable opsonin t., a t. for opsonic activity of antibody in the absence of effect of heat-labile complement.

Thompson's t., the urine, in a case of gonorrhea, is passed into two glasses; if the gonococci and gonorrheal threads are found only in the first glass the probability is that the process is limited to the anterior urethra. SYN two-glass t.

Thormählen's t., a t. for melanin; the suspected liquid is treated with sodium nitroprusside, caustic potash, and acetic acid; if melanin is present, the solution takes on a deep blue color.

Thorn t., a putative t. of adrenal cortical function; stimulation of a normally functioning adrenal cortex by the adrenocorticotrophic hormone is followed by a reduction in the number of circulating eosinophils and lymphocytes and an increase in the excretion of uric acid. The t. lacks sufficient specificity and is rarely used.

three-glass t., the bladder is emptied by passing urine into a series of 3-ounce test tubes, and the contents of the first and the last are examined; the first tube contains the washings from the anterior urethra, the second, material from the bladder, and the last, material from the posterior urethra, prostate, and seminal vesicles. SYN Valentine's t.

thymol turbidity t., precipitation of abnormal proportions of albumin and globulin from the serum of patients with liver disease by addition of thymol. Although popular in the past it has been superseded by quantitative determination of specific proteins and direct measurement of liver enzymes. SYN Maclagan's t., Maclagan's thymol turbidity t.

thyroid-stimulating hormone stimulation t., TSH stimulating t., a t. that measures the uptake of ^{131}I in the thyroid gland before and after administration of thyroid-stimulating hormone; useful in distinguishing primary hyperthyroidism (increased TSH serum concentration) from secondary or tertiary hyperthyroidism (low TSH serum concentrations).

thyroid suppression t., a thyroid function t. used to diagnose difficult cases of hyperthyroidism, now largely replaced by the thyrotropin-releasing hormone stimulation t.; triiodothyronine is administered for a week to 10 days, and a reduction of its uptake by the thyroid gland to less than half of the initial uptake is a normal response. SYN Werner's t.

thyrotropin-releasing hormone stimulation t., TRH stimulation t., a t. of pituitary response to injection of thyrotropin-releasing hormone, which normally stimulates pituitary secretion of thyroid-stimulating hormone (TSH, thyrotropin), used primarily to distinguish pituitary from hypothalamic causes of thyroid disorders; TSH does not rise in cases of pituitary dysfunction, but does rise in cases of hypothalamic disorders.

tilt t., any measurement of response during tilting of the body usually head up but also head down. The t. may be monitored by catheterization, echocardiography, electrophysiologic measurements, electrocardiography, or mechanocardiography.

tine t., SEE tuberculin t.

titratable acidity t., the number of milliliters of 0.1 N NaOH required to neutralize a 24-hr specimen of urine.

tolbutamide t., a t. to detect insulin-producing tumors; after a 1-g intravenous dose of tolbutamide, plasma insulin and glucose are measured at intervals up to 3 hr; higher insulin responses and lower glucose values characterize patients with such tumors.

tone decay t., the sounding of a continuous tone at threshold for

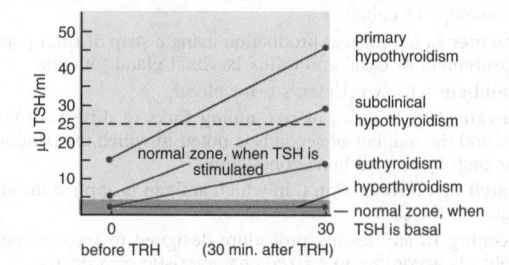

changes in concentration of thyroid-stimulating hormone in serum after intravenous injection of thyrotropin-releasing hormone

1 min; if the intensity must be increased by more than 5 dB for continued perception, it may be a sign of retrocochlear damage.

Töpfer's t., an obsolete t. for free hydrochloric acid in the gastric contents; dimethylaminoazobenzene is used as the indicator.

total catecholamine t., a fluorometric determination of catecholamines in 24-hr urine specimens; elevated values are seen in patients with pheochromocytoma and neuroblastoma; spurious elevations may be seen due to excretion products of medication containing adrenaline, tetracyclines, quinidine, and some antihypertensive agents; false-positive elevations may be seen in persons with extensive burns, in vigorous exercise, or in progressive muscular dystrophy.

tourniquet t., SEE capillary fragility t., Rumpel-Leede t.

TPHA t., SYN Treponema pallidum hemagglutination t.

TPI t., SYN Treponema pallidum immobilization t.

Trendelenburg's t., a t. of the valves of the leg veins; the leg is raised above the level of the heart until the veins are empty and is then rapidly lowered; in varicosity and incompetence of the valves the veins will at once become distended, but placement of a touriquet around the leg will prevent distention of veins below the incompetent perforators or valves below the tourniquet.

Treponema pallidum hemagglutination t., a highly sensitive and specific t. for the serologic diagnosis of syphilis; tanned sheep red blood cells are coated with the antigen of *Treponema pallidum* and, following absorption of nonspecific patient serum antibody, a positive reaction with tanned sheep red blood cells and patient serum indicates the presence of specific antibody for *Treponema pallidum* in patient serum. SYN TPHA t.

Treponema pallidum immobilization t., TPH t., a t. for syphilis in which an antibody other than Wassermann antibody is present in the serum of a syphilitic patient, which in the presence of complement causes the immobilization of actively motile *Treponema pallidum* obtained from testes of a rabbit infected with syphilis. SYN TPI t., *Treponema pallidum* immobilization reaction.

triiodothyronine uptake t., a t. of thyroid function in which triiodothyronine (T_3) is added to a patient's serum *in vitro* to measure the relative affinities of serum proteins and of an added competitive substance for T3; higher T3 uptakes are associated with hyperthyroidism. SYN T_3 uptake t.

tuberculin t., application of the skin t. to the diagnosis of infection by *Mycobacterium tuberculosis* in which tuberculin or its "purified" protein derivative serves as an antigen (allergen); injection of graduated doses of tuberculin or of purified protein derivative into the skin, most often by means of a needle and syringe (Mantoux t.) or by means of tines (tine t.); t. material may also be applied by means of a "patch" in which it is absorbed but this method (patch t.) is viewed as being less reliable; the t. is read on the basis of induration and erythema, the former being considered the more diagnostic of infection with the tubercle bacillus (*M. tuberculosis*); the t. does not distinguish between infection in a resistant person without disease and an individual with clinical manifestations of disease.

T_3 uptake t., SYN triiodothyronine uptake t.

two-glass t., SYN Thompson's t.

two-step exercise t., a t. used mainly for coronary insufficiency;

significant depression of RS-T in the electrocardiogram is considered abnormal and suggests coronary insufficiency.

two-tail t., a statistical t. based on the assumption that the data are distributed in both directions from some central value.

Tzanck t., the examination of fluid from a bullous lesion for Tzanck cells (altered epithelial cells, rounded and devoid of intercellular attachments). The periphery of these cells is basophilic and the nucleus is spherical and enlarged with prominent nucleoli. They are characteristic of lesions due to varicella, herpes zoster, herpes simplex, and pemphigus vulgaris.

urea clearance t., a t. of renal function based on urea clearance.

urease t., (1) a t. for urea based on the conversion of urea into ammonium carbonate by the enzyme urease; **(2)** a t. for the production of urease, used for identification of *cryptococci* and *Heilcobacter pylori.*

urecholine supersensitivity t., urodynamic t. that tries to elicit an abnormal cystometrogram after subcutaneous injection of a drug, urecholine. Subcutaneous injection of urecholine may increase detrusor pressure response during filling in patients with some types of neuropathic bladder.

urinary concentration t., a t. of renal tubular function whereby the patient is dehydrated for a measured period of time and the specific gravity of the urine is subsequently determined.

vaginal cornification t., a t. for estrogenic activity, in which the appearance of cornified epithelial cells in a vaginal smear of a test animal is an indication of the action of an estrogen.

vaginal mucification t., a t. for progestational activity; stimulation of mucus production by the vaginal epithelium in rats, guinea pigs, or mice by progestogens.

Valentine's t., SYN three-glass t.

Valsalva t., the heart is monitored by ECG, pressure recording, or other methods while the patient performs the Valsalva maneuver; the heart becomes smaller in normal persons but may dilate in the patient with impaired myocardial reserve; there is a characteristic complex sequence of cardiocirculatory events, departure from which indicates disease or malfunction.

van Deen's t., SYN Almén's t. for blood.

van den Bergh's t., a t. for bile pigments (bilirubin) by reaction with diazotized sulfanilic acid (diazo reaction).

van der Velden's t., a t. for free hydrochloric acid, the presence of which turns an added solution of methylene blue from violet to green.

vanillylmandelic acid t., a t. for catecholamine-secreting tumors (pheochromocytoma and neuroblastoma) performed on a 24-hr urine specimen; it is based on the fact that vanillylmandelic acid is the major urinary metabolite of norepinephrine and epinephrine. SYN 3-methoxy-4-hydroxymandelic acid t., VMA t.

VDRL t., a flocculation t. for syphilis, using cardiolipin-lecithin-cholesterol antigen as developed by the Venereal Disease Research Laboratory of the United States Public Health Service.

vitality t., a group of thermal and electrical t.'s used to aid in assessment of dental pulp health. SYN pulp t.

vitamin C t., SYN capillary fragility t.

VMA t., SYN vanillylmandelic acid t.

Volhard's t., a t. for renal function: the patient drinks 1500 ml of water on an empty stomach; if the patient was not dehydrated beforehand and the kidneys are normal, this fluid will be excreted by the end of 4 hr, with specific gravity of the urine being from 1.001 to 1.004.

Vollmer t., a tuberculin patch t.

Wada t., unilateral internal carotid injection of amobarbital to determine the laterality of speech; injection on the dominant side causes transient aphasia or mutism; used prior to surgical treatment of epilepsy.

Waldenström's t., a t. for porphyrin in the urine; 2 ml of urine are mixed with an equal amount of 2% dimethyl-*p*-aminobenzaldehyde in 50/100 HCl. A red color appears if urobilinogen (Ehrlich's benzaldehyde reaction) or porphobilinogen is present.

Wang's t., a quantitative t. for indican, which is transformed into indigo-sulfuric acid and then titrated by a solution of potassium permanganate.

washout t., a means of estimating renal obstruction by the rate of disappearance of excreted radioactive material from the kidney.

Wassermann t., a complement-fixation t. used in the diagnosis of syphilis; originally the "antigen" was an extract of liver from a syphilitic fetus, but later the active substance, referred to as cardiolipin, was found to be present in normal tissues, including heart, and has been identified as a diphosphatidylglycerol. SYN Wassermann reaction.

water-drinking t., a t. of the assessment of open-angle glaucoma, measuring intraocular pressure after drinking a quart of water in five minutes.

Watson-Schwartz t., a qualitative screening t. for diagnosis of acute intermittent porphyria by the addition of Ehrlich's reagent and saturated sodium acetate to the urine; a pink or red color indicates the presence of porphobilinogen or urobilinogen; the former indicates porphyria, the latter does not; therefore, positive results require further differential extraction with butanol and chloroform to eliminate false-positive results due to urobilinogen.

Weber's t. for hearing, the application of a vibrating tuning fork to one of several points in the midline of the head or face, to ascertain in which ear the sound is heard best by bone conduction, that ear being the affected one if the sound-conducting apparatus (middle ear) is at fault (positive t.), but probably the normal one if the neurosensory apparatus is diseased (negative t.).

Webster's t., a t. for trinitrotoluene in the urine.

Weil-Felix t., a t. for the presence and type of rickettsial disease based on the agglutination of X-strains of *Proteus vulgaris* with suspected rickettsia in a patient's blood serum. SYN Weil-Felix reaction.

Werner's t., SYN thyroid suppression t.

Wheeler-Johnson t., cystosine or uracil when treated with bromine yields dialuric acid which gives a green color with excess of barium hydroxide.

Wormley's t., a t. for alkaloids, by treating the solution with picric acid or a dilute iodine-potassium-iodide solution, the presence of alkaloids being shown by a color reaction.

Wurster's t., a t. for tyrosine; the substance is dissolved in boiling water and quinone is added; if tyrosine is present a ruby-colored reaction takes place, the solution changing to brown after a few hours.

x^2 t., SYN chi-square t.

Xiphophorus t., SYN swordfish t.

xylose t., a laboratory aid in diagnosing alimentary or essential pentosuria, conditions in which xylose (a pentose) is excreted; the xylose may be identified by rapid reduction of Benedict's solution, by nonfermentation by yeasts, or by a positive Bial's t. for pentose.

Yvon's t., (1) for alkaloids; to the suspected solution is added a mixture of bismuth subnitrate, potassium iodide, and hydrochloric acid in water; a positive reaction is indicated by the appearance of a red color; **(2)** for acetanilid in the urine; the suspected fluid is extracted with chloroform and heated with yellow nitrate of mercury; if acetanilid is present, the fluid will be green.

Zimmermann t., SYN Zimmermann *reaction.*

Zondek-Aschheim t., SYN Aschheim-Zondek t.

Zsigmondy's t., SYN Lange's t.

---

tes·ta (tes'tă). **1.** SYN eggshell. **2.** In protozoology, usually termed test; an envelope of certain forms of ameboid protozoa, consisting of various earthy materials cemented to a chitinous base (as in the testate rhizopods of the subclass Testacealobosia) or the calcareous, siliceous, organic, or strontium sulfate skeletons in the rhizopod subclass Foraminifera. **3.** In botany, the outer, sometimes the only, coat of a seed. [L. shell]

Tes·ta·ce·a·lo·bo·sia (tes-tā'shē-ă-lō-bō'zē-ă). A subclass of the subphylum Sarcodina (amebae), in which the cells are provided with a firm chitinous envelope, often containing earthy material, with an opening through which the pseudopodia are protruded. [L. *testa,* shell]

tes·tal·gia (tes-tal'jē-ă). SYN orchialgia. [testis + G. *algos,* pain]

test·cross (test'kros). Crossing of an unknown genotype to a recessive homozygote so that the phenotype of the progeny corresponds directly to the chromosomes carried by the parents of unknown genotype. SYN backcross (2).

tes·tec·to·my (tes-tek'tō-mē). SYN orchiectomy. [testis + G. G. *ektomē*, excision]

tes·tes (tes'tēz). Plural of testis. [L.]

tes·ti·cle (tes'tĭ-kl). SYN testis. [L. *testiculus*, dim. of *testis*]

tes·tic·u·lar (tes-tik'yū-lăr). Relating to the testes.

tes·tic·u·lus (tes-tik'yū-lŭs). SYN testis. [L.]

test·ing. SEE test.

  bench t., t. of a device against specifications in a simulated (nonliving) environment.

  genetic t., SYN DNA diagnostics.

  histocompatibility testing, a testing system for HLA antigens, of major importance in transplantation.

  reality testing, in psychiatry and psychology, the ego function by which the objective or real world and one's subjectively sensed relationship to it are evaluated and appreciated; the ability to distinguish internal from external events.

  susceptibility t., the determination of the ability of an antibiotic to kill or inhibit the growth of bacteria.

tes·tis, pl. **tes·tes** (tes'tis, -tēz) [NA]. One of the two male reproductive glands, located in the cavity of the scrotum. SYN didymus, genital gland (1), male gonad, orchis, testicle, testiculus. [L.]

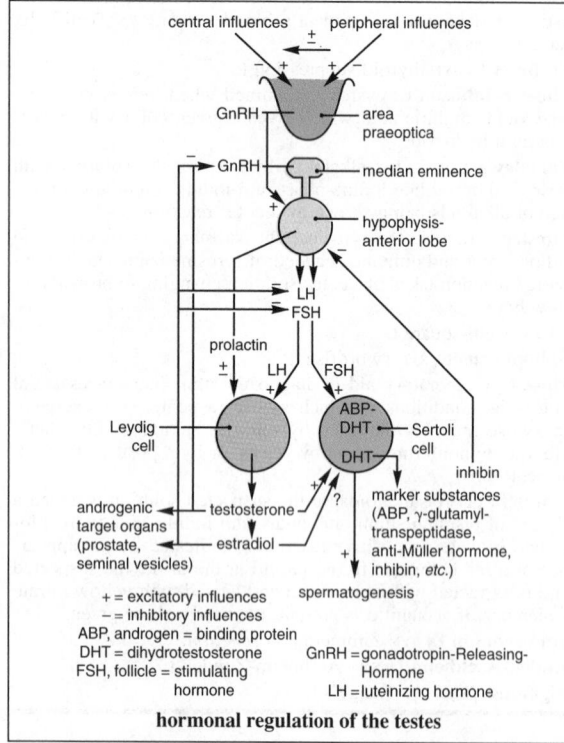

hormonal regulation of the testes

  cryptorchid t., SYN undescended t.

  ectopic t., a variant of undescended t. wherein testicular position is outside the usual pathway of descent. SEE ALSO testis *ectopia*.

  movable t., a condition in which there is a tendency in the t. to ascend to the upper part of the scrotum or into the inguinal canal.

  retractile t., a t. that periodically disappears from the scrotum, as contrasted with an undescended t.

  undescended t., a t. that has failed to descend into the scrotum; there are palpable and unpalpable (impalpable) variants. SYN cryptorchid t.

tes·ti·tis (tes-tī'tis). SYN orchitis.

test let·ter. SEE test types.

tes·toid (tes'toyd). **1.** SYN androgenic. **2.** SYN androgen. [testis + G. *eidos*, resemblance]

tes·to·lac·tone (tes-tō-lak'tōn). D-Homo-17α-oxa-1,4-androstadiene-3,17-dione; an androgenic agent used as an antineoplastic agent for treatment of mammary carcinoma.

tes·tos·ter·one (tes-tos'tĕ-rōn). 17β-Hydroxy-4-androstene-3-one; the most potent naturally occurring androgen, formed in greatest quantities by the interstitial cells of the testes, and possibly secreted also by the ovary and adrenal cortex; may be produced in nonglandular tissues from precursors such as androstenedione; used in the treatment of hypogonadism, cryptorchism, certain carcinomas, and menorrhagia.

  t. cypionate, a preparation with the same actions and uses as t. propionate, but with a prolonged duration of action.

  t. enanthate, a preparation with the same actions and uses as t., but with a prolonged duration of action, being administered in oil.

  t. phenylpropionate, an alternate preparation for the propionate.

  t. propionate, a preparation that has an action similar to but more pronounced and prolonged than that of t.; used in the treatment of undescended testes and in menorrhagia.

test sym·bols. SEE test types.

test types. Letters of various sizes used to test visual acuity.

  Jaeger's t. t., type of different sizes used for testing the acuity of near vision.

  point system t. t., a near-vision test chart in which the various test types are multiples of a point (1/72 inch), lower-case letters being one-half the designated point size; reading 4-point at 16 inches is normal, and is designated N-4.

  Snellen's t. t., square black symbols employed in testing the acuity of distant vision; the letters vary in size in such a way that each one subtends a visual angle of 5' at a particular distance.

△**tetan-.** SEE tetano-.

te·ta·nia (te-tā'nē-ă). Obsolete synonym for tetan.

  t. gas'trica, SYN gastric *tetany*.

  t. gravida'rum, tetany in pregnant women.

  t. neonato'rum, SYN neonatal *tetany*.

  t. parathyreopri'va, SYN parathyroid *tetany*.

te·tan·ic (te-tan'ik). **1.** Relating to or marked by a sustained muscular contraction, as in tetanus. **2.** An agent, such as strychnine, that in poisonous doses produces tonic muscular spasm. [G. *tetanikos*]

te·tan·i·form (te-tan'i-fōrm). SYN tetanoid (1).

tet·a·nig·e·nous (tet-ă-nij'ĕ-nŭs). Causing tetanus or tetaniform spasms. [tetanus + G. *-gen*, producing]

tet·a·nil·la (tet-ă-nil'ă). **1.** SYN fibrillary *myoclonia*. **2.** SYN tetany. [Mod. L. dim. of L. *tetanus*]

tet·a·nism (tet'ă-nizm). SYN neonatal *tetany*.

tet·a·ni·za·tion (tet'ă-ni-zā'shŭn). **1.** The act of tetanizing the muscles. **2.** A condition of tetaniform spasm.

tet·a·nize (tet'ă-nīz). To stimulate a muscle by a rapid series of stimuli so that the individual muscular responses (contractions) are fused into a sustained contraction; to cause tetanus (2) in a muscle.

△**tetano-, tetan-.** Combining forms denoting tetanus, tetany. [G. *tetanos*, convulsive tension]

tet·a·node (tet'ă-nōd). Denoting the quiet interval between the recurrent tonic spasms in tetanus. [G. *tetanōdēs*]

tet·a·noid (tet'ă-noyd). **1.** Resembling or of the nature of tetanus. SYN tetaniform. **2.** Resembling tetany. [tetano- + G. *eidos*, resemblance]

tet·a·no·ly·sin (tet-ă-nol'i-sin). A hemolytic principle, elaborated by *Clostridium tetani*, which seems to have no role in the etiology of tetanus.

tet·a·nom·e·ter (tet-ă-nom'ĕ-ter). An instrument for measuring the force of tonic muscular spasms. [tetano- + G. *metron*, measure]

tet·a·no·mo·tor (tet'ă-nō-mō'ter). An instrument by means of which tonic spasms are produced by the mechanical irritation of a hammer striking the motor nerve of the muscle affected. [tetano- + L. *motor,* a mover]

tet·a·no·spas·min (tet'ă-nō-spaz'min). The neurotoxin of *Clostridium tetani,* which causes the characteristic signs and symptoms of tetanus; chief action is on the anterior horn cells, and the spasms seem to be due to action at inhibitory synapses.

tet·a·no·toxin (tet'ă-nō-tok'sin). SYN tetanus *toxin.* [tetano- + G. *toxikon,* poison]

tet·a·nus (tet'ă-nŭs). **1.** A disease marked by painful tonic muscular contractions, caused by the neurotropic toxin (tetanospasmin) of *Clostridium tetani* acting upon the central nervous system. **2.** A sustained muscular contraction caused by a series of nerve stimuli repeated so rapidly that the individual muscular responses are fused; producing a sustained tetanic contraction. SEE emprosthotonos, opisthotonos, pleurothotonos. [L. fr. G. *tetanos,* convulsive tension]

acoustic t., experimental t. induced by a faradic current, the speed of which is estimated by the pitch of the vibrations.

anodal closure t. (ACTe), obsolete term for a tetanic muscular contraction occurring during the time the circuit is closed, the current then running, while the positive pole is applied.

anodal duration t. (ADTe, AnDTe), obsolete term for the period of muscular contraction occurring at the anode when the electric circuit is closed.

anodal opening t., obsolete term for a tonic contraction in a muscle, to which the anode is applied, when the circuit is opened.

t. anti'cus, SYN emprosthotonos.

apyretic t., SYN tetany.

benign t., a disorder marked by intermittent tonic muscular contractions of the extremities, especially the hands and feet (carpopedal spasm), accompanied by paresthesias and, when severe, by crowing respirations due to laryngospasm and seizures; results from hypocalcemia, caused by various disorders, including gastrointestinal abnormalities. SYN intermittent cramp (2).

cathodal closure t. (CCTe), obsolete term for a tetanic muscular contraction occurring during the time the circuit is closed, the current then running, while the negative pole is applied.

cathodal duration t. (CaDTe), obsolete term for a tetanic contraction occurring on application of the cathode or negative pole, while the circuit is closed.

cathodal opening t., obsolete term for a tonic contraction in a muscle, to which the cathode is applied; when the circuit is opened, the contraction is suddenly interrupted.

cephalic t., a type of local tetanus that follows wounds to the face and head; after a brief incubation (1–2 days) the facial and ocular muscles become paretic yet undergo repeated tetanic spasms. The throat and tongue muscles may also be affected. SYN cerebral t., head t., hydrophobic t., rose cephalic t., Rose's cephalic t.

cerebral t., SYN cephalic t.

complete t., t. (2) in which stimuli to a particular muscle are repeated so rapidly that decrease of tension between stimuli cannot be detected.

t. dorsa'lis, SYN opisthotonos.

drug t., tonic spasms caused by strychnine or other tetanic. SYN toxic t.

generalized t., the most common type of t., often with trismus as its initial manifestation; the muscles of the head, neck, trunk and limbs become persistently contracted, and then painful paroxysmal tonic contractions (tetanic seizures) are superimposed; the high mortality rate (50%) is due to asphyxia or cardiac failure.

head t., SYN cephalic t.

hydrophobic t., SYN cephalic t.

imitative t., conversion hysteria that resembles t.

incomplete t., t. (2) in which each stimulus causes a contraction to be initiated when the muscle has only partly relaxed from the previous contraction.

intermittent t., SYN tetany.

local t., the most benign type of t.; the muscles in close proximity to an infected wound develop persistent involuntary contractions, often with transient, intense superimposed spasms trig-

gered by various stimuli. The more distal upper extremity muscles are most often affected; gradual but complete recovery is typical.

neonatal t., SYN t. neonatorum.

t. neonatorum (nē-ō-nā'tōr-ŭm), t. occurring in newborn infants, usually due to infection of umbilical area with *Clostridium tetani,* often a result of ritualistic practices; has high fatality rate (about 60%). SYN neonatal t.

t. posti'cus, SYN opisthotonos.

postpartum t., SYN puerperal t.

puerperal t., t. occurring during the puerperium from infection of the obstetric wound. SYN postpartum t., uterine t.

Ritter's opening t., the tetanic contraction that occasionally occurs when a strong current, passing through a long stretch of nerve, is suddenly interrupted.

rose cephalic t., SYN cephalic t.

Rose's cephalic t., SYN cephalic t.

toxic t., SYN drug t.

traumatic t., t. following infection of a wound.

uterine t., SYN puerperal t.

tet·a·ny (tet'ă-nē). A clinical neurological syndrome characterized by muscle twitches, cramps, and carpopedal spasm, and when severe, laryngospasm and seizures; these findings reflect irritability of the central and peripheral nervous systems, usually resulting from low serum levels of ionized calcium or, rarely, magnesium. Causes include hyperventilation, hypoparathyroidism, rickets, and uremia. SYN apyretic tetanus, intermittent cramp (1), intermittent tetanus, tetanilla (2). [G. *tetanos,* tetanus]

t. of alkalosis, t. due to a loss of acid from the body or an increase in alkali, resulting in a reduction of ionized calcium in plasma and body fluids, *e.g.,* hyperventilation t. (loss of CO_2), gastric t. (loss of HCl by vomiting), or injection or ingestion of excessive amounts of sodium bicarbonate.

duration t. (DT), a tonic spasm occurring in degenerated muscles upon application of a strong galvanic current.

epidemic t., SYN rheumatic t.

gastric t., t. associated with a gastric disorder, especially with loss of HCl by vomiting. SYN tetania gastrica.

grass t., a highly fatal disease of cows and sheep occurring generally during the first two weeks in the spring after the animals have been out on lush pastures; it is characterized by convulsions, hypomagnesemia, and usually hypocalcemia. SYN wheat pasture poisoning.

hyperventilation t., t. caused by forced overbreathing, due to a reduction in CO_2 in the blood.

hypoparathyroid t., SYN parathyroid t.

infantile t., t. of infants occurring usually in rickets, due to dietary deficiency of vitamin D.

latent t., a rather vague disorder recognized more in Europe than in the U.S. consisting of a number of nonspecific complaints, including generalized weakness, hand and foot cramping, distal paresthesia, anxiety, and depression. Some think it is a "normocalcemic tetany"; others consider it "chronic hyperventilation syndrome." Typically with certain provoking procedures (*e.g.,* limb ischemia, hyperventilation) in which case, obvious tetany develops. SEE Trousseau's *sign,* Chvostek's *sign,* Erb *sign.* SYN crytotetany, spasmophilia.

manifest t., t. from any cause in which neuromuscular hyperexcitability are clearly evident, as opposed to latent t. SYN symptomatic t.

neonatal t., hypocalcemic t. occurring in neonates or young infants, due to transient functional hypoparathyroidism in consumption of cow's milk (high phosphorus content). SYN myotonia neonatorum, tetania neonatorum, tetanism.

parathyroid t., t. due to lack of parathyroid function, spontaneous or following excision of the parathyroid glands. SYN hypoparathyroid t., parathyroprival t., tetania parathyreopriva.

parathyroprival t., SYN parathyroid t.

phosphate t., t. due to the ingestion of an excess of alkaline phosphates (Na_2HPO_4 or K_2HPO_4); most commonly produced experimentally in animals by the injection of alkaline phosphate, which reduces the ionized calcium of the blood.

forms of tetany in adults

form, name	etiology, concomitant phenomena
I. hypocalcemic tetanies	
1. parathyrogenous	postoperative (1–3 days after removal of epithelial corpuscles = parathyroprival tetany) or idiopathic hypoparathyroidism
2. recalcification t.	calcium avidity after operative removal of an epithelial corpuscle adenoma
3. enterogenous and primary calcium deficiency t.	severe calcium resorption difficulty or deficient diet
4. toxic-conditioned t.	chemical binding of blood calcium by oxalates, fluorides, citrate infusion, etc.
5. kidney-conditioned t.	hyperphosphatemia (through kidney insufficiency)
6. in pseudo-hypoparathyroidism	genetic defect; frequently with brachymetacarpia and -tarsia, dwarfism
II. normocalcemic tetanies	
1. idiopathic t.	frequently in neurasthenics and psychopaths (pseudo-t.), with attacks during the best psychological conditions; despite normocalcemia, resolved by injection of calcium
2. hyperventilation t.	respiratory alkalosis (reduced calcium ionization)
3. in infectious diseases and pharmacologic poisoning	primarily: guanidine, adrenaline, caffeine, morphine
4. cerebrally conditioned t.	lesion (trauma, tumor, encephalitis), definite hypothalamus structures
5. Mg deficiency	extreme Mg deficiency in the organism
6. stomach t., chloriprivic t.	hypochloremia and alkalosis after vomiting (e.g., pyloric stenosis)
7. pregnancy t.	hyperemesis, gestosis

postoperative t., parathyroid t. caused by injury to or excision of the parathyroids during thyroid removal.

recurrent t., a simple autosomal recessive trait in Scottish terrier dogs, characterized by arching of the back and a stiff-legged gait due to overflexed hindlimbs and abducted forelimbs. SYN Scotch cramp.

rheumatic t., an acute epidemic form of t., of several weeks' duration, occurring chiefly in winter. SYN epidemic t.

symptomatic t., SYN manifest t.

transport t., an acute disease seen in cattle and sheep during and shortly after shipping; it appears most often in females in advanced pregnancy and is believed to be precipitated by stress, lack of food and water, and perhaps heat. SYN railroad disease, railroad sickness.

△**tetra-.** Four (properly affixed to words derived from G. roots). [G. *tetra-,* four]

tet·ra·a·me·lia (tet′ră-ă-mē′lē-ă). Absence of upper and lower limbs. [tetra- + G. *a-* priv. + *melos,* limb]

tet·ra·ba·sic (tet-ră-bā′sik). Denoting an acid having four acid groups and thereby being able to neutralize four equivalents of base.

tet·ra·ben·a·zine (tet′ră-ben′ă-zen). 2-Oxo-3-isobutyl-9,10-dimethoxy-1,2,3,4,6,7-hexahydro-11b*H*-benzo[α]quinolizine; formerly used as a tranquilizer; resembles reserpine in its actions but duration of effect is shorter.

tet·ra·bo·ric ac·id (tet′ră-bōr′ik). Perboric or pyroboric acid. SYN pyroboric acid.

tet·ra·bra·chi·us (tet′ră-brā′kē-ŭs). An individual with four arms. [tetra- + G. *brachiōn,* arm]

tet·ra·bro·mo·phe·nol·phthal·ein so·di·um (tet′ră-brō′mō-fē′nol-thal′ēn, -ē-in). The sodium salt of a brominated dye; it was used early in the development of cholecystography.

tet·ra·caine hy·dro·chlo·ride (tet′ră-kān). 2-(Dimethylamino)-ethyl *p*-(butylamino)benzoate monohydrochloride; a highly potent local anesthetic used for spinal, nerve block, and topical anesthesia.

tet·ra·chi·rus (tet′ră-kī′rŭs). A malformed individual having four hands. [tetra- + G. *cheir,* hand]

tet·ra·chlor·eth·y·lene (tet′ră-klōr-eth′i-lēn). An anthelmintic against hookworm and other nematodes. SYN carbon dichloride, ethylene tetrachloride, tetrachloroethylene.

tet·ra·chlor·me·thi·a·zide (tet′ră-klōr-me-thī′ă-zīd). 6-chloro-3,4-dihydro-3-trichloromethyl-2*H*-1,2,4 -benzothiadiazine-7-sulfonamide 1,1-dioxide; a diuretic of the thiazide type. SYN teclothiazide.

tet·ra·chlo·ro·eth·ane (tet′ră-klōr-ō-eth′ăn). Cl_2HC—$CHCl_2$; acetylene tetrachloride; a nonflammable solvent for fats, oils, waxes, resins, etc.; used in the manufacture of paint and varnish removers, photographic films, lacquers, and insecticides. Its toxicity exceeds that of chloroform and carbon tetrachloride, and produces narcosis, liver damage, kidney damage, and gastroenteritis. SYN cellon.

tet·ra·chlo·ro·eth·yl·ene (tet′ră-klōr-ō-eth′i-lēn). SYN tetrachlorethylene.

tet·ra·chlo·ro·meth·ane (tet′tră-klōr-ō-meth′ăn). SYN *carbon* tetrachloride.

tet·ra·coc·cus, pl. **tet·ra·coc·ci** (tet′ră-kok′ŭs, -kok′sī). A spherical bacterium that divides in two planes and characteristically forms groups of four cells. [tetra- + G. *kokkos,* berry]

tet·ra·co·sac·tide, tet·ra·co·sac·tin (tet′ră-kō-sak′tid, -tin). SYN cosyntropin.

n-**tet·ra·co·sa·no·ic ac·id** (tet′ră-kō-să-nō′ik). SYN lignoceric acid.

tet·ra·crot·ic (tet′ră-krot′ik). Denoting a pulse curve with four upstrokes in the cycle. [tetra- + G. *krotos,* a striking]

tet·ra·cus·pid (tet-ră-kŭs′pid). Having four cusps. SYN quadricuspid.

tet·ra·cy·cline (tet-ră-sī′klēn, -klin). A broad spectrum antibiotic (a naphthacene derivative), the parent of oxytetracycline, prepared from chlortetracycline and also obtained from the culture filtrate of several species of *Streptomyces;* also available as t. hydrochloride and t. phosphate complex. T. fluorescence has been used in studies of growing tumors and calcium deposition in developing bone and teeth.

tet·rad. 1. A collection of four things having something in common such as a deformity with four features *e.g.,* Fallot's tetralogy. SYN tetralogy. 2. In chemistry, a quadrivalent element. 3. In heredity, a bivalent chromosome that divides into four during meiosis. [G. *tetras* (*tetrad-*), the number four]

Fallot's t., SYN *tetralogy* of Fallot.

narcoleptic t., the clinical syndrome of narcolepsy, cataplexy, sleep paralysis, and hypnagogic hallucinations.

tet·ra·dac·tyl (tet-ră-dak′til). Having only four fingers or toes on a hand or foot. SYN quadridigitate. [tetra- + G. *daktylos,* finger or toe]

tet·ra·dec·a·no·ic ac·id (tet′ră-dek-ă-nō′ik). SYN myristic acid.

12-*O*-tet·ra·dec·a·no·yl·phor·bol 13-ac·e·tate (TPA) (tet′ră-dek′ă-nō-il-fōr′bol). A double ester of phorbol found in croton oil; a cocarcinogen or tumor promoter.

te·trad·ic (te-trad′ik). Relating to a tetrad.

tet·ra·do·tox·in (TTX) (tet′rŏ-dō-tok′sin). A potent neurotoxin found in the liver and ovaries of the Japanese pufferfish, *Sphoeroides rubripes*, other species of pufferfish, and certain newts; produces axonal blocks of the preganglionic cholinergic fibers and the somatic motor nerves. T. blocks voltage-gated Na channels in excitable tissues.

tet·ra·eth·yl·am·mo·ni·um chlo·ride (tet-ră-eth′il-ă-mō′nē-ŭm). $(C_2H_5)_4N^+Cl^-$; a quaternary ammonium compound that partially blocks transmission of impulses through parasympathetic and sympathetic ganglia; its clinical usefulness is limited; formerly used as an antihypertensive drug.

tet·ra·eth·yl·lead (tet′ră-eth′i-led). $Pb(C_2H_5)_4$; tetraethylplumbane; an anti-knock compound added to motor fuel; has a toxic action causing anorexia, nausea, vomiting, diarrhea, tremors, muscular weakness, insomnia, irritability, nervousness, and anxiety; death may occur. SYN lead tetraethyl.

tet·ra·eth·yl·mon·o·thi·o·no·py·ro·phos·phate (tet-ră-eth′il-mon-ō-thī′ō-nō-pī-rō-fos′fāt). An anticholinesterase agent used in the treatment of glaucoma.

tet·ra·eth·yl py·ro·phos·phate (TEPP) (tet′ră-eth′il). $Et_4P_2O_7$; $[(EtO)_2PO]_2O$; an organic phosphoric compound used as an insecticide; a potent irreversible cholinesterase inhibitor.

tet·ra·eth·yl·thi·u·ram di·sul·fide (tet′ră-eth-il-thī′yū-ram). SYN disulfiram.

tet·ra·gas·trin (tet-ră-gas′trin). **1.** A tetrapeptide (Trp-Met-Asp-Phe-NH_2) used to test the secretion of digestive juice. **2.** A pterin derivative that is a required cofactor for a number of enzymes; *e.g.*, in the conversion of L-phenylalanine to L-tyrosine; the inability to synthesize tetrahydrobiopterin is associated with forms of malignant hyperphenylalaninemia.

tet·ra·gly·cine hy·dro·per·i·o·dide (tet-ră-glī′sēn hī′drō-per-ī′ō-dīd). $(NH_2CH_2COOH)_4HI·1¼I_2$; dissolves in water to the extent of 380 g per liter; used for the emergency disinfection of drinking water in amounts to yield 8 p.p.m. of active iodine.

tet·ra·gon, tet·ra·go·num (tet′ră-gon, tet′ră-gō′nŭm). Quadrangle; a figure having four sides. [tetra- + G. *gōnia*, angle]
  t. lumba′le, a quadrangular space bounded laterally by the obliquus externus abdominis muscle, medially by the erector spinae, above by the serratus posterior inferior, and below by the internal abdominal oblique muscle.

tet·ra·go·nus (tet′ră-gō′nŭs). Obsolete term for platysma *muscle*.

tet·ra·hy·dric (tet-ră-hī′drik). Denoting a compound containing four ionizable hydrogen atoms (four acid groups).

△**tetrahydro-.** Prefix denoting attachment of four hydrogen atoms; *e.g.*, tetrahydrofolate, H_4folate.

tet·ra·hy·dro·can·nab·i·nol (THC) (tet′ră-hī′drō-kă-nab′i-nol). $C_{21}H_{30}O_2$; the $Δ^1$-3,4-*trans* isomer and the $Δ^6$-3,4-*trans* isomer are believed to be the active isomers present in *Cannabis*, having been isolated from marijuana. SEE ALSO cannabis, dronabinol.

5,6,7,8-tet·ra·hy·dro·fo·late de·hy·dro·gen·ase (tet′ră-hī-drō-fō′lāt). SYN dihydrofolate reductase.

tet·ra·hy·dro·fo·late meth·yl·trans·fer·ase (tet′ră-hī-drō-fōl′āt). SYN *methionine* synthase.

tet·ra·hy·dro·fo·lic ac·id (FH₄) (tet′ră-hī-drō-fōl′ik). The active coenzyme form of folic acid; participates in one-carbon metabolism. SYN coenzyme F.

tet·ra·hy·droz·o·line hy·dro·chlo·ride (tet-ră-hī-droz′ō-lēn). A sympathomimetic agent related to ephedrine, used as a topical nasal and conjunctival decongestant; excessive amounts may convert an acute congestion into a chronic reactive hyperemia.

Tet·ra·hy·me·na pyr·i·for·mis (tet-ră-hī′mē-nă pir-i-fōr′mis). A ciliate belonging to a large group characterized by three membranes on one side of the buccal cavity and one on the other; it somewhat resembles the paramecium and, like it, is readily cultured and used extensively for experimental studies. [tetra- + G. *hymēn*, membrane]

tet·ra·i·o·do·phe·nol·phthal·ein so·di·um (tet′ră-ī-ō′dō-fē′nol-thal′ĕn, -thal′ē-in). SYN iodophthalein.

te·tral·o·gy (te-tral′ō-jē). SYN tetrad (1). [G. *tetralogia*]
  Eisenmenger's t., SYN Eisenmenger's *complex*.

t. of Fallot, a set of congenital cardiac defects including ventricular septal defect, pulmonic valve stenosis or infundibular stenosis, and dextroposition of the aorta so that it overrides the ventricular septum and receives venous as well as arterial blood. Right ventricular hypertrophy is considered part of the tetralogy although it is reactive to the other defects. SYN Fallot's tetrad.

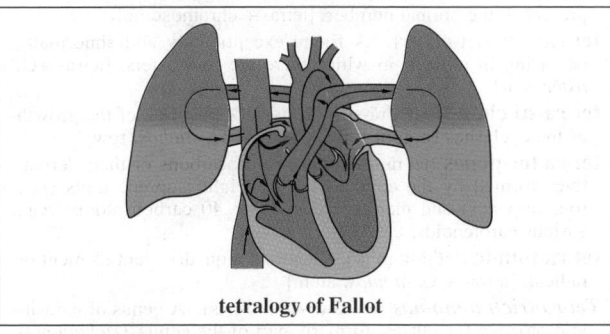

tetralogy of Fallot

tet·ra·mas·tia (tet′ră-mas′tē-ă). Presence of four breasts on an individual. [tetra- + G. *mastos*, breast]

tet·ra·mas·ti·gote (tet-ră-mas′ti-gōt). A protozoan or other microorganism possessing four flagella. [tetra- + G. *mastix*, whip]

tet·ra·mas·tous (tet′ră-mas′tŭs). Having four breasts.

te·tram·e·lus (tĕ-tram′ĕ-lŭs). Conjoined twins possessing four arms (tetrabrachius), or four legs (tetrascelus). SEE conjoined *twins*, under *twin*. [tetra- + G. *melos*, limb]

Tet·ra·me·res (tet-ram′ĕ-rēz). A genus of stomach-infecting parasitic nematodes (family Spiruridae) of birds. When filled with eggs, the female worm is enormously enlarged and has a globular, blood-red appearance. Species include *T. americana*, found in the proventriculus of chickens (sometimes severely pathogenic in young chicks), turkeys, grouse, and quail, and transmitted by infected cockroaches and grasshoppers, and *T. fissispina*, found in the proventriculum of ducks, geese, wild waterfowl, pigeons, and doves but rarely in gallinaceous birds. [see tetrameric]

tet·ra·mer·ic, te·tram·er·ous (tet′ră-mer′ik, tĕ-tram′ĕ-rŭs). Having four parts, or parts arranged in groups of four, or capable of existing in four forms. [tetra- + G. *meros*, part]

1,2,9,10-te·tra·meth·ox·y·a·por·phine. SYN glaucine.

tet·ra·meth·yl·am·mo·ni·um io·dide (tet-ră-meth′il-ă-mō′nē-ŭm). $(CH_3)_4NI_3$; dissolves in water to the extent of 0.25 gm per liter; used for the emergency disinfection of drinking water.

tet·ra·meth·yl·di·ar·sine (tet-ră-meth′il-dī-ar′sēn). SYN cacodyl.

tet·ra·meth·yl·pu·tres·cine (tet-ră-meth′il-pyū-tres′ēn). A derivative of putrescine, $C_8H_{20}N_2$, similar in its action to muscarine.

tet·ra·ni·trol (tet-ră-nī′trol). SYN erythrityl tetranitrate.

tet·ra·nu·cle·o·tide (tet′ră-nū′klē-ō-tīd). A compound of four nucleotides; once thought to represent the actual structure of nucleic acid (tetranucleotide theory).

tet·ra·ot·us (tet′ră-ō′tus). SYN tetrotus.

tet·ra·pa·re·sis (tet′ră-pă-rē′sis). Weakness of all four extremities. SYN quadriparesis.

tet·ra·pep·tide (tet′ră-pep′tīd). A compound of four amino acids in peptide linkage.

tet·ra·pe·ro·me·lia (tet′ră-pē-rō-mē′lē-ă). Peromelia involving all four extremities. [tetra- + G. *peros*, maimed, + *melos*, limb]

tet·ra·pho·co·me·lia (tet′ră-fō-kō-mē′lē-ă). Phocomelia involving all four limbs.

tet·ra·ple·gia (tet′ră-plē′jē-ă). SYN quadriplegia. [tetra- + G. *plēgē*, stroke]

tet·ra·ple·gic (tet′ră-plē′jik). SYN quadriplegic.

tet·ra·ploid (tet′ră-ployd). SEE polyploidy. [G. *tetraploos*, fourfold, + *eidos*, form]

tet·ra·pus (tet′ră-pŭs). A malformed individual with four feet. [G. *tetrapous*, fr. tetra- + *pous*, foot]

tet·ra·pyr·role (tet′ră-pir′ōl). A molecule containing four pyrrole nuclei; *e.g.*, porphyrin.

te

tet·ra·sac·cha·ride (tet′ră-sak′ă-rīd). A sugar containing four molecules of a monosaccharide; *e.g.,* stachyose.

te·tras·ce·lus (te-tras′ĕ-lŭs). A malformed individual with four legs. [tetra- + G. *skelos,* leg]

tet·ra·so·mic (tet′ră-sō′mik). Relating to a cell nucleus in which one chromosome is represented four times while all others are present in the normal number. [tetra- + chromosome]

tet·ras·ter (tet-ras′ter). A figure exceptionally and abnormally occurring in mitosis, in which there are four asters. [tetra- +G. *astēr,* star]

tet·ra·sti·chi·a·sis (tet′ră-sti-kī′ă-sis). Duplication of the growth of the eyelashes (in four rows). [tetra- + G. *stichos,* row]

tet·ra·ter·penes (tet′ră-ter′pēnz). Hydrocarbons or their derivatives formed by the condensation of eight isoprene units (*i.e.,* four terpenes) and therefore containing 40 carbon atoms; *e.g.,* various carotenoids.

tet·ra·tom·ic (tet′ră-tom′ik). Denoting a quadrivalent element or radical. [tetra- + G. *atomos,* atom]

Tet·ra·trich·o·mo·nas (tet′ră-tri-kom′ŏ-nas). A genus of parasitic protozoan flagellates, formerly part of the genus *Trichomonas* but now separated into a distinct genus by the presence of four anterior and one trailing flagella, a pelta, and a disc-shaped parabasal body. SEE *Trichomonas.* [tetra- + *Trichomonas*]

T. o′vis, a species that occurs in the cecum or rumen of domestic sheep.

tet·ra·va·lent (tet′ră-vā′lent). SYN quadrivalent. [tetra- + L. *valentia,* strength]

tet·ra·zole (tet′ră-zōl). The compound CN_4H_2 with the structure of tetrazolium.

tet·ra·zo·li·um (tet′ră-zō′lē-ŭm). Any of a group of organic salts having the general structure which on reduction (cleaving the 2,3 bond) yields a colored insoluble formazan; used as a reagent in oxidative enzyme histochemistry.

nitroblue t. (NBT), a pale yellow dye that is converted on reduction to colored formazans in the histochemical demonstration of dehydrogenases; used in hematology for staining of neutrophils to help indicate the presence of bacterial infections.

tet·rose (tet′rōs). A monosaccharide containing only four carbon atoms in the main chain; *e.g.,* erythrose, threose, erythrulose.

te·tro·tus (te-trō′tŭs). A malformed individual with four ears, four eyes, two faces, and two almost separate heads. SYN tetraotus. [tetra- + G. *ous* (*ōt*-), ear]

te·trox·ide (te-trok′sīd). An oxide containing four oxygen atoms; *e.g.,* OsO_4.

tet·ter (tet′er). An outmoded colloquial term, popularly applied to ringworm and eczema, and occasionally applied to other eruptions. [A.S. *teter*]

branny t., (1) SYN dandruff. **(2)** SYN *seborrhea capitis.*

crusted t., SYN impetigo.

dry t., obsolete colloquialism for eczema.

honeycomb t., obsolete term for favus.

humid t., SYN wet t.

milk t., obsolete term for *crusta* lactea.

moist t., SYN wet t.

scaly t., obsolete colloquialism for eczema.

wet t., outmoded term for a moist eczematous dermatitis. SYN humid t., moist t.

Teutleben, F.E.K. von, German anatomist, 1842–?. SEE T.'s *ligament.*

tex·ti·form (teks′tĭ-fōrm). Weblike. [L. *textum,* something woven]

tex·tur·al (teks′chŭr-ăl). Relating to the texture of the tissues.

tex·ture (teks′chŭr). The composition or structure of a tissue or organ. [L. *textura,* fr. *texo,* pp. *textus,* to weave]

tex·tus (teks′tŭs). A tissue. [L.]

TGC Abbreviation for time-varied gain *control;*time-gain *compensation.*

TGE Abbreviation for transmissible *gastroenteritis* of swine.

TGF Abbreviation for transforming growth *factors,* under *factor.*

TGFα Abbreviation for transforming growth *factor* α.

TGFβ Abbreviation for transforming growth *factor* β.

Th Abbreviation for T helper *cells,* under *cell.*

Th Symbol for thorium.

Thal, Alan P., U.S. surgeon, *1925. SEE T. *procedure.*

△**thalam-.** SEE thalamo-.

thal·a·mec·to·my (thal-ă-mek′tō-mē). SEE chemothalamectomy. [thalamus + G. *ektomē,* excision]

thal·a·men·ce·phal·ic (thal′ă-men-se-fal′ik). Relating to the thalamencephalon.

thal·a·men·ceph·a·lon (thal′ă-men-sef′ă-lon). That part of the diencephalon comprising the thalamus and its associated structures. [thalamus + G. *enkephalos,* brain]

tha·lam·ic (tha-lam′ik). Relating to the thalamus.

△**thalamo-, thalam-.** The thalamus. [G. *thalamos,* bedroom (thalamus)]

thal·a·mo·cor·ti·cal (thal′ă-mō-kōr′ti-kăl). Relating to the efferent connections of the thalamus with the cerebral cortex.

thal·a·mo·len·tic·u·lar (thal′ă-mō-len-tik′yū- lăr). Relating to the thalamus, usually the dorsal thalamus, and the lenticular nucleus (putamen and globus pallidus).

thal·a·mot·o·my (thal-ă-mot′ō-mē). Destruction of a selected portion of the thalamus by stereotaxy for the relief of pain, involuntary movements, epilepsy, and, rarely, emotional disturbances; produces few, if any, neurological deficits or undesirable personality changes. [thalamus + G. *tomē,* incision]

thal·a·mus, pl. **thal·a·mi** (thal′ă-mŭs, -mī) [NA]. The large, ovoid mass of gray matter that forms the larger dorsal subdivision of the diencephalon; it is placed medial to the internal capsule and the body and tail of the caudate nucleus. Its medial aspect forms the dorsal half of the lateral wall of the third ventricle; its dorsal surface can be subdivided into a lateral triangle forming the floor of the body (central part) of the lateral ventricle, and a medial triangle covered by the velum interpositum; its taillike caudal part curves ventralward around the posterolateral aspect of the cerebral peduncle and ends in the lateral geniculate body. The t. is composed of a large number of anatomically and functionally distinct cell groups or nuclei, usually classified as 1) sensory relay nuclei (ventral posterior nucleus, lateral and medial geniculate body) each receiving a modally specific sensory conduction system and in turn projecting each to the corresponding primary sensory area of the cortex; 2) "secondary" relay nuclei (ventral intermediate nucleus and ventral anterior nucleus) receiving fibers from the medial segment of the globus pallidus, the contralateral deep cerebellar nuclei (*i.e.,* cerebellothalamic fibers) and the pars reticulata of the substantia nigra which project to various regions of the motor cortex; 3) a nucleus associated with the limbic system: the composite anterior nucleus receiving the mamillothalamic tract and projecting to the fornicate gyrus; 4) association nuclei (medial dorsal nucleu, lateral nucleus including the large pulvinar) each projecting to a particular large expanse of association cortex; 5) the midline and intralaminar nuclei or "nonspecific" nuclei (centromedian nucleus, central lateral nucleus, paracentral nucleus, nucleus reuniens). [G. *thalamos,* a bed, a bedroom]

dorsal t., the large part of the diencephalon located dorsal to the hypothalamus and excluding the subthalamus and the medial and lateral geniculate bodies (sometime the latter two are collectively called the metathalamus); the dorsal t. includes the major motor and somatosensory relay nuclei, nuclei that project to association areas, and the intralaminar nuclei.

thal·as·se·mia, thal·as·sa·ne·mia (thal-ă-sē′mē-ă, thă-las-ă-nē′mē-ă). Any of a group of inherited disorders of hemoglobin metabolism in which there is impaired synthesis of one or more of the polypeptide chains of globin; several genetic types exist, and the corresponding clinical picture may vary from barely detectable hematologic abnormality to severe and fatal anemia. [G. *thalassa,* the sea, + *haima,* blood]

α **t.,** t. due to one of two or more genes that depress (severely or moderately) synthesis of α-globin chains by the chromosome with the abnormal gene. Heterozygous state: severe type, t. minor with 5 to 15% of Hb Barts at birth, only traces of Hb Barts in adult; mild type, 1 to 2% of Hb Barts at birth, not detectable in adult. Homozygous state: severe type, erythroblastosis fetalis and fetal death, only Hb Barts and Hb H present; mild type not clinically defined. SEE ALSO *hemoglobin* H.

A₂ t., β t., heterozygous state.

β t., t. due to one of two or more genes that depress (partially or completely) synthesis of β-globin chains by the chromosome bearing the abnormal gene. Heterozygous state (A₂ t.): t. minor with Hb A₂ increased, Hb F normal or variably increased, Hb A normal or slightly reduced. Homozygous state: t. major with Hb A reduced to very low but variable levels, Hb F very high level.

β-δ t., t. due to a gene that depresses synthesis of both β- and δ-globin chains by the chromosome bearing the abnormal gene. Heterozygous state: t. minor with Hb F comprising 5 to 30% of total hemoglobin but distributed unevenly among cells, Hb A₂ reduced or normal. Homozygous state: moderate anemia with only Hb F present, no Hb A or Hb A₂. SYN F t.

F t., SYN β-δ t.

t. interme′dia, a clinical variant of t. characterized by an intermediate degree of severity. These patients have severe anemia but usually do not require regular blood transfusions. Intermedia disorders represented a heterogeneous group of genetic disorders and may include cases with homozygous or heterozygous abnormalities in the β-globin chain gene.

α **t. interme′dia,** SEE *hemoglobin* H.

Lepore t. [MIM*142000.0020 and others], t. syndrome due to production of abnormally structured Lepore hemoglobin. Heterozygous state: t. minor with about 10% of Hb Lepore, Hb F moderately increased, Hb A₂ normal. Homozygous state: t. major with only Hb F and Hb Lepore produced, no Hb A or Hb A₂.

t. ma′jor [MIM*141800-142310 passim], the syndrome of severe anemia resulting from the homozygous state of one of the t. genes or one of the hemoglobin Lepore genes with onset, in infancy or childhood, of pallor, icterus, weakness, splenomegaly, cardiac enlargement, thinning of inner and outer tables of skull, microcytic hypochromic anemia with poikilocytosis, anisocytosis, stippled cells, target cells, and nucleated erythrocytes; types of hemoglobin are variable and depend on the gene involved. SYN Cooley's anemia, primary erythroblastic anemia.

t. mi′nor [MIM*141800-142310 passim], the heterozygous state of a t. gene or a hemoglobin Lepore gene; usually asymptomatic and quite variable hematologically, with target cells, mild hypochromic microcytosis, and often slightly reduced hemoglobin level with slightly increased erythrocyte count; types of hemoglobin are variable and depend on the gene involved.

tha·las·so·pho·bia (thal′ă-sō-fō′bē-ă, thă-las′ō-). Morbid fear of the sea. [G. *thalassa,* the sea, + *phobos,* fear]

tha·las·so·po·sia (thal′ă-sō-pō′zē-ă, thă-las′ō-). SYN mariposia. [G. *thalassa,* the sea, + *posis,* drinking]

tha·las·so·ther·a·py (thal′ă-sō-thār′ă-pē). Treatment of disease by exposure to sea air, by sea bathing, or by a sea voyage. [G. *thalassa,* the sea]

tha·lid·o·mide (thă-lid′ō-mīd). α-Phthalimidoglutarimide; *N*-phthalylglutamimide; *N*-(2,6-dioxo-3-(piperidyl)phthalimide; a hypnotic drug which, if taken in early pregnancy, may cause the birth of infants with phocomelia and other defects; occasionally used for the treatment of pyoderma gangrenosun.

thal·lic (thal′lik). Denoting conidia produced with no enlargement or growth after delimitation by septa in the hypha (thallus); the entire parent cell becomes an arthroconidium.

thal·li·um (Tl) (thal′ē-ŭm). A white metallic element, atomic no. 81, atomic wt. 204.3833; ²⁰¹Tl (half-life equal to 3.038 days) is used to scan the myocardium. [G. *thallos,* a green shoot (it gives a green line in the spectrum)]

t.-201 (²⁰¹Tl), the radioisotope of t. used widely for myocardial nuclear imaging; it is also taken up by certain tumors.

Thal·lo·phy·ta (thă-lof′i-tă). In older classification systems, a primary division of the plant kingdom whose members, with a few exceptions, were devoid of true roots, stems, and leaves; it included bacteria, fungi, and algae. [G. *thallos,* a green shoot, + *phyton,* plant]

thal·lo·phyte (thal′ō-fīt). A member of the division Thallophyta.

thal·lo·spore (thal′ō-spōr). Obsolete term for a reproductive asexual type of spore formed as an integral part of the thallus or

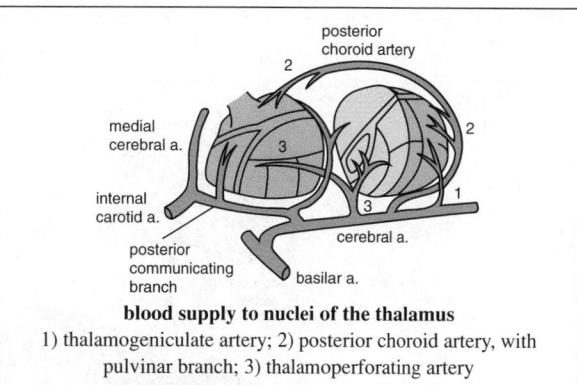

blood supply to nuclei of the thalamus
1) thalamogeniculate artery; 2) posterior choroid artery, with pulvinar branch; 3) thalamoperforating artery

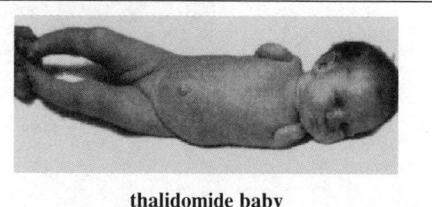

thalidomide baby

mycelium, in contrast to a conidium formed on a specialized hypha. [G. *thallos,* a green twig, + *sporos,* seed]

thal·lo·tox·i·co·sis (thal′ō-tok-si-kō′sis). Poisoning by thallium; marked by stomatitis, gastroenteritis, peripheral and retrobulbar neuritis, endocrine disorders, and alopecia. [thallium + G. *toxikon,* poison, + *-osis,* condition]

thal·lus (thal′ŭs). A simple plant or fungus body which is devoid of roots, stems, and leaves. The vegatative growth of a fungus. [G. *thallos,* a young shoot]

thanato-. Death. SEE ALSO necro-. [G. *thanatos,* death]

than·a·to·bi·o·log·ic (than′ă-tō-bī-ō-loj′ik). Relating to the processes involved in life and death. [thanato- + G. *bios,* life, + *logos,* study]

than·a·to·gno·mon·ic (than′ă-tō-nō-mon′ik). Of fatal prognosis, indicating the approach of death. [thanato- + G. *gnōmē,* a sign]

than·a·tog·ra·phy (than-ă-tog′ră-fē). **1.** A description of one's symptoms and thoughts while dying. **2.** A treatise on death. [thanato- + G. *graphē,* a writing]

than·a·toid (than′ă-toyd). **1.** Resembling death. **2.** Deadly. [thanato- + G. *eidos,* resemblance]

than·a·tol·o·gy (than-ă-tol′ō-jē). The branch of science concerned with the study of death and dying. [thanato- + G. *logos,* study]

than·a·to·ma·nia (than′ă-tō-mā′nē-ă). Illness or death resulting from belief in the efficacy of magic; a phenomenon observed among those primitive societies or illiterate and superstitious people who believe in the power of evil spirits, spells, curses, and individuals over one's bodily processes, with such belief and resulting fear manifesting itself as psychosomatic illness and even death. [thanato- + G. *mania,* frenzy]

than·a·to·phid·ia (than′ă-tō-fid′ē-ă). Venomous snakes. [thanato- + G. *ophidion,* dim. of *ophis,* a serpent]

than·a·to·pho·bia (than′ă-tō-fō′bē-ă). Morbid fear of death. [thanato- + G. *phobos,* fear]

than·a·to·phor·ic (than′ă-tō-fōr′ik). Leading to death. [thanato- + G. *phoros,* bearing]

than·a·top·sy (than′ă-top-sē). SYN autopsy (1). [thanato- + G. *opsis,* view]

than·a·tos (than′ă-tos). In psychoanalysis, the death principle, representing all instinctual tendencies toward senescence and death. See also entries under instinct. Cf. eros. [G. death]

th

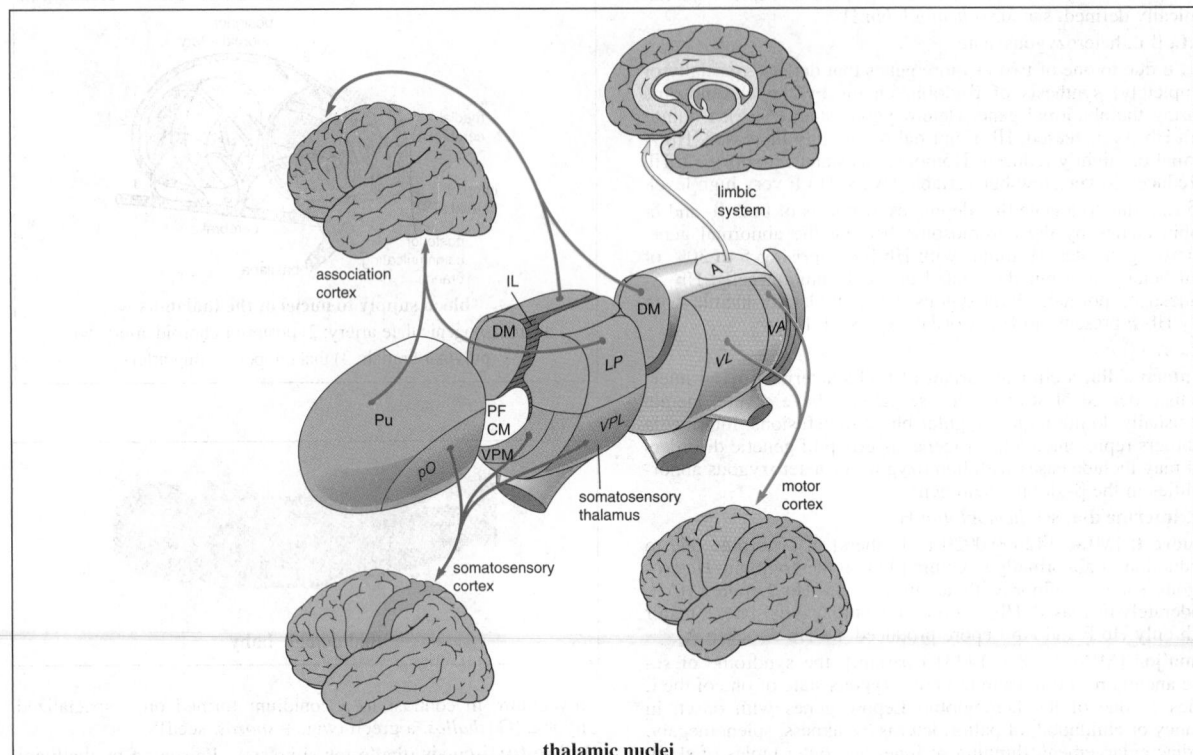

thalamic nuclei

schematic view of principal *thalamic nuclei* and their cortical projections; nuclei colored *blue* contain somatosensory projections; pO, posterior nucleus, VPM and VPL, ventroposterior medial and lateral nuclei (ventrobasal complex); IL, intralaminar nuclei; A, anterior n.; VL and VA, ventrolateral and ventroanterior nuclei with entrances from cerebellum or pallidum; DM, dorsomedial n., LP, lateral posterior n.; Pu = pulvinar; PF and CM, parafascicular and centromedian nuclei

Thane, Sir George D., English anatomist, 1850–1930. SEE T.'s *method*.

thau·mat·ro·py (thaw-mat′rō-pē). The transformation of one form of tissue into another. [G. *thauma* (*thaumat*-), a wonder, + *tropē*, a turning]

Thayer, J.D. SEE T.-Martin *medium*, *agar*.

THC Abbreviation for tetrahydrocannabinol.

Thd Symbol for ribothymidine.

thea (thē-ă). SYN tea. [Mod. L.]

the·a·ism (thē′ă-izm). SYN theinism.

the·a·ter (thē′ă-ter). **1.** A large room for lectures and demonstrations; sometimes applied to an operating room equipped for observation by persons other than the surgical team. **2.** Any operating room or suite of such rooms. [G. *theatron*, a place for seeing, theater, fr. *theomai*, to look at]

the·ba·ic (thē-bā′ik). Relating to or derived from opium. [L. *Thebaicus*, relating to Thebes, whence opium was formerly obtained]

the·ba·ine (thē-bā′ēn, -in). $C_{19}H_{21}NO_3$; an alkaloid obtained from opium (0.3 to 1.5%); it resembles strychnine in its action, causing tetanic convulsions. SYN paramorphine.

Thebesius, Adam C., German physician, 1686–1732. SEE thebesian *foramina*, under *foramen*, thebesian *valve*, thebesian *veins*, under *vein*.

the·ca, pl. **the·cae** (thē′kă, thē′sē). A sheath or capsule. [G. *thēkē*, a box]

t. cor′dis, SYN pericardium.

t. exter′na, SYN *tunica* externa thecae folliculi.

t. follic′uli, the wall of a vesicular ovarian follicle. SEE ALSO *tunica* externa, *tunica* interna thecae folliculi.

t. inter′na, SYN *tunica* interna thecae folliculi.

t. ten′dinis, SYN synovial tendon *sheath*.

t. vertebra′lis, SYN *dura mater* of spinal cord.

the·cal (thē′kăl). Relating to a sheath, especially a tendon sheath. [see theca]

the·ci·tis (thē-sī′tis). Inflammation of the sheath of a tendon. [G. *thēkē*, box (sheath), + -*itis*, inflammation]

thec·o·dont (thē′kō-dont). Having the teeth inserted in alveoli. [G. *thēkē*, box, + *odous* (*odont*-), tooth]

the·co·ma (thē-kō′mă). A neoplasm derived from ovarian mesenchyme, consisting chiefly of spindle-shaped cells that frequently contain small droplets of fat; gross features generally resemble those of a granulosa cell tumor, *i.e.*, firm, yellow, encapsulated mass, ordinarily about 10 cm or less in diameter, but it tends to be less malignant; it may form considerable quantities of estrogens, thereby resulting in precocious development of secondary sexual features in prepubertal girls, or hyperplasia of the endometrium in older patients. SYN theca cell tumor. [G. *thēkē*, box (theca), + -*oma*, tumor]

the·co·ma·to·sis (thē′kō-mă-tō′sis). A stromal hyperplasia or increase in the number of connective tissue elements of an ovary.

the·co·steg·no·sia, the·co·steg·no·sis (thē′kō-steg-nō′sē-ă, -nō′sis). Constriction of a tendon sheath. [G. *thēkē*, box (sheath), + *stegnōsis*, a narrowing]

Theden, Johann C.A., German surgeon, 1714–1797. SEE T.'s *method*.

Theile, Friedrich W., German anatomist, 1801–1879. SEE T.'s *canal*, *glands*, under *gland*, *muscle*.

Theiler, Max, South African microbiologist in the U.S. and Nobel laureate, 1899–1972. SEE T.'s *disease*, *virus*.

Thei·ler·ia (thī-lēr′ē-ă). A genus of piroplasmid sporozoan protozoa (family Theileriidae, order Piroplasmida, class Sporozoea) that are tick-borne parasites and among the most important pathogens of domestic animals; they multiply asexually in lymphocytes or other cells and then invade the erythrocytes, where they remain without multiplying until ingested by a transmitting tick. SYN *Cytauxzoon.* [A. *Theiler*]

T. annula'ta, a species that causes Mediterranean or tropical theileriosis in cattle.

T. bo'vis, SYN *T. parva bovis.*

T. fe'lis, a highly pathogenic species that causes theileriosis in domestic cats and bobcats. SYN *Cytauxzoon felis.*

T. hir'ci, a species that causes malignant theileriosis in sheep and goats.

T. lawren'cei, SYN *T. parva lawrencei.*

T. mu'tans, a species that causes benign bovine theileriosis in Africa and the Carribbean; occasionally causes fatal disease in cattle.

T. orienta'lis, a bovine species found worldwide which, in some regions, has been reported to cause clinical disease in cattle. SYN *T. sergenti.*

T. par'va, a species now divided into three subspecies: *T. parva bovis, T. parva lawrencei,* and *T. parva parva.*

T. par'va bo'vis, a parasite causing Rhodesian malignant theileriosis in cattle. SYN *T. bovis.*

T. par'va lawren'cei, a parasite of the wild African buffalo (*Syncerus caffer*); it is highly pathogenic to cattle, causing Corridor disease. SYN *T. lawrencei.*

T. par'va par'va, a highly pathogenic parasite causing East Coast fever in cattle.

T. sergen'ti, SYN *T. orientalis.*

T. taurotra'gi, a species that causes benign bovine theileriosis, and is infective to sheep and goats; transmitted by *Rhipicephalus pulchellus* in Africa.

thei·le·ri·a·sis (thī-le-rī'ă-sis). SYN theileriosis.

Thei·le·ri·i·dae (thī-lē'rē-i-dē). A family of sporozoan protozoa which, combined with the family Babesiidae, comprises the order Piroplasmida; it consists of one recognized genus, *Theileria,* transmitted by ixodid ticks; some species are highly pathogenic to domestic and wild ruminants, causing theileriosis.

thei·le·ri·o·sis (thī-lēr-ē-ō'sis). Protozoan disease of cattle, sheep, and goats caused by infection with protozoan of the genus *Theileria,* and transmitted by ixodid ticks. SYN theileriasis.

benign bovine t., t. in cattle, a protozoan disease caused either by *Theileria mutans* (transmitted by ticks of the genus *Amblyomma* in Africa and the Caribbean) or by *T. taurotragi* (transmitted by the ticks *Rhipicephalus appendiculatus* and *R. pulchellus* in Africa).

malignant ovine and caprine t., a highly pathogenic protozoan disease of sheep and goats in southeastern Europe, northern Africa, and the Near and Middle East; it is caused by *Theileria hirci* and transmitted by the tick *Hyalomma anatolicum anatolicum.*

Mediterranean t., SYN tropical t.

Rhodesian malignant t., a highly pathogenic protozoan disease of cattle in Zimbabwe caused by *Theileria parva bovis* and transmitted by the tick *Rhipicephalus appendiculatus.* SEE ALSO kaodzera.

tropical t., a highly pathogenic protozoan disease of cattle in northern Africa, southern Europe, the Near and Middle East, and central Asia; caused by *Theileria annulata* and transmitted by ticks of the genus *Hyalomma.* SYN Mediterranean t.

the·in (thē'in, tē'in). SYN caffeine.

the·in·ism, the·ism (thē'i-nizm; thē'izm, tē'-). Chronic poisoning resulting from immoderate tea-drinking, marked by palpitation, insomnia, nervousness, headache, and dyspepsia. SYN theaism. [Mod. L. *thea,* tea]

⚠**thel-.** SEE thelo-.

the·lar·che (the-lar'kē). The beginning of development of the breasts in the female. [thel- + G. *archē,* beginning]

The·la·zia (the-lā'zē-ă). The eye worms, a genus of spiruroid nematodes that inhabit the lacrimal ducts and surface of the eyes of various domestic and wild animals, but rarely man; a number of species have been reported from wild birds. Cyclic development occurs in muscoid flies; infective larvae emerge from the

fly mouthparts while the fly is feeding on or near the eyes of the host. [G. *thēlazō,* to suck]

T. californien'sis, a species occurring in the tear ducts, conjunctival sac, or under the nictitating membrane of dogs, coyotes, black bears, sheep, deer, jack rabbits, cats, and occasionally humans in the western and southwestern U.S.; heavy infections cause photophobia, lacrimation, eyelid edema, conjunctivitis, and even blindness.

T. callipae'da, a species reported from man in Southeast Asia and California; the worm, embedded in a subconjunctival tumor or swimming in the aqueous humor after penetrating the corneoscleral limbus, causes pain, photophobia, and tearing.

thel·a·zi·a·sis (thē-lă-zī'ă-sis, thel-ă-). Infection with nematodes of the genus *Thelazia.*

the·le (thē'lē). SYN nipple. [G.]

the·le·plas·ty (thē'lē-plas-tē). SYN mammillaplasty. [thel- + G. *plastos,* formed]

the·li·um, pl. **the·lia** (thē'lē-ŭm, -lē-ă). **1.** A nipple-like structure. **2.** A cellular layer. **3.** SYN nipple. [Mod. L., fr. G. *thēlē,* nipple]

⚠**thelo-, thel-.** The nipples. Cf. mamil-. [G. *thēlē*]

the·lon·cus (thē-long'kŭs). A neoplasm involving the nipple. [thelo- + G. *onkos,* a mass]

the·lor·rha·gia (thē-lō-rā'jē-ă). Bleeding from the nipple. [thelo- + G. *rhēgnymi,* to burst forth]

the·nad (thē'nad). Toward the thenar or lateral side of the palm of the hand. [G. *thenar,* the palm of the hand, + L. *ad,* to]

the·nal (thē'năl). SYN thenar (2).

the·nal·dine (thē-nal'dēn). Thenophenopiperidine; 1-methyl-4-*N*-2-thenylanilinopiperidine; an antihistaminic and antipruritic agent (as the tartrate).

the·nar (thē'nar). **1** [NA]. SYN thenar *eminence.* **2.** Applied to any structure in relation with the thenar eminence or its underlying collective components. SYN thenal. [G. the palm of the hand]

the·nen (thē'nen). Relating only to the palm, specifically to the radial side. [G. *thenar,* palm, + *en,* in]

then·yl (then'il). The radical of 2-methylthiophene, (SC_4H_3)-CH_2-. Cf. thienyl.

then·yl·di·a·mine hy·dro·chlo·ride (then-il-dī'ă-mēn). $C_{14}H_{19}N_3S \cdot HCl$; 2-[(2-Dimethylaminoethyl)-3-thenylamino]-pyridine hydrochloride; an antihistaminic.

Theobald Smith, SEE Smith.

the·o·bro·ma (thē-ō-brō'mă). SYN cacao. [G. *theos,* a god, + *brōma,* food]

t. oil, the fat obtained from the wasted seed of *Theobroma cacao* (family Sterculiaceae); it contains the glycerides of stearic, palmitic, oleic, arichidic, and linoleic acids; used as a base for suppositories and ointments and, in operative dentistry, as a lubricant and protective. SYN cacao butter, cocoa butter, cacao oil.

the·o·bro·mine (thē-ō-brō'mēn). 3,7-Dimethyl-2,6-dihydroxypurine; 3,7-di-methylxanthine; an alkaloid resembling caffeine in its action, prepared from the dried ripe seed of *Theobroma cacao* or made synthetically; formerly used widely as a diuretic, myocardial stimulant, dilator of coronary arteries, and smooth muscle relaxant. Compounds with calcium gluconate, calcium salicylate, sodium acetate, sodium lactate, and sodium salicylate have been listed.

the·o·ma·nia (thē-ō-mā'nē-ă). A delusion in which one believes that he or she is God. [G. *theos,* god, + *mania,* frenzy]

the·o·pho·bia (thē-ō-fō'bē-ă). Morbid fear of God. [G. *theos,* god, + *phobos,* fear]

the·o·phyl·line (the-of'i-lēn, -lin). 1,3-Dimethylxanthine; an alkaloid found with caffeine in tea leaves (commercial t. is prepared synthetically); a smooth muscle relaxant, diuretic, cardiac stimulant, and vasodilator; used in bronchial asthma and other forms of chronic obstructive pulmonary disease.

t. aminoisobutanol, SYN ambuphylline.

t. calcium salicylate, a mixture of calcium t. and sodium salicylate in molecular proportion; has the same actions and uses as t.

th

t. ethanolamine, t. monoethanolamine, with the same actions and uses as t.

t. ethylenediamine, SYN aminophylline.

t. isopropanolamine, has the same actions and uses as aminophylline, but a more rapid onset and a longer duration of action.

t. sodium acetate, a mixture of t. sodium and sodium acetate, with 60% of t.; has the same uses as t.

t. sodium glycinate, equilibrium mixture containing t. sodium and glycine in approximately molecular proportions, buffered with an additional mole of glycine; similar in action and uses to aminophylline but more stable in air, and less irritating to the gastric mucosa.

the·o·rem (thē′ō-rem). A proposition that can be proved, and so is established as a law or principle. SEE ALSO law, principle, rule.

Bayes t., the impacts of new data on the evidential merits of competing scientific hypotheses are compared by computing for each the product of the antecedent plausibility (the prior probability) and the likelihood of the current data given that hypothesis (the conditional probability) and rescaling them so that their total is unity (the rescaled values being posterior probabilities). SEE ALSO diagnostic *sensitivity*, diagnostic *specificity*, predictive *value*.

Bernoulli's t., SYN Bernoulli's *law*.

central limit t., the sum (or average) of n realizations of the same process, provided only that it has a finite variance, will approach the gaussian distribution as n becomes indefinitely large. This theory provides a broad warrant for the use of normal theory even for nongaussian data. In the form stated here, it constitutes the classical version; more general versions allow serious relaxation of the usual assumptions.

Gibbs' t., substances that lower the surface tension of the pure dispersion medium tend to collect in its surface, whereas substances that raise the surface tension tend to remain out of the surface film.

THEORY

the·o·ry (thē′ōr-ē). A reasoned explanation of known facts or phenomena that serves as a basis of investigation by which to reach the truth. SEE ALSO hypothesis, postulate. [G. *theōria,* a beholding, speculation, theory, fr. *theōros,* a beholder]

adsorption t. of narcosis, that a drug becomes concentrated at the surface of the cell as a result of adsorption, and thus alters permeability and metabolism.

Altmann's t., a t. that protoplasm consists of granular particles (called bioblasts) that are clustered and enclosed in indifferent matter.

Arrhenius-Madsen t., that the reaction of an antigen with its antibody is a reversible reaction, the equilibrium being determined according to the law of mass action by the concentrations of the reacting substances.

atomic t., that chemical compounds are formed by the union of atoms in certain definite proportions; in its modern form, first advanced in 1803 by John Dalton.

Baeyer's t., that carbon bonds are set at fixed angles (109° 28′) and that those carbon rings are most stable that least distort those angles; for this reason, planar rings composed of 5 or 6 carbon atoms (*e.g.,* cyclopentane, benzene) are more common than rings containing less than 5 or more than 6 carbon atoms.

balance t., in social psychology, a t. which assumes that steady and unsteady states can be specified for cognitive units, such as an individual and his or her attitudes or acts, and that such units tend to seek steady states (balance); *e.g.,* balance exists when both parts of a unit are evaluated the same, but disequilibrium arises when both parts are not evaluated the same, which causes either cognitive reevaluation of the parts or their segregation. SEE ALSO cognitive dissonance t., consistency *principle*.

beta-oxidation-condensation t., that the two carbon fragments

split from the fatty acid molecule by beta-oxidation are converted to acetic acid and then condensed to acetoacetic acid.

Bohr's t., that spectrum lines are produced 1) by the quantized emission of radiant energy when electrons drop from an orbit of a higher to one of a lower energy level, or 2) by absorption of radiation when an electron rises from a lower to a higher energy level.

Bordeau t., Bordeu t., SEE de Bordeau t.

Bowman's t., that the urine is formed by passive filtration through the glomeruli and secretion by the epithelium of the tubules, the water and salts being separated from the plasma in the former situation, the urea and other urinary constituents in the latter. Parts of this t. are now known to be wrong.

Brønsted t., that an acid is a substance, charged or uncharged, liberating hydrogen ions in solution, and that a base is a substance that removes them from solution (*e.g.,* NH_4^+, CH_3COOH, and HSO_4^- are acids; NH_3, CH_3COO^-, and SO_4^- are bases); useful in the concept of weak electrolytes and buffers. Cf. Brønsted *acid*, Brønsted *base*.

Burn and Rand t., that stimulation of sympathetic fibers results first in the production of acetylcholine in the postganglionic nerve endings, which then release norepinephrine to act on the active site of the effector cell.

Cannon-Bard t., the view that the feeling aspect of emotion and the pattern of emotional behavior are controlled by the hypothalamus.

Cannon's t., SYN emergency t.

catastrophe t., a branch of mathematics dealing with large changes in the total system that may result from a small change in a critical variable in the system; an example is the change in the physical properties of H_2O as the temperature reaches zero or 100° C; many applications of catastrophe t. occur in clinical medicine and in epidemiology.

cellular immune t., a concept, put forth by Elie Metchnikoff, that cells, not antibodies, were responsible for the immune response of an organism.

celomic metaplasia t. of endometriosis, that endometrial tissue arises directly from the peritoneal mesothelium.

chaos t., a branch of mathematics dealing with events and processes that cannot be predicted precisely on the basis of conventional mathematical t.'s or laws; some biological processes, *e.g.,* spread of malignant disease, appear to conform to chaos t., at least sometimes.

chemiosmotic t., A hypothesis proposing that cellular energy requiring processes such as ATP synthesis and ion pumping may be driven by a pH and membrane potential gradient; proposed by Peter Mitchell in 1961.

cloacal t., the belief sometimes held by neurotic adults or children that a child is born, as a stool is passed, from a common opening.

clonal deletion t., the elimination of certain T cell populations in the thymus that have receptors for self-antigens. SEE immunologic *tolerance*.

clonal selection t., a t. which states that each lymphocyte has membrane bound immunoglobulin receptors specific for a particular antigen and once the receptor is engaged, proliferation of the cell occurs such that a clone of antibody producing cells (plasma cell) is produced.

cognitive dissonance t., a t. of attitude formation and behavior describing a motivational state that exists when an individual's cognitive elements (attitudes, perceived behaviors, etc.) are inconsistent with each other, such as the espousal of the Ten Commandments concurrent with the belief that it is all right to cheat on one's taxes; a t. which indicates that persons try to achieve consistency (consonance) and avoid dissonance which, when it arises, may be coped with by changing one's attitudes, rationalizing, selective perception, and other means. SEE ALSO balance t., consistency *principle*.

Cohnheim's t., that neoplasms originate from various cell rests, *i.e.,* embryonic cells thought to persist in various sites after the development of the fetal organs and tissues. SYN emigration t.

colloid t. of narcosis, that coagulation or flocculation of protein causes dehydration and reduction of metabolism.

darwinian t., the t. of the origin of species and of the development of higher organisms from lower forms through natural selection (survival of the fittest in the struggle for existence), and of the evolution of humans from an ancestor common to himself and the apes.

de Bordeau t., that each organ of the body manufactured a specific humor which it secreted into the bloodstream.

decay t., a t. of forgetting based on the premise that an engram or memory trace dissipates progressively with time during the interval when it is not activated.

Dieulafoy's t., an obsolete t. that appendicitis is always the result of the transformation of the appendicular canal into a closed cavity.

dipole t., a t. in which the activation current of the heart is conceived as a single net moving dipole, the positive pole leading.

duplicity t. of vision, that the cones of the retina function in bright light and the rods function in dim light.

Ehrlich's t., Ehrlich's side-chain t., SEE side-chain t.

t. of electrolytic dissociation, SEE Arrhenius *doctrine*.

emergency t., a t. of the emotions, advanced by W.B. Cannon, that animal and human organisms respond to emergency situations by increased sympathetic nervous system activity including an increased catecholamine production with associated increases in blood pressure, heart and respiratory rates, and skeletal muscle blood flow. SEE ALSO relaxation *response*. SYN Cannon's t.

emigration t., SYN Cohnheim's t.

enzyme inhibition t. of narcosis, that narcotics inhibit respiratory enzymes by suppression of the formation of high energy phosphate bonds within the cell.

Flourens' t., that thought is a process depending upon the action of the entire cerebrum.

Frerichs' t., that uremia represents a toxic condition caused by ammonium carbonate, which is formed as the result of the action of a plasma enzyme on the increased amounts of urea.

Freud's t., a comprehensive t. of how personality is formed and develops in normal and emotionally disturbed individuals; *e.g.,* that an attack of conversion hysteria is due to a psychic trauma which was not adequately reacted to at the time it was received, and persists as an affect memory. SEE ALSO psychoanalysis.

game t., the branch of mathematical logic concerned with the range of possible reactions to a particular strategy; each reaction can be assigned a probability and each reaction can lead to a counter-reaction by the "adversary" in the game. Used mainly in systems analysis, game t. has some applications in disease surveillance and control; it is one of the underlying t.'s in clinical decision analysis.

gastrea t., SYN Haeckel's gastrea t.

gate-control t., a theory to explain the mechanism of pain; small fiber afferent stimuli, particularly pain, entering the substantia gelatinosa can be modulated by large fiber afferent stimuli and descending spinal pathways so that their transmission to ascending spinal pathways is blocked (gated). SYN gate-control hypothesis.

germ t., the t., now a doctrine, that infectious diseases are due to the presence and functional activity of microorganisms within the body.

germ layer t., the concept that young embryos differentiate three primary germ layers (ectoderm, mesoderm, and endoderm), each of which has the potentiality of forming different characteristic structures and organs in the developing body.

gestalt t., SEE gestaltism.

Haeckel's gastrea t., that the two-layered gastrula is the ancestral form of all multicellular animals. SYN gastrea t.

Helmholtz t. of accommodation, that the ciliary muscle relaxes for near vision and allows the anterior aspect of the lens to become more convex.

Helmholtz t. of color vision, SYN Young-Helmholtz t. of color vision.

Helmholtz-Gibbs t., SEE Gibbs-Helmholtz *equation*.

Helmholtz t. of hearing, SYN resonance t. of hearing.

hematogenous t. of endometriosis, that endometrial tissue is carried, like metastases of a malignant tumor, through the blood stream.

Hering's t. of color vision, that there are three opponent visual processes: blue-yellow, red-green, and white-black.

humoral t., SEE humoral *doctrine*.

hydrate microcrystal t. of anesthesia, a t. of narcosis pertaining to nonhydrogen-bonding agents; postulates the interaction of the molecules of the anesthetic drug with water molecules in the brain. SYN Pauling's t.

implantation t. of the production of endometriosis, that, at the time of menstruation, cells of the uterine mucosa pass through the fallopian tubes and escape into the pelvic cavity where they implant themselves on the peritoneum.

incasement t., SYN preformation t.

information t., in the behavioral sciences, a system for studying the communication process through the detailed analysis, often mathematical, of all aspects of the process including the encoding, transmission, and decoding of signals; not concerned in any direct sense with the meaning of a message.

instructive t., a t. that states that an antibody learns or acquires its specificity after contact with a particular antigen.

James-Lange t., that bodily changes, such as tachycardia or sweating, precede rather than follow the conscious perception of an emotion and by themselves evoke the emotional feeling.

kern-plasma relation t., enunciated by Hertwig (1903) that a definite relation as to size normally exists in every cell between the mass of nuclear material and that of the protoplasm. [Ger. *kern,* kernel, nucleus]

Knoop's t., that the catabolism of fatty acids occurs in stages in each of which there is a loss of two carbon atoms as a result of oxidation at the β-carbon atom, *e.g.,*

$$C_6H_5\overset{\beta}{-}CH_2\overset{\alpha}{-}CH_2-COOH \rightarrow C_6H_5-COOH.$$

Ladd-Franklin t., SYN molecular dissociation t.

lamarckian t., that acquired characteristics may be transmitted to the descendants and that experience, and not biology alone, can change and thereby influence genetic transmission.

learning t., any of several prominent theories designed to explain learning, especially those promulgated by Pavlov, Thorndike, Guthrie, Hull, Kohler, Spence, Miller, Skinner, and their modern followers. SEE ALSO conditioning.

libido t., Freud's t. that humans psychic life results mainly from instinctual or libidinal needs and the attempts to satisfy them.

Liebig's t., that the hydrocarbons that oxidize readily and burn are aliments that produce the greatest quantity of animal heat.

lipoid t. of narcosis, that narcotic efficiency parallels the coefficient of partition between oil and water, and that lipoids in the cell and on the cell membrane absorb the drug because of this affinity. SYN Meyer-Overton t. of narcosis.

lymphatic dissemination t. of endometriosis, that endometrial tissue is transmitted by the lymphatic channels.

mass action t., that large areas of brain tissue function as a whole in learned or intelligent action.

t. of medicine, the science, as distinguished from the art, or practice, of medicine.

membrane expansion t., that adsorption of anesthetics into membranes so alters membrane volume and/or configuration that membrane function is affected in such a way as to produce anesthesia.

Metchnikoff's t., the phagocytic t., that the body is protected against infection by the leukocytes and other cells that engulf and destroy the invading microorganisms.

Meyer-Overton t. of narcosis, SYN lipoid t. of narcosis.

miasma t. (mī-az′mă), an explanation of the origin of epidemics, based on the false notion that they were caused by air of bad quality, *e.g.,* emanating from rotting vegetation in marshes or swamps.

migration t., obsolete t. that sympathetic ophthalmia is caused by a migration of the pathogenic agent through the lymph channels of the optic nerve.

Miller's chemicoparasitic t., that dental caries is caused by microorganisms of the mouth fermenting dietary carbohydrates and producing acids that demineralize the teeth.

mnemic t., SYN mnemic *hypothesis.*

molecular dissociation t., a t., pertaining to color vision, that gray is the earliest of color sensations, from which are derived, by molecular change, two paired substances that, respectively, detect yellow and blue, and that the yellow gives rise to paired substances for detection of red and green. SYN Ladd-Franklin t.

monophyletic t., SYN monophyletism.

myoelastic t., a t. stating that sound of the human voice is produced by vibrations of the vocal cords resulting from folding upward due to air pressure below, and subsequent movement downward due to elastic tension of cords.

myogenic t., that cardiac movements are due mainly to stimuli originating in the heart muscle itself and that the heart does not act solely in response to nerve stimulation.

Nernst's t., that the passage of an electric current through the tissues causes a dissociation of the ions, with consequent concentration of salts in the solution bathing the cell membranes, the electric stimulus being thereby effected.

neurochronaxic t., t. stating that variations in pitch of the human voice are produced by active muscular contractions synchronized with cycles per second of pitch, no longer believed to be true.

Ollier's t., a t. of compensatory growth; after resection of the articular extremity of a bone, the articular cartilage of the other bone entering into the structure of the joint takes on an increased growth.

omega-oxidation t., that the oxidation of fatty acids commences at the CH_3 group, *i.e.,* the terminal or omega-group; beta-oxidation then proceeds at both ends of the fatty acid chain.

overproduction t., SYN Weigert's *law.*

oxygen deprivation t. of narcosis, that narcotics inhibit oxidation, which causes the cell to be narcotized.

Pauling's t., SYN hydrate microcrystal t. of anesthesia.

permeability t. of narcosis, that the permeability of the cell membrane is decreased by narcotic concentrations of aliphatic and other central nervous system depressants.

phlogiston t., SEE phlogiston.

pithecoid t., the t. of human's descent with the ape from a common ancestor. SEE ALSO darwinian t.

place t., a t. of pitch perception which states that the perception of the pitch of a sound depends upon the level or region of the basilar membrane of the cochlea which is set into vibration by the sound waves. SEE ALSO resonance t. of hearing.

Planck's t., SYN quantum t.

polyphyletic t., SYN polyphyletism.

preformation t., archaic t. that the embryo was fully formed in miniature within a gamete at the time of conception. SEE ALSO homunculus. SYN emboitement, incasement t.

quantum t., that energy can be emitted, transmitted, and absorbed only in discrete quantities (quanta), so that atoms and subatomic particles can exist only in certain energy states. SYN Planck's t.

recapitulation t., the t. formulated by E.H. Haeckel that individuals in their embryonic development pass through stages similar in general structural plan to the stages their species passed through in its evolution; more technically phrased, the t. that ontogeny is an abbreviated recapitulation of phylogeny. SYN biogenetic law, law of biogenesis, Haeckel's law, law of recapitulation.

Reed-Frost t. of epidemics, a mathematical t. to explain how epidemics originate and continue.

reed instrument t., a no longer tenable t. stating that in human voice production the larynx functions in a manner similar to a reed musical instrument.

reentry t., that extrasystoles are due to reentry of an impulse initiated by the sinus impulse, to which the extrasystole is coupled, into the ectopic focus.

resonance t. of hearing, that the basilar membrane of the cochlea acts as a resonating structure, recording low tones from its apical turns and high tones from its basal turns. SYN Helmholtz t. of hearing.

Ribbert's t., that a neoplasm may result when a reduction in

tension (exerted by adjacent tissues) leads to conditions favorable to uncontrolled growth of cell rests.

Semon-Hering t., SYN mnemic *hypothesis.*

sensorimotor t., in the developmental t. of Piaget, the postulation that during the first 18 months of life there occurs a transformation of action into thought; at first there is a gradual shift from inborn to acquired behavior, then from body-centered to object-centered activity, ultimately permitting intentional behavior and inventive thinking.

side-chain t., Ehrlich postulated that cells contained surface extensions or side chains (haptophores) that bind to the antigenic determinants of a toxin (toxophores); after a cell is stimulated, the haptophores are released into the circulation and become the antibodies. SEE ALSO receptor. SYN Ehrlich's postulate.

somatic mutation t. of cancer, that cancer is caused by a mutation or mutations in the body cells (as opposed to germ cells), especially nonlethal mutations associated with increased proliferation of the mutant cells.

Spitzer's t., an interpretation of the partitioning of the heart of mammalian embryos primarily on the basis of recapitulations of the adult structural pattern of lower forms; most frequently cited in relation to the partitioning of the truncus arteriosus to form ascending aorta and pulmonary trunk, which is achieved by the phylogenetic development of the lungs.

stringed instrument t., a no longer tenable t. stating that in human voice production the vocal cords function in a manner similar to the strings in a stringed musical instrument.

surface tension t. of narcosis, that substances which lower the surface tension of water pass more readily into the cell and cause narcosis by decreasing metabolism.

telephone t., a t. of pitch perception which states that the cochlea possesses no faculty of sound analysis, but that the frequency of the impulses transmitted over the auditory nerve fibers corresponds to the frequency of the sound vibrations, and is the sole basis for pitch discrimination; a t. no longer tenable.

thermodynamic t. of narcosis, that the interposition of narcotic molecules in nonaqueous cellular phase causes changes that interfere with facilitation of ionic exchange.

two-sympathin t., a t., now obsolete, advanced by Cannon and Rosenblueth that two different types of substances (sympathin E and I) diffuse into circulation when adrenergic nerves are stimulated, although the mediator itself is the same.

van't Hoff's t., that substances in dilute solution obey the gas laws. Cf. van't Hoff's *law.*

Warburg's t., that the development of cancer is due to irreversible damage to the respiratory mechanism of cells, leading to the selective multiplication of cells with increased glycolytic metabolism, both aerobic and anaerobic.

Wollaston's t., a t. that the semidecussation of the optic nerves at the chiasm is proved by the homonymous hemianopia seen in brain lesions.

Young-Helmholtz t. of color vision, a t. that there are three color-perceiving elements in the retina: red, green, and blue. Perception of other colors arises from the combined stimulation of these elements; deficiency or absence of any one of these elements results in inability to perceive that color and a misperception of any other color of which it forms a part. SYN Helmholtz t. of color vision.

---

the·o·ther·a·py (thē-ō-thār′ă-pē). Treatment of disease by prayer or religious exercises. [G. *theos,* god, + *therapeia,* therapy]

thèque (tek). A nest or aggregation of nevocytes in the epidermis. [Fr. a small box]

ther·a·peu·sis (thār-ă-pyū′sis). 1. SYN therapeutics. 2. SYN therapy.

ther·a·peu·tic (thār-ă-pyū′tik). Relating to therapeutics or to the treatment, remediating, or curing of a disorder or disease. [G. *therapeutikos*]

ther·a·peu·tics (thār-ă-pyū′tiks). The practical branch of medicine concerned with the treatment of disease or disorder. SYN therapeusis (1), therapia (2). [G. *therapeutikē,* medical practice]

ray t., obsolete term for radiotherapy.

suggestive t., treatment of disease or disorder by means of suggestion.

ther·a·peu·tist (thār-ă-pyū′tist).   One skilled in therapeutics.

the·ra·pia (thār-ă-pē′ă). **1.** SYN therapy. **2.** SYN therapeutics.   [L. fr. G. *therapeia,* therapy]

t. mag′na sterili′sans, Ehrlich's concept that an infectious disease, especially one of protozoal origin, can be cured by one large dose of a suitable remedy, large enough to sterilize all the tissues and to destroy the microorganism contained therein.

ther·a·pist (thār′ă-pist).   One professionally trained and/or skilled in the practice of a particular type of therapy.

THERAPY

ther·a·py (thār′ă-pē). **1.** The treatment of disease or disorder by various methods. SEE ALSO therapeutics. **2.** In psychiatry, and clinical psychology, a short term for psychotherapy. SEE ALSO psychotherapy, psychiatry, psychology, psychoanalysis. SYN therapeusis (2), therapia (1).   [G. *therapeia,* medical treatment]

alkali t., SEE alkalitherapy.

analytic t., short term for psychoanalytic t.

anticoagulant t., the use of anticoagulant drugs to reduce or prevent intravascular or intracardiac clotting.

antisense t., use of antisense DNA for the inhibition of translation of a specific gene product for therapeutic purposes.

autoserum t., t. with serum obtained from the patient's own blood.

aversion t., a form of behavior t. that pairs an unpleasant stimulus with undesirable behavior(s) so that the patient learns to avoid the latter. SEE ALSO aversive *training.*

behavior t., an offshoot of psychotherapy involving the use of procedures and techniques associated with research in the fields of conditioning and learning for the treatment of a variety of psychological conditions; distinguished from psychotherapy because specific symptoms (*e.g.,* phobia, enuresis, high blood pressure) are selected as the target for change, planned interventions or remedial steps to extinguish or modify these symptoms are then employed, and the progress of changes is continuously and quantitatively monitored. SEE systematic *desensitization.* SYN conditioning t.

client-centered t., a system of nondirective psychotherapy based on the assumption that the client (patient) both has the internal resources to improve and is in the best position to resolve his or her own personality dysfunction, provided that the therapist can establish a permissive, accepting, and genuine atmosphere in which the client feels free to discuss problems and to obtain insight into them in order to achieve self-actualization.

cognitive t., any of a variety of techniques in psychotherapy that utilizes guided self-discovery, imaging, self-instruction, symbolic modeling, and related forms of explicitly elicited cognitions as the principal mode of treatment.

collapse t., the surgical treatment of pulmonary tuberculosis whereby the diseased lung is placed, totally or partially, temporarily or permanently, in a nonfunctional respiratory state of retraction and immobilization. Now rarely performed except in drug resistant TB, such as with AIDS.

conditioning t., SYN behavior t.

conjoint t., a type of t. in which a therapist sees the two spouses, or parent and child, or other partners together in joint sessions.

convulsive t., SYN electroshock t.

cytoreductive t., t. with the intention of reducing the number of cells in a lesion, usually a malignancy.

depot t., injection of a drug together with a substance that slows the release and prolongs the action of the drug.

diathermic t., treatment of various lesions by diathermy.

electroconvulsive t. (ECT), SYN electroshock t.

electroshock t. (ECT), a form of treatment of mental disorders in which convulsions are produced by the passage of an electric current through the brain. SYN convulsive t., electroconvulsive t.

electrotherapeutic sleep t., treatment by inducing sleep by means of nonconvulsive electric stimulation of the brain.

extended family t., a type of family t. that involves family members outside the nuclear family and who are closely associated with it and affect it.

family t., a type of group psychotherapy in which a family in conflict meets as a group with the therapist and explores its relationships and processes; focus is on the resolution of current interactions between members rather than on individual members.

fever t., SEE pyrotherapy.

foreign protein t., SYN protein shock t.

functional orthodontic t., SYN functional jaw *orthopedics.*

gene t., the process of inserting a gene into an organism to replace or repair gene function to treat a disease or genetic defect.

> Alterations of somatic or germ-line DNA to correct or prevent disease. Multiple animal experiments have demonstrated the feasibility of somatic gene therapy, in which functional DNA sequences are inserted into cells which lack or bear faulty versions of a particular gene. Vectors include modified viruses (e.g., adenovirus) and liposomes. In some cases, cells are removed from the body, treated with modified DNA, cultured, and returned to the body. The first human trial of somatic therapy took place in 1990, with melanoma patients. Germ-line therapy inserts specific genes directly into the DNA of sperm, eggs, or embryos, producing heritable alterations of the genome. Experimenters have inserted human DNA into germ cells of pigs, mice, and other laboratory animals, creating chimeras, but experiments with human germ cells are under federal ban.

geriatric t., SYN gerontotherapy.

gestalt t., a type of psychotherapy, used with individuals or groups, that emphasizes treatment of the person as a whole: the individual's biological component parts and their organic functioning, perceptual configuration, and interrelationships with the external world; it focuses on the sensory awareness of the person's immediate experiences rather than on past recollections or future expectations, employing role playing and other techniques to promote the patient's growth process and to develop the individual's full potential.

heterovaccine t., t. with a vaccine obtained from organisms not directly concerned with the disorder being treated.

hormone replacement t., in females, treatment with sex hormones for a number for reasons, including menopause, partial or full hysterectomy, or amenorrhea.

> In women, treatment with sex hormones is indicated for a number of reasons, including menopause, partial or full hysterectomy, or amenorrhea. After menopause, conjugated estrogens, estradiol, or estrone sulfate are given to reduce pain during intercourse, limit blood vessel effects, and prevent loss of bone mass. After radical hysterectomy, conjugated estrogens are given for similar reasons. After menopause or partial hysterectomy, progestin is administered at the same time to offset an increased risk of endometrial cancer. In some amenorrheas, estrogen is given to restore menses; if the therapy is unsuccessful, this may indicate the presence of pathology, for instance, pituitary tumor. Benefits for postmenopausal women include a lowered risk of heart attack (estrogen lowers LDL and raises HDL levels), and prevention of osteoporosis, since the rate of bone loss is directly linked to a drop in estrogen levels (see perimenopause). Medical opinion about the hazard posed by such therapy remains divided. Some studies have indicated increased incidence of breast

th

cancer; however, a comprehensive 1992 review of the literature contradicted this finding.

---

hyperbaric oxygen t., treatment in which oxygen is provided in a sealed chamber at an ambient pressure greater than 1 atmosphere. SEE ALSO hyperbaric *oxygenation.*

implosive t., a type of behavior t. using implosion.

individual t., SYN dyadic *psychotherapy.*

inhalation t., therapeutic use of gases or aerosols by inhalation.

insulin coma t., SEE insulin coma *treatment.*

interstitial t., radiation t. by means of radioactive seeds or needles implanted directly into the tissues to be irradiated.

intralesional t., t. by injection directly into a lesion, as in corticosteroid injections into skin lesions.

maintenance drug t., in chemotherapy, systematic dosage at a level that maintains protection against exacerbation.

marital t., SYN marriage t.

marriage t., a type of family t. that involves both husband and wife and focuses on the marital relationship as it affects the individual personalities, behaviors, and psychopathologies of the partners; the rationale for this method is the assumption that emotional or psychopathological processes within the family structure and in the social matrix of the marriage perpetuate individual pathological personality structures, which find expression in the disturbed marriage and are aggravated by the feedback between partners. SYN marital t.

microwave t., SYN microkymatotherapy.

milieu t., psychiatric treatment employing manipulation of the social environment for the benefit of the patient; *e.g.,* using the day-to-day experiences of patients living in a ward as the stimuli for discussion and therapeutic change.

myofunctional t., t. of malocclusion and other dental and speech disorders utilizing muscular exercises of the tongue and lips; most often intended to alter a tongue thrust swallowing pattern.

nonspecific t., the injection of a foreign protein, typhoid vaccine, etc., to induce fever in the treatment of certain diseases, especially those of a parasyphilitic nature. SYN phlogotherapy.

occupational t. (OT), therapeutic use of self-care, work, and recreational activities to increase independent function, enhance development, and prevent disability; may include adaptation of tasks or environment to achieve maximum independence and optimum quality of life.

orthodontic t., SEE orthodontics.

orthomolecular t., treatment designed to remedy deficiencies in any of the normal chemical constituents of the body.

oxygen t., treatment in which an increased concentration of oxygen is made available for breathing, through a nasal catheter, tent, chamber, or mask.

parenteral t., t. introduced usually by a needle through some other route than the alimentary canal.

photoradiation t., SYN photoradiation.

physical t. (PT), (1) treatment of pain, disease, or injury by physical means; SYN physiotherapy. **(2)** the health profession concerned with promotion of health, with prevention of physical disabilities, with evaluation and rehabilitation of persons disabled by pain, disease, or injury, and with treatment by physical therapeutic measures as opposed to medical, surgical, or radiologic measures.

plasma t., treatment with plasma.

play t., a type of t. used with children in which they can express or reveal their problems and fantasies by playing with dolls or other toys, drawing, etc.

proliferation t., rehabilitation of an incompetent structure (ligament or tendon) by the induced proliferation of new cells; accomplished by injecting an irritating substance into the loose ligament or tendon, the resulting scar formation and contracture serving to tighten up the ligament or tendon as scar tissue proliferates.

protein shock t., the injection of a foreign protein to induce fever as a means of treating certain diseases. SYN foreign protein t.

psychedelic t., psychiatric t. utilizing psychedelic drugs.

psychoanalytic t., SYN psychoanalysis (1).

pulse t., a short, intensive course of pharmacotherapy, usually given at intervals such as weekly or monthly; often used in chemotherapy of malignancy.

quadrangular t., marriage t. involving the husband and wife and their respective therapists.

radiation t., treatment with x-rays or radionuclides. SEE radiation *oncology.*

radium beam t., SYN teleradium t.

rational t., therapeutic procedures introduced by Albert Ellis and based on the premise that lack of information or illogical thought patterns are basic causes of a patient's difficulties; it is assumed that the patient can be assisted in overcoming his or her problems by a direct, prescriptive, advice-giving approach by the therapist.

reflex t., treatment of some morbid condition by exciting a reflex action, as in the household treatment of nosebleed by a piece of ice applied to the cervical spine. SYN reflexotherapy.

replacement t., t. designed to compensate for a lack or deficiency arising from inadequate nutrition, from certain dysfunctions (*e.g.,* glandular hyposecretion), or from losses (*e.g.,* hemorrhage); replacement may be physiological or may entail administration of a substitute (*e.g.,* a synthetic estrogen in place of estradiol).

root canal t., dental t. for damaged pulp by removal of the pulp and sterilization and filling of the root canal.

rotation t., teletherapy in which a desirable radiation dose distribution is achieved by rotating the patient or machine about an axis passing through the center of the tumor.

sclerosing t., SYN sclerotherapy.

serum t., SYN serotherapy.

shock t., SEE shock *treatment.*

social t., a psychiatric rehabilitative t. to improve a patient's social functioning.

social network t., a type of t. involving the assembling of all persons emotionally or functionally important to the patient for the purpose of affecting behavioral change in the patient.

solar t., treatment of disease by exposure to sunlight.

specific t., t. aimed at the cause(s) of a disease process, as opposed to symptomatic therapy.

substitution t., replacement t., particularly when replacement is not physiological but entails administration of a substitute.

substitutive t., SYN allopathy.

teleradium t., therapeutic use of radium rays, the source of which is a quantity of radium at a distance from the patient. SYN radium beam t.

thyroid t., the treatment of hypothyroidism.

total push t., the application of all available t.'s to the treatment of a psychiatric patient in a hospital setting.

ultrasonic t., t. for musculoskeletal disease using ultrasonic waves to produce heat.

viral t., the use of genetically altered virus particles for delivering genes to specific sites for the purpose of t.

x-ray t., radiation t. using x-rays; sometimes used ironically to refer to excessive use of diagnostic radiation.

---

ther·en·ceph·a·lous (thĕr'en-sef'ă-lŭs, -ther-). Denoting a skull in which the angle at the hormion, formed by lines converging from the inion and nasion, measures from 116°to 129°. [G. *thēr,* wild beast, + *enkephalos,* brain]

the·ri·a·ca (thē-rī'ă-kă). A mixture containing a great number of ingredients, used in the Middle Ages and believed to possess antidotal and curative powers to an almost miraculous degree. [L. antidote to snake bite, fr. G. *thēriakos,* pertaining to wild beasts]

the·ri·at·rics (thĕr-ē-at'riks). The medical treatment of animals in a zoo or menagerie. [G. *thērion,* beast, + *iatrikē,* medical treatment]

△**therio-.** Animals. [G. *thēr, thērion,* beast]

the·ri·o·gen·o·log·ic, the·ri·o·gen·o·log·i·cal (thē'rē-ō-jen-ō-loj'ik, -loj'i-kăl). Pertaining to theriogenology.

the·ri·o·gen·ol·o·gy (thĕr'ē-ō-jen-ol'ōjē). The study of reproduction in animals, especially domestic animals; includes the study of obstetrics and genital diseases in male and female animals, as well as the physiology of animal reproduction. [therio- + G. *genos* birth, + *logos,* study]

the·ri·o·mor·phism (thēr′ē-ō-mōr′fizm). Ascription of animal characteristics to human beings. Cf. anthropomorphism. [therio- + *morphē,* form]

therm. A unit of heat used indiscriminately for: 1) a small calorie, 2) a large calorie, 3) 1000 large calories, 4) 100,000 British thermal units. [G. *thermē,* heat]

⌂ **therm-.** SEE thermo-.

ther·ma·co·gen·e·sis (ther′mă-kō-jen′ĕ-sis). The elevation of body temperature by drug action. [G. *thermē,* heat, + *pharmakon,* drug, + *genesis,* production]

ther·mal (ther′măl). Pertaining to heat.

ther·mal·ge·sia (ther-mal-jē′zē-ă). High sensibility to heat; pain caused by a slight degree of heat. SYN thermoalgesia. [therm- + G. *algēsis,* sense of pain]

ther·mal·gia (ther-mal′jē-ă). Burning pain. SEE ALSO causalgia. [therm- + G. *algos,* pain]

therm·an·al·ge·sia (therm′an-al-jē′zē-ă). SYN thermoanesthesia. [therm- + analgesia]

therm·an·es·the·sia (therm′an-es-thē′zē-ă). SYN thermoanesthesia.

ther·ma·tol·o·gy (ther-mă-tol′ō-jē). The branch of therapeutics concerned with the application of heat. SEE ALSO thermotherapy. [therm- + G. *logos,* study]

ther·me·lom·e·ter (ther-mĕ-lom′ĕ-ter). An electric thermometer, especially used for recording slight variations of temperature. [therm- + electric + G. *metron,* measure]

therm·es·the·sia (therm-es-thē′zē-ă). SYN thermoesthesia.

therm·es·the·si·om·e·ter (therm′es-thē-zē-om′ĕ-ter). SYN thermoesthesiometer.

therm·is·tor (ther′mis-ter, -tōr). A device for determining temperature; also may be used to monitor control of temperature. [G. *thermē,* heat]

⌂ **thermo-, therm-.** Heat. [G. *thermē,* heat; *thermos,* warm or hot]

ther·mo·ac·id·o·philes (ther′mō-as-id-ō-fīlz). Archaebacteria that grow in hot sulfur springs at low pH.

ther·mo·al·ge·sia (ther′mō-al-jē′zē-ă). SYN thermalgesia.

ther·mo·an·al·ge·sia (ther′mō-an′al-jē′zē-ă). SYN thermoanesthesia.

ther·mo·an·es·the·sia (ther′mō-an-es-thē′zē-ă). Loss of the temperature sense or of the ability to distinguish between heat and cold; insensibility to heat or to temperature changes. SYN ardanesthesia, thermalgesia, thermanesthesia, thermoanalgesia. [thermo- + G. *an-* priv. + *aisthēsis,* sensation]

ther·mo·cau·ter·ec·to·my (ther′mō-kaw-ter-ek′tō-mē). Removal of tissue by thermocautery. [thermocautery + G. *ektomē,* excision]

ther·mo·cau·tery (ther′mō-kaw′ter-ē). The use of an actual cautery, such as an electrocautery. [thermo- + G. *kautērion,* branding iron (cautery)]

ther·mo·chem·is·try (ther-mō-kem′is-trē). The interrelation of chemical action and heat.

ther·mo·chro·ic (ther-mō-krō′ik). **1.** Relating to thermochrose. **2.** Exerting a selective action on heat rays.

ther·moch·ro·ism (ther-mok′rō-izm). SYN thermochrosis.

ther·mo·chrose (ther′mō-krōz). The property possessed by heat rays of reflection, refraction, and absorption, similar to that of light rays. SYN thermochrosy. [thermo- + G. *chrōsis,* coloring]

ther·mo·chro·sis (ther-mō-krō′sis). The selective action of certain substances on radiant heat, absorbing some of the rays, reflecting or transmitting others. SYN thermochroism. [thermo- + G. *chrōsis,* coloring]

ther·moch·ro·sy (ther-mok′rŏ-sē). SYN thermochrose.

ther·mo·co·ag·u·la·tion (ther′mō-kō-ag-yū-lā′shŭn). The process of converting tissue into a gel by heat.

ther·mo·cou·ple (ther-mō-kŭp′l). A device for measuring slight

changes in temperature, consisting of two wires of different metals, one wire being kept at a certain low temperature, the other in the tissue or other material whose temperature is to be measured; a thermoelectric current is set up which is measured by a potentiometer. SYN thermojunction.

ther·mo·cur·rent (ther-mō-ker′ent). A current of thermoelectricity.

ther·mo·dif·fu·sion (ther′mō-di-fyū′zhŭn). Diffusion of fluids, either gaseous or liquid, as influenced by the temperature of the fluid.

ther·mo·di·lu·tion (ther′mō-di-lū′shŭn). Reduction in temperature in a liquid that occurs when it is introduced into a colder liquid; the volume of the latter liquid can be calculated from the amount of rise in its temperature.

ther·mo·du·ric (ther-mō-dū′rik). Resistant to the effects of exposure to high temperature; used especially with reference to microorganisms. [thermo- + L. *durus,* hard, enduring]

ther·mo·dy·nam·ics (ther′mō-dī-nam′iks). **1.** The branch of physicochemical science concerned with heat and energy and their conversions one into the other involving mechanical work. **2.** The study of the flow of heat. [thermo- + G. *dynamis,* force]

ther·mo·e·lec·tric (ther′mō-ē-lek′trik). Relating to thermoelectricity.

ther·mo·e·lec·tric·i·ty (ther′mō-ē-lek-tris′i-tē). An electrical current generated in a thermopile.

ther·mo·es·the·sia (ther′mō-es-thē′zē-ă). The ability to distinguish differences of temperature. SYN temperature sense, thermal sense, thermic sense, thermesthesia. [thermo- + G. *aisthēsis,* sensation]

ther·mo·es·the·si·om·e·ter (ther′mō-es-thē′zē-om′ĕ-ter). An instrument for testing the temperature sense, consisting of a metal disk with thermometer attached, by which the exact temperature of the disk at the time of application may be known. SYN thermesthesiometer. [thermo- + G. *aisthēsis,* sensation, + *metron,* measure]

ther·mo·ex·ci·to·ry (ther′mō-ek-sī′tŏ-rē). Stimulating the production of heat.

ther·mo·gen·e·sis (ther′mō-jen′ĕ-sis). The production of heat; specifically the physiologic process of heat production in the body. [thermo- + G. *genesis,* production]

ther·mo·ge·net·ic, ther·mo·gen·ic (ther′mō-je-net′ik, -jen′ik). **1.** Relating to thermogenesis. SYN thermogenous. **2.** SYN calorigenic (2).

ther·mo·gen·ics (ther-mō-jen′iks). The science of heat production.

ther·mo·gen·in (ther-mō-jen′in). A protein found in brown adipose tissue that acts as a thermogenic uncoupling protein of oxidative phosphorylation; it allows thermogenesis in this type of tissue.

ther·mog·e·nous (ther-moj′ĕ-nŭs). SYN thermogenetic (1).

ther·mo·gram (ther′mō-gram). **1.** A regional temperature map of the surface of a part of the body, obtained by infrared sensing device; it measures radiant heat, and thus subcutaneous blood flow, if the environment is constant. **2.** The record made by a thermograph. [thermo- + G. *gramma,* a writing]

ther·mo·graph (ther′mō-graf). An instrument or device used in producing a thermogram. [thermo- + G. *graphō,* to write]

th

ther·mog·ra·phy (ther-mog′ră-fē). The technique for making a thermogram.

infrared t., measurement of the regional skin temperature with an infrared sensing device.

liquid crystal t., measurement of the regional skin temperature by contact with a flexible plate containing liquid crystals that change color with changes in temperature.

ther·mo·hy·per·al·ge·sia (ther′mō-hī′per-al-jē′zē-ă). Excessive thermalgesia. [thermo- + G. *hyper,* over, *algēsis,* sense of pain]

ther·mo·hy·per·es·the·sia (ther′mō-hī′per-es-thē′zē-ă). Very acute thermoesthesia or temperature sense; exaggerated perception of hot and cold. [thermo- + G. *hyper,* over, + *aisthēsis,* sensation]

ther·mo·hyp·es·the·sia (ther-mō-hip′es-thē′zē-ă, -hī′pes-thē′zē-ă). Diminished perception of temperature differences. SYN thermohypoesthesia. [thermo- + G. *hypo,* under, + *aisthēsis,* sensation]

ther·mo·hy·po·es·the·sia (ther-mō-hī′pō-es-thē′zē-ă). SYN thermohypesthesia.

ther·mo·in·hib·i·to·ry (ther′mō-in-hib′i-tōr-ē). Inhibiting or arresting thermogenesis.

ther·mo·in·te·gra·tor (ther-mō-in′tĕ-grā-ter, -tōr). Any device for assessing the effective warmth or coldness of an environment as it might be experienced by a living organism, taking into account radiation and convection as well as conduction. Conceived of as a thermal model of an organism, the device usually consists of a standard object (*e.g.,* sphere, cylinder), the surface temperature of which is measured while it is being heated internally at a standard rate.

ther·mo·junc·tion (ther-mō-jŭngk′shŭn). SYN thermocouple.

ther·mo·ker·a·to·plas·ty (ther-mō-ker′ă-tō-plas-tē). A procedure in which the application of heat shrinks the collagen of the corneal stroma and flattens the cornea in the area of heat application. This tends to make the eye less myopic. SEE refractive *keratoplasty.* [thermo- + G. *keras,* horn, + *plassō,* to form]

ther·mo·la·bile (ther-mō-lā′bĭl, -bil). Subject to alteration or destruction by heat. [thermo- + L. *labilis,* perishable]

ther·mo·lamp (ther′mō-lamp). SYN heat *lamp.*

ther·mol·o·gy (ther-mol′ō-jē). The science of heat. SYN thermotics. [thermo- + G. *logos,* study]

ther·mol·y·sis (ther-mol′i-sis). 1. Loss of body heat by evaporation, radiation, etc. 2. Chemical decomposition by heat. [thermo- + G. *lysis,* dissolution]

ther·mo·lyt·ic (ther-mō-lit′ik). 1. Relating to thermolysis. 2. An agent promoting heat dissipation.

ther·mo·mas·sage (ther′mō-mă-sahzh′). Combination of heat and massage in physical therapy.

ther·mom·e·ter (ther-mom′ĕ-ter). An instrument for indicating the temperature of any substance; usually a sealed vacuum tube containing mercury, which expands with heat and contracts with cold, its level accordingly rising or falling in the tube, with the exact degree of variation of level being indicated by a scale. SEE ALSO scale. [thermo- + G. *metron,* measure]

air t., SEE gas t.

axilla t., t. used by placing it in the armpit, with arm held closely to the side. SYN axillary t.

axillary t., SYN axilla t.

clinical t., a small, self-registering t., consisting of a simple scaled glass tube containing mercury, used for taking the temperature of the body.

differential t., SYN thermoscope.

gas t., a t. filled with dry air or a gas, the expansion or increased pressure of which indicates the degree of heat; used to measure high temperatures.

resistance t., a device measuring temperature by the change of the electrical resistance of a metal wire. SYN resistance pyrometer.

self-registering t., a t. in which the maximum or minimum temperature, during the period of observation, is registered by means of a special appliance; in the clinical t. only the highest temperature is registered, usually by a steel bar above the column

of mercury or by a segment of the mercury separated from the main column by a bubble of air; after the maximum temperature is registered, the bar or segment of mercury remains in place as the column of mercury contracts.

spirit t., a t. filled with alcohol, used to measure extreme degrees of cold.

surface t., a t. in the form of a disk or strip that indicates the temperature of the portion of the skin to which it is applied.

wet and dry bulb t., SYN psychrometer.

ther·mo·met·ric (ther-mō-met′rik). Relating to thermometry or to a thermometer reading.

ther·mom·e·try (ther-mom′ĕ-trē). The measurement of temperature. [thermo- + G. *metron,* measure]

ther·mo·neu·ro·sis (ther′mō-nū-rō′sis). Elevation of the temperature of the body due to an emotional influence.

ther·mo·nu·cle·ar (ther-mō-nū′klē-er). Pertaining to nuclear reactions brought about by nuclear fusion; (*e.g.,* the fusion of hydrogen to helium at temperatures of over 100,000,000°C). (the reaction in the "hydrogen bomb").

ther·mo·pen·e·tra·tion (ther′mō-pen-ĕ-trā′shŭn). SYN medical *diathermy.*

ther·mo·phile, ther·mo·phil (ther′mō-fīl, -fil). An organism that thrives at a temperature of 50°C or higher. [thermo- + G. *phileō,* to love]

ther·mo·phil·ic (ther-mō-fil′ik). Pertaining to a thermophile.

ther·mo·pho·bia (ther-mō-fō′bē-ă). Morbid fear of heat. [thermo- + G. *phobos,* fear]

ther·mo·phore (ther′mō-fōr). 1. An arrangement for applying heat to a part; consists of a water heater, a tube conveying hot water to a coil, and another tube conducting the water back to the heater. 2. A flat bag containing certain salts that produce heat when moistened; used as a substitute for the hot-water bag. [thermo- + G. *phoros,* bearing]

ther·mo·phy·lic (ther-mō-fī′lik). Resistant to heat, denoting certain microorganisms. [thermo- + G. *phylaxis,* protection]

ther·mo·pile (ther′mō-pīl). A thermoelectric battery, consisting usually of a series of bars of antimony and bismuth joined together, that generates a thermoelectric current when the junctions are heated; used as a thermoscope. SYN thermoelectric pile. [thermo- + pile]

ther·mo·plac·en·tog·ra·phy (ther′mō-plă-sen-tog′ră-fē). Obsolete method for determination of placental position by detection of infrared rays from the large amounts of blood flowing through the placenta. [thermo- + L. *placenta,* placenta, + G. *graphō,* to write]

Ther·mo·plas·ma (ther′mō-plaz′mă). A genus of bacteria (order Mycoplasmatales) which possess the same characteristics as the organisms in the genus *Mycoplasma* except that the thermoplasmas do not require sterol for growth, have an optimal temperature of 55 to 59°C, have an optimal pH of 1.0 to 2.0, and reproduce by budding. The type species is *T. acidophilum.* [thermo- + G. *plasma,* something formed]

T. acidoph′ilum, a species found in a coal refuse pile which had undergone self-heating; it is also found in acid hot springs; it is the type species of the genus *T.*

ther·mo·plas·ma, pl. **ther·mo·plas·ma·ta** (ther′mō-plaz′mă, -plaz′mah-tă). A vernacular term used to refer to any member of the genus *Thermoplasma.*

ther·mo·plas·tic (ther-mō-plas′tik). A classification for materials that can be made soft by the application of heat and harden upon cooling.

ther·mo·ple·gia (ther-mō-plē′jē-ă). A rarely used term for sunstroke. [thermo- + G. *plēgē,* stroke]

ther·mo·re·cep·tor (ther′mō-rē-sep′ter, -tōr). A receptor that is sensitive to heat.

ther·mo·reg·u·la·tion (ther′mō-reg-yū-lā′shŭn). Temperature control, as by a thermostat.

ther·mo·reg·u·la·tor (ther-mō-reg′yū-lā-ter, -tōr). SYN thermostat.

ther·mo·scope (ther′mō-skōp). An instrument for indicating slight differences of temperature, without registering or recording them. SYN differential thermometer. [thermo- + G. *skopeō*, to view]

ther·mo·set (ther′mō-set). A classification for materials that become hardened or cured by the application of heat.

ther·mo·sta·bile, ther·mo·sta·ble (ther-mō-stā′bil, -stā′bl). Not readily subject to alteration or destruction by heat. [thermo- + L. *stabilis*, stable]

ther·mo·stat (ther′mō-stat). An apparatus for the automatic regulation of heat, as in an incubator. SYN thermoregulator. [thermo- + G. *statos*, standing]

ther·mo·ste·re·sis (ther′mō-stĕ-rē′sis). The abstraction or deprivation of heat. [thermo- + G. *sterēsis*, deprivation, loss]

ther·mo·stro·muhr (ther-mō-strom′ūr). A stromuhr that consists of a heating element between two thermocouples, which are applied to the outside of a vessel; blood flow is calculated from the difference in temperatures recorded by the proximal and distal thermocouples.

ther·mo·sys·tal·tic (ther′mō-sis-tal′tik). Relating to thermosystaltism. [thermo- + G. *systaltikos*, contractile]

ther·mo·sys·tal·tism (ther-mō-sis′tal-tizm). Contraction, as of the muscles, under the influence of heat. [see thermosystaltic]

ther·mo·tac·tic, ther·mo·tax·ic (ther-mō-tak′tik, tak′sik). Relating to thermotaxis.

ther·mo·tax·is (ther-mō-tak′sis). **1.** Reaction of living protoplasm to the stimulus of heat. Cf. thermotropism. **2.** Regulation of the temperature of the body. [thermo- + G. *taxis*, orderly arrangement]

    negative t., repulsion of a plant or animal from heat.

    positive t., attraction of a plant or animal to heat.

ther·mo·ther·a·py (ther′mō-thār′ă-pē). Treatment of disease by therapeutic application of heat. [thermo- + G. *therapeia*, treatment]

ther·mot·ic (ther-mot′ik). Relating to thermotics.

ther·mot·ics (ther-mot′iks). SYN thermology. [G. *thermotēs*, heat]

ther·mo·to·nom·e·ter (ther′mō-tō-nom′ĕ-ter). An instrument for measuring the degree of thermosystaltism, or muscular contraction under the influence of heat. [thermo- + G. *tonos*, tone, tension, + *metron*, measure]

ther·mot·ro·pism (ther-mot′rō-pizm). The motion by a part of an organism (*e.g.*, leaves or stems) toward or away from a source of heat. Cf. thermotaxis. [thermo- + G. *tropē*, a turning]

the·roid (thē′royd). Resembling an animal in instincts or propensities. [G. *thēr*, a wild beast, + *eidos*, resemblance]

the·rol·o·gy (thē-rol′ō-jē). The study of mammals. [G. *thēr*, a wild beast, + *logos*, study]

the·sau·ris·mo·sis (thē-saw-riz-mō′sis). Rarely used term for a metabolic disorder in which a substance accumulates or is stored in certain cells, usually in large amounts. [G. *thēsauros*, store, storehouse, + G. *-osis*, condition]

the·sau·ris·mot·ic (thē′saw-riz-mot′ik). Pertaining to thesaurismosis.

the·sau·ro·sis (thē-saw-rō′sis). Abnormal or excessive storage in the body of normal or foreign substances. [G. *thēsauros*, store, storehouse]

the·sis, pl. **the·ses** (thē′sis, -sēz). **1.** An essay on a medical topic prepared by the graduating student. **2.** A proposition submitted by the candidate for a doctoral degree in some universities, which must be sustained by argument against any objections offered. **3.** Any theory or hypothesis advanced as a basis for discussion. [G. a placing, a position, thesis]

the·ta (θ, Θ) (thā′ta). **1.** 8th Letter in the Greek alphabet. **2.** Symbol for angle; the eighth in a series; denotes the position of a substituent located on the eighth atom from the carboxyl or other functional group.

the·tins (thē′tinz). Methyl sulfonium compounds, abundant in marine algae, in which the *S*-methyl group is "active," and that therefore act as methyl donors in some plants; *e.g.*, dimethylpropriothetin, $(CH_3)_2S^+–CH_2–CH_2–COO^-$.

THF Abbreviation for tetrahydrofolate. SEE 5,6,7,8-

tetrahydrofolate dehydrogenase, tetrahydrofolate methyltransferase.

△**thia-.** The replacement of carbon by sulfur in a ring or chain. Cf. thio-. [G. *theion*]

thi·a·ben·da·zole (thī-ă-ben′dă-zōl). 2-(4-Thiazolyl)-benzimidazole; a broad spectrum anthelmintic especially useful against *Strongyloides stercoralis* and, with corticosteroids, against *Trichinella* infection (trichina worm).

thi·a·bu·ta·zide (thī-ă-byū′tă-zīd). SYN buthiazide.

thi·a·cet·a·zone (thī-ă-set′ă-zōn, -ă-se′tă-zōn). SYN amithiozone.

thi·al·bar·bi·tal (thī-al-bar′bi-tawl). 5-Allyl-5-(2-cyclohexen-1-yl)-2-thiobarbituric acid; an ultra-short acting thiobarbiturate for induction of general anesthesia by intravenous injection; used as the sodium salt.

thi·am·bu·to·sine (thī-am-byū′tō-sēn). 4-Butoxy-4′-(dimethylamino)thiocarbanilide; an antileprotic agent.

thi·a·min (thī′ă-min). A heat-labile and water-soluble vitamin contained in milk, yeast, synthesized; in the germ and husk of grains, also artificially synthesized; essential for growth; a deficiency of t. is associated with beriberi and Wernicke-Korsakoff's syndrome. SYN aneurine, antiberiberi factor, antiberiberi vitamin, antineuritic factor, antineuritic vitamin, thiamine, vitamin B_1. [*thia-* + vitamin]

    t. hydrochloride, a coenzyme used in the prevention of beriberi and other conditions associated with a deficiency of t. in the diet. SYN aneurine hydrochloride.

    t. mononitrate, same action as t. hydrochloride.

    t. pyridinylase, an enzyme catalyzing transfer of a pyridine or other bases into the position of the pyrimidine in t.; *e.g.,* t. reacting with pyridine produces heteropyrithiamin and 4-methyl-5-(2′-hydroxyethyl)-thiazole. SYN pyrimidine transferase, thiaminase I.

    t. pyrophosphate (TPP), the diphosphoric ester of t., a coenzyme of several (de)carboxylases, transketolases, and α-oxoacid dehydrogenases. SYN aneurine pyrophosphate, cocarboxylase, diphosphothiamin.

thi·am·i·nase (thī-am′i-nās). **1.** An enzyme present in raw fish that destroys thiamin and may produce thiamin deficiency in animals on a diet largely composed of raw fish. **2.** A hydrolase cleaving thiamin into a pyrimidine moiety (*i.e.,* 2-methyl-4-amino-5-hydroxymethylpyrimidine) and a thiazole moiety (*i.e.,* 4-methyl-5-(2′-hydroxyethyl)-thiazole); the pyrimidine moiety may appear in the urine as pyramin. SYN t. II.

    t. I, SYN *thiamin* pyridinylase.

    t. II, SYN thiaminase (2).

thi·a·mine (thī′ă-min, -mēn). SYN thiamin.

thi·am·phen·i·col (thī-am-fen′i-kol). dextrosulphenidol; D-(+)-*threo*-2,2-dichloro-*N*-[β-hydroxy-α-(hydroxymethyl)-*p*-(methylsulfonyl)phenethyl]acetamide; an antibiotic with uses and toxicity similar to those of chloramphenicol. SYN thiophenicol.

thi·am·y·lal so·di·um (thī-am′i-lawl). Sodium 5-allyl-5-(1-methylbutyl)-2-thiobarbiturate; a short-acting barbiturate, prepared as a mixture with sodium bicarbonate, used intravenously to produce anesthesia of short duration.

Thi·a·ra (thī-ah′ră). A widespread genus of operculate snails (family Thiaridae, subclass Prosobranchiata) found in fresh and brackish waters, chiefly in tropical and subtropical Africa and Asia. *T. tuberculata* is one of the initial intermediate hosts of the human lung fluke, *Paragonimus westermani*, and of several fish-borne heterophyid flukes of man and fish-eating mammals.

thi·a·zides (thī′ă-zīdz). Abbreviated form of benzothiadiazides.

thi·a·zin (thī′ă-zin). $C_{12}H_{10}SN_2$; Iminothiodiphenylimine; parent substance of a family of biological blue dyes; *e.g.,* methylene blue, thionin, toluidine blue.

thi·a·zol·sul·fone (thī-ă-zol-sŭl′fōn). 2-Amino-5-sulfanylthiazole; it has the same uses as glucosulfone sodium, but is less toxic and also less effective in the treatment of leprosy.

thick·ness (thik′nes). **1.** The measure of the depth of something, as opposed to its length or width. **2.** A layer or stratum.

    Breslow's t., maximal t. of a primary cutaneous melanoma measured in tissue sections from the top of the epidermal granular layer, or from the ulcer base (if the tumor is ulcerated), to the bottom of the tumor; metastatic rates correlate closely with tumor t.

thi·el. SYN sulfhydryl.

thi·e·mia (thī-ē'mē-ă). The presence of sulfur in the circulating blood. [G. *theion,* sulfur, + *haima,* blood]

thi·e·na·my·cin (thī'-en-mī-sin). The first member of a family of des-thia-carbapenem nucleus antibiotics having a thioethylamine side-chain on the enamine portion of the fused 5-membered ring.

thi·e·nyl (thī'en-il). The radical of thiophene, SC_4H_3-. Cf. thenyl.

thi·e·nyl·al·a·nine (thī'ĕ-nil-al'ă-nēn). 3-(3-Thienyl)alanine; a compound structurally similar to phenylalanine that inhibits the growth of *Escherichia coli,* presumably by competitive inhibition of enzymes for which L-phenylalanine is the substrate.

Thier, Carl Jörg, German physician. SEE Weyers-T. *syndrome.*

Thiers, Joseph, French physician, *1885. SEE Achard-T. *syndrome.*

Thiersch, Karl, German surgeon, 1822–1895. SEE T. *graft;* T.'s *canaliculi,* under *canaliculus, method, operation;* Ollier-T. *graft.*

thi·eth·yl·per·a·zine ma·le·ate (thī-eth'il-per'ă-zēn). 2-Ethylmercapto-10-3-(1-methyl-4-piperazinyl)propyl phenothiazine dimaleate; an antiemetic agent used to control nausea and vomiting associated with vertigo, the administration of general anesthetics, and with several other clinical conditions; it also has weak hypotensive, spasmolytic, antihistaminic, and hypothermic actions.

thigh (thī). The part of the inferior limb, between the hip and the knee.

driver's t., sciatic neuropathy due to pressure on the nerve produced by the long-continued use of the accelerator pedal in driving a vehicle.

Heilbronner's t., in cases of organic paralysis, flattening and broadening of the t., when the patient lies supine on a hard mattress; absent in hysterical paralysis.

thig·mes·the·sia (thig-mes-thē'zē-ă). Sensibility to touch. [G. *thigma,* touch, + *aisthēsis,* sensation]

thig·mo·tax·is (thig-mō-tak'sis). A form of barotaxis; denoting the reaction of plant or animal protoplasm to contact with a solid body. Cf. thigmotropism. [G. *thigma,* touch, + *taxis,* orderly arrangement]

thig·mot·ro·pism (thig-mot'rō-pizm). A movement toward or away from a touch stimulus on the part of a portion of an organism, such as leaves or tendrils. Cf. thigmotaxis. [G. *thigma,* touch, + *tropē,* a turning]

thi·mer·o·sal (thī-mer'ō-săl). [(*o*-carboxyphenyl)thio]-ethylmercury sodium salt; an antiseptic. SYN thiomersal, thiomersalate.

think·ing. The act of reasoning.

abstract t., t. in terms of concepts and general principles (*e.g.,* perceiving a table and a chair as furniture), as contrasted with concrete t.

archaic-paralogical t., SYN prelogical t.

concrete t., t. of objects or ideas as specific items rather than as an abstract representation of a more general concept, as contrasted with abstract t. (*e.g.,* perceiving a chair and a table as individual useful items and not as members of the general class, furniture).

creative t., productive t., with novel rather than routine elements and results.

magical t., the irrational equating of t. with doing.

prelogical t., a concrete type of t., characteristic of children and primitives, to which schizophrenic persons are sometimes said to regress. SYN archaic-paralogical t., prelogical mind.

think·ing through. The psychological process of understanding, with insight, one's own behavior.

thin·ning (thin'ing). Causing a decrease in viscosity by chemical means, as by the addition of a solvent, or by mechanical means, as in shear t.

shear t., decreasing the viscosity of a polymer or macromolecule or gel by increasing the rate of shear; not ordinarily a function of time. SEE ALSO thixotropy.

☍thio-. Prefix denoting the replacement of oxygen by sulfur in a compound. Cf. thia-. [G. *theion,* sugar]

thi·o·ac·id (thī-ō-as'id). An organic acid in which one or more of the oxygen atoms have been replaced by sulfur atoms; *e.g.,* thiosulfuric acid. SYN sulfacid, sulfoacid (1).

thi·o·al·co·hol (thī-ō-al'kō-hol). SYN mercaptan (1).

thi·o·am·ide (thī-ō-am'īd). An amide in which S replaces O.

thi·o·ate (thī'ō-āt). A salt or ester of a -thioic acid.

thi·o·bar·bi·tu·rates (thī'ō-bar-bich'yūr-āts). Hypnotics of the barbiturate group, *e.g.,* thiopental, in which the oxygen atom at carbon-2 is replaced by sulfur.

thi·o·car·bam·ide (thī-ō-kar'bă-mīd). SYN thiourea.

thi·o·car·lide (thī-ō-kar'līd). 4,4'-Di(isoamyloxy)-thiocarbanilide; a synthetic compound whose molecule contains the three antituberculous groups *p*-aminosalicylic acid, *p*-aminobenzaldehyde thiosemicarbazone, and the thiocarbamide group; an antitubercular agent.

thi·o·chrome (thī'ō-krōm). A fluorescent compound, $C_{12}H_{14}N_4OS$, produced by the oxidation of thiamin; used in methods for detection and determination of thiamin.

thi·oc·tic ac·id (thī-ok'tik). SYN lipoic acid.

thi·o·cy·a·nate (thī-ō-sī'ă-nāt). A salt of thiocyanic acid. SYN rhodanate, sulfocyanate.

thi·o·cy·an·ic ac·id (thī-ō-sī-an'ik). HS–CN; hydrogen thiocyanate. SYN rhodanic acid, sulfocyanic acid.

thi·o·dep·si·pep·tide (thī-ō-dep'-sē-pep-tīd). Peptides that also contain one or more acylated thiol groups (*e.g.,* of cysteine). [thio- + G. *depseō,* to knead, blend, + peptide]

thi·o·di·phen·yl·a·mine (thī'ō-dī-fen'il-am'ēn). SYN phenothiazine.

thi·o·es·ter (thī-ō-es'ter). An acylated thiol; RCOSR'; *e.g.,* acetyl-CoA. SYN acylmercaptan.

thi·o·es·ter·ase (thī-ō-es-ter-ās). An enzyme that hydrolyzes thioesters; *e.g.,* the deacylating activity at the end of fatty acid biosynthesis that releases palmitate. SYN thiolesterase.

thi·o·es·ters (thī'ō-es'-terz). In enzymology, an ester where the oxygen bridging the substrate or product carbonyl carbon and the enzyme is replaced by a sulphur (usually through a cys residue); a high energy intermediate in many enzymes.

thi·o·eth·a·nol·a·mine ace·tyl·trans·fer·ase (thī'ō-eth-ă-nol'ă-mēn). An enzyme transferring acetyl from acetyl-CoA to the sulfur atom of thioethanolamine, thus producing coenzyme A and *S*-acetylthioethanolamine. SYN thiotransacetylase B.

thi·o·e·ther (thī-ō-ē'ther). An organic sulfide; an ether in which the oxygen is replaced by sulfur; R–S–R'

thi·o·fla·vine S (thī-ō-flā'vin) [C.I. 49010]. A methylated and sulfonated derivative of primulin; a yellowish dye used in fluorescence microscopy as a vital stain.

thi·o·fla·vin T (thī-ō-flā'vin) [C.I. 49005]. A yellow thiazole dye, $C_{17}H_{19}N_2SCl$, used in histopathology as a fluorochrome for hyaline and amyloid.

thi·o·fu·ran (thī'ō-fūr'an). SYN thiophene.

thi·o·glu·co·si·dase (thī-ō-glū'kō-si-dās). An enzyme in mustard seed that converts thioglycosides into thiols plus sugars. SYN myrosinase, sinigrase, sinigrinase.

thi·o·glyc·er·ol (thī-ō-glis'er-ol). SYN monothioglycerol.

thi·o·gly·co·late, thi·o·gly·col·late (thī-ō-glī'kō-lāt). A salt or ester of thioglycolic acid; frequently used in bacterial media to reduce their oxygen content so as to create favorable conditions for the growth of anaerobes; the t. will also inactivate any mercurial that might be carried over with the inoculum.

thi·o·gly·col·ic ac·id (thī'ō-glī-kol'ik). $HSCH_2COOH$; used as a reagent for the detection of metals such as iron, molybdenum, silver, and tin; the ammonium and sodium salts are used in home permanents, the calcium salt as a depilatory. SYN mercaptoacetic acid.

thi·o·gua·nine (thī-ō-gwah'nēn). 2-Aminopurine-6-thiol; an antineoplastic agent used for leukemias and nephrosis.

☍-thioic ac·id. Suffix denoting the radical, –C(S)OH or –C(O)-SH, the sulfur analog of a carboxylic acid, *i.e.,* a thiocarboxylic acid.

thi·o·ki·nase (thī-ō-kī′nās). Group term for enzymes that form acyl-CoA compounds from the corresponding fatty acids and CoA; the bond is through the sulfur atom of the CoA.

thi·ol (thī′ol). 1. The monovalent radical –SH when attached to carbon; a hydrosulfide; a mercaptan. 2. A mixture of sulfurated and sulfonated petroleum oils purified with ammonia; used in the treatment of skin diseases.

thi·o·lase (thī′ō-lās). SYN *acetyl-CoA* acetyltransferase.

thi·ole (thī′ōl). SYN thiophene.

thi·ol·es·ter·ase. SYN thioesterase.

thi·ol·his·ti·dyl·be·ta·ine (thī′ol-his′ti-dil-bē′tă-ēn). SYN ergothioneine.

thi·ol·trans·a·cet·y·lase A (thī′ol-trans-ă-set′i-lās). SYN dihydrolipoamide acetyltransferase.

thi·ol·y·sis (thī-ol′i-sis). The cleavage of a chemical bond with the addition of coenzyme A to one part; analogous to hydrolysis and phosphorolysis.

thi·o·mer·sal (thī-ō-mer′săl). SYN thimerosal.

thi·o·mer·sa·late (thī-ō-mer′să-lāt). SYN thimerosal.

thi·o·meth·yl·a·den·o·sine (thī′ō-meth′il-ă-den′ō-sēn). SYN methylthioadenosine.

β-thi·o·nase (thī′ō-nās). SYN cystathionine β-synthase.

☐**-thione.** Suffix denoting the radical =C=S, the sulfur analog of a ketone, *i.e.,* a thiocarbonyl group.

thi·o·nein (thī′ō-nēn). The apoprotein of metallothionein.

thi·o·ne·ine (thī′ō-ne′in). SYN ergothioneine.

thi·on·ic (thī-on′ik). Relating to sulfur.

thi·o·nine (thī′ō-nin) [C.I. 52000]. amidophenthiazine; a dark green powder, giving a purple solution in water; useful as a basic stain in histology for chromatin and mucin because of its metachromatic properties. SYN Lauth's violet.

☐**thiono-.** Prefix sometimes used for thioxo-.

thi·o·pan·ic ac·id (thī-ō-pan′ik). SYN pantoyltaurine.

thi·o·pen·tal so·di·um (thī-ō-pen′tawl). Sodium 5-ethyl-5-(1-methylbutyl)-2-thiobarbiturate; an ultra-short-acting barbiturate administered intravenously or rectally for induction of anesthesia.

thi·o·phene (thī-ō-fēn). The fundamental ring compound. SYN thiofuran, thiole.

thi·o·phe·ni·col (thī-ō-fen′i-kol). SYN thiamphenicol.

thi·o·pro·pa·zate hy·dro·chlo·ride (thī-ō-prō′pă-zāt). 2-Chloro-10-{3-[4-(2-acetoxyethyl)piperazinyl]-propyl}phenothiazine dihydrochloride; a phenothiazine derivative related chemically and pharmacologically to prochlorperazine and perphenazine; an antipsychotic.

thi·o·pro·per·a·zine (thī-ō-prō-per′ă-zēn). N,N-Dimethyl-10-[3-(4-methyl-1-piperazinyl)propyl]phenothiazine-2-sulfonamide; an antiemetic and antianxiety agent.

thi·o·re·dox·in (thī-ō-rē-doks′in). A protein that participates in the oxidation-reduction reactions associated with the biosynthesis of deoxyribonucleotides.
   t. reductase, a flavoprotein that uses NADPH to re-reduce t. in the formation of deoxyribonucleotides.

thi·o·rid·a·zine hy·dro·chlo·ride (thī-ō-rid′ă-zēn). 10-[2-(1-Methyl-2-piperidylethyl)-2-(methylthio)phenothiazine monohydrochloride; an antipsychotic with action similar to that of chlorpromazine.

thi·o·sem·i·car·ba·zide (thī′ō-sem′ē-kar′bă-zīd). One of the group of thiosemicarbazones with a tuberculostatic action; used as a reagent in the detection of metals.

thi·o·sem·i·car·ba·zone (thī′ō-sem′ē-kar′bă-zōn). 1. A compound containing the thiosemicarbazide radical, =N—NH—C(S)—NH₂. 2. One of a group of tuberculostatic drugs that includes thiosemicarbazide, benzaldehyde thiosemicarbazone, and 4-aminoacetylbenzaldehyde thiosemicarbazone.

thi·o·sul·fate (thī-ō-sŭl′fāt). S₂O₃⁼; the anion of thiosulfuric acid; elevated in individuals with a molybdenum cofactor deficiency.
   t. cyanide transsulfurase, SYN t. sulfurtransferase.
   t. sulfurtransferase, a transferase that catalyzes the formation of

thiocyanate and sulfite from cyanide and t. SYN rhodanese, t. cyanide transsulfurase, t. thiotransferase.
   t. thiotransferase, SYN t. sulfurtransferase.

thi·o·sul·fur·ic ac·id (thī′ō-sŭl-fyūr′ik). H₂S₂O₃; sulfuric acid in which an atom of oxygen has been replaced by one of sulfur.

thi·o·te·pa (thī-ō-tep′ă). SYN triethylenethiophosphoramide.

thi·o·thix·ene (thī-ō-thik′sēn). N,N-Dimethyl-9-[3-(4-methyl-i-piperazinyl)propylidene]thioxanthene-2-sulfonamide; an antipsychotic.

thi·o·trans·a·cet·y·lase B (thī′ō-trans-ă-set′i-lās). SYN thioethanolamine acetyltransferase.

2-thi·o·u·ra·cil (thī-ō-yūr′ă-sil). 2-Mercapto-4-pyrimidinone; a rare component of transfer RNA's; a thioamide derivative that inhibits the synthesis of thyroid hormones; hence, a goitrogen.

4-thi·o·u·ra·cil. Uracil with S replacing O in position 4, isomeric with 2-thiouracil; a rare component of transfer RNA's.

thi·o·u·rea (thī′ō-yū-rē′ă). SC(NH₂)₂; an antithyroid compound of the thioamide group, with the same actions and uses as thiouracil. Several derivatives of t. are useful in the treatment of leprosy. SYN thiocarbamide.

thi·o·xan·thene (thī-ō-zan′thēn). A class of tricyclic compounds resembling phenothiazine, but with the central ring nitrogen replaced by a carbon atom; current use emphasizes the antipsychotic and antiemetic properties of this class.

☐**thioxo-.** Prefix indicating =S in a thioketone.

thi·ox·o·lone (thī-ok′sō-lōn). 6-Hydroxy-1,3-benzoxathiol-2-one; an antiseborrheic.

THIP. α-(4,5,6,7-tetrahydroisoxazolo[5,4-c] pyridin-3-ol; an agonist at γ-aminobutyric acid (GABA) type A receptors. Unlike other agonists of this type, upon systemic administration THIP penetrates the blood-brain barrier and is used as a pharmacological tool to explore GABA receptor function in the brain and spinal cord.

thi·phen·a·mil hy·dro·chlo·ride (thī-fen′ă-mil). Diphenylthioacetic acid S-(2-diethylaminoethyl) ester hydrochloride; an anticholinergic drug.

thirst. A desire to drink associated with uncomfortable sensations in the mouth and pharynx. [A.S. *thurst*]
   false t., t. that is not satisfied by drinking or taking water; t. associated with a dry mouth but not with a bodily need for water. SYN pseudodipsia.
   insensible t., SYN hypodipsia.
   morbid t., SYN dipsesis.
   subliminal t., SYN hypodipsia.
   true t., t. that can be satisfied by drinking water.

Thiry, Ludwig, Austrian physiologist, 1817–1897. SEE T.'s *fistula;* T.-Vella *fistula.*

thix·o·la·bile (thik-sō-lā′bil, -bīl). Susceptible to thixotropy.

thix·o·tro·pic (thik-sō-trop′ik). Pertaining to, or characterized by, thixotropy.

thix·ot·ro·py (thik-sot′rō-pē). The property of certain gels of becoming less viscous when shaken or subjected to shearing forces and returning to the original viscosity upon standing (*e.g.,* synovial fluid, ferrous hydroxide gel); a characteristic of a system exhibiting a decrease in viscosity with an increase in the rate of shear, usually a function of time. SYN reclotting phenomenon. [G. *thixis,* a touching, + *tropē,* turning]

Thoma, Richard, German histologist, 1847–1923. SEE T.'s *ampulla, fixative, laws,* under *law.*

Thomas, Hugh Owen, British surgeon, 1834–1891. SEE T. *splint.*

Thompson, Sir Henry, English surgeon, 1820–1904. SEE T.'s *test.*

Thomsen, Asmus J., Danish physician, 1815–1896. SEE T.'s *disease.*

Thomson, F.H., English physician, 1867–1938. SEE T.'s *sign.*

Thomson, Matthew Sidney, English dermatologist, *1894. SEE Rothmund-T. *syndrome.*

thon·zo·ni·um bro·mide (thon-zō′nē-ŭm). Hexadecyl[2-[(p-methoxybenzyl)-2-pyrimidinylamino]ethyl]dimethylammonium bromide; a surface-active agent used in ear drops and aerosols.

thon·zyl·a·mine hy·dro·chlo·ride (thon-zil′ă-mēn). 2-[(2-Dimethylaminoethyl)(p-methoxybenzyl)amino]pyrimidine hydrochloride; an antihistamine.

⊘**thorac-.** SEE thoraco-.

tho·ra·cal (thor′ă-kăl). SYN thoracic.

tho·ra·cal·gia (thōr-ă-kal′jē-ă). Pain in the chest. SYN thoracodynia. [thoraco- + G. algos, pain]

tho·ra·cen·te·sis (thōr′ă-sen-tē′sis). Paracentesis of the pleural cavity. SYN pleuracentesis, pleurocentesis, thoracocentesis. [thoraco- + G. kentēsis, puncture]

tho·rac·ic (thō-ras′ik). Relating to the thorax. SYN thoracal.

⊘**thoracico-.** SEE thoraco-.

tho·rac·i·co·ab·dom·i·nal (thŏ-ras′i-kō-ab-dom′i-năl). SYN thoracoabdominal.

tho·rac·i·co·a·cro·mi·al (thor-as′i-kō-ā-krō′mē-al). SYN thoracoacromial.

tho·rac·i·co·hu·mer·al (thŏ-ras′i-kō-hyū′mer-ăl). Relating to the thorax and the humerus.

⊘**thoraco-, thorac-, thoracico-.** The chest (thorax). [G. thōrax]

tho·ra·co·ab·dom·i·nal (thōr′ă-kō-ab-dom′i-năl). Relating to the thorax and the abdomen. SYN thoracicoabdominal.

tho·ra·co·a·cro·mi·al (thōr′ă-kō-ă-krō′mē-ăl). Relating to the acromion and the thorax; denoting especially the thoracoacromial artery. SYN acromiothoracic, thoracicoacromial.

tho·ra·co·ce·los·chi·sis (thōr′ă-kō-sē-los′ki-sis). A congenital fissure of the trunk embracing both the thoracic and abdominal cavities. SYN thoracogastroschisis. [thoraco- + G. koilia, belly, + schisis, fissure]

tho·ra·co·cen·te·sis (thōr′ă-kō-sen-tē′sis). SYN thoracentesis.

tho·ra·co·cyl·lo·sis (thōr′ă-kō-si-lō′sis). A deformity of the chest. [thoraco- + G. kyllōsis, a crippling]

tho·ra·co·cyr·to·sis (thōr′ă-kō-ser-tō′sis). Abnormally wide curvature of the chest wall. [thoraco- + G. kyrtōsis, a being crooked]

tho·ra·co·del·phus (thōr′ă-kō-del′fŭs). SYN thoradelphus.

tho·ra·co·dor·sal (thor-ak-ō-dōr′sal). Relating to the external posterior chest wall, denoting especially an artery, vein, and nerve.

tho·ra·co·dyn·ia (thōr′ă-kō-din′ē-ă). SYN thoracalgia. [thoraco- + G. odynē, pain]

tho·ra·co·gas·tros·chi·sis (thōr′ă-kō-gas-tros′ki-sis). SYN thoracoceloschisis. [thoraco- + G. gastēr, belly, + schisis, fissure]

tho·ra·co·graph (thōr′ă-kō-graf). An obsolete term for an instrument for determining the horizontal contour of the chest. [thoraco- + G. graphō, to record]

tho·ra·co·lap·a·rot·o·my (thōr′ă-kō-lap-ă-rot′ō-mē). Exposure of diaphragmatic region by an incision that opens both thorax and abdomen (thoraco-abdominal incision). [thoraco- + laparotomy]

tho·ra·co·lum·bar (thōr′ă-kō-lŭm′bar). 1. Relating to the thoracic and lumbar portions of the vertebral column. 2. Relating to the origins of the sympathetic division of the autonomic nervous system. SEE autonomic nervous system.

tho·ra·col·y·sis (thōr′ă-kol′i-sis). Breaking up of pleural adhesions. [thoraco- + G. lysis, dissolution]

tho·ra·com·e·lus (thōr′ă-kom′ě-lŭs). Unequal conjoined twins in which the parasite, often only a single arm or leg, is attached to the thorax of the autosite. SEE conjoined twins, under twin. [thoraco- + G. melos, limb]

tho·ra·com·e·ter (thōr′ă-kom′ě-ter). An instrument for measuring the circumference of the chest or its variations in respiration. [thoraco- + G. metron, measure]

tho·ra·co·my·o·dyn·ia (thōr′ă-kō-mī-ō-din′ē-ă). Pain in the muscles of the chest wall. [thoraco- + G. mys, muscle, + odynē, pain]

tho·ra·cop·a·gus (thōr-ă-kop′ă-gŭs). Conjoined twins with fusion in the thoracic region. SEE conjoined twins, under twin. SYN synthorax. [thoraco- + G. pagos, something fastened]

tho·ra·co·par·a·ceph·a·lus (thōr′ă-kō-par-ă-sef′ă-lŭs). Unequal conjoined twins in which a rudimentary parasitic head is attached to the thorax of the autosite. SEE conjoined twins, under twin. [thoraco- + G. para, beside, + kephalē, head]

tho·ra·cop·a·thy (thōr-ă-kop′ă-thē). Any disease of the thoracic organs or tissues. [thoraco- + G. pathos, suffering]

tho·ra·co·plas·ty (thōr′ă-kō-plas-tē). An operation that reduces intra-thoracic space. [thoraco- + G. plastos, formed]

conventional t., resection of ribs to allow inward retraction of the chest wall to reduce size of the pleural space; may be used in the treatment of empyema.

tho·ra·co·pneu·mo·plas·ty (thōr′ă-kō-nū′mō-plas-tē). Plastic surgery of the chest in which the lung is also involved. [thoraco- + G. pneumōn, lung, + plastos, formed]

tho·ra·cos·chi·sis (thōr-ă-kos′ki-sis). Congenital fissure of the chest wall. [thoraco- + G. schisis, fissure]

tho·ra·co·scope (thō-rak′ō-skōp). A scope for viewing intrathoracic structures; may be video-assisted. [thoraco- + G. skopeō, to view]

tho·ra·cos·co·py (thōr-ă-kos′kŏ-pē). Examination of the pleural cavity with an endoscope. SYN pleuroscopy. [thoraco- + G. skopeō, to view]

tho·ra·co·ste·no·sis (thōr′ă-kō-stě-nō′sis). Narrowness of the chest. [thoraco- + G. stenōsis, narrowing]

tho·ra·cos·to·my (thōr-ă-kos′tō-mē). Establishment of an opening into the chest cavity, as for the drainage of an empyema. [thoraco- + G. stoma, mouth]

tho·ra·cot·o·my (thōr-ă-kot′ō-mē). Incision into the chest wall. SYN pleurotomy. [thoraco- + G. tomē, incision]

tho·ra·del·phus (thōr-ă-del′fŭs). Duplicitas posterior in which, from the navel upward, the conjoined twins are fused into one. SEE conjoined twins, under twin. SYN thoracodelphus. [thoraco- + G. adelphos, brother]

tho·rax, gen. **tho·ra·cis,** pl. **tho·ra·ces** (thō′raks, thō′ră-sis, -rā′sēz) [NA]. The upper part of the trunk between the neck and the abdomen; it is formed by the 12 thoracic vertebrae, the 12 pairs of ribs, the sternum, and the muscles and fasciae attached to these; below it is separated from the abdomen by the diaphragm; it contains the chief organs of the circulatory and respiratory systems, as distinguished from the abdomen which encloses those of the digestive apparatus. [L. fr. G. thōrax, breastplate, the chest, fr. thōrēssō, to arm]

barrel-shaped t., increased antero-posterior dimension of the t., so that lateral and antero-posterior dimensions are about equal, due to hyperinflation of the lungs. Seen in patients with emphysema.

Peyrot's t., an obliquely oval deformity of the chest in cases of a very large pleural effusion.

tho·ri·um (Th) (thōr′ē-ŭm). A radioactive metallic element; atomic no. 90, atomic wt. 232.0381. ^{232}Th, the only naturally occurring nuclide, with a half-life of 14×10^9 years, is used in colloidal form in electron microscopy as a stain for acid mucopolysaccharides. [Thor, Norse god of thunder]

Thormählen, Johann, 19th century German physician. SEE T.'s test.

Thorn, George W., U.S. physician. *1906. SEE T. test; T.'s syndrome.

thorn (thōrn). In anatomy, a thornlike or spinous structure.

dendritic t.'s, SYN dendritic spines, under spine.

penis t.'s, SYN penis spines, under spine.

thorn ap·ple. SYN Datura stramonium.

Thornwaldt, Gustavus Ludwig. SEE Tornwaldt.

thor·ough·bred (ther′ō-bred). A breed of light horses used for racing purposes; often used erroneously for purebred.

thor·ough-pin (ther′ō-pin). Synovial distention of the sheath of the flexor perforans tendon of the horse, causing a swelling on each side of the hollow of the hock.

thought broad·cast·ing (thot brod′kas′ting). The delusion of experiencing one's thoughts, as they occur, as being broadcast from one's head to the external world where other people can hear them.

thought in·ser·tion (thot in-ser′shŭn). The delusion that one's thoughts are not really one's own but are being placed into one's mind by an external force.

thought with·draw·al (thot with-draw′ăl). The delusion that one's thoughts have been removed from one's head resulting in a diminished number of thoughts remaining.

Thr Symbol for threonine or its radical forms.

thread (thred). **1.** A fine strand of suture material. **2.** A filamentous structure. [M.E., fr. A.S. *thraed*]

Simonart's t.'s, SYN amniotic *bands,* under *band.*

terminal t., SYN terminal *filum.*

thread·worm (thred′werm). Common name for species of the genus *Strongyloides;* sometimes applied to any of the smaller parasitic nematodes.

thre·on·ic ac·id (thrē-on′ik). The acid derived by oxidation of the CHO group of threose to COOH; a product of the oxidation of ascorbic acid by hypoiodite.

thre·o·nine (T, Thr) (thrē′ō-nēn). $CH_3CH(OH)–CH(NH_3)^+COO^-$; 2-amino-3-hydroxybutyric acid; the L-isomer is one of the naturally occurring amino acids, included in the structure of most proteins, and nutritionally essential in the diet of man and other mammals.

t. deaminase, SYN t. dehydratase.

t. dehydratase, an enzyme catalyzing the anaerobic deamination of L-t. to 2-ketobutyric acid and ammonia; a central step in t. catabolism. SYN serine deaminase, t. deaminase.

thre·ose (thrē′ōs). An aldotetrose; one of the two aldoses (the other is erythrose) containing four carbon atoms.

thresh·old (thresh′ōld). **1.** The point at which a stimulus first produces a sensation. **2.** The lower limit of perception of a stimulus. **3.** The minimal stimulus that produces excitation of any structure; *e.g.,* the minimal stimulus eliciting a motor response. **4.** SYN limen. [A.S. *therxold*]

absolute t., the lowest limit of any perception whatever. Cf. differential t. SYN stimulus t.

achromatic t., SYN visual t.

auditory t., the intensity of any barely perceptible sound.

brightness difference t., the smallest difference that can be perceived as a difference in brightness. SYN light difference (2).

t. of consciousness, the lowest point at which a stimulus sensation can be perceived.

convulsant t., the smallest amount of stimulation, electric current, or drug required to induce a convulsion.

differential t., the lowest limit at which two stimuli can be differentiated. SYN threshold differential.

displacement t., the least distinguishable break in the contour of a line.

double-point t., the least degree of separation of two points applied to the body surface that permits of their being felt as two.

erythema t., the dose at which erythema of the skin is produced by irradiation with ultraviolet, gamma, or x-rays.

fibrillation t., least intensity of an electrical stimulus that will initiate fibrillation.

galvanic t., SYN rheobase.

t. of island of Reil, SYN *limen* insulae.

light differential t., the smallest difference in light intensity that can be appreciated.

minimum light t., SYN visual t.

t. of nose, SYN *limen* nasi.

pain t., the smallest intensity of a painful stimulus at which the subject perceives pain.

phenotypic t., a quantitative genetic trait with a continuous distribution termed its liability may generate two kinds of phenotype, according to whether the liability lies above or below some critical t. at about which a radical change in behavior occurs. For instance, blood uric acid level is a liability with an approximately gaussian distribution. At a critical point of chemical saturation (the t. crystallization occurs and the resulting gout or nongout is a t. trait.

relational t., the smallest degree of difference between two stimuli that permits them to be perceived as different.

renal t., concentration of plasma substance above which the substance appears in the urine.

stimulus t., SYN absolute t.

swallowing t., (1) the moment that the act of swallowing begins after the mastication of food; **(2)** the critical moment of reflex action initiated by minimum stimulation, prior to the act of deglutition.

visual t., t. of visual sensation, the minimal light intensity evoking a visual sensation. SYN achromatic t., minimum light t.

thrill. A vibration accompanying a cardiac or vascular murmur that can be palpated. SEE ALSO fremitus.

diastolic t., a t. felt over the precordium or over a blood vessel during ventricular diastole.

hydatid t., the peculiar trembling or vibratory sensation felt on palpation of a hydatid cyst. SYN Blatin's syndrome, hydatid fremitus.

presystolic t., a t. immediately preceding the ventricular contraction, that is sometimes felt on palpation over the apex of the heart.

systolic t., a t. felt over the precordium or over a blood vessel during ventricular systole.

thrix (thriks). SYN hair. [G.]

t. annula′ta, SYN ringed *hair.*

throat (thrōt). **1.** The fauces and pharynx. SYN gullet. **2.** The anterior aspect of the neck. SYN jugulum. **3.** Any narrowed entrance into a hollow part. [A.S. *throtu*]

sore t., a condition characterized by pain or discomfort on swallowing; it may be due to any of a variety of inflammations of the tonsils, pharynx, or larynx.

throb. 1. To pulsate. **2.** A beating or pulsation.

△**thromb-.** SEE thrombo-.

throm·base (throm′bās). SYN thrombin.

throm·bas·the·ni·a (throm-bas-thē′nē-ă). An abnormality of platelets characteristic of Glanzmann's t. SEE ALSO Bernard-Soulier *syndrome.* SYN thromboasthenia. [thromb- + G. *astheneia,* weakness]

Glanzmann's t. [MIM*273800], a hemorrhagic diathesis of autosomal recessive inheritance in almost all cases, characterized by normal or prolonged bleeding time, normal coagulation time, defective clot retraction, normal platelet count but morphologic or functional abnormality of platelets; several different kinds of platelet abnormalities have been described; defect in platelet membrane glycoprotein IIb-IIIa complex. SYN constitutional thrombopathy, Glanzmann's disease, hereditary hemorrhagic t.

hereditary hemorrhagic t., SYN Glanzmann's t.

throm·bec·to·my (throm-bek′tō-mē). The excision of a thrombus. [thromb- + G. *ektomē,* excision]

throm·bi (throm′bī). Plural of thrombus.

throm·bin. 1. An enzyme (proteinase), formed in shed blood, that converts fibrinogen into fibrin by hydrolyzing peptides (and amides and esters) of L-arginine; formed from prothrombin by the action of prothrombinase (factor Xa, another proteinase). **2.** A sterile protein substance prepared from prothrombin of bovine origin through interaction with thromboplastin in the presence of calcium; causes clotting of whole blood, plasma, or a fibrinogen solution; used as a topical hemostatic for capillary bleeding with or without fibrin foam in general and plastic surgical procedures. SYN factor IIa, fibrinogenase, thrombase, thrombosin.

human t., t. obtained from human plasma by precipitation with suitable salts and organic solvents; same uses as t.

throm·bin·o·gen (throm-bin′ō-jen). SYN prothrombin.

throm·bi·no·gen·e·sis (throm′bi-nō-jen′ĕ-sis). Thrombin production.

△**thrombo-, thromb-.** Blood clot; coagulation; thrombin. [G. *thrombos,* clot (thrombus)]

throm·bo·an·gi·tis (throm′bō-an-ji-ī′tis). Inflammation of the intima of a blood vessel, with thrombosis. [thrombo- + G. *angeion,* vessel, + *-itis,* inflammation]

t. oblit′erans, inflammation of the entire wall and connective tissue surrounding medium-sized arteries and veins, especially of the legs of young and middle-aged men; associated with throm-

th

botic occlusion and commonly resulting in gangrene. SYN Buerger's disease, Winiwarter-Buerger disease.

throm·bo·ar·te·ri·tis (throm′bō-ar-ter-ī′tis). Arterial inflammation with thrombus formation.

throm·bo·as·the·nia (throm′bō-as-thē′nē-ă). SYN thrombasthenia.

throm·bo·blast (throm′bō-blast). SYN megakaryocyte. [thrombo- + G. *blastos,* germ]

throm·bo·clas·tic (throm-bō-klas′tik). SYN thrombolytic.

throm·bo·cyst, throm·bo·cys·tis (throm′bō-sist, -sis′tis). A membranous sac enclosing a thrombus. [thrombo- + G. *kystis,* a bladder]

throm·bo·cy·tas·the·nia (throm′bō-sī-tas-thē′nē-ă). A term for a group of hemorrhagic disorders in which the platelets may be only slightly reduced in number, or even within the normal range, but are morphologically abnormal, or are lacking in factors that are effective in the coagulation of blood. [thrombocyte + G. *astheneia,* weakness]

throm·bo·cyte (throm′bō-sīt). SYN platelet. [thrombo- + G. *kytos,* cell]

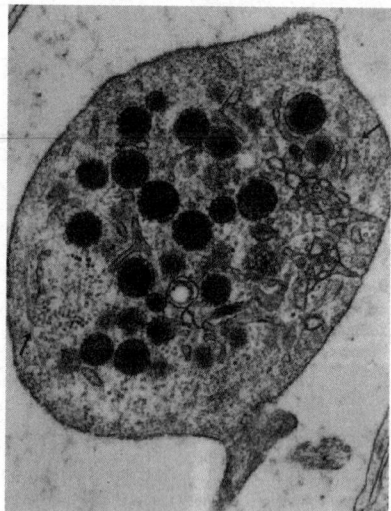

thrombocyte (or platelet)
note granulation in center (granulomere) and microtubules in the periphery (hyalomere)

throm·bo·cy·the·mia (throm′bō-sī-thē′mē-ă). SYN thrombocytosis. [thrombocyte + G. *haima,* blood]

throm·bo·cy·tin (throm-bō-sī′tin). SYN serotonin.

throm·bo·cy·top·a·thy (throm′bō-sī-top′ă-thē). General term for any disorder of the coagulating mechanism that results from dysfunction of the blood platelets. [thrombocyte + G. *pathos,* suffering]

throm·bo·cy·to·pe·nia (throm′bō-sī-tō-pē′nē-ă). A condition in which there is an abnormally small number of platelets in the circulating blood. SYN thrombopenia. [thrombocyte + G. *penia,* poverty]

autoimmune neonatal t., isoimmune neotal thrombocytopenia

canine infectious cyclic t., an infection of dogs with the rickettsia *Ehrlichia platys* characterized by recurrent cyclic t.

essential t., a primary form of t., in contrast to secondary forms that are associated with metastatic neoplasms, tuberculosis, and leukemia involving the bone marrow, or with direct suppression of bone marrow by the use of chemical agents, or with other conditions.

immune t., t. associated with antiplatelet antibodies. SEE isoimmune neonatal t., autoimmune neonatal t.

isoimmune neonatal t., immune t. resulting from maternal-fetal platelet incompatibility.

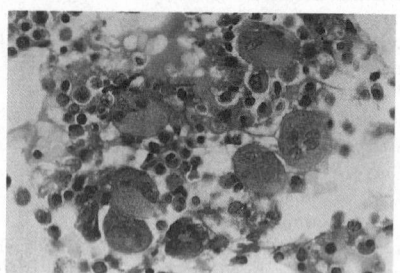

essential thrombocytopenia
a reactive increase of erythrocytes and megacaryocytes

throm·bo·cy·to·poi·e·sis (throm′bō-sī-tō-poy-ē′sis). The process of formation of thrombocytes or platelets. [thrombocyte + G. *poiēsis,* a making]

throm·bo·cy·to·sis (throm′bō-sī-tō′sis). An increase in the number of platelets in the circulating blood. SYN thrombocythemia. [thrombocyte + G. *-osis,* condition]

throm·bo·e·las·to·gram (throm′bō-ē-las′tō-gram). Registration of coagulation process by a thromboelastograph.

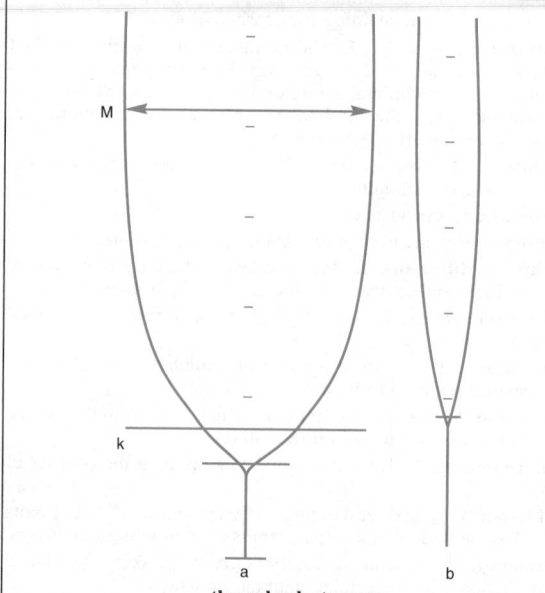

thromboelastogram
a) normal; b) in thrombocytopenia; coagulation time lengthened because of delayed formation of coagulants (k); maximal amplitude (M) is clearly reduced

throm·bo·e·las·to·graph (throm′bō-ē-las′tō-graf). Apparatus for registering elastic variations of a thrombus during the process of coagulation. [thromb- + G. *elastreō,* to push, + *graphō,* to write]

throm·bo·em·bo·lec·to·my (throm′bō-em-bō-lek′tō-mē). Extraction of an embolic thrombus. [thrombo- + G. *embolos,* embolus, + *ektomē,* excision]

throm·bo·em·bo·lism (throm′bō-em′bō-lizm). Embolism from a thrombus. [thrombo- + G. *embolismos,* embolism]

throm·bo·end·ar·ter·ec·to·my (throm′bō-end-ar-ter-ek′tō-mē). An operation that involves opening an artery, removing an occluding thrombus along with the intima and atheromatous material, and leaving a clean, fresh plane internal to the adventitia. [thrombo- + endarterectomy]

throm·bo·en·do·car·di·tis (throm′bō-en′dō-kar-dī′tis). SYN nonbacterial thrombotic *endocarditis*.

throm·bo·gen (throm′bō-jen). SYN prothrombin. [thrombo- + G. -gen, producing]

throm·bo·gene (throm′bō-jēn). SYN *factor* V.

throm·bo·gen·ic (throm-bō-jen′ik). **1.** Relating to thrombogen. **2.** Causing thrombosis or coagulation of the blood.

throm·boid (throm′boyd). Resembling a thrombus. [thrombo- + G. *eidos*, resemblance]

throm·bo·kat·i·ly·sin (throm′bō-kat-i-lī′sin). SYN *factor* VIII.

throm·bo·ki·nase (throm-bō-kī′nās). SYN thromboplastin.

throm·bol·ic (throm-bol′ik). Relating to a thrombolus.

throm·bo·lus (throm′bō-lŭs). An embolus composed of agglutinated platelets. [thrombo- + G. *embolos*, embolus]

throm·bo·lym·phan·gi·tis (throm′bō-lim-fan-jī′tis). Inflammation of a lymphatic vessel with the formation of a lymph clot.

throm·bol·y·sis (throm-bol′i-sis). Fluidifying or dissolving of a thrombus. [thrombo- + G. *lysis*, a dissolving]

throm·bo·lyt·ic (throm-bō-lit′ik). Breaking up or dissolving a thrombus. SYN thromboclastic.

throm·bo·mod·u·lin (throm′bō-mo-dū-lin). A glycoprotein present in the plasma membrane of endothelial cells that binds thrombin; participates in an additional regulatory mechanism in coagulation. [thrombo- + odulate + -in]

throm·bon. An all-inclusive term for circulating thrombocytes (blood platelets) and the cellular forms from which they arise (thromboblasts or megakaryocytes). It is analogous to erythron and leukon of the red and white blood cells, respectively.

throm·bo·ne·cro·sis (throm′bō-ne-krō′sis). Necrosis of the walls of a blood vessel, with thrombosis in the lumen.

throm·bop·a·thy (throm-bop′ă-thē). A nonspecific term applied to disorders of blood platelets resulting in defective thromboplastin, without obvious change in the appearance or number of platelets. [thrombo- + G. *pathos*, disease]

    constitutional t., SYN Glanzmann's *thrombasthenia*.

throm·bo·pe·nia (throm-bō-pē′nē-ă). SYN thrombocytopenia.

throm·bo·phil·ia (throm-bō-fil′ē-ă). A disorder of the hemopoietic system in which there is a tendency to the occurrence of thrombosis. [thrombo- + G. *philos*, fond]

throm·bo·phle·bi·tis (throm′bō-flĕ-bī′tis). Venous inflammation with thrombus formation. [thrombo- + G. *phleps*, vein, + -*itis*, inflammation]

    t. mi′grans, creeping or slowly advancing t., appearing in first one vein and then another.

    t. sal′tans, t. occurring in the same vein, but at a distance from the original lesion, or appearing suddenly in a distant vein.

throm·bo·plas·tid (throm-bō-plas′tid). **1.** SYN platelet. **2.** A nucleated spindle cell in submammalian blood. [thrombo- + G. *plastos*, formed]

throm·bo·plas·tin (throm-bō-plas′tin). A substance present in tissues, platelets, and leukocytes necessary for the coagulation of blood; in the presence of calcium ions t. is necessary for the conversion of prothrombin to thrombin, an important step in coagulation of blood. It is now generally believed that t. activity may be developed through blood (intrinsic) or tissue (extrinsic) systems. Tissue t. (factor III) interacts with factor VII and calcium to activate factor X; active factor X combines with factor V in the presence of calcium and phospholipid to produce t. activity (also commonly called t.). SYN platelet tissue factor, thrombokinase, thrombozyme, tissue factor, zymoplastic substance.

throm·bo·plas·tin·o·gen (throm′bō-plas-tin′ō-jen). SYN *factor* VIII.

throm·bo·plas·tin·o·ge·nase (throm′bō-plas-tin′ō-jĕ-nās, -ti-noj′ĕ-nās). An enzyme in blood that catalyzes the conversion of inactive thromboplastinogen to thromboplastin.

throm·bo·plas·tin·o·ge·ne·mia (throm′bō-plas-tin′ō-jĕ-nē′mē-ă). The presence of thromboplastinogen in the circulating blood. [thromboplastinogen + G. *haima*, blood]

throm·bo·poi·e·sis (throm′bō-poy-ē′sis). Precisely, the process of a clot forming in blood, but generally used with reference to the formation of blood platelets (thrombocytes). [thrombo- + G. *poiēsis*, a making]

throm·bosed (throm′bōsd). **1.** Clotted. **2.** Denoting a blood vessel that is the seat of thrombosis.

throm·bo·ses (throm-bō′sēz). Plural of thrombosis.

throm·bo·sin (throm′bō-sin). SYN thrombin.

throm·bo·sis, pl. **throm·bo·ses** (throm-bō′sis, -sēz). Formation or presence of a thrombus; clotting within a blood vessel which may cause infarction of tissues supplied by the vessel. [G. *thrombōsis*, a clotting, fr. *thrombos*, clot]

    atrophic t., t. due to feebleness of the circulation, as in marasmus. SYN marantic t., marasmic t.

    cerebral t., clotting of blood in a cerebral vessel.

    compression t., t. due to arrest of the circulation in a vessel by compression, as from a tumor.

    coronary t., coronary occlusion by thrombus formation, usually the result of atheromatous changes in the arterial wall and usually leading to myocardial infarction.

    creeping t., a gradually increasing t. involving one section of a vein after another in continuity.

    dilation t., t. due to slowed circulation consequent upon dilation of a vein.

    effort-induced t., SYN Paget-von Schrötter *syndrome*.

    marantic t., marasmic t., SYN atrophic t.

    mural t., the formation of a thrombus in contact with the endocardial lining of a cardiac chamber, or a large blood vessel, if not occlusive.

    placental t., t. of the veins of the uterus at the placental site.

    plate t., platelet t., t. due to an abnormal accumulation of platelets.

    posttraumatic arterial t., posttraumatic venous t., intravascular clotting due to injury to a vessel wall.

throm·bo·sta·sis (throm-bos′tă-sis). Local arrest of the circulation by thrombosis. [thrombo- + G. *stasis*, a standing]

throm·bo·sthe·nin (throm-bō-sthe′nin). SYN platelet *actomyosin.*

throm·bot·ic (throm-bot′ik). Relating to, caused by, or characterized by thrombosis.

throm·bo·to·nin (throm-bō-tō′nin). SYN serotonin.

throm·box·ane (throm′bok-zān). Homo-11a-oxaprostane (2*R-trans*)-3-heptyltetrahydro-2-octyl-2*H*-pyran; the formal parent of the thromboxanes; prostanoic acid in which the –COOH has been reduced to –CH₃ and an oxygen atom has been inserted between carbons 11 and 12.

throm·box·anes (throm′bok-zānz). A group of compounds, included in the eicosanoids, formally based on thromboxane, but with the terminal COOH group present; biochemically related to the prostaglandins and formed from them through a series of steps involving the formation of an endoperoxide (an O–O bridge between carbons 9 and 11 in the prostaglandins) by a cyclooxygenase, followed by a rearrangement (catalyzed by thromboxane synthase) that inserts one of the two oxygen atoms between carbons 11 and 12, leaving the other still bridging carbons 9 and 11. T. are so named from their influence on platelet aggregation and the formation of the oxygen-containing six-membered ring (pyran or oxane). Like the prostaglandins, individual t. (abbreviated TX) are designated by letters (A, B, C, etc.) and subscripts indicating structural features.

throm·bo·zyme (throm′bō-zīm). SYN thromboplastin.

throm·bus, pl. **throm·bi** (throm′bŭs, -bī). A clot in the cardiovascular systems formed during life from constituents of blood; it may be occlusive or attached to the vessel or heart wall without obstructing the lumen (mural t.). [L. fr. G. *thrombos*, a clot]

    agglutinative t., SYN hyaline t.

    agonal t., a heart clot formed during the act of dying after prolonged heart failure.

    antemortem t., a clot formed in the circulation during life.

    ball t., an antemortem t. found in the left or right atrium usually in certain cases of mitral stenosis.

    ball-valve t., ball t. intermittently occluding the mitral or tricuspid orifice.

th

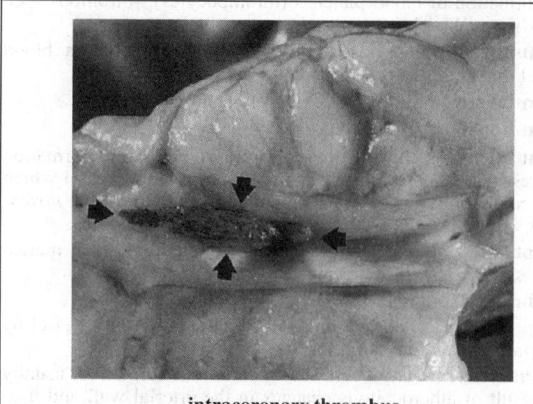
intracoronary thrombus

bile t., an intracanalicular deposit of bile, usually a result of obstruction to bile drainage.

fibrin t., a t. formed by repeated deposits of fibrin from the circulating blood; it usually does not completely occlude the vessel.

globular t., one of a number of thrombi of varying size, from a pea to a walnut, within the heart cavity, connected by a delicate fibrinous network.

hyaline t., a translucent colorless plug, partly or wholly filling a capillary or small artery or vein, formed by agglutination of red blood corpuscles. SYN agglutinative t.

infective t., a t. formed in septic phlebitis.

laminated t., a t. formed gradually by clotting of the blood in successive layers.

marantic t., marasmic t., a t. formed in cases of marasmus or general debility.

mixed t., a laminated t., the layers of different ages being of different color or consistency. SYN stratified t.

mural t., a t. formed on and attached to a diseased patch of endocardium, not on a valve or on one side of a large blood vessel. SEE ALSO parietal t.

obstructive t., a t. due to obstruction in the vessel from compression or other cause.

pale t., SYN white t.

parietal t., an arterial t. adhering to one side of the wall of the vessel. SEE ALSO mural t.

postmortem t., a clot formed within the heart or in a blood vessel after death.

propagated t., SEE creeping *thrombosis.*

red t., a t. formed rapidly by the coagulation of stagnating blood, composed mainly of red blood cells rather than platelets.

secondary t., a t. formed about an embolus as a nucleus.

stratified t., SYN mixed t.

valvular t., a parietal t. that projects into the lumen of the vessel.

white t., t. of opaque dull white color composed essentially of blood platelets. SYN pale t.

thrush (thrŭsh). **1.** Infection of the oral tissues with *Candida albicans;* often an opportunistic infection in people with AIDS or people suffering from other conditions that depress the immune system. **2.** A rare foul-smelling infective process of the horse's foot, involving the frog and sole; the affected parts degenerate and soften, and a black exudate is present; generally occurs when horses are made to stand in wet, unhygienic stalls. [fr. the thrush fungus, *Candida albicans*]

thu·ja (thū′jă, -yă). The fresh tops of *Thuja occidentalis* (family Pinaceae), an ornamental evergreen tree of eastern North America, a source of cedar leaf oil; has been used internally as an expectorant, emmenagogue, and anthelmintic, and externally as a mild counterirritant. SYN thuya. [G. *thyia,* an African tree with sweet-smelling wood]

t. oil, SYN cedar leaf oil.

thu·jol (thū′jol). SYN thujone.

thu·jone (thū′jōn). $C_{10}H_{16}O$; the chief constituent of cedar leaf oil; a stimulant similar to camphor. SYN absinthol, tanacetol, tanacetone, thujol, thuyol, thuyone.

thu·li·um (Tm) (thū′lē-ŭm). A metallic element of the lanthanide series, atomic no. 69, atomic wt. 168.93421. [L. *Thule,* the earliest name for Scandinavia]

thumb (thŭmb). The first digit on the radial side of the hand. SYN digitus primus [NA], pollex [NA], first finger. [A.S. *thuma*]

bifid t., a congenital malformed t. where the distal phalanx is divided.

gamekeeper's t., chronic radial subluxation of the metacarpophalangeal joint of the t.

hitchhiker t.'s, malposition of the t.'s which as a result of shortness of the first metacarpal stand at right angles to the radial border of the hand and in the same place as it; a characteristic sign of diastrophic dwarfism.

tennis t., tendinitis with calcification in the tendon of the long flexor of the t. (flexor pollicis longus) caused by friction and strain as in tennis playing, but also occurring in other exercises in which the t. is subject to repeated pressure or strain.

thumb·print·ing (thŭm′print-ing). A radiographic sign of intestinal ischemia associated with hematoma formation edema in the bowel wall; the thickened and edematous tissues encroach on the air- or contrast-filled lumen radiographically.

thumps (thŭmps). **1.** Spasmodic contractions of the diaphragm, or hiccups, occasionally seen in animals. **2.** In swine, a type of irregular jerky breathing seen in swine influenza, in severely anemic pigs, and in young pigs when ascarid larvae are migrating through the tissues.

thus (thŭs, thūs). SYN olibanum. [L. incense]

thu·ya (thū′yă). SYN thuja.

thu·yol, thu·yone (thū′yol, thū′yōn). SYN thujone.

Thy Abbreviation for thymine.

Thygeson, Phillips, U.S. ophthalmologist, *1903. SEE T.'s *disease.*

thy·la·ci·tis (thī-lă-sī′tis). Inflammation of the sebaceous glands of the skin. [G. *thylax,* bag, + *-itis,* inflammation]

△**thym-.** SEE thymo-.

thyme (tīm). The dried leaves and flowering tops of *Thymus vulgaris* (family Labiatae), used as a condiment; it contains a volatile oil (t. oil) and is a source of thymol. [G. *thymon,* thyme]

t. oil, oil of t., a volatile oil distilled from the flowering plants of *Thymus vulgaris* or *T. zygis;* a flavoring agent.

thy·mec·to·my (thī-mek′tō-mē). Removal of the thymus gland. [thymus + G. *ektomē,* excision]

thy·mel·co·sis (thī-mel-kō′sis). Obsolete term for suppuration of the thymus gland. [thymus + G. *helkōsis,* ulceration]

△**thymi-.** SEE thymo-.

△**-thymia.** Mind, soul, emotions. SEE ALSO thymo- (2). [G. *thymos,* the mind or heart as the seat of strong feelings or passion]

thy·mic (thī′mik). Relating to the thymus gland.

thy·mic ac·id. SYN thymol. [see thyme]

thy·mi·co·lym·phat·ic (thī′mi-kō-lim-fat′ik). Relating to the thymus and the lymphatic system.

thy·mi·dine (dThd) (thī′mi-dēn). 1-(2-deoxyribosyl)thymine; one of the four major nucleosides in DNA (the others being deoxyadenosine, deoxycytidine, and deoxyguanosine). SYN deoxythymidine, thymine deoxyribonucleoside.

t. phosphorylase, phosphorylase that catalyzes the phosphorolysis of t.; *i.e.,* thymidine and P_i react to form thymine and 2-deoxy-D-ribose 1-phosphate.

tritiated t., t. containing the hydrogen radionuclide, tritium (H); used as a marker to measure and localize by radioautography the synthesis of DNA, into which it is incorporated.

thy·mi·dine 5′-di·phos·phate (dTDP). Thymidine esterified at its 5′ position with diphosphoric acid.

thy·mi·dine 5′-mono·phos·phate (dTMP). SYN thymidylic acid.

thy·mi·dine 5′-tri·phos·phate (dTTP). Thymidine esterified at its 5′ position with triphosphoric acid; the immediate precursor of thymidylic acid in DNA.

thy·mi·dyl·ate syn·thase (thī-mi-dil′āt). An enzyme catalyzing conversion of deoxyuridine 5′-monophosphate to thymidine 5′-monophosphate, the methyl group coming from N^5,N^{10}- methylenetetrahydrofolate.

thy·mi·dyl·ic ac·id (thī′mi-dil′ik). A major constituent of DNA. SYN thymidine 5′-monophosphate, thymine nucleotide.

thy·min (thī′min). SEE thymopoietin.

thy·mine (Thy) (thī′mēn, -min). 5-Methyluracil; a constituent of thymidylic acid and DNA; elevated in hyperuracil-thyminuria.
 t. deoxyribonucleoside, SYN thymidine.
 t. deoxyribonucleotide, SYN deoxythymidylic acid.
 t. nucleotide, SYN thymidylic acid.

thy·mi·nu·ria (thī-mēn-ūr′ē-ă). SEE hyperuracil thyminuria.

thy·mi·tis (thī-mī′tis). Inflammation of the thymus gland.

△**thymo-, thym-, thymi-.** **1.** The thymus. [G. *thymos*] **2.** Mind, soul, emotions. [G. *thymos*, the mind or heart as the seat of strong feelings or passions] **3.** Wart, warty. [G. *thymos, thymion*]

thy·mo·cyte (thī′mō-sīt). A cell that develops in the thymus, seemingly from a stem cell of bone marrow and of fetal liver, and is the precursor of the thymus-derived lymphocyte (T lymphocyte) that effects cell-mediated (delayed type) sensitivity. [thymus + G. *kytos*, cell]

thy·mo·gen·ic (thī-mō-jen′ik). Of affective origin. [G. *thymos*, mind, + *genesis*, origin]

thy·mo·ki·net·ic (thī′mō-ki-net′ik). Activating the thymus gland. [thymus + G. *kinēsis*, movement]

thy·mol (thī′mol). $C_{10}H_{14}O$; 1-methyl-3-hydroxy-4-isopropylbenzene; a phenol present in the volatile oil of *Thymus vulgaris* (thyme), *Monarda punctata* (horsemint), and other volatile oils; used externally and internally as an antiseptic, as a deodorizer of offensive discharges, and as a specific for ancylostomiasis. SYN thyme camphor, thymic acid.
 t. blue [C.I. 52025], a dye used as an acid-base indicator, with a pK value at 1.7 and another at 8.9; red at pH values below 1.2, yellow between 2.8 and 8.0, and blue above 9.6.
 t. iodide, $C_{20}H_{24}I_2O_2$; has been used as a substitute for iodoform in skin diseases, wounds, ulcers, purulent rhinitis, otitis, etc.

thy·mo·ma (thī-mō′mă). A neoplasm in the anterior mediastinum, originating from thymic tissue, usually benign, and frequently encapsulated; occasionally invasive, but metastases are extremely rare; histologically consists of any type of thymic epithelial cell as well as lymphocytes that are usually abundant. Malignant lymphoma that involves the thymus, *e.g.*, Hodgkin's disease, should not be regarded as t. [thymus + G. *-oma*, tumor]

thy·mo·nu·cle·ase (thī-mō-nū′klē-ās). SYN *deoxyribonuclease* I.

thy·mo·poi·et·in (thī′mō-poy-ē′tin). Formerly called thymin; a polypeptide hormone that induces differentiation of lymphocytes to thymocytes. SEE ALSO thymic lymphopoietic *factor*.

thy·mo·pri·val, thy·mo·priv·ic, thy·mo·pri·vous (thī-mō-prī′văl, -priv′ik, -prī′vŭs). Relating to or marked by premature atrophy or removal of the thymus. [thymus + L. *privus*, deprived of]

thy·mo·sin (thī′mō-sin). A polypeptide hormone that restores T cell fucntion in a thymectomized animal. SEE ALSO thymic lymphopoietic *factor*.

thy·mox·a·mine (thī-mok′să-mēn). SYN moxisylyte.

thy·mus, pl. **thy·mi, thy·mus·es** (thī′mŭs, thī′mī). **1** [NA]. A primary lymphoid organ, located in the superior mediastinum and lower part of the neck, that is necessary in early life for the normal development of immunological function. It reaches its greatest relative weight shortly after birth and its greatest absolute weight at puberty; it then begins to involute, and much of the lymphoid tissue is replaced by fat. The t. consists of two irregularly shaped parts united by a connective tissue capsule. Each part is partially subdivided by connective tissue septa into lobules, 0.5 to 2 mm in diameter, which consist of an inner medullary portion, continuous with the medullae of adjacent lobules, and an outer cortical portion. It is supplied by the inferior thyroid and internal thoracic arteries, and its nerves are derived from the vagus and sympathetic nerves. **2.** The t. of the calf or lamb. SYN thymus gland. [G. *thymos*, excrescence, sweetbread]

△**thyr-.** SEE thyro-.

△**thyreo-.** Obsolete spelling for thyro-.

△**thyro-, thyr-.** The thyroid gland. [see thyroid]

thy·ro·a·ce·tic ac·id (thī′rō-ă-sē′tik). A degradation product of thyronine (alanine side chain reduced to acetic acid), itself a degradation product (or precursor) of thyroxine.

thy·ro·ad·e·ni·tis (thī′rō-ad-ĕ-nī′tis). SYN thyroiditis. [thyro- + G. *adēn*, gland, + *-itis*, inflammation]

thy·ro·a·pla·sia (thī′rō-ă-plā′zē-ă). Anomalies observed in individuals with congenital defects of the thyroid gland and deficiency of its secretion. [thyro- + G. *a-* priv. + *plasis*, a molding]

thy·ro·ar·y·te·noid (thī′rō-ar′i-tē′noyd). Relating to the thyroid and arytenoid cartilages. SEE thyroarytenoid *muscle*.

thy·ro·cal·ci·to·nin (thī′rō-kal-si-tō′nin). SYN calcitonin.

thy·ro·car·di·ac (thī-rō-kar′dē-ak). Affecting the heart as a result of hypo- or hyperthyroidism.

thy·ro·cele (thī′rō-sēl). A tumor of the thyroid gland, such as a goiter. [thyro- + G. *kēlē*, tumor]

thy·ro·cer·vi·cal (thī′rō-ser′vi-kăl). Relating to the thyroid gland and the neck, denoting an arterial trunk.

thy·ro·col·loid (thī-rō-kol′oyd). A colloid substance in the thyroid gland.

thy·ro·ep·i·glot·tic (thī′rō-ep-i-glot′ik). Relating to the thyroid cartilage and the epiglottis.

thy·ro·fis·sure (thī′rō-fish′er). SYN laryngofissure.

thy·ro·gen·ic, thy·rog·e·nous (thī-rō-jen′ik, -roj′ĕ-nŭs). Of thyroid gland origin. [thyroid + G. *-gen*, producing]

thy·ro·glob·u·lin (thī-rō-glob′yū-lin). **1.** A thyroid hormone-containing protein, usually stored in the colloid within the thyroid follicles; biosynthesis of thyroid hormone entails iodination of the L-tyrosyl moieties of this protein and the combination of two iodotyrosines to form thyroxine, the fully iodinated thyronine; secretion of thyroid hormone requires proteolytic degradation of t., with the attendant release of free hormone; a defect in t. will lead to hypothyroidism. SYN iodoglobulin, thyroprotein (1). **2.** A substance obtained by the fractionation of thyroid glands from the hog, *Sus scrofa*, containing not less than 0.7% of total iodine; used as a thyroid hormone in the treatment of hypothyroidism.

thy·ro·glos·sal (thī-rō-glos′ăl). Relating to the thyroid gland and the tongue, denoting especially an embryological duct. SYN thyrolingual.

thy·ro·hy·al (thī-rō-hī′ăl). The greater cornu of the hyoid bone.

thy·ro·hy·oid (thī-rō-hī′oyd). Relating to the thyroid cartilage and the hyoid bone. SEE thyrohyoid *muscle*.

thy·roid (thī′royd). **1.** Resembling a shield; denoting a gland (thyroid gland) and a cartilage of the larynx (thyroid cartilage) having such a shape. **2.** The cleaned, dried, and powdered t. gland obtained from one of the domesticated animals used for food and containing 0.17 to 0.23% of iodine; used in the treatment of hypothyroidism, cretinism and myxedema, in certain cases of obesity, and in skin disorders. [G. *thyreoeidēs*, fr. *thyreos*, an oblong shield, + *eidos*, form]
 accessory t., SYN accessory thyroid *gland*.

thy·roi·dea (thī-roy′dē-ă). SYN thyroid *gland*.
 t. accesso′ria, t. i′ma, SYN accessory thyroid *gland*.

thy·roid·ec·to·my (thī-roy-dek′tō-mē). Removal of the thyroid gland. [thyroid + G. *ektomē*, excision]
 "chemical" t., jargon for the reduction of thyroid function produced by the administration of antithyroid drugs. SEE ALSO radiothyroidectomy.
 near-total t., removal of nearly all of each thyroid lobe leaving unresected only a small portion of gland adjacent to the entrance of the recurrent laryngeal nerve into the larynx.
 subtotal t., removal of most but not all of each lobe of the thyroid.

thy·roid·ism (thī′roy-dizm). Obsolete designation for: **1.** SYN hyperthyroidism. **2.** Poisoning by overdoses of a thyroid extract.

th

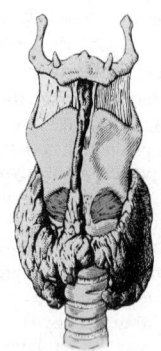

thyroid adenoma
thyroid gland with pyramidal lobe extending to the hyoid bone

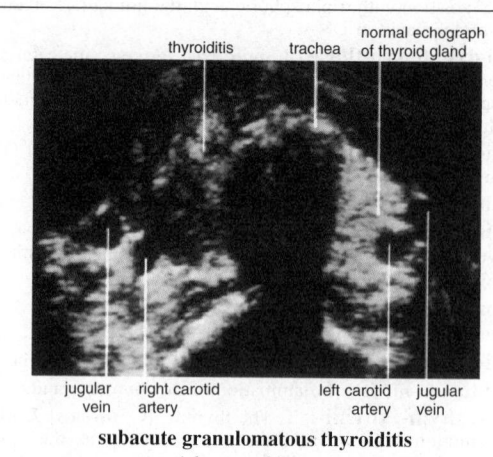

subacute granulomatous thyroiditis
(ultrasound image)

thy·roid·i·tis (thī-roy-dī'tis). Inflammation of the thyroid gland. SYN thyroadenitis. [thyroid + G. -*itis,* inflammation]

autoimmune t., SYN Hashimoto's t.

chronic atrophic t., replacement of the thyroid gland by fibrous tissue, the commonest cause of myxedema in older persons.

chronic fibrous t., SYN Riedel's t.

chronic lymphadenoid t., SYN Hashimoto's t.

chronic lymphocytic t., SYN Hashimoto's t.

de Quervain's t., SYN subacute granulomatous t.

focal lymphocytic t., focal infiltration of the thyroid by lymphocytes and plasma cells. SEE ALSO Hashimoto's t.

giant cell t., SYN subacute granulomatous t.

giant follicular t., a variant of Hashimoto's t. in which lymphocytic infiltrate in thyroid has formed into giant follicles.

Hashimoto's t., diffuse infiltration of the thyroid gland with lymphocytes, resulting in diffuse goiter, progressive destruction of the parenchyma and hypothyroidism. SYN autoimmune t., chronic lymphadenoid t., chronic lymphocytic t., Hashimoto's disease, Hashimoto's struma, lymphadenoid goiter, lymphocytic t., struma lymphomatosa.

ligneous t., SYN Riedel's t.

lymphocytic t., SYN Hashimoto's t.

parasitic t., chronic South American trypanosomiasis with involvement of the thyroid gland, causing myxedema.

Riedel's t., a rare fibrous induration of the thyroid gland, with adhesion to adjacent structures, which may cause tracheal compression. SYN chronic fibrous t., ligneous struma, ligneous t., Riedel's disease, Riedel's struma.

subacute granulomatous t., t. with round cell (usually lymphocytes) infiltration, destruction of thyroid cells, epithelial giant cell proliferation, and evidence of regeneration; thought by some to be a reflection of a systemic infection and not an example of true chronic t. SYN de Quervain's t., giant cell t.

subacute lymphocyte t., a subacute variant of Hashimoto's t.

thy·roi·dol·o·gy (thī-roy-dol'ō-jē). The study of the thyroid gland, both normal and pathological. [thyroid + G. *logos,* study]

thy·roid·o·to·my (thī'roy-dot'ō-mē). SYN laryngofissure. [thyroid + G. *tomē,* incision]

thy·ro·in·tox·i·ca·tion. SYN hyperthyroidism.

thy·ro·la·ryn·ge·al (thī'rō-lă-rin'jē-ăl). Relating to the thyroid gland or cartilage and the larynx.

thy·ro·lib·er·in (thī-rō-lib'er-in). A tripeptide hormone from the hypothalamus, which stimulates the anterior lobe of the hypophysis to release thyrotropin; L-pyroglutamyl-L-histidyl-L-prolinamide. SYN thyroid-stimulating hormone-releasing factor, thyrotropin-releasing hormone. [thyrotropin + L. *libero,* to free, + -in]

thy·ro·lin·gual (thī'rō-ling'gwăl). SYN thyroglossal. [thyro- + L. *lingua,* tongue]

thy·ro·lyt·ic (thī-rō-lit'ik). Causing destruction of thyroid gland cells. [thyro- + G. *lytikos,* dissolving]

thy·ro·meg·a·ly (thī-rō-meg'ă-lē). Enlargement of the thyroid gland. [thyro- + G. *megas,* large]

thy·ro·nine (thī'rō-nēn, -nin). $HOC_6H_4-O-C_6H_4-CH_2-CHNH_2-COOH$; an amino acid with a diphenyl ether group in the side chain; occurs in proteins only in the form of iodinated derivatives (iodothyronines), such as thyroxine.

thy·ro·pal·a·tine (thī-rō-pal'ă-tīn). Denoting the palatopharyngeus muscle.

thy·ro·par·a·thy·roid·ec·to·my (thī'rō-par-ă-thī'roy-dek'tō-mē). Excision of thyroid and parathyroid glands.

thy·rop·a·thy (thī-rop'ă-thē). A disorder of the thyroid gland. [thyro- + G. *pathos,* suffering]

thy·ro·per·ox·i·dase (thī-rō-per-oks'i-dās). A protein that participates in iodine metabolism in the thyroid follicle or in the follicular space; it utilized H_2O_2 to produce I^+.

thy·ro·pha·ryn·ge·al (thī-rō-fă-rin'jē-ăl). Denoting the thyropharyngeal portion of the inferior pharyngeal constrictor muscle.

thy·ro·plas·ty. A surgical method of restoring vocal quality by altering the geometry of the thyroid cartilage. [thyro- + G. *plastos,* formed]

thy·ro·pri·val (thī-rō-prī'văl). Relating to thyroprivia, denoting hypothyroidism produced by disease or thyroidectomy. SYN thyroprivic, thyroprivous. [thyro- + L. *privus,* deprived of]

thy·ro·priv·ia (thī-rō-priv'ē-ă). A state characterized by reduced activity of the thyroid.

thy·ro·priv·ic, thy·ro·pri·vous (thī-rō-priv'ik, -priv'ŭs). SYN thyroprival.

thy·ro·pro·tein (thī-rō-prō'tēn). **1.** SYN thyroglobulin (1). **2.** An iodinated protein, usually casein, that has thyroxine activity.

thy·rop·to·sis (thī-rop-tō'sis). Downward dislocation of the thyroid gland. [thyro- + G. *ptōsis,* a falling]

thy·rot·o·my (thī'rot'ō-mē). **1.** Any cutting operation on the thyroid gland. **2.** SYN laryngofissure. [thyro- + G. *tomē,* a cutting]

thy·ro·tox·ic (thī-rō-tok'sik). Denoting thyrotoxicosis.

thy·ro·tox·i·co·sis (thī'rō-tok-si-kō'sis). The state produced by excessive quantities of endogenous or exogenous thyroid hormone. [thyro- + G. *toxikon,* poison, + -*osis,* condition]

apathetic t., chronic t., presenting as cardiac disease or as a wasting syndrome, with weakness of proximal muscles and depression but with few of the more typical clinical manifestations of t.

t. medicamento'sa, a hyperthyroid state resulting from excessive doses of thyroid hormone preparation.

thy·ro·tox·in (thī-rō-tok'sin). **1.** A hypothetical substance formerly believed to be an abnormal product of diffusely hyperplastic thyroid glands in persons with Graves' disease, and presumed to be the cause of the distinctive signs and symptoms of that condition (in contrast to simple hyperthyroidism). **2.** A complement-fixing antigenic factor associated with certain diseases of the thyroid gland. SEE ALSO thyrotoxic complement-fixation *factor*. **3.** Rarely used term referring to any material toxic to thyroidal tissue.

thy·ro·troph (thī′rō-trof). A cell in the anterior lobe of the pituitary that produces thyrotropin.

thy·ro·tro·phic (thī-rō-trof′ik). SYN thyrotropic. [thyro- + G. *trophē*, nourishment]

thy·rot·ro·phin (thī-rot′rō-fin, thī-rō-trō′fin). SYN thyrotropin.

thy·ro·tro·pic (thī-rō-trop′ik). Stimulating or nurturing the thyroid gland. SYN thyrotrophic. [thyro- + G. *tropē*, a turning]

thy·rot·ro·pin (thī-rot′rō-pin, thī-rō-trō′pin). A glycoprotein hormone produced by the anterior lobe of the hypophysis which stimulates the growth and function of the thyroid gland; it also is used as a diagnostic test to differentiate primary and secondary hypothyroidism. SYN thyroid-stimulating hormone, thyrotrophin, thyrotropic hormone. [for thyrotrophin, fr. thyro- + G. *throphē*, nourishment; corrupted to -tropin, and reanalyzed as fr. G. tropē, a turning]

thy·rox·ine (T₄), thy·rox·in (thī-rok′sēn, -sin). 3,3′,5,5′-Tetraiodothyronine β-[(3,5-diiodo-4-hydroxyphenoxy)-3,5-diiodophenyl]alanine; the L-isomer is the active iodine compound existing normally in the thyroid gland and extracted therefrom in crystalline form for therapeutic use; also prepared synthetically; used for the relief of hypothyroidism, cretinism, and myxedema.

labeled t., SYN radioactive t.

radioactive t., t. in which a radioisotope of iodine (^{125}I or ^{131}I) is incorporated into its molecule; used in experiments tracing the metabolism of t. SYN labeled t., radiolabeled t., radiothyroxin.

radiolabeled t., SYN radioactive t.

t. sodium, a preparation obtained by the action of a limited amount of sodium carbonate upon t.; it contains between 61 and 65% of iodine. SEE *sodium* levothyroxine, *sodium* liothyronine.

Thys·a·no·so·ma ac·ti·noi·des (this-ă-nō-sō′mă ak-ti-noyd′ēz). Fringed tapeworm of sheep, a relatively short, thick tapeworm (family Anocephalidae) in which the posterior borders of the proglottids are fringed. It inhabits the small intestine, but often invades the bile ducts and causes many livers to be condemned for human food. It is essentially nonpathogenic and is common in stock-raising countries, where it infects a wide variety of ruminants; oribatid mites are probably the vectors.

TI. The delay time between the inverting pulse and the "read" pulse in the inversion recovery experiment, in magnetic resonance imaging.

Ti Symbol for titanium.

TIA Abbreviation for transient ischemic *attack*.

tib·ia, gen. and pl. **tib·i·ae** (tib′ē-ă, tib′ē-ē) [NA]. The medial and larger of the two bones of the leg, articulating with the femur, fibula, and talus. SYN shank bone (2), shin bone. [L. the large shinbone]

saber t., deformity of the t. occurring in tertiary syphilis or yaws, the bone having a marked forward convexity as a result of the formation of gummas and periostitis.

t. val′ga, SYN *genu* valgum.

t. va′ra, SYN *genu* varum.

tib·i·ad (tib′ē-ad). In a direction toward the tibia. [tibia + L. *ad,* to]

tib·i·al (tib′ē-ăl). Relating to the tibia or to any structure named from it; also denoting the medial or tibial aspect of the lower limb. SYN tibialis [NA]. [L. *tibialis*]

tib·i·a·le pos·ti·cum (tib-ē-ā′lē pos-tī′kŭm). SYN *os* tibiale posterius.

tib·i·al·gia (tib′ē-al′jē-ă). Pain in the shin. [tibia + G. *algos,* pain]

tib·i·a·lis (tib-ē-ā′lis) [NA]. SYN tibial. [L.]

⌂**tibio-.** The tibia. [L. *tibia,* the large shinbone]

tib·i·o·cal·ca·ne·an (tib′ē-ō-kal-kā′nē-an). Relating to the tibia and the calcaneus.

tib·i·o·fas·ci·a·lis (tib-ē-ō-fas-ē-ā′lis). See entries under musculus tibiofascialis.

tib·i·o·fem·o·ral (tib-ē-ō-fem′ŏ-răl). Relating to the tibia and the femur.

tib·i·o·fib·u·lar (tib-ē-ō-fib′yū-lăr). Relating to both tibia and fibula; denotes especially the joints and ligaments between the two bones. SYN peroneotibial, tibioperoneal.

tib·i·o·na·vic·u·lar (tib-ē-ō-na-vik′yū-lăr). Relating to the tibia and the navicular bone of the tarsus. SYN tibioscaphoid.

tib·i·o·per·o·ne·al (tib′ē-ō-per′ō-nē′ăl). SYN tibiofibular.

tib·i·o·scaph·oid (tib′ē-ō-skaf′oyd). SYN tibionavicular.

tib·i·o·tar·sal (tib-ē-ō-tar′săl). Relating to the tarsal bones and the tibia. SYN tarsotibial.

tic (tik). Habitual, repeated contraction of certain muscles, resulting in stereotyped individualized actions that can be voluntarily suppressed for only brief periods, *e.g.,* clearing the throat, sniffing, pursing the lips, excessive blinking; especially prominent when the person is under stress; there is no known pathologic substrate. SEE ALSO spasm. SYN Brissaud's disease, habit chorea, habit spasm. [Fr.]

convulsive t., SYN facial t.

t. de pensée (dě pahn-sā′), the habit of involuntarily giving expression to any thought that comes to mind. [Fr. of thought]

t. douloureux (dū-lū-rě′), SYN trigeminal *neuralgia.* [Fr. painful]

facial t., involuntary twitching of the facial muscles, sometimes unilateral. SYN Bell's spasm, convulsive t., facial spasm, histrionic spasm, mimic convulsion, mimic spasm, mimic t., palmus (1), prosopospasm.

glossopharyngeal t., SYN glossopharyngeal *neuralgia.*

habit t., a habitual repetition of some grimace, shrug of the shoulder, twisting or jerking of the head, or the like.

local t., a t. of very limited extent, as the winking of an eye or a twitch of a finger.

mimic t., SYN facial t.

psychic t., a gesture or exclamation made under the influence of an irresistible morbid impulse.

rotatory t., SYN spasmodic *torticollis.*

spasmodic t., a disorder in which sudden spasmodic coordinated movements of certain muscles or groups of physiologically related muscles occur at irregular intervals. SYN Henoch's chorea.

ti·car·cil·lin di·so·di·um (tī-kar-sil′in). The disodium salt of 6-(α-carboxy-α-thien-3-ylacetamido)penicillanic acid; a bactericidal antibiotic useful in treating *Pseudomonas aeruginosa* infections and similar in effect to carbenicillin disodium.

tick (tik). An acarine of the families Ixodidae (hard t.'s) or Argasidae (soft t.'s), which contain many bloodsucking species that are important pests of man and domestic birds and mammals, and that probably exceed all other arthropods in the number and variety of disease agents that they transmit. T.'s are differentiated from the much smaller true mites by possession of an armed hypostome and a pair of tracheal spiracular openings located behind the basal segment of the third or fourth pair of walking legs; the larva (seed t.) has six legs, and after molting appears as an eight-limbed nymph. Some important t.'s are *Amblyomma americanum* (Lone Star t.) and *A. hebraeum* (South African bont t.); *Argas persicus* (adobe, fowl, or Persian t.) and *A. reflexus* (pigeon t.); *Boophilus* (cattle t.'s); *Dermacentor albopictus* (horse or winter t.), *D. andersoni* (Rocky Mountain, spotted-fever, or wood t.), *D. nitens* (tropical horse t.), *D. occidentalis* (Pacific or wood t.), and *D. variabilis* (American dog t.); *Haemaphysalis chordeilis* (bird t.) and *H. laporis-palustris*(rabbit t.); *Ixodes pacificus* (California black-legged t.), *I. pilosus* (paralysis t.), *I. ricinus* (castor bean t.), and *I. scapularis* (black-legged or shoulder t.); *Ornithodoros coriaceus* (pajaroello t.) and *O. moubata* (African relapsing fever or tampan t.); and *Rhipicephalus everti* (African red t.), *R. sanguineus* (brown dog t.), and *R. simus* (black-pitted t.).

tick·ling (tik′ling). Denoting a peculiar itching or tingling sensation caused by excitation of surface nerves, as of the skin by light stroking.

ti·cryn·a·fen (tī-krin′ă-fen). [2,3-Dichloro-4-(2-thenoyl)-phenoxy]acetic acid; an antihypertensive diuretic and uricosuric agent; its clinical use is associated with an unusually high incidence of hepatitis; no longer used clinically.

ti

t.i.d. Abbreviation for L. *ter in die*, three times a day.

tid·al (tī′dăl). Relating to or resembling the tides, alternately rising and falling.

tide (tīd). An alternate rise and fall, ebb and flow, or an increase or a decrease. [A.S. *tīd*, time]

acid t., a temporary increase in the acidity of the urine occurring during fasting. SYN acid wave.

alkaline t., a period of urinary neutrality or even alkalinity after meals due to withdrawal of hydrogen ion for the purpose of secretion of the highly acid gastric juice. SYN alkaline wave.

fat t., an increase in the fat content of blood and lymph following a meal.

Tièche, Max, Swiss dermatologist, 1878–1938. SEE Jadassohn-T. *nevus.*

Tiedemann, Friedrich, German anatomist, 1781–1861. SEE T.'s *gland, nerve.*

Tier·fell·nae·vus (tēr′fel-nē-vŭs). SYN bathing trunk *nevus.* [Ger. a nevus simulating the pelt of an animal]

Tietze, Alexander, German surgeon, 1864–1927. SEE T.'s *syndrome.*

tig·late (tig′lāt). A salt or ester of tiglic acid.

tig·li·an (tig′lē-ăn). Original trivial name for the saturated form of phorbol. [fr. *Croton tiglium* (Euphorbiaceae)]

tig·lic ac·id (tig′lik). $CH_3CH=C(CH_3)COOH$; (*E*)-2-Methyl-2-butenoic acid; *trans*-2,3-dimethyl-acrylic acid; an unsaturated fatty acid present in glycerides in croton oil.

ti·glyl-CoA (tig′lil). $CH_3-CH=C(CH_3)-COSCoA$; an intermediate in the degradation of L-isoleucine. SYN tiglyl-coenzyme A.

ti·glyl-coen·zyme A. SYN tiglyl-CoA.

ti·gre·ti·er (tē-grĕ-ty-ā′). A form of saltatory chorea or dancing mania occurring in certain parts of Abyssinia. [Fr.]

ti·groid (tī′groyd). SEE chromophil *substance.* [G. *tigroidēs,* fr. *tigris,* tiger, + *eidos,* appearance]

ti·grol·y·sis (tī-grol′i-sis). SYN chromatolysis. [tigroid + G. *lysis,* dissolution]

Tillaux, Paul J., French surgeon, 1834–1904. SEE *spiral* of T.

til·or·one (til′or-ōn). A small synthetic molecule used to induce interferon in mice.

TILS Abbreviation for tumor-infiltrating *lymphocytes,* under *lymphocyte.*

tim·bre (tam′br, tim′br). The distinguishing quality of a sound, by which one may determine its source. SYN tone color. [Fr.]

time (t) (tīm). **1.** That relation of events which is expressed by the terms past, present, and future, and measured by units such as minutes, hours, days, months, or years. **2.** A certain period during which something definite or determined is done. SYN tempus (2). [A.S. *tima*]

activated clotting t. (ACT), the most common test used for coagulation t. in cardiovascular surgery.

activated partial thromboplastin t. (aPTT), the t. needed for plasma to form a fibrin clot following the addition of calcium and a phospholipid reagent; used to evaluate the intrinsic clotting system.

A-H conduction t., SEE atrioventricular *conduction.*

association t., t. elapsing between a stimulus and the verbalized response to it.

biologic t., the concept that our appreciation of t. varies with age and is governed by the neural organization of the individual; it obeys a logarithmic rather than an arithmetic law.

bleeding t., the t. interval between the appearance of the first drop of blood and the removal of the last drop following puncture of the ear lobe or the finger, usually 1 to 3 minutes; it is prolonged in cases of thrombocytopenia, diminished prothrombin, phosphorus poisoning, or chloroform poisoning, and in some liver diseases; it is normal in hemophilia. Since the earlier techniques were not well controlled, better controlled modifications such as that of Ivy are now employed to determine the bleeding t.

circulation t., the t. taken for the blood to pass through a given circuit of the vascular system, *e.g.,* the pulmonary or systemic circulation, from one arm to another, from arm to tongue, or from arm to lung; it is measured by the injection into an arm vein of a substance, such as sodium dehydrocholate, ether, fluorescein, histamine, or a radium salt, which can be detected when it arrives at another point in the vascular system.

clot retraction t., the t. required for a blood clot to separate from the tube wall and express serum, usually completed in 18 to 24 hours, but retarded or absent in persons with thrombocytopenic purpura.

clotting t., SYN coagulation t.

coagulation t., the t. required for blood to coagulate; prolonged in hemophilia and in the presence of obstructive jaundice, some anemias and leukemias, and some of the infectious diseases. SYN clotting t.

euglobulin clot lysis t., a measure of the ability of plasminogen activators and plasmin to lyse a clot; normally, clot lysis is determined by the balance of factors which activate fibrinolysis (plasminogen activators and plasmin) and those which inhibit lysis; in certain conditions (*e.g.,* carcinoma or hepatic insufficiency) activating factors predominate and can be measured by noting the t. it takes the euglobulin fraction of plasma (excluding inhibitors of fibrinolysis) to clot.

fading t., the t. required for a constant stimulus applied to a fixed area of the peripheral visual field to stop.

t. of flight, the t. for a photon created by annihilation of a positron-electron pair to reach a detector; since annihilation photons are created in pairs and travel in opposite directions at about 3×10^{10} cm/sec, measurement of the difference in arrival t. at detectors with sub-nanosecond resolution allows calculation of the location of the event; the basic physics of positron emission tomography.

forced expiratory t. (FET), the t. taken to expire a given volume or a given fraction of vital capacity during measurement of forced vital capacity; subscripts specify the exact parameters measured.

half-t., SEE half-time.

H-R conduction t., SEE intraventricular *conduction.*

H-V conduction t., SEE intraventricular *conduction.*

inertia t., the interval elapsing between the reception of the stimulus from a nerve and the contraction of the muscle.

intra-atrial conduction t., the total duration of electrical activity of the atria in one cardiac cycle.

left ventricular ejection t. (LVET), the t. measured clinically from onset to incisural notch of the carotid or other pulse; properly the time of ejection of blood from the left ventricle beginning with aortic valve opening and ending with aortic valve closure.

P-A conduction t., SEE atrioventricular *conduction.*

partial thromboplastin t. (PTT), SEE activated partial thromboplastin t.

P-H conduction t., SEE atrioventricular *conduction.*

prothrombin t. (PT), the t. required for clotting after thromboplastin and calcium are added in optimal amounts to blood of normal fibrinogen content; if prothrombin is diminished, the clotting t. increases; used to evaluate the extrinsic clotting system. SEE ALSO prothrombin *test.*

reaction t., the interval between the presentation of a stimulus and the responsive reaction to it.

recognition t., the interval between the application of a stimulus and the recognition of its nature.

relaxation t. (τ), the time required for the substrate in an enzymatic or chemical reaction to fall to 1/e of its initial value.

repetition t. (TR), in magnetic resonance imaging, the t. between repetitions of the pulse sequence.

rise t., the t. required for a pulse or echo to rise from 10% to 90% of its peak amplitude.

running t., the t. during which an activity (*e.g.,* chromatography development) occurs.

Russell's viper venom clotting t., a clotting t. determination performed on citrated platelet-poor plasma using Russell's viper *venom* as an activating agent. This allows activation of factor X directly without the need for other coagulation factors and is used to confirm factor X defects. SEE ALSO Stypven time *test.*

sensation t., the minimal t. a visual image must be exposed in order to be perceived.

sinoatrial conduction t. (SACT), the t. required for an impulse to travel from sinus node to atrium; estimated indirectly during reset nodus sinuatrialis period by halving the average interval from the premature beat to the following normal sinus beat of the atrium.

sinoatrial recovery t. (SART), interval from the last paced P wave to the first succeeding spontaneous P wave (after 2 to 5 minutes of right atrial pacing at 120 to 140 beats per minute, and when expressed as percentage of control cycle length, it normally ranges from 115 to 159%).

survival t., (1) the period elapsing between the completion or institution of any procedure and death; **(2)** the life-span of biologically or physically marked erythrocytes or other cells.

thrombin t., the t. needed for a fibrin clot to form after the addition of thrombin to citrated plasma; prolonged thrombin t. is seen in patients receiving heparin therapy.

tissue thromboplastin inhibition t., a test used to identify lupus anticoagulant; the thromboplastin source used in the prothrombin test is diluted to increase sensitivity to inhibitors.

utilization t., the minimum duration of a stimulus of rheobasic strength that is just sufficient to produce excitation. SYN temps utile.

TIMI Acronym for *t*hrombolysis *i*n *m*yocardial *i*nfarction; a large multicenter controlled clinical trial.

tim·no·don·ic ac·id (tim-nō-don'ok). A 20-carbon fatty acid with five *cis* double bonds located on carbons 5, 8, 11, 14, and 17; an important component of fish oils; a precursor to the 3-series prostaglandins *e.g.,* PGE₃.

ti·mo·lol ma·le·ate (tī'mō-lōl). (-)-1-(*tert*-Butylamino)-3-[(4-morpholino-1,2,5-thiadiazol-3-yl)oxy]-2-propanol maleate; a β-adrenergic blocking agent used in the treatment of hypertension and used in eyedrops in the treatment of chronic open-angle glaucoma.

tin (Sn) (tin). A metallic element, atomic no. 50, atomic wt. 118.710. SYN stannum. [AS, tin]

t. oxide, SYN stannic oxide.

tin-113 (¹¹³Sn). A radioisotope of tin with a physical half-life of 115.1 days; used in the manufacture of radionuclide generators for the production of indium-113m.

tinct. Abbreviation of L. *tinctura,* tincture.

tinc·ta·ble (tingk'tă-bl). Stainable.

tinc·tion (tingk'shŭn). **1.** A stain; a preparation for staining. **2.** The act of staining. [L. *tingo,* pp. *tinctus,* to dye]

tinc·to·ri·al (tingk-tōr'ē-ăl). Relating to coloring or staining. [L. *tinctorius,* fr. *tingo,* to dye]

tinc·tu·ra, gen. and pl. **tinc·tu·rae** (tingk-tū'ră, -rē). SYN tincture. [L. a dyeing, fr. *tingo,* pp. *tinctus,* to dye]

tinc·tu·ra·tion (tingk-chū-rā'shŭn). The making of a tincture from a crude drug.

tinc·ture (tingk'chŭr). An alcoholic or hydroalcoholic solution prepared from vegetable materials or from chemical substances; most t.'s are prepared by percolation or by maceration. The proportions of drug represented in the different t.'s are not uniform, but vary according to the established standards for each. T.'s of potent drugs essentially represent the activity of 10 g of the drug in each 100 ml of t., the potency being adjusted after assay; most other t.'s represent 20 g of drug in each 100 ml of t. Compound t.'s are made according to long-established formulas. SYN tinctura. [see *tinctura*]

alcoholic t., a t. made with undiluted alcohol.

ammoniated t., a t. made with ammoniated alcohol.

belladonna t., a green hydroalcoholic mobile liquid containing the alkaloids atropine and scopolamine and other substances extracted from the leaves of *Atropa belladonna,* the botanical source for these anticholinergic drugs. The t. allows for gradual titration of dose by counting drops of the preparation ingested. Formerly widely used in ulcer therapy or the symptomatic treatment of diarrhea, alone or in combination with antacids and insoluble clays.

digitalis t., an hydroalcoholic solution containing the glycosides of the leaves of the foxglove (digitalis) plant *Digitalis purpurea* or *D. lanata.* Although digitalis preparations are used exten-

sively, they are currently used as the pure glycosides, digoxin and digitoxin. The t. was formerly widely used but was standardized by bioassay using frogs, cats, or pigeons.

ethereal t., a class of preparations consisting of 10% percolations of drugs in a menstruum of ether 1 and alcohol 2.

glycerinated t., a t. made with diluted alcohol to which glycerin is added to facilitate the extraction or to preserve the preparation.

green soap t., a liquid preparation containing potassium soaps and alcohol; frequently advocated in skin cleansing, particularly after exposure to plant toxins such as poison ivy.

hydroalcoholic t., a t. made with diluted alcohol in various proportions with water.

tine (tīn). **1.** In dentistry, the slender, pointed end of an explorer. **2.** An instrument used to introduce antigen, such as tuberculin into the skin, and usually containing several individual t.'s. [A.S. *tind,* a prong]

tin·ea (tin'ē-ă). A fungus infection (dermatophytosis) of the keratin component of hair, skin, or nails. Genera of fungi causing such infection are *Microsporum, Trichophyton,* and *Epidermophyton.* SYN ringworm, serpigo (1). [L. worm, moth]

t. amianta'cea, an inflammatory condition of the scalp in which heavy scales extend onto the hairs and bind the proximal portions together; it is not caused by a fungus. SYN pityriasis amiantacea.

t. bar'bae, t. of the beard, occurring as a follicular infection or as a granulomatous lesion; the primary lesions are papules and pustules. SYN barber's itch, folliculitis barbae, ringworm of beard, t. sycosis, trichophytosis barbae.

t. cap'itis, a common form of fungus infection of the scalp caused by various species of *Microsporum* and *Trichophyton* on or within hair shafts, occurring almost exclusively in children and characterized by irregularly placed and variously sized patches of apparent baldness because of hairs breaking off at the surface of the scalp, scaling, black dots (see black-dot *ringworm*), and occasionally erythema and pyoderma. SYN ringworm of scalp, trichophytosis capitis.

t. circina'ta, SYN t. corporis.

t. cor'poris, a well-defined, scaling, macular eruption of dermatophytosis that frequently forms annular lesions and may appear on any part of the body. SYN ringworm of body, t. circinata, trichophytosis corporis.

t. cru'ris, a form of t. imbricata occurring in the genitocrural region, including the inner side of the thighs, the perineal region, and the groin. SYN dhobie itch, eczema marginatum, jock itch, ringworm of genitocrural region, t. inguinalis, trichophytosis cruris.

t. favo'sa, SYN favus.

t. glabro'sa, ringworm or fungus infection of the hairless skin.

t. imbrica'ta, an eruption consisting of a number of concentric rings of overlapping scales forming papulosquamous patches scattered over the body; it occurs in tropical climates and is caused by the fungus *Trichophyton concentricum.* SYN herpes desquamans, Malabar itch, Oriental ringworm, scaly ringworm, t. tropicalis, Tokelau ringworm.

t. inguina'lis, SYN t. cruris.

t. ke'rion, an inflammatory fungus infection of the scalp and beard, marked by pustules and a boggy infiltration of the surrounding parts; most commonly caused by *Microsporum audouinii.* SYN Celsus kerion.

t. ma'nus, ringworm of the hand, usually referring to infections of the palmar surface. SEE ALSO t. corporis.

t. ni'gra, a fungus infection due to *Exophiala werneckii,* marked by dark lesions giving a spattered appearance and occurring most commonly on the palms of the hands. SYN pityriasis nigra.

t. pe'dis, dermatophytosis of the feet, especially of the skin between the toes, and the nails, caused by one of the dermatophytes, usually a species of *Trichophyton* or *Epidermophyton;* the disease consists of small vesicles, fissures, scaling, maceration, and eroded areas between the toes and on the plantar surface of the foot; other skin areas may be involved. SYN athlete's foot, dermatomycosis pedis, Hong Kong foot, Hong Kong toe, ringworm of foot.

t. profun'da, SYN Majocchi *granulomas,* under *granuloma.*

t. syco'sis, SYN t. barbae.

ti

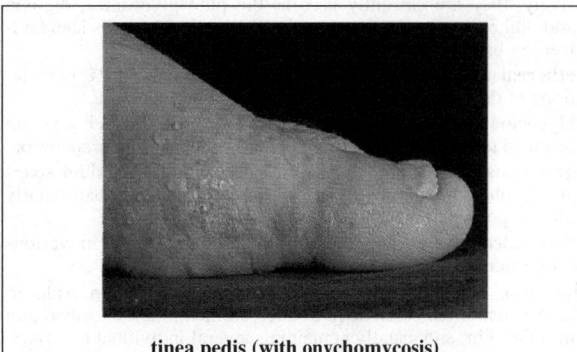

tinea pedis (with onychomycosis)

t. tonsu′rans, t. capitis or t. corporis caused by *Trichophyton tonsurans;* characterized by small plaques and fewer broken off hairs than in t. capitis caused by other species. SYN porrigo furfurans.

t. tropica′lis, SYN t. imbricata.

t. un′guium, ringworm of the nails due to a dermatophyte.

t. versic′olor, an eruption of tan or brown branny patches on the skin of the trunk, often appearing white, in contrast with hyperpigmented skin after exposure to the summer sun; caused by growth of *Malassezia furfur* in the stratum corneum with minimal inflammatory reaction. SYN pityriasis versicolor.

Tinel, Jules, French neurologist, 1879–1952. SEE T.'s *sign.*

tin·foil (tin′foyl). **1.** Tin rolled into extremely thin sheets. **2.** A base metal foil used as a separating material, as between the cast and denture base material during flasking and curing procedures.

tin·gi·bil·i·ty (tin′ji-bil′i-tē). The property of being tingible.

tin·gi·ble (tin′ji-bl). Capable of being stained. [L. *tingo,* to dye]

tin·gle (ting′gl). To feel a peculiar pricking sensation.

tin·gling. A pricking type of paresthesia.

distal t. on percussion (dis′tăl ting′ling on per-kŭsh′un), A term sometimes used for Tinel's *sign.*

ti·nid·a·zole (ti-nid′ă-zōl). 1-[2-(Ethylsulfonyl)ethyl]-2-methyl-5-nitroimidazole; an antiprotozoal agent.

tin·ni·tus (ti-nī′tŭs). Noises (ringing, whistling, booming, etc.) in the ears. [L. a jingling, fr. *tinnio,* pp. *tinnitus,* to jingle, clink]

t. au′rium, sensation of sound in one or both ears usually associated with disease in the middle ear, the inner ear, or the central auditory apparatus. SYN syrigmus, tympanophonia (1), tympanophony.

t. cere′bri, subjective sensation of noise in head rather than ears.

clicking t., an objective clicking sound in the ear in cases of chronic catarrhal otitis media; it may be audible to the bystander as well as to the patient and is supposed to be due to an opening and closing of the mouth of the eustachian tube, or to a rhythmical spasm of the velum palati.

Leudet's t., a dry spasmodic click, audible also through the otoscope, heard in catarrhal inflammation of the eustachian tube; caused by reflex spasm of the tensor palati muscle.

tint. A shade of color varying according to the amount of white admixed with the pigment. [L. *tingo,* pp. *tinctus,* to dye]

ti·o·con·a·zole (tī-ō-kon′ă-zōl). 1-[2,4-Dichloro-β-[(2-chloro-3-thenyl)-oxy]phenethyl]imidazole; an antifungal agent.

tip. **1.** A point; a more or less sharp extremity. **2.** A separate, but attached, piece of the same or another structure, forming the extremity of a part.

t. of auricle, a point projecting upward and posteriorly from the free outcurved margin of the helix a little posterior to its upper end. SYN apex auriculae [NA], apex satyri, Woolner's t.

t. of elbow, SYN olecranon.

t. of nose, anteriormost pointed end of external nose. SYN apex nasi [NA].

t. of posterior horn, SYN *apex* of the posterior horn.

root t., SYN t. of tooth root.

t. of tongue, the anterior extreme of the tongue which can be

made pointed for sensing or probing and which rests against the lingual aspect of the incisor teeth. SYN apex linguae [NA].

t. of tooth root, the tip of a tooth root, the part farthest from the incisal or occlusal side. SYN apex radicis dentis [NA], root apex, root t.

Woolner's t., SYN t. of auricle.

tip·ping. A tooth movement in which the angulation of the long axis of the tooth is altered.

ti·pren·o·lol hy·dro·chlo·ride (tip-ren′ō-lol). (±)-1-(Isopropylamino)-3-[*o*-(methylthio)phenoxy]-2-propanol hydrochloride; a β-receptor blocking agent.

TIPS Acronym for transjugular intrahepatic portosystemic *shunt.*

tir·ing (tīr′ing). SYN cerclage. [Eng. tire]

Tiselius, Arne, Swedish biochemist and Nobel laureate, 1902–1971. SEE T. *apparatus,* electrophoresis *cell.*

Tis·si·er·el·la prae·acu·ta. SYN *Bacteroides praeacutus.*

Tissot, Jules, early 20th century French physiologist. SEE T. *spirometer.*

tis·sue (tish′ū). A collection of similar cells and the intercellular substances surrounding them. There are four basic tissues in the body: 1) epithelium; 2) the connective tissues, including blood, bone, and cartilage; 3) muscle tissue; and 4) nerve tissue. [Fr. *tissu,* woven, fr. L. *texo,* to weave]

adenoid t., SYN lymphatic t.

adipose t., a connective t. consisting chiefly of fat cells surrounded by reticular fibers and arranged in lobular groups or along the course of one of the smaller blood vessels. SYN fat (1), fatty t. (1), white fat (1).

areolar t., loose, irregularly arranged connective t. that consists of collagenous and elastic fibers, a protein polysaccharide ground substance, and connective t. cells (fibroblasts, macrophages, mast cells, and sometimes fat cells, plasma cells, leukocytes, and pigment cells).

bone t., SYN osseous t.

brown adipose t., SYN brown *fat.*

cancellous t., latticelike or spongy osseous t.

cardiac muscle t., SEE cardiac *muscle.*

cartilaginous t., SEE cartilage.

cavernous t., SYN erectile t.

chondroid t., **(1)** in an adult, t. resembling cartilage; SYN fibrohyaline t., pseudocartilage. **(2)** in an embryo, an early stage in cartilage formation.

chromaffin t., a cellular t., vascular and well supplied with nerves, made up chiefly of chromaffin cells; it is found in the medulla of the suprarenal glands and, in smaller collections, in the paraganglia.

connective t., the supporting or framework t. of the animal body, formed of fibrous and ground substance with more or less numerous cells of various kinds; it is derived from the mesenchyme, and this in turn from the mesoderm; the varieties of connective t. are: areolar or loose; adipose; dense, regular or irregular, white fibrous; elastic; mucous; and lymphoid t.; cartilage; and bone; the blood and lymph may be regarded as connective t.'s the ground substance of which is a liquid. SYN interstitial t., tela conjunctiva.

dartoic t., t. resembling tunica dartos.

elastic t., a form of connective t. in which the elastic fibers predominate; it constitutes the ligamenta flava of the vertebrae and the ligamentum nuchae, especially of quadrupeds; it occurs also in the walls of the arteries and of the bronchial tree, and connects the cartilages of the larynx. SYN elastica (2), tela elastica.

epithelial t., SEE epithelium.

erectile t., a t. with numerous vascular spaces that may become engorged with blood. SYN cavernous t.

fatty t., **(1)** SYN adipose t. **(2)** in some animals, brown *fat.*

fibrohyaline t., SYN chondroid t. (1).

fibrous t., a t. composed of bundles of collagenous white fibers between which are rows of connective t. cells; the tendons, ligaments, aponeuroses, and some of the membranes, such as the dura mater.

Gamgee t., a thick layer of absorbent cotton between two layers of absorbent gauze, used in surgical dressings.

gelatinous t., SYN mucous connective t.

gingival t.'s, SEE gingiva.

granulation t., vascular connective t. forming granular projections on the surface of a healing wound, ulcer, or inflamed t. surface. SEE ALSO granulation.

gut-associated lymphoid t. (GALT) (lim'fōid), lymphoid t. of the gastrointestinal tract that is especially rich in B cells. This t. is responsible for localized immunity to pathogens such as bacteria, viruses, and parasites.

Haller's vascular t., SYN vascular *lamina* of choroid.

hard t., (1) t. that has become mineralized; **(2)** t. having a firm intercellular substance, *e.g.,* cartilage and bone.

hemopoietic t., t. in which there is a development of blood cells or other formed elements.

indifferent t., undifferentiated, nonspecialized, embryonic t.

interstitial t., SYN connective t.

investing t.'s, the t.'s covering or enclosing a structure.

islet t., SYN *islets* of Langerhans, under *islet.*

lymphatic t., lymphoid t., a three-dimensional network of reticular fibers and cells the meshes of which are occupied in varying degrees of density with lymphocytes; there is nodular, diffuse, and loose lymphatic t. SYN adenoid t.

mesenchymal t., embryonic connective tissue. SEE mesenchyme.

mesonephric t., intermediate mesoderm situated in the thoracic and lumbar regions of the embryo or fetus; it evolves into the mesonephros and associated structures.

metanephrogenic t., t. derived from the intermediate mesoderm caudal to mesonephric levels and concerned with the formation of the nephrons of the metanephros.

mucous connective t., a type of connective t. little differentiated beyond the mesenchymal stage; its ground substance of glycoproteins is abundant and contains fine collagenous fibers and fibroblasts; in its most characteristic form, it appears in the umbilical cord as Wharton's jelly. SYN gelatinous t.

multilocular adipose t., SYN brown *fat.*

muscular t., a t. characterized by the ability to contract upon stimulation; its three varieties are skeletal, cardiac, and smooth. SEE muscle. SYN flesh (2).

myeloid t., bone marrow consisting of the developmental and adult stages of erythrocytes, granulocytes, and megakaryocytes in a stroma of reticular cells and fibers, with sinusoidal vascular channels.

nasion soft t., the outer point of intersection between the nasion-sella line and the soft tissue profile.

nephrogenic t., the t. from which the pronephros, mesonephros, and metanephros develop.

nervous t., a highly differentiated t. composed of nerve cells, nerve fibers, dendrites, and a supporting t. (neuroglia).

nodal t., SEE atrioventricular *node,* sinuatrial *node.*

osseous t., a connective t., the matrix of which consists of collagen fibers and ground substance and in which are deposited calcium salts (phosphate, carbonate, and some fluoride) in the form of an apatite. SYN bone t.

osteogenic t., a connective t. with the property of forming osseous t.

osteoid t., osseous t. prior to calcification.

periapical t., the structures adjacent to a root apex, particularly the periodontal ligament and bone.

reticular t., retiform t., a t. in which the argyrophilic collagenous fibers form a network and that usually has a network of reticular cells associated with the fibers.

rubber t., a thin sheet of rubber used as a cover in surgical dressings.

skeletal muscle t., SEE skeletal *muscle.*

smooth muscle t., SEE smooth *muscle.*

subcutaneous t., a layer of loose, irregular, connective t. immediately beneath the skin and closely attached to the corium by coarse fibrous bands, the retinacula cutis; it contains fat cells except in the auricles, eyelids, penis, and scrotum.

tis·sue-trim·ming. SYN border *molding.*

tis·su·lar (tish'yū-lăr). Relating or pertaining to a tissue.

ti·ta·ni·um (Ti) (tī-tā'nē-ŭm). A metallic element, atomic no. 22, atomic wt. 47.88. [*Titans,* in G. myth., sons of Earth]

t. dioxide, TiO_2; contains not less than 99.0% and not more than 100.5% of TiO_2, calculated on the dry basis; used in creams and powders as a protectant against external irritations and solar rays.

ti·ter (tī'ter). The standard of strength of a volumetric test solution; the assay value of an unknown measure by volumetric means. [Fr. *titre,* standard]

TITh Abbreviation for 3,5,3'-triiodothyronine.

tit·il·la·tion (tit-i-lā'shŭn). The act or sensation of tickling. [L. *titillatio,* fr. *titillo,* pp. *-atus,* to tickle]

ti·tin (tī'tin). A very large fibrous protein that connects thick myosin filaments to Z discs in the sarcomere.

ti·trant (tī'trant). In chemistry, the solution that is added (titrated with) in a titration.

ti·trate (tī'trāt). To analyze volumetrically by a solution (the titrant) of known strength to an end point.

ti·tra·tion (tī-trā'shŭn). Volumetric analysis by means of the addition of definite amounts of a test solution to a solution of the substance being assayed. [Fr. *titre,* standard]

colorimetric t., a t. in which the end point is marked by a color change.

formol t., a method of titrating the amino groups of amino acids, by adding formaldehyde to the neutral solution; the formaldehyde reacts with the NH_3^+ group, liberating an equivalent quantity of H^+, which may then be estimated by t. with NaOH.

potentiometric t., a t. during which the pH is continually measured with some value of the pH serving as end point.

tit·u·ba·tion (tit-yū-bā'shŭn). **1.** A staggering or stumbling in trying to walk. **2.** A tremor or shaking of the head, of cerebellar origin. [L. *titubo,* pp. *-atus,* to stagger]

Tizzoni, Guido, Italian physician, 1853–1932. SEE Tizzoni's *stain.*

Tl Symbol for thallium.

^{201}Tl Abbreviation for *thallium*-201.

TLC Abbreviation for thin-layer *chromatography;* total lung *capacity.*

TLE Abbreviation for thin-layer *electrophoresis.*

TLV Abbreviation for threshold limit *value.*

TM Abbreviation for transcendental meditation.

Tm Symbol for thulium; transport *maximum* or tubular *maximum.*

TMD Abbreviation for temporomandibular joint *dysfunction.*

TMJ Colloquial abbreviation for temporomandibular joint *dysfunction.*

TM-mode. SYN M-mode.

TMP Abbreviation for ribothymidylic acid; trimethoprim; sometimes for deoxyribothymidylic acid.

T-my·co·plas·ma. SYN *Ureaplasma.*

Tn Abbreviation for ocular *tension.*

TNF Abbreviation for tumor necrosis *factor.*

TNM Abbreviation for tumor-node-metastasis. SEE TNM *staging.*

TNT Abbreviation for trinitrotoluene.

TO Abbreviation for Theiler's Original, Theiler's original strain of mouse encephalomyelitis virus.

to·bac·co (tō-bak'ō). A South American herb, *Nicotiana tabacum,* that has large ovate to lanceolate leaves and terminal clusters of tubular white or pink flowers. T. leaves contain 2 to 8% of nicotine and are the source of smoking and chewing t.

wild t., SYN lobelia.

to·bra·my·cin (tō-brǎ-mī'sin). An aminoglycoside antibiotic produced by *Streptomyces tenebrarius,* having bactericidal effects and used mainly in the treatment of *Pseudomonas* infections.

to·cai·nide hy·dro·chlo·ride (tō-kā'nīd). 2-Amino-2',6'-propionoxylidide hydrochloride; an oral antiarrhythmic agent, similar in action to lidocaine, used in the treatment of ventricular arrhythmias.

to

to·cam·phyl (tō-kam′fil). *p*,α-Dimethylbenzyl camphorate, diethanolamine salt; a choleretic.

⚠**toco-.** Childbirth. [G. *tokos,* birth]

to·co·chro·ma·nol-3 (tō′kō-krō′mă-nol). An α-tocotrienol. SEE tocotrienol.

toc·o·dy·na·graph (tō-kō-dī′nă-graf, tok-ō-). A recording of the force of uterine contractions. SYN tocograph. [toco- + G. *dynamis,* force, + *graphē,* a writing]

toc·o·dy·na·mom·e·ter (tō′kō-dī-nă-mom′ĕ-ter, tok′ō-). An instrument for measuring the force of uterine contractions. SYN tocometer. [toco- + G. *dynamis,* force, + *metron,* measure]

toc·o·graph (tō′kō-graf). SYN tocodynagraph.

to·cog·ra·phy (tō-kog′ră-fē). The process of recording uterine contractions. [toco- + G. *graphō,* to write]

to·col (tō′kol). Fundamental unit of the tocopherols; 6-phytylhydroquinone (see structure *A*, in figure) becomes, in the chromanol form, 2-methyl-2-(4,8,12-trimethyltridecyl)chroman-6-ol (structure *B*, in figure).

to·col·o·gy (tō-kol′ō-jē). SYN obstetrics. [toco- + G. *logos,* study]

to·co·lyt·ic (tō-kō-lit′ik). Denoting any pharmacological agent used to arrest uterine contractions; often used in an attempt to arrest premature labor contractions *e.g.,* ritodrine. [G. *tokos,* childbirth, labor, + *lysis,* loosening]

to·com·e·ter (tō-kom′ĕ-ter). SYN tocodynamometer.

to·coph·er·ol (T) (tō-kof′er-ōl). **1.** Name given to vitamin E by its discoverer, but now a generic term for vitamin E and compounds chemically related to it, with or without biological activity; similar in chemical structure and properties to vitamins K and coenzyme Q. **2.** A methylated tocol or methylated tocotrienol.

mixed t.'s concentrate, a source of vitamin E, obtained by vacuum distillation of edible vegetable oils or their by-products.

α-to·coph·er·ol (α-T). 2,5,7,8-tetramethyl-2-(4′,8′,12′-trimethyltridecyl)-6-chromanol; 5,7,8-trimethyltocol; a light yellow, viscous, odorless, oily liquid that deteriorates on exposure to light, is obtained from wheat germ oil or by synthesis, biologically exhibits the most vitamin E activity of the α-tocopherol's, and is an antioxidant retarding rancidity by interfering with the autoxidation of fats. Prepared from natural phytol, it is called 2-*ambo*-α-tocopherol; from synthetic phytol, *all-rac*-α-tocopherol or *synt*-α-tocopherol; also available are *d*-α-tocopheryl acetate, *dl*-α-tocopheryl acetate, *d*-α-tocopheryl acid succinate, and *d*-α-tocopheryl acetate concentrate. One of several forms of vitamin E. SYN vitamin E (1).

β-to·coph·er·ol (β-T). 5,8-Dimethyltocol; a lower homolog of α-tocopherol, that contains one less methyl group in the aromatic nucleus and is less active biologically; accompanies α-T and γ-β-tocopherol

γ-to·coph·er·ol (γ-T). 7,8-Dimethyltocol; a form biologically less active than α-γ-tocopherol

to·coph·er·ol·qui·none (TQ) (tō-kof′er-ol-kwī′nōn). An oxidized tocopherol, formed from the isomeric 2-methyl-2-phytyl-6-chromenol with methyl groups in one or more of positions 5,7, and 8, by migration of H atom from 6-OH to C-4, which yields a 1,4-benzoquinone. Abbreviated TQ and preceded by α-, β-, etc., as in the tocopherols, to indicate degree of methylation. SYN tocopherylquinone.

to·coph·er·yl·qui·none (tō-kof′er-il-kwī′nōn). SYN tocopherol-quinone.

toc·o·pho·bia (tō′kō-fō′bē-ă, tok′ō-). Morbid dread of childbirth. [toco- + G. *phobos,* fear]

to·co·qui·none (tō-kō-kwī′nōn). Class name for the 2,3,5-trimethyl-6-multiprenyl-1,4-benzoquinones.

to·co·tri·en·ol (tō-kō-trī′en-ol). A tocol with three double bonds in the side chain, *i.e.,* with three additional double bonds in the phytyl chain, thus a 6-(3′,7′,11′,15′-tetramethyl-2′,6′,10′,14′-hexadecatetraenyl)-1,4-hydroquinone or a 2-methyl-2-(4,8,12-trimethyltrideca-3,7,11-trienyl)chroman-6-ol. The natural products carry methyls at one or more of positions 5, 7, and 8 on the chromanol and are thus identical, except for the unsaturation in the phytyl-like side chain, to the tocopherols; also analogous is the cyclization to form a chromanol derivative and oxidation to form the tocotrienolquinones (or chromenols). Abbreviated T-*n*

(hydroquinone form) or TQ-*n* (quinone form) and preceded by α-, β-, etc., as in the tocopherols, to indicate degree of methylation (the *n* indicates the number of intact isoprene or prenyl units remaining in the chromanol or chromenol form). T. terminology is used to indicate relationships to tocols and tocoenols (vitamin E-like), the chromanol terminology to indicate relationship to the isoprenoidal compounds of the vitamin K and coenzyme Q series.

to·co·tri·en·ol·qui·none (tō-kō-trī′en-ol-kwī′nōn). A tocotrienol in which the hydroquinone has been oxidized to a quinone (the chromanol has become a chromenol); the t.'s carry α, β, γ, and δ prefixes in accordance with the degree of methylation, as do the tocotrienols.

TOCP Abbreviation for triorthocresyl phosphate.

Tod, David, British surgeon, 1794–1856. SEE T.'s *muscle.*

Todaro, Francesco, Italian anatomist, 1839–1918. SEE T.'s *tendon.*

Todd, Robert B., English physician, 1809–1860. SEE T.'s *paralysis,* postepileptic *paralysis.*

toe (tō). One of the digits of the feet. SYN digitus pedis [NA]. [A.S. *ta*]

great t., SYN hallux.

hammer t., permanent flexion at the midphalangeal joint of one or more of the t.'s.

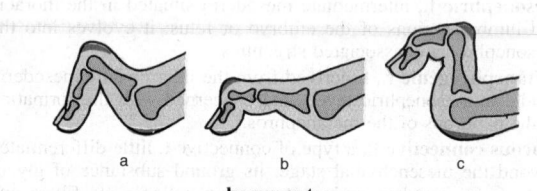

hammer toe
a) at the proximal midphalangeal joint; b) at the distal midphalangeal joint; c) claw toe

Hong Kong t., SYN *tinea* pedis.

Morton's t., a particular form of metatarsalgia caused by enlargement of the digital nerve. Cf. Morton's *syndrome.*

painful t., SYN *hallux* dolorosus.

seedy t., a condition of the hoof wall in the t. region of horses, characterized by loss of substance and change in character of the horn, most often as a sequela of mild chronic laminitis. SYN dystrophia ungulae, hollow wall.

stiff t., SYN *hallux* rigidus.

webbed t.'s, syndactyly involving the toes.

toe-crack (tō′krak′). SEE sand-crack.

toe-drop (tō′drop). Inability to dorsiflex the toes, usually due to paralysis of the toe extensor muscles.

toe·nail (tō′nāl). SEE nail.

ingrowing t., SYN ingrown *nail.*

to·fen·a·cin hy·dro·chlo·ride (tō-fen′ă-sin). *N*-Methyl-2-[(*o*-methyl-α-phenylbenzyl)oxy]ethylamine hydrochloride; an anticholinergic drug.

To·ga·vir·i·dae (tō-gă-vir′i-dē). A family of viruses that includes the following genera: *Alphavirus,* which includes eastern equine encephalitis, western equine encephalitis, and Venezuelan equine encephalitis virus, the rubella virus (*Rubivirus*), hog cholera virus, related cattle and pig viruses of the genus *Pestivirus,* and the equine arteritis virus *Arterivirus.* Virions are 60 to 70 nm in diameter, enveloped, and ether-sensitive; the capsid is of icosahedral symmetry, containing probably 32 capsomeres; genomes contain single-stranded positive sense RNA.

to·ga·vi·rus (tō′gă-vī′rŭs). Any virus of the family Togaviridae. [L. *toga,* garment covering, + virus]

toi·let (toy-let′). **1.** Cleansing of the obstetrical patient after childbirth or of a wound after an operation preparatory to the application of the dressing. **2.** In dentistry, cavity debridement, the final step before placing a restoration in a tooth whereby the cavity is cleaned and all debris is removed. [Fr. *toilette*]

pulmonary t., cleansing of the trachea and bronchial tree.

Toison, J., French histologist, 1858–1950. SEE T.'s *stain*.

△**toko-.** SEE toco-.

to·laz·a·mide (tō-laz'ă-mīd). 1-(Hexahydro-1*H*-azeprin-1-yl)-3-(*p*-tolylsulfonyl)urea; an oral hypoglycemic agent similar in use to tolbutamide.

to·laz·o·line hy·dro·chlo·ride (tō-laz'ō-lēn). 2-Benzyl-2-imidazoline hydrochloride; an adrenergic α-receptor blocking agent used to augment blood flow in peripheral vascular disorders.

tol·bu·ta·mide (tol-byū'tă-mīd). 1-Butyl-3-*p*-tolylsulfonylurea; an orally active hypoglycemic agent used in the management of adult-onset diabetes mellitus; it appears to stimulate the synthesis and release of endogenous insulin from functional islets; available as t. sodium for injection.

tol·cy·cla·mide (tol-sī'klă-mīd). SYN glycyclamide.

Toldt, Karl, Austrian anatomist, 1840–1920. SEE T.'s *fascia, membrane;* white *line* of T.

tol·er·ance (tol'er-ăns). **1.** The ability to endure or be less responsive to a stimulus, especially over a period of continued exposure. **2.** The power of resisting the action of a poison or of taking a drug continuously or in large doses without injurious effects. [L. *tolero*, pp. *-atus*, to endure]

acoustic t., the maximum sound pressure level that can be experienced without producing pain or permanent defect of hearing in a normal individual.

cross t., the resistance to one or several effects of a compound as a result of t. developed to a pharmacologically similar compound.

frustration t., the level of an individual's ability to withstand frustration without developing inadequate modes of response, such as "going to pieces" emotionally.

high dose t., the induction of t. by exposure to high doses of antigen.

immunologic t., lack of immune response to antigen. Theories of t. induction include clonal deletion and clonal anergy. In clonal deletion, the actual clone of cells is eliminated whereas in clonal anergy the cells are present but nonfunctional. SYN immunological t., immunotolerance, nonresponder t.

immunologic high dose t. (im'mū-nō-loj'ik), induction of tolerance by exposure to large amounts of protein antigens.

immunological t., SYN immunologic t.

impaired glucose t., excessive levels of blood glucose developing after carbohydrate-rich meal or test dosage of glucose (usually 75 grams). Not necessarily diagnostic of diabetes mellitus.

individual t., t. to a drug that the person has never received before.

nonresponder t., SYN immunologic t.

pain t., the greatest intensity of painful stimulation that an individual is able to tolerate.

species t., the insensitivity to a particular drug exhibited by a particular species.

split t., SYN immune *deviation*.

vibration t., the maximum vibratory or oscillatory movements that an individual can experience and bear without pain; the limit of t. is a function of amplitude and frequency of the vibration and varies with the direction of application.

tol·er·ant (tol'er-ănt). Having the property of tolerance.

tol·er·o·gen (tol'er-ō-jen). A substance that produces immunological tolerance.

tol·er·o·gen·ic (tol'er-ō-jen'ik). Producing immunologic tolerance.

tol·hex·a·mide (tol-hek'să-mīd). SYN glycyclamide.

tol·met·in (tol'met-in). 1-Methyl-5-*p*-toluoylpyrrole-2-acetic acid; an anti-inflammatory drug used in the treatment of rheumatoid arthritis.

tol·naf·tate (tol-naf'tāt). *o*-2-Naphthyl *m,N*-dimethylthiocarbanilate; a topical antifungal agent.

to·lo·ni·um chlo·ride (tō-lō'nē-ŭm). 3-Amino-7-dimethylami-no-2-methylphenazothionium chloride; the medicinal grade of toluidine blue O, used as an antiheparin compound.

Tolosa, E., 20th century Spanish neurosurgeon. SEE T.-Hunt *syndrome*.

tol·pro·pa·mine (tol-prō'pă-mēn). *N,N*-Dimethyl-3-phenyl-3-*p*-tolylpropylamine; a topical antipruritic agent.

tol·u·ene (tol'yū-ēn). A colorless liquid obtained by the dry distillation of tolu and other resinous bodies, and also derived from coal tar; its physical and chemical properties resemble those of benzene. Used in explosives and dyes, and in the extraction of various principles from plants. SYN methylbenzene, toluol.

to·lu·ic ac·id (tō-lū'ik). $CH_3C_6H_4COOH$; Methylbenzoic acid; an oxidation product of xylene.

to·lu·i·dine (tō-lū'i-dēn, -din). Aminotoluene; one of three isomeric substances, $CH_3C_6H_4NH_2$, derived from toluene.

alkaline t. blue O, t. blue O in borax solution, used with heat on semithick sections of epoxy embedded tissues.

t. blue O [C.I. 52040], , a blue basic dye, $C_{15}H_{16}N_3SCl$, used as an antibacterial agent, as a nuclear stain, and to stain metachromatically certain structures (*e.g.,* the granules in mast cells which are believed to contain heparin and cartilage matrix which is rich in chondroitin sulfate), and in electrophoresis to stain RNA, RNase, and mucopolysaccharides; it also antagonizes the anticoagulant action of heparin. SEE ALSO tolonium chloride.

tol·u·ol (tol'ū-ol). SYN toluene.

tol·u·o·yl (tol-ū'ō-il). $CH_3C_6H_4CO-$; the radical of toluic acid.

tol·u·yl·ene red (tol-ū'i-lēn). SYN neutral red.

tol·yl (tol'il). $CH_3C_6H_4-$; the univalent radical of toluene.

Toma's sign. See under sign.

△**-tome. 1.** A cutting instrument, the first element in the compound usually indicating the part that the instrument is designed to cut. **2.** Segment, part, section. **3.** Tomography. **4.** Surgery. [G. *tomos,* cutting, sharp; a cutting (section or segment)]

to·men·tum, to·men·tum ce·re·bri (tō-men'tŭm, tō-men'tŭm ser'ĕ-brī). The numerous small blood vessels passing between the cerebral surface of the pia mater and the cortex of the brain. [L. a stuffing for cushions]

Tomes, Sir Charles S., English dentist, 1846–1928. SEE T.'s *processes,* under *process.*

Tomes, Sir John, English dentist and anatomist, 1815–1895. SEE T.'s *fibers,* under *fiber,* granular *layer.*

Tommaselli, Salvatore, Italian physician, 1834–1906. SEE T.'s *disease.*

to·mo·gram (tō'mō-gram). A radiograph obtained by tomography. [G. *tomos,* a cutting (section) + *gramma,* a writing]

to·mo·graph (tō'mō-graf). The radiographic equipment used in tomography. [G. *tomos,* a cutting (section), + *graphō,* to write]

to·mog·ra·phy (tō-mog'ră-fē). Making a radiographic image of a selected plane by means of reciprocal linear or curved motion of the x-ray tube and film cassette; images of all other planes are blurred ("out of focus") by being relatively displaced on the film. SYN conventional t., planigraphy, planography, sectional radiography, stratigraphy.

computed t. (CT), imaging anatomical information from a cross-sectional plane of the body, each image generated by a computer synthesis of x-ray transmission data obtained in many different directions in a given plane. SYN computerized axial t.

Developed in 1967 by British electronics engineer Godfrey Hounsfield, CT has revolutionized diagnostic medicine. Hounsfield linked x-ray sensors to a computer and worked out a mathematical technique called algebraic reconstruction for assembling images from transmission data. In 1973, the Mayo Clinic began operating the first machine in the U.S. Early machines yielded digital images with at least 100 times the clarity of normal x-rays. Subsequently, the speed and accuracy of machines has improved many times over. CT scans reveal both bone and soft tissues, including organs, muscles, and tumors. Image tones can be adjusted to highlight tissues of similar density, and, through graphics software, the data from multiple cross-sections can be assembled into 3-D imag-

to

es. CT aids diagnosis and surgery or other treatment, including radiation therapy, in which effective dosage is highly dependent on the precise density, size, and location of a tumor.

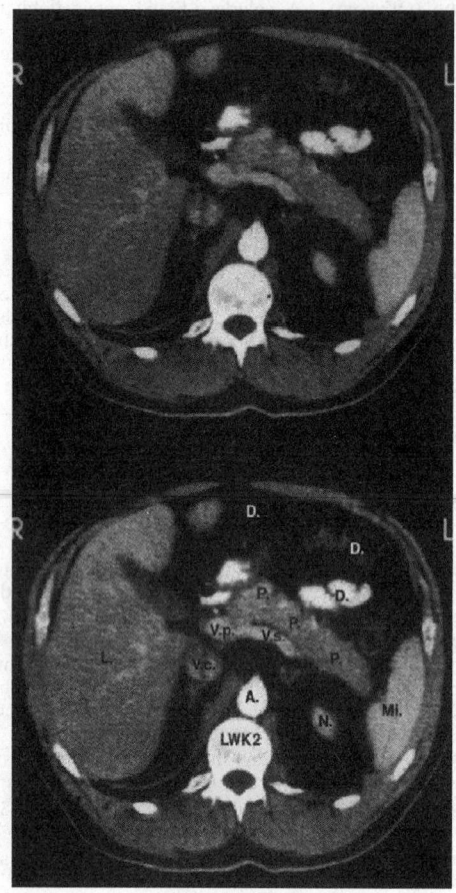

computed tomography

computed tomogram of the upper stomach; view is looking toward the head, from below; taken at the level of the 2nd lumbar vertabra

A = aorta	N = upper pole of left kidney
D = intestinal bends	P = pancreas
L = liver and gallbladder	Vc = lower vena cava
M = spleen	Vp = portal vein with opening of the splenic vein

computerized axial t. (CAT), SYN computed t.

conventional t., SYN tomography.

dynamic computed t., computed t. with rapid injection of contrast medium, usually with sequential scans at only one or a few levels; used to enhance the vascular compartment. SYN dynamic CT.

helical computed t., SYN spiral computed t.

high resolution computed t. (HRCT), computed t. with narrow collimation to reduce volume-averaging and an edge-enhancing reconstruction algorithm to sharpen the image, sometimes with a restricted field of view to minimize the size of pixels in the region imaged; used particularly for lung imaging.

hypocycloidal t., body section radiography using a complex film and tube motion with a pattern resembling a three-leaf clover.

nuclear magnetic resonance t., SYN magnetic resonance *imaging.*

positron emission t. (PET), tomographic images formed by computer analysis of photons detected from annihilation of posi-

trons emitted by radionucldes incorporated into biochemical substances; the images, often quantitated with a color scale, show the uptake and distribution of the substances in the tissue, permitting analysis and localization of metabolic and physiological function.

Because the half-lives of the radionuclides are so short (20 minutes to 2 hours), and the equipment expensive, PET is rarely used in a clinical setting. But since its development in the mid-1970s, it has proved the most important tool yet devised for experimental investigation of the living brain, whether healthy, traumatized, or diseased. With CT and MRI, it represents a new generation of computer imaging techniques that have revolutionized medicine and physiology.

single photon emission computed t. (SPECT), tomographic imaging of metabolic and physiological functions in tissues, the image being formed by computer synthesis of photons of a single energy emitted by radionuclides administered in suitable form to the patient.

spiral computed t., computed t. in which the x-ray tube continuously revolves around the patient, who is simultaneously moved longitudinally; computer interpolation allows reconstruction of standard transverse scans or images in any preferred plane. SYN helical computed t., helical CT, spiral CT.

trispiral t., hypocycloidal t. that allows a much thinner and more uniform plane of focus; used especially for inner ear t.

to·mo·lev·el (tō′mō-lev-el). Obsolete term for the level at which tomography is performed.

to·mo·ma·nia (tō-mō-mā′nē-ă). An irrational desire to use operative procedures by a doctor or a patient. [G. *tomos,* cutting, + *mania,* frenzy]

⌂-tomy. A cutting operation. SEE ALSO -ectomy. [G. *tomē,* incision]

ton·a·pha·sia (tōn-ă-fā′zē-ă). Loss, through cerebral lesion, of the ability to remember tunes. [G. *tonos,* tone, + *a-* priv. + *phasis,* speech]

tone (tōn). 1. A musical sound. 2. The character of the voice expressing an emotion. 3. The tension present in resting muscles. 4. Firmness of the tissues; normal functioning of all the organs. 5. To perform toning. [G. *tonos,* tone, or a tone]

affective t., emotional t., SYN feeling t.

feeling t., the mental state (pleasure, repugnance, etc.) that accompanies every act or thought. SYN affective t., emotional t., affectivity.

fundamental t., the component of lowest frequency in a complex t.

heart t.'s, SYN heart *sounds,* under *sound.*

Traube's double t., a double sound heard on auscultation over the femoral vessels in cases of aortic and tricuspid insufficiency.

ton·er (tō′ner). A solution used in toning.

tongue (tŭng). 1. A mobile mass of muscular tissue covered with mucous membrane, occupying the cavity of the mouth and forming part of its floor, constituting also by its posterior portion the anterior wall of the pharynx. It bears the organ of taste and assists in mastication, deglutition, and articulation. SYN lingua (1) [NA], glossa. 2. A tongue-like structure. SYN lingua (2) [NA]. [A.S. *tunge*]

baked t., the dry blackish t. noted when patients with typhoid fever or other disorders are allowed to become dehydrated.

bald t., SYN atrophic *glossitis.*

beet-t., sometimes used of the t. in pellagra, where intense erythema appears, first at the tip, then along the edges, and finally over the dorsum; there may be pain and increased elevation; the shiny appearance results from edema, not atrophy, except in chronic pellagra.

bifid t., a structural defect of the t. in which the extremity is divided longitudinally for a greater or lesser distance. SEE diglossia. SYN cleft t.

black t., black to yellowish brown discoloration of the dorsum of the t. due to staining by exogenous material such as the components of tobacco; usually superimposed on hairy t. (2) in canines.

a disorder associated with a deficency of nicotinic acid. SYN lingua nigra, melanoglossia, nigrities linguae.

t. of cerebellum, SYN *lingula* of cerebellum.

cleft t., SYN bifid t.

coated t., a t. with a whitish layer on its upper surface, composed of epithelial debris, food particles, and bacteria; often an indication of indigestion or of fever. SYN furred t.

dotted t., one in which each separate papilla is capped with a whitish deposit. SYN stippled t.

fissured t., a painless condition of the t. characterized by numerous grooves or furrows on the dorsal surface. SYN grooved t., lingua fissurata, lingua plicata, scrotal t.

furred t., SYN coated t.

geographic t., idiopathic, asymptomatic erythematous circinate macules, often bounded peripherally by a white band, as a result of atrophy of the filiform papillae; with time the lesions resolve, coalesce, and change in distribution; frequently associated with fissured t.'s. SYN benign migratory glossitis, erythema migrans, erythema migrans linguae, glossitis areata exfoliativa, lingua dissecta, lingua geographica, pityriasis linguae.

grooved t., SYN fissured t.

hairy t., a t. with abnormal elongation of the filiform papillae, resulting in a thickened furry appearance. SYN glossotrichia, trichoglossia.

hobnail t., interstitial glossitis with hypertrophy and verrucous changes in papillae; seen in some cases of late acquired syphilis.

magenta t., purplish red coloration of the t., with edema and flattening of the filiform papillae, occurring in riboflavin deficiency. Cf. cyanosis.

mandibular t., SYN *lingula* of mandible.

raspberry t., strawberry t. that is a dark red color.

red strawberry t., clinical manifestation of Kawasaki's *disease.*

scrotal t., SYN fissured t.

smoker's t., obsolete term for leukoplakia.

stippled t., SYN dotted t.

strawberry t., a t. with a whitish coat through which the enlarged fungiform papillae project as red points, characteristic of scarlet fever and of mucocutaneous lymph node syndrome.

wooden t. of cattle, SYN actinobacillosis.

tongue crib. An appliance used to control visceral (infantile) swallowing and tongue thrusting and to encourage the mature or somatic tongue posture and function.

tongue‑swal·low·ing. A slipping back of the tongue against the pharynx, causing choking.

tongue thrust. The infantile pattern of the suckle‑swallow movement in which the tongue is placed between the incisor teeth or the alveolar ridges during the initial stage of swallowing, resulting sometimes in an anterior open bite.

tongue‑tie. SYN ankyloglossia.

ton·ic (ton′ik). **1.** In a state of continuous unremitting action; denoting especially a muscular contraction. **2.** Invigorating; increasing physical or mental tone or strength. **3.** A remedy purported to restore enfeebled function and promote vigor and a sense of well being; qualified, according to the organ or system on which they are presumed to act, as cardiac, digestive, hematic, vascular, nervine, uterine, general, etc. [G. *tonikos,* fr. *tonos,* tone]

bitter t., a t. of bitter taste, such as quinine, gentian, quassia, etc., which acts chiefly by stimulating the appetite and improving digestion.

tonic t., sustained contractures of skeletal muscle as occur during convulsions.

to·nic·i·ty (tō‑nis′i‑tē). **1.** A state of normal tension of the tissues by virtue of which the parts are kept in shape, alert, and ready to function in response to a suitable stimulus. In the case of muscle, it refers to a state of continuous activity or tension beyond that related to the physical properties; *i.e.,* it is active resistance to stretch; in skeletal muscle it is dependent upon the efferent innervation. SYN tonus. **2.** The osmotic pressure or tension of a solution, usually relative to that of blood. SEE ALSO isotonicity. [G. *tonos,* tone]

coatings of the tongue

underlying illness	clinical symptoms	other findings
nonspecific mouth infection	whitish coating (scales)	connected with reduced nutrient intake in gastritis and enteritis and with fever
oral candidiasis	whitish, membranous specks; difficult to remove, with red edges	evidence of *Candida albicans* in smear
scarlet fever	opaque white coating with redness at tip and edges of tongue	angina, exanthema, evidence of β‑hemolytic streptococci in throat culture
diphtheria	grayish white membranous coating, sickly‑sweet odor	coating difficult to remove, under‑layer bleeds easily; general symptoms
typhus	gray‑white tongue with bright‑red edges	infection by *Salmonella typhi;* general symptoms
uremia	lumpy brown coating on tongue	kidney failure

ton·i·co·clon·ic (ton‑i‑kō‑klon′ik). Both tonic and clonic, referring to muscular spasms. SYN tonoclonic.

to·nin (tō′nin). An enzyme converting angiotensin I to angiotensin II, thus similar to or identical with angiotensin‑converting enzyme.

ton·ing (tōn′ing). The replacing of a silver deposit with one of gold in an impregnated histologic section, by treatment with a solution of gold chloride.

ton·i·tro·pho·bia (tō′ni‑trō‑fō′bē‑ă). SYN brontophobia. [L. *tonitrus,* thunder, + G. *phobos,* fear]

♳**tono‑.** Tone, tension, pressure. [G. *tonos*]

ton·o·clon·ic (ton‑ō‑klon′ik). SYN tonicoclonic.

ton·o·fi·bril (ton‑ō‑fī′bril). One of a system of fibers found in the cytoplasm of epithelial cells. SEE cytoskeleton. SYN epitheliofibril, tenofibril.

ton·o·fil·a·ment (ton‑ō‑fil′ă‑ment). A structural cytoplasmic protein, of a class known as intermediate filaments, bundles of which together form a tonofibril; a t. is made up of a variable number or related proteins, keratins, and is found in all epithelial cells, but is particularly well developed in the epidermis.

ton·o·graph (ton′ō‑graf, tō′nō‑). A recording tonometer. [tono‑ + G. *graphō,* to write]

to·nog·ra·phy (tō‑nog′ră‑fē). Continuous measurement of intra‑

to

ocular pressure by means of a recording tonometer, in order to determine the facility of aqueous outflow.

to·nom·e·ter (tō-nom'ĕ-ter). **1.** An instrument for determining pressure or tension, especially an instrument for determining ocular tension. **2.** A vessel for equilibrating a liquid (*e.g.*, blood) with a gas, usually at a controlled temperature; originally so named because it was used with a very small gas/blood ratio to allow the gas to approach blood oxygen tension and thus serve as a measure of it; now commonly used with a very large gas/blood ratio to adjust the blood to the oxygen pressure of the gas. SYN aerotonometer (2). [tono- + G. *metron*, measure]

applanation t., an instrument for determining ocular tension by application of a small flat disk to the cornea.

Gärtner's t., an apparatus for estimating the blood pressure by noting the force, expressed by the height of a column of mercury, needed to arrest pulsation in a finger encircled by a compressing ring.

Goldmann's applanation t., an applanation t. that flattens only 3 sq mm of cornea, used with a slitlamp.

Mackay-Marg t., a recording electronic applanation t.

Mueller electronic t., a Schiötz type t. that electronically indicates the extent of corneal indentation; may also have an attached recorder for continuous pressure readings (tonography).

pneumatic t., a recording applanation t. operated by compressed gas.

Schiötz t., an instrument that measures ocular tension by indicating the ease with which the cornea is indented.

to·nom·e·try (tō-nom'ĕ-trē). **1.** Measurement of the tension of a part, *e.g.*, intravascular tension or blood pressure. **2.** Measurement of ocular tension.

ton·o·phant (tō'nō-fant, ton'ō-). An instrument for visualizing sound waves. [tono- + G. *phainō*, to appear]

ton·o·plast (tō'nō-plast, ton'ō-). An intracellular structure or vacuole. [tono- + G. *plastos*, formed]

to·nos·cil·lo·graph (tō-nos'i-lō-graf). An instrument that produces graphic records of arterial and capillary pressures as well as of individual pulse characters. [tono- + L. *oscillo*, to swing, + G. *graphō*, to write]

to·no·top·ic (tō-nō-top'ik). Denoting a spatial arrangement of structures such that certain tone frequencies are transmitted, as in the auditory pathway. [tono- + G. *topos*, place]

to·no·tro·pic (tō-nō-trop'ik). Denoting the shortening of the resting length of a muscle. [G. *tonikos, tonos*, tone, + *tropos*, a turning]

ton·sil (ton'sil). **1.** Any collection of lymphoid tissue. **2.** SYN palatine t. [L. *tonsilla*, a stake, in pl. the tonsils]

cerebellar t., a rounded lobule on the undersurface of each cerebellar hemisphere, continuous medially with the uvula of the cerebellar vermis. SYN tonsilla cerebelli [NA], amygdala cerebelli.

eustachian t., SYN tubal t.

faucial t., SYN palatine t.

Gerlach's t., SYN tubal t.

laryngeal t.'s, SYN *folliculi* lymphatici laryngei, under *folliculus*.

lingual t., a collection of lymphoid follicles on the posterior or pharyngeal portion of the dorsum of the tongue. SYN tonsilla lingualis [NA].

Luschka's t., SYN pharyngeal t.

palatine t., a large oval mass of lymphoid tissue embedded in the lateral wall of the oral pharynx on either side between the pillars of the fauces. SYN tonsilla palatina [NA], tonsilla [NA], faucial t., tonsil (2).

pharyngeal t., a collection of more or less closely aggregated lymphoid nodules on the posterior wall and roof of the nasopharynx, the hypertrophy of which constitutes the morbid condition called adenoids. SYN tonsilla pharyngealis [NA], tonsilla adenoidea [✶] [NA], Luschka's gland (1), Luschka's t., third t.

submerged t., a faucial t. that is flat and lying below the level of the pillars of the fauces.

third t., SYN pharyngeal t.

tubal t., a collection of lymphoid nodules near the pharyngeal opening of the auditory tube. SYN tonsilla tubaria [NA], eustachian t., Gerlach's t.

ton·sil·la, pl. **ton·sil·lae** (ton-sil'ă, -ē) [NA]. SYN palatine *tonsil.* [L. (see tonsil)]

t. adenoi′dea [NA], [✶]official alternate term for pharyngeal *tonsil.*

t. cerebel′li [NA], SYN cerebellar *tonsil.*

t. intestina′lis, SEE Peyer's *patches*, under *patch.*

t. lingua′lis [NA], SYN lingual *tonsil.*

t. palati′na [NA], SYN palatine *tonsil.*

t. pharyngea′lis [NA], SYN pharyngeal *tonsil.*

t. tuba′ria [NA], SYN tubal *tonsil.*

ton·sil·lar, ton·sil·lary (ton'si-lăr, ton'si-lă-rē). Relating to a tonsil, especially the palatine tonsil. SYN amygdaline (3).

ton·sil·lec·to·my (ton'si-lek'tō-mē). Removal of the entire tonsil. [tonsil + G. *ektomē*, excision]

ton·sil·lith (ton'si-lith). SYN tonsillolith.

ton·sil·li·tis (ton'si-lī'tis). Inflammation of a tonsil, especially of the palatine tonsil. [tonsil + G. *-itis*, inflammation]

lacunar t., inflammation of the mucous membrane lining the tonsillar crypts.

Vincent's t., angina limited chiefly to the tonsils, caused by Vincent's organisms (bacillus and spirillum).

△tonsillo-. Tonsil. [L. *tonsilla*]

ton·sil·lo·lith (ton-sil'ō-lith). A calcareous concretion in a distended tonsillar crypt. SYN tonsillar calculus, tonsillith. [tonsillo- + G. *lithos*, stone]

ton·sil·lop·a·thy (ton'si-lop'ă-thē). Disease of the tonsil. [tonsillo- + G. *pathos*, suffering]

ton·sil·lo·tome (ton-sil'ō-tōm). An instrument, sometimes modelled after a guillotine, for use in cutting away a portion or all of a hypertrophied tonsil. [tonsillo- + G. *tomos*, cutting]

ton·sil·lot·o·my (ton'si-lot'ō-mē). The cutting away of a portion or all of a hypertrophied faucial tonsil. [tonsillo- + G. *tomē*, incision]

to·nus (tō'nŭs). SYN tonicity (1). [L., fr. G. *tonos*]

baseline t., intrauterine pressure between contractions during labor.

myogenic t., contraction of a muscle caused by intrinsic properties of the muscle or by its intrinsic innervation.

neurogenic t., contraction of a muscle caused by the influence of its extrinsic nerve supply.

Tooth, Howard H., English physician, 1856–1925. Tooth, pl. teeth. SEE Charcot-Marie-T. *disease.* SYN dens (1) [NA].

TOOTH

tooth, pl. **teeth** (tūth, tēth). One of the hard conical structures set in the alveoli of the upper and lower jaws, used in mastication and assisting in articulation. A t. is a dermal structure composed of dentin and encased in cementum on the anatomic root and enamel on its anatomic crown. It consists of a root buried in the alveolus, a neck covered by the gum, and a crown, the exposed portion. In the center is the pulp cavity filled with a connective tissue reticulum containing a jelly-like substance (dental pulp) and blood vessels and nerves that enter through a canal at the apex of the root. The 20 deciduous teeth or primary teeth appear between the sixth and ninth and the 24th month of life; these exfoliate and are replaced by the 32 permanent teeth appearing between the fifth and seventh year and the 17th to 23rd year. There are four kinds of teeth: incisor, canine, premolar, and molar. [A.S. *tōth*]

acrylic resin t., a t. made of acrylic resin.

anatomic teeth, artificial teeth that duplicate the anatomic forms of natural teeth.

ankylosed t., SEE dental *ankylosis.*

anterior teeth, the central incisor, lateral incisor, and cuspid teeth, which comprise the organs for incision and are located in the front portion of the jaws. SYN oral teeth.

t. arrangement, (1) The placement of teeth on a denture base with definite objectives in mind. **(2)** The setting of teeth on temporary bases.

auditory teeth, tooth-shaped formations or ridges occurring on the vestibular lip of the limbus lamina spiralis of the cochlear duct. SYN dentes acustici [NA], Corti's auditory teeth, Huschke's auditory teeth.

baby t., SYN deciduous t.

back teeth, all teeth posterior to the canines.

bicuspid t., SYN premolar t.

buck t., an anterior t. in labioversion.

canine t., a t. having a crown of thick conical shape and a long, slightly flattened conical root; there are two canine teeth in each jaw, one on either side adjacent to the distal surface of the lateral incisors, in both the deciduous and the permanent dentition. SYN dens caninus [NA], canine (3), cuspid t., cuspidate t., cuspid (2), dens angularis, dens cuspidatus, eye t.

carnassial t., (1) a t. adapted to shear flesh; **(2)** the last upper premolar or first lower molar t. of certain carnivores.

cheek t., SYN molar t.

Corti's auditory teeth, SYN auditory teeth.

crossbite teeth, posterior teeth designed to permit the modified cusps of the upper teeth to be positioned in the fossae of the lower teeth.

cuspid t., cuspidate t., SYN canine t.

cuspless t., (1) a t. devoid of cusp formation; **(2)** severe abrasion of an occlusal surface; **(3)** a type of artificial denture t.

cutting teeth, the maxillary and mandibular anterior teeth.

dead t., a misnomer for pulpless t.

deciduous t., a t. of the first set of teeth, comprising 20 in all, that erupts between the mean ages of 6 and 28 months of life. SYN dens deciduus [NA], baby t., deciduous dentition, dens lacteus, first dentition, milk t., primary dentition, primary t., temporary t.

devitalized t., a misnomer for a pulpless t.

extruded teeth, SEE *extrusion* of a tooth.

eye t., SYN canine t.

fluoridated teeth, teeth exposed to fluorine salts during odontogenesis.

fused teeth, teeth joined by dentin as a result of embryological fusion or juxtaposition of two adjacent tooth germs.

geminated teeth, a developmental anomaly arising from the attempted division of one t. bud, resulting in incomplete formation of two teeth and usually manifest as a bifid crown upon a single root.

ghost t., a t. with reduced radiodensity seen in regional odontodysplasia.

green t., green to brown discoloration of the primary teeth associated with erythroblastosis fetalis and caused by deposition of hemoglobin pigments in the developing teeth.

Horner's teeth, incisor teeth having a horizontal hypoplastic groove.

Huschke's auditory teeth, SYN auditory teeth.

Hutchinson's teeth, the teeth of congenital syphilis in which the incisal edge is notched and narrower than the cervical area. SEE ALSO Hutchinson's crescentic *notch.* SYN notched teeth, screwdriver teeth, syphilitic teeth.

impacted t., (1) a t. whose normal eruption is prevented by adjacent teeth or bone; **(2)** a t. that has been driven into the alveolar process or surrounding tissue as a result of trauma.

incisor t., a t. with a chisel-shaped crown and a single conical tapering root; there are four of these teeth in the anterior part of each jaw, in both the deciduous and the permanent dentitions. SYN dens incisivus [NA].

metal insert teeth, prosthetic teeth containing metal cutting surfaces in the occlusal surfaces.

migrating teeth, teeth which are changing position under natural forces.

milk t., SYN deciduous t.

molar t., a t. having a somewhat quadrangular crown with four

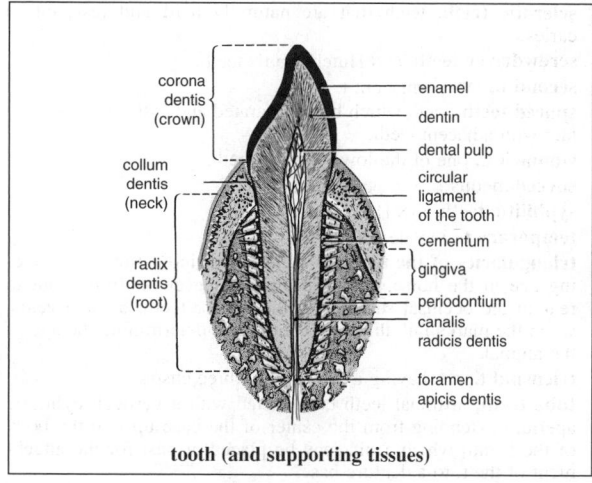

corona dentis (crown) — enamel — dentin — dental pulp
collum dentis (neck) — circular ligament of the tooth
radix dentis (root) — cementum — gingiva — periodontium — canalis radicis dentis — foramen apicis dentis

tooth (and supporting tissues)

or five cusps on the grinding surface; the root is bifid in the lower jaw, but there are three conical roots in the upper jaw; there are six molars in each jaw, three on either side behind the premolars in the permanent dentition; in the deciduous dentition there are but four molars in each jaw, two on either side behind the canines. SYN dens molaris [NA], cheek t., molar (2), multicuspid t.

mottled t., SEE mottled *enamel.*

multicuspid t., SYN molar t.

natal t., a predeciduous supernumerary t. present at birth.

neonatal t., a t. erupting up to 30 days after birth.

nonanatomic teeth, (1) teeth with occlusal surfaces not based on anatomic forms; **(2)** artificial teeth so designed that the occlusal surfaces are not copied from natural forms, but rather are given forms which in the opinion of the designer seem more nearly to fulfill the requirements of mastication, tissue tolerance, etc.

nonvital t., a t. with a nonvital pulp.

normally posed t., a t. in correct spatial relationship with its antagonist.

notched teeth, SYN Hutchinson's teeth.

oral teeth, SYN anterior teeth.

pegged t., a conical t. whose sides converge from the cervical to the incisal region.

permanent t., one of the 32 teeth belonging to the second or permanent dentition; eruption of the permanent teeth begins from the fifth to the seventh year, and is not completed until the seventeenth to the twenty-third year, when the last of the wisdom teeth appears. SYN dens permanens [NA], dens succedaneus, second t., secondary dentition, succedaneous dentition, succedaneous t.

perpetually growing t., a physiologic phenomenon whereby the t. continually or constantly grows, calcifies, and erupts; *e.g.,* the rat incisor t. SYN persistently growing t.

persistently growing t., SYN perpetually growing t.

plastic teeth, artificial teeth constructed of synthetic resins.

posterior teeth, the bicuspid and molar teeth which comprise the organs of mastication and are located in the back part of the jaws.

premolar t., a t. usually having two tubercles or cusps on the grinding surface and a flattened root, single in the lower jaw and upper second premolar, and furrowed in the upper first premolar. There are four premolars in each jaw, two on either side between the canine and the molars; there are no premolars in the deciduous dentition. SYN dens premolaris [NA], bicuspid t., dens bicuspidus.

primary t., SYN deciduous t.

protruding teeth, teeth extending beyond the normal contour of the dental arches; usually in an anterior direction.

pulpless t., a t. with a nonvital or necrotic pulp, or one from which the pulp has been extirpated.

to

sclerotic teeth, teeth that are naturally hard and resistant to caries.

screwdriver teeth, SYN Hutchinson's teeth.

second t., SYN permanent t.

spaced teeth, teeth which have separated and lost proximal contact with adjacent teeth.

stomach t., one of the lower canine teeth.

succedaneous t., SYN permanent t.

syphilitic teeth, SYN Hutchinson's teeth.

temporary t., SYN deciduous t.

triangularity of the teeth, a well-marked indication of advancing age in the horse, shown by increasing depth from front to rear in the occlusal surfaces of the incisor teeth; at nine years, when the marks fail, this sign is of use in determining the age of the animal.

tricuspid t., a t. having a crown with three cusps.

tube teeth, artificial teeth constructed with a vertical, cylindric aperture extending from the center of the base up into the body of the t. into which a pin may be placed or cast for the attachment of the t. to a denture base.

Turner's t., enamel hypoplasia involving a solitary permanent t.; related to infection in the primary t. that preceded it or to trauma during odontogenesis.

unerupted t., (1) a t. prior to emergence; **(2)** a t. unable to break out or emerge from the dental alveolar tissues into the oral cavity.

vital t., a t. with a living pulp.

wisdom t., SYN third *molar.*

wolf t., a rudimentary first premolar t. of the horse, usually appearing in the upper jaw.

zero degree teeth, prosthetic teeth having no cusp angles in relation to the horizontal.

---

tooth·ache (tūth′āk). Pain in a tooth due to the condition of the pulp or periodontal ligament resulting from caries, infection, or trauma. SYN dentalgia, odontalgia, odontodynia.

tooth-borne. A term used to describe a prosthesis or part of a prosthesis which depends entirely upon the abutment teeth for support.

△**top-.** SEE topo-.

top·ag·no·sis (top-ag-nō′sis). Inability to localize tactile sensations. SYN topoanesthesia. [top- + G. *a-* priv. + *gnōsis,* recognition]

to·pal·gia (tō-pal′jē-ă). Pain localized in one spot; a symptom occurring in neuroses whereby localized pain, without evident organic basis, is experienced. [top- + G. *algos,* pain]

top·es·the·sia (top′es-thē′zē-ă). The ability to localize a light touch applied to any part of the skin. [top- + G. *aisthēsis,* sensation]

Töpfer, Alfred E., German physician, *1858. SEE T.'s *test.*

to·pha·ceous (tō-fā′shŭs). Sandy; gritty; pertaining to or manifesting the features of a tophus. [L. *tophaceus*]

to·phi (tō′fī). Plural of tophus.

to·phus, pl. **to·phi** (tō′fŭs, tō′fī). **1.** SEE gouty t. **2.** A salivary calculus, or tartar. [L. a calcareous deposit from springs, tufa]

gouty t., a deposit of uric acid and urates in periarticular fibrous tissue, cartilage of the external ear, or kidney, in gout. SYN arthritic calculus, uratoma.

top·i·ca (top′i-kă). Remedies for local external use. [neut. pl. of Mod. L. *topicus,* local]

top·i·cal (top′i-kăl). Relating to a definite place or locality; local. [G. *topikos,* fr. *topos,* place]

Topinard, Paul, French anthropologist, 1830–1912. SEE T.'s facial *angle, line.*

to·pis·tic (tō-pis′tik). Denoting an anatomically defined region in the nervous system. [G. *topos,* place]

△**topo-, top-.** Place, topical. [G. *topos*]

top·o·an·es·the·sia (top′ō-an-es-thē′zē-ă, tō′pō-). SYN topagnosis. [topo- + anesthesia]

top·og·no·sis, top·og·no·sia (top-og-nō′sis, -nō′zē-ă). Recogni-

tion of the location of a sensation; in the case of touch, topesthesia. [topo- + G. *gnōsis,* knowledge]

top·o·gom·e·ter (top-ō-gom′ĕ-ter). A movable fixation target attached to the front of a keratometer, used in fitting contact lenses to measure the curvatures of the cornea in its peripheral zones. [topo- + G. *gonia,* angle, + *metron,* measure]

to·pog·ra·phy (tō-pog′ră-fē). In anatomy, the description of any part of the body, especially in relation to a definite and limited area of the surface. [topo- + G. *graphē,* a writing]

to·po·i·so·mer·ase (tō′pō-i-som′er-ās). A type of enzyme converting (isomerizing) one topological version of DNA into another; acts by catalyzing the breakage and reformation of DNA phosphodiester linkages. [topo- + isomerase]

Topolanski, Alfred, Austrian ophthalmologist, 1861–1960. SEE T.'s *sign.*

to·pol·o·gy (tō-pol′ō-jē). **1.** SYN regional *anatomy.* **2.** The study of the dimensions of personality. [topo- + G. *logos,* study]

top·o·nar·co·sis (top′ō-nar-kō′sis). A localized cutaneous anesthesia. [topo- + narcosis]

top·o·nym (tō′pō-nim). A regional term; one designating a region as distinguished from the name of a structure, system, or organ. [topo- + G. *onyma,* name]

to·pon·y·my (tō-pon′i-mē). Topical or regional nomenclature, as distinguished from organonymy. [topo- + G. *onyma,* name]

top·o·path·o·gen·e·sis (tō′pō-path-ō-jen′ĕ-sis). Topography of lesions related to their pathogenesis. [topo- + pathogenesis]

top·o·pho·bia (tō-pō-fō′bē-ă). A neurotic dread of or related to a particular place or locality. [topo- + G. *phobos,* fear]

top·o·phy·lax·is (tō′pō-fī-lak′sis). Prevention of arsphenamine shock by a tourniquet applied to the limb above the site of injection and its slow release five or six minutes later. [topo- + G. *phylaxis,* protection]

top·o·scope (top′ō-skōp). An apparatus to project the electrical activity of the cerebral cortex as a spatial coordinate visual system. [topo- + G. *skopeō,* to view]

top·o·therm·es·the·si·om·e·ter (top′ō-therm′es-the-zē-om′ĕ-ter). A device for determining the temperature sense in different parts of the surface. [topo- + G. *thermē,* heat, + *aisthēsis,* sensation, + *metron,* measure]

TORCH Acronym for *t*oxoplasmosis, *o*ther infections, *r*ubella, *c*ytomegalorvirus infection, and *h*erpes simplex. SEE TORCH *syndrome.*

tor·cu·lar he·roph·i·li (tōr′kyū-lăr hĕ-rof′i-lī). Archaic term for *confluence* of sinuses. [L. wine-press of *Herophilus,* fr. *torqueo,* to twist]

Torek, Franz J.A., U.S. surgeon, 1861–1938. SEE T. *operation.*

to·ric (tō′rik). Relating to, or having the curvature of, a torus.

Torkildsen, Arne, 20th century Norwegian neurosurgeon. SEE T. *shunt.*

Tornwaldt, Gustavus Ludwig, German physician, 1843–1910. SEE T.'s *abscess, cyst, disease, syndrome.*

to·rose, to·rous (tō′rōs, -rŭs). Bulging; knobby. [L. *torosus,* fleshy, fr. *torus,* a knot, bulge]

tor·pent (tōr′pent). **1.** SYN torpid. **2.** A benumbing agent. [L. *torpeo,* pres. p. *-ens,* to be sluggish]

tor·pid (tōr′pid). Inactive; sluggish. SYN torpent (1). [L. *torpidus,* fr. *torpeo,* to be sluggish]

tor·pid·i·ty (tōr-pid′i-tē). SYN torpor.

tor·por (tōr′per, pōr). Inactivity, sluggishness. SYN torpidity. [L. sluggishness, numbness]

t. ret′inae, an obsolete term for a form of nyctalopia, the retina responding only to bright luminous stimuli.

torque (T) (tōrk). **1.** A rotatory force. **2.** In dentistry, a torsion force applied to a tooth to produce or maintain crown or root movement. [L. *torqueo,* to twist]

torr (tōr). A unit of pressure sufficient to support a 1-mm column of mercury at 0°C against the standard acceleration of gravity at 45° north latitude (980.621 cm/sec²); equivalent to 1333.224 dynes/cm², 1.333224 millibars, 1.35951 cm H_2O, 133.3224 newtons/m² (or Pa); one standard atmosphere equals 760 t. [Evangelista *Torricelli.*]

Torre, Douglas P., U.S. dermatologist, *1919. SEE T.'s *syndrome;* Muir-Torre *syndrome.*

tor·re·fac·tion (tōr-ē-fak′shŭn). Parching or drying by heat; a pharmaceutical operation for rendering drugs friable. [L. *torre-facio,* pp. *-factus,* to make dry by heat, fr. *torreo,* to parch]

tor·re·fy (tōr′ē-fī). To parch.

Torricelli, Evangelista, Italian scientist, 1608–1647. SEE torr.

torsade de pointes (tōr-săd dĕ pwant′). "Twisting of the points" a form of ventricular tachycardia nearly always due to medications and characterized by a long QT interval and a "short-long-short" sequence in the beat preceding its onset. The QRS complexes during this rhythm tend to show a series of complexes points up followed by complexes points down often with a narrow waist between. At one time referred to as "cardiac ballet". [Fr. *torsade,* fringe, twist, or coil, + *pointe,* point or tip (euphonious for "wave burst")]

tor·si·om·e·ter (tōr-si-om′ĕ-ter). An obsolete term for an instrument for measuring ocular torsion, cycloductions, and cyclophorias.

tor·sion (tōr′shŭn). **1.** A twisting or rotation of a part upon its long axis. **2.** Twisting of the cut end of an artery to arrest hemorrhage. **3.** Rotation of the eye around its anteroposterior axis. SEE ALSO intorsion, extorsion, dextrotorsion, levotorsion. [L. *torsio,* fr. *torqueo,* to twist]

  t. of appendage, t. of testis or epididymis

  extravaginal t., high t. above insertion of tunica vaginalis.

  intravaginal t., t. below insertion of tunica vaginalis. SEE bell clapper *deformity.*

  perinatal t., tends to be extravaginal type.

  t. of testis, rotation producing ischemia of testis.

  t. testis, SYN spermatic *cord.*

  t. of a tooth, rotation of a tooth in its socket.

tor·sion·om·e·ter (tōr-shŭn-om′ĕ-ter). A device for measuring the degree of rotation of the spinal column.

tor·si·ver·sion (tōr-si-ver′shŭn). A malposition of a tooth in which it is rotated on its long axis. SYN torsive occlusion, torsoclusion (2).

tor·so (tōr′sō). The trunk; the body without relation to head or extremities. [It.]

tor·so·clu·sion (tōr′sō-klū-zhŭn). **1.** Acupressure performed by entering the needle in the tissues parallel with the artery, then turning it so that it crosses the artery transversely, and passing it into the tissues on the opposite side of the vessel. **2.** SYN torsiversion. [L. *torqueo,* to twist, + *claudo* or *cludo,* to close]

tor·ti·col·lar (tōr-ti-kol′ăr). Relating to or marked by torticollis.

tor·ti·col·lis (tōr-ti-kol′is). A contraction, often spasmodic, of the muscles of the neck, chiefly those supplied by the spinal accessory nerve; the head is drawn to one side and usually rotated so that the chin points to the other side. SYN accessory cramp, collum distortum, loxia, wry neck, wryneck. [L. *tortus,* twisted, + *collum,* neck]

  congenital t., t. due to a unilateral fibrous tumor in the sternocleidomastoid muscle, present at birth as a swelling that may subside or may lead to t. by shortening of the muscle.

  dermatogenic t., painful stiff neck with limitation of motion due to extensive skin lesion in the area.

  dystonic t., SYN spasmodic t.

  fixed t., persistent contracture of cervical muscles on one side.

  hysterical t., t. believed to be psychosomatic in etiology. SEE hysteria.

  intermittent t., SYN t. spastica.

  labyrinthine t., t. due to vestibular disorder.

  ocular t., t. incident to paralysis of an extraocular muscle, especially an oblique muscle.

  psychogenic t., spasmodic contractions of the neck muscles, of psychosomatic origin. SEE ALSO spasmodic t.

  rheumatic t., SYN symptomatic t.

  spasmodic t., a disorder of unknown cause, manifested as a restricted dystonia, localized to some of the neck muscles, especially the sternomastoid and trapezius; occurs in adults and tends to progress slowly; the head movements increase with standing

and walking and decrease with contractual stimuli, *e.g.,* touching the chin or neck. SYN dystonic t., rotatory spasm, rotatory tic.

  t. spas′tica, stiff neck due to spasm of the neck muscles. SYN intermittent t.

  spurious t., stiffness of the neck due to caries, malformation, or fracture of the cervical vertebrae.

  symptomatic t., stiff neck due to cervical or neck myositis, chiefly of the sternocleidomastoid, occurring especially in children. SYN rheumatic t.

tor·ti·pel·vis (tōr-ti-pel′vis). Twisted pelvis.

tor·tu·ous (tōr′chū-ŭs). Having many curves; full of turns and twists. [L. *tortuosus,* fr. *torqueo,* to twist]

tor·u·lo·ma (tōr-yū-lō′mă). SYN cryptococcoma. [fr. *Torula,* old name for *Cryptococcus,* + G. *-oma,* tumor]

Tor·u·lop·sis (tōr-ū-lop′sis). A genus of yeasts with smaller blastoconidia (2 to 4 nm) with a wide attachment to the parent cell; the species *T. glabrata* is the causative agent of torulopsosis, usually in compromised hosts.

tor·u·lop·so·sis (tōr-ū-lop′sō-sis). An usually opportunistic infection caused by *Torulopsis glabrata* and seen in patients with severe underlying disease or in immunocompromised patients; the pattern of disease may be bronchopulmonary, genitourinary, or septicemic.

tor·u·lus, pl. **tor·u·li** (tōr′yū-lŭs, -lī). A minute elevation or papilla. [L. dim. of *torus,* a protuberance, swelling]

  tor′uli tact′iles [NA], SYN tactile *elevations,* under *elevation.*

to·rus, pl. **to·ri** (tō′rŭs, tō′rī). **1.** A geometrical figure formed by the revolution of a circle round the base of any of its arcs, such as the convex molding at the base of a pillar. **2** [NA]. A rounded swelling, such as that caused by a contracting muscle. [L. swelling, knot, bulge]

  t. fronta′lis, a slight prominence on the frontal bone at the root of the nose.

  t. levator′ius [NA], SYN levator *cushion.*

  mandibular t., t. mandibula′ris, an exostosis protruding from the lingual aspect of the mandible, usually opposite the premolar teeth.

  t. ma′nus, archaic term for the carpal bones.

  t. occipita′lis, an occasional ridge near the superior nuchal line of the occipital bone.

  palatine t., t. palati′nus, an exostosis protruding from the midline of the hard palate.

  t. tuba′rius [NA], a ridge in the naso-pharyngeal wall posterior to the opening of the auditory (eustachian) tube, caused by the projection of the cartilaginous portion of this tube. SYN eustachian cushion, tubal prominence.

  t. ureter′icus, SYN interureteric *fold.*

  t. uteri′nus, a transverse ridge on the back part of the cervix of the uterus, formed by the junction of the rectouterine folds.

TOS Abbreviation for thoracic outlet *syndrome.*

tos·yl (tō′sil). Toluenesulfonyl radical, widely used to block amino groups in the course of organic syntheses of drugs and other biologically active compounds.

tos·yl·ate (tō′si-lāt). USAN-approved contraction for *p*-toluenesulfonate.

to·tem (tō′tem). An object (usually an animal or plant) serving as the emblem of a family or clan and often as a reminder of its ancestry; something that serves as a revered symbol. [Amer. Indian]

to·tem·ism (tō′tem-izm). Belief in a kinship with, or a mystical relationship between, a group or individual and a totem.

to·tem·is·tic (tō-tem-is′tik). Relating to totemism.

to·tip·o·ten·cy, to·tip·o·tence (tō-ti-pō′ten-sē, tō-tip′ō-tens). The ability of a cell to differentiate into any type of cell and thus form a new organism or regenerate any part of an organism; *e.g.,* a fertilized ovum, or a small excised portion of a *Planaria,* which is capable of regenerating a complete new organism. [L. *totus,* entire, + *potentia,* power]

to·tip·o·tent, to·ti·po·ten·tial (tō-tip′ŏ-tent, tō′ti-pō-ten′shăl). Relating to totipotency.

touch (tŭch). **1.** The sense by which slight contact with the skin or mucous membrane is appreciated. SYN tactile sense. **2.** Digital examination. [Fr. *toucher*]

royal t., a touching of a patient by the king, which was thought to be curative; usually applied to patients with scrofula, but also done with patients with enlarged lymph glands (buboes) of plague.

Touraine, Albert, French dermatologist, 1883–1961. SEE Christ-Siemens-Touraine *syndrome.*

Tourette. SEE Gilles de la Tourette.

Tournay, Auguste, French ophthalmologist, 1878–1969. SEE T. *sign.*

tour·ni·quet (tūr′ni-ket). An instrument for temporarily arresting the flow of blood to or from a distal part by pressure applied with an encircling device. [Fr. fr. *tourner,* to turn]

Dupuytren's t., an instrument for compression on the abdominal aorta.

Esmarch t., a narrow hard rubber t. with a chain fastener. SYN Esmarch bandage.

Rummel t., a t. fashioned by passing an umbilical tape around a vessel and bringing both ends through a short red rubber catheter. The t. can be tightened and secured with a perpendicularly placed hemostat at the end of the catheter farthest from the vessel.

Tourtual, Kaspar, Prussian anatomist, 1802–1865. SEE T.'s *membrane, sinus.*

Touton, Karl, German dermatologist, *1858. SEE T. giant *cell.*

Tovell, Ralph M., U.S. anesthesiologist, 1901–1967. SEE T. *tube.*

Towne, E.B., U.S. otolaryngologist, 1883–1957. SEE T. *projection,* projection *radiograph, view.*

⚠**tox-.** SEE toxico-.

tox·al·bu·mins (toks-al-byū′minz). Phytotoxins that inhibit protein synthesis.

tox·a·ne·mia (tok-să-nē′mē-ă). Anemia resulting from the effects of a hemolytic poison. [G. *toxikon,* poison, + anemia]

tox·a·phene (tok′să-fēn). A chlorinated hydrocarbon insecticide.

Tox·as·ca·ris le·o·ni·na (tok-sas′kă-ris lē-ō-nī′nă). An ascarid nematode of the dog that differs from *Toxocara* in that the larvae do not migrate through the lungs; the entire developmental cycle occurs in the gut. This parasite has been found in humans in a few instances and is a cause of visceral larva migrans in children, though less frequently implicated than is *Toxocara canis.* [G. *toxon,* bow, + *Ascaris*]

tox·e·mia (tok-sē′mē-ă). **1.** Clinical manifestations observed during certain infectious diseases, assumed to be caused by toxins and other noxious substances elaborated by the infectious agent; in certain infections by Gram-negative bacteria, endotoxins probably play a role when the bacterial cell wall breaks down, releasing the complex lipopolysaccharide; however, the role of other bacterial substances is unclear, except in the case of the specific exotoxins such as those of diphtheria and tetanus. **2.** The clinical syndrome caused by toxic substances in the blood. **3.** A lay term referring to the hypertensive disorders of pregnancy. SYN toxicemia. [G. *toxikon,* poison, + *haima,* blood]

pregnancy t. of sheep, a disease of preparturient ewes characterized primarily by impaired nervous function; the primary predisposing cause is undernutrition in late pregnancy. SYN ovine acetonemia.

tox·e·mic (tok-sē′mik). Pertaining to, affected by, or manifesting the features of toxemia.

⚠**toxi-.** SEE toxico-.

tox·ic (tok′sik). **1.** SYN poisonous. **2.** Pertaining to a toxin. [G. *toxikon,* an arrow-poison]

tox·i·cant (tok′si-kant). **1.** SYN poisonous. **2.** Any poisonous agent, specifically an alcoholic or other poison, causing symptoms of what is popularly called intoxication.

tox·i·ce·mia (tok-si-sē′mē-ă). SYN toxemia.

tox·ic·i·ty (tok-sis′i-tē). The state of being poisonous.

oxygen t., a body disturbance resulting from breathing high partial pressures of oxygen; characterized by visual and hearing abnormalities, unusual fatigue while breathing, muscular twitching, anxiety, confusion, incoordination, and convulsions; al-

though the mechanism for development of the condition is obscure, a disruption of enzymatic activity is likely, perhaps as a result of free radical formation. SYN oxygen poisoning.

⚠**toxico-, tox-, toxi-, toxo-.** Poison, toxin. [G. *toxikon,* bow, hence (arrow) poison]

Tox·i·co·den·dron (tok′si-kō-den′dron). A genus of poisonous plants (family Anacardiaceae) comprising those members of the genus *Rhus* with smooth fruits and foliage that contain urushiol, which produces a contact dermatitis (rhus dermatitis); species include poison ivy (*T. radicans*), poison oak (*T. diversilobum*), and poison sumac (*T. vernix*) [toxico- + G. *dendron,* tree]

tox·i·co·der·ma (tok′si-kō-der′mă). Any skin disease caused by a poison or by a toxin-producing microorganism. SYN toxicodermatosis. [toxico- + G. *derma,* skin]

tox·i·co·der·ma·ti·tis (tok′si-kō-der′mă-tī′tis). Inflammation of the skin caused by the action of a poison.

tox·i·co·der·ma·to·sis (tok′si-kō-der′mă-tō′sis). SYN toxicoderma.

tox·i·co·gen·ic (tok′si-kō-jen′ik). **1.** Producing a poison. **2.** Caused by a poison. [toxico- + G. *-gen,* producing]

tox·i·coid (tok′si-koyd). Having an action like that of a poison; temporarily poisonous. [toxico- + G. *eidos,* resemblance]

tox·i·co·log·ic (tok′si-kō-loj′ik). Relating to toxicology.

tox·i·col·o·gist (tok-si-kol′ŏ-jist). A specialist or expert in toxicology.

tox·i·col·o·gy (tok-si-kol′ŏ-jē). The science of poisons, including their source, chemical composition, action, tests, and antidotes. [toxico- + G. *logos,* study]

tox·i·co·path·ic (tok′si-kō-path′ik). Denoting any morbid state caused by the action of a poison.

tox·i·co·pho·bia (tok′si-kō-fō′bē-ă). Morbid fear of being poisoned. SYN toxiphobia. [toxico- + G. *phobos,* fear]

tox·i·co·sis (tok-si-kō′sis). Any disease of toxic origin. SYN systemic poisoning. [toxico- + G. *-osis,* condition]

endogenic t., SYN autointoxication.

exogenic t., any disease caused by a poison introduced from without and not generated within the body.

slaframine t., a disease of horses and cattle caused by ingestion of forages infected with the fungus *Rhizoctonia leguminicola,* which produces the toxic alkaloid slaframine, and characterized by profuse salivation. SEE ALSO slaframine.

thyroid t., SYN triiodothyronine t.

triiodothyronine t., T₃ t., hyperthyroidism resulting from excessive circulating 3,5,3′-triiodothyronine. SYN thyroid t.

tox·if·er·ines (tok-sif′er-ēnz). The most potent group of the curare alkaloids; the principle source is *Strychnos toxifera.*

tox·if·er·ous (tok-sif′er-ŭs). SYN poisonous. [toxi- + L. *fero,* to bear]

tox·i·gen·ic (tok-si-jen′ik). SYN toxinogenic.

tox·i·ge·nic·i·ty (tok′si-jĕ-nis′i-tē). SYN toxinogenicity.

tox·il·ic ac·id (tok-sil′ik). SYN maleic acid.

tox·in (tok′sin). A noxious or poisonous substance that is formed or elaborated either as an integral part of the cell or tissue, as an extracellular product (exotoxin), or as a combination of the two, during the metabolism and growth of certain microorganisms and some higher plant and animal species. [G. *toxikon,* poison]

animal t., SYN zootoxin.

anthrax t., a culture filtrate of *Bacillus anthracis* containing an exotoxin with at least three different antigenically distinct components: edema factor, lethal factor, and protective antigen. SYN Bacillus anthracis t.

Bacillus anthracis t., SYN anthrax t.

bacterial t., any intracellular or extracellular t. formed in or elaborated by bacterial cells.

bee t., the t. delivered by a bee sting; contains three active principles: biogenic amines, active peptides, and certain hydrolytic enzymes.

botulinus t., a potent neurotoxin from *Clostridium botulinum.* SYN botulin, botulismotoxin.

cholera t., SEE *Vibrio cholerae.*

cobra t., SYN cobrotoxin.

Crotalus t., the t. of rattlesnake.

diagnostic diphtheria t., SYN Schick test t.

Dick test t., SYN streptococcus erythrogenic t.

dinoflagellate t., a potent neurotoxin that is thought to act similarly to botulinus t. by impairing the synthesis or the release of acetylcholine.

diphtheria t., SEE *Corynebacterium diphtheriae.*

erythrogenic t., SYN streptococcus erythrogenic t.

extracellular t., SYN exotoxin.

intracellular t., SYN endotoxin.

normal t., a t. solution holding exactly 100 lethal doses in 1 ml.

plant t., SYN phytotoxin.

scarlet fever erythrogenic t., SYN streptococcus erythrogenic t.

Schick test t., *Corynebacterium diphtheriae* t. diluted so that the inoculated dose (0.1 or 0.2 ml) will contain $\frac{1}{50}$ th of guinea pig minimal lethal dose. SEE ALSO Schick *test.* SYN diagnostic diphtheria t.

streptococcus erythrogenic t., a culture filtrate of lysogenized group A strains of β-hemolytic streptococci, erythrogenic when inoculated into the skin of susceptible persons, and neutralized by antibodies that appear during scarlet fever convalescence; three immunological types (A, B, and C) are recognized. SYN Dick test t., erythrogenic t., scarlet fever erythrogenic t.

tetanus t., the neurotropic, heat-labile exotoxin of *Clostridium tetani* and the cause of tetanus; it has been isolated as a crystalline protein (molecular weight 67,000), is one of the most poisonous substances known, and seems to function by blocking inhibitory synaptic impulses. SYN tetanotoxin.

tox·in·ic (tok-sin′ik). Relating to a toxin.

tox·i·no·gen·ic (tok′si-nō-jen′ik). Producing a toxin, said of an organism. SYN toxigenic. [toxin + G. -*gen,* producing]

tox·i·no·ge·nic·i·ty (tok′si-nō-jĕ-nis′i-tē). The capacity to produce toxin. SYN toxigenicity.

tox·i·nol·o·gy (tok′si-nol′ō-jē). The study of toxins, in a restricted sense, with reference to the relatively unstable proteinaceous substances of microbial, plant, or animal origins. [toxin + G. *logos,* study]

tox·i·no·sis (tok-si-nō′sis). Any disease or lesion caused by the action of a toxin. SYN toxonosis. [toxin + G. -*osis,* condition]

tox·i·path·ic (tok-si-path′ik). Relating to any diseased state caused by a poison, *e.g.,* neuritis or hepatitis caused by arsenic.

tox·ip·a·thy (tok-sip′ă-thē). Any disease due to poisoning, especially chronic poisoning. [toxi- + G. *pathos,* suffering]

tox·i·pho·bia (tok-si-fō′bē-ă). SYN toxicophobia.

tox·is·ter·ol (tok-sis′ter-ol). A toxic substance formed by excessive irradiation of ergosterol or calciferol.

toxo-. SEE toxico-.

Tox·o·ca·ra (tok′sō-kar′ă). A genus of ascarid nematodes, chiefly found in carnivores, that cause toxocariasis. [G. *toxon,* bow, + *kara,* head]

T. ca′nis, the common ascarid species in the small intestine of the dog, where prenatal infection is a common mode of infection of pups; it is also reported in cats, wolves, foxes, coyotes, and badgers; the second-stage larva is the most frequent cause of visceral larva migrans in the liver of children.

T. mys′tax, a common ascarid species of cats, but not reported from dogs; prenatal infection of kittens does not occur, infection being by infective eggs, which hatch in the intestine, releasing second-stage larvae, which then undergo migration through the heart, lung, trachea, mouth, and gut, as with *Ascaris lumbricoides* in man; mice and other vertebrates, and also some invertebrates (*e.g.,* earthworms, cockroaches) may serve as transport hosts, in which the migrating larvae encyst in the tissues.

tox·o·ca·ri·a·sis (tok′sō-kă-rī′ă-sis). Infection with nematodes of the genus *Toxocara;* parenterally migrating larvae, chiefly of *Toxocara canis,* may cause visceral larva migrans; ocular involvement results in either a solitary granuloma in the retina, peripheral inflammatory masses, or chronic endophthalmitis.

tox·oid (tok′soyd). A toxin that has been treated (commonly with formaldehyde) so as to destroy its toxic property but retain its antigenicity, *i.e.,* its capability of stimulating the production of antitoxin antibodies and thus of producing an active immunity. For specific toxoids, see entries under vaccine. SYN anatoxin. [toxin + G. *eidos,* resemblance]

tox·on, tox·one (tok′sŏn, tok′sōn). A hypothetical bacterial product, of feeble toxicity and weak affinity for antitoxin.

tox·o·neme (tok′sō-nēm). SYN rhoptry. [G. *toxon,* bow, + *nema,* thread]

tox·o·no·sis (tok-sō-nō′sis). SYN toxinosis. [toxo- + G. *nosos,* disease]

tox·o·phil, tox·o·phile (tok′sō-fil, -fīl). Susceptible to the action of a poison; having an affinity for toxins. [toxo- + G. *philos,* fond]

tox·o·phore (tok′sō-fōr). Denoting the atomic group of the toxin molecule which carries the poisonous principle. [toxo- + G. *phoros,* bearing]

tox·oph·o·rous (tok-sof′ăr-ŭs). Relating to the toxophore group of the toxin molecule.

Tox·o·plas·ma gon·dii (tok-sō-plaz′mă gon′dē-ī). An abundant, widespread sporozoan species (family Toxoplasmatidae) that is an intracellular, nonhost-specific parasite in a great variety of vertebrates. It develops its sexual cycle, leading to oocyst production, exclusively in cats and other felids; proliferative stages (tachyzoites) and tissue cysts (containing bradyzoites) develop in a wide variety of animal species that acquire the infection from ingestion of oocysts, tissue cysts from infected meat, or by transplacental migration, leading to infection in utero. [G. *toxon,* bow or arc, + *plasma,* anything formed]

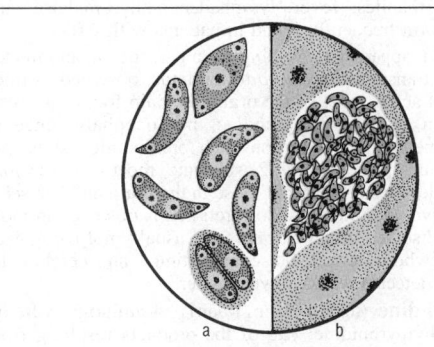

Toxoplasma gondii
a) freely swimming in liquid; b) colony (cyst) in the brain

Tox·o·plas·mat·i·dae (tok′sō-plaz-mat′i-dē). A family of coccidian sporozoa including the genera *Toxoplasma* and *Frankelia,* characterized by endodyogeny and by the presence of cysts (sometimes termed pseudocysts) containing bradyzoites in parenteral cells of the host; schizonts and gamonts are produced in intestinal cells, and gamonts give rise to oocysts. Final hosts of *Toxoplasma* are cats and other felids; final hosts of *Frankelia* are unknown.

tox·o·plas·mo·sis (tok′sō-plaz-mō′sis). Disease caused by the protozoan parasite *Toxoplasma gondii* which can produce abortion in sheep, encephalitis in mink, and a variety of syndromes in humans. Prenatally acquired human infection can result in the presence of abnormalities such as microcephalus or hydrocephalus at birth, the development of jaundice with hepatosplenomegaly or meningoencephalitis in early childhood, or the delayed appearance of ocular lesions such as chorioretinitis in later childhood. Postnatally acquired human infections typically remain subclinical; if clinical disease does occur, symptoms include fever, lymphadenopathy, headache, myalgia, and fatigue, with eventual recovery, except in the immunocompromised patient where fatal encephalitis often develops.

acquired t. in adults, a form of t. that may result in fever, encephalomyelitis, chorioretinopathy, maculopapular rash, arthralgia, myalgia, myocarditis, and pneumonitis; a lymphadenopathic form seems to be more prevalent in adults, and such

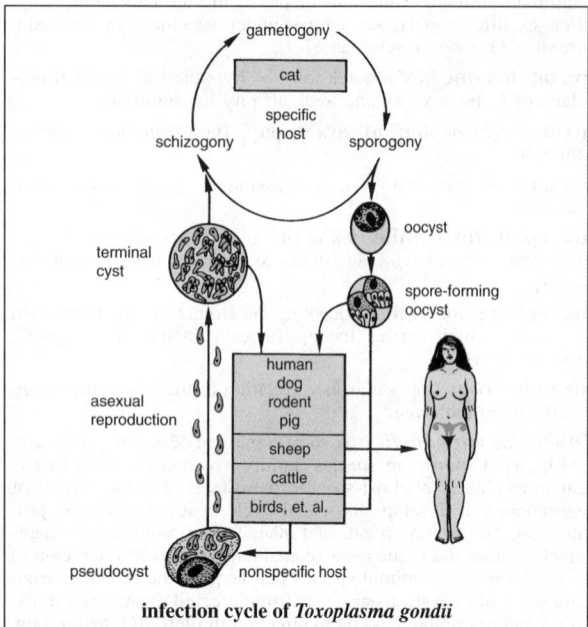

infection cycle of *Toxoplasma gondii*

Diagram labels: gametogony, cat, specific host, schizogony, sporogony, oocyst, terminal cyst, spore-forming oocyst, asexual reproduction, human dog rodent pig, sheep, cattle, birds, et. al., pseudocyst, nonspecific host

persons may manifest fever, lymphadenopathy, malaise, and headache, a form frequently found in patients with AIDS.

congenital t., t. apparently resulting from parasites in an infected mother being transmitted *in utero* to the fetus, observed as three syndromes: 1) acute, most of the organs contain foci of necrosis in association with fever, jaundice, hydrocephaly, encephalomyelitis, pneumonitis, cutaneous rash, ophthalmic lesions, hepatomegaly, and splenomegaly; 2) subacute, most of the lesions are partly healed or calcified, but those in the brain and eye seem to remain active, inasmuch as chorioretinitis is observed in more than 80% of diseased infants; 3) chronic, usually not recognized during the newborn period, but chorioretinitis and cerebral lesions may be detected weeks to years later.

tox·o·py·rim·i·dine (toks′ō-pi-rim′i-dēn). 4-amino-5-hydroxymethyl-2-methylpyrimidine; one of the products resulting from the hydrolysis of thiamin by thiaminase and appearing in the urine; a competitive inhibitor of pyridoxal. SYN pyramin, pyramine.

Toynbee, Joseph, English otologist, 1815–1866. SEE T.'s *corpuscles*, under *corpuscle, muscle, tube.*

TPA Abbreviation for tissue plasminogen *activator*; 12-*O*-tetradecanoylphorbol 13-acetate.

TPN Abbreviation for total parenteral *nutrition.*

TPN, TPNH Abbreviation for triphosphopyridine nucleotide and its reduced form (the oxidized form is TPN$^+$).

TPP Abbreviation for *thiamin* pyrophosphate.

TPR. Abbreviation for total peripheral *resistance.*

TQ Abbreviation for tocopherolquinone.

TR Abbreviation for repetition *time.*

tr. Abbreviation for L. *tinctura,* or tincture.

tra·bec·u·la, gen. and pl. **tra·bec·u·lae** (tră-bek′yū-lă, -lē). **1.** One of the supporting bundles of fibers traversing the substance of a structure, usually derived from the capsule or one of the fibrous septa. **2.** A small piece of the spongy substance of bone usually interconnected with other similar pieces. **3.** In histopathology, a band of neoplastic tissue two or more cells wide. [L. dim. of *trabs,* a beam]

anterior chamber t., tissue at the angle of the anterior chamber through which aqueous humor exits from the eye.

arachnoid t., fine, delicate strands composed of fibroblast and extracellular collagen that traverse the subarachnoid space between the arachnoid mater, which is attached to the dura, and the pia mater, which is adherent to the surface of the brain.

trabec′ulae car′neae [NA], muscular bundles on the lining walls of the ventricles of the heart. SYN columnae carneae, Rathke's bundles.

trabeculae of corpora cavernosa, fibromuscular bands and cords given off from the fibrous envelopes and septum of the corpora cavernosa penis and that separate the cavernous veins. SYN trabeculae corporum cavernosorum [NA].

trabec′ulae cor′poris spongio′si pe′nis [NA], SYN trabeculae of corpus spongiosum.

trabec′ulae cor′porum cavernoso′rum [NA], SYN trabeculae of corpora cavernosa.

trabeculae of corpus spongiosum, the fibrous bands interlacing between the vascular spaces of the corpus spongiosum and glans penis. SYN trabeculae corporis spongiosi penis [NA].

trabec′ulae cra′nii, a pair of chondrification centers in the base of the embryonic cartilaginous neurocranium, lying in front of the developing hypophysis; they become the sella turcica.

trabec′ulae lie′nis [NA], ☆official alternate term for trabeculae of spleen.

septomarginal t., one of the trabeculae carneae in the right ventricle of the heart; it carries part of the right branch of the A-V bundle from the septum to the anterior papillary muscle on the opposite wall of the ventricle. SYN t. septomarginalis [NA], moderator band, Reil's band (1).

t. septomargina′lis [NA], SYN septomarginal t.

trabeculae of spleen, small fibrous bands given off from the capsule of the spleen and constituting the framework of that organ. SYN trabeculae lienis☆ [NA], trabeculae splenicae.

trabec′ulae sple′nicae, SYN trabeculae of spleen.

t. tes′tis, SYN *septula* of testis, under *septulum.*

tra·bec·u·lar (tră-bek′yū-lăr). Relating to or containing trabeculae. SYN trabeculate.

tra·bec·u·late (-yū-lāt). SYN trabecular.

tra·bec·u·la·tion (tră-bek′yū-lā′shŭn). **1.** The occurrence of trabeculae in the walls of an organ or part. **2.** The process of forming trabeculae, as in spongy bone.

tra·bec·u·lec·to·my (tră-bek′yū-lek′tō-mē). A filtering operation for glaucoma by creation of a fistula between the anterior chamber of the eye and the subconjunctival space, through a subscleral excision of a portion of the trabecular meshwork. [trabecula + G. *ektomē,* excision]

tra·bec·u·lo·plas·ty (tră-bek′yū-lō-plas-tē). Photocoagulation of the trabecular meshwork of the eye using the laser in the treatment of glaucoma.

laser t., an operation for glaucoma in which laser energy is applied to trabecular meshwork.

> a procedure in which a laser (usually argon) is used to create small openings in the trabecular network of the eye. This improves the flow of the aqueous humor and relieves pressure owed to open-angle glaucoma, although by what precise mechanism is not known. LTP has proven effective with only certain types of glaucoma (especially capsular and pigmentary glaucomas), and is sometimes used in conjunction with laser iridotomy. Investigations into laser treatments of open-angle glaucoma began in the early 1970s, but not until the late 1980s was LTP adopted as a standard treatment for the condition, with a 2-year success rate of over 70% (dropping to 50% after 5 years). LTP lessens chances of postoperative infection and hemorrhaging, and can be performed on an outpatient basis. LTP joins other laser techniques that have radically altered eye surgery since their advent.

tra·bec·u·lot·o·my (tră-bek-yū-lot′ō-mē). Surgical opening of the sinus venosus sclerae (canal of Schlemm) to treat glaucoma. [trabekula + G. *tomē,* incision]

trace (trās). **1.** Evidence of the former existence, influence, or action of an object, phenomenon, or event. **2.** An extremely small amount or barely discernible indication of something.

memory t., SEE engram.

trac·er (trā′ser). **1.** An element or compound containing atoms that can be distinguished from their normal counterparts by physical means (*e.g.,* radioactivity assay or mass spectrography) and can thus be used to follow (trace) the metabolism of the normal substances. **2.** A colored substance (*e.g.,* a dye) used as a t. to follow the flow of water. **3.** An instrument used in dissecting out nerves and blood vessels. **4.** A mechanical device with a marking point attached to one jaw and a graph plate or tracing plate attached to the other jaw; used to record the direction and extent of movements of the mandible. SEE ALSO tracing (2). [M.E. track, fr. O. Fr. *tracier,* to make one's way, fr. L. *traho,* pp. *tractum,* to draw, + *-er,* agent suffix]

trache-. SEE tracheo-.

tra·chea, pl. **tra·che·ae** (trā′kē-ă, -kē-ē) [NA]. The air tube extending from the larynx into the thorax (level of the fifth or sixth thoracic vertebra) where it bifurcates into the right and left main bronchi. The t. is composed of from 16 to 20 rings of hyaline cartilage connected by a membrane (annular ligament); posteriorly, the rings are deficient for one-fifth to one-third of their circumference, the interval forming the membranous wall being closed by a fibrous membrane containing smooth muscular fibers. Internally, the mucosa is composed of a pseudostratified ciliated columnar epithelium with mucous goblet cells; numerous small mixed mucous and serous glands occur, the ducts of which open to the surface of the epithelium. SYN windpipe. [G. *tracheia artēria,* rough artery]

saber-sheath t., a type of tracheal collapse seen in chronic obstructive pulmonary disease in which there is an increase in the outer posterior tracheal dimension with side-to-side narrowing involving the lower 2/3 of the trachea.

scabbard t., a deformity of the t. caused by flattening and approximation of the lateral walls, producing more or less pronounced stenosis.

tra·che·al (trā′kē-ăl). Relating to the trachea.

tra·che·al·gia (trā-kē-al′jē-ă). Pain in the trachea. [trachea + G. *algos,* pain]

tra·che·a·lis. SEE trachealis *muscle.*

tra·che·i·tis (trā-kē-ī′tis). Inflammation of the lining membrane of the trachea. SYN trachitis. [trachea + G. *-itis,* inflammation]

trachel-. SEE trachelo-.

trach·e·lag·ra (trak-ě-lag′ră). A gouty or rheumatic affection of the muscles of the neck, producing torticollis. [trachel- + G. *agra,* seizure]

trach·e·la·lis (trak-ě-lā′lis). Archaic term for longissimus capitis *muscle.*

trach·e·lec·to·my (trak-ě-lek′tō-mē). SYN cervicectomy. [trachel- + G. *ektomē,* excision]

trach·e·le·ma·to·ma (trak′ě-lē-mă-tō′mă). A hematoma of the neck. [trachel- + hematoma]

trach·e·li·an (tră-kē′lē-an). Archaic term for cervical. [G. *trachēlos,* neck]

trach·e·lism, trach·e·lis·mus (trak′ě-lizm, -liz′mŭs). A bending backward of the neck, such as sometimes ushers in an epileptic attack. [G. *trachēlismos,* a seizing by the throat]

trach·e·li·tis (trak-ě-lī′tis). SYN cervicitis.

trachelo-, trachel-. Neck. [G. *trachēlos*]

trach·e·lo·cele (trak′ě-lō-sēl). SYN tracheocele. [trachelo- + G. *kēlē,* tumor, hernia]

trach·e·lo·cyr·to·sis (trak′ě-lō-ser-tō′sis). SYN tuberculous *spondylitis.* [trachelo- + G. *kyrtos,* bent]

trach·e·lo·dyn·ia (trak′ě-lō-din′ē-ă). SYN cervicodynia. [trachelo- + G. *odynē,* pain]

trach·e·lo·ky·pho·sis (trak′ě-lō-kī-fō′sis). SYN tuberculous *spondylitis.* [trachelo- + G. *kyphōsis,* hump-back]

trach·e·lol·o·gy (trak-ě-lol′ō-jē). The study of the neck and its injuries and diseases. [trachelo- + G. *logos,* study]

trach·e·lo·mas·toid (trak′ě-lō-mas′toyd). Archaic term for longissimus capitis *muscle.*

trach·e·lo·my·i·tis (trak′ě-lō-mī-ī′tis). Obsolete term for inflammation of the muscles of the neck. [trachelo- + G. *mys,* muscle, + *-itis,* inflammation]

trach·e·lo·oc·cip·i·ta·lis (trak′ě-lō-ok-sip′i-tā′lis). Archaic term for semispinalis capitis *muscle.*

trach·e·lo·pa·nus (trak′ě-lō-pā′nŭs). **1.** Swelling of the lymphatic vessels of the neck. **2.** Lymphatic engorgement of the cervix uteri. [trachelo- + L. *panus,* tumor, swelling]

trach·e·lo·pex·ia, trach·e·lo·pexy (trak′ě-lō-pek′sē-ă, -pek-sē). Surgical fixation of the cervix uteri. [trachelo- + G. *pēxis,* fixation]

trach·e·lo·phy·ma (trak′ě-lō-fī′mă). A tumor or swelling of the neck. [trachelo- + G. *phyma,* tumor]

trach·e·lo·plas·ty (trak′ě-lō-plas-tē). Rarely used term for plastic surgery of the cervix uteri. [trachelo- + G. *plastos,* formed]

trach·e·lor·rha·phy (trak-ě-lōr′ă-fē). Repair by suture of a laceration of the cervix uteri. SYN Emmet's operation. [trachelo- + G. *rhaphē,* suture]

trach·e·los (trak′ě-los). Archaic term for collum. [G. *trachēlos*]

trach·e·los·chi·sis (trak-ě-los′ki-sis). Congenital fissure in the neck. [trachelo- + G. *schisis,* fissure]

trach·e·lot·o·my (trak-ě-lot′ō-mē). SYN cervicotomy. [trachelo- + G. *tomē,* incision]

tracheo-, trache-. The trachea. [see trachea]

tra·che·o·aer·o·cele (trā′kē-ō-ār′ō-sēl). An air cyst in the neck caused by distention of a tracheocele. [tracheo- + G. *aēr,* air, + *kēlē,* hernia]

tra·che·o·bil·i·ary (trā′kē-ō-bil′ē-ār-ē). Relating to the trachea or bronchi and the biliary duct system.

tra·che·o·bron·che·o·pa·thia os·te·o·plas·ti·ca. a benign submucoid tumor or series of tumors that ossify near the tracheal walls.

tra·che·o·bron·chi·al (trā′kē-ō-brong′kē-ăl). Relating to both trachea and bronchi, denoting especially a set of lymph nodes.

tra·che·o·bron·chi·tis (trā′kē-ō-brong-kī′tis). Inflammation of the mucous membrane of the trachea and bronchi.

tra·che·o·bron·cho·meg·a·ly (trā′kē-ō-brong′kō-meg′ă-lē). Gross widening of the trachea and main bronchi, usually congenital. SYN Mounier-Kuhn syndrome. [tracheo- + bronchus + G. *megas,* large]

tra·che·o·bron·chos·co·py (trā′kē-ō-brong-kos′kŏ-pē). Inspection of the interior of the trachea and bronchi. [tracheo- + bronchus, + G. *skopeō,* to view]

tra·che·o·cele (trā′kē-ō-sēl). A protrusion of the mucous membrane through a defect in the wall of the trachea. SYN trachelocele. [tracheo- + G. *kēlē,* hernia]

tra·che·o·e·soph·a·ge·al (trā′kē-ō-ē-sof′ă-jē′ăl). Relating to the trachea and the esophagus.

tra·che·o·la·ryn·ge·al (trā′kē-ō-lă-rin′jē-ăl). Relating to the trachea and the larynx.

tra·che·o·ma·la·cia (trā′kē-ō-mă-lā′shē-ă). Degeneration of elastic and connective tissue of the trachea. [tracheo- + G. *malakia,* softness]

tra·che·o·meg·a·ly (trā′kē-ō-meg′ă-lē). An abnormally dilated trachea which may, like bronchiectasis, result from infection or prolonged positive pressure ventilation. [tracheo- + G. *megas* (*megal-*), large]

tra·che·o·path·ia, tra·che·op·a·thy (trā′kē-ō-path′ē-ă, -op′ă-thē). Any disease of the trachea. [tracheo- + G. *pathos,* disease]

t. osteoplas′tica, a rare disease characterized by cartilaginous and bony growths in the trachea and bronchi which produce sessile polyps and plaques projecting into and partly obstructing the lumina.

tra·che·o·pha·ryn·ge·al (trā′kē-ō-fă-rin′jē-ăl). Relating to both trachea and pharynx; denoting an occasional band of muscular fibers passing from the inferior constrictor of the pharynx to the trachea.

tra·che·o·pho·ne·sis (trā′kē-ō-fō-nē′sis). Auscultation of the heart sounds at the sternal notch. [tracheo- + G. *phōnēsis,* a sounding]

tra·che·oph·o·ny (trā-kē-of′ō-nē). The hollow voice sound heard in auscultating over the trachea. SEE ALSO bronchophony. [tracheo- + G. *phōnē,* voice]

tra·che·o·plas·ty (trā′kē-ō-plas-tē). Plastic surgery of the trachea. [tracheo- + G. *plastos,* formed]

tra·che·or·rha·gia (trā-kē-ō-rā′jē-ă). Hemorrhage from the mucous membrane of the trachea. [tracheo- + G. *rhēgnymi,* to burst forth]

tra·che·os·chi·sis (trā-kē-os′ki-sis). A fissure into the trachea. [tracheo- + G. *schisis,* fissure]

tra·che·o·scope (trā′kē-ō-skōp). An instrument used in tracheoscopy.

tra·che·o·scop·ic (trā-kē-ō-skop′ik). Relating to tracheoscopy.

tra·che·os·co·py (trā-kē-os′kŏ-pē). Inspection of the interior of the trachea. [tracheo- + G. *skopeō,* to examine]

tra·che·o·ste·no·sis (trā′kē-ō-stě-nō′sis). Narrowing of the lumen of the trachea. [tracheo- + G. *stenōsis,* constriction]

tra·che·os·to·ma (trā′kē-os′tō-mă). Permanent opening into the trachea through the neck; generally applied to such an opening after or laryngectomy. [tracheo- + G. *stoma,* mouth]

tra·che·os·to·my (trā′kē-os′tō-mē). SYN tracheotomy. [tracheo- + G. *stoma,* mouth]

tra·che·o·tome (trā′kē-ō-tōm). A knife used in the operation of tracheotomy.

tra·che·ot·o·my (trā-kē-ot′ō-mē). The operation of opening into the trachea, usually intended to be temporary. SYN tracheostomy. [tracheo- + G. *tomē,* incision]

tra·chi·tis (trā-kī′tis). SYN tracheitis.

tra·cho·ma (tră-kō′mă). Chronic contagious microbial inflammation, with hypertrophy, of the conjunctiva, marked by the formation of minute grayish or yellowish translucent granules caused by *Chlamydia trachomatis.* SYN Egyptian ophthalmia, granular lids, granular ophthalmia. [G. *trachōma,* fr. *trachys,* rough, harsh]

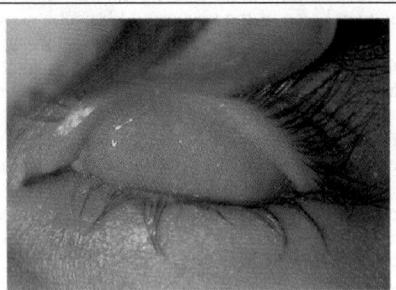

trachoma
note whitish follicles on the inner eyelid

follicular t., the ordinary form of t. marked by the presence of granulations on the conjunctiva. SYN granular t.

granular t., SYN follicular t.

tra·chom·a·tous (tră-kō′mă-tŭs). Relating to or suffering from trachoma.

tra·chy·chro·mat·ic (trak-i-krō-mat′ik). Denoting a nucleus with very deeply staining chromatin. [G. *trachys,* rough, + *chrōmatikos,* chromatic]

tra·chy·o·nych·ia (trak′ē-ō-nik′ē-ă). Rough-surfaced nails. [G. *trachys,* rough, + *onyx, onychos,* nail, + suffix -*ia,* condition]

tra·chy·pho·nia (trak′ē-fō′nē-ă). Roughness of voice. [G. *trachys,* rough, + *phōnē,* voice]

trac·ing (trās′ing). 1. Any graphic display of electrical or mechanical cardiovascular events, *e.g.,* electrocardiogram, phlebogram. SEE ALSO curve. 2. In dentistry, a line or lines, scribed on a table or plate by a pointed instrument, representing a record of movements of the mandible; may be extraoral (made outside the oral cavity) or intraoral (made within the oral cavity).

arrow point t., SYN needle point t.

cephalometric t., an overlay drawing or t. of the teeth, facial bones, and anthropometric landmarks made directly from a cephalometric radiograph and used as a basis for cephalometric analysis.

Gothic arch t., SYN needle point t.

needle point t., a t. of mandibular movements made by means of a device attached to the opposing arches; its shape resembles that of an arrowhead or a Gothic arch, and when the instrument's marking point is at the apex of the arch, the jaws are considered to be in centric relation. SYN arrow point t., Gothic arch t., Gothic arch, stylus t.

stylus t., SYN needle point t.

TRACT

tract (trakt). An elongated area, *e.g.,* path, track, way. SEE ALSO fascicle. SYN tractus. [L. *tractus,* a drawing out]

alimentary t., SYN digestive t.

anterior corticospinal t., SYN anterior pyramidal t.

anterior pyramidal t., uncrossed fibers forming a small bundle in the pyramidal t. SEE pyramidal t. SYN tractus corticospinalis anterior [NA], tractus pyramidalis anterior [NA], anterior corticospinal t., anterior pyramidal fasciculus, direct pyramidal t., fasciculus corticospinalis anterior, fasciculus pyramidalis anterior, Türck's bundle, Türck's column, Türck's t.

anterior spinocerebellar t., a bundle of fibers originating in the base of the posterior horn and zona intermedia throughout lumbosacral segments of the spinal cord, crossing to the opposite side and ascending in a peripheral position in the ventral half of the lateral funiculus. In its ascent through the rhombencephalon, the tract curves sharply dorsalward along the rostral border of the trigeminal motor nucleus, entering the cerebellum in a caudal direction over the dorsal surface of the superior cerebellar peduncle, and terminating as mossy fibers in the granular layer of the cortex of the cerebellar vermis. The bundle conveys proprioceptive and exteroceptive information largely from the opposite lower extremity. SYN tractus spinocerebellaris anterior [NA], Gowers' column, Gowers' t., ventral spinocerebellar t.

anterior spinothalamic t., the more anterior or ventral part of the spinothalamic t. that is involved in tactile sensation. SEE spinothalamic t. SYN tractus spinothalamicus anterior [NA], ventral spinothalamic t.

Arnold's t., SYN temporopontine t.

association t., SEE association *system.*

auditory t., SYN lateral *lemniscus.*

Burdach's t., SYN cuneate *fasciculus.*

central tegmental t., a large fiber bundle passing longitudinally through the central mesencephalic and pontine tegmentum, distinguished from adjacent longitudinal groups of fiber-fascicles of the reticular formation by a more compact composition. In transverse sections of the mesencephalon the bundle occupies a large triangular area lateral to the medial longitudinal fasciculus; farther caudally it expands ventralward and finally passes over the lateral side of the (inferior) olivary nucleus, becoming part of the latter's fiber capsule. The bundle contains fibers from the mesencephalic tegmentum and regions surrounding the central gray substance descending to the olivary nucleus; it also includes numerous fibers ascending from the medullary, pontine, and mesencephalic reticular formation to the thalamus and subthalamus region. SYN tractus tegmentalis centralis [NA], central tegmental fasciculus, tractus centralis tegmenti.

cerebellorubral t., that component of the superior cerebellar peduncle (brachium conjunctivum) which distributes fibers within the red nucleus of the opposite side. SYN tractus cerebellorubralis [NA].

cerebellothalamic t., that component of the superior cerebellar peduncle (brachium conjunctivum) which originates in the cerebellar nuclei, crosses completely in the decussation of the brachia conjunctiva, bypasses the red nucleus, and terminates in parts of the ventral anterior, ventral intermediate, ventral posterolateral, and central lateral nuclei of the thalamus. SYN tractus cerebello-thalamicus [NA], dentatothalamic t.

Collier's t., SYN medial longitudinal *fasciculus.*

comma t. of Schultze, SYN semilunar *fasciculus.*

corticobulbar t., collective term for those fibers (corticonuclear fibers) which separate from the corticospinal tract in the course of the latter's descent through the pons and medulla oblongata. Fibers of this t. innervate the motor nuclei of the trigeminal, facial, and hypoglossal nerves (perhaps also the nucleus ambiguus), directly and by way of interneurons in the lateral part of the rhombencephalic tegmentum. No direct supranuclear cortical innervation of the motor nuclei innervating the external eye muscles (oculomotor, trochlear, abducens) has been identified. Fibers of the corticobulbar t. also project into the formatio reticularis (*i.e.,* corticoreticular fibers) and terminate upon sensory relay nuclei (*e.g.,* gracile and cuneate nuclei, nucleus spinalis trigeminalis and nucleus solitarius). SYN tractus corticobulbaris.

corticopontine t., collective term for the multitude of fibers which, originating in all of the major subdivisions of the cerebral cortex, descend in the internal capsule and crus cerebri to terminate in the nuclei of the ventral part of the pons. Individual components of this massive fiber system are indicated, according to their origin in the cerebral cortex, as the frontopontine t., parietopontine t., occipitopontine t., and temporopontine t. SYN tractus corticopontini [NA].

corticospinal t., SYN pyramidal t.

crossed pyramidal t., SYN lateral pyramidal t.

cuneocerebellar t., the nerve fiber system originating from the accessory cuneate nucleus and entering the cerebellum as a component of the restiform body, the larger part of the inferior cerebellar peduncle.

dead t.'s, dentin areas characterized by degenerated odontoblastic processes; may result from injury caused by caries, attrition, erosion, or cavity preparation.

deiterospinal t., SYN vestibulospinal t.

dentatothalamic t., SYN cerebellothalamic t.

descending t. of trigeminal nerve, SYN spinal t. of trigeminal nerve.

digestive t., the passage leading from the mouth to the anus through the pharynx, esophagus, stomach, and intestine. SYN alimentary canal, alimentary t., digestive tube, tubus digestorius.

direct pyramidal t., SYN anterior pyramidal t.

dorsolateral t., SYN dorsolateral *fasciculus.*

fastigiobulbar t., a fiber bundle originating in the fastigial nucleus (nucleus tecti) of both sides, passing out of the cerebellum in the inferior cerebellar peduncle (corpus restiforme), and distributing its fibers to the vestibular nuclei and other cell groups in the medulla oblongata. Prominent crossed fibers loop over the dorsal surface of the superior cerebellar peduncle before turning ventrally, forming the uncinate bundle of Russell. SYN tractus fastigiobulbaris.

Flechsig's t., SYN posterior spinocerebellar t.

frontopontine t., a large group of fibers arising from the frontal lobe of the cerebral hemisphere, especially the precentral gyrus, descending in the capsula interna, farther caudally composing the medial part of the crus cerebri in which they extend caudalward to end in the gray matter (pontine nuclei) of the ventral part of the pons. SYN tractus frontopontinus [NA].

frontotemporal t., SYN uncinate *fasciculus.*

gastrointestinal t., (G.I. t.) the stomach, small intestine, and large intestine; often used as a synonym of digestive t.

geniculocalcarine t., SYN optic *radiation.*

genital t., the genital passages of the urogenital apparatus. SYN genital duct.

t. of Goll, SYN *fasciculus* gracilis.

Gowers' t., SYN anterior spinocerebellar t.

habenulointerpeduncular t., SYN retroflex *fasciculus.*

habenulopeduncular t., SYN tractus habenulopeduncularis.

Hoche's t., SEE semilunar *fasciculus.*

hypothalamohypophysial t., SYN supraopticohypophysial t.

iliopubic t., thickened inferior margin of the transversalis fascia seen as a fibrous band running parallel and posterior (deep) to the inguinal ligament, contributing to the posterior wall of the inguinal canal as it bridges the external iliac-femoral vessels from the iliopectineal arch to the superior pubic ramus. It marks the inferior edge of the deep inguinal ring and the medial margin of the femoral canal. Seen only when the inguinal region is viewed from its internal aspect, it is a useful landmark in laparoscopy of this region, as for repair of inguinal herniae. SYN deep crural arch, Thompson's ligament.

iliotibial t., a fibrous reinforcement of the fascia lata on the lateral surface of the thigh, extending from the crest of the ilium to the lateral condyle of the tibia. SYN tractus iliotibialis [NA], iliotibial band, Maissiat's band.

James t.'s, SYN James *fibers,* under *fiber.*

lateral corticospinal t., SYN lateral pyramidal t.

lateral pyramidal t., those fibers of the pyramidal t. that cross to the opposite side in the pyramidal decussation and descend in the dorsal half of the lateral funiculus of the spinal cord; they are distributed throughout the length of the spinal cord to interneurons of the zona intermedia of the spinal gray matter. SEE pyramidal t. SYN tractus corticospinalis lateralis [NA], tractus pyramidalis lateralis, crossed pyramidal t., fasciculus corticospinalis lateralis, fasciculus pyramidalis lateralis, lateral corticospinal t., lateral pyramidal fasciculus.

lateral spinothalamic t., the dorsal part of the spinothalamic t., which conveys impulses associated with pain and temperature sensation. SEE spinothalamic t. SYN tractus spinothalamicus lateralis [NA].

Lissauer's t., SYN dorsolateral *fasciculus.*

Loewenthal's t., SYN tectospinal t.

mamillothalamic t., SYN mamillothalamic *fasciculus.*

Marchi's t., SYN tectospinal t.

mesencephalic t. of trigeminal nerve, located alongside the central substance of the midbrain and composed of primary sensory fibers, the cells of origin of which compose the mesencephalic nucleus of the trigeminus. SYN tractus mesencephalicus nervi trigemini [NA].

Monakow's t., SYN rubrospinal t.

t. of Münzer and Wiener, SYN tectopontine t.

nerve t., a bundle or group of nerve fibers in the brain or spinal cord.

occipitocollicular t., SYN occipitotectal t.

occipitopontine t., a group of fibers originating in the occipital lobe of the cerebral hemisphere and descending in the internal capsule and lateral part of the crus cerebri to the pontine nuclei or ventral part of the pons. SYN tractus occipitopontinus [NA].

occipitotectal t., the system of nerve fibers by which the occipital cortex projects to the superior colliculus. SYN occipitocollicular t.

olfactory t., a nervelike, white band composed primarily of nerve fibers originating from the mitral cells and tufted cells of the olfactory bulb but also containing the scattered cells of the anterior olfactory nucleus. The t. is closely applied to the ventral surface of the frontal lobe, and attaches itself to the base of the cerebral hemisphere at the olfactory trigone, beyond which it extends in the form of the olfactory striae which distribute their fibers to the olfactory tubercle and, in largest number, to the olfactory cortex on and around the uncus of the parahippocampal gyrus. SEE ALSO olfactory *nerves,* under *nerve.* SYN tractus olfactorius [NA], olfactory peduncle.

olivocerebellar t., a large group of loosely arranged fiber fascicles emerging from the hilus of the olivary nucleus, crossing to the opposite side of the medulla oblongata through the stratum interolivare lemnisci and the contralateral olive, and joining the restiform body, the larger part of the contralateral inferior cerebellar peduncle; its fibers terminate in all parts of the cerebellar cortex as climbing fibers. SYN tractus olivocerebellaris [NA].

olivocochlear t., SEE olivocochlear *bundle.*

olivospinal t., a slender bundle of nerve fibers in the peripheral zone of the lateral funiculus of the spinal cord, composed of spino-olivary fibers more likely than olivospinal fibers. SYN Helweg's bundle.

optic t., the continuation of the optic nerve fibers beyond (behind) the latter's hemidecussation in the optic chiasm; each of

tr

the two symmetrical optic t.'s is composed of fibers originating from the temporal half of the retina of the ipsilateral eye and a nearly equal number of fibers from the nasal half of the contralateral retina; it forms a compact, somewhat flattened fiber band passing caudolaterally alongside the base of the hypothalamus and over the basal surface of the crus cerebri; most of its fibers terminate in the lateral geniculate body; a smaller number of fibers enter the brachium of the superior colliculus, to terminate in the superior colliculus and the pretectal region. SYN tractus opticus [NA].

parietopontine t., a system of fibers originating in the parietal lobe of the cerebral hemisphere which descend in the internal capsule and lateral part of the crus cerebri to terminate in the pontine nuclei or ventral part of the pons. SYN tractus parietopontinus [NA].

posterior spinocerebellar t., a compact bundle of heavily myelinated, thick fibers at the periphery of the dorsal half of the lateral funiculus of the spinal cord, originating in the ipsilateral thoracic nucleus (column of Clarke) and ascending by way of the inferior cerebellar peduncle. Terminals end as mossy fibers in the granular layer of the cortex of the cerebellar vermis. The bundle conveys largely proprioceptive information originating from the annulospiral nerve endings surrounding muscle spindles and from Golgi tendon organs. SYN tractus spinocerebellaris posterior [NA], Flechsig's t.

prepyramidal t., SYN rubrospinal t.

pyramidal t., a massive bundle of fibers originating from pyramidal cells of various sizes in the fifth layer of the precentral motor (area 4), the premotor area (area 6), and to a lesser extent from the postcentral gyrus. Cells of origin in area 4 include the gigantopyramidal cells of Betz. Fibers from these cortical regions descend through the internal capsule, the middle third of the crus cerebri, and the ventral part of the pons to emerge on the ventral surface of the medulla oblongata as the pyramis. Continuing caudally, most of the fibers cross to the opposite side in the pyramidal decussation and descend in the dorsal half of the lateral funiculus of the spinal cord as the lateral pyramidal t., which distributes its fibers throughout the length of the spinal cord to interneurons of the zona intermedia of the spinal gray matter. In the (extremity-related) spinal cord enlargements, fibers also pass directly to motoneuronal groups that innervate distal extremity muscles subserving particular hand-and-finger or foot-and-toe movements. The uncrossed fibers form a small bundle, the anterior pyramidal t., which descends in the anterior funiculus of the spinal cord and terminates in synaptic contact with interneurons in the medial half of the anterior horn on both sides of the spinal cord. Interruption of the pyramidal tract at or below its cortical origin causes impairment of movement in the opposite body-half, especially severe in the arm and leg; characterized by muscular weakness, spasticity and hyperreflexia, and a loss of discrete finger and hand movements. Babinski's sign is associated with this condition of hemiplegia. SYN tractus corticospinalis [NA], tractus pyramidalis [NA], corticospinal t.

respiratory t., the air passages from the nose to the pulmonary alveoli, through the pharynx, larynx, trachea, and bronchi.

reticulospinal t., collective term denoting a variety of fiber tracts descending to the spinal cord from the reticular formation of the pons and medulla oblongata. Part of these fibers conduct impulses from the neural mechanisms regulating autonomic functions to the corresponding somatic and visceral motor neurons of the spinal cord; others form links in nonpyramidal motor mechanisms affecting muscle tonus, reflex activity, and somatic movement. SYN tractus reticulospinalis [NA].

rubrobulbar t., (1) that component of the rubrospinal t. which distributes its fibers to lateral parts of the rhombencephalic tegmentum rather than the spinal cord; (2) uncrossed rubro-olivary fibers.

rubroreticular t., fibers that pass from the red nucleus to the reticular formation of the pons and medulla.

rubrospinal t., a somatotopically organized fiber bundle, relatively small in humans, arising from the red nucleus, immediately crossing in the ventral tegmental decussation, descending near the lateral surface of the brainstem into the lateral funiculus of the spinal cord at the ventral border of the lateral pyramidal t.

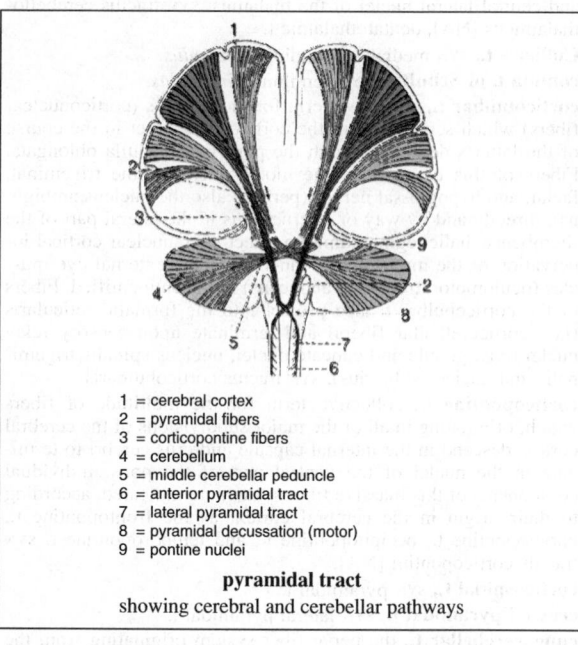

1 = cerebral cortex
2 = pyramidal fibers
3 = corticopontine fibers
4 = cerebellum
5 = middle cerebellar peduncle
6 = anterior pyramidal tract
7 = lateral pyramidal tract
8 = pyramidal decussation (motor)
9 = pontine nuclei

pyramidal tract
showing cerebral and cerebellar pathways

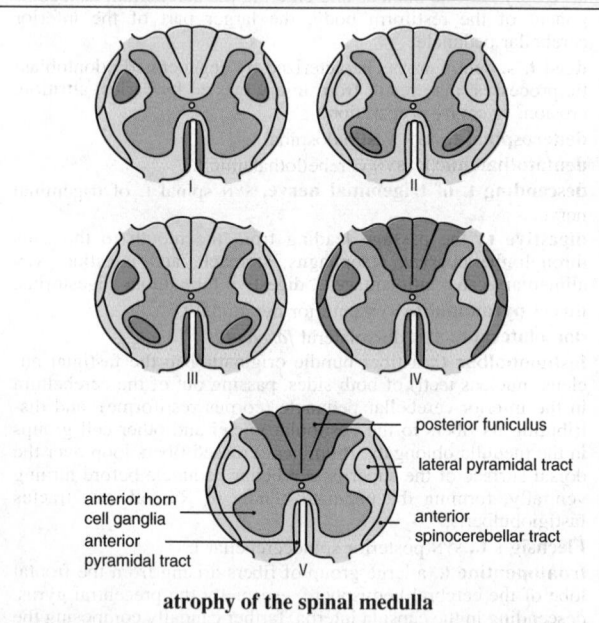

posterior funiculus

lateral pyramidal tract

anterior horn
cell ganglia

anterior

anterior
spinocerebellar tract

anterior
pyramidal tract

atrophy of the spinal medulla

It terminates in the zona intermedia of the spinal cord where its distribution coincides with that of the lateral pyramidal t.; in contrast to the latter it appears not to have direct connections with spinal motor neurons. Impulses conveyed by this t. indirectly increase flexor muscle tone. SYN tractus rubrospinalis [NA], Monakow's bundle, Monakow's t., prepyramidal t.

t. of Schütz, SYN dorsal longitudinal *fasciculus*.

sensory t., SEE lemniscus.

septomarginal t., SEE semilunar *fasciculus*.

solitary t., a slender, compact fiber bundle extending longitudinally through the dorsolateral region of the medullary tegmentum, surrounded by the nucleus of the solitary t., below the obex decussating over the central canal, and descending over some distance into the upper cervical segments of the spinal cord. It is composed of primary sensory fibers that enter with the vagus, glossopharyngeal, and facial nerves, and in part convey information from stretch receptors and chemoreceptors in the walls of the cardiovascular, respiratory, and intestinal tracts; in rostral parts of the tract impulses are generated by the receptor cells of the taste buds in the mucosa of the tongue. Its fibers are distributed to the nucleus of the solitary tract. SYN tractus solitarius [NA], fasciculus rotundus, fasciculus solitarius, funiculus solitarius, Gierke's respiratory bundle, Krause's respiratory bundle, round fasciculus, solitary bundle, solitary fasciculus.

sphincteroid t. of ileum, SYN basal *sphincter.*

spinal t., any one of a multitude of fiber bundles ascending or descending in the spinal cord.

spinal t. of trigeminal nerve, a compact fiber bundle, comma-shaped on transverse section, composed of primary sensory fibers of the portio major of the trigeminal nerve, descending from the level of the entrance of the trigeminus in the upper pons down through the dorsolateral region of the rhombencephalic tegmentum along the lateral side of the descending or spinal nucleus of the trigeminus, emerging on the dorsolateral surface of the lower medulla oblongata as the tuberculum cinereum, and continuing as far as the second cervical segment of the spinal cord. Its fibers are distributed to the descending or spinal nucleus of the trigeminus. SYN tractus spinalis nervi trigemini [NA], descending t. of trigeminal nerve, tractus descendens nervi trigemini.

spinocerebellar t.'s, SEE anterior spinocerebellar t., posterior spinocerebellar t.

spinocervicothalamic t., a t. composed of axons that originate from laminae III-V, ascend ipsilaterally to the lateral cervical nucleus (LCN) where they synapse, LCN neurons project to the contralateral thalamus via the medial lemniscus.

spino-olivary t., multiple spinal tracts terminating in the accessory olivary nuclei. SEE olivospinal t.

spinoreticular t., SYN spinoreticular *fibers,* under *fiber.*

spinotectal t., the relatively small component of the spinothalamic t. that terminates in the intermediate and deep layers of the superior colliculus and in parts of the periaqueductal gray. SYN tractus spinotectalis [NA].

spinothalamic t., a large ascending fiber bundle in the ventral half of the lateral funiculus of the spinal cord, arising from cells in the posterior horn at all levels of the cord, which cross within their segments of origin in the white commissure. In their contralateral ascent, the bundle is intermingled with numerous intersegmental fibers. The spinothalamic t. continues from the spinal cord into the brainstem, occupying a ventrolateral position and issuing numerous fibers to the rhombencephalic and mesencephalic reticular formation, to the lateral part of the central gray substance of the mesencephalon, and to the deep and intermediate layers of the superior colliculus; the relatively few fibers (10 to 20%) that remain form the true spinothalamic t. which enters the diencephalon and ends in the nucleus ventralis posterior (caudal part) and intralaminar nuclei of the thalamus. In its ascent in the spinal cord the t. is composed of a dorsal part, the lateral spinothalamic t., which conveys impulses associated with pain and temperature sensation, and a more ventral part, the anterior spinsothalamic t., involved in tactile sensation. SYN lemniscus spinalis [NA], spinal lemniscus, tractus spinothalamicus.

spiral foraminous t., openings in the cochlear area of the bottom of the internal acoustic meatus through which the fibers of the cochlear nerve leave the bony labyrinth to enter the cranial cavity. SYN tractus spiralis foraminosus [NA].

Spitzka's marginal t., SYN dorsolateral *fasciculus.*

sulcomarginal t., collective term for those fiber t.'s which descend in the anterior funiculus of the spinal cord along the wall of the anterior median fissure: tectospinal t., medial longitudinal fasciculus, and anterior pyramidal t.

supraopticohypophysial t., a bundle of unmyelinated fibers originating from all cells of the supraoptic nucleus and an estimated 20% of those of the paraventricular nucleus of the hypothalamus, which extend through the infundibulum and pituitary stalk to their endings in the posterior lobe of the hypophysis; the fibers convey neurosecretory substances, vasopressin and oxytocin, which are stored in (and can be released into the circulating blood from) their terminals. SEE ALSO hypophysis, neurosecretion. SYN tractus supraopticohypophysialis [NA], hypothalamo-hypophysial t.

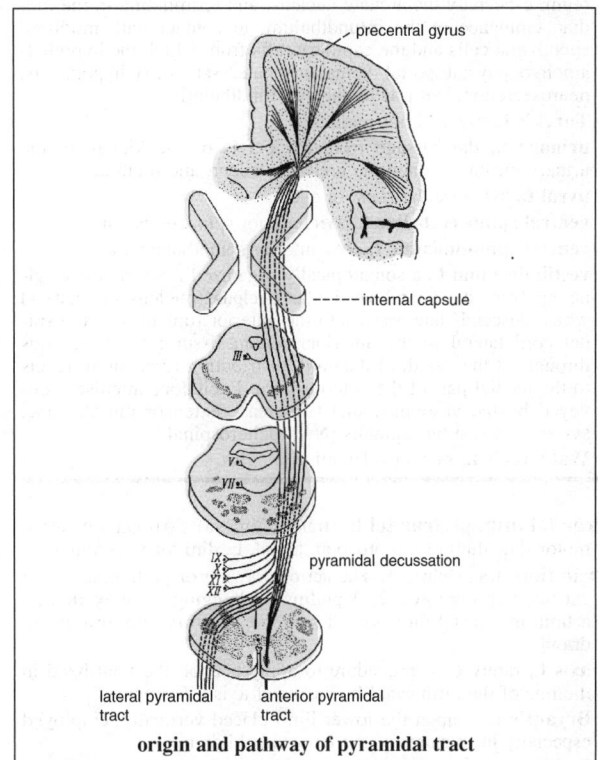

origin and pathway of pyramidal tract

tectobulbar t., fibers originating in the deep layers of the superior colliculus and accompanying the tectospinal t. but, unlike the latter, terminating in medial regions of the pontine and medullary tegmentum. SYN tractus tectobulbaris.

tectopontine t., a fiber bundle arising in the superior colliculus, passing caudoventrally on the same side along the medial side of the lateral lemniscus, issuing fibers terminating in the lateral zone of the mesencephalic tegmentum, and ending in the lateral part of the gray matter of the ventral part of the pons. SYN t. of Münzer and Wiener, tractus tectopontinus.

tectospinal t., a bundle of thick, heavily myelinated fibers originating in the deep layers of the superior colliculus, crossing to the opposite side in the dorsal tegmental decussation, descending along the median plane, between the medial longitudinal fasciculus dorsally, the medial lemniscus ventrally, into the anterior funiculus of the spinal cord. The t. ends in the medial region of the anterior horn of the cervical spinal cord, and appears to be involved in head movements during visual and auditory tracking. Throughout its course in the brainstem it is accompanied by fibers of the tectobulbar t. SYN tractus tectospinalis [NA], Held's bundle, Loewenthal's bundle, Loewenthal's t., Marchi's t., predorsal bundle.

temporofrontal t., SYN uncinate *fasciculus.*

temporopontine t., a fiber group originating in the cerebral cortex of the temporal lobe, particularly the superior and middle temporal gyri, following the sublenticular limb of the internal capsule into the lateral margin of the crus cerebri in which it descends to its termination in the pontine nuclei or the ventral part of the pons. SYN tractus temporopontinus [NA], Arnold's bundle, Arnold's t.

trigeminothalamic t., general term designating projections from the spinal trigeminal and principal sensory nuclei of the trigeminal nerve to the thalamus; divided into a ventral trigeminothalamic t. (spinal trigeminal nucleus projections to the contralateral ventral posteromedial nucleus - VPM) and a dorsal trigeminothalamic t. (principal sensory nucleus projections to the ipsilateral VPM); SEE ALSO trigeminal *lemniscus.*

tuberoinfundibular t., a system of fine, unmyelinated fibers apparently originating from small-celled nuclei of the tuber cinereum, especially the arcuate nucleus, and terminating in the median eminence of the infundibulum, in contact with modified ependymal cells and the capillary tufts from which the hypothalamohypophysial portal veins originate. SEE ALSO hypophysis, neurosecretion. SYN tractus tuberoinfundibularis.

Türck's t., SYN anterior pyramidal t.

urinary t., the passage from the pelvis of the kidney to the urinary meatus through the ureters, bladder, and urethra.

uveal t., SYN vascular *tunic* of eye.

ventral spinocerebellar t., SYN anterior spinocerebellar t.

ventral spinothalamic t., SYN anterior spinothalamic t.

vestibulospinal t., a somatopically organized fiber bundle originating from the lateral vestibular nucleus (nucleus of Deiters) which descends uncrossed into the anterior funiculus of the spinal cord lateral to the anterior median fissure; the t. extends throughout the length of the cord, distributing fibers at all levels to the medial part of the anterior horn. Excitatory impulses conveyed by the vestibulospinal t. increase extensor muscle tone. SYN tractus vestibulospinalis [NA], deiterospinal t.

Waldeyer's t., SYN dorsolateral *fasciculus.*

---

trac·tel·lum, pl. **trac·tel·la** (trak-tel′ŭm, -ă). An anterior locomotor flagellum of a protozoon. [Mod. L. dim. of L. *tractus*]

trac·tion (trak′shŭn). **1.** The act of drawing or pulling, as by an elastic or spring force. **2.** A pulling or dragging force exerted on a limb in a distal direction. [L. *tractio,* fr. *traho,* pp. *tractus,* to draw]

axis t., rarely used procedure to apply t. upon the fetal head in the line of the birth canal by means of axis t. forceps.

Bryant's t., t. upon the lower limb placed vertically, employed especially in fractures of the femur in children.

Buck's t., SYN Buck's *extension.*

external t., a pulling force created by using fixed anchorage (*e.g.,* a headcap or bed frame) outside the oral cavity; principally used in the management of midfacial fractures.

halo t., application of skeletal t. to the head by means of a halo device.

intermaxillary t., SYN maxillomandibular t.

internal t., a pulling force created by using one of the cranial bones, above the point of fracture, for anchorage.

isometric t., t. in which the length of the limb does not change.

isotonic t., t. in which the amount of force does not change.

maxillomandibular t., a pulling force developed by using elastic or wire ligatures and interdental wiring or splints, or both. SYN intermaxillary t.

Russell t., an improvement of Buck's extension that permits the resultant vector of the applied traction force to be changed, for fractures of the femur.

Sayre's suspension t., spinal t. obtained by vertical suspension of the patient by means of a head halter.

skeletal t., t. pull on a bone structure mediated through pin or wire inserted into the bone to reduce a fracture of long bones. SYN skeletal extension.

skin t., t. on an extremity by means of adhesive tape or other types of strapping applied to the limb.

trac·tor (trak′ter, tōr). An instrument for exerting traction upon, or pulling out, an organ or structure. [Mod. L. a drawer, see traction]

Lowsley t., a slender curved instrument with flexible blades at its tip, which can be opened or closed by rotation at the proximal end of the t.; it is passed per urethram into the bladder and used to retract the prostate gland downward into the operative field in the initial stages of perineal prostatectomy.

Syms t., a collapsible rubber bag attached to the extremity of a tube; the tube is introduced into the bladder through the perineal wound and the bag is inflated; traction produced draws the enlarged prostate into the wound where it is more accessible.

Young prostatic t., a short, straight tubular instrument with blades at its tip, which can be rotated open and closed; it is passed into the prostatic urethra, through a prostatotomy incision made during the later stages of open perineal prostatectomy, with

its tip into the bladder; direct traction on the instrument brings the prostate gland down into the operative field where enucleation can be more easily performed.

trac·tot·o·my (trak-tot′ō-mē). Interruption of a nerve tract in the brainstem or spinal cord. [L. *tractus,* tract, + G. *tomē,* incision]

anterolateral t., SYN anterolateral *cordotomy.*

intramedullary t., SYN trigeminal t.

pyramidal t., may be mesencephalic (pedunculotomy or crusotomy), medullary (medullary pyramidotomy), or spinal (spinal pyramidotomy).

Schwartz t., a medullary spinothalamic t.

Sjöqvist t., SYN trigeminal t.

spinal t., SYN anterolateral *cordotomy.*

spinothalamic t., may be spinal (cordotomy), medullary (Schwartz t.), or mesencephalic (Walker t.).

trigeminal t., division of the descending fibers of the trigeminal tract in the medulla. SYN intramedullary t., Sjöqvist t.

Walker t., a mesencephalic spinothalamic t.

TRACTUS

---

trac·tus, gen. and pl. **trac·tus** (trak′tŭs). SYN tract. [L. a drawing, drawing out, extent, tract, fr. *traho,* pp. *tractus,* to draw]

t. centra′lis tegmen′ti, SYN central tegmental *tract.*

t. cerebellorubra′lis [NA], SYN cerebellorubral *tract.*

t. cerebellothalam′icus [NA], SYN cerebellothalamic *tract.*

t. corticobulba′ris, SYN corticobulbar *tract.*

t. corticoponti′ni [NA], SYN corticopontine *tract.*

t. corticospina′lis [NA], SYN pyramidal *tract.*

t. corticospina′lis ante′rior [NA], SYN anterior pyramidal *tract.*

t. corticospina′lis latera′lis [NA], SYN lateral pyramidal *tract.*

t. descen′dens ner′vi trigem′ini, SYN spinal *tract* of trigeminal nerve.

t. dorsolatera′lis [NA], SYN dorsolateral *fasciculus.*

t. fastigiobulba′ris, SYN fastigiobulbar *tract.*

t. frontoponti′nus [NA], SYN frontopontine *tract.*

t. habenulopeduncula′ris, SYN habenulopeduncular *tract.*

t. iliotibia′lis [NA], SYN iliotibial *tract.*

t. mesencephal′icus ner′vi trigem′ini [NA], SYN mesencephalic *tract* of trigeminal nerve.

t. occipitoponti′nus [NA], SYN occipitopontine *tract.*

t. olfacto′rius [NA], SYN olfactory *tract.*

t. olivocerebella′ris [NA], SYN olivocerebellar *tract.*

t. op′ticus [NA], SYN optic *tract.*

t. parietoponti′nus [NA], SYN parietopontine *tract.*

t. pyramida′lis [NA], SYN pyramidal *tract.*

t. pyramida′lis ante′rior [NA], SYN anterior pyramidal *tract.*

t. pyramida′lis latera′lis [NA], SYN lateral pyramidal *tract.*

t. reticulospina′lis [NA], SYN reticulospinal *tract.*

t. rubrospina′lis [NA], SYN rubrospinal *tract.*

t. solita′rius [NA], SYN solitary *tract.*

t. spina′lis ner′vi trigem′ini [NA], SYN spinal *tract* of trigeminal nerve.

t. spinocerebella′ris ante′rior [NA], SYN anterior spinocerebellar *tract.*

t. spinocerebella′ris poste′rior [NA], SYN posterior spinocerebellar *tract.*

t. spinotecta′lis [NA], SYN spinotectal *tract.*

t. spinothalam′icus, SYN spinothalamic *tract.*

t. spinothalam′icus ante′rior [NA], SYN anterior spinothalamic *tract.*

t. spinothalam′icus latera′lis [NA], SYN lateral spinothalamic *tract.*

t. spira′lis foramino′sus [NA], SYN spiral foraminous *tract.*

t. supraopticohypophysia′lis [NA], SYN supraopticohypophysial *tract.*

t. tectobulba′ris, SYN tectobulbar *tract.*

t. tectoponti′nus, SYN tectopontine *tract.*

t. tectospina′lis [NA], SYN tectospinal *tract.*

t. tegmenta′lis centra′lis [NA], SYN central tegmental *tract.*

t. temporoponti′nus [NA], SYN temporopontine *tract.*

t. tuberoinfundibula′ris, SYN tuberoinfundibular *tract.*

t. vestibulospina′lis [NA], SYN vestibulospinal *tract.*

---

traf·fick·ing (traf′ik-ing). SYN processing (1).

trag·a·canth, trag·a·can·tha (trag′ă-kanth, -kan′thă; -santh). A gummy exudation from *Astragalus* species, including *A. gummifer,* shrubs of the eastern end of the Mediterranean; it occurs as bands or strings of a tough gummy substance, forming a jellylike mucilage with 50 parts of water; used as a demulcent and excipient in emulsions and suspensions. [G. *tragakantha,* a gum-producing shrub, fr. *tragos,* goat, + *akanthos,* thorn]

tra·gal (trā′găl). Relating to the tragus.

tra·gi (trā′jī). **1.** Plural of tragus. **2** [NA]. The hairs growing at the entrance to the external acoustic meatus.

tra·gi·cus. SEE tragicus *muscle.*

trag·i·on (trā′jē-on). A cephalometric point in the notch just above the tragus of the ear; it lies 1 to 2 mm below the spine of the helix, which can be palpated.

trag·o·mas·chal·ia (trag-ō-mas-kal′ē-ă). Bromidrosis of the axillae. [G. *tragomaschalos,* with smelling armpits, fr. *tragos,* goat, + *maschalē,* the axilla]

trag·o·pho·nia, tra·goph·o·ny (trag′ō-fō′nē-ă, tră-gof′ō-nē). SYN egophony. [G. *tragos,* goat, + *phōnē,* voice]

tra·gus, pl. **tra·gi** (trā′gŭs, -jī). **1** [NA]. A tonguelike projection of the cartilage of the auricle in front of the opening of the external acoustic meatus and continuous with the cartilage of this canal. SYN antilobium, hircus (3). **2.** SEE tragi (2). [G. *tragos,* goat, in allusion to the hairs growing on the part, like a goatee]

accessory t., small nodules present at birth, anterior to the tragus, derived from first branchial arch remnants and often containing central cartilage.

train·ing (trān′ing). An organized system of education, instruction, or discipline.

assertive t., a form of behavior modification or therapy in which a client is taught to feel free to make legitimate demands and refusals in situations which previously elicited diffident responses. SYN assertive conditioning.

aversive t., a form of behavior t. or modification in which a noxious event is used to punish or extinguish undesirable behavior. SEE ALSO aversion *therapy.* SYN aversive conditioning.

avoidance t., SYN avoidance *conditioning.*

escape t., SYN escape *conditioning.*

toilet t., t. directed at teaching a child proper control of bladder and bowel functions; in psychoanalytic personality theory, it is believed that the attitudes of both parent and child concerning this t. may have important psychological implications for the child's later development.

trait (trāt). A qualitative characteristic; a discrete attribute as contrasted with metrical character. A t. is amenable to segregation rather than quantitative analysis; it is an attribute of phenotype, not of genotype. [Fr. from L. *tractus,* a drawing out, extension]

Bombay t., SEE Bombay *phenomenon.*

categorical t., in genetics, a feature that can conveniently and effectively be analyzed by sorting into classes either because there is no satisfactory way of measuring it (as with blood groups) or because it falls into natural classes so that the variation among classes far exceeds that within classes (*e.g.,* the phenotypic effects of many enzyme polymorphisms); existence of categories suggests but does not prove the operation of a major, simple, underlying cause. SYN qualitative t.

chromosomal t., a t. dependent on a recurrent chromosomal aberration.

codominant t., SEE codominant.

dominant t., (1) an outstanding mental or physical characteristic; SEE *dominance* of traits. **(2)** SEE *dominance* of traits.

dominant lethal t., t., expressed in the phenotype if present in the genotype, that precludes having descendants. All such cases are necessarily sporadic and must represent new mutations as the usual methods of classical genetics provide no means of demonstrating any genetic component whatsoever, except for tenuous arguments such as advanced paternal age. Molecular biology may help although the methods may be tedious; if there is an epistatic gene that may mask the trait, the logic is more tractable, though complex.

galtonian t., a quantitative genetic t. due to contributions from many more of less equally important loci that resembles a continuous t.

intermediate t., a measurable t. in which there is some evidence of the operation of a simple major cause, but in which the variation within the putative categories is such as to cause overlap and hence ambiguity in classification of any particular reading.

liminal t., SYN threshold t.

marker t., a t. that may be of little importance in itself but which by association, linkage, or other means facilitates the detection, anticipation, or understanding of a disease or (for genetic diseases) the localization of the causative gene on the karyotype.

mendelian t., a categorical t. that segregates in accordance with a single-locus genetic system.

nonpenetrant t., a genetic t. that is not phenotypically manifest because of non-genetic factors it therefore does not include recessivity, epistasis, hypostasis, or parastasis but does include environmental factors and pure random effects such as lyonization.

penetrant t., a t. that in the appropriate genotypes is phenotypically manifest; strictly, it is the t. that is penetrant, not the gene. SEE penetrance.

qualitative t., SYN categorical t.

recessive t., (1) SEE *dominance* of traits. SEE *dominance* of traits.

sickle cell t., the heterozygous state of the gene for hemoglobin S in sickle cell anemia.

threshold t., a t. that falls into natural groups that originate not in categorically distinct causes but in whether or not the outcome attains critical values; *e.g.,* gallstones may result from a categorical cause or from unusual levels of causal factors that themselves show no evidence of grouping. SYN liminal t.

tra·jec·tor (tră-jek′ter, -tōr). An instrument for locating the course of a bullet in a wound. [L. fr. *tra-jicio,* pp. *-jectus,* to throw over or across]

tram·a·dol (tră′mă-dol). An analgesic drug whose mechanism of action is unusual in that one optical isomer exerts typical opioid-type effects and the other isomer interacts with the reuptake and/or release of norepinephrine and serotonin in nerve terminals.

tra·maz·o·line hy·dro·chlo·ride (tră-maz′ō-lēn). 2-[(5,6,7,8-Tetrahydro-1-naphthyl)amino]-2-imidazoline hydrochloride; an adrenergic and sympathomimetic agent used for nasal decongestion.

trance (trans). An altered state of consciousness as in hypnosis, catalepsy, or ecstasy. [L. *trans-eo,* to go across]

death t., a condition of suspended animation, marked by unconsciousness and barely perceptible respiration and heart action.

induced t., the artificially induced state of hypnosis or of somnambulistic t.

somnambulistic t., a state of somnambulism, paralysis, anesthesia, or catalepsy induced by suggestion in major hypnosis.

tran·ex·am·ic ac·id (tran-eks-am′ik). *trans*-4(Aminomethyl)-cyclohexanecarboxylic acid; a competitive inhibitor of plasminogen activation and of plasmin; used in hemophilia to reduce or prevent hemorrhage.

tran·quil·iz·er (trang′kwi-lī-zer). A drug that promotes tranquility by calming, soothing, quieting, or pacifying without sedating or depressant effects.

major t., SYN antipsychotic *agent.*

minor t., SYN antianxiety *agent.*

△**trans-. 1.** Prefix denoting across, through, beyond; opposite of *cis-.* **2.** In genetics, denoting the location of two genes on opposite chromosomes of a homologous pair. **3.** In organic chemistry, a form of geometric isomerism in which the atoms attached to two carbon atoms, joined by double bonds, are located on opposite sides of the molecule. **4.** In biochemistry, a prefix to a group name in an enzyme name or a reaction denoting transfer of that group from one compound to another; *e.g.,* transformylase (transfers a formyl group), transpeptidation. [L. *trans,* through, across]

trans·a·cet·y·lase (trans-ă-set′i-lās). SYN acetyltransferase.

trans·a·cet·y·la·tion (trans′ă-set-i-lā′shŭn). Transfer of an acetyl group (CH₃CO–), from one compound to another; such reactions, usually involving formation of acetyl-CoA, occur notably in the initiation of the tricarboxylic acid cycle by the transfer of an acetyl group to oxaloacetate to form citrate.

trans·ac·tion (tranz-ak′shŭn). **1.** Interaction arising from the encounter of two or more persons. **2.** In transactional analysis, the unit of analysis involving a social stimulus and a response.

trans·ac·yl·as·es (trans-as′i-lā-sez). SYN acyltransferases.

trans·ac·yl·a·tion (trans-as′il-ā′shŭn). The reversible transfer of acyl groups.

trans·al·dol·ase (trans-al′dō-lās). Dihydroxyacetonetransferase; glycerone-transferase; transferase interconverting sedoheptulose 7-phosphate and D-glyceraldehyde 3-phosphate to D-erythrose 4-phosphate and D-fructose 6-phosphate; part of the pentose phosphate pathway. SEE ALSO transketolase.

trans·al·do·la·tion (trans′al-dō-lā′shŭn). A reaction involving the transfer of an aldol group (CH₂OH–CO–CHOH–) from one compound to another; such reactions generally involve the sugar phosphates and occur in the phosphogluconate oxidation pathway of carbohydrate catabolism.

trans·a·mi·da·tion (trans-am′i-dā-shŭn). The transfer of NH₂ from an amide moiety (*e.g.,* from glutamine) to another molecule.

trans·am·i·di·nas·es (trans-am′i-di-nās-ez). SYN amidinotransferases.

trans·am·i·di·na·tion (trans-am′i-di-nā′shŭn). A reaction involving the transfer of an amidine group (NH₂C=NH) from one compound to another; the amidine donor is generally L-arginine and the reaction is of significance in the biosynthesis of creatine.

trans·am·i·nas·es (trans-am′i-nās-ez). SYN aminotransferases.

trans·am·i·na·tion (trans-am′i-nā′shŭn). The reaction between an amino acid and an α-keto acid through which the amino group is transferred from the former to the latter; in certain cases the reaction may be between an amino acid and an aldehyde (*e.g.,* glutamate with glutamate semialdehyde via ornithine transaminase).

trans·an·i·ma·tion (trans-an′i-mā′shŭn). Resuscitation of a stillborn infant. [trans- + L. *anima,* breath, life]

trans·au·di·ent (trans-aw′dē-ent). Permeable to sound waves. [trans- + L. *audio,* pres. p. *audiens,* to hear]

trans·ca·lent (trans-kā′lent). SYN diathermanous. [trans- + L. *caleo,* to be warm]

trans·cap·si·da·tion (trans-kap-si-dā′shŭn). The phenomenon whereby the adenovirus capsid of the SV40 adenovirus "hybrid" is replaced by the capsid of another type of adenovirus; extended to include a similar phenomenon in other viruses.

trans·car·bam·o·y·las·es (trans-kar-bam′ō-i-lā-sez). SYN carbamoyltransferases.

trans·car·bam·o·yl·a·tion (trans-kar-bam′ō-il-ā′shŭn). The transfer of carbamoyl moiety from one molecule to another; *e.g.,* the reaction catalyzed by ornithine transcarbamoylase in the urea cycle.

trans·car·box·yl·as·es (trans-kar-boks′i-lās-ez). SYN carboxyltransferases.

tran·scen·den·tal med·i·ta·tion (tranz′en-den-tal med′ĭ-tā-shŭn). A form of meditation practiced over 2500 years ago in Eastern cultures and which was recently made popular in the West by Maharishi Mahesh Yogi as a means to help increase energy, reduce stress, and have a positive effect on mental and physical health; it involves the person sitting upright for 20 minutes, with eyes closed, and silently speaking a mantra (a key stimulus word used uniquely by each individual to return to the proper meditative state) whenever thought occurs.

trans·co·bal·a·mins (trans-kō-bal′ă-minz). Substances included in "R binder," the name given a family of cobalamin-binding proteins; deficiencies have been associated with low serum cobalamin levels, and can lead to megaloblastic anemia.

trans·con·dy·lar (trans-kon′di-lăr). Across or through the condyles; denoting the line of bone incision in Carden's amputation.

trans·cor·ti·cal (tranz-kōr′ti-kăl). **1.** Across or through the cortex of the brain, ovary, kidney, or other organ. **2.** From one part of the cerebral cortex to another; denoting the various association tracts.

trans·cor·tin (trans-kōr′tin). An α₂-globulin in blood that binds cortisol and corticosterone; the principle corticosteroid-binding protein in the plasma. SYN corticosteroid-binding globulin, corticosteroid-binding protein.

tran·scrip·tase (tran-skrip′tās). A polymerase associated with the process of transcription; especially the DNA-dependent RNA polymerase. [L. *transcribo,* pp. *transcriptum,* to copy, + -ase]
reverse t., RNA-dependent DNA polymerase, present in virions of RNA tumor viruses.

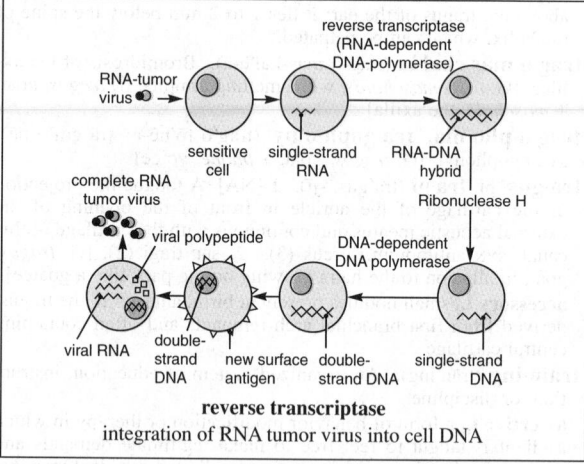

reverse transcriptase
integration of RNA tumor virus into cell DNA

tran·scrip·tion (tran-skrip′shŭn). Transfer of genetic code information from one kind of nucleic acid to another, especially with reference to the process by which a base sequence of messenger RNA is synthesized (by an RNA polymerase) on a template of complementary DNA.
reverse t., reversal of the normal pattern of t. (from DNA to RNA); the effective means is the viral enzyme reverse transcriptase.

trans·cu·ta·ne·ous (trans-kyū-tā′nē-ŭs). SYN percutaneous.

trans·cy·to·sis (trans-sī-tō′sis). A mechanism for transcellular transport in which a cell encloses extracellular material in an invagination of the cell membrane to form a vesicle (endocytosis), then moves the vesicle across the cell to eject the material through the opposite cell membrane by the reverse process (exocytosis). The transport mechanism by which most proteins reach the Golgi apparatus or the plasma membrane; the vesicles targeted toward lysosomes and secretory storage granules appear to be coated with clathrin. SYN cytopempsis, vesicular transport.

trans·der·mic (trans-der′mik). SYN percutaneous.

trans·duce (trans-dūs′). To effect transduction.

trans·duc·er (trans-dū′ser). A device designed to convert energy from one form to another. [see transduction]
piezoelectric t., a t. that converts electric into mechanical energy and vice versa, used in ultrasound diagnosis or therapy.
ultrasound t., a piezoelectric t. used in diagnostic ultrasound.

trans·duc·in (trans-dū′sin). A protein that binds guanine nucleotides (*i.e.,* a G protein), found in retinal rods and cones, that plays a major role in signal transduction; in vertebrate rod cells it acts as a link of the photolysis of rhodopsin to the activation of cGMP phosphodiesterase.

trans·duc·tant (trans-dŭk′tănt). A cell that has acquired a new character by means of transduction; may be *complete*, with integration of the transferred genetic fragment into its genome, or *abortive*, in which case the genetic fragment is not integrated and passes to only one of the two daughter cells on division.

trans·duc·tion (trans-dŭk′shŭn). **1.** Transfer of genetic material (and its phenotypic expression) from one cell to another by viral infection. **2.** A form of genetic recombination in bacteria. **3.** Conversion of energy from one form to another. [trans- + L. *duco*, pp. *ductus*, to lead across]

abortive t., t. in which the genetic fragment from the donor bacterium is not integrated in the genome of the recipient bacterium, and, when the latter divides, is transmitted to only one of the daughter cells.

complete t., t. in which the transferred genetic fragment is fully integrated in the genome of the recipient bacterium.

general t., t. in which the transducing bacteriophage is able to transfer any gene of the donor bacterium.

high frequency t., specialized t. in which the donor bacterium contains not only the transducing, defective probacteriophage but also nondefective prophage that serves as "helper" virus, enabling most of the defective prophage particles to develop sufficiently to function as transducing agents.

low frequency t., specialized t. in which only a small portion of the prophage particles, because of their defectiveness, are able to develop sufficiently to serve as effective transducing agents.

specialized t., t. in which the bacteriophage strain is able to transfer only some, or only one, of the donor bacterium genes. SYN specific t.

specific t., SYN specialized t.

tran·sec·tion (tran-sek′shŭn). **1.** A cross section. **2.** Cutting across. SYN transsection. [trans- + L. *seco*, pp. *sectus*, to cut]

trans·eth·moi·dal (trans′eth-moy′dăl). Across or through the ethmoid bone.

trans·fec·tion (trans-fek′shŭn). A method of gene transfer utilizing infection of a cell with nucleic acid (as from a retrovirus) resulting in subsequent viral replication in the transfected cell. [trans- + in*fection*]

trans·fer. **1.** Process of removal or transferral. **2.** A condition in which learning in one situation influences learning in another situation; a carry-over of learning which may be positive in effect, as when learning one behavior facilitates the learning of something else, or may be negative, as when one habit interferes with the acquisition of a later one. SYN transmission (1). [L. *trans-fero*, to bear across]

cavernous t. of portal vein, replacement of the portal vein by a number of collateral channels, a consequence of thrombosis.

embryo t., after *in vitro* artificial insemination, the fertilized ovum is transferred at the blastocyst stage to the recipient's uterus or oviduct.

Fourier t., a mathematical technique to express a time-varying function or signal into components at different frequencies, giving the phase and amplitude of each; used in computed tomography and magnetic resonance image reconstruction transformation.

group t., the t. of a functional moiety from one molecule to another.

linear energy t. (LET), the amount of energy deposited by radiation per unit length of travel, expressed in keV per micron; protons, neutrons, and alpha particles have much higher LET than gamma or x-rays. A property of radiation considered in radiation protection. SEE relative biological effectiveness.

trans·fer·ase. A class of enzymes that move a chemical group from one compound to another.

trans·fer·as·es (trans′fer-ās-ez). Enzymes (EC class 2) transferring: one-carbon groups (2.1, including methyltransferases, 2.1.1; formyltransferases, 2.1.2; carboxyl- and carbamoyltransferases, 2.1.3, and amidinotransferases, 2.1.4); acyl residues (acyltransferases, 2.3); glycosyl residues (glycosyltransferases, 2.4, including hexosyltransferases, 2.4.1, and pentosyltransferases, 2.4.2); alkyl or aryl groups (2.5); nitrogenous groups (2.6); phos-

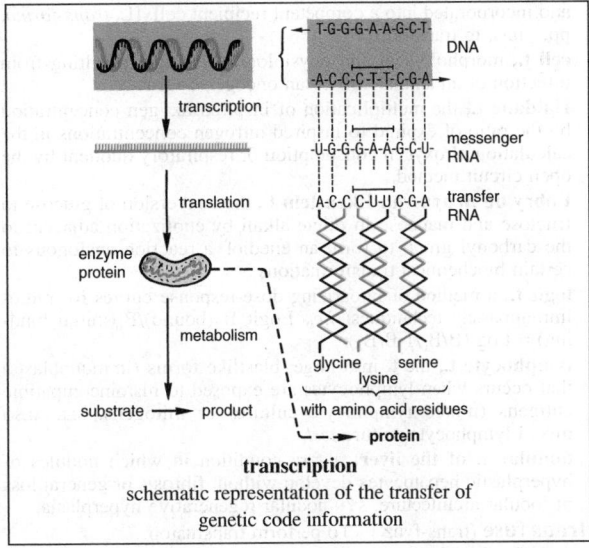

transcription
schematic representation of the transfer of genetic code information

phorus-containing groups (2.7, phosphotransferases); and sulfur-containing groups (2.8, including sulfurtransferases, 2.8.1; sulfotransferases, 2.8.2; and CoA-transferases, 2.8.3). SYN transferring enzymes.

terminal t., enzymes that covalently add nucleotides to the 3′ end of polynucleic acids; *e.g.,* DNA nucleotidylexotransferase.

trans·fer·ence (trans-fer′ens). **1.** Conveyance of an object from one place to another. **2.** Shifting of symptoms from one side of the body to the other, as seen in certain cases of conversion hysteria. **3.** Displacement of affect from one person or one idea to another; in psychoanalysis, generally applied to the projection of feelings, thoughts, and wishes onto the analyst, who has come to represent some person from the patient's past.

counter t., SEE countertransference.

extrasensory thought t., SYN telepathy.

negative t., t. characterized by predominantly hostile feelings on the part of the patient toward the analyst.

passive t., the passage of an immunity or allergic susceptibility by the injection of serum of an animal or individual who has acquired an active immunity to the disease.

positive t., t. characterized by predominantly friendly, respectful, and positive feelings on the part of the patient toward the analyst.

trans·fer·ence love. Love expressed by the patient for the psychoanalyst as a manifestation of transference (3).

trans·fer·rin (trans-fer′in). **1.** A non-heme β_1-globulin of the plasma, capable of associating reversibly with up to 1.25 μg of iron per g, and acting therefore as an iron-transporting protein. **2.** A glycoprotein, found in mammalian milk (lactoferrin) and egg white (conalbumin, ovotransferrin), that binds and transports iron (Fe^{3+}). [trans- + L. *ferrum*, iron, + -ia]

trans·fer-RNA. See entries under ribonucleic acid.

trans·fix (trans′fiks). To pierce with a sharp instrument. [L. *trans-figo*, pp. *-fixus*, to pierce through, fr. *figo*, to fasten]

trans·fix·ion (trans-fĭk′shŭn). A maneuver in amputation in which the knife is passed from side to side through the soft parts, close to the bone, and the muscles are then divided from within outward. [L. *transfixio* (see transfix)]

trans·form·ant (trans-fōr′mănt). A bacterium that has received genetic material (and its phenotypic expression) from another bacterium by means of transformation.

trans·for·ma·tion (trans-fōr-mā′shŭn). **1.** SYN metamorphosis. **2.** A change of one tissue into another, as cartilage into bone. **3.** In metals, a change in phase and physical properties in the solid state caused by heat treatment. **4.** In microbial genetics, transfer of genetic information between bacteria by means of "naked" intracellular DNA fragments derived from bacterial donor cells and incorporated into a competent recipient cell. [L. *trans-formo,* pp. *-atus,* to transform]

cell t., morphological and physiological changes resulting from infection of an animal cell by an oncogenic virus.

Haldane t., the multiplication of inspired oxygen concentration by the ratio of expired to inspired nitrogen concentrations in the calculation of oxygen consumption or respiratory quotient by the open circuit method.

Lobry de Bruyn-van Ekenstein t., the conversion of glucose to fructose and mannose in dilute alkali by enolization adjacent to the carbonyl group to form an enediol, a reaction analogous to certain biochemical transformations.

logit t., a method of linearizing dose-response curves for radio-immunoassay techniques; *i.e.,* Logit B (bound)/B$_0$(initial binding) = Log (B/B$_0$/1-B/B$_0$).

lymphocyte t., the t. into large, blastlike forms (immunoblasts) that occurs when lymphocytes are exposed to histoincompatible antigens (mixed lymphocyte culture) or mitogens. SEE ALSO mixed lymphocyte culture *test.*

nodular t. of the liver, a rare condition in which nodules of hyperplastic hepatocytes develop without fibrosis or general loss of lobular architecture. SYN nodular regenerative hyperplasia.

trans·fuse (trans-fyūz′). To perform transfusion.

trans·fu·sion (trans-fyū′zhŭn). 1. Transfer of blood or blood component of an individual (donor) to another individual (receptor). 2. Intravascular injection of physiologic saline solution. [L. *trans-fundo,* pp. *-fusus,* to pour from one vessel to another]

arterial t., direct t. from an artery of the donor into an artery of the receptor.

direct t., t. of blood from the donor to the receptor, either through a tube connecting their blood or by suturing the vessels together. SYN immediate t.

drip t., t. slow enough to measure by drops.

exchange t., removal of most of a patient's blood followed by introduction of an equal amount from donors. SYN exsanguination t., substitution t., total t.

exsanguination t., SYN exchange t.

fetomaternal t., passage of fetal blood into maternal circulation.

immediate t., SYN direct t.

indirect t., t. into a patient of blood previously obtained from a donor and stored in a suitable container. SYN mediate t.

intrauterine t., to treat erythroblastosis fetalis, Rh-negative blood is placed into the peritoneal cavity of the fetus.

mediate t., SYN indirect t.

peritoneal t., the injection of saline solution or other fluid into the peritoneal cavity.

placental t., return to the newborn via the umbilical vessels some of the fetal placental blood.

reciprocal t., an attempt to confer immunity by transfusing blood taken from a donor into a receiver suffering from the same affection, the balance being maintained by transfusing an equal amount from the receiver to the donor.

subcutaneous t., an infusion of absorbable solutions beneath the skin.

substitution t., SYN exchange t.

total t., SYN exchange t.

twin-twin t., direct vascular anastomosis, arterial or venous, between the placental circulations of twins.

trans·gene (trans′gēn). A newly introduced gene.

trans·gen·ic (trans-jen′ik). Referring to an organism in which new DNA has been introduced into the germ cells by injection into the nucleus of the ovum.

trans·gen·ic mice (tranz′jen-ik). Mice that have a piece of foreign lincor DNA integrated into their genome.

trans·glu·co·syl·ase (trans-glū′kō-si-lās). SYN glucosyltransferase.

trans·glu·ta·min·ase (trans-glū-ta-min-ās). A group of enzymes that catalyze the calcium-dependent acyl transfer reaction in which the amide moiety of peptide-bound glutaminyl residues serve as acyl donor; a specific t. covalently cross-links fibrin molecules between glutamine and the ε-amino group of a lysyl residue, thus producing a more stable fibrin clot; another t. par-

ticipates in the formation of the chemically resistant envelope of the stratum corneum during terminal differentiation of keratinocytes.

trans·gly·co·si·da·tion (trans-glī-ko-sid′ā-shŭn). The transfer of a glycosidically bound sugar to another molecule.

trans·gly·co·syl·ase (trans-glī′kō-si-lās). SYN glycosyltransferase.

trans·hi·a·tal (trans-hī-ā′tăl). By way of a hiatus; said of a surgical procedure.

tran·sient (trans′shĕnt, -sē-ĕnt). 1. Short-lived; passing; not permanent; said of a disease or an attack. 2. A short-lived cardiac sound having little duration (less than 0.12 second) as distinct from a murmur; *e.g.,* first, second, third, and fourth heart sounds, clicks, and opening snaps. [L. *transeo,* pres. p. *transiens,* to cross over]

trans·il·i·ac (tran-sil′ē-ak). Extending from one ilium or iliac crest or spine to the other.

tran·sil·i·ent (tran-sil′yent, -zil-). Jumping across; passing over; pertaining to those cortical association fibers in the brain that pass from one convolution to another nonadjacent one. [L. *trans-silio,* to leap across, fr. *salio,* to leap]

trans·il·lu·mi·na·tion (trans-i-lū′mi-nā′shŭn). Method of examination by the passage of light through tissues or a body cavity. [trans- + L. *illumino,* pp. *-atus,* to light up]

trans·in·su·lar (tranz-in′sū-lăr). Across the insula or island of Reil.

trans·is·chi·ac (trans-is′kē-ak). Extending from one ischium to the other.

trans·isth·mi·an (trans-is′mē-an). Across any isthmus; specifically, across the isthmus of the fornicate gyrus, denoting the gyrus transitivus.

tran·si·tion (tran-sish′ŭn, -zish′ŭn). 1. Passage from one condition or one part to another. 2. In polynucleic acid, replacement of a purine base by another purine base or a pyrimidine base by a different pyrimidine. [L. *transitio,* fr. *transeo,* pp. *-itus,* to go across]

cervicothoracic t., the junction between the last cervical vertebra and first thoracic vertebra.

isomeric t., the t. of a nuclear isomer to a lower quantum state; *e.g.,* $^{131m}Xe \rightarrow$ $^{131}Xe + \gamma.$

tran·si·tion·al (tran-sish′ŭn-ăl, -zish-). Relating to or marked by a transition; transitory.

trans·ke·tol·ase (trans-kē′tō-lās). A transferase bringing about the reversible interconversion of sedoheptulose 7-phosphate and D-glyceraldehyde 3-phosphate to produce D-ribose 5-phosphate and D-xylulose 5-phosphate, and also other similar reactions, such as hydroxypyruvate and an aldehyde into CO_2 and an extended hydroxypyruvate; a part of the nonoxidative phase of the pentose phosphate pathway. SEE ALSO transaldolase. SYN glycolaldehydetransferase.

trans·ke·to·la·tion (trans′kē-tō-lā′shŭn). A reaction involving the transfer of a ketole group (HOCH$_2$CO–) from one compound to another.

trans·la·tion (trans-lā′shŭn). 1. A change or conversion into another form. 2. The rather complex process by which messenger RNA, transfer RNA, and ribosomes effect the production of protein from amino acids, the specificity of synthesis being controlled by the base sequences of the messenger RNA. 3. In dentistry, the movement of a tooth through alveolar bone without change in axial inclination. [L. *translatio,* a transferring, fr. *trans- fero,* pp. *-latus,* to carry across]

nick t., a technique in which a bacterial DNA polymerase is used to degrade a single strand of DNA that has been nicked and then to resynthesize that strand, often with labeled nucleoside triphosphates.

trans·lo·ca·tion (trans-lō-kā′shŭn). 1. Transposition of two segments between nonhomologous chromosomes as a result of abnormal breakage and refusion of reciprocal segments. 2. Transport of a metabolite across a biomembrane. [trans- + L. *location,* placement, fr. *loco,* to place]

balanced t., t. of the long arm of an acrocentric chromosome to another chromosome; an individual with a balanced t. has a normal diploid genome and is clinically normal but has a chromosome count of 45 and as a result of asymmetrical meiosis may have children lacking the genes on the translocated sigment or have them in trisomy.

group t., a form of active transport across a biomembrane in which the transporting molecule is altered in the course of the transport.

reciprocal t., t. without demonstrable loss of genetic material.

robertsonian t., t. in which the centromeres of two acrocentric chromosomes appear to have fused, forming an abnormal chromosome consisting of the long arms of two different chromosomes; if the t. is balanced, the individual is clinically normal but a carrier of the t.; if the t. is unbalanced, the individual is trisomic for the long arm of a chromosome. SYN centric fusion. [W.R.B. *Robertson,* U.S. geneticist, *1881]

unbalanced t., condition resulting from fertilization of a gamete containing a t. chromosome by a normal gamete; if this abnormality is compatible with life, the individual would have 46 chromosomes but a segment of the t. chromosome would be represented three times in each cell and a partial or complete trisomic state would exist.

trans·lu·cent (trans-lū′sent). Partially transparent; permitting light to pass through diffusely. [L. *translucens,* fr. trans- + *luceo,* to shine through]

trans·mem·brane (trans-mem′brān). Through or across a membrane.

trans·meth·yl·ase (trans-meth′i-lās). SYN methyltransferase.

trans·meth·yl·a·tion (trans′meth-i-lā′shŭn). Transfer of a methyl group from one compound to another; *e.g.,* L-homocysteine is converted to L-methionine by the transfer to the latter of a methyl group. SEE *methionine* synthase.

trans·mi·gra·tion (trans-mī-grā′shŭn). Movement from one site to another; may entail the crossing of some usually limiting barrier, as in the passage of blood cells through the walls of the vessels (diapedesis). [L. *trans-migro,* pp. *-atus,* to remove from one place to another]

ovular t., the passage of an ovum from one ovary into the fallopian tube of the other side; **external ovular t., direct ovular t.** occurs when the ovum passes across the pelvic cavity; **internal ovular t., indirect ovular t.** when the ovum crosses the uterine cavity and so enters the tube of the opposite side.

trans·mis·si·ble (trans-mis′i-bl). Capable of being transmitted (carried across) from one person to another, as a t. disease, an infectious or contagious disease.

trans·mis·sion (trans-mish′ŭn). **1.** SYN transfer. **2.** The conveyance of disease from one person to another. **3.** The passage of a nerve impulse across an anatomic cleft, as in autonomic or central nervous system synapses and at neuromuscular junctions, by activation of a specific chemical mediator that stimulates or inhibits the structure across the synapse. SEE neurohumoral t. **4.** In general, passage of energy through a material. [L. *transmissio,* a sending across]

duplex t., the passage of impulses in both directions through a nerve trunk.

horizontal t., t. of infectious agents from an infected individual to a susceptible contemporary, in contradistinction to vertical t.

iatrogenic t., t. of infectious agents due to medical interference (*e.g.,* t. by contaminated needles).

neurohumoral t., a process by which a presynaptic cell, upon excitation, releases a specific chemical agent (a neurotransmitter) to cross a synapse to stimulate or inhibit the postsynaptic cell. SYN neurotransmission.

transovarial t. (trans′ō-vă-rē-al), passage of parasites or infective agents from the maternal body to eggs within the ovaries; commonly used to describe certain arthropods, to explain the ability of larvae of the next generation to transmit disease pathogens, as with the infection of larval mites or ticks with rickettsiae or viruses.

transstadial t., passage of a microbial parasite, such as a virus or rickettsia, from one developmental stage (stadium) of the host to its subsequent stage or stages, particularly as seen in mites. SEE ALSO transovarial t.

vertical t., (1) t. of a virus (*e.g.,* RNA tumor virus) by means of

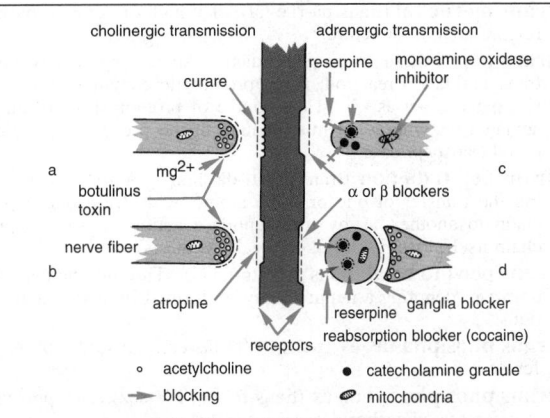

transmission (and inhibition) of impulses
a) cholinergic transmission, at motor endplate, b) at smooth muscle synapse, c) direct adrenergic transmission, d) indirect adrenergic transmission

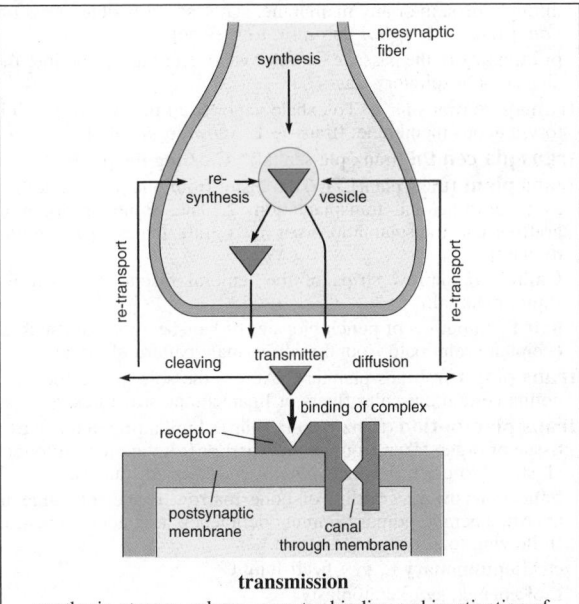

transmission
synthesis, storage, release, receptor-binding and inactivation of transmitter at point of contact between presynaptic fiber and postsynaptic neuron

the genetic apparatus of a cell in which the viral genome is integrated; **(2)** for infectious agents in general, t. of an agent from an individual to its offspring. *i.e.,* from one generation to the next. Cf. horizontal t.

trans·mu·ral (trans-myū′răl). Through any wall, as of the body or of a cyst or any hollow structure. [trans- + L. *murus,* wall]

trans·mu·ta·tion (trans-myū-tā′shŭn). A change; transformation. SYN conversion (1). [L. *trans-muto,* pp. *-atus,* to change, transmute]

trans·oc·u·lar (trans-ok′yū-lăr). Across the eye.

tran·so·nance (trans′ō-nans). Transmission of a sound arising in one organ through another. [trans- + L. *sonans,* sounding]

tran·son·ic (tran-son′ik). In ultrasound, describes a region of a relatively unattenuating medium. A distinction should be made between a t. region and an acoustic echo. [trans- + sonic]

tr

trans·pa·ri·e·tal (trans-pă-rī′ĕ-tăl). Through or across a parietal region, area, or structure.

trans·pep·ti·dase (trans-pep′ti-dās). An enzyme catalyzing a transpeptidation reaction; many proteolytic enzymes (*e.g.,* trypsin, papain) act as t.'s in the course of proteolysis, forming an acylated enzyme as an intermediate in the process; *e.g.,* γ-glutamyl transpeptidase.

trans·pep·ti·da·tion (trans′pep-ti-dā′shŭn). A reaction involving the transfer of one or more amino acids from one peptide chain to another, as by transpeptidase action, or of a peptide chain itself, as in bacterial cell wall synthesis.

trans·per·i·to·ne·al (trans′per-i-tō-nē′ăl). Through the peritoneum; *e.g.,* denoting a nephrectomy performed by abdominal section.

trans·phos·pha·tas·es (trans-fos′fă-tās-ez). SYN phosphotransferases.

trans·phos·pho·ryl·as·es (trans-fos-fōr′i-lā-sez). SEE phosphotransferases, phosphorylases, kinase.

trans·phos·pho·ryl·a·tion (trans′fos-fōr-i-lā′shŭn). A reaction involving the transfer of a phosphoric group from one compound to another, often with the involvement of ATP, as by the action of a phosphotransferase or kinase.

tran·spir·a·ble (trans-pī′ră-bl). Capable of transpiring or being transpired.

tran·spi·ra·tion (trans-pi-rā′shŭn). Passage of watery vapor through the skin or any membrane. SEE ALSO insensible *perspiration*. [trans- + L. *spiro,* pp. *-atus,* to breathe]

pulmonary t., the passage of water vapor from the blood into the air via the respiratory tract.

tran·spire (trans-pīr′). To exhale vapor from the skin or respiratory mucous membrane. [trans- + L. *spiro,* to breathe]

trans·pla·cen·tal (tranz-pla-sen′tăl). Crossing the placenta.

trans·plant (tranz′plant). **1.** To transfer from one part to another, as in grafting and transplantation. **2.** The tissue or organ in grafting and transplantation. SEE ALSO graft. [trans- + L. *planto,* to plant]

Gallie's t., narrow strips of the femoral fascia lata used for suture material.

hair t., autografts of punch biopsies of hair-bearing skin, such as occipital scalp, onto frontal scalp in male pattern alopecia.

trans·plan·tar (trans-plan′tar). Across the sole of the foot; denoting certain muscular fibers or ligamentous structures.

trans·plan·ta·tion (tranz-plan-tā′shŭn). Implanting in one part a tissue or organ taken from another part or from another individual. SEE ALSO graft. [L. *trans-planto,* pp. *-atus,* to transplant]

bone marrow t., grafting of bone marrow tissue; of value in aplastic anemia, primary immunodeficiency, and acute leukemia (following total body irradiation).

cardiopulmonary t., SYN heart-lung t.

t. of cornea, SYN keratoplasty.

corneal t., SYN keratoplasty.

heart t., replacement of a severely damaged heart by: 1) a healthy donated heart from a victim of trauma or other morbid process not incompatible with t.; 2) an artificial heart.

heart-lung t., usually done for irreversible pulmonary hypertension. SYN cardiopulmonary t.

pancreaticoduodenal t., a technically feasible t. including both the duodenum and pancreas.

renal t., t. of a kidney from a compatible donor to restore kidney function in a recipient suffering from renal failure.

tendon t., (1) insertion of a slip from the tendon of a sound muscle into the tendon of a paralyzed muscle; **(2)** replacement of a length of tendon by a free graft.

tooth t., the transfer of a tooth from one alveolus to another.

trans·pleu·ral (trans-plū′răl). Through the pleura or across the pleural cavity; on the other side of the pleura.

trans·port (trans′pōrt). The movement or transference of biochemical substances in biologic systems. [L. *transporto,* to carry over, fr. trans- + *porto,* to carry]

active t., the passage of ions or molecules across a cell membrane, not by passive diffusion but by an energy-consuming

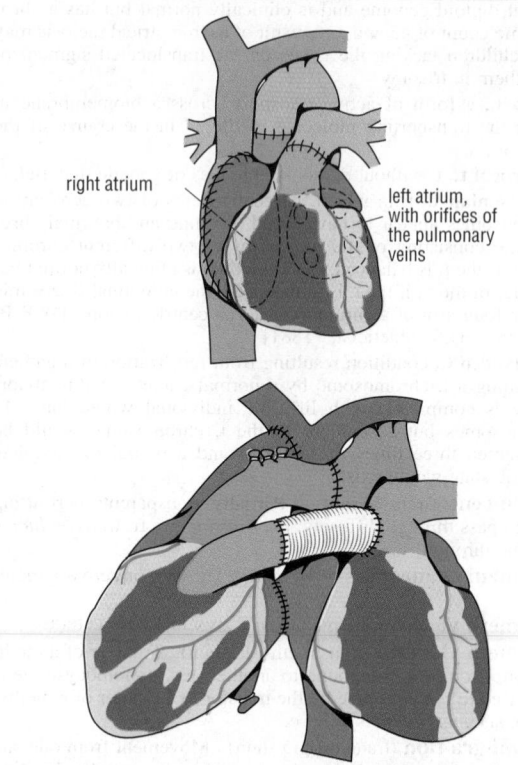

heart transplant

top, <u>orthotopic transplant</u>. The position of the anastomoses between the transplant and the aorta and pulmonary artery is clearly seen. The anastomosis of both atria with existing atrial tissue of the patient is shown by dotted line. *bottom,* <u>heterotopic transplant</u>. The donor's heart is transplanted piggy-back into the right side of patient's thorax.

right atrium

left atrium, with orifices of the pulmonary veins

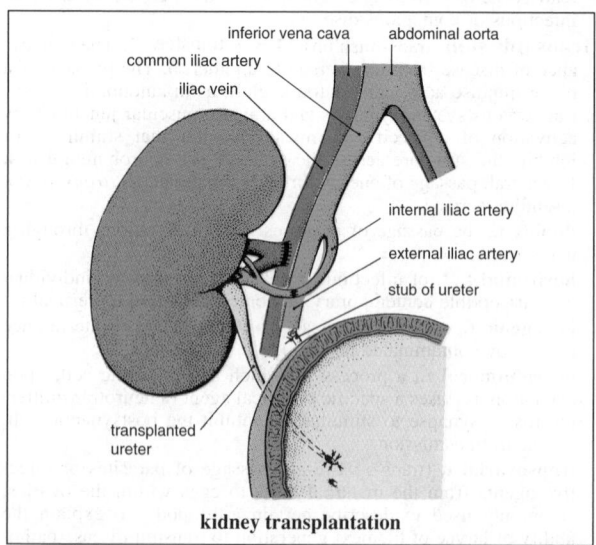

inferior vena cava
abdominal aorta
common iliac artery
iliac vein
internal iliac artery
external iliac artery
stub of ureter
transplanted ureter

kidney transplantation

process at the expense of catabolic processes proceeding within the cell; in active t., movement takes place against an electrochemical gradient.

axoplasmic t., transport by way of flow of axoplasm toward cell soma (retrograde) or toward axon terminal (anterograde).

facilitated t., the protein-mediated t. of a compound across a biomembrane that is not ion-driven; a saturable t. system. SYN passive t.

hydrogen t., the transfer of hydrogen from one metabolite (hydrogen donor) to another (hydrogen acceptor) through the action of an enzyme system; the donor is thus oxidized and the acceptor reduced.

paracellular t., solvent movement across an epithelial cell layer through the tight junctions between cells. Cf. transcellular t.

passive t., SYN facilitated t.

transcellular t., solute movement across an epithelial cell layer through the cells. Cf. paracellular t.

vesicular t., SYN transcytosis.

trans·pos·ase (tranz-pōz′ās). An enzyme that is required for transposition of DNA segments. [L. *trans-pono,* pp. *transpositum,* to set across, transfer, + -ase]

trans·pose (tranz-pōz). To transfer one tissue or organ to the place of another and *vice versa.* [L. *trans-pono,* pp. *-positus,* to place across, transfer]

trans·po·si·tion (tranz-pō-zish′ŭn). **1.** Removal from one place to another; metathesis. **2.** The condition of being transposed to the wrong side of the body, as in t. of the viscera, in which the viscera are located opposite their normal position; *e.g.,* the liver on the left, the apex of the heart on the right. **3.** Positioning of teeth out of their normal sequence in an arch.

t. of arterial stems, SYN t. of the great vessels.

corrected t. of the great vessels, anatomically or physiologically corrected malposition of the great arteries. In anatomically corrected t., they arise from the correct ventricles but have an abnormal relation to each other (actually a malposition rather than a t.) In physiologically or functionally corrected t., the aorta arises from a systemic ventricle that has the morphologic characteristics of a right ventricle, and the pulmonary artery arises from a "venous" ventricle that has the morphologic characteristics of a left ventricle.

t. of the great vessels, congenital malformation in which the aorta arises from the morphologic right ventricle and the pulmonary artery from the morphologic left ventricle resulting in two separate and parallel circulations. The condition is lethal unless some communication exists between the systemic and pulmonic circulation after birth; otherwise, unoxygenated venous blood inappropriately enters the systemic circulation, and oxygenated pulmonary venous blood is inappropriately directed to the pulmonary circulation. The life sustaining communication may be an intra-atrial passage or a patent ductus arteriosus. SYN t. of arterial stems.

penoscrotal t., SYN webbed *penis.*

trans·po·son (trans-pō′son). A segment of DNA (*e.g.,* an R-factor gene) which has a repeat of an insertion sequence element at each end that can migrate from one plasmid to another within the same bacterium, to a bacterial chromosome, or to a bacteriophage; the mechanism of transposition seems to be independent of the host's usual recombination mechanism. SEE jumping *gene.* [L. *transpono,* pp. *transpositum,* to transfer, + -on]

trans·sec·tion (trans-sek′shŭn). SYN transection.

trans·seg·men·tal (trans-seg-men′tăl). Across or through a segment.

trans·sep·tal (trans-sep′tăl). Across or through a septum; on the other side of a septum.

trans·sex·u·al (trans-sek′shū-ăl). **1.** A person with the external genitalia and secondary sexual characteristics of one sex, but whose personal identification and psychosocial configuration is that of the opposite sex; a study of morphologic, genetic, and gonadal structure may be genitally congruent or incongruent. **2.** Denoting or relating to such a person. **3.** Relating to medical and surgical procedures designed to alter a patient's external sexual characteristics so that they resemble those of the opposite sex.

trans·sex·u·al·ism (tranz-sek′shū-ă-lizm). **1.** The state of being a transsexual. **2.** The desire to change one's anatomic sexual characteristics to conform physically with one's perception of self as a member of the opposite sex.

trans·sphe·noi·dal (trans-sfē-noy′dăl). Through or across the sphenoid bone.

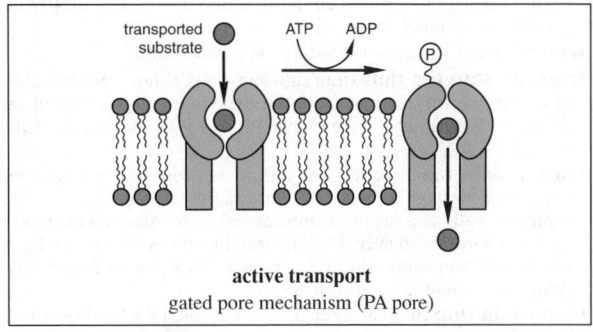

active transport
gated pore mechanism (PA pore)

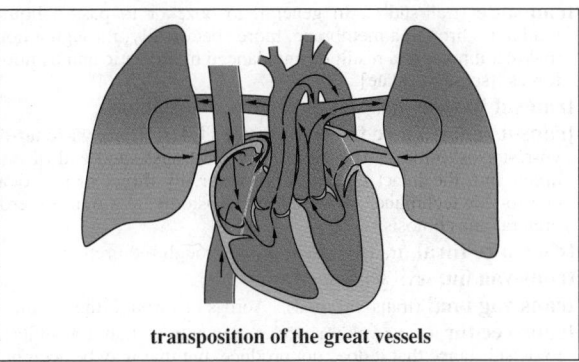

transposition of the great vessels

trans·-splic·ing (trans-splīs′ing). Formation of spliced products containing portions of two different transcripts.

trans·sul·fu·rase (trans-sŭl′fer-ās). Descriptive term applied to the enzymes catalyzing, among others, the following reactions involving sulfur-containing compounds: 1) cystathionine → cysteine + α-ketobutyrate + NH₃ (cystathionine γ-lyase); 2) cystathionine → homocysteine + pyruvate + NH₃ (cystathionine β-lyase); 3) cystine → thiocysteine + pyruvate + NH₃ (cystathionine γ-lyase); 4) cystathionine → serine + homocysteine (cystathionine synthase). SYN transulfurase.

trans·sul·fur·a·tion (trans-sŭl′fer-ā′shŭn). The exchange of sulfur, or sulfur, containing moiety, between two different compounds.

trans·syn·ap·tic (trans-si-nap′tik). Indicating transmission of a nerve impulse across a synapse.

trans·ten·to·ri·al (trans-ten-tōr′ē-ăl). Passing across or through either the tentorial notch or tentorium cerebelli.

trans·tha·lam·ic (trans-tha-lam′ik). Passing across the thalamus.

trans·ther·mia (trans-ther′mē-ă). SYN diathermy. [trans- + G. *thermē,* heat]

trans·tho·rac·ic (trans-thōr-as′ik). Passing through the thoracic cavity.

trans·tho·ra·cot·o·my (trans-thōr′ă-kot′ō-mē). A surgical pro-

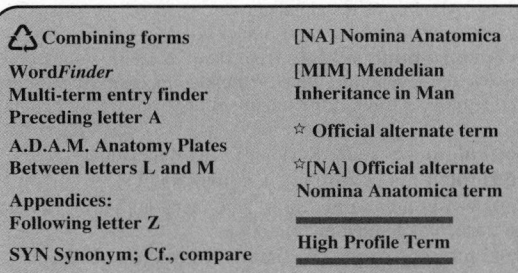

cedure carried out through an incision into the chest wall. [trans- + thorax + G. *tomē,* incision]

trans·thy·ret·in (trans-thī'rē-tin). SYN prealbumin.

tran·sub·stan·ti·a·tion (tran'sŭb-stan-shē-ā'shŭn). Substitution of one tissue for another, as in the experimental patching of an artery with peritoneal membrane. [trans- + L. *substantia,* substance]

tran·su·date (tran'sū-dāt). Any fluid (solvent and solute) that has passed through a presumably normal membrane, such as the capillary wall, as a result of imbalanced hydrostatic and osmotic forces; characteristically low in protein unless there has been secondary concentration. Cf. exudate. SYN transudation (2). [trans- + L. *sudo,* pp. *-atus,* to sweat]

tran·su·da·tion (tran-sū-dā'shŭn). 1. Passage of a fluid or solute through a membrane by a hydrostatic or osmotic pressure gradient. 2. SYN transudate. [see transudate]

tran·sude (tran-sūd'). In general, to ooze or to pass a liquid gradually through a membrane, more specifically, through a normal membrane, as a result of imbalanced hydrostatic and osmotic forces. [see transudate]

tran·sul·fu·rase (tran-sŭl'fer-ās). SYN transsulfurase.

trans·u·re·ter·o·u·re·ter·os·to·my (TUU) (tranz-yū-rē'ter-ō-yū-rē-ter-os'tō-mē). Anastomosis of the transsected end of one ureter into the intact contralateral ureter, by direct or elliptical end-to-side technique. SEE ureteroureterostomy. SYN transureteroureteral anastomosis.

trans·u·re·thral (trans-yū-rē'thrăl). Through the urethra.

trans·vaa·lin. SYN *scillaren* A.

trans·vag·i·nal (trans-vaj'i-năl). Across or through the vagina.

trans·vec·tor (trans-vek'tŏr, tōr). An animal that transmits a toxic substance that it does not produce, but that may be accumulated from animal (dinoflagellate) or plant (algae) sources; *e.g.,* filter-feeding mollusks.

trans·ver·sa·lis (trans-ver-sā'lis) [NA]. Transverse, denotes especially a fascia. SYN transverse, transverse. [L.]

trans·verse (trans-vers'). Crosswise; lying across the long axis of the body or of a part. SYN transversalis [NA], transversus [NA]. [L. *transversus*]

trans·ver·sec·to·my (trans-ver-sek'tō-mē). Resection of the transverse process of a vertebra. [transverse + G. *ektomē,* excision]

trans·ver·sion (trans-ver'zhŭn). 1. Substitution in DNA and RNA of a pyrimidine for a purine, or vice-versa, by mutation. 2. In dentistry, the eruption of a tooth in a position normally occupied by another; transposition of a tooth.

trans·ver·so·cos·tal (trans-ver'sō-kos'tăl). SYN costotransverse.

trans·ver·so·u·re·thra·lis (trans-ver-sō-yū-rē-thrā'lis). Denoting the transverse fibers of the sphincter urethrae muscle, arising from the arch of the pubes.

trans·ver·sus (trans-ver'sŭs) [NA]. SYN transverse. [L. fr. *trans,* across, + *verto,* pp. *versus,* to turn]

trans·ves·tism (trans-ves'tizm). The practice of dressing or masquerading in the clothes of the opposite sex; especially the adoption of feminine mannerisms and costume by a male. SYN transvestitism. [trans- + L. *vestio,* to dress]

trans·ves·tite (trans-ves'tīt). A person who practices transvestism.

trans·ves·ti·tism (trans-ves'ti-tizm). SYN transvestism.

Trantas, Alexios, Greek ophthalmologist, 1867–1960. SEE T.'s *dots,* under *dot;* Horner-T. *dots,* under *dot.*

tran·yl·cyp·ro·mine sul·fate (tran-il-sip'rō-mēn). (+)-*trans*-2-Phenylcyclopropylamine sulfate; a monoamine oxidase inhibitor; an antidepressant used in the treatment of severe mental depression.

tra·pe·zi·al (tra-pē'zē-ăl). Relating to any trapezium.

tra·pe·zi·form (tra-pē'zi-form). SYN trapezoid (1).

tra·pe·zi·o·met·a·car·pal (tra-pē'zē-ō-met'ă-kar'păl). Relating to the trapezium and the metacarpus.

tra·pe·zi·um, pl. **tra·pe·zia, tra·pe·zi·ums** (tra-pē'zē-ŭm, -ă). 1. A four-sided geometrical figure having no two sides parallel. 2. The lateral (radial) bone in the distal row of the carpus; it

articulates with the first and second metacarpals, scaphoid, and trapezoid bones. SYN os trapezium [NA], greater multangular bone, os multangulum majus, trapezium bone. [G. *trapezoin,* a table or counter, a trapezium, dim. of *trapeza,* a table, fr. *tra-* (= *tetra-*), four, + *pous* (*pod-*), foot]

tra·pe·zi·us (tra-pē'zē-ŭs). SYN trapezius *muscle.*

trap·e·zoid (trap'ĕ-zoyd). 1. Resembling a trapezium. SYN trapeziform. 2. A geometrical figure resembling a trapezium except that two of its opposite sides are parallel. 3. SYN trapezoid *bone.* 4. SYN trapezoid *body.* [G. *trapeza,* table, + *eidos,* resemblance]

trap·i·dil (trap'ĭ-dil). *N,N*-Diethyl-5-methyl-[1,2,4]triazolo-[1,5-a]pyrimidin-7-amine; an antagonist and selective synthesis inhibitor of thromboxane A_2; used to prevent cerebral vasospasm.

Trapp, Julius, Russian pharmacist, 1815–1908. SEE T.'s *formula;* T.-Häser *formula.*

Traube, Ludwig, German physician and pathologist, 1818–1876. SEE T.'s *bruit, corpuscle, dyspnea, plugs,* under *plug,* semilunar *space, sign,* double *tone;* T.-Hering *curves,* under *curve, waves,* under *wave.*

Traugott, Carl, German internist, *1885. SEE Staub-T. *effect.*

△**traum-.** SEE traumato-.

trau·ma, pl. **trau·ma·ta, trau·mas** (traw'mă, -mă-tă). An injury, physical or mental. SYN traumatism. [G. wound]

birth t., (1) physical injury to an infant during its delivery; (2) the supposed emotional injury, inflicted by events incident to birth, upon an infant which allegedly appears in symbolic form in patients with mental illness.

t. from occlusion, a reversible lesion in the periodontium caused by excessive movement of teeth.

occlusal t., abnormal occlusal stresses capable of producing or which have produced pathologic changes in the tooth and its surrounding structures.

psychic t., an upsetting experience precipitating or aggravating an emotional or mental disorder.

trau·mas·the·nia (traw-mas-thē'nē-ă). Nervous exhaustion following an injury. [traum- + G. *astheneia,* weakness]

trau·ma·ta (traw'mă-tă). Plural of trauma.

trau·mat·ic (traw-mat'ik). Relating to or caused by trauma. [G. *traumatikos*]

trau·ma·tism (traw'mă-tizm). SYN trauma.

trau·ma·tize (traw'mă-tīz). To cause or inflict trauma. [G. *traumatizō,* to wound]

△**traumato-, traumat-, traum-.** Wound, injury. [G. *trauma*]

trau·ma·tol·o·gy (traw-mă-tol'ō-jē). The branch of surgery concerned with the injured. [traumato- + G. *logos,* study]

trau·ma·to·ne·sis (traw'mă-tō-nē'sis, -ton'ē-sis). Surgical repair of an accidental wound. [traumato- + G. *nēis,* a spinning]

trau·ma·top·a·thy (traw-mă-top'ă-thē). Any pathologic condition resulting from violence or wounds. [traumato- + G. *pathos,* suffering]

trau·ma·top·nea (traw'mă-top-nē'ă). Passage of air in and out through a wound of the chest wall. [traumato- + G. *pnoē,* breath]

trau·ma·to·py·ra (traw'mă-tō-pī'ră). Obsolete synonym of traumatic *fever.* [traumato- + G. *pyr,* fire, fever]

trau·ma·to·sep·sis (traw'mă-tō-sep'sis). Infection of a wound; septicemia following a wound. [traumato- + G. *sēpsis,* putrefaction]

trau·ma·to·ther·a·py (traw'mă-tō-thār'ă-pē). Treatment of trauma or the result of injury.

Trautmann, Moritz F., German otologist, 1832–1902. SEE T.'s triangular *space.*

tra·verse (trav'ers). In computed tomography, one complete linear movement of the gantry across the object being scanned, as occurred in the original translate and rotate CT machines. [M.E., fr. O.Fr., fr. L.L. *transverso,* fr. L. *trans-verto,* to turn across]

tray (trā). A flat receptacle with raised edges.

acrylic resin t., a plastic impression t. used in dentistry; usually fashioned for the individual patient from an autopolymerizing acrylic resin.

annealing t., an electrically heated, thermostatically controlled device used to drive off the protective NH_3 gas coating from the surface of cohesive gold foil.

impression t., a receptacle used to carry and confine plastic impression material when making an impression of oral structures.

traz·o·done hy·dro·chlo·ride (traz′ō-dōn). 2-[3-[4-(*m*-Chlorophenyl)-1-piperazinyl]propyl]-*s*-triazolo[4,3-*a*]pyridin-3(2*H*)one monohydrochloride; an antidepressant structurally unrelated to other antidepressants.

Treacher Collins. SEE Collins.

trea·cle (trē′kl). **1.** Molasses, a viscid syrup that drains from sugar-refining molds. **2.** A saccharine fluid. **3.** Formerly, a remedy for poison, hence any effective remedy. SEE ALSO theriaca. [M.E. *triacle,* antidote, fr. L. *theriaca,* antidote to snake bite, fr. G. *thēriakos,* pertaining to wild beasts]

treat (trēt). To manage a disease by medicinal, surgical, or other measures; to care for a patient medically or surgically. [Fr. *traiter,* fr. L. *tracto,* to drag, handle, perform]

treat·ment (trēt′ment). Medical or surgical management of a patient. SEE ALSO therapy, therapeutics. [Fr. *traitement* (see treat)]

active t., a therapeutic substance or course intended to ameliorate the basic disease problem, as opposed to supportive or palliative t. Cf. causal t.

Carrel's t., t. of wound surfaces by intermittent flushing with Dakin's solution. SYN Dakin-Carrel t.

causal t., t. aimed at reversing the causal factor in a disease.

conservative t., a course of therapeutic action designed to avoid harm, with less possibility of benefit than more risky actions.

Dakin-Carrel t., SYN Carrel's t.

dietetic t., treatment of a clinical condition with a specific diet.

empiric t., a t. based on experience, usually without adequate data to support its use.

endodontic t., SYN root canal t.

Goeckerman t., a t. for psoriasis; the involved areas are painted with a solution of coal tar, or are covered with crude coal tar ointment and subsequently irradiated with ultraviolet (UVB).

heat t., in dentistry, a method of controlled temperature handling of metals so as to change the microscopic structure and thus the physical properties. SEE ALSO temper, anneal.

insulin coma t., rarely used t. of major mental illness by means of hypoglycemic coma induced by insulin.

insulin shock t., formerly used t. for serious mental disorders in which the patient was given insulin to induce a seizure; supplanted by electroshock *therapy.*

isoserum t., therapeutic use of serum taken from a person having or having had the same disease as the patient under treatment.

Kenny's t., a method for the t. of anterior poliomyelitis; the affected parts are wrapped in woolen cloth wrung out with hot water; after the acute stage of the disease has passed, the limbs are passively exercised to reeducate the paralyzed muscles.

light t., SYN phototherapy.

medical t., t. of disease by hygienic and pharmacologic remedies, as distinguished from invasive surgical procedures.

Mitchell's t., t. of mental illness by rest, nourishing diet, and a change of environment. SYN Weir Mitchell t.

moral t., a type of milieu therapy utilized in the 19th century, emphasizing religious doctrine and benevolent guidance in activities of daily living; as such it was a form of psychotherapy as opposed to somatic t.'s such as bloodletting and purging.

Nauheim t., t. of certain cardiac affections by baths in water through which carbonic acid gas is bubbling, followed by resisting exercises. SYN Nauheim bath, Schott t. [*Bad Nauheim,* W. Germany]

palliative t., t. to alleviate symptoms without curing the disease.

preventive t., SYN prophylactic t.

prophylactic t., the institution of measures designed to protect a person from an attack of a disease to which he has been, or is liable to be exposed. SYN preventive t.

root canal t., (1) the means by which painful or diseased teeth, in which the pulp is involved, are restored to a healthy state; **(2)** removal of a normal, diseased, or dead pulp by biochemical and mechanical means, enlargement and sterilization of the root ca-

nal, followed by filling the canal, to effect healing of diseased periapical tissues; **(3)** the diagnosis and t. of diseases of the pulp and their sequelae. SYN endodontic t.

Schott t., SYN Nauheim t.

shock t., SEE electroshock *therapy.*

solar t., syn xref to solar therapy.

symptomatic t., therapy aimed at relieving symptoms without necessarily affecting the basic underlying cause(s) of the symptoms.

Tallerman t., use of special apparatus to administer dry heat to rheumatic disorders, traumatic sprains, etc.

thymus t., t. of disease by administration of extracts of thymus gland.

Tweed edgewise t., SEE edgewise *appliance.*

Weir Mitchell t., SYN Mitchell's t.

tre·ha·la (trē-hah′lă). A saccharine substance containing trehalose and resembling manna, excreted by a parasitic beetle, *Larinus maculatus.* [Fr., fr. Turk. *tigala,* fr. Pers. *tīghāl*]

tre·ha·lase (trē-hă′lās). A glycosidase secreted in the duodenum that hydrolyzes α-glycosidic 1,1 bonds; an absence or deficiency of this enzyme will lead to deficient digestion of trehalose (autosomal recessive).

tre·ha·lose (trē′hă-lōs). A nonreducing disaccharide, (α-D-glucosido)-α-D-glucoside, contained in trehala; also found in fungi, such as *Amanita muscaria;* elevated in individuals with a trehalase deficiency. SYN mycose.

Treitz, Wenzel, Bohemian pathologist, 1819–1872. SEE T.'s *arch;* T.'s *fascia, fossa;* T.'s *hernia, ligament, muscle.*

Trélat, Ulysse, French surgeon, 1828–1890. SEE T.'s *stools,* under *stool;* Leser-T. *sign;* T.'s *sign.*

tre·ma (trē′mă). **1.** SYN foramen. **2.** SYN vulva. [G. *trēma,* a hole]

Trem·a·to·da (trem′ă-tō′dă). A class in the phylum Platyhelminthes (the flatworms), consisting of flukes with a leaf-shaped body and two muscular suckers, and an acelomate parenchyma-filled body cavity. Circulatory system and sense organs are not present, but an incomplete alimentary canal is found (lacking an anus). Flukes of interest to human or veterinary medicine are members of the order Digenea, with complete life cycles involving embryonic multiplication in a mollusk first intermediate host. The other order, Monogenea, consists chiefly of parasites of fish that have a simpler pattern of direct development on a single host. [G. *trēmatōdēs,* full of holes, fr. *trēma,* a hole, + *eidos,* appearance]

trem·a·tode, trem·a·toid (trem′ă-tōd, trem′ă-toyd). **1.** Common name for a fluke of the class Trematoda. **2.** Relating to a fluke of the class Trematoda.

trem·bles (trem′blz). An intoxication of cattle, caused by eating white snakeroot, *Eupatorium urticaefolium,* or the rayless goldenrod; the active agent is a higher alcohol, tremetol, which intoxicated cows eliminate in their milk, causing milk sickness when ingested by humans. [L. *tremulus,* trembling, fr. *tremo,* to tremble]

trem·b′ling. The shaking or quaking of a tremor.

trem·el·loid, trem·el·lose (trem′ĕ-loyd, -lōs). Jelly-like. [L. *tremulus,* trembling]

trem·o·gram (trem′ō-gram). The graphic representation of a tremor taken by means of the tremograph or kymograph. SYN tremorgram.

trem·o·graph (trem′ō-graf). An apparatus for making a graphic record of a tremor. [L. *tremor,* a shaking, + G. *graphō,* to write]

trem·o·la·bile (trem-ō-lā′bil, -bīl). Inactivated or destroyed by shaking. [L. *tremor,* a shaking, + *labilis,* perishable]

trem·o·pho·bia (trem-ō-fō′bē-ă). Morbid fear of trembling. [L. *tremor,* trembling, + G. *phobos,* fear]

trem·or (trem′er, -ōr). **1.** Repetitive, often regular, oscillatory movements caused by alternate, or synchronous, but irregular contraction of opposing muscle groups; usually involuntary. **2.** Minute ocular movement occurring during fixation on an object. SYN trepidation (1). [L. a shaking]

action t., SYN intention t.

alcoholic withdrawal t., intention t. present in the withdrawal period of one of two types: 1) a t. of greater than 8 Hz, with continuous antagonistic muscle activity, and 2) a t. of less than 8 Hz, with intermittent spontaneous antagonistic muscle activity.

alternating t., a form of hyperkinesia characterized by regular, symmetrical, to-and-fro movements (at about 4 per second) that are produced by patterned, alternating contraction of muscles and their antagonists.

alternative t., a coarse, low frequency (3–8 Hz) pathologic t. produced by alternating contraction of muscles and their antagonists; seen with Parkinson disease and kinetic predominant action t.

arsenical t., a t. caused by chronic poisoning by arsenic.

t. ar′tuum, trembling of the extremities, especially of the hands.

ataxic t., SYN intention t.

benign essential t., SYN heredofamilial t.

coarse t., a t. in which the amplitude is large and the oscillations are usually irregular and slow.

continuous t., SYN persistent t.

epidemic t., SYN avian infectious *encephalomyelitis.*

essential t., an action t. of 4–8 Hz frequency that usually begins in early adult life and is limited to the upper limbs and head; called familial when it appears in several family members.

familial t., SYN heredofamilial t.

fine t., a t. in which the amplitude is small and the frequency is usually greater than 12 Hz.

flapping t., SYN asterixis.

head t.'s, SYN head-nodding.

heredofamilial t. [MIM*190300], a benign t. inherited as a dominant character; it may be a rapid oscillation resembling that seen in thyrotoxicosis, a coarse t. during rest and inhibited by a voluntary effort, or one which appears only upon movement. SYN benign essential t., familial t.

hysterical t., usually a coarse, irregular t. limited to one limb. SYN psychogenic t.

intention t., a t. that occurs during the performance of precise voluntary movements, caused by disorders of the cerebellum or its connections. SYN action t., ataxic t., kinetic t., volitional t. (2).

kinetic t., SYN intention t.

mercurial t., a t. caused by chronic mercury poisoning.

metallic t., a t. caused by poisoning with metal.

t. opiophago′rum, a t. occurring in opium addicts.

passive t., SYN resting t.

persistent t., a t. that is constant, whether the subject is at rest or moving. SYN continuous t.

physiologic t., fine t., 8–13 Hz frequency, which is a normal phenomenon.

pill-rolling t., resting t. of the thumb and fingers seen in Parkinson disease.

postural t., t. present when the limbs or trunk are kept in certain positions and when they are moved actively, usually due to near-synchronous rhythmic bursts in opposing muscle groups. SYN static t.

t. potato′rum, a t. occurring in the subjects of chronic alcoholism.

progressive cerebellar t., SYN Hunt's *syndrome* (1).

psychogenic t., SYN hysterical t.

resting t., a coarse, rhythmic t. 3–5 Hz frequency, usually confined to hands and forearms, that appears when the limbs are relaxed, and disappears with active limb movements; characteristic of Parkinson disease. SYN passive t.

saturnine t., a t. caused by chronic lead poisoning.

senile t., an essential t. that becomes symptomatic in elderly adults.

static t., SYN postural t.

t. ten′dinum, SYN *subsultus* tendinum.

volitional t., (1) a t. that can be arrested by a strong effort of the will; **(2)** SYN intention t.

trem·or·gram (trem′ōr-gram). SYN tremogram.

trem·or·ine (trem′er-ēn). A chemical which in the laboratory produces a tremor resembling parkinsonian tremor and is used to produce experimental parkinsonism.

trem·o·sta·ble (trem-ō-stā′bl). Not subject to alteration or destruction by being shaken. [L. *tremor,* a shaking, + *stabilis,* stable]

trem·u·lor (trem′yū-ler, -lōr). An instrument for giving vibratory massage.

trem·u·lous (trem′yū-lŭs). Characterized by tremor.

Trenaunay, Paul, French physician, *1875. SEE Klippel-T.-Weber *syndrome.*

Trendelenburg, Friedrich, German surgeon, 1844–1924. SEE T.'s *operation, position;* reverse T. *position;* T.'s *sign, symptom, test.*

trend of thought. Thinking with a tendency toward or centering on a particular idea with a particular affect.

tre·pan (trē-pan′). SYN trephine. [G. *trypanon,* a borer]

trep·a·na·tion (trep-ă-nā′shŭn). SYN trephination.

corneal t., t. of cornea, SYN keratoplasty.

treph·i·na·tion (tref-i-nā′shŭn). Removal of a circular piece ("button") of cranium by a trephine. SYN trepanation.

tre·phine (trē-fīn′, -fēn′). **1.** A cylindrical or crown saw used for the removal of a disc of bone, especially from the skull, or of other firm tissue as that of the cornea. **2.** To remove a disc of bone or other tissue by means of a t. SYN trepan. [contrived fr. L. *tres fines,* three ends]

treph·o·cyte (tref′ō-sīt). SYN trophocyte. [G. *trephō,* to nourish, + *kytos,* cell]

trep·i·dant (trep′i-dant). Marked by tremor. [L. *trepidans,* pres. p. of *trepido,* to tremble, to be agitated]

trep·i·da·tio cor·dis (trep-i-dā′shē-ō kōr′dis). SYN palpitation.

trep·i·da·tion (trep-i-dā′shŭn). **1.** SYN tremor. **2.** Anxious fear. [L. *trepidatio,* fr. *trepido,* to tremble, to be agitated]

Trep·o·ne·ma (trep-ō-nē′mă). A genus of anaerobic bacteria (order Spirochaetales) consisting of cells, 3 to 8 μm in length, with acute, regular, or irregular spirals and no obvious protoplasmic structure. A terminal filament may be present. They stain with difficulty except with Giemsa's stain or silver impregnation. Some species are pathogenic and parasitic for humans and other animals, generally producing local lesions in tissues. The type species is *T. pallidum.* [G. *trepō,* to turn, + *nēma,* thread]

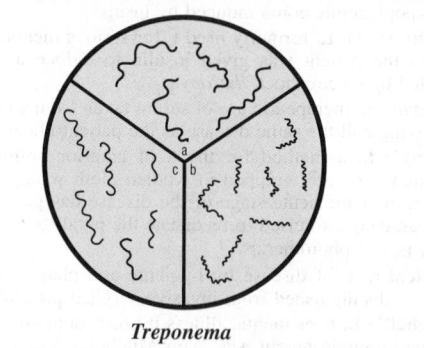

Treponema
a) *Borrelia;* b) *Treponema;* c) *Leptospira*

T. cara′teum, a species that causes pinta, or carate.

T. cunic′uli, a species which causes spirochetosis in rabbits.

T. dentico′la, cultivatable species that does not ferment carbohydrates and can be isolated from the oral cavity of humans.

T. genita′lis, a nonpathogenic species found on the genitalia of humans.

T. hyodysente′riae, an enteropathogenic species that causes swine dysentery.

T. muco′sum, a species found in pyorrhea alveolaris; it possesses pyogenic properties.

T. pal′lidum, a species that causes syphilis in humans; this organism can be experimentally transmitted to anthropoid apes and to rabbits; it is the type species of the genus *T.*

T. perten′ue, a species that causes yaws; patients with this disease give positive results in serologic screening tests for syphilis.

trep·o·ne·ma·to·sis (trep′ō-nē-mă-tō′sis). SYN treponemiasis.

trep·o·neme (trep′ō-nēm). A vernacular term used to refer to any member of the genus *Treponema*.

trep·o·ne·mi·a·sis (trep′ō-nē-mī′ă-sis). Infection caused by *Treponema*. SYN treponematosis.

trep·o·ne·mi·ci·dal (trep′ō-nē′mi-sī′dăl). Destructive to any species of *Treponema*, but usually with reference to *T. pallidum*. SYN antitreponemal. [*Treponema* + L. *caedo*, to kill]

trep·pe (trep′eh). A phenomenon in cardiac muscle first observed by H.P. Bowditch; if a number of stimuli of the same intensity are sent into the muscle after a quiescent period, the first few contractions of the series show a successive increase in amplitude (strength). SYN staircase phenomenon. [Ger. *Treppe*, staircase]

Tresilian, Frederick J., English physician, 1862–1926. SEE T.'s *sign*.

tre·sis (trē′sis). SYN perforation. [G. *trēsis*, a boring]

tret·i·noin (tret′i-nō-in). All-*trans*-retinoic acid; a keratolytic agent. SEE retinoic acid.

Treves, Sir Frederick, English surgeon, 1853–1923. SEE T.'s *fold*.

Treves, Norman, U.S. surgeon, 1894–1964. SEE Stewart-T. *syndrome*.

Trevor, David, 20th century British orthopedic surgeon. SEE T.'s *disease*.

TRF Abbreviation for thyrotropin-releasing *factor*.

TRH Abbreviation for thyrotropin-releasing *hormone*.

△**tri-.** Three. Cf. tris-. [L. and G.]

tri·a·ce·tic ac·id (trī-ă-sē′tik). $CH_3COCH_2COCH_2COOH$; 3,5-Dioxohexanoic acid; formed by condensation of acetyl and malonyl CoA's in the course of fatty acid synthesis.

tri·ac·e·tin (trī-as′ĕ-tin). Used as a solvent of basic dyes, as a fixative in perfumery, and as a topical antifungal agent. SYN glyceryl triacetate, triacetylglycerol.

tri·a·ce·tyl·glyc·er·ol (trī-as′i-til-glis′er-ol). SYN triacetin.

tri·a·ce·tyl·o·le·an·do·my·cin (trī-as′ĕ-til-ō′lē-an-dō-mī′sin). SYN troleandomycin.

tri·ac·yl·glyc·er·ol (trī-as′il-glis′er-ol). Glycerol esterified at each of its three hydroxyl groups by a fatty (aliphatic) acid; *e.g.*, tristearoylglycerol. SYN fat (4), triglyceride.

    t. lipase, the fat-splitting enzyme in pancreatic juice; it hydrolyzes t. to produce a diacylglycerol and a fatty acid anion; a deficiency of the hepatic enzyme results in hypercholesterolemia and hypertriglyceridemia. SYN steapsin, tributyrase, tributyrinase.

tri·ad (trī′ad). **1.** A collection of three things having something in common. **2.** The transverse tubule and the terminal cisternae on each side of it in skeletal muscle fibers. **3.** SYN portal t. **4.** The father, mother, and child relationship projectively experienced in group psychotherapy. [G. *trias* (*triad*-), the number 3, fr. *treis*, three]

    acute compression t., the rising venous pressure, falling arterial pressure, and decreased heart sounds of pericardial tamponade. SYN Beck's t.

    Beck's t., SYN acute compression t.

    Bezold's t., diminished perception of the deeper tones, retarded bone conduction, and negative Rinne's test, pointing, in the absence of objective signs, to otosclerosis.

    Charcot's t., (1) in multiple (disseminated) sclerosis, the three symptoms: nystagmus, tremor, and scanning speech; (2) combination of jaundice, fever, and upper abdominal pain that occurs as a result of cholangitis.

    Fallot's t., SYN *trilogy* of Fallot.

    hepatic t., SYN portal t.

    Hull's t., the association of diastolic gallop, anasarca, and small pulse pressure.

    Hutchinson's t., parenchymatous keratitis, labyrinthine disease, and Hutchinson's teeth, significant of congenital syphilis.

    Kartagener's t., SYN Kartagener's *syndrome*.

    portal t., branches of the portal vein, hepatic artery, and the

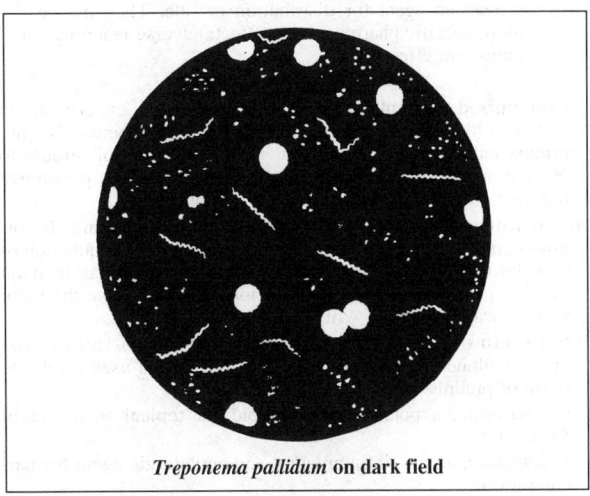

***Treponema pallidum* on dark field**

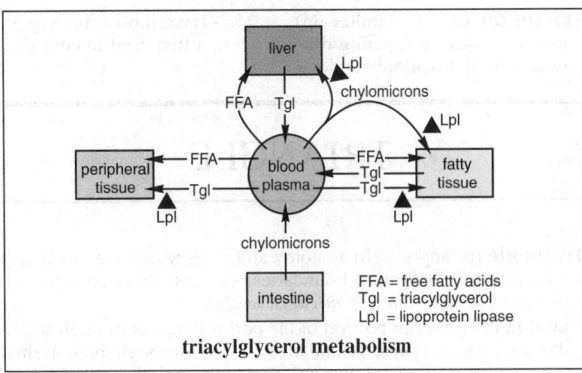

triacylglycerol metabolism

biliary ducts bound together in the perivascular fibrous capsule or portal tract as they ramify within the substance of the liver. SYN hepatic t., triad (3).

    Saint's t., the concurrence of hiatal hernia, diverticulosis, and cholelithiasis.

tri·age (trē′ahzh). Medical screening of patients to determine their relative priority for treatment; the separation of a large number of casualties, in military or civilian disaster medical care, into three groups: 1) those who cannot be expected to survive even with treatment; 2) those who will recover without treatment; 3) the highest priority group, those who will not survive without treatment. [Fr. sorting]

tri·al. a test or experiment, usually conducted under specific conditions.

    clinical t., an internationally recognized research protocol designed to evaluate the efficacy or safety of drugs, vaccines, or other therapeutic agents, and to produce scientifically valid results.

    Four phases of trial are distinguished. Phase I trials usually involve fewer than 100 healthy volunteers who are exposed to a new drug or vaccine. Studies may attempt to gauge adverse reactions, optimal dose, and best route of administration. Phase II trials generally involve 200–500 volunteers randomly assigned to control and study groups. These are pilot efficacy studies, with emphasis on immunogenicity in the case of vaccines, and on relative efficacy and safety in the case of drugs. Phase III trials, often multicenter, involve thousands of volunteers, randomly assigned to control and study groups. The aim is to generate statistically relevant data. Phase IV trials are conducted after a national drug registration authority (in the U.S., the Food and Drug Administration) has approved an agent for distribution or sale. They may explore specific pharmacologic effect, adverse reactions, or long-term effects.

randomized controlled t., an epidemiological experiment in which subjects in a population are allocated randomly into groups, called "experimental" or "study" and "control" groups to receive or not receive an experimental therapeutic or preventive regimen, procedure, maneuver, or intervention.

tri·al and er·ror. The apparently random, haphazard, hit-or-miss exploratory activity which often precedes the acquisition of new information or adjustments; it may be overt, as in a rat running in a maze, or covert (vicarious), as when one thinks of various ways of coping with a situation.

tri·am·cin·o·lone (trī-am-sin′ō-lōn). 9α-Fluoro-16α-hydroxyprednisolone; a glucocorticoid with actions and uses similar to those of prednisolone.

t. acetonide, a potent glucocorticoid for topical treatment of dermatoses.

t. diacetate, an anti-inflammatory and antiallergic agent for parenteral use.

tri·a·me·lia (trī′ă-mē′lē-ă). Absence of three limbs. [tri- + G. *a*-priv. + *melos,* limb]

tri·am·ter·ene (trī-am′ter-ēn). 2,4,7-Triamino-6-phenylpteridine; a potassium sparing diuretic agent, often used in combination with hydrochlorthiazide.

TRIANGLE

tri·an·gle (trī′ang-gl). In anatomy and surgery, a three-sided area with arbitrary or natural boundaries. SEE ALSO trigonum. [L. *triangulum,* fr. *tri-,* three, + *angulus,* angle]

anal t., the posterior portion of the perineal region through which the anal canal opens; bounded by a line through both isehial tuberosities, the sacrotuberous ligaments and the coccyx. SYN regio analis [NA], anal region.

anterior t. of neck, the area of the neck bounded by the mandible, the anterior border of the sternocleidomastoid muscle, and the anterior midline of the neck; it is subdivided into carotid, muscular, submandibular, and submental t.'s. SYN anterior region of neck, regio cervicalis anterior, trigonum cervicale anterius.

Assézat's t., a t. formed by lines connecting the nasion with the alveolar and nasal point; used to indicate prognathism in comparative craniology.

auricular t., a t. formed by the base of the auricle and by lines drawn from the true tip of the auricle to the extremities of the base.

t. of auscultation, space bounded by the lower border of the trapezius, the latissimus dorsi, and the medial margin of the scapula, where the absence of musculature allows respiratory sounds to be heard clearly with a stethoscope.

axillary t., a triangular area embracing the medial aspect of the arm, the axilla, and the pectoral region which is one of the seats of predilection for the petechial initial rash of smallpox.

Béclard's t., area bounded by the posterior border of the hyoglossus muscle, the posterior belly of the digastric and the greater horn of the hyoid bone.

Bonwill t., an equilateral t. formed by lines from the contact points of the lower central incisors, or the medial line of the residual ridge of the mandible, to the condyle on either side and from one condyle to the other.

Bryant's t., in fracture of the neck of the femur to determine upward displacement of the trochanter, lines are drawn on the body to form a t.: line *a* is drawn around the body at the level of the anterior superior iliac spines; line *b,* perpendicular to line *a,* is drawn to the great trochanter of the femur; line *c* is drawn from the trochanter to the iliac spine; upward displacement is measured along line *b.* SYN iliofemoral t.

Burger's t., a scalene t. representing the frontal plane electrocar-

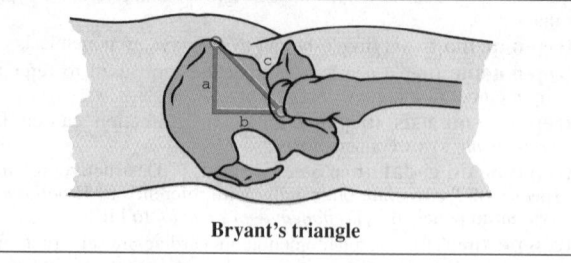
Bryant's triangle

diographic leads comparable to but more accurate than Einthoven's t. SEE Einthoven's t.

Burow's t., a t. of skin and subcutaneous fat excised so that a pedicle flap can be advanced without buckling the adjacent tissue.

Calot's t., t. bounded by the cystic artery, cystic duct, and hepatic duct; its dissection early in cholecystectomy safeguards essential structures, should there be anatomic variations from the norm.

cardiohepatic t., SYN cardiohepatic *angle.*

carotid t., a space bounded by the superior belly of the omohyoid muscle, anterior border of the sternocleidomastoid, and posterior belly of the digastric; it contains the bifurcation of the common carotid artery. SYN trigonum caroticum [NA], fossa carotica, Gerdy's hyoid fossa, Malgaigne's fossa, Malgaigne's t., superior carotid t.

cephalic t., a t. on the cranium formed by lines connecting the metopion, the pogonion, and the occipital point.

cervical t., any of the t.'s of the neck.

Codman's t., in radiology, the interface between growing bone tumor and normal bone, presenting as an incomplete triangle formed by periosteum.

crural t., an area of predilection for the petechial initial rash of smallpox; it occupies the lower abdominal, inguinal, and genital regions and the inner aspects of the thighs, the base of the t. traversing the umbilicus.

deltoideopectoral t., SYN infraclavicular *fossa.*

digastric t., SYN submandibular t.

Einthoven's t., an imaginary equilateral t. with the heart at its center, its equal sides representing the three standard limb leads of the electrocardiogram.

Elaut's t., t. formed by the iliac arteries and the promontory of the sacrum.

t. of elbow, SYN cubital *fossa.*

facial t., a t. formed by lines connecting the basion, the prosthion, and the nasion.

Farabeuf's t., the t. formed by the internal jugular and facial veins and the hypoglossal nerve.

femoral t., a triangular space at the upper part of the thigh, bounded by the sartorius and adductor longus muscles and the inguinal ligament, with a floor formed laterally by the iliopsoas muscle and medially by the pectineus muscle; the branches of the femoral nerve are distributed within the femoral t.; it is bisected by the femoral vessels, which enter the adductor canal at its apex. SYN trigonum femorale [NA], fossa scarpae major, Scarpa's t., subinguinal t.

t. of fillet, SYN lemniscal *trigone.*

frontal t., a t. bounded above by the maximum frontal diameter and laterally by lines joining the extremities of this diameter with the glabella.

Garland's t., a triangular area of relative resonance in the lower back near the spine, found in the same side as a pleural effusion.

Gombault's t., SEE semilunar *fasciculus.*

Grocco's t., a triangular patch of dullness at the base of the chest alongside the spinal column, on the side opposite a pleural effusion. SYN paravertebral t.

Grynfeltt's t., a triangular space bounded above by the end of the last rib and the serratus posterior inferior muscle, anteriorly by the internal oblique, and posteriorly by the quadratus lumborum; lumbar hernia occurs in this space. SYN Lesshaft's t.

Hesselbach's t., SYN inguinal t.

iliofemoral t., SYN Bryant's t.

inferior carotid t., SYN muscular t.

inferior occipital t., a t. with its apex at the external occipital protuberance; its base is formed by a line joining the two mastoid processes.

infraclavicular t., SYN infraclavicular *fossa.*

inguinal t., the triangular area in the lower abdominal wall bounded by the inguinal ligament below, the border of the rectus abdominis medially and the inferior epigastric vessels (lateral umbilical fold) laterally. It is the site of direct inguinal hernia. SYN trigonum inguinale [NA], Hesselbach's t., inguinal trigone.

interscalene t., SYN scalene *hiatus.*

Killian's t., the triangular-shaped area of the cervical esophagus bordered by the oblique fibers of the inferior constrictor muscle of the pharynx and the transverse fibers of the cricopharyngeus muscle through which Zenker's diverticulum occurs, and the A-V nodal triangle between the coronary sinus orifice and the ventricular crest. SYN laimer t.

Koch's t., a triangular area of the wall of the right atrium of the heart, that marks the situation of the atrioventricular node.

Labbé's t., an area bounded below by a horizontal line touching the lower edge of the cartilage of the left ninth rib, laterally by the line of the false ribs, and to the right side by the liver; here the stomach is normally in contact with the abdominal wall.

laimer t., SYN Killian's t.

Langenbeck's t., a t. formed by lines drawn from the anterior superior iliac spine to the surface of the great trochanter and to the surgical neck of the femur; a penetrating wound in this area probably involves the joint.

Lesser's t., the space between the bellies of the digastric muscle and the hypoglossal nerve.

Lesshaft's t., SYN Grynfeltt's t.

Lieutaud's t., SYN *trigone* of bladder.

lumbar t., an area in the posterior abdominal wall bounded by the edges of the latissimus dorsi and external oblique muscles and the iliac crest; herniations occasionally occur here. SYN trigonum lumbale [NA], Petit's lumbar t.

lumbocostoabdominal t., an irregular area bounded by the serratus posterior inferior, obliquus externus, obliquus internus, and erector spinae muscles.

Macewen's t., SYN suprameatal t.

Malgaigne's t., SYN carotid t.

Marcille's t., an area bounded by the medial border of the psoas major, the lateral margin of the vertebral column, and the iliolumbar ligament below; it is crossed by the obturator nerve.

muscular t., the t. bounded by the sternocleidomastoid muscle, the superior belly of the omohyoid muscle, and the anterior midline of the neck; the infrahyoid muscles occupy most of it. SYN trigonum musculare [NA], trigonum omotracheale [NA], inferior carotid t., omotracheal t., tracheal t.

occipital t., a t. of the neck bounded by the trapezius, the sternocleidomastoid, and the omohyoid muscles. SEE ALSO inferior occipital t.

omoclavicular t., SYN supraclavicular t.

omotracheal t., SYN muscular t.

palatal t., a triangular area bounded by the greatest transverse diameter of the palate and by lines converging from its extremities to the alveolar point. SYN trigonum palati.

paravertebral t., SYN Grocco's t.

Petit's lumbar t., SYN lumbar t.

Philippe's t., SEE semilunar *fasciculus.*

Pirogoff's t., a t. formed by the intermediate tendon of the digastric muscle, the posterior border of the mylohyoid muscle, and the hypoglossal nerve.

posterior t. of neck, the region of the neck bounded by the sternocleidomastoid muscle, the trapezius muscle, and the upper border of the clavicle, including the omoclavicular triangle. SYN lateral region of neck, regio cervicalis lateralis, trigonum cervicale posterius.

pubourethral t., a t. in the perineum bounded by the transversus perinei, the ischiocavernosus, and the bulbocavernosus muscles.

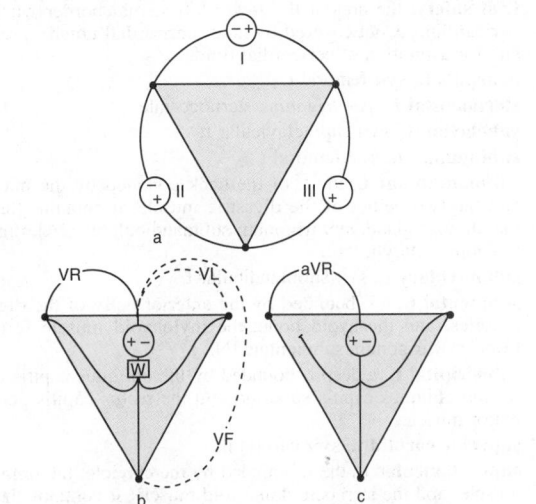

Einthoven's triangle (with various configurations)
a: bipolar limb leads (I, II, III); b: unipolar limb leads, with Wilson's electrode (W), from the right arm (VR), from the left arm (VL), or foot (VF), with corresponding switch of exploring electrode (dotted lines); c: unipolar limb leads (Goldberger's) from the right arm (aVR), from the left arm (aVL), or foot (aVF), with corresponding switch of the exploring electrode and interruption of the reference electrode (not shown)

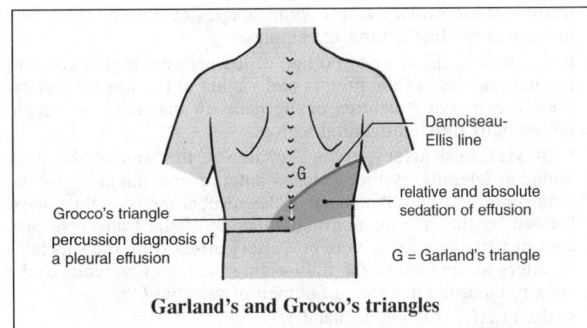

Garland's and Grocco's triangles

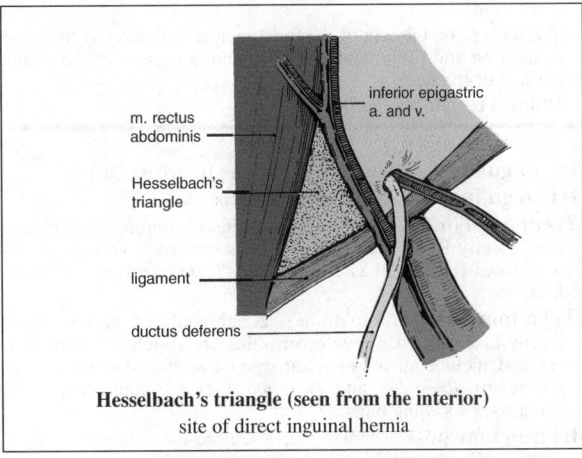

Hesselbach's triangle (seen from the interior)
site of direct inguinal hernia

Reil's t., SYN lemniscal *trigone.*

sacral t., the surface area over the sacrum.

t. of safety, the area at the lower left sternal border where the pericardium is not covered by lung (pericardial notch); preferred site for aspiration of pericardial fluid.

Scarpa's t., SYN femoral t.

sternocostal t., SYN *trigonum* sternocostale.

subclavian t., SYN supraclavicular t.

subinguinal t., SYN femoral t.

submandibular t., the t. of the neck bounded by the mandible and the two bellies of the digastric muscle; it contains the submandibular gland. SYN trigonum submandibulare [NA], digastric t., submaxillary t.

submaxillary t., SYN submandibular t.

submental t., a t. bounded by the anterior belly of the digastric muscles, and the hyoid bone; the mylohyoid muscle forms its floor. SYN trigonum submentale [NA].

suboccipital t., a deep t. bounded by the obliquus capitis inferior, the obliquus capitis superior, and the rectus capitis posterior major muscles.

superior carotid t., SYN carotid t.

supraclavicular t., the t. bounded by the clavicle, the omohyoid muscle, and the sternocleidomastoid muscle; it contains the subclavian artery and vein. SYN fossa supraclavicularis major [NA], trigonum omoclaviculare [NA], greater supraclavicular fossa, omoclavicular t., subclavian t.

suprameatal t., a t. formed by the root of the zygomatic arch, the posterior wall of the bony external acoustic meatus, and an imaginary line connecting the extremities of the first two lines; used as a guide in mastoid operations. SYN Macewen's t.

tracheal t., SYN muscular t.

Tweed t., a t. defined by facial and dental landmarks on a lateral cephalometric film, using the Frankfort horizontal plane as a base and intended for use as a guide in the evaluation and planning of orthodontic treatment.

umbilicomammillary t., a t. with its apex at the umbilicus and its base at the line joining the nipples.

urogenital t., the anterior portion of the perineal region containing the openings of the urethra and vagina in the female and the urethra and root structures of the penis in the male. SYN regio urogenitalis [NA], urogenital region.

t. of vertebral artery, triangular area in the root of the neck bounded laterally by the scalenus anterior and medially by the longus coli muscles; the two muscles meet at the triangle's apex, formed by the anterior (carotid) tubercle of the transverse process of vertebra C6; the vertebral artery arises from the subclavian artery at the base of the t., bisecting the t. as it ascends to the apex to enter the transverse foramen of vertebra C6.

vesical t., SYN *trigone* of bladder.

Ward's t., an area of diminished density in the trabecular pattern of the neck of the femur evident by x-ray as well as by direct inspection.

Weber's t., on the sole of the foot, an area indicated by the heads of the first and fifth metatarsal bone and the center of the plantar surface of the heel.

Wilde's t., SYN *pyramid* of light.

---

tri·an·gu·la·ris. SEE triangular *muscle*. [L. triangular]

tri·an·gu·lum (trī-ang'gū-lŭm). SEE triangle. [L.]

Tri·at·o·ma (trī-ă-tō'mă). A genus of insects (subfamily Triatominae, family Reduviidae) that includes important vectors of *Trypanosoma cruzi,* such as *T. dimidiata, T. infestans,* and *T. maculata.*

Tri·a·tom·i·nae (trī-ă-tō'mi-nē). A subfamily of insects (family Reduviidae, suborder Heteroptera) that are vertebrate bloodsuckers and include such important disease vector species as *Panstrongylus, Rhodnius,* and *Triatoma;* they are commonly called conenose or kissing bugs.

tri·a·zo·lam (trī-ā'zō-lam). un; 8-Chloro-6-(*o*-chlorophenyl)-1-methyl-4*H*-*s*-triazolo[4,3-*a*][1,4]benzodiazepine; a short-acting benzodiazepine derivative used as a sedative and hypnotic.

tri·az·o·lo·gua·nine (trī'ă-zol-ō-gwah'nēn). SYN 8-azaguanine.

trib·ade (trib'ād). A lesbian, especially one who obtains sexual

pleasure by rubbing her external genitalia against those of another woman. [G. *tribō,* to rub]

trib·a·dism, trib·a·dy (trib'ād-izm, -ā-dē). Lesbianism, particularly as practiced by a tribade. [G. *tribō,* to rub]

tri·ba·sic (trī-bā'sik). Having three titratable hydrogen atoms; denoting an acid with a basicity of 3.

tri·bas·i·lar (trī-bas'i-lăr). Having three bases.

tribe (trīb). In biological classification, an occasionally used division between the family and the genus; often the same as the subfamily. [L. *tribus*]

tri·bol·o·gy (tri-bol'ŏ-jē). The study of friction and its effects in biological systems, especially in regard to articulated surfaces of the skeleton. [G. *tribō,* to rub, + *logos,* study]

tri·bo·lu·mi·nes·cence (trib'ō-lū-mi-nes'ens). Luminosity produced by friction. [G. *tribō,* to rub, + luminescence]

tri·bra·chia (trī-brā'kē-ă). Condition seen in conjoined twins when the fusion has merged the adjacent arms to form a single one, so that there are only three arms for the two bodies. SEE conjoined *twins,* under *twin.* [tri- + G. *brachiōn,* arm]

tri·bra·chi·us (trī-brā'kē-ŭs). Conjoined twins exhibiting tribrachia.

tri·bro·mo·eth·a·nol (trī-brō-mō-eth'ă-nol). Br_3C—CH_2OH; formerly used as a basal anesthetic agent administered rectally.

tri·brom·sa·lan (trī-brom'să-lan). 3,4′,5-Tribromosalicylanilide; a disinfectant used in soaps.

tri·bu·ty·rase (trī-byū'ti-rās). SYN *triacylglycerol* lipase.

tri·bu·tyr·in (trī-byū'ti-rin). A synthetic substrate for lipase assays. SYN glyceryl tributyrate, tributyrylglycerol.

tri·bu·tyr·in·ase (trī-byū'ti-ri-nās). SYN *triacylglycerol* lipase.

tri·bu·tyr·yl·glyc·er·ol (trī-byū'ti-ril-glis'er-ol). SYN tributyrin.

TRIC Acronym for *tr*achoma and *i*nclusion *c*onjunctivitis. SEE TRIC *agents,* under *agent.*

tri·cal·ci·um phos·phate (trī-kal'sē-ŭm). SYN tribasic *calcium* phosphate.

tri·ceph·a·lus (trī-sef'ă-lŭs). Fetus with three heads. [tri- + G. *kephalē,* head]

tri·ceps (trī'seps). Three-headed; denoting especially two muscles: t. brachii and t. surae. SEE muscle. [L. fr. *tri-,* three, + *caput,* head]

△**trich-.** SEE tricho-.

trich·al·gia (trik-al'jē-ă). Pain produced by touching the hair. SYN trichodynia. [trich- + G. *algos,* pain]

trich·an·gi·on (trik-an'jē-on). SYN telangion. [trich- + G. *angeion,* vessel]

trich·a·tro·phia (trik-ă-trō'fē-ă). Atrophy of the hair bulbs, with brittleness, splitting, and falling out of hair. [trich- + G. *atrophia,* atrophy]

trich·aux·is (trik-awk'sis). Excessive growth of hair in length and quantity. [trich- + G. *auxis,* increase]

△**trichi-.** SEE tricho-.

△**-trichia.** Condition or type of hair. [G. *thrix* (*trich-*), hair, + *-ia,* condition]

tri·chi·a·sis (trī-kī'ă-sis). A condition in which the hair adjacent to a natural orifice turns inward and causes irritation; *e.g.,* in inversion of an eyelid (entropion), eyelashes irritate the eye. SYN trichoma, trichomatosis. [trich- + G. *-iasis,* condition]

trich·i·lem·mo·ma (trik'i-le-mō'mă). A benign tumor derived from outer root sheath epithelium of a hair follicle, consisting of cells with pale-staining cytoplasm containing glycogen; multiple t.'s are present on the face in Cowden's disease. SYN tricholemmoma. [trichi- + G. *lemma,* husk, + *-ōma,* tumor]

Tri·chi·na (tri-kī'nă). Old name for a genus of nematode worms, correctly called *Trichinella.*

tri·chi·na, pl. **tri·chi·nae** (tri-kī'nă, -nē). A larval worm of the genus *Trichinella;* the infective form in pork. [Mod. L., fr. G. *thrix* (*trich-*), a hair]

Trich·i·nel·la (trik'i-nel'ă). A nematode genus in the aphasmid group that causes trichinosis in man and carnivores. [Mod. L. fr. trichina + dim. suffix *ella*]

T. spira'lis, the pork or trichina worm, a species of parasites that cause trichinosis, found in most regions of the world but more frequently in the Northern Hemisphere; transmission occurs as a result of ingesting raw or inadequately cooked meat (especially pork) that contains encysted larvae which develop into adults that survive in the jejunum and ileum for approximately six weeks; the female worm is viviparous, and bears approximately 1500 embryonic larvae that are laid deep in the mucosa so that they are picked up in the submucosal capillaries and are transported via the liver to the heart, lungs, and systemic circulation; eventually the larvae break out of the body capillaries, penetrate a muscle fiber, coil, and encyst, thereby inducing the strong sensitization, pain, fever, edema, and eosinophilic reaction characteristic of trichinosis.

trich·i·nel·li·a·sis (trik'i-nel-ī'ă-sis). SYN trichinosis.

Trich·i·nel·li·cae (tri-ki-nel'i-kē). SYN Trichinelloidea.

Trich·i·nel·loi·dea (trik'i-nel-oy'dē-ă). A superfamily of nematodes, including the following roundworms that are parasitic in man: *Trichinella spiralis*, the trichina worm (family Trichinellidae); *Trichuris trichiura*, the human whipworm; *Capillaria hepatica*, the capillary liver worm; and *C. philippinensis* (family Trichuridae). SYN Trichinellicae.

trich·i·nel·lo·sis (trik'i-nel-ō'sis). SYN trichinosis.

trich·i·ni·a·sis (trik-i-nī'ă-sis). SYN trichinosis.

trich·i·nif·er·ous (trik-i-nif'ĕ-rŭs). Containing trichina worms.

trich·i·ni·za·tion (trik'i-ni-zā'shŭn). Infection with trichina worms.

tri·chi·no·scope (trik'i-nō-skōp). A magnifying glass used in the examination of meat suspected of being trichinous. [trichina + G. *skopeō*, to view]

trich·i·no·sis (trik-i-nō'sis). The disease resulting from ingestion of raw or inadequately cooked pork (or bear or walrus meat in Alaska) that contains encysted larvae of the nematode parasite *Trichinella spiralis*. The initial symptoms of human disease are abdominal pain, cramping, and diarrhea, associated with the development of the parasites in the small intestine. Once the resultant larval parasites migrate and invade muscular tissue, a second set of symptoms is manifest, including facial and periorbital edema, myalgia, fever, pruritus, urticaria, conjunctivitis, and signs of myocarditis. SYN trichinelliasis, trichinellosis, trichiniasis. [*Trichinella* (trichina) + G. *-osis*, condition]

tri·chi·nous (trik'i-nŭs). Infected with trichina worms.

trich·i·on (trik'ē-on). A cephalometric point at the midpoint of the hairline at the top of the forehead. [G. *thrix*, hair]

trich·ite (trik'īt). SYN trichocyst.

tri·chi·tis (tri-kī'tis). Inflammation of the hair bulbs. [trich- + G. *-itis*, inflammation]

tri·chlo·ral (trī-klōr'ăl). SYN *m*-chloral.

tri·chlor·fon (trī-klōr'fon). $C_4H_8Cl_3O_4P$; an organophosphorus compound effective against immature and mature stages of *Schistosoma haematobium*, but ineffective against other species of *Schistosoma* in humans. SYN metrifonate.

tri·chlo·ride (trī-klōr'īd). A chloride having three chlorine atoms in the molecule; *e.g.*, PCl_3.

tri·chlor·me·thi·a·zide (trī-klōr-me-thī'ă-zīd). 6-Chloro-3-(dichloromethyl)-3,4-dihydro-2*H*-1,2,4-benzothiadiazine-7-sulfonamide; an orally effective benzothiazide diuretic and antihypertensive agent.

tri·chlor·meth·ine (trī-klōr-meth'ēn). 2,2',2''-Trichlorotriethylamine hydrochloride; tris(2-chloroethyl)amine hydrochloride; a nitrogen mustard used in the treatment of leukemia.

tri·chlo·ro·a·ce·tic ac·id (trī-klōr'ō-ă-sē'tik). CCl_3COOH; used as an astringent antiseptic in 1 to 5% solution or as an escharotic for venereal and other warts; a widely used protein precipitant.

tri·chlo·ro·eth·ane (trī-klōr-ō-eth'ān). CH_3CCl_3; 1,1,1-Trichloroethane; an industrial solvent with pronounced inhalation anesthetic activity. SYN methylchloroform.

tri·chlo·ro·eth·a·nol (trī-klōr-ō-eth'ă-nol). CCl_3CH_2OH; 2,2,2-Trichloroethanol; a hypnotic and sedative; as a metabolite of chloral hydrate, it contributes to the depressant activity of chloral hydrate. SYN trichloroethyl alcohol.

tri·chlo·ro·eth·ene (trī-klōr-ō-eth'ēn). SYN trichloroethylene.

tri·chlo·ro·eth·yl al·co·hol (trī-klōr-ō-eth'il). SYN trichloroethanol.

tri·chlo·ro·eth·yl·ene (trī-klōr-ō-eth'i-lēn). $ClCH=CCl_2$; an analgesic and inhalation anesthetic used in minor surgical operations and in obstetrical practice; administration requires that only nonrebreathing circuits be used because of the toxicity of dichloracetylene resulting from interaction of t. with soda lime. SYN ethinyl trichloride, trichloroethene.

tri·chlo·ro·flu·o·ro·meth·ane (trī-klōr'ō-flūr-ō-meth'ān). CCl_3F; a propellant used for aerosol sprays; has anesthetic and arrhythmogenic activity if inhaled in high concentration. SYN trichloromonofluoromethane.

tri·chlo·ro·meth·ane (trī-klōr-ō-meth'ān). SYN chloroform.

tri·chlo·ro·mon·o·flu·o·ro·meth·ane (trī-klōr-ō-mon'ō-flūr-ō-meth'ān). SYN trichlorofluoromethane.

tri·chlo·ro·phe·nol (trī-klōr-ō-fē'nol). 2,4,5-Trichlorophenol or 2,4,6-trichlorophenol; used as an antiseptic, disinfectant, and fungicide.

(2,4,5-tri·chlo·ro·phen·oxy) ace·tic ac·id (2,4,5-T) (trī-klōr-ō-fe-nok'sē). A herbicide and defoliant synthesized by condensation of chloracetic acid and 2,4,5-trichlorophenol, used as the principal constituent of Agent Orange.

ⵕtricho-, trich-, trichi-. The hair; a hairlike structure. [G. *thrix* (*trich-*)]

trich·o·be·zoar (trik-ō-bē'zōr). A hair cast in the stomach or intestinal tract, common in cats. SYN hair ball, pilobezoar. [tricho- + bezoar]

Trich·o·ceph·a·lus (trik-ō-sef'ă-lŭs). Incorrect name for *Trichuris*. [tricho- + G. *kephalē*, head]

trich·o·chrome (trī'kō-krōm). Yellow-orange and violet natural pigments related to melanins; partly responsible for the red and auburn colors of human hair. [tricho- + G. *chrōma*, color]

trich·o·cla·sia, tri·choc·la·sis (trik-ō-klā'zē-ă, tri-kok'lă-sis). SYN *trichorrhexis* nodosa. [tricho- + G. *klasis*, breaking off]

trich·o·cryp·to·sis (trik'ō-krip-tō'sis). Any disease of the hair follicles. [tricho- + G. *kryptos*, concealed]

trich·o·cyst (trik'ō-sist). One of a number of structures, in the form of minute elongated cysts, arranged radially around the periphery of a protozoan cell and containing fluid which when discharged serves for offense or defense; found in ciliates, such as *Paramecium* species. SYN trichite. [tricho- + G. *kystis*, bladder]

Trich·o·dec·tes (trik-ō-dek'tēz). A genus of biting lice that includes the species *T. canis* (*T. latus*), the biting louse of dogs that commonly serves as an intermediate host for the dog tapeworm, *Dipylidium caninum*, as well as the species *T. climax* (*Bovicola caprae*), *T. parumpilosus* (*B. equi*), *T. scalaris* (*B. bovis*), and *T. sphaerocephalus* (*B. ovis*). SEE ALSO *Bovicola*, *Damalinia*. [tricho- + G. *dektēs*, a beggar]

Trich·o·der·ma (trik-ō-der'mă). A genus of fungi in soil that furnishes the antibiotic gliotoxin. Has produced rare opportunistic infections. [tricho- + G. *derma*, skin]

trich·o·dis·co·ma (trik'ō-dis-kō'mă). Dominantly inherited or nonfamilial elliptical parafollicular mesenchymal hamartomas. SYN haarscheibe tumor.

trich·o·dyn·ia (trik-ō-din'ē-ă). SYN trichalgia. [tricho- + G. *odynē*, pain]

trich·o·dys·tro·phy (trik'ō-dis-trō-fē). Defective nutrition of hair, often culminating in alopecia. May be acquired or congenital; the latter often with metabolic or other birth defects. [tricho- + G. prefix *dys-*, abnormal, + *trophē*, growth]

trich·o·ep·i·the·li·o·ma (trik'ō-ep-i-thē-lē-ō'mă) [MIM* 132700]. Multiple small benign nodules, occurring mostly on the skin of the face, derived from basal cells of hair follicles enclosing small keratin cysts; frequent autosomal dominant inheritance. SYN acanthoma adenoides cysticum, Brooke's tumor, epithelioma adenoides cysticum, hereditary multiple t. [tricho- + epithelioma]

acquired t., SYN dilated *pore*.

desmoplastic t., a solitary, hard, annular, centrally depressed papule, occurring usually in women on the face, consisting of dermal strands of basaloid cells and small keratinous cysts within sclerotic desmoplastic stroma.

hereditary multiple t., SYN trichoepithelioma.

trich·o·es·the·sia (trik′ō-es-thē′zē-ă). **1.** The sensation felt when a hair is touched. **2.** A form of paresthesia in which there is a sensation as of a hair on the skin, on the mucous membrane of the mouth, or on the conjunctiva. [tricho- + G. *aisthēsis,* sensation]

trich·o·fol·lic·u·lo·ma (trik′ō-fol-ik-yū-lō′mă). A usually solitary tumor or hamartoma in which multiple abortive hair follicles open into a central cyst or space opening on the skin surface. [tricho- + L. *folliculus,* fountain, spring, + G. *-oma,* tumor]

trich·o·gen (trik′o-jen). An agent that promotes the growth of hair. [tricho- + G. *-gen,* producing]

tri·chog·e·nous (tri-koj′ĕ-nŭs). Promoting the growth of the hair.

trich·o·glos·sia (trik-ō-glos′ē-ă). SYN hairy *tongue.* [tricho- + G. *glōssa,* tongue]

trich·o·hy·a·lin (trik-ō-hī′ă-lin). A substance of the nature of keratohyalin found in the developing inner root sheath of the hair follicle.

trich·oid (trik′oyd). Hairlike. [tricho- + G. *eidos,* resemblance]

trich·o·lem·mo·ma (trik′ō-le-mō′mă). SYN trichilemmoma.

trich·o·lith (trik′ō-lith). A concretion on the hair; the lesion of piedra. [tricho- + G. *lithos,* stone]

trich·o·lo·gia (trik-ō-lō′jē-ă). A nervous habit of plucking at the hair. SYN trichology (2). [G. *trichologeō,* to pluck hairs, fr. tricho- + *lego,* to pick out, gather]

tri·chol·o·gy (tri-kol′ō-jē). **1.** The study of the anatomy, growth, and diseases of the hair. [tricho- + G. *logos,* study] **2.** SYN trichologia. [G. *trichologeo,* fr. tricho- + *legō,* to pick out]

tri·cho·ma (tri-kō′mă). SYN trichiasis. [tricho- + G. *-oma,* tumor]

tri·cho·ma·tose (tri-kō′mă-tōs). SYN trichomatous.

tri·cho·ma·to·sis (tri-kō′mă-tō′sis). SYN trichiasis.

tri·chom·a·tous (tri-kō′mă-tŭs). Relating to or suffering from trichoma. SYN trichomatose.

trich·o·meg·a·ly (trik′ō-meg′ă-lē). Congenital condition characterized by abnormally long eyelashes; associated with dwarfism. [tricho- + G. *megas,* large]

trich·o·mo·na·cide (trik-ō-mō′nă-sīd). An agent that is destructive to *Trichomonas* organisms.

trich·o·mon·ad (trik-ō-mō′nad). Common name for members of the family Trichomonadidae.

Trich·o·mo·nad·i·dae (trik′ō-mō-nad′i-dē). A family of protozoan flagellates that includes the genus *Trichomonas.*

Trich·o·mon·as (trik-ō-mō′nas). A genus of parasitic protozoan flagellates (subfamily Trichomonidinae, family Trichomonadidae) causing trichomoniasis in humans, other primates, and birds. Specificity is more marked for its precise microhabitat than for host species. The genus has been divided into several genera: *Trichomonas, Pentatrichomonas, Tetratrichomonas,* and *Tritrichomonas.* [tricho- + G. *monas,* single (unit)]

T. bucca′lis, SYN *T. tenax.*

T. foe′tus, former name for *Tritrichomonas foetus.*

T. galli′nae, the species that causes avian trichomoniasis; the pigeon is the natural host, but the organism also occurs in turkeys, chickens, doves, hawks, falcons, and other birds; infection is most serious in young domestic pigeons, who acquire it from pigeon milk produced in the pigeon crop; other birds are infected from contaminated water or by feeding on infected birds.

T. gallina′rum, former name for *Tetratrichomonas gallinarium.*

T. hom′inis, former name for *Pentatrichomonas hominis.*

T. o′vis, former name for *Tetratrichomonas ovis.*

T. su′is, former name for *Tritrichomonas suis.*

T. te′nax, a species that lives as a commensal in the mouth of humans and other primates, especially in the tartar around the teeth or in the defects of carious teeth; there is no evidence of direct pathogenesis, but it is frequently associated with pyogenic organisms in pus pockets or at the base of teeth. SYN *T. buccalis.*

T. vagina′lis, a species frequently found in the vagina and ure-thra of women and in the urethra and prostate gland of men (the only known natural hosts), in whom it causes trichomoniasis vaginitis; considerable differences in pathogenicity exists among various strains of this species.

trich·o·mo·ni·a·sis (trik′ō-mō-nī′ă-sis). Disease caused by infection with a species of protozoan of the genus *Trichomonas* or related genera; often used to designate t. vaginitis.

avian t., t. occurring in the upper digestive tract in a variety of birds and caused by *Trichomonas gallinae;* it causes necrotic ulceration in the mouth, esophagus, crop, and proventriculus, frequently with rapid weight loss and death.

bovine t., a venereal infection in cattle caused by *Tritrichomonas foetus;* in the bull, the infection is usually asymptomatic, the organisms being present in small or moderate numbers, chiefly in the preputial sheath; infection in the female may result in delayed conception, abortion early in pregnancy, or pyometra; transmission occurs during copulation or by artificial insemination from infected bulls.

t. vagini′tis, acute vaginitis or urethritis caused by infection with *Trichomonas vaginalis,* which does not invade the mucosa or the tissue but provokes an inflammatory reaction; infection is venereal or by other forms of contact; widespread infection in human populations is usually asymptomatic but may produce vaginitis, with vaginal and vulvar pruritis, leukorrhea with frothy watery discharge, and (rarely) purulent urethritis in males.

trich·o·my·ce·to·sis (trik′ō-mī-sē-tō′sis). SYN trichomycosis.

trich·o·my·co·sis (trik′ō-mī-kō′sis). Formerly used to mean any disease of the hair caused by a fungus; presently synonymous with trichonocardiosis or t. axillaris. In present usage, t. is a misnomer because the causative agent of the disease is a nocardia (an entity intermediate between fungus and bacterium) or *Corynebacterium* and not a true fungus. SYN trichomycetosis. [tricho- + G. *mykēs,* fungus, + *-osis,* condition]

t. axilla′ris, *Corynebacterium* infection of axillary and pubic hairs with development of yellow (flava), black (nigra), or red (rubra) concretions around the hair shafts; frequently asymptomatic. SYN lepothrix, Paxton's disease, t. chromatica, t. nodosa, t. nodularis, t. palmellina, trichonocardiosis axillaris, trichonodosis.

t. chromat′ica, SYN t. axillaris.

t. nodo′sa, SYN t. axillaris.

t. nodula′ris, SYN t. axillaris.

t. palmelli′na, SYN t. axillaris.

t. pustulo′sa, any parasitic disease of the hair marked by pustule formation at the orifices of the hair follicles.

trich·o·no·car·di·o·sis (trik′ō-nō-kar′dē-ō′sis). An infection of hair shafts, especially of the axillary and pubic regions, with nocardiae. Yellow, red, or black concretions develop around the infected hair shafts and contain the causative agent and, frequently, micrococci; the micrococci probably account for the variety of the colors of the concretions and for the resultant varieties of t. which have been described. SEE ALSO trichomycosis, *trichomycosis* axillaris. [tricho- + *Nocardia* + G. *-osis,* condition]

t. axilla′ris, SYN *trichomycosis* axillaris.

trich·o·no·do·sis (trik′ō-nō-dō′sis). SYN *trichomycosis* axillaris. [tricho- + L. *nodus,* node (swelling), + G. *-osis,* condition]

trich·o·no·sis (trik′ō-nō′sis). SYN trichopathy.

tri·cho·no·sus (tri-kon′ō-sŭs). SYN trichopathy. [tricho- + G. *nosos,* disease]

t. versic′olor, SYN ringed *hair.*

trich·o·path·ic (trik-ō-path′ik). Relating to any disease of the hair.

trich·o·path·o·pho·bia (trik′ō-path-ō-fō′bē-ă). Excessive worry regarding disease of the hair, its color, or abnormalities of its growth. [tricho- + G. *pathos,* suffering, + *phobos,* fear]

tri·chop·a·thy (tri-kop′ă-thē). Any disease of the hair. SYN trichonosis, trichonosus, trichosis. [tricho- + G. *pathos,* suffering]

trich·o·pha·gia (trik-ō-fāj′ē-a). The eating of hair or wool.

tri·choph·a·gy (tri-kof′ă-jē). Habitual biting of the hair. [tricho- + G. *phagein,* to eat]

trich·o·pho·bia (trik-ō-fō′bē-ă). Morbid disgust caused by the sight of loose hairs on clothing or elsewhere. [tricho- + G. *phobos,* fear]

trich·o·phyt·ic (trik-ō-fit'ik). Relating to trichophytosis.

trich·o·phy·tid (tri-kof'i-tid, trik-ō-fi'tid). An eruption remote from the site of infection, which is the expression of allergic response to *Trichophyton* infection. [tricho- + G. *phyton,* plant, + *-id* (1)]

tri·choph·y·tin (tri-kof'i-tin). An extract of cultures of several species of *Trichophyton,* the ringworm fungus. Formerly used in the diagnosis and treatment of a number of varieties of ringworm infection; now used only as a measure of general immune response in a compromised person.

trich·o·phy·to·be·zoar (trik'ō-fi'tō-be'zōr). A mixed hair and food ball, consisting of vegetable fibers, seeds and skins of fruits, and animal hair that are matted together to form a ball in the stomach of man or animals, especially ruminants. SYN phytotrichobezoar. [tricho- + G. *phyton,* plant, + bezoar]

Trich·o·phy·ton (tri-kof'i-tŏn). A genus of pathogenic fungi causing dermatophytosis in humans and animals; species may be anthropophilic, zoophilic, or geophilic, and attack the hair, skin, and nails, and are characterized by their growth in hair. Endothrix species grow from the skin into the hair follicle, penetrate the shaft, and grow into it, producing rows of arthroconidia as the hyphae septate; there is no growth on the external surface of the shaft. Ectothrix species are of two kinds, large spored and small spored. In both, the fungus grows into the hair follicle, surrounds the hair shaft, and penetrates it, but continues to grow both within and outside the hair shaft, producing arthroconidia externally. [tricho- + G. *phyton,* plant]

T. concen'tricum, an anthropophilic species which is the causative agent of tinea imbricata; it closely resembles the branching mycelium of *T. schoenleinii.*

T. equi'num, a zoophilic species causing ectothrix infections of hair in horses, from which humans may also be infected; it requires nicotinic acid for growth.

T. megnin'ii, an anthropophilic ectothrix species of dermatophyte with spores in chains, causing infection in man; it requires histidine, which differentiates it from *Microsporum gallinae.*

T. mentagrophy'tes, a zoophilic small-spored ectothrix species that causes infection of the hair, skin, and nails; it is a cause of ringworm in dogs, horses, rabbits, mice, rats, chinchillas, foxes, and man (especially tinea pedis with severe inflammation, and tinea cruris).

T. ru'brum, a widely distributed anthropophilic species that causes persistent infections of the skin, especially tinea pedis and tinea cruris, and in the nails that are unusually resistant to therapy; it rarely invades the hair, where it is ectothrix in nature; occasional subcutaneous and systemic infections have been reported.

T. schoenlei'nii, an anthropophilic endothrix species of dermatophyte causing favus in man; it is endemic throughout Eurasia and Africa and, because of travel, is seen more frequently in the Western Hemisphere; it produces tunnels within the hair shaft which are filled with air bubbles after the hyphae disintegrate.

T. sim'ii, a zoophilic species that causes infection in rhesus monkeys, dogs, and man; most infections have had their origin in India.

T. ton'surans, an anthropophilic endothrix species that causes epidemic dermatophytosis in Europe, South America, and the U.S.; it infects some animals and requires thiamin for growth. It is the most common cause of tinea capitis in the U.S., forming black dots where hair breaks off at the skin surface.

T. verrucos'um, a zoophilic species that causes ringworm in cattle, from which man can become infected.

T. viola'ceum, an anthropophilic species that causes black-dot ringworm or favus infection of the scalp; hair infection is of the endothrix type; usually found in South America, Europe, Asia, and Africa.

trich·o·phyt·o·sis (trik'ō-fī-tō'sis). Superficial fungus infection caused by species of *Trichophyton.* [tricho- + G. *phyton,* plant, + *-osis,* condition]

t. bar'bae, SYN *tinea* barbae.

t. cap'itis, SYN *tinea* capitis.

t. cor'poris, SYN *tinea* corporis.

t. cru'ris, SYN *tinea* cruris.

t. un'guium, fungus infection of the nail plates. SEE ALSO onychomycosis.

Trich·o·pleu·ris (trik'-ō-plū'ris). A genus of biting lice that infest ruminants, *e.g., T. lipeuroides* and *T. parallelus* in American deer; considered by some to be a subgenus of *Damalinia.* [tricho- + G. *pleura,* rib, side]

tri·chop·o·li·o·dys·tro·phy. SYN kinky-hair *disease.*

trich·o·po·li·o·sis (trik'ō-pō-lē-ō'sis). SYN poliosis. [tricho- + G. *polios,* gray, + *-osis,* condition]

Tri·chop·tera (tri-kop'ter-ă). An order of insects in which the aquatic larvae (caddis flies) construct a protective case (caddis) of bits of submerged material in a highly specific form; commonly found attached under stones in freshwater streams. The adult caddis flies, having hairy wings, shed their hairs and epithelia, causing hay fever-like (allergic) symptoms in sensitive people. [tricho- + G. *pteron,* wing]

trich·o·pti·lo·sis (trik'ō-ti-lō'sis, tri-kop-ti-lō'sis). A condition of splitting of the shaft of the hair, giving it a feathery appearance. [tricho- + G. *ptilōsis,* plumage, + *-osis,* condition]

trich·or·rhex·is (trik-ō-rek'sis). A condition in which the hairs tend to readily break or split. [tricho- + G. *rhēxis,* a breaking]

t. invagina'ta, SYN bamboo *hair.*

t. nodo'sa, a congenital or acquired condition in which minute nodes are formed in the hair shafts; splitting and breaking, complete or incomplete, may occur at these points or nodes. SYN clastothrix, nodositas crinium, trichoclasia, trichoclasis.

tri·chos·chi·sis (tri-kos'ki-sis). The presence of broken or split hairs. SEE ALSO trichorrhexis. [tricho- + G. *schisis,* a cleaving]

tri·chos·co·py (tri-kos'kŏ-pē). Examination of the hair. [tricho- + G. *skopeō,* to examine]

tri·cho·sis (tri-kō'sis). SYN trichopathy. [tricho- + G. *-osis,* condition]

t. carun'culae, a growth of hair on the lacrimal caruncle.

t. sensiti'va, hyperesthesia of the hairy parts.

t. seto'sa, coarseness of the hair.

trich·o·so·ma·tous (trik-ō-sō'mă-tŭs). Having flagella with a small body; denoting certain protozoan organisms. SEE *Trichomonas.* [tricho- + G. *sōma,* body]

Tri·cho·spo·ron (tri-kos'pō-ron, trik-ō-spōr'on). A genus of imperfect fungi that possess branching septate hyphae with arthroconidia and blastoconidia; these organisms are part of the normal flora of the intestinal tract of humans. *T. beigelii* is the causative agent of white piedra or trichosporosis and fatal fungemia in immunocompromised patients. [tricho- + G. *sporos,* seed (spore)]

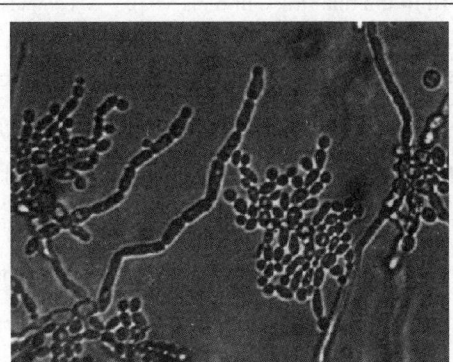

Trichosporon cutaneum

trich·o·spor·o·no·sis (trik'ō-spor-o-nō'sis). Systemic infection by *Trichosporan beigelii;* marked by fever or pneumonia with a high mortality; seen in neutropenic patients. Local infection with *T. beigelii* is white piedra, also known as trichosporosis.

trich·o·spo·ro·sis (trik'ō-spō-rō'sis). SYN white *piedra*. [*Trichosporon* + G. *-osis,* condition]

trich·o·sta·sis spi·nu·lo·sa (tri-kos'tă-sis spī'nū-lō'să). A condition in which hair follicles are blocked with a keratin plug containing lanugo hairs. [tricho- + G. *stasis,* a standing; L. *spinulosus,* thorny]

trich·o·stron·gyle (trik-ō-stron'jil). Common name for members of the family Trichostrongylidae.

Trich·o·stron·gyl·i·dae (trik'ō-stron-jil'i-dē). A family of nematodes (order Strongylida or, in older terminology, Strongylata); includes the important genera *Cooperia, Ostertagia, Haemonchus, Trichostrongylus, Nematodirus,* and *Hippostrongylus.* SEE *Trichostrongylus.*

trich·o·stron·gy·lo·sis (trik'ō-stron-ji-lō'sis). Infection with nematodes of the genus *Trichostrongylus.*

Trich·o·stron·gy·lus (trik-ō-stron'ji-lŭs). The hairworm, or bankrupt or black scour worm; an economically important genus (about 30 species) of small slender nematodes (family Trichostrongylidae) that inhabit the small intestine, in some cases the stomach, of a variety of herbivorous animals and gallinaceous birds. They burrow into the mucosa and suck blood; in large numbers they do serious damage, especially to young hosts. [tricho- + G. *strongylos,* round]

T. ax'ei, the most common species in cattle, occurring also in the abomasum of sheep, horses, antelope, bison, llama, and deer, and in the stomach of pigs and horses.

T. capric'ola, a species that occurs in the small intestine and abomasum of sheep, goats, deer, and pronghorn.

T. colubrifor'mis, a species that occurs in anterior portions of the small intestine and sometimes in the abomasum of sheep, goats, cattle, camels, and some wild ruminants, and in the stomach of primates (including humans), rabbits, and squirrels; it is distributed worldwide and is common in the U.S., especially in sheep.

T. longispicula'ris, a species found in the small intestine of cattle, sheep, and goats; it is distributed worldwide but uncommon in the U.S.

T. ten'uis, a species that is a widespread pathogenic parasite of the ceca and small intestines of fowl, including ducks, geese, turkeys, pheasants, and partridges.

T. vitri'nus, a species that is an important pathogen of lambs, found chiefly in the duodenum of sheep, camels, rabbits, and goats but also reported from humans and pigs.

Trich·o·the·ci·um (tri-kō-thē'sē-ŭm). A genus of imperfect fungi generally considered a common saprophyte.

trich·o·thi·o·dys·tro·phy (trik'ō-thī'ō-dis'trō-fē) [MIM* 234050]. Congenital fragile hair with multiple fractures resulting from low sulfur-containing amino acid (cysteine) content of the hair, mental impairment, and short stature. [tricho- + thio- + G. *dys,* bad, + *trophē,* nourishment]

trich·o·til·lo·ma·nia (trik'ō-til-ō-mā'nē-ă). A compulsion to pull out one's own hair. [tricho- + G. *tillo,* pull out, + *mania,* insanity]

tri·chot·o·my (tri-kot'ō-mē). A division into three parts. [G. *trichia,* threefold, + *tomē,* a cutting]

trich·o·tox·in (trik'ō-tok'sin). A cytotoxin having an injurious effect specifically for ciliated epithelium.

tri·chot·ro·phy (tri-kot'rō-fē). Nutrition of the hair. [tricho- + G. *trophē,* nourishment]

tri·chro·ic (trī-krō'ik). Relating to or marked by trichroism.

tri·chro·ism (trī'krō-izm). The property of some crystals of emitting different colors in three different directions. [G. *trichroos,* three-colored, fr. tri- + *chroa,* color]

tri·chro·mat (trī-krō'mat). A person who sees three primary colors; hence, one with normal color vision. [tri- + G. *chrōma,* color]

tri·chro·mat·ic (trī-krō-mat'ik). **1.** Having, or relating to, the three primary colors, red, green, and blue. **2.** Capable of perceiving the three primary colors; having normal color vision. SYN trichromic.

tri·chro·ma·tism (trī-krō'mă-tizm). The state of being trichromatic. [tri- + G. *chrōma,* color]

anomalous t., a defect in color perception in which there appears to be an abnormality or deficiency in one of the three primary pigments of the retinal cones. SEE protanomaly, deuteranomaly, tritanomaly.

tri·chro·ma·top·sia (trī-krō'mă-top'sē-ă). Normal color vision; the ability to perceive the three primary colors. [tri- + G. *chrōma,* color, + *opsis,* vision]

tri·chro·mic (trī-krō'mik). SYN trichromatic.

trich·ter·brust (tricht'er-brŭst). SYN *pectus* excavatum. [Ger. *Trichterbrust,* funnel chest]

trich·u·ri·a·sis (tri-kū-rī'ă-sis). Infection with nematodes of the genus *Trichuris.* In humans, intestinal parasitization by *T. trichiura* is usually asymptomatic and not associated with peripheral eosinophilia; in massive infections it frequently induces diarrhea or rectal prolapse.

Trich·u·ris (tri-kū'ris). A genus of aphasmid nematodes (sometimes improperly termed *Trichocephalus*) related to the trichina worm, *Trichinella spiralis,* and having a body with a slender, elongated, anterior portion threaded into the mucosa of the colon or large intestine of the host and a thick posterior portion bearing reproductive organs and their products. *T.* contains about 70 species, all in mammals. [tricho- + G. *oura,* tail]

T. trichiu'ra, the whipworm of humans, a species that causes trichuriasis; the body is filiform and slender in the anterior three-fifths, and more robust posteriorly; females are 4 or 5 cm long, males are shorter (with coiled caudal extremity and a single eversible spicule); eggs are barrel-shaped, 50 to 56 by 20 to 22 μm, with double shell and translucent knobs at each of the two poles; humans are the only susceptible hosts and usually acquire infection by direct finger-to-mouth contact or by ingestion of soil, water, or food that contains larvated eggs (development in the soil takes 3 to 6 weeks under proper conditions of warmth and moisture, hence distribution is chiefly tropical); larvae escape from eggs in the ileum, mature in approximately a month, and then pass directly into the cecum without undergoing a parenteral migration as occurs with *Ascaris lumbricoides;* adults may persist for 2 to 7 years.

tri·cip·i·tal (trī-sip'i-tăl). Having three heads; denoting a triceps muscle.

tri·clo·bi·so·ni·um chlo·ride (trī'klō-bi-sō'nē-ŭm). Hexamethylenebis[dimethyl[1-methyl-3-(2,2,6-trimethylcyclohexyl)propyl]ammonium chloride]; a bisquaternary ammonium compound used topically in the treatment of superficial infections of the skin and vagina; a cationic antiseptic effective against both Gram-negative and Gram-positive organisms. It is inactivated by soap and pH changes.

tri·clo·fen·ol pi·per·a·zine (trī-klō'fen-ol). Bis(2,4,5-trichlorophenol) piperazine; an anthelmintic.

tri·clo·fos (trī'klō-fōs). A phosphorylated derivative of chloral hydrate, which is hydrolyzed to chloral hydrate in the body and produces characteristic sedative-hypnotic properties.

tri·corn (trī'kōrn). **1.** One of the lateral ventricles of the brain. **2.** SYN tricornute. [tri- + L. *cornu,* horn]

tri·cor·nute (trī-kōr'nūt). Having three cornua or horns. SYN tricorn (2). [tri- + L. *cornutus,* horned, fr. *cornu,* a horn]

tri·cre·sol (trī-krē'sol). SYN cresol.

tri·crot·ic (trī-krot'ik). Thrice-beating; marked by three waves in the arterial pulse tracing. SYN tricrotous. [tri- + G. *krotos,* a beat]

tri·cro·tism (trī'krō-tizm). The condition of being tricrotic.

tri·cro·tous (trī'krō-tŭs). SYN tricrotic.

Tric·u·la (trik'yū-lă). A genus of operculate freshwater snails related to *Oncomelania* (the *Schistosoma japonicum* intermediate hosts) of the subfamily triculinae, family Hydrobiidae, subclass Prosobranchiata; it includes *T. aperta,* intermediate host of *Schistosoma mekongi.*

tri·cus·pid, tri·cus·pi·dal, tri·cus·pi·date (trī-kŭs'pid, -kŭs'pi-dăl, -kŭs'pi-dāt). **1.** Having three points, prongs, or cusps, as the tricuspid valve of the heart. **2.** Having three tubercles or cusps, as the second upper molar tooth (occasionally) and the upper third molar (usually). SYN tritubercular.

tri·cy·cla·mol chlo·ride (trī-sī'klă-mol). SYN procyclidine methochloride.

tri·dac·ty·lous (trī-dak'ti-lŭs). SYN tridigitate.

tri·dent (trī'dent). SYN tridentate.

tri·den·tate (trī-den'tāt). Three-toothed; three-pronged. SYN trident. [tri- + L. *dentatus,* toothed]

tri·der·mic (trī-der'mik). Relating to or derived from the three primary germ layers of the embryo: ectoderm, endoderm, and mesoderm. [tri- + G. *derma,* skin]

tri·der·mo·ma (trī-der-mō'mă). SYN triphyllomatous *teratoma.* [tri- + G. *derma,* skin, + -*oma,* tumor]

tri·dig·i·tate (trī-dij'i-tāt). Having three fingers or three toes on one hand or foot. SYN tridactylous. [tri- + L. *digitus,* digit]

tri·di·hex·eth·yl chlo·ride (trī'dī-heks-eth'il). 3-Diethylamino-1-phenyl-1-cyclohexyl 1-propanol ethylchloride; an anticholinergic drug.

trid·y·mite (trid'i-mīt). A form of silica used in dental casting investment. [fr. G. *tridymos,* threefold]

trid·y·mus (trid'ĭ-mŭs). SYN triplet (1). [L. fr. G. *tridymos,* threefold]

tri·el·con (trī-el'kon). A long, three-jawed forceps for the extraction of foreign bodies from wounds or canals. [tri- + G. *helkō,* to draw]

tri·en·tine hy·dro·chlo·ride (trī'en-tēn). $C_6H_{18}N_4 \cdot 2HCl$; a chelating agent used to remove excess copper from the body in Wilson's disease. SYN triethylenetetramine dihydrochloride.

tri·eth·a·nol·a·mine (trī'eth-ă-nol'ă-mēn). A mixture of mono-, di-, and triethanolamine, used as an emulsifying agent in the preparation of medicated ointments and lotions and as an aid in the absorption of such medicaments through the skin.

tri·eth·yl·ene gly·col (trī-eth'i-lēn). $C_6H_{14}O_4$; 2,2'-Ethylenedioxybis(ethanol); used in the vapor state as an air-sterilizing agent; toxic to bacteria, fungi, and viruses in very low concentrations in air; variations in the humidity of the air limit the germicidal effectiveness.

tri·eth·yl·ene·mel·a·mine (TEM) (trī-eth'i-lēn-mel'ă-mēn). 2,4,6-Tris(ethyleneimino)-*s*-triazine; an antineoplastic agent chemically related to the nitrogen mustards; used in the treatment of leukemia.

tri·eth·yl·ene·phos·phor·a·mide (TEPA) (trī-eth'i-lēn-fos-fōr'ă-mīd). A drug with the same actions and uses as triethylenemelamine in the treatment of leukemias.

tri·eth·yl·ene·tet·ra·mine di·hy·dro·chlo·ride (trī-eth'i-lēn-tet'ră-am'ēn). SYN trientine hydrochloride.

tri·eth·yl·ene·thi·o·phos·phor·a·mide (trī-eth'i-lēn-thī'ō-fos-fōr'ă-mīd). Tris(1-aziridinyl)phosphine sulfide; an alkylating agent used for the palliative treatment of malignant diseases such as leukemia, lymphoma, and carcinoma. SYN thiotepa.

tri·fa·cial (trī-fā'shăl). Denoting the fifth pair of cranial nerves, the trigeminal nerves. [tri- + L. *facies,* face]

tri·fid (trī'fid). Split into three. [L. *trifidus,* three-cleft]

tri·flu·o·per·a·zine hy·dro·chlo·ride (trī'flū-ō-per'ă-zēn). 10-[3-(4-Methyl-1-piperazinyl)propyl]-2-(trifluoromethyl)-phenothiazine hydrochloride; an antipsychotic.

tri·flu·o·ro·ace·tyl (trī-flur'ō-as'ē-til). A group used to protect amino moieties of amino acid and peptides during peptide synthesis.

2,2,2-tri·flu·o·ro·ethyl vi·nyl (trī-flūr-ō-eth'il). SYN fluroxene.

5-tri·flu·o·ro·meth·yl·de·ox·y·u·ri·dine (trī-flūr'ō-meth'il-dē-ok-si-yū'ri-dēn). A pyrimidine analogue used topically in the treatment of herpes simplex keratitis.

tri·flu·per·i·dol hy·dro·chlo·ride (trī-flū-per'i-dol). 4'-Fluoro-4-[4-hydroxy-4-(α,α,α-trifluoro-*m*-tolyl)piperidino]-butyrophenone hydrochloride; a tranquilizer.

tri·flu·pro·ma·zine hy·dro·chlo·ride (trī-flū-prō'mă-zēn). 10-[3-(Dimethylamino)propyl]-2-trifluoromethylphenothiazine hydrochloride; an antipsychotic closely related chemically and pharmacologically to chlorpromazine.

tri·flur·i·dine (trī-flūr'i-dēn). 2'-Deoxy-5-(trifluoromethyl)-uridine; an antiviral agent used in eye drops to treat herpes simplex infections of the eye.

tri·fo·cal (trī'fō-kăl). Having three foci. SEE trifocal *lens.*

tri·fo·li·o·sis (trī-fō-lē-ō'sis). A form of photosensitization that occurs in horses, cattle, sheep, and pigs from eating several types

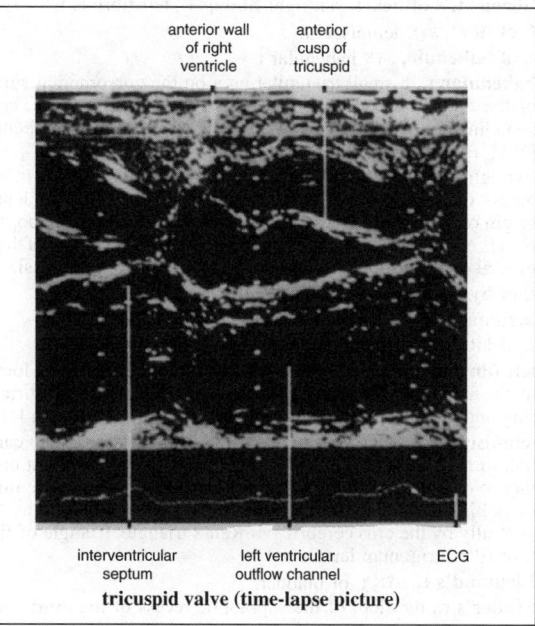

anterior wall of right ventricle · anterior cusp of tricuspid · interventricular septum · left ventricular outflow channel · ECG

tricuspid valve (time-lapse picture)

of clover and alfalfa. SYN clover disease, trefoil dermatitis. [L. *trifolium,* trefoil, clover]

tri·fur·ca·tion (trī-fŭr-kā'shŭn). **1.** A division into three branches. **2.** The area where the tooth roots divide into three distinct portions. [tri- + L. *furca,* fork]

tri·gas·tric (trī-gas'trik). Having three bellies; denoting a muscle with two tendinous interruptions. [tri- + G. *gastēr,* belly]

tri·gem·i·nal (trī-jem'i-năl). Relating to the fifth cranial or trigeminus nerve. SYN trigeminus. [L. *trigeminus,* threefold]

tri·gem·i·nus (trī-jem'i-nŭs). SYN trigeminal. [L. threefold, fr. tri- + *geminus,* twin]

tri·gem·i·ny (trī-jem'i-nē). SYN trigeminal *rhythm.* [L. *trigeminus,* threefold]

trig·e·nol·line (trig-ĕ-nol'ēn). SYN trigonelline.

trig·ger (trig'er). Term describing a system in which a relatively small input turns on a relatively large output, the magnitude of which is unrelated to the magnitude of the input.

ECG t., use of the electrocardiogram, usually the R wave, to control electronically some recording or imaging apparatus. SEE cardiac *gating.* SYN EKG t.

EKG t., SYN ECG t.

tri·glyc·er·ide (trī-glis'er-īd). SYN triacylglycerol.

tri·go·na (trī-gō'nă). Plural of trigonum. [L.]

trig·o·nal (trig'ō-năl). Triangular; relating to a trigonum.

tri·gone (trī'gōn). **1.** SYN trigonum. **2.** The first three dominant cusps (protocone, paracone, and metacone), taken collectively, of an upper molar tooth. [L. *trigonum,* fr. G. *trigōnon,* triangle]

t. of auditory nerve, the slight prominence of the floor of the lateral recess of the fourth ventricle, corresponding to the underlying cochlear and vestibular nuclei. SYN acoustic tubercle, trigonum acustici.

t. of bladder, a triangular smooth area at the base of the bladder between the openings of the two ureters and that of the urethra. SYN trigonum vesicae [NA], Lieutaud's body, Lieutaud's triangle, Lieutaud's t., vesical triangle.

cerebral t., SYN fornix.

collateral t., a triangular prominence of the floor of the lateral ventricle at the transition between occipital and temporal horn, continuous rostrally with the collateral eminence and, like the latter, caused by the deep penetration of the collateral sulcus from the ventral surface of the temporal lobe. SYN trigonum collaterale [NA], t. of lateral ventricle, trigonum ventriculi, ventricular t.

deltoideopectoral t., SYN infraclavicular *fossa.*

tr

fibrous t.'s of heart, SEE right fibrous t., left fibrous t.

t. of fillet, SYN lemniscal t.

t. of habenula, SYN habenular t.

habenular t., a small triangular area on the dorsomedial surface of the thalamus at the caudal end of the medullary stria, corresponding to the underlying habenula. SYN trigonum habenulae [NA], t. of habenula.

hypoglossal t., a slight elevation in the floor of the inferior recess of the fourth ventricle, beneath which is the nucleus of origin of the twelfth cranial nerve. SYN trigonum nervi hypoglossi [NA], eminentia hypoglossi, hypoglossal eminence, t. of hypoglossal nerve, trigonum hypoglossi, tuberculum hypoglossi.

t. of hypoglossal nerve, SYN hypoglossal t.

inguinal t., SYN inguinal *triangle.*

t. of lateral ventricle, SYN collateral t.

left fibrous t., the part of the fibrous skeleton of the heart located in the interval between the left side of the left atrioventricular ring and the aortic ring. SYN trigonum fibrosum sinistrum [NA].

lemniscal t., a triangular area on the lateral surface of the caudal half of the mesencephalon, bordered caudally by the slight prominence of the lateral lemniscus, dorsally by the base of the inferior colliculus and the brachium of the superior colliculus, and ventrally by the crus cerebri. SYN Reil's triangle, triangle of fillet, t. of fillet, trigonum lemnisci.

Lieutaud's t., SYN t. of bladder.

Müller's t., the floor of the supraoptic recess of the third ventricle.

olfactory t., a grayish triangular area corresponding to the attachment of the olfactory peduncle ("olfactory nerve" or olfactory tract) to the base of the brain, at the anterior border of the anterior perforated substance. SYN trigonum olfactorium [NA].

right fibrous t., part of the fibrous skeleton of the heart located between the aortic fibrous ring and rings surrounding the right and left atrioventricular ostia. SYN trigonum fibrosum dextrum [NA].

vagal t., a prominence in the floor of the inferior fovea of the fourth ventricle that overlies the dorsal motor nucleus of the vagus. SYN trigonum nervi vagi [NA], ala cinerea, ashen wing, gray wing, t. of vagus nerve, va'gi eminentia.

t. of vagus nerve, SYN vagal t.

ventricular t., SYN collateral t.

vertebrocostal t., a triangular area in the diaphragm near the lateral arcuate ligament that is devoid of muscle fibers; it is covered by pleura superiorly and by peritoneum inferiorly. SYN Bochdalek's gap, trigonum lumbocostale.

trig·o·nel·line (trig-ō-nel'ēn). *N*-methylnicotinic acid; the methyl betaine of nicotinic acid; a product of the metabolism of nicotinic acid; excreted in the urine. SYN caffearine, trigenolline.

tri·go·nid (trī-gon'id, -gō'nid). The first three dominant cusps, taken collectively, of a lower molar tooth. SEE ALSO trigone. [see *trigonum*]

tri·go·ni·tis (trī'gō-nī'tis). Inflammation of the urinary bladder, localized in the trigone. [trigone + G. *-itis,* inflammation]

trig·o·no·ce·phal·ic (trig'ō-nō-se-fal'ik). Pertaining to trigonocephaly.

trig·o·no·ceph·a·ly (trig'ō-nō-sef'ă-lē, trī'gō-nō-). Malformation characterized by a triangular configuration of the skull, due in part to premature synostosis of the cranial bones with compression of the cerebral hemispheres. [trigone + G. *kephalē,* head]

tri·go·num, pl. **tri·go·na** (trī-gō'nŭm, -nă). Any triangular area. SEE triangle. SYN trigone (1). [L., fr. G. *trigōnon,* a triangle]

t. acus'tici, SYN *trigone* of auditory nerve.

t. carot'icum [NA], SYN carotid *triangle.*

t. cerebra'le, SYN fornix (2).

t. cervica'le, any one of the triangles of the neck. SYN t. colli.

t. cervica'le ante'rius, SYN anterior *triangle* of neck.

t. cervica'le poste'rius, SYN posterior *triangle* of neck.

t. collatera'le [NA], SYN collateral *trigone.*

t. col'li, SYN t. cervicale.

t. deltoideopectora'le, SYN infraclavicular *fossa.*

t. femora'le [NA], SYN femoral *triangle.*

trigo'na fibro'sa cor'dis, SEE right fibrous *trigone,* left fibrous *trigone.*

t. fibro'sum dex'trum [NA], SYN right fibrous *trigone.*

t. fibro'sum sinis'trum [NA], SYN left fibrous *trigone.*

t. haben'ulae [NA], SYN habenular *trigone.*

t. hypoglos'si, SYN hypoglossal *trigone.*

t. inguina'le [NA], SYN inguinal *triangle.*

t. lemnis'ci, SYN lemniscal *trigone.*

t. lumba'le [NA], SYN lumbar *triangle.*

t. lumbocosta'le, SYN vertebrocostal *trigone.*

t. muscula're [NA], SYN muscular *triangle.*

t. ner'vi hypoglos'si [NA], SYN hypoglossal *trigone.*

t. ner'vi va'gi [NA], SYN vagal *trigone.*

t. olfacto'rium [NA], SYN olfactory *trigone.*

t. omoclavicula're [NA], SYN supraclavicular *triangle.*

t. omotrachea'le [NA], ✭official alternate term for muscular *triangle.*

t. pala'ti, SYN palatal *triangle.*

t. sternocosta'le, a muscular defect in the diaphragm between the costal and the sternal portions. SYN Larrey's cleft, sternocostal triangle.

t. submandibula're [NA], SYN submandibular *triangle.*

t. submenta'le [NA], SYN submental *triangle.*

t. ventric'uli, SYN collateral *trigone.*

t. vesi'cae [NA], SYN *trigone* of bladder.

tri·hex·o·syl·cer·a·mide. SYN globotriaosylceramide.

tri·hex·y·phen·i·dyl hy·dro·chlo·ride (trī-heks'ē-fen'ĭ-dil). A synthetic anticholinergic agent reputed to exert a higher degree of anticholinergic activity in the brain as compared with peripheral parasympathetic neuroeffector junctions. Widely used in the treatment of parkinsonism secondary to idiopathic or neuroleptic-induced parkinsonism.

tri·hy·brid (trī-hī'brid). The offspring of parents which that in three mendelian characters. [tri- + L. *hybrida,* hybrid]

tri·hy·dric (trī-hī'drik). Denoting a chemical compound containing three replaceable hydrogen atoms.

tri·hy·drox·y·es·trin (trī'hī-drok'sē-es'trin). SYN estriol.

tri·in·i·od·y·mus (trī-in'i-od'i-mŭs). A grossly malformed fetus with three heads, joined at the occiput, and a single body. [tri- + G. *inion,* nape of the neck, + *didymos,* twin]

tri·i·o·dide (trī-ī'ō-did, -dīd). An iodide with three atoms of iodine in the molecule; *e.g.,* KI_3.

tri·i·o·do·meth·ane (trī-ī'ō-dō-meth'ān). SYN iodoform.

3,5,3'-tri·i·o·do·thy·ro·nine (TITh, T₃) (trī-ī'ō-dō-thī'rō-nēn). A thyroid hormone normally synthesized in smaller quantities than thyroxine; present in blood and in thyroid gland and exerts the same biological effects as thyroxine but, on a molecular basis, is more potent and the onset of its effect is more rapid.

tri·ke·to·hy·drin·dene hy·drate (trī-kē-tō-hī'drin-dēn). Former name for ninhydrin.

tri·ke·to·pu·rine (trī-kē-tō-pyūr'ēn). SYN uric acid.

tri·labe (trī'lāb). A three-pronged forceps for removal of foreign bodies from the bladder. [tri- + G. *labē,* a handle, hold]

tri·lam·i·nar (trī-lam'i-nar). Having three laminae.

tri·lat·er·al (tri-lat'ĕ-răl). Having three sides.

tri·lo·bate, tri·lobed (trī-lō'bāt, trī'lobd). Having three lobes.

tri·loc·u·lar (trī-lok'yū-lăr). Having three cavities or cells.

tril·o·gy (tril'ō-jē). A triad of related entities. [G. *trilogia,* fr. tri- + *logos,* study, discourse]

t. of Fallot, a set of congenital defects including pulmonic stenosis, atrial septal defect, and right ventricular hypertrophy. SYN Fallot's triad.

tri·lo·stane (trī'lō-stān). 4α,5-Epoxy-3,17β-dihydroxy-5α-androst-2-ene-2-carbonitrile; an adrenal steroid inhibitor used for amelioration of adrenal hyperfunction in Cushing's syndrome.

tri·mas·ti·gote (trī-mas'ti-gōt). Having three flagella, as observed in certain protozoan organisms. [tri- + G. *mastix,* whip]

tri·mep·ra·zine tar·trate (trī-mep'ră-zēn). 10-[3-(Dimethylamino)-2-methylpropyl]phenothiazine tartrate; a phenothiazine compound related chemically and pharmacologically to promazine but with a more pronounced histamine-antagonizing action; used for the symptomatic relief of pruritus.

trim·er (trī'mer). A compound, complex, or structure made up of three components.

tri·mes·ter (trī'mes-ter, trī-mes'ter). A period of 3 months; one-third of the length of a pregnancy. [L. *trimestris,* of three-month duration]

tri·met·a·phan cam·sy·late (trī-met'ă-fan). SYN trimethaphan camsylate.

tri·me·taz·i·dine (trī-me-taz'i-dēn). 1-(2,3,4-Trimethoxybenzyl)piperazine; a coronary vasodilator.

tri·meth·a·di·one (trī'meth-ă-dī'ōn). 3,5,5-trimethyl-2,4-oxazolidinedione; an anticonvulsant used for the treatment of absence seizures (petit mal) and psychomotor epilepsy. SYN troxidone.

tri·meth·a·phan cam·sy·late (trī-meth'ă-fan). *d*-1,3-dibenzyldecahydro-2-oxoimidazo[*c*]thieno[1,2-α]thiolium camphorsulfonate; a ganglionic blocking agent that produces vasodilation of brief duration; used in surgery, particularly neurosurgery, to produce a relatively bloodless operative field (controlled hypotension). SYN trimetaphan camsylate.

tri·meth·i·di·um meth·o·sul·fate (trī-me-thid'ē-ŭm meth-ō-sŭl'fāt). (+)-[*N*-Methyl-*N*-(γ-trimethylammoniumpropyl)]-1,8,8-t rimethyl-3-azabicyclo[3.2.1]octane dimethosulfate; a quaternary ammonium compound that blocks ganglionic transmission at sympathetic and parasympathetic ganglia; used in the treatment of severe hypertension.

tri·meth·o·benz·a·mide hy·dro·chlo·ride (trī'meth-ō-ben'ză-mīd). *N*-[(2-Dimethylaminoethoxy)benzyl]-3,4,5-trimethoxybenzamide hydrochloride; an antiemetic.

tri·meth·o·prim (trī-meth'ō-prim). 2,4-Diamino-5-(3,4,5-trimethoxybenzyl)pyrimidine; an antimicrobial agent that potentiates the effect of sulfonamides and sulfones.

tri·meth·o·prim-sul·fa·meth·ox·a·zole. A drug combination consisting of a dihydrofolate reductase inhibitor (trimethoprim) and a sulfonamide antibacterial drug (sulfamethoxazole). The drug combination is synergistic as the drugs interfere with two successive steps in the formation/utilization of folic acid by microorganisms. Used to treat many infectious diseases.

tri·meth·yl·a·mine (trī-meth'il-am'ēn). N(CH₃)₃; a degradation product, often by putrefaction, of nitrogenous plant and animal substances such as beet sugar residue or herring brine; in the body, it probably results from decomposition of choline.

tri·meth·yl·am·i·nur·ia (trī-meth'il-am-i-nūr'ē-ă). Increased excretion of trimethylamine in urine and sweat, with characteristic offensive, fishy body odor.

tri·meth·yl·car·bin·ol (trī-meth'il-kar'bin-ol). Tertiary butyl alcohol. SEE *butyl* alcohol.

tri·meth·yl·ene (trī-meth'il-ēn). SYN cyclopropane.

tri·meth·yl·eth·yl·ene (trī-meth-il-eth'il-ēn). SYN amylene.

tri·meth·yl·glyc·ine (trī-meth'il-glī'cēn). SYN betaine.

tri·meth·yl·gly·co·coll an·hy·dride (trī-meth'il-glī'kō-kol). SYN betaine.

Nᵉ-tri·meth·yl·ly·sine (trī-meth-il-lī-sēn). An amino acid residue found in a number of proteins by the action of *S*-adenosyl-L-methionine on L-lysyl residues; upon release by proteolysis, *N*ᵉ-trimethyllysine becomes the precursor of carnitine.

tri·meth·y·lo·mel·a·mine (trī'meth-i-lō-mel'ă-mēn). (*s*-Triazine-2,4,6-triyltriimino)trimethanol; an antineoplastic agent.

tri·met·o·zine (trī-met'ō-zēn). 4-(3,4,5-Trimethoxybenzoyl)morpholine; an antianxiety agent.

tri·me·trex·ate (trī-me-treks'āt). 2,4-Diamino-5-methyl-6-[(3,4,5-trimethoxyanilino)methyl]quinazoline; an antineoplastic agent and antiprotozoal orphan drug used in the treatment of *Pneumocystis carinii* pneumonia in AIDS patients.

tri·mip·ra·mine (trī-mip'ră-mēn). 5-[3-(Dimethylamino)-2-methylpropyl]-10,11-dihydro-5*H*-dibenz[*b,f*]azepine; an antidepressant.

tri·mor·phic (trī-mōr'fik). SYN trimorphous.

tri·mor·phism (trī-mōr'fizm). Existence under three forms, as

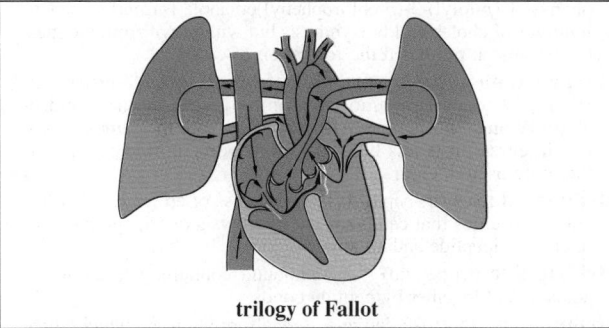

trilogy of Fallot

in holometabolous insects that pass through larval, pupal, and imago stages. [tri- + G. *morphē,* form]

tri·mor·phous (trī-mōr'fŭs). Existing under three forms; marked by trimorphism. SYN trimorphic.

tri·ni·tro·cel·lu·lose (trī'nī-trō-sel'yū-lōs). A constituent of soluble guncotton; used in the preparation of collodion and of pyroxylin.

tri·ni·tro·glyc·er·in (trī'nī-trō-glis'ě-rin). SYN nitroglycerin.

tri·ni·tro·tol·u·ene (TNT) (trī'nī-trō-tol'yū-ēn). CH₃C₆H₂(NO₂)₃; an explosive made by the nitrification of toluene; it causes gastric and intestinal disturbances and dermatitis in workers in munition factories. SYN trinitrotoluol.

tri·ni·tro·tol·u·ol (trī'nī-trō-tol'yū-ol). SYN trinitrotoluene.

tri·nu·cle·o·tide (trī-nū'klē-ō-tīd). A combination of three adjacent nucleotides, free or in a polynucleotide or nucleic acid molecule; often used with specific reference to the unit (codon or anticodon) specifying a particular amino acid in expression of the genetic code.

tri·o·ki·nase (trī-ō-kī'nās). A phosphotransferase catalyzing the phosphorylation of D-glyceraldehyde by ATP to produce D-glyceraldehyde 3-phosphate and ADP; participates in a step in D-fructose metabolism. SYN triosekinase.

tri·ol (trī-ol). A compound containing three hydroxyl groups; *e.g.,* glycerol.

tri·o·le·in (trī-ō'lē-in). SYN olein.

tri·oph·thal·mos (trī-of-thal'mos). Conjoined twins with fusion in the facial region such that the eyes on the joined sides have merged to form a single one; a variety of opodidymus. SEE conjoined *twins,* under *twin.* [tri- + G. *ophthalmos,* eye]

tri·or·chism (trī-ōr'kizm). Condition of having three testes.

tri·orth·o·cres·yl phos·phate (trī'-ōr-thō-kres'il fos'fāt). A triaryl phosphate; produces a delayed neurotoxicity. An infamous incident occurred when it appeared as an adulterant in Jamaica ginger and was responsible for thousands of cases of paralysis during the Prohibition era.

tri·ose (trī'ōs). A three-carbon monosaccharide; *e.g.,* glyceraldehyde and dihydroxyacetone.

tri·ose·ki·nase (trī'ōs-kī'nās). SYN triokinase.

tri·ose·phos·phate isom·er·ase (trī'ōs-fos'fāt). An isomerizing enzyme that catalyzes the reversible interconversion of D-glyceraldehyde 3-phosphate and dihydroxyacetone phosphate, a reaction of importance in glycolysis and gluconeogenesis; a deficiency of this enzyme will result in hemolytic anemia and severe neurological deficits. SYN phosphotriose isomerase.

tri·o·tus (trī-ō'tŭs). Diprosopus in which three ears are present. [tri- + G. *ous,* ear]

tri·ox·ide (trī-oks'īd). A molecule containing three atoms of oxygen. SYN teroxide.

tri·ox·sa·len (trī-ok'să-len). 4,5,8-Trimethylpsoralen; 2,5,9-trimethyl-7*H*-furo[3,2-g][1]benzopyrano-7-one; an orally effective pigmenting, photosensitizing agent; used as a tanning agent and in the treatment of vitiligo.

tri·ox·y·meth·yl·ene (trī'ok-sē-meth'i-lēn). SYN paraformaldehyde.

tri·pal·mi·tin (trī-pal'mi-tin). SYN palmitin.

tri·par·a·nol (trī-par'ă-nol). 1-[*p*-(2-Diethylaminoethoxy)-

phenyl]-1-(*p*-tolyl)-2-(*p*-chlorophenyl)ethanol; formerly used as inhibitor of cholesterol biosynthesis but withdrawn from the market because it promoted the formation of cataracts.

tri·pel·en·na·mine hy·dro·chlo·ride (trī-pĕ-len′ă-mēn). 2-[Benzyl[2-(dimethylamino)ethyl]amino]pyridine monohydrochloride; an antihistamine. Also available, with the same actions, is t. h. citrate; it is less bitter than the hydrochloride salt, and is therefore used in elixir.

tri·pep·tid·ases (trī-pep′ti-dās-es). A class of enzymes of different specificities that catalyzes the hydrolysis of tripeptides, producing a dipeptide and an amino acid.

tri·pep·tide (trī-pep′tīd). A compound containing three amino acids linked together by peptide bonds.

tri·pha·lan·gia (trī-fă-lan′jē-ă). Malformation in which three phalanges are present in the thumb or great toe. [tri- + phalanx]

tri·phos·pha·tase (trī-fos′fă-tās). SYN adenosine triphosphatase.

tri·phos·pho·pyr·i·dine nu·cle·o·tide (TPN, TPNH) (trī-fos′fō-pir′i-dēn). Former name for nicotinamide adenine dinucleotide phosphate.

Tripier, Léon, French surgeon, 1842–1891. SEE T.'s *amputation.*

tri·plant (trī′plant). SEE triplant *implant.*

tri·ple·gia (trī-plē′jē-ă). Paralysis of an upper and a lower extremity and of the face, or of both extremities on one side and of one on the other. [tri- + G. *plēgē,* stroke]

trip·let. 1. One of three children delivered at the same birth. SYN tridymus. **2.** A set of three similar objects, as a compound lens in a microscope, formed of three planoconvex lenses. **3.** SYN codon.

nonsense t., (1) a trinucleotide (codon) in which a base change to a termination codon results in premature termination of the growing polypeptide chain and, consequently, incomplete protein molecules; **(2)** a termination codon.

trip·lo·blas·tic (trip-lō-blas′tik). Formed of three primary germ layers (ectoderm, mesoderm, endoderm), or containing tissue derived from all three layers. [G. *triploos,* threefold, + *blastos,* germ]

trip·loid (trip′loyd). Pertaining to or characteristic of triploidy. [tri- + -ploid]

trip·loi·dy (trip′loy-dē). The presence of three haploid sets of chromosomes, instead of two, in all cells; results in fetal or neonatal death.

trip·lo·pia (trip-lō′pē-ă). Visual defect in which three images of the same object are seen. SYN triple vision. [G. *triploos,* triple, + *opsis,* sight]

tri·pod (trī′pod). **1.** Three-legged. **2.** A stand having three legs or supports. [G. *tripous,* fr. tri- + *pous,* foot]

Haller's t., SYN celiac *trunk.*

vital t., the brain, the heart, and the lungs, regarded as the three organs essential to life.

tri·po·dia (trī-pō′dē-ă). Condition seen in conjoined twins when fusion has merged the lower extremities on the joined sides to form a single foot, so that there are only three feet for the two bodies. SEE conjoined *twins,* under *twin.* [tri- + G. *pous,* foot]

tri·prol·i·dine hy·dro·chlo·ride (trī-prol′i-dēn). *trans*-2-[3-(1-Pyrrolidinyl)-1-(*p*-tolyl)propenyl]pyridine hydrochloride; an antihistaminic used in the management of allergic and pruritic conditions.

tri·pro·so·pus (trī′prō-sō′pŭs). Fetus with three heads fused, leaving only parts of three faces. [tri- + G. *prosōpon,* face]

trip·sis (trip′sis). **1.** SYN trituration (1). **2.** SYN massage. [G. a rubbing]

tri·que·trous (trī-kwē′trŭs, -kwet-). Triangular. [L. *triquetrus,* three-cornered]

tri·que·trum (trī-kwē′trŭm, -kwet-). SYN triquetral *bone.* [L. *triquetrus,* three-cornered]

tri·ra·di·al, tri·ra·di·ate (trī-rā′dē-ăl, trī-rā′dē-āt). Radiating in three directions.

tri·ra·di·us (trī-rā′dē-ŭs). In dermatoglyphics, the figure at the base of each finger in the palm, produced by rows of papillae running in three directions so as to form a triangle. SYN Galton's delta (2).

Tris Abbreviation for tris(hydroxymethyl)aminomethane and tris(hydroxymethyl)methylamine; used as a trivial name.

⟁**tris-.** Chemical prefix indicating three of the substituents that follow, independently linked. Cf. tri-.

tri·sac·cha·ride (trī-sak′ă-rīd). A carbohydrate containing three monosaccharide residues, *e.g.,* raffinose.

tris(hy·drox·y·meth·yl·)a·mi·no·meth·ane (Tris). SYN tromethamine.

tris(hy·drox·y·meth·yl)meth·yl·a·mine (Tris). SYN tromethamine.

tris·kai·dek·a·pho·bia (tris′kī-dek-ă-fō′bē-ă). Superstitious dread of the number thirteen. [G. *triskaideka,* thirteen, + *phobos,* fear]

tris·mic (triz′mik). Relating to or marked by trismus.

tris·moid (triz′moyd). **1.** Resembling trismus. **2.** Trismus nascentium, formerly regarded as a distinct variety due to pressure on the occiput during birth. [trismus + G. *eidos,* resemblance]

tris·mus (triz′mŭs). Persistent contraction of the masseter muscles due to failure of central inhibition; often the initial manifestation of generalized tetanus. SYN *Ankylostoma* (2), lock-jaw, lockjaw. [L. fr. G. *trismos,* a creaking, rasping]

t. capistra′tus, congenital adhesion of the cheeks to the gums.

t. dolorif′icus, SYN trigeminal *neuralgia.*

t. nascen′tium, stiffness of the jaw muscles in neonates, usually as the beginning of tetanus neonatorum. SYN t. neonatorum.

t. neonato′rum, SYN t. nascentium.

t. sardon′icus, SYN risus caninus.

tri·so·mic (trī-sō′mik). Relating to trisomy.

tri·so·my (trī′sō-mē). The state of an individual or cell with an extra chromosome instead of the normal pair of homologous chromosomes; in humans, the state of a cell containing 47 normal chromosomes. For various types of trisomy syndrome, see under syndrome. [tri- + (chromo)some]

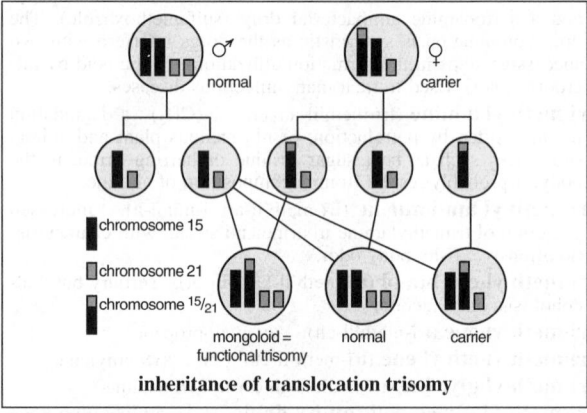

inheritance of translocation trisomy

tri·splanch·nic (trī-splangk′nik). Relating to the three visceral cavities: skull, thorax, and abdomen. [tri- + G. *splanchnon,* viscus]

tri·ste·a·rin (trī-stē′ă-rin). SYN stearin.

tri·stich·ia (trī-stik′i-ă). Presence of three rows of eyelashes. [G. *tristichos,* in three rows, fr. *tri-,* three, + *stichos,* row]

tri·sul·cate (trī-sŭl′kāt). Marked by three grooves.

tri·ta·nom·a·ly (trī′tă-nom′ă-lē). A type of partial color deficiency due to a deficiency or abnormality of blue-sensitive retinal cones. [G. *tritos,* third, + *anōmalia,* irregularity]

trit·an·o·pia (trī′tă-nō′pē-ă). Deficient color perception in which there is an absence of blue-sensitive pigment in the retinal cones. [G. *tritos,* third, + *an-* priv. + *ōps,* eye]

tri·ter·penes (trī-ter′pēnz). Hydrocarbons or their derivatives formed by the condensation of six isoprene units (equivalent to three terpene units) and containing, therefore, 30 carbon atoms; *e.g.,* squalene, certain steroids, cardiac glycosides.

trit·i·at·ed (trit′ē-ā-ted). Containing atoms of tritium (hydrogen-3) in the molecule.

tri·ti·ce·o·glos·sus (tri-tish′ē-ō-glos′ŭs). SEE *musculus* triticeoglossus. [L. *triticeum*, + G. *glōssa*, tongue]

tri·ti·ceous (tri-tish′ŭs). Resembling or shaped like a grain of wheat. [L. *triticeus*, fr. *triticum*, a grain of wheat]

tri·tic·e·um (tri-tish′ē-ŭm). SYN triticeal *cartilage*. [L. *triticeus*, triticeous, like a grain of wheat]

trit·i·um (T, *t*) (trit′ē-ŭm, trish′-). SYN hydrogen-3.

tri·to·cal·ine (trit-ō-kal′ēn). SYN tritoqualine.

trit·o·qual·ine (trit-ō-kwal′ēn). 7-amino-4,5,6-triethoxy-3-(5,6,7,8-tetrahydro-4-methoxy-6-methyl-1,3-dioxolo[4,5-*g*]-isoquinolin-5-yl)phthalide; an antihistaminic. SYN tritocaline.

Tri·trich·o·mon·as (trī′trīk-ō-mō′nas). A genus of parasitic protozoan flagellates, formerly part of the genus *Trichomonas* but now separated as a distinct genus by the absence of a pelta and the presence of three anterior flagella. Species include *T. foetus*, which causes bovine trichomoniasis, and *T. suis*, which occurs in the nasal passages, stomach, cecum, and colon of pigs. SEE ALSO *Trichomonas*. [G. *tri-*, three, + *Trichomonas*]

tri·tu·ber·cu·lar (trī-tū-ber′kyū-lăr). SYN tricuspid (2).

trit·u·ra·ble (trit′yū-ră-bl). Capable of being triturated.

trit·u·rate (trit′yū-rāt). **1.** To accomplish trituration. **2.** A triturated substance.

    tablet t., a compressed tablet of a medicated powder dispersed with milk sugar.

trit·u·ra·tion (trit-yū-rā′shŭn). **1.** The act of reducing a drug to a fine powder and incorporating it thoroughly with sugar of milk by rubbing the two together in a mortar. SYN tripsis (1). **2.** Mixing of dental amalgam in a mortar and pestle or with a mechanical device. [L. *trituratio*, fr. *trituro*, to thresh, fr. *tero*, pp. *tritus*, to rub]

tri·tyl (trī′til). The triphenylmethyl radical, Ph₃C–.

tri·va·lence, tri·va·len·cy (trī-vā′lens, -len-sē). The property of being trivalent.

tri·va·lent (trī-vā′lent). Having the combining power (valence) of 3.

tri·valve (trī′valv). Provided with three valves, as a speculum with three diverging blades.

triv·i·al name. A name of a chemical, no part of which is necessarily used in a systematic sense; *i.e.,* it gives little or no indication as to chemical structure. Such names are common for drugs, hormones, proteins, and other biologicals, and are used by the general public. They may not be officially sanctioned, in contrast to nonproprietary names, but may be adopted as official nonproprietary names as a result of widespread usage. Examples are water, aspirin, chlorophyll, heme, methotrexate, folic acid, caffeine, thyroxine, epinephrine, barbital, etc.; also common abbreviations for chemically defined substances, such as ACTH, MSH, BAL, DDT, which are spoken as such and not in terms of the words they represent. The distinction between trivial and semitrivial names is seldom made; thus tetrahydrofolate, methylglycine, glucosamine, etc., are often termed trivial even though each contains a systematic part that is used in the correct systematic sense (tetrahydro for four hydrogen atoms, methyl for a –CH₃ group, amine for –NH₂ in the above). Trivial names are often assigned arbitrarily to chemical compounds, especially from natural sources, before the chemical structures, hence systematic names can be assigned; also, they afford useful shortenings of long systematic names even when these can be stated (although most such shortenings turn out to be semisystematic, as they incorporate some portion of the systematic name).

tri·zon·al (trī-zō′năl). Having, or arranged in, three zones or layers.

tRNA Abbreviation for transfer RNA.

tro·car (trō′kar). An instrument for withdrawing fluid from a cavity, or for use in paracentesis; it consists of a metal tube (cannula) into which fits an obturator with a sharp three-cornered tip, which is withdrawn after the instrument has been pushed into the cavity; the name t. is usually applied to the obturator alone, the entire instrument being designated t. and cannula. [Fr. *trocart*, fr. *trois*, three, + *carre*, side (of a sword blade)]

    Hasson t., a blunt t. inserted into the peritoneal cavity after making a small celiotomy; and used for insufflation and introduction of a laparoscope.

troch Abbreviation for trochiscus.

tro·chan·ter (trō-kan′ter). One of the bony prominences developed from independent osseous centers near the upper extremity of the femur; there are two in man, three in the horse. [G. *trochantēr*, a runner, fr. *trechō*, to run]

    greater t., a strong process at the proximal and lateral part of the shaft of the femur, overhanging the root of the neck; it gives attachment to the gluteus medius and minimus, piriformis, obturator internus and externus, and gemelli muscles. SYN t. major [NA].

    lesser t., a pyramidal process projecting from the medial and proximal part of the shaft of the femur at the line of junction of the shaft and the neck; it receives the insertion of the psoas major and iliacus (iliopsoas) muscles. SYN t. minor [NA], small t., trochantin.

    t. ma′jor [NA], SYN greater t.

    t. mi′nor [NA], SYN lesser t.

    small t., SYN lesser t.

    t. ter′tius [NA], SYN gluteal *tuberosity*.

    third t., an occasional process at the proximal end of the lateral lip of the linea aspera of the femur, about on a level with the lesser t., giving insertion to the greater part of the gluteus maximus muscle. SEE ALSO gluteal *tuberosity*.

tro·chan·ter·i·an, tro·chan·ter·ic (trō-kan-ter′ē-an, -ter′ik). Relating to a trochanter; especially the trochanter major.

tro·chan·ter·plas·ty (trō-kan′ter-plas-tē). Plastic surgery of the trochanters and neck of the femur. [trochanter + G. *plastos*, formed]

tro·chan·tin (trō-kan′tin). SYN lesser *trochanter*.

tro·chan·tin·i·an (trō-kan-tin′ē-an). Relating to the trochanter minor.

tro·che (trōk, trō′kē). A small, disk-shaped or rhombic body composed of solidifying paste containing an astringent, antiseptic, or demulcent drug, used for local treatment of the mouth or throat, the t. being held in the mouth until dissolved. The vehicle or base of the t. is usually sugar, made adhesive by admixture with acacia or tragacanth, fruit paste, made from black or red currants, confection of rose, or balsam of tolu. SYN lozenge, morsulus, pastil (2), pastille, trochiscus. [L. *trochiscus*]

tro·chis·cus (troch), pl. **tro·chis·ci** (trō-kis′kŭs). SYN troche. [L., fr. G. *trochiskos*, a small wheel, a lozenge, fr. *trochos*, a wheel]

troch·lea, pl. **troch·le·ae** (trok′lē-ă, -lē-ē) [NA]. **1.** A structure serving as a pulley. **2.** A smooth articular surface of bone upon which another glides. **3.** A fibrous loop in the orbit, near the nasal process of the frontal bone, through which passes the tendon of the superior oblique muscle of the eye. [L. pulley, fr. G. *trochileia*, a pulley, fr. *trechō*, to run]

    t. fem′oris, SYN patellar *surface* of femur.

    t. fibula′ris calca′nei [NA], ☆official alternate term for peroneal t. of calcaneus.

    t. hu′meri [NA], SYN t. of humerus.

    t. of humerus, the grooved surface at the lower end of the humerus articulating with the trochlear notch of the ulna. SYN t. humeri [NA], pulley of humerus.

    t. muscula′ris [NA], SYN muscular *pulley*.

    peroneal t. of calcaneus, a projection from the lateral side of the calcaneus between the tendons of the peroneus longus and brevis. SYN t. peronealis [NA], t. fibularis calcanei☆ [NA], peroneal pulley, processus trochlearis, spina peronealis, trochlear process.

    t. peronea′lis [NA], SYN peroneal t. of calcaneus.

    t. phalan′gis [NA], ☆official alternate term for *head* of phalanx, *head* of phalanx.

    t. ta′li [NA], SYN t. of the talus.

    t. of the talus, the rounded articular surface of the talus articulating with the distal ends of the tibia and fibula. SYN t. tali [NA], pulley of talus.

troch·le·ar (trok′lē-ar). **1.** Relating to a trochlea, especially the trochlea of the superior oblique muscle of the eye. SYN trochlearis (1). **2.** SYN trochleiform.

troch·le·ar·i·form (trok-lē-ar'i-fōrm). SYN trochleiform.

troch·le·ar·is (trok-lē-ā'ris). **1.** SYN trochlear (1). **2.** SYN trochleiform. [L.]

troch·le·i·form (trok'lē-i-fōrm). Pulley-shaped. SYN trochlear (2), trochleariform, trochlearis (2).

troch·o·car·dia (trok-ō-kar'dē-ă). Rotary displacement of the heart around its axis. [G. *trochos,* wheel, + *kardia,* heart]

tro·choid (trō'koyd). Revolving; rotating; denoting a revolving or wheel-like articulation. [G. *trochōdēs,* fr. *trochos,* wheel, + *eidos,* resemblance]

tro·chor·i·zo·car·dia (trō-kōr-ī'zō-kar'dē-ă). Combined trochocardia and horizocardia.

Trog·lo·tre·ma sal·min·co·la (trog-lō-trē'mă sal-mingk'ō-lă). SYN *Nanophyetus salmincola.*

Troisier, Charles-Emile, French physician, 1844–1919. SEE T.'s *ganglion, node.*

tro·la·mine (trō'lă-mēn). USAN-approved contraction for triethanolamine, N(CH₂CH₂OH)₃.

tro·land (trō'land). A unit of visual stimulation at the retina equal to the illumination per square millimeter of pupil received from a surface of 1 lux brightness. [L.T. *Troland,* U.S. physicist, 1889–1932]

Trolard, Paulin, French anatomist, 1842–1910. SEE T.'s *vein.*

tro·le·an·do·my·cin (trō'lē-an-dō-mī'sin). The triacetyl ester of oleandomycin, a macrolide antibiotic, with a potency of not less than 760 μg per mg; an orally effective antibiotic for infections produced by Gram-positive, penicillin-resistant bacteria. SYN triacetyloleandomycin.

trol·ni·trate phos·phate (trol-nī'trāt). Triethanolamine trinitrate diphosphate; an organic nitrate with mild but persistent vasodilator action on smooth muscle of the smaller vessels of postarteriolar vascular beds; used to prevent attacks of angina pectoris.

Tröltsch, Anton F. von, German otologist, 1829–1890. SEE T.'s *corpuscles,* under *corpuscle, fold, pockets,* under *pocket, recesses,* under *recess.*

Trom·bic·u·la (trom-bik'yū-lă). The chigger mite, a genus of mites (family Trombiculidae) whose larvae (chiggers, red bugs) include pests of humans and other animals, and vectors of rickettsiai and probably viral diseases.

T. akamu'shi, SYN *Leptotrombidium akamushi.*

T. alfredduge'si, a species common in second growth and grassy brush areas of the Americas; the larvae attack humans (as well as reptiles, birds, and wild and domestic animals), causing an intensely itching dermatitis.

T. delien'sis, SEE *Leptotrombidium, Leptotrombidium akamushi.*

trom·bic·u·li·a·sis (trom-bik-yū-lī'ă-sis). Infestation by mites of the genus *Trombicula.*

trom·bic·u·lid (trom-bik'yū-lid). Common name for members of the family Trombiculidae.

Trom·bic·u·li·dae (trom-bik-ū-lī'dē). A family of mites whose larvae (redbugs, rougets, harvest mites, scrub mites, or chiggers) are parasitic on vertebrates and whose nymphs and adults are bright red and free-living, living on insect eggs or minute organisms in the soil. The six-legged larvae are barely visible red or orange parasites that attach to the skin for a few days to a month, producing an exceedingly irritating reaction. In the Orient, trombiculid chiggers of the genus *Leptotrombidium* transmit tsutsugamushi disease caused by *Rickettsia tsutsugamushi,* which is transovarially transmitted in these mites.

Trom·bi·di·i·dae (trom-bi-dī'i-dē). A family of mites that formerly included the subfamily Trombiculinae, now raised to the family Trombiculidae (including the vectors of tsutsugamushi disease). T. larvae are characteristically parasitic on insects, not on vertebrates as with the larvae of Trombiculidae.

tro·meth·a·mine (trō-meth'ă-mēn). H₂N–C(CH₂OH)₃; 2-amino-2-(hydroxymethyl)-1,3-propanediol; a weakly basic compound used as an alkalizing agent and as a buffer in enzymic reactions. SYN tris(hydroxymethyl)aminomethane, tris(hydroxymethyl)-methylamine.

Trömner, Ernest L.O., German neurologist, *1868. SEE T.'s *reflex.*

tro·na (trō'nă). A native sodium carbonate.

tro·pa·ic ac·id (trō-pā'ik). SYN tropic acid.

tro·pane (trō'pān). **1.** A bicyclic hydrocarbon, the fundamental structure of tropine, atropine, and other physiologically active substances. **2.** In plural form, a class of alkaloids containing the t. (1) structure.

tro·pate (trō'pāt). A salt or ester of tropic acid.

tro·pe·ic ac·id (trō-pē'ik). SYN tropic acid.

tro·pe·ine (trō'pē-in). An ester of tropine; either a naturally occurring alkaloid or prepared synthetically.

tro·pen·tane (trō-pen'tān). 1-Phenylcyclopentanecarboxylic acid 3α-tropanyl ester hydrochloride; an antispasmodic with anticholinergic properties.

tro·pe·o·lins (trō-pē'ō-linz). A group of azo dyes used as indicators; *e.g.,* methyl orange. [G. *tropaios,* pertaining to a turning or change, fr. *tropē,* a turn]

△**troph-.** SEE tropho-.

troph·ec·to·derm (trof-ek'tō-derm). Outermost layer of cells in the mammalian blastodermic vesicle, which will make contact with the endometrium and take part in establishing the embryo's means of receiving nutrition; the cell layer from which the trophoblast differentiates. [troph- + ectoderm]

tro·phe·sic (trō-fē'sik). Pertaining to trophesy.

troph·e·sy (trof'ě-sē). The results of any disorder of the trophic nerves.

tro·phic (trof'ik, trō'fik). **1.** Relating to or dependent upon nutrition. **2.** Resulting from interruption of nerve supply. [G. *trophē,* nourishment]

△**-trophic.** Nutrition. Cf. -tropic. [G. *trophē,* nourishment]

tro·phic·i·ty (trō-fis'i-tē). A trophic influence or condition. SYN trophism (1).

tro·phism (trof'izm). **1.** SYN trophicity. **2.** SYN nutrition (1). [G. *trophē,* nourishment]

△**tropho-, troph-.** Food, nutrition. [G. *trophē,* nourishment]

troph·o·blast (trof'ō-blast, trō'fō-blast). The mesectodermal cell layer covering the blastocyst that erodes the uterine mucosa and through which the embryo receives nourishment from the mother; the cells do not enter into the formation of the embryo itself, but contribute to the formation of the placenta. The t. develops processes that later receive a core of vascular mesoderm and are then known as the chorionic villi; the t. soon becomes two-layered, differentiating into the syncytiotrophoblast, an outer layer consisting of a multinucleated protoplasmic mass (syncytium), and the cytotrophoblast, the inner layer next to the mesoderm in which the cells retain their membranes. SYN chorionic ectoderm. [tropho- + G. *blastos,* germ]

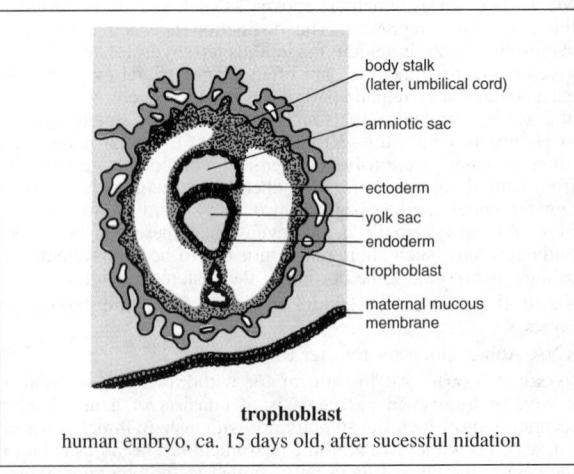

trophoblast
human embryo, ca. 15 days old, after successful nidation

plasmodial t., SYN syncytiotrophoblast.

syncytial t., SYN syncytiotrophoblast.

troph·o·blas·tic (trō-fō-blas′tik). Relating to the trophoblast.

troph·o·blas·to·ma (trof′ō-blas-tō′mă). Obsolete term for choriocarcinoma.

troph·o·chro·ma·tin (trof-ō-krō′mă-tin). SYN trophochromidia. [tropho- + G. *chrōma,* color]

troph·o·chro·mid·ia (trof′ō-krō-mid′ē-ă). Nongerminal or vegetative extranuclear masses of chromatin, found in certain protozoan forms; *e.g.,* the macronucleus of certain ciliates, such as *Paramecium.* SYN trophochromatin.

troph·o·cyte (trof′ō-sīt). A cell that supplies nourishment; *e.g.,* Sertoli cells in the seminiferous tubules. SYN trephocyte. [tropho- + G. *kytos,* cell]

troph·o·derm (trof′ō-derm). The trophectoderm, or trophoblast, together with the vascular mesodermal layer underlying it. SEE ALSO serosa (2). [tropho- + G. *derma,* skin]

troph·o·der·ma·to·neu·ro·sis (trof′ō-der′mă-tō-nū-rō′sis). Cutaneous trophic changes due to neural involvement.

troph·o·dy·nam·ics (trof′ō-dī-nam′iks). The dynamics of nutrition or metabolism. SYN nutritional energy. [tropho- + G. *dynamis,* power]

troph·o·neu·ro·sis (trof′ō-nū-rō′sis). A trophic disorder, such as atrophy, hypertrophy, or a skin eruption, occurring as a consequence of disease or injury of the nerves of the part. [tropho- + G. *neuron,* nerve, + *-osis,* condition]

facial t., SYN facial *hemiatrophy.*

lingual t., SYN lingual *hemiatrophy.*

muscular t., SYN amyotrophic lateral *sclerosis.*

Romberg's t., SYN facial *hemiatrophy.*

troph·o·neu·rot·ic (trof-ō-nū-rot′ik). Relating to a trophoneurosis.

troph·o·nu·cle·us (trof-ō-nū′klē-ŭs). SYN macronucleus (2).

troph·o·plast (trof′ō-plast). SYN plastid (1). [tropho- + G. *plastos,* formed]

troph·o·spon·gia (trof′ō-spon′jē-ă). **1.** Canalicular structures described by A.F. Holmgren in the protoplasm of certain cells. **2.** Vascular endometrium of the uterus between the myometrium and the trophoblast. [tropho- + G. *spongia,* a sponge]

troph·o·tax·is (trof-ō-tak′sis). SYN trophotropism. [tropho- + G. *taxis,* arrangement]

troph·o·tro·pic (trof-ō-trop′ik). Relating to trophotropism.

tro·phot·ro·pism (trō-fot′rō-pizm). Chemotaxis of living cells in relation to nutritive material; it may be positive (toward nutritive material) or negative (away from nutritive material). SYN trophotaxis. [tropho- + G. *tropē,* a turning]

troph·o·zo·ite (trof-ō-zō′īt). The ameboid, vegetative, asexual form of certain Sporozoea, such as the schizont of the plasmodia of malaria and related parasites. [tropho- + G. *zōon,* animal]

△**-trophy.** Food, nutrition. [G. *trophē,* nourishment]

tro·pia (trō′pē-ă). Abnormal deviation of the eye. SEE strabismus. [G. *tropē,* a turning]

△**-tropic.** A turning toward, having an affinity for. Cf. -trophic. [G. *tropē,* a turning]

tro·pic ac·id (trop′ik). HOCH₂CH(C₆H₅)COOH; α-phenylhydracrylic acid; 2-phenyl-3-hydroxypropionic acid; a constituent of atropine and of scopolamine, in which it is esterified through its COOH to the 3-CHOH of tropine. SYN tropaic acid, tropeic acid.

tro·pic·a·mide (trō-pik′ă-mīd). *N*-Ethyl-2-phenyl-*N*-4-pyridylmethyl)hydracrylamide; an anticholinergic agent used to effect a rapid and brief mydriasis for eye examinations.

tro·pine (trō′pēn). 3α-Tropanol; 3α-hydroxytropane; the major constituent of atropine and scopolamine, from which it is obtained on hydrolysis.

t. mandelate, SYN homatropine.

t. tropate, SYN atropine.

tro·pism (trō′pizm). The phenomenon, observed in living organisms, of moving toward (**positive t.**) or away from (**negative t.**) a focus of light, heat, or other stimulus; usually applied to the movement of a portion of the organism as opposed to taxis, the movement of an entire organism. [G. *tropē,* a turning]

viral t., the specificity of a virus for a particular host tissue, determined in part by the interaction of viral surface structures with host cell-surface receptors.

tro·po·col·la·gen (trō-pō-kol′ă-jen, trop′ō-). The fundamental units of collagen fibrils, consisting of three helically arranged polypeptide chains.

trop·o·e·las·tin (trō-pō-ē-las′tin). The precursor to elastin; t. does not contain desmosine or isodesmosine cross links.

tro·pom·e·ter (trō-pom′ĕ-ter). Any instrument for measuring the degree of rotation or torsion, as of the eyeball or the shaft of a long bone. [G. *tropē,* a turning, + *metron,* measure]

tro·po·my·o·sin (trō-pō-mī′ō-sin). A fibrous protein extractable from muscle; sometimes specified as t. B to distinguish it from t. A (paramyosin) prominent in mollusks.

tro·po·nin (trō′pō-nin). A globular protein of muscle that binds to tropomyosin and has considerable affinity for calcium ions; a central regulatory protein of muscle contraction. T. T binds to tropomyosin; T. I inhibits F-actin-myosin interactions; T. C is a calcium-binding protein and has a key role in muscle contraction.

trough (trawf). A long, narrow, shallow channel or depression.

gingival t., the formation of a crater as a result of destruction of interdental tissues so that, in effect, there exists a labial and lingual curtain of gingiva with no interproximal connection at all.

Langmuir t., a t. with a movable surface barrier for studying the compression of surface films.

synaptic t., the depression of the surface of the striated muscle fiber that accommodates the motor endplate.

Trousseau, Armand, French physician, 1801–1867. SEE T.'s *point, sign, spot, syndrome;* T.-Lallemand *bodies,* under *body.*

trox·e·ru·tin (troks′ē-rū-tin). 7,3′,4′-Tris[*O*-(2-hydroxyethyl)]-rutin; used for treatment of venous disorders.

trox·i·done (trok′si-dōn). SYN trimethadione.

Trp Symbol for tryptophan and its radicals.

trun·cal (trŭng′kăl). Relating to the trunk of the body or to any arterial or nerve trunk, etc.

trun·cate (trŭng′kāt). Truncated; cut across at right angles to the long axis, or appearing to be so cut. [L. *trunco,* pp. *-atus,* to maim, cut off]

trun·cus, gen. and pl. **trun·ci** (trŭng′kŭs, -kī). SYN trunk. [L. stem, trunk]

t. arterio′sus, the common arterial trunk opening out of both ventricles in early fetal life, later destined to be divided into aorta and pulmonary artery by development of the spiral septum.

t. arterio′sus commu′nis, SEE t. arteriosus.

t. fascicula′ris atrioventricula′ris, SYN *trunk* of atrioventricular bundle. SEE ALSO conducting *system* of heart.

t. brachiocepha′licus [NA], SYN brachiocephalic *trunk.*

t. bronchiomediastina′lis [NA], SYN bronchomediastinal *trunk.*

t. celi′acus [NA], SYN celiac *trunk.*

t. cor′poris callo′si [NA], SYN *trunk* of corpus callosum.

t. costocervica′lis [NA], SYN costocervical *trunk.*

t. infe′rior plex′us brachia′lis [NA], SYN inferior *trunk* of brachial plexus.

trun′ci intestina′les [NA], SYN intestinal *trunks,* under *trunk.*

t. jugula′ris [NA], SYN jugular lymphatic *trunk.*

t. linguofacia′lis [NA], SYN linguofacial *trunk.*

trun′ci lumba′les [NA], SYN lumbar *trunks,* under *trunk.*

t. lum′bosacra′lis [NA], SYN lumbosacral *trunk.*

t. me′dius plex′us brachia′lis [NA], SYN middle *trunk* of brachial plexus.

persistent t. arterio′sus, a congenital cardiovascular deformity resulting from failure of development of the spiral septum and consisting of a common arterial trunk opening out of both ventricles, the pulmonary arteries being given off from the ascending common trunk.

trun′ci plex′us brachia′lis [NA], SYN *trunks* of brachial plexus, under *trunk.*

t. pulmona′lis [NA], SYN pulmonary *trunk.*

t. subcla′vius [NA], SYN subclavian lymphatic *trunk*.

t. supe′rior plex′us brachia′lis [NA], SYN superior *trunk* of brachial plexus.

t. sympath′icus [NA], SYN sympathetic *trunk*.

t. thyrocervica′lis [NA], SYN thyrocervical *trunk*.

t. vaga′lis [NA], SYN vagal *trunk*.

Trunecek, Karel, Czechoslovakian physician, *1865. SEE T.'s *sign*.

trunk (trŭnk). **1.** The body (trunk or torso), excluding the head and extremities. **2.** A primary nerve, vessel, or collection of tissue before its division. **3.** A large collecting lymphatic vessel. SYN truncus. [L. *truncus*]

accessory nerve t., part of the accessory nerve formed within the cranial cavity by the union of the cranial and spinal roots, which then divides within the jugular foramen into internal and external branches, the former uniting with the vagus, the latter exiting the foramen as in independent branch which is commonly considered to be the accessory nerve.

t. of atrioventricular bundle, the singular initial portion (stem) of the atrioventricular bundle which passes from the atrioventricular node into the right trigone of the fibrous skeleton of the heart and along the periphery of the membranous interventricular septum; upon reaching the muscular interventricular septum, the t. terminates by dividing into the right and left crura of the atrioventricular bundle. SYN truncus fascicularis atrioventricularis.

t.'s of brachial plexus, the superior, middle, and inferior trunks; they divide distally to form the cords (fasciculi) of the plexus. SYN trunci plexus brachialis [NA].

brachiocephalic t., *origin*, arch of aorta; *branches*, right subclavian and right common carotid; occasionally it gives off the thyroidea ima. SYN truncus brachiocephalicus [NA].

bronchomediastinal t., a lymphatic vessel arising from the union of the efferent lymphatics from the tracheo-bronchial and mediastinal nodes on either side. On the left side, it may be largely replaced by direct drainage into the thoracic duct. SYN truncus bronchiomediastinalis [NA].

celiac t., *origin*, abdominal aorta just below diaphragm; *branches*, left gastric, common hepatic, splenic. SYN truncus celiacus [NA], arteria celiaca, celiac artery, celiac axis, Haller's tripod.

t. of corpus callosum, the main arched portion of the corpus callosum. SYN truncus corporis callosi [NA].

costocervical t., a short artery that arises from the subclavian artery on each side and divides into deep cervical and superior intercostal branches, the latter dividing usually to form the first and second posterior intercostal arteries. SYN truncus costocervicalis [NA], costocervical artery.

inferior t. of brachial plexus, the nerve bundle formed by the union of the ventral rami of the eighth cervical and first thoracic nerves; it provides fibers to the posterior and medial cords (fasciculi) of the brachial plexus. SYN truncus inferior plexus brachialis [NA].

intestinal t.'s, the vessels conveying lymph from the lower part of the liver, the stomach, spleen, pancreas, and small intestine; they discharge into the cisterna chyli and are sometimes duplicated. SYN trunci intestinales [NA].

jugular lymphatic t., lymphatic vessel on each side, conveying the lymph from the head and neck; that on the right side empties into the right lymphatic duct, that on the left into the thoracic duct. SYN truncus jugularis [NA], jugular duct.

linguofacial t., the common t. by which the lingual and facial arteries frequently arise from the external carotid artery. SYN truncus linguofacialis [NA].

lumbar t.'s, two lymphatic ducts conveying lymph from the lower limbs, pelvic viscera and walls, large intestine, kidneys, and suprarenal glands; they discharge into the cisterna chyli. SYN trunci lumbales [NA].

lumbosacral t., a large nerve, formed by the union of the fifth lumbar and first sacral nerves, with a branch from the fourth lumbar nerve, which enters into the formation of the sacral plexus. SYN truncus lumbosacralis [NA].

middle t. of brachial plexus, the continuation of the ventral ramus of the seventh cervical nerve; it contributes fibers to the posterior and lateral cords (fasciculi) of the brachial plexus. SYN truncus medius plexus brachialis [NA].

nerve t., a collection of funiculi or bundles of nerve fibers enclosed in a connective tissue sheath, the epineurium.

pulmonary t., *origin*, right ventricle of heart; *distribution*, it divides into the right pulmonary artery and the left pulmonary artery, which enter the corresponding lungs and branch along with the segmental bronchi. SYN truncus pulmonalis [NA], arteria pulmonalis, pulmonary artery, venous artery.

subclavian lymphatic t., it is formed by the union of the vessels draining the lymph nodes of either upper limb, emptying into the thoracic duct at the root of the neck on the left or into the right lymphatic duct. SYN truncus subclavius [NA], subclavian duct.

superior t. of brachial plexus, the nerve bundle formed by the union of the ventral rami of the fifth and sixth cervical nerves and some fibers from the fourth; it contributes fibers to the posterior and lateral cords (fasciculi) of the brachial plexus. SYN truncus superior plexus brachialis [NA].

sympathetic t., one of the two long ganglionated nerve strands alongside the vertebral column that extend from the base of the skull to the coccyx; they are connected to each spinal nerve by gray rami and receive fibers from the spinal cord through white rami connecting with the thoracic and upper lumbar spinal nerves. SYN truncus sympathicus [NA], gangliated cord.

thoracoacromial t., SYN thoracoacromial *artery*.

thyrocervical t., a short arterial t. arising from the subclavian artery, giving rise to the suprascapular (which may instead arise directly from the subclavian artery) and terminating by dividing into the ascending cervical and inferior thyroid arteries. SYN truncus thyrocervicalis [NA], thyroid axis.

vagal t., one of the two nerve bundles, anterior and posterior, into which the esophageal plexus continues as it passes through the diaphragm. SYN truncus vagalis [NA].

tru·sion (trū′zhŭn). Displacement of a body, *e.g.*, a tooth, from an initial position. [L. *trudo*, pp. *trusus*, to thrust]

truss (trŭs). An appliance designed to prevent the return of a reduced hernia or the increase in size of an irreducible hernia; it consists of a pad attached to a belt and kept in place by a spring or straps. [Fr. *trousser*, to tie up, to pack]

Try Former abbreviation for tryptophan.

try-in (trī′in). Preliminary insertion of a complete denture wax-up (trial denture), of a partial denture casting, or of a finished restoration to determine the fit, esthetics, maxillomandibular relation, etc.

try·pan blue (trī′pan, trip′) [C.I. 23850]. An acid azo dye, $C_{34}H_{34}N_6O_{14}S_4Na_4$, used for vital staining of the reticuloendothelial system, uriniferous tubules, and cells in tissue culture, and as an experimental teratogen; formerly used as a trypanocide.

try·pan·i·ci·dal (tri-pan-i-sī′dăl). SYN trypanocidal.

try·pan·i·cide (tri-pan′i-sīd). SYN trypanocide.

tryp·a·nid (trip′ă-nid). SYN trypanosomatid.

try·pan·o·ci·dal (tri-pan′ō-sī′dăl, trip′ă-nō-). Destructive to trypanosomes. SYN trypanicidal.

try·pan·o·cide (tri-pan′ō-sīd, trip′ă-nō-). An agent that kills trypanosomes. SYN trypanicide, trypanosomicide. [trypanosome + L. *caedo*, to kill]

Try·pan·o·plas·ma (tri-pan-ō-plaz′mă, trip′ă-nō-). A genus of flagellate Protozoa (family Cryptobiidae), the members of which have a body of varying shape, an undulating membrane, and a flagellum projecting from either extremity; parasitic in the blood of fishes. [G. *trypanon*, auger, + *plasma*, anything formed]

Try·pan·o·so·ma (tri-pan′ō-sō′mă, trip′ă-nō-). A genus of asexual digenetic protozoan flagellates (family Trypanosomatidae) that have a spindle-shaped body with an undulating membrane on one side, a single anterior flagellum, and a kinetoplast; they are parasitic in the blood plasma of many vertebrates (only a few being pathogenic) and as a rule have an intermediate host, a bloodsucking invertebrate, such as a leech, tick, or insect; pathogenic species cause trypanosomiasis in humans and a number of other diseases in domestic animals. [G. *trypanon*, an auger, + *sōma*, body]

T. a′vium, a species that occurs in owls, crows, and other birds;

various bloodsucking arthropods are the vectors, including mosquitoes, black flies, and hippoboscids; this species was reported under a large number of names now considered to be physiologic strains of the species.

T. bru′cei, a species now divided into three subspecies: *T. brucei brucei, T. brucei rhodesiense,* and *T. brucei gambiense.*

T. bru′cei bru′cei, a subspecies causing nagana in Africa; it produces fatal disease in camels, acute disease in equines, dogs, and cats, and chronic disease in swine, cattle, sheep, and goats; it is transmitted primarily by tsetse flies of the genus *Glossina.* In wild African ungulates the infection is widespread but rarely fatal.

T. bru′cei gambien′se, a subspecies causing Gambian trypanosomiasis; transmitted by tsetse flies, especially *Glossina palpalis.* SYN *T. gambiense, T. hominis, T. ugandense.*

T. bru′cei rhodesien′se, a subspecies causing Rhodesian trypanosomiasis; it is transmitted by tsetse flies, especially *Glossina morsitans;* various game animals can act as reservoir hosts. SYN *T. rhodesiense.*

T. congolen′se, a species transmitted primarily by tsetse flies of the genus *Glossina* and causing nagana in Africa, with anemia as a prominent feature; most domestic mammals (cattle, sheep, goats, equines, camels, dogs, and cats) are highly susceptible to infection, with the resultant disease taking an acute to chronic course with or without recovery; swine are more resistant, with clinical disease running a mild course.

T. cru′zi, a species that causes South American trypanosomiasis and is endemic in Mexico and various countries of Central and South America; transmission and infection are common only where the triatomine bug vector defecates while taking blood, as the bug feces contains the infective agents that are scratched into the skin or brought in contact with mucosal surfaces. Trypomastigotes are found in the blood, and amastigotes occur intracellularly in clusters or colonies in the tissues; heart muscle fibers and cells of many other organs are attacked, the organisms not being restricted to macrophages as in visceral leishmaniasis; humans, dogs, cats, house rats, armadillos, bats, certain monkeys, and opossums are the usual vertebrate hosts; vectors are members of the family Triatominae. Also known as *Schizotrypanum cruzi,* a distinct generic designation widely used in the endemic regions. SYN *T. escomelis, T. triatomae.*

T. dimor′phon, an African species found in horses, cattle, sheep, goats, pigs, and dogs, formerly thought to be the same as *T. congolense* but now recognized as a distinct and more pathogenic species in cattle, sheep, and dogs; it is spread by tsetse flies across central Africa.

T. equi′num, a species that causes mal de caderas of horses in Central and South America; except for being akinetoplastic, it is transmitted mechanically by bloodsucking flies.

T. equiper′dum, a species that causes dourine.

T. escome′lis, SYN *T. cruzi.*

T. ev′ansi, a parasite chiefly of cattle, camels, horses, and dogs, causing surra and murrina; it is transmitted mechanically by tabanid and other bloodsucking flies. SYN *T. hippicum.*

T. gambien′se, SYN *T. brucei gambiense.*

T. hip′picum, SYN *T. evansi.*

T. hom′inis, SYN *T. brucei gambiense.*

T. igno′tum, old name for *T. simiae.*

T. lew′isi, species that is a worldwide nonpathogenic parasite in the blood of rats widely used for laboratory study; it is transmitted by the rat flea, *Nosopsyllus fasciatus.*

T. melopha′gium, a nonpathogenic species (related to *T. theileri*) found in sheep throughout the world, and probably in goats as well; the vector is *Melophagus ovinus.*

T. range′li, a species that parasitizes a wide variety of mammals, including humans, in South America and is transmitted by the triatomid bugs *Rhodnius prolixus* and *Tiratoma dimidiata,* and probably others; it is apparently nonpathogenic but may be pathogenic in the bug host.

T. rhodesien′se, SYN *T. brucei rhodesiense.*

T. simi′ae, a species normally found in warthogs; it is highly pathogenic in pigs and camels, and is transmitted cyclically by tsetse flies and mechanically by bloodsucking flies.

T. su′is, a species pathogenic for swine in Africa; it is transmitted by tsetse flies.

T. thei′leri, a large, relatively nonpathogenic species found in African antelopes and in cattle in many parts of the world; the parasites are spread by bloodsucking tabanid horseflies.

T. triatom′ae, SYN *T. cruzi.*

T. uganden′se, SYN *T. brucei gambiense.*

T. vi′vax, a species causing nagana in cattle, sheep, and goats in Africa, and trypanosomiasis in cattle and water buffalo in South America; it is transmitted cyclically by tsetse flies (*Glossina* spp.) in Africa and presumably mechanically by bloodsucking flies in South America.

try·pan·o·so·mat·id (trī-pan′ō-sō-mat′id). Common name for a member of the family Trypanosomatidae. SYN trypanid.

Try·pan·o·so·mat·i·dae (trī-pan′ō-sō-mat′i-dē). A protozoan family of hemoflagellates (order Kinetoplastida, class Zoomastigophorea, subphylum Mastigophora); asexual blood and/or tissue parasites of leeches, insects, and vertebrates and sap inhabitants of plants, characterized by a rounded or elongate form, a single nucleus, elongate mitochondrion (its position in relation to the nucleus is a characteristic of each genus), and an anteriorly directed single flagellum (in some genera, it borders an undulating membrane). T. includes the genera *Crithidia, Herpetomonas, Leptomonas,* and *Blastocrithidia,* all of which are monogenetic and found in insects, and *Phytomonas* (found in plants), *Endotrypanum, Leishmania,* and *Trypanosoma,* all of which are digenetic; *Leishmania* and *Trypanosoma* include important pathogens of man and animals. Many trypanosomes pass through developmental or life cycle stages similar to the body forms characteristic of the genera; these forms include amastigote, choanomastigote, opisthomastigote, promastigote, epimastigote, and trypomastigote.

try·pan·o·some (tri-pan′ō-sōm, trip′ă-nō-). Common name for any member of the genus *Trypanosoma* or of the family Trypanosomatidae. [G. *trypanon,* an auger, + *sōma,* body]

try·pan·o·so·mi·a·sis (tri-pan′ō-sō-mī′ă-sis, trip′ă-nō-). Any disease caused by a trypanosome.

acute t., SYN Rhodesian t.

African t., a serious endemic disease in tropical Africa, of two types: Gambian or West African t. and Rhodesian or East African t.

American t., SEE South American t.

chronic t., SYN Gambian t.

Cruz t., SYN South American t.

East African t., SYN Rhodesian t.

Gambian t., a chronic disease of humans caused by *Trypanosoma brucei gambiense* in northern and sub-Saharan Africa from Senegal east to Sudan and Uganda; characterized by splenomegaly, drowsiness, an uncontrollable urge to sleep, and the development of psychotic changes; basal ganglia and cerebellar involvement commonly lead to chorea and athetosis; the terminal phase of the disease is characterized by wasting, anorexia, and emaciation that gradually leads to coma and death, usually from intercurrent infection. SYN chronic African sleeping sickness, chronic t., West African sleeping sickness, West African t.

Rhodesian t., a disease of humans caused by *Trypanosoma brucei rhodesiense* in eastern Africa from Ethiopia and Uganda south to Zimbabwe; it is clinically similar to Gambian t. but of

---

♺ **Combining forms**	**[NA]** Nomina Anatomica
Word*Finder*	**[MIM]** Mendelian
Multi-term entry finder	**Inheritance in Man**
Preceding letter A	
A.D.A.M. Anatomy Plates	☆ **Official alternate term**
Between letters L and M	
	☆**[NA] Official alternate**
Appendices:	**Nomina Anatomica term**
Following letter Z	
	High Profile Term
SYN Synonym; Cf., compare	

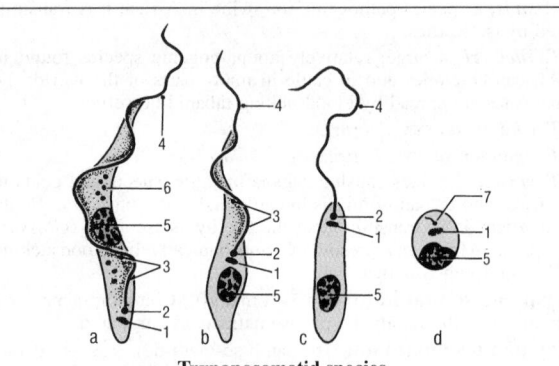

Trypanosomatid species

a) trypomastigote or trypanosome form; b) epimastigote or *Crithidia* form; c) promastigote or *Leptomonas* form; (only in *Leishmania*) d) amastigote or *Leishmania* form; 1) kinetoplast; 2) base of flagellum; 3) undulating membrane with flagellum; 4) free flagellum; 5) nucleus; 6) cytoplasmic granules; and 7) vestigial flagellum

shorter duration and more acute in form; patients suffer repeated episodes of pyrexia, become anemic, and die commonly from cardiac failure. SYN acute African sleeping sickness, acute t., East African sleeping sickness, East African t.

South American t., t. caused by Trypanosoma (or *Schizotrypanum) cruzi* and transmitted by certain species of reduviid (triatomine) bugs. In its acute form, it is seen most frequently in young children, with swelling of the skin at the site of entry, most often the face, and regional lymph node enlargement; in its chronic form it can assume several aspects, commonly cardiomyopathy, but megacolon and megaesophagus also occur; natural reservoirs include dogs, armadillos, rodents, and other domestic, domiciliated, and wild mammals. SYN Chagas' disease, Chagas-Cruz disease, Cruz t.

West African t., SYN Gambian t.

try·pan·o·so·mic (tri-pan-ō-sō'mik, trip'ă-nō-). Relating to trypanosomes, especially denoting infection by such organisms.

try·pan·o·so·mi·cide (tri-pan'ō-sō'mi-sīd). SYN trypanocide.

try·pan·o·so·mid (tri-pan'ō-sō-mid). A skin lesion resulting from immunologic changes from trypanosome disease. [trypanosome + G. *-id* (1)]

try·pan red (trī'pan, trip'). [C.I. 22850]. An azo dye formerly used in the treatment of trypanosomiasis.

tryp·ar·sa·mide (trī-par'să-mīd). Sodium *N*-carbamylmethyl-*p*-aminobenzenearsonate; used in the treatment of trypanosomic and spirochetal infections, especially neurosyphilis, and the late stages of African sleeping sickness.

tryp·o·mas·ti·gote (trip-ō-mas'ti-gōt). Term to replace the older term, "trypanosome stage," which was often confused with the flagellate genus *Trypanosoma*. It denotes the stage (infective stage for South American trypanosomiasis and African trypanosomiasis, and the only stage found in man in the latter illness) in which the flagellum arises from a posteriorly located kinetoplast and emerges from the side of the body, with an undulating membrane running along the length of the body. [G. *trypanon*, auger, + *mastix*, whip]

tryp·sin (trip'sin). A proteolytic enzyme formed in the small intestine from trypsinogen by the action of enteropeptidase; a serine proteinase that hydrolyzes peptides, amides, esters, etc., at bonds of the carboxyl groups of L-arginyl or L-lysyl residues; it also produces the meromyosins.

crystallized t., a purified preparation of the pancreatic enzyme; used as an adjunct to surgery for débridement of necrotic wounds and ulcers.

tryp·sin·o·gen, tryp·so·gen (trip-sin'ō-jen, trip'sō-jen). An inactive protein secreted by the pancreas that is converted into trypsin by the action of enteropepsinase. SYN protrypsin.

trypt·a·mine (trip'tă-mēn, -min). 3-(2-Aminoethyl)indole; a decarboxylation product of L-tryptophan that occurs in plants and certain foods (*e.g.,* cheese). It raises the blood pressure through vasoconstrictor action, by the release of norepinephrine at postganglionic sympathetic nerve endings, and is believed to be one of the agents responsible for hypertensive episodes following therapy with monoamine oxidase inhibitors (*e.g.,* pargyline hydrochloride).

trypt·a·mine-stro·phan·thi·din (trip'ta-mēn-strō-fan'thi-din). A semisynthetic cardiac glycoside that is a condensation product of strophanthidin and tryptamine; given orally, it has a rapid onset and short duration of cardiac action.

tryp·tic (trip'tik). Relating to trypsin, as t. digestion.

tryp·tone (trip'tōn). A peptone produced by proteolytic digestion with trypsin.

tryp·to·ne·mia (trip-tō-nē'mē-ă). The presence of tryptone in the circulating blood.

tryp·to·phan (Trp, W) (trip'tō-fan). 2-Amino-3-(3-indolyl)-propionic acid; the L-isomer is a component of proteins; a nutritionally essential amino acid.

t. decarboxylase, SYN aromatic D-amino-acid decarboxylase.

t. desmolase, SYN t. synthase.

t. 2,3-dioxygenase, an oxidoreductase catalyzing the reaction of L-t. and O_2 to produce L-*N*-formylkynurenine; an adaptive enzyme, the level (in the liver) being controlled by adrenal hormones; a step in t. catabolism; also, a step in the synthesis of NAD^+ from t. SYN pyrrolase, t. oxygenase, t. pyrrolase, tryptophanase (1).

t. oxygenase, SYN t. 2,3-dioxygenase.

t. pyrrolase, SYN t. 2,3-dioxygenase.

t. synthase, a nonmammalian hydro-lyase condensing L-serine indole-3-glycerol phosphate to produce L-tryptophan and glyceraldehyde phosphate; pyridoxal phosphate is required; it will also react L-serine with indole. SYN t. desmolase, t. synthetase.

t. synthetase, SYN t. synthase.

tryp·to·pha·nase (trip'to-fă-nās). **1.** SYN *tryptophan* 2,3-dioxygenase. **2.** An enzyme found in bacteria that catalyzes the cleavage of L-tryptophan to indole, pyruvic acid, and ammonia; pyridoxal phosphate is a coenzyme.

tryp·to·pha·nu·ria (trip'tō-fă-nū'rē-ă). Enhanced urinary excretion of tryptophan.

t. with dwarfism [MIM*276100], a syndrome of dwarfism, mental defect, cutaneous photosensitivity, and gait disturbance associated with t.; autosomal recessive inheritance.

tset·se (tset'sē, tsē'tsē). SEE *Glossina*. [S. African native name]

TSH Abbreviation for thyroid-stimulating *hormone*.

TSH-RF Abbreviation for thyroid-stimulating hormone-releasing *factor.*

TSI Abbreviation for thyroid-stimulating *immunoglobulins,* under *immunoglobulin.*

TSS Abbreviation for toxic shock *syndrome.*

TSTA Abbreviation for tumor-specific transplantation *antigens,* under *antigen.*

TTP Abbreviation for ribothymidine 5'-triphosphate.

TTP-HUS Abbreviation for thrombotic thrombocytopenic purpura and hemolytic uremic syndrome. SEE thrombotic thrombocytopenic *purpura,* hemolytic uremic *syndrome.*

TTX Abbreviation for tetradotoxin.

T.U. Abbreviation for toxic *unit* or toxin *unit.*

tu·a·mi·no·hep·tane (tū'am-i-nō-hep'tān). 2-Aminoheptane; a sympathomimetic volatile amine, used by inhalation as a nasal decongestant; available also as t. sulfate, with the same actions, and more potent as a vasoconstrictor than ephedrine.

tu·ba, gen. and pl. **tu·bae** (tū'bă, tū'bē). SYN tube. [L. a straight trumpet]

t. acus'tica, SYN auditory *tube.*

t. auditi'va [NA], SYN auditory *tube.*

t. audito'ria [NA], ☆official alternate term for auditory *tube,* auditory *tube.*

t. eustachia'na, t. eusta'chii, SYN auditory *tube.*

t. fallopia′na, t. fallo′pii, SYN uterine *tube.*

t. uteri′na [NA], SYN uterine *tube.*

tub·age (tū′baj). Introduction of a tube into a canal. SEE ALSO intubation.

tub·al (tū′băl). Relating to a tube, especially the uterine tube.

tu·ba·tor·sion (tū-bă-tōr′shŭn). SYN tubotorsion.

tub·ba, tub·bae (tŭb′ă, tŭb′bē). SYN foot *yaws.*

TUBE

tube (tūb). **1.** A hollow cylindrical structure or canal. **2.** A hollow cylinder or pipe. SYN tuba. [L. *tubus*]

Abbott's t., SYN Miller-Abbott t.

air t., the trachea, or a bronchus or any of its branches conveying air to the lungs.

auditory t., a tube leading from the tympanic cavity to the nasopharynx; it consists of an osseous (posterolateral) portion at the tympanic end, and a fibrocartilaginous (anteromedial) portion at the pharyngeal end; where the two portions join, in the region of the sphenopetrosal fissure, is the narrowest portion of the tube (isthmus); the auditory t. enables equalization of pressure within the tympanic cavity with ambient air pressure, referred to commonly as "popping of the ears". SYN tuba auditiva [NA], tuba auditoria✶ [NA], eustachian t., guttural duct, otopharyngeal t., otosalpinx, pharyngotympanic t., salpinx (2), tuba acustica, tuba eustachiana, tuba eustachii.

Babcock t., a t. in which milk, after treatment with sulfuric acid, is centrifuged and its fat content then determined in a graduated neck.

Bouchut's t., a short cylindrical t. used in intubation of the larynx.

Bourdon t., a curved and partially flattened t. that tends to straighten out in proportion to internal pressure; used as a transducer to move the pointer of an aneroid manometer.

bronchial t.'s, SYN bronchia.

Cantor t., a long, single-lumen intestinal t. with a sealed rubber bag tip; mercury is injected into the rubber bag with a needle and syringe.

cardiac t., the primitive tubular heart in the embryo, before its division into chambers.

Carlen's t., a double lumen flexible endobronchial t. used for bronchospirometry, for isolation of one lung to prevent contamination or secretions from the contralateral lung, or for ventilation of one lung.

cathode ray t. (CRT), an evacuated t. containing a beam of electrons which can be deflected to various parts of a fluorescent screen; used in the cathode ray oscilloscope.

Celestin t., a plastic t. introduced through a tumor in the esophagus; it permits maintenance of swallowing certain substances when the lesion is unresectable.

Coolidge t., an x-ray t., in which the cathode consists of a tungsten wire spiral surrounded by a focusing cup; the tungsten spiral is heated by an electric current; the quantity and quality of the x-rays so generated are regulated by varying the temperature of the cathode and the voltage between cathode and anode.

Crookes-Hittorf t., a simple evacuated t. containing a cathode, that emitted x-rays from the glass envelope when a current was passed through it; the type used by Roentgen to discover x-rays.

digestive t., SYN digestive *tract.*

drainage t., a t. introduced into a wound or cavity to facilitate removal of a fluid.

Durham's t., a jointed tracheotomy t.

empyema t., a rubber drainage t., piercing a sheet rubber shield, passed through the chest wall in order to drain an empyema.

endobronchial t., a single or double lumen t. with an inflatable cuff at the distal end that, after being passed through the larynx and trachea, is positioned so that ventilation is restricted to one lung; a single lumen t. is placed in the main stem bronchus of the lung; a double lumen t. is positioned at the tracheal carina to permit ventilation of either or both lungs.

endotracheal t., SYN tracheal t.

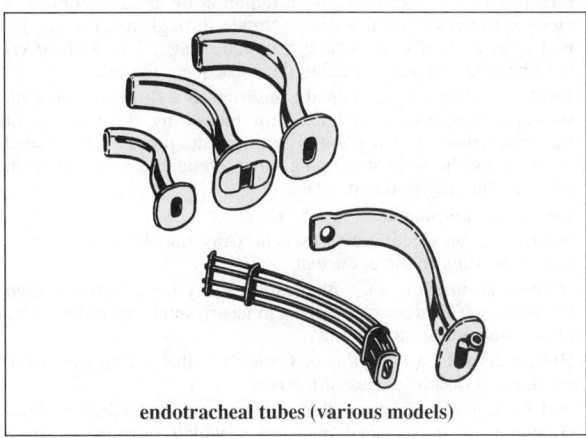

endotracheal tubes (various models)

eustachian t., SYN auditory t.

fallopian t., SYN uterine t.

feeding t., a flexible t. passed through the oral pharynx and into the esophagus and stomach, through which liquid food is fed.

Ferrein's t., SYN convoluted *tubule* of kidney.

field emission t., an x-ray t. that uses a cold cathode, relying on the t. voltage to pull electrons from it to the anode.

Geiger-Müller t., SEE Geiger-Müller *counter.*

germ t., a young hypha growing out of a yeast cell or spore, the beginning of a mycelium; also used as a rapid test for differentiating *Candida albicans* from other *Candida* species.

Haldane t., a t. for securing human alveolar air samples; consisting of a narrow hosepipe with a mouthpiece from which a t. is attached for the withdrawal of expired air at the end of a sudden, maximal expiration.

intratracheal t., SYN tracheal t.

Levin t., a t. introduced through the nose into the upper alimentary canal, to facilitate intestinal decompression.

Martin's t., a drainage t. with a cross piece near the extremity to keep it from slipping out of a cavity.

medullary t., SYN neural t.

Miescher's t.'s, elongate fusiform or cylindrical bodies forming the encapsulated cystic intramuscular stage of the protozoan *Sarcocystis.*

Miller-Abbott t., a t. with two lumens, one ending in a small collapsible balloon and the other in a metallic tip with numerous perforations; used for intestinal decompression. SYN Abbott's t.

molybdenum target t., an x-ray t. with an anode surface made of molybdenum instead of tungsten, used in mammography.

Moss t., (1) a triple-lumen, nasogastric, feeding-decompression t., that utilizes a gastric balloon to occlude cardioesophageal junction, with simultaneous esophageal aspiration and intragastric feeding; (2) a double-lumen, gastric lavage t., that provides continuous delivery of saline via a small bore, with simultaneous aspiration of fluid and some particles via a large bore.

nasogastric t., a stomach t. passed through the nose.

nasotracheal t., a tracheal t. inserted through the nasal passages.

nephrostomy t., a t. placed in the renal collecting system for drainage, diagnostic tests, or removal of calculi. May be placed through a percutaneous route or during an open surgical procedure.

neural t., the epithelial t. formed from the neuroectoderm of the early embryo by the closure of the neural groove; by complex processes of cell proliferation and organization the neural t. develops into the spinal cord and brain. SYN medullary t.

O'Dwyer's t., a metal t. formerly used for intubation of the larynx in diphtheria.

orotracheal t., a tracheal t. inserted through the mouth.

tu

otopharyngeal t., SYN auditory t.

pharyngotympanic t., SYN auditory t.

photomultiplier t., a detector which amplifies a signal (by as much as 10^6) of electromagnetic radiation by an acceleration of electrons released from a photocathode through a series of dynodes; as each electron strikes a dynode stage, 3 to 4 electrons are liberated and accelerated to the subsequent dynode.

Pitot t., a stationary L-shaped t. inserted in a fluid stream, with its opening upstream, and used for measuring the velocity of fluid movement at that point in terms of the pressure developed in the t. by the fluid impinging on it, compared to a second t. opening laterally or downstream.

pus t., SYN pyosalpinx.

rectifier t., an electronic t., used in x-ray transformers, to convert alternating to direct current.

Rehfuss stomach t., a t. with a calibrated syringe, formerly used for aspiration of stomach contents in gastric analysis; replaced by plastic disposable stomach t.'s.

Robertshaw t., a variation of Carlen's t. that eliminates some mechanical disadvantages of the latter.

roll t., a modification of the plate culture; a seeded medium containing agar is placed in a test t. which is rolled or spun horizontally until the medium solidifies evenly on the interior of the t.

rotating anode t., a modern x-ray t., in which heat buildup is distributed through a larger volume by rotating the target.

Ruysch's t., a minute tubular cavity opening in the lower and anterior portion of each surface of the nasal septum; best seen in the early fetal period when it is associated with the vomeronasal organ (Jacobson's organ).

Ryle's t., a thin rubber t., with about the lumen of a no. 8 catheter, and an olive-tipped extremity, used in the giving of a test meal.

Sengstaken-Blakemore t., a t. with three lumens, one for drainage of the stomach and two for inflation of attached gastric and esophageal balloons; used for emergency treatment of bleeding esophageal varices.

Southey's t.'s, obsolete cannulas of small, almost capillary, caliber, thrust by a trocar into the subcutaneous tissues to drain the fluid of anasarca.

stomach t., a flexible t. passed into the stomach for lavage or feeding.

T t., a self-retaining t. with side extensions, shaped like a T.

test t., a t. of thin glass closed at one end, used in the examination of urine and other chemical operations, for bacterial cultures, etc.

thoracostomy t., a t. placed through the heart wall that drains the pleural space.

Tovell t., an armored tracheal t. with a wire spiral embedded in the wall to prevent obstruction of the lumen when the t. is compressed and kinking when the t. is bent at a sharp angle.

Toynbee's t., a t. by which an otologist can listen to the sounds in a patient's ear during politzerization.

tracheal t., a flexible t. inserted nasally, orally, or through a tracheotomy into the trachea to provide an airway, as in tracheal intubation. SYN endotracheal t., intratracheal t.

tracheotomy t., a curved t. used to keep the opening free after tracheotomy. May be metal or plastic.

tympanostomy t., a small t. inserted through the tympanic membrane after myringotomy to aerate the middle ear; often used for serous otitis media.

uterine t., one of the t.'s leading on either side from the upper or outer extremity of the ovary, which is largely enveloped by its expanded infunclibulum, to the fundus of the uterus; it consists of infundibulum, ampulla, isthmus, and uterine parts. SYN salpinx uterina [NA], tuba uterina [NA], salpinx (1)✶, fallopian t., gonaduct (2), oviduct, tuba fallopiana, tuba fallopii.

vacuum t., a glass t. from which the air has been removed, containing two or more electrodes, between which passes an electrical current or spark; used in the production of x-rays, or to control circuits. Previously in wide use, the vacuum t. has been supplanted by transistors in electronic circuits.

Venturi t., a t. with a specially streamlined constriction to minimize energy losses in the fluid flowing through it while maximizing the fall in pressure in the constriction in accordance with Bernoulli's law; the basis of the Venturi meter.

Wangensteen t., SYN Wangensteen *suction.*

x-ray t., SEE x-ray.

---

tu·bec·to·my (tū-bek′tō-mē). SYN salpingectomy. [L. *tuba*, tube, + G. *ektomē*, excision]

tu·ber, pl. **tu·bera** (tū′ber, tū′ber-ă). **1** [NA]. A localized swelling; a knob. **2.** A short, fleshy, thick, underground stem of plants, such as the potato. [L. protuberance, swelling]

t. ante′rius, SYN t. cinereum.

ashen t., SYN t. cinereum.

calcaneal t., SYN calcaneal *tuberosity.*

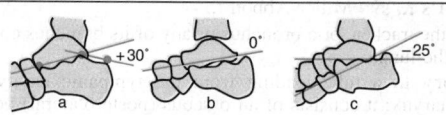

angle of calcaneal tuber
a) normal condition and with fractured calcaneus and no dislocation; b) with dislocation, but without affecting the ankle joint; and c) with multiple fractures

t. calca′nei [NA], SYN calcaneal *tuberosity.*

t. cal′cis, SYN calcaneal *tuberosity.*

t. cine′reum [NA], a prominence of the base of the hypothalamus, bordered caudally by the mamillary bodies, rostrally by the optic chiasm, and laterally by the optic tract, extending ventrally into the infundibulum and hypophysial stalk. SYN ashen t., gray t., t. anterius.

t. coch′leae, SYN *promontory* of tympanic cavity.

t. cor′poris callo′si, SYN *splenium* corporis callosi.

t. dorsa′le, SYN t. vermis.

eustachian t., a slight projection from the labyrinthine wall of the middle ear below the fenestra vestibuli (ovalis).

frontal t., SYN frontal *eminence.*

t. fronta′le [NA], SYN frontal *eminence.*

gray t., SYN t. cinereum.

t. ischiad′icum [NA], SYN ischial *tuberosity.*

t. of ischium, SYN ischial *tuberosity.*

t. maxil′lae [NA], SYN maxillary *tuberosity.*

omental t., SYN t. omentale.

t. omenta′le [NA], **(1)** an eminence on the visceral surface of the left hepatic lobe to the left of the fossa for the ductus venosus; **(2)** a bulge on the anterior surface of the body of the pancreas to the left of the superior mesenteric vessels. SYN omental t.

parietal t., SYN parietal *eminence.*

t. parieta′le [NA], SYN parietal *eminence.*

t. ra′dii, SYN radial *tuberosity.*

t. val′vulae, SYN t. vermis.

t. of vermis, SYN t. vermis.

t. ver′mis [NA], the posterior division of the inferior vermis of the cerebellum located between the folium and the pyramis. SYN t. dorsale, t. of vermis, t. valvulae.

t. zygomat′icum, SYN articular *tubercle* of temporal bone.

tu·ber·cle (tū′ber-kl). **1.** A nodule, especially in an anatomical, not pathologic, sense. SYN tuberculum [NA]. **2.** A circumscribed, rounded, solid elevation on the skin, mucous membrane, or surface of an organ. SYN tuberculum [NA]. **3.** A slight elevation from the suface of a bone giving attachment to a muscle or ligament. SYN tuberculum [NA]. **4.** In dentistry, a small elevation arising on the surface of a tooth. **5.** A granulomatous lesion due to infection by *Mycobacterium tuberculosis.* Although somewhat variable in size (0.5 to 2 or 3 mm in diameter) and in the proportions of various histologic components, t.'s tend to be fairly well circumscribed, spheroidal, firm lesions that usually consist of three irregularly outlined but moderately distinct zones: 1) an inner focus of necrosis, coagulative at first, and then becoming caseous; 2) a middle zone that consists of a fairly dense accumulation of large mononuclear phagocytes (macrophages), frequently arranged somewhat radially (with reference to the necrotic material) resembling an epithelium, and hence termed epithelioid cells—multinucleated giant cells of Langhans type may also be present; 3) an outer zone of numerous lymphocytes, and a few monocytes and plasma cells. In instances where healing has begun, a fourth zone of fibrous tissue may form at the periphery. Morphologically indistinguishable lesions may occur in diseases caused by other agents; many observers use the term nonspecifically, *i.e.*, with reference to any such granuloma; others use "tubercle" only for tuberculous lesions, and then designate those of undetermined causes as epithelioid-cell granulomas. [L. *tuberculum*, dim. of *tuber*, a swelling]

accessory t., SYN accessory *process.*

acoustic t., SYN *trigone* of auditory nerve.

adductor t., the prominence above the medial epicondyle of the femur to which the tendon of the adductor magnus attaches. SYN tuberculum adductorium [NA].

amygdaloid t., a projection from the roof of the anterior end-portion of the temporal horn of the lateral ventricle, marking the location of the amygdaloid nucleus.

anatomical t., SYN postmortem *wart.*

anterior t. of atlas, a conical protuberance on the anterior surface of the arch of the atlas. SYN tuberculum anterius atlantis [NA].

anterior t. of cervical vertebrae, the anterior projection from the transverse process. SYN tuberculum anterius vertebrarum cervicalium.

t. of anterior scalene muscle, SYN scalene t.

anterior thalamic t., a prominence at the anterior extremity of the thalamus which corresponds to the nuclei anteriores. SYN tuberculum anterius thalami [NA], anterior t. of thalamus.

anterior t. of thalamus, SYN anterior thalamic t.

articular t. of temporal bone, articular eminence of the temporal bone which bounds the mandibular fossa anteriorly; it forms the anterior root of the zygomatic process; it is enclosed by the articular capsule of the temporomandibular joint with the articular fossa; the head of the mandible (and intervening articular disc) move onto the articular t. to allow full depression of mandible (opening of mouth). SYN tuberculum articulare ossis temporalis [NA], articular eminence of temporal bone, eminentia articularis ossis temporalis, tuber zygomaticum.

ashen t., SYN *tuberculum* cinereum.

auricular t., a small projection from the upper end of the posterior portion of the incurved free margin of the helix. SYN tuberculum auriculae [NA], darwinian t., tuberculum superius.

calcaneal t., the projection, often double, on the inferior aspect of the calcaneus at the anterior end of the area for attachment of the long plantar ligament. SYN tuberculum calcanei [NA].

Carabelli t., a small t., resembling a supernumerary cusp, found occasionally on the lingual surface of the mesiolingual cusp of a permanent maxillary first molar.

carotid t., the anterior t. of the transverse process of the sixth cervical vertebra, against which the carotid artery may be compressed by the finger. SYN tuberculum caroticum [NA], Chassaignac's t.

caseous t., SYN soft t.

Chassaignac's t., SYN carotid t.

conoid t., the prominence near the lateral end of the inferior surface of the clavicle that gives attachment to the conoid ligament. SYN tuberculum conoideum [NA], conoid process.

corniculate t., a rounded eminence on the posterior part of the aryepiglottic fold, formed by the underlying corniculate cartilages. SYN tuberculum corniculatum [NA], Santorini's t.

crown t., SYN dental t.

t. of cuneate nucleus, the bulbous rostral extremity of the fasciculus cuneatus corresponding to the position of the cuneate nucleus, lying lateral to the clava and separated from the tuberculum cinereum on its lateral side by the posterior lateral sulcus. SYN

tuberculum nuclei cuneati [NA], tuberculum cuneatum, wedge-shaped t.

cuneiform t., a rounded eminence on the posterior part of the aryepiglottic fold, formed by the underlying cuneiform cartilage. SYN tuberculum cuneiforme [NA], Wrisberg's t.

darwinian t., SYN auricular t.

dental t., a small elevation on some portions of a crown produced by an extra formation of enamel. SYN tuberculum dentis [NA], crown t., t. of tooth, tuberculum coronae.

dissection t., SYN postmortem *wart.*

dorsal t. of radius, a small prominence on the dorsal aspect of the distal end of the radius lateral to the groove for the extensor pollicis longus tendon; it serves as a trochlea or pulley for the tendon. SYN tuberculum dorsale [NA], Lister's t.

epiglottic t., a convexity at the lower part of the epiglottis over the upper part of the thyroepiglottic ligament. SYN tuberculum epiglotticum [NA], cushion of epiglottis.

fibrous t., a t. in which fibroblasts proliferate about the periphery (and into the cellular zones), eventually resulting in a rim or wall of cellular fibrous tissue or collagenous material around the t.

genial t., SYN mental *spine.*

genital t., the median elevation just cephalic to the urogenital orifice of an embryo; it is the primordium of the penis of the male or the clitoris of the female. SYN phallic t.

Gerdy's t., a t. on the lateral side of the upper end of the tibia giving attachment to the iliotibial tract and some fibers of the tibialis anterior muscle.

Ghon's t., calcification seen in pulmonary parenchyma (usually mid-lung area) and hilar nodes resulting from earlier, usually childhood, infection with tuberculosis. SYN Ghon's complex, Ghon's focus, Ghon's primary lesion.

gracile t., SYN t. of gracile nucleus.

t. of gracile nucleus, the somewhat expanded upper end of the gracile fasciculus, corresponding to the position of the gracile nucleus. SYN tuberculum nuclei gracilis [NA], clava, gracile t., t. of nucleus gracilis, tuberculum gracile.

gray t., SYN *tuberculum* cinereum.

greater t. of humerus, the larger of the two t.'s next to the head of the humerus; it gives attachment to the supraspinatus, infraspinatus, and teres minor muscles. SYN tuberculum majus humeri [NA], greater tuberosity of humerus.

hard t., a t. lacking necrosis.

hyaline t., a form of fibrous t. in which the cellular fibrous tissue and collagenous fibers become altered and merged into a fairly homogeneous, acellular, deeply acidophilic, firm mass.

iliac t., SYN t. of iliac crest.

t. of iliac crest, a prominence on the outer lip of the iliac crest about 5 cm behind the anterior superior iliac spine. SYN tuberculum iliacum [NA], iliac t.

inferior thyroid t., a slight lateral projection from the lower margin of the lamina of the thyroid cartilage on either side, at the inferior end of the oblique line. SYN tuberculum thyroideum inferius [NA].

infraglenoid t., a rough surface below the glenoid cavity of the scapula, giving attachment to the long tendon of the triceps. SYN tuberculum infraglenoidale [NA], infraglenoid tuberosity.

intercolumnar t., SEE subfornical *organ.*

intercondylar t., one of two projections, medial and lateral, springing from the central lip of each articular surface of the tibia on either side of the intercondylar eminence. SYN tuberculum intercondylare [NA].

intervenous t., the slight projection on the wall of the right atrium between the orifices of the venae cavae. SYN tuberculum intervenosum [NA], Lower's t.

jugular t., an oval elevation on the cerebral surface of the lateral part of the occipital bone, on either side of the foramen magnum above the hypoglossal canal. SYN tuberculum jugulare [NA].

labial t., the slight projection on the free edge of the center of the upper lip at the lower extent of the philtrum. SYN tuberculum labii superioris [NA], procheilon, prochilon, t. of upper lip.

lateral t. of posterior process of talus, the prominence lateral to

tu

the groove for the flexor hallucis longus tendon. SYN tuberculum laterale processus posterioris tali [NA].

lesser t. of humerus, the anterior of the two tubercles of the neck of the humerus on which the subscapularis is inserted. SYN tuberculum minus humeri [NA], lesser tuberosity of humerus.

Lisfranc's t., SYN scalene t.

Lister's t., SYN dorsal t. of radius.

Lower's t., SYN intervenous t.

mamillary t., SYN mamillary *process.*

mamillary t. of hypothalamus, SYN mamillary *body.*

marginal t., SYN marginal t. of zygomatic bone.

marginal t. of zygomatic bone, a prominence on the temporal border of the zygomatic bone to which the temporal fascia is attached. SYN tuberculum marginale ossis zygomatici [NA], marginal t.

medial t. of posterior process of talus, the eminence medial to the sulcus for the flexor hallucis longus tendon. SYN tuberculum mediale processus posterioris tali [NA].

mental t., a paired eminence on the mental protuberance of the mandible. SYN tuberculum mentale [NA], eminentia symphysis.

Montgomery's t.'s, elevated reddened areolar glands, usually associated with pregnancy.

Morgagni's t., SYN cuneiform *cartilage.*

Müller's t., a median protuberance projecting into the embryonic urogenital sinus from its dorsal wall; it is formed from the fused caudal ends of the paramesonephric ducts and is the first evidence of the embryonic uterus and vagina. SYN sinus t.

nuchal t., SYN *vertebra* prominens.

t. of nucleus gracilis, SYN t. of gracile nucleus.

obturator t., one of two processes, anterior and posterior, on the margin of the pubic portion of the obturator foramen, bounding the termination of the obturator groove. SYN tuberculum obturatorium [NA].

olfactory t., a small, oval area at the base of the cerebral hemisphere, between the diverging medial and lateral olfactory striae, in the anteromedial part of the anterior perforated substance; it is formed by a small area of allocortex characterized by the presence of the islands of Calleja. Corresponding to a much more prominent structure in nonprimate mammals (especially rodents and insectivores), the olfactory tubercle receives fibers from the olfactory bulb by way of the intermediate olfactory stria; it has efferent connections with the hypothalamus and the mediodorsal nucleus of the thalamus. SYN tuberculum olfactorium.

orbital t. of zygomatic bone, a small elevation on the orbital surface of the zygomatic bone, just within the orbital margin, about 1 cm below the zygomaticofrontal suture; it gives attachment to the lateral check ligament, the lateral palpebral ligament, and the suspensory ligament of the eyeball. SYN eminentia orbitalis ossis zygomatici [NA], orbital eminence of zygomatic bone, Whitnall's t.

phallic t., SYN genital t.

pharyngeal t., a projection from the undersurface of the basilar portion of the occipital bone, giving attachment to the fibrous raphe of the pharynx. SYN tuberculum pharyngeum [NA].

posterior t. of atlas, a protuberance of the posterior extremity of the arch of the atlas, a rudiment of the spinous process giving attachment to the musculus rectus capitis posterior minor muscle. SYN tuberculum posterius atlantis [NA].

posterior t. of cervical vertebrae, a posterior projection from the transverse processes. SYN tuberculum posterius vertebrarum cervicalium.

postmortem t., SYN postmortem *wart.*

Princeteau's t., a slight prominence on the temporal bone near the apex of the petrous part where the superior petrosal sinus commences.

prosector's t., SYN postmortem *wart.*

pterygoid t., a slight prominence on the posterior surface of the medial pterygoid plate, inferior and to the medial side of the pterygoid canal.

pubic t., a small projection at the anterior extremity of the crest of the pubis about 2 cm from the symphysis. SYN tuberculum pubicum [NA], pubic spine, spina pubis.

t. of rib, the knob on the posterior surface of a rib, at the junction of its neck and shaft, which articulates with the transverse process of the vertebra, whch corresponds in number to the rib, forming a costotransverse joint. SYN tuberculum costae [NA].

Rolando's t., SYN *tuberculum* cinereum.

t. of saddle, SYN *tuberculum* sellae.

Santorini's t., SYN corniculate t.

scalene t., a small spine on the inner edge of the first rib, giving attachment to the scalenus anterior muscle. SYN tuberculum musculi scaleni anterioris [NA], Lisfranc's t., scalene t. of Lisfranc, t. of anterior scalene muscle.

scalene t. of Lisfranc, SYN scalene t.

t. of scaphoid bone, a projection at the inferior lateral angle of the scaphoid (navicular) bone; it can be felt at the root of the thumb. SYN tuberculum ossis scaphoidei [NA].

sebaceous t., SYN milium.

sinus t., SYN Müller's t.

soft t., a t. showing caseous necrosis. SYN caseous t.

superior thyroid t., a blunt projection on the lamina of the thyroid cartilage on either side at the superior end of the oblique line. SYN tuberculum thyroideum superius [NA].

supraglenoid t., a rough surface above the glenoid cavity of the scapula, giving attachment to the tendon of the long head of the biceps within the articular cavity of the shoulder joint. SYN tuberculum supraglenoidale [NA].

supratragic t., a small elevation often present on the edge of the upper tragus. SYN tuberculum supratragicum [NA].

t. of tooth, SYN dental t.

t. of trapezium, a prominent ridge on the trapezium forming the lateral border of the groove in which runs the tendon of the flexor carpi radialis. SYN tuberculum ossis trapezii [NA], oblique ridge of trapezium.

t. of upper lip, SYN labial t.

wedge-shaped t., SYN t. of cuneate nucleus.

Whitnall's t., SYN orbital t. of zygomatic bone.

Wrisberg's t., SYN cuneiform t.

⌂**tubercul-.** SEE tuberculo-.

tu·ber·cu·la (tū-ber′kyū-lă). Plural of tuberculum.

tu·ber·cu·lar, tu·ber·cu·late, tu·ber·cu·lat·ed (tū-ber′kyū-lăr, -lāt, -lăt-ed). Pertaining to or characterized by tubercles or small nodules. Cf. tuberculous.

tu·ber·cu·la·tion (tū-ber-kyū-lā′shŭn). **1.** The formation of tubercles or nodules. SYN tuberculization. **2.** The arrangement of tubercles or nodules in a part.

tu·ber·cu·lid (tū-ber′kyū-lid). A lesion of the skin or mucous membrane resulting from hypersensitivity to mycobacterial antigens disseminated from a distant site of active tuberculosis. [tubercul- + G. -id (1)]

nodular t., SYN *erythema* induratum.

papular t., SYN *lichen* scrofulosorum.

papulonecrotic t., dusky-red papules followed by crusting and ulceration primarily on the extremities and predominantly in young adults with a deep focus of tuberculosis or with a history of preceding infection. SYN tuberculosis cutis follicularis disseminata, tuberculosis papulonecrotica.

rosacea-like t., SYN granulomatous *rosacea.*

tu·ber·cu·lin (tū-ber′kyū-lin). **1.** A glycerin-broth culture of *Mycobacterium tuberculosis* evaporated to $\frac{1}{10}$ volume at 100°C and filtered; introduced by Robert Koch for the treatment of tuberculosis but now used chiefly for diagnostic tests; originally known as Koch's old t. (OT) or Koch's original t. **2.** One or another of a relatively large number of extracts of *Mycobacterium tuberculosis* cultures, different from OT and now obsolete.

Koch's old t. (OT), Koch's original t., SEE tuberculin (1).

purified protein derivative of t. (PPD), purified t. containing the active protein fraction; the t. from which it is prepared differs from t. (1) chiefly in that the bacteria are grown in a synthetic rather than in a broth medium.

tu·ber·cu·li·tis (tū-ber-kyū-lī′tis). Inflammation of any tubercle. [tubercul- + G. -itis, inflammation]

tu·ber·cu·li·za·tion (tū-ber′kyū-li-zā′shŭn). SYN tuberculation (1).

tuberculo-, tubercul-. A tubercle, tuberculosis. [L. *tuberculum,* tubercle]

tu·ber·cu·lo·cele (tū-ber′kyū-lō-sēl). Tuberculosis of the testes. [tuberculo- + G. *kēlē,* tumor, hernia]

tu·ber·cu·lo·che·mo·ther·a·peu·tic (tū-ber′kyū-lō-kē′mō-ther-ă-pyū′tik). Relating to the treatment of tuberculosis by tuberculostatic or tuberculocidal drugs.

tu·ber·cu·lo·ci·dal (tū-ber′kyū-lō-sī′dăl). Destructive to the tubercle bacillus.

tu·ber·cu·lo·der·ma (tū-ber′kyū-lō-der′mă). **1.** Any tubercular process of the skin. **2.** The cutaneous manifestation of tuberculosis.

tu·ber·cu·lo·fi·broid (tū-ber′kyū-lō-fī′broyd). A discrete, well-circumscribed, usually spheroidal, moderately to extremely firm, encapsulated nodule that is formed during the process of healing in a focus of tuberculous granulomatous inflammation.

tu·ber·cu·loid (tū-ber′kyū-loyd). Resembling tuberculosis or a tubercle. [tuberculo- + G. *eidos,* resemblance]

tu·ber·cu·lo·ma (tū-ber-kyū-lō′mă). A rounded tumorlike but non-neoplastic mass, usually in the lungs or brain, due to localized tuberculous infection. [tuberculo- + G. *-oma,* tumor]

tu·ber·cu·lo·pro·tein (tū-ber′kyū-lō-prō′tēn). Any one, or a mixture of any or all of the proteins present in the body of the tubercle bacillus, all of which have been found to possess certain properties of tuberculin.

tu·ber·cu·lo·sis (TB) (tū-ber-kyū-lō′sis). A specific disease caused by the presence of *Mycobacterium tuberculosis,* which may affect almost any tissue or organ of the body, the most common seat of the disease being the lungs; the anatomical lesion is the tubercle, which can undergo caseation necrosis; local symptoms vary according to the part affected; general symptoms are those of sepsis: hectic fever, sweats, and emaciation; often progressive with high mortality if not treated. Has in recent years proved to be an opportunistic infection of people with compromised immune systems, including those with AIDS. There is also a high incidence among IV drug abusers. [tuberculo- + G. *-osis,* condition]

acute t., a rapidly fatal disease due to the general dissemination of tubercle bacilli in the blood, resulting in the formation of miliary tubercles in various organs and tissues, and producing symptoms of profound toxemia. SYN acute miliary t., disseminated t.

acute miliary t., SYN acute t.

adult t., SYN secondary t.

aerogenic t., infection with the *Mycobacterium tuberculosis* spread by inhalation of infected droplets.

anthracotic t., SYN pneumoconiosis.

arrested t., SYN healed t.

attenuated t., a mild chronic form marked by caseous tubercles of the skin and the occurrence of cold abscesses.

basal t., t. of the basilar portions of the lungs.

cerebral t., (1) SYN tuberculous *meningitis.* **(2)** cerebral tuberculoma.

childhood t., initial (primary) infection with *Mycobacterium tuberculosis,* characterized by pneumonic lesions in middle parts of lungs, rarely cavitary, with rapid spread to lymph nodes in hilar and paratracheal areas; more often seen in childhood, but pattern is not limited to children.

childhood type t., SYN primary t.

cutaneous t., pathologic lesions of the skin caused by *Mycobacterium tuberculosis.* SYN dermal t., t. cutis.

t. cu′tis, SYN cutaneous t.

t. cu′tis follicula′ris dissemina′ta, SYN papulonecrotic *tuberculid.*

t. cu′tis lupo′sa, SYN *lupus* vulgaris.

t. cu′tis orificia′lis, any tuberculous lesion in or about the mouth or anus. SYN t. ulcerosa.

t. cu′tis verruco′sa, a tuberculous skin lesion having a warty surface with a chronic inflammatory base seen on the hands in adults and lower extremities in children, with marked hypersensitivity to tuberculous antigens. SEE ALSO postmortem *wart.* SYN lupus papillomatosus, lupus verrucosus, tuberculous wart, verrucous scrofuloderma.

dermal t., SYN cutaneous t.

disseminated t., SYN acute t.

enteric t., a complication of cavitary pulmonary t. usually resulting from expectoration and swallowing of bacilli that then infect areas of the digestive tract where there is relative stasis or abundant lymphoid tissue. SEE ALSO tuberculous *enteritis.*

exudative t., a stage of infection with *Mycobacterium tuberculosis* causing severe edema and cellular inflammatory reaction without much necrosis or fibrosis.

general t., SYN miliary t.

healed t., a scar or a calcified, fibrous, or caseous nodule in the lung pleura, lymph node, or other organ, resulting from previous t. that has regressed; reactivation is possible. SYN arrested t., inactive t.

inactive t., SYN healed t.

miliary t., a general dissemination of tubercle bacilli with the production of countless minute discrete tubercles in various organs and tissues; evident in the lung as numerous tiny densities on the radiograph. SYN general t.

open t., pulmonary t., tuberculous ulceration, or other form in which the tubercle bacilli are present in the excretions or secretions; in the lung, usually the result of cavity formation.

t. papulonecrot′ica, SYN papulonecrotic *tuberculid.*

postprimary t., SYN secondary t.

primary t., first infection by *Mycobacterium tuberculosis,* typically seen in children but also occurs in adults, characterized in the lungs by the formation of a primary complex consisting of small peripheral pulmonary focus with spread to hilar or paratracheal lymph nodes; may cavitate or heal with scarring or may progress. SYN childhood type t.

pulmonary t., t. of the lungs.

reinfection t., SYN secondary t.

secondary t., t. found in adults and characterized by lesions near the apex of an upper lobe, which may cavitate or heal with scarring without spreading to lymph nodes; theoretically, secondary t. may be due to exogenous reinfection or to reactivation of a dormant endogenous infection. SYN adult t., postprimary t., reinfection t.

t. ulcero′sa, SYN t. cutis orificialis.

tu·ber·cu·lo·stat (tū-ber′kyū-lō-stat). A tuberculostatic agent.

tu·ber·cu·lo·stat·ic (tū-ber′kyū-lō-stat′ik). Relating to an agent that inhibits the growth of tubercle bacilli. [tuberculo- + G. *statikos,* causing to stand]

tu·ber·cu·lous (tū-ber′kyū-lŭs). Relating to or affected by tuberculosis. Cf. tubercular.

TUBERCULUM

tu·ber·cu·lum, pl. **tu·ber·cu·la** (tū-ber′kyū-lŭm, -lă) [NA]. SYN tubercle (1), tubercle (2), tubercle (3). **2.** A circumscribed, rounded, solid elevation on the skin, mucous membrane, or surface of an organ. **3.** A slight elevation from the surface of a bone giving attachment to a muscle or ligament. [L. dim. of *tuber,* a knob, swelling, tumor]

t. adducto′rium [NA], SYN adductor *tubercle.*

t. ante′rius atlan′tis [NA], SYN anterior *tubercle* of atlas.

t. ante′rius thal′ami [NA], SYN anterior thalamic *tubercle.*

t. ante′rius vertebra′rum cervica′lium, SYN anterior *tubercle* of cervical vertebrae.

t. arthrit′icum, (1) SYN Heberden's *nodes,* under *node.* **(2)** any gouty concretion in or around a joint.

t. articula′re os′sis tempora′lis [NA], SYN articular *tubercle* of temporal bone.

t. auric′ulae [NA], SYN auricular *tubercle.*

t. calca′nei [NA], SYN calcaneal *tubercle.*

tu

t. carot′icum [NA], SYN carotid *tubercle*.

t. cine′reum, a longitudinal prominence on the dorsolateral surface of the medulla oblongata along the lateral border of the t. cuneatum; it is the surface profile of the spinal tract of trigeminal nerve, continuous caudally with the dorsolateral fasciculus (Lissauer's tract). SYN ashen tubercle, gray tubercle, Rolando's tubercle.

t. conoi′deum [NA], SYN conoid *tubercle*.

t. cornicula′tum [NA], SYN corniculate *tubercle*.

t. coro′nae, SYN dental *tubercle*.

t. cos′tae [NA], SYN *tubercle* of rib.

t. cunea′tum, SYN *tubercle* of cuneate nucleus.

t. cuneifor′me [NA], SYN cuneiform *tubercle*.

t. den′tis [NA], SYN dental *tubercle*.

tuber′cula doloro′sa, obsolete term for multiple cutaneous myomas or neuromas which are painful on pressure.

t. dorsa′le [NA], SYN dorsal *tubercle* of radius.

t. epiglot′ticum [NA], SYN epiglottic *tubercle*.

t. grac′ile, SYN *tubercle* of gracile nucleus.

t. hypoglos′si, SYN hypoglossal *trigone*.

t. ili′acum [NA], SYN *tubercle* of iliac crest.

t. im′par, a small median protuberance on the floor of the oral cavity of the embryo between the mandibular and hyoid arches, which plays a minor role in the development of the tongue. SYN median tongue bud.

t. infraglenoida′le [NA], SYN infraglenoid *tubercle*.

t. intercondyla′re [NA], SYN intercondylar *tubercle*.

t. interveno′sum [NA], SYN intervenous *tubercle*.

t. jugula′re [NA], SYN jugular *tubercle*.

t. la′bii superio′ris [NA], SYN labial *tubercle*.

t. latera′le proces′sus posterio′ris ta′li [NA], SYN lateral *tubercle* of posterior process of talus.

t. ma′jus hu′meri [NA], SYN greater *tubercle* of humerus.

t. mal′lei, SYN lateral *process* of malleus.

t. margina′le os′sis zygomat′ici [NA], SYN marginal *tubercle* of zygomatic bone.

t. media′le proces′sus posterio′ris ta′li [NA], SYN medial *tubercle* of posterior process of talus.

t. menta′le [NA], SYN mental *tubercle*.

t. mi′nus hu′meri [NA], SYN lesser *tubercle* of humerus.

t. mus′culi scale′ni anterio′ris [NA], SYN scalene *tubercle*.

t. nu′clei cunea′ti [NA], SYN *tubercle* of cuneate nucleus.

t. nu′clei gra′cilis [NA], SYN *tubercle* of gracile nucleus.

t. obturato′rium [NA], SYN obturator *tubercle*.

t. olfacto′rium, SYN olfactory *tubercle*.

t. os′sis scaphoi′dei [NA], SYN *tubercle* of scaphoid bone.

t. os′sis trape′zii [NA], SYN *tubercle* of trapezium.

t. pharyn′geum [NA], SYN pharyngeal *tubercle*.

t. poste′rius atlan′tis [NA], SYN posterior *tubercle* of atlas.

t. poste′rius vertebra′rum cervica′lium, SYN posterior *tubercle* of cervical vertebrae.

t. pu′bicum [NA], SYN pubic *tubercle*.

t. seba′ceum, SYN milium.

t. sel′lae [NA], the slight elevation in front of the pituitary fossa (sella turcica) on the body of the sphenoid bone. SYN tubercle of saddle.

t. sep′ti na′rium, a flat elevation on the septum in each naris opposite the anterior end of the middle concha; it is due to an aggregation of glands.

t. supe′rius, SYN auricular *tubercle*.

t. supraglenoida′le [NA], SYN supraglenoid *tubercle*.

t. supratra′gicum [NA], SYN supratragic *tubercle*.

t. syphilit′icum, gumma of the skin.

t. thyroi′deum infe′rius [NA], SYN inferior thyroid *tubercle*.

t. thyroi′deum supe′rius [NA], SYN superior thyroid *tubercle*.

---

tu·ber·if·er·ous (tū-ber-if′er-ŭs). SYN tuberous. [tuber + L. *ferro,* to bear]

tu·ber·ose (tū′ber-ōs). SYN tuberous.

tu·ber·os·i·tas (tū′ber-os′i-tas). SYN tuberosity. [LL., fr. L. *tuberosus,* full of lumps, fr. *tuber,* a knob]

t. coracoi′dea, SYN coracoid *tuberosity*.

t. costa′lis, SYN *impression* for costoclavicular ligament.

t. deltoi′dea [NA], SYN deltoid *tuberosity*.

t. glu′tea [NA], SYN gluteal *tuberosity*.

t. ili′aca [NA], SYN iliac *tuberosity*.

t. masseter′ica [NA], SYN masseteric *tuberosity*.

t. mus′culi serra′ti anterio′ris [NA], SYN *tuberosity* for serratus anterior muscle.

t. os′sis cuboi′dei [NA], SYN *tuberosity* of cuboid bone.

t. os′sis metatarsa′lis pri′mi [NA], SYN *tuberosity* of first metatarsal.

t. os′sis metatarsa′lis quin′ti [NA], SYN *tuberosity* of fifth metatarsal.

t. os′sis navicula′ris [NA], SYN *tuberosity* of navicular bone.

t. phalan′gis dista′lis [NA], SYN *tuberosity* of distal phalanx.

t. pterygoi′dea [NA], SYN pterygoid *tuberosity*.

t. ra′dii [NA], SYN radial *tuberosity*.

t. sacra′lis [NA], SYN sacral *tuberosity*.

t. tib′iae [NA], SYN tibial *tuberosity*.

t. ul′nae [NA], SYN *tuberosity* of ulna.

t. unguicula′ris, SYN *tuberosity* of distal phalanx.

tu·ber·os·i·ty (tū′ber-os′i-tē). A large tubercle or rounded elevation, especially from the surface of a bone. SYN tuberositas.

bicipital t., SYN radial t.

calcaneal t., the posterior extremity of the calcaneus, or os calcis, forming the projection of the heel. SYN tuber calcanei [NA], calcaneal tuber, tuber calcis.

coracoid t., the conoid tubercle and trapezoid line of the coracoid process of the scapula, giving attachment to the two parts of the coracoclavicular ligament: the conoid and trapezoid ligaments. SYN tuberositas coracoidea.

costal t., SYN *impression* for costoclavicular ligament.

t. of cuboid bone, a slight eminence on the lateral surface of the cuboid bone, capped with an articular facet for a sesamoid bone in the tendon of the peroneus longus muscle. SYN tuberositas ossis cuboidei [NA].

deltoid t., a rough elevation about the middle of the lateral side of the shaft of the humerus, giving attachment to the deltoid muscle. SYN tuberositas deltoidea [NA], deltoid crest, deltoid eminence, deltoid impression.

t. of distal phalanx, a roughened raised surface of horseshoe shape on the palmar surface of the distal end of the terminal or ungual phalanx of each finger and toe, which serves to support the pulp of the digit. SYN tuberositas phalangis distalis [NA], tuberositas unguicularis, ungual t.

t. of fifth metatarsal, a tubercle at the base of this bone to the posterior part of which is attached the tendon of the peroneus brevis muscle. SYN tuberositas ossis metatarsalis quinti [NA].

t. of first metatarsal, a tubercle at the base of the bone to which is attached the tendon of the peroneus longus muscle. SYN tuberositas ossis metatarsalis primi [NA].

gluteal t., the point of insertion on the upper portion of the shaft of the femur of the greater part of the gluteus maximus muscle; when markedly developed this t. is called the third trochanter. SYN trochanter tertius [NA], tuberositas glutea [NA], crista glutea, gluteal crest, gluteal ridge.

greater t. of humerus, SYN greater *tubercle* of humerus.

iliac t., a rough area above the auricular surface on the medial aspect of the ala of the ilium, giving attachment to the posterior sacroiliac ligament. SYN tuberositas iliaca [NA].

infraglenoid t., SYN infraglenoid *tubercle*.

ischial t., the rough bony projection at the junction of the lower end of the body of the ischium and its ramus; this is a weight-bearing point in the sitting position; provides attachment for the sacrotuberous ligament and is the site of origin of the hamstring muscles. SYN tuber ischiadicum [NA], tuber of ischium.

lateral femoral t., SYN lateral *epicondyle* of femur.

lesser t. of humerus, SYN lesser *tubercle* of humerus.

masseteric t., a roughened surface on the external aspect of the angle of the mandible, giving attachment to fibers of the masseter muscle. SYN tuberositas masseterica [NA].

maxillary t., the bulging lower extremity of the posterior surface of the body of the maxilla, behind the root of the last molar tooth. SYN tuber maxillae [NA], eminentia maxillae☆ [NA], maxillary eminence.

medial femoral t., SYN medial *epicondyle* of femur.

t. of navicular bone, a rounded eminence on the medial surface of the navicular bone, giving attachment to a part of the tendon of the tibialis posterior muscle. SYN tuberositas ossis navicularis [NA], scaphoid t.

pterygoid t., a roughened area on the internal aspect of the mandible, giving attachment to fibers of the medial pterygoid muscle. SYN tuberositas pterygoidea [NA].

radial t., an oval projection from the medial surface of the radius just distal to the neck, giving attachment on its posterior half to the tendon of the biceps. SYN tuberositas radii [NA], bicipital t., tuber radii, t. of radius.

t. of radius, SYN radial t.

sacral t., a rough prominence on the lateral surface of the sacrum posterior to the auricular surface for attachment of posterior sacroiliac ligaments. SYN tuberositas sacralis [NA].

scaphoid t., SYN t. of navicular bone.

t. for serratus anterior muscle, a rough oval area, about the middle of the outer surface and lower border of the second rib, for the attachment of the serratus anterior muscle. SYN tuberositas musculi serrati anterioris [NA].

tibial t., an oval elevation on the anterior surface of the tibia about 3 cm distal to the articular surface, giving attachment at its distal part to the patellar ligament. SYN tuberositas tibiae [NA].

t. of ulna, a prominence at the lower border of the anterior surface of the coronoid process, giving attachment to the brachialis muscle. SYN tuberositas ulnae [NA].

ungual t., SYN t. of distal phalanx.

tu·ber·ous (tū′ber-ŭs). Knobby, lumpy, or nodular; presenting many tubers or tuberosities. SYN tuberiferous, tuberose. [L. *tuberosus*]

△**tubo-.** Tubular, a tube. SEE ALSO salpingo-. [L. *tubus, tuba,* tube]

tu·bo·ab·dom·i·nal (tū′bō-ab-dom′i-năl). Relating to a uterine (fallopian) tube and the abdomen.

tu·bo·cu·ra·rine chlo·ride (tū′bō-kūr-ar′ēn). $C_{38}H_{44}Cl_2N_2O_6$·-$5H_2O$; *d*-Tubocurarine chloride; an alkaloid (obtained from the stems of *Chondodendron*, particularly *C. tomentosum*) that blocks the action of acetylcholine at the myoneural junction by occupying the receptors competitively; also blocks ganglionic transmission and releases histamine; used to produce muscular relaxation during surgical operations.

tu·bo·lig·a·men·tous (tū′bō-lig-ă-men′tŭs). Relating to the uterine (fallopian) tube and the broad ligament of the uterus.

tu·bo·o·var·i·an (tū′bō-ō-vā′rē-an). Relating to the uterine (fallopian) tube and the ovary.

tu·bo·o·var·i·ec·to·my (tū′bō-ō-var-ē-ek′to-mĭ). SYN salpingo-oophorectomy.

tu·bo·o·va·ri·tis (tū′bō-ō-va-rī′tis). SYN salpingo-oophoritis.

tu·bo·per·i·to·ne·al (tū′bō-per-i-tō-nē′ăl). Relating to the uterine (fallopian) tubes and the peritoneum.

tu·bo·plas·ty (tū′bō-plas-tē). SYN salpingoplasty.

tu·bo·tor·sion (tū′bō-tōr-shŭn). Twisting of a tubular structure, such as an oviduct. SYN tubatorsion. [tubo- + L. *torsio,* torsion]

tu·bo·tym·pan·ic, tu·bo·tym·pa·nal (tū′bō-tim-pan′ik, -tim′pă-năl). Relating to the auditory (eustachian) tube and the tympanic cavity of the ear.

tu·bo·u·ter·ine (tū′bō-ū′ter-in). Relating to a uterine (fallopian) tube and the uterus.

tu·bo·vag·i·nal (tū-bō-vaj′i-năl). Relating to a uterine (fallopian) tube and the vagina.

tu·bu·lar (tū′byū-lăr). Relating to or of the form of a tube or tubule. SYN tubuliform.

tu·bu·la·ture (tu′byū-lă-chūr). The short neck of a retort.

tu·bule (tū′byūl). A small tube. SYN tubulus. [L. *tubulus,* dim. of *tubus,* tube]

Albarran y Dominguez' t.'s, SYN Albarran's *glands,* under *gland.*

collecting t., SYN straight seminiferous t.

connecting t., a narrow arching t. of the kidney joining the distal convoluted t. and the collecting t.

convoluted t. of kidney, the highly convoluted segments of the nephron in the renal labyrinth comprising the proximal convoluted tubule, which leads from Bowman's capsule to the descending limb of Henle's loop, and the distal convoluted t., which leads from the ascending limb of Henle's loop to the collecting tube. SYN tubulus renalis contortus [NA], Ferrein's tube, tubulus contortus (1).

convoluted seminiferous t., one of two or three twisted curved t.'s in each lobule of the testis, in which spermatogenesis occurs. SYN tubulus seminiferus contortus [NA], tubulus contortus (2).

dental t.'s, SYN *canaliculi* dentales, under *canaliculus.*

dentinal t.'s, SYN *canaliculi* dentales, under *canaliculus.*

discharging t., a urinary t. formed by the union of several collecting t.'s and terminating as a papillary duct.

Henle's t.'s, the straight portions of the uriniferous t.'s that form Henle's loop, distinguished as the descending and ascending t.'s of Henle.

Kobelt's t.'s, remnants of the mesonephric t.'s in the female, contained within the epoöphoron. SYN wolffian t.'s.

malpighian t.'s, in insects, slender tubular or hairlike excretory structures that emerge from the alimentary canal between the mesenteron (midgut) and proctodeum (hindgut) in a region frequently termed the pylorus; they vary in number from 1 to over 100, and may be assorted in equally sized bundles in some insects.

mesonephric t., an excretory t. of the mesonephros. SYN segmental t.

metanephric t., an excretory unit of the metanephros or permanent kidney.

paragenital t.'s, remnants of embryonic mesonephric t.'s, some of which form the paradidymis.

pronephric t., an excretory unit of the pronephros, present only in vestigial form in human embryos.

segmental t., SYN mesonephric t.

seminiferous t., the tubulus seminiferus contortus; or the tubulus seminiferus rectus.

Skene's t.'s, the embryonic urethral glands which are the female homologue of the prostate.

spiral t., the segment of urinary t. coming next after the proximal convoluted t.

straight t., (1) one of the straight t.'s of the kidney, present in the medulla and pars radiata of the cortex; **(2)** SYN straight seminiferous t.

straight seminiferous t., the continuation of the t. seminiferus contortus which becomes straight just before entering the mediastinum to form the rete testis. SYN tubulus renalis rectus [NA], tubulus seminiferus rectus [NA], collecting t., straight t. (2), tubulus rectus (1), tubulus rectus (2), vasa recta (2).

T t., the transverse t. that passes from the sarcolemma across a myofibril of striated muscle; it is the intermediate t. of the triad.

uriniferous t., the functional unit of the kidney, composed of a long convoluted portion (nephron) and an intrarenal collecting duct.

wolffian t.'s, SYN Kobelt's t.'s.

tu·bu·li (tū′byū-lī). Plural of tubulus.

tu·bu·li·form (tū′byū-li-fōrm). SYN tubular.

tu·bu·lin (tū′byū-lin). A protein subunit of microtubules; it is a dimer composed of two globular polypeptides, α-tubulin and β-tubulin. SEE ALSO dynein.

t.-tyrosine ligase, an enzyme that covalently links a tyrosine to the C-terminal glutamyl residue of t., coupled with the hydrolysis of ATP to ADP and P_i; this is a unique posttranslational modification that may have a significant role in cytoskeletal traffic and design.

tu·bu·li·za·tion (tū′byū-li-zā′shŭn). Enclosing the joined ends of a divided nerve, after neurorrhaphy, in a cylinder of paraffin or

tu

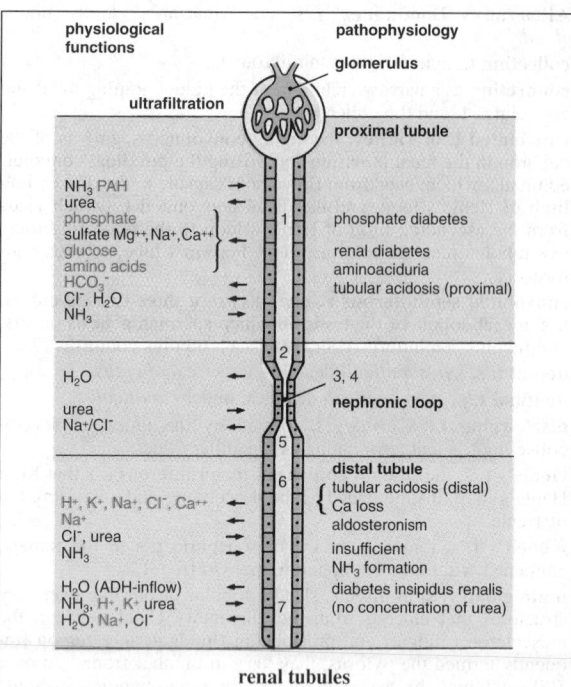

physiological functions / pathophysiology

ultrafiltration

glomerulus

proximal tubule

NH₃ PAH
urea
phosphate
sulfate Mg++, Na+, Ca++
glucose
amino acids
HCO₃⁻
Cl⁻, H₂O
NH₃

phosphate diabetes

renal diabetes
aminoaciduria
tubular acidosis (proximal)

H₂O
urea
Na+/Cl⁻

3, 4
nephronic loop

distal tubule
tubular acidosis (distal)
Ca loss
aldosteronism

insufficient
NH₃ formation
diabetes insipidus renalis
(no concentration of urea)

H+, K+, Na+, Cl⁻, Ca++
Na+
Cl⁻, urea
NH₃

H₂O (ADH-inflow)
NH₃, H+, K+ urea
H₂O, Na+, Cl⁻

renal tubules

functions and pathology; active resorption and secretion processes in *blue letters*; numbers 1–7 correspond to figure shown under *nephron*

of some slowly absorbable material to keep the surrounding tissues from pushing in and preventing union.

tu·bu·lo·cyst (tū′byū-lō-sist). A cyst formed by the dilation of any occluded canal or tube. SYN tubular cyst.

tu·bu·lo·der·moid (tū′byū-lō-der′moyd). A dermoid cyst arising from a persistent embryonal tubular structure.

tu·bu·lo·neo·gen·e·sis (tū-byū-lō-nē′ō-jen′ĕ-sis). The formation of new tubules; usually refers to proliferation of tubules in renal tumors such as Wilms' tumor or mesoblastic nephroma. [tubule + neogenesis]

tu·bu·lo·rac·e·mose (tū′byū-lō-ras′ĕ-mōs). Denoting a gland of combined tubular and racemose structure.

tu·bu·lor·rhex·is (tū′byū-lō-rek′sis). A pathologic process characterized by necrosis of the epithelial lining in localized segments of renal tubules, with focal rupture or loss of the basement membrane. [tubule + G. *rhēxis,* a breaking]

tu·bu·lose, tu·bu·lous (tū′byū-lōs, -lŭs). Having many tubules.

tu·bu·lus, pl. **tu·bu·li** (tū′byū-lŭs, -lī). SYN tubule. [L. dim. of *tubus,* a pipe]

tu′buli bilif′eri, SYN biliary *ductules,* under *ductule.*

t. contor′tus, (1) SYN convoluted *tubule* of kidney. (2) SYN convoluted seminiferous *tubule.*

tu′buli denta′les, SYN *canaliculi* dentales, under *canaliculus.*

tu′buli epooph′ori, SYN transverse *ductules* of epoöphoron, under *ductule.*

tu′buli galactoph′ori, SYN lactiferous *ducts,* under *duct.*

tu′buli lactif′eri, SYN lactiferous *ducts,* under *duct.*

tu′buli parooph′ori, SYN *ductuli* paroöphori, under *ductulus.*

t. rec′tus, (1) SYN straight seminiferous *tubule.* (2) SYN straight seminiferous *tubule.*

t. rena′lis contor′tus [NA], SYN convoluted *tubule* of kidney.

t. rena′lis rec′tus [NA], SYN straight seminiferous *tubule.*

t. seminife′rus contor′tus [NA], SYN convoluted seminiferous *tubule.*

t. seminif′erus rec′tus [NA], SYN straight seminiferous *tubule.*

t. transver′sus, a tubular invagination of the sarcolemma of skeletal or cardiac muscle fibers that surrounds myofibrils as the intermediate element of the triad; involved in transmitting the action potential from the sarcolemma to the interior of the myofibril.

tu·bus, pl. **tu·bi** (tū′bŭs, -bī). A tube or canal. [L.]

t. digesto′rius, SYN digestive *tract.*

t. medulla′ris, SYN central *canal.*

t. vertebra′lis, SYN vertebral *canal.*

Tucker, Ervin Alden, U.S. obstetrician, 1862–1902. SEE T.-McLean *forceps.*

tuft (tŭft). A cluster, clump, or bunch, as of hairs.

enamel t., a group of structures representing defects in tooth mineralization that extend from the dentino-enamel junction into the enamel to about one-half its thickness.

malpighian t., SYN glomerulus (2).

synovial t.'s, SYN synovial *villi,* under *villus.*

tuft·sin (tuf′sin). A tetrapeptide derived from the Fc region of an immunoglobulin. Tuftsin enhances macrophage functions. [*Tufts* University + -in]

tug, tug·ging (tŭg, tŭg′ing). A pulling or dragging movement or sensation.

tracheal t., (1) a downward pull of the trachea, manifested by a downward movement of the thyroid cartilage, synchronous with the action of the heart and symptomatic of aneurysm of the aortic arch; the sign is elicited most easily by drawing the cricoid cartilage upward with the thumb and forefinger while the patient sits with head thrown back and mouth closed; (2) a jerky type of inspiration seen when the intercostal muscles and the sternocostal parts of the diaphragm are paralyzed by deep general anesthesia or muscle relaxants; due to the unopposed action of the crura pulling on the dome of the diaphragm and thence on the pericardium, lung roots, and tracheobronchial tree during each inspiration.

tu·la·re·mia (tū-lă-rē′mē-ă). A disease caused by *Francisella tularensis* and transmitted to humans from rodents through the bite of a deer fly, *Chrysops discalis,* and other bloodsucking insects; can also be acquired directly through the bite of an infected animal or through handling of an infected animal carcass; symptoms, similar to those of undulant fever and plague, consist of a prolonged intermittent or remittent fever and often swelling and suppuration of the lymph nodes draining the site of infection; rabbits are an important reservoir host. SYN deer-fly disease, deer-fly fever, Pahvant Valley fever, Pahvant Valley plague, rabbit fever. [*Tulare,* Lake and County, CA, + G. *haima,* blood]

glandular t., t. with predominant lymph node infection as main manifestation.

pulmonary t., t. affecting the lungs; tularemic *pneumonia.* SYN pulmonic t.

pulmonic t., SYN pulmonary t.

tulle gras (tūl-grä′). A dressing for wounds, used chiefly in France, comprised of wide-mesh curtain net cut into squares and impregnated with soft paraffin (98 parts), balsam of Peru (1 part), and olive oil (1 part). [Fr. oily net]

Tulp (Tulpius), Nicholas (Nicolaus), Dutch anatomist, 1593–1674. SEE T.'s *valve.*

tu·me·fa·cient (tū-mĕ-fā′shent). Causing or tending to cause swelling. [L. *tume-facio,* to cause to swell, fr. *tumeo,* to swell]

tu·me·fac·tion (tū-mĕ-fak′shŭn). **1.** A swelling. SYN tumentia. **2.** SYN tumescence. [see tumefacient]

tu·me·fy (tū′mĕ-fī). To swell or to cause to swell.

tu·men·tia (tū-men′shē-ă). SYN tumefaction (1). [L. fr. *tumeo,* to swell]

tu·mes·cence (tū-mes′ens). The condition of being or becoming tumid. SYN tumefaction (2), turgescence. [L. *tumesco,* to begin to swell]

tu·mes·cent (tū-mes′ent). Denoting tumescence. SYN turgescent.

tu·mid (tū′mid). Swollen, as by congestion, edema, hyperemia. SYN turgid. [L. *tumidus*]

TUMOR

tu·mor (tū′mŏr). **1.** Any swelling or tumefaction. **2.** SYN neoplasm. **3.** One of the four signs of inflammation (t., calor, dolor, rubor) enunciated by Celsus. [L. *tumor*, a swelling]

acinar cell t., a solid and cystic t. of the pancreas, occurring in young women; t. cells contain zymogen granules.

acute splenic t., acute splenitis, enlargement, and softening of the spleen, usually due to bacteremia or severe bacterial toxemia.

adenoid t., adenoma, or neoplasm with glandlike spaces.

adenomatoid t., a small benign t. of the male epididymis and female genital tract, consisting of fibrous tissue or smooth muscle enclosing anastomosing glandlike spaces containing acid mucopolysaccharide lined by flattened cells that have ultra-structural characteristics of mesothelial cells. SYN adenofibromyoma, adenoleiomyofibroma, angiomatoid t., benign mesothelioma of genital tract, Recklinghausen's t.

adenomatoid odontogenic t., a benign epithelial odontogenic t. appearing radiographically as a well-circumscribed radiolucent-radiopaque lesion usually surrounding the crown of an impacted tooth in an adolescent or young adult; characterized histologically by columnar cells organized in a duct-like configuration interspersed with spindle-shaped cells and amyloid-like deposition that gradually undergoes dystrophic calcification. SYN adenoameloblastoma, ameloblastic adenomatoid t.

adipose t., SYN lipoma.

ameloblastic adenomatoid t., SYN adenomatoid odontogenic t.

amyloid t., SYN nodular *amyloidosis*.

angiomatoid t., SYN adenomatoid t.

aortic body t., SYN chemodectoma.

Bednar t., SYN pigmented *dermatofibrosarcoma protuberans*.

benign t., a t. that does not form metastases and does not invade and destroy adjacent normal tissue. SYN innocent t.

blood t., term sometimes used to denote an aneurysm, hemorrhagic cyst, or hematoma.

borderline t., a neoplasm of the ovary, usually arising in young women, composed of complex epithelial hyperplasia without stromas invasion; may recur if incompletely removed surgically, but is clinically less aggressive than carcinoma. SYN low malignant potential t.

Brenner t., a relatively infrequent benign neoplasm of the ovary, consisting chiefly of fibrous tissue that contains nests of cells resembling transitional type epithelium, as well as glandlike structures that contain mucin; origin is controversial, but it may arise from Walthard's cell rest; ordinarily found incidentally in ovaries removed for other reasons, especially in postmenopausal women.

Brooke's t., SYN trichoepithelioma.

brown t., a mass of fibrous tissue containing hemosiderin-pigmented macrophages and multinucleated giant cells, replacing and expanding part of a bone in primary hyperparathyroidism.

t. burden, The total mass of tumor tissue carried by a patient with cancer.

Buschke-Löwenstein t., SYN giant *condyloma*.

calcifying epithelial odontogenic t., a benign epithelial odontogenic neoplasm derived from the stratum intermedium of the enamel organ; a painless, slowly growing, mixed radiolucent-radiopaque lesion characterized histologically by cords of polyhedral epithelial cells, deposits of amyloid, and spherical calcifications. SYN Pindborg t.

carcinoid t., a usually small, slow-growing neoplasm composed of islands of rounded, oxyphilic, or spindle-shaped cells of medium size, with moderately small vesicular nuclei, and covered by intact mucosa with a yellow cut surface; neoplastic cells are frequently palisaded at the periphery of the small groups, and the latter have a tendency to infiltrate surrounding tissue. Such neoplasms occur anywhere in the gastrointestinal tract (and in the lungs and other sites), with approximately 90% in the appendix and the remainder chiefly in the ileum, but also in the stomach,

other parts of the small intestine, the colon, and the rectum; those of the appendix and small t.'s seldom metastasize, but reported incidences of metatases from other primary sites and from t.'s exceeding 2.0 cm in diameter vary from 25 to 75%; lymph nodes in the abdomen and the liver may be conspicuously involved, but metastases above the diaphragm are rare. SEE ALSO carcinoid *syndrome*. SYN argentaffinoma.

carotid body t., SYN chemodectoma.

cellular t., a t. composed mainly of closely packed cells.

cerebellopontine angle t., SYN acoustic *schwannoma*.

chemoreceptor t., SYN chemodectoma.

chromaffin t., SYN chromaffinoma.

Codman's t., chondroblastoma of the proximal humerus.

collision t., two originally separate t.'s, especially a carcinoma and a sarcoma, that appear to have developed by chance in close proximity, so that an area of mingling exists. SEE ALSO carcinosarcoma.

connective t., any t. of the connective tissue group, such as osteoma, fibroma, sarcoma.

dermal duct t., a benign small t. derived from the intradermal part of eccrine sweat gland ducts occurring often on the head and neck.

dermoid t., SYN dermoid *cyst*.

desmoid t., SYN desmoid (2).

dysembryoplastic neuroepithelial t., a rare low grade neoplasm most frequently seen in children and associated with seizures and cortical dysplasia; the often multinodular, multicystic t. is comprised of an oligodendroglial-like background with accompanying neurons.

eighth nerve t., SYN acoustic *schwannoma*.

embryonal t., embryonic t., a neoplasm, usually malignant, which arises during intrauterine or early postnatal development from an organ rudiment or immature tissue; it forms immature structures characteristic of the part from which it arises, and may form other tissues as well. The term includes neuroblastoma and Wilms' t., and is also used to include certain neoplasms presenting in later life, this usage being based on the belief that such t.'s arise from embryonic rests. SEE ALSO teratoma. SYN embryoma.

embryonal t. of ciliary body, SYN embryonal *medulloepithelioma*.

endocervical sinus t., malignant germ cell t. commonly found in the ovary. The t. arises from primitive germ cells and develops into extra-embryonic tissue resembling the yolk sac. SYN yolk sac carcinoma.

endodermal sinus t., a malignant neoplasm occurring in the gonads, in sacrococcygeal teratomas, and in the mediastinum; produces α-fetoprotein and is thought to be derived from primitive endodermal cells. SYN yolk sac t.

endometrioid t., a t. of the ovary containing epithelial or stromal elements resembling t.'s of the endometrium.

Erdheim t., SYN craniopharyngioma.

Ewing's t., a malignant neoplasm which occurs usually before the age of 20 years, about twice as frequently in males, and in about 75% of patients involves bones of the extremities, including the shoulder girdle, with a predilection for the metaphysis; histologically, there are conspicuous foci of necrosis in association with irregular masses of small, regular, rounded, or ovoid cells (2 to 3 times the diameter of erythrocytes), with very scanty cytoplasm. SYN endothelial myeloma, Ewing's sarcoma.

fecal t., SYN coproma.

fibroid t., old term for certain fibromas and leiomyomas.

giant cell t. of bone, a soft, reddish brown, sometimes malignant, osteolytic t. composed of multinucleated giant cells and ovoid or spindle-shaped cells, occurring most frequently in an end of a long tubular bone of young adults. SYN giant cell myeloma, osteoclastoma.

giant cell t. of tendon sheath, a nodule, possibly inflammatory in nature, arising commonly from the flexor sheath of the fingers and thumb; composed of fibrous tissue, lipid- and hemosiderin-containing macrophages, and multinucleated giant cells. SYN localized nodular tenosynovitis.

glomus t. [MIM*138000], an unusual vascular neoplasm composed of specialized pericytes (sometimes termed glomus cells), usually in single encapsulated nodular masses which may be several millimeters in diameter and occur almost exclusively in the skin; it is exquisitely tender and may be so painful that patients voluntarily immobilize an extremity, sometimes leading to atrophy of muscles; multiple glomus t.'s occur, sometimes with autosomal dominant inheritance. SEE ALSO glomangioma.

glomus jugulare t., SYN chemodectoma.

Godwin t., SYN benign lymphoepithelial *lesion.*

granular cell t., a microscopically specific, generally benign t., often involving peripheral nerves in skin, mucosa, or connective tissue, derived from Schwann cells; the abundant cytoplasm contains lysosomal granules, the cells infiltrate between adjacent tissues although growth is slow, and adjacent surface epithelium may show hyperplasia.

granulosa cell t., a benign or malignant t. of the ovary arising from the membrana granulosa of the graafian follicle and frequently secreting estrogen; it is soft, solid, white or yellow, and consists of small round cells sometimes enclosing Call-Exner bodies; larger lipid-containing cells may be present. SYN folliculoma (1).

Grawitz' t., old eponym for renal *adenocarcinoma.*

Gubler's t., a fusiform swelling on the wrist in lead palsy.

haarscheibe t., SYN trichodiscoma. [Ger. *Haar,* hair, + *Scheibe,* disk]

heterologous t., a t. composed of a tissue unlike that from which it springs.

hilar cell t. of ovary, a small benign masculinizing ovarian t. derived from hilar cells, which resemble Leydig cells of the testis.

histoid t., old term for a t. composed of a single type of differentiated tissue.

homologous t., a t. composed of tissue of the same sort as that from which it springs.

Hürthle cell t., a neoplasm of the thyroid gland composed of polyhedral acidophilic cells, thought by some to be oncocytes; it may be benign or malignant, the behavior of the latter depending on the general microscopic pattern, whether follicular, papillary, or undifferentiated. SEE ALSO Hürthle cell *adenoma.* SYN Hürthle cell carcinoma.

hylic t., SYN hyloma.

innocent t., SYN benign t.

interstitial cell t. of testis, SYN Leydig cell *adenoma.*

Koenen's t., SYN periungual *fibroma.*

Krukenberg's t., a metastatic carcinoma of the ovary, usually bilateral and secondary to a mucous carcinoma of the stomach, which contains signet-ring cells filled with mucus.

Landschutz t., a transplantable, possibly isoantigenic, highly virulent neoplasm which can be grown in any strain of mice; the host is killed in a few days by what is apparently an anaplastic carcinoma.

Lindau's t., SYN hemangioblastoma.

low malignant potential t., SYN borderline t.

malignant t., a t. that invades surrounding tissues, is usually capable of producing metastases, may recur after attempted removal, and is likely to cause death of the host unless adequately treated. SEE ALSO cancer.

malignant mixed müllerian t. (MMMT), SYN mixed mesodermal t.

melanotic neuroectodermal t. of infancy, a benign neoplasm of neuroectodermal origin that most often involves the anterior maxilla of infants in the first year of life. It presents clinically as a rapidly growing blue-black lesion producing a destructive radiolucency; histologically, it is characterized by small round undifferentiated t. cells interspersed with larger polyhedral melanin-producing cells arranged in an alveolar configuration. SYN melanoameloblastoma, pigmented ameloblastoma, pigmented epulis, progonoma of jaw, retinal anlage t.

Merkel cell t., a rare malignant cutaneous t. seen in sun-exposed skin of elderly patients composed of dermal nodules of small round cells with scanty cytoplasm in a trabecular pattern; the tumor cells contain cytoplasmic dense core granules resembling neurosecretory granules seen in Merkel cells. SYN primary neuroendocrine carcinoma of the skin, trabecular carcinoma.

mesonephroid t., SYN mesonephroma.

mixed t., a t. composed of two or more varieties of tissue.

mixed mesodermal t., a sarcoma of the body of the uterus arising in older women, composed of more than one mesenchymal tissue, especially including striated muscle cells. SYN malignant mixed müllerian t.

mixed t. of salivary gland, a t. composed of salivary gland epithelium and fibrous tissue with mucoid or cartilaginous areas. SYN pleomorphic adenoma.

mixed t. of skin, SYN chondroid *syringoma.*

mucoepidermoid t., SYN mucoepidermoid *carcinoma.*

Nelson t., a pituitary t. causing the symptoms of Nelson *syndrome.*

oil t., SYN lipogranuloma.

oncocytic hepatocellular t., SYN fibrolamellar liver cell *carcinoma.*

organoid t., a t. of complex structure, glandular in origin, containing epithelium, connective tissue, etc.

Pancoast t., an adenocarcinoma of a lung apex causing Pancoast syndrome. SYN superior pulmonary sulcus t.

papillary t., SYN papilloma.

paraffin t., SYN paraffinoma.

pearl t., obsolete term for cholesteatoma.

phantom t., accumulation of fluid in the interlobar spaces of the lung, secondary to congestive heart failure, radiologically simulating a neoplasm.

phyllodes t., a spectrum of neoplasms consisting of a mixture of benign epithelium and stroma with variable cellularity and cytologic abnormalities, ranging from benign phyllodes t. to cytosarcoma phyllodes; most often involves the breast.

pilar t. of scalp, a solitary t. of the scalp in elderly women that may ulcerate; microscopically resembles squamous cell carcinoma composed of glycogen-rich clear cells, but is benign. SYN proliferating tricholemmal cyst.

Pindborg t., SYN calcifying epithelial odontogenic t.

Pinkus t., SYN fibroepithelioma.

placental site trophoblastic t., a t. usually arising in the uterus of parous women during reproductive years. Histologically, the t. consists of a predominance of intermediate trophoblastic cells with fibrinoid material and vascular invasion.

pontine angle t., a t. in the angle formed by the cerebellum and the lateral pons, often refers to an acoustic schwannoma.

potato t. of neck, a firm nodular mass in the neck, usually a carotid body t. (chemodectoma).

Pott's puffy t., a circumscribed swelling of the scalp indicating an underlying osteitis of the skull or an extradural abscess.

pregnancy t., SYN *granuloma* gravidarum.

primitive neuroectodermal t., a designation used to refer to a group of morphologically similar embryonal neoplasms that arise in intracranial and peripheral sites of the nervous system and which may show various degrees of cellular differentiation; includes medulloblastoma, pineoblastoma, etc.

ranine t., SYN ranula (2).

Rathke's pouch t., SYN craniopharyngioma.

Recklinghausen's t., SYN adenomatoid t.

retinal anlage t., SYN melanotic neuroectodermal t. of infancy.

Rous t., SYN Rous *sarcoma.*

sand t., SYN psammomatous *meningioma.*

Sertoli cell t., SYN androblastoma (1).

solitary fibrous t., a benign t. of fibrous tissue which usually arises in the pleural space on other sites. SYN benign mesothelioma.

squamous odontogenic t., a benign epithelial odontogenic t. thought to arise from the epithelial cell rests of Malassez; appears clinically as a radiolucent lesion closely associated with the tooth root and histologically as islands of squamous epithelium enclosed by a peripheral layer of flattened cells.

sugar t., a benign clear cell t. of the lung containing abundant glycogen.

superior pulmonary sulcus t., SYN Pancoast t.

teratoid t., SYN teratoma.

theca cell t., SYN thecoma.

transmissible venereal t., SYN canine venereal *granuloma*.

triton t., a peripheral nerve t. with striated muscle differentiation, seen most often in neurofibromatosis; named after Masson's theory of transformation of motor nerve fibers into muscle in triton salamanders.

turban t., cylindroma of the scalp which, when overgrown, may resemble a turban.

villous t., SYN villous *papilloma*.

Warthin's t., SYN adenolymphoma.

Wilms' t., a malignant renal t. of young children, composed of small spindle cells and various other types of tissue, including tubules and, in some cases, structures resembling fetal glomeruli, and striated muscle and cartilage. Often inherited as an autosomal dominant trait [MIM*194070, *194080, *194090]. SYN adenomyosarcoma, embryoma of the kidney, nephroblastoma.

wing-beating t., a coarse, irregular t. that is most prominent when the limbs are held outstretched, reminiscent of a bird flapping its wings; due to up and down excursion of arm at abducted shoulder. Seen mainly with Wilson's disease.

Yaba t., a poxvirus-induced neoplasm of monkeys caused by the Yaba monkey virus, a member of the family Poxviridae; tumor-like growths occur chiefly on the head and limbs; the natural disease has been reported only in Africa in monkeys kept outdoors.

yolk sac t., SYN endodermal sinus t.

Zollinger-Ellison t., a non-beta cell t. of pancreatic islets causing the Zollinger-Ellison syndrome.

tu·mor·af·fin (tū′mŏr-af′in). SYN oncotropic. [tumor + L. *affinis,* related to]

tu·mor·i·ci·dal (tū′mŏr-i-sī′dăl). Denoting an agent destructive to tumors. [tumor + L. *caedo,* to kill]

tu·mor·i·gen·e·sis (tū′mŏr-i-jen′ĕ-sis). Production of a new growth or growths. [tumor + G. *genesis,* origin]

foreign body t., induction of malignant tumors in tissues by nonviable, nonabsorable solid material not known to contain a chemical carcinogen.

tu·mor·i·gen·ic (tū′mŏr-i-jen′ik). Causing or producing tumors.

tu·mor·lets (tū′mŏr-lets). Minute foci of atypical bronchiolar epithelial hyperplasia that are found multifocally; although now considered benign, they were once believed to be precursors of carcinoma.

tu·mor·ous (tū′mŏr-ŭs). Swollen; tumor-like; protuberant.

tu·mul·tus cor·dis (tū-mŭl′tŭs kŏr′dis). Palpitation and irregular action of the heart.

Tun·ga pen·e·trans (tŭng′ă pen′ĕ-tranz). A member of the flea family, Tungidae, commonly known as chigger flea, sand flea, chigoe, or jiggers; the minute female penetrates the skin, frequently under the toenails; as she becomes distended with eggs to about pea size, a painful ulcer with inflammation develops at the site. SYN *Sarcopsylla penetrans.*

tun·gi·a·sis (tŭng-ī′ă-sis). Infestation with sand fleas (*Tunga penetrans*)

Tung·i·dae (tŭng′i-dē). A family of fleas containing the jigger or chigoe flea species, *Tunga penetrans.*

tung·state (tŭng′stāt). An anionic form of tungsten.

calcium t., a phosphor with a high stopping power for x-rays that was formerly used widely in fluoroscopic screens and intensifying screens for radiography.

tung·sten (W) (tŭng′sten). A metallic element, atomic no. 74, atomic wt. 183.85. SYN wolfram, wolframium. [Swed. *tung,* heavy, + *sten,* stone]

t. carbide, one of the hardest known materials, used as an abrasive and in the manufacture of dental cutting instruments.

tu·nic (tū′nik). Coat or covering; one of the enveloping layers of a part, especially one of the coats of a blood vessel or other tubular structure. SYN tunica [NA]. [L. *tunica*]

Bichat's t., the tunica intima of the blood vessels.

Brücke's t., SYN *tunica* nervea.

fibrous t. of corpus spongiosum, SYN *tunica* albuginea of corpus spongiosum.

fibrous t. of eye, the outer layer of the eyeball composed of the sclera and cornea. SYN tunica fibrosa bulbi [NA], tunica externa oculi.

mucosal t.'s, mucous t.'s, SYN mucosa.

muscular t.'s, SEE muscular *coat*.

muscular t. of gallbladder, muscular t. of the gallbladder, consisting of layers of smooth muscle fibers coursing in various directions immediately external to the mucosa of the gallbladder.

nervous t. of eyeball, SYN retina.

serous t., SYN serosa.

vascular t. of eye, the vascular, pigmentary, or middle coat of the eye, comprising the choroid, ciliary body, and iris. SYN tunica vasculosa bulbi [NA], Haller's tunica vasculosa, tunica vasculosa oculi, uvea, uveal tract.

TUNICA

tu·ni·ca, pl. **tu·ni·cae** (tū′ni-kă, -kē) [NA]. SYN tunic. [L. a coat]

t. abdomina′lis, the aponeurosis of the abdominal muscles of quadrupeds.

t. adventi′tia [NA], SYN adventitia.

t. albugin′ea [NA], a dense white collagenous tunic surrounding a structure.

t. albuginea of corpora cavernosi, a strong, fibrous membrane enveloping the corpora cavernosa penis. SYN t. albuginea corporum cavernosorum [NA].

t. albugin′ea cor′poris spongio′si [NA], SYN t. albuginea of corpus spongiosum.

t. albugin′ea cor′porum cavernoso′rum [NA], SYN t. albuginea of corpora cavernosi.

t. albuginea of corpus spongiosum, the thick layer of fibrous tissue surrounding the corpus spongiosum penis; it is thinner than the corresponding layer around each corpus cavernosum. SYN t. albuginea corporis spongiosi [NA], fibrous tunic of corpus spongiosum.

t. albugin′ea oc′uli, SYN sclera.

t. albugin′ea tes′tis [NA], SYN t. albuginea of testis.

t. albuginea of testis, a thick white fibrous membrane forming the outer coat of the testis. SYN t. albuginea testis [NA], peridydimis.

t. car′nea, SYN dartos *fascia*.

t. conjuncti′va [NA], SYN conjunctiva.

t. conjuncti′va bul′bi [NA], SYN bulbar *conjunctiva*.

t. conjuncti′va palpebra′rum [NA], SYN palpebral *conjunctiva*.

t. dar′tos [NA], SYN dartos *fascia*. SEE ALSO *dartos* muliebris.

t. elas′tica, t. media of large arteries.

t. exter′na [NA], **(1)** the outer of two or more enveloping layers of any structure; **(2)** specifically, the outer fibroelastic coat of a blood or lymph vessel. SYN t. extima.

t. exter′na oc′uli, SYN fibrous *tunic* of eye.

t. exter′na the′cae follic′uli, the external fibrous layer of the theca of a well-developed vesicular ovarian follicle; the cells and fibers are arranged in a concentric fashion. SYN theca externa.

t. ex′tima, SYN t. externa.

t. fibro′sa [NA], SYN fibrous *capsule*.

t. fibro′sa bul′bi [NA], SYN fibrous *tunic* of eye.

t. fibro′sa hep′atis [NA], SYN fibrous *capsule* of liver (2).

t. fibro′sa lie′nis [NA], ⍟official alternate term for fibrous *capsule* of spleen, fibrous *capsule* of spleen.

t. fibro′sa re′nis, SYN fibrous *capsule* of kidney.

t. fibro′sa sple′nis [NA], SYN fibrous *capsule* of spleen.

tu′nicae funic′uli spermat′ici [NA], SYN *coverings* of spermatic cord, under *covering*.

Haller's t. vasculosa, SYN vascular *tunic* of eye.

t. inter′na bul′bi [NA], SYN retina.

t. inter′na the′cae follic′uli, the inner cellular and vascular layer of the vesicular ovarian follicle; there is evidence that the epithelioid cells produce estrogen and contribute to the formation of the corpus luteum after ovulation. SYN theca interna.

t. in′tima [NA], the innermost coat of a blood or lymphatic vessel; it consists of endothelium, usually a thin fibroelastic subendothelial layer, and an inner elastic membrane or longitudinal fibers.

t. me′dia [NA], the middle, usually muscular, coat of an artery or other tubular structure. SYN media (1).

t. muco′sa [NA], SYN mucosa.

t. muco′sa bronchio′rum [NA], SYN mucosa of bronchi.

t. muco′sa cavita′tis tym′pani [NA], SYN mucosa of tympanic cavity.

t. muco′sa co′li [NA], SYN mucosa of *colon*.

t. muco′sa duc′tus deferen′tis [NA], SYN *mucosa* of ductus deferens.

t. muco′sa esoph′agi [NA], SYN esophageal *mucosa*.

t. muco′sa gas′trica [ventric′uli] [NA], SYN gastric *mucosa*.

t. muco′sa intesti′ni ten′uis [NA], SYN *mucosa* of small intestine.

t. muco′sa laryn′gis [NA], SYN laryngeal *mucosa*.

t. muco′sa lin′guae [NA], SYN lingual *mucosa*.

t. muco′sa na′si [NA], SYN nasal *mucosa*.

t. muco′sa o′ris [NA], SYN oral *mucosa*.

t. muco′sa pharyn′gis [NA], SYN pharyngeal *mucosa*.

t. muco′sa tra′cheae [NA], SYN tracheal *mucosa*.

t. muco′sa tu′bae auditi′vae [NA], SYN *mucosa* of auditory tube.

t. muco′sa tu′bae uteri′nae [NA], SYN *mucosa* of uterine tube.

t. muco′sa ure′teris [NA], SYN *mucosa* of ureter.

t. muco′sa ure′thrae femini′nae [NA], SYN *mucosa* of female urethra.

t. muco′sa u′teri [NA], SYN endometrium.

t. muco′sa vagi′nae [NA], SYN vaginal *mucosa*.

t. muco′sa vesi′cae bilia′ris [NA], SYN *mucosa* of gallbladder.

t. muco′sa vesi′cae fel′leae [NA], ⋆official alternate term for *mucosa* of gallbladder, *mucosa* of gallbladder.

t. muco′sa vesi′cae urina′riae [NA], SYN *mucosa* of urinary bladder.

t. muco′sa vesic′ulae semina′lis [NA], SYN *mucosa* of seminal vesicle.

t. muscula′ris [NA], SYN muscular *coat*.

t. muscula′ris bronchio′rum [NA], SYN muscular *coat* of bronchi.

t. muscula′ris co′li [NA], SYN muscular *coat* of colon.

t. muscula′ris duc′tus deferen′tis [NA], SYN muscular *coat* of ductus deferens.

t. muscula′ris esoph′agi [NA], SYN muscular *coat* of esophagus.

t. muscula′ris gas′trica [NA], SYN muscular *coat* of stomach.

t. muscula′ris intesti′ni ten′uis [NA], SYN muscular *coat* of small intestine.

t. muscula′ris pharyn′gis [NA], SYN muscular *coat* of pharynx.

t. muscula′ris rec′ti [NA], SYN muscular *coat* of rectum.

t. muscula′ris tra′cheae [NA], SYN muscular *coat* of trachea.

t. muscula′ris tu′bae uteri′nae [NA], SYN muscular *coat* of uterine tube.

t. muscula′ris ure′teris [NA], SYN muscular *coat* of ureter.

t. muscula′ris ure′thrae femini′nae [NA], SYN muscular *coat* of female urethra.

t. muscula′ris u′teri [NA], SYN myometrium.

t. muscula′ris vagi′nae [NA], SYN muscular *coat* of vagina.

t. muscula′ris ventric′uli, ⋆official alternate term for muscular *coat* of stomach.

t. muscula′ris vesi′cae bilia′ris [NA], SYN muscular *coat* of gallbladder.

t. muscula′ris vesi′cae fel′leae [NA], ⋆official alternate term for muscular *coat* of gallbladder.

t. muscula′ris vesi′cae urina′riae [NA], SYN muscular *coat* of urinary bladder.

t. ner′vea, an older term, formerly used to designate the retina exclusive of the layer of rods and cones. SYN Brücke's tunic.

t. pro′pria, the special envelope of a part as distinguished from the peritoneal or other investment common to several parts.

t. pro′pria co′rii, SYN *stratum* reticulare corii.

t. pro′pria lie′nis, SYN fibrous *capsule* of spleen.

t. reflex′a, the reflected layer of the t. vasculosa testis that lines the scrotum.

t. sclerot′ica, SYN sclera.

t. sero′sa [NA], SYN serosa.

t. sero′sa co′li [NA], SYN *serosa* of colon.

t. sero′sa gas′trica [NA], SYN *serosa* of stomach.

t. sero′sa hep′atis [NA], SYN *serosa* of liver.

t. sero′sa intesti′ni ten′uis [NA], SYN *serosa* of small intestine.

t. sero′sa peritone′i [NA], SYN serous *layer* of peritoneum.

t. sero′sa tu′bae uteri′nae [NA], SYN *serosa* of uterine tube.

t. sero′sa u′teri [NA], SYN perimetrium, *serosa* of uterus.

t. sero′sa ventric′uli [NA], ⋆official alternate term for *serosa* of stomach.

t. sero′sa vesi′cae bilia′ris [NA], SYN *serosa* of gallbladder.

t. sero′sa vesi′cae fel′leae [NA], ⋆official alternate term for *serosa* of gallbladder.

t. sero′sa vesi′cae urina′riae [NA], SYN *serosa* of urinary bladder.

t. submuco′sa, SYN submucosa.

t. vagina′lis commu′nis, SYN internal spermatic *fascia*.

t. vagina′lis tes′tis [NA], the serous sheath of the testis and epididymis, derived from the peritoneum; it consists of outer parietal and inner visceral serous layers.

t. vasculo′sa, any vascular layer.

t. vasculo′sa bul′bi [NA], SYN vascular *tunic* of eye.

t. vasculo′sa len′tis, a nutrient vascular layer enveloping the lens of the eye in the fetus.

t. vasculo′sa oc′uli, SYN vascular *tunic* of eye.

t. vasculo′sa tes′tis, the vascular layer enveloping the testis beneath the t. albuginea.

t. vit′rea, SYN posterior limiting *layer* of cornea.

---

tun·nel (tŭn′ĕl). An elongated passageway, usually open at both ends.

aortico-left ventricular t., congenital connection between the aorta above exit of coronary arteries and the left ventricle.

carpal t., the passageway deep to the transverse carpal ligament between tubercles of the scaphoid and trapezoid bones on the radial side and the pisiform and hook of the hamate on the ulnar side, through which the median nerve and the flexor tendons of the fingers and thumb pass; compression of the median nerve may occur here (carpal tunnel syndrome). SYN canalis carpi [NA], carpal canal (1).

Corti's t., the spiral canal in the organ of Corti, formed by the outer and inner pillar cells or rods of Corti; it is filled with fluid and occasionally crossed by nonmedullated nerve fibers. SYN Corti's canal.

Tuohy, Edward B., 20th century U.S. anesthesiologist. SEE T. *needle*.

tu·ran·ose (tūr′ă-nōs). 3-*O*-α-D-Glucopyranosyl-D-fructose; a reducing disaccharide.

Tur·ba·trix (ter-bā′triks). A genus of free-living nematodes in the family Cephalobidae; it includes the species *T. aceti* (the vinegar eel), found in old vinegar or in rotting fruits and vegetables. [L. *turbare,* to disturb]

tur·bid (ter′bid). Cloudy, as by sediment or insoluble matter in a solution. [L. *turbidus,* confused, disordered]

tur·bi·dim·e·ter (ter-bi-dim′ĕ-ter). An instrument for measuring turbidity.

tur·bi·di·met·ric (ter′bid-i-met′rik). Pertaining to the measurement of turbidity.

tur·bi·dim·e·try (ter-bi-dim′ĕ-trē). A method for determining the concentration of a substance in a solution by the degree of cloudiness or turbidity it causes or by the degree of clarification it induces in a turbid solution. [turbidity + G. *metron*, measure]

tur·bid·i·ty (ter-bid'i-tē). The quality of being turbid, of losing transparency because of sediment or insoluble matter. [L. *turbiditas*, fr. *turbidus*, turbid]

tur·bi·nal (ter'bi-năl). SYN turbinated *body* (1).

tur·bi·nate (ter'bi-nāt). A bone shaped like a top, especially referring to turbinated bones. SEE inferior nasal *concha*, middle nasal *concha*, superior nasal *concha*, supreme nasal *concha*.

tur·bi·nat·ed (ter'bi-nāt-ed). Scroll-shaped. [L. *turbinatus*, shaped like a top]

tur·bi·nec·to·my (ter'bi-nek'tō-mē). Surgical removal of a turbinated bone. [turbinate + G. *ektomē*, excision]

tur·bi·no·tome (ter'bi-nō-tōm). An instrument for use in turbinotomy or turbinectomy.

tur·bi·not·o·my (ter'bi-not'ō-mē). Incision into or excision of a turbinated body. [turbinate + G. *tomē*, incision]

Türck, Ludwig, Austrian neurologist, 1810–1868. SEE T.'s *bundle, column, degeneration, tract.*

Turcot syn·drome. See under syndrome.

tur·ges·cence (ter-jes'ens). SYN tumescence. [L. *turgesco*, to begin to swell, fr. *turgeo*, to swell]

tur·ges·cent (ter-jes'ent). SYN tumescent.

tur·gid (ter'jid). SYN tumid. [L. *turgidus*, swollen, fr. *turgeo*, to swell]

tur·gom·e·ter (ter-gom'ĕ-ter). A device for measuring turgor, or turgescence, particularly of the skin. [turgor + G. *metron*, measure]

tur·gor (ter'gōr). Fullness. [L., fr. *turgeo*, to swell]
  t. vita'lis, the normal fullness of the capillaries.

tu·ris·ta (tū-rēs'tă). Term for traveler's *diarrhea*, of Mexican derivation. [Sp. tourist]

Türk, Siegmund, 20th century Swiss ophthalmologist. SEE Ehrlich-T. *line.*

Türk, Wilhelm, Austrian hematologist, 1871–1916. SEE T. *cell;* T.'s *leukocyte.*

tur·key red (ter'kē). SYN madder.

tur·mer·ic (ter'mer-ik). Curcuma.

turn (tern). To revolve or cause to revolve; specifically, to change the position of the fetus within the uterus to convert a malpresentation into a presentation permitting normal delivery. [A.S. *tyrnan*]

Turner, George Grey, English surgeon, 1877–1951. SEE Grey T.'s *sign.*

Turner, Henry H., U.S. endocrinologist, 1892–1970. SEE T.'s *syndrome.*

Turner, Joseph G., English dentist, †1955. SEE T.'s *tooth.*

Turner, Sir William, English anatomist, 1832–1916. SEE intraparietal *sulcus* of Turner, Turner's *sulcus.*

turn·o·ver (tern'ō-ver). The quantity of a material metabolized or processed, usually within a given length of time.

tur·pen·tine (ter'pen-tīn). An oleoresin from *Pinus palustris* and other species of *Pinus;* source of t. oil and a constituent of stimulating ointments. [G. *terebinthinos*, pertaining to *terebinthos*, the terebinth tree]
  Canada t., SYN Canada *balsam.*
  Chian t., an exudation from *Pistacia terebinthus*, a small tree of Chios and regions eastward; on exposure to air it thickens and forms translucent yellow masses similar to mastic.
  larch t., a transparent, yellowish, thick liquid, the oleoresin obtained from *Larix europaea* (family Pinaceae). SYN Venice t.
  Venice t., SYN larch t.
  white t., t. from *Pinus palustris.*

tur·pen·tine oil. A volatile oil, distilled from turpentine, that has been used as a diuretic, carminative, vermifuge, expectorant, rubefacient, and counterirritant. SYN oleum terebinthinae, turpentine spirit.
  rectified t. o., obtained by treating t. o. with sodium hydroxide, and redistilling; used externally as a counterirritant.

tur·pen·tine spir·it. SYN turpentine oil.

turps (terps). Popular name for turpentine oil.

tur·ri·ceph·a·ly (tūr-i-sef'ă-lē). SYN oxycephaly. [L. *turris*, tower, + G. *kephalē*, head]

tu·run·da, pl. **tu·run·dae** (tū-rŭn'dă, -dē). A surgical tent, gauze drain, or tampon. [L.]

tush, tusk (tŭsh, tŭsk). A canine tooth in the horse, pig, or muskdeer; an incisor in the elephant and walrus.

tus·sal (tŭs'ăl). SYN tussive.

tus·sic·u·lar (tŭ-sik'yū-lăr). SYN tussive. [L. *tussicularis*, fr. *tussicula*, a slight cough, dim. of *tussis*, cough]

tus·sic·u·la·tion (tŭ-sik'yū-lā'shŭn). A hacking cough.

tus·si·gen·ic (tus'ĭ-jen'ik). Causing cough. [L. *tussis*, cough, + *-gen*, producing]

tus·sis (tŭs'is). A cough. [L.]

tus·sive (tŭs'siv). Relating to a cough. SYN tussal, tussicular. [L. *tussis*, a cough]

tu·ta·men, pl. **tu·ta·mi·na** (tū-tā'men, -tā'mi-nă). Any defensive or protective structure. [L. protection]
  tuta'mina cer'ebri, the scalp, cranium, and cerebral meninges.
  tuta'mina oc'uli, the eyebrows, eyelids, and eyelashes.

Tuttle, James P., U.S. surgeon, 1857–1913. SEE T.'s *proctoscope.*

TUU Abbreviation for transureteroureterostomy.

TVG Abbreviation for time-varied *gain.*

Tweed, Charles H., U.S. orthodontist, 1895–1970. SEE T. edgewise *treatment, triangle.*

tweez·ers (twē'zerz). An instrument with pincers that are squeezed together to grasp or extract fine structures. [A.S. *twisel*, fork]

twig. One of the finer terminal branches of an artery; a small branch or small ramus. [A.S.]

twi·light (twī'līt). **1.** Figuratively, a faint light. **2.** Pertaining to faint or indistinct mental perception, as in twilight *state.* [A.S. *twi-*, two]

twin. **1.** One of two children born at one birth. **2.** Double; growing in pairs. [A.S. *getwin*, double]

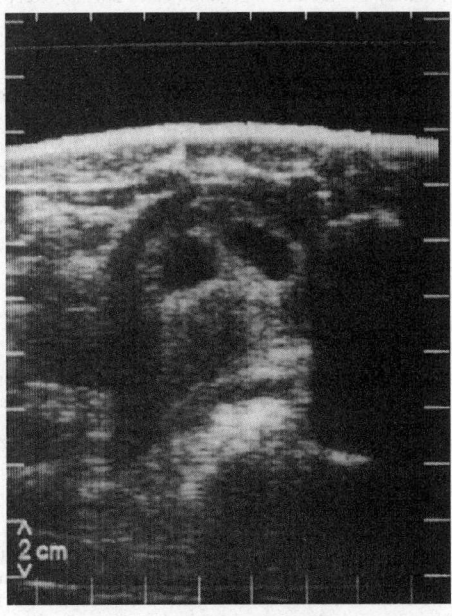

twins
sonogram of twins *in utero* (8th week): an embryo with moving heart is apparent in both amniotic sacs

allantoidoangiopagous t.'s, unequal monochorial t.'s with fu-

classification of conjoined twins		
Terata catadidyma	Terata anadidyma	Terata ancatadidyma
joined by lower part of body, or twins single in lower body and double in upper body	single in upper body and double in lower body, or joined by some body part	united at midpoint of body
a) pygopagus back to back, coccyx and sacrum fused	a) cephalopagus fused in the cranial vault	a) thoracopagus attached along part of thoracic wall; thoracic and abdominal organs may be abnormal
b) ischiopagus inferior parts of coccyx and sacrum fused; separate vertebral columns lying in same axis	b) syncephalus fused at the face; may also be joined by thorax (cephalo-thoracopagus)	b) omphalopagus attached from umbilicus to xiphoid cartilage
c) dicephalus two separate heads on one body	c) dipygus single head, thorax, and/or abdomen; pelvis, external genitalia, and limbs are duplicate	c) rachipagus attached at the vertebral column above the sacrum
d) diprosopus two faces with one head and one body		

sion of their allantoic vessels within the placenta; the lesser t. is essentially a parasite on the placental circulation of the larger t.

conjoined t.'s, monozygotic t.'s with varying extent of union and different degrees of residual duplication. The various types of union are named by the use of a prefix designating the region that is united and adding the suffix *-pagus,* meaning fused (*e.g.,* craniopagus, thoracopagus); the various types of residual duplication are named by designating the parts duplicated and adding the suffix *-didymus,* or *-dymus,* meaning twin (*e.g.,* cephalodidymus, cephalodymus).

conjoined asymmetrical t.'s, SYN conjoined unequal t.'s.

conjoined equal t.'s, conjoined t.'s in which both members are approximately of the same size, and nearly normal except for the areas of fusion. SYN conjoined symmetrical t.'s.

conjoined symmetrical t.'s, SYN conjoined equal t.'s.

conjoined unequal t.'s, conjoined t.'s in which one member is nearly normal (host or autosite) and the other (parasite) is small, incomplete, and dependent for its nutrition upon the more nearly normal member. SYN conjoined asymmetrical t.'s.

dichorial t.'s, SYN dizygotic t.'s.

diovular t.'s, SYN dizygotic t.'s.

dizygotic t.'s, t.'s derived from two separate zygotes. SYN dichorial t.'s, diovular t.'s, fraternal t.'s, heterologous t.'s.

enzygotic t.'s, SYN monozygotic t.'s.

fraternal t.'s, SYN dizygotic t.'s.

heterologous t.'s, SYN dizygotic t.'s.

identical t.'s, SYN monozygotic t.'s.

incomplete conjoined t.'s, conjoined t.'s, the two components of which equal one another but are less than entire individuals.

monoamniotic t.'s, t.'s within a common amnion; such t.'s are monovular in origin and may be conjoined.

monochorial t.'s, SYN monozygotic t.'s.

monovular t.'s, SYN monozygotic t.'s.

monozygotic t.'s, t.'s resulting from a single fertilized ovum that at an early stage of development becomes separated into independently growing cell aggregations giving rise to two individuals of the same sex and identical genetic constitution. SYN enzygotic t.'s, identical t.'s, monochorial t.'s, monovular t.'s, uniovular t.'s.

omphaloangiopagous t.'s, obsolete term for allantoidoangiopagous t.'s.

parasitic t., the smaller of unequal conjoined t.'s.

placental parasitic t., SYN omphalosite.

polyzygotic t.'s, t.'s resulting from fertilization of more than two ova discharged in a single ovulating cycle.

Siamese t.'s, originally, a much publicized conjoined pair of t.'s (xiphopagus) from Siam in the 19th century; this term has since come into general lay usage for any type of conjoined t.'s, but is incorrect.

uniovular t.'s, SYN monozygotic t.'s.

twinge (twinj). A sudden momentary sharp pain.

twin·ning. Production of equivalent structures by division; the tendency of divided parts to assume symmetrical relations.

twitch. **1.** To jerk spasmodically. **2.** A momentary spasmodic contraction of a muscle fiber. [A.S. *twiccian*]

Twort, Frederick W., British bacteriologist, 1877–1950. SEE T. *phenomenon;* T.-d'Herelle *phenomenon.*

TX Abbreviation for individual thromboxanes, designated by capital letters with subscripts indicating structural features.

ty·ba·mate (tī'bă-māt). 2-(Hydroxymethyl)-2-methylpentyl butylcarbamate carbamate; a tranquilizer related to meprobamate.

ty·le (tī'lē). SYN callosity. [G. *tylē,* a swelling, a callus]

ty·lec·to·my (tī-lek'tō-mē). Surgical removal of a localized swelling or tumor. SEE ALSO lumpectomy. [G. *tylē,* lump, + *ektomē,* excision]

tyl·i·on, pl. **tyl·ia** (til'ē-on, -lē-ă; tī'lē-on). A craniometric point at the middle of the anterior edge of the chiasmatic groove. [G. a small pin, dim. of *tylē,* a lump]

ty·lo·ma (tī-lō'mă). SYN callosity. [G. a callus]

t. conjuncti'vae, localized keratinization of the conjunctiva, occurring in xerosis of the conjunctiva.

ty·lo·sis, pl. **ty·lo·ses** (tī-lō'sis, -sēz). Formation of a callosity (tyloma). [G. a becoming callous]

t. cilia'ris, SYN pachyblepharon.

t. ling'uae, leukoplakia of the tongue.

t. palma'ris et planta'ris, SYN palmoplantar *keratoderma.*

ty·lot·ic (tī-lot'ik). Relating to or marked by tylosis.

ty·lox·a·pol (tī-lok'să-pol). Oxyethylated *tert*-octylphenol formaldehyde polymer; a detergent and mucolytic agent used as an aerosol to liquify sputum.

ty·maz·o·line (tī-maz'ō-lēn). 2-[(Thymyloxy)methyl]-2-imidazoline; a nasal decongestant.

tympan-. SEE tympano-.

tym·pa·nal (tim'pă-năl). **1.** SYN tympanic (1). **2.** Resonant. **3.** SYN tympanitic (2).

tym·pa·nec·to·my (tim′pă-nek′tō-mē). Excision of the tympanic membrane. [tympan- + G. *ektomē,* excision]

tym·pan·ia (tim-pan′ē-ă). SYN tympanites.

tym·pan·ic (tim-pan′ik). **1.** Relating to the tympanic cavity or membrane. SYN tympanal (1). **2.** Resonant. **3.** SYN tympanitic (2).

tym·pan·i·chord (tim-pan′i-kōrd). SYN *chorda* tympani.

tym·pan·i·chor·dal (tim-pan-i-kōr′dăl). Relating to the chorda tympani nerve.

tym·pa·nic·i·ty (tim′pă-nis′i-tē). The quality of being tympanic or drumlike in tone.

tym·pa·nism (tim′pă-nizm). SYN tympanites.

tym·pa·ni·tes (tim-pă-nī′tēz). Swelling of the abdomen from gas in the intestinal or peritoneal cavity. SYN meteorism, tympania, tympanism. [L. fr. G. *tympanitēs,* an edema in which the belly is stretched like a drum, *tympanon*]

uterine t., SYN physometra.

tym·pa·nit·ic (tim-pă-nit′ik). **1.** Referring to tympanites. SYN tympanous. **2.** Denoting the quality of sound elicited by percussing over the inflated intestine or a large pulmonary cavity. SYN tympanal (3), tympanic (3).

tym·pa·ni·tis (tim-pă-nī′tis). SYN myringitis.

⌂**tympano-, tympan-, tympani-.** Tympanum, tympanites. [G. *tympanon,* drum]

tym·pa·no·cen·te·sis (tim′pă-nō-sen-tē′sis). Puncture of the tympanic membrane with a needle to aspirate middle ear fluid. [tympano- + G. *kentēsis,* puncture]

tym·pa·no·eu·sta·chian (tim′pă-nō-ū-stā′shŭn, -stā′kē-an). Relating to the tympanic cavity and the auditory tube.

tym·pa·no·hy·al (tim′pă-nō-hī′ăl). Pertaining to the relationship between the tympanic cavity and the hyoid arch.

tym·pa·no·mal·le·al (tim′pă-nō-mal′ē-ăl). Relating to the tympanic membrane and the malleus.

tym·pa·no·man·dib·u·lar (tim′pă-nō-man-dib′yū-lăr). Relating to the tympanic cavity and the mandible.

tym·pa·no·mas·toid (tim′pă-nō-mas′toyd). Relating to the tympanic cavity and the mastoid cells.

tym·pa·no·mas·toid·i·tis (tim′pă-nō-mas-toy-dī′tis). Inflammation of the middle ear and the mastoid cells.

tym·pa·no·me·a·to·mas·toid·ec·to·my (tim′pă-nō-mē′ă-tō-mas-toy-dek′tō-mē). SYN radical *mastoidectomy.*

tym·pa·no·pho·nia, tym·pa·noph·o·ny (tim′pă-nō-fō′nē-ă, tim′pă-nof′ō-nē). **1.** SYN *tinnitus* aurium. **2.** SYN autophony. [tympano- + G. *phōne,* sound]

tym·pa·no·plas·ty (tim′pă-nō-plas-tē). Operative correction of a damaged middle ear. [tympano- + G. *plassō,* to form]

tym·pa·no·squa·mo·sal (tim′pă-nō-skwā-mō′săl). Relating to the tympanic and squamous parts of the temporal bone. SYN squamotympanic.

tym·pa·no·sta·pe·di·al (tim′pă-nō-stā-pē′dē-ăl). Relating to the tympanic cavity and the stapes.

tym·pan·os·to·my (tim-pan-os′tō-mē). SYN myringotomy. [tympano- + G. *ostium,* mouth]

tym·pa·no·tem·po·ral (tim′pă-nō-tem′pō-răl). Relating to the tympanic cavity and the temporal region or bone.

tym·pa·not·o·my (tim′pă-not′-ō-mē). SYN myringotomy. [tympano- + G. *tomē,* incision]

tym·pa·nous (tim′pă-nŭs). SYN tympanitic (1).

tym·pa·num, pl. **tym·pa·na, tym·pa·nums** (tim′pă-nŭm, tim′pă-nă). SYN tympanic *cavity.* [L., fr. G. *tympanon,* a drum]

tym·pa·ny (tim′pă-nē). A low-pitched, resonant, drumlike note obtained by percussing the surface of a large air-containing space, such as the distended abdomen or the thorax with or without pneumothorax. SYN tympanitic resonance.

Skoda's t., SYN skodaic *resonance.*

Tyndall, John, English physicist, 1820–1893. SEE T. *effect;* tyndallization; T. *phenomenon.*

tyn·dal·li·za·tion (tin′dăl-i-zā′shŭn). SYN fractional *sterilization.* [John *Tyndall*]

type (tīp). **1.** The usual form, or a composite form, that all others of the class resemble more or less closely; a model, denoting

especially a disease or a symptom complex giving the stamp or characteristic to a class. SEE ALSO constitution, habitus, personality. **2.** In chemistry, a substance in which the arrangement of the atoms in a molecule may be taken as representative of other substances in that class. [G. *typos,* a mark, a model]

basic personality t., (1) an individual's unique, covert, or underlying personality propensities, whether or not they are behaviorally manifest or overt; **(2)** personality characteristics of an individual which are also shared by a majority of the members of a social group.

blood t., SEE blood type.

buffalo t., term used to describe the distribution of a fat deposit seen posteriorly over the upper thoracic vertebrae; seen in hyperadrenocorticalism (Cushing's *syndrome*). SYN buffalo hump.

nomenclatural t., the constituent element of a taxon to which the name of the taxon is permanently attached; the t. of a species is preferably a strain (in special cases it may be a description, a preserved specimen or preparation, or an illustration); the t. of a genus is a species; and the t. of an order, family, or tribe is the genus on whose name the name of the higher taxon is based.

test t., SEE test types.

wild t., a gene, phenotype, or genotype that is overwhelmingly common among those possible at a locus of interest, and therefore presumably not harmful.

ty·phin·ia (tī-fin′ē-ă). SYN relapsing *fever.* [G. *typhos,* smoke, stupor arising from fever]

⌂**typhl-.** SEE typhlo-.

typh·lec·ta·sis (tif-lek′tă-sis). Dilation of the cecum. [G. *typhlon,* cecum, + *ektasis,* a stretching out]

typh·lec·to·my (tif-lek′tō-mē). SYN cecectomy.

typh·len·ter·i·tis (tif′len-ter-ī′tis). SYN cecitis.

typh·li·tis (tif′lī′tis). SYN cecitis.

⌂**typhlo-, typhl-. 1.** The cecum. SEE ALSO ceco-. [G. cecum] **2.** Blindness. [G. *typhlos,* blind]

typh·lo·dic·li·di·tis (tif-lō-dik-li-dī′tis). Inflammation of the ileocecal valve. [G. *typhlon,* cecum, + *diklis (diklid-),* double-folding (of doors), + *-itis,* inflammation]

typh·lo·em·py·e·ma (tif′lō-em-pī-ē′mă). Presence of an abscess following typhlitis. [G. *typhlon,* cecum, + *empyēma,* abscess]

typh·lo·en·ter·i·tis (tif′lō-en-ter-ī′tis). SYN cecitis.

typh·lo·li·thi·a·sis (tif′lō-li-thī′ă-sis). Presence of fecal concretions in the cecum. [G. *typhlon,* cecum, + *lithos,* stone]

typh·lol·o·gy (tif-lol′ō-jē). An obsolete term for the branch of science concerned with the causes and prevention of blindness, and the rehabilitation of those afflicted. [G. *typhlos,* blind, + *logos,* study]

typh·lo·meg·a·ly (tif′lō-meg′ă-lē). Old term for enlargement of the cecum. [G. *typhlon,* cecum, + *megas (megal-),* large]

typh·lon (tif′lon). SYN cecum (1). [G.]

typh·lo·pexy, typh·lo·pex·ia (tif′lō-pek-sē, tif-lō-pek′sē-ă). SYN cecopexy.

typh·lor·rha·phy (tif-lōr′ă-fē). SYN cecorrhaphy.

typh·lo·sis (tif-lō′sis). SYN blindness. [G. *typhlos,* blind]

typh·los·to·my (tif-los′tō-mē). SYN cecostomy.

typh·lot·o·my (tif-lot′ō-mē). SYN cecotomy.

⌂**typho-.** Typhus, typhoid. [G. *typhos,* smoke, dullness]

ty·phoid (tī′foyd). **1.** Typhus-like; stuporous from fever. **2.** SYN typhoid *fever.* [typhus + G. *eidos,* resemblance]

abdominal t., SYN typhoid *fever.*

ambulatory t., SYN walking t.

apyretic t., t. fever in which the temperature does not rise more than a degree or two.

bilious t. of Griesinger, SYN relapsing *fever.*

equine t., SYN equine viral *arteritis.*

fowl t., a septicemic disease of chickens and turkeys, caused by *Salmonella gallinarum;* some human infections with this organism have been reported.

latent t., SYN walking t.

provocation t., an accelerated onset of t. fever, sometimes of unusual severity, resulting from typhoid-paratyphoid A and B (T.A.B.) vaccination late in the incubation period.

walking t., t. fever without much prostration, the patient being up and around and sometimes working. SYN ambulatory t., latent t.

ty·phoi·dal (tī-foyd'ăl). Relating to or resembling typhoid fever.

ty·phol·y·sin (tī-fol'i-sin). A hemolysin formed by *Salmonella typhi*.

ty·pho·ma·nia (tī-fō-mā'nē-ă). A muttering delerium characteristic of that in typhoid fever and typhus. [typho- + G. *mania,* frenzy]

ty·pho·sep·sis (tī-fō-sep'sis). SYN typhoid *septicemia.*

ty·phous (tī'fŭs). Relating to typhus.

ty·phus (tī'fŭs). A group of acute infectious and contagious diseases, caused by rickettsiae that are transmitted by arthropods, and occurring in two principal forms: epidemic t. and endemic (murine) t. Also called jail, camp, or ship fever. SYN camp fever (1), jail fever, ship fever. [G. *typhos,* smoke, stupor]

Australian tick t., rarely fatal form of t. caused by the *Rickettsia australis,* seen in eastern Australia, transmitted by tick bite, and characterized by severe headache and conjunctivitis. Reservoir is in rodents and marsupials. SYN Queensland tick t.

canine t., SYN Stuttgart *disease.*

endemic t., SYN murine t.

epidemic t., t. caused by *Rickettsia prowazekii* and spread by body lice; marked by high fever, mental and physical depression, and a macular and papular eruption; lasts for about two weeks and occurs when large crowds are brought together and personal hygiene is at a low ebb; recrudescences can occur. SYN hospital fever, louse-borne t., prison fever t.

European t., epidemic, louse-born typhus fever, due to infection with *Rickettsia prowazekii.*

exanthematous t., t. fever with the usual petechial skin lesions seen in that disease.

flea-borne t., SYN murine t.

Indian tick t., SYN boutonneuse *fever.*

louse-borne t., SYN epidemic t.

Manchurian t., tick transmitted infection with *Rickettsia sibirica.* SEE ALSO Korean hemorrhagic *fever.*

Mexican t., infection with *Rickettsia typhi (mooseri)* causing a syndrome similar to epidemic t., but spread from rats to man by the rat flea (Xenopsylla (polyplax) cheopis). Spread from rat to rat by the rat louse (Polyplax spinulosa). Most common form of t. in the United State. It has various geographical names based on region in which it was observed.

mite t., SYN tsutsugamushi *disease.*

mite-born t., SYN rickettsialpox.

t. mit'ior, a mild or abortive t.

murine t., a milder form of epidemic t. caused by *Rickettsia typhi* and transmitted to humans by rat or mouse fleas. SYN Congolian red fever, endemic t., flea-borne t., red fever, red fever of the Congo.

North Queensland tick t., t. caused by *Rickettsia australis.*

prison fever t., SYN epidemic t.

Queensland tick t., SYN Australian tick t.

recrudescent t., SYN Brill-Zinsser *disease.*

Sao Paulo t., infection with *Rickettsia rickettsii;* spread by tick bite. SEE ALSO Rocky Mountain spotted *fever.*

scrub t., SYN tsutsugamushi *disease.*

shop t., a mild form of t. occurring in urban areas, reported in Mediterranean areas. SYN urban t.

Siberian tick t., tick-borne rickettsiosis caused by infection with *Rickettsia sibirica.*

tick t., SYN boutonneuse *fever.*

tropical t., SYN tsutsugamushi *disease.*

urban t., SYN shop t.

typ·ing (tīp'ing). Classification according to type. [see type]

bacteriophage t., a microbiological procedure, of epidemiological importance, for distinguishing types within a seemingly homogeneous bacterial species or strain by the use of type-specific bacteriophage.

HLA t., tests done in order to determine if a patient has antibodies against a potential donor's HLA antigens. The presence of antibodies means that a particular graft will be rapidly rejected. Also used to establish paternity and in forensic medicine.

Tyr Symbol for tyrosine and its radicals.

ty·ra·mi·nase (tī'ră-mi-nās, tir'ă-). SYN *amine* oxidase (flavin-containing).

ty·ra·mine (tī'ră-mēn, tir'ă-). 4-Hydroxyphenylethylamine; decarboxylated tyrosine, a sympathomimetic amine having an action in some respects resembling that of epinephrine; present in ergot, mistletoe, ripe cheese, beers, red wines, and putrefied animal matter; elevated in individuals with tyrosinemia type II.

t. oxidase, SYN *amine* oxidase (flavin-containing).

tyr·an·nism (tir'ă-nizm). A form of sadism characterized by a lust for domination and cruelty, with subsequent humiliation of the partner. [G. *tyrannos,* a tyrant]

ty·rem·e·sis (tī-rem'ĕ-sis). Vomiting of curdy material by infants. SYN tyrosis (1). [G. *tyros,* cheese, + *emesis,* vomiting]

ty·ro·ci·din, ty·ro·ci·dine (tī-rō-sī'din). An antibacterial cyclopeptide obtained from *Bacillus brevis.* SEE ALSO tyrothricin.

Tyrode, Maurice V., U.S. pharmacologist, 1878–1930. SEE T.'s *solution.*

ty·rog·e·nous (tī-roj'ĕ-nŭs). Produced by, or originating in, cheese. [G. *tyros,* cheese, + G. -gen, producing]

Ty·rog·ly·phus lon·gi·or (tī-rog'li-fŭs lon'gē-ōr, tī'rō-glif'ŭs). SYN *Tyrophagus putrescentiae.* [G. *tyros,* cheese, + *glyphē* carving]

ty·roid (tī'royd). Cheesy; caseous. [G. *tyrōdēs,* fr. *tyros,* cheese, + *eidos,* resemblance]

ty·ro·ke·to·nu·ria (tī'rō-kē-tō-nū'rē-ă). The urinary excretion of ketonic metabolites of tyrosine, such as *p*-hydroxyphenylpyruvic acid.

ty·ro·ma (tī-rō'mă). A caseous tumor. [G. *tyros,* cheese, + -ōma, tumor]

ty·ro·pa·no·ate so·di·um (tī'rō-pă-nō'āt). 3-Butyramido-α-ethyl-2,4,6-triiodohydrocinnamic acid, sodium salt; an oral contrast medium for cholecystography.

Ty·roph·a·gus pu·tres·cen·ti·ae (tī-rof'ă-gŭs pyū'tre-sen'tē-ē). One of the grain mite species that cause various forms of dermatitis resulting from infestation by grain mites in food and produce, which sensitizes and causes dermatitis in storage and handling personnel. SYN *Tyroglyphus longior.* [G. *tyros,* cheese, + *phagō,* to eat]

ty·ro·sin·ase (tī'rō-si-nās, tir'ō-). SYN monophenol monooxygenase (1).

β-ty·ro·sin·ase. SYN *tyrosine* phenol-lyase.

ty·ro·sine (Tyr, Y) (tī'rō-sēn, -sin). 2-Amino-3-(4-hydroxyphenyl)propionic acid; 3-(4-hydroxyphenyl)alanine; the L-isomer is an α-amino acid present in most proteins.

t. aminotransferase, an enzyme that catalyzes the reversible reaction of L-t. and α-ketoglutarate producing *p*-hydroxyphenylpyruvate and L-glutamate; this enzyme catalyzes a step in L-phenylalanine and L-tyrosine catabolism; a deficiency of this enzyme is associated with tyrosinemia II. SYN t. transaminase.

t. iodinase, a postulated enzyme in the thyroid catalyzing iodination of t., a reaction important in the eventual biosynthesis of thyroxine. SEE ALSO peroxidases.

t. kinase, an enzyme that phosphorylates tyrosyl residues on certain proteins; many are products of viral oncogenes; a number of receptors (*e.g.,* receptors for epidermal growth factor, insulin, etc.) have this enzymatic activity; a misnomer, since the physiological substrate is not t. but tyrosyl residues in a protein.

t. phenol-lyase, an enzyme catalyzing the hydrolysis of L-tyrosine to phenol, pyruvate, and NH_3. SYN β-tyrosinase.

t. transaminase, SYN t. aminotransferase.

ty·ro·si·ne·mia (tī'rō-si-nē'mē-ă) [MIM*276600, *276700, and *276710]. A disorder consisting of elevated blood concentrations of tyrosine, enhanced urinary excretion of tyrosine and tyrosyl compounds, hepatosplenomegaly, nodular cirrhosis of the liver, multiple renal tubular reabsorptive defects, and vitamin D-resistant rickets; autosomal recessive inheritance. SYN hypertyrosinemia. [tyrosine + G. *haima,* blood]

ty·ro·si·no·sis (tī'rō-si-nō'sis) [MIM*276800]. A very rare, possibly heritable disorder of tyrosine metabolism that may be caused by defective formation of *p*-hydroxyphenylpyruvic acid oxidase or of tyrosine transaminase; characterized by enhanced urinary excretion of *p*-hydroxyphenylpyruvic acid and of other tyrosyl metabolites upon ingestion of tyrosine or proteins containing that amino acid. [tyrosine + G. *-osis,* condition]

ty·ro·si·nu·ria (tī'rō-si-nū're-ă). The excretion of tyrosine in the urine. [tyrosine + G. *ouron,* urine]

ty·ro·sis (tī-rō'sis). **1.** SYN tyremesis. **2.** SYN caseation. [G. *tyros,* cheese]

ty·ro·sy·lu·ria (tī'rō-si-lū're-ă). Enhanced urinary excretion of certain metabolites of tyrosine, such as *p*-hydroxyphenylpyruvic acid; present in tyrosinosis, scurvy, pernicious anemia, and other diseases.

ty·ro·thri·cin (tī-rō-thrī'sin). An antibacterial mixture obtained from peptone cultures of *Bacillus brevis;* bactericidal and bacteriostatic, and active against Gram-positive bacteria. It yields the crystalline antibacterial agents gramicidin and tyrocidin; the gramicidin component is a polypeptide containing L-tryptophan, D-leucine, D-valine, L-valine, L-alanine, glycine, and an aminoethanol; the tyrocidin component is a cyclopolypeptide containing tyrosine, ornithine, and several other amino acids.

ty·ro·tox·ism (tī-rō-tok'sizm). Poisoning by cheese or any milk product. [G. *tyros,* cheese, + *toxikon,* poison]

Tyrrell, Frederick, English anatomist and surgeon, 1797–1843. SEE T.'s *fascia.*

Tyson, Edward, English anatomist, 1649–1708. SEE T.'s *glands,* under *gland.*

Tyz·ze·ria (tī-ze're-ă). A genus of coccidia (family Eimeriidae) in which the oocyst contains eight naked sporozoites. Important species are *T. anseris,* a relatively nonpathogenic species found in the small intestine of domestic and wild geese, whistling swans, and certain wild ducks, and *T. perniciosa,* which occurs in the small intestine of the domestic duck in North America and Europe, and is pathogenic in ducklings.

Tzanck, Arnault, Russian dermatologist, 1886–1954. SEE T. *cells,* under *cell, test.*

Tz

υ. **1.** Upsilon, 20th letter of the Greek alphabet. **2.** Symbol for kinematic *viscosity*.

U **1.** Abbreviation for unit. **2.** Symbol for kilurane; uranium; uridine in polymers; uracil; internal *energy*; urinary concentration, followed by subscripts indicating location and chemical species.

ubi·hy·dro·qui·none (yū′bi-hī-drō-quī′nōn). SYN ubiquinol.

ubi·qui·nol (H₂Q, Q-H₂) (yū′bi-kwī′nol, yū-bik′wi-nol). The reduction product of a ubiquinone. SYN ubihydroquinone.

ubi·qui·none (yū′bi-kwī′nōn, yū-bik′wi-nōn). A 2,3-dimethoxy-5-methyl-1,4-benzoquinone with a multiprenyl side chain; a mobile component of electron transport. SEE ALSO coenzyme Q.

ubi·qui·none-6 (-Q₆). Ubiquinone-30; coenzyme Q₆; 2,3-Dimethoxy-5-methyl-6-hexaprenyl-1,4 benzoquinone.

ubi·qui·none-10 (-Q₁₀). Ubiquinone-50; coenzyme Q₁₀; 2,3-Dimethoxy-5-methyl-6-decaprenyl-1,4-benzoquinone.

ubiq·ui·tin (yū-bik′kwi-tin). A small (76 amino acid residues) protein found in all cells of higher organisms and one whose structure has changed minimally during evolutionary history; involved in at least two processes; histone modification and intracellular protein breakdown.

ud·der (ŭd′er). The large complex of mammary glands of the cow and other ungulates. [A.S., *ūder*]

UDP Abbreviation for *uridine* 5′-diphosphate.

UDP-*N*-ace·tyl·glu·co·sam·ine:ly·so·som·al en·zyme *N*-ace·tyl·glu·co·sam·in·yl-1-phos·pho·trans·fer·ase. An enzyme that participates in the posttranslational modification of a number of lysosomal proteins; a deficiency or defect in this enzyme results in two forms of mucolipidoses, I-cell disease, and pseudo-Hurler polydystrophy.

UDPG Abbreviation for uridine diphosphoglucose.

UDPGal Abbreviation for uridine diphosphogalactose.

UDPga·lac·tose. Uridine diphosphogalactose.

UDPga·lac·tose 4-ep·i·mer·ase. SYN UDPglucose 4-epimerase.

UDPGlc Abbreviation for uridine diphosphoglucose.

UDP-GlcUA Abbreviation for uridine diphosphoglucuronic acid.

UDPglu·cose. SYN uridine diphosphoglucose.

UDPglu·cose 4-ep·i·mer·ase. An enzyme that catalyzes the reversible Walden inversion of UDPglucose to UDPgalactose; a deficiency of this enzyme is associated with one type of galactosemia. SYN UDPgalactose 4-epimerase, uridine diphosphoglucose 4-epimerase.

UDPglu·cose-hex·ose-1-phos·phate uri·dyl·yl·trans·fer·-ase. An enzyme that catalyzes the reversible reaction of α-D-glucose 1-phosphate UDPgalactose to produce UDPglucose and α-D-galactose 1-phosphate. SEE ALSO UDPglucose 4-epimerase. SYN hexose-1-phosphate uridylyltransferase, phosphogalactoisomerase.

UDPglu·cur·o·nate-bil·i·ru·bin·glu·cu·ron·o·side glu·cu·-ron·o·syl·trans·fer·ase. SYN UDPglucuronate-bilirubin glucuronosyltransferase.

UDPglu·cur·o·nate-bil·i·ru·bin glu·cu·ron·o·syl·trans·-fer·ase. Hepatic transferases that catalyze the transfer of the glucuronic moiety of UDP-glucuronic acid to bilirubin or bilirubin glucuronide, thus producing UDP and either bilirubin-glucoronoside or bilirubin bisglucuronoside, respectively; these bile conjugates are then secreted into the bile. SYN UDPglucuronate-bilirubinglucuronoside glucuronosyltransferase.

UDP·xy·lose. A pyrophosphate group links the 5′ position of uridine and the 1-position of D-xylose; formed by the decarboxylation of UDPglucuronic acid; required for the synthesis of proteoglycans; inhibits UDPglucose dehydrogenase.

Uehlinger, E., Swiss pathologist, *1899. SEE Meyenburg-Altherr-U. *syndrome.*

UFA Abbreviation for unesterified free *fatty acid.*

Uffelmann, Jules, German physician, 1837–1894. SEE U.'s *reagent.*

UGI Abbreviation for upper gastrointestinal series.

Uhl, Henry S.M., S. internist, *1921. SEE U. *anomaly.*

Uhthoff, Wilhelm, German ophthalmologist, 1853–1927. SEE U.'s *sign;* Uhthoff *symptom.*

UIP Abbreviation for usual interstitial *pneumonia* of Liebow.

ukam·bin (ū-kam′bin). An African arrow poison from plants of the family Apocynaceae; a heart poison resembling digitalis or strophanthus in its action.

ULCER

ul·cer (ŭl′ser). A lesion on the surface of the skin or on a mucous surface, caused by superficial loss of tissue, usually with inflammation. A wound with superficial loss of tissue from trauma is not primarily an u., but may become ulcerated if infection occurs. SYN ulcus. [L. *ulcus* (*ulcer-*), a sore, ulcer]

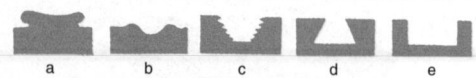

characteristic forms of ulcers
a) carcinomic ulcer, hard, up-turned margin; b) rodent ulcer, slightly raised margin; c) "septic" ulcer, stepped margin; d) tuberculous ulcer, undermined margin; and e) ulcer in tertiary syphilis, as if stamped out

acute decubitus u., a severe form of bedsore, of neutrophic origin, occurring in hemiplegia or paraplegia.

Aden u., the lesion occurring in cutaneous leishmaniasis.

amputating u., an u. encircling a limb.

anastomotic u., an u. of jejunum, after gastroenterostomy.

atonic u., an u. that shows little or no tendency to heal.

Buruli u., an u. of the skin, with widespread necrosis of subcutaneous fat, due to infection with *Mycobacterium ulcerans;* occurs in Uganda in persons living on the Nile river banks. [*Buruli,* district in Uganda]

chiclero u., lesion of the pinna of the ear due to cutaneous *leishmaniasis,* usually *Leishmania mexicana;* seen in workers harvesting chicle plants in Central America. SYN bay sore. [Sp. chicle farmer, fr. *chicle,* fr. Nahuatl *chictli*]

chrome u., an u. produced by exposure to chromium compounds. SYN tanner's u.

chronic u., a longstanding u. with fibrous scar tissue in the floor of the u.

cockscomb u., an u. that may occur in association with condylomata acuminata.

cold u., a small gangrenous u. on the extremities; due to defective circulation.

constitutional u., an u. due to systemic disease, such as tuberculosis. SYN symptomatic u.

corrosive u., SYN noma.

creeping u., SYN serpiginous u.

Curling's u., an u. of the duodenum in a patient with extensive superficial burns, intracranial lesions, or severe bodily injury. SYN stress u.'s.

decubitus u.'s, a chronic u. that appears in pressure areas of skin overlying a bony prominence in debilitated patients confined to bed or otherwise immobilized, due to a circulatory defect. SYN bedsore, decubital gangrene, hospital gangrene, nosocomial gangrene, pressure gangrene, pressure sore, sloughing phagedena, ulcus hypostaticum.

dendritic corneal u., keratitis caused by herpes simplex virus.

dental u., an u. on the oral mucuous membrane caused by biting or by rubbing against the edge of a broken tooth.

diphtheritic u., an u. covered with a gray adherent membrane, caused by *Corynebacterium diphtheriae.*

distention u., an u. of the intestine in the dilated part above a stricture.

elusive u., SYN Hunner's u.

fascicular u., a localized vascularization of the cornea to the site of a corneal u.

Fenwick-Hunner u., SYN Hunner's u.

Gaboon u., a form of tropical u. affecting the residents of this region; it resembles a syphilitic u., especially in the appearance of its scar. [*Gaboon,* a region in Africa]

gastric u., an u. of the stomach.

gravitational u., a chronic u. of the leg with impaired healing because of the dependent position of the extremity and the incompetence of the valves of the varicosed veins; the venous return stagnates and creates hypoxemia. SEE ALSO varicose u.

groin u., SYN *granuloma* inguinale tropicum.

gummatous u., lesion of the skin occurring in late syphilis.

hard u., SYN chancre.

healed u., an u. covered by epithelial regeneration, beneath which there may be scarring and absence of glands or appendages.

herpetic u., u. caused by herpes simplex virus.

Hunner's u., a focal and often multiple lesion involving all layers of the bladder wall in chronic interstitial cystitis; the surface epithelium is destroyed by inflammation and the initially pale lesion cracks and bleeds with distention of the bladder. SYN elusive u., Fenwick-Hunner u.

hypopyon u., (1) an advancing central suppurative u. of the cornea; SEE ALSO hypopyon. **(2)** a corneal u. with pus in the anterior chamber;

indolent u., a chronic u., with hard elevated edges and few or no granulations, and showing no tendency to heal.

inflamed u., an u. with a purulent discharge and inflamed borders.

Kurunegala u.'s, SYN *pyosis* tropica. [*Kurunegala,* a district in Sri Lanka]

Lipschütz' u., a simple acute ulceration of the vulva or lower vagina of nonvenereal origin. SYN ulcus vulvae acutum.

lupoid u., an u. resembling that of cutaneous tuberculosis.

Mann-Williamson u., SEE Mann-Williamson *operation.*

marginal ring u. of cornea, a slowly advancing intermittent u. involving the circumference of the corneal margin.

Marjolin's u., well-differentiated but aggressive squamous cell carcinoma occurring in cicatricial tissue at the epidermal edge of a sinus draining underlying osteomyelitis.

Meleney's u., undermining u. of the skin and subcutaneous tissues, usually following an operation, caused by a synergistic interaction between microaerophilic nonhemolytic streptococci and aerobic hemolytic staphylococci. SYN Meleney's gangrene, progressive bacterial synergistic gangrene.

Mooren's u., chronic inflammation of the peripheral cornea that slowly progresses centrally with corneal thinning and sometimes perforation.

Oriental u., the lesion occurring in cutaneous leishmaniasis. SYN Oriental sore.

penetrating u., an u. extending into deeper tissues of an organ.

peptic u., an u. of the alimentary mucosa, usually in the stomach or duodenum, exposed to acid gastric secretion.

perambulating u., SYN phagedenic u.

perforated u., an u. extending through the wall of an organ.

perforating u. of foot, a round, deep, trophic u. of the sole of the foot, following disease or injury, in any part of its course from the center to the periphery of the nerve supplying the part. SYN mal perforant.

phagedenic u., a rapidly spreading u. attended by the formation of extensive sloughing. SYN perambulating u., sloughing u., ulcus ambulans.

phlegmonous u., a u. accompanied by inflammation of the neighboring tissues.

pudendal u., SYN *granuloma* inguinale.

recurrent aphthous u.'s, SYN aphtha (2).

ring u. of cornea, inflammation of the greater part or the whole of the corneal periphery.

rodent u., obsolete term for a slowly enlarging ulcerated basal cell carcinoma, usually on the face.

Saemisch's u., a form of serpiginous keratitis, frequently accompanied by hypopyon.

serpent u. of cornea, SYN serpiginous *keratitis.*

serpiginous u., an u. extending on one side while healing at the opposite edge, forming an undulating margin. SYN creeping u.

serpiginous corneal u., serpentine ulceration of the cornea, due to infection, most often with *Streptococcus pneumoniae.*

simple u., a local, not constitutional, u. not accompanied by marked pain or inflammation.

sloughing u., SYN phagedenic u.

soft u., SYN chancroid.

stasis u., SYN varicose u.

stercoral u., an u. of the colon due to pressure and irritation of retained fecal masses.

steroid u., an u., usually on the leg or foot, developing from a wound in patients undergoing long-term steroid therapy; results from the wound-healing inhibitory effects characteristic of steroids.

stomal u., an intestinal u. occurring after gastrojejunostomy in the jejunal mucosa near the opening (stoma) between the stomach and the jejunum.

stress u.'s, SYN Curling's u.

Sutton's u., a solitary, deep, painful u. of the buccal or genital mucous membrane.

symptomatic u., SYN constitutional u.

syphilitic u., (1) SYN chancre. **(2)** any ulceration caused by a syphilitic infection.

Syriac u., Syrian u., old names for diphtheria.

tanner's u., SYN chrome u.

transparent u. of the cornea, obsolete term for an u. of the cornea, occurring usually in children, that heals without opacity.

trophic u., u. resulting from cutaneous sensory denervation. SEE ALSO perforating u. of foot. SYN trophic gangrene.

tropical u., (1) the lesion occurring in cutaneous leishmaniasis; **(2)** tropical phagedenic ulceration caused by a variety of microorganisms, including mycobacteria; common in northern Nigeria. SYN tropical sore.

undermining u., a chronic cutaneous u. with overhanging margins; due to hemolytic streptococci or other bacteria.

varicose u., the loss of skin surface in the drainage area of a varicose vein, usually in the leg, resulting from stasis and infection. SYN stasis u.

venereal u., SYN chancroid.

Zambesi u., an u., usually single, about 3 cm in diameter, on the foot or leg, occurring in laborers in the Zambesi Delta; it has a sloughing surface, but does not spread and produces no constitutional symptoms or glandular enlargement; it is associated with the presence of a spirillum and a large fusiform bacillus; one attack seems to confer a partial immunity.

---

ul·ce·ra (ŭl′ser-ă). Plural of ulcus.

ul·cer·ate (ŭl′ser-āt). To form an ulcer.

ul·cer·at·ed (ŭl′ser-āt-ed). Having undergone ulceration.

ul·cer·a·tion (ŭl-ser-ā′shŭn). 1. The formation of an ulcer. 2. An ulcer or aggregation of ulcers.

lip and leg u., SYN ulcerative *dermatosis.*

tracheal u., erosion of the tracheal mucous membrane with, in some cases, exposure of the rings, at the site at which a cuffed tracheostomy tube has been present for some time.

ul·cer·a·tive (ŭl′ser-ă-tiv). Relating to, causing, or marked by an ulcer or ulcers.

ul·cer·o·gen·ic (ŭl′ser-ō-jen′ik). Ulcer-producing.

ul·cer·o·glan·du·lar (ŭl′ser-ō-gland′yū-lăr). Denoting a local ulceration at a site of infection followed by regional or generalized lymphadenopathy.

ul·cer·o·mem·bra·nous (ŭl′ser-ō-mem′bră-nŭs). Relating to or characterized by ulceration and the formation of a false membrane.

ul·cer·ous (ŭl′ser-ŭs). Relating to, affected with, or containing an ulcer. [L. *ulcerosus*]

ul·cus, pl. **ul·ce·ra** (ŭl′kŭs, ŭl′ser-ă). SYN ulcer. [L.]

u. am′bulans, SYN phagedenic *ulcer.*

u. hypostat′icum, SYN decubitus *ulcer.*

u. tere′brans, obsolete term for an invasive basal cell carcinoma, usually around the eye, nose, or ear, and extending to underlying bony tissue.

u. vene′reum, (1) SYN chancre. **(2)** SYN chancroid.

u. vul′vae acu′tum, SYN Lipschütz′ *ulcer.*

ule-. SEE ulo-.

ulec·to·my (yū-lek′tō-mē). Obsolete synonym for cicatrectomy. [G. *oulē*, scar, + *ektomē*, excision]

ule·gy·ri·a (yū-lē-jī′rē-ă). A defect of the cerebral cortex characterized by narrow and distorted gyri; may be congenital or the result of scars. [G. *oulē*, scar, + *gyros*, ring]

uler·y·the·ma (ū′ler-i-thē′mă). Scarring with erythema. [G. *oulē*, scar, + *erythēma*, redness of the skin]

u. ophryog′enes, folliculitis of the eyebrows resulting in scarring and alopecia.

u. sycosifor′me, SYN lupoid *sycosis.*

ulet·omy (yū-let′ō-mē). Obsolete synonym for cicatricotomy. [G. *oulē*, scar, + *tomē*, incision]

u·lex eu·ro·pae·us (ū-leks ū′o-pā-ŭs). A lectin that reacts specifically with α-L-fucose, used as a marker for endothelial cells in paraffin sections.

Ullmann, Emerich, Hungarian surgeon, 1861–1937. SEE U.'s *line, syndrome.*

Ullrich, Otto, German physician, 1894–1957. SEE Morquio-U. *disease.*

ul·na, gen. and pl. **ul·nae** (ŭl′nă, ŭl′nē) [NA]. The medial and larger of the two bones of the forearm. SYN cubitus (2) [NA]. [L. elbow, arm, fr. G. *ōlenē*]

ul·nad (ŭl′nad). In a direction toward the ulna. [ulna + L. *ad,* to]

ul·nar (ŭl′năr). Relating to the ulna, or to any of the structures (artery, nerve, etc.) named from it; relating to the ulnar or medial aspect of the upper limb. SYN ulnaris [NA].

ul·na·ris (ŭl-nā′ris) [NA]. SYN ulnar. [Mod. L.]

ul·nen (ŭl′nen). Relating to the ulna independent of other structures. [ulna + G. *en,* in]

ul·no·car·pal (ŭl′nō-kar′păl). Relating to the ulna and the carpus, or to the ulnar side of the wrist.

ul·no·ra·di·al (ŭl′nō-rā′dē-ăl). Relating to both ulna and radius; denoting the two articulations, ligaments, etc., between them.

ulo-, ule-. 1. Scar, scarring. [G. *oulē*] **2.** obsolete the gums. SEE ALSO gingivo-. [G. *oulon*] **3.** Curly. [G. *oulo-, ouli-,* woolly.]

ulo·der·ma·ti·tis (ū′lō-der-mă-tī′tis). Inflammation of the skin resulting in destruction of tissue and the formation of scars. [G. *oulē*, scar, + *derma,* skin, + *-itis,* inflammation]

uloid (yū′loyd). **1.** Resembling a scar. **2.** A scarlike lesion due to a degenerative process in deeper layers of skin. [G. *oulē*, scar + *eidos,* resemblance]

ulot·o·my (yū-lot′ō-mē). Obsolete term for cicatricotomy. [G. *oulē*, scar, + *tomē*, incision]

ulot·ri·chous (yū-lot′ri-kŭs). Having curly hair. Cf. leiotrichous. [G. *oulotrichos,* curly haired, fr. *oulos,* wooly, + *thrix (trich-),* hair]

ul·ti·mo·bran·chi·al (ŭl′ti-mō-brang′kē-ăl). In embryology, re-

lating to the caudal pharyngeal pouch. [L. *ultimus,* last, + G. *branchia,* gills]

ul·ti·mum mo·ri·ens (ŭl′ti-mŭm mōr′ī-enz). The right atrium of the heart, said to contract after the rest of the heart is still. [L. the last thing dying]

ultra-. Excess, exaggeration, beyond. [L. beyond]

ul·tra·brach·y·ce·phal·ic (ŭl-tră-brak-ē-se-fal′ik). Denoting an extremely short skull, one with an index of at least 90.

ul·tra·cen·tri·fu·ga·tion (ŭl-tră-sen′tri-fyū-gā-shŭn). The process of subjecting to an ultracentrifuge.

ul·tra·cen·tri·fuge (ŭl-tră-sen′-tri-fyūj). A high-speed centrifuge (up to 100,000 rpm) by means of which large molecules, *e.g.,* of protein or nucleic acids, are caused to sediment at practicable rates; used for determinations of molecular weights, separation of large molecules, criteria of homogeneity of large molecules, conformational studies, etc.

ul·tra·cy·to·stome (ŭl-tră-sī′tō-stōm). Former name for micropore. [ultra- + G. *kytos,* cell, + *stoma,* mouth]

ul·tra·di·an (ŭl-trā′dē-ăn). Relating to biologic variations or rhythms occurring in cycles more frequent than every 24 hours. Cf. circadian, infradian. [ultra- + L. *dies,* day]

ul·tra·dol·i·cho·ce·phal·ic (ŭl-tră-dol-i-kō-se-fal′ik). Denoting a very long skull, one with a cephalic index of less than 65.

ul·tra·fil·ter (ŭl′tră-fil-ter). A semipermeable membrane (collodion, fish bladder, or filter paper impregnated with gels) used as a filter to separate colloids and large molecules from water and small molecules, which pass through.

ul·tra·fil·tra·tion (ŭl′tră-fil-trā′shŭn). Filtration through a semipermeable membrane or any filter that separates colloid solutions from crystalloids or separates particles of different size in a colloid mixture.

ul·tra·li·ga·tion (ŭl-tră-lī-gā′shŭn). Ligation of a blood vessel beyond the point where a branch is given off.

ul·tra·mi·cro·scope (ŭl-tră-mī′krō-skōp). A microscope that utilizes refracted light for visualizing objects not visible with the ordinary microscope when direct light is used.

ul·tra·mi·cro·scop·ic (ŭl′tră-mī-krō-skop′ik). SYN submicroscopic.

ul·tra·mi·cro·tome (ŭl-tră-mī′krō-tōm). A microtome used in cutting sections 0.1 μm thick, or less, for electron microscopy.

ul·tra·mi·crot·o·my (ŭl′tră-mī-krot′ō-mē). The cutting of ultrathin sections for electron microscopy by use of an ultramicrotome.

ul·tra·son·ic (ŭl-tră-son′ik). Relating to energy waves similar to those of sound but of higher frequencies (above 30,000 Hz). [ultra- + L. *sonus,* sound]

ul·tra·son·ics (ŭl-tră-son′iks). The science and technology of ultrasound, its characteristics and phenomena.

ul·tra·son·o·gram (ŭl-tră-son′ō-gram). The image obtained by ultrasonography. SEE ALSO echogram. SYN sonogram.

ul·tra·son·o·graph (ŭl′tră-son′ō-graf). Computerized instrument used to create an image using ultrasound. SYN sonograph. [ultra- + L. *sonus,* sound, + G. *graphō,* to write]

ul·tra·so·nog·ra·pher (ŭl′tră-sŏ-nog′ră-fer). A person who performs and interprets ultrasonographic examinations. SYN echographer, sonographer.

ul·tra·so·nog·ra·phy (ŭl′tră-sŏ-nog′ră-fē). The location, measurement, or delineation of deep structures by measuring the reflection or transmission of high frequency or ultrasonic waves. Computer calculation of the distance to the sound-reflecting or absorbing surface plus the known orientation of the sound beam gives a two-dimensional image. SEE ALSO ultrasound. SYN echography, sonography. [ultra- + L. *sonus,* sound, + G. *graphō,* to write]

Doppler u., application of the Doppler effect in ultrasound to detect movement of scatterers (usually red blood cells) by the analysis of the change in frequency of the returning echoes.

In many instances, ultrasound has supplanted x-radiography as the imaging method of choice, because it poses no risk to patients, is noninvasive, and of moderate cost.

Doppler-corrected ultrasound enables real-time viewing of tissues, blood flow, and organs that cannot be obtained by any other method. It has proved a boon to cardiology, greatly aiding evaluations of cardiovascular patients, and to obstetrics, where it is used for fetal monitoring.

duplex u., the combination of real-time and Doppler u.

endovaginal u., pelvic u. using a probe inserted into the vagina.

gray-scale u., the display of the ultrasound echo amplitude or signal intensity as different shades of gray, improving image quality compared to the obsolete black and white presentation.

real-time u., rapid serial ultrasound images produced using a phased array or scanning transducer; produces a video display of organ motion, such as heart valve or fetal motion.

ul·tra·son·o·sur·gery (ŭl′tră-son-ō-ser′jer-ē). Use of ultrasound techniques to disrupt cells, tissues, or tracts, particularly in the central nervous system.

ul·tra·sound (ŭl′tră-sownd). Sound having a frequency greater than 30,000 Hz.

diagnostic u., the use of u. to obtain images for medical diagnostic purposes, employing frequencies ranging from 1.6 to about 10 MHz.

obstetric u., use of diagnostic u. during pregnancy.

ul·tra·struc·ture (ŭl-tră-strŭk′chŭr). Structures or particles seen with the electron microscope. SYN fine structure.

ul·tra·therm (ŭl′tră-therm). A short-wave diathermy machine. [ultra- + G. *thermē,* heat]

ul·tra·vi·o·let (ŭl-tră-vī′ō-let). Denoting electromagnetic rays at higher frequency than the violet end of the visible spectrum.

u. A (UVA), u. radiation from 320 to 400 nm that causes skin tanning but is very weakly sunburn-producing and carcinogenic.

u. B (UVB), u. radiation from 290 to 320 nm that most effectively causes sunburning and tanning; excessive UVB exposure is a cause of cancer of fair skin.

u. C (UVC), u. radiation from 200 to 290 nm; UVC in sunlight does not reach the surface of the earth; germicidal and mercury arc lamps may cause sunburn and photokeratitis.

extravital u., having wavelengths of 2900 to 1850 Å.

intravital u., having wavelengths of 3900 to 3200 Å.

vital u., rays necessary or helpful to normal growth; they promote calcium metabolism, are antirachitic in action, and have wavelengths between 3200 and 2900 Å.

ul·tra·vi·rus (ŭl′tră-vī′rŭs). SYN virus (2).

ul·tro·mo·tiv·i·ty (ŭl′trō-mō-tiv′i-tē). Power of spontaneous movement. [L. *ultro,* beyond, on one's own part + L. *motio,* movement]

ulu·la·tion (ū-lū-lā′shŭn). Rarely used term for the inarticulate crying of emotionally disturbed persons. [L. *ululo,* pp. *-atus,* to howl]

Uly′sses, Latin form of Greek mythological character. SEE Ulysses *syndrome.*

um·bil·i·cal (ŭm-bil′i-kăl). Relating to the umbilicus. SYN omphalic.

um·bil·i·cate, um·bil·i·cat·ed (ŭm-bil′i-kāt, -kāt-ed). Of navel shape; pitlike; dimpled. [L. *umbilicatus*]

um·bil·i·ca·tion (ŭm-bil-i-kā′shŭn). **1.** A pit or navel-like depression. **2.** Formation of a depression at the apex of a papule, vesicle, or pustule.

um·bil·i·cus, pl. **um·bil·i·ci** (ŭm-bil′i-kŭs, ŭm-bi-lī-kŭs; -i-sī, -lī′ kī) [NA]. The pit in the center of the abdominal wall marking the point where the umbilical cord entered in the fetus. SYN belly button, navel. [L. navel]

um·bo, gen. **um·bo·nis,** pl. **um·bo·nes** (ŭm′bō, -bō-nis, -bō-nēs). **1** [NA]. A projecting point of a surface. **2.** SYN u. of tympanic membrane. [L. boss of a shield, a knob]

u. membra′nae tym′pani [NA], SYN u. of tympanic membrane.

u. of tympanic membrane, the projection on the inner surface of the tympanic membrane at the end of the manubrium of the malleus; this corresponds to the most depressed point of the membrane, viewed laterally, that is commonly called the umbo. SYN u. membranae tympani [NA], umbo (2).

UMP Abbreviation for *uridine* 5′-monophosphate.

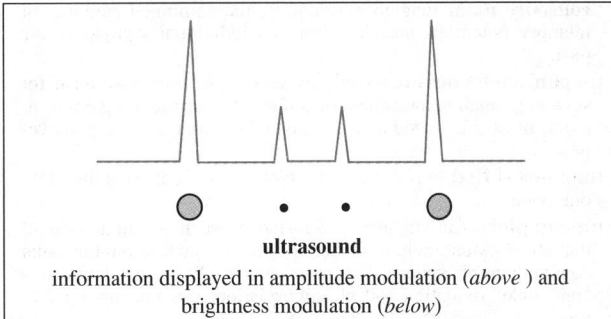

ultrasound

information displayed in amplitude modulation (*above*) and brightness modulation (*below*)

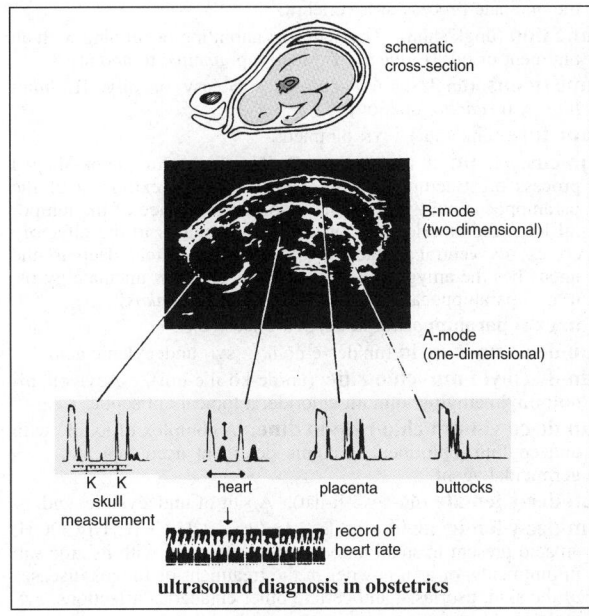

schematic cross-section

B-mode (two-dimensional)

A-mode (one-dimensional)

K K skull measurement

heart

placenta

buttocks

record of heart rate

ultrasound diagnosis in obstetrics

UMP syn·thase. SYN uridylic acid.

un-. 1. Not, akin to L. *in-* and G. *a-, an-.* **2.** Reversal, removal, release, deprivation. **3.** An intensive action. [M.E.]

un·cal (ŭng′kăl). Denoting or relating to the uncus.

un·ci (ŭn′sī). Plural of uncus.

un·cia (ŭn′sē-ă). An ounce. [L. a twelfth part, an ounce]

un·ci·form (ŭn′si-fōrm). SYN uncinate. [L. *uncus,* hook, + *forma,* form]

un·ci·for·me (ŭn-si-fōr′mē). SYN hamate *bone.* [Mod. L. unciform]

Un·ci·nar·ia (ŭn-si-nar′ē-ă). A genus of nematode hookworms that infect various mammals. Species include *U. stenocephala,* the European hookworm of dogs, cats, and various wild carnivores, also found in North America, where it is much less common than *Ancylostoma caninum,* though it has been implicated in human cutaneous larva migrans. [LL. *uncinus,* a hook]

un·ci·na·ri·a·sis (ŭn′si-nă-rī′ă-sis). SYN ancylostomiasis.

un·ci·nate (ŭn′si-nāt). **1.** Hooklike or hook-shaped. **2.** Relating to an uncus or, specifically, to the u. gyrus (2) or a process of the pancreas or of a vertebra. SYN unciform. [L. *uncinatus*]

un·ci·na·tum (ŭn-si-nā′tŭm). SYN hamate *bone.*

un·ci·pres·sure (ŭn′si-presh-ŭr). Arrest of hemorrhage from a cut artery by pressure with a blunt hook. [L. *uncus,* hook]

un·com·ple·ment·ed (ŭn-kom′plĕ-men-ted). Not united with complement and therefore inactive.

un·con·scious (ŭn-kon′shŭs). **1.** Not conscious. **2.** In psychoanalysis, the psychic structure comprising the drives and feelings of which one is unaware. SYN insensible (1).

collective u., in Jungian psychology, the combined engrams or memory potentials inherited from an individual's phylogenetic past.

un·con·scious·ness (ŭn-kon'shŭs-ness). An imprecise term for severely impaired awareness of self and the surrounding environment; most often used as a synonym for coma or unresponsiveness.

un·co-os·si·fied (ŭn-kō-os'i-fīd). Not co-ossified; not united into one bone.

un·cou·plers (ŭn-kŭp'lerz). Substances such as dinitrophenol that allow oxidation in mitochondria to proceed without the usual concomitant phosphorylation to produce ATP; these poisons thus "uncouple" oxidation and phosphorylation. SYN uncoupling factors.

un·co·ver·te·bral (ŭn-kō-ver'tĕ-brăl). Pertaining to or affecting the uncinate process of a vertebra.

unc·tion (ŭngk'shŭn). The action of anointing or rubbing with an ointment or oil. [L. unctio, fr. ungo, pp. unctus, to anoint]

unc·tu·ous (ŭngk'shū-ŭs, -chū-ŭs). Greasy or oily. [L. unctuosus, fr. unctio, unction]

unc·ture (ŭnk'chūr). SYN ointment.

un·cus, pl. **un·ci** (ŭn'kŭs, ŭn'sī) [NA]. **1.** Any hook-shaped process or structure. **2.** The anterior, hooked extremity of the parahippocampal gyrus on the basomedial surface of the temporal lobe; the anterior face of the u. corresponds to the olfactory cortex, its ventral surface to the entorhinal area; deep to the uncus lies the amygdala (amygdaloid body). SYN uncinate gyrus, u. gyri parahippocampalis. [L. a hook, fr. G. onkos]
u. gy'ri parahippocampa'lis, SYN uncus (2).

un·dec·e·no·ic ac·id (ŭn'des-ĕ-nō'ik). SYN undecylenic acid.

un·de·co·yl·i·um chlo·ride (ŭn-de-kō-il'ē-ŭm). Acylcolaminoformylmethylpyridinium chloride; a topical antiseptic.

un·de·co·yl·i·um chlo·ride-io·dine. A complex of iodine with undecoylium chloride; a cationic detergent used topically as a germicidal agent.

un·dec·y·len·ate (ŭn-des'i-li-nāt). A salt of undecylenic acid.

un·dec·y·len·ic ac·id (ŭn-des-i-len'ik). CH₂CH(CH₂)₈COOH; an acid present in small amounts in sweat; used with its zinc salt in ointments, or as a powder in the treatment of fungus diseases of the skin, psoriasis, and certain other cutaneous affections. SYN undecenoic acid.

un·der·a·chieve·ment (ŭn'der-ă-chēv'ment). Failure to achieve as well as one's abilities would seem to allow.

un·der·a·chiev·er (ŭn'der-ă-chēv'er). One who manifests underachievement.

un·der·bite (ŭn'der-bīt). A nontechnical term applied to mandibular underdevelopment or to excessive maxillary development.

un·der·cut (ŭn'der-kŭt). **1.** That portion of a tooth that lies between the survey line (height of contour) and the gingivae. **2.** The contour of a cross-section of a residual ridge or dental arch which would prevent the insertion of a denture. **3.** The contour of a flasking stone which interlocks in such a way as to prevent the separation of the parts.

un·der·drive pac·ing (ŭn'der-drīv pās'ing). Electrical stimulation of the heart at a rate lower than that of an existing tachycardia; designed to capture the heart between beats, *i.e.,* to interrupt a reentry pathway in order to terminate the tachycardia.

un·der·nu·tri·tion (ŭn'der-nū-tri'shŭn). A form of malnutrition resulting from a reduced supply of food or from inability to digest, assimilate, and utilize the necessary nutrients.

un·der·sens·ing (un'der-sen'sing). Non-sensing of the intracardiac atrial or ventricular depolarization signal by a pacemaker.

un·der·shoot (un'der-shūt). A temporary decrease below the final steady-state value that may occur immediately following the removal of an influence that had been raising that value, *i.e.,* overshoot in a negative direction.

un·der·stain (un'der-stān). To stain less deeply than usual.

un·der·ven·ti·la·tion (ŭn'der-ven-ti-lā'shŭn). SYN hypoventilation.

un·der·wind·ing (ŭn'der-wīnd'ing). The effect of negative supercoiling on a structure of DNA.

Underwood, Michael, English pediatrician, 1737–1820. SEE U.'s *disease.*

un·dif·fer·en·ti·at·ed (ŭn'dif-er-en'shē-ā-ted). Not differentiated; *e.g.,* primitive, embryonic, immature, or having no special structure or function.

un·dine (ŭn'dēn, -dīn). A small glass flask that was used in irrigation of the conjunctiva. [Mod. L. undina, fr. L. unda, wave]

un·din·ism (ŭn'di-nizm). A condition in which sexual thoughts are aroused by water, urine, and urination. [Mod. L. undina, fr. L. unda, wave]

un·di·ver·sion (ŭn-di-ver'shŭn). Surgical restoration of continuity in any organ system, the flow through which had previously been diverted; *e.g.,* between the upper urinary tract and bladder after supravesical urinary diversion.

un·do·ing (ŭn-dū'ing). In psychology and psychiatry, an unconscious defense mechanism by which one symbolically acts out in reverse some earlier unacceptable behavior.

un·du·late (ŭn'dū-lāt). Having an irregular, wavy border; denoting the shape of a bacterial colony. [Mod. L. undula, dim. of unda, wave]

un·du·li·po·di·um, pl. **un·du·li·po·dia** (ŭn'dū-li-pō'dē-um, -ă). A flexible whiplike intracellular extension of many eukaryotic cells, with a characteristic nine-fold symmetry, an arrangement of nine paired peripheral microtubules and one central pair, often termed 9 + 2 symmetry; it appears to grow out from a basal body (kinetosome) in the cell and is a fundamental component of the eukaryotic cell. Both the cilium and the eukaryotic flagellum (not the bacterial flagellum which lacks the 9 + 2 pattern) are considered u. [LL. undulo, to move in waves, fr. L. unda, wave, + Mod.L. podium, fr. G. podion, dim. of pous, foot]

ung Abbreviation of L. unguentum, ointment.

un·gual (ŭng'gwăl). Relating to a nail or the nails. SYN unguinal. [L. unguis, nail]

un·guent (ŭng'gwent). SYN ointment. [L. unguentum]

un·gues (ŭng'gwēz). Plural of unguis.

Un·guic·u·la·ta (ŭng-gwik-yū-lā'tă). A division of Mammalia including all mammals having nails or claws, as distinguished from the Ungulata. [L. unguiculus, nail or claw]

un·guic·u·late (ŭng-gwik'yū-lāt). Having nails or claws, as distinguished from hooves.

un·guic·u·lus (ŭn-gwik'yū-lŭs). A small nail or claw. [L. dim. of unguis, nail]

un·gui·nal (ŭng'gwi-năl). SYN ungual.

un·guis, pl. **un·gues** (ŭng'gwis, -gwēz) [NA]. SYN nail. [L.]
u. adun'cus, SYN ingrown *nail.*
u. a'vis, SYN *calcar* avis.
Haller's u., SYN *calcar* avis.
u. incarna'tus, SYN ingrown *nail.*

Un·gu·la·ta (ŭng-gyū-lā'tă). A division of Mammalia containing the mammals with hooves, as distinguished from the Unguiculata.

un·gu·late (ŭng'gyū-lāt). Having hooves. [L. ungulatus, fr. ungula, hoof]

un·gu·li·grade (ŭng'gyū-li-grād). Walking on hooves, as by horses, pigs, and ruminants. [L. ungula, a hoof, + gradus, a step]

⌂**uni-.** One, single, not paired; corresponds to G. *mono-.* [L. *unus*]

u·ni·ar·tic·u·lar (yū-nē-ar-tik'yū-lăr). SYN monarticular.

uni·ax·i·al (yū-nē-ak'sē-ăl). Having but one axis; growing chiefly in one direction.

uni·bas·al (yū-ni-bā'săl). Having but one base.

Un·i·blue A (yū'nē-blū) [C.I. 14553]. A protein stain used in electrophoresis.

uni·cam·er·al, uni·cam·er·ate (yū-nē-kam'ĕ-răl, -kam'ĕ-rāt). SYN monolocular.

uni·cel·lu·lar (yū-ni-sel'yū-lăr). Composed of but one cell, as in the protozoons; for such u. organisms capable of undertaking life processes independently of other cells, the term acellular is also used.

u·ni·cen·tral (yū-ni-sen'trăl). Having a single center, as of growth or of ossification.

uni·corn (yū′nē-kōrn). SYN unicornous.

uni·cor·nous (yū′ni-kōr′nŭs). Having but one horn, or cornu. SYN unicorn. [L. *unicornis,* fr. uni- + *cornu,* horn]

uni·cus·pid, uni·cus·pi·date (yū-ni-kŭs′pid, -kŭs′pi-dāt). Having only one cusp, as a canine tooth.

uni·fa·mil·i·al (yū′nē-fa-mil′ē-ăl). Relating to or occurring in a single family; denoting especially a nervous disease attacking several of the children in the same family in which no hereditary trait is apparent.

uni·fla·gel·late (yū-ni-flaj′ĕ-lāt). SYN monotrichous.

uni·fo·rate (yū-ni-fō′rāt). Having but one foramen, pore, or opening of any kind.

uni·form (yū′ni-fōrm). **1.** Having but one form; not variable in form. **2.** Of the same form or shape as another structure or object. [L. *uniformis,* fr. uni- + *forma,* form]

uni·ger·mi·nal (yū-ni-jer′mi-năl). Relating to a single germ or ovum, *e.g.,* monozygotic. SYN monogerminal, monozygotic, monozygous.

uni·glan·du·lar (yū-ni-glan′dū-lăr). Involving, relating to, or containing but one gland.

uni·lam·i·nar, uni·lam·i·nate (yū-ni-lam′i-năr, -lam′i-nāt). Having but one layer or lamina.

uni·lat·e·ral (yū-ni-lat′ĕ-răl). Confined to one side only.

uni·lo·bar (yū-ni-lō′băr). Having but one lobe.

uni·lo·cal (yū-ni-lō′kăl). Strictly, denoting a trait in which the genetic component is contributed exclusively by one locus; in practice, any trait in which the contribution from one locus is so large that the data are readily interpreted as mendelian.

uni·loc·u·lar (yū-ni-lok′yū-lăr). Having but one compartment or cavity, as in a fat cell. [uni- + L. *loculus,* compartment]

uni·mo·lec·u·lar (yū′ni-mō-lek′yū-lăr). Denoting a single molecule. SYN monomolecular.

uni·nu·cle·ar, uni·nu·cle·ate (yū-ni-nū′klē-ăr, -nū′klē-āt). Having but one nucleus. Cf. mononuclear.

uni·oc·u·lar (yū-ni-ok′yū-lăr). **1.** Relating to one eye only. **2.** Having vision in only one eye.

un·ion (yūn′yŭn). **1.** The joining or amalgamation of two or more bodies. **2.** The structural adhesion or growing together of the edges of a wound. [L. *unus,* one]

autogenous u., in dentistry, the u. of two pieces of metal without solder.

faulty u., SYN fibrous u.

fibrous u., u. of fracture by fibrous tissue. SEE nonunion. SYN faulty u.

primary u., SYN *healing* by first intention.

secondary u., SYN *healing* by second intention.

vicious u., u. of the ends of a broken bone resulting in a deformity or a crooked limb; frequently used interchangeably with faulty u. SYN malunion.

uni·o·val, uni·ov·u·lar (yū-nē-ō′văl, -ov′yū-lăr). Relating to or formed from a single ovum.

uni·pen·nate (yū-ni-pen′āt). **1.** Having a feather arrangement on one side; resembling one-half of a feather. **2.** Denoting certain muscles with fibers running at an acute angle from one side of a tendon. SYN demipenniform. [uni- + L. *penna,* feather]

uni·po·lar (yū-ni-pō′lăr). **1.** Having but one pole; denoting a nerve cell from which the branches project from one side only. **2.** Situated at one extremity only of a cell.

uni·port (yū′ni-pōrt). Transport of a molecule or ion through a membrane by a carrier mechanism (uniporter), without known coupling to any other molecule or ion transport. Cf. antiport, symport. [uni- + L. *porto,* to carry]

uni·port·er (yū′ni-pōrt-er). A protein that mediates the transport of one molecule or ion through a membrane without known coupling to the transport of any other molecule or ion.

uni·po·tent (yū′ni-pō′tent). Referring to those cells that produce a single type of daughter cell; *e.g.,* a u. stem cell. Cf. pluripotent *cells,* under cell.

uni·sep·tate (yū-ni-sep′tāt). Having but one septum or partition.

UNIT

unit (U) (yū′nit). **1.** One; a single person or thing. **2.** A standard of measure, weight, or any other quality, by multiplications or fractions of which a scale or system is formed. **3.** A group of persons or things considered as a whole because of mutual activities or functions. **4.** SYN international u. [L. *unus,* one]

absolute u., a u. whose value is constant regardless of place or time and not derived from dependent on gravitation.

alexin u., SYN complement u.

Allen-Doisy u., the quantity of estrogen capable of producing in a spayed mouse a characteristic change in the vaginal epithelium, namely, disappearance of leukocytes and appearance of cornified cells, as determined by a vaginal smear; equal approximately to one-half of an estrone u. SYN mouse u.

alpha u.'s, cytoplasmic glycogen granules arranged in rosettes.

amboceptor u., SYN hemolysin u.

androgen u. (international), the androgenic activity of 100 μg (0.1 mg) of crystalline androsterone as assayed by the comb growth response in capons.

Ångström u. (Å), SEE Ångström.

antigen u., the smallest amount of antigen that, in the presence of specific antiserum, will fix 1 complement u.

antitoxin u., a u. expressing the strength or activity of an antitoxin; in general, determined with reference to a preserved standard preparation of antitoxin. SEE ALSO L *doses,* under *dose.*

antivenene u., the amount of antivenum which, injected in the ear vein, will protect 1 g weight of rabbit against a fatal dose of snake venom.

atomic mass u. (amu), a u. of mass by definition equal to $\frac{1}{12}$ of the mass of an atom of carbon-12, which equals $1.6605402 \times 10^{-27}$ kg; in terms of energy, 1 amu equals 931.49432 MeV. Cf. dalton.

base u.'s, the fundamental u.'s of length, mass, time, electric current, thermodynamic temperature, amount of substance, and luminous intensity in the International System of Units (SI); the names and symbols of the u.'s for these quantities are meter (m), kilogram (kg), second (s), ampere (A), kelvin (K), mole (mol), and candela (cd). SEE ALSO International System of Units.

Bethesda u., a measure of inhibitor activity: the amount of inhibitor that will inactivate 50% or 0.5 unit of a coagulation factor during the incubation period. [*Bethesda,* MD]

biological standard u., a specific quantity of biologically active reference material (antibiotic, antitoxin, enzyme, hormone, vitamin, etc.).

bird u., a u. of prolactin activity: the minimal quantity of the hormone which will cause a certain increase in weight of the crop gland of pigeons.

Bodansky u., that amount of phosphatase that liberates 1 mg of phosphorus as inorganic phosphate during the first hour of incubation with a buffered substrate containing sodium β-glycerophosphate.

British thermal u. (BTU), the quantity of heat required to raise one pound of water from 3.9°C to 4.4°C; equal to 251.996 calories or to 1055.056 joules. SYN u. of heat (2).

capon u., amount of androgen needed to produce an increase in the capon comb surface of 20%. SYN capon-comb u.

capon-comb u., SYN capon u.

cat u., the dose of a drug (per kilogram of body weight of cat) which is just large enough to kill a cat when administered intravenously; was applied in the standardization of digitalis materials.

centimeter-gram-second u. (CGS, cgs), CGS u., cgs u., an absolute u. of the centimeter-gram-second system.

chlorophyll u., the number of chlorophyll molecules required to reduce one molecule of carbon dioxide by photosynthesis.

chorionic gonadotropin u. (international), the specific gonadotropic activity of 0.1 mg of the standard preparation of chorionic

un

gonadotropin originating from the urine or placentas of pregnant women.

Clauberg u., SEE Clauberg *test*.

complement u., the smallest amount (highest dilution) of complement that will cause hemolysis of a u. of red blood cells in the presence of a hemolysin u. SYN alexin u.

Corner-Allen u., a u. of progestational activity, measured in rabbits; the minimum dose which, divided into five equal daily portions, produces on the sixth day the uterine changes characteristic of the eighth day of normal pregnancy; the u. has about the same potency as the international u.

coronary care u. (CCU), a group of beds within a hospital set aside for the care of patients having or suspected of having myocardial infarction.

corpus luteum hormone u., SYN progesterone u.

critical care u. (CCU), SYN intensive care u.

CT u., a unit of x-ray attenuation in each picture element of the CT image. SEE Hounsfield u.

Dam u., a u. of activity of vitamin K; the smallest amount of vitamin K, per gram of chick per day, capable of producing normal coagulability in the blood of K-avitaminotic chicks after 3 days of oral administration.

digitalis u. (international), the activity of 0.1 g of the international standard powdered digitalis.

diphtheria antitoxin u., the antitoxin activity of 0.0628 mg standard diphtheria antitoxin.

dog u., the amount of adrenal cortical extract per kilogram of body weight which, given daily, will maintain an adrenalectomized dog in good condition for 7 to 10 days.

electromagnetic u. (emu), the u. in an absolute system (CGS) of u.'s utilizing the magnetic effects of current; *e.g.,* abampere, abfarad, abhenry, abohm, abvolt.

electrostatic u. (esu), the u. in an absolute system (CGS) of u.'s utilizing static electricity; *e.g.,* statampere, statcoulomb, statfarad, stathenry, statvolt.

u. of energy, (1) CGS system: erg, joule; **(2)** MKS system: newton-meter (joule); **(3)** FPS system: foot-poundal; **(4)** gravitational u.: gram-centimeter, gram-meter, kilogram-meter, footpound; **(5)** SI: joule.

equine gonadotropin u. (international), the specific gonadotropic activity of 0.25 mg of standard preparation of the gonadotropic principle of pregnant mares' serum.

estradiol benzoate u. (international), the estrogenic activity of 0.1 μg of a standard preparation of estradiol benzoate.

estrone u. (international), the estrogenic activity of 0.1 μg (0.0001 mg) of a standard preparation of crystalline estrone.

Fishman-Lerner u., a u. of serum acid phosphatase activity based upon measurement of the amount of phenol released from a phenylphosphate substrate.

Florey u., SYN Oxford u.

foot-pound-second u. (FPS, fps), FPS u., fps u., an absolute u. of the foot-pound-second system.

u. of force, (1) CGS system: dyne; **(2)** FPS system: poundal; **(3)** MKS system: newton; **(4)** SI: newton.

gravitational u.'s (G), of energy: gram-centimeter, gram-meter, kilogram-meter, and foot-pound.

G u. of streptomycin, SEE streptomycin u.'s.

u. of heat, (1) calorie (gram calorie; kilocalorie) **(2)** SYN British thermal u. **(3)** SYN joule.

hemolysin u., hemolytic u., the smallest quantity (highest dilution) of inactivated immune serum (hemolysin) that will sensitize the standard suspension of erythrocytes so that the standard complement will cause complete hemolysis. SYN amboceptor u.

heparin u., the quantity of heparin required to keep 1 ml of cat's blood fluid for 24 hr at 0°C; it is equivalent approximately to 0.002 mg of pure heparin. SYN Howell u.

Holzknecht u. (H), an obsolete u. of x-ray dosage equal to one-fifth of the erythema dose.

Hounsfield u., a normalized index of x-ray attenuation based on a scale of -1000 (air) to +1000 (bone), with water being 0; used in CT imaging.

Howell u., SYN heparin u.

insulin u. (international), the activity contained in $\frac{1}{22}$ mg of the international standard of zinc-insulin crystals.

intensive care u. (ICU), a hospital facility for provision of intensive nursing and medical care of critically ill patients, characterized by high quality and quantity of continuous nursing and medical supervision and by use of sophisticated monitoring and resuscitative equipment; may be organized for the care of specific patient groups, *e.g.,* neonatal or newborn ICU, neurological ICU, pulmonary ICU. SYN critical care u.

u. of intermedin, a u. based upon the action of the hormone in causing the expansion of the melanophores in a hypophysectomized frog; equal to 1 μg of alkali-treated USP Posterior-pituitary Reference Standard.

international u. (IU), the amount of a substance, such as a drug, hormone, vitamin, enzyme, etc., that produces a specific effect as defined by an international body and accepted internationally; *e.g.,* for an enzyme it is μmole of product formed (or substrate consumed) per minute. SYN unit (4).

International System of U.'s, SEE International System of Units.

Jenner-Kay u., that amount of phosphatase that liberates 1 mg of phosphorus; approximately 2 Bodansky u.'s or 1 King u.

Karmen u., a formerly used enzyme u. for aminotransferase activity; a change of 0.001 in the absorbance of NADH/min.

Kienböck's u. (X), an obsolete u. of x-ray dosage equivalent to $\frac{1}{10}$ the erythema dose.

King u., the quantity of phosphatase that, acting upon disodium phenylphosphate in excess, at pH 9 for 30 min, liberates 1 mg of phenol. SYN King-Armstrong u.

King-Armstrong u., SYN King u.

u. of length, (1) metric system and SI: meter; **(2)** CGS system: centimeter; **(3)** variable in the English system: inch for short distances, foot for moderate distances and for elevation, mile for long distances.

u. of light, SEE candela, lux.

L u. of streptomycin, SEE streptomycin u.'s.

u. of luminous flux, SEE lumen.

u. of luminous intensity, SEE candela.

lung u., (1) a respiratory bronchiole together with the alveolar ducts and sacs and pulmonary alveoli into which the respiratory bronchiole leads; **(2)** considered by some to include the terminal bronchiole and its subdivisions, and called a pulmonary *acinus*.

u. of luteinizing activity (international), SYN progesterone u.

u. of magnetic field intensity, SEE gauss, tesla.

u. of magnetic flux intensity, SEE gauss, tesla.

u. of mass, (1) metric system: gram; **(2)** SI: kilogram; **(3)** english system: pound.

meter-kilogram-second u., MKS u., mks u., an absolute u. of the meter-kilogram-second system.

motor u., a single somatic motor neuron and the group of muscle fibers innervated by it.

mouse u. (m.u.), SYN Allen-Doisy u.

u. of ocular convergence, SYN meter *angle*.

ostiomeatal u., SYN ostiomeatal *complex*.

Oxford u., the minimum amount of penicillin which will prevent the growth of *Staphylococcus aureus* over an area 26 mm in diameter in a standard culture medium; 1 u. equals 0.6 μg of crystalline sodium salt of penicillin. SYN Florey u.

u. of oxytocin, the oxytocic activity of 0.5 mg of the USP Posterior-pituitary Reference Standard; 1 mg of synthetic oxytocin corresponds to 500 IU.

u. of penicillin (international), the penicillin activity of 0.6 μg of penicillin G.

phosphatase u., SEE Bodansky u., King u.

physiologic u., (1) the ultimate (hypothetical) vital u. of protoplasm, as conceived by Spencer; **(2)** the smallest division of an organ that will perform its function; *e.g.,* the uriniferous tubule.

practical u.'s, u.'s of magnitudes convenient for use in the practical applications of electricity; as originally defined they were absolute u.'s (multiples of CGS electromagnetic u.'s); they include the ampere, coulomb, farad, henry, joule, ohm, volt, and watt.

u. of progestational activity (international), SEE progesterone u.

progesterone u. (international), the progestational activity of 1 mg of u. of progestational activity (international); standard preparation of pure progesterone. SEE ALSO Clauberg *test,* Corner-Allen u. SYN corpus luteum hormone u., u. of luteinizing activity.

prolactin u. (international), the specific lactogenic activity contained in 0.1 mg of the standard preparation of the lactogenic substance of the anterior pituitary gland.

u. of radioactivity, SEE Becquerel.

riboflavin u., potency usually expressed in terms of weight of pure riboflavin. SEE ALSO Sherman-Bourquin u. of vitamin B_2. SYN vitamin B_2 u.

roentgen u., SEE Roentgen.

Schwann cell u., a single Schwann cell and all of the axons lying in troughs indenting its surface; this u. regarded as an unmyelinated fiber in the peripheral nervous system.

Sherman u., u. of vitamin C, minimum protective dose; the minimum amount of vitamin C which, fed daily, will protect a 300-g guinea pig from scurvy for 90 days; equivalent to 0.5 to 0.6 mg of ascorbic acid.

Sherman-Bourquin u. of vitamin B_2, the amount of vitamin B_2 required in the diet daily to sustain an average weekly gain of 3 g for 8 weeks in standard test rats; one u. is equivalent to 1 to 7 µg (0.001 to 0.007 mg) of riboflavin, depending on the deficiency diet used in the above assay.

Sherman-Munsell u., a rat growth u.; the daily amount of vitamin A which sustains a rate of gain amounting to 3 g a week in standard test rats.

SI u.'s, SEE base u.'s, International System of Units.

Somogyi u., a measure of the level of activity of amylase in blood serum, as analyzed by means of the Somogyi method (the most frequently used procedure); one u. is equivalent to 1 mg of reducing sugar liberated as glucose per 100 ml of serum, when an aliquot of the latter is mixed with a standard starch substrate (plus sodium chloride for maximal activation) and incubated for a standard time; normal range is 80 to 150 u.'s, but values are usually not regarded as clinically significant unless they are greater than 200.

S u. of streptomycin, SEE streptomycin u.'s.

Steenbock u., a u. of vitamin D; the total amount of vitamin D which will produce within 10 days a narrow line of calcium deposit in the rachitic metaphyses of the distal ends of the radii and ulnae of standard rachitic rats.

streptomycin u.'s, (1) g u.: equals 1 g of the crystalline material or about 1,000,000 S u.'s; **(2)** l u.: equal to 1000 S u.'s; **(3)** s u.: the amount of streptomycin which will inhibit the growth of a standard strain of *Escherichia coli* in 1 ml of nutrient broth or other suitable medium.

Svedberg u. (S), a sedimentation constant of 1×10^{-13} seconds.

tetanus antitoxin u., the antitoxin activity of 0.3094 mg of standard tetanus antitoxin.

thiamin chloride u., thiamin hydrochloride u. (international).

thiamin hydrochloride u. (international), the antineuritic activity of 0.003 mg of the standard crystalline vitamin B_1 hydrochloride. SYN vitamin B_1 hydrochloride u.

u. of thyrotrophic activity, the activity of an amount of an extract of the anterior lobe of the hypophysis which, given daily for 5 days, will cause the thyroid of a guinea pig (weighing 200 g) to reach a weight of 600 mg.

Todd u., the u. in which the results of testing for antistreptolysin O (ASO) are expressed. It denotes the reciprocal of the highest dilution of test serum at which there continues to be neutralization of a standard preparation of the streptococcal enzyme streptolysin O.

toxic u. (T.U.), a u. formerly synonymous with minimal lethal dose but which, because of the instability of toxins, is now measured in terms of the quantity of standard antitoxin with which the toxin combines. SEE ALSO L *doses,* under *dose,* minimal lethal *dose.* SYN toxin u.

toxin u. (T.U.), SYN toxic u.

USP u., a u. as defined and adopted by the *United States Pharmacopeia.*

u. of vasopressin, the pressor activity of 0.5 mg of the USP Posterior-pituitary Reference Standard; 1 mg of synthetic vasopressin corresponds to 600 IU.

vitamin A u. (international), the specific biologic activity of 0.3 µg of vitamin A (alcohol form). SEE ALSO Sherman-Munsell u.

vitamin B_2 u., SYN riboflavin u.

vitamin B_6 u., potency expressed in terms of weight of pure crystalline pyridoxine.

vitamin B_1 hydrochloride u., SYN thiamin hydrochloride u.

vitamin C u. (international), the vitamin C activity of 0.05 mg of the standard crystalline levoascorbic acid; 1 mg of crystalline vitamin C provides 20 USP u.'s. SEE ALSO Sherman u.

vitamin D u. (international), the antirachitic activity contained in 0.025 µg of a preparation of crystalline vitamin D_3 (activated 7-dehydrocholesterol). SEE ALSO Steenbock u.

vitamin E u., potency usually expressed in terms of weight of pure α-tocopherol.

vitamin K u., SEE Dam u.

volume u. (VU), a u. of a logarithmic scale for expressing the power level of a complex audio-frequency electrical signal, such as that transmitting music or speech; the power in volume u.'s equals the decibels of power above a reference level of one milliwatt, as measured with an appropriate meter.

u. of wavelength, SEE Ångström, nanometer.

u. of weight, SEE u. of mass.

Wood u.'s, a simplified measurement of pulmonary vascular resistance that uses pressures instead of more complicated u.'s measured by subtracting pulmonary capillary wedge pressure from the mean pulmonary arterial pressure and dividing by cardiac output in liters per minute.

u. of work, SEE u. of energy.

Uni·ted States Adopt·ed Names (USAN). Designation for nonproprietary names (for drugs) adopted by the USAN Council in cooperation with the manufacturers concerned; the designation USAN is applicable only to nonproprietary names coined since June 1961.

Uni·ted States Phar·ma·co·pe·ia (USP). SEE Pharmacopeia.

Uni·ted States Pub·lic Health Ser·vice (USPHS). A bureau of the Department of Health and Human Services, served by a corps of medical officers presided over by the Surgeon General, concerned with scientific research, domestic and insular quarantine, administration of government hospitals, publication of sanitary reports, and statistics; associated with it are the National Institutes of Health, Centers for Disease Control and Prevention, and other units.

uni·va·lence, uni·va·len·cy (yū-ni-vā′lens, -vā′len-sē). SYN monovalence.

uni·va·lent (yū-ni-vā′lent). SYN monovalent (1).

un·med·ul·lat·ed (ŭn-med′yū-lā-ted). SYN unmyelinated.

un·my·e·li·nat·ed (ŭn-mī′ĕ-li-nā-ted). Denoting nerve fibers (axons) lacking a myelin sheath. SYN amyelinated, amyelinic, nonmedullated, nonmyelinated, unmedullated.

Unna, Paul G., German dermatologist and staining expert, 1850–1929. SEE U.'s *disease, mark, stain;* U.-Pappenheim *stain;* U.-Taenzer *stain.*

un·of·fi·cial (ŭn-ŏ-fish′ăl). Denoting a drug that is not listed in the United States Pharmacopeia or the National Formulary.

un·phys·i·o·log·ic (ŭn-fis′ē-ō-loj′ik). Pertaining to conditions in the organism which are abnormal; can be used to refer to subjecting the body to abnormal amounts of substances normally present.

un·san·i·tary (ŭn-san′i-tār-ē). SYN insanitary.

un·sat·u·rat·ed (ŭn-sach′ŭr-āt-ed). **1.** Not saturated; denoting a solution in which the solvent is capable of dissolving more of the solute. **2.** Denoting a chemical compound in which all the affinities are not satisfied, so that still other atoms or radicals may be added to it. **3.** In organic chemistry, denoting compounds containing double and/or triple bonds.

un·sex (ŭn′seks). To castrate; to deprive of the gonads.

un·sound·ness (ŭn-sownd′nes). In a horse, any deviation in form or function from the normal that interferes with the animal's usefulness.

un·stri·at·ed (ŭn-strī′āt-ed). Without striations; not striped; denoting the structure of the smooth or involuntary muscles.

un·thrifty (ŭn-thrif′tē). In animals, denoting a failure to grow or develop normally as a result of disease.

Unverricht, Heinrich, German physician, 1853–1912. SEE U.'s *disease.*

UPJ Abbreviation for ureteropelvic *junction.*

up·reg·u·la·tion. Opposite of down-regulation.

up·si·loid (ŭp′si-loyd). SYN hypsiloid.

up·si·lon (up′si-lon). 20th Letter in the Greek alphabet.

up·stream (ŭp′strēm). Refers to nucleic acid base sequences proceeding the opposite direction from expression.

up·take (ŭp′tāk). The absorption by a tissue of some substance, food material, mineral, etc. and its permanent or temporary retention.

Ura Abbreviation for uracil.

ura·chal (yūr′ă-kăl). Relating to the urachus.

ura·chus (yūr′ă-kŭs). That portion of the reduced allantoic stalk between the apex of the bladder and the umbilicus median umbilical ligament; postnatally, the u. is normally merely a fibrous cord, but occasionally the old allantoic lumen may persist as a vesicoumbilical fistula. [G. *ourachos,* the urinary canal of a fetus]

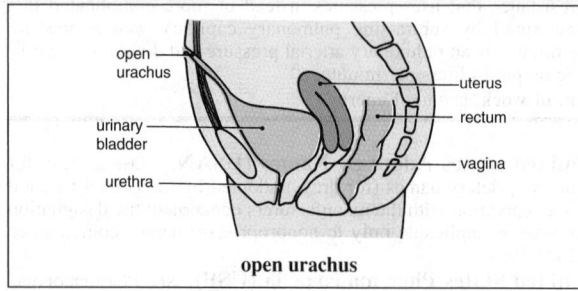

open urachus — uterus — urinary bladder — rectum — urethra — vagina

open urachus

ura·cil (Ura, U) (yūr′ă-sil). 2,4-Dioxopyrimidine; 2,4-(1*H*,3*H*)-pyrimidinedione; a pyrimidine (base) present in ribonucleic acid.

u. dehydrogenase, an oxidoreductase catalyzing oxidation of uracil to barbituric acid; also oxidizes thymine. SYN u. oxidase.

u. mustard, 5-[bis(2-chloroethyl)amino]uracil; an alkylating antineoplastic agent. SYN uramustine.

u. oxidase, SYN u. dehydrogenase.

u. phosphoribosyltransferase, SEE phosphoribosyltransferase.

ura·cil·-6-car·box·yl·ic ac·id. SYN orotic acid.

Ur·a·go·ga (yūr′ă-gō-gă). A genus of tropical plants (family Rubiaceae). *U. ipecacuanha* (*Cephaelis ipecacuanha*) is the source of Rio or Brazilian ipecac; *U. acuminata* (*C. acuminata*) is the source of Cartagena, Nicaragua, or Panama ipecac. SYN *Cephaelis.*

ur·a·mus·tine (yūr-ă-mŭs′tēn). SYN *uracil* mustard.

ura·nin (yū′ră-nin). SYN *fluorescein* sodium.

ura·ni·nite (yū-ran′i-nīt). SYN pitchblende.

△**uranisco-.** SEE urano-.

ura·nis·co·chasm (yū-ră-nis′kō-kazm). SYN uranoschisis. [uranisco- + G. *chasma,* cleft]

ura·nis·co·ni·tis (yū′ră-nis-kō-nī′tis). SYN palatitis.

ura·nis·co·plas·ty (yū′ră-nis′kō-plas-tē). SYN palatoplasty. [uranisco- + G. *plassō,* to form]

ura·nis·cor·rha·phy (yū′ră-nis-kōr′ă-fē). SYN palatorrhaphy. [uranisco- + G. *rhaphē,* suture]

ura·nis·cus (yū′ră-nis′kŭs). SYN palate. [G. *ouraniskos,* roof of the mouth, dim. of *ouranos,* sky]

ura·ni·um (U) (yū-rā′nē-ŭm). A radioactive metallic element, atomic no. 92, atomic wt. 238.0289, occurring mainly in pitchblende and notable for its two isotopes: ^{238}U and ^{235}U (99.2745% and 0.720%, respectively, the rest being made up by ^{234}U), ^{235}U

being the first substance ever shown capable of supporting a self-sustaining chain reaction. [G. myth. character, *Uranus*]

△**urano-, uranisco-.** The hard palate. [G. *ouranos,* sky vault, *ouraniskos,* roof of mouth (palate)]

ura·no·plas·ty (yū′ră-nō-plas-tē). SYN palatoplasty.

ura·nor·rha·phy (yū′ră-nōr′ă-fē). SYN palatorrhaphy. [urano- + G. *rhaphē,* suture]

ura·nos·chi·sis (yū′ră-nos′ki-sis). Cleft of the hard palate. SYN uraniscochasm. [urano- + G. *schisis,* fissure]

ura·no·staph·y·lo·plas·ty (yū′ră-nō-staf′i-lō-plas-tē). Repair of a cleft of both hard and soft palate. SYN uranostaphylorrhaphy. [urano- + G. *staphylē,* uvula, + *plassō,* to form]

ura·no·staph·y·lor·rha·phy (yū′ră-nō-staf-i-lōr′ă-fē). SYN uranostaphyloplasty.

ura·no·staph·y·los·chi·sis (yū′ră-nō-staf′i-los′ki-sis). Cleft of the soft and hard palates. SYN uranoveloschisis. [urano- + G. *staphylē,* uvula, + *schisis,* fissure]

ura·no·ve·los·chi·sis (yū′ră-nō-vĕ-los′ki-sis). SYN uranostaphyloschisis.

ura·nyl (yūr′ă-nil). The ion, UO_2^{2+} usually found in such salts as uranyl nitrate, $UO_2(NO_3)_2$; uranyl acetate, $UO_2(CH_3COO)_2$, is used in electron microscopy.

urap·i·dil (ū-ră′pĭ-dil). An antihypertensive agent which acts by influencing serotonin receptors.

ura·ro·ma (yū′ră-rō′mă). A spicy, aromatic odor of the urine. [G. *ouron,* urine, + *arōma,* spice]

urar·thri·tis (yū-rar-thrī′tis). Gouty inflammation of a joint. [urate + arthritis]

urate (yūr′āt). A salt of uric acid.

u. oxidase, a copper-containing, oxygen-requiring oxidoreductase that oxidizes uric acid; used in the clinical diagnosis of increased uric acid levels. SYN uricase.

ura·te·mia (yū-rā-tē′mē-ă). The presence of urates, especially sodium urate, in the blood. [urate + G. *haima,* blood]

ur·ate·ri·bo·nu·cle·o·tide phos·pho·ryl·ase (yūr′āt-rī-bō-nū′klē-ō-tīd). A ribosyltransferase that reacts urate D-ribonucleotide with orthophosphate to produce urate plus D-ribose 1-phosphate.

urat·ic (yū-rat′ik). Pertaining to a urate or to urates.

ura·tol·y·sis (yū-ră-tol′i-sis). The decomposition or solution of urates. [urate + G. *lysis,* solution]

ura·to·ly·tic (yū′ră-tō-lit′ik). Causing the decomposition, or solution and removal of urates, from the tissues.

ura·to·ma (yū-ră-tō′mă). SYN gouty *tophus.* [urate + G. *-oma,* tumor]

ura·to·sis (yū-ră-tō′sis). Any morbid condition due to the presence of urates in the blood or tissues.

ura·tu·ria (yū-rā-tū′rē-ă). The passage of an increased amount of urates in the urine. [urate + G. *ouron,* urine]

Urbach, Erich, U.S. dermatologist, 1893–1946. SEE U.-Wiethe *disease.*

Urban, Jerome A., S. surgeon, *1914. SEE U.'s *operation.*

ur·ce·i·form (yūr-sē′i-fōrm). Pitcher-shaped. SYN urceolate. [L. *urceus,* pitcher, + *forma,* form]

ur·ce·o·late (yūr′sē-ō-lāt). SYN urceiform. [L. *urceolus,* dim. of *urceus,* pitcher]

Urd Abbreviation for uridine.

ur·de·fens·es (ūr′dē-fens-ez). Fundamental beliefs essential for human psychological integrity; *e.g.,* religion, science.

△**ure-, urea-, ureo-.** Urea; urine. SEE ALSO urin-, uro-. [G. *ouron,* urine]

urea (yū-rē′ă). NH_2-CO-NH_2; carbonyldiamide; the chief end product of nitrogen metabolism in mammals, formed in the liver, by means of the Krebs-Henseleit cycle, and excreted in normal adult human urine in the amount of about 32 g a day (about 6⁄7 of the nitrogen excreted from the body). It may be obtained artificially by heating a solution of ammonium cyanate. It occurs as colorless or white prismatic crystals, without odor but with a cooling saline taste, is soluble in water, and forms salts with acids; has been used as a diuretic in kidney function tests, and topically for various dermatitides. [G. *ouron,* urine]

u. peroxide, $CH_4N_2O \cdot H_2O_2$; a white crystalline compound used in an aqueous solution as an oxidizing mouthwash.

u. stibamine, a u. derivative of stibanilic acid, used in the treatment of kala azar and certain other tropical diseases.

ure·a·gen·e·sis (yū-rē-ă-jen'ĕ-sis). Formation of urea, usually referring to the metabolism of amino acids to urea. SYN ureapoiesis. [urea + G. *genesis,* production]

ure·al (yū-rē'ăl). Relating to or containing urea. SYN ureic.

Ure·a·plas·ma (yū-rē'ă-plaz'mă). A genus of microaerophilic to anaerobic, nonmotile bacteria (family Mycoplasmataceae) containing Gram-negative, predominantly coccoidal to coccobacillary elements, approximately 0.3 μm in diameter, which frequently grow in short filaments; colonies are generally small, 20 to 30 μm in diameter, and are normally without zones of surface growth. These organisms hydrolyze urea with production of ammonia, and are found in the human genitourinary tract, occasionally in the pharynx and rectum. In males, they are associated with nongonococcal urethritis and prostatitis; in females, with genitourinary tract infections and reproductive failure. The type species is *U. urealyticum.* SYN T-mycoplasma.

U. urealy'ticum, a species that has been isolated from the respiratory tract and central nerve system of newborns. It causes infections of the genitourinary tract, particularly urethritis. Thought to be sexually transmitted and transmitted from mother to infant.

ure·a·poi·e·sis (yū-rē'ă-poy-ē'sis). SYN ureagenesis. [urea + G. *poiēsis,* a making]

ure·ase (yūr'ē-ās). An enzyme that catalyzes the hydrolysis of urea to carbon dioxide and ammonia; used as an antitumor enzyme; it is present in intestinal bacterial and accounts for most of the ammonia generated from urea in mammals.

urec·chy·sis (yū-rek'i-sis). Obsolete term for extravasation of urine into the tissues. [G. *ouron,* urine, + *ekchysis,* a pouring out]

ure·de·ma (yū-re-dē'mă). Edema due to infiltration of urine into the subcutaneous tissues. [G. *ouron,* urine, + *oidēma,* swelling]

ure·do (yū-rē'dō). **1.** SYN urticaria. **2.** A burning sensation in the skin. [L. a blight, a burning itch, fr. *uro,* pp. *ustus,* to burn]

ure·ic (yū-rē'ik). SYN ureal.

ure·ide (yūr'ē-īd). Any compound of urea in which one or more of its hydrogen atoms have been substituted by acid radicals.

3-ure·i·do·hy·dan·to·in (u-rē'i-dō-hī'dan-tō-in). SYN allantoin.

3-ure·i·do·i·so·bu·tyr·ic ac·id (yū-rē'i-dō-ī'sō-byū-tir'ik). $H_2NCONH–CH_2CH(CH_3)COOH$; an intermediate in thymine catabolism.

3-ure·i·do·pro·pi·on·ic ac·id (yū-rē'i-dō-prō-pi-on'ik). H_2N-CONH–CH_2CH_2COOH; an intermediate in uracil catabolism.

ure·i·do·suc·cin·ic ac·id (yū-rē'i-dō-sŭk-sin'ik). $NH_2CONHCH$ (COOH)CH_2COOH; *N*-carbamoylaspartic acid; a precursor of the pyrimidines. SYN *N*-carbamoylaspartic.

urel·co·sis (yū-rel-kō'sis). Ulceration of any part of the urinary tract. [G. *ouron,* urine, + *helkōsis,* ulceration]

ure·mia (yū-rē'mē-ă). **1.** An excess of urea and other nitrogenous waste in the blood. **2.** The complex of symptoms due to severe persisting renal failure that can be relieved by dialysis. SYN azotemia. [G. *ouron,* urine, + *haima,* blood]

hypercalcemic u., u. due to renal failure caused by hypercalcemia with nephrocalcinosis.

ure·mic (yū-rē'mik). Relating to uremia.

ure·mi·gen·ic (yū-rē-mi-jen'ik). **1.** Of uremic origin or causation. **2.** Causing or resulting in uremia.

ureo-. SEE ure-.

ure·o·tele (yūr'ē-ō-tēl). An organism that is ureotelic; *e.g.,* primates.

ure·o·tel·ia (yūr'ē-ō-tēl'ē-a). The process or type of nitrogen excretion in which urea is the primary end product. [urea + G. *telos,* end, outcome, + -ia]

ure·o·tel·ic (yūr'ē-ō-tel'ik). Excreting nitrogen primarily in the form of urea. [ureo- + G. *telos,* end]

ur·er·y·thrin (yūr-er'i-thrin). SYN uroerythrin.

ure·si·es·the·sia (yū-rē'si-es-thē'zē-ă). The desire to urinate. SYN uriesthesia. [G. *ourēsis,* a urinating, + *aisthēsis,* sensation]

ure·sis (yū-rē'sis). SYN urination. [G. *ourēsis*]

ure·ter (yū-rē'ter, yū'rē-ter) [NA]. The thick-walled tube that conducts the urine from the renal pelvis to the bladder; it consists of an abdominal part and a pelvic part, is lined with transitional epithelium surrounded by smooth muscle, both circular and longitudinal, and is covered externally by a tunica adventitia. [G. *ourētēr,* urinary canal]

curlicue u., term given to the radiographic appearance of an opacified u., herniated through the sciatic foramen; a very rare condition.

ectopic u., opens somewhere other than the bladder wall.

postcaval u., congenital defect where the right u. passes deep to the inferior vena cava on its descent to the bladder.

retrocaval u., in urography, the medial deviation of the right u. in the rare circumstance in which it passes behind the inferior vena cava before entering the pelvis.

retroiliac u., congenital defect where the u. passes deep to the iliac artery.

ure·ter·al (yū-rē'tĕ-răl). Relating to the ureter. SYN ureteric.

ure·ter·al·gia (yū-rē-ter-al'jē-ă). Pain in the ureter. [ureter + G. *algos,* pain]

ure·ter·cys·to·scope (yū-rē'ter-sis'tō-skōp). SYN ureterocystoscope.

ure·ter·ec·ta·sia (yū-rē'ter-ek-tā'zē-ă). Dilation of a ureter. [ureter + G. *ektasis,* a stretching out]

ure·ter·ec·to·my (yū-rē-ter-ek'tō-mē). Excision of a segment or all of a ureter. [ureter + G. *ektomē,* excision]

ure·ter·ic (yū-rē-ter'ik). SYN ureteral.

ure·ter·i·tis (yū-rē-ter-ī'tis). Inflammation of a ureter.

△ureter-. The ureter. [G. *ourētēr,* urinary canal]

ure·ter·o·cal·i·cos·to·my (yū-rē'ter-kal-ĭ-kos'-tō- mē). Anastomosis of ureter to lower-pole collecting system of kidney after amputation of a portion of lower-pole parenchyma. [uretero- + G. *kalyx,* cup of a flower, + *stoma,* mouth]

ure·ter·o·cele (yū-rē'ter-ō-sēl). Saccular dilatation of the terminal portion of the ureter which protrudes into the lumen of the urinary bladder, probably due to a congenital stenosis of the ureteral meatus. [uretero- + G. *kēlē,* hernia]

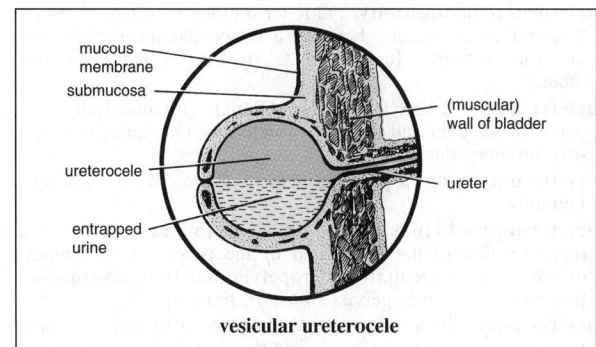

vesicular ureterocele

ure·ter·o·ce·lor·ra·phy (yū-rē'ter-ō-se-lōr'ă-fē). Excision and suturing of a ureterocele performed through an open cystotomy incision. [ureterocele + G. *raphē,* suture]

ure·ter·o·co·lic (yū-rē'ter-ō-kol'ik). Relating to the ureter and the colon, especially to an anastomosis for lesions of the lower urinary tract.

ure·ter·o·co·los·to·my (yū-rē'ter-ō-kō-los'tō-mē). Implantation of the ureter into the colon. [uretero- + G. *kolon,* colon, + *stoma,* mouth]

ure·ter·o·cys·to·scope (yū-rē'ter-ō-sis'tō-skōp). A cystoscope with an attachment for catheterization of the ureters; the catheter is passed into the ureter when its orifice is brought into view with the cystoscope. SYN uretercystoscope. [uretero- + G. *kystis,* bladder, + *skopeō,* to view]

ure·ter·o·cys·tos·to·my (yū-rē'ter-ō-sis-tos'tō-mē). SYN ureteroneocystostomy. [uretero- + G. *kystis,* bladder, + *stoma,* mouth]

ur

ure·ter·o·en·ter·ic (yū-rē′ter-ō-en-ter′ik). Relating to a ureter and the intestine.

ure·ter·o·en·ter·os·to·my (yū-rē′ter-ō-en-ter-os′tō-mē). Formation of an opening between a ureter and the intestine. [uretero- + G. *enteron,* intestine, + *stoma,* mouth]

ure·ter·og·ra·phy (yū-rē′ter-og′ră-fē). Radiography of the ureter after the direct injection of contrast medium. [uretero- + G. *graphē,* a writing]

ure·ter·o·hy·dro·ne·phro·sis (yū-rē′ter-ō-hī′drō-nef-rō′sis). Hydronephrosis also involving the ureters.

ure·ter·o·il·e·o·ne·o·cys·tos·to·my (yū-rē′ter-ō-il′ē-ō-nē′ō-sis-tos′tō-mē). Restoration of the continuity of the urinary tract by anastomosis of the upper segment of a partially destroyed ureter to a segment of ileum, the lower end of which is then implanted into the bladder. [uretero- + ileum + G. *neos,* new, + *hystis,* bladder, + *stoma,* mouth]

ure·ter·o·il·e·os·to·my (yū-rē′ter-ō-il-ē-os′tō-mē). Implantation of a ureter into an isolated segment of ileum which drains through an abdominal stoma. [uretero- + ileum + G. *stoma,* mouth]

ure·ter·o·li·thi·a·sis (yū-rē′ter-ō-li-thī′ă-sis). The formation or presence of a calculus or calculi in one or both ureters. [uretero-lith + G. *-iasis,* condition]

ure·ter·o·li·thot·o·my (yū-rē′ter-ō-li-thot′ō-mē). Removal of a stone lodged in a ureter. [ureterolith + G. *tomē,* incision]

ure·ter·ol·y·sis (yū′rē-ter-ol′i-sis). Surgical freeing of the ureter from surrounding disease or adhesions. [uretero- + G. *lysis,* a loosening]

ure·ter·o·ne·o·cys·tos·to·my (yū-rē′ter-ō-nē′ō-sis-tos′tō-mē). An operation whereby a ureter is implanted into the bladder. SYN ureterocystostomy. [uretero- + G. *neos,* new, + *kystis,* bladder, + *stoma,* mouth]

ure·ter·o·ne·phrec·to·my (yū-rē′ter-ō-nĕ-frek′tō-mē). SYN nephroureterectomy. [uretero- + G. *nephros,* kidney, + *ektomē,* excision]

ure·ter·op·a·thy (yū-rē′ter-op′ă-thē). Disease of the ureter. [uretero- + G. *pathos,* suffering]

ure·ter·o·plas·ty (yū-rē′ter-ō-plas-tē). Surgical reconstruction of the ureters. [uretero- + G. *plastos,* formed]

ure·ter·o·proc·tos·to·my (yū-rē′ter-ō-prok-tos′tō-mē). Establishment of an opening between a ureter and the rectum. SYN ureterorectostomy. [uretero- + G. *prōktos,* rectum, + *stoma,* mouth]

ure·ter·o·py·e·li·tis (yū-rē′ter-ō-pī-ĕ-lī′tis). Inflammation of the pelvis of a kidney and its ureter. [uretero- + G. *pyelos,* pelvis, + *-itis,* inflammation]

ure·ter·o·py·e·log·ra·phy (yū-rē′ter-ō-pī′ĕ-log′ră-fē). SYN pyelography.

ure·ter·o·py·e·lo·plas·ty (yū-rē′ter-ō-pī′ĕ-lō-plas-tē). Surgical reconstruction of the ureter and of the pelvis of the kidney, usually for congenital ureteropelvic junction obstruction. [uretero- + G. *pyelos,* pelvis, + *plastos,* formed]

ure·ter·o·py·e·los·to·my (yū-rē′ter-ō-pī-ĕ-los′tō-mē). Formation of a junction of the ureter and the renal pelvis. [uretero- + pelvis, + *stoma,* mouth]

ure·ter·o·py·o·sis (yū-rē′ter-ō-pī-ō′sis). An accumulation of pus in the ureter. [uretero- + G. *pyōsis,* suppuration]

ure·ter·o·rec·tos·to·my (yū-rē′ter-ō-rek-tos′tō-mē). SYN ureteroproctostomy.

ure·ter·or·rha·gia (yū-rē′ter-ō-rā′jē-ă). Hemorrhage from a ureter. [uretero- + G. *rhēgnymi,* to burst forth]

ure·ter·or·rha·phy (yū-rē-ter-ōr′ă-fē). Suture of a ureter. [uretero- + G. *rhaphē,* suture]

ure·ter·o·scope (yū-rē′ter-o-skōp). An optical device passed in a retrograde fashion through the bladder up into the ureter to inspect the ureteral lumen.

ure·ter·o·sig·moid (yū-rē′ter-ō-sig′moyd). Relating to the ureter and the sigmoid colon, especially to an anastomosis between the two.

ure·ter·o·sig·moi·dos·to·my (yū-rē′ter-ō-sig-moy-dos′tō-mē). Implantation of the ureter into the sigmoid colon.

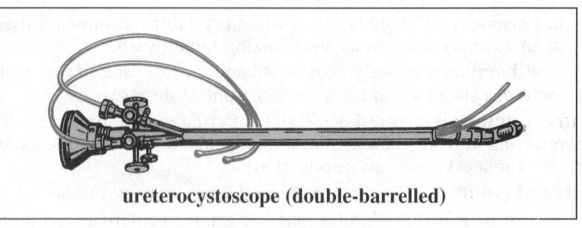
ureterocystoscope (double-barrelled)

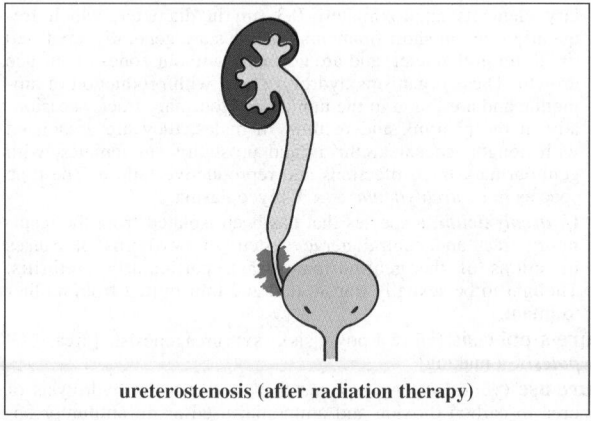
ureterostenosis (after radiation therapy)

ure·ter·o·sten·o·sis (yū-rē′ter-ō-ste-nō′sis). Stricture of a ureter. [uretero- + G. *stenōsis,* a narrowing]

ure·ter·os·to·my (yū-rē-ter-os′tō-mē). Establishment of an external opening into the ureter. [uretero- + G. *stoma,* mouth]

cutaneous loop u., SYN cutaneous u.

cutaneous u., a stoma constructed of ureter at skin level for drainage of urine. This may be an end stoma or a loop stoma. Usually performed because of distal obstruction. SYN cutaneous loop u.

ure·ter·ot·o·my (yū-rē-ter-ot′ō-mē). Incision and stenting of a narrow ureter. [uretero- + G. *tomē,* incision]

ure·ter·o·tri·go·no·en·ter·os·to·my (yū-rē′ter-ō-tri-gō′nō-en-ter-os′tō-mē). Implantation of a ureter and its portion of the trigone of the bladder into the intestine. [uretero-, + trigone (of bladder), + enterostomy]

ure·ter·o·u·re·ter·al (yū-rē′ter-ō-yū-re′ter-ăl). Relating to two segments of the same ureter or to both ureters, especially an artificial anastomosis between them.

ure·ter·o·u·re·ter·os·to·my (yū-rē′ter-ō-yū-rē′ter-os′tō-mē). Establishment of an anastomosis between the two ureters or between two segments of the same ureter. SEE transureteroureterostomy.

ure·ter·o·ves·i·cal (yū-rē′ter-ō-ves′i-kăl). Relating to the ureter and the bladder, specifically the junction of ureter with bladder.

ure·ter·o·ves·i·cos·to·my (yū-rē′ter-ō-ves-i-kos′tō-mē). Surgical joining of a ureter to the bladder. [uretero- + L. *vesica,* bladder, + *stoma,* mouth]

ure·than, ure·thane (yū′rĕ-than, -thān). $NH_2COOC_2H_5$; has antimitotic activity; formerly used medically as a hypnotic, but now more often used as an anesthetic for laboratory animals. SYN ethyl carbamate.

⌂**urethr-.** SEE urethro-.

ure·thra (yū-rē′thră). A canal leading from the bladder, discharging the urine externally. SYN urogenital canal. [G. *ourēthra*]

anterior u., the portion of u. distal to urogenital diaphragm (external sphincter).

female u., a canal about 4 cm long passing from the bladder, in close relation with the anterior wall of the vagina and having a long axis that parallels that of the vagina, opening in the vestibule of the vagina posterior to the clitoris and anterior to the vaginal orifice. SYN u. feminina [NA], u. muliebris.

u. femini′na [NA], SYN female u.

male u., a canal about 20 cm in length opening at the extremity of the glans penis; it gives passage to the spermatic fluid as well as the urine. SYN u. masculina [NA], u. virilis.

u. masculi′na [NA], SYN male u.

membranous u., SYN membranous *part* of male urethra.

u. mulie′bris, SYN female u.

penile u., SYN spongy u.

posterior u., the portion of u. posterior to the urogenital diaphram (external sphincter).

prostatic u., the prostatic part of the male urethra, about 2.5 cm in length, that traverses the prostate; it includes the seminal colliculus, and the ejaculatory and prostatic ducts open into it. SYN pars prostatica urethrae [NA].

spongy u., the portion of the male urethra, about 15 cm in length, which traverses the corpus spongiosum. SYN pars spongiosa urethrae masculinae [NA], pars cavernosa, penile u., spongy part of the male urethra.

u. viri′lis, SYN male u.

ure·thral (yū-rē′thrăl). Relating to the urethra.

ure·thral·gia (yū-rē-thral′jē-ă). Pain in the urethra. SYN urethrodynia. [urethr- + G. *algos,* pain]

ure·threc·to·my (yūr-ĕ-threk′tō-mē). Excision of a segment or the entire urethra. [urethr- + G. *ektomē,* excision]

ure·threm·or·rha·gia (yū-rē′threm-ō-rā′jē-ă). Bleeding from the urethra. SYN urethrorrhagia. [urethr- + G. *haima,* blood, + *rhēgnymi,* to burst forth]

ure·thrism, ure·thris·mus (yū′rē-thrizm, -thriz′mŭs). Irritability or spasmodic stricture of the urethra. SYN urethrospasm.

ure·thri·tis (yū-rē-thrī′tis). Inflammation of the urethra. [ureth- + G. *-itis,* inflammation]

anterior u., inflammation of the portion of the urethra anterior to the triangular ligament.

follicular u., chronic u. with nodular lymphocytic infiltrations in the mucosa. SYN granular u.

gonorrheal u., infection of the urethra usually in association with a purulent discharge due to *Neisseria gonorrhoeae.*

granular u., SYN follicular u.

nongonococcal u., u. not resulting from gonococcal infection; venereally transmitted *Chlamydia trachomatis* is the most common cause.

nonspecific u., u. not resulting from gonococcal, chlamydial, or other specific infectious agents. SYN simple u.

u. petrif′icans, u., sometimes of gouty origin, in which there is a deposit of calcareous matter in the wall of the urethra.

posterior u., inflammation of the membranous and prostatic portions of the urethra.

simple u., SYN nonspecific u.

specific u., obsolete term for gonorrhea.

u. vene′rea, obsolete term for gonorrhea.

△urethro-, urethr-. The urethra. [G. *ourēthra*]

ure·thro·bul·bar (yū-rē′thrō-bŭl′băr). SYN bulbourethral.

ure·thro·cele (yū-rē′thrō-sēl). Prolapse of the female urethra. [urethro- + G. *kēlē,* tumor, hernia]

ure·thro·cys·to·me·trog·ra·phy (yū-rē′thrō-sis′tō-me-trog′ră-fē). SYN urethrocystometry. [urethro- + G. *kystis,* bladder, + *metron, measure,* + *skopeō,* to view]

ure·thro·cys·tom·e·try (yū-rē′thrō-sis-tom′ĕ-trē). A procedure that simultaneously measures pressures in urinary bladder and urethra. SYN urethrocystometrography. [urethro- + G. *kystis,* bladder, + *metron,* measure]

ure·thro·cys·to·pexy (yū-rē′thrō-sis′tō-pek-sē). Fixation of urethra and bladder for stress incontinence. SYN urethropexy. [urethro- + G. *kystis,* bladder, + *pēxis,* fixation]

ure·thro·dyn·ia (yū-rē-thrō-din′ē-ă). SYN urethralgia. [urethro- + G. *odynē,* pain]

ure·throg·ra·phy (yū-rē-throg′ră-fē). Contrast radiography of the male or female urethra, by retrograde injection or during

voiding of contrast medium in the bladder (cystourethrogram). [urethra + G. *graphō,* to write]

ure·throm·e·ter (yū-rē-throm′ĕ-ter). An instrument for measuring the caliber of the urethra. [urethro- + G. *metron,* measure]

ure·thro·pe·nile (yū-rē′thrō-pē′nīl). Relating to the urethra and the penis.

ure·thro·per·i·ne·al (yū-rē′thrō-pĕ-rī-nē′ăl). Relating to the urethra and the perineum.

ureth·ro·per·i·ne·o·scro·tal (yū-rē′thrō-pe-rī-nē-ō-skrō′tăl). Relating to the urethra, perineum, and scrotum.

ure·thro·pexy (yū-rē′thrō-pek-sē). SYN urethrocystopexy. [urethro- + G. *pēxis,* fixation]

ure·thro·plasty (yū-rē′thrō-plas-tē). Surgical reconstruction of the urethra. [urethro- + G. *plastos,* formed]

cecil u., a staged urethral reconstructive procedure wherein the urethral portion of the penis is left buried in the scrotum after urethroplasty at the first stage because of inadequate ventral skin cover.

ure·thro·pros·ta·tic (yū-rē′thrō-pros-tat′ik). Relating to the urethra and the prostate.

ure·thro·rec·tal (yū-rē′thrō-rek′tăl). Relating to the urethra and the rectum.

ure·thror·rha·gia (yū-rē-thrō-rā′jē-ă). SYN urethremorrhagia.

ure·thror·rha·phy (yū-rē-thrōr′ă-fē). Suture of the urethra. [urethro- + G. *rhaphē,* suture]

ure·thror·rhea (yū-rē-thrō-rē′ă). An abnormal discharge from the urethra. [urethro- + G. *rhoia,* a flow]

ure·thro·scope (yū-rē′thrō-skōp). An instrument for viewing the interior of the urethra. [urethro- + G. *skopeō,* to view]

ure·thro·scop·ic (yū-rē-thrō-skop′ik). Relating to the urethroscope or to urethroscopy.

ure·thros·co·py (yū-rē-thros′kŏ-pē). Inspection of the urethra with a urethroscope.

ure·thro·spasm (yū-rē′thrō-spazm). SYN urethrism.

ure·thro·stax·is (yū-rē′thrō-stak′sis). Oozing of blood from the urethra. [urethro- + G. *staxis,* trickling]

ure·thro·ste·no·sis (yū-rē′thrō-ste-nō′sis). Stricture of the urethra. [urethro- + G. *stenōsis,* a narrowing]

ure·thros·to·my (yū-rē-thros′tō-mē). Surgical formation of a permanent opening between the urethra and the skin. [urethro- + G. *stoma,* mouth]

perineal u., formation of a permanent opening into the bulbous portion of the urethra through a perineal skin incision.

ure·thro·tome (yū-rē′thrō-tōm). An instrument for dividing a stricture of the urethra. [urethro- + G. *tomos,* cutting]

ure·throt·o·my (yū-rē-throt′ō-mē). Surgical incision of a stricture of the urethra. [urethro- + G. *tomē,* incision]

external u., u. via an external opening in the perineum or penile skin. SYN perineal u.

internal u., u. by means of an instrument passed through the urethra.

perineal u., SYN external u.

ure·thro·vag·i·nal (yū-rē′thrō-vaj′i-năl). Relating to the urethra and the vagina.

ure·thro·ves·i·cal (yū-rē′thrō-ves′i-kăl). Relating to the urethra and bladder.

ure·thro·ves·i·co·pexy (yū-rē′thrō-ves′i-kŏ-pek-sē). Surgical suspension of the urethra and the base of the bladder from the posterior surface of the pubic symphysis (or anterior abdominal wall or Cooper's ligament) for correction of urinary stress incontinence. [urethro- + L. *vesica,* bladder, + G. *pexis,* fixation]

△-uretic. Urine. [G. *ourētikos,* relating to the urine]

URF Abbreviation for unidentified *reading frame*; uterine relaxing *factor.*

ur·gen·cy (er′jen-sē). A strong desire to void.

motor u., u. from overactive detrusor function.

sensory u., u. due to vesicourethral hypersensitivity.

ur·gi·nea (er-jin′ē-ă). The bulbs of *Urginea indica* (Indian squill) and *Urginea maritima* (white or Mediterranean squill);

the source of squill. [L. *urgeo*, to press, referring to the shape of the seeds]

ur·hi·dro·sis (yŭr-hi-drō'sis). SYN uridrosis.

⌂**uri-, uric-, urico-.** Uric acid. [G. *ouron*, urine]

uri·an (yūr'ē-ăn). SYN urochrome.

uric (yūr'ik). Relating to urine.

uric ac·id. 2,6,8-trioxypurine; white crystals, poorly soluble, contained in solution in the urine of mammals and in solid form in the urine of birds and reptiles; sometimes solidified in small masses as stones or crystals or in larger concretions as calculi; with sodium and other bases it forms urates; elevated levels associated with gout. SYN lithic acid, triketopurine.

u. a. oxidase, SEE *urate* oxidase.

uri·case (yūr'i-kās). SYN *urate* oxidase.

⌂**urico-.** SEE uri-.

uri·col·y·sis (yūr-i-kol'i-sis). Decomposition of uric acid. [urico- + G. *lysis*, a loosening]

uri·co·lyt·ic (yūr'i-kō-lit'ik). Relating to or effecting the hydrolysis of uric acid.

uri·cos·o·me (yūr-ik'ō-sōm). A microbody rich in urate oxidase.

uri·co·su·ria (yū'ri-kō-sū'rē-ă). Excessive amounts of uric acid in the urine. [urico- + G. *ouron*, urine]

uri·co·su·ric (yū'ri-kō-sū'rik). Tending to increase the excretion of uric acid.

uri·co·tele (ūr'ik-ō-tēl). An organism that is uricotelic; *e.g.,* birds and land-dwelling reptiles.

uri·co·tel·ia (yūr-ik'ō-tēl-ē-a). The process or type of nitrogen excretion in which uric acid is the chief excretion product. [uric (acid) + G. *telos*, end, outcome, + -ia]

uri·co·tel·ic (yūr'i-kō-tel'ik). Producing uric acid as the chief excretory product of nitrogen metabolism. [urico- + G. *telos*, end]

uri·dine (Urd) (yūr'i-dēn). Uracil ribonucleoside; one of the major nucleosides in RNAs; as the pyrophosphate (UDP, UDPG, etc.), u. is active in sugar metabolism. SYN 1-β-D-ribofuranosyluracil.

cyclic u. 3′,5′-monophosphate (cUMP), a cyclic nucleotide involved in metabolic regulation; inhibits the growth of some tumors.

u. 5′-diphosphate (UDP), uridine 5′-pyrophosphate; a condensation product of uridine and pyrophosphoric acid. SEE ALSO UDP.

u. 5′-monophosphate (UMP), SYN uridylic acid.

u. phosphorylase, a ribosyltransferase that catalyzes the reaction of uridine with orthophosphate to produce uracil and α-D-ribose 1-phosphate.

u. 5′-triphosphate (UTP), u. esterified with triphosphoric acid at its 5′-position; the immediate precursor of uridylic acid residues in RNA.

uri·dine di·phos·pho·ga·lac·tose (UDPGal) (yūr'i-dēn-dī-fos'fō-gă-lak'tōs). A pyrophosphate group links the 5′-position of uridine and the 1 position of D-galactose.

u. d. 4-epimerase, SEE UDPglucose 4-epimerase.

uri·dine di·phos·pho·glu·cose (UDPG, UDPGlc) (yūr'i-dēn-dī-fos'fō-glū'kōs). A pyrophosphate group links the 5′-position of uridine and the 1-position of D-glucose; an intermediate in glycogen biosynthesis. SYN UDPglucose.

u. d. 4-epimerase, SYN UDPglucose 4-epimerase.

uri·dine di·phos·pho·glu·cu·ron·ic ac·id (UDP-GlcUA) (yūr'i-dēn-dī-fos'fō-glū-kū-ron'ik). Uridine diphosphoglucose in which the 6 CH₂OH of the glucose has been oxidized to COOH (has become a glucuronyl residue); participates in the formation of conjugates of bilirubin or drugs such as aspirin.

uri·dine di·phos·pho·xylose. SYN xylose.

uri·dro·sis (yū-ri-drō'sis). The excretion of urea or uric acid in the sweat. SYN sudor urinosus, urhidrosis. [uri- + G. *hidrōs*, sweat]

u. crystalli′na, SYN urea *frost*.

uri·dyl·ic ac·id (yūr-i-dil'ik). Uridine esterified by phosphoric acid on one or more sugar hydroxyl groups; UMP is typically uridine 5′-monophosphate; 2′ and 3′ derivatives also occur; pre-

cursor for the biosynthesis of other pyrimidine nucleotides. SYN UMP synthase, uridine 5′-monophosphate.

u. a. synthase, a bifunctional enzyme that contains the activities of both orotate phosphoribosyltransferase and orotidine-5′-monophosphate decarboxylase; catalyzes a key step in pyrimidine biosynthesis; a deficiency of this enzyme leads to orotic aciduria.

uri·dyl·trans·fer·ase (yūr'i-dil-trans'fer-ās). UDPglucose-hexose-1-phosphate; uridylyltransferase.

uri·es·the·sia (yūri-es-thē′zē-ă). SYN uresiesthesia.

⌂**urin-, urino-.** Urine. SEE ALSO ure-, uro-. [G. *ouron*]

uri·nal (yū'rin-ăl). A vessel into which urine is passed.

uri·nal·y·sis (yū-ri-nal'i-sis). Analysis of the urine.

uri·nary (yūr'i-nār-ē). Relating to urine.

uri·nate (yūr'i-nāt). To pass urine. SYN micturate.

uri·na·tion (yūr'i-nā'shŭn). The passing of urine. SYN miction, micturition (1), uresis.

stuttering u., the passage of urine in jets caused by intermittent spasmodic contraction of the bladder.

urine (yūr'in). The fluid and dissolved substances excreted by the kidney. [L. *urina*; G. *ouron*]

ammoniacal u., SYN ammoniuria.

black u., the dark u. of melanuria or hemoglobinuria.

chylous u., u. of a milky appearance, containing chyle. SYN milky u.

cloudy u., u. with a cloudy appearance, usually due to pus, crystals, bacteria, blood, or free fat globules. SYN nebulous u.

crude u., pale u. of low specific gravity, with very little sediment.

febrile u., dark colored, concentrated u. of strong odor, passed by one suffering from fever. SYN feverish u.

feverish u., SYN febrile u.

gouty u., u. of a high color containing uric acid in excess.

honey u., obsolete term for *diabetes* mellitus.

maple syrup u., SEE maple syrup urine *disease*.

milky u., SYN chylous u.

nebulous u., SYN cloudy u.

residual u., u. remaining in the bladder at the end of micturition in cases of prostatic obstruction, bladder atony, etc.

uri·ne·mia (yūr-i-nē′mē-ă). Obsolete term for uremia.

uri·nif·er·ous (yūr-i-nif′ĕ-rŭs). Conveying urine; denoting the tubules of the kidney. [urine + L. *fero*, to carry]

uri·nif·ic (yūr-i-nif'ik). SYN uriniparous. [urine + L. *facio*, to make]

uri·nip·a·rous (yūr-i-nip′ă-rŭs). Producing or excreting urine; denoting the malpighian bodies and certain tubules in the renal cortex. SYN urinific. [urine + L. *pario*, to produce]

⌂**urino-.** SEE urin-.

uri·no·gen·i·tal (yūr'i-nō-jen'i-tăl). SYN genitourinary.

uri·nog·e·nous (yūr-i-noj′ĕ-nŭs). **1.** Producing or excreting urine. **2.** Of urinary origin. SYN urogenous.

uri·no·ma (yūr'i-nō'mă). A cystic collection of extravasated urine.

uri·nom·e·ter (yūr-i-nom′ĕ-ter). A hydrometer for determining the specific gravity of the urine. SYN urogravimeter, urometer. [urine + G. *metron*, measure]

uri·nom·e·try (yūr-i-nom′ĕ-trē). The determination of the specific gravity of the urine.

uri·nos·co·py (yūr-i-nos′kŏ-pē). SYN uroscopy.

uri·no·sex·u·al (yūr-i-nō-sek'shū-ăl). SYN genitourinary.

uri·nous (yūr'i-nŭs). Relating to or of the nature of urine.

uri·po·sia (yūr-i-pō′sē-ă). Urine-drinking. [urine + G. *posis*, drinking]

uri·tis (yū-rī′tis). SYN *dermatitis* ambustionis. [L. *uro*, pp. *ustus*, to singe, burn, + G. *-itis*, inflammation]

⌂**uro-.** Urine. SEE ALSO ure-, urin-. [G. *ouron*]

uro·am·mo·ni·ac (yū-rō-ă-mo'nē-ak). Relating to uric acid and ammonia; denoting a variety of urinary calculus.

uro·an·the·lone (yū-rō-an'thĕ-lōn). SYN urogastrone.

uro·bi·lin (yūr-ō-bī′lin, -bil'in). A uroporphyrin; an acyclic tetra-

urine

in general		organic components (in mg/24 hr., unless otherwise noted)	
quantity (in ml/24hr.)	500–2000	acetone bodies	10–100
specific weight	1.010–1.025	amino acids, total (g/24 hr.)	1.3–3.2
solid matter (g/24hr., 100% dry residue)	40–60	amino acids, free (g/24 hr.)	0.35–1.20
freezing point lowered (°C)	0.1–2.5	amino acid N	40–130
osmolality (mosm/l)	50–1400	creatine ♂	10–190
pH	4.8–7.5	creatine ♀	10–270
total acidity (mval/24 hr.)	50–60	creatinine	500–2500
acidity (by titration)	20–60	diazo bodies	traces
total nitrogen (g/24 hr.)	7–17	fatty acids	8–50
amino acid–N (% of total N)	<2	bile pigments	
ammonia (NH_4^+)–N	4.6	bilirubin	0.02–1.9
creatinine–N	3.7	urobilinogen	0.05–2.5
uric acid–N	1.6	bile acid (g/24 hr., as glyco and as taurocholic acid)	5–10
urea–N	82.7	glucoronic acid	200–600
inorganic components (in mg/24 hr., unless otherwise noted)		uric acid	80–1000
ammonia	0.3–1.2	urea (g/24 hr.)	12–30
calcium	130–330	hippuric acid (g/24 hr.)	1.0–2.5
chloride (g/24 hr.)	4.3–8.5	hydroxyindoleacetic acid	1.0–14.7
iron	0.4–0.15	indican	4.0–20.0
iodine	0.02–0.5	indoxylsulfuric acid	15–100
potassium (g/24 hr.)	1.4–3.1	lactic acid	100–600
copper	0.03–0.07	oxal acid	10–25
magnesium	60.7–200	porphyrins	
sodium (g/24 hr.)	2.8–5.0	aminolevulinic acid	1.5–7.0
phosphorus, total (g/24 hr.)	0.8–2.0	coproporphorin	0.02–0.2
sulphur, total (g/24 hr.)	1.24–1.50	porphyrobilinogen	0.4–2.4
sulphur, inorganic (g/24 hr.)	1.07–1.30	uroporphyrin	0.004–0.02
sulphur, neutral (g/24 hr.)	0.05–0.08	proteins	10–100
sulphur, esterized (g/24 hr.)	0.08–0.10	purine bases (g/24 hr.)	0.2–0.5
zinc	0.14–0.70	citric acid	150–1200
		sugar (reducing substances)	500–1500
		galactose	3–25
		glucose	15–130
		lactose	0–90

pyrrole that is one of the natural breakdown products of heme via choleglobin, verdohemochrome, biliverdin, bilirubin, and *d*-urobilinogen; a urinary pigment that gives a varying orange-red coloration to urine according to its degree of oxidation. SYN urohematin, urohematoporphyrin.

uro·bi·lin IX-α. SYN mesobilene.

uro·bi·li·ne·mia (yū′rō-bil-i-nē′mē-ă). The presence of urobilins in the blood.

uro·bi·lin·o·gen (yūr-ō-bī-lin′ō-jen). Precursor of urobilin.

uro·bi·lin·o·gen IXα. SYN mesobilane.

uro·bi·lin·u·ria (yū′rō-bil-i-nū′rē-ă). The presence in the urine of urobilins in excessive amount, formed mainly from hemoglobin.

uro·can·ase (yū′rō-kă-nās). SYN *urocanate* hydratase.

ur·o·can·ate (yūr′ō-kă-nāt). A salt or ester of urocanic acid.

u. hydratase, an enzyme catalyzing the reaction of water with urocanic acid to produce 4-imidazolone-5-propionic acid, a step in L-histidine catabolism; this enzyme is absent in cases of urocanic aciduria. SYN urocanase.

uro·can·ic ac·id (yū′rō-kan′ik). 4-Imidazoleacrylic acid; an acid derived from the oxidative deamination of L-histidine; present in sweat and in dog's urine; elevated levels are observed in cases of urocanate hydratase deficiency.

uro·can·ic ac·i·du·ria (ūr′ō-kan′ik-as′id-yūr′ē-a). Elevated levels of urocanic acid in the urine.

uro·can·i·case (yūr-ō-kan′i-kās). One of a group of at least three enzymes that convert urocanic acid to glutamic acid.

uro·cele (yū′rō-sēl). Extravasation of urine into the scrotal sac. [uro- + G. *kēlē*, hernia]

uroch·er·as (yū-rok′er-as). **1.** SYN gravel. **2.** SYN uropsammus (2). [uro- + G. *cheras*, gravel (an incorrect form of *cherados*, gravel)]

uro·che·sia (yū-rō-kē′zē-ă). Passage of urine from the anus. [uro- + G. *chezō*, to defecate]

uro·chrome (yūr′ō-krōm). The principal pigment of urine, a compound of urobilin and a peptide of unknown structure. SYN urian.

uro·chro·mo·gen (yūr-ō-krō′mō-jen). Originally, a body in the urine that, on taking up oxygen, formed urochrome; now, probably urobilinogen.

uro·cris·ia (yū-rō-kris′ē-ă, -kriz′ē-ă). **1.** SYN urocrisis. **2.** Obsolete term for diagnosis based upon the results of a urinary examination. [uro- + G. *krinō*, to separate, judge]

uro·cri·sis (yū′rō-krī′sis). **1.** Obsolete term for the critical stage of a disease accompanied by a copious discharge of urine. **2.** Severe pain in any of the urinary organs or passages occurring in tabes dorsalis. SYN urocrisia (1). [uro- + G. *krisis*, crisis]

ur

uro·cy·a·nin (yū′rō-sī′ă-nin). An indigo blue pigment sometimes observed in the urine in certain diseases, especially scarlet fever. SYN uroglaucin. [uro- + G. *kyanos,* a blue substance]

uro·cy·an·o·gen (yū-rō-sī-an′ō-jen). A blue pigment sometimes observed in the urine in cases of cholera.

uro·cy·a·no·sis (yū′rō-sī-ă-nō′sis). A bluish discoloration of the urine in indicanuria.

uro·cyst (yū′rō-sist). SYN urinary *bladder.* [uro- + G. *kystis,* bladder]

uro·cys·tic (yū′rō-sis′tik). Relating to the urinary bladder.

uro·cys·tis (yū′rō-sis′tis). SYN urinary *bladder.*

uro·dy·na·mics (yū′rō-dī-nam′iks). The study of the storage of urine within, and the flow of urine through and from, the urinary tract. [uro- + G. *dynamis,* force]

uro·dyn·ia (yūr-ō-din′ē-ă). Pain on urination. [uro- + G. *odynē,* pain]

uro·en·ter·one (yūr-ō-en′ter-ōn). SYN urogastrone.

uro·er·y·thrin (yū-rō-er′i-thrin). A urinary pigment that gives a pink color to deposits of urates; presumably derived from melanin. SYN purpurin (1), urerythrin.

uro·fla·vin (yūr-ō-flā′vin). A fluorescent product of riboflavin catabolism, or perhaps riboflavin itself, found in mammalian urine and feces.

uro·flow·me·ter (yū-rō′flō-mē-ter). A device that measures urine flow rates during micturition, including these parameters: peak flow rate, average flow rate, voided volume, and time of voiding.

ur·o·fol·li·tro·pin (yūr-ō-fol′i-trō-pin). A preparation of gonadotropin extracted from the urine of postmenopausal women, used in conjunction with human chorionic gonadotropin to induce ovulation. SEE ALSO menotropins.

uro·fus·co·hem·a·tin (yū-rō-fŭs-kō-hē′mă-tin). A brownish red pigment found in the urine in a case of leprosy.

uro·gas·trone (yūr-ō-gas′trōn). A fluorescent pigment extracted from urine; an inhibitor of gastric secretion and motility. Cf. enterogastrone. SYN anthelone U, anthelone, uroanthelone, uroenterone.

uro·gen·i·tal (yū′rō-jen′i-tăl). SYN genitourinary.

urog·e·nous (yū-roj′ĕ-nŭs). SYN urinogenous.

uro·glau·cin (yū-rō-glaw′sin). SYN urocyanin. [uro- + G. *glaukos,* bluish gray]

ur·o·go·nad·o·tro·pin (yūr′ō-gō-nad-ō-trō′pin). SEE human menopausal *gonadotropin.*

uro·graf·fin (yūr-ō-graf′fin). A mixture of salts of diatrizoic acid used to form density gradients.

uro·gram (yūr′ō-gram). The radiographic record obtained by urography.

urog·ra·phy (yū-rog′ră-fē). Radiography of any part (kidneys, ureters, or bladder) of the urinary tract. SEE ALSO pyelography. [uro- + G. *graphō,* to write]

   antegrade u., radiography following percutaneous injection of contrast agent with a needle or catheter into the renal calices or pelvis (antegrade pyelography), or into the urinary bladder (antegrade cystography).

   cystoscopic u., SYN retrograde u.

   intravenous u., excretory u., radiography of kidneys, ureters, and bladder following injection of contrast medium into a peripheral vein.

   retrograde u., radiography of the urinary tract following injection of contrast medium directly into the bladder, ureter, or renal pelvis. SYN cystoscopic u.

uro·gra·vim·e·ter (yū′rō-gră-vim′ĕ-ter). SYN urinometer. [uro- + L. *gravis,* heavy, + G. *metron,* measure]

uro·hem·a·tin (yūr-ō-hēm′ă-tin). SYN urobilin.

uro·hem·a·to·por·phy·rin (yūr′ō-hēm′ă-tō-pōr′fi-rin). SYN urobilin.

uro·hep·a·rin (yūr-ō-hep′ă-rin). An inactive form of heparin excreted in the urine.

uro·hy·per·ten·sin (yūr′ō-hī-per-ten′sin). A pressor substance derived from the urine.

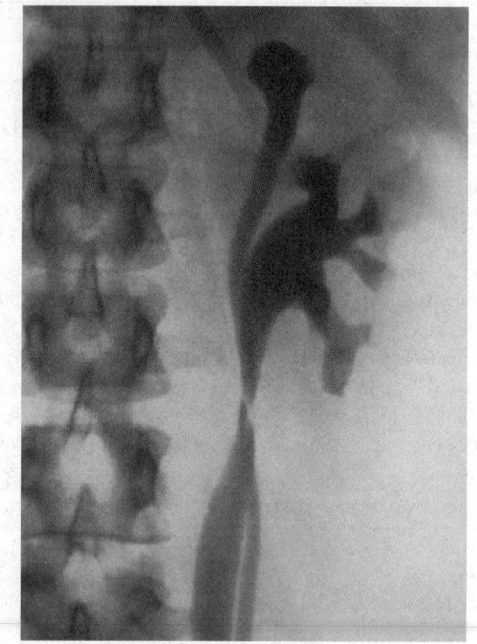

antegrade urography (pyelography)
postpartum pyelogram of patient with pyelonephritis gravidarum showing double formation of left renal pelvis and ureter

uro·ki·nase (yūr-ō-kī′nās). SYN plasminogen *activator.*

uro·lag·nia (yūr-ō-lag′nē-ă). Sexual stimulation occasioned by the sight of a person urinating. [uro- + G. *lagneia,* lust]

uro·leu·cin·ic ac·id, uro·leu·cic ac·id (yū′rō-lū-sin′ik, yū-rō-lū′sik). An aromatic compound, $C_9H_{10}O_5$, excreted in the urine of persons with alcaptonuria.

uro·lith (yū′rō-lith). SYN urinary *calculus.* [uro- + G. *lithos,* stone]

uro·li·thi·a·sis (yū-rō-li-thī′ă-sis). Presence of calculi in the urinary system.

uro·lith·ic (yū-rō-lith′ik). Relating to urinary calculi.

uro·li·thol·o·gy (yū′rō-li-thol′ō-jē). The branch of medicine concerned with the formation, composition, effects, and removal of urinary calculi. [uro- + G. *lithos,* stone, + *logos,* study]

uro·log·ic, uro·log·i·cal (yū-rō-loj′ik, i-kăl). Relating to urology.

urol·o·gist (yū-rol′ō-jist). A specialist in urology.

urol·o·gy (yū-rol′ō-jē). The medical specialty concerned with the study, diagnosis, and treatment of diseases of the genitourinary tract. [uro- + G. *logos,* study]

uro·lu·te·in (yū-rō-lū′tē-in). Name given to yellow pigment in the urine. SEE urochrome, uroporphyrin (1).

uro·mel·a·nin (yūr-ō-mel′ă-nin). A black pigment occasionally found in the urine, possibly a decomposition product of urochrome.

urom·e·ter (yū-rom′ĕ-ter). SYN urinometer.

uron·cus (yū-rong′kŭs). A urinary cyst; a circumscribed area of extravasation of urine. [uro- + G. *onkos,* mass (tumor)]

uro·ne·phro·sis (yū′rō-ne-frō′sis). SYN hydronephrosis.

uron·ic ac·ids (yū-ron′ik). Acids derived from monosaccharides by oxidation of the primary alcohol group ($-CH_2OH$) farthest removed from the carbonyl group to a carboxyl group ($-COOH$); *e.g.,* glucuronic acid.

uro·nos·co·py (yū-rō-nos′kŏ-pē). SYN uroscopy.

urop·a·thy (yū-rop′ă-thē). Any disorder involving the urinary tract. [uro- + G. *pathos,* suffering]

obstructive u., any pathologic condition, anatomic or functional, of the urinary tract caused by obstruction.

uro·phan·ic (yūr-ō-fan′ik). Appearing in the urine; denoting any constituent, normal or pathologic, of the urine. [uro- + G. *phainō,* to appear]

uro·phe·in (yū-rō-fē′in). A grayish pigment occasionally found in the urine, possibly identical with urobilin. [uro- + G. *phaios,* gray]

uro·poi·e·sis (yū′rō-poy-ē′sis). The production or secretion and excretion of urine. [uro- + G. *poiēsis,* a making]

uro·poi·e·tic (yū′rō-poy-et′ik). Relating or pertaining to uropoiesis.

uro·por·phy·rin (yūr-ō-pōr′fi-rin). **1.** Porphyrin excreted in the urine in porphyrinuria; *e.g.,* urobilin. **2.** Class name for all porphyrins containing 4 acetic acid groups and 4 propionic acid groups in positions 1 through 8. SEE ALSO porphyrinogens.

u. I, porphin-1,3,5,7-tetraacetic acid-2,4,6,8-tetrapropionic acid; formed by the action of light on uroporphyrinogen I; elevated levels observed in certain porphyrias.

u. III, porphin-1,3,5,8-tetraacetic acid-2,4,6,7-tetrapropionic acid; formed by the action of light on uroporphyrinogen III; elevated levels observed in certain porphyrias.

ur·o·por·phy·rin·o·gen (yūr′ō-pōr-fi-rin′ō-jen). SEE porphyrinogens.

u. decarboxylase, an enzyme that participates in heme biosynthesis; it catalyzes the decarboxylation of u. III to produce coproporphyrinogen III; it also acts on u. I; a deficiency of this enzyme will result in either porphyria cutanea tarda or hepatoerythropoietic porphyria.

u. III cosynthase, an enzyme in heme biosynthesis that participates in the formation of u. III; a deficiency of this protein results in congenital erythropoietic porphyria.

uro·psam·mus (yū-rō-sam′ŭs). **1.** SYN gravel. **2.** Any inorganic or uratic urinary sediment. SYN urocheras (2). [uro- + G. *psammos,* sand]

urop·ter·in (yū-rop′ter-in). SYN urothion.

uro·pur·pur·in (yūr-ō-pŭr′pūr-in). A purple pigment in the urine.

ur·o·ra·di·ol·o·gy (yū′rō-rā-dē-ol′ŏ-jē). The study of the radiology of the urinary tract.

uro·rec·tal (yū′rō-rek′tăl). Relating to the urinary tract and rectum.

uro·ro·se·in (yūr-ō-rō′zē-in). A chromogen in the urine that forms a red color on the addition of nitric acid; normally exists in very minute quantities but is increased in tuberculosis and other wasting diseases, and is related to ingestion of indole compounds.

uro·ru·bin (yūr-ō-rū′bin). A red pigment in urine made more visible by treatment with hydrochloric acid.

uro·ru·bro·hem·a·tin (yūr′ō-rū-brō-hē′mă-tin). A reddish pigment occasionally present in the urine in various chronic diseases.

uros·che·sis (yū-ros′kē-sis). **1.** Retention of urine. **2.** Suppression of urine. [uro- + G. *schesis,* a checking]

uro·scop·ic (yūr-ō-skop′ik). Relating to uroscopy.

uros·co·py (yū-ros′kŏ-pē). Examination of the urine, usually by means of a microscope. SYN urinoscopy, uronoscopy. [uro- + G. *skopeō,* to view]

uro·sem·i·ol·o·gy (yū′rō-sem-ē-ol′ō-jē). The study of the urine as an aid to diagnosis. [uro- + G. *sēmeion,* a sign, + *logos,* study]

uro·sep·sin (yūr-ō-sep′sin). A substance formed by the decomposition of urine, supposed to be the cause of septic poisoning after urinary extravasation.

uro·sep·sis (yūr-ō-sep′sis). **1.** Sepsis resulting from the decomposition of extravasated urine. **2.** Sepsis from obstruction of infected urine. [uro- + G. *sēpsis,* decomposition]

uro·spec·trin (yūr-ō-spek′trin). A pigment found in the urine, possibly the same as urobilin.

u·ro·the·li·um (yū-rō-thē′lē-ŭm). The epithelial lining of the urinary tract. [uro- + epithelium]

ur·o·thi·on (yūr-ō-thī′on). A sulfur-containing pteridine derivative isolated from urine. SYN uropterin.

ur·o·thor·ax (yūr-ō-thōr′aks). The presence of urine in the thoracic cavity, usually following complex multiple organ injuries.

uro·xan·thin (yūr-ō-zan′thin). SYN indican (2).

urox·in (yū-rok′sin). SYN alloxantin.

ur·ti·ca (er-tī′kă, er′ti-). The herb, *Urtica dioica* (family Urticaceae); a weed, the leaves of which produce a stinging sensation when touching the skin. It has been used as a diuretic and hemostatic in metrorrhagia, epistaxis, and hematemesis. SYN nettle. [L. a nettle, fr. *uro,* pp. *ustus,* to burn]

ur·ti·cant (er′ti-kant). Producing a wheal or other similar itching agent. [L. *urtica,* nettle; see urtica]

ur·ti·car·ia (er′ti-kar′i-ă). An eruption of itching wheals, usually of systemic origin; it may be due to a state of hypersensitivity to foods or drugs, foci of infection, physical agents (heat, cold, light, friction), or psychic stimuli. SYN hives (1), uredo (1), urtication (3). [L. *urtica*]

acute u., SYN febrile u.

u. acu′ta, SYN febrile u.

u. bullo′sa, an eruption of wheals capped with subepidermal vesicles. SYN u. vesiculosa.

cholinergic u., a form of physical or non-allergic u. initiated by heat (*e.g.,* hot baths, physical exercise, pyrexia, exposure to sun or to a warm room) or by excitement; the rather distinctive lesions consist of pruritic areas 1 to 2 mm in diameter surrounded by bright red macules. SYN heat u.

chronic u., a form of u. in which the wheals recur frequently, or persist. SYN u. chronica.

u. chron′ica, SYN chronic u.

cold u., wheal formation that develops after exposure to lowered temperatures, with or without demonstrable passive-transfer antibodies. SYN congelation u.

u. confer′ta, a form of u. in which the wheals are aggregated in a group.

congelation u., SYN cold u.

u. endem′ica, u. epidem′ica, u. caused by the nettling hairs of certain caterpillars.

u. facti′tia, SYN dermatographism.

factitious u., SYN dermatographism.

febrile u., u. accompanied by slight constitutional symptoms. SYN acute u., u. acuta, u. febrilis.

u. febri′lis, SYN febrile u.

giant u., SYN angioedema.

heat u., SYN cholinergic u.

u. hemorrhag′ica, u. bullosa in which the serous exudate contains blood.

u. maculo′sa, a chronic form of u. with lesions of a red color and little edema.

u. medicamento′sa, an urticarial form of drug eruption.

papular u., a sensitivity reaction to insect bites, especially human and pet fleas, seen mostly in young children as wheals followed by papules on exposed areas. SYN lichen urticatus, prurigo infantilis, u. papulosa.

u. papulo′sa, SYN papular u.

u. per′stans, a form of chronic u. in which the wheals persist unchanged for long periods; includes urticarial vasculitis.

u. pigmento′sa, cutaneous mastocytosis resulting from an excess of mast cells in the superficial dermis, producing a chronic eruption characterized by flat or slightly elevated brownish papules which urticate when stroked. The disease in children frequently involutes spontaneously whereas resolution is rare with adult onset and there may be systemic lesions.

urticaria u., SYN diffuse cutaneous *mastocytosis.*

pressure u., u. of unknown etiology occurring after local pressure on the skin.

solar u., a form of u. resulting from exposure to specific light spectra; *e.g.,* sunlight; some patients have passive-transfer antibodies and others do not.

u. subcuta′nea, u. in which itching is present without the wheals.

u. tubero′sa, SYN angioedema.

u. vesiculo′sa, SYN u. bullosa.

vibratory u., a form of u. that occurs in response to vibratory stimuli.

ur·ti·car·i·al, ur·ti·car·i·ous (er-ti-kar′ē-ăl, -kar′ē-ŭs). Relating to or marked by urticaria.

ur·ti·cate (er′ti-kāt). **1.** To perform urtication. **2.** Marked by the presence of wheals. [L. *urticatus*]

ur·ti·ca·tion (er-ti-kā′shŭn). **1.** Whipping with nettles to induce counterirritation, formerly used in the treatment of peripheral paralysis. **2.** A burning sensation resembling that produced by urticaria or resulting from nettle poisoning. **3.** SYN urticaria. [L. *urticatio*]

uru·shi·ol (ū′rū-shē-ōl). A mixture of nonvolatile hydrocarbons, derivatives of catechol with unsaturated C_{15} or C_{17} side chains, constituting the active allergen of the irritant oil of poison ivy, *Toxicodendron radicans*, poison oak, *T. diversilobum*, and the Asiatic laquer tree, *T. verniciferum*. [Jap. *urushi*, lac, + L. *oleum*, oil]

u. oxidase, SYN laccase.

USAN Abbreviation for United States Adopted Names.

Usher, Barney, Canadian dermatologist, *1899. SEE Senear-U. *disease, syndrome*.

Usher, Charles Howard, English ophthalmologist, 1865–1942. SEE U.'s *syndrome*.

USP Abbreviation for United States Pharmacopeia. SEE Pharmacopeia.

USPHS Abbreviation for United States Public Health Service.

us·ti·lag·i·nism (ŭs-ti-laj′i-nizm). Poisoning by *Ustilago maydis* (corn smut), which produces burning, itching, hyperemia, acrocyanosis, and edema of the extremities; resembles ergotism, pellagra, or infantile acrocynia.

Us·ti·la·go (ŭs-ti-lā′gō). A genus of smuts (order Ustilaginales). [L. a kind of thistle, fr. *ustio*, a burning]

U. may′dis, a species that resembles ergot of rye in its metabolic action; its black spores on the ears of corn are dispersed by wind and can cause contamination of laboratory cultures. SYN corn ergot, corn smut, U. zeae.

U. ze′ae, SYN *U. maydis.*

us·tu·la·tion (ŭs-tyū-lā′shŭn). **1.** Separation of compounds by heat, as in the process of freeing ores from sulfur by roasting. **2.** Drying of a drug by heat to prepare it for pulverization. [L. *ustulo*, pp. *-atus*, to scorch]

usur·pa·tion (yū-ser-pā′shŭn). Assumption of pacemaker function of the heart by a subsidiary focus as a result of its own increased automaticity; *e.g.,* accelerated junctional pacemaker takes command when it exceeds the sinus rate. [L. *usurpo*, pp. *-atus*, to seize]

uta (ū′tă). A mild form of New World or American cutaneous leishmaniasis caused by *Leishmania peruana*, occurring in the high Andean valleys of Peru and Bolivia, and characterized by numerous small dermal lesions occurring almost exclusively on exposed skin surfaces; the dog is an important reservoir. Unlike all other forms of American cutaneous leishmaniasis, this disease is found at high elevations (2000 to 2500 m) in barren open country, rather than in lowland tropical forests. [Sp.]

△**uter-.** SEE utero-.

uter·ec·to·my (yū-tĕ-rek′tō-mē). SYN hysterectomy.

uter·ine (yū′ter-in, yū′ter-īn). Relating to the uterus.

uter·is·mus (yū-tĕ-riz′mŭs). Obsolete term for painful spasmodic contraction of the uterus. [uter- + L. *-ismus*, action or condition, fr. G. *-ismos*]

uter·i·tis (yū-tĕ-rī′tis). SYN metritis.

in utero (in yū′ter-ō). Within the womb; not yet born. [L.]

△**utero-, uter-.** The uterus. SEE ALSO hystero- (1), metra-, metro-. [L. *uterus*]

uter·o·ab·dom·i·nal (yū′ter-ō-ab-dom′i-năl). Relating to the uterus and the abdomen. SYN uteroventral.

uter·o·cer·vi·cal (yū′ter-ō-ser′vi-kăl). Relating to the cervix of the uterus.

uter·o·cys·tos·to·my (yū′ter-ō-sis-tos′tō-mē). Formation of a communication between the uterus (cervix) and the bladder. [utero- + G. *kystis*, bladder, + *stoma*, mouth]

uter·o·fix·a·tion (yū′ter-ō-fik-sā′shŭn). SYN hysteropexy.

uter·o·lith (yū′ter-ō-lith). SYN uterine *calculus*. [utero- + G. *lithos*, stone]

uter·om·e·ter (yū-ter-om′ĕ-ter). SYN hysterometer.

uter·o·o·var·i·an (yū′ter-ō-ō-văr′ē-an). Relating to the uterus and an ovary.

uter·o·pa·ri·e·tal (yū′ter-ō-pa-rī′ĕ-tăl). Relating to the uterus and the abdominal wall.

uter·o·pel·vic (yū′ter-ō-pel′vik). Relating to the uterus and the pelvis.

uter·o·pexy (yū′ter-ō-pek-sē). SYN hysteropexy.

uter·o·pla·cen·tal (yū′ter-ō-pla-sen′tăl). Relating to the uterus and the placenta.

uter·o·plas·ty (yū′ter-ō-plas-tē). Plastic surgery of the uterus. SYN hysteroplasty, metroplasty. [utero- + G. *plastos*, formed]

uter·o·sa·cral (yū′ter-ō-sā′krăl). Relating to the uterus and the sacrum.

uter·o·sal·pin·gog·ra·phy (yū′ter-ō-sal-pin-gog′ră-fē). SYN hysterosalpingography.

uter·o·scope (yū′ter-ō-skōp). SYN hysteroscope.

uter·os·co·py (yū-ter-os′kŏ-pē). SYN hysteroscopy.

uter·ot·o·my (yū-ter-ot′ō-mē). SYN hysterotomy.

uter·o·ton·ic (yū′ter-ō-ton′ik). **1.** Giving tone to the uterine muscle. **2.** An agent that overcomes relaxation of the muscular wall of the uterus. [utero- + G. *tonos*, tone, tension]

uter·o·trop·ic (yū′ter-ō-trō′pik). Causing an effect on the uterus.

uter·o·tub·al (yū′ter-ō-tū′băl). Pertaining to the uterus and the uterine tubes.

uter·o·tu·bog·ra·phy (yū′ter-ō-tū-bog′ră-fē). SYN hysterosalpingography.

uter·o·vag·i·nal (yū-ter-ō-vaj′i-năl). Relating to the uterus and the vagina.

uter·o·ven·tral (yū′ter-ō-ven′trăl). SYN uteroabdominal. [utero- + L. *venter*, belly]

uter·o·ver·dine (yū′ter-ō-ver′din). Biliverdin from dog placenta.

uter·o·ves·i·cal (yū′ter-ō-ves′i-kăl). Relating to the uterus and the urinary bladder.

uter·us, pl. **uteri** (yū′ter-ŭs, yū′ter-ī) [NA]. The hollow muscular organ in which the impregnated ovum is developed into the child; it is about 7.5 cm in length in the nonpregnant woman, and consists of a main portion (body) with an elongated lower part (neck), at the extremity of which is the opening (os). The upper rounded portion of the u., opposite the os, is the fundus, at each extremity of which is the horn marking the part where uterine tube joins the u. and through which the ovum reaches the uterine cavity after leaving the ovary. The organ is supported in the pelvic cavity by the broad ligaments, round ligaments, cardinal ligaments, and rectouterine and vesicouterine folds or ligaments. SYN metra, womb. [L.]

u. acol′lis, a u. with atresia or absence of the cervix.

anomalous u., a malformed u. caused by abnormal development or fusion of the paramesonephric ducts.

arcuate u., a u. with a depression at the fundus; an incomplete u. bicornis. SYN u. arcuatus.

u. arcua′tus, SYN arcuate u.

bicornate u., a u. that is more or less completely divided into two lateral horns as a result of imperfect fusion of the paramesonephric ducts; it differs from septate u., in which there is no external mark of separation; in u. bicornis, the cervix may be single (u. bicornate unicollis) or double (u. bicornate bicollis). SYN bifid u., u. bicornis, u. bifidus.

u. bicornate bicollis, SEE bicornate u.

u. bicornate unicollis, SEE bicornate u.

u. bicor′nis, SYN bicornate u.

bifid u., SYN bicornate u.

u. bi′fidus, SYN bicornate u.

biforate u., septate u. in which the cervix is divided into two by a septum. SYN double-mouthed u., u. biforis.

u. bifor′is, SYN biforate u.

u. bilocula′ris, SYN septate u.

u. biparti′tus, SYN septate u.

bipartite u., SYN septate u.

capped u., a condition of tonic contraction of the fundus musculature of the u.

cordiform u., an incomplete u. bicornis with a wedge-shaped depression at the fundus. SYN heart-shaped u., u. cordiformis.

u. cordiform′is, SYN cordiform u.

Couvelaire u., extravasation of blood into the uterine musculature and beneath the uterine peritoneum in association with severe forms of abruptio placentae. SYN uteroplacental apoplexy.

u. didel′phys, double u. with double cervix and double vagina; due to failure of the paramesonephric ducts to unite. [G. *di-*, two, + *delphys,* womb]

double-mouthed u., SYN biforate u.

duplex u., any u. with double lumen (u. didelphys, u. bicornis bicollis, or septate u.). SYN u. duplex.

u. du′plex, SYN duplex u.

gravid u., the condition of the u. in pregnancy.

heart-shaped u., SYN cordiform u.

incudiform u., u. bicornis in which the fundus between the two cornua is broad and flat. SYN triangular u., u. incudiformis, u. triangularis.

u. incudiform′is, SYN incudiform u.

masculine u., SYN prostatic *utricle*.

u. masculi′nus, SYN prostatic *utricle*.

one-horned u., obsolete term for unicorn u.

u. parvicol′lis, a u. of normal size with an abnormal, disproportionately small cervix.

septate u., a u. divided into two cavities by an anteroposterior septum. SYN bipartite u., u. bilocularis, u. bipartitus, u. septus.

u. sep′tus, SYN septate u.

subseptate u., an incomplete u. septus. SYN u. subseptus.

u. subsep′tus, SYN subseptate u.

triangular u., SYN incudiform u.

u. triangula′ris, SYN incudiform u.

unicorn u., a u. in which only one lateral half exists, the other half being undeveloped or absent. SYN u. unicornis.

u. unicor′nis, SYN unicorn u.

UTI Abbreviation for urinary tract *infection*.

util·i·ty. In biomedical ethics and clinical decision analysis, the satisfaction or economic advantage gained from the outcome that results from a particular decision.

UTP Abbreviation for *uridine 5′-triphosphate.*

utri·cle (yū′tri-kl). The larger of the two membranous sacs in the vestibule of the labyrinth, lying in the elliptical recess; from it arise the semicircular ducts. SYN utriculus [NA], sacculus communis.

prostatic u., a minute pouch in the prostate opening on the summit of the seminal colliculus, the analogue of the uterus and vagina in the female, being the remains of the fused caudal ends of the paramesonephric ducts. SYN utriculus prostaticus [NA], masculine uterus, Morgagni's sinus (2), sinus pocularis, uterus masculinus, vagina masculina, vesica prostatica, Weber's organ.

utric·u·lar (yū-trik′yū-lăr). Relating to or resembling a utricle.

utric·u·li (yū-trik′yū-lī). Plural of utriculus.

utric·u·li·tis (yū-trik-yū-lī′tis). **1.** Inflammation of the internal ear. **2.** Inflammation of the prostaticutricle. [utriculus + G. *-itis,* inflammation]

utric·u·lo·sac·cu·lar (yū-trik′yū-lō-sak′yū-lăr). Relating to the utricle and the saccule of the labyrinth, denoting especially a duct connecting the two structures.

utric·u·lus, pl. **utric·u·li** (yū-trik′yū-lŭs, -lī) [NA]. SYN utricle. SEE ALSO vestibular *organ.* [L. dim. of *uter,* leather bag]

u. prostat′icus [NA], SYN prostatic *utricle.*

utri·form (yū′tri-fōrm). Shaped like a leather bottle (wineskin). [L. *uter,* a skin bag, + *forma,* form]

UV, uv. Abbreviation for ultraviolet.

UVA Abbreviation for *ultraviolet* A.

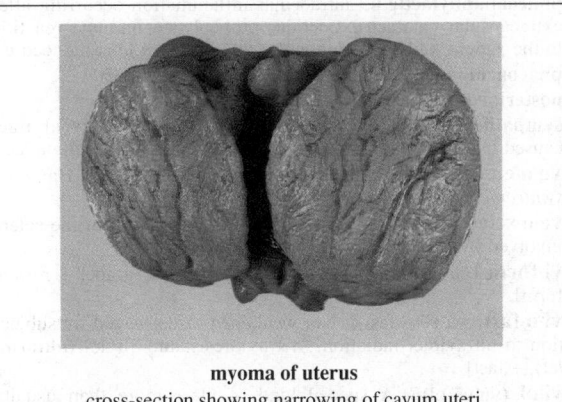

myoma of uterus
cross-section showing narrowing of cavum uteri

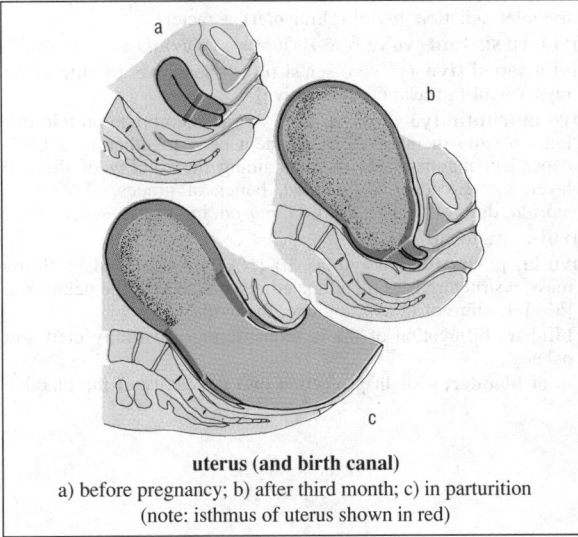

uterus (and birth canal)
a) before pregnancy; b) after third month; c) in parturition
(note: isthmus of uterus shown in red)

uvae·for·mis (yū-vē-fōr′mis). SYN vascular *lamina* of choroid. [L. *uva,* grape, + *forma,* form]

uva ur·si (ū′vă er′sī). The dried leaves of *Arctostaphylos uva-ursi* (family Ericaceae), bearberry, mountain box, a common plant of the north temperate zone; contains antiseptic glycosides, arbutin, methylarbutin, and tannins; has been used in chronic inflammations of the urinary tract. [L. *uva,* grape + *ursus,* bear]

UVB Abbreviation for *ultraviolet* B.

UVC Abbreviation for *ultraviolet* C.

uvea (yū′vē-ă). SYN vascular *tunic* of eye. [L. *uva,* grape]

uve·al (yū′vē-ăl). Relating to the uvea.

UVEB Abbreviation for unifocal ventricular ectopic beat.

uve·it·ic (yū-vē-it′ik). Relating to the uvea.

uve·i·ti·des (yū-vē-it′i-dēz). Plural of uveitis.

uve·i·tis, pl. **uve·i·ti·des** (yū-vē-ī′tis, -it′ĭ-dēz). Inflammation of the uveal tract: iris, ciliary body, and choroid. [uvea + G. *-itis,* inflammation]

anterior u., inflammation involving the ciliary body and iris.

Förster's u., syphilitic inflammation, with diffuse nodules involving the choroid and retinal vasculitis.

Fuchs' u., SYN heterochromic u.

heterochromic u., anterior uveitis and depigmentation of the iris. SYN Fuchs' u.

intermediate u., a u. that is neither anterior nor posterior but tends to involve the pars plana and the ciliary body.

lens-induced u., SYN phacoanaphylactic u.

uv

phacoanaphylactic u., intraocular inflammation occurring after extracapsular cataract extraction; probably an immune reaction to the patient's liberated lenticular proteins. SYN lens-induced u.

phacogenic u., u. secondary to hypermature cataract.

posterior u., SYN choroiditis.

sympathetic u., a bilateral inflammation of the uveal tract caused by a perforating wound of one eye that injures the uvea.

uve·o·en·ceph·a·li·tis (yū′vē-ō-en-sef-ă-lī′tis). SYN Harada's *syndrome.*

uve·o·scle·ri·tis (yū′vē-ō-sklē-rī′tis). Inflammation of the sclera involved by extension from the uvea.

uvi·form (yū′vi-fōrm). SYN botryoid. [L. *uva,* grape, + *forma,* form]

uvi·o·fast (yū′vē-ō-fast). Not weakened or destroyed by subjection to ultraviolet radiation. SYN uvioresistant. [uviol (*ultraviolet*), + fast]

uvi·ol (yū′vē-ol). A special kind of glass more than usually transparent to ultraviolet or actinic rays, *e.g.,* crystallinequartz. [*ultraviolet*]

uvi·om·e·ter (yū-vē-om′ĕ-ter). An instrument for measuring ultraviolet radiation. [uviol (*ultraviolet*), + meter]

uvi·o·re·sis·tant (yū′vē-ō-rē-zis′tant). SYN uviofast.

uvi·o·sen·si·tive (yū′vē-ō-sen′si-tiv). Sensitive to ultraviolet rays. [uviol (*ultraviolet*) + sensitive]

uvo·mor·u·lin (yū-vō-mō′rū-lin). A transmembrane protein that links plasma membranes of adjacent cells together in a Ca^{2+}-dependent manner; aids in maintaining the rigidity of the cell layer. SYN E-cadherin. [L. *uva,* bunch of grapes, + Mod. L. *morula,* dim. of L. *morum,* fr. G. *moron,* mulberry, + -in]

♲**uvul-.** SEE uvulo-.

uvu·la, pl. **uvu·li** (yū′vyū-lă, -lī) [NA]. An appendant fleshy mass; a structure bearing a fancied resemblance to the palatine u. [Mod. L. dim. of L. *uva,* a grape, the uvula]

bifid u., bifurcation of the u., constituting a partially cleft soft palate.

u. of bladder, a slight projection into the cavity of the bladder, usually more prominent in old men, just behind the urethral opening, marking the location of the middle lobe of the prostate. SYN u. vesicae [NA], Lieutaud's u.

u. cerebel′li, SYN u. vermis.

Lieutaud's u., SYN u. of bladder.

u. palati′na [NA], SYN palatine u.

palatine u., a conical projection from the posterior edge of the middle of the soft palate, composed of connective tissue containing a number of racemose glands, and some muscular fibers (uvulae muscle). SYN u. palatina [NA], pendulous palate.

u. ver′mis [NA], a triangular elevation on the vermis of the cerebellum, lying between the two tonsils anterior to the pyramis. SYN u. cerebelli.

u. vesi′cae [NA], SYN u. of bladder.

uvu·lap·to·sis (yū′vyū-lap-tō′sis). SYN uvuloptosis.

uvu·lar (yū′vyū-lăr). Relating to the uvula.

uvu·la·ris (yū′vyū-lā′ris). SYN uvulae *muscle.*

uvu·la·tome (yū′vyū-lă-tōm). SYN uvulotome.

uvu·lec·to·my (yū-vyū-lek′tō-mē). Excision of the uvula. SYN staphylectomy. [uvula + G. *ektomē,* excision]

uvu·li·tis (yū-vyū-lī′tis). Inflammation of the uvula.

♲**uvulo-, uvul-.** The uvula, usually the uvula palatina. SEE ALSO staphylo-. [L. *uvula*]

uvu·lo·pal·a·to·pha·ryn·go·plas·ty (-pal′ă-tō-fa-rin′gō-plas-tē). SYN palatopharyngoplasty.

uvu·lo·pal·a·to·plas·ty (yū′vyū-lō-pal′ă-tō-plas-tē). SYN palatopharyngoplasty.

uvu·lop·to·sis (yū′vyū-lop-tō′sis). Relaxation or elongation of the uvula. SYN falling palate, staphylodialysis, staphyloptosis, uvulaptosis. [uvulo- + G. *ptōsis,* a falling]

uvu·lo·tome (yū′vyū-lō-tōm). An instrument for cutting the uvula. SYN uvulatome.

uvu·lot·o·my (yū-vyū-lot′ō-mē). Any cutting operation on the uvula. [uvulo- + G. *tomē,* a cutting]

V 1. Abbreviation for vision or visual *acuity*; volt; with subscript 1, 2, 3, etc., the abbreviation for unipolar electrocardiogram leads. **2.** Symbol for vanadium; valine; volume, frequently with subscripts denoting location, chemical species, and/or conditions.

V̇ 1. Symbol for gas flow, frequently with subscripts indicating location and chemical species. SEE flow (3). **2.** Symbol for ventilation (3), frequently with a subscript. See entries under ventilation (3). [volume + overdot denoting time derivative]

V$_D$. Symbol for physiologic dead *space*.

V$_T$. Symbol for tidal *volume*.

V̇$_A$. Symbol for alveolar *ventilation*.

V$_{max}$ Symbol for maximum *velocity*.

V̇$_{O_2}$ Symbol for oxygen *consumption*.

V̇$_{CO_2}$ Symbol for carbon dioxide *elimination*.

v 1. Abbreviation for volt; initial rate velocity; velocity; *vel* [L, or]. **2.** As a subscript, refers to venous *blood*.

v̄. As a subscript, refers to mixed venous (pulmonary arterial) blood.

V-A Abbreviation for ventriculoatrial.

VAC Abbreviation for ventriculoatrial *conduction*.

vac·cen·ic ac·id (vak-sen′ik). CH$_3$(CH$_2$)$_5$CH=CH(CH$_2$)$_9$COOH; *n-trans*-11-octadecenoic acid; an unsaturated fatty acid of which both *cis* and *trans* isomers are found in butter and other animal fats.

vac·ci·na (vak-sin′ă). SYN vaccinia.

vac·ci·nal (vak′si-năl). Relating to vaccine or vaccination.

vac·ci·nate (vak′si-nāt). To administer a vaccine.

vac·ci·na·tion (vak′si-nā′shŭn). The act of administering a vaccine.

vac·ci·na·tor (vak′si-nā-tŏr). **1.** A person who vaccinates. SYN vaccinist. **2.** A scarifier or other instrument used in vaccination.

VACCINE

---

vac·cine (vak′sēn, vak-sēn′). Originally, the live v. (vaccinia, cowpox) virus inoculated in the skin as prophylaxis against smallpox and obtained from the skin of calves inoculated with seed virus. Usage has extended the meaning to include essentially any preparation intended for active immunological prophylaxis; *e.g.,* preparations of killed microbes of virulent strains or living microbes of attenuated (variant or mutant) strains; or microbial, fungal, plant, protozoal, or metazoan derivatives or products. Method of administration varies according to the v., inoculation being the most common, but ingestion is preferred in some instances and nasal spray is used occasionally. SYN vaccinum. [L. *vaccinus,* relating to a cow]

adjuvant v., a v. that contains an adjuvant; most often the antigen (immunogen) is included in a water-in-oil emulsion (Freund incomplete type adjuvant), or is adsorbed onto an inorganic gel (alum, aluminum hydroxide or phosphate).

aqueous v., a v. having a liquid vehicle (*e.g.,* physiological salt solution) as distinguished from an emulsion.

attenuated v. (a-ten′ū-āt′id), live pathogens that have lost their virulence but are still capable of inducing a protective immune response to the virulent forms of the pathogen, *e.g.,* Sabin polio v.

autogenous v., a v. made from a culture of the patient's own bacteria.

bacillus Calmette-Guérin v., SYN BCG v.

BCG v., a suspension of an attenuated strain (bacillus Calmette-Guérin) of *Mycobacterium tuberculosis*, bovine type, which is inoculated into the skin for tuberculosis prophylaxis. SYN bacillus Calmette-Guérin v., Calmette-Guérin v., tuberculosis v.

vaccine	
newborns	BCG (especially with high risk of TB infection)
3 and 5 months	diphtheria-tetanus* (2X), together with polio oral vaccine
15 months	measles/mumps (live vaccine)
18 months	renewal of diphtheria-tetanus; 3rd dose of polio vaccine
6–7 yrs.	renewal of diphtheria-tetanus
10–14 yrs.	rubella (live vaccine; for girls, before menarche)
every 5–10 yrs.	tetanus booster
every 8–10 yrs.	oral polio vaccine

* in some circumstances combined with whooping cough vaccine (usually avoided because of danger of complications)

brucella strain 19 v., a live bacterial v. prepared from an attenuated variant strain of *Brucella abortus* (strain 19); used for vaccinating cattle against brucellosis.

Calmette-Guérin v., SYN BCG v.

cholera v., an inactivated suspension of Inaba and Ogawa strains of *Vibrio cholerae* grown either on agar or in broth and preserved with phenol.

crystal violet v., SEE hog cholera v.'s.

diphtheria toxoid, tetanus toxoid, and pertussis v. (DTP), a v. available in three forms: 1) diphtheria and tetanus toxoids plus pertussis v. (DTP); 2) tetanus and diphtheria toxoids, adult type (Td); and 3) tetanus toxoid (T); used for active immunization against diphtheria, tetanus, and whooping cough.

duck embryo origin v. (DEV), SEE rabies v.

Flury strain v., SEE rabies v., Flury strain egg-passage.

foot-and-mouth disease virus v.'s, v.'s either of inactivated virus from infected cattle tongue epithelium or, more recently, of live virus attenuated by embryonated egg or mouse passage and propagated in tissue culture.

***Haemophilus influenzae* type B v.,** a conjugate of oligosaccharides of the capsular antigen of *H. influenzae* type B and diphtheria CRM protein.

Haffkine's v., (1) a killed culture of *Vibrio cholerae* in two strengths, a weaker one for the initial inoculation and a stronger one for the second inoculation 7 to 10 days after the first; **(2)** a killed plague bacillus (*Yersinia pestis*) v.

hepatitis B v., a formalin-inactivated v. prepared from the surface antigen (HBsAg) of the hepatitis B virus; the antigen can be obtained from the plasma of human carriers of the virus; purified HBsAg for immunization is also prepared by recombinant DNA technology.

heterogenous v., v. that is not autogenous, but is prepared from the same species of bacterium.

high-egg-passage v., HEP v., SEE rabies v., Flury strain egg-passage.

hog cholera v.'s, v.'s either of virus from blood of infected swine, inactivated with crystal violet, or live virus attenuated in rabbits or tissue culture and frequently used in conjunction with hog cholera virus antiserum.

human diploid cell v. (HDCV), an iodinated virus vaccine used for protection against rabies vaccine usually prepared in the human diploid cell WI-38. SYN human diploid cell rabies v.

human diploid cell rabies v. (HDCV), SYN human diploid cell v.

inactivated poliovirus v. (IPV), SEE poliovirus v.'s (2).

va

influenza virus v.'s, influenza virus grown in embryonated eggs and inactivated, usually by the addition of formalin; both whole virus and subunit preparations containing hemagglutinins and neuraminidase are used; because of the marked and progressive antigenic variation of the influenza viruses, the strains included are regularly changed following various outbreaks of influenza in order to include most recently isolated epidemic strains of both type A influenza and type B influenza.

live v., v. prepared from living, attenuated organisms.

live oral poliovirus v., SEE poliovirus v.'s (2).

low-egg-passage v., LEP v., SEE rabies v., Flury strain egg-passage.

measles, mumps, and rubella v. (MMR), a combination of live attenuated measles, mumps, and rubella viruses in an aqueous suspension; used for immunization against the respective diseases.

measles virus v., v. containing live, attenuated strains of measles virus prepared in chick embryo cell culture. SEE measles, mumps, and rubella v.

multivalent v., SYN polyvalent v.

mumps virus v., v. containing live, attenuated mumps virus prepared in chick embryo cell cultures. SEE measles, mumps, and rubella v.

oil v., SEE adjuvant v.

oral poliovirus v. (OPV), SEE poliovirus v.'s (2).

Pasteur v., SEE rabies v.

pertussis v., SEE diphtheria toxoid, tetanus toxoid, and pertussis v.

plague v., v. (licensed for use in the U.S.) prepared from cultures of *Yersinia pestis*, inactivated with formaldehyde, and preserved with 0.5% phenol; injections are made intramuscularly, and booster inoculations are recommended every 6 to 12 months while individuals remain in an area of risk; live, attenuated bacterial and chemical fraction v.'s are also available.

pneumococcal v., v. comprised of purified capsular polysaccharide antigen from 23 types of *Streptococcus pneumoniae* (representing those types responsible for most of the reported pneumococcal diseases in the U.S.).

poliomyelitis v.'s, SYN poliovirus v.'s.

poliovirus v.'s, (1) inactivated poliovirus v. (IPV), an aqueous suspension of inactivated strains of poliomyelitis virus (types 1, 2, and 3) used by injection; has largely been replaced by the oral v.; SEE Salk v. **(2)** oral poliovirus v. (OPV), an aqueous suspension of live, attenuated strains of poliomyelitis virus (types 1, 2, and 3) given orally for active immunization against poliomyelitis. SEE Sabin v. SYN poliomyelitis v.'s.

polyvalent v., a v. prepared from cultures of two or more strains of the same species or microorganism. SYN multivalent v.

rabies v., a v. introduced by Pasteur as a method of treatment for the bite of a rabid animal: daily (14 to 21) injections of virus that increased serially from noninfective to fully infective "fixed" virus were given to render the central nervous system refractory to infection by virulent virus; this v., with but slight modification (*e.g.,* Semple v.), was used for many years but had the serious defect that the large quantity of heterologous nervous tissue inoculated along with the virus occasionally gave rise to an allergic (immunological) demyelinization. It was replaced, in the case of humans, by rabies v. of duck embryo origin (DEV), prepared from embryonated duck eggs infected with "fixed" virus and inactivated with β-propiolactone. At the present time DEV has been replaced by human diploid cell v. (HDCV) which is gronw in WI-38 cells; it has a low incidence of adverse reactions and requires fewer injections.

rabies v., Flury strain egg-passage, (1) high-egg-passage (HEP) v.: living Flury strain rabies virus at the 180th to 190th level egg passage (embryonate eggs), used for vaccination of cattle and cats; **(2)** low-egg-passage (LEP) v.: at the 40th to 50th passage level, containing 10^3 to 10^4 mouse LD_{50}; nonpathogenic in dogs but retains some pathogenicity for cattle and cats.

rickettsia v., attenuated, SEE typhus v.

Rocky Mountain spotted fever v., suspension of inactivated *Rickettsia rickettsii* prepared by growing the rickettsiae in the embryonate yolk sac of fowl eggs.

rubella virus v., live, a live virus v. prepared from duck embryo or human diploid cell culture infected with rubella virus; administered as a single subcutaneous injection. SEE measles, mumps, and rubella v.

Sabin v., an orally administered v. containing live, attenuated strains of poliovirus. SEE poliovirus v.'s.

Salk v., the original poliovirus v., composed of virus propagated in monkey kidney tissue culture and inactivated. SEE poliovirus v.'s.

Semple v., a modification of the original (Pasteur) rabies v., formerly widely used in the U.S., prepared from rabbit nerve tissue, inactivated with phenol and administered in 14 to 21 daily injections; has variable potency and is associated with a high incidence of postvaccinal demyelination.

smallpox v., v. of live vaccinia virus suspensions prepared from cutaneous vaccinial lesions of calves (calf lymph) or chick embryo origin.

split-virus v., SEE subunit v.

staphylococcus v., a suspension of organisms from cultures of one or more strains of *Staphylococcus;* used for furunculosis, acne, and other suppurative conditions.

stock v., a v. made from a stock microbial strain, in contradistinction to an autogenous v.

subunit v., a v. which, through chemical extraction, is free of viral nucleic acid and contains only specific protein subunits of a given virus; such v.'s are relatively free of the adverse reactions (*e.g.,* influenza virus) associated with v.'s containing the whole virion.

T.A.B. v., SYN typhoid-paratyphoid A and B v.

tetanus v., SEE diphtheria toxoid, tetanus toxoid, and pertussis v.

tuberculosis v., SYN BCG v.

typhoid v., a suspension of *Salmonella typhi* inactivated either by heat or by chemical (acetone) with an added preservative; in the U.S., the combined typhoid and paratyphoid A and B v.'s have been largely replaced by the monovalent typhoid v. because of the lack of evidence of effectiveness of paratyphoid A and paratyphoid B ingredients.

typhoid-paratyphoid A and B v., a suspension of killed typhoid and paratyphoid A and B bacilli. SEE ALSO typhoid v. SYN T.A.B. v.

typhus v., a formaldehyde-inactivated suspension of *Rickettsia prowazekii* grown in embryonated eggs; effective against louse-borne (epidemic) typhus; primary immunization consists of two subcutaneous injections 4 or more weeks apart; booster doses are required every 6 to 12 months, as long as the possibility of exposure exists. A v. containing living rickettsiae of an attenuated strain of *R. prowazekii* has also been used.

whooping-cough v., SEE diphtheria toxoid, tetanus toxoid, and pertussis v.

yellow fever v., a living, attenuated strain (17D) of yellow fever virus propagated in embryonated fowl eggs. **(2)** a suspension of dried mouse brain infected with French neurotropic (Dakar) strain of yellow fever virus, administered topically by the scratch method; not officially recommended in the United States because of meningoencephalitic reactions.

vac·cin·ia (vak-sin′ē-ă). An infection, primarily local and limited to the site of inoculation, induced in man by inoculation with the vaccinia virus in order to confer resistance to smallpox. On about the third day after this vaccination, papules form at the site of inoculation which become transformed into umbilicated vesicles and later pustules; they then dry up, and the scab falls off on about the 21st day, leaving a pitted scar; in some cases there are more or less marked constitutional disturbances. SYN primary reaction, vaccina, variola vaccine, variola vaccinia, variola vaccinia. [L. *vaccinus,* relating to a cow, fr. *vacca,* a cow]

v. gangreno′sa, SYN progressive v.

generalized v., secondary lesions of the skin following vaccination which may occur in subjects with previously healthy skin but are more common in the case of traumatized skin, especially in the case of eczema (eczema vaccinatum). In the latter instance, generalized v. may result from mere contact with a vaccinated person. Secondary vaccinial lesions may also occur following transfer of virus from the vaccination to another site by means of the fingers.

progressive v., a severe or even fatal form of v. occurring chiefly in subjects with an immunologic deficiency or dyscrasia and characterized by progressive enlargement of the initial and also of secondary lesions. SYN v. gangrenosa.

v. vaccin′ia, SYN vaccinia.

vac·cin·i·al (vak-sin′ē-ăl). Relating to vaccinia.

vac·cin·i·form (vak-sin′i-fōrm). Resembling vaccinia.

vac·ci·nist (vak′si-nist). SYN vaccinator (1).

vac·cin·i·za·tion (vak′sin-i-zā′shŭn). Vaccination repeated at short intervals until it will no longer take.

vac·cin·o·gen (vak-sin′-ō-jen). A source of vaccine, such as an inoculated heifer.

vac·ci·nog·e·nous (vak-si-noj′ĕ-nŭs). Producing vaccine, or relating to the production of vaccine.

vac·ci·noid (vak′si-noyd). Resembling vaccinia.

vac·ci·no·style (vak′si-nō-stīl). A pointed instrument used in vaccination.

vac·ci·num (vak′si-nŭm). SYN vaccine. [L.]

in vac·uo (in vak′yū-ō). In a vacuum, *e.g.,* under reduced pressure. [L.]

vac·u·o·lar (vak-yū-ō′lăr). Relating to or resembling a vacuole.

vac·u·o·late, vac·u·o·lat·ed (vak′yū-ō-lāt, -lāt′ed). Having vacuoles.

vac·u·o·la·tion (vak′yū-ō-lā′shŭn). 1. Formation of vacuoles. 2. The condition of having vacuoles. SYN vacuolization.

vac·u·ole (vak′yū-ōl). 1. A minute space in any tissue. 2. A clear space in the substance of a cell, sometimes degenerative in character, sometimes surrounding an englobed foreign body and serving as a temporary cell stomach for the digestion of the body. [Mod. L. *vacuolum,* dim. of L. *vacuum,* an empty space]

autophagic v., SYN cytolysosome.

contractile v., a cavity formed by the accumulation of fluid in the ectoplasm of a protozoan; after increasing for a time it empties itself externally by a sudden contraction; it functions as an osmoregulatory mechanism for water balance, especially in freshwater protozoans.

digestive v., SYN secondary *lysosomes,* under *lysosome.*

parasitophorous v., a v. formed by layers of endoplasmic reticulum around an intracellular parasite which may serve to isolate the parasite and enclose it for lysozymal attack.

vac·u·o·li·za·tion (vak′yū-ō-li-zā′shŭn). SYN vacuolation.

vac·u·ome (vak′yū-ōm). A system of vacuoles that can be stained with neutral red in the living cell. [vacuole + G. *-oma,* tumor]

vac·u·tome (vak′yū-tōm). Electrodermatome that applies suction to the skin to raise it before an advancing blade, usually for taking a split-thickness skin graft. [vacuum + G. *tomē,* a cutting]

vac·u·um (vak′ūm). An empty space, one practically exhausted of air or gas. [L. ntr. of *vacuus,* empty]

va·dum (vā′dŭm). An occasional elevation from the bottom of a cerebral sulcus nearly obliterating it for a short distance. [L. a ford]

va·gal (vā′găl). Relating to the vagus nerve.

va·gec·to·my (vā-jek′tō-mē). Surgical removal of a segment of a vagus nerve.

va·gi (vā′gī, -jī). Plural of vagus.

vagin-. SEE vagino-.

va·gi·na, gen. and pl. **va·gi·nae** (vă-jī′nă, -nē). 1. SYN sheath (1). 2 [NA]. The genital canal in the female, extending from the uterus to the vulva. [L. sheath, the vagina]

bipartite v., SYN septate v.

v. bul′bi [NA], SYN fascial *sheath* of eyeball.

v. carot′ica [NA], SYN carotid *sheath.*

v. cellulo′sa, the connective tissue sheath of a nerve or muscle (perineurium or perimysium, respectively).

v. commu′nis musculo′rum flexo′rum [NA], SYN common flexor *sheath.*

v. exter′na ner′vi op′tici [NA], SYN external *sheath* of optic nerve.

vagi′nae fibro′sae digito′rum ma′nus [NA], SYN fibrous digital *sheaths* of hand, under *sheath.* SEE annular *part* of fibrous digital sheath, cruciform *part* of fibrous digital sheath.

vagi′nae fibro′sae digito′rum pe′dis [NA], SYN fibrous digital *sheaths* of foot, under *sheath.* SEE annular *part* of fibrous digital sheath, cruciform *part* of fibrous digital sheath.

v. fibro′sa ten′dinis [NA], SYN fibrous tendon *sheath.*

v. inter′na ner′vi op′tici [NA], SYN internal *sheath* of optic nerve.

v. intertubercula′ris, SYN intertubercular *sheath.*

v. masculi′na, SYN prostatic *utricle.*

v. muco′sa ten′dinis, SYN synovial tendon *sheath.*

v. mus′culi rec′ti abdo′minis [NA], SYN rectus *sheath.*

vagi′nae ner′vi op′tici, sheaths of the optic nerve, formed by extensions of the central meninges. SEE internal *sheath* of optic nerve, external *sheath* of optic nerve.

v. oc′uli, SYN fascial *sheath* of eyeball.

v. proces′sus styloi′dei [NA], SYN *sheath* of styloid process.

septate v., a bipartite v. caused by the presence of a more or less complete longitudinal septum. SYN bipartite v.

vagi′nae synovia′les digito′rum ma′nus [NA], SYN synovial *sheaths* of digits of hand, under *sheath.*

vagi′nae synovia′les digito′rum pe′dis [NA], SYN synovial *sheaths* of digits of foot, under *sheath.*

v. synovia′lis ten′dinis [NA], SYN synovial tendon *sheath.*

v. synovia′lis troch′leae, SYN tendon *sheath* of superior oblique muscle.

v. ten′dinis mus′culi extenso′ris car′pi ulna′ris [NA], SYN tendon *sheath* of extensor carpi ulnaris muscle.

v. ten′dinis mus′culi extenso′ris dig′iti min′imi [NA], SYN tendon *sheath* of extensor digiti minimi muscle.

v. ten′dinis mus′culi extenso′ris hal′lucis lon′gi [NA], SYN tendon *sheath* of extensor hallucis longus muscle.

v. ten′dinis mus′culi extenso′ris pol′licis lon′gi [NA], SYN tendon *sheath* of extensor pollicis longus muscle.

v. ten′dinis mus′culi flexo′ris car′pi radia′lis [NA], SYN tendon *sheath* of flexor carpi radialis muscle.

v. ten′dinis mus′culi flexo′ris hal′lucis lon′gi [NA], SYN tendon *sheath* of flexor hallucis longus muscle.

v. ten′dinis mus′culi flexo′ris pol′licis lon′gi [NA], SYN tendon *sheath* of flexor pollicis longus muscle.

v. ten′dinis mus′culi obli′qui superio′ris [NA], SYN tendon *sheath* of superior oblique muscle.

v. ten′dinis mus′culi perone′i lon′gi planta′ris [NA], SYN plantar tendon *sheath* of peroneus longus muscle.

v. ten′dinis mus′culi tibia′lis anterio′ris [NA], SYN tendon *sheath* of tibialis anterior muscle.

v. ten′dinis mus′culi tibia′lis posterio′ris [NA], SYN tendon *sheath* of tibialis posterior muscle.

v. ten′dinum mus′culi extenso′ris digito′rum pe′dis lon′gi [NA], SYN tendon *sheath* of extensor digitorum longus muscle of foot.

⌂ Combining forms	**[NA] Nomina Anatomica**
Word*Finder*	**[MIM] Mendelian**
Multi-term entry finder	**Inheritance in Man**
Preceding letter A	
A.D.A.M. Anatomy Plates	**☆ Official alternate term**
Between letters L and M	
	☆[NA] Official alternate
Appendices:	**Nomina Anatomica term**
Following letter Z	
	High Profile Term
SYN Synonym; Cf., compare	

va

v. ten'dinum mus'culi flexo'ris digito'rum pe'dis lon'gi [NA], SYN tendon *sheath* of flexor digitorum longus muscle of foot.

v. ten'dinum musculo'rum abducto'ris lon'gi et extenso'ris bre'vis pol'licis [NA], SYN tendon *sheath* of abductor pollicis longus and extensor pollicis brevis muscles.

v. ten'dinum musculo'rum extenso'ris digitor'um et extenso'ris in'dicis [NA], SYN tendon *sheath* of extensor digitorum and extensor indicis muscles.

v. ten'dinum musculo'rum extenso'rum car'pi radia'lium [NA], SYN tendon *sheath* of extensor carpi radialis muscles.

v. ten'dinum musculo'rum fibula'rium commu'nis, ☆official alternate term for common peroneal tendon *sheath*.

v. ten'dinum musculo'rum peroneo'rum commu'nis [NA], SYN common peroneal tendon *sheath*.

vagi'nae vaso'rum, SYN vascular *sheaths,* under *sheath*.

vag·i·nal (vaj'i-năl). Relating to the vagina or to any sheath. [Mod. L. *vaginalis*]

va·gi·na·pexy (va-jī'nă-pek-sē). SYN vaginofixation.

vag·i·nate (vaj'i-nāt). 1. To ensheathe; to enclose in a sheath. 2. Ensheathed; provided with a sheath.

vag·i·nec·to·my (vaj-i-nek'tō-mē). Excision of the vagina or a segment thereof. SYN colpectomy. [vagina + G. *ektomē,* excision]

vag·i·nism (vaj'i-nizm). SYN vaginismus.

vag·i·nis·mus (vaj-i-niz'mŭs). Painful spasm of the vagina preventing intercourse. SYN vaginism, vulvismus. [vagina + L. *-ismus,* action, condition]

  posterior v., spasmodic stenosis of the vagina caused by contraction of the levator ani muscle.

vag·i·ni·tis, pl. **vag·i·ni·ti·des** (vaj-i-nī'tis, -nī'ti-dēz). Inflammation of the vagina. [vagina + G. *-itis,* inflammation]

  adhesive v., inflammation of vaginal mucosa with adhesions of the vaginal walls to each other. SYN v. adhesiva.

  v. adhesi'va, SYN adhesive v.

  amebic v., v. caused by *Entamoeba histolytica.*

  atrophic v., thinning and atrophy of the vaginal epithelium usually resulting from diminished estrogen stimulation; a common occurrence in postmenopausal women.

  v. cys'tica, SYN v. emphysematosa.

  desquamative inflammatory v., an acute inflammation of the vagina of unknown cause, characterized by grayish pseudomembrane, free discharge, and easy bleeding on trauma; the discharge contains pus and immature epithelial cells, although estrogen levels are normal.

  v. emphysemato'sa, v. characterized by accumulation of gas in small connective tissue spaces lined by foreign-body giant cells. SYN pachyvaginitis cystica, v. cystica.

  Gardnerella v., SYN bacterial *vaginosis.*

  granular v., a condition of cattle manifested by the appearance of small, spherical, transparent nodules in the mucosa of the vagina of cows and of the penis of bulls; the mucosa is reddened and a mucopurulent exudate appears on the affected surfaces; it is a non specific hyperplastic response of the lymphatic tissue of these areas to an irritant or an antigen.

  nonspecific v., SYN bacterial *vaginosis.*

  pinworm v., v. caused by *Enterobius vermicularis.*

  senile v., atrophic v. resulting from withdrawal of estrogen stimulation of mucosa, often assuming the form of adhesive v. SYN v. senilis.

  v. seni'lis, SYN senile v.

♻**vagino-, vagin-.** The vagina. SEE ALSO colpo-. [L. *vagina,* sheath]

vag·i·no·ab·dom·i·nal (vaj'i-nō-ab-dom'i-năl). Relating to the vagina and the abdomen.

vag·i·no·cele (vaj'i-nō-sēl). SYN colpocele (1).

vag·i·no·dyn·ia (vaj'i-nō-din'ē-ă). Vaginal pain. SYN colpodynia.

vag·i·no·fix·a·tion (vaj'i-nō-fik-sā'shŭn). Suture of a relaxed and prolapsed vagina to the abdominal wall. SYN colpopexy, vaginapexy, vaginopexy.

vag·i·no·hys·ter·ec·to·my (vaj'i-nō-his-ter-ek'tō-mē). SYN vaginal *hysterectomy.*

vag·i·no·la·bi·al (vaj'i-nō-lā'bē-ăl). Relating to the vagina and the pudendal labia.

vag·i·no·my·co·sis (vaj'i-nō-mī-kō'sis). Vaginal infection due to a fungus. SYN colpomycosis.

vag·i·nop·a·thy (vaj-i-nop'ă-thē). Any diseased condition of the vagina. SYN colpopathy. [vagino- + G. *pathos,* suffering]

vag·i·no·per·i·ne·al (vaj'i-nō-per-i-nē'ăl). Relating to or involving the vagina and perineum.

vag·i·no·per·i·ne·o·plas·ty (vaj'i-nō-per-i-nē'ō-plas-tē). Plastic surgery of the perineum involving the vagina. SYN colpoperineoplasty. [vagino- + perineum, + G. *plastos,* formed]

vag·i·no·per·i·ne·or·rha·phy (vaj'i-nō-per-i-nē-ōr'ă-fē). Repair of a lacerated vagina and perineum. SYN colpoperineorrhaphy. [vagino- + perineum, + G. *rhaphē,* suture]

vag·i·no·per·i·ne·ot·o·my (vaj'i-nō-per-i-nē-ot'ō-mē). Division of the posterior aspect of the vagina and adjacent portion of the perineum to facilitate childbirth. [vagino- + perineum, + G. *tomē,* incision]

vag·i·no·per·i·to·ne·al (vaj'i-nō-per-i-tō-nē'ăl). Relating to the vagina and the peritoneum.

vag·i·no·pexy (vaj'i-nō-pek-sē). SYN vaginofixation.

vag·i·no·plas·ty (vaj'i-nō-plas-tē). Plastic surgery of the vagina. SYN colpoplasty. [vagino- + G. *plastos,* formed]

vag·i·nos·co·py (vaj-i-nos'kŏ-pē). Inspection of the vagina, usually with an instrument.

vag·in·o·sis. Disease of the vagina.

  bacterial v., infection of the vagina of humans that may be caused by *Gardnerella vaginalis.* Characterized by excessive, sometimes malodorous, discharge. SYN *Gardnerella* vaginitis, nonspecific vaginitis.

vag·i·not·o·my (vaj-i-not'ō-mē). A cutting operation in the vagina. SYN coleotomy (2), colpotomy.

vag·i·no·ves·i·cal (vaj'i-nō-ves'i-kăl). Relating to the vagina and the urinary bladder.

vag·i·no·vul·var (vaj'i-nō-vŭl'văr). Relating to the vagina and the vulva.

Vag·in·u·lus ple·be·i·us (vaj-i-nū'lŭs plē'bē-ē-ŭs). The slug vector of *Angiostrongylus costaricensis.*

va·gi·tus uter·i·nus (va-jī'tŭs yū-ter-ī'nŭs). Crying of the fetus while still within the uterus, possible when the membranes have been ruptured and air has entered the uterine cavity. [L. fr. *vagio,* to squall; L. fr. *uterus,* womb]

♻**vago-.** The vagus nerve. [L. *vagus*]

va·go·ac·ces·so·ri·us (vā-gō-ak-ses-sō'rē-ŭs). The vagus and the cranial root (accessory portion) of the accessory nerve, regarded as one nerve. SEE accessory *nerve.*

va·go·glos·so·pha·ryn·ge·al (vā'gō-glos'ō-fă-rin'jē-ăl). Relating to the vagus and glossopharyngeal nerves; denoting their contiguous or common nuclei of origin and termination and regions innervated by both nerves such as the musculature of the pharynx.

va·gol·y·sis (vā-gol'i-sis). Surgical destruction of the vagus nerve. [vago- + G. *lysis,* a loosening]

va·go·lyt·ic (vā-gō-lit'ik). 1. Pertaining to or causing vagolysis. 2. A therapeutic or chemical agent that has inhibitory effects on the vagus nerve. 3. Denoting an agent having such effects.

va·go·mi·met·ic (vā'gō-mi-met'ik). Mimicking the action of the efferent fibers of the vagus nerve.

va·got·o·my (vā-got'ō-mē). Division of the vagus nerve. [vago- + G. *tomē,* incision]

va·go·to·nia (vā-gō-tō'nē-ă). Archaic designation for a condition in which the parasympathetic autonomic system is reputedly overactive. SYN parasympathotonia, sympathetic imbalance. [vago- + G. *tonos,* strain]

va·go·ton·ic (vā-gō-ton'ik). Relating to or marked by vagotonia.

va·go·tro·pic (vā-gō-trop'ik). Attracted by, hence acting upon, the vagus nerve. [vago- + G. *tropos,* turning]

va·go·va·gal (vā'gō-vā'găl). Pertaining to a process that utilizes both afferent and efferent vagal fibers.

va·gus, gen. and pl. **va·gi** (vā'gŭs; vā'gī, -jī). SYN vagus *nerve.*

[L. wandering, so-called because of the wide distribution of the nerve]

Val Symbol for valine and its radicals.

va·lence, va·len·cy (vā'lens, -len-sē). The combining power of one atom of an element (or a radical), that of the hydrogen atom being the unit of comparison, determined by the number of electrons in the outer shell of the atom (v. electrons); *e.g.,* in HCl, chlorine is monovalent; in H_2O, oxygen is bivalent; in NH_3, nitrogen is trivalent. [L. *valentia,* strength]

negative v., the number of v. electrons an atom can take up.

positive v., the number of v. electrons an atom can give up.

va·lent (vā'lent). Possessing valence.

Valentin, Gabriel G., German-Swiss physiologist, 1810–1883. SEE V.'s *corpuscles,* under *corpuscle, ganglion, nerve.*

Valentine, Ferdinand C., U.S. surgeon, 1851–1909. SEE V.'s *position, test.*

va·lep·o·tri·ates (val'ē-pō'trē-āts). A class of iridoid alkaloids from *Valeriana* sp. and *Kentranthus* sp.; *e.g.,* the drug valtratum is a member of this class.

val·er·ate (val'ĕ-rāt). A salt of valeric acid; some are used in modern medicine. SYN valerianate.

va·le·ri·an (vă-lēr'ē-an). **1.** The rhizome and roots of *Valeriana officinalis* (family Valerianaceae), a herb native in southern Europe and northern Asia, cultivated also in Great Britain and the U.S.; has been used as a sedative in hysteria and at the menopause. **2.** Referring to a class of terpene alkaloids obtained from v. (1). SYN vandal root.

va·le·ri·a·nate (vă-lē'rē-ă-nāt). SYN valerate.

va·le·ric ac·id (vă-lēr'ik, vă-ler'ik). $CH_3(CH_2)_3COOH$; normal aliphatic acid; distilled from valerian; some of its salts are used in medicine; found in human colon. SYN pentanoic acid.

va·leth·a·mate bro·mide (vă-leth'ă-māt). 2-Diethylaminoethyl 3-methyl-2-phenylvalerate methylbromide; an anticholinergic agent.

val·e·tu·di·nar·i·an (val'ĕ-tū-di-nār'ē-ăn). **1.** An invalid or person in chronically poor health. **2.** One whose chief concern is his/her invalidism or poor health. [L. *valetudinarius,* sickly]

val·e·tu·di·nar·i·an·ism (val'ĕ-tū-di-nār'ē-ăn-izm). A weak or infirm state due to invalidism.

val·goid (val'goyd). Relating to valgus; knock-kneed; suffering from talipes valgus. [L. *valgus,* bowlegged, + G. *eidos,* resemblance]

val·gus (val'gŭs). Bent or twisted outward away from the midline or body; modern accepted usage, particularly in orthopedics, erroneously transposes the meaning of varus to v., as in *genu* valgum (knock-knee). [Mod. L. turned outward, fr. L. bowlegged]

val·id. Effective; producing the desired result; verifiably correct. [L. *valeo,* to be strong]

val·i·da·tion (val-i-dā'shŭn). The act or process of making valid.

consensual v., the confirmation of the experience or judgment of one person by another.

va·lid·i·ty (vă-lid'i-tē). An index of how well a test or procedure in fact measures what it purports to measure; an objective index by which to describe how valid a test or procedure is.

concurrent v., an index of criterion-related v. used to predict performance in a real-life situation given at about the same time as the test or procedure; the extent to which the index from one test correlates with that of a nonidentical test or index; *e.g.,* how well a score on an aptitude test correlates with the score on an intelligence test.

construct v., the extent to which a test or procedure appears to measure a higher order, inferred theoretical construct, or trait in contrast to measuring a more limited, specific dimension; *e.g.,* a sychrony in the scores on the Stanford-Binet Test, on a test of information processing, and the rate of glucose metabolism in the brain all are indices of intelligence.

content v., the extent to which the items of a test or procedure are in fact a representative sample of that which is to be measured; *e.g.,* items relating to ability in arithmetic and defining words are appropriate content for an intelligence test.

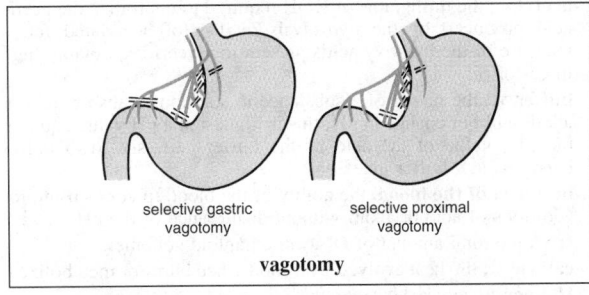

selective gastric vagotomy   selective proximal vagotomy

vagotomy

criterion-related v., the degree of effectiveness with which performance on a test or procedure predicts performance in a real-life situation; *e.g.,* a good correlation between a score on an intelligence test such as the Scholastic Aptitude Test and one's 4-year college grade point average.

face v., the extent to which the items of a test or procedure appear superficially to sample that which is to be measured.

predictive v., criterion-related v. used to predict performance in a real-life task at a future time. SEE construct v., criterion-related v.

va·line (Val, V) (val'in). $(CH_3)_2CHCH(NH_3)^+COO^-$; 2-Amino-3-methylbutanoic acid; the L-isomer is a constituent of most proteins; a nutritionally essential amino acid.

va·lin·o·my·cin (val'ĭ-nō-mī-sin). Cyclododecadepsipeptides ionophore antibiotic derived from *Streptomyces fulvissius;* a 36-membered ring structure consisting of 3 moles each of L-valine, D-α-hydroxyisovaleric acid, D-valine and L-lactic acid linked alternately. The material is used as an insecticide and nematocide.

val·la (val'ă). Plural of vallum.

val·late (val'āt). Bordered with an elevation, as a cupped structure; denoting especially certain lingual papillae. SEE ALSO circumvallate. [L. *vallo,* pp. *-atus,* to surround with, fr. *vallum,* a rampart]

val·lec·u·la, pl. **val·lec·u·lae** (vă-lek'yū-lă, -lē) [NA]. A crevice or depression on any surface. SYN valley. [L. dim. of *vallis,* valley]

v. cerebel'li [NA], a deep hollow on the inferior surface of the cerebellum, between the hemispheres, containing the medulla oblongata and the falx cerebelli. SYN vallis.

epiglottic v., a depression immediately posterior to the root of the tongue between the median and lateral glossoepiglottic folds on either side. SYN v. epiglottica [NA].

v. epiglot'tica [NA], SYN epiglottic v.

v. syl'vii, SYN lateral cerebral *fossa.*

v. un'guis, SYN *sulcus* matricis unguis.

Valleix, François L. I., French physician, 1807–1855. SEE V.'s *points,* under *point.*

val·ley (val'ē). SYN vallecula.

val·lis (val'is). SYN *vallecula* cerebelli. [L. valley]

val·lum, pl. **val·la** (val'ŭm, -ă). **1** [NA]. Any raised, more or less circular ridge. **2.** The slightly raised outer wall of the circular depression, or fossa, surrounding a vallate papilla of the tongue. [L. a rampart, fr. *vallus,* a stake]

v. un'guis [NA], SYN nail *fold.*

val·meth·a·mide (val-meth'ă-mīd). SYN valnoctamide.

val·noc·ta·mide (val-nok'tă-mīd). 2-ethyl-3-methylvaleramide; an antianxiety agent. SYN valmethamide.

val·oid (val'oyd). SYN equivalent *extract.* [L. *valeo,* to be strong]

val·pro·ic ac·id (val-prō'ik). $C_8H_{16}O_2$; 2-Propylvaleric acid; an anticonvulsant used to treat seizure disorders; also used as the sodium salt, valproate sodium.

Valsalva, Antonio M., Italian anatomist, 1666–1723. SEE *aneurysm* of sinus of V.; V.'s *antrum, ligaments,* under *ligament;* V. *maneuver;* V.'s *muscle, sinus; teniae* of V., under *tenia;* V. *test.*

val·ue (val'yū). A particular quantitative determination. For v.'s not given below, see the specific name. SEE ALSO index, number. [M.E., fr. O.Fr., fr. L. *valeo,* to be of value]

va

acetyl v., the milligrams of KOH required to neutralize the acetic acid produced by the hydrolysis of 1 g of acetylated fat; a measure of the hydroxy acids present in glycerides; notably high in castor oil.

buffer v., the power of a substance in solution to absorb acid or alkali without change in pH; this is highest at a pH value equal to the pK_a value of the acid of the buffer pair. SEE ALSO buffer *capacity*. SYN buffer index.

buffer v. of the blood, the ability of the blood to compensate for additions of acid or alkali without disturbance of the pH.

C v., the total amount of DNA in a haploid genome.

caloric v., the heat evolved by a food when burnt or metabolized.

Hehner v., SYN Hehner *number*.

homing v., in a cybernetic system such as homeostasis, that v. of a trait of interest that the restorative forces are directed towards maintaining.

iodine v., SYN iodine *number*.

maturation v., an indicator of the level of maturation attained by vaginal epithelium and used as a factor in cytohormonal evaluation from the maturation index by valuing the parabasal cells at 0.0, the intermediate cells at 0.5, and the superficial cells at 1.0; for special investigations, subtypes of a major cell can be given different v.'s.

normal v.'s, a set of laboratory test v.'s used to characterize apparently healthy individuals; now replaced by reference v.'s.

pH v., SEE Ph.

phenotypic v., in quantitative genetics, the metrical quantity of some trait associated with a particular phenotype.

predictive v., an expresion of the likelihood that a given test result correlates with the presence or absence of disease. A positive predictive v. is the ratio of patients with the disease who test positive to the entire population of individuals with a positive test result; a negative predictive v. is the ratio of patients without the disease who test negative to the entire population of individuals with a negative test.

R_f v., SEE R_f.

reference v.'s, a set of laboratory test v.'s obtained from an individual or group in a defined state of health; this term replaces normal v.'s, since it is based on a defined state of health rather than on apparent health.

thiocyanogen v., SYN thiocyanogen *number*.

threshold limit v. (TLV), the maximum concentration of a chemical recommended by the American Conference of Government Industrial Hygienists for repeated exposure without adverse health effects on workers.

val·va, pl. **val·vae** (val′vă, -vē) [NA]. SYN valve. [L. one leaf of a double door]

v. aor′tae [NA], SYN aortic *valve*.

v. atrioventricula′ris dex′tra [NA], SYN tricuspid *valve*.

v. atrioventricula′ris sinis′tra [NA], SYN mitral *valve*.

v. ileoceca′lis [NA], SYN ileocecal *valve*.

v. mitra′lis, SYN mitral *valve*.

v. tricuspida′lis, SYN tricuspid *valve*.

v. trun′ci pulmona′lis [NA], SYN pulmonary *valve*.

val·val, val·var (val′văl, val′văr). Relating to a valve.

val·vate (val′vāt). Relating to or provided with a valve. SYN valvular.

valve (valv). **1.** A fold of the lining membrane of a canal or other hollow organ serving to retard or prevent a reflux of fluid. **2.** Any reduplication of tissue or flaplike structure resembling a v. SEE ALSO valvule, plica. SYN valva [NA]. [L. *valva*]

Amussat's v., SYN spiral *fold* of cystic duct.

anal v.'s, delicate crescent-shaped mucosal folds that pass between the lower ends of neighboring anal columns; the small pocket thus formed is an anal sinus. SYN valvulae anales [NA], Morgagni's v.'s.

anterior urethral v., a crescentic horizontal fold in the proximal spongy urethra.

aortic v., the v. between the left ventricle and the ascending aorta, consisting of three fibrous semilunar cusps (valvules), located in the adult in anterior, right posterior, and left posterior

positions; they are named, however, in accordance with their embryonic derivation in which the anteriorly-located cusp is the right cusp (above which the right coronary artery arises), the left posteriorly-positioned cusp is designated as the left cusp (above which the left coronary artery arises), and the right posteriorly-positioned cusp is designated as the posterior or non-coronary cusp. SYN valva aortae [NA].

atrioventricular v.'s, SEE tricuspid v., mitral v.

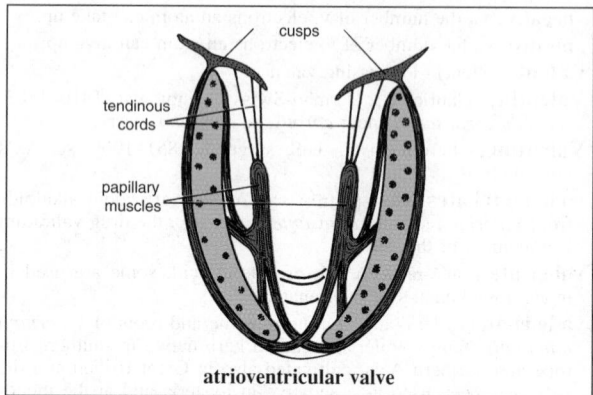

atrioventricular valve

A-V v.'s, abbreviation for the cardiac atrioventricular valves; the mitral and tricuspid valves.

ball v., any of a variety of prosthetic cardiac v.'s comprised of a ball within a retaining cage affixed to the orifice; when appropriately sized, used in aortic, mitral, or tricuspid position.

Bauhin's v., SYN ileocecal v.

Béraud's v., a small fold in the interior of the lacrimal sac at its junction with the lacrimal duct. SYN Krause's v.

Bianchi's v., SYN lacrimal *fold*.

bicuspid v., SYN mitral v.

bi-leaflet v., a low profile mechanical heart v. that is less obstructive to outflow, especially in small size.

Bjork-Shiley v., a low profile tilting disc mechanical heart v.

Bochdalek's v., a fold of mucous membrane in the lacrimal canaliculus at the lacrimal punctum. SYN Foltz' valvule.

Braune's v., a fold of mucous membrane at the junction of the esophagus with the stomach.

Carpentier-Edwards v., a bioprosthetic v. made from preserved porcine aortic v.'s.

caval v., SYN v. of inferior vena cava.

congenital v., an abnormal lining fold obstructing a passage; *e.g.,* of a mucous membrane in the urethra.

coronary v., SYN v. of coronary sinus.

v. of coronary sinus, a delicate fold of endocardium at the opening of the coronary sinus into the right atrium. SYN valvula sinus coronarii [NA], coronary v., thebesian v.

eustachian v., SYN v. of inferior vena cava.

v. of foramen ovale, a fold projecting into the left atrium from the margin of the foramen ovale in the fetus; when, with beginning inspiration, the blood pressure within the left atrium increases, the valve closes and its edges become adherent to the margin of the foramen ovale, occluding it. SYN valvula foraminis ovalis [NA], falx septi [NA], v. of oval foramen.

Gerlach's v., SYN v. of vermiform appendix.

Guérin's v., SYN v. of navicular fossa.

Hasner's v., SYN lacrimal *fold*.

Heister's v., SYN spiral *fold* of cystic duct.

Heyer-Pudenz v., a v. used in the shunting procedure for hydrocephaly; consisting of a catheter-v. system in which the ventricular catheter leads the cerebrospinal fluid into a one-way pump through which the cerebrospinal fluid passes down the distal catheter into the right atrium of the heart.

Hoboken's v.'s, the flangelike protrusions into the lumen of the umbilical arteries where they are twisted or kinked in their course through the umbilical cord.

Houston's v.'s, SYN transverse rectal *folds,* under *fold.*

Huschke's v., SYN lacrimal *fold.*

ileocecal v., the bilabial prominence of the terminal ileum into the large intestine at the cecocolic junction as seen in cadavers; in the living individual it appears as a truncated cone with a star-shaped orifice. SYN valva ileocecalis [NA], Bauhin's v., ileocecal eminence, ileocolic v., Tulp's v., Tulpius' v., v. of Varolius.

ileocolic v., SYN ileocecal v.

v. of inferior vena cava, an endocardial fold extending from the anterior inferior margin of the inferior vena cava to the anterior part of the limbus fossa ovalis. SYN valvula venae cavae inferioris [NA], caval v., eustachian v., sylvian v.

Kerckring's v.'s, SYN *plicae* circulares, under *plica.*

Kohlrausch's v.'s, SYN transverse rectal *folds,* under *fold.*

Krause's v., SYN Béraud's v.

left atrioventricular v., SYN mitral v.

Mercier's v., an occasional fold of mucosa of the bladder partially occluding the ureteral orifice.

mitral v., the v. closing the orifice between the left atrium and left ventricle of the heart; its two cusps are called anterior and posterior. SYN valva atrioventricularis sinistra [NA], bicuspid v., left atrioventricular v., valva mitralis, valvula bicuspidalis.

Morgagni's v.'s, SYN anal v.'s.

nasal v., the variable aperture between the nasal septum and the moveable inferior margin of the lower lateral nasal cartilage.

v. of navicular fossa, a fold of mucous membrane sometimes found in the root of the navicular fossa of the urethra. SYN valvula fossae navicularis [NA], Guérin's fold, Guérin's v.

nonrebreathing v., a type of v. that prevents mixture of inhaled and exhaled gases.

O'Beirne's v., SYN rectosigmoid *sphincter.*

v. of oval foramen, SYN v. of foramen ovale.

parachute mitral v., congenital deformity of the mitral v. characterized by the presence of a single papillary muscle from which the chordae of both v. leaflets divide; thus the resemblance to a parachute; the condition often produces a stenosis as the combined result of the tugging action of the chordae on and the subsequent narrowing between the leaflets. SYN parachute deformity.

porcine v., SYN tissue v.

posterior urethral v.'s, anomalous folds occurring at the level of the seminal colliculus. SYN Amussat's valvula.

prosthetic v.'s, v.'s used to replace human v.'s. They are divided into mechanical and tissue v.'s. The tissue is divided into homografts and heterografts. There are many different types of prosthetic v.'s, including the Saint Jude v., Hancock v., Starr-Edwards v., and Carpentier-Edwards v.

pulmonary v., the v. at the entrance to the pulmonary trunk from the right ventricle; it consists of semilunar cusps (valvules) which are usually arranged in the adult in right anterior, left anterior, and posterior positions; however, they are named in accordance with their embryonic derivation; thus the posteriorly-located cusp is designated as the left cusp, the right anteriorly-located cusp is designated the right cusp and the left anteriorly-positioned cusp is called the anterior cusp. SYN valva trunci pulmonalis [NA], pulmonic v., v. of pulmonary trunk.

v. of pulmonary trunk, SYN pulmonary v.

pulmonic v., SYN pulmonary v.

pyloric v., SYN pyloric *constriction.*

rectal v.'s, SYN transverse rectal *folds,* under *fold.*

reducing v., a v. designed to lower the pressure of a gas coming from a cylinder containing compressed gas under high pressure.

right atrioventricular v., SYN tricuspid v.

Rosenmüller's v., SYN lacrimal *fold.*

semilunar v., (1) a heart v. comprised of a set of three semilunar cusps (valvules); hence both the aortic and pulmonary valves are semilunar v.'s. SYN valvula semilunaris [NA].

spiral v. of cystic duct, SYN spiral *fold* of cystic duct.

Starr-Edwards v., a cage and ball artificial cardiac valve with high reliability and durability.

sylvian v., SYN v. of inferior vena cava.

Tarin's v., SYN inferior medullary *velum.*

Terrien's v., a valvelike fold between the gallbladder and the cystic duct; the first ridge of the spiral fold of the cystic duct.

thebesian v., SYN v. of coronary sinus.

tilting disc v., a variety of prosthetic cardiac v. composed of one or two discs within a retaining device.

tissue v., a prosthetic cardiac v. derived from the pig heart, which is preserved and sterilized with glutaraldehyde, and permanently sutured to a shape-retaining artificial strut; in appropriate sizes, it can replace any natural heart v. SYN porcine v.

tricuspid v., the v. closing the orifice between the right atrium and right ventricle of the heart; its three cusps are called anterior, posterior, and septal. SYN valva atrioventricularis dextra [NA], right atrioventricular v., valva tricuspidalis, valvula tricuspidalis.

Tulp's v., Tulpius' v., SYN ileocecal v.

urethral v.'s, folds in the urethral mucous membrane. SEE ALSO anterior urethral v., posterior urethral v.'s.

v. of Varolius, SYN ileocecal v.

venous v., a fold of the lining layer of a vein to prevent a reflux of blood. SYN valvula venosa (2).

v. of vermiform appendix, a fold of mucous membrane, simulating a v., sometimes found at the origin of the vermiform appendix. SYN Gerlach's v., valvula processus vermiformis.

vesicoureteral v., a lock mechanism in the wall of the intravesical portion of the ureter that normally prevents urinary reflux.

v. of Vieussens, a prominent v. in the great cardiac vein where it turns around the obtuse margin to become the coronary sinus.

Vieussens' v., SYN superior medullary *velum.*

valve·less (valv′les). Without valves; denoting certain veins, such as the portal, that are not provided with valves as are most of the veins.

val·vi·form (val′vi-fōrm). Valve-shaped.

val·vo·plas·ty (val′vō-plas-tē). Surgical reconstruction of a deformed cardiac valve, for the relief of stenosis or incompetence. SYN valvuloplasty. [valve + G. *plastos,* formed]

val·vot·o·my (val-vot′ō-mē). **1.** Cutting through a stenosed cardiac valve to relieve the obstruction. SYN valvulotomy. **2.** Incision of a valvular structure. [valve + G. *tomē,* incision]

mitral v., deliberate incision or enlargement by inserting a finger in the mitral valve due to mitral stenosis.

rectal v., cutting through rectal folds that are too rigid or large.

val·vu·la, pl. **val·vu·lae** (val′vyū-lă, -lē) [NA]. SYN valvule. [Mod. L. dim. of *valva*]

Amussat's v., SYN posterior urethral *valves,* under *valve.*

val′vulae ana′les [NA], SYN anal *valves,* under *valve.*

v. bicuspida′lis, SYN mitral *valve.*

val′vulae conniven′tes, SYN *plicae* circulares, under *plica.*

v. fora′minis ova′lis [NA], SYN *valve* of foramen ovale.

v. fos′sae navicula′ris [NA], SYN *valve* of navicular fossa.

Gerlach's v., SYN trabecular *reticulum.*

v. lymphat′ica [NA], SYN lymphatic *valvule.*

v. proces′sus vermifor′mis, SYN *valve* of vermiform appendix.

v. pylor′i, SYN pyloric *constriction.*

valvulae pylo′ri, SYN pyloric *constriction.*

v. semiluna′ris [NA], SYN semilunar *valve.*

v. semiluna′ris ante′rior val′vae trun′ci pulmona′lis, anterior semilunar cusp of the pulmonary valve.

v. semiluna′ris dex′tra val′vae aor′tae, right semilunar cusp of the aortic valve.

v. semiluna′ris dex′tra val′vae trun′ci pulmona′lis, right semilunar cusp of the pulmonary valve.

v. semiluna′ris poste′rior val′vae aor′tae, posterior semilunar cusp of the aortic valve.

v. semiluna′ris sinis′tra val′vae aor′tae, left semilunar cusp of the aortic valve.

v. semiluna′ris sinis′tra val′vae trun′ci pulmona′lis, left semilunar cusp of the pulmonary valve.

v. semiluna′ris tari′ni, SYN inferior medullary *velum.*

v. si′nus corona′rii [NA], SYN *valve* of coronary sinus.

v. spiral′is, SYN spiral *fold* of cystic duct.

va

v. tricuspida′lis, SYN tricuspid *valve.*

v. ve′nae ca′vae inferio′ris [NA], SYN *valve* of inferior vena cava.

v. veno′sa, (1) in the embryo, one of the pair of valves at the opening from the sinus venosus into the right atrium; **(2)** [NA], SYN venous *valve.*

v. vestib′uli, obsolete term for v. venosa (1).

val·vu·lar (val′vyū-lăr). SYN valvate.

val·vule (val′vūl). A valve, especially one of small size. SYN valvula [NA]. [L. *valvula*]

Foltz′ v., SYN Bochdalek's *valve.*

lymphatic v., one of the delicate semilunar valves found in lymphatic vessels; they are usually paired and similar in structure to venous valves and occur at close intervals along the vessel wall. SYN valvula lymphatica [NA].

val·vu·li·tis (val-vyū-lī′tis). Inflammation of a valve, especially a heart valve. [Mod. L. *valvula,* valve, + G. *-itis,* inflammation]

rheumatic v., v. characterized in the acute stage by small fibrin vegetations along the lines of closure and by Aschoff bodies in the cusps; in the chronic stage, it is characterized by scarring, commissural adhesion, and stenosis and/or regurgitation.

val·vu·lo·plas·ty (val′vyū-lō-plas′tē). SYN valvoplasty.

val·vu·lo·tome (val′vyū-lō-tōm). An instrument for sectioning a valve.

val·vu·lot·o·my (val-vyū-lot′ō-mē). SYN valvotomy (1).

val·yl (val′il). The radical of valine.

Van, van. For some names with this prefix not found below, see the principal part of the name.

van·a·date (van′ă-dāt). A salt of vanadic acid.

va·na·dic ac·id (vă-nad′ik). An acid, H_3VO_4, derived from vanadium, forming salts with various bases.

va·na·di·um (V) (vă-nā′dē-ŭm). A metallic element, atomic no. 23, atomic wt. 50.9415; a bioelement, its deficiency can result in abnormal bone growth and a rise in cholesterol and triacylglycerol levels. [*Vanadis,* Scand. goddess]

v. group, Those elements resembling vanadium in chemical and metallurgical properties; included with vanadium are niobium and tantalum.

va·na·di·um group. See under vanadium.

van Bogaert, Ludo, 20th century Belgian neurologist. SEE Canavan-v. B.-Bertrand *disease;* v. B. *encephalitis.*

van Buchem, Francis Steven Peter, Dutch internist, *1897. SEE Van B.'s *syndrome.*

van Buren, William H., U.S. surgeon, 1819–1883. SEE van B. *sound;* van B.'s *disease.*

van·co·my·cin (van-kō-mī′sin). An antibiotic isolated from cultures of *Nocardia orientalis,* bactericidal and bacteriostatic against Gram-positive organisms; available as the hydrochloride.

van Creveld, S., Dutch pediatrician, *1894. SEE Ellis-van C. *syndrome.*

van·dal root (van′dăl). SYN valerian.

van Deen, Izaak A., Dutch physiologist, 1804–1869. SEE van D.'s *test.*

van den Bergh, A.A.H., Dutch physician, 1869–1943. SEE van den B.'s *test.*

van der Kolk, Jacobus L.C.S., Dutch physician, 1797–1862. SEE van der K.'s *law.*

van der Spieghel. SEE Spigelius.

van der Velden, Reinhardt, German physician, 1851–1903. SEE van der V.'s's *test.*

van der Waals, Johannes D., Dutch physicist and Nobel laureate, 1837–1923. SEE van der W.'s *forces,* under *force.*

van Ekenstein, W.A., 19th century scientist. SEE Lobry de Bruyn-van E. *transformation.*

van Ermengen, Emile P., Belgian bacteriologist, 1851–1932. SEE van E.'s *stain.*

van Gieson, Ira, U.S. histologist and bacteriologist, 1865–1913. SEE van G.'s *stain.*

van Helmont, Jean B., Flemish physician and chemist, 1577–1644. SEE van H.'s *mirror.*

van Horne (Hoorne, Hoorn, Heurenius), Jan (Johannes), Dutch anatomist, 1621–1670. SEE van H.'s *canal.*

va·nil·la (vă-nil′ă). The cured, full-grown, unripe fruit of *Vanila planifolia* (Mexican or Bourbon v.) or of *v. tahitensis* (Tahiti v.), orchids (family Orchidaceae) native to Mexico and cultivated in other tropical countries; a flavoring agent. [Sp. *vainilla,* little pod]

va·nil·late (vă-nil′āt). A compound of vanillic acid; $C_8H_8O_4$.

va·nil·lic ac·id (vă-nil′ik). $CH_3O–C_6H_3(OH)COOH$; Methylprotocatechuic acid; 4-hydroxy-3-methoxybenzoic acid; a flavoring agent.

va·nil·lin (vă-nil′in). Methylprotocatechuic aldehyde; vanillic aldehyde; 4-hydroxy-3-methoxybenzaldehyde; obtained from vanilla and also prepared synthetically; a flavoring agent; used to detect ornithine, sugar alcohols, phenols, and certain sterols.

va·nil·lism (vă-nil′izm). **1.** Symptoms of irritation of the skin, nasal mucous membrane, and conjunctiva from which workers with vanilla sometimes suffer. **2.** Infestation of the skin by sarcoptiform mites found in vanilla pods.

va·nil·lyl·man·del·ic ac·id (VMA) (van′i-lil-man-del′ik, vă-nil′il-). Misnomer for 4-hydroxy-3-methoxymandelic acid (α,3-dihydroxy-2-methoxybenzeneacetic acid); the major urinary metabolite of adrenal and sympathetic catecholamines (*e.g.,* from both epinephrine and norepinephrine); elevated in most patients with pheochromocytoma.

Van Slyke, Donald D., U.S. biochemist, 1883–1971. SEE slyke; Van S. *apparatus;* Van S.'s *formula.*

van′t Hoff, Jacobus H., Dutch chemist and Nobel laureate, 1852–1911. SEE van′t H.'s *equation, law, theory;* Le Belvan′t H. *rule.*

va·por (vā′per). **1.** Molecules in the gaseous phase of a solid or liquid substance exposed to a gas. **2.** A visible emanation of fine particles of a liquid. **3.** A medicinal preparation to be administered by inhalation. [L. steam]

anesthetic v., the gaseous phase of a liquid anesthetic with sufficient partial pressure at room temperature to produce general anesthesia when inhaled.

va·por·i·za·tion (vă-pōr-i-zā′shŭn). **1.** The change of a solid or liquid to a state of vapor. **2.** The therapeutic application of a vapor.

va·por·ize (vā′-per-īz). **1.** To convert a solid or liquid into a vapor. **2.** To apply a vapor therapeutically.

va·por·iz·er (vā′per-īz-er). **1.** An apparatus for reducing medicated liquids to a state of vapor suitable for inhalation or application to accessible mucous membranes. SEE ALSO nebulizer, atomizer. **2.** A device for volatizing liquid anesthetics.

flow-over v., a device for vaporization of a liquid anesthetic by causing gases to pass over the anesthetic or over material saturated with the anesthetic.

temperature-compensated v., a v. of liquid anesthetics with graduated settings calibrated to deliver a known constant concentration of a specific anesthetic despite changes in inflow volume and despite cooling brought about by vaporization.

va·por·tho·rax (vāp-er-thō′raks). The existence of large water vapor bubbles in the pleural space between the lungs and the chest wall in an unprotected person exposed to altitudes above 63,000 ft., where the barometric pressure is less than 47 mm Hg and where water at body temperature vaporizes from the liquid state.

va·po·ther·a·py (vā′pō-thār′ă-pē). Treatment of disease by means of vapor or spray.

V̇a/Q̇ Abbreviation for ventilation/perfusion *ratio.*

Vaquez, Louis H., French physician, 1860–1936. SEE V.'s *disease.*

var·i·a·bil·i·ty (vār′ē-ă-bil′i-tē). **1.** The capability of being variable. **2.** In genetics, the potential or actual differences, either quantitative or qualitative, in phenotype among individuals.

baseline v. of fetal heart rate, the beat-to-beat changes in fetal heart rate as recorded on a graph.

var·i·a·ble (vār′ē-ă-bl). **1.** That which is inconstant, which can or does change, as contrasted with a constant. **2.** Deviating from the type in structure, form, physiology, or behavior. [L. *vario,* to vary, change, differ]

continuous v., a v. that may take on any value in an interval or intervals (its domain).

continuous random v., continuous v. that may randomly assume any value in its domain but any particular value has no probability of occurring, only a probability density.

dependent v., in experiments, a v. that is influenced by or dependent upon changes in the independent v.; *e.g.,* the amount of a written passage retained (dependent v.) as a function of the different numbers of minutes (independent v.) allowed to study the passage.

discrete v., a v. that may assume only a countable (usually finite) number of values.

discrete random v., a random v. that may assume a countable number of values, each with a probability strictly greater than zero.

independent v., a characteristic being measured or observed that is hypothesized to influence another event or manifestation (the dependent v.) within a defined area of relationships under study; that is, the independent v. is not influenced by the event or manifestation, but may cause it or contribute to its variation. SEE dependent v.

intermediate v., a v. in a causal pathway that causes variation in the dependent v. and is itself caused to vary by the independent v.

intervening v., an event, such as an attitude or emotion, inferred to occur within an organism between the stimulation and response in such a way as to influence or determine the response.

mixed discrete-continuous random v., a random v. that may assume some values with probabilities and others with probability densities. For example, in a 35-year-old man with familial polyposis of the colon, the distribution of time until malignant disease occurs consists of a probability that he already has cancer (which would be assigned the waiting time 0), a probability density of developing it in the future and a probability that he will die of some other cause before he develops cancer.

moderator v., a v. that interacts by virtue of being antecedent or intermediate in the causal pathway.

random v., a v. that may assume a set of values, each with fixed probabilities or probability densities (its distribution), in such a way that the total probability assigned to the distribution is unity; the random v. may be discrete, continuous, or mixed discrete-continuous.

var·i·ance (vār′ē-ans). **1.** The state of being variable, different, divergent, or deviate; a degree of deviation. **2.** A measure of the variation shown by a set of observations, defined as the sum of squares of deviations from the mean, divided by the number of degrees of freedom in the set of observations.

ball v., swelling and changes in shape and consistency of the ball in a ball-valve prosthesis, especially in one replacing the aortic valve.

var·i·ant (vār′ē-ant). **1.** That which, or one who, is variable. **2.** Having the tendency to alter or change, exhibit variety or diversity, not conform, or differ from the type.

inherited albumin v.'s [MIM*103600], types of human serum albumin, distinguished by characteristic mobility patterns on electrophoresis; each type is due to a mutation of a gene controlling albumin synthesis; the mutant genes are codominant with the normal gene for albumin A, and the group forms a system of genetic polymorphism; types include: albumin b (slow), found occasionally in persons of European ancestry; albumin Ghent (fast), found first at Ghent, Belgium; albumin Mexico (slow), found in Indians of Mexico and the southwestern United States; albumin Naskapi (fast), found in the Naskapi and other Indians of northern North America; and albumin Reading (fast), found first at Reading, England.

L-phase v.'s, bacterial v.'s which do not have rigid cell walls but which may contain varying amounts of cell wall material; they are spherical to coccobacillary in shape and vary in size from small bodies that pass through filters which retain bacteria to bodies that are larger than the bacterial form; they are Gram-negative and resistant to penicillin; some revert to the bacterial

phase upon removal of the inducing substance, whereas others do not; the v.'s differ greatly from the parent bacterial cells in mode of reproduction, physiology, growth requirements, and individual and colonial morphology; they are generally considered to be nonpathogenic, even if derived from a pathogenic bacterium. [L. fr. Lister Institute]

var·i·ate (vār′ē-ăt). A measurable quantity capable of taking on a number of values; may be binary (*i.e.,* capable of taking on two values in a certain interval of values), continuous (*i.e.,* capable of taking on all values in a certain interval of real values), or discrete (*i.e.,* capable of taking on a limited number of values in a certain interval of real values).

var·i·a·tion (vār-ē-ā′shŭn). Deviation from the type, especially the parent type, in structure, form, physiology, or behavior. [L. *variatio,* fr. *vario,* to change, vary]

beat-to-beat v. of fetal heart rate, v. of fetal heart rate measured in changes in the QRS-QRS interval from heart beat to heart beat; measured with electronic internal fetal heart rate monitors.

continuous v., a series of very slight v.'s.

var·i·ca·tion (vār-i-kā′shŭn). Formation or presence of varices.

var·i·ce·al (vār-ĭ-sē′ăl, vă-ris′ē-ăl). Of or pertaining to a varix.

var·i·cel·la (vār-i-sel′ă). An acute contagious disease, usually occurring in children, caused by the varicella-zoster virus, a member of the family Herpesviridae, and marked by a sparse eruption of papules, which become vesicles and then pustules, like that of smallpox although less severe and varying in stages, usually with mild constitutional symptoms; incubation period is about 14 to 17 days. SYN chickenpox, waterpox. [Mod. L. dim. of *variola*]

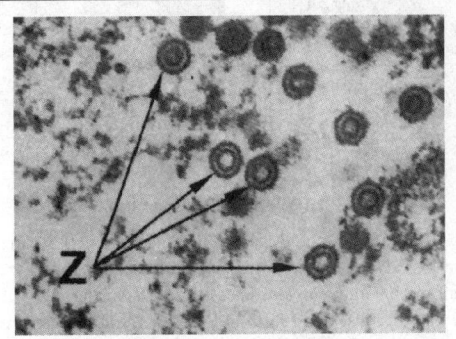

varicella-zoster viruses
(in the nucleus of an epidermal cell)

v. gangreno′sa, gangrenous ulceration of v. lesions with or without secondary infection, occurring mainly in children with severe underlying disease.

var·i·cel·la·tion (vār-i-sĕ-lā′shŭn). Inoculation with the virus of chickenpox as a means of protection against that disease.

var·i·cel·li·form (vār-ĭ-sel′ĭ-fōrm). Resembling varicella. SYN varicelloid.

var·i·cel·loid (vār-ĭ-sel′oyd). SYN varicelliform.

va·ri·ces (vār′i-sēz). Plural of varix.

var·i·ci·form (vār′ĭ-si-fōrm, vă-ris′ĭ-fōrm). Resembling a varix. SYN cirsoid, varicoid.

△**varico-.** A varix, varicose, varicosity. [L. *varix,* a dilated vein]

var·i·co·bleph·a·ron (var′i-kō-blef′ă-ron). A varicosity of the eyelid. [varico- + G. *blepharon,* eyelid]

var·i·co·cele (vār′i-kō-sēl). A condition manifested by abnormal dilation of the veins of the spermatic cord, caused by incompetent valves in the internal spermatic vein and resulting in impaired drainage of blood into the spermatic cord veins when the patient assumes the upright position. SYN cirsocele, pampinocele. [varico- + G. *kēlē,* tumor, hernia]

ovarian v., a varicose condition of the pampiniform plexus in the

va

broad ligament of the uterus. SYN tubo-ovarian v., utero-ovarian v.

symptomatic v., a v. caused by obstruction of the internal spermatic vein, usually at the level of the renal vein and usually due to invasive renal cell carcinoma, characterized by failure of the dilated veins in the spermatic cord to empty when the patient assumes a recumbent position.

tubo-ovarian v., SYN ovarian v.

utero-ovarian v., SYN ovarian v.

var·i·co·ce·lec·to·my (văr′i-kō-sē-lek′tō-mē). Operation for the correction of a varicocele by ligature and excision and by ligation of the dilated veins. [varicocele + G. *ektomē*, excision]

var·i·cog·ra·phy (văr′ĭ-kog′ră-fē). Radiography of the veins after injection of contrast medium into varicose veins. [varico- + G. *graphō*, to write]

var·i·coid (văr′i-koyd). SYN variciform.

var·i·com·pha·lus (văr-i-kom′fă-lŭs). A swelling formed by varicose veins at the umbilicus. [varico- + G. *omphalos*, navel]

var·i·co·phle·bi·tis (văr′i-kō-flĕ-bī′tis). Inflammation of varicose veins. [varico- + G. *phleps*, vein, + -*itis*, inflammation]

var·i·cose (văr′i-kōs). Relating to, affected with, or characterized by varices or varicosis.

var·i·co·sis, pl. **var·i·cos·es** (văr-i-kō′sis, -sēz). A dilated or varicose state of a vein or veins. [varico- + G. -*osis*, condition]

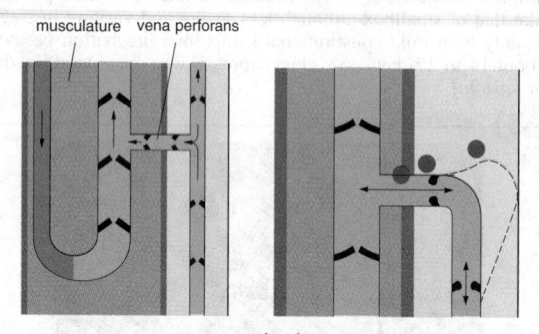

varicosis
a) model of normal, non-dilated veins: the venous bloodstream is guided by valves into the deeper vein system; b) varicose development: peripheral veins become dilated, impairing the efficiency of the valves; a back and forth blood flow results, causing ectasia of the surface veins beyond the fascia lata

var·i·cos·i·ty (văr-i-kos′i-tē). A varix or varicose condition.

var·i·cot·o·my (văr-i-kot′ō-mē). An operation for varicose veins by subcutaneous incision. [varico- + G. *tomē*, a cutting]

va·ric·u·la (vă-rik′yū-lă). A varicose condition of the veins of the conjunctiva. SYN conjunctival varix. [L. dim. of *varix*]

var·i·cule (văr′i-kyūl). A small varicose vein ordinarily seen in the skin; may be associated with venous stars, venous lakes, or larger varicose veins. [L. *varicula*, dim. of *varix*]

va·ri·eg·a·tion (ver′ē-a-gā′shŭn). The diversification or alteration of a phenotype produced by a change in the genotype during somatic development.

va·ri·o·la (vă-rī′ō-lă). SYN smallpox. [Med. L. dim of L. *varius*, spotted]

v. benig′na, SYN varioloid (2).

v. hemorrha′gica, SYN hemorrhagic *smallpox*.

v. ma′jor, SYN smallpox.

v. malig′na, malignant smallpox, usually of the hemorrhagic form. SYN malignant smallpox.

v. milia′ris, a form of varioloid in which the eruption consists of miliary vesicles without the formation of pustules.

v. mi′nor, SYN alastrim.

v. pemphigo′sa, a form of smallpox in which the eruption consists of pemphigus-like blebs.

v. si′ne eruptio′ne, an abortive form of smallpox in which the disease subsides without the appearance of any eruption, or at most a few papules that never go on to pustulation.

v. vaccine, v. vaccin′ia, SYN vaccinia.

v. ve′ra, simple smallpox of ordinary severity in the unvaccinated.

v. verruco′sa, a mild or abortive form of varioloid, the eruption of which consists mainly of papules, with occasionally minute vesicles at the apices, which persist for a time as wartlike lesions. SYN wartpox.

va·ri·o·lar (vă-rī′ō-lăr). Relating to smallpox. SYN variolic, variolous.

var·i·o·late (văr′ē-ō-lāt). **1.** To inoculate with smallpox. **2.** Pitted or scarred, as if by smallpox.

var·i·o·la·tion (văr′ē-ō-lā′shŭn). The obsolete process of inoculating a susceptible person with material from a vesicle of a patient with smallpox. SYN variolization.

var·i·ol·ic (văr-ē-ol′ik). SYN variolar.

var·i·ol·i·form (vă-rī′ō-li-fōrm, văr-ē-ō′li-fōrm). SYN varioloid (1). [variola + L. *forma*, form]

var·i·o·li·za·tion (văr′ē-ō-li-zā′shŭn). SYN variolation.

va·ri·o·loid (văr′ē-ō-loyd). **1.** Resembling smallpox. SYN varioliform. **2.** A mild form of smallpox occurring in persons who are relatively resistant, usually as a result of a previous vaccination. SYN modified smallpox, varicelloid smallpox, variola benigna. [variola + G. *eidos*, resemblance]

va·ri·o·lous (vă-rī′ō-lŭs). SYN variolar.

va·ri·o·lo·vac·cine (vă-rī′ō-lō-vak′sēn). A vaccine obtained from the eruption following inoculation of a heifer with smallpox from the human.

var·ix, pl. **va·ri·ces** (văr′iks, văr′i-sēz). **1.** A dilated vein. **2.** An enlarged and tortuous vein, artery, or lymphatic vessel. [L. *varix* (*varic-*), a dilated vein]

v. anastomot′icus, SYN aneurysmal v.

aneurysmal v., dilation and tortuosity of a vein resulting from an acquired communication with an adjacent artery. SYN Pott's aneurysm, v. anastomoticus.

cirsoid v., SYN cirsoid *aneurysm*.

conjunctival v., SYN varicula.

esophageal varices, longitudinal venous varices at the lower end of the esophagus as a result of portal hypertension; they are superficial and liable to ulceration and massive bleeding.

gelatinous v., a lumpy or nodular condition of the umbilical cord.

lymph v., the formation of varices or cysts in the lymph nodes in consequence of obstruction in the efferent lymphatics.

turbinal v., a condition of permanent dilation of the veins of the turbinated bodies, especially of the inferior turbinate.

var·nish (den·tal). Solutions of natural resins and gums in a suitable solvent, of which a thin coating is applied over the surfaces of the cavity preparations before placement of restorations, used as a protective agent for the tooth against constituents of restorative materials. SYN cavity liner, vernix.

Varolius (Varolio), Constantius (Costanzio), Italian anatomist and physician, 1543–1575. SEE ileal *sphincter; valve* of V.; *pons* varolii.

var·us (vā′rŭs). Bent or twisted inward toward the midline of the limb or body; modern accepted usage, particularly in orthopedics, erroneously transposes the meaning of valgus to v., as in *genu* varum (bowleg). [Mod. L. bent inward, fr. L. knock-kneed]

vas, gen. **va·′sis,** pl. **va·sa,** gen. and pl. **va·so·rum** (vas, vā′sis, vā′să, vā-sō′rŭm) [NA]. A duct or canal conveying any liquid, such as blood, lymph, chyle, or semen. SEE ALSO vessel. [L. a vessel, dish]

v. aber′rans hep′atis, pl. **va·sa aberran′tia hep′atis,** blind and/or atrophic bile duct remnants in the fibrous appendix and in the capsule of the liver at the margins of the left lobe and the groove for the inferior vena cava.

v. aberrans of Roth, an occasional diverticulum of the rete testis or of the efferent ductules of the testis.

vasa aberran′tes, SYN aberrant *ductules*, under *ductule*.

v. af'ferens, pl. **va'sa afferen'tia** [NA], SYN afferent glomerular *arteriole*.

v. anastomot'icum [NA], SYN anastomosing *vessel*.

va'sa aur'is inter'nae [NA], SYN *vessels* of internal ear, under *vessel*.

va'sa bre'via, SYN short gastric *arteries*, under *artery*.

v. capilla're [NA], SYN capillary (2). SEE blood *capillary*, lymph *capillary*.

va'sa chylif'era, chyle vessels. SEE lacteal (2).

v. collatera'le [NA], SYN collateral *vessel*.

v. def'erens, pl. **va'sa deferen'tia**, SYN *ductus* deferens.

v. ef'ferens, pl. **va'sa efferen'tia** [NA], (1) a vein carrying blood away from a part; SYN efferent lymphatic. (2) SYN efferent glomerular *arteriole*. (3) SYN efferent *ductules* of testis, under *ductule*.

Ferrein's vasa aberrantia, biliary canaliculi that are not connected with hepatic lobules.

Haller's v. aberrans, SYN inferior aberrant *ductule*.

va'sa lymphat'ica [NA], SYN lymph *vessels*, under *vessel*.

v. lympha'ticum, SYN lymphatic (3).

v. lympha'ticum affe'rens [NA], SYN afferent *lymphatic*.

v. lympha'ticum effe'rens [NA], SYN efferent *lymphatic*.

v. lympha'ticum profun'dum [NA], SYN deep lymphatic *vessel*.

v. lympha'ticum superficia'le [NA], SYN superficial lymphatic *vessel*.

va'sa nervor'um [NA], blood vessels supplying nerves.

va'sa pre'via, umbilical vessels presenting in advance of the fetal head, usually traversing the membranes and crossing the internal cervical os.

v. prom'inens duc'tus cochlea'ris [NA], a blood vessel in the substance of the spiral prominence of the cochler duct.

va'sa rec'ta, (1) straight vessels into which the efferent arteriole of the juxtamedullary glomeruli breaks up; they form a leash of vessels which, arising at the bases of the pyramids, run through the renal medulla toward the apex of each pyramid, then reverse direction in a hairpin turn, and run straight back again toward the base of the pyramid as venae rectae; (2) SYN straight seminiferous *tubule*. SYN arteriolae rectae [NA].

va'sa sanguin'ea ret'inae [NA], SYN retinal *blood vessels*, under *blood vessel*.

v. spira'le [NA], a blood vessel, larger than its fellows, running in the tympanic layer of the basilar membrane just beneath the tunnel of Corti.

va'sa vaso'rum [NA], small arteries distributed to the outer and middle coats of the larger blood vessels, and their corresponding veins. SYN vessels of vessels.

va'sa vortico'sa, SYN vortex *veins*, under *vein*.

⌂**vas-.** A vas, blood vessel. SEE ALSO vasculo-, vaso-. [L. *vas*]

va·sa (vā'să). Plural of vas.

va·sal (vā'săl). Relating to a vas or to vasa.

vas·cu·lar (vas'kyū-lăr). Relating to or containing blood vessels. [L. *vasculum*, a small vessel, dim. of *vas*]

vas·cu·lar·i·ty (vas-kyū-lar'i-tē). The condition of being vascular.

vas·cu·lar·i·za·tion (vas'kyū-lăr-i-zā'shŭn). The formation of new blood vessels in a part. SYN arterialization (3).

vas·cu·lar·ized (vas-kyū-lăr-īzd). Rendered vascular by the formation of new vessels.

vas·cu·la·ture (vas'kyū-lă-chūr). The vascular network of an organ.

vas·cu·li·tis (vas-kyū-lī'tis). SYN angiitis.

cutaneous v., an acute form of v. which may affect the skin only, but also may involve other organs, with a polymorphonuclear infiltrate in the walls of and surrounding small (dermal) vessels. Nuclear fragments are formed by karyorrhexis of the neutrophils. SEE ALSO leukocytoclastic v. SYN allergic angiitis, hypersensitivity v.

hypersensitivity v., SYN cutaneous v.

hypocomplementemic v. (hī'pō-com'ple-men-tem-ik), SYN urticarial v.

leukocytoclastic v. (lū'kō-sī-tō-klas-tik), cutaneous acute v. characterized clinically by palpable purpura, especially of the legs, and histologically by exudation of the neutrophils and sometimes fibrin around dermal venules, with nuclear dust and extravasation of red cells; may be limited to the skin or involve other tissues as in Henoch-Schönlein purpura. SEE ALSO cutaneous v. [G. *leukos*, white, + *kytos*, cell, + *klastos*, broken, fr. *klao*, to break]

livedo v. (liv'ē-dō), hyaline degeneration of the walls of small dermal blood vessels with occlusion seen with cryoglobulinemia or in atrophie blanche.

nodular v., chronic or recurrent nodular lesions of subcutaneous tissue, especially of the legs of older women, with lobular panniculitis, granulomatous inflammation with multinucleated giant cells, focal necrosis, and obliterative inflammation of the small blood vessels, resembling erythema induratum but without evidence of associated tuberculosis.

urticarial v., cutaneous lesions resembling urticaria but lasting more than 24 hours, with biopsy findings of leukocytoclastic v. and variable systemic changes, usually with hypocomplementemia. SYN hypocomplementemic v.

⌂**vasculo-.** A blood vessel. SEE ALSO vas-, vaso-. [L. *vasculum,* a small vessel, dim. of *vas*]

vas·cu·lo·car·di·ac (vas'kyū-lō-kar'dē-ak). SYN cardiovascular.

vas·cu·lo·gen·e·sis (vas'kyū-lō-jen'ĕ-sis). Formation of the vascular system. [vasculo- + G. *genesis,* production]

vas·cu·lo·mo·tor (vas'kū-lō-mō'ter). SYN vasomotor.

vas·cu·lo·my·e·li·nop·a·thy (vas'kyū-lō-mī-ĕ-li-nop'ă-thē). Small cerebral vessel vasculopathy with subsequent perivascular demyelination, presumably due to circulating immune complexes.

vas·cu·lop·a·thy (vas-kyū-lop'ă-thē). Any disease of the blood vessels. [vasculo- + G. *pathos,* disease]

vas·cu·lum, pl. **vas·cu·la** (vas'kyū-lŭm, -lă). A small vessel. [L. dim of *vas,* a vessel]

va·sec·to·my (va-sek'tō-mē). Excision of a segment of the vas deferens, performed in association with prostatectomy, or to produce sterility. SYN deferentectomy. [vas- + G. *ektomē,* excision]

vas·i·fac·tion (vas-i-fak'shŭn). SYN angiopoiesis.

vas·i·fac·tive (vas-i-fak'tiv). SYN angiopoietic.

vas·i·form (vas'i-fōrm). Having the shape of a vas or tubular structure.

vas·i·tis (va-sī'tis). SYN deferentitis.

vas·i·tis no·do·sa (va-sī'tis nō-dō'sa). An inflammatory condition of the vas deferens characterized by the presence of numerous epithelium-lined spaces with the muscularis and adventitia, often containing spermatozoa; usually seen after vasectomy, and may clinically and microscopically mimic adenocarcinoma. SEE ALSO *vas* deferens.

⌂**vaso-.** Vas, blood vessel. SEE ALSO vas-, vasculo-. [L. *vas,* a vessel]

va·so·ac·tive (vā-sō-ak'tiv, vas-ō-). Influencing the tone and caliber of blood vessels.

va·so·con·stric·tion (vā'sō-kon-strik'shŭn, vas'ō-). Narrowing of the blood vessels.

active v., reduced caliber of a vessel caused by increased tonus in the smooth muscle in its walls.

passive v., reduced caliber of a vessel caused by decreased intraluminal pressure.

va·so·con·stric·tive (vā'sō-kon-strik'tiv, vas'ō-). 1. Causing narrowing of the blood vessels. 2. SYN vasoconstrictor (1).

va·so·con·stric·tor (vā'sō-kon-strik'ter, vas'ō-). 1. An agent that causes narrowing of the blood vessels. SYN vasoconstrictive (2). 2. A nerve, stimulation of which causes vascular constriction.

va·so·den·tin (vā-sō-den'tin, vas-ō-). Dentin in which the primitive capillaries have remained uncalcified and so are wide enough to give passage to the formed elements of the blood. SYN vascular dentin.

va·so·de·pres·sion (vā'sō-dē-presh'ŭn, vas'ō). Reduction of tone in blood vessels with vasodilation and resulting lowered blood pressure.

va

va·so·de·pres·sor (vā′sō-dē-pres′er, vas′ō). **1.** Producing vaso-depression. **2.** An agent that produces vasodepression.

va·so·di·la·ta·tion (vā′sō-dil-ă-tā′shŭn, vas′ō-). SYN vasodila-tion.

va·so·di·la·tion (vā′sō-dī-lā′shŭn, vas-ō-). widening of the lu-men of blood vessels. SYN vasodilatation.

active v., v. caused by decrease in tonus of smooth muscle in the wall of a vessel.

passive v., v. related to increased pressure in lumen of a vessel.

va·so·di·la·tive (vā′sō-dī-lā′tiv, vas′ō-). **1.** Causing dilation of the blood vessels. **2.** SYN vasodilator (1).

va·so·di·la·tor (vā′sō-dī-lā′ter, vas′ō-). **1.** An agent that causes dilation of the blood vessels. SYN vasodilative (2). **2.** A nerve, stimulation of which results in dilation of the blood vessels.

va·so·ep·i·did·y·mos·to·my (vā′sō-ep-i-did-i-mos′tō-mē, vas′ō-). Surgical anastomosis of the vasa deferentia to the epididy-mis, to bypass an obstruction at the level of the mid to distal epididymis or proximal vas. [vaso- + epididymis + G. *stoma*, mouth]

va·so·fac·tive (vā-sō-fak′tiv, vas-ō-). SYN angiopoietic.

va·so·for·ma·tion (vā-sō-fōr-mā′shŭn, vas-ō-). SYN angiopoie-sis.

va·so·for·ma·tive (vā-sō-fōr′mă-tiv, vas-ō-). SYN angiopoietic.

va·so·gan·gli·on (vā-sō-gang′glē-on, vas-ō-). A mass of blood vessels.

va·sog·ra·phy (vā-sog′ră-fē). Radiography of the vas deferens to determine patency, by injecting contrast medium into its lumen either transurethrally or by open vasotomy. [vas + G. *graphō*, to write]

va·so·hy·per·ton·ic (vā′sō-hī-per-ton′ik, vas′ō-). Relating to in-creased arteriolar tension or vasoconstriction. [vaso- + G. *hyper*, over, + *tonos*, tone]

va·so·hy·po·ton·ic (vā′sō-hī-po-ton′ik, vas′ō-). Relating to re-duced arteriolar tension or vasodilation. [vaso- + G. *hypo*, under, + *tonos*, tone]

va·so·in·hib·i·tor (vā′sō-in-hib′i-ter, vas′ō-). An agent that re-stricts or prevents the functioning of the vasomotor nerves.

va·so·in·hib·i·to·ry (vā′sō-in-hib′i-tōr-ē, vas′ō-). Restraining vasomotor action.

va·so·la·bile (vā-sō-lā′bil, -bīl, vas-ō-). Characterizing the condi-tion in which there is lability or active vasomotion of blood vessels.

va·so·li·ga·tion (vā′sō-li-gā′shŭn, vas′ō-). Ligation of the vas deferens, usually after its division.

va·so·mo·tion (vā-sō-mō′shŭn, vas-ō-). Change in caliber of a blood vessel. SYN angiokinesis.

va·so·mo·tor (vā-sō-mō′ter, vas-ō-). **1.** Causing dilation or con-striction of the blood vessels. **2.** Denoting the nerves which have this action. SYN angiokinetic, vasculomotor.

va·so·neu·rop·a·thy (vā′sō-nū-rop′ă-thē, vas′ō-). Any disease involving both the nerves and blood vessels. [vaso- + G. *neuron*, nerve, + *pathos*, suffering]

va·so·neu·ro·sis (vā′sō-nū-rō′sis, vas′ō-). SYN vasomotor *neuro-sis*.

va·so·or·chi·dos·to·my (vā′sō-ōr-ki-dos′tō-mē, vas′ō-). Re-establishment of the interrupted seminiferous channels by uniting the tubules of the epididymis or of the rete testis to the divided end of the vas deferens. [vaso- + G. *orchis*, testis, + *stoma*, mouth]

va·so·pa·ral·y·sis (vā′sō-pă-ral′i-sis, vas′ō-). Paralysis, atonia, or hypotonia of blood vessels. SYN angiohypotonia, angioparaly-sis.

va·so·pa·re·sis (vā′sō-pă-rē′sis, -par′ē-sis, vas′ō-). A mild de-gree of vasoparalysis. SYN angioparesis, vasomotor paralysis. [vaso- + G. *paresis*, weakness]

va·so·pres·sin (VP) (vā-sō-pres′in, vas-ō-). A nonapeptide neu-rohypophysial hormone related to oxytocin and vasotocin; syn-thetically prepared or obtained from the posterior lobe of the pituitary of healthy domestic animals. In pharmacological doses v. causes contraction of smooth muscle, notably that of all blood vessels; large doses may produce cerebral or coronary arterial

spasm. SYN antidiuretic hormone, antidiuretin, Pitressin. [vaso- + L. *premo*, pp. *pressum*, to press down, + -in]

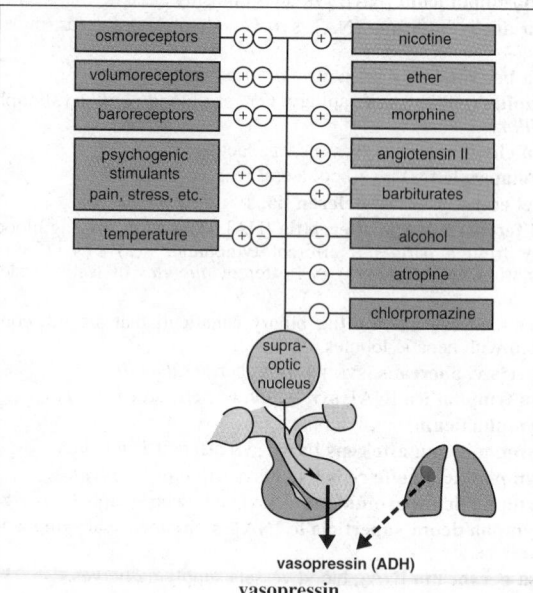

vasopressin

regulation of ADH secretion: effects of various neural and mechanical factors on the supraoptic nucleus (+ = stimulation, – = inhibition); note that some malignant neoplasms (e.g., bronchogenic carcinoma) may also secrete ADH

arginine v. (AVP), [8-arginine]vasopressin; [Arg^8]vasopressin; v. containing an arginyl residue in position 8 (as in chickens and most mammals, including man); porcine v. has a lysyl residue at position 8. All are vasopressors. SYN argipressin.

va·so·pres·sor (vā-sō-pres′er, vas′ō-). **1.** Producing vasocon-striction and a rise in blood pressure, usually understood to be systemic arterial pressure unless otherwise specified. **2.** An agent that has this effect.

va·so·punc·ture (vā-sō-pŭnk′chūr, vas-ō-). The act of punctur-ing a vessel with a needle.

va·so·re·flex (vā-sō-rē′fleks, vas′ō-). A reflex that influences the caliber of blood vessels.

va·so·re·lax·a·tion (vā′sō-rē-lak-sā′shŭn, vas-ō). Reduction in tension of the walls of the blood vessels.

va·so·sec·tion (vā-sō-sek′shŭn, vas-ō-). SYN vasotomy.

va·so·sen·so·ry (vā-sō-sen′ser-ē, vas-ō-). **1.** Relating to sensa-tion in the blood vessels. **2.** Denoting sensory nerve fibers inner-vating blood vessels.

va·so·spasm (vā′sō-spazm, vas′ō-). Contraction or hypertonia of the muscular coats of the blood vessels. SYN angiohypertonia, angiospasm.

va·so·spas·tic (vā-sō-spas′tik, vas-ō-). Relating to or character-ized by vasospasm. SYN angiospastic.

va·so·stim·u·lant (va-sō-stim′yŭ-lant, vas-ō-). **1.** Exciting vasomotor action. **2.** An agent that excites the vasomotor nerves to action. **3.** SYN vasotonic (2).

va·sos·to·my (vā-sos′tō-mē). Establishment of an artificial open-ing into the deferent duct. [vaso- + G. *stoma*, mouth]

va·so·throm·bin (vā-sō-throm′bin, vas-ō-). Thrombin derived from the lining cells of the blood vessels.

va·so·to·cin (vā-sō-tō′sin, vas-ō-). A nonapeptide hormone of the neurohypophysis of subvertebrates, with activities similar to that of vasopressin and oxytocin; chemically identical with hu-man vasopressin except for an isoleucyl residue at position 3; thus [3-isoleucine]vasopressin or [Ile^3]vasopressin. [vaso, pressin + oxy*tocin*]

arginine v., v. with arginyl residue at position 8 (identical with arginine oxytocin). SEE ALSO arginine *vasopressin.*

va·sot·o·my (vă-sot'ŏ-mē). Incision into or division of the vas deferens. SYN vasosection. [vaso- + G. *tomē,* incision]

va·so·to·nia (vā-sō-tō'nē-ă, vas-ō-). The tone of blood vessels, particularly the arterioles. SYN angiotonia. [vaso- + G. *tonos,* tone]

va·so·ton·ic (vā-sō-ton'ik, vas-ō-). **1.** Relating to vascular tone. SYN angiotonic. **2.** An agent that increases vascular tension. SYN vasostimulant (3).

va·so·tro·phic (vā-sō-trof'ik, vas-ō-). Relating to the nutrition of the blood vessels or the lymphatics. [vaso- + G. *trophē,* nourishment]

va·so·tro·pic (vā-sō-trō'pik, vas-ō-). Tending to act on the blood vessels. [vaso- + G. *tropē,* a turning]

va·so·va·gal (vā-sō-vā'găl, vas-ō-). Relating to the action of the vagus nerve upon the blood vessels.

va·so·va·sos·to·my (vā'sō-vă-sos'tō-mē, vas'ō-). Surgical anastomosis of vasa deferentia, to restore fertility in a previously vasectomized male. [vaso- + vaso- + G. *stoma,* mouth]

va·so·ve·sic·u·lec·to·my (vā'sō-vě-sik-yū-lek'tō-mē, vas'ō-). Excision of the vas deferens and seminal vesicles. [vaso- + L. *vesicula,* vesicle, + G. *ektomē,* excision]

vas·tus (vas'tŭs). Great. SEE vastus intermedius *muscle,* vastus lateralis *muscle,* vastus medialis *muscle.* [L.]

VATER Acronym for *v*ertebral defects, *a*nal atresia, *t*racheoesophageal fistula with *e*sophageal atresia, and *r*adial and *r*enal anomalies. SEE VATER *complex.*

Vater, Abraham, German anatomist and botanist, 1684–1751. SEE V.'s *ampulla, corpuscles,* under *corpuscle, fold;* V.-Pacini *corpuscles,* under *corpuscle.*

VATS Abbreviation for video-assisted thoracic *surgery.*

vault (vawlt). A part resembling an arched roof or dome, *e.g.,* the pharyngeal v. or fornix, the non-muscular upper part of the nasopharynx; the palatine v., arch of the plate; v. of the vagina, fornix of vagina. [thr. O. Fr., fr. L. *volvo,* pp. *volutus,* to turn round]

  cranial v., SYN neurocranium.

V-bends. V-shaped bends incorporated in an archwire, usually placed mesially or distally to the canines (cuspids) and used as a "dead" area of wire through which torquing bends may be placed.

VC Abbreviation for colored *vision;* vital *capacity.*

VCUG Abbreviation for voiding cystourethrogram.

VDRL Abbreviation for Venereal Disease Research Laboratories. SEE VDRL *test.*

vec·tion (vek'shŭn). Transference of the agents of disease from an infected to an uninfected individual by a vector. [L. *vectio,* conveyance]

vec·tis (vek'tis). An instrument resembling one of the blades of an obstetrical forceps, used as an aid in delivery by making leverage on the presenting part of the fetus. [L. a lever or bar]

vec·tor (vek'ter, tōr). **1.** An invertebrate animal (*e.g.,* tick, mite, mosquito, bloodsucking fly) capable of transmitting an infectious agent among vertebrates. **2.** Anything (*e.g.,* velocity, mechanical force, electromotive force) having magnitude, direction, and sense; it can be represented by a straight line of appropriate length and direction. **3.** The net electrical axis of the heart (represented by an arrow) whose length is proportional to the magnitude of the electrical force, whose direction gives the direction of the force, and whose tip represents the positive pole of the force. **4.** DNA such as a chromosome or plasmid that autonomously replicates in a cell to which another DNA segment may be inserted and be itself replicated as in cloning. **5.** SYN recombinant v. [L. *vector,* a carrier]

  biological v., a v., such as the *Anopheles* mosquito for malarial agents or the tsetse fly for agents of African sleeping sickness, in which the agent multiplies prior to being transmitted to another host.

  cloning v., an autonomously replicating plasmid or phage with regions that are not essential for its propagation in bacteria and into which foreign DNA can be inserted; this foreign DNA is

replicated and propagated as if it were a normal component of the v.

  expression v., a v. (plasmid, yeast, or animal virus genome) used experimentally to introduce foreign genetic material into a propagatable host cell in order to replicate and amplify the foreign DNA sequences as a recombinant molecule (recombinant DNA cloning of sequences).

  instantaneous v., the resultant v. of the heart's action currents at any given moment, usually represented as an arrow of appropriate direction and magnitude.

  manifest v., projection of a spatial cardiac v. on a single plane.

  mean v., a single cardiac v. representing the average of all v.'s present during a given time interval. SYN mean manifest v.

  mean manifest v., SYN mean v.

  mechanical v., a v. that conveys pathogens to a susceptible individual without essential biological development of the pathogens in the v., as in the transfer of septic organisms on the feet or mouth parts of the housefly.

  recombinant v., a v. into which a foreign DNA has been inserted. SYN vector (5).

  retroviral v., a specially constructed retrovirus containing one or more genes to correct certain genetic disorders.

  shuttle v., a v. (4) that contains both bacterial and eukaryotic replication signals; thus, replication can occur in both types of cells.

  spatial v., a cardiac v. represented in more than one plane simultaneously; two- or three-dimensional orientation of a v.

vec·tor-borne (vek'ter-bōrn). Denoting a disease or infection that is transmitted by an invertebrate vector.

vec·tor·car·di·o·gram (vek'tōr-kar'dē-ō-gram). A graphic representation of the magnitude and direction of the heart's action currents in the form of vector loops.

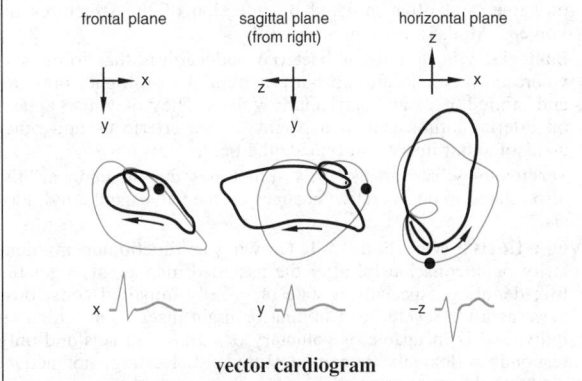

vector cardiogram
normal scale ECG leads, as well as QRS and T vector loops in a vectorcardiogram (black line = adult; red line = child; thick dot = vector .02 secs after beginning of ventricular stimulation)

vec·tor·car·di·og·ra·phy (vek'tōr-kar-dē-og'ră-fē). **1.** A variant of electrocardiography in which the heart's activation currents are represented by vector loops. **2.** The study and interpretation of vectorcardiograms.

  spatial v., three-dimensional v. in which vector loops are inscribed in frontal, sagittal, and horizontal planes.

vec·to·ri·al (vek-tōr'ē-ăl). Relating in any way to a vector.

vec·tors. Recombinant DNA systems especially suited for production of large quantities of specific proteins in bacterial, yeast, insect, or mammalian cell systems.

ve·cu·ro·ni·um bro·mide (ve-kyū-rō'nē-ŭm). 1-[3,17-Bis-(acetyloxy)-2-(1-piperidinyl)androstan-16-yl]-1-methylpiperidinium; a nondepolarizing neuromuscular relaxant with a relatively short duration of action; a monoquaternary homologue of pancuronium.

VEE Abbreviation for Venezuelan equine *encephalomyelitis.*

veg·a·ly·sen (ve'ga-lī'sen). SYN hexamethonium chloride.

veg·an (veg'an). A strict vegetarian; *i.e.,* one who consumes no animal or dairy products of any type. Cf. vegetarian.

veg·e·ta·ble (vej'tă-bl, vej'ĕ-tă-bl). **1.** A plant, specifically one used for food. **2.** Relating to plants, as distinguished from animals or minerals. SYN vegetal (1). [M.E., fr. L. *vegetabilis* (see vegetation)]

veg·e·tal (vej'ĕ-tăl). **1.** SYN vegetable (2). **2.** Denoting the vital functions common to plants and animals, such as respiration, metabolism, growth, generation, etc., distinguished from those peculiar to animals, such as conscious sensation and the mental faculties.

veg·e·tal·i·ty (vej-ĕ-tal'i-tē). The aggregate of the vital functions common to both plants and animals.

veg·e·tar·i·an (vej-ĕ-tār'ē-ăn). One whose diet is restricted to foods of vegetable origin, excluding primarily animal meats. Cf. vegan.

lacto-v., a v. who consumes dairy products but does not eat animal flesh or eggs.

lacto-ovo-v., a v. who consumes dairy products and eggs but does not eat animal flesh.

ovo-v., a v. who consumes eggs but does not consume dairy products nor animal flesh.

pesco-v., a v. who consumes dairy products, eggs, and fish, but does not consume other animal flesh.

semi-v., a v. who consumes dairy products, eggs, chicken, and fish, but does not consume other animal flesh.

veg·e·tar·i·an·ism (vej-ĕ-tār'ē-ăn-izm). The practice as to diet of a vegetarian.

veg·e·ta·tion (vej-ĕ-tā'shŭn). **1.** The process of growth in plants. **2.** A condition of sluggishness, comparable to the inactivity of plant life. **3.** A growth or excrescence of any sort. **4.** Specifically, a clot, composed largely of fused blood platelets, fibrin, and sometimes microorganisms, adherent to a diseased heart orifice or valve, and often initiated by infection of the structures involved. [Mod. L. *vegetatio,* growth]

bacterial v.'s, lesions of bacterial endocarditis that form anywhere on the endocardium but preferentially on higher pressure and injured areas and particularly valves. They may also appear on arterial intima and in a patent ductus arteriosus and other areas of shunt inside and outside the heart.

verrucous v.'s, wart-like v.'s sometimes due to endocarditis, also related to degenerative changes on the valves and amyloidosis.

veg·e·ta·tive (vej'ĕ-tā-tiv). **1.** Growing or functioning involuntarily or unconsciously, after the assumed manner of vegetable life; denoting especially a state of grossly impaired consciousness, as after severe head trauma or brain disease, in which an individual is incapable of voluntary or purposeful acts and only responds reflexively to painful stimuli. **2.** Resting; not active; denoting the stage of a cell or its nucleus in which the process of karyokinesis is quiescent. [see vegetation]

veg·e·to·an·i·mal (vej'ĕ-tō-an'i-măl). Relating to both plants and animals.

ve·hi·cle (vē'hi-kl). **1.** An excipient or a menstruum; a substance, usually without therapeutic action, used as a medium to give bulk for the administration of medicines. **2.** An inanimate substance (*e.g.,* food, milk, dust, clothing, instrument) by which or upon which an infectious agent passes from an infected to a susceptible host; v.'s consequently act as important sources of infection. [L. *vehiculum,* a conveyance, fr. *veho,* to carry]

veil (vāl). **1.** SYN velum (1). **2.** SYN caul (1). [L. *velum*]

aqueduct v., a membrane obstructing the sylvian aqueduct, causing a noncommunicating hydrocephalus.

Jackson's v., SYN Jackson's *membrane*.

Sattler's v., a diffuse edema of the corneal epithelium that may develop after wearing contact lenses.

Veil·lo·nel·la (vā'yō-nel'ă). A genus of nonmotile, nonsporeforming, anaerobic bacteria (family Veillonellaceae) containing small (0.3 to 0.5 μm in diameter), Gram-negative cocci which occur as diplococci and in masses. Carbon dioxide is required for growth, and carbohydrates are not fermented. These organisms are parasitic in the mouth and the intestinal and respiratory tracts of humans and other animals. They produce serologically specific endotoxins (lipopolysaccharides) which induce pyrogenicity and the Schwarzman phenomenon in rabbits. The type species is *V. parvula.* [Adrien *Veillon,* French bacteriologist, 1864–1931]

V. alcales'cens subsp. *alcales'cens,* a subspecies found primarily in the mouth of humans but occasionally in the buccal cavity of rabbits and rats; it is the type subspecies of the species *V. alcalescens.*

V. alcales'cens subsp. *cri'ceti,* a subspecies found in the mouth of hamsters.

V. alcales'cens subsp. *dis'par,* a subspecies found in the mouth and respiratory tract of humans.

V. alcales'cens subsp. *rat'ti,* a subspecies found in the mouth and intestinal contents of rats.

V. alcales'ens, a species found in the saliva of humans and other animals.

V. atypica, SYN *V. parvula* subsp. *atypica.*

V. par'vula, a species found normally as a harmless parasite in the natural cavities, especially the mouth and digestive tract, of humans and other animals; it is the types species of the genus *V.*

V. par'vula subsp. *atyp'ica,* a subspecies found in the buccal cavity of rats and humans. SYN *V. atypica.*

V. par'vula subsp. *par'vula,* a subspecies found in the mouth or the intestinal or respiratory tract of humans; it is the type subspecies of the species *V. parvula.*

V. par'vula subsp. *roden'tium,* a subspecies found in the buccal cavity and intestinal tract of hamsters, rats, and rabbits. SYN *V. rodentium.*

V. rodentium, SYN *V. parvula* subsp. *rodentium.*

Veil·lo·nel·la·ce·ae (vā'yō-nĕ-lā'sē-ē). A family of nonmotile, nonsporeforming, anaerobic bacteria (order Eubacteriales) containing Gram-negative (with a tendency to resist decolorization) cocci which vary in diameter from small (0.3 to 0.5 μm) to large (2.5 μm). Characteristically, they occur in pairs; single cells, masses, or chains may also occur, but the chains may show gaps illustrating the basic diplococcal arrangement. These organisms are chemoorganotrophic; they may or may not ferment carbohydrates. They are parasites of homothermic animals such as humans, ruminants, rodents, and pigs, and are primarily found in the alimentary tract. The type genus is *Veillonella.*

VEIN

vein (vān). A blood vessel carrying blood toward the heart; all the veins except the pulmonary carry dark or oxygenated blood. SYN vena [NA]. [L. *vena*]

accessory cephalic v., a variable v. that passes along the radial border of the forearm to join the cephalic v. near the elbow. SYN vena cephalica accessoria [NA].

accessory hemiazygos v., formed by the union of the fourth to seventh left posterior intercostal v.'s, passes along the side of the bodies of the fifth, sixth, and seventh thoracic vertebrae, then crosses the midline behind the aorta, esophagus, and thoracic duct, and empties into the azygos v., sometimes in common with the hemiazygos v. SYN vena hemiazygos accessoria [NA], vena azygos minor superior.

accessory saphenous v., an occasional v. running in the thigh parallel to the great saphenous v. which it joins just before the latter empties into the femoral v. SYN vena saphena accessoria [NA].

accessory vertebral v., a v. that accompanies the vertebral v. but passes through the foramen of the transverse process of the seventh cervical vertebra and opens independently into the brachiocephalic v. SYN vena vertebralis accessoria [NA].

accompanying v., SYN *vena* comitans.

accompanying v. of hypoglossal nerve, SYN *vena* comitans nervi hypoglossi.

anastomotic v.'s, SEE inferior anastomotic v., superior anastomotic v.

angular v., a short v. at the medial angle of the eye, formed by the supraorbital and supratrochlear v.'s and continuing as the facial v. SYN vena angularis [NA].

anonymous v.'s, obsolete term for brachiocephalic v.'s.

anterior auricular v., one of several v.'s draining the auricle and acoustic meatus and emptying into the retromandibular v. SYN venae auriculares anterior [NA], vena preauricularis.

anterior cardiac v.'s, two or three small v.'s in the anterior wall of the right ventricle opening directly into the right atrium independently of the coronary sinus. SYN venae cordis anteriores [NA].

anterior cardinal v.'s, SEE cardinal v.'s.

anterior cerebral v., a small v. that parallels the anterior cerebral artery and drains into the basal v. SYN vena cerebri anterior [NA].

anterior facial v., SYN facial v.

anterior intercostal v.'s, tributaries to the musculophrenic or internal thoracic v.'s from the anterior portions of intercostal spaces. SYN venae intercostales anteriores [NA].

anterior jugular v., it arises below the chin from v.'s draining the lower lip and mental region, descends the anterior portion of the neck superficially, and terminates in the external jugular v. at the lateral border of the scalenus anterior muscle. SYN vena jugularis anterior [NA].

anterior labial v.'s, tributaries of the femoral or external pudendal v.'s draining the mons pubis and anterior labia majora. SYN venae labiales anteriores [NA].

anterior pontomesencephalic v., SYN *vena* pontomesencephalica anterior.

anterior scrotal v.'s, tributaries of the femoral or exteranl pudendal v.'s drainign the anterior aspect of the scrotum and the skin and dartos fascia of the shaft and base of the penis. SYN venae scrotales anteriores [NA].

anterior v. of septum pellucidum, v. draining the anterior part of the transparent septum; it empties into the superior thalamostriate v. SYN vena septi pellucidi anterior [NA].

anterior tibial v.'s, the venae comitantes of the anterior tibial artery which empty into the popliteal v. SYN venae tibiales anteriores [NA].

anterior vertebral v., the small v. that accompanies the ascending cervical artery; it opens below into the vertebral v. SYN vena vertebralis anterior [NA].

appendicular v., the tributary of the ileocolic v. that accompanies the appendicular artery. SYN vena appendicularis [NA].

aqueous v., a tributary of the anterior ciliary v. which receives aqueous humor from the sinus venosus sclerae.

arciform v.'s of kidney, SYN arcuate v.'s of kidney.

arcuate v.'s of kidney, v.'s that parallel the arcuate arteries, receive blood from interlobular v.'s and straight venules, and terminate in interlobar v.'s. SYN venae arcuatae renis [NA], arciform v.'s of kidney.

arterial v., so called because it ramifies like an artery (portal v.) or because, while proceeding from the heart like an artery, it contains unoxygenated blood, like a v. (pulmonary artery). SYN vena arteriosa.

ascending lumbar v., paired, vertical v. of the posterior abdominal wall, adjacent and parallel to the vertebral column, posterior to the origin of the psoas major muscle; it connects the common iliac, iliolumbar, and lumbar v.'s in the paravertebral line, the right v. joining the right subcostal v. to form the azygos v., the left v. uniting with the left subcostal v. to form the hemiazygos v. SYN vena lumbalis ascendens [NA].

auricular v.'s, SEE anterior auricular v., posterior auricular v.

axillary v., a continuation of the basilic and brachial v.'s running from the lower border of the teres major muscle to the outer border of the first rib where it becomes the subclavian v. SYN vena axillaris [NA].

azygos v., arises from the merger of the right ascending lumbar v. with the right subcostal v. and often a communication with the inferior vena cava; ascends through the aortic hiatus of the diaphragm or its right crus; it runs along the right side of the thoracic vertebral bodies in the posterior mediastinum, and terminates by arching anteriorly over the root of the right lung to enter the posterior aspect of the superior vena cava. SYN vena azygos [NA], azygos (2), vena azygos major.

basal v.'s, SEE basal v. of Rosenthal, common basal v., inferior basal v., superior basal v.

basal v. of Rosenthal, a large v. passing caudally and dorsally along the medial surface of the temporal lobe from which it receives tributaries; it empties into the great cerebral v. (of Galen) from the lateral side. SYN vena basalis [NA], Rosenthal's v.

basilic v., arises from the ulnar side of the dorsal venous network of the hand; it curves around the medial side of the forearm, communicates with the cephalic v. via the median cubital v., and passes up the medial side of the arm to join the axillary v. SYN vena basilica [NA].

basivertebral v., one of a number of v.'s in the spongy substance of the bodies of the vertebrae, emptying into the anterior internal vertebral venous plexus. SYN vena basivertebralis [NA].

Baumgarten's v.'s, nonobliterated remnants of the vena umbilicalis.

Boyd communicating perforation v.'s, a v. connecting the superficial and deep venous system in the anteromedial calf.

brachial v.'s, venae comitantes of the brachial artery which empty into the axillary v. SYN venae brachiales [NA].

brachiocephalic v.'s, formed by the union of the internal jugular and subclavian v.'s; other tributaries of the right brachiocephalic v. are the right vertebral and internal thoracic v.'s, and the right lymphatic duct; other tributaries of the left brachiocephalic v. are the left vertebral, internal thoracic, superior intercostal, thyroidea ima, and various anterior pericardial, bronchial, mediastinal v.'s, and the thoracic duct. SYN venae brachiocephalicae [NA].

Breschet's v.'s, SYN diploic v.

bronchial v.'s, many v.'s running in front of and behind the bronchi and uniting into two main trunks which empty on the right side into the azygos v., on the left into the accessory hemiazygos or the left superior intercostal v. SYN venae bronchiales [NA].

Browning's v., SYN inferior anastomotic v.

v. of bulb of penis, a tributary of the internal pudendal v. that drains the bulb of the penis. SYN vena bulbi penis [NA].

Burow's v., (**1**) an occasional v. passing from the inferior epigastric, sometimes receiving a tributary from the urinary bladder, which empties into the portal v.; (**2**) one of the renal v.'s.

capillary v., SYN venule.

cardiac v.'s, SEE anterior cardiac v.'s, great cardiac v., middle cardiac v., *venae* cordis minimae, under *vena*.

cardinal v.'s, the major systemic venous channels in adult primitive vertebrates and in the embryos of higher vertebrates; the **anterior cardinal v.'s** are the major drainage channels from the cephalic part of the body, and the **posterior cardinal v.'s**, from the caudal part; the **common cardinal v.'s**, formed by the anastomosis of the anterior and posterior cardinal v.'s, are the main systemic return channels to the heart; in the older literature, sometimes called Cuvier's ducts.

v.'s of caudate nucleus, SYN *venae* nuclei caudati, under *vena*.

cavernous v.'s of penis, the cavernous venous spaces in the erectile tissue of the penis. SYN venae cavernosae penis [NA].

central v.'s of liver, the terminal branches of the hepatic v.'s that lie centrally in the hepatic lobules and receive blood from the liver sinusoids. SYN venae centrales hepatis [NA], Krukenberg's v.'s.

central v. of retina, formed by union of the retinal v.'s and accompanies the artery of the same name in the optic nerve. SYN vena centralis retinae [NA].

central v. of suprarenal gland, the single draining v. of the gland; it receives a number of medullary v.'s; on the right side it empties directly into the inferior vena cava and on the left into the left renal v. SYN vena centralis glandulae suprarenalis [NA].

cephalic v., arises at the radial border of the dorsal venous rete of the hand, passes upward in front of the elbow and along the lateral side of the arm; it empties into the upper part of the axillary v. SYN vena cephalica [NA].

ve

cerebellar v.'s, the v.'s draining the cerebellum. SEE inferior v.'s of cerebellar hemisphere, superior v.'s of cerebellar hemisphere, petrosal v., precentral cerebellar v., inferior v. of vermis, superior v. of vermis. SYN venae cerebelli [NA], v.'s of cerebellum.

v.'s of cerebellum, SYN cerebellar v.'s.

cerebral v.'s, SEE anterior cerebral v., deep middle cerebral v., great cerebral v., superficial middle cerebral v.

cervical v., SEE deep cervical v.

choroid v., SEE inferior choroid v., superior choroid v.

choroid v.'s of eye, SYN vortex v.'s.

ciliary v.'s, several small v.'s, anterior and posterior, coming from the ciliary body. SYN venae ciliares [NA].

circumflex v.'s, SEE deep circumflex iliac v., superficial circumflex iliac v., lateral circumflex femoral v.'s, medial circumflex femoral v.'s.

v. of cochlear aqueduct, SYN v. of cochlear canaliculus.

v. of cochlear canaliculus, it drains the cochlea, sacculus, and part of the utricules, and empties into the superior bulb of the jugular v. by accompanying the perilymphatic duct through the cochlear canaliculus. SYN vena aqueductus cochleae [NA], v. of cochlear aqueduct, vena canaliculi cochleae.

Cockett communicating perforating v.'s, mid-thigh perforation v.'s that connect the deep and superficial venous systems.

colic v.'s, SEE right colic v., middle colic v., left colic v.

common basal v., the tributary to the inferior pulmonary v. (right and left) that receives blood from the superior and inferior basal v.'s. SYN vena basalis communis [NA].

common cardinal v.'s, SEE cardinal v.'s.

common facial v., a short vessel formed by the union of the facial v. and the retromandibular v., emptying into the jugular v.; considered to be a continuation of the facial v. in the NA. SYN vena facialis communis.

common iliac v., formed by the union of the external and internal iliac v.'s at the brim of the pelvis and passes upward behind the internal iliac artery to the right side of the body of the fifth lumbar vertebra where it unites with its fellow of the opposite side to form the inferior vena cava; the left common iliac v. is submitted to a pulsating compression by the right common iliac artery against the vertebral column which may result in partial obstruction of the v. SYN vena iliaca communis [NA].

companion v., SYN *vena* comitans.

companion v.'s, SYN *venae* comitantes, under *vena*.

condylar emissary v., a v. that connects the sigmoid sinus and the external vertebral venous plexuses through the condylar canal of the occipital bone. SYN vena emissaria condylaris [NA], emissarium condyloideum.

conjunctival v.'s, the v.'s of the conjunctiva which drain primarily to the ophthalmic v.'s. SYN venae conjunctivales [NA].

coronary v., SYN left gastric v.

v. of corpus striatum, SYN superior thalamostriate v.

costoaxillary v., one of a number of anastomotic v.'s connecting the intercostal v.'s of the first to seventh intercostal spaces with the lateral thoracic or the thoracoepigastric v.

cutaneous v., SYN superficial v.

Cuvier's v.'s, the common cardinal v.'s of the embryo. SEE cardinal v.'s.

cystic v., v.'s, usually anterior and posterior, which drain the neck of the gallbladder and cystic duct, along which they pass to enter the right branch of the portal v.; they communicate extensively with surrounding v.'s of the stomach, duodenum and pancreas. SYN vena cystica [NA].

deep cerebral v.'s, the numerous v.'s draining the deep structures of the cerebral hemispheres; they empty into the tributaries of the great cerebral v. SYN venae cerebri profundae [NA].

deep cervical v., large v. running with the artery of the same name between the semispinalis capitis and semispinalis cervicis draining the deep muscles at the back of the neck and emptying into the brachiocephalic or the vertebral v. SYN vena cervicalis profunda [NA].

deep circumflex iliac v., corresponds to the artery of the same name, and empties, near or in a common trunk with the inferior

epigastric v., into the external iliac v. SYN vena circumflexa iliaca profunda [NA].

deep v.'s of clitoris, the v.'s that pass from the dorsum of the clitoris to join the vesical plexus. SYN venae profundae clitoridis [NA].

deep dorsal v. of clitoris, a tributary of the vesical venous plexus; it runs a course deep to the fascia on the dorsum of the clitoris. SYN vena dorsalis clitoridis profunda [NA].

deep dorsal v. of penis, a vein on the dorsum of the penis deep to the fascia of the penis; it is a tributary to the prostatic venous plexus. SYN vena dorsalis penis profunda [NA].

deep epigastric v., SYN inferior epigastric v.

deep facial v., the communicating v. that passes from the pterygoid venous plexus of the infratemporal fossa to the facial v.; it is devoid of valves. SYN vena faciei profunda [NA].

deep femoral v., the v. that accompanies the deep femoral artery, receiving perforating v.'s from the lateral and posterior aspects of the thigh. It joins the femoral v. in the femoral triangle, usually in common with the medial and lateral circumflex femoral v.'s. SYN vena profunda femoris [NA].

deep lingual v., the principle v. of the tongue that accompanies the deep lingual artery and joins the lingual v. It drains the body and apex of the tongue, running posteriorly near the median plane; they are often visible through the mucosa on the underside of the tongue, to each side of the frenulum. SYN vena profunda linguae [NA].

deep middle cerebral v., the v. that accompanies the middle cerebral artery in the depths of the lateral sulcus and empties into the basal v. of Rosenthal. SYN vena cerebri media profunda [NA].

deep v. of penis, the v. deep to the deep fascia on the dorsum of the penis. It enters the prostatic plexus by passing through a gap between the arcuate pubic ligament and the transverse perineal ligament. SYN vena profunda penis [NA].

deep temporal v.'s, v.'s corresponding to the arteries of the same name; they empty into the pterygoid venous plexus. SYN venae temporales profundae [NA].

digital v.'s, SEE dorsal digital v.'s of foot, palmar digital v.'s, plantar digital v.'s.

diploic v., one of the v.'s in the diploë of the cranial bones, connected with the cerebral sinuses by emissary v.'s; the main diploic v.'s are the frontal, anterior temporal, posterior temporal, and occipital. SYN vena diploica [NA], Breschet's v., Dupuytren's canal.

dorsal callosal v., SYN *vena* corporis callosi dorsalis.

dorsal v.'s of clitoris, SEE deep dorsal v. of clitoris, superficial dorsal v.'s of clitoris.

dorsal v. of corpus callosum, SYN *vena* corporis callosi dorsalis.

dorsal digital v.'s of foot, they receive intercapitular v.'s from the plantar venous arch, join to form four common dorsal digital v.'s, and terminate in the dorsal venous arch. SYN venae digitales dorsales pedis [NA], dorsal digital v.'s of toes.

dorsal digital v.'s of toes, SYN dorsal digital v.'s of foot.

dorsal lingual v., multiple tributaries of the lingual v. draining the dorsum of the tongue, becoming increasingly larger toward the root of the tongue. SYN venae dorsales linguae [NA].

dorsal metacarpal v.'s, three v.'s on the dorsum of the hand draining blood from the four medial digits into the dorsal venous network of the hand. SYN venae metacarpeae dorsales [NA].

dorsal metatarsal v.'s, v.'s arising from the dorsal digital v.'s forming the dorsal venous arch of the foot. SYN venae metatarseae dorsales [NA].

dorsal v.'s of penis, SEE deep dorsal v. of penis, superficial dorsal v.'s of penis.

dorsal scapular v., the vena comitans of the descending scapular artery; it is a tributary to the subclavian or the external jugular v. SYN vena scapularis dorsalis [NA].

dorsispinal v.'s, v.'s forming a plexus around the neural arches and processes of the vertebrae.

emissary v., one of the channels of communication between the venous sinuses of the dura mater and the v.'s of the diploë and the scalp. SEE ALSO condylar emissary v., mastoid emissary v., occipital emissary v., parietal emissary v. SYN vena emissaria [NA], emissarium, emissary (2).

epigastric v.'s, SEE inferior epigastric v., superficial epigastric v., superior epigastric v.'s.

episcleral v.'s, a series of small venules in the sclera close to the corneal margin that empty into the anterior ciliary v.'s. SYN venae episclerales [NA].

esophageal v.'s, series of v.'s draining the submucous venous plexus of the esophagus; proceding inferiorly from the cervical portion of the esophagus, they drain to the inferior thyroid v., the superior intercostal v.'s, the azygos, accessory hemiazygos and hemiazygos v.'s, all of which are ultimately tributaries of the superior vena cava; the most inferior esophageal v.'s, from the cardiac portion of the esophagus, drain via the esophageal branches of the left gastric v., a tributary of the portal v. Thus, the submucosal v.'s of the inferior esophagus form a portocaval anastomoses, and are subject to the formation of varicosities in portal hypertension. SYN venae esophageae [NA].

ethmoidal v.'s, v.'s that accompany the anterior and posterior ethmoidal arteries and pass into the superior ophthalmic v.; they drain the ethmoidal sinuses. SYN venae ethmoidales [NA].

external iliac v., a direct continuation of the femoral v. superior to the inguinal ligament, uniting with the internal iliac v. to form the common iliac v. SYN vena iliaca externa [NA].

external jugular v., superficial v. formed inferior to the parotid gland by the junction of the posterior auricular v. and the retromandibular v., and passes down the side of the neck crossing to the sternocleidomastoid muscle vertically to empty into the subclavian v. SYN vena jugularis externa [NA].

external nasal v.'s, several vessels that drain the external nose, emptying into the angular or facial v. SYN venae nasales externae [NA].

external pudendal v.'s, these correspond to the arteries of the same name; they empty into the great saphenous v. or directly into the femoral v., and receive the superficial dorsal v. of the penis (clitoris) and the anterior scrotal (or labial) v.'s. SYN venae pudendae externae [NA].

v.'s of eyelids, SYN palpebral v.'s.

facial v., a continuation of the angular v. at the medial angle of the eye; it passes diagonally downward and outward, uniting with the retromandibular v. below the border of the lower jaw before emptying into the internal jugular v. SYN anterior facial v., vena facialis anterior, vena facialis.

femoral v., a continuation of the popliteal v., it accompanies the femoral artery through the adductor canal and into the femoral triangle where it lies with in the femoral sheath; it becomes the external iliac v. as it passes deep to inguinal ligament. SYN vena femoralis [NA].

fibular v.'s, SYN peroneal v.'s.

frontal v.'s, (1) the superficial v.'s draining the frontal cortex and emptying into the superior sagittal sinus; (2) SYN supratrochlear v.'s.

v.'s of Galen, (1) SYN internal cerebral v.'s. (2) SEE great cerebral v. SEE great cerebral v.

gastric v.'s, SEE short gastric v.'s, right gastric v., left gastric v.

gastroepiploic v.'s, SEE right gastroepiploic v., left gastroepiploic v.

gluteal v.'s, SEE inferior gluteal v.'s, superior gluteal v.'s.

great cardiac v., begins at the apex of the heart (where it anastomoses with the middle cardiac v.), runs first with the anterior interventricular artery as it ascends the anterior interventricular groove, then turns to the left as it approaches or reaches the coronary groove to run with the circumflex branch of the left coronary artery; it merges with the oblique v. of the left atrium to form the coronary sinus. SYN vena cordis magna [NA], left coronary v., vena cardiaca magna.

great cerebral v., SYN great cerebral v. of Galen.

great cerebral v. of Galen, a large, unpaired v. formed by the junction of the two internal cerebral v.'s in the caudal part of the tela choroidea of the third ventricle; it passes caudally between the splenium of the corpus callosum and the pineal gland, curving dorsally to merge with the inferior sagittal sinus to form the straight sinus. SYN vena cerebri magna [NA], great cerebral v., great v. of Galen.

great v. of Galen, SYN great cerebral v. of Galen.

great saphenous v., formed by the union of the dorsal v. of the great toe and the dorsal venous arch of the foot, ascends in front of the medial malleolus, behind the medial condyle of the femur, and traverses the saphenois hiatus in the fascia lata to empty into the femoral v. in the upper part of the femoral triangle. SYN vena saphena magna [NA], large saphenous v., long saphenous v.

hemiazygos v., formed by the merger of the left ascending lumbar v. with the left subcostal v. or a communication fromthe inferior vena cava, it pierces the left crus of the diaphragm, ascends along the left side of the bodies of the lower thoracic vertebrae, opposite the eighth vertebra, crosses the midline behind the aorta, thoracic duct, and esophagus, and empties into the azygos v., sometimes in common with the accessory hemiazygos v. SYN vena hemiazygos [NA], vena azygos minor inferior.

hemorrhoidal v.'s, obsolete term for rectal v.'s. SEE inferior rectal v.'s, middle rectal v.'s, superior rectal v.

hepatic v.'s, the v.'s that drain the liver; they collect blood from the central v.'s and terminate in three large v.'s opening into the inferior vena cava below the diaphragm and several small inconstant v.'s entering the vena cava at more inferior levels. SYN venae hepaticae [NA].

hepatic portal v., SYN portal v.

highest intercostal v., the v. draining the first intercostal space into either the vertebral or the brachiocephalic v. SYN vena intercostalis suprema [NA], supreme intercostal v.

hypogastric v., obsolete term for internal iliac v.

ileal v.'s, SEE jejunal and ileal v.'s.

ileocolic v., a large tributary of the superior mesenteric v. that runs parallel to the ileocolic artery and drains the terminal ileum, appendix, cecum, and the lower part of the ascending colon. SYN vena ileocolica [NA].

iliac v.'s, SEE common iliac v., external iliac v., internal iliac v., deep circumflex iliac v., superficial circumflex iliac v.

iliolumbar v., accompanying the artery of the same name, anastomosing with the lumbar and deep circumflex iliac v.'s, and emptying into the internal iliac v. SYN vena iliolumbalis [NA].

inferior anastomotic v., an inconstant v. that passes from the superficial middle cerebral v. posteriorly over the lateral aspect of the temporal lobe to enter the transverse sinus. SYN vena anastomotica inferior [NA], Browning's v., Labbé's v.

inferior basal v., tributary to the common basal v. draining the medial and posterior part of the inferior lobe in each lung. SYN vena basalis inferior [NA].

inferior cardiac v., SYN middle cardiac v.

inferior v.'s of cerebellar hemisphere, several v.'s draining the inferior portion of the cerebellar hemispheres; they terminate in the petrosal v. SYN venae hemispherii cerebelli inferiores [NA].

inferior cerebral v.'s, numerous cerebral v.'s that drain the undersurface of the cerebral hemispheres and empty into the cavernous and transverse sinuses. SYN venae cerebri inferiores [NA].

inferior choroid v., a small v. draining the lower part of the choroid plexus of the lateral ventricle into the basal v. SYN vena choroidea inferior [NA].

inferior epigastric v., corresponds to the artery of the same name and empties into the external iliac v. just proximal to the inguinal ligament. SYN vena epigastrica inferior [NA], deep epigastric v.

v.'s of inferior eyelid, SYN inferior palpebral v.'s.

inferior gluteal v.'s, the venae comitantes of the inferior gluteal artery uniting at the sciatic foramen to form a common trunk which empties into the internal iliac v. SYN venae gluteae inferiores [NA].

inferior hemorrhoidal v.'s, obsolete term for inferior rectal v.'s.

inferior labial v., a tributary of the facial v. draining the lower lip. SYN vena labialis inferior [NA].

inferior laryngeal v., the v. passing from the lower part of the larynx to the plexus thyroideus impar. SYN vena laryngea inferior [NA].

inferior mesenteric v., a continuation of the superior rectal v. at the brim of the pelvis, ascending to the left of the aorta behind the peritoneum and emptying into the splenic v. or into the superior mesenteric v. or rarely in the angle between these v.'s. SYN vena mesenterica inferior [NA].

inferior ophthalmic v., arises from the inferior palpebral and lacrimal v.'s and divides into two terminal branches, one of which runs to the pterygoid plexus while the other joins the superior ophthalmic v. or empties into the cavernous sinus. SYN vena ophthalmica inferior [NA].

inferior palpebral v.'s, v.'s of inferior eyelid; v.'s originatin gin the inferior eyelid and emptying into the angular v. SYN venae palpebrales inferiores [NA], v.'s of inferior eyelid.

inferior phrenic v., the v. that drains the substance of the diaphragm and empties on the right side into the inferior vena cava, on the left side into the left suprarenal v.; often a second v. on the left side passes transversely across the diaphragm anterior to the esophageal hiatus to enter the inferior vena cava. SYN vena phrenica inferior [NA].

inferior rectal v.'s, v.'s that pass to the internal pudendal v. from the inferior rectal venous plexus around the anal canal. SYN venae rectales inferiores [NA].

inferior thalamostriate v.'s, v.'s draining the thalamus and striate body exiting the anterior perforated substance; tributary to the basal v. SYN venae thalamostriatae inferiores [NA], striate v.'s, venae striatae.

inferior thyroid v., unpaired v. formed by v.'s from the isthmus and lateral lobe of the thyroid gland and from the plexus thyroideus impar; it terminates in the left brachiocephalic v. SYN vena thyroidea inferior [NA], vena thyroidea ima.

inferior ventricular v., SYN *vena* ventricularis inferior.

inferior v. of vermis, a v. draining part of the inferior part of the cerebellum; it courses on the inferior surface of the vermis and terminates in the straight sinus. SYN vena vermis inferior [NA].

infrasegmental v.'s, SYN pars intersegmentalis [NA]. SEE intersegmental v.'s.

innominate v.'s, obsolete term for brachiocephalic v.'s.

innominate cardiac v.'s, the small superficial v.'s of the heart. SYN Vieussens' v.'s.

insular v.'s, SYN *venae* insulares, under *vena*.

intercapitular v.'s, the v.'s connecting the dorsal and palmar v.'s in the hand, or the dorsal and plantar v.'s in the foot. SYN venae intercapitales [NA].

intercostal v.'s, SEE anterior intercostal v.'s, posterior intercostal v.'s, highest intercostal v., left superior intercostal v.

interlobar v.'s of kidney, the v.'s in the kidney that parallel the interlobar arteries, receiving blood from arcuate v.'s, and terminate in the renal v. SYN venae interlobares renis [NA].

interlobular v.'s of kidney, they parallel the interlobular arteries and drain the peritubular capillary plexus, emptying into the arcuate v.'s. SYN venae interlobulares renis [NA].

interlobular v.'s of liver, the terminal branches of the portal v. that course in the portal canals between the conceptual liver lobules and empty into the liver sinusoids. SYN venae interlobulares hepatis [NA].

intermediate antebrachial v., SYN median antebrachial v.

intermediate basilic v., the medial branch of the median antebrachial v. which joins the basilic v. SYN vena intermedia basilica [NA], median basilic v., vena mediana basilica.

intermediate cephalic v., the lateral branch of the median antebrachial v. that joins the cephalic v. near the elbow. SYN vena intermedia cephalica [NA], median cephalic v., vena mediana cephalica.

intermediate cubital v., SYN median cubital v.

intermediate v. of forearm, SYN median antebrachial v.

internal auditory v.'s, SYN labyrinthine v.'s.

internal cerebral v.'s, paired v.'s passing caudally near the midline in the tela choroidea of the third ventricle, formed by the union of the choroid v., thalamostriate (terminal) v., and v. of septum pellucidum, and uniting caudally so as to form the great cerebral v. SYN venae cerebri internae [NA], v.'s of Galen (1).

internal iliac v., runs from the upper border of the greater sciatic notch to the brim of the pelvis where it joins the external iliac v. to form the common iliac v.; it drains most of the territory supplied by the internal iliac artery. SYN vena iliaca interna [NA].

internal jugular v., main venouus structure of the neck, formed as a continuation of the sigmoid sinus of the dura mater, contained within the carotid sheath as it descends the neck uniting, behind the sternoclavicular joint, with the subclavian v. to form the brachiocephalic v. SYN vena jugularis interna [NA].

internal pudendal v., a tributary of the internal iliac v. that accompanies the internal pudendal artery as a single or double vessel. It drains the perineum. SYN vena pudenda interna [NA].

internal thoracic v., venae comitantes of each artery of the same name, fusing into one at the upper part of the thorax and emptying into the brachiocephalic v. of the same side; receive drainage of anterior chest wall. SYN vena thoracica interna [NA].

intersegmental v., a v. receiving blood from adjacent bronchopulmonary segments; it emerges from the inferior margin of a segment to become a tributary of a branch of a pulmonary v. SYN infrasegmental part, intersegmental part of pulmonary vein, pars infrasegmentalis.

intervertebral v., one of numerous v.'s accompanying the spinal nerves through the intervertebral foramina, draining spinal cord and vertebral venous plexuses, and emptying in the neck into the vertebral v., in the thorax into the intercostal v.'s, in the lumbar and sacral regions into the lumbar and sacral v.'s. SYN vena intervertebralis [NA].

intrasegmental v.'s, a v. emerging from the bronchopulmonary segment it drains; a tributary to a branch of a pulmonary v. SYN pars intrasegmentalis [NA], intrasegmental part.

jejunal and ileal v.'s, the v.'s that drain the jejunum and ileum; they terminate in the superior mesenteric v. SYN venae jejunales et ilei [NA].

jugular v.'s, SEE anterior jugular v., external jugular v., internal jugular v. SEE ALSO posterior anterior jugular v.

key v., a deep-seated, dilated v. causing a "spider burst" on the surface.

v.'s of kidney, the tributaries of the renal v. that drain the kidney; they parallel the arteries in the kidney and consist of interlobular, arcuate, and interlobar v.'s. SYN venae renis [NA].

v.'s of knee, the v.'s that accompany the genicular arteries; they drain blood from the structures around the knee, terminating in the popliteal v. SYN venae genus [NA].

Krukenberg's v.'s, SYN central v.'s of liver.

Labbé's v., SYN inferior anastomotic v.

labial v.'s, SEE anterior labial v.'s, posterior labial v.'s, inferior labial v., superior labial v.

labyrinthine v.'s, one or more v.'s accompanying the labyrinthine artery; they drain the internal ear, pass out through the internal acoustic meatus, and empty into the transverse sinus or the inferior petrosal sinus. SYN venae labyrinthi [NA], internal auditory v.'s.

lacrimal v., small v. which it drains the lacrimal gland, passing posteriorly through the orbit with the lacrimal artery to empty into the superior ophthalmic v. SYN vena lacrimalis [NA].

large v., a v., such as the inferior vena cava, characterized by having a reduced or absent tunica media and an adventitia with large bundles of longitudinally disposed smooth muscle.

large saphenous v., SYN great saphenous v.

laryngeal v.'s, SEE inferior laryngeal v., superior laryngeal v.

Latarget's v., SYN prepyloric v.

lateral atrial v., SYN *vena* atrii lateralis.

lateral circumflex femoral v.'s, the v.'s that accompany the lateral circumflex femoral artery, usually terminating in the femoral v. SYN venae circumflexae femoris laterales [NA].

lateral direct v.'s, SYN *venae* directae laterales, under *vena*.

lateral v. of lateral ventricle, SYN *vena* atrii lateralis.

v. of lateral recess of fourth ventricle, SYN *vena* recessus lateralis ventriculi quarti.

lateral sacral v.'s, several v.'s that receive the drainage of the sacral venous plexus and sacral intervertebral v.'s then accompany the corresponding artery and empty into the internal iliac v. on each side. SYN venae sacrales laterales [NA].

lateral thoracic v., a tributary of the axillary v. that drains the lateral thoracic wall and communicates with the thoracoepigastric and intercostal v.'s. SYN vena thoracica lateralis [NA].

left colic v., a tributary of the inferior mesenteric v. that accompanies the left colic artery and drains the left flexure and descending colon. SYN vena colica sinistra [NA].

left coronary v., SYN great cardiac v.

left gastric v., arises from a union of v.'s from both surfaces of the cardia of the stomach and an esophageal tributary from the cardiac portion of the esophagus; it runs in the lesser omentum and empties into the portal v. SEE ALSO esophageal v.'s. SYN vena gastrica sinistra [NA], coronary v., vena coronaria ventriculi.

left gastroepiploic v., the v. that accompanies the left gastroepiploic artery along the greater curvature of the stomach; it empties into the splenic v. SYN vena gastro-omentalis sinistra [NA], left gastroomental v.

left gastroomental v., SYN left gastroepiploic v.

left hepatic v.'s, v.'s draining the lateral segments [II & III] of the left lobe of the liver which join to form a single or paired trunk of variable size which usually (90% of the time) merges with that formed by the middle hepatic v.'s prior to entering the terminal portion of the superior vena cava. SYN venae hepaticae sinistrae [NA].

left inferior pulmonary v., the v. returning oxygenated blood from the inferior lobe of the left lung to the left atrium. SYN vena pulmonalis inferior sinistra [NA].

left ovarian v., begins as the pampiniform plexus at the hilum of the ovary and empties into the left renal v. SYN vena ovarica sinistra [NA].

left superior intercostal v., the v. formed by the union of the left second, third, and fourth intercostal v.'s; it passes forward across the arch of the aorta to empty into the left brachiocephalic v. and frequently communicates also with the accessory hemiazygos v. SYN vena intercostalis superior sinistra [NA].

left superior pulmonary v., the v. returning oxygenated blood from the left superior lobe of the lung to the left atrium. SYN vena pulmonalis superior sinistra [NA].

left suprarenal v., the v. from the hilum of the left suprarenal gland that passes downward to open into the left renal v.; it usually is joined by the left inferior phrenic v. SYN vena suprarenalis sinistra [NA].

left testicular v., v. conveying blood from the left testis, originating as the pampiniform plexus and entering the left renal v. SYN vena testicularis sinistra [NA].

left umbilical v., the v. that returns the blood from the placenta to the fetus; traversing the umbilical cord, it enters the fetal body at the umbilicus and passes thence into the liver, where it is joined by the portal v.; its blood then flows by way of the ductus venosus and the inferior vena cava to the right atrium. SYN vena umbilicalis sinistra [NA].

levoatrio-cardinal v., the communication of a systemic v. with the left atrium, other than a left superior vena cava or coronary sinus; may be the right superior vena cava.

lingual v., receives blood from the tongue, sublingual and submandibular glands, and muscles of the floor of the mouth; empties into the internal jugular or the facial v. SYN vena lingualis [NA].

long saphenous v., SYN great saphenous v.

long thoracic v., incorrect term for lateral thoracic v.

lumbar v.'s, five in number, these v.'s accompany the lumbar arteries, drain the posterior body wall and the lumbar vertebral venous plexuses, and terminate anteriorly as follows: the first and second in the ascending lumbar v., the third and fourth in the inferior vena cava, and the fifth in the iliolumbar v.; all communicate via the ascending lumbar v.'s. SYN venae lumbales [NA].

Marshall's oblique v., SYN oblique v. of left atrium.

masseteric v.'s, plexiform v.'s accompanying the masseteric artery that empty into the pterygoid venous plexus.

mastoid emissary v., the vein that connects the sigmoid sinus with the occipital vein or one of the tributaries of the external jugular vein by way of the mastoid foramen. SYN vena emissaria mastoidea [NA], emissarium mastoideum.

maxillary v., the posterior continuation of the pterygoid plexus; it joins the superficial temporal vein to form the retromandibular vein. SYN vena maxillaris [NA].

Mayo's v., SYN prepyloric v.

medial atrial v., SYN vena atrii medialis.

medial circumflex femoral v.'s, the venae comitantes that parallel the medial circumflex femoral artery. SYN venae circumflexae femoris mediales [NA].

medial v. of lateral ventricle, SYN vena atrii medialis.

median antebrachial v., it begins at the base of the dorsum of the thumb, curves around the radial side, ascends the middle of the forearm, and just below the bend of the elbow divides into the intermediate basilic and intermediate cephalic v.'s; sometimes it divides lower down, one branch going to the basilic v., the other to the intermediate v. of the elbow. SYN vena intermedia antebrachii [NA], intermediate antebrachial v., intermediate v. of forearm, median v. of forearm, vena mediana antebrachii.

median basilic v., SYN intermediate basilic v.

median cephalic v., SYN intermediate cephalic v.

median cubital v., a v. which passes across the anterior aspect of the elbow from the cephalic v. to the basilic v.; commonly this v. is replaced by intermediate basilic and intermediate cephalic v.'s. The median cubital v. is often used for venipuncture. SYN vena intermedia cubiti [NA], intermediate cubital v., vena mediana cubiti.

median v. of forearm, SYN median antebrachial v.

median v. of neck, a v. occasionally present due to fusion of the two anterior jugular v.'s.

median sacral v., an unpaired v. accompanying the middle sacral artery receiving blood from the sacral venous plexus and emptying into the left common iliac v. SYN vena sacralis mediana [NA].

mediastinal v.'s, several small v.'s from the mediastinum emptying into the brachiocephalic v.'s or the superior vena cava. SYN venae mediastinales [NA].

medium v., a v. characterized by having a thinner wall and larger lumen than its corresponding artery, and a media with small bundles of circular muscle separated by considerable connective tissue; valves also occur.

v.'s of medulla oblongata, SYN venae medullae oblongatae, under vena.

meningeal v.'s, v.'s that accompany the meningeal arteries; they communicate with venous sinuses and diploic v.'s and drain into regional v.'s outside the cranial vault. SYN venae meningeae [NA].

mesencephalic v.'s, SYN venae mesencephalicae, under vena.

mesenteric v.'s, SEE inferior mesenteric v., superior mesenteric v.

metacarpal v.'s, SEE dorsal metacarpal v.'s, palmar metacarpal v.'s.

middle cardiac v., begins at the apex of the heart (where it anastomoses with the great cardiac v.), and ascends within the posterior interventricular sulcus to the coronary sinus. SYN vena cordis media [NA], inferior cardiac v.

middle colic v., the tributary of the superior mesenteric v. that carries drainage of the transverse colon and accompanies the middle colic artery. SYN vena colica media [NA].

middle hemorrhoidal v.'s, obsolete term for middle rectal v.'s.

middle hepatic v.'s, v.'s draining the central portion of the liver (the superior anterior segment [VIII] and the left side of the inferior anterior segment [V] of the right lobe and the medial segment [IV] of the left lobe) which join to form a trunk that merges with that of the left hepatic v.'s about 90% of the time prior to entering the left side of the inferior vena cava. SYN venae hepaticae mediae [NA].

middle meningeal v.'s, the venae comitantes of the middle meningeal artery that empty into the pterygoid plexus. SYN venae meningeae mediae [NA].

middle rectal v.'s, several v.'s that pass from the rectal venous plexus (in which they anastomose with the superior rectal v.'s) to the internal iliac v., which ultimately drains into the inferior vena cava. Since the superior rectal v.'s ultimately drain into the portal v., the middle retal v.'s participate in a portocaval anastomosis, and the rectal venous plexus is subject to varicosities during portal hypertension. SYN venae rectales mediae [NA].

middle temporal v., it arises near the lateral angle of the eye and

ve

joins the superficial temporal v.'s to form the retromandibular v. SYN vena temporalis media [NA].

middle thyroid v., it passes from the thyroid gland across the common carotid artery with the inferior thyroid arteries to empty into the internal jugular v. SYN vena thyroidea media [NA].

musculophrenic v.'s, the v.'s that accompany the musculophrenic artery and drain blood from the upper abdominal wall, and anterior portions of the lower intercostal spaces and the diaphragm. SYN venae musculophrenicae [NA].

nasofrontal v., the v. located in the anterior medial part of the orbit that connects the superior ophthalmic v. with the angular v. SYN vena nasofrontalis [NA].

oblique v. of left atrium, a small v. on the posterior wall of the left atrium which merges with the great cardiac v. to form the coronary sinus; it is developed from the left common cardinal v., and occasionally persists as a left superior vena cava. SYN vena obliqua atrii sinistri [NA], Marshall's oblique v.

obturator v., formed by the union of tributaries draining the hip joint and the obturator and adductor muscles of the thigh; it enters the pelvis by the obturator canal as venae comitantes of the obturator artery and empties into the internal iliac v. SYN vena obturatoria [NA].

occipital v., drains the occipital region and empties into the internal jugular v. or the suboccipital plexus. SYN vena occipitalis [NA].

occipital cerebral v.'s, the superior cerebral v.'s draining the occipital cortex and emptying into the superior sagittal sinus and the transverse sinus. SYN venae occipitales [NA].

occipital emissary v., an inconstant vessel perforating the squama of the occipital bone to connect the occipital v.'s with the confluens sinuum. SYN vena emissaria occipitalis [NA], emissarium occipitale.

v. of olfactory gyrus, SYN *vena gyri olfactorii*.

ophthalmic v.'s, SEE inferior ophthalmic v., superior ophthalmic v.

ovarian v.'s, SEE right ovarian v., left ovarian v.

palatine v., drains the palatine regions and empties into the facial v. SYN vena palatina [NA].

palmar digital v.'s, paired venae comitantes of the proper and common digital arteries that empty into the superficial palmar venous arch. SYN venae digitales palmares [NA].

palmar metacarpal v.'s, v.'s emptying into the deep venous arch from which the radial and ulnar v.'s arise. SYN venae metacarpeae palmares [NA].

palpebral v.'s, v.'s draining the superior eyelid posteriorly as tributaries of the superior ophthalmic v. SYN venae palpebrales [NA], v.'s of eyelids.

pancreatic v.'s, v.'s draining the pancreas, emptying into the splenic v. and the superior mesenteric v. SYN venae pancreaticae [NA].

pancreaticoduodenal v.'s, v.'s that accompany the superior and inferior pancreaticoduodenal arteries, emptying into the superior mesenteric or portal v. SYN venae pancreaticoduodenales [NA].

paraumbilical v.'s, several small v.'s arising from cutaneous v.'s about the umbilicus running along the round ligament of the liver, and terminating as accessory portal v.'s in the substance of this organ; they constitute a portocaval anastomosis and are subject to varicosity druign portal hypertension; varicose paraumbilical v.'s form the "caput medussae". SYN venae paraumbilicales [NA], Sappey's v.'s.

parietal v.'s, the superficial v.'s draining the parietal cerebral cortex and emptying into the superior sagittal sinus. SYN venae parietales [NA].

parietal emissary v., the v. that connects the superior sagittal sinus with the tributaries of the superficial temporal v. and other v.'s of the scalp. SYN vena emissaria parietalis [NA], emissarium parietale, Santorini's v.

parotid v.'s, branches draining part of the parotid gland and emptying into the retromandibular v. SYN venae parotidea [NA], posterior parotid v.'s.

pectoral v.'s, v.'s draining the pectoral muscles and emptying directly into the subclavian v. SYN venae pectorales [NA].

peduncular v.'s, SYN *venae pedunculares*, under *vena*.

perforating v.'s, the v.'s that accompany the perforating arteries from the profunda femoris artery; they drain blood from the vastus lateralis and hamstring muscles and terminate in the profunda femoris v. SYN venae perforantes [NA].

pericardiacophrenic v.'s, the v.'s accompanying the pericardiacophrenic artery and emptying into the brachiocephalic v.'s or superior vena cava. SYN venae pericardiacophrenicae [NA].

pericardial v.'s, several small v.'s from the pericardium emptying into the brachiocephalic v.'s or superior vena cava. SYN venae pericardiacae [NA].

peroneal v.'s, venae comsitantes of the peroneal artery; they join the posterior tibial v.'s to enter the popliteal v. SYN venae peroneae [NA], venae fibulares☆ [NA], fibular v.'s.

petrosal v., a short trunk formed by the union of four or five cerebellar and pontine v.'s opposite the middle cerebellar peduncle; it terminates in the superior petrosal sinus. SEE ALSO superior petrosal *sinus*, inferior petrosal *sinus*. SYN vena petrosa [NA].

pharyngeal v.'s, several v.'s from the pharyngeal venous plexus emptying into the internal jugular v. SYN venae pharyngeae [NA].

phrenic v.'s, SEE inferior phrenic v., superior phrenic v.'s.

plantar digital v.'s, drain the plantar and distal dorsal aspects (nail beds) of the toes and pass back to form four metatarsal v.'s that in turn empty into the plantar venous arch. SYN venae digitales plantares [NA].

plantar metatarsal v.'s, v.'s receiving the plantar digital v.'s and draining in turn into the deep plantar venous arch, which empties into the medial and lateral plantar v.'s. SYN venae metatarseae plantares [NA].

v.'s of pons, SYN pontine v.'s.

pontine v.'s, several v.'s running transversely on the pons to join the petrosal v. SYN venae pontis [NA], v.'s of pons.

popliteal v., formed at the lower border of the popliteus muscle by the union of the anterior and posterior tibial v.'s, ascends through the popliteal space where it receives the lesser saphenous v. and passes through the adductor hiatus, entering the adductor canal as the femoral v. SYN vena poplitea [NA].

portal v., a wide short v. formed by the superior mesenteric and splenic v. posterior to the neck of the pancreas, ascending in front of the inferior vena cava, and dividing at the right end of the porta hepatis into right and left branches, which ramify within the liver. SYN vena portae hepatis [NA], hepatic portal v., vena portalis.

posterior anterior jugular v., a variable tributary of the external jugular v. arising in the upper posterior part of the neck.

posterior auricular v., drains the region posterior to the ear then merges with the retromandibular v. to form the external jugular v. SYN vena auricularis posterior [NA].

posterior cardinal v.'s, SEE cardinal v.'s.

posterior facial v., SYN retromandibular v.

v. of posterior horn, SYN *vena cornus posterioris*.

posterior intercostal v.'s, v.'s draining the intercostal spaces posteriorly; those of the first 1-C space drain into the brachiocephalic v.'s; from spaces 2–3 they drain into right and left superior intercostal v.'s; from the fourth to the eleventh spaces on the right they are tributaries of the azygos v.; on the left they empty into either the hemiazygos or accessory hemiazygos v.'s. SYN venae intercostales posteriores [NA].

posterior labial v.'s, they pass posteriorly from the labia majora and minora to the internal pudendal v.'s. SYN venae labiales posteriores [NA].

posterior v. of left ventricle, arises on the diaphragmatic surface of the heart near the apex, runs to the left and parallel to the posterior interventricular sulcus, and empties in the coronary sinus. SYN vena posterior ventriculi sinistri [NA].

posterior marginal v., SYN *vena corporis callosi dorsalis*.

posterior parotid v.'s, SYN parotid v.'s.

posterior pericallosal v., SYN *vena corporis callosi dorsalis*.

posterior scrotal v.'s, v.'s from the posteriro aspect of the scrotum to the internal pudendal v.'s. SYN venae scrotales posteriores [NA].

posterior v. of septum pellucidum, v. draining the posterior part of the transparent septum; it empties into the superior thalamostriate v. SYN vena septi pellucidi posterior [NA].

posterior tibial v.'s, venae comitantes of the posterior tibial artery that join those of the anterior tibial artery to form the popliteal v. SYN venae tibiales posteriores [NA].

precentral cerebellar v., an unpaired v. originating in the precentral cerebellar fissure passing anterior and superior to the culmen on its way to terminate in the great cerebral v. SYN vena precentralis cerebelli [NA].

prefrontal v.'s, SYN *venae* prefrontales, under *vena*.

prepyloric v., a tributary of the right gastric v. that passes anterior to the pylorus at its junction with the duodenum. SYN vena prepylorica [NA], Latarget's v., Mayo's v.

v. of pterygoid canal, a v. accompanying the nerve and artery through the pterygoid canal and emptying into the pharyngeal venous plexus. SYN vena canalis pterygoidei [NA], vidian v.

pudendal v.'s, SEE external pudendal v.'s, internal pudendal v.

pulmonary v.'s, four v.'s, two on each side, conveying oxygenated blood from the lungs to the left atrium of the heart. Those from the left lung and the inferior v. from the right lung are lobar v.'s, each draining a single lobe with the corresponding name; the right superior pulmonary v. drains both the superior and middle lobes of the right lung. SEE ALSO left inferior pulmonary v., left superior pulmonary v., right inferior pulmonary v., right superior pulmonary v. SYN venae pulmonales [NA].

pyloric v., SYN right gastric v.

radial v.'s, venae comitantes of the raidal artery continuing from those of the radial aspect of the deep palmar arch, draining into the venae comitantes of the brachial artery in the cubital fossa. SYN venae radiales [NA].

renal v.'s, large v.'s formed at the renal hilus by the merger of the segmental v.'s anterior to the corresponding arteries; they open at right angles into the inferior vena cava at the level of the second lumbar vertebra. The left renal v. receives the left suprarenal v. and the left gonadal v., and passes through the angle between the abdominal aorta and superior mesenteric artery where it may be compressed. SYN venae renales [NA].

retromandibular v., it is formed by the union of the superficial temporal and maxillary v.'s in front of the ear, runs posterior to the ramus of the mandible through the parotid gland, and unites with the posterior auricular v. to form the external jugular v.; it usually has a large communicating branch with the facial v. SYN vena retromandibularis [NA], posterior facial v., temporomaxillary v., vena facialis posterior.

Retzius' v.'s, portacaval anastomoses formed from v.'s in the walls of retroperitoneal viscera, such as the ascending and descending colon, passing to the tributaries of the inferior vena cava in the posterior body wall instead of those of the portal v. SYN Ruysch's v.'s.

right colic v., the v. that parallels the right colic artery and drains blood from the ascending colon and right colic flexure. SYN vena colica dextra [NA].

right gastric v., it receives v.'s from both surfaces of the upper portion of the stomach, runs to the right along the lesser curvature of the stomach, and empties into the portal v. SYN vena gastrica dextra [NA], pyloric v.

right gastroepiploic v., a tributary of the superior mesenteric v. that parallels the right gastroepiploic artery along the greater curvature of the stomach. SYN vena gastro-omentalis dextra [NA], right gastroomental v.

right gastroomental v., SYN right gastroepiploic v.

right hepatic v.'s, v.'s draining much of the right lobe of the liver (posterior segments [VI & VII] and part of the inferior anterior segment [V]) which merge to form a single or sometimes double trunk, draining into the right side of the suprahepatic portion of the inferior vena cava (between the superior surface of the liver and the diaphragm); when single, it is the largest v. of the liver. SYN venae hepaticae dextrae [NA].

right inferior pulmonary v., the v. returning oxygenated blood from the inferior lobe of the right lung to the left atrium. SYN vena pulmonalis inferior dextra [NA].

right ovarian v., begins as the pampiniform plexus at the hilum

of the ovary and opens into the inferior vena cava. SYN vena ovarica dextra [NA].

right superior intercostal v., a tributary of the azygos v. formed by the union of the right second, third, and fourth posterior intercostal v.'s. SYN vena intercostalis superior dextra [NA].

right superior pulmonary v., the v. returning oxygenated blood from the superior and middle lobes of the right lung to the left atrium. SYN vena pulmonalis superior dextra [NA].

right suprarenal v., the short v. that passes from the hilum of the right suprarenal to the inferior vena cava. SYN vena suprarenalis dextra [NA].

right testicular v., begins as the pampiniform plexus and ascends to joint the inferior vena cava. SYN vena testicularis dextra [NA].

Rosenthal's v., SYN basal v. of Rosenthal.

Ruysch's v.'s, SYN Retzius' v.'s.

sacral v.'s, SEE lateral sacral v.'s, median sacral v.

Santorini's v., SYN parietal emissary v.

saphenous v.'s, SEE accessory saphenous v., great saphenous v., small saphenous v.

Sappey's v.'s, SYN paraumbilical v.'s.

scleral v.'s, small v.'s draining the sclera; they are tributaries to the anterior ciliary v.'s. SYN venae sclerales [NA].

scrotal v.'s, SEE anterior scrotal v.'s, posterior scrotal v.'s.

v. of septum pellucidum, SEE anterior v. of septum pellucidum, posterior v. of septum pellucidum.

short gastric v.'s, small vessels that drain the fundus and left portion of the stomach wall and empty into the splenic v. SYN venae gastricae breves [NA].

short saphenous v., SYN small saphenous v.

sigmoid v.'s, the several tributaries of the inferior mesenteric v. that drain the sigmoid colon. SYN venae sigmoideae [NA].

small v., a v. in which the three tunics are poorly defined and thin; longitudinal elastic networks occur and the smooth muscle of the media, which is circularly arranged, may be incomplete or in one or two layers.

small cardiac v., an inconstant vessel, accompanying the right coronary artery in the coronary sulcus, from the right margin of the right ventricle, and emptying into the coronary sinus or the middle cardiac v. SYN vena cordis parva [NA].

smallest cardiac v.'s, SYN *venae* cordis minimae, under *vena*.

small saphenous v., arises on the lateral side of the foot from a union of the dorsal v. of the little toe with the dorsal venous arch, ascends behind the lateral malleolus, along the lateral border of the calcanean tendon and then through the middle of the calf to the lower portion of the popliteal space where it empties into the popliteal v. SYN vena saphena parva [NA], short saphenous v.

spermatic v., SEE right testicular v., left testicular v.

spinal v.'s, the v.'s that drain the spinal cord; they form a plexus on the surface of the cord from which v.'s pass along the spinal roots to the internal vertebral venous plexus. SYN venae spinales [NA].

spiral v. of modiolus, the v. running a spiral course in the modiolus of the cochlea; it is tributary to both the labyrinthine v. and the v. of the cochlear canaliculus. SYN vena spiralis modioli [NA].

splenic v., arises by the union of several small v.'s at the hilum on the anterior surface of the spleen with the short gastric and left gastroepiploic v.'s; passes backward through the splenorenal ligament to the left kidney, then runs behind the upper border of the pancreas to the neck of the pancreas where it joins the superior mesenteric v. to form the portal v. SYN vena splenica [NA], vena lienalis.

stellate v.'s, SYN *venulae* stellatae, under *venula*.

Stensen's v.'s, SYN vortex v.'s.

sternocleidomastoid v., it arises in the sternocleidomastoid muscle and accompanies the sternocleidomastoid branch of the occipital artery; it drains into the internal jugular or superior thyroid v. SYN vena sternocleidomastoidea [NA].

striate v.'s, SYN inferior thalamostriate v.'s.

vein strip′per, an instrument used to remove a vein by tying the

ve

vein at one end and pulling it, tearing its branches, and thus, stripping it out of the body.

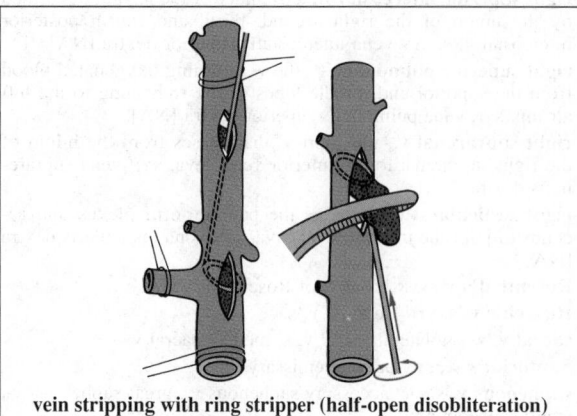

vein stripping with ring stripper (half-open disobliteration)

stylomastoid v., it drains the tympanic cavity, traverses the facial canal exiting via the stylomastoid foramen, and empties into the retromandibular v. SYN vena stylomastoidea [NA].

subclavian v., the direct continuation of the axillary v. at the lateral border of the first rib; it passes medially to join the internal jugular v. and form the brachiocephalic v. on each side. SYN vena subclavia [NA].

subcutaneous v.'s of abdomen, the network of superficial v.'s of the abdominal wall that empty into the thoracoepigastric, superficial epigastric, or superior epigastric v.'s and form portocaval anastomoses through their communications with the paraumbilical v.'s. SYN venae subcutaneae abdominis [NA].

sublingual v., v. which accompanies the sublingual artery in the floor of the mouth, lateral to the hypoglossal nerve; it may join the deep lingual v. to form the lingual v., or join the vena comitans nerve hypoglossi. SYN vena sublingualis [NA].

submental v., a v. situated below the chin, anastomosing with the sublingual v., connecting with the anterior jugular v., and emptying into the facial v. SYN vena submentalis [NA].

superficial v., one of a number of v.'s that course in the subcutaneous tissue and empty into deep v.'s; they form prominent systems of vessels in the limbs and are usually not accompanied by arteries. SYN vena cutanea [NA], cutaneous v.

superficial cerebral v.'s, the v.'s on the superficial surface of the cerebral hemispheres; they comprise three groups: superior, middle, and inferior. SYN venae cerebri superficiales [NA].

superficial circumflex iliac v., corresponding to the artery of the same name, emptying usually into the great saphenous v., or sometimes into the femoral v. SYN vena circumflexa iliaca superficialis [NA].

superficial dorsal v.'s of clitoris, a pair of v.'s on the dorsum of the clitoris, tributary to the external pudendal v. on either side. SYN venae dorsales clitoridis superficiales [NA].

superficial dorsal v.'s of penis, a pair of v.'s on the dorsum of the penis superficial to the fascia penis; they are tributaries of the external pudendal v.'s on each side. SYN venae dorsales penis superficiales [NA].

superficial epigastric v., drains the lower and medial part of the anterior abdominal wall and empties into the great saphenous v. SYN vena epigastrica superficialis [NA].

superficial middle cerebral v., a large v. passing along the line of the sylvian fissure to join the cavernous sinus; it communicates with the superior sagittal sinus and transverse sinus via the superior and inferior anastomotic v.'s, respectively. SYN vena cerebri media superficialis [NA].

superficial temporal v.'s, v.'s that pass from the temporal region to join the maxillary v. to form the retromandibular v. SYN venae temporales superficiales [NA].

superior anastomotic v., a large communicating v. between the superficial middle cerebral v. and the superior sagittal sinus; it passes upward from the lateral sulcus, often following the line of the central sulcus (Rolando's fissure). SYN vena anastomotica superior [NA], Trolard's v.

superior basal v., tributary to the common basal v. draining the lateral and anterior part of the inferior lobe of each lung. SYN vena basalis superior [NA].

superior v.'s of cerebellar hemisphere, several v.'s draining the superior part of the cerebellar hemispheres; they terminate in the superior petrosal sinus or the petrosal v. SYN venae hemispherii cerebelli superiores [NA].

superior cerebral v.'s, numerous (8 to 10) v.'s that drain the dorsal convexity of the cortical hemisphere and empty into the superior sagittal sinus, curving rostrally in passing through the subdural space so as to enter the sinus at an acute forward angle. SYN venae cerebri superiores [NA].

superior choroid v., a tortuous v. that follows the choroid plexus of the lateral ventricle and unites with the superior thalamostriate v. and the anterior v. of the transparent septum to form the internal cerebral v. SYN vena choroidea superior [NA].

superior epigastric v.'s, the venae comitantes of the artery of the same name, tributaries of the internal thoracic v. SYN venae epigastricae superiores [NA].

v.'s of superior eyelid, SYN superior palpebral v.'s.

superior gluteal v.'s, the v.'s that accompany the superior gluteal artery, entering the pelvis as two v.'s which unite into one and empty into the internal iliac v. SYN venae gluteae superiores [NA].

superior hemorrhoidal v., outmoded term for superior rectal v.

superior intercostal v., SEE left superior intercostal v., right superior intercostal v.

superior labial v., v.'s taking blood from the upper lip and discharging into the facial v. SYN vena labialis superior [NA].

superior laryngeal v., vein which accompanies the superior laryngeal artery and empties into the superior thyroid vein. SYN vena laryngea superior [NA].

superior mesenteric v., begins at the ileum in the right iliac fossa, ascends in the root of the mesentery, and unites behind the pancreas with the splenic v. to form the hepatic portal v. SYN vena mesenterica superior [NA].

superior ophthalmic v., begins anteriorly from the nasofrontal v., passes along the upper part of the medial wall of the orbit, passes through the superior orbital fissure, to empty into the cavernous sinus. SYN vena ophthalmica superior [NA].

superior palpebral v.'s, v.'s draining the superior eyelid anteriorly into the angular v. SYN venae palpebrales superiores [NA], v.'s of superior eyelid.

superior phrenic v.'s, small v.'s that drain the upper surface of the diaphragm; they are tributaries of the azygos and hemiazygos v.'s. SYN venae phrenicae superiores [NA].

superior rectal v., it drains the greater part of the rectal venous plexus, and ascends between the layers of the mesorectum to the brim of the pelvis, where it becomes the inferior mesenteric v. As a tributary of the portal v., it forms a portocaval anastomosis with the middle and inferior rectal v.'s (caval tributaries) via the rectal venous plexus. SYN vena rectalis superior [NA].

superior thalamostriate v., a long v. passing forward in the groove between the thalamus and caudate nucleus, covered by the lamina affixa, receiving the transverse caudate v.'s along its lateral side, and joining at the caudal wall of Monro's foramen with the choroidal v. and v. of septum pellucidum to form the internal cerebral v. SYN vena terminalis [NA], vena thalamostriata superior [NA], terminal v., v. of corpus striatum.

superior thyroid v., receives blood from the upper part of the thyroid gland and larynx, accompanies the artery of the same name, and empties into the internal jugular v. SYN vena thyroidea superior [NA].

superior v. of vermis, a v. draining part of the superior part of the cerebellum; it runs on the superior surface of the vermis to terminate in the internal cerebral v. SYN vena vermis superior [NA].

supraorbital v., drains the front of the scalp and unites with the supratrochlear v.'s to form the angular v. SYN vena supraorbitalis [NA].

suprarenal v.'s, SEE right suprarenal v., left suprarenal v.

suprascapular v., v. that accompanies the suprascapular artery and empties into the external jugular v. SYN vena suprascapularis [NA], transverse v. of scapula, vena transversa scapulae.

supratrochlear v.'s, several v.'s that drain the front part of the scalp and unite with the supraorbital v. to form the angular v. SYN venae supratrochleares [NA], frontal v.'s (2), venae frontales (2), venae frontales (1).

supreme intercostal v., SYN highest intercostal v.

surface thalamic v.'s, SYN *venae* directae laterales, under *vena.*

temporal v.'s, SEE middle temporal v., deep temporal v.'s, superficial temporal v.'s.

v.'s of temporomandibular joint, several small tributaries to the retromandibular v. from the temporomandibular joint. SYN venae articulares temporomandibulares.

temporomaxillary v., SYN retromandibular v.

terminal v., SYN superior thalamostriate v.

testicular v.'s, SEE right testicular v., left testicular v.

thalamostriate v.'s, SEE inferior thalamostriate v.'s, superior thalamostriate v.

thebesian v.'s, SYN *venae* cordis minimae, under *vena.*

thoracic v.'s, SEE internal thoracic v., lateral thoracic v.

thoracoacromial v., corresponding to the artery of the same name, empties into the axillary v., sometimes by a common trunk with the cephalic v. SYN vena thoracoacromialis [NA], thoracic axis (2).

thoracoepigastric v., one of two v.'s, sometimes a single v., arising from the region of the superficial epigastric v. and opening into the axillary or the lateral thoracic v., thus forming an anastomotic or collateral pathway between tributaries of the inferior and superior venae cavae. SYN vena thoracoepigastrica [NA].

thymic v.'s, a number of small v.'s from the thymus emptying into the left brachiocephalic v. SYN venae thymicae [NA].

thyroid v.'s, SEE inferior thyroid v., middle thyroid v., superior thyroid v., *plexus* thyroideus impar.

tracheal v.'s, several small venous trunks from the trachea, emptying into the brachiocephalic v.'s or the superior vena cava. SYN venae tracheales [NA].

transverse cervical v.'s, venae comitantes of the corresponding arteries, emptying into the external jugular v. or sometimes into the subclavian v. SYN venae transversae colli [NA], transverse v.'s of neck.

transverse v. of face, SYN transverse facial v.

transverse facial v., a tributary of the superficial temporal or retromandibular v.'s, anastomosing with the facial v. SYN vena transversa faciei [NA], transverse v. of face.

transverse v.'s of neck, SYN transverse cervical v.'s.

transverse v. of scapula, SYN suprascapular v.

Trolard's v., SYN superior anastomotic v.

tympanic v.'s, v.'s exiting from the tympanic cavity through the petrotympanic fissure with the chorda tympani and emptying into the retromandibular v. SYN venae tympanicae [NA].

ulnar v.'s, venae comitantes of the ulnar artery, continuing from those of the superficial palmar arch and joining with those of the radial artery to form the brachial veins in the cubital fossa. SYN venae ulnares [NA].

umbilical v., SEE left umbilical v.

v. of uncus, SYN *vena* unci.

uterine v.'s, two v.'s on each side which arise from the uterine venous plexus, pass through a part of the broad ligament and then through a peritoneal fold, and empty into the internal iliac v. SYN venae uterinae [NA].

varicose v.'s, permanent dilation and tortuosity of v.'s, most commonly seen in the legs, probably as a result of congenitally incomplete valves; there is a predisposition to varicose v.'s among persons in occupations requiring long periods of standing, and in pregnant women.

vertebral v., a v. derived from tributaries (venae comitantes) which run through the foramina in the transverse processes of the first six cervical vertebrae and form a plexus around the vertebral artery; it empties as a single trunk into the brachiocephalic v.'s. SYN vena vertebralis [NA].

v.'s of vertebral column, includes the internal and external

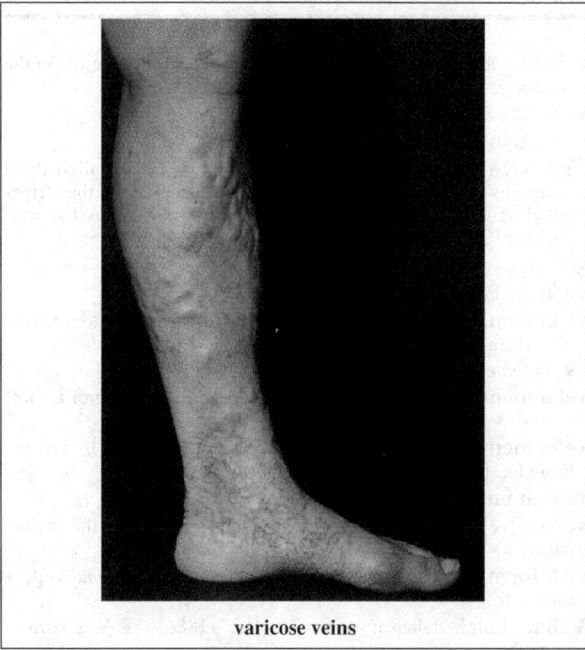

varicose veins

vertebral venous plexuses, the basivertebral v.'s, and the anterior and posterior spinal v.'s. SYN venae columnae vertebralis [NA].

Vesalius' v., the emissary v. passing through the foramen venosum.

vesical v.'s, v.'s that drain the vesical venous plexus; they join the internal iliac v.'s. SYN venae vesicales [NA].

vestibular v.'s, v.'s draining the saccule and utricle; they are tributaries of both the labyrinthine v.'s and the v. of the vestibular aqueduct. SYN venae vestibulares [NA].

v. of vestibular aqueduct, a small v. accompanying the endolymphatic duct; it drains much of the vestibular portion of the labyrinth and terminates in the inferior petrosal sinus. SYN vena aqueductus vestibuli [NA].

v. of vestibular bulb, the v. draining the bulb of the vestibule; a tributary of the internal pudendal v. SYN vena bulbi vestibuli [NA].

vidian v., SYN v. of pterygoid canal.

Vieussens' v.'s, SYN innominate cardiac v.'s.

vitelline v., a v. returning blood from the yolk sac to the embryo. SYN vena vitellina.

vortex v.'s, several v.'s (usually four) from the vascular tunic formed of v.'s accompanying the posterior ciliary arteries and the ciliary body; then drain into the superior or inferior ophthalmic

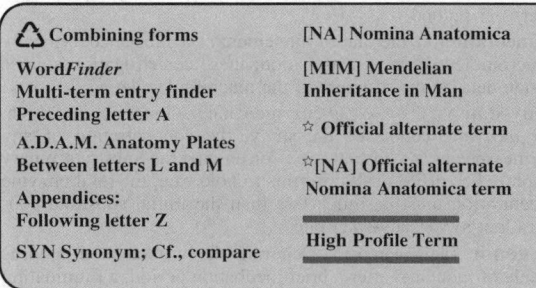

♻ **Combining forms**	**[NA] Nomina Anatomica**
Word*Finder* **Multi-term entry finder** Preceding letter A	**[MIM] Mendelian Inheritance in Man**
A.D.A.M. Anatomy Plates Between letters L and M	☆ **Official alternate term**
Appendices: Following letter Z	☆**[NA] Official alternate Nomina Anatomica term**
SYN Synonym; Cf., compare	**High Profile Term**

ve

v. SYN venae vorticosae [NA], venae choroideae oculi[★] [NA], choroid v.'s of eye, Stensen's v.'s, vasa vorticosa, vorticose v.'s. **vorticose v.'s,** SYN vortex v.'s.

veined (vānd). Marked by veins or lines resembling veins on the surface.

vein·let (vān'let). SYN venule.

vein strip·'per. See under vein.

Ve·jo·vis (vē-jō'vis). A genus of scorpions (the so-called devil scorpions of North America), including *V. spinigerus*, the stripe-tailed devil scorpion; *V. carolinianus*, the southern devil scorpion; and *V. flavus*, the slender devil scorpion.

vel (vel). or [L. or]

ve·la (vē'lă). Plural of velum.

ve·la·men, pl. **ve·lam·i·na** (vē-lā'men, vě-lam'i-nă). SYN velum (1). [L. a veil]

v. **vul'vae,** hypertrophy of the labia minora.

vel·a·men·tous (vel-ă-men'tŭs). Expanded in the form of a sheet or veil. SYN veliform.

vel·a·men·tum, pl. **vel·a·men·ta** (vel'ă-men'tŭm, -tă). SYN velum (1). [L. a cover]

ve·lam·i·na (vě-lam'i-nă). Plural of velamen.

ve·lar (vē'lăr). Relating to any velum, especially the velum palati.

ve·li·form (vel'i-fōrm). SYN velamentous. [L. *velum,* veil, + *forma,* form]

Vella, Luigi, Italian physiologist, 1825–1886. SEE V.'s *fistula;* Thiry-V. *fistula.*

vel·li·cate (vel'i-kāt). To twitch or contract spasmodically; said especially of fibrillary muscular spasms. [L. *vellico,* pp. *-atus,* to pluck, to twitch, fr. *vello,* to deprive of hair, pluck]

vel·li·ca·tion (vel'i-kā'shŭn). A fibrillary muscular spasm.

vel·lus (vel'ŭs). **1.** Fine nonpigmented hair covering most of the body. **2.** A structure that is fleecy or soft and woolly in appearance. [L. fleece]

v. **oli'vae inferio'ris,** a stratum of nerve fibers surrounding the inferior olive.

ve·loc·i·ty (v) (vě-los'i-tē). Rate and direction of movement; specifically, distance traveled or quantity converted per unit time in a given direction. Cf. speed. [L. *velocitas,* fr. *velox (veloc-),* quick, swift]

initial v., the rate of a reaction, *e.g.,* an enzyme-catalyzed reaction, at the early stages of the reaction such that the product(s) concentrations have not risen to a level to significantly affect the observable rate; typically, initial v.'s are observed when less than 10% of the reaction's approach toward equilibrium has occurred. SYN initial rate.

maximum v. (V_{max}), (1) the maximum rate of an enzyme-catalyzed reaction that can be achieved by progressively increasing the substrate concentration at a given enzyme concentration; in cases of substrate inhibition, V_{max} is an extrapolated value in the absence of such inhibition; Cf. Michaelis-Menten *equation.* **(2)** the maximum initial rate of shortening of a myocardial fiber that can be obtained under zero load; used to evaluate the contractility of the fiber.

nerve conduction v., the rate of impulse conduction in a peripheral nerve or its various component fibers, generally expressed in meters per second.

sedimentation v., the rate of movement of a substance, typically a macromolecule, in centrifugation; these centrifugation studies provide data on the structure of the macromolecule.

steady-state v., the v. of an enzyme-catalyzed reaction in which, over the time course of the study, the concentration of any enzyme species is constant (*i.e.,* for an enzyme-substrate binary complex, ES, d[ES]/dt≡00; for this to hold true, the total enzyme concentration must be much less than the initial substrate concentration. SYN steady-state rate.

vel·o·gen·ic (vel-ō-jen'ik). Denoting the virulence of a virus capable of inducing, after a brief incubation period, a fulminating and often lethal disease in embryonic, immature, and adult hosts;

used in characterizing Newcastle disease virus. [L. *velox,* rapid, + G. *-gen,* producing]

ve·lo·no·ski·as·co·py (vē'lō-nō-ski-as'kŏ-pē). An obsolete subjective test for ametropia in which a thin rod is moved across the pupil while a distant light source is fixed; the shadow of the rod moves with the rod in myopia, and in the opposite direction in hyperopia. [G. *velonē (belonē),* needle, + skiascopy]

vel·o·pha·ryn·ge·al (vē'lō-fă-rin'jē-ăl). Pertaining to the soft palate (velum palatinum) and the posterior nasopharyngeal wall.

ve·lo·syn·the·sis (vē'lō-sin'thě-sis). SYN palatorrhaphy.

Velpeau, Alfred A.L.M., French surgeon, 1795–1867. SEE V.'s *bandage, canal, fossa, hernia.*

ve·lum, pl. **ve·la** (vē'lŭm, -lă). **1.** Any structure resembling a veil or curtain. SYN veil (1), velamen, velamentum. **2.** SYN caul (1). **3.** SYN greater *omentum.* **4.** Any serous membrane or membranous envelope or covering. [L. veil, sail]

anterior medullary v., SYN superior medullary v.

inferior medullary v., a thin sheet of white matter, hidden by the cerebellar tonsil, attached along the peduncle of the flocculus and, at and near the midline, to the nodulus of the vermis; it is continuous caudally with the epithelial lamina and choroid plexus of the fourth ventricle. SYN v. medullare inferius [NA], posterior medullary v., Tarin's valve, valvula semilunaris tarini, v. semilunare, v. tarini.

v. **interpos'itum,** SYN choroid *tela* of third ventricle.

v. **medulla're infe'rius** [NA], SYN inferior medullary v.

v. **medulla're supe'rius** [NA], SYN superior medullary v.

v. **palati'num** [NA], [★]official alternate term for soft *palate,* soft *palate.*

v. **pen'dulum pala'ti,** SYN soft *palate.*

posterior medullary v., SYN inferior medullary v.

v. **semiluna're,** SYN inferior medullary v.

superior medullary v., the thin layer of white matter stretching between the two superior cerebellar peduncles, forming the roof of the superior recess of the fourth ventricle. SYN v. medullare superius [NA], anterior medullary v., Vieussens' valve.

v. **tari'ni,** SYN inferior medullary v.

v. **termina'le,** SYN *lamina* terminalis of cerebrum.

transverse v., a fold in the dorsal wall of the embryonic brain at the boundary between the telencephalon and diencephalon. SYN v. transversum.

v. **transver'sum,** SYN transverse v.

v. **triangula're,** SYN choroid *tela* of third ventricle.

VENA

ve·na, gen. and pl. **ve·nae** (vē'nă, -nē) [NA]. SYN vein. [L.]

v. **ad'vehens**, pl. **ve'nae advehen'tes,** collective term for a series of branching channels in the early embryo receiving blood from the umbilical and/or vitelline venous systems and passing the mixed blood to the sinusoids of the liver; they become terminal branches of the hepatic portal vein. SYN v. afferentes hepatis.

v. **afferen'tes hepa'tis,** SYN v. advehens.

v. **anastomot'ica infe'rior** [NA], SYN inferior anastomotic *vein.*

v. **anastomot'ica supe'rior** [NA], SYN superior anastomotic *vein.*

v. **angula'ris** [NA], SYN angular *vein.*

v. **appendicula'ris** [NA], SYN appendicular *vein.*

v. **aqueduc'tus coch'leae** [NA], SYN *vein* of cochlear canaliculus.

v. **aqueduc'tus vestib'uli** [NA], SYN *vein* of vestibular aqueduct.

ve'nae arcua'tae re'nis [NA], SYN arcuate *veins* of kidney, under *vein.*

v. **arterio'sa,** SYN arterial *vein.*

ve'nae articula'res temporomandibula'res, SYN *veins* of temporomandibular joint, under *vein.*

v. **a'trii latera'lis** [NA], a vein draining deep portions of the temporal and parietal lobes; it runs in the lateral wall of the lateral ventricle to terminate in the superior thalamostriate vein.

SYN v. ventriculi lateralis lateralis [NA], lateral atrial vein, lateral vein of lateral ventricle.

v. a'trii media'lis [NA], a vein that drains deep portions of the parietal and occipital lobes; it runs in the medial wall of the lateral ventricle to empty into the internal cerebral vein or the great cerebral vein. SYN v. ventriculi lateralis medialis [NA], medial atrial vein, medial vein of lateral ventricle.

v. auricula'ris ante'rior [NA], SYN anterior auricular *vein*.

v. auricula'ris poste'rior [NA], SYN posterior auricular *vein*.

v. axilla'ris [NA], SYN axillary *vein*.

v. az'ygos [NA], SYN azygos *vein*.

v. az'ygos ma'jor, SYN azygos *vein*.

v. az'ygos mi'nor infe'rior, SYN hemiazygos *vein*.

v. az'ygos mi'nor supe'rior, SYN accessory hemiazygos *vein*.

v. basa'lis [NA], SYN basal *vein* of Rosenthal.

v. basa'lis commu'nis [NA], SYN common basal *vein*.

v. basa'lis infe'rior [NA], SYN inferior basal *vein*.

v. basa'lis supe'rior [NA], SYN superior basal *vein*.

v. basil'ica [NA], SYN basilic *vein*.

v. basivertebra'lis [NA], SYN basivertebral *vein*.

Billroth's venae cavernosae, SYN venae cavernosae of spleen.

ve'nae brachia'les [NA], SYN brachial *veins*, under *vein*.

ve'nae brachiocephal'icae [NA], SYN brachiocephalic *veins*, under *vein*.

ve'nae bronchia'les [NA], SYN bronchial *veins*, under *vein*.

v. bul'bi pe'nis [NA], SYN *vein* of bulb of penis.

v. bul'bi vestib'uli [NA], SYN *vein* of vestibular bulb.

v. canalic'uli coch'leae, SYN *vein* of cochlear canaliculus.

v. cana'lis pterygoi'dei [NA], SYN *vein* of pterygoid canal.

v. cardi'aca mag'na, SYN great cardiac *vein*.

v. ca'va infe'rior [NA], SYN inferior v. cava.

v. ca'va supe'rior [NA], SYN superior v. cava.

ve'nae caverno'sae pe'nis [NA], SYN cavernous *veins* of penis, under *vein*.

ve'nae centra'les hep'atis [NA], SYN central *veins* of liver, under *vein*.

v. centra'lis glan'dulae suprarena'lis [NA], SYN central *vein* of suprarenal gland.

v. centra'lis ret'inae [NA], SYN central *vein* of retina.

v. cephal'ica [NA], SYN cephalic *vein*.

v. cephal'ica accesso'ria [NA], SYN accessory cephalic *vein*.

ve'nae cerebel'li [NA], SYN cerebellar *veins*, under *vein*.

ve'nae cerebel'li inferio'res, SEE inferior *veins* of cerebellar hemisphere, under *vein*.

ve'nae cerebel'li superio'res, SEE superior *veins* of cerebellar hemisphere, under *vein*.

v. cer'ebri ante'rior [NA], SYN anterior cerebral *vein*.

ve'nae cer'ebri inferio'res [NA], SYN inferior cerebral *veins*, under *vein*.

ve'nae cer'ebri inter'nae [NA], SYN internal cerebral *veins*, under *vein*.

v. cer'ebri mag'na [NA], SYN great cerebral *vein* of Galen.

v. cer'ebri me'dia profun'da [NA], SYN deep middle cerebral *vein*.

v. cer'ebri me'dia superficia'lis [NA], SYN superficial middle cerebral *vein*.

ve'nae cer'ebri profun'dae [NA], SYN deep cerebral *veins*, under *vein*.

ve'nae cer'ebri superficia'les [NA], SYN superficial cerebral *veins*, under *vein*.

ve'nae cer'ebri superio'res [NA], SYN superior cerebral *veins*, under *vein*.

v. cervica'lis profun'da [NA], SYN deep cervical *vein*.

ve'nae choroi'deae oc'uli [NA], ✫official alternate term for vortex *veins*, under *vein*.

v. choroi'dea infe'rior [NA], SYN inferior choroid *vein*.

v. choroi'dea supe'rior [NA], SYN superior choroid *vein*.

ve'nae cilia'res [NA], SYN ciliary *veins*, under *vein*.

ve'nae circumflex'ae fem'oris latera'les [NA], SYN lateral circumflex femoral *veins*, under *vein*.

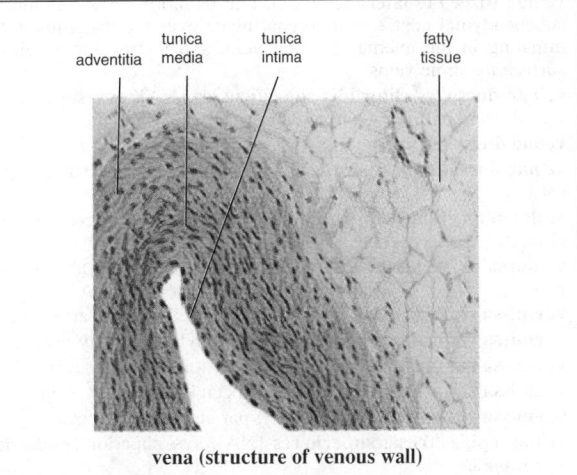

vena (structure of venous wall)

ve'nae circumflex'ae fem'oris media'les [NA], SYN medial circumflex femoral *veins*, under *vein*.

v. circumflex'a ili'aca profun'da [NA], SYN deep circumflex iliac *vein*.

v. circumflex'a ili'aca superficia'lis [NA], SYN superficial circumflex iliac *vein*.

v. col'ica dex'tra [NA], SYN right colic *vein*.

v. col'ica me'dia [NA], SYN middle colic *vein*.

v. col'ica sinis'tra [NA], SYN left colic *vein*.

ve'nae colum'nae vertebra'lis [NA], SYN *veins* of vertebral column, under *vein*.

v. com'itans [NA], a vein accompanying another structure. SYN accompanying vein, companion vein.

v. com'itans ner'vi hypoglos'si [NA], runs with the hypoglossal nerve below and lateral to the hyoglossus muscle, emptying usually into the lingual vein. SYN accompanying vein of hypoglossal nerve.

ve'nae comitan'tes [NA], a pair of veins, occasionally more, that closely accompany an artery in such a manner that the pulsations of the artery aid venous return. SYN companion veins.

ve'nae conjunctiva'les [NA], SYN conjunctival *veins*, under *vein*.

ve'nae cor'dis anterio'res [NA], SYN anterior cardiac *veins*, under *vein*.

v. cor'dis mag'na [NA], SYN great cardiac *vein*.

v. cor'dis me'dia [NA], SYN middle cardiac *vein*.

ve'nae cor'dis min'imae [NA], numerous small valveless venous channels that open directly into the chambers of the heart from the capillary bed in the cardiac wall, enabling a form of collateral circulation unique to the heart. SYN smallest cardiac veins, thebesian veins.

v. cor'dis par'va [NA], SYN small cardiac *vein*.

v. cor'nus posterio'ris [NA], a small vein draining the surface region of the posterior horn of the lateral ventricle; it is a tributary to the great cerebral vein. SYN vein of posterior horn.

v. corona'ria ventric'uli, SYN left gastric *vein*.

v. cor'poris callo'si dorsa'lis [NA], it originates on the superior surface of the corpus callosum and runs posteriorly to terminate in the great cerebral vein. SYN dorsal callosal vein, dorsal vein of corpus callosum, posterior marginal vein, posterior pericallosal vein.

v. cuta'nea [NA], SYN superficial *vein*.

v. cys'tica [NA], SYN cystic *vein*.

ve'nae digita'les dorsa'les pe'dis [NA], SYN dorsal digital *veins* of foot, under *vein*.

ve'nae digita'les palma'res [NA], SYN palmar digital *veins*, under *vein*.

ve'nae digita'les planta'res [NA], SYN plantar digital *veins*, under *vein*.

v. diplo'ica [NA], SYN diploic *vein*.

ve

ve'nae direc'tae latera'les [NA], one or more veins running a subependymal course in a coronal plane over the thalamus, terminating in the internal cerebral vein. SYN lateral direct veins, surface thalamic veins.

ve'nae dorsa'les clitor'idis superficia'les [NA], SYN superficial dorsal veins of clitoris, under vein.

venae dorsa'les lin'guae [NA], SYN dorsal lingual vein.

ve'nae dorsa'les pe'nis superficia'les [NA], SYN superficial dorsal veins of penis, under vein.

v. dorsa'lis clitor'idis profun'da [NA], SYN deep dorsal vein of clitoris.

v. dorsa'lis pe'nis profun'da [NA], SYN deep dorsal vein of penis.

v. emissa'ria, pl. ve'nae emissa'riae [NA], SYN emissary vein.

v. emissa'ria condyla'ris [NA], SYN condylar emissary vein.

v. emissa'ria mastoi'dea [NA], SYN mastoid emissary vein.

v. emissa'ria occipita'lis [NA], SYN occipital emissary vein.

v. emissa'ria parieta'lis [NA], SYN parietal emissary vein.

ve'nae epigas'tricae superio'res [NA], SYN superior epigastric veins, under vein.

v. epigas'trica infe'rior [NA], SYN inferior epigastric vein.

v. epigas'trica superficia'lis [NA], SYN superficial epigastric vein.

ve'nae episclera'les [NA], SYN episcleral veins, under vein.

ve'nae esopha'geae [NA], SYN esophageal veins, under vein.

ve'nae ethmoida'les [NA], SYN ethmoidal veins, under vein.

v. facia'lis, SYN facial vein.

v. facia'lis ante'rior, SYN facial vein.

v. facia'lis commu'nis, SYN common facial vein.

v. facia'lis poste'rior, SYN retromandibular vein.

v. facie'i profun'da [NA], SYN deep facial vein.

v. femora'lis [NA], SYN femoral vein.

ve'nae fibula'res [NA], *official alternate term for peroneal veins, under vein, peroneal veins, under vein.

ve'nae fronta'les, (1) [NA], SYN supratrochlear veins, under vein. (2) SYN supratrochlear veins, under vein.

v. gas'trica dex'tra [NA], SYN right gastric vein.

ve'nae gas'tricae bre'ves [NA], SYN short gastric veins, under vein.

v. gas'trica sinis'tra [NA], SYN left gastric vein.

v. gastro-omenta'lis dex'tra [NA], SYN right gastroepiploic vein.

v. gastro-omenta'lis sinis'tra [NA], SYN left gastroepiploic vein.

ve'nae ge'nus [NA], SYN veins of knee, under vein.

ve'nae glu'teae inferio'res [NA], SYN inferior gluteal veins, under vein.

ve'nae glu'teae superio'res [NA], SYN superior gluteal veins, under vein.

v. gy'ri olfacto'rii [NA], a tributary of the basal vein which drains the medial olfactory stria. SYN vein of olfactory gyrus.

v. hemiaz'ygos [NA], SYN hemiazygos vein.

v. hemiaz'ygos accesso'ria [NA], SYN accessory hemiazygos vein.

ve'nae hemisphe'rii cerebel'li inferio'res [NA], SYN inferior veins of cerebellar hemisphere, under vein.

ve'nae hemisphe'rii cerebel'li superio'res [NA], SYN superior veins of cerebellar hemisphere, under vein.

ve'nae hemorrhoida'les inferio'res, outmoded term for inferior rectal veins, under vein.

ve'nae hemorrhoida'les me'diae, outmoded term for middle rectal veins, under vein.

v. hemorrhoida'lis supe'rior, outmoded term for superior rectal vein.

ve'nae hepat'icae [NA], SYN hepatic veins, under vein.

ve'nae hepat'icae dex'trae [NA], SYN right hepatic veins, under vein.

ve'nae hepat'icae me'diae [NA], SYN middle hepatic veins, under vein.

ve'nae hepat'icae sinis'trae [NA], SYN left hepatic veins, under vein.

v. hypogas'trica, obsolete term for internal iliac vein.

v. ileocol'ica [NA], SYN ileocolic vein.

v. ili'aca commu'nis [NA], SYN common iliac vein.

v. ili'aca exter'na [NA], SYN external iliac vein.

v. ili'aca inter'na [NA], SYN internal iliac vein.

v. iliolumba'lis [NA], SYN iliolumbar vein.

inferior v. cava (IVC), receives the blood from the lower limbs and the greater part of the pelvic and abdominal organs; it begins at the level of the fifth lumbar vertebra on the right side by the merger of the right and left common iliac veins, pierces the diaphragm at the level of the eighth thoracic vertebra, and empties into the posteroinferior aspect of the right atrium of the heart. SYN v. cava inferior [NA], postcava.

v. innomina'ta, archaic term for brachiocephalic veins, under vein.

ve'nae insula'res [NA], veins draining the cortex of the insula, tributaries to the deep middle cerebral vein. SYN insular veins.

ve'nae intercapita'les [NA], SYN intercapitular veins, under vein.

ve'nae intercosta'les anterio'res [NA], SYN anterior intercostal veins, under vein.

ve'nae intercosta'les posterio'res [NA], SYN posterior intercostal veins, under vein.

v. intercosta'lis supe'rior dex'tra [NA], SYN right superior intercostal vein.

v. intercosta'lis supe'rior sinis'tra [NA], SYN left superior intercostal vein.

v. intercosta'lis supre'ma [NA], SYN highest intercostal vein.

ve'nae interloba'res re'nis [NA], SYN interlobar veins of kidney, under vein.

ve'nae interlobula'res hep'atis [NA], SYN interlobular veins of liver, under vein.

ve'nae interlobula'res re'nis [NA], SYN interlobular veins of kidney, under vein.

v. interme'dia antebra'chii [NA], SYN median antebrachial vein.

v. interme'dia basil'ica [NA], SYN intermediate basilic vein.

v. interme'dia cephal'ica [NA], SYN intermediate cephalic vein.

v. interme'dia cu'biti [NA], SYN median cubital vein.

v. intervertebra'lis [NA], SYN intervertebral vein.

ve'nae jejuna'les et il'ei [NA], SYN jejunal and ileal veins, under vein.

v. jugula'ris ante'rior [NA], SYN anterior jugular vein.

v. jugula'ris exter'na [NA], SYN external jugular vein.

v. jugula'ris inter'na [NA], SYN internal jugular vein.

ve'nae labia'les anterio'res [NA], SYN anterior labial veins, under vein.

ve'nae labia'les posterio'res [NA], SYN posterior labial veins, under vein.

v. labia'lis infe'rior [NA], SYN inferior labial vein.

v. labia'lis supe'rior [NA], SYN superior labial vein.

ve'nae labyrin'thi [NA], SYN labyrinthine veins, under vein.

v. lacrima'lis [NA], SYN lacrimal vein.

v. laryn'gea infe'rior [NA], SYN inferior laryngeal vein.

v. laryn'gea supe'rior [NA], SYN superior laryngeal vein.

v. liena'lis, SYN splenic vein.

v. lingua'lis [NA], SYN lingual vein.

ve'nae lumba'les [NA], SYN lumbar veins, under vein.

v. lumba'lis ascen'dens [NA], SYN ascending lumbar vein.

v. mamma'ria inter'na, obsolete term for internal thoracic vein.

v. maxilla'ris, pl. ve'nae maxilla'res [NA], SYN maxillary vein.

v. media'na antebra'chii, SYN median antebrachial vein.

v. media'na basil'ica, SYN intermediate basilic vein.

v. media'na cephal'ica, SYN intermediate cephalic vein.

v. media'na cu'biti, SYN median cubital vein.

ve'nae mediastina'les [NA], SYN mediastinal veins, under vein.

ve'nae medul'lae oblonga'tae [NA], several veins draining the medulla oblongata; they are tributaries of the anterior spinal vein and the petrosal vein. SYN veins of medulla oblongata.

ve'nae menin'geae [NA], SYN meningeal veins, under vein.

ve'nae menin'geae me'diae [NA], SYN middle meningeal veins, under vein.

ve'nae mesencephal'icae [NA], several veins draining the mesencephalon; the posterior ones are tributaries to the great cerebral vein; the lateral ones are tributaries to the basal vein. SYN mesencephalic veins.

v. mesenter'ica infe'rior [NA], SYN inferior mesenteric *vein.*

v. mesenter'ica supe'rior [NA], SYN superior mesenteric *vein.*

ve'nae metacar'peae dorsa'les [NA], SYN dorsal metacarpal *veins,* under *vein.*

ve'nae metacar'peae palma'res [NA], SYN palmar metacarpal *veins,* under *vein.*

ve'nae metatar'seae dorsa'les [NA], SYN dorsal metatarsal *veins,* under *vein.*

ve'nae metatar'seae planta'res [NA], SYN plantar metatarsal *veins,* under *vein.*

ve'nae mus'culophren'icae [NA], SYN musculophrenic *veins,* under *vein.*

ve'nae nasa'les exter'nae [NA], SYN external nasal *veins,* under *vein.*

v. nasofronta'lis [NA], SYN nasofrontal *vein.*

ve'nae nu'clei cauda'ti [NA], small veins from the caudate nucleus draining into the superior thalamostriate vein. SYN veins of caudate nucleus.

v. obli'qua a'trii sinis'tri [NA], SYN oblique *vein* of left atrium.

v. obturato'ria, pl. **ve'nae obturato'riae** [NA], SYN obturator *vein.*

ve'nae occipita'les [NA], SYN occipital cerebral *veins,* under *vein.*

v. occipita'lis [NA], SYN occipital *vein.*

v. ophthal'mica infe'rior [NA], SYN inferior ophthalmic *vein.*

v. ophthal'mica supe'rior [NA], SYN superior ophthalmic *vein.*

v. ova'rica dex'tra [NA], SYN right ovarian *vein.*

v. ova'rica sinis'tra [NA], SYN left ovarian *vein.*

v. palati'na [NA], SYN palatine *vein.*

ve'nae palpebra'les [NA], SYN palpebral *veins,* under *vein.*

ve'nae palpebra'les inferio'res [NA], SYN inferior palpebral *veins,* under *vein.*

ve'nae palpebra'les superio'res [NA], SYN superior palpebral *veins,* under *vein.*

ve'nae pancreat'icae [NA], SYN pancreatic *veins,* under *vein.*

ve'nae pancreat'icoduodena'les [NA], SYN pancreaticoduodenal *veins,* under *vein.*

ve'nae paraumbilica'les [NA], SYN paraumbilical *veins,* under *vein.*

ve'nae parieta'les [NA], SYN parietal *veins,* under *vein.*

ve'nae parotid'ea [NA], SYN parotid *veins,* under *vein.*

ve'nae pectora'les [NA], SYN pectoral *veins,* under *vein.*

ve'nae peduncula'res [NA], small tributaries of the basal vein from the cerebral peduncle. SYN peduncular veins.

ve'nae perforan'tes [NA], SYN perforating *veins,* under *vein.*

ve'nae pericardi'acae [NA], SYN pericardial *veins,* under *vein.*

ve'nae pericardiacophren'icae [NA], SYN pericardiacophrenic *veins,* under *vein.*

ve'nae perone'ae [NA], SYN peroneal *veins,* under *vein.*

v. petro'sa [NA], SYN petrosal *vein.*

ve'nae pharyn'geae [NA], SYN pharyngeal *veins,* under *vein.*

ve'nae phren'icae superio'res [NA], SYN superior phrenic *veins,* under *vein.*

v. phren'ica infe'rior, pl. **ve'nae phren'icae inferio'res** [NA], SYN inferior phrenic *vein.*

ve'nae pon'tis [NA], SYN pontine *veins,* under *vein.*

v. pontomesencephal'ica ante'rior [NA], a vein in the midline of the interpeduncular fossa on the superior and anterior aspects of the pons; it communicates with the basal vein superiorly and the petrosal vein inferiorly. SYN anterior pontomesencephalic vein.

v. poplit'ea [NA], SYN popliteal *vein.*

v. por'tae hep'atis [NA], SYN portal *vein.*

v. porta'lis, SYN portal *vein.*

v. poste'rior ventric'uli sinis'tri [NA], SYN posterior *vein* of left ventricle.

v. preauricula'ris, SYN anterior auricular *vein.*

v. precentra'lis cerebel'li [NA], SYN precentral cerebellar *vein.*

ve'nae prefronta'les [NA], the superficial veins draining the prefrontal cerebral cortex and emptying into the superior sagittal sinus. SYN prefrontal veins.

v. prepylo'rica [NA], SYN prepyloric *vein.*

ve'nae profun'dae clitor'idis [NA], SYN deep *veins* of clitoris, under *vein.*

v. profun'da fem'oris [NA], SYN deep femoral *vein.*

v. profun'da lin'guae [NA], SYN deep lingual *vein.*

v. profun'da pe'nis [NA], SYN deep *vein* of penis.

ve'nae puden'dae exter'nae [NA], SYN external pudendal *veins,* under *vein.*

v. puden'da inter'na [NA], SYN internal pudendal *vein.*

ve'nae pulmona'les [NA], SYN pulmonary *veins,* under *vein.*

v. pulmona'lis infe'rior dex'tra [NA], SYN right inferior pulmonary *vein.*

v. pulmona'lis infe'rior sinis'tra [NA], SYN left inferior pulmonary *vein.*

v. pulmona'lis supe'rior dex'tra [NA], SYN right superior pulmonary *vein.*

v. pulmona'lis supe'rior sinis'tra [NA], SYN left superior pulmonary *vein.*

ve'nae radia'les [NA], SYN radial *veins,* under *vein.*

v. reces'sus latera'lis ventric'uli quar'ti [NA], a small vein originating in the cerebellar tonsil, coursing by the lateral recess of the fourth ventricle on its way to terminate in the petrosal vein. SYN vein of lateral recess of fourth ventricle.

ve'nae rec'tae, the ascending limbs of the vasa rectae in the renal medulla.

ve'nae recta'les inferio'res [NA], SYN inferior rectal *veins,* under *vein.*

ve'nae recta'les me'diae [NA], SYN middle rectal *veins,* under *vein.*

v. recta'lis supe'rior [NA], SYN superior rectal *vein.*

ve'nae rena'les [NA], SYN renal *veins,* under *vein.*

ve'nae re'nis [NA], SYN *veins* of kidney, under *vein.*

v. retromandibula'ris [NA], SYN retromandibular *vein.*

v. re'vehens, pl. **ve'nae revehen'tes,** veins in the embryo, passing from the sinusoid vessels in the liver to the inferior v. cava, that develop into the hepatic veins.

ve'nae sacra'les latera'les [NA], SYN lateral sacral *veins,* under *vein.*

v. sacra'lis media'na [NA], SYN median sacral *vein.*

v. saphe'na accesso'ria [NA], SYN accessory saphenous *vein.*

v. saphe'na mag'na [NA], SYN great saphenous *vein.*

v. saphe'na par'va [NA], SYN small saphenous *vein.*

v. scapula'ris dorsa'lis [NA], SYN dorsal scapular *vein.*

ve'nae sclera'les [NA], SYN scleral *veins,* under *vein.*

ve'nae scrota'les anterio'res [NA], SYN anterior scrotal *veins,* under *vein.*

ve'nae scrota'les posterio'res [NA], SYN posterior scrotal *veins,* under *vein.*

v. sep'ti pellu'cidi ante'rior [NA], SYN anterior *vein* of septum pellucidum.

v. sep'ti pellu'cidi poste'rior [NA], SYN posterior *vein* of septum pellucidum.

ve'nae sigmoi'deae [NA], SYN sigmoid *veins,* under *vein.*

ve'nae spina'les [NA], SYN spinal *veins,* under *vein.*

v. spira'lis modi'oli [NA], SYN spiral *vein* of modiolus.

venae cavernosae of spleen, small tributaries of the splenic vein in the pulp of the spleen. SYN Billroth's venae cavernosae.

v. sple'nica [NA], SYN splenic *vein.*

ve'nae stella'tae, SYN *venulae stellatae,* under *venula.*

v. sternocleidomastoi'dea [NA], SYN sternocleidomastoid *vein.*

ve'nae stria'tae, SYN inferior thalamostriate *veins,* under *vein.*

v. stylomastoi'dea [NA], SYN stylomastoid *vein.*

v. subcla'via [NA], SYN subclavian *vein.*

ve'nae subcuta'neae abdom'inis [NA], SYN subcutaneous *veins* of abdomen, under *vein.*

v. sublingua'lis [NA], SYN sublingual *vein.*

v. submenta′lis [NA], SYN submental *vein*.

superior v. cava, returns blood from the head and neck, upper limbs, and thorax to the posterosuperior aspect of the right atrium; formed in the superior mediastinum by union of the two brachiocephalic veins. SYN v. cava superior [NA], precava.

v. supraorbita′lis [NA], SYN supraorbital *vein*.

v. suprarena′lis dex′tra [NA], SYN right suprarenal *vein*.

v. suprarena′lis sinis′tra [NA], SYN left suprarenal *vein*.

v. suprascapula′ris [NA], SYN suprascapular *vein*.

ve′nae supratrochlea′res [NA], SYN supratrochlear *veins*, under *vein*.

ve′nae tempora′les profun′dae [NA], SYN deep temporal *veins*, under *vein*.

ve′nae tempora′les superficia′les [NA], SYN superficial temporal *veins*, under *vein*.

v. tempora′lis me′dia [NA], SYN middle temporal *vein*.

v. termina′lis [NA], SYN superior thalamostriate *vein*.

v. testicula′ris dex′tra [NA], SYN right testicular *vein*.

v. testicula′ris sinis′tra [NA], SYN left testicular *vein*.

ve′nae thalamostria′tae inferio′res [NA], SYN inferior thalamostriate *veins*, under *vein*.

v. thalamostria′ta supe′rior [NA], SYN superior thalamostriate *vein*.

v. thora′cica inter′na, pl. **ve′nae thora′cicae inter′nae** [NA], SYN internal thoracic *vein*.

v. thora′cica latera′lis [NA], SYN lateral thoracic *vein*.

v. thoracoacromia′lis [NA], SYN thoracoacromial *vein*.

v. thoracoepigas′trica, pl. **ve′nae thoracoepigas′tricae** [NA], SYN thoracoepigastric *vein*.

ve′nae thy′micae [NA], SYN thymic *veins*, under *vein*.

v. thyroi′dea i′ma, SYN inferior thyroid *vein*.

v. thyroi′dea infe′rior [NA], SYN inferior thyroid *vein*.

v. thyroi′dea me′dia [NA], SYN middle thyroid *vein*.

v. thyroi′dea supe′rior [NA], SYN superior thyroid *vein*.

ve′nae tibia′les anterio′res [NA], SYN anterior tibial *veins*, under *vein*.

ve′nae tibia′les posterio′res [NA], SYN posterior tibial *veins*, under *vein*.

ve′nae trachea′les [NA], SYN tracheal *veins*, under *vein*.

ve′nae transver′sae col′li [NA], SYN transverse cervical *veins*, under *vein*.

v. transver′sa facie′i [NA], SYN transverse facial *vein*.

v. transver′sa scap′ulae, SYN suprascapular *vein*.

ve′nae tympan′icae [NA], SYN tympanic *veins*, under *vein*.

ve′nae ulna′res [NA], SYN ulnar *veins*, under *vein*.

v. umbilica′lis sinis′tra [NA], SYN left umbilical *vein*.

v. un′ci [NA], a vein draining the uncus into the inferior cerebral vein of the same side. SYN vein of uncus.

ve′nae uteri′nae [NA], SYN uterine *veins*, under *vein*.

v. ventricula′ris infe′rior [NA], vein draining the deep white matter of the superior and lateral portions of the temporal lobe; it begins in the body of the lateral ventricle and exits from the choroid fissure of the inferior horn where it joins the basal vein. SYN inferior ventricular vein.

v. ventric′uli latera′lis latera′lis [NA], SYN v. atrii lateralis.

v. ventric′uli latera′lis media′lis [NA], SYN v. atrii medialis.

v. ver′mis infe′rior [NA], SYN inferior *vein* of vermis.

v. ver′mis supe′rior [NA], SYN superior *vein* of vermis.

v. vertebra′lis [NA], SYN vertebral *vein*.

v. vertebra′lis accesso′ria [NA], SYN accessory vertebral *vein*.

v. vertebra′lis ante′rior [NA], SYN anterior vertebral *vein*.

ve′nae vesica′les [NA], SYN vesical *veins*, under *vein*.

ve′nae vestibula′res [NA], SYN vestibular *veins*, under *vein*.

v. vitelli′na, SYN vitelline *vein*.

ve′nae vortico′sae [NA], SYN vortex *veins*, under *vein*.

ve·na·ca·vog·ra·phy (vē′nă-kā-vog′ră-fē). Angiography of a vena cava. SYN cavography.

ve·na·tion (vē-nā′shŭn). The arrangement and distribution of veins. [L. *vena*, vein]

△**vene-. 1.** The veins, venous. SEE ALSO veno-. [L. *vena*, vein] **2.** Combining form relating to venom. [L. *venenum*, poison]

ve·nec·ta·sia (ve-nek-tā′sē-ă). SYN phlebectasia.

ve·nec·to·my (ve-nek′tō-mē). SYN phlebectomy.

ve·neer (vĕ-nēr′). **1.** A thin surface layer laid over a base of common material. **2.** In dentistry, a layer of tooth-colored material, usually porcelain or acrylic resin, attached to and covering the surface of a metal crown or natural tooth structure. [Fr. *fournir*, to furnish]

ven·e·na·tion (ven-ĕ-nā′shŭn, vē-nĕ-). Poisoning, as from a sting or bite. [L. *veneno*, pp. *-atus*, to poison, fr. *venenum*, poison]

ven·e·nif·er·ous (ven-ĕ-nif′ĕ-rŭs). Conveying poison, as through a sting or bite. [L. *venenifer*, fr. *venenum*, poison, + *fero*, to carry]

ven·e·no·sal·i·vary (ven′ĕ-nō-sal′i-vār-ē). Secreting a poisonous saliva, said of venomous reptiles. SYN venomosalivary.

ven·e·nos·i·ty (ven-ĕ-nos′i-tē). The state of containing poison or being poisonous. [L. *venenosus*, poisonous]

ven·e·nous (ven′ĕ-nŭs). SYN poisonous. [L. *venenosus*]

ve·ne·re·al (ve-nēr′ē-ăl). Relating to or resulting from sexual intercourse. [L. *Venus* (*vener*-), goddess of love]

ve·ne·re·ol·o·gy (ve-nēr-ē-ol′ō-jē). The study of venereal disease. [venereal (disease) + G. *logos*, study]

ve·ne·re·o·pho·bia (ve-nēr′ē-ō-fō′bē-ă). Morbid fear of venereal disease. [venereal (disease) + G. *phobos*, fear]

ven·e·sec·tion (ven-ē-sek′shŭn). SYN phlebotomy. [L. *vena*, vein, + *sectio*, a cutting]

△**veni-.** SEE veno-.

ven·in (ven′in). Any poisonous substance found in snake venom. [see venom]

ven·i·punc·ture (ven′i-pŭnk-chŭr, vē′ni-). The puncture of a vein, usually to withdraw blood or inject a solution.

Venn, John, English logician and philosopher, 1834–1923. SEE Venn *diagram*.

△**veno-, veni-.** The veins. SEE ALSO vene- (1). [L. *vena*]

ve·no·cly·sis (vē-nok′li-sis). SYN phleboclysis. [veno- + G. *klysis*, a washing out]

ve·no·fi·bro·sis (vē′nō-fī-brō′sis). SYN phlebosclerosis.

ve·no·gram (vē′nō-gram). **1.** Radiograph of opacified veins. **2.** SYN phlebogram. [veno- + G. *gramma*, a writing]

ve·nog·ra·phy (vē-nog′ră-fē). Radiographic demonstration of a vein, after the injection of contrast medium. SYN phlebography (2). [veno- + G. *graphō*, to write]

splenic portal v., SYN splenoportography.

transosseous v., radiographic demonstration of veins that drain a bone's marrow, by injection of contrast medium into the marrow at an appropriate point, as in vertebral v. or azygography by rib injection.

vertebral v., radiographic demonstration of the epidural venous plexus by injection of contrast medium into the spinous process.

ven·om (ven′ŏm). A poisonous fluid secreted by snakes, spiders, scorpions, etc. [M. Eng. and O. Fr. *venim*, fr. L. *venenum*, poison]

kokoi v., a potent neurotoxin found in the frog *Phyllobates bicolor;* it is a nonprotein compound with a molecular weight of approximately 400, and is lethal in microgram quantities.

Russell's viper v., a v. used as a coagulant in the arrest of hemorrhage from accessible sites in hemophilia.

ven·o·mo·sal·i·vary (ven′ō-mō-sal′i-var-ē). SYN venenosalivary.

ve·no·mo·tor (vē′nō-mō′ter). Causing change in the caliber of a vein. [veno- + L. *motor*, a move]

ve·no·per·i·to·ne·os·to·my (vē′nō-per-i-tō-nē-os′tō-mē). An obsolete operation involving insertion of the cut end of the saphenous vein into the peritoneal cavity in cases of ascites; the vein is inverted so that the valves prevent regurgitation of blood into the cavity while the ascitic fluid flows into the vein. [veno- + peritoneum + G. *stoma*, mouth]

ve·no·pres·sor (vē-nō-pres′er). Relating to the venous blood pressure and consequently the volume of venous supply to the right side of the heart.

ve·no·scle·ro·sis (vē′nō-skle-rō′sis). SYN phlebosclerosis.

ve·nose (vē′nŏs). Having veins; veiny. [L. *venosus*]

ve·no·si·nal (vē′nō-sī′năl). Pertaining to the vena cava and the atrial sinus of the heart.

ve·nos·i·ty (vē-nos′i-tē). **1.** A venous state; a condition in which the bulk of the blood is in the veins at the expense of the arteries. **2.** The unaerated condition of venous blood.

ve·nos·ta·sis (vē-nō-stā′sis, vē-nos′tă-sis). SYN phlebostasis. [veno- + G. *stasis*, a standing]

ve·no·stat (vē′nō-stat). Any instrument for arresting venous bleeding. [veno- + G. *statos*, standing, stationary]

ve·nos·to·my (vē-nos′tō-mē). SYN cutdown.

ve·not·o·my (vē-not′ō-mē). SYN phlebotomy.

ve·nous (vē′nŭs). Relating to a vein or to the veins. SYN phleboid (2). [L. *venosus*]

ve·nous re·turn. The blood returning to the heart via the great veins and coronary sinus.

ve·no·ve·nos·to·my (vē′nō-vē-nos′tō-mē). The formation of an anastomosis between two veins. SYN phlebophlebostomy. [veno- + veno- + G. *stoma*, mouth]

vent. An opening into a cavity or canal, especially one through which the contents of such a cavity are discharged, as the anus. [O. Fr. *fente*, a chink, cleft]

ven·ter (ven′ter). **1.** SYN abdomen. **2** [NA]. SYN belly (2). **3.** One of the great cavities of the body. **4.** The uterus. [L. *venter (ventr-)*, belly]

v. ante′rior mus′culi digas′trici [NA], SYN anterior *belly* of digastric muscle.

v. fronta′lis mus′culi occipitofronta′lis [NA], SYN frontal *belly* of occipitofrontalis muscle.

v. infe′rior mus′culi omohyoi′dei [NA], SYN inferior *belly* of omohyoid *muscle*.

v. occipita′lis mus′culi occipitofron′talis [NA], SYN occipital *belly* of occipitofrontalis muscle.

v. poste′rior mus′culi digas′trici [NA], SYN posterior *belly* of digastric muscle.

v. propen′dens, (1) anteversion of the uterus; **(2)** a pendulous abdomen.

v. supe′rior mus′culi omohyoi′dei [NA], SYN superior *belly* of omohyoid muscle.

ven·ti·late (ven′ti-lāt). To aerate, or oxygenate, the blood in the pulmonary capillaries. SYN air (2), atmosphere (1). [L. *ventilo*, pp. -*atus*, to fan, fr. *ventus*, the wind]

ven·ti·la·tion (ven-ti-lā′shŭn). **1.** Replacement of air or other gas in a space by fresh air or gas. **2.** Movement of gas(es) into and out of the lungs. SYN oxidative metabolism, respiration (2). **3** (V̇). In physiology, the tidal exchange of air between the lungs and the atmosphere that occurs in breathing. SEE ALSO respiration. [see ventilate]

alveolar v. (V̇ₐ), the volume of gas expired from the alveoli to the outside of the body per minute; calculated as the respiratory frequency (f) multiplied by the difference between tidal volume and the dead space ($V_T - V_D$); units: ml/min BTPS.

artificial v., application of mechanically or manually generated pressures, usually positive, to gas(es) in or about the airway as a means of producing gas exchange between the lungs and surrounding atmosphere. SYN artificial respiration.

assist-control v., artificial respiration in which inspiration is produced automatically after a set interval if the person has not already begun to inspire. Cf. assisted v., controlled v.

assisted v., application of mechanically or manually generated positive pressure to gas(es) in or about the airway during inhalation as a means of augmenting movement of gases into the lungs. SYN assisted respiration.

continuous positive pressure v. (CPPV), SYN controlled mechanical v.

controlled v., intermittent application of mechanically or manually generated positive pressure to gas(es) in or about the airway

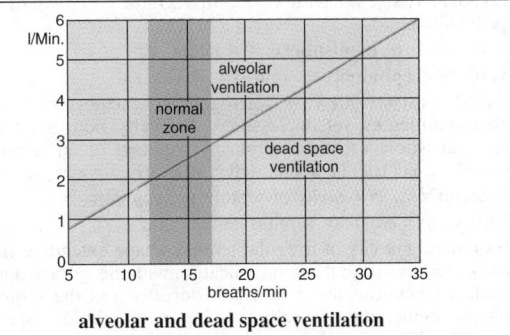

alveolar and dead space ventilation
depending on the number of breaths taken (respiratory frequency), with a constant tidal volume of 6 L

as a means of forcing gases into the lungs in the absence of spontaneous ventilatory efforts. SYN controlled respiration.

controlled mechanical v. (CMV), artificial v. in which all inspirations are provided by positive pressure applied to the airway. SYN continuous positive pressure breathing, continuous positive pressure v., intermittent positive pressure breathing, intermittent positive pressure v.

intermittent mandatory v. (IMV), mechanical application of positive pressure at a predetermined frequency to the airway to increase tidal volume.

intermittent positive pressure v. (IPPV), SYN controlled mechanical v.

manual v., intermittent manual compression of a gas-filled reservoir bag to force gases into a patient's lungs and thus maintain oxygenation and carbon dioxide elimination during apnea or hypoventilation.

maximum voluntary v. (MVV), the volume of air breathed when an individual breathes as deeply and as quickly as possible for a given time (*e.g.,* 15 sec.). SYN maximum breathing capacity.

mechanical v., use of automatically cycling devices to generate airway pressures; employed in assisted or controlled v.

pulmonary v., respiratory minute volume, *i.e.,* the total volume of gas per minute inspired (V_I) or expired (V_E) expressed in liters per minute; differs from alveolar v. by including the exchange of dead space gas.

spontaneous intermittent mandatory v. (SIMV), intermittent mandatory v. spontaneously initiated by the patient, to increase tidal volume, and subsequently synchronized with patient's respiratory cycle. SYN synchronized intermittent mandatory v.

synchronized intermittent mandatory v. (SIMV), SYN spontaneous intermittent mandatory v.

wasted v., that part of the pulmonary v. which is ineffective in exchanging oxygen and carbon dioxide with pulmonary capillary blood; calculated as physiologic dead space multiplied by respiratory frequency.

ven·ti·la·tion/per·fu·sion mis·match. An imbalance between alveolar ventilation and pulmonary capillary blood flow.

vent·plant. An endo-osseous implant, usually made of titanium, utilized to provide support and fixation for a dental prosthesis by means of projections through the mucosa; also used to designate a family of implants.

ven·trad (ven′trad). Toward the ventral aspect; opposed to dorsad. [L. *venter*, belly, + *ad*, to]

ven·tral (ven′trăl). **1.** Pertaining to the belly or to any venter. **2.** SYN anterior (1). **3.** In veterinary anatomy, the undersurface of an animal; often used to indicate the position of one structure relative to another, *i.e.,* situated nearer the undersurface of the body. SYN ventralis [NA]. [L. *ventralis*]

ven·tra·lis (ven-trā′lis) [NA]. SYN ventral. [L.]

ven·tri·cle (ven′tri-kl). A normal cavity, as of the brain or heart. SYN ventriculus (2). [L. *ventriculus*, dim. of *venter*, belly]

Arantius' v., SYN *calamus* scriptorius.

cerebral v.'s, SEE lateral v., fourth v., third v., *cavity* of septum pellucidum.

v. of cerebral hemisphere, SYN lateral v.

v. of diencephalon, SYN third v.

double outlet right v., a heterogeneous category of congenital abnormalities as yet unclassified. Basically both great arteries arise in whole or in part from the right v. or an infundibular chamber. Ventricular septal defect is nearly always present.

Duncan's v., SYN *cavity* of septum pellucidum.

fifth v., SYN *cavity* of septum pellucidum.

fourth v., a cavity of irregular tentlike shape extending from the obex rostralward to its communication with the sylvian aqueduct, enclosed between the cerebellum dorsally and the rhombence-phalic tegmentum ventrally, having a rhomboid-shaped floor (rhomboid fossa) and a tentlike roof which in its caudal part is formed by the tela choroidea and the posterior medullary velum, in its middle part by the white matter of the cerebellum, and in its narrowing rostral part (recessus superior) by the anterior medullary velum. The fourth v. reaches its greatest width at the ponto-medullary transition, where it expands laterally behind the cerebellar peduncles into the spoutlike lateral recess, and its greatest height at the fastigial recess, which reaches up into the cerebellar white matter. Direct communication of the brain's v. system and the subarachnoid space is established at the level of the fourth v. by a median opening in the tela choroidea, the medial aperture of Magendie's foramen, which opens into the cerebellomedullary cistern, and on both sides by the lateral aperture or foramen of Luschka, which connects the lateral recess with the interpeduncular cistern. SYN ventriculus quartus [NA], v. of rhombencephalon.

v.'s of heart, one of the two lower chambers of the heart. SYN ventriculus cordis [NA].

laryngeal v., the recess in each lateral wall of the larynx between the vestibular and vocal folds and into which the layrngeal sacculus opens. SYN ventriculus laryngis [NA], laryngeal sinus, Morgagni's sinus (3), Morgagni's v., sinus laryngeus.

lateral v., a cavity shaped somewhat like a horseshoe in conformity with the general shape of the hemisphere; each lateral v. communicates with the third v. through the interventricular foramen of Monro, and expands from there forward into the frontal lobe as the anterior horn as well as caudally over the thalamus as the central part or cella media which, behind the thalamus, curves ventrally and laterally, then forward into the temporal lobe as the inferior horn; from the apex of the curve a variably sized posterior horn extends back into the white matter of the occipital lobe. The large choroid plexus of the lateral v. invades the cella media and the inferior horn (but not the anterior and posterior horn) from the medial side. SYN ventriculus lateralis [NA], v. of cerebral hemisphere.

left v., the lower chamber on the left side of the heart that receives the arterial blood from the left atrium and drives it by the contraction of its walls into the aorta. SYN ventriculus sinister [NA].

Morgagni's v., SYN laryngeal v.

v. of rhombencephalon, SYN fourth v.

right v., the lower chamber on the right side of the heart which receives the venous blood from the right atrium and drives it by the contraction of its walls into the pulmonary artery. SYN ventriculus dexter [NA].

single v., congenital absence or near total absence of the ventricular septum.

sixth v., SYN Verga's v.

sylvian v., SYN *cavity* of septum pellucidum.

v. of Sylvius, SYN *cavity* of septum pellucidum.

terminal v., a dilation of the central canal of the spinal cord at the tip of the medullary cone. SYN ventriculus terminalis [NA].

third v., a narrow, vertically oriented, irregularly quadrilateral cavity in the midplane, extending from the lamina terminalis to the rostral opening of the mesencephalic aqueduct. This v. communicates at its rostrodorsal corner with each of the two lateral v.'s through the left and right interventricular foramen of Monro. Its narrow roof is formed by the tela choroidea which is attached on either side to the tenia thalami; its lateral wall by the medial

surface of the thalamus and, below the hypothalamic sulcus, by the hypothalamus which also forms its floor. In lateral profile, the third v. exhibits a number of recesses: in its floor, from before backward, 1) the preoptic recess in the acute angle between the base of the lamina terminalis and the dorsum of the optic chiasm, 2) the infundibular recess extending ventrally into the infundibulum but (in humans) not into the hypophysial stalk, and 3) the mamillary or inframamillary recess caused by the protrusion of the mamillary bodies into the v. From its dorsocaudal corner, the pineal recess extends caudally into the pineal stalk. SYN ventriculus tertius [NA], diacele, v. of diencephalon.

Verga's v., an inconstant, horizontal, slitlike space between the posterior one-third of the corpus callosum and the underlying commissura fornicis (commissura hippocampi; psalterium) resulting from failure of these two commissural plates to fuse completely during fetal development; like the cavity of the septum pellucidum, the space is not a true v. in the sense that it did not develop from the central canal of the neural tube. SYN cavum psalterii, cavum vergae, sixth v.

Vieussens' v., SYN *cavity* of septum pellucidum.

Wenzel's v., SYN *cavity* of septum pellucidum.

ven·tri·cose (ven′tri-kōs). Bulging or swollen on one side or unequally.

ven·tric·u·lar (ven-trik′yū-lăr). Relating to a ventricle, in any sense. SYN ventricularis (1).

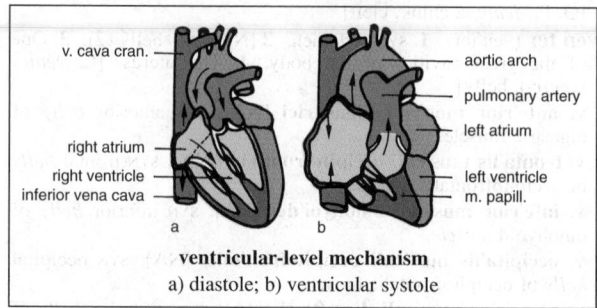

ventricular-level mechanism
a) diastole; b) ventricular systole

Labels: v. cava cran.; aortic arch; pulmonary artery; right atrium; left atrium; right ventricle; left ventricle; inferior vena cava; m. papill.; a; b

ven·tric·u·lar·is (ven-trik′yū-lā′ris). **1.** SYN ventricular. **2.** SYN thyroepiglottic *muscle.* [Mod. L. fr. L. *ventriculus*]

ven·tric·u·lar·i·za·tion (ven-trik′yū-lar-i-zā′shŭn). Transformation of an atrial phenomenon to simulate a ventricular one, especially of the atrial (or venous) pulse tracing in tricuspid regurgitation.

ven·tric·u·lar pon·der·ance (pon′der-ans). a semiobsolete electrocardiographic term suggesting that one ventricle is either larger or thicker than the other.

ven·tric·u·li·tis (ven-trik-yū-lī′tis). Inflammation of the ventricles of the brain. [ventricle + G. *-itis,* inflammation]

⌂**ventriculo-.** A ventricle. [L. *ventriculus*]

ven·tric·u·lo·a·tri·al (**V-A**) (ven-trik′yū-lō-ā′trē-ăl). Relating to both ventricles and atria, especially to the sequential passage of conduction in the retrograde direction from ventricle to atrium.

ven·tric·u·lo·cis·ter·nos·to·my (ven-trik′yū-lō-sis′ter-nos′tō-mē). An artificial opening between the ventricles of the brain and the cisterna magna. SEE ALSO shunt (2). [ventriculo- + L. *cisterna,* cistern, + G. *stoma,* mouth]

ven·tric·u·log·ra·phy (ven-trik-yū-log′ră-fē). **1.** Radiograph demonstration of the cerebral ventricles by direct injection of air or contrast medium; developed and described by Dandy in 1918. Cf. pneumoencephalography. **2.** Demonstration of the contractility of the cardiac ventricles by recording serially the distribution of intravenously injected radionuclide or that of radiographic contrast medium injected through an intracardiac catheter. **3.** Visualization by roentgenography of a cardiac ventricle by injection of radiopaque contrast material. [ventriculo- + G. *graphē,* a writing]

radionuclide v., SYN radionuclide *angiocardiography.* SEE ventriculography.

ven·tric·u·lo·mas·toi·dos·to·my (ven-trik′yū-lō-mas′toy-dos′ tō-mē). Operation for the establishment of a communication between the lateral cerebral ventricle and the mastoid antrum by means of a polythene tube for the relief of hydrocephalus. SEE ALSO shunt (2). [ventriculo- + mastoid, + G. *stoma,* mouth]

ven·tric·u·lo·nec·tor (ven-trik′yū-lō-nek′ter, -tōr). SYN atrioventricular *bundle.* [ventriculo- + L. *necto,* to join]

ven·tric·u·lo·pha·sic (ven-trik′yū-lō-fā′zik). Influenced by ventricular contraction; applied to the atrial rhythm when this is modified by ventricular contraction; in v. sinus arrhythmia in complete A-V block the sinus impulse immediately following a ventricular contraction usually appears sooner than expected.

ven·tric·u·lo·plas·ty (ven-trik′yū-lō-plas-tē). Any surgical procedure to repair a defect of one of the ventricles of the heart. [ventriculo- + G. *plastos,* formed]

ven·tric·u·lo·punc·ture (ven-trik′yū-lō-pŭnk′chūr). Insertion of a needle into a ventricle.

ven·tric·u·los·co·py (ven-trik-yū-los′kŏ-pē). Direct inspection of a ventricle with an endoscope. [ventriculo- + G. *skopeō,* to view]

ven·tric·u·los·to·my (ven-trik-yū-los′tō-mē). Establishment of an opening in a ventricle, usually from the third ventricle to the subarachnoid space to relieve hydrocephalus. SEE ALSO shunt (2). [ventriculo- + G. *stoma,* mouth]

third v., an operation to establish an opening from the third ventricle to the prechiasmal and interpeduncular cisterns (Stookey-Scarff operation) or from the third ventricle to the interpeduncular cistern (Dandy operation).

ven·tric·u·lo·sub·a·rach·noid (ven-trik′yū-lō-sŭb-ă-rak′noyd). Relating to the space occupied by the cerebrospinal fluid. [ventriculo- + subarachnoid]

ven·tric·u·lot·o·my (ven-trik-yū-lot′ō-mē). Incision into a ventricle; *e.g.,* into the cerebral third ventricle for the relief of hydrocephalus or into a cardiac ventricle to surgically correct an abnormality.. [ventriculo- + G. *tomē,* incision]

ven·tric·u·lus, pl. **ven·tric·u·li** (ven-trik′yū-lŭs, -lī). **1** [NA]. ☆official alternate term for stomach. **2** [NA]. SYN ventricle. **3.** The enlarged posterior portion of the mesenteron of the insect alimentary canal, in which digestion occurs. [L. dim. of *venter,* belly]

v. cor′dis [NA], SYN *ventricles* of heart, under *ventricle.*

v. dex′ter [NA], SYN right *ventricle.*

v. laryn′gis [NA], SYN laryngeal *ventricle.*

v. latera′lis [NA], SYN lateral *ventricle.*

v. quar′tus [NA], SYN fourth *ventricle.*

v. quin′tus, SYN *cavity* of septum pellucidum.

v. sinis′ter [NA], SYN left *ventricle.*

v. termina′lis [NA], SYN terminal *ventricle.*

v. ter′tius [NA], SYN third *ventricle.*

ven·tri·duct (ven′tri-dŭkt). To draw toward the abdomen. [L. *venter,* belly, + *duco,* pp. *ductus,* to lead]

ven·tri·duc·tion (ven-tri-dŭk′shŭn). Drawing toward the abdomen or abdominal wall.

ventro-. Ventral. [L. *venter,* belly]

ven·tro·cys·tor·rha·phy (ven′trō-sis-tōr′ă-fē). SYN cystopexy. [ventro- + G. *kystis,* cyst, + *rhaphē,* suture]

ven·tro·dor·sad (ven-trō-dōr′sad). In a direction from the venter to the dorsum.

ven·tro·in·gui·nal (ven′trō-ing′gwi-năl). Relating to the abdomen and the groin.

ven·tro·lat·er·al (ven-trō-lat′ĕ-răl). Both ventral and lateral, *i.e.,* to the front and to the side.

ven·tro·me·di·an (ven-trō-mē′dē-an). Relating to the midline of the ventral surface.

ven·trop·to·sis (ven-trō-tō′sis, -tō′sē-ă). SYN gastroptosis. [ventro- + G. *ptōsis,* a falling]

ven·tros·co·py (ven-tros′kŏ-pē). SYN peritoneoscopy. [ventro- + G. *skopeō,* to view]

ven·trot·o·my (ven-trot′ō-mē). SYN celiotomy. [ventro- + G. *tomē,* incision]

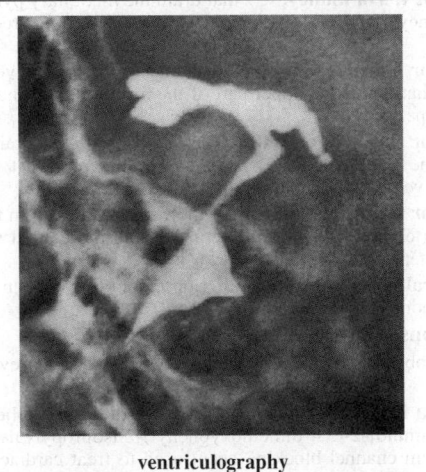
ventriculography

Venturi, Giovanni B., Italian physicist, 1746–1822. SEE V. *effect, meter, tube.*

ven·u·la, pl. **ven·u·lae** (ven′yū-lă, -lē) [NA]. SYN venule. [L. dim. of *vena,* vein]

v. macula′ris infe′rior [NA], SYN inferior macular *venule.*

v. macula′ris supe′rior [NA], SYN superior macular *venule.*

v. media′lis ret′inae [NA], SYN medial *venule* of retina.

v. nasa′lis ret′inae infe′rior [NA], SYN inferior nasal *venule* of retina.

v. nasa′lis ret′inae supe′rior [NA], SYN superior nasal *venule* of retina.

ven′ulae rec′tae re′nis [NA], SYN straight *venules* of kidney, under *venule.*

ven′ulae stella′tae [NA], the star-shaped groups of venules in the renal cortex. SYN stellate veins, stellate venules, stellulae verheyenii, venae stellatae, Verheyen's stars.

v. tempora′lis ret′inae infe′rior [NA], SYN inferior temporal *venule* of retina.

v. tempora′lis ret′inae supe′rior [NA], SYN superior temporal *venule* of retina.

ven·u·lar (ven′yū-lăr). Pertaining to venules. SYN venulous.

ven·ule (ven′yūl, vē′nūl). A venous radicle continuous with a capillary. SYN venula [NA], capillary vein, veinlet.

high endothelial postcapillary v.'s, v.'s in the lymph nodes, tonsils, and Peyer's patches that have a high-walled endothelium through which blood lymphocytes migrate into the lymphatic parenchyma.

inferior macular v., a small tributary of the central vein of the retina that drains the lower part of the macula. SYN venula macularis inferior [NA].

inferior nasal v. of retina, the small vein that passes from the inferior medial (nasal) part of the retina to join the central vein. SYN venula nasalis retinae inferior [NA].

inferior temporal v. of retina, the small vein that passes from the lower lateral (temporal) part of the retina to enter the central vein. SYN venula temporalis retinae inferior [NA].

medial v. of retina, the small vein that passes from the part of the retina between the macula and the optic disk to join the central vein. SYN venula medialis retinae [NA].

nasal v.'s of retina, SEE inferior nasal v. of retina, superior nasal v. of retina.

pericytic v.'s, SYN postcapillary v.'s.

postcapillary v.'s, the microvasculature immediately following the capillaries, ranging in size from 10 to 50 μm, and characterized by investment of pericytes; they are the site of extravasation of blood cells, are particularly sensitive to histamine, and are believed to be important in blood-interstitial fluid exchanges. SYN pericytic v.'s.

stellate v.'s, SYN *venulae* stellatae, under *venula.*

ve

straight v.'s of kidney, v.'s that drain the medullary pyramids of the kidney; they open into arcuate veins. SYN venulae rectae renis [NA].

superior macular v., a small tributary of the central vein of the retina that drains the upper part of the macula. SYN venula macularis superior [NA].

superior nasal v. of retina, the small vein that drains blood from the upper medial (nasal) part of the retina; it joins the central vein. SYN venula nasalis retinae superior [NA].

superior temporal v. of retina, the v. that passes from the upper lateral (temporal) part of the retina to join the central vein. SYN venula temporalis retinae superior [NA].

temporal v.'s of retina, SEE inferior temporal v. of retina, superior temporal v. of retina.

ven·u·lous (ven′yū-lŭs). SYN venular.

VER Abbreviation for visual evoked response. SEE evoked response.

ve·rap·a·mil (ver-ap′ă-mil). 5-[(3,4-dimethoxyphenethyl)-methylamino]-2-(3,4-dimethoxyphenyl)-2-isopropylvaleronitrile; a calcium channel blocking agent used to treat cardiac arrhythmias and angina pectoris. SYN iproveratril.

ve·rat·ric ac·id (vĕ-rat′rik). $C_9H_{10}O_4$; 3,4-Dimethoxybenzoic acid; obtained by methylation and subsequent oxidation of protocatechuic acid; present in the seeds of *Schoenocaulon officinale (Sabadilla officinarum)*.

ver·a·tri·dine (ver-ă-trī′dēn). 4,9-Epoxycevane-3,4,12,14,-16,17,20-heptol 3-(3,4-dimethoxybenzoate); 3-veretroyl-veracevine; an alkaloid derived from *Veratrum viridae* and *V. album*. Probably responsible for antihypertensive properties of this class of alkaloids.

ver·a·trine (ver′ă-trēn, -trin). A mixture of alkaloids from the seeds of *Schoenocaulon officinale (Sabadilla officinarum)* (family Liliaceae), including cevine, cevadine, cevadilline, sabadine, and veratridine; a powder of acrid taste, intensely irritating to the nasal mucous membrane, that has been used as an anodyne counterirritant in neuralgias and arthritis.

Ve·ra·trum (vĕ-rā′trŭm). A genus of toxic liliaceous plants. [L. hellebore]

V. al′bum, the rhizome has emetic and cathartic actions.

V. vir′ide, the dried rhizome and roots contain therapeutically important alkaloids (cevadine, veratridine, jervine, pseudojervine, rubijervine, and several ester alkaloids of the base germine) used in the treatment of hypertensive disorders.

ver·big·er·a·tion (ver-bij-er-ā′shŭn). Constant repetition of meaningless words or phrases; seen in schizophrenia. SYN catalogia, cataphasia, oral stereotypy. [L. *verbum*, word, + *gero*, to carry about]

ver·bo·ma·nia (ver-bō-mā′nē-ă). An abnormal talkativeness; a psychotic flow of speech. [L. *verbum*, word, + G. *mania*, frenzy]

ver·di·gris (ver′di-grēs, -gris, -grē). Cupric acetate (normal). [O. Fr. *verd*, green, *de*, of, *Gris*, Greeks]

ver·dine (ver′din). SYN biliverdin.

ver·do·glo·bin (ver-dō-glō′bin). Obsolete term for choleglobin.

ver·do·he·mo·chrome (ver-dō-hē′mō-krōm). An intermediate stage in hemoglobin degradation to yield the bile pigments, *i.e.,* hemoglobin yields choleglobin (verdohemoglobin) and the loss of globin leaves v., the precursor of biliverdin.

ver·do·he·mo·glo·bin (ver′dō-hē-mō-glō′bin). SYN choleglobin.

ver·do·per·ox·i·dase (ver′dō-per-oks′i-dās). A peroxidase, occurring in leukocytes, that contains a greenish ferriheme; responsible for the peroxidase activity of pus.

Verga, Andrea, Italian neurologist, 1811–1895. SEE V.'s *ventricle; cavum* vergae.

verge (verj). An edge or margin.

anal v., the transitional zone between the moist, hairless, modified skin of the anal canal and the perianal skin.

ver·gence (ver′jens). A disjunctive movement of the eyes in which the fixation axes are not parallel, as in convergence or divergence. [L. *vergo*, to incline, to turn]

v. of lens, the reciprocal of the principal focal distance used as a measure of the divergence or convergence of parallel rays.

ver·ge·ture (ver′jĕ-chūr). SYN striae cutis distensae, under *stria*. [Fr. wheal, mark of a lash, fr. L. *virga*, rod, switch]

Verheyen, Philippe, Flemish anatomist, 1648–1710. SEE V.'s stars, under *star; stellulae* verheyenii, under *stellula*.

Verhoeff, Frederick H., U.S. ophthalmologist, 1874–1968. SEE V.'s elastic tissue *stain*.

Ver·mes (ver′mēz). Archaic term for a subkingdom of the animal kingdom containing worms and wormlike organisms; an unnatural division no longer in taxonomic use. [L. *vermis*, worm]

⚠**vermi-.** A worm; wormlike. [L. *vermis*]

ver·mi·ci·dal (ver′mi-sī′dăl). Destructive to worms; specifically, destructive to parasitic intestinal worms. [vermi- + L. *caedo*, to kill]

ver·mi·cide (ver′mi-sīd). An agent that kills intestinal parasitic worms. [vermi- + L. *caedo*, to kill]

ver·mic·u·lar (ver-mik′yū-lăr). Relating to, resembling, or moving like a worm. [L. *vermiculus*, dim. of *vermis*, worm]

ver·mic·u·la·tion (ver-mik-yū-lā′shŭn). A wormlike movement, as in peristalsis.

ver·mi·cule (ver′mi-kūl). 1. A small worm or wormlike organism or structure. 2. SYN ookinete. [L. *vermiculus*, a small worm]

ver·mic·u·lose, ver·mic·u·lous (ver-mik′yū-lōs, -lŭs). 1. Wormy; infected with worms or larvae. 2. Wormlike. SEE ALSO vermiform.

ver·mic·u·lus (ver-mik′yū-lŭs). SEE vermicule. [L. dim. of *vermis*, worm]

ver·mi·form (ver′mi-fōrm). Worm-shaped; resembling a worm in form, denoting especially the appendix of the cecum. SEE ALSO lumbricoid, scolecoid (2). [vermi- + L. *forma*, form]

ver·mif·u·gal (ver-mif′yū-găl). SYN anthelmintic (2). [vermi- + L. *fugo*, to chase away]

ver·mi·fuge (ver′mi-fūj). SYN anthelmintic (1). [vermi- + L. *fugo*, to chase away]

ver·mil·ion (ver-mil′yon) [C.I. 77766]. A red pigment made from cinnabar or red mercuric sulfide.

ver·mil·ion·ec·to·my (ver-mil-yon-ek′tō-mē). Excision of the vermilion border. [vermilion border + G. *ektomē*, cutting out]

ver·min (ver′min). Parasitic insects, such as lice and bedbugs. [L. *vermis*, a worm]

ver·mi·nal (ver′mi-năl). SYN verminous.

ver·mi·na·tion (ver-mi-nā′shŭn). 1. The production or breeding of worms or larvae. 2. Infestation with vermin.

ver·min·ous (ver′mi-nŭs). Relating to, caused by, or infested with worms, larvae, or vermin. SYN verminal. [L. *verminosus*, wormy]

ver·mis, pl. **ver·mes** (ver′mis, -mēz). 1. A worm; any structure or part resembling a worm in shape. 2 [NA]. The narrow middle zone between the two hemispheres of the cerebellum; the portion projecting above the level of the hemispheres on the upper surface is called the superior v.; the lower portion, sunken between the two hemispheres and forming the floor of the vallecula, is the inferior v. [L. worm]

ver·mix (ver′miks). SYN vermiform *appendix*.

Verner, John, U.S. internist, *1927. SEE V.-Morrison *syndrome*.

Vernet, Maurice, French neurologist, *1887. SEE V.'s *syndrome*.

Verneuil, Aristide A., French surgeon, 1823–1895. SEE V.'s *neuroma; hidradenitis* axillaris of V.

Vernier, Pierre, French mathematician, 1580–1637. SEE V. *acuity*.

ver·nix (ver′niks). SYN varnish (dental). [Mod. L.]

v. caseo′sa, the fatty substance, consisting of desquamated epithelial cells, lanugo hairs, and sebaceous matter, which covers the skin of the fetus.

Verocay, José, Czechoslovakian pathologist, 1876–1927. SEE V. *bodies*, under *body*.

Ver·on·al (ver′ō-nal). SYN barbital.

ver·ru·ca, pl. **ver·ru·cae** (vĕ-rū′kă, -kē). A flesh-colored growth characterized by circumscribed hypertrophy of the papillae of the corium, with thickening of the malpighian, granular, and keratin layers of the epidermis, caused by human papilloma virus; also applied to epidermal verrucous tumors of nonviral etiology. SYN verruga, wart. [L.]

v. acumina′ta, obsolete term for *condyloma* acuminatum.

v. digita′ta, a wart in which the papillae project like fingers; they occur in groups, often on the scalp. SYN digitate wart.

v. filifor′mis, a wart composed of a single or many greatly elongated papillae; appears more commonly on the face and neck. SYN filiform wart.

v. gla′bra, a smooth wart.

v. molluscifor′mis, SYN condyloma.

v. necrogen′ica, SYN postmortem *wart.*

v. perua′na, v. peruvia′na, SYN *verruca* peruana.

v. pla′na, a smooth, flat, flesh-colored wart of small size, occurring in groups, seen especially on the face of the young; often associated with common warts of the hands, due to human papilloma virus, commonly, types 3 and 10. SYN flat wart, plane wart, v. plana juvenilis.

v. pla′na juveni′lis, SYN v. plana.

v. pla′na seni′lis, SYN actinic *keratosis.*

v. planta′ris, SYN plantar *wart.*

seborrheic v., SYN seborrheic *keratosis.*

v. seni′lis, SYN actinic *keratosis.*

v. sim′plex, SYN v. vulgaris.

v. vulga′ris, a keratotic papilloma of the epidermis which occurs most frequently in young persons as a result of localized infection by human papilloma virus, usually types 2 and 4; the lesions are of variable duration, eventually undergoing spontaneous regression, and are both exophytic and endophytic, with hyperkeratosis, parakeratosis, hypergranulosis, koilocytosis, and papillomatosis. SYN common wart, infectious warts, v. simplex, viral wart.

ver·ru·ci·form (vĕ-rū′si-fōrm). Wart-shaped. [L. *verruca,* wart, + *forma,* form]

ver·ru·cose (vĕ-rū′kōs). Resembling a wart; denoting wartlike elevations. SYN verrucous. [L. *verrucosus*]

ver·ru·co·sis (ver-ū-kō′sis). A condition marked by the appearance of multiple warts. [L. *verruca,* wart, + G. *-osis,* condition]

lymphostatic v., SYN mossy *foot.*

ver·ru·cous (vĕ-rū′kŭs). SYN verrucose.

ver·ru·ga (vĕ-rū′gă). SYN verruca. [Sp.]

v. perua′na, a late, eruptive stage of bartonellosis; characterized by soft conical or pedunculated vascular papules anywhere on the skin or mucous membranes from miliary size to several centimeters, resolving without scars after a few months. SYN hemorrhagic pian, Peruvian wart, verruca peruana, verruca peruviana.

ver·si·col·or (ver-si-kŏl′ŏr). Variegated; marked by a variety of color. [L. particolored, fr. *verso,* to turn, twist, + *color,* color]

ver·sion (ver′zhŭn, -shŭn). **1.** Displacement of the uterus, with tilting of the entire organ without bending upon itself; such displacement may be anteversion, retroversion, or lateroversion. **2.** Change of position of the fetus in the uterus, occurring spontaneously or effected by manipulation. **3.** SYN inclination. **4.** Conjugate rotation of the eyes in the same direction; such rotation may be dextroversion, levoversion, supraversion, or infraversion. [L. *verto,* pp. *versus,* to turn]

bimanual v., turning of the baby *in utero,* performed by the hands acting upon both extremities of the fetus; it may be external v. or combined v. SYN bipolar v.

bipolar v., SYN bimanual v.

Braxton Hicks v., obsolete term for internal v. of the fetus, substituting the breech for the head as the leading pole.

cephalic v., v. in which the fetus is turned so that the head presents; can be external cephalic v. or internal cephalic v. SEE ALSO external cephalic v., internal cephalic v.

combined v., bipolar v. by means of one hand in the vagina, the other on the abdominal wall.

external cephalic v., v. performed entirely by external manipulation. SEE ALSO cephalic v.

internal cephalic v., v. performed by means of one hand within the vagina. SEE ALSO cephalic v.

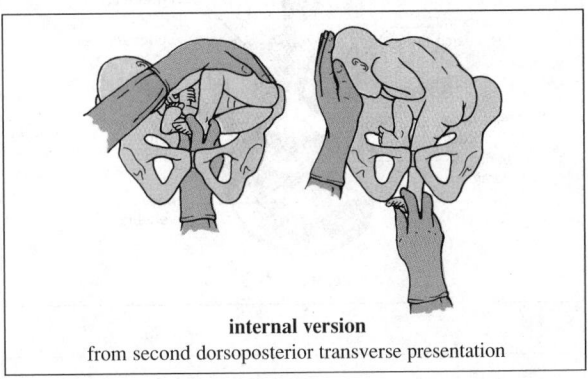

internal version
from second dorsoposterior transverse presentation

pelvic v., v. by means of which a transverse or oblique presentation is converted into a pelvic presentation by manipulating the buttocks of the fetus.

podalic v., a manual procedure that results in a podalic extraction.

postural v., nonmanual v. obtained by changing the position of the mother.

Potter's v., obsolete term for a v. in which both feet are brought down until the buttocks are delivered, the back is then rotated to an anterior position, the arms and shoulders are delivered by twisting and downward movements.

spontaneous v., turning of the fetus effected by the unaided contraction of the uterine muscle.

Wright's v., a cephalic v. employed in cases of shoulder presentation when the shoulders are pushed upward while the breech is moved toward the center of the uterus by the other hand; the head is then guided into the pelvis.

ver·te·bra, gen. and pl. **ver·te·brae** (ver′tĕ-bră, -brē) [NA]. One of the segments of the spinal column; in man there are usually 33 vertebrae, 7 cervical, 12 thoracic, 5 lumbar, 5 sacral (fused into one bone, the sacrum), and 4 coccygeal (fused into one bone, the coccyx). [L. joint, fr. *verto,* to turn]

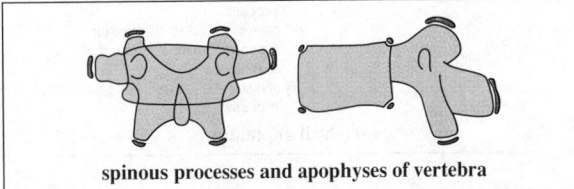

spinous processes and apophyses of vertebra

basilar v., the lowest lumbar v.

block vertebrae, congenitally fused and hypoplastic vertebral bodies which, on radiographs, give the appearance of a more or less solid bony mass. SEE Klippel-Feil *syndrome.*

butterfly v., a hemivertebra or sagittally cleft v. that has a butterfly configuration on frontal radiographs; congenital in origin.

caudal vertebrae, the vertebrae that form the skeleton of the tail.

cervical vertebrae, the seven segments of the vertebral column located in the neck. SYN vertebrae cervicales [NA].

ver′tebrae cervica′les [NA], SYN cervical vertebrae.

ver′tebrae coccyg′eae [NA], SYN coccygeal vertebrae.

coccygeal vertebrae, [Co-1–Co-4]; the four terminal segments of the vertebral column, usually fused to form the coccyx. SYN vertebrae coccygeae [NA], tail vertebrae.

codfish vertebrae, exaggeration of the concavity of the upper and lower end plates of the vertebrae, as demonstrated radiographically in various types of osteopenia.

ve

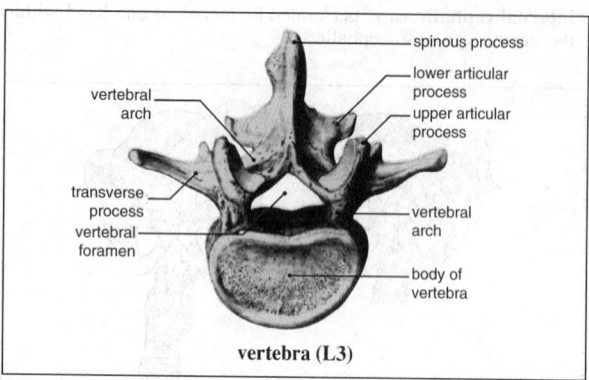

vertebra (L3)

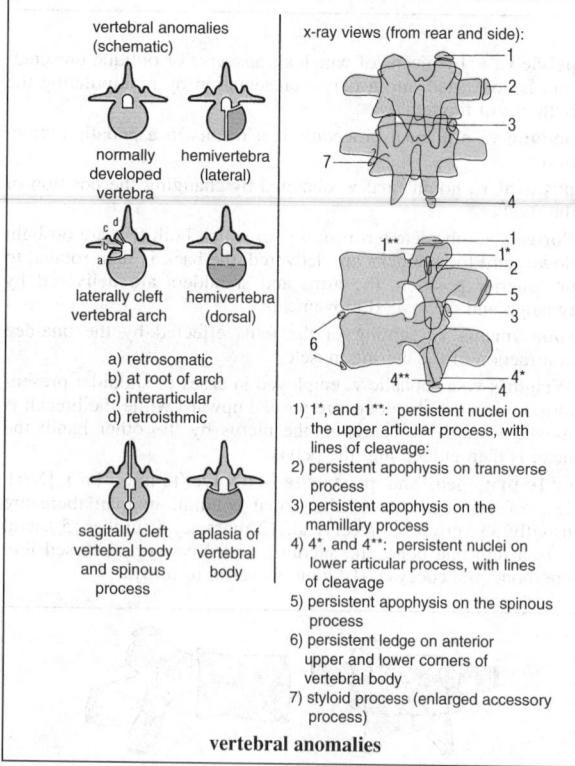

vertebral anomalies (schematic)

normally developed vertebra

hemivertebra (lateral)

laterally cleft vertebral arch

hemivertebra (dorsal)

a) retrosomatic
b) at root of arch
c) interarticular
d) retroisthmic

sagitally cleft vertebral body and spinous process

aplasia of vertebral body

x-ray views (from rear and side):

1) 1*, and 1**: persistent nuclei on the upper articular process, with lines of cleavage
2) persistent apophysis on transverse process
3) persistent apophysis on the mamillary process
4) 4*, and 4**: persistent nuclei on lower articular process, with lines of cleavage
5) persistent apophysis on the spinous process
6) persistent ledge on anterior upper and lower corners of vertebral body
7) styloid process (enlarged accessory process)

vertebral anomalies

cranial v., a segment of the skull regarded as homologous with a segment of the vertebral column.

v. denta′ta, SYN axis (5).

dorsal vertebrae, [L1–L4] an archaic term for thoracic vertebrae.

false vertebrae, the fused vertebral segments of the sacrum and coccyx. SYN vertebrae spuriae.

hourglass vertebrae, the radiographic appearance of some vertebrae in osteogenesis imperfecta tarda.

H-shape vertebrae, sharply delimited depression of the central portion of the endplates of the vertebrae, producing a stocky "H" shape on radiographs, as in sickle cell anemia.

ivory v., a radiographically dense v., usually from metastatic disease, especially lymphoma when solitary.

ver′tebrae lumba′les [NA], SYN lumbar vertebrae.

lumbar vertebrae, the vertebrae, usually five in number, located in the lumbar region of the back. SYN vertebrae lumbales [NA].

v. mag′na, SYN sacrum.

odontoid v., SYN axis (5).

picture frame v., radiographically diminished density of trabecular bone with relative preservation of the cortex, a sign of osteopenia.

v. pla′na, spondylitis with reduction of vertebral body to a thin disk.

v. prom′inens [NA], the v. in the cervicothoracic region which has the most prominent spinous process (seventh cervical v. in 70% of the cases, sixth in 20%, and first thoracic v. in 10%). SYN nuchal tubercle.

rugger jersey v., appearance of a vertebral body with horizontal sclerotic bands adjacent to the endplates; associated with renal osteodystrophy.

sacral vertebrae, [S1–S5] the segments of the vertebral column, usually five in number, that fuse to form the sacrum. SYN vertebrae sacrales [NA].

ver′tebrae sacra′les [NA], SYN sacral vertebrae.

ver′tebrae spu′riae, SYN false vertebrae.

tail vertebrae, SYN coccygeal vertebrae.

thoracic vertebrae, [T1–T12] the segments of the vertebral column, usually twelve, which articulate with ribs to form part of the thoracic cage. SYN vertebrae thoracicae [NA].

ver′tebrae thora′cicae [NA], SYN thoracic vertebrae.

toothed v., SYN axis (5).

true v., any one of the cervical, thoracic, or lumbar vertebrae. SYN v. vera.

v. ve′ra, SYN true v.

ver·te·bral (ver′tĕ-brăl). Relating to a vertebra or the vertebrae.

ver·te·bra·ri·um (ver-tĕ-brā′rē-ŭm). SYN vertebral *column*. [Mod. L.]

Ver·te·bra·ta (ver-tĕ-brah′tă, -brā′tă). The vertebrates, a major division of the phylum Chordata, consisting of those animals with a dorsal hollow nerve cord enclosed in a cartilaginous or bony spinal column; includes several classes of fishes, and the amphibians, reptiles, birds, and mammals. SYN Craniata. [L. *vertebratus*, jointed]

ver·te·brate (ver′tĕ-brāt). **1.** Having a vertebral column. **2.** An animal having vertebrae.

notochordal v., a lower v. in which the notochord persists, unossified, in adult life.

ver·te·brat·ed (ver′tĕ-brāt-ed). Jointed; composed of segments arranged longitudinally as in certain instruments.

ver·te·brec·to·my (ver′tĕ-brek′tō-mē). Resection of a vertebral body. [vertebra + G. *ektomē*, excision]

△**vertebro-.** A vertebra, vertebral. [L. *vertebra*]

ver·te·bro·ar·te·ri·al (ver′tĕ-brō-ar-tēr′ē-ăl). Relating to a vertebra and an artery, or to the vertebral artery.

ver·te·bro·chon·dral (ver′tĕ-brō-kon′drăl). Denoting the three false ribs (eighth, ninth, and tenth), which are connected with the vertebrae at one extremity and the costal cartilages at the other, these cartilages not articulating directly with the sternum. SYN vertebrocostal (2). [vertebro- + G. *chondros*, cartilage]

ver·te·bro·cos·tal (ver′tĕ-brō-kos′tăl). **1.** SYN costovertebral. **2.** SYN vertebrochondral. [vertebro- + L. *costa*, rib]

ver·te·bro·fem·o·ral (ver-tĕ-brō-fem′ŏ-răl). Relating to the vertebrae and the femur.

ver·te·bro·il·i·ac (ver′tĕ-brō-il′ē-ak). Relating to the vertebrae and the ilium.

ver·te·bro·sa·cral (ver-tĕ-brō-sā′krăl). Relating to the vertebrae and the sacrum.

ver·te·bro·ster·nal (ver′tĕ-brō-ster′năl). SYN sternovertebral.

ver·tex, pl. **ver·ti·ces** (ver′teks, ver′ti-sēz). **1** [NA]. The topmost point of the vault of the skull, a landmark in craniometry. **2.** In obstetrics, the portion of the fetal head bounded by the planes of the trachelobregmatic and biparietal diameters, with the posterior fontanel at the apex. [L. whirl, whorl]

v. cor′dis, SYN apex of heart.

v. of cornea, the central part of the cornea, slightly thinner than the peripheral part. SYN v. corneae [NA].

v. cor′neae [NA], SYN v. of cornea.

ver·ti·cal (ver′ti-kăl). **1.** Relating to the vertex, or crown of the head. **2.** Perpendicular. **3.** Denoting any plane or line that passes longitudinally through the body in the anatomical position. SYN verticalis [NA].

ver·ti·ca·lis (ver-ti-kā'lis) [NA]. SYN vertical. [L.]

ver·ti·ces (ver'ti-sēz). Plural of vertex.

ver·ti·cil (ver'ti-sil). A collection of similar parts radiating from a common axis. SYN vortex (1), whorl (4). [L. *verticillus*, the whirl of a spindle, dim. of *vertex*, a whirl]

ver·ti·cil·late (ver'ti-sil'āt). Disposed in the form of a verticil.

Ver·ti·cil·li·um (ver-ti-sil'ē-ŭm). A genus of hyphomycetous fungi often found in clinical specimens as contaminants. They are occasionally found in the meatus in cases of otitis externa, but are of doubtful pathogenicity. [L. *verticillus,* the whirl of a spindle]

ver·ti·co·men·tal (ver-ti-kō-men'tăl). Relating to the crown of the head and the chin; denoting a diameter in craniometry.

ver·tig·i·nous (ver-tij'i-nŭs). Relating to or suffering from vertigo.

ver·ti·go (ver'ti-gō, ver-tī'gō). **1.** A sensation of spinning or whirling motion. V. implies a definite sensation of rotation of the subject or of objects about the subject in any plane. **2.** Imprecisely used as a general term to describe dizziness. [L. *vertigo* (*vertigin-*), dizziness, fr. *verto,* to turn]

v. ab au're lae'so, v. dependent upon chronic middle ear lesions.

auditory v., SYN Ménière's *disease.*

aural v., (1) v. caused by disease of the internal ear or pressure of cerumen on the drum membrane. **(2)** nonspecific term for v. caused by labyrinthine disorders.

benign paroxysmal postural v., a recurrent, brief form of postural v. occurring in clusters; believed to result from displaced remnants of utricular otoconia. SYN cupulolithiasis.

benign positional v., brief attacks of paroxysmal v. and nystagmus that occur solely with certain head movements or positions, *e.g.,* with neck extension; due to labyrinthine dysfunction. SYN positional v. of Bárány, postural v. (1).

Charcot's v., SYN tussive *syncope.*

chronic v., SYN *status* vertiginosus.

endemic paralytic v., SYN vestibular *neuronitis.*

epidemic v., SYN vestibular *neuronitis.*

gastric v., v. symptomatic of disease of the stomach. SYN Trousseau's syndrome (1).

height v., dizziness experienced when looking down from a great height or in looking up at a high building or cliff. SYN vertical v. (1).

horizontal v., dizziness experienced on lying down.

hysterical v., a sensation of dizziness, as from a whirling motion, whose etiology is psychosomatic.

labyrinthine v., SYN Ménière's *disease.*

laryngeal v., SYN tussive *syncope.*

lateral v., dizziness caused by watching the telegraph poles and fences from the window of a fast-moving vehicle.

mechanical v., v. caused by continued rotation or vibration of the body.

nocturnal v., a feeling of falling when dropping off to sleep.

ocular v., dizziness attributed to refractive errors or imbalance of the extrinsic muscles.

organic v., v. due to brain damage.

paralyzing v., SYN vestibular *neuronitis.*

physiologic v., SYN space *sickness.*

positional v. of Bárány, SYN benign positional v.

postural v., (1) SYN benign positional v. **(2)** light-headedness that appears particularly in elderly people with change of position, usually from lying or sitting to standing; due to orthostatic hypotension.

sham-movement v., dizziness accompanied by an impression that the body is rotating or that objects are rotating about the body. SYN gyrosa.

vertical v., (1) SYN height v. **(2)** dizziness experienced when standing upright.

ver·tom·e·ter (ver-tom'ĕ-ter). SYN lensometer. [vertex + G. *metron,* measure]

ver·u·mon·ta·ni·tis (ver'ū-mon-tă-nī'tis). SYN colliculitis. [see verumontanum]

ver·u·mon·ta·num (ver-ū-mon-tā'nŭm). SYN seminal *colliculus.* [L. *veru,* a spit, + *montanus,* mountainous]

ve·sa·li·a·num (ve-sā'lē-ā'nŭm). SYN os vesalianum.

Vesalius (We·sal, Vesal), Andreas (Andre), Flemish anatomist, 1514–1564. SEE V.'s *bone, foramen, vein.*

⌂**vesic-.** SEE vesico-.

ve·si·ca, gen. and pl. **ve·si·cae** (vě sī' kă, vě sī' sē; -kē). **1** [NA]. SYN bladder. **2.** Any hollow structure or sac, normal or pathologic, containing a serous fluid. [L.]

v. bilia'ris [NA], SYN gallbladder.

v. fel'lea [NA], ✳official alternate term for gallbladder.

v. prostat'ica, SYN prostatic *utricle.*

v. urina'ria [NA], SYN urinary *bladder.*

ves·i·cal (ves'i-kăl). Relating to any bladder, but usually the urinary bladder.

ves·i·cant (ves'i-kănt). An agent that produces a vesicle. SYN blister agent, epispastic, vesicatory.

ves·i·cate (ves'i-kāt). To form a vesicle.

ves·i·ca·tion (ves-i-kā'shŭn). SYN vesiculation (1).

ves·i·ca·to·ry (ves'i-kă-tōr-ē). SYN vesicant.

ves·i·cle (ves'i-kl). **1.** SYN vesicula. **2.** A small (less than 0.5 cm) circumscribed elevation of the skin containing fluid. SEE ALSO bleb, blister, bulla. **3.** A small sac containing liquid or gas. [L. *vesicula,* a blister, dim. of *vesica,* bladder]

acoustic v., SYN auditory v.

acrosomal v., a v. derived from the Golgi apparatus during spermiogenesis whose limiting membrane adheres to the nuclear envelope; together with the acrosomal granule within, it spreads in a thin layer over the pole of the nucleus to form the acrosomal cap.

air v.'s, SYN pulmonary *alveolus.*

allantoic v., the hollow portion of the allantois.

amniocardiac v., the rostral portion of the most primitive intraembryonic celom.

auditory v., one of the paired sacs of invaginated ectoderm that develop into the membranous labyrinth of the internal ear. SYN acoustic v., otic v.

Baer's v., obsolete term for vesicular ovarian *follicle.*

blastodermic v., SYN blastocyst.

cerebral v., each of the three divisions of the early embryonic brain (prosencephalon, mesencephalon, and rhombencephalon). SYN encephalic v., primary brain v.

cervical v., an abnormally persisting vestige of the cervical sinus or its associated branchial grooves.

coated v., a v. that has its biomembrane coated with the protein clathrin. It is involved in the transport of proteins from one membrane site to another.

encephalic v., SYN cerebral v.

forebrain v., SYN prosencephalon.

germinal v., archaic term for the nucleus of the ovum.

hindbrain v., SYN rhombencephalon.

lens v., in the embryo, the ectodermal invagination that forms opposite the optic cup; it is the primordium of the lens of the eye. SYN lenticular v.

lenticular v., SYN lens v.

malpighian v.'s, the minute air-filled v.'s on the surface of an expanded lung.

midbrain v., SYN mesencephalon.

ocular v., SYN ophthalmic v.

ophthalmic v., in the embryo, one of the paired evaginations from the ventrolateral walls of the forebrain from which the sensory and pigment layers of the retina develop. SYN vesicula ophthalmica [NA], ocular v., optic v.

optic v., SYN ophthalmic v.

otic v., SYN auditory v.

pinocytotic v., a v., a fraction of a micrometer in diameter, containing fluid or solute being ingested into a cell by endocytosis. SEE ALSO pinocytosis.

ve

primary brain v., SYN cerebral v.

seminal v., one of two folded, sacculated, glandular structures which is a diverticulum of the ductus deferens; its secretion is one of the components of the semen; it normally does not store spermatozoa as was thought historically. SYN glandula seminalis [NA], vesicula seminalis [NA], gonecyst, gonecystis, seminal capsule, seminal gland.

synaptic v.'s, the small (average diameter 30 nm), intracellular, membrane-bound v.'s near the presynaptic membrane of a synaptic junction, containing the transmitter substance which, in chemical synapses, mediates the passage of nerve impulses across the junction. SEE ALSO synapse.

telencephalic v., paired diverticula arising from the prosencephalon, from which the forebrain develops.

umbilical v., SYN yolk *sac.*

⌂**vesico-, vesic-.** A vesica, vesicle. SEE ALSO vesiculo-. [L. *vesica,* bladder]

ves·i·co·ab·dom·i·nal (ves'i-kō-ab-dom'i-năl). Relating to the urinary bladder and the abdominal wall.

ves·i·co·bul·lous (ves'i-kō-bŭl'ŭs). Denoting an eruption of variously sized lesions containing fluid.

ves·i·co·cele (ves'i-kō-sēl). SYN cystocele.

ves·i·co·cer·vi·cal (ves'i-kō-ser'vi-kăl). Relating to the urinary bladder and the cervix of the uterus.

ves·i·coc·ly·sis (ves'i-kok'li-sis). Washing out, or lavage, of the urinary bladder. [vesico- + G. *klysis,* a washing out]

ves·i·co·in·tes·ti·nal (ves'i-kō-in-tes'ti-năl). Relating to the urinary bladder and the intestine; *e.g.,* vesicointestinal fistula.

ves·i·co·lith·i·a·sis (ves'i-kō-li-thī'ă-sis). SYN cystolithiasis. [vesico- + G. *lithos,* stone, + *-iasis,* condition]

ves·i·co·pros·ta·tic (ves'i-kō-pros-tat'ik). Relating to the bladder and the prostate gland.

ves·i·co·pu·bic (ves'i-kō-pyū'bik). Relating to the bladder and the os pubis.

ves·i·co·pus·tu·lar (ves'i-kō-pŭs'tyū-lăr). Pertaining to a vesicopustule. SYN vesiculopustular (1).

ves·i·co·pus·tule (ves'i-kō-pŭs'tyūl). A vesicle which is developing pus formation.

ves·i·co·rec·tal (ves'i-kō-rek'tăl). Relating to the bladder and the rectum.

ves·i·co·rec·tos·to·my (ves'i-kō-rek-tos'tō-mē). Surgical urinary tract diversion by anastomosis of the posterior bladder wall to the rectum. [vesico- + rectum + G. *stoma,* mouth]

ves·i·co·sig·moid (ves'i-kō-sig'moyd). Relating to the bladder and the sigmoid colon.

ves·i·co·sig·moi·dos·to·my (ves'i-kō-sig-moy-dos'tō-mē). Operative formation of a communication between the bladder and the sigmoid colon. [vesico- + sigmoid + G. *stoma,* mouth]

ves·i·co·spi·nal (ves'i-kō-spī'năl). Relating to the urinary bladder and the spinal cord; denoting the neural mechanisms that control retention and evacuation of urine by the bladder, located in the second lumbar and second sacral segment, respectively, of the spinal cord.

ves·i·cos·to·my (ves'i-kos'tō-mē). SYN cystostomy. [vesico- + G. *stoma,* mouth]

ves·i·cot·o·my (ves'i-kot'ō-mē). SYN cystotomy.

ves·i·co·um·bi·li·cal (ves'i-kō-ŭm-bil'i-kăl). Relating to the urinary bladder and the umbilicus. SYN omphalovesical.

ves·i·co·u·re·ter·al (ves'i-kō-yū-rē'ter-ăl). Relating to the bladder and the ureters.

ves·i·co·u·re·thral (ves'i-kō-yū-rē'thrăl). Relating to the bladder and the urethra.

ves·i·co·u·ter·ine (ves'i-kō-yū'ter-in). Relating to the bladder and the uterus.

ves·i·co·u·ter·o·vag·i·nal (ves'i-kō-yū'ter-ō-vaj'i-năl). Relating to the bladder, uterus, and vagina.

ves·i·co·vag·i·nal (ves-i-kō-vaj'i-năl). Relating to the bladder and vagina.

ves·i·co·vag·i·no·rec·tal (ves'i-kō-vaj'i-nō-rek'tăl). Relating to the bladder, vagina, and rectum.

ves·i·co·vis·cer·al (ves'i-kō-vis'er-ăl). Relating to the urinary bladder and any other adjacent organ or viscus.

ve·sic·u·la, gen. and pl. **ve·sic·u·lae** (vě-sik'yū-lă, -lē). A small bladder or bladder-like structure. SYN vesicle (1). [L. blister, vesicle, dim. of *vesica,* bladder]

v. fel'lis, SYN gallbladder.

v. ophthal'mica [NA], SYN ophthalmic *vesicle.*

v. semina'lis [NA], SYN seminal *vesicle.*

v. umbilica'lis, SYN yolk *sac.*

ve·sic·u·lar (vě-sik'yū-lăr). **1.** Relating to a vesicle. **2.** Characterized by or containing vesicles. SYN vesiculate (2), vesiculated, vesiculose, vesiculous.

ve·sic·u·late (vě-sik'yū-lāt). **1.** To become vesicular. **2.** SYN vesicular (2).

ve·sic·u·lat·ed (vě-sik'yū-lāt-ed). SYN vesicular (2).

ve·sic·u·la·tion (vě-sik'yū-lā'shŭn). **1.** The formation of vesicles. SYN blistering, vesication. **2.** SYN inflation. **3.** Presence of a number of vesicles.

ve·sic·u·lec·to·my (vě-sik'yū-lek'tō-mē). Resection of a portion or all of each of the seminal vesicles. [L. *vesicula,* vesicle, + G. *ektomē,* excision]

ve·sic·u·li·form (vě-sik'yū-li-fōrm). Resembling a vesicle.

ve·sic·u·li·tis (vě-sik'yū-lī'tis). Inflammation of any vesicle; especially of a seminal vesicle. [L. *vesicula,* vesicle, + G. *-itis,* inflammation]

⌂**vesiculo-.** A vesicle. [L. *vesicula,* vesicle, dim. of *vesica,* bladder]

ve·sic·u·lo·bron·chi·al (vě-sik'yū-lō-brong'kē-ăl). Denoting an auscultatory sound having both a vesicular and a bronchial quality.

ve·sic·u·lo·cav·ern·ous (vě-sik'yū-lō-kav'er-nŭs). Both vesicular and cavernous; denoting: **1.** An auscultatory sound having both a vesicular and a cavernous quality; **2.** The structure of certain neoplasms.

ve·sic·u·log·ra·phy (vě-sik-yū-log'ră-fī). Radiographic contrast study of the seminal vesicles. [vesiculo- + G. *graphō,* to write]

ve·sic·u·lo·pap·u·lar (vě-sik'yū-lō-pap'yū-lăr). Pertaining to or consisting of a combination of vesicles and papules, or of papules becoming increasingly edematous with sufficient collection of fluid to form vesicles.

ve·sic·u·lo·pros·ta·ti·tis (vě-sik'yū-lō-pros'tă-tī'tis). Inflammation of the bladder and prostate. [vesiculo- + prostate + G. *-itis,* inflammation]

ve·sic·u·lo·pus·tu·lar (vě-sik'yū-lō-pŭs'tyū-lăr). **1.** SYN vesicopustular. **2.** Pertaining to a mixed eruption of vesicles and pustules.

ve·si·cu·lose (vě-sik'yū-lōs). SYN vesicular (2).

ve·sic·u·lot·o·my (vě-sik-yū-lot'ō-mē). Surgical incision of the seminal vesicles. [vesiculo- + G. *tomē,* incision]

ve·sic·u·lo·tu·bu·lar (vě-sik'yū-lō-tū'byū-ler). Denoting an auscultatory sound having both a vesicular and a tubular quality.

ve·sic·u·lo·tym·pan·ic (vě-sik'yū-lō-tim-pan'ik). Denoting a percussion sound having both a vesicular and a tympanic quality.

ve·sic·u·lous (vě-sik'yū-lŭs). SYN vesicular (2).

Ve·si·cu·lo·vi·rus (vě-sik'yū-lō-vī'rŭs). A genus of viruses (family Rhabdoviridae) that includes the vesicular stomatitis virus (of cattle) and related viruses.

vesp. (ves'per). Abbreviation for L. *vesper,* evening. [L. evening]

ves·sel (ves'ĕl). A structure conveying or containing a fluid, especially a liquid. SEE ALSO vas. [O. Fr. fr. L. *vascellum,* dim. of *vas*]

absorbent v.'s, SYN lymph v.'s.

afferent v., (1) any artery conveying blood to a part; (2) SYN afferent glomerular *arteriole.* (3) SYN afferent *lymphatic.*

anastomosing v., a v. that establishes a connection between arteries, between veins, or between lymph v.'s. SYN vas anastomoticum [NA].

blood v., SEE blood vessel.

capillary v., SYN capillary (2). SEE blood *capillary,* lymph *capillary.*

chyle v., SYN lacteal (2).

collateral v., (1) a branch of an artery running parallel with the parent trunk; (2) a v. that runs in parallel with another v., nerve, or other long structure. SYN vas collaterale [NA].

deep lymphatic v., one of the v.'s that drain lymph from the deep structures of the body; they tend to follow the courses of blood v.'s to reach regional lymph nodes. SYN vas lymphaticum profundum [NA].

efferent v., SYN efferent glomerular *arteriole.*

v.'s of internal ear, blood v.'s of the internal ear, consisting of the labyrinthine artery and its branches and the labyrinthine veins and their tributaries. SYN vasa auris internae [NA].

lacteal v., SYN lacteal (2).

lymph v.'s, the v.'s that convey the lymph; they anastomose freely with each other. SYN vasa lymphatica [NA], absorbent v.'s, lymphatic v.'s, lymphatics.

lymphatic v.'s, SYN lymph v.'s.

nutrient v., SYN nutrient *artery.*

superficial lymphatic v., one of the lymphatic v.'s that lie in the skin and subcutaneous tissues; they join the deep lymphatic v.'s. SYN vas lymphaticum superficiale [NA].

v.'s of vessels, SYN *vasa* vasorum, under *vas.*

vitelline v.'s, SEE vitelline *artery,* vitelline *vein.*

ves·tib·u·la (ves-tib'yū-lă). Plural of vestibulum.

ves·tib·u·lar (ves-tib'yū-lăr). Relating to a vestibule, especially the vestibule of the ear. SYN vestibularis [NA].

ves·ti·bu·la·ris (ves-tib-yū-lā'ris) [NA]. SYN vestibular, vestibular. [L.]

ves·tib·u·late (ves-tib'yū-lăt). Possessing a vestibule.

ves·ti·bule (ves'ti-būl). 1. A small cavity or a space at the entrance of a canal. 2. Specifically, the central, somewhat ovoid, cavity of the osseous labyrinth communicating with the semicircular canals posteriorly and the cochlea anteriorly. SYN vestibulum [NA]. [L. *vestibulum*]

aortic v., the anterosuperior portion of the left ventricle of the heart immediately below the aortic orifice, having fibrous walls and affording room for the segments of the closed aortic valve. SYN Sibson's aortic v., vestibulum aortae.

buccal v., that part of the oral vestibule related to the cheek.

esophagogastric v., SYN gastroesophageal v.

gastroesophageal v., the dilated aboral portion of the esophagus, just above the cardiac orifice; usually it corresponds to the lumen of abdominal part of the esophagus although its relation to the diaphragm is variable. SYN esophagogastric v.

labial v., that part of the oval vestibule related to the lips.

v. of larynx, the upper part of the laryngeal cavity from the superior aperture to the vestibular folds, bounded anteriorly by the epiglottis, laterally by themucosa overlying the quadrangular membranes and posteriorly by the mucosa overlying the arytenoid cartilages and arytenoideus muscle. SYN vestibulum laryngis [NA], atrium glottidis, superior laryngeal cavity.

v. of mouth, SYN oral v.

v. of nose, the anterior part of the nasal cavity, especially that enclosed by cartilage. SYN vestibulum nasi [NA].

v. of omental bursa, the upper part of the bursa omentalis, just within the epiploic foramen (of Winslow), behind the caudate lobe of the liver. SYN vestibulum bursae omentalis [NA].

oral v., that part of the mouth bounded anteriorly and laterally by the lips and the cheeks, posteriorly and medially by the teeth and/or gums, and above and below by the reflections of the mucosa from the lips and cheeks to the gums. SYN vestibulum oris [NA], buccal cavity, v. of mouth.

Sibson's aortic v., SYN aortic v.

v. of vagina, the space behind the glans clitoridis and between the labia minora, containing the openings of the vagina, urethra, and ducts of the greater vestibular glands. SYN vestibulum vaginae [NA], vaginal introitus, vestibulum pudendi.

ves·tib·u·li·tis. An inflammation of the vulvar vestibule and the periglandular and subepithelial stroma characterized by burning sensation and painful coitus.

⬦**vestibulo-.** Vestibule, vestibulum. [L. *vestibulum*]

ves·tib·u·lo·cer·e·bel·lum (ves-tib'yū-lō-ser-ĕ-bel'ŭm). Those regions of the cerebellar cortex whose predominant afferent fibers arise from the ganglion vestibulare and the vestibular nuclei; structures included under this term are nodulus, flocculus, ventral parts of the uvula and small ventral parts of the lingula. SYN archeocerebellum. [vestibulo- + L. *cerebellum*]

ves·tib·u·lo·co·chle·ar (ves-tib'yū-lō-kok'lē-ăr). 1. Relating to the vestibulum and cochlea of the ear. 2. SYN statoacoustic.

ves·tib·u·lop·a·thy (ves-tib'ū-lop'a-thē). Any abnormality of the vestibular apparatus, *e.g.,* Ménière's disease.

idiopathic bilateral v., slowly progressive disorder affecting young to middle-aged adults, manifested as gait unsteadiness (especially when visual cues are absent) and oscillopsia, unaccompanied by vertigo and hearing loss.

ves·tib·u·lo·plas·ty (ves-tib'yū-lō-plas-tē). Any of a series of surgical procedures designed to restore alveolar ridge height by lowering muscles attaching to the buccal, labial, and lingual aspects of the jaws. [vestibulo- + G. *plassō,* to form]

ves·tib·u·lo·spi·nal (ves-tib'yū-lō-spī'năl). SEE vestibulospinal *tract.*

ves·tib·u·lot·o·my (ves-tib'yū-lot'ō-mē). Operation for an opening into the vestibule of the labyrinth. [vestibulo- + G. *tomē,* incision]

ves·tib·u·lo·u·re·thral (ves-tib'yū-lō-ū-rē'thrăl). Relating to the vestibule of the vagina and urethra.

ves·tib·u·lum, pl. **ves·tib·u·la** (ves-tib'yū-lŭm, -lă) [NA]. SYN vestibule. [L. antechamber, entrance court]

v. aor'tae, SYN aortic *vestibule.*

v. bur'sae omenta'lis [NA], SYN *vestibule* of omental bursa.

v. laryn'gis [NA], SYN *vestibule* of larynx.

v. na'si [NA], SYN *vestibule* of nose.

v. o'ris [NA], SYN oral *vestibule.*

v. puden'di, SYN *vestibule* of vagina.

v. vagi'nae [NA], SYN *vestibule* of vagina.

ves·tige (ves'tij). A trace or a rudimentary structure; the degenerated remains of any structure which occurs as an entity in the embryo or fetus. SYN vestigium. [L. *vestigium*]

v. of processus vaginalis, incompletely obliterated remnants of the vaginal process of the peritoneum remaining in the spermatic cord. SYN vestigium processus vaginalis [NA], v. of vaginal process.

v. of vaginal process, SYN v. of processus vaginalis.

ves·tig·i·al (ves-tij'ē-ăl). Relating to a vestige.

ves·tig·i·um, pl. **ves·tig·ia** (ves-tij'ē-ŭm, -ă). SYN vestige. [L. footprint (trace), fr. *vestigo,* to track, trace]

v. proces'sus vagina'lis [NA], SYN *vestige* of processus vaginalis.

ve·su·vin (vĕ-sū'vin) [C.I. 21000]. SYN Bismarck brown Y. [*Vesuvius,* volcano in Italy]

vet·er·i·nar·i·an (vet'ĕ-rin-ār'ē-ăn). A person who holds an academic degree in veterinary medicine; a licensed practitioner of veterinary medicine. [see veterinary]

Vet·er·i·nar·i·an's Oath. The official oath of the veterinary profession, adopted by the American Veterinary Medical Association in 1954: "Being admitted to the profession of veterinary medicine, I solemnly dedicate myself and the knowledge I possess to the benefit of society, to the conservation of our livestock resources and to the relief of suffering of animals. I will practice my profession conscientiously with dignity. The health of my patients, the best interest of their owners, and the welfare of my fellow man, will be my primary considerations. I will, at all times, be humane and temper pain with anesthesia where indicated. I will not use my knowledge contrary to the laws of humanity, nor in contravention to the ethical code of my profession. I will uphold and strive to advance the honor and noble traditions of the veterinary profession. These pledges I make freely in the eyes of God and upon my honor."

vet·er·i·nary (vet'ĕ-rin-ār-ē). Relating to the diseases of animals. [L. *veterinarius,* fr. *veterina,* beast of burden]

VHDL Abbreviation for very high density lipoprotein. SEE lipoprotein.

via, pl. **vi·ae** (vī′ă, vī′ē; vē′ă). Any passage in the body, as the intestine, the vagina, etc. [L. way, road]

vi·a·bil·i·ty (vī-ă-bil′i-tē). Capability of living; the state of being viable; usually connotes a fetus that has reached 500 g in weight and 20 gestational weeks. [Fr. *viabilité* fr. L. *vita,* life]

vi·a·ble (vī′ă-bl). Capable of living; denoting a fetus sufficiently developed to live outside of the uterus. [Fr. fr. *vie,* life, fr. L. *vita*]

vi·al (vī′ăl). A small bottle or receptacle for holding liquids, including medicines. SYN phial. [G. *phialē,* a drinking cup]

vi·bes·ate (vī′bĕ-sāt). A mixture of polvinate and malrosinol in organic solvent and a propellant; a modified polyvinyl plastic used as a topical spray for wounds.

vi·bra·tion (vī-brā′shŭn). **1.** A shaking. **2.** A to-and-fro movement, as in oscillation. [L. *vibratio,* fr. *vibro,* pp. *-atus,* to quiver, shake]

vi·bra·tive (vī′bră-tiv). SYN vibratory.

vi·bra·tor (vī′brā-ter, tōr). An instrument used for imparting vibrations.

vi·bra·to·ry (vī′bră-tōr-ē). Marked by vibrations. SYN vibrative.

Vib·rio (vib′rē-ō). A genus of motile (occasionally nonmotile), nonsporeforming, aerobic to facultatively anaerobic, Gram-negative bacteria (family Spirillaceae) containing short (0.5 to 3.0 μm), curved or straight rods which occur singly or which are occasionally united into S-shapes or spirals. Motile cells contain a single polar flagellum; in some species, two or more flagella occur in one polar tuft. Some of these organisms are saprophytes in salt and fresh water and in soil; others are parasites or pathogens. The type species is *V. cholerae.* [L. *vibro,* to vibrate]

V. alginolyt′icus, a species associated with wound and ear infections, and with bacteremia in immunocompromised and in burn patients.

V. chol′erae, a species that produces a soluble exotoxin (permeability factor) and is the cause of cholera in man; it is the type species of the genus *V.* SYN cholera bacillus, comma bacillus, Koch's bacillus (2).

V. fe′tus, former name for *Campylobacter fetus.*

V. fluvia′lis, a species, similar to strains of *Aeromonas,* associated with diarrheal disease in humans.

V. furnis′sii, an aerogenic strain, similar to *V. fluvialis,* associated with diarrheal disease and outbreaks of gastroenteritis.

V. hol′lisae, species which can cause dysentery in humans.

V. metschniko′vii, a species causing acute enteric disease in chickens and other avian species; also isolated from human stool.

V. mim′icus, a sucrose-negative strain, similar to *V. cholerae,* isolated from human stool in diarrheal disease and from human ear infections.

V. parahaemolyt′icus, a marine species that causes gastroenteritis and bloody diarrhea, usually from eating contaminated shellfish.

V. sputo′rum, former name for *Campylobacter sputorum.*

V. vulnif′icus, a species capable of causing cutaneous lesions in an cirrhotic or immunocompromised patient; usually contracted from contaminated oysters; also a cause of wound infections, especially those associated with handling of shellfish.

vib·rio (vib′rē-ō). A member of the genus *Vibrio.*

El Tor v., a bacterium regarded as a biovar of *V. cholerae.* It was originally isolated from six pilgrims who died of dysentery or gangrene of the colon at the Tor quarantine station on the Sinai Peninsula.

Nasik v., an organism differing from the cholera v., being shorter and stouter and less comma-shaped; its cultures are very toxic to laboratory animals on intravenous injections.

vib·ri·on sep·tique (vē-brē-on′ sep-tēk′). SYN *Clostridium septicum.* [Fr. septic vibrio]

vib·ri·o·sis, pl. **vib·ri·o·ses** (vib-rē-ō′sis). Infection caused by species of bacteria of the genus *Vibrio.*

vi·bris·sa, gen. and pl. **vi·bris·sae** (vī-bris′ă, vī-bris′ē) [NA]. One of the hairs growing at the nares, or vestibule of the nose. [L. found only in pl. *vibrissae,* fr. *vibro,* to quiver]

vi·bris·sal (vib-ris′ăl). Relating to the vibrissae.

vi·bro·car·di·o·gram (vī′brō-kar′dē-ō-gram). A graphic record of chest vibrations produced by hemodynamic events of the cardiac cycle; the record provides an indirect, externally recorded measurement of isovolumic contraction and ejection times. [L. *vibro,* to shake, + G. *kardia,* heart, + *gramma,* a drawing]

vi·bro·mas·seur (vī′brō-ma-ser′). A type of vibrator for giving vibratory massage.

vi·bro·ther·a·peu·tics (vī′brō-thār-ă-pyū′tiks). SYN vibratory *massage.*

Vi·bur·num pru·ni·fo·li·um (vī-bur′num prū-′nī-fō′lē-ŭm). A medication derived from the root bark of *Viburnum prunifolium* (family Caprifoliaceae); contains viburnin; bitter resin; tannin; sugar; citric, malic, oxalic and valeric acids. Formerly used as a smooth muscle relaxant/antispasmodic (uterine).

vi·car·i·ous (vī-ker′ē-ŭs). Acting as a substitute; occurring in an abnormal situation. [L. *vicarius,* from *vicis,* supplying place of]

Vicat, L.J., French engineer, 1786–1861. SEE V. *needle.*

vi·cine (vī′sēn). 2,5-Diamino-4,6-diketopyrimidine-3-β-D-glucoside; a glucoside occurring in akta, a weed which contaminates *Lathyrus sativus* and is thought by some to be responsible for the symptoms of lathyrism. [*Vicia* (genus name) + -ine]

Vicq d'Azyr, Félix, French anatomist, 1748–1794. SEE V. d''s *bundle, centrum* semiovale, *foramen.*

Vic·to·ria blue. Any of several blue diphenylnaphthylmethane derivatives; used as a stain in histology. [Queen *Victoria*]

Vic·to·ria or·ange. An alkaline salt of dinitrocresol; a reddish yellow stain formerly used in histology.

Vidal, Jean Baptiste Emile, French dermatologist, 1825–1893. SEE V.'s *disease.*

vi·dar·a·bine (vī-der′ă-bēn). 9-β-D-Arabinofuranosyladenine monohydrate; a purine nucleoside obtained from fermentation cultures of *Streptomyces antibioticus* and used to treat herpes simplex infections.

vid·e·o·ker·a·to·scope (vid′ē-ō-ker′ah-tō-skōp). A keratoscope fitted with a video camera.

vid·i·an (vid′ē-an). Named after or described by Vidius.

Vidius (Vidus), Guidi (Guido), Italian anatomist and physician, 1500–1569. SEE vidian *artery,* vidian *canal,* vidian *nerve,* vidian *vein.*

Vierra, J.P., 20th century Brazilian dermatologist. SEE V.'s *sign.*

Vieussens, Raymond de, French anatomist, 1641–1715. SEE V.'s *annulus, ansa, centrum, foramina,* under *foramen, ganglia,* under *ganglion, isthmus, limbus, loop, ring; valve* of V.; V.'s *valve, veins,* under *vein, ventricle.*

view (vyū). SYN projection.

axial v., SYN axial *projection.*

base v., SYN submentovertex *radiograph.*

Caldwell v., SYN Caldwell *projection.*

half axial v., SYN Towne *projection.*

long axis v., in echocardiography, a projection parallel to the interventricular septum of the heart; four-chamber view.

Stenvers v., SYN Stenvers *projection.*

Towne v., SYN Towne *projection.*

verticosubmental v., SYN axial *projection.*

Waters' v., SYN Waters' *projection.*

vig·a·bat·rin (vī-gă′bă-trin). An irreversible inhibitor of γ-aminobutyric acid transaminase, a degradative enzyme for γ-aminobutyric acid (GABA), the inhibitory neurotransmitter. The drug intensifies the effects of GABA and thus inhibition of the central nervous system; used as an antiepileptic agent.

vig·il (vij′il). A state of wakefulness or sleeplessness. [L. *vigilia,* wakefulness, alertness, fr. *vigeo,* to be active, to rouse]

coma v., SYN akinetic *mutism.*

vig·il·am·bu·lism (vij-i-lam′byū-lizm). A condition of unconsciousness regarding one's surroundings, with automatism, resembling somnambulism but occurring in the waking state. [L. *vigil,* awake, alert, + *ambulo,* to walk about]

vig·i·lance (vij′i-lans). An attentiveness, alertness, or watchfulness for whatever may occur. [L. *vigilantia,* wakefulness]

vil·li (vil′ī). Plural of villus.

vil·lin (vil′in). An actin-binding protein that, at low calcium ion concentrations, nucleates polymerization of actin filaments; micromolar Ca^{2+} causes villin to sever actin filaments into short fragments.

vil·li·tis. SYN villositis.

vil·lo·ma (vi-lō′mă). SYN papilloma.

vil·lose (vil′ōs). SYN villous (2).

vil·lo·si·tis (vil-ō-sī′tis). Inflammation of the villous surface of the placenta. SYN villitis. [villous + G. -itis inflammation]

vil·los·i·ty (vi-los′i-tē). Shagginess; an aggregation of villi.

vil·lous (vil′ŭs). 1. Relating to villi. 2. Shaggy; covered with villi. villose.

vil·lus, pl. **vil·li** (vil′ŭs, vil′ī). 1. A projection from the surface, especially of a mucous membrane. If the projection is minute, as from a cell surface, it is termed a microvillus. 2. An elongated dermal papilla projecting into an intraepidermal vesicle or cleft. SEE festooning. [L. shaggy hair (of beasts)]

anchoring v., a chorionic v. that is attached to the decidua basalis.

arachnoid villi, tufted prolongations of pia-arachnoid that protrude through the meningeal layer of the dura mater and have a thin limiting membrane; collections of arachnoid v. form arachnoid granulations that lie in venous lacunae at the margin of the superior sagittal sinus; the spongy tissue of the a. v. contains tubules that serve as one-way valves for transfer of cerebrospinal fluid from the subarachnoid space to the venous system. Both a. v. and the granulations formed from them are major sites of fluid transfer. SEE ALSO arachnoid *granulations*, under *granulation*.

chorionic villi, vascular processes of the chorion of the embryo entering into the formation of the placenta.

floating v., SYN free v.

free v., a chorionic v. that is not attached to the decidua basalis, but is "free" in the maternal blood of the intervillous spaces. SYN floating v.

intestinal villi, projections (0.5 to 1.5 mm in length) of the mucous membrane of the intestine; they are leaf-shaped in the duodenum and become shorter, more finger-shaped, and sparser in the ileum. SYN villi intestinales [NA].

vil′li intestina′les [NA], SYN intestinal villi.

vil′li pericardi′aci, SYN pericardial villi.

pericardial villi, minute filiform projections from the surface of the serous pericardium. SYN villi pericardiaci.

peritoneal villi, villi on the surface of the peritoneum. SYN villi peritoneales.

vil′li peritonea′les, SYN peritoneal villi.

pleural villi, shaggy appendages on the pleura in the neighborhood of the costomediastinal sinus. SYN villi pleurales.

vil′li pleura′les, SYN pleural villi.

primary v., the first stage of chorionic v. development, with columns of cytotrophoblastic cells covered by syncytiotrophoblast.

secondary v., an intermediate stage of chorionic v. development following invasion by a connective tissue core.

synovial villi, small vascular processes given off from a synovial membrane. SYN villi synoviales [NA], synovial fringe, synovial tufts.

vil′li synovia′les [NA], SYN synovial villi.

tertiary v., the definitive chorionic v. with a vascular core separated from maternal blood by connective tissue, cytotrophoblast, and syncytiotrophoblast.

vil·lus·ec·to·my (vil-ŭs-ek′tō-mē). SYN synovectomy. [villus + G. ektomē, excision]

vi·men·tin (vī-men′tin). The major polypeptide that co-polymerizes with other subunits to form the intermediate filament cytoskeleton of mesenchymal cells; they may have a role in maintaining the internal organization of certain cells. SEE ALSO desmins.

vin·blas·tine sul·fate (vin-blas′tēn). A dimeric alkaloid obtained from *Vinca rosea*. It arrests mitosis in metaphase (although vincristine is more active in this respect) and exhibits greater antimetabolic activity than does vincristine; used in the treatment of Hodgkin's disease, choriocarcinoma, acute and chronic leukemias, and other neoplastic diseases; blocks microtubule assembly. SYN vincaleucoblastine.

vin·ca·leu·co·blas·tine (ving′kă-lū-kō-blas′tēn). SYN vinblastine sulfate.

Vin·ca ro·sea (ving′kă rō′zē-ă). A species of myrtle (family Myrtaceae) used in various parts of the world as a home remedy; two active dimeric alkaloids obtained from this plant are vinblastine and vincristine. SYN periwinkle.

Vincent, Henri, French physician, 1862–1950. SEE V.'s *angina, bacillus, disease, infection,* white *mycetoma, spirillum, tonsillitis.*

vin·cris·tine sul·fate (vin-kris′tēn). A dimeric alkaloid obtained from *Vinca rosea;* its antineoplastic activity is similar to that of vinblastine, but no cross-resistance develops between these two agents, and it is more useful than vinblastine in lymphocytic lymphosarcoma and acute leukemia. SYN leurocristine.

vin·cu·lin (ving′kū-lin). A protein associated with actin microfilaments; found in intercalated discs of cardiac muscle and focal adhesion plaques; may have a role in how a tumor virus causes pleiotropic effects of transformation. [L. *vinculum*, bond, fr. *vincio*, to bind + -in]

vin·cu·lum, pl. **vin·cu·la** (ving′kū-lŭm, -lă) [NA]. A frenum, frenulum, or ligament. [L. a fetter, fr. *vincio*, to bind]

v. bre′ve [NA], SYN short v. SEE ALSO vincula of tendons.

v. lin′guae, SYN lingual *frenulum.*

vin′cula lin′gulae cerebell′i, small lateral prolongations of the lingula of the vermis of the cerebellum resting on the dorsal surface of the superior cerebellar peduncle. SYN alae lingulae cerebelli.

long v., a long, threadlike band that extends from the dorsal surface of each of the flexor tendons of a digit to the proximal phalanx. SYN v. longum [NA].

v. lon′gum [NA], SYN long v. SEE ALSO vincula of tendons.

v. prepu′tii, SYN *frenulum* of prepuce.

short v., a triangular band that extends from the dorsal surface of each of the flexor tendons of a digit to the capsule of the nearby interphalangeal joint and to the phalanx proximal to the insertion of the tendon. SYN v. breve [NA].

vin′cula ten′dinum [NA], SYN vincula of tendons. SEE ALSO short v., long v.

vincula of tendons, fibrous bands that extend from the flexor tendons of the fingers and toes to the capsules of the interphalangeal joints and to the phalanges; they convey small vessels to the tendons. SYN vincula tendinum [NA], synovial frena, synovial frenula.

vin·de·sine (vin′dĕ-sēn). Synthetic derivative of vinblastine which shares antineoplastic properties with the latter agent. Used in the treatment of childhood lymphocytic leukemia.

Vineberg, Arthur M., Canadian thoracic surgeon, *1903. SEE V. *procedure.*

vin·e·gar (vin′ĕ-găr). Impure dilute acetic acid, made from wine, cider, malt, etc. SYN acetum. [Fr. *vinaigre,* fr. *vin,* wine, + *aigre,* sour]

pyroligneous v., SYN wood v.

wood v., pyracetic acid; impure acetic acid produced by the destructive distillation of pine tar and wood. SYN pyroligneous v.

vi·nic (vī′nik). Relating to or derived from wine. [L. *vinum,* wine]

vi·nous (vī′nŭs). Relating to, containing, or of the nature of wine.

Vinson, Porter P., U.S. surgeon, 1890–1959. SEE Plummer-V. *syndrome.*

vi·nyl (vī′nil). The hydrocarbon radical, CH$_2$=CH–. SYN ethenyl.

v. carbinol, SYN *allyl* alcohol.

v. chloride, a substance used in the plastics industry and suspected of being a potent carcinogen in humans. SYN chloroethylene.

vi·nyl·ben·zene (vī′nil-ben′zēn). SYN styrene.

vi·nyl·ene (vī′nil-ēn). The bivalent radical, –CH=CH–. SYN ethenylene.

vi·nyl ether. SYN divinyl ether.

vi·nyl·i·dene (vī-nil′i-dēn). The bivalent radical, H$_2$C=C=.

vi

RNA viruses									
nucleic acid core	capsid symmetry	virion: envelope	ether sensitivity	number of capsomeres	size of virus particle (nm)[a]	molecular weight of nucleic acid in virion (x10^6)	nucleic acid: physical type	number of genes (approx.)	family
RNA	icosa-hedral	absent	resistant	32	20–30	2–2.8	SS	12	Picornaviridae
				?[b]	60–80	12–19	DS segmented	40	Reoviridae
		present	sensitive	32?	40–70	4	SS	15	Togaviridae
	unknown or complex	present	sensitive		50–300	3–5	SS segmented	15	Arenaviridae
					80–130	9	SS	30	Coronaviridae
					~100	7–10	SS segmented	50	Retroviridae
	helical	present	sensitive		90–100	6–7	SS segmented	15	Bunyaviridae
					80–120	4	SS segmented	15	Orthomyxoviridae
					130–300	5–8	SS	30	Paramyxoviridae
					70 x 175	3–4	SS	20	Rhabdoviridae

classification according to chemical and physical properties; [a] diameter or diameter x length; [b] Reoviruses have an outer and inner capsid, the inner apparently of 32 capsomeres, but the number in the outer is not yet clearly known (perhaps as high as 92); SS, single stranded; DS, double stranded

vi·o·la·ceous (vī-ō-lā′shŭs). Denoting a purple discoloration, usually of the skin. [L. *viola*, violet]

vi·o·let (vī′ō-let). The color evoked by wavelengths of the visible spectrum shorter than 450 nm. For individual violet dyes, see the specific name. [L. *viola*]

  Hoffman's v., dahlia.

  visual v., SYN iodopsin.

vi·o·my·cin (vī-ō-mī′sin). $C_{23}H_{36}N_{12}O_8$; an antibiotic agent obtained from *Streptomyces puniceus* var. *floridae;* active against acid-fast bacteria, including strains of tubercle bacilli resistant to streptomycin; may produce vestibular damage and deafness.

vi·os·ter·ol (vī-os′ter-ōl). SYN ergocalciferol.

VIP Abbreviation for vasoactive intestinal *polypeptide*.

vi·per (vī′per). A member of the snake family Viperidae. [L. *vipera*, serpent, snake]

  Russell's v., characteristically marked, highly venomous snake (*Vipera russelli*) of southeastern Asia. The venom is coagulant in action and is used locally in a 1:10,000 solution for the arrest of hemorrhage in hemophilia.

Vi·per·i·dae (vī-per′i-dē). A family of poisonous Old World snakes, the true vipers, comprised of about 50 species and characterized by two relatively long caniculated fangs at the front of the upper jaw which are attached to movable bones, allowing them to be erect during the bite when the mouth is open, and folded into a palate skin fold when the jaws are shut. [L. *vipera*, viper]

vi·po·ma (vi-pō′mă). An endocrine tumor, usually originating in the pancreas, which produces a vasoactive intestinal polypeptide believed to cause profound cardiovascular and electrolyte changes with vasodilatory hypotension, watery diarrhea, hypokalemia, and dehydration. [*v*asoactive *i*ntestinal *p*olypeptide + G. *-ōma*, tumor]

Vipond, French physician. SEE V.'s *sign*.

vip·ryn·i·um em·bo·nate (vip-rin′ē-ŭm em′bō-nāt). SYN pyrvinium pamoate.

vir·a·gin·i·ty (vir′ă-jin′i-tē). Presence of pronounced masculine psychological qualities in a woman. [L. *virago* (*viragin*-), a female warrior]

vi·ral (vī′răl). Of, pertaining to, or caused by a virus.

Virchow, Rudolf, German pathologist and politician, 1821–1902. SEE V.'s *angle, cells,* under *cell, corpuscles,* under *corpuscle, crystals,* under *crystal, disease, law, node, psammoma;* V.-Holder *angle;* V.-Hassall *bodies,* under *body;* V.-Robin *space.*

vi·re·mia (vī-rē′mē-ă). The presence of a virus in the bloodstream. [virus + G. *haima*, blood]

vi·res (vī′rēz). Plural of vis.

vir·ga (vir′gă). SYN penis. [L. a rod]

vir·gin (ver′jin). 1. A person who has never had sexual intercourse. 2. Unused; uncontaminated. SYN virginal (2). [L. *virgo* (*virgin*-), maiden]

vir·gin·al (ver′ji-năl). 1. Relating to a virgin. 2. SYN virgin (2). [L. *virginalis*]

vir·gin·i·ty (ver-jin′i-tē). The virgin state. [L. *virginitas*]

vir·go·phre·nia (ver-gō-frē′nē-ă). The receptive, capacious, and retentive mind of youth. [L. *virgo*, maiden, + G. *phrēn*, mind]

vir·i·ci·dal (vī-ri-sī′dă). SYN virucidal.

vir·i·cide (vī′ri-sīd). SYN virucide.

△**-viridae.** A virus family. [L. *vir*, fr. *virus*, venom]

vir·ile (vir′il). 1. Relating to the male sex. 2. Manly, strong, masculine. 3. Possessing masculine traits. [L. *virilis*, masculine, fr. *vir*, a man]

vir·i·les·cence (vir-i-les′ens). Assumption of male characteristics by the female.

vi·ril·ia (vi-ril′ē-ă). The male sexual organs. [L. ntr. pl. of *virilis*, virile]

vir·i·lism (vir′i-lizm). Possession of mature masculine somatic characteristics by a girl, woman, or prepubescent male; may be present at birth or may appear later, depending on its cause; may be relatively mild (e.g., hirsutism) or severe and is commonly the result of gonadal or adrenocortical dysfunction, or of androgenic therapy. [L. *virilis*, masculine]

  adrenal v., v. produced by excessive or abnormal secretory patterns of adrenocortical steroids. SYN adrenal virilizing syndrome.

vi·ril·i·ty (vi-ril′i-tē). The condition or quality of being virile. [L. *virilitas*, manhood, fr. *vir*, man]

vir·i·li·za·tion (vir′i-li-zā′shŭn). Production or acquisition of virilism.

vir·i·liz·ing (vir′i-līz-ing). Causing virilism.

△**-virinae.** A subfamily of viruses.

vi·ri·on (vī′rē-on, vir′ē-on). The complete virus particle that is structurally intact and infectious.

vi·rip·o·tent (vir-i-pō′tent, vĭ-rip′ō-tent). Obsolete term denoting a sexually mature male. [L. *viripotens*, fr. *vir*, man, + *potens*, having power]

vi·roid (vī′royd). An infectious pathogen of plants that is smaller

viral embryopathy			
virus infections during pregnancy and the possible consequences for the child (embryopathy, fetopathy, perinatal infection)			
virus	symptoms of infection during 1st to 14th wk. of pregnancy	symptoms of infection from 15th wk. to birth	symptoms of infection shortly before birth, or perinatal
cytomegalo-virus	miscarriage, microcephaly	encephalitis, hepato-splenomegaly, chorioretinitis, premature birth, thrombocytopenia, minimal cerebral damage	cytomegaly
rubella	miscarriage, heart defects, cataract, microphthalmos, hearing deficiency, etc.	encephalitis, hepatosplenomegaly, thrombocytepenis, premature birth	—
measles	microcephaly, heart defects, anal atresia, etc.	fetal death, premature birth	measles
herpes simplex I and II	isolated cases: microph-thalmos, microcephaly chorioretinitis	—	generalized herpes infection, fatal encephalitis
varicella-zoster	isolated cases: eye deformation, cerebral damage	encephalitis, exanthema, premature birth	generalized varicella
coxsackie B	—	—	encephalitis, myocarditis, hepatitis
mumps	isolated cases: miscarriage	—	—
lymphocytic choriomeningitis	miscarriage (?)	isolated cases: encephalitis, chorioretinitis	—
hepatitis B	—	—	hepatitis (partly chronic)
hepatitis C	—	—	hepatitis
poliomyelitis	miscarriage	fetal death premature birth	poliomyelitis

than a virus (MW 75,000-100,000) and differs from one in that it consists only of single-stranded closed circular RNA, lacking a protein covering (capsid); replication does not depend on a helper virus, but is mediated by host cell enzymes. [virus + G. *eidos*, resemblance]

vi·rol·o·gist (vī-rol′ō-jist). A specialist in virology.

vi·rol·o·gy (vī-rol′ō-jē, vi-). The study of viruses and of virus disease. [virus + G. *logos*, study]

vi·ro·pex·is (vī-rō-pek′sis). Binding of virus to a cell and subsequent absorption (engulfment) of virus particles by that cell. [viro- + G. *pēxis*, fixation]

vi·ru·ci·dal (vī-rŭ-sī′dăl). Destructive to a virus. SYN viricidal.

vi·ru·cide (vī-rŭ-sīd). An agent active against virus infections. SYN viricide. [virus + L. *caedo*, to kill]

vi·ru·co·pria (vī-rŭ-kō′prē-ă). Presence of virus in feces. [virus + G. *kopros*, feces]

vir·u·lence. The disease-evoking power of a pathogen; numerically expressed as the ratio of the number of cases of overt infection to the total number infected, as determined by immunoassay. [L. *virulentia*, fr. *virulentus*, poisonous]

vir·u·lent (vir′ū-lent). Extremely toxic, denoting a markedly pathogenic microorganism. [L. *virulentus*, poisonous]

vir·u·lif·er·ous (vī-rŭ-lif′er-ŭs). Conveying virus.

vir·u·ria (vī-rū′rē-ă). Presence of viruses in the urine. [virus + G. *ouron*, urine]

VIRUS

vi·rus, pl. **vi·rus·es** (vī′rŭs). **1.** Formerly, the specific agent of an infectious disease. **2.** Specifically, a term for a group of infectious agents which with few exceptions are capable of passing through fine filters that retain most bacteria, are usually not visible through the light microscope, lack independent metabolism, and are incapable of growth or reproduction apart from living cells. They have a prokaryotic genetic apparatus but differ sharply from bacteria in other respects. The complete particle usually contains only DNA or RNA, not both, and is usually covered by a protein shell or capsid that protects the nucleic acid. They range in size from 15 mm up to several hundred mm. Classification of v.'s depends upon characteristics of virions as well as upon mode of transmission, host range, symptomatology, and other factors. For v.'s not listed below, see the specific name. SYN filtrable v., ultravirus. **3.** Relating to or caused by a v., as a virus disease. [L. poison]

2060 v., a strain of common cold v.; early isolate of *Rhinovirus*. SYN JH v.

Abelson murine leukemia v., a retrovirus belonging to the Type C retrovirus group subfamily (family Oncovirinae) which is associated with leukemia and produces *in vitro* transformation of mouse cells.

adeno-associated v. (AAV), SYN *Dependovirus.*

adenoidal-pharyngeal-conjunctival v., SYN adenovirus.

adenosatellite v., SYN *Dependovirus.*

African horse sickness v., a v. of the genus *Orbivirus*, in the family Reoviridae; the cause of African horse sickness.

African swine fever v., a DNA v. related to the family Iridoviridae and the etiologic agent of African swine fever.

AIDS-related v. (ARV), obsolete term for human immunodeficiency v.

Akabane v., a v. of the genus *Bunyavirus*, family Bunyaviridae, causing abortion in cattle and congenital arthrogryposis and hydranencephaly in bovine fetuses in Israel, Japan, and Australia; it is transmitted by mosquitoes.

Aleutian mink disease v., a v. of the genus *Parvovirus* causing Aleutian mink disease.

amphotropic v., an oncornavirus that does not produce disease in its natural host but does replicate in tissue culture cells of the host species and also in cells from other species.

animal viruses, v.'s occurring in man and other animals, causing inapparent infection or producing disease.

A-P-C v., SYN adenovirus.

Argentine hemorrhagic fever v. (ar-jen-tēn'), a member of the Arenaviridae.

attenuated v., a variant strain of a pathogenic v., so modified as to excite the production of protective antibodies, yet not producing the specific disease.

Aujeszky's disease v., SYN pseudorabies v.

Australian X disease v., SYN Murray Valley encephalitis v.

avian encephalomyelitis v., a v. of the genus *Enterovirus* (family Picornaviridae) causing avian infectious encephalomyelitis in young chicks.

avian erythroblastosis v., SYN avian leukosis-sarcoma *complex* (2).

avian infectious laryngotracheitis v., a herpesvirus causing avian infectious laryngotracheitis.

avian influenza v., a type A influenza v. (genus *Influenzavirus*) that causes fowl plague. SYN fowl plague v.

avian leukosis-sarcoma v., SYN avian leukosis-sarcoma *complex* (2).

avian lymphomatosis v., (1) SYN avian leukosis-sarcoma *complex* (2). **(2)** SYN avian neurolymphomatosis v.

avian myeloblastosis v., SYN avian leukosis-sarcoma *complex* (2).

avian neurolymphomatosis v., the herpesvirus that causes avian lymphomatosis (Marek's disease); is distinct from those causing other forms of leukosis. SYN avian lymphomatosis v. (2), fowl neurolymphomatosis v., Marek's disease v.

avian pneumoencephalitis v., SYN Newcastle disease v.

avian sarcoma v., SYN avian leukosis-sarcoma *complex* (2).

avian viral arthritis v., a v. of the genus *Reovirus*, family Reoviridae, causing tenosynovitis and arthritis in chickens.

B v., a herpesvirus, in the family Herpesviridae, affecting Old World monkeys, that is very similar morphologically to herpes simplex v.; fatal infection may occur in humans following the bite of an infected monkey, although other modes of transmission have also been documented. SYN monkey B v.

B19 v., a human parvovirus associated with arthritis and arthralgia and a number of specific clinical entities, including erythema infectiosum and aplastic crisis in the presence of hemolytic anemia.

bacterial v., a v. which "infects" bacteria; a bacteriophage.

Bittner v. (bit'ner), SYN mammary tumor v. of mice.

BK v., a human polyomavirus, in the family Papovaviridae, of worldwide distribution which produces infections that are usually subclinical in immunocompetent individuals. [initials of patient from whom first isolated]

bluecomb v., SYN transmissible turkey enteritis v.

bluetongue v., a v. of the genus *Orbivirus*, in the family Reoviridae; the agent of bluetongue in sheep.

Bolivian hemorrhagic fever v., a member of the Arenavirus group of single-stranded RNA viruses also known as Machupo v.; primary reservoir in rodents; produces multiple abnormalities in coagulation system including widespread capillary leak syndrome, which can be fatal.

Borna disease v., an unclassified RNA v. that is the cause of Borna disease, a disease of horses. SYN enzootic encephalomyelitis v.

Bornholm disease v., SYN epidemic pleurodynia v.

bovine ephemeral fever v., a rhabdovirus causing bovine ephemeral fever in cattle.

bovine immunodeficiency v., a lentivirus causing lymphocytosis in cattle.

bovine leukemia v. (BLV), a type C retrovirus in the subfamily Retrovirinae, commonly infecting cattle, especially dairy cows; in a small proportion of infected cattle, it will cause enzootic bovine leukosis. SYN bovine leukosis v.

bovine leukosis v., SYN bovine leukemia v.

bovine papular stomatitis v., a poxvirus of the genus *Parapox-virus*, reported from North America, Africa and Europe, causing bovine papular stomatitis. SYN papular stomatitis v. of cattle.

bovine respiratory syncytial v., a pneumovirus causing an emerging disease in young cattle characterized by pneumonia, interstitial pulmonary edema, and emphysema; sheep are also susceptible to the v.

bovine virus diarrhea v., a v. of the genus *Pestivirus*, in the family Togaviridae, causing bovine v. diarrhea; New York, Oregon, and Indiana strains of the v. are recognized. SYN mucosal disease v.

Bunyamwera v., a serologic group of the genus *Bunyavirus*, composed of over 150 v. types in the family Bunyaviridae. [*Bunyamwera*, Uganda, where first isolated]

Bwamba v., a genus of viruses in the family Bunyaviridae; a serologic group of the genus *Bunyavirus;* associated with cases of Bwamba fever in Uganda. [*Bwamba*, forest in Uganda where first isolated]

CA v., abbreviation for croup-associated v.

California v., a serologic group of the genus *Bunyavirus*, comprising over 14 strains including La Crosse and Tahyna v., and the type strain, California v., which causes encephalitis, chiefly in the age group 4 to 14 years.

camelpox v., an orthopoxvirus causing camelpox in camels.

canarypox v., a poxvirus of the genus *Avipoxvirus* causing a fatal disease of canaries, and also infecting sparrows.

canine distemper v., an RNA v. of the genus *Morbillivirus*, a member of the family Paramyxoviridae, that causes canine distemper. SYN dog distemper v.

Capim viruses, a serologic group of the genus *Bunyavirus*, the type species of which is Capim v.

caprine arthritis-encephalomyelitis v., a lentivirus causing caprine arthritis-encephalomyelitis in goats.

Caraparu v., a species of C group *Bunyavirus* and an agent of bunyavirus encephalitis.

cat distemper v., SYN feline panleukopenia v.

cattle plague v., SYN rinderpest v.

Catu v., an arbovirus of the genus *Bunyavirus*, of the family Bunyaviridae; an agent of bunyavirus encephalitis.

CELO v., a v. with characteristics of adenovirus, and similar to quail bronchitis v. SYN chicken embryo lethal orphan v.

Central European tick-borne encephalitis v., one of the v.'s of the tick-borne encephalitis complex of group B arboviruses (genus *Flavivirus*); the causative agent of tick-borne encephalitis (Central European subtype).

C group viruses, a serologic group of the genus *Bunyavirus* (formerly called group C arboviruses), composed of 12 species including Caraparu, Murutucu, and Oriboca v.

Chagres v., a v. in the family Bunyaviridae, an agent of bunyavirus encephalitis.

chicken embryo lethal orphan v., SYN CELO v.

chickenpox v., SYN varicella-zoster v.

chikungunya v., a mosquito-transmitted arbovirus of the genus *Alphavirus* (family Togaviridae) found in parts of Africa and in India, Thailand, and Malaysia; causes a febrile illness with joint pains. [named for the "bent up" position of persons so infected]

Coe v., a v. serologically identical with the A-21 strain of coxsackievirus; the cause of a common cold-like disease in military recruits.

cold v., SYN common cold v.

Colorado tick fever v., a v. of the genus *Orbivirus*, from the family Reoviridae, found in the Rocky Mountain region of the United States and transmitted by the tick, *Dermacentor andersoni;* it causes Colorado tick fever.

Columbia S. K. v., a strain of encephalomyocarditis v.

common cold v., any of the numerous strains of v. etiologically associated with the common cold, chiefly the rhinoviruses, but also strains of adenovirus, *Coxsackievirus*, ECHO v., and parainfluenza v. SYN cold v.

contagious ecthyma (pustular dermatitis) v. of sheep, the poxvirus of the genus *Parapoxvirus* causing contagious ecthyma (pustular dermatitis) of sheep. SYN soremouth v.

contagious pustular stomatitis v., SYN horsepox v.

cowpox v., a v. of the genus *Orthopoxvirus* that causes cowpox.

Coxsackie v., SEE Coxsackievirus.

Crimean-Congo hemorrhagic fever v., a v. of the genus *Nairovirus* (family Bunyaviridae) from Africa and the southern USSR, carried by ticks (*Hyalomma* and *Amblyomma*) and found in human blood; the cause of Crimean-Congo hemorrhagic fever.

croup-associated v. (CA v.), parainfluenza v. type 2. SEE parainfluenza viruses.

cytopathogenic v., a v. whose multiplication leads to degenerative changes in the host cell. SEE ALSO cytopathic *effect*.

defective v., a v. particle that contains insufficient nucleic acid to provide for production of all essential viral components; consequently, infectious v. is not produced except under certain conditions (*e.g.,* when the host cell is infected with a "helper" v. also).

delta v., SYN hepatitis delta v.

dengue, a v. of the genus *Flavivirus,* about 50 nm in diameter; the etiologic agent of dengue in humans and also occurring in monkeys and chimpanzees, usually as inapparent infection; four serotypes are recognized; transmission is effected by mosquitoes of the genus *Aedes.*

distemper v., SEE canine distemper v., feline panleukopenia v.

DNA v., a major group of animal v.'s in which the core consists of deoxyribonucleic acid (DNA); it includes parvoviruses, papovaviruses, adenoviruses, herpesviruses, poxviruses, and other unclassified DNA v.'s. SYN deoxyvirus.

dog distemper v., SYN canine distemper v.

duck hepatitis v., a DNA v. of the genus *Hepadnavirus,* in the family Hepadnaviridae, causing v. hepatitis of ducks.

duck influenza v., an influenza A v., a member of the family Orthomyxoviridae, distinct from human influenza A strains on bases of hemagglutination-inhibition.

duck plague v., a herpesvirus that causes duck plague.

eastern equine encephalomyelitis v., a v. of the genus *Alphavirus* (formerly group A arbovirus), in the family Togaviridae, occurring in the eastern United States; it is normally present in certain wild birds as an inapparent infection, but is capable of causing eastern equine encephalomyelitis in horses and humans following transfer by the bites of culicine mosquitoes. SYN EEE v.

EB v., SYN Epstein-Barr v.

Ebola v., a v. morphologically similar to but antigenically distinct from Marburg v., in the family Filoviridae, which causes viral hemorrhagic fever. SYN viral hemorrhagic fever v.

ECBO v., former name for early isolates of bovine enteroviruses. SYN enteric cytopathogenic bovine orphan v.

ECHO v., an enterovirus belonging to the Picornaviridae, isolated from humans; while there are many inapparent infections, certain of the several serotypes are associated with fever and aseptic meningitis, and some appear to cause mild respiratory disease. SYN echovirus, enteric cytopathogenic human orphan v.

ECMO v., simian picornavirus recovered from monkey kidney cells and stools. SYN enteric cytopathogenic monkey orphan v.

ecotropic v., an oncornavirus that does not produce disease in its natural host but does replicate in tissue culture cells derived from the host species.

ECSO v., a picornavirus isolated from outbreaks of enteritis in swine, but not known to be a natural pathogen. SYN enteric cytopathogenic swine orphan v.

ectromelia v., SYN infectious ectromelia v.

EEE v., SYN eastern equine encephalomyelitis v.

EMC v., SYN encephalomyocarditis v.

emerging viruses, in epidemiology, a class of viruses that have long infected humans or animals but now have the opportunity to attain epidemic proportions due to human encroachment on tropical rainforests, increased international travel, burgeoning populations in less developed countries, and, possibly, global warming. About two dozen viruses have been termed emergent, including hemorrhagic viruses such as Ebola, Marburg, and Hantaan; the rabies-like viruses Mokola and Duvenhage; rodent-borne Jinin and Lassa virus; and mosquito-borne dengue. Virologists speculate that the strain of HIV that causes AIDS may also fall into this category, having entered humans through contact

with monkeys in central Africa, possibly having existed among monkey populations for some 50,000 years.

encephalitis v., any one of a variety of v.'s that cause encephalitis.

encephalomyocarditis v., a picornavirus, probably of rodents, isolated from blood and stools of humans, other primates, pigs, and rabbits; occasionally causes febrile illness with central nervous system involvement in humans, and an often fatal myocarditis in chimpanzees, monkeys and pigs; strains of this v. include Columbia S. K. v. and Mengo v. SYN EMC v.

enteric viruses, v.'s of the genus Enterovirus.

enteric cytopathogenic bovine orphan v., SYN ECBO v.

enteric cytopathogenic human orphan v., SYN ECHO v.

enteric cytopathogenic monkey orphan v., SYN ECMO v.

enteric cytopathogenic swine orphan v., SYN ECSO v.

enteric orphan viruses, enteroviruses isolated from humans and other animals, "orphan" implying lack of known association with disease when isolated; many v.'s of the group are now known to be pathogenic; they include ECBO viruses, ECHO viruses, and ECSO viruses.

enzootic encephalomyelitis v., SYN Borna disease v.

ephemeral fever v., a rhabdovirus that causes ephemeral fever of cattle.

epidemic gastroenteritis v., a RNA v., about 27 nm in diameter, which has not been cultured *in vitro;* it is the cause of epidemic nonbacterial gastroenteritis; at least five antigenically distinct serotypes have been recognized, including the Norwalk agent. These viruses are probably classified with the Caliciviruses in the family Caliciviridae. SYN gastroenteritis v. type A.

epidemic keratoconjunctivitis v., an adenovirus (type 8) causing epidemic keratoconjunctivitis, especially among shipyard workers, and also associated with outbreaks of swimming pool conjunctivitis.

epidemic myalgia v., SYN epidemic pleurodynia v.

epidemic parotitis v., SYN mumps v.

epidemic pleurodynia v., a v. of *Enterovirus* coxsackievirus type B, in the family Picornaviridae, that causes epidemic pleurodynia. SYN Bornholm disease v., epidemic myalgia v.

epizootic hemorrhagic disease of deer v., an orbivirus causing epizootic hemorrhagic disease of deer.

Epstein-Barr v. (EBV), a herpesvirus that causes infectious mononucleosis and is also found in cell cultures of Burkitt's lymphoma; associated with nasopharyngeal carcinoma. SYN EB v., human herpesvirus 4.

equine abortion v., SYN equine rhinopneumonitis v.

equine arteritis v., a v. of the genus *Pestivirus,* a member of the family Togaviridae, that causes equine viral arteritis and, frequently, abortion; probably the most common cause of equine influenza. SYN infectious arteritis v. of horses.

equine coital exanthema v., a herpesvirus causing coital exanthema in male and female horses.

equine encephalosis v., an orbivirus causing equine encephalosis in horses.

equine infectious anemia v., caused by a retrovirus, of the Lentivirinae subfamily, and the cause of equine infectious anemia. SYN swamp fever v.

equine influenza viruses, strains of influenza v. type A which cause horse influenza; there are several subtypes.

♻ Combining forms	[NA] Nomina Anatomica
Word*Finder* **Multi-term entry finder** Preceding letter A	**[MIM] Mendelian** **Inheritance in Man**
A.D.A.M. Anatomy Plates **Between letters L and M**	☆ **Official alternate term**
Appendices: **Following letter Z**	☆**[NA] Official alternate** **Nomina Anatomica term**
SYN Synonym; Cf., compare	**High Profile Term**

equine rhinopneumonitis v., a herpesvirus reported in the U.S. Europe, and South Africa, causing equine rhinopneumonitis and equine virus abortion. SYN equine abortion v.

FA v., a strain of mouse encephalomyelitis v.

feline immunodeficiency v. (FIV), a lentivirus causing acquired immunodeficiency in cats.

feline leukemia v. (FeLV), a retrovirus of the Oncornovirinae subfamily causing many proliferative (neoplastic) and degenerative (blastopenic) diseases in domestic cats, including lymphosarcoma, thymic atrophy, immune complex glomerulonephritis, fetal abortions and resorptions, and several myeloproliferative and myelodegenerative conditions; it also causes immunosuppression in infected cats.

feline panleukopenia v., a v. of the genus *Parvovirus* that causes panleukopenia; the v. infects all Felidae, raccoons and mink, but not dogs or other Canidae. SYN cat distemper v., panleukopenia v. of cats.

feline rhinotracheitis v., a herpesvirus that causes feline viral rhinotracheitis.

fibromatosis v. of rabbits, SYN rabbit fibroma v.

fibrous bacterial viruses, SYN filamentous bacterial viruses.

filamentous bacterial viruses, deoxyribonucleoproteins that "infect" and replicate in Gram-negative bacteria having sex pili and that, unlike bacteriophage, are released from infected bacteria without damage to the cell; they seem to be of two kinds, one of which has a specificity for F pili and the other for I pili. SYN fibrous bacterial viruses.

filtrable v., SYN virus (2).

fixed v., rabies v. whose virulence for rabbits has been stabilized by numerous passages through this experimental host. SEE ALSO street v.

Flury strain rabies v., SEE rabies v., Flury strain.

FMD v., SYN foot-and-mouth disease v.

foamy viruses, retroviruses of the subfamily Spumavirinae, found in primates and other mammals; so named because of lacelike changes produced in monkey kidney cells; syncytia are also produced. SYN foamy agents.

foot-and-mouth disease v., a picornavirus of the genus *Rhinovirus* causing foot-and-mouth disease of cattle, swine, sheep, goats, and wild ruminants; it has wide distribution throughout Africa and Asia, causing serious economic losses; the v. is spread by contamination of the animal environment with infected saliva and excreta. SYN FMD v.

fowl erythroblastosis v., SYN avian leukosis-sarcoma *complex* (2).

fowl lymphomatosis v., SYN avian leukosis-sarcoma *complex* (2).

fowl myeloblastosis v., SYN avian leukosis-sarcoma *complex* (2).

fowl neurolymphomatosis v., SYN avian neurolymphomatosis v.

fowl plague v., SYN avian influenza v.

fowlpox v., a v. of the genus *Avipoxvirus* causing fowlpox and avian diphtheria.

fox encephalitis v., SYN canine *adenovirus* 1.

Friend v., a strain of the splenic group of mouse leukemia v.'s, related to Moloney and Rauscher v.'s. SYN Friend leukemia v., Swiss mouse leukemia v.

Friend leukemia v., SYN Friend v.

GAL v., a v. with characteristics of adenovirus, not known to be associated with natural disease. SYN gallus adeno-like v.

gallus adeno-like v., SYN GAL v.

gastroenteritis v. type A, SYN epidemic gastroenteritis v.

gastroenteritis v. type B, SYN rotavirus.

German measles v., SYN rubella v.

Germiston v., a virus in the genus *Bunyavirus*, family Bunyaviridae

goatpox v., a v. of the genus *Capripoxvirus;* the cause of goatpox.

Graffi's v., a mouse myeloleukemia v. from filtrates of transplantable tumors; possibly related to Gross' v.

green monkey v., SYN Marburg v.

Gross' v., a strain of mouse leukemia v. SYN Gross' leukemia v.

Gross' leukemia v., SYN Gross' v.

Guama v., a serologic group of the genus *Bunyavirus*, composed of 6 species including Catu v., and the type strain, Guama v.

Guaroa v., a v. of the Bunyamwera group of the genus *Bunyavirus*, and an agent of bunyavirus encephalitis.

HA1 v., SYN hemadsorption v. type 1. SEE parainfluenza viruses.

HA2 v., SYN hemadsorption v. type 2. SEE parainfluenza viruses.

hand-foot-and-mouth disease v., the v. causing hand-foot-and-mouth disease; chiefly type A16 but also types A4, A5, A7, A9, or A10 *Entervirus* coxsackievirus.

Hantaan v., a v. of the family Bunyaviridae that causes Korean hemorrhagic fever.

hard pad v., the v. causing hard pad disease, probably canine distemper v., but sometimes not recovered.

helper v., a v. whose replication renders it possible for a defective v. or a virusoid (also present in the host cell) to develop into fully infectious agent.

hemadsorption v. type 1, parainfluenza v. type 3. SEE parainfluenza viruses. SYN HA1 v.

hemadsorption v. type 2, parainfluenza v. type 1. SEE parainfluenza viruses. SYN HA2 v.

hepatitis A v. (HAV), an RNA virus in the family Picornaviridae; the causative agent of viral hepatitis type A. SYN infectious hepatitis v.

hepatitis B v. (HBV), a DNA virus in the family Hepadnaviridae; the causative agent of viral hepatitis type B. SYN serum hepatitis v.

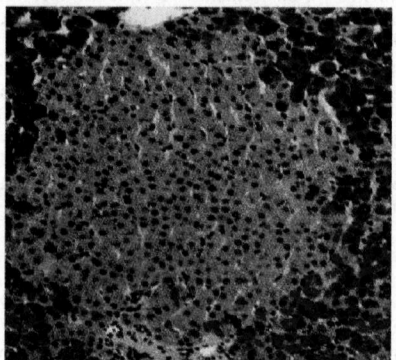

viral hepatitis, type B
viral antigen (HBAg) in serum of patient with chronic active hepatitis B

hepatitis C v. (HCV), a non-A, non-B RNA v. causing post-transfusion hepatitis; it appears to be a member of the family Flaviviridae.

hepatitis delta v. (HDV), a small "defective" RNA v., similar to viroids and virusoids, that requires the presence of hepatitis B v. for replication. The clinical course is variable but is usually more severe than other hepatitides. SYN delta agent, delta antigen, delta v.

hepatitis E v. (HEV), a RNA v., possibly a Calcivirus, that is the principal cause of enterically transmitted, waterborne, or epidemic non A, non B hepatitis occurring primarily in Asia or Africa.

herpes v., SEE herpesvirus.

herpes simplex v. (HSV), SEE *herpes* simplex.

herpes zoster v., SYN varicella-zoster v.

hog cholera v., an RNA virus of the genus *Pestivirus*, in the family Togaviridae, that causes hog cholera. SYN swine fever v.

horsepox v., the poxvirus causing horsepox. SYN contagious pustular stomatitis v.

human immunodeficiency v. (HIV), human T-cell lymphotropic v. type III; a cytopathic retrovirus (subfamily Lentvirinae, family Retroviridae) that is about 100 nm in diameter, has a lipid envelope, and has a characteristic dense cylindrical nucleoid containing core proteins and genomic RNA; it is the etiologic agent of acquired immunodeficiency syndrome (AIDS). Formerly or also known as the lymphadenopathy v. (LAV) or the human T-cell lymphotropic v. type III (HTLV-III). Identified in 1984 by Luc Montagnier and colleagues. RNA; it is the etiologic agent of acquired immunodeficiency syndrome (AIDS). SYN lymphadenopathy-associated v.

human papilloma v. (HPV), an icosahedral DNA v., 55 nm in diameter, of the genus *Papillomavirus,* family Papovaviridae; certain types cause cutaneous and genital warts in humans, including verruca vulgaris and condyloma acuminatum; other types are associated with severe cervical intraepithelial neoplasia and anogenital and laryngeal carcinomas. Over 70 types have been characterized on the basis of DNA relatedness. SYN infectious papilloma v.

> HPV infection has emerged as a major public health problem, especially for women. Eighty percent of cervical cancer is attributable to HPV infection, and some 25% of all irregularities seen on Pap smears are also believed to be owed to the presence of the virus, which is often otherwise asymptomatic. Some 40% of HIV-positive women present with severe cervical dysplasia caused by HPV, which in many cases proceeds to fatal cancer with an aggressiveness not commonly seen among non–HIV-positive women. A significant number of AIDS patients who are homosexual men also display anal dysplasia and squamous cell carcinomas due to HPV. The risk of contracting the virus goes up with the number of sexual partners. Some protection is conveyed by diaphragms and condoms.

human T-cell lymphoma/leukemia v. (HTLV), a group of viruses (subfamily Oncovirinae, family Retroviridae) that are lymphotropic with a selective affinity for the helper/inducer cell subset of T lymphocytes and that are associated with adult T-cell leukemia and lymphoma. SYN human T-cell lymphotropic v.

human T-cell lymphotropic v., SYN human T-cell lymphoma/leukemia v.

human T lymphotrophic v., a virus that has a predilection for human lymphoid cells.

Ibaraki v., a v. of cattle in Japan, closely related to the bluetongue v.

IBR v., SYN infectious bovine rhinotracheitis v.

v. III of rabbits, obsolete name for a latent herpesvirus infection of rabbits. [the third strain isolated, used for study]

Ilhéus v., a v. of the genus *Flavivirus* (group B arbovirus) first isolated in Brazil, later found in Colombia, Central America, and the Caribbean; the cause of Ilhéus encephalitis and Ilhéus fever.

inclusion conjunctivitis viruses, former name for *Chlamydia trachomatis.*

infantile gastroenteritis v., SYN rotavirus.

infectious arteritis v. of horses, SYN equine arteritis v.

infectious bovine rhinotracheitis v., a herpesvirus causing infectious bovine rhinotracheitis. SYN IBR v.

infectious bronchitis v. (IBV), an RNA v. of the family Coronaviridae and the type species of the genus *Coronavirus,* causing infectious avian bronchitis, being most pathogenic in chicks up to about 4 weeks of age; not to be confused with avian infectious laryngotracheitis v.

infectious bursal disease v., a birnavirus causing infectious bursal disease in chickens.

infectious ectromelia v., a virus belonging to the family Poxviridae morphologically similar to vaccinia v., which occurs as a latent infection in laboratory mice, but which may be activated by stresses such as irradiation and transport to cause disease; inoculation into the footpad results in edema and necrosis. SYN ectromelia v., mousepox v., pseudolymphocytic choriomeningitis v.

infectious hepatitis v., SYN hepatitis A v.

infectious papilloma v., SYN human papilloma v.

infectious porcine encephalomyelitis v., SYN Teschen disease v.

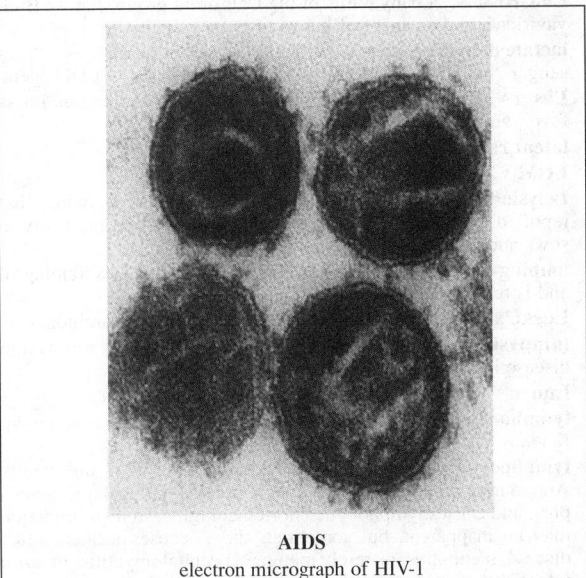

AIDS
electron micrograph of HIV-1

influenza viruses, v.'s of the family Orthomyxoviridae which cause influenza and influenza-like infections of humans and other animals; v.'s included are influenza v. types A and B of the genus *Influenzavirus,* causing, respectively, influenza A and B, and influenza v. type C, which probably belongs to a separate genus and causes influenza C.

insect viruses, v.'s pathogenic for insects.

iridescent v., an insect virus in the family Iridoviridae.

Jamestown Canyon v., a member of the California group of arboviruses (family Bunyaviridae) which has been associated with a mild febrile illness in humans in North America.

Japanese B encephalitis v., a v. of the genus *Flavivirus* (group B arbovirus) occurring particularly in Japan but probably widespread throughout Southeast Asia; the v. is normally present in humans, especially in children, as an inapparent infection, but may cause febrile response and sometimes encephalitis; it may cause encephalitis in horses and abortion in pigs; wild birds are probably the natural hosts and culicine mosquitoes the vectors. SYN Russian autumn encephalitis v.

JC v., a human polyomavirus, family Papovaviridae, of worldwide distribution which produces infections that are usually subclinical in immunocompetent individuals, but is associated with progressive multifocal leukoencephalopathy in immuno-suppressed individuals. [initials of patient from whom first isolated]

JH v., SYN 2060 v. [*Johns Hopkins* University, where first isolated]

Junin v., a v. of the Tacaribe complex of arboviruses, genus *Arenavirus,* and the cause of Argentinian hemorrhagic fever; also isolated from mites and rodents.

K v., a polyomavirus, family Papovaviridae, that causes pneumonia in young mice by various routes of inoculation.

Kelev strain rabies v., SEE rabies v., Kelev strain.

Kilham rat v., a v. of the genus *Parvovirus* causing inapparent infection in rats; also recoverable from rat tumors. SYN latent rat v.

Kisenyi sheep disease v., a v., in the family Bunyaviridae, that is probably the same as Nairobi sheep disease v.

Koongol viruses, a serologic group of the genus *Bunyavirus,* comprising two species, Koongol (type species) and Wongal v.

Korean hemorrhagic fever v., SEE Hantavirus.

Kyasanur Forest disease v., a group B arbovirus, in the family Flaviviridae, isolated from monkeys in India and capable of causing Kyasanur Forest disease in humans; the v. is spread by monkeys and birds having mild infections; the vectors are probably species of the tick *Haemaphysalis.*

vi

La Crosse v., a bunyavirus of the California group, family Bunyaviridae, and an agent of bunyavirus encephalitis.

lactate dehydrogenase v., a togavirus present perhaps as a "passenger" in various transplantable mouse tumors. SYN LDH agent.

Lassa v., an arenavirus, family Arenaviridae, that causes Lassa fever, an actue febrile disease with a high mortality.

latent rat v., SYN Kilham rat v.

LCM v., SYN lymphocytic choriomeningitis v.

Lelystad v., an arterivirus causing a new disease in swine, first reported in 1987 and characterized by abortion and infertility in sows and respiratory problems in piglets.

louping-ill v., a v. of the genus *Flavivirus* that causes louping ill and is transmitted by the hard tick *Ixodes ricinus*.

Lucké's v., a herpesvirus associated with Lucké's carcinoma.

lumpyskin disease v., a capripoxvirus causing lumpyskin disease in cattle.

Lunyo v., an atypical strain of Rift Valley fever v.

lymphadenopathy-associated v. (LAV), SYN human immunodeficiency v.

lymphocytic choriomeningitis v., an RNA v. of the family Arenaviridae that infects mice, man, monkeys, dogs, and guinea pigs, and causes lymphocytic choriomeningitis; in man, infection may be inapparent, but sometimes the v. causes influenza-like disease, meningitis, or rarely meningoencephalomyelitis; *in utero* infections of mice establish a type of immunological tolerance. SYN LCM v.

lymphogranuloma venereum v., former name for *Chlamydia trachomatis*.

Machupo v., a v. of the Tacaribe complex (genus *Arenavirus*, family Arenaviridae); the cause of Bolivian hemorrhagic fever.

maedi v., a retrovirus (subfamily Lentivirinae) that is the cause of maedi; it is very similar to the visna v. SYN medi v., progressive pneumonia v.

malignant catarrhal fever v., a herpesvirus of wide distribution causing malignant catarrhal fever of cattle; sheep and wildebeests harbor inapparent infections and may transmit the v. to cattle.

Maloney leukemia v. (mā-lō'nē), a retrovirus associated with leukemia in rodents.

mammary cancer v. of mice, SYN mammary tumor v. of mice.

mammary tumor v. of mice, member of the retrovirus subfamily Oncornavirinae, antigenically distinct from the murine leukemia-sarcoma complex, that is associated with adenocarcinomatous tumors of the mammary gland, commonly latent in wild and laboratory mice and causing cancer only in genetically susceptible strains under certain hormonal influences. SYN Bittner agent, Bittner v., Bittner's milk factor, mammary cancer v. of mice, milk factor, mouse mammary tumor v.

Marburg v., an RNA-containing v., genus *Filovirus* in the family Filoviridae, first recognized at Marburg University (Germany), where it was the cause of a highly fatal hemorrhagic fever among handlers and laboratory workers of green monkeys. SYN green monkey v.

Marek's disease v., SYN avian neurolymphomatosis v.

marmoset v., a herpesvirus obtained repeatedly from throat swabs and tissues of New World monkeys.

masked v., a v. ordinarily occurring in the host in a noninfective state, but which may be activated and demonstrated by special procedures such as blind passage in experimental animals.

Mason-Pfizer v., a D-type retrovirus in the subfamily Oncornaviridae that was isolated from a mammary carcinoma of a rhesus monkey.

Mayaro v., a v. of the genus *Alphavirus*, family Togaviridae, causing epidemics of undifferentiated type fever in South America.

measles v., an RNA v. of the genus *Morbillivirus*, family Paramyxoviridae, that causes measles in man and is transmitted via the respiratory tract; possesses hemagglutinating, hemadsorbing, and hemolyzing properties. SYN rubeola v.

medi v., SYN maedi v.

Mengo v., a strain of encephalomyocarditis v.

milker's nodule v., a virus in the family Poxviridae.

mink enteritis v., a parvovirus that causes enteritis of mink.

MM v., a strain of encephalomyocarditis v.

Mokola v., a rabies related v. of the genus *Lyssavirus*, family Rhabdoviridae, first isolated from shrews (*Crocidura* spp.) in Nigeria, which has caused fatal neurological disease in man and cats in Africa.

molluscum contagiosum v., the poxvirus causing molluscum contagiosum of humans.

Moloney's v., a lymphoid leukemia retrovirus of mice, in the subfamily Oncovirinae, isolated originally during propagation of S 37 mouse sarcoma.

monkey B v., SYN B v.

monkeypox v., a v. of the genus *Orthopoxvirus* causing monkeypox.

mouse encephalomyelitis v., a v. of the genus *Enterovirus*, family Picornaviridae, normally associated with inapparent infections and found in the intestinal tracts of infected mice, occasionally causing mouse encephalomyelitis in experimentally inoculated susceptible mice. SYN mouse poliomyelitis v.

mouse hepatitis v., a coronavirus, in the family Coronaviridae, that in the presence of *Eperythrozoon coccoides* causes fatal hepatitis in newly weaned mice; otherwise causes inapparent infection.

mouse leukemia viruses, retroviruses of the murine leukemia-sarcoma complex that produce leukemia and sometimes lymphosarcomas in mice, including the Abelron, Gross, Moloney, Friend, and Rauscher strains of v.; they have been isolated from inbred mice having high incidence of spontaneous lymphoid leukemia.

mouse mammary tumor v., SYN mammary tumor v. of mice.

mouse parotid tumor v., SYN polyoma v.

mouse poliomyelitis v., SYN mouse encephalomyelitis v.

mousepox v., SYN infectious ectromelia v.

mouse thymic v., an unclassified ether-sensitive v., 75 to 100 nm in diameter, that causes necrosis of the thymus in young mice.

mucosal disease v., SYN bovine virus diarrhea v.

mumps v., a v. of the genus *Paramyxovirus*, family Paramyxoviridae, causing parotitis in man, sometimes with complications of orchitis, oophoritis, pancreatitis, meningoencephalitis and others, and transmitted by infectious salivary secretions. SYN epidemic parotitis v.

murine sarcoma v., a seemingly defective retrovirus that produces sarcomas in mice when growing in the presence of a "helper" v.; *e.g.,* mouse leukemia v.

Murray Valley encephalitis v., a group B arbovirus of the genus *Flavivirus* that causes Murray Valley encephalitis; it is transmitted by *Culex* mosquitoes, and also infects birds and horses. SYN Australian X disease v., MVE v.

Murutucu v., a C group mosquito-borne v. of the genus *Bunyavirus*, which has caused undifferentiated type fever in Brazil and French Guiana.

MVE v., SYN Murray Valley encephalitis v.

myxomatosis v., SYN rabbit myxoma v.

Nairobi sheep disease v., an unclassified arbovirus of the family Bunyaviridae causing Nairobi sheep disease, transmitted by the tick, *Rhipicephalus appendiculatus;* it is a serologic group of v.'s morphologically like *Bunyavirus* but antigenically unrelated to it.

naked v., a v. consisting only of a nucleocapsid; *i.e.,* one that does not possess an enclosing envelope.

ND v., SYN Newcastle disease v.

Nebraska calf scours v., the bovine rotavirus. SEE rotavirus.

Neethling v., SEE lumpyskin disease v.

negative strand v., a v. the genome of which is a strand of RNA that is complementary to messenger RNA; negative strand v.'s also carry RNA polymerases necessary for the synthesis of messenger RNA.

Negishi v., one of the group B arboviruses (genus *Flavivirus*) of the tick-borne encephalitis complex, isolated from fatal infections in Japan.

neonatal calf diarrhea v., one of two v.'s causing neonatal calf diarrhea; a reovirus-like v. is associated with disease in newborn calves, and a coronavirus is associated with disease in calves over 5 days of age.

neurotropic v., a v. that has an affinity for nervous tissue, *e.g.,* poliomyelitis v., neurotropic v. variant of yellow fever, and the "fixed" v. of rabies.

Newcastle disease v., a v. of the genus *Paramyxovirus* causing Newcastle disease in chickens and, to a lesser extent, in turkeys and other birds; it may occasionally infect laboratory and poultry workers, causing conjunctivitis and lymphadenitis. SYN avian pneumoencephalitis v., ND v.

non-A, non-B hepatitis v., term used to group any of a number of viruses, other than A or B, which cause hepatitis in humans.

nonoccluded v., a v. not inclosed in an inclusion body, usually with reference to an insect v.

Norwalk v., a v. associated with acute viral gastroenteritis and probably belonging to the calicivirus group.

occluded v., a v. inclosed in an inclusion body, usually with reference to an insect v.

Omsk hemorrhagic fever v., a v. of the genus *Flavivirus* causing Omsk hemorrhagic fever.

oncogenic v., a v. of one of the two groups of tumor-inducing v.'s: the RNA tumor v.'s (subfamily Oncovirinae), which are well defined and rather homogeneous, or the DNA v.'s, which are more diverse. SYN tumor v.

O'nyong-nyong v., a v. of the genus *Alphavirus*, in the family Togaviridae, found in Uganda, Kenya, and Congo, which causes O'nyong-nyong fever.

orf v., a parapoxvirus causing orf in sheep and goats and sometimes humans.

Oriboca v., a C group v. of the genus *Bunyavirus*, and an agent of bunyavirus encephalitis.

ornithosis v., former name for *Chlamydia psittaci*.

orphan viruses, v.'s, such as the enteric orphan v.'s, which when originally found were not specifically associated with disease; a number of these have since been shown to be pathogenic.

Pacheco's parrot disease v., probably a v. of the family Herpesviridae, possibly related to the v. of infectious laryngotracheitis. SYN parrot v. (2).

panleukopenia v. of cats, SYN feline panleukopenia v.

pantropic v., the ordinary strain of yellow fever v., as distinguished from the neurotropic strain; has an affinity for different tissues.

papilloma v. (pap-i-lō′mă), SYN *Papillomavirus*.

pappataci fever viruses, SYN phlebotomus fever viruses.

papular stomatitis v. of cattle, SYN bovine papular stomatitis v.

parainfluenza viruses, v.'s of the genus *Paramyxovirus*, of four types: type 1 (hemadsorption v. type 2), which includes sendai v., causes acute laryngotracheitis in children and occasionally adults; type 2 (croup-associated v.) is associated especially with acute laryngotracheitis or croup in young children and minor upper respiratory infections in adults; type 3 (hemadsorption v. type 1; shipping fever v.) has been isolated from small children with pharyngitis, bronchiolitis, and pneumonia, and causes occasional respiratory infection in adults; bovine strains have been isolated from cattle with shipping fever, and the v. has also been isolated from sheep; type 4 has been isolated from a very few children with minor respiratory illness.

paravaccinia v., SYN pseudocowpox v.

parrot v., (1) obsolete term for *Chlamydia psittaci*; **(2)** SYN Pacheco's parrot disease v.

Patois v., a serologic group of the genus *Bunyavirus*, comprising 4 species.

peste des petits ruminants v., a morbillivirus causing peste des petits ruminants in sheep and goats.

pharyngoconjunctival fever v., one of several types of adenoviruses associated with outbreaks of fever and pharyngitis, sometimes with conjunctivitis, especially in service recruits and people in boarding schools.

phlebotomus fever viruses, an unclassified serologic group of arboviruses morphologically like *Bunyavirus* but antigenically unrelated, transmitted by *Phlebotomus papatasi* (sandfly) and

---

oncogenic viruses

DNA viruses

papovaviridae

rabbit	papillomavirus
mouse	polyoma virus (PV)
ape[1]	simian virus 40 (SV)

adenoviridae

ape, cattle, bird	adenovirus
human[1]	subgroups A, B, C, D

herpesviridae

human[1]	herpes simplex virus
human[2]	Epstein-Barr virus
ape	herpesvirus saimiri and ateles
rabbit	herpesvirus sylvilagus
fowl	Marek disease virus
frog	Lucke herpesvirus

hepadnaviridae

human	hepatitis-B virus

RNA viruses

retroviridae (with reverse transcriptase)
B-type

mouse	Bittner-virus (MTV)
ape	Mason-Pfizer mammatumor-virus
(human?)	B-type particles in mother's milk

C-type

bird	leukemia virus (AMV)
	Rous sarcoma virus (RSV)
	reticuloendotheliosis virus (REV)
mouse	leukemia virus (MLV)
	sarcoma virus (MSV)
cat	leukemia virus (FeLV)
	sarcoma virus (FeSV)
hamster	leukemia virus (HaLV)
snake	Russel viper sarcoma virus (ViSV)
human	human T-cell lymphoma virus (HTLV I and II)

[1] isolated from host organism, but without producing tumors in host

[2] cofactor for formation of tumor

---

causing phlebotomus fever; there are 20 strains, including Icoarachi and Itaporanga. SYN pappataci fever viruses, sandfly fever viruses.

plant viruses, v.'s pathogenic to higher plants.

pneumonia v. of mice, an RNA v. of the genus *Pneumovirus*, a member of the family Paramyxoviridae, occurring normally as latent infection in laboratory mice, but capable of activation by serial intranasal passage and causing pneumonia. SYN PVM v.

poliomyelitis v., the picornavirus (genus *Enterovirus*) causing poliomyelitis in humans; the route of infection is the alimentary tract, but the v. may enter the bloodstream and nervous system, sometimes causing paralysis of the limbs and, rarely, encephalitis; many infections are inapparent; serologic types 1, 2, and 3 are recognized, type 1 being responsible for most paralytic poliomyelitis and most epidemics. SYN poliovirus hominis, poliovirus.

polyoma v., a papovavirus (genus *Polyomavirus*) which normally occurs in inapparent infections in laboratory and wild mice, but after growth on tissue culture is capable of producing parotid

vi

tumors in mice and sarcomas in hamsters as well as tumors in other laboratory animals. SYN mouse parotid tumor v.

porcine epidemic diarrhea v., a coronavirus causing porcine epidemic diarrhea in pigs.

porcine hemagglutinating encephalomyelitis v., a coronavirus causing vomiting, wasting, and encephalomyelitis in young pigs.

porcine sarcoma v., a retrovirus causing sarcoma in swine.

Powassan v., a v. of the genus *Flavivirus* (family Flaviviridae), transmitted by ixodid ticks and causing Powassan encephalitis in children; also capable of producing meningoencephalomyelitis in rabbits and children. [*Powassan,* Canada, where first isolated]

progressive pneumonia v., SYN maedi v.

pseudocowpox v., a v. of the genus *Parapoxvirus* that causes pseudocowpox in humans and cattle; it is closely related to orf v. and papular stomatitis v. SYN paravaccinia v.

pseudolymphocytic choriomeningitis v., SYN infectious ectromelia v.

pseudorabies v., a herpesvirus causing pseudorabies in swine. SYN Aujeszky's disease v.

psittacosis v., former name for *Chlamydia psittaci.*

PVM v., SYN pneumonia v. of mice.

quail bronchitis v., a v., similiar to an adenovirus, closely related antigenically to CELO v.

Quaranfil v., an ungrouped arbovirus isolated from human blood and from herons.

rabbit fibroma v., a poxvirus of the genus *Leporipoxvirus,* closely related to vaccinia and myxoma v.'s, that causes Shope fibroma. SYN fibromatosis v. of rabbits, Shope fibroma v.

rabbit myxoma v., the poxvirus of the genus *Leporipoxvirus* causing myxomatosis of rabbits. SYN myxomatosis v.

rabbitpox v., an orthopoxvirus that causes epidemics of pox in laboratory rabbits; immunologically, it is closely related to vaccinia v. but is more virulent in rabbits.

rabies v., a large bullet-shaped v. of the genus *Lyssavirus,* in the family Rhabdoviridae, that is the causative agent of rabies.

rabies v., Flury strain, a v. isolated from human brain, attenuated (fixed) by serial propagation in nonmammalian hosts, and subsequently established in chick embryo culture.

rabies v., Kelev strain, an attenuated, embryonate fowl egg-passaged strain.

rat sialodacryoadenitis v., a coronavirus causing sialodacryoadenitis in rats.

Rauscher leukemia v., an RNA retrovirus associated with leukemia in rodents; similar to Friend v. SYN Rauscher's v.

Rauscher's v., SYN Rauscher leukemia v.

REO v., SYN respiratory enteric orphan v.

respiratory enteric orphan v., a nonenveloped icosahedral virus whose genome consists of double stranded RNA, belonging to the family Reoviridae, frequently found in both the respiratory and enteric tract. SYN REO v.

respiratory syncytial v., an RNA v. of the genus *Pneumovirus,* in the family Paramyxoviridae, with a tendency to form syncytia in tissue culture, that causes minor respiratory infection with rhinitis and cough in adults, but is capable of causing severe bronchitis and bronchopneumonia in young children; first isolated from chimpanzees with respiratory disease. SYN chimpanzee coryza agent, Rs v.

Rida v., a variant of the scrapie agent.

Rift Valley fever v., a v. of the genus Phlebovirus (family Bunyaviridae) that occurs in central and southern Africa in sheep, goats, and cattle, causing abortions and severe febrile disease, especially in young lambs; humans, especially herdsmen and veterinarians, who may become infected through close contact with infected animals, developing a dengue-like disease; the v. also infects buffaloes, camels and antelopes; it is mosquito-borne, but also probably infects by contact and respiratory tract.

rinderpest v., an RNA v. of the genus *Morbillivirus,* causing rinderpest; it is closely related to the measles and canine distemper v.'s. SYN cattle plague v.

RNA v., a group of v.'s in which the core consists of RNA; a major group of animal v.'s that includes the families Picornaviridae, Reoviridae, Togaviridae, Flaviviridae, Bunyaviridae, Arenaviridae, Paramyxoviridae, Retroviridae, Coronaviridae, Orthomyxoviridae, and Rhabdoviridae. SYN ribovirus.

RNA tumor viruses, v.'s of the subfamily Oncovirinae.

Ross River v., a mosquito-borne alphavirus, family Togaviridae, that causes epidemic polyarthritis.

Rous-associated v. (RAV), a leukemia v. of the leukosis-sarcoma complex which by phenotypic mixing with a defective (noninfectious) strain of Rous sarcoma v. effects production of infectious sarcoma v. with envelope antigenicity of the RAV.

Rous sarcoma v. (RSV), a sarcoma-producing v. of the avian leukosis-sarcoma complex identified by Rous in 1911.

Rs v., SYN respiratory syncytial v.

Rubarth's disease v., SYN canine *adenovirus* 1.

rubella v., an RNA v. of the genus *Rubivirus;* the agent causing rubella (German measles) in humans. SYN German measles v.

rubeola v., SYN measles v.

Russian autumn encephalitis v., SYN Japanese B encephalitis v.

Russian spring-summer encephalitis v., SYN tick-borne encephalitis v.

Salisbury common cold viruses, strains of rhinovirus of historical interest because of early studies that established the viral etiology of common colds.

salivary v., a highly species-specific herpesvirus (cytomegalovirus) with particular affinity for the salivary gland tissue. SYN salivary gland v.

salivary gland v., SYN salivary v.

sandfly fever viruses, SYN phlebotomus fever viruses.

San Miguel sea lion v., a calicivirus, family Caliciviridae, first isolated from sea lions on San Miguel island off the California coast, which is indistinguishable from the vesicular exanthema of swine v. both biophysically and clinically in terms of the vesicular disease syndrome that it produces in swine.

Sendai v., a parainfluenza v. type 1 reported to cause pneumonia in pigs; also used extensively to effect fusion of tissue culture cells.

serum hepatitis v., SYN hepatitis B v.

sheep-pox v., a poxvirus of the genus *Capripoxvirus* causing sheep-pox.

shipping fever v., parainfluenza v. type 3. SEE parainfluenza viruses.

Shope fibroma v., SYN rabbit fibroma v.

Shope papilloma v., a papillomavirus infecting wild cottontail rabbits. SEE Shope *papilloma.*

Simbu v., a serologic group of the genus *Bunyavirus,* comprising a number of species including the type strain, Simbu v.

simian v. (SV), any of a number of v.'s, belonging to various families, isolated from monkeys or from cultures of monkey cells. SYN vacuolating v.

simian v. 40, SYN simian vacuolating v. No. 40.

simian hemorrhagic fever v., an arterivirus causing simian hemorrhagic fever in macaque monkeys.

simian vacuolating v. No. 40 (SV40), a small (40 to 45 nm) DNA v. of the genus *Polyomavirus,* family Papovaviridae; the cause of seemingly inapparent infections in monkeys, especially rhesus, and a common contaminant of monkey cell cultures; the v. may cause inapparent infection in humans and may be excreted in stools of children for several weeks; it can produce fibrosarcoma in suckling hamsters, and transformation may occur in human diploid cells; it may also form "hybrid" v. in cells also infected with certain adenoviruses. SYN simian v. 40.

Sindbis v., the type species of the genus *Alphavirus,* in the family Togaviridae, usually transmitted by mosquitoes of the genus Culex; and causative agent of Sindbis fever. [village in Egypt where first isolated]

slow v., a v., or a virus-like agent, etiologically associated with a disease having a long incubation period of months to years with a gradual onset frequently terminating in severe illness and/or death.

smallpox v., SYN variola v.

snowshoe hare v., a member of the California group of arboviruses (family Bunyaviridae) causing fever, severe headache, and nausea in humans in North America.

soremouth v., SYN contagious ecthyma (pustular dermatitis) v. of sheep.

Spondweni v., an arbovirus of the genus *Flavivirus* isolated from mosquitoes in Africa; may cause disease in humans.

St. Louis encephalitis v., a group B arbovirus, in the family Flaviviridae, occurring in the U.S., Trinidad, and Panama; normally present as inapparent infection in humans, but sometimes a cause of encephalitis; the v. has been isolated from birds in Panama and from several mosquito species, especially *Psorophora.*

street v., an isolate of rabies v. from a naturally infected domestic animal.

swamp fever v., SYN equine infectious anemia v.

swine encephalitis v., a coronavirus, in the family Coronaviridae, that causes swine encephalitis.

swine fever v., SYN hog cholera v.

swine influenza viruses, strains of influenza v. type A which cause influenza of swine and can infect humans.

swinepox v., a poxvirus distinct from vaccinia v. and the cause of swinepox; the pig louse plays an important role in transmission.

swine vesicular disease v., a porcine enterovirus causing vesicular disease in swine.

Swiss mouse leukemia v., SYN Friend v.

Tacaribe v., the type v. of the Tacaribe complex of v.'s (arenaviruses), isolated from bats and mosquitoes in Trinidad.

Tahyna v., a California group arbovirus, in the family Bunyaviridae, from central Europe, known to infect humans.

temperate v., referring to a phage that does not lyse its host immediately but may persist in latent form and eventually lyse its host. SEE lysogeny.

Teschen disease v., a picornavirus causing Teschen disease of pigs; the v. is normally a harmless inhabitant of the intestinal tract, but virulent strains cause epizootics of the disease. SYN infectious porcine encephalomyelitis v.

Tete viruses, a serologic group of the genus *Bunyavirus*, comprising a number of types.

TGE v., SYN transmissible gastroenteritis v. of swine.

Theiler's original v., SYN Theiler's mouse encephalomyelitis v.

Theiler's v., SYN Theiler's mouse encephalomyelitis v.

Theiler's mouse encephalomyelitis v., a virus in the family Picornaviridae. SYN Theiler's original v., Theiler's v.

tick-borne v., SYN tick-borne encephalitis v.

tick-borne encephalitis v., an arbovirus of the genus *Flavivirus* that occurs in Central Europe and the USSR in two subtypes, causing two forms of encephalitis in humans: tick-borne encephalitis (Central European subtype) and tick-borne encephalitis (Eastern subtype); the vectors are ticks of the genus *Ixodes*. SYN Russian spring-summer encephalitis v., tick-borne v.

TO v., theiler's original v. SEE mouse encephalomyelitis v.

trachoma v., former name for *Chlamydia trachomatis.*

transmissible gastroenteritis v. of swine, a coronavirus that causes transmissible gastroenteritis of swine. SYN TGE v.

transmissible turkey enteritis v., a coronavirus causing bluecomb disease of turkeys. SYN bluecomb v.

tumor v., SYN oncogenic v.

turkey meningoencephalitis v., a v. of the genus *Flavivirus* causing paralysis and enteritis in turkeys in Israel.

turkey rhinotracheitis v., a pneumovirus causing rhinotracheitis in turkeys and swollen head syndrome in chickens.

Turlock v., an unclassified serologic group of arboviruses morphologically like *Bunyavirus* but antigenically unrelated to it.

Umbre v., an arbovirus related serologically to the Turlock v.

vaccine v., SEE vaccine.

vaccinia v., the poxvirus (genus *Orthopoxvirus*) used in the immunization of people against variola (smallpox), usually causing a local reaction but sometimes generalized vaccinia, especially in children; the v. is closely related serologically to the v.'s of variola and cowpox, but certain differences have been demonstrated which indicate that they are perhaps distinct but closely related strains of a variola-vaccinia-cowpox complex; the lineage of vaccinia v. is uncertain, and it is very unlikely that it descended from Jenner's original v. SYN poxvirus officinalis.

vacuolating v., SYN simian v.

varicella-zoster v., a herpesvirus, morphologically identical to herpes simplex v., that causes varicella (chickenpox) and herpes zoster in man; varicella results from a primary infection with the v.; herpes zoster results from secondary invasion by the same v. or by reactivation of infection which in many instances has been latent for many years. SYN chickenpox v., herpes zoster v., human herpesvirus 3.

variola v., a poxvirus of the genus *Orthopoxvirus*, the pathogen of smallpox in humans. SYN smallpox v.

VEE v., SYN Venezuelan equine encephalomyelitis v.

Venezuelan equine encephalomyelitis v., a group A arbovirus of the genus *Alphavirus*, family Togaviridae, occurring in Venezuela and several other South American countries, in Panama and Trinidad, and occasionally the United States causing Venezuelan equine encephalomyelitis in horses and humans; it seems to be more viscerotropic than neurotropic; the v. is transmitted by Culex mosquitoes. SYN VEE v.

vesicular exanthema of swine v., a calicivirus causing vesicular exanthema of swine. SEE ALSO San Miguel sea lion v.

vesicular stomatitis v., an RNA v. of the genus *Vesiculovirus*, in the family Rhabdoviridae, causing vesicular stomatitis in horses, cattle, sheep, and pigs. SYN VS v.

viral hemorrhagic fever v., SYN Ebola v.

visceral disease v., SYN cytomegalovirus.

visna v., an RNA v. (subfamily Lentivirinae) that causes visna; it is closely related antigenically to the similar maedi v.

VS v., SYN vesicular stomatitis v.

WEE v., SYN western equine encephalomyelitis v.

Wesselsbron disease v., a mosquito-borne group B arbovirus of the genus *Flavivirus* causing Wesselsbron fever.

western equine encephalomyelitis v., a group A arbovirus of the genus *Alphavirus*, family Togaviridae, occurring in the western United States and parts of South America; it occurs naturally, usually as a symptomless infection in birds, but causes western equine encephalomyelitis in horses and humans following transfer by the bites of mosquitoes, chiefly *Culex tarsalis*. SYN WEE v.

West Nile v., SYN West Nile encephalitis v.

West Nile encephalitis v., caused by a virus in the family Flaviviridae. SYN West Nile v.

xenotropic v., a retrovirus that does not produce disease in its natural host and replicates only in tissue culture cells derived from a different species.

Yaba v., a poxvirus from the family Poxviridae, distinct from monkeypox v., that causes Yaba tumors in monkeys. SYN Yaba monkey v.

Yaba monkey v., SYN Yaba v.

yellow fever v., an arbovirus, the type species of the genus *Flavivirus*, in the family Flaviviridae, endemic in tropical Africa south of the Sahara and in tropical South America, occasionally spreading to countries outside these areas; it is the cause of yellow fever of humans and other primates; the v. exists in wild primates, and probably also in edentates, marsupials, and rodents, and is transmitted to humans by *Aedes Aegypti* and the *Haemagogus* complex of tree-top mosquitoes which feed on arboreal mammals.

Zika v., a mosquito-borne virus of the genus *Flavivirus* (family Flaviviridae), found in parts of Africa and in Malaysia, that causes Zika fever. [*Zika*, forest in Uganda, where first isolated]

△**-virus.** A genus of viruses.

vi·rus·oid (vī′rŭs-oyd). A plant pathogen resembling a viroid but having a much larger circular or linear RNA segment and a capsid; it is a satellite agent requiring RNA of an associated virus (helper virus) for replication. [virus + G. *eidos*, resembling]

vi·rus shed·ding. Excretion of virus by any route from the infected host; route and duration of excretion vary according to the pathogenesis of the infection or disease.

vis, pl. **vi·res** (vis, vī′rēs). Force, energy, or power. [L. force]

v. conserva′trix, the inherent power in the organism resisting the effects of injury.

v. a fron′te, a force acting from in front; an obstructive, restraining, or impeding force.

v. a ter′go, a force acting from behind; a pushing or accelerating force.

v. vi′tae, v. vita′lis, SYN vitalism.

vis·cance (vis′kans). A measure of the energy dissipation due to a flow in a viscous system. In medicine and physiology, usually a measure of the energy dissipation in the flow of liquids, sols, or gels within cells and tissues, or of fluids (e.g., blood, respiratory gases) in tubes. The v. is the pressure gradient from one end to the other of the flow path when unit flow occurs. The relationship between viscosity and v. is of the same nature as that between specific resistance, or resistivity, of a conductor material and the resistance of a particular conductor made from that material.

vis·cera (vis′er-ă). Plural of viscus. SYN vitals.

vis·cer·ad (vis′er-ad). In a direction toward the viscera. [viscera + L. *ad,* to]

vis·cer·al (vis′er-ăl). Relating to the viscera. SYN splanchnic.

vis·cer·al·gia (vis-er-al′jē-ă). Pain in any viscera. [viscera + G. *algos,* pain]

vis·cer·i·mo·tor (vis′er-i-mō′ter). SYN visceromotor.

⚠ **viscero-.** The viscera. SEE ALSO splanchno-. [L. *viscus,* pl. *viscera,* the internal organs]

vis·cer·o·cra·ni·um (vis′er-ō-krā′nē-ŭm). That part of the skull derived from the embryonic pharyngeal arches; it comprises the facial bones of the facial skeleton (under *bone*) and is distinct from that part of the skull which forms the neurocranium or braincase. SYN cranium viscerale, visceral cranium, jaw skeleton, splanchnocranium. [viscero- + cranium]

cartilaginous v., those elements of the fetal skull derived from the second and succeeding pharyngeal arch cartilages.

membranous v., membranous bones, developed in the fetal skull, that overlie maxillary and mandibular components of the first pharyngeal arch cartilage.

vis·cer·o·gen·ic (vis′er-ō-jen′ik). Of visceral origin; denoting a number of sensory and other reflexes. [viscero- + G. *-gen,* producing]

vis·cer·o·graph (vis′er-ō-graf). An instrument for recording the mechanical activity of the viscera. [viscero- + G. *graphō,* to write]

vis·cer·o·in·hib·i·to·ry (vis′er-ō-in-hib′i-tōr-ē). Restricting or arresting the functional activity of the viscera.

vis·cer·o·meg·a·ly (vis′er-ō-meg′ă-lē). Abnormal enlargement of the viscera, such as may be seen in acromegaly and other disorders. SYN organomegaly, splanchnomegaly. [viscero- + G. *megas,* large]

vis·cer·o·mo·tor (vis′er-ō-mō′ter). 1. Relating to or controlling movement in the viscera; denoting the autonomic nerves innervating the viscera, especially the intestines. 2. Denoting a movement having a relation to the viscera; referring to reflex muscular contractions of the abdominal wall in cases of visceral disease. SYN viscerimotor.

vis·cer·o·pa·ri·e·tal (vis′er-ō-pă-rī′ĕ-tăl). Relating to the viscera and the wall of the abdomen. [viscero- + L. *paries,* wall]

vis·cer·o·per·i·to·ne·al (vis′er-ō-per-i-tō-nē′ăl). Relating to the peritoneum and the abdominal viscera.

vis·cer·o·pleu·ral (vis′er-ō-plū′răl). Relating to the pleural and the thoracic viscera. SYN pleurovisceral.

vis·cer·op·to·sis, vis·cer·op·to·sia (vis′er-op-tō′sis, -tō′sē-ă). Descent of the viscera from their normal positions. SYN splanchnoptosis, splanchnoptosia. [viscero- + G. *ptōsis,* a falling]

vis·cer·o·sen·so·ry (vis′er-ō-sen′sōr-ē). Relating to the sensory innervation of internal organs.

vis·cer·o·skel·e·tal (vis′er-ō-skel′ĕ-tăl). Relating to the visceroskeleton. SYN splanchnoskeletal.

vis·cer·o·skel·e·ton (vis′er-ō-skel′ĕ-tŏn). 1. Any bony formation in an organ, as in the heart, tongue, or penis of certain animals; the term also includes, according to some anatomists,

the cartilaginous rings of the trachea and bronchi. 2. The bony framework protecting the viscera, such as the ribs and sternum, the pelvic bones, and the anterior portion of the skull. SYN splanchnoskeleton, visceral skeleton.

vis·cer·o·so·mat·ic (vis′er-ō-sō-mat′ik). Relating to the viscera and the body. SYN splanchnosomatic. [viscero- + G. *sōma,* body]

vis·cer·o·tome (vis′er-ō-tōm). An instrument by means of which a section of an organ, *e.g.,* the liver, can be removed from a cadaver for examination without performing a general autopsy. [viscero- + G. *tomos,* cutting]

vis·cer·ot·o·my (vis-er-ot′ō-mē). Dissection of the viscera by incision, especially postmortem. [viscero- + G. *tomē,* incision]

vis·cer·o·to·nia (vis′er-ō-tō′nē-ă). Personality traits of love of food, sociability, general relaxation, friendliness, and affection. [viscero- + G. *tonos,* tone]

vis·cer·o·tro·phic (vis′er-ō-trof′ik). Relating to any trophic change determined by visceral conditions. [viscero- + G. *trophē,* nourishment]

vis·cer·o·tro·pic (vis′er-ō-trop′ik). Affecting the viscera. [L. *viscero* internal organs, + G. *tropē,* a turning]

vis·cid (vis′id). Sticky; glutinous. [L. *viscidus,* stick, fr. *viscum,* birdlime]

vis·cid·i·ty (vi-sid′i-tē). Stickiness; adhesiveness.

vis·ci·do·sis (vis-i-dō′sis). SYN cystic *fibrosis.*

vis·co·e·las·tic·i·ty (vis′kō-ē-las-tis′i-tē). The property of a viscous material that also shows elasticity.

vis·com·e·ter (vis-kom′ĕ-ter). SYN viscosimeter.

vis·co·sim·e·ter (vis-kō-sim′ĕ-ter). An apparatus for determining the viscosity of a fluid; in medicine, usually of the blood. SYN viscometer.

vis·co·sim·e·try (vis-kō-sim′ĕ-trē). Determination of the viscosity of a fluid, such as the blood. [viscosity + G. *metron,* measure]

vis·cos·i·ty (vis-kos′i-tē). In general, the resistance to flow or alteration of shape by any substance as a result of molecular cohesion; most frequently applied to liquids as the resistance of a fluid to flow because of a shearing force. [L. *viscositas,* fr. *viscosus,* viscous]

absolute v., force per unit area applied tangentially to a fluid, causing unit rate of displacement of parallel planes separated by a unit distance; units in CGS system: poise.

anomalous v., the viscous behavior of nonhomogenous fluids or suspensions, *e.g.,* blood, in which the apparent v. increases as flow or shear rate decreases toward zero.

apparent v., the v. calculated from Poiseuille's law at any particular flow and tube diameter; it is used for suspensions, such as blood, that exhibit anomalous v. and the Fahraeus-Lindqvist effect.

dynamic v. (μ), the internal or molecular frictional resistance of a fluid by Newton's law of v. as the ratio of the applied force per unit area to the relative velocity of adjacent fluid layers (produced by the force).

kinematic v. (ν, υ), a measure used in studies of fluid flow; the dynamic viscosity, μ, in poises divided by the density of the material; units: stokes.

newtonian v., the v. characteristics of a newtonian fluid.

relative v., the ratio of the v. of a solution or dispersion to the v. of the solvent or continuous phase.

vis·co·tox·ins (vis′kō-toks′ins). A class of phytotoxins that have a hypotensive activity and slow the heart beat.

vis·cous (vis′kŭs). Sticky; marked by high viscosity. [see viscid, viscosity]

vis·cum (vis′kŭm). 1. The berries of *Viscum album* (family Loranthaceae), a parasitic plant growing on apple, pear, and other trees; has been used as an oxytocic. SYN mistletoe. 2. Herbage of *Phoradendron flavescens,* American mistletoe; has been used as an oxytocic and emmenagogue.

vis·cus, pl. **vis·cera** (vis′kŭs, vis′er-ă). An organ of the digestive, respiratory, urogenital, and endocrine systems as well as the spleen, the heart, and great vessels; hollow and multilayered walled organs studied in splanchnology. [L. the soft parts, internal organs]

vis·ile (viz'il). **1.** An obsolete term denoting the type of mental imagery in which one recalls most readily that which has been seen. Cf. audile, motile. **2.** A person with such mental imagery. **3.** SYN visual.

vi·sion (vizh'ŭn). The act of seeing. SEE ALSO sight. [L. *visio,* fr. *video,* pp. *visus,* to see]

achromatic v., SYN achromatopsia.

binocular v., v. with a single image, by both eyes simultaneously.

blue v., SYN cyanopsia.

central v., v. stimulated by an object imaged on the fovea centralis. SYN direct v.

chromatic v., SYN chromatopsia.

colored v. (VC), SYN chromatopsia.

cone v., SYN photopic v.

direct v., SYN central v.

double v., SYN diplopia.

facial v., sensing the proximity of objects by the nerves of the face, presumed in the case of the blind and also in sighted persons who are blindfolded or in darkness.

green v., SYN chloropsia.

halo v., a condition in which colored or luminous rings are seen around lights.

haploscopic v., stereoscopic v. produced by the haploscope, or mirror-type stereoscope.

indirect v., SYN peripheral v.

multiple v., SYN polyopia.

night v., SYN scotopic v.

oscillating v., SYN oscillopsia.

peripheral v., v. resulting from retinal stimulation beyond the macula. SYN indirect v.

photopic v., v. when the eye is light-adapted. SEE light *adaptation,* light-adapted *eye.* SYN cone v., photopia.

red v., SYN erythropsia.

rod v., SYN scotopic v.

scotopic v., v. when the eye is dark-adapted. SEE ALSO dark *adaptation,* dark-adapted *eye.* SYN night v., rod v., scotopia, twilight v.

stereoscopic v., the single perception of a slightly different image from each eye. SYN stereopsis.

subjective v., visual impressions that arise centrally and do not originate with ocular stimuli.

tinted v., SYN chromatopsia.

triple v., SYN triplopia.

tubular v., a constriction of the visual field, as though one were looking through a hollow cylinder or tube. SYN tunnel v.

tunnel v., SYN tubular v.

twilight v., SYN scotopic v.

yellow v., SYN xanthopsia.

vis·na (vis'nă). A chronic meningoencephalitis of sheep, occurring almost exclusively in Iceland caused by a "slow virus" (subfamily Lentivirinae); it is now considered that v. and maedi are two histopathological and clinical manifestations of the same viral infection.

vi·su·al (vizh'ū-ăl). **1.** Relating to vision. **2.** Denoting a person who learns and remembers more readily through sight than through hearing. SYN visile (3). [Late L. *visualis,* fr. *visus,* vision]

functional v. loss, an apparent loss of visual acuity or visual field with no substantiating physical signs; often due to a natural concern about visual loss combined with suggestibility and a fear of the worst; best treated with reassurance.

vi·su·al·ize (vizh'ū-ă-līz). To picture in the mind or to perceive; commonly misused by ascribing to the technique the act of making visible.

vi·su·o·au·di·tory (vizh'yū-ō-aw'di-tōr-ē). Relating to both vision and hearing; denoting nerves connecting the centers for these senses.

vi·su·og·no·sis (vizh'yū-og-nō'sis). Recognition and understanding of visual impressions. [L. *visus,* vision, + G. *gnōsis,* knowledge]

vis·u·o·mo·tor (viz'yū-ō-mō'ter). Denoting the ability to synchronize visual information with physical movement, *e.g.,* driving a car or playing a video game of skill.

vi·su·o·psy·chic (vizh'yū-ō-sī'kik). Pertaining to the portion of the cerebral cortex concerned with the integration of visual impressions. [L. *visus,* vision, + G. *psychē,* mind]

vi·su·o·sen·so·ry (vizh'yū-ō-sen'sōr-ē). Pertaining to the perception of visual stimuli.

vis·u·o·spa·tial (viz'yū-ō-spā'shăl). Denoting the ability to comprehend and conceptualize visual representations and spatial relationships in learning and performing a task.

vi·su·scope (viz'yū-skōp). A modified ophthalmoscope that projects a black star on the patient's fundus.

vi·tal (vīt-ăl). Relating to life. [L. *vitalis,* fr. *vita,* life]

vi·tal·ism (vīt'ăl-izm). The theory that animal functions are dependent upon a special form of energy or force, the vital force, distinct from the physical forces. SYN vis vitae, vis vitalis. [L. *vitalis,* pertaining to life]

vi·tal·is·tic (vīt'ă-lis'tik). Pertaining to vitalism.

vi·tal·i·ty (vīt-al'i-tē). Vital force or energy.

vi·tal·ize (vīt'ăl-īz). To endow with vital force.

vi·ta·lom·e·ter (vī-tă-lom'ĕ-ter). An electrical device for determining the vitality of the tooth pulp.

vi·tal red [C.I. 23570]. Trisodium salt of a sulfonated diazo dye (a ditolyl group diazotized to sulfonated aminonaphthalene residues), used as a vital stain. SYN brilliant vital red.

vi·tals (vīt'ălz). SYN viscera.

vi·ta·mer (vī'tă-mer). One of two or more similar compounds capable of fulfilling a specific vitamin function in the body; *e.g.,* niacin, niacinamide.

VITAMIN

vi·ta·min (vīt'ă-min). One of a group of organic substances, present in minute amounts in natural foodstuffs, that are essential to normal metabolism; insufficient amounts in the diet may cause deficiency diseases. [L. *vita,* life, + amine]

classification of vitamins		
with coenzyme function	without coenzyme function	vitamin-like agents
vit. B$_1$	vit. A*	vit. F
vit. B$_2$	vit. C	vit. T (carnitine)
vit. B$_6$	vit. D*	flavonoids
vit. B$_{12}$	vit. E*	mesoinositol
vit. K*		
biotin		
folic acid		
α-lipoic acid		
pantothenic acid		
*lipolytic		

v. A, (1) any β-ionone derivative, except provitamin A carotenoids, possessing qualitatively the biological activity of retinol; deficiency interferes with the production and resynthesis of rhodopsin, thereby causing night blindness, and produces a keratinizing metaplasia of epithelial cells that may result in xerophthalmia, keratosis, susceptibility to infections, and retarded growth; **(2)** the original v. A, now known as retinol. SYN axerophthol.

v. A₁, SYN retinol.

v. A₂, SYN dehydroretinol.

v. A₁ acid, SYN retinoic acid.

v. A₁ alcohol, SYN retinol.

v. A aldehyde, SYN retinaldehyde.

v. A₂ aldehyde, SYN dehydroretinaldehyde.

antiberiberi v., SYN thiamin.

antihemorrhagic v., SYN v. K.

antineuritic v., SYN thiamin.

antirachitic v.'s, ergocalciferol (v. D₂) and cholecalciferol (v. D₃).

antiscorbutic v., SYN ascorbic acid.

antisterility v., SYN v. E (2).

v. B, a group of water-soluble substances originally considered as one v.

v. B₁, SYN thiamin.

v. B₂, (1) SYN riboflavin. **(2)** obsolete term for a complex of folic acid, nicotinic acid, nicotinamide, pantothenic acid, and riboflavin.

v. B₃, (1) obsolete term for nicotinamide and/or nicotinic acid; **(2)** obsolete term for pantothenic acid.

v. B₄, (1) once believed to be a factor necessary for nutrition of the chick, now identified simply as certain essential amino acids and/or adenine; **(2)** obsolete term for adenine.

v. B₅, once used to describe biological activities now ascribed to pantothenic acid or nicotinic acid.

v. B₆, pyridoxine and related compounds (pyridoxal; pyridoxamine).

v. B₁₂, generic descriptor for compounds exhibiting the biological activity of cyanocobalamin (cyanocob(III)alamin); the antianemia factor of liver extract that contains cobalt, a cyano group, and corrin in a cobamide structure. Several substances with similar formulas and with the characteristic hematinic action have been isolated and designated: B₁₂ₐ, hydroxocobalamin; B₁₂ᵦ, aquacobalamin; B₁₂ᵧ, nitritocobalamin; B₁₂ᵣ, cob(II)alamin; B₁₂ₛ, cob(I)alamin; B₁₂ᵢᵢᵢ, factors A and V₁ₐ (cobyric acid), and pseudovitamin B₁₂. Vitamins B₁₂ₐ and B₁₂ᵦ are known to be tautomeric compounds; B₁₂ᵦ has been obtained from cultures of *Streptomyces aureofaciens;* B₁₂ᵧ has been obtained from cultures of *Streptomyces griseus* and is distinguishable from B₁₂ by differences in its absorption spectrum. The physiologically active v. B₁₂ coenzymes are methylcobalamin and deoxyadenosinecobalamine. A deficiency of v. B₁₂ is often associated with certain methylmalonic acidurias. SYN animal protein factor, antianemic factor, antipernicious anemia factor (1), erythrocyte maturation factor, maturation factor, methylcobalamin.

v. Bₜ, SYN carnitine.

v. Bₓ, SYN *p*-aminobenzoic acid.

v. B complex, a pharmaceutical term applied to drug products containing a mixture of the B v.'s, usually B₁, B₂, B₃, B₅, and B₆.

v. Bᴄ conjugase, an enzyme catalyzing the hydrolysis of the pteroylpolyglutamic acids to pteroylmonoglutamic acid, with consequent increase in vitamin activity; v. Bᴄ is an obsolete term for folic acid.

v. B₁₂ with intrinsic factor concentrate, a combination of v. B₁₂ with suitable preparations of the mucosa of the stomach or intestine of domestic animals used for food by humans.

v. C, SYN ascorbic acid.

coagulation v., obsolete term for v. K.

v. D, generic descriptor for all steroids exhibiting the biological activity of ergocalciferol or cholecalciferol, the antirachitic v.'s popularly called the "sun-ray v.'s." They promote the proper utilization of calcium and phosphorus, thereby producing growth in young children, together with proper bone and tooth formation; the sulfate, a water-soluble conjugate, is found in the aqueous phase of human milk; v. D₁ is a 1:1 mixture of lumisterol and v. D₂.

v. D₂, SYN ergocalciferol.

v. D₃, SYN cholecalciferol.

v. E, (1) SYN α-tocopherol. **(2)** generic descriptor of tocol and tocotrienol derivatives possessing the biological activity of α-tocopherol; contained in various oils (wheat germ, cotton-seed,

palm, rice) and whole grain cereals where it constitutes the nonsaponifiable fraction, also in animal tissue (liver, pancreas, heart) and lettuce; deficiency produces resorption or abortion in female rats and sterility in males. SYN antisterility factor, antisterility v., fertility v.

v. F, term sometimes applied to the essential unsaturated fatty acids, linoleic, linolenic, and arachidonic acids.

fat-soluble v.'s, those v.'s, soluble in fat solvents (nonpolar solvents) and relatively insoluble in water, marked in chemical structure by the presence of large hydrocarbon moieties in the molecule; *e.g.,* v.'s A, D, E, K.

fertility v., SYN v. E (2).

v. G, obsolete term for riboflavin.

v. H, SYN biotin. [Ger, H for *Haut,* skin]

v. K, generic descriptor for compounds with the biological activity of phylloquinone; fat-soluble, thermostable compounds found in alfalfa, hog liver, fish meal, and vegetable oils, essential for the formation of normal amounts of prothrombin. SYN antihemorrhagic factor, antihemorrhagic v.

v. K₁, v. K₁(20), SYN phylloquinone.

v. K₂, v. K₂(30), SYN menaquinone-6.

v. K₂(35), SYN menaquinone-7.

v. K₃, SYN menadione.

v. K₄, SYN menadiol diacetate.

v. K₅, 4-amino-2-methyl-1-naphthol; an antihemorrhagic v.

microbial v., a substance necessary for the growth of certain microorganisms, *e.g.,* biotin, *p*-aminobenzoic acid.

v. P, a mixture of bioflavonoids extracted from plants (especially citrus fruits). It reduces the permeability and fragility of capillaries and is useful in the treatment of certain cases of purpura that are resistant to v. C therapy. SEE ALSO hesperidin, quercetin, rutin. SYN capillary permeability factor, citrin, permeability v.

permeability v., SYN v. P.

v. PP, SYN nicotinic acid.

v. U, term given to a factor in fresh cabbage juice that encourages the healing of peptic ulcer; (3-amino-3-carboxypropyl)-dimethylsulfonium chloride; a methionine derivative.

---

vi·tel·lar·i·um (vit′ĕl-lar′ē-ŭm). In cestodes and trematodes, a common chamber receiving vitelline (yolk) material from the two vitelline ducts; the yolk material then passes into the ootype to surround the ovum with nutritive vitelline granules that are enclosed by a characteristically formed eggshell. SYN vitelline reservoir.

vi·tel·li·form (vī-tel′i-fōrm). Relating to or resembling the yolk of an egg.

vi·tel·lin (vī-tel′in). A lipophosphoprotein combined with lecithin in the yolk of egg. SYN lipovitellin, ovovitellin.

vi·tel·line (vī-tel′in, -ēn). Relating to the vitellus. SEE yolk *sac.*

vi·tel·lo·gen·e·sis (vī-tel′lō-jen′ĕ-sis, vī′tĕ-lō-). Formation of the yolk and its accumulation in the yolk sac. [L. *vitellus,* yolk, + G. *genesis,* production]

vi·tel·lo·gen·in (vī′tel-ō-jen′in). An egg yolk precursor protein; production is stimulated by estrogens. [L. *vitellus,* egg yolk, + *-gen* + *-in*]

vi·tel·lo·lu·te·in (vī-tel-ō-lū′tē-in). Lutein from the yolk of egg.

vitel·lo·ru·bin (vī-tel-ō-rū″bin). A reddish pigment from the yolk of egg.

vi·tel·lose (vī-tel′ōs). A protein fragment from vitellin.

vi·tel·lus (vī-tel′ŭs). SYN yolk (1). [L.]

v. o′vi, yolk of egg; used in pharmacy for emulsifying oils and camphors.

vi·ti·a·tion (vish-ē-ā′shŭn). A change that impairs utility or reduces efficiency. [L. *vitiatio* fr. *vitio,* pp. *vitiatus,* to corrupt, fr. *vitium,* vice]

vit·i·lig·i·nes (vit-i-lij′i-nēz). Plural of vitiligo.

vit·i·lig·i·nous (vit-i-lij′i-nŭs). Relating to or characterized by vitiligo.

vit·i·li·go, pl. **vit·i·lig·i·nes** (vit-i-lī′gō, vit-i-lij′i-nēz). The appearance on otherwise normal skin of nonpigmented white patches of varied sizes, often symmetrically distributed and usually bordered by hyperpigmented areas; hair in the affected areas is usually, but not always, white. Epidermal melanocytes are completely lost in depigmented areas by an autoimmune process. SYN acquired leukoderma, acquired leukopathia, leukasmus. [L. a skin eruption, fr. *vitium*, blemish, vice]

v. cap'itis, obsolete term for *alopecia* areata.

Cazenave's v., obsolete term for *alopecia* areata.

Celsus' v., obsolete term for *alopecia* areata.

v. i'ridis, small white patches in brown irides.

vit·i·li·goi·dea (vit′i-lī-goy′dē-ă). Obsolete term for xanthoma. [vitiligo + G. *eidos*, appearance]

vit·rec·to·my (vi-trek′tō-mē). Removal of the vitreous by means of an instrument which simultaneously removes vitreous by suction and cutting, and replaces it with saline or some other fluid. [vitreous + G. *ektomē*, excision]

anterior v., removal of the central vitreous gel.

posterior v., removal of the posterior cortical vitreous; sometimes the preretinal membranes are removed.

vit·re·in (vit′rē-in). A collagen-like protein that, with hyaluronic acid, accounts for the gel state of the vitreous humor. SYN vitrosin.

vit·re·i·tis (vit-rē-ī′tis). Inflammation of the corpus vitreum. SYN hyalitis. [L. *vitreus*, glassy, + G. *-itis*, inflammation]

vitreo-. Vitreous. [L. *vitreus*, glassy]

vit·re·o·den·tin (vit′rē-ō-den′tin). Dentin of a particularly brittle character.

vit·re·o·ret·i·nal (vit′rē-ō-ret′i-năl). Pertaining to the retina and the vitreous body.

vit·re·o·ret·i·nop·a·thy (vit′rē-ō-ret′i-nop′ă-thē). Retinopathy with vitreous complications.

exudative v. [MIM*193220], a familial, slowly progressive ocular disease; characterized by posterior vitreous detachment, vitreous membranes, heterotopia of macula, retinal detachment, neovascularization, and recurrent hemorrhage.

vit·re·ous (vit′rē-ŭs). **1.** Glassy; resembling glass. **2.** SYN vitreous *body.* [L. *vitreus*, glassy, fr. *vitrum*, glass]

persistent anterior hyperplastic primary v., a unilateral congenital abnormality occurring in full-term infants; characterized by a retrolental fibrovascular membrane formed by persistent primary v. with remnants of the hyaloid artery and tunica vasculosa lentis; associated with leukokoria, microphthalmos, shallow anterior chamber, and elongated ciliary processes.

persistent posterior hyperplastic primary v., a unilateral congenital anomaly in full-term infants; associated with a congenital retinal fold and a v. membranous stalk containing remnants of the hyaloid artery.

primary v., the v. first formed in the embryo between the optic cup and the lens vesicle, and later vascularized by the hyaloid artery and its branches.

secondary v., avascular v. formed around the primary v.

tertiary v., v. fibrils derived from the neuroepithelium of the ciliary body and forming the ciliary zonule.

vit·re·um (vit′rē-ŭm). SYN vitreous *body.* [L. ntr. of *vitreus*, glassy]

vit·ri·fi·ca·tion (vit′ri-fi-kā′shŭn). Conversion of dental porcelain (frit) to a glassy substance by heat and fusion. [L. *vitrium*, glassy, + *facio*, to make]

vit·ri·ol (vit′rē-ol). Any of the various salts of sulfuric acid, *e.g.*, blue v. (cupric sulfate), green v. (ferrous sulfate), white v. (zinc sulfate). [L. *vitreolus*, glassy]

vit·ro·sin (vit′rō-sin). SYN vitrein.

vi·var·i·um, pl. **vi·var·ia** (vī-var′ē-ŭm, -ă). Quarters in which animals are housed, particularly animals used in medical research. [L. *vivarius*, pertaining to living creatures]

vivi-. Living. [L. *vivus*, alive]

viv·i·di·al·y·sis (viv′i-dī-al′i-sis). Removal by dialysis, as by lavage of peritoneal cavity.

viv·i·dif·fu·sion (viv′i-di-fyū′zhŭn). Archaic term for a method by which circulating blood may be submitted to dialysis outside the body and returned to the circulation without exposure to the air or to any noxious influences; the principle used in the performance of renal dialysis with the artificial kidney. [vivi- + diffusion]

viv·i·fi·ca·tion (viv′i-fi-kā′shŭn). SYN revivification (2). [L. *vivifico*, pp. *-atus*, fr. *vivus*, alive, + *facio*, to make]

viv·i·par·i·ty (viv′i-pār′i-tē). The quality or state of being viviparous, *i.e.*, producing offspring that are living at the time of birth. SYN zoogony.

vi·vip·a·rous (vī-vip′ă-rŭs). Giving birth to living young, in distinction to oviparous. SYN zoogonous. [vivi- + L. *pario*, to bear]

viv·i·per·cep·tion (viv′i-per-sep′shŭn). Observation of the vital processes in the organism without the aid of vivisection. [vivi- + perception]

viv·i·sect (viv-i-sekt′). To practice vivisection.

viv·i·sec·tion (viv-i-sek′shŭn). Any cutting operation on a living animal for purposes of experimentation; often extended to denote any form of animal experimentation. [vivi- + section]

viv·i·sec·tion·ist, viv·i·sec·tor (vi-vi-sek′shŭn-ist, -tōr; vi-vi-sek′tŏr). One who practices vivisection.

in vi·vo (in vē′vō). In the living body, referring to a process or reaction occurring therein. Cf. *in vitro*. [L. in the living being]

Vladimiroff, Vladimir D., Russian surgeon, 1837–1903. SEE Mikulicz-V. *amputation;* V.-Mikulicz *amputation.*

VLDL Abbreviation for very low density lipoprotein. SEE lipoprotein.

VMA Abbreviation for vanillylmandelic acid.

V-max. SEE V_{max}.

VMC Abbreviation for void metal composite.

V.M.D. Abbreviation for Doctor of Veterinary Medicine.

V-MI Abbreviation for Volpe-Manhold *Index.*

vo·cal (vō′kăl). Pertaining to the voice or the organs of speech. [L. *vocalis*]

Vogel's law. See under law.

Voges, Otto, German physician, *1867. SEE V.-Proskauer *reaction.*

Vogt, Alfred, Swiss ophthalmologist, 1879–1943. SEE V.-Koyanagi *syndrome.*

Vogt, Cécile, German neurologist, 1875–1962. SEE V. *syndrome.*

Vogt, Heinrich, German neurologist, *1875. SEE Spielmeyer-V. *disease.*

Vogt, Karl, German physiologist, 1817–1895. SEE V.'s *angle.*

Vogt, Oskar, German neurologist, 1870–1959. SEE V. *syndrome.*

Vogt ceph·a·lo·dac·ty·ly. SYN type II *acrocephalosyndactyly.*

Vohwinkel, 20th Century German dermatologist. SEE Vohwinkel *syndrome.*

voice (voys). The sound made by air passing out through the larynx and upper respiratory tract, the vocal folds being approximated. SYN vox. [L. *vox*]

amphoric v., a v. sound having a hollow, blowing character, heard over a pulmonary cavity when the patient speaks or whispers. SYN amphorophony.

bronchial v., SYN bronchophony.

cavernous v., the hollow or metallic v. sound heard over a pulmonary cavity.

epigastric v., the delusion of a v. proceeding from the epigastrium.

eunuchoid v., high pitched v. in the adult male resembling the v. of an immature boy; usually functional in origin.

myxedema v., the forced, rough, raucous v. of subjects of myxedema, probably due to myxedematous thickening of the vocal folds.

void (voyd). To evacuate urine or feces.

flow v., in magnetic resonance imaging, the absence of signal from blood whose activated protons leave a region before their magnetization is measured. SEE ALSO signal v.

signal v., in magnetic resonance imaging, a region emitting no radiofrequency signal, either because there are no activated protons in the region (such as flowing blood) or because a different element predominates, particularly calcium.

VO

void met·al com·pos·ite (VMC). A porous metal structure that enables tissue growth within the openings to establish long-term attachment between prosthesis and tissue.

Voigt, Christian A., Austrian anatomist, 1809–1890. SEE V.'s *lines*, under *line*.

vol. Abbreviation for [L.] *volatilis*, volatile.

vo·la (vō′lă). Palm of the hand or sole of the foot. [L.]

vo·lar (vō′lăr). Referring to the vola; denoting either the palm of the hand or sole of the foot. SYN volaris [NA].

vo·la·ris (vō-lā′ris) [NA]. SYN volar, volar.

vol·a·tile (vol.) (vol′ă-til). **1.** Tending to evaporate rapidly. **2.** Tending toward violence, explosiveness, or rapid change. [L. *volatilis*, fr. *volo*, to fly]

vol·a·til·i·za·tion (vol′ă-til-i-zā′shŭn). SYN evaporation. [fr. L. *volatilis*, volatile, fr. *volo*, pp. *volatus*, to fly]

vol·a·til·ize (vol′ă-til-īz). SYN evaporate.

Volhard, Franz, German physician, 1872–1950. SEE V.'s *test*.

vo·li·tion (vō-lish′ŭn). The conscious impulse to perform any act or to abstain from its performance; voluntary action. [L. *volo*,, to wish]

vo·li·tion·al (vo-lish′ŭn-ăl). Done by an act of will; relating to volition.

Volkmann, Alfred W., German physiologist, 1800–1877. SEE V.'s *canals*, under *canal*.

Volkmann, Richard, German surgeon, 1830–1889. SEE V.'s *cheilitis*, *contracture*, *spoon*.

vol·ley (vol′ē). A synchronous group of impulses induced simultaneously by artificial stimulation of either nerve fibers or muscle fibers. [Fr. *volée*, fr. L. *volo*, to fly]

Vollmer, Herman, U.S. pediatrician, 1896–1959. SEE V. *test*.

Volpe, Anthony R., U.S. dentist, *1932. SEE V.-Manhold *Index*.

Volpe-Manhold In·dex (V-MI). See under index.

vol·sel·la (vol-sel′ă). SYN vulsella *forceps*. [see vulsella]

volt (v, V) (vōlt). The unit of electromotive force; the electromotive force that will produce a current of 1 ampere in a circuit that has a resistance of 1 ohm; *i.e.*, joule per coulomb. [Allesandro *Volta*, It. physicist, 1745–1827]

volt·age (vōl′tej). Electromotive force, pressure, or potential expressed in volts.

vol·ta·ic (vōl-tā′ik). SYN galvanic.

vol·ta·ism (vōl′tă-izm). SYN galvanism.

vol·tam·e·ter (vōl-tam′ĕ-ter). An apparatus for measuring the strength of a galvanic current by its electrolytic action. [volt + G. *metron*, measure]

volt·am·pere (vōlt′am-pēr). A unit of electrical power; the product of 1 volt by 1 ampere; equivalent to 1 watt or ¹⁄₁₀₀₀ kilowatt.

volt·me·ter (vōlt′mē-ter). An apparatus for measuring the electromotive force or difference of potential.

Voltolini, Friedrich E.R., German laryngologist, 1819–1889. SEE V.'s *disease*.

vol·ume (V) (vol′yŭm). Space occupied by matter, expressed usually in cubic millimeters, cubic centimeters, liters, etc. SEE water. SEE ALSO capacity. [L. *volumen*, something rolled up, scroll, fr. *volvo*, to roll]

atomic v., the atomic weight of an element divided by its density in the solid state; the v. of the gram-atomic weight of a solid element.

v. averaging, in computed tomography or magnetic resonance imaging, the effect of expressing the average density of a voxel as a pixel in the image; the greater the slice thickness, the more averaging is necessary, with loss in density resolution.

closing v. (CV), the lung v. at which the flow from the lower parts of the lungs becomes severely reduced or stops during expiration, presumably because of airway closure; measured by the sharp rise in expiratory concentration of a tracer gas that had been inspired at the beginning of a breath that started from residual volume.

distribution v., the v. throughout which an added tracer substance appears to have been evenly distributed, calculated by dividing the amount of tracer added by its concentration after equilibration.

end-diastolic v., the amount of blood in the ventricle immediately before a cardiac contraction begins; a measurement of cardiac filling between beats, related to diastolic function.

end-systolic v., the amount of blood in the ventricle at the end of the cardiac ejection period and immediately preceding the beginning of ventricular relaxation; a measurement of the adequacy of cardiac emptying, related to systolic function.

expiratory reserve v. (ERV), the maximal v. of air (about 1000 ml) that can be expelled from the lungs after a normal expiration. SYN reserve air, supplemental air.

extracellular fluid v. (ECFV), the fraction of body wate rnot in cells; about 25% of body weight. It consists of plasma water (4.5% of body weight), water between cells (interstitial waterlymph, 11.5% of body weight), water in dense bone and connective tissue (7.5% of body weight) and water secretions. See entries under See transcellular water, about 1.5% of body weight..

forced expiratory v. (FEV), the maximal v. that can be expired in a specific time interval when starting from maximal inspiration.

inspiratory reserve v. (IRV), the maximal v. of air that can be inspired after a normal inspiration; the inspiratory capacity less the tidal v. SYN complemental air.

mean corpuscular v. (MCV), the average v. of red cells, calculated from the hematocrit and the red cell count, in erythrocyte indices.

minute v., the v. of any gas or fluid moved per minute; *e.g.,* cardiac output or the respiratory minute v.

packed cell v., the v. of the blood cells in a sample of blood after it has been centrifuged in the hematocrit; normally, it amounts to 45% of the blood sample.

partial v., the actual v. occupied by one species of molecule or particle in a solution; the reciprocal of the density of the molecule.

residual v. (RV), the v. of air remaining in the lungs after a maximal expiratory effort. SYN residual air, residual capacity.

respiratory minute v. (RMV), the minute v. of breathing; the product of tidal v. times the respiratory frequency. SEE pulmonary *ventilation*.

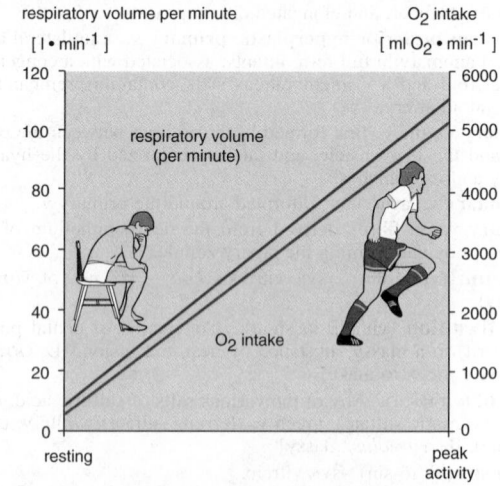

respiratory volume (per minute)
oxygen intake and respiratory volume per minute of a 160 lb. (70 kg.) man, resting and at peak activity

resting tidal v., the tidal v. under normal conditions, *i.e.,* in the absence of exercise or other conditions that stimulate breathing.

standard v., the v. of an ideal gas at standard temperature and pressure, approximately 22.414 liters.

stroke v., the v. pumped out of one ventricle of the heart in a single beat. SYN stroke output.

tidal v. (V$_T$), the v. of air that is inspired or expired in a single breath during regular breathing. SYN tidal air.

vol·ume·nom·e·ter (vol′yū-mĕ-nom′ĕ-ter). A device for determining the volume of a solid by measuring the amount of liquid it displaces. SYN volumometer. [volume + G. *metron,* measure]

vol·u·met·ric (vol-yū-met′rik). Relating to measurement by volume.

vol·u·mom·e·ter (vol-yū-mom′ĕ-ter). SYN volumenometer.

vol·un·tary (vol′ŭn-tār-ē). Relating or acting in obedience to the will; not obligatory. [L. *voluntarius,* fr. *voluntas,* will, fr. *volo,* to wish]

vo·lup·tu·ous (vō-lŭp′tyū-ŭs). Causing or caused by sensual pleasure; given to gratification of the senses. [L. *voluptuosus,* fr. *voluptas,* pleasure]

vo·lute (vō-lūt). Rolled up; convoluted. [L. *voluta,* a scroll, fr. *volvo,* pp. *volutus,* to roll]

vol·u·tin (vol′ū-tin). A nucleoprotein complex found as cytoplasmic granules in certain bacteria, yeasts, and protozoa (such as trypanosome flagellates) which serves as food reserves. SYN volutin granules.

Vol·vox (vol′voks). A genus of highly organized colonial green flagellates of the class Phytomastigophorea. [L. *volvo,* to roll]

vol·vu·lo·sis (vol-vū-lō′sis). SYN onchocerciasis.

vol·vu·lus (vol′vyū-lŭs). A twisting of the intestine causing obstruction. [L. *volvo,* to roll]

cecal v., rotation and twisting of the cecum toward the left upper quadrant, with ascending colon obstruction; associated with a cecum on a long mesentery.

gastric v., twisting of the stomach that may result in obstruction and impairment of the blood supply to the organ; it can occur in paraesophageal hernia and occasionally in eventration of the diaphragm.

sigmoid v., relatively common location of v., with obstruction either proximal or distal to the sigmoid segment.

vo·mer, gen. **vo·me·ris** (vō′mer, vō′mer-is) [NA]. A flat bone of trapezoidal shape forming the inferior and posterior portion of the nasal septum; it articulates with the sphenoid, ethmoid, two maxillae, and two palatine bones. [L. ploughshare]

v. cartilagin′eus, SYN *cartilago* vomeronasalis.

vo·mer·ine (vō′mer-ēn). Relating to the vomer.

vom·er·o·bas·i·lar (vō′mer-ō-bas′i-lăr). Relating to the vomer and the base of the skull.

vom·er·o·na·sal (vō′mer-ō-nā′săl). Relating to the vomer and the nasal bone.

vom·i·ca (vom′i-kă). **1.** Profuse expectoration of purulent matter. SYN vomicus. **2.** Obsolete term for a pulmonary cavity containing pus. [L. an ulcer, boil, fr. *vomo,* to vomit]

vom·i·cose (vom′i-kōs). Profusely suppurating, as by many ulcers. [L. *vomica,* an ulcer]

vom·i·cus (vom′i-kŭs). SYN vomica (1). [L.]

vom·it. 1. To eject matter from the stomach through the mouth. **2.** Vomitus; the matter so ejected. SYN vomitus (2). [L. *vomo,* pp. *vomitus,* to vomit]

Barcoo v., attacks of nausea and vomiting accompanied by bulimia affecting those living in the interior of the southern part of Australia.

bilious v., v. containing large amounts of bile suggestive of bowel obstruction distal to the papilla of Vater.

black v., the coffee-ground-colored material that is vomited, specifically, in severe yellow fever. SEE ALSO coffee-ground v. SYN vomitus niger.

coffee-ground v., v. consisting of fresh or old blood. SEE ALSO black v.

vom·it·ing (vom′i-ting). The ejection of matter from the stomach through the esophagus and mouth. SYN emesis (1), vomition, vomitus (1).

cerebral v., v. due to intracranial disease, especially elevated intracranial pressure.

dry v., SYN retching.

---

causes of vomiting

functional causes

psychogenic, pregnancy, functional esophageal illness

organic causes

esophagus: tumors, infections, stenoses, diverticular, mediastinal tumors, incl. bronchial carcinoma

stomach: acute gastritis, ulcer, stenosis by scars or tumors (postsurgical gastroatonia) pylorospasm (in children)

small and large intestines: acute gastroenteritis, mechanical ileus, obstruction

liver, gall bladder, pancreas: infections, gall stones, tumors

peritoneum: acute peritonitis (diffuse and local)

extraabdominal diseases

cerebral: meningitis, encephalitis, Ménière's disease, migranes, glaucoma, tumors, skull-brain injury, bleeding, hypertonic crises

disturbances of metabolism: diabetic precoma lactacidosis, uremia, thyreotoxicosis, Addison's disease

exogenous causes

numerous drugs (digitalis, cytostasis, antibiotics, opiates, etc.)

intoxications (mushroom poisoning, alcohol, etc.)

---

epidemic v., v. caused by Norwalk virus, a 27 nm RNA virus in the family Caliciviridae frequently occurring in a group of people (*e.g.,* in a school or small community) suddenly and without prodromal illness or malaise, is intense while it lasts, but ceases abruptly after a few hours or a day or so; symptoms are headache, abdominal pain, giddiness, and diarrhea in most of the cases, and extreme prostration in about 75%. SYN epidemic nausea.

fecal v., vomitus with appearance and/or odor of feces suggestive of long standing and distal small bowel or colonic obstruction. SYN copremesis, stercoraceous v.

morning v., v. occurring on rising or immediately after breakfast in some women during early pregnancy.

pernicious v., uncontrollable v.

v. of pregnancy, v. occurring in the early months of pregnancy.

projectile v., expulsion of the contents of the stomach with great force.

psychogenic v., v. associated with emotional distress and anxiety.

retention v., v. due to mechanical obstruction, usually hours after ingestion of a meal.

stercoraceous v., SYN fecal v.

vo·mi·tion (vō-mish′ŭn). SYN vomiting. [L. *vomitio,* fr. *vomo,* to vomit]

vom·i·tu·ri·tion (vom′i-tū-rish′ŭn). SYN retching.

vom·i·tus (vom′i-tŭs). **1.** SYN vomiting. **2.** SYN vomit (2). [L. a vomiting, vomit]

v. cruen′tes, SYN hematemesis.

v. mari′nus, SYN seasickness.

v. ni′ger, SYN black *vomit.*

von. Often abbreviated to v. For names with this prefix not found here, see under the principal part of the name.

von Bruns, SEE Bruns.

von Ebner, Victor, Austrian histologist, 1842–1925. SEE Ebner's *glands,* under *gland;* Ebner's *reticulum;* imbrication *lines* of von E., under *line;* incremental *lines* of von E. under *line.*

von Economo, Constantin, Austrian neurologist, 1876–1931. SEE von E.'s *disease.*

von Hippel, Eugen, German ophthalmologist, 1867–1939. SEE von H.-Lindau *syndrome.*

von Kossa, Julius, 19th century Austro-Hungarian pathologist. SEE von K. *stain.*

VO

von Linné, SEE Linné.

von Meyenburg (von māy'en-berg), SEE Meyenburg.

von Schrötter, Leopold, Austrian laryngologist, 1837-1908. SEE Paget-von S. *syndrome.*

von Willebrand, E.A., Finnish physician, 1870–1949. SEE von W.'s *disease.*

Voorhoeve, N., Dutch radiologist, 1879–1927. SEE V.'s *disease.*

vor·tex, pl. **vor·ti·ces** (vōr'teks, vōr'ti-sēz). **1.** SYN verticil. **2.** SYN whorl (5). **3.** SYN v. lentis. [L. whirlpool, whorl, fr. *verto* or *vorto,* to turn around]

v. coccy′geus, a spiral arrangement of coarse hairs sometimes present over the region of the coccyx. SYN coccygeal whorl.

v. cor′dis [NA], SYN v. of heart.

Fleischer's v., SYN *cornea* verticillata.

v. of heart, a spiral arrangement of muscular fibers at the apex of the heart. SYN v. cordis [NA], whorl (2).

v. len′tis, one of the stellar figures on the surface of the lens of the eye. SYN vortex (3).

vor′tices pilo′rum [NA], SYN hair *whorls,* under *whorl.*

Vor·ti·cel·la (vōr-ti-sel′ă). A genus of Ciliata of the order Peritrichida, of bell shape and with a spiral of cilia around the adoral zone; various free-living species have been found at times in the feces, urine, and mucous discharges. [Mod. L. dim. of L. *vortex,* a whorl]

vor·ti·ces (vōr′ti-sēz). Plural of vortex.

vor·ti·cose (vōr′ti-kōs). Arranged in a whorl. [L. *vorticosus,* fr. *vortex,* a whorl]

Vossius, Adolf, German pathologist, 1855–1925. SEE V.'s lenticular *ring.*

vox (voks). SYN voice. [L.]

v. cholera′ica, a peculiar, hoarse, almost inaudible voice of a sufferer in the last stage of Asiatic cholera.

vox·el (vok′sel). A contraction for volume element, which is the basic unit of CT or MR reconstruction; represented as a pixel in the display of the CT or MR image.

voy·eur (vwah-yer′). One who practices voyeurism.

voy·eur·ism (vwah-yer′izm). The practice of obtaining sexual pleasure by looking, especially at the naked body or genitals of another or at erotic acts between others. SYN scopophilia. [Fr. *voir,* to see]

VP Abbreviation for vasopressin; variegate *porphyria.*

VR Abbreviation for vocal *resonance.*

VS Abbreviation for volumetric *solution.*

VU Abbreviation for volume *unit.*

vul·ga·ris (vŭl-gā′ris). Ordinary; of the usual type. [L. fr. *vulgus,* a crowd]

Vulpian, Edme F.A., French physician, 1826–1887. SEE V.'s *atrophy.*

vul·sel·la, vul·sel·lum (vŭl-sel′ă, -lŭm). SYN vulsella *forceps.* [L. pincers, fr. *vello,* pp. *vulsus,* to pluck]

vul·va, pl. **vul·′vae** (vŭ′vă). [NA] The external genitalia of the female, comprised of the mons pubis, the labia majora and minora, the clitoris, the vestibule of the vagina and its glands, and the opening of the urethra and of the vagina. SYN pudendum femininum [NA], cunnus, pudendum muliebre, trema (2). [L. a wrapper or covering, seed covering, womb, fr. *volvo,* to roll]

vul·var, vul·val (vŭl′văr, vŭl′văl). Relating to the vulva.

vul·vec·to·my (vŭl-vek′tō-mē). Excision (either partial, complete, or radical) of the vulva. [vulva + G. *ektomē,* excision]

vul·vis·mus (vŭl-viz′mŭs). SYN vaginismus.

vul·vi·tis (vŭl-vī′tis). Inflammation of the vulva. [vulva + G. *-itis,* inflammation]

chronic atrophic v., an inflammation of atrophic vulvar skin, usually with severe pruritus.

chronic hypertrophic v., swelling of the vulval tissues due to lymphatic obstruction; in some cases it may be caused by filariasis, with induration or ulceration of the skin. SYN elephantiasis vulvae.

follicular v., inflammation of the vulvar follicles.

leukoplakic v., SYN *leukoplakia* vulvae.

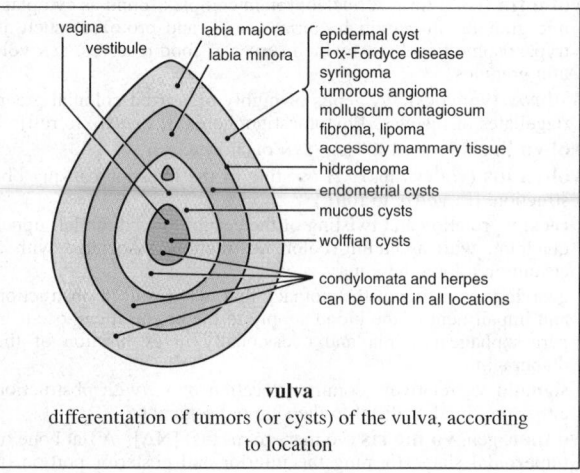

vulva
differentiation of tumors (or cysts) of the vulva, according to location

vulvo-. The vulva. [L. *vulva*]

vul·vo·cru·ral (vŭl′vō-krū′răl). Relating to the vulva and the clitoris.

vul·vo·dyn·ia. Chronic vulvar discomfort with complaints of burning and superficial irritation.

vul·vo·u·ter·ine (vŭl-vō-yū′ter-in). Relating to the vulva and the uterus.

vul·vo·vag·i·nal (vŭl-vō-vaj′i-năl). Relating to the vulva and the vagina.

vul·vo·vag·i·ni·tis (vŭl′vō-vaj-i-nī′tis). Inflammation of both vulva and vagina.

Vve·den·skii. Alternative surname of Wedensky, Nikolai I.

V-Y plas·ty. SYN V-Y *flap.*

W Symbol for tungsten; watt; tryptophan.

Waage, P., Norwegian chemist, 1833–1900. SEE Guldberg-W. *law.*

Waaler, Erik, 20th century Norwegian biologist. SEE Rose-W. *test.*

Waardenburg, Petrus Johannes, Dutch ophthalmologist, 1886–1979. SEE W. *syndrome.*

Wachendorf, Eberhard J., German botanist and anatomist, 1702–1758. SEE W.'s *membrane.*

Wachstein, Max, U.S. histologist and pathologist, 1905–1965. SEE W.-Meissel *stain* for calcium-magnesium-ATPase.

Wachter, Herman J.G., German pathologist, *1878. SEE Bracht-W. *lesion.*

Wada, J.A., 20th century Japanese-Canadian neurologist. SEE W. *test.*

wad·ding (wahd′ing). Carded cotton or wool in sheets, used for surgical dressings.

Waddington, C. H., British embryologist and geneticist, 1905–1975. SEE waddingtonian *homeostasis.*

wad·dle (wod′l). SYN waddling *gait.*

wa·fer (wā′fer). A thin sheet of dried flour paste, used to enclose a powder, the wafer being moistened and folded over the drug, so that it can be swallowed without taste. [M.E., fr. O.Fr. *waufre,* fr. Germanic]

Wagner, Hans, Swiss ophthalmologist, *1905. SEE W.'s *disease, syndrome.*

Wagstaffe, William, English surgeon, 1843–1910. SEE W.'s *fracture.*

waist (wāst). The portion of the trunk between the ribs and the pelvis. [A.S. *waext*]

w. of the heart, an obsolete term for the middle segment of the cardiac silhouette, on the chest x-ray, containing the pulmonary salient.

Walcher, Gustav A., German obstetrician, 1856–1935. SEE W. *position.*

Waldenström, Jan G., Swedish physician, *1906. SEE W.'s *macroglobulinemia, purpura, syndrome, test.*

Waldeyer (Waldeyer-Hartz), Heinrich G. von, German anatomist and pathologist, 1836–1921. SEE W.'s *fossae,* under *fossa, glands,* under *gland,* zonal *layer,* throat *ring, sheath, space, tract.*

walk. 1. To move on foot. **2.** The characteristic manner in which one moves on foot. SEE ALSO gait. [M.E. *walken,* fr. O.E. *wealcen,* to roll]

Walker, A. Earl, U.S. neurologist, *1907. SEE W. *tractotomy;* Dandy-W. *syndrome.*

Walker, J.T. Ainslie, English chemist, 1868–1930. SEE Rideal-W. *coefficient, method.*

Walker, James, British gynecologist, *1916. SEE W.'s *chart.*

Walker car·ci·no·ma. See under carcinoma.

Walker car·ci·no·sar·co·ma. See under carcinosarcoma.

walk·ing (wo′king). Characteristic of sequential movement or progression in steps.

chromosome w., sequential isolation of overlapping sequences of DNA (*i.e.,* clones) with this procedure large regions of the chromosome can be spanned. SYN overlap hybridization.

wall (wawl). An investing part enclosing a cavity such as the chest or abdomen, or covering a cell or any anatomical unit. A wall, as of the chest, abdomen, or any hollow organ. SYN paries [NA]. [L. *vallum*]

anterior w. of middle ear, SYN anterior w. of tympanic cavity.

anterior w. of stomach, the part of the gastric w. that faces the peritoneal cavity. SYN paries anterior gastris [NA].

anterior w. of tympanic cavity, it contains the carotid canal and the opening of the auditory tube. SYN paries caroticus cavi tympani [NA], anterior w. of middle ear, carotid w. of middle ear.

anterior w. of vagina, it is somewhat shorter than the posterior w. and at its upper end is penetrated by the cervix of the uterus. SYN paries anterior vaginae [NA].

axial w.'s of the pulp chambers, the w.'s parallel with the long axis of a tooth: the mesial, distal, buccal, and lingual w.'s.

carotid w. of middle ear, SYN anterior w. of tympanic cavity.

cavity w., one of the surfaces bounding a cavity.

cell w., the outer layer or membrane of some animal and plant cells; in the latter it is mainly cellulose.

chest w., in respiratory physiology, the total system of structures outside the lungs that move as a part of breathing; it includes the rib cage, diaphragm, abdominal w., and abdominal contents. SYN thoracic w.

enamel w., in dentistry, the part of the w. of a cavity consisting of enamel.

external w. of cochlear duct, the w. that faces the outer side of the cochlea. SYN paries externus ductus cochlearis [NA].

hollow w., SYN seedy *toe.*

inferior w. of orbit, SYN *floor* of orbit.

inferior w. of tympanic cavity, SYN *floor* of tympanic cavity.

jugular w. of middle ear, SYN *floor* of tympanic cavity.

labyrinthine w. of middle ear, SYN medial w. of tympanic cavity.

lateral w. of middle ear, SYN lateral w. of tympanic cavity.

lateral w. of orbit, a triangular w. of the orbit formed by the zygomatic bone, the greater wing of the sphenoid bone, and a small part of the frontal bone; posteriorly it is bounded by the superior and inferior orbital fissures. SYN paries lateralis orbitae [NA].

lateral w. of tympanic cavity, the wall formed mainly by the tympanic membrane. SYN paries membranaceus cavi tympani [NA], lateral w. of middle ear, membranous w. of middle ear.

mastoid w. of middle ear, SYN posterior w. of tympanic cavity.

medial w. of middle ear, SYN medial w. of tympanic cavity.

medial w. of orbit, the thin, rectangular w. of the orbit formed by the orbital plate of the ethmoid, lacrimal, frontal and a small part of the sphenoid bones; the fossa for the lacrimal sac lies at its anterior limit. SYN paries medialis orbitae [NA].

medial w. of tympanic cavity, a bony layer separating the middle from the internal ear or labyrinth; it contains the fenestra vestibuli and the fenestra cochleae. SYN paries labyrinthicus cavi tympani [NA], labyrinthine w. of middle ear, medial w. of middle ear.

membranous w. of middle ear, SYN lateral w. of tympanic cavity.

membranous w. of trachea, the part of the tracheal w. posteriorly that is not reinforced by tracheal cartilages. SYN paries membranaceus tracheae [NA].

w. of nail, SYN nail *fold.*

parietal w., the body w. or the somatopleure from which it is formed.

posterior w. of middle ear, SYN posterior w. of tympanic cavity.

posterior w. of stomach, that part of the gastric w. that faces the omental bursa. SYN paries posterior gastris [NA].

posterior w. of tympanic cavity, it contains the opening into the mastoid antrum. SYN paries mastoideus cavi tympani [NA], mastoid w. of middle ear, posterior w. of middle ear.

posterior w. of vagina, it is longer than the anterior w. and has a low ridge in the midline throughout most of its length. SYN paries posterior vaginae [NA].

pulpal w., (1) one of the w.'s of the pulp cavity; **(2)** the w. of a cavity preparation adjacent to the pulp space; *e.g.,* mesial pulpal w.

splanchnic w., the w. of one of the viscera or the splanchnopleure from which it is formed.

superior w. of orbit, SYN *roof* of orbit.

tegmental w. of middle ear, SYN *roof* of tympanic cavity.

thoracic w., SYN chest w.

wa

tympanic w. of cochlear duct, the wall that separates the cochlear duct from the scala tympani; it consists of the osseous spiral lamina and the basilar membrane. SYN paries tympanicus ductus cochlearis [NA], membrana spiralis☆ [NA], spiral membrane.

vestibular w. of cochlear duct, SYN vestibular *membrane*.

Wallenberg, Adolf, German physician, 1862–1949. SEE W.'s *syndrome*.

Waller, Augustus V., English physiologist, 1816–1870. SEE wallerian *degeneration*, wallerian *law*.

wal·le·ri·an (waw-ler′ē-an). Relating to or described by A.V. Waller.

wall-eye (wawl′ī). **1.** SYN exotropia. **2.** Absence of color in the iris, or leukoma of the cornea.

Walthard, Max, Swiss gynecologist, 1867–1933. SEE W.'s cell *rest*.

Walther, August F., German anatomist, 1688–1746. SEE W.'s *dilator, canals,* under *canal, ducts,* under *duct, ganglion, plexus*.

wan·der·ing (wahn′der-ing). Moving about; not fixed; abnormally motile. [A.S. *wandrian,* to wander]

Wang, Chung T., Chinese pathologist, 1889–1931. SEE W.'s *test*.

Wangensteen, Owen H., U.S. surgeon, 1898–1981. SEE W. *drainage, suction, tube*.

Wang·i·el·la (wang-gē-el′ǎ). A dematiaceous genus of fungi characterized by phialides without collarettes, a black yeastlike colony with yeast forms, and later hyphae; the fungi grow well at 40°C. *W. dermatitidis* is an etiological agent of phaeohyphomycosis.

war·ble (war′bl). Small swelling in the skin on the back of cattle caused by the presence of larvae of *Hypoderma bovis* or *H. lineatum,* the so-called warble flies. [M. Sw. *varbulde,* boil]

Warburg, Otto, German biochemist and Nobel laureate, 1883–1970. SEE W.'s *apparatus,* respiratory *enzyme,* old yellow *enzyme, theory;* W.-Lipmann-Dickens-Horecker *shunt;* Barcroft-W. *apparatus, technique*.

Ward, Frederick O., British osteologist, 1818–1877. SEE w.W.'s *triangle*.

Ward, O.C., 20th century pediatrician. SEE Romano-W. *syndrome*.

ward (wōrd). A large room or hall in a hospital containing a number of beds. SEE ALSO unit. [A.S. *weard*]

Wardrop, James, British surgeon, 1782–1869. SEE W.'s *disease, method*.

war·fa·rin so·di·um (war′fǎ-rin). [[3-(α-Acetonylbenzyl)-2-oxo-2*H*-1-benzopyran-4-yl]oxy]sodium; an anticoagulant with the same actions as dicumarol; also used as a rodenticide; also available as the potassium salt, with the same actions and uses. [*W*isconsin *A*lumni *R*esearch *F*oundation + coum*arin*]

warm-blood·ed (wărm′blŭd-ed). SYN homeothermic.

Warren, Dean, U.S. surgeon, *1924. SEE W. *shunt*.

wart (wōrt). SYN verruca.

anatomical w., SYN postmortem w.

asbestos w., SYN asbestos *corn*.

cattle w.'s, SYN infectious *papilloma* of cattle.

common w., SYN *verruca* vulgaris.

digitate w., SYN *verruca* digitata.

fig w., obsolete term for *condyloma* acuminatum.

filiform w., SYN *verruca* filiformis.

flat w., SYN *verruca* plana.

fugitive w., a transitory w.; one that does not persist.

genital w., SYN *condyloma* acuminatum.

Henle's w.'s, SYN Hassall-Henle *bodies,* under *body*.

infectious w.'s, SYN *verruca* vulgaris.

moist w., obsolete term for *condyloma* acuminatum.

mosaic w., plantar growth of numerous closely aggregated w.'s forming a mosaic appearance, frequently caused by human papilloma virus type 2.

necrogenic w., SYN postmortem w.

Peruvian w., SYN *verruca* peruana.

pitch w., a precancerous keratotic epidermal tumor, common among workers in pitch and coal tar derivatives. SEE pitch-worker's *cancer*.

plane w., SYN *verruca* plana.

plantar w., a w. on the sole, often painful; usually caused by human papilloma virus type 1. SYN verruca plantaris.

pointed w., obsolete term for *condyloma* acuminatum.

postmortem w., a tuberculous warty growth (tuberculosis cutis verrucosa) on the hand of one who performs postmortem examinations. SYN anatomical tubercle, anatomical w., dissection tubercle, necrogenic w., postmortem tubercle, prosector's tubercle, prosector's w., verruca necrogenica.

prosector's w., SYN postmortem w.

seborrheic w., SYN seborrheic *keratosis*.

senile w., SYN actinic *keratosis*.

soft w., SYN skin *tag*.

soot w., the precancerous lesion of chimney sweep's cancer.

telangiectatic w., SYN angiokeratoma.

tuberculous w., SYN *tuberculosis* cutis verrucosa.

venereal w., SYN *condyloma* acuminatum.

viral w., SYN *verruca* vulgaris.

Wartenberg, Robert, German neurologist, 1887–1956. SEE W.'s *symptom*.

Warthin, Aldred S., U.S. pathologist, 1866–1931. SEE W.'s *tumor;* W.-Finkeldey *cells,* under *cell;* W.-Starry silver *stain*.

wart·pox (wōrt′poks). SYN *variola* verrucosa.

warty (wōrt′ē). Relating to or covered with warts.

wash (wosh). A solution used to clean or bathe a part. For types of w.'s, see the specific term; *e.g.,* eyewash, mouthwash.

Wasmann, Adolphus, 19th century German anatomist. SEE W.'s *glands,* under *gland*.

Wassermann, August P. von, German bacteriologist, 1866–1925. SEE W. *antibody, reaction, test;* provocative W. *test*.

Wassermann-fast. A term used to designate a case in which the Wassermann reaction remains positive despite all treatment.

wast·ing (wāst′ing). **1.** SYN emaciation. **2.** Denoting a disease characterized by emaciation.

salt w., inappropriately large renal excretion of salt despite the apparent need of the body to retain it.

wa·ter (wah′ter). **1.** H_2O; a clear, odorless, tasteless liquid, solidifying at 32°F (0°C and R), and boiling at 212°F (100°C, 80°R), that is present in all animal and vegetable tissues and dissolves more substances than any other liquid. SEE volume. **2.** Euphemism for urine. **3.** A pharmacopeial preparation of a clear saturated aqueous solution (unless otherwise specified) of volatile oils, or other aromatic or volatile substances, prepared by processes involving distillation or solution (agitation followed by filtration). SYN aromatic w. [A.S. *waeter*]

w. of adhesion, w. held by molecular attraction in contact with solid surfaces, but not forming an essential part of their constitution.

alkaline w., a w. that contains appreciable amounts of the bicarbonates of calcium, lithium, potassium, or sodium.

aromatic w., SYN water (3).

baryta w., a saturated aqueous solution of barium hydroxide; used as an alkaline reagent.

bitter w., a natural mineral w. containing Epsom salt.

black w., SYN *azoturia* of horses.

bound w., w. held to colloids and other substances and not removed by simple filtration.

bromine w., a w. containing the bromides of magnesium, potassium, or sodium in therapeutic amounts.

calcic w., a w. containing appreciable quantities of calcium salts in solution.

carbonated w., carbonic w., w. that contains a considerable amount of carbonic acid in solution.

carbon dioxide-free w., purified w. that has been boiled vigorously for 5 minutes or more.

chalybeate w., a w. that contains salts of iron in appreciable quantities.

chlorine w., a w. that contains the chlorides of sodium, potassium, calcium, and magnesium in varying amounts.

w. of combustion, SYN w. of metabolism.

w. of constitution, w. held by a unit of structure as an essential part of its constitution, though not an ingredient of its molecules. SEE w. of crystallization.

w. of crystallization, w. of constitution that unites with certain salts and is essential to their arrangement in crystalline form; e.g., $CuSO_4 \cdot 5H_2O$.

deionized w., w. purified by passing through ion-exchange columns.

distilled w., w. purified by distillation.

earthy w., a w. containing a large amount of mineral matter, chiefly sulfate, in solution.

free w., w. in the body that can be removed by ultrafiltration and in which substances can be dissolved.

gentian aniline w., gentian violet with saturated aniline w., a more effective stain than simple gentian violet.

hard w., w. containing ions, such as Mg^{2+} and Ca^{2+}, that form insoluble salts with fatty acids so that ordinary soap will not lather in it.

heavy w., D_2O; w. in which the hydrogen atoms are deuterium, or heavy hydrogen (^2H), with physical properties that differ noticeably from those of ordinary w.; an elevated presence will cause a decrease in metabolic activity; used as a moderator in nuclear reactors because of its capacity to absorb neutrons. SYN deuterium oxide.

indifferent w., a mineral w. containing only a small quantity of saline matter.

w. for injection, w. purified by distillation for the preparation of products for parenteral use.

lime w., calcium hydroxide solution; a saturated solution prepared by mixing 3 g of calcium hydroxide in a liter of purified cool w. Undissolved calcium hydroxide is allowed to precipitate and the solution is dispensed without agitation; lime w. is a common ingredient in lotions and is used internally extensively in veterinary medicine.

w. of metabolism, the w. formed in the body by oxidation of the hydrogen of the food, the greatest amount being produced in the metabolism of fat (about 117 g/100 g of fat). SYN w. of combustion.

mineral w., w. that contains appreciable amounts of certain salts, which give it therapeutic properties.

potable w., a w. fit for drinking, being free from contamination and not containing a sufficient quantity of saline material to be regarded as a mineral w.

purified w., w. obtained by distillation or deionization.

saline w., a w. that contains neutral salts (chlorides, bromides, iodides, sulfates) in appreciable amounts.

Selters w., Seltzer w., a mineral w. containing carbonates of sodium, calcium, and magnesium, and chloride of sodium. [Nieder *Selters,* a mineral spring in Prussia]

soft w., w. lacking those ions, such as Mg^{2+} and Ca^{2+}, that form insoluble salts with fatty acids, so that ordinary soap will lather easily in it.

sulfate w., a w. holding in solution appreciable quantities of the sulfates of calcium, magnesium, or sodium.

sulfur w., w. containing hydrogen sulfide or the metallic sulfides.

total body w. (TBW), the sum of intracellular w. and extracellular w. (volume). About 60% of body weight.

transcellular w., that fraction of extracellular w. in cerebrospinal, digestive, epithelial, introcular, pleural, sweat, and synovial secretions; about 1.5% of body weight.

wa·ter·fall (wah'ter-fawl). A term used to describe flow in vascular beds where lateral pressure tending to collapse vessels greatly exceeds venous pressure. Flow is independent of venous pressure and occurs only when arterial pressure exceeds lateral pressure; likened to flow making a waterfall from a sluice or spillway over a dam, with arterial pressure being height of water behind the dam, lateral pressure being spillway height, and venous pressure being height of outflow stream below the dam. SYN sluice.

Waterhouse, Rupert, British physician, 1873–1958. SEE W.-Friderichsen *syndrome.*

wa·ter·pox (wah'ter-poks). SYN varicella.

Waters, Charles Alexander, U.S. radiologist, 1888-1961. SEE W.'s view *radiograph.*

Waters, Edward G., U.S. obstetrician and gynecologist, *1898. SEE W.'s *operation.*

wa·ters (wah'ters). Colloquialism for amniotic *fluid.*

bag of w., See entries under bag.

false w., a leakage of fluid prior to or in beginning labor, before the rupture of the amnion.

wa·ter·shed. 1. The area of marginal blood flow at the extreme periphery of a vascular bed. 2. Slopes in the abdominal cavity, formed by projections of the lumbar vertebrae and the pelvic brim that determine the direction in which a free effusion will gravitate when the body is in a supine position.

Waterston, David J., British thoracic and pediatric surgeon, *1910. SEE W. *operation, shunt.*

Watson, C.J., U.S. physician, born 1901, Professor and Chairman of Medicine at the University of Minnesota from 1942 to 1966. He made major contributions in the study of liver disease and porphyria. SEE Watson-Schwartz *test.*

Watson, James D., U.S. geneticist and Nobel laureate, *1928. SEE W.-Crick *helix.*

Watsonius wat·soni (waht'sō'nē-ŭs waht-sō'nī). An amphistome intestinal fluke of primates in West Africa and Singapore.

watt (W) (waht). The SI unit of electrical power; the power available when the current is 1 ampere and the electromotive force is 1 volt; equal to 1 joule (10^7 ergs) per second or 1 voltampere. [James *Watt,* Scot. engineer, 1736–1819]

wave (wāv). **1.** A movement of particles in an elastic body, whether solid or fluid, whereby an advancing series of alternate elevations and depressions, or expansions and condensations, is produced. **2.** The elevation of the pulse, felt by the finger, or represented graphically in the curved line of the sphygmograph. **3.** The complete cycle of changes in the level of a source of energy that is repetitively varying with respect to time; in the electrocardiogram and the electroencephalogram the w. is essentially a voltage-time graph. SEE ALSO rhythm. [A.S. *wafian,* to fluctuate]

A w., (1) the initial negative deflection in the electroretinogram, presumably reflecting retinal photoreceptor activity; (2) an atrial deflection in an electrocardiogram recorded from within the atrium of the heart; (3) the first positive deflection of the atrial and venous pulses due to atrial systole.

acid w., SYN acid *tide.*

alkaline w., SYN alkaline *tide.*

alpha w., SYN alpha *rhythm.*

arterial w., a w. in the jugular phlebogram due to transmission of carotid artery pulsation.

B w., the initial positive deflection in the electroretinogram, possibly arising from the inner nuclear layer of the retina.

beta w., SYN beta *rhythm.*

brain w., colloquialism for electroencephalogram.

C w., a monophasic positive deflection in the electroretinogram arising in the pigment epithelium of the retina.

c w., w. in the venous and atrial pulses occurring during isovolumic ventricular contraction in which the closed atrioventricular valves (mitral and tricuspid) are abruptly displaced into the atria with a creation of a pressure transient.

cannon w., an exaggerated A w. in the jugular pulse caused by right atrial contraction occurring after ventricular contraction has closed the tricuspid valve, as in ventricular premature beats and in complete A-V block.

D w., a positive or negative deflection in the electroretinogram occurring when a light stimulus is removed (off-response).

delta w., (1) a premature upstroke of the QRS complex due to an atrial ventricular bypass tract as in WPW syndrome; (2) SYN delta *rhythm.*

dicrotic w., the second rise in the tracing of a dicrotic pulse. SYN recoil w.

wa

electrocardiographic w., a deflection of special shape and extent in the electrocardiogram representing the electric activity of a portion of the heart muscle.

excitation w., a w. of altered electrical conditions that is propagated along a muscle fiber preparatory to its contraction.

F w.'s, ff w.'s, the w.'s of atrial flutter usually best seen in ECG leads 2, 3, and AVF. (A small f indicates atrial fibrillation). SYN fibrillary w.'s, fibrillatory w.'s, flutter-fibrillation w.'s.

fibrillary w.'s, SYN F w.'s.

fibrillatory w.'s, SYN F w.'s.

flat top w.'s, activity in the electroencephalogram having a pattern suggesting a flat top; these w.'s are often found in temporal lobe discharges.

fluid w., a sign of free fluid in the abdominal cavity; percussion on one side of the abdomen transmits a w. that is felt on the opposite side.

flutter-fibrillation w.'s, SYN F w.'s.

microelectric w.'s, SYN microwaves.

overflow w., the descending w. of the sphygmogram from the apex to the first anacrotic break.

P w., the first complex of the electrocardiogram, representing depolarization of the atria; if the P w. is retrograde or ectopic in axis or form, it is labeled P′.

percussion w., the main positive w. of an arterial pulse tracing.

postextrasystolic T w., the modified T w. of the beat immediately following an extrasystole.

pulse w., the progressive expansion of the arteries occurring with each contraction of the left ventricle of the heart.

Q w., the initial deflection of the QRS complex when such deflection is negative (downward).

R w., the first positive (upward) deflection of the QRS complex in the electrocardiogram; successive upward deflections within the same QRS complex are labeled R′, R″, etc.

random w.'s, w.'s in the electroencephalogram which occur paroxysmally and asynchronously.

recoil w., SYN dicrotic w.

retrograde P w., the P w. pattern in the electrocardiogram representing retrograde depolarization of the atria, the impulse spreading from the A-V junction or the lower atrium upward.

S w., a negative (downward) deflection of the QRS complex following an R w; successive downward deflections within the same QRS complex are labeled S′, S″, etc.

sonic w.'s, audible sound w.'s, as distinguished from ultrasonic w.'s.

supersonic w.'s, SEE supersonic.

T w., the next deflection in the electrocardiogram following the QRS complex; represents ventricular repolarization.

theta w., SYN theta *rhythm*.

tidal w., the w. between the percussion w. and the dicrotic w. in the downward limb of the arterial pulse tracing.

Traube-Hering w.'s, SYN Traube-Hering *curves*, under *curve.*

U w., a positive w. following the T w. of the electrocardiogram.

ultrasonic w.'s, the periodic configuration of energy produced by sound having a frequency greater than 30,000 Hz.

V w., a large pressure w. visible in recordings from either atrium or its incoming veins, normally produced by venous return but becoming very large when blood regurgitates through the A-V valve beyond the chamber from which the recording is made.

x w., the w. in the atrial or venous pulse curves produced when ventricular ejection moves the floors of the atria toward the ventricular apices.

y w., the w. in the atrial and venous pulse curves reflecting rapid filling of the ventricles just after the atrioventricular valves open.

wave·length (Λ) (wāv′length). The distance from one point on a wave (frequently shaped like a sine curve) to the next point in the same phase; *i.e.,* from peak to peak or from trough to trough.

wave·num·ber (σ) (wāv′nŭm-ber). The number of waves per centimeter (cm^{-1}), used to simplify the large and unwieldy numbers heretofore used to designate frequency.

wave·shape (wāv′shāp). SYN wave *form.*

wax (waks). **1.** A thick, tenacious substance, plastic at room temperature, secreted by bees for building the cells of their honeycomb. SYN beeswax, cera. **2.** Any substance with physical properties similar to those of beeswax, of animal, vegetable, or mineral origin (oils, lipids, or fats that are solids at room temperature). **3.** Esters of high-molecular-weight fatty acids with monohydric or dihydric alcohols (aliphatic or cyclic), that are solid at room temperature. Often accompanied by free fatty acids. [A.S. *weax*]

animal w., beeswax, spermaceti, and any w. derived from the animal kingdom.

baseplate w., a hard pink w. used in dentistry for making occlusion rims.

bleached w., SYN white w.

bone w., a mixture of antiseptic agents, oil, and w. used to stop bleeding by plugging bone cavities or haversian canals. SYN Horsley's bone w.

boxing w., w. used for boxing impressions. SEE ALSO boxing.

Brazil w., SYN carnauba w.

carnauba w., a w. obtained from the Brazilian w. palm, *Copernica cerifera;* used in pharmaceuticals to coat medicaments in sustained release preparations and surfaces of tablets; used in waxes for wood and metal. SYN Brazil w., palm w.

casting w., any soft solid w. used in dentistry for patterns of all types and for many other purposes; most are basically paraffin but are modified by addition of gum dammar, carnauba w., or other ingredients, to meet various requirements. SYN inlay w.

Chinese w., (1) a vegetable w.; (2) a w. secreted by a scale insect, *Coccus ceriferus* or *C. pela,* and deposited in the twigs of a species of ash tree; used in China to make candles and also medicinally.

ear w., SYN cerumen.

earth w., SYN ceresin.

emulsifying w., a washable ointment base consisting of a mixture of cetostearyl alcohol, sodium lauryl sulfate, and water.

grave w., SYN adipocere.

Horsley's bone w., SYN bone w.

inlay w., SYN casting w.

Japan w., a vegetable w. derived from *Rhus succedanea* and *Toxicodendron verniciferum.*

mineral w., (1) SYN paraffin w. (2) SYN ceresin. (3) a mineral substance whose physical properties are similar to wax.

montan w., a mineral w. extracted from lignite. [L. *montanus,* of a mountain, fr. *mons,* mountain]

palm w., SYN carnauba w.

paraffin w., a w. derived from petroleum. SYN mineral w. (1).

vegetable w., palm w. or any w. derived from plants such as the bayberry.

white w., yellow w. bleached by being rolled very thin and exposed to the light and air, or bleached by chemical oxidants; same uses as yellow w. SYN bleached w., white beeswax.

wool w., SYN adeps lanae.

yellow w., a yellowish, solid, brittle substance prepared from the honeycomb of the bee, *Apis mellifera;* the chief constituent is myricin (myricyl palmitate); others are cerotic acid (cerin), melissic acid, heptacosane, and hentriacontane; used in the preparation of ointments, cerates, plasters, and suppositories.

wax·ing, wax·ing-up (wak′sing). The contouring of a pattern in wax, generally applied to the shaping in wax of the contours of a trial denture or a crown prior to casting in metal.

Way, Stanley, British obstetrician-gynecologist. SEE Stanley Way *procedure.*

Wb Symbol for weber.

WBC Abbreviation for white blood *cell.*

WDLL Abbreviation for well-differentiated lymphocytic *lymphoma.*

wean (wēn). To implement weaning. [A.S. *wenian*]

wean·ing (wēn′ing). **1.** Permanent deprivation of breast milk and commencement of nourishment with other food. SYN ablactation. **2.** Gradual withdrawal of a patient from dependency on a life support system or other form of therapy.

wean·ling (wēn′ling). A young animal that has become adjusted to food other than its mother's milk.

wear (wār). Wasting or deterioration caused by friction.

occlusal w., attritional loss of substance on opposing occlusal units or surfaces. SEE ALSO abrasion (3).

web (wĕb). A tissue or membrane bridging a space. SEE ALSO tela. [A.S.]

esophageal w., a cribriform or w. formation in the esophagus caused by an irregular atrophy.

w. of fingers/toes, one of the folds of skin, or rudimentary web, between the fingers and toes. SYN interdigital folds, plica inter-digitalis.

terminal w., a network of actin filaments in the apical end of columnar epithelial cells that anchor in the zonula adherens.

web·bing (web′ing). Congenital condition apparent when adjacent structures are joined by a broad band of tissue not normally present to such a degree.

Weber, Ernst H., German physiologist and anatomist, 1795–1878. SEE W.'s *experiment, glands,* under *gland, law, paradox, test* for hearing; Fechner-Weber *law;* W.-Fechner *law.*

Weber, Frederick Parkes, English physician, 1863–1962. SEE W.-Christian *disease;* W.-Cockayne *syndrome;* Rendu-Osler-W. *syndrome;* Sturge-Kalischer-W. *syndrome;* Sturge-W. *disease, syndrome;* Klippel-Trenaunay-W. *syndrome.*

Weber, Sir Hermann, English physician, 1823–1918. SEE Weber's *sign;* Weber's *syndrome.*

Weber, Moritz I., German anatomist, 1795–1875. SEE W.'s *organ.*

Weber, Wilhelm E., German physicist, 1804–1891. SEE W.'s *point, triangle.*

we·ber (Wb) (web′er). SI unit of magnetic flux, equal to volt-seconds (V·s). [Wilhelm E. Weber]

Webster, John, English chemist, 1878–1927. SEE W.'s *test.*

Webster, John C., U.S. gynecologist, 1863–1950. SEE W.'s *operation.*

Wechsler, David, U.S. psychologist, *1896. SEE W. intelligence *scales,* under *scale;* W.-Bellevue *scale.*

wed·del·lite (hwed′del-īte). Ca$(O_2C–CO_2)\cdot 2H_{a2}O$; a dihydrate of calcium oxalate; found in renal calculi. Cf. whewellite. [for *Weddell Sea,* after James Weddell, Eng. navigator, + -ite]

Wedensky (Vve·den·skii), Nikolai I., Russian neurophysiologist, 1852–1922. SEE W. *effect, facilitation, inhibition.*

wedge (wej). A solid body having the shape of an acute-angled triangular prism. [A.S. *weeg*]

dental w., a double inclined plane used for separating the teeth, maintaining the separation once obtained, or holding a matrix in place.

WEE Abbreviation for western equine *encephalomyelitis.*

Weeks, John E., U.S. ophthalmologist, 1853–1949. SEE W.'s *bacillus;* Koch-W. *bacillus.*

Wegener, Friedrich, German pathologist, 1907–1990. SEE W.'s *granulomatosis.*

Wegner, Friedrich R.G., German pathologist, 1843–1917. SEE W.'s *disease, line.*

Weibel, Ewald R., 20th century Swiss physician. SEE W.-Palade *bodies,* under *body.*

Weichselbaum, Anthony, Austrian pathologist, 1845–1920. SEE W.'s *coccus;* Fraenkel-W. *pneumococcus.*

Weidel, Hugo, Austrian chemist, 1849–1899. SEE W.'s *reaction.*

Weigert, Carl, German pathologist, 1845–1904. SEE W.'s *law,* iodine *solution.* See entries under stain.

weight (wāt). The product of the force of gravity, defined internationally as 9.80665 m/s^2, times the mass of the body. [A.S. *gewiht*]

apothecaries' w., an obsolescent system of w.'s based upon the w. of a grain of wheat. Has been used for centuries in weighing medicines and precious metals (Troy measure). Some drugs which have been available for long periods are still often designated as grains (*e.g.,* 5 grains of aspirin, 1/2 grain of codeine, 1/100 grain nitroglycerin). This w. system has been largely su-perseded by the metric system (based on grams). One grain is the equivalent of 64.8 milligrams. One scruple contains 20 grains; one dram contains 60 grains; one apothecary ounce contains 8 drams (480 grains); one apothecary pound contains 12 ounces (5760 grains).

atomic w. (at wt, AW), the mass in grams of 1 mol (6.02×10^{23}, atoms) of an atomic species; the mass of an atom of a chemical element in relation to the mass of an atom of carbon-12 (^{12}C), which is set equal to 12.000, thus a ratio and therefore dimensionless (although the actual mass, numerically the same, is sometimes expressed in daltons); not necessarily the w. of any individual atom of an element, since most elements are made up of several isotopes of different masses; *e.g.,* the atomic w. of chlorine is 35.4527, because it is composed of ^{35}Cl and ^{37}Cl in proportions that give an average of 35.4527. SEE ALSO molecular w.

birth w., in humans, the first w. of an infant obtained within less than the first 60 completed minutes after birth; a full-size infant is one weighing 2500 g or more; a low birth w. is less than 2500 g.

combining w., SYN gram *equivalent.*

dry w., the w. of material remaining after removing the water (*e.g.,* after heating above 100°C).

equivalent w., SYN gram *equivalent.*

gram-atomic w., atomic w. expressed in grams. Cf. mole.

gram-molecular w., molecular w. expressed in grams. Cf. mole.

molecular w. (mol wt, MW), the sum of the atomic w.'s of all the atoms constituting a molecule; the mass of a molecule relative to the mass of a standard atom, now ^{12}C (taken as 12.000). Relative molecular mass (M_r) is the mass relative to the dalton and has no units. SEE ALSO atomic w. SYN molecular mass, molecular weight ratio, relative molecular mass.

weight·less·ness (wāt′les-nes). The psychophysiologic effect of zero gravity, as experienced by someone falling freely in a vacuum (*e.g.,* astronauts in a stable orbit). A temporary state of simulated w. can be achieved during powered flight within the earth's atmosphere by traversing an inverted parabolic curve where gravitational pull and centrifugal force cancel each other out.

Weil, Adolf, German physician, 1848–1916. SEE W.'s *disease;* Larrey-W. *disease.*

Weil, Edmund, Austrian physician, 1880–1922. SEE W.-Felix *reaction, test.*

Weil, Ludwig A., German dentist, 1849–1895. SEE W.'s basal *layer,* basal *zone.*

Weill, Georges, French ophthalmologist, 1866–1952. SEE W.-Marchesani *syndrome.*

Weill, Jean A., French physician, *1903. SEE Leri-W. *disease, syndrome.*

Weinberg, Michel, French pathologist, 1868–1940. SEE W.'s *reaction.*

Weinberg, Wilhelm, German physician, 1862–1937. SEE Hardy-W. *equilibrium, law.*

Weingrow's re·flex. See under reflex.

Weir, Robert F., U.S. surgeon, 1838–1927. SEE W.'s *operation.*

Weir Mitchell. SEE Mitchell.

Weisbach, Albin, Austrian anthropologist, 1837–1914. SEE W.'s *angle.*

Weismann, August Friedrich Leopold, German biologist, 1834–1914. SEE weismannism.

weis·mann·ism (vīs′man-izm). theory of the noninheritance of acquired characteristics.

Weiss, Nathan, Austrian physician, 1851–1883. SEE W.'s *sign.*

Weiss, Soma, U.S. physician, 1898–1942. SEE Charcot-W.-Baker *syndrome;* Mallory-W. *lesion, syndrome, tear.*

Weitbrecht, Josias, German-Russian anatomist in St. Petersburg, 1702–1747. SEE W.'s *cartilage, cord, fibers,* under *fiber, foramen, ligament; apparatus* ligamentosus weitbrechti.

Welander, Lisa, Swedish neurologist, *1909. SEE Kugelberg-W. *disease;* Wohlfart-Kugelberg-W. *disease.*

We

Welch, William H., U.S. pathologist, 1850–1934. SEE W.'s *bacillus.*

Welcker, Hermann, German anthropologist and anatomist, 1822–1898. SEE W.'s *angle.*

Wells, G.C., 20th century British dermatologist. SEE W.'s *syndrome.*

Wells, Michael Vernon, 20th century English physician. SEE Muckle-W. *syndrome.*

welt (wĕlt). SYN wheal. [O.E. *waelt*]

wen (wĕn). Old term for pilar *cyst.* [A.S.]

Wenckebach, Karel F., Dutch internist, 1864–1940. SEE W. *block, period, phenomenon.*

Wenzel, Joseph, German anatomist and physiologist, 1768–1808. SEE W.'s *ventricle.*

Wepfer, Johann J., 1620–1695. SEE W.'s *glands,* under *gland.*

Werdnig, Guido, Austrian neurologist, 1862–1919. SEE W.-Hoffmann *disease;* Werdnig-Hoffmann muscular *atrophy.*

WERL HOF. Paul G., German physician, 1699–1767. SEE Werlhof's *disease.*

Wermer, Paul, U.S. internist, 1898–1975.

Wernekinck (Werneking), Friedrich C.G., German anatomist and physician, 1798–1835. SEE W.'s *commissure, decussation.*

Werner, F.F., early 20th century German chemist. SEE W.'s *test.*

Werner, Otto, German physician, *1879. SEE W.'s *syndrome.*

Wernicke, Karl, German neurologist, 1848–1905. SEE W.'s *aphasia, area, center, disease, encephalopathy, field, radiation, reaction, region, sign, syndrome, zone;* W.-Korsakoff *encephalopathy, syndrome.*

Wertheim, Ernst, Austrian gynecologist, 1864–1920. SEE W.'s *operation.*

Werther, J., 20th century German physician. SEE W.'s *disease.*

West, Charles, English physician, 1816–1898. SEE W.'s *syndrome.*

West. John B., Australian-U.S. pulmonary physiologist, *1928.

Westberg, Friedrich, 19th century German physician. SEE W.'s *space.*

Westergren, Alf, Swedish physician, *1891. SEE W. *method.*

West·ern blot, West·ern blot·ting. SYN Western blot *analysis.* SEE immunoblot.

Westphal, Karl F.O., German neurologist, 1833–1890. SEE W.'s *disease, phenomenon, pseudosclerosis,* pupillary *reflex, sign;* W.-Erb *sign;* W.-Piltz *phenomenon;* W.-Strümpell *pseudosclerosis;* Edinger-W. *nucleus;* Erb-W. *sign;* Strümpell-W. *disease.*

Wetzel, Norman C., U.S. pediatrician, *1897. SEE W. *grid.*

Wever, Ernest Glen, U.S. psychologist, *1902. SEE W.-Bray *phenomenon.*

Weyers, Helmut, 20th century German pediatrician. SEE W.-Thier *syndrome.*

Wharton, Thomas, English anatomist and physician, 1614–1673. SEE W.'s *duct, jelly.*

wheal (hwēl). A circumscribed, evanescent papule or irregular plaque of edema of the skin, appearing as an urticarial lesion, slightly reddened, often changing in size and shape and extending to adjacent areas, and usually accompanied by intense itching; produced by intradermal injection or test, or by exposure to allergenic substances in susceptible persons; also encountered in dermatitis herpetiformis (Darier's sign). SYN hives (2), welt. [A.S. *hwēle*]

wheat germ oil (hwēt jerm). An oil obtained by expression from the germ of the wheat seed, *Triticum aestivum* (family Gramineae); one of the richest sources of natural vitamin E; used as a nutritional supplement.

Wheatstone, Charles, English physicist, 1802–1875. SEE W.'s *bridge.*

wheel (hwēl). A circular frame or disk designed to revolve around an axis.

Burlew w., SYN Burlew *disk.*

Wheeler, Henry Lord, U.S. chemist, 1867–1914. SEE Wheeler-Johnson *test.*

Wheeler, John M., U.S. ophthalmologist, 1879–1938. SEE W. *method.*

Wheeler-Johnson test. See under test.

Wheelhouse, Claudius G., English surgeon, 1826–1909. SEE W.'s *operation.*

wheeze (hwēz). **1.** To breathe with difficulty and noisily. **2.** A whistling, squeaking, musical, or puffing sound made by air passing through the fauces, glottis, or narrowed tracheobronchial airways in difficult breathing. [A.S. *hwēsan*]

asthmatoid w., a puffing or musical sound heard in front of the patient's open mouth in a case of foreign body in the trachea or a bronchus.

whelp (hwelp). The act of a female dog (bitch) giving birth to puppies. [A.S.]

whe·wel·lite (hwa'wel-īt). $Ca(O_2C–CO_2)\cdot H_2O$; a monohydrate of calcium oxalate; found in renal calculi. Cf. weddellite. [William *Whewell,* Eng. philosopher, + -ite]

whey (hwā). The watery part of milk remaining after the separation of the casein. SYN serum lactis. [A.S. *hwaeg*]

alum w., w. produced by curdling milk by means of powdered alum.

w. protein, SEE whey *protein.*

whip·lash (hwip'lash). SEE whiplash *injury.*

Whipple, Allen O., U.S. surgeon, 1881–1963. SEE W.'s *operation.*

Whipple, George H., U.S. pathologist and Nobel laureate, 1878–1976. SEE W.'s *disease.*

whip·worm (hwip'werm). SEE *Trichuris trichiura.*

whis·ky, whis·key (hwis'kē). An alcoholic liquid obtained by the distillation of the fermented mash of wholly or partly malted cereal grains, containing 47 to 53% by volume of C_2H_5OH, at 15.56°C; it must have been stored in charred wood containers for not less than 2 years. The various grains used in the manufacture of w. are barley, maize, rye, and wheat. [Gael, *usquebaugh,* water of life]

whis·per (hwis'per). To speak without phonation, as with an open posterior glottis. [A.S. *hwisprian*]

whis·tle (hwis'l). **1.** A sharp, shrill sound made by forcing air through a narrow opening. **2.** An instrument for producing a w. [A.S. *hwistle*]

Galton's w., a cylindrical w., attached to a compressible bulb, with a screw attachment that changes the note; used to test the hearing.

White, Paul Dudley, U.S. cardiologist, 1886–1973. SEE Lee-W. *method;* Wolff-Parkinson-W. *syndrome.*

white (hwīt). The color resulting from commingling of all the rays of the spectrum; the color of chalk or of snow. SYN albicans (1). [A.S. *hwīt*]

w. of eye, the visible portion of the sclera.

Whitehead, Walter, English surgeon, 1840–1913. SEE W. *deformity;* W.'s *operation.*

white·head (hwīt'hed). **1.** SYN milium. **2.** SYN closed *comedo.*

white·pox (hwīt'poks). SYN alastrim.

whites (hwīts). Colloquialism for leukorrhea or blennorrhea.

whit·ing (hwīt'ing). Chalk ($CaCO_3$) used for polishing metals or plastic appliances.

whit·loc·kite (hwit'lok-īt). SYN tribasic *calcium* phosphate. [Herbert P. *Whitlock,* Am. mineralogist, + -ite]

whit·low (hwit'lō). SYN felon. [M.E. *whitflawe*]

herpetic w., painful herpes simplex virus infection of a finger from direct inoculation of the unprotected perionychial fold, often accompanied by lymphangitis and regional adenopathy, lasting up to several weeks; most common in physicians, dentists, and nurses as a result of exposure to the virus in a patient's mouth.

melanotic w., SYN subungual *melanoma.*

thecal w., suppurative lesion of distal phalanx; may involve tendon sheath and bone.

Whitman, Royal, U.S. surgeon, 1857–1946. SEE W.'s *frame.*

Whitmore, Alfred, English surgeon, 1876–1946. SEE W.'s *bacillus, disease.*

Whitnall, Samuel E., English anatomist, 1876–1952. SEE W.'s *tubercle.*

WHO Abbreviation for World Health Organization.

whoop (hoop). The loud sonorous inspiration in pertussis with which the paroxysm of coughing terminates, due to spasm of the larynx (glottis).

systolic w., SYN systolic *honk.*

whorl (hwerl). **1.** A turn of the spiral cochlea of the ear. **2.** SYN *vortex* of heart. **3.** A turn of a concha nasalis. **4.** SYN verticil. **5.** An area of hair growing in a radial manner suggesting whirling or twisting. SYN vortex (2). SEE hair w.'s. **6.** One of the distinguishing patterns comprising Galton's system of classification of fingerprints. SYN digital w.

coccygeal w., SYN *vortex* coccygeus.

digital w., SYN whorl (6).

hair w.'s, a spiral arrangement of the hairs, as at the crown of the head. SYN vortices pilorum [NA].

whorled (hwerld). Marked by or arranged in whorls. SEE ALSO vorticose, turbinate, convoluted, verticillate.

Wickham, Louis-Frédéric, French dermatologist, 1861–1913. SEE W.'s *striae,* under *stria.*

Widal, Georges F.I., French physician, 1862–1929. SEE W.'s *reaction, syndrome;* Gruber-W. *reaction;* Hayem-W. *syndrome.*

wid·ow's peak. A sharp point of hair growth in the midline of the anterior scalp margin, usually resulting from recession of hair of the temple areas, or occurring as a congenital configuration of scalp hair.

width (width, with). Wideness; the distance from one side of an object or area to the other.

orbital w., the distance between the dacryon and the farthest point on the anterior edge of the outer border of the orbit (Broca), or between the latter point and the junction of the frontolacrimal suture and the posterior edge of the lacrimal groove.

window w., the range of CT numbers (in Hounsfield units) included in the gray scale video display of the CT image, ranging from 1 to 2000 or 3000, depending on the type of machine. SEE ALSO window *level.*

Wiedemann, Hans Rudolf, German pediatrician, *1915. SEE Beckwith-W. *syndrome.*

Wiener, H. SEE *tract* of Münzer and W.

Wigand, J. Heinrich, German obstetrician and gynecologist, 1766–1817. SEE W. *maneuver.*

Wilde, Sir William R.W., Irish oculist and otologist, 1815–1876. SEE W.'s *cords,* under *cord, triangle.*

Wilder, Helenor C., 20th century U.S. scientist. SEE W.'s *stain* for reticulum.

Wilder, Joseph, U.S. neuropsychiatrist, *1895. SEE W.'s *law* of initial value.

Wilder, William H., U.S. ophthalmologst, 1860–1935. SEE W.'s *sign.*

Wildermuth, Hermann A., German psychiatrist, 1852–1907. SEE W.'s *ear.*

Wildervanck, L.S., 20th century Dutch geneticist. SEE W. *syndrome.*

wild·fire (wīld'fīr). SYN fogo selvagem.

Wilhelmy, Ludwig F., German scientist, 1812–1864. SEE W. *balance.*

Wilkie, David P.D., Scottish surgeon, 1882–1938. SEE W.'s *artery, disease.*

Wilkinson, Daryl Sheldon, 20th century English dermatologist. SEE Sneddon-W. *disease.*

Willebrand, E.A. von. SEE von Willebrand.

Willett, J. Abernethy, English obstetrician, †1932. SEE W.'s *forceps.*

Willi, Heinrich, 20th century Swiss pediatrician. SEE Prader-W. *syndrome.*

Williams, Anna, U.S. bacteriologist, 1863–1955. SEE W.'s *stain;* Park-W. *bacillus, fixative.*

Williams, J.C.P., 20th century New Zealand cardiologist. SEE W. *syndrome.*

Williamson, Carl S., U.S. surgeon, 1896–1952. SEE Mann-W. *operation, ulcer.*

Willis, Thomas, English physician, 1621–1675. SEE W.'s *centrum* nervosum, *cords,* under *cord, pancreas, paracusis, pouch; circle* of W.; *accessorius* willisii; *chordae* willisii, under *chorda.*

Williston, Samuel Wendell, U.S. paleontologist, 1852–1918. SEE W.'s *law.*

wil·low (wil'ō). A tree of the genus *Salix;* the bark of several species, especially *S. fragilis,* is a source of salicin. [A.S. *welig*]

Wilms, Max, German surgeon, 1867–1918. SEE W.'s *tumor.*

Wilson, Clifford, English physician, *1906. SEE Kimmelstiel-W. *disease, syndrome.*

Wilson, Frank Norman, U.S. cardiologist, 1890–1952. SEE W. *block.*

Wilson, James, English anatomist, physiologist, and surgeon, 1765–1821. SEE W.'s *muscle.*

Wilson, Miriam G., U.S. pediatrician, *1922. SEE W.-Mikity *syndrome.*

Wilson, Samuel A. Kinnier, English neurologist, 1878–1937. SEE W.'s *disease, syndrome.*

Wilson, Sir William J.E., English dermatologist, 1809–1884. SEE W.'s *disease, lichen.*

Wilson's meth·od. See under method.

wind·age (win'dej). Internal injury with no surface lesion, caused by collision with the pressure of compressed air or with an object propelled by compressed air.

wind-broken (wind'brō-ken). Heaving; said of a horse.

wind·burn (wind'bern). Erythema of the face due to exposure to wind.

wind·gall (wind'gawl). A soft, pulpy swelling in the neighborhood of the fetlock joint of the horse, varying in size from a pinhead to a large hen's egg.

win·dow (win'dō). SYN fenestra.

aortic w., obsolete term for a radiolucent region below the aortic arch on a left anterior oblique chest radiograph, formed by the bifurcation of the trachea and crossed by the left pulmonary artery.

aorticopulmonary w., SYN aortic septal *defect.*

aortic-pulmonic w., SYN aortopulmonary w.

aortopulmonary w., the indentation of the left side of the mediastinum by the lung partially interposed between the aortic arch and the left pulmonary artery, seen on frontal radiographs of the chest. SYN aortic-pulmonic w.

cochlear w., SYN *fenestra* cochleae.

lung w., CT settings of w. level and width appropriate to showing lung detail; soft tissues are white or nearly so.

mediastinal w., CT settings of w. level and width appropriate to showing soft tissue structures; the lungs become black at these settings. SYN soft tissue w.

oval w., SYN *fenestra* vestibuli.

round w., SYN *fenestra* cochleae.

soft tissue w., SYN mediastinal w.

Combining forms
WordFinder
Multi-term entry finder
Preceding letter A
A.D.A.M. Anatomy Plates
Between letters L and M
Appendices:
Following letter Z
SYN Synonym; Cf., compare

[NA] Nomina Anatomica
[MIM] Mendelian Inheritance in Man
☆ Official alternate term
☆[NA] Official alternate Nomina Anatomica term
High Profile Term

tachycardia w., in paroxysmal tachycardia of the reentry type, the interval of time (the window) between the earliest and latest premature activation that can excite the paroxysm.

vestibular w., SYN *fenestra* vestibuli.

wind·pipe (wind′pīp). SYN trachea.

wind·puffs (wind′pŭfs). An affliction of horses marked by a collection of synovial fluid between the tendons of the legs, particularly just above the fetlock joint, the prominence appearing on both sides of the tendon; most common in hard-worked animals and may end in lameness.

wind-suck·ing. A more severe form of crib-biting where air is ingested abnormally and forcefully by swallowing. SEE aerophagia.

wine (wīn). **1.** The fermented juice of the grape. SYN vinous liquor. **2.** A group of preparations consisting of a solution of one or more medicinal substances in w., usually white w. because of its comparative freedom from tannin. There are no official w.'s. [Fr. *vin;* L. *vinum*]

high w., the strong spirit obtained by rectification or redistillation of low w. in making whisky.

low w., the first weak distillate obtained from the mash in the process of making whisky.

red w., claret, an alcoholic liquor made by fermenting grapes, the fruit of *Vitis vinifera*, with their skins (which imparts color); has been used as a tonic.

sherry w., a w. of amber color, obtained originally from Jerez, Spain, containing about 20% alcohol; used in preparation of medicinal w.'s.

wing. 1. The anterior appendage of a bird. **2.** In anatomy, ala. SYN ala (1).

angel's w., a deformity in which both scapulae project conspicuously. SEE ALSO winged *scapula.*

ashen w., SYN vagal *trigone.*

w. of crista galli, a small lateral expansion of the ethmoid bone from the front of the crista galli on each side that articulates with the frontal bone and forms the foramen cecum. SYN ala cristae galli [NA], alar process.

gray w., SYN vagal *trigone.*

greater w. of sphenoid bone, strong squamous processes extending in a broad superolateral curve from the body of the sphenoid bone. The greater w. presents these suraces (facies): 1) cerebral surface: forms anterior third of the floor of the lateral portions of the middle cranial fossa; 2) temporal surface: forms the deepest portion of the temporal fossa; 3) infratemporal surface, forms the "roof" of the infratemporal fossa; 4) orbital surface: forms posterolateral wall of orbit. The greater w. forms the inferior border of the supraorbital fissure, and is perforated at its root by foramina rotundum ovale, and spinosum and the pterygoid canal. SYN ala major ossis sphenoidalis [NA], ala temporalis.

w. of ilium, the upper flaring portion of the ilium. SYN ala ossis ilii [NA].

Ingrassia's w., SYN lesser w. of sphenoid bone.

lesser w. of sphenoid bone, one of a bilateral pair of triangular, pointed plates extending laterally from the anterolateral body of the sphenoid bone. Forming the posteriormost portion of the floor of the anterior cranial fossa, their sharp posterior edge forms the sphenoidal ridge separating anterior and middle cranial fossae. The medial end of the lesser w. attaches to the body by means of two pedicles, thus forming the optic canal. The w. itself forms the superior margin of the supraorbital fissure. SYN ala minor ossis sphenoidalis [NA], ala orbitalis, Ingrassia's apophysis, Ingrassia's w.

w. of nose, the outer more or less flaring wall of each nostril. SYN ala nasi [NA], pinna nasi.

w. of sacrum, the upper surface of the lateral part of the sacrum adjacent to the body. SYN ala sacralis [NA].

w. of vomer, an everted lip on either side of the upper border of the vomer, between which fits the rostrum of the sphenoid bone. SYN ala vomeris [NA].

Winiwarter, Felix von, German surgeon, 1852–1931. SEE W.-Buerger *disease.*

wink (wink). To close and open the eyes rapidly; an involuntary act by which the tears are spread over the conjunctiva, keeping it moist. [A.S. *wincian*]

Winkler, Max, Swiss physician, 1875–1952. SEE W.'s *disease.*

Winslow, Jacob B., Danish anatomist, physicist, and surgeon in Paris, 1669–1760. SEE W.'s *foramen, ligament, pancreas, stars,* under *star; stellulae* winslowii, under *stellula.*

Winterbottom, Thomas M., English physician, 1765–1859. SEE W.'s *sign.*

win·ter·green oil (win′ter-grēn). SYN *methyl* salicylate.

Winternitz, Wilhelm, Austrian physician, 1835–1917. SEE W.'s *sound.*

Wintersteiner, Hugo, Austrian ophthalmologist, 1865–1918. SEE W. *rosettes,* under *rosette.*

wire (wīr). Slender and pliable rod or thread of metal.

arch w., SYN archwire.

guide w., SEE guidewire.

Kirschner's w., an apparatus for skeletal traction in long bone fracture. SYN Kirschner's apparatus.

ligature w., a soft thin w. of stainless steel used in dentistry to tie an archwire to band attachments or brackets.

separating w., a w., usually of soft brass, used to gain separation between teeth. SEE ALSO separation (2).

wrought w., a w. formed by drawing a cast structure through a die into a desired shape and size; used in dentistry for partial denture clasps and orthodontic appliances.

wir·ing (wīr′ing). Fastening together the ends of a broken bone by wire sutures.

circumferential w., fixation of mandibular fractures by passing wires around a section of bone with the ends exiting into the oral cavity; *i.e.,* circummandibular and circumzygomatic w.

continuous loop w., the formation of wire loops on both maxillary and mandibular teeth, for the placement of intermaxillary elastics; used in reduction and fixation of fractures. SYN Stout's w.

craniofacial suspension w., a method of w. using areas of bones not contiguous with the oral cavity for the support of fractured jaw segments (*e.g.,* pyriform aperture, zygomatic arch, zygomatic process of the frontal bone).

Gilmer w., a method of intermaxillary fixation in which single opposing teeth are wired circumferentially, and the wires are twisted together.

Ivy loop w., placement of a wire around two adjacent teeth to provide an attachment for intermaxillary elastics.

perialveolar w., fixing a splint to the maxillary arch by passing a wire through the alveolar process from the buccal plate to the palate.

pyriform aperture w., a method of w. using the nasal bones at the area of the pyriform aperture for the stabilization of fractures of the jaw.

Stout's w., SYN continuous loop w.

Wirsung, Johann G., German anatomist in Padua, 1600–1643. SEE W.'s *canal, duct.*

wiry (wīr′ē). Resembling or having the feel of a wire; filiform and hard; denoting a variety of pulse.

Wiskott, Arthur, 20th century German pediatrician. SEE W.-Aldrich *syndrome.*

Wissler, Hans, Swiss pediatrician, *1906. SEE W.'s *syndrome.*

Wistar, Caspar, U.S. biologist, 1760–1818, after whom the Wistar Institute is named. SEE W. *rats,* under *rat.*

witch ha·zel (wich hāz′l). SYN hamamelis.

with·draw·al (with-draw′ăl). **1.** The act of removal or retreating. **2.** A psychological and/or physical syndrome caused by the abrupt cessation of the use of a drug in an habituated individual. **3.** The therapeutic process of discontinuing a drug so as to avoid w. (2). **4.** A pattern of behavior observed in schizophrenia and depression, characterized by a pathological retreat from interpersonal contact and social involvement and leading to self-preoccupation.

with·ers (with′erz). The region of the back of an animal, particularly of the horse, which lies between the shoulder blades. [A.S. *wither,* against]

fistulous w., a fistula, caused by bacterial infection, of the w.

wit·kop. A favoid condition of the scalp seen in South Africans.

wit·zel·sucht (vit′sel-zŭkht). A morbid tendency to pun, make poor jokes, and tell pointless stories, while being oneself inordinately entertained thereby. [Ger. *witzeln,* to affect wit, + *Sucht,* mania]

wob·ble (wah′bl). In molecular biology, unorthodox pairing between the base at the 5′ end of an anticodon and the base that pairs with it (in the 3′-position of the codon); thus, the anticodon 3′-UCU-5′ may pair with 5′-AGA-3′ (normal or Watson-Crick pairing) or with 5′-AGG-3′ (wobble). Wobble pairings can occur between the unusual base hypoxanthine and adenine, uracil, or cytosine, between uracil and guanine, and between guanine and uracil, when in the 5′-position of an anticodon. SEE ALSO wobble *base.*

Wohl·fahr·tia (vōl-far′tē-ă). A genus of larviparous dipterous fleshflies (family Sarcophagidae), of which some species' larvae breed in ulcerated surfaces and flesh wounds of humans and animals. Important species include *W. magnifica,* a widely distributed obligatory fleshfly whose tissue-destroying maggots invade wounds or head cavities of domestic animals and humans; *W. nuba,* a facultative fleshfly of Old World distribution, also found in head wounds or head cavities but not in dermal sores; and *W. vigil* (*W. opaca*), which produces cutaneous myiasis in human infants in the northern U.S. and southern Canada by larvae that penetrate the skin and cause infected, boil-like, or furuncular lesions; mink and fox pups in fur farms, and probably rabbits and rodents, are attacked by this species. [P. *Wohlfahrt,* Ger. medical writer, †1726]

wohl·fahr·ti·o·sis (vōl-far-tē-ō′sis). Infection of animals and humans with larvae of flies of the genus *Wohlfahrtia.*

Wohlfart, Gunnar, Swedish neurologist, 1910–1961. SEE W.-Kugelberg-Welander *disease.*

Wolf, A., 20th century U.S. pathologist. SEE W.-Orton *bodies,* under *body.*

Wolfe, John R., Scottish ophthalmologist, 1824–1904. SEE W.'s *method;* W. *graft;* W.-Krause *graft.*

Wolff, Kaspar F., German embryologist in Russia, 1733–1794. SEE wolffian *body;* wolffian *cyst;* wolffian *duct;* wolffian *rest;* wolffian *ridge;* wolffian *tubules,* under *tubule.*

Wolff, Julius, German anatomist, 1836–1902. SEE Wolff's *law.*

Wolff, Louis, U.S. cardiologist, 1898–1972. SEE W.-Chaikoff *block, effect;* W.-Parkinson-White *syndrome.*

wolff·i·an (wulf′ē-an). Relating to or described by Kaspar Wolff.

Wölfler, Anton, Bohemian surgeon, 1850–1917. SEE W.'s *gland.*

wolf·ram, wolf·ram·i·um (wulf′ram, wulf-ram′ē-ŭm). SYN tungsten. [from *wolframite*]

Wolfring, Emilj F. von, Polish ophthalmologist, 1832–1906. SEE W.'s *glands,* under *gland.*

wolfs·bane (wulfs′bān). SEE aconite.

Wolinel·la (wō-li-nel′ah). Genus of Gram-negative, microaerophilic bacteria with helical to curved cell; exhibits motility by a single polar flagellum. Isolated from the gingival sulcus and from root canal infections in humans, and from the bovine rumen. Type species is *Wolinella succinogenes.*

Wollaston, William H., English physician and physicist, 1766–1828. SEE W.'s *doublet, theory.*

Wolman, Moshe, 20th century Israeli neuropathologist, *1914. SEE W.'s *disease, xanthomatosis.*

womb (woom). SYN uterus. [A.S. the belly]

falling of the w., SYN *prolapse* of the uterus.

Wood, Robert, U.S. physicist, 1868–1955. SEE W.'s *glass, lamp, light.*

Wood. Paul SEE Wood *units,* under *unit.*

wood al·co·hol (wud). SYN *methyl* alcohol.

wood wool. A specially prepared, not compressed, wood fiber used for surgical dressings.

wool (wul). The hair of the sheep; sometimes, when defatted, used as a surgical dressing. SYN lana.

w. alcohols, Wool wax alcohols prepared by saponification of the grease of sheep wool and separation of the fraction that contains cholesterol (not less than 30%) and other alcohols; used to prepare w. ointment.

w. fat, The purified, anhydrous, fatlike substance obtained from the wool of sheep. SEE ALSO adeps lanae.

hydrous w. fat, SYN adeps lanae.

wool al·co·hols. See under wool.

Woolf, B., 20th-century British biochemist. SEE W.-Lineweaver-Burk *plot.*

wool fat. See under wool.

Woolner, Thomas, English sculptor, 1826–1892. SEE W.'s *tip.*

word sal·ad (werd sal′ăd). A jumble of meaningless and unrelated words emitted by persons with certain kinds of schizophrenia.

Woringer, M.M.F., 20th century French dermatologist. SEE Woringer-Kolopp *disease.*

work (work). **1.** Physical and/or mental effort to achieve a result. **2.** That which is accomplished when a force acts against resistance to produce motion.

work·ing out (werk′ing). In psychoanalysis, the state in the treatment process in which the patient's personal history and psychodynamics are uncovered.

work·ing through. In psychoanalysis, the process of obtaining additional insight and personality changes in a patient through repeated and varied examination of a conflict or problem; the interactions between free association, resistance, interpretation, and working out constitute the fundamental facets of this process.

work·sta·tion (werk′stā′shŭn). A computer or television monitor with controls for studying and manipulating graphical or clinical images.

World Health Or·ga·ni·za·tion (WHO). A unit of the United Nations devoted to international health problems.

Worm, Ole, Danish anatomist, 1588–1654. SEE wormian *bones,* under *bone.*

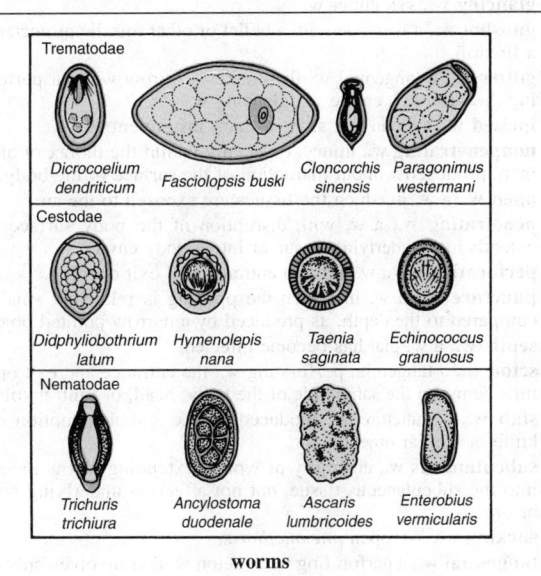

worms
eggs of various species

worm (werm). **1.** In anatomy, any structure resembling a w., *e.g.,* the midline part of the cerebellum. **2.** SYN lyssa (1). **3.** Term once used to designate any member of the invertebrate group or former subkingdom Vermes, a collective term no longer used taxonomically; now commonly used to designate any member of the separate phyla Annelida (the segmented or true w.'s), the Nematoda (roundworms), and the Platyhelminthes (flatworms). Important species include *Dracunculus medinensis* (dragon, guinea, Medina, or serpent w.), *Enterobius vermicularis* (seat w. or pinworm), *Haemonchus contortus* (stomach, barberpole, or twisted stomach w.), *Loa loa* (African eye w.), *Moniliformis* (phylum Acanthocephala, thorny-headed w.'s), *Oxyspirura mansoni* (Manson's eye w.), *Oxyuris* (animal pinworm), *Pentastomida* (tongue w.), *Stephanurus dentatus* (kidney or lard w. of swine), *Strongylus* (palisade w.), *Syngamus trachea* (gapeworm or forked w.), *Thelazia* (eye w.), *Trichinella spiralis* (pork or trichina w.), and *Trichostrongylus* (hairworm, or bankrupt or black scour w.). For some types of w.'s not listed as subentries here (because they are usually written as one word), see the full name. [A.S. *wyrm*]

caddis w., aquatic larva in the insect order Trichoptera.

fleece w., SYN wool *maggot*.

Manson's eye w., SYN *Oxyspirura mansoni.*

meal w., the larva of beetles of the genus *Tenebrio;* both larvae and adults are important pests, destroying flour, meal, and other cereal products; they are also intermediate hosts of nematodes of the genus *Gongylonema*, and of various tapeworms of the genus *Hymenolepis.*

worm bark. SYN andira.

wor·mi·an (werm′ē-an). Relating to or described by Ole Worm.

Wormley, Theodore G., U.S. chemist, 1826–1897. SEE W.'s *test.*

worm·seed (werm′sēd). **1.** Santonica. **2.** SYN chenopodium.

worm·wood (werm′wud). SYN absinthium.

wort (wŏrt). **1.** A suffix in the popular names of many plants, such as liverwort, lungwort, woundwort, etc. **2.** An infusion of malt. [A.S. *wyrt,* a plant]

Worth, Claud, British ophthalmologist, 1869–1936. SEE W.'s *amblyoscope.*

Woulfe, Peter, English chemist, 1727–1803. SEE W.'s *bottle.*

wound (wūnd). **1.** Trauma to any of the tissues of the body, especially that caused by physical means and with interruption of continuity. **2.** A surgical incision. [O.E. *wund*]

abraded w., SYN abrasion (1).

avulsed w., a w. caused by or resulting from avulsion.

crease w., SYN gutter w.

glancing w., SYN gutter w.

gunshot w., a w. made with a bullet or other missile projected by a firearm.

gutter w., a tangential w. that makes a furrow without perforating the skin. SYN crease w., glancing w.

incised w., a clean cut, as by a sharp instrument.

nonpenetrating w., injury, especially within the thorax or abdomen, produced without disruption of the surface of the body.

open w., a w. in which the tissues are exposed to the air.

penetrating w., a w. with disruption of the body surface that extends into underlying tissue or into a body cavity.

perforating w., a w. with an entrance and exit opening.

puncture w., a w. in which the opening is relatively small as compared to the depth, as produced by a narrow pointed object.

septic w., a w. that has become infected.

seton w., a tangential perforating w., the entrance and exit openings being on the same side of the body, head, or limb involved.

stab w., a puncture w. produced by the stabbing motion of a knife or similar object.

subcutaneous w., an injury or wound extending below the skin into the subcutaneous tissue, but not affecting underlying bones or organs.

sucking w., SYN open *pneumothorax.*

tangential w., a perforating w. or seton w. that involves only one side of the part.

W-plas·ty. Surgery to prevent the contracture of a straight-line scar; the edges of the wound are trimmed in the shape of a W, or a series of W's, and closed in a zig-zag manner. SYN W procedure.

W.r. Abbreviation for Wassermann *reaction.*

Wrᵃ Abbreviation for Wright *antigens,* under *antigen.* See low frequency blood groups, Blood Groups appendix.

wrap (rap). A cover, particularly one that enfolds or encloses.

cardiac muscle wrap, SYN cardiomyoplasty.

wreath (rēth). A structure resembling a twisted or entwined band or a garland. [A.S. *wraeth,* a bandage]

ciliary w., SYN *corona* ciliaris.

Wright, Basil Martin, 20th century British physician. SEE W. *respirometer.*

Wright, James Homer, U.S. pathologist, 1871–1928. SEE W.'s *stain.*

Wright, Marmaduke Burr, U.S. obstetrician, 1803–1879. SEE W.'s *version.*

wright·ine (rīt′ēn). SYN conessine.

wrin·kle (ring′kl). A furrow, fold, or crease in the skin, particularly with increasing occurrence as a result of sun exposure or, in perioral skin, cigarette smoking; associated with degeneration of dermal elastic tissue.

Wrisberg, Heinrich A., German anatomist and gynecologist, 1739–1808. SEE W.'s *cartilage, ganglia,* under *ganglion, ligament, nerve, tubercle.*

wrist (rist). The proximal segment of the hand consisting of the carpal bones and the associated soft parts. SYN carpus (1) [NA]. [A.S. wrist joint, ankle joint]

w.-drop, Paralysis of the extensors of the wrist and fingers; most often caused by lesion of the radial nerve. SYN carpoptosis, carpoptosia, drop hand.

wrist-drop. See under wrist.

wry·neck (rī′nek). SYN torticollis.

Wuch·er·e·ria (vū-ker-e′rē-ă). A genus of filarial nematodes (family Onchocercidae, superfamily Filarioidea) characterized by adult forms that live chiefly in lymphatic vessels and produce large numbers of embryos or microfilariae that circulate in the bloodstream (microfilaremia), often appearing in the peripheral blood at regular intervals. The extreme form of this infection (wuchereriasis or filariasis) is elephantiasis or pachydermia.

W. bancrof′ti, the bancroftian filaria, a species endemic in South Pacific islands, coastal China, India, and Burma, and throughout tropical Africa and northeastern South America (including certain Caribbean islands); transmitted to humans (apparently the only definitive host) by mosquitoes, especially *Culex quinquefasciatus* and *Aedes pseudoscutellaris,* but also by several other species of *Culex, Aedes, Anopheles,* and *Mansonia,* depending on the specific geographic area; adults are white, 40–100 mm cylindroid, threadlike worms, and the microfilariae are ensheathed, with rounded anterior end and tapered, nonnucleated tail; the adult worms inhabit the larger lymphatic vessels (*e.g.,* in the extremities (especially lower), breasts, spermatic cord, and retroperitoneal tissues) and the sinuses of lymph nodes (*e.g.,* the popliteal, femoral, and inguinal groups, and also the epitrochlear and axillary nodes), where they sometimes cause temporary obstruction to the flow of lymph and slight or moderate degrees of inflammation.

W. mala′yi, former name for *Brugia malayi.*

wu·cher·e·ri·a·sis (vū′ker-ē-rī′ă-sis). Infection with worms of the genus *Wuchereria.* SEE ALSO filariasis.

Wurster, Casimir, German chemist, 1856–1913. SEE W.'s *reagent, test.*

Wyburn-Mason, Roger, British physician. SEE Wyburn-Mason *syndrome.*

Wyman. Jeffries, U.S. biochemist, *1901. SEE Monod-Wyman-Changeux *model.*

X Symbol for Kienböck's *unit*; reactance; xanthosine; halogen atom; unspecified amino acid; reactance.

Xaa Symbol for unspecified amino acid.

Xan Abbreviation for xanthine.

xan·chro·mat·ic (zan-krō-mat′ik). SYN xanthochromatic.

xanth-. SEE xantho-.

xan·the·las·ma (zan-thĕ-laz′mă). SYN x. palpebrarum. [xanth- + G. *elasma*, a beaten metal plate]

generalized x., xanthoma planum of the neck, trunk, extremities, and eyelids in patients with normal plasma lipid levels.

x. palpebra′rum, soft yellow-orange plaques on the eyelids or medial canthus, the most common form of xanthoma; may be associated with low-density lipoproteins, especially in younger adults. SYN xanthelasma, xanthoma palpebrarum.

xan·them·a·tin (zan-thĕm′ă-tin). A yellow substance derived from hematin by treating with nitric acid.

xan·the·mia (zan-thē′mē-ă). SYN carotenemia. [xanth- + G. *haima*, blood]

xan·thene (zan′thēn). **1.** The basic structure of many natural products, drugs, dyes (*e.g.*, fluorescein, pyronin, eosins), indicators, pesticides, antibiotics, etc. **2.** A class of molecules based upon x. (1).

xan·thic (zan′thik). **1.** Yellow or yellowish in color. **2.** Relating to xanthine.

xan·thi·dy·lic ac·id (zan′thi-dil-ik). SYN *xanthosine* 5′-monophosphate.

xan·thine (Xan) (zan′thēn). 2,6-Dioxopurine; 2,6(1*H*,3*H*)-purinedione; oxidation product of guanine and hypoxanthine, precursor of uric acid; occurs in many organs and in the urine, occasionally forming urinary calculi; elevated in molybdenum cofactor deficiency and in xanthinuria.

x. dehydrogenase, an oxidoreductase oxidizing x. to urate with NAD$^+$ as the oxidant; lower activity in individuals with a deficiency of molybdenum cofactor.

x. nucleotide, SYN *xanthosine* 5′-monophosphate.

x. oxidase, a flavoprotein containing molybdenum; an oxidoreductase catalyzing the reaction of x., O_2, and H_2O to produce urate and superoxide; also oxidizes hypoxanthine, some other purines and pterins, and aldehydes. A lower activity is observed in molybdenum cofactor deficiency. SYN hypoxanthine oxidase, Schardinger enzyme.

x. ribonucleoside, SYN xanthosine.

xan·thi·nol ni·a·cin·ate, xan·thi·nol nic·o·tin·ate (zan′thi-nōl). 7-[2-Hyroxy-3-[(2-hydroxyethyl)methylamino]propyl]-theophylline compound with nicotinic acid; a peripheral vasodilator.

xan·thi·nu·ria (zan-thi-nū′rē-ă). **1.** Excretion of abnormally large amounts of xanthine in the urine. **2.** A disorder [MIM*278300] resulting from defective synthesis of xanthine oxidase, characterized by urinary excretion of xanthine in place of uric acid, hypouricemia, and, in some cases, the formation of xanthine stones; autosomal recessive inheritance. SYN xanthiuria, xanthuria. [xanthine + G. *ouron*, urine]

xan·thism (zan′thizm) [MIM*278400]. A pigmentary anomaly of blacks, characterized by red or yellow-red hair color, copper-red skin, and often by dilution of iris pigment. SYN rufous albinism. [G. *xanthos*, yellowish]

xan·thi·u·ria (zan-thē-yū′rē-ă). SYN xanthinuria.

xantho-, xanth-. Yellow, yellowish. [G. *xanthos*]

xan·tho·as·tro·cy·to·ma (zan′thrō-as′trō-sī-tō- mă). SYN pleomorphic x. [xantho + astrocytoma]

pleomorphic x., a rare variant of astrocytoma usually presenting early in life with seizures. The tumor is superficially located and composed of pleomorphic glial cells, lipidized astrocytes, and perivascular lymphocytes. SYN xanthoastrocytoma.

xan·tho·choria (zan-thō-kroy′ă). SYN xanthochromia.

xan·tho·chro·mat·ic (zan′thō-krō-mat′ik). Yellow-colored. SYN xanchromatic, xanthochromic.

xan·tho·chro·mia (zan-thō-krō′mē-ă). The occurrence of patch-es of yellow color in the skin, resembling xanthoma, but without the nodules or plates. SYN cholesteroderma, xanthochroia, xanthoderma (1), xanthopathy, yellow disease, yellow skin (1). [xantho- + G. *chrōma*, color]

xan·tho·chro·mic (zan-thō-krō′mik). SYN xanthochromatic.

xan·thoch·ro·ous (zan-thok′rō-ŭs). Light-skinned; Having a fair yellowish complexion; blond. [xantho- + G. *chroa*, complexion]

xan·tho·der·ma (zan-thō-der′mă). **1.** SYN xanthochromia. **2.** Any yellow coloration of the skin. SYN yellow skin (2). [xantho- + G. *derma*, skin]

xan·tho·dont (zan′thō-dont). One who has yellow teeth. [xantho- + G. *odous*, tooth]

xan·tho·gran·u·lo·ma (zan′thō-gran′yū-lō′mă). A peculiar infiltration of retroperitoneal tissue by lipid macrophages, occurring most commonly in women.

juvenile x., single or multiple reddish to yellow papules or nodules, usually found in young children, consisting of dermal infiltration by histiocytes and Touton giant cells, with increasing fibrosis. SYN nevoxanthoendothelioma.

necrobiotic x., a cutaneous and subcutaneous x. with focal necrosis, presenting as multiple large, sometimes ulcerated, red to yellow granulomatous nodules with giant cells (often around the eyes) associated with paraproteinemia (usually monoclonal gammopathy).

xan·tho·gran·u·lo·ma·tous (zan′thō-gran′yū-lō′mă-tŭs). Relating to, of the nature of, or affected by xanthogranuloma.

xan·tho·ma (zan-thō′mă). A yellow nodule or plaque, especially of the skin, composed of lipid-laden histiocytes. [xantho- + G. -*oma*, tumor]

x. diabetico′rum, eruptive x. associated with severe diabetes.

x. dissemina′tum, a rare benign normolipemic disorder of adults with coalescent cutaneous x.'s composed of non-X histiocytes on flexural surfaces, often with mild diabetes insipidus.

eruptive x., the sudden appearance of groups of 1–4 mm waxy yellow or yellowish-brown papules with an erythematous halo, especially over extensors of the elbows and knees, and on the back and buttocks of patients with severe hyperlipemia, often familial or more rarely in severe diabetes.

fibrous x., SEE fibroxanthoma.

x. mul′tiplex, SYN xanthomatosis.

x. palpebra′rum, SYN *xanthelasma* palpebrarum.

x. pla′num, a form marked by the occurrence of yellow flat bands or minimally palpable rectangular plates in the corium, either normolipemic or associated with type IIa or III hyperlipoproteinemia.

tendinous x., x. involving tendons, ligaments, and fascia, forming deep, smooth, sometimes painful nodules beneath normal-appearing freely movable skin of the extremities; associated with abnormal lipid metabolism, commonly familial increased β lipoproteins or obstructive liver disease.

x. tubero′sum, xanthomatosis associated with familial type II, and occasionally type III, hyperlipoproteinemia. SYN x. tuberosum simplex.

x. tubero′sum sim′plex, SYN x. tuberosum.

verrucous x., histocytosis Y; a papilloma of the oral mucosa and skin in which squamous epithelium covers connective tissue papillae filled with large foamy histiocytes. SYN histiocytosis Y.

xan·tho·ma·to·sis (zan′thō-mă-tō′sis). Widespread xanthomas, especially on the elbows and knees, that sometimes affect mucous membranes and are sometimes associated with metabolic disturbances. SYN cholesterosis cutis, lipid granulomatosis, lipoid granulomatosis, xanthoma multiplex.

biliary x., x. with hypercholesterolemia, resulting from biliary cirrhosis. SYN Rayer's disease.

x. bul′bi, ulcerative fatty degeneration of the cornea after injury.

cerebrotendinous x. [MIM*213700], a disorder with deposition of cholestanol in the brain and other tissues and high levels in plasma but with normal cholesterol level; characterized by progressive cerebellar ataxia beginning after puberty, juvenile cataracts, spinal cord involvement, and tendinous or tuberous xantho-

xa

mata; autosomal recessive inheritance. Probably due to a defect in hepatic mitochondrial 26-hydroxylase in bile acid biosynthesis. SYN cerebrotendinous cholesterinosis.

chronic idiopathic x., vague or indefinite term for inherited abnormalities of lipid metabolism leading to xanthoma formation (*e.g.,* primary familial xanthomatosis).

familial hypercholesteremic x., SYN type II familial *hyperlipoproteinemia.*

normal cholesteremic x., SYN Hand-Schüller-Christian *disease.*

Wolman's x., SEE cholesterol ester storage *disease.*

xan·thom·a·tous (zan-thō′mă-tŭs). Relating to xanthoma.

Xan·tho·mo·nas (zan-thō-mō′as). Genus of the family Pseudomonadaceae; aerobic, Gram-negative, chemoorganotrophic, straight bacilli which exhibit motility by flagella. Type species is *Xanthomonas campestris.*

X. maltophil′ia, a species found primarily in clinical specimens but also in water, milk, and frozen food. Frequent cause of infections in hospitalized and immunocompromised humans. SYN *Pseudomonas maltophilia.*

xan·thop·a·thy (zan-thop′ă-thē). SYN xanthochromia. [xantho- + G. *pathos,* suffering]

xan·tho·phyll (zan′thō-fil). (3*R*,3′*R*,6′*R*)-β,ε-carotene-3′,3′-diol; oxygenated derivative of carotene; a yellow plant pigment, occurring also in egg yolk and corpus luteum. SYN lutein (2), luteol, luteole.

xan·tho·pro·te·ic (zan-thō-prō′tē-ik). Relating to xanthoprotein.

xan·tho·pro·te·ic ac·id. A noncrystallizable yellow substance derived from proteins upon treatment with nitric acid.

xan·tho·pro·tein (zan-thō-prō′tēn). The yellow product formed upon treating protein with hot nitric acid, probably from nitration of phenyl groups.

xan·thop·sia (zan-thop′sē-ă). A condition in which objects appear yellow; may occur in picric acid and santonin poisoning, in jaundice, and in digitalis intoxication. SYN yellow vision. [xantho- + G. *opsis,* vision]

xan·thop·sy·dra·cia (zan-thop-si-drā′sē-ă). An eruption of small yellow pustules. [G. *xanthos,* yellow + *psydrax,* a blister on the tip of the tongue]

xan·tho·puc·cine (zan-thō-pŭk′sēn). SYN canadine.

xan·tho·sine (X, Xao) (zan′thō-sēn, -sin). 9-β-D-ribosylxanthine; the deamination product of guanosine (O replacing –NH₂). SYN xanthine ribonucleoside.

x. 5′-monophosphate (XMP), the monophosphoric ester of x. An intermediate in GMP biosynthesis. SYN xanthidylic acid, xanthine nucleotide, xanthylic acid.

x. 5′-triphosphate (XTP), x. with a triphosphoric acid esterified at its 5′ position.

xan·tho·sis (zan-thō′sis). A yellowish discoloration of degenerating tissues, especially seen in malignant neoplasms. [xantho- + G. *-osis,* condition]

xan·thous (zan′thŭs). Yellowish; yellow-colored. [G. *xanthos,* yellow]

xanth·u·ren·ic ac·id (zan-thū-rēn′ik). 4,8-Dihydroxyquinoline-2-carboxylic acid; 4,8-dihydroquinaldic acid; the sulfur-yellow crystals form a red compound with Millon reagent, or an intensely green one with ferrous sulfate; excreted in the urine of pyridoxine-deficient animals after the ingestion of tryptophan, and of rats fed almost exclusively with fibrin.

xan·thu·ria (zan-thū′rē-ă). SYN xanthinuria.

xan·thyl (zan′thil). A radical consisting of xanthine minus a hydrogen atom.

xan·thyl·ic (zan-thil′ik). Relating to xanthine.

xan·thyl·ic ac·id. SYN *xanthosine* 5′-monophosphate.

Xao Symbol for xanthosine.

Xe Symbol for xenon.

¹³³Xe. Symbol for xenon-133.

△**xeno-.** Strange; foreign material; parasite. SEE hetero-, allo-. [G. *xenos,* guest, host, stranger, foreign]

xen·o·bi·ot·ic (zen′ō-bī-ot′ik). A pharmacologically, endocrinologically, or toxicologically active substance not endogenously produced and therefore foreign to an organism.

xen·o·di·ag·no·sis (zen′ō-dī-ag-nō′sis). **1.** A method of diagnosing acute or early *Trypanosoma cruzi* infection (Chagas' disease) in humans. Infection-free (laboratory-reared) triatomine bugs are fed on the suspected person and the trypanosome is identified by microscopic examination of the intestinal contents of the bug after a suitable incubation period. **2.** A similar method of biological diagnosis based upon experimental exposure of a parasite-free normal host capable of allowing the organism in question to multiply, enabling it to be more easily and reliably detected.

xen·o·gen·e·ic (zen′ō-jĕ-nē′ik). Heterologous, with respect to tissue grafts, especially when donor and recipient belong to widely separated species. SYN xenogenic (2), xenogenous (2). [xeno- + G. *-gen,* producing]

xen·o·gen·ic (zen-ō-jen′ik). **1.** Originating outside of the organism, or from a foreign substance that has been introduced into the organism. SYN xenogenous (1). **2.** SYN xenogeneic. [xeno- + G. *-gen,* producing]

xe·nog·e·nous (zĕ-noj′ĕ-nŭs). **1.** SYN xenogenic (1). **2.** SYN xenogeneic.

xen·o·graft (zen′ō-graft). A graft transferred from an animal of one species to one of another species. SYN heterograft, heterologous graft, heteroplastic graft, heterospecific graft, interspecific graft, xenogeneic graft.

xe·non (Xe) (zē′non). A gaseous element, atomic no. 54, atomic wt. 131.29; present in minute proportion (0.087 ppm) in the dry atmosphere; produces general anesthesia in concentrations of 70 vol.%. [G. *xenos,* a stranger]

xe·non-133 (¹³³Xe). A radioisotope of xenon with a gamma emission at 81 keV and a physical half-life of 5.243 days; used in the study of pulmonary function and organ blood flow.

xen·o·par·a·site (zen-ō-par′ă-sīt). An ecoparasite that becomes pathogenic in consequence of weakened resistance on the part of its host.

xen·o·pho·bia (zen-ō-fō′bē-ă). Morbid fear of strangers. [xeno- + G. *phobos,* fear]

xen·o·pho·nia (zen-ō-fō′nē-ă). A speech defect marked by an alteration in accent and intonation. [xeno- + G. *phōnē,* voice]

xen·oph·thal·mia (zen′of-thal′mē-ă). An obsolete term for inflammation excited by the presence of a foreign body in the eye.

Xen·o·psyl·la (zen-op-sil′ă). The rat flea; a genus of fleas parasitic on the rat and involved in the transmission of bubonic plague. The species *X. cheopis* serves as a potent vector of *Yersinia pestis,* largely because its gut becomes "blocked" by a mass of *Y. pestis* cells which prevents the flea from feeding normally, so that it is inclined to attack man and other hosts; it is an important source of infection in traditional epidemic areas such as India. *X. astia* and *X. braziliensis* are also efficient vectors of plague. [xeno- + G. *psylla,* flea]

xen·yl (zen′il). A radical consisting of biphenyl minus a hydrogen atom.

xe·ran·sis (zē-ran′sis). A gradual loss of moisture in the tissues. [G. *xēransis,* fr. *xēros,* dry]

xe·ran·tic (zē-ran′tik). Denoting xeransis.

xe·ra·sia (zē-rā′zē-ă). A condition of the hair characterized by dryness and brittleness. [G. *xērasia,* fr. *xēros,* dry]

△**xero-.** Dry. [G. *xeros*]

xer·o·chi·lia (zēr-ō-kī′lē-ă). Dryness of lips. [xero- + G. *cheilos,* lip]

xe·ro·der·ma (zēr′ō-der′mă). A mild form of ichthyosis characterized by excessive dryness of the skin due to slight increase of the horny layer and diminished water content of the stratum corneum from decreased perspiration, wind, or low humidity; seen with aging, atopic dermatitis, vitamin A deficiency, etc. [xero- + G. *derma,* skin]

x. pigmento′sum [MIM*278700], an eruption of exposed skin occurring in childhood and characterized by photosensitivity with severe sunburn in infancy and the development of numerous pigmented spots resembling freckles, larger atrophic lesions eventually resulting in glossy white thinning of the skin surrounded by telangiectases, and multiple solar keratoses which undergo malignant change at an early age; results from several rare autosomal recessive disorders in which DNA repair process-

differential diagnosis of xeroderma pigmentosum					
groups	later skin cancer	neurological problems	ultraviolet tolerance	endonuclease (ultraviolet-specific)	remarks
1. typical isolated x.p.	+	−	reduced	reduced	multiple alleles?
2. cases of xeroderma	+	−	normal	normal	
3. DeSanctis-Cacchione syndrome	+	++	reduced	reduced	compensation with in hybridized double-nuclei cells
4. pigmented xerodermoid	+	−	reduced	normal	possible deficiency in postreplicational repair?
5. actinic skin damage	+		?	normal	

es are defective, so that they are more liable to chromosome breaks and cancerous change when exposed to ultraviolet light. Severe ophthalmic and neurologic abnormalities are also found.

xe·ro·gram (zē′rō-gram). SYN xeroradiograph.

xe·rog·ra·phy (zēr-og′ră-fē). SYN xeroradiography.

xe·ro·ma (zē-rō′mă). SYN xerophthalmia.

xe·ro·mam·mog·ra·phy (zēr′ō-mam-og′ră-fē). Examination of the breast by xeroradiography.

xe·ro·me·nia (zēr-ō-mē′nē-ă). Obsolete term for occurrence of the usual constitutional symptoms at the menstrual period without any show of blood. [xero- + G. *mēniaia*, menses]

xe·ro·myc·te·ria (zēr′ō-mik-tēr′ē-ă). Extreme dryness of the nasal mucous membrane. [xero- + G. *myktēr*, the nose]

xe·ron·o·sus (zē-ron′ō-sŭs). SYN xerosis. [xero- + G. *nosos*, disease]

xe·ro·pha·gia, xe·roph·a·gy (zēr-ō-fā′jē-ă, zēr-of′ă-jē). The eating of dry foodstuffs; subsisting on a dry diet. [xero- + G. *phagō*, to eat]

xe·roph·thal·mia (zēr-of-thal′mē-ă). Excessive dryness of the conjunctiva and cornea, which lose their luster and become keratinized; may be due to local disease or to a systemic deficiency of vitamin A. SYN conjunctivitis arida, xeroma, xerophthalmus. [xero- + G. *ophthalmos*, eye]

xe·roph·thal·mus (zēr′of-thal′mŭs). SYN xerophthalmia.

xe·ro·ra·di·o·graph (zē-rō-rā′dē-ō-graf). The permanent record made by xeroradiography. SYN xerogram.

xe·ro·ra·di·og·ra·phy (zē′rō-rā′dē-og′ră-fē). Radiography using a specially coated charged plate instead of x-ray film, developing with a dry powder rather than liquid chemicals, and transferring the powder image onto paper for a permanent record; edge enhancement is inherent. SYN xerography.

xe·ro·sis (zē-rō′sis). Pathologic dryness of the skin (xeroderma), the conjunctiva (xerophthalmia), or mucous membranes. SYN xeronosus. [xero- + G. *-osis*, condition]

x. parenchymato′sus, superficial drying of the conjunctiva due to diffuse scarring, with closure of the lacrimal gland openings.

xe·ro·sto·mia (zēr′ō-stō′mē-ă). A dryness of the mouth, having a varied etiology, resulting from diminished or arrested salivary secretion, or asialism. [xero- + G. *stoma*, mouth]

xe·ro·tes (zē-rō′tēz). Dryness. [G. *xērotēs*]

xe·ro·tic (zē-rot′ik). Dry; affected with xerosis.

xe·ro·trip·sis (zēr-ō-trip′sis). Dry friction. [xero- + G. *tripsis*, a rubbing, fr. *tribō*, to rub]

Xg blood group. See Blood Groups appendix.

X-in·ac·ti·va·tion. SYN lyonization.

xiph-. SEE xipho-.

xiph·i·ster·nal (zif-i-ster′năl). Relating to the xiphoid process.

xiph·i·ster·num (zif′i-ster′nŭm). SYN xiphoid *process*. [xiphoid + G. *sternon*, chest]

xipho-, xiph-, xiphi-. Xiphoid, usually the processus xyphoideus. [G. *xiphos*, sword]

xiph·o·cos·tal (zif′ō-kos′tăl). Relating to the xiphoid process and the ribs. [xipho- + L. *costa*, rib]

xiph·o·dyn·ia (zif-ō-din′ē-ă). Pain of a neuralgic character, in the region of the xiphoid cartilage. SEE ALSO hypersensitive xiphoid *syndrome*. SYN xiphoidalgia. [xipho- + G. *odynē*, pain]

xi·phoid (zif′oyd). Sword-shaped; applied especially to the xiphoid process. SYN ensiform, gladiate, mucronate. [xipho- + G. *eidos*, appearance]

xi·phoi·dal·gia (zif-oy-dal′jē-ă). SYN xiphodynia. [xiphoid + G. *algos*, pain]

xi·phoi·di·tis (zif′oy-dī′tis). Inflammation of the xiphoid process of the sternum. [xiphoid + G. *-itis*, inflammation]

xi·phop·a·gus (zi-fop′ă-gŭs). Conjoined twins united in the region of the xiphoid process of the sternum. SEE conjoined *twins*, under *twin*. [xipho- + G. *pagos*, something fixed]

X-linked. Pertaining to genes borne on the X chromosome. Commonly but erroneously used synonymously with sex-linked, which would also comprise Y-linked traits.

XMP Abbreviation for *xanthosine* 5′-monophosphate.

x-o-mat (eks′ō-mat). A trade name (of Kodak) that has become the generic designation of an automatic processor for x-ray films.

x-ra·di·a·tion. Radiant energy from an x-ray tube. SEE ALSO x-ray.

x-ray. 1. The ionizing electromagnetic radiation emitted from a highly evacuated tube, resulting from the excitation of the inner orbital electrons by the bombardment of the target anode with a stream of electrons from a heated cathode. **2.** Ionizing electromagnetic radiation produced by the excitation of the inner orbital electrons of an atom by other processes, such as nuclear delay and its sequelae. **3.** A radiograph. SYN roentgen ray.

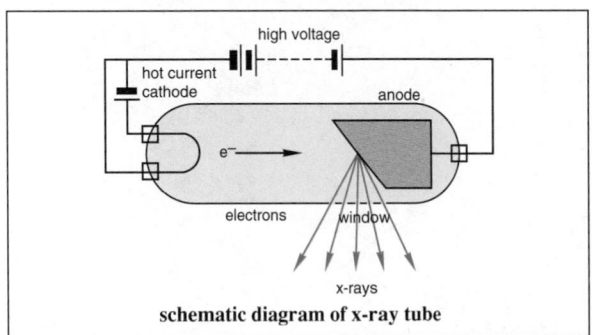

schematic diagram of x-ray tube

XTP Abbreviation for *xanthosine* 5′-triphosphate.

Xy Abbreviation for xylose.

Xyl Abbreviation for xylose.

xyl-, xylo-. Wood, woody; xylose, xylene. [G. *xylon*]

xy·la·zine (zī′lă-zēn). A sedative/hypnotic/anesthetic widely used in veterinary medicine and in laboratory animals.

xy·lene (zī′lēn). SYN xylol.

x. cyanol FF [C.I. 43535], an acidic triphenylmethane dye used for histochemical staining of hemoglobin peroxidase and as a tracking dye for DNA sequencing in electrophoresis.

xy·le·nol (zī′lĕ-nol). $(CH_3)_2C_6H_3OH$; occurring in six isomeric forms; used in the manufacture of coal tar disinfectants and synthetic resins. SYN dimethylphenol.

xy·li·dine (zī′li-dēn). $(CH_3)_2C_6H_3NH_2$; aminoxylene; aminodimethylbenzene; used as a reagent and in the manufacture of dyes.

xy·li·tol (zī′li-tol). $HOCH_2(CHOH)_5CH_2OH$; an optically inactive sugar alcohol; often used as a sugar substitute in diabetic diets; the synthesis of x. from L-xylulose is blocked in individuals with idiopathic pentosuria.

xy·li·tol de·hy·dro·gen·ase. SYN *xylulose* reductase.

△**xylo-.** SEE xyl-.

xy·lo·bi·ose (zī′lō-bī′ōs). A disaccharide of two xylose residues linked β1→4, both in pyranose rings.

xy·loi·din (zī-loy′din). SYN pyroxylin.

xy·lo·ke·tose (zī-lō-kē′tōs). SYN xylulose.

xy·lol (zī′lol). $C_6H_4(CH_3)_2$; a volatile liquid obtained from coal tar, having physical and chemical properties similar to those of benzene; it occurs as three isomers; *m*-, *o*-, and *p*-xylol; used as a solvent, in the manufacture of chemicals and synthetic fibers, and in histology as a clearing agent. SYN dimethylbenzene, xylene.

xy·lo·met·az·o·line hy·dro·chlo·ride (zī′lō-mĕ-taz′ō-lēn). 2-(4′-*tert*-Butyl-2′,6′-dimethylphenylmethyl)imidazoline hydrochloride; a sympathomimetic drug used as a nasal decongestant.

xy·lon·ic ac·id (zi′lon-ik). A mild oxidation product of xylose.

xy·lo·py·ra·nose (zī-lō-pir′ă-nōs). Xylose in pyranose form.

xy·lose (Xy, Xyl) (zī′lōs). An aldopentose, isomeric with ribose, obtained by fermentation or hydrolysis of naturally occurring carbohydrate substances, *e.g.*, in wood fiber. An important dietary component for herbivores. The D-isomer is wood or beechwood sugar. SYN uridine diphosphoxylose.

xy·lu·lose (zī′lū-lōs). *threo*-pentulose; a 2-ketopentose. L-Xylulose appears in the urine in cases of essential pentosuria; it is also an intermediate in the glucuronate pathway. SYN xyloketose.

x. 5-phosphate, the D-isomer is an intermediate in the pentose phosphate pathway and in transketolization.

x. reductase, an enzyme that reversibly converts x. to xylitol using either NADH (D-x. reductase) or NADPH (L-x. reductase); a deficiency of the L-form is seen in individuals with essential pentosuria. SYN xylitol dehydrogenase.

L-xy·lu·lo·su·ria (zī′lū-lō-sū′rē-ă). SYN essential *pentosuria*.

xy·lyl (zī′lil). The radical consisting of xylene (xylol) minus a hydrogen atom.

x. bromide, $CH_3C_6H_4CH_2Br$; the *o*-, *m*-, and *p*-forms are powerful lacrimators.

xy·lyl·ene (zī′li-lēn). The radical consisting of xylene (xylol) minus two hydrogen atoms.

xy·ro·spasm (zī′rō-spazm). SYN shaving *cramp*. [G. *xyron*, razor, fr. *xyō*, to scrape]

xys·ma (ziz′mă). Membranous shreds in the feces. [G. filings, shavings, fr. *xyō*, to scrape]

Y Symbol for yttrium; tyrosine; pyrimidine nucleoside.

y⁺. SEE system (5).

YAC Abbreviation for yeast artificial *chromosomes*, under *chromosome*.

yang (yang). SEE yin-yang.

yang·go·na (yang′gō-nă). SYN yaqona.

ya·qo·na (ya′kōnă). A Fijian drink made from the powdered root of *Piper methysticum* (family Piperaceae); excessive drinking of it causes a state of hyperexcitability and a loss of power in the legs; chronic intoxication induces roughening of the skin and a state of debility. SEE ALSO methysticum. SYN kava (2), yanggona. [Fijian name]

yaw (yau). An individual lesion of the eruption of yaws.

    mother y., a large granulomatous lesion, considered to be the initial lesion in yaws, most commonly present on the hand, leg, or foot. SYN buba madre, frambesioma, mamanpian, protopianoma.

yawn (yaun). **1.** To gape. **2.** An involuntary opening of the mouth, usually accompanied by a movement of respiration; it may be a sign of drowsiness or of vital depression, as after hemorrhage, but is often caused by suggestion. [A.S. *gānian*]

yawn·ing. The act of producing a yawn. SYN oscitation.

yaws (yawz). An infectious tropical disease caused by *Treponema pertenue* and characterized by the development of crusted granulomatous ulcers on the extremities; may involve bone, but, unlike syphilis, does not produce central nervous system or cardiovascular pathology. SEE ALSO nonvenereal *syphilis.* SYN Amboyna button, boubas, bubas, Charlouis' disease, frambesia tropica, granuloma tropicum, mycosis framboesioides, pian, polypapilloma (2), rupia (2), zymotic papilloma. [of Caribbean origin; similar to Calinago yaya, the disease]

    bosch y., SYN *pian* bois.

    bush y., SYN *pian* bois.

    crab y., SYN foot y.

    foot y., y. of the feet with keratoderma of the palms and soles and ulcer formation. SYN crab y., dumas, tubba, tubbae.

    forest y., SYN *pian* bois.

    guinea corn y., a form of y. in which the lesions resemble grains of Indian corn.

    ringworm y., round, scaling, and crusted lesions that resemble ringworm.

Yb Symbol for ytterbium.

year·ling (yēr′ling). An animal between one and two years of age; generally applied to horses and cattle.

years of po·ten·tial life lost. Measure of the relative impact of various diseases and lethal forces on society, computed by estimating the years that people would have lived if they had not died prematurely from injury, cancer, heart disease, etc.

yeast (yēst). A general term denoting true fungi of the family Saccharomycetaceae that are widely distributed in substrates that contain sugars (such as fruits), and in soil, animal excreta, the vegetative parts of plants, etc. Because of their ability to ferment carbohydrates, some y.'s are important to the brewing and baking industries. [A.S. *gyst*]

    brewers' y., y. produced by *Saccharomyces cerevisiae;* a by-product from the brewing of beer.

    compressed y., the moist living cells of *Saccharomyces cerevisiae* combined with a starchy or absorbent base.

    cultivated y., a form of y. propagated by culture and used in breadmaking, brewing, etc.

    dried y., the dry cells of a suitable strain of *Saccharomyces cerevisiae;* brewers' dried y., debittered brewers' dried y., or primary dried y. are the sources of dried y.; it contains not less than 45% of protein, and in 1 g not less than 0.3 mg of nicotinic acid, 0.04 mg riboflavin, and 0.12 mg thiamin hydrochloride; used as a dietary supplement.

    primary dried y., a source of dried y.; obtained from suitable

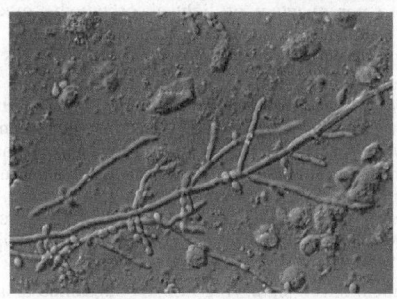

yeast (microscopic finding of urine)

strains of *Saccharomyces cerevisiae* grown in media other than those required for the production of beer.

    wild y., any of the uncultivated forms of y.'s, useless as ferments and sometimes pathogenic.

yel·low (yel′ō). A color occupying a position in the spectrum between green and orange. For individual yellow dyes see specific name. [A.S. *geolu*]

    corralin y., the sodium salt of rosolic acid.

    indicator y., a compound formed in the bleaching of rhodopsin by light; it is chrome y. at pH 3.3–4.0 and pale y. at pH 9.0–10.0.

    tumeric yellow, SYN curcumin.

    visual y., SYN all-*trans*-retinal.

yel·low root. SYN hydrastis.

yer·ba san·ta (yer′bă san′tă). SYN eriodictyon. [Sp. sacred herb]

Yer·sin·ia (yer-sin′ē-ă). A genus of motile and nonmotile, nonsporeforming bacteria (family Enterobacteriaceae) containing Gram-negative, unencapsulated, ovoid to rod-shaped cells. These organisms are nonmotile at 37°C, but some species are motile at temperatures below 30°C; motile cells are peritrichous. Citrate is not used as a sole source of carbon. These organisms are parasitic on humans and other animals. The type species is *Y. pestis.* [A. J. E. Yersin, Swiss bacteriologist, 1862–1943]

    Y. enterocolit′ica, a species that causes yersiniosis in humans; it is found in the feces and lymph nodes of sick and healthy animals, including humans, in material likely to be contaminated with feces, and in the cadavers of cattle, rabbits, hares, dogs, guinea pigs, horses, monkeys, pigs, and sheep.

    Y. frederikse′nii, reclassified from *Y. enterocolitica;* rare cause of enterocolitis in humans.

    Y. interme′dia, reclassified from *Y. enterocolitica;* rare cause of enterocolitis in humans.

    Y. kristense′nii, reclassified from *Y. enterocolitica;* pathogenicity uncertain.

    Y. pes′tis, a species causing plague in humans, rodents, and many other mammalian species, and transmitted from rat to rat and from rat to man by the rat flea, *Xenopsylla;* it is the type species of the genus *Y.* SYN Kitasato's bacillus, *Pasteurella pestis,* plague bacillus.

    Y. pseudotuberculo′sis, a species causing pseudotuberculosis in birds, rodents, and rarely in humans. SYN *Pasteurella pseudotuberculosis.*

yer·sin·i·o·sis (yer-sin-ē-ō′sis). A common human infectious disease caused by *Yersinia enterocolitica* and marked by diarrhea, enteritis, pseudoappendicitis, ileitis, erythema nodosum, and sometimes septicemia or acute arthritis.

    pseudotubercular y., SYN pseudotuberculosis.

yield (yēld). The amount or quantity produced or returned, often measured as a percent of the starting material; *e.g.,* a y. in an enzyme preparation is equal to the units of enzyme activity recovered at the end of the preparation divided by the total units observed in the starting material.

yi

quantum y. (φ), the number of molecules transformed (*e.g.,* via a reaction) per quantum of light absorbed; the inverse of the quantum requirement. SYN quantum efficiency.

yin-yang (yin'yang). In ancient Chinese thought, the concept of two complementary and opposing influences, Yin and Yang, underlying and controlling all nature, the aim of Chinese medicine being to produce proper balance between them. Used in modern terms to characterize any dualistic, reciprocal control system in which one influence tends to promote things that the opposing influence tends to inhibit, and vice versa; *e.g.,* the yin-yang hypothesis of biological control in which cyclic GMP and cyclic AMP are supposed to act in this dualistic, reciprocal way in controlling cellular functions.

△**-yl.** Chemical suffix signifying that the substance is a radical by loss of an H atom (*e.g.,* alkyl, methyl, phenyl) or OH group (*e.g.,* acyl, acetyl, carbamoyl).

△**-ylene.** Chemical suffix denoting a bivalent hydrocarbon radical (*e.g.,* methylene, $-CH_2-$) or possessing a double bond (*e.g.,* ethylene, $CH_2=CH_2$).

yl·ides (il'idz). A class of compounds in which a positively charged negative element from group V or VI of the periodic table (*e.g.,* N, O, S, P) is bonded to a carbon atom having an unshared pair of electrons; ylides have been observed in a number of enzyme-catalyzed reactions.

Y-link·age. The state of a genetic factor (gene) being borne on the Y chromosome. This idea is analogous with X-linkage but since the Y chromosome does not fully take part in chiasma formation and recombination, it not amenable to analysis by conventional linkage methods. Little is known about its content. There is a gene for the H-Y antigen, and indirect arguments suggest that there is a principle that determines the formation of the testis and masculinization of the fetus but its localization, though narrowing the limits, remains elusive.

yo·gurt, yo·ghurt (yō'gert). Fermented, partially evaporated, whole milk prepared by maintaining it at 50°C for 12 hours after the addition of a mixed culture of *Lactobacillus bulgaricus*, *L. acidophilus*, and *Streptococcus lactis;* used as a food. [Turkish]

yo·him·bine (yō-him'bēn). An alkaloid, the active principle of yohimbe, the bark of *Corynanthe yohimbi* (family Rubiaceae); it produces a competitive blockade, of limited duration, of adrenergic α-receptors; has also been used for its alleged aphrodisiac properties.

yoke (yōk). SYN jugum (1). [A.S. *geoc*]
　alveolar y., SYN *jugum* alveolare.

yolk (yōk, yōlk). **1.** One of the types of nutritive material stored in the ovum for the nutrition of the embryo; y. is particularly abundant and conspicuous in the eggs of birds. SYN vitellus. **2.** Fatty material found in the wool of sheep; when extracted and purified, it becomes lanolin. [A.S. *geolca; geolu,* yellow]
　white y., y. consisting of much finer particles than those of yellow y.; thin layers of it lie between the zones of yellow y. and form the latebra.
　yellow y., the chief constituent of the y. in a bird's egg; it consists of relatively coarse particles of stored food materials and is laid down in concentric zones with interposed thin layers of white y.

Yorke's au·to·lyt·ic re·ac·tion. See under reaction.

Young, Hugh H., U.S. urologist, 1870–1945. SEE Y. prostatic *tractor.*

Young, Thomas, English physician and physicist, 1773–1829. SEE Y.'s *modulus, rule;* Y.-Helmholtz *theory* of color vision.

Young, William John, 20th century Australian biochemist. SEE Harden-Y. *ester.*

YPLL Abbreviation for years of potential life lost.

yp·sil·i·form (ip'si-li-fōrm). SYN hypsiloid. [G. *ypsilon, upsilon,* the letter u or y, + L. *forma,* form]

yt·ter·bi·um (Yb) (i-ter'bē-ŭm). A metallic element of the lanthanide group; atomic no. 70, atomic wt. 173.04. [169]Yb, with a half-life of 32.03 days, has been used in cisternography and in brain scans. [*Ytterby,* village in Sweden]

yt·tri·um (Y) (it're-ŭm). A metallic element, atomic no. 39, atomic wt. 88.90585. [*Ytterby,* village in Sweden]

yt·tri·um-90. An artificial radioactive isotope with a physical half-life of 2.67 days which decays with the emission of a 2.282 Mev β particle; used as an implant in pituitary ablation.

Yvon, Paul, French physician and chemist, 1848–1913. SEE Y.'s *test.*

Z Abbreviation for benzyloxycarbonyl (carbobenzoxy); atomic *number*; symbol for an amino acid that is either glutamic acid, glutamine, or a substance that yields glutamic acid on acid hydrolysis of peptides (*e.g.,* 4-carboxyglutamate or 5-oxoproline); carbobenzoxy; in italics, zusammen.

Z_{O_2} Symbol for microliters of oxygen taken up per hour by 10^8 spermatozoa; can vary as a function of temperature.

z. Abbreviation for zepto-.

Zaffaroni, Alejandro, Uruguayan-U.S. chemist and biochemist, *1923. SEE Zaffaroni *system.*

Zaglas, John, 19th century anatomist's assistant in Edinburgh. SEE Z.'s *ligament.*

Zahn, Friedrich W., German pathologist, 1845–1904. SEE Z.'s *infarct; lines* of Z., under *line; striae* of Z. under *stria.*

Zambusch, Leo von, 20th century German physician. SEE generalized pustular *psoriasis* of Z.

Zappert, Julius, Austrian physician, 1867–1942. SEE Z. counting *chamber.*

zea (zē´ă). The styles and stigmas of *Zea mays* (family Gramineae), Indian corn; formerly used as a diuretic and antispasmodic. SYN cornsilk, stigmata maydis. [Mod. L. maize]

ze·ral·e·none (zē´ă-ral-en-ōn). One of the resorcylic acid lactones; used in veterinary medicine as an anabolic.

ze·a·tin (zē´ă-tin). 6-(*trans*-4-Hydroxy-3-methyl-2-butenylamino)purine; a cytokinin first isolated from kernels of sweet corn. SYN maize factor.

ze·a·xan·thin (zē´ă-zan´thin). β,β-carotene-3,3′-diol; a carotene found in corn, fruits, seeds, and egg yolk; isomeric with xanthophyll. SYN zeaxanthol. [Mod. L. *Zea,* Indian corn, fr. L. *zea,* grain + G. *xanthos,* yellow, + -in]

ze·ax·an·thol (zē-ă-za-thol). SYN zeaxanthin.

Zeeman, Pieter, Dutch physicist and Nobel laureate, 1865–1943. SEE Z. *effect.*

ZEEP Abbreviation for zero end-expiratory *pressure.*

ze·in (zē´in). A prolamine present in maize; it lacks chiefly the amino acids L-tryptophan and L-lysine, and is low in cysteine content.

Zeis, Eduard, Dresden ophthalmologist, 1807–1868. SEE Z.'s *glands,* under *gland;* zeisian *sty.*

zeis·i·an (zīs´ē-ăn). Relating to or described by Eduard Zeis.

Zeit·geist (zīt´gīst). In psychology, the climate of opinion, conventions of thought, covert influences, and unquestioned assumptions that are implicit in a given culture, the arts, or science at any point in time, and in which the individual operates and thus is influenced. [Ger. *zeit,* time, + *geist,* spirit]

Zellweger, Hans U., U.S. pediatrician, *1909. SEE Z. *syndrome.*

ze·lo·pho·bia (zē-lō-fō´bē-ă). Morbid fear of jealousy. [G. *zēlos,* zeal, + *phobos,* fear]

ze·lo·typ·ia (zē-lō-tip´ē-ă). Excessive zeal, carried to the point of morbidity, in the advocacy of any cause. [G. *zēlotypia;* rivalry, envy, fr. *zēlos,* zeal, + *typtō,* to strike]

Zenker, Friedrich A., German pathologist, 1825–1898. SEE Z.'s *degeneration, diverticulum, fixative, necrosis, paralysis;* formol-Z. *fixative.*

ze·o·lite (zē´ō-līt). A naturally occurring hydrated sodium aluminum silicate, $Na_2O·Al_2O_3·(SiO_2)_x·(H_2O)_x$, used for softening of ha rd water by exchanging its Na^+ for the Ca^{2+} of the water; thus z. is an ion exchanger. Some synthetic ion exchangers are termed synthetic z.'s, although there is no chemical relationship.

ze·o·scope (zē´ō-skōp). A device for determining the alcoholic content of a liquid by ascertaining its exact boiling point. [G. *zeō,* to boil, + *skopeō,* to examine]

zep·to- (**z.**). Prefix used in the SI and metric systems to signify 10^{-21}.

ze·ro (zē´rō). **1.** The figure 0, indicating the absence of magnitude, or nothing. **2.** In thermometry, the point from which the figures on the scale start in one or the other direction; in the Celsius and Réaumur scales, z. indicates the freezing point for distilled water; in the Fahrenheit scale, it is 32° below the freezing point of water. [Sp. fr. Ar. *sifr,* cipher]

absolute z., the lowest possible temperature, that at which the form of translational motion constituting heat is assumed no longer to exist, determined as −273.15°C or 0 Kelvin.

ze·ro grav·i·ty (zē-rō-grav´i-tē). A physical state existing in space or at a time in flight when the centrifugal thrust of a parabolic glide or turn exactly counteracts the force of gravity.

ze·ta (zāt´a). **1.** 6th Letter of the Greek alphabet, ζ **2.** In chemistry, denotes the sixth in a series, *e.g.,* the sixth carbon from a functional group. **3.** Symbol for electrokinetic potential.

ze·ta·crit (zā´tă-krit). The packed cell volume produced by vertical centrifugation of blood in capillary tubes, allowing controlled compaction and dispersion of red blood cells; read with a hematocrit to produce the zeta sedimentation ratio.

ze·ta·pro·tein. SYN fibronectins.

zeug·ma·tog·ra·phy (zūg-mă-tog´ră-fē). Term coined by Lauterbur in 1972 for the joining of a magnetic field and spatially defined radiofrequency field gradients to generate a two-dimensional display of proton density and relaxation times in tissues, the first nuclear magnetic resonance image. [G. *zeugma,* that which joins together]

zi·do·vu·dine (zī-dō´vū-dēn). $C_{10}H_{13}N_5O_4$; a thymidine analogue that is an inhibitor of *in vitro* replication of HIV virus, the causative agent of AIDS and ARC, and is used in the management of these diseases. SYN azidothymidine.

Ziegler, S. Louis, U.S. ophthalmologist, 1861–1925.

Ziehen, Georg T., German psychiatrist, 1862–1950. SEE Z.-Oppenheim *disease.*

Ziehl, Franz, German bacteriologist, 1857–1926. SEE Z.'s *stain;* Z.-Neelsen *stain.*

Ziemann, Hans R.P., German pathologist, *1865. SEE Z.'s *dots,* under *dot, stippling.*

Zieve, Leslie, U.S. physician, *1915. SEE Z.'s *syndrome.*

Zimmerlin, Franz, Swiss physician, 1858–1932. SEE Z.'s *atrophy.*

Zimmermann, Karl W., German histologist, 1861–1935. SEE Z.'s *corpuscle, granule,* elementary *particle;* polkissen of Z.

Zimmermann, Wilhelm, German physician, *1910. SEE Z. *reaction, test.*

zinc (Zn) (zingk). A metallic element, atomic no. 30, atomic wt. 65.39; an essential bioelement; a number of salts of z. are used in medicine; a cofactor in many proteins. [Ger. *Zink*]

z. acetate, $Zn(C_2H_3O_2)2H_2O$; an emetic, styptic, and astringent.

z. caprylate, a topical antifungal compound.

z. chloride, $ZnCl_2$; formerly used as a caustic for the removal of cutaneous cancers, nevi, etc., and in weak solution in the treatment of gonorrhea and conjunctivitis. SYN butter of zinc.

z. gelatin, z. oxide, gelatin, glycerin, and purified water; used topically as a protectant.

z. iodide, ZnI_2; has been used as an antiseptic and astringent.

medicinal z. peroxide, a mixture of z. peroxide, z. carbonate, and z. hydroxide; a topical disinfectant, astringent, and deodorant.

z. oxide, ZnO; used as a protective in ointment, as a dusting powder; also used in paint as a substitute for lead carbonate. SYN flowers of zinc, z. white.

z. oxide and eugenol, used as a base material beneath metallic dental restorations and as a temporary filling material or impression material; setting and hardening result from complex reactions between the powder and the eugenol.

z. permanganate, action is similar to that of potassium permanganate, but more astringent; used in urethritis, by injection or douche in a 1:4000 solution.

z. peroxide, ZnO_2; a yellowish white powder, insoluble in water

zi

and decomposed by acids; used in pharmaceutical preparations. SYN z. superoxide.

z. phenolsulfonate, used as an intestinal antiseptic and locally as an astringent in chronic inflammation of the mucous membranes. SYN z. sulfocarbolate.

z. phosphide, Zn_3P_2; used as a bait poison for the extermination of rats and mice.

z. stearate, a z. compound with variable proportions of stearic and palmitic acids; a water-repellent, protective agent used in powders and ointments in the treatment of eczema, acne, and other skin diseases.

z. sulfate, $ZnSO_4 \cdot 7H_2O$; used as a local astringent in the treatment of gonorrhea, indolent ulcers, conjunctivitis, and various skin diseases, and internally as an emetic.

z. sulfocarbolate, SYN z. phenolsulfonate.

z. superoxide, SYN z. peroxide.

z. undecylenate, z. undecenoate, $[CH_2=CH(CH_2)_8COO]_2Zn$; the z. salt of undecylenic acid; used in the treatment of fungal and other affections of the skin, including psoriasis.

z. white, SYN z. oxide.

zinc-65 (^{65}**Zn**). A radioactive zinc isotope that decays mainly by K-capture with a half-life of 243.8 days; used as a tracer in studies of zinc metabolism.

zinc·if·er·ous (zing-kif'er-ŭs). Containing zinc.

zinc·oid (zing'koyd). Relating to or resembling zinc. [G. *eidos,* resemblance]

zin·gi·ber (zin'ji-ber). SYN ginger.

Zinn, Johann G., German anatomist, 1727–1759. SEE Z.'s *artery, vascular circle, corona, ligament, membrane, ring, tendon, zonule.*

Zinsser, Hans, U.S. bacteriologist and immunologist, 1878–1940. SEE Brill-Z. *disease.*

zir·co·ni·um (Zr) (zir-kō'nē-ŭm). A metallic element, atomic no. 40, atomic wt. 91.224; widely distributed in nature, but never found in quantity in any one place. [*zircon,* a mineral, fr. Ar. *zarkūn,* cinnabar, Pers, *zargun,* goldlike]

zir·co·ni·um ox·ide. Used as a coating for the skin in dermatologic pharmaceuticals and as a pigment in paints.

zm. Abbreviation for zeptometer.

Zn Symbol for zinc.

^{65}**Zn.** Abbreviation for zinc-65.

⌂**zo-.** SEE ZOO-.

zo·ac·an·tho·sis (zō'ă-kan-thō'sis). A cutaneous eruption due to introduction into the human skin of hair, bristles, stingers, etc., of lower animals. [G. *zōon,* animal, + acanthosis]

zo·am·y·lin (zō-am'i-lin). Former term for glycogen. [G. *zōē,* life, + *amylon,* starch]

zo·an·throp·ic (zō-an-throp'ik). Relating to or marked by zoanthropy.

zo·an·thro·py (zō-an'thrō-pē). A delusion that one is an animal, such as a dog. [G. *zōon,* animal, + *anthrōpos,* man]

zo·et·ic (zō-et'ik). Relating to life. [G. *zōē,* life]

zo·ic (zō'ik). Relating to living things; having life. [G. *zōikos,* relating to an animal]

zo·ite (zō'īt). SYN sporozoite. [G. *zōon,* animal]

Zollinger, Robert M., U.S. surgeon, *1903. SEE Z.-Ellison *syndrome, tumor.*

Zöllner, Johann F., German physicist, 1834–1882. SEE Z.'s *lines,* under *line.*

Zol·pi·dem (zol'pē-dĕm). A sedative/hypnotic drug useful for treating anxiety and resembling benzodiazepines in its pharmacology but differing somewhat in chemical structure. Unlike benzodiazepines, Z. lacks prominent anticonvulsant properties, and less tolerance may develop with its use.

zo·me·pir·ac so·di·um (zō-mĕ-pir'ak). Sodium 5-(*p*-chlorodoenzoyl)-1,4-dimethylpyrrole-2-acet ate dihydrate; an analgesic anti-inflammatory agent, no longer marketed.

zo·na, pl. **zo·nae** (zō'nă, zō'nē). **1.** SYN zone. **2.** SYN *herpes* zoster. [L. fr. G. *zōnē,* a girdle, one of the zones of the sphere]

z. arcua'ta, SYN arcuate *zone.*

z. cilia'ris, SYN ciliary *zone.*

z. coro'na, SYN costal *fringe.*

z. dermat'ica, a ridge of thickened skin surrounding the protrusion in spina bifida.

z. epitheliosero'sa, the membranous ring, within the z. dermatica, surrounding the protrusion in spina bifida.

z. facia'lis, herpes zoster involving the face.

z. fascicula'ta, the layer of radially arranged cell cords in the cortical portion of the suprarenal gland, between the z. glomerulosa and z. reticularis; secretes cortisol and dehydroepiandrosterone.

z. glomerulo'sa, the outer layer of the cortex of the suprarenal gland just beneath the capsule; secretes aldosterone.

z. hemorrhoida'lis, SYN hemorrhoidal *zone.*

z. ig'nea, SYN *herpes* zoster.

z. incer'ta [NA], a flat, obliquely disposed plate of gray matter in the subthalamic region situated between the thalamic fasciculus (tegmental field H_1 of Forel) and the lenticular fasciculus (tegmental field H_2). Medially, cells of this nucleus are adjacent to the prerubral area (tegmental field H) and, laterally, they are continuous with the reticular nucleus of the thalamus. Z. i. is a derivative of the ventral thalamus; it receives afferents from the precentral motor cortex and the cerebellum.

z. medullovasculo'sa, the fissured segment of the spinal cord that dorsally closes the sac in meningomyelocele.

z. ophthal'mica, herpes zoster in the distribution of the ophthalmic nerve.

z. orbicula'ris [NA], fibers of the articular capsule of the hip joint encircling the neck of the femur. SYN orbicular zone, ring ligament, zonular band.

z. pectina'ta, SYN pectinate *zone.*

z. pellu'cida, a layer consisting of microvilli of the oocyte, cellular processes of follicular cells, and an intervening substance rich in glycoprotein; it appears homogeneous and translucent under the light microscope. SYN pellucid zone.

z. perfora'ta, SYN *foramina* nervosa, under *foramen.*

z. pupilla'ris, SYN pupillary *zone.*

z. radia'ta, SYN z. striata.

z. reticula'ris, the inner layer of the cortex of the adrenal gland, where the cell cords anastomose in a netlike fashion.

z. serpigino'sa, SYN *herpes* zoster.

z. stria'ta, the thickened cell membrane of the ovum in forms, such as certain amphibia, in which it appears radially striated under the light microscope; with the electron microscope the striations can be seen to be microvilli. SYN membrana striata, striated membrane, z. radiata.

z. tec'ta, SYN arcuate *zone.*

z. vasculo'sa, SYN vascular *zone.*

zon·al (zō'năl). Relating to a zone.

zo·na·ry (zō'nar-ē). Relating to or having the form of a zone or belt.

zon·ate (zō'nāt). Zoned; ringed; having concentric layers of differing texture or pigmentation.

Zondek, Bernhardt, German obstetrician and gynecologist, 1891–1966. SEE Aschheim-Z. *test.*

ZONE

zone (zōn). A segment; any encircling or beltlike structure, either external or internal, longitudinal or transverse. SEE ALSO area, band, region, space, spot. SYN zona (1). [L. *zona*]

abdominal z.'s, SYN abdominal *regions,* under *region.*

androgenic z., (1) SYN X z. (1). **(2)** SYN fetal reticularis (2). SYN fetal adrenal *cortex.* [Named in the belief (as yet unsubstantiated) that the cells within this zone secrete androgens.]

arcuate z., the inner third of the basilar membrane of the cochlear duct extending from the tympanic lip of the osseous spiral lamina to the outer pillar cell of the spiral organ (of Corti). SYN zona arcuata, zona tecta.

Barnes' z., the lower fourth of the pregnant uterus, attachment of the placenta to any part of which may cause dangerous hemorrhage. SYN cervical z.

cervical z., SYN Barnes' z.

cervical z. of tooth, SYN *neck* of tooth.

ciliary z., the outer, wider z. of the anterior surface of the iris, separated from the pupillary z. by the collarette. SYN zona ciliaris.

comfort z., the temperature range between 28°C and 30°C at which the naked body is able to maintain the heat balance without either shivering or sweating; in the clothed body the range is from 13°C to 21°C.

z.'s of discontinuity, concentric z.'s of varying optical density in the lens of the eye, as seen in slitlamp biomicroscopy.

dolorogenic z., SYN trigger *point.*

entry z., the area of the dorsal funiculus of the spinal cord, medial to the tip of the posterior horn, in which the entering fibers of the posterior nerve root divide into ascending and descending branches.

ependymal z., SYN ependymal *layer.*

epileptogenic z., a cortical region which on stimulation reproduces the patient's spontaneous seizure or aura.

equivalence z., in a precipitin reaction, the z. in which neither antibody nor antigen is in excess. SEE ALSO precipitation. SYN equivalence point.

erogenous z.'s, erotogenic z.'s, areas of the body such as genitals and nipples which elicit sexual arousal when stimulated.

fetal z., SYN fetal adrenal *cortex.*

gingival z., that portion of the oral mucosa which surrounds the teeth and is firmly attached to the underlying alveolar bone.

Golgi z., (1) part of the cytoplasm occupied by the Golgi apparatus; (2) in secretory cells of exocrine glands, a z. between the nucleus and the luminal surface.

grenz z. (grents), in histopathology, a narrow layer beneath the epidermis that is not infiltrated or involved in the same way as are the lower layers of the dermis. [Ger. *Grenze,* borderline, boundary]

Head's z.'s, SYN Head's *lines,* under *line.*

hemorrhoidal z., the part of the anal canal that contains the rectal venous plexus. SYN annulus hemorrhoidalis, zona hemorrhoidalis.

interpalpebral z., the exposed area of the cornea and sclera between the lids of the open eye.

intertubular z., the dentinal matrix which lies between z.'s of peritubular dentin; it is less calcified and contains larger collagen fibers than does peritubular dentin.

isoelectric z., the range of H− ion concentration (pH) over which isoelectric precipitation occurs.

isopycnic z., the region in density gradient centrifugation having the same density as the buoyant density of the macromolecule.

language z., a large area of the cerebral cortex on the left side (in right-handed persons) considered by some to embrace all the centers of memories and associations connected with language.

latent z., that portion of the cerebral cortex, the stimulation of which produces no movement and a lesion of which produces no symptoms; mainly the more anterior areas of the frontal lobes.

Lissauer's marginal z., SYN dorsolateral *fasciculus.*

Looser's z.'s, SYN Looser's *lines,* under *line.*

mantle z., (1) SYN mantle *layer.* (2) a layer of small B lymphocytes surrounding the paler-staining germinal centers of lymphoid follicles.

Marchant's z., the area on the sphenoid and occipital bones at the base of the skull from which the dura mater is readily detached.

marginal z., SYN marginal *layer.*

motor z., that portion of the cerebral cortex, primarily the posterior region of the frontal lobe, near the central sulcus, which when stimulated produces a movement and when injured produces spasticity or paralysis.

neutral z., in dentistry, the potential space between the lips and cheeks on one side and the tongue on the other; natural or artificial teeth in this z. are subject to equal and opposite forces from the surrounding musculature.

nucleolar z., SYN nucleolar *organizer.*

Obersteiner-Redlich z., the narrow line along the course of a nerve (or nerve root) where the Schwann cells and connective tissue that support its axons are replaced by glia cells. The z. marks the true boundary between the central and the peripheral nervous system. Usually located at or near the surface of the spinal cord or brainstem, it can extend (*e.g.,* in the eighth nerve) several millimeters out along the nerve. SYN Obersteiner-Redlich line.

orbicular z., SYN *zona* orbicularis.

pectinate z., the outer two-thirds of the basilar membrane of the cochlear duct. SYN zona pectinata.

pellucid z., SYN *zona* pellucida.

peritubular z., the dentinal matrix surrounding the odontoblastic process; it is more highly calcified and contains finer collagen fibers than does the rest of the dentinal matrix.

polar z., the region in the vicinity of an electrode applied to the body. SEE ALSO electrotonus.

protective z., the time in the cardiac cycle, immediately following the vulnerable period, during which a second stimulus will prevent the initiation of ventricular fibrillation by a previous stimulus applied during the vulnerable period, probably by blocking a reentrant pathway.

pupillary z., the central region of the anterior surface of the iris located between the collarette and the pupillary margin. SYN zona pupillaris.

reflexogenic z., the area or z. where stimulation will elicit a given reflex.

secondary X z., an adrenocortical z., situated in the inner zona fasciculata, that appears upon postpubertal gonadectomy in some male rodents, most notably the mouse; the development of this z. is believed to be stimulated by pituitary gonadotropins.

segmental z., in a young embryo, the thickened dorsal portion of the undifferentiated paraxial mesoderm which becomes metamerically divided to form the mesodermal somites. SYN segmental plate.

Spitzka's marginal z., SYN dorsolateral *fasciculus.*

subplasmalemmal dense z., SYN corneocyte *envelope.*

sudanophobic z., a z. of cells, at the periphery of the zona fasciculata in the adrenal cortex of the rat, that is not stained by Sudan dyes.

tender z.'s, SYN Head's *lines,* under *line.*

thymus-dependent z., SYN paracortex.

trabecular z., SYN trabecular *reticulum.*

transformation z., z. on the cervix at which squamous epithelium and columnar epithelium meet; changes location in response to a woman's hormonal status.

transitional z., (1) the equatorial region of the lens of the eye where the anterior epithelial cells become transformed into lens fibers; (2) that portion of a scleral contact lens between the corneal and scleral sections.

trigger z., SYN trigger *point.*

trophotropic z. of Hess, an area in the hypothalamus concerned with rewarding bodily sensations.

vascular z., an area in the external acoustic meatus where a number of minute blood vessels enter from the mastoid bone. SYN spongy spot, zona vasculosa.

vermilion z., vermilion transitional z., SYN vermilion *border.*

Weil's basal z., SYN Weil's basal *layer.*

Wernicke's z., SYN Wernicke's *center.*

z. 1, 2, 3, 4 of West, in pulmonary physiology, defines the levels in a vertical lung according to the relationships of alveolar gas pressure, capillary blood pressure, and pulmonary venous pressure.

X z., (1) a transient adrenocortical z. present in some rodents at birth, most notably in mice, situated between the zona reticularis and the adrenal medulla; it degenerates in males with the secretion at puberty and in females during their first pregnancy; it slowly enlarges in unmated females after puberty and does not

ZO

degenerate until middle age; the X z. appears to secrete no hormone; SYN androgenic z. (1). **(2)** misnomer for the fetal adrenal *cortex* of primates. SYN fetal reticularis (3).

zo·nes·the·sia (zōn-es-thē′zē-ă). A sensation as if a cord were drawn around the body, constricting it. SYN cincture sensation, girdle sensation, strangalesthesia. [G. *zōnē*, girdle, + *aisthēsis*, sensation]

zo·nif·u·gal (zō-nif′yū-găl). Passing from within any region outward; as in mapping out an area of disturbed sensation, when the stimulus is first applied to the affected region and is carried into the area where sensation is normal. [L. *zona*, zone, + *fugio*, to flee]

zon·ing (zōn′ing). The occurrence of a stronger reaction in a lesser amount of suspected serum, observed sometimes in serologic tests used in the diagnosis of syphilis, and probably the result of high antibody titer.

zo·nip·e·tal (zō-nip′ĕ-tăl). Passing from without toward and into any region; as in mapping out an area of disturbed sensation, when the stimulus begins in a normal area and is carried into the affected region. [L. *zona*, zone, + *peto*, to seek]

zon·og·ra·phy (zō-nog′ră-fē). A form of tomography with a relatively thick plane of focus; especially used in renal radiography. [zone + G. *graphō*, to write]

zo·no·skel·e·ton (zō′nō-skel′ĕ-tŏn). The proximal skeletal segments of the limbs, *i.e.*, scapula, clavicle, hip *bone*. [L. *zona*, zone, + skeleton]

zo·nu·la, pl. **zo·nu·lae** (zō′nyū-lă, zon′yū-; -lē) [NA]. SYN zonule. [L. dim. of *zona*, zone]

z. adhe′rens, a belt-like desmosomal attachment between columnar epithelial cells, upon which filaments attach. SYN intermediate junction.

z. cilia′ris [NA], SYN ciliary *zonule*.

z. occlu′dens, tight junctions formed by the fusion of integral proteins of the lateral cell membranes of adjacent epithelial cells, limiting transepithelial permeability.

zo·nu·lar (zō′nyū-lăr, zon′yū-). Relating to a zonula.

zon·ule (zō′nyūl, zon′yūl). A small zone. SYN zonula [NA].

ciliary z., a series of delicate meridional fibers arising from the inner surface of the orbiculus ciliaris that run in bundles between, and in a very thin layer over, the ciliary processes; at the inner border of the corona, the fibers diverge into two groups that are attached to the capsule on the anterior and posterior surfaces of the lens close to the equator; the spaces between these two layers of fibers are filled with aqueous humor. SYN zonula ciliaris [NA], apparatus suspensorius lentis, suspensory ligament of lens, Zinn's z.

Zinn's z., SYN ciliary z.

zo·nu·li·tis (zō-nyū-lī′tis). Assumed inflammation of the zonule of Zinn, or suspensory ligament of the lens of the eye. [zonule + G. *-itis*, inflammation]

zo·nu·lol·y·sis, zo·nu·ly·sis (zō′nyū-lol′i-sis, -lī′sis). Dissolution of the zonula ciliaris by enzymes (α-chymotrypsin) to facilitate surgical removal of a cataract. SYN Barraquer's method. [zonule + G. *lysis*, dissolution]

⌂zoo-, zo-. Animal, animal life. [G. *zōon*]

zo·o·an·thro·po·no·sis (zō′ō-an′thrō-pō-nō′sis). A zoonosis normally maintained by humans but which can be transmitted to other vertebrates (*e.g.*, amebiasis to dogs, tuberculosis). Cf. anthropozoonosis, amphixenosis. [zoo- + G. *anthrōpos*, man, + *nosos*, disease]

zo·o·blast (zō′-ō-blast). An animal cell. [zoo- + G. *blastos*, germ]

zo·o·chrome (zō′ō-krōm). A naturally occurring animal pigment; includes human pigments. [zoo- + G. *derma*, skin]

zo·o·der·mic (zō-ō-der′mik). Relating to the skin of an animal. [zoo- + G. *derma*, skin]

zo·o·e·ras·tia (zō′ō-ĕ-ras′tē-ă). SYN bestiality. [zoo- + G. *erastēs*, lover]

zo·o·ful·vin (zō′ō-fŭl′vin). A yellow pigment obtained from the feathers of certain birds.

zo·o·gen·e·sis (zō-ō-jen′ĕ-sis). The doctrine of animal production or generation. [zoo- + G. *genesis*, origin]

zo·o·ge·og·ra·phy (zō′ō-jē-og′ră-fē). The geography of animals; the study of the distribution of animals on the earth's surface.

zo·o·glea (zō-og′lē-ă, zō-ō-glē′ă). In bacteriology, an old term for a mass of bacteria held together by a clear gelatinous substance. [zoo- + G. *glia*, glue]

zo·og·o·nous (zō-oj′ŏ-nŭs). SYN viviparous.

zo·og·o·ny (zō-oj′ŏ-nē). SYN viviparity.

zo·o·graft (zō′ō-graft). A graft of tissue from an animal to a human. SYN animal graft, zooplastic graft.

zo·o·graft·ing (zō-ō-graft′ing). SYN zooplasty.

zo·oid (zō′oyd). **1.** Resembling an animal; an organism or object with an animal-like appearance. **2.** An animal cell capable of independent existence or movement, as the ovum or a spermatozoon, or the segment of a tapeworm. **3.** An individual of a colonial invertebrate, such as a coral. [G. *zoōdēs*, fr. *zōon*, animal, + *eidos*, resemblance]

zo·o·lag·nia (zō-ō-lag′nē-ă). Sexual attraction toward animals. [zoo- + G. *lagneia*, lust]

zo·o·lite, zo·o·lith (zō′ō-līt, zō-ō-lith). A petrified animal. [zoo- + G. *lithos*, stone]

zo·ol·o·gist (zō-ol′ō-jist). One who specializes in zoology.

zo·ol·o·gy (zō-ol′ō-jē). The biology of animals. [zoo- + G. *logos*, study]

zoom (zūm). The action of a varifocal lens system in a camera or microscope that maintains an object in focus while approaching it or receding from it; this effect may be obtained by moving two or more of the lens components at rates bearing a linear relation to one another.

zo·o·ma·nia (zō-ō-mā′nē-ă). An excessive, abnormal love of animals. [zoo- + G. *mania*, frenzy]

zo·o·mar·ic ac·id (zō′ō-mer-ik). SYN palmitoleic acid.

Zo·o·mas·tig·i·na (zō′ō-mas-ti-jī′nă). SYN Zoomastigophorea. [zoo- + G. *mastix*, whip]

Zo·o·mas·ti·go·pho·ras·i·da (zō′ō-mas-ti-gō-fō-ras′i-dă). SYN Zoomastigophorea.

Zo·o·mas·ti·go·pho·rea (zō′ō-mas-ti-gō-fō′rē-ă). A class of flagellates (superclass Mastigophora) within the phylum Sarcomastigophora (flagellate and ameboid protozoans), of animallike as opposed to plantlike characteristics. Chromatophores are absent; one to many flagella are found, although they may be absent in ameboid forms; sexuality is known in some groups. It includes many human parasites such as the trypanosomes and trichomonads, as well as a number of other parasitic and symbiotic forms. SYN Zoomastigina, Zoomastigophorasida. [zoo- + G. *mastix*, whip, + *phoros*, bearing]

zo·om·y·lus (zō-om′i-lŭs). Obsolete term for dermoid *cyst*. [zoo- + G. *mylos*, stone]

Zoon, Johannes Jacobus, Dutch dermatologist, *1902. SEE *balanitis* of Z.; Z.'s *erythroplasia*.

zo·o·no·sis (zō-ō-nō′sis). An infection or infestation shared in nature by humans and other animals that are the normal or usual host; a disease of humans acquired from an animal source. SEE ALSO anthropozoonosis, cyclozoonosis, metazoonosis, saprozoonosis, zooanthroponosis. [zoo- + G. *nosos*, disease]

direct z., a z. transmitted between animal and humans from an infected to a susceptible host by contact, by airborne droplets or droplet nuclei, or by some vehicle of transmission; the agent requires a single vertebrate host for completion of its life cycle and does not develop or show significant change during transmission; may include anthropozoonoses (rabies), zooanthroponoses (amebiasis), and amphixenoses (certain streptococcoses).

zo·o·not·ic (zō′ō-not′ik). Relating to a zoonosis.

zo·o·par·a·site (zō-ō-par′ă-sīt). An animal parasite; an animal existing as a parasite.

zo·o·pa·thol·o·gy (zō-ō-pă-thol′ō-jē). The study or science of diseases of the lower animals.

zo·oph·a·gous (zō-of′ă-gŭs). SYN carnivorous. [G. *zōophagos*, fr. *zōon*, animal, + *phagein*, to eat]

zo·o·phile (zō′ō-fīl). **1.** A lover of animals; especially one more fond of animals than of people. **2.** One opposed to any animal experimentation; an antivivisectionist. [zoo- + G. *philos,* fond]

zo·o·phil·ia (zō-ō-fil′ē-ă). SYN zoophilism.

zo·o·phil·ic (zō-ō-fil′ik). **1.** Relating to or displaying zoophilism. **2.** Animal-seeking or animal-preferring; denoting preference of a parasite for an animal host over a human. [zoo- + G. *philos,* fond, loving]

zo·oph·i·lism (zō-of′i-lizm). Fondness for animals, especially an extravagant fondness for them. SYN zoophilia.

erotic z., the deriving of sexual pleasure by patting or stroking animals.

zo·o·pho·bia (zō-ō-fō′bē-ă). Morbid fear of animals. [zoo- + G. *phobos,* fear]

zo·o·phyte (zō′ō-fīt). An animal that resembles a plant, such as the sponges or sea anemones. [zoo- + G. *phyton,* plant]

zo·o·plas·ty (zō′ō-plas-tē). Grafting of tissue from an animal to a human. SYN zoografting.

zo·o·sa·dism (zō-ō-sā′dizm). Sexual pleasure from cruelty to animals.

zo·os·mo·sis (zō-os-mō′sis). The process of osmosis in living tissues. [G. *zōos,* living, + osmosis]

zo·o·sperm·ia (zō-ō-sper′mē-ă). The presence of live spermatozoa in the ejaculated semen. [G. *zoon,* living, + *sperma,* seed, + -ia]

zo·o·ster·ol (zō′ō-stēr′ol). An animal sterol.

zo·o·tech·nics (zō-ō-tek′niks). The art of managing domestic or captive animals, including handling, breeding, and keeping. [zoo- + G. *technē,* art]

zo·ot·ic (zō-ot′ik). Pertaining to animals other than humans.

zo·o·tox·in (zō-ōtok′sin). A substance, resembling the bacterial toxins in its antigenic properties, found in the fluids of certain animals; *e.g.,* in snake venom, the secretions of poisonous insects, eel-blood. SYN animal toxin.

zo·o·tro·phic (zō-ō-trof′ik). Relating to or serving for the nutrition of the lower animals. [zoo- + Gr. *trophē,* nourishment]

zor·ub·i·cin (zō-rū-bĭ-sin). Semisynthetic derivative of daunorubicin; also similar to doxorubicin. Like those agents, zorubicin exerts significant myocardial toxicity. Used as an antineoplastic in breast cancer.

zos·ter (zos′ter). SYN *herpes* zoster. [G. *zōstēr,* a girdle]

geniculate z. (jen-i′kyu-lāt zos′ter), SYN *herpes* zoster oticus.

zos·ter·i·form (zos-ter′i-fōrm). SYN zosteroid.

zos·ter·oid (zos′ter-oyd). Resembling herpes zoster. SYN zosteriform. [zoster + G. *eidos,* resemblance]

zox·a·zo·la·mine (zok-să-zō′lă-mēn). 2-Amino-5-chlorobenzoxazole; a centrally acting skeletal muscle relaxant that is no longer used because of its hepatic toxicity.

Z-plas·ty. Surgery to elongate a contracted scar or to rotate tension 90°; the middle line of a Z-shaped incision is made along the line of greatest tension or contraction, and triangular flaps are raised on opposite sides of the two ends and transposed. SYN Z procedure.

Zr Symbol for zirconium.

Zsigmondy, Richard, Austro-German chemist and Nobel laureate, 1865–1929. SEE Z.'s *test;* brownian-Z. *movement.*

ZSR Abbreviation for zeta sedimentation *ratio.*

zuc·ker·guss·le·ber (zuk′er-gus-lā-ber). SYN frosted *liver.* [Ger. *Zuckerguss,* sugar frosting, + *Leber,* liver]

Zuckerkandl, Emil, Austrian anatomist, 1849–1910. SEE Z.'s *bodies,* under *body, convolution, fascia; organs* of Z., under *organ.*

zu·sam·men (Z) (zu-sam′men). **1.** SYN cis- (4). **2.** A form of geometric isomerism with regards to carbon-carbon double bonds in which all four moieties attached to the carbons are different. If the substituents with the higher ranking (based on established rules) are on the same side of the double bond, *Z* is used. SEE entgegen. [Ger. together]

zwie·back (zwī′bak). Sweetened bread which has been baked twice, preferred for infant feeding during teething. [Ger. twice-baked]

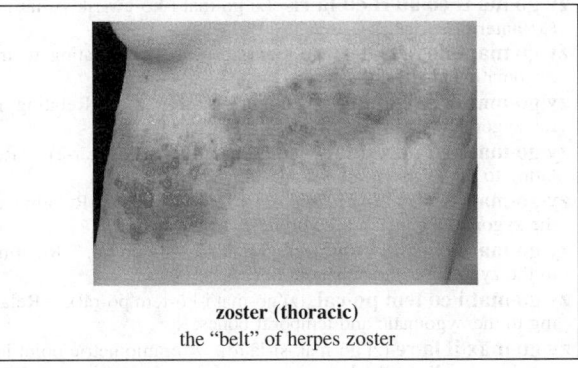

zoster (thoracic)
the "belt" of herpes zoster

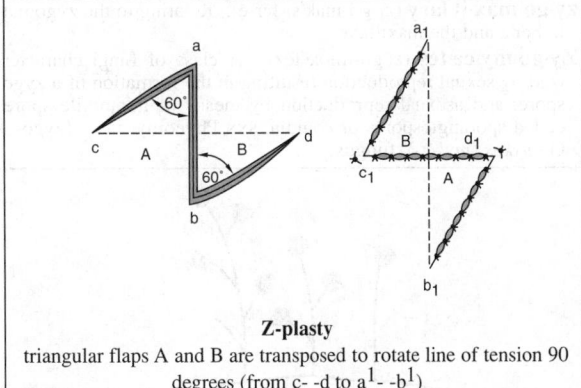

Z-plasty
triangular flaps A and B are transposed to rotate line of tension 90 degrees (from c- -d to a^1- -b^1)

Zwis·chen·fer·ment (tsvish′en-fer-ment′). SYN glucose-6-phosphate dehydrogenase. [Ger. *zwischen,* between, + *Ferment,* fermentation]

zwit·ter·gents (tsvit′er-jents). Detergents that are zwitterionic; often used as surfactants and in the release of proteins from biomembranes. SYN zwitterionic detergent. [*zwitter*ion + deter*gent*]

zwit·ter·i·on·ic (tsvit′er-ī-on′ik). Denoting a substance with the properties of a zwitterion; *e.g.,* at pH value of 6.11, alanine is z.

zwit·ter·i·ons (tsvit′er-ī-onz). SYN dipolar *ions,* under ion. SEE ALSO zwitter *hypothesis.* [Ger. *Zwitter,* hermaphrodite, mongrel + ion]

zyg-. SEE zygo-.

zy·gal (zī′găl). Relating to or shaped like a zygon or yoke; H-shaped.

zyg·a·poph·y·ses (-sēz). Articular processes in vertebra.

zyg·a·poph·y·si·al, zyg·a·poph·y·se·al (zī′gă-pō-fiz′ē-ăl, zī-gă-pof′i-se′ăl). Relating to a zygapophysis or articular process of a vertebra.

zyg·a·poph·y·sis, pl. **zyg·a·poph·y·ses** (zī′gă-pof′i-sis, -sēz) [NA]. official alternate term for articular *process,* articular *process.* [G. *zygon,* yoke, + *apophysis,* offshoot]

zyg·i·on (zig′ē-on). In cephalometrics and craniometrics, the most lateral point of the zygomatic arch. [G. a later form of *zygon,* yoke]

zygo-, zyg-. A yoke, a joining. [G. *zygon,* yoke, *zygōsis,* a joining]

zy·go·ma (zī-gō′mă). **1.** SYN zygomatic *bone.* **2.** SYN zygomatic *arch.* [G. a bar, bolt, the os jugale, fr. *zygon,* yoke]

zy·go·mat·ic (zī′gō-mat′ik). Relating to the zygomatic bone.

zygomatico-. Zygomatic; Relating usually to the zygomatic bone. SEE zygo-. [G. *zygōma*]

zy·go·mat·i·co·au·ric·u·lar (zī′gō-mat′i-kō-aw-rik′yū-lăr). Relating to the zygomatic bone and the auricle.

zy

zy·go·ma·ti·co·au·ri·cu·la·ris (zī′gō-mat′i-kō-aw-rik′yū-lār′is). SYN anterior auricular *muscle*.

zy·go·mat·i·co·fa·cial (zī′gō-mat′i-kō-fā′shăl). Relating to the zygomatic bone and the face.

zy·go·mat·i·co·fron·tal (zī′gō-mat′i-kō-fron′tăl). Relating to the zygomatic and frontal bones.

zy·go·mat·i·co·max·il·lary (zī′gō-mat′i-kō-mak′si-lār-ē). Relating to the zygomatic bone and the maxilla.

zy·go·mat·i·co·or·bi·tal (zī′gō-mat′i-kō-ōr′bi-tăl). Relating to the zygomatic bone and the orbit.

zy·go·mat·i·co·sphe·noid (zī′gō-mat′i-kō-sfē′noyd). Relating to the zygomatic and sphenoid bones.

zy·go·mat·i·co·tem·po·ral (zī′gō-mat′i-kō-tem′pŏ-răl). Relating to the zygomatic and temporal bones.

zy·go·max·il·la·re (zī′gō-mak-si-lā′rē). A craniometric point located externally at the lowest extent of the zygomaticomaxillary suture. SYN key ridge, zygomaxillary point.

zy·go·max·il·lary (zī-gō-mak′si-lār-ē). Relating to the zygomatic bone and the maxilla.

Zy·go·my·ce·tes (zī′gō-mī-sē′tēz). A class of fungi characterized by sexual reproduction resulting in the formation of a zygospore, and asexual reproduction by means of nonmotile spores called sporangiospores or conidia. SYN Phycomycetes. [zygo- + G. *mykēs* (*mykēt-*), fungus]

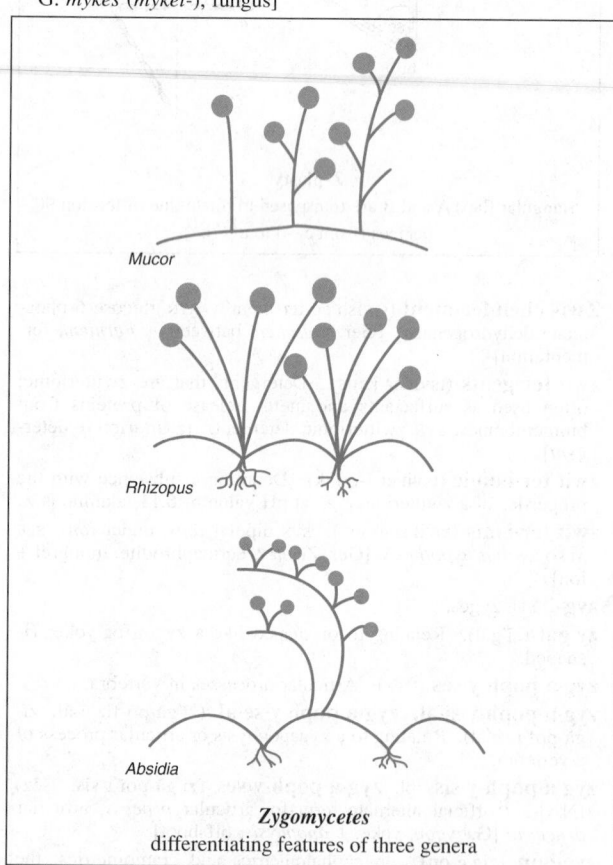

Mucor

Rhizopus

Absidia

Zygomycetes
differentiating features of three genera

zy·go·my·co·sis (zī′gō-mī-kō′sis). A fungous infection associated with species in various genera of the class Zygomycetes, *e.g., Absidia, Mortierella, Mucor, Rhizopus.* The genera *Conidiobolus* and *Basidiobolus* have species that are also causative agents. SYN mucormycosis, phycomycetosis, phycomycosis.

zy·gon (zī′gon). The short crossbar connecting the branches of a zygal fissure. [G. crossbar, yoke]

zy·go·ne·ma (zī-g-ō-nē′mă). SYN zygotene. [zygo- + G. *nēma,* thread]

zy·go·po·di·um (zī-gō-pō′dē-ŭm). The distal intermediate segment of the limb skeleton, *i.e.,* radius and ulna, tibia and fibula. [zygo- + G. *podion,* small foot]

zy·go·sis (zī-gō′sis). True conjugation or sexual union of two unicellular organisms, consisting essentially in the fusion of the nuclei of the two cells. [G. a joining]

zy·gos·i·ty (zī-gos′i-tē). The nature of the zygotes from which individuals are derived; *e.g.,* whether by separation of the division of one zygote (monozygotic), in which case they will be genetically identical, or from two separate fertilized ova (dizygotic).

zy·go·sperm (zī′gō-sperm). SYN zygospore. [zygo- + G. *sperma,* seed]

zy·go·spore (zī′gō-spōr). Among the Phycomycetes, a thick-walled sexual spore arising from fusion of two morphologically identical structures, generally hyphal tips, bearing nuclei of opposite mating types (gametangia). SYN zygosperm.

zy·gote (zī′gōt). **1.** The diploid cell resulting from union of a sperm and an ovum. Cf. conceptus. **2.** The individual that develops from a fertilized ovum. [G. *zygōtos,* yoked]

zy·go·tene (zī′gō-tēn). The stage of prophase in meiosis in which precise point for point pairing of homologous chromosomes begins. SYN zygonema. [zygo- + G. *tainia* (L. *taenia*), band]

zy·got·ic (zī-got′ik). Pertaining to a zygote, or to zygosis.

zy·go·to·blast (zī-gō′tō-blast). SYN sporozoite. [G. *zygōtos,* yoked, + *blastos,* germ]

zy·go·to·mere (zī-gō′tō-mēr). SYN sporoblast. [G. *zygōtos,* yoked, + *meros,* part]

zym-. SEE zymo-.

zy·mase (zī′mās). **1.** Obsolete term for a mixture of enzymes. **2.** Specifically, the intracellular enzymes of yeast that promotes alcoholic fermentation.

zymo-, zym-. Fermentation, enzymes. [G. *zymē,* leaven]

zy·mo·deme (zī′mō-dēm). An isoenzyme pattern, as identified by isoenzyme electrophoresis. [zymo- + G. *dēmos,* populace]

zy·mo·gen (zī′mō-jen). SYN proenzyme.

zy·mo·gen·e·sis (zī-mō-jen′ĕ-sis). Transformation of a proenzyme (zymogen) into an active enzyme. [zymo- + G. *genesis,* production]

zy·mo·gen·ic (zī-mō-jen′ik). **1.** Relating to a zymogen or to zymogenesis. SYN zymogenous. **2.** Causing fermentation.

zy·mog·e·nous (zī-moj′ĕ-nŭs). SYN zymogenic (1).

zy·mo·gram (zī′mō-gram). Strips of paper, gels, etc. in which the locations of enzymes, separated electrophoretically or by other means, are demonstrated by histochemical methods. [zymo- + G. *gramma,* something written]

zy·mo·hex·ase (zī-mō-heks′ās). Obsolete term for fructose-bisphosphate aldolase.

zy·mol·o·gist (zī-mol′ō-jist). Obsolete term for enzymologist.

zy·mol·o·gy (zī-mol′ō-jē). Obsolete term for enzymology.

zy·mo·san (zī′mō-san). A carbohydrate (glucose polymer) obtained from the walls of yeast cells that interferes with complement.

zy·mo·scope (zī′mō-skōp). An instrument measuring CO_2 evolved and, therefore, the fermenting power of yeast. [zymo- + G. *skopeō,* to view]

zy·mos·ter·ol (zī-mos′ter-ol). 5α-Cholesta-8,24-dien-3β-ol; an intermediate in the biosynthesis of cholesterol from lanosterol.

zy·xin (ziks′in). A cytoplasmic protein found in a number of distinct types of adherens junctions; it may play a role in the organization of membrane-cytoskeletal attachments.

ZZ. SEE ZZ genotype.

APPENDICES

APPENDICES

CONTENTS TO THE APPENDICES

Appendices

TABLE OF ELEMENTS AND THEIR ATOMIC WEIGHTS

Element	Symbol	Atomic Number	Atomic Weight	Element	Symbol	Atomic Number	Atomic Weight
Actinium	Ac	89	227.0278*	Mendelevium	Md	101	258.10*
Aluminum	Al	13	26.981539	Mercury	Hg	80	200.59
Americium	Am	95	243.0614*	Molybdenum	Mo	42	95.94
Antimony	Sb	51	121.75	Neodymium	Nd	60	144.24
Argon	Ar	18	39.948	Neon	Ne	10	20.1797
Arsenic	As	33	74.92159	Neptunium	Np	93	237.0482*
Astatine	At	85	209.9871*	Nickel	Ni	28	58.69
Barium	Ba	56	137.327	Niobium	Nb	41	92.90638
Berkelium	Bk	97	247.0703*	Nitrogen	N	7	14.00674
Beryllium	Be	4	9.012182	Nobelium	No	102	259.1009*
Bismuth	Bi	83	208.98037	Osmium	Os	76	190.2
Boron	B	5	10.811	Oxygen	O	8	15.9994
Bromine	Br	35	79.904	Palladium	Pd	46	106.42
Cadmium	Cd	48	112.411	Phosphorus	P	15	30.973762
Calcium	Ca	20	40.078	Platinum	Pt	78	195.08
Californium	Cf	98	251.0796*	Plutonium	Pu	94	244.0642*
Carbon	C	6	12.011	Polonium	Po	84	208.9824*
Cerium	Ce	58	140.115	Potassium	K	19	39.0983
Cesium	Cs	55	132.90543	Praseodymium	Pr	59	140.90765
Chlorine	Cl	17	35.4527	Promethium	Pm	61	144.9127*
Chromium	Cr	24	51.9961	Protactinium	Pa	91	231.0359*
Cobalt	Co	27	58.93320	Radium	Ra	88	226.0254*
Copper	Cu	29	63.546	Radon	Rn	86	222.0176*
Curium	Cm	96	247.0703*	Rhenium	Re	75	186.207
Dysprosium	Dy	66	162.50	Rhodium	Rh	45	102.90550
Einsteinium	Es	99	252.083*	Rubidium	Rb	37	85.4678
Erbium	Er	68	167.26	Ruthenium	Ru	44	101.07
Europium	Eu	63	151.965	Samarium	Sm	62	150.36
Fermium	Fm	100	257.0951*	Scandium	Sc	21	44.955910
Fluorine	F	9	18.9984032	Selenium	Se	34	78.96
Francium	Fr	87	223.0197*	Silicon	Si	14	28.0855
Gadolinium	Gd	64	157.25	Silver	Ag	47	107.8682
Gallium	Ga	31	69.723	Sodium	Na	11	22.989768
Germanium	Ge	32	72.61	Strontium	Sr	38	87.62
Gold	Au	79	196.96654	Sulfur	S	16	32.066
Hafnium	Hf	72	178.49	Tantalum	Ta	73	180.9479
Helium	He	2	4.002602	Technetium	Tc	43	97.9072*
Holmium	Ho	67	164.93032	Tellurim	Te	52	127.60
Hydrogen	H	1	1.00794	Terbium	Tb	65	158.92534
Indium	In	49	114.82	Thallium	Tl	81	204.3833
Iodine	I	53	126.90447	Thorium	Th	90	232.0381
Iridium	Ir	77	192.22	Thulium	Tm	69	168.93421
Iron	Fe	26	55.947	Tin	Sn	50	118.710
Krypton	Kr	36	83.80	Titanium	Ti	22	47.88
Lanthanum	La	57	138.9055	Tungsten	W	74	183.85
Lawrencium	Lr	103	262.11*	Unnilquadium	Unq	104	216.11*
Lead	Pb	82	207.2	Unnilpentium	Unp	105	262.114*
Lithium	Li	3	6.941	Unnihexium	Unh	106	263.118*
Lutetium	Lu	71	174.967	Unnilseptium	Uns	107	262.12*
Magnesium	Mg	12	24.3050	Uranium	U	92	238.0289
Manganese	Mn	25	54.93805	Vanadium	V	23	50.9415

Element	Symbol	Atomic Number	Atomic Weight	Element	Symbol	Atomic Number	Atomic Weight
Xenon	Xe	54	131.29	Zinc	Zn	30	65.39
Ytterbium	Yb	70	173.04	Zirconium	Zr	40	91.224
Yttrium	Y	39	88.90585				

*Relative atomic mass of the isotope of that element with the longest known half-life.

From Budavari et al., Eds. The Merck index: an encyclopedia of chemicals, drugs and biologicals. 11th ed. New Jersey: Merck & Co. Inc., 1989.

Appendices

COMPARATIVE TEMPERATURE SCALES

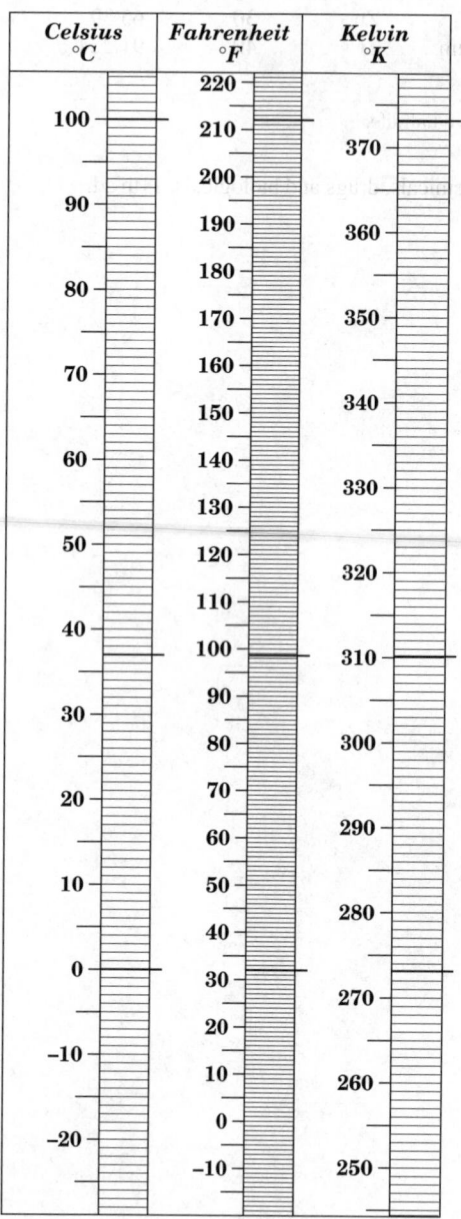

To convert Celsius or Fahrenheit to Kelvin:

    C to K: add 273.16
    10°C to K: 10 + 273.16 = 283.16 K

    F to K: convert to C, add 273.16
    63°F = 17.2°C + 273.16 = 290.36 K

To convert Fahrenheit to Celsius, Celsius to Fahrenheit:

Above 0°C or 32°F

    F to C: subtract 32, multiply by 5, divide by 9
    63°F to C: 63 – 32 = 31 × 5 = 155 ÷ 9 = 17.2°C

    C to F: multiply by 9, divide by 5, add 32
    37°C to F: 37 × 9 = 333 ÷ 5 = 66.6 + 32 = 98.6°F

TEMPERATURE EQUIVALENTS

	Celsius to Fahrenheit				Fahrenheit to Celsius					
°C	°F	°C	°F		°F	°C	°F	°C	°F	°C
− 50	− 58.0	49	120.0		− 50	− 46.7	99	37.2	157	69.4
− 40	− 40.0	50	122.0		− 40	− 40.0	100	37.7	158	70.0
− 35	− 31.0	51	123.8		− 35	− 37.2	101	38.3	159	70.5
− 30	− 22.0	52	125.6		− 30	− 34.4	102	38.8	160	71.1
− 25	− 13.0	53	127.4		− 25	− 31.7	103	39.4	161	71.6
− 20	− 4.0	54	129.2		− 20	− 28.9	104	40.0	162	72.2
− 15	5.0	55	131.0		− 15	− 26.6	105	40.5	163	72.7
− 10	14.0	56	132.8		− 10	− 23.3	106	41.1	164	73.3
− 5	23.0	57	134.6		− 5	− 20.6	107	41.6	165	73.8
0	**32.0**	58	136.4		0	− 17.7	108	42.2	166	74.4
1	33.8	59	138.2		1	− 17.2	109	42.7	167	75.0
2	35.6	60	140.0		5	− 15.0	110	43.3	168	75.5
3	37.4	61	141.8		10	− 12.2	111	43.8	169	76.1
4	39.2	62	143.6		15	− 9.4	112	44.4	170	76.6
5	41.0	63	145.4		20	− 6.6	113	45.0	171	77.2
6	42.8	64	147.2		25	− 3.8	114	45.5	172	77.7
7	44.6	65	149.0		30	− 1.1	115	46.1	173	78.3
8	46.4	66	150.8		31	− 0.5	116	46.6	174	78.8
9	48.2	67	152.6		**32**	**0**	117	47.2	175	79.4
10	50.0	68	154.4		33	0.5	118	47.7	176	80.0
11	51.8	69	156.2		34	1.1	119	48.3	177	80.5
12	53.6	70	158.0		35	1.6	120	48.8	178	81.1
13	55.4	71	159.8		36	2.2	121	49.4	179	81.6
14	57.2	72	161.6		37	2.7	122	50.0	180	82.2
15	59.0	73	163.4		38	3.3	123	50.5	181	82.7
16	60.8	74	165.2		39	3.8	124	51.1	182	83.3
17	62.6	75	167.0		40	4.4	125	51.6	183	83.8
18	64.4	76	168.8		41	5.0	126	52.2	184	84.4
19	66.2	77	170.6		42	5.5	127	52.7	185	85.0
20	68.0	78	172.4		43	6.1	128	53.3	186	85.5
21	69.8	79	174.2		44	6.6	129	53.8	187	86.1
22	71.6	80	176.0		45	7.2	130	54.4	188	86.6
23	73.4	81	177.8		46	7.7	131	55.0	189	87.2
24	75.2	82	179.6		47	8.3	132	55.5	190	87.7
25	77.0	83	181.4		48	8.8	133	56.1	191	88.3
26	78.8	84	183.2		49	9.4	134	56.6	192	88.8
27	80.6	85	185.0		50	10.0	135	57.2	193	89.4
28	82.4	86	186.8		55	12.7	136	57.7	194	90.0
29	84.2	87	188.6		60	5.5	137	58.3	195	90.5
30	86.0	88	190.4		65	18.3	138	58.8	196	91.1
31	87.8	89	192.2		70	21.1	139	59.4	197	91.6
32	89.6	90	194.0		75	23.8	140	60.0	198	92.2
33	91.4	91	195.8		80	26.6	141	60.5	199	92.7
34	93.2	92	197.6		85	29.4	142	61.1	200	93.3
35	95.0	93	199.4		86	30.0	143	61.6	201	93.8
36	96.8	94	201.2		87	30.5	144	62.2	202	94.4
37	**98.6**	95	203.0		88	31.0	145	62.7	203	95.0
38	100.4	96	204.8		89	31.6	146	63.3	204	95.5
39	102.2	97	206.6		90	32.2	147	63.8	205	96.1
40	104.0	98	208.4		91	32.7	148	64.4	206	96.6
41	105.8	99	210.2		92	33.3	149	65.0	207	97.2
42	107.6	**100**	**212.0**		93	33.8	150	65.5	208	97.7
43	109.4	101	213.8		94	34.4	151	66.1	209	98.3
44	111.2	102	215.6		95	35.0	152	66.6	210	98.8
45	113.0	103	217.4		96	35.5	153	67.2	211	99.4
46	114.8	104	219.2		97	36.1	154	67.7	**212**	**100.0**
47	116.6	105	221.0		98	36.6	155	68.3	213	100.5
48	118.4	106	222.8		**98.6**	**37.0**	156	68.8	214	101.1

WEIGHTS & MEASURES

Scale of the Metric System and SI

Prefix	Symbol	Power	Multiple or Submultiple
exa-	E	10^{18}	1,000,000,000,000,000,000
peta-	P	10^{15}	1,000,000,000,000,000
tera-	T	10^{12}	1,000,000,000,000
giga-	G	10^{9}	1,000,000,000
mega-	M	10^{6}	1,000,000
kilo-	k	10^{3}	1,000
hecto-	h	10^{2}	100
deca-	da	10^{1}	10
UNIT			1
deci-	d	10^{-1}	0.1
centi-	c	10^{-2}	0.01
milli-	m	10^{-3}	0.001
micro-	μ	10^{-6}	0.000001
nano-	n	10^{-9}	0.000000001
pico-	p	10^{-12}	0.000000000001
femto-	f	10^{-15}	0.000000000000001
atto-	a	10^{-18}	0.000000000000000001

SI Base Units

Quantity	Name	Symbol
length	meter	m
mass*	kilogram†	kg
time	second	s
electric current	ampere	A
thermodynamic temperature	kelvin‡	K
luminous intensity	candela	cd
amount of substance	mole	mol

* In commercial and everyday use, "weight" usually means mass; *e.g.*, when speaking of a person's weight, the quanity referred to is mass.

† For historic reasons, kilogram is the only base unit with a prefix. Multiples and submultiples of the kilogram are formed by attaching the appropriate prefix to the stem word "gram" (*e.g.*, milligram) and the appropriate prefix symbol to the symbol "g" (*e.g.*, mg.).

‡The degree Celsius (°C) is still widely accepted usage for expressing temperature and temperature intervals. Celsius (formerly centigrade) *temperature* is converted to kelvin (K) thermodynamic temperature by adding 273.16 to the Celsius scale. For *temperature interval*, 1°C equals K.

Some SI Derived Units
Expressed in Terms of Base Units

Quantity	Name	Symbol
area	square meter	m^2
volume*	cubic meter	m^3
specific volume	cubic meter per kilogram	m^3/kg
speed, velocity	meter per second	m/s
acceleration	meter per second squared	m/s^2
mass density	kilogram per cubic meter	kg/m^3
concentration	mole per cubic meter	mol/m^3
luminance	candela per square meter	cd/m^2

*Liter (L, l). 10^{-3} m^3, is regarded as a special name for the cubic decimeter, which is preferred for high accuracy measurement.

Some SI Derived Units with Special Names

Quanity	Name	Symbol	Expression
Frequency	hertz	Hz	s^{-1}
force	newton	N	$m\ kg\ s^{-2}$
pressure, stress	pascal	Pa	$m^{-1}\ kg\ s^{-2}$
energy	joule	J	$m^2\ kg\ s^{-2}$
power	watt	W	$m^2\ kg\ s^{-3}$
quantity of electricity, electric charge	coulomb	C	$s\ A$
electric potential, electromotive force	volt	V	$m^2\ kg\ s^{-3}\ A^{-1}$
capacitance	farad	F	$m^{-2}\ kg^{-1}s^4\ A^2$
electrical resistance	ohm	Ω	$m^2\ kg^{-2}\ A^{-2}$
electrical conductance	siemens	S	$m^{-2}\ kg\ s^{-2}\ A^{-1}$
magnetic flux	weber	Wb	$m^2\ kg\ s^{-2}\ A^{-1}$
magnetic flux density	tesla	T	$kg\ s^{-2}\ A^{-1}$
activity of radionuclide	becquerel*	Bq	s^{-1}
absorbed dose of radiation	gray†	Gy	$m^2\ s^{-2}$
exposure (x and γ radiation)	coulomb per kilogram‡	C kg	$kg^{-1}\ s\ A$

*Replacing the curie (Ci), 3.7×10^{10} s^{-1}.

†Replacing the rad (rad), 10^{-2} J kg^{-1}.

‡Replacing the roentgen (R), 2.58×10^{-4} C kg^{-1}.

Measures of Length

Micrometers	Millimeters	Centimeters	Meters	Kilometers	Miles	Yards	Feet	Inches
1	0.001	10^{-4}						0.000039
10^3	**1**	10^{-1}					0.00328	0.03937
10^4	10	**1**	0.01			0.0109	0.03281	0.3937
254,000	25.4	2.54	0.0254			0.0278	0.0833	**1**
	304.8	30.48	0.3048			0.333	**1**	12
10^6	10^3	10^2	**1**	0.001	0.0006213	1.0936	3.2808	39.37
914,400	914.40	91.44	0.9144	0.009	0.0005681	**1**	3	36
10^9	10^6	10^5	10^3	**1**	0.6215	1093.6121	3280.8	
			1609.0	1.609	**1**	1760.0	5280.0	

To convert:

Millimeters to inches: multiply by 10, divide by 254
Inches to millimeters: multiply by 254, divide by 10

Centimeters to feet: multiply by 10, divide by 307
Feet to centimeters: multiply by 307, divide by 10

Meters to yards: multiply by 70, divide by 64
Yards to meters: multiply by 64, divide by 70

Kilometers to miles: multiply by 5, divide by 8
Miles to kilometers: multiply by 8, divide by 5

Measures of Mass (Weight)

Avoirdupois Weights

				Metric Equivalents		
Grains	Drams	Ounces	Pounds	Milligrams	Grams	Kilograms
1	0.0366	0.0023	0.00014	64.8	0.0648	0.000065
27.34	**1**	0.0625	0.0039		1.772	0.001772
437.5	16	**1**	0.0625		28.350	0.028350
7,000	256	16	**1**		453.5924	0.453592
0.0154				**1**	0.001	
15.4324	0.5648	0.0353	0.002205	1000	**1**	0.001
15,432.358	564.32	35.27	2.2046		1000	**1**

To convert (approximately):

Kilograms to pounds: multiply by 1000, divide by 454
Pounds to kilograms: multiply by 454, divide 1000

Grams to ounces: multiply by 20, divide by 567
Ounces to grams: multiply by 567, divide by 20

Apothecaries' Weights

					Metric Equivalents		
Grains	Scruples	Drams	Ounces	Pounds	Milligrams	Grams	Kilograms
1	0.05	0.0167	0.0021	0.00017	64.8	0.0648	0.000065
20	**1**	0.333	0.042	0.0035		1.296	0.001296
60	3	**1**	0.125	0.0104		3.888	0.000389
480	24	8	**1**	0.0833		31.103	0.031103
5,760	288	96	12	**1**		373.2418	0.373242
0.0154						0.001	
15.4324		0.2576	0.0322	0.0027	1000	**1**	0.001
15,432.358		257.2	32.15	2.6792		1000	**1**

Measures of Capacity

Apothecaries' Measures

						Metric Equivalents	
Minims	Fluid Drams	Fluid Ounces	Pints	Quarts	Gallons	Liters	Milliliters
1	0.0166	0.002	0.00013			0.0006	0.06161
60	**1**	0.125	0.0078	0.0039		0.0037	3.6967
480	8	**1**	0.0625	0.0312	0.0078	0.0296	29.5737
7,680	128	16	**1**	0.5	0.125	0.4732	473.166
15,360	256	32	2	**1**	0.25	0.9464	946.358
61,440	1024	128	8	4	**1**	3.7854	3785.434
16,230	270.52	33.8418	2.1134	1.0567	0.2642	**1**	1000
16.23	0.2705	0.0338	0.00212	0.00106	0.000265	0.001	**1**

To convert (approximately):

Liters to gallons: multiply by 264, divide by 1000
Gallons to liters: divide by 264, multiply by 1000

Liters to pints: multiply by 21, divide by 10
Pints to liters: multiply by 10, divide by 21

Approximate Household Measures and Weights*

Teaspoons	Tablespoons	Cups or Glases	Drams	Fluid Ounces	Milliliters	Grams
1			1	0.125	5	5
3	**1**		4	0.50	15	15
48	16	**1**	64	8	237	240

*A drop is a measure of uncertain quantity, depending on the nature of the liquid as well as the shape of the container and of the opening from which the liquid falls. One drop of water is roughly equivalent to 1 minim.

SYMBOLS

Angles, Triangles, and Circles

$\wedge$ above • diastolic blood pressure (anesthesa records) • elevated • enlarged • improved • increased • superior (position) • upper

$\vee$ below • decreased • deficiency • deficit • depressed • deteriorated • diminished • down • inferior (position) • lower • systolic blood pressure (anesthesia records)

$>$ causes • demonstrates • distal • followed by • derived from • greater than • indicates • larger than • leads to • more severe than • produces • radiates to • radiating to • results in • reveals • shows • to • toward • worse than • yields

$<$ caused by • derived from • less severe than • less than • produced by • proximal • smaller than

$\angle$ angle • flexion • flexor

$\angle_E$ angle of entry

$\angle_X$ angle of exit

$\llcorner$ factorial product • right lower quadrant

$\ulcorner$ right upper quadrant

$\urcorner$ left upper quadrant

$\lrcorner$ left lower quadrant

Δ anion gap • centrad prism • change • delta gap • heat • increment • occipital triangle • prism diopter • temperature (anesthesia records)

$\Delta+$ time interval

ΔA change in absorbance

ΔdB difference in decibels

ΔP change in (intraocular) pressure

ΔpH change in pH

Δt time interval

ΔH, H'sΔ Hesselbach's triangle

$\bigcirc$ respiration (anesthesia records)

$\female$ female • female sex

$\male$ male • male sex

Ⓐ, ⓐx axilla (temperature)

Ⓗ, ⓗ hypodermic • hypodermically

Ⓘ𝖬 intramuscular • intramuscularly

Ⓘ𝖵 intravenous • intravenously

Ⓛ left

Ⓜ murmur

ⓜ by mouth • mouth (temperature) • murmur

$\sqrt{}$ⓜ factitial murmur

Ⓞ by mouth • oral • orally

Ⓡ rectal • rectally • rectum (temperature) • right

Ⓧ end of anesthesia (anesthesia records) • end of operation

Arrows

$\uparrow$ above • elevated • elevation • enlarged • gas • greater than • improved • increase • increased • increases • more than • rising • superior (position) • up • upper

$\uparrow$g increasing • rising

$\uparrow$V increase due to in vivo effect (lab)

$\downarrow$ below • decrease • decreased • deficiency • deficit • depressed • depression • deteriorated • deteriorating • diminished • diminution • down • falling • inferior (position) • less than • low • lower • normal plantar reflex • precipitate • precipitates

$\downarrow$g decreasing • diminishing • falling • lowering

$\downarrow$V decrease due to in vivo effect (lab)

$\nearrow$ deviated • displaced • increasing

$\searrow$ decreasing

$\rightarrow$ approaches limit of • causes • demonstrates • direction of flow or reaction • distal • due to • followed by • indicates • leads to • produces • radiating to • results in • reveals • shows • to • to right • toward • yields

$\leftarrow$ caused by • derived from • direction of flow or reaction • due to • produced by • resulting from • secondary to • to left

$\uparrow\uparrow$ extensor response (Babinski sign) • positive Babinski • testes undescended

$\downarrow\downarrow$ down bilaterally • plantar response (Babinski sign) • testes descended

$\uparrow\downarrow$ reversible reaction • up and down

$\leftrightarrows, \rightleftharpoons$ reversible (chemical) reaction

Genetic Symbols

☐ male

○ female

◊ sex unspecified

☐─○ mating

☐─○ consanguinity

☐ⱼ○ illegitimacy

I☐ⱼ○ parents and offspring, in
II☐ ○ generations

☐○ dizygotic twins

☐○ monozygotic twins

④ ③ number of children of sex indicated

☐○ adopted individuals

☿ abortion or stillbirth, sex unspecified

☐ ○ normal individuals

☐ ♀ individual died without leaving offspring

☐ⱼ○ no issue

■ ● affected individuals

↗■ ↗● proband or propositus

☐ examined professionally • normal for trait

☐ not examined • dubiously reported to have trait

☐ not examined • reliably reported to have trait

◼ ◑ heterozygotes for autosomal recessive

⊙ carrier of sex-linked recessive

⊠ ⊘ death

Numbers

0 completely absent (pulse) • no response (reflexes)

+1, 1+ markedly impaired (pulse)

1+ low normal or somewhat diminished (reflexes) •
slight reaction or trace (lab tests)

+2, 2+ moderately impaired (pulse)

2+ average or normal (reflexes) • noticable reaction
or trace (lab tests)

+3, 3+ slightly impaired (pulse)

3+ moderate reaction (lab tests) • more brisk than
average (reflexes)

+4, 4+ normal (pulse)

4+ hyperactive (reflexes) • large amount (lab tests) •
pronounced reaction (lab tests) • very brisk
(reflexes)

$\dot{1}$ bowel movement (numeral indicates number of
stools in a given period)

1x once • one time

2x, x2 twice • two times

3x etc. three times, etc.

Arabic	Roman
0	
1	I, i
2	II, ii
3	III, iii
4	IV, iv
5	V, v
6	VI, vi
7	VII, vii
8	VIII, viii
9	IX, ix
10	X, x
11	XI, xi
12	XII, xii
13	XIII, xiii
14	XIV, xiv
15	XV
16	XVI

Arabic	Roman
17	XVII
18	XVIII
19	XIX
20	XX
30	XXX
40	XL
50	L
60	LX
70	LXX
80	LXXX
90	XC
100	C
1,000	M
5,000	$\overline{V}$
10,000	$\overline{X}$
100,000	$\overline{C}$
1,000,000	$\overline{M}$

Plus, Minus, and Equivalencies

+   acid (reaction) • added to • convex lens • decreased or diminished (reflexes) • excess • less than 50% inhibition of hemolysis (Wassermann) • low normal (reflexes) • markedly impaired (pulse) • mild (severity) • plus • plus (slightly more than stated amount) • positive (lab tests) • present • slight reaction or trace (lab) • sluggish (reflexes) • somewhat diminished (reflexes)

(+)   significant • uncommon or uncertain mode of inheritance

(+)**ive**   positive

+ **to** ++   slight pain

++   average (reflexes) • 50% inhibition of hemolysis (Wassermann) • moderate (pain, severity) • moderately impaired (pulse) • normally active (reflexes) *also* ‡ • noticeable reaction or trace (lab tests)

+++   increased reflexes • 75% inhibition of hemolysis (Wassermann) • moderate amount • moderate reaction (lab tests) • moderately hyperactive (reflexes) • moderately severe (pain, severity) • more brisk than average (reflexes) • slightly impaired (pulse)

++++   complete inhibition of hemolysis (Wassermann) • large amount (lab tests) • markedly hyperactive reflexes • markedly severe (pain, severity) • normal (pulse) • pronounced reaction (lab test) • very brisk (reflexes)

−   absent • alkaline (reaction) • concave lens • deficiency • deficient • minus • negative (lab test) • none • subtract • without

(−)   insignificant

±   doubtful • either positive or negative • equivocal (reflexes, qualitative tests) • flicker (reflexes) • indefinite • more or less • plus or minus • possibly significant • questionable • suggestive • variable • very slight (reaction, severity, trace) • with or without

(±)   possibly significant

± to +   minimal pain

∓   minus or plus

‡   moderate (severity) • normally active (reflexes) *also* ++

fracture • gauge • number • pound(s) • weight

~   about • approximate • approximately • proportionate to

≈   approximately equal • nearly equal to

=   equal • equals • equal to

≠   does not equal • not equal • not equal to • unequal

⌣   combined with

⌀   equivalent

⊘   not equivalent to

≡   identical • identical with

≢   not identical • not identical with

≑   nearly equal to

≐   approximately equal

≅   approximately • approximately equals • congruent to

≐   approaches

⊥   equilateral

≜   equiangular

>   greater than

<   less than

≯   not greater than

≮   not less than

≥, ⩾   greater than or equal to

≤, ⩽   less than or equal to

Primes, Checks, and Dots

?   doubtful • equivocal (reflexes) • flicker (reflexes) *also* ± • not tested (severity) • possible • questionable • question of • suggested • suggestive (severity) • unknown

!   factorial product

†   death • deceased

/   divided by • either meaning • extension • extensor • fraction • of • per • to

′   foot • hour • univalent

″   bivalent • ditto • inch • minute • second ($\frac{1}{60}$ degree)

‴   line ($\frac{1}{12}$ inch) • trivalent

√   check • observe for • urine • voided (urine)

√·   urine and defecation • voided and bowels moved

√c̄   check with

√d	checked • observed	°	degree • measurement ($1/_{260}$ of circle) • severity (burns, wounds) • temperature • time (hour)
√g, √ing	checking	:	is to • ratio
√qs	voided sufficient quanity	⋯	no data (in given category)
√	radical root	∴	therefore
$\sqrt[2]{}$	square root	∵	because • since
$\sqrt[3]{}$	cube root	::	as • equality between ratios • proportion • porportionate to
*	birth • multiplication sign (genetics) • not verified • presumed • supposed		

Statistical Symbols

α	probability of Type I error • significance level	s	sample standard deviation
β	probability of Type II error	s^2	sample variance
$1-\beta$	power of statistical test	SE	standard error of estimate
$nCk; \binom{n}{k}$	binomial coefficient • number of combination of n things taken k at a time	σ	population standard deviation
		σ^2	population variance
χ^2	chi-squared statistic	$\sigma_{\text{diff.}}$	standard error of difference between scores
E	expected frequency in cell of contingency table	$\sigma_{\text{est.}}$	standard error of estimate
$E(X)$	expected value of random variable X	$\sigma_{\text{meas.}}$	standard error of measurement
F	F statistic (variance ratio)	$\sum_{i=1}^{n} x_i, \Sigma_i \overset{n}{=} x_i$	$x_1 + x_2 + \ldots + x_n$
f	frequency	t	Student's t statistic • Student's test variable
H_0	null hypothesis	θ	latent trait
H_1	alternative hypothesis	U	Mann-Whitney rank sum statistic
μ	population mean	W	Wilcoxson rank sum statistic
N	population size	$\overline{X}$	sample mean
n	sample size	$|x|$	absolute value of x
$n!$	n factorial	$\sqrt{x}$	square root of x
O	observed frequency in a contingency table	z	standard score
ϕ	ability continuum • phi coefficient	$=$	equal
P	probability	$\neq$	not equal
p	probability of success in independent trials	$\approx$	approximately equal
$P(A)$	probability that event A ocurrs	$>$	greater than
$P(A\backslash B)$	conditional probability that A occurs given that B has occurred	$\not>$	not greater than
		$<$	less than
r	sample correlation coefficient, usually the Pearson product-moment correlation	$\not<$	not less than
r^2	coefficient of determination	$\geq, \geqslant$	greater than or equal to
r_s	Spearman rank correlation coefficient	$\leq, \leqslant$	less than or equal to
ρ	population correlation coefficient	∞	infinity

From Stedman's abbreviations, acronyms & symbols. Baltimore: Williams & Wilkins, 1992.

Appendices

LABORATORY REFERENCE RANGE VALUES

Show-Hong Duh, Ph.D., D.A.B.C.C., Department of Pathology,
University of Maryland School of Medicine, Baltimore, MD.

Gladys Alonsozana, M.D., Department of Pathology,
University of Maryland School of Medicine, Baltimore, MD.

Reference range values are for apparently healthy individuals and often overlap significantly with values for persons who are sick. Actual values may vary significantly due to differences in assay methodologies and standardization. Institutions may also set up their own reference ranges based on the particular populations that they serve, thus there can be regional differences. Consequently, values reported by individual laboratories may differ from those listed in this appendix.

All values are given in conventional and SI units. However, where the SI units have not been widely accepted, conventional units are used. In case of the heterogenous nature of the materials measured or uncertainty of the exact molecular weight of the compounds, the SI system cannot be followed, and mass per volume is used as the unit of concentration.

Abbreviations:

ACD, acid-citrate-dextrose; **CHF**, congestive heart failure; **Cit**, citrate; **CNS**, central nervous system; **CSF**, cerebrospinal fluid; **cyclic AMP**, adenosine 3': 5'- cyclic phosphate; **EDTA**, ethylenediaminetetraacetic acid; **HDL**, high-density lipoprotein; **Hep**, heparin; **LDL-C**, low-density lipoprotein-cholesterol; **Ox**, oxalate; **RBC**, red blood cell(s); **RIA**, radioimmunoassay; **SD**, standard deviation

References:

Reference Intervals. In *Tietz Textbook of Clinical Chemistry*. 2nd ed., C.A. Burtis and E.R. Ashwood, Eds. Philadelphia, W.B. Saunders Co., 1994.

Hematologic Values. In *Clinical Hematology and Fundamentals of Hemostasis*. 2nd ed., D.M. Harmening, Ed. Philadelphia, F.A. Davis Co., 1992.

National Cholesterol Education Program: Report of the expert panel on detection, evaluation, and treatment of high blood cholesterol in adults. *Arch. Intern. Med.* 1988; 148:36-69.

Clinical Chemistry Laboratory: *Reference Range Values in Clinical Chemistry*. Professional services manual. Baltimore, Department of Pathology, University of Maryland Medical System, 1993.

Triglyceride, High Density Lipoprotein, and Coronary Heart Disease. National Institute of Health Consensus Statement, NIH Consensus Development Conference, 1992, Volume 10, Number 2.

Tests	Conventional Units	SI Units
Acetaminophen, serum or plasma (Hep or EDTA)		
Therapeutic	10–30 µg/mL	66–199 µmol/L
Toxic	>200 µg/mL	>1324 µmol/L
Acetone		
Serum		
Qualitative	Negative	Negative
Quantitative	0.3–2.0 mg/dL	3–20 mg/L
Urine		
Qualitative	Negative	Negative
Acid hemolysis test (Ham)	No hemolysis	No hemolysis
Adrenocorticotropin (ACTH), plasma		
6 AM	10–80 pg/mL	10–80 ng/L
6 PM	<50 pg/mL	<50 ng/L
Alanine aminotransferase (see Transaminase)		
Albumin		
Serum		
Adult	3.5–5.0 g/dL	35–50 g/L
>60 y	3.4–4.8 g/dL	34–48 g/L
	Avg. of 0.3 g/dL higher in upright individuals	Avg. of 3 g/L higher in upright individuals
Urine		
Qualitative	Negative	Negative
Quantitative	10–100 mg/24 h	10–100 mg/24 h
CSF	10–30 mg/dL	100–300 mg/L
*Aldolase, serum	0–11 U/L (30°C)	0–11 U/L (30°C)
Aldosterone		
Serum		
Supine	3–10 ng/dL	0.08–0.3 nmol/L
Standing		
Male	6–22 ng/dL	0.17–0.61 nmol/L
Female	5–30 ng/dL	0.14–0.8 nmol/L
Urine	3–20 µg/24 h	8.3–55 nmol/24 h
Alpha amino nitrogen		
Serum	3.0–5.5 mg/dL	2.1–3.9 mmol/L
Urine	50–200 mg/24 h	3.6–14.3 nmol/24 h
Amikacin, serum or plasma (EDTA)		
Therapeutic		
Peak	25–35 µg/mL	43–60 µmol/L
Trough		
Less severe infection	1–4 µg/mL	1.7–6.8 µmol/L
Life-threatening infection	4–8 µg/mL	6.8–13.7 µmol/L
Toxic		
Peak	>35–40 µg/mL	>60–68 µmol/L
Trough	>10–15 µg/mL	>17–26 µmol/L
∂-Aminolevulinic acid, urine	1.3–7.0 mg/24 h	10–53 µmol/24 h

*Test values are method dependent.

Tests	Conventional Units		SI Units	
Amitriptyline, serum or plasma (Hep or EDTA); trough (≥12 h after dose)				
Therapeutic	120–250 ng/mL		433–903 nmol/L	
Toxic	>500 ng/mL		>1805 nmol/L	
Ammonia nitrogen				
Plasma	15–45 µg/dL		11–32 µmol/L	
Urine	140–1500 mg/d		10–107 mmol/d	
*Amylase				
Serum	25–125 mIU/mL		25–125 U/L	
Urine	1–17 U/h		1–17 U/h	
Amylase/creatinine clearance ratio	1–4%		0.01–0.04	
Anion gap	8–16 mEq/L		8–16 mmol/L	
Arsenic				
Whole blood (Hep)	0.2–6.2 µg/dL		0.03–0.83 µmol/L	
Chronic poisoning	10–50 µg/dL		1.33–6.65 µmol/L	
Acute poisoning	60–930 µg/dL		7.98–124 µmol/L	
Urine, 24 h	5–50 µg/d		0.07–0.67 µmol/d	
Ascorbic acid, blood	0.4–1.5 mg/dL		23–85 µmol/L	
Aspartate aminotransferase (see Transaminase)				
Base excess, blood	0 ± 2 mEq/L		0 ± 2 mmol/L	
Bicarbonate, serum	23–29 mEq/L		23–29 mmol/L	
Bile acids, serum	0.3–3.0 mg/dL		3.0–30.0 mg/L	
*Bilirubin				
Serum				
Adults				
Conjugated	0.0–0.3 mg/dL		0–5 µmol/L	
Unconjugated	0.01–1.1mg/dL		0–19 µmol/L	
Delta	0–0.2 mg/dL		0–3 µmol/L	
Total	0.2–1.3 mg/L		3–22 µmol/L	
Neonates				
Conjugated	0–0.6 mg/dL		0–10 µmol/L	
Unconjugated	0.6–10.5 mg/dL		10–180 µmol/L	
Total	1.0–10.5 mg/dL		1.7–180 µmol/L	
Urine, qualitative	Negative		Negative	

Bone marrow, differential cell count	Range (%)	Average (%)	Range	Average
Myeloblasts	0.3–5.0	2.0	0.003–0.05	0.02
Promyelocytes	1.0–8.0	5.0	0.01–0.08	0.05
Myelocytes				
Neutrophilic	5.0–19.0	12.0	0.05–0.19	0.12
Eosinophilic	0.5–3.0	1.5	0.005–0.03	0.015
Basophilic	0.0–0.5	0.3	0.00–0.005	0.003
Metamyelocytes	13.0–32.0	22.0	0.13–0.32	0.22
Polymorphonuclear neutrophils	7.0–30.0	20.0	0.07–0.30	0.20
Polymorphonuclear eosinophils	0.5–4.0	2.0	0.005–0.04	0.02
Polymorphonuclear basophils	0.0–0.7	0.2	0.00–0.007	0.002
Lymphocytes	3.0–17.0	10.0	0.03–0.17	0.10

*Test values are method dependent.

Tests	Conventional Units		SI Units	
Plasma cells	0.0–2.0	0.4	0.00–0.02	0.004
Monocytes	0.5–5.0	2.0	0.005–0.05	0.02
Reticulum cells	0.1–2.0	0.2	0.001–0.02	0.002
Megakaryocytes	0.3–3.0	0.4	0.003–0.03	0.004
Pronormoblasts	1.0–8.0	4.0	0.01–0.08	0.04
Normoblasts	7.0–32.0	18.0	0.07–0.32	0.18
Cadmium, whole blood (Hep)	0.1–0.5 μg/dL		0.89–4.45 nmol/L	
Toxic	10–300 μg/dL		0.89–26.70 μmol/L	
Cadmium, urine, 24 h	<15 μg/d		<0.13 μmol/d	
Calcium, serum	8.4–10.2 mg/dL		2.1–2.6 mmol/L	
	(Slightly higher in children)		(Slightly higher in children)	
Calcium, ionized, serum	4.65–5.28 mg/dL		1.16–1.32 mmol/L	
Calcium, urine				
Low calcium diet	<150 mg/24 h		<3.8 nmol/24 h	
Usual diet; trough	<250 mg/24 h		<6.3 nmol/24 h	
Carbamazepine, serum or plasma (Hep or EDTA)				
Therapeutic	8–12 μg/mL		34–51 μmol/L	
Toxic	>15 μg/mL		>63 μmol/L	
Carbon dioxide, total, serum/ plasma (Hep)	22–29 mmol/L (lower in children)		Same	
Carbon dioxide tension (PCO$_2$), blood	35–45mm Hg		35–45 mm Hg	
Carbon monoxide as carboxyhemoglobin (HbCO), whole blood (EDTA)				
Nonsmokers	0.5–1.5% total Hb		0.005–0.015 HbCO fraction	
Smokers				
1–2 packs/d	4–5% total Hb		0.04–0.05 HbCO fraction	
>2 packs/d	8–9% total Hb		0.08–0.09 HbCO fraction	
Toxic	>20% total Hb		>0.20 HbCO fraction	
Lethal	>50% total Hb		>0.5 HbCO fraction	
Carotene, serum	40–200 μg/dL		0.74–3.72 μmol/L	
*Catecholamines, urine				
Epinephrine	<10 μg/24 h		<55 nmol/24 h	
Norepinephrine	<100 μg/24 h		<590 nmol/24 h	
Total free catecholamines	4–126 μg/24 h		24–745 nmol/24 h (as norepinephrine)	
Total metanephrines	0.1–1.6 mg/24 h		0.5–8.1 μmol/24 h (as metanephrine)	
Cell counts (Coulter)				
Erythrocytes				
Males	4.7–6.1 × 10^6/μL		4.7–6.1 × 10^{12}/L	
Females	4.2–5.4 × 10^6/μL		4.2–5.4 × 10^{12}/L	
Children (varies with age)	3.8–5.5 × 10^6/μL		3.8–5.5 × 10^{12}/L	
Leukocytes				
Total	4.8–10.8 × 10^3/μL		4.8–10.8 × 10^9/L	
Differential	*Percentage*	*Absolute*		
Myelocytes	0	0/μL	0/L	
Band neutrophils	3–5	150–400/μL	150–400 × 10^6/L	
Segmented neutrophils	54–62	3000–5800/μL	3000–5800 × 10^6/L	

*Test values are method dependent.

Appendices

Tests	Conventional Units		SI Units
Lymphocytes	25–33	1500–3000/μL	1500–3000 × 10⁶/L
Monocytes	3-7	300–500/μL	300–500 × 10⁶/L
Eosinophils	1–3	50–250/μL	50–250 × 10⁶/L
Basophils	0-0.75	15–50/μL	15–50 × 10⁶/L
Platelets	150–450 × 10³/μL		150–450 × 10⁹/L
Reticulocytes	25,000–75,000/μL		25–75 × 10⁹/L
	0.5–1.5% of erythrocytes		
Cells, CSF	<5/μL (all mononucleocytes)		Same
*Ceruloplasmin, serum	23–44 mg/dL		230–440 mg/L
Chloramphenicol, serum or plasma (Hep or EDTA); trough			
Therapeutic	10–25 μg/mL		31–77 μmol/L
Toxic	>25 μg/mL		>77 μmol/L
Chloride			
Serum	96–106 mmol/L		96–106 mmol/L
Sweat			
Normal	0–30 mmol/L		Same
Cystic fibrosis	60–200 mmol/L		Same
Urine, 24 h (vary greatly with Cl intake)			
Infant	2–10 mmol/d		Same
Child	14–50 mmol/d		Same
Adults	110–250 mmol/d		Same
CSF	120–130 mmol/L (20 mmol/L higher than serum)		Same
Cholesterol, serum	Recommended desirable range: <200 mg/dL		Recommended desirable range: <5.2 mmol/L
	Borderline range: 200–239 mg/dL		Borderline range: 5.2–6.2 mmol/L
Cholinesterase			
Serum	0.5–1.3 pH units		0.5–1.3 pH units
Erythrocytes	0.5–1.0 pH unit		0.5–1.0 pH unit
*Chorionic gonadotropin, β-subunit (β-hCG)			
Serum or plasma (EDTA)			
Male and nonpregnant female	<3.0IU/L		<3.0 IU/L
Female, post-conception			
7-10 d	>3.0 IU/L		Same
30 d	100–5000 IU/L		Same
40 d	>2000 IU/L		Same
10 wk	50,000–140,000 IU/L		Same
14 wk	10,000–50,000 IU/L		Same
Trophoblastic disease	>100,000 IU/L		Same
Urine, 24 h			
Male and nonpregnant female	0 IU/d		Same
Pregnancy (wk)			
6th	13,000 U/d (mean)		Same
8th	30,000 U/d (mean)		Same
12-14th	105,000 U/d (mean)		Same
16th	46,000 U/d (mean)		Same
Thereafter	5,000–20,000 U/d (mean)		Same

*Test values are method dependent.

Tests	Conventional Units	SI Units
Clonazepam, serum or plasma (Hep or EDTA); trough		
Therapeutic	15–60 ng/mL	48–190 nmol/L
Toxic	>80 ng/mL	>254 nmol/L
Coagulation tests		
Antithrombin III (synthetic substrate)	80–120% of normal	0.8–1.2 of normal
Bleeding time (Duke)	0–6 min	0–6 min
Bleeding time (Ivy)	1–6 min	1–6 min
Bleeding time (template)	2.3–9.5 min	2.3–9.5 min
Clot retraction, qualitative	Begins in 30–60 min	Begins in 30–60 min
	Complete in 24 h	Complete in 24 h
Coagulation time (Lee-White)	5–15 min (glass tubes)	5–15 min (glass tubes)
	19–60 min (siliconized tubes)	19–60 min (siliconized tubes)
Cold hemolysin test (Donath-Landsteiner)	No hemolysis	No hemolysis
Complement components		
Total hemolytic complement activity, plasma (EDTA)	75–160 U/mL or >33% of plasma CH50	75–160 kU/L Fraction of CH50 : >0.33
Total complement decay rate (functional), plasma (EDTA)	10–20% Deficiency: >50%	Fraction decay rate: 0.10–0.20 >0.50
$C1_q$, serum	5.1–7.9 mg/dL	51–79 mg/L
$C1_r$, serum	2.2–4.6 mg/dL	22–46 mg/L
$C1_s$(C1 esterase), serum	2.1–4.1 mg/dL	21–41 mg/L
C2, serum	1.9–2.5 mg/dL	19–25 mg/L
C3, serum	83–177 mg/dL	830–1770 mg/L
C4, serum	12–36 mg/dL	120–360 mg/L
C5, serum	3.8–9.0 mg/dL	38–90 mg/L
C6, serum	4.0–7.2 mg/dL	40–72 mg/L
C7, serum	4.9–7.0 mg/dL	49–70 mg/L
C8, serum	4.3–6.3 mg/dL	43–63 mg/L
C9, serum	4.7–6.9 mg/dL	47–69 mg/L
Coombs' test		
Direct	Negative	Negative
Indirect	Negative	Negative
Copper		
Serum		
Males	70–140 μg/dL	11–22 μmol/L
Females	85–155 μg/dL	13–24 μmol/L
Urine 0–50 μg/24 h	0–0.80 μmol/24 h	
Corpuscular values of erythrocytes (values are for adults; in children, values vary with age)		
Mean corpuscular hemoglobin (MCH)	27–31 pg	0.42–0.48 fmol

Tests	Conventional Units	SI Units
Mean corpuscular hemoglobin concentration (MCHC)	33–37 g/dL	330–370 g/L
Mean corpuscular volume (MCV)	80-96 μ^3	80-96 fL
Cortisol		
Plasma		
8 AM	5–23 µg/dL	138–635 nmol/L
4 PM	3–16 µg/dL	82–441 nmol/L
10 PM	<50% of 8 AM value	<0.5 of 8 AM value
Free, urine	10–100 µg/24 h	27.6–276 mmol/24 h
Creatine		
Serum	0.2–0.8 mg/dL	15–61 µmol/L
Urine		
Males	0–40 mg/24 h	0–0.30 mmol/24 h
Females	0–100 mg/24 h	0– 0.76 mmol/24 h
	(Higher in children and pregnant women)	(Higher in children and pregnant women)
*†Creatine kinase, serum (CK, CPK)		
White		
Male	60–320 U/L (37°C)	60–320 U/L (37°C)
Female	50–200 U/L (37°C)	50–200 U/L (37°C)
Black		
Male	130–450 U/L (37°C)	130–450 U/L (37°C)
Female	60–270 U/L (37°C)	60–270 U/L (37°C)
*Creatine kinase MB isoenzyme, serum	0–5 ng/mL	0–5 µg/L
*Creatinine		
Serum or plasma, adult		
Male	0.7–1.3 mg/dL	62–115 µmol/L
Female	0.6–1.1 mg/dL	53–97 µmol/L
Urine		
Male	14–26 mg/kg body weight/24 h	0.12–0.23 mmol/kg body weight/24h
Female	11–20 mg/kg body weight/24 h	0.10–0.18 mmol/kg body weight/24 h
*Creatinine clearance, enzymatic		
Males	90–139 mL/min/1.73 m²	0.87–1.34 mL/s/m²
Females	80–125 mL/min/1.73 m²	0.77–1.2 mL/s/m²
Cryoglobulins, serum	0	0
Cyanide		
Serum		
Nonsmokers	0.004 mg/L	0.15 µmol/L
Smokers	0.006 mg/L	0.23 µmol/L
Nitroprusside therapy	0.01–0.06 mg/L	0.38–2.30 µmol/L
Toxic	>0.1 mg/L	>3.84 µmol/L
Whole blood (Ox)		
Nonsmokers	0.016 mg/L	0.61 µmol/L
Smokers	0.041 mg/L	1.57 µmol/L
Nitroprusside therapy	0.05–0.5 mg/L	1.92–19.20 µmol/L
Toxic	>1 mg/L	>38.40 µmol/L

*Test values are method dependent.
†Test values are race dependent.

Tests	Conventional Units	SI Units
Cyclic AMP		
Plasma (EDTA)		
Males	4.6–8.6 ng/mL	14–26 nmol/L
Females	4.3–7.6 ng/mL	13–23 nmol/L
Urine, 24 h	0.3–3.6 mg/d	1.0–10.9 μmol/d or
	or 0.29–2.1 mg/g creatinine	100–723 μmol/mol creatinine
Cystine or cysteine, urine, qualitative	Negative	Negative
*C-Peptide, serum	0.78–1.89 ng/mL	0.26–0.62 nmol/L
*C-Reactive protein, serum		
Cord blood	1–35 μg/dL	10–350 μg/L
Adult	6.8–820 μg/dL	68–8200 μg/L
*≠Cyclosporine, whole blood		
Therapeutic, trough	100–200 ng/mL	83–166 nmol/L
Dehydroepiandrosterone, urine	<15% of total 17–ketosteroids	<15% of total 17–ketosteroids
Males	0.2–2.0 mg/24 h	0.7–6.9 μmol/24 h
Females	0.2–1.8 mg/24 h	0.7–6.2 μmol/24 h
Desipramine, serum or plasma (Hep or EDTA); trough (12 h after dose)		
Therapeutic	75–300 ng/mL	281–1125 nmol/L
Toxic	>400 ng/mL	>1500 nmol/L
Diazepam, serum or plasma (Hep or EDTA); trough		
Therapeutic	100–1000 ng/mL	0.35–3.51 μmol/L
Toxic	>5000 ng/mL	>17.55 μmol/L
Digitoxin, serum or plasma (Hep or EDTA); 6 h after dose		
Therapeutic	20–35 ng/mL	26–46 nmol/L
Toxic	>45 ng/mL	>59 nmol/L
Digoxin, serum or plasma (Hep or EDTA); 12 h after dose		
Therapeutic		
CHF	0.8–1.5 ng/mL	1.0–1.9 nmol/L
Arrhythmias	1.5–2.0 ng/mL	1.9–2.6 nmol/L
Toxic		
Adult	>2.5 ng/mL	>3.2 nmol/L
Child	>3.0 ng/mL	>3.8 nmol/L
Disopyramide, serum or plasma (Hep or EDTA); trough		
Therapeutic arrhythmias		
Atrial	2.8–3.2 μg/mL	8.3–9.4 μmol/L
Ventricular	3.3–7.5 μg/mL	9.7–22 μmol/L
Toxic	>7 μg/mL	>20.7 μmol/L
Doxepin, serum or plasma (Hep or EDTA); trough (≥ 12 h after dose)		

*Test values are method dependent.
≠ Actual therapeutic range should be adjusted for individual patient.
‡Assuming a mixture of estrone, estradioles, and estriol in a molecular proportion of 2:1:2.

Tests	Conventional Units	SI Units
Therapeutic	30–150 ng/mL	107–537 nmol/L
Toxic	>500 ng/mL	>1790 nmol/L
Electrophoresis, CSF	Predominantly albumin	Predominantly albumin
Estrogens, urine		
Males		
Estrone	3–8 µg/24 h	11–30 nmol/24 h
Estradiol	0–6 µg/24 h	0–22 nmol/24 h
Estriol	1–11 µg/24 h	3–38 nmol/24 h
‡Total	4–25 µg/24 h	14–90 nmol/24 h
Females		
Estrone	4–31 µg/24 h	15–115 nmol/24 h
Estradiol	0–14 µg/24 h	0–51 nmol/24 h
Estriol	0–72 µg/24 h	0–250 nmol/24 h
‡Total	5–100 µg/24 h	18–360 nmol/24 h
	(Markedly increased during pregnancy)	(Markedly increased during pregnancy)
Ethanol, whole blood (Ox) or serum		
Depression of CNS	>100 mg/dL	>21.7 mmol/L
Fatalities reported	>400 mg/dL	>86.8 mmol/L
Ethosuximide, serum or plasma (Hep or EDTA); trough		
Therapeutic	40–100 µg/mL	283–708 µmol/L
Toxic	>150 µg/mL	>1062 µmol/L
Euglobulin lysis time	2–6 h at 37°C	2–6 h at 37°C
Factor VIII and other coagulation factors	70–150% of normal	0.70–1.5 of normal
Fibrin split products (Thrombo–Wellco test)	<10 µg/mL	<10mg/L
Fibrinogen	200–400 mg/dL	5.9–11.7 µmol/L
Fibrinolysins	0	0
Partial thromboplastin time, activated (APTT)	20–35 sec	20–35 sec
Prothrombin consumption	Over 80% consumed in 1 h	Over 0.80 consumed in 1 h
Prothrombin content	100% (calculated from prothrombin time)	1.0 (calculated from prothrombin time)
Prothrombin time (one stage)	12.0–14.0 sec	12.0–14.0 sec
Tourniquet test	Ten or fewer petechiae in a 2.5 cm circle after 5 min	Ten or fewer petechiae in a 2.5 cm circle after 5 min
Fat, fecal, F, 72 h		
Infant, breast–fed	<1 g/d	Same
0–6 y	<2 g/d	Same
Adult	<7 g/d	Same
Adult (fat–free diet)	<4 g/d	Same
§Fatty acids, total, serum	190–420 mg/dL	7–15 mmol/L
Nonesterified, serum	8–25 mg/dL	0.30–0.90 mmol/L
Ferritin, serum		
Males	20–250 ng/mL	20–250 µg/L
Females	10–120 ng/mL (higher if postmenopausal)	10–120 µg/L (higher if postmenopausal)

‡ Assuming a mixture of estrone, estradioles, and estriol in a molecular proportion of 2:1:2.

§ "Fatty acids" include a mixture of different aliphatic acids of varying molecular weight; a mean molecular weight of 284 daltons has been assumed.

Tests	Conventional Units	SI Units
Ferritin values of <20 ng/mL (20 µg/L) have been reported to be generally associated with depleted iron stores		
Fibrinogen, plasma	200–400 mg/dL	5.9–11.7 µmol/L
Fluoride		
Plasma (Hep)	0.01–0.2 µg/mL	0.5–10.5 µmol/L
Urine	0.2–1.1 µg/mL	10.5–57.9 µmol/L
Urine, occupational exposure	<8 µg/mL	<421 µmol/L
Folate, serum	2.2–17.3 ng/mL	5.0–39.2 nmol/L
Erythrocytes	169–707 ng/mL	451–1602 nmol/L
*Follicle-stimulating hormone (FSH), serum		
Males		
Folicular phase	2.0–17.7 mIU/L	2.0–17.7 IU/L
Midcycle	3.6–16.0 IU/L	3.6–16.0 IU/L
Gastrin, serum		
Males	<100 pg/mL	<100 ng/L
Females	<75 pg/mL	<75 ng/L
Gentamicin, serum or plasma (EDTA)		
Therapeutic		
Peak		
Less severe infection	5–8 µg/mL	10.4–16.7 µmol/L
Severe infection	8–10 µg/mL	16.7–20.9 µmol/L
Trough		
Less severe infection	<1 µg/mL	<2.1 µmol/L
Moderate infection	<2 µg/mL	<4.2 µmol/L
Severe infection	<2–4 µg/mL	<4.2–8.4 µmol/L
Toxic		
Peak	>10–12 µg/mL	>21–25 µmol/L
Trough	>2–4 µg/mL	>4.2–8.4 µmol/L
Glucose (fasting)		
Blood	60–100 mg/dL	3.33–5.55 mmol/L
Plasma or serum	70–115 mg/dL	3.89–6.38 mmol/L
Glucose, 2 h postprandial, serum	<120 mg/dL	<6.7 mmol/L
Glucose, urine		
Quantitative	<500 mg/24 h	<2.8 mmol/24 h
Qualitative	Negative	Negative
Glucose, CSF	50–75 mg/dL (20 mg/dL less than serum)	2.8–4.2 mmol/L (1.1 mmol/L less than serum)
*Glucose-6-phosphate dehydrogenase (G-6-PD) in erythrocytes, whole blood (ACD, EDTA, or Hep)	12.1 ± 2.1 U/g Hb (SD) 351 ± 60.6 U/10^12 RBC 4.11 ± 0.71 U/mL RBC	0.78 ± 0.13 mU/mol Hb 0.35 ± 0.06 nU/RBC 4.11 ± 0.71 kU/L RBC
*γ-Glutamyltransferase		
Males	≤50 U/L (37°C)	≤50 U/L (37°C)
Females	≤30 U/L (37°C)	≤30 U/L (37°C)
Glutethimide, serum		
Therapeutic	2–6 µg/mL	9–28 µmol/L
Toxic	>5 µg/mL	>23 µmol/L
Growth hormone, serum	0–10 ng/mL	0–10 µg/L

*Test values are method dependent.

Appendices

Tests	Conventional Units	SI Units
Haptoglobin, serum	26–185 mg/dL	260–1850 mg/L
Haptoglobin (as hemoglobin binding capacity)	40–336 mg/dL	0.4–36 g/L
HDL-cholesterol (HDL-C), serum or plasma (EDTA)	Recommended desirable range: >40 mg/dL	Recommended desirable range: >1.04 mmol/L
Borderline: 35–40 mg/dL		
Hematocrit		
Males	42–52%	0.42–0.52
Females	37–47%	0.37–0.47
Newborn	53–65%	0.53–0.65
Children (varies with age)	30–43%	0.30–0.43
Hemoglobin (Hb)		
Males	14.0–18.0 g/dL	2.17–2.79 mmol/L
Females	12.0–16.0 g/dL	1.86–2.48 mmol/L
Newborn	17.0–23.0 g/dL	2.64–3.57 mmol/L
Children (varies with age)	11.2–16.5 g/dL	1.74–2.56 mmol/L
Hemoglobin, fetal	≥1 y old: <2% of total Hb	≥1 y old: <2% of total Hb
Hemoglobin, plasma	0–5.0 mg/dL	0–0.8 μmol/L
Hemoglobin and myoglobin, urine, qualitative	Negative	Negative
Hemoglobin electrophoresis, whole blood (EDTA, Cit or Hep)		
HbA	96–98.6%	0.96–0.986 Hb fraction
HbA$_{1c}$	5.3–7.5%	0.053–0.075 Hb fraction
HbA$_2$	1.5–3.5%	0.015–0.035 Hb fraction
HbF	<2%	<0.02 Hb fraction
Homogentisic acid, urine, qualitative	Negative	Negative
*Hydroxybutyric dehydrogenase serum (HBD)	0–180 mU/mL (30°C)	0–180 U/L (30°C)
17-Hydroxycorticosteroids, plasma	8–18 μg/dL	0.22–0.50 μmol/L
Urine		
Males	3–9 mg/24 h	8.3–25 μmol/24 h (as cortisol)
Females	2–8 mg/24 h	5.5–22 μmol/24 h (as cortisol)
5-Hydroxyindoleacetic acid, urine		
Qualitative	Negative	Negative
Quantitative	2–6 mg/24 h	10.4–31.2 μmol/24 h
Imipramine, serum or plasma (Hep or EDTA); trough (≥12 h after dose)		
Therapeutic	125–250 ng/mL	446–893 nmol/L
Toxic	>500 ng/mL	>1785 nmol/L
*Immunoglobulins, serum		
IgG	723–1685 mg/dL	7.2–16.9 g/L
IgA	69–382 mg/dL	0.69–3.8 g/L
IgM	63–277 mg/dL	0.63–2.8 g/L
IgD	0–8 mg/dL	0–80 mg/L
IgE	0–380 IU/mL	0–380 kIU/L
Immunoglobulin G (IgG), CSF	0.5–6.1 mg/dL	0.5–6.1 g/L

*Test values are method dependent.

Tests	Conventional Units	SI Units
Insulin, plasma (fasting)	5–25 µU/mL	36–179 pmol/L
*Iron, serum		
Males	65–170 µg/dL	11.6–30.4 µmol/L
Females	50–170 µg/dL	9.0–30.4 µmol/L
Iron binding capacity, serum		
Total 250–450 mg/24 h	45–81 µmol/L	43–73
Saturation	20–55%	0.20–0.55
Ketosteroids, urine		
Males	8–20 mg/24 h	28–70 µmol/24 h
Females	6–15 mg/24 h (decrease with age)	21–52 µmol/24 h (decrease with age)
L-Lactate		
Plasma (NaF)		
Venous	4.5–19.8 mg/dL	0.5–2.2 mmol/L
Arterial	4.5–14.4 mg/dL	0.5–1.6 mmol/L
Whole blood (Hep), at bed rest		
Venous	8.1–15.3 mg/dL	0.9–1.7 mmol/L
Arterial	3–7 mg/dL	0.36–0.75 mmol/L
Urine, 24 h	496–1982 mg/d	5.5–22 mmol/d
CSF	<25.5 mg/dL	<2.8 mmol/L
*Lactate dehydrogenase (LDH)		
Total (L→P), 37°C, serum		
Newborn	290–775 U/L	Same
Neonate	545–2000 U/L	Same
Infant	180–430 U/L	Same
Child	110–295 U/L	Same
Adult	100–190 U/L	Same
>60 y	110–210 U/L	Same
*Isoenzymes, serum by agarose gel electrophoresis		
Fraction 1	14–26% of total	0.14–0.26 fraction of total
Fraction 2	29–39% of total	0.29–0.39 fraction of total
Fraction 3	20–26% of total	0.20–0.26 fraction of total
Fraction 4	8–16% of total	0.08–0.16 fraction of total
Fraction 5	6–16% of total	0.06–0.16 fraction of total
*Lactate dehydrogenase, CSF	10% of serum value	0.10 fraction of serum value
LDL-cholesterol (LDL–C), calculated, serum or plasma (EDTA)	Recommended desirable range for adults: <130 mg/dL	<3.37 mmol/L
Lead,		
Whole blood (Hep)	<10 µg/dL	<0.48 µmol/L
Urine, 24 h	<80 µg/d <0.39 µmol/d	
Lecithin–sphingomyelin (L/S) ratio, amniotic fluid	2.0–5.0 indicates probable fetal lung maturity; > 3.5 in diabetics	Same
*Leucine aminopeptidase, serum	14–40 mU/mL (30°C)	14–40 U/L (30°C)
Lidocaine, serum or plasma (Hep or EDTA); 45 min after bolus dose		
Therapeutic	1.5–6.0 µg/mL	6.4–26 µmol/L
Toxic		

*Test values are method dependent.

Tests	Conventional Units	SI Units
CNS, cardiovascular depression	6–8 µg/mL	26–34.2 µmol/L
Seizures, obtundation, decreased cardiac output	>8 µg/mL	>34.2 µmol/L
*Lipase, serum	23–208 U/L (37°C)	23–208 U/L (37°C)
Lithium, serum or plasma (Hep or EDTA); 12 h after last dose		
Therapeutic	0.6–1.2 mEq/L	0.6–1.2 mmol/L
Toxic	>2 mEq/L	>2 mmol/L
Lorazepam, serum or plasma (Hep or EDTA), therapeutic	50–240 ng/mL	156–746 nmol/L
*Luteinizing hormone (LH), serum		
Males	0.9–10.6 mIU/mL	0.9–10.6 IU/L
Females		
Follicular phase	1.1–11.1 mIU/mL	1.1–11.1 IU/L
Midcycle peak	17.5–72.9 mIU/mL	17.5–72.9 IU/L
Luteal phase	0.4–15.1 mIU/mL	0.4–15.1 IU/L
Postmenopausal	6.8–46.6 mIU/mL	6.8–46.6 IU/L
Magnesium		
Serum	1.3–2.1 mEq/L	0.65–1.05 mmol/L
	1.6–2.5 mg/dL	16–25 mg/L
Urine	6.0–10.0 mEq/24 h	3.0–5.0 mmol/24 h
Mercury		
Whole blood (EDTA)	0.6–59 µg/L	<0.29 µmol/L
Urine, 24 h	<20 µg/d	<0.1 µmol/d
Toxic	>150 µg/d	>0.75 µmol/d
Metanephrines (see Catecholamines)		
Methemoglobin (MetHb, hemoglobin), whole blood (EDTA, Hep or ACD)	0.06–0.24 g/dL or 0.78 ± 0.37% of total Hb (SD)	9.3–37.2 µmol/L or Mass fraction of total Hb: 0.008 ± 0.0037 (SD)
Methotrexate, serum or plasma (Hep or EDTA)		
Therapeutic	Variable	Variable
Toxic		
post IV infusion	24 h <5 µmol/L	Same
48 h	<0.5 µmol/L	Same
72 h	<0.05 µmol/L	Same
Myelin basic protein, CSF	<2.5 mg/mL	<2.5 µg/L
Nortriptyline, serum or plasma (Hep or EDTA); trough (≥12 h after dose)		
Therapeutic	50–150 ng/mL	190–570 nmol/L
Toxic	>500 ng/mL	>1900 nmol/L
*5′-Nucleotidase, serum	2–17 U/L	2–17 U/L

*Test values are method dependent.

Tests	Conventional Units	SI Units
N-Acetylprocainamide, serum or plasma (Hep or EDTA); trough		
Therapeutic	5–30 µg/mL	18–108 µmol/L
Toxic	>40 µg/mL	>144 µmol/L
Occult blood, feces, random	Negative (<2 mL blood/150 g stool/d)	Negative (<13.3 mL blood/kg stool/d)
Qualitative, urine, random	Negative	Negative
Osmolality		
Serum	275–295 mOsm/kg serum water	285–295 mmol/kg serum water
Urine	50–1200 mOsm/kg water	38–1400 mmol/kg water
Ratio, urine/serum	1.0–3.0, 3.0–4.7 after 12 h fluid restriction	Same
Osmotic fragility of erythrocytes	Begins in 0.45–0.39% NaCl Complete in 0.33– 0.30% NaCl	Begins in 77–67 mmol/L NaCl Complete in 56–51 mmol/L NaCl
Oxazepam, serum or plasma (Hep or EDTA), therapeutic	0.2–1.4 µg/mL	0.70–4.9 µmol/L
Oxygen, blood		
Capacity	16–24 vol% (varies with hemoglobin)	7.14–10.7 mmol/L (varies with hemoglobin)
Content		
Arterial	15–23 vol%	6.69–10.3 mmol/L
Venous	10–16 vol%	4.46–7.14 mmol/L
Saturation		
Arterial and capillary	95–98% of capacity	0.95–0.98 of capacity
Venous	60–85% of capacity	0.60–0.85 of capacity
Tension		
pO_2 arterial and capillary	83–108 mm Hg	Same
Venous	35–45 mm Hg	Same
P50, blood	25–29 mm Hg (adjusted to pH 7.4)	3.33–3.86 kPa
Pentobarbital, serum or plasma (Hep or EDTA); trough		
Therapeutic		
Hypnotic	1–5 µg/mL	4–22 µmol/L
Therapeutic coma	20–50 µg/mL	88–221 µmol/L
Toxic	>10 µg/mL	>44 µmol/L
pH		
Blood, arterial	7.35–7.45	7.35–7.45
Urine	4.6–8.0 (depends on diet)	Same
Phenacetin, plasma (EDTA)		
Therapeutic	1–30 µg/mL	6–167 µmol/L
Toxic	50–250 µg/mL	279–1395 µmol/L
Phenobarbital, serum or plasma (Hep or EDTA); trough		
Therapeutic	15–40 µg/mL	65–170 µmol/L
Toxic		
Slowness, ataxia, nystagmus	35–80 µg/mL	151–345 µmol/L
Coma with reflexes	65–117 µg/mL	280–504 µmol/L

Appendices

Tests	Conventional Units	SI Units
Coma without reflexes	>100 µg/mL	>430 µmol/L
Phenolsulfonphthalein excretion (PSP), urine	28–51% in 15 min	0.28–0.51 in 15 min
	13–24% in 30 min	0.13–0.24 in 30 min
	9–17% in 60 min	0.09–0.17 in 60 min
	3–10% in 2 h	0.03–0.10 in 2 hr
	(After injection of 1 mL PSP intravenously)	(After injection of 1 mL PSP intravenously)
Phenylalanine, serum	0.8–1.8 mg/dL	48–109 µmol/L
Phenylpyruvic acid, urine, qualitative	Negative	Negative
Phenytoin, serum or plasma (Hep or EDTA); trough		
Therapeutic	10–20 µg/mL	40–79 µmol/L
Toxic	>20 µg/mL	>79 µmol/L
*Phosphatase, acid, prostatic, serum		
RIA	<3.0 ng/mL	<3.0 µg/L
*Phosphatase, alkaline		
Leukocyte	Total score: 14–100	Total score: 14–100
Serum (ALP)	20–90 mU/mL (30˚C)	20–90 U/L (30˚C)
	(Values are higher in children)	(Values are higher in children)
Phosphate, inorganic, serum		
Adults	2.7–4.5 mg/dL	0.87–1.45 mmol/L
Children	4.5–5.5 mg/dL	1.45–1.78 mmol/L
Phosphatidylglycerol (PG), amniotic fluid		
Fetal immaturity	Absent	Same
Fetal maturity	Present	Same
Phospholipids, serum	125–275 mg/dL	1.25–2.75 g/L
Phosphorus, urine	0.4–1.3 g/24 h	12.9–42 mmol/24 h
Porphobilinogen, urine		
Qualitative	Negative	Negative
Quantitative	<2.0 mg/24 h	<9 µmol/24 h
Porphyrins, urine		
Coproporphyrin	34–230 µg/24 h	52–351 nmol/24 h
Uroporphyrin	<50 µg/24 h	<60 nmol/24 h
Potassium, plasma (Hep)		
Males	3.5–4.5 mEq/L	3.5–4.5 mmol/L
Females	3.4–4.4 mEq/L	3.4–4.4 mmol/L
Potassium		
Serum		
Premature		
Cord	5.0–10.2 mEq/L	5.0–10.2 mmol/L
48 h	3.0–6.0 mEq/L	3.0–6.0 mmol/L
Newborn, cord	5.6–12.0 mEq/L	5.6–12.0 mmol/L
Newborn	3.7–5.9 mEq/L	3.7–5.9 mmol/L
Infant	4.1–5.3 mEq/L	4.1–5.3 mmol/L
Child	3.4–4.7 mEq/L	3.4–4.7 mmol/L
Adult	3.5–5.1 mEq/L	3.5–5.1 mmol/L
Urine, 24 h	25–125 mEq/d, varies with diet	25–125 mmol/d; varies with diet
CSF	70% of plasma level or 2.5–3.2 mEq/L; rises with plasma hyperosmolality	0.70 of plasma level or 2.5–3.2 mmol/L; rises with plasma hyperosmolality

*Test values are method dependent.

Tests	Conventional Units	SI Units
Pregnanediol, urine		
Males	0–1.9 mg/24 h	0–5.9 µmol/24 h
Females		
Follicular phase	<2.6 mg/24 h	<8 µmol/24 h
Luteal phase	2.6–10.6 mg/24 h	8–33 µmol/24 h
Postmenopausal phase	0.2–1.0 mg/24 h	6.2–3.1 µmol/24 h
Pregnanetriol, urine	0.4–2.5 mg/24 h in adults	1.2–7.5 µmol/24 h in adults
Pressure, CSF	70–180 mm H_2O	Same
Primidone, serum or plasma		
(Hep or EDTA);		
trough		
Therapeutic	5–12 µg/mL	23–55 µmol/L
Toxic	>15 µg/mL	>69 µmol/L
Procainamide, serum or plasma		
(Hep or EDTA);		
trough		
Therapeutic	4–10 µg/mL	17–42 µmol/L
Toxic (also consider effect of		
metabolite (NAPA))	>10–12 µg/mL	>42–51 µmol/L
Prolactin, serum		
Males	1.58–23.12 ng/mL	1.58–23.12 µg/L
Females	<0.6–27.33 ng/mL	<0.6–27.33 µg/L
Propoxyphene, plasma (EDTA)		
Therapeutic	0.1–0.4 µg/mL	0.3–1.2 µmol/L
Toxic	>0.5 µg/mL	>1.5 µmol/L
Propranolol, serum or plasma		
(Hep or EDTA);		
trough		
Therapeutic	50–100 ng/mL	193–386 nmol/L
*Protein, serum		
Total	6.4–8.3 g/dL	64–83 g/L
Albumin	3.9–5.1 g/dL	39–51 g/L
Globulin		
α_1	0.2–0.4 g/dL	2–4 g/L
α_2	0.5–0.9 g/dL	5–9 g/L
β	0.6–1.1 g/dL	6–11 g/L
γ	0.7–1.7 g/dL	7–17 g/L
Protein		
Urine		
Qualitative	Negative	Negative
Quantitative	50–80 mg/24 h (at rest)	Same
CSF, total	15–40 mg/dL	150–400 mg/dL
Protoporphyrin, free,		
erythrocyte	17–77 µg/dL packed RBC	0.3–1.37 µmol/L packed RBC
Pyruvate, blood	0.3–0.9 mg/dL	34–103 µmol/L
Quinidine, serum or plasma		
(Hep or EDTA);		
trough		
Therapeutic	2–5 µg/mL	6–15 µmol/L
Toxic	>6 µg/mL	>18 µmol/L

*Test values are method dependent.

Tests	Conventional Units	SI Units
Salicylates, serum or plasma (Hep or EDTA); trough		
Therapeutic	150–300 µg/mL	1.09–2.17 mmol/L
Toxic	>500 µg/mL	>3.62 mmol/L
Sedimentation rate		
Wintrobe		
Males	0–10 mm in 1 h	0–5 mm/h
Females	0–20 mm in 1 h	0–15 mm/H
Westergren		
Males	0–15 mm in 1 h	0–15 mm/h
Females	0–20 mm in 1 h	0–20 mm/h
Sodium		
Serum or plasma (Hep)		
Premature		
Cord	116–140 mEq/L	116–140 mmol/L
48 h	128–148 mEq/L	128–148 mmol/L
Newborn, cord	126–166 mEq/L	126–166 mmol/L
Newborn	134–144 mEq/L	134–144 mmol/L
Infant	139–146 mEq/L	139–146 mmol/L
Child	138–145 mEq/L	138–145 mmol/L
Adult	136–146 mEq/L	136–146 mmol/L
Urine, 24 h	40–220 mEq/d (diet dependent)	40–220 mmol/d (diet dependent)
Sweat		
Normal	10–40 mEq/L	10–40 mmol/L
Cystic fibrosis	70–190 mEq/L	70–190 mmol/L
Specific gravity	1.002–1.030	1.002–1.030
Sulfates, inorganic, serum	0.8–1.2 mg/dL	83–125 µmol/L
*Testosterone, plasma		
Males	300–1000 ng/dL	10.4–34.7 nmol/L
Females	20–75 ng/dL	0.69–2.6 nmol/L
Pregnant females	3–4 times the adult level	Same
Theophylline, serum or plasma (Hep or EDTA)		
Therapeutic		
Bronchodilator	8–20 µg/mL	44–111 µmol/L
Prem. apnea	6–13 µg/mL	33–72 µmol/L
Toxic	>20 µg/mL	>110 µmol/L
Thiocyanate		
Serum or plasma (EDTA)		
Nonsmoker	1–4 µg/mL	17–69 µmol/L
Smoker	3–12 µg/mL	52–206 µmol/L
Therapeutic after nitroprusside infusion	6–29 µg/mL	103–499 µmol/L
Urine		
Nonsmoker	1–4 mg/d	17–69 µmol/d
Smoker	7–17 mg/d	120–292 µmol/d
Thiopental, serum or plasma (Hep or EDTA); trough		
Hypnotic	1.0–5.0 µg/mL	4.1–20.7 µmol/L
Coma	30–100 µg/mL	124–413 µmol/L

*Test values are method dependent.

Tests	Conventional Units	SI Units
Anesthesia	7–130 µg/mL	29–536 µmol/L
Toxic concentration	>10 µg/mL	>41 µmol/L
*Thyroid-stimulating hormone (TSH), serum	0.32–5 µIU/L	0.32–5 mIU/L
Thyroxine (T₄) serum	5–12 µg/dL (varies with age, higher in children and pregnant women)	65–155 nmol/L (varies with age, higher in children and pregnant women)
Thyroxine, free, serum	0.8–2.3 ng/dL	10.3–31 pmol/L
Thyroxine binding globulin (TBG), serum (as thyroxine)	1.5–3.4 mg/dL	15–34 mg/L
Tobramycin, serum or plasma (Hep or EDTA)		
Therapeutic		
Peak		
Less severe infection	5–8 µg/mL	11–17 µmol/L
Severe infection	8–10 µg/mL	17–21 µmol/L
Trough		
Less severe infection	<1 µg/mL	<2 µmol/L
Moderate infection	<2 µg/mL	<4 µmol/L
Severe infection	<2–4 µg/mL	<4–9 µmol/L
Toxic		
Peak	>10–12 µg/mL	>21–26 µmol/L
Trough	>2–4 µg/mL	>4–9 µmol/L
*Transaminase, serum		
AST (asparate aminotransferase, SGOT)	5–40 U/L (37˚C)	Same
ALT (alanine aminotransferase, SGPT)	7–56 U/L (37˚C)	Same
Transferrin, serum		
Newborn	130–275 mg/dL	1.30–2.75 g/L
Adult	220–400 mg/dL	2.20–4.00 g/L
>60 y	180–380 mg/dL	1.80–3.80 g/L
Triglycerides, serum, fasting		
Males	40–160 mg/dL	0.45–1.81 mmol/L
Females	35–135 mg/dL	0.4–1.53 mmol/L
Triiodothyronine, total (T₃) serum	150–250 ng/dL	1.54–3.08 nmol/L
*Triiodothyronine (T₃) uptake, resin (T₃RU)	24–34% uptake	0.24–0.34 uptake
Uric acid		
Serum, enzymatic		
Male	4.5–8.0 mg/dL	0.27–0.47 mmol/L
Female	2.5–6.2 mg/dL	0.15–0.37 mmol/L
Child	2.0–5.5 mg/dL	0.12–0.32 mmol/L
*Urine	250–750 mg/24 h (with normal diet)	1.48–4.43 mmol/24 h (with normal diet)
Urea nitrogen, serum	7–18 mg/dL	2.5–6.4 mmol Urea/L
Urea nitrogen/creatinine ratio, serum	12:1 to 20:1	48–80 urea/creatinine mole ratio
Urobilinogen, urine	0.1–0.8 Ehrlich unit/2 h	Same
	0.5–4.0 mg/24 h	Same

*Test values are method dependent.

Tests	Conventional Units	SI Units
Valproic acid, serum or plasma (Hep or EDTA); trough		
Therapeutic	50–100 µg/mL	347–693 µmol/L
Toxic	>100 µg/mL	>693 µmol/L
Vancomycin, serum or plasma (Hep or EDTA); trough		
Therapeutic		
Peak	20–40 µg/mL	14–28 µmol/L
Trough	5–10 µg/mL	3–7 µmol/L
Toxic	>80–100 µg/mL	>55–69 µmol/L
Vanillylmandelic acid (VMA), urine (4-hydroxy-3-methoxymandelic acid)	1.4–6.5 mg/24 h	7–33 µmol/d
Viscosity, serum	1.4–1.8 times water	1.4–1.8 times water
Vitamin A, serum	30–80 µg/dL	1.05–2.8 µmol/L
Vitamin B_{12}, serum	100–700 pg/mL	74–516 pmol/L
Vitamin E, serum		
Normal	5–18 µg/mL	11.6–46.4 µmol/L
Therapeutic	30–50 µg/mL	69.6–116 µmol/L
Zinc, serum	70–150 µg/mL	10.7–22.9 µmol/L

BLOOD GROUPS

John Moulds, MT(ASCP)SBP, President and C.O.O., Gamma Biologicals, Houston, TX.

In this appendix, and in the related terms defined in the dictionary proper, blood group is used to refer to an entire blood group system consisting of heritable antigens whose specificity is controlled by a series of allelic genes. Most blood components, i.e., erythrocytes, leukocytes, platelets or plasma protein, possess heritable antigens that have been identified as belonging to systems. Traditionally, blood group is used predominantly in reference to erythrocyte antigens. The terms blood type and phenotype are used to refer to a specific reaction pattern to testing antisera within a system. The term blood group factor is used to refer to a specific antigen within a system. This usage is not universal. It should be noted that in current literature, a single system may be referred to in the plural (i.e., ABO blood groups) and the term blood group may be assigned to a single phenotype (i.e., blood group A).

Each blood group is defined in terms of reaction to the original antisera with which the system was discovered, with modification or extension as required by the discovery of additional antisera proven to be related to the same system. A new blood group antigen or factor can be defined by showing that it is detected by an antiserum with reactions different from those of previously known antisera. If it is shown that the new antigen is genetically independent of known blood group systems, it may qualify as a prototype antigen for a new blood group. Alternatively, if it can be shown that the new antigen is controlled by a gene allelic to one of the known blood group genes, it is assigned to the blood group system of its alleles.

In the blood group definitions, emphasis has been placed on identification of symbols for genes, antigens, antisera, and phenotypes. These often appear in the literature without specification that they refer to a blood group. Attention is called to the general convention, followed here, that symbols for genes and genotypes are set in italics, whereas symbols for gene products or antigens, antisera, and phenotypes are set in Roman type. In the Rh-Hr terminology for the Rh blood group, Roman type is used to designate antigen substances, and boldface type is used to designate serological factors and their corresponding antibodies. These are in wide use but are not consistently followed by all authors.

Nomenclature

The designation of blood group systems and antigens has been based upon alphabetical assignment of names or initials of first antibody producer, reactive or nonreactive red cell source or derivation of name, location or discovering institution. The International Society of Blood Transfusion (ISBT) developed a Working Party on Terminology of Red Cell Surface Antigens to establish a uniform nomenclature, while not modifying historical designations and guidelines. Part of the Working Party's charge is to review periodically the available data and report additions, alterations, or deletions to those blood group antigens considered extinct. In addition, the Working Party developed a nomenclature coding system, based on order of discovery of the blood group systems, to aid in the computerization of data. Reports of the Working Party are published in Vox Sanguinis (1990; 58:152–169, 1993; 65:77–80).

Currently, there are 22 blood group systems. Each system is serologically, immunochemically, and genetically proven to be products of distinct independent genes. The Rh system has 47 separate antigens while others (i.e., P, Xg, Hh, and Kx systems) have only one antigen associated with the system. Table 1 lists the approved system names, abbreviated symbol, and numerical designation developed by the ISBT. For clinical considerations, the ABO and Rh are of most importance; others are useful for genetic linkage or red cell membrane protein studies.

In addition to the defined blood group systems, there are other blood group antigens that fail, as of yet, to fit the system criteria. Some are loosely associated by serological and immunochemical reactivity but insufficient data exist to classify them as a system. Hence they are referred to as collections (Table 2).

A second set of antigens occurring with a high incidence in the random population are collectively referred to as high incidence or public antigens. These occur in almost all individuals but are absent in a few. The antibodies usually have been found in the serum of patients lacking the antigen who have become immunized by transfusion or pregnancy. There are 11 distinct high incidence antigens and some of the symbols applied to public antigens include: Vel, Lan, At^a, Jr^a and JMH.

The third set of erythrocyte antigens, each defined by a specific antiserum, are uncommon, and each is found only in members of a very few families. Because of their rarity, they are often referred to as low incidence or private antigens. The antibodies usually have been found in the serum of patients who have received transfusions or in mothers of infants with Hemolytic Disease of the Newborn (HDN). They are often named for the family in which they were first discovered. There are 36 distinct low incidence antigens, and some symbols assigned to the private antigens are: By, Sw^a, Bi^a, Hey, NFLD, RAS, HJK and ELO.

Table 1. Designation of Blood Group Systems

System Name	Symbol	System No.	No. Antigens	System Name	Symbol	System No.	No. Antigens
ABO	ABO	001	4	Xg	XG	012	1
MNS	MNS	002	37	Scianna	SC	013	3
P	P1	003	1	Dombrock	DO	014	5
Rh	RH	004	47	Colton	CO	015	3
Lutheran	LU	005	18	Landsteiner-Weiner	LW	016	3
Kell	KEL	006	21	Chido/Rogers	CH/RG	017	9
Lewis	LE	007	3	Hh	H	018	1
Duffy	FY	008	6	Kx	XK	019	1
Kidd	JK	009	3	Gerbich	GE	020	7
Diego	DI	010	2	Cromer	CR	021	10
Yt	YT	011	2	Knops	KN	022	5

Table 2. Designations of Collections

Collection Name	Symbol	No.	No.of Associated Antigens
Indian	IN	203	2
Cost	COST	205	2
Ii	I	207	2
Er	ER	208	2
		209	3
		210	2
Wright	WR	211	2

DIAGNOSIS RELATED GROUPS (DRGs)

RG	DRG Description
1	Craniotomy, Age Greater than 17 Except for Trauma
2	Craniotomy for Trauma, Age Greater than 17
3	Craniotomy, Age 0–17
4	Spinal Procedures
5	Extracranial Vascular Procedures
6	Carpal Tunnel Release
7	Peripheral and Cranial Nerve and Other Nervous System Procedures with CC
8	Peripheral and Cranial Nerve and Other Nervous System Procedures without CC
9	Spinal Disorders and Injuries
10	Nervous System Neoplasms with CC
11	Nervous System Neoplasms without CC
12	Degenerative Nervous System Disorders
13	Multiple Sclerosis and Cerebellar Ataxia
14	Specific Cerebrovascular Disorders Except Transient Ischemic Attack
15	Transient Ischemic Attack and Precerebral Occlusions
16	Nonspecific Cerebrovascular Disorders with CC
17	Nonspecific Cerebrovascular Disorders without CC
18	Cranial and Peripheral Nerve Disorders with CC
19	Cranial and Peripheral Nerve Disorders without CC
20	Nervous System Infection Except Viral Meningitis
21	Viral Meningitis
22	Hypertensive Encephalopathy
23	Nontraumatic Stupor and Coma
24	Seizure and Headache, Age Greater than 17 with CC
25	Seizure and Headache, Age Greater than 17 without CC
26	Seizure and Headache, Age 0–17
27	Traumatic Stupor and Coma, Coma Greater than One Hour
28	Traumatic Stupor and Coma, Coma Less than One Hour, Age Greater than 17 with CC
29	Traumatic Stupor and Coma, Coma Less than One Hour, Age Greater than 17 without CC
30	Traumatic Stupor and Coma, Coma Less than One Hour, Age 0–17
31	Concussion, Age Greater than 17 with CC

DRG	DRG Description
32	Concussion, Age Greater than 17 without CC
33	Concussion, Age 0–17
34	Other Disorders of Nervous System with CC
35	Other Disorders of Nervous System without CC
36	Retinal Procedures
37	Orbital Procedures
38	Primary Iris Procedures
39	Lens Procedures with or without Vitrectomy
40	Extraocular Procedures except Orbit, Age Greater than 17
41	Extraocular Procedures Except Orbit, Age 0–17
42	Intraocular Procedures Except Retina, Iris and Lens
43	Hyphema
44	Acute Major Eye Infections
45	Neurological Eye Disorders
46	Other Disorders of the Eye, Age Greater than 17 with CC
47	Other Disorders of the Eye, Age Greater than 17 without CC
48	Other Disorders of the Eye, Age 0–17
49	Major Head and Neck Procedures
50	Sialoadenectomy
51	Salivary Gland Procedures Except Sialoadenectomy
52	Cleft Lip and Palate Repair
53	Sinus and Mastoid Procedures, Age Greater than 17
54	Sinus and Mastoid Procedures, Age 0–17
55	Miscellaneous Ear, Nose, Mouth and Throat Procedures
56	Rhinoplasty
57	T and A Procedures Except Tonsillectomy and/or Adenoidectomy Only, Age Greater than 17
58	T and A Procedures Except Tonsillectomy and/or Adenoidectomy Only, Age 0–17
59	Tonsillectomy and/or Adenoidectomy Only, Age Greater than 17
60	Tonsillectomy and/or Adenoidectomy Only, Age 0–17
61	Myringotomy with Tube Insertion, Age Greater than 17
62	Myringotomy with Tube Insertion, Age 0–17

63 Other Ear, Nose, Mouth and Throat OR Procedures

64 Ear, Nose, Mouth and Throat Malignancy

65 Dysequilibrium

66 Epistaxis

67 Epiglottitis

68 Otitis Media and URI, Age Greater than 17 with CC

69 Otitis Media and URI, Age Greater than 17 without CC

70 Otitis Media and URI, Age 0–17

71 Laryngotracheitis

72 Nasal Trauma and Deformity

73 Other Ear, Nose, Mouth and Throat Diagnoses, Age Greater than 17

74 Other Ear, Nose, Mouth and Throat Diagnoses, Age 0–17

75 Major Chest Procedures

76 Other Respiratory System OR Procedures with CC

77 Other Respiratory System OR Procedures without CC

78 Pulmonary Embolism

79 Respiratory Infections and Inflammations, Age Greater than 17 with CC

80 Respiratory Infections and Inflammations, Age Greater than 17 without CC

81 Respiratory Infections and Inflammations, Age 0–17

82 Respiratory Neoplasms

83 Major Chest Trauma with CC

84 Major Chest Trauma without CC

85 Pleural Effusion with CC

86 Pleural Effusion without CC

87 Pulmonary Edema and Respiratory Failure

88 Chronic Obstructive Pulmonary Disease

89 Simple Pneumonia and Pleurisy, Age Greater than 17 with CC

90 Simple Pneumonia and Pleurisy, Age Greater than 17 without CC

91 Simple Pneumonia and Pleurisy, Age 0–17

92 Interstitial Lung Disease with CC

93 Interstitial Lung Disease without CC

94 Pneumothorax with CC

95 Pneumothorax without CC

96 Bronchitis and Asthma, Age Greater than 17 with CC

97 Bronchitis and Asthma, Age Greater than 17 without CC

98 Bronchitis and Asthma, Age 0–17

99 Respiratory Signs and Symptoms with CC

100 Respiratory Signs and Symptoms without CC

101 Other Respiratory System Diagnoses with CC

102 Other Respiratory System Diagnoses without CC

103 Heart Transplant

104 Cardiac Valve Procedures with Cardiac Catheterization

105 Cardiac Valve Procedures without Cardiac Catheterization

106 Coronary Bypass with Cardiac Catheterization

107 Coronary Bypass without Cardiac Catheterization

108 Other Cardiothoracic Procedures

109 No Longer Valid

110 Major Cardiovascular Procedures with CC

111 Major Cardiovascular Procedures without CC

112 Percutaneous Cardiovascular Procedures

113 Amputation for Circulatory System Disorders Except Upper Limb and Toe

114 Upper Limb and Toe Amputation for Circulatory System Disorders

115 Permanent Cardiac Pacemaker Implant with Acute Myocardial Infarction, Heart Failure or Shock

116 Other Permanent Cardiac Pacemaker Implant or AICD Lead or Generator Procedure

117 Cardiac Pacemaker Revision Except Device Replacement

118 Cardiac Pacemaker Device Replacement

119 Vein Ligation and Stripping

120 Other Circulatory System OR Procedures

121 Circulatory Disorders with Acute Myocardial Infarction and Cardiovascular Complication, Discharged Alive

122 Circulatory Disorders with Acute Myocardial Infarction without Cardiovascular Complication, Discharged Alive

123 Circulatory Disorders with Acute Myocardial Infarction, Expired

124 Circulatory Disorders Except Acute Myocardial Infarction with Cardiac Catheterization and Complex Diagnosis

125 Circulatory Disorders Except Acute Myocardial Infarction with Cardiac Catheterization without Complex Diagnosis

126 Acute and Subacute Endocarditis

127 Heart Failure and Shock

128 Deep Vein Thrombophlebitis

129 Cardiac Arrest, Unexplained

130 Peripheral Vascular Disorders with CC

131 Peripheral Vascular Disorders without CC

132 Atherosclerosis with CC

133 Atherosclerosis without CC

134 Hypertension

135 Cardiac Congenital and Valvular Disorders, Age Greater than 17 with CC

136 Cardiac Congenital and Valvular Disorders, Age Greater than 17 without CC

137 Cardiac Congenital and Valvular Disorders, Age 0–17

138 Cardiac Arrhythmia and Conduction Disorders with CC

139 Cardiac Arrhythmia and Conduction Disorders without CC

140 Angina Pectoris

141 Syncope and Collapse with CC

142 Syncope and Collapse without CC

143 Chest Pain

144 Other Circulatory System Diagnoses with CC

145 Other Circulatory System Diagnoses without CC

146 Rectal Resection with CC

147 Rectal Resection without CC

148 Major Small and Large Bowel Procedures with CC

149 Major Small and Large Bowel Procedures without CC

150 Peritoneal Adhesiolysis with CC

151 Peritoneal Adhesiolysis without CC

152 Minor Small and Large Bowel Procedures with CC

153 Minor Small and Large Bowel Procedures without CC

154 Stomach, Esophageal and Duodenal Procedures, Age Greater than 17 with CC

155 Stomach, Esophageal and Duodenal Procedures, Age Greater than 17 without CC

156 Stomach, Esophageal and Duodenal Procedures, Age 0–17

157 Anal and Stomal Procedures with CC

158 Anal and Stomal Procedures without CC

159 Hernia Procedures Except Inguinal and Femoral, Age Greater than 17 with CC

160 Hernia Procedures Except Inguinal and Femoral, Age Greater than 17 without CC

161 Inguinal and Femoral Hernia Procedures, Age Greater than 17 with CC

162 Inguinal and Femoral Hernia Procedures, Age Greater than 17 without CC

163 Hernia Procedures, Age 0–17

164 Appendectomy with Complicated Principal Diagnosis with CC

165 Appendectomy with Complicated Principal Diagnosis without CC

166 Appendectomy without Complicated Principal Diagnosis with CC

167 Appendectomy without Complicated Principal Diagnosis without CC

168 Mouth Procedures with CC

169 Mouth Procedures without CC

170 Other Digestive System OR Procedures with CC

171 Other Digestive System OR Procedures without CC

172 Digestive Malignancy with CC

173 Digestive Malignancy without CC

174 GI Hemorrhage with CC

175 GI Hemorrhage without CC

176 Complicated Peptic Ulcer

177 Uncomplicated Peptic Ulcer with CC

178 Uncomplicated Peptic Ulcer without CC

179 Inflammatory Bowel Disease

180 GI Obstruction with CC

181 GI Obstruction without CC

182 Esophagitis, Gastroenteritis and Miscellaneous Digestive Disorders, Age Greater than 17 with CC

183 Esophagitis, Gastroenteritis and Miscellaneous Digestive Disorders, Age Greater than 17 without CC

184 Esophagitis, Gastroenteritis and Miscellaneous Digestive Disorders, Age 0–17

185 Dental and Oral Diseases Except Extractions and Restorations, Age Greater than 17

186 Dental and Oral Diseases Except Extractions and Restorations, Age 0–17

187 Dental Extractions and Restorations

188 Other Digestive System Diagnoses, Age Greater than 17 with CC

189 Other Digestive System Diagnoses, Age Greater than 17 without CC

190 Other Digestive System Diagnoses, Age 0–17

191 Pancreas, Liver and Shunt Procedures with CC

192 Pancreas, Liver and Shunt Procedures without CC

193 Biliary Tract Procedures Except Only Cholecystectomy with or without Common Duct Exploration with CC

194 Biliary Tract Procedures Except Only Cholecystectomy with or without Common Duct Exploration without CC

195 Cholecystectomy with Common Duct Exploration with CC

196 Cholecystectomy with Common Duct Exploration without CC

197 Cholecystectomy Except by Laparoscope without Common Duct Exploration with CC

198 Cholecystectomy Except by Laparoscope without Common Duct Exploration without CC

199 Hepatobiliary Diagnostic Procedure for Malignancy

200 Hepatobiliary Diagnostic Procedure for Nonmalignancy

201 Other Hepatobiliary or Pancreas OR Procedures

202 Cirrhosis and Alcoholic Hepatitis

203 Malignancy of Hepatobiliary System or Pancreas

204 Disorders of Pancreas Except Malignancy

205 Disorders of Liver Except Malignancy, Cirrhosis and Alcoholic Hepatitis with CC

206 Disorders of Liver Except Malignancy, Cirrhosis and Alcoholic Hepatitis without CC

207 Disorders of the Biliary Tract with CC

208 Disorders of the Biliary Tract without CC

209 Major Joint and Limb Reattachment Procedures of Lower Extremity

210 Hip and Femur Procedures Except Major Joint Procedures, Age Greater than 17 with CC

211 Hip and Femur Procedures Except Major Joint Procedures, Age Greater than 17 without CC

212 Hip and Femur Procedures Except Major Joint Procedures, Age 0–17

213 Amputation For Musculoskeletal System and Connective Tissue Disorders

214 Back and Neck Procedures with CC

215 Back and Neck Procedures without CC

216 Biopsies of Musculoskeletal System and Connective Tissue

217 Wound Debridement and Skin Graft Except Hand for Musculoskeletal and Connective Tissue Disorders

218 Lower Extremity and Humerus Procedures Except Hip, Foot and Femur, Age Greater than 17 with CC

219 Lower Extremity and Humerus Procedures Except Hip, Foot and Femur, Age Greater than 17 without CC

220 Lower Extremity and Humerus Procedures Except Hip, Foot and Femur, Age 0–17

221 Knee Procedures with CC

222 Knee Procedures without CC

223 Major Shoulder/Elbow Procedures or Other Upper Extremity Procedures with CC

224 Major Shoulder/Elbow Procedures or Other Upper Extremity Procedures without CC

225 Foot Procedures

226 Soft Tissue Procedures with CC

227 Soft Tissue Procedures without CC

228 Major Thumb or Joint Procedures or Other Hand or Wrist Procedures with CC

229 Major Thumb or Joint Procedures or Other Hand or Wrist Procedures without CC

230 Local Excision and Removal of Internal Fixation Devices of Hip and Femur

231 Local Excision and Removal of Internal Fixation Devices Except Hip and Femur

232 Arthroscopy

233 Other Musculoskeletal System and Connective Tissue OR Procedures with CC

234 Other Musculoskeletal System and Connective Tissue OR Procedures without CC

235 Fractures of Femur

236 Fractures of Hip and Pelvis

237 Sprains, Strains and Dislocations of Hip, Pelvis and Thigh

238 Osteomyelitis

239 Pathological Fractures and Musculoskeletal and Connective Tissue Malignancy

240 Connective Tissue Disorders with CC

241 Connective Tissue Disorders without CC

242 Septic Arthritis

243 Medical Back Problems

244 Bone Diseases and Specific Arthropathies with CC

245 Bone Diseases and Specific Arthropathies without CC

246 Nonspecific Arthropathies

247 Signs and Symptoms of Musculoskeletal System and Connective Tissue

248 Tendonitis, Myositis and Bursitis

249 Aftercare, Musculoskeletal System and Connective Tissue

250 Fractures, Sprains, Strains and Dislocations of Forearm, Hand and Foot, Age Greater than 17 with CC

251 Fractures, Sprains, Strains and Dislocations of Forearm, Hand and Foot, Age Greater than 17 without CC

252 Fractures, Sprains, Strains and Dislocations of Forearm, Hand and Foot, Age 0–17

253 Fractures, Sprains, Strains and Dislocations of Upper Arm and Lower Leg Except Foot, Age Greater than 17 with CC

254 Fractures, Sprains, Strains and Dislocations of Upper Arm and Lower Leg Except Foot, Age Greater than 17 without CC

255 Fractures, Sprains, Strains and Dislocations of Upper Arm and Lower Leg Except Foot, Age 0–17

256 Other Musculoskeletal System and Connective Tissue Diagnoses

257 Total Mastectomy for Malignancy with CC

258 Total Mastectomy for Malignancy without CC

259 Subtotal Mastectomy for Malignancy with CC

260 Subtotal Mastectomy for Malignancy without CC

261 Breast Procedure for Nonmalignancy Except Biopsy and Local Excision

262 Breast Biopsy and Local Excision for Nonmalignancy

263 Skin Grafts and/or Debridement for Skin Ulcer or Cellulitis with CC

264 Skin Grafts and/or Debridement for Skin Ulcer or Cellulitis without CC

265 Skin Grafts and/or Debridement Except for Skin Ulcer or Cellulitis with CC

266 Skin Grafts and/or Debridement Except for Skin Ulcer or Cellulitis without CC

267 Perianal and Pilonidal Procedures

268 Skin, Subcutaneous Tissue and Breast Plastic Procedures

269 Other Skin, Subcutaneous Tissue and Breast Procedures with CC

270 Other Skin, Subcutaneous Tissue and Breast Procedures without CC

271 Skin Ulcers

272 Major Skin Disorders with CC

273 Major Skin Disorders without CC

274 Malignant Breast Disorders with CC

275 Malignant Breast Disorders without CC

276 Nonmalignant Breast Disorders

277 Cellulitis, Age Greater than 17 with CC

278 Cellulitis, Age Greater than 17 without CC

279 Cellulitis, Age 0–17

280 Trauma to Skin, Subcutaneous Tissue and Breast, Age Greater than 17 with CC

281 Trauma to Skin, Subcutaneous Tissue and Breast, Age Greater than 17 without CC

282 Trauma to Skin, Subcutaneous Tissue and Breast, Age 0–17

283 Minor Skin Disorders with CC

284 Minor Skin Disorders without CC

285 Amputation of Lower Limb for Endocrine, Nutritional and Metabolic Disorders

286 Adrenal and Pituitary Procedures

287 Skin Grafts and Wound Debridement for Endocrine, Nutritional and Metabolic Disorders

288 OR Procedures for Obesity

289 Parathyroid Procedures

290 Thyroid Procedures

291 Thyroglossal Procedures

292 Other Endocrine, Nutritional and Metabolic OR Procedures with CC

293 Other Endocrine, Nutritional and Metabolic OR Procedures without CC

294 Diabetes, Age Greater than 35

295 Diabetes, Age 0–35

296 Nutritional and Miscellaneous Metabolic Disorders, Age Greater than 17 with CC

297 Nutritional and Miscellaneous Metabolic Disorders, Age Greater than 17 without CC

298 Nutritional and Miscellaneous Metabolic Disorders, Age 0–17

299 Inborn Errors of Metabolism

300 Endocrine Disorders with CC

301 Endocrine Disorders without CC

302 Kidney Transplant

303 Kidney, Ureter and Major Bladder Procedures for Neoplasm

304 Kidney, Ureter and Major Bladder Procedures for Neoplasms with CC

305 Kidney, Ureter and Major Bladder Procedures for Neoplasms without CC

306 Prostatectomy with CC

307 Prostatectomy without CC

Appendices

308 Minor Bladder Procedures with CC

309 Minor Bladder Procedures without CC

310 Transurethral Procedures with CC

311 Transurethral Procedures without CC

312 Urethral Procedures, Age Greater than 17 with CC

313 Urethral Procedures, Age Greater than 17 without CC

314 Urethral Procedures, Age 0–17

315 Other Kidney and Urinary Tract OR Procedures

316 Renal Failure

317 Admission for Renal Dialysis

318 Kidney and Urinary Tract Neoplasms with CC

319 Kidney and Urinary Tract Neoplasms without CC

320 Kidney and Urinary Tract Infections, Age Greater than 17 with CC

321 Kidney and Urinary Tract Infections, Age Greater than 17 without CC

322 Kidney and Urinary Tract Infections, Age 0–17

323 Urinary Stones with CC and/or ESW Lithotripsy

324 Urinary Stones without CC

325 Kidney and Urinary Tract Signs and Symptoms, Age Greater than 17 with CC

326 Kidney and Urinary Tract Signs and Symptoms, Age Greater than 17 without CC

327 Kidney and Urinary Tract Signs and Symptoms, Age 0–17

328 Urethral Stricture, Age Greater than 17 with CC

329 Urethral Stricture, Age Greater than 17 without CC

330 Urethral Stricture, Age 0–17

331 Other Kidney and Urinary Tract Diagnoses, Age Greater than 17 with CC

332 Other Kidney and Urinary Tract Diagnoses, Age Greater than 17 without CC

333 Other Kidney and Urinary Tract Diagnoses, Age 0–17

334 Major Male Pelvic Procedures with CC

335 Major Male Pelvic Procedures without CC

336 Transurethral Prostatectomy with CC

337 Transurethral Prostatectomy without CC

338 Testes Procedures for Malignancy

339 Testes Procedures for Nonmalignancy, Age Greater than 17

340 Testes Procedures for Nonmalignancy, Age 0–17

341 Penis Procedures

342 Circumcision, Age Greater than 17

343 Circumcision, Age 0–17

344 Other Male Reproductive System OR Procedures for Malignancy

345 Other Male Reproductive System OR Procedures Except for Malignancy

346 Malignancy of Male Reproductive System with CC

347 Malignancy of Male Reproductive System without CC

348 Benign Prostatic Hypertrophy with CC

349 Benign Prostatic Hypertrophy without CC

350 Inflammation of the Male Reproductive System

351 Sterilization, Male

352 Other Male Reproductive System Diagnoses

353 Pelvic Evisceration, Radical Hysterectomy and Radical Vulvectomy

354 Uterine and Adnexal Procedures for Nonovarian/Adnexal Malignancy with CC

355 Uterine and Adnexal Procedures for Nonovarian/Adnexal Malignancy without CC

356 Female Reproductive System Reconstructive Procedures

357 Uterine and Adnexal Procedures for Ovarian or Adnexal Malignancy

358 Uterine and Adnexal Procedures for Nonmalignancy with CC

359 Uterine and Adnexal Procedures for Nonmalignancy without CC

360 Vagina, Cervix and Vulva Procedures

361 Laparoscopy and Incisional Tubal Interruption

362 Endoscopic Tubal Interruption

363 D and C, Conization and Radioimplant for Malignancy

364 D and C, Conization Except for Malignancy

365 Other Female Reproductive System OR Procedures

366 Malignancy of Female Reproductive System with CC

367 Malignancy of Female Reproductive System without CC

368 Infections of Female Reproductive System

369 Menstrual and Other Female Reproductive System Disorders

370 Cesarean Section with CC

371 Cesarean Section without CC

372 Vaginal Delivery with Complicating Diagnoses

373 Vaginal Delivery without Complicating Diagnoses

374 Vaginal Delivery with Sterilization and/or D and C

375 Vaginal Delivery with OR Procedure Except Sterilization and/or D and C

376 Postpartum and Postabortion Diagnoses without OR Procedure

377 Postpartum and Postabortion Diagnoses with OR Procedure

378 Ectopic Pregnancy

379 Threatened Abortion

380 Abortion without D and C

381 Abortion with D and C, Aspiration Curettage or Hysterotomy

382 False Labor

383 Other Antepartum Diagnoses with Medical Complications

384 Other Antepartum Diagnoses without Medical Complications

385 Neonates, Died or Transferred to Another Acute Care Facility

386 Extreme Immaturity or Respiratory Distress Syndrome of Neonate

387 Prematurity with Major Problems

388 Prematurity without Major Problems

389 Full Term Neonate with Major Problems

390 Neonate with Other Significant Problems

391 Normal Newborn

392 Splenectomy, Age Greater than 17

393 Splenectomy, Age 0–17

394 Other OR Procedures of the Blood and Blood-Forming Organs

395 Red Blood Cell Disorders, Age Greater than 17

396 Red Blood Cell Disorders, Age 0–17

397 Coagulation Disorders

398 Reticuloendothelial and Immunity Disorders with CC

399 Reticuloendothelial and Immunity Disorders without CC

400 Lymphoma and Leukemia with Major OR Procedures

401 Lymphoma and Nonacute Leukemia with Other OR Procedure with CC

402 Lymphoma and Nonacute Leukemia with Other OR Procedure without CC

403 Lymphoma and Nonacute Leukemia with CC

404 Lymphoma and Nonacute Leukemia without CC

405 Acute Leukemia without Major OR Procedure, Age 0–17

406 Myeloproliferative Disorders or Poorly Differentiated Neoplasms with Major OR Procedures with CC

407 Myeloproliferative Disorders or Poorly Differentiated Neoplasms with Major OR Procedures without CC

408 Myeloproliferative Disorders or Poorly Differentiated Neoplasms with Other OR Procedures

409 Radiotherapy

410 Chemotherapy without Acute Leukemia as Secondary Diagnosis

411 History of Malignancy without Endoscopy

412 History of Malignancy with Endoscopy

413 Other Myeloproliferative Disorders or Poorly Differentiated Neoplasm Diagnoses with CC

414 Other Myeloproliferative Disorders or Poorly Differentiated Neoplasm Diagnoses without CC

415 OR Procedure for Infectious and Parasitic Diseases

416 Septicemia, Age Greater than 17

417 Septicemia, Age 0–17

418 Postoperative and Posttraumatic Infections

419 Fever of Unknown Origin, Age Greater than 17 with CC

420 Fever of Unknown Origin, Age Greater than 17 without CC

421 Viral Illness, Age Greater than 17

422 Viral Illness and Fever of Unknown Origin, Age 0–17

423 Other Infectious and Parasitic Diseases Diagnoses

424 OR Procedures with Principal Diagnosis of Mental Illness

425 Acute Adjustment Reactions and Disturbances of Psychosocial Dysfunction

426 Depressive Neuroses

427 Neuroses Except Depressive

428 Disorders of Personality and Impulse Control

429 Organic Disturbances and Mental Retardation

430 Psychoses

431 Childhood Mental Disorders

432 Other Mental Disorder Diagnoses

433 Alcohol/Drug Abuse or Dependence, Left against Medical Advice

434 Alcohol/Drug Abuse or Dependence, Detoxification or Other Symptomatic Treatment with CC

435 Alcohol/Drug Abuse or Dependence, Detoxification or Other Symptomatic Treatment without CC

436 Alcohol/Drug Dependence with Rehabilitation Therapy

Appendices

437 Alcohol/Drug Dependence with Combined Rehabilitation and Detoxification Therapy

438 No Longer Valid

439 Skin Grafts for Injuries

440 Wound Debridements for Injuries

441 Hand Procedures for Injuries

442 Other OR Procedures for Injuries with CC

443 Other OR Procedures for Injuries without CC

444 Traumatic Injury, Age Greater than 17 with CC

445 Traumatic Injury, Age Greater than 17 without CC

446 Traumatic Injury, Age 0–17

447 Allergic Reactions, Age Greater than 17

448 Allergic Reactions, Age 0–17

449 Poisoning and Toxic Effects of Drugs, Age Greater than 17 with CC

450 Poisoning and Toxic Effects of Drugs, Age Greater than 17 without CC

451 Poisoning and Toxic Effects of Drugs, Age 0–17

452 Complications of Treatment with CC

453 Complications of Treatment without CC

454 Other Injury, Poisoning and Toxic Effect Diagnoses with CC

455 Other Injury, Poisoning and Toxic Effect Diagnoses without CC

456 Burns, Transferred to Another Acute Care Facility

457 Extensive Burns without OR Procedure

458 Nonextensive Burns with Skin Graft

459 Nonextensive Burns with Wound Debridement or Other OR Procedure

460 Nonextensive Burns without OR Procedure

461 OR Procedures with Diagnoses of Other Contact with Health Services

462 Rehabilitation

463 Signs and Symptoms with CC

464 Signs and Symptoms without CC

465 Aftercare with History of Malignancy as Secondary Diagnosis

466 Aftercare without History of Malignancy as Secondary Diagnosis

467 Other Factors Influencing Health Status

468 Extensive OR Procedure Unrelated to Principal Diagnosis

469 Principal Diagnosis Invalid as Discharge Diagnosis

470 Ungroupable

471 Bilateral or Multiple Major Joint Procedures of Lower Extremity

472 Extensive Burns with OR Procedure

473 Acute Leukemia without Major OR Procedure, Age Greater than 17

474 No Longer Valid

475 Respiratory System Diagnosis with Ventilator Support

476 Prostatic OR Procedure Unrelated to Principal Diagnosis

477 Nonextensive OR Procedure Unrelated to Principal Diagnosis

478 Other Vascular Procedures with CC

479 Other Vascular Procedures without CC

480 Liver Transplant

481 Bone Marrow Transplant

482 Tracheostomy for Face, Mouth and Neck Diagnosis

483 Tracheostomy Except for Face, Mouth and Neck Diagnoses

484 Craniotomy for Multiple Significant Trauma

485 Limb Reattachment, Hip and Femur Procedures for Multiple Significant Trauma

486 Other OR Procedures for Multiple Significant Trauma

487 Other Multiple Significant Trauma

488 HIV with Extensive OR Procedure

489 HIV with Major Related Condition

490 HIV with or without Other Related Condition

491 Major Joint and Limb Reattachment Procedures of Upper Extremity

492 Chemotherapy with Acute Leukemia as Secondary Diagnosis

493 Laparoscopic Cholecystectomy without Common Duct Exploration with CC

494 Laparoscopic Cholecystectomy without Common Duct Exploration without CC

CERTIFIED REGIONAL POISON CENTERS

As of October 1994

ALABAMA

Regional Poison Control Center
The Children's Hospital of Alabama
1600-7th Avenue South
Birmingham, AL 35233-1711
(205) 939-9201,
(800) 292-6678
(AL only) or
(205) 933-4050

ARIZONA

Arizona Poison and Drug Information Center
Arizona Health Sciences Center;
Room #3204-K
1501 N. Campbell Avenue
Tucson, AZ 85724
(800) 362-0101 (AZ only),
(602) 626-6016

Samaritan Regional Poison Center
Teleservices Department
1441 North 12th Street
Phoenix, AZ 85006
(602) 253-3334

CALIFORNIA

Fresno Regional Poison Control Center
Valley Children's Hospital
3141 N. Millbrook, IN31
Fresno, CA 93703
(800) 346-5922 (Central CA only) or
(209) 445-1222

San Diego Regional Poison Center
UCSD Medical Center
200 West Arbor Drive
San Diego, CA 92103-8925
(619) 543-6000,
(800) 876-4766 (in 619 area code only)

San Francisco Bay Area Regional Poison Control Center
San Francisco General Hospital
1001 Potrero Avenue, Building 80,
Room 230
San Francisco, CA 94110
(800) 523-2222

Santa Clara Valley Medical Center Regional Poison Center
Valley Health Center, Suite 310
San Jose, CA 95128
(408) 885-6000,
(800) 662-9886 (CA only)

University of California, Davis, Medical Center Regional Poison Control Center
2315 Stockton Boulevard
Sacramento, CA 95817
(916) 734-3692;
(800) 342-9293 (Northern CA only)

COLORADO

Rocky Mountain Poison and Drug Center
645 Bannock Street
Denver, CO 80204
(303) 629-1123

DISTRICT OF COLUMBIA

National Capital Poison Center
3201 New Mexico Avenue, NW,
Suite 310
Washington, DC 20007
(202) 625-3333;
(202) 362-8563 (TTY)

FLORIDA

The Florida Poison Information Center and Toxicology Resource Center
Tampa General Hospital
Post Office Box 1289
Tampa, FL 33601
(813) 253-4444 (Tampa);
(800) 282-3171 (FL)

GEORGIA

Georgia Poison Center
Grady Memorial Hospital
80 Butler Street, SE
PO Box 26066
Atlanta, GA 30335-3801
(800) 282-5846 (GA only);
(404) 616-9000

INDIANA

Indiana Poison Center
Methodist Hospital of Indiana
1701 N. Senate Boulevard
PO Box 1367
Indianapolis, IN 46206-1367
(800) 382-9097 (IN only);
(317) 929-2323

MARYLAND

Maryland Poison Center
20 N. Pine Street
Baltimore, MD 21201
(410) 528-7701,
(800) 492-2414 (MD only)

National Capital Poison Center
(DC suburbs only)
3201 New Mexico Avenue, NW,
Suite 310
Washington, DC 20016
Emergency Numbers: (202) 625-3333;
(202) 362-8563 (TTY)

MASSACHUSETTS

Massachusetts Poison Control System
300 Longwood Avenue
Boston, MA 02115
(617) 232-2120,
(800) 682-9211

MICHIGAN

Poison Control Center
Children's Hospital of Michigan
3901 Beaubien Boulevard
Detroit, MI 48201
(313) 745-5711

MINNESOTA

Hennepin Regional Poison Center
Hennepin County Medical Center
701 Park Avenue
Minneapolis, MN 55415
(612) 347-3141,
Petline: (612) 337-7387,
TDD (612) 337-7474

Minnesota Regional Poison Center
St. Paul-Ramsey Medical Center
640 Jackson Street
St. Paul, MN 55101
(612) 221-2113

MISSOURI

Cardinal Glennon Children's Hospital Regional Poison Center
1465 S. Grand Boulevard
St. Louis, MO 63104
(314) 772-5200,
(800) 366-8888

MONTANA

Rocky Mountain Poison and Drug Center
645 Bannock Street
Denver, CO 80204
(303) 629-1123

NEBRASKA

The Poison Center
8301 Dodge Street
Omaha, NE 68114
(402) 390-5555 (Omaha),
(800) 955-9119 (NE & WY)

NEW JERSEY

New Jersey Poison Information and Education System
201 Lyons Avenue
Newark, NJ 07112
(800) 962-1253

NEW MEXICO

New Mexico Poison and Drug Information Center
University of New Mexico
Albuquerque, NM 87131-1076
(505) 843-2551,
(800) 432-6866 (NM only)

NEW YORK

Hudson Valley Poison Center
Nyack Hospital
160 N. Midland Avenue
Nyack, NY 10960
(800) 336-6997,
(914) 353-1000

Long Island Regional Poison Control Center
Winthrop University Hospital
259 First Street
Mineola, NY 11501
(516) 542-2323, 2324, 2325, 3813

New York City Poison Control Center
NYC Department of Health
455 First Avenue, Room 123
New York, NY 10016
(212) 340-4494,
(212) P-O-I-S-O-N-S,
TDD (212) 689-9014

OHIO

Central Ohio Poison Center
700 Children's Drive
Columbus, OH 43205-2696
(614) 228-1323,
(800) 682-7625,
(614) 228-2272
(TTY), (614) 461-2012

Cincinnati Drug & Poison Information Center and Regional Poison Control System
231 Bethesda Avenue, ML 144
Cincinnati, OH 45267-0144
(513) 558-5111,
(800) 872-5111 (OH only)

OREGON

Oregon Poison Center
Oregon Health Sciences University
3181 SW Sam Jackson Park Road
Portland, OR 97201
(503) 494-8968,
(800) 452-7165 (OR only)

PENNSYLVANIA

Central Pennsylvania Poison Center
University Hospital
Milton S. Hershey Medical Center
Hershey, PA 17033
(800) 521-6110

The Poison Control Center serving the greater Philadelphia metropolitan area
One Children's Center
Philadelphia, PA 19104-4303
(215) 386-2100

Pittsburgh Poison Center
3705 Fifth Avenue
Pittsburgh, PA 15213
(412) 681-6669

RHODE ISLAND

Rhode Island Poison Center
593 Eddy Street
Providence, RI 02903
(401) 277-5727

TEXAS

North Texas Poison Center
5201 Harry Hines Boulevard
PO Box 35926
Dallas, TX 75235
(214) 590-5000, Texas Watts
(800) 441-0040

Texas State Poison Center
The University of Texas Medical Branch
Galveston, TX 77550-2780
(409) 765-1420 (Galveston),
(713) 654-1701 (Houston)

UTAH

Utah Poison Control Center
410 Chipeta Way, Suite 230
Salt Lake City, UT 84108
(801) 581-2151,
(800) 456-7707 (UT only)

VIRGINIA

Blue Ridge Poison Center
Box 67
Blue Ridge Hospital
Charlottesville, VA 22901
(804) 924-5543,
(800) 451-1428

National Capital Poison Center
(Northern VA only)
3201 New Mexico Avenue, NW, Suite 310
Washington, DC 20016
(202) 625-3333;
(202) 362-8563 (TTY)

WEST VIRGINIA

West Virginia Poison Center
3110 MacCorkle Avenue, SE
Charleston, WV 25304
(800) 642-3625 (WV only),
(304) 348-4211

WYOMING

The Poison Center
8301 Dodge Street
Omaha, NE 68114
(402) 390-5555 (Omaha),
(800) 955-9119 (NE & WY)

CENTERS FOR DISEASE CONTROL

Universal Precautions to Prevent Transmission of HIV

Since medical history and examination cannot reliably identify all patients infected with HIV or other blood-borne pathogens, blood and body-fluid precautions should be consistently used for *all* patients. This approach, previously recommended by CDC, and referred to as "universal blood and body-fluid precautions" or "universal precautions," should be used in the care of *all* patients, especially including those in emergency-care settings in which the risk of blood exposure is increased and the infection status of the patient is usually unknown.

1. All health-care workers should routinely use appropriate barrier precautions to prevent skin and mucous-membrane exposure when contact with blood or other body fluids of any patient is anticipated. Gloves should be worn for touching blood and body fluids, mucous membranes, or non-intact skin of all patients, for handling items or surfaces soiled with blood or body fluids, and for performing venipuncture and other vascular access procedures. Gloves should be changed after contact with each patient. Masks and protective eyewear or face shields should be worn during procedures that are likely to generate droplets of blood or other body fluids to prevent exposure of mucous membranes of the mouth, nose and eyes. Gowns or aprons should be worn during procedures that are likely to generate splashes of blood or other body fluids.

2. Hands and other skin surfaces should be washed immediately and thoroughly if contaminated with blood or other body fluids. Hands should be washed immediately after gloves are removed.

3. All health-care workers should take precautions to prevent injuries caused by needles, scalpels, and other sharp instruments or devices during procedures; when cleaning used instruments; during disposal of used needles; and when handling sharp instruments after procedures. To prevent needlestick injuries, needles should not be recapped, purposely bent or broken by hand, removed from disposable syringes, or otherwise manipulated by hand. After they are used, disposable syringes and needles, scalpel blades, and other sharp items should be placed in puncture-resistant containers for disposal; the puncture-resistant containers should be located as close as practical to the use area. Large-bore reusable needles should be placed in a puncture-resistant container for transport to the reprocessing area.

4. Although saliva has not been implicated in HIV transmission, to minimize the need for emergency mouth-to-mouth resuscitation, mouthpieces, resuscitation bags, or other ventilation devices should be available for use in areas in which the need for resuscitation is predictable.

5. Health-care workers who have exudative lesions or weeping dermatitis should refrain from all direct patient care and from handling patient-care equipment until the condition resolves.

6. Pregnant health-care workers are not known to be at greater risk of contracting HIV infection than health-care workers who are not pregnant; however, if a health-care worker develops HIV infection during pregnancy, the infant is at risk of infection resulting from perinatal transmission. Because of this risk, pregnant health-care workers should be especially familiar with and strictly adhere to precautions to minimize the risk of HIV transmission.

Precautions for Invasive Procedures

In this document, an invasive procedure is defined as surgical entry into tissues, cavities, or organs or repair of major traumatic injuries 1) in an operating or delivery room, emergency department, or outpatient setting, including both physicians' and dentists' offices; 2) cardiac catheterization and angiographic procedures; 3) a vaginal or cesarean delivery or other invasive obstetric procedure during which bleeding may occur; or 4) the manipulation, cutting, or removal of any oral or perioral tissues, including tooth structure, during which bleeding occurs or the potential for bleeding exists. The universal blood and body-fluid precautions listed above, combined with the precautions listed below, should be the minimum precautions for *all* such invasive procedures.

1. All health-care workers who participate in invasive procedures must routinely use appropriate barrier precautions to prevent skin and mucous-membrane contact with blood and other body fluids of all patients. Gloves and surgical masks must be worn for all invasive procedures. Protective eyewear or face shields should be worn for procedures that commonly result in the generation of droplets, splashing of blood or other body fluids, or the generation of bone chips. Gowns or aprons made of materials that provide an effective barrier should be worn during invasive procedures that are likely to result in the splashing of blood or other body fluids. All health-care workers who perform or assist in vaginal or cesarean deliveries should wear gloves and gowns when handling the placenta or the infant until blood and amniotic fluid have been removed from the infant's skin and should wear gloves during post-delivery care of the umbilical cord.

2. If a glove is torn or a needlestick or other injury occurs, the glove should be removed and a new glove used as promptly as patient safety permits; the needle or instrument involved in the incident should also be removed from the sterile field.

Precautions for Dentistry

Blood, saliva, and gingival fluid from *all* dental patients should be considered infective. Special emphasis should be placed on the following precautions for preventing transmission of blood-borne pathogens in dental practice in both institutional and non-institutional settings.

1. In addition to wearing gloves for contact with oral mucous membranes of all patients, all dental workers should wear surgical masks and protective eyewear or chin-length plastic face shields during dental procedures in which splashing or spattering of blood, saliva, or gingival fluids is likely. Rubber dams, high-speed evacuation, and proper patient positioning, when appropriate, should be utilized to minimize generation of droplets and spatter.

2. Handpieces should be sterilized after use with each patient, since blood, saliva, or gingival fluid of patients may be aspirated into the handpiece or waterline. Handpieces that cannot be sterilized should at least be flushed, the outside surface cleaned and wiped with a suitable chemical germicide, and then rinsed. Handpieces should be flushed at the beginning of the day and after use with each patient. Manufacturers' recommendations should be followed for use and maintenance of waterlines and check valves and for flushing of handpieces. The same precautions should be used for ultrasonic scalers and air/water syringes.

3. Blood and saliva should be thoroughly and carefully cleaned from material that has been used in the mouth (e.g., impression materials, bite registration), especially before polishing and grinding intra-oral devices. Contaminated materials, impressions, and intra-oral devices should also be cleaned and disinfected before being handled in the dental laboratory and before they are placed in the patient's mouth. Because of the increasing variety of dental materials used intra-orally, dental workers should consult with manufacturers as to the stability of specific materials when using disinfection procedures.

4. Dental equipment and surfaces that are difficult to disinfect (e.g., light handles or x-ray-unit heads) and that may become contaminated should be wrapped with impervious-backed paper, aluminum foil, or clear plastic wrap. The coverings should be removed and discarded, and clean coverings should be put in place after use with each patient.

Precautions for Autopsies or Morticians' Services

In addition to the universal blood and body-fluid precautions listed above, the following precautions should be used by persons performing postmortem procedures:

1. All persons performing or assisting in postmortem procedures should wear gloves, masks, protective eyewear, gowns, and waterproof aprons.

2. Instruments and surfaces contaminated during postmortem procedures should be decontaminated with an appropriate chemical germicide.

Precautions for Dialysis

Patients with end-stage renal disease who are undergoing maintenance dialysis and who have HIV infection can be dialyzed in hospital-based or free-standing dialysis units using conventional infection-control precautions. Universal blood and body-fluid precautions should be used when dialyzing *all* patients.

Strategies for disinfecting the dialysis fluid pathways of the hemodialysis machine are targeted to control bacterial contamination and generally consist of using 500–750 parts per million (ppm) of sodium hypochlorite (household bleach) for 30-40 minutes or 1.5%–2.0% formaldehyde overnight. In addition, several chemical germicides formulated to disinfect dialysis machines are commercially available. None of these protocols or procedures need to be changed for dialyzing patients infected with HIV.

Patients infected with HIV can be dialyzed by either hemodialysis or peritoneal dialysis and do not need to be isolated from other patients. The type of dialysis treatment (i.e., hemodialysis or peritoneal dialysis) should be based on the needs of the patient. The dialyzer may be discarded after each use. Alternatively, centers that reuse dialyzers (i.e., a specific single-use dialyzer is issued to a specific patient, removed, cleaned, disinfected, and reused several times on the same patient only) may include HIV-infected patients in the dialyzer-reuse program. An individual dialyzer must never be used on more than one patient.

Precautions for Laboratories

Blood and other body fluids from *all* patients should be considered infective. To supplement the universal blood and body-fluid precautions listed above, the following precautions are recommended for health-care workers in clinical laboratories.

1. All specimens of blood and body fluids should be put in a well-constructed container with a secure lid to prevent leaking during transport. Care should be taken when collecting each specimen to avoid contaminating the outside of the container and of the laboratory form accompanying the specimen.

2. All persons processing blood and body-fluid specimens (e.g., removing tops from vacuum tubes) should wear gloves. Masks and protective eyewear should be worn if mucous-membrane contact with blood or body fluids is anticipated. Gloves should be changed and hands washed after completion of specimen processing.

3. For routine procedures, such as histologic and pathologic studies or microbiologic culturing, a biological safety cabinet is not necessary. However, biological safety cabinets (Class I or II) should be used whenever procedures are conducted that have a high potential for generating droplets. These include activities such as blending, sonicating, and vigorous mixing.

4. Mechanical pipetting devices should be used for manipulating all liquids in the laboratory. Mouth pipetting must not be done.

5. Use of needles and syringes should be limited to situations in which there is no alternative, and the recommendations for preventing injuries with needles outlined under universal precautions should be followed.

6. Laboratory work surfaces should be decontaminated with an appropriate chemical germicide after a spill of blood or other body fluids and when work activities are completed.

7. Contaminated materials used in laboratory tests should be decontaminated before reprocessing or be placed in bags and disposed of in accordance with institutional policies for disposal of infective waste.

8. Scientific equipment that has been contaminated with blood or other body fluids should be decontaminated and cleaned before being repaired in the laboratory or transported to the manufacturer.

9. All persons should wash their hands after completing laboratory activities and should remove protective clothing before leaving the laboratory.

Implementation of universal blood and body-fluid precautions for *all* patients eliminates the need for warning labels on specimens since blood and other body fluids from all patients should be considered infective.

Courtesy of the Centers for Disease Control, Atlanta, GA.

Appendices

AIDS RESOURCES

CALIFORNIA

AIDS Education/Services for the Deaf, Greater Los Angeles Council on Deafness
6565 Sunset Boulevard, Ste. 415
Hollywood, CA 90028
(213) 962-0874,
(213) 962-0870 (TTY/TDD),
(213) 962-0895 (FAX)

California Aids Clearinghouse
P.O. Box 1830
Santa Cruz, CA 95061-1830
(408) 438-4822,
(408) 438-3618 (FAX)

Multicultural Training Resource Center, Multicultural AIDS Resource Center
1540 Market Street, Ste. 320
San Francisco, CA 94702
(415) 861-2142

National Native American AIDS Prevention Center
3515 Grand Avenue, Ste. 100
Oakland, CA 94610
(510) 444-2051,
(800) 283-2437,
(510) 444-1593 (FAX)

Project Inform
1965 Market Street
Ste. 220
San Francisco, CA 94103
(415) 558-8669,
(800) 334-7422,
(415) 558-0684 (FAX)

Ron Shipton HIV Information Center, West Hollywood Library County of Los Angeles Public Library
715 North San Vicente Boulevard West
Hollywood, CA 90069
(310) 652-5340,
(310) 652-2580 (FAX)

U.S. Department of Veterans Affairs, AIDS Information Center
c/o Library Service (142D)
Veterans Affairs Medical Center
4150 Clement Street
San Francisco, CA 94121
(415) 221-4810, extension 3305,
(700) 470-3305 (FTS),
(415) 750-6919 (FAX)

COLORADO

National Conference of State Legislatures
1560 Broadway, Ste. 700
Denver, CO 80202-5140
(303) 830-2200,
(303) 863-2054 (publications orders),
(303) 863-8003 (FAX)

GEORGIA

AID Atlanta
1438 West Peachtree Street
Atlanta, GA 30309
(404) 872-0600,
(404) 885-6799 (FAX)

ILLINOIS

Kupona Network
4611 South Ellis Avenue
Chicago, IL 60653
(312) 536-3000,
(312) 536-8355 (FAX)

MARYLAND

AIDS Clinic Trials Information Service
P.O. Box 6003
Rockville, MD 20849-6003
(301) 217-0023 (international),
(800) TRIALS-A (1-800-874-2572),
(800) 243-7012 (TTY/TDD),
(301) 738-6616 (FAX)

CDC Business Responds to AIDS Resource Service
P.O. Box 6003
Rockville, MD 20849-6003
(800) 458-5231,
(800) 243-7012 (TTY/TDD),
(301) 738-6616 (FAX)

CDC National AIDS Clearinghouse
P.O. Box 6003
Rockville, MD 20849-6003
(301) 217-0023 (international),
(800) 458-5231,
(800) 243-7012 (TTY/TDD),
(301) 738-6616 (FAX)

National Agricultural Library, U.S. Department of Agriculture
Beltsville, MD 20705
(301) 504-6400

National Clearinghouse for Alcohol and Drug Information, Center for Substance Abuse Prevention, Substance Abuse and Mental Health Services Administration
P.O. Box 2345
Rockville, MD 20847-2345
(301) 468-2600,
(800) 729-6686,
(301) 230-2867 (TTY/TDD),
(800) 487-7889 (TTY/TDD)

National Library of Medicine
8600 Rockville Pike
Bethesda, MD 20894
(301) 496-6308 (public information)

MISSOURI

Good Samaritan Project
3030 Walnut Street
Kansas City, MO 64108
(816) 561-8784,
(800) 234-TEENS
(TEENS TAP National Hotline),
(816) 531-7199 (FAX)

NEW JERSEY

National Pediatric HIV Resource Center, Children's Hospital of New Jersey
15 South Ninth Street
Newark, NJ 07107
(201) 269-8251,
(800) 362-0071,
(201) 485-7769 (FAX)

Recording for the Blind
20 Roszel Road
Princeton, NJ 08540
(609) 452-0606,
(800) 221-4792

NEW YORK

American Civil Liberties Union Foundation, AIDS Project
132 West 43rd Street
New York, NY 10036
(212) 944-9800, extension 545,
(212) 869-9061 (FAX)

American Foundation for AIDS Research
733 Third Avenue, 12th Floor
New York, NY 10017
(212) 682-7440,
(212) 682-9812 (FAX)

Foundation Center
79 Fifth Avenue
New York, NY 10003-3076
(212) 620-4230

Gay Men's Health Crisis
129 West 20th Street
New York, NY 10011-0022
(212) 337-3553,
(212) 645-7470 (TTY/TDD),
(212) 337-3656 (FAX)

Hastings Center
255 Elm Road
Briarcliff Manor, NY 10510
(914) 762-8500,
(914) 762-2124 (FAX)

Hemophilia and AIDS/HIV Network for the Dissemination of Information, The National Hemophilia Foundation
110 Greene Street, Ste. 303
New York, NY 10012
(212) 431-8541,
(800) 42-HANDI,
(212) 431-0906 (FAX)

HIV Resource Library, Bureau of HIV Prevention Services, New York City Department of Health
125 Worth Street, Box A/1
New York, NY 10013
(212) 788-4280

Monroe Community College, AIDS Resource Library
1000 East Henrietta Road
Building 2, Room 315
Rochester, NY 14623
(716) 292-2309,
(716) 424-1402 (FAX)

Planned Parenthood Federation of America
810 Seventh Avenue
New York, NY 10019
(212) 541-7800,
(800) 669-0156 (publication orders)

Sex Information and Education Council of the U.S.
130 West 42nd Street, Ste. 2500
New York, NY 10036
(212) 819-9770

NORTH CAROLINA

Access to Respite Care and Help, National Resource Center for Crisis Nurseries and Respite Care Services
800 Eastowne Drive, Ste. 105
Chapel Hill, NC 27514
(919) 490-5577,
(800) 473-1727,
(919) 490-4905 (FAX)

CDC National AIDS Hotline
P.O. Box 13827
Research Triangle Park, NC 27709
(800) 342-AIDS,
(800) 344-7432 (Spanish),
(800) 243-7889 (TTY/TDD)

PENNSYLVANIA

AIDS Information Network
32 North Third Street
Philadelphia, PA 19106
(215) 922-5120,
(215) 922-7999 (TTY/TDD),
(215) 922-6762 (FAX)

TEXAS

Center for Health Policy Development, Hispanic Health Resource Center
6905 Alamo Downs Parkway
San Antonio, TX 78238-4519
(512) 520-8020,
(800) 847-7212,
(512) 520-9522 (FAX)

Funding Information Center, Texas Department of Health, Reprographics and Library Services Division
1100 West 49th Street
Austin, TX 78756-3199
(512) 458-7684,
(512) 458-7683 (FAX)

Texas Respite Resource Network
519 West Houston Street
San Antonio, TX 78207-3198
(210) 228-2794,
(210) 228-2797 (FAX)

VIRGINIA

National Center for Education in Maternal and Child Health
2000 15th Street North, Ste. 701
Arlington, VA 22201
(703) 524-7802,
(703) 524-9335 (FAX)

National School Boards Association, HIV/AIDS Education Project
1680 Duke Street
Alexandria, VA 22314
(703) 838-6722,
(703) 683-7590 (FAX)

WASHINGTON

Seattle Treatment Education Project
127 Broadway East, Ste. 200
Seattle, WA 98102
(206) 329-4857,
(800) 869-7837,
(206) 325-2689 (shared FAX)

WASHINGTON D.C.

American Civil Liberties Union Foundation, National Prison Project
1875 Connecticut Avenue, N.W., Ste. 410
Washington, DC 20009
(202) 234-4830,
(202) 234-4890 (FAX)

Americans for a Sound AIDS/HIV Policy
P.O. Box 17433
Washington, DC 20041-0433
(703) 471-7350,
(703) 471-8409 (FAX)

Center for Population Options
1025 Vermont Avenue, N.W., Ste. 210
Washington, DC 20005
(202) 347-5700

Center for Women's Policy Studies, National Resource Center on Women and AIDS
2000 P Street, N.W., Ste. 508
Washington, DC 20036
(202) 872-1770

Intergovernmental Health Policy Project, AIDS Project Center, George Washington University
2021 K Street, N.W., Ste. 800
Washington, DC 20006
(202) 872-1445,
(202) 785-0014 (FAX)

National Association of People with AIDS
1413 K Street, N.W., Eighth Floor
Washington, DC 20005
(202) 898-0414,
(202) 898-0435 (FAX),
(703) 998-3144 (BBS)

National Coalition of Hispanic Health and Human Services Organizations
1501 16th Street, N.W.
Washington, DC 20036
(202) 387-7000,
(202) 797-4353 (FAX)

National Council of La Raza
810 First Street, N.E., Ste. 300
Washington, DC 20002-4205
(202) 289-1380,
(202) 289-8173 (FAX)

National Information Center on Deafness, Gallaudet University
800 Florida Avenue, N.E.
Washington, DC 20002
(202) 651-5051,
(202) 651-5052 (TTY/TDD),
(202) 651-5054 (FAX)

National Leadership Coalition on AIDS
1730 M Street, N.W., Ste. 905
Washington, DC 20036
(202) 429-0930,
(202) 452-8845 (publications orders),
(202) 872-1977 (FAX)

National Library Service for the Blind and Physically Handicapped, Library of Congress
Washington, DC 20542
(202) 707-5100,
(202) 707-0744 (TTY/TDD),
(202) 707-0712 (FAX)

National Reference Center for Bioethics Literature, Kennedy Institute of Ethics, Georgetown University
Washington, DC 20057-1065
(202) 687-6770,
(800) MED-ETHX

Office of Minority Health Resource Center, Office of Minority Health, Public Health Service, U.S. Department of Health and Human Services
P.O. Box 37337
Washington, DC 20013-7337
(301) 587-1938,
(800) 444-6472

AIDS HOTLINES

National AIDS Hotline   1-800-342-AIDS

Alabama 1-800-228-0469	Kentucky 1-800-342-AIDS	Ohio 1-800-332-2437
Alaska 1-800-478-2437	Louisiana 1-800-992-4379	Oklahoma 1-800-342-AIDS
Arizona 1-800-352-3792	Maine 1-800-851-2437	Oregon 1-800-777-2437
Arkansas 1-800-364-2437	Maryland 1-800-638-6252	Pennsylvania 1-800-662-6080
California (No.) 1-800-367-2437	Massachusetts 1-800-235-2331	Puerto Rico 1-800-981-5721
California (So.) 1-800-922-2437	Michigan 1-800-872-2437	Rhode Island 1-800-726-3010
Colorado 1-800-252-2437	Minnesota 1-800-248-2437	South Carolina 1-800-322-2437
Connecticut 1-800-203-1234	Mississippi 1-800-826-2961	South Dakota 1-800-592-1861
Delaware 1-800-422-0429	Missouri 1-800-533-2437	Tennessee 1-800-525-2437
D.C. 1-202-332-2437	Montana 1-800-233-6668	Texas 1-800-299-2437
Florida 1-800-352-2437	Nebraska 1-800-782-2437	Utah 1-800-366-2437
Georgia 1-800-551-2728	Nevada 1-800-842-2437	Vermont 1-800-882-2437
Hawaii 1-800-321-1555	New Hampshire 1-800-752-2437	Virginia 1-800-533-4148
Idaho 1-800-677-2437	New Jersey 1-800-624-2377	Virgin Islands 1-809-773-2437
Illinois 1-800-243-2437	New Mexico 1-800-545-2437	Washington 1-800-272-2437
Indiana 1-800-848-2437	New York 1-800-541-2437	West Virginia 1-800-642-8244
Iowa 1-800-445-2437	North Carolina 1-800-342-AIDS	Wisconsin 1-800-334-2437
Kansas 1-800-342-AIDS	North Dakota 1-800-472-2180	Wyoming 1-800-327-3577

Many of these numbers are only available within a specific state or designated area codes.

AIDS EDUCATION AND TRAINING CENTERS

Serving six counties in Southern California (Riverside, San Bernardino, Los Angeles, Orange, Ventura, and Santa Barbara):
    University of Southern California
    AIDS ETC.
    1420 San Pablo Street, B207
    Los Angeles, CA 90033
    Jerry Gates
    (213) 342-1846,
    (213) 221-1235 (FAX)

Serving Nevada, Arizona, Hawaii, and California (excluding the six counties noted above):
    Western AIDS ETC
    5110 East Clinton Way, Ste. 115
    Fresno, CA 93727-2098
    Clark Jones
    (209) 252-2851,
    (209) 454-8012 (FAX)

Serving Washington, Alaska, Montana, Idaho, and Oregon:
University of Washington AIDS ETC
    10001 Broadway, Ste. 217
    Mail Stop ZH-20
    Seattle, WA 98122
    Ann Downer
    (206) 720-4250,
    (206) 720-4218 (FAX)

Serving Ohio, Michigan, Kentucky, and Tennessee:
    The Ohio State University, East Central AIDS ETC,
    Department of Family Medicine
    1314 Kinnear Road, Area 300
    Columbus, OH 43212
    Lawrence Gabel
    (614) 292-1400,
    (614) 292-4056 (FAX)

Serving New York and the Virgin Islands: Columbia University, School of Public Health AIDS ETC
    600 West 168th Street
    New York, NY 10032
    Cheryl Healton
    (212) 305-3616,
    (212) 305-6832 (FAX)

Serving Alabama, Georgia, North Carolina, and South Carolina:
    Emory University, Emory AIDS Training Network
    735 Gatewood Road, N.E.
    Atlanta, GA 30322
    Kathleen Miner
    (404) 727-2929,
    (404) 727-4562 (FAX)

Serving Arkansas, Louisiana, and Mississippi:
    Louisiana State University, Delta Region AIDS ETC
    1542 Tulane Avenue
    New Orleans, LA 70112
    William Brandon
    (504) 568-3855,
    (504) 568-7893 (FAX)

Serving North Dakota, South Dakota, Utah, Colorado, New Mexico, Nebraska, Kansas, and Wyoming:
University of Colorado Mountain Plains Regional AIDS ETC
    4200 East Ninth Avenue, Box A-096
    Denver, CO 80262
    Lorraine Adams
    (303) 355-1301,
    (303) 355-1448 (FAX)

Serving Iowa, Minnesota, Wisconsin, Illinois, Indiana, and Missouri:
    University of Illinois at Chicago, Midwest AIDS Training and Education Center
    808 South Wood Street (M/C 779)
    Chicago, IL 60612
    Nathan Linsk
    (312) 996-1373 or 1426,
    (312) 413-4184 (FAX)

Serving Pennsylvania:
    University of Pittsburgh, Graduate School of Public Health, Pennsylvania AIDS ETC
    130 DeSoto Street, Room A425
    Pittsburgh, PA 15261
    Linda Frank-Hertweck
    (412) 624-1895,
    (412) 624-4767 (FAX)

Serving Florida:
    Florida AIDS ETC
    P.O. Box 016960 (D-90)
    Miami, FL 33101
    Leonard Hoenig
    (305) 549-7836,
    (305) 324-4931 (FAX)

Serving Connecticut, Maine, Massachusetts, New Hampshire, Rhode Island, and Vermont:
    University of Massachusetts, New England AIDS ETC
    55 Lake Avenue North
    Worcester, MA 01655
    Donna Gallagher
    (508) 856-3255,
    (508) 856-6128 (FAX)

Serving Texas and Oklahoma:
The University of Texas AIDS ETC
1200 Herman Pressler Street
P.O. Box 20186
Houston, TX 77225
Richard Grimes
(713) 794-4075,
(713) 794-4877 (FAX)

Serving New Jersey:
University of Medicine and Dentistry of New Jersey AIDS
ETC, Office of Continuing Education
30 Bergen Street
Newark, NJ 07107
Charles McKinney
(201) 456-3690,
(201) 456-7128 (FAX)

Serving the metropolitan Washington, D.C., area (including
the Maryland counties of Montgomery, Prince Georges,
Calvert, Charles, and Frederick and the Virginia counties of
Arlington, Fairfax, Loudoun, Prince William, and Stafford):
District of Columbia AIDS ETC, Howard University
Hospital
Department of Medicine, Ste. 5C
2041 Georgia Avenue, N.W.
Washington, D.C. 20060
Margaret Kadree
(202) 865-6641, (202) 745-3731 (FAX)
Sylvia Silver
(202) 994-2945,
(202) 994-1791 (FAX)

Serving West Virginia, Delaware, Virginia (excluding the five
counties noted above), and Maryland (excluding the five counties noted above):
Mid-Atlantic AIDS ETC
P.O. Box 49
MCV Station
Richmond, VA 23298-0049
(804) 786-2210,
(804) 371-0495 (FAX)

Serving Puerto Rico:
University of Puerto Rico
Medical Sciences Campus
GPO 36-5067, Room 745A
Rio Piedras, PR 00936-5067
Angel Bravo
(809) 759-6528,
(809) 764-2470 (FAX)